2017

D1444119

ICD-10-CM

FOR HOSPITALS

INCLUDES NETTER'S ANATOMY ART

Carol J. Buck
MS, CPC, CCS-P

Former Program Director
Medical Secretary Programs
Northwest Technical College
East Grand Forks, Minnesota

ELSEVIER

ELSEVIER

3251 Riverport Lane
St. Louis, Missouri 63043

2017 ICD-10-CM HOSPITAL EDITION

ISBN: 978-0-323-43121-7

Notice

Knowledge and best practice in this field are constantly changing. As new research and experience broaden our understanding, changes in research methods, professional practices, or medical treatment may become necessary.

Practitioners and researchers must always rely on their own experience and knowledge in evaluating and using any information, methods, compounds, or experiments described herein. In using such information or methods they should be mindful of their own safety and the safety of others, including parties for whom they have a professional responsibility.

With respect to any drug or pharmaceutical products identified, readers are advised to check the most current information provided (i) on procedures featured or (ii) by the manufacturer of each product to be administered, to verify the recommended dose or formula, the method and duration of administration, and contraindications. It is the responsibility of practitioners, relying on their own experience and knowledge of their patients, to make diagnoses, to determine dosages and the best treatment for each individual patient, and to take all appropriate safety precautions.

To the fullest extent of the law, neither the Publisher nor the authors, contributors, or editors, assume any liability for any injury and/or damage to persons or property as a matter of products liability, negligence or otherwise, or from any use or operation of any methods, products, instructions, or ideas contained in the material herein.

Library of Congress Cataloging-in-Publication Data
Names: Buck, Carol J., author.
Title: 2017 ICD-10-CM for hospitals / Carol J. Buck.
Other titles: ICD-10-CM for hospitals
Description: Professional edition. | St. Louis, Missouri : Elsevier, [2017]
|
  Includes index. | Preceded by 2016 ICD-10-CM for hospitals / Carol J.
  Buck. Professional edition. [2015].
Identifiers: LCCN 2016016060 | ISBN 9780323431217 (pbk.)
Subjects: | MESH: International statistical classification of diseases and
  related health problems. 10th revision. Clinical modification. |
  Disease--classification | International Classification of Diseases |
  Medical Records | Forms and Records Control--methods
Classification: LCC RB115 | NLM WB 15 | DDC 616.001/2--dc23 LC record available at
https://lccn.loc.gov/2016016060

Director, Private Sector Education & Professional/References: Jeanne R. Olson
Content Development Manager: Luke Held
Associate Content Development Specialist: Anna Miller
Publishing Services Manager: Jeffrey Patterson
Project Manager: Lisa A. P. Bushey
Design Manager: Julia Dummitt

Printed in the United States of America

Last digit is the print number: 9 8 7 6 5 4 3 2 1

Working together
to grow libraries in
developing countries

www.elsevier.com • www.bookaid.org

DEDICATION

To all the brave medical coders who transitioned the nation into a new coding system.
Decades of waiting finally concluded with the implementation of I-10,
and you have been the pioneers leading the way.

With greatest appreciations for your efforts!

Carol J. Buck, MS, CPC, CCS-P

DEVELOPMENT OF THIS EDITION

Query Team

Patricia Cordy Henricksen, MS, CHCA, CPC-I, CPC, CCP-P, ASC-PM
Auditing and Coding Educator
Soterion Medical Services
Lexington, Kentucky

Jackie L. Grass, CPC
Coding and Reimbursement Specialist
Grand Forks, North Dakota

Kathleen Buchda, CPC, CPMA
Revenue Recognition
New Richmond, Wisconsin

Editorial Consultant

Jenna Price, CPC-A
President
Price Editorial Services, LLC
St. Louis, Missouri

Elsevier/MC Strategies Revenue Cycle, Coding and Compliance Staff

"Experts in providing e-learning on revenue cycle, coding and compliance."

Deborah Neville, RHIA, CCS-P
Director

Lynn-Marie D. Wozniak, MS, RHIT
Content Manager

Sandra L. Macica, MS, RHIA, CCS, ROCC
Content Manager

CONTENTS

ICD-10-CM

Guide to Using the 2017 ICD-10-CM for Hospitals   vi
Symbols and Conventions   viii
Guide to the 2017 Updates   xiii

Part I Introduction   1

ICD-10-CM Official Guidelines for Coding and
    Reporting   1
Netter's Anatomy Illustrations   49

Part II Alphabetic Index   81

Index to Diseases and Injuries   81
Table of Neoplasms   465
Table of Drugs and Chemicals   493
External Cause of Injuries Index   589

Part III Tabular List of Diseases and Injuries   633

Chapter 1   Certain Infectious and Parasitic
        Diseases (A00-B99)   634

Chapter 2   Neoplasms (C00-D49)   669

Chapter 3   Diseases of the Blood and Blood-
        Forming Organs and Certain
        Disorders Involving the Immune
        Mechanism (D50-D89)   720

Chapter 4   Endocrine, Nutritional and Metabolic
        Diseases (E00-E89)   731

Chapter 5   Mental, Behavioral and
        Neurodevelopmental Disorders
        (F01-F99)   757

Chapter 6   Diseases of the Nervous System
        (G00-G99)   784

Chapter 7   Diseases of the Eye and Adnexa
        (H00-H59)   809

Chapter 8   Diseases of the Ear and Mastoid Process
        (H60-H95)   854

Chapter 9   Diseases of the Circulatory System
        (I00-I99)   867

Chapter 10 Diseases of the Respiratory System
        (J00-J99)   917

Chapter 11 Diseases of the Digestive System
        (K00-K95)   935

Chapter 12 Diseases of the Skin and Subcutaneous
        Tissue (L00-L99)   962

Chapter 13 Diseases of the Musculoskeletal System
        and Connective Tissue
        (M00-M99)   986

Chapter 14 Diseases of the Genitourinary System
        (N00-N99)   1091

Chapter 15 Pregnancy, Childbirth and the
        Puerperium (O00-O9A)   1113

Chapter 16 Certain Conditions Originating in the
        Perinatal Period (P00-P96)   1159

Chapter 17 Congenital Malformations,
        Deformations and Chromosomal
        Abnormalities (Q00-Q99)   1173

Chapter 18 Symptoms, Signs and Abnormal Clinical
        and Laboratory Findings, Not
        Elsewhere Classified
        (R00-R99)   1194

Chapter 19 Injury, Poisoning and Certain Other
        Consequences of External Causes
        (S00-T88)   1217

Chapter 20 External Causes of Morbidity
        (V00-Y99)   1516

Chapter 21 Factors Influencing Health Status
        and Contact with Health Services
        (Z00-Z99)   1602

GUIDE TO USING THE 2017 ICD-10-CM FOR HOSPITALS

Medical coding has long been a part of the health care profession. Through the years medical coding systems have become more complex and extensive. Today, medical coding is an intricate and immense process that is present in every health care setting. The increased use of electronic submissions for health care services only increases the need for coders who understand the coding process.

2017 ICD-10-CM for Hospitals, Professional Edition was developed to help meet the needs of coding professionals at all levels by offering a comprehensive coding text at a reasonable price.

All material strictly adheres to the latest government versions available at the time of printing. Updates from the *Definitions of Medicare Code Edits* (MCE) will be posted to the companion website (www. codingupdates.com) when available.

Illustrations and Items

The ICD-10-CM Tabular List contains illustrations, pictures, and items to assist you in understanding difficult terminology, diseases/conditions, or coding in a specific category. Items are always printed in ▒▒▒▒▒ ink so that the added material is not mistaken for official notations or instructions. ▒▒▒▒ ink is used for other annotations in the text. Your ideas on what other descriptions or illustrations should be in future editions of this text are always appreciated.

Instructional Notations

Includes Notes

Includes

The word 'Includes' appears immediately under certain categories to further define, or give examples of, the content of the category.

Excludes Notes

The ICD-10-CM has two types of excludes notes. Each note has a different definition for use, but they are both similar in that they indicate that codes excluded from each other are independent of each other.

Excludes1

A type 1 Excludes note is a pure excludes. It means "NOT CODED HERE!" An Excludes1 note indicates that the code excluded should never be used at the same time as the code above the Excludes1 note. An Excludes1 is for use when two conditions cannot occur together, such as a congenital form versus an acquired form of the same condition.

Excludes2

A type 2 Excludes note represents "NOT INCLUDED HERE." An Excludes2 note indicates that the condition excluded is not part of the condition it is excluded from but a patient may have both conditions at the same time. When an Excludes2 note appears under a code, it is acceptable to use both the code and the excluded code together.

Code First/Use Additional Code notes (etiology/manifestation paired codes)

Certain conditions have both an underlying etiology and multiple body system manifestations due to the underlying etiology. For such conditions the ICD-10-CM has a coding convention that requires the underlying condition be sequenced first, followed by the manifestation. Wherever such a combination exists, there is a "use additional code" note at the etiology code, and a "code first" note at the manifestation code. These instructional notes indicate the proper sequencing order of the codes, etiology followed by manifestation.

In most cases the manifestation codes will have in the code title, "in diseases classified elsewhere." Codes with this title are a component of the etiology/manifestation convention. The code title indicates that it is a manifestation code. "In diseases classified elsewhere" codes are never permitted to be used as first-listed or principal diagnosis codes. They must be used in conjunction with an underlying condition code, and they must be listed following the underlying condition.

Use additional

The words indicate an instructional note that another code may be needed.

Code first

The words indicate an instructional note that directs the coder to sequence the underlying condition before the manifestation.

Code also

A "code also" note instructs that two codes may be required to fully describe a condition, but the sequencing of the two codes is discretionary, depending on the severity of the conditions and the reason for the encounter.

Unspecified

The highlight indicates that although the code is valid as a principal (first-listed) diagnosis, it is not as specific as other codes without the highlight.

7th characters and placeholder X

For codes less than 6 characters that require a 7th character a placeholder X should be assigned for all characters less than 6. The 7th character must always be the 7th character of a code.

Annotated

Throughout the manual, revisions, additions, and deleted codes or words are indicated by the following symbols:

◄▥▥▥ **Revised:** Revisions within the line or code from the previous edition are indicated by the arrow.

◄ **New:** Additions to the previous edition are indicated by the triangle.

~~deleted~~ **Deleted:** Deletions from the previous edition are struck through.

ICD-10-CM Tabular List Symbols

● **Use Additional Character(s):** The red stop sign cautions that the code requires additional character(s) to ensure the greatest specificity.

X For codes less than 6 characters that require a 7th character, a placeholder X should be assigned for all characters less than 6. The 7th character must always be the 7th character of a code.

● **Unacceptable Principal Diagnosis:** These codes have a blue dot before them and give additional information or describe the circumstances affecting the health care encounter but are unacceptable as principal diagnosis in the *Definitions of Medicare Code Edits* (MCE) for inpatient admission.

OGCR The ***Official Guidelines for Coding and Reporting*** symbol includes the placement of a portion of a guideline as that guideline pertains to the code by which it is located. The complete OGCR are located in Part I.

🔗🔗 Indicates **complications and comorbidities and major complications and comorbidities** according to the *Medicare Severity Diagnosis Related Groups (MS-DRGs), Definitions Manual.*

(Ex) Indicates exclusions to complications and comorbidities (CC) and major complications and comorbidities (MCC) for both primary and secondary diagnoses, according to the *Medicare Severity Diagnosis Related Groups (MS-DRGs), Definitions Manual.*

PDX as its own CC/MCC Indicates a combination code that when assigned as the Principal Diagnosis, it includes a condition that also qualifies as a CC/MCC according to the *Medicare Severity Diagnosis Related Groups (MS-DRGs), Definitions Manual.*

🔗 HAC is a **Hospital-Acquired Condition** that, when present as a secondary diagnosis in an inpatient setting, is a higher cost, higher volume, or both and results in a higher MS-DRG assignment according to the *Medicare Severity Diagnosis Related Groups (MS-DRGs), Definitions Manual.*

▯ **Manifestation Code:** Describes the manifestation of an underlying disease, not the disease itself, and therefore should not be assigned as a principal diagnosis, according to the *Definitions of Medicare Code Edits* (MCE).

Age conflict: The *Definitions of Medicare Code Edits* (MCE) detects inconsistencies between a patient's age and diagnosis. For example, a 5-year-old patient with benign prostatic hypertrophy or a 78-year-old pregnant female.

The diagnosis is clinically and virtually impossible in a patient of the stated age. Therefore, either the diagnosis or the age is presumed to be incorrect. There are four age categories for diagnoses in the *Definitions of Medicare Code Edits* (MCE):

N • Newborn. Age of 0 years; a subset of diagnoses intended only for newborns and neonates (e.g., fetal distress, perinatal jaundice).

P • Pediatric. Age range is 0-17 years inclusive (e.g., Reye's syndrome, routine child health exam).

M • Maternity. Age range is 12-55 years inclusive (e.g., diabetes in pregnancy, antepartum pulmonary complication).

A • Adult. Age range is 15-124 years inclusive (e.g., senile delirium, mature cataract).

♀♂ **Sex conflict:** *Definitions of Medicare Code Edits* (MCE) detects inconsistencies between a patient's sex and any diagnosis or procedure on the patient's record. For example, a male patient with cervical cancer (diagnosis) or a female patient with a prostatectomy (procedure). In both instances, the indicated diagnosis or the procedure conflicts with the stated sex of the patient. Therefore, either the patient's diagnosis, procedure, or sex is presumed to be incorrect.

Coding Clinic Identifies the year, quarter, and page number that presents information about an ICD-10-CM code in the American Hospital Association's *Coding Clinic®* for ICD-10-CM.

Visit codingupdates.com for the full list of 2017 Present on Admission codes.

SYMBOLS AND CONVENTIONS

ICD-10-CM Tabular

Use Additional Character(s): The red stop sign cautions you that the code requires additional character(s) to ensure greatest specificity.

Placeholder X: The red X reminds you that for codes less than 6 characters that require a 7th character, a placeholder X should be assigned to all characters less than 6.

Volume 1, Tabular List

● K22 **Other diseases of esophagus**

    Excludes2   esophageal varices (I85.-)

X ● V00.01 **Pedestrian on foot injured in collision with roller-skater**

A02.20 **Localized salmonella infection, unspecified**

Unspecified: These codes are for use when the information in the medical record is insufficient to assign a more specific code. For those categories for which an unspecified code is not provided, the "other specified" code may represent both other and unspecified.

Unacceptable Principal Diagnosis: These codes have a blue dot before them and are not permitted as a first-listed or principal diagnosis. They must be assigned in conjunction with an underlying condition code, and they must be listed following the underlying condition.

● B95.0 **Streptococcus, group A, as the cause of diseases classified elsewhere**

A48.3 **Toxic shock syndrome**

    Use additional code to identify the organism (B95, B96)

Use additional code: Located at the etiology code and directs you to assign a manifestation code.

Code first indicates the etiology code is to be first-listed before the manifestation code.

B39 **Histoplasmosis**

    Code first associated AIDS (B20)

Notes define terms or give coding instructions.

E34.0 **Carcinoid syndrome**

    Note: May be used as an additional code to identify functional activity associated with a carcinoid tumor.

Codes or index entries are for purposes of illustration only and may not be current.

OGCR Section I.C.6.B.5.

Neoplasm Related Pain Code G89.3 is assigned to pain documented as being related, associated or due to cancer, primary or secondary malignancy, or tumor. This code is assigned regardless of whether the pain is acute or chronic.

OGCR: The *Official Guidelines for Coding and Reporting* are placed near the codes to which they refer and are highlighted.

I70.2   **Atherosclerosis of native arteries of the extremities**
Mönckeberg's (medial) sclerosis

Use additional code, if applicable, to identify chronic total occlusion of artery of extremity (I70.92)

code, if applicable, directs the coder to other conditions that may be appropriate to report.

The word "and" should be interpreted to mean either "and" or "or" when it appears in a statement.

I74   **Arterial embolism and thrombosis**
  Includes   embolic infarction
embolic occlusion
thrombotic infarction
thrombotic occlusion

Bold typeface is used on all codes and titles.

I83.001   **Varicose veins of unspecified lower extremity with ulcer of thigh**

"with" should be interpreted to mean "associated with" or "due to."

K73.2   **Chronic active hepatitis, not elsewhere classified**

"not elsewhere classified" or **NEC** identifies a code that is assigned only when the information at hand specifies a condition for which no more specific code is available.

"not otherwise specified" or **NOS** is equivalent to unspecified.

W13.9   **Fall from, out of or through building, not otherwise specified**

Codes or index entries are for purposes of illustration only and may not be current.

Excludes1 means "NOT CODED HERE!" An Excludes1 note indicates that the code excluded should never be assigned at the same time as the code above the Excludes1 note.

Includes: This note appears immediately under a three-character code title to further define, or give examples of, the content.

Codes titled "other" or "other specified" are for use when the information in the medical record provides detail for which a specific code does not exist.

Pediatric Age, Ø-17, according to the *Definitions of Medicare Code Edits* (MCE).

Females Only according to the *Definitions of Medicare Code Edits* (MCE).

M19 Other and unspecified osteoarthritis
Excludes1   polyarthritis (M15.-)
Excludes2   arthrosis of spine (M47.-)
                 hallux rigidus (M2Ø.2)
                 osteoarthritis of spine (M47.-)

A06 Amebiasis
Includes   infection due to Entamoeba histolytica

E26.Ø1 Conn's syndrome
         Code also adrenal adenoma (D35.Ø)

E25.8 Other adrenogenital disorders

O00.2 Ovarian pregnancy   M

P02.20 Newborn (suspected to be) affected by unspecified morphological and functional abnormalities of placenta   N

L21.Ø Seborrhea capitis   P
         Cradle cap

G30.1 Alzheimer's disease with late onset   A

B37.3 Candidiasis of vulva and vagina ♀

C6Ø.1 Malignant neoplasm of glans penis ♂

Excludes2 represents "NOT INCLUDED HERE." An Excludes2 note indicates that the condition excluded is not part of the condition represented by the code, but a patient may have both conditions at the same time and it is acceptable to use both the code and the excluded code together, when appropriate.

Code also instructs that two codes may be required to fully describe a condition, but this note does not provide sequencing direction.

Maternity DX (Diagnosis) for ages 12-55 according to the *Definitions of Medicare Code Edits* (MCE).

Newborn, Age Ø, according to the *Definitions of Medicare Code Edits* (MCE).

Adult Age, 15-124, according to the *Definitions of Medicare Code Edits* (MCE).

Males Only according to the *Definitions of Medicare Code Edits* (MCE).

Manifestation according to the *Definitions of Medicare Code Edits* (MCE).

▶ H22 *Disorders of iris and ciliary body in diseases classified elsewhere*
     Code first *underlying disease, such as:*
          gout (M1A-, M10.-)

G14 **Postpolio syndrome**
     Includes   Postpolio myelitic syndrome
     Excludes1 sequelae of poliomyelitis (B91)

T81.512 **Adhesions due to foreign body accidentally left in body following kidney dialysis** 🔗 ◀

Hospital-Acquired Condition according to the *Medicare Severity Diagnosis Related Groups (MS-DRGs).*

Major Complication/ Comorbidity (MCC) according to the *Medicare Severity Diagnosis Related Groups (MS-DRGs).*

R57.1 **Hypovolemic shock** 🔗

B25.1 **Cytomegaloviral hepatitis** 🔗 ◀

Complication/ Comorbidity (CC) according to the *Medicare Severity Diagnosis Related Groups (MS-DRGs).*

Coding Clinic identifies the year, quarter, and page number that presents information about an ICD-10-PCS code in the American Hospital Association's *Coding Clinic®.*

B96.5 **Pseudomonas (aeruginosa) (mallei) (pseudomallei) as the cause of diseases classified elsewhere**
     ▶ **Coding Clinic: 2015, Q1, P18**

Codes or index entries are for purposes of illustration only and may not be current.

Alphabetic Index

Main terms are in **bold** typeface.

Aberrant (congenital) —*see also* Malposition, congenital
    adrenal gland Q89.1

Etiology code first followed by the manifestation code in **brackets**. The code in brackets is always to be sequenced second.

Amyloid heart (disease) E85.4 *[I43]*

"**see**" indicates another term should be referenced.

Amylophagia —*see* Pica

Angiofibroma —*see also* Neoplasm, benign, by site

"**see also**" follows a main term and instructs that there is another main term that may also be referenced.

Appendicitis (pneumococcal) (retrocecal) K37
    with
        perforation or rupture K35.2
        peritoneal abscess K35.3

A default code is listed next to the main term and represents that condition most commonly associated with the main term. If a condition is documented in a medical record without any additional information, such as acute or chronic, the default code should be assigned.

CHAPTER 1

CERTAIN INFECTIOUS AND PARASITIC DISEASES (A00-B99)

A40 Streptococcal sepsis
   Code first
Revised   postprocedural streptococcal sepsis (T81.4-)

A41 Other sepsis
   Code first
Revised   postprocedural sepsis (T81.4-)
Deleted   **Excludes1**   sepsis NOS (A41.9)

New   **A92.5 Zika virus disease**
New   Zika virus fever
New   Zika virus infection
New   Zika NOS

      B17.9 Acute viral hepatitis, unspecified
New   Acute infectious hepatitis NOS

B18 Chronic viral hepatitis
New   **Includes**   Carrier of viral hepatitis
   B18.1 Chronic viral hepatitis B without delta-agent
New   Carrier of viral hepatitis B
   B18.2 Chronic viral hepatitis C
New   Carrier of viral hepatitis C
   B18.8 Other chronic viral hepatitis
New   Carrier of other viral hepatitis
   B18.9 Chronic viral hepatitis, unspecified
New   Carrier of unspecified viral hepatitis

CHAPTER 2

NEOPLASMS (C00-D49)

C00 Malignant neoplasm of lip
C01 Malignant neoplasm of base of tongue
C02 Malignant neoplasm of other and unspecified parts of tongue
C03 Malignant neoplasm of gum
C04 Malignant neoplasm of floor of mouth
C05 Malignant neoplasm of palate
C06 Malignant neoplasm of other and unspecified parts of mouth
C07 Malignant neoplasm of parotid gland
C08 Malignant neoplasm of other and unspecified major salivary glands
C09 Malignant neoplasm of tonsil
C10 Malignant neoplasm of oropharynx
C11 Malignant neoplasm of nasopharynx
C12 Malignant neoplasm of pyriform sinus
C13 Malignant neoplasm of hypopharynx
C14 Malignant neoplasm of other and ill-defined sites in the lip, oral cavity and pharynx
      Use additional code to identify:
Revised   history of tobacco dependence (Z87.891)

MALIGNANT NEOPLASM OF DIGESTIVE ORGANS (C15-C26)

New   **Excludes2**   gastrointestinal stromal tumors (C49.A-)
C25 Malignant neoplasm of pancreas
New   Code also exocrine pancreatic insufficiency (K86.81)
C32 Malignant neoplasm of larynx
C33 Malignant neoplasm of trachea
C34 Malignant neoplasm of bronchus and lung
C39 Malignant neoplasm of other and ill-defined sites in the respiratory system and intrathoracic organs
      Use additional code to identify:
Revised   history of tobacco dependence (Z87.891)

New   **C49.A Gastrointestinal stromal tumor**
New   **C49.A0 Gastrointestinal stromal tumor, unspecified site**
New   **C49.A1 Gastrointestinal stromal tumor of esophagus**
New   **C49.A2 Gastrointestinal stromal tumor of stomach**
New   **C49.A3 Gastrointestinal stromal tumor of small intestine**
New   **C49.A4 Gastrointestinal stromal tumor of large intestine**
New   **C49.A5 Gastrointestinal stromal tumor of rectum**
New   **C49.A9 Gastrointestinal stromal tumor of other sites**

C61 Malignant neoplasm of prostate
New   Use additional code to identify:
New   hormone sensitivity status (Z19.1-Z19.2)
New   rising PSA following treatment for malignant neoplasm of prostate (R97.21)

Revised   **C7A.094 Malignant carcinoid tumor of the foregut unspecified**
Revised   **C7A.095 Malignant carcinoid tumor of the midgut unspecified**
Revised   **C7A.096 Malignant carcinoid tumor of the hindgut unspecified**

C78 Secondary malignant neoplasm of respiratory and digestive organs
Deleted   **Excludes1**   lymph node metastases (C77.0)
New   **Excludes2**   lymph node metastases (C77.0)
      C78.89 Secondary malignant neoplasm of other digestive organs
New   Code also exocrine pancreatic insufficiency (K86.81)

C79 Secondary malignant neoplasm of other and unspecified sites
Deleted   **Excludes1**   lymph node metastases (C77.0)
New   **Excludes2**   lymph node metastases (C77.0)

Revised	C81.1	Nodular sclerosis Hodgkin lymphoma
New		Nodular sclerosis classical Hodgkin lymphoma
Revised	C81.10	Nodular sclerosis Hodgkin lymphoma, unspecified site
Revised	C81.11	Nodular sclerosis Hodgkin lymphoma, lymph nodes of head, face, and neck
Revised	C81.12	Nodular sclerosis Hodgkin lymphoma, intrathoracic lymph nodes
Revised	C81.13	Nodular sclerosis Hodgkin lymphoma, intra-abdominal lymph nodes
Revised	C81.14	Nodular sclerosis Hodgkin lymphoma, lymph nodes of axilla and upper limb
Revised	C81.15	Nodular sclerosis Hodgkin lymphoma, lymph nodes of inguinal region and lower limb
Revised	C81.16	Nodular sclerosis Hodgkin lymphoma, intrapelvic lymph nodes
Revised	C81.17	Nodular sclerosis Hodgkin lymphoma, spleen
Revised	C81.18	Nodular sclerosis Hodgkin lymphoma, lymph nodes of multiple sites
Revised	C81.19	Nodular sclerosis Hodgkin lymphoma, extranodal and solid organ sites
Revised	C81.2	Mixed cellularity Hodgkin lymphoma
New		Mixed cellularity classical Hodgkin lymphoma
Revised	C81.20	Mixed cellularity Hodgkin lymphoma, unspecified site
Revised	C81.21	Mixed cellularity Hodgkin lymphoma, lymph nodes of head, face, and neck
Revised	C81.22	Mixed cellularity Hodgkin lymphoma, intrathoracic lymph nodes
Revised	C81.23	Mixed cellularity Hodgkin lymphoma, intra-abdominal lymph nodes
Revised	C81.24	Mixed cellularity Hodgkin lymphoma, lymph nodes of axilla and upper limb
Revised	C81.25	Mixed cellularity Hodgkin lymphoma, lymph nodes of inguinal region and lower limb
Revised	C81.26	Mixed cellularity Hodgkin lymphoma, intrapelvic lymph nodes
Revised	C81.27	Mixed cellularity Hodgkin lymphoma, spleen
Revised	C81.28	Mixed cellularity Hodgkin lymphoma, lymph nodes of multiple sites
Revised	C81.29	Mixed cellularity Hodgkin lymphoma, extranodal and solid organ sites
Revised	C81.3	Lymphocyte depleted Hodgkin lymphoma
New		Lymphocyte depleted classical Hodgkin lymphoma
Revised	C81.30	Lymphocyte depleted Hodgkin lymphoma, unspecified site
Revised	C81.31	Lymphocyte depleted Hodgkin lymphoma, lymph nodes of head, face, and neck
Revised	C81.32	Lymphocyte depleted Hodgkin lymphoma, intrathoracic lymph nodes
Revised	C81.33	Lymphocyte depleted Hodgkin lymphoma, intra-abdominal lymph nodes
Revised	C81.34	Lymphocyte depleted Hodgkin lymphoma, lymph nodes of axilla and upper limb
Revised	C81.35	Lymphocyte depleted Hodgkin lymphoma, lymph nodes of inguinal region and lower limb
Revised	C81.36	Lymphocyte depleted Hodgkin lymphoma, intrapelvic lymph nodes
Revised	C81.37	Lymphocyte depleted Hodgkin lymphoma, spleen
Revised	C81.38	Lymphocyte depleted Hodgkin lymphoma, lymph nodes of multiple sites
Revised	C81.39	Lymphocyte depleted Hodgkin lymphoma, extranodal and solid organ sites
Revised	C81.4	Lymphocyte-rich Hodgkin lymphoma
New		Lymphocyte-rich classical Hodgkin lymphoma
Revised	C81.40	Lymphocyte-rich Hodgkin lymphoma, unspecified site
Revised	C81.41	Lymphocyte-rich Hodgkin lymphoma, lymph nodes of head, face, and neck
Revised	C81.42	Lymphocyte-rich Hodgkin lymphoma, intrathoracic lymph nodes
Revised	C81.43	Lymphocyte-rich Hodgkin lymphoma, intra-abdominal lymph nodes
Revised	C81.44	Lymphocyte-rich Hodgkin lymphoma, lymph nodes of axilla and upper limb
Revised	C81.45	Lymphocyte-rich Hodgkin lymphoma, lymph nodes of inguinal region and lower limb
Revised	C81.46	Lymphocyte-rich Hodgkin lymphoma, intrapelvic lymph nodes
Revised	C81.47	Lymphocyte-rich Hodgkin lymphoma, spleen
Revised	C81.48	Lymphocyte-rich Hodgkin lymphoma, lymph nodes of multiple sites
Revised	C81.49	Lymphocyte-rich Hodgkin lymphoma, extranodal and solid organ sites
Revised	C81.7	Other Hodgkin lymphoma
New		Other classical Hodgkin lymphoma
Revised	C81.70	Other Hodgkin lymphoma, unspecified site
Revised	C81.71	Other Hodgkin lymphoma, lymph nodes of head, face, and neck
Revised	C81.72	Other Hodgkin lymphoma, intrathoracic lymph nodes
Revised	C81.73	Other Hodgkin lymphoma, intra-abdominal lymph nodes
Revised	C81.74	Other Hodgkin lymphoma, lymph nodes of axilla and upper limb
Revised	C81.75	Other Hodgkin lymphoma, lymph nodes of inguinal region and lower limb
Revised	C81.76	Other Hodgkin lymphoma, intrapelvic lymph nodes
Revised	C81.77	Other Hodgkin lymphoma, spleen
Revised	C81.78	Other Hodgkin lymphoma, lymph nodes of multiple sites
Revised	C81.79	Other Hodgkin lymphoma, extranodal and solid organ sites
	C94.20	Acute megakaryoblastic leukemia not having achieved remission
Revised		Acute megakaryoblastic leukemia with failed remission

	D00.0	Carcinoma in situ of lip, oral cavity and pharynx
		Use additional code to identify:
Revised		history of tobacco dependence (Z87.891)
	D01.3	Carcinoma in situ of anus and anal canal
New		Anal intraepithelial neoplasia III [AIN III]
New		Severe dysplasia of anus
New		**Excludes1** anal intraepithelial neoplasia I and II [AIN I and AIN II] (K62.82)
	D02	Carcinoma in situ of middle ear and respiratory system
		Use additional code to identify:
Revised		history of tobacco dependence (Z87.891)

D07.5   Carcinoma in situ of prostate

Revised **Excludes1**   dysplasia (mild) (moderate) of prostate (N42.3-)

New   prostatic intraepithelial neoplasia II [PIN II] (N42.3-)

Revised **D10.3   Benign neoplasm of other and unspecified parts of mouth**

D16.4   Benign neoplasm of bones of skull and face

Deleted **Excludes1**   benign neoplasm of lower jaw bone (D16.5)

New **Excludes2**   benign neoplasm of lower jaw bone (D16.5)

D27   Benign neoplasm of ovary

Revised **Excludes2**   corpus albicans cyst (N83.2-)
Revised   corpus luteum cyst (N83.1-)
Revised   follicular (atretic) cyst (N83.0-)
Revised   graafian follicle cyst (N83.0-)
Revised   ovarian cyst NEC (N83.2-)
Revised   ovarian retention cyst (N83.2-)

Revised **D3A.094   Benign carcinoid tumor of the foregut, unspecified**

Revised **D3A.095   Benign carcinoid tumor of the midgut, unspecified**

Revised **D3A.096   Benign carcinoid tumor of the hindgut, unspecified**

Revised **D46.2   Refractory anemia with excess of blasts [RAEB]**

New **D47.Z2   Castleman disease**
New   Code also if applicable human herpesvirus 8 infection (B10.89)

New **Excludes2**   Kaposi's sarcoma (C46-)

D49.2   Neoplasm of unspecified behavior of bone, soft tissue, and skin

Revised **Excludes1**   neoplasm of unspecified behavior of skin of genital organs (D49.59)

New **D49.51   Neoplasm of unspecified behavior of kidney**

New **D49.511   Neoplasm of unspecified behavior of right kidney**

New **D49.512   Neoplasm of unspecified behavior of left kidney**

New **D49.519   Neoplasm of unspecified behavior of unspecified kidney**

New **D49.59   Neoplasm of unspecified behavior of other genitourinary organ**

CHAPTER 3

DISEASES OF THE BLOOD AND BLOOD-FORMING ORGANS AND CERTAIN DISORDERS INVOLVING THE IMMUNE MECHANISM (D50-D89)

D61.81   Pancytopenia

Deleted **Excludes1**   pancytopenia (due to) (with) myelodysplastic syndromes (D46.-)

New **Excludes2**   pancytopenia (due to) (with) myelodysplastic syndromes (D46.-)

D64.81   Anemia due to antineoplastic chemotherapy

Deleted **Excludes1**   anemia in neoplastic disease (D63.0)

New **Excludes2**   anemia in neoplastic disease (D63.0)

D68.62   Lupus anticoagulant syndrome

Revised **Excludes1**   lupus anticoagulant (LAC) finding without diagnosis (R76.0)

D76   Other specified diseases with participation of lymphoreticular and reticulohistiocytic tissue

New **Excludes1**   histiocytic medullary reticulosis (C96.9)
New   leukemic reticuloendotheliosis (C91.4-)
New   lipomelanotic reticulosis (I89.8)
Deleted   leukemic reticuloendotheliosis or reticulosis (C91.4-)
Deleted   lipomelanotic reticuloendotheliosis or reticulosis (I89.8)
New   malignant reticulosis (C86.0)
New   nonlipid reticuloendotheliosis (C96.0)

Revised **D78.2   Postprocedural hemorrhage of the spleen following a procedure**

Revised **D78.21   Postprocedural hemorrhage of the spleen following a procedure on the spleen**

Revised **D78.22   Postprocedural hemorrhage of the spleen following other procedure**

New **D78.3   Postprocedural hematoma and seroma of the spleen following a procedure**

New **D78.31   Postprocedural hematoma of the spleen following a procedure on the spleen**

New **D78.32   Postprocedural hematoma of the spleen following other procedure**

New **D78.33   Postprocedural seroma of the spleen following a procedure on the spleen**

New **D78.34   Postprocedural seroma of the spleen following other procedure**

New **D89.4   Mast cell activation syndrome and related disorders**

New **Excludes1**   aggressive systemic mastocytosis (C96.2)
New   cutaneous mastocytosis (Q82.2)
New   indolent systemic mastocytosis (D47.0)
New   malignant mastocytoma (C96.2)
New   mast cell leukemia (C94.3-)
New   mastocytoma (D47.0)
New   systemic mastocytosis associated with a clonal hematologic non-mast cell lineage disease (SM-AHNMD) (D47.0)

New **D89.40   Mast cell activation, unspecified**
New   Mast cell activation disorder, unspecified
New   Mast cell activation syndrome, NOS

New **D89.41   Monoclonal mast cell activation syndrome**

New **D89.42   Idiopathic mast cell activation syndrome**

New **D89.43   Secondary mast cell activation**
New   Secondary mast cell activation syndrome
New   Code also underlying etiology, if known

New **D89.49   Other mast cell activation disorder**
New   Other mast cell activation syndrome

CHAPTER 4

ENDOCRINE, NUTRITIONAL AND METABOLIC DISEASES (E00-E89)

E08   Diabetes mellitus due to underlying condition

Revised   Use additional code to identify control using:
New   insulin (Z79.4)
New   oral antidiabetic drugs (Z79.84)
New   oral hypoglycemic drugs (Z79.84)

    E08.32   Diabetes mellitus due to underlying condition with mild nonproliferative diabetic retinopathy

New   One of the following 7th characters is to be assigned to codes in subcategory E08.32 to designate laterality of the disease:

New   1   right eye
New   2   left eye
New   3   bilateral
New   9   unspecified eye

    E08.33   Diabetes mellitus due to underlying condition with moderate nonproliferative diabetic retinopathy

New   One of the following 7th characters is to be assigned to codes in subcategory E08.33 to designate laterality of the disease:

New   1   right eye
New   2   left eye
New   3   bilateral
New   9   unspecified eye

    E08.34   Diabetes mellitus due to underlying condition with severe nonproliferative diabetic retinopathy

New   One of the following 7th characters is to be assigned to codes in subcategory E08.34 to designate laterality of the disease:

New   1   right eye
New   2   left eye
New   3   bilateral
New   9   unspecified eye

    E08.35   Diabetes mellitus due to underlying condition with proliferative diabetic retinopathy

New   One of the following 7th characters is to be assigned to codes in subcategory E08.35 to designate laterality of the disease:

New   1   right eye
New   2   left eye
New   3   bilateral
New   9   unspecified eye

New   **E08.352   Diabetes mellitus due to underlying condition with proliferative diabetic retinopathy with traction retinal detachment involving the macula**

New   **E08.353   Diabetes mellitus due to underlying condition with proliferative diabetic retinopathy with traction retinal detachment not involving the macula**

New   **E08.354   Diabetes mellitus due to underlying condition with proliferative diabetic retinopathy with combined traction retinal detachment and rhegmatogenous retinal detachment**

New   **E08.355   Diabetes mellitus due to underlying condition with stable proliferative diabetic retinopathy**

New   **E08.37   Diabetes mellitus due to underlying condition with diabetic macular edema, resolved following treatment**

New   One of the following 7th characters is to be assigned to code E08.37 to designate laterality of the disease:

New   1   right eye
New   2   left eye
New   3   bilateral
New   9   unspecified eye

E09   Drug or chemical induced diabetes mellitus

Revised   Use additional code to identify control using:
New   insulin (Z79.4)
New   oral antidiabetic drugs (Z79.84)
New   oral hypoglycemic drugs (Z79.84)

    E09.32   Drug or chemical induced diabetes mellitus with mild nonproliferative diabetic retinopathy

New   One of the following 7th characters is to be assigned to codes in subcategory E09.32 to designate laterality of the disease:

New   1   right eye
New   2   left eye
New   3   bilateral
New   9   unspecified eye

    E09.33   Drug or chemical induced diabetes mellitus with moderate nonproliferative diabetic retinopathy

New   One of the following 7th characters is to be assigned to codes in subcategory E09.33 to designate laterality of the disease:

New   1   right eye
New   2   left eye
New   3   bilateral
New   9   unspecified eye

    E09.34   Drug or chemical induced diabetes mellitus with severe nonproliferative diabetic retinopathy

New   One of the following 7th characters is to be assigned to codes in subcategory E09.34 to designate laterality of the disease:

New   1   right eye
New   2   left eye
New   3   bilateral
New   9   unspecified eye

E09.35 **Drug or chemical induced diabetes mellitus with proliferative diabetic retinopathy**

New

One of the following 7th characters is to be assigned to codes in subcategory E09.35 to designate laterality of the disease:

1	right eye
2	left eye
3	bilateral
9	unspecified eye

New *New* *New* *New*

New **E09.352** **Drug or chemical induced diabetes mellitus with proliferative diabetic retinopathy with traction retinal detachment involving the macula**

New **E09.353** **Drug or chemical induced diabetes mellitus with proliferative diabetic retinopathy with traction retinal detachment not involving the macula**

New **E09.354** **Drug or chemical induced diabetes mellitus with proliferative diabetic retinopathy with combined traction retinal detachment and rhegmatogenous retinal detachment**

New **E09.355** **Drug or chemical induced diabetes mellitus with stable proliferative diabetic retinopathy**

New **E09.37** **Drug or chemical induced diabetes mellitus with diabetic macular edema, resolved following treatment**

New

One of the following 7th characters is to be assigned to code E09.37 to designate laterality of the disease:

1	right eye
2	left eye
3	bilateral
9	unspecified eye

New *New* *New* *New*

E10.32 **Type 1 diabetes mellitus with mild nonproliferative diabetic retinopathy**

New

One of the following 7th characters is to be assigned to codes in subcategory E10.32 to designate laterality of the disease:

1	right eye
2	left eye
3	bilateral
9	unspecified eye

New *New* *New* *New*

E10.33 **Type 1 diabetes mellitus with moderate nonproliferative diabetic retinopathy**

New

One of the following 7th characters is to be assigned to codes in subcategory E10.33 to designate laterality of the disease:

1	right eye
2	left eye
3	bilateral
9	unspecified eye

New *New* *New* *New*

E10.34 **Type 1 diabetes mellitus with severe nonproliferative diabetic retinopathy**

New

One of the following 7th characters is to be assigned to codes in subcategory E10.34 to designate laterality of the disease:

1	right eye
2	left eye
3	bilateral
9	unspecified eye

New *New* *New* *New*

E10.35 **Type 1 diabetes mellitus with proliferative diabetic retinopathy**

New

One of the following 7th characters is to be assigned to codes in subcategory E10.35 to designate laterality of the disease:

1	right eye
2	left eye
3	bilateral
9	unspecified eye

New *New* *New* *New*

New **E10.352** **Type 1 diabetes mellitus with proliferative diabetic retinopathy with traction retinal detachment involving the macula**

New **E10.353** **Type 1 diabetes mellitus with proliferative diabetic retinopathy with traction retinal detachment not involving the macula**

New **E10.354** **Type 1 diabetes mellitus with proliferative diabetic retinopathy with combined traction retinal detachment and rhegmatogenous retinal detachment**

New **E10.355** **Type 1 diabetes mellitus with stable proliferative diabetic retinopathy**

New **E10.37** **Type 1 diabetes mellitus with diabetic macular edema, resolved following treatment**

One of the following 7th characters is to be assigned to code E10.37 to designate laterality of the disease:

1	right eye
2	left eye
3	bilateral
9	unspecified eye

New *New* *New* *New*

E11 **Type 2 diabetes mellitus**

Revised Use additional code to identify control using:
New insulin (Z79.4)
New oral antidiabetic drugs (Z79.84)
New oral hypoglycemic drugs (Z79.84)

E11.32 **Type 2 diabetes mellitus with mild nonproliferative diabetic retinopathy**

New

One of the following 7th characters is to be assigned to codes in subcategory E11.32 to designate laterality of the disease:

1	right eye
2	left eye
3	bilateral
9	unspecified eye

New *New* *New* *New*

E11.33 **Type 2 diabetes mellitus with moderate nonproliferative diabetic retinopathy**

New

One of the following 7th characters is to be assigned to codes in subcategory E11.33 to designate laterality of the disease:

New	1 right eye
New	2 left eye
New	3 bilateral
New	9 unspecified eye

E11.34 **Type 2 diabetes mellitus with severe nonproliferative diabetic retinopathy**

New

One of the following 7th characters is to be assigned to codes in subcategory E11.34 to designate laterality of the disease:

New	1 right eye
New	2 left eye
New	3 bilateral
New	9 unspecified eye

E11.35 **Type 2 diabetes mellitus with proliferative diabetic retinopathy**

New

One of the following 7th characters is to be assigned to codes in subcategory E11.35 to designate laterality of the disease:

New	1 right eye
New	2 left eye
New	3 bilateral
New	9 unspecified eye

New **E11.352** **Type 2 diabetes mellitus with proliferative diabetic retinopathy with traction retinal detachment involving the macula**

New **E11.353** **Type 2 diabetes mellitus with proliferative diabetic retinopathy with traction retinal detachment not involving the macula**

New **E11.354** **Type 2 diabetes mellitus with proliferative diabetic retinopathy with combined traction retinal detachment and rhegmatogenous retinal detachment**

New **E11.355** **Type 2 diabetes mellitus with stable proliferative diabetic retinopathy**

New **E11.37** **Type 2 diabetes mellitus with diabetic macular edema, resolved following treatment**

New

One of the following 7th characters is to be assigned to code E11.37 to designate laterality of the disease:

New	1 right eye
New	2 left eye
New	3 bilateral
New	9 unspecified eye

E13 **Other specified diabetes mellitus**

Revised	Use additional code to identify control using:
New	insulin (Z79.4)
New	oral antidiabetic drugs (Z79.84)
New	oral hypoglycemic drugs (Z79.84)
New	**Excludes1** type 1 diabetes mellitus (E10.-)

E13.32 **Other specified diabetes mellitus with mild nonproliferative diabetic retinopathy**

New

One of the following 7th characters is to be assigned to codes in subcategory E13.32 to designate laterality of the disease:

New	1 right eye
New	2 left eye
New	3 bilateral
New	9 unspecified eye

E13.33 **Other specified diabetes mellitus with moderate nonproliferative diabetic retinopathy**

New

One of the following 7th characters is to be assigned to codes in subcategory E13.33 to designate laterality of the disease:

New	1 right eye
New	2 left eye
New	3 bilateral
New	9 unspecified eye

E13.34 **Other specified diabetes mellitus with severe nonproliferative diabetic retinopathy**

New

One of the following 7th characters is to be assigned to codes in subcategory E13.34 to designate laterality of the disease:

New	1 right eye
New	2 left eye
New	3 bilateral
New	9 unspecified eye

E13.35 **Other specified diabetes mellitus with proliferative diabetic retinopathy**

New

One of the following 7th characters is to be assigned to codes in subcategory E13.35 to designate laterality of the disease:

New	1 right eye
New	2 left eye
New	3 bilateral
New	9 unspecified eye

New **E13.352** **Other specified diabetes mellitus with proliferative diabetic retinopathy with traction retinal detachment involving the macula**

New **E13.353** **Other specified diabetes mellitus with proliferative diabetic retinopathy with traction retinal detachment not involving the macula**

New		E13.354	Other specified diabetes mellitus with proliferative diabetic retinopathy with combined traction retinal detachment and rhegmatogenous retinal detachment
New		E13.355	Other specified diabetes mellitus with stable proliferative diabetic retinopathy
New	E13.37		Other specified diabetes mellitus with diabetic macular edema, resolved following treatment
New			One of the following 7th characters is to be assigned to code E13.37 to designate laterality of the disease:

New	1 right eye
New	2 left eye
New	3 bilateral
New	9 unspecified eye

	E16.0	Drug-induced hypoglycemia without coma
New		**Excludes 1** diabetes with hypoglycemia without coma (E09.692)
	E16.1	Other hypoglycemia
New		**Excludes 1** diabetes with hypoglycemia (E08.649, E10.649, E11.649, E13.649)
	E16.2	Hypoglycemia, unspecified
New		**Excludes 1** diabetes with hypoglycemia (E08.649, E10.649, E11.649, E13.649)

	E29	Testicular dysfunction
Revised		**Excludes 1** Klinefelter's syndrome (Q98.0-Q98.1, Q98.4)

	E66.2	Morbid (severe) obesity with alveolar hypoventilation
New		Obesity hypoventilation syndrome (OHS)

	E78.0	Pure hypercholesterolemia
Deleted		Familial hypercholesterolemia
Deleted		Fredrickson's hyperlipoproteinemia, type IIa
Deleted		Hyperbetalipoproteinemia
Deleted		Hyperlipidemia, Group A
Deleted		Low-density-lipoprotein-type [LDL] hyperlipoproteinemia
New	E78.00	Pure hypercholesterolemia, unspecified
New		Fredrickson's hyperlipoproteinemia, type IIa
New		Hyperbetalipoproteinemia
New		Low-density-lipoprotein-type [LDL] hyperlipoproteinemia
New	E78.01	Familial hypercholesterolemia

	E84	Cystic fibrosis
New		Code also exocrine pancreatic insufficiency (K86.81)

	E85.0	Non-neuropathic heredofamilial amyloidosis
Deleted		Familial Mediterranean fever

	E86	Volume depletion
New		Use additional code(s) for any associated disorders of electrolyte and acid-base balance (E87.-)

	E88.42	MERRF syndrome
Revised		Code also progressive myoclonic epilepsy (G40.3-)
Revised	E89.81	Postprocedural hemorrhage of an endocrine system organ or structure following a procedure
Revised		E89.810 Postprocedural hemorrhage of an endocrine system organ or structure following an endocrine system procedure
Revised		E89.811 Postprocedural hemorrhage of an endocrine system organ or structure following other procedure
New	E89.82	Postprocedural hematoma and seroma of an endocrine system organ or structure
New		E89.820 Postprocedural hematoma of an endocrine system organ or structure following an endocrine system procedure
New		E89.821 Postprocedural hematoma of an endocrine system organ or structure following other procedure
New		E89.822 Postprocedural seroma of an endocrine system organ or structure following an endocrine system procedure
New		E89.823 Postprocedural seroma of an endocrine system organ or structure following other procedure

CHAPTER 5

MENTAL, BEHAVIORAL AND NEURODEVELOPMENTAL DISORDERS (F01-F99)

	F01.50	Vascular dementia without behavioral disturbance
New		Major neurocognitive disorder without behavioral disturbance
	F01.51	Vascular dementia with behavioral disturbance
New		Major neurocognitive disorder due to vascular disease, with behavioral disturbance
New		Major neurocognitive disorder with aggressive behavior
New		Major neurocognitive disorder with combative behavior
New		Major neurocognitive disorder with violent behavior

	F02	Dementia in other diseases classified elsewhere
		Code first the underlying physiological condition, such as:
New		dementia with Parkinsonism (G31.83)
New		Huntington's disease (G10)
New		prion disease (A81.9)
New		traumatic brain injury (S06.-)
New		**Includes** Major neurocognitive disorder in other diseases classified elsewhere
Deleted		**Excludes 1** dementia with Parkinsonism (G31.83)

	F02.80	**Dementia in other diseases classified elsewhere without behavioral disturbance**
New		Major neurocognitive disorder in other diseases classified elsewhere
	F02.81	**Dementia in other diseases classified elsewhere with behavioral disturbance**
New		Major neurocognitive disorder in other diseases classified elsewhere with aggressive behavior
New		Major neurocognitive disorder in other diseases classified elsewhere with combative behavior
New		Major neurocognitive disorder in other diseases classified elsewhere with violent behavior
	F06.1	**Catatonic disorder due to known physiological condition**
New		Catatonia associated with another mental disorder
New		Catatonia NOS
	F10.10	**Alcohol abuse, uncomplicated**
New		Alcohol use disorder, mild
	F10.14	**Alcohol abuse with alcohol-induced mood disorder**
New		Alcohol use disorder, mild, with alcohol-induced bipolar or related disorder
New		Alcohol use disorder, mild, with alcohol-induced depressive disorder
	F10.20	**Alcohol dependence, uncomplicated**
New		Alcohol use disorder, moderate
New		Alcohol use disorder, severe
	F10.22	**Alcohol dependence with intoxication**
		Acute drunkenness (in alcoholism)
Deleted		**Excludes1** alcohol dependence with withdrawal (F10.23-)
New		**Excludes2** alcohol dependence with withdrawal (F10.23-)
	F10.23	**Alcohol dependence with withdrawal**
Deleted		**Excludes1** alcohol dependence with intoxication (F10.22-)
New		**Excludes2** alcohol dependence with intoxication (F10.22-)
	F10.24	**Alcohol dependence with alcohol-induced mood disorder**
New		Alcohol use disorder, moderate, with alcohol-induced bipolar or related disorder
New		Alcohol use disorder, moderate, with alcohol-induced depressive disorder
New		Alcohol use disorder, severe, with alcohol-induced bipolar or related disorder
New		Alcohol use disorder, severe, with alcohol-induced depressive disorder
	F10.26	**Alcohol dependence with alcohol-induced persisting amnestic disorder**
New		Alcohol use disorder, moderate, with alcohol-induced major neurocognitive disorder, amnestic-confabulatory type
New		Alcohol use disorder, severe, with alcohol-induced major neurocognitive disorder, amnestic-confabulatory type

	F10.27	**Alcohol dependence with alcohol-induced persisting dementia**
New		Alcohol use disorder, moderate, with alcohol-induced major neurocognitive disorder, nonamnestic-confabulatory type
New		Alcohol use disorder, severe, with alcohol-induced major neurocognitive disorder, nonamnestic-confabulatory type
	F10.288	**Alcohol dependence with other alcohol-induced disorder**
New		Alcohol use disorder, moderate, with alcohol-induced mild neurocognitive disorder
New		Alcohol use disorder, severe, with alcohol-induced mild neurocognitive disorder
	F10.94	**Alcohol use, unspecified with alcohol-induced mood disorder**
New		Alcohol-induced bipolar or related disorder, without use disorder
New		Alcohol-induced depressive disorder, without use disorder
	F10.959	**Alcohol use, unspecified with alcohol-induced psychotic disorder, unspecified**
New		Alcohol-induced psychotic disorder without use disorder
	F10.96	**Alcohol use, unspecified with alcohol-induced persisting amnestic disorder**
New		Alcohol-induced major neurocognitive disorder, amnestic-confabulatory type, without use disorder
	F10.97	**Alcohol use, unspecified with alcohol-induced persisting dementia**
New		Alcohol-induced major neurocognitive disorder, nonamnestic-confabulatory type, without use disorder
	F10.980	**Alcohol use, unspecified with alcohol-induced anxiety disorder**
New		Alcohol-induced anxiety disorder, without use disorder
	F10.981	**Alcohol use, unspecified with alcohol-induced sexual dysfunction**
New		Alcohol-induced sexual dysfunction, without use disorder
	F10.982	**Alcohol use, unspecified with alcohol-induced sleep disorder**
New		Alcohol-induced sleep disorder, without use disorder
	F10.988	**Alcohol use, unspecified with other alcohol-induced disorder**
New		Alcohol-induced mild neurocognitive disorder, without use disorder
	F11.10	**Opioid abuse, uncomplicated**
		Opioid use disorder, mild
	F11.14	**Opioid abuse with opioid-induced mood disorder**
New		Opioid use disorder, mild, with opioid-induced depressive disorder

F11.20 **Opioid dependence, uncomplicated**
New   Opioid use disorder, moderate
New   Opioid use disorder, severe
F11.24 **Opioid dependence with opioid-induced mood disorder**
New   Opioid use disorder, moderate, with opioid-induced depressive disorder

   F11.921 **Opioid use, unspecified with intoxication delirium**
New   Opioid-induced delirium
F11.94 **Opioid use, unspecified with opioid-induced mood disorder**
New   Opioid-induced depressive disorder, without use disorder

   F11.981 **Opioid use, unspecified with opioid-induced sexual dysfunction**
New   Opioid-induced sexual dysfunction, without use disorder
   F11.982 **Opioid use, unspecified with opioid-induced sleep disorder**
New   Opioid-induced sleep disorder, without use disorder
   F11.988 **Opioid use, unspecified with other opioid-induced disorder**
New   Opioid-induced anxiety disorder, without use disorder

F12.10 **Cannabis abuse, uncomplicated**
New   Cannabis use disorder, mild

   F12.188 **Cannabis abuse with other cannabis-induced disorder**
New   Cannabis use disorder, mild, with cannabis-induced sleep disorder
F12.2 **Cannabis dependence**
   F12.20 **Cannabis dependence, uncomplicated**
New   Cannabis use disorder, moderate
New   Cannabis use disorder, severe

   F12.288 **Cannabis dependence with other cannabis-induced disorder**
New   Cannabis use disorder, moderate, with cannabis-induced sleep disorder
New   Cannabis use disorder, severe, with cannabis-induced sleep disorder
New   Cannabis withdrawal

   F12.959 **Cannabis use, unspecified with psychotic disorder, unspecified**
New   Cannabis-induced psychotic disorder, without use disorder

   F12.980 **Cannabis use, unspecified with anxiety disorder**
New   Cannabis-induced anxiety disorder, without use disorder
   F12.988 **Cannabis use, unspecified with other cannabis-induced disorder**
New   Cannabis-induced sleep disorder, without use disorder

F13.10 **Sedative, hypnotic or anxiolytic abuse, uncomplicated**
New   Sedative, hypnotic, or anxiolytic use disorder, mild
F13.14 **Sedative, hypnotic or anxiolytic abuse with sedative, hypnotic or anxiolytic-induced mood disorder**
New   Sedative, hypnotic, or anxiolytic use disorder, mild, with sedative, hypnotic, or anxiolytic-induced bipolar or related disorder
New   Sedative, hypnotic, or anxiolytic use disorder, mild, with sedative, hypnotic, or anxiolytic-induced depressive disorder

F13.23 **Sedative, hypnotic or anxiolytic dependence with withdrawal**
New   Sedative, hypnotic, or anxiolytic use disorder, moderate
New   Sedative, hypnotic, or anxiolytic use disorder, severe
   F13.232 **Sedative, hypnotic or anxiolytic dependence with withdrawal with perceptual disturbance**
New   Sedative, hypnotic, or anxiolytic withdrawal with perceptual disturbances
   F13.239 **Sedative, hypnotic or anxiolytic dependence with withdrawal, unspecified**
New   Sedative, hypnotic, or anxiolytic withdrawal without perceptual disturbances
F13.24 **Sedative, hypnotic or anxiolytic dependence with sedative, hypnotic or anxiolytic-induced mood disorder**
New   Sedative, hypnotic, or anxiolytic use disorder, moderate, with sedative, hypnotic, or anxiolytic-induced bipolar or related disorder
New   Sedative, hypnotic, or anxiolytic use disorder, moderate, with sedative, hypnotic, or anxiolytic-induced depressive disorder
New   Sedative, hypnotic, or anxiolytic use disorder, severe, with sedative, hypnotic, or anxiolytic-induced bipolar or related disorder
New   Sedative, hypnotic, or anxiolytic use disorder, severe, with sedative, hypnotic, or anxiolytic-induced depressive disorder
F13.27 **Sedative, hypnotic or anxiolytic dependence with sedative, hypnotic or anxiolytic-induced persisting dementia**
New   Sedative, hypnotic, or anxiolytic use disorder, moderate, with sedative, hypnotic, or anxiolytic-induced major neurocognitive disorder
New   Sedative, hypnotic, or anxiolytic use disorder, severe, with sedative, hypnotic, or anxiolytic-induced major neurocognitive disorder

F13.288   **Sedative, hypnotic or anxiolytic dependence with other sedative, hypnotic or anxiolytic-induced disorder**
New   Sedative, hypnotic, or anxiolytic use disorder, moderate, with sedative, hypnotic, or anxiolytic-induced mild neurocognitive disorder
New   Sedative, hypnotic, or anxiolytic use disorder, severe, with sedative, hypnotic, or anxiolytic-induced mild neurocognitive disorder

F13.921   **Sedative, hypnotic or anxiolytic use, unspecified with intoxication delirium**
New   Sedative, hypnotic, or anxiolytic-induced delirium

F13.94   **Sedative, hypnotic or anxiolytic use, unspecified with sedative, hypnotic or anxiolytic-induced mood disorder**
New   Sedative, hypnotic, or anxiolytic-induced bipolar or related disorder, without use disorder
New   Sedative, hypnotic, or anxiolytic-induced depressive disorder, without use disorder

F13.959   **Sedative, hypnotic or anxiolytic use, unspecified with sedative, hypnotic or anxiolytic-induced psychotic disorder, unspecified**
New   Sedative, hypnotic, or anxiolytic-induced psychotic disorder, without use disorder

F13.97   **Sedative, hypnotic or anxiolytic use, unspecified with sedative, hypnotic or anxiolytic-induced persisting dementia**
New   Sedative, hypnotic, or anxiolytic-induced major neurocognitive disorder, without use disorder

F13.980   **Sedative, hypnotic or anxiolytic use, unspecified with sedative, hypnotic or anxiolytic-induced anxiety disorder**
New   Sedative, hypnotic, or anxiolytic-induced anxiety disorder, without use disorder

F13.981   **Sedative, hypnotic or anxiolytic use, unspecified with sedative, hypnotic or anxiolytic-induced sexual dysfunction**
New   Sedative, hypnotic, or anxiolytic-induced sexual dysfunction disorder, without use disorder

F13.982   **Sedative, hypnotic or anxiolytic use, unspecified with sedative, hypnotic or anxiolytic-induced sleep disorder**
New   Sedative, hypnotic, or anxiolytic-induced sleep disorder, without use disorder

F13.988   **Sedative, hypnotic or anxiolytic use, unspecified with other sedative, hypnotic or anxiolytic-induced disorder**
New   Sedative, hypnotic, or anxiolytic-induced mild neurocognitive disorder

F14.10   **Cocaine abuse, uncomplicated**
New   Cocaine use disorder, mild

F14.14   **Cocaine abuse with cocaine-induced mood disorder**
New   Cocaine use disorder, mild, with cocaine-induced bipolar or related disorder
New   Cocaine use disorder, mild, with cocaine-induced depressive disorder

F14.188   **Cocaine abuse with other cocaine-induced disorder**
New   Cocaine use disorder, mild, with cocaine-induced obsessive-compulsive or related disorder

F14.20   **Cocaine dependence, uncomplicated**
New   Cocaine use disorder, moderate
New   Cocaine use disorder, severe

F14.24   **Cocaine dependence with cocaine-induced mood disorder**
New   Cocaine use disorder, moderate, with cocaine-induced bipolar or related disorder
New   Cocaine use disorder, moderate, with cocaine-induced depressive disorder
New   Cocaine use disorder, severe, with cocaine-induced bipolar or related disorder
New   Cocaine use disorder, severe, with cocaine-induced depressive disorder

F14.288   **Cocaine dependence with other cocaine-induced disorder**
New   Cocaine use disorder, moderate, with cocaine-induced obsessive-compulsive or related disorder
New   Cocaine use disorder, severe, with cocaine-induced obsessive-compulsive or related disorder

F14.94   **Cocaine use, unspecified with cocaine-induced mood disorder**
New   Cocaine-induced bipolar or related disorder, without use disorder
New   Cocaine-induced depressive disorder, without use disorder

New

F14.959 **Cocaine use, unspecified with cocaine-induced psychotic disorder, unspecified**
Cocaine-induced psychotic disorder, without use disorder

New

F14.980 **Cocaine use, unspecified with cocaine-induced anxiety disorder**
Cocaine-induced anxiety disorder, without use disorder

New

F14.981 **Cocaine use, unspecified with cocaine-induced sexual dysfunction**
Cocaine-induced sexual dysfunction, without use disorder

New

F14.982 **Cocaine use, unspecified with cocaine-induced sleep disorder**
Cocaine-induced sleep disorder, without use disorder

New

F14.988 **Cocaine use, unspecified with other cocaine-induced disorder**
Cocaine-induced obsessive-compulsive or related disorder

New

F15.10 **Other stimulant abuse, uncomplicated**
Amphetamine type substance use disorder, mild

New

Other or unspecified stimulant use disorder, mild

New

F15.122 **Other stimulant abuse with intoxication with perceptual disturbance**
Amphetamine or other stimulant use disorder, mild, with amphetamine or other stimulant intoxication, with perceptual disturbances

New

F15.129 **Other stimulant abuse with intoxication, unspecified**
Amphetamine or other stimulant use disorder, mild, with amphetamine or other stimulant intoxication, without perceptual disturbances

New

F15.14 **Other stimulant abuse with stimulant-induced mood disorder**
Amphetamine or other stimulant use disorder, mild, with amphetamine or other stimulant-induced bipolar or related disorder

New

Amphetamine or other stimulant use disorder, mild, with amphetamine or other stimulant-induced depressive disorder

New

F15.188 **Other stimulant abuse with other stimulant-induced disorder**
Amphetamine or other stimulant use disorder, mild, with amphetamine or other stimulant-induced obsessive-compulsive or related disorder

F15.20 **Other stimulant dependence, uncomplicated**

New

Amphetamine type substance use disorder, moderate

New

Amphetamine type substance use disorder, severe

New

Other or unspecified stimulant use disorder, moderate

New

Other or unspecified stimulant use disorder, severe

F15.222 **Other stimulant dependence with intoxication with perceptual disturbance**

New

Amphetamine or other stimulant use disorder, moderate, with amphetamine or other stimulant intoxication, with perceptual disturbances

New

Amphetamine or other stimulant use disorder, severe, with amphetamine or other stimulant intoxication, with perceptual disturbances

F15.229 **Other stimulant dependence with intoxication, unspecified**

New

Amphetamine or other stimulant use disorder, moderate, with amphetamine or other stimulant intoxication, without perceptual disturbances

Amphetamine or other stimulant use disorder, severe, with amphetamine or other stimulant intoxication, without perceptual disturbances

F15.23 **Other stimulant dependence with withdrawal**

New

Amphetamine or other stimulant withdrawal

F15.24 **Other stimulant dependence with stimulant-induced mood disorder**

New

Amphetamine or other stimulant use disorder, moderate, with amphetamine or other stimulant-induced bipolar or related disorder

New

Amphetamine or other stimulant use disorder, moderate, with amphetamine or other stimulant-induced depressive disorder

New

Amphetamine or other stimulant use disorder, severe, with amphetamine or other stimulant-induced bipolar or related disorder

New

Amphetamine or other stimulant use disorder, severe, with amphetamine or other stimulant-induced depressive disorder

F15.288   **Other stimulant dependence with other stimulant-induced disorder**

New

Amphetamine or other stimulant use disorder, moderate, with amphetamine or other stimulant-induced obsessive-compulsive or related disorder

New

Amphetamine or other stimulant use disorder, severe, with amphetamine or other stimulant-induced obsessive-compulsive or related disorder

F15.921   **Other stimulant use, unspecified with intoxication delirium**

New

Amphetamine or other stimulant-induced delirium

F15.929   **Other stimulant use, unspecified with intoxication, unspecified**

New

Caffeine intoxication

F15.93   **Other stimulant use, unspecified with withdrawal**

New

Caffeine withdrawal

F15.94   **Other stimulant use, unspecified with stimulant-induced mood disorder**

New

Amphetamine or other stimulant-induced bipolar or related disorder, without use disorder

New

Amphetamine or other stimulant-induced depressive disorder, without use disorder

F15.959   **Other stimulant use, unspecified with stimulant-induced psychotic disorder, unspecified**

New

Amphetamine or other stimulant-induced psychotic disorder, without use disorder

F15.980   **Other stimulant use, unspecified with stimulant-induced anxiety disorder**

New

Amphetamine or other stimulant-induced anxiety disorder, without use disorder

New

Caffeine-induced anxiety disorder, without use disorder

F15.981   **Other stimulant use, unspecified with stimulant-induced sexual dysfunction**

New

Amphetamine or other stimulant-induced sexual dysfunction, without use disorder

F15.982   **Other stimulant use, unspecified with stimulant-induced sleep disorder**

New

Amphetamine or other stimulant-induced sleep disorder, without use disorder

New

Caffeine-induced sleep disorder, without use disorder

F15.988   **Other stimulant use, unspecified with other stimulant-induced disorder**

New

Amphetamine or other stimulant-induced obsessive-compulsive or related disorder, without use disorder

F16.10   **Hallucinogen abuse, uncomplicated**

New   Other hallucinogen use disorder, mild
New   Phencyclidine use disorder, mild

F16.14   **Hallucinogen abuse with hallucinogen-induced mood disorder**

New

Other hallucinogen use disorder, mild, with other hallucinogen-induced bipolar or related disorder

New

Other hallucinogen use disorder, mild, with other hallucinogen-induced depressive disorder

New

Phencyclidine use disorder, mild, with phencyclidine-induced bipolar or related disorder

New

Phencyclidine use disorder, mild, with phencyclidine-induced depressive disorder

F16.20   **Hallucinogen dependence, uncomplicated**

New

Other hallucinogen use disorder, moderate

New   Other hallucinogen use disorder, severe
New   Phencyclidine use disorder, moderate
New   Phencyclidine use disorder, severe

F16.24   **Hallucinogen dependence with hallucinogen-induced mood disorder**

New

Other hallucinogen use disorder, moderate, with other hallucinogen-induced bipolar or related disorder

New

Other hallucinogen use disorder, moderate, with other hallucinogen-induced depressive disorder

New

Other hallucinogen use disorder, severe, with other hallucinogen-induced bipolar or related disorder

New

Other hallucinogen use disorder, severe, with other hallucinogen-induced depressive disorder

New

Phencyclidine use disorder, moderate, with phencyclidine-induced bipolar or related disorder

New

Phencyclidine use disorder, moderate, with phencyclidine-induced depressive disorder

New

Phencyclidine use disorder, severe, with phencyclidine-induced bipolar or related disorder

New

Phencyclidine use disorder, severe, with phencyclidine-induced depressive disorder

	F16.921 Hallucinogen use, unspecified with intoxication with delirium
New	Other hallucinogen intoxication delirium
	F16.94 Hallucinogen use, unspecified with hallucinogen-induced mood disorder
New	Other hallucinogen-induced bipolar or related disorder, without use disorder
New	Other hallucinogen-induced depressive disorder, without use disorder
New	Phencyclidine-induced bipolar or related disorder, without use disorder
New	Phencyclidine-induced depressive disorder, without use disorder
	F16.959 Hallucinogen use, unspecified with hallucinogen-induced psychotic disorder, unspecified
New	Other hallucinogen-induced psychotic disorder, without use disorder
New	Phencyclidine-induced psychotic disorder, without use disorder
	F16.980 Hallucinogen use, unspecified with hallucinogen-induced anxiety disorder
New	Other hallucinogen-induced anxiety disorder, without use disorder
New	Phencyclidine-induced anxiety disorder, without use disorder
	F17.200 Nicotine dependence, unspecified, uncomplicated
New	Tobacco use disorder, mild
New	Tobacco use disorder, moderate
New	Tobacco use disorder, severe
	F17.203 Nicotine dependence unspecified, with withdrawal
New	Tobacco withdrawal
	F18.10 Inhalant abuse, uncomplicated
New	Inhalant use disorder, mild
	F18.14 Inhalant abuse with inhalant-induced mood disorder
New	Inhalant use disorder, mild, with inhalant-induced depressive disorder
	F18.17 Inhalant abuse with inhalant-induced dementia
New	Inhalant use disorder, mild, with inhalant-induced major neurocognitive disorder
	F18.188 Inhalant abuse with other inhalant-induced disorder
New	Inhalant use disorder, mild, with inhalant-induced mild neurocognitive disorder

	F18.20 Inhalant dependence, uncomplicated
New	Inhalant use disorder, moderate
New	Inhalant use disorder, severe
	F18.24 Inhalant dependence with inhalant-induced mood disorder
New	Inhalant use disorder, moderate, with inhalant-induced depressive disorder
New	Inhalant use disorder, severe, with inhalant-induced depressive disorder
	F18.27 Inhalant dependence with inhalant-induced dementia
New	Inhalant use disorder, moderate, with inhalant-induced major neurocognitive disorder
New	Inhalant use disorder, severe, with inhalant-induced major neurocognitive disorder
	F18.288 Inhalant dependence with other inhalant-induced disorder
New	Inhalant use disorder, moderate, with inhalant-induced mild neurocognitive disorder
New	Inhalant use disorder, severe, with inhalant-induced mild neurocognitive disorder
	F18.94 Inhalant use, unspecified with inhalant-induced mood disorder
	Inhalant-induced depressive disorder
	F18.97 Inhalant use, unspecified with inhalant-induced persisting dementia
New	Inhalant-induced major neurocognitive disorder
	F18.988 Inhalant use, unspecified with other inhalant-induced disorder
New	Inhalant-induced mild neurocognitive disorder
	F19.10 Other psychoactive substance abuse, uncomplicated
New	Other (or unknown) substance use disorder, mild
	F19.14 Other psychoactive substance abuse with psychoactive substance-induced mood disorder
New	Other (or unknown) substance use disorder, mild, with other (or unknown) substance-induced bipolar or related disorder
New	Other (or unknown) substance use disorder, mild, with other (or unknown) substance-induced depressive disorder
	F19.17 Other psychoactive substance abuse with psychoactive substance-induced persisting dementia
New	Other (or unknown) substance use disorder, mild, with other (or unknown) substance-induced major neurocognitive disorder

	F19.188	**Other psychoactive substance abuse with other psychoactive substance-induced disorder**
New		Other (or unknown) substance use disorder, mild, with other (or unknown) substance-induced mild neurocognitive disorder
New		Other (or unknown) substance use disorder, mild, with other (or unknown) substance-induced obsessive-compulsive or related disorder
	F19.20	**Other psychoactive substance dependence, uncomplicated**
New		Other (or unknown) substance use disorder, moderate
New		Other (or unknown) substance use disorder, severe
	F19.24	**Other psychoactive substance dependence with psychoactive substance-induced mood disorder**
New		Other (or unknown) substance use disorder, moderate, with other (or unknown) substance-induced bipolar or related disorder
New		Other (or unknown) substance use disorder, moderate, with other (or unknown) substance-induced depressive disorder
New		Other (or unknown) substance use disorder, severe, with other (or unknown) substance-induced bipolar or related disorder
New		Other (or unknown) substance use disorder, severe, with other (or unknown) substance-induced depressive disorder
	F19.27	**Other psychoactive substance dependence with psychoactive substance-induced persisting dementia**
New		Other (or unknown) substance use disorder, moderate, with other (or unknown) substance-induced major neurocognitive disorder
New		Other (or unknown) substance use disorder, severe, with other (or unknown) substance-induced major neurocognitive disorder
	F19.288	**Other psychoactive substance dependence with other psychoactive substance-induced disorder**
New		Other (or unknown) substance use disorder, moderate, with other (or unknown) substance-induced mild neurocognitive disorder
New		Other (or unknown) substance use disorder, severe, with other (or unknown) substance-induced mild neurocognitive disorder
New		Other (or unknown) substance use disorder, moderate, with other (or unknown) substance-induced obsessive-compulsive or related disorder
New		Other (or unknown) substance use disorder, severe, with other (or unknown) substance-induced obsessive-compulsive or related disorder

	F19.921	**Other psychoactive substance use, unspecified with intoxication with delirium**
New		Other (or unknown) substance-induced delirium
	F19.94	**Other psychoactive substance use, unspecified with psychoactive substance-induced mood disorder**
New		Other (or unknown) substance-induced bipolar or related disorder, without use disorder
New		Other (or unknown) substance-induced depressive disorder, without use disorder
	F19.959	**Other psychoactive substance use, unspecified with psychoactive substance-induced psychotic disorder, unspecified**
New		Other or unknown substance-induced psychotic disorder, without use disorder
	F19.97	**Other psychoactive substance use, unspecified with psychoactive substance-induced persisting dementia**
New		Other (or unknown) substance-induced major neurocognitive disorder, without use disorder
	F19.980	**Other psychoactive substance use, unspecified with psychoactive substance-induced anxiety disorder**
New		Other (or unknown) substance-induced anxiety disorder, without use disorder
	F19.981	**Other psychoactive substance use, unspecified with psychoactive substance-induced sexual dysfunction**
New		Other (or unknown) substance-induced sexual dysfunction, without use disorder
	F19.982	**Other psychoactive substance use, unspecified with psychoactive substance-induced sleep disorder**
New		Other (or unknown) substance-induced sleep disorder, without use disorder
	F19.988	**Other psychoactive substance use, unspecified with other psychoactive substance-induced disorder**
New		Other (or unknown) substance-induced mild neurocognitive disorder, without use disorder
New		Other (or unknown) substance-induced obsessive-compulsive or related disorder, without use disorder
	F20.3	**Undifferentiated schizophrenia**
Revised		**Excludes2** post-schizophrenic depression (F32.89)

	F32.8	**Other depressive episodes**
Deleted		Atypical depression
Deleted		Post-schizophrenic depression
Deleted		Single episode of 'masked' depression NOS
New	**F32.81**	**Premenstrual dysphoric disorder**
New		**Excludes1** premenstrual tension syndrome (N94.3)
New	**F32.89**	**Other specified depressive episodes**
New		Atypical depression
New		Post-schizophrenic depression
New		Single episode of 'masked' depression NOS

	F34.1	**Dysthymic disorder**
New		Persistent depressive disorder
	F34.8	**Other persistent mood [affective] disorders**
New	**F34.81**	**Disruptive mood dysregulation disorder**
New	**F34.89**	**Other specified persistent mood disorders**

	F42	**Obsessive-compulsive disorder**
Deleted		Anancastic neurosis
Deleted		Obsessive-compulsive neurosis
New	**F42.2**	**Mixed obsessional thoughts and acts**
New	**F42.3**	**Hoarding disorder**
New	**F42.4**	**Excoriation (skin-picking) disorder**
New		**Excludes1** factitial dermatitis (L98.1)
New		other specified behavioral and emotional disorders with onset usually occurring in early childhood and adolescence (F98.8)
New	**F42.8**	**Other obsessive-compulsive disorder**
New		Anancastic neurosis
New		Obsessive-compulsive neurosis
New	**F42.9**	**Obsessive-compulsive disorder, unspecified**

	F43.8	**Other reactions to severe stress**
New		Other specified trauma and stressor-related disorder
	F43.9	**Reaction to severe stress, unspecified**
New		Trauma and stressor-related disorder, NOS

	F44.0	**Dissociative amnesia**
New		**Excludes1** dissociative amnesia with dissociative fugue (F44.1)
	F44.1	**Dissociative fugue**
		Dissociative amnesia with dissociative fugue

	F45.1	**Undifferentiated somatoform disorder**
New		Somatic symptom disorder
	F45.21	**Hypochondriasis**
New		Illness anxiety disorder

	F50.0	**Anorexia nervosa**
Revised		**Excludes1** psychogenic loss of appetite (F50.89)
	F50.8	**Other eating disorders**
Deleted		Pica in adults
Deleted		Psychogenic loss of appetite
New	**F50.81**	**Binge eating disorder**
New	**F50.89**	**Other specified eating disorder**
New		Pica in adults
New		Psychogenic loss of appetite

	F52.0	**Hypoactive sexual desire disorder**
Deleted		Anhedonia (sexual)
New		Sexual anhedonia
	F52.22	**Female sexual arousal disorder**
Deleted		Frigidity
	F52.32	**Male orgasmic disorder**
New		Delayed ejaculation

	F52.6	**Dyspareunia not due to a substance or known physiological condition**
New		Genito-pelvic pain penetration disorder
Revised		**Excludes2** dyspareunia (due to a known physiological condition) (N94.1-)

	F60.5	**Obsessive-compulsive personality disorder**
Revised		**Excludes2** obsessive-compulsive disorder (F42-)

	F64.0	**Transsexualism**
New		Gender identity disorder in adolescence and adulthood
New		Gender dysphoria in adolescents and adults
Revised	**F64.1**	**Dual role transvestism**
Deleted		Dual role transvestism
Deleted		Transvestism
	F64.2	**Gender identity disorder of childhood**
New		Gender dysphoria in children
Revised		**Excludes1** gender identity disorder in adolescence and adulthood (F64.0)

	F80.0	**Phonological disorder**
New		Speech-sound disorder
	F80.8	**Other developmental disorders of speech or language**
New	**F80.82**	**Social pragmatic communication disorder**
New		**Excludes1** Asperger's syndrome (F84.5)
New		autistic disorder (F84.0)

	F84.0	**Autistic disorder**
New		Autism spectrum disorder

	F88	**Other disorders of psychological development**
New		Global developmental delay
New		Other specified neurodevelopmental disorder
	F89	**Unspecified disorder of psychological development**
New		Neurodevelopmental disorder NOS

	F91.8	**Other conduct disorders**
New		Other specified conduct disorder
New		Other specified disruptive disorder
	F91.9	**Conduct disorder, unspecified**
New		Disruptive disorder NOS

	F95.0	**Transient tic disorder**
New		Provisional tic disorder

	F98	**Other behavioral and emotional disorders with onset usually occurring in childhood and adolescence**
Revised		**Excludes2** obsessive-compulsive disorder (F42-)
	F98.4	**Stereotyped movement disorders**
Revised		**Excludes2** compulsions in obsessive-compulsive disorder (F42-)

CHAPTER 6

DISEASES OF THE NERVOUS SYSTEM (G00-G99)

	G00.1	**Pneumococcal meningitis**
New		Meningitis due to Streptococcal pneumoniae
	G31.84	**Mild cognitive impairment, so stated**
Revised		**Excludes1** cognitive deficits following (sequelae of) cerebral hemorrhage or infarction (I69.01-, I69.11-, I69.21-, I69.31-, I69.81-, I69.91-)

	G40	Epilepsy and recurrent seizures
Deleted		**Excludes1** hippocampal sclerosis (G93.81)
Deleted		mesial temporal sclerosis (G93.81)
Deleted		temporal sclerosis (G93.81)
Deleted		Todd's paralysis (G83.8)
New		**Excludes2** hippocampal sclerosis (G93.81)
New		mesial temporal sclerosis (G93.81)
New		temporal sclerosis (G93.81)
New		Todd's paralysis (G83.84)

G56.0 Carpal tunnel syndrome
New G56.03 Carpal tunnel syndrome, bilateral upper limbs

G56.1 Other lesions of median nerve
New G56.13 Other lesions of median nerve, bilateral upper limbs

G56.2 Lesion of ulnar nerve
New G56.23 Lesion of ulnar nerve, bilateral upper limbs

G56.3 Lesion of radial nerve
New G56.33 Lesion of radial nerve, bilateral upper limbs

G56.4 Causalgia of upper limb
New G56.43 Causalgia of bilateral upper limbs

G56.8 Other specified mononeuropathies of upper limb
New G56.83 Other specified mononeuropathies of bilateral upper limbs

G56.9 Unspecified mononeuropathy of upper limb
New G56.93 Unspecified mononeuropathy of bilateral upper limbs

G57.0 Lesion of sciatic nerve
New G57.03 Lesion of sciatic nerve, bilateral lower limbs

G57.1 Meralgia paresthetica
New G57.13 Meralgia paresthetica, bilateral lower limbs

G57.2 Lesion of femoral nerve
New G57.23 Lesion of femoral nerve, bilateral lower limbs

G57.3 Lesion of lateral popliteal nerve
New G57.33 Lesion of lateral popliteal nerve, bilateral lower limbs

G57.4 Lesion of medial popliteal nerve
New G57.43 Lesion of medial popliteal nerve, bilateral lower limbs

G57.5 Tarsal tunnel syndrome
New G57.53 Tarsal tunnel syndrome, bilateral lower limbs

G57.6 Lesion of plantar nerve
New G57.63 Lesion of plantar nerve, bilateral lower limbs

G57.7 Causalgia of lower limb
New G57.73 Causalgia of bilateral lower limbs

G57.8 Other specified mononeuropathies of lower limb
New G57.83 Other specified mononeuropathies of bilateral lower limbs

G57.9 Unspecified mononeuropathy of lower limb
New G57.93 Unspecified mononeuropathy of bilateral lower limbs

G61.8 Other inflammatory polyneuropathies
New G61.82 Multifocal motor neuropathy
New MMN

G89 Pain, not elsewhere classified
Revised **Excludes2** pain from prosthetic devices, implants, and grafts (T82.84, T83.84, T84.84, T85.84-)

G97 Intraoperative and postprocedural complications and disorders of nervous system, not elsewhere classified
Revised G97.5 Postprocedural hemorrhage of a nervous system organ or structure following a procedure
Revised G97.51 Postprocedural hemorrhage of a nervous system organ or structure following a nervous system procedure
Revised G97.52 Postprocedural hemorrhage of a nervous system organ or structure following other procedure
New G97.6 Postprocedural hematoma and seroma of a nervous system organ or structure following a procedure
New G97.61 Postprocedural hematoma of a nervous system organ or structure following a nervous system procedure
New G97.62 Postprocedural hematoma of a nervous system organ or structure following other procedure
New G97.63 Postprocedural seroma of a nervous system organ or structure following a nervous system procedure
New G97.64 Postprocedural seroma of a nervous system organ or structure following other procedure

CHAPTER 7

DISEASES OF THE EYE AND ADNEXA (H00-H59)

H34.81 Central retinal vein occlusion
New One of the following 7th characters is to be assigned to codes in subcategory H34.81 to designate the severity of the occlusion:

New 0 with macular edema
New 1 with retinal neovascularization
New 2 stable
New Old central retinal vein occlusion

H34.83 Tributary (branch) retinal vein occlusion
New One of the following 7th characters is to be assigned to codes in subcategory H34.83 to designate the severity of the occlusion:

New 0 with macular edema
New 1 with retinal neovascularization
New 2 stable
New Old tributary (branch) retinal vein occlusion

	H35.31	Nonexudative age-related macular degeneration
New		Dry age-related macular degeneration
New		One of the following 7th characters is to be assigned to codes in subcategory H35.31 to designate the stage of the disease:

New	Ø	stage unspecified
New	1	early dry stage
New	2	intermediate dry stage
New	3	advanced atrophic without subfoveal involvement
New		advanced dry stage
New	4	advanced atrophic with subfoveal involvement

New	H35.311	Nonexudative age-related macular degeneration, right eye
New	H35.312	Nonexudative age-related macular degeneration, left eye
New	H35.313	Nonexudative age-related macular degeneration, bilateral
New	H35.319	Nonexudative age-related macular degeneration, unspecified eye
	H35.32	Exudative age-related macular degeneration
New		Wet age-related macular degeneration
New		One of the following 7th characters is to be assigned to codes in subcategory H35.32 to designate the stage of the disease:

New	Ø	stage unspecified
New	1	with active choroidal neovascularization
New	2	with inactive choroidal neovascularization
New		with involuted or regressed neovascularization
New	3	with inactive scar

New	H35.321	Exudative age-related macular degeneration, right eye
New	H35.322	Exudative age-related macular degeneration, left eye
New	H35.323	Exudative age-related macular degeneration, bilateral
New	H35.329	Exudative age-related macular degeneration, unspecified eye
	H40.11	Primary open-angle glaucoma
New	H40.111	Primary open-angle glaucoma, right eye
New	H40.112	Primary open-angle glaucoma, left eye
New	H40.113	Primary open-angle glaucoma, bilateral
New	H40.119	Primary open-angle glaucoma, unspecified eye

	H42	**Glaucoma in diseases classified elsewhere**
Revised	**Excludes1**	glaucoma (in) onchocerciasis (B73.02)
Deleted		diabetes mellitus (E08.39, E09.39, E10.39, E11.39, E13.39)
Deleted		onchocerciasis (B73.02)
Revised		glaucoma (in) syphilis (A52.71)
Revised		glaucoma (in) tuberculous (A18.59)
New	**Excludes2**	glaucoma (in) diabetes mellitus (E08.39, E09.39, E10.39, E11.39, E13.39)

	H53.0	Amblyopia ex anopsia
New	**H53.04**	Amblyopia suspect
New	H53.041	Amblyopia suspect, right eye
New	H53.042	Amblyopia suspect, left eye
New	H53.043	Amblyopia suspect, bilateral
New	H53.049	Amblyopia suspect, unspecified eye

	H59	**Intraoperative and postprocedural complications and disorders of eye and adnexa, not elsewhere classified**
Revised	**H59.3**	Postprocedural hemorrhage, hematoma, and seroma of eye and adnexa following other procedure
Revised	H59.31	Postprocedural hemorrhage of eye and adnexa following an ophthalmic procedure
Revised	H59.311	Postprocedural hemorrhage of right eye and avdnexa following an ophthalmic procedure
Revised	H59.312	Postprocedural hemorrhage of left eye and adnexa following an ophthalmic procedure
Revised	H59.313	Postprocedural hemorrhage of eye and adnexa following an ophthalmic procedure, bilateral
Revised	H59.319	Postprocedural hemorrhage of unspecified eye and adnexa following an ophthalmic procedure
Revised	H59.32	Postprocedural hemorrhage of eye and adnexa following other procedure
Revised	H59.321	Postprocedural hemorrhage of right eye and adnexa following other procedure
Revised	H59.322	Postprocedural hemorrhage of left eye and adnexa following other procedure
Revised	H59.323	Postprocedural hemorrhage of eye and adnexa following other procedure, bilateral
Revised	H59.329	Postprocedural hemorrhage of unspecified eye and adnexa following other procedure
New	H59.33	Postprocedural hematoma of eye and adnexa following an ophthalmic procedure
New	H59.331	Postprocedural hematoma of right eye and adnexa following an ophthalmic procedure
New	H59.332	Postprocedural hematoma of left eye and adnexa following an ophthalmic procedure
New	H59.333	Postprocedural hematoma of eye and adnexa following an ophthalmic procedure, bilateral
New	H59.339	Postprocedural hematoma of unspecified eye and adnexa following an ophthalmic procedure
New	H59.34	Postprocedural hematoma of eye and adnexa following other procedure
New	H59.341	Postprocedural hematoma of right eye and adnexa following other procedure
New	H59.342	Postprocedural hematoma of left eye and adnexa following other procedure
New	H59.343	Postprocedural hematoma of eye and adnexa following other procedure, bilateral
New	H59.349	Postprocedural hematoma of unspecified eye and adnexa following other procedure

New		H59.35	Postprocedural seroma of eye and adnexa following an ophthalmic procedure
New			H59.351 Postprocedural seroma of right eye and adnexa following an ophthalmic procedure
New			H59.352 Postprocedural seroma of left eye and adnexa following an ophthalmic procedure
New			H59.353 Postprocedural seroma of eye and adnexa following an ophthalmic procedure, bilateral
New			H59.359 Postprocedural seroma of unspecified eye and adnexa following an ophthalmic procedure
New		H59.36	Postprocedural seroma of eye and adnexa following other procedure
New			H59.361 Postprocedural seroma of right eye and adnexa following other procedure
New			H59.362 Postprocedural seroma of left eye and adnexa following other procedure
New			H59.363 Postprocedural seroma of eye and adnexa following other procedure, bilateral
New			H59.369 Postprocedural seroma of unspecified eye and adnexa following other procedure

CHAPTER 8

DISEASES OF THE EAR AND MASTOID PROCESS (H60-H95)

	H65	**Nonsuppurative otitis media**
	H66	**Suppurative and unspecified otitis media**
		Use additional code to identify:
New		history of tobacco dependence (Z87.891)

	H90	**Conductive and sensorineural hearing loss**	
New		H90.A	Conductive and sensorineural hearing loss with restricted hearing on the contralateral side
New		H90.A1	Conductive hearing loss, unilateral, with restricted hearing on the contralateral side
New			H90.A11 Conductive hearing loss, unilateral, right ear with restricted hearing on the contralateral side
New			H90.A12 Conductive hearing loss, unilateral, left ear with restricted hearing on the contralateral side
New		H90.A2	Sensorineural hearing loss, unilateral, with restricted hearing on the contralateral side
New			H90.A21 Sensorineural hearing loss, unilateral, right ear, with restricted hearing on the contralateral side
New			H90.A22 Sensorineural hearing loss, unilateral, left ear, with restricted hearing on the contralateral side

New			H90.A3 Mixed conductive and sensorineural hearing loss, unilateral with restricted hearing on the contralateral side
New			H90.A31 Mixed conductive and sensorineural hearing loss, unilateral, right ear with restricted hearing on the contralateral side
New			H90.A32 Mixed conductive and sensorineural hearing loss, unilateral, left ear with restricted hearing on the contralateral side
	H93	**Other disorders of ear, not elsewhere classified**	
New		H93.A	Pulsatile tinnitus
New			H93.A1 Pulsatile tinnitus, right ear
New			H93.A2 Pulsatile tinnitus, left ear
New			H93.A3 Pulsatile tinnitus, bilateral
New			H93.A9 Pulsatile tinnitus, unspecified ear
	H95	**Intraoperative and postprocedural complications and disorders of ear and mastoid process, not elsewhere classified**	
Revised		H95.4	Postprocedural hemorrhage of ear and mastoid process following a procedure
Revised			H95.41 Postprocedural hemorrhage of ear and mastoid process following a procedure on the ear and mastoid process
Revised			H95.42 Postprocedural hemorrhage of ear and mastoid process following other procedure
New		H95.5	Postprocedural hematoma and seroma of ear and mastoid process following a procedure
New			H95.51 Postprocedural hematoma of ear and mastoid process following a procedure on the ear and mastoid process
New			H95.52 Postprocedural hematoma of ear and mastoid process following other procedure
New			H95.53 Postprocedural seroma of ear and mastoid process following a procedure on the ear and mastoid process
New			H95.54 Postprocedural seroma of ear and mastoid process following other procedure

CHAPTER 9 DISEASES OF THE CIRCULATORY SYSTEM (I00-I99)

This chapter contains the following blocks:

Revised	I10-I16	Hypertensive diseases

HYPERTENSIVE DISEASES (I10-I16)

		Use additional code to identify:
Revised		history of tobacco dependence (Z87.891)
New		**Excludes2** hypertensive disease complicating pregnancy, childbirth and the puerperium (O10-O11, O13-O16)

New	**I16**	**Hypertensive crisis**	
New		Code also any identified hypertensive disease (I10-I15)	
New		I16.0	**Hypertensive urgency**
New		I16.1	**Hypertensive emergency**
New		I16.9	**Hypertensive crisis, unspecified**

ISCHEMIC HEART DISEASES (I20-I25)

Revised Use additional code to identify presence of hypertension (I10-I16)

I20 **Angina pectoris**
Use additional code to identify:
Revised history of tobacco dependence (Z87.891)

I20.8 **Other forms of angina pectoris**
New Stable angina

I21 **ST elevation (STEMI) and non-ST elevation (NSTEMI) myocardial infarction**

I22 **Subsequent ST elevation (STEMI) and non-ST elevation (NSTEMI) myocardial infarction**

I25 **Chronic ischemic heart disease**
Use additional code to identify:
Revised history of tobacco dependence (Z87.891)

I42 **Cardiomyopathy**
Deleted **Excludes1** ischemic cardiomyopathy (I25.5)
Deleted peripartum cardiomyopathy (O90.3)
New **Excludes2** ischemic cardiomyopathy (I25.5)
New peripartum cardiomyopathy (O90.3)

I50 **Heart failure**
Deleted **Excludes1** cardiac arrest (I46.-)
New **Excludes2** cardiac arrest (I46.-)

I50.9 **Heart failure, unspecified**
Deleted **Excludes1** fluid overload (E87.70)
New **Excludes2** fluid overload (E87.70)

CEREBROVASCULAR DISEASES (I60-I69)

Revised Use additional code to identify presence of:
history of tobacco dependence (Z87.891)

I60 **Nontraumatic subarachnoid hemorrhage**
Deleted **Excludes1** sequelae of subarachnoid hemorrhage (I69.0-)
New **Excludes2** sequelae of subarachnoid hemorrhage (I69.0-)

I60.2 **Nontraumatic subarachnoid hemorrhage from anterior communicating artery**
Deleted I60.20 Nontraumatic subarachnoid hemorrhage from unspecified anterior communicating artery
Deleted I60.21 Nontraumatic subarachnoid hemorrhage from right anterior communicating artery
Deleted I60.22 Nontraumatic subarachnoid hemorrhage from left anterior communicating artery

I61 **Nontraumatic intracerebral hemorrhage**
Deleted **Excludes1** sequelae of intracerebral hemorrhage (I69.1-)
New **Excludes2** sequelae of intracerebral hemorrhage (I69.1-)

I62 **Other and unspecified nontraumatic intracranial hemorrhage**
Deleted **Excludes1** sequelae of intracerebral hemorrhage (I69.2)
New **Excludes2** sequelae of intracranial hemorrhage (I69.2)

I63 **Cerebral infarction**
New Use additional code, if known, to indicate National Institutes of Health Stroke Scale (NIHSS) score (R29.7-)
Deleted **Excludes1** sequelae of cerebral infarction (I69.3-)
New **Excludes2** sequelae of cerebral infarction (I69.3-)
New **I63.013** **Cerebral infarction due to thrombosis of bilateral vertebral arteries**

I63.03 **Cerebral infarction due to thrombosis of carotid artery**
New **I63.033** **Cerebral infarction due to thrombosis of bilateral carotid arteries**
New **I63.113** **Cerebral infarction due to embolism of bilateral vertebral arteries**
New **I63.133** **Cerebral infarction due to embolism of bilateral carotid arteries**
New **I63.213** **Cerebral infarction due to unspecified occlusion or stenosis of bilateral vertebral arteries**
New **I63.233** **Cerebral infarction due to unspecified occlusion or stenosis of bilateral carotid arteries**
New **I63.313** **Cerebral infarction due to thrombosis of bilateral middle cerebral arteries**
New **I63.323** **Cerebral infarction due to thrombosis of bilateral anterior arteries**
New **I63.333** **Cerebral infarction to thrombosis of bilateral posterior arteries**
New **I63.343** **Cerebral infarction to thrombosis of bilateral cerebellar arteries**
New **I63.413** **Cerebral infarction due to embolism of bilateral middle cerebral arteries**
New **I63.423** **Cerebral infarction due to embolism of bilateral anterior cerebral arteries**
New **I63.433** **Cerebral infarction due to embolism of bilateral posterior cerebral arteries**
New **I63.443** **Cerebral infarction due to embolism of bilateral cerebellar arteries**
New **I63.513** **Cerebral infarction due to unspecified occlusion or stenosis of bilateral middle arteries**

New		I63.523	Cerebral infarction due to unspecified occlusion or stenosis of bilateral anterior arteries
New		I63.533	Cerebral infarction due to unspecified occlusion or stenosis of bilateral posterior arteries
New		I63.543	Cerebral infarction due to unspecified occlusion or stenosis of bilateral cerebellar arteries

	I67		Other cerebrovascular diseases
Deleted		**Excludes1**	sequelae of the listed conditions (I69.8)
New		**Excludes2**	sequelae of the listed conditions (I69.8)
New		I69.010	Attention and concentration deficit following nontraumatic subarachnoid hemorrhage
New		I69.011	Memory deficit following nontraumatic subarachnoid hemorrhage
New		I69.012	Visuospatial deficit and spatial neglect following nontraumatic subarachnoid hemorrhage
New		I69.013	Psychomotor deficit following nontraumatic subarachnoid hemorrhage
New		I69.014	Frontal lobe and executive function deficit following nontraumatic subarachnoid hemorrhage
New		I69.015	Cognitive social or emotional deficit following nontraumatic subarachnoid hemorrhage
New		I69.018	Other symptoms and signs involving cognitive functions following nontraumatic subarachnoid hemorrhage
New		I69.019	Unspecified symptoms and signs involving cognitive functions following nontraumatic subarachnoid hemorrhage
New		I69.110	Attention and concentration deficit following nontraumatic intracerebral hemorrhage
New		I69.111	Memory deficit following nontraumatic intracerebral hemorrhage
New		I69.112	Visuospatial deficit and spatial neglect following nontraumatic intracerebral hemorrhage
New		I69.113	Psychomotor deficit following nontraumatic intracerebral hemorrhage
New		I69.114	Frontal lobe and executive function deficit following nontraumatic intracerebral hemorrhage
New		I69.115	Cognitive social or emotional deficit following nontraumatic intracerebral hemorrhage
New		I69.118	Other symptoms and signs involving cognitive functions following nontraumatic intracerebral hemorrhage
New		I69.119	Unspecified symptoms and signs involving cognitive functions following nontraumatic intracerebral hemorrhage

		I69.123	Fluency disorder following nontraumatic intracerebral hemorrhage
Revised			Stuttering following nontraumatic intracerebral hemorrhage
	I69.21		Cognitive deficits following other nontraumatic intracranial hemorrhage
New		I69.210	Attention and concentration deficit following other nontraumatic intracranial hemorrhage
New		I69.211	Memory deficit following other nontraumatic intracranial hemorrhage
New		I69.212	Visuospatial deficit and spatial neglect following other nontraumatic intracranial hemorrhage
New		I69.213	Psychomotor deficit following other nontraumatic intracranial hemorrhage
New		I69.214	Frontal lobe and executive function deficit following other nontraumatic intracranial hemorrhage
New		I69.215	Cognitive social or emotional deficit following other nontraumatic intracranial hemorrhage
New		I69.218	Other symptoms and signs involving cognitive functions following other nontraumatic intracranial hemorrhage
New		I69.219	Unspecified symptoms and signs involving cognitive functions following other nontraumatic intracranial hemorrhage
		I69.223	Fluency disorder following other nontraumatic intracerebral hemorrhage
Revised			Stuttering following other nontraumatic intracranial hemorrhage
New		I69.310	Attention and concentration deficit following cerebral infarction
New		I69.311	Memory deficit following cerebral infarction
New		I69.312	Visuospatial deficit and spatial neglect following cerebral infarction
New		I69.313	Psychomotor deficit following cerebral infarction
New		I69.314	Frontal lobe and executive function deficit following cerebral infarction
New		I69.315	Cognitive social or emotional deficit following cerebral infarction
New		I69.318	Other symptoms and signs involving cognitive functions following cerebral infarction
New		I69.319	Unspecified symptoms and signs involving cognitive functions following cerebral infarction

	I69.323	Fluency disorder following cerebral infarction
Revised		Stuttering following cerebral infarction
New	I69.810	Attention and concentration deficit following other cerebrovascular disease
New	I69.811	Memory deficit following other cerebrovascular disease
New	I69.812	Visuospatial deficit and spatial neglect following other cerebrovascular disease
New	I69.813	Psychomotor deficit following other cerebrovascular disease
New	I69.814	Frontal lobe and executive function deficit following other cerebrovascular disease
New	I69.815	Cognitive social or emotional deficit following other cerebrovascular disease
New	I69.818	Other symptoms and signs involving cognitive functions following other cerebrovascular disease
New	I69.819	Unspecified symptoms and signs involving cognitive functions following other cerebrovascular disease
	I69.823	Fluency disorder following other cerebrovascular disease
Revised		Stuttering following other cerebrovascular disease
New	I69.910	Attention and concentration deficit following unspecified cerebrovascular disease
New	I69.911	Memory deficit following unspecified cerebrovascular disease
New	I69.912	Visuospatial deficit and spatial neglect following unspecified cerebrovascular disease
New	I69.913	Psychomotor deficit following unspecified cerebrovascular disease
New	I69.914	Frontal lobe and executive function deficit following unspecified cerebrovascular disease
New	I69.915	Cognitive social or emotional deficit following unspecified cerebrovascular disease
New	I69.918	Other symptoms and signs involving cognitive functions following unspecified cerebrovascular disease
New	I69.919	Unspecified symptoms and signs involving cognitive functions following unspecified cerebrovascular disease
	I69.923	Fluency disorder following unspecified cerebrovascular disease
Revised		Stuttering following unspecified cerebrovascular disease

	I70	Atherosclerosis
Revised		Use additional code to identify: history of tobacco dependence (Z87.891)
	I72	Other aneurysm
New		**Excludes2** dissection of precerebral artery, congenital (nonruptured) (Q28.1)
New	I72.5	Aneurysm of other precerebral arteries
New		Aneurysm of basilar artery (trunk)
New		**Excludes2** aneurysm of carotid artery (I72.0)
New		aneurysm of vertebral artery (I72.6)
New		dissection of carotid artery (I77.71)
New		dissection of other precerebral arteries (I77.75)
New		dissection of vertebral artery (I77.74)
New	I72.6	Aneurysm of vertebral artery
New		**Excludes2** dissection of vertebral artery (I77.74)
	I74	Arterial embolism and thrombosis
Revised		**Excludes2** mesenteric embolism and thrombosis (K55.0-)
New	I77.70	Dissection of unspecified artery
	I77.74	Dissection of vertebral artery
New		**Excludes2** aneurysm of vertebral artery (I72.6)
New	I77.75	Dissection of other precerebral arteries
New		Dissection of basilar artery (trunk)
New		**Excludes2** aneurysm of carotid artery (I72.0)
New		aneurysm of other precerebral arteries (I72.5)
New		aneurysm of vertebral artery (I72.6)
New		dissection of carotid artery (I77.71)
New		dissection of vertebral artery (I77.74)
New	I77.76	Dissection of artery of upper extremity
New	I77.77	Dissection of artery of lower extremity
Revised	I77.79	Dissection of other specified artery
	I82	Other venous embolism and thrombosis
Revised		**Excludes2** mesenteric (K55.0-)
Deleted	I83.1	Varicose veins of lower extremities with inflammation
		Stasis dermatitis
New	I87.2	Venous insufficiency (chronic) (peripheral)
		Stasis dermatitis
New		**Excludes1** stasis dermatitis with varicose veins of lower extremities (I83.1-, I83.2-)
	I89	Other noninfective disorders of lymphatic vessels and lymph nodes
Revised		**Excludes1** chylocele, tunica vaginalis (nonfilarial) NOS (N50.89)
	I96	Gangrene, not elsewhere classified
Revised		**Excludes1** gangrene in diabetes mellitus (E08-E13 with .52)

Revised	I97.6			Postprocedural hemorrhage, hematoma and seroma of a circulatory system organ or structure following a procedure
Revised		I97.61		Postprocedural hemorrhage of a circulatory system organ or structure following a circulatory system procedure
Revised			I97.610	Postprocedural hemorrhage of a circulatory system organ or structure following a cardiac catheterization
Revised			I97.611	Postprocedural hemorrhage of a circulatory system organ or structure following cardiac bypass
Revised			I97.618	Postprocedural hemorrhage of a circulatory system organ or structure following other circulatory system procedure
Revised		I97.62		Postprocedural hemorrhage, hematoma and seroma of a circulatory system organ or structure following other procedure
New			I97.620	Postprocedural hemorrhage of a circulatory system organ or structure following other procedure
New			I97.621	Postprocedural hematoma of a circulatory system organ or structure following other procedure
New			I97.622	Postprocedural seroma of a circulatory system organ or structure following other procedure
New		I97.63		Postprocedural hematoma of a circulatory system organ or structure following a circulatory system procedure
New			I97.630	Postprocedural hematoma of a circulatory system organ or structure following a cardiac catheterization
New			I97.631	Postprocedural hematoma of a circulatory system organ or structure following cardiac bypass
New			I97.638	Postprocedural hematoma of a circulatory system organ or structure following other circulatory system procedure
New		I97.64		Postprocedural seroma of a circulatory system organ or structure following a circulatory system procedure
New			I97.640	Postprocedural seroma of a circulatory system organ or structure following a cardiac catheterization
New			I97.641	Postprocedural seroma of a circulatory system organ or structure following cardiac bypass
New			I97.648	Postprocedural seroma of a circulatory system organ or structure following other circulatory system procedure
Revised			I97.820	Postprocedural cerebrovascular infarction following cardiac surgery
Revised			I97.821	Postprocedural cerebrovascular infarction following other surgery

CHAPTER 10

DISEASES OF THE RESPIRATORY SYSTEM (J00-J99)

	J31		Chronic rhinitis, nasopharyngitis and pharyngitis
	J32		Chronic sinusitis
	J33		Nasal polyp
	J35		Chronic diseases of tonsils and adenoids
	J37		Chronic laryngitis and laryngotracheitis
	J38		Diseases of vocal cords and larynx, not elsewhere classified
	J40		Bronchitis, not specified as acute or chronic
	J41		Simple and mucopurulent chronic bronchitis
	J42		Unspecified chronic bronchitis
	J43		Emphysema
	J44		Other chronic obstructive pulmonary disease
			Use additional code to identify:
Revised			history of tobacco dependence (Z87.891)
Deleted			**Excludes1** lung diseases due to external agents (J60-J70)
New			**Excludes2** lung diseases due to external agents (J60-J70)

	J45		Asthma
	J47		Bronchiectasis
			Use additional code to identify:
Revised			history of tobacco dependence (Z87.891)
		J47.0	Bronchiectasis with acute lower respiratory infection
New			Use additional code to identify the infection
	J81		Pulmonary edema
			Use additional code to identify:
Revised			history of tobacco dependence (Z87.891)
		J84.89	Other specified interstitial pulmonary diseases
Deleted			Organizing pneumonia due to known underlying cause
Revised		J95.83	Postprocedural hemorrhage of a respiratory system organ or structure following a procedure
Revised		J95.830	Postprocedural hemorrhage of a respiratory system organ or structure following a respiratory system procedure
Revised		J95.831	Postprocedural hemorrhage of a respiratory system organ or structure following other procedure
New		J95.86	Postprocedural hematoma and seroma of a respiratory system organ or structure following a procedure
New		J95.860	Postprocedural hematoma of a respiratory system organ or structure following a respiratory system procedure
New		J95.861	Postprocedural hematoma of a respiratory system organ or structure following other procedure
New		J95.862	Postprocedural seroma of a respiratory system organ or structure following a respiratory system procedure
New		J95.863	Postprocedural seroma of a respiratory system organ or structure following other procedure

	J98	**Other respiratory disorders**
		Use additional code to identify:
Revised		history of tobacco dependence (Z87.891)
	J98.5	**Diseases of mediastinum, not elsewhere classified**
Deleted		Fibrosis of mediastinum
Deleted		Hernia of mediastinum
Deleted		Retraction of mediastinum
Deleted		Mediastinitis
New	**J98.51**	**Mediastinitis**
New		*Code first underlying condition, if applicable, such as postoperative mediastinitis (T81.-)*
New	**J98.59**	**Other diseases of mediastinum, not elsewhere classified**
New		Fibrosis of mediastinum
New		Hernia of mediastinum
New		Retraction of mediastinum

CHAPTER 11

DISEASES OF THE DIGESTIVE SYSTEM (K00-K95)

	K02	**Dental caries**
New	**Includes**	caries of dentine
New		dental cavities
New		early childhood caries
New		pre-eruptive caries
New		recurrent caries (dentino enamel junction) (enamel) (to the pulp)
	K02.52	**Dental caries on pit and fissure surface penetrating into dentin**
New		Primary dental caries, cervical origin
	K04.0	**Pulpitis**
Deleted		Reversible pulpitis
Deleted		Irreversible pulpitis
New	**K04.01**	**Reversible pulpitis**
New	**K04.02**	**Irreversible pulpitis**
	K05	**Gingivitis and periodontal diseases**
		Use additional code to identify:
Revised		history of tobacco dependence (Z87.891)
	K05.00	**Acute gingivitis, plaque induced**
New		Plaque induced gingival disease
	K05.1	**Chronic gingivitis**
New		Pregnancy associated gingivitis
New		*Code first, if applicable, diseases of the digestive system complicating pregnancy (O99.61-)*
New	**K05.211**	**Aggressive periodontitis, localized, slight**
New	**K05.212**	**Aggressive periodontitis, localized, moderate**
New	**K05.213**	**Aggressive periodontitis, localized, severe**
New	**K05.219**	**Aggressive periodontitis, localized, unspecified severity**
New	**K05.221**	**Aggressive periodontitis, generalized, slight**
New	**K05.222**	**Aggressive periodontitis, generalized, moderate**
New	**K05.223**	**Aggressive periodontitis, generalized, severe**
New	**K05.229**	**Aggressive periodontitis, generalized, unspecified severity**

New	**K05.311**	**Chronic periodontitis, localized, slight**
New	**K05.312**	**Chronic periodontitis, localized, moderate**
New	**K05.313**	**Chronic periodontitis, localized, severe**
New	**K05.319**	**Chronic periodontitis, localized, unspecified severity**
New	**K05.321**	**Chronic periodontitis, generalized, slight**
New	**K05.322**	**Chronic periodontitis, generalized, moderate**
New	**K05.323**	**Chronic periodontitis, generalized, severe**
New	**K05.329**	**Chronic periodontitis, generalized, unspecified severity**
	K05.5	**Other periodontal diseases**
New		Combined periodontic-endodontic lesion
New		Narrow gingival width (of periodontal soft tissue)
New	**K06.3**	**Horizontal alveolar bone loss**
	K06.8	**Other specified disorders of gingiva and edentulous alveolar ridge**
New		Vertical ridge deficiency
	K08.8	**Other specified disorders of teeth and supporting structures**
Deleted		Enlargement of alveolar ridge NOS
Deleted		Irregular alveolar process
Deleted		Toothache NOS
New	**K08.81**	**Primary occlusal trauma**
New	**K08.82**	**Secondary occlusal trauma**
New	**K08.89**	**Other specified disorders of teeth and supporting structures**
New		Enlargement of alveolar ridge NOS
New		Insufficient anatomic crown height
New		Insufficient clinical crown length
New		Irregular alveolar process
New		Toothache NOS

	K11	**Diseases of salivary glands**
	K12	**Stomatitis and related lesions**
	K13	**Other diseases of lip and oral mucosa**
	K14	**Diseases of tongue**
		Use additional code to identify:
Revised		history of tobacco dependence (Z87.891)

	K35.3	**Acute appendicitis with localized peritonitis**
Revised		Acute appendicitis with or without perforation or rupture with peritonitis NOS

NONINFECTIVE ENTERITIS AND COLITIS (K50-K52)

Revised	**Excludes1**	megacolon (K59.3-)
	K52.2	**Allergic and dietetic gastroenteritis and colitis**
New	**Excludes2**	allergic eosinophilic colitis (K52.82)
New		allergic eosinophilic esophagitis (K20.0)
New		allergic eosinophilic gastritis (K52.81)
New		allergic eosinophilic gastroenteritis (K52.81)
New		food protein-induced proctocolitis (K52.82)
New	**K52.21**	**Food protein-induced enterocolitis syndrome**
New		Use additional code for hypovolemic shock, if present (R57.1)
New	**K52.22**	**Food protein-induced enteropathy**
	K52.29	**Other allergic and dietetic gastroenteritis and colitis**
New		Food hypersensitivity gastroenteritis or colitis
New		Immediate gastrointestinal hypersensitivity

New	K52.3	Indeterminate colitis
New		Colonic inflammatory bowel disease unclassified (IBDU)
New		**Excludes1** unspecified colitis (K52.9)
	K52.81	Eosinophilic gastritis or gastroenteritis
		Eosinophilic enteritis
Deleted		**Excludes1** eosinophilic esophagitis (K20.0)
New		**Excludes2** eosinophilic esophagitis (K20.0)
	K52.82	Eosinophilic colitis
New		Allergic proctocolitis
New		Food-induced eosinophilic proctocolitis
New		Food protein-induced proctocolitis
New		Milk protein-induced proctocolitis
New	K52.83	Microscopic colitis
New		K52.831 Collagenous colitis
New		K52.832 Lymphocytic colitis
New		K52.838 Other microscopic colitis
New		K52.839 Microscopic colitis, unspecified
	K52.89	Other specified noninfective gastroenteritis and colitis
Deleted		Collagenous colitis
Deleted		Lymphocytic colitis
Deleted		Microscopic colitis (collagenous or lymphocytic)
	K55.0	Acute vascular disorders of intestine
Deleted		Acute fulminant ischemic colitis
Deleted		Acute intestinal infarction
Deleted		Acute small intestine ischemia
Deleted		Necrosis of intestine
Deleted		Subacute ischemic colitis
New	K55.01	Acute (reversible) ischemia of small intestine
New		K55.011 Focal (segmental) acute (reversible) ischemia of small intestine
New		K55.012 Diffuse acute (reversible) ischemia of small intestine
New		K55.019 Acute (reversible) ischemia of small intestine, extent unspecified
New	K55.02	Acute infarction of small intestine
New		Gangrene of small intestine
New		Necrosis of small intestine
New		K55.021 Focal (segmental) acute infarction of small intestine
New		K55.022 Diffuse acute infarction of small intestine
New		K55.029 Acute infarction of small intestine, extent unspecified
New	K55.03	Acute (reversible) ischemia of large intestine
New		Acute fulminant ischemic colitis
New		Subacute ischemic colitis
New		K55.031 Focal (segmental) acute (reversible) ischemia of large intestine
New		K55.032 Diffuse acute (reversible) ischemia of large intestine
New		K55.039 Acute (reversible) ischemia of large intestine, extent unspecified
New	K55.04	Acute infarction of large intestine
New		Gangrene of large intestine
New		Necrosis of large intestine
New		K55.041 Focal (segmental) acute infarction of large intestine
New		K55.042 Diffuse acute infarction of large intestine
New		K55.049 Acute infarction of large intestine, extent unspecified

New	K55.05	Acute (reversible) ischemia of intestine, part unspecified
New		K55.051 Focal (segmental) acute (reversible) ischemia of intestine, part unspecified
New		K55.052 Diffuse acute (reversible) ischemia of intestine, part unspecified
New		K55.059 Acute (reversible) ischemia of intestine, part and extent unspecified
New	K55.06	Acute infarction of intestine, part unspecified
New		Acute intestinal infarction
New		Gangrene of intestine
New		Necrosis of intestine
New		K55.061 Focal (segmental) acute infarction of intestine, part unspecified
New		K55.062 Diffuse acute infarction of intestine, part unspecified
New		K55.069 Acute infarction of intestine, part and extent unspecified
New	K55.3	Necrotizing enterocolitis
New		**Excludes1** necrotizing enterocolitis of newborn (P77.-)
New		**Excludes2** necrotizing enterocolitis due to Clostridium difficile (A04.7)
New	K55.30	Necrotizing enterocolitis, unspecified
New		Necrotizing enterocolitis, NOS
New	K55.31	Stage 1 necrotizing enterocolitis
New		Necrotizing enterocolitis without pneumatosis, without perforation
New	K55.32	Stage 2 necrotizing enterocolitis
New		Necrotizing enterocolitis with pneumatosis, without perforation
New	K55.33	Stage 3 necrotizing enterocolitis
New		Necrotizing enterocolitis with perforation
New		Necrotizing enterocolitis with pneumatosis and perforation
New	K58.1	Irritable bowel syndrome with constipation
New	K58.2	Mixed irritable bowel syndrome
New	K58.8	Other irritable bowel syndrome
	K59.0	Constipation
New		Use additional code for adverse effect, if applicable, to identify drug (T36-T50 with fifth or sixth character 5)
New	K59.03	Drug induced constipation
New		Use additional code for adverse effect, if applicable, to identify drug (T36-T50 with fifth or sixth character 5)
New	K59.04	Chronic idiopathic constipation
New		Functional constipation
New	K59.09	Other constipation
New		Chronic constipation
	K59.3	Megacolon, not elsewhere classified
Deleted		Toxic colon
New	K59.31	Toxic megacolon
New	K59.39	Other megacolon
New		Megacolon NOS

K72   Hepatic failure, not elsewhere classified

Deleted   **Includes**   acute hepatitis NEC, with hepatic failure
Deleted   **Excludes1** viral hepatitis with hepatic coma
                               (B15-B19)

New   **Excludes2** viral hepatitis with hepatic coma
                               (B15-B19)

K72.0   Acute and subacute hepatic failure
New   Acute non-viral hepatitis NOS

K75.0   Abscess of liver
New   **Excludes2** acute or subacute hepatitis NOS
                               (B17.9)
New   acute or subacute non-viral
                               hepatitis (K72.0)
New   chronic hepatitis NEC (K73.8)

K76.7   Hepatorenal syndrome
Revised   **Excludes1** postprocedural hepatorenal
                               syndrome (K91.83)

K85   Acute pancreatitis

Deleted   **Includes**   abscess of pancreas
Deleted   acute necrosis of pancreas
Deleted   gangrene of (gangrenous) pancreas
Deleted   hemorrhagic pancreatitis
Deleted   infective necrosis of pancreas
Deleted   suppurative pancreatitis

New   **K85.00   Idiopathic acute pancreatitis without necrosis or infection**

New   **K85.01   Idiopathic acute pancreatitis with uninfected necrosis**

New   **K85.02   Idiopathic acute pancreatitis with infected necrosis**

New   **K85.10   Biliary acute pancreatitis without necrosis or infection**

New   **K85.11   Biliary acute pancreatitis with uninfected necrosis**

New   **K85.12   Biliary acute pancreatitis with infected necrosis**

New   **K85.20   Alcohol induced acute pancreatitis without necrosis or infection**

New   **K85.21   Alcohol induced acute pancreatitis with uninfected necrosis**

New   **K85.22   Alcohol induced acute pancreatitis with infected necrosis**

New   **K85.30   Drug induced acute pancreatitis without necrosis or infection**

New   **K85.31   Drug induced acute pancreatitis with uninfected necrosis**

New   **K85.32   Drug induced acute pancreatitis with infected necrosis**

New   **K85.80   Other acute pancreatitis without necrosis or infection**

New   **K85.81   Other acute pancreatitis with uninfected necrosis**

New   **K85.82   Other acute pancreatitis with infected necrosis**

New   **K85.90   Acute pancreatitis without necrosis or infection, unspecified**

New   **K85.91   Acute pancreatitis with uninfected necrosis, unspecified**

New   **K85.92   Acute pancreatitis with infected necrosis, unspecified**

K86.0   Alcohol-induced chronic pancreatitis
New   Code also exocrine pancreatic insufficiency
                 (K86.81)
Revised   **Excludes2** alcohol induced acute pancreatitis
                               (K85.2-)

K86.1   Other chronic pancreatitis
New   Code also exocrine pancreatic insufficiency
                 (K86.81)

K86.8   Other specified diseases of pancreas
Deleted   Aseptic pancreatic necrosis
Deleted   Atrophy of pancreas
Deleted   Calculus of pancreas
Deleted   Cirrhosis of pancreas
Deleted   Fibrosis of pancreas
Deleted   Pancreatic fat necrosis
Deleted   Pancreatic infantilism
Deleted   Pancreatic necrosis NOS

New   **K86.81   Exocrine pancreatic insufficiency**
New   **K86.89   Other specified diseases of pancreas**
New   Aseptic pancreatic necrosis, unrelated
                 to acute pancreatitis
New   Atrophy of pancreas
New   Calculus of pancreas
New   Cirrhosis of pancreas
New   Fibrosis of pancreas
New   Pancreatic fat necrosis, unrelated to
                 acute pancreatitis
New   Pancreatic infantilism
New   Pancreatic necrosis NOS, unrelated to
                 acute pancreatitis

K90.0   Celiac disease
New   Celiac disease with steatorrhea
Deleted   Idiopathic steatorrhea
New   Code also exocrine pancreatic insufficiency
                 (K86.81)

K90.4   Other malabsorption due to intolerance
Deleted   Malabsorption due to intolerance to
                 carbohydrate
Deleted   Malabsorption due to intolerance to fat
Deleted   Malabsorption due to intolerance to protein
Deleted   Malabsorption due to intolerance to starch

New   **K90.41   Non-celiac gluten sensitivity**
New   Gluten sensitivity NOS
New   Non-celiac gluten sensitive enteropathy

New   **K90.49   Malabsorption due to intolerance, not elsewhere classified**
New   Malabsorption due to intolerance to
                 carbohydrate
New   Malabsorption due to intolerance to fat
New   Malabsorption due to intolerance to
                 protein
New   Malabsorption due to intolerance to
                 starch

Revised **K91.61   Intraoperative hemorrhage and hematoma of a digestive system organ or structure complicating a digestive system procedure**

Revised **K91.84   Postprocedural hemorrhage of a digestive system organ or structure following a procedure**

Revised   **K91.840   Postprocedural hemorrhage of a digestive system organ or structure following a digestive system procedure**

Revised   **K91.841   Postprocedural hemorrhage of a digestive system organ or structure following other procedure**

New   K91.87   Postprocedural hematoma and seroma of a digestive system organ or structure following a procedure

New   K91.870   Postprocedural hematoma of a digestive system organ or structure following a digestive system procedure

New   K91.871   Postprocedural hematoma of a digestive system organ or structure following other procedure

New   K91.872   Postprocedural seroma of a digestive system organ or structure following a digestive system procedure

New   K91.873   Postprocedural seroma of a digestive system organ or structure following other procedure

CHAPTER 12

DISEASES OF THE SKIN AND SUBCUTANEOUS TISSUE (L00-L99)

L02.2   Cutaneous abscess, furuncle and carbuncle of trunk

Revised   **Excludes2**   abscess of breast (N61.1)

L03.211   Cellulitis of face

New   **Excludes2**   abscess of orbit (H05.01-)

Revised   cellulitis of orbit (H05.01-)

New   L03.213   Periorbital cellulitis
New   Preseptal cellulitis

L03.31   Cellulitis of trunk

Revised   **Excludes2**   cellulitis of breast NOS (N61.0)

L05.01   Pilonidal cyst with abscess
Deleted   Parasacral dimple with abscess
New   **Excludes2**   congenital sacral dimple (Q82.6)
New   parasacral dimple (Q82.6)

L05.91   Pilonidal cyst without abscess
Deleted   Parasacral dimple
New   **Excludes2**   congenital sacral dimple (Q82.6)
New   parasacral dimple (Q82.6)

DERMATITIS AND ECZEMA (L20-L30)

Revised   **Excludes2**   stasis dermatitis (I87.2)

L30   Other and unspecified dermatitis
Revised   **Excludes2**   stasis dermatitis (I87.2)

L50.2   Urticaria due to cold and heat
New   **Excludes2**   familial cold urticaria (M04.2)

L70   Acne
Revised   L70.5   Acné excoriée
New   Acné excoriée des jeunes filles

Revised   L76.2   Postprocedural hemorrhage of skin and subcutaneous tissue following a procedure

Revised   L76.21   Postprocedural hemorrhage of skin and subcutaneous tissue following a dermatologic procedure

Revised   L76.22   Postprocedural hemorrhage of skin and subcutaneous tissue following other procedure

New   L76.3   Postprocedural hematoma and seroma of skin and subcutaneous tissue following a procedure

New   L76.31   Postprocedural hematoma of skin and subcutaneous tissue following a dermatologic procedure

New   L76.32   Postprocedural hematoma of skin and subcutaneous tissue following other procedure

New   L76.33   Postprocedural seroma of skin and subcutaneous tissue following a dermatologic procedure

New   L76.34   Postprocedural seroma of skin and subcutaneous tissue following other procedure

L82   Seborrheic keratosis
New   **Includes**   basal cell papilloma

L89.521   Pressure ulcer of left ankle, stage 1
Revised   Pressure pre-ulcer skin changes limited to persistent focal edema, left ankle

L98.1   Factitial dermatitis
New   **Excludes1**   Excoriation (skin-picking) disorder (F42.4)

L98.7   Excessive and redundant skin and subcutaneous tissue
New   Loose or sagging skin following bariatric surgery weight loss
New   Loose or sagging skin following dietary weight loss
New   Loose or sagging skin, NOS
New   **Excludes2**   acquired excess or redundant skin of eyelid (H02.3-)
New   congenital excess or redundant skin of eyelid (Q10.3)
New   skin changes due to chronic exposure to nonionizing radiation (L57.-)

CHAPTER 13

DISEASES OF THE MUSCULOSKELETAL SYSTEM AND CONNECTIVE TISSUE (M00-M99)

This chapter contains the following blocks:

New	M04	Autoinflammatory syndromes
New	M97	Periprosthetic fracture around internal prosthetic joint

AUTOINFLAMMATORY SYNDROMES (M04)

New   M04   Autoinflammatory syndromes
New   **Excludes2**   Crohn's disease (K50.-)
New   M04.1   Periodic fever syndromes
New   Familial Mediterranean fever
New   Hyperimmunoglobin D syndrome
New   Mevalonate kinase deficiency
New   Tumor necrosis factor receptor associated periodic syndrome [TRAPS]
New   M04.2   Cryopyrin-associated periodic syndromes
New   Chronic infantile neurological, cutaneous and articular syndrome [CINCA]
New   Familial cold autoinflammatory syndrome
New   Familial cold urticaria
New   Muckle-Wells syndrome
New   Neonatal onset multisystemic inflammatory disorder [NOMID]

New	**M04.8 Other autoinflammatory syndromes**	
New	Blau syndrome	
New	Deficiency of interleukin 1 receptor antagonist [DIRA]	
New	Majeed syndrome	
New	Periodic fever, aphthous stomatitis, pharyngitis, and adenopathy syndrome [PFAPA]	
New	Pyogenic arthritis, pyoderma gangrenosum, and acne syndrome [PAPA]	
New	**M04.9 Autoinflammatory syndrome, unspecified**	
	M1A Chronic gout	
Deleted	**Excludes1** acute gout (M10.-)	
New	**Excludes2** acute gout (M10.-)	
	M10 Gout	
Deleted	Gout NOS	
Deleted	**Excludes1** chronic gout (M1A.-)	
New	**Excludes2** chronic gout (M1A.-)	
	M20.1 Hallux valgus (acquired)	
Deleted	Bunion	
New	**Excludes2** bunion (M21.6-)	
	M21.1 Varus deformity, not elsewhere classified	
Revised	**Excludes1** metatarsus varus (Q66.22)	
	M21.6 Other acquired deformities of foot	
Revised	**Excludes2** deformities of toe (acquired) (M20.1-M20.6-)	
New	**M21.61 Bunion**	
New	**M21.611 Bunion of right foot**	
New	**M21.612 Bunion of left foot**	
New	**M21.619 Bunion of unspecified foot**	
New	**M21.62 Bunionette**	
New	**M21.621 Bunionette of right foot**	
New	**M21.622 Bunionette of left foot**	
New	**M21.629 Bunionette of unspecified foot**	
New	**M25.5 Pain in joint**	
New	**M25.54 Pain in joints of hand**	
New	**M25.541 Pain in joints of right hand**	
New	**M25.542 Pain in joints of left hand**	
New	**M25.549 Pain in joints of unspecified hand**	
New	Pain in joints of hand NOS	
New	**M26.601 Right temporomandibular joint disorder, unspecified**	
New	**M26.602 Left temporomandibular joint disorder, unspecified**	
New	**M26.603 Bilateral temporomandibular joint disorder, unspecified**	
New	**M26.609 Unspecified temporomandibular joint disorder, unspecified side**	
New	Temporomandibular joint disorder NOS	
New	**M26.611 Adhesions and ankylosis of right temporomandibular joint**	
New	**M26.612 Adhesions and ankylosis of left temporomandibular joint**	
New	**M26.613 Adhesions and ankylosis of bilateral temporomandibular joint**	
New	**M26.619 Adhesions and ankylosis of temporomandibular joint, unspecified side**	

New	**M26.621 Arthralgia of right temporomandibular joint**	
New	**M26.622 Arthralgia of left temporomandibular joint**	
New	**M26.623 Arthralgia of bilateral temporomandibular joint**	
New	**M26.629 Arthralgia of temporomandibular joint, unspecified side**	
New	**M26.631 Articular disc disorder of right temporomandibular joint**	
New	**M26.632 Articular disc disorder of left temporomandibular joint**	
New	**M26.633 Articular disc disorder of bilateral temporomandibular joint**	
New	**M26.639 Articular disc disorder of temporomandibular joint, unspecified side**	
	M48.5 Collapsed vertebra, not elsewhere classified	
New	Compression fracture of vertebra NOS	
	M50.02 Cervical disc disorder with myelopathy, mid-cervical region	
Deleted	C4-C5 disc disorder with myelopathy	
Deleted	C5-C6 disc disorder with myelopathy	
Deleted	C6-C7 disc disorder with myelopathy	
	M50.020 Cervical disc disorder with myelopathy, mid-cervical region, unspecified level	
	M50.021 Cervical disc disorder at C4-C5 level with myelopathy	
	C4-C5 disc disorder with myelopathy	
	M50.022 Cervical disc disorder at C5-C6 level with myelopathy	
	C5-C6 disc disorder with myelopathy	
	M50.023 Cervical disc disorder at C6-C7 level with myelopathy	
	C6-C7 disc disorder with myelopathy	
	M50.12 Cervical disc disorder with radiculopathy, mid-cervical region	
Deleted	C4-C5 disc disorder with radiculopathy	
Deleted	C5 radiculopathy due to disc disorder	
Deleted	C5-C6 disc disorder with radiculopathy	
Deleted	C6 radiculopathy due to disc disorder	
Deleted	C6-C7 disc disorder with radiculopathy	
Deleted	C7 radiculopathy due to disc disorder	
New	**M50.120 Mid-cervical disc disorder, unspecified**	
New	**M50.121 Cervical disc disorder at C4-C5 level with radiculopathy**	
New	C4-C5 disc disorder with radiculopathy	
New	C5 radiculopathy due to disc disorder	
New	**M50.122 Cervical disc disorder at C5-C6 level with radiculopathy**	
New	C5-C6 disc disorder with radiculopathy	
New	C6 radiculopathy due to disc disorder	
New	**M50.123 Cervical disc disorder at C6-C7 level with radiculopathy**	
New	C6-C7 disc disorder with radiculopathy	
New	C7 radiculopathy due to disc disorder	

	M50.22	**Other cervical disc displacement, mid-cervical region**
Deleted		Other C4-C5 cervical disc displacement
Deleted		Other C5-C6 cervical disc displacement
Deleted		Other C6-C7 cervical disc displacement
New	**M50.220**	**Other cervical disc displacement, mid-cervical region, unspecified level**
New	**M50.221**	**Other cervical disc displacement at C4-C5 level**
New		Other C4-C5 cervical disc displacement
New	**M50.222**	**Other cervical disc displacement at C5-C6 level**
New		Other C5-C6 cervical disc displacement
New	**M50.223**	**Other cervical disc displacement at C6-C7 level**
New		Other C6-C7 cervical disc displacement
	M50.32	**Other cervical disc degeneration, mid-cervical region**
Deleted		Other C4-C5 cervical disc displacement
Deleted		Other C5-C6 cervical disc displacement
Deleted		Other C6-C7 cervical disc displacement
New	**M50.320**	**Other cervical disc degeneration, mid-cervical region, unspecified level**
New	**M50.321**	**Other cervical disc degeneration at C4-C5 level**
New		Other C4-C5 cervical disc degeneration
New	**M50.322**	**Other cervical disc degeneration at C5-C6 level**
New		Other C5-C6 cervical disc degeneration
New	**M50.323**	**Other cervical disc degeneration at C6-C7 level**
New		Other C6-C7 cervical disc degeneration
	M50.82	**Other cervical disc disorders, mid-cervical region**
Deleted		Other C4-C5 cervical disc disorders
Deleted		Other C5-C6 cervical disc disorders
Deleted		Other C6-C7 cervical disc disorders
New	**M50.820**	**Other cervical disc disorders, mid-cervical region, unspecified level**
New	**M50.821**	**Other cervical disc disorders at C4-C5 level**
New		Other C4-C5 cervical disc disorders
New	**M50.822**	**Other cervical disc disorders at C5-C6 level**
New		Other C5-C6 cervical disc disorders
New	**M50.823**	**Other cervical disc disorders at C6-C7 level**
New		Other C6-C7 cervical disc disorders
	M50.92	**Cervical disc disorder, unspecified, mid-cervical region**
Deleted		C4-C5 cervical disc disorder, unspecified
Deleted		C5-C6 cervical disc disorder, unspecified
Deleted		C6-C7 cervical disc disorder, unspecified
New	**M50.920**	**Unspecified cervical disc disorder, mid-cervical region, unspecified level**
New	**M50.921**	**Unspecified cervical disc disorder at C4-C5 level**
New		Unspecified C4-C5 cervical disc disorder

New	**M50.922**	**Unspecified cervical disc disorder at C5-C6 level**
New		Unspecified C5-C6 cervical disc disorder
New	**M50.923**	**Unspecified cervical disc disorder at C6-C7 level**
New		Unspecified C6-C7 cervical disc disorder
	M62.5	**Muscle wasting and atrophy, not elsewhere classified**
New	**Excludes1**	sarcopenia (M62.84)
	M62.81	**Muscle weakness (generalized)**
New	**Excludes1**	muscle weakness in sarcopenia (M62.84)
	M62.84	**Sarcopenia**
New		Age-related sarcopenia
New		*Code first underlying disease, if applicable, such as:*
New		disorders of myoneural junction and muscle disease in diseases classified elsewhere (G73.-)
New		other and unspecified myopathies (G72.-)
New		primary disorders of muscles (G71.-)
	M71.5	**Other bursitis, not elsewhere classified**
Revised	**Excludes2**	bursitis of shoulder (M75.5) bursitis of tibial collateral [Pellegrini-Stieda] (M76.4-)
	M84.7	**Nontraumatic fracture, not elsewhere classified**
New	**M84.75**	**Atypical femoral fracture**
New		The appropriate 7th character is to be added to each code from M84.75:
New		A initial encounter for fracture
New		D subsequent encounter for fracture with routine healing
New		G subsequent encounter for fracture with delayed healing
New		K subsequent encounter for fracture with nonunion
New		P subsequent encounter for fracture with malunion
New		S sequela
New	**M84.750**	**Atypical femoral fracture, unspecified**
New	**M84.751**	**Incomplete atypical femoral fracture, right leg**
New	**M84.752**	**Incomplete atypical femoral fracture, left leg**
New	**M84.753**	**Incomplete atypical femoral fracture, unspecified leg**
New	**M84.754**	**Complete transverse atypical femoral fracture, right leg**
New	**M84.755**	**Complete transverse atypical femoral fracture, left leg**
New	**M84.756**	**Complete transverse atypical femoral fracture, unspecified leg**
New	**M84.757**	**Complete oblique atypical femoral fracture, right leg**
New	**M84.758**	**Complete oblique atypical femoral fracture, left leg**
New	**M84.759**	**Complete oblique atypical femoral fracture, unspecified leg**
	M90	**Osteopathies in diseases classified elsewhere**
Revised	**Excludes1**	diabetes mellitus (E08-E13 with .69-)

	M96 Intraoperative and postprocedural complications and disorders of musculoskeletal system, not elsewhere classified
New	**Excludes2** periprosthetic fracture around internal prosthetic joint (M97.-)
Revised	**M96.83 Postprocedural hemorrhage of a musculoskeletal structure following a procedure**
Revised	**M96.830 Postprocedural hemorrhage of a musculoskeletal structure following a musculoskeletal system procedure**
Revised	**M96.831 Postprocedural hemorrhage of a musculoskeletal structure following other procedure**
New	**M96.84 Postprocedural hematoma and seroma of a musculoskeletal structure following a procedure**
New	**M96.840 Postprocedural hematoma of a musculoskeletal structure following a musculoskeletal system procedure**
New	**M96.841 Postprocedural hematoma of a musculoskeletal structure following other procedure**
New	**M96.842 Postprocedural seroma of a musculoskeletal structure following a musculoskeletal system procedure**
New	**M96.843 Postprocedural seroma of a musculoskeletal structure following other procedure**

New	**PERIPROSTHETIC FRACTURE AROUND INTERNAL PROSTHETIC JOINT (M97)**
New	**M97 Periprosthetic fracture around internal prosthetic joint**
New	**Excludes2** fracture of bone following insertion of orthopedic implant, joint prosthesis or bone plate (M96.6-)
New	breakage (fracture) of prosthetic joint (T84.01-)
New	The appropriate 7th character is to be added to each code from category M97:
New	A initial encounter
New	D subsequent encounter
New	S sequela
New	**M97.0 Periprosthetic fracture around internal prosthetic hip joint**
New	**M97.01 Periprosthetic fracture around internal prosthetic right hip joint**
New	**M97.02 Periprosthetic fracture around internal prosthetic left hip joint**
New	**M97.1 Periprosthetic fracture around internal prosthetic knee joint**
New	**M97.11 Periprosthetic fracture around internal prosthetic right knee joint**
New	**M97.12 Periprosthetic fracture around internal prosthetic left knee joint**
New	**M97.2 Periprosthetic fracture around internal prosthetic ankle joint**
New	**M97.21 Periprosthetic fracture around internal prosthetic right ankle joint**
New	**M97.22 Periprosthetic fracture around internal prosthetic left ankle joint**
New	**M97.3 Periprosthetic fracture around internal prosthetic shoulder joint**
New	**M97.31 Periprosthetic fracture around internal prosthetic right shoulder joint**
New	**M97.32 Periprosthetic fracture around internal prosthetic left shoulder joint**

New	**M97.4 Periprosthetic fracture around internal prosthetic elbow joint**
New	**M97.41 Periprosthetic fracture around internal prosthetic right elbow joint**
New	**M97.42 Periprosthetic fracture around internal prosthetic left elbow joint**
New	**M97.8 Periprosthetic fracture around other internal prosthetic joint**
New	Periprosthetic fracture around internal prosthetic finger joint
New	Periprosthetic fracture around internal prosthetic spinal joint
New	Periprosthetic fracture around internal prosthetic toe joint
New	Periprosthetic fracture around internal prosthetic wrist joint
New	Use additional code to identify the joint (Z96.6-)
New	**M97.9 Periprosthetic fracture around unspecified internal prosthetic joint**

CHAPTER 14

DISEASES OF THE GENITOURINARY SYSTEM (N00-N99)

Revised	**N10 Acute pyelonephritis**
Revised	Acute tubulo-interstitial nephritis
New	**N13.0 Hydronephrosis with ureteropelvic junction obstruction**
New	Hydronephrosis due to acquired occlusion of ureteropelvic junction
New	**Excludes2** Hydronephrosis with ureteropelvic junction obstruction due to calculus (N13.2)
Revised	**N13.6 Pyonephrosis**
	Conditions in N13.0-N13.5 with infection
	N36.0 Urethral fistula
New	**Excludes1** urethroscrotal fistula (N50.89)
	N36.8 Other specified disorders of urethra
New	**Excludes1** congenital urethrocele (Q64.7)
New	female urethrocele (N81.0)
	N39.42 Incontinence without sensory awareness
New	Insensible (urinary) incontinence
	N39.49 Other specified urinary incontinence
New	**N39.491 Coital incontinence**
New	**N39.492 Postural (urinary) incontinence**
	N40 Benign prostatic hyperplasia
Deleted	**Includes** benign prostatic hyperplasia
New	enlarged prostate
Revised	**N40.0 Benign prostatic hyperplasia without lower urinary tract symptoms**
Revised	**N40.1 Benign prostatic hyperplasia with lower urinary tract symptoms**
	N42.3 Dysplasia of prostate
Deleted	Prostatic intraepithelial neoplasia I (PIN I)
Deleted	Prostatic intraepithelial neoplasia II (PIN II)
Deleted	**Excludes1** prostatic intraepithelial neoplasia III (PIN III) (D07.5)
New	**N42.30 Unspecified dysplasia of prostate**
New	**N42.31 Prostatic intraepithelial neoplasia**
New	PIN
New	Prostatic intraepithelial neoplasia I (PIN I)
New	Prostatic intraepithelial neoplasia II (PIN II)
New	**Excludes1** prostatic intraepithelial neoplasia III (PIN III) (D07.5)
New	**N42.32 Atypical small acinar proliferation of prostate**
New	**N42.39 Other dysplasia of prostate**

	N50.8	**Other specified disorders of male genital organs**
Deleted		Atrophy of scrotum, seminal vesicle, spermatic cord, tunica vaginalis and vas deferens
Deleted		Edema of scrotum, seminal vesicle, spermatic cord, testis, tunica vaginalis and vas deferens
Deleted		Hypertrophy of scrotum, seminal vesicle, spermatic cord, testis, tunica vaginalis and vas deferens
Deleted		Ulcer of scrotum, seminal vesicle, spermatic cord, testis, tunica vaginalis and vas deferens
Deleted		Chylocele, tunica vaginalis (nonfilarial) NOS
Deleted		Urethroscrotal fistula
Deleted		Stricture of spermatic cord, tunica vaginalis, and vas deferens
New	**N50.81**	**Testicular pain**
New	**N50.811**	**Right testicular pain**
New	**N50.812**	**Left testicular pain**
New	**N50.819**	**Testicular pain, unspecified**
New	**N50.82**	**Scrotal pain**
New	**N50.89**	**Other specified disorders of the male genital organs**
New		Atrophy of scrotum, seminal vesicle, spermatic cord, tunica vaginalis and vas deferens
New		Chylocele, tunica vaginalis (nonfilarial) NOS
New		Edema of scrotum, seminal vesicle, spermatic cord, tunica vaginalis and vas deferens
New		Hypertrophy of scrotum, seminal vesicle, spermatic cord, tunica vaginalis and vas deferens
New		Stricture of spermatic cord, tunica vaginalis, and vas deferens
New		Ulcer of scrotum, seminal vesicle, spermatic cord, testis, tunica vaginalis and vas deferens
New		Urethroscrotal fistula
Revised	**N52.3**	**Postprocedural erectile dysfunction**
New	**N52.35**	**Erectile dysfunction following radiation therapy**
New	**N52.36**	**Erectile dysfunction following interstitial seed therapy**
New	**N52.37**	**Erectile dysfunction following prostate ablative therapy**
New		Erectile dysfunction following cryotherapy
New		Erectile dysfunction following other prostate ablative therapies
New		Erectile dysfunction following ultrasound ablative therapies
Revised	**N52.39**	**Other and unspecified postprocedural erectile dysfunction**
	N61	**Inflammatory disorders of breast**
Deleted		Abscess (acute) (chronic) (nonpuerperal) of areola
Deleted		Abscess (acute) (chronic) (nonpuerperal) of breast
Deleted		Carbuncle of breast
Deleted		Infective mastitis (acute) (subacute) (nonpuerperal)
Deleted		Mastitis (acute) (subacute) (nonpuerperal) NOS
New	**N61.0**	**Mastitis without abscess**
New		Infective mastitis (acute) (nonpuerperal) (subacute)
New		Mastitis (acute) (nonpuerperal) (subacute) NOS
New		Cellulitis (acute) (nonpuerperal) (subacute) of breast NOS
New		Cellulitis (acute) (nonpuerperal) (subacute) of nipple NOS

New	**N61.1**	**Abscess of the breast and nipple**
New		Abscess (acute) (chronic) (nonpuerperal) of areola
New		Abscess (acute) (chronic) (nonpuerperal) of breast
New		Carbuncle of breast
New		Mastitis with abscess
	N64.1	**Fat necrosis of breast**
Revised		Code first breast necrosis due to breast graft (T85.898)
	N81	**Female genital prolapse**
Revised	Excludes1	prolapse and hernia of ovary and fallopian tube (N83.4-)
New	**N83.00**	**Follicular cyst of ovary, unspecified side**
New	**N83.01**	**Follicular cyst of right ovary**
New	**N83.02**	**Follicular cyst of left ovary**
New	**N83.10**	**Corpus luteum cyst of ovary, unspecified side**
New	**N83.11**	**Corpus luteum cyst of right ovary**
New	**N83.12**	**Corpus luteum cyst of left ovary**
	N83.20	**Unspecified ovarian cysts**
New	**N83.201**	**Unspecified ovarian cyst, right side**
New	**N83.202**	**Unspecified ovarian cyst, left side**
New	**N83.209**	**Unspecified ovarian cyst, unspecified side**
New		Ovarian cyst, NOS
New	**N83.291**	**Other ovarian cyst, right side**
New	**N83.292**	**Other ovarian cyst, left side**
New	**N83.299**	**Other ovarian cyst, unspecified side**
New	**N83.311**	**Acquired atrophy of right ovary**
New	**N83.312**	**Acquired atrophy of left ovary**
New	**N83.319**	**Acquired atrophy of ovary, unspecified side**
New		Acquired atrophy of ovary, NOS
New	**N83.321**	**Acquired atrophy of right fallopian tube**
New	**N83.322**	**Acquired atrophy of left fallopian tube**
New	**N83.329**	**Acquired atrophy of fallopian tube, unspecified side**
New		Acquired atrophy of fallopian tube, NOS
New	**N83.331**	**Acquired atrophy of right ovary and fallopian tube**
New	**N83.332**	**Acquired atrophy of left ovary and fallopian tube**
New	**N83.339**	**Acquired atrophy of ovary and fallopian tube, unspecified side**
New		Acquired atrophy of ovary and fallopian tube, NOS
New	**N83.40**	**Prolapse and hernia of ovary and fallopian tube, unspecified side**
New		Prolapse and hernia of ovary and fallopian tube, NOS

New		N83.41	Prolapse and hernia of right ovary and fallopian tube
New		N83.42	Prolapse and hernia of left ovary and fallopian tube
New			N83.511 Torsion of right ovary and ovarian pedicle
New			N83.512 Torsion of left ovary and ovarian pedicle
New			N83.519 Torsion of ovary and ovarian pedicle, unspecified side
New			Torsion of ovary and ovarian pedicle, NOS
New			N83.521 Torsion of right fallopian tube
New			N83.522 Torsion of left fallopian tube
New			N83.529 Torsion of fallopian tube, unspecified side
New			Torsion of fallopian tube, NOS

N83.6 **Hematosalpinx**
Revised   **Excludes1**   tubal pregnancy (O00.1-)

N90.6 **Hypertrophy of vulva**
Deleted   Hypertrophy of labia
New   N90.60   Unspecified hypertrophy of vulva
New   Unspecified hypertrophy of labia
New   N90.61   Childhood asymmetric labium majus enlargement
New   CALME
New   N90.69   Other specified hypertrophy of vulva
New   Other specified hypertrophy of labia

New   N93.1   **Pre-pubertal vaginal bleeding**

New   N94.10   Unspecified dyspareunia
New   N94.11   Superficial (introital) dyspareunia
New   N94.12   Deep dyspareunia
New   N94.19   Other specified dyspareunia

N94.3 **Premenstrual tension syndrome**
New   **Excludes1**   Premenstrual dysphoric disorder (F32.81)

Revised   N99.113   **Postprocedural anterior bulbous urethral stricture**

New   N99.115   **Postprocedural fossa navicularis urethral stricture**

N99.5 **Complications of stoma of urinary tract**
Revised   **Excludes2**   mechanical complication of urinary catheter (T83.0-)

Revised   N99.52   **Complication of incontinent external stoma of urinary tract**
Revised   N99.520   **Hemorrhage of incontinent external stoma of urinary tract**
Revised   N99.521   **Infection of incontinent external stoma of urinary tract**
Revised   N99.522   **Malfunction of incontinent external stoma of urinary tract**
New   N99.523   **Herniation of incontinent stoma of urinary tract**
New   N99.524   **Stenosis of incontinent stoma of urinary tract**
Revised   N99.528   **Other complication of incontinent external stoma of urinary tract**

Revised   N99.53   **Complication of continent stoma of urinary tract**
Revised   N99.530   **Hemorrhage of continent stoma of urinary tract**
Revised   N99.531   **Infection of continent stoma of urinary tract**
Revised   N99.532   **Malfunction of continent stoma of urinary tract**
New   N99.533   **Herniation of continent stoma of urinary tract**
New   N99.534   **Stenosis of continent stoma of urinary tract**
Revised   N99.538   **Other complication of continent stoma of urinary tract**

Revised   N99.82   **Postprocedural hemorrhage of a genitourinary system organ or structure following a procedure**
Revised   N99.820   **Postprocedural hemorrhage of a genitourinary system organ or structure following a genitourinary system procedure**
Revised   N99.821   **Postprocedural hemorrhage of a genitourinary system organ or structure following other procedure**

New   N99.84   **Postprocedural hematoma and seroma of a genitourinary system organ or structure following a procedure**
New   N99.840   **Postprocedural hematoma of a genitourinary system organ or structure following a genitourinary system procedure**
New   N99.841   **Postprocedural hematoma of a genitourinary system organ or structure following other procedure**
New   N99.842   **Postprocedural seroma of a genitourinary system organ or structure following a genitourinary system procedure**
New   N99.843   **Postprocedural seroma of a genitourinary system organ or structure following other procedure**

CHAPTER 15

PREGNANCY, CHILDBIRTH AND THE PUERPERIUM (O00-O9A)

Revised   Use additional code from category Z3A, Weeks of gestation, to identify the specific week of the pregnancy, if known.

O00.0 **Abdominal pregnancy**
New   O00.00   **Abdominal pregnancy without intrauterine pregnancy**
New   Abdominal pregnancy NOS
New   O00.01   **Abdominal pregnancy with intrauterine pregnancy**

O00.1 **Tubal pregnancy**
New   O00.10   **Tubal pregnancy without intrauterine pregnancy**
New   Tubal pregnancy NOS
New   O00.11   **Tubal pregnancy with intrauterine pregnancy**

	O00.2	Ovarian pregnancy		
New		O00.20	Ovarian pregnancy without intrauterine pregnancy
New			Ovarian pregnancy NOS
New		O00.21	Ovarian pregnancy with intrauterine pregnancy
New	O00.8	Other ectopic pregnancy	
New		O00.80	Other ectopic pregnancy without intrauterine pregnancy
New			Other ectopic pregnancy NOS
New		O00.81	Other ectopic pregnancy with intrauterine pregnancy
New	O00.9	Ectopic pregnancy, unspecified	
New		O00.90	Unspecified ectopic pregnancy without intrauterine pregnancy
New			Ectopic pregnancy NOS
New		O00.91	Unspecified ectopic pregnancy with intrauterine pregnancy
Revised	O09.1	Supervision of pregnancy with history of ectopic pregnancy	
Revised		O09.10	Supervision of pregnancy with history of ectopic pregnancy, unspecified trimester
Revised		O09.11	Supervision of pregnancy with history of ectopic pregnancy, first trimester
Revised		O09.12	Supervision of pregnancy with history of ectopic pregnancy, second trimester
Revised		O09.13	Supervision of pregnancy with history of ectopic pregnancy, third trimester
New	O09.A	Supervision of pregnancy with history of molar pregnancy	
New		O09.A0	Supervision of pregnancy with history of molar pregnancy, unspecified trimester
New		O09.A1	Supervision of pregnancy with history of molar pregnancy, first trimester
New		O09.A2	Supervision of pregnancy with history of molar pregnancy, second trimester
New		O09.A3	Supervision of pregnancy with history of molar pregnancy, third trimester
		O09.81	Supervision of pregnancy resulting from assisted reproductive technology
New			**Excludes2** gestational carrier status (Z33.3)
New	O11.4	Pre-existing hypertension with pre-eclampsia, complicating childbirth	
New	O11.5	Pre-existing hypertension with pre-eclampsia, complicating the puerperium	
New		O12.04	Gestational edema, complicating childbirth
New		O12.05	Gestational edema, complicating the puerperium
New		O12.14	Gestational proteinuria, complicating childbirth
New		O12.15	Gestational proteinuria, complicating the puerperium
New		O12.24	Gestational edema with proteinuria, complicating childbirth
New		O12.25	Gestational edema with proteinuria, complicating the puerperium

	O13	Gestational [pregnancy-induced] hypertension without significant proteinuria		
New		Includes	transient hypertension of pregnancy
New	O13.4	Gestational [pregnancy-induced] hypertension without significant proteinuria, complicating childbirth	
New	O13.5	Gestational [pregnancy-induced] hypertension without significant proteinuria, complicating the puerperium	
New		O14.04	Mild to moderate pre-eclampsia, complicating childbirth
New		O14.05	Mild to moderate pre-eclampsia, complicating the puerperium
New		O14.14	Severe pre-eclampsia complicating childbirth
New		O14.15	Severe pre-eclampsia, complicating the puerperium
New		O14.24	HELLP syndrome, complicating childbirth
New		O14.25	HELLP syndrome, complicating the puerperium
New		O14.94	Unspecified pre-eclampsia, complicating childbirth
New		O14.95	Unspecified pre-eclampsia, complicating the puerperium
Revised	O15.0	Eclampsia complicating pregnancy	
Revised		O15.00	Eclampsia complicating pregnancy, unspecified trimester
Revised		O15.02	Eclampsia complicating pregnancy, second trimester
Revised		O15.03	Eclampsia complicating pregnancy, third trimester
Revised	O15.1	Eclampsia complicating labor	
Revised	O15.2	Eclampsia complicating the puerperium	
New	O16.4	Unspecified maternal hypertension, complicating childbirth	
New	O16.5	Unspecified maternal hypertension, complicating the puerperium	
Revised	O24.0	Pre-existing type 1 diabetes mellitus, in pregnancy, childbirth and the puerperium	
Revised		O24.01	Pre-existing type 1 diabetes mellitus, in pregnancy
Revised			O24.011	Pre-existing type 1 diabetes mellitus, in pregnancy, first trimester
Revised			O24.012	Pre-existing type 1 diabetes mellitus, in pregnancy, second trimester
Revised			O24.013	Pre-existing type 1 diabetes mellitus, in pregnancy, third trimester
Revised			O24.019	Pre-existing type 1 diabetes mellitus, in pregnancy, unspecified trimester
Revised		O24.02	Pre-existing type 1 diabetes mellitus, in childbirth
Revised		O24.03	Pre-existing type 1 diabetes mellitus, in the puerperium
Revised	O24.1	Pre-existing type 2 diabetes mellitus, in pregnancy, childbirth and the puerperium	

Revised	O24.11	Pre-existing type 2 diabetes mellitus, in pregnancy
Revised	O24.111	Pre-existing type 2 diabetes mellitus, in pregnancy, first trimester
Revised	O24.112	Pre-existing type 2 diabetes mellitus, in pregnancy, second trimester
Revised	O24.113	Pre-existing type 2 diabetes mellitus, in pregnancy, third trimester
Revised	O24.119	Pre-existing type 2 diabetes mellitus, in pregnancy, unspecified trimester
Revised	O24.12	Pre-existing type 2 diabetes mellitus, in childbirth
Revised	O24.13	Pre-existing type 2 diabetes mellitus, in the puerperium
New	O24.415	Gestational diabetes mellitus in pregnancy, controlled by oral hypoglycemic drugs
New		Gestational diabetes mellitus in pregnancy, controlled by oral antidiabetic drugs
New	O24.425	Gestational diabetes mellitus in childbirth, controlled by oral hypoglycemic drugs
New		Gestational diabetes mellitus in childbirth, controlled by oral antidiabetic drugs
New	O24.435	Gestational diabetes mellitus in puerperium, controlled by oral hypoglycemic drugs
New		Gestational diabetes mellitus in puerperium, controlled by oral antidiabetic drugs

O33.7 Maternal care for disproportion due to other fetal deformities

New
One of the following 7th characters is to be assigned to code O33.7. 7th character 0 is for single gestations and multiple gestations where the fetus is unspecified. 7th characters 1 through 9 are for cases of multiple gestations to identify the fetus for which the code applies. The appropriate code from category O30, Multiple gestation, must also be assigned when assigning code O33.7 with a 7th character of 1 through 9.

New	0	not applicable or unspecified
New	1	fetus 1
New	2	fetus 2
New	3	fetus 3
New	4	fetus 4
New	5	fetus 5
New	9	other fetus

O34.0 Maternal care for congenital malformation of uterus

New Maternal care for double uterus
New Maternal care for uterus bicornis

New	O34.211	Maternal care for low transverse scar from previous cesarean delivery
New	O34.212	Maternal care for vertical scar from previous cesarean delivery
New		Maternal care for classical scar from previous cesarean delivery
New	O34.219	Maternal care for unspecified type scar from previous cesarean delivery
New	O34.29	Maternal care due to uterine scar from other previous surgery
New		Maternal care due to uterine scar from other transmural uterine incision
	O42.02	Full-term premature rupture of membranes, onset of labor within 24 hours of rupture
Revised		Premature rupture of membranes at or after 37 completed weeks of gestation, onset of labor within 24 hours of rupture
	O42.12	Full-term premature rupture of membranes, onset of labor more than 24 hours following rupture
Revised		Premature rupture of membranes at or after 37 completed weeks of gestation, onset of labor more than 24 hours following rupture
	O42.92	Full-term premature rupture of membranes, unspecified as to length of time between rupture and onset of labor
Revised		Premature rupture of membranes at or after 37 completed weeks of gestation, unspecified as to length of time between rupture and onset of labor
Revised	O44.0	Complete placenta previa NOS or without hemorrhage
Deleted		Low implantation of placenta specified as without hemorrhage
New		Placenta previa NOS
Revised	O44.00	Complete placenta previa NOS or without hemorrhage, unspecified trimester
Revised	O44.01	Complete placenta previa NOS or without hemorrhage, first trimester
Revised	O44.02	Complete placenta previa NOS or without hemorrhage, second trimester
Revised	O44.03	Complete placenta previa NOS or without hemorrhage, third trimester
Revised	O44.1	Complete placenta previa with hemorrhage
Deleted		Complete placenta previa with hemorrhage
Deleted		Low implantation of placenta, NOS or with hemorrhage
Deleted		Marginal placenta previa, NOS or with hemorrhage
Deleted		Partial placenta previa, NOS or with hemorrhage
Deleted		Total placenta previa, NOS or with hemorrhage
Revised	O44.10	Complete placenta previa with hemorrhage, unspecified trimester
Revised	O44.11	Complete placenta previa with hemorrhage, first trimester
Revised	O44.12	Complete placenta previa with hemorrhage, second trimester
Revised	O44.13	Complete placenta previa with hemorrhage, third trimester

New		O44.2	Partial placenta previa without hemorrhage
			Marginal placenta previa, NOS or without hemorrhage
New		O44.20	Partial placenta previa NOS or without hemorrhage, unspecified trimester
New		O44.21	Partial placenta previa NOS or without hemorrhage, first trimester
New		O44.22	Partial placenta previa NOS or without hemorrhage, second trimester
New		O44.23	Partial placenta previa NOS or without hemorrhage, third trimester
New	O44.3		Partial placenta previa with hemorrhage
New			Marginal placenta previa with hemorrhage
New		O44.30	Partial placenta previa with hemorrhage, unspecified trimester
New		O44.31	Partial placenta previa with hemorrhage, first trimester
New		O44.32	Partial placenta previa with hemorrhage, second trimester
New		O44.33	Partial placenta previa with hemorrhage, third trimester
New	O44.4		Low lying placenta NOS or without hemorrhage
New			Low implantation of placenta NOS or without hemorrhage
New		O44.40	Low lying placenta NOS or without hemorrhage, unspecified trimester
New		O44.41	Low lying placenta NOS or without hemorrhage, first trimester
New		O44.42	Low lying placenta NOS or without hemorrhage, second trimester
New		O44.43	Low lying placenta NOS or without hemorrhage, third trimester
New	O44.5		Low lying placenta with hemorrhage
New			Low implantation of placenta with hemorrhage
New		O44.50	Low lying placenta with hemorrhage, unspecified trimester
New		O44.51	Low lying placenta with hemorrhage, first trimester
New		O44.52	Low lying placenta with hemorrhage, second trimester
New		O44.53	Low lying placenta with hemorrhage, third trimester
New		O70.20	Third degree perineal laceration during delivery, unspecified
New		O70.21	Third degree perineal laceration during delivery, IIIa
New			Third degree perineal laceration during delivery with less than 50% of external anal sphincter (EAS) thickness torn
New		O70.22	Third degree perineal laceration during delivery, IIIb
New			Third degree perineal laceration during delivery with more than 50% external anal sphincter (EAS) thickness torn
New		O70.23	Third degree perineal laceration during delivery, IIIc
New			Third degree perineal laceration during delivery with both external anal sphincter (EAS) and internal anal sphincter (IAS) torn
Revised		O99.33	Tobacco use disorder complicating pregnancy, childbirth, and the puerperium
New			Smoking complicating pregnancy, childbirth, and the puerperium
New			Use additional code from category F17 to identify type of tobacco nicotine dependence

	O99.6		Diseases of the digestive system complicating pregnancy, childbirth and the puerperium
New		**Excludes2**	hemorrhoids in pregnancy (O22.4-)
	O99.82		Streptococcus B carrier state complicating pregnancy, childbirth and the puerperium
New		**Excludes1**	Carrier of streptococcus group B (GBS) in a nonpregnant woman (Z22.33Ø)

CHAPTER 16

CERTAIN CONDITIONS ORIGINATING IN THE PERINATAL PERIOD (P00-P96)

NEWBORN AFFECTED BY MATERNAL FACTORS AND BY COMPLICATIONS OF PREGNANCY, LABOR, AND DELIVERY (P00–P04)

Revised			**Note:** These codes are for use when the listed maternal conditions are specified as the cause of confirmed morbidity or potential morbidity which have their origin in the perinatal period (before birth through the first 28 days after birth).
Revised	P00		Newborn affected by maternal conditions that may be unrelated to present pregnancy
New		**Excludes2**	encounter for observation of newborn for suspected diseases and conditions ruled out (Z05.-)
New			newborn affected by maternal complications of pregnancy (P01.-)
Revised		P00.0	Newborn affected by maternal hypertensive disorders
Revised			Newborn affected by maternal conditions classifiable to O1Ø-O11, O13-O16
Revised		P00.1	Newborn affected by maternal renal and urinary tract diseases
Revised			Newborn affected by maternal conditions classifiable to NØØ-N39
Revised		P00.2	Newborn affected by maternal infectious and parasitic diseases
Revised			Newborn affected by maternal infectious disease classifiable to AØØ-B99, JØ9 and J1Ø
Revised		P00.3	Newborn affected by other maternal circulatory and respiratory diseases
Revised			Newborn affected by maternal conditions classifiable to IØØ-I99, JØØ-J99, Q2Ø-Q34 and not included in P00.0, P00.2
Revised		P00.4	Newborn affected by maternal nutritional disorders
Revised			Newborn affected by maternal disorders classifiable to E4Ø-E64
Revised		P00.5	Newborn affected by maternal injury
Revised			Newborn affected by maternal conditions classifiable to O9A.2-
Revised		P00.6	Newborn affected by surgical procedure on mother
Revised			Newborn affected by amniocentesis
Revised		P00.7	Newborn affected by other medical procedures on mother, not elsewhere classified
Revised			Newborn affected by radiation to mother
Revised		P00.8	Newborn affected by other maternal conditions
Revised		P00.81	Newborn affected by periodontal disease in mother
Revised		P00.89	Newborn affected by other maternal conditions
Revised			Newborn affected by conditions classifiable to T8Ø-T88
Revised			Newborn affected by maternal genital tract or other localized infections
Revised			Newborn affected by maternal systemic lupus erythematosus
Revised		P00.9	Newborn affected by unspecified maternal condition

Revised	**P01**	**Newborn affected by maternal complications of pregnancy**
New		**Excludes2** encounter for observation of newborn for suspected diseases and conditions ruled out (Z05.-)
Revised	**P01.0**	**Newborn affected by incompetent cervix**
Revised	**P01.1**	**Newborn affected by premature rupture of membranes**
Revised	**P01.2**	**Newborn affected by oligohydramnios**
Revised	**P01.3**	**Newborn affected by polyhydramnios**
Revised		Newborn affected by hydramnios
Revised	**P01.4**	**Newborn affected by ectopic pregnancy**
Revised		Newborn affected by abdominal pregnancy
Revised	**P01.5**	**Newborn affected by multiple pregnancy**
Revised		Newborn affected by triplet (pregnancy)
Revised		Newborn affected by twin (pregnancy)
Revised	**P01.6**	**Newborn affected by maternal death**
Revised	**P01.7**	**Newborn affected by malpresentation before labor**
Revised		Newborn affected by breech presentation before labor
Revised		Newborn affected by external version before labor
Revised		Newborn affected by face presentation before labor
Revised		Newborn affected by transverse lie before labor
Revised		Newborn affected by unstable lie before labor
Revised	**P01.8**	**Newborn affected by other maternal complications of pregnancy**
Revised	**P01.9**	**Newborn affected by maternal complication of pregnancy, unspecified**
Revised	**P02**	**Newborn affected by complications of placenta, cord and membranes**
New		**Excludes2** encounter for observation of newborn for suspected diseases and conditions ruled out (Z05.-)
Revised	**P02.0**	**Newborn affected by placenta previa**
Revised	**P02.1**	**Newborn affected by other forms of placental separation and hemorrhage**
Revised		Newborn affected by abruptio placenta
Revised		Newborn affected by accidental hemorrhage
Revised		Newborn affected by antepartum hemorrhage
Revised		Newborn affected by damage to placenta from amniocentesis, cesarean delivery or surgical induction
Revised		Newborn affected by maternal blood loss
Revised		Newborn affected by premature separation of placenta
Revised	**P02.2**	**Newborn affected by other and unspecified morphological and functional abnormalities of placenta**
Revised	**P02.20**	**Newborn affected by unspecified morphological and functional abnormalities of placenta**
Revised	**P02.29**	**Newborn affected by other morphological and functional abnormalities of placenta**
Revised		Newborn affected by placental dysfunction
Revised		Newborn affected by placental infarction
Revised		Newborn affected by placental insufficiency
Revised	**P02.3**	**Newborn affected by placental transfusion syndromes**
Revised		Newborn affected by placental and cord abnormalities resulting in twin-to-twin or other transplacental transfusion
Revised	**P02.4**	**Newborn affected by prolapsed cord**
Revised	**P02.5**	**Newborn affected by other compression of umbilical cord**
Revised		Newborn affected by umbilical cord (tightly) around neck
Revised		Newborn affected by entanglement of umbilical cord
Revised		Newborn affected by knot in umbilical cord
Revised	**P02.6**	**Newborn affected by other and unspecified conditions of umbilical cord**
Revised	**P02.60**	**Newborn affected by unspecified conditions of umbilical cord**
Revised	**P02.69**	**Newborn affected by other conditions of umbilical cord**
Revised		Newborn affected by short umbilical cord
		Newborn affected by vasa previa
Revised	**P02.7**	**Newborn affected by chorioamnionitis**
Revised		Newborn affected by amnionitis
Revised		Newborn affected by membranitis
Revised		Newborn affected by placentitis
Revised	**P02.8**	**Newborn affected by other abnormalities of membranes**
Revised	**P02.9**	**Newborn affected by abnormality of membranes, unspecified**
Revised	**P03**	**Newborn affected by other complications of labor and delivery**
New		**Excludes2** encounter for observation of newborn for suspected diseases and conditions ruled out (Z05.-)
Revised	**P03.0**	**Newborn affected by breech delivery and extraction**
Revised	**P03.1**	**Newborn affected by other malpresentation, malposition and disproportion during labor and delivery**
Revised		Newborn affected by contracted pelvis
Revised		Newborn affected by conditions classifiable to O64-O66
Revised		Newborn affected by persistent occipitoposterior
Revised		Newborn affected by transverse lie
Revised	**P03.2**	**Newborn affected by forceps delivery**
Revised	**P03.3**	**Newborn affected by delivery by vacuum extractor [ventouse]**
Revised	**P03.4**	**Newborn affected by Cesarean delivery**
Revised	**P03.5**	**Newborn affected by precipitate delivery**
Revised		Newborn affected by rapid second stage
Revised	**P03.6**	**Newborn affected by abnormal uterine contractions**
Revised		Newborn affected by conditions classifiable to O62.-, except O62.3
Revised		Newborn affected by hypertonic labor
Revised		Newborn affected by uterine inertia
Revised	**P03.8**	**Newborn affected by other specified complications of labor and delivery**
Revised	**P03.81**	**Newborn affected by abnormality in fetal (intrauterine) heart rate or rhythm**
Revised	**P03.810**	**Newborn affected by abnormality in fetal (intrauterine) heart rate or rhythm before the onset of labor**
Revised	**P03.811**	**Newborn affected by abnormality in fetal (intrauterine) heart rate or rhythm during labor**
Revised	**P03.819**	**Newborn affected by abnormality in fetal (intrauterine) heart rate or rhythm, unspecified as to time of onset**

Revised	P03.89		**Newborn affected by other specified complications of labor and delivery**
Revised			Newborn affected by abnormality of maternal soft tissues
Revised			Newborn affected by conditions classifiable to O60-O75 and by procedures used in labor and delivery not included in P02.- and P03.0-P03.6
Revised			Newborn affected by induction of labor
Revised	P03.9		**Newborn affected by complication of labor and delivery, unspecified**
Revised	P04		**Newborn affected by noxious substances transmitted via placenta or breast milk**
New		**Excludes2**	congenital malformations (Q00-Q99) encounter for observation of newborn for suspected diseases and conditions ruled out (Z05.-)
Revised	P04.0		**Newborn affected by maternal anesthesia and analgesia in pregnancy, labor and delivery**
			Newborn affected by reactions and intoxications from maternal opiates and tranquilizers administered during labor and delivery
Revised	P04.1		**Newborn affected by other maternal medication**
Revised			Newborn affected by cancer chemotherapy
Revised			Newborn affected by cytotoxic drugs
Revised	P04.2		**Newborn affected by maternal use of tobacco**
			Newborn affected by exposure in utero to tobacco smoke
Revised	P04.3		**Newborn affected by maternal use of alcohol**
	P04.4		**Newborn affected by maternal use of drugs of addiction**
Revised			
Revised		P04.41	**Newborn affected by maternal use of cocaine**
Revised		P04.49	**Newborn affected by maternal use of other drugs of addiction**
Revised			**Excludes2** newborn affected by maternal anesthesia and analgesia (P04.0)
Revised	P04.5		**Newborn affected by maternal use of nutritional chemical substances**
Revised	P04.6		**Newborn affected by maternal exposure to environmental chemical substances**
Revised	P04.8		**Newborn affected by other maternal noxious substances**
Revised	P04.9		**Newborn affected by maternal noxious substance, unspecified**
	P05.0		**Newborn light for gestational age**
New			Weight below but length above 10th percentile for gestational age
New		P05.09	**Newborn light for gestational age, 2500 grams and over**
New			Newborn light for gestational age, other
	P05.1		**Newborn small for gestational age**
New			Weight and length below 10th percentile for gestational age
New		P05.19	**Newborn small for gestational age, other**
New			Newborn small for gestational age, 2500 grams and over

	P07		**Disorders of newborn related to short gestation and low birth weight, not elsewhere classified**
Deleted		**Excludes1**	low birth weight due to slow fetal growth and fetal malnutrition (P05.-)
	P07.0		**Extremely low birth weight newborn**
New		**Excludes1**	low birth weight due to slow fetal growth and fetal malnutrition (P05.-)
	P07.1		**Other low birth weight newborn**
New		**Excludes1**	low birth weight due to slow fetal growth and fetal malnutrition (P05.-)
	P96.5		**Complication to newborn due to (fetal) intrauterine procedure**
Revised		**Excludes2**	newborn affected by amniocentesis (P00.6)

CHAPTER 17

CONGENITAL MALFORMATIONS, DEFORMATIONS AND CHROMOSOMAL ABNORMALITIES (Q00-Q99)

	Q25.1		**Coarctation of aorta**
New			Stenosis of aorta
	Q25.2		**Atresia of aorta**
New		Q25.21	**Interruption of aortic arch**
New			Atresia of aortic arch
New		Q25.29	**Other atresia of aorta**
New			Atresia of aorta
	Q25.4		**Other congenital malformations of aorta**
Deleted			Absence of aorta
Deleted			Aneurysm of sinus of Valsalva (ruptured)
Deleted			Aplasia of aorta
Deleted			Congenital aneurysm of aorta
Deleted			Congenital malformations of aorta
Deleted			Congenital dilatation of aorta
Deleted			Double aortic arch [vascular ring of aorta]
Deleted			Hypoplasia of aorta
Deleted			Persistent convolutions of aortic arch
Deleted			Persistent right aortic arch
New		Q25.40	**Congenital malformation of aorta unspecified**
New		Q25.41	**Absence and aplasia of aorta**
New		Q25.42	**Hypoplasia of aorta**
New		Q25.43	**Congenital aneurysm of aorta**
			Congenital aneurysm of aortic root
			Congenital aneurysm of aortic sinus
New		Q25.44	**Congenital dilation of aorta**
New		Q25.45	**Double aortic arch**
			Vascular ring of aorta
New		Q25.46	**Tortuous aortic arch**
			Persistent convolutions of aortic arch
New		Q25.47	**Right aortic arch**
			Persistent right aortic arch
New		Q25.48	**Anomalous origin of subclavian artery**
New		Q25.49	**Other congenital malformations of aorta**
	Q52.12		**Longitudinal vaginal septum**
Deleted			Longitudinal vaginal septum with or without obstruction
New		Q52.120	**Longitudinal vaginal septum, nonobstructing**
New		Q52.121	**Longitudinal vaginal septum, obstructing, right side**

New		Q52.122	**Longitudinal vaginal septum, obstructing, left side**
New		Q52.123	**Longitudinal vaginal septum, microperforate, right side**
New		Q52.124	**Longitudinal vaginal septum, microperforate, left side**
New		Q52.129	**Other and unspecified longitudinal vaginal septum**
New		Q66.21	**Congenital metatarsus primus varus**
New		Q66.22	**Congenital metatarsus adductus**
			Congenital metatarsus varus
New	Q82.6	**Congenital sacral dimple**	
New		Parasacral dimple	
New		**Excludes2**	pilonidal cyst with abscess (L05.01)
New			pilonidal cyst without abscess (L05.91)
New		Q87.82	**Arterial tortuosity syndrome**

CHAPTER 18

SYMPTOMS, SIGNS AND ABNORMAL CLINICAL AND LABORATORY FINDINGS, NOT ELSEWHERE CLASSIFIED (R00-R99)

	R00	**Abnormalities of heart beat**	
Deleted		**Excludes1**	specified arrhythmias (I47-I49)
New		**Excludes2**	specified arrhythmias (I47-I49)
	R01.1	**Cardiac murmur, unspecified**	
New		Systolic murmur NOS	

SYMPTOMS AND SIGNS INVOLVING THE DIGESTIVE SYSTEM AND ABDOMEN (R10-R19)

Deleted		**Excludes1**	congenital or infantile pylorospasm (Q40.0)
Deleted			gastrointestinal hemorrhage (K92.0-K92.2)
Deleted			intestinal obstruction (K56.-)
Deleted			newborn gastrointestinal hemorrhage (P54.0-P54.3)
Deleted			newborn intestinal obstruction (P76.-)
Deleted			pylorospasm (K31.3)
Deleted			signs and symptoms involving the urinary system (R30-R39)
Deleted			symptoms referable to female genital organs (N94.-)
Deleted			symptoms referable to male genital organs (N48-N50)
New		**Excludes2**	congenital or infantile pylorospasm (Q40.0)
New			gastrointestinal hemorrhage (K92.0-K92.2)
New			intestinal obstruction (K56.-)
New			newborn gastrointestinal hemorrhage (P54.0-P54.3)
New			newborn intestinal obstruction (P76.-)
New			pylorospasm (K31.3)
New			signs and symptoms involving the urinary system (R30-R39)
New			symptoms referable to female genital organs (N94.-)
New			symptoms referable to male genital organs (N48-N50)
	R11	**Nausea and vomiting**	
Revised		**Excludes1**	psychogenic vomiting (F50.89)

New	R29.7	**National Institutes of Health Stroke Scale (NIHSS) score**	
New		*Code first* the type of cerebral infarction (I63-)	
New	R29.70	**NIHSS score 0-9**	
New		R29.700	**NIHSS score 0**
New		R29.701	**NIHSS score 1**
New		R29.702	**NIHSS score 2**
New		R29.703	**NIHSS score 3**
New		R29.704	**NIHSS score 4**
New		R29.705	**NIHSS score 5**
New		R29.706	**NIHSS score 6**
New		R29.707	**NIHSS score 7**
New		R29.708	**NIHSS score 8**
New		R29.709	**NIHSS score 9**
New	R29.71	**NIHSS score 10-19**	
New		R29.710	**NIHSS score 10**
New		R29.711	**NIHSS score 11**
New		R29.712	**NIHSS score 12**
New		R29.713	**NIHSS score 13**
New		R29.714	**NIHSS score 14**
New		R29.715	**NIHSS score 15**
New		R29.716	**NIHSS score 16**
New		R29.717	**NIHSS score 17**
New		R29.718	**NIHSS score 18**
New		R29.719	**NIHSS score 19**
New	R29.72	**NIHSS score 20-29**	
New		R29.720	**NIHSS score 20**
New		R29.721	**NIHSS score 21**
New		R29.722	**NIHSS score 22**
New		R29.723	**NIHSS score 23**
New		R29.724	**NIHSS score 24**
New		R29.725	**NIHSS score 25**
New		R29.726	**NIHSS score 26**
New		R29.727	**NIHSS score 27**
New		R29.728	**NIHSS score 28**
New		R29.729	**NIHSS score 29**
New	R29.73	**NIHSS score 30-39**	
New		R29.730	**NIHSS score 30**
New		R29.731	**NIHSS score 31**
New		R29.732	**NIHSS score 32**
New		R29.733	**NIHSS score 33**
New		R29.734	**NIHSS score 34**
New		R29.735	**NIHSS score 35**
New		R29.736	**NIHSS score 36**
New		R29.737	**NIHSS score 37**
New		R29.738	**NIHSS score 38**
New		R29.739	**NIHSS score 39**
New	R29.74	**NIHSS score 40-42**	
New		R29.740	**NIHSS score 40**
New		R29.741	**NIHSS score 41**
New		R29.742	**NIHSS score 42**
New	R31.21	**Asymptomatic microscopic hematuria**	
New		AMH	
New	R31.29	**Other microscopic hematuria**	
	R39.19	**Other difficulties with micturition**	
New		R39.191	**Need to immediately re-void**
New		R39.192	**Position dependent micturition**
New		R39.198	**Other difficulties with micturition**
New		R39.82	**Chronic bladder pain**

SYMPTOMS AND SIGNS INVOLVING COGNITION, PERCEPTION, EMOTIONAL STATE AND BEHAVIOR (R40-R46)

Deleted — **Excludes1** symptoms and signs constituting part of a pattern of mental disorder (F01-F99)

New — **Excludes2** symptoms and signs constituting part of a pattern of mental disorder (F01-F99)

R40.2 Coma

Revised — **Note:** One code from each subcategory R40.21-R40-23 is required to complete the coma scale

R40.24 Glasgow coma scale, total score

Deleted — Use codes R40.21- through R40.23- only when the individual score(s) are documented

New — Note: Assign a code from subcategory R40.24, when only the total coma score is documented

New — The following appropriate 7th character is to be added to subcategory R40.24-:

New Ø	unspecified time
New 1	in the field [EMT or ambulance]
New 2	at arrival to emergency department
New 3	at hospital admission
New 4	24 hours or more after hospital admission

R41.84 Other specified cognitive deficit

New — **Excludes1** cognitive deficits as sequelae of cerebrovascular disease (I69.01-, I69.11-, I69.21-, I69.31-, I69.81-, I69.91-)

R46.81 Obsessive-compulsive behavior

Revised — **Excludes1** obsessive-compulsive disorder (F42-)

R50.82 Postprocedural fever

Revised — **Excludes1** postprocedural infection (T81.4-)

R53.1 Weakness

New — **Excludes1** sarcopenia (M62.84)

R54 Age-related physical debility

New — **Excludes1** sarcopenia (M62.84)

R63.0 Anorexia

Revised — **Excludes1** loss of appetite of nonorganic origin (F50.89)

R65.2 Severe sepsis

Revised — *Code first underlying infection, such as:* infection following a procedure (T81.4-)

R68.84 Jaw pain

Revised — **Excludes1** temporomandibular joint arthralgia (M26.62-)

ABNORMAL FINDINGS ON EXAMINATION OF BLOOD, WITHOUT DIAGNOSIS (R70-R79)

Deleted — **Excludes1** abnormalities (of)(on):

Deleted — abnormal findings on antenatal screening of mother (O28.-)

Deleted — coagulation hemorrhagic disorders (D65-D68)

Deleted — lipids (E78.-)

Deleted — platelets and thrombocytes (D69.-)

Deleted — white blood cells classified elsewhere (D70-D72)

Deleted — diagnostic abnormal findings classified elsewhere - see Alphabetical Index

Deleted — hemorrhagic and hematological disorders of newborn (P50-P61)

New — **Excludes2** abnormal findings on antenatal screening of mother (O28.-)

New — abnormalities of lipids (E78.-)

New — abnormalities of platelets and thrombocytes (D69.-)

New — abnormalities of white blood cells classified elsewhere (D70-D72)

New — coagulation hemorrhagic disorders (D65-D68)

New — diagnostic abnormal findings classified elsewhere —*see* Alphabetical Index

New — hemorrhagic and hematological disorders of newborn (P50-P61)

New — **R73.03 Prediabetes**
New — Latent diabetes

New — **R73.09 Other abnormal glucose**
Deleted — Latent diabetes
Deleted — Prediabetes

R78.81 Bacteremia

Revised — **Excludes1** sepsis-code to specified infection

R82.7 Abnormal findings on microbiological examination of urine

Deleted — Positive culture findings of urine

New — **R82.71 Bacteriuria**

New — **R82.79 Other abnormal findings on microbiological examination of urine**

New — Positive culture findings of urine

R93.4 Abnormal findings on diagnostic imaging of urinary organs

Deleted — Filling defect of bladder found on diagnostic imaging

Deleted — Filling defect of kidney found on diagnostic imaging

Deleted — Filling defect of ureter found on diagnostic imaging

Deleted — **Excludes1** hypertrophy of kidney (N28.81)

New — **Excludes2** hypertrophy of kidney (N28.81)

New — **R93.41 Abnormal radiologic findings on diagnostic imaging of renal pelvis, ureter, or bladder**

New — Filling defect of bladder found on diagnostic imaging

New — Filling defect of renal pelvis found on diagnostic imaging

New — Filling defect of ureter found on diagnostic imaging

New	R93.42		Abnormal radiologic findings on diagnostic imaging of kidney
New		R93.421	Abnormal radiologic findings on diagnostic imaging of right kidney
New		R93.422	Abnormal radiologic findings on diagnostic imaging of left kidney
New		R93.429	Abnormal radiologic findings on diagnostic imaging of unspecified kidney
New	R93.49		Abnormal radiologic findings on diagnostic imaging of other urinary organs
New	R97.20		Elevated prostate specific antigen [PSA]
New	R97.21		Rising PSA following treatment for malignant neoplasm of prostate

CHAPTER 19

INJURY, POISONING AND CERTAIN OTHER CONSEQUENCES OF EXTERNAL CAUSES (S00-T88)

	S00.8		Superficial injury of other parts of head
New			Superficial injuries of face [any part]
New		S02.101	Fracture of base of skull, right side
New		S02.102	Fracture of base of skull, left side
New		S02.109	Fracture of base of skull, unspecified side
Revised		S02.110	Type I occipital condyle fracture, unspecified side
Revised		S02.111	Type II occipital condyle fracture, unspecified side
Revised		S02.112	Type III occipital condyle fracture, unspecified side
Revised		S02.118	Other fracture of occiput, unspecified side
New		S02.11A	Type I occipital condyle fracture, right side
New		S02.11B	Type I occipital condyle fracture, left side
New		S02.11C	Type II occipital condyle fracture, right side
New		S02.11D	Type II occipital condyle fracture, left side
New		S02.11E	Type III occipital condyle fracture, right side
New		S02.11F	Type III occipital condyle fracture, left side
New		S02.11G	Other fracture of occiput, right side
New		S02.11H	Other fracture of occiput, left side
New	S02.30		Fracture of orbital floor, unspecified side
New	S02.31		Fracture of orbital floor, right side
New	S02.32		Fracture of orbital floor, left side
Revised		S02.400	Malar fracture, unspecified side
Revised		S02.401	Maxillary fracture, unspecified side
Revised		S02.402	Zygomatic fracture, unspecified side
New		S02.40A	Malar fracture, right side
New		S02.40B	Malar fracture, left side
New		S02.40C	Maxillary fracture, right side
New		S02.40D	Maxillary fracture, left side
New		S02.40E	Zygomatic fracture, right side
New		S02.40F	Zygomatic fracture, left side
Revised		S02.600	Fracture of unspecified part of body of mandible, unspecified side
New		S02.601	Fracture of unspecified part of body of right mandible
New		S02.602	Fracture of unspecified part of body of left mandible
New		S02.610	Fracture of condylar process of mandible, unspecified side
New		S02.611	Fracture of condylar process of right mandible
New		S02.612	Fracture of condylar process of left mandible
New		S02.620	Fracture of subcondylar process of mandible, unspecified side
New		S02.621	Fracture of subcondylar process of right mandible
New		S02.622	Fracture of subcondylar process of left mandible
New		S02.630	Fracture of coronoid process of mandible, unspecified side
New		S02.631	Fracture of coronoid process of right mandible
New		S02.632	Fracture of coronoid process of left mandible
New		S02.640	Fracture of ramus of mandible, unspecified side
New		S02.641	Fracture of ramus of right mandible
New		S02.642	Fracture of ramus of left mandible
New		S02.650	Fracture of angle of mandible, unspecified side
New		S02.651	Fracture of angle of right mandible
New		S02.652	Fracture of angle of left mandible
New		S02.670	Fracture of alveolus of mandible, unspecified side
New		S02.671	Fracture of alveolus of right mandible
New		S02.672	Fracture of alveolus of left mandible
New	S02.80		Fracture of other specified skull and facial bones, unspecified side
New	S02.81		Fracture of other specified skull and facial bones, right side
New	S02.82		Fracture of other specified skull and facial bones, left side
New	S03.00		Dislocation of jaw, unspecified side
New	S03.01		Dislocation of jaw, right side
New	S03.02		Dislocation of jaw, left side
New	S03.03		Dislocation of jaw, bilateral side

New	S03.40	**Sprain of jaw, unspecified side**	
New	S03.41	**Sprain of jaw, right side**	
New	S03.42	**Sprain of jaw, left side**	
New	S03.43	**Sprain of jaw, bilateral side**	
	S06.0	**Concussion**	
Revised		**Excludes1** concussion with other intracranial injuries classified in subcategories S06.1- to S06.6- , S06.81- and S06.82- code to specified intracranial injury	
Deleted		~~S06.0X2~~ ~~Concussion with loss of consciousness of 31 minutes to 59 minutes~~	
Deleted		~~S06.0X3~~ ~~Concussion with loss of consciousness of 1 hour to 5 hours 59 minutes~~	
Deleted		~~S06.0X4~~ ~~Concussion with loss of consciousness of 6 hours to 24 hours~~	
Deleted		~~S06.0X5~~ ~~Concussion with loss of consciousness greater than 24 hours with return to pre-existing conscious level~~	
Deleted		~~S06.0X6~~ ~~Concussion with loss of consciousness greater than 24 hours without return to pre-existing conscious level with patient surviving~~	
Deleted		~~S06.0X7~~ ~~Concussion with loss of consciousness of any duration with death due to brain injury prior to regaining consciousness~~	
Deleted		~~S06.0X8~~ ~~Concussion with loss of consciousness of any duration with death due to other cause prior to regaining consciousness~~	
	S06.89	**Other specified intracranial injury**	
New		**Excludes1** concussion (S06.0X-)	
	S06.9	**Unspecified intracranial injury**	
New		Traumatic brain injury NOS	
New		**Excludes1** conditions classifiable to S06.0- to S06.8-code to specified intracranial injury	
	S34.101	**Unspecified injury to L₁ level of lumbar spinal cord**	
New		Unspecified injury to lumbar spinal cord level 1	
	S34.102	**Unspecified injury to L₂ level of lumbar spinal cord**	
New		Unspecified injury to lumbar spinal cord level 2	
	S34.103	**Unspecified injury to L₃ level of lumbar spinal cord**	
New		Unspecified injury to lumbar spinal cord level 3	
	S34.104	**Unspecified injury to L₄ level of lumbar spinal cord**	
New		Unspecified injury to lumbar spinal cord level 4	
	S34.105	**Unspecified injury to L₅ level of lumbar spinal cord**	
New		Unspecified injury to lumbar spinal cord level 5	

	S34.111	**Complete lesion of L₁ level of lumbar spinal cord**	
New		Complete lesion of lumbar spinal cord level 1	
	S34.112	**Complete lesion of L₂ level of lumbar spinal cord**	
New		Complete lesion of lumbar spinal cord level 2	
	S34.113	**Complete lesion of L₃ level of lumbar spinal cord**	
New		Complete lesion of lumbar spinal cord level 3	
	S34.114	**Complete lesion of L₄ level of lumbar spinal cord**	
New		Complete lesion of lumbar spinal cord level 4	
	S34.115	**Complete lesion of L₅ level of lumbar spinal cord**	
New		Complete lesion of lumbar spinal cord level 5	
	S34.121	**Incomplete lesion of L₁ level of lumbar spinal cord**	
New		Incomplete lesion of lumbar spinal cord level 1	
	S34.122	**Incomplete lesion of L₂ level of lumbar spinal cord**	
New		Incomplete lesion of lumbar spinal cord level 2	
	S34.123	**Incomplete lesion of L₃ level of lumbar spinal cord**	
New		Incomplete lesion of lumbar spinal cord level 3	
	S34.124	**Incomplete lesion of L₄ level of lumbar spinal cord**	
New		Incomplete lesion of lumbar spinal cord level 4	
	S34.125	**Incomplete lesion of L₅ level of lumbar spinal cord**	
New		Incomplete lesion of lumbar spinal cord level 5	
Revised	S49.031	**Salter-Harris Type III physeal fracture of upper end of humerus, right arm**	
Revised	S49.032	**Salter-Harris Type III physeal fracture of upper end of humerus, left arm**	
Revised	S49.039	**Salter-Harris Type III physeal fracture of upper end of humerus, unspecified arm**	
Revised	S49.13	**Salter-Harris Type III physeal fracture of lower end of humerus**	
Revised	S49.131	**Salter-Harris Type III physeal fracture of lower end of humerus, right arm**	
Revised	S49.132	**Salter-Harris Type III physeal fracture of lower end of humerus, left arm**	
Revised	S49.139	**Salter-Harris Type III physeal fracture of lower end of humerus, unspecified arm**	
Revised	S54.8X	**Injury of other nerves at forearm level**	
Revised	S54.8X1	**Injury of other nerves at forearm level, right arm**	
Revised	S54.8X2	**Injury of other nerves at forearm level, left arm**	
Revised	S54.8X9	**Injury of other nerves at forearm level, unspecified arm**	

New   **S92.0**   **Fracture of calcaneus**
New   **Excludes2**   Physeal fracture of calcaneus (S99.0-)
New   **S92.3**   **Fracture of metatarsal bone(s)**
New   **Excludes2**   Physeal fracture of metatarsal (S99.1-)
New   **S92.4**   **Fracture of great toe**
    Excludes2   Physeal fracture of phalanx of toe (S99.2-)
New   **S92.5**   **Fracture of lesser toe(s)**
    Excludes2   Physeal fracture of phalanx of toe (S99.2-)
New   **S92.8**   **Other fracture of foot, except ankle**
New   **S92.81**   **Other fracture of foot**
     Sesamoid fracture of foot
New   **S92.811**   **Other fracture of right foot**
New   **S92.812**   **Other fracture of left foot**
New   **S92.819**   **Other fracture of unspecified foot**

  S99   **Other and unspecified injuries of ankle and foot**
Deleted   The appropriate 7th character is to be added to each code from subcategories S99

Deleted   A   initial encounter
Deleted   D   subsequent encounter
Deleted   S   sequela

New   **S99.0**   **Physeal fracture of calcaneus**
New   The appropriate 7th character is to be added to each code from subcategories S99.0

New A   initial encounter for closed fracture
New B   initial encounter for open fracture
New D   subsequent encounter for fracture with routine healing
New G   subsequent encounter for fracture with delayed healing
New K   subsequent encounter for fracture with nonunion
New P   subsequent encounter for fracture with malunion
New S   sequela

New   **S99.00**   **Unspecified physeal fracture of calcaneus**
New   **S99.001**   **Unspecified physeal fracture of right calcaneus**
New   **S99.002**   **Unspecified physeal fracture of left calcaneus**
New   **S99.009**   **Unspecified physeal fracture of unspecified calcaneus**
New   **S99.01**   **Salter-Harris Type I physeal fracture of calcaneus**
New   **S99.011**   **Salter-Harris Type I physeal fracture of right calcaneus**
New   **S99.012**   **Salter-Harris Type I physeal fracture of left calcaneus**
New   **S99.019**   **Salter-Harris Type I physeal fracture of unspecified calcaneus**
New   **S99.02**   **Salter-Harris Type II physeal fracture of calcaneus**
New   **S99.021**   **Salter-Harris Type II physeal fracture of right calcaneus**
New   **S99.022**   **Salter-Harris Type II physeal fracture of left calcaneus**
New   **S99.029**   **Salter-Harris Type II physeal fracture of unspecified calcaneus**

New   **S99.03**   **Salter-Harris Type III physeal fracture of calcaneus**
New   **S99.031**   **Salter-Harris Type III physeal fracture of right calcaneus**
New   **S99.032**   **Salter-Harris Type III physeal fracture of left calcaneus**
New   **S99.039**   **Salter-Harris Type III physeal fracture of unspecified calcaneus**
New   **S99.04**   **Salter-Harris Type IV physeal fracture of calcaneus**
New   **S99.041**   **Salter-Harris Type IV physeal fracture of right calcaneus**
New   **S99.042**   **Salter-Harris Type IV physeal fracture of left calcaneus**
New   **S99.049**   **Salter-Harris Type IV physeal fracture of unspecified calcaneus**
New   **S99.09**   **Other physeal fracture of calcaneus**
New   **S99.091**   **Other physeal fracture of right calcaneus**
New   **S99.092**   **Other physeal fracture of left calcaneus**
New   **S99.099**   **Other physeal fracture of unspecified calcaneus**

New   **S99.1**   **Physeal fracture of metatarsal**
New   The appropriate 7th character is to be added to each code from subcategories S99.1

New A   initial encounter for closed fracture
New B   initial encounter for open fracture
New D   subsequent encounter for fracture with routine healing
New G   subsequent encounter for fracture with delayed healing
New K   subsequent encounter for fracture with nonunion
New P   subsequent encounter for fracture with malunion
New S   sequela

New   **S99.10**   **Unspecified physeal fracture of metatarsal**
New   **S99.101**   **Unspecified physeal fracture of right metatarsal**
New   **S99.102**   **Unspecified physeal fracture of left metatarsal**
New   **S99.109**   **Unspecified physeal fracture of unspecified metatarsal**
New   **S99.11**   **Salter-Harris Type I physeal fracture of metatarsal**
New   **S99.111**   **Salter-Harris Type I physeal fracture of right metatarsal**
New   **S99.112**   **Salter-Harris Type I physeal fracture of left metatarsal**
New   **S99.119**   **Salter-Harris Type I physeal fracture of unspecified metatarsal**
New   **S99.12**   **Salter-Harris Type II physeal fracture of metatarsal**
New   **S99.121**   **Salter-Harris Type II physeal fracture of right metatarsal**
New   **S99.122**   **Salter-Harris Type II physeal fracture of left metatarsal**
New   **S99.129**   **Salter-Harris Type II physeal fracture of unspecified metatarsal**

New   S99.13   Salter-Harris Type III physeal fracture of metatarsal

New   S99.131   Salter-Harris Type III physeal fracture of right metatarsal

New   S99.132   Salter-Harris Type III physeal fracture of left metatarsal

New   S99.139   Salter-Harris Type III physeal fracture of unspecified metatarsal

New   S99.14   Salter-Harris Type IV physeal fracture of metatarsal

New   S99.141   Salter-Harris Type IV physeal fracture of right metatarsal

New   S99.142   Salter-Harris Type IV physeal fracture of left metatarsal

New   S99.149   Salter-Harris Type IV physeal fracture of unspecified metatarsal

New   S99.19   Other physeal fracture of metatarsal

New   S99.191   Other physeal fracture of right metatarsal

New   S99.192   Other physeal fracture of left metatarsal

New   S99.199   Other physeal fracture of unspecified metatarsal

New   S99.2   Physeal fracture of phalanx of toe

New   The appropriate 7th character is to be added to each code from subcategories S99.2

New   A   initial encounter for closed fracture
New   B   initial encounter for open fracture
New   D   subsequent encounter for fracture with routine healing
New   G   subsequent encounter for fracture with delayed healing
New   K   subsequent encounter for fracture with nonunion
New   P   subsequent encounter for fracture with malunion
New   S   sequela

New   S99.20   Unspecified physeal fracture of phalanx of toe

New   S99.201   Unspecified physeal fracture of phalanx of right toe

New   S99.202   Unspecified physeal fracture of phalanx of right toe

New   S99.209   Unspecified physeal fracture of phalanx of unspecified toe

New   S99.21   Salter-Harris Type I physeal fracture of phalanx of toe

New   S99.211   Salter-Harris Type I physeal fracture of phalanx of right toe

New   S99.212   Salter-Harris Type I physeal fracture of phalanx of left toe

New   S99.219   Salter-Harris Type I physeal fracture of phalanx of unspecified toe

New   S99.22   Salter-Harris Type II physeal fracture of phalanx of toe

New   S99.221   Salter-Harris Type II physeal fracture of phalanx of right toe

New   S99.222   Salter-Harris Type II physeal fracture of phalanx of left toe

New   S99.229   Salter-Harris Type II physeal fracture of phalanx of unspecified toe

New   S99.23   Salter-Harris Type III physeal fracture of phalanx of toe

New   S99.231   Salter-Harris Type III physeal fracture of phalanx of right toe

New   S99.232   Salter-Harris Type III physeal fracture of phalanx of left toe

New   S99.239   Salter-Harris Type III physeal fracture of phalanx of unspecified toe

New   S99.24   Salter-Harris Type IV physeal fracture of phalanx of toe

New   S99.241   Salter-Harris Type IV physeal fracture of phalanx of right toe

New   S99.242   Salter-Harris Type IV physeal fracture of phalanx of left toe

New   S99.249   Salter-Harris Type IV physeal fracture of phalanx of unspecified toe

New   S99.29   Other physeal fracture of phalanx of toe

New   S99.291   Other physeal fracture of phalanx of right toe

New   S99.292   Other physeal fracture of phalanx of left toe

New   S99.299   Other physeal fracture of phalanx of unspecified toe

New   S99.8   Other specified injuries of ankle and foot

New   The appropriate 7th character is to be added to each code from subcategory S99.8

New   A   initial encounter
New   D   subsequent encounter
New   S   sequela

New   S99.9   Unspecified injury of ankle and foot

New   The appropriate 7th character is to be added to each code from subcategory S99.9

New   A   initial encounter
New   D   subsequent encounter
New   S   sequela

T17.32   Food in larynx
Revised   Bones in larynx

T61   Toxic effect of noxious substances eaten as seafood
    Excludes1   allergic reaction to food, such as:
Deleted   gastroenteritis (noninfective) (K52.2)
New   food protein-induced enterocolitis syndrome (K52.21)
New   food protein-induced enteropathy (K52.22)
New   gastroenteritis (noninfective) (K52.29)

T62   Toxic effect of other noxious substances eaten as food
    Excludes1   allergic reaction to food, such as:
Deleted   gastroenteritis (noninfective) (K52.2)
New   food protein-induced enterocolitis syndrome (K52.21)
New   food protein-induced enteropathy (K52.22)
New   gastroenteritis (noninfective) (K52.29)

T78.05   Anaphylactic reaction due to tree nuts and seeds
Deleted   Excludes1   anaphylactic reaction due to peanuts (T78.01)
New   Excludes2   anaphylactic reaction due to peanuts (T78.01)

	T78.1	**Other adverse food reactions, not elsewhere classified**	
Revised		Use additional code to identify the type of reaction, if applicable	
Revised		**Excludes2** allergic and dietetic gastroenteritis and colitis (K52.29)	
New		food protein-induced enterocolitis syndrome (K52.21)	
New		food protein-induced enteropathy (K52.22)	
	T78.4	**Other and unspecified allergy**	
		Excludes1 specified types of allergic reaction such as:	
Revised		allergic diarrhea (K52.29)	
Revised		allergic gastroenteritis and colitis (K52.29)	
New		food protein-induced enterocolitis syndrome (K52.21)	
New		food protein-induced enteropathy (K52.22)	
	T80.1	**Vascular complications following infusion, transfusion and therapeutic injection**	
Revised		**Excludes2** vascular complications specified as due to prosthetic devices, implants and grafts (T82.8-, T83.8-, T84.8-, T85.8-)	
	T80.2	**Infections following infusion, transfusion and therapeutic injection**	
Revised		**Excludes2** postprocedural infections (T81.4-)	
		T80.21 **Infection due to central venous catheter**	
New		Infection due to pulmonary artery catheter (Swan-Ganz catheter)	
		T80.211 **Bloodstream infection due to central venous catheter**	
New		Bloodstream infection due to pulmonary artery catheter	
		T80.212 **Local infection due to central venous catheter**	
New		Local infection due to pulmonary artery catheter	
		T80.218 **Other infection due to central venous catheter**	
New		Other infection due to pulmonary artery catheter	
		T80.219 **Unspecified infection due to central venous catheter**	
New		Unspecified infection due to pulmonary artery catheter	
	T80.6	**Other serum reactions**	
Revised		**Excludes2** serum hepatitis (B16-B19)	
		T81.12 **Postprocedural septic shock**	
Revised		Postprocedural endotoxic shock resulting from a procedure, not elsewhere classified	
Revised		Postprocedural gram-negative shock resulting from a procedure, not elsewhere classified	
	T81.7	**Vascular complications following a procedure, not elsewhere classified**	
Revised		**Excludes2** embolism due to prosthetic devices, implants and grafts (T82.8-, T83.81, T84.8-, T85.1-)	

Revised	**T82.81**	**Embolism due to cardiac and vascular prosthetic devices, implants and grafts**	
Revised		T82.817 **Embolism due to cardiac prosthetic devices, implants and grafts**	
Revised		T82.818 **Embolism due to vascular prosthetic devices, implants and grafts**	
Revised	**T82.82**	**Fibrosis due to cardiac and vascular prosthetic devices, implants and grafts**	
Revised		T82.827 **Fibrosis due to cardiac prosthetic devices, implants and grafts**	
Revised		T82.828 **Fibrosis due to vascular prosthetic devices, implants and grafts**	
Revised	**T82.83**	**Hemorrhage due to cardiac and vascular prosthetic devices, implants and grafts**	
Revised		T82.837 **Hemorrhage due to cardiac prosthetic devices, implants and grafts**	
Revised		T82.838 **Hemorrhage due to vascular prosthetic devices, implants and grafts**	
Revised	**T82.84**	**Pain due to cardiac and vascular prosthetic devices, implants and grafts**	
Revised		T82.847 **Pain due to cardiac prosthetic devices, implants and grafts**	
Revised		T82.848 **Pain due to vascular prosthetic devices, implants and grafts**	
Revised	**T82.85**	**Stenosis due to cardiac and vascular prosthetic devices, implants and grafts**	
New		T82.855 **Stenosis of coronary artery stent**	
New		In-stent stenosis (restenosis) of coronary artery stent	
New		Restenosis of coronary artery stent	
New		T82.856 **Stenosis of peripheral vascular stent**	
New		In-stent stenosis (restenosis) of peripheral vascular stent	
New		Restenosis of peripheral vascular stent	
Revised		T82.857 **Stenosis of other cardiac prosthetic devices, implants and grafts**	
Revised		T82.858 **Stenosis of other vascular prosthetic devices, implants and grafts**	
Revised	**T82.86**	**Thrombosis of cardiac and vascular prosthetic devices, implants and grafts**	
Revised		T82.867 **Thrombosis due to cardiac prosthetic devices, implants and grafts**	
Revised		T82.868 **Thrombosis due to vascular prosthetic devices, implants and grafts**	
Revised	**T83.0**	**Mechanical complication of urinary catheter**	
Revised		T83.01 **Breakdown (mechanical) of urinary catheter**	
New		T83.011 **Breakdown (mechanical) of indwelling urethral catheter**	
New		T83.012 **Breakdown (mechanical) of nephrostomy catheter**	
Revised		T83.018 **Breakdown (mechanical) of other urinary catheter**	
New		Breakdown (mechanical) of Hopkins catheter	
New		Breakdown (mechanical) of ileostomy catheter	
New		Breakdown (mechanical) urostomy catheter	

Revised	**T83.02**	**Displacement of urinary catheter**
Revised		Malposition of urinary catheter
New	**T83.021**	**Displacement of indwelling urethral catheter**
New	**T83.022**	**Displacement of nephrostomy catheter**
Revised	**T83.028**	**Displacement of other urinary catheter**
New		Displacement of Hopkins catheter
New		Displacement of ileostomy catheter
New		Displacement of urostomy catheter
Revised	**T83.03**	**Leakage of urinary catheter**
New	**T83.031**	**Leakage of indwelling urethral catheter**
New	**T83.032**	**Leakage of nephrostomy catheter**
Revised	**T83.038**	**Leakage of other urinary catheter**
New		Leakage of Hopkins catheter
New		Leakage of ileostomy catheter
New		Leakage of urostomy catheter
Revised	**T83.09**	**Other mechanical complication of urinary catheter**
Revised		Obstruction (mechanical) of urinary catheter
Revised		Perforation of urinary catheter
Revised		Protrusion of urinary catheter
New	**T83.091**	**Other mechanical complication of indwelling urethral catheter**
New	**T83.092**	**Other mechanical complication of nephrostomy catheter**
Revised	**T83.098**	**Other mechanical complication of other urinary catheter**
New		Other mechanical complication of Hopkins catheter
New		Other mechanical complication of ileostomy catheter
New		Other mechanical complication of urostomy catheter
	T83.110	**Breakdown (mechanical) of urinary electronic stimulator device**
New	**Excludes2**	Breakdown (mechanical) of electrode (lead) for sacral nerve neuro-stimulator (T85.111)
New		Breakdown (mechanical) of implanted electronic sacral neuro-stimulator, pulse generator or receiver (T85.113)
Revised	**T83.111**	**Breakdown (mechanical) of implanted urinary sphincter**
Revised	**T83.112**	**Breakdown (mechanical) of indwelling ureteral stent**

New	**T83.113**	**Breakdown (mechanical) of other urinary stents**
New		Breakdown (mechanical) of ileal conduit stent
New		Breakdown (mechanical) of nephroureteral stent
	T83.120	**Displacement of urinary electronic stimulator device**
New	**Excludes2**	Displacement of electrode (lead) for sacral nerve neuro-stimulator (T85.121)
New		Displacement of implanted electronic sacral neuro-stimulator, pulse generator or receiver (T85.123)
Revised	**T83.121**	**Displacement of implanted urinary sphincter**
Revised	**T83.122**	**Displacement of indwelling ureteral stent**
New	**T83.123**	**Displacement of other urinary stents**
New		Displacement of ileal conduit stent
New		Displacement of nephroureteral stent
	T83.190	**Other mechanical complication of urinary electronic stimulator device**
New	**Excludes2**	Other mechanical complication of electrode (lead) for sacral nerve neuro-stimulator (T85.191)
New		Other mechanical complication of implanted electronic sacral neuro-stimulator, pulse generator or receiver (T85.193)
Revised	**T83.191**	**Other mechanical complication of implanted urinary sphincter**
Revised	**T83.192**	**Other mechanical complication of indwelling ureteral stent**
New	**T83.193**	**Other mechanical complication of other urinary stent**
New		Other mechanical complication of ileal conduit stent
New		Other mechanical complication of nephroureteral stent

New	T83.24	**Erosion of graft of urinary organ**
New	T83.25	**Exposure of graft of urinary organ**
	T83.32	**Displacement of intrauterine contraceptive device**
New		Missing string of intrauterine contraceptive device
Revised	T83.410	**Breakdown (mechanical) of implanted penile prosthesis**
New		Breakdown (mechanical) of penile prosthesis cylinder
New		Breakdown (mechanical) of penile prosthesis pump
New		Breakdown (mechanical) of penile prosthesis reservoir
New	T83.411	**Breakdown (mechanical) of implanted testicular prosthesis**
Revised	T83.420	**Displacement of implanted penile prosthesis**
New		Displacement of penile prosthesis cylinder
New		Displacement of penile prosthesis pump
New		Displacement of penile prosthesis reservoir
New	T83.421	**Displacement of implanted testicular prosthesis**
Revised	T83.490	**Other mechanical complication of implanted penile prosthesis**
New		Other mechanical complication of penile prosthesis cylinder
New		Other mechanical complication of penile prosthesis pump
New		Other mechanical complication of penile prosthesis reservoir
New	T83.491	**Other mechanical complication of implanted testicular prosthesis**
Revised	T83.51	**Infection and inflammatory reaction due to urinary catheter**
New	T83.510	**Infection and inflammatory reaction due to cystostomy catheter**
New	T83.511	**Infection and inflammatory reaction due to indwelling urethral catheter**
New	T83.512	**Infection and inflammatory reaction due to nephrostomy catheter**
New	T83.518	**Infection and inflammatory reaction due to other urinary catheter**
New		Infection and inflammatory reaction due to Hopkins catheter
New		Infection and inflammatory reaction due to ileostomy catheter
New		Infection and inflammatory reaction due to urostomy catheter

New	T83.590	**Infection and inflammatory reaction due to implanted urinary neurostimulation device**
New		**Excludes2** Infection and inflammatory reaction due to electrode lead of sacral nerve neurostimulator (T85.732)
New		Infection and inflammatory reaction due to pulse generator or receiver of sacral nerve neurostimulator (T85.734)
New	T83.591	**Infection and inflammatory reaction due to implanted urinary sphincter**
New	T83.592	**Infection and inflammatory reaction due to indwelling ureteral stent**
New	T83.593	**Infection and inflammatory reaction due to other urinary stents**
New		Infection and inflammatory reaction due to ileal conduit stents
New		Infection and inflammatory reaction due to nephroureteral stent
New	T83.598	**Infection and inflammatory reaction due to other prosthetic device, implant and graft in urinary system**
New	T83.61	**Infection and inflammatory reaction due to implanted penile prosthesis**
New		Infection and inflammatory reaction due to penile prosthesis cylinder
New		Infection and inflammatory reaction due to penile prosthesis pump
New		Infection and inflammatory reaction due to penile prosthesis reservoir
New	T83.62	**Infection and inflammatory reaction due to implanted testicular prosthesis**
New	T83.69	**Infection and inflammatory reaction due to other prosthetic device, implant and graft in genital tract**
Revised	T83.711	**Erosion of implanted vaginal mesh to surrounding organ or tissue**
Revised		Erosion of implanted vaginal mesh into pelvic floor muscles
New	T83.712	**Erosion of implanted urethral mesh to surrounding organ or tissue**
New		Erosion of implanted female urethral sling
New		Erosion of implanted male urethral sling
New		Erosion of implanted urethral mesh into pelvic floor muscles

New		T83.713	**Erosion of implanted urethral bulking agent to surrounding organ or tissue**
New		T83.714	**Erosion of implanted ureteral bulking agent to surrounding organ or tissue**
Revised		T83.718	**Erosion of other implanted mesh to organ or tissue**
New		T83.719	**Erosion of other prosthetic materials to surrounding organ or tissue**
	T83.72		**Exposure of implanted mesh and other prosthetic materials into surrounding organ or tissue**
New			Extrusion of implanted mesh
Revised		T83.721	**Exposure of implanted vaginal mesh into vagina**
Revised			Exposure of implanted vaginal mesh through vaginal wall
New		T83.722	**Exposure of implanted urethral mesh into urethra**
New			Exposure of implanted female urethral sling
New			Exposure of implanted male urethral sling
New			Exposure of implanted urethral mesh through urethral wall
New		T83.723	**Exposure of implanted urethral bulking agent into urethra**
New		T83.724	**Exposure of implanted ureteral bulking agent into ureter**
Revised		T83.728	**Exposure of other implanted mesh into organ or tissue**
New		T83.729	**Exposure of other prosthetic materials into organ or tissue**
New	T83.79		**Other specified complications due to other genitourinary prosthetic materials**
	T83.8		**Other specified complications of genitourinary prosthetic devices, implants and grafts**
Revised		T83.81	**Embolism due to genitourinary prosthetic devices, implants and grafts**
Revised		T83.82	**Fibrosis due to genitourinary prosthetic devices, implants and grafts**
Revised		T83.83	**Hemorrhage due to genitourinary prosthetic devices, implants and grafts**
Revised		T83.84	**Pain due to genitourinary prosthetic devices, implants and grafts**
Revised		T83.85	**Stenosis due to genitourinary prosthetic devices, implants and grafts**
Revised		T83.86	**Thrombosis due to genitourinary prosthetic devices, implants and grafts**
Deleted	T84.04		~~Periprosthetic fracture around internal prosthetic joint~~
Deleted		**Excludes2**	breakage (fracture) of prosthetic joint (T84.01)
Deleted		T84.040	~~Periprosthetic fracture around internal prosthetic right hip joint~~
Deleted		T84.041	~~Periprosthetic fracture around internal prosthetic left hip joint~~
Deleted		T84.042	~~Periprosthetic fracture around internal prosthetic right knee joint~~
Deleted		T84.043	~~Periprosthetic fracture around internal prosthetic left knee joint~~

Deleted		T84.048	~~Periprosthetic fracture around other internal prosthetic joint~~
Deleted			Use additional code to identify the joint (Z96.6-)
Deleted		T84.049	~~Periprosthetic fracture around unspecified internal prosthetic joint~~
Revised		T85.110	**Breakdown (mechanical) of implanted electronic neurostimulator of brain electrode (lead)**
Revised		T85.111	**Breakdown (mechanical) of implanted electronic neurostimulator of peripheral nerve electrode (lead)**
New			Breakdown of electrode (lead) for cranial nerve neurostimulators
New			Breakdown of electrode (lead) for gastric neurostimulator
New			Breakdown of electrode (lead) for sacral nerve neurostimulator
New			Breakdown of electrode (lead) for vagal nerve neurostimulators
Revised		T85.112	**Breakdown (mechanical) of implanted electronic neurostimulator of spinal cord electrode (lead)**
New		T85.113	**Breakdown (mechanical) of implanted electronic neurostimulator, generator**
New			Breakdown (mechanical) of implanted electronic neurostimuator generator, brain, peripheral, gastric, spinal
New			Breakdown (mechanical) of implanted electronic sacral neurostimulator, pulse generator or receiver
Revised		T85.120	**Displacement of implanted electronic neurostimulator of brain electrode (lead)**
Revised		T85.121	**Displacement of implanted electronic neurostimulator of peripheral nerve electrode (lead)**
New			Displacement of electrode (lead) for cranial nerve neurostimulators
New			Displacement of electrode (lead) for gastric neurostimulator
New			Displacement of electrode (lead) for sacral nerve neurostimulator
New			Displacement of electrode (lead) for vagal nerve neurostimulators
Revised		T85.122	**Displacement of implanted electronic neurostimulator of spinal cord electrode (lead)**

New **T85.123 Displacement of implanted electronic neurostimulator, generator**

New Displacement of implanted electronic neurostimulator generator, brain, peripheral, gastric, spinal

New Displacement of implanted electronic sacral neurostimulator, pulse generator or receiver

Revised **T85.190 Other mechanical complication of implanted electronic neurostimulator of brain electrode (lead)**

Revised **T85.191 Other mechanical complication of implanted electronic neurostimulator of peripheral nerve electrode (lead)**

New Other mechanical complication of electrode (lead) for cranial nerve neurostimulators

New Other mechanical complication of electrode (lead) for gastric neurostimulator

New Other mechanical complication of electrode (lead) for sacral nerve neurostimulator

New Other mechanical complication of electrode (lead) for vagal nerve neurostimulators

Revised **T85.192 Other mechanical complication of implanted electronic neurostimulator of spinal cord electrode (lead)**

New **T85.193 Other mechanical complication of implanted electronic neurostimulator, generator**

New Other mechanical complication of implanted electronic neurostimulator generator, brain, peripheral, gastric, spinal

New Other mechanical complication of implanted electronic sacral neurostimulator, pulse generator or receiver

Revised **T85.610 Breakdown (mechanical) of cranial or spinal infusion catheter**

New Breakdown (mechanical) of epidural infusion catheter

New Breakdown (mechanical) of intrathecal infusion catheter

New Breakdown (mechanical) of subarachnoid infusion catheter

New Breakdown (mechanical) of subdural infusion catheter

New **T85.615 Breakdown (mechanical) of other nervous system device, implant or graft**

New Breakdown (mechanical) of intrathecal infusion pump

Revised **T85.620 Displacement of cranial or spinal infusion catheter**

New Displacement of epidural infusion catheter

New Displacement of intrathecal infusion catheter

New Displacement of subarachnoid infusion catheter

New Displacement of subdural infusion catheter

New **T85.625 Displacement of other nervous system device, implant or graft**

New Displacement of intrathecal infusion pump

Revised **T85.630 Leakage of cranial or spinal infusion catheter**

New Leakage of epidural infusion catheter

New Leakage of intrathecal infusion catheter

New Leakage of subdural infusion catheter

New Leakage of subarachnoid infusion catheter

New **T85.635 Leakage of other nervous system device, implant or graft**

New Leakage of intrathecal infusion pump

Revised **T85.690 Other mechanical complication of cranial or spinal infusion catheter**

New Other mechanical complication of epidural infusion catheter

New Other mechanical complication of intrathecal infusion catheter

New Other mechanical complication of subarachnoid infusion catheter

New Other mechanical complication of subdural infusion catheter

New **T85.695 Other mechanical complication of other nervous system device, implant or graft**

New Other mechanical complication of intrathecal infusion pump

New **T85.73 Infection and inflammatory reaction due to nervous system devices, implants and graft**

New **T85.730 Infection and inflammatory reaction due to ventricular intracranial (communicating) shunt**

New **T85.731 Infection and inflammatory reaction due to implanted electronic neurostimulator of brain, electrode (lead)**

New	T85.732	**Infection and inflammatory reaction due to implanted electronic neurostimulator of peripheral nerve, electrode (lead)**
New		Infection and inflammatory reaction due to electrode (lead) for cranial nerve neurostimulators
New		Infection and inflammatory reaction due to electrode (lead) for gastric neurostimulator
New		Infection and inflammatory reaction due to electrode (lead) for sacral nerve neurostimulators
New		Infection and inflammatory reaction due to electrode (lead) for vagal nerve neurostimulators
New	T85.733	**Infection and inflammatory reaction due to implanted electronic neurostimulator of spinal cord, electrode (lead)**
New	T85.734	**Infection and inflammatory reaction due to implanted electronic neurostimulator, generator**
New		Generator pocket infection
New	T85.735	**Infection and inflammatory reaction due to cranial or spinal infusion catheter**
New		Infection and inflammatory reaction due to epidural catheter
New		Infection and inflammatory reaction due to intrathecal infusion catheter
New		Infection and inflammatory reaction due to subarachnoid catheter
New		Infection and inflammatory reaction due to subdural catheter
New	T85.738	**Infection and inflammatory reaction due to other nervous system device, implant or graft**
New		Infection and inflammatory reaction due to intrathecal infusion pump
New	T85.810	**Embolism due to nervous system prosthetic devices, implants and grafts**
New	T85.818	**Embolism due to other internal prosthetic devices, implants and grafts**
New	T85.820	**Fibrosis due to nervous system prosthetic devices, implants and grafts**
New	T85.828	**Fibrosis due to other internal prosthetic devices, implants and grafts**
New	T85.830	**Hemorrhage due to nervous system prosthetic devices, implants and grafts**
New	T85.838	**Hemorrhage due to other internal prosthetic devices, implants and grafts**

New	T85.840	**Pain due to nervous system prosthetic devices, implants and grafts**
New	T85.848	**Pain due to other internal prosthetic devices, implants and grafts**
New	T85.850	**Stenosis due to nervous system prosthetic devices, implants and grafts**
New	T85.858	**Stenosis due to other internal prosthetic devices, implants and grafts**
New	T85.860	**Thrombosis due to nervous system prosthetic devices, implants and grafts**
New	T85.868	**Thrombosis due to other internal prosthetic devices, implants and grafts**
	T85.89	**Other specified complication of internal prosthetic devices, implants and grafts, not elsewhere classified**
New		Erosion or breakdown of subcutaneous device pocket
New	T85.890	**Other specified complication of nervous system prosthetic devices, implants and grafts**
New	T85.898	**Other specified complication of other internal prosthetic devices, implants and grafts**
New	T88.53	**Unintended awareness under general anesthesia during procedure**
New		**Excludes2** personal history of unintended awareness under general anesthesia (Z92.84)

CHAPTER 20

EXTERNAL CAUSES OF MORBIDITY (V00-Y99)

This chapter contains the following blocks:

New	X50	Overexertion and strenuous or repetitive movements
Revised	X92-Y09	Assault

TRANSPORT ACCIDENTS (V00-V99)

Deleted **Note:** This section is structured in 12 groups. Those relating to land transport accidents (V01-V89) reflect the victim's mode of transport and are subdivided to identify the victim's 'counterpart' or the type of event. The vehicle of which the injured person is an occupant is identified in the first two characters since it is seen as the most important factor to identify for prevention purposes. A transport accident is one in which the vehicle involved must be moving or running or in use for transport purposes at the time of the accident.

New **Note:** This section is structured in 12 groups. Those relating to land transport accidents (V00-V89) reflect the victim's mode of transport and are subdivided to identify the victim's 'counterpart' or the type of event. The vehicle of which the injured person is an occupant is identified in the first two characters since it is seen as the most important factor to identify for prevention purposes. A transport accident is one in which the vehicle involved must be moving or running or in use for transport purposes at the time of the accident.

Revised   **Note:** Definitions related to transport accidents:

Revised   (a) A transport accident (V00-V99) is any accident involving a device designed primarily for, or used at the time primarily for, conveying persons or good from one place to another.

Revised   (e) A pedestrian is any person involved in an accident who was not at the time of the accident riding in or on a motor vehicle, railway train, streetcar or animal-drawn or other vehicle, or on a pedal cycle or animal. This includes, a person changing a tire, working on a parked car, or a person on foot. It also includes the user of a pedestrian conveyance such as a baby-stroller, ice-skates, skis, sled, roller skates, a skateboard, nonmotorized or motorized wheelchair, motorized mobility scooter, or nonmotorized scooter.

Revised   (h) A person on the outside of a vehicle is any person being transported by a vehicle but not occupying the space normally reserved for the driver or passengers, or the space intended for the transport of property. This includes a person travelling on the bodywork, bumper, fender, roof, running board or step of a vehicle, as well as, hanging on the outside of the vehicle.

Revised   (k) A motorcycle is a two-wheeled motor vehicle with one or two riding saddles and sometimes with a third wheel for the support of a sidecar. The sidecar is considered part of the motorcycle. This includes a moped, motor scooter, or motorized bicycle.

Revised   (n) A car [automobile] is a four-wheeled motor vehicle designed primarily for carrying up to 7 persons. A trailer being towed by the car is considered part of the car. It does not include a van or minivan—see definition (o)

Revised   (t) A special vehicle mainly used on industrial premises is a motor vehicle designed primarily for use within the buildings and premises of industrial or commercial establishments. This includes battery-powered airport passenger vehicles or baggage/mail trucks, forklifts, coal-cars in a coal mine, logging cars and trucks used in mines or quarries.

Revised   (w) A special all-terrain vehicle is a motor vehicle of special design to enable it to negotiate over rough or soft terrain, snow or sand. Examples of special design are high construction, special wheels and tires, tracks, and support on a cushion of air. This includes snow mobiles, all-terrain vehicles (ATV), and dune buggies. It does not include passenger vehicle designated as sport utility vehicles (SUV).

Deleted   ~~V47.01 Driver of sport utility vehicle injured in collision with fixed or stationary object in nontraffic accident~~

Deleted   ~~V47.02 Driver of other type car injured in collision with fixed or stationary object in nontraffic accident~~

Deleted   ~~V47.11 Passenger of sport utility vehicle injured in collision with fixed or stationary object in nontraffic accident~~

Deleted   ~~V47.12 Passenger of other type car injured in collision with fixed or stationary object in nontraffic accident~~

Deleted   ~~V47.31 Unspecified occupant of sport utility vehicle injured in collision with fixed or stationary object in nontraffic accident~~

Deleted   ~~V47.32 Unspecified occupant of other type car injured in collision with fixed or stationary object in nontraffic accident~~

Deleted   ~~V47.51 Driver of sport utility vehicle injured in collision with fixed or stationary object in traffic accident~~

Deleted   ~~V47.52 Driver of other type car injured in collision with fixed or stationary object in traffic accident~~

Deleted   ~~V47.61 Passenger of sport utility vehicle injured in collision with fixed or stationary object in traffic accident~~

Deleted   ~~V47.62 Passenger of other type car injured in collision with fixed or stationary object in traffic accident~~

Deleted   ~~V47.91 Unspecified occupant of sport utility vehicle injured in collision with fixed or stationary object in traffic accident~~

Deleted   ~~V47.92 Unspecified occupant of other type car injured in collision with fixed or stationary object in traffic accident~~

EXPOSURE TO INANIMATE MECHANICAL FORCES (W20-W49)

Revised   **Excludes1** assault (X92-Y09)

W25 Contact with sharp glass
  Excludes2 glass embedded in skin (W45)

Revised   **W26 Contact with other sharp objects**
New   **Excludes2** sharp object(s) embedded in skin (W45)
New   **W26.2 Contact with edge of stiff paper**
    Paper cut
New   **W26.8 Contact with other sharp object(s), not elsewhere classified**
New   Contact with tin can lid
New   **W26.9 Contact with unspecified sharp object(s)**

W45 Foreign body or object entering through skin
New   **Includes** foreign body or object embedded in skin
    nail embedded in skin
Revised   **Excludes2** contact with other sharp object(s) (W26.-)
Deleted   ~~W45.1 Paper entering through skin~~
Deleted   ~~Paper cut~~
Deleted   ~~W45.2 Lid of can entering through skin~~

W89 Exposure to man-made visible and ultraviolet light
Deleted   **Excludes2** exposure to sunlight (X32)
New   **Excludes1** exposure to sunlight (X32)

X32 Exposure to sunlight
Deleted   **Excludes1** radiation-related disorders of the skin and subcutaneous tissue (L55-L59)

X39.0 Exposure to natural radiation
Revised   **Excludes1** contact with and (suspected) exposure to radon and other naturally occuring radiation (Z77.123)

OVEREXERTION AND STRENUOUS OR REPETITIVE MOVEMENTS (X50)
New

New   **X50 Overexertion and strenuous or repetitive movements**
New   The appropriate 7th character is to be added to each code from category X50

New A	initial encounter
New D	subsequent encounter
New S	sequela

New   **X50.0 Overexertion from strenuous movement or load**
New   Lifting heavy objects
New   Lifting weights
New   **X50.1 Overexertion from prolonged static or awkward postures**
New   Prolonged bending
New   Prolonged kneeling
New   Prolonged reaching
New   Prolonged sitting
New   Prolonged standing
New   Prolonged twisting
New   Static bending
New   Static kneeling
New   Static reaching
New   Static sitting
New   Static standing
New   Static twisting

New	X50.3	Overexertion from repetitive movements
New		Use of hand as hammer
New		**Excludes2** Overuse from prolonged static or awkward postures (X50.1)
New	X50.9	Other and unspecified overexertion or strenuous movements or postures
New		Contact pressure
New		Contact stress
Deleted		ASSAULT (X92-Y08)
New		ASSAULT (X92-Y09)

MISADVENTURES TO PATIENTS DURING SURGICAL AND MEDICAL CARE (Y62-Y69)

New	**Excludes1**	surgical and medical procedures as the cause of abnormal reaction of the patient, without mention of misadventure at the time of the procedure (Y83-Y84)
Deleted	**Excludes2**	surgical and medical procedures as the cause of abnormal reaction of the patient, without mention of misadventure at the time of the procedure (Y83-Y84)

MEDICAL DEVICES ASSOCIATED WITH ADVERSE INCIDENTS IN DIAGNOSTIC AND THERAPEUTIC USE (Y70-Y82)

Deleted	**Excludes1**	misadventure to patients during surgical and medical care, classifiable to (Y62-Y69)
Deleted		later complications following use of medical devices without breakdown or malfunctioning of device (Y83-Y84)
New	**Excludes2**	breakdown or malfunctioning of medical device (after implantation) (during procedure) (ongoing use) (Y70-Y82)
New		later complications following use of medical devices without breakdown or malfunctioning of device (Y83-Y84)
New		misadventure to patients during surgical and medical care, classifiable to (Y62-Y69)
New		surgical and other medical procedures as the cause of abnormal reaction of the patient, or of later complication, without mention of misadventure at the time of the procedure (Y83-Y84)

SURGICAL AND OTHER MEDICAL PROCEDURES AS THE CAUSE OF ABNORMAL REACTION OF THE PATIENT, OR OF LATER COMPLICATION, WITHOUT MENTION OF MISADVENTURE AT THE TIME OF THE PROCEDURE (Y83-Y84)

New	**Excludes2**	breakdown or malfunctioning of medical device (after implantation) (during procedure) (ongoing use) (Y70-Y82)
Revised	Y92.4	Street, highway and other paved roadways as the place of occurrence of the external cause
New	Y93.85	Activity, choking game
New		Activity, blackout game
New		Activity, fainting game
New		Activity, pass out game

CHAPTER 21

FACTORS INFLUENCING HEALTH STATUS AND CONTACT WITH HEALTH SERVICES (Z00-Z99)

This chapter contains the following blocks:

Deleted	Z20-Z28	Persons with potential health hazards related to communicable diseases
New	Z19	Hormone sensitivity malignancy status
New	Z20-Z29	Persons with potential health hazards related to communicable diseases

	Z01.411	Encounter for gynecological examination (general) (routine) with abnormal findings
New		Use additional code to identify any abnormal findings
	Z01.419	Encounter for gynecological examination (general) (routine) without abnormal findings
Deleted		Use additional code to identify any abnormal findings
New Z05		Encounter for observation and evaluation of newborn for suspected diseases and conditions ruled out
New		This category is to be used for newborns, within the neonatal period (the first 28 days of life), who are suspected of having an abnormal condition unrelated to exposure from the mother or the birth process, but without signs or symptoms, and which, after examination and observation, is ruled out.
New	**Excludes2**	newborn observation for suspected condition, related to exposure from the mother or birth process (P00-P04)
New	Z05.0	Observation and evaluation of newborn for suspected cardiac condition ruled out
New	Z05.1	Observation and evaluation of newborn for suspected infectious condition ruled out
New	Z05.2	Observation and evaluation of newborn for suspected neurological condition ruled out
New	Z05.3	Observation and evaluation of newborn for suspected respiratory condition ruled out
New	Z05.4	Observation and evaluation of newborn for suspected genetic, metabolic or immunologic condition ruled out
New	Z05.41	Observation and evaluation of newborn for suspected genetic condition ruled out
New	Z05.42	Observation and evaluation of newborn for suspected metabolic condition ruled out
New	Z05.43	Observation and evaluation of newborn for suspected immunologic condition ruled out
New	Z05.5	Observation and evaluation of newborn for suspected gastrointestinal condition ruled out
New	Z05.6	Observation and evaluation of newborn for suspected genitourinary condition ruled out
New	Z05.7	Observation and evaluation of newborn for suspected skin, subcutaneous, musculoskeletal and connective tissue condition ruled out
New	Z05.71	Observation and evaluation of newborn for suspected skin and subcutaneous tissue condition ruled out
New	Z05.72	Observation and evaluation of newborn for suspected musculoskeletal condition ruled out
New	Z05.73	Observation and evaluation of newborn for suspected connective tissue condition ruled out
New	Z05.8	Observation and evaluation of newborn for other specified suspected condition ruled out
New	Z05.9	Observation and evaluation of newborn for unspecified suspected condition ruled out
	Z12.4	Encounter for screening for malignant neoplasm of cervix
Deleted	**Excludes1**	encounter for screening for human papillomavirus (Z11.51)
New	**Excludes2**	encounter for screening for human papillomavirus (Z11.51)

New		**HORMONE SENSITIVITY MALIGNANCY STATUS (Z19)**	

New   **Z19   Hormone sensitivity malignancy status**

New   **Code first** malignant neoplasm —*see* Table of Neoplasms, by site, malignant

New   **Z19.1   Hormone sensitive malignancy status**

New   **Z19.2   Hormone resistant malignancy status**

New   Castrate resistant prostate malignancy status

Deleted   **PERSONS WITH POTENTIAL HEALTH HAZARDS RELATED TO COMMUNICABLE DISEASES (Z20-Z28)**

New   **PERSONS WITH POTENTIAL HEALTH HAZARDS RELATED TO COMMUNICABLE DISEASES (Z20-Z29)**

Z22   Carrier of infectious disease

New   **Excludes2**   carrier of viral hepatitis (B18.-)

            Z22.330   Carrier of Group B streptococcus

New   **Excludes1**   Carrier of streptococcus group B (GBS) complicating pregnancy, childbirth and the puerperium (O99.82-)

Deleted   ~~Z22.5   Carrier of viral hepatitis~~

Deleted   ~~Z22.50   Carrier of unspecified viral hepatitis~~

Deleted   ~~Z22.51   Carrier of viral hepatitis B~~

Deleted   ~~Hepatitis B surface antigen [HBsAg] carrier~~

Deleted   ~~Z22.52   Carrier of viral hepatitis C~~

Deleted   ~~Z22.59   Carrier of other viral hepatitis~~

New   **Z29   Encounter for other prophylactic measures**

New   **Excludes1**   desensitization to allergens (Z51.6)

New   prophylactic surgery (Z40.-)

New   **Z29.1   Encounter for prophylactic immunotherapy**

New   Encounter for administration of immunoglobulin

New   **Z29.11   Encounter for prophylactic immunotherapy for respiratory syncytial virus (RSV)**

New   **Z29.12   Encounter for prophylactic antivenin**

New   **Z29.13   Encounter for prophylactic Rho(D) immune globulin**

New   **Z29.14   Encounter for prophylactic rabies immune globin**

New   **Z29.3   Encounter for prophylactic fluoride administration**

New   **Z29.8   Encounter for other specified prophylactic measures**

New   **Z29.9   Encounter for prophylactic measures, unspecified**

New   **Z30.015   Encounter for initial prescription of vaginal ring hormonal contraceptive**

New   **Z30.016   Encounter for initial prescription of transdermal patch hormonal contraceptive device**

New   **Z30.017   Encounter for initial prescription of implantable subdermal contraceptive**

New   **Z30.018   Encounter for initial prescription of other contraceptives**

New   Encounter for initial prescription of barrier contraception

New   Encounter for initial prescription of diaphragm

New   **Z30.44   Encounter for surveillance of vaginal ring hormonal contraceptive device**

New   **Z30.45   Encounter for surveillance of transdermal patch hormonal contraceptive device**

New   **Z30.46   Encounter for surveillance of implantable subdermal contraceptive**

New   Encounter for checking, reinsertion or removal of implantable subdermal contraceptive

New   **Z30.49   Encounter for surveillance of other contraceptives**

New   Encounter for surveillance of barrier contraception

New   Encounter for surveillance of diaphragm

New   **Z31.7   Encounter for procreative management and counseling for gestational carrier**

New   **Excludes1**   pregnant state, gestational carrier (Z33.3)

        Z33.1   Pregnant state, incidental

New   **Excludes1**   pregnant state, gestational carrier (Z33.3)

New   **Z33.3   Pregnant state, gestational carrier**

New   **Excludes1**   encounter for procreative management and counseling for gestational carrier (Z31.7)

    Z3A   Weeks of gestation

Revised   **Note:** Codes from category Z3A are for use, only on the maternal record, to indicate the weeks of gestation of the pregnancy, if known.

                Z45.01   Encounter for adjustment and management of cardiac pacemaker

New   Encounter for adjustment and management of cardiac resynchronization therapy pacemaker (CRT-P)

                Z45.02   Encounter for adjustment and management of automatic implantable cardiac defibrillator

New   Encounter for adjustment and management of cardiac resynchronization therapy defibrillator (CRT-D)

Revised   **Z51   Encounter for other aftercare and medical care**

New   **Z51.6   Encounter for desensitization to allergens**

New   **Z53.3   Procedure converted to open procedure**

New   **Z53.31   Laparoscopic surgical procedure converted to open procedure**

New   **Z53.32   Thoracoscopic surgical procedure converted to open procedure**

New   **Z53.33   Arthroscopic surgical procedure converted to open procedure**

New   **Z53.39   Other specified procedure converted to open procedure**

Z77   Other contact with and (suspected) exposures hazardous to health

Revised   **Excludes2**   newborn affected by noxious substances transmitted via placenta or breast milk (P04.-)

Z79   Long term (current) drug therapy

New   **Excludes2**   long term (current) use of oral antidiabetic drugs (Z79.84)

New   long term (current) use of oral hypoglycemic drugs (Z79.84)

New   **Z79.84**   **Long term (current) use of oral hypoglycemic drugs**

New   Long term (current) use of oral antidiabetic drugs

New   **Excludes2**   long term (current) use of insulin (Z79.4)

   Z79.891   **Long term (current) use of opiate analgesic**

Revised   **Excludes1**   methodone use NOS (F11.9-)

New   **Z83.42**   **Family history of familial hypercholesterolemia**

New   **Z84.82**   **Family history of sudden infant death syndrome**

New   Family history of SIDS

Z85   Personal history of malignant neoplasm

Use additional code to identify:

Revised   history of tobacco dependence (Z87.891)

Z85.8   **Personal history of malignant neoplasms of other organs and systems**

Revised   Conditions classifiable to C00-C14, C40-C49, C69-C75, C7A.098, C76-C79

   Z86.00   **Personal history of in-situ neoplasm**

New   Conditions classifiable to D00-D09

   Z86.001   **Personal history of in-situ neoplasm of cervix uteri**

New   Personal history of cervical intraepithelial neoplasia III [CIN III]

   Z86.008   **Personal history of in-situ neoplasm of other site**

New   Personal history of vaginal intraepithelial neoplasia III [VAIN III]

New   Personal history of vulvar intraepithelial neoplasia III [VIN III]

   Z87.41   **Personal history of dysplasia of the female genital tract**

New   **Excludes1**   personal history of intraepithelial neoplasia III of female genital tract (Z87.001, Z87.008)

   Z90.41   **Acquired absence of pancreas**

New   Code also exocrine pancreatic insufficiency (K86.81)

New   **Z92.84**   **Personal history of unintended awareness under general anesthesia**

New   **Excludes2**   unintended awareness under general anesthesia during procedure (T88.53)

   Z95.0   **Presence of cardiac pacemaker**

New   Presence of cardiac resynchronization therapy (CRT-P) pacemaker

New   **Excludes1**   adjustment or management of cardiac device (Z45.0-)

   Z95.1   **Presence of aortocoronary bypass graft**

New   Presence of coronary artery bypass graft

   Z95.810   **Presence of automatic (implantable) cardiac defibrillator**

New   Presence of cardiac resynchronization therapy defibrillator (CRT-D)

New   Presence of cardioverter-defribillator (ICD)

   Z97.5   **Presence of (intrauterine) contraceptive device**

Revised   **Excludes1**   checking, reinsertion or removal of implantable subdermal contraceptive (Z30.46)

New   checking, reinsertion or removal of intrauterine contraceptive device (Z30.43-)

   Z98.89   **Other specified postprocedural states**

Deleted   Personal history of surgery, not elsewhere classified

New   **Z98.890**   **Other specified postprocedural states**

New   Personal history of surgery, not elsewhere classified

New   **Z98.891**   **History of uterine scar from previous surgery**

New   **Excludes1**   Maternal care due to uterine scar from previous surgery (O34.2-)

   Z99.2   **Dependence on renal dialysis**

Deleted   **Excludes1**   noncompliance with renal dialysis (Z91.15)

New   **Excludes2**   noncompliance with renal dialysis (Z91.15)

Introduction

ICD-10-CM Official Guidelines for Coding and Reporting 2017

Narrative changes appear in bold text
Items <u>underlined</u> have been moved within the guidelines since the 2016 version
***Italics* are used to indicate revisions to heading changes**

The Centers for Medicare and Medicaid Services (CMS) and the National Center for Health Statistics (NCHS), two departments within the U.S. Federal Government's Department of Health and Human Services (DHHS) provide the following guidelines for coding and reporting using the International Classification of Diseases, 10th Revision, Clinical Modification (ICD-10-CM). These guidelines should be used as a companion document to the official version of the ICD-10-CM as published on the NCHS website. The ICD-10-CM is a morbidity classification published by the United States for classifying diagnoses and reason for visits in all health care settings. The ICD-10-CM is based on the ICD-10, the statistical classification of disease published by the World Health Organization (WHO).

These guidelines have been approved by the four organizations that make up the Cooperating Parties for the ICD-10-CM: the American Hospital Association (AHA), the American Health Information Management Association (AHIMA), CMS, and NCHS.

These guidelines are a set of rules that have been developed to accompany and complement the official conventions and instructions provided within the ICD-10-CM itself. The instructions and conventions of the classification take precedence over guidelines. These guidelines are based on the coding and sequencing instructions in the Tabular List and Alphabetic Index of ICD-10-CM, but provide additional instruction. Adherence to these guidelines when assigning ICD-10-CM diagnosis codes is required under the Health Insurance Portability and Accountability Act (HIPAA). The diagnosis codes (Tabular List and Alphabetic Index)

have been adopted under HIPAA for all healthcare settings. A joint effort between the healthcare provider and the coder is essential to achieve complete and accurate documentation, code assignment, and reporting of diagnoses and procedures. These guidelines have been developed to assist both the healthcare provider and the coder in identifying those diagnoses that are to be reported. The importance of consistent, complete documentation in the medical record cannot be overemphasized. Without such documentation accurate coding cannot be achieved. The entire record should be reviewed to determine the specific reason for the encounter and the conditions treated.

The term encounter is used for all settings, including hospital admissions. In the context of these guidelines, the term provider is used throughout the guidelines to mean physician or any qualified health care practitioner who is legally accountable for establishing the patient's diagnosis. Only this set of guidelines, approved by the Cooperating Parties, is official.

The guidelines are organized into sections. Section I includes the structure and conventions of the classification and general guidelines that apply to the entire classification, and chapter-specific guidelines that correspond to the chapters as they are arranged in the classification. Section II includes guidelines for selection of principal diagnosis for non-outpatient settings. Section III includes guidelines for reporting additional diagnoses in non-outpatient settings. Section IV is for outpatient coding and reporting. It is necessary to review all sections of the guidelines to fully understand all of the rules and instructions needed to code properly.

ICD-10-CM Official Guidelines for Coding and Reporting

Section I. Conventions, general coding guidelines and chapter specific guidelines

A. Conventions for the ICD-10-CM
  1. The Alphabetic Index and Tabular List
  2. Format and Structure:
  3. Use of codes for reporting purposes
  4. Placeholder character
  5. 7th Characters
  6. Abbreviations
     a. Alphabetic Index abbreviations
     b. Tabular List abbreviations
  7. Punctuation
  8. Use of "and"
  9. Other and Unspecified codes
     a. "Other" codes
     b. "Unspecified" codes
  10. Includes Notes
  11. Inclusion terms
  12. Excludes Notes
     a. Excludes1
     b. Excludes2
  13. Etiology/manifestation convention ("code first", "use additional code" and "in diseases classified elsewhere" notes)
  14. "And"
  15. "With"
  16. "See" and "See Also"
  17. "Code also note"
  18. Default codes
  19. Code assignment and Clinical Criteria
B. General Coding Guidelines
  1. Locating a code in the ICD-10-CM
  2. Level of Detail in Coding
  3. Code or codes from A00.0 through T88.9, Z00-Z99.8
  4. Signs and symptoms
  5. Conditions that are an integral part of a disease process
  6. Conditions that are not an integral part of a disease process
  7. Multiple coding for a single condition
  8. Acute and Chronic Conditions
  9. Combination Code
  10. Sequela (Late Effects)
  11. Impending or Threatened Condition
  12. Reporting Same Diagnosis Code More than Once
  13. Laterality
  14. Documentation for BMI, *Depth of* Non-pressure ulcers, Pressure Ulcer Stages, Coma Scale, and *NIH Stroke Scale*
  15. Syndromes
  16. Documentation of Complications of Care
  17. Borderline Diagnosis
  18. Use of Sign/Symptom/Unspecified Codes
C. Chapter-Specific Coding Guidelines
  1. Chapter 1: Certain Infectious and Parasitic Diseases (A00-B99)
     a. Human Immunodeficiency Virus (HIV) Infections
     b. Infectious agents as the cause of diseases classified to other chapters
     c. Infections resistant to antibiotics
     d. Sepsis, Severe Sepsis, and Septic Shock
     e. Methicillin Resistant *Staphylococcus aureus* (MRSA) Conditions
     f. Zika virus infection
  2. Chapter 2: Neoplasms (C00-D49)
     a. Treatment directed at the malignancy
     b. Treatment of secondary site
     c. Coding and sequencing of complications
     d. Primary malignancy previously excised
     e. Admissions/Encounters involving chemotherapy, immunotherapy and radiation therapy
     f. Admission/encounter to determine extent of malignancy
     g. Symptoms, signs, and abnormal findings listed in Chapter 18 associated with neoplasms
     h. Admission/encounter for pain control/management
     i. Malignancy in two or more noncontiguous sites
     j. Disseminated malignant neoplasm, unspecified
     k. Malignant neoplasm without specification of site
     l. Sequencing of neoplasm codes
     m. Current malignancy versus personal history of malignancy
     n. Leukemia, Multiple Myeloma, and Malignant Plasma Cell Neoplasms in remission versus personal history
     o. Aftercare following surgery for neoplasm
     p. Follow-up care for completed treatment of a malignancy
     q. Prophylactic organ removal for prevention of malignancy
     r. Malignant neoplasm associated with transplanted organ
  3. Chapter 3: Disease of the blood and blood-forming organs and certain disorders involving the immune mechanism (D50-D89)
  4. Chapter 4: Endocrine, Nutritional, and Metabolic Diseases (E00-E89)
     a. Diabetes mellitus
  5. Chapter 5: Mental, Behavioral and Neurodevelopmental disorders (F01 – F99)
     a. Pain disorders related to psychological factors
     b. Mental and behavioral disorders due to psychoactive substance use
  6. Chapter 6: Diseases of the Nervous System (G00-G99)
     a. Dominant/nondominant side
     b. Pain - Category G89
  7. Chapter 7: Diseases of the Eye and Adnexa (H00-H59)
     a. Glaucoma
  8. Chapter 8: Diseases of the Ear and Mastoid Process (H60-H95)
  9. Chapter 9: Diseases of the Circulatory System (I00-I99)
     a. Hypertension
     b. Atherosclerotic Coronary Artery Disease and Angina
     c. Intraoperative and Postprocedural Cerebrovascular Accident
     d. Sequelae of Cerebrovascular Disease
     e. Acute myocardial infarction (AMI)

10. Chapter 10: Diseases of the Respiratory System (J00-J99)
    a. Chronic Obstructive Pulmonary Disease [COPD] and Asthma
    b. Acute Respiratory Failure
    c. Influenza due to certain identified influenza viruses
    d. Ventilator associated Pneumonia
11. Chapter 11: Diseases of the Digestive System (K00-K95)
12. Chapter 12: Diseases of the Skin and Subcutaneous Tissue (L00-L99)
    a. Pressure ulcer stage codes
13. Chapter 13: Diseases of the Musculoskeletal System and Connective Tissue (M00-M99)
    a. Site and laterality
    b. Acute traumatic versus chronic or recurrent musculoskeletal conditions
    c. Coding of Pathologic Fractures
    d. Osteoporosis
14. Chapter 14: Diseases of Genitourinary System (N00-N99)
    a. Chronic kidney disease
15. Chapter 15: Pregnancy, Childbirth, and the Puerperium (O00-O9A)
    a. General Rules for Obstetric Cases
    b. Selection of OB Principal or First-listed Diagnosis
    c. Pre-existing conditions versus conditions due to the pregnancy
    d. Pre-existing hypertension in pregnancy
    e. Fetal Conditions Affecting the Management of the Mother
    f. HIV Infection in Pregnancy, Childbirth and the Puerperium
    g. Diabetes mellitus in pregnancy
    h. Long term use of insulin and oral hypoglycemics
    i. Gestational (pregnancy induced) diabetes
    j. Sepsis and septic shock complicating abortion, pregnancy, childbirth and the puerperium
    k. Puerperal sepsis
    l. Alcohol and tobacco use during pregnancy, childbirth and the puerperium
    m. Poisoning, toxic effects, adverse effects and underdosing in a pregnant patient
    n. Normal Delivery, Code O80
    o. The Peripartum and Postpartum Periods
    p. Code O94, Sequelae of complication of pregnancy, childbirth, and the puerperium
    q. Termination of Pregnancy and Spontaneous abortions
    r. Abuse in a pregnant patient
16. Chapter 16: Certain Conditions Originating in the Perinatal Period (P00-P96)
    a. General Perinatal Rules
    b. Observation and Evaluation of Newborns for Suspected Conditions not Found
    c. Coding Additional Perinatal Diagnoses
    d. Prematurity and Fetal Growth Retardation
    e. Low birth weight and immaturity status
    f. Bacterial Sepsis of Newborn
    g. Stillbirth

17. Chapter 17: Congenital malformations, deformations, and chromosomal abnormalities (Q00-Q99)
18. Chapter 18: Symptoms, signs, and abnormal clinical and laboratory findings, not elsewhere classified (R00-R99)
    a. Use of symptom codes
    b. Use of a symptom code with a definitive diagnosis code
    c. Combination codes that include symptoms
    d. Repeated falls
    e. Coma scale
    f. Functional quadriplegia
    g. SIRS due to Non-Infectious Process
    h. Death NOS
    i. NIHSS Stroke Scale
19. Chapter 19: Injury, poisoning, and certain other consequences of external causes (S00-T88)
    a. Application of 7th Characters in Chapter 19
    b. Coding of Injuries
    c. Coding of Traumatic Fractures
    d. Coding of Burns and Corrosions
    e. Adverse Effects, Poisoning, Underdosing and Toxic Effects
    f. Adult and child abuse, neglect and other maltreatment
    g. Complications of care
20. Chapter 20: External Causes of Morbidity (V00-Y99)
    a. General External Cause Coding Guidelines
    b. Place of Occurrence Guideline
    c. Activity Code
    d. Place of Occurrence, Activity, and Status Codes Used with other External Cause Code
    e. If the Reporting Format Limits the Number of External Cause Codes
    f. Multiple External Cause Coding Guidelines
    g. Child and Adult Abuse Guideline
    h. Unknown or Undetermined Intent Guideline
    i. Sequelae (Late Effects) of External Cause Guidelines
    j. Terrorism Guidelines
    k. External cause status
21. Chapter 21: Factors influencing health status and contact with health services (Z00-Z99)
    a. Use of Z codes in any healthcare setting
    b. Z Codes indicate a reason for an encounter
    c. Categories of Z Codes

Section II. Selection of Principal Diagnosis

A. Codes for symptoms, signs, and ill-defined conditions
B. Two or more interrelated conditions, each potentially meeting the definition for principal diagnosis
C. Two or more diagnoses that equally meet the definition for principal diagnosis
D. Two or more comparative or contrasting conditions
E. A symptom(s) followed by contrasting/comparative diagnoses
F. Original treatment plan not carried out
G. Complications of surgery and other medical care
H. Uncertain Diagnosis

I. Admission from Observation Unit
  1. Admission Following Medical Observation
  2. Admission Following Post-Operative Observation
J. Admission from Outpatient Surgery
K. Admissions/Encounters for Rehabilitation

Section III. Reporting Additional Diagnoses

A. Previous conditions
B. Abnormal findings
C. Uncertain Diagnosis

Section IV. Diagnostic Coding and Reporting Guidelines for Outpatient Services

A. Selection of first-listed condition
  1. Outpatient Surgery
  2. Observation Stay
B. Codes from A00.0 through T88.9, Z00-Z99
C. Accurate reporting of ICD-10-CM diagnosis codes
D. Codes that describe symptoms and signs
E. Encounters for circumstances other than a disease or injury
F. Level of Detail in Coding
  1. ICD-10-CM codes with 3, 4, 5, 6, or 7 characters
  2. Use of full number of characters required for a code
G. ICD-10-CM code for the diagnosis, condition, problem, or other reason for encounter/visit
H. Uncertain diagnosis
I. Chronic diseases
J. Code all documented conditions that coexist
K. Patients receiving diagnostic services only
L. Patients receiving therapeutic services only
M. Patients receiving preoperative evaluations only
N. Ambulatory surgery
O. Routine outpatient prenatal visits
P. Encounters for general medical examinations with abnormal findings
Q. Encounters for routine health screenings

Appendix I: Present on Admission Reporting Guidelines

Section I. Conventions, general coding guidelines and chapter specific guidelines

The conventions, general guidelines and chapter-specific guidelines are applicable to all health care settings unless otherwise indicated. The conventions and instructions of the classification take precedence over guidelines.

A. Conventions for the ICD-10-CM

The conventions for the ICD-10-CM are the general rules for use of the classification independent of the guidelines. These conventions are incorporated within the Alphabetic Index and Tabular List of the ICD-10-CM as instructional notes.

  1. **The Alphabetic Index and Tabular List**
     The ICD-10-CM is divided into the Alphabetic Index, an alphabetical list of terms and their corresponding code, and the Tabular List, a structured list of codes divided into chapters based on body system or condition. The Alphabetic Index consists of the following parts: the Index of Diseases and Injury, the Index of External Causes of Injury, the Table of Neoplasms and the Table of Drugs and Chemicals.
     See Section I.C2. General guidelines
     See Section I.C.19. Adverse effects, poisoning, underdosing and toxic effects

  2. **Format and Structure:**
     The ICD-10-CM Tabular List contains categories, subcategories and codes. Characters for categories, subcategories and codes may be either a letter or a number. All categories are 3 characters. A three-character category that has no further subdivision is equivalent to a code. Subcategories are either 4 or 5 characters. Codes may be 3, 4, 5, 6 or 7 characters. That is, each level of subdivision after a category is a subcategory. The final level of subdivision is a code. Codes that have applicable 7th characters are still referred to as codes, not subcategories. A code that has an applicable 7th character is considered invalid without the 7th character.
     The ICD-10-CM uses an indented format for ease in reference

  3. **Use of codes for reporting purposes**
     For reporting purposes only codes are permissible, not categories or subcategories, and any applicable 7th character is required.

  4. **Placeholder character**
     The ICD-10-CM utilizes a placeholder character "X". The "X" is used as a placeholder at certain codes to allow for future expansion. An example of this is at the poisoning, adverse effect and underdosing codes, categories T36-T50. Where a placeholder exists, the X must be used in order for the code to be considered a valid code.

  5. **7th Characters**
     Certain ICD-10-CM categories have applicable 7th characters. The applicable 7th character is required for all codes within the category, or as the notes in the Tabular List instruct. The 7th character must always be the 7th character in the data field. If a code that requires a 7th character is not 6 characters, a placeholder X must be used to fill in the empty characters.

  6. **Abbreviations**
     a. **Alphabetic Index abbreviations**
        NEC "Not elsewhere classifiable"
           This abbreviation in the Alphabetic Index represents "other specified". When a specific code is not available for a condition the Alphabetic Index directs the coder to the "other specified" code in the Tabular List.
        NOS "Not otherwise specified"
           This abbreviation is the equivalent of unspecified.

b. **Tabular List abbreviations**
NEC "Not elsewhere classifiable"
This abbreviation in the Tabular List represents "other specified". When a specific code is not available for a condition, the Tabular List includes an NEC entry under a code to identify the code as the "other specified" code.
NOS "Not otherwise specified"
This abbreviation is the equivalent of unspecified.

7. **Punctuation**
[ ] Brackets are used in the Tabular List to enclose synonyms, alternative wording or explanatory phrases. Brackets are used in the Alphabetic Index to identify manifestation codes.
( ) Parentheses are used in both the Alphabetic Index and Tabular List to enclose supplementary words that may be present or absent in the statement of a disease or procedure without affecting the code number to which it is assigned. The terms within the parentheses are referred to as nonessential modifiers. The nonessential modifiers in the Alphabetic Index to Diseases apply to subterms following a main term except when a nonessential modifier and a subentry are mutually exclusive, the subentry takes precedence. For example, in the ICD-10-CM Alphabetic Index under the main term Enteritis, "acute" is a nonessential modifier and "chronic" is a subentry. In this case, the nonessential modifier "acute" does not apply to the subentry "chronic".
: Colons are used in the Tabular List after an incomplete term which needs one or more of the modifiers following the colon to make it assignable to a given category.

8. **Use of "and".**
See Section I.A.14. Use of the term "And"

9. **Other and Unspecified codes**
a. **"Other" codes**
Codes titled "other" or "other specified" are for use when the information in the medical record provides detail for which a specific code does not exist. Alphabetic Index entries with NEC in the line designate "other" codes in the Tabular List. These Alphabetic Index entries represent specific disease entities for which no specific code exists so the term is included within an "other" code.

b. **"Unspecified" codes**
Codes titled "unspecified" are for use when the information in the medical record is insufficient to assign a more specific code. For those categories for which an unspecified code is not provided, the "other specified" code may represent both other and unspecified.
See Section I.B.18 Use of Signs/Symptom/Unspecified Codes

10. **Includes Notes**
This note appears immediately under a three-character code title to further define, or give examples of, the content of the category.

11. **Inclusion terms**
List of terms is included under some codes. These terms are the conditions for which that code is to be used. The terms may be synonyms of the code title, or, in the case of "other specified" codes, the terms are a list of the various conditions assigned to that code. The inclusion terms are not necessarily exhaustive. Additional terms found only in the Alphabetic Index may also be assigned to a code.

12. **Excludes Notes**
The ICD-10-CM has two types of excludes notes. Each type of note has a different definition for use but they are all similar in that they indicate that codes excluded from each other are independent of each other.

a. **Excludes1**
A type 1 Excludes note is a pure excludes note. It means "NOT CODED HERE!" An Excludes1 note indicates that the code excluded should never be used at the same time as the code above the Excludes1 note. An Excludes1 is used when two conditions cannot occur together, such as a congenital form versus an acquired form of the same condition.

An exception to the Excludes1 definition is the circumstance when the two conditions are unrelated to each other. If it is not clear whether the two conditions involving an Excludes1 note are related or not, query the provider. For example, code F45.8, Other somatoform disorders, has an Excludes1 note for "sleep related teeth grinding (G47.63)," because "teeth grinding" is an inclusion term under F45.8. Only one of these two codes should be assigned for teeth grinding. However psychogenic dysmenorrhea is also an inclusion term under F45.8, and a patient could have both this condition and sleep related teeth grinding. In this case, the two conditions are clearly unrelated to each other, and so it would be appropriate to report F45.8 and G47.63 together.

b. **Excludes2**
A Type 2 Excludes note represents "Not included here." An excludes2 note indicates that the condition excluded is not part of the condition represented by the code, but a patient may have both conditions at the same time. When an Excludes2 note appears under a code, it is acceptable to use both the code and the excluded code together, when appropriate.

13. **Etiology/manifestation convention ("code first", "use additional code" and "in diseases classified elsewhere" notes)**
Certain conditions have both an underlying etiology and multiple body system manifestations

due to the underlying etiology. For such conditions, the ICD-10-CM has a coding convention that requires the underlying condition be sequenced first, **if applicable,** followed by the manifestation. Wherever such a combination exists, there is a "use additional code" note at the etiology code, and a "code first" note at the manifestation code. These instructional notes indicate the proper sequencing order of the codes, etiology followed by manifestation.

In most cases the manifestation codes will have in the code title, "in diseases classified elsewhere." Codes with this title are a component of the etiology/ manifestation convention. The code title indicates that it is a manifestation code. "In diseases classified elsewhere" codes are never permitted to be used as first-listed or principal diagnosis codes. They must be used in conjunction with an underlying condition code and they must be listed following the underlying condition. See category F02, Dementia in other diseases classified elsewhere, for an example of this convention.

There are manifestation codes that do not have "in diseases classified elsewhere" in the title. For such codes, there is a "use additional code" note at the etiology code and a "code first" note at the manifestation code and the rules for sequencing apply.

In addition to the notes in the Tabular List, these conditions also have a specific Alphabetic Index entry structure. In the Alphabetic Index both conditions are listed together with the etiology code first followed by the manifestation codes in brackets. The code in brackets is always to be sequenced second.

An example of the etiology/manifestation convention is dementia in Parkinson's disease. In the Alphabetic Index, code G20 is listed first, followed by code F02.80 or F02.81 in brackets. Code G20 represents the underlying etiology, Parkinson's disease, and must be sequenced first, whereas codes F02.80 and F02.81 represent the manifestation of dementia in diseases classified elsewhere, with or without behavioral disturbance.

"Code first" and "Use additional code" notes are also used as sequencing rules in the classification for certain codes that are not part of an etiology/manifestation combination.

See Section I.B.7. Multiple coding for a single condition.

14. **"And"**
The word "and" should be interpreted to mean either "and" or "or" when it appears in a title.

For example, cases of "tuberculosis of bones", "tuberculosis of joints" and "tuberculosis of bones and joints" are classified to subcategory A18.0, Tuberculosis of bones and joints.

15. **"With"**
The word "with" should be interpreted to mean "associated with" or "due to" when it appears in a code title, the Alphabetic Index, or an instructional note in the Tabular List. **The**

classification presumes a causal relationship between the two conditions linked by these terms in the Alphabetic Index or Tabular List. These conditions should be coded as related even in the absence of provider documentation explicitly linking them, unless the documentation clearly states the conditions are unrelated. For conditions not specifically linked by these relational terms in the classification, provider documentation must link the conditions in order to code them as related.

The word "with" in the Alphabetic Index is sequenced immediately following the main term, not in alphabetical order.

16. **"See" and "See Also"**
The "see" instruction following a main term in the Alphabetic Index indicates that another term should be referenced. It is necessary to go to the main term referenced with the "see" note to locate the correct code.

A "see also" instruction following a main term in the Alphabetic Index instructs that there is another main term that may also be referenced that may provide additional Alphabetic Index entries that may be useful. It is not necessary to follow the "see also" note when the original main term provides the necessary code.

17. **"Code also" note**
A "code also" note instructs that two codes may be required to fully describe a condition, but this note does not provide sequencing direction.

18. **Default codes**
A code listed next to a main term in the ICD-10-CM Alphabetic Index is referred to as a default code. The default code represents that condition that is most commonly associated with the main term, or is the unspecified code for the condition. If a condition is documented in a medical record (for example, appendicitis) without any additional information, such as acute or chronic, the default code should be assigned.

19. **Code assignment and Clinical Criteria**
The assignment of a diagnosis code is based on the provider's diagnostic statement that the condition exists. The provider's statement that the patient has a particular condition is sufficient. Code assignment is not based on clinical criteria used by the provider to establish the diagnosis.

B. **General Coding Guidelines**
1. **Locating a code in the ICD-10-CM**
To select a code in the classification that corresponds to a diagnosis or reason for visit documented in a medical record, first locate the term in the Alphabetic Index, and then verify the code in the Tabular List. Read and be guided by instructional notations that appear in both the Alphabetic Index and the Tabular List.

It is essential to use both the Alphabetic Index and Tabular List when locating and assigning a code. The Alphabetic Index does not always provide the full code. Selection of the full code, including laterality and any applicable 7th character can only be done in the Tabular List. A dash (-) at the end of an Alphabetic Index entry indicates that additional characters are required. Even if a dash is not included at the Alphabetic Index entry, it is necessary to refer to the Tabular List to verify that no 7th character is required.

2. **Level of Detail in Coding**
   Diagnosis codes are to be used and reported at their highest number of characters available.

   ICD-10-CM diagnosis codes are composed of codes with 3, 4, 5, 6 or 7 characters. Codes with three characters are included in ICD-10-CM as the heading of a category of codes that may be further subdivided by the use of fourth and/or fifth characters and/or sixth characters, which provide greater detail.

   A three-character code is to be used only if it is not further subdivided. A code is invalid if it has not been coded to the full number of characters required for that code, including the 7th character, if applicable.

3. **Code or codes from A00.0 through T88.9, Z00-Z99.8**
   The appropriate code or codes from A00.0 through T88.9, Z00-Z99.8 must be used to identify diagnoses, symptoms, conditions, problems, complaints or other reason(s) for the encounter/visit.

4. **Signs and symptoms**
   Codes that describe symptoms and signs, as opposed to diagnoses, are acceptable for reporting purposes when a related definitive diagnosis has not been established (confirmed) by the provider. Chapter 18 of ICD-10-CM, Symptoms, Signs, and Abnormal Clinical and Laboratory Findings, Not Elsewhere Classified (codes R00.0 - R99) contains many, but not all codes for symptoms.

   See Section I.B.18 Use of Signs/Symptom/ Unspecified Codes

5. **Conditions that are an integral part of a disease process**
   Signs and symptoms that are associated routinely with a disease process should not be assigned as additional codes, unless otherwise instructed by the classification.

6. **Conditions that are not an integral part of a disease process**
   Additional signs and symptoms that may not be associated routinely with a disease process should be coded when present.

7. **Multiple coding for a single condition**
   In addition to the etiology/manifestation convention that requires two codes to fully describe a single condition that affects multiple body systems, there are other single conditions that also require more than one code. "Use additional code" notes are found in the Tabular List at codes that are not part of an etiology/manifestation pair where a secondary code is useful to fully describe

a condition. The sequencing rule is the same as the etiology/manifestation pair, "use additional code" indicates that a secondary code should be added.

For example, for bacterial infections that are not included in chapter 1, a secondary code from category B95, Streptococcus, Staphylococcus, and Enterococcus, as the cause of diseases classified elsewhere, or B96, Other bacterial agents as the cause of diseases classified elsewhere, may be required to identify the bacterial organism causing the infection. A "use additional code" note will normally be found at the infectious disease code, indicating a need for the organism code to be added as a secondary code.

"Code first" notes are also under certain codes that are not specifically manifestation codes but may be due to an underlying cause. When there is a "code first" note and an underlying condition is present, the underlying condition should be sequenced first.

"Code, if applicable, any causal condition first," notes indicate that this code may be assigned as a principal diagnosis when the causal condition is unknown or not applicable. If a causal condition is known, then the code for that condition should be sequenced as the principal or first-listed diagnosis.

Multiple codes may be needed for sequela, complication codes and obstetric codes to more fully describe a condition. See the specific guidelines for these conditions for further instruction.

8. **Acute and Chronic Conditions**
   If the same condition is described as both acute (subacute) and chronic, and separate subentries exist in the Alphabetic Index at the same indentation level, code both and sequence the acute (subacute) code first.

9. **Combination Code**
   A combination code is a single code used to classify:
   Two diagnoses, or
   A diagnosis with an associated secondary process (manifestation)
   A diagnosis with an associated complication
   Combination codes are identified by referring to subterm entries in the Alphabetic Index and by reading the inclusion and exclusion notes in the Tabular List.

   Assign only the combination code when that code fully identifies the diagnostic conditions involved or when the Alphabetic Index so directs. Multiple coding should not be used when the classification provides a combination code that clearly identifies all of the elements documented in the diagnosis. When the combination code lacks necessary specificity in describing the manifestation or complication, an additional code should be used as a secondary code.

10. **Sequela (Late Effects)**
    A sequela is the residual effect (condition produced) after the acute phase of an illness or injury has terminated. There is no time limit on when a sequela code can be used. The residual may

be apparent early, such as in cerebral infarction, or it may occur months or years later, such as that due to a previous injury. Examples of sequela include: scar formation resulting from a burn, deviated septum due to a nasal fracture, and infertility due to tubal occlusion from old tuberculosis. Coding of sequela generally requires two codes sequenced in the following order: the condition or nature of the sequela is sequenced first. The sequela code is sequenced second.

An exception to the above guidelines are those instances where the code for the sequela is followed by a manifestation code identified in the Tabular List and title, or the sequela code has been expanded (at the fourth, fifth or sixth character levels) to include the manifestation(s). The code for the acute phase of an illness or injury that led to the sequela is never used with a code for the late effect.

See Section I.C.9. Sequelae of cerebrovascular disease
See Section I.C.15. Sequelae of complication of pregnancy, childbirth and the puerperium
See Section I.C.19. Application of 7th characters for Chapter 19

11. **Impending or Threatened Condition**
Code any condition described at the time of discharge as "impending" or "threatened" as follows:

If it did occur, code as confirmed diagnosis.

If it did not occur, reference the Alphabetic Index to determine if the condition has a subentry term for "impending" or "threatened" and also reference main term entries for "Impending" and for "Threatened."

If the subterms are listed, assign the given code.

If the subterms are not listed, code the existing underlying condition(s) and not the condition described as impending or threatened.

12. **Reporting Same Diagnosis Code More than Once**
Each unique ICD-10-CM diagnosis code may be reported only once for an encounter. This applies to bilateral conditions when there are no distinct codes identifying laterality or two different conditions classified to the same ICD-10-CM diagnosis code.

13. **Laterality**
Some ICD-10-CM codes indicate laterality, specifying whether the condition occurs on the left, right or is bilateral. If no bilateral code is provided and the condition is bilateral, assign separate codes for both the left and right side. If the side is not identified in the medical record, assign the code for the unspecified side.

When a patient has a bilateral condition and each side is treated during separate encounters, assign the "bilateral" code (as the condition still exists on both sides), including for the encounter to treat the first side. For the second encounter for treatment after one side has previously been treated and the condition no longer exists on that side, assign the appropriate unilateral code for the side where the condition still exists (e.g., cataract surgery performed on each eye in separate encounters). The bilateral code would

not be assigned for the subsequent encounter, as the patient no longer has the condition in the previously-treated site. If the treatment on the first side did not completely resolve the condition, then the bilateral code would still be appropriate.

14. **Documentation for BMI,** *Depth of* **Non-pressure ulcers, Pressure Ulcer Stages, Coma Scale,** *and NIH Stroke Scale*
For the Body Mass Index (BMI), depth of non-pressure chronic ulcers, pressure ulcer stage**, coma scale, and NIH stroke scale (NIHSS) codes,** code assignment may be based on medical record documentation from clinicians who are not the patient's provider (i.e., physician or other qualified healthcare practitioner legally accountable for establishing the patient's diagnosis), since this information is typically documented by other clinicians involved in the care of the patient (e.g., a dietitian often documents the BMI, a nurse often documents the pressure ulcer stages**, and an emergency medical technician often documents the coma scale**). However, the associated diagnosis (such as overweight, obesity, **acute stroke,** or pressure ulcer) must be documented by the patient's provider. If there is conflicting medical record documentation, either from the same clinician or different clinicians, the patient's attending provider should be queried for clarification.

The BMI**, coma scale, and NIHSS** codes should only be reported as secondary diagnoses.

15. **Syndromes**
Follow the Alphabetic Index guidance when coding syndromes. In the absence of Alphabetic Index guidance, assign codes for the documented manifestations of the syndrome. Additional codes for manifestations that are not an integral part of the disease process may also be assigned when the condition does not have a unique code.

16. **Documentation of Complications of Care**
Code assignment is based on the provider's documentation of the relationship between the condition and the care or procedure, **unless otherwise instructed by the classification.** The guideline extends to any complications of care, regardless of the chapter the code is located in. It is important to note that not all conditions that occur during or following medical care or surgery are classified as complications. There must be a cause-and-effect relationship between the care provided and the condition, and an indication in the documentation that it is a complication. Query the provider for clarification, if the complication is not clearly documented.

17. **Borderline Diagnosis**
If the provider documents a "borderline" diagnosis at the time of discharge, the diagnosis is coded as confirmed, unless the classification provides a specific entry (e.g., borderline diabetes). If a borderline condition has a specific index entry in ICD-10-CM, it should be coded as such. Since

borderline conditions are not uncertain diagnoses, no distinction is made between the care setting (inpatient versus outpatient). Whenever the documentation is unclear regarding a borderline condition, coders are encouraged to query for clarification.

18. **Use of Sign/Symptom/Unspecified Codes**

Sign/symptom and "unspecified" codes have acceptable, even necessary, uses. While specific diagnosis codes should be reported when they are supported by the available medical record documentation and clinical knowledge of the patient's health condition, there are instances when signs/symptoms or unspecified codes are the best choices for accurately reflecting the healthcare encounter. Each healthcare encounter should be coded to the level of certainty known for that encounter.

If a definitive diagnosis has not been established by the end of the encounter, it is appropriate to report codes for sign(s) and/or symptom(s) in lieu of a definitive diagnosis. When sufficient clinical information isn't known or available about a particular health condition to assign a more specific code, it is acceptable to report the appropriate "unspecified" code (e.g., a diagnosis of pneumonia has been determined, but not the specific type). Unspecified codes should be reported when they are the codes that most accurately reflect what is known about the patient's condition at the time of that particular encounter. It would be inappropriate to select a specific code that is not supported by the medical record documentation or conduct medically unnecessary diagnostic testing in order to determine a more specific code.

C. **Chapter-Specific Coding Guidelines**

In addition to general coding guidelines, there are guidelines for specific diagnoses and/or conditions in the classification. Unless otherwise indicated, these guidelines apply to all health care settings. Please refer to Section II for guidelines on the selection of principal diagnosis.

1. **Chapter 1: Certain Infectious and Parasitic Diseases (A00-B99)**

a. **Human Immunodeficiency Virus (HIV) Infections**

1) **Code only confirmed cases**

Code only confirmed cases of HIV infection/illness. This is an exception to the hospital inpatient guideline Section II, H.

In this context, "confirmation" does not require documentation of positive serology or culture for HIV; the provider's diagnostic statement that the patient is HIV positive, or has an HIV-related illness is sufficient.

2) **Selection and sequencing of HIV codes**

(a) **Patient admitted for HIV-related condition**

If a patient is admitted for an HIV-related condition, the principal diagnosis should be B20,

Human immunodeficiency virus [HIV] disease followed by additional diagnosis codes for all reported HIV-related conditions.

(b) **Patient with HIV disease admitted for unrelated condition**

If a patient with HIV disease is admitted for an unrelated condition (such as a traumatic injury), the code for the unrelated condition (e.g., the nature of injury code) should be the principal diagnosis. Other diagnoses would be B20 followed by additional diagnosis codes for all reported HIV-related conditions.

(c) **Whether the patient is newly diagnosed**

Whether the patient is newly diagnosed or has had previous admissions/encounters for HIV conditions is irrelevant to the sequencing decision.

(d) **Asymptomatic human immunodeficiency virus**

Z21, Asymptomatic human immunodeficiency virus [HIV] infection status, is to be applied when the patient without any documentation of symptoms is listed as being "HIV positive," "known HIV," "HIV test positive," or similar terminology. Do not use this code if the term "AIDS" is used or if the patient is treated for any HIV-related illness or is described as having any condition(s) resulting from his/her HIV positive status; use B20 in these cases.

(e) **Patients with inconclusive HIV serology**

Patients with inconclusive HIV serology, but no definitive diagnosis or manifestations of the illness, may be assigned code R75, Inconclusive laboratory evidence of human immunodeficiency virus [HIV].

(f) **Previously diagnosed HIV-related illness**

Patients with any known prior diagnosis of an HIV-related illness should be coded to B20. Once a patient has developed an HIV-related illness, the patient should always be assigned code B20 on every subsequent admission/encounter. Patients previously diagnosed with any HIV illness (B20) should never be assigned to R75 or Z21, Asymptomatic human immunodeficiency virus [HIV] infection status.

(g) **HIV Infection in Pregnancy, Childbirth and the Puerperium**

During pregnancy, childbirth or the puerperium, a patient admitted (or presenting for a health care encounter) because of an HIV-related illness should receive a principal diagnosis code of O98.7-, Human immunodeficiency [HIV] disease complicating pregnancy, childbirth and the puerperium, followed by B20 and the code(s) for the HIV-related illness(es). Codes from Chapter 15 always take sequencing priority.

Patients with asymptomatic HIV infection status admitted (or presenting for a health care encounter) during pregnancy, childbirth, or the puerperium should receive codes of O98.7- and Z21.

(h) Encounters for testing for HIV
If a patient is being seen to determine his/her HIV status, use code Z11.4, Encounter for screening for human immunodeficiency virus [HIV]. Use additional codes for any associated high risk behavior.

If a patient with signs or symptoms is being seen for HIV testing, code the signs and symptoms. An additional counseling code Z71.7, Human immunodeficiency virus [HIV] counseling, may be used if counseling is provided during the encounter for the test.

When a patient returns to be informed of his/her HIV test results and the test result is negative, use code Z71.7, Human immunodeficiency virus [HIV] counseling.

If the results are positive, see previous guidelines and assign codes as appropriate.

b. Infectious agents as the cause of diseases classified to other chapters
Certain infections are classified in chapters other than Chapter 1 and no organism is identified as part of the infection code. In these instances, it is necessary to use an additional code from Chapter 1 to identify the organism. A code from category B95, Streptococcus, Staphylococcus, and Enterococcus as the cause of diseases classified to other chapters, B96, Other bacterial agents as the cause of diseases classified to other chapters, or B97, Viral agents as the cause of diseases classified to other chapters, is to be used as an additional code to identify the organism. An instructional note will be found at the infection code advising that an additional organism code is required.

c. Infections resistant to antibiotics
Many bacterial infections are resistant to current antibiotics. It is necessary to identify all infections documented as antibiotic resistant. Assign a code from category Z16, Resistance to antimicrobial drugs, following the infection code only if the infection code does not identify drug resistance.

d. Sepsis, Severe Sepsis, and Septic Shock
   1) Coding of Sepsis and Severe Sepsis
      (a) Sepsis
For a diagnosis of sepsis, assign the appropriate code for the underlying systemic infection. If the type of infection or causal organism is not further specified, assign code A41.9, Sepsis, unspecified organism.

A code from subcategory R65.2, Severe sepsis, should not be assigned unless severe sepsis or an associated acute organ dysfunction is documented.

      (i) Negative or inconclusive blood cultures and sepsis
Negative or inconclusive blood cultures do not preclude a diagnosis of sepsis in patients with clinical evidence of the condition, however, the provider should be queried.

      (ii) Urosepsis
The term urosepsis is a nonspecific term. It is not to be considered synonymous with sepsis. It has no default code in the Alphabetic Index. Should a provider use this term, he/she must be queried for clarification.

      (iii) Sepsis with organ dysfunction
If a patient has sepsis and associated acute organ dysfunction or multiple organ dysfunction (MOD), follow the instructions for coding severe sepsis.

      (iv) Acute organ dysfunction that is not clearly associated with the sepsis
If a patient has sepsis and an acute organ dysfunction, but the medical record documentation indicates that the acute organ dysfunction is related to a medical condition other than the sepsis, do not assign a code from subcategory R65.2, Severe sepsis. An acute organ dysfunction must be associated with the sepsis in order to assign the severe sepsis code. If the documentation is not clear as to whether an acute organ dysfunction is related to the sepsis or another medical condition, query the provider.

      (b) Severe sepsis
The coding of severe sepsis requires a minimum of 2 codes: first a code for the underlying systemic infection, followed by a code from subcategory R65.2, Severe sepsis. If the causal organism is not documented, assign code A41.9, Sepsis, unspecified organism, for the infection. Additional code(s) for the associated acute organ dysfunction are also required.

Due to the complex nature of severe sepsis, some cases may require querying the provider prior to assignment of the codes.

   2) Septic shock
      (a) Septic shock generally refers to circulatory failure associated with severe sepsis, and therefore, it represents a type of acute organ dysfunction.
For all cases of septic shock, the code for the systemic infection should be sequenced first, followed by code R65.21, Severe sepsis with septic shock or code T81.12, Postprocedural septic shock. Any additional codes for the other acute organ dysfunctions should also be assigned. As noted in the sequencing instructions in the Tabular List, the code for septic shock cannot be assigned as a principal diagnosis.

3) Sequencing of severe sepsis

If severe sepsis is present on admission, and meets the definition of principal diagnosis, the underlying systemic infection should be assigned as principal diagnosis followed by the appropriate code from subcategory R65.2 as required by the sequencing rules in the Tabular List. A code from subcategory R65.2 can never be assigned as a principal diagnosis.

When severe sepsis develops during an encounter (it was not present on admission) the underlying systemic infection and the appropriate code from subcategory R65.2 should be assigned as secondary diagnoses.

Severe sepsis may be present on admission but the diagnosis may not be confirmed until sometime after admission. If the documentation is not clear whether severe sepsis was present on admission, the provider should be queried.

4) Sepsis and severe sepsis with a localized infection

If the reason for admission is both sepsis or severe sepsis and a localized infection, such as pneumonia or cellulitis, a code(s) for the underlying systemic infection should be assigned first and the code for the localized infection should be assigned as a secondary diagnosis. If the patient has severe sepsis, a code from subcategory R65.2 should also be assigned as a secondary diagnosis. If the patient is admitted with a localized infection, such as pneumonia, and sepsis/severe sepsis doesn't develop until after admission, the localized infection should be assigned first, followed by the appropriate sepsis/severe sepsis codes.

5) Sepsis due to a postprocedural infection

(a) Documentation of causal relationship

As with all postprocedural complications, code assignment is based on the provider's documentation of the relationship between the infection and the procedure.

(b) Sepsis due to a postprocedural infection

For such cases, the postprocedural infection code, such as, T80.2, Infections following infusion, transfusion, and therapeutic injection, T81.4, Infection following a procedure, T88.0, Infection following immunization, or O86.0, Infection of obstetric surgical wound, should be coded first, followed by the code for the specific infection. If the patient has severe sepsis the appropriate code from subcategory R65.2 should also be assigned with the additional code(s) for any acute organ dysfunction.

(c) Postprocedural infection and postprocedural septic shock

In cases where a postprocedural infection has occurred and has resulted in severe sepsis the code for the precipitating complication such as code T81.4, Infection following a procedure, or O86.0, Infection of obstetrical surgical wound should be coded first followed by code R65.20, Severe sepsis

without septic shock. A Code for the systemic infection should also be assigned.

If a postprocedural infection has resulted in postprocedural septic shock, the code for the precipitating complication such as code T81.4, Infection following a procedure, or O86.0, Infection of obstetrical surgical wound should be coded first followed by code T81.12-, Postprocedural septic shock. A code for the systemic infection should also be assigned.

6) Sepsis and severe sepsis associated with a noninfectious process (condition)

In some cases a noninfectious process (condition), such as trauma, may lead to an infection which can result in sepsis or severe sepsis. If sepsis or severe sepsis is documented as associated with a noninfectious condition, such as a burn or serious injury, and this condition meets the definition for principal diagnosis, the code for the noninfectious condition should be sequenced first, followed by the code for the resulting infection. If severe sepsis is present, a code from subcategory R65.2 should also be assigned with any associated organ dysfunction(s) codes. It is not necessary to assign a code from subcategory R65.1, Systemic inflammatory response syndrome (SIRS) of non-infectious origin, for these cases.

If the infection meets the definition of principal diagnosis it should be sequenced before the non-infectious condition. When both the associated non-infectious condition and the infection meet the definition of principal diagnosis either may be assigned as principal diagnosis.

Only one code from category R65, Symptoms and signs specifically associated with systemic inflammation and infection, should be assigned. Therefore, when a non-infectious condition leads to an infection resulting in severe sepsis, assign the appropriate code from subcategory R65.2, Severe sepsis. Do not additionally assign a code from subcategory R65.1, Systemic inflammatory response syndrome (SIRS) of non-infectious origin.

See Section I.C.18. SIRS due to non-infectious process

7) Sepsis and septic shock complicating abortion, pregnancy, childbirth, and the puerperium

See Section I.C.15. Sepsis and septic shock complicating abortion, pregnancy, childbirth and the puerperium

8) Newborn sepsis

See Section I.C.16. f. Bacterial sepsis of Newborn

e. Methicillin Resistant Staphylococcus aureus (MRSA) Conditions

1) Selection and sequencing of MRSA codes

(a) Combination codes for MRSA infection

When a patient is diagnosed with an infection that is due to methicillin resistant *Staphylococcus aureus* (MRSA), and that infection has a combination code that includes the causal organism (e.g., sepsis, pneumonia) assign the appropriate combination code for the condition (e.g., code A41.02, Sepsis due to Methicillin resistant Staphylococcus aureus or code J15.212, Pneumonia due to Methicillin resistant Staphylococcus aureus). Do not assign code B95.62, Methicillin resistant Staphylococcus aureus infection as the cause of diseases classified elsewhere, as an additional code because the combination code includes the type of infection and the MRSA organism. Do not assign a code from subcategory Z16.11, Resistance to penicillins, as an additional diagnosis.

See Section C.1. for instructions on coding and sequencing of sepsis and severe sepsis.

(b) Other codes for MRSA infection

When there is documentation of a current infection (e.g., wound infection, stitch abscess, urinary tract infection) due to MRSA, and that infection does not have a combination code that includes the causal organism, assign the appropriate code to identify the condition along with code B95.62, Methicillin resistant Staphylococcus aureus infection as the cause of diseases classified elsewhere for the MRSA infection. Do not assign a code from subcategory Z16.11, Resistance to penicillins.

(c) Methicillin susceptible Staphylococcus aureus (MSSA) and MRSA colonization

The condition or state of being colonized or carrying MSSA or MRSA is called colonization or carriage, while an individual person is described as being colonized or being a carrier. Colonization means that MSSA or MSRA is present on or in the body without necessarily causing illness. A positive MRSA colonization test might be documented by the provider as "MRSA screen positive" or "MRSA nasal swab positive".

Assign code Z22.322, Carrier or suspected carrier of Methicillin resistant Staphylococcus aureus, for patients documented as having MRSA colonization. Assign code Z22.321, Carrier or suspected carrier of Methicillin susceptible Staphylococcus aureus, for patient documented as having MSSA colonization. Colonization is not necessarily indicative of a disease process or as the cause of a specific condition the patient may have unless documented as such by the provider.

(d) MRSA colonization and infection

If a patient is documented as having both MRSA colonization and infection during a hospital admission, code Z22.322, Carrier or suspected carrier of Methicillin resistant Staphylococcus aureus, and a code for the MRSA infection may both be assigned.

f. Zika virus infections

1) Code only confirmed cases

Code only a confirmed diagnosis of Zika virus (A92.5, Zika virus disease) as documented by the provider. This is an exception to the hospital inpatient guideline Section II, H.

In this context, "confirmation" does not require documentation of the type of test performed; the physician's diagnostic statement that the condition is confirmed is sufficient. This code should be assigned regardless of the stated mode of transmission.

If the provider documents "suspected", "possible" or "probable" Zika, do not assign code A92.5. Assign a code(s) explaining the reason for encounter (such as fever, rash, or joint pain) or Z20.828, Contact with and (suspected) exposure to other viral communicable diseases.

2. **Chapter 2: Neoplasms (C00-D49)**
General guidelines
Chapter 2 of the ICD-10-CM contains the codes for most benign and all malignant neoplasms. Certain benign neoplasms, such as prostatic adenomas, may be found in the specific body system chapters. To properly code a neoplasm it is necessary to determine from the record if the neoplasm is benign, in-situ, malignant, or of uncertain histologic behavior. If malignant, any secondary (metastatic) sites should also be determined.

Primary malignant neoplasms overlapping site boundaries

A primary malignant neoplasm that overlaps two or more contiguous (next to each other) sites should be classified to the subcategory/ code .8 ('overlapping lesion'), unless the combination is specifically indexed elsewhere. For multiple neoplasms of the same site that are not contiguous such as tumors in different quadrants of the same breast, codes for each site should be assigned.

Malignant neoplasm of ectopic tissue

Malignant neoplasms of ectopic tissue are to be coded to the site of origin mentioned, e.g., ectopic pancreatic malignant neoplasms involving the stomach are coded to pancreas, unspecified (C25.9).

The neoplasm table in the Alphabetic Index should be referenced first. However, if the histological term is documented, that term should be referenced first, rather than going immediately to the Neoplasm Table, in order to determine which column in the Neoplasm Table is appropriate. For example, if the documentation indicates "adenoma," refer to the term in the Alphabetic Index to review the entries under this term and the instructional note to "see also neoplasm, by site, benign." The table provides the proper code based on the type of neoplasm and the site. It is important to select the proper column in the table that corresponds to the type of neoplasm. The Tabular List should then be referenced to verify that the correct code has been selected from the table and that a more specific site code does not exist.

See Section I.C.21. Factors influencing health status and contact with health services, Status, for information regarding Z15.0, codes for genetic susceptibility to cancer.

a. Treatment directed at the malignancy
If the treatment is directed at the malignancy, designate the malignancy as the principal diagnosis.

The only exception to this guideline is if a patient admission/encounter is solely for the administration of chemotherapy, immunotherapy or radiation therapy, assign the appropriate Z51.— code as the first-listed or principal diagnosis, and the diagnosis or problem for which the service is being performed as a secondary diagnosis.

b. Treatment of secondary site
When a patient is admitted because of a primary neoplasm with metastasis and treatment is directed toward the secondary site only, the secondary neoplasm is designated as the principal diagnosis even though the primary malignancy is still present.

c. Coding and sequencing of complications
Coding and sequencing of complications associated with the malignancies or with the therapy thereof are subject to the following guidelines:

1) Anemia associated with malignancy
When admission/encounter is for management of an anemia associated with the malignancy, and the treatment is only for anemia, the appropriate code for the malignancy is sequenced as the principal or first-listed diagnosis followed by the appropriate code for the anemia (such as code D63.0, Anemia in neoplastic disease).

2) Anemia associated with chemotherapy, immunotherapy and radiation therapy
When the admission/encounter is for management of an anemia associated with an adverse effect of the administration of chemotherapy or immunotherapy and the only treatment is for the anemia, the anemia code is sequenced first followed by the appropriate codes for the neoplasm and the adverse effect (T45.1X5, Adverse effect of antineoplastic and immunosuppressive drugs).

When the admission/encounter is for management of an anemia associated with an adverse effect of radiotherapy, the anemia code should be sequenced first, followed by the appropriate neoplasm code and code Y84.2, Radiological procedure and radiotherapy as the cause of abnormal reaction of the patient, or of later complication, without mention of misadventure at the time of the procedure.

3) Management of dehydration due to the malignancy
When the admission/encounter is for management of dehydration due to the malignancy and only the dehydration is being treated (intravenous rehydration), the dehydration is sequenced first, followed by the code(s) for the malignancy.

4) Treatment of a complication resulting from a surgical procedure
When the admission/encounter is for treatment of a complication resulting from a surgical procedure, designate the complication as the principal or first-listed diagnosis if treatment is directed at resolving the complication.

d. Primary malignancy previously excised
When a primary malignancy has been previously excised or eradicated from its site and there is no further treatment directed to that site and there is no evidence of any existing primary malignancy, a code from category Z85, Personal history of malignant neoplasm, should be used to indicate the former site of the malignancy. Any mention of extension, invasion, or metastasis to another site is coded as a secondary malignant neoplasm to that site. The secondary site may be the principal or first-listed with the Z85 code used as a secondary code.

e. Admissions/Encounters involving chemotherapy, immunotherapy and radiation therapy

1) Episode of care involves surgical removal of neoplasm
When an episode of care involves the surgical removal of a neoplasm, primary or secondary site, followed by adjunct chemotherapy or radiation treatment during the same episode of care, the code for the neoplasm should be assigned as principal or first-listed diagnosis.

2) Patient admission/encounter solely for administration of chemotherapy, immunotherapy and radiation therapy
If a patient admission/encounter is solely for the administration of chemotherapy, immunotherapy or radiation therapy assign code Z51.0, Encounter for antineoplastic radiation therapy, or Z51.11, Encounter for antineoplastic chemotherapy, or Z51.12, Encounter for antineoplastic immunotherapy as the first-listed or principal diagnosis. If a patient receives more than one of these therapies during the same admission more than one of these codes may be assigned, in any sequence.

The malignancy for which the therapy is being administered should be assigned as a secondary diagnosis.

3) Patient admitted for radiation therapy, chemotherapy or immunotherapy and develops complications
When a patient is admitted for the purpose of radiotherapy, immunotherapy or chemotherapy and develops complications such as uncontrolled nausea and vomiting or dehydration, the principal or first-listed diagnosis is Z51.0, Encounter for antineoplastic radiation therapy, or Z51.11, Encounter for antineoplastic chemotherapy, or Z51.12, Encounter for antineoplastic immunotherapy followed by any codes for the complications.

f. Admission/encounter to determine extent of malignancy
When the reason for admission/encounter is to determine the extent of the malignancy, or for a procedure such as paracentesis or thoracentesis, the primary malignancy or appropriate metastatic site is designated as the principal or first-listed diagnosis, even though chemotherapy or radiotherapy is administered.

g. Symptoms, signs, and abnormal findings listed in Chapter 18 associated with neoplasms

Symptoms, signs, and ill-defined conditions listed in Chapter 18 characteristic of, or associated with, an existing primary or secondary site malignancy cannot be used to replace the malignancy as principal or first-listed diagnosis, regardless of the number of admissions or encounters for treatment and care of the neoplasm.

See section I.C.21. Factors influencing health status and contact with health services, Encounter for prophylactic organ removal.

h. Admission/encounter for pain control/management

See Section I.C.6. for information on coding admission/encounter for pain control/management.

i. Malignancy in two or more noncontiguous sites

A patient may have more than one malignant tumor in the same organ. These tumors may represent different primaries or metastatic disease, depending on the site. Should the documentation be unclear, the provider should be queried as to the status of each tumor so that the correct codes can be assigned.

j. Disseminated malignant neoplasm, unspecified

Code C80.0, Disseminated malignant neoplasm, unspecified, is for use only in those cases where the patient has advanced metastatic disease and no known primary or secondary sites are specified. It should not be used in place of assigning codes for the primary site and all known secondary sites.

k. Malignant neoplasm without specification of site

Code C80.1, Malignant (primary) neoplasm, unspecified, equates to Cancer, unspecified. This code should only be used when no determination can be made as to the primary site of a malignancy. This code should rarely be used in the inpatient setting.

l. Sequencing of neoplasm codes

1) Encounter for treatment of primary malignancy

If the reason for the encounter is for treatment of a primary malignancy, assign the malignancy as the principal/first-listed diagnosis. The primary site is to be sequenced first, followed by any metastatic sites.

2) Encounter for treatment of secondary malignancy

When an encounter is for a primary malignancy with metastasis and treatment is directed toward the metastatic (secondary) site(s) only, the metastatic site(s) is designated as the principal/first-listed diagnosis. The primary malignancy is coded as an additional code.

3) Malignant neoplasm in a pregnant patient

When a pregnant woman has a malignant neoplasm, a code from subcategory O9A.1-, Malignant neoplasm complicating pregnancy, childbirth, and the puerperium, should be sequenced first, followed by the appropriate code from Chapter 2 to indicate the type of neoplasm.

4) Encounter for complication associated with a neoplasm

When an encounter is for management of a complication associated with a neoplasm, such as dehydration, and the treatment is only for the complication, the complication is coded first, followed by the appropriate code(s) for the neoplasm.

The exception to this guideline is anemia. When the admission/encounter is for management of an anemia associated with the malignancy, and the treatment is only for anemia, the appropriate code for the malignancy is sequenced as the principal or first-listed diagnosis followed by code D63.0, Anemia in neoplastic disease.

5) Complication from surgical procedure for treatment of a neoplasm

When an encounter is for treatment of a complication resulting from a surgical procedure performed for the treatment of the neoplasm, designate the complication as the principal/first-listed diagnosis. See guideline regarding the coding of a current malignancy versus personal history to determine if the code for the neoplasm should also be assigned.

6) Pathologic fracture due to a neoplasm

When an encounter is for a pathological fracture due to a neoplasm, and the focus of treatment is the fracture, a code from subcategory M84.5, Pathological fracture in neoplastic disease, should be sequenced first, followed by the code for the neoplasm.

If the focus of treatment is the neoplasm with an associated pathological fracture, the neoplasm code should be sequenced first, followed by a code from M84.5 for the pathological fracture.

m. Current malignancy versus personal history of malignancy

When a primary malignancy has been excised but further treatment, such as an additional surgery for the malignancy, radiation therapy or chemotherapy is directed to that site, the primary malignancy code should be used until treatment is completed.

When a primary malignancy has been previously excised or eradicated from its site, there is no further treatment (of the malignancy) directed to that site, and there is no evidence of any existing primary malignancy, a code from category Z85, Personal history of malignant neoplasm, should be used to indicate the former site of the malignancy.

See Section I.C.21. Factors influencing health status and contact with health services, History (of)

n. Leukemia, Multiple Myeloma, and Malignant Plasma Cell Neoplasms in remission versus personal history

The categories for leukemia, and category C90, Multiple myeloma and malignant plasma cell neoplasms, have codes indicating whether or not the leukemia has achieved remission. There are also codes Z85.6, Personal history of leukemia, and Z85.79, Personal history of other malignant neoplasms of lymphoid, hematopoietic and related tissues. If the documentation is unclear, as to whether the leukemia has achieved remission, the provider should be queried.

See Section I.C.21. Factors influencing health status and contact with health services, History (of)

o. Aftercare following surgery for neoplasm
See Section I.C.21. Factors influencing health status and contact with health services, Aftercare

p. Follow-up care for completed treatment of a malignancy
See Section I.C.21. Factors influencing health status and contact with health services, Follow-up

q. Prophylactic organ removal for prevention of malignancy
See Section I.C. 21, Factors influencing health status and contact with health services, Prophylactic organ removal

r. Malignant neoplasm associated with transplanted organ
A malignant neoplasm of a transplanted organ should be coded as a transplant complication. Assign first the appropriate code from category T86.-, Complications of transplanted organs and tissue, followed by code C80.2, Malignant neoplasm associated with transplanted organ. Use an additional code for the specific malignancy.

3. Chapter 3: Disease of the blood and blood-forming organs and certain disorders involving the immune mechanism (D50-D89)
Reserved for future guideline expansion

4. Chapter 4: Endocrine, Nutritional, and Metabolic Diseases (E00-E89)

a. Diabetes mellitus
The diabetes mellitus codes are combination codes that include the type of diabetes mellitus, the body system affected, and the complications affecting that body system. As many codes within a particular category as are necessary to describe all of the complications of the disease may be used. They should be sequenced based on the reason for a particular encounter. Assign as many codes from categories E08 – E13 as needed to identify all of the associated conditions that the patient has.

1) Type of diabetes
The age of a patient is not the sole determining factor, though most type 1 diabetics develop the condition before reaching puberty. For this reason type 1 diabetes mellitus is also referred to as juvenile diabetes.

2) Type of diabetes mellitus not documented
If the type of diabetes mellitus is not documented in the medical record the default is E11.-, Type 2 diabetes mellitus.

3) Diabetes mellitus and the use of insulin oral hypoglycemics
If the documentation in a medical record does not indicate the type of diabetes but does indicate that the patient uses insulin, code E11, Type 2 diabetes mellitus, should be assigned. Code Z79.4, Long-term (current) use of insulin, **or Z79.84, Long term (current) use of oral hypoglycemic drugs,** should also be assigned to indicate that the patient uses insulin **or hypoglycemic drugs**. Code Z79.4 should not be assigned if insulin is given temporarily to bring a type 2 patient's blood sugar under control during an encounter.

4) Diabetes mellitus in pregnancy and gestational diabetes
See Section I.C.15. Diabetes mellitus in pregnancy.
See Section I.C.15. Gestational (pregnancy induced) diabetes

5) Complications due to insulin pump malfunction

(a) Underdose of insulin due to insulin pump failure
An underdose of insulin due to an insulin pump failure should be assigned to a code from subcategory T85.6, Mechanical complication of other specified internal and external prosthetic devices, implants and grafts, that specifies the type of pump malfunction, as the principal or first-listed code, followed by code T38.3X6-, Underdosing of insulin and oral hypoglycemic [antidiabetic] drugs. Additional codes for the type of diabetes mellitus and any associated complications due to the underdosing should also be assigned.

(b) Overdose of insulin due to insulin pump failure
The principal or first-listed code for an encounter due to an insulin pump malfunction resulting in an overdose of insulin, should also be T85.6-, Mechanical complication of other specified internal and external prosthetic devices, implants and grafts, followed by code T38.3X1-, Poisoning by insulin and oral hypoglycemic [antidiabetic] drugs, accidental (unintentional).

6) Secondary diabetes mellitus
Codes under categories E08, Diabetes mellitus due to underlying condition, E09, Drug or chemical induced diabetes mellitus and E13, Other specified diabetes mellitus, identify complications/manifestations associated with secondary diabetes mellitus. Secondary diabetes is always caused by another condition or event (e.g., cystic fibrosis, malignant neoplasm of pancreas, pancreatectomy, adverse effect of drug, or poisoning).

(a) Secondary diabetes mellitus and the use of insulin or hypoglycemic drugs
For patients who routinely use insulin **or hypoglycemic drugs,** code Z79.4, Long-term (current) use of insulin, **or Z79.84, Long term (current) use of oral hypoglycemic drugs** should also be assigned. Code Z79.4 should not be assigned if insulin is given temporarily to bring a patient's blood sugar under control during an encounter.

(b) Assigning and sequencing secondary diabetes codes and its causes
The sequencing of the secondary diabetes codes in relationship to codes for the cause of the diabetes is based on the Tabular List instructions for categories E08, E09 and E13.

(i) **Secondary diabetes mellitus due to pancreatectomy** For postpancreatectomy diabetes mellitus (lack of insulin due to the surgical removal of all or part of the pancreas), assign code E89.1, Postprocedural hypoinsulinemia. Assign a code from category E13 and a code from subcategory Z90.41-, Acquired absence of pancreas, as additional codes.

(ii) **Secondary diabetes due to drugs** Secondary diabetes may be caused by an adverse effect of correctly administered medications, poisoning or sequela of poisoning.

See section I.C.19.e for coding of adverse effects and poisoning, and section I.C.20 for external cause code reporting.

5. **Chapter 5: Mental, Behavioral and Neurodevelopmental disorders (F01 – F99)**

a. **Pain disorders related to psychological factors**
Assign code F45.41, for pain that is exclusively related to psychological disorders. As indicated by the Excludes 1 note under category G89, a code from category G89 should not be assigned with code F45.41

Code F45.42, Pain disorders with related psychological factors, should be used with a code from category G89, Pain, not elsewhere classified, if there is documentation of a psychological component for a patient with acute or chronic pain.
See Section I.C.6. Pain

c. **Mental and behavioral disorders due to psychoactive substance use**

1) **In Remission**
Selection of codes for "in remission" for categories F10-F19, Mental and behavioral disorders due to psychoactive substance use (categories F10-F19 with -.21) requires the provider's clinical judgment. The appropriate codes for "in remission" are assigned only on the basis of provider documentation (as defined in the Official Guidelines for Coding and Reporting).

2) **Psychoactive Substance Use, Abuse And Dependence**
When the provider documentation refers to use, abuse and dependence of the same substance (e.g. alcohol, opioid, cannabis, etc.), only one code should be assigned to identify the pattern of use based on the following hierarchy:
- If both use and abuse are documented, assign only the code for abuse
- If both abuse and dependence are documented, assign only the code for dependence
- If use, abuse and dependence are all documented, assign only the code for dependence
- If both use and dependence are documented, assign only the code for dependence.

3) **Psychoactive Substance Use**
As with all other diagnoses, the codes for psychoactive substance use (F10.9-, F11.9-, F12.9-, F13.9-, F14.9-, F15.9-, F16.9-) should only be assigned based on provider documentation and when they meet the definition of a reportable diagnosis (see Section III, Reporting Additional Diagnoses). The codes are to be used only when the psychoactive substance use is associated with a mental or behavioral disorder, and such a relationship is documented by the provider.

6. **Chapter 6: Diseases of the Nervous System (G00-G99)**

a. **Dominant/nondominant side**
Codes from category G81, Hemiplegia and hemiparesis, and subcategories, G83.1, Monoplegia of lower limb, G83.2, Monoplegia of upper limb, and G83.3, Monoplegia, unspecified, identify whether the dominant or nondominant side is affected. Should the affected side be documented, but not specified as dominant or nondominant, and the classification system does not indicate a default, code selection is as follows:
- For ambidextrous patients, the default should be dominant.
- If the left side is affected, the default is non-dominant.
- If the right side is affected, the default is dominant.

b. **Pain - Category G89**

1) **General coding information**
Codes in category G89, Pain, not elsewhere classified, may be used in conjunction with codes from other categories and chapters to provide more detail about acute or chronic pain and neoplasm-related pain, unless otherwise indicated below.

If the pain is not specified as acute or chronic, post-thoracotomy, postprocedural, or neoplasm-related, do not assign codes from category G89.

A code from category G89 should not be assigned if the underlying (definitive) diagnosis is known, unless the reason for the encounter is pain control/management and not management of the underlying condition.

When an admission or encounter is for a procedure aimed at treating the underlying condition (e.g., spinal fusion, kyphoplasty), a code for the underlying condition (e.g., vertebral fracture, spinal stenosis) should be assigned as the principal diagnosis. No code from category G89 should be assigned.

(a) **Category G89 Codes as Principal or First-Listed Diagnosis**
Category G89 codes are acceptable as principal diagnosis or the first-listed code:
- When pain control or pain management is the reason for the admission/encounter (e.g., a patient with displaced intervertebral disc, nerve impingement and severe back pain presents for injection of steroid into the spinal canal). The underlying cause of the pain

should be reported as an additional diagnosis, if known.

- When a patient is admitted for the insertion of a neurostimulator for pain control, assign the appropriate pain code as the principal or first-listed diagnosis. When an admission or encounter is for a procedure aimed at treating the underlying condition and a neurostimulator is inserted for pain control during the same admission/encounter, a code for the underlying condition should be assigned as the principal diagnosis and the appropriate pain code should be assigned as a secondary diagnosis.

(b) Use of Category G89 Codes in Conjunction with Site Specific Pain Codes

(i) Assigning Category G89 and Site-Specific Pain Codes

Codes from category G89 may be used in conjunction with codes that identify the site of pain (including codes from chapter 18) if the category G89 code provides additional information. For example, if the code describes the site of the pain, but does not fully describe whether the pain is acute or chronic, then both codes should be assigned.

(ii) Sequencing of Category G89 Codes with Site-Specific Pain Codes

The sequencing of category G89 codes with site-specific pain codes (including chapter 18 codes), is dependent on the circumstances of the encounter/admission as follows:

- If the encounter is for pain control or pain management, assign the code from category G89 followed by the code identifying the specific site of pain (e.g., encounter for pain management for acute neck pain from trauma is assigned code G89.11, Acute pain due to trauma, followed by code M54.2, Cervicalgia, to identify the site of pain).
- If the encounter is for any other reason except pain control or pain management, and a related definitive diagnosis has not been established (confirmed) by the provider, assign the code for the specific site of pain first, followed by the appropriate code from category G89.

2) Pain due to devices, implants and grafts
See Section I.C.19. Pain due to medical devices

3) Postoperative Pain

The provider's documentation should be used to guide the coding of postoperative pain, as well as *Section III. Reporting Additional Diagnoses* and *Section IV. Diagnostic Coding and Reporting in the Outpatient Setting.*

The default for post-thoracotomy and other postoperative pain not specified as acute or chronic is the code for the acute form.

Routine or expected postoperative pain immediately after surgery should not be coded.

(a) Postoperative pain not associated with specific postoperative complication

Postoperative pain not associated with a specific postoperative complication is assigned to the appropriate postoperative pain code in category G89.

(b) Postoperative pain associated with specific postoperative complication

Postoperative pain associated with a specific postoperative complication (such as painful wire sutures) is assigned to the appropriate code(s) found in Chapter 19, Injury, poisoning, and certain other consequences of external causes. If appropriate, use additional code(s) from category G89 to identify acute or chronic pain (G89.18 or G89.28).

4) Chronic pain

Chronic pain is classified to subcategory G89.2. There is no time frame defining when pain becomes chronic pain. The provider's documentation should be used to guide use of these codes.

5) Neoplasm Related Pain

Code G89.3 is assigned to pain documented as being related, associated or due to cancer, primary or secondary malignancy, or tumor. This code is assigned regardless of whether the pain is acute or chronic.

This code may be assigned as the principal or first-listed code when the stated reason for the admission/encounter is documented as pain control/pain management. The underlying neoplasm should be reported as an additional diagnosis.

When the reason for the admission/encounter is management of the neoplasm and the pain associated with the neoplasm is also documented, code G89.3 may be assigned as an additional diagnosis. It is not necessary to assign an additional code for the site of the pain.

See Section I.C.2 for instructions on the sequencing of neoplasms for all other stated reasons for the admission/encounter (except for pain control/pain management).

6) Chronic pain syndrome

Central pain syndrome (G89.0) and chronic pain syndrome (G89.4) are different than the term "chronic pain," and therefore codes should only be used when the provider has specifically documented this condition.

See Section I.C.5. Pain disorders related to psychological factors

7. Chapter 7: Diseases of the Eye and Adnexa (H00-H59)

a. Glaucoma

1) Assigning Glaucoma Codes

Assign as many codes from category H40, Glaucoma, as needed to identify the type of glaucoma, the affected eye, and the glaucoma stage.

2) Bilateral glaucoma with same type and stage

When a patient has bilateral glaucoma and both eyes are documented as being the same type and stage, and there is a code for bilateral glaucoma, report only the code for the type of glaucoma, bilateral, with the seventh character for the stage.

When a patient has bilateral glaucoma and both eyes are documented as being the same type and stage, and the classification does not provide a code for bilateral glaucoma (i.e. subcategories H40.10, H40.11 and H40.20) report only one code for the type of glaucoma with the appropriate seventh character for the stage.

3) Bilateral glaucoma stage with different types or stages

When a patient has bilateral glaucoma and each eye is documented as having a different type or stage, and the classification distinguishes laterality, assign the appropriate code for each eye rather than the code for bilateral glaucoma.

When a patient has bilateral glaucoma and each eye is documented as having a different type, and the classification does not distinguish laterality (i.e. subcategories H40.10, H40.11 and H40.20), assign one code for each type of glaucoma with the appropriate seventh character for the stage.

When a patient has bilateral glaucoma and each eye is documented as having the same type, but different stage, and the classification does not distinguish laterality (i.e. subcategories H40.10, H40.11 and H40.20), assign a code for the type of glaucoma for each eye with the seventh character for the specific glaucoma stage documented for each eye.

4) Patient admitted with glaucoma and stage evolves during the admission

If a patient is admitted with glaucoma and the stage progresses during the admission, assign the code for highest stage documented.

5) Indeterminate stage glaucoma

Assignment of the seventh character "4" for "indeterminate stage" should be based on the clinical documentation. The seventh character "4" is used for glaucomas whose stage cannot be clinically determined. This seventh character should not be confused with the seventh character "0", unspecified, which should be assigned when there is no documentation regarding the stage of the glaucoma.

8. **Chapter 8: Diseases of the Ear and Mastoid Process (H60-H95)**

Reserved for future guideline expansion

9. **Chapter 9: Diseases of the Circulatory System (I00-I99)**

a. **Hypertension**

The classification presumes a causal relationship between hypertension and heart involvement and between hypertension and kidney involvement, as the two conditions are linked by the term "with" in the Alphabetic Index. These conditions should be coded as related even in the absence of provider documentation explicitly linking them, unless the documentation clearly states the conditions are unrelated.

For hypertension and conditions not specifically linked by relational terms such as "with," "associated with" or "due to" in the classification, provider documentation must link the conditions in order to code them as related.

1) **Hypertension with Heart Disease**

Hypertension with heart conditions classified to I50.- or I51.4-I51.9, are assigned to, a code from category I11, Hypertensive heart disease. Use an additional code from category I50, Heart failure, to identify the type of heart failure in those patients with heart failure.

The same heart conditions (I50.-, I51.4-I51.9) with hypertension are coded separately **if the provider has specifically documented a different cause**. Sequence according to the circumstances of the admission/encounter.

2) **Hypertensive Chronic Kidney Disease**

Assign codes from category I12, Hypertensive chronic kidney disease, when both hypertension and a condition classifiable to category N18, Chronic kidney disease (CKD), are present. **CKD should not be coded as hypertensive if the physician has specifically documented a different cause.**

The appropriate code from category N18 should be used as a secondary code with a code from category I12 to identify the stage of chronic kidney disease.

See Section I.C.14. Chronic kidney disease.

If a patient has hypertensive chronic kidney disease and acute renal failure, an additional code for the acute renal failure is required.

3) **Hypertensive Heart and Chronic Kidney Disease**

Assign codes from combination category I13, Hypertensive heart and chronic kidney disease, when **there is hypertension with both heart and kidney involvement.** If heart failure is present, assign an additional code from category I50 to identify the type of heart failure.

The appropriate code from category N18, Chronic kidney disease, should be used as a secondary code with a code from category I13 to identify the stage of chronic kidney disease.

See Section I.C.14. Chronic kidney disease.

The codes in category I13, Hypertensive heart and chronic kidney disease, are combination codes that include hypertension, heart disease and chronic kidney disease. The Includes note at I13 specifies that the conditions included at I11 and I12 are included together in I13. If a patient has hypertension, heart disease and chronic kidney disease then a code from I13 should be used, not individual codes for hypertension, heart disease and chronic kidney disease, or codes from I11 or I12.

For patients with both acute renal failure and chronic kidney disease an additional code for acute renal failure is required.

4) Hypertensive Cerebrovascular Disease

For hypertensive cerebrovascular disease, first assign the appropriate code from categories I60-I69, followed by the appropriate hypertension code.

5) Hypertensive Retinopathy

Subcategory H35.Ø, Background retinopathy and retinal vascular changes, should be used with a code from category I1Ø – I15, Hypertensive disease to include the systemic hypertension. The sequencing is based on the reason for the encounter.

6) Hypertension, Secondary

Secondary hypertension is due to an underlying condition. Two codes are required: one to identify the underlying etiology and one from category I15 to identify the hypertension. Sequencing of codes is determined by the reason for admission/ encounter.

7) Hypertension, Transient

Assign code RØ3.Ø, Elevated blood pressure reading without diagnosis of hypertension, unless patient has an established diagnosis of hypertension. Assign code O13.-, Gestational [pregnancy-induced] hypertension without significant proteinuria, or O14.-, Pre-eclampsia, for transient hypertension of pregnancy.

8) Hypertension, Controlled

This diagnostic statement usually refers to an existing state of hypertension under control by therapy. Assign the appropriate code from categories I1Ø-I15, Hypertensive diseases.

9) Hypertension, Uncontrolled

Uncontrolled hypertension may refer to untreated hypertension or hypertension not responding to current therapeutic regimen. In either case, assign the appropriate code from categories I1Ø-I15, Hypertensive diseases.

10) Hypertensive Crisis

Assign a code from category I16, Hypertensive crisis, for documented hypertensive urgency, hypertensive emergency or unspecified hypertensive crisis. Code also any identified hypertensive disease (I1Ø-I15). The sequencing is based on the reason for the encounter.

b. Atherosclerotic Coronary Artery Disease and Angina

ICD-10-CM has combination codes for atherosclerotic heart disease with angina pectoris. The subcategories for these codes are I25.11, Atherosclerotic heart disease of native coronary artery with angina pectoris and I25.7, Atherosclerosis of coronary artery bypass graft(s) and coronary artery of transplanted heart with angina pectoris.

When using one of these combination codes it is not necessary to use an additional code for angina pectoris. A causal relationship can be assumed in a patient with both atherosclerosis and angina pectoris, unless the documentation indicates the angina is due to something other than the atherosclerosis.

If a patient with coronary artery disease is admitted due to an acute myocardial infarction (AMI), the AMI should be sequenced before the coronary artery disease.

See Section I.C.9. Acute myocardial infarction (AMI)

c. Intraoperative and Postprocedural Cerebrovascular Accident

Medical record documentation should clearly specify the cause-and-effect relationship between the medical intervention and the cerebrovascular accident in order to assign a code for intraoperative or postprocedural cerebrovascular accident.

Proper code assignment depends on whether it was an infarction or hemorrhage and whether it occurred intraoperatively or postoperatively. If it was a cerebral hemorrhage, code assignment depends on the type of procedure performed.

d. Sequelae of Cerebrovascular Disease

1) Category I69, Sequelae of Cerebrovascular disease

Category I69 is used to indicate conditions classifiable to categories I60-I67 as the causes of sequela (neurologic deficits), themselves classified elsewhere. These "late effects" include neurologic deficits that persist after initial onset of conditions classifiable to categories I60-I67. The neurologic deficits caused by cerebrovascular disease may be present from the onset or may arise at any time after the onset of the condition classifiable to categories I60-I67.

Codes from category I69, Sequelae of cerebrovascular disease, that specify hemiplegia, hemiparesis and monoplegia identify whether the dominant or nondominant side is affected. Should the affected side be documented, but not specified as dominant or nondominant, and the classification system does not indicate a default, code selection is as follows:

- For ambidextrous patients, the default should be dominant.
- If the left side is affected, the default is non-dominant.
- If the right side is affected, the default is dominant.

2) Codes from category I69 with codes from I60-I67

Codes from category I69 may be assigned on a health care record with codes from I60-I67, if the patient has a current cerebrovascular disease and deficits from an old cerebrovascular disease.

3) Codes from category I69 and Personal history of transient ischemic attack (TIA) and cerebral infarction (Z86.73)

Codes from category I69 should not be assigned if the patient does not have neurologic deficits.

See Section I.C.21. 4. History (of) for use of personal history codes

e. Acute myocardial infarction (AMI)

1) ST elevation myocardial infarction (STEMI) and non ST elevation myocardial infarction (NSTEMI)

The ICD-10-CM codes for acute myocardial infarction (AMI) identify the site, such as anterolateral wall or true posterior wall. Subcategories I21.0-I21.2 and code I21.3 are used for ST elevation myocardial infarction (STEMI). Code I21.4, Non-ST elevation (NSTEMI) myocardial infarction, is used for non ST elevation myocardial infarction (NSTEMI) and nontransmural MIs.

If NSTEMI evolves to STEMI, assign the STEMI code. If STEMI converts to NSTEMI due to thrombolytic therapy, it is still coded as STEMI.

For encounters occurring while the myocardial infarction is equal to, or less than, four weeks old, including transfers to another acute setting or a postacute setting, and the myocardial infarction **meets the definition for "other diagnoses" (see Section III, Reporting Additional Diagnoses)**, codes from category I21 may continue to be reported. For encounters after the 4 week time frame and the patient is still receiving care related to the myocardial infarction, the appropriate aftercare code should be assigned, rather than a code from category I21. For old or healed myocardial infarctions not requiring further care, code I25.2, Old myocardial infarction, may be assigned.

2) Acute myocardial infarction, unspecified

Code I21.3, ST elevation (STEMI) myocardial infarction of unspecified site, is the default for unspecified acute myocardial infarction. If only STEMI or transmural MI without the site is documented, assign code I21.3.

3) AMI documented as nontransmural or subendocardial but site provided

If an AMI is documented as nontransmural or subendocardial, but the site is provided, it is still coded as a subendocardial AMI.

See Section I.C.21.3 for information on coding status post administration of tPA in a different facility within the last 24 hours.

4) Subsequent acute myocardial infarction

A code from category I22, Subsequent ST elevation (STEMI) and non ST elevation (NSTEMI) myocardial infarction, is to be used when a patient who has suffered an AMI has a new AMI within the 4 week time frame of the initial AMI. A code from category I22 must be used in conjunction with a code from category I21. The sequencing of the I22 and I21 codes depends on the circumstances of the encounter.

10. Chapter 10: Diseases of the Respiratory System (J00-J99)

a. Chronic Obstructive Pulmonary Disease [COPD] and Asthma

1) Acute exacerbation of chronic obstructive bronchitis and asthma

The codes in categories J44 and J45 distinguish between uncomplicated cases and those in acute exacerbation. An acute exacerbation is a worsening or a decompensation of a chronic condition. An acute exacerbation is not equivalent to an infection superimposed on a chronic condition, though an exacerbation may be triggered by an infection.

b. Acute Respiratory Failure

1) Acute respiratory failure as principal diagnosis

A code from subcategory J96.0, Acute respiratory failure, or subcategory J96.2, Acute and chronic respiratory failure, may be assigned as a principal diagnosis when it is the condition established after study to be chiefly responsible for occasioning the admission to the hospital, and the selection is supported by the Alphabetic Index and Tabular List. However, chapter-specific coding guidelines (such as obstetrics, poisoning, HIV, newborn) that provide sequencing direction take precedence.

2) Acute respiratory failure as secondary diagnosis

Respiratory failure may be listed as a secondary diagnosis if it occurs after admission, or if it is present on admission, but does not meet the definition of principal diagnosis.

3) Sequencing of acute respiratory failure and another acute condition

When a patient is admitted with respiratory failure and another acute condition, (e.g., myocardial infarction, cerebrovascular accident, aspiration pneumonia), the principal diagnosis will not be the same in every situation. This applies whether the other acute condition is a respiratory or nonrespiratory condition. Selection of the principal diagnosis will be dependent on the circumstances of admission. If both the respiratory failure and the other acute condition are equally responsible for occasioning the admission to the hospital, and there are no chapter-specific sequencing rules, the guideline regarding two or more diagnoses that equally meet the definition for principal diagnosis *(Section II, C.)* may be applied in these situations.

If the documentation is not clear as to whether acute respiratory failure and another condition are equally responsible for occasioning the admission, query the provider for clarification.

c. Influenza due to certain identified influenza viruses

Code only confirmed cases of influenza due to certain identified influenza viruses (category J09), and due to other identified influenza virus (category J10). This is an exception to the hospital inpatient guideline Section II, H. (Uncertain Diagnosis).

In this context, "confirmation" does not require documentation of positive laboratory testing specific for avian or other novel influenza A or other identified influenza virus. However, coding should be based on the provider's diagnostic statement that the patient has avian influenza, or other novel influenza A, for category J09, or has another particular identified strain of influenza, such as H1N1 or H3N2, but not identified as novel or variant, for category J1Ø.

If the provider records "suspected" or "possible" or "probable" avian influenza, or novel influenza, or other identified influenza, then the appropriate influenza code from category J11, Influenza due to unidentified influenza virus, should be assigned. A code from category JØ9, Influenza due to certain identified influenza viruses, should not be assigned nor should a code from category J1Ø, Influenza due to other identified influenza virus.

d. Ventilator associated Pneumonia
1) Documentation of Ventilator associated Pneumonia
As with all procedural or postprocedural complications, code assignment is based on the provider's documentation of the relationship between the condition and the procedure.

Code J95.851, Ventilator associated pneumonia, should be assigned only when the provider has documented ventilator associated pneumonia (VAP). An additional code to identify the organism (e.g., Pseudomonas aeruginosa, code B96.5) should also be assigned. Do not assign an additional code from categories J12-J18 to identify the type of pneumonia.

Code J95.851 should not be assigned for cases where the patient has pneumonia and is on a mechanical ventilator and the provider has not specifically stated that the pneumonia is ventilator-associated pneumonia. If the documentation is unclear as to whether the patient has a pneumonia that is a complication attributable to the mechanical ventilator, query the provider.

2) Ventilator associated Pneumonia Develops after Admission
A patient may be admitted with one type of pneumonia (e.g., code J13, Pneumonia due to Streptococcus pneumonia) and subsequently develop VAP. In this instance, the principal diagnosis would be the appropriate code from categories J12-J18 for the pneumonia diagnosed at the time of admission. Code J95.851, Ventilator associated pneumonia, would be assigned as an additional diagnosis when the provider has also documented the presence of ventilator associated pneumonia.

11. Chapter 11: Diseases of the Digestive System (KØØ-K95)
Reserved for future guideline expansion

12. Chapter 12: Diseases of the Skin and Subcutaneous Tissue (LØØ-L99)
a. Pressure ulcer stage codes
1) Pressure ulcer stages
Codes from category L89, Pressure ulcer, identify the site of the pressure ulcer as well as the stage of the ulcer.

The ICD-10-CM classifies pressure ulcer stages based on severity, which is designated by stages 1-4, unspecified stage and unstageable.

Assign as many codes from category L89 as needed to identify all the pressure ulcers the patient has, if applicable.

2) Unstageable pressure ulcers
Assignment of the code for unstageable pressure ulcer (L89.--Ø) should be based on the clinical documentation. These codes are used for pressure ulcers whose stage cannot be clinically determined (e.g., the ulcer is covered by eschar or has been treated with a skin or muscle graft) and pressure ulcers that are documented as deep tissue injury but not documented as due to trauma. This code should not be confused with the codes for unspecified stage (L89.--9). When there is no documentation regarding the stage of the pressure ulcer, assign the appropriate code for unspecified stage (L89.--9).

3) Documented pressure ulcer stage
Assignment of the pressure ulcer stage code should be guided by clinical documentation of the stage or documentation of the terms found in the Alphabetic Index. For clinical terms describing the stage that are not found in the Alphabetic Index, and there is no documentation of the stage, the provider should be queried.

4) Patients admitted with pressure ulcers documented as healed
No code is assigned if the documentation states that the pressure ulcer is completely healed.

5) Patients admitted with pressure ulcers documented as healing
Pressure ulcers described as healing should be assigned the appropriate pressure ulcer stage code based on the documentation in the medical record. If the documentation does not provide information about the stage of the healing pressure ulcer, assign the appropriate code for unspecified stage.

If the documentation is unclear as to whether the patient has a current (new) pressure ulcer or if the patient is being treated for a healing pressure ulcer, query the provider.

For ulcers that were present on admission but healed at the time of discharge, assign the code for the site and stage of the pressure ulcer at the time of admission.

6) Patient admitted with pressure ulcer evolving into another stage during the admission
If a patient is admitted with a pressure ulcer at one stage and it progresses to a higher stage, **two separate codes should be assigned: one code for the site and stage of the ulcer on admission and a second code for the same ulcer site and the highest stage reported during the stay.**

13. Chapter 13: Diseases of the Musculoskeletal System and Connective Tissue (MØØ-M99)
a. Site and laterality
Most of the codes within Chapter 13 have site and laterality designations. The site represents the bone, joint or the muscle involved. For some conditions where more than one bone, joint or

muscle is usually involved, such as osteoarthritis, there is a "multiple sites" code available. For categories where no multiple site code is provided and more than one bone, joint or muscle is involved, multiple codes should be used to indicate the different sites involved.

1) Bone versus joint

For certain conditions, the bone may be affected at the upper or lower end, (e.g., avascular necrosis of bone, M87, Osteoporosis, M80, M81). Though the portion of the bone affected may be at the joint, the site designation will be the bone, not the joint.

b. Acute traumatic versus chronic or recurrent musculoskeletal conditions

Many musculoskeletal conditions are a result of previous injury or trauma to a site, or are recurrent conditions. Bone, joint or muscle conditions that are the result of a healed injury are usually found in chapter 13. Recurrent bone, joint or muscle conditions are also usually found in chapter 13. Any current, acute injury should be coded to the appropriate injury code from chapter 19. Chronic or recurrent conditions should generally be coded with a code from chapter 13. If it is difficult to determine from the documentation in the record which code is best to describe a condition, query the provider.

c. Coding of Pathologic Fractures

7th character A is for use as long as the patient is receiving active treatment for the fracture. While the patient may be seen by a new or different provider over the course of treatment for a pathological fracture, assignment of the 7th character is based on whether the patient is undergoing active treatment and not whether the provider is seeing the patient for the first time.

7th character, D is to be used for encounters after the patient has completed active treatment. The other 7th characters, listed under each subcategory in the Tabular List, are to be used for subsequent encounters for **routine care of fractures during the healing and recovery phase as well as** treatment of problems associated with the healing, such as malunions, nonunions, and sequelae.

Care for complications of surgical treatment for fracture repairs during the healing or recovery phase should be coded with the appropriate complication codes.

See Section I.C.19. Coding of traumatic fractures.

d. Osteoporosis

Osteoporosis is a systemic condition, meaning that all bones of the musculoskeletal system are affected. Therefore, site is not a component of the codes under category M81, Osteoporosis without current pathological fracture. The site codes under category M80, Osteoporosis with current pathological fracture, identify the site of the fracture, not the osteoporosis.

1) Osteoporosis without pathological fracture

Category M81, Osteoporosis without current pathological fracture, is for use for patients with osteoporosis who do not currently have a pathologic fracture due to the osteoporosis, even if they have had a fracture in the past. For patients with a history of osteoporosis fractures, status code Z87.310, Personal history of (healed) osteoporosis fracture, should follow the code from M81.

2) Osteoporosis with current pathological fracture

Category M80, Osteoporosis with current pathological fracture, is for patients who have a current pathologic fracture at the time of an encounter. The codes under M80 identify the site of the fracture. A code from category M80, not a traumatic fracture code, should be used for any patient with known osteoporosis who suffers a fracture, even if the patient had a minor fall or trauma, if that fall or trauma would not usually break a normal, healthy bone.

14. Chapter 14: Diseases of Genitourinary System (N00-N99)

a. Chronic kidney disease

1) Stages of chronic kidney disease (CKD)

The ICD-10-CM classifies CKD based on severity. The severity of CKD is designated by stages 1-5. Stage 2, code N18.2, equates to mild CKD; stage 3, code N18.3, equates to moderate CKD; and stage 4, code N18.4, equates to severe CKD. Code N18.6, End stage renal disease (ESRD), is assigned when the provider has documented end-stage-renal disease (ESRD).

If both a stage of CKD and ESRD are documented, assign code N18.6 only.

2) Chronic kidney disease and kidney transplant status

Patients who have undergone kidney transplant may still have some form of chronic kidney disease CKD because the kidney transplant may not fully restore kidney function. Therefore, the presence of CKD alone does not constitute a transplant complication. Assign the appropriate N18 code for the patient's stage of CKD and code Z94.0, Kidney transplant status. If a transplant complication such as failure or rejection or other transplant complication is documented, see section I.C.19.g for information on coding complications of a kidney transplant. If the documentation is unclear as to whether the patient has a complication of the transplant, query the provider.

3) Chronic kidney disease with other conditions

Patients with CKD may also suffer from other serious conditions, most commonly diabetes mellitus and hypertension. The sequencing of the CKD code in relationship to codes for other contributing conditions is based on the conventions in the Tabular List.

See I.C.9. Hypertensive chronic kidney disease.
See I.C.19. Chronic kidney disease and kidney transplant complications.

15. Chapter 15: Pregnancy, Childbirth, and the Puerperium (O00-O9A)

a. General Rules for Obstetric Cases

1) Codes from chapter 15 and sequencing priority

Obstetric cases require codes from chapter 15, codes in the range O00-O9A, Pregnancy, Childbirth, and the Puerperium. Chapter 15 codes have sequencing priority over codes from other chapters. Additional codes from other chapters may be used in conjunction with chapter 15 codes to further specify conditions. Should the provider document that the pregnancy is incidental to the encounter, then code Z33.1, Pregnant state, incidental, should be used in place of any chapter 15 codes. It is the provider's responsibility to state that the condition being treated is not affecting the pregnancy.

2) Chapter 15 codes used only on the maternal record

Chapter 15 codes are to be used only on the maternal record, never on the record of the newborn.

3) Final character for trimester

The majority of codes in Chapter 15 have a final character indicating the trimester of pregnancy. The timeframes for the trimesters are indicated at the beginning of the chapter. If trimester is not a component of a code it is because the condition always occurs in a specific trimester, or the concept of trimester of pregnancy is not applicable. Certain codes have characters for only certain trimesters because the condition does not occur in all trimesters, but it may occur in more than just one.

Assignment of the final character for trimester should be based on the provider's documentation of the trimester (or number of weeks) for the current admission/encounter. This applies to the assignment of trimester for pre-existing conditions as well as those that develop during or are due to the pregnancy. The provider's documentation of the number of weeks may be used to assign the appropriate code identifying the trimester.

Whenever delivery occurs during the current admission, and there is an "in childbirth" option for the obstetric complication being coded, the "in childbirth" code should be assigned.

4) Selection of trimester for inpatient admissions that encompass more than one trimester

In instances when a patient is admitted to a hospital for complications of pregnancy during one trimester and remains in the hospital into a subsequent trimester, the trimester character for the antepartum complication code should be assigned on the basis of the trimester when the complication developed, not the trimester of the discharge. If the condition developed prior to the current admission/encounter or represents a pre-existing condition, the trimester character for the trimester at the time of the admission/encounter should be assigned.

5) Unspecified trimester

Each category that includes codes for trimester has a code for "unspecified trimester." The "unspecified trimester" code should rarely be used, such as when the documentation in the record is insufficient to determine the trimester and it is not possible to obtain clarification.

6) 7th character for Fetus Identification

Where applicable, a 7th character is to be assigned for certain categories (O31, O32, O33.3 - O33.6, O35, O36, O40, O41, O60.1, O60.2, O64, and O69) to identify the fetus for which the complication code applies.

Assign 7th character "0":
- For single gestations
- When the documentation in the record is insufficient to determine the fetus affected and it is not possible to obtain clarification.
- When it is not possible to clinically determine which fetus is affected.

b. Selection of OB Principal or First-listed Diagnosis

1) Routine outpatient prenatal visits

For routine outpatient prenatal visits when no complications are present, a code from category Z34, Encounter for supervision of normal pregnancy, should be used as the first-listed diagnosis. These codes should not be used in conjunction with chapter 15 codes.

2) *Supervision of High-Risk Pregnancy*

Codes from category O09, Supervision of high-risk pregnancy, are intended for use only during the prenatal period. For complications during the labor or delivery episode as a result of a high-risk pregnancy, assign the applicable complication codes from Chapter 15. If there are no complications during the labor or delivery episode, assign code O80, Encounter for full-term uncomplicated delivery.

For routine prenatal outpatient visits for patients with high-risk pregnancies, a code from category O09, Supervision of high-risk pregnancy, should be used as the first-listed diagnosis. Secondary chapter 15 codes may be used in conjunction with these codes if appropriate.

3) Episodes when no delivery occurs

In episodes when no delivery occurs, the principal diagnosis should correspond to the principal complication of the pregnancy which necessitated the encounter. Should more than one complication exist, all of which are treated or monitored, any of the complications codes may be sequenced first.

4) When a delivery occurs

When an obstetric patient is admitted and delivers during that admission, the condition that prompted the admission should be sequenced as the principal diagnosis. If multiple conditions prompted the admission, sequence the one most related to the delivery as the principal

diagnosis. A code for any complication of the delivery should be assigned as an additional diagnosis. In cases of cesarean delivery, if the patient was admitted with a condition that resulted in the performance of a cesarean procedure, that condition should be selected as the principal diagnosis. If the reason for the admission was unrelated to the condition resulting in the cesarean delivery, the condition related to the reason for the admission should be selected as the principal diagnosis.

5) Outcome of delivery

A code from category Z37, Outcome of delivery, should be included on every maternal record when a delivery has occurred. These codes are not to be used on subsequent records or on the newborn record.

c. Pre-existing conditions versus conditions due to the pregnancy

Certain categories in Chapter 15 distinguish between conditions of the mother that existed prior to pregnancy (pre-existing) and those that are a direct result of pregnancy. When assigning codes from Chapter 15, it is important to assess if a condition was pre-existing prior to pregnancy or developed during or due to the pregnancy in order to assign the correct code.

Categories that do not distinguish between pre-existing and pregnancy-related conditions may be used for either. It is acceptable to use codes specifically for the puerperium with codes complicating pregnancy and childbirth if a condition arises postpartum during the delivery encounter.

d. Pre-existing hypertension in pregnancy

Category O10, Pre-existing hypertension complicating pregnancy, childbirth and the puerperium, includes codes for hypertensive heart and hypertensive chronic kidney disease. When assigning one of the O10 codes that includes hypertensive heart disease or hypertensive chronic kidney disease, it is necessary to add a secondary code from the appropriate hypertension category to specify the type of heart failure or chronic kidney disease.

See Section I.C.9. Hypertension.

e. Fetal Conditions Affecting the Management of the Mother

1) Codes from categories O35 and O36

Codes from categories O35, Maternal care for known or suspected fetal abnormality and damage, and O36, Maternal care for other fetal problems, are assigned only when the fetal condition is actually responsible for modifying the management of the mother, i.e., by requiring diagnostic studies, additional observation, special care, or termination of pregnancy. The fact that the fetal condition exists does not justify assigning a code from this series to the mother's record.

2) In utero surgery

In cases when surgery is performed on the fetus, a diagnosis code from category O35, Maternal care for known or suspected fetal abnormality and damage, should be assigned identifying the fetal condition. Assign the appropriate procedure code for the procedure performed.

No code from Chapter 16, the perinatal codes, should be used on the mother's record to identify fetal conditions. Surgery performed in utero on a fetus is still to be coded as an obstetric encounter.

f. HIV Infection in Pregnancy, Childbirth and the Puerperium

During pregnancy, childbirth or the puerperium, a patient admitted because of an HIV-related illness should receive a principal diagnosis from subcategory O98.7-, Human immunodeficiency [HIV] disease complicating pregnancy, childbirth and the puerperium, followed by the code(s) for the HIV-related illness(es).

Patients with asymptomatic HIV infection status admitted during pregnancy, childbirth, or the puerperium should receive codes of O98.7- and Z21, Asymptomatic human immunodeficiency virus [HIV] infection status.

g. Diabetes mellitus in pregnancy

Diabetes mellitus is a significant complicating factor in pregnancy. Pregnant women who are diabetic should be assigned a code from category O24, Diabetes mellitus in pregnancy, childbirth, and the puerperium, first, followed by the appropriate diabetes code(s) (E08-E13) from Chapter 4.

h. Long term use of insulin and oral hypoglycemics

Code Z79.4, Long-term (current) use of insulin, or **code Z79.84, Long-term (current) use of oral hypoglycemic drugs,** should also be assigned if the diabetes mellitus is being treated with insulin **or oral medications. If the patient is treated with both oral medications and insulin, only the code for insulin-controlled should be assigned.**

i. Gestational (pregnancy induced) diabetes

Gestational (pregnancy induced) diabetes can occur during the second and third trimester of pregnancy in women who were not diabetic prior to pregnancy. Gestational diabetes can cause complications in the pregnancy similar to those of pre-existing diabetes mellitus. It also puts the woman at greater risk of developing diabetes after the pregnancy. Codes for gestational diabetes are in subcategory O24.4, Gestational diabetes mellitus. No other code from category O24, Diabetes mellitus in pregnancy, childbirth, and the puerperium, should be used with a code from O24.4.

The codes under subcategory O24.4 include diet controlled, insulin controlled, **and controlled by oral hypoglycemic drugs.** If a patient with gestational diabetes is treated with both diet and insulin, only the code for insulin-controlled is required. **If a patient with gestational diabetes is treated with both diet and oral hypoglycemic medications, only the code for "controlled by oral hypoglycemic drugs" is required.** Code Z79.4, Long-term (current) use of insulin **or code Z79.84, Long-term (current) use of oral hypoglycemic drugs,** should not be assigned with codes from subcategory O24.4.

An abnormal glucose tolerance in pregnancy is assigned a code from subcategory O99.81, Abnormal glucose complicating pregnancy, childbirth, and the puerperium.

j. **Sepsis and septic shock complicating abortion, pregnancy, childbirth and the puerperium**

When assigning a chapter 15 code for sepsis complicating abortion, pregnancy, childbirth, and the puerperium, a code for the specific type of infection should be assigned as an additional diagnosis. If severe sepsis is present, a code from subcategory R65.2, Severe sepsis, and code(s) for associated organ dysfunction(s) should also be assigned as additional diagnoses.

k. **Puerperal sepsis**

Code O85, Puerperal sepsis, should be assigned with a secondary code to identify the causal organism (e.g., for a bacterial infection, assign a code from category B95-B96, Bacterial infections in conditions classified elsewhere). A code from category A40, Streptococcal sepsis, or A41, Other sepsis, should not be used for puerperal sepsis. If applicable, use additional codes to identify severe sepsis (R65.2-) and any associated acute organ dysfunction.

l. **Alcohol and tobacco use during pregnancy, childbirth and the puerperium**

1) **Alcohol use during pregnancy, childbirth and the puerperium**

Codes under subcategory O99.31, Alcohol use complicating pregnancy, childbirth, and the puerperium, should be assigned for any pregnancy case when a mother uses alcohol during the pregnancy or postpartum. A secondary code from category F10, Alcohol related disorders, should also be assigned to identify manifestations of the alcohol use.

2) **Tobacco use during pregnancy, childbirth and the puerperium**

Codes under subcategory O99.33, Smoking (tobacco) complicating pregnancy, childbirth, and the puerperium, should be assigned for any pregnancy case when a mother uses any type of tobacco product during the pregnancy or postpartum. A secondary code from category F17, Nicotine dependence, should also be assigned to identify the type of nicotine dependence.

m. **Poisoning, toxic effects, adverse effects and underdosing in a pregnant patient**

A code from subcategory O9A.2, Injury, poisoning and certain other consequences of external causes complicating pregnancy, childbirth, and the puerperium, should be sequenced first, followed by the appropriate injury, poisoning, toxic effect, adverse effect or underdosing code, and then the additional code(s) that specifies the condition caused by the poisoning, toxic effect, adverse effect or underdosing.

See Section I.C.19. Adverse effects, poisoning, underdosing and toxic effects.

n. **Normal Delivery, Code O80**

1) **Encounter for full term uncomplicated delivery**

Code O80 should be assigned when a woman is admitted for a full-term normal delivery and delivers a single, healthy infant without any complications antepartum, during the delivery, or postpartum during the delivery episode. Code O80 is always a principal diagnosis. It is not to be used if any other code from chapter 15 is needed to describe a current complication of the antenatal, delivery, or perinatal period. Additional codes from other chapters may be used with code O80 if they are not related to or are in any way complicating the pregnancy.

2) **Uncomplicated delivery with resolved antepartum complication**

Code O80 may be used if the patient had a complication at some point during the pregnancy, but the complication is not present at the time of the admission for delivery.

3) **Outcome of delivery for O80**

Z37.0, Single live birth, is the only outcome of delivery code appropriate for use with O80.

o. **The Peripartum and Postpartum Periods**

1) **Peripartum and Postpartum periods**

The postpartum period begins immediately after delivery and continues for six weeks following delivery. The peripartum period is defined as the last month of pregnancy to five months postpartum.

2) **Peripartum and postpartum complication**

A postpartum complication is any complication occurring within the six-week period.

3) **Pregnancy-related complications after 6 week period**

Chapter 15 codes may also be used to describe pregnancy-related complications after the peripartum or postpartum period if the provider documents that a condition is pregnancy related.

4) **Admission for routine postpartum care following delivery outside hospital**

When the mother delivers outside the hospital prior to admission and is admitted for routine postpartum care and no complications are noted, code Z39.0, Encounter for care and examination of mother immediately after delivery, should be assigned as the principal diagnosis.

5) Pregnancy associated cardiomyopathy
Pregnancy associated cardiomyopathy, code O90.3, is unique in that it may be diagnosed in the third trimester of pregnancy but may continue to progress months after delivery. For this reason, it is referred to as peripartum cardiomyopathy. Code O90.3 is only for use when the cardiomyopathy develops as a result of pregnancy in a woman who did not have pre-existing heart disease.

p. Code O94, Sequelae of complication of pregnancy, childbirth, and the puerperium
1) Code O94
Code O94, Sequelae of complication of pregnancy, childbirth, and the puerperium, is for use in those cases when an initial complication of a pregnancy develops a sequelae requiring care or treatment at a future date.

2) After the initial postpartum period
This code may be used at any time after the initial postpartum period.

3) Sequencing of Code O94
This code, like all sequela codes, is to be sequenced following the code describing the sequelae of the complication.

q. Termination of Pregnancy and Spontaneous abortions
1) Abortion with Liveborn Fetus
When an attempted termination of pregnancy results in a liveborn fetus assign code Z33.2, Encounter for elective termination of pregnancy and a code from category Z37, Outcome of Delivery.

2) Retained Products of Conception following an abortion
Subsequent encounters for retained products of conception following a spontaneous abortion or elective termination of pregnancy are assigned the appropriate code from category O03, Spontaneous abortion, or codes O07.4, Failed attempted termination of pregnancy without complication and Z33.2, Encounter for elective termination of pregnancy. This advice is appropriate even when the patient was discharged previously with a discharge diagnosis of complete abortion.

3) Complications leading to abortion
Codes from Chapter 15 may be used as additional codes to identify any documented complications of the pregnancy in conjunction with codes in categories in O07 and O08.

r. Abuse in a pregnant patient
For suspected or confirmed cases of abuse of a pregnant patient, a code(s) from subcategories O9A.3, Physical abuse complicating pregnancy, childbirth, and the puerperium, O9A.4, Sexual abuse complicating pregnancy, childbirth, and the puerperium, and O9A.5, Psychological abuse complicating pregnancy, childbirth, and the puerperium, should be sequenced first, followed by the appropriate codes (if applicable) to identify any associated current injury due to physical abuse, sexual abuse, and the perpetrator of abuse.
See Section I.C.19. Adult and child abuse, neglect and other maltreatment.

16. Chapter 16: Certain Conditions Originating in the Perinatal Period (P00-P96)
For coding and reporting purposes the perinatal period is defined as before birth through the 28th day following birth. The following guidelines are provided for reporting purposes

a. General Perinatal Rules
1) Use of Chapter 16 Codes
Codes in this chapter are never for use on the maternal record. Codes from Chapter 15, the obstetric chapter, are never permitted on the newborn record. Chapter 16 codes may be used throughout the life of the patient if the condition is still present.

2) Principal Diagnosis for Birth Record
When coding the birth episode in a newborn record, assign a code from category Z38, Liveborn infants according to place of birth and type of delivery, as the principal diagnosis. A code from category Z38 is assigned only once, to a newborn at the time of birth. If a newborn is transferred to another institution, a code from category Z38 should not be used at the receiving hospital.

A code from category Z38 is used only on the newborn record, not on the mother's record.

3) Use of Codes from other Chapters with Codes from Chapter 16
Codes from other chapters may be used with codes from chapter 16 if the codes from the other chapters provide more specific detail. Codes for signs and symptoms may be assigned when a definitive diagnosis has not been established. If the reason for the encounter is a perinatal condition, the code from chapter 16 should be sequenced first.

4) Use of Chapter 16 Codes after the Perinatal Period
Should a condition originate in the perinatal period, and continue throughout the life of the patient, the perinatal code should continue to be used regardless of the patient's age.

5) Birth process or community acquired conditions
If a newborn has a condition that may be either due to the birth process or community acquired and the documentation does not indicate which it is, the default is due to the birth process and the code from Chapter 16 should be used. If the condition is community-acquired, a code from Chapter 16 should not be assigned.

6) Code all clinically significant conditions
All clinically significant conditions noted on routine newborn examination should be coded. A condition is clinically significant if it requires:
- clinical evaluation; or
- therapeutic treatment; or
- diagnostic procedures; or

- extended length of hospital stay; or
- increased nursing care and/or monitoring; or
- has implications for future health care needs

Note: The perinatal guidelines listed above are the same as the general coding guidelines for "additional diagnoses", except for the final point regarding implications for future health care needs. Codes should be assigned for conditions that have been specified by the provider as having implications for future health care needs.

b. Observation and Evaluation of Newborns for Suspected Conditions not Found

1) **Assign a code from category Z05, Observation and evaluation of newborns and infants for suspected conditions ruled out, to identify those instances when a healthy newborn is evaluated for a suspected condition that is determined after study not to be present. Do not use a code from category Z05 when the patient has identified signs or symptoms of a suspected problem; in such cases code the sign or symptom.**

2) **A code from category Z05 may also be assigned as a principal or first-listed code for readmissions or encounters when the code from category Z38 code no longer applies. Codes from category Z05 are for use only for healthy newborns and infants for which no condition after study is found to be present.**

3) **Z05 on a birth record**

   A code from category Z05 is to be used as a secondary code after the code from category Z38, Liveborn infants according to place of birth and type of delivery.

c. Coding Additional Perinatal Diagnoses

1) **Assigning codes for conditions that require treatment**

Assign codes for conditions that require treatment or further investigation, prolong the length of stay, or require resource utilization.

2) **Codes for conditions specified as having implications for future health care needs**

Assign codes for conditions that have been specified by the provider as having implications for future health care needs.

Note: This guideline should not be used for adult patients.

d. Prematurity and Fetal Growth Retardation

Providers utilize different criteria in determining prematurity. A code for prematurity should not be assigned unless it is documented. Assignment of codes in categories P05, Disorders of newborn related to slow fetal growth and fetal malnutrition, and P07, Disorders of newborn related to short gestation and low birth weight, not elsewhere classified, should be based on the recorded birth weight and estimated gestational age. Codes from category P05 should not be assigned with codes from category P07.

When both birth weight and gestational age are available, two codes from category P07 should be assigned, with the code for birth weight sequenced before the code for gestational age.

e. Low birth weight and immaturity status

Codes from category P07, Disorders of newborn related to short gestation and low birth weight, not elsewhere classified, are for use for a child or adult who was premature or had a low birth weight as a newborn and this is affecting the patient's current health status.

See Section I.C.21. Factors influencing health status and contact with health services, Status.

f. Bacterial Sepsis of Newborn

Category P36, Bacterial sepsis of newborn, includes congenital sepsis. If a perinate is documented as having sepsis without documentation of congenital or community acquired, the default is congenital and a code from category P36 should be assigned. If the P36 code includes the causal organism, an additional code from category B95, Streptococcus, Staphylococcus, and Enterococcus as the cause of diseases classified elsewhere, or B96, Other bacterial agents as the cause of diseases classified elsewhere, should not be assigned. If the P36 code does not include the causal organism, assign an additional code from category B96. If applicable, use additional codes to identify severe sepsis (R65.2-) and any associated acute organ dysfunction.

g. Stillbirth

Code P95, Stillbirth, is only for use in institutions that maintain separate records for stillbirths. No other code should be used with P95. Code P95 should not be used on the mother's record.

17. **Chapter 17: Congenital malformations, deformations, and chromosomal abnormalities (Q00-Q99)**

Assign an appropriate code(s) from categories Q00-Q99, Congenital malformations, deformations, and chromosomal abnormalities when a malformation/deformation or chromosomal abnormality is documented. A malformation/deformation/or chromosomal abnormality may be the principal/first-listed diagnosis on a record or a secondary diagnosis.

When a malformation/deformation/or chromosomal abnormality does not have a unique code assignment, assign additional code(s) for any manifestations that may be present.

When the code assignment specifically identifies the malformation/deformation/or chromosomal abnormality, manifestations that are an inherent component of the anomaly should not be coded separately. Additional codes should be assigned for manifestations that are not an inherent component.

Codes from Chapter 17 may be used throughout the life of the patient. If a congenital malformation or deformity has been corrected, a personal history code should be used to identify the history of the malformation or deformity. Although present at birth, malformation/deformation/or chromosomal abnormality may not be identified until later in life. Whenever the condition is diagnosed by the physician, it is appropriate to assign a code from codes Q00-Q99.

For the birth admission, the appropriate code from category Z38, Liveborn infants, according to place of birth and type of delivery, should be sequenced as the principal diagnosis, followed by any congenital anomaly codes, Q00-Q99.

18. **Chapter 18: Symptoms, signs, and abnormal clinical and laboratory findings, not elsewhere classified (R00-R99)**
Chapter 18 includes symptoms, signs, abnormal results of clinical or other investigative procedures, and ill-defined conditions regarding which no diagnosis classifiable elsewhere is recorded. Signs and symptoms that point to a specific diagnosis have been assigned to a category in other chapters of the classification.

a. **Use of symptom codes**
Codes that describe symptoms and signs are acceptable for reporting purposes when a related definitive diagnosis has not been established (confirmed) by the provider.

b. **Use of a symptom code with a definitive diagnosis code**
Codes for signs and symptoms may be reported in addition to a related definitive diagnosis when the sign or symptom is not routinely associated with that diagnosis, such as the various signs and symptoms associated with complex syndromes. The definitive diagnosis code should be sequenced before the symptom code.

Signs or symptoms that are associated routinely with a disease process should not be assigned as additional codes, unless otherwise instructed by the classification.

c. **Combination codes that include symptoms**
ICD-10-CM contains a number of combination codes that identify both the definitive diagnosis and common symptoms of that diagnosis. When using one of these combination codes, an additional code should not be assigned for the symptom.

d. **Repeated falls**
Code R29.6, Repeated falls, is for use for encounters when a patient has recently fallen and the reason for the fall is being investigated.

Code Z91.81, History of falling, is for use when a patient has fallen in the past and is at risk for future falls. When appropriate, both codes R29.6 and Z91.81 may be assigned together.

e. **Coma scale**
The coma scale codes (R40.2-) can be used in conjunction with traumatic brain injury codes, acute cerebrovascular disease or sequelae of cerebrovascular disease codes. These codes are primarily for use by trauma registries, but they may be used in any setting where this information is collected. **The coma scale may also be used to assess the status of the central nervous system for other non-trauma conditions, such as monitoring patients in the intensive care unit regardless of medical condition.** The coma scale codes should be sequenced after the diagnosis code(s).

These codes, one from each subcategory, are needed to complete the scale. The 7th character indicates when the scale was recorded. The 7th character should match for all three codes.

At a minimum, report the initial score documented on presentation at your facility. This may be a score from the emergency medicine technician (EMT) or in the emergency department. If desired, a facility may choose to capture multiple coma scale scores.

Assign code R40.24, Glasgow coma scale, total score, when only the total score is documented in the medical record and not the individual score(s).

f. **Functional quadriplegia**
Functional quadriplegia (code R53.2) is the lack of ability to use one's limbs or to ambulate due to extreme debility. It is not associated with neurologic deficit or injury, and code R53.2 should not be used for cases of neurologic quadriplegia. It should only be assigned if functional quadriplegia is specifically documented in the medical record.

g. **SIRS due to Non-Infectious Process**
The systemic inflammatory response syndrome (SIRS) can develop as a result of certain non-infectious disease processes, such as trauma, malignant neoplasm, or pancreatitis. When SIRS is documented with a noninfectious condition, and no subsequent infection is documented, the code for the underlying condition, such as an injury, should be assigned, followed by code R65.10, Systemic inflammatory response syndrome (SIRS) of non-infectious origin without acute organ dysfunction, or code R65.11, Systemic inflammatory response syndrome (SIRS) of non-infectious origin with acute organ dysfunction. If an associated acute organ dysfunction is documented, the appropriate code(s) for the specific type of organ dysfunction(s) should be assigned in addition to code R65.11. If acute organ dysfunction is documented, but it cannot be determined if the acute organ dysfunction is associated with SIRS or due to another condition (e.g., directly due to the trauma), the provider should be queried.

h. **Death NOS**
Code R99, Ill-defined and unknown cause of mortality, is only for use in the very limited circumstance when a patient who has already died is brought into an emergency department or other healthcare facility and is pronounced dead upon arrival. It does not represent the discharge disposition of death.

i. **NIHSS Stroke Scale**
The NIH stroke scale (NIHSS) codes (R29.7- -) can be used in conjunction with acute stroke codes (I63) to identify the patient's neurological status and the severity of the stroke. The stroke scale codes should be sequenced after the acute stroke diagnosis code(s).

At a minimum, report the initial score documented. If desired, a facility may choose to capture multiple stroke scale scores.

See Section I.B.14. for information concerning the medical record documentation that may be used for assignment of the NIHSS codes.

19. **Chapter 19: Injury, poisoning, and certain other consequences of external causes (S00-T88)**

a. **Application of 7th Characters in Chapter 19**

Most categories in chapter 19 have a 7th character requirement for each applicable code. Most categories in this chapter have three 7th character values (with the exception of fractures): A, initial encounter, D, subsequent encounter and S, sequela. Categories for traumatic fractures have additional 7th character values. While the patient may be seen by a new or different provider over the course of treatment for an injury, assignment of the 7th character is based on whether the patient is undergoing active treatment and not whether the provider is seeing the patient for the first time.

For complication codes, active treatment refers to treatment for the condition described by the code, even though it may be related to an earlier precipitating problem. For example, code T84.50XA, Infection and inflammatory reaction due to unspecified internal joint prosthesis, initial encounter, is used when active treatment is provided for the infection, even though the condition relates to the prosthetic device, implant or graft that was placed at a previous encounter.

7th character "A", initial encounter is used **for each encounter where** the patient is receiving active treatment for the condition.

7th character "D" subsequent encounter is used for encounters after the patient has **completed** active treatment of the condition and is receiving routine care for the condition during the healing or recovery phase.

The aftercare Z codes should not be used for aftercare for conditions such as injuries or poisonings, where 7th characters are provided to identify subsequent care. For example, for aftercare of an injury, assign the acute injury code with the 7th character "D" (subsequent encounter).

7th character "S", sequela, is for use for complications or conditions that arise as a direct result of a condition, such as scar formation after a burn. The scars are sequelae of the burn. When using 7th character "S", it is necessary to use both the injury code that precipitated the sequela and the code for the sequela itself. The "S" is added only to the injury code, not the sequela code. The 7th character "S" identifies the injury responsible for the sequela. The specific type of sequela (e.g. scar) is sequenced first, followed by the injury code.

See Section I.B.10. Sequelae, (Late Effects)

b. **Coding of Injuries**

When coding injuries, assign separate codes for each injury unless a combination code is provided, in which case the combination code is assigned. Code T07, Unspecified multiple injuries should not be assigned in the inpatient setting unless information for a more specific code is not available. Traumatic injury codes (S00-T14.9) are not to be used for normal, healing surgical wounds or to identify complications of surgical wounds.

The code for the most serious injury, as determined by the provider and the focus of treatment, is sequenced first.

1) **Superficial injuries**

Superficial injuries such as abrasions or contusions are not coded when associated with more severe injuries of the same site.

2) **Primary injury with damage to nerves/ blood vessels**

When a primary injury results in minor damage to peripheral nerves or blood vessels, the primary injury is sequenced first with additional code(s) for injuries to nerves and spinal cord (such as category S04), and/or injury to blood vessels (such as category S15). When the primary injury is to the blood vessels or nerves, that injury should be sequenced first.

c. **Coding of Traumatic Fractures**

The principles of multiple coding of injuries should be followed in coding fractures. Fractures of specified sites are coded individually by site in accordance with both the provisions within categories S02, S12, S22, S32, S42, S49, S52, S59, S62, S72, S79, S82, S89, S92 and the level of detail furnished by medical record content.

A fracture not indicated as open or closed should be coded to closed. A fracture not indicated whether displaced or not displaced should be coded to displaced.

More specific guidelines are as follows:

1) **Initial vs. Subsequent Encounter for Fractures**

Traumatic fractures are coded using the appropriate 7th character for initial encounter (A, B, C) **for each encounter where** the patient is receiving active treatment for the fracture. The appropriate 7th character for initial encounter should also be assigned for a patient who delayed seeking treatment for the fracture or nonunion.

Fractures are coded using the appropriate 7th character for subsequent care for encounters after the patient has completed active treatment of the fracture and is receiving routine care for the fracture during the healing or recovery phase.

Care for complications of surgical treatment for fracture repairs during the healing or recovery phase should be coded with the appropriate complication codes.

Care of complications of fractures, such as malunion and nonunion, should be reported with the appropriate 7th character for subsequent care with nonunion (K, M, N,) or subsequent care with malunion (P, Q, R).

Malunion/nonunion: The appropriate 7th character for initial encounter should also be assigned for a patient who delayed seeking treatment for the fracture or nonunion.

The open fracture designations in the assignment of the 7th character for fractures of the forearm, femur and lower leg, including ankle are based on the Gustilo open fracture classification. When the Gustilo classification type is not specified for an open fracture, the 7th character for open fracture type I or II should be assigned (B, E, H, M, Q).

A code from category M80, not a traumatic fracture code, should be used for any patient with known osteoporosis who suffers a fracture, even if the patient had a minor fall or trauma, if that fall or trauma would not usually break a normal, healthy bone.

See Section I.C.13. Osteoporosis.

The aftercare Z codes should not be used for aftercare for traumatic fractures. For aftercare of a traumatic fracture, assign the acute fracture code with the appropriate 7th character.

2) Multiple fractures sequencing

Multiple fractures are sequenced in accordance with the severity of the fracture.

d. Coding of Burns and Corrosions

The ICD-10-CM makes a distinction between burns and corrosions. The burn codes are for thermal burns, except sunburns, that come from a heat source, such as a fire or hot appliance. The burn codes are also for burns resulting from electricity and radiation. Corrosions are burns due to chemicals. The guidelines are the same for burns and corrosions.

Current burns (T20-T25) are classified by depth, extent and by agent (X code). Burns are classified by depth as first degree (erythema), second degree (blistering), and third degree (full-thickness involvement). Burns of the eye and internal organs (T26-T28) are classified by site, but not by degree.

1) Sequencing of burn and related condition codes

Sequence first the code that reflects the highest degree of burn when more than one burn is present.

   a. When the reason for the admission or encounter is for treatment of external multiple burns, sequence first the code that reflects the burn of the highest degree.

   b. When a patient has both internal and external burns, the circumstances of admission govern the selection of the principal diagnosis or first-listed diagnosis.

   c. When a patient is admitted for burn injuries and other related conditions such as smoke inhalation and/or respiratory failure, the circumstances of admission govern the selection of the principal or first-listed diagnosis.

2) Burns of the same local site

Classify burns of the same local site (three-character category level, T20-T28) but of different degrees to the subcategory identifying the highest degree recorded in the diagnosis.

3) Non-healing burns

Non-healing burns are coded as acute burns.

Necrosis of burned skin should be coded as a non-healed burn.

4) Infected Burn

For any documented infected burn site, use an additional code for the infection.

5) Assign separate codes for each burn site

When coding burns, assign separate codes for each burn site. Category T30, Burn and corrosion, body region unspecified is extremely vague and should rarely be used.

6) Burns and Corrosions Classified According to Extent of Body Surface Involved

Assign codes from category T31, Burns classified according to extent of body surface involved, or T32, Corrosions classified according to extent of body surface involved, when the site of the burn is not specified or when there is a need for additional data. It is advisable to use category T31 as additional coding when needed to provide data for evaluating burn mortality, such as that needed by burn units. It is also advisable to use category T31 as an additional code for reporting purposes when there is mention of a third-degree burn involving 20 percent or more of the body surface.

Categories T31 and T32 are based on the classic "rule of nines" in estimating body surface involved: head and neck are assigned nine percent, each arm nine percent, each leg 18 percent, the anterior trunk 18 percent, posterior trunk 18 percent, and genitalia one percent. Providers may change these percentage assignments where necessary to accommodate infants and children who have proportionately larger heads than adults, and patients who have large buttocks, thighs, or abdomen that involve burns.

7) Encounters for treatment of sequela of burns

Encounters for the treatment of the late effects of burns or corrosions (i.e., scars or joint contractures) should be coded with a burn or corrosion code with the 7th character "S" for sequela.

8) Sequelae with a late effect code and current burn

When appropriate, both a code for a current burn or corrosion with 7th character "A" or "D" and a burn or corrosion code with 7th character "S" may be assigned on the same record (when both a current burn and sequelae of an old burn exist). Burns and corrosions do not heal at the same rate and a current healing wound may still exist with sequela of a healed burn or corrosion.

See Section I.B.10. Sequela, (Late Effects)

9) Use of an external cause code with burns and corrosions

An external cause code should be used with burns and corrosions to identify the source and intent of the burn, as well as the place where it occurred.

e. Adverse Effects, Poisoning , Underdosing and Toxic Effects

Codes in categories T36-T65 are combination codes that include the substance that was taken as well as the intent. No additional external cause code is required for poisonings, toxic effects, adverse effects and underdosing codes.

1) Do not code directly from the Table of Drugs

Do not code directly from the Table of Drugs and Chemicals. Always refer back to the Tabular List.

2) Use as many codes as necessary to describe

Use as many codes as necessary to describe completely all drugs, medicinal or biological substances.

3) If the same code would describe the causative agent

If the same code would describe the causative agent for more than one adverse reaction, poisoning, toxic effect or underdosing, assign the code only once.

4) If two or more drugs, medicinal or biological substances

If two or more drugs, medicinal or biological substances are reported, code each individually unless a combination code is listed in the Table of Drugs and Chemicals.

5) The occurrence of drug toxicity is classified in ICD-10-CM as follows:

(a) Adverse Effect

When coding an adverse effect of a drug that has been correctly prescribed and properly administered, assign the appropriate code for the nature of the adverse effect followed by the appropriate code for the adverse effect of the drug (T36-T50). The code for the drug should have a 5th or 6th character "5" (for example T36.0X5-) Examples of the nature of an adverse effect are tachycardia, delirium, gastrointestinal hemorrhaging, vomiting, hypokalemia, hepatitis, renal failure, or respiratory failure.

(b) Poisoning

When coding a poisoning or reaction to the improper use of a medication (e.g., overdose, wrong substance given or taken in error, wrong route of administration), first assign the appropriate code from categories T36-T50. The poisoning codes have an associated intent as their 5th or 6th character (accidental, intentional self-harm, assault and undetermined). **If the intent of the poisoning is unknown or unspecified, code the intent as accidental intent. The undetermined intent is only for use if the documentation in the record specifies that the intent cannot be determined.** Use additional code(s) for all manifestations of poisonings.

If there is also a diagnosis of abuse or dependence of the substance, the abuse or dependence is assigned as an additional code.

Examples of poisoning include:

(i) Error was made in drug prescription Errors made in drug prescription or in the administration of the drug by provider, nurse, patient, or other person.

(ii) Overdose of a drug intentionally taken If an overdose of a drug was intentionally taken or administered and resulted in drug toxicity, it would be coded as a poisoning.

(iii) Nonprescribed drug taken with correctly prescribed and properly administered drug. If a nonprescribed drug or medicinal agent was taken in combination with a correctly prescribed and properly administered drug, any drug toxicity or other reaction resulting from the interaction of the two drugs would be classified as a poisoning.

(iv) Interaction of drug(s) and alcohol. When a reaction results from the interaction of a drug(s) and alcohol, this would be classified as poisoning.

See Section I.C.4. if poisoning is the result of insulin pump malfunctions.

(c) Underdosing

Underdosing refers to taking less of a medication than is prescribed by a provider or a manufacturer's instruction. For underdosing, assign the code from categories T36-T50 (fifth or sixth character "6").

Codes for underdosing should never be assigned as principal or first-listed codes. If a patient has a relapse or exacerbation of the medical condition for which the drug is prescribed because of the reduction in dose, then the medical condition itself should be coded.

Noncompliance (Z91.12-, Z91.13-) or complication of care (Y63.6-Y63.9) codes are to be used with an underdosing code to indicate intent, if known.

(d) Toxic Effects

When a harmful substance is ingested or comes in contact with a person, this is classified as a toxic effect. The toxic effect codes are in categories T51-T65.

Toxic effect codes have an associated intent: accidental, intentional self-harm, assault and undetermined.

f. Adult and child abuse, neglect and other maltreatment

Sequence first the appropriate code from categories T74.- (Adult and child abuse, neglect and other maltreatment, confirmed) or T76.- (Adult and child abuse, neglect and other maltreatment, suspected) for abuse, neglect and other maltreatment, followed by any accompanying mental health or injury code(s).

If the documentation in the medical record states abuse or neglect it is coded as confirmed (T74.-). It is coded as suspected if it is documented as suspected (T76.-).

For cases of confirmed abuse or neglect an external cause code from the assault section (X92-**Y09**) should be added to identify the cause of any physical injuries. A perpetrator code (Y07) should be added when the perpetrator of the abuse is known. For suspected cases of abuse or neglect, do not report external cause or perpetrator code.

If a suspected case of abuse, neglect or mistreatment is ruled out during an encounter code Z04.71, Encounter for examination and observation following alleged physical adult abuse, ruled out, or code Z04.72, Encounter for examination and observation following alleged child physical abuse, ruled out, should be used, not a code from T76.

If a suspected case of alleged rape or sexual abuse is ruled out during an encounter code Z04.41, Encounter for examination and observation following alleged **adult rape** or code Z04.42, Encounter for examination and observation following alleged **child** rape, should be used, not a code from T76.

See Section I.C.15. Abuse in a pregnant patient.

g. Complications of care

1) General guidelines for complications of care

(a) Documentation of complications of care

See Section I.B.16. for information on documentation of complications of care.

2) Pain due to medical devices

Pain associated with devices, implants or grafts left in a surgical site (for example painful hip prosthesis) is assigned to the appropriate code(s) found in Chapter 19, Injury, poisoning, and certain other consequences of external causes. Specific codes for pain due to medical devices are found in the T code section of the ICD-10-CM. Use additional code(s) from category G89 to identify acute or chronic pain due to presence of the device, implant or graft (G89.18 or G89.28).

3) Transplant complications

(a) Transplant complications other than kidney

Codes under category T86, Complications of transplanted organs and tissues, are for use for both complications and rejection of transplanted organs. A transplant complication code is only assigned if the complication affects the function of the transplant organ. Two codes are required to fully describe a transplant complication: the appropriate code from category T86 and a secondary code that identifies the complication.

Pre-existing conditions or conditions that develop after the transplant are not coded as complications unless they affect the function of the transplanted organs.

See I.C.21. for transplant organ removal status
See I.C.2. for malignant neoplasm associated with transplanted organ.

(b) Kidney transplant complications

Patients who have undergone kidney transplant may still have some form of chronic kidney disease (CKD) because the kidney transplant may not fully restore kidney function. Code T86.1- should be assigned for documented complications of a kidney transplant, such as transplant failure or rejection or other transplant complication. Code T86.1- should not be assigned for post kidney transplant patients who have chronic kidney (CKD) unless a transplant complication such as transplant failure or rejection is documented. If the documentation is unclear as to whether the patient has a complication of the transplant, query the provider.

Conditions that affect the function of the transplanted kidney, other than CKD, should be assigned a code from subcategory T86.1, Complications of transplanted organ, Kidney, and a secondary code that identifies the complication.

For patients with CKD following a kidney transplant, but who do not have a complication such as failure or rejection, *see section I.C.14. Chronic kidney disease and kidney transplant status.*

4) Complication codes that include the external cause

As with certain other T codes, some of the complications of care codes have the external cause included in the code. The code includes the nature of the complication as well as the type of procedure that caused the complication. No external cause code indicating the type of procedure is necessary for these codes.

5) Complications of care codes within the body system chapters

Intraoperative and postprocedural complication codes are found within the body system chapters with codes specific to the organs and structures of that body system. These codes should be sequenced first, followed by a code(s) for the specific complication, if applicable.

20. Chapter 20: External Causes of Morbidity (V00-Y99)

The external causes of morbidity codes should never be sequenced as the first-listed or principal diagnosis.

External cause codes are intended to provide data for injury research and evaluation of injury prevention strategies. These codes capture how the injury or health condition happened (cause), the intent (unintentional or accidental; or intentional, such as suicide or assault), the place where the event occurred the activity of the patient at the time of the event, and the person's status (e.g., civilian, military).

There is no national requirement for mandatory ICD-10-CM external cause code reporting. Unless a provider is subject to a state-based external cause code reporting mandate or these codes are required by a particular payer, reporting of ICD-10-CM codes in Chapter 20, External Causes of Morbidity, is not required. In the absence of a mandatory reporting requirement, providers are encouraged to voluntarily report external cause codes, as they provide valuable data for injury research and evaluation of injury prevention strategies.

a. General External Cause Coding Guidelines

1) Used with any code in the range of A00.0-T88.9, Z00-Z99

An external cause code may be used with any code in the range of A00.0-T88.9, Z00-Z99, classification that is a health condition due to an external cause. Though they are most applicable to injuries, they are also valid for use with such things as infections or diseases due to an external source, and other health conditions, such as a heart attack that occurs during strenuous physical activity.

2) External cause code used for length of treatment

Assign the external cause code, with the appropriate 7th character (initial encounter, subsequent encounter or sequela) for each encounter for which the injury or condition is being treated.

Most categories in chapter 20 have a 7th character requirement for each applicable code. Most categories in this chapter have three 7th character values: A, initial encounter, D, subsequent encounter and S, sequela. While the patient may be seen by a new or different provider over the course of treatment for an injury or condition, assignment of the 7th character for external cause should match the 7th character of the code assigned for the associated injury or condition for the encounter.

3) Use the full range of external cause codes

Use the full range of external cause codes to completely describe the cause, the intent, the place of occurrence and if applicable, the activity of the patient at the time of the event, and the patient's status, for all injuries, and other health conditions due to an external cause.

4) Assign as many external cause codes as necessary

Assign as many external cause codes as necessary to fully explain each cause. If only one external code can be recorded, assign the code most related to the principal diagnosis.

5) The selection of the appropriate external cause code

The selection of the appropriate external cause code is guided by the Alphabetic Index of External Causes and by Inclusion and Exclusion notes in the Tabular List.

6) External cause code can never be a principal diagnosis

An external cause code can never be a principal (first-listed) diagnosis.

7) Combination external cause codes

Certain of the external cause codes are combination codes that identify sequential events that result in an injury, such as a fall which results in striking against an object. The injury may be due to either event or both. The combination external cause code used should correspond to the sequence of events regardless of which caused the most serious injury.

8) No external cause code needed in certain circumstances

No external cause code from Chapter 20 is needed if the external cause and intent are included in a code from another chapter (e.g. T36.0X1- Poisoning by penicillins, accidental (unintentional)).

b. Place of Occurrence Guideline

Codes from category Y92, Place of occurrence of the external cause, are secondary codes for use after other external cause codes to identify the location of the patient at the time of injury or other condition.

Generally, a place of occurrence code is assigned only once, at the initial encounter for treatment. However, in the rare instance that a new injury occurs during hospitalization, an additional place of occurrence code may be assigned. No 7th characters are used for Y92. Only one code from Y92 should be recorded on a medical record.

Do not use place of occurrence code Y92.9 if the place is not stated or is not applicable.

c. Activity Code

Assign a code from category Y93, Activity code, to describe the activity of the patient at the time the injury or other health condition occurred.

An activity code is used only once, at the initial encounter for treatment. Only one code from Y93 should be recorded on a medical record.

The activity codes are not applicable to poisonings, adverse effects, misadventures or sequela.

Do not assign Y93.9, Unspecified activity, if the activity is not stated.

A code from category Y93 is appropriate for use with external cause and intent codes if identifying the activity provides additional information about the event.

d. Place of Occurrence, Activity, and Status Codes Used with other External Cause Code

When applicable, place of occurrence, activity, and external cause status codes are sequenced after the main external cause code(s). Regardless of the number of external cause codes assigned, there should be only one place of occurrence code, one activity code, and one external cause status code assigned to an encounter.

GUIDELINES (ICD-10-CM)

e. If the Reporting Format Limits the Number of External Cause Codes

If the reporting format limits the number of external cause codes that can be used in reporting clinical data, report the code for the cause/intent most related to the principal diagnosis. If the format permits capture of additional external cause codes, the cause/intent, including medical misadventures, of the additional events should be reported rather than the codes for place, activity, or external status.

f. Multiple External Cause Coding Guidelines

More than one external cause code is required to fully describe the external cause of an illness or injury. The assignment of external cause codes should be sequenced in the following priority:

If two or more events cause separate injuries, an external cause code should be assigned for each cause. The first-listed external cause code will be selected in the following order:

External codes for child and adult abuse take priority over all other external cause codes.

See Section I.C.19., Child and Adult abuse guidelines.

External codes for terrorism events take priority over all other external cause codes except child and adult abuse.

External cause codes for cataclysmic events take priority over all other external cause codes except child and adult abuse and terrorism.

External cause codes for transport accidents take priority over all other external cause codes except cataclysmic events, child and adult abuse and terrorism.

Activity and external cause status codes are assigned following all causal (intent) external cause codes.

The first-listed external cause code should correspond to the cause of the most serious diagnosis due to an assault, accident, or self-harm, following the order of hierarchy listed above.

g. Child and Adult Abuse Guideline

Adult and child abuse, neglect and maltreatment are classified as assault. Any of the assault codes may be used to indicate the external cause of any injury resulting from the confirmed abuse.

For confirmed cases of abuse, neglect and maltreatment, when the perpetrator is known, a code from Y07, Perpetrator of maltreatment and neglect, should accompany any other assault codes.

See Section I.C.19. Adult and child abuse, neglect and other maltreatment

h. Unknown or Undetermined Intent Guideline

If the intent (accident, self-harm, assault) of the cause of an injury or other condition is unknown or unspecified, code the intent as accidental intent. All transport accident categories assume accidental intent.

1) Use of undetermined intent

External cause codes for events of undetermined intent are only for use if the documentation in the record specifies that the intent cannot be determined.

i. Sequelae (Late Effects) of External Cause Guidelines

1) Sequelae external cause codes

Sequela are reported using the external cause code with the 7th character "S" for sequela. These codes should be used with any report of a late effect or sequela resulting from a previous injury.

See Section I.B.10. Sequela, (Late Effects)

2) Sequela external cause code with a related current injury

A sequela external cause code should never be used with a related current nature of injury code.

3) Use of sequela external cause codes for subsequent visits

Use a late effect external cause code for subsequent visits when a late effect of the initial injury is being treated. Do not use a late effect external cause code for subsequent visits for follow-up care (e.g., to assess healing, to receive rehabilitative therapy) of the injury when no late effect of the injury has been documented.

j. Terrorism Guidelines

1) Cause of injury identified by the Federal Government (FBI) as terrorism

When the cause of an injury is identified by the Federal Government (FBI) as terrorism, the first-listed external cause code should be a code from category Y38, Terrorism. The definition of terrorism employed by the FBI is found at the inclusion note at the beginning of category Y38. Use additional code for place of occurrence (Y92.-). More than one Y38 code may be assigned if the injury is the result of more than one mechanism of terrorism.

2) Cause of an injury is suspected to be the result of terrorism

When the cause of an injury is suspected to be the result of terrorism a code from category Y38 should not be assigned. Suspected cases should be classified as assault.

3) Code Y38.9, Terrorism, secondary effects

Assign code Y38.9, Terrorism, secondary effects, for conditions occurring subsequent to the terrorist event. This code should not be assigned for conditions that are due to the initial terrorist act.

It is acceptable to assign code Y38.9 with another code from Y38 if there is an injury due to the initial terrorist event and an injury that is a subsequent result of the terrorist event.

k. External cause status

A code from category Y99, External cause status, should be assigned whenever any other external cause code is assigned for an encounter, including an Activity code, except for the events noted below. Assign a code from category Y99, External cause status, to indicate the work status of the person at the time the event occurred. The status code indicates whether the event occurred during military activity, whether a non-military person was at work, whether an individual including a student or volunteer was involved in a non-work activity at the time of the causal event.

A code from Y99, External cause status, should be assigned, when applicable, with other external cause codes, such as transport accidents and falls. The external cause status codes are not applicable to poisonings, adverse effects, misadventures or late effects.

Do not assign a code from category Y99 if no other external cause codes (cause, activity) are applicable for the encounter.

An external cause status code is used only once, at the initial encounter for treatment. Only one code from Y99 should be recorded on a medical record.

Do not assign code Y99.9, Unspecified external cause status, if the status is not stated.

21. **Chapter 21: Factors influencing health status and contact with health services (Z00-Z99)**
    Note: The chapter specific guidelines provide additional information about the use of Z codes for specified encounters.

    a. Use of Z codes in any healthcare setting
    Z codes are for use in any healthcare setting. Z codes may be used as either a first-listed (principal diagnosis code in the inpatient setting) or secondary code, depending on the circumstances of the encounter. Certain Z codes may only be used as first-listed or principal diagnosis.

    b. Z Codes indicate a reason for an encounter
    Z codes are not procedure codes. A corresponding procedure code must accompany a Z code to describe any procedure performed.

    c. Categories of Z Codes
    1) Contact/Exposure
    Category Z20 indicates contact with, and suspected exposure to, communicable diseases. These codes are for patients who do not show any sign or symptom of a disease but are suspected to have been exposed to it by close personal contact with an infected individual or are in an area where a disease is epidemic.

    Category Z77, Other contact with and (suspected) exposures hazardous to health, indicates contact with and suspected exposures hazardous to health.

    Contact/exposure codes may be used as a first-listed code to explain an encounter for testing, or, more commonly, as a secondary code to identify a potential risk.

    2) Inoculations and vaccinations
    Code Z23 is for encounters for inoculations and vaccinations. It indicates that a patient is being seen to receive a prophylactic inoculation against a disease. Procedure codes are required to identify the actual administration of the injection and the type(s) of immunizations given. Code Z23 may be used as a secondary code if the inoculation is given as a routine part of preventive health care, such as a well-baby visit.

    3) Status
    Status codes indicate that a patient is either a carrier of a disease or has the sequelae or residual of a past disease or condition. This includes such things as the presence of prosthetic or mechanical devices resulting from past treatment. A status code is informative, because the status may affect the course of treatment and its outcome. A status code is distinct from a history code. The history code indicates that the patient no longer has the condition.

    A status code should not be used with a diagnosis code from one of the body system chapters, if the diagnosis code includes the information provided by the status code. For example, code Z94.1, Heart transplant status, should not be used with a code from subcategory T86.2, Complications of heart transplant. The status code does not provide additional information. The complication code indicates that the patient is a heart transplant patient.

    For encounters for weaning from a mechanical ventilator, assign a code from subcategory J96.1, Chronic respiratory failure, followed by code Z99.11, Dependence on respirator [ventilator] status.

    The status Z codes/categories are:
    Z14   Genetic carrier
    Genetic carrier status indicates that a person carries a gene, associated with a particular disease, which may be passed to offspring who may develop that disease. The person does not have the disease and is not at risk of developing the disease.
    Z15   Genetic susceptibility to disease Genetic susceptibility indicates that a person has a gene that increases the risk of that person developing the disease.

    Codes from category Z15 should not be used as principal or first-listed codes. If the patient has the condition to which he/she is susceptible, and that condition is the reason for the encounter, the code for the current condition should be sequenced first. If the patient is being seen for follow-up after completed treatment for this condition, and the condition no longer exists, a follow-up code should be sequenced first, followed by the appropriate personal history and genetic susceptibility codes. If the purpose of the encounter is genetic counseling associated with procreative management, code Z31.5, Encounter for genetic counseling, should be assigned as the first-listed code, followed by a code from category Z15. Additional codes should be assigned for any applicable family or personal history.
    Z16   Resistance to antimicrobial drugs
    This code indicates that a patient has a condition that is resistant to antimicrobial drug treatment. Sequence the infection code first.

Z17 Estrogen receptor status
Z18 Retained foreign body fragments
Z19 Hormone sensitivity malignancy status
Z21 Asymptomatic HIV infection status This code indicates that a patient has tested positive for HIV but has manifested no signs or symptoms of the disease.
Z22 Carrier of infectious disease Carrier status indicates that a person harbors the specific organisms of a disease without manifest symptoms and is capable of transmitting the infection.
Z28.3 Underimmunization status
Z33.1 Pregnant state, incidental This code is a secondary code only for use when the pregnancy is in no way complicating the reason for visit. Otherwise, a code from the obstetric chapter is required.
Z66 Do not resuscitate

This code may be used when it is documented by the provider that a patient is on do not resuscitate status at any time during the stay.

Z67 Blood type
Z68 Body mass index (BMI)
As with all other secondary diagnosis codes, the BMI codes should only be assigned when they meet the definition of a reportable diagnosis (see Section III, Reporting Additional Diagnoses).
Z74.01 Bed confinement status
Z76.82 Awaiting organ transplant status
Z78 Other specified health status

Code Z78.1, Physical restraint status, may be used when it is documented by the provider that a patient has been put in restraints during the current encounter. Please note that this code should not be reported when it is documented by the provider that a patient is temporarily restrained during a procedure.

Z79 Long-term (current) drug therapy

Codes from this category indicate a patient's continuous use of a prescribed drug (including such things as aspirin therapy) for the long-term treatment of a condition or for prophylactic use. It is not for use for patients who have addictions to drugs. This subcategory is not for use of medications for detoxification or maintenance programs to prevent withdrawal symptoms in patients with drug dependence (e.g., methadone maintenance for opiate dependence). Assign the appropriate code for the drug dependence instead.

Assign a code from Z79 if the patient is receiving a medication for an extended period as a prophylactic measure (such as for the prevention of deep vein thrombosis) or as treatment of a chronic condition (such as arthritis) or a disease requiring a lengthy course of treatment (such as cancer). Do not assign a code from category Z79 for medication being administered for a brief period of time to treat an acute illness or injury (such as a course of antibiotics to treat acute bronchitis).

Z88 Allergy status to drugs, medicaments and biological substances Except: Z88.9, Allergy status to unspecified drugs, medicaments and biological substances status
Z89 Acquired absence of limb
Z90 Acquired absence of organs, not elsewhere classified
Z91.0- Allergy status, other than to drugs and biological substances
Z92.82 Status post administration of tPA (rtPA) in a different facility within the last 24 hours prior to admission to a current facility Assign code Z92.82, Status post administration of tPA (rtPA) in a different facility within the last 24 hours prior to admission to current facility, as a secondary diagnosis when a patient is received by transfer into a facility and documentation indicates they were administered tissue plasminogen activator (tPA) within the last 24 hours prior to admission to the current facility. This guideline applies even if the patient is still receiving the tPA at the time they are received into the current facility. The appropriate code for the condition for which the tPA was administered (such as cerebrovascular disease or myocardial infarction) should be assigned first. Code Z92.82 is only applicable to the receiving facility record and not to the transferring facility record.
Z93 Artificial opening status
Z94 Transplanted organ and tissue status
Z95 Presence of cardiac and vascular implants and grafts
Z96 Presence of other functional implants
Z97 Presence of other devices
Z98 Other postprocedural states

Assign code Z98.85, Transplanted organ removal status, to indicate that a transplanted organ has been previously removed. This code should not be assigned for the encounter in which the transplanted organ is removed. The complication necessitating removal of the transplant organ should be assigned for that encounter.

See section I.C.19. for information on the coding of organ transplant complications.

Z99 Dependence on enabling machines and devices, not elsewhere classified

Note: Categories Z89-Z90 and Z93-Z99 are for use only if there are no complications or malfunctions of the organ or tissue replaced, the amputation site or the equipment on which the patient is dependent.

4) History (of)
There are two types of history Z codes, personal and family. Personal history codes explain a

patient's past medical condition that no longer exists and is not receiving any treatment, but that has the potential for recurrence, and therefore may require continued monitoring.

Family history codes are for use when a patient has a family member(s) who has had a particular disease that causes the patient to be at higher risk of also contracting the disease.

Personal history codes may be used in conjunction with follow-up codes and family history codes may be used in conjunction with screening codes to explain the need for a test or procedure. History codes are also acceptable on any medical record regardless of the reason for visit. A history of an illness, even if no longer present, is important information that may alter the type of treatment ordered.

The history Z code categories are:

Z80	Family history of primary malignant neoplasm
Z81	Family history of mental and behavioral disorders
Z82	Family history of certain disabilities and chronic diseases (leading to disablement)
Z83	Family history of other specific disorders
Z84	Family history of other conditions
Z85	Personal history of malignant neoplasm
Z86	Personal history of certain other diseases
Z87	Personal history of other diseases and conditions
Z91.4-	Personal history of psychological trauma, not elsewhere classified
Z91.5	Personal history of self-harm
Z91.8-	Other specified personal risk factors, not elsewhere classified Exception: Z91.83, Wandering in diseases classified elsewhere
Z92	Personal history of medical treatment Except: Z92.0, Personal history of contraception Except: Z92.82, Status post administration of tPA (rtPA) in a different facility within the last 24 hours prior to admission to a current facility

5) Screening

Screening is the testing for disease or disease precursors in seemingly well individuals so that early detection and treatment can be provided for those who test positive for the disease (e.g., screening mammogram).

The testing of a person to rule out or confirm a suspected diagnosis because the patient has some sign or symptom is a diagnostic examination, not a screening. In these cases, the sign or symptom is used to explain the reason for the test.

A screening code may be a first-listed code if the reason for the visit is specifically the screening exam. It may also be used as an additional code if the screening is done during an office visit for other health problems. A screening code is not necessary if the screening is inherent to a routine examination, such as a pap smear done during a routine pelvic examination.

Should a condition be discovered during the screening then the code for the condition may be assigned as an additional diagnosis.

The Z code indicates that a screening exam is planned. A procedure code is required to confirm that the screening was performed.

The screening Z codes/categories:

Z11	Encounter for screening for infectious and parasitic diseases
Z12	Encounter for screening for malignant neoplasms
Z13	Encounter for screening for other diseases and disorders Except: Z13.9, Encounter for screening, unspecified
Z36	Encounter for antenatal screening for mother

6) Observation

There are **three** observation Z code categories. They are for use in very limited circumstances when a person is being observed for a suspected condition that is ruled out. The observation codes are not for use if an injury or illness or any signs or symptoms related to the suspected condition are present. In such cases the diagnosis/symptom code is used with the corresponding external cause code.

The observation codes are to be used as principal diagnosis only. **The only exception to this is when the principal diagnosis is required to be a code from category Z38, Liveborn infants according to place of birth and type of delivery. Then a code from category Z05, Encounter for observation and evaluation of newborn for suspected diseases and conditions ruled out, is sequenced after the Z38 code.** Additional codes may be used in addition to the observation code, but only if they are unrelated to the suspected condition being observed.

Codes from subcategory Z03.7 Encounter for suspected maternal and fetal conditions ruled out, may either be used as a first-listed or as an additional code assignment depending on the case. They are for use in very limited circumstances on a maternal record when an encounter is for a suspected maternal or fetal condition that is ruled out during that encounter (for example, a maternal or fetal condition may be suspected due to an abnormal test result). These codes should not be used when the condition is confirmed. In those cases, the confirmed condition should be coded. In addition, these codes are not for use if an illness or any signs or symptoms related to the suspected condition or problem are present. In such cases the diagnosis/symptom code is used.

GUIDELINES (ICD-10-CM)

Additional codes may be used in addition to the code from subcategory Z03.7, but only if they are unrelated to the suspected condition being evaluated.

Codes from subcategory Z03.7 may not be used for encounters for antenatal screening of mother. *See Section I.C.21. Screening.*

For encounters for suspected fetal condition that are inconclusive following testing and evaluation, assign the appropriate code from category O35, O36, O40 or O41.

The observation Z code categories:

Z03 Encounter for medical observation for suspected diseases and conditions ruled out

Z04 Encounter for examination and observation for other reasons Except: Z04.9, Encounter for examination and observation for unspecified reason

Z05 Encounter for observation and evaluation of newborn for suspected diseases and conditions ruled out

7) Aftercare

Aftercare visit codes cover situations when the initial treatment of a disease has been performed and the patient requires continued care during the healing or recovery phase, or for the long-term consequences of the disease. The aftercare Z code should not be used if treatment is directed at a current, acute disease. The diagnosis code is to be used in these cases.

Exceptions to this rule are codes Z51.0, Encounter for antineoplastic radiation therapy, and codes from subcategory Z51.1, Encounter for antineoplastic chemotherapy and immunotherapy. These codes are to be first-listed, followed by the diagnosis code when a patient's encounter is solely to receive radiation therapy, chemotherapy, or immunotherapy for the treatment of a neoplasm. If the reason for the encounter is more than one type of antineoplastic therapy, code Z51.0 and a code from subcategory Z51.1 may be assigned together, in which case one of these codes would be reported as a secondary diagnosis.

The aftercare Z codes should also not be used for aftercare for injuries. For aftercare of an injury, assign the acute injury code with the appropriate 7th character (for subsequent encounter).

The aftercare codes are generally first-listed to explain the specific reason for the encounter. An aftercare code may be used as an additional code when some type of aftercare is provided in addition to the reason for admission and no diagnosis code is applicable. An example of this would be the closure of a colostomy during an encounter for treatment of another condition.

Aftercare codes should be used in conjunction with other aftercare codes or diagnosis codes to provide better detail on the specifics of an aftercare encounter visit, unless otherwise directed by the classification. Should a patient receive multiple types of antineoplastic therapy during the same encounter, code Z51.0, Encounter for antineoplastic radiation therapy, and codes from subcategory Z51.1, Encounter for antineoplastic chemotherapy and immunotherapy, may be used together on a record. The sequencing of multiple aftercare codes depends on the circumstances of the encounter.

Certain aftercare Z code categories need a secondary diagnosis code to describe the resolving condition or sequelae. For others, the condition is included in the code title.

Additional Z code aftercare category terms include fitting and adjustment, and attention to artificial openings.

Status Z codes may be used with aftercare Z codes to indicate the nature of the aftercare. For example code Z95.1, Presence of aortocoronary bypass graft, may be used with code Z48.812, Encounter for surgical aftercare following surgery on the circulatory system, to indicate the surgery for which the aftercare is being performed. A status code should not be used when the aftercare code indicates the type of status, such as using Z43.0, Encounter for attention to tracheostomy, with Z93.0, Tracheostomy status.

The aftercare Z category/codes:

Z42 Encounter for plastic and reconstructive surgery following medical procedure or healed injury

Z43 Encounter for attention to artificial openings

Z44 Encounter for fitting and adjustment of external prosthetic device

Z45 Encounter for adjustment and management of implanted device

Z46 Encounter for fitting and adjustment of other devices

Z47 Orthopedic aftercare

Z48 Encounter for other postprocedural aftercare

Z49 Encounter for care involving renal dialysis

Z51 Encounter for other aftercare **and medical care**

8) Follow-up

The follow-up codes are used to explain continuing surveillance following completed treatment of a disease, condition, or injury. They imply that the condition has been fully treated and no longer exists. They should not be confused with aftercare codes, or injury codes with a 7th character for subsequent encounter, that explain ongoing care of a healing condition or its sequelae. Follow-up codes may be used in conjunction with history codes to provide the full picture of the healed condition and its treatment. The follow-up code is sequenced first, followed by the history code.

A follow-up code may be used to explain multiple visits. Should a condition be found to have recurred on the follow-up visit, then the diagnosis code for the condition should be assigned in place of the follow-up code.

The follow-up Z code categories:

Z08   Encounter for follow-up examination after completed treatment for malignant neoplasm

Z09   Encounter for follow-up examination after completed treatment for conditions other than malignant neoplasm

Z39   Encounter for maternal postpartum care and examination

9) Donor

Codes in category Z52, Donors of organs and tissues, are used for living individuals who are donating blood or other body tissue. These codes are only for individuals donating for others, not for self-donations. They are not used to identify cadaveric donations.

10) Counseling

Counseling Z codes are used when a patient or family member receives assistance in the aftermath of an illness or injury, or when support is required in coping with family or social problems. They are not used in conjunction with a diagnosis code when the counseling component of care is considered integral to standard treatment.

The counseling Z codes/categories:

Z30.0-   Encounter for general counseling and advice on contraception

Z31.5   Encounter for genetic counseling

Z31.6-   Encounter for general counseling and advice on procreation

Z32.2   Encounter for childbirth instruction

Z32.3   Encounter for childcare instruction

Z69   Encounter for mental health services for victim and perpetrator of abuse

Z70   Counseling related to sexual attitude, behavior and orientation

Z71   Persons encountering health services for other counseling and medical advice, not elsewhere classified

Z76.81   Expectant mother prebirth pediatrician visit

11) Encounters for Obstetrical and Reproductive Services

See Section I.C.15. Pregnancy, Childbirth, and the Puerperium, for further instruction on the use of these codes.

Z codes for pregnancy are for use in those circumstances when none of the problems or complications included in the codes from the Obstetrics chapter exist (a routine prenatal visit or postpartum care). Codes in category Z34, Encounter for supervision of normal pregnancy, are always first listed and are not to be used with any other code from the OB chapter.

Codes in category Z3A, Weeks of gestation, may be assigned to provide additional information about the pregnancy. **Category Z3A codes should not be assigned for pregnancies with abortive outcomes (categories O00-O08), elective termination of pregnancy (code Z33.32), nor for postpartum conditions, as category Z3A is not applicable to**

these conditions. The date of the admission should be used to determine weeks of gestation for inpatient admissions that encompass more than one gestational week.

The outcome of delivery, category Z37, should be included on all maternal delivery records. It is always a secondary code. Codes in category Z37 should not be used on the newborn record.

Z codes for family planning (contraceptive) or procreative management and counseling should be included on an obstetric record either during the pregnancy or the postpartum stage, if applicable.

Z codes/categories for obstetrical and reproductive services:

Z30   Encounter for contraceptive management

Z31   Encounter for procreative management

Z32.2   Encounter for childbirth instruction

Z32.3   Encounter for childcare instruction

Z33   Pregnant state

Z34   Encounter for supervision of normal pregnancy

Z36   Encounter for antenatal screening of mother

Z3A   Weeks of gestation

Z37   Outcome of delivery

Z39   Encounter for maternal postpartum care and examination

Z76.81   Expectant mother prebirth pediatrician visit

12) Newborns and Infants

See Section I.C.16. Newborn (Perinatal) Guidelines, for further instruction on the use of these codes.

Newborn Z codes/categories:

Z76.1   Encounter for health supervision and care of foundling

Z00.1-   Encounter for routine child health examination

Z38   Liveborn infants according to place of birth and type of delivery

13) Routine and administrative examinations

The Z codes allow for the description of encounters for routine examinations, such as, a general check-up, or, examinations for administrative purposes, such as, a pre-employment physical. The codes are not to be used if the examination is for diagnosis of a suspected condition or for treatment purposes. In such cases the diagnosis code is used. During a routine exam, should a diagnosis or condition be discovered, it should be coded as an additional code. Pre-existing and chronic conditions and history codes may also be included as additional codes as long as the examination is for administrative purposes and not focused on any particular condition.

Some of the codes for routine health examinations distinguish between "with" and "without" abnormal findings. Code assignment depends on the information that is known at the time the encounter is being coded. For example, if no abnormal findings were found during the examination, but the encounter is being coded before test results are back, it is acceptable to assign the code for "without abnormal findings." When assigning a code for "with abnormal findings," additional code(s) should be assigned to identify the specific abnormal finding(s).

Pre-operative examination and pre-procedural laboratory examination Z codes are for use only in those situations when a patient is being cleared for a procedure or surgery and no treatment is given.

The Z codes/categories for routine and administrative examinations:

Z00	Encounter for general examination without complaint, suspected or reported diagnosis
Z01	Encounter for other special examination without complaint, suspected or reported diagnosis
Z02	Encounter for administrative examination Except: Z02.9, Encounter for administrative examinations, unspecified
Z32.0-	Encounter for pregnancy test

14) Miscellaneous Z codes

The miscellaneous Z codes capture a number of other health care encounters that do not fall into one of the other categories. Certain of these codes identify the reason for the encounter; others are for use as additional codes that provide useful information on circumstances that may affect a patient's care and treatment.

Prophylactic Organ Removal

For encounters specifically for prophylactic removal of an organ (such as prophylactic removal of breasts due to a genetic susceptibility to cancer or a family history of cancer), the principal or first-listed code should be a code from category Z40, Encounter for prophylactic surgery, followed by the appropriate codes to identify the associated risk factor (such as genetic susceptibility or family history).

If the patient has a malignancy of one site and is having prophylactic removal at another site to prevent either a new primary malignancy or metastatic disease, a code for the malignancy should also be assigned in addition to a code from subcategory Z40.0, Encounter for prophylactic surgery for risk factors related to malignant neoplasms. A Z40.0 code should not be assigned if the patient is having organ removal for treatment of a malignancy, such as the removal of the testes for the treatment of prostate cancer.

Miscellaneous Z codes/categories:

Z28	Immunization not carried out Except: Z28.3, Underimmunization status
Z29	**Encounter for other prophylactic measures**
Z40	Encounter for prophylactic surgery
Z41	Encounter for procedures for purposes other than remedying health state Except: Z41.9, Encounter for procedure for purposes other than remedying health state, unspecified

Z53	Persons encountering health services for specific procedures and treatment, not carried out
Z55	Problems related to education and literacy
Z56	Problems related to employment and unemployment
Z57	Occupational exposure to risk factors
Z58	Problems related to physical environment
Z59	Problems related to housing and economic circumstances
Z60	Problems related to social environment
Z62	Problems related to upbringing
Z63	Other problems related to primary support group, including family circumstances
Z64	Problems related to certain psychosocial circumstances
Z65	Problems related to other psychosocial circumstances
Z72	Problems related to lifestyle **Note: These codes should be assigned only when the documentation specifies that the patient has an associated problem**
Z73	Problems related to life management difficulty
Z74	Problems related to care provider dependency Except: Z74.01, Bed confinement status
Z75	Problems related to medical facilities and other health care
Z76.0	Encounter for issue of repeat prescription
Z76.3	Healthy person accompanying sick person
Z76.4	Other boarder to healthcare facility
Z76.5	Malingerer [conscious simulation]
Z91.1-	Patient's noncompliance with medical treatment and regimen
Z91.83	Wandering in diseases classified elsewhere
Z91.89	Other specified personal risk factors, not elsewhere classified

15) Nonspecific Z codes

Certain Z codes are so non-specific, or potentially redundant with other codes in the classification, that there can be little justification for their use in the inpatient setting. Their use in the outpatient setting should be limited to those instances when there is no further documentation to permit more precise coding. Otherwise, any sign or symptom or any other reason for visit that is captured in another code should be used.

Nonspecific Z codes/categories:

Z02.9	Encounter for administrative examinations, unspecified
Z04.9	Encounter for examination and observation for unspecified reason
Z13.9	Encounter for screening, unspecified

Z41.9   Encounter for procedure for purposes other than remedying health state, unspecified

Z52.9   Donor of unspecified organ or tissue

Z86.59   Personal history of other mental and behavioral disorders

Z88.9   Allergy status to unspecified drugs, medicaments and biological substances status

Z92.0   Personal history of contraception

16) Z Codes That May Only be Principal/First-Listed Diagnosis

The following Z codes/categories may only be reported as the principal/first-listed diagnosis, except when there are multiple encounters on the same day and the medical records for the encounters are combined:

Z00   Encounter for general examination without complaint, suspected or reported diagnosis
         Except: Z00.6

Z01   Encounter for other special examination without complaint, suspected or reported diagnosis

Z02   Encounter for administrative examination

Z03   Encounter for medical observation for suspected diseases and conditions ruled out

Z04   Encounter for examination and observation for other reasons

Z33.2   Encounter for elective termination of pregnancy

Z31.81   Encounter for male factor infertility in female patient

Z31.83   Encounter for assisted reproductive fertility procedure cycle

Z31.84   Encounter for fertility preservation procedure

Z34   Encounter for supervision of normal pregnancy

Z39   Encounter for maternal postpartum care and examination

Z38   Liveborn infants according to place of birth and type of delivery

Z42   Encounter for plastic and reconstructive surgery following medical procedure or healed injury

Z51.0   Encounter for antineoplastic radiation therapy

Z51.1-   Encounter for antineoplastic chemotherapy and immunotherapy

Z52   Donors of organs and tissues Except: Z52.9, Donor of unspecified organ or tissue

Z76.1   Encounter for health supervision and care of foundling

Z76.2   Encounter for health supervision and care of other healthy infant and child

Z99.12   Encounter for respirator [ventilator] dependence during power failure

Section II. Selection of Principal Diagnosis

The circumstances of inpatient admission always govern the selection of principal diagnosis. The principal diagnosis is defined in the Uniform Hospital Discharge Data Set (UHDDS) as "that condition established after study to be chiefly responsible for occasioning the admission of the patient to the hospital for care."

The UHDDS definitions are used by hospitals to report inpatient data elements in a standardized manner. These data elements and their definitions can be found in the July 31, 1985, Federal Register (Vol. 50, No, 147), pp. 31038-40.

Since that time the application of the UHDDS definitions has been expanded to include all nonoutpatient settings (acute care, short term, long term care and psychiatric hospitals; home health agencies; rehab facilities; nursing homes, etc). **The UHDDS definitions also apply to hospice services (all levels of care).**

In determining principal diagnosis, coding conventions in the ICD-10-CM, the Tabular List and Alphabetic Index take precedence over these official coding guidelines.

(See Section I.A., Conventions for the ICD-10-CM)

The importance of consistent, complete documentation in the medical record cannot be overemphasized. Without such documentation the application of all coding guidelines is a difficult, if not impossible, task.

A. **Codes for symptoms, signs, and ill-defined conditions**

Codes for symptoms, signs, and ill-defined conditions from Chapter 18 are not to be used as principal diagnosis when a related definitive diagnosis has been established.

B. **Two or more interrelated conditions, each potentially meeting the definition for principal diagnosis.**

When there are two or more interrelated conditions (such as diseases in the same ICD-10-CM chapter or manifestations characteristically associated with a certain disease) potentially meeting the definition of principal diagnosis, either condition may be sequenced first, unless the circumstances of the admission, the therapy provided, the Tabular List, or the Alphabetic Index indicate otherwise.

C. **Two or more diagnoses that equally meet the definition for principal diagnosis**

In the unusual instance when two or more diagnoses equally meet the criteria for principal diagnosis as determined by the circumstances of admission, diagnostic workup and/or therapy provided, and the Alphabetic Index, Tabular List, or another coding guidelines does not provide sequencing direction, any one of the diagnoses may be sequenced first.

D. **Two or more comparative or contrasting conditions.**

In those rare instances when two or more contrasting or comparative diagnoses are documented as "either/or" (or similar terminology), they are coded as if the diagnoses were confirmed and the diagnoses are sequenced according to the circumstances of the admission. If no further determination can be made as to which diagnosis should be principal, either diagnosis may be sequenced first.

E. A symptom(s) followed by contrasting/ comparative diagnoses
GUIDELINE HAS BEEN DELETED EFFECTIVE OCTOBER 1, 2014

F. Original treatment plan not carried out
Sequence as the principal diagnosis the condition, which after study occasioned the admission to the hospital, even though treatment may not have been carried out due to unforeseen circumstances.

G. Complications of surgery and other medical care
When the admission is for treatment of a complication resulting from surgery or other medical care, the complication code is sequenced as the principal diagnosis. If the complication is classified to the T80-T88 series and the code lacks the necessary specificity in describing the complication, an additional code for the specific complication should be assigned.

H. Uncertain Diagnosis
If the diagnosis documented at the time of discharge is qualified as "probable", "suspected", "likely", "questionable", "possible", or "still to be ruled out", or other similar terms indicating uncertainty, code the condition as if it existed or was established. The bases for these guidelines are the diagnostic workup, arrangements for further workup or observation, and initial therapeutic approach that correspond most closely with the established diagnosis.

Note: This guideline is applicable only to inpatient admissions to short-term, acute, long-term care and psychiatric hospitals.

I. Admission from Observation Unit

1. Admission Following Medical Observation
When a patient is admitted to an observation unit for a medical condition, which either worsens or does not improve, and is subsequently admitted as an inpatient of the same hospital for this same medical condition, the principal diagnosis would be the medical condition which led to the hospital admission.

2. Admission Following Post-Operative Observation
When a patient is admitted to an observation unit to monitor a condition (or complication) that develops following outpatient surgery, and then is subsequently admitted as an inpatient of the same hospital, hospitals should apply the Uniform Hospital Discharge Data Set (UHDDS) definition of principal diagnosis as "that condition established after study to be chiefly responsible for occasioning the admission of the patient to the hospital for care."

J. Admission from Outpatient Surgery
When a patient receives surgery in the hospital's outpatient surgery department and is subsequently admitted for continuing inpatient care at the same hospital, the following guidelines should be followed in selecting the principal diagnosis for the inpatient admission:
- If the reason for the inpatient admission is a complication, assign the complication as the principal diagnosis.
- If no complication, or other condition, is documented as the reason for the inpatient admission, assign the reason for the outpatient surgery as the principal diagnosis.
- If the reason for the inpatient admission is another condition unrelated to the surgery, assign the unrelated condition as the principal diagnosis.

K. Admissions/Encounters for Rehabilitation
When the purpose for the admission/encounter is rehabilitation, sequence first the code for the condition for which the service is being performed. For example, for an admission/encounter for rehabilitation for right-sided dominant hemiplegia following a cerebrovascular infarction, report code I69.351, Hemiplegia and hemiparesis following cerebral infarction affecting right dominant side, as the first-listed or principal diagnosis.

If the condition for which the rehabilitation service is no longer present, report the appropriate aftercare code as the first-listed or principal diagnosis. For example, if a patient with severe degenerative osteoarthritis of the hip, underwent hip replacement and the current encounter/ admission is for rehabilitation, report code Z47.1, Aftercare following joint replacement surgery, as the first-listed or principal diagnosis.

See Section I.C.21.c.7, Factors influencing health states and contact with health services, Aftercare.

Section III. Reporting Additional Diagnoses

GENERAL RULES FOR OTHER (ADDITIONAL) DIAGNOSES
For reporting purposes the definition for "other diagnoses" is interpreted as additional conditions that affect patient care in terms of requiring:

clinical evaluation; or
therapeutic treatment; or
diagnostic procedures; or
extended length of hospital stay; or
increased nursing care and/or monitoring.

The UHDDS item #11-b defines Other Diagnoses as "all conditions that coexist at the time of admission, that develop subsequently, or that affect the treatment received and/or the length of stay. Diagnoses that relate to an earlier episode which have no bearing on the current hospital stay are to be excluded." UHDDS definitions

GUIDELINES (ICD-10-CM)

apply to inpatients in acute care, short-term, long term care and psychiatric hospital setting. The UHDDS definitions are used by acute care short-term hospitals to report inpatient data elements in a standardized manner. These data elements and their definitions can be found in the July 31, 1985, Federal Register (Vol. 50, No, 147), pp. 31038-40.

Since that time the application of the UHDDS definitions has been expanded to include all nonoutpatient settings (acute care, short term, long term care and psychiatric hospitals; home health agencies; rehab facilities; nursing homes, etc). **The UHDDS definitions also apply to hospice services (all levels of care).**

The following guidelines are to be applied in designating "other diagnoses" when neither the Alphabetic Index nor the Tabular List in ICD-10-CM provide direction. The listing of the diagnoses in the patient record is the responsibility of the attending provider.

A. Previous conditions

If the provider has included a diagnosis in the final diagnostic statement, such as the discharge summary or the face sheet, it should ordinarily be coded. Some providers include in the diagnostic statement resolved conditions or diagnoses and status-post procedures from previous admission that have no bearing on the current stay. Such conditions are not to be reported and are coded only if required by hospital policy.

However, history codes (categories Z80-Z87) may be used as secondary codes if the historical condition or family history has an impact on current care or influences treatment.

B. Abnormal findings

Abnormal findings (laboratory, x-ray, pathologic, and other diagnostic results) are not coded and reported unless the provider indicates their clinical significance. If the findings are outside the normal range and the attending provider has ordered other tests to evaluate the condition or prescribed treatment, it is appropriate to ask the provider whether the abnormal finding should be added.

Please note: This differs from the coding practices in the outpatient setting for coding encounters for diagnostic tests that have been interpreted by a provider.

C. Uncertain Diagnosis

If the diagnosis documented at the time of discharge is qualified as "probable", "suspected", "likely", "questionable", "possible", or "still to be ruled out" or other similar terms indicating uncertainty, code the condition as if it existed or was established. The bases for these guidelines are the diagnostic workup, arrangements for further workup or observation, and initial therapeutic approach that correspond most closely with the established diagnosis.

Note: This guideline is applicable only to inpatient admissions to short-term, acute, long-term care and psychiatric hospitals.

Section IV. Diagnostic Coding and Reporting Guidelines for Outpatient Services

These coding guidelines for outpatient diagnoses have been approved for use by hospitals/ providers in coding and reporting hospital-based outpatient services and provider-based office visits. **Guidelines in Section I, Conventions, general coding guidelines and chapter-specific guidelines, should also be applied for outpatient services and office visits.**

Information about the use of certain abbreviations, punctuation, symbols, and other conventions used in the ICD-10-CM Tabular List (code numbers and titles), can be found in Section IA of these guidelines, under "Conventions Used in the Tabular List." Section I.B. contains general guidelines that apply to the entire classification. Section I.C. contains chapter-specific guidelines that correspond to the chapters as they are arranged in the classification. Information about the correct sequence to use in finding a code is also described in Section I.

The terms encounter and visit are often used interchangeably in describing outpatient service contacts and, therefore, appear together in these guidelines without distinguishing one from the other.

Though the conventions and general guidelines apply to all settings, coding guidelines for outpatient and provider reporting of diagnoses will vary in a number of instances from those for inpatient diagnoses, recognizing that:

The Uniform Hospital Discharge Data Set (UHDDS) definition of principal diagnosis **does not apply to hospital-based outpatient services and provider-based office visits.**

Coding guidelines for inconclusive diagnoses (probable, suspected, rule out, etc.) were developed for inpatient reporting and do not apply to outpatients.

A. Selection of first-listed condition

In the outpatient setting, the term first-listed diagnosis is used in lieu of principal diagnosis.

In determining the first-listed diagnosis the coding conventions of ICD-10-CM, as well as the general and disease specific guidelines take precedence over the outpatient guidelines.

Diagnoses often are not established at the time of the initial encounter/visit. It may take two or more visits before the diagnosis is confirmed.

The most critical rule involves beginning the search for the correct code assignment through the Alphabetic Index. Never begin searching initially in the Tabular List as this will lead to coding errors.

1. Outpatient Surgery

When a patient presents for outpatient surgery (same day surgery), code the reason for the surgery as the first-listed diagnosis (reason for the encounter), even if the surgery is not performed due to a contraindication.

2. Observation Stay

When a patient is admitted for observation for a medical condition, assign a code for the medical condition as the first-listed diagnosis.

When a patient presents for outpatient surgery and develops complications requiring admission to observation, code the reason for the surgery as the first reported diagnosis (reason for the encounter), followed by codes for the complications as secondary diagnoses.

B. Codes from A00.0 through T88.9, Z00-Z99
The appropriate code(s) from A00.0 through T88.9, Z00-Z99 must be used to identify diagnoses, symptoms, conditions, problems, complaints, or other reason(s) for the encounter/visit.

C. Accurate reporting of ICD-10-CM diagnosis codes
For accurate reporting of ICD-10-CM diagnosis codes, the documentation should describe the patient's condition, using terminology which includes specific diagnoses as well as symptoms, problems, or reasons for the encounter. There are ICD-10-CM codes to describe all of these.

D. Codes that describe symptoms and signs
Codes that describe symptoms and signs, as opposed to diagnoses, are acceptable for reporting purposes when a diagnosis has not been established (confirmed) by the provider. Chapter 18 of ICD-10-CM, Symptoms, Signs, and Abnormal Clinical and Laboratory Findings Not Elsewhere Classified (codes R00-R99) contain many, but not all codes for symptoms.

E. Encounters for circumstances other than a disease or injury
ICD-10-CM provides codes to deal with encounters for circumstances other than a disease or injury. The Factors Influencing Health Status and Contact with Health Services codes (Z00-Z99) are provided to deal with occasions when circumstances other than a disease or injury are recorded as diagnosis or problems.
See Section I.C.21. Factors influencing health status and contact with health services.

F. Level of Detail in Coding
1. ICD-10-CM codes with 3, 4, 5, 6 or 7 characters
ICD-10-CM is composed of codes with 3, 4, 5, 6 or 7 characters. Codes with three characters are included in ICD-10-CM as the heading of a category of codes that may be further subdivided by the use of fourth, fifth, sixth or seventh characters to provide greater specificity.
2. Use of full number of characters required for a code
A three-character code is to be used only if it is not further subdivided. A code is invalid if it has not been coded to the full number of characters required for that code, including the 7th character, if applicable.

G. ICD-10-CM code for the diagnosis, condition, problem, or other reason for encounter/visit
List first the ICD-10-CM code for the diagnosis, condition, problem, or other reason for encounter/visit shown in the medical record to be chiefly responsible for the services provided. List additional codes that describe any coexisting conditions. In some cases the first-listed diagnosis may be a symptom when a diagnosis has not been established (confirmed) by the physician.

H. Uncertain diagnosis
Do not code diagnoses documented as "probable", "suspected," "questionable," "rule out," or "working diagnosis" or other similar terms indicating uncertainty. Rather, code the condition(s) to the highest degree of certainty for that encounter/visit, such as symptoms, signs, abnormal test results, or other reason for the visit.
Please note: This differs from the coding practices used by short-term, acute care, long-term care and psychiatric hospitals.

I. Chronic diseases
Chronic diseases treated on an ongoing basis may be coded and reported as many times as the patient receives treatment and care for the condition(s)

J. Code all documented conditions that coexist
Code all documented conditions that coexist at the time of the encounter/visit, and require or affect patient care treatment or management. Do not code conditions that were previously treated and no longer exist. However, history codes (categories Z80-Z87) may be used as secondary codes if the historical condition or family history has an impact on current care or influences treatment.

K. Patients receiving diagnostic services only
For patients receiving diagnostic services only during an encounter/visit, sequence first the diagnosis, condition, problem, or other reason for encounter/visit shown in the medical record to be chiefly responsible for the outpatient services provided during the encounter/visit. Codes for other diagnoses (e.g., chronic conditions) may be sequenced as additional diagnoses.

For encounters for routine laboratory/radiology testing in the absence of any signs, symptoms, or associated diagnosis, assign Z01.89, Encounter for other specified special examinations. If routine testing is performed during the same encounter as a test to evaluate a sign, symptom, or diagnosis, it is appropriate to assign both the Z code and the code describing the reason for the non-routine test.

For outpatient encounters for diagnostic tests that have been interpreted by a physician, and the final report is available at the time of coding, code any confirmed or definitive diagnosis(es) documented in the interpretation. Do not code related signs and symptoms as additional diagnoses.
Please note: This differs from the coding practice in the hospital inpatient setting regarding abnormal findings on test results.

L. Patients receiving therapeutic services only
For patients receiving therapeutic services only during an encounter/visit, sequence first the diagnosis, condition, problem, or other reason for encounter/visit shown in the medical record to be chiefly responsible for the outpatient services provided during the encounter/visit. Codes for other diagnoses (e.g., chronic conditions) may be sequenced as additional diagnoses.

The only exception to this rule is that when the primary reason for the admission/encounter is chemotherapy or radiation therapy, the appropriate Z code for the service is listed first, and the diagnosis or problem for which the service is being performed listed second.

M. Patients receiving preoperative evaluations only

For patients receiving preoperative evaluations only, sequence first a code from subcategory Z01.81, Encounter for pre-procedural examinations, to describe the pre-op consultations. Assign a code for the condition to describe the reason for the surgery as an additional diagnosis. Code also any findings related to the pre-op evaluation.

N. Ambulatory surgery

For ambulatory surgery, code the diagnosis for which the surgery was performed. If the postoperative diagnosis is known to be different from the preoperative diagnosis at the time the diagnosis is confirmed, select the postoperative diagnosis for coding, since it is the most definitive.

O. Routine outpatient prenatal visits

See Section I.C.15. Routine outpatient prenatal visits.

P. Encounters for general medical examinations with abnormal findings

The subcategories for encounters for general medical examinations, Z00.0-, provide codes for with and without abnormal findings. Should a general medical examination result in an abnormal finding, the code for general medical examination with abnormal finding should be assigned as the first-listed diagnosis. **An examination with abnormal findings refers to a condition/diagnosis that is newly identified or a change in severity of a chronic condition (such as uncontrolled hypertension, or an acute exacerbation of chronic obstructive pulmonary disease) during a routine physical examination.** A secondary code for the abnormal finding should also be coded.

Q. Encounters for routine health screenings

See Section I.C.21. Factors influencing health status and contact with health services, Screening

Appendix I
Present on Admission Reporting Guidelines

Introduction

These guidelines are to be used as a supplement to the *ICD-10-CM Official Guidelines for Coding and Reporting* to facilitate the assignment of the Present on Admission (POA) indicator for each diagnosis and external cause of injury code reported on claim forms (UB-04 and 837 Institutional).

These guidelines are not intended to replace any guidelines in the main body of the *ICD-10-CM Official Guidelines for Coding and Reporting*. The POA guidelines are not intended to provide guidance on when a condition should be coded, but rather, how to apply the POA indicator to the final set of diagnosis codes that have been assigned in accordance with Sections I, II, and III of the official coding guidelines. Subsequent to the assignment of the ICD-10-CM codes, the POA indicator should then be assigned to those conditions that have been coded.

As stated in the Introduction to the ICD-10-CM Official Guidelines for Coding and Reporting, a joint effort between the healthcare provider and the coder is essential to achieve complete and accurate documentation, code assignment, and reporting of diagnoses and procedures. The importance of consistent, complete documentation in the medical record cannot be overemphasized. Medical record documentation from any provider involved in the care and treatment of the patient may be used to support the determination of whether a condition was present on admission or not. In the context of the official coding guidelines, the term "provider" means a physician or any qualified healthcare practitioner who is legally accountable for establishing the patient's diagnosis.

These guidelines are not a substitute for the provider's clinical judgment as to the determination of whether a condition was/was not present on admission. The provider should be queried regarding issues related to the linking of signs/symptoms, timing of test results, and the timing of findings.

Please see the CDC website for the detailed list of ICD-10-CM codes that do not require the use of a POA indicator (ftp://ftp.cdc.gov/pub/Health_Statistics/NCHS/Publications/ICD10CM/2017/). The conditions on this exempt list represent categories and/or codes for circumstances regarding the healthcare encounter or factors influencing health status that do not represent a current disease or injury or are always present on admission.

General Reporting Requirements

All claims involving inpatient admissions to general acute care hospitals or other facilities that are subject to a law or regulation mandating collection of present on admission information.

Present on admission is defined as present at the time the order for inpatient admission occurs—conditions that develop during an outpatient encounter, including emergency department, observation, or outpatient surgery, are considered as present on admission.

POA indicator is assigned to principal and secondary diagnoses (as defined in Section II of the Official Guidelines for Coding and Reporting) and the external cause of injury codes.

Issues related to inconsistent, missing, conflicting or unclear documentation must still be resolved by the provider.

If a condition would not be coded and reported based on UHDDS definitions and current official coding guidelines, then the POA indicator would not be reported.

Reporting Options

Y - Yes

N - No

U - Unknown

W - Clinically undetermined

Unreported/Not used - (Exempt from POA reporting)

Reporting Definitions

Y = present at the time of inpatient admission

N = not present at the time of inpatient admission

U = documentation is insufficient to determine if condition is present on admission

W = provider is unable to clinically determine whether condition was present on admission or not

Timeframe for POA Identification and Documentation

There is no required timeframe as to when a provider (per the definition of "provider" used in these guidelines) must identify or document a condition to be present on admission. In some clinical situations, it may not be possible for a provider to make a definitive diagnosis (or a condition may not be recognized or reported by the patient) for a period of time after admission. In some cases it may be several days before the provider arrives at a definitive diagnosis. This does not mean that the condition was not present on admission. Determination of whether the condition was present on admission or not will be based on the applicable POA guideline as identified in this document, or on the provider's best clinical judgment.

If at the time of code assignment the documentation is unclear as to whether a condition was present on admission or not, it is appropriate to query the provider for clarification.

Assigning the POA Indicator

Condition is on the "Exempt from Reporting" list

Leave the "present on admission" field blank if the condition is on the list of ICD-10-CM codes for which this field is not applicable. This is the only circumstance in which the field may be left blank.

POA Explicitly Documented

Assign Y for any condition the provider explicitly documents as being present on admission.

Assign N for any condition the provider explicitly documents as not present at the time of admission.

Conditions diagnosed prior to inpatient admission

Assign "Y" for conditions that were diagnosed prior to admission (example: hypertension, diabetes mellitus, asthma)

Conditions diagnosed during the admission but clearly present before admission

Assign "Y" for conditions diagnosed during the admission that were clearly present but not diagnosed until after admission occurred.

Diagnoses subsequently confirmed after admission are considered present on admission if at the time of admission they are documented as suspected, possible, rule out, differential diagnosis, or constitute an underlying cause of a symptom that is present at the time of admission.

Condition develops during outpatient encounter prior to inpatient admission

Assign Y for any condition that develops during an outpatient encounter prior to a written order for inpatient admission.

Documentation does not indicate whether condition was present on admission

Assign "U" when the medical record documentation is unclear as to whether the condition was present on admission. "U" should not be routinely assigned and used only in very limited circumstances. Coders are encouraged to query the providers when the documentation is unclear.

Documentation states that it cannot be determined whether the condition was or was not present on admission

Assign "W" when the medical record documentation indicates that it cannot be clinically determined whether or not the condition was present on admission.

Chronic condition with acute exacerbation during the admission

If a single code identifies both the chronic condition and the acute exacerbation, see POA guidelines pertaining to **codes that contain multiple clinical concepts**.

If a single code only identifies the chronic condition and not the acute exacerbation (e.g., acute exacerbation of chronic leukemia), assign "Y."

Conditions documented as possible, probable, suspected, or rule out at the time of discharge

If the final diagnosis contains a possible, probable, suspected, or rule out diagnosis, and this diagnosis was based on signs, symptoms or clinical findings suspected at the time of inpatient admission, assign "Y."

If the final diagnosis contains a possible, probable, suspected, or rule out diagnosis, and this diagnosis was based on signs, symptoms or clinical findings that were not present on admission, assign "N".

Conditions documented as impending or threatened at the time of discharge

If the final diagnosis contains an impending or threatened diagnosis, and this diagnosis is based on symptoms or clinical findings that were present on admission, assign "Y".

If the final diagnosis contains an impending or threatened diagnosis, and this diagnosis is based on symptoms or clinical findings that were not present on admission, assign "N".

Acute and Chronic Conditions

Assign "Y" for acute conditions that are present at time of admission and N for acute conditions that are not present at time of admission.

Assign "Y" for chronic conditions, even though the condition may not be diagnosed until after admission.

If a single code identifies both an acute and chronic condition, see the POA guidelines for codes **that contain multiple clinical concepts.**

Codes **That Contain Multiple Clinical Concepts**

Assign "N" if at least one of the clinical concepts included in the code was not present on admission (e.g., COPD with acute exacerbation and the exacerbation was not present on admission; gastric ulcer that does not start bleeding until after admission; asthma patient develops status asthmaticus after admission).

Assign "Y" if all of the **clinical concepts included in the code** were present on admission (e.g., **duodenal ulcer that perforates prior to admission**).

For infection codes that include the causal organism, assign "Y" if the infection (or signs of the infection) **were** present on admission, even though the culture results may not be known until after admission (e.g., patient is admitted with pneumonia and the provider documents Pseudomonas as the causal organism a few days later).

Same Diagnosis Code for Two or More Conditions

When the same ICD-10-CM diagnosis code applies to two or more conditions during the same encounter (e.g. two separate conditions classified to the same ICD-10-CM diagnosis code):

Assign "Y" if all conditions represented by the single ICD-10-CM code were present on admission (e.g. bilateral unspecified age-related cataracts).

Assign "N" if any of the conditions represented by the single ICD-10-CM code was not present on admission (e.g. traumatic secondary and recurrent hemorrhage and seroma is assigned to a single code T79.2, but only one of the conditions was present on admission).

Obstetrical conditions

Whether or not the patient delivers during the current hospitalization does not affect assignment of the POA indicator. The determining factor for POA assignment is whether the pregnancy complication or obstetrical condition described by the code was present at the time of admission or not.

If the pregnancy complication or obstetrical condition was present on admission (e.g., patient admitted in preterm labor), assign "Y".

If the pregnancy complication or obstetrical condition was not present on admission (e.g., 2nd degree laceration during delivery, postpartum hemorrhage that occurred during current hospitalization, fetal distress develops after admission), assign "N".

If the obstetrical code includes more than one diagnosis and any of the diagnoses identified by the code were not present on admission assign "N".

(e.g., Category O11, Pre-existing hypertension with pre-eclampsia)

GUIDELINES (ICD-10-CM)

47

Perinatal conditions

Newborns are not considered to be admitted until after birth. Therefore, any condition present at birth or that developed in utero is considered present at admission and should be assigned "Y". This includes conditions that occur during delivery (e.g., injury during delivery, meconium aspiration, exposure to streptococcus B in the vaginal canal).

Congenital conditions and anomalies

Assign "Y" for congenital conditions and anomalies except for categories Q00-Q99, Congenital anomalies, which are on the exempt list. Congenital conditions are always considered present on admission.

External cause of injury codes

Assign "Y" for any external cause code representing an external cause of morbidity that occurred prior to inpatient admission (e.g., patient fell out of bed at home, patient fell out of bed in emergency room prior to admission).

Assign "N" for any external cause code representing an external cause of morbidity that occurred during inpatient hospitalization (e.g., patient fell out of hospital bed during hospital stay, patient experienced an adverse reaction to a medication administered after inpatient admission).

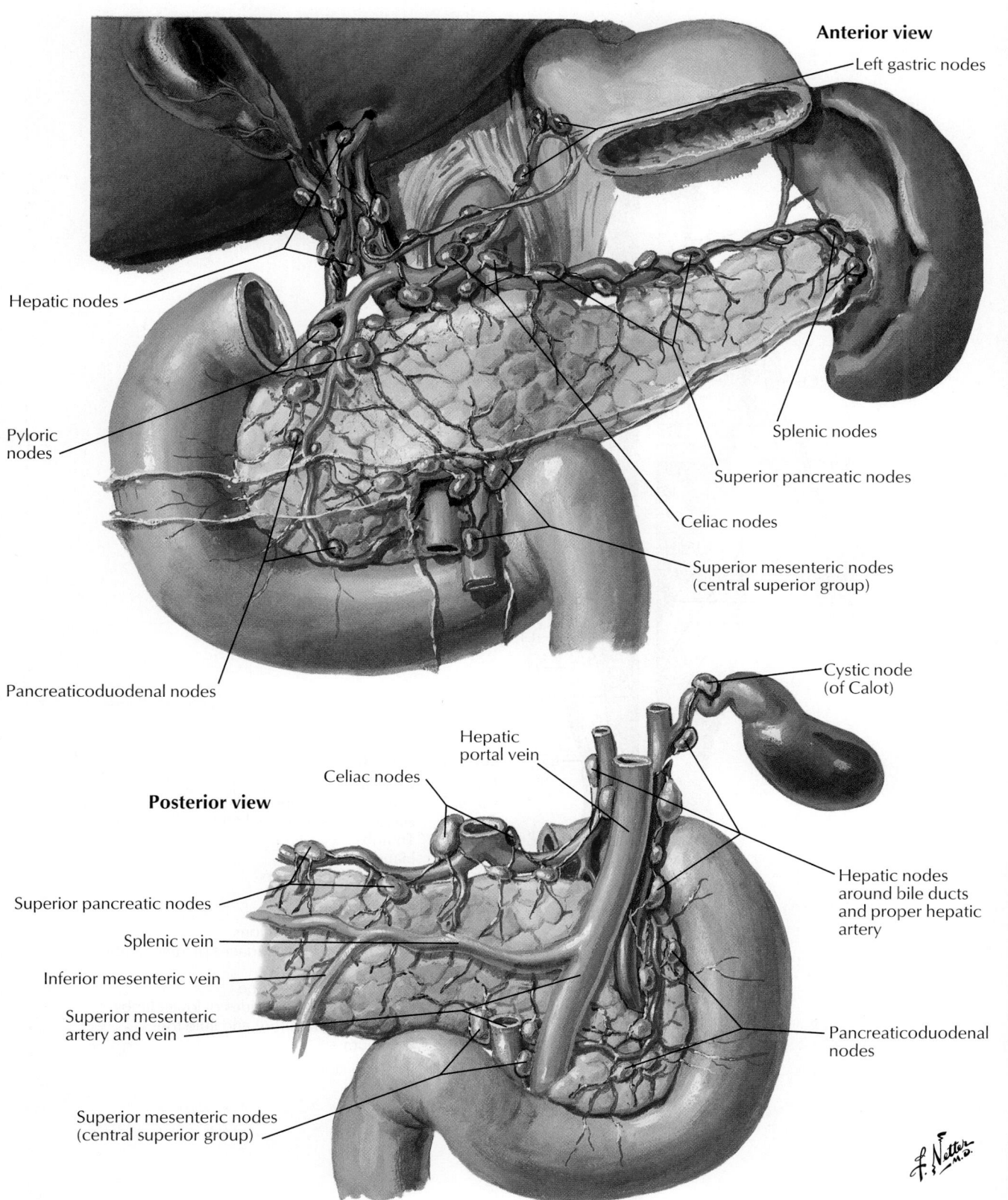

Anterior view

Left gastric nodes

Hepatic nodes

Pyloric nodes

Pancreaticoduodenal nodes

Splenic nodes

Superior pancreatic nodes

Celiac nodes

Superior mesenteric nodes (central superior group)

Posterior view

Celiac nodes

Hepatic portal vein

Cystic node (of Calot)

Hepatic nodes around bile ducts and proper hepatic artery

Superior pancreatic nodes

Splenic vein

Inferior mesenteric vein

Superior mesenteric artery and vein

Superior mesenteric nodes (central superior group)

Pancreaticoduodenal nodes

Plate 315 Lymph Vessels and Nodes of Pancreas. (Netter: Atlas of Human Anatomy, 4 ed, 2006, Saunders.)

Dermatome pattern

Levels of principal dermatomes

C5	Clavicles
C5, 6, 7	Lateral parts of upper limbs
C8; T1	Medial sides of upper limbs
C6	Thumb
C6, 7, 8	Hand
C8	Ring and little fingers
T4	Level of nipples
T10	Level of umbilicus
T12	Inguinal or groin regions
L1, 2, 3, 4	Anterior and inner surfaces of lower limbs
L4, 5; S1	Foot
L4	Medial side of great toe
L5; S1, 2	Outer and posterior sides of lower limbs
S1	Lateral margin of foot and little toe
S2, 3, 4	Perineum

Plate 164   Dermatomes. (Netter: Atlas of Human Anatomy, 4 ed, 2006, Saunders.)

Female: frontal section

- Peritoneum
- Body of bladder
- Fundus of bladder
- Interureteric crest
- Left ureteric orifice
- Trigone of bladder
- Neck of bladder
- Paravesical endopelvic fascia and vesical venous plexus
- Vesical fascia
- Tendinous arch of levator ani muscle
- Obturator internus muscle
- Levator ani muscle
- Tendinous arch of pelvic fascia
- Urethra
- Sphincter urethrae muscle
- Perineal membrane
- Inferior pubic ramus
- Crus of clitoris and ischiocavernosus muscle
- Bulb of vestibule and bulbospongiosus muscle
- Deep perineal (investing or Gallaudet's) fascia
- Superficial perineal (Colles') fascia

- Round ligament of uterus
- Vagina

Male: frontal section

- Peritoneum
- Body of bladder
- Fundus of bladder
- Ductus (vas) deferens
- Interureteric crest
- Right ureteric orifice
- Trigone of bladder
- Neck of bladder
- Paravesical endopelvic fascia and vesical venous plexus
- Tendinous arch of levator ani muscle
- Uvula of bladder
- Obturator internus muscle
- Levator ani muscle
- Capsule of prostate
- Prostate and prostatic urethra
- Seminal colliculus
- Bulbourethral (Cowper's) gland
- Perineal membrane and sphincter urethrae muscle
- Bulbous portion of spongy urethra
- Corpus spongiosum and bulbospongiosus muscle
- Deep perineal (investing or Gallaudet's) fascia

- Internal urethral sphincter
- Tendinous arch of pelvic fascia
- Anterior recess of ischio-anal fossa
- Inferior pubic ramus
- Crus of penis and ischiocavernosus muscle
- Superficial perineal (Colles') fascia

Plate 366 Urinary Bladder: Female and Male. (Netter: Atlas of Human Anatomy, 4 ed, 2006, Saunders.)

Sites of ectopic implantation

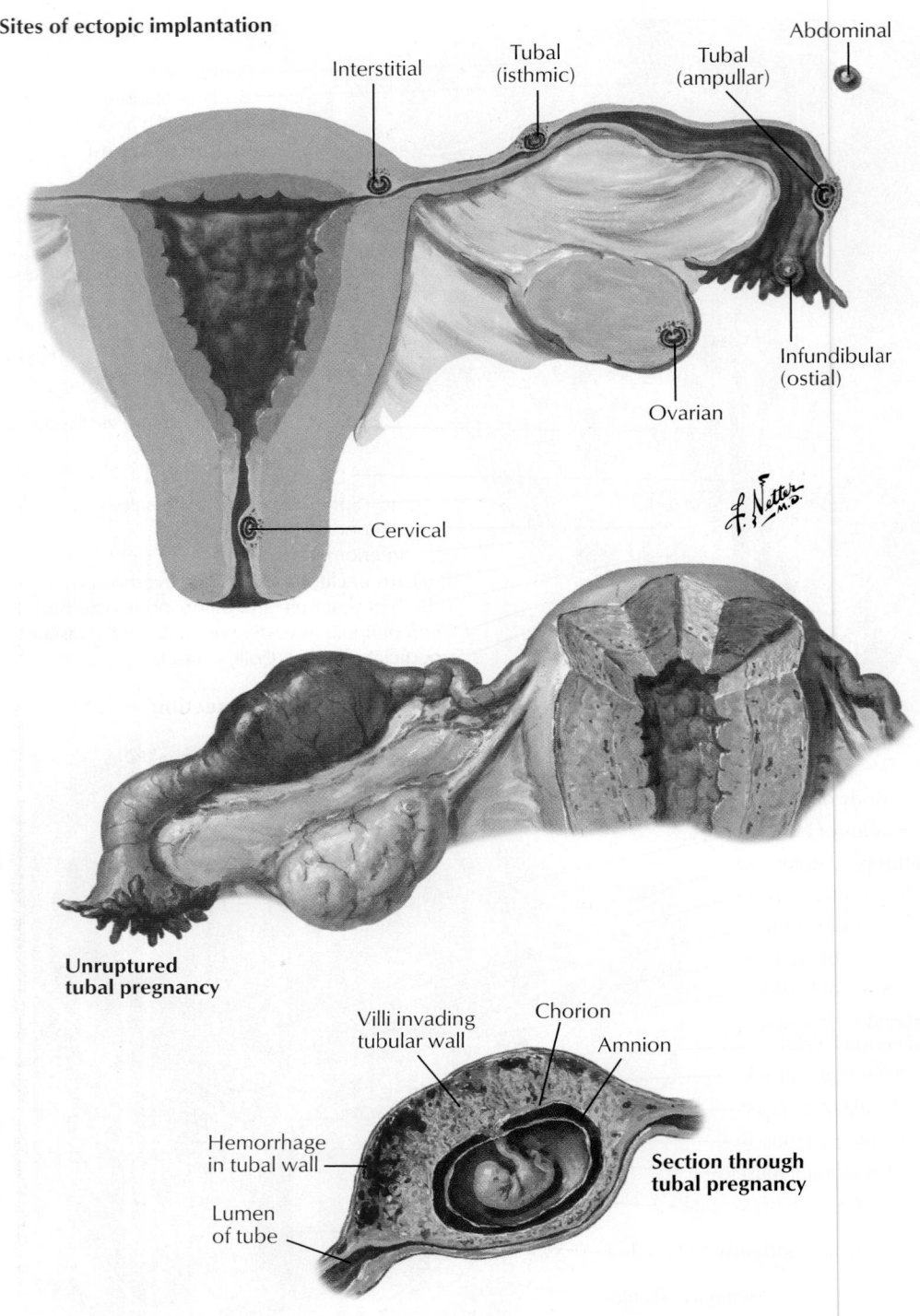

Interstitial

Tubal (isthmic)

Tubal (ampullar)

Abdominal

Infundibular (ostial)

Ovarian

Cervical

Unruptured tubal pregnancy

Villi invading tubular wall

Chorion

Amnion

Hemorrhage in tubal wall

Lumen of tube

Section through tubal pregnancy

Plate 375 Ectopic Pregnancy. (Netter: Atlas of Human Anatomy, 4 ed, 2006, Saunders.)

Skin of penis

Superficial fascia of penis (Colles' fascia)

Deep (Buck's) fascia of penis

Testicular artery

Ductus deferens

Artery to ductus deferens

Genital branch of genitofemoral nerve

Pampiniform (venous) plexus

Epididymis

Appendix of epididymis

Appendix of testis

Testis (covered by visceral layer of tunica vaginalis)

Parietal layer of tunica vaginalis

Superficial inguinal ring

External spermatic fascia

Cremaster muscle and fascia

Septum of scrotum (formed by dartos fascia)

Superficial (dartos) fascia of scrotum

Skin of scrotum

Superficial (dartos) fascia of scrotum

External spermatic fascia

Cremaster muscle and fascia

Internal spermatic fascia

Parietal layer of tunica vaginalis

Epididymis

Testis (covered by visceral layer of tunica vaginalis)

Skin of scrotum

Plate 387 Scrotum and Contents. (Netter: Atlas of Human Anatomy, 4 ed, 2006, Saunders.)

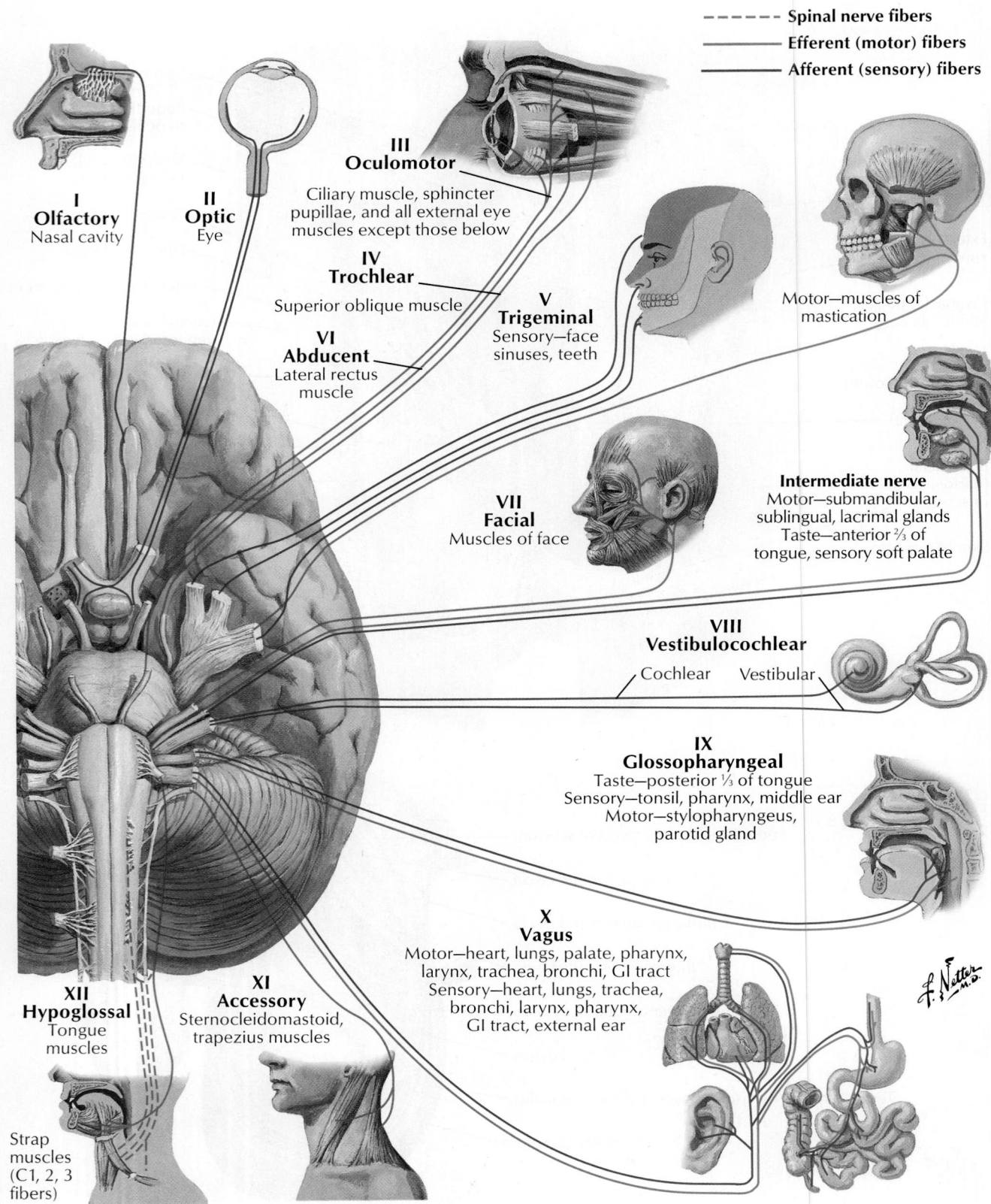

- - - - - Spinal nerve fibers
——— Efferent (motor) fibers
——— Afferent (sensory) fibers

I
Olfactory
Nasal cavity

II
Optic
Eye

III
Oculomotor
Ciliary muscle, sphincter pupillae, and all external eye muscles except those below

IV
Trochlear
Superior oblique muscle

V
Trigeminal
Sensory—face sinuses, teeth

Motor—muscles of mastication

VI
Abducent
Lateral rectus muscle

VII
Facial
Muscles of face

Intermediate nerve
Motor—submandibular, sublingual, lacrimal glands
Taste—anterior ⅔ of tongue, sensory soft palate

VIII
Vestibulocochlear
Cochlear   Vestibular

IX
Glossopharyngeal
Taste—posterior ⅓ of tongue
Sensory—tonsil, pharynx, middle ear
Motor—stylopharyngeus, parotid gland

X
Vagus
Motor—heart, lungs, palate, pharynx, larynx, trachea, bronchi, GI tract
Sensory—heart, lungs, trachea, bronchi, larynx, pharynx, GI tract, external ear

XII
Hypoglossal
Tongue muscles

Strap muscles (C1, 2, 3 fibers)

XI
Accessory
Sternocleidomastoid, trapezius muscles

Plate 118 Cranial Nerves (Motor and Sensory Distribution): Schema. (Netter: Atlas of Human Anatomy, 4 ed, 2006, Saunders.)

Superior view

- Supratrochlear nerve
- Medial rectus muscle
- Superior oblique muscle
- Infratrochlear nerve
- Nasociliary nerve
- Trochlear nerve (IV)
- Common tendinous ring
- Ophthalmic nerve (V₁)
- Optic nerve (II)
- Internal carotid artery and nerve plexus
- Oculomotor nerve (III)
- Trochlear nerve (IV)
- Abducent nerve (VI)
- Tentorium cerebelli

- Medial branch } Supraorbital nerve
- Lateral branch
- Levator palpebrae superioris muscle
- Superior rectus muscle
- Lacrimal gland
- Lacrimal nerve
- Lateral rectus muscle
- Frontal nerve
- Maxillary nerve (V₂)
- Meningeal branch of maxillary nerve
- Mandibular nerve (V₃)
- Lesser petrosal nerve
- Meningeal branch of mandibular nerve
- Greater petrosal nerve
- Trigeminal (semilunar) ganglion
- Tentorial (meningeal) branch of ophthalmic nerve

Superior view:
levator palpebrae superioris, superior rectus, and superior oblique muscles partially cut away

- Supratrochlear nerve (cut)
- Supraorbital nerve branches (cut)
- Infratrochlear nerve
- Anterior ethmoidal nerve
- Optic nerve (II)
- Posterior ethmoidal nerve
- Superior branch of oculomotor nerve (III) (cut)
- Nasociliary nerve
- Internal carotid plexus
- Trochlear nerve (IV) (cut)
- Oculomotor nerve (III)
- Abducent nerve (VI)

- Long ciliary nerves
- Short ciliary nerves
- Lacrimal nerve
- Ciliary ganglion
- Parasympathetic root of ciliary ganglion (from inferior branch of oculomotor nerve)
- Sympathetic root of ciliary ganglion (from internal carotid plexus)
- Sensory root of ciliary ganglion (from nasociliary nerve)
- Branches to inferior and medial rectus muscles
- Abducent nerve (VI)
- Inferior branch of oculomotor nerve (III)
- Lacrimal nerve
- Frontal nerve (cut)
- Ophthalmic nerve (V₁)

Plate 86   Nerves of Orbit. (Netter: Atlas of Human Anatomy, 4 ed, 2006, Saunders.)

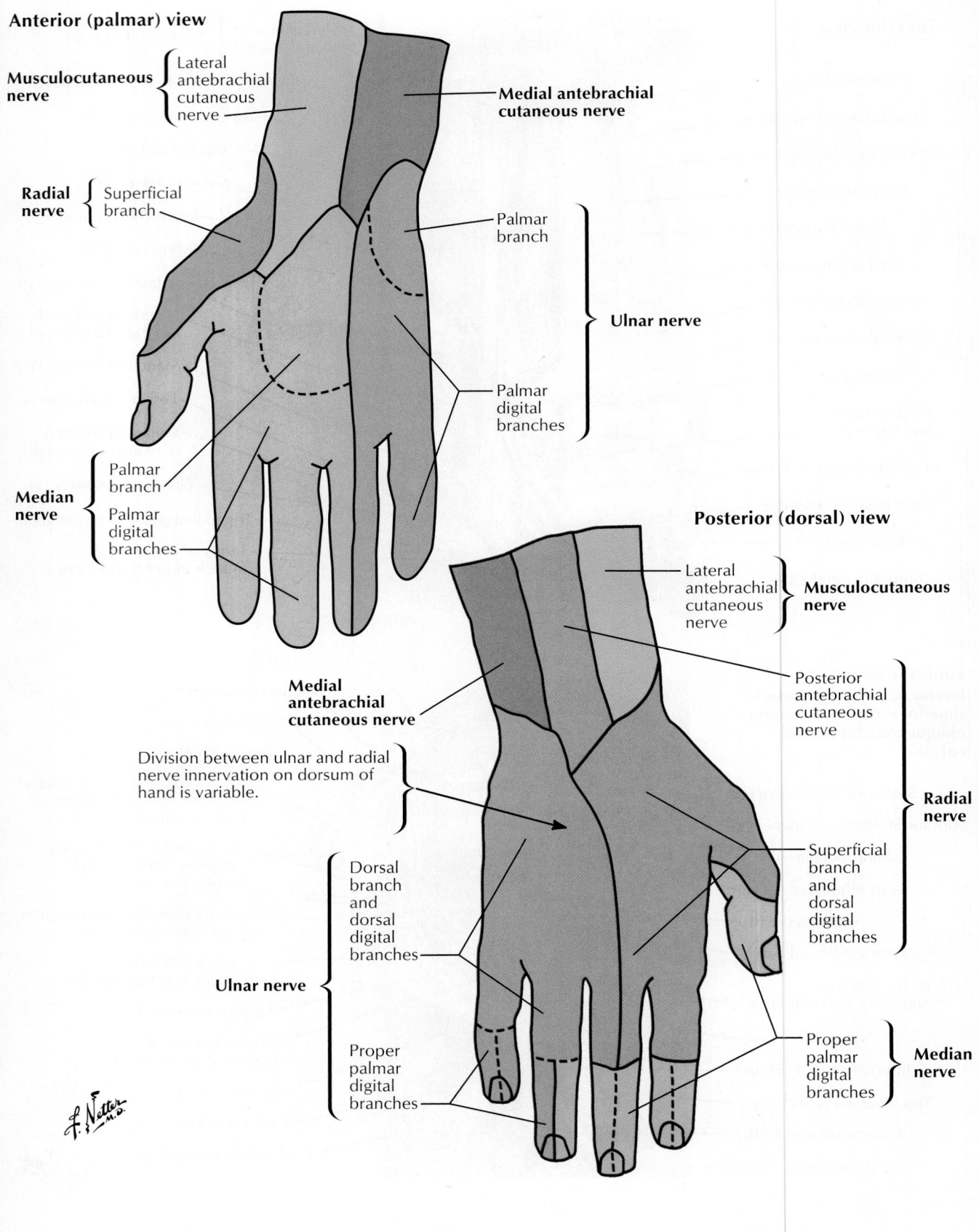

Anterior (palmar) view

Musculocutaneous nerve { Lateral antebrachial cutaneous nerve

Medial antebrachial cutaneous nerve

Radial nerve { Superficial branch

Palmar branch

Ulnar nerve

Palmar digital branches

Median nerve { Palmar branch / Palmar digital branches

Posterior (dorsal) view

Lateral antebrachial cutaneous nerve — **Musculocutaneous nerve**

Posterior antebrachial cutaneous nerve

Radial nerve

Medial antebrachial cutaneous nerve

Division between ulnar and radial nerve innervation on dorsum of hand is variable.

Superficial branch and dorsal digital branches

Dorsal branch and dorsal digital branches

Ulnar nerve

Proper palmar digital branches

Proper palmar digital branches — **Median nerve**

Plate 472 Cutaneous Innervation of Wrist and Hand. (Netter: Atlas of Human Anatomy, 4 ed, 2006, Saunders.)

Anterior view

Deltoid muscle

Coracobrachialis muscle

Biceps brachii muscle
  Short head (*cut*)
  Long head (*cut*)

Musculocutaneous nerve

Brachialis muscle

Biceps brachii muscle (*cut*) and tendon

Lateral antebrachial cutaneous nerve (from musculocutaneous nerve)

Radial nerve
  Deep branch
  Superficial branch

Supinator muscle

Brachioradialis muscle

Radial artery

Pronator teres muscle (*partially cut*)

Median nerve

Flexor pollicis longus muscle

Flexor carpi radialis tendon (*cut*)

Flexor retinaculum (transverse carpal ligament)

Superficial branch of radial nerve

Recurrent (motor) branch of median nerve to thenar muscles

Common palmar digital branches of median nerve

Proper palmar digital branches of median nerve

Intercostobrachial nerve

Medial brachial cutaneous nerve

Radial nerve

Ulnar nerve

Medial antebrachial cutaneous nerve

Median nerve

Brachial artery

Bicipital aponeurosis

Humeral head (*cut*)
Ulnar head
} Pronator teres muscle

Flexor carpi radialis muscle (*cut*)

Humeroulnar head
Radial head
} Flexor digitorum superficialis muscle (*cut*)

Flexor digitorum profundus muscle

Flexor carpi ulnaris muscle

Ulnar artery and nerve

Dorsal branch of ulnar nerve

Flexor digitorum superficialis tendons (*cut*)

Deep palmar branch of ulnar artery and deep branch of ulnar nerve

Superficial branch of ulnar nerve

Superficial palmar arch (*cut*)

Common palmar digital branch of ulnar nerve

Communicating branch of median nerve with ulnar nerve

Proper palmar digital branches of ulnar nerve

F. Netter, M.D.

Plate 473   Arteries and Nerves of Upper Limb. (Netter: Atlas of Human Anatomy, 4 ed, 2006, Saunders.)

Lateral cutaneous branch of subcostal nerve

Inguinal ligament (Poupart's)

Superficial circumflex iliac vein

Femoral branches of genitofemoral nerve

Lateral femoral cutaneous nerve

Saphenous opening (fossa ovalis)

Fascia lata

Anterior cutaneous branches of femoral nerve

Patellar nerve plexus

Branches of lateral sural cutaneous nerve (from common fibular [peroneal] nerve)

Deep fascia of leg (crural fascia)

Superficial fibular (peroneal) nerve
Medial dorsal cutaneous branch

Intermediate dorsal cutaneous branch

Small saphenous vein and lateral dorsal cutaneous nerve (from sural nerve)

Lateral dorsal digital nerve and vein of 5th toe

Dorsal metatarsal veins

Dorsal digital nerves and veins

Superficial epigastric vein

Ilioinguinal nerve (scrotal branch) (usually passes through superficial inguinal ring)

Genital branch of genitofemoral nerve

Femoral vein

Superficial external pudendal vein

Accessory saphenous vein

Great saphenous vein

Cutaneous branches of obturator nerve

Infrapatellar branch of saphenous nerve

Saphenous nerve (terminal branch of femoral nerve)

Great saphenous vein

Dorsal digital nerves

Dorsal venous arch

Dorsal digital nerve and vein of medial side of great toe

Dorsal digital branch of deep fibular (peroneal) nerve

Plate 544   Superficial Nerves and Veins of Lower Limb: Anterior View. (Netter: Atlas of Human Anatomy, 4 ed, 2006, Saunders.)

Lateral cutaneous branch of iliohypogastric nerve

Iliac crest

Medial clunial nerves (from dorsal rami of S1, 2, 3)

Superior clunial nerves (from dorsal rami of L1, 2, 3)

Inferior clunial nerves (from posterior femoral cutaneous nerve)

Perforating cutaneous nerve (from dorsal rami of S1, 2, 3)

Branches of posterior femoral cutaneous nerve

Branches of lateral femoral cutaneous nerve

Accessory saphenous vein

Branch of femoral cutaneous nerve

Branch of cutaneous branch of femoral nerve

Terminal branches of posterior femoral cutaneous nerve

Great saphenous vein

Lateral sural cutaneous nerve (from common fibular [peroneal] nerve)

Small saphenous vein

Sural communicating nerve

Branches of saphenous nerve

Medial sural cutaneous nerve (from tibial nerve)

Sural nerve

Lateral calcaneal branches of sural nerve

Medial calcaneal branches of tibial nerve

Lateral dorsal cutaneous nerve (continuation of sural nerve)

Plantar cutaneous branches of medial plantar nerve

Plantar cutaneous branches of lateral plantar nerve

Plate 545 Superficial Nerves and Veins of Lower Limb: Posterior View. (Netter: Atlas of Human Anatomy, 4 ed, 2006, Saunders.)

Superficial dissections

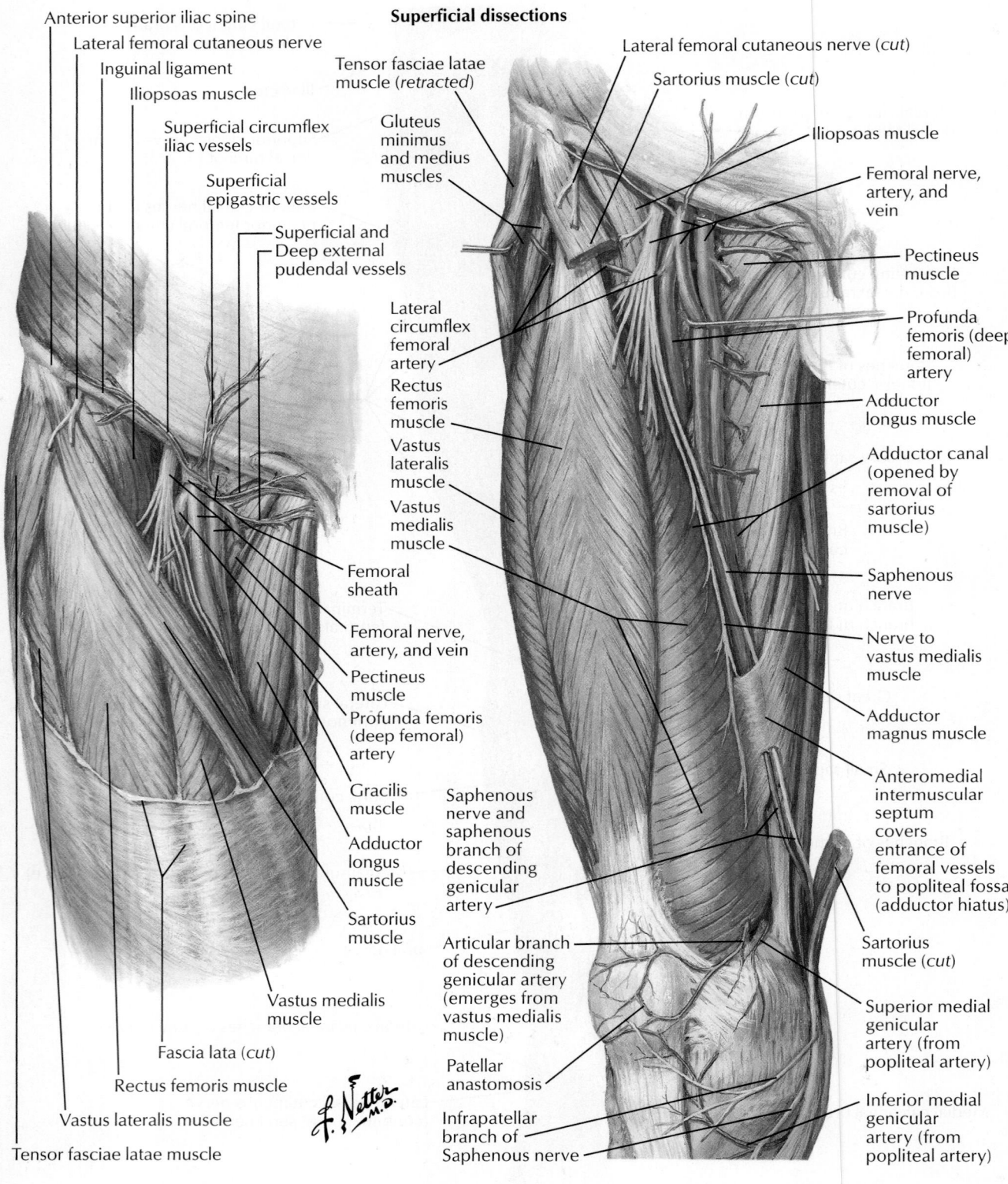

Anterior superior iliac spine

Lateral femoral cutaneous nerve

Inguinal ligament

Iliopsoas muscle

Superficial circumflex iliac vessels

Superficial epigastric vessels

Superficial and Deep external pudendal vessels

Tensor fasciae latae muscle (*retracted*)

Gluteus minimus and medius muscles

Lateral circumflex femoral artery

Rectus femoris muscle

Vastus lateralis muscle

Vastus medialis muscle

Femoral sheath

Femoral nerve, artery, and vein

Pectineus muscle

Profunda femoris (deep femoral) artery

Gracilis muscle

Adductor longus muscle

Sartorius muscle

Saphenous nerve and saphenous branch of descending genicular artery

Articular branch of descending genicular artery (emerges from vastus medialis muscle)

Patellar anastomosis

Infrapatellar branch of Saphenous nerve

Vastus medialis muscle

Fascia lata (*cut*)

Rectus femoris muscle

Vastus lateralis muscle

Tensor fasciae latae muscle

Lateral femoral cutaneous nerve (*cut*)

Sartorius muscle (*cut*)

Iliopsoas muscle

Femoral nerve, artery, and vein

Pectineus muscle

Profunda femoris (deep femoral) artery

Adductor longus muscle

Adductor canal (opened by removal of sartorius muscle)

Saphenous nerve

Nerve to vastus medialis muscle

Adductor magnus muscle

Anteromedial intermuscular septum covers entrance of femoral vessels to popliteal fossa (adductor hiatus)

Sartorius muscle (*cut*)

Superior medial genicular artery (from popliteal artery)

Inferior medial genicular artery (from popliteal artery)

Plate 500 Arteries and Nerves of Thigh: Anterior Views. (Netter: Atlas of Human Anatomy, 4 ed, 2006, Saunders.)

Deep dissection

Deep circumflex iliac artery

Lateral femoral cutaneous nerve

Sartorius muscle (cut)

Iliopsoas muscle

Tensor fasciae latae muscle (retracted)

Gluteus medius and minimus muscles

Femoral nerve

Rectus femoris muscle (cut)

Ascending, transverse and descending branches of Lateral circumflex femoral artery

Medial circumflex femoral artery

Pectineus muscle (cut)

Profunda femoris (deep femoral) artery

Perforating branches

Adductor longus muscle (cut)

Vastus lateralis muscle

Vastus intermedius muscle

Rectus femoris muscle (cut)

Saphenous nerve

Anteromedial intermuscular septum (opened)

Vastus medialis muscle

Quadriceps femoris tendon

Patella and patellar anastomosis

Medial patellar retinaculum

Patellar ligament

External iliac artery and vein

Inguinal ligament (Poupart's)

Femoral artery and vein (cut)

Pectineus muscle (cut)

Obturator canal

Obturator externus muscle

Adductor longus muscle (cut)

Anterior branch and Posterior branch of obturator nerve

Quadratus femoris muscle

Adductor brevis muscle

Branches of posterior branch of obturator nerve

Adductor magnus muscle

Gracilis muscle

Cutaneous branch of obturator nerve

Femoral artery and vein (cut)

Descending genicular artery
Articular branch
Saphenous branch

Adductor hiatus

Sartorius muscle (cut)

Adductor magnus tendon

Adductor tubercle on medial epicondyle of femur

Superior medial genicular artery (from popliteal artery)

Infrapatellar branch of Saphenous nerve

Inferior medial genicular artery (from popliteal artery)

Plate 5Ø1   Arteries and Nerves of Thigh: Posterior View. (Netter: Atlas of Human Anatomy, 4 ed, 2006, Saunders.)

61

Deep dissection

Superior clunial nerves

Gluteus maximus muscle (*cut*)

Medial clunial nerves

Inferior gluteal artery and nerve

Pudendal nerve

Nerve to obturator internus
(and superior gemellus)

Posterior femoral
cutaneous nerve

Sacrotuberous ligament

Ischial tuberosity

Inferior clunial nerves (*cut*)

Adductor magnus muscle

Gracilis muscle

Sciatic nerve

Muscular branches of sciatic nerve

Semitendinosus muscle (*retracted*)

Semimembranosus muscle

Sciatic nerve

Articular branch

Adductor hiatus

Popliteal vein and artery

Superior medial genicular artery

Medial epicondyle of femur

Tibial nerve

Gastrocnemius muscle (medial head)

Medial sural cutaneous nerve

Small saphenous vein

Iliac crest

Gluteal aponeurosis and
gluteus medius muscle (*cut*)

Superior gluteal artery and nerve

Gluteus minimus muscle

Tensor fasciae latae muscle

Piriformis muscle

Gluteus medius muscle (*cut*)

Superior gemellus muscle

Greater trochanter of femur

Obturator internus muscle

Inferior gemellus muscle

Gluteus maximus muscle (*cut*)

Quadratus femoris muscle

Medial circumflex femoral
artery

Vastus lateralis muscle
and iliotibial tract

Adductor minimus part of
adductor magnus muscle

1st perforating artery (from
profunda femoris artery)

Adductor magnus muscle

2nd and 3rd perforating arteries
(from profunda femoris artery)

4th perforating artery (from
profunda femoris artery)

Long head (*retracted*) ⎫ Biceps femoris
Short head ⎭ muscle

Superior lateral genicular artery

Common fibular (peroneal) nerve

Plantaris muscle

Gastrocnemius muscle (lateral head)

Lateral sural cutaneous nerve

NETTER'S ANATOMY ILLUSTRATIONS

Plate 502 Arteries and Nerves of Thigh: Posterior View. (Netter: Atlas of Human Anatomy, 4 ed, 2006, Saunders.)

62

Horizontal section

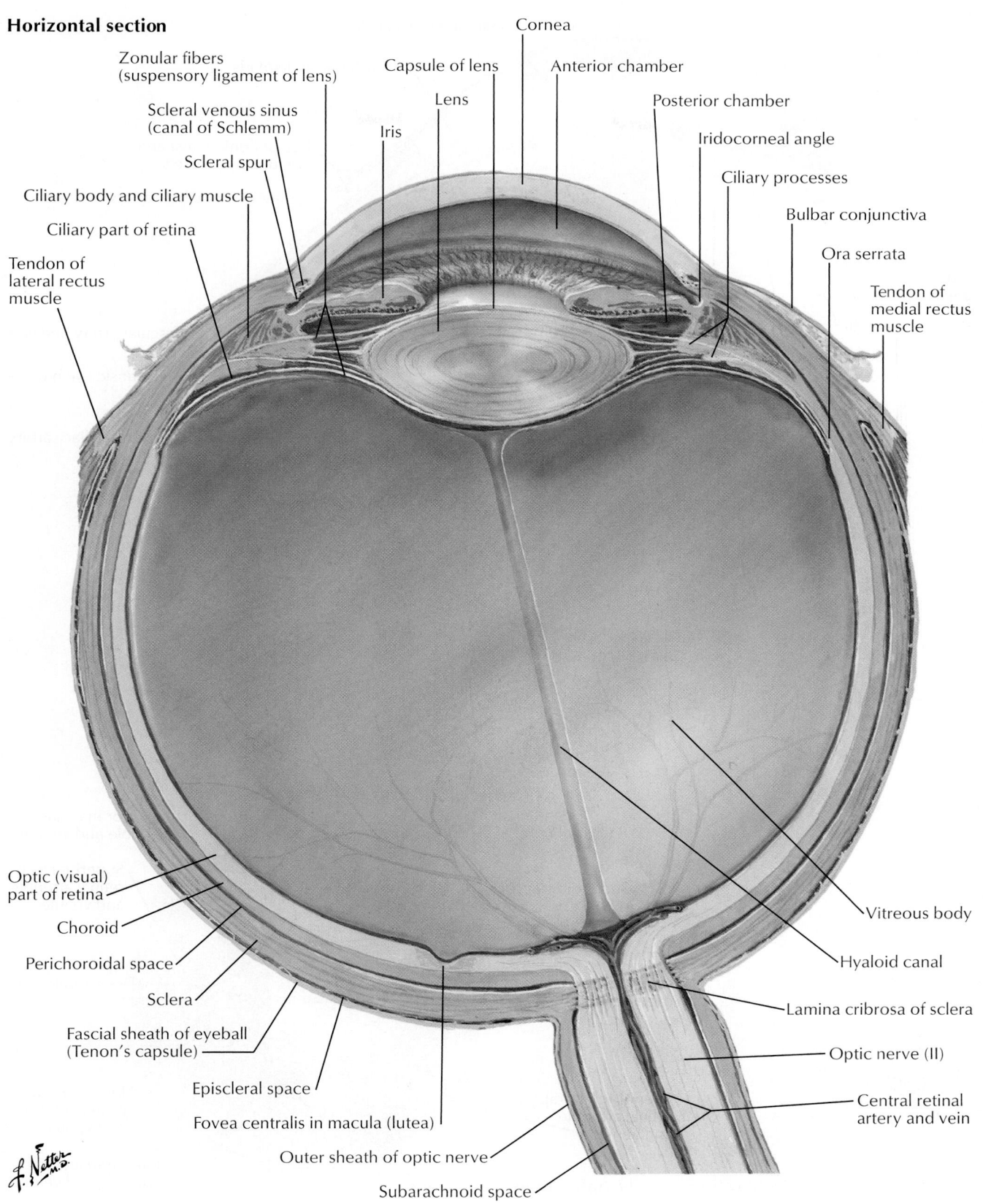

Zonular fibers (suspensory ligament of lens)

Scleral venous sinus (canal of Schlemm)

Scleral spur

Ciliary body and ciliary muscle

Ciliary part of retina

Tendon of lateral rectus muscle

Capsule of lens

Lens

Iris

Cornea

Anterior chamber

Posterior chamber

Iridocorneal angle

Ciliary processes

Bulbar conjunctiva

Ora serrata

Tendon of medial rectus muscle

Optic (visual) part of retina

Choroid

Perichoroidal space

Sclera

Fascial sheath of eyeball (Tenon's capsule)

Episcleral space

Fovea centralis in macula (lutea)

Outer sheath of optic nerve

Subarachnoid space

Vitreous body

Hyaloid canal

Lamina cribrosa of sclera

Optic nerve (II)

Central retinal artery and vein

Plate 87   Eyeball. (Netter: Atlas of Human Anatomy, 4 ed, 2006, Saunders.)

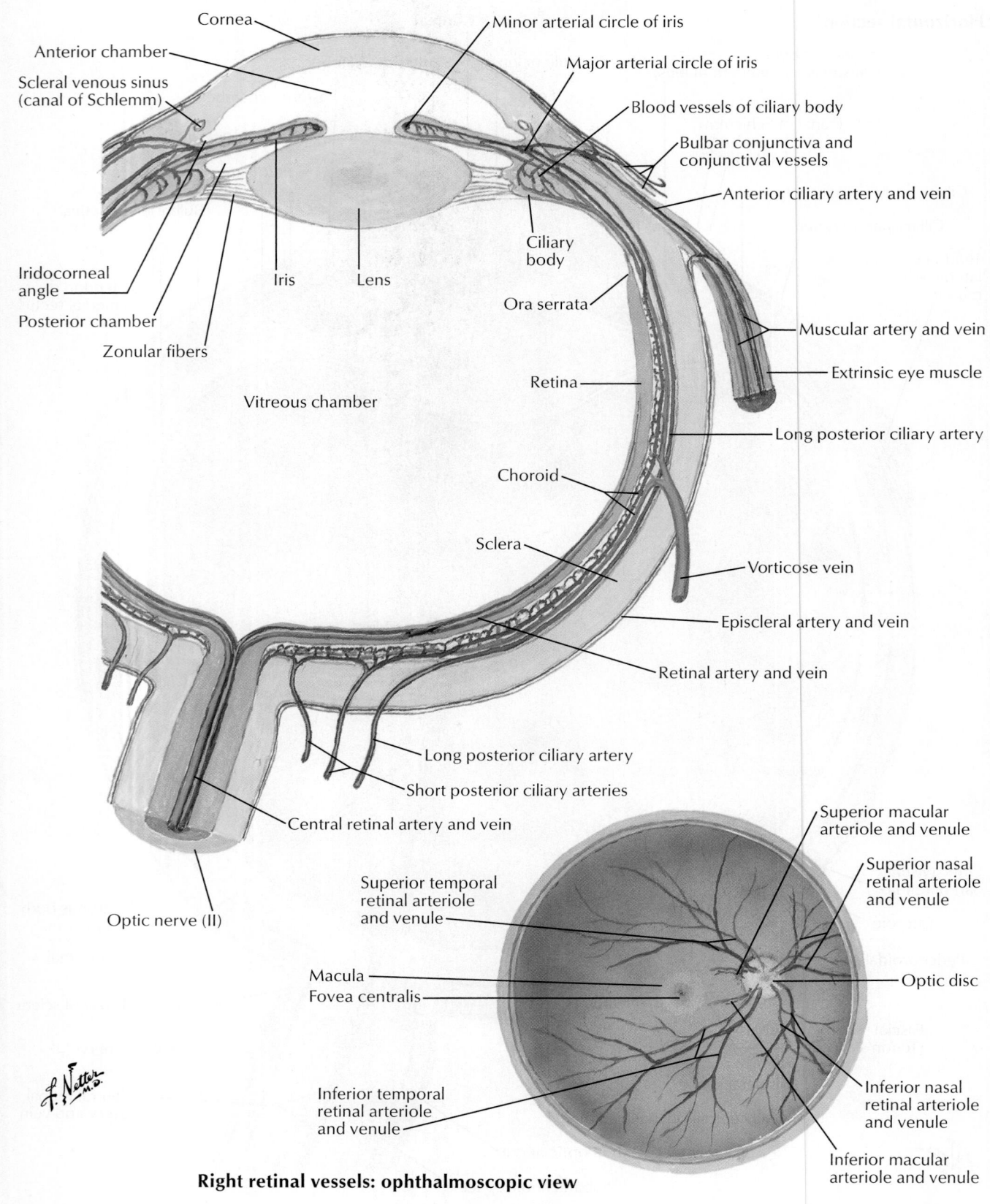

Cornea

Minor arterial circle of iris

Anterior chamber

Major arterial circle of iris

Scleral venous sinus
(canal of Schlemm)

Blood vessels of ciliary body

Bulbar conjunctiva and
conjunctival vessels

Anterior ciliary artery and vein

Iridocorneal
angle

Iris

Lens

Ciliary
body

Ora serrata

Muscular artery and vein

Posterior chamber

Extrinsic eye muscle

Zonular fibers

Retina

Long posterior ciliary artery

Vitreous chamber

Choroid

Sclera

Vorticose vein

Episcleral artery and vein

Retinal artery and vein

Long posterior ciliary artery

Short posterior ciliary arteries

Central retinal artery and vein

Optic nerve (II)

Superior macular
arteriole and venule

Superior nasal
retinal arteriole
and venule

Superior temporal
retinal arteriole
and venule

Macula

Fovea centralis

Optic disc

Inferior temporal
retinal arteriole
and venule

Inferior nasal
retinal arteriole
and venule

Inferior macular
arteriole and venule

Right retinal vessels: ophthalmoscopic view

Plate 90   Intrinsic Arteries and Veins of Eye. (Netter: Atlas of Human Anatomy, 4 ed, 2006, Saunders.)

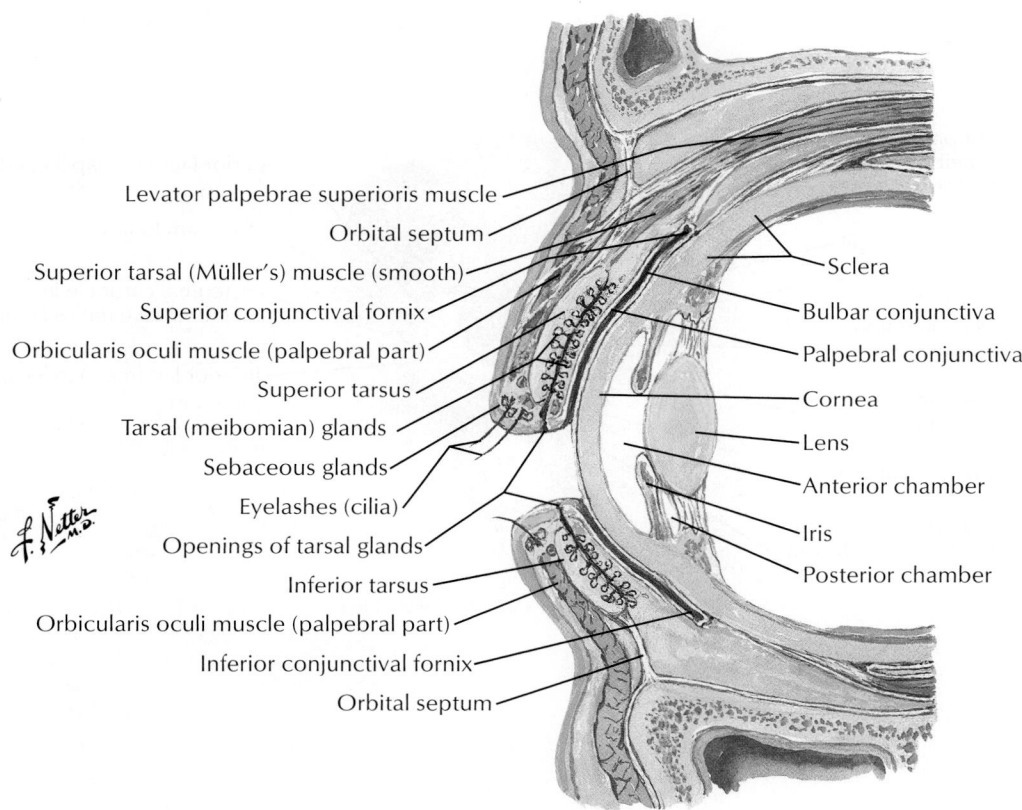

Levator palpebrae superioris muscle
Orbital septum
Superior tarsal (Müller's) muscle (smooth)
Superior conjunctival fornix
Orbicularis oculi muscle (palpebral part)
Superior tarsus
Tarsal (meibomian) glands
Sebaceous glands
Eyelashes (cilia)
Openings of tarsal glands
Inferior tarsus
Orbicularis oculi muscle (palpebral part)
Inferior conjunctival fornix
Orbital septum

Sclera
Bulbar conjunctiva
Palpebral conjunctiva
Cornea
Lens
Anterior chamber
Iris
Posterior chamber

Plate 81, Middle   Eyelids. (Netter: Atlas of Human Anatomy, 4 ed, 2006, Saunders.)

Superior palpebral conjunctiva: tarsal (meibomian) glands shining through

Seen through cornea { Pupil
Iris

Corneoscleral junction (corneal limbus)

Bulbar conjunctiva over sclera

Inferior conjunctival fornix

Inferior palpebral conjunctiva: tarsal glands shining through

Superior lacrimal papilla and punctum

Plica semilunaris

Lacrimal caruncle in lacrimal lake (lacus lacrimalis)

Inferior lacrimal papilla and punctum

Plate 81, Upper Eyelid. (Netter: Atlas of Human Anatomy, 4 ed, 2006, Saunders.)

Orbital part of lacrimal gland

Palpebral part of lacrimal gland

Excretory ducts of lacrimal gland

Plica semilunaris

Lacrimal caruncle

Inferior lacrimal papilla and punctum

Superior lacrimal papilla and punctum

Lacrimal canaliculi

Lacrimal sac

Nasolacrimal duct

Opening of nasolacrimal duct

Frontal bone (cut away)

Orbital part of lacrimal gland

Palpebral part of lacrimal gland

Excretory ducts of lacrimal gland

Plica semilunaris and lacrimal lake

Lacrimal caruncle

Inferior lacrimal papilla and punctum

Opening of nasolacrimal duct

Superior lacrimal papilla and punctum

Lacrimal canaliculi

Lacrimal sac

Nasolacrimal duct

Middle nasal concha

Nasal cavity

Inferior nasal concha (cut)

Inferior nasal meatus

Plate 82   Lacrimal Apparatus. (Netter: Atlas of Human Anatomy, 4 ed, 2006, Saunders.)

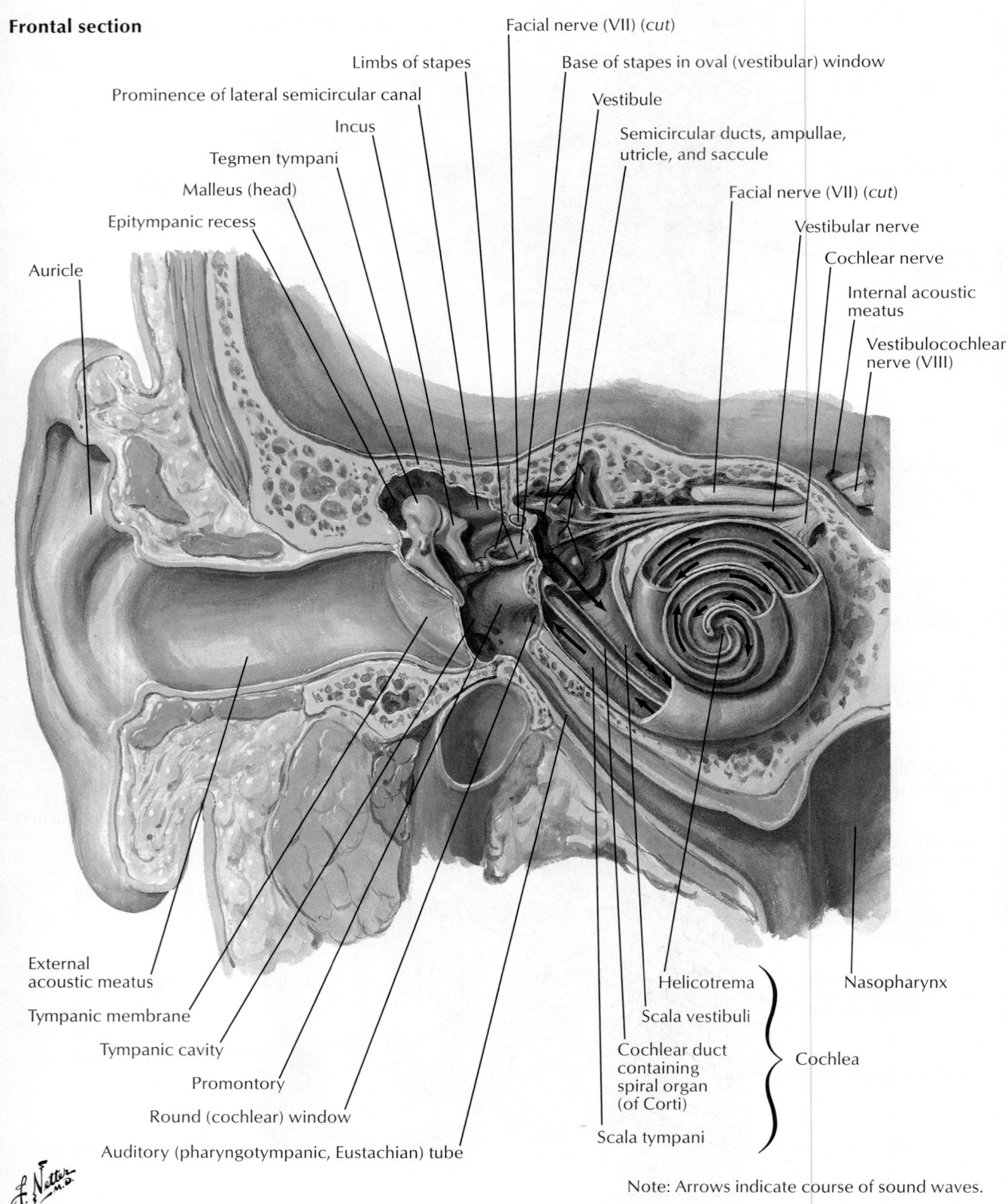

Facial nerve (VII) (*cut*)

Limbs of stapes

Base of stapes in oval (vestibular) window

Prominence of lateral semicircular canal

Vestibule

Incus

Semicircular ducts, ampullae, utricle, and saccule

Tegmen tympani

Malleus (head)

Facial nerve (VII) (*cut*)

Epitympanic recess

Vestibular nerve

Auricle

Cochlear nerve

Internal acoustic meatus

Vestibulocochlear nerve (VIII)

External acoustic meatus

Tympanic membrane

Tympanic cavity

Promontory

Round (cochlear) window

Auditory (pharyngotympanic, Eustachian) tube

Helicotrema

Scala vestibuli

Cochlear duct containing spiral organ (of Corti)

Scala tympani

Cochlea

Nasopharynx

Note: Arrows indicate course of sound waves.

Plate 92 Pathway of Sound Reception. (Netter: Atlas of Human Anatomy, 4 ed, 2006, Saunders.)

Medial wall of tympanic cavity: lateral view

Mastoid antrum

Prominence of lateral semicircular canal

Prominence of facial canal

Geniculum (geniculate ganglion) of facial nerve

Greater petrosal nerve

Base of stapes in fossa of oval (vestibular) window

Limbs of stapes

Pyramidal eminence

Chorda tympani nerve (cut)

Mastoid cells

Tendon of stapedius muscle

Fossa of round (cochlear) window

Facial nerve (VII) in stylomastoid foramen

Jugular fossa

Tympanic cells

Tensor tympani muscle (tendon cut)

Auditory (pharyngotympanic, Eustachian) tube

Levator veli palatini muscle

Promontory with tympanic nerve (of Jacobson) and plexus under mucosa

Internal carotid artery

Plate 94 Tympanic Cavity. (Netter: Atlas of Human Anatomy, 4 ed, 2006, Saunders.)

Otoscopic view of right tympanic membrane

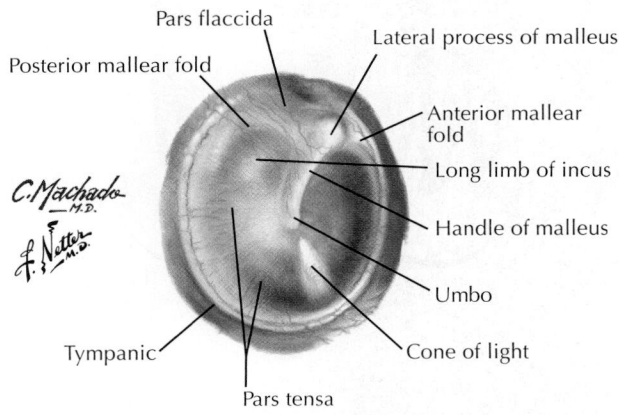

Pars flaccida

Posterior mallear fold

Lateral process of malleus

Anterior mallear fold

Long limb of incus

Handle of malleus

Umbo

Cone of light

Tympanic

Pars tensa

Plate 93 Tympanic Cavity. (Netter: Atlas of Human Anatomy, 4 ed, 2006, Saunders.)

Dissected right bony labyrinth (otic capsule): membranous labyrinth removed

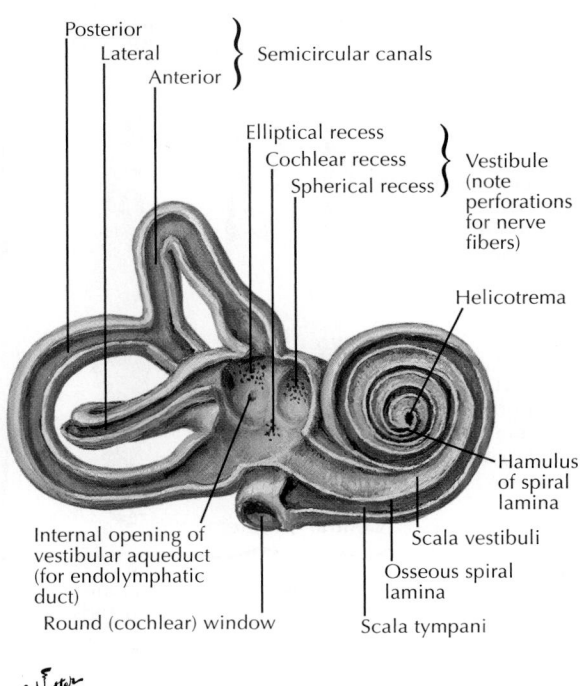

Posterior

Lateral

Anterior

Semicircular canals

Elliptical recess

Cochlear recess

Spherical recess

Vestibule (note perforations for nerve fibers)

Helicotrema

Hamulus of spiral lamina

Scala vestibuli

Osseous spiral lamina

Scala tympani

Internal opening of vestibular aqueduct (for endolymphatic duct)

Round (cochlear) window

Plate 95 Bony Membranous Labyrinth. (Netter: Atlas of Human Anatomy, 4 ed, 2006, Saunders.)

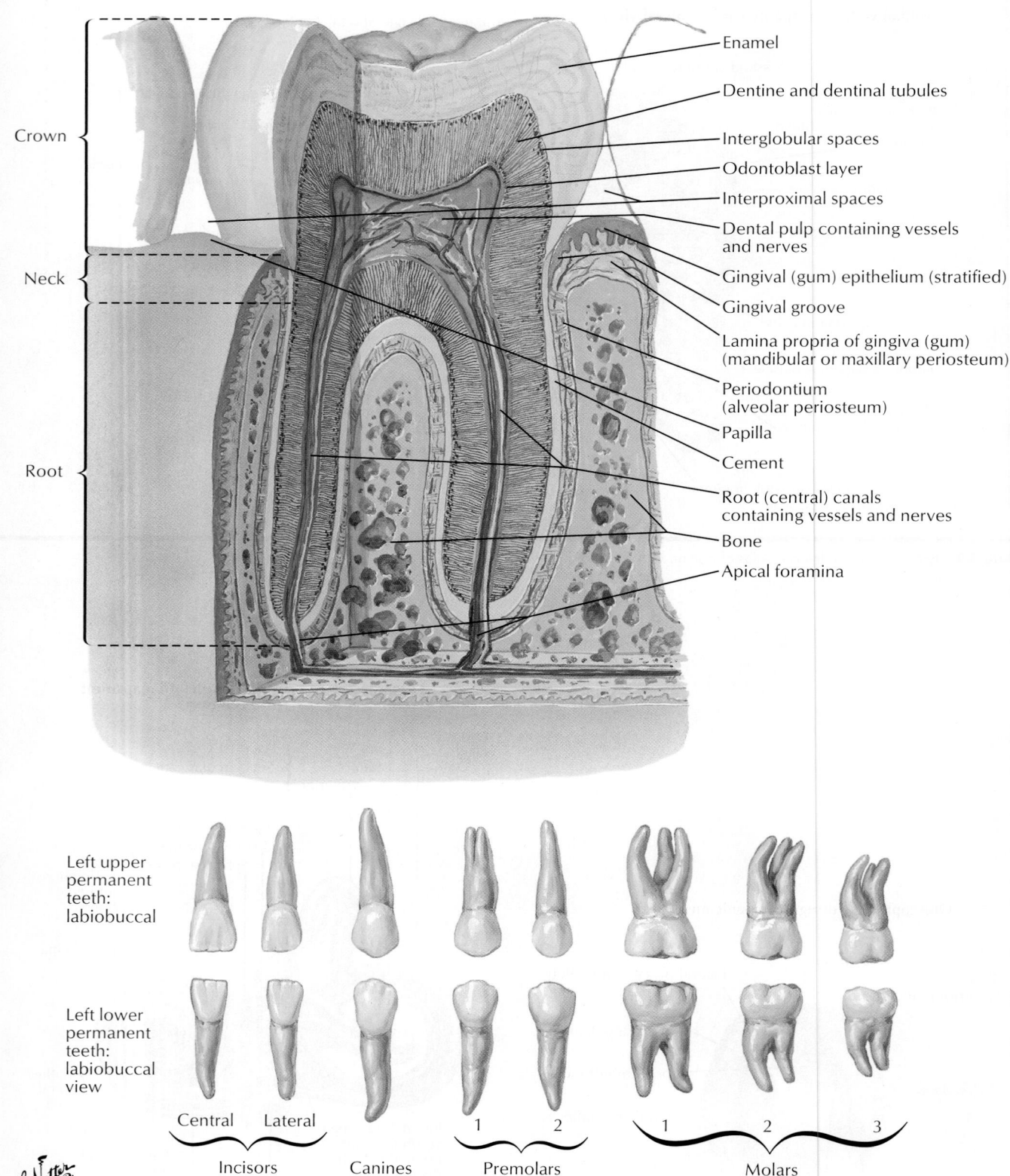

Enamel

Dentine and dentinal tubules

Interglobular spaces

Odontoblast layer

Interproximal spaces

Dental pulp containing vessels and nerves

Gingival (gum) epithelium (stratified)

Gingival groove

Lamina propria of gingiva (gum) (mandibular or maxillary periosteum)

Periodontium (alveolar periosteum)

Papilla

Cement

Root (central) canals containing vessels and nerves

Bone

Apical foramina

Crown

Neck

Root

Left upper permanent teeth: labiobuccal

Left lower permanent teeth: labiobuccal view

Central   Lateral

Incisors

Canines (cuspids)

1   2

Premolars

1   2   3

Molars

Plate 57   Teeth. (Netter: Atlas of Human Anatomy, 4 ed, 2006, Saunders.)

Tongue

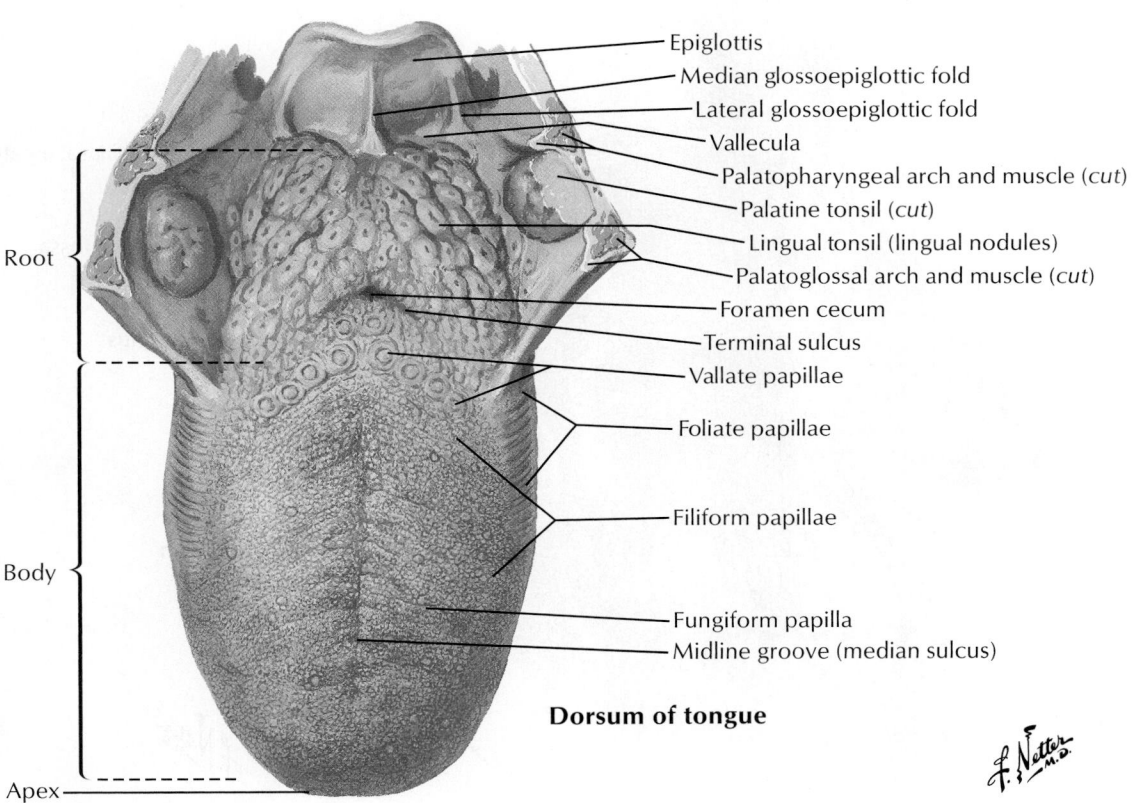

Epiglottis

Median glossoepiglottic fold

Lateral glossoepiglottic fold

Vallecula

Palatopharyngeal arch and muscle (*cut*)

Palatine tonsil (*cut*)

Lingual tonsil (lingual nodules)

Palatoglossal arch and muscle (*cut*)

Foramen cecum

Terminal sulcus

Vallate papillae

Foliate papillae

Filiform papillae

Fungiform papilla

Midline groove (median sulcus)

Root

Body

Apex

Dorsum of tongue

Plate 58   Tongue. (Netter: Atlas of Human Anatomy, 4 ed, 2006, Saunders.)

71

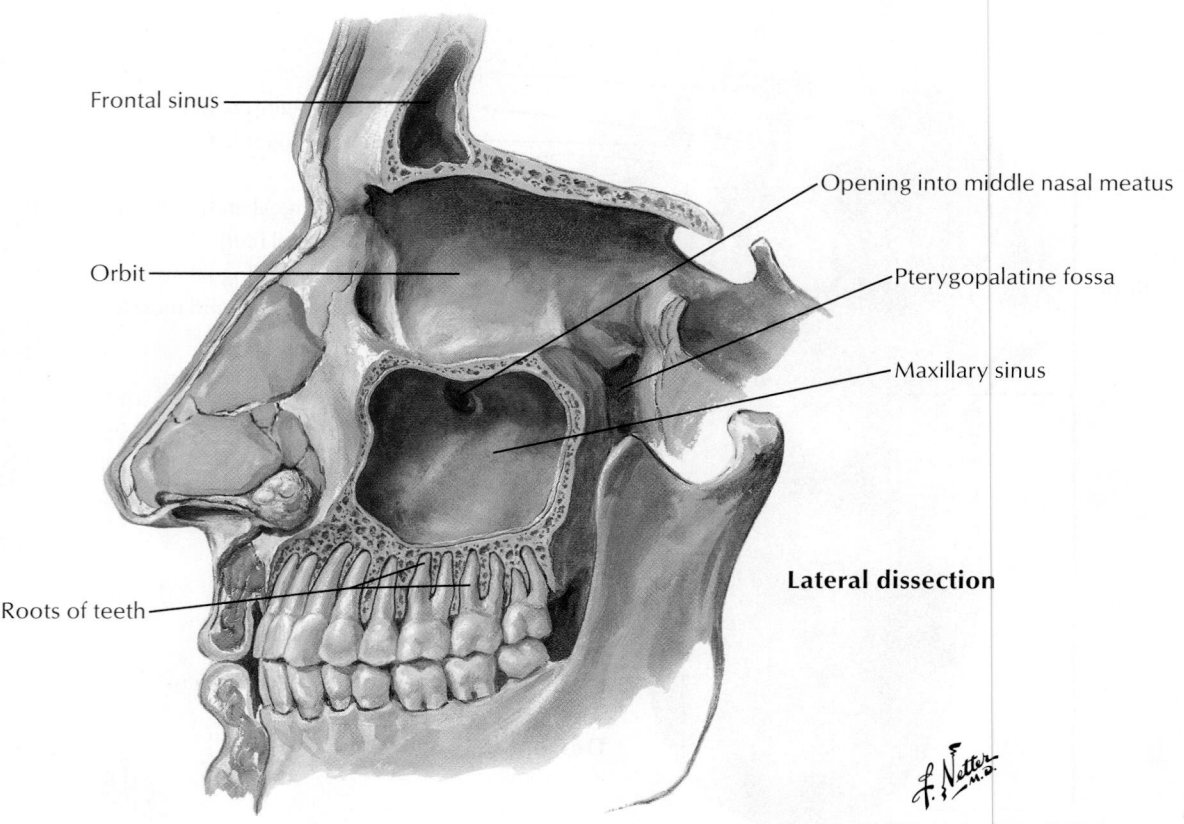

Frontal sinus

Opening into middle nasal meatus

Orbit

Pterygopalatine fossa

Maxillary sinus

Roots of teeth

Lateral dissection

Plate 49 Paranasal Sinuses. (Netter: Atlas of Human Anatomy, 4 ed, 2006, Saunders.)

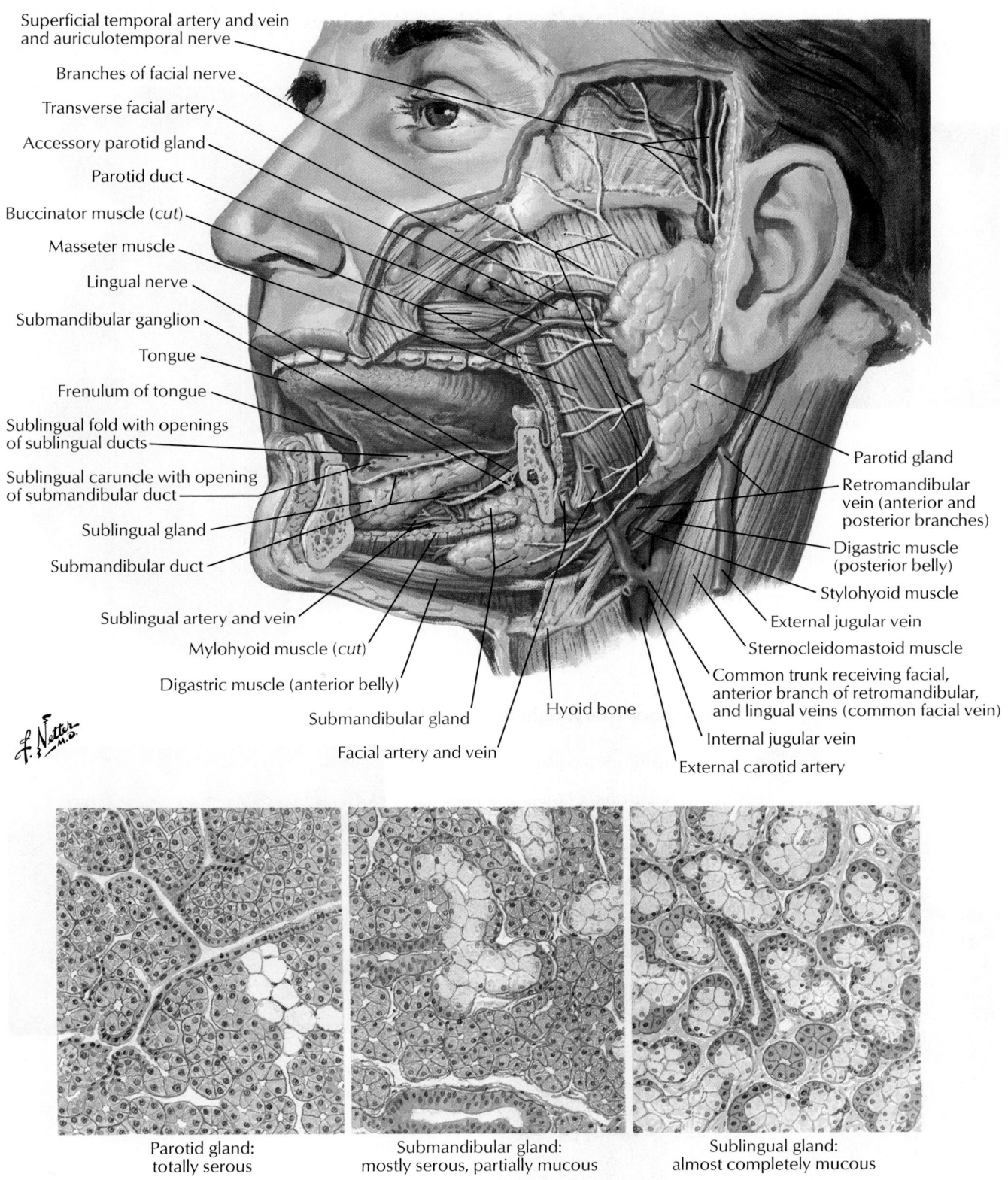

Superficial temporal artery and vein and auriculotemporal nerve

Branches of facial nerve

Transverse facial artery

Accessory parotid gland

Parotid duct

Buccinator muscle (*cut*)

Masseter muscle

Lingual nerve

Submandibular ganglion

Tongue

Frenulum of tongue

Sublingual fold with openings of sublingual ducts

Sublingual caruncle with opening of submandibular duct

Sublingual gland

Submandibular duct

Sublingual artery and vein

Mylohyoid muscle (*cut*)

Digastric muscle (anterior belly)

Submandibular gland

Facial artery and vein

Hyoid bone

Parotid gland

Retromandibular vein (anterior and posterior branches)

Digastric muscle (posterior belly)

Stylohyoid muscle

External jugular vein

Sternocleidomastoid muscle

Common trunk receiving facial, anterior branch of retromandibular, and lingual veins (common facial vein)

Internal jugular vein

External carotid artery

Parotid gland: totally serous

Submandibular gland: mostly serous, partially mucous

Sublingual gland: almost completely mucous

Plate 61   Salivary Glands. (Netter: Atlas of Human Anatomy, 4 ed, 2006, Saunders.)

Coronary Arteries: Arteriographic Views

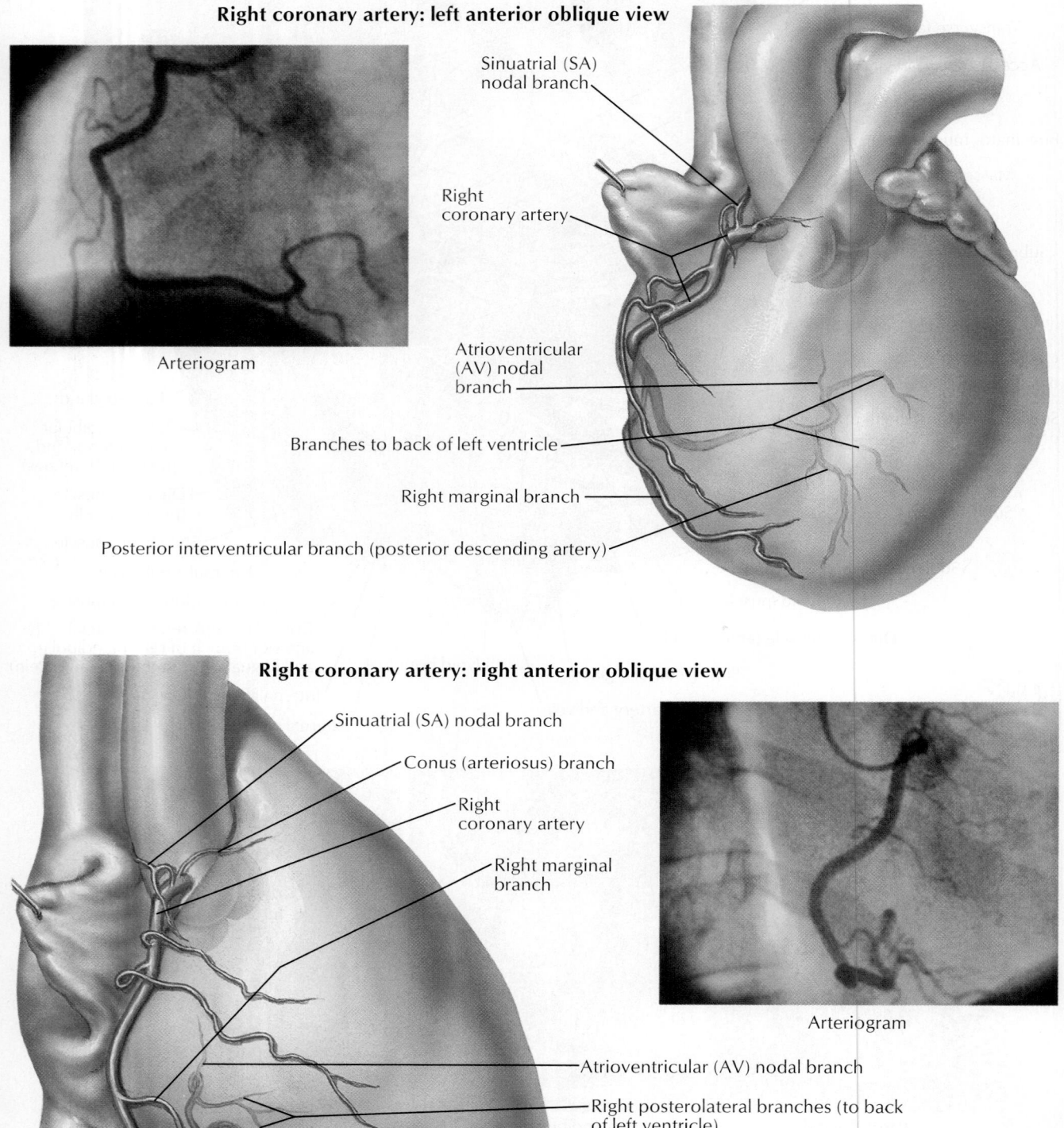

Right coronary artery: left anterior oblique view

Arteriogram

Sinuatrial (SA) nodal branch

Right coronary artery

Atrioventricular (AV) nodal branch

Branches to back of left ventricle

Right marginal branch

Posterior interventricular branch (posterior descending artery)

Right coronary artery: right anterior oblique view

Sinuatrial (SA) nodal branch

Conus (arteriosus) branch

Right coronary artery

Right marginal branch

Arteriogram

Atrioventricular (AV) nodal branch

Right posterolateral branches (to back of left ventricle)

Posterior interventricular branch (posterior descending artery)

Plate 218 Coronary Arteries: Arteriographic Views. (Netter: Atlas of Human Anatomy, 4 ed, 2006, Saunders.)

Left coronary artery: left anterior oblique view

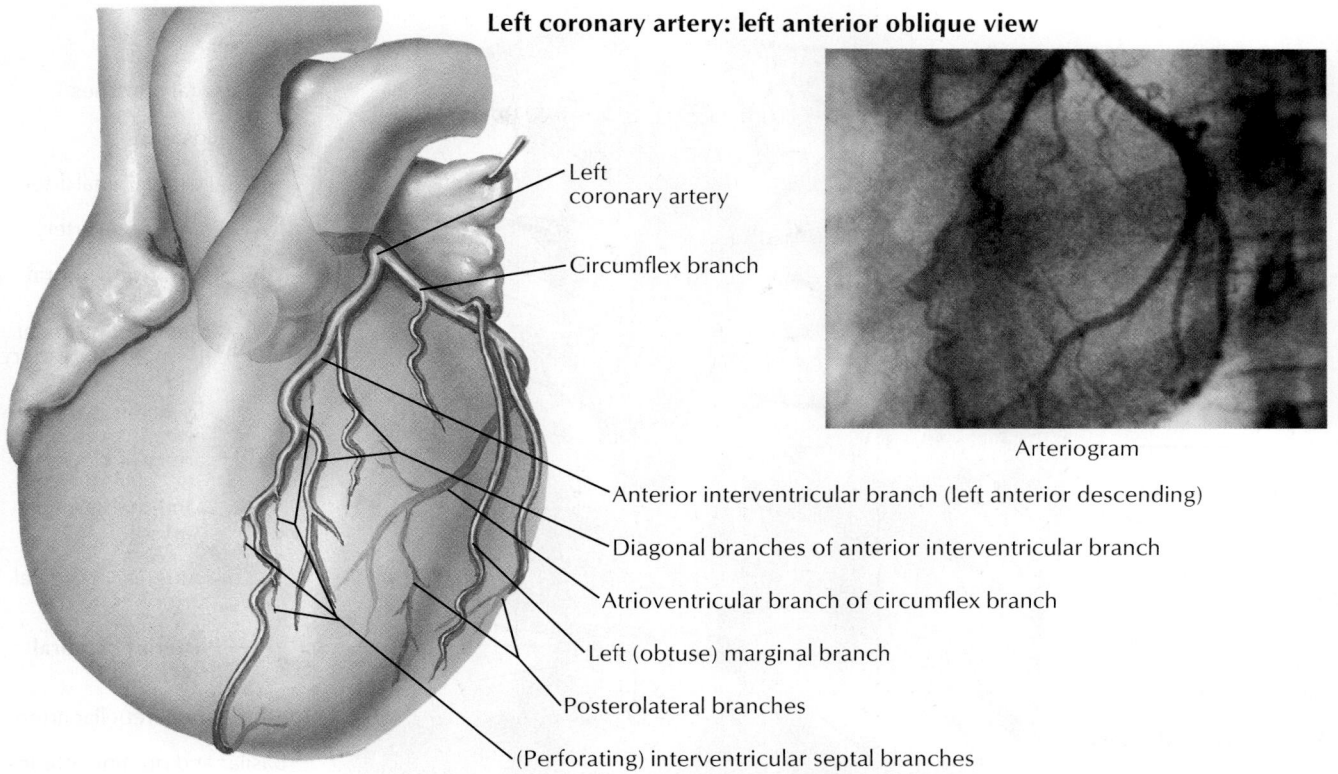

Left coronary artery

Circumflex branch

Arteriogram

Anterior interventricular branch (left anterior descending)

Diagonal branches of anterior interventricular branch

Atrioventricular branch of circumflex branch

Left (obtuse) marginal branch

Posterolateral branches

(Perforating) interventricular septal branches

Left coronary artery: right anterior oblique view

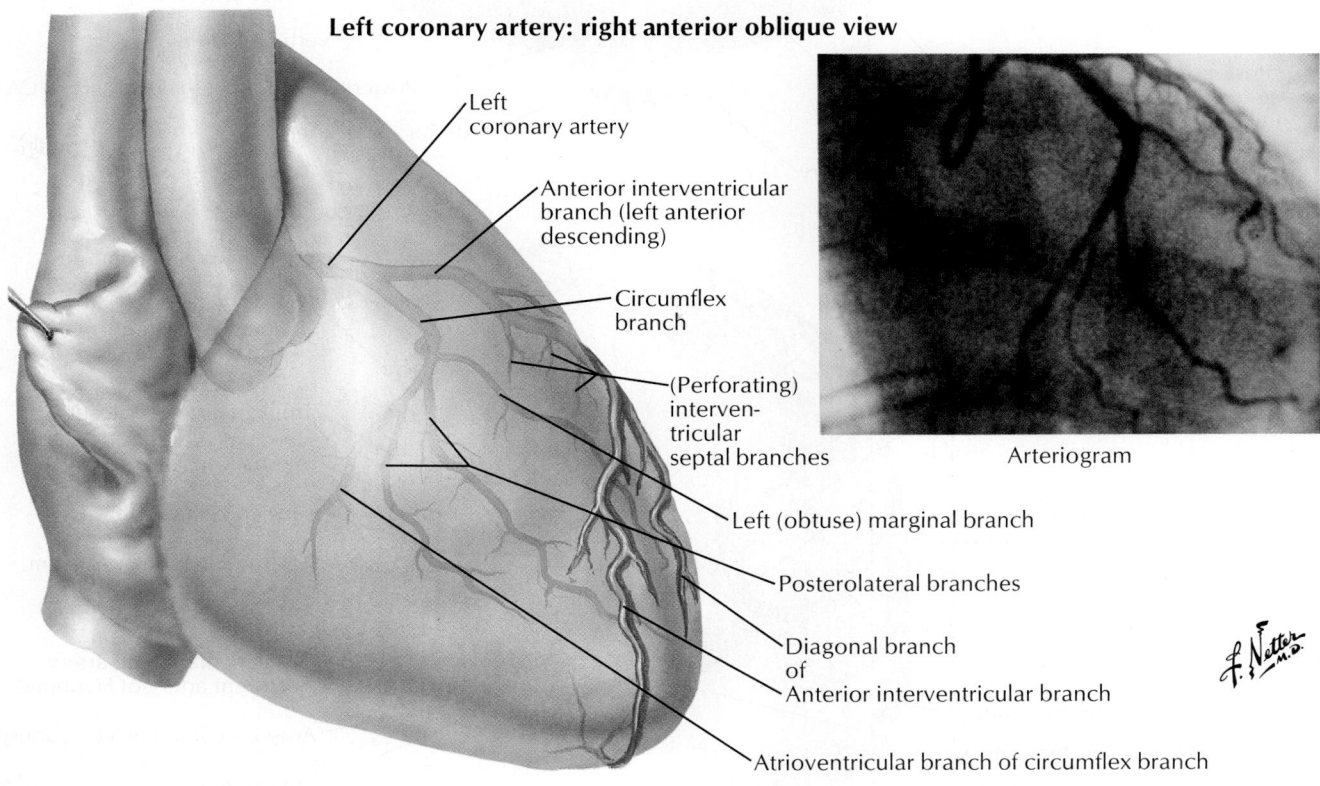

Left coronary artery

Anterior interventricular branch (left anterior descending)

Circumflex branch

(Perforating) interventricular septal branches

Arteriogram

Left (obtuse) marginal branch

Posterolateral branches

Diagonal branch of Anterior interventricular branch

Atrioventricular branch of circumflex branch

Plate 219   Coronary Arteries: Arteriographic Views. (Netter: Atlas of Human Anatomy, 4 ed, 2006, Saunders.)

Corpus callosum

Anterolateral central
(lenticulostriate) arteries

Lateral frontobasal
(orbitofrontal) artery

Prefrontal artery

Precentral (pre-Rolandic)
and central (Rolandic)
sulcal arteries

Anterior parietal
(postcentral sulcal)
artery

Posterior parietal
artery

Branch to
angular gyrus

Temporal branches
(anterior, middle,
and posterior)

Middle cerebral artery
and branches
(deep in lateral cerebral
[Sylvian] sulcus)

Anterior communicating artery

Posterior communicating artery

Anterior inferior cerebellar artery (AICA)

Posterior spinal artery

Paracentral artery

Medial frontal branches

Pericallosal artery

Callosomarginal artery

Polar frontal artery

**Anterior cerebral
arteries**

Medial frontobasal
(orbitofrontal) artery

Distal medial striate
artery (recurrent
artery of Heubner)

Internal carotid
artery

Anterior choroidal
artery

**Posterior cerebral
artery**

Superior cerebellar artery

Basilar and pontine arteries

Labyrinthine (internal
acoustic) artery

Vertebral artery

Posterior inferior cerebellar artery (PICA)

Anterior spinal artery

Falx cerebri

Corpus striatum
(caudate and lentiform nuclei)

Anterolateral central
(lenticulostriate) arteries

Insula (island of Reil)

Limen of insula

Precentral (pre-Rolandic),
central (Rolandic) sulcal,
and parietal arteries

Lateral cerebral (Sylvian) sulcus

Temporal branches of
middle cerebral artery

Temporal lobe

Middle cerebral artery

Internal carotid artery

Callosomarginal arteries
and
Pericallosal arteries
(branches of anterior
cerebral arteries)

Trunk of corpus callosum

Internal capsule

Septum pellucidum

Rostrum of corpus callosum

Anterior cerebral arteries

Distal medial striate artery
(recurrent artery of Heubner)

Anterior communicating artery

Optic chiasm

Plate 141   Arteries of Brain: Frontal View and Section. (Netter: Atlas of Human Anatomy, 4 ed, 2006, Saunders.)

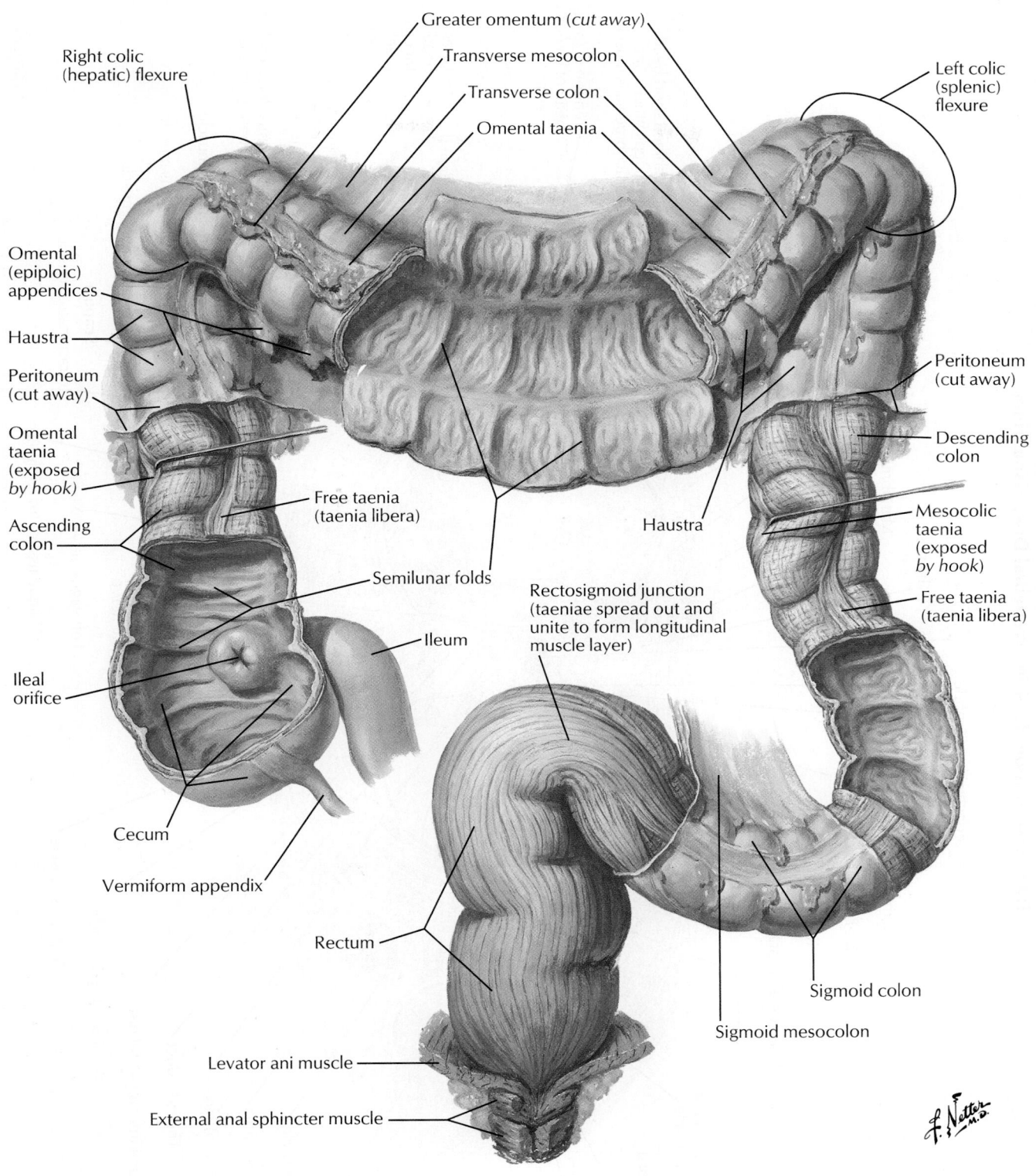

Greater omentum (*cut away*)

Transverse mesocolon

Transverse colon

Omental taenia

Right colic (hepatic) flexure

Left colic (splenic) flexure

Omental (epiploic) appendices

Haustra

Peritoneum (cut away)

Omental taenia (exposed *by hook*)

Ascending colon

Ileal orifice

Free taenia (taenia libera)

Semilunar folds

Ileum

Haustra

Peritoneum (cut away)

Descending colon

Mesocolic taenia (exposed *by hook*)

Free taenia (taenia libera)

Cecum

Vermiform appendix

Rectosigmoid junction (taeniae spread out and unite to form longitudinal muscle layer)

Rectum

Sigmoid colon

Sigmoid mesocolon

Levator ani muscle

External anal sphincter muscle

Plate 284 Mucosa and Musculature of Large Intestine. (Netter: Atlas of Human Anatomy, 4 ed, 2006, Saunders.)

Transverse Section: T3–4 Intervertebral Disc, Manubrium

Plate 244

T3–4

Superior tracheobronchial lymph node

Trachea

Superior vena cava

Right phrenic nerve

Thymus

Manubrium

Arch of aorta

Internal thoracic artery and vein

Pectoralis major muscle

Pectoralis minor muscle

Axillary fossa

Combined short head of biceps brachii and coracobrachialis muscles

Tendon of long head of biceps brachii muscle

Shaft of humerus

Lateral head of triceps brachii muscle

Long head of triceps brachii muscle

Left latissimus dorsi tendon (inserting onto humerus)

Teres major muscle

Subscapularis muscle

Teres minor muscle

Scapula

Infraspinatus muscle

Left lung

Ribs

Arch of azygos vein

Right lung

Intercostal muscles

Serratus anterior muscle

Tendon of long head of biceps brachii muscle

Latissimus dorsi tendon

Shaft of humerus

Deltoid muscle

Long head of triceps brachii muscle

Teres major muscle

Teres minor muscle

Scapula

Esophagus

Thoracic duct

T3–4 intervertebral disc

Rhomboid muscle

Trapezius muscle

Spinal cord

Left recurrent laryngeal nerve

Left vagus nerve (X)

Oblique fissure (of left lung)

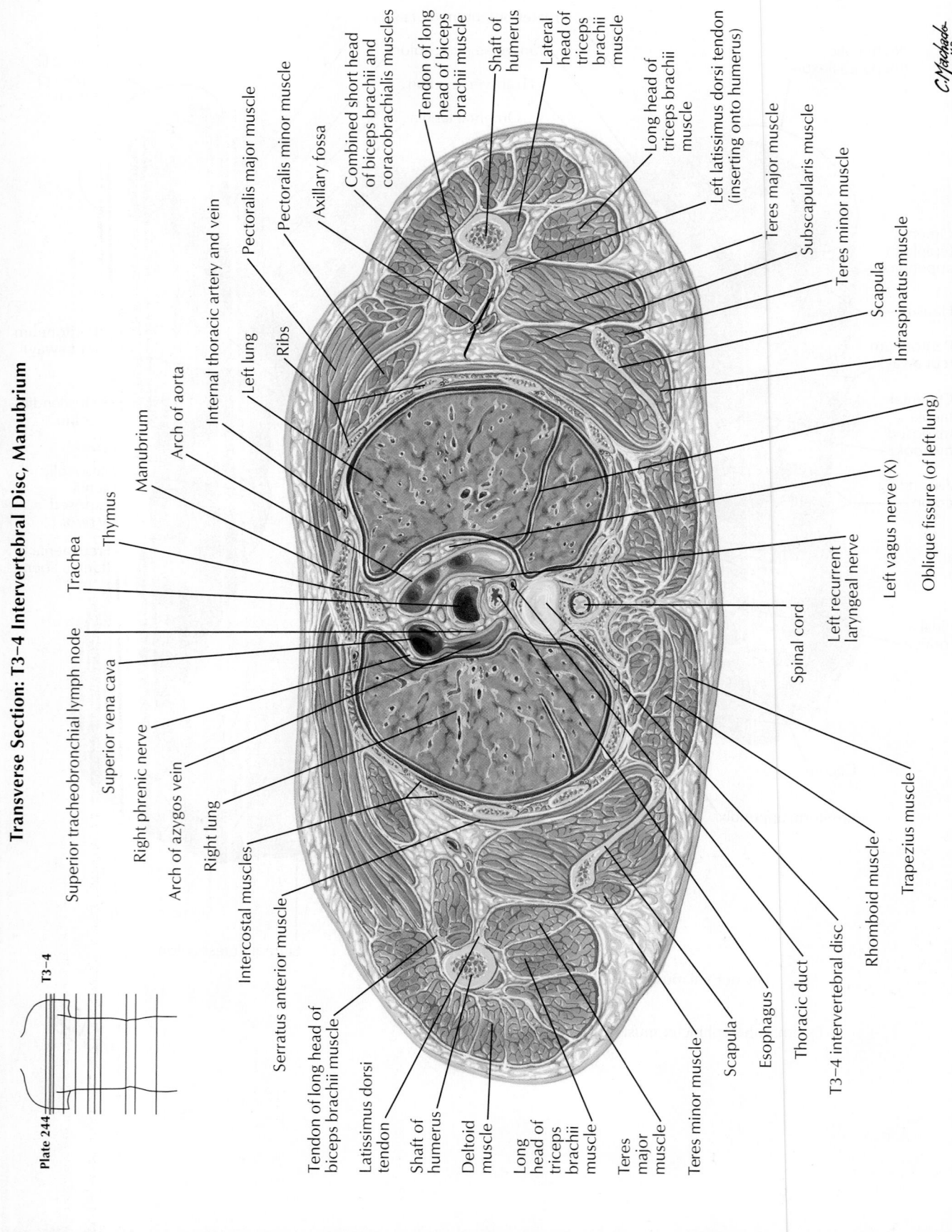

C. Machado ___M.D.

Plate 244 Cross Section of Thorax at T3-4 Disc Level. (Netter: Atlas of Human Anatomy, 4 ed, 2006, Saunders.)

Right knee in extension: posterior view

Posterior cruciate ligament

Anterior cruciate ligament

Posterior meniscofemoral ligament

Lateral condyle of femur (articular surface)

Popliteus tendon

Fibular collateral ligament

Lateral meniscus

Head of fibula

Adductor tubercle on medial epicondyle of femur

Medial condyle of femur (articular surface)

Medial meniscus

Tibial collateral ligament

Medial condyle of tibia

NETTER'S ANATOMY ILLUSTRATIONS

Plate 509   Knee: Cruciate and Collateral Ligaments. (Netter: Atlas of Human Anatomy, 4 ed, 2006, Saunders.)

Paramedian (sagittal) dissection

Ureter

Uterine (fallopian) tube

Ovary

Ligament of ovary

Round ligament of uterus

Broad ligament (*cut*)

Superior pubic ramus (*cut*)

Inferior pubic ramus (*cut*)

Ischiocavernosus muscle

Body of clitoris

Labia minora

Labium majus

Rectouterine pouch (of Douglas)

Peritoneum (*cut edge*)

Vesicouterine pouch

Rectum

Ureter

Urinary bladder

Vagina

Pelvic diaphragm (levator ani muscle)

Deep transverse perineal muscle (*cut*)

External anal sphincter muscle

Median (sagittal) section

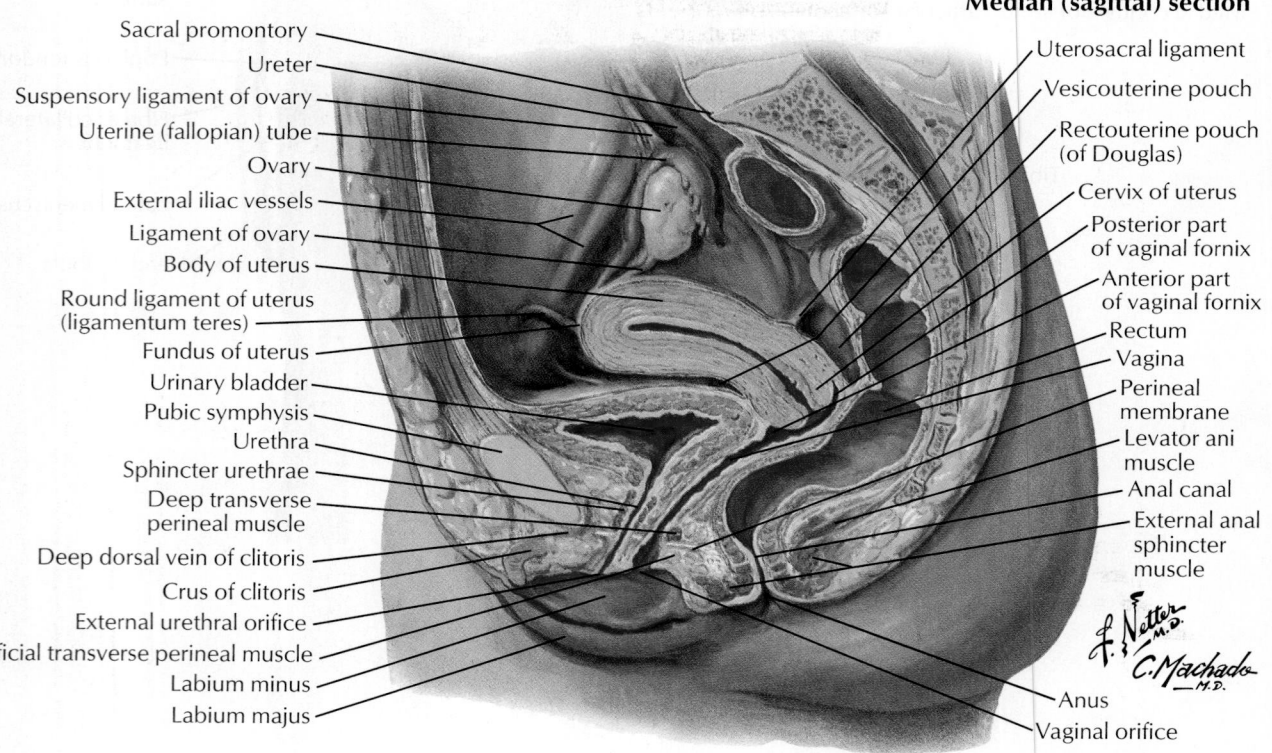

Sacral promontory

Ureter

Suspensory ligament of ovary

Uterine (fallopian) tube

Ovary

External iliac vessels

Ligament of ovary

Body of uterus

Round ligament of uterus (ligamentum teres)

Fundus of uterus

Urinary bladder

Pubic symphysis

Urethra

Sphincter urethrae

Deep transverse perineal muscle

Deep dorsal vein of clitoris

Crus of clitoris

External urethral orifice

Superficial transverse perineal muscle

Labium minus

Labium majus

Uterosacral ligament

Vesicouterine pouch

Rectouterine pouch (of Douglas)

Cervix of uterus

Posterior part of vaginal fornix

Anterior part of vaginal fornix

Rectum

Vagina

Perineal membrane

Levator ani muscle

Anal canal

External anal sphincter muscle

Anus

Vaginal orifice

Plate 360 Pelvic Viscera and Perineum: Female. (Netter: Atlas of Human Anatomy, 4 ed, 2006, Saunders.)

Alphabetic Index

ICD-10-CM INDEX TO DISEASES AND INJURIES

A

Aarskog's syndrome Q87.1
Abandonment —*see* Maltreatment
Abasia (-astasia) (hysterical) F44.4
Abderhalden-Kaufmann-Lignac syndrome (cystinosis) E72.04
Abdomen, abdominal —*see also* condition
  acute R10.0
  angina K55.1
  muscle deficiency syndrome Q79.4
Abdominalgia —*see* Pain, abdominal
Abduction contracture, hip or other joint —*see* Contraction, joint
Aberrant (congenital) —*see also* Malposition, congenital
  adrenal gland Q89.1
  artery (peripheral) Q27.8
    basilar NEC Q28.1
    cerebral Q28.3
    coronary Q24.5
    digestive system Q27.8
    eye Q15.8
    lower limb Q27.8
    precerebral Q28.1
    pulmonary Q25.79
    renal Q27.2
    retina Q14.1
    specified site NEC Q27.8
    subclavian Q27.8
    upper limb Q27.8
    vertebral Q28.1
  breast Q83.8
  endocrine gland NEC Q89.2
  hepatic duct Q44.5
  pancreas Q45.3
  parathyroid gland Q89.2
  pituitary gland Q89.2
  sebaceous glands, mucous membrane, mouth, congenital Q38.6
  spleen Q89.09
  subclavian artery Q27.8
  thymus (gland) Q89.2
  thyroid gland Q89.2
  vein (peripheral) NEC Q27.8
    cerebral Q28.3
    digestive system Q27.8
    lower limb Q27.8
    precerebral Q28.1
    specified site NEC Q27.8
    upper limb Q27.8
Aberration
  distantial —*see* Disturbance, visual
  mental F99
Abetalipoproteinemia E78.6
Abiotrophy R68.89
Ablatio, ablation
  retinae —*see* Detachment, retina
Ablepharia, ablepharon Q10.3
Abnormal, abnormality, abnormalities —*see also* Anomaly
  acid-base balance (mixed) E87.4
  albumin R77.0
  alphafetoprotein R77.2
  alveolar ridge K08.9
  anatomical relationship Q89.9
  apertures, congenital, diaphragm Q79.1
  auditory perception H93.29-
    diplacusis —*see* Diplacusis
    hyperacusis —*see* Hyperacusis
    recruitment —*see* Recruitment, auditory
    threshold shift —*see* Shift, auditory threshold
  autosomes Q99.9
    fragile site Q95.5
  basal metabolic rate R94.8
  biosynthesis, testicular androgen E29.1
  bleeding time R79.1

Abnormal, abnormality, abnormalities — (*Continued*)
  blood level (of)
    cobalt R79.0
    copper R79.0
    iron R79.0
    lithium R78.89
    magnesium R79.0
    mineral NEC R79.0
    zinc R79.0
  blood pressure
    elevated R03.0
    low reading (nonspecific) R03.1
  blood sugar R73.09
  blood-gas level R79.81
  bowel sounds R19.15
    absent R19.11
    hyperactive R19.12
  brain scan R94.02
  breathing R06.9
  caloric test R94.138
  cerebrospinal fluid R83.9
    cytology R83.6
    drug level R83.2
    enzyme level R83.0
    hormones R83.1
    immunology R83.4
    microbiology R83.5
    nonmedicinal level R83.3
    specified type NEC R83.8
  chemistry, blood R79.9
    C-reactive protein R79.82
    drugs —*see* Findings, abnormal, in blood
    gas level R79.81
    minerals R79.0
    pancytopenia D61.818
    PTT R79.1
    specified NEC R79.89
    toxins —*see* Findings, abnormal, in blood
  chest sounds (friction) (rales) R09.89
  chromosome, chromosomal Q99.9
    with more than three X chromosomes, female Q97.1
    analysis result R89.8
      bronchial washings R84.8
      cerebrospinal fluid R83.8
      cervix uteri NEC R87.89
      nasal secretions R84.8
      nipple discharge R89.8
      peritoneal fluid R85.89
      pleural fluid R84.8
      prostatic secretions R86.8
      saliva R85.89
      seminal fluid R86.8
      sputum R84.8
      synovial fluid R89.8
      throat scrapings R84.8
      vagina R87.89
      vulva R87.89
      wound secretions R89.8
    dicentric replacement Q93.2
    ring replacement Q93.2
    sex Q99.8
      female phenotype Q97.9
        specified NEC Q97.8
      male phenotype Q98.9
        specified NEC Q98.8
      structural male Q98.6
    specified NEC Q99.8
  clinical findings NEC R68.89
  coagulation D68.9
    newborn, transient P61.6
    profile R79.1
    time R79.1
  communication —*see* Fistula
  conjunctiva, vascular H11.41-
  coronary artery Q24.5
  cortisol-binding globulin E27.8
  course, eustachian tube Q17.8

Abnormal, abnormality, abnormalities — (*Continued*)
  creatinine clearance R94.4
  cytology
    anus R85.619
      atypical squamous cells cannot exclude high grade squamous intraepithelial lesion (ASC-H) R85.611
      atypical squamous cells of undetermined significance (ASC-US) R85.610
      cytologic evidence of malignancy R85.614
      high grade squamous intraepithelial lesion (HGSIL) R85.613
      human papillomavirus (HPV) DNA test
        high risk positive R85.81
        low risk postive R85.82
      inadequate smear R85.615
      low grade squamous intraepithelial lesion (LGSIL) R85.612
      satisfactory anal smear but lacking transformation zone R85.616
      specified NEC R85.618
      unsatisfactory smear R85.615
    female genital organs —*see* Abnormal, Papanicolaou (smear)
  dark adaptation curve H53.61
  dentofacial NEC —*see* Anomaly, dentofacial
  development, developmental Q89.9
    central nervous system Q07.9
  diagnostic imaging
    abdomen, abdominal region NEC R93.5
    biliary tract R93.2
    bladder R93.41 ◀
    breast R92.8
    central nervous system NEC R90.89
    cerebrovascular NEC R90.89
    coronary circulation R93.1
    digestive tract NEC R93.3
    gastrointestinal (tract) R93.3
    genitourinary organs R93.8
    head R93.0
    heart R93.1
    intrathoracic organ NEC R93.8
    kidney R93.42- ◀
    limbs R93.6
    liver R93.2
    lung (field) R91.8
    musculoskeletal system NEC R93.7
    renal pelvis R93.41 ◀
    retroperitoneum R93.5
    site specified NEC R93.8
    skin and subcutaneous tissue R93.8
    skull R93.0
    ~~urinary organs R93.4~~
    urinary organs specified NEC R93.49 ◀
    ureter R93.41 ◀
  direction, teeth, fully erupted M26.30
  ear ossicles, acquired NEC H74.39-
    ankylosis —*see* Ankylosis, ear ossicles
    discontinuity —*see* Discontinuity, ossicles, ear
    partial loss —*see* Loss, ossicles, ear (partial)
  Ebstein Q22.5
  echocardiogram R93.1
  echoencephalogram R90.81
  echogram —*see* Abnormal, diagnostic imaging
  electrocardiogram [ECG] [EKG] R94.31
  electroencephalogram [EEG] R94.01
  electrolyte —*see* Imbalance, electrolyte
  electromyogram [EMG] R94.131
  electro-oculogram [EOG] R94.110
  electrophysiological intracardiac studies R94.39
  electroretinogram [ERG] R94.111
  erythrocytes
    congenital, with perinatal jaundice D58.9
  feces (color) (contents) (mucus) R19.5

◀ New   ◀═ Revised   ~~deleted~~ Deleted

Abnormal, abnormality, abnormalities —
(Continued)
finding —see Findings, abnormal, without
diagnosis
fluid
amniotic —see Abnormal, specimen,
specified
cerebrospinal —see Abnormal,
cerebrospinal fluid
peritoneal —see Abnormal, specimen,
digestive organs
pleural —see Abnormal, specimen,
respiratory organs
synovial —see Abnormal, specimen,
specified
thorax (bronchial washings) (pleural
fluid) —see Abnormal, specimen,
respiratory organs
vaginal —see Abnormal, specimen, female
genital organs
form
teeth K00.2
uterus —see Anomaly, uterus
function studies
auditory R94.120
bladder R94.8
brain R94.09
cardiovascular R94.30
ear R94.128
endocrine NEC R94.7
eye NEC R94.118
kidney R94.4
liver R94.5
nervous system
central NEC R94.09
peripheral NEC R94.138
pancreas R94.8
placenta R94.8
pulmonary R94.2
special senses NEC R94.128
spleen R94.8
thyroid R94.6
vestibular R94.121
gait —see Gait
hysterical F44.4
gastrin secretion E16.4
globulin R77.1
cortisol-binding E27.8
thyroid-binding E07.89
glomerular, minor —see also N00-N07 with
fourth character .0 N05.0
glucagon secretion E16.3
glucose tolerance (test) (non-fasting)
R73.09
gravitational (G) forces or states (effect of)
T75.81
hair (color) (shaft) L67.9
specified NEC L67.8
hard tissue formation in pulp (dental)
K04.3
head movement R25.0
heart
rate R00.9
specified NEC R00.8
shadow R93.1
sounds NEC R01.2
hemoglobin (disease) —see also Disease,
hemoglobin D58.2
trait —see Trait, hemoglobin, abnormal
histology NEC R89.7
immunological findings R89.4
in serum R76.9
specified NEC R76.8
increase in appetite R63.2
involuntary movement —see Abnormal,
movement, involuntary
jaw closure M26.51
karyotype R89.8
kidney function test R94.4
knee jerk R29.2
leukocyte (cell) (differential) NEC D72.9

Abnormal, abnormality, abnormalities —
(Continued)
liver
loss of
height R29.890
weight R63.4
mammogram NEC R92.8
calcification (calculus) R92.1
microcalcification R92.0
Mantoux test R76.11
movement (disorder) —see also Disorder,
movement
head R25.0
involuntary R25.9
fasciculation R25.3
of head R25.0
spasm R25.2
specified type NEC R25.8
tremor R25.1
myoglobin (Aberdeen) (Annapolis) R89.7
neonatal screening P09
oculomotor study R94.113
palmar creases Q82.8
Papanicolaou (smear)
anus R85.619
atypical squamous cells cannot
exclude high grade squamous
intraepithelial lesion (ASC-H)
R85.611
atypical squamous cells of undetermined
significance (ASC-US) R85.610
cytologic evidence of malignancy
R85.614
high grade squamous intraepithelial
lesion (HGSIL) R85.613
human papillomavirus (HPV)
DNA test
high risk positive R85.81
low risk postive R85.82
inadequate smear R85.615
low grade squamous intraepithelial
lesion (LGSIL) R85.612
satisfactory anal smear but lacking
transformation zone R85.616
specified NEC R85.618
unsatisfactory smear R85.615
bronchial washings R84.6
cerebrospinal fluid R83.6
cervix R87.619
atypical squamous cells cannot
exclude high grade squamous
intraepithelial lesion (ASC-H)
R87.611
atypical squamous cells of undetermined
significance (ASC-US) R87.610
cytologic evidence of malignancy
R87.614
high grade squamous intraepithelial
lesion (HGSIL) R87.613
inadequate smear R87.615
low grade squamous intraepithelial
lesion (LGSIL) R87.612
non-atypical endometrial cells
R87.618
satisfactory cervical smear but
lacking transformation zone
R87.616
specified NEC R87.618
thin preparaton R87.619
unsatisfactory smear R87.615
nasal secretions R84.6
nipple discharge R89.6
peritoneal fluid R85.69
pleural fluid R84.6
prostatic secretions R86.6
saliva R85.69
seminal fluid R86.6
sites NEC R89.6
sputum R84.6
synovial fluid R89.6
throat scrapings R84.6

Abnormal, abnormality, abnormalities —
(Continued)
Papanicolaou (smear) (Continued)
vagina R87.629
atypical squamous cells cannot
exclude high grade squamous
intraepithelial lesion (ASC-H)
R87.621
atypical squamous cells of
undetermined significance
(ASC-US) R87.620
cytologic evidence of malignancy
R87.624
high grade squamous intraepithelial
lesion (HGSIL) R87.623
inadequate smear R87.625
low grade squamous intraepithelial
lesion (LGSIL) R87.622
specified NEC R87.628
thin preparation R87.629
unsatisfactory smear R87.625
vulva R87.69
wound secretions R89.6
partial thromboplastin time (PTT) R79.1
pelvis (bony) —see Deformity, pelvis
percussion, chest (tympany) R09.89
periods (grossly) —see Menstruation
phonocardiogram R94.39
plantar reflex R29.2
plasma
protein R77.9
specified NEC R77.8
viscosity R70.1
pleural (folds) Q34.0
posture R29.3
product of conception O02.9
specified type NEC O02.89
prothrombin time (PT) R79.1
pulmonary
artery, congenital Q25.79
function, newborn P28.89
test results R94.2
pulsations in neck R00.2
pupillary H21.56-
function (reaction) (reflex) —see Anomaly,
pupil, function
radiological examination —see Abnormal,
diagnostic imaging
red blood cell (s) (morphology) (volume)
R71.8
reflex —see Reflex
renal function test R94.4
response to nerve stimulation R94.130
retinal correspondence H53.31
retinal function study R94.111
rhythm, heart —see also Arrhythmia
saliva —see Abnormal, specimen, digestive
organs
scan
kidney R94.4
liver R93.2
thyroid R94.6
secretion
gastrin E16.4
glucagon E16.3
semen, seminal fluid —see Abnormal,
specimen, male genital organs
serum level (of)
acid phosphatase R74.8
alkaline phosphatase R74.8
amylase R74.8
enzymes R74.9
specified NEC R74.8
lipase R74.8
triacylglycerol lipase R74.8
shape
gravid uterus —see Anomaly, uterus
sinus venosus Q21.1
size, tooth, teeth K00.2
spacing, tooth, teeth, fully erupted
M26.30

Abnormal, abnormality, abnormalities —
(Continued)
specimen
digestive organs (peritoneal fluid) (saliva)
R85.9
cytology R85.69
drug level R85.2
enzyme level R85.0
histology R85.7
hormones R85.1
immunology R85.4
microbiology R85.5
nonmedicinal level R85.3
specified type NEC R85.89
female genital organs (secretions) (smears)
R87.9
cytology R87.69
cervix R87.619
human papillomavirus (HPV) DNA
test
high risk positive R87.810
low risk positive R87.820
inadequate (unsatisfactory) smear
R87.615
non-atypical endometrial cells
R87.618
specified NEC R87.618
vagina R87.629
human papillomavirus (HPV) DNA
test
high risk positive R87.811
low risk positive R87.821
inadequate (unsatisfactory) smear
R87.625
vulva R87.69
drug level R87.2
enzyme level R87.0
histological R87.7
hormones R87.1
immunology R87.4
microbiology R87.5
nonmedicinal level R87.3
specified type NEC R87.89
male genital organs (prostatic secretions)
(semen) R86.9
cytology R86.6
drug level R86.2
enzyme level R86.0
histological R86.7
hormones R86.1
immunology R86.4
microbiology R86.5
nonmedicinal level R86.3
specified type NEC R86.8
nipple discharge —see Abnormal,
specimen, specified
respiratory organs (bronchial washings)
(nasal secretions) (pleural fluid)
(sputum) R84.9
cytology R84.6
drug level R84.2
enzyme level R84.0
histology R84.7
hormones R84.1
immunology R84.4
microbiology R84.5
nonmedicinal level R84.3
specified type NEC R84.8
specified organ, system and tissue NOS
R89.9
cytology R89.6
drug level R89.2
enzyme level R89.0
histology R89.7
hormones R89.1
immunology R89.4
microbiology R89.5
nonmedicinal level R89.3
specified type NEC R89.8
synovial fluid —see Abnormal, specimen,
specified

Abnormal, abnormality, abnormalities —
(Continued)
specimen (Continued)
thorax (bronchial washings) (pleural
fluids) —see Abnormal, specimen,
respiratory organs
vagina (secretion) (smear) R87.629
vulva (secretion) (smear) R87.69
wound secretion —see Abnormal,
specimen, specified
spermatozoa —see Abnormal, specimen, male
genital organs
sputum (amount) (color) (odor) R09.3
stool (color) (contents) (mucus) R19.5
bloody K92.1
guaiac positive R19.5
synchondrosis Q78.8
thermography —see also Abnormal,
diagnostic imaging R93.8
thyroid-binding globulin E07.89
tooth, teeth (form) (size) K00.2
toxicology (findings) R78.9
transport protein E88.09
tumor marker NEC R97.8
ultrasound results —see Abnormal, diagnostic
imaging
umbilical cord complicating delivery O69.9
urination NEC R39.198 ◀▥
urine (constituents) R82.90
bile R82.2
cytological examination R82.8
drugs R82.5
fat R82.0
glucose R81
heavy metals R82.6
hemoglobin R82.3
histological examination R82.8
ketones R82.4
microbiological examination (culture)
R82.79 ◀▥
myoglobin R82.1
positive culture R82.79 ◀▥
protein —see Proteinuria
specified substance NEC R82.99
chromoabnormality NEC R82.91
substances nonmedical R82.6
uterine hemorrhage —see Hemorrhage,
uterus
vectorcardiogram R94.39
visually evoked potential (VEP) R94.112
white blood cells D72.9
specified NEC D72.89
X-ray examination —see Abnormal,
diagnostic imaging
Abnormity (any organ or part) —see Anomaly
Abocclusion M26.29
hemolytic disease (newborn) P55.1
incompatibility reaction ABO —see
Complication (s), transfusion,
incompatibility reaction, ABO
Abolition, language R48.8
Aborter, habitual or recurrent —see Loss (of),
pregnancy, recurrent
Abortion (complete) (spontaneous) O03.9
with
retained products of conception - see
Abortion, incomplete
attempted (elective) (failed) O07.4
complicated by O07.30
afibrinogenemia O07.1
cardiac arrest O07.36
chemical damage of pelvic organ (s)
O07.34
circulatory collapse O07.31
cystitis O07.38
defibrination syndrome O07.1
electrolyte imbalance O07.33
embolism (air) (amniotic fluid) (blood
clot) (fat) (pulmonary) (septic)
(soap) O07.2
endometritis O07.0

Abortion (Continued)
attempted (Continued)
complicated by (Continued)
genital tract and pelvic infection O07.0
hemolysis O07.1
hemorrhage (delayed) (excessive) O07.1
infection
genital tract or pelvic O07.0
urinary tract tract O07.38
intravascular coagulation O07.1
laceration of pelvic organ(s) O07.34
metabolic disorder O07.33
oliguria O07.32
oophoritis O07.0
parametritis O07.0
pelvic peritonitis O07.0
perforation of pelvic organ(s) O07.34
renal failure or shutdown O07.32
salpingitis or salpingo-oophoritis O07.0
sepsis O07.37
shock O07.31
specified condition NEC O07.39
tubular necrosis (renal) O07.32
uremia O07.32
urinary tract infection O07.38
venous complication NEC O07.35
embolism (air) (amniotic fluid) (blood
clot) (fat) (pulmonary) (septic)
(soap) O07.2
complicated (by) (following) O03.80
afibrinogenemia O03.6
cardiac arrest O03.86
chemical damage of pelvic organ (s) O03.84
circulatory collapse O03.81
cystitis O03.88
defibrination syndrome O03.6
electrolyte imbalance O03.83
embolism (air) (amniotic fluid) (blood
clot) (fat) (pulmonary) (septic) (soap)
O03.7
endometritis O03.5
genital tract and pelvic infection O03.5
hemolysis O03.6
hemorrhage (delayed) (excessive) O03.6
infection
genital tract or pelvic O03.5
urinary tract O03.88
intravascular coagulation O03.6
laceration of pelvic organ (s) O03.84
metabolic disorder O03.83
oliguria O03.82
oophoritis O03.5
parametritis O03.5
pelvic peritonitis O03.5
perforation of pelvic organ (s) O03.84
renal failure or shutdown O03.82
salpingitis or salpingo-oophoritis O03.5
sepsis O03.87
shock O03.81
specified condition NEC O03.89
tubular necrosis (renal) O03.82
uremia O03.82
urinary tract infection O03.88
venous complication NEC O03.85
embolism (air) (amniotic fluid) (blood
clot) (fat) (pulmonary) (septic)
(soap) O03.7
failed —see Abortion, attempted
habitual or recurrent N96
with current abortion —see categories
O03-O06
without current pregnancy N96
care in current pregnancy O26.2-
incomplete (spontaneous) O03.4
complicated (by) (following) O03.30
afibrinogenemia O03.1
cardiac arrest O03.36
chemical damage of pelvic organ (s)
O03.34
circulatory collapse O03.31
cystitis O03.38

◀ New　　◀▥ Revised　　~~deleted~~ Deleted

Abortion *(Continued)*
  incomplete *(Continued)*
    complicated *(Continued)*
      defibrination syndrome O03.1
      electrolyte imbalance O03.33
      embolism (air) (amniotic fluid) (blood clot) (fat) (pulmonary) (septic) (soap) O03.2
      endometritis O03.0
      genital tract and pelvic infection O03.0
      hemolysis O03.1
      hemorrhage (delayed) (excessive) O03.1
      infection
        genital tract or pelvic O03.0
        urinary tract O03.38
      intravascular coagulation O03.1
      laceration of pelvic organ (s) O03.34
      metabolic disorder O03.33
      oliguria O03.32
      oophoritis O03.0
      parametritis O03.0
      pelvic peritonitis O03.0
      perforation of pelvic organ (s) O03.34
      renal failure or shutdown O03.32
      salpingitis or salpingo-oophoritis O03.0
      sepsis O03.37
      shock O03.31
      specified condition NEC O03.39
      tubular necrosis (renal) O03.32
      uremia O03.32
      urinary infection O03.38
      venous complication NEC O03.35
        embolism (air) (amniotic fluid) (blood clot) (fat) (pulmonary) (septic) (soap) O03.2
  induced (encounter for) Z33.2
    complicated by O04.80
      afibrinogenemia O04.6
      cardiac arrest O04.86
      chemical damage of pelvic organ (s) O04.84
      circulatory collapse O04.81
      cystitis O04.88
      defibrination syndrome O04.6
      electrolyte imbalance O04.83
      embolism (air) (amniotic fluid) (blood clot) (fat) (pulmonary) (septic) (soap) O04.7
      endometritis O04.5
      genital tract and pelvic infection O04.5
      hemolysis O04.6
      hemorrhage (delayed) (excessive) O04.6
      infection
        genital tract or pelvic O04.5
        urinary tract O04.88
      intravascular coagulation O04.6
      laceration of pelvic organ (s) O04.84
      metabolic disorder O04.83
      oliguria O04.82
      oophoritis O04.5
      parametritis O04.5
      pelvic peritonitis O04.5
      perforation of pelvic organ (s) O04.84
      renal failure or shutdown O04.82
      salpingitis or salpingo-oophoritis O04.5
      sepsis O04.87
      shock O04.81
      specified condition NEC O04.89
      tubular necrosis (renal) O04.82
      uremia O04.82
      urinary tract infection O04.88
      venous complication NEC O04.85
        embolism (air) (amniotic fluid) (blood clot) (fat) (pulmonary) (septic) (soap) O04.7
  missed O02.1
  spontaneous —*see* Abortion (complete) (spontaneous)
  threatened O20.0
  threatened (spontaneous) O20.0

Abortion *(Continued)*
  tubal O00.10
    with intrauterine pregnancy O00.11
Abortus fever A23.1
Aboulomania F60.7
Abrami's disease D59.8
Abramov-Fiedler myocarditis (acute isolated myocarditis) I40.1
Abrasion T14.8
  abdomen, abdominal (wall) S30.811
  alveolar process S00.512
  ankle S90.51-
  antecubital space —*see* Abrasion, elbow
  anus S30.817
  arm (upper) S40.81-
  auditory canal —*see* Abrasion, ear
  auricle —*see* Abrasion, ear
  axilla —*see* Abrasion, arm
  back, lower S30.810
  breast S20.11-
  brow S00.81
  buttock S30.810
  calf —*see* Abrasion, leg
  canthus —*see* Abrasion, eyelid
  cheek S00.81
    internal S00.512
  chest wall —*see* Abrasion, thorax
  chin S00.81
  clitoris S30.814
  cornea S05.0-
  costal region —*see* Abrasion, thorax
  dental K03.1
  digit (s)
    foot —*see* Abrasion, toe
    hand —*see* Abrasion, finger
  ear S00.41-
  elbow S50.31-
  epididymis S30.813
  epigastric region S30.811
  epiglottis S10.11
  esophagus (thoracic) S27.818
    cervical S10.11
  eyebrow —*see* Abrasion, eyelid
  eyelid S00.21-
  face S00.81
  finger (s) S60.41-
    index S60.41-
    little S60.41-
    middle S60.41-
    ring S60.41-
  flank S30.811
  foot (except toe (s) alone) S90.81-
    toe —*see* Abrasion, toe
  forearm S50.81-
    elbow only —*see* Abrasion, elbow
  forehead S00.81
  genital organs, external
    female S30.816
    male S30.815
  groin S30.811
  gum S00.512
  hand S60.51-
  head S00.91
    ear —*see* Abrasion, ear
    eyelid —*see* Abrasion, eyelid
    lip S00.511
    nose S00.31
    oral cavity S00.512
    scalp S00.01
    specified site NEC S00.81
  heel —*see* Abrasion, foot
  hip S70.21-
  inguinal region S30.811
  interscapular region S20.419
  jaw S00.81
  knee S80.21-
  labium (majus) (minus) S30.814
  larynx S10.11
  leg (lower) S80.81-
    knee —*see* Abrasion, knee
    upper —*see* Abrasion, thigh

Abrasion *(Continued)*
  lip S00.511
  lower back S30.810
  lumbar region S30.810
  malar region S00.81
  mammary —*see* Abrasion, breast
  mastoid region S00.81
  mouth S00.512
  nail
    finger —*see* Abrasion, finger
    toe —*see* Abrasion, toe
  nape S10.81
  nasal S00.31
  neck S10.91
    specified site NEC S10.81
    throat S10.11
  nose S00.31
  occipital region S00.01
  oral cavity S00.512
  orbital region —*see* Abrasion, eyelid
  palate S00.512
  palm —*see* Abrasion, hand
  parietal region S00.01
  pelvis S30.810
  penis S30.812
  perineum
    female S30.814
    male S30.810
  periocular area —*see* Abrasion, eyelid
  phalanges
    finger —*see* Abrasion, finger
    toe —*see* Abrasion, toe
  pharynx S10.11
  pinna —*see* Abrasion, ear
  popliteal space —*see* Abrasion, knee
  prepuce S30.812
  pubic region S30.810
  pudendum
    female S30.816
    male S30.815
  sacral region S30.810
  scalp S00.01
  scapular region —*see* Abrasion, shoulder
  scrotum S30.813
  shin —*see* Abrasion, leg
  shoulder S40.21-
  skin NEC T14.8
  sternal region S20.319
  submaxillary region S00.81
  submental region S00.81
  subungual
    finger (s) —*see* Abrasion, finger
    toe (s) —*see* Abrasion, toe
  supraclavicular fossa S10.81
  supraorbital S00.81
  temple S00.81
  temporal region S00.81
  testis S30.813
  thigh S70.31-
  thorax, thoracic (wall) S20.91
    back S20.41-
    front S20.31-
  throat S10.11
  thumb S60.31-
  toe (s) (lesser) S90.416
    great S90.41-
  tongue S00.512
  tooth, teeth (dentifrice) (habitual) (hard tissues) (occupational) (ritual) (traditional) K03.1
  trachea S10.11
  tunica vaginalis S30.813
  tympanum, tympanic membrane —*see* Abrasion, ear
  uvula S00.512
  vagina S30.814
  vocal cords S10.11
  vulva S30.814
  wrist S60.81-
Abrism —*see* Poisoning, food, noxious, plant

Abruptio placentae O45.9-
  with
    afibrinogenemia O45.01-
    coagulation defect O45.00-
      specified NEC O45.09-
    disseminated intravascular coagulation O45.02-
    hypofibrinogenemia O45.01-
    specified NEC O45.8-
Abruption, placenta —see Abruptio placentae
Abscess (connective tissue) (embolic) (fistulous) (infective) (metastatic) (multiple) (pernicious) (pyogenic) (septic) L02.91
  with
    diverticular disease (intestine) K57.80
      with bleeding K57.81
      large intestine K57.20
        with
          bleeding K57.21
          small intestine K57.40
            with bleeding K57.41
        small intestine K57.00
          with
            bleeding K57.01
            large intestine K57.40
              with bleeding K57.41
    lymphangitis - code by site under Abscess
  abdomen, abdominal
    cavity K65.1
    wall L02.211
  abdominopelvic K65.1
  accessory sinus —see Sinusitis
  adrenal (capsule) (gland) E27.8
  alveolar K04.7
    with sinus K04.6
  ambebic A06.4
    brain (and liver or lung abscess) A06.6
    genitourinary tract A06.82
    liver (without mention of brain or lung abscess) A06.4
    lung (and liver) (without mention of brain abscess) A06.5
    specified site NEC A06.89
    spleen A06.89
  anerobic A48.0
  ankle —see Abscess, lower limb
  anorectal K61.2
  antecubital space —see Abscess, upper limb
  antrum (chronic) (Highmore) —see Sinusitis, maxillary
  anus K61.0
  apical (tooth) K04.7
    with sinus (alveolar) K04.6
  appendix K35.3
  areola (acute) (chronic) (nonpuerperal) N61.1 ◀
    puerperal, postpartum or gestational —see Infection, nipple
  arm (any part) —see Abscess, upper limb
  artery (wall) I77.89
  atheromatous I77.2
  auricle, ear —see Abscess, ear, external
  axilla (region) L02.41-
    lymph gland or node L04.2
  back (any part, except buttock) L02.212
  Bartholin's gland N75.1
    with
      abortion —see Abortion, by type complicated by, sepsis
      ectopic or molar pregnancy O08.0
      following ectopic or molar pregnancy O08.0
  Bezold's —see Mastoiditis, acute
  bilharziasis B65.1
  bladder (wall) —see Cystitis, specified type NEC
  bone (subperiosteal) —see also Osteomyelitis, specified type NEC
    accessory sinus (chronic) —see Sinusitis
    chronic or old —see Osteomyelitis, chronic
    jaw (lower) (upper) M27.2

Abscess (Continued)
  bone (Continued)
    mastoid —see Mastoiditis, acute, subperiosteal
    petrous —see Petrositis
    spinal (tuberculous) A18.01
      nontuberculous —see Osteomyelitis, vertebra
  bowel K63.0
  brain (any part) (cystic) (otogenic) G06.0
    amebic (with abscess of any other site) A06.6
    gonococcal A54.82
    pheomycotic (chromomycotic) B43.1
    tuberculous A17.81
  breast (acute) (chronic) (nonpuerperal) N61.1 ◀
    newborn P39.0
    puerperal, postpartum, gestational —see Mastitis, obstetric, purulent
  broad ligament N73.2
    acute N73.0
    chronic N73.1
  Brodie's (localized) (chronic) M86.8X-
  bronchi J98.09
  buccal cavity K12.2
  bulbourethral gland N34.0
  bursa M71.00
    ankle M71.07-
    elbow M71.02-
    foot M71.07-
    hand M71.04-
    hip M71.05-
    knee M71.06-
    multiple sites M71.09
    pharyngeal J39.1
    shoulder M71.01-
    specified site NEC M71.08
    wrist M71.03-
  buttock L02.31
  canthus —see Blepharoconjunctivitis
  cartilage —see Disorder, cartilage, specified type NEC
  cecum K35.3
  cerebellum, cerebellar G06.0
    sequelae G09
  cerebral (embolic) G06.0
    sequelae G09
  cervical (meaning neck) L02.11
    lymph gland or node L04.0
  cervix (stump) (uteri) —see Cervicitis
  cheek (external) L02.01
    inner K12.2
  chest J86.9
    with fistula J86.0
    wall L02.213
  chin L02.01
  choroid —see Inflammation, chorioretinal
  circumtonsillar J36
  cold (lung) (tuberculous) —see also Tuberculosis, abscess, lung
    articular —see Tuberculosis, joint
  colon (wall) K63.0
  colostomy K94.02
  conjunctiva —see Conjunctivitis, acute
  cornea H16.31-
  corpus
    cavernosum N48.21
    luteum —see Oophoritis
  Cowper's gland N34.0
  cranium G06.0
  cul-de-sac (Douglas') (posterior) —see Peritonitis, pelvic, female
  cutaneous —see Abscess, by site
  dental K04.7
    with sinus (alveolar) K04.6
  dentoalveolar K04.7
    with sinus K04.6
  diaphragm, diaphragmatic K65.1
  Douglas' cul-de-sac or pouch —see Peritonitis, pelvic, female
  Dubois A50.59

Abscess (Continued)
  ear (middle) —see also Otitis, media, suppurative
    acute —see Otitis, media, suppurative, acute
    external H60.0-
  entamebic —see Abscess, amebic
  enterostomy K94.12
  epididymis N45.4
  epidural G06.2
    brain G06.0
    spinal cord G06.1
  epiglottis J38.7
  epiploon, epiploic K65.1
  erysipelatous —see Erysipelas
  esophagus K20.8
  ethmoid (bone) (chronic) (sinus) J32.2
  external auditory canal —see Abscess, ear, external
  extradural G06.2
    brain G06.0
      sequelae G09
    spinal cord G06.1
  extraperitoneal K68.19
  eye —see Endophthalmitis, purulent
  eyelid H00.03-
  face (any part, except ear, eye and nose) L02.01
  fallopian tube —see Salpingitis
  fascia M72.8
  fauces J39.1
  fecal K63.0
  femoral (region) —see Abscess, lower limb
  filaria, filarial —see Infestation, filarial
  finger (any) —see also Abscess, hand
    nail —see Cellulitis, finger
  foot L02.61-
  forehead L02.01
  frontal sinus (chronic) J32.1
  gallbladder K81.0
  genital organ or tract
    female (external) N76.4
    male N49.9
      multiple sites N49.8
      specified NEC N49.8
  gestational mammary O91.11-
  gestational subareolar O91.11-
  gingival —see Peridontitis, aggressive, localized ◀
  gland, glandular (lymph) (acute) —see Lymphadenitis, acute
  gluteal (region) L02.31
  gonorrheal —see Gonococcus
  groin L02.214
  gum —see Peridontitis, aggressive, localized ◀
  hand L02.51-
  head NEC L02.811
    face (any part, except ear, eye and nose) L02.01
  heart —see Carditis
  heel —see Abscess, foot
  helminthic —see Infestation, helminth
  hepatic (cholangitic) (hematogenic) (lymphogenic) (pylephlebitic) K75.0
    amebic A06.4
  hip (region) —see Abscess, lower limb
  ileocecal K35.3
  ileostomy (bud) K94.12
  iliac (region) L02.214
    fossa K35.3
  infraclavicular (fossa) —see Abscess, upper limb
  inguinal (region) L02.214
    lymph gland or node L04.1
  intestine, intestinal NEC K63.0
    rectal K61.1
  intra-abdominal —see also Abscess, peritoneum K65.1
    ~~postoperative T81.4~~
    ~~retroperitoneal K68.11~~
    postprocedural T81.43 ◀
    retroperitoneal K68.11 ◀
  intra-muscular, postprocedural T81.42 ◀

◀ New ◀═ Revised ~~deleted~~ Deleted

Abscess *(Continued)*
intracranial G06.0
intramammary —*see* Abscess, breast
intraorbital —*see* Abscess, orbit
intraperitoneal K65.1
intrasphincteric (anus) K61.4
intraspinal G06.1
intratonsillar J36
ischiorectal (fossa) K61.3
jaw (bone) (lower) (upper) M27.2
joint —*see* Arthritis, pyogenic or pyemic
spine (tuberculous) A18.01
nontuberculous —*see* Spondylopathy,
infective
kidney N15.1
with calculus N20.0
with hydronephrosis N13.6
puerperal (postpartum) O86.21
knee —*see also* Abscess, lower limb
joint M00.9
labium (majus) (minus) N76.4
lacrimal
caruncle —*see* Inflammation, lacrimal,
passages, acute
gland —*see* Dacryoadenitis
passages (duct) (sac) —*see* Inflammation,
lacrimal, passages, acute
lacunar N34.0
larynx J38.7
lateral (alveolar) K04.7
with sinus K04.6
leg (any part) —*see* Abscess, lower limb
lens H27.8
lingual K14.0
tonsil J36
lip K13.0
Littre's gland N34.0
liver (cholangitic) (hematogenic)
(lymphogenic) (pylephlebitic)
(pyogenic) K75.0
amebic (due to Entamoeba histolytica)
(dysenteric) (tropical) A06.4
with
brain abscess (and liver or lung
abscess) A06.6
lung abscess A06.5
loin (region) L02.211
lower limb L02.41-
lumbar (tuberculous) A18.01
nontuberculous L02.212
lung (miliary) (putrid) J85.2
with pneumonia J85.1
due to specified organism (*see*
Pneumonia, in (due to))
amebic (with liver abscess) A06.5
with
brain abscess A06.6
pneumonia A06.5
lymph, lymphatic, gland or node (acute) —*see
also* Lymphadenitis, acute
mesentery I88.0
malar M27.2
mammary gland —*see* Abscess, breast
marginal, anus K61.0
mastoid —*see* Mastoiditis, acute
maxilla, maxillary M27.2
molar (tooth) K04.7
with sinus K04.6
premolar K04.7
sinus (chronic) J32.0
mediastinum J85.3
meibomian gland —*see* Hordeolum
meninges G06.2
mesentery, mesenteric K65.1
mesosalpinx —*see* Salpingitis
mons pubis L02.215
mouth (floor) K12.2
muscle —*see* Myositis, infective
myocardium I40.0
nabothian (follicle) —*see* Cervicitis
nasal J32.9
nasopharyngeal J39.1

Abscess *(Continued)*
navel L02.216
newborn P38.9
with mild hemorrhage P38.1
without hemorrhage P38.9
neck (region) L02.11
lymph gland or node L04.0
nephritic —*see* Abscess, kidney
nipple N61.1 ◄▦
associated with
lactation —*see* Pregnancy, complicated
by ◄▦
pregnancy —*see* Pregnancy, complicated
by
nose (external) (fossa) (septum) J34.0
sinus (chronic) —*see* Sinusitis
omentum K65.1
operative wound T81.40 ◄▦
orbit, orbital —*see* Cellulitis, orbit
otogenic G06.0
ovary, ovarian (corpus luteum) —*see*
Oophoritis
oviduct —*see* Oophoritis
palate (soft) K12.2
hard M27.2
palmar (space) —*see* Abscess, hand
pancreas (duct) —*see* Pancreatitis, acute
parafrenal N48.21
parametric, parametrium N73.2
acute N73.0
chronic N73.1
paranephric N15.1
parapancreatic —*see* Pancreatitis, acute
parapharyngeal J39.0
pararectal K61.1
parasinus —*see* Sinusitis
parauterine (*see also* Disease, pelvis,
inflammatory) N73.2
paravaginal —*see* Vaginitis
parietal region (scalp) L02.811
parodontal —*see* Peridontitis, aggressive,
localized ◄▦
parotid (duct) (gland) K11.3
region K12.2
pectoral (region) L02.213
pelvis, pelvic
female —*see* Disease, pelvis, inflammatory
male, peritoneal K65.1
penis N48.21
gonococcal (accessory gland) (periurethral)
A54.1
perianal K61.0
periapical K04.7
with sinus (alveolar) K04.6
periappendicular K35.3
pericardial I30.1
pericecal K35.3
pericemental —*see* Peridontitis, aggressive,
localized ◄▦
pericholecystic —*see* Cholecystitis, acute
pericoronal —*see* Peridontitis, aggressive,
localized ◄▦
peridental —*see* Peridontitis, aggressive,
localized ◄▦
perimetric —*see also* Disease, pelvis,
inflammatory N73.2
perinephric, perinephritic —*see* Abscess,
kidney
perineum, perineal (superficial) L02.215
urethra N34.0
periodontal (parietal) —*see* Peridontitis,
aggressive, localized ◄▦
apical K04.7
periosteum, periosteal —*see also*
Osteomyelitis, specified type NEC
with osteomyelitis —*see also* Osteomyelitis,
specified type NEC
acute —*see* Osteomyelitis, acute
chronic —*see* Osteomyelitis, chronic
peripharyngeal J39.0
peripleuritic J86.9
with fistula J86.0

Abscess *(Continued)*
periprostatic N41.2
perirectal K61.1
perirenal (tissue) —*see* Abscess, kidney
perisinuous (nose) —*see* Sinusitis
peritoneum, peritoneal (perforated)
(ruptured) K65.1
with appendicitis K35.3
pelvic
female —*see* Peritonitis, pelvic, female
male K65.1
postoperative T81.43 ◄▦
puerperal, postpartum, childbirth O85
tuberculous A18.31
peritonsillar J36
perityphlic K35.3
periureteral N28.89
periurethral N34.0
gonococcal (accessory gland) (periurethral)
A54.1
periuterine —*see also* Disease, pelvis,
inflammatory N73.2
perivesical —*see* Cystitis, specified type NEC
petrous bone —*see* Petrositis
phagedenic NOS L02.91
chancroid A57
pharynx, pharyngeal (lateral) J39.1
pilonidal L05.01
pituitary (gland) E23.6
pleura J86.9
with fistula J86.0
popliteal —*see* Abscess, lower limb
postcecal K35.3
postlaryngeal J38.7
postnasal J34.0
postoperative (any site) T81.40 ◄▦
retroperitoneal K68.11
postpharyngeal J39.0
posttonsillar J36
post-typhoid A01.09
pouch of Douglas —*see* Peritonitis, pelvic,
female
premammary —*see* Abscess, breast
prepatellar —*see* Abscess, lower limb
prostate N41.2
gonococcal (acute) (chronic) A54.22
psoas muscle K68.12
puerperal - code by site under Puerperal,
abscess
pulmonary —*see* Abscess, lung
pulp, pulpal (dental) K04.01 ◄▦
irreversible K04.02 ◄
reversible K04.01 ◄
rectovaginal septum K63.0
rectovesical —*see* Cystitis, specified type NEC
rectum K61.1
renal —*see* Abscess, kidney
retina —*see* Inflammation, chorioretinal
retrobulbar —*see* Abscess, orbit
retrocecal K65.1
retrolaryngeal J38.7
retromammary —*see* Abscess, breast
retroperitoneal NEC K68.19
postprocedural K68.11
retropharyngeal J39.0
retrouterine —*see* Peritonitis, pelvic, female
retrovesical —*see* Cystitis, specified type NEC
root, tooth K04.7
with sinus (alveolar) K04.6
round ligament —*see also* Disease, pelvis,
inflammatory N73.2
rupture (spontaneous) NOS L02.91
sacrum (tuberculous) A18.01
nontuberculous M46.28
salivary (duct) (gland) K11.3
scalp (any part) L02.811
scapular —*see* Osteomyelitis, specified type
NEC
sclera —*see* Scleritis
scrofulous (tuberculous) A18.2
scrotum N49.2

◄ New   ◄▦ Revised   ~~deleted~~ Deleted

Abscess *(Continued)*
  seminal vesicle N49.0
  septal, dental K04.7
    with sinus (alveolar) K04.6
  serous —*see* Periostitis
  shoulder (region) —*see* Abscess, upper limb
  sigmoid K63.0
  sinus (accessory) (chronic) (nasal) —*see also*
    Sinusitis
    intracranial venous (any) G06.0
  Skene's duct or gland N34.0
  skin —*see* Abscess, by site
  specified site NEC L02.818
  spermatic cord N49.1
  sphenoidal (sinus) (chronic) J32.3
  spinal cord (any part) (staphylococcal) G06.1
    tuberculous A17.81
  spine (column) (tuberculous) A18.01
    epidural G06.1
    nontuberculous —*see* Osteomyelitis,
      vertebra
  spleen D73.3
    amebic A06.89
  stitch T81.48 ◄▥
  subarachnoid G06.2
    brain G06.0
    spinal cord G06.1
  subareolar —*see* Abscess, breast
  subcecal K35.3
  subcutaneous —*see also* Abscess, by site
    pheomycotic (chromomycotic) B43.2
    postprocedural T81.41 ◄
  subdiaphragmatic K65.1
  subdural G06.2
    brain G06.0
      sequelae G09
    spinal cord G06.1
  subgaleal L02.811
  subhepatic K65.1
  sublingual K12.2
    gland K11.3
  submammary —*see* Abscess, breast
  submandibular (region) (space) (triangle) K12.2
    gland K11.3
  submaxillary (region) L02.01
    gland K11.3
  submental L02.01
    gland K11.3
  subperiosteal —*see* Osteomyelitis, specified
    type NEC
  subphrenic K65.1
    postoperative T81.43 ◄▥
  suburethral N34.0
  sudoriparous L75.8
  supraclavicular (fossa) —*see* Abscess, upper
    limb
  suprapelvic, acute N73.0
  suprarenal (capsule) (gland) E27.8
  sweat gland L74.8
  tear duct —*see* Inflammation, lacrimal,
    passages, acute
  temple L02.01
  temporal region L02.01
  temporosphenoidal G06.0
  tendon (sheath) M65.00
    ankle M65.07-
    foot M65.07-
    forearm M65.03-
    hand M65.04-
    lower leg M65.06-
    pelvic region M65.05-
    shoulder region M65.01-
    specified site NEC M65.08
    thigh M65.05-
    upper arm M65.02-
  testis N45.4
  thigh —*see* Abscess, lower limb
  thorax J86.9
    with fistula J86.0
  throat J39.1
  thumb —*see also* Abscess, hand
    nail —*see* Cellulitis, finger

Abscess *(Continued)*
  thymus (gland) E32.1
  thyroid (gland) E06.0
  toe (any) —*see also* Abscess, foot
    nail —*see* Cellulitis, toe
  tongue (staphylococcal) K14.0
  tonsil (s) (lingual) J36
  tonsillopharyngeal J36
  tooth, teeth (root) K04.7
    with sinus (alveolar) K04.6
    supporting structures NEC —*see*
      Peridontitis, aggressive, localized ◄▥
  trachea J39.8
  trunk L02.219
    abdominal wall L02.211
    back L02.212
    chest wall L02.213
    groin L02.214
    perineum L02.215
    umbilicus L02.216
  tubal —*see* Salpingitis
  tuberculous —*see* Tuberculosis, abscess
  tubo-ovarian —*see* Salpingo-oophoritis
  tunica vaginalis N49.1
  umbilicus L02.216
  upper
    limb L02.41-
    respiratory J39.8
  urethral (gland) N34.0
  urinary N34.0
  uterus, uterine (wall) —*see also* Endometritis
    ligament —*see also* Disease, pelvis,
      inflammatory N73.2
    neck —*see* Cervicitis
  uvula K12.2
  vagina (wall) —*see* Vaginitis
  vaginorectal —*see* Vaginitis
  vas deferens N49.1
  vermiform appendix K35.3
  vertebra (column) (tuberculous) A18.01
    nontuberculous —*see* Osteomyelitis,
      vertebra
  vesical —*see* Cystitis, specified type NEC
  vesico-uterine pouch —*see* Peritonitis, pelvic,
    female
  vitreous (humor) —*see* Endophthalmitis,
    purulent
  vocal cord J38.3
  von Bezold's —*see* Mastoiditis, acute
  vulva N76.4
  vulvovaginal gland N75.1
  web space —*see* Abscess, hand
  wound T81.40 ◄▥
  wrist —*see* Abscess, upper limb
Absence (of) (organ or part) (complete or
  partial)
  adrenal (gland) (congenital) Q89.1
    acquired E89.6
  albumin in blood E88.09
  alimentary tract (congenital) Q45.8
    upper Q40.8
  alveolar process (acquired) —*see* Anomaly,
    alveolar
  ankle (acquired) Z89.44-
  anus (congenital) Q42.3
    with fistula Q42.2
  aorta (congenital) Q25.41 ◄▥
  appendix, congenital Q42.8
  arm (acquired) Z89.20-
    above elbow Z89.22-
      congenital (with hand present) —*see*
        Agenesis, arm, with hand present
      and hand —*see* Agenesis, forearm,
        and hand
    below elbow Z89.21-
      congenital (with hand present) —*see*
        Agenesis, arm, with hand present
      and hand —*see* Agenesis, forearm,
        and hand
    congenital —*see* Defect, reduction, upper
      limb

Absence *(Continued)*
  arm *(Continued)*
    shoulder (following explantation of
      shoulder joint prosthesis) (joint) (with
      or without presence of antibiotic-
      impregnated cement spacer) Z89.23-
      congenital (with hand present) —*see*
        Agenesis, arm, with hand present
  artery (congenital) (peripheral) Q27.8
    brain Q28.3
    coronary Q24.5
    pulmonary Q25.79
    specified NEC Q27.8
    umbilical Q27.0
  atrial septum (congenital) Q21.1
  auditory canal (congenital) (external) Q16.1
  auricle (ear), congenital Q16.0
  bile, biliary duct, congenital Q44.5
  bladder (acquired) Z90.6
    congenital Q64.5
  bowel sounds R19.11
  brain Q00.0
    part of Q04.3
  breast (s) (and nipple (s)) (acquired) Z90.1-
    congenital Q83.8
  broad ligament Q50.6
  bronchus (congenital) Q32.4
  canaliculus lacrimalis, congenital Q10.4
  cerebellum (vermis) Q04.3
  cervix (acquired) (with uterus) Z90.710
    with remaining uterus Z90.712
    congenital Q51.5
  chin, congenital Q18.8
  cilia (congenital) Q10.3
    acquired —*see* Madarosis
  clitoris (congenital) Q52.6
  coccyx, congenital Q76.49
  cold sense R20.8
  congenital
    lumen —*see* Atresia
    organ or site NEC —*see* Agenesis
    septum —*see* Imperfect, closure
  corpus callosum Q04.0
  cricoid cartilage, congenital Q31.8
  diaphragm (with hernia), congenital Q79.1
  digestive organ (s) or tract, congenital Q45.8
    acquired NEC Z90.49
    upper Q40.8
  ductus arteriosus Q28.8
  duodenum (acquired) Z90.49
    congenital Q41.0
  ear, congenital Q16.9
    acquired H93.8-
    auricle Q16.0
    external Q16.0
    inner Q16.5
    lobe, lobule Q17.8
    middle, except ossicles Q16.4
      ossicles Q16.3
    ossicles Q16.3
  ejaculatory duct (congenital) Q55.4
  endocrine gland (congenital) NEC Q89.2
    acquired E89.89
  epididymis (congenital) Q55.4
    acquired Z90.79
  epiglottis, congenital Q31.8
  esophagus (congenital) Q39.8
    acquired (partial) Z90.49
  eustachian tube (congenital) Q16.2
  extremity (acquired) Z89.9
    congenital Q73.0
    knee (following explantation of knee joint
      prosthesis) (joint) (with or without
      presence of antibiotic-impregnated
      cement spacer) Z89.52-
    lower (above knee) Z89.619
      below knee Z89.51-
    upper —*see* Absence, arm
  eye (acquired) Z90.01
    congenital Q11.1
    muscle (congenital) Q10.3

Absence *(Continued)*
eyeball (acquired) Z90.01
eyelid (fold) (congenital) Q10.3
  acquired Z90.01
face, specified part NEC Q18.8
fallopian tube (s) (acquired) Z90.79
  congenital Q50.6
family member (causing problem in home)
    NEC —*see also* Disruption, family Z63.32
femur, congenital —*see* Defect, reduction,
    lower limb, longitudinal, femur
fibrinogen (congenital) D68.2
  acquired D65
finger (s) (acquired) Z89.02-
  congenital —*see* Agenesis, hand
foot (acquired) Z89.43-
  congenital —*see* Agenesis, foot
forearm (acquired) —*see* Absence, arm, below
    elbow
gallbladder (acquired) Z90.49
  congenital Q44.0
gamma globulin in blood D80.1
  hereditary D80.0
genital organs
  acquired (female) (male) Z90.79
  female, congenital Q52.8
    external Q52.71
    internal NEC Q52.8
  male, congenital Q55.8
genitourinary organs, congenital NEC
  female Q52.8
  male Q55.8
globe (acquired) Z90.01
  congenital Q11.1
glottis, congenital Q31.8
hand and wrist (acquired) Z89.11-
  congenital —*see* Agenesis, hand
head, part (acquired) NEC Z90.09
heat sense R20.8
hip (following explantation of hip joint
    prosthesis) (joint) (with or without
    presence of antibiotic-impregnated
    cement spacer) Z89.62-
hymen (congenital) Q52.4
ileum (acquired) Z90.49
  congenital Q41.2
immunoglobulin, isolated NEC D80.3
  IgA D80.2
  IgG D80.3
  IgM D80.4
incus (acquired) —*see* Loss, ossicles, ear
  congenital Q16.3
inner ear, congenital Q16.5
intestine (acquired) (small) Z90.49
  congenital Q41.9
    specified NEC Q41.8
  large Z90.49
    congenital Q42.9
      specified NEC Q42.8
iris, congenital Q13.1
jejunum (acquired) Z90.49
  congenital Q41.1
joint
  acquired
    hip (following explantation of hip
      joint prosthesis) (with or without
      presence of antibiotic-impregnated
      cement spacer) Z89.62-
    knee (following explantation of knee
      joint prosthesis) (with or without
      presence of antibiotic-impregnated
      cement spacer) Z89.52-
    shoulder (following explantation of
      shoulder joint prosthesis) (with
      or without presence of antibiotic-
      impregnated cement spacer)
      Z89.23-
  congenital NEC Q74.8
kidney (s) (acquired) Z90.5
  congenital Q60.2
    bilateral Q60.1
    unilateral Q60.0

Absence *(Continued)*
knee (following explantation of knee joint
    prosthesis) (joint) (with or without
    presence of antibiotic-impregnated
    cement spacer) Z89.52-
labyrinth, membranous Q16.5
larynx (congenital) Q31.8
  acquired Z90.02
leg (acquired) (above knee) Z89.61-
  below knee (acquired) Z89.51-
  congenital —*see* Defect, reduction, lower
    limb
lens (acquired) —*see also* Aphakia
  congenital Q12.3
  post cataract extraction Z98.4-
limb (acquired) —*see* Absence, extremity
lip Q38.6
liver (congenital) Q44.7
lung (fissure) (lobe) (bilateral) (unilateral)
    (congenital) Q33.3
  acquired (any part) Z90.2
menstruation —*see* Amenorrhea
muscle (congenital) (pectoral) Q79.8
  ocular Q10.3
neck, part Q18.8
neutrophil —*see* Agranulocytosis
nipple (s) (with breast (s)) (acquired) Z90.1-
  congenital Q83.2
nose (congenital) Q30.1
  acquired Z90.09
organ
  of Corti, congenital Q16.5
  or site, congenital NEC Q89.8
    acquired NEC Z90.89
osseous meatus (ear) Q16.4
ovary (acquired)
  bilateral Z90.722
  congenital
    bilateral Q50.02
    unilateral Q50.01
  unilateral Z90.721
oviduct (acquired)
  bilateral Z90.722
  congenital Q50.6
  unilateral Z90.721
pancreas (congenital) Q45.0
  acquired Z90.410
    complete Z90.410
    partial Z90.411
    total Z90.410
parathyroid gland (acquired) E89.2
  congenital Q89.2
patella, congenital Q74.1
penis (congenital) Q55.5
  acquired Z90.79
pericardium (congenital) Q24.8
pituitary gland (congenital) Q89.2
  acquired E89.3
prostate (acquired) Z90.79
  congenital Q55.4
pulmonary valve Q22.0
punctum lacrimale (congenital) Q10.4
radius, congenital —*see* Defect, reduction,
    upper limb, longitudinal, radius
rectum (congenital) Q42.1
  with fistula Q42.0
  acquired Z90.49
respiratory organ NOS Q34.9
rib (acquired) Z90.89
  congenital Q76.6
sacrum, congenital Q76.49
salivary gland (s), congenital Q38.4
scrotum, congenital Q55.29
seminal vesicles (congenital) Q55.4
  acquired Z90.79
septum
  atrial (congenital) Q21.1
  between aorta and pulmonary artery Q21.4
  ventricular (congenital) Q20.4
sex chromosome
  female phenotype Q97.8
  male phenotype Q98.8

Absence *(Continued)*
skull bone (congenital) Q75.8
  with
    anencephaly Q00.0
    encephalocele —*see* Encephalocele
    hydrocephalus Q03.9
      with spina bifida —*see* Spina
        bifida, by site, with
        hydrocephalus
    microcephaly Q02
spermatic cord, congenital Q55.4
spine, congenital Q76.49
spleen (congenital) Q89.01
  acquired Z90.81
sternum, congenital Q76.7
stomach (acquired) (partial) Z90.3
  congenital Q40.2
superior vena cava, congenital
    Q26.8
teeth, tooth (congenital) K00.0
  acquired (complete) K08.109
    class I K08.101
    class II K08.102
    class III K08.103
    class IV K08.104
    due to
      caries K08.139
        class I K08.131
        class II K08.132
        class III K08.133
        class IV K08.134
      periodontal disease K08.129
        class I K08.121
        class II K08.122
        class III K08.123
        class IV K08.124
      specified NEC K08.199
        class I K08.191
        class II K08.192
        class III K08.193
        class IV K08.194
      trauma K08.119
        class I K08.111
        class II K08.112
        class III K08.113
        class IV K08.114
    partial K08.409
      class I K08.401
      class II K08.402
      class III K08.403
      class IV K08.404
      due to
        caries K08.439
          class I K08.431
          class II K08.432
          class III K08.433
          class IV K08.434
        periodontal disease K08.429
          class I K08.421
          class II K08.422
          class III K08.423
          class IV K08.424
        specified NEC K08.499
          class I K08.491
          class II K08.492
          class III K08.493
          class K08.494
        trauma K08.419
          class I K08.411
          class II K08.412
          class III K08.413
          class IV K08.414
tendon (congenital) Q79.8
testis (congenital) Q55.0
  acquired Z90.79
thumb (acquired) Z89.01-
  congenital —*see* Agenesis, hand
thymus gland Q89.2
thyroid (gland) (acquired) E89.0
  cartilage, congenital Q31.8
  congenital E03.1

Absence *(Continued)*
  toe (s) (acquired) Z89.42-
    with foot —*see* Absence, foot and
      ankle
    congenital —*see* Agenesis, foot
    great Z89.41-
  tongue, congenital Q38.3
  trachea (cartilage), congenital Q32.1
  transverse aortic arch, congenital
    Q25.49 ◄▥
  tricuspid valve Q22.4
  umbilical artery, congenital Q27.0
  upper arm and forearm with hand present,
    congenital —*see* Agenesis, arm, with
    hand present
  ureter (congenital) Q62.4
    acquired Z90.6
  urethra, congenital Q64.5
  uterus (acquired) Z90.710
    with cervix Z90.710
    with remaining cervical stump
      Z90.711
    congenital Q51.0
  uvula, congenital Q38.5
  vagina, congenital Q52.0
  vas deferens (congenital) Q55.4
    acquired Z90.79
  vein (peripheral) congenital NEC
    Q27.8
    cerebral Q28.3
    digestive system Q27.8
    great Q26.8
    lower limb Q27.8
    portal Q26.5
    precerebral Q28.1
    specified site NEC Q27.8
    upper limb Q27.8
  vena cava (inferior) (superior), congenital
    Q26.8
  ventricular septum Q20.4
  vertebra, congenital Q76.49
  vulva, congenital Q52.71
  wrist (acquired) Z89.12-
Absorbent system disease I87.8
Absorption
  carbohydrate, disturbance K90.49 ◄▥
  chemical —*see* Table of Drugs and
    Chemicals
    through placenta (newborn) P04.9
      environmental substance P04.6
      nutritional substance P04.5
      obstetric anesthetic or analgesic drug
        P04.0
  drug NEC —*see* Table of Drugs and
    Chemicals
    addictive
      through placenta (newborn) P04.49
        cocaine P04.41
    medicinal
      through placenta (newborn) P04.1
    through placenta (newborn) P04.1
      obstetric anesthetic or analgesic drug
        P04.0
  fat, disturbance K90.49 ◄▥
    pancreatic K90.3
  noxious substance —*see* Table of Drugs and
    Chemicals
  protein, disturbance K90.49 ◄▥
  starch, disturbance K90.49 ◄▥
  toxic substance —*see* Table of Drugs and
    Chemicals
  uremic —*see* Uremia
Abstinence symptoms, syndrome
  alcohol F10.239
    with delirium F10.231
  cocaine F14.23
  neonatal P96.1
  nicotine —*see* Dependence, drug, nicotine,
    with, withdrawal
  opioid F11.93
    with dependence F11.23

Abstinence symptoms, syndrome *(Continued)*
  psychoactive NEC F19.939
    with
      delirium F19.931
      dependence F19.239
        with
          delirium F19.231
          perceptual disturbance F19.232
        uncomplicated F19.230
      perceptual disturbance F19.932
    uncomplicated F19.930
  sedative F13.939
    with
      delirium F13.931
      dependence F13.239
        with
          delirium F13.231
          perceptual disturbance F13.232
        uncomplicated F13.230
      perceptual disturbance F13.932
    uncomplicated F13.930
  stimulant NEC F15.93
    with dependence F15.23
Abulia R68.89
Abulomania F60.7
Abuse
  adult —*see* Maltreatment, adult
    as reason for
      couple seeking advice (including
        offender) Z63.0
  alcohol (non-dependent) F10.10
    with
      anxiety disorder F10.180
      intoxication F10.129
        with delirium F10.121
        uncomplicated F10.120
      mood disorder F10.14
      other specified disorder F10.188
      psychosis F10.159
        delusions F10.150
        hallucinations F10.151
      sexual dysfunction F10.181
      sleep disorder F10.182
      unspecified disorder F10.19
    counseling and surveillance Z71.41
  amphetamine (or related substance) —*see*
    Abuse, drug, stimulant NEC
  analgesics (non-prescribed) (over the counter)
    F55.8
  antacids F55.0
  antidepressants —*see* Abuse, drug,
    psychoactive NEC
  anxiolytic —*see* Abuse, drug, sedative
  barbiturates —*see* Abuse, drug, sedative
  caffeine —*see* Abuse, drug, stimulant NEC
  cannabis, cannabinoids —*see* Abuse, drug,
    cannabis
  child —*see* Maltreatment, child
  cocaine —*see* Abuse, drug, cocaine
  drug NEC (non-dependent) F19.10
    with sleep disorder F19.182
    amphetamine type —*see* Abuse, drug,
      stimulant NEC
    analgesics (non-prescribed) (over the
      counter) F55.8
    antacids F55.0
    antidepressants —*see* Abuse, drug,
      psychoactive NEC
    anxiolytics —*see* Abuse, drug, sedative
    barbiturates —*see* Abuse, drug, sedative
    caffeine —*see* Abuse, drug, stimulant NEC
    cannabis F12.10
      with
        anxiety disorder F12.180
        intoxication F12.129
          with
            delirium F12.121
            perceptual disturbance
              F12.122
          uncomplicated F12.120
        other specified disorder F12.188

Abuse *(Continued)*
  drug NEC *(Continued)*
    cannabis *(Continued)*
      with *(Continued)*
        psychosis F12.159
          delusions F12.150
          hallucinations F12.151
        unspecified disorder F12.19
    cocaine F14.10
      with
        anxiety disorder F14.180
        intoxication F14.129
          with
            delirium F14.121
            perceptual disturbance F14.122
          uncomplicated F14.120
        mood disorder F14.14
        other specified disorder F14.188
        psychosis F14.159
          delusions F14.150
          hallucinations F14.151
        sexual dysfunction F14.181
        sleep disorder F14.182
        unspecified disorder F14.19
    counseling and surveillance Z71.51
    hallucinogen F16.10
      with
        anxiety disorder F16.180
        flashbacks F16.183
        intoxication F16.129
          with
            delirium F16.121
            perceptual disturbance F16.122
          uncomplicated F16.120
        mood disorder F16.14
        other specified disorder F16.188
        perception disorder, persisting F16.183
        psychosis F16.159
          delusions F16.150
          hallucinations F16.151
        unspecified disorder F16.19
    hashish —*see* Abuse, drug, cannabis
    herbal or folk remedies F55.1
    hormones F55.3
    hypnotics —*see* Abuse, drug, sedative
    inhalant F18.10
      with
        anxiety disorder F18.180
        dementia, persisting F18.17
        intoxication F18.129
          with delirium F18.121
          uncomplicated F18.120
        mood disorder F18.14
        other specified disorder F18.188
        psychosis F18.159
          delusions F18.150
          hallucinations F18.151
        unspecified disorder F18.19
    laxatives F55.2
    LSD —*see* Abuse, drug, hallucinogen
    marihuana —*see* Abuse, drug, cannabis
    morphine type (opioids) —*see* Abuse, drug,
      opioid
    opioid F11.10
      with
        intoxication F11.129
          with
            delirium F11.121
            perceptual disturbance F11.122
          uncomplicated F11.120
        mood disorder F11.14
        other specified disorder F11.188
        psychosis F11.159
          delusions F11.150
          hallucinations F11.151
        sexual dysfunction F11.181
        sleep disorder F11.182
        unspecified disorder F11.19
    PCP (phencyclidine) (or related
      substance) —*see* Abuse, drug,
      hallucinogen

◄ New   ◄▥ Revised   ~~deleted~~ Deleted

Abuse *(Continued)*
  drug NEC *(Continued)*
    psychoactive NEC F19.10
      with
        amnestic disorder F19.16
        anxiety disorder F19.180
        dementia F19.17
        intoxication F19.129
          with
            delirium F19.121
            perceptual disturbance F19.122
          uncomplicated F19.120
        mood disorder F19.14
        other specified disorder F19.188
        psychosis F19.159
          delusions F19.150
          hallucinations F19.151
        sexual dysfunction F19.181
        sleep disorder F19.182
        unspecified disorder F19.19
    sedative, hypnotic or anxiolytic F13.10
      with
        anxiety disorder F13.180
        intoxication F13.129
          with delirium F13.121
          uncomplicated F13.120
        mood disorder F13.14
        other specified disorder F13.188
        psychosis F13.159
          delusions F13.150
          hallucinations F13.151
        sexual dysfunction F13.181
        sleep disorder F13.182
        unspecified disorder F13.19
    solvent —*see* Abuse, drug, inhalant
    steroids F55.3
    stimulant NEC F15.10
      with
        anxiety disorder F15.180
        intoxication F15.129
          with
            delirium F15.121
            perceptual disturbance F15.122
          uncomplicated F15.120
        mood disorder F15.14
        other specified disorder F15.188
        psychosis F15.159
          delusions F15.150
          hallucinations F15.151
        sexual dysfunction F15.181
        sleep disorder F15.182
        unspecified disorder F15.19
    tranquilizers —*see* Abuse, drug, sedative
    vitamins F55.4
  hallucinogens —*see* Abuse, drug, hallucinogen
  hashish —*see* Abuse, drug, cannabis
  herbal or folk remedies F55.1
  hormones F55.3
  hypnotic —*see* Abuse, drug, sedative
  inhalant —*see* Abuse, drug, inhalant
  laxatives F55.2
  LSD —*see* Abuse, drug, hallucinogen
  marihuana —*see* Abuse, drug, cannabis
  morphine type (opioids) —*see* Abuse, drug, opioid
  non-psychoactive substance NEC F55.8
    antacids F55.0
    folk remedies F55.1
    herbal remedies F55.1
    hormones F55.3
    laxatives F55.2
    steroids F55.3
    vitamins F55.4
  opioids —*see* Abuse, drug, opioid
  PCP (phencyclidine) (or related substance) — *see* Abuse, drug, hallucinogen
  physical (adult) (child) —*see* Maltreatment
  psychoactive substance —*see* Abuse, drug, psychoactive NEC

Abuse *(Continued)*
  psychological (adult) (child) —*see* Maltreatment
  sedative —*see* Abuse, drug, sedative
  sexual —*see* Maltreatment
  solvent —*see* Abuse, drug, inhalant
  steroids F55.3
  vitamins F55.4
Acalculia R48.8
  developmental F81.2
Acanthamebiasis (with) B60.10
  conjunctiva B60.12
  keratoconjunctivitis B60.13
  meningoencephalitis B60.11
  other specified B60.19
Acanthocephaliasis B83.8
Acanthocheilonemiasis B74.4
Acanthocytosis E78.6
Acantholysis L11.9
Acanthosis (acquired) (nigricans) L83
  benign Q82.8
  congenital Q82.8
  seborrheic L82.1
    inflamed L82.0
  tongue K14.3
Acapnia E87.3
Acarbia E87.2
Acardia, acardius Q89.8
Acardiacus amorphus Q89.8
Acardiotrophia I51.4
Acariasis B88.0
  scabies B86
Acarodermatitis (urticarioides) B88.0
Acarophobia F40.218
Acatalasemia, acatalasia E80.3
Acathisia (drug induced) G25.71
Accelerated atrioventricular conduction I45.6
Accentuation of personality traits (type A) Z73.1
Accessory (congenital)
  adrenal gland Q89.1
  anus Q43.4
  appendix Q43.4
  atrioventricular conduction I45.6
  auditory ossicles Q16.3
  auricle (ear) Q17.0
  biliary duct or passage Q44.5
  bladder Q64.79
  blood vessels NEC Q27.9
    coronary Q24.5
  bone NEC Q79.8
  breast tissue, axilla Q83.1
  carpal bones Q74.0
  cecum Q43.4
  chromosome (s) NEC (nonsex) Q92.9
    with complex rearrangements NEC Q92.5
      seen only at prometaphase Q92.8
    13 —*see* Trisomy, 13
    18 —*see* Trisomy, 18
    21 —*see* Trisomy, 21
    partial Q92.9
    sex
      female phenotype Q97.8
  coronary artery Q24.5
  cusp (s), heart valve NEC Q24.8
    pulmonary Q22.3
  cystic duct Q44.5
  digit (s) Q69.9
  ear (auricle) (lobe) Q17.0
  endocrine gland NEC Q89.2
  eye muscle Q10.3
  eyelid Q10.3
  face bone (s) Q75.8
  fallopian tube (fimbria) (ostium) Q50.6
  finger (s) Q69.0
  foreskin N47.8
  frontonasal process Q75.8

Accessory *(Continued)*
  gallbladder Q44.1
  genital organ (s)
    female Q52.8
      external Q52.79
      internal NEC Q52.8
    male Q55.8
  genitourinary organs NEC Q89.8
    female Q52.8
    male Q55.8
  hallux Q69.2
  heart Q24.8
    valve NEC Q24.8
      pulmonary Q22.3
  hepatic ducts Q44.5
  hymen Q52.4
  intestine (large) (small) Q43.4
  kidney Q63.0
  lacrimal canal Q10.6
  leaflet, heart valve NEC Q24.8
  ligament, broad Q50.6
  liver Q44.7
    duct Q44.5
  lobule (ear) Q17.0
  lung (lobe) Q33.1
  muscle Q79.8
  navicular of carpus Q74.0
  nervous system, part NEC Q07.8
  nipple Q83.3
  nose Q30.8
  organ or site not listed —*see* Anomaly, by site
  ovary Q50.31
  oviduct Q50.6
  pancreas Q45.3
  parathyroid gland Q89.2
  parotid gland (and duct) Q38.4
  pituitary gland Q89.2
  preauricular appendage Q17.0
  prepuce N47.8
  renal arteries (multiple) Q27.2
  rib Q76.6
    cervical Q76.5
  roots (teeth) K00.2
  salivary gland Q38.4
  sesamoid bones Q74.8
    foot Q74.2
    hand Q74.0
  skin tags Q82.8
  spleen Q89.09
  sternum Q76.7
  submaxillary gland Q38.4
  tarsal bones Q74.2
  teeth, tooth K00.1
  tendon Q79.8
  thumb Q69.1
  thymus gland Q89.2
  thyroid gland Q89.2
  toes Q69.2
  tongue Q38.3
  tooth, teeth K00.1
  tragus Q17.0
  ureter Q62.5
  urethra Q64.79
  urinary organ or tract NEC Q64.8
  uterus Q51.2
  vagina Q52.10
  valve, heart NEC Q24.8
    pulmonary Q22.3
  vertebra Q76.49
  vocal cords Q31.8
  vulva Q52.79
Accident
  birth —*see* Birth, injury
  cardiac —*see* Infarct, myocardium
  cerebral I63.9
  cerebrovascular (embolic) (ischemic) (thrombotic) I63.9
    aborted I63.9
    hemorrhagic —*see* Hemorrhage, intracranial, intracerebral

Accident (Continued)
　cerebrovascular (Continued)
　　old (without sequelae) Z86.73
　　　with sequelae (of) —see Sequelae,
　　　　infarction, cerebral
　　coronary —see Infarct, myocardium
　　craniovascular I63.9
　　vascular, brain I63.9
Accidental —see condition
Accommodation (disorder) —see also condition
　hysterical paralysis of F44.89
　insufficiency of H52.4
　paresis —see Paresis, of accommodation
　spasm —see Spasm, of accommodation
Accouchement —see Delivery
Accreta placenta O43.21-
Accretio cordis (nonrheumatic) I31.0
Accretions, tooth, teeth K03.6
Acculturation difficulty Z60.3
Accumulation secretion, prostate N42.89
Acephalia, acephalism, acephalus, acephaly
　Q00.0
Acephalobrachia monster Q89.8
Acephalochirus monster Q89.8
Acephalogaster Q89.8
Acephalostomus monster Q89.8
Acephalothorax Q89.8
Acerophobia F40.298
Acetonemia R79.89
　in Type 1 diabetes E10.10
　　with coma E10.11
Acetonuria R82.4
Achalasia (cardia) (esophagus) K22.0
　congenital Q39.5
　pylorus Q40.0
　sphincteral NEC K59.8
Ache (s) —see Pain
Acheilia Q38.6
Achillobursitis —see Tendinitis, Achilles
Achillodynia —see Tendinitis, Achilles
Achlorhydria, achlorhydric (neurogenic)
　K31.83
　anemia D50.8
　diarrhea K31.83
　psychogenic F45.8
　secondary to vagotomy K91.1
Achluophobia F40.228
Acholia K82.8
Acholuric jaundice (familial)
　(splenomegalic) —see also Spherocytosis
　acquired D59.8
Achondrogenesis Q77.0
Achondroplasia (osteosclerosis congenita)
　Q77.4
Achroma, cutis L80
Achromat (ism), achromatopsia (acquired)
　(congenital) H53.51
Achromia, congenital —see Albinism
Achromia parasitica B36.0
Achylia gastrica K31.89
　psychogenic F45.8
Acid
　burn —see Corrosion
　deficiency
　　amide nicotinic E52
　　ascorbic E54
　　folic E53.8
　　nicotinic E52
　　pantothenic E53.8
　intoxication E87.2
　peptic disease K30
　phosphatase deficiency E83.39
　stomach K30
　　psychogenic F45.8
Acidemia E87.2
　argininosuccinic E72.22
　isovaleric E71.110
　metabolic (newborn) P19.9
　　first noted before onset of labor P19.0
　　first noted during labor P19.1
　　noted at birth P19.2

Acidemia (Continued)
　methylmalonic E71.120
　pipecolic E72.3
　propionic E71.121
Acidity, gastric (high) K30
　psychogenic F45.8
Acidocytopenia —see Agranulocytosis
Acidocytosis D72.1
Acidopenia —see Agranulocytosis
Acidosis (lactic) (respiratory) E87.2
　in Type 1 diabetes E10.10
　　with coma E10.11
　kidney, tubular N25.89
　lactic E87.2
　metabolic NEC E87.2
　　with respiratory acidosis E87.4
　　late, of newborn P74.0
　mixed metabolic and respiratory,
　　newborn P84
　newborn P84
　renal (hyperchloremic) (tubular)
　　N25.89
　respiratory E87.2
　　complicated by
　　　metabolic
　　　　acidosis E87.4
　　　　alkalosis E87.4
Aciduria
　argininosuccinic E72.22
　glutaric (type I) E72.3
　　type II E71.313
　　type III E71.5-
　orotic (congenital) (hereditary) (pyrimidine
　　deficiency) E79.8
　　anemia D53.0
Acladiosis (skin) B36.0
Aclasis, diaphyseal Q78.6
Acleistocardia Q21.1
Aclusion —see Anomaly, dentofacial,
　malocclusion
Acne L70.9
　artificialis L70.8
　atrophica L70.2
　cachecticorum (Hebra) L70.8
　conglobata L70.1
　cystic L70.0
　decalvans L66.2
　excoriée des jeunes filles L70.5
　excoriée (des jeunes filles) L70.5 ◀
　frontalis L70.2
　indurata L70.0
　infantile L70.4
　keloid L73.0
　lupoid L70.2
　necrotic, necrotica (miliaris) L70.2
　neonatal L70.4
　nodular L70.0
　occupational L70.8
　picker's L70.5
　pustular L70.0
　rodens L70.2
　rosacea L71.9
　specified NEC L70.8
　tropica L70.3
　varioliformis L70.2
　vulgaris L70.0
Acnitis (primary) A18.4
Acosta's disease T70.29
Acoustic —see condition
Acousticophobia F40.298
Acquired —see also condition
　immunodeficiency syndrome (AIDS) B20
Acrania Q00.0
Acroangiodermatitis I78.9
Acroasphyxia, chronic I73.89
Acrobystitis N47.7
Acrocephalopolysyndactyly Q87.0
Acrocephalosyndactyly Q87.0
Acrocephaly Q75.0
Acrochondrohyperplasia —see Syndrome,
　Marfan's

Acrocyanosis I73.8
　newborn P28.2
　　meaning transient blue hands and feet -
　　　omit code
Acrodermatitis L30.8
　atrophicans (chronica) L90.4
　continua (Hallopeau) L40.2
　enteropathica (hereditary) E83.2
　Hallopeau's L40.2
　infantile papular L44.4
　perstans L40.2
　pustulosa continua L40.2
　recalcitrant pustular L40.2
Acrodynia —see Poisoning, mercury
Acromegaly, acromegalia E22.0
Acromelalgia I73.81
Acromicria, acromikria Q79.8
Acronyx L60.0
Acropachy, thyroid —see Thyrotoxicosis
Acroparesthesia (simple) (vasomotor) I73.89
Acropathy, thyroid —see Thyrotoxicosis
Acrophobia F40.241
Acroposthitis N47.7
Acroscleriasis, acroscleroderma,
　acrosclerosis —see Sclerosis, systemic
Acrosphacelus I96
Acrospiroma, eccrine —see Neoplasm, skin,
　benign
Acrostealgia —see Osteochondropathy
Acrotrophodynia —see Immersion
ACTH ectopic syndrome E24.3
Actinic —see condition
Actinobacillosis, actinobacillus A28.8
　mallei A24.0
　muris A25.1
Actinomyces israelii (infection) —see
　Actinomycosis
Actinomycetoma (foot) B47.1
Actinomycosis, actinomycotic A42.9
　with pneumonia A42.0
　abdominal A42.1
　cervicofacial A42.2
　cutaneous A42.89
　gastrointestinal A42.1
　pulmonary A42.0
　sepsis A42.7
　specified site NEC A42.89
Actinoneuritis G62.82
Action, heart
　disorder I49.9
　irregular I49.9
　　psychogenic F45.8
Activated protein C resistance D68.51
Activation ◀
　mast cell (disorder) (syndrome) D89.40 ◀
　　idiopathic D89.42 ◀
　　monoclonal D89.41 ◀
　　secondary D89.43 ◀
　　specified type NEC D89.49 ◀
Active —see condition
Acute —see also condition
　abdomen R10.0
　gallbladder —see Cholecystitis, acute
Acyanotic heart disease (congenital) Q24.9
Acystia Q64.5
Adair-Dighton syndrome (brittle bones and
　blue sclera, deafness) Q78.0
Adamantinoblastoma —see Ameloblastoma
Adamantinoma —see also Cyst, calcifying
　odontogenic
　long bones C40.90
　　lower limb C40.2-
　　upper limb C40.0-
　malignant C41.1
　　jaw (bone) (lower) C41.1
　　　upper C41.0
　tibial C40.2-
Adamantoblastoma —see Ameloblastoma
Adams-Stokes (-Morgagni) disease or
　syndrome I45.9
Adaption reaction —see Disorder, adjustment

Addiction —see also Dependence F19.20
  alcohol, alcoholic (ethyl) (methyl) (wood)
      (without remission) F10.20
    with remission F10.21
  drug —see Dependence, drug
  ethyl alcohol (without remission) F10.20
    with remission F10.21
  heroin —see Dependence, drug, opioid
  methyl alcohol (without remission) F10.20
    with remission F10.21
  methylated spirit (without remission) F10.20
    with remission F10.21
  morphine(-like substances) —see
      Dependence, drug, opioid
  nicotine —see Dependence, drug, nicotine
  opium and opioids —see Dependence, drug,
      opioid
  tobacco —see Dependence, drug, nicotine
Addisonian crisis E27.2
Addison's
  anemia (pernicious) D51.0
  disease (bronze) or syndrome E27.1
    tuberculous A18.7
  keloid L94.0
Addison-Biermer anemia (pernicious) D51.0
Addison-Schilder complex E71.528
Additional —see also Accessory
  chromosome (s) Q99.8
    21 —see Trisomy, 21
    sex —see Abnormal, chromosome, sex
Adduction contracture, hip or other joint —see
    Contraction, joint
Adenitis —see also Lymphadenitis
  acute, unspecified site L04.9
  axillary I88.9
    acute L04.2
    chronic or subacute I88.1
  Bartholin's gland N75.8
  bulbourethral gland —see Urethritis
  cervical I88.9
    acute L04.0
    chronic or subacute I88.1
  chancroid (Hemophilus ducreyi) A57
  chronic, unspecified site I88.1
  Cowper's gland —see Urethritis
  due to Pasteurella multocida (p. septica) A28.0
  epidemic, acute B27.09
  gangrenous L04.9
  gonorrheal NEC A54.89
  groin I88.9
    acute L04.1
    chronic or subacute I88.1
  infectious (acute) (epidemic) B27.09
  inguinal I88.9
    acute L04.1
    chronic or subacute I88.1
  lymph gland or node, except mesenteric I88.9
    acute —see Lymphadenitis, acute
    chronic or subacute I88.1
  mesenteric (acute) (chronic) (nonspecific)
      (subacute) I88.0
  parotid gland (suppurative) —see
      Sialoadenitis
  salivary gland (any) (suppurative) —see
      Sialoadenitis
  scrofulous (tuberculous) A18.2
  Skene's duct or gland —see Urethritis
  strumous, tuberculous A18.2
  subacute, unspecified site I88.1
  sublingual gland (suppurative) —see
      Sialoadenitis
  submandibular gland (suppurative) —see
      Sialoadenitis
  submaxillary gland (suppurative) —see
      Sialoadenitis
  tuberculous —see Tuberculosis, lymph gland
  urethral gland —see Urethritis
  Wharton's duct (suppurative) —see
      Sialoadenitis
Adenoacanthoma —see Neoplasm, malignant,
    by site

Adenoameloblastoma —see Cyst, calcifying
    odontogenic
Adenocarcinoid (tumor) —see Neoplasm,
    malignant, by site
Adenocarcinoma —see also Neoplasm,
    malignant, by site
  acidophil
    specified site —see Neoplasm, malignant,
        by site
    unspecified site C75.1
  adrenal cortical C74.0-
  alveolar —see Neoplasm, lung, malignant
  apocrine
    breast —see Neoplasm, breast, malignant
    in situ
      breast D05.8-
      specified site NEC —see Neoplasm, skin,
          in situ
      unspecified site D04.9
    specified site NEC —see Neoplasm, skin,
        malignant
    unspecified site C44.99
  basal cell
    specified site —see Neoplasm, skin,
        malignant
    unspecified site C08.9
  basophil
    specified site —see Neoplasm, malignant,
        by site
    unspecified site C75.1
  bile duct type C22.1
    liver C22.1
    specified site NEC —see Neoplasm,
        malignant, by site
    unspecified site C22.1
  bronchiolar —see Neoplasm, lung, malignant
  bronchioloalveolar —see Neoplasm, lung,
      malignant
  ceruminous C44.29-
  cervix, in situ (see also Carcinoma, cervix
      uteri, in situ) D06.9
  chromophobe
    specified site —see Neoplasm, malignant,
        by site
    unspecified site C75.1
  diffuse type
    specified site —see Neoplasm, malignant,
        by site
    unspecified site C16.9
  duct
    infiltrating
      with Paget's disease —see Neoplasm,
          breast, malignant
      specified site —see Neoplasm,
          malignant, by site
      unspecified site (female) C50.91-
        male C50.92-
    specified site —see Neoplasm, malignant,
        by site
    unspecified site
      female C56.9
      male C61
  eosinophil
    specified site —see Neoplasm, malignant,
        by site
    unspecified site C75.1
  follicular
    with papillary C73
    moderately differentiated C73
    specified site —see Neoplasm, malignant,
        by site
    trabecular C73
    unspecified site C73
    well differentiated C73
  Hurthle cell C73
  in
    adenomatous
      polyposis coli C18.9
    infiltrating duct
      with Paget's disease —see Neoplasm,
          breast, malignant

Adenocarcinoma (Continued)
  infiltrating duct (Continued)
    specified site —see Neoplasm, malignant,
        by site
    unspecified site (female) C50.91-
      male C50.92-
  inflammatory
    specified site —see Neoplasm, malignant,
        by site
    unspecified site (female) C50.91-
      male C50.92-
  intestinal type
    specified site —see Neoplasm, malignant,
        by site
    unspecified site C16.9
  intracystic papillary
  intraductal
    breast D05.1-
    noninfiltrating
      breast D05.1-
    papillary
      with invasion
        specified site —see Neoplasm,
            malignant, by site
        unspecified site (female) C50.91-
          male C50.92-
      breast D05.1-
      specified site NEC —see Neoplasm, in
          situ, by site
      unspecified site D05.1-
    specified site NEC —see Neoplasm, in
        situ, by site
    unspecified site D05.1-
  papillary
    with invasion
      specified site —see Neoplasm,
          malignant, by site
      unspecified site (female) C50.91-
        male C50.92-
    breast D05.1-
    specified site —see Neoplasm, in situ,
        by site
    unspecified site D05.1-
    specified site NEC —see Neoplasm, in situ,
        by site
    unspecified site D05.1-
  islet cell
    with exocrine, mixed
      specified site —see Neoplasm,
          malignant, by site
      unspecified site C25.9
    pancreas C25.4
    specified site NEC —see Neoplasm,
        malignant, by site
    unspecified site C25.4
  lobular
    in situ
      breast D05.0-
      specified site NEC —see Neoplasm, in
          situ, by site
      unspecified site D05.0-
    specified site —see Neoplasm, malignant,
        by site
    unspecified site (female) C50.91-
      male C50.92-
  mucoid —see also Neoplasm, malignant, by site
    cell
      specified site —see Neoplasm,
          malignant, by site
      unspecified site C75.1
  nonencapsulated sclerosing C73
  papillary
    with follicular C73
    follicular variant C73
    intraductal (noninfiltrating)
      with invasion
        specified site —see Neoplasm,
            malignant, by site
        unspecified site (female) C50.91-
          male C50.92-
      breast D05.1-

Adenocarcinoma (Continued)
  papillary (Continued)
    intraductal (Continued)
      specified site NEC —see Neoplasm, in situ, by site
      unspecified site D05.1-
    serous
      specified site —see Neoplasm, malignant, by site
      unspecified site C56.9
    papillocystic
      specified site —see Neoplasm, malignant, by site
      unspecified site C56.9
    pseudomucinous
      specified site —see Neoplasm, malignant, by site
      unspecified site C56.9
    renal cell C64-
    sebaceous —see Neoplasm, skin, malignant, by site
    serous —see also Neoplasm, malignant, by site
      papillary
        specified site —see Neoplasm, malignant, by site
        unspecified site C56.9
    sweat gland —see Neoplasm, skin, malignant
    water-clear cell C75.0
Adenocarcinoma-in-situ —see also Neoplasm, in situ, by site
  breast D05.9-
Adenofibroma
  clear cell —see Neoplasm, benign, by site
  endometrioid D27.9
    borderline malignancy D39.10
    malignant C56-
  mucinous
    specified site —see Neoplasm, benign, by site
    unspecified site D27.9
  papillary
    specified site —see Neoplasm, benign, by site
    unspecified site D27.9
  prostate —see Enlargement, enlarged, prostate
  serous
    specified site —see Neoplasm, benign, by site
    unspecified site D27.9
  specified site —see Neoplasm, benign, by site
  unspecified site D27.9
Adenofibrosis
  breast —see Fibroadenosis, breast
  endometrioid N80.0
Adenoiditis (chronic) J35.02
  with tonsillitis J35.03
  acute J03.90
    recurrent J03.91
    specified organism NEC J03.80
      recurrent J03.81
    staphylococcal J03.80
      recurrent J03.81
    streptococcal J03.00
      recurrent J03.01
Adenoids —see condition
Adenolipoma —see Neoplasm, benign, by site
Adenolipomatosis, Launois-Bensaude E88.89
Adenolymphoma
  specified site —see Neoplasm, benign, by site
  unspecified site D11.9
Adenoma —see also Neoplasm, benign, by site
  acidophil
    specified site —see Neoplasm, benign, by site
    unspecified site D35.2
  acidophil-basophil, mixed
    specified site —see Neoplasm, benign, by site
    unspecified site D35.2

Adenoma (Continued)
  adrenal (cortical) D35.00
    clear cell D35.00
    compact cell D35.00
    glomerulosa cell D35.00
    heavily pigmented variant D35.00
    mixed cell D35.00
  alpha-cell
    pancreas D13.7
    specified site NEC —see Neoplasm, benign, by site
    unspecified site D13.7
  alveolar D14.30
  apocrine
    breast D24-
    specified site NEC —see Neoplasm, skin, benign, by site
    unspecified site D23.9
  basal cell D11.9
  basophil
    specified site —see Neoplasm, benign, by site
    unspecified site D35.2
  basophil-acidophil, mixed
    specified site —see Neoplasm, benign, by site
    unspecified site D35.2
  beta-cell
    pancreas D13.7
    specified site NEC —see Neoplasm, benign, by site
    unspecified site D13.7
  bile duct D13.4
    common D13.5
    extrahepatic D13.5
    intrahepatic D13.4
    specified site NEC —see Neoplasm, benign, by site
    unspecified site D13.4
  black D35.00
  bronchial D38.1
    cylindroid type —see Neoplasm, lung, malignant
  ceruminous D23.2-
  chief cell D35.1
  chromophobe
    specified site —see Neoplasm, benign, by site
    unspecified site D35.2
  colloid
    specified site —see Neoplasm, benign, by site
    unspecified site D34
  duct
  eccrine, papillary —see Neoplasm, skin, benign
  endocrine, multiple
    single specified site —see Neoplasm, uncertain behavior, by site
    two or more specified sites D44-
    unspecified site D44.9
  endometrioid —see also Neoplasm, benign
    borderline malignancy —see Neoplasm, uncertain behavior, by site
  eosinophil
    specified site —see Neoplasm, malignant, by site
    unspecified site D35.2
  fetal
    specified site —see Neoplasm, benign, by site
    unspecified site D34
  follicular
    specified site —see Neoplasm, benign, by site
    unspecified site D34
  hepatocellular D13.4
  Hurthle cell D34
  islet cell
    pancreas D13.7
    specified site NEC —see Neoplasm, benign, by site
    unspecified site D13.7

Adenoma (Continued)
  liver cell D13.4
  macrofollicular
    specified site —see Neoplasm, benign, by site
    unspecified site D34
  malignant, malignum —see Neoplasm, malignant, by site
  microcystic
    pancreas D13.6 ◀▥
    specified site NEC —see Neoplasm, benign, by site
    unspecified site D13.6 ◀▥
  microfollicular
    specified site —see Neoplasm, benign, by site
    unspecified site D34
  mucoid cell
    specified site —see Neoplasm, benign, by site
    unspecified site D35.2
  multiple endocrine
    single specified site —see Neoplasm, uncertain behavior, by site
    two or more specified sites D44-
    unspecified site D44.9
  nipple D24-
  papillary —see also Neoplasm, benign, by site
    eccrine —see Neoplasm, skin, benign, by site
  Pick's tubular
    specified site —see Neoplasm, benign, by site
    unspecified site
      female D27.9
      male D29.20
  pleomorphic
    carcinoma in —see Neoplasm, salivary gland, malignant
      specified site —see Neoplasm, malignant, by site
      unspecified site C08.9
  polypoid —see also Neoplasm, benign
    adenocarcinoma in —see Neoplasm, malignant, by site
    adenocarcinoma in situ —see Neoplasm, in situ, by site
  prostate —see Neoplasm, benign, prostate
  rete cell D29.20
  sebaceous —see Neoplasm, skin, benign
  Sertoli cell
    specified site —see Neoplasm, benign, by site
    unspecified site
      female D27.9
      male D29.20
  skin appendage —see Neoplasm, skin, benign
  sudoriferous gland —see Neoplasm, skin, benign
  sweat gland —see Neoplasm, skin, benign
  testicular
    specified site —see Neoplasm, benign, by site
    unspecified site
      female D27.9
      male D29.20
  tubular —see also Neoplasm, benign, by site
    adenocarcinoma in —see Neoplasm, malignant, by site
    adenocarcinoma in situ —see Neoplasm, in situ, by site
    Pick's
      specified site —see Neoplasm, benign
      unspecified site
        female D27.9
        male D29.20
  tubulovillous —see also Neoplasm, benign, by site
    adenocarcinoma in —see Neoplasm, malignant, by site
    adenocarcinoma in situ —see Neoplasm, in situ, by site

◀ New   ◀▥ Revised   ~~deleted~~ Deleted

Adenoma *(Continued)*
  villous —*see* Neoplasm, uncertain behavior,
      by site
    adenocarcinoma in —*see* Neoplasm,
        malignant, by site
    adenocarcinoma in situ —*see* Neoplasm, in
        situ, by site
    water-clear cell D35.1
Adenomatosis
  endocrine (multiple) E31.20
    single specified site —*see* Neoplasm,
        uncertain behavior, by site
  erosive of nipple D24-
  pluriendocrine —*see* Adenomatosis,
      endocrine
  pulmonary D38.1
    malignant —*see* Neoplasm, lung,
        malignant
  specified site —*see* Neoplasm, benign, by site
  unspecified site D12.6
Adenomatous
  goiter (nontoxic) E04.9
    with hyperthyroidism —*see* Hyper-
        thyroidism, with, goiter, nodular
    toxic —*see* Hyperthyroidism, with, goiter,
        nodular
Adenomyoma —*see also* Neoplasm, benign, by
    site
  prostate —*see* Enlarged, prostate
Adenomyometritis N80.0
Adenomyosis N80.0
Adenopathy (lymph gland) R59.9
  generalized R59.1
  inguinal R59.0
  localized R59.0
  mediastinal R59.0
  mesentery R59.0
  syphilitic (secondary) A51.49
  tracheobronchial R59.0
    tuberculous A15.4
      primary (progressive) A15.7
  tuberculous —*see also* Tuberculosis, lymph
      gland
    tracheobronchial A15.4
      primary (progressive) A15.7
Adenosalpingitis —*see* Salpingitis
Adenosarcoma —*see* Neoplasm, malignant, by
    site
Adenosclerosis I88.8
Adenosis (sclerosing) **breast** —*see*
    Fibroadenosis, breast
Adenovirus, as cause of disease classified
    elsewhere B97.0
Adentia (complete) (partial) —*see* Absence,
    teeth
Adherent —*see also* Adhesions
  labia (minora) N90.89
  pericardium (nonrheumatic) I31.0
    rheumatic I09.2
  placenta (with hemorrhage) O72.0
    without hemorrhage O73.0
  prepuce, newborn N47.0
  scar (skin) L90.5
  tendon in scar L90.5
Adhesions, adhesive (postinfective) K66.0
  with intestinal obstruction K56.5
  abdominal (wall) —*see* Adhesions,
      peritoneum
  appendix K38.8
  bile duct (common) (hepatic) K83.8
  bladder (sphincter) N32.89
  bowel —*see* Adhesions, peritoneum
  cardiac I31.0
    rheumatic I09.2
  cecum —*see* Adhesions, peritoneum
  cervicovaginal N88.1
    congenital Q52.8
    postpartal O90.89
      old N88.1
  cervix N88.1
  ciliary body NEC —*see* Adhesions, iris

Adhesions, adhesive *(Continued)*
  clitoris N90.89
  colon —*see* Adhesions, peritoneum
  common duct K83.8
  congenital —*see also* Anomaly, by site
    fingers —*see* Syndactylism, complex,
        fingers
    omental, anomalous Q43.3
    peritoneal Q43.3
    tongue (to gum or roof of mouth)
        Q38.3
  conjunctiva (acquired) H11.21-
    congenital Q15.8
  cystic duct K82.8
  diaphragm —*see* Adhesions, peritoneum
  due to foreign body —*see* Foreign body
  duodenum —*see* Adhesions, peritoneum
  ear
    middle H74.1-
  epididymis N50.89 ◄▥
  epidural —*see* Adhesions, meninges
  epiglottis J38.7
  eyelid H02.59
  female pelvis N73.6
  gallbladder K82.8
  globe H44.89
  heart I31.0
    rheumatic I09.2
  ileocecal (coil) —*see* Adhesions, peritoneum
  ileum —*see* Adhesions, peritoneum
  intestine —*see also* Adhesions, peritoneum
    with obstruction K56.5
  intra-abdominal —*see* Adhesions, peritoneum
  iris H21.50-
    anterior H21.51-
    goniosynechiae H21.52-
    posterior H21.54-
    to corneal graft T85.898 ◄▥
  joint —*see* Ankylosis
    knee M23.8X
    temporomandibular M26.61- ◄▥
  labium (majus) (minus), congenital Q52.5
  liver —*see* Adhesions, peritoneum
  lung J98.4
  mediastinum J98.59 ◄▥
  meninges (cerebral) (spinal) G96.12
    congenital Q07.8
    tuberculous (cerebral) (spinal) A17.0
  mesenteric —*see* Adhesions, peritoneum
  nasal (septum) (to turbinates) J34.89
  ocular muscle —*see* Strabismus, mechanical
  omentum —*see* Adhesions, peritoneum
  ovary N73.6
    congenital (to cecum, kidney or omentum)
        Q50.39
  paraovarian N73.6
  pelvic (peritoneal)
    female N73.6
      postprocedural N99.4
    male —*see* Adhesions, peritoneum
    postpartal (old) N73.6
    tuberculous A18.17
  penis to scrotum (congenital) Q55.8
  periappendiceal —*see also* Adhesions,
      peritoneum
  pericardium (nonrheumatic) I31.0
    focal I31.8
    rheumatic I09.2
    tuberculous A18.84
  pericholecystic K82.8
  perigastric —*see* Adhesions, peritoneum
  periovarian N73.6
  periprostatic N42.89
  perirectal —*see* Adhesions, peritoneum
  perirenal N28.89
  peritoneum, peritoneal (postinfective)
      (postprocedural) K66.0
    with obstruction (intestinal) K56.5
    congenital Q43.3
    pelvic, female N73.6
      postprocedural N99.4

Adhesions, adhesive *(Continued)*
  peritoneum, peritoneal *(Continued)*
    postpartal, pelvic N73.6
    to uterus N73.6
  peritubal N73.6
  periureteral N28.89
  periuterine N73.6
  perivesical N32.89
  perivesicular (seminal vesicle) N50.89 ◄▥
  pleura, pleuritic J94.8
    tuberculous NEC A15.6
  pleuropericardial J94.8
  postoperative (gastrointestinal tract)
      K66.0
    with obstruction K91.3
    due to foreign body accidentally left
        in wound —*see* Foreign body,
        accidentally left during a procedure
    pelvic peritoneal N99.4
    urethra —*see* Stricture, urethra,
        postprocedural
    vagina N99.2
  postpartal, old (vulva or perineum) N90.89
  preputial, prepuce N47.5
  pulmonary J98.4
  pylorus —*see* Adhesions, peritoneum
  sciatic nerve —*see* Lesion, nerve, sciatic
  seminal vesicle N50.89 ◄▥
  shoulder (joint) —*see* Capsulitis, adhesive
  sigmoid flexure —*see* Adhesions, peritoneum
  spermatic cord (acquired) N50.89 ◄▥
    congenital Q55.4
  spinal canal G96.12
  stomach —*see* Adhesions, peritoneum
  subscapular —*see* Capsulitis, adhesive
  temporomandibular M26.61- ◄▥
  tendinitis —*see also* Tenosynovitis, specified
      type NEC
    shoulder —*see* Capsulitis, adhesive
  testis N44.8
  tongue, congenital (to gum or roof of mouth)
      Q38.3
    acquired K14.8
  trachea J39.8
  tubo-ovarian N73.6
  tunica vaginalis N44.8
  uterus N73.6
    internal N85.6
    to abdominal wall N73.6
  vagina (chronic) N89.5
    postoperative N99.2
  vitreomacular H43.82-
  vitreous H43.89
  vulva N90.89
Adiaspiromycosis B48.8
Adie (-Holmes) **pupil or syndrome** —*see*
    Anomaly, pupil, function, tonic pupil
Adiponecrosis neonatorum P83.8
Adiposis —*see also* Obesity
  cerebralis E23.6
  dolorosa E88.2
Adiposity —*see also* Obesity
  heart —*see* Degeneration, myocardial
  localized E65
Adiposogenital dystrophy E23.6
Adjustment
  disorder —*see* Disorder, adjustment
  implanted device —*see* Encounter (for),
      adjustment (of)
  prosthesis, external —*see* Fitting
  reaction —*see* Disorder, adjustment
Administration of tPA (rtPA) in a different
    facility within the last 24 hours prior to
    admission to current facility Z92.82
Admission (for) —*see also* Encounter (for)
  adjustment (of)
    artificial
      arm Z44.00-
        complete Z44.01-
        partial Z44.02-
      eye Z44.2

Admission *(Continued)*
  adjustment *(Continued)*
    artificial *(Continued)*
      leg Z44.10-
        complete Z44.11-
        partial Z44.12-
    brain neuropacemaker Z46.2
      implanted Z45.42
    breast
      implant Z45.81
      prosthesis (external) Z44.3
    colostomy belt Z46.89
    contact lenses Z46.0
    cystostomy device Z46.6
    dental prosthesis Z46.3
    device NEC
      abdominal Z46.89
      implanted Z45.89
        cardiac Z45.09
          defibrillator (with synchronous
            cardiace pacemaker) Z45.02
          pacemaker (cardiac
            resynchronization therapy
            (CRT-P)) Z45.018 ◀▥
            pulse generator Z45.010
          resynchronization therapy
            defibrillator (CRT-D) Z45.02 ◀
      hearing device Z45.328
        bone conduction Z45.320
        cochlear Z45.321
      infusion pump Z45.1
      nervous system Z45.49
        CSF drainage Z45.41
        hearing device —*see* Admission,
          adjustment, device, implanted,
          hearing device
        neuropacemaker Z45.42
        visual substitution Z45.31
      specified NEC Z45.89
      vascular access Z45.2
      visual substitution Z45.31
    nervous system Z46.2
      implanted —*see* Admission,
        adjustment, device, implanted,
        nervous system
    orthodontic Z46.4
    prosthetic Z44.9
      arm —*see* Admission, adjustment,
        artificial, arm
      breast Z44.3
      dental Z46.3
      eye Z44.2
      leg —*see* Admission, adjustment,
        artificial, leg
      specified type NEC Z44.8
    substitution
      auditory Z46.2
        implanted —*see* Admission,
          adjustment, device, implanted,
          hearing device
      nervous system Z46.2
        implanted —*see* Admission,
          adjustment, device, implanted,
          nervous system
      visual Z46.2
        implanted Z45.31
    urinary Z46.6
    hearing aid Z46.1
      implanted —*see* Admission, adjustment,
        device, implanted, hearing device
    ileostomy device Z46.89
    intestinal appliance or device NEC Z46.89
    neuropacemaker (brain) (peripheral nerve)
      (spinal cord) Z46.2
      implanted Z45.42
    orthodontic device Z46.4
    orthopedic (brace) (cast) (device) (shoes)
      Z46.89
    pacemaker (cardiac resynchronization
      therapy (CRT-P)) ◀▥
      cardiac Z45.018
        pulse generator Z45.010

Admission *(Continued)*
  adjustment *(Continued)*
    pacemaker *(Continued)*
      nervous system Z46.2
        implanted Z45.42
    portacath (port-a-cath) Z45.2
    prosthesis Z44.9
      arm —*see* Admission, adjustment,
        artificial, arm
      breast Z44.3
      dental Z46.3
      eye Z44.2
      leg —*see* Admission, adjustment,
        artificial, leg
      specified NEC Z44.8
    spectacles Z46.0
  aftercare *(see also* Aftercare) Z51.89
    postpartum
      immediately after delivery Z39.0
      routine follow-up Z39.2
    radiation therapy (antineoplastic) Z51.0
  attention to artificial opening (of) Z43.9
    artificial vagina Z43.7
    colostomy Z43.3
    cystostomy Z43.5
    enterostomy Z43.4
    gastrostomy Z43.1
    ileostomy Z43.2
    jejunostomy Z43.4
    nephrostomy Z43.6
    specified site NEC Z43.8
      intestinal tract Z43.4
      urinary tract Z43.6
    tracheostomy Z43.0
    ureterostomy Z43.6
    urethrostomy Z43.6
  breast augmentation or reduction Z41.1
  breast reconstruction following mastectomy
    Z42.1
  change of
    dressing (nonsurgical) Z48.00
    neuropacemaker device (brain) (peripheral
      nerve) (spinal cord) Z46.2
      implanted Z45.42
    surgical dressing Z48.01
  circumcision, ritual or routine (in absence of
    diagnosis) Z41.2
  clinical research investigation (control)
    (normal comparison) (participant) Z00.6
  contraceptive management Z30.9
  cosmetic surgery NEC Z41.1
  counseling *(see also* Counseling)
    dietary Z71.3
    gestational carrier Z31.7 ◀
    HIV Z71.7
    human immunodeficiency virus Z71.7
    nonattending third party Z71.0
    procreative management NEC Z31.69
  delivery, full-term, uncomplicated O80
    cesarean, without indication O82
  desensitization to allergens Z51.6 ◀
  dietary surveillance and counseling Z71.3
  ear piercing Z41.3
  examination at health care facility (adult) —
    see also Examination Z00.00
    with abnormal findings Z00.01
    clinical research investigation (control)
      (normal comparison) (participant)
      Z00.6
    dental Z01.20
      with abnormal findings Z01.21
    donor (potential) Z00.5
    ear Z01.10
      with abnormal findings NEC Z01.118
    eye Z01.00
      with abnormal findings Z01.01
    general, specified reason NEC Z00.8
    hearing Z01.10
      with abnormal findings NEC Z01.118
    postpartum checkup Z39.2
    psychiatric (general) Z00.8
      requested by authority Z04.6

Admission *(Continued)*
  examination at health care facility *(Continued)*
    vision Z01.00
      with abnormal findings Z01.01
  fitting (of)
    artificial
      arm —*see* Admission, adjustment,
        artificial, arm
      eye Z44.2
      leg —*see* Admission, adjustment,
        artificial, leg
    brain neuropacemaker Z46.2
      implanted Z45.42
    breast prosthesis (external) Z44.3
    colostomy belt Z46.89
    contact lenses Z46.0
    cystostomy device Z46.6
    dental prosthesis Z46.3
    dentures Z46.3
    device NEC
      abdominal Z46.89
      nervous system Z46.2
        implanted —*see* Admission,
          adjustment, device, implanted,
          nervous system
      orthodontic Z46.4
      prosthetic Z44.9
        breast Z44.3
        dental Z46.3
        eye Z44.2
      substitution
        auditory Z46.2
          implanted —*see* Admission,
            adjustment, device, implanted,
            hearing device
        nervous system Z46.2
          implanted —*see* Admission,
            adjustment, device, implanted,
            nervous system
        visual Z46.2
          implanted Z45.31
    hearing aid Z46.1
    ileostomy device Z46.89
    intestinal appliance or device NEC Z46.89
    neuropacemaker (brain) (peripheral nerve)
      (spinal cord) Z46.2
      implanted Z45.42
    orthodontic device Z46.4
    orthopedic device (brace) (cast) (shoes)
      Z46.89
    prosthesis Z44.9
      arm —*see* Admission, adjustment,
        artificial, arm
      breast Z44.3
      dental Z46.3
      eye Z44.2
      leg —*see* Admission, adjustment,
        artificial, leg
      specified type NEC Z44.8
    spectacles Z46.0
  follow-up examination Z09
  intrauterine device management Z30.431
    initial prescription Z30.014
  mental health evaluation Z00.8
    requested by authority Z04.6
  observation —*see* Observation
  Papanicolaou smear, cervix Z12.4
    for suspected malignant neoplasm Z12.4
  plastic and reconstructive surgery following
    medical procedure or healed injury
    NEC Z42.8
  plastic surgery, cosmetic NEC Z41.1
  postpartum observation
    immediately after delivery Z39.0
    routine follow-up Z39.2
  poststerilization (for restoration) Z31.0
    aftercare Z31.42
  procreative management Z31.9
  prophylactic (measure) —*see also* Encounter,
    prophylactic measures ◀▥
    organ removal Z40.00
      breast Z40.01
      ovary Z40.02

◀ New   ◀▥ Revised   ~~deleted~~ Deleted

Admission *(Continued)*
  prophylactic *(Continued)*
    organ removal *(Continued)*
      specified organ NEC Z40.09
      testes Z40.09
    vaccination Z23
  psychiatric examination (general) Z00.8
    requested by authority Z04.6
  radiation therapy (antineoplastic) Z51.0
  reconstructive surgery following medical
      procedure or healed injury NEC Z42.8
  removal of
    cystostomy catheter Z43.5
    drains Z48.03
    dressing (nonsurgical) Z48.00
    implantable subdermal contraceptive
        Z30.46 ◀
    intrauterine contraceptive device Z30.432
    neuropacemaker (brain) (peripheral nerve)
        (spinal cord) Z46.2
      implanted Z45.42
    staples Z48.02
    surgical dressing Z48.01
    sutures Z48.02
    ureteral stent Z46.6
  respirator [ventilator] use during power
      failure Z99.12
  restoration of organ continuity
      (poststerilization) Z31.0
    aftercare Z31.42
  sensitivity test —*see also* Test, skin
    allergy NEC Z01.82
    Mantoux Z11.1
  tuboplasty following previous sterilization
      Z31.0
    aftercare Z31.42
  vasoplasty following previous sterilization
      Z31.0
    aftercare Z31.42
  vision examination Z01.00
    with abnormal findings Z01.01
  waiting period for admission to other facility
      Z75.1
Adnexitis (suppurative) —*see*
    Salpingo-oophoritis
Adolescent X-linked adrenoleukodystrophy
    E71.521
Adrenal (gland) —*see* condition
Adrenalism, tuberculous A18.7
Adrenalitis, adrenitis E27.8
  autoimmune E27.1
  meningococcal, hemorrhagic A39.1
Adrenarche, premature E27.0
Adrenocortical syndrome —*see* Cushing's,
    syndrome
Adrenogenital syndrome E25.9
  acquired E25.8
  congenital E25.0
  salt loss E25.0
Adrenogenitalism, congenital E25.0
Adrenoleukodystrophy E71.529
  neonatal E71.511
  X-linked E71.529
    Addison only phenotype E71.528
    Addison-Schilder E71.528
    adolescent E71.521
    adrenomyeloneuropathy E71.522
    childhood cerebral E71.520
    other specified E71.528
Adrenomyeloneuropathy E71.522
Adventitious bursa —*see* Bursopathy, specified
    type NEC
Adverse effect —*see* Table of Drugs and
    Chemicals, categories T36-T50, with 6th
    character 5
Advice —*see* Counseling
Adynamia (episodica) (hereditary) (periodic)
    G72.3
Aeration lung imperfect, newborn —*see*
    Atelectasis
Aerobullosis T70.3
Aerocele —*see* Embolism, air

Aerodermectasia
  subcutaneous (traumatic) T79.7
Aerodontalgia T70.29
Aeroembolism T70.3
Aerogenes capsulatus infection A48.0
Aero-otitis media T70.0
Aerophagy, aerophagia (psychogenic) F45.8
Aerophobia F40.228
Aerosinusitis T70.1
Aerotitis T70.0
Affection —*see* Disease
Afibrinogenemia —*see also* Defect, coagulation
    D68.8
  acquired D65
  congenital D68.2
  following ectopic or molar pregnancy O08.1
  in abortion —*see* Abortion, by type,
      complicated by, afibrinogenemia
  puerperal O72.3
African
  sleeping sickness B56.9
  tick fever A68.1
  trypanosomiasis B56.9
    gambian B56.0
    rhodesian B56.1
Aftercare —*see also* Care Z51.89
  following surgery (for) (on)
    amputation Z47.81
    attention to
      drains Z48.03
      dressings (nonsurgical) Z48.00
        surgical Z48.01
      sutures Z48.02
    circulatory system Z48.812
    delayed (planned) wound closure Z48.1
    digestive system Z48.815
    explantation of joint prosthesis (staged
        procedure)
      hip Z47.32
      knee Z47.33
      shoulder Z47.31
    genitourinary system Z48.816
    joint replacement Z47.1
    neoplasm Z48.3
    nervous system Z48.811
    oral cavity Z48.814
    organ transplant
      bone marrow Z48.290
      heart Z48.21
      heart-lung Z48.280
      kidney Z48.22
      liver Z48.23
      lung Z48.24
      multiple organs NEC Z48.288
      specified NEC Z48.298
    orthopedic NEC Z47.89
    planned wound closure Z48.1
    removal of internal fixation device Z47.2
    respiratory system Z48.813
    scoliosis Z47.82
    sense organs Z48.810
    skin and subcutaneous tissue Z48.817
    specified body system
      circulatory Z48.812
      digestive Z48.815
      genitourinary Z48.816
      nervous Z48.811
      oral cavity Z48.814
      respiratory Z48.813
      sense organs Z48.810
      skin and subcutaneous tissue Z48.817
      teeth Z48.814
    specified NEC Z48.89
    spinal Z48.89
    teeth Z48.814
  fracture — code to fracture with seventh
      character D
  involving
    removal of
      drains Z48.03
      dressings (nonsurgical) Z48.00

Aftercare *(Continued)*
  involving *(Continued)*
    removal of *(Continued)*
      staples Z48.02
      surgical dressings Z48.01
      sutures Z48.02
    neuropacemaker (brain) (peripheral nerve)
        (spinal cord) Z46.2
      implanted Z45.42
    orthopedic NEC Z47.89
    postprocedural —*see* Aftercare, following
        surgery
After-cataract —*see* Cataract, secondary
Agalactia (primary) O92.3
  elective, secondary or therapeutic O92.5
Agammaglobulinemia (acquired (secondary))
    (nonfamilial) D80.1
  with
    immunoglobulin-bearing B-lymphocytes
        D80.1
    lymphopenia D81.9
  autosomal recessive (Swiss type) D80.0
  Bruton's X-linked D80.0
  common variable (CVAgamma) D80.1
  congenital sex-linked D80.0
  hereditary D80.0
  lymphopenic D81.9
  Swiss type (autosomal recessive) D80.0
  X-linked (with growth hormone deficiency)
      (Bruton) D80.0 ◀▥
Aganglionosis (bowel) (colon) Q43.1
Age (old) —*see* Senility
Agenesis
  adrenal (gland) Q89.1
  alimentary tract (complete) (partial) NEC
      Q45.8
    upper Q40.8
  anus, anal (canal) Q42.3
    with fistula Q42.2
  aorta Q25.41 ◀▥
  appendix Q42.8
  arm (complete) Q71.0-
    with hand present Q71.1-
  artery (peripheral) Q27.9
    brain Q28.3
    coronary Q24.5
    pulmonary Q25.79
    specified NEC Q27.8
    umbilical Q27.0
  auditory (canal) (external) Q16.1
  auricle (ear) Q16.0
  bile duct or passage Q44.5
  bladder Q64.5
  bone Q79.9
  brain Q00.0
    part of Q04.3
  breast (with nipple present) Q83.8
    with absent nipple Q83.0
  bronchus Q32.4
  canaliculus lacrimalis Q10.4
  carpus —*see* Agenesis, hand
  cartilage Q79.9
  cecum Q42.8
  cerebellum Q04.3
  cervix Q51.5
  chin Q18.8
  cilia Q10.3
  circulatory system, part NOS Q28.9
  clavicle Q74.0
  clitoris Q52.6
  coccyx Q76.49
  colon Q42.9
    specified NEC Q42.8
  corpus callosum Q04.0
  cricoid cartilage Q31.8
  diaphragm (with hernia) Q79.1
  digestive organ (s) or tract (complete)
      (partial) NEC Q45.8
    upper Q40.8
  ductus arteriosus Q28.8
  duodenum Q41.0

Agenesis *(Continued)*
  ear Q16.9
    auricle Q16.0
    lobe Q17.8
  ejaculatory duct Q55.4
  endocrine (gland) NEC Q89.2
  epiglottis Q31.8
  esophagus Q39.8
  eustachian tube Q16.2
  eye Q11.1
    adnexa Q15.8
  eyelid (fold) Q10.3
  face
    bones NEC Q75.8
    specified part NEC Q18.8
  fallopian tube Q50.6
  femur —*see* Defect, reduction, lower limb,
      longitudinal, femur
  fibula —*see* Defect, reduction, lower limb,
      longitudinal, fibula
  finger (complete) (partial) —*see* Agenesis,
      hand
  foot (and toes) (complete) (partial) Q72.3-
  forearm (with hand present) —*see* Agenesis,
      arm, with hand present
      and hand Q71.2-
  gallbladder Q44.0
  gastric Q40.2
  genitalia, genital (organ (s))
    female Q52.8
      external Q52.71
      internal NEC Q52.8
    male Q55.8
  glottis Q31.8
  hair Q84.0
  hand (and fingers) (complete) (partial) Q71.3-
  heart Q24.8
    valve NEC Q24.8
      pulmonary Q22.0
  hepatic Q44.7
  humerus —*see* Defect, reduction, upper limb
  hymen Q52.4
  ileum Q41.2
  incus Q16.3
  intestine (small) Q41.9
    large Q42.9
      specified NEC Q42.8
  iris (dilator fibers) Q13.1
  jaw M26.09
  jejunum Q41.1
  kidney (s) (partial) Q60.2
    bilateral Q60.1
    unilateral Q60.0
  labium (majus) (minus) Q52.71
  labyrinth, membranous Q16.5
  lacrimal apparatus Q10.4
  larynx Q31.8
  leg (complete) Q72.0-
    with foot present Q72.1-
    lower leg (with foot present) —*see*
        Agenesis, leg, with foot present
        and foot Q72.2-
  lens Q12.3
  limb (complete) Q73.0
    lower —*see* Agenesis, leg
    upper —*see* Agenesis, arm
  lip Q38.0
  liver Q44.7
  lung (fissure) (lobe) (bilateral) (unilateral)
      Q33.3
  mandible, maxilla M26.09
  metacarpus —*see* Agenesis, hand
  metatarsus —*see* Agenesis, foot
  muscle Q79.8
    eyelid Q10.3
    ocular Q15.8
  musculoskeletal system NEC Q79.8
  nail (s) Q84.3
  neck, part Q18.8
  nerve Q07.8
  nervous system, part NEC Q07.8

Agenesis *(Continued)*
  nipple Q83.2
  nose Q30.1
  nuclear Q07.8
  organ
    of Corti Q16.5
    or site not listed —*see* Anomaly, by site
  osseous meatus (ear) Q16.1
  ovary
    bilateral Q50.02
    unilateral Q50.01
  oviduct Q50.6
  pancreas Q45.0
  parathyroid (gland) Q89.2
  parotid gland (s) Q38.4
  patella Q74.1
  pelvic girdle (complete) (partial) Q74.2
  penis Q55.5
  pericardium Q24.8
  pituitary (gland) Q89.2
  prostate Q55.4
  punctum lacrimale Q10.4
  radioulnar —*see* Defect, reduction, upper
      limb
  radius —*see* Defect, reduction, upper limb,
      longitudinal, radius
  rectum Q42.1
    with fistula Q42.0
  renal Q60.2
    bilateral Q60.1
    unilateral Q60.0
  respiratory organ NEC Q34.8
  rib Q76.6
  roof of orbit Q75.8
  round ligament Q52.8
  sacrum Q76.49
  salivary gland Q38.4
  scapula Q74.0
  scrotum Q55.29
  seminal vesicles Q55.4
  septum
    atrial Q21.1
    between aorta and pulmonary artery
        Q21.4
    ventricular Q20.4
  shoulder girdle (complete) (partial) Q74.0
  skull (bone) Q75.8
    with
      anencephaly Q00.0
      encephalocele —*see* Encephalocele
      hydrocephalus Q03.9
        with spina bifida —*see* Spina bifida, by
            site, with hydrocephalus
      microcephaly Q02
  spermatic cord Q55.4
  spinal cord Q06.0
  spine Q76.49
  spleen Q89.01
  sternum Q76.7
  stomach Q40.2
  submaxillary gland (s) (congenital) Q38.4
  tarsus —*see* Agenesis, foot
  tendon Q79.8
  testicle Q55.0
  thymus (gland) Q89.2
  thyroid (gland) E03.1
    cartilage Q31.8
  tibia —*see* Defect, reduction, lower limb,
      longitudinal, tibia
  tibiofibular —*see* Defect, reduction, lower
      limb, specified type NEC
  toe (and foot) (complete) (partial) —*see*
      Agenesis, foot
  tongue Q38.3
  trachea (cartilage) Q32.1
  ulna —*see* Defect, reduction, upper limb,
      longitudinal, ulna
  upper limb —*see* Agenesis, arm
  ureter Q62.4
  urethra Q64.5
  urinary tract NEC Q64.8

Agenesis *(Continued)*
  uterus Q51.0
  uvula Q38.5
  vagina Q52.0
  vas deferens Q55.4
  vein (s) (peripheral) Q27.9
    brain Q28.3
    great NEC Q26.8
    portal Q26.5
  vena cava (inferior) (superior) Q26.8
  vermis of cerebellum Q04.3
  vertebra Q76.49
  vulva Q52.71
Ageusia R43.2
Agitated —*see* condition
Agitation R45.1
Aglossia (congenital) Q38.3
Aglossia-adactylia syndrome Q87.0
Aglycogenosis E74.00
Agnosia (body image) (other senses) (tactile)
      R48.1
  developmental F88
  verbal R48.1
    auditory R48.1
      developmental F80.2
    developmental F80.2
  visual (object) R48.3
Agoraphobia F40.00
  with panic disorder F40.01
  without panic disorder F40.02
Agrammatism R48.8
Agranulocytopenia —*see* Agranulocytosis
Agranulocytosis (chronic) (cyclical) (genetic)
      (infantile) (periodic) (pernicious) (*see also*
      Neutropenia) D70.9
  congenital D70.0
  cytoreductive cancer chemotherapy sequela
      D70.1
  drug-induced D70.2
    due to cytoreductive cancer chemotherapy
        D70.1
  due to infection D70.3
  secondary D70.4
    drug-induced D70.2
      due to cytoreductive cancer
          chemotherapy D70.1
Agraphia (absolute) R48.8
  with alexia R48.0
  developmental F81.81
Ague (dumb) —*see* Malaria
Agyria Q04.3
Ahumada-del Castillo syndrome E23.0
Aichomophobia F40.298
AIDS (related complex) B20
Ailment heart —*see* Disease, heart
Ailurophobia F40.218
Ainhum (disease) L94.6
AIN —*see* Neoplasia, intraepithelial, anal ◀
AIPHI (acute idiopathic pulmonary hemorrhage
      in infants (over 28 days old)) R04.81
Air
  anterior mediastinum J98.2
  compressed, disease T70.3
  conditioner lung or pneumonitis J67.7
  embolism (artery) (cerebral) (any site) T79.0
    with ectopic or molar pregnancy O08.2
    due to implanted device NEC —*see*
        Complications, by site and type,
        specified NEC
    following
      abortion —*see* Abortion by type,
          complicated by, embolism
      ectopic or molar pregnancy O08.2
    infusion, therapeutic injection or
        transfusion T80.0
    in pregnancy, childbirth or puerperium —
        see Embolism, obstetric
    traumatic T79.0
  hunger, psychogenic F45.8
  rarefied, effects of —*see* Effect, adverse, high
      altitude
  sickness T75.3

◀ New   ◀▥ Revised   ~~deleted~~ Deleted

Airplane sickness T75.3
Akathisia (drug-induced) (treatment- induced) G25.71
  neuroleptic induced (acute) G25.71
Akinesia R29.898
Akinetic mutism R41.89
Akureyri's disease G93.3
Alactasia, congenital E73.0
Alagille's syndrome Q44.7
Alastrim B03
Albers-Schönberg syndrome Q78.2
Albert's syndrome —see Tendinitis, Achilles
Albinism, albino E70.30
  with hematologic abnormality E70.339
    Chédiak-Higashi syndrome E70.330
    Hermansky-Pudlak syndrome E70.331
    other specified E70.338
  I E70.320
  II E70.321
  ocular E70.319
    autosomal recessive E70.311
    other specified E70.318
    X-linked E70.310
  oculocutaneous E70.329
    other specified E70.328
    tyrosinase (ty) negative E70.320
    tyrosinase (ty) positive E70.321
  other specified E70.39
Albinismus E70.30
Albright (-McCune)(-Sternberg) syndrome Q78.1
Albuminous —see condition
Albuminuria, albuminuric (acute) (chronic) (subacute) —see also Proteinuria R80.9
  complicating pregnancy —see Proteinuria, gestational
    with
      gestational hypertension —see Pre-eclampsia
      pre-existing hypertension —see Hypertension, complicating pregnancy, pre-existing, with, pre-eclampsia
  gestational —see Proteinuria, gestational
    with
      gestational hypertension —see Pre-eclampsia
      pre-existing hypertension —see Hypertension, complicating pregnancy, pre-existing, with, pre-eclampsia
  orthostatic R80.2
  postural R80.2
  pre-eclamptic —see Pre-eclampsia
  scarlatinal A38.8
Albuminurophobia F40.298
Alcaptonuria E70.29
Alcohol, alcoholic, alcohol-induced
  addiction (without remission) F10.20
    with remission F10.21
  amnestic disorder, persisting F10.96
    with dependence F10.26
  anxiety disorder F10.980 ◀
  bipolar and related disorder F10.94 ◀
  brain syndrome, chronic F10.97
    with dependence F10.27
  cardiopathy I42.6
  counseling and surveillance Z71.41
    family member Z71.42
  delirium (acute) (tremens) (withdrawal) F10.231
    with intoxication F10.921
      in
        abuse F10.121
        dependence F10.221
  dementia F10.97
    with dependence F10.27
  depressive disorder F10.94 ◀
  deterioration F10.97
    with dependence F10.27

Alcohol, alcoholic, alcohol-induced (Continued)
  hallucinosis (acute) F10.951
    in
      abuse F10.151
      dependence F10.251
  insanity F10.959
  intoxication (acute) (without dependence) F10.129
    with
      delirium F10.121
      dependence F10.229
        with delirium F10.221
        uncomplicated F10.220
      uncomplicated F10.120
  jealousy F10.988
  Korsakoff's, Korsakov's, Korsakow's F10.26
  liver K70.9
    acute —see Disease, liver, alcoholic, hepatitis
  major neurocognitive disorder, amnestic-confabulatory type F10.96 ◀
  major neurocognitive disorder, nonamnestic-confabulatory type F10.97 ◀
  mania (acute) (chronic) F10.959
  mild neurocognitive disorder F10.988 ◀
  paranoia, paranoid (type) psychosis F10.950
  pellagra E52
  poisoning, accidental (acute) NEC —see Table of Drugs and Chemicals, alcohol, poisoning
  psychosis —see Psychosis, alcoholic
  psychotic disorder F10.959 ◀
  sexual dysfunction F10.981 ◀
  sleep disorder F10.982 ◀
  withdrawal (without convulsions) F10.239
    with delirium F10.231
Alcoholism (chronic) (without remission) F10.20
  with
    psychosis —see Psychosis, alcoholic
      remission F10.21
  Korsakov's F10.96
    with dependence F10.26
Alder (-Reilly) anomaly or syndrome (leukocyte granulation) D72.0
Aldosteronism E26.9
  familial (type I) E26.02
  glucocorticoid-remediable E26.02
  primary (due to (bilateral) adrenal hyperplasia) E26.09
  primary NEC E26.09
  secondary E26.1
  specified NEC E26.89
Aldosteronoma D44.10
Aldrich(-Wiskott) syndrome (eczema-thrombocytopenia) D82.0
Alektorophobia F40.218
Aleppo boil B55.1
Aleukemic —see condition Aleukia
  congenital D70.0
  hemorrhagica D61.9
    congenital D61.09
  splenica D73.1
Alexia R48.0
  developmental F81.0
  secondary to organic lesion R48.0
Algoneurodystrophy M89.00
  ankle M89.07-
  foot M89.07-
  forearm M89.03-
  hand M89.04-
  lower leg M89.06-
  multiple sites M89.0-
  shoulder M89.01-
  specified site NEC M89.08
  thigh M89.05-
  upper arm M89.02-
Algophobia F40.298
Alienation, mental —see Psychosis
Alkalemia E87.3

Alkalosis E87.3
  metabolic E87.3
    with respiratory acidosis E87.4
  respiratory E87.3
Alkaptonuria E70.29
Allen-Masters syndrome N83.8
Allergy, allergic (reaction) (to) T78.40
  air-borne substance NEC (rhinitis) J30.89
  alveolitis (extrinsic) J67.9
    due to
      Aspergillus clavatus J67.4
      Cryptostroma corticale J67.6
      organisms (fungal, thermophilic actinomycete) growing in ventilation (air conditioning) systems J67.7
      specified type NEC J67.8
  anaphylactic reaction or shock T78.2
  angioneurotic edema T78.3
  animal (dander) (epidermal) (hair) (rhinitis) J30.81
  bee sting (anaphylactic shock) —see Toxicity, venom, arthropod, bee
  biological —see Allergy, drug
  colitis —see also Colitis, allergic K52.29 ◀▥
  dander (animal) (rhinitis) J30.81
  dandruff (rhinitis) J30.81
  dental restorative material (existing) K08.55
  dermatitis —see Dermatitis, contact, allergic
  diathesis —see History, allergy
  drug, medicament & biological (any) (external) (internal) T78.40
    correct substance properly administered —see Table of Drugs and Chemicals, by drug, adverse effect
    wrong substance given or taken NEC (by accident) —see Table of Drugs and Chemicals, by drug, poisoning
  due to pollen J30.1
  dust (house) (stock) (rhinitis) J30.89
    with asthma —see Asthma, allergic extrinsic
  eczema —see Dermatitis, contact, allergic
  epidermal (animal) (rhinitis) J30.81
  feathers (rhinitis) J30.89
  food (any) (ingested) NEC T78.1
    anaphylactic shock —see Shock, anaphylactic, due to food
    dermatitis —see Dermatitis, due to, food
    dietary counseling and surveillance Z71.3
    in contact with skin L23.6
    rhinitis J30.5
    status (without reaction) Z91.018
      eggs Z91.012
      milk products Z91.011
      peanuts Z91.010
      seafood Z91.013
      specified NEC Z91.018
  gastrointestinal —see also specific type of allergic reaction ◀▥
    meaning colitis —see also Colitis, allergic) K52.29 ◀
    meaning gastroenteritis —see also Gastroenteritis, allergic) K52.29 ◀
    meaning other adverse food reaction not elsewhere classified T78.1 ◀
  grain J30.1
  grass (hay fever) (pollen) J30.1
    asthma —see Asthma, allergic extrinsic
  hair (animal) (rhinitis) J30.81
  history (of) —see History, allergy
  horse serum —see Allergy, serum
  inhalant (rhinitis) J30.89
    pollen J30.1
  kapok (rhinitis) J30.89
  medicine —see Allergy, drug
  milk protein —see also Allergy, food Z91.011 ◀▥
    anaphylactic reaction T78.07 ◀
    dermatitis L27.2 ◀
    enterocolitis syndrome K52.21 ◀
    enteropathy K52.22 ◀
    gastroenteritis K52.29 ◀

Allergy, allergic (Continued)
  milk protein (Continued)
    gastroesophageal reflux —see also Reaction,
        adverse, food) K21.9 ◄
      with esophagitis K21.0 ◄
    proctocolitis K52.82 ◄]
  nasal, seasonal due to pollen J30.1
  pneumonia J82
  pollen (any) (hay fever) J30.1
    asthma —see Asthma, allergic extrinsic
  primrose J30.1
  primula J30.1
  proctocolitis K52.82 ◄
  purpura D69.0
  ragweed (hay fever) (pollen) J30.1
    asthma —see Asthma, allergic extrinsic
  rose (pollen) J30.1
  seasonal NEC J30.2
  Senecio jacobae (pollen) J30.1
  serum —see also Reaction, serum T80.69
    anaphylactic shock T80.59
  shock (anaphylactic) T78.2
    due to
      administration of blood and blood
          products T80.51
      adverse effect of correct medicinal
          substance properly administered
          T88.6
      immunization T80.52
      serum NEC T80.59
      vaccination T80.52
  specific NEC T78.49
  tree (any) (hay fever) (pollen) J30.1
    asthma —see Asthma, allergic extrinsic
  upper respiratory J30.9
  urticaria L50.0
  vaccine —see Allergy, serum
  wheat —see Allergy, food
Allescheriasis B48.2
Alligator skin disease Q80.9
Allocheiria, allochiria R20.8
Almeida's disease —see
    Paracoccidioidomycosis
Alopecia (hereditaria) (seborrheica) L65.9
  androgenic L64.9
    drug-induced L64.0
    specified NEC L64.8
  areata L63.9
    ophiasis L63.2
    specified NEC L63.8
    totalis L63.0
    universalis L63.1
  cicatricial L66.9
    specified NEC L66.8
  circumscripta L63.9
  congenital, congenitalis Q84.0
  due to cytotoxic drugs NEC L65.8
  mucinosa L65.2
  postinfective NEC L65.8
  postpartum L65.0
  premature L64.8
  specific (syphilitic) A51.32
  specified NEC L65.8
  syphilitic (secondary) A51.32
  totalis (capitis) L63.0
  universalis (entire body) L63.1
  X-ray L58.1
Alpers' disease G31.81
Alpine sickness T70.29
Alport syndrome Q87.81
ALTE (apparent life threatening event) in
    newborn and infant R68.13
Alteration (of), Altered
  awareness, transient R40.4
  awareness ◄
    transient R40.4 ◄
    unintended under general anesthesia,
        during procedure T88.53 ◄
  mental status R41.82
  pattern of family relationships affecting child
      Z62.898

Alteration (of), Altered (Continued)
  sensation
    following
      cerebrovascular disease I69.998
        cerebral infarction I69.398
        intracerebral hemorrhage I69.198
        nontraumatic intracranial hemorrhage
            NEC I69.298
        specified disease NEC I69.898
        subarachnoid hemorrhage I69.098
Alternating —see condition
Altitude, high (effects) —see Effect, adverse,
    high altitude
Aluminosis (of lung) J63.0
Alveolitis
  allergic (extrinsic) —see Pneumonitis,
      hypersensitivity
  due to
    Aspergillus clavatus J67.4
    Cryptostroma corticale J67.6
  fibrosing (cryptogenic) (idiopathic) J84.112
  jaw M27.3
  sicca dolorosa M27.3
Alveolus, alveolar —see condition
Alymphocytosis D72.810
  thymic (with immunodeficiency) D82.1
Alymphoplasia, thymic D82.1
Alzheimer's disease or sclerosis —see Disease,
    Alzheimer's
Amastia (with nipple present) Q83.8
  with absent nipple Q83.0
Amathophobia F40.228
Amaurosis (acquired) (congenital) —see also
    Blindness
  fugax G45.3
  hysterical F44.6
  Leber's congenital H35.50
  uremic —see Uremia
Amaurotic idiocy (infantile) (juvenile) (late) E75.4
Amaxophobia F40.248
Ambiguous genitalia Q56.4
Amblyopia (congenital) (ex anopsia) (partial)
    (suppression) H53.00-
  anisometropic —see Amblyopia, refractive
  deprivation H53.01-
  hysterical F44.6
  nocturnal —see also Blindness, night
    vitamin A deficiency E50.5
  refractive H53.02-
  strabismic H53.03-
  suspect H53.04- ◄
  tobacco H53.8
  toxic NEC H53.8
  uremic —see Uremia
Ameba, amebic (histolytica) —see also Amebiasis
  abscess (liver) A06.4
Amebiasis A06.9
  with abscess —see Abscess, amebic
  acute A06.0
  chronic (intestine) A06.1
    with abscess —see Abscess, amebic
  cutaneous A06.7
  cutis A06.7
  cystitis A06.81
  genitourinary tract NEC A06.82
  hepatic —see Abscess, liver, amebic
  intestine A06.0
  nondysenteric colitis A06.2
  skin A06.7
  specified site NEC A06.89
Ameboma (of intestine) A06.3
Amelia Q73.0
  lower limb —see Agenesis, leg
  upper limb —see Agenesis, arm
Ameloblastoma —see also Cyst, calcifying
    odontogenic
  long bones C40.9-
    lower limb C40.2-
    upper limb C40.0-
  malignant C41.1
    jaw (bone) (lower) C41.1
      upper C41.0
  tibial C40.2-

Amelogenesis imperfecta K00.5
  nonhereditaria (segmentalis) K00.4
Amenorrhea N91.2
  hyperhormonal E28.8
  primary N91.0
  secondary N91.1
Amentia —see Disability, intellectual
  Meynert's (nonalcoholic) F04
American
  leishmaniasis B55.2
  mountain tick fever A93.2
Ametropia —see Disorder, refraction
AMH (asymptomatic microscopic hematuria)
    R31.21 ◄
Amianthosis J61
Amimia R48.8
Amino-acid disorder E72.9
  anemia D53.0
Aminoacidopathy E72.9
Aminoaciduria E72.9
Amnes (t)ic syndrome (post-traumatic) F04
  induced by
    alcohol F10.96
      with dependence F10.26
    psychoactive NEC F19.96
      with
        abuse F19.16
        dependence F19.26
    sedative F13.96
      with dependence F13.26
Amnesia R41.3
  anterograde R41.1
  auditory R48.8
  dissociative F44.0
    with dissociative fugue F44.1 ◄
  hysterical F44.0
  postictal in epilepsy —see Epilepsy
  psychogenic F44.0
  retrograde R41.2
  transient global G45.4
Amnion, amniotic —see condition
Amnionitis —see Pregnancy, complicated by
Amok F68.8
Amoral traits F60.89
Amphetamine (or other stimulant) —
    induced ◄
  anxiety disorder F15.980 ◄
  bipolar and related disorder F15.94 ◄
  delirium F15.921 ◄
  depressive disorder F15.94 ◄
  obsessive-compulsive and related disorder
      F15.988 ◄
  psychotic disorder F15.959 ◄
  sexual dysfunction F15.981 ◄
  sleep disorder F15.982 ◄
  stimulant withdrawal F15.23 ◄
Ampulla
  lower esophagus K22.8
  phrenic K22.8
Amputation —see also Absence, by site,
    acquired
  neuroma (postoperative) (traumatic) —see
      Complications, amputation stump,
      neuroma
  stump (surgical)
    abnormal, painful, or with complication
        (late) —see Complications,
        amputation stump
    healed or old NOS Z89.9
  traumatic (complete) (partial)
    arm (upper) (complete) S48.91-
      at
        elbow S58.01-
          partial S58.02-
        shoulder joint (complete) S48.01-
          partial S48.02-
      between
        elbow and wrist (complete) S58.11-
          partial S58.12-
        shoulder and elbow (complete) S48.11-
          partial S48.12-
      partial S48.92-

◄ New   ◄▥ Revised   deleted Deleted

Amputation (Continued)
  traumatic (Continued)
    breast (complete) S28.21-
      partial S28.22-
    clitoris (complete) S38.211
      partial S38.212
    ear (complete) S08.11-
      partial S08.12-
    finger (complete) (metacarpophalangeal)
        S68.11-
      index S68.11-
      little S68.11-
      middle S68.11-
      partial S68.12-
        index S68.12-
        little S68.12-
        middle S68.12-
        ring S68.12-
      ring S68.11-
      thumb —see Amputation, traumatic,
        thumb
      transphalangeal (complete) S68.61-
        index S68.61-
        little S68.61-
        middle S68.61-
        partial S68.62-
          index S68.62-
          little S68.62-
          middle S68.62-
          ring S68.62-
        ring S68.61-
    foot (complete) S98.91-
      at ankle level S98.01-
        partial S98.02-
      midfoot S98.31-
        partial S98.32-
      partial S98.92-
    forearm (complete) S58.91-
      at elbow level (complete) S58.01-
        partial S58.02-
      between elbow and wrist (complete)
        S58.11-
        partial S58.12-
      partial S58.92-
    genital organ (s) (external)
      female (complete) S38.211
        partial S38.212
      male
        penis (complete) S38.221
          partial S38.222
        scrotum (complete) S38.231
          partial S38.232
        testes (complete) S38.231
          partial S38.232
    hand (complete) (wrist level) S68.41-
      finger (s) alone —see Amputation,
        traumatic, finger
      partial S68.42-
      thumb alone —see Amputation,
        traumatic, thumb
      transmetacarpal (complete) S68.71-
        partial S68.72-
    head
      ear —see Amputation, traumatic, ear
      nose (partial) S08.812
        complete S08.811
      part S08.89
      scalp S08.0
    hip (and thigh) (complete) S78.91-
      at hip joint (complete) S78.01-
        partial S78.02-
      between hip and knee (complete) S78.11-
        partial S78.12-
      partial S78.92-
    labium (majus) (minus) (complete) S38.21-
      partial S38.21-
    leg (lower) S88.91-
      at knee level S88.01-
        partial S88.02-
      between knee and ankle S88.11-
        partial S88.12-
      partial S88.92-

Amputation (Continued)
  traumatic (Continued)
    nose (partial) S08.812
      complete S08.811
    penis (complete) S38.221
      partial S38.222
    scrotum (complete) S38.231
      partial S38.232
    shoulder —see Amputation, traumatic, arm
      at shoulder joint —see Amputation,
        traumatic, arm, at shoulder joint
    testes (complete) S38.231
      partial S38.232
    thigh —see Amputation, traumatic, hip
    thorax, part of S28.1
      breast —see Amputation, traumatic,
        breast
    thumb (complete) (metacarpophalangeal)
        S68.01-
      partial S68.02-
      transphalangeal (complete) S68.51-
        partial S68.52-
    toe (lesser) S98.13-
      great S98.11-
        partial S98.12-
      more than one S98.21-
        partial S98.22-
      partial S98.14-
    vulva (complete) S38.211
      partial S38.212
Amputee (bilateral) (old) Z89.9
Amsterdam dwarfism Q87.1
Amusia R48.8
  developmental F80.89
Amyelencephalus, amyelencephaly Q00.0
Amyelia Q06.0
Amygdalitis —see Tonsillitis
Amygdalolith J35.8
Amyloid heart (disease) E85.4 [I43]
Amyloidosis (generalized) (primary) E85.9
  with lung involvement E85.4 [J99]
  familial E85.2
  genetic E85.2
  heart E85.4 [I43]
  hemodialysis-associated E85.3
  liver E85.4 [K77]
  localized E85.4
  neuropathic heredofamilial E85.1
  non-neuropathic heredofamilial E85.0
  organ limited E85.4
  Portuguese E85.1
  pulmonary E85.4 [J99]
  secondary systemic E85.3
  skin (lichen) (macular) E85.4 [L99]
  specified NEC E85.8
  subglottic E85.4 [J99]
Amylopectinosis (brancher enzyme deficiency)
    E74.03
Amylophagia —see Pica
Amyoplasia congenita Q79.8
Amyotonia M62.89
  congenita G70.2
Amyotrophia, amyotrophy, amyotrophic G71.8
  congenita Q79.8
  diabetic —see Diabetes, amyotrophy
  lateral sclerosis G12.21
  neuralgic G54.5
  spinal progressive G12.21
Anacidity, gastric K31.83
  psychogenic F45.8
Anaerosis of newborn P28.89
Analbuminemia E88.09
Analgesia —see Anesthesia
Analphalipoproteinemia E78.6
Anaphylactic
  purpura D69.0
  shock or reaction —see Shock, anaphylactic
Anaphylactoid shock or reaction —see Shock,
    anaphylactic
Anaphylactoid syndrome of pregnancy
    O88.01-

Anaphylaxis —see Shock, anaphylactic
Anaplasia cervix —see also Dysplasia, cervix
    N87.9
Anaplasmosis, human A77.49
Anarthria R47.1
Anasarca R60.1
  cardiac —see Failure, heart, congestive
  lung J18.2
  newborn P83.2
  nutritional E43
  pulmonary J18.2
  renal N04.9
Anastomosis
  aneurysmal —see Aneurysm
  arteriovenous ruptured brain I60.8
  intestinal K63.89
    complicated NEC K91.89
      involving urinary tract N99.89
  retinal and choroidal vessels (congenital)
    Q14.8
Anatomical narrow angle H40.03-
Ancylostoma, ancylostomiasis (braziliense)
    (caninum) (ceylanicum) (duodenale) B76.0
  Necator americanus B76.1
Andersen's disease (glycogen storage) E74.09
Anderson-Fabry disease E75.21
Andes disease T70.29
Andrews' disease (bacterid) L08.89
Androblastoma
  benign
    specified site —see Neoplasm, benign, by
      site
    unspecified site
      female D27.9
      male D29.20
  malignant
    specified site —see Neoplasm, malignant,
      by site
    unspecified site
      female C56.9
      male C62.90
  specified site —see Neoplasm, uncertain
      behavior, by site
  tubular
    with lipid storage
      specified site —see Neoplasm, benign,
        by site
      unspecified site
        female D27.9
        male D29.20
    specified site —see Neoplasm, benign, by site
    unspecified site
      female D27.9
      male D29.20
  unspecified site
    female D39.10
    male D40.10
Androgen insensitivity syndrome —see also
    Syndrome, androgen insensitivity E34.50
Androgen resistance syndrome —see also
    Syndrome, androgen insensitivity
    E34.50
Android pelvis Q74.2
  with disproportion (fetopelvic) O33.3
    causing obstructed labor O65.3
Androphobia F40.290
Anectasis, pulmonary (newborn) —see
    Atelectasis
Anemia (essential) (general) (hemoglobin
    deficiency) (infantile) (primary)
    (profound) D64.9
  with (due to) (in)
    disorder of
      anaerobic glycolysis D55.2
        pentose phosphate pathway D55.1
      koilonychia D50.9
    achlorhydric D50.8
    achrestic D53.1
    Addison (-Biermer) (pernicious) D51.0
    agranulocytic —see Agranulocytosis
    amino-acid-deficiency D53.0

Anemia (Continued)
  aplastic D61.9
    congenital D61.09
    drug-induced D61.1
    due to
      drugs D61.1
      external agents NEC D61.2
      infection D61.2
      radiation D61.2
    idiopathic D61.3
    red cell (pure) D60.9
      chronic D60.0
      congenital D61.01
      specified type NEC D60.8
      transient D60.1
    specified type NEC D61.89
    toxic D61.2
  aregenerative
    congenital D61.09
  asiderotic D50.9
  atypical (primary) D64.9
  Baghdad spring D55.0
  Balantidium coli A07.0
  Biermer's (pernicious) D51.0
  blood loss (chronic) D50.0
    acute D62
  bothriocephalus B70.0 [D63.8]
  brickmaker's B76.9 [D63.8]
  cerebral I67.89
  childhood D58.9
  chlorotic D50.8
  chronic
    blood loss D50.0
    hemolytic D58.9
      idiopathic D59.9
    simple D53.9
  chronica congenita aregenerativa D61.09
  combined system disease NEC D51.0 [G32.0]
    due to dietary vitamin B12 deficiency
      D51.3 [G32.0]
  complicating pregnancy, childbirth
    or puerperium —see Pregnancy,
    complicated by (management affected
    by), anemia
  congenital P61.4
    aplastic D61.09
    due to isoimmunization NOS P55.9
    dyserythropoietic, dyshematopoietic D64.4
    following fetal blood loss P61.3
    Heinz body D58.2
    hereditary hemolytic NOS D58.9
    pernicious D51.0
    spherocytic D58.0
  Cooley's (erythroblastic) D56.1
  cytogenic D51.0
  deficiency D53.9
    2, 3 diphosphoglycurate mutase D55.2
    2, 3 PG D55.2
    6 phosphogluconate dehydrogenase D55.1
    6-PGD D55.1
    amino-acid D53.0
    combined B12 and folate D53.1
    enzyme D55.9
      drug-induced (hemolytic) D59.2
      glucose-6-phosphate dehydrogenase
        (G6PD) D55.0
      glycolytic D55.2
      nucleotide metabolism D55.3
      related to hexose monophosphate
        (HMP) shunt pathway NEC D55.1
      specified type NEC D55.8
    erythrocytic glutathione D55.1
    folate D52.9
      dietary D52.0
      drug-induced D52.1
    folic acid D52.9
      dietary D52.0
      drug-induced D52.1
    G SH D55.1
    G6PD D55.0
    GGS-R D55.1

Anemia (Continued)
  deficiency (Continued)
    glucose-6-phosphate dehydrogenase D55.0
    glutathione reductase D55.1
    glyceraldehyde phosphate dehydrogenase
      D55.2
    hexokinase D55.2
    iron D50.9
      secondary to blood loss (chronic) D50.0
    nutritional D53.9
      with
        poor iron absorption D50.8
        specified deficiency NEC D53.8
    phosphofructo-aldolase D55.2
    phosphoglycerate kinase D55.2
    PK D55.2
    protein D53.0
    pyruvate kinase D55.2
    transcobalamin II D51.2
    triose-phosphate isomerase D55.2
    vitamin B12 NOS D51.9
      dietary D51.3
      due to
        intrinsic factor deficiency D51.0
        selective vitamin B12 malabsorption
          with proteinuria D51.1
      pernicious D51.0
      specified type NEC D51.8
  Diamond-Blackfan (congenital hypoplastic)
    D61.01
  dibothriocephalus B70.0 [D63.8]
  dimorphic D53.1
  diphasic D53.1
  Diphyllobothrium (Dibothriocephalus) B70.0
    [D63.8]
  due to (in) (with)
    antineoplastic chemotherapy D64.81
    blood loss (chronic) D50.0
      acute D62
    chemotherapy, antineoplastic D64.81
    chronic disease classified elsewhere NEC
      D63.8
    chronic kidney disease D63.1
    deficiency
      amino-acid D53.0
      copper D53.8
      folate (folic acid) D52.9
        dietary D52.0
        drug-induced D52.1
      molybdenum D53.8
      protein D53.0
      zinc D53.8
    dietary vitamin B12 deficiency D51.3
    disorder of
      glutathione metabolism D55.1
      nucleotide metabolism D55.3
    drug —see Anemia, by type —see also Table
      of Drugs and Chemicals
    end stage renal disease D63.1
    enzyme disorder D55.9
    fetal blood loss P61.3
    fish tapeworm (D latum) infestation B70.0
      [D63.8]
    hemorrhage (chronic) D50.0
      acute D62
    impaired absorption D50.9
    loss of blood (chronic) D50.0
      acute D62
    myxedema E03.9 [D63.8]
    Necator americanus B76.1 [D63.8]
    prematurity P61.2
    selective vitamin B12 malabsorption with
      proteinuria D51.1
    transcobalamin II deficiency D51.2
  Dyke-Young type (secondary) (symptomatic)
    D59.1
  dyserythropoietic (congenital) D64.4
  dyshematopoietic (congenital) D64.4
  Egyptian B76.9 [D63.8]
  elliptocytosis —see Elliptocytosis
  enzyme-deficiency, drug-induced D59.2

Anemia (Continued)
  epidemic —see also Ancylostomiasis B76.9
    [D63.8]
  erythroblastic
    familial D56.1
    newborn —see also Disease, hemolytic P55.9
    of childhood D56.1
  erythrocytic glutathione deficiency D55.1
  erythropoietin-resistant anemia (EPO
    resistant anemia) D63.1
  Faber's (achlorhydric anemia) D50.9
  factitious (self-induced blood letting) D50.0
  familial erythroblastic D56.1
  Fanconi's (congenital pancytopenia) D61.09
  favism D55.0
  fish tapeworm (D. latum) infestation B70.0
    [D63.8]
  folate (folic acid) deficiency D52.9
  glucose-6-phosphate dehydrogenase (G6PD)
    deficiency D55.0
  glutathione-reductase deficiency D55.1
  goat's milk D52.0
  granulocytic —see Agranulocytosis
  Heinz body, congenital D58.2
  hemolytic D58.9
    acquired D59.9
      with hemoglobinuria NEC D59.6
      autoimmune NEC D59.1
      infectious D59.4
      specified type NEC D59.8
      toxic D59.4
    acute D59.9
      due to enzyme deficiency specified type
        NEC D55.8
      Lederer's D59.1
    autoimmune D59.1
      drug-induced D59.0
    chronic D58.9
      idiopathic D59.9
    cold type (secondary) (symptomatic) D59.1
    congenital (spherocytic) —see
      Spherocytosis
    due to
      cardiac conditions D59.4
      drugs (nonautoimmune) D59.2
        autoimmune D59.0
      enzyme disorder D55.9
        drug-induced D59.2
      presence of shunt or other internal
        prosthetic device D59.4
    familial D58.9
    hereditary D58.9
      due to enzyme disorder D55.9
        specified type NEC D55.8
      specified type NEC D58.8
    idiopathic (chronic) D59.9
    mechanical D59.4
    microangiopathic D59.4
    nonautoimmune D59.4
      drug-induced D59.2
    nonspherocytic
      congenital or hereditary NEC D55.8
        glucose-6-phosphate dehydrogenase
          deficiency D55.0
        pyruvate kinase deficiency D55.2
        type
          I D55.1
          II D55.2
      type
        I D55.1
        II D55.2
    secondary D59.4
      autoimmune D59.1
    specified (hereditary) type NEC D58.8
    Stransky-Regala type —see also
      Hemoglobinopathy D58.8
    symptomatic D59.4
      autoimmune D59.1
    toxic D59.4
    warm type (secondary) (symptomatic)
      D59.1

◀ New   ◀⦚ Revised   ~~deleted~~ Deleted

Anemia *(Continued)*
  hemorrhagic (chronic) D50.0
    acute D62
  Herrick's D57.1
  hexokinase deficiency D55.2
  hookworm B76.9 *[D63.8]*
  hypochromic (idiopathic) (microcytic)
    (normoblastic) D50.9
    due to blood loss (chronic) D50.0
      acute D62
    familial sex-linked D64.0
    pyridoxine-responsive D64.3
    sideroblastic, sex-linked D64.0
  hypoplasia, red blood cells D61.9
    congenital or familial D61.01
  hypoplastic (idiopathic) D61.9
    congenital or familial (of childhood)
      D61.01
  hypoproliferative (refractive) D61.9
  idiopathic D64.9
    aplastic D61.3
    hemolytic, chronic D59.9
  in (due to) (with)
    chronic kidney disease D63.1
    end stage renal disease D63.1
    failure, kidney (renal) D63.1
    neoplastic disease —*see also* Neoplasm
      D63.0
  intertropical —*see also* Ancylostomiasis D63.8
  iron deficiency D50.9
    secondary to blood loss (chronic) D50.0
      acute D62
    specified type NEC D50.8
  Joseph-Diamond-Blackfan (congenital
    hypoplastic) D61.01
  Lederer's (hemolytic) D59.1
  leukoerythroblastic D61.82
  macrocytic D53.9
    nutritional D52.0
    tropical D52.8
  malarial (*see also* Malaria) B54 *[D63.8]*
  malignant (progressive) D51.0
  malnutrition D53.9
  marsh (*see also* Malaria) B54 *[D63.8]*
  Mediterranean (with other
    hemoglobinopathy) D56.9
  megaloblastic D53.1
    combined B12 and folate deficiency
      D53.1
    hereditary D51.1
    nutritional D52.0
    orotic aciduria D53.0
    refractory D53.1
    specified type NEC D53.1
  megalocytic D53.1
  microcytic (hypochromic) D50.9
    due to blood loss (chronic) D50.0
      acute D62
    familial D56.8
  microdrepanocytosis D57.40
  microelliptopoikilocytic (Rietti-Greppi-
    Micheli) D56.9
  miner's B76.9 *[D63.8]*
  myelodysplastic D46.9
  myelofibrosis D75.81
  myelogenous D64.89
  myelopathic D64.89
  myelophthisic D61.82
  myeloproliferative D47.Z9
  newborn P61.4
    due to
      ABO (antibodies, isoimmunization,
        maternal/fetal incompatibility)
        P55.1
      Rh (antibodies, isoimmunization,
        maternal/fetal incompatibility)
        P55.0
    following fetal blood loss P61.3
    posthemorrhagic (fetal) P61.3
  nonspherocytic hemolytic —*see* Anemia,
    hemolytic, nonspherocytic

Anemia *(Continued)*
  normocytic (infectional) D64.9
    due to blood loss (chronic) D50.0
      acute D62
    myelophthisic D61.82
  nutritional (deficiency) D53.9
    with
      poor iron absorption D50.8
      specified deficiency NEC D53.8
    megaloblastic D52.0
  of prematurity P61.2
  orotaciduric (congenital) (hereditary) D53.0
  osteosclerotic D64.89
  ovalocytosis (hereditary) —*see* Elliptocytosis
  paludal —*see also* Malaria B54 *[D63.8]*
  pernicious (congenital) (malignant)
    (progressive) D51.0
  pleochromic D64.89
    of sprue D52.8
  posthemorrhagic (chronic) D50.0
    acute D62
    newborn P61.3
  postoperative (postprocedural)
    due to (acute) blood loss D62
      chronic blood loss D50.0
    specified NEC D64.9
  postpartum O90.81
  pressure D64.89
  progressive D64.9
    malignant D51.0
    pernicious D51.0
  protein-deficiency D53.0
  pseudoleukemica infantum D64.89
  pure red cell D60.9
    congenital D61.01
  pyridoxine-responsive D64.3
  pyruvate kinase deficiency D55.2
  refractory D46.4
    with
      excess of blasts D46.20
        1 (RAEB 1) D46.21
        2 (RAEB 2) D46.22
        in transformation (RAEB T) —*see*
          Leukemia, acute myeloblastic
      hemochromatosis D46.1
      sideroblasts (ring) (RARS) D46.1
    without ring sideroblasts, so stated D46.0
    without sideroblasts without excess of
      blasts D46.0
    megaloblastic D53.1
    sideroblastic D46.1
    sideropenic D50.9
  Rietti-Greppi-Micheli D56.9
  scorbutic D53.2
  secondary to
    blood loss (chronic) D50.0
      acute D62
    hemorrhage (chronic) D50.0
      acute D62
  semiplastic D61.89
  sickle-cell —*see* Disease, sickle-cell
  sideroblastic D64.3
    hereditary D64.0
    hypochromic, sex-linked D64.0
    pyridoxine-responsive NEC D64.3
    refractory D46.1
    secondary (due to)
      disease D64.1
      drugs and toxins D64.2
    specified type NEC D64.3
  sideropenic (refractory) D50.9
    due to blood loss (chronic) D50.0
      acute D62
  simple chronic D53.9
  specified type NEC D64.89
  spherocytic (hereditary) —*see* Spherocytosis
  splenic D64.89
  splenomegalic D64.89
  stomatocytosis D58.8
  syphilitic (acquired) (late) A52.79 *[D63.8]*
  target cell D64.89

Anemia *(Continued)*
  thalassemia D56.9
  thrombocytopenic —*see* Thrombocytopenia
  toxic D61.2
  tropical B76.9 *[D63.8]*
    macrocytic D52.8
  tuberculous A18.89 *[D63.8]*
  vegan D51.3
  vitamin
    B6-responsive D64.3
    B12 deficiency (dietary) pernicious D51.0
  von Jaksch's D64.89
  Witts' (achlorhydric anemia) D50.8
Anemophobia F40.228
Anencephalus, anencephaly Q00.0
Anergasia —*see* Psychosis, organic
Anesthesia, anesthetic R20.0
  complication or reaction NEC —*see also*
    Complications, anesthesia T88.59
    due to
      correct substance properly
        administered —*see* Table of Drugs
        and Chemicals, by drug, adverse
        effect
      overdose or wrong substance given —*see*
        Table of Drugs and Chemicals, by
        drug, poisoning
      unintended awareness under general
        anesthesia during procedure
        T88.53 ◀
        personal history of Z92.84 ◀
  cornea H18.81-
  dissociative F44.6
  functional (hysterical) F44.6
  hyperesthetic, thalamic G89.0
  hysterical F44.6
  local skin lesion R20.0
  sexual (psychogenic) F52.1
  shock (due to) T88.2
  skin R20.0
  testicular N50.9
Anetoderma (maculosum) (of) L90.8
  Jadassohn-Pellizzari L90.2
  Schweniger-Buzzi L90.1
Aneurin deficiency E51.9
Aneurysm (anastomotic) (artery) (cirsoid)
  (diffuse) (false) (fusiform) (multiple)
  (saccular) I72.9
  abdominal (aorta) I71.4
    ruptured I71.3
    syphilitic A52.01
  aorta, aortic (nonsyphilitic) I71.9
    abdominal I71.4
      ruptured I71.3
    arch I71.2
      ruptured I71.1
    arteriosclerotic I71.9
      ruptured I71.8
    ascending I71.2
      ruptured I71.1
    congenital Q25.43 ◀▥
    descending I71.9
      abdominal I71.4
        ruptured I71.3
      ruptured I71.8
      thoracic I71.2
        ruptured I71.1
    root Q25.43 ◀
    ruptured I71.8
    sinus, congenital Q25.43 ◀▥
    syphilitic A52.01
    thoracic I71.2
      ruptured I71.1
    thoracoabdominal I71.6
      ruptured I71.5
    thorax, thoracic (arch) I71.2
      ruptured I71.1
    transverse I71.2
      ruptured I71.1
    valve (heart) —*see also* Endocarditis, aortic
      I35.8

Aneurysm *(Continued)*
  arteriosclerotic I72.9
    cerebral I67.1
      ruptured —*see* Hemorrhage, intracranial,
        subarachnoid
  arteriovenous (congenital) —*see also*
    Malformation, arteriovenous
    acquired I77.0
      brain I67.1
      coronary I25.41
      pulmonary I28.0
    brain Q28.2
      ruptured I60.8
    peripheral —*see* Malformation,
      arteriovenous, peripheral
    precerebral vessels Q28.0
    specified site NEC —*see also* Malformation,
      arteriovenous
      acquired I77.0
  basal —*see* Aneurysm, brain
  basilar (trunk) I72.5 ◀
  berry (congenital) (nonruptured) I67.1
    ruptured I60.7
  brain I67.1
    arteriosclerotic I67.1
      ruptured —*see* Hemorrhage, intracranial,
        subarachnoid
    arteriovenous (congenital) (nonruptured)
      Q28.2
      acquired I67.1
        ruptured I60.8
      ruptured I60.8
    berry (congenital) (nonruptured) I67.1
      ruptured —*see also* Hemorrhage,
        intracranial, subarachnoid I60.7
    congenital Q28.3
      aorta (root) (sinus) Q25.43 ◀
      ruptured I60.7
    meninges I67.1
      ruptured I60.8
    miliary (congenital) (nonruptured) I67.1
      ruptured —*see also* Hemorrhage,
        intracranial, subarachnoid I60.7
    mycotic I33.0
    ruptured —*see* Hemorrhage, intracranial,
      subarachnoid
    syphilitic (hemorrhage) A52.05
  cardiac (false) —*see also* Aneurysm, heart I25.3
  carotid artery (common) (external) I72.0
    internal (intracranial) I67.1
      extracranial portion I72.0
    ruptured into brain I60.0-
    syphilitic A52.09
      intracranial A52.05
  cavernous sinus I67.1
    arteriovenous (congenital) (nonruptured)
      Q28.3
      ruptured I60.8
  celiac I72.8
  central nervous system, syphilitic A52.05
  cerebral —*see* Aneurysm, brain
  chest —*see* Aneurysm, thorax
  circle of Willis I67.1
    congenital Q28.3
      ruptured I60.6
    ruptured I60.6
  common iliac artery I72.3
  congenital (peripheral) Q27.8
    aorta (root) (sinus) Q25.43 ◀
    brain Q28.3
      ruptured I60.7
    coronary Q24.5
    digestive system Q27.8
    lower limb Q27.8
    pulmonary Q25.79
    retina Q14.1
    specified site NEC Q27.8
    upper limb Q27.8
  conjunctiva —*see* Abnormality, conjunctiva,
    vascular
  conus arteriosus —*see* Aneurysm, heart

Aneurysm *(Continued)*
  coronary (arteriosclerotic) (artery) I25.41
    arteriovenous, congenital Q24.5
    congenital Q24.5
    ruptured —*see* Infarct, myocardium
    syphilitic A52.06
    vein I25.89
  cylindroid (aorta) I71.9
    ruptured I71.8
    syphilitic A52.01
  ductus arteriosus Q25.0
  endocardial, infective (any valve) I33.0
  femoral (artery) (ruptured) I72.4
  gastroduodenal I72.8
  gastroepiploic I72.8
  heart (wall) (chronic or with a stated duration
    of over 4 weeks) I25.3
    valve —*see* Endocarditis
  hepatic I72.8
  iliac (common) (artery) (ruptured) I72.3
  infective I72.9
    endocardial (any valve) I33.0
  innominate (nonsyphilitic) I72.8
    syphilitic A52.09
  interauricular septum —*see* Aneurysm, heart
  interventricular septum —*see* Aneurysm,
    heart
  intrathoracic (nonsyphilitic) I71.2
    ruptured I71.1
    syphilitic A52.01
  lower limb I72.4
  lung (pulmonary artery) I28.1
  mediastinal (nonsyphilitic) I72.8
    syphilitic A52.09
  miliary (congenital) I67.1
    ruptured —*see* Hemorrhage, intracerebral,
      subarachnoid, intracranial
  mitral (heart) (valve) I34.8
  mural —*see* Aneurysm, heart
  mycotic I72.9
    endocardial (any valve) I33.0
    ruptured, brain —*see* Hemorrhage,
      intracerebral, subarachnoid
  myocardium —*see* Aneurysm, heart
  neck I72.0
  pancreaticoduodenal I72.8
  patent ductus arteriosus Q25.0
  peripheral NEC I72.8
    congenital Q27.8
      digestive system Q27.8
      lower limb Q27.8
      specified site NEC Q27.8
      upper limb Q27.8
  popliteal (artery) (ruptured) I72.4
  ~~precerebral, congenital (nonruptured)~~
    ~~Q28.1~~
  precerebral ◀
    congenital (nonruptured) Q28.1 ◀
    specified site, NEC I72.5 ◀
  pulmonary I28.1
    arteriovenous Q25.72
      acquired I28.0
    syphilitic A52.09
    valve (heart) —*see* Endocarditis,
      pulmonary
  racemose (peripheral) I72.9
    congenital —*see* Aneurysm,
      congenital
  radial I72.1
  Rasmussen NEC A15.0
  renal (artery) I72.2
  retina —*see also* Disorder, retina,
    microaneurysms
    congenital Q14.1
    diabetic —*see* Diabetes, microaneurysms,
      retinal
  sinus of Valsalva Q25.49 ◀⃫
  specified NEC I72.8
  spinal (cord) I72.8
    syphilitic (hemorrhage) A52.09
  splenic I72.8

Aneurysm *(Continued)*
  subclavian (artery) (ruptured) I72.8
    syphilitic A52.09
  superior mesenteric I72.8
  syphilitic (aorta) A52.01
    central nervous system A52.05
    congenital (late) A50.54 *[I79.0]*
    spine, spinal A52.09
  thoracoabdominal (aorta) I71.6
    ruptured I71.5
    syphilitic A52.01
  thorax, thoracic (aorta) (arch) (nonsyphilitic)
    I71.2
    ruptured I71.1
    syphilitic A52.01
  traumatic (complication) (early), specified
    site —*see* Injury, blood vessel
  tricuspid (heart) (valve) I07.8
  ulnar I72.1
  upper limb (ruptured) I72.1
  valve, valvular —*see* Endocarditis
  visceral NEC I72.8
  venous —*see also* Varix I86.8
    congenital Q27.8
      digestive system Q27.8
      lower limb Q27.8
      specified site NEC Q27.8
      upper limb Q27.8
  ventricle —*see* Aneurysm, heart
  vertebral artery I72.6 ◀
  visceral NEC I72.8
Angelman syndrome Q93.5
Anger R45.4
Angiectasis, angiectopia I99.8
Angiitis I77.6
  allergic granulomatous M30.1
  hypersensitivity M31.0
  necrotizing M31.9
    specified NEC M31.8
  nervous system, granulomatous I67.7
Angina (attack) (cardiac) (chest) (heart)
    (pectoris) (syndrome) (vasomotor) I20.9
  with
    atherosclerotic heart disease —*see*
      Arteriosclerosis, coronary (artery)
    documented spasm I20.1
  abdominal K55.1
  accelerated —*see* Angina, unstable
  agranulocytic —*see* Agranulocytosis
  angiospastic —*see* Angina, with documented
    spasm
  aphthous B08.5
  crescendo —*see* Angina, unstable
  croupous J05.0
  cruris I73.9
  de novo effort —*see* Angina, unstable
  diphtheritic, membranous A36.0
  equivalent I20.8
  exudative, chronic J37.0
  following acute myocardial infarction
    I23.7
  gangrenous diphtheritic A36.0
  intestinal K55.1
  Ludovici K12.2
  Ludwig's K12.2
  malignant diphtheritic A36.0
  membranous J05.0
    diphtheritic A36.0
    Vincent's A69.1
  mesenteric K55.1
  monocytic —*see* Mononucleosis, infectious
  of effort —*see* Angina, specified NEC
  phlegmonous J36
    diphtheritic A36.0
  post-infarctional I23.7
  pre-infarctional —*see* Angina, unstable
  Prinzmetal —*see* Angina, with documented
    spasm
  progressive —*see* Angina, unstable
  pseudomembranous A69.1
  pultaceous, diphtheritic A36.0

◀ New   ◀⃫ Revised   ~~deleted~~ Deleted

Angina *(Continued)*
  spasm-induced —*see* Angina, with
    documented spasm
  specified NEC I20.8
  stable I20.8 ◀▥
  stenocardia —*see* Angina, specified NEC
  stridulous, diphtheritic A36.2
  tonsil J36
  trachealis J05.0
  unstable I20.0
  variant —*see* Angina, with documented
    spasm
  Vincent's A69.1
  worsening effort —*see* Angina, unstable
Angioblastoma —*see* Neoplasm, connective
  tissue, uncertain behavior
Angiocholecystitis —*see* Cholecystitis, acute
Angiocholitis —*see also* Cholecystitis, acute K83.0
Angiodysgenesis spinalis G95.19
Angiodysplasia (cecum) (colon) K55.20
  with bleeding K55.21
  duodenum (and stomach) K31.819
    with bleeding K31.811
  stomach (and duodenum) K31.819
    with bleeding K31.811
Angioedema (allergic) (any site) (with urticaria)
  T78.3
  hereditary D84.1
Angioendothelioma —*see* Neoplasm, uncertain
  behavior, by site
  benign D18.00
    intra-abdominal D18.03
    intracranial D18.02
    skin D18.01
    specified site NEC D18.09
  bone —*see* Neoplasm, bone, malignant
  Ewing's —*see* Neoplasm, bone, malignant
Angioendotheliomatosis C85.8-
Angiofibroma —*see also* Neoplasm, benign, by
  site
  juvenile
    specified site —*see* Neoplasm, benign, by
      site
    unspecified site D10.6
Angiohemophilia (A) (B) D68.0
Angioid streaks (choroid) (macula) (retina)
  H35.33
Angiokeratoma —*see* Neoplasm, skin, benign
  corporis diffusum E75.21
Angioleiomyoma —*see* Neoplasm, connective
  tissue, benign
Angiolipoma —*see also* Lipoma
  infiltrating —*see* Lipoma
Angioma —*see also* Hemangioma, by site
  capillary I78.1
  hemorrhagicum hereditaria I78.0
  intra-abdominal D18.03
  intracranial D18.02
  malignant —*see* Neoplasm, connective tissue,
    malignant
  plexiform D18.00
    intra-abdominal D18.03
    intracranial D18.02
    skin D18.01
    specified site NEC D18.09
  senile I78.1
  serpiginosum L81.7
  skin D18.01
  specified site NEC D18.09
  spider I78.1
  stellate I78.1
  venous Q28.3
Angiomatosis Q82.8
  bacillary A79.89
  encephalotrigeminal Q85.8
  hemorrhagic familial I78.0
  hereditary familial I78.0
  liver K76.4
Angiomyolipoma —*see* Lipoma
Angiomyoliposarcoma —*see* Neoplasm,
  connective tissue, malignant

Angiomyoma —*see* Neoplasm, connective
  tissue, benign
Angiomyosarcoma —*see* Neoplasm, connective
  tissue, malignant
Angiomyxoma —*see* Neoplasm, connective
  tissue, uncertain behavior
Angioneurosis F45.8
Angioneurotic edema (allergic) (any site) (with
  urticaria) T78.3
  hereditary D84.1
Angiopathia, angiopathy I99.9
  cerebral I67.9
    amyloid E85.4 [I68.0]
  diabetic (peripheral) —*see* Diabetes,
    angiopathy
  peripheral I73.9
    diabetic —*see* Diabetes, angiopathy
    specified type NEC I73.89
  retinae syphilitica A52.05
  retinalis (juvenilis)
    diabetic —*see* Diabetes, retinopathy
    proliferative —*see* Retinopathy,
      proliferative
Angiosarcoma —*see also* Neoplasm, connective
  tissue, malignant
  liver C22.3
Angiosclerosis —*see* Arteriosclerosis
Angiospasm (peripheral) (traumatic) (vessel)
  I73.9
  brachial plexus G54.0
  cerebral G45.9
  cervical plexus G54.2
  nerve
    arm —*see* Mononeuropathy, upper limb
      axillary G54.0
      median —*see* Lesion, nerve, median
      ulnar —*see* Lesion, nerve, ulnar
    axillary G54.0
    leg —*see* Mononeuropathy, lower limb
    median —*see* Lesion, nerve, median
    plantar —*see* Lesion, nerve, plantar
    ulnar —*see* Lesion, nerve, ulnar
Angiospastic disease or edema I73.9
Angiostrongyliasis
  due to
    Parastrongylus
      cantonensis B83.2
      costaricensis B81.3
  intestinal B81.3
Anguillulosis —*see* Strongyloidiasis
Angulation
  cecum —*see* Obstruction, intestine
  coccyx (acquired) —*see also* subcategory
    M43.8
    congenital NEC Q76.49
  femur (acquired) —*see also* Deformity, limb,
    specified type NEC, thigh
    congenital Q74.2
  intestine (large) (small) —*see* Obstruction,
    intestine
  sacrum (acquired) —*see also* subcategory M43.8
    congenital NEC Q76.49
  sigmoid (flexure) —*see* Obstruction, intestine
  spine —*see* Dorsopathy, deforming, specified
    NEC
  tibia (acquired) —*see also* Deformity, limb,
    specified type NEC, lower leg
    congenital Q74.2
  ureter N13.5
    with infection N13.6
  wrist (acquired) —*see also* Deformity, limb,
    specified type NEC, forearm
    congenital Q74.0
Angulus infectiosus (lips) K13.0
Anhedonia R45.84
  sexual F52.0 ◀
Anhidrosis L74.4
~~Anhydration, anhydremia E86.0~~
  ~~with~~
    ~~hypernatremia E87.0~~
    ~~hyponatremia E87.1~~

Anhydration E86.0 ◀
Anhydremia E86.0
  ~~with~~
    ~~hypernatremia E87.0~~
    ~~hyponatremia E87.1~~
Anidrosis L74.4
Aniridia (congenital) Q13.1
Anisakiasis (infection) (infestation) B81.0
Anisakis larvae infestation B81.0
Aniseikonia H52.32
Anisocoria (pupil) H57.02
  congenital Q13.2
Anisocytosis R71.8
Anisometropia (congenital) H52.31
Ankle —*see* condition
Ankyloblepharon (eyelid) (acquired) —*see also*
  Blepharophimosis
  filiforme (adnatum) (congenital) Q10.3
  total Q10.3
Ankyloglossia Q38.1
Ankylosis (fibrous) (osseous) (joint) M24.60
  ankle M24.67-
  arthrodesis status Z98.1
  cricoarytenoid (cartilage) (joint) (larynx) J38.7
  dental K03.5
  ear ossicles H74.31-
  elbow M24.62-
  foot M24.67-
  hand M24.64-
  hip M24.65-
  incostapedial joint (infectional) —*see*
    Ankylosis, ear ossicles
  jaw (temporomandibular) M26.61- ◀▥
  knee M24.66-
  lumbosacral (joint) M43.27
  postoperative (status) Z98.1
  produced by surgical fusion, status Z98.1
  sacro-iliac (joint) M43.28
  shoulder M24.61-
  spine (joint) —*see also* Fusion, spine
    spondylitic —*see* Spondylitis, ankylosing
  surgical Z98.1
  temporomandibular M26.61- ◀▥
  tooth, teeth (hard tissues) K03.5
  wrist M24.63-
Ankylostoma —*see* Ancylostoma
Ankylostomiasis —*see* Ancylostomiasis
Ankylurethria —*see* Stricture, urethra
Annular —*see also* condition
  detachment, cervix N88.8
  organ or site, congenital NEC —*see* Distortion
  pancreas (congenital) Q45.1
Anodontia (complete) (partial) (vera) K00.0
  acquired K08.10
Anomaly, anomalous (congenital) (unspecified
  type) Q89.9
  abdominal wall NEC Q79.59
  acoustic nerve Q07.8
  adrenal (gland) Q89.1
  Alder (-Reilly) (leukocyte granulation) D72.0
  alimentary tract Q45.9
    upper Q40.9
  alveolar M26.70
    hyperplasia M26.79
      mandibular M26.72
      maxillary M26.71
    hypoplasia M26.79
      mandibular M26.74
      maxillary M26.73
    ridge (process) M26.79
    specified NEC M26.79
  ankle (joint) Q74.2
  anus Q43.9
  aorta (arch) NEC Q25.40 ◀▥
    coarctation (preductal) (postductal) Q25.1
  aortic cusp or valve Q23.9
  appendix Q43.8
  apple peel syndrome Q41.1
  aqueduct of Sylvius Q03.0
    with spina bifida —*see* Spina bifida, with
      hydrocephalus

Anomaly, anomalous *(Continued)*
arm Q74.0
arteriovenous NEC
  coronary Q24.5
  gastrointestinal Q27.33
    acquired —*see* Angiodysplasia
artery (peripheral) Q27.9
  basilar NEC Q28.1
  cerebral Q28.3
  coronary Q24.5
  digestive system Q27.8
  eye Q15.8
  great Q25.9
    specified NEC Q25.8
  lower limb Q27.8
  peripheral Q27.9
    specified NEC Q27.8
  pulmonary NEC Q25.79
  renal Q27.2
  retina Q14.1
  specified site NEC Q27.8
  subclavian Q27.8
    origin Q25.48 ◄
  umbilical Q27.0
  upper limb Q27.8
  vertebral NEC Q28.1
aryteno-epiglottic folds Q31.8
atrial
  bands or folds Q20.8
  septa Q21.1
atrioventricular
  excitation I45.6
  septum Q21.0
auditory canal Q17.8
auricle
  ear Q17.8
    causing impairment of hearing
      Q16.9
  heart Q20.8
Axenfeld's Q15.0
back Q89.9
band
  atrial Q20.8
  heart Q24.8
  ventricular Q24.8
Bartholin's duct Q38.4
biliary duct or passage Q44.5
bladder Q64.70
  absence Q64.5
  diverticulum Q64.6
  exstrophy Q64.10
    cloacal Q64.12
    extroversion Q64.19
    specified type NEC Q64.19
    supravesical fissure Q64.11
  neck obstruction Q64.31
  specified type NEC Q64.79
bone Q79.9
  arm Q74.0
  face Q75.9
  leg Q74.2
  pelvic girdle Q74.2
  shoulder girdle Q74.0
  skull Q75.9
    with
      anencephaly Q00.0
      encephalocele —*see* Encephalocele
      hydrocephalus Q03.9
        with spina bifida —*see* Spina bifida,
          by site, with hydrocephalus
      microcephaly Q02
brain (multiple) Q04.9
  vessel Q28.3
breast Q83.9
broad ligament Q50.6
bronchus Q32.4
bulbus cordis Q21.9
bursa Q79.9
canal of Nuck Q52.4
canthus Q10.3
capillary Q27.9

Anomaly, anomalous *(Continued)*
cardiac Q24.9
  chambers Q20.9
    specified NEC Q20.8
  septal closure Q21.9
    specified NEC Q21.8
  valve NEC Q24.8
    pulmonary Q22.3
cardiovascular system Q28.8
carpus Q74.0
caruncle, lacrimal Q10.6
cascade stomach Q40.2
cauda equina Q06.3
cecum Q43.9
cerebral Q04.9
  vessels Q28.3
cervix Q51.9
Chédiak-Higashi(-Steinbrinck) (congenital
    gigantism of peroxidase granules)
    E70.330
cheek Q18.9
chest wall Q67.8
  bones Q76.9
chin Q18.9
chordae tendineae Q24.8
choroid Q14.3
  plexus Q07.8
chromosomes, chromosomal Q99.9
  D (1) —*see* condition, chromosome 13
  E (3) —*see* condition, chromosome 18
  G —*see* condition, chromosome 21
  sex
    female phenotype Q97.8
    gonadal dysgenesis (pure) Q99.1
    Klinefelter's Q98.4
    male phenotype Q98.9
    Turner's Q96.9
  specified NEC Q99.8
cilia Q10.3
circulatory system Q28.9
clavicle Q74.0
clitoris Q52.6
coccyx Q76.49
colon Q43.9
common duct Q44.5
communication
  coronary artery Q24.5
  left ventricle with right atrium Q21.0
concha (ear) Q17.3
connection
  portal vein Q26.5
  pulmonary venous Q26.4
    partial Q26.3
    total Q26.2
  renal artery with kidney Q27.2
cornea (shape) Q13.4
coronary artery or vein Q24.5
cranium —*see* Anomaly, skull
cricoid cartilage Q31.8
cystic duct Q44.5
dental
  alveolar —*see* Anomaly, alveolar
  arch relationship M26.20
    specified NEC M26.29
dentofacial M26.9
  alveolar —*see* Anomaly, alveolar
  dental arch relationship M26.20
    specified NEC M26.29
  functional M26.50
    specified NEC M26.59
  jaw-cranial base relationship M26.10
    asymmetry M26.12
      maxillary M26.11
    specified type NEC M26.19
  jaw size M26.00
    macrogenia M26.05
    mandibular
      hyperplasia M26.03
      hypoplasia M26.04
    maxillary
      hyperplasia M26.01
      hypoplasia M26.02

Anomaly, anomalous *(Continued)*
dentofacial *(Continued)*
  jaw size *(Continued)*
    microgenia M26.06
    specified type NEC M26.09
  malocclusion M26.4
    dental arch relationship NEC M26.29
    jaw-cranial base relationship —*see*
      Anomaly, dentofacial, jaw-cranial
      base relationship
    jaw size —*see* Anomaly, dentofacial, jaw
      size
  specified type NEC M26.89
  temporomandibular joint M26.60- ◄▥
    adhesions M26.61- ◄▥
    ankylosis M26.61- ◄▥
    arthralgia M26.62- ◄▥
    articular disc M26.63- ◄▥
    specified type NEC M26.69
  tooth position, fully erupted M26.30
    specified NEC M26.39
dermatoglyphic Q82.8
diaphragm (apertures) NEC Q79.1
digestive organ (s) or tract Q45.9
  lower Q43.9
  upper Q40.9
distance, interarch (excessive) (inadequate)
    M26.25
distribution, coronary artery Q24.5
ductus
  arteriosus Q25.0
  botalli Q25.0
duodenum Q43.9
dura (brain) Q04.9
  spinal cord Q06.9
ear (external) Q17.9
  causing impairment of hearing Q16.9
  inner Q16.5
  middle (causing impairment of hearing)
    Q16.4
    ossicles Q16.3
Ebstein's (heart) (tricuspid valve) Q22.5
ectodermal Q82.9
Eisenmenger's (ventricular septal defect)
    Q21.8
ejaculatory duct Q55.4
elbow Q74.0
endocrine gland NEC Q89.2
epididymis Q55.4
epiglottis Q31.8
esophagus Q39.9
eustachian tube Q17.8
eye Q15.9
  anterior segment Q13.9
    specified NEC Q13.89
  posterior segment Q14.9
    specified NEC Q14.8
  ptosis (eyelid) Q10.0
  specified NEC Q15.8
eyebrow Q18.8
eyelid Q10.3
  ptosis Q10.0
face Q18.9
  bone(s) Q75.9
fallopian tube Q50.6
fascia Q79.9
femur NEC Q74.2
fibula NEC Q74.2
finger Q74.0
fixation, intestine Q43.3
flexion (joint) NOS Q74.9
  hip or thigh Q65.89
foot NEC Q74.2
  varus (congenital) Q66.3
foramen
  Botalli Q21.1
  ovale Q21.1
forearm Q74.0
forehead Q75.8
form, teeth K00.2
fovea centralis Q14.1

◄ New   ◄▥ Revised   ~~deleted~~ Deleted

Anomaly, anomalous *(Continued)*
frontal bone —*see* Anomaly, skull
gallbladder (position) (shape) (size) Q44.1
Gartner's duct Q52.4
gastrointestinal tract Q45.9
genitalia, genital organ (s) or system
    female Q52.9
        external Q52.70
        internal NOS Q52.9
    male Q55.9
        hydrocele P83.5
        specified NEC Q55.8
genitourinary NEC
    female Q52.9
    male Q55.9
Gerbode Q21.0
glottis Q31.8
granulation or granulocyte, genetic
    (constitutional) (leukocyte) D72.0
gum Q38.6
gyri Q07.9
hair Q84.2
hand Q74.0
hard tissue formation in pulp K04.3
head —*see* Anomaly, skull
heart Q24.9
    auricle Q20.8
    bands or folds Q24.8
    fibroelastosis cordis I42.4
    obstructive NEC Q22.6
    patent ductus arteriosus (Botalli) Q25.0
    septum Q21.9
        auricular Q21.1
        interatrial Q21.1
        interventricular Q21.0
            with pulmonary stenosis or atresia,
                dextraposition of aorta and
                hypertrophy of right ventricle
                Q21.3
        specified NEC Q21.8
        ventricular Q21.0
            with pulmonary stenosis or atresia,
                dextraposition of aorta and
                hypertrophy of right ventricle
                Q21.3
    tetralogy of Fallot Q21.3
    valve NEC Q24.8
        aortic
            bicuspid valve Q23.1
            insufficiency Q23.1
            stenosis Q23.0
                subaortic Q24.4
        mitral
            insufficiency Q23.3
            stenosis Q23.2
        pulmonary Q22.3
            atresia Q22.0
            insufficiency Q22.2
            stenosis Q22.1
                infundibular Q24.3
                subvalvular Q24.3
        tricuspid
            atresia Q22.4
            stenosis Q22.4
    ventricle Q20.8
heel NEC Q74.2
Hegglin's D72.0
hemianencephaly Q00.0
hemicephaly Q00.0
hemicrania Q00.0
hepatic duct Q44.5
hip NEC Q74.2
hourglass stomach Q40.2
humerus Q74.0
hydatid of Morgagni
    female Q50.5
    male (epididymal) Q55.4
        testicular Q55.29
hymen Q52.4
hypersegmentation of neutrophils, hereditary
    D72.0

Anomaly, anomalous *(Continued)*
hypophyseal Q89.2
ileocecal (coil) (valve) Q43.9
ileum Q43.9
ilium NEC Q74.2
integument Q84.9
    specified NEC Q84.8
interarch distance (excessive) (inadequate)
    M26.25
intervertebral cartilage or disc Q76.49
intestine (large) (small) Q43.9
    with anomalous adhesions, fixation or
        malrotation Q43.3
iris Q13.2
ischium NEC Q74.2
jaw —*see* Anomaly, dentofacial
    alveolar —*see* Anomaly, alveolar
jaw-cranial base relationship —*see*
        Anomaly, dentofacial, jaw-cranial
        base relationship
jejunum Q43.8
joint Q74.9
    specified NEC Q74.8
Jordan's D72.0
kidney(s) (calyx) (pelvis) Q63.9
    artery Q27.2
    specified NEC Q63.8
Klippel-Feil (brevicollis) Q76.1
knee Q74.1
labium (majus) (minus) Q52.70
labyrinth, membranous Q16.5
lacrimal apparatus or duct Q10.6
larynx, laryngeal (muscle) Q31.9
    web (bed) Q31.0
lens Q12.9
leukocytes, genetic D72.0
    granulation (constitutional) D72.0
lid (fold) Q10.3
ligament Q79.9
    broad Q50.6
    round Q52.8
limb Q74.9
    lower NEC Q74.2
        reduction deformity —*see* Defect,
            reduction, lower limb
    upper Q74.0
lip Q38.0
liver Q44.7
    duct Q44.5
lower limb NEC Q74.2
lumbosacral (joint) (region) Q76.49
    kyphosis —*see* Kyphosis, congenital
    lordosis —*see* Lordosis, congenital
lung (fissure) (lobe) Q33.9
mandible —*see* Anomaly, dentofacial
maxilla —*see* Anomaly, dentofacial
May (-Hegglin) D72.0
meatus urinarius NEC Q64.79
meningeal bands or folds Q07.9
    constriction of Q07.8
    spinal Q06.9
meninges Q07.9
    cerebral Q04.8
    spinal Q06.9
meningocele Q05.9
mesentery Q45.9
metacarpus Q74.0
metatarsus NEC Q74.2
middle ear Q16.4
    ossicles Q16.3
mitral (leaflets) (valve) Q23.9
    insufficiency Q23.3
    specified NEC Q23.8
    stenosis Q23.2
mouth Q38.6
Müllerian —*see also* Anomaly, by site
    uterus NEC Q51.818
multiple NEC Q89.7
muscle Q79.9
    eyelid Q10.3
musculoskeletal system, except limbs Q79.9

Anomaly, anomalous *(Continued)*
myocardium Q24.8
nail Q84.6
narrowness, eyelid Q10.3
nasal sinus (wall) Q30.8
neck (any part) Q18.9
nerve Q07.9
    acoustic Q07.8
    optic Q07.8
nervous system (central) Q07.9
nipple Q83.9
nose, nasal (bones) (cartilage) (septum)
    (sinus) Q30.9
    specified NEC Q30.8
ocular muscle Q15.8
omphalomesenteric duct Q43.0
opening, pulmonary veins Q26.4
optic
    disc Q14.2
    nerve Q07.8
opticociliary vessels Q13.2
orbit (eye) Q10.7
organ Q89.9
    of Corti Q16.5
origin
    artery
        innominate Q25.8
        pulmonary Q25.79
        renal Q27.2
        subclavian Q25.48 ◄▥
osseous meatus (ear) Q16.1
ovary Q50.39
oviduct Q50.6
palate (hard) (soft) NEC Q38.5
pancreas or pancreatic duct Q45.3
papillary muscles Q24.8
parathyroid gland Q89.2
paraurethral ducts Q64.79
parotid (gland) Q38.4
patella Q74.1
Pelger-Huët (hereditary hyposegmentation)
    D72.0
pelvic girdle NEC Q74.2
pelvis (bony) NEC Q74.2
    rachitic E64.3
penis (glans) Q55.69
pericardium Q24.8
peripheral vascular system Q27.9
Peter's Q13.4
pharynx Q38.8
pigmentation L81.9
    congenital Q82.8
pituitary (gland) Q89.2
pleural (folds) Q34.0
portal vein Q26.5
    connection Q26.5
position, tooth, teeth, fully erupted M26.30
    specified NEC M26.39
precerebral vessel Q28.1
prepuce Q55.69
prostate Q55.4
pulmonary Q33.9
    artery NEC Q25.79
    valve Q22.3
        atresia Q22.0
        insufficiency Q22.2
        specified type NEC Q22.3
        stenosis Q22.1
            infundibular Q24.3
            subvalvular Q24.3
    venous connection Q26.4
        partial Q26.3
        total Q26.2
pupil Q13.2
    function H57.00
        anisocoria H57.02
        Argyll Robertson pupil H57.01
        miosis H57.03
        mydriasis H57.04
        specified type NEC H57.09
        tonic pupil H57.05-

Anomaly, anomalous (*Continued*)
pylorus Q40.3
radius Q74.0
rectum Q43.9
reduction (extremity) (limb)
 femur (longitudinal) —*see* Defect,
  reduction, lower limb, longitudinal,
  femur
 fibula (longitudinal) —*see* Defect,
  reduction, lower limb, longitudinal,
  fibula
 lower limb —*see* Defect, reduction, lower
  limb
 radius (longitudinal) —*see* Defect,
  reduction, upper limb, longitudinal,
  radius
 tibia (longitudinal) —*see* Defect, reduction,
  lower limb, longitudinal, tibia
 ulna (longitudinal) —*see* Defect, reduction,
  upper limb, longitudinal, ulna
 upper limb —*see* Defect, reduction, upper
  limb
refraction —*see* Disorder, refraction
renal Q63.9
 artery Q27.2
 pelvis Q63.9
  specified NEC Q63.8
respiratory system Q34.9
 specified NEC Q34.8
retina Q14.1
rib Q76.6
 cervical Q76.5
Rieger's Q13.81
rotation —*see* Malrotation
 hip or thigh Q65.89
round ligament Q52.8
sacroiliac (joint) NEC Q74.2
sacrum NEC Q76.49
 kyphosis —*see* Kyphosis, congenital
 lordosis —*see* Lordosis, congenital
saddle nose, syphilitic A50.57
salivary duct or gland Q38.4
scapula Q74.0
scrotum —*see* Malformation, testis and
  scrotum
sebaceous gland Q82.9
seminal vesicles Q55.4
sense organs NEC Q07.8
sex chromosomes NEC —*see also* Anomaly,
  chromosomes
 female phenotype Q97.8
 male phenotype Q98.9
shoulder (girdle) (joint) Q74.0
sigmoid (flexure) Q43.9
simian crease Q82.8
sinus of Valsalva Q25.49 ◄▥
skeleton generalized Q78.9
skin (appendage) Q82.9
skull Q75.9
 with
  anencephaly Q00.0
  encephalocele —*see* Encephalocele
  hydrocephalus Q03.9
   with spina bifida —*see* Spina bifida, by
    site, with hydrocephalus
  microcephaly Q02
specified organ or site NEC Q89.8
spermatic cord Q55.4
spine, spinal NEC Q76.49
 column NEC Q76.49
  kyphosis —*see* Kyphosis, congenital
  lordosis —*see* Lordosis, congenital
 cord Q06.9
 nerve root Q07.8
spleen Q89.09
 agenesis Q89.01
stenonian duct Q38.4
sternum NEC Q76.7
stomach Q40.3
submaxillary gland Q38.4
tarsus NEC Q74.2

Anomaly, anomalous (*Continued*)
tendon Q79.9
testis —*see* Malformation, testis and
  scrotum
thigh NEC Q74.2
thorax (wall) Q67.8
 bony Q76.9
throat Q38.8
thumb Q74.0
thymus gland Q89.2
thyroid (gland) Q89.2
 cartilage Q31.8
tibia NEC Q74.2
 saber A50.56
toe Q74.2
tongue Q38.3
tooth, teeth K00.9
 eruption K00.6
 position, fully erupted M26.30
 spacing, fully erupted M26.30
trachea (cartilage) Q32.1
tragus Q17.9
tricuspid (leaflet) (valve) Q22.9
 atresia or stenosis Q22.4
 Ebstein's Q22.5
Uhl's (hypoplasia of myocardium, right
  ventricle) Q24.8
ulna Q74.0
umbilical artery Q27.0
union
 cricoid cartilage and thyroid cartilage
  Q31.8
 thyroid cartilage and hyoid bone
  Q31.8
 trachea with larynx Q31.8
upper limb Q74.0
urachus Q64.4
ureter Q62.8
 obstructive NEC Q62.39
  cecoureterocele Q62.32
  orthotopic ureterocele Q62.31
urethra Q64.70
 absence Q64.5
 double Q64.74
 fistula to rectum Q64.73
 obstructive Q64.39
  stricture Q64.32
 prolapse Q64.71
 specified type NEC Q64.79
urinary tract Q64.9
uterus Q51.9
 with only one functioning horn Q51.4
uvula Q38.5
vagina Q52.4
valleculae Q31.8
valve (heart) NEC Q24.8
 coronary sinus Q24.5
 inferior vena cava Q24.8
 pulmonary Q22.3
 sinus coronario Q24.5
 venae cavae inferioris Q24.8
vas deferens Q55.4
vascular Q27.9
 brain Q28.3
 ring Q25.45 ◄▥
vein (s) (peripheral) Q27.9
 brain Q28.3
 cerebral Q28.3
 coronary Q24.5
 developmental Q28.3
 great Q26.9
  specified NEC Q26.8
vena cava (inferior) (superior) Q26.9
venous —*see* Anomaly, vein (s)
venous return Q26.8
ventricular
 bands or folds Q24.8
 septa Q21.0
vertebra Q76.49
 kyphosis —*see* Kyphosis, congenital
 lordosis —*see* Lordosis, congenital

Anomaly, anomalous (*Continued*)
vesicourethral orifice Q64.79
vessel (s) Q27.9
 optic papilla Q14.2
 precerebral Q28.1
vitelline duct Q43.0
vitreous body or humor Q14.0
vulva Q52.70
wrist (joint) Q74.0
Anomia R48.8
Anonychia (congenital) Q84.3
 acquired L60.8
Anophthalmos, anophthalmus (congenital)
  (globe) Q11.1
 acquired Z90.01
Anopia, anopsia H53.46-
 quadrant H53.46-
Anorchia, anorchism, anorchidism Q55.0
Anorexia R63.0
 hysterical F44.89
 nervosa F50.00
  atypical F50.9
  binge-eating type F50.2
   with purging F50.02
  restricting type F50.01
Anorgasmy, psychogenic (female)
  F52.31
 male F52.32
Anosmia R43.0
 hysterical F44.6
 postinfectional J39.8
Anosognosia R41.89
Anosteoplasia Q78.9
Anovulatory cycle N97.0
Anoxemia R09.02
 newborn P84
Anoxia (pathological) R09.02
 altitude T70.29
 cerebral G93.1
  complicating
   anesthesia (general) (local) or other
    sedation T88.59
    in labor and delivery O74.3
    in pregnancy O29.21-
    postpartum, puerperal O89.2
   delivery (cesarean) (instrumental)
    O75.4
  during a procedure G97.81
  newborn P84
  resulting from a procedure G97.82
 due to
  drowning T75.1
  high altitude T70.29
 heart —*see* Insufficiency, coronary
 intrauterine P84
 myocardial —*see* Insufficiency, coronary
 newborn P84
 spinal cord G95.11
 systemic (by suffocation) (low content in
   atmosphere) —*see* Asphyxia,
   traumatic
Anteflexion —*see* Anteversion
Antenatal
 care (normal pregnancy) Z34.90
 screening (encounter for) of mother
  Z36
Antepartum —*see* condition
Anterior —*see* condition
Antero-occlusion M26.220
Anteversion
 cervix —*see* Anteversion, uterus
 femur (neck), congenital Q65.89
 uterus, uterine (cervix) (postinfectional)
   (postpartal, old) N85.4
  congenital Q51.818
  in pregnancy or childbirth —*see* Pregnancy,
    complicated by
Anthophobia F40.228
Anthracosilicosis J60
Anthracosis (lung) (occupational) J60
 lingua K14.3

◄ New ◄▥ Revised ~~deleted~~ Deleted

Anthrax A22.9
  with pneumonia A22.1
  cerebral A22.8
  colitis A22.2
  cutaneous A22.0
  gastrointestinal A22.2
  inhalation A22.1
  intestinal A22.2
  meningitis A22.8
  pulmonary A22.1
  respiratory A22.1
  sepsis A22.7
  specified manifestation NEC A22.8
Anthropoid pelvis Q74.2
  with disproportion (fetopelvic) O33.0
Anthropophobia F40.10
  generalized F40.11
Antibodies, maternal (blood group) —see
      Isoimmunization, affecting management
      of pregnancy
  anti-D —see Isoimmunization, affecting
      management of pregnancy, Rh
      newborn P55.0
Antibody
  anticardiolipin R76.0
    with
      hemorrhagic disorder D68.312
      hypercoagulable state D68.61
  antiphosphatidylglycerol R76.0
    with
      hemorrhagic disorder D68.312
      hypercoagulable state D68.61
  antiphosphatidylinositol R76.0
    with
      hemorrhagic disorder D68.312
      hypercoagulable state D68.61
  antiphosphatidylserine R76.0
    with
      hemorrhagic disorder D68.312
      hypercoagulable state D68.61
  antiphospholipid R76.0
    with
      hemorrhagic disorder D68.312
      hypercoagulable state D68.61
Anticardiolipin syndrome D68.61
Anticoagulant, circulating (intrinsic) —see also -
      Disorder, hemorrhagic D68.318
  drug-induced (extrinsic) —see also - Disorder,
      hemorrhagic D68.32
  iatrogenic D68.32 ◀
Antidiuretic hormone syndrome E22.2
Antimonial cholera —see Poisoning,
      antimony
Antiphospholipid
  antibody
    with hemorrhagic disorder D68.312
    syndrome D68.61
Antisocial personality F60.2
Antithrombinemia —see Circulating
      anticoagulants
Antithromboplastinemia D68.318
Antithromboplastinogenemia D68.318
Antitoxin complication or reaction —see
      Complications, vaccination
Antlophobia F40.228
Antritis J32.0
  maxilla J32.0
    acute J01.00
      recurrent J01.01
  stomach K29.60
    with bleeding K29.61
Antrum, antral —see condition
Anuria R34
  calculous (impacted) (recurrent) —see also
      Calculus, urinary N20.9
  following
    abortion —see Abortion by type
        complicated by, renal failure
    ectopic or molar pregnancy O08.4
  newborn P96.0
  postprocedural N99.0

Anuria (Continued)
  postrenal N13.8
  traumatic (following crushing) T79.5
Anus, anal —see condition
Anusitis K62.89
Anxiety F41.9
  depression F41.8
  episodic paroxysmal F41.0
  generalized F41.1
  hysteria F41.8
  neurosis F41.1
  panic type F41.0
  reaction F41.1
  separation, abnormal (of childhood) F93.0
  specified NEC F41.8
  state F41.1
Aorta, aortic —see condition
Aortectasia —see Ectasia, aorta
  with aneurysm —see Aneurysm, aorta
Aortitis (nonsyphilitic) (calcific) I77.6
  arteriosclerotic I70.0
  Doehle-Heller A52.02
  luetic A52.02
  rheumatic —see Endocarditis, acute,
      rheumatic
  specific (syphilitic) A52.02
  syphilitic A52.02
    congenital A50.54 [I79.1]
Apathetic thyroid storm —see Thyrotoxicosis
Apathy R45.3
Apeirophobia F40.228
Apepsia K30
  psychogenic F45.8
Aperistalsis, esophagus K22.0
Apertognathia M26.29
Apert's syndrome Q87.0
Aphagia R13.0
  psychogenic F50.9
Aphakia (acquired) (postoperative) H27.0-
  congenital Q12.3
Aphasia (amnestic) (global) (nominal)
      (semantic) (syntactic) R47.01
  acquired, with epilepsy (Landau-Kleffner
      syndrome) —see Epilepsy, specified
      NEC
  auditory (developmental) F80.2
  developmental (receptive type) F80.2
    expressive type F80.1
    Wernicke's F80.2
  following
    cerebrovascular disease I69.920
      cerebral infarction I69.320
      intracerebral hemorrhage I69.120
      nontraumatic intracranial hemorrhage
          NEC I69.220
      specified disease NEC I69.820
      subarachnoid hemorrhage I69.020
  primary progressive G31.01 [F02.80]
    with behavioral disturbance G31.01
        [F02.81]
  progressive isolated G31.01 [F02.80]
    with behavioral disturbance G31.01
        [F02.81]
  sensory F80.2
  syphilis, tertiary A52.19
  Wernicke's (developmental) F80.2
Aphonia (organic) R49.1
  hysterical F44.4
  psychogenic F44.4
Aphthae, aphthous —see also condition
  Bednar's K12.0
  cachectic K14.0
  epizootic B08.8
  fever B08.8
  oral (recurrent) K12.0
  stomatitis (major) (minor) K12.0
  thrush B37.0
  ulcer (oral) (recurrent) K12.0
    genital organ (s) NEC
      female N76.6
      male N50.89 ◀▥
    larynx J38.7

Apical —see condition
Apiphobia F40.218
Aplasia —see also Agenesis
  abdominal muscle syndrome Q79.4
  alveolar process (acquired) —see Anomaly,
      alveolar
    congenital Q38.6
  aorta (congenital) Q25.41 ◀▥
  axialis extracorticalis (congenita) E75.29
  bone marrow (myeloid) D61.9
    congenital D61.01
  brain Q00.0
    part of Q04.3
  bronchus Q32.4
  cementum K00.4
  cerebellum Q04.3
  cervix (congenital) Q51.5
  congenital pure red cell D61.01
  corpus callosum Q04.0
  cutis congenita Q84.8
  erythrocyte congenital D61.01
  extracortical axial E75.29
  eye Q11.1
  fovea centralis (congenital) Q14.1
  gallbladder, congenital Q44.0
  iris Q13.1
  labyrinth, membranous Q16.5
  limb (congenital) Q73.8
    lower —see Defect, reduction, lower limb
    upper —see Agenesis, arm
  lung, congenital (bilateral) (unilateral) Q33.3
  pancreas Q45.0
  parathyroid-thymic D82.1
  Pelizaeus-Merzbacher E75.29
  penis Q55.5
  prostate Q55.4
  red cell (with thymoma) D60.9
    acquired D60.9
      due to drugs D60.9
    adult D60.9
    chronic D60.0
    congenital D61.01
    constitutional D61.01
    due to drugs D60.9
    hereditary D61.01
    of infants D61.01
    primary D61.01
    pure D61.01
      due to drugs D60.9
    specified type NEC D60.8
    transient D60.1
  round ligament Q52.8
  skin Q84.8
  spermatic cord Q55.4
  spleen Q89.01
  testicle Q55.0
  thymic, with immunodeficiency D82.1
  thyroid (congenital) (with myxedema)
      E03.1
  uterus Q51.0
  ventral horn cell Q06.1
Apnea, apneic (of) (spells) R06.81
  newborn NEC P28.4
    obstructive P28.4
    sleep (central) (obstructive) (primary)
        P28.3
  prematurity P28.4
  sleep G47.30
    central (primary) G47.31
      in conditions classified elsewhere
          G47.37
    obstructive (adult) (pediatric) G47.33
    primary central G47.31
    specified NEC G47.39
Apneumatosis, newborn P28.0
Apocrine metaplasia (breast) —see Dysplasia,
      mammary, specified type NEC
Apophysitis (bone) —see also
      Osteochondropathy
  calcaneus M92.8
  juvenile M92.9

Apoplectiform convulsions (cerebral ischemia) I67.82
Apoplexia, apoplexy, apoplectic
  adrenal A39.1
  heart (auricle) (ventricle) —see Infarct, myocardium
  heat T67.0
  hemorrhagic (stroke) —see Hemorrhage, intracranial
  meninges, hemorrhagic —see Hemorrhage, intracranial, subarachnoid
  uremic N18.9 [I68.8]
Appearance
  bizarre R46.1
  specified NEC R46.89
  very low level of personal hygiene R46.0
Appendage
  epididymal (organ of Morgagni) Q55.4
  intestine (epiploic) Q43.8
  preauricular Q17.0
  testicular (organ of Morgagni) Q55.29
Appendicitis (pneumococcal) (retrocecal) K37
  with
    perforation or rupture K35.2
    peritoneal abscess K35.3
    peritonitis NEC K35.3
      generalized (with perforation or rupture) K35.2
      localized (with perforation or rupture) K35.3
  acute (catarrhal) (fulminating) (gangrenous) (obstructive) (retrocecal) (suppurative) K35.80
    with
      peritoneal abscess K35.3
      peritonitis NEC K35.3
        generalized (with perforation or rupture) K35.2
        localized (with perforation or rupture) K35.3
      specified NEC K35.89
  amebic A06.89
  chronic (recurrent) K36
  exacerbation —see Appendicitis, acute
  gangrenous —see Appendicitis, acute
  healed (obliterative) K36
  interval K36
  neurogenic K36
  obstructive K36
  recurrent K36
  relapsing K36
  subacute (adhesive) K36
  subsiding K36
  suppurative —see Appendicitis, acute
  tuberculous A18.32
Appendicopathia oxyurica B80
Appendix, appendicular —see also condition
  epididymis Q55.4
  Morgagni
    female Q50.5
    male (epididymal) Q55.4
    testicular Q55.29
  testis Q55.29
Appetite
  depraved —see Pica
  excessive R63.2
  lack or loss —see also Anorexia R63.0
    nonorganic origin F50.89 ◄▥
    psychogenic F50.89 ◄▥
  perverted (hysterical) —see Pica
Apple peel syndrome Q41.1
Apprehension state F41.1
Apprehensiveness, abnormal F41.9
Approximal wear K03.0
Apraxia (classic) (ideational) (ideokinetic) (ideomotor) (motor) (verbal) R48.2
  following
    cerebrovascular disease I69.990
      cerebral infarction I69.390
      intracerebral hemorrhage I69.190

Apraxia (Continued)
  following (Continued)
    cerebrovascular disease (Continued)
      nontraumatic intracranial hemorrhage NEC I69.290
      specified disease NEC I69.890
      subarachnoid hemorrhage I69.090
    oculomotor, congenital H51.8
Aptyalism K11.7
Apudoma —see Neoplasm, uncertain behavior, by site
Aqueous misdirection H40.83-
Arabicum elephantiasis —see Infestation, filarial
Arachnitis —see Meningitis
Arachnodactyly —see Syndrome, Marfan's
Arachnoiditis (acute) (adhesive) (basal) (brain) (cerebrospinal) —see Meningitis
Arachnophobia F40.210
Arboencephalitis, Australian A83.4
Arborization block (heart) I45.5
ARC (AIDS-related complex) B20
Arches —see condition
Arcuate uterus Q51.810
Arcuatus uterus Q51.810
Arcus (cornea) senilis —see Degeneration, cornea, senile
Arc-welder's lung J63.4
Areflexia R29.2
Areola —see condition
Argentaffinoma —see also Neoplasm, uncertain behavior, by site
  malignant —see Neoplasm, malignant, by site
  syndrome E34.0
Argininemia E72.21
Arginosuccinic aciduria E72.22
Argyll Robertson phenomenon, pupil or syndrome (syphilitic) A52.19
  atypical H57.09
  nonsyphilitic H57.09
Argyria, argyriasis
  conjunctival H11.13-
  from drug or medicament —see Table of Drugs and Chemicals, by substance
Argyrosis, conjunctival H11.13-
Arhinencephaly Q04.1
Ariboflavinosis E53.0
Arm —see condition
Arnold-Chiari disease, obstruction or syndrome (type II) Q07.00
  with
    hydrocephalus Q07.02
      with spina bifida Q07.03
    spina bifida Q07.01
      with hydrocephalus Q07.03
  type III —see Encephalocele
  type IV Q04.8
Aromatic amino-acid metabolism disorder E70.9
  specified NEC E70.8
Arousals, confusional G47.51
Arrest, arrested
  cardiac I46.9
    complicating
      abortion —see Abortion, by type, complicated by, cardiac arrest
      anesthesia (general) (local) or other sedation —see Table of Drugs and Chemicals, by drug
        in labor and delivery O74.2
        in pregnancy O29.11-
        postpartum, puerperal O89.1
      delivery (cesarean) (instrumental) O75.4
    due to
      cardiac condition I46.2
      specified condition NEC I46.8
    intraoperative I97.71-
    newborn P29.81
    postprocedural I97.12-
      obstetric procedure O75.4

Arrest, arrested (Continued)
  cardiorespiratory —see Arrest, cardiac
  circulatory —see Arrest, cardiac
  deep transverse O64.0
  development or growth
    bone —see Disorder, bone, development or growth
    child R62.50
    tracheal rings Q32.1
  epiphyseal
    complete
      femur M89.15-
      humerus M89.12-
      tibia M89.16-
      ulna M89.13-
    forearm M89.13-
      specified NEC M89.13-
      ulna —see Arrest, epiphyseal, by type, ulna
    lower leg M89.16-
      specified NEC M89.168
      tibia —see Arrest, epiphyseal, by type, tibia
    partial
      femur M89.15-
      humerus M89.12-
      tibia M89.16-
      ulna M89.13-
    specified NEC M89.18
  granulopoiesis —see Agranulocytosis
  growth plate —see Arrest, epiphyseal
  heart —see Arrest, cardiac
  legal, anxiety concerning Z65.3
  physeal —see Arrest, epiphyseal
  respiratory R09.2
    newborn P28.81
  sinus I45.5
  spermatogenesis (complete) —see Azoospermia
    incomplete —see Oligospermia
  transverse (deep) O64.0
Arrhenoblastoma
  benign
    specified site —see Neoplasm, benign, by site
    unspecified site
      female D27.9
      male D29.20
  malignant
    specified site —see Neoplasm, malignant, by site
    unspecified site
      female C56.9
      male C62.90
  specified site —see Neoplasm, uncertain behavior, by site
  unspecified site
    female D39.10
    male D40.10
Arrhythmia (auricle)(cardiac) (juvenile) (nodal) (reflex)(sinus)(supraventricular) (transitory)(ventricle) I49.9
  block I45.9
  extrasystolic I49.49
  newborn
    bradycardia P29.12
    occurring before birth P03.819
      before onset of labor P03.810
      during labor P03.811
    tachycardia P29.11
  psychogenic F45.8
  specified NEC I49.8
  vagal R55
  ventricular re-entry I47.0
Arrillaga-Ayerza syndrome (pulmonary sclerosis with pulmonary hypertension) I27.0
Arsenical pigmentation L81.8
  from drug or medicament —see Table of Drugs and Chemicals
Arsenism —see Poisoning, arsenic

◄ New   ◄▥ Revised   ~~deleted~~ Deleted

Arterial —*see* condition
Arteriofibrosis —*see* Arteriosclerosis
Arteriolar sclerosis —*see* Arteriosclerosis
Arteriolith —*see* Arteriosclerosis
Arteriolitis I77.6
  necrotizing, kidney I77.5
  renal —*see* Hypertension, kidney
Arteriolosclerosis —*see* Arteriosclerosis
Arterionephrosclerosis —*see* Hypertension,
  kidney
Arteriopathy I77.9
Arteriosclerosis, arteriosclerotic (diffuse)
    (obliterans) (of) (senile) (with calcification)
    I70.90
  aorta I70.0
  arteries of extremities —*see* Arteriosclerosis,
    extremities
  brain I67.2
  bypass graft
    coronary —*see* Arteriosclerosis, coronary,
      bypass graft
    extremities —*see* Arteriosclerosis,
      extremities, bypass graft
  cardiac —*see* Disease, heart, ischemic,
    atherosclerotic
  cardiopathy —*see* Disease, heart, ischemic,
    atherosclerotic
  cardiorenal —*see* Hypertension, cardiorenal
  cardiovascular —*see* Disease, heart, ischemic,
    atherosclerotic
  carotid —*see also* Occlusion, artery, carotid
    I65.2-
  central nervous system I67.2
  cerebral I67.2
  cerebrovascular I67.2
  coronary (artery) I25.10
    bypass graft I25.810
      with
        angina pectoris I25.709
          with documented spasm I25.701
          specified type NEC I25.708
          unstable I25.700
        ischemic chest pain I25.709
      autologous artery I25.810
        with
          angina pectoris I25.729
            with documented spasm I25.721
            specified type I25.728
            unstable I25.720
          ischemic chest pain I25.729
      autologous vein I25.810
        with
          angina pectoris I25.719
            with documented spasm I25.711
            specified type I25.718
            unstable I25.710
          ischemic chest pain I25.719
      nonautologous biological I25.810
        with
          angina pectoris I25.739
            with documented spasm I25.731
            specified type I25.738
            unstable I25.730
          ischemic chest pain I25.739
      specified type NEC I25.810
        with
          angina pectoris I25.799
            with documented spasm I25.791
            specified type I25.798
            unstable I25.790
          ischemic chest pain I25.799
    due to
      calcified coronary lesion (severely) I25.84
      lipid rich plaque I25.83
    native vessel
      with
        angina pectoris I25.119
          with documented spasm I25.111
          specified type NEC I25.118
          unstable I25.110
        ischemic chest pain I25.119

Arteriosclerosis, arteriosclerotic (Continued)
  coronary (Continued)
    transplanted heart I25.811
      bypass graft I25.812
        with
          angina pectoris I25.769
           with documented spasm
            I25.761
           specified type I25.768
           unstable I25.760
          ischemic chest pain I25.769
      native coronary artery I25.811
        with
          angina pectoris I25.759
           with documented spasm I25.751
           specified type I25.758
           unstable I25.750
          ischemic chest pain I25.759
  extremities (native arteries) I70.209
    bypass graft I70.309
      autologous vein graft I70.409
        leg I70.409
          with
            gangrene (and intermittent
              claudication, rest pain and
              ulcer) I70.469
            intermittent claudication
              I70.419
            rest pain (and intermittent
              claudication) I70.429
        bilateral I70.403
          with
            gangrene (and intermittent
              claudication, rest pain
              and ulcer) I70.463
            intermittent claudication
              I70.413
            rest pain (and intermittent
              claudication) I70.423
          specified type NEC I70.493
        left I70.402
          with
            gangrene (and intermittent
              claudication, rest pain
              and ulcer) I70.462
            intermittent claudication
              I70.412
            rest pain (and intermittent
              claudication) I70.422
            ulceration (and intermittent
              claudication and rest
              pain) I70.449
              ankle I70.443
              calf I70.442
              foot site NEC I70.445
              heel I70.444
              lower leg NEC I70.448
              midfoot I70.444
              thigh I70.441
          specified type NEC I70.492
        right I70.401
          with
            gangrene (and intermittent
              claudication, rest pain
              and ulcer) I70.461
            intermittent claudication
              I70.411
            rest pain (and intermittent
              claudication) I70.421
            ulceration (and intermittent
              claudication and rest
              pain) I70.439
              ankle I70.433
              calf I70.432
              foot site NEC I70.435
              heel I70.434
              lower leg NEC I70.438
              midfoot I70.434
              thigh I70.431
          specified type NEC I70.491
        specified type NEC I70.499

Arteriosclerosis, arteriosclerotic (Continued)
  extremities (Continued)
    bypass graft (Continued)
      autologous vein graft (Continued)
        specified NEC I70.408
          with
            gangrene (and intermittent
              claudication, rest pain and
              ulcer) I70.468
            intermittent claudication I70.418
            rest pain (and intermittent
              claudication) I70.428
            ulceration (and intermittent
              claudication and rest pain)
              I70.45
        specified type NEC I70.498
      leg I70.309
        with
          gangrene (and intermittent
            claudication, rest pain and
            ulcer) I70.369
          intermittent claudication I70.319
          rest pain (and intermittent
           claudication) I70.329
      bilateral I70.303
        with
          gangrene (and intermittent
            claudication, rest pain and
            ulcer) I70.363
          intermittent claudication I70.313
          rest pain (and intermittent
           claudication) I70.323
        specified type NEC I70.393
      left I70.302
        with
          gangrene (and intermittent
            claudication, rest pain and
            ulcer) I70.362
          intermittent claudication I70.312
          rest pain (and intermittent
           claudication) I70.322
          ulceration (and intermittent
           claudication and rest pain)
           I70.349
           ankle I70.343
           calf I70.342
           foot site NEC I70.345
           heel I70.344
           lower leg NEC I70.348
           midfoot I70.344
           thigh I70.341
        specified type NEC I70.392
      right I70.301
        with
          gangrene (and intermittent
            claudication, rest pain and
            ulcer) I70.361
          intermittent claudication I70.311
          rest pain (and intermittent
           claudication) I70.321
          ulceration (and intermittent
           claudication and rest pain)
           I70.339
           ankle I70.333
           calf I70.332
           foot site NEC I70.335
           heel I70.334
           lower leg NEC I70.338
           midfoot I70.334
           thigh I70.331
        specified type NEC I70.391
      specified type NEC I70.399
    nonautologous biological graft I70.509
      leg I70.509
        with
          gangrene (and intermittent
           claudication, rest pain and
           ulcer) I70.569
          intermittent claudication I70.519
          rest pain (and intermittent
           claudication) I70.529

Arteriosclerosis, arteriosclerotic *(Continued)*
  extremities *(Continued)*
    bypass graft *(Continued)*
      nonautologous biological graft
        (Continued)
        leg *(Continued)*
          bilateral I70.503
            with
              gangrene (and intermittent
                claudication, rest pain
                and ulcer) I70.563
              intermittent claudication
                I70.513
              rest pain (and intermittent
                claudication) I70.523
              specified type NEC I70.593
          left I70.502
            with
              gangrene (and intermittent
                claudication, rest pain
                and ulcer) I70.562
              intermittent claudication
                I70.512
              rest pain (and intermittent
                claudication)
                I70.522
              ulceration (and intermittent
                claudication and rest
                pain) I70.549
                ankle I70.543
                calf I70.542
                foot site NEC I70.545
                heel I70.544
                lower leg NEC I70.548
                midfoot I70.544
                thigh I70.541
              specified type NEC I70.592
          right I70.501
            with
              gangrene (and intermittent
                claudication, rest pain
                and ulcer) I70.561
              intermittent claudication
                I70.511
              rest pain (and intermittent
                claudication) I70.521
              ulceration (and intermittent
                claudication and rest
                pain) I70.539
                ankle I70.533
                calf I70.532
                foot site NEC I70.535
                heel I70.534
                lower leg NEC I70.538
                midfoot I70.534
                thigh I70.531
              specified type NEC I70.591
          specified type NEC I70.599
        specified NEC I70.508
          with
            gangrene (and intermittent
              claudication, rest pain and
              ulcer) I70.568
            intermittent claudication
              I70.518
            rest pain (and intermittent
              claudication) I70.528
            ulceration (and intermittent
              claudication and rest pain)
              I70.55
          specified type NEC I70.598
      nonbiological graft I70.609
        leg I70.609
          with
            gangrene (and intermittent
              claudication, rest pain and
              ulcer) I70.669
            intermittent claudication
              I70.619
            rest pain (and intermittent
              claudication) I70.629

Arteriosclerosis, arteriosclerotic *(Continued)*
  extremities *(Continued)*
    bypass graft *(Continued)*
      nonbiological graft *(Continued)*
        leg *(Continued)*
          bilateral I70.603
            with
              gangrene (and intermittent
                claudication, rest
                pain and ulcer)
                I70.663
              intermittent claudication
                I70.613
              rest pain (and intermittent
                claudication) I70.623
              specified type NEC I70.693
          left I70.602
            with
              gangrene (and intermittent
                claudication, rest
                pain and ulcer)
                I70.662
              intermittent claudication
                I70.612
              rest pain (and intermittent
                claudication) I70.622
              ulceration (and intermittent
                claudication and rest
                pain) I70.649
                ankle I70.643
                calf I70.642
                foot site NEC I70.645
                heel I70.644
                lower leg NEC I70.648
                midfoot I70.644
                thigh I70.641
              specified type NEC I70.692
          right I70.601
            with
              gangrene (and intermittent
                claudication, rest pain
                and ulcer) I70.661
              intermittent claudication
                I70.611
              rest pain (and intermittent
                claudication) I70.621
              ulceration (and intermittent
                claudication and rest
                pain) I70.639
                ankle I70.633
                calf I70.632
                foot site NEC I70.635
                heel I70.634
                lower leg NEC I70.638
                midfoot I70.634
                thigh I70.631
              specified type NEC I70.691
          specified NEC I70.608
            with
              gangrene (and intermittent
                claudication, rest pain and
                ulcer) I70.668
              intermittent claudication
                I70.618
              rest pain (and intermittent
                claudication) I70.628
              ulceration (and intermittent
                claudication and rest pain)
                I70.65
            specified type NEC I70.698
        specified graft NEC I70.709
          leg I70.709
            with
              gangrene (and intermittent
                claudication, rest pain and
                ulcer) I70.769
              intermittent claudication
                I70.719
              rest pain (and intermittent
                claudication) I70.729

Arteriosclerosis, arteriosclerotic *(Continued)*
  extremities *(Continued)*
    bypass graft *(Continued)*
      specified graft NEC *(Continued)*
        leg *(Continued)*
          bilateral I70.703
            with
              gangrene (and intermittent
                claudication, rest pain
                and ulcer) I70.763
              intermittent claudication
                I70.713
              rest pain (and intermittent
                claudication) I70.723
              specified type NEC I70.793
          left I70.702
            with
              gangrene (and intermittent
                claudication, rest pain
                and ulcer) I70.762
              intermittent claudication
                I70.712
              rest pain (and intermittent
                claudication) I70.722
              ulceration (and intermittent
                claudication and rest
                pain) I70.749
                ankle I70.743
                calf I70.742
                foot site NEC I70.745
                heel I70.744
                lower leg NEC I70.748
                midfoot I70.744
                thigh I70.741
              specified type NEC I70.792
          right I70.701
            with
              gangrene (and intermittent
                claudication, rest pain
                and ulcer) I70.761
              intermittent claudication
                I70.711
              rest pain (and intermittent
                claudication) I70.721
              ulceration (and intermittent
                claudication and rest
                pain) I70.739
                ankle I70.733
                calf I70.732
                foot site NEC I70.735
                heel I70.734
                lower leg NEC I70.738
                midfoot I70.734
                thigh I70.731
              specified type NEC I70.791
          specified type NEC I70.799
        specified NEC I70.708
          with
            gangrene (and intermittent
              claudication, rest pain and
              ulcer) I70.768
            intermittent claudication
              I70.718
            rest pain (and intermittent
              claudication) I70.728
            ulceration (and intermittent
              claudication and rest pain)
              I70.75
          specified type NEC I70.798
      specified NEC I70.308
        with
          gangrene (and intermittent
            claudication, rest pain and
            ulcer) I70.368
          intermittent claudication I70.318
          rest pain (and intermittent
            claudication) I70.328
          ulceration (and intermittent
            claudication and rest pain)
            I70.35
        specified type NEC I70.398

◀ New   ◀▥ Revised   ~~deleted~~ Deleted

Arteriosclerosis, arteriosclerotic (*Continued*)
  extremities (*Continued*)
    leg I70.209
      with
        gangrene (and intermittent
            claudication, rest pain and ulcer)
            I70.269
        intermittent claudication I70.219
        rest pain (and intermittent
            claudication) I70.229
      bilateral I70.203
        with
          gangrene (and intermittent
              claudication, rest pain and
              ulcer) I70.263
          intermittent claudication I70.213
          rest pain (and intermittent
              claudication) I70.223
          specified type NEC I70.293
      left I70.202
        with
          gangrene (and intermittent
              claudication, rest pain and
              ulcer) I70.262
          intermittent claudication I70.212
          rest pain (and intermittent
              claudication) I70.222
          ulceration (and intermittent
              claudication and rest pain)
              I70.249
            ankle I70.243
            calf I70.242
            foot site NEC I70.245
            heel I70.244
            lower leg NEC I70.248
            midfoot I70.244
            thigh I70.241
          specified type NEC I70.292
      right I70.201
        with
          gangrene (and intermittent
              claudication, rest pain and
              ulcer) I70.261
          intermittent claudication I70.211
          rest pain (and intermittent
              claudication) I70.221
          ulceration (and intermittent
              claudication and rest pain)
              I70.239
            ankle I70.233
            calf I70.232
            foot site NEC I70.235
            heel I70.234
            lower leg NEC I70.238
            midfoot I70.234
            thigh I70.231
          specified type NEC I70.291
        specified type NEC I70.299
    specified site NEC I70.208
      with
        gangrene (and intermittent
            claudication, rest pain and ulcer)
            I70.268
        intermittent claudication I70.218
        rest pain (and intermittent
            claudication) I70.228
        ulceration (and intermittent
            claudication and rest pain) I70.25
      specified type NEC I70.298
  generalized I70.91
  heart (disease) —*see* Arteriosclerosis,
      coronary (artery)
  kidney —*see* Hypertension, kidney
  medial —*see* Arteriosclerosis, extremities
  mesenteric (artery) K55.1
  Mönckeberg's —*see* Arteriosclerosis,
      extremities
  myocarditis I51.4
  peripheral (of extremities) —*see*
      Arteriosclerosis, extremities
  pulmonary (idiopathic) I27.0

Arteriosclerosis, arteriosclerotic (*Continued*)
  renal (arterioles) —*see also* Hypertension,
      kidney
    artery I70.1
  retina (vascular) I70.8 [H35.0-]
  specified artery NEC I70.8
  spinal (cord) G95.19
  vertebral (artery) I67.2
Arteriospasm I73.9
Arteriovenous —*see* condition
Arteritis I77.6
  allergic M31.0
  aorta (nonsyphilitic) I77.6
    syphilitic A52.02
  aortic arch M31.4
  brachiocephalic M31.4
  brain I67.7
    syphilitic A52.04
  cerebral I67.7
    in
      diseases classified elsewhere I68.2
      systemic lupus erythematosus M32.19
    listerial A32.89
    syphilitic A52.04
    tuberculous A18.89
  coronary (artery) I25.89
    rheumatic I01.8
      chronic I09.89
    syphilitic A52.06
  cranial (left) (right), giant cell M31.6
  deformans —*see* Arteriosclerosis
  giant cell NEC M31.6
    with polymyalgia rheumatica M31.5
  necrosing or necrotizing M31.9
    specified NEC M31.8
  nodosa M30.0
  obliterans —*see* Arteriosclerosis
  pulmonary I28.8
  rheumatic —*see* Fever, rheumatic
  senile —*see* Arteriosclerosis
  suppurative I77.2
  syphilitic (general) A52.09
    brain A52.04
    coronary A52.06
    spinal A52.09
  temporal, giant cell M31.6
  young female aortic arch syndrome M31.4
Artery, arterial —*see also* condition
  abscess I77.89
  single umbilical Q27.0
Arthralgia (allergic) —*see also* Pain, joint
  in caisson disease T70.3
  temporomandibular M26.62
Arthritis, arthritic (acute) (chronic)
    (nonpyogenic) (subacute) M19.90
  allergic —*see* Arthritis, specified form NEC
  ankylosing (crippling) (spine) —*see also*
      Spondylitis, ankylosing
    sites other than spine —*see* Arthritis,
        specified form NEC
  atrophic —*see* Osteoarthritis
    spine —*see* Spondylitis, ankylosing
  back —*see* Spondylopathy, inflammatory
  blennorrhagic (gonococcal) A54.42
  Charcot's —*see* Arthropathy, neuropathic
    diabetic —*see* Diabetes, arthropathy,
        neuropathic
    syringomyelic G95.0
  chylous (filarial) —*see also* category M01
      B74.9
  climacteric (any site) NEC —*see* Arthritis,
      specified form NEC
  crystal (-induced) —*see* Arthritis, in, crystals
  deformans —*see* Osteoarthritis
  degenerative —*see* Osteoarthritis
  due to or associated with
    acromegaly E22.0
    brucellosis —*see* Brucellosis
    caisson disease T70.3
    diabetes —*see* Diabetes, arthropathy
    dracontiasis —*see also* category M01 B72

Arthritis, arthritic (*Continued*)
  due to or associated with (*Continued*)
    enteritis NEC
      regional —*see* Enteritis, regional
    erysipelas —*see also* category M01 A46
    erythema
      epidemic A25.1
      nodosum L52
    filariasis NOS B74.9
    glanders A24.0
    helminthiasis —*see also* category M01 B83.9
    hemophilia D66 [M36.2]
    Henoch-(Schönlein) purpura D69.0 [M36.4]
    human parvovirus —*see also* category M01
        B97.6
    infectious disease NEC —*see* category M01
    leprosy (*see also* category M01) —*see also*
        Leprosy A30.9
    Lyme disease A69.23
    mycobacteria —*see also* category M01
        A31.8
    parasitic disease NEC —*see also* category
        M01 B89
    paratyphoid fever (*see also* category M01)
        —*see also* Fever, paratyphoid A01.4
    rat bite fever —*see also* category M01
        A25.1
    regional enteritis —*see* Enteritis, regional
    respiratory disorder NOS J98.9
    serum sickness —*see also* Reaction, serum
        T80.69
    syringomyelia G95.0
    typhoid fever A01.04
  epidemic erythema A25.1
  febrile —*see* Fever, rheumatic
  gonococcal A54.42
  gouty (acute) —*see* Gout ◄ⅢⅢ
  in (due to)
    acromegaly —*see also* subcategory
        M14.8- E22.0
    amyloidosis —*see also* subcategory
        M14.8- E85.4
    bacterial disease —*see also* subcategory
        M01 A49.9
    Behçet's syndrome M35.2
    caisson disease —*see also* subcategory
        M14.8- T70.3
    coliform bacilli (Escherichia coli) —*see*
        Arthritis, in, pyogenic organism NEC
    crystals M11.9
      dicalcium phosphate —*see* Arthritis, in,
          crystals, specified type NEC
      hydroxyapatite M11.0-
      pyrophosphate —*see* Arthritis, in,
          crystals, specified type NEC
      specified type NEC M11.80
        ankle M11.87-
        elbow M11.82-
        foot joint M11.87-
        hand joint M11.84-
        hip M11.85-
        knee M11.86-
        multiple sites M11.8-
        shoulder M11.81-
        vertebrae M11.88
        wrist M11.83-
    dermatoarthritis, lipoid E78.81
    dracontiasis (dracunculiasis) —*see also*
        category M01 B72
    endocrine disorder NEC —*see also*
        subcategory M14.8- E34.9
    enteritis, infectious NEC —*see also* category
        M01 A09
      specified organism NEC —*see also*
          category M01 A08.8
    erythema
      multiforme —*see also* subcategory
          M14.8- L51.9
      nodosum —*see also* subcategory
          M14.8- L52
    gout —*see* Gout ◄ⅢⅢ

Arthritis, arthritic *(Continued)*
  in *(Continued)*
    helminthiasis NEC —*see also* category M01
      B83.9
    hemochromatosis —*see also* subcategory
      M14.8- E83.118
    hemoglobinopathy NEC D58.2 *[M36.3]*
    hemophilia NEC D66 *[M36.2]*
    Hemophilus influenzae M00.8- *[B96.3]*
    Henoch(-Schönlein) purpura D69.0 *[M36.4]*
    hyperparathyroidism NEC —*see also*
      subcategory M14.8- E21.3
    hypersensitivity reaction NEC T78.49
      [M36.4]
    hypogammaglobulinemia —*see also*
      subcategory M14.8- D80.1
    hypothyroidism NEC —*see also*
      subcategory M14.8- E03.9
    infection —*see* Arthritis, pyogenic or
      pyemic
      spine —*see* Spondylopathy, infective
    infectious disease NEC —*see* category M01
    leprosy —*see also* category M01 A30.9
    leukemia NEC C95.9- *[M36.1]*
    lipoid dermatoarthritis E78.81
    Lyme disease A69.23
    Mediterranean fever, familial —*see also*
      subcategory M14.8- M04.1 ◀▦
    Meningococcus A39.83
    metabolic disorder NEC —*see also*
      subcategory M14.8- E88.9
    multiple myelomatosis C90.0- *[M36.1]*
    mumps B26.85
    mycosis NEC —*see also* category M01 B49
    myelomatosis (multiple) C90.0- *[M36.1]*
    neurological disorder NEC G98.0
    ochronosis —*see also* subcategory
      M14.8- E70.29
    O'nyong-nyong —*see also* category M01
      A92.1
    parasitic disease NEC —*see also* category
      M01 B89
    paratyphoid fever —*see also* category M01
      A01.4
    Pseudomonas —*see* Arthritis, pyogenic,
      bacterial NEC
    psoriasis L40.50
    pyogenic organism NEC —*see* Arthritis,
      pyogenic, bacterial NEC
    Reiter's disease —*see* Reiter's disease
    respiratory disorder NEC —*see also*
      subcategory M14.8- J98.9
    reticulosis, malignant —*see also*
      subcategory M14.8- C86.0
    rubella B06.82
    Salmonella (arizonae) (cholerae-suis)
      (enteritidis) (typhimurium)
      A02.23
    sarcoidosis D86.86
    specified bacteria NEC —*see* Arthritis,
      pyogenic, bacterial NEC
    sporotrichosis B42.82
    syringomyelia G95.0
    thalassemia NEC D56.9 *[M36.3]*
    tuberculosis —*see* Tuberculosis, arthritis
    typhoid fever A01.04
    urethritis, Reiter's —*see* Reiter's disease
    viral disease NEC —*see also* category M01
      B34.9
  infectious or infective —*see also* Arthritis,
    pyogenic or pyemic
    spine —*see* Spondylopathy, infective
  juvenile M08.90
    with systemic onset —*see* Still's disease
    ankle M08.97-
    elbow M08.92-
    foot joint M08.97-
    hand joint M08.94-
    hip M08.95-
    knee M08.96-
    multiple site M08.99

Arthritis, arthritic *(Continued)*
  juvenile *(Continued)*
    pauciarticular M08.40
      ankle M08.47-
      elbow M08.42-
      foot joint M08.47-
      hand joint M08.44-
      hip M08.45-
      knee M08.46-
      shoulder M08.41-
      vertebrae M08.48
      wrist M08.43-
    psoriatic L40.54
    rheumatoid —*see* Arthritis, rheumatoid,
      juvenile
    shoulder M08.91-
    specified type NEC M08.80
      ankle M08.87-
      elbow M08.82-
      foot joint M08.87-
      hand joint M08.84-
      hip M08.85-
      knee M08.86-
      multiple site M08.89
      shoulder M08.81-
      specified joint NEC M08.88
      vertebrae M08.88
      wrist M08.83-
    vertebra M08.98
    wrist M08.93-
  meaning osteoarthritis —*see* Osteoarthritis
  meningococcal A39.83
  menopausal (any site) NEC —*see* Arthritis,
    specified form NEC
  mutilans (psoriatic) L40.52
  mycotic NEC —*see also* category M01 B49
  neuropathic (Charcot) —*see* Arthropathy,
    neuropathic
    diabetic —*see* Diabetes, arthropathy,
      neuropathic
    nonsyphilitic NEC G98.0
    syringomyelic G95.0
  ochronotic —*see also* subcategory
    M14.8- E70.29
  palindromic (any site) —*see* Rheumatism,
    palindromic
  pneumococcal M00.10
    ankle M00.17-
    elbow M00.12-
    foot joint —*see* Arthritis, pneumococcal,
      ankle
    hand joint M00.14-
    hip M00.15-
    knee M00.16-
    multiple site M00.19
    shoulder M00.11-
    vertebra M00.18
    wrist M00.13-
  postdysenteric —*see* Arthropathy,
    postdysenteric
  postmeningococcal A39.84
  postrheumatic, chronic —*see* Arthropathy,
    postrheumatic, chronic
  primary progressive —*see also* Arthritis,
    specified form NEC
    spine —*see* Spondylitis, ankylosing
  psoriatic L40.50
  purulent (any site except spine) —*see*
    Arthritis, pyogenic or pyemic
    spine —*see* Spondylopathy, infective
  pyogenic or pyemic (any site except spine)
    M00.9
    bacterial NEC M00.80
      ankle M00.87-
      elbow M00.82-
      foot joint —*see* Arthritis, pyogenic,
        bacterial NEC, ankle
      hand joint M00.84-
      hip M00.85-
      knee M00.86-
      multiple site M00.89

Arthritis, arthritic *(Continued)*
  pyogenic or pyemic *(Continued)*
    bacterial NEC *(Continued)*
      shoulder M00.81-
      vertebra M00.88
      wrist M00.83-
    pneumococcal —*see* Arthritis,
      pneumococcal
    spine —*see* Spondylopathy, infective
    staphylococcal —*see* Arthritis,
      staphylococcal
    streptococcal —*see* Arthritis, streptococcal
      NEC
      pneumococcal —*see* Arthritis,
        pneumococcal
  reactive —*see* Reiter's disease
  rheumatic —*see also* Arthritis, rheumatoid
    acute or subacute —*see* Fever, rheumatic
  rheumatoid M06.9
    with
      carditis —*see* Rheumatoid, carditis
      endocarditis —*see* Rheumatoid, carditis
      heart involvement NEC —*see*
        Rheumatoid, carditis
      lung involvement —*see* Rheumatoid,
        lung
      myocarditis —*see* Rheumatoid, carditis
      myopathy —*see* Rheumatoid, myopathy
      pericarditis —*see* Rheumatoid, carditis
      polyneuropathy —*see* Rheumatoid,
        polyneuropathy
      rheumatoid factor —*see* Arthritis,
        rheumatoid, seropositive
      splenoadenomegaly and leukopenia —
        see Felty's syndrome
      vasculitis —*see* Rheumatoid, vasculitis
      visceral involvement NEC —*see*
        Rheumatoid, arthritis, with
        involvement of organs NEC
    juvenile (with or without rheumatoid
      factor) M08.00
      ankle M08.07-
      elbow M08.02-
      foot joint M08.07-
      hand joint M08.04-
      hip M08.05-
      knee M08.06-
      multiple site M08.09
      shoulder M08.01-
      vertebra M08.08
      wrist M08.03-
    seronegative M06.00
      ankle M06.07-
      elbow M06.02-
      foot joint M06.07-
      hand joint M06.04-
      hip M06.05-
      knee M06.06-
      multiple sites M06.09
      shoulder M06.01-
      vertebra M06.08
      wrist M06.03-
    seropositive M05.9
      without organ involvement M05.70
        ankle M05.77-
        elbow M05.72-
        foot joint M05.77-
        hand joint M05.74-
        hip M05.75-
        knee M05.76-
        multiple sites M05.79
        shoulder M05.71-
        vertebra —*see* Spondylitis, ankylosing
        wrist M05.73-
    specified NEC M05.80
      ankle M05.87-
      elbow M05.82-
      foot joint M05.87-
      hand joint M05.84-
      hip M05.85-
      knee M05.86-

Arthritis, arthritic (Continued)
  rheumatoid (Continued)
    specified NEC (Continued)
      multiple sites M05.89
      shoulder M05.81-
      vertebra —see Spondylitis, ankylosing
      wrist M05.83-
    specified type NEC M06.80
      ankle M06.87-
      elbow M06.82-
      foot joint M06.87-
      hand joint M06.84-
      hip M06.85-
      knee M06.86-
      multiple site M06.89
      shoulder M06.81-
      vertebra M06.88
      wrist M06.83-
    spine —see Spondylitis, ankylosing
  rubella B06.82
  scorbutic —see also subcategory M14.8- E54
  senile or senescent —see Osteoarthritis
  septic (any site except spine) —see Arthritis,
    pyogenic or pyemic
  spine —see Spondylopathy, infective
  serum (nontherapeutic) (therapeutic) —see
    Arthropathy, postimmunization
  specified form NEC M13.80
    ankle M13.87-
    elbow M13.82-
    foot joint M13.87-
    hand joint M13.84-
    hip M13.85-
    knee M13.86-
    multiple site M13.89
    shoulder M13.81-
    specified joint NEC M13.88
    wrist M13.83-
  spine —see also Spondylopathy,
    inflammatory
    infectious or infective NEC —see
      Spondylopathy, infective
    Marie-Strümpell —see Spondylitis,
      ankylosing
    pyogenic —see Spondylopathy, infective
    rheumatoid —see Spondylitis, ankylosing
    traumatic (old) —see Spondylopathy,
      traumatic
    tuberculous A18.01
  staphylococcal M00.00
    ankle M00.07-
    elbow M00.02-
    foot joint —see Arthritis, staphylococcal,
      ankle
    hand joint M00.04-
    hip M00.05-
    knee M00.06-
    multiple site M00.09
    shoulder M00.01-
    vertebra M00.08
    wrist M00.03-
  streptococcal NEC M00.20
    ankle M00.27-
    elbow M00.22-
    foot joint —see Arthritis, streptococcal,
      ankle
    hand joint M00.24-
    hip M00.25-
    knee M00.26-
    multiple site M00.29
    shoulder M00.21-
    vertebra M00.28
    wrist M00.23-
  suppurative —see Arthritis, pyogenic or
    pyemic
  syphilitic (late) A52.16
    congenital A50.55 [M12.80]
  syphilitica deformans (Charcot) A52.16
  temporomandibular M26.69
  toxic of menopause (any site) —see Arthritis,
    specified form NEC

Arthritis, arthritic (Continued)
  transient —see Arthropathy, specified form
    NEC
  traumatic (chronic) —see Arthropathy,
    traumatic
  tuberculous A18.02
    spine A18.01
  uratic —see Gout ◄‖‖
  urethritica (Reiter's) —see Reiter's disease
  vertebral —see Spondylopathy, inflammatory
  villous (any site) —see Arthropathy, specified
    form NEC
Arthrocele —see Effusion, joint
Arthrodesis status Z98.1
Arthrodynia —see also Pain, joint
Arthrodysplasia Q74.9
Arthrofibrosis, joint —see Ankylosis
Arthrogryposis (congenital) Q68.8
  multiplex congenita Q74.3
Arthrokatadysis M24.7
Arthropathy (see also Arthritis) M12.9
  Charcot's —see Arthropathy, neuropathic
    diabetic —see Diabetes, arthropathy,
      neuropathic
    syringomyelic G95.0
  cricoarytenoid J38.7
  crystal(-induced) —see Arthritis, in, crystals
  diabetic NEC —see Diabetes, arthropathy
  distal interphalangeal, psoriatic L40.51
  enteropathic M07.60
    ankle M07.67-
    elbow M07.62-
    foot joint M07.67-
    hand joint M07.64-
    hip M07.65-
    knee M07.66-
    multiple site M07.69
    shoulder M07.61-
    vertebra M07.68
    wrist M07.63-
  following intestinal bypass M02.00
    ankle M02.07-
    elbow M02.02-
    foot joint M02.07-
    hand joint M02.04-
    hip M02.05-
    knee M02.06-
    multiple site M02.09
    shoulder M02.01-
    vertebra M02.08
    wrist M02.03-
  gouty —see also Gout ◄‖‖
    in (due to)
      Lesch-Nyhan syndrome E79.1 [M14.8-]
      sickle-cell disorders D57- [M14.8-]
  hemophilic NEC D66 [M36.2]
    in (due to)
      hyperparathyroidism NEC E21.3 [M14.8-]
      metabolic disease NOS E88.9 [M14.8-]
  in (due to)
    acromegaly E22.0 [M14.8-]
    amyloidosis E85.4 [M14.8-]
    blood disorder NOS D75.9 [M36.3]
    diabetes —see Diabetes, arthropathy
    endocrine disease NOS E34.9 [M14.8-]
    erythema
      multiforme L51.9 [M14.8-]
      nodosum L52 [M14.8-]
    hemochromatosis E83.118 [M14.8-]
    hemoglobinopathy NEC D58.2 [M36.3]
    hemophilia NEC D66 [M36.2]
    Henoch-Schönlein purpura D69.0 [M36.4]
    hyperthyroidism E05.90 [M14.8-]
    hypothyroidism E03.9 [M14.8-]
    infective endocarditis I33.0 [M12.80]
    leukemia NEC C95.9- [M36.1]
    malignant histiocytosis C96.A [M36.1]
    metabolic disease NOS E88.9 [M14.8-]
    multiple myeloma C90.0- [M36.1]
    neoplastic disease NOS (see also Neoplasm)
      D49.9 [M36.1]

Arthropathy (Continued)
  hemochromatosis (Continued)
    nutritional deficiency —see also
      subcategory M14.8- E63.9
    psoriasis NOS L40.50
    sarcoidosis D86.86
    syphilis (late) A52.77
      congenital A50.55 [M12.80]
    thyrotoxicosis —see also subcategory
      M14.8- E05.90
    ulcerative colitis K51.90 [M07.60]
    viral hepatitis (postinfectious) NEC B19.9
      [M12.80]
    Whipple's disease —see also subcategory
      M14.8- K90.81
  Jaccoud —see Arthropathy, postrheumatic,
    chronic
  juvenile —see Arthritis, juvenile
    psoriatic L40.54
  mutilans (psoriatic) L40.52
  neuropathic (Charcot) M14.60
    ankle M14.67-
    diabetic —see Diabetes, arthropathy,
      neuropathic
    elbow M14.62-
    foot joint M14.67-
    hand joint M14.64-
    hip M14.65-
    knee M14.66-
    multiple site M14.69
    nonsyphilitic NEC G98.0
    shoulder M14.61-
    syringomyelic G95.0
    vertebra M14.68
    wrist M14.63-
  osteopulmonary —see Osteoarthropathy,
    hypertrophic, specified NEC
  postdysenteric M02.10
    ankle M02.17-
    elbow M02.12-
    foot joint M02.17-
    hand joint M02.14-
    hip M02.15-
    knee M02.16-
    multiple site M02.19
    shoulder M02.11-
    vertebra M02.18
    wrist M02.13-
  postimmunization M02.20
    ankle M02.27-
    elbow M02.22-
    foot joint M02.27-
    hand joint M02.24-
    hip M02.25-
    knee M02.26-
    multiple site M02.29
    shoulder M02.21-
    vertebra M02.28
    wrist M02.23-
  postinfectious NEC B99 [M12.80]
    in (due to)
      enteritis due to Yersinia enterocolitica
        A04.6 [M12.80]
      syphilis A52.77
      viral hepatitis NEC B19.9
        [M12.80]
  postrheumatic, chronic (Jaccoud)
    M12.00
    ankle M12.07-
    elbow M12.02-
    foot joint M12.07-
    hand joint M12.04-
    hip M12.05-
    knee M12.06-
    multiple site M12.09
    shoulder M12.01-
    specified joint NEC M12.08
    vertebrae M12.08
    wrist M12.03-
  psoriatic NEC L40.59
    interphalangeal, distal L40.51

A

Arthropathy (Continued)
　reactive M02.9
　　in (due to)
　　　infective endocarditis I33.0 [M02.9]
　　specified type NEC M02.80
　　　ankle M02.87-
　　　elbow M02.82-
　　　foot joint M02.87-
　　　hand joint M02.84-
　　　hip M02.85-
　　　knee M02.86-
　　　multiple site M02.89
　　　shoulder M02.81-
　　　vertebra M02.88
　　　wrist M02.83-
　specified form NEC M12.80
　　ankle M12.87-
　　elbow M12.82-
　　foot joint M12.87-
　　hand joint M12.84-
　　hip M12.85-
　　knee M12.86-
　　multiple site M12.89
　　shoulder M12.81-
　　specified joint NEC M12.88
　　vertebrae M12.88
　　wrist M12.83-
　syringomyelic G95.0
　tabes dorsalis A52.16
　tabetic A52.16
　transient —see Arthropathy, specified form
　　NEC
　traumatic M12.50
　　ankle M12.57-
　　elbow M12.52-
　　foot joint M12.57-
　　hand joint M12.54-
　　hip M12.55-
　　knee M12.56-
　　multiple site M12.59
　　shoulder M12.51-
　　specified joint NEC M12.58
　　vertebrae M12.58
　　wrist M12.53-
Arthropyosis —see Arthritis, pyogenic or pyemic
Arthrosis (deformans) (degenerative)
　　(localized) —see also Osteoarthritis
　　M19.90
　spine —see Spondylosis
Arthus' phenomenon or reaction T78.41
　due to
　　drug —see Table of Drugs and Chemicals,
　　　by drug
Articular —see condition
Articulation, reverse (teeth) M26.24
Artificial
　insemination complication —see
　　Complications, artificial, fertilization
　opening status (functioning) (without
　　complication) Z93.9
　　anus (colostomy) Z93.3
　　colostomy Z93.3
　　cystostomy Z93.50
　　　appendico-vesicostomy Z93.52
　　　cutaneous Z93.51
　　　specified NEC Z93.59
　　enterostomy Z93.4
　　gastrostomy Z93.1
　　ileostomy Z93.2
　　intestinal tract NEC Z93.4
　　jejunostomy Z93.4
　　nephrostomy Z93.6
　　specified site NEC Z93.8
　　tracheostomy Z93.0
　　ureterostomy Z93.6
　　urethrostomy Z93.6
　　urinary tract NEC Z93.6
　　vagina Z93.8
　vagina status Z93.8
Arytenoid —see condition
Asbestosis (occupational) J61

ASC-H (atypical squamous cells cannot exclude
　　high grade squamous intraepithelial lesion
　　on cytologic smear)
　anus R85.611
　cervix R87.611
　vagina R87.621
ASC-US (atypical squamous cells of
　　undetermined significance on cytologic
　　smear)
　anus R85.610
　cervix R87.610
　vagina R87.620
Ascariasis B77.9
　with
　　complications NEC B77.89
　　intestinal complications B77.0
　　pneumonia, pneumonitis B77.81
Ascaridosis, ascaridiasis —see Ascariasis
Ascaris (infection) (infestation)
　　(lumbricoides) —see Ascariasis
Ascending —see condition
Aschoff's bodies —see Myocarditis,
　　rheumatic
Ascites (abdominal) R18.8
　cardiac I50.9
　chylous (nonfilarial) I89.8
　　filarial —see Infestation, filarial
　due to
　　cirrhosis, alcoholic K70.31
　　hepatitis
　　　alcoholic K70.11
　　　chronic active K71.51
　　S. japonicum B65.2
　heart I50.9
　malignant R18.0
　pseudochylous R18.8
　syphilitic A52.74
　tuberculous A18.31
Aseptic —see condition
Asherman's syndrome N85.6
Asialia K11.7
Asiatic cholera —see Cholera
Asimultagnosia (simultanagnosia)
　　R48.3
Askin's tumor —see Neoplasm, connective
　　tissue, malignant
Asocial personality F60.2
Asomatognosia R41.4
Aspartylglucosaminuria E77.1
Asperger's disease or syndrome F84.5
Aspergilloma —see Aspergillosis
Aspergillosis (with pneumonia) B44.9
　bronchopulmonary, allergic B44.81
　disseminated B44.7
　generalized B44.7
　pulmonary NEC B44.1
　　allergic B44.81
　　invasive B44.0
　specified NEC B44.89
　tonsillar B44.2
Aspergillus (flavus) (fumigatus) (infection)
　　(terreus) —see Aspergillosis
Aspermatogenesis —see Azoospermia
Aspermia (testis) —see Azoospermia
Asphyxia, asphyxiation (by) R09.01
　antenatal P84
　birth P84
　bunny bag —see Asphyxia, due to,
　　mechanical threat to breathing, trapped
　　in bed clothes
　crushing S28.0
　drowning T75.1
　gas, fumes, or vapor —see Table of Drugs and
　　Chemicals
　inhalation —see Inhalation
　intrauterine P84
　local I73.00
　　with gangrene I73.01
　mucus —see also Foreign body, respiratory
　　tract, causing asphyxia
　newborn P84

Asphyxia, asphyxiation (Continued)
　pathological R09.01
　postnatal P84
　　mechanical —see Asphyxia, due to,
　　　mechanical threat to breathing
　prenatal P84
　reticularis R23.1
　strangulation —see Asphyxia, due to,
　　mechanical threat to breathing
　submersion T75.1
　traumatic T71.9
　　due to
　　　crushed chest S28.0
　　　foreign body (in) —see Foreign body,
　　　　respiratory tract, causing asphyxia
　　　low oxygen content of ambient air T71.20
　　　　due to
　　　　　being trapped in
　　　　　　low oxygen environment T71.29
　　　　　　in car trunk T71.221
　　　　　　　circumstances undetermined
　　　　　　　　T71.224
　　　　　　　done with intent to harm by
　　　　　　　　another person T71.223
　　　　　　　　self T71.222
　　　　　　in refrigerator T71.231
　　　　　　　circumstances undetermined
　　　　　　　　T71.234
　　　　　　　done with intent to harm by
　　　　　　　　another person T71.233
　　　　　　　　self T71.232
　　　cave-in T71.21
　　mechanical threat to breathing
　　　(accidental) T71.191
　　　circumstances undetermined T71.194
　　　done with intent to harm by
　　　　another person T71.193
　　　　self T71.192
　　　hanging T71.161
　　　　circumstances undetermined
　　　　　T71.164
　　　　done with intent to harm by
　　　　　another person T71.163
　　　　　self T71.162
　　　plastic bag T71.121
　　　　circumstances undetermined
　　　　　T71.124
　　　　done with intent to harm by
　　　　　another person T71.123
　　　　　self T71.122
　　　smothering
　　　　in furniture T71.151
　　　　　circumstances undetermined
　　　　　　T71.154
　　　　　done with intent to harm by
　　　　　　another person T71.153
　　　　　　self T71.152
　　　　under
　　　　　another person's body T71.141
　　　　　　circumstances undetermined
　　　　　　　T71.144
　　　　　　done with intent to harm
　　　　　　　T71.143
　　　　　pillow T71.111
　　　　　　circumstances undetermined
　　　　　　　T71.114
　　　　　　done with intent to harm by
　　　　　　　another person T71.113
　　　　　　　self T71.112
　　　trapped in bed clothes T71.131
　　　　circumstances undetermined
　　　　　T71.134
　　　　done with intent to harm by
　　　　　another person T71.133
　　　　　self T71.132
　vomiting, vomitus —see Foreign body,
　　respiratory tract, causing asphyxia
Aspiration
　amniotic (clear) fluid (newborn) P24.10
　　with
　　　pneumonia (pneumonitis) P24.11
　　　respiratory symptoms P24.11

◀ New　◀ⅢⅢ Revised　deleted Deleted

Aspiration *(Continued)*
  blood
    newborn (without respiratory symptoms)
        P24.20
      with
        pneumonia (pneumonitis) P24.21
        respiratory symptoms P24.21
      specified age NEC —*see* Foreign body,
          respiratory tract
  bronchitis J69.0
  food or foreign body (with asphyxiation) —
      see Asphyxia, food
  liquor (amnii) (newborn) P24.10
    with
      pneumonia (pneumonitis) P24.11
      respiratory symptoms P24.11
  meconium (newborn) (without respiratory
      symptoms) P24.00
    with
      pneumonitis (pneumonitis) P24.01
      respiratory symptoms P24.01
  milk (newborn) (without respiratory
      symptoms) P24.30
    with
      pneumonia (pneumonitis) P24.31
      respiratory symptoms P24.31
    specified age NEC—*see* Foreign body,
        respiratory tract
  mucus —*see also* Foreign body, by site,
      causing asphyxia
    newborn P24.10
      with
        pneumonia (pneumonitis) P24.11
        respiratory symptoms P24.11
  neonatal P24.9
    specific NEC (without respiratory
        symptoms) 24.80
      with
        pneumonia (pneumonitis) P24.81
        respiratory symptoms P24.81
  newborn P24.9
    specific NEC (without respiratory
        symptoms) P24.80
      with
        pneumonia (pneumonitis) P24.81
        respiratory symptoms P24.81
  pneumonia J69.0
  pneumonitis J69.0
  syndrome of newborn —*see* Aspiration, by
      substance, with pneumonia
  vernix caseosa (newborn) P24.80
    with
      pneumonia (pneumonitis) P24.81
      respiratory symptoms P24.81
  vomitus —*see also* Foreign body, respiratory
      tract
    newborn (without respiratory symptoms)
        P24.30
      with
        pneumonia (pneumonitis)
            P24.31
        respiratory symptoms P24.31
Asplenia (congenital) Q89.01
  postsurgical Z90.81
Assam fever B55.0
Assault, sexual —*see* Maltreatment
Assmann's focus NEC A15.0
Astasia (-abasia) (hysterical) F44.4
Asteatosis cutis L85.3
Astereognosia, astereognosis R48.1
Asterixis R27.8
  in liver disease K71.3
Asteroid hyalitis —*see* Deposit, crystalline
Asthenia, asthenic R53.1
  cardiac —*see also* Failure, heart I50.9
    psychogenic F45.8
  cardiovascular —*see also* Failure, heart
      I50.9
    psychogenic F45.8
  heart —*see also* Failure, heart I50.9
    psychogenic F45.8

Asthenia, asthenic *(Continued)*
  hysterical F44.4
  myocardial —*see also* Failure, heart
      I50.9
    psychogenic F45.8
  nervous F48.8
  neurocirculatory F45.8
  neurotic F48.8
  psychogenic F48.8
  psychoneurotic F48.8
  psychophysiologic F48.8
  reaction (psychophysiologic) F48.8
  senile R54
Asthenopia —*see also* Discomfort, visual
  hysterical F44.6
  psychogenic F44.6
Asthenospermia —*see* Abnormal, specimen,
    male genital organs
Asthma, asthmatic (bronchial) (catarrh)
    (spasmodic) J45.909
  with
    chronic obstructive bronchitis
        J44.9
      with
        acute lower respiratory infection J44.0
        exacerbation (acute) J44.1
    chronic obstructive pulmonary disease
        J44.9
      with
        acute lower respiratory infection
            J44.0
        exacerbation (acute) J44.1
    exacerbation (acute) J45.901
    hay fever —*see* Asthma, allergic extrinsic
    rhinitis, allergic —*see* Asthma, allergic
        extrinsic
    status asthmaticus J45.902
  allergic extrinsic J45.909
    with
      exacerbation (acute) J45.901
      status asthmaticus J45.902
  atopic —*see* Asthma, allergic extrinsic
  cardiac —*see* Failure, ventricular, left
  cardiobronchial I50.1
  childhood J45.909
    with
      exacerbation (acute) J45.901
      status asthmaticus J45.902
  chronic obstructive J44.9
    with
      acute lower respiratory infection
          J44.0
      exacerbation (acute) J44.1
  collier's J60
  cough variant J45.991
  detergent J69.8
  due to
    detergent J69.8
    inhalation of fumes J68.3
  eosinophilic J82
  extrinsic, allergic —*see* Asthma, allergic
      extrinsic
  grinder's J62.8
  hay —*see* Asthma, allergic extrinsic
  heart I50.1
  idiosyncratic —*see* Asthma, nonallergic
  intermittent (mild) J45.20
    with
      exacerbation (acute) J45.21
      status asthmaticus J45.22
  intrinsic, nonallergic —*see* Asthma,
      nonallergic
  Kopp's E32.8
  late-onset J45.909
    with
      exacerbation (acute) J45.901
      status asthmaticus J45.902
  mild intermittent J45.20
    with
      exacerbation (acute) J45.21
      status asthmaticus J45.22

Asthma, asthmatic *(Continued)*
  mild persistent J45.30
    with
      exacerbation (acute) J45.31
      status asthmaticus J45.32
  Millar's (laryngismus stridulus) J38.5
  miner's J60
  mixed J45.909
    with
      exacerbation (acute) J45.901
      status asthmaticus J45.902
  moderate persistent J45.40
    with
      exacerbation (acute) J45.41
      status asthmaticus J45.42
  nervous —*see* Asthma, nonallergic
  nonallergic (intrinsic) J45.909
    with
      exacerbation (acute) J45.901
      status asthmaticus J45.902
  persistent
    mild J45.30
      with
        exacerbation (acute) J45.31
        status asthmaticus J45.32
    moderate J45.40
      with
        exacerbation (acute) J45.41
        status asthmaticus J45.42
    severe J45.50
      with
        exacerbation (acute) J45.51
        status asthmaticus J45.52
  platinum J45.998
  pneumoconiotic NEC J64
  potter's J62.8
  predominantly allergic J45.909
  psychogenic F54
  pulmonary eosinophilic J82
  red cedar J67.8
  Rostan's I50.1
  sandblaster's J62.8
  sequoiosis J67.8
  severe persistent J45.50
    with
      exacerbation (acute) J45.51
      status asthmaticus J45.52
  specified NEC J45.998
  stonemason's J62.8
  thymic E32.8
  tuberculous —*see* Tuberculosis, pulmonary
  Wichmann's (laryngismus stridulus) J38.5
  wood J67.8
Astigmatism (compound) (congenital) H52.20-
  irregular H52.21-
  regular H52.22-
Astraphobia F40.220
Astroblastoma
  specified site —*see* Neoplasm, malignant, by
      site
  unspecified site C71.9
Astrocytoma (cystic)
  anaplastic
    specified site —*see* Neoplasm, malignant,
        by site
    unspecified site C71.9
  fibrillary
    specified site —*see* Neoplasm, malignant,
        by site
    unspecified site C71.9
  fibrous
    specified site —*see* Neoplasm, malignant,
        by site
    unspecified site C71.9
  gemistocytic
    specified site —*see* Neoplasm, malignant,
        by site
    unspecified site C71.9
  juvenile
    specified site —*see* Neoplasm, malignant,
        by site
    unspecified site C71.9

A

Astrocytoma *(Continued)*
  pilocytic
    specified site —*see* Neoplasm, malignant,
      by site
    unspecified site C71.9
  piloid
    specified site —*see* Neoplasm, malignant,
      by site
    unspecified site C71.9
  protoplasmic
    specified site —*see* Neoplasm, malignant,
      by site
    unspecified site C71.9
  specified site NEC —*see* Neoplasm,
    malignant, by site
  subependymal D43.2
    giant cell
      specified site —*see* Neoplasm, uncertain
        behavior, by site
      unspecified site D43.2
    specified site —*see* Neoplasm, uncertain
      behavior, by site
    unspecified site D43.2
  unspecified site C71.9
Astroglioma
  specified site —*see* Neoplasm, malignant, by
    site
  unspecified site C71.9
Asymbolia R48.8
Asymmetry —*see also* Distortion
  between native and reconstructed breast
    N65.1
  face Q67.0
  jaw (lower) —*see* Anomaly, dentofacial, jaw-
    cranial base relationship, asymmetry
Asynergia, asynergy R27.8
  ventricular I51.89
Asystole (heart) —*see* Arrest, cardiac
At risk
  for falling Z91.81
Ataxia, ataxy, ataxic R27.0
  acute R27.8
  brain (hereditary) G11.9
  cerebellar (hereditary) G11.9
    with defective DNA repair G11.3
    alcoholic G31.2
    early-onset G11.1
    in
      alcoholism G31.2
      myxedema E03.9 [G13.2]
      neoplastic disease —*see also* Neoplasm
        D49.9 [G32.81] ◄ⅧⅢ
      specified disease NEC G32.81
    late-onset (Marie's) G11.2
  cerebral (hereditary) G11.9
  congenital nonprogressive G11.0
  family, familial —*see* Ataxia, hereditary
  following
    cerebrovascular disease I69.993
      cerebral infarction I69.393
      intracerebral hemorrhage I69.193
      nontraumatic intracranial hemorrhage
        NEC I69.293
      specified disease NEC I69.893
      subarachnoid hemorrhage I69.093
  Friedreich's (heredofamilial) (cerebellar)
    (spinal) G11.1
  gait R26.0
    hysterical F44.4
  general R27.8
  gluten M35.9 [G32.81]
    with celiac disease K90.0 [G32.81]
  hereditary G11.9
    with neuropathy G60.2
    cerebellar —*see* Ataxia, cerebellar
    spastic G11.4
    specified NEC G11.8
    spinal (Friedreich's) G11.1
  heredofamilial —*see* Ataxia, hereditary
  Hunt's G11.1
  hysterical F44.4

Ataxia, ataxy, ataxic *(Continued)*
  locomotor (progressive) (syphilitic) (partial)
    (spastic) A52.11
    diabetic —*see* Diabetes, ataxia
  Marie's (cerebellar) (heredofamilial) (late-
    onset) G11.2
  nonorganic origin F44.4
  nonprogressive, congenital G11.0
  psychogenic F44.4
  Roussy-Lévy G60.0
  Sanger-Brown's (hereditary) G11.2
  spastic hereditary G11.4
  spinal
    hereditary (Friedreich's) G11.1
    progressive (syphilitic) A52.11
  spinocerebellar, X-linked recessive G11.1
  telangiectasia (Louis-Bar) G11.3
Ataxia-telangiectasia (Louis-Bar) G11.3
Atelectasis (massive) (partial) (pressure)
    (pulmonary) J98.11
  newborn P28.10
    due to resorption P28.11
    partial P28.19
    primary P28.0
    secondary P28.19
  primary (newborn) P28.0
  tuberculous —*see* Tuberculosis, pulmonary
Atelocardia Q24.9
Atelomyelia Q06.1
Atheroembolism
  of
    extremities
      lower I75.02-
      upper I75.01-
    kidney I75.81
    specified NEC I75.89
Atheroma, atheromatous —*see also*
    Arteriosclerosis I70.90
  aorta, aortic I70.0
    valve —*see also* Endocarditis, aortic I35.8
  aorto-iliac I70.0
  artery —*see* Arteriosclerosis
  basilar (artery) I67.2
  carotid (artery) (common) (internal) I67.2
  cerebral (arteries) I67.2
  coronary (artery) I25.10
    with angina pectoris —*see* Arteriosclerosis,
      coronary (artery)
  degeneration —*see* Arteriosclerosis
  heart, cardiac —*see* Disease, heart, ischemic,
    atherosclerotic
  mitral (valve) I34.8
  myocardium, myocardial —*see* Disease, heart,
    ischemic, atherosclerotic
  pulmonary valve (heart) —*see also*
    Endocarditis, pulmonary I37.8
  tricuspid (heart) (valve) I36.8
  valve, valvular —*see* Endocarditis
  vertebral (artery) I67.2
Atheromatosis —*see* Arteriosclerosis
Atherosclerosis —*see also* Arteriosclerosis
  coronary
    artery I25.10
      with angina pectoris —*see*
        Arteriosclerosis, coronary (artery),
      due to
        calcified coronary lesion (severely)
          I25.84
        lipid rich plaque I25.83
    transplanted heart I25.811
      bypass graft I25.812
        with angina pectoris —*see*
          Arteriosclerosis, coronary (artery)
      native coronary artery I25.811
        with angina pectoris —*see*
          Arteriosclerosis, coronary (artery)
Athetosis (acquired) R25.8
  bilateral (congenital) G80.3
  congenital (bilateral) (double) G80.3
  double (congenital) G80.3
  unilateral R25.8

Athlete's
  foot B35.3
  heart I51.7
Athrepsia E41
Athyrea (acquired) —*see also* Hypothyroidism
  congenital E03.1
Atonia, atony, atonic
  bladder (sphincter) (neurogenic) N31.2
  capillary I78.8
  cecum K59.8
    psychogenic F45.8
  colon —*see* Atony, intestine
  congenital P94.2
  esophagus K22.8
  intestine K59.8
    psychogenic F45.8
  stomach K31.89
    neurotic or psychogenic F45.8
  uterus (during labor) O62.2
    with hemorrhage (postpartum) O72.1
    postpartum (with hemorrhage) O72.1
      without hemorrhage O75.89
Atopy —*see* History, allergy
Atransferrinemia, congenital E88.09
Atresia, atretic
  alimentary organ or tract NEC Q45.8
    upper Q40.8
  ani, anus, anal (canal) Q42.3
    with fistula Q42.2
  aorta (ring) Q25.29 ◄ⅧⅢ
  aortic (orifice) (valve) Q23.0
    arch Q25.21 ◄ⅧⅢ
    congenital with hypoplasia of ascending
      aorta and defective development of
      left ventricle (with mitral stenosis)
      Q23.4
    in hypoplastic left heart syndrome Q23.4
  aqueduct of Sylvius Q03.0
    with spina bifida —*see* Spina bifida, with
      hydrocephalus
  artery NEC Q27.8
    cerebral Q28.3
    coronary Q24.5
    digestive system Q27.8
    eye Q15.8
    lower limb Q27.8
    pulmonary Q25.5
    specified site NEC Q27.8
    umbilical Q27.0
    upper limb Q27.8
  auditory canal (external) Q16.1
  bile duct (common) (congenital) (hepatic)
    Q44.2
    acquired —*see* Obstruction, bile duct
  bladder (neck) Q64.39
    obstruction Q64.31
  bronchus Q32.4
  cecum Q42.8
  cervix (acquired) N88.2
    congenital Q51.828
    in pregnancy or childbirth —*see* Anomaly,
      cervix, in pregnancy or childbirth
      causing obstructed labor O65.5
  choana Q30.0
  colon Q42.9
    specified NEC Q42.8
  common duct Q44.2
  cricoid cartilage Q31.8
  cystic duct Q44.2
    acquired K82.8
      with obstruction K82.0
  digestive organs NEC Q45.8
  duodenum Q41.0
  ear canal Q16.1
  ejaculatory duct Q55.4
  epiglottis Q31.8
  esophagus Q39.0
    with tracheoesophageal fistula Q39.1
  eustachian tube Q17.8
  fallopian tube (congenital) Q50.6
    acquired N97.1

Atresia, atretic *(Continued)*
  follicular cyst N83.0- ◀▥
  foramen of
    Luschka Q03.1
      with spina bifida —*see* Spina bifida, with
        hydrocephalus
    Magendie Q03.1
      with spina bifida —*see* Spina bifida, with
        hydrocephalus
  gallbladder Q44.1
  genital organ
    external
      female Q52.79
      male Q55.8
    internal
      female Q52.8
      male Q55.8
  glottis Q31.8
  gullet Q39.0
    with tracheoesophageal fistula Q39.1
  heart valve NEC Q24.8
    pulmonary Q22.0
    tricuspid Q22.4
  hymen Q52.3
    acquired (postinfective) N89.6
  ileum Q41.2
  intestine (small) Q41.9
    large Q42.9
      specified NEC Q42.8
  iris, filtration angle Q15.0
  jejunum Q41.1
  lacrimal apparatus Q10.4
  larynx Q31.8
  meatus urinarius Q64.33
  mitral valve Q23.2
    in hypoplastic left heart syndrome
      Q23.4
  nares (anterior) (posterior) Q30.0
  nasopharynx Q34.8
  nose, nostril Q30.0
    acquired J34.89
  organ or site NEC Q89.8
  osseous meatus (ear) Q16.1
  oviduct (congenital) Q50.6
    acquired N97.1
  parotid duct Q38.4
    acquired K11.8
  pulmonary (artery) Q25.5
    valve Q22.0
  pulmonic Q22.0
  pupil Q13.2
  rectum Q42.1
    with fistula Q42.0
  salivary duct Q38.4
    acquired K11.8
  sublingual duct Q38.4
    acquired K11.8
  submandibular duct Q38.4
    acquired K11.8
  submaxillary duct Q38.4
    acquired K11.8
  thyroid cartilage Q31.8
  trachea Q32.1
  tricuspid valve Q22.4
  ureter Q62.10
    pelvic junction Q62.11
    vesical orifice Q62.12
  ureteropelvic junction Q62.11
  ureterovesical orifice Q62.12
  urethra (valvular) Q64.39
    stricture Q64.32
  urinary tract NEC Q64.8
  uterus Q51.818
    acquired N85.8
  vagina (congenital) Q52.4
    acquired (postinfectional) (senile)
      N89.5
  vas deferens Q55.3
  vascular NEC Q27.8
    cerebral Q28.3
    digestive system Q27.8

Atresia, atretic *(Continued)*
  vascular NEC *(Continued)*
    lower limb Q27.8
    specified site NEC Q27.8
    upper limb Q27.8
    vein NEC Q27.8
      digestive system Q27.8
      great Q26.8
      lower limb Q27.8
      portal Q26.5
      pulmonary Q26.3
      specified site NEC Q27.8
      upper limb Q27.8
    vena cava (inferior) (superior) Q26.8
  vesicourethral orifice Q64.31
  vulva Q52.79
    acquired N90.5
Atrichia, atrichosis —*see* Alopecia
Atrophia —*see also* Atrophy
  cutis senilis L90.8
    due to radiation L57.8
  gyrata of choroid and retina H31.23
  senilis R54
    dermatological L90.8
      due to radiation (nonionizing) (solar)
        L57.8
  unguium L60.3
    congenita Q84.6
Atrophie blanche (en plaque) (de Milian) L95.0
Atrophoderma, atrophodermia (of) L90.9
  diffusum (idiopathic) L90.4
  maculatum L90.8
    et striatum L90.8
      due to syphilis A52.79
    syphilitic A51.39
  neuriticum L90.8
  Pasini and Pierini L90.3
  pigmentosum Q82.1
  reticulatum symmetricum faciei L66.4
  senile L90.8
    due to radiation (nonionizing) (solar) L57.8
  vermiculata (cheeks) L66.4
Atrophy, atrophic (of)
  adrenal (capsule) (gland) E27.49
    primary (autoimmune) E27.1
  alveolar process or ridge (edentulous) K08.20
  anal sphincter (disuse) N81.84
  appendix K38.8
  arteriosclerotic —*see* Arteriosclerosis
  bile duct (common) (hepatic) K83.8
  bladder N32.89
    neurogenic N31.8
  blanche (en plaque) (of Milian) L95.0
  bone (senile) NEC —*see also* Disorder, bone,
      specified type NEC
    due to
      tabes dorsalis (neurogenic) A52.11
  brain (cortex) (progressive) G31.9
    frontotemporal circumscribed G31.01
      [F02.80]
      with behavioral disturbance G31.01
        [F02.81]
    senile NEC G31.1
  breast N64.2
    obstetric —*see* Disorder, breast, specified
      type NEC
  buccal cavity K13.79
  cardiac —*see* Degeneration, myocardial
  cartilage (infectional) (joint) —*see* Disorder,
      cartilage, specified NEC
  cerebellar —*see* Atrophy, brain
  cerebral —*see* Atrophy, brain
  cervix (mucosa) (senile) (uteri) N88.8
    menopausal N95.8
  Charcot-Marie-Tooth G60.0
  choroid (central) (macular) (myopic) (retina)
      H31.10-
    diffuse secondary H31.12-
    gyrate H31.23
    senile H31.11-
  ciliary body —*see* Atrophy, iris

Atrophy, atrophic *(Continued)*
  conjunctiva (senile) H11.89
  corpus cavernosum N48.89
  cortical —*see* Atrophy, brain
  cystic duct K82.8
  Déjérine-Thomas G23.8
  disuse NEC —*see* Atrophy, muscle
  Duchenne-Aran G12.21
  ear H93.8-
  edentulous alveolar ridge K08.20
  endometrium (senile) N85.8
    cervix N88.8
  enteric K63.89
  epididymis N50.89 ◀▥
  eyeball —*see* Disorder, globe, degenerated
      condition, atrophy
  eyelid (senile) —*see* Disorder, eyelid,
      degenerative
  facial (skin) L90.9
  fallopian tube (senile) N83.32- ◀▥
    with ovary N83.33- ◀▥
  fascioscapulohumeral (Landouzy- Déjérine)
      G71.0
  fatty, thymus (gland) E32.8
  gallbladder K82.8
  gastric K29.40
    with bleeding K29.41
  gastrointestinal K63.89
  glandular I89.8
  globe H44.52-
  gum —*see also* Recession, gingival K06.0 ◀▥
  hair L67.8
  heart (brown) —*see* Degeneration, myocardial
  hemifacial Q67.4
    Romberg G51.8
  infantile E41
    paralysis, acute —*see* Poliomyelitis,
      paralytic
  intestine K63.89
  iris (essential) (progressive) H21.26-
    specified NEC H21.29
  kidney (senile) (terminal) —*see also* Sclerosis,
      renal N26.1
    congenital or infantile Q60.5
      bilateral Q60.4
      unilateral Q60.3
    hydronephrotic —*see* Hydronephrosis
  lacrimal gland (primary) H04.14-
    secondary H04.15-
  Landouzy-Déjérine G71.0
  laryngitis, infective J37.0
  larynx J38.7
  Leber's optic (hereditary) H47.22
  lip K13.0
  liver (yellow) K72.90
    with coma K72.91
    acute, subacute K72.00
      with coma K72.01
    chronic K72.10
      with coma K72.11
  lung (senile) J98.4
  macular (dermatological) L90.8
    syphilitic, skin A51.39
      striated A52.79
  mandible (edentulous) K08.20
    minimal K08.21
    moderate K08.22
    severe K08.23
  maxilla K08.20
    minimal K08.24
    moderate K08.25
    severe K08.26
  muscle, muscular (diffuse) (general)
      (idiopathic) (primary) M62.50
    ankle M62.57-
    Duchenne-Aran G12.21
    foot M62.57-
    forearm M62.53-
    hand M62.54-
    infantile spinal G12.0
    lower leg M62.56-

Atrophy, atrophic *(Continued)*
  muscle, muscular *(Continued)*
    multiple sites M62.59
    myelopathic —*see* Atrophy, muscle,
      spinal
    myotonic G71.11
    neuritic G58.9
    neuropathic (peroneal) (progressive)
      G60.0
    pelvic (disuse) N81.84
    peroneal G60.0
    progressive (bulbar) G12.21
      adult G12.1
      infantile (spinal) G12.0
      spinal G12.9
        adult G12.1
        infantile G12.0
    pseudohypertrophic G71.0
    shoulder region M62.51-
    specified site NEC M62.58
    spinal G12.9
      adult form G12.1
      Aran-Duchenne G12.21
      childhood form, type II G12.1
      distal G12.1
      hereditary NEC G12.1
      infantile, type I (Werdnig- Hoffmann)
        G12.0
      juvenile form, type III (Kugelberg-
        Welander) G12.1
      progressive G12.21
      scapuloperoneal form G12.1
      specified NEC G12.8
    syphilitic A52.78
    thigh M62.55-
    upper arm M62.52-
  myocardium —*see* Degeneration,
    myocardial
  myometrium (senile) N85.8
    cervix N88.8
  myopathic NEC —*see* Atrophy, muscle
  myotonia G71.11
  nail L60.3
  nasopharynx J31.1
  nerve —*see also* Disorder, nerve
    abducens —*see* Strabismus, paralytic, sixth
      nerve
    accessory G52.8
    acoustic or auditory —*see* subcategory
      H93.3
    cranial G52.9
      eighth (auditory) —*see* subcategory
        H93.3
      eleventh (accessory) G52.8
      fifth (trigeminal) G50.8
      first (olfactory) G52.0
      fourth (trochlear) —*see* Strabismus,
        paralytic, fourth nerve
      second (optic) H47.20
      sixth (abducens) —*see* Strabismus,
        paralytic, sixth nerve
      tenth (pneumogastric) (vagus) G52.2
      third (oculomotor) —*see* Strabismus,
        paralytic, third nerve
      twelfth (hypoglossal) G52.3
    hypoglossal G52.3
    oculomotor —*see* Strabismus, paralytic,
      third nerve
    olfactory G52.0
    optic (papillomacular bundle)
      syphilitic (late) A52.15
        congenital A50.44
    pneumogastric G52.2
    trigeminal G50.8
    trochlear —*see* Strabismus, paralytic,
      fourth nerve
    vagus (pneumogastric) G52.2
  neurogenic, bone, tabetic A52.11
  nutritional E41
  old age R54
  olivopontocerebellar G23.8

Atrophy, atrophic *(Continued)*
  optic (nerve) H47.20
    glaucomatous H47.23-
    hereditary H47.22
    primary H47.21-
    specified type NEC H47.29-
    syphilitic (late) A52.15
      congenital A50.44
  orbit H05.31-
  ovary (senile) N83.31- ◀▥
    with fallopian tube N83.33- ◀▥
  oviduct (senile) —*see* Atrophy, fallopian tube
  palsy, diffuse (progressive) G12.22
  pancreas (duct) (senile) K86.89 ◀▥
  parotid gland K11.0
  pelvic muscle N81.84
  penis N48.89
  pharynx J39.2
  pluriglandular E31.8
    autoimmune E31.0
  polyarthritis M15.9
  prostate N42.89
  pseudohypertrophic (muscle) G71.0
  renal —*see also* Sclerosis, renal N26.1
  retina, retinal (postinfectional) H35.89
  rhinitis J31.0
  salivary gland K11.0
  scar L90.5
  sclerosis, lobar (of brain) G31.09 *[F02.80]*
    with behavioral disturbance G31.09
      [F02.81]
  scrotum N50.89 ◀▥
  seminal vesicle N50.89 ◀▥
  senile R54
    due to radiation (nonionizing) (solar) L57.8
  skin (patches) (spots) L90.9
    degenerative (senile) L90.8
    due to radiation (nonionizing) (solar) L57.8
    senile L90.8
  spermatic cord N50.89 ◀▥
  spinal (acute) (cord) G95.89
    muscular —*see* Atrophy, muscle, spinal
    paralysis G12.20
      acute —*see* Poliomyelitis, paralytic
      meaning progressive muscular atrophy
        G12.21
  spine (column) —*see* Spondylopathy,
    specified NEC
  spleen (senile) D73.0
  stomach K29.40
    with bleeding K29.41
  striate (skin) L90.6
    syphilitic A52.79
  subcutaneous L90.9
  sublingual gland K11.0
  submandibular gland K11.0
  submaxillary gland K11.0
  Sudeck's —*see* Algoneurodystrophy
  suprarenal (capsule) (gland) E27.49
    primary E27.1
  systemic affecting central nervous system
    in
      myxedema E03.9 *[G13.2]*
      neoplastic disease —*see also* Neoplasm
        D49.9 *[G13.1]*
      specified disease NEC G13.8
  tarso-orbital fascia, congenital Q10.3
  testis N50.0
  thenar, partial —*see* Syndrome, carpal tunnel
  thymus (fatty) E32.8
  thyroid (gland) (acquired) E03.4
    with cretinism E03.1
    congenital (with myxedema) E03.1
  tongue (senile) K14.8
    papillae K14.4
  trachea J39.8
  tunica vaginalis N50.89 ◀▥
  turbinate J34.89
  tympanic membrane (nonflaccid) H73.82-
    flaccid H73.81-
  upper respiratory tract J39.8

Atrophy, atrophic *(Continued)*
  uterus, uterine (senile) N85.8
    cervix N88.8
    due to radiation (intended effect)
      N85.8
      adverse effect or misadventure
        N99.89
  vagina (senile) N95.2
  vas deferens N50.89 ◀▥
  vascular I99.8
  vertebra (senile) —*see* Spondylopathy,
    specified NEC
  vulva (senile) N90.5
  Werdnig-Hoffmann G12.0
  yellow —*see* Failure, hepatic
Attack, attacks
  with alteration of consciousness (with
    automatisms) —*see* Epilepsy,
    localization-related, symptomatic, with
    complex partial seizures
  without alteration of consciousness —
    see Epilepsy, localization-related,
    symptomatic, with simple partial seizures
  Adams-Stokes I45.9
  akinetic —*see* Epilepsy, generalized, specified
    NEC
  angina —*see* Angina
  atonic —*see* Epilepsy, generalized, specified
    NEC
  benign shuddering G25.83
  cataleptic —*see* Catalepsy
  coronary —*see* Infarct, myocardium
  cyanotic, newborn P28.2
  drop NEC R55
  epileptic —*see* Epilepsy
  heart —*see* infarct, myocardium
  hysterical F44.9
  jacksonian —*see* Epilepsy, localization-
    related, symptomatic, with simple
    partial seizures
  myocardium, myocardial —*see* Infarct,
    myocardium
  myoclonic —*see* Epilepsy, generalized,
    specified NEC
  panic F41.0
  psychomotor —*see* Epilepsy, localization-
    related, symptomatic, with complex
    partial seizures
  salaam —*see* Epilepsy, spasms
  schizophreniform, brief F23
  shuddering, benign G25.83
  Stokes-Adams I45.9
  syncope R55
  transient ischemic (TIA) G45.9
    specified NEC G45.8
  unconsciousness R55
    hysterical F44.89
  vasomotor R55
  vasovagal (paroxysmal) (idiopathic) R55
Attention (to)
  artificial
    opening (of) Z43.9
      digestive tract NEC Z43.4
        colon Z43.3
        ilium Z43.2
        stomach Z43.1
      specified NEC Z43.8
      trachea Z43.0
      urinary tract NEC Z43.6
        cystostomy Z43.5
        nephrostomy Z43.6
        ureterostomy Z43.6
        urethrostomy Z43.6
      vagina Z43.7
  colostomy Z43.3
  cystostomy Z43.5
  deficit disorder or syndrome F98.8
    with hyperactivity —*see* Disorder,
      attention-deficit hyperactivity
  gastrostomy Z43.1
  ileostomy Z43.2

◀ New   ◀▥ Revised   ~~deleted~~ Deleted

Attention (Continued)
    jejunostomy Z43.4
    nephrostomy Z43.6
    surgical dressings Z48.01
    sutures Z48.02
    tracheostomy Z43.0
    ureterostomy Z43.6
    urethrostomy Z43.6
Attrition
    gum —*see also* Recession, gingival K06.0 ◄▥
    tooth, teeth (excessive) (hard tissues) K03.0
Atypical, atypism —*see also* condition
    cells (on cytolgocial smear) (endocervical)
        (endometrial) (glandular)
        cervix R87.619
        vagina R87.629
    cervical N87.9
    endometrium N85.9
        hyperplasia N85.00
    parenting situation Z62.9
Auditory —*see* condition
Aujeszky's disease B33.8
Aurantiasis, cutis E67.1
Auricle, auricular —*see also* condition
    cervical Q18.2
Auriculotemporal syndrome G50.8
Austin Flint murmur (aortic insufficiency)
    I35.1
Australian
    Q fever A78
    X disease A83.4
Autism, autistic (childhood) (infantile) F84.0
    atypical F84.9
    spectrum disorder F84.0 ◄
Autodigestion R68.89
Autoerythrocyte sensitization (syndrome)
    D69.2
Autographism L50.3
Autoimmune
    disease (systemic) M35.9
    inhibitors to clotting factors D68.311
    lymphoproliferative syndrome [ALPS]
        D89.82
    thyroiditis E06.3
Autointoxication R68.89
Automatism G93.89
    with temporal sclerosis G93.81
    epileptic —*see* Epilepsy, localization- related,
        symptomatic, with complex partial
        seizures

Automatism (Continued)
    paroxysmal, idiopathic —*see* Epilepsy,
        localization-related, symptomatic, with
        complex partial seizures
Autonomic, autonomous
    bladder (neurogenic) N31.2
    hysteria seizure F44.5
Autosensitivity, erythrocyte D69.2
Autosensitization, cutaneous L30.2
Autosome —*see* condition by chromosome
    involved
Autotopagnosia R48.1
Autotoxemia R68.89
Autumn —*see* condition
Avellis' syndrome G46.8
Aversion
    oral R63.3
        newborn P92.-
        nonorganic origin F98.2
    sexual F52.1
Aviator's
    disease or sickness —*see* Effect, adverse, high
        altitude
    ear T70.0
Avitaminosis (multiple) —*see also* Deficiency,
    vitamin E56.9
    B E53.9
        with
            beriberi E51.11
            pellagra E52
    B2 E53.0
    B6 E53.1
    B12 E53.8
    D E55.9
        with rickets E55.0
    G E53.0
    K E56.1
    nicotinic acid E52
AVNRT (atrioventricular nodal re-entrant
    tachycardia) I47.1
AVRT (atrioventricular nodal re-entrant
    tachycardia) I47.1
Avulsion (traumatic)
    blood vessel —*see* Injury, blood vessel
    bone —*see* Fracture, by site
    cartilage —*see also* Dislocation, by site
        symphyseal (inner), complicating delivery
            O71.6
    external site other than limb —*see* Wound,
        open, by site

Avulsion (Continued)
    eye S05.7-
    head (intracranial)
        external site NEC S08.89
        scalp S08.0
    internal organ or site —*see* Injury, by site
    joint —*see also* Dislocation, by site
        capsule —*see* Sprain, by site
    kidney S37.06-
    ligament —*see* Sprain, by site
    limb —*see also* Amputation, traumatic,
        by site
        skin and subcutaneous tissue —*see* Wound,
            open, by site
    muscle —*see* Injury, muscle
    nerve (root) —*see* Injury, nerve
    scalp S08.0
    skin and subcutaneous tissue —*see* Wound,
        open, by site
    spleen S36.032
    symphyseal cartilage (inner), complicating
        delivery O71.6
    tendon —*see* Injury, muscle
    tooth S03.2
Awareness of heart beat R00.2
Axenfeld's
    anomaly or syndrome Q15.0
    degeneration (calcareous) Q13.4
Axilla, axillary —*see also* condition
    breast Q83.1
Axonotmesis —*see* Injury, nerve
Ayerza's disease or syndrome (pulmonary
    artery sclerosis with pulmonary
    hypertension) I27.0
Azoospermia (organic) N46.01
    due to
        drug therapy N46.021
        efferent duct obstruction N46.023
        infection N46.022
        radiation N46.024
        specified cause NEC N46.029
        systemic disease N46.025
Azotemia R79.89
    meaning uremia N19
Aztec ear Q17.3
Azygos
    continuation inferior vena cava Q26.8
    lobe (lung) Q33.1

B

Baastrup's disease —*see* Kissing spine
Babesiosis B60.0
Babington's disease (familial hemorrhagic telangiectasia) I78.0
Babinski's syndrome A52.79
Baby
  crying constantly R68.11
  floppy (syndrome) P94.2
Bacillary —*see* condition
Bacilluria R82.71 ◀▥
Bacillus —*see also* Infection, bacillus
  abortus infection A23.1
  anthracis infection A22.9
  coli infection —*see also* Escherichia coli B96.20
  Flexner's A03.1
  mallei infection A24.0
  Shiga's A03.0
  suipestifer infection —*see* Infection, salmonella
Back —*see* condition
Backache (postural) M54.9
  sacroiliac M53.3
  specified NEC M54.89
Backflow —*see* Reflux
Backward reading (dyslexia) F81.0
Bacteremia R78.81
  with sepsis —*see* Sepsis
Bactericholia —*see* Cholecystitis, acute
Bacterid, bacteride (pustular) L40.3
Bacterium, bacteria, bacterial
  agent NEC, as cause of disease classified elsewhere B96.89
  in blood —*see* Bacteremia
  in urine —*see* Bacteriuria
Bacteriuria, bacteruria R82.71 ◀▥
  asymptomatic R82.71 ◀▥
Bacteroides
  fragilis, as cause of disease classified elsewhere B96.6
Bad
  heart —*see* Disease, heart
  trip
    due to drug abuse —*see* Abuse, drug, hallucinogen
    due to drug dependence —*see* Dependence, drug, hallucinogen
Baelz's disease (cheilitis glandularis apostematosa) K13.0
Baerensprung's disease (eczema marginatum) B35.6
Bagasse disease or pneumonitis J67.1
Bagassosis J67.1
Baker's cyst —*see* Cyst, Baker's
Bakwin-Krida syndrome (metaphyseal dysplasia) Q78.5
Balancing side interference M26.56
Balanitis (circinata) (erosiva) (gangrenosa) (phagedenic) (vulgaris) N48.1
  amebic A06.82
  candidal B37.42
  due to Haemophilus ducreyi A57
  gonococcal (acute) (chronic) A54.09
  xerotica obliterans N48.0
Balanoposthitis N47.6
  gonococcal (acute) (chronic) A54.09
  ulcerative (specific) A63.8
Balanorrhagia —*see* Balanitis
Balantidiasis, balantidiosis A07.0
Bald tongue K14.4
Baldness —*see also* Alopecia
  male-pattern —*see* Alopecia, androgenic
Balkan grippe A78
Balloon disease —*see* Effect, adverse, high altitude
Balo's disease (concentric sclerosis) G37.5
Bamberger-Marie disease —*see* Osteoarthropathy, hypertrophic, specified type NEC
Bancroft's filariasis B74.0

Band (s)
  adhesive —*see* Adhesions, peritoneum
  anomalous or congenital —*see also* Anomaly, by site
    heart (atrial) (ventricular) Q24.8
    intestine Q43.3
    omentum Q43.3
  cervix N88.1
  constricting, congenital Q79.8
  gallbladder (congenital) Q44.1
  intestinal (adhesive) —*see* Adhesions, peritoneum
  obstructive
    intestine K56.5
    peritoneum K56.5
  periappendiceal, congenital Q43.3
  peritoneal (adhesive) —*see* Adhesions, peritoneum
  uterus N73.6
    internal N85.6
  vagina N89.5
Bandemia D72.825
Bandl's ring (contraction), complicating delivery O62.4
Bangkok hemorrhagic fever A91
Bang's disease (brucella abortus) A23.1
Bankruptcy, anxiety concerning Z59.8
Bannister's disease T78.3
  hereditary D84.1
Banti's disease or syndrome (with cirrhosis) (with portal hypertension) K76.6
Bar, median, prostate —*see* Enlargement, enlarged, prostate
Barcoo disease or rot —*see* Ulcer, skin
Barlow's disease E54
Barodontalgia T70.29
Baron Münchausen syndrome —*see* Disorder, factitious
Barosinusitis T70.1
Barotitis T70.0
Barotrauma T70.29
  odontalgia T70.29
  otitic T70.0
  sinus T70.1
Barraquer (-Simons) disease or syndrome (progressive lipodystrophy) E88.1
Barré-Guillain disease or syndrome G61.0
Barré-Liéou syndrome (posterior cervical sympathetic) M53.0
Barrel chest M95.4
Barrett's
  disease —*see* Barrett's, esophagus
  esophagus K22.70
    with dysplasia K22.719
      high grade K22.711
      low grade K22.710
    without dysplasia K22.70
  syndrome —*see* Barrett's, esophagus
  ulcer K22.10
    with bleeding K22.11
    without bleeding K22.10
Barth syndrome E78.71
Bársony (-Polgár) (-Teschendorf) syndrome (corkscrew esophagus) K22.4
Bartholinitis (suppurating) N75.8
  gonococcal (acute) (chronic) (with abscess) A54.1
Bartonellosis A44.9
  cutaneous A44.1
  mucocutaneous A44.1
  specified NEC A44.8
  systemic A44.0
Barton's fracture S52.56-
Bartter's syndrome E26.81
Basal —*see* condition
Basan's (hidrotic) ectodermal dysplasia Q82.4
Baseball finger —*see* Dislocation, finger
Basedow's disease (exophthalmic goiter) —*see* Hyperthyroidism, with, goiter
Basic —*see* condition
Basilar —*see* condition

Bason's (hidrotic) ectodermal dysplasia Q82.4
Basopenia —*see* Agranulocytosis
Basophilia D72.824
Basophilism (cortico-adrenal) (Cushing's) (pituitary) E24.0
Bassen-Kornzweig disease or syndrome E78.6
Bat ear Q17.5
Bateman's
  disease B08.1
  purpura (senile) D69.2
Bathing cramp T75.1
Bathophobia F40.248
Batten (-Mayou) disease E75.4
  retina E75.4 [H36]
Batten-Steinert syndrome G71.11
Battered —*see* Maltreatment
Battey Mycobacterium infection A31.0
Battle exhaustion F43.0
Battledore placenta O43.19-
Baumgarten-Cruveilhier cirrhosis, disease or syndrome K74.69
Bauxite fibrosis (of lung) J63.1
Bayle's disease (general paresis) A52.17
Bazin's disease (primary) (tuberculous) A18.4
Beach ear —*see* Swimmer's, ear
Beaded hair (congenital) Q84.1
Béal conjunctivitis or syndrome B30.2
Beard's disease (neurasthenia) F48.8
Beat (s)
  atrial, premature I49.1
  ectopic I49.49
  elbow —*see* Bursitis, elbow
  escaped, heart I49.49
  hand —*see* Bursitis, hand
  knee —*see* Bursitis, knee
  premature I49.40
    atrial I49.1
    auricular I49.1
    supraventricular I49.1
Beau's
  disease or syndrome —*see* Degeneration, myocardial
  lines (transverse furrows on fingernails) L60.4
Bechterev's syndrome —*see* Spondylitis, ankylosing
Beck's syndrome (anterior spinal artery occlusion) I65.8
Becker's
  cardiomyopathy I42.8
  disease
    idiopathic mural endomyocardial disease I42.3
    myotonia congenita, recessive form G71.12
  dystrophy G71.0
  pigmented hairy nevus D22.5
Beckwith-Wiedemann syndrome Q87.3
Bed confinement status Z74.01
Bed sore —*see* Ulcer, pressure, by site
Bedbug bite (s) —*see* Bite (s), by site, superficial, insect
Bedclothes, asphyxiation or suffocation by —*see* Asphyxia, traumatic, due to, mechanical, trapped
Bednar's
  aphthae K12.0
  tumor —*see* Neoplasm, malignant, by site
Bedridden Z74.01
Bedsore —*see* Ulcer, pressure, by site
Bedwetting —*see* Enuresis
Bee sting (with allergic or anaphylactic shock) —*see* Toxicity, venom, arthropod, bee
Beer drinker's heart (disease) I42.6
Begbie's disease (exophthalmic goiter) —*see* Hyperthyroidism, with, goiter
Behavior
  antisocial
    adult Z72.811
    child or adolescent Z72.810
  disorder, disturbance —*see* Disorder, conduct
  disruptive —*see* Disorder, conduct

◀ New   ◀▥ Revised   ~~deleted~~ Deleted

Behavior *(Continued)*
drug seeking Z76.5 ◄▥
inexplicable R46.2
marked evasiveness R46.5
obsessive-compulsive R46.81
overactivity R46.3
poor responsiveness R46.4
self-damaging (life-style) Z72.89
sleep-incompatible Z72.821
slowness R46.4
specified NEC R46.89
strange (and inexplicable) R46.2
suspiciousness R46.5
type A pattern Z73.1
undue concern or preoccupation with stressful events R46.6
verbosity and circumstantial detail obscuring reason for contact R46.7
Behcet's disease or syndrome M35.2
Behr's disease —*see* Degeneration, macula
Beigel's disease or morbus (white piedra) B36.2
Bejel A65
Bekhterev's syndrome —*see* Spondylitis, ankylosing
Belching —*see* Eructation
Bell's
mania F30.8
palsy, paralysis G51.0
infant or newborn P11.3
spasm G51.3
Bence Jones albuminuria or proteinuria NEC R80.3
Bends T70.3
Benedikt's paralysis or syndrome G46.3
Benign *(see also* condition)
prostatic hyperplasia —*see* Hyperplasia, prostate
Bennett's fracture (displaced) S62.21-
Benson's disease —*see* Deposit, crystalline
Bent
back (hysterical) F44.4
nose M95.0
congenital Q67.4
Bereavement (uncomplicated) Z63.4
Bergeron's disease (hysterical chorea) F44.4
Berger's disease —*see* Nephropathy, IgA
Beriberi (dry) E51.11
heart (disease) E51.12
polyneuropathy E51.11
wet E51.12
involving circulatory system E51.11
Berlin's disease or edema (traumatic) S05.8X-
Berlock (berloque) dermatitis L56.2
Bernard-Horner syndrome G90.2
Bernard-Soulier disease or thrombopathia D69.1
Bernhardt (-Roth) disease —*see* Mononeuropathy, lower limb, meralgia paresthetica
Bernheim's syndrome —*see* Failure, heart, congestive
Bertielliasis B71.8
Berylliosis (lung) J63.2
Besnier-Boeck (-Schaumann) disease —*see* Sarcoidosis
Besnier's
lupus pernio D86.3
prurigo L20.0
Bestiality F65.89
Best's disease H35.50
Beta-mercaptolactate-cysteine disulfiduria E72.09
Betalipoproteinemia, broad or floating E78.2
Betting and gambling Z72.6
pathological (compulsive) F63.0
Bezoar T18.9
intestine T18.3
stomach T18.2
Bezold's abscess —*see* Mastoiditis, acute
Bianchi's syndrome R48.8

Bicornate or bicornis uterus Q51.3
in pregnancy or childbirth O34.0- ◄▥
causing obstructed labor O65.5
Bicuspid aortic valve Q23.1
Biedl-Bardet syndrome Q87.89
Bielschowsky (-Jansky) disease E75.4
Biermer's (pernicious) anemia or disease D51.0
Biett's disease L93.0
Bifid (congenital)
apex, heart Q24.8
clitoris Q52.6
kidney Q63.8
nose Q30.2
patella Q74.1
scrotum Q55.29
toe NEC Q74.2
tongue Q38.3
ureter Q62.8
uterus Q51.3
uvula Q35.7
Biforis uterus (suprasimplex) Q51.3
Bifurcation (congenital)
gallbladder Q44.1
kidney pelvis Q63.8
renal pelvis Q63.8
rib Q76.6
tongue, congenital Q38.3
trachea Q32.1
ureter Q62.8
urethra Q64.74
vertebra Q76.49
Big spleen syndrome D73.1
Bigeminal pulse R00.8
Bilateral —*see* condition
Bile
duct —*see* condition
pigments in urine R82.2
Bilharziasis —*see also* Schistosomiasis
chyluria B65.0
cutaneous B65.3
galacturia B65.0
hematochyluria B65.0
intestinal B65.1
lipemia B65.9
lipuria B65.0
oriental B65.2
piarhemia B65.9
pulmonary NOS B65.9 *[J99]*
pneumonia B65.9 *[J17]*
tropical hematuria B65.0
vesical B65.0
Biliary —*see* condition
Bilirubin metabolism disorder E80.7
specified NEC E80.6
Bilirubinemia, familial nonhemolytic E80.4
Bilirubinuria R82.2
Biliuria R82.2
Bilocular stomach K31.2
Binswanger's disease I67.3
Biparta, bipartite
carpal scaphoid Q74.0
patella Q74.1
vagina Q52.10
Bird
face Q75.8
fancier's disease or lung J67.2
Birt-Hogg-Dube syndrome Q87.89
Birth
complications in mother —*see* Delivery, complicated
compression during NOS P15.9
defect —*see* Anomaly
immature (less than 37 completed weeks) — *see* Preterm, newborn
extremely (less than 28 completed weeks) —*see* Immaturity, extreme
inattention, at or after —*see* Maltreatment, child, neglect
injury NOS P15.9
basal ganglia P11.1
brachial plexus NEC P14.3

Birth *(Continued)*
injury NOS *(Continued)*
brain (compression) (pressure) P11.2
central nervous system NOS P11.9
cerebellum P11.1
cerebral hemorrhage P10.1
external genitalia P15.5
eye P15.3
face P15.4
fracture
bone P13.9
specified NEC P13.8
clavicle P13.4
femur P13.2
humerus P13.3
long bone, except femur P13.3
radius and ulna P13.3
skull P13.0
spine P11.5
tibia and fibula P13.3
intracranial P11.2
laceration or hemorrhage P10.9
specified NEC P10.8
intraventricular hemorrhage P10.2
laceration
brain P10.1
by scalpel P15.8
peripheral nerve P14.9
liver P15.0
meninges
brain P11.1
spinal cord P11.5
nerve
brachial plexus P14.3
cranial NEC (except facial) P11.4
facial P11.3
peripheral P14.9
phrenic (paralysis) P14.2
paralysis
facial nerve P11.3
spinal P11.5
penis P15.5
rupture
spinal cord P11.5
scalp P12.9
scalpel wound P15.8
scrotum P15.5
skull NEC P13.1
fracture P13.0
specified type NEC P15.8
spinal cord P11.5
spine P11.5
spleen P15.1
sternomastoid (hematoma) P15.2
subarachnoid hemorrhage P10.3
subcutaneous fat necrosis P15.6
subdural hemorrhage P10.0
tentorial tear P10.4
testes P15.5
vulva P15.5
lack of care, at or after —*see* Maltreatment, child, neglect
neglect, at or after —*see* Maltreatment, child, neglect
palsy or paralysis, newborn, NOS (birth injury) P14.9
premature (infant) —*see* Preterm, newborn
shock, newborn P96.89
trauma —*see* Birth, injury
weight
4000 grams to 4499 grams P08.1
4500 grams or more P08.0
low (2499 grams or less) —*see* Low, birthweight
extremely (999 grams or less) —*see* Low, birthweight, extreme
Birthmark Q82.5
Bisalbuminemia E88.09
Biskra's button B55.1

Bite (s) (animal) (human)
  abdomen, abdominal
    wall S31.159
      with penetration into peritoneal cavity
        S31.659
      epigastric region S31.152
        with penetration into peritoneal cavity
          S31.652
      left
        lower quadrant S31.154
          with penetration into peritoneal
            cavity S31.654
        upper quadrant S31.151
          with penetration into peritoneal
            cavity S31.651
      periumbilic region S31.155
        with penetration into peritoneal cavity
          S31.655
      right
        lower quadrant S31.153
          with penetration into peritoneal
            cavity S31.653
        upper quadrant S31.150
          with penetration into peritoneal
            cavity S31.650
      superficial NEC S30.871
        insect S30.861
  alveolar (process) —see Bite, oral cavity
  amphibian (venomous) —see Venom, bite,
    amphibian
  animal —see also Bite, by site
    venomous —see Venom
  ankle S91.05-
    superficial NEC S90.57-
      insect S90.56-
  antecubital space —see Bite, elbow
  anus S31.835
    superficial NEC S30.877
      insect S30.867
  arm (upper) S41.15-
    lower —see Bite, forearm
    superficial NEC S40.87-
      insect S40.86-
  arthropod NEC —see Venom, bite,
    arthropod
  auditory canal (external) (meatus) —
    see Bite, ear
  auricle, ear —see Bite, ear
  axilla —see Bite, arm
  back —see also Bite, thorax, back
    lower S31.050
      with penetration into retroperitoneal
        space S31.051
      superficial NEC S30.870
        insect S30.860
  bedbug —see Bite (s), by site, superficial,
    insect
  breast S21.05-
    superficial NEC S20.17-
      insect S20.16-
  brow —see Bite, head, specified site NEC
  buttock S31.805
    left S31.825
    right S31.815
    superficial NEC S30.870
      insect S30.860
  calf —see Bite, leg
  canaliculus lacrimalis —see Bite, eyelid
  canthus, eye —see Bite, eyelid
  centipede —see Toxicity, venom, arthropod,
    centipede
  cheek (external) S01.45-
    internal —see Bite, oral cavity
    superficial NEC S00.87
      insect S00.86
  chest wall —see Bite, thorax
  chigger B88.0
  chin —see Bite, head, specified site
    NEC
  clitoris —see Bite, vulva
  costal region —see Bite, thorax

Bite (Continued)
  digit (s)
    hand —see Bite, finger
    toe —see Bite, toe
  ear (canal) (external) S01.35-
    superficial NEC S00.47-
      insect S00.46-
  elbow S51.05-
    superficial NEC S50.37-
      insect S50.36-
  epididymis —see Bite, testis
  epigastric region —see Bite, abdomen
  epiglottis —see Bite, neck, specified site
    NEC
  esophagus, cervical S11.25
    superficial NEC S10.17
      insect S10.16
  eyebrow —see Bite, eyelid
  eyelid S01.15-
    superficial NEC S00.27-
      insect S00.26-
  face NEC —see Bite, head, specified site
    NEC
  finger (s) S61.259
    with
      damage to nail S61.359
    index S61.258
      with
        damage to nail S61.358
      left S61.251
        with
          damage to nail S61.351
      right S61.250
        with
          damage to nail S61.350
      superficial NEC S60.478
        insect S60.46-
    little S61.25-
      with
        damage to nail S61.35-
      superficial NEC S60.47-
        insect S60.46-
    middle S61.25-
      with
        damage to nail S61.35-
      superficial NEC S60.47-
        insect S60.46-
    ring S61.25-
      with
        damage to nail S61.35-
      superficial NEC S60.47-
        insect S60.46-
    superficial NEC S60.479
      insect S60.469
    thumb —see Bite, thumb
  flank —see Bite, abdomen, wall
  flea —see Bite, by site, superficial,
    insect
  foot (except toe (s) alone) S91.35-
    superficial NEC S90.87-
      insect S90.86-
    toe —see Bite, toe
  forearm S51.85-
    elbow only —see Bite, elbow
    superficial NEC S50.87-
      insect S50.86-
  forehead —see Bite, head, specified site
    NEC
  genital organs, external
    female S31.552
      superficial NEC S30.876
        insect S30.866
      vagina and vulva —see Bite, vulva
    male S31.551
      penis —see Bite, penis
      scrotum —see Bite, scrotum
      superficial NEC S30.875
        insect S30.865
      testes —see Bite, testis
  groin —see Bite, abdomen, wall
  gum —see Bite, oral cavity

Bite (Continued)
  hand S61.45-
    finger —see Bite, finger
    superficial NEC S60.57-
      insect S60.56-
    thumb —see Bite, thumb
  head S01.95
    cheek —see Bite, cheek
    ear —see Bite, ear
    eyelid —see Bite, eyelid
    lip —see Bite, lip
    nose —see Bite, nose
    oral cavity —see Bite, oral cavity
    scalp —see Bite, scalp
    specified site NEC S01.85
      superficial NEC S00.87
        insect S00.86
    superficial NEC S00.97
      insect S00.96
    temporomandibular area —see Bite, cheek
  heel —see Bite, foot
  hip S71.05-
    superficial NEC S70.27-
      insect S70.26-
  hymen S31.45
  hypochondrium —see Bite, abdomen, wall
  hypogastric region —see Bite, abdomen, wall
  inguinal region —see Bite, abdomen, wall
  insect —see Bite, by site, superficial, insect
  instep —see Bite, foot
  interscapular region —see Bite, thorax, back
  jaw —see Bite, head, specified site NEC
  knee S81.05-
    superficial NEC S80.27-
      insect S80.26-
  labium (majus) (minus) —see Bite, vulva
  lacrimal duct —see Bite, eyelid
  larynx S11.015
    superficial NEC S10.17
      insect S10.16
  leg (lower) S81.85-
    ankle —see Bite, ankle
    foot —see Bite, foot
    knee —see Bite, knee
    superficial NEC S80.87-
      insect S80.86-
    toe —see Bite, toe
    upper —see Bite, thigh
  lip S01.551
    superficial NEC S00.571
      insect S00.561
  lizard (venomous) —see Venom, bite, reptile
  loin —see Bite, abdomen, wall
  lower back —see Bite, back, lower
  lumbar region —see Bite, back, lower
  malar region —see Bite, head, specified site
    NEC
  mammary —see Bite, breast
  marine animals (venomous) —see Toxicity,
    venom, marine animal
  mastoid region —see Bite, head, specified site
    NEC
  mouth —see Bite, oral cavity
  nail
    finger —see Bite, finger
    toe —see Bite, toe
  nape —see Bite, neck, specified site NEC
  nasal (septum) (sinus) —see Bite, nose
  nasopharynx —see Bite, head, specified site
    NEC
  neck S11.95
    involving
      cervical esophagus —see Bite,
        esophagus, cervical
      larynx —see Bite, larynx
      pharynx —see Bite, pharynx
      thyroid gland S11.15
      trachea —see Bite, trachea
    specified site NEC S11.85
      superficial NEC S10.87
        insect S10.86

◀ New   ◀▥ Revised   ~~deleted~~ Deleted

Bite (Continued)
  neck (Continued)
    superficial NEC S10.97
      insect S10.96
    throat S11.85
      superficial NEC S10.17
        insect S10.16
  nose (septum) (sinus) S01.25
    superficial NEC S00.37
      insect S00.36
  occipital region —see Bite, scalp
  oral cavity S01.552
    superficial NEC S00.572
      insect S00.562
  orbital region —see Bite, eyelid
  palate —see Bite, oral cavity
  palm —see Bite, hand
  parietal region —see Bite, scalp
  pelvis S31.050
    with penetration into retroperitoneal space
      S31.051
    superficial NEC S30.870
      insect S30.860
  penis S31.25
    superficial NEC S30.872
      insect S30.862
  perineum
    female —see Bite, vulva
    male —see Bite, pelvis
  periocular area (with or without lacrimal
      passages) —see Bite, eyelid
  phalanges
    finger —see Bite, finger
    toe —see Bite, toe
  pharynx S11.25
    superficial NEC S10.17
      insect S10.16
  pinna —see Bite, ear
  poisonous —see Venom
  popliteal space —see Bite, knee
  prepuce —see Bite, penis
  pubic region —see Bite, abdomen, wall
  rectovaginal septum —see Bite, vulva
  red bug B88.0
  reptile NEC —see also Venom, bite,
      reptile
    nonvenomous —see Bite, by site
    snake —see Venom, bite, snake
  sacral region —see Bite, back, lower
  sacroiliac region —see Bite, back, lower
  salivary gland —see Bite, oral cavity
  scalp S01.05
    superficial NEC S00.07
      insect S00.06
  scapular region —see Bite, shoulder
  scrotum S31.35
    superficial NEC S30.873
      insect S30.863
  sea-snake (venomous) —see Toxicity, venom,
      snake, sea snake
  shin —see Bite, leg
  shoulder S41.05-
    superficial NEC S40.27-
      insect S40.26-
  snake —see also Venom, bite, snake
    nonvenomous —see Bite, by site
  spermatic cord —see Bite, testis
  spider (venomous) —see Toxicity, venom,
      spider
    nonvenomous —see Bite, by site,
      superficial, insect
  sternal region —see Bite, thorax, front
  submaxillary region —see Bite, head,
      specified site NEC
  submental region —see Bite, head, specified
      site NEC
  subungual
    finger (s) —see Bite, finger
    toe —see Bite, toe
  superficial —see Bite, by site, superficial
  supraclavicular fossa S11.85

Bite (Continued)
  supraorbital —see Bite, head, specified site
    NEC
  temple, temporal region —see Bite, head,
      specified site NEC
  temporomandibular area —see Bite, cheek
  testis S31.35
    superficial NEC S30.873
      insect S30.863
  thigh S71.15-
    superficial NEC S70.37-
      insect S70.36-
  thorax, thoracic (wall) S21.95
    back S21.25-
      with penetration into thoracic cavity
        S21.45-
    breast —see Bite, breast
    front S21.15-
      with penetration into thoracic cavity
        S21.35-
    superficial NEC S20.97
      back S20.47-
      front S20.37-
      insect S20.96
        back S20.46-
        front S20.36-
  throat —see Bite, neck, throat
  thumb S61.05-
    with
      damage to nail S61.15-
    superficial NEC S60.37-
      insect S60.36-
  thyroid S11.15
    superficial NEC S10.87
      insect S10.86
  toe (s) S91.15-
    with
      damage to nail S91.25-
    great S91.15-
      with
        damage to nail S91.25-
    lesser S91.15-
      with
        damage to nail S91.25-
    superficial NEC S90.47-
      great S90.47-
      insect S90.46-
        great S90.46-
  tongue S01.552
  trachea S11.025
    superficial NEC S10.17
      insect S10.16
  tunica vaginalis —see Bite, testis
  tympanum, tympanic membrane —see Bite,
      ear
  umbilical region S31.155
  uvula —see Bite, oral cavity
  vagina —see Bite, vulva
  venomous —see Venom
  vocal cords S11.035
    superficial NEC S10.17
      insect S10.16
  vulva S31.45
    superficial NEC S30.874
      insect S30.864
  wrist S61.55-
    superficial NEC S60.87-
      insect S60.86-
Biting, cheek or lip K13.1
Biventricular failure (heart) I50.9
Björck (-Thorson) syndrome (malignant
    carcinoid) E34.0
Black
  death A20.9
  eye S00.1-
  hairy tongue K14.3
  heel (foot) S90.3-
  lung (disease) J60
  palm (hand) S60.22-
Blackfan-Diamond anemia or syndrome
    (congenital hypoplastic anemia) D61.01

Blackhead L70.0
Blackout R55
Bladder —see condition
Blast (air) (hydraulic) (immersion) (underwater)
  blindness S05.8X-
  injury
    abdomen or thorax —see Injury, by site
    ear (acoustic nerve trauma) —see Injury,
      nerve, acoustic, specified type NEC
    syndrome NEC T70.8
Blastoma —see Neoplasm, malignant, by site
  pulmonary —see Neoplasm, lung, malignant
Blastomycosis, blastomycotic B40.9
  Brazilian —see Paracoccidioidomycosis
  cutaneous B40.3
  disseminated B40.7
  European —see Cryptococcosis
  generalized B40.7
  keloidal B48.0
  North American B40.9
  primary pulmonary B40.0
  pulmonary B40.2
    acute B40.0
    chronic B40.1
  skin B40.3
  South American —see Paracoccidioidomycosis
  specified NEC B40.89
Bleb (s) R23.8
  emphysematous (lung) (solitary) J43.9
  endophthalmitis H59.43
  filtering (vitreous), after glaucoma surgery
    Z98.83
  inflamed (infected), postprocedural H59.40
    stage 1 H59.41
    stage 2 H59.42
    stage 3 H59.43
  lung (ruptured) J43.9
    congenital —see Atelectasis
    newborn P25.8
  subpleural (emphysematous) J43.9
Blebitis, postprocedural H59.40
  stage 1 H59.41
  stage 2 H59.42
  stage 3 H59.43
Bleeder (familial) (hereditary) —see Hemophilia
Bleeding —see also Hemorrhage
  anal K62.5
  anovulatory N97.0
  atonic, following delivery O72.1
  capillary I78.8
    puerperal O72.2
  contact (postcoital) N93.0
  due to uterine subinvolution N85.3
  ear —see Otorrhagia
  excessive, associated with menopausal onset
    N92.4
  familial —see Defect, coagulation
  following intercourse N93.0
  gastrointestinal K92.2
  hemorrhoids —see Hemorrhoids
  intermenstrual (regular) N92.3
    irregular N92.1
  intraoperative —see Complication,
    intraoperative, hemorrhage
  irregular N92.6
  menopausal N92.4
  newborn, intraventricular —see
    Newborn, affected by, hemorrhage,
    intraventricular
  nipple N64.59
  nose R04.0
  ovulation N92.3
  postclimacteric N95.0
  postcoital N93.0
  postmenopausal N95.0
  postoperative —see Complication,
    postprocedural, hemorrhage
  preclimacteric N92.4
  pre-pubertal vaginal N93.1 ◄
  puberty (excessive, with onset of menstrual
    periods) N92.2

Bleeding *(Continued)*
  rectum, rectal K62.5
    newborn P54.2
  tendencies —*see* Defect, coagulation
  throat R04.1
  tooth socket (post-extraction) K91.840
  umbilical stump P51.9
  uterus, uterine NEC N93.9
    climacteric N92.4
    dysfunctional of functional N93.8
    menopausal N92.4
    preclimacteric or premenopausal N92.4
    unrelated to menstrual cycle N93.9
  vagina, vaginal (abnormal) N93.9
    dysfunctional or functional N93.8
    newborn P54.6
    pre-pubertal N93.1 ◀
  vicarious N94.89
Blennorrhagia, blennorrhagic —*see* Gonorrhea
Blennorrhea (acute) (chronic) —*see also*
    Gonorrhea
  inclusion (neonatal) (newborn) P39.1
  lower genitourinary tract (gonococcal)
    A54.00
  neonatorum (gonococcal ophthalmia)
    A54.31
Blepharelosis —*see* Entropion
Blepharitis (angularis) (ciliaris) (eyelid)
    (marginal) (nonulcerative) H01.009
  herpes zoster B02.39
  left H01.006
    lower H01.005
    upper H01.004
  right H01.003
    lower H01.002
    upper H01.001
  squamous H01.029
    left H01.026
      lower H01.025
      upper H01.024
    right H01.023
      lower H01.022
      upper H01.021
  ulcerative H01.019
    left H01.016
      lower H01.015
      upper H01.014
    right H01.013
      lower H01.012
      upper H01.011
Blepharochalasis H02.30
  congenital Q10.0
  left H02.36
    lower H02.35
    upper H02.34
  right H02.33
    lower H02.32
    upper H02.31
Blepharoclonus H02.59
Blepharoconjunctivitis H10.50-
  angular H10.52-
  contact H10.53-
  ligneous H10.51-
Blepharophimosis (eyelid) H02.529
  congenital Q10.3
  left H02.526
    lower H02.525
    upper H02.524
  right H02.523
    lower H02.522
    upper H02.521
Blepharoptosis H02.40-
  congenital Q10.0
  mechanical H02.41-
  myogenic H02.42-
  neurogenic H02.43-
  paralytic H02.43-
Blepharopyorrhea, gonococcal A54.39
Blepharospasm G24.5
  drug induced G24.01
Blighted ovum O02.0

Blind —*see also* Blindness
  bronchus (congenital) Q32.4
  loop syndrome K90.2
    congenital Q43.8
  sac, fallopian tube (congenital) Q50.6
  spot, enlarged —*see* Defect, visual field,
    localized, scotoma, blind spot area
  tract or tube, congenital NEC —*see* Atresia,
    by site
Blindness (acquired) (congenital) (both eyes)
    H54.0
  blast S05.8X-
  color —*see* Deficiency, color vision
  concussion S05.8X-
  cortical H47.619
    left brain H47.612
    right brain H47.611
  day H53.11
  due to injury (current episode) S05.9-
    sequelae — code to injury with seventh
      character S
  eclipse (total) —*see* Retinopathy, solar
  emotional (hysterical) F44.6
  face H53.16
  hysterical F44.6
  legal (both eyes) (USA definition) H54.8
  mind R48.8
  night H53.60
    abnormal dark adaptation curve H53.61
    acquired H53.62
    congenital H53.63
    specified type NEC H53.69
    vitamin A deficiency E50.5
  one eye (other eye normal) H54.40
    left (normal vision on right) H54.42
      low vision on right H54.12
    low vision, other eye H54.10
    right (normal vision on left) H54.41
      low vision on left H54.11
  psychic R48.8
  river B73.01
  snow —*see* Photokeratitis
  sun, solar —*see* Retinopathy, solar
  transient —*see* Disturbance, vision, subjective,
    loss, transient
  traumatic (current episode) S05.9-
  word (developmental) F81.0
    acquired R48.0
    secondary to organic lesion R48.0
Blister (nonthermal)
  abdominal wall S30.821
  alveolar process S00.522
  ankle S90.52-
  antecubital space —*see* Blister, elbow
  anus S30.827
  arm (upper) S40.82-
  auditory canal —*see* Blister, ear
  auricle —*see* Blister, ear
  axilla —*see* Blister, arm
  back, lower S30.820
  beetle dermatitis L24.89
  breast S20.12-
  brow S00.82
  calf —*see* Blister, leg
  canthus —*see* Blister, eyelid
  cheek S00.82
    internal S00.522
  chest wall —*see* Blister, thorax
  chin S00.82
  costal region —*see* Blister, thorax
  digit (s)
    foot —*see* Blister, toe
    hand —*see* Blister, finger
  due to burn —*see* Burn, by site, second degree
  ear S00.42-
  elbow S50.32-
  epiglottis S10.12
  esophagus, cervical S10.12
  eyebrow —*see* Blister, eyelid
  eyelid S00.22-
  face S00.82

Blister *(Continued)*
  fever B00.1
  finger (s) S60.429
    index S60.42-
    little S60.42-
    middle S60.42-
    ring S60.42-
  foot (except toe (s) alone) S90.82-
    toe —*see* Blister, toe
  forearm S50.82-
    elbow only —*see* Blister, elbow
  forehead S00.82
  fracture - omit code
  genital organ
    female S30.826
    male S30.825
  gum S00.522
  hand S60.52-
  head S00.92
    ear —*see* Blister, ear
    eyelid —*see* Blister, eyelid
    lip S00.521
    nose S00.32
    oral cavity S00.522
    scalp S00.02
    specified site NEC S00.82
  heel —*see* Blister, foot
  hip S70.22-
  interscapular region S20.429
  jaw S00.82
  knee S80.22-
  larynx S10.12
  leg (lower) S80.82-
    knee —*see* Blister, knee
    upper —*see* Blister, thigh
  lip S00.521
  malar region S00.82
  mammary —*see* Blister, breast
  mastoid region S00.82
  mouth S00.522
  multiple, skin, nontraumatic R23.8
  nail
    finger —*see* Blister, finger
    toe —*see* Blister, toe
  nasal S00.32
  neck S10.92
    specified site NEC S10.82
    throat S10.12
  nose S00.32
  occipital region S00.02
  oral cavity S00.522
  orbital region —*see* Blister, eyelid
  palate S00.522
  palm —*see* Blister, hand
  parietal region S00.02
  pelvis S30.820
  penis S30.822
  periocular area —*see* Blister, eyelid
  phalanges
    finger —*see* Blister, finger
    toe —*see* Blister, toe
  pharynx S10.12
  pinna —*see* Blister, ear
  popliteal space —*see* Blister, knee
  scalp S00.02
  scapular region —*see* Blister, shoulder
  scrotum S30.823
  shin —*see* Blister, leg
  shoulder S40.22-
  sternal region S20.329
  submaxillary region S00.82
  submental region S00.82
  subungual
    finger (s) —*see* Blister, finger
    toe (s) —*see* Blister, toe
  supraclavicular fossa S10.82
  supraorbital S00.82
  temple S00.82
  temporal region S00.82
  testis S30.823
  thermal —*see* Burn, second degree, by site

◀ New   ◀️ Revised   ~~deleted~~ Deleted

Blister (Continued)
 thigh S70.32-
 thorax, thoracic (wall) S20.92
  back S20.42-
  front S20.32-
 throat S10.12
 thumb S60.32-
 toe (s) S90.42-
  great S90.42-
 tongue S00.522
 trachea S10.12
 tympanum, tympanic membrane —see Blister,
  ear
 upper arm —see Blister, arm (upper)
 uvula S00.522
 vagina S30.824
 vocal cords S10.12
 vulva S30.824
 wrist S60.82-
Bloating R14.0
Bloch-Sulzberger disease or syndrome Q82.3
Block, blocked
 alveolocapillary J84.10
 arborization (heart) I45.5
 arrhythmic I45.9
 atrioventricular (incomplete) (partial) I44.30
  with atrioventricular dissociation I44.2
  complete I44.2
   congenital Q24.6
  congenital Q24.6
  first degree I44.0
  second degree (types I and II) I44.1
  specified NEC I44.39
  third degree I44.2
  types I and II I44.1
 auriculoventricular —see Block,
  atrioventricular
 bifascicular (cardiac) I45.2
 bundle-branch (complete) (false) (incomplete)
  I45.4
  bilateral I45.2
  left I44.7
   with right bundle branch block I45.2
   hemiblock I44.60
    anterior I44.4
    posterior I44.5
   incomplete I44.7
    with right bundle branch block I45.2
  right I45.10
   with
    left bundle branch block I45.2
    left fascicular block I45.2
   specified NEC I45.19
  Wilson's type I45.19
 cardiac I45.9
 conduction I45.9
  complete I44.2
 fascicular (left) I44.60
  anterior I44.4
  posterior I44.5
  right I45.0
  specified NEC I44.69
 foramen Magendie (acquired) G91.1
  congenital Q03.1
   with spina bifida —see Spina bifida, by
    site, with hydrocephalus
 heart I45.9
  bundle branch I45.4
   bilateral I45.2
  complete (atrioventricular) I44.2
  congenital Q24.6
  first degree (atrioventricular) I44.0
  second degree (atrioventricular) I44.1
  specified type NEC I45.5
  third degree (atrioventricular) I44.2
 hepatic vein I82.0
 intraventricular (nonspecific) I45.4
  bundle branch
   bilateral I45.2
 kidney N28.9
  postcystoscopic or postprocedural N99.0

Block, blocked (Continued)
 Mobitz (types I and II) I44.1
 myocardial —see Block, heart
 nodal I45.5
 organ or site, congenital NEC —see Atresia,
  by site
 portal (vein) I81
 second degree (types I and II) I44.1
 sinoatrial I45.5
 sinoauricular I45.5
 third degree I44.2
 trifascicular I45.3
 tubal N97.1
 vein NOS I82.90
 Wenckebach (types I and II) I44.1
Blockage —see Obstruction
Blocq's disease F44.4
Blood
 constituents, abnormal R78.9
 disease D75.9
 donor —see Donor, blood
 dyscrasia D75.9
  with
   abortion —see Abortion, by type,
    complicated by, hemorrhage
   ectopic pregnancy O08.1
   molar pregnancy O08.1
  following ectopic or molar pregnancy
   O08.1
  newborn P61.9
  puerperal, postpartum O72.3
 flukes NEC —see Schistosomiasis
 in
  feces K92.1
   occult R19.5
  urine —see Hematuria
 mole O02.0
 occult in feces R19.5
 pressure
  decreased, due to shock following injury
   T79.4
  examination only Z01.30
  fluctuating I99.8
  high —see Hypertension
   borderline R03.0
   incidental reading, without diagnosis of
    hypertension R03.0
  low —see also Hypotension
   incidental reading, without diagnosis of
    hypotension R03.1
 spitting —see Hemoptysis
 staining cornea —see Pigmentation, cornea,
  stromal
 transfusion
  reaction or complication —see
   Complications, transfusion
  type
   A (Rh positive) Z67.10
    Rh negative Z67.11
   AB (Rh positive) Z67.30
    Rh negative Z67.31
   B (Rh positive) Z67.20
    Rh negative Z67.21
   O (Rh positive) Z67.40
    Rh negative Z67.41
   Rh (positive) Z67.90
    negative Z67.91
 vessel rupture —see Hemorrhage
 vomiting —see Hematemesis
Blood-forming organs, disease D75.9
Bloodgood's disease —see Mastopathy,
 cystic
Bloom (-Machacek)(-Torre) syndrome
 Q82.8
Blount's disease or osteochondrosis —see
 Osteochondrosis, juvenile, tibia
Blue
 baby Q24.9
 diaper syndrome E72.09
 dome cyst (breast) —see Cyst, breast
 dot cataract Q12.0

Blue (Continued)
 nevus D22.9
 sclera Q13.5
  with fragility of bone and deafness Q78.0
 toe syndrome I75.02-
Blueness —see Cyanosis
Blues, postpartal O90.6
 baby O90.6
Blurring, visual H53.8
Blushing (abnormal) (excessive) R23.2
BMI —see Body, mass index
Boarder, hospital NEC Z76.4
 accompanying sick person Z76.3
 healthy infant or child Z76.2
 foundling Z76.1
Bockhart's impetigo L01.02
Bodechtel-Guttman disease (subacute
 sclerosing panencephalitis) A81.1
Boder-Sedgwick syndrome (ataxia-
 telangiectasia) G11.3
Body, bodies
 Aschoff's —see Myocarditis, rheumatic
 asteroid, vitreous —see Deposit, crystalline
 cytoid (retina) —see Occlusion, artery, retina
 drusen (degenerative) (macula) (retinal) —see
  also Degeneration, macula, drusen
  optic disc —see Drusen, optic disc
 foreign —see Foreign body
 loose
  joint, except knee —see Loose, body, joint
   knee M23.4-
  sheath, tendon —see Disorder, tendon,
   specified type NEC
 mass index (BMI)
  adult
   19 or less Z68.1
   20.0-20.9 Z68.20
   21.0-21.9 Z68.21
   22.0-22.9 Z68.22
   23.0-23.9 Z68.23
   24.0-24.9 Z68.24
   25.0-25.9 Z68.25
   26.0-26.9 Z68.26
   27.0-27.9 Z68.27
   28.0-28.9 Z68.28
   29.0-29.9 Z68.29
   30.0-30.9 Z68.30
   31.0-31.9 Z68.31
   32.0-32.9 Z68.32
   33.0-33.9 Z68.33
   34.0-34.9 Z68.34
   35.0-35.9 Z68.35
   36.0-36.9 Z68.36
   37.0-37.9 Z68.37
   38.0-38.9 Z68.38
   39.0-39.9 Z68.39
   40.0-44.9 Z68.41
   45.0-49.9 Z68.42
   50.0-59.9 Z68.43
   60.0-69.9 Z68.44
   70 and over Z68.45
  pediatric
   5th percentile to less than 85th percentile
    for age Z68.52
   85th percentile to less than 95th
    percentile for age Z68.53
   greater than or equal to ninety-fifth
    percentile for age Z68.54
   less than fifth percentile for age Z68.51
 Mooser's A75.2
 rice —see also Loose, body, joint
  knee M23.4-
 rocking F98.4
Boeck's
 disease or sarcoid —see Sarcoidosis
 lupoid (miliary) D86.3
Boerhaave's syndrome (spontaneous
 esophageal rupture) K22.3
Boggy
 cervix N88.8
 uterus N85.8

Boil —see also Furuncle, by site
  Aleppo B55.1
  Baghdad B55.1
  Delhi B55.1
  lacrimal
    gland —see Dacryoadenitis
    passages (duct) (sac) —see Inflammation,
      lacrimal, passages, acute
  Natal B55.1
  orbit, orbital —see Abscess, orbit
  tropical B55.1
Bold hives —see Urticaria
Bombé, iris —see Membrane, pupillary
Bone —see condition
Bonnevie-Ullrich syndrome —see also Turner's
  syndrome Q87.1 ◀▥
Bonnier's syndrome —see subcategory H81.8
Bonvale dam fever T73.3
Bony block of joint —see Ankylosis
BOOP (bronchiolitis obliterans organized
  pneumonia) J84.89
Borderline
  diabetes mellitus R73.03 ◀▥
  hypertension R03.0
  osteopenia M85.8-
  pelvis, with obstruction during labor O65.1
  personality F60.3
Borna disease A83.9
Bornholm disease B33.0
Boston exanthem A88.0
Botalli, ductus (patent) (persistent) Q25.0
Bothriocephalus latus infestation B70.0
Botulism (foodborne intoxication) A05.1
  infant A48.51
  non-foodborne A48.52
  wound A48.52
Bouba —see Yaws
Bouchard's nodes (with arthropathy) M15.2
Bouffée délirante F23
Bouillaud's disease or syndrome (rheumatic
  heart disease) I01.9
Bourneville's disease Q85.1
Boutonniere deformity (finger) —see
  Deformity, finger, boutonniere
Bouveret (-Hoffmann) syndrome (paroxysmal
  tachycardia) I47.9
Bovine heart —see Hypertrophy, cardiac
Bowel —see condition
Bowen's
  dermatosis (precancerous) —see Neoplasm,
    skin, in situ
  disease —see Neoplasm, skin, in situ
  epithelioma —see Neoplasm, skin, in situ
  type
    epidermoid carcinoma-in-situ —see
      Neoplasm, skin, in situ
    intraepidermal squamous cell carcinoma —
      see Neoplasm, skin, in situ
Bowing
  femur —see also Deformity, limb, specified
    type NEC, thigh
    congenital Q68.3
  fibula —see also Deformity, limb, specified
    type NEC, lower leg
    congenital Q68.4
  forearm —see Deformity, limb, specified type
    NEC, forearm
  leg (s), long bones, congenital Q68.5
  radius —see Deformity, limb, specified type
    NEC, forearm
  tibia —see also Deformity, limb, specified type
    NEC, lower leg
    congenital Q68.4
Bowleg (s) (acquired) M21.16-
  congenital Q68.5
  rachitic E64.3
Boyd's dysentery A03.2
Brachial —see condition
Brachycardia R00.1
Brachycephaly Q75.0
Bradley's disease A08.19

Bradyarrhythmia, cardiac I49.8
Bradycardia (sinoatrial) (sinus) (vagal) R00.1
  neonatal P29.12
  reflex G90.09
  tachycardia syndrome I49.5
Bradykinesia R25.8
Bradypnea R06.89
Bradytachycardia I49.5
Brailsford's disease or osteochondrosis —see
  Osteochondrosis, juvenile, radius
Brain —see also condition
  death G93.82
  syndrome —see Syndrome, brain
Branched-chain amino-acid disorder E71.2
Branchial —see condition
  cartilage, congenital Q18.2
Branchiogenic remnant (in neck) Q18.0
Brandt's syndrome (acrodermatitis
  enteropathica) E83.2
Brash (water) R12
Bravais-jacksonian epilepsy —see Epilepsy,
  localization-related, symptomatic, with
  simple partial seizures
Braxton Hicks contractions —see False, labor
Brazilian leishmaniasis B55.2
BRBPR K62.5
Break, retina (without detachment) H33.30-
  with retinal detachment —see Detachment,
    retina
  horseshoe tear H33.31-
  multiple H33.33-
  round hole H33.32-
Breakdown
  device, graft or implant —see also
    Complications, by site and type,
    mechanical T85.618
    arterial graft NEC —see Complication,
      cardiovascular device, mechanical,
      vascular
    breast (implant) T85.41
    catheter NEC T85.618
      cystostomy T83.010
      dialysis (renal) T82.41
        intraperitoneal T85.611
      Hopkins T83.018 ◀
      ileostomy T83.018 ◀
      infusion NEC T82.514
        cranial T85.610 ◀
        epidural T85.610 ◀
        intrathecal T85.610 ◀
        spinal T85.610 ◀▥
        subarachnoid T85.610 ◀
        subdural T85.610 ◀
      urinary (indwelling) T83.018
      nephrostomy T83.012 ◀
      urethral indwelling T83.011 ◀
      urinary NEC T83.018 ◀
      urostomy T83.018 ◀
    electronic (electrode) (pulse generator)
      (stimulator)
      bone T84.310
      cardiac T82.119
        electrode T82.110
        pulse generator T82.111
        specified type NEC T82.118
      nervous system —see Complication,
        prosthetic device, mechanical,
        electronic nervous system stimulator
      urinary —see Complication,
        genitourinary, device, urinary,
        mechanical
    fixation, internal (orthopedic) NEC —see
      Complication, fixation device,
      mechanical
    gastrointestinal —see Complications,
      prosthetic device, mechanical,
      gastrointestinal device
    genital NEC T83.418
      intrauterine contraceptive device T83.31
      penile prosthesis (cylinder) (implanted)
        (pump) (resevoir) T83.410 ◀▥
      testicular prosthesis T83.411 ◀

Breakdown (Continued)
  device, graft or implant (Continued)
    heart NEC —see Complication,
      cardiovascular device, mechanical
    intrathecal infusion pump T85.615 ◀
    joint prosthesis —see Complications...,
      joint prosthesis, internal, mechanical,
      by site
    nervous system, specified device NEC
      T85.615 ◀
    ocular NEC —see Complications, prosthetic
      device, mechanical, ocular device
    orthopedic NEC —see Complication,
      orthopedic, device, mechanical
    specified NEC T85.618
    subcutaneous device pocket ◀
      nervous system prosthetic device,
        implant, or graft T85.890 ◀
      other internal prosthetic device, implant,
        or graft T85.898 ◀
    sutures, permanent T85.612
      used in bone repair —see Complications,
        fixation device, internal
        (orthopedic), mechanical
    urinary NEC T83.118 ◀▥
      graft T83.21
      sphincter, implanted T83.111 ◀
      stent (ileal conduit) (nephroureteral)
        T83.113 ◀
      ureteral indwelling T83.112 ◀
    vascular NEC —see Complication,
      cardiovascular device, mechanical
    ventricular intracranial shunt T85.01
  nervous F48.8
  perineum O90.1
  respirator J95.850
    specified NEC J95.859
  ventilator J95.850
    specified NEC J95.859
Breast —see also condition
  buds E30.1
    in newborn P96.89
  dense R92.2
  nodule N63
Breath
  foul R19.6
  holder, child R06.89
  holding spell R06.89
  shortness R06.02
Breathing
  labored —see Hyperventilation
  mouth R06.5
    causing malocclusion M26.5
  periodic R06.3
    high altitude G47.32
Breathlessness R06.81
Breda's disease —see Yaws
Breech presentation (mother) O32.1
  causing obstructed labor O64.1
  footling O32.8
    causing obstructed labor O64.8
  incomplete O32.8
    causing obstructed labor O64.8
Breisky's disease N90.4
Brennemann's syndrome I88.0
Brenner
  tumor (benign) D27.9
    borderline malignancy D39.1-
    malignant C56
    proliferating D39.1
Bretonneau's disease or angina A36.0
Breus' mole O02.0
Brevicollis Q76.49
Brickmakers' anemia B76.9 [D63.8]
Bridge, myocardial Q24.5
Bright red blood per rectum (BRBPR) K62.5
Bright's disease —see also Nephritis
  arteriosclerotic —see Hypertension, kidney
Brill (-Zinsser) disease (recrudescent typhus)
  A75.1
  flea-borne A75.2
  louse-borne A75.1

◀ New   ◀▥ Revised   ~~deleted~~ Deleted

Brill-Symmers' disease C82.90
Brion-Kayser disease —see Fever, parathyroid
Briquet's disorder or syndrome F45.0
Brissaud's
    infantilism or dwarfism E23.0
    motor-verbal tic F95.2
Brittle
    bones disease Q78.0
    nails L60.3
        congenital Q84.6
Broad —see also condition
    beta disease E78.2
    ligament laceration syndrome N83.8
Broad- or floating-betalipoproteinemia E78.2
Brock's syndrome (atelectasis due to enlarged
    lymph nodes) J98.19
Brocq-Duhring disease (dermatitis
    herpetiformis) L13.0
Brodie's abscess or disease M86.8X-
Broken
    arches —see also Deformity, limb, flat foot
    arm (meaning upper limb) —see Fracture, arm
    back —see Fracture, vertebra
    bone —see Fracture
    implant or internal device —see
        Complications, by site and type,
        mechanical
    leg (meaning lower limb) —see Fracture, leg
    nose S02.2
    tooth, teeth —see Fracture, tooth
Bromhidrosis, bromidrosis L75.0
Bromidism, bromism G92
    chronic (dependence) F13.20
    due to
        correct substance properly administered —
            see Table of Drugs and Chemicals, by
            drug, adverse effect
        overdose or wrong substance given or
            taken —see Table of Drugs and
            Chemicals, by drug, poisoning
Bromidrosiphobia F40.298
Bronchi, bronchial —see condition
Bronchiectasis (cylindrical) (diffuse) (fusiform)
    (localized) (saccular) J47.9
    with
        acute
            bronchitis J47.0
            lower respiratory infection J47.0
        exacerbation (acute) J47.1
    congenital Q33.4
    tuberculous NEC —see Tuberculosis,
        pulmonary
Bronchiolectasis —see Bronchiectasis
Bronchiolitis (acute) (infective) (subacute) J21.9
    with
        bronchospasm or obstruction J21.9
        influenza, flu or grippe —see Influenza,
            with, respiratory manifestations NEC
    chemical (chronic) J68.4
        acute J68.0
    chronic (fibrosing) (obliterative) J44.9
    due to
        external agent —see Bronchitis, acute, due to
        human metapneumovirus J21.1
        respiratory syncytial virus J21.0
        specified organism NEC J21.8
    fibrosa obliterans J44.9
    influenzal —see Influenza, with, respiratory
        manifestations NEC
    obliterans J42
        with organizing pneumonia (BOOP) J84.89
    obliterative (chronic) (subacute) J44.9
        due to chemicals, gases, fumes or vapors
            (inhalation) J68.4
        due to fumes or vapors J68.4
    respiratory, interstitial lung disease J84.115
Bronchitis (diffuse) (fibrinous) (hypostatic)
    (infective) (membranous) J40
    with
        influenza, flu or grippe —see Influenza,
            with, respiratory manifestations NEC

Bronchitis (Continued)
    with (Continued)
        obstruction (airway) (lung) J44.9
        tracheitis (15 years of age and above) J40
            acute or subacute J20.9
            chronic J42
            under 15 years of age J20.9
    acute or subacute (with bronchospasm or
        obstruction) J20.9
        with
            bronchiectasis J47.0
            chronic obstructive pulmonary disease
                J44.0
        chemical (due to gases, fumes or vapors)
            J68.0
        due to
            fumes or vapors J68.0
            Haemophilus influenzae J20.1
            Mycoplasma pneumoniae J20.0
            radiation J70.0
            specified organism NEC J20.8
            Streptococcus J20.2
            virus
                coxsackie J20.3
                echovirus J20.7
                parainfluenzae J20.4
                respiratory syncytial J20.5
                rhinovirus J20.6
            viral NEC J20.8
    allergic (acute) J45.909
        with
            exacerbation (acute) J45.901
            status asthmaticus J45.902
    arachidic T17.528
    aspiration (due to fumes or vapors) J68.0
    asthmatic J45.9
        chronic J44.9
            with
                acute lower respiratory infection J44.0
                exacerbation (acute) J44.1
    capillary —see Pneumonia, broncho
    caseous (tuberculous) A15.5
    Castellani's A69.8
    catarrhal (15 years of age and above) J40
        acute —see Bronchitis, acute
        chronic J41.0
        under 15 years of age J20.9
    chemical (acute) (subacute) J68.0
        chronic J68.4
        due to fumes or vapors J68.0
            chronic J68.4
    chronic J42
        with
            airways obstruction J44.9
            tracheitis (chronic) J42
        asthmatic (obstructive) J44.9
        catarrhal J41.0
        chemical (due to fumes or vapors) J68.4
        due to
            chemicals, gases, fumes or vapors
                (inhalation) J68.4
            radiation J70.1
            tobacco smoking J41.0
        emphysematous J44.9
        mucopurulent J41.1
        non-obstructive J41.0
        obliterans J44.9
        obstructive J44.9
        purulent J41.1
        simple J41.0
    croupous —see Bronchitis, acute
    due to gases, fumes or vapors (chemical)
        J68.0
    emphysematous (obstructive) J44.9
    exudative —see Bronchitis, acute
    fetid J41.1
    grippal —see Influenza, with, respiratory
        manifestations NEC
    in those under 15 years age —see Bronchitis,
        acute
    chronic —see Bronchitis, chronic

Bronchitis (Continued)
    influenzal —see Influenza, with, respiratory
        manifestations NEC
    mixed simple and mucopurulent J41.8
    moulder's J62.8
    mucopurulent (chronic) (recurrent) J41.1
        acute or subacute J20.9
        simple (mixed) J41.8
    obliterans (chronic) J44.9
    obstructive (chronic) (diffuse) J44.9
    pituitous J41.1
    pneumococcal, acute or subacute J20.2
    pseudomembranous, acute or subacute —see
        Bronchitis, acute
    purulent (chronic) (recurrent) J41.1
        acute or subacute —see Bronchitis, acute
    putrid J41.1
    senile (chronic) J42
    simple and mucopurulent (mixed) J41.8
    smokers' J41.0
    spirochetal NEC A69.8
    subacute —see Bronchitis, acute
    suppurative (chronic) J41.1
        acute or subacute —see Bronchitis, acute
    tuberculous A15.5
    under 15 years of age —see Bronchitis, acute
        chronic —see Bronchitis, chronic
    viral NEC, acute or subacute —see also
        Bronchitis, acute J20.8
Bronchoalveolitis J18.0
Bronchoaspergillosis B44.1
Bronchocele meaning goiter E04.0
Broncholithiasis J98.09
    tuberculous NEC A15.5
Bronchomalacia J98.09
    congenital Q32.2
Bronchomycosis NOS B49 [J99]
    candidal B37.1
Bronchopleuropneumonia —see Pneumonia,
    broncho
Bronchopneumonia —see Pneumonia, broncho
Bronchopneumonitis —see Pneumonia,
    broncho
Bronchopulmonary —see condition
Bronchopulmonitis —see Pneumonia, broncho
Bronchorrhagia (see Hemoptysis)
Bronchorrhea J98.09
    acute J20.9
    chronic (infective) (purulent) J42
Bronchospasm (acute) J98.01
    with
        bronchiolitis, acute J21.9
        bronchitis, acute (conditions in J20) —see
            Bronchitis, acute
    due to external agent —see condition,
        respiratory, acute, due to
    exercise induced J45.990
Bronchospirochetosis A69.8
    Castellani A69.8
Bronchostenosis J98.09
Bronchus —see condition
Brontophobia F40.220
Bronze baby syndrome P83.8
Brooke's tumor —see Neoplasm, skin, benign
Brown enamel of teeth (hereditary) K00.5
Brown's sheath syndrome H50.61-
Brown-Séquard disease, paralysis or
    syndrome G83.81
Bruce sepsis A23.0
Brucellosis (infection) A23.9
    abortus A23.1
    canis A23.3
    dermatitis A23.9
    melitensis A23.0
    mixed A23.8
    sepsis A23.9
        melitensis A23.0
        specified NEC A23.8
    suis A23.2
Bruck-de Lange disease Q87.1
Bruck's disease —see Deformity, limb

Brugsch's syndrome Q82.8
Bruise (skin surface intact) —*see also* Contusion
  with
     open wound —*see* Wound, open
   internal organ —*see* Injury, by site
   newborn P54.5
   scalp, due to birth injury, newborn P12.3
   umbilical cord O69.5
Bruit (arterial) R09.89
   cardiac R01.1
Brush burn —*see* Abrasion, by site
Bruton's X-linked agammaglobulinemia D80.0
Bruxism
   psychogenic F45.8
   sleep related G47.63
Bubbly lung syndrome P27.0
Bubo I88.8
   blennorrhagic (gonococcal) A54.89
   chancroidal A57
   climatic A55
   due to Haemophilus ducreyi A57
   gonococcal A54.89
   indolent (nonspecific) I88.8
   inguinal (nonspecific) I88.8
     chancroidal A57
     climatic A55
     due to H. ducreyi A57
     infective I88.8
   scrofulous (tuberculous) A18.2
   soft chancre A57
   suppurating —*see* Lymphadenitis, acute
   syphilitic (primary) A51.0
     congenital A50.07
   tropical A55
   virulent (chancroidal) A57
Bubonic plague A20.0
Bubonocele —*see* Hernia, inguinal
Buccal —*see* condition
Buchanan's disease or osteochondrosis M91.0
Buchem's syndrome (hyperostosis corticalis)
   M85.2
Bucket-handle fracture or tear (semilunar
   cartilage) —*see* Tear, meniscus
Budd-Chiari syndrome (hepatic vein
   thrombosis) I82.0
Budgerigar fancier's disease or lung
   J67.2
Buds
   breast E30.1
     in newborn P96.89
Buerger's disease (thromboangiitis obliterans)
   I73.1
Bulbar —*see* condition
Bulbus cordis (left ventricle) (persistent)
   Q21.8
Bulimia (nervosa) F50.2
   atypical F50.9
   normal weight F50.9
Bulky
   stools R19.5
   uterus N85.2
Bulla (e) R23.8
   lung (emphysematous) (solitary) J43.9
     newborn P25.8
Bullet wound —*see also* Wound, open
   fracture - code as Fracture, by site
   internal organ —*see* Injury, by site
Bundle
   branch block (complete) (false)
     (incomplete) —*see* Block, bundle-branch
   of His —*see* condition
Bunion M21.61- ◀▥
   tailor's M21.62- ◀
Bunionette M21.62- ◀
Buphthalmia, buphthalmos (congenital) Q15.0
Burdwan fever B55.0
Bürger-Grütz disease or syndrome E78.3
Buried
   penis (congenital) Q55.64
     acquired N48.83
   roots K08.3

Burke's syndrome K86.89 ◀▥
Burkitt
   cell leukemia C91.0-
   lymphoma (malignant) C83.7-
     small noncleaved, diffuse C83.7-
     spleen C83.77
     undifferentiated C83.7-
   tumor C83.7-
   type
     acute lymphoblastic leukemia C91.0-
     undifferentiated C83.7-
Burn (electricity) (flame) (hot gas, liquid or hot
   object) (radiation) (steam) (thermal) T30.0
   abdomen, abdominal (muscle) (wall)
     T21.02
     first degree T21.12
     second degree T21.22
     third degree T21.32
   above elbow T22.039
     first degree T22.139
     left T22.032
       first degree T22.132
       second degree T22.232
       third degree T22.332
     right T22.031
       first degree T22.131
       second degree T22.231
       third degree T22.331
     second degree T22.239
     third degree T22.339
   acid (caustic) (external) (internal) —*see*
     Corrosion, by site
   alimentary tract NEC T28.2
     esophagus T28.1
     mouth T28.0
     pharynx T28.0
   alkaline (caustic) (external) (internal) —*see*
     Corrosion, by site
   ankle T25.019
     first degree T25.119
     left T25.012
       first degree T25.112
       second degree T25.212
       third degree T25.312
       multiple with foot —*see* Burn, lower, limb,
         multiple, ankle and foot
     right T25.011
       first degree T25.111
       second degree T25.211
       third degree T25.311
     second degree T25.219
     third degree T25.319
   anus —*see* Burn, buttock
   arm (lower) (upper) —*see* Burn, upper,
     limb
   axilla T22.049
     first degree T22.149
     left T22.042
       first degree T22.142
       second degree T22.242
       third degree T22.342
     right T22.041
       first degree T22.141
       second degree T22.241
       third degree T22.341
     second degree T22.249
     third degree T22.349
   back (lower) T21.04
     first degree T21.14
     second degree T21.24
     third degree T21.34
     upper T21.03
       first degree T21.13
       second degree T21.23
       third degree T21.33
   blisters - code as Burn, second degree, by site
   breast (s) —*see* Burn, chest wall
   buttock (s) T21.05
     first degree T21.15
     second degree T21.25
     third degree T21.35

Burn (*Continued*)
   calf T24.039
     first degree T24.139
     left T24.032
       first degree T24.132
       second degree T24.232
       third degree T24.332
     right T24.031
       first degree T24.131
       second degree T24.231
       third degree T24.331
     second degree T24.239
     third degree T24.339
   canthus (eye) —*see* Burn, eyelid
   caustic acid or alkaline —*see* Corrosion, by
     site
   cervix T28.3
   cheek T20.06
     first degree T20.16
     second degree T20.26
     third degree T20.36
   chemical (acids) (alkalines) (caustics) (external)
     (internal) —*see* Corrosion, by site
   chest wall T21.01
     first degree T21.11
     second degree T21.21
     third degree T21.31
   chin T20.03
     first degree T20.13
     second degree T20.23
     third degree T20.33
   colon T28.2
   conjunctiva (and cornea) —*see* Burn, cornea
   cornea (and conjunctiva) T26.1-
     chemical —*see* Corrosion, cornea
   corrosion (external) (internal) —*see*
     Corrosion, by site
   deep necrosis of underlying tissue - code as
     Burn, third degree, by site
   dorsum of hand T23.069
     first degree T23.169
     left T23.062
       first degree T23.162
       second degree T23.262
       third degree T23.362
     right T23.061
       first degree T23.161
       second degree T23.261
       third degree T23.361
     second degree T23.269
     third degree T23.369
   due to ingested chemical agent —*see*
     Corrosion, by site
   ear (auricle) (external) (canal) T20.01
     first degree T20.11
     second degree T20.21
     third degree T20.31
   elbow T22.029
     first degree T22.129
     left T22.022
       first degree T22.122
       second degree T22.222
       third degree T22.322
     right T22.021
       first degree T22.121
       second degree T22.221
       third degree T22.321
     second degree T22.229
     third degree T22.329
   epidermal loss - code as Burn, second degree,
     by site
   erythema, erythematous - code as Burn, first
     degree, by site
   esophagus T28.1
   extent (percentage of body surface)
     less than 10 percent T31.0
     10-19 percent T31.10
       with 0-9 percent third degree burns
         T31.10
       with 10-19 percent third degree burns
         T31.11

◀ New   ▥ Revised   ~~deleted~~ Deleted

Burn *(Continued)*
 extent *(Continued)*
  20-29 percent T31.20
   with 0-9 percent third degree burns T31.20
   with 10-19 percent third degree burns T31.21
   with 20-29 percent third degree burns T31.22
  30-39 percent T31.30
   with 0-9 percent third degree burns T31.30
   with 10-19 percent third degree burns T31.31
   with 20-29 percent third degree burns T31.32
   with 30-39 percent third degree burns T31.33
  40-49 percent T31.40
   with 0-9 percent third degree burns T31.40
   with 10-19 percent third degree burns T31.41
   with 20-29 percent third degree burns T31.42
   with 30-39 percent third degree burns T31.43
   with 40-49 percent third degree burns T31.44
  50-59 percent T31.50
   with 0-9 percent third degree burns T31.50
   with 10-19 percent third degree burns T31.51
   with 20-29 percent third degree burns T31.52
   with 30-39 percent third degree burns T31.53
   with 40-49 percent third degree burns T31.54
   with 50-59 percent third degree burns T31.55
  60-69 percent T31.60
   with 0-9 percent third degree burns T31.60
   with 10-19 percent third degree burns T31.61
   with 20-29 percent third degree burns T31.62
   with 30-39 percent third degree burns T31.63
   with 40-49 percent third degree burns T31.64
   with 50-59 percent third degree burns T31.65
   with 60-69 percent third degree burns T31.66
  70-79 percent T31.70
   with 0-9 percent third degree burns T31.70
   with 10-19 percent third degree burns T31.71
   with 20-29 percent third degree burns T31.72
   with 30-39 percent third degree burns T31.73
   with 40-49 percent third degree burns T31.74
   with 50-59 percent third degree burns T31.75
   with 60-69 percent third degree burns T31.76
   with 70-79 percent third degree burns T31.77
  80-89 percent T31.80
   with 0-9 percent third degree burns T31.80
   with 10-19 percent third degree burns T31.81
   with 20-29 percent third degree burns T31.82
   with 30-39 percent third degree burns T31.83
   with 40-49 percent third degree burns T31.84

Burn *(Continued)*
 extent *(Continued)*
  80-89 percent T31.80 *(Continued)*
   with 50-59 percent third degree burns T31.85
   with 60-69 percent third degree burns T31.86
   with 70-79 percent third degree burns T31.87
   with 80-89 percent third degree burns T31.88
  90 percent or more T31.90
   with 0-9 percent third degree burns T31.90
   with 10-19 percent third degree burns T31.91
   with 20-29 percent third degree burns T31.92
   with 30-39 percent third degree burns T31.93
   with 40-49 percent third degree burns T31.94
   with 50-59 percent third degree burns T31.95
   with 60-69 percent third degree burns T31.96
   with 70-79 percent third degree burns T31.97
   with 80-89 percent third degree burns T31.98
   with 90 percent or more third degree burns T31.99
 extremity —*see* Burn, limb
 eye (s) and adnexa T26.4-
  with resulting rupture and destruction of eyeball T26.2-
  conjunctival sac —*see* Burn, cornea
  cornea —*see* Burn, cornea
  lid —*see* Burn, eyelid
  periocular area —*see* Burn, eyelid
  specified site NEC T26.3-
 eyeball —*see* Burn, eye
 eyelid (s) T26.0-
  chemical —*see* Corrosion, eyelid
 face —*see* Burn, head
 finger T23.029
  first degree T23.129
  left T23.022
   first degree T23.122
   second degree T23.222
   third degree T23.322
  multiple sites (without thumb) T23.039
   with thumb T23.049
    first degree T23.149
    left T23.042
     first degree T23.142
     second degree T23.242
     third degree T23.342
    right T23.041
     first degree T23.141
     second degree T23.241
     third degree T23.341
    second degree T23.249
    third degree T23.349
   first degree T23.139
   left T23.032
    first degree T23.132
    second degree T23.232
    third degree T23.332
   right T23.031
    first degree T23.131
    second degree T23.231
    third degree T23.331
   second degree T23.239
   third degree T23.339
  right T23.021
   first degree T23.121
   second degree T23.221
   third degree T23.321
  second degree T23.229
  third degree T23.329
 flank —*see* Burn, abdominal wall

Burn *(Continued)*
 foot T25.029
  first degree T25.129
  left T25.022
   first degree T25.122
   second degree T25.222
   third degree T25.322
  multiple with ankle —*see* Burn, lower, limb, multiple, ankle and foot
  right T25.021
   first degree T25.121
   second degree T25.221
   third degree T25.321
  second degree T25.229
  third degree T25.329
 forearm T22.019
  first degree T22.119
  left T22.012
   first degree T22.112
   second degree T22.212
   third degree T22.312
  right T22.011
   first degree T22.111
   second degree T22.211
   third degree T22.311
  second degree T22.219
  third degree T22.319
 forehead T20.06
  first degree T20.16
  second degree T20.26
  third degree T20.36
 fourth degree - code as Burn, third degree, by site
 friction —*see* Burn, by site
 from swallowing caustic or corrosive substance NEC —*see* Corrosion, by site
 full thickness skin loss - code as Burn, third degree, by site
 gastrointestinal tract NEC T28.2
  from swallowing caustic or corrosive substance T28.7
 genital organs
  external
   female T21.07
    first degree T21.17
    second degree T21.27
    third degree T21.37
   male T21.06
    first degree T21.16
    second degree T21.26
    third degree T21.36
  internal T28.3
   from caustic or corrosive substance T28.8
 groin —*see* Burn, abdominal wall
 hand (s) T23.009
  back —*see* Burn, dorsum of hand
  finger —*see* Burn, finger
  first degree T23.109
  left T23.002
   first degree T23.102
   second degree T23.202
   third degree T23.302
  multiple sites with wrist T23.099
   first degree T23.199
   left T23.092
    first degree T23.192
    second degree T23.292
    third degree T23.392
   right T23.091
    first degree T23.191
    second degree T23.291
    third degree T23.391
   second degree T23.299
   third degree T23.399
  palm —*see* Burn, palm
  right T23.001
   first degree T23.101
   second degree T23.201
   third degree T23.301

Burn *(Continued)*
  hand *(Continued)*
    second degree T23.209
    third degree T23.309
    thumb —*see* Burn, thumb
  head (and face) (and neck) T20.00
    cheek —*see* Burn, cheek
    chin —*see* Burn, chin
    ear —*see* Burn, ear
    eye (s) only —*see* Burn, eye
    first degree T20.10
    forehead —*see* Burn, forehead
    lip —*see* Burn, lip
    multiple sites T20.09
      first degree T20.19
      second degree T20.29
      third degree T20.39
    neck —*see* Burn, neck
    nose —*see* Burn, nose
    scalp —*see* Burn, scalp
    second degree T20.20
    third degree T20.30
  hip (s) —*see* Burn, thigh
  inhalation —*see* Burn, respiratory tract
    caustic or corrosive substance (fumes) —*see* Corrosion, respiratory tract
  internal organ (s) T28.40
    alimentary tract T28.2
      esophagus T28.1
    eardrum T28.41
    esophagus T28.1
    from caustic or corrosive substance (swallowing) NEC —*see* Corrosion, by site
    genitourinary T28.3
    mouth T28.0
    pharynx T28.0
    respiratory tract —*see* Burn, respiratory tract
    specified organ NEC T28.49
  interscapular region —*see* Burn, back, upper
  intestine (large) (small) T28.2
  knee T24.029
    first degree T24.129
    left T24.022
      first degree T24.122
      second degree T24.222
      third degree T24.322
    right T24.021
      first degree T24.121
      second degree T24.221
      third degree T24.321
    second degree T24.229
    third degree T24.329
  labium (majus) (minus) —*see* Burn, genital organs, external, female
  lacrimal apparatus, duct, gland or sac —*see* Burn, eye, specified site NEC
  larynx T27.0
    with lung T27.1
  leg (s) (lower) (upper) —*see* Burn, lower, limb
  lightning —*see* Burn, by site
  limb (s)
    lower (except ankle or foot alone) —*see* Burn, lower, limb
    upper —*see* Burn, upper limb
  lip (s) T20.02
    first degree T20.12
    second degree T20.22
    third degree T20.32
  lower
    back —*see* Burn, back
    limb T24.009
      ankle —*see* Burn, ankle
      calf —*see* Burn, calf
      first degree T24.109
      foot —*see* Burn, foot
      hip —*see* Burn, thigh
      knee —*see* Burn, knee

Burn *(Continued)*
  lower *(Continued)*
    limb *(Continued)*
      left T24.002
        first degree T24.102
        second degree T24.202
        third degree T24.302
      multiple sites, except ankle and foot T24.099
        ankle and foot T25.099
          first degree T25.199
          left T25.092
            first degree T25.192
            second degree T25.292
            third degree T25.392
          right T25.091
            first degree T25.191
            second degree T25.291
            third degree T25.391
          second degree T25.299
          third degree T25.399
        first degree T24.199
        left T24.092
          first degree T24.192
          second degree T24.292
          third degree T24.392
        right T24.091
          first degree T24.191
          second degree T24.291
          third degree T24.391
        second degree T24.299
        third degree T24.399
      right T24.001
        first degree T24.101
        second degree T24.201
        third degree T24.301
      second degree T24.209
      thigh —*see* Burn, thigh
      third degree T24.309
      toe —*see* Burn, toe
  lung (with larynx and trachea) T27.1
  mouth T28.0
  neck T20.07
    first degree T20.17
    second degree T20.27
    third degree T20.37
  nose (septum) T20.04
    first degree T20.14
    second degree T20.24
    third degree T20.34
  ocular adnexa —*see* Burn, eye
  orbit region —*see* Burn, eyelid
  palm T23.059
    first degree T23.159
    left T23.052
      first degree T23.152
      second degree T23.252
      third degree T23.352
    right T23.051
      first degree T23.151
      second degree T23.251
      third degree T23.351
    second degree T23.259
    third degree T23.359
  partial thickness - code as Burn, unspecified degree, by site
  pelvis —*see* Burn, trunk
  penis —*see* Burn, genital organs, external, male
  perineum
    female —*see* Burn, genital organs, external, female
    male —*see* Burn, genital organs, external, male
  periocular area —*see* Burn, eyelid
  pharynx T28.0
  rectum T28.2
  respiratory tract T27.3
    larynx —*see* Burn, larynx
    specified part NEC T27.2
    trachea —*see* Burn, trachea

Burn *(Continued)*
  sac, lacrimal —*see* Burn, eye, specified site NEC
  scalp T20.05
    first degree T20.15
    second degree T20.25
    third degree T20.35
  scapular region T22.069
    first degree T22.169
    left T22.062
      first degree T22.162
      second degree T22.262
      third degree T22.362
    right T22.061
      first degree T22.161
      second degree T22.261
      third degree T22.361
    second degree T22.269
    third degree T22.369
  sclera —*see* Burn, eye, specified site NEC
  scrotum —*see* Burn, genital organs, external, male
  shoulder T22.059
    first degree T22.159
    left T22.052
      first degree T22.152
      second degree T22.252
      third degree T22.352
    right T22.051
      first degree T22.151
      second degree T22.251
      third degree T22.351
    second degree T22.259
    third degree T22.359
  stomach T28.2
  temple —*see* Burn, head
  testis —*see* Burn, genital organs, external, male
  thigh T24.019
    first degree T24.119
    left T24.012
      first degree T24.112
      second degree T24.212
      third degree T24.312
    right T24.011
      first degree T24.111
      second degree T24.211
      third degree T24.311
    second degree T24.219
    third degree T24.319
  thorax (external) —*see* Burn, trunk
  throat (meaning pharynx) T28.0
  thumb (s) T23.019
    first degree T23.119
    left T23.012
      first degree T23.112
      second degree T23.212
      third degree T23.312
    multiple sites with fingers T23.049
      first degree T23.149
      left T23.042
        first degree T23.142
        second degree T23.242
        third degree T23.342
      right T23.041
        first degree T23.141
        second degree T23.241
        third degree T23.341
      second degree T23.249
      third degree T23.349
    right T23.011
      first degree T23.111
      second degree T23.211
      third degree T23.311
    second degree T23.219
    third degree T23.319
  toe T25.039
    first degree T25.139
    left T25.032
      first degree T25.132
      second degree T25.232
      third degree T25.332

◀ New   ◀═ Revised   ~~deleted~~ Deleted

Burn (Continued)
  toe (Continued)
    right T25.031
      first degree T25.131
      second degree T25.231
      third degree T25.331
    second degree T25.239
    third degree T25.339
  tongue T28.0
  tonsil (s) T28.0
  trachea T27.0
    with lung T27.1
  trunk T21.00
    abdominal wall —see Burn, abdominal wall
    anus —see Burn, buttock
    axilla —see Burn, upper limb
    back —see Burn, back
    breast —see Burn, chest wall
    buttock —see Burn, buttock
    chest wall —see Burn, chest wall
    first degree T21.10
    flank —see Burn, abdominal wall
    genital
      female —see Burn, genital organs, external, female
      male —see Burn, genital organs, external, male
    groin —see Burn, abdominal wall
    interscapular region —see Burn, back, upper
    labia —see Burn, genital organs, external, female
    lower back —see Burn, back
    penis —see Burn, genital organs, external, male
    perineum
      female —see Burn, genital organs, external, female
      male —see Burn, genital organs, external, male
    scapula region —see Burn, scapular region
    scrotum —see Burn, genital organs, external, male
    second degree T21.20
    specified site NEC T21.09
      first degree T21.19
      second degree T21.29
      third degree T21.39
    testes —see Burn, genital organs, external, male
    third degree T21.30
    upper back —see Burn, back, upper
    vulva —see Burn, genital organs, external, female
  unspecified site with extent of body surface involved specified
    less than 10 percent T31.0
    10-19 percent (0-9 percent third degree) T31.10
      with 10-19 percent third degree T31.11
    20-29 percent (0-9 percent third degree) T31.20
      with
        10-19 percent third degree T31.21
        20-29 percent third degree T31.22
    30-39 percent (0-9 percent third degree) T31.30
      with
        10-19 percent third degree T31.31
        20-29 percent third degree T31.32
        30-39 percent third degree T31.33
    40-49 percent (0-9 percent third degree) T31.40
      with
        10-19 percent third degree T31.41
        20-29 percent third degree T31.42
        30-39 percent third degree T31.43
        40-49 percent third degree T31.44

Burn (Continued)
  unspecified site with extent of body surface involved specified (Continued)
    50-59 percent (0-9 percent third degree) T31.50
      with
        10-19 percent third degree T31.51
        20-29 percent third degree T31.52
        30-39 percent third degree T31.53
        40-49 percent third degree T31.54
        50-59 percent third degree T31.55
    60-69 percent (0-9 percent third degree) T31.60
      with
        10-19 percent third degree T31.61
        20-29 percent third degree T31.62
        30-39 percent third degree T31.63
        40-49 percent third degree T31.64
        50-59 percent third degree T31.65
        60-69 percent third degree T31.66
    70-79 percent (0-9 percent third degree) T31.70
      with
        10-19 percent third degree T31.71
        20-29 percent third degree T31.72
        30-39 percent third degree T31.73
        40-49 percent third degree T31.74
        50-59 percent third degree T31.75
        60-69 percent third degree T31.76
        70-79 percent third degree T31.77
    80-89 percent (0-9 percent third degree) T31.80
      with
        10-19 percent third degree T31.81
        20-29 percent third degree T31.82
        30-39 percent third degree T31.83
        40-49 percent third degree T31.84
        50-59 percent third degree T31.85
        60-69 percent third degree T31.86
        70-79 percent third degree T31.87
        80-89 percent third degree T31.88
    90 percent or more (0-9 percent third degree) T31.90
      with
        10-19 percent third degree T31.91
        20-29 percent third degree T31.92
        30-39 percent third degree T31.93
        40-49 percent third degree T31.94
        50-59 percent third degree T31.95
        60-69 percent third degree T31.96
        70-79 percent third degree T31.97
        80-89 percent third degree T31.98
        90-99 percent third degree T31.99
  upper limb T22.00
    above elbow —see Burn, above elbow
    axilla —see Burn, axilla
    elbow —see Burn, elbow
    first degree T22.10
    forearm —see Burn, forearm
    hand —see Burn, hand
    interscapular region —see Burn, back, upper
    multiple sites T22.099
      first degree T22.199
      left T22.092
        first degree T22.192
        second degree T22.292
        third degree T22.392
      right T22.091
        first degree T22.191
        second degree T22.291
        third degree T22.391
      second degree T22.299
      third degree T22.399
    scapular region —see Burn, scapular region
    second degree T22.20
    shoulder —see Burn, shoulder
    third degree T22.30
    wrist —see Burn, wrist
  uterus T28.3
  vagina T28.3

Burn (Continued)
  vulva —see Burn, genital organs, external, female
  wrist T23.079
    first degree T23.179
    left T23.072
      first degree T23.172
      second degree T23.272
      third degree T23.372
    multiple sites with hand T23.099
      first degree T23.199
      left T23.092
        first degree T23.192
        second degree T23.292
        third degree T23.392
      right T23.091
        first degree T23.191
        second degree T23.291
        third degree T23.391
      second degree T23.299
      third degree T23.399
    right T23.071
      first degree T23.171
      second degree T23.271
      third degree T23.371
    second degree T23.279
    third degree T23.379
Burnett's syndrome E83.52
Burning
  feet syndrome E53.9
  sensation R20.8
  tongue K14.6
Burn-out (state) Z73.0
Burns' disease or osteochondrosis —see Osteochondrosis, juvenile, ulna
Bursa —see condition
Bursitis M71.9
  Achilles —see Tendinitis, Achilles
  adhesive —see Bursitis, specified NEC
  ankle —see Enthesopathy, lower limb, ankle, specified type NEC
  calcaneal —see Enthesopathy, foot, specified type NEC
  collateral ligament, tibial —see Bursitis, tibial collateral
  due to use, overuse, pressure —see also Disorder, soft tissue, due to use, specified type NEC
    specified NEC —see Disorder, soft tissue, due to use, specified NEC
  Duplay's M75.0
  elbow NEC M70.3-
    olecranon M70.2-
  finger —see Disorder, soft tissue, due to use, specified type NEC, hand
  foot —see Enthesopathy, foot, specified type NEC
  gonococcal A54.49
  gouty —see Gout ◀▥
  hand M70.1-
  hip NEC M70.7-
    trochanteric M70.6-
  infective NEC M71.10
    abscess —see Abscess, bursa
    ankle M71.17-
    elbow M71.12-
    foot M71.17-
    hand M71.14-
    hip M71.15-
    knee M71.16-
    multiple sites M71.19
    shoulder M71.11-
    specified site NEC M71.18
    wrist M71.13-
  ischial —see Bursitis, hip
  knee NEC M70.5-
    prepatellar M70.4-
  occupational NEC —see also Disorder, soft tissue, due to, use
  olecranon —see Bursitis, elbow, olecranon
  pharyngeal J39.1

Bursitis (Continued)
  popliteal —see Bursitis, knee
  prepatellar M70.4-
  radiohumeral M77.8
  rheumatoid M06.20
    ankle M06.27-
    elbow M06.22-
    foot joint M06.27-
    hand joint M06.24-
    hip M06.25-
    knee M06.26-
    multiple site M06.29
    shoulder M06.21-
    vertebra M06.28
    wrist M06.23-
  scapulohumeral —see Bursitis, shoulder
  semimembranous muscle (knee) —see
    Bursitis, knee
  shoulder M75.5-
    adhesive —see Capsulitis, adhesive
  specified NEC M71.50
    ankle M71.57-
    due to use, overuse or pressure —see
      Disorder, soft tissue, due to, use
    elbow M71.52-
    foot M71.57-
    hand M71.54-

Bursitis (Continued)
  specified NEC (Continued)
    hip M71.55-
    knee M71.56-
    shoulder —see Bursitis, shoulder
    specified site NEC M71.58
    tibial collateral M76.4-
    wrist M71.53-
  subacromial —see Bursitis, shoulder
  subcoracoid —see Bursitis, shoulder
  subdeltoid —see Bursitis, shoulder
  syphilitic A52.78
  Thornwaldt, Tornwaldt J39.2
  tibial collateral M76.4- ◀▥
  toe —see Enthesopathy, foot, specified type
    NEC
  trochanteric (area) —see Bursitis, hip,
    trochanteric
  wrist —see Bursitis, hand
Bursopathy M71.9
  specified type NEC M71.80
    ankle M71.87-
    elbow M71.82-
    foot M71.87-
    hand M71.84-
    hip M71.85-
    knee M71.86-

Bursopathy (Continued)
  specified type NEC (Continued)
    multiple sites M71.89
    shoulder M71.81-
    specified site NEC M71.88
    wrist M71.83-
Burst stitches or sutures (complication of
  surgery) T81.31
  external operation wound T81.31
  internal operation wound T81.32
Buruli ulcer A31.1
Bury's disease L95.1
Buschke's
  disease B45.3
  scleredema —see Sclerosis, systemic
Busse-Buschke disease B45.3
Buttock —see condition
Button
  Biskra B55.1
  Delhi B55.1
  oriental B55.1
Buttonhole deformity (finger) —see Deformity,
  finger, boutonniere
Bwamba fever A92.8
Byssinosis J66.0
Bywaters' syndrome T79.5

B

◀ New   ◀▥ Revised   ~~deleted~~ Deleted

C

Cachexia R64
  cancerous R64
  cardiac —*see* Disease, heart
  dehydration E86.0
    with
      hypernatremia E87.0
      hyponatremia E87.1
  due to malnutrition R64
  exophthalmic —*see* Hyperthyroidism
  heart —*see* Disease, heart
  hypophyseal E23.0
  hypopituitary E23.0
  lead —*see* Poisoning, lead
  malignant R64
  marsh —*see* Malaria
  nervous F48.8
  old age R54
  paludal —*see* Malaria
  pituitary E23.0
  renal N28.9
  saturnine —*see* Poisoning, lead
  senile R54
  Simmonds' E23.0
  splenica D73.0
  strumipriva E03.4
  tuberculous NEC —*see* Tuberculosis
Café au lait spots L81.3
Caffeine-induced ◀
  anxiety disorder F15.980 ◀
  sleep disorder F15.982 ◀
Caffey's syndrome Q78.8
Caisson disease T70.3
Cake kidney Q63.1
Caked breast (puerperal, postpartum) O92.79
Calabar swelling B74.3
Calcaneal spur —*see* Spur, bone, calcaneal
Calcaneo-apophysitis M92.8
Calcareous —*see* condition
Calcicosis J62.8
Calciferol (vitamin D) deficiency E55.9
  with rickets E55.0
Calcification
  adrenal (capsule) (gland) E27.49
    tuberculous E35 [B90.8]
  aorta I70.0
  artery (annular) —*see* Arteriosclerosis
  auricle (ear) —*see* Disorder, pinna, specified
    type NEC
  basal ganglia G23.8
  bladder N32.89
    due to Schistosoma hematobium
      B65.0
  brain (cortex) —*see* Calcification, cerebral
  bronchus J98.09
  bursa M71.40
    ankle M71.47-
    elbow M71.42-
    foot M71.47-
    hand M71.44-
    hip M71.45-
    knee M71.46-
    multiple sites M71.49
    shoulder M75.3-
    specified site NEC M71.48
    wrist M71.43-
  cardiac —*see* Degeneration, myocardial
  cerebral (cortex) G93.89
    artery I67.2
  cervix (uteri) N88.8
  choroid plexus G93.89
  conjunctiva —*see* Concretion, conjunctiva
  corpora cavernosa (penis) N48.89
  cortex (brain) —*see* Calcification, cerebral
  dental pulp (nodular) K04.2
  dentinal papilla K00.4
  fallopian tube N83.8
  falx cerebri G96.19
  gallbladder K82.8
  general E83.59

Calcification (Continued)
  heart —*see also* Degeneration, myocardial
    valve —*see* Endocarditis
  idiopathic infantile arterial (IIAC) Q28.8
  intervertebral cartilage or disc
    (postinfective) —*see* Disorder, disc,
    specified NEC
  intracranial —*see* Calcification, cerebral
  joint —*see* Disorder, joint, specified type NEC
  kidney N28.89
    tuberculous N29 [B90.1]
  larynx (senile) J38.7
  lens —*see* Cataract, specified NEC
  lung (active) (postinfectional) J98.4
    tuberculous B90.9
  lymph gland or node (postinfectional) I89.8
    tuberculous —*see also* Tuberculosis, lymph
      gland B90.8
  mammographic R92.1
  massive (paraplegic) —*see* Myositis,
    ossificans, in, quadriplegia
  medial —*see* Arteriosclerosis, extremities
  meninges (cerebral) (spinal) G96.19
  metastatic E83.59
  Mönckeberg's —*see* Arteriosclerosis,
    extremities
  muscle M61.9
    due to burns —*see* Myositis, ossificans, in,
      burns
    paralytic —*see* Myositis, ossificans, in,
      quadriplegia
    specified type NEC M61.40
      ankle M61.47-
      foot M61.47-
      forearm M61.43-
      hand M61.44-
      lower leg M61.46-
      multiple sites M61.49
      pelvic region M61.45-
      shoulder region M61.41-
      specified site NEC M61.48
      thigh M61.45-
      upper arm M61.42-
  myocardium, myocardial —*see* Degeneration,
    myocardial
  ovary N83.8
  pancreas K86.89 ◀▥
  penis N48.89
  periarticular —*see* Disorder, joint, specified
    type NEC
  pericardium —*see also* Pericarditis I31.1
  pineal gland E34.8
  pleura J94.8
    postinfectional J94.8
    tuberculous NEC B90.9
  pulpal (dental) (nodular) K04.2
  sclera H15.89
  spleen D73.89
  subcutaneous L94.2
  suprarenal (capsule) (gland) E27.49
  tendon (sheath) —*see also* Tenosynovitis,
    specified type NEC
    with bursitis, synovitis or tenosynovitis —
      see Tendinitis, calcific
  trachea J39.8
  ureter N28.89
  vitreous —*see* Deposit, crystalline
Calcified —*see* Calcification
Calcinosis (interstitial) (tumoral) (universalis)
  E83.59
  with Raynaud's phenomenon, esophageal
    dysfunction, sclerodactyly,
    telangiectasia (CREST syndrome) M34.1
  circumscripta (skin) L94.2
  cutis L94.2
Calciphylaxis —*see also* Calcification, by site
  E83.59
Calcium
  deposits —*see* Calcification, by site
  metabolism disorder E83.50
  salts or soaps in vitreous —*see* Deposit,
    crystalline

Calciuria R82.99
Calculi —*see* Calculus
Calculosis, intrahepatic —*see* Calculus, bile
  duct
Calculus, calculi, calculous
  ampulla of Vater —*see* Calculus, bile duct
  anuria (impacted) (recurrent) —*see also*
    Calculus, urinary N20.9
  appendix K38.1
  bile duct (common) (hepatic) K80.50
    with
      calculus of gallbladder —*see* Calculus,
        gallbladder and bile duct
      cholangitis K80.30
        with
          cholecystitis —*see* Calculus, bile
            duct, with cholecystitis
          obstruction K80.31
        acute K80.32
          with
            chronic cholangitis K80.36
              with obstruction K80.37
            obstruction K80.33
        chronic K80.34
          with
            acute cholangitis K80.36
              with obstruction K80.37
            obstruction K80.35
      cholecystitis (with cholangitis) K80.40
        with obstruction K80.41
        acute K80.42
          with
            chronic cholecystitis K80.46
              with obstruction K80.47
            obstruction K80.43
        chronic K80.44
          with
            acute cholecystitis K80.46
              with obstruction K80.47
            obstruction K80.45
      obstruction K80.51
  biliary —*see also* Calculus, gallbladder
    specified NEC K80.80
      with obstruction K80.81
  bilirubin, multiple —*see* Calculus,
    gallbladder
  bladder (encysted) (impacted) (urinary)
    (diverticulum) N21.0
  bronchus J98.09
  calyx (kidney) (renal) —*see* Calculus, kidney
  cholesterol (pure) (solitary) —*see* Calculus,
    gallbladder
  common duct (bile) —*see* Calculus, bile duct
  conjunctiva —*see* Concretion, conjunctiva
  cystic N21.0
    duct —*see* Calculus, gallbladder
  dental (subgingival) (supragingival)
    K03.6
  diverticulum
    bladder N21.0
    kidney N20.0
  epididymis N50.89 ◀▥
  gallbladder K80.20
    with
      bile duct calculus —*see* Calculus,
        gallbladder and bile duct
      cholecystitis K80.10
        with obstruction K80.11
        acute K80.00
          with
            chronic cholecystitis K80.12
              with obstruction K80.13
            obstruction K80.01
        chronic K80.10
          with
            acute cholecystitis K80.12
              with obstruction K80.13
            obstruction K80.11
      specified NEC K80.18
        with obstruction K80.19
    obstruction K80.21

Calculus, calculi, calculous *(Continued)*
  gallbladder and bile duct K80.70
    with
      cholecystitis K80.60
        with obstruction K80.61
        acute K80.62
          with
            chronic cholecystitis K80.66
              with obstruction K80.67
            obstruction K80.63
          chronic K80.64
          with
            acute cholecystitis K80.66
              with obstruction K80.67
            obstruction K80.65
        obstruction K80.71
  hepatic (duct) —*see* Calculus, bile duct
  hepatobiliary K80.80
    with obstruction K80.81
  ileal conduit N21.8
  intestinal (impaction) (obstruction) K56.49
  kidney (impacted) (multiple) (pelvis)
      (recurrent) (staghorn) N20.0
    with calculus, ureter N20.2
    congenital Q63.8
  lacrimal passages —*see* Dacryolith
  liver (impacted) —*see* Calculus, bile duct
  lung J98.4
  mammographic R92.1
  nephritic (impacted) (recurrent) —*see*
      Calculus, kidney
  nose J34.89
  pancreas (duct) K86.89 ◀▥
  parotid duct or gland K11.5
  pelvis, encysted —*see* Calculus, kidney
  prostate N42.0
  pulmonary J98.4
  pyelitis (impacted) (recurrent) N20.0
    with hydronephrosis N13.2
  pyelonephritis (impacted) (recurrent) —*see*
      category N20
    with hydronephrosis N13.2
  renal (impacted) (recurrent) —*see* Calculus,
      kidney
  salivary (duct) (gland) K11.5
  seminal vesicle N50.89 ◀▥
  staghorn —*see* Calculus, kidney
  Stensen's duct K11.5
  stomach K31.89
  sublingual duct or gland K11.5
    congenital Q38.4
  submandibular duct, gland or region K11.5
  submaxillary duct, gland or region K11.5
  suburethral N21.8
  tonsil J35.8
  tooth, teeth (subgingival) (supragingival)
      K03.6
  tunica vaginalis N50.89 ◀▥
  ureter (impacted) (recurrent) N20.1
    with calculus, kidney N20.2
      with hydronephrosis N13.2
        with infection N13.6
  urethra (impacted) N21.1
  urinary (duct) (impacted) (passage) (tract)
      N20.9
    with hydronephrosis N13.2
      with infection N13.6
    in (due to)
    lower N21.9
      specified NEC N21.8
  vagina N89.8
  vesical (impacted) N21.0
  Wharton's duct K11.5
  xanthine E79.8 *[N22]*
Calicectasis N28.89
Caliectasis N28.89
California
  disease B38.9
  encephalitis A83.5
Caligo cornea —*see* Opacity, cornea, central
Callositas, callosity (infected) L84

Callus (infected) L84
  bone —*see* Osteophyte
    excessive, following fracture - code as
      Sequelae of fracture
CALME (childhood asymmetric labium majus
    enlargement) N90.61 ◀
Calorie deficiency or malnutrition —*see also*
    Malnutrition E46
Calvé-Perthes disease —*see* Legg-Calve-Perthes
    disease
Calvé's disease —*see* Osteochondrosis, juvenile,
    spine
Calvities —*see* Alopecia, androgenic
Cameroon fever —*see* Malaria
Camptocormia (hysterical) F44.4
Camurati-Engelmann syndrome Q78.3
Canal —*see also* condition
  atrioventricular common Q21.2
Canaliculitis (lacrimal) (acute) (subacute) H04.33-
  Actinomyces A42.89
  chronic H04.42-
Canavan's disease E75.29
Canceled procedure (surgical) Z53.9
  because of
    contraindication Z53.09
      smoking Z53.01
    left against medical advice (AMA) Z53.21
    patient's decision Z53.20
      for reasons of belief or group pressure
        Z53.1
      specified reason NEC Z53.29
    specified reason NEC Z53.8
Cancer —*see also* Neoplasm, by site, malignant
  bile duct type, liver C22.1
  blood —*see* Leukemia
  breast —*see also* Neoplasm, breast, malignant
      C50.91-
  hepatocellular C22.0
  lung —*see also* Neoplasm, lung, malignant
      C34.90-
  ovarian —*see also* Neoplasm, ovary,
      malignant C56.9-
  unspecified site (primary) C80.1
Cancer (o)phobia F45.29
Cancerous —*see* Neoplasm, malignant, by site
Cancrum oris A69.0
Candidiasis, candidal B37.9
  balanitis B37.42
  bronchitis B37.1
  cheilitis B37.83
  congenital P37.5
  cystitis B37.41
  disseminated B37.7
  endocarditis B37.6
  enteritis B37.82
  esophagitis B37.81
  intertrigo B37.2
  lung B37.1
  meningitis B37.5
  mouth B37.0
  nails B37.2
  neonatal P37.5
  onychia B37.2
  oral B37.0
  osteomyelitis B37.89
  otitis externa B37.84
  paronychia B37.2
  perionyxis B37.2
  pneumonia B37.1
  proctitis B37.82
  pulmonary B37.1
  pyelonephritis B37.49
  sepsis B37.7
  skin B37.2
  specified site NEC B37.89
  stomatitis B37.0
  systemic B37.7
  urethritis B37.41
  urogenital site NEC B37.49
  vagina B37.3
  vulva B37.3
  vulvovaginitis B37.3

Candidid L30.2
Candidosis —*see* Candidiasis
Candiru infection or infestation B88.8
Canities (premature) L67.1
  congenital Q84.2
Canker (mouth) (sore) K12.0
  rash A38.9
Cannabinosis J66.2
Cannabis induced ◀
  anxiety disorder F12.980 ◀
  psychotic disorder F12.959 ◀
  sleep disorder F12.988 ◀
Canton fever A75.9
Cantrell's syndrome Q87.89
Capillariasis (intestinal) B81.1
  hepatic B83.8
Capillary —*see* condition
Caplan's syndrome —*see* Rheumatoid, lung
Capsule —*see* condition
Capsulitis (joint) —*see also* Enthesopathy
  adhesive (shoulder) M75.0-
  hepatic K65.8
  labyrinthine —*see* Otosclerosis, specified NEC
  thyroid E06.9
Caput
  crepitus Q75.8
  medusae I86.8
  succedaneum P12.81
Car sickness T75.3
Carapata (disease) A68.0
Carate —*see* Pinta
Carbon lung J60
Carbuncle L02.93
  abdominal wall L02.231
  anus K61.0
  auditory canal, external —*see* Abscess, ear,
      external
  auricle ear —*see* Abscess, ear, external
  axilla L02.43-
  back (any part) L02.232
  breast N61.1 ◀▥
  buttock L02.33
  cheek (external) L02.03
  chest wall L02.233
  chin L02.03
  corpus cavernosum N48.21
  ear (any part) (external) (middle) —*see*
      Abscess, ear, external
  external auditory canal —*see* Abscess, ear,
      external
  eyelid —*see* Abscess, eyelid
  face NEC L02.03
  femoral (region) —*see* Carbuncle, lower limb
  finger —*see* Carbuncle, hand
  flank L02.231
  foot L02.63-
  forehead L02.03
  genital —*see* Abscess, genital
  gluteal (region) L02.33
  groin L02.234
  hand L02.53-
  head NEC L02.831
  heel —*see* Carbuncle, foot
  hip —*see* Carbuncle, lower limb
  kidney —*see* Abscess, kidney
  knee —*see* Carbuncle, lower limb
  labium (majus) (minus) N76.4
  lacrimal
    gland —*see* Dacryoadenitis
    passages (duct) (sac) —*see* Inflammation,
        lacrimal, passages, acute
  leg —*see* Carbuncle, lower limb
  lower limb L02.43-
  malignant A22.0
  navel L02.236
  neck L02.13
  nose (external) (septum) J34.0
  orbit, orbital —*see* Abscess, orbit
  palmar (space) —*see* Carbuncle, hand
  partes posteriores L02.33
  pectoral region L02.233
  penis N48.21

◀ New   ◀▥ Revised   ~~deleted~~ Deleted

Carbuncle *(Continued)*
 perineum L02.235
 pinna —*see* Abscess, ear, external
 popliteal —*see* Carbuncle, lower limb
 scalp L02.831
 seminal vesicle N49.0
 shoulder —*see* Carbuncle, upper limb
 specified site NEC L02.838
 temple (region) L02.03
 thumb —*see* Carbuncle, hand
 toe —*see* Carbuncle, foot
 trunk L02.239
  abdominal wall L02.231
  back L02.232
  chest wall L02.233
  groin L02.234
  perineum L02.235
  umbilicus L02.236
 umbilicus L02.236
 upper limb L02.43-
 urethra N34.0
 vulva N76.4
Carbunculus —*see* Carbuncle
Carcinoid (tumor) —*see* Tumor, carcinoid
Carcinoidosis E34.0
Carcinoma (malignant) —*see also* Neoplasm, by
   site, malignant
 acidophil
  specified site —*see* Neoplasm, malignant,
    by site
  unspecified site C75.1
 acidophil-basophil, mixed
  specified site —*see* Neoplasm, malignant,
    by site
  unspecified site C75.1
 adnexal (skin) —*see* Neoplasm, skin,
   malignant
 adrenal cortical C74.0-
 alveolar —*see* Neoplasm, lung, malignant
  cell —*see* Neoplasm, lung, malignant
 ameloblastic C41.1
  upper jaw (bone) C41.0
 apocrine
  breast —*see* Neoplasm, breast, malignant
  specified site NEC —*see* Neoplasm, skin,
    malignant
  unspecified site C44.99
 basal cell (pigmented) (*see also* Neoplasm,
   skin, malignant) C44.91
  fibro-epithelial —*see* Neoplasm, skin,
    malignant
  morphea —*see* Neoplasm, skin, malignant
  multicentric —*see* Neoplasm, skin, malignant
 basaloid
 basal-squamous cell, mixed —*see* Neoplasm,
   skin, malignant
 basophil
  specified site —*see* Neoplasm, malignant,
    by site
  unspecified site C75.1
 basophil-acidophil, mixed
  specified site —*see* Neoplasm, malignant,
    by site
  unspecified site C75.1
 basosquamous —*see* Neoplasm, skin, malignant
 bile duct
  with hepatocellular, mixed C22.0
  liver C22.1
  specified site NEC —*see* Neoplasm,
    malignant, by site
  unspecified site C22.1
 branchial or branchiogenic C10.4
 bronchial or bronchogenic —*see* Neoplasm,
   lung, malignant
 bronchiolar —*see* Neoplasm, lung, malignant
 bronchioloalveolar —*see* Neoplasm, lung,
   malignant
 C cell
  specified site —*see* Neoplasm, malignant,
    by site
  unspecified site C73
 ceruminous C44.29-

Carcinoma *(Continued)*
 cervix uteri
  in situ D06.9
   endocervix D06.0
   exocervix D06.1
   specified site NEC D06.7
 chorionic
  specified site —*see* Neoplasm, malignant,
    by site
  unspecified site
   female C58
   male C62.90
 chromophobe
  specified site —*see* Neoplasm, malignant,
    by site
  unspecified site C75.1
 cloacogenic
  specified site —*see* Neoplasm, malignant,
    by site
  unspecified site C21.2
 diffuse type
  specified site —*see* Neoplasm, malignant,
    by site
  unspecified site C16.9
 duct (cell)
  with Paget's disease —*see* Neoplasm,
    breast, malignant
  infiltrating
   with lobular carcinoma (in situ)
    specified site —*see* Neoplasm,
      malignant, by site
    unspecified site (female) C50.91-
     male C50.92-
   specified site —*see* Neoplasm,
     malignant, by site
   unspecified site (female) C50.91-
    male C50.92-
 ductal
  with lobular
   specified site —*see* Neoplasm,
     malignant, by site
   unspecified site (female) C50.91-
    male C50.92-
 ductular, infiltrating
  specified site —*see* Neoplasm, malignant,
    by site
  unspecified site (female) C50.91-
   male C50.92-
 embryonal
  liver C22.7
 endometrioid
  specified site —*see* Neoplasm, malignant,
    by site
  unspecified site
   female C56.9
   male C61
 eosinophil
  specified site —*see* Neoplasm, malignant,
    by site
  unspecified site C75.1
 epidermoid —*see also* Neoplasm, skin
   malignant
  in situ, Bowen's type —*see* Neoplasm, skin,
    in situ
 fibroepithelial, basal cell —*see* Neoplasm,
   skin, malignant
 follicular
  with papillary (mixed) C73
  moderately differentiated C73
  pure follicle C73
  specified site —*see* Neoplasm, malignant,
    by site
  trabecular C73
  unspecified site C73
  well differentiated C73
 generalized, with unspecified primary site
   C80.0
 glycogen-rich —*see* Neoplasm, breast,
   malignant
 granulosa cell C56-
 hepatic cell C22.0

Carcinoma *(Continued)*
 hepatocellular C22.0
  with bile duct, mixed C22.0
  fibrolamellar C22.0
 hepatocholangiolitic C22.0
 Hurthle cell C73
 in
  adenomatous
   polyposis coli C18.9
  pleomorphic adenoma —*see* Neoplasm,
    salivary glands, malignant
  situ —*see* Carcinoma-in-situ
 infiltrating
  duct
   with lobular
    specified site —*see* Neoplasm,
      malignant, by site
    unspecified site (female) C50.91-
     male C50.92-
   with Paget's disease —*see* Neoplasm,
     breast, malignant
   specified site —*see* Neoplasm,
     malignant
   unspecified site (female) C50.91-
    male C50.92-
  ductular
   specified site —*see* Neoplasm,
     malignant
   unspecified site (female) C50.91-
    male C50.92-
  lobular
   specified site —*see* Neoplasm,
     malignant
   unspecified site (female) C50.91-
    male C50.92-
 inflammatory
  specified site —*see* Neoplasm, malignant
  unspecified site (female) C50.91-
   male C50.92-
 intestinal type
  specified site —*see* Neoplasm, malignant,
    by site
  unspecified site C16.9
 intracystic
  noninfiltrating —*see* Neoplasm, in situ,
    by site
 intraductal (noninfiltrating)
  with Paget's disease —*see* Neoplasm,
    breast, malignant
  breast D05.1-
  papillary
   with invasion
    specified site —*see* Neoplasm,
      malignant, by site
    unspecified site (female) C50.91-
     male C50.92-
   breast D05.1-
   specified site NEC —*see* Neoplasm,
     in situ, by site
   unspecified site (female) D05.1-
  specified site NEC —*see* Neoplasm,
    in situ, by site
  unspecified site (female) D05.1-
 intraepidermal —*see* Neoplasm, in situ
  squamous cell, Bowen's type —*see*
    Neoplasm, skin, in situ
 intraepithelial —*see* Neoplasm, in situ,
   by site
  squamous cell —*see* Neoplasm, in situ,
    by site
 intraosseous C41.1
  upper jaw (bone) C41.0
 islet cell
  with exocrine, mixed
   specified site —*see* Neoplasm,
     malignant, by site
   unspecified site C25.9
  pancreas C25.4
  specified site NEC —*see* Neoplasm,
    malignant, by site
  unspecified site C25.4

Carcinoma *(Continued)*
juvenile, breast —*see* Neoplasm, breast,
malignant
large cell
small cell
specified site —*see* Neoplasm,
malignant, by site
unspecified site C34.90
Leydig cell (testis)
specified site —*see* Neoplasm, malignant,
by site
unspecified site
female C56.9
male C62.90
lipid-rich (female) C50.91-
male C50.92-
liver cell C22.0
liver NEC C22.7
lobular (infiltrating)
with intraductal
specified site —*see* Neoplasm,
malignant, by site
unspecified site (female) C50.91-
male C50.92-
noninfiltrating
breast D05.0-
specified site NEC —*see* Neoplasm, in
situ, by site
unspecified site D05.0-
specified site —*see* Neoplasm, malignant,
by site
unspecified site (female) C50.91-
male C50.92-
medullary
with
amyloid stroma
specified site —*see* Neoplasm,
malignant, by site
unspecified site C73
lymphoid stroma
specified site —*see* Neoplasm,
malignant, by site
unspecified site (female) C50.91-
male C50.92-
Merkel cell C4A.9
anal margin C4A.51
anal skin C4A.51
canthus C4A.1-
ear and external auricular canal C4A.2-
external auricular canal C4A.2-
eyelid, including canthus C4A.1-
face C4A.30
specified NEC C4A.39
hip C4A.7-
lip C4A.0
lower limb, including hip C4A.7-
neck C4A.4
nodal presentation C7B.1
nose C4A.31
overlapping sites C4A.8
perianal skin C4A.51
scalp C4A.4
secondary C7B.1
shoulder C4A.6-
skin of breast C4A.52
trunk NEC C4A.59
upper limb, including shoulder C4A.6-
visceral metastatic C7B.1
metastatic —*see* Neoplasm, secondary
metatypical —*see* Neoplasm, skin, malignant
morphea, basal cell —*see* Neoplasm, skin,
malignant
mucoid
cell
specified site —*see* Neoplasm,
malignant, by site
unspecified site C75.1
neuroendocrine —*see also* Tumor,
neuroendocrine
high grade, any site C7A.1
poorly differentiated, any site C7A.1

Carcinoma *(Continued)*
nonencapsulated sclerosing C73
noninfiltrating
intracystic —*see* Neoplasm, in situ, by site
intraductal
breast D05.1-
papillary
breast D05.1-
specified site NEC —*see* Neoplasm, in
situ, by site
unspecified site D05.1-
specified site —*see* Neoplasm, in situ,
by site
unspecified site D05.1-
lobular
breast D05.0-
specified site NEC —*see* Neoplasm, in
situ, by site
unspecified site (female) D05.0-
oat cell
specified site —*see* Neoplasm, malignant,
by site
unspecified site C34.90
odontogenic C41.1
upper jaw (bone) C41.0
papillary
with follicular (mixed) C73
follicular variant C73
intraductal (noninfiltrating)
with invasion
specified site —*see* Neoplasm,
malignant, by site
unspecified site (female) C50.91-
male C50.92-
breast D05.1-
specified site NEC —*see* Neoplasm, in
situ, by site
unspecified site D05.1-
serous
specified site —*see* Neoplasm,
malignant, by site
surface
specified site —*see* Neoplasm,
malignant, by site
unspecified site C56.9
unspecified site C56.9
papillocystic
specified site —*see* Neoplasm, malignant,
by site
unspecified site C56.9
parafollicular cell
specified site —*see* Neoplasm, malignant,
by site
unspecified site C73
pilomatrix —*see* Neoplasm, skin, malignant
pseudomucinous
specified site —*see* Neoplasm, malignant,
by site
unspecified site C56.9
renal cell C64-
Schmincke —*see* Neoplasm, nasopharynx,
malignant
Schneiderian
specified site —*see* Neoplasm, malignant,
by site
unspecified site C30.0
sebaceous —*see* Neoplasm, skin, malignant
secondary —*see also* Neoplasm, secondary,
by site
Merkel cell C7B.1
secretory, breast —*see* Neoplasm, breast,
malignant
serous
papillary
specified site —*see* Neoplasm,
malignant, by site
unspecified site C56.9
surface, papillary
specified site —*see* Neoplasm,
malignant, by site
unspecified site C56.9

Carcinoma *(Continued)*
Sertoli cell
specified site —*see* Neoplasm, malignant,
by site
unspecified site C62.90
female C56.9
male C62.90
skin appendage —*see* Neoplasm, skin,
malignant
small cell
fusiform cell
specified site —*see* Neoplasm,
malignant, by site
unspecified site C34.90
intermediate cell
specified site —*see* Neoplasm,
malignant, by site
unspecified site C34.90
large cell
specified site —*see* Neoplasm,
malignant, by site
unspecified site C34.90
solid
with amyloid stroma
specified site —*see* Neoplasm,
malignant, by site
unspecified site C73
microinvasive
specified site —*see* Neoplasm,
malignant, by site
unspecified site C53.9
sweat gland —*see* Neoplasm, skin,
malignant
theca cell C56.-
thymic C37
unspecified site (primary) C80.1
water-clear cell C75.0
Carcinoma-in-situ —*see also* Neoplasm, in situ,
by site
breast NOS D05.9-
specified type NEC D05.8-
epidermoid —*see also* Neoplasm, in situ, by
site
with questionable stromal invasion
cervix D06.9
specified site NEC —*see* Neoplasm, in
situ, by site
unspecified site D06.9
Bowen's type —*see* Neoplasm, skin,
in situ
intraductal
breast D05.1-
specified site NEC —*see* Neoplasm, in situ,
by site
unspecified site D05.1-
lobular
with
infiltrating duct
breast (female) C50.91-
male C50.92-
specified site NEC —*see* Neoplasm,
malignant
unspecified site (female) C50.91-
male C50.92-
intraductal
breast D05.8-
specified site NEC —*see* Neoplasm, in
situ, by site
unspecified site (female) D05.8-
breast D05.0-
specified site NEC —*see* Neoplasm, in situ,
by site
unspecified site D05.0-
squamous cell —*see also* Neoplasm, in situ,
by site
with questionable stromal invasion
cervix D06.9
specified site NEC —*see* Neoplasm, in
situ, by site
unspecified site D06.9
Carcinomaphobia F45.29

◀ New   ◀▥ Revised   ~~deleted~~ Deleted

Carcinomatosis C80.0
  peritonei C78.6
  unspecified site (primary) (secondary) C80.0
Carcinosarcoma —see Neoplasm, malignant, by site
  embryonal —see Neoplasm, malignant, by site
Cardia, cardial —see condition
Cardiac —see also condition
  death, sudden —see Arrest, cardiac
  pacemaker
    in situ Z95.0
    management or adjustment Z45.018
  tamponade I31.4
Cardialgia —see Pain, precordial
Cardiectasis —see Hypertrophy, cardiac
Cardiochalasia K21.9
Cardiomalacia I51.5
Cardiomegalia glycogenica diffusa E74.02 [I43]
Cardiomegaly —see also Hypertrophy, cardiac
  congenital Q24.8
  glycogen E74.02 [I43]
  idiopathic I51.7
Cardiomyoliposis I51.5
Cardiomyopathy (familial) (idiopathic) I42.9
  alcoholic I42.6
  amyloid E85.4 [I43]
  arteriosclerotic —see Disease, heart, ischemic, atherosclerotic
  beriberi E51.12
  cobalt-beer I42.6
  congenital I42.4
  congestive I42.0
  constrictive NOS I42.5
  dilated I42.0
  due to
    alcohol I42.6
    beriberi E51.12
    cardiac glycogenosis E74.02 [I43]
    drugs I42.7
    external agents NEC I42.7
    Friedreich's ataxia G11.1
    myotonia atrophica G71.11 [I43]
    progressive muscular dystrophy G71.0
  glycogen storage E74.02 [I43]
  hypertensive —see Hypertension, heart
  hypertrophic (nonobstructive) I42.2
    obstructive I42.1
      congenital Q24.8
  in
    Chagas' disease (chronic) B57.2
      acute B57.0
    sarcoidosis D86.85
  ischemic I25.5
  metabolic E88.9 [I43]
    thyrotoxic E05.90 [I43]
      with thyroid storm E05.91 [I43]
  newborn I42.8
    congenital I42.4
  nutritional E63.9 [I43]
    beriberi E51.12
  obscure of Africa I42.8
  peripartum O90.3
  postpartum O90.3
  restrictive NEC I42.5
  rheumatic I09.0
  secondary I42.9
  stress induced I51.81
  takotsubo I51.81
  thyrotoxic E05.90 [I43]
    with thyroid storm E05.91 [I43]
  toxic NEC I42.7
  tuberculous A18.84
  viral B33.24
Cardionephritis —see Hypertension, cardiorenal
Cardionephropathy —see Hypertension, cardiorenal
Cardionephrosis —see Hypertension, cardiorenal
Cardiopathia nigra I27.0

Cardiopathy —see also Disease, heart I51.9
  idiopathic I42.9
  mucopolysaccharidosis E76.3 [I52]
Cardiopericarditis —see Pericarditis
Cardiophobia F45.29
Cardiorenal —see condition
Cardiorrhexis —see Infarct, myocardium
Cardiosclerosis —see Disease, heart, ischemic, atherosclerotic
Cardiosis —see Disease, heart
Cardiospasm (esophagus) (reflex) (stomach) K22.0
  congenital Q39.5
    with megaesophagus Q39.5
Cardiostenosis —see Disease, heart
Cardiosymphysis I31.0
Cardiovascular —see condition
Carditis (acute) (bacterial) (chronic) (subacute) I51.89
  meningococcal A39.50
  rheumatic —see Disease, heart, rheumatic
  rheumatoid —see Rheumatoid, carditis
  viral B33.20
Care (of) (for) (following)
  child (routine) Z76.2
  family member (handicapped) (sick)
    creating problem for family Z63.6
    provided away from home for holiday relief Z75.5
    unavailable, due to
      absence (person rendering care) (sufferer) Z74.2
      inability (any reason) of person rendering care Z74.2
  foundling Z76.1
  holiday relief Z75.5
  improper —see Maltreatment
  lack of (at or after birth) (infant) —see Maltreatment, child, neglect
  lactating mother Z39.1
  palliative Z51.5
  postpartum
    immediately after delivery Z39.0
    routine follow-up Z39.2
  respite Z75.5
  unavailable, due to
    absence of person rendering care Z74.2
    inability (any reason) of person rendering care Z74.2
  well-baby Z76.2
Caries
  bone NEC A18.03
  dental (dentino enamel junction) (early childhood) (of dentine) (pre-eruptive) (recurrent) (to the pulp) K02.9 ◄▥
    arrested (coronal) (root) K02.3
    chewing surface
      limited to enamel K02.51
      penetrating into dentin K02.52
      penetrating into pulp K02.53
    coronal surface
      chewing surface
        limited to enamel K02.51
        penetrating into dentin K02.52
        penetrating into pulp K02.53
      pit and fissure surface
        limited to enamel K02.51
        penetrating into dentin K02.52
        penetrating into pulp K02.53
      smooth surface
        limited to enamel K02.61
        penetrating into dentin K02.62
        penetrating into pulp K02.63
    pit and fissure surface
      limited to enamel K02.51
      penetrating into dentin K02.52
      penetrating into pulp K02.53
    primary, cervical origin K02.52 ◄
    root K02.7

Caries (Continued)
  dental (Continued)
    smooth surface
      limited to enamel K02.61
      penetrating into dentin K02.62
      penetrating into pulp K02.63
    external meatus —see Disorder, ear, external, specified type NEC
  hip (tuberculous) A18.02
  initial (tooth)
    chewing surface K02.51
    pit and fissure surface K02.51
    smooth surface K02.61
  knee (tuberculous) A18.02
  labyrinth —see subcategory H83.8
  limb NEC (tuberculous) A18.03
  mastoid process (chronic) —see Mastoiditis, chronic
  tuberculous A18.03
  middle ear —see subcategory H74.8
  nose (tuberculous) A18.03
  orbit (tuberculous) A18.03
  ossicles, ear —see Abnormal, ear ossicles
  petrous bone —see Petrositis
  root (dental) (tooth) K02.7
  sacrum (tuberculous) A18.01
  spine, spinal (column) (tuberculous) A18.01
  syphilitic A52.77
    congenital (early) A50.02 [M90.80]
  tooth, teeth —see Caries, dental
  tuberculous A18.03
  vertebra (column) (tuberculous) A18.01
Carious teeth —see Caries, dental
Carneous mole O02.0
Carnitine insufficiency E71.40
Carotid body or sinus syndrome G90.01
Carotidynia G90.01
Carotinemia (dietary) E67.1
Carotinosis (cutis) (skin) E67.1
Carpal tunnel syndrome —see Syndrome, carpal tunnel
Carpenter's syndrome Q87.0
Carpopedal spasm —see Tetany
Carr-Barr-Plunkett syndrome Q97.1
Carrier (suspected) of
  amebiasis Z22.1
  bacterial disease NEC Z22.39
    diphtheria Z22.2
    intestinal infectious NEC Z22.1
      typhoid Z22.0
    meningococcal Z22.31
    sexually transmitted Z22.4
    specified NEC Z22.39
    staphylococcal (Methicillin susceptible) Z22.321
      Methicillin resistant Z22.322
    streptococcal Z22.338
      group B Z22.330
        complicating pregnancy or delivery O99.82- ◄
  typhoid Z22.0
  cholera Z22.1
  diphtheria Z22.2
  gastrointestinal pathogens NEC Z22.1
  genetic Z14.8
    cystic fibrosis Z14.1
    hemophilia A (asymptomatic) Z14.01
      symptomatic Z14.02
  gestational, pregnant Z33.1 ◄
  gonorrhea Z22.4
  HAA (hepatitis Australian-antigen) B18.8 ◄▥
  HB (c)(s)-AG B18.1 ◄▥
  hepatitis (viral) B18.9 ◄▥
    Australia-antigen (HAA) B18.8 ◄▥
    B surface antigen (HBsAg) B18.1 ◄▥
      with acute delta- (super)infection B17.0
    C B18.2 ◄▥
    specified NEC B18.8 ◄▥
  human T-cell lymphotropic virus type-1 (HTLV-1) infection Z22.6

Carrier of *(Continued)*
  infectious organism Z22.9
    specified NEC Z22.8
  meningococci Z22.31
  Salmonella typhosa Z22.0
  serum hepatitis —*see* Carrier, hepatitis
  staphylococci (Methicillin susceptible) Z22.321
    Methicillin resistant Z22.322
  streptococci Z22.338
    group B Z22.330
      complicating pregnancy or delivery
        O99.82- ◄
  syphilis Z22.4
  typhoid Z22.0
  venereal disease NEC Z22.4
Carrion's disease A44.0
Carter's relapsing fever (Asiatic) A68.1
Cartilage —*see* condition
Caruncle (inflamed)
  conjunctiva (acute) —*see* Conjunctivitis, acute
  labium (majus) (minus) N90.89
  lacrimal —*see* Inflammation, lacrimal,
    passages
  myrtiform N89.8
  urethral (benign) N36.2
Cascade stomach K31.2
Caseation lymphatic gland (tuberculous) A18.2
Cassidy (-Scholte) syndrome (malignant
    carcinoid) E34.0
Castellani's disease A69.8
Castration, traumatic, male S38.231
Casts in urine R82.99
Cat
  cry syndrome Q93.4
  ear Q17.3
  eye syndrome Q92.8
Catabolism, senile R54
Catalepsy (hysterical) F44.2
  schizophrenic F20.2
Cataplexy (idiopathic) —*see* - Narcolepsy
Cataract (cortical) (immature) (incipient) H26.9
  with
    neovascularization —*see* Cataract,
      complicated
  age-related —*see* Cataract, senile
  anterior
    and posterior axial embryonal Q12.0
    pyramidal Q12.0
  associated with
    galactosemia E74.21 [H28]
    myotonic disorders G71.19 [H28]
  blue Q12.0
  central Q12.0
  cerulean Q12.0
  complicated H26.20
    with
      neovascularization H26.21-
      ocular disorder H26.22-
      glaucomatous flecks H26.23-
  congenital Q12.0
  coraliform Q12.0
  coronary Q12.0
  crystalline Q12.0
  diabetic —*see* Diabetes, cataract
  drug-induced H26.3-
  due to
    ocular disorder —*see* Cataract, complicated
    radiation H26.8
  electric H26.8
  extraction status Z98.4-
  glass-blower's H26.8
  heat ray H26.8
  heterochromic —*see* Cataract, complicated
  hypermature —*see* Cataract, senile,
    morgagnian type
  in (due to)
    chronic iridocyclitis —*see* Cataract,
      complicated
    diabetes —*see* Diabetes, cataract
    endocrine disease E34.9 [H28]
    eye disease —*see* Cataract, complicated

Cataract *(Continued)*
  in (due to) *(Continued)*
    hypoparathyroidism E20.9 [H28]
    malnutrition-dehydration E46 [H28]
    metabolic disease E88.9 [H28]
    myotonic disorders G71.19 [H28]
    nutritional disease E63.9 [H28]
  infantile —*see* Cataract, presenile
  irradiational —*see* Cataract, specified NEC
  juvenile —*see* Cataract, presenile
  malnutrition-dehydration E46 [H28]
  morgagnian —*see* Cataract, senile,
    morgagnian type
  myotonic G71.19 [H28]
  myxedema E03.9 [H28]
  nuclear
    embryonal Q12.0
    sclerosis —*see* Cataract, senile, nuclear
  presenile H26.00-
    combined forms H26.06-
    cortical H26.01-
    lamellar —*see* Cataract, presenile, cortical
    nuclear H26.03-
    specified NEC H26.09
    subcapsular polar (anterior) H26.04-
      posterior H26.05-
    zonular —*see* Cataract, presenile, cortical
  secondary H26.40
    Soemmering's ring H26.41-
    specified NEC H26.49-
    to eye disease —*see* Cataract, complicated
  senile H25.9
    brunescens —*see* Cataract, senile, nuclear
    combined forms H25.81-
    coronary —*see* Cataract, senile, incipient
    cortical H25.01-
    hypermature —*see* Cataract, senile,
      morgagnian type
    incipient (mature) (total) H25.09-
      cortical —*see* Cataract, senile, cortical
      subcapsular —*see* Cataract, senile,
        subcapsular
    morgagnian type (hypermature) H25.2-
    nuclear (sclerosis) H25.1-
    polar subcapsular (anterior) (posterior) —
      see Cataract, senile, incipient
    punctate —*see* Cataract, senile, incipient
    specified NEC H25.89
    subcapsular polar (anterior) H25.03-
      posterior H25.04-
  snowflake —*see* Diabetes, cataract
  specified NEC H26.8
  toxic —*see* Cataract, drug-induced
  traumatic H26.10-
    localized H26.11-
    partially resolved H26.12-
    total H26.13-
  zonular (perinuclear) Q12.0
Cataracta —*see also* Cataract
  brunescens —*see* Cataract, senile, nuclear
  centralis pulverulenta Q12.0
  cerulea Q12.0
  complicata —*see* Cataract, complicated
  congenita Q12.0
  coralliformis Q12.0
  coronaria Q12.0
  diabetic —*see* Diabetes, cataract
  membranacea
    accreta —*see* Cataract, secondary
    congenita Q12.0
  nigra —*see* Cataract, senile, nuclear
  sunflower —*see* Cataract, complicated
Catarrh, catarrhal (acute) (febrile) (infectious)
    (inflammation) (*see also* condition) J00
  bronchial —*see* Bronchitis
  chest —*see* Bronchitis
  chronic J31.0
  due to congenital syphilis A50.03
  enteric —*see* Enteritis
  eustachian H68.009
  fauces —*see* Pharyngitis

Catarrh, catarrhal *(Continued)*
  gastrointestinal —*see* Enteritis
  gingivitis K05.00
    nonplaque induced K05.01
    plaque induced K05.00
  hay —*see* Fever, hay
  intestinal —*see* Enteritis
  larynx, chronic J37.0
  liver B15.9
    with hepatic coma B15.0
  lung —*see* Bronchitis
  middle ear, chronic —*see* Otitis, media,
    nonsuppurative, chronic, serous
  mouth K12.1
  nasal (chronic) —*see* Rhinitis
  nasobronchial J31.1
  nasopharyngeal (chronic) J31.1
    acute J00
  pulmonary —*see* Bronchitis
  spring (eye) (vernal) —*see* Conjunctivitis,
    acute, atopic
  summer (hay) —*see* Fever, hay
  throat J31.2
  tubotympanal —*see also* Otitis, media,
    nonsuppurative
    chronic —*see* Otitis, media,
      nonsuppurative, chronic, serous
Catatonia (schizophrenic) F20.2
Catatonic
  disorder due to known physiologic condition
    F06.1
  schizophrenia F20.2
  stupor R40.1
Cat-scratch —*see also* Abrasion
  disease or fever A28.1
Cauda equina —*see* condition
Cauliflower ear M95.1-
Causalgia (upper limb) G56.4-
  lower limb G57.7-
Cause
  external, general effects T75.89
Caustic burn —*see* Corrosion, by site
Cavare's disease (familial periodic paralysis)
    G72.3
Cave-in, injury
  crushing (severe) —*see* Crush
  suffocation —*see* Asphyxia, traumatic, due to
    low oxygen, due to cave-in
Cavernitis (penis) N48.29
Cavernositis N48.29
Cavernous —*see* condition
Cavitation of lung —*see also* Tuberculosis,
    pulmonary
  nontuberculous J98.4
Cavities, dental —*see* Caries, dental
Cavity
  lung —*see* Cavitation of lung
  optic papilla Q14.2
  pulmonary —*see* Cavitation of lung
Cavovarus foot, congenital Q66.1
Cavus foot (congenital) Q66.7
  acquired —*see* Deformity, limb, foot, specified
    NEC
Cazenave's disease L10.2
Cecitis K52.9
  with perforation, peritonitis, or rupture K65.8
Cecum —*see* condition
Celiac
  artery compression syndrome I77.4
  disease (with steatorrhea) K90.0 ◄▬
  infantilism K90.0
Cell (s), cellular —*see also* condition
  in urine R82.99
Cellulitis (diffuse) (phlegmonous) (septic)
    (suppurative) L03.90
  abdominal wall L03.311
  anaerobic A48.0
  ankle —*see* Cellulitis, lower limb
  anus K61.0
  arm —*see* Cellulitis, upper limb
  auricle (ear) —*see* Cellulitis, ear

◄ New   ◄▬ Revised   ~~deleted~~ Deleted

Cellulitis (Continued)
axilla L03.11-
back (any part) L03.312
breast (acute) (nonpuerperal) (subacute) N61.0 ◄
nipple N61.0 ◄
broad ligament
acute N73.0
buttock L03.317
cervical (meaning neck) L03.221
cervix (uteri) —see Cervicitis
cheek (external) L03.211
internal K12.2
chest wall L03.313
chronic L03.90
clostridial A48.0
corpus cavernosum N48.22
digit
finger —see Cellulitis, finger
toe —see Cellulitis, toe
Douglas' cul-de-sac or pouch
acute N73.0
drainage site (following operation) T81.48 ◄▦
ear (external) H60.1-
eosinophilic (granulomatous) L98.3
erysipelatous —see Erysipelas
external auditory canal —see Cellulitis, ear
eyelid —see Abscess, eyelid
face NEC L03.211
finger (intrathecal) (periosteal)
(subcutaneous) (subcuticular) L03.01-
foot —see Cellulitis, lower limb
gangrenous —see Gangrene
genital organ NEC
female (external) N76.4
male N49.9
multiple sites N49.8
specified NEC N49.8
gluteal (region) L03.317
gonococcal A54.89
groin L03.314
hand —see Cellulitis, upper limb
head NEC L03.811
face (any part, except ear, eye and nose) L03.211
heel —see Cellulitis, lower limb
hip —see Cellulitis, lower limb
jaw (region) L03.211
knee —see Cellulitis, lower limb
labium (majus) (minus) —see Vulvitis
lacrimal passages —see Inflammation, lacrimal, passages
larynx J38.7
leg —see Cellulitis, lower limb
lip K13.0
lower limb L03.11-
toe —see Cellulitis, toe
mouth (floor) K12.2
multiple sites, so stated L03.90
nasopharynx J39.1
navel L03.316
newborn P38.9
with mild hemorrhage P38.1
without hemorrhage P38.9
neck (region) L03.221
nipple (acute) (nonpuerperal) (subacute) N61.0 ◄
nose (septum) (external) J34.0
orbit, orbital H05.01-
palate (soft) K12.2
pectoral (region) L03.313
pelvis, pelvic (chronic)
female —see also Disease, pelvis, inflammatory N73.2
acute N73.0
following ectopic or molar pregnancy O08.0
male K65.0
penis N48.22
perineal, perineum L03.315
periorbital L03.213 ◄

Cellulitis (Continued)
perirectal K61.1
peritonsillar J36
periurethral N34.0
periuterine —see also Disease, pelvis, inflammatory N73.2
acute N73.0
pharynx J39.1
preseptal L03.213 ◄
rectum K61.1
retroperitoneal K68.9
round ligament
acute N73.0
scalp (any part) L03.811
scrotum N49.2
seminal vesicle N49.0
shoulder —see Cellulitis, upper limb
specified site NEC L03.818
submandibular (region) (space) (triangle) K12.2
gland K11.3
submaxillary (region) K12.2
gland K11.3
thigh —see Cellulitis, lower limb
thumb (intrathecal) (periosteal)
(subcutaneous) (subcuticular) —see
Cellulitis, finger
toe (intrathecal) (periosteal) (subcutaneous)
(subcuticular) L03.03-
tonsil J36
trunk L03.319
abdominal wall L03.311
back (any part) L03.312
buttock L03.317
chest wall L03.313
groin L03.314
perineal, perineum L03.315
umbilicus L03.316
tuberculous (primary) A18.4
umbilicus L03.316
upper limb L03.11-
axilla —see Cellulitis, axilla
finger —see Cellulitis, finger
thumb —see Cellulitis, finger
vaccinal T88.0
vocal cord J38.3
vulva —see Vulvitis
wrist —see Cellulitis, upper limb
Cementoblastoma, benign —see Cyst, calcifying odontogenic
Cementoma —see Cyst, calcifying odontogenic
Cementoperiostitis —see Periodontitis
Cementosis K03.4
Central auditory processing disorder H93.25
Central pain syndrome G89.0
Cephalematocele, cephal (o)hematocele
newborn P52.8
birth injury P10.8
traumatic —see Hematoma, brain
Cephalematoma, cephalhematoma (calcified)
newborn (birth injury) P12.0
traumatic —see Hematoma, brain
Cephalgia, cephalalgia —see also Headache
histamine G44.009
intractable G44.001
not intractable G44.009
trigeminal autonomic (TAC) NEC G44.099
intractable G44.091
not intractable G44.099
Cephalic —see condition
Cephalitis —see Encephalitis
Cephalocele —see Encephalocele
Cephalomenia N94.89
Cephalopelvic —see condition
Cerclage (with cervical incompetence) in
pregnancy —see Incompetence, cervix, in pregnancy
Cerebellitis —see Encephalitis
Cerebellum, cerebellar —see condition
Cerebral —see condition
Cerebritis —see Encephalitis

Cerebro-hepato-renal syndrome Q87.89
Cerebromalacia —see Softening, brain
sequelae of cerebrovascular disease I69.398
Cerebroside lipidosis E75.22
Cerebrospasticity (congenital) G80.1
Cerebrospinal —see condition
Cerebrum —see condition
Ceroid-lipofuscinosis, neuronal E75.4
Cerumen (accumulation) (impacted) H61.2-
Cervical —see also condition
auricle Q18.2
dysplasia in pregnancy —see Abnormal, cervix, in pregnancy or childbirth
erosion in pregnancy —see Abnormal, cervix, in pregnancy or childbirth
fibrosis in pregnancy —see Abnormal, cervix, in pregnancy or childbirth
fusion syndrome Q76.1
rib Q76.5
shortening (complicating pregnancy) O26.87-
Cervicalgia M54.2
Cervicitis (acute) (chronic) (nonvenereal)
(senile (atrophic)) (subacute) (with ulceration) N72
with
abortion —see Abortion, by type
complicated by genital tract and pelvic infection
ectopic pregnancy O08.0
molar pregnancy O08.0
chlamydial A56.09
gonococcal A54.03
herpesviral A60.03
puerperal (postpartum) O86.11
syphilitic A52.76
trichomonal A59.09
tuberculous A18.16
Cervicocolpitis (emphysematosa) (see also Cervicitis) N72
Cervix —see condition
Cesarean delivery, previous, affecting
management of pregnancy O34.219 ◄▦
classical (vertical) scar O34.212 ◄
low transverse scar O34.211 ◄
Céstan (-Chenais) paralysis or syndrome G46.3
Céstan-Raymond syndrome I65.8
Cestode infestation B71.9
specified type NEC B71.8
Cestodiasis B71.9
Chabert's disease A22.9
Chacaleh E53.8
Chafing L30.4
Chagas' (-Mazza) disease (chronic) B57.2
with
cardiovascular involvement NEC B57.2
digestive system involvement B57.30
megacolon B57.32
megaesophagus B57.31
other specified B57.39
megacolon B57.32
megaesophagus B57.31
myocarditis B57.2
nervous system involvement B57.40
meningitis B57.41
meningoencephalitis B57.42
other specified B57.49
specified organ involvement NEC B57.5
acute (with) B57.1
cardiovascular NEC B57.0
myocarditis B57.0
Chagres fever B50.9
Chairridden Z74.09
Chalasia (cardiac sphincter) K21.9
Chalazion H00.19
left H00.16
lower H00.15
upper H00.14
right H00.13
lower H00.12
upper H00.11

Chalcosis —*see also* Disorder, globe,
    degenerative, chalcosis
    cornea —*see* Deposit, cornea
    crystalline lens —*see* Cataract, complicated
    retina H35.89
Chalicosis (pulmonum) J62.8
Chancre (any genital site) (hard) (hunterian)
    (mixed) (primary) (seronegative)
    (seropositive) (syphilitic) A51.0
    congenital A50.07
    conjunctiva NEC A51.2
    Ducrey's A57
    extragenital A51.2
    eyelid A51.2
    lip A51.2
    nipple A51.2
    Nisbet's A57
    of
        carate A67.0
        pinta A67.0
        yaws A66.0
    palate, soft A51.2
    phagedenic A57
    simple A57
    soft A57
        bubo A57
        palate A51.2
    urethra A51.0
    yaws A66.0
Chancroid (anus) (genital) (penis) (perineum)
    (rectum) (urethra) (vulva) A57
Chandler's disease (osteochondritis dissecans,
    hip) —*see* Osteochondritis, dissecans,
    hip
Change (s) (in) (of) —*see also* Removal
    arteriosclerotic —*see* Arteriosclerosis
    bone —*see also* Disorder, bone
        diabetic —*see* Diabetes, bone change
    bowel habit R19.4
    cardiorenal (vascular) —*see* Hypertension,
        cardiorenal
    cardiovascular —*see* Disease, cardiovascular
    circulatory I99.9
    cognitive (mild) (organic) R41.89
    color, tooth, teeth
        during formation K00.8
        posteruptive K03.7
    contraceptive device Z30.433
    corneal membrane H18.30
        Bowman's membrane fold or rupture
            H18.31-
        Descemet's membrane
            fold H18.32-
            rupture H18.33-
    coronary —*see* Disease, heart, ischemic
    degenerative, spine or vertebra —*see*
        Spondylosis
    dental pulp, regressive K04.2
    dressing (nonsurgical) Z48.00
        surgical Z48.01
    heart —*see* Disease, heart
    hip joint —*see* Derangement, joint, hip
    hyperplastic larynx J38.7
    hypertrophic
        nasal sinus J34.89
        turbinate, nasal J34.3
        upper respiratory tract J39.8
    indwelling catheter Z46.6
    inflammatory —*see also* Inflammation
        sacroiliac M46.1
    job, anxiety concerning Z56.1
    joint —*see* Derangement, joint
    life —*see* Menopause
    mental status R41.82
    minimal (glomerular) —*see also* N00-N07
        with fourth character .0 N05.0
    myocardium, myocardial —*see*
        Degeneration, myocardial - of life —*see*
        Menopause
    pacemaker Z45.018
        pulse generator Z45.010

Change (*Continued*)
    personality (enduring) F68.8
        due to (secondary to)
            general medical condition F07.0
        secondary (nonspecific) F60.89
    regressive, dental pulp K04.2
    renal —*see* Disease, renal
    retina H35.9
        myopic H44.2-
    sacroiliac joint M53.3
    senile —*see also* condition R54
    sensory R20.8
    skin R23.9
        acute, due to ultraviolet radiation L56.9
            specified NEC L56.8
        chronic, due to nonionizing radiation L57.9
            specified NEC L57.8
        cyanosis R23.0
        flushing R23.2
        pallor R23.1
        petechiae R23.3
        specified change NEC R23.8
        swelling —*see* Mass, localized
        texture R23.4
    trophic
        arm —*see* Mononeuropathy, upper limb
        leg —*see* Mononeuropathy, lower limb
    vascular I99.9
    vasomotor I73.9
    voice R49.9
        psychogenic F44.4
        specified NEC R49.8
Changing sleep-work schedule, affecting sleep
    G47.26
Changuinola fever A93.1
Chapping skin T69.8
Charcot-Marie-Tooth disease, paralysis or
    syndrome G60.0
Charcot's
    arthropathy —*see* Arthropathy, neuropathic
    cirrhosis K74.3
    disease (tabetic arthropathy) A52.16
    joint (disease) (tabetic) A52.16
        diabetic —*see* Diabetes, with, arthropathy
        syringomyelic G95.0
    syndrome (intermittent claudication) I73.9
CHARGE association Q89.8
Charley-horse (quadriceps) M62.831
    traumatic (quadriceps) S76.11-
Charlouis' disease —*see* Yaws
Cheadle's disease E54
Checking (of)
    cardiac pacemaker (battery) (electrode (s))
        Z45.018
        pulse generator Z45.010
    implantable subdermal contraceptive Z30.46 ◄
    intrauterine contraceptive device Z30.431
Check-up —*see* Examination
Chédiak-Higashi (-Steinbrinck) syndrome
    (congenital gigantism of peroxidase
    granules) E70.330
Cheek —*see* condition
Cheese itch B88.0
Cheese-washer's lung J67.8
Cheese-worker's lung J67.8
Cheilitis (acute) (angular) (catarrhal) (chronic)
    (exfoliative) (gangrenous) (glandular)
    (infectional) (suppurative) (ulcerative)
    (vesicular) K13.0
    actinic (due to sun) L56.8
        other than from sun L59.8
    candidal B37.83
Cheilodynia K13.0
Cheiloschisis —*see* Cleft, lip
Cheilosis (angular) K13.0
    with pellagra E52
    due to
        vitamin B2 (riboflavin) deficiency E53.0
Cheiromegaly M79.89
Cheiropompholyx L30.1
Cheloid —*see* Keloid

Chemical burn —*see* Corrosion, by site
Chemodectoma —*see* Paraganglioma,
    nonchromaffin
Chemosis, conjunctiva —*see* Edema,
    conjunctiva
Chemotherapy (session) (for)
    cancer Z51.11
    neoplasm Z51.11
Cherubism M27.8
Chest —*see* condition
Cheyne-Stokes breathing (respiration) R06.3
Chiari's
    disease or syndrome (hepatic vein
        thrombosis) I82.0
    malformation
        type I G93.5
        type II —*see* Spina bifida
    net Q24.8
Chicago disease B40.9
Chickenpox —*see* Varicella
Chiclero ulcer or sore B55.1
Chigger (infestation) B88.0
Chignon (disease) B36.8
    newborn (from vacuum extraction) (birth
        injury) P12.1
Chilaiditi's syndrome (subphrenic
    displacement, colon) Q43.3
Chilblain (s) (lupus) T69.1
Child
    custody dispute Z65.3
Childbirth —*see* Delivery
Childhood
    cerebral X-linked adrenoleukodystrophy
        E71.520
    period of rapid growth Z00.2
Chill (s) R68.83
    with fever R50.9
    without fever R68.83
    congestive in malarial regions B54
Chilomastigiasis A07.8
Chimera 46,XX/46,XY Q99.0
Chin —*see* condition
Chinese dysentery A03.9
Chionophobia F40.228
Chitral fever A93.1
Chlamydia, chlamydial A74.9
    cervicitis A56.09
    conjunctivitis A74.0
    cystitis A56.01
    endometritis A56.11
    epididymitis A56.19
    female
        pelvic inflammatory disease A56.11
        pelviperitonitis A56.11
    orchitis A56.19
    peritonitis A74.81
    pharyngitis A56.4
    proctitis A56.3
    psittaci (infection) A70
    salpingitis A56.11
    sexually-transmitted infection NEC A56.8
    specified NEC A74.89
    urethritis A56.01
    vulvovaginitis A56.02
Chlamydiosis —*see* Chlamydia
Chloasma (skin) (idiopathic) (symptomatic)
    L81.1
    eyelid H02.719
        hyperthyroid E05.90 [*H02.719*]
            with thyroid storm E05.91 [*H02.719*]
        left H02.716
            lower H02.715
            upper H02.714
        right H02.713
            lower H02.712
            upper H02.711
Chloroma C92.3-
Chlorosis D50.9
    Egyptian B76.9 [*D63.8*]
    miner's B76.9 [*D63.8*]
Chlorotic anemia D50.8

◄ New   ◄▦ Revised   ~~deleted~~ Deleted

Chocolate cyst (ovary) N80.1
Choked
  disc or disk —*see* Papilledema
  on food, phlegm, or vomitus NOS —*see*
      Foreign body, by site
  while vomiting NOS —*see* Foreign body, by
      site
Chokes (resulting from bends) T70.3
Choking sensation R09.89
Cholangiectasis K83.8
Cholangiocarcinoma
  with hepatocellular carcinoma, combined
      C22.0
  liver C22.1
  specified site NEC —*see* Neoplasm,
      malignant, by site
  unspecified site C22.1
Cholangiohepatitis K83.8
  due to fluke infestation B66.1
Cholangiohepatoma C22.0
Cholangiolitis (acute) (chronic) (extrahepatic)
      (gangrenous) (intrahepatic) K83.0
  paratyphoidal —*see* Fever, paratyphoid
  typhoidal A01.09
Cholangioma D13.4
  malignant —*see* Cholangiocarcinoma
Cholangitis (ascending) (primary) (recurrent)
      (sclerosing) (secondary) (stenosing)
      (suppurative) K83.0
  with calculus, bile duct —*see* Calculus, bile
      duct, with cholangitis
  chronic nonsuppurative destructive K74.3
Cholecystectasia K82.8
Cholecystitis K81.9
  with
    calculus, stones in
      bile duct (common) (hepatic) —
          see Calculus, bile duct, with
          cholecystitis
      cystic duct —*see* Calculus, gallbladder,
          with cholecystitis
      gallbladder —*see* Calculus, gallbladder,
          with cholecystitis
      choledocholithiasis —*see* Calculus, bile
          duct, with cholecystitis
      cholelithiasis —*see* Calculus, gallbladder,
          with cholecystitis
  acute (emphysematous) (gangrenous)
      (suppurative) K81.0
    with
      calculus, stones in
        cystic duct —*see* Calculus,
            gallbladder, with cholecystitis,
            acute
        gallbladder —*see* Calculus,
            gallbladder, with cholecystitis,
            acute
        choledocholithiasis —*see* Calculus, bile
            duct, with cholecystitis, acute
        cholelithiasis —*see* Calculus,
            gallbladder, with cholecystitis,
            acute
      chronic cholecystitis K81.2
        with gallbladder calculus K80.12
          with obstruction K80.13
  chronic K81.1
    with acute cholecystitis K81.2
      with gallbladder calculus K80.12
        with obstruction K80.13
  emphysematous (acute) —*see* Cholecystitis,
      acute
  gangrenous —*see* Cholecystitis, acute
  paratyphoidal, current A01.4
  suppurative —*see* Cholecystitis, acute
  typhoidal A01.09
Cholecystolithiasis —*see* Calculus, gallbladder
Choledochitis (suppurative) K83.0
Choledocholith —*see* Calculus, bile duct
Choledocholithiasis (common duct) (hepatic
      duct) —*see* Calculus, bile duct
  cystic —*see* Calculus, gallbladder
  typhoidal A01.09

Cholelithiasis (cystic duct) (gallbladder)
      (impacted) (multiple) —*see* Calculus,
      gallbladder
  bile duct (common) (hepatic) —*see* Calculus,
      bile duct
  hepatic duct —*see* Calculus, bile duct
  specified NEC K80.80
    with obstruction K80.81
Cholemia —*see also* Jaundice
  familial (simple) (congenital) E80.4
  Gilbert's E80.4
Choleperitoneum, choleperitonitis K65.3
Cholera (Asiatic) (epidemic) (malignant) A00.9
  antimonial —*see* Poisoning, antimony
  classical A00.0
  due to Vibrio cholerae 01 A00.9
    biovar cholerae A00.0
    biovar eltor A00.1
    el tor A00.1
  el tor A00.1
Cholerine —*see* Cholera
Cholestasis NEC K83.1
  with hepatocyte injury K71.0
  due to total parenteral nutrition (TPN) K76.89
  pure K71.0
Cholesteatoma (ear) (middle) (with reaction)
      H71.9-
  attic H71.0-
  external ear (canal) H60.4-
  mastoid H71.2-
  postmastoidectomy cavity (recurrent) —*see*
      Complications, postmastoidectomy,
      recurrent cholesteatoma
  recurrent (postmastoidectomy) —*see*
      Complications, postmastoidectomy,
      recurrent cholesteatoma
  tympanum H71.1-
Cholesteatosis, diffuse H71.3-
Cholesteremia E78.00 ◀▥
Cholesterin in vitreous —*see* Deposit, crystalline
Cholesterol
  deposit
    retina H35.89
    vitreous —*see* Deposit, crystalline
  elevated (high) E78.00 ◀▥
    with elevated (high) triglycerides E78.2
    screening for Z13.220
  imbibition of gallbladder K82.4
Cholesterolemia (essential) (pure) E78.00 ◀▥
  familial E78.01 ◀
  hereditary E78.01 ◀
Cholesterolosis, cholesterosis (gallbladder)
      K82.4
  cerebrotendinous E75.5
Cholocolic fistula K82.3
Choluria R82.2
Chondritis M94.8X9
  aurical H61.03-
  costal (Tietze's) M94.0
  external ear H61.03-
  patella, posttraumatic —*see* Chondromalacia,
      patella
  pinna H61.03-
  purulent M94.8X-
  tuberculous NEC A18.02
    intervertebral A18.01
Chondroblastoma —*see also* Neoplasm, bone,
      benign
  malignant —*see* Neoplasm, bone, malignant
Chondrocalcinosis M11.20
  ankle M11.27-
  elbow M11.22-
  familial M11.10
    ankle M11.17-
    elbow M11.12-
    foot joint M11.17-
    hand joint M11.14-
    hip M11.15-
    knee M11.16-
    multiple site M11.19
    shoulder M11.11-

Chondrocalcinosis (*Continued*)
  familial (*Continued*)
    vertebrae M11.18
    wrist M11.13-
  foot joint M11.27-
  hand joint M11.24-
  hip M11.25-
  knee M11.26-
  multiple site M11.29
  shoulder M11.21-
  specified type NEC M11.20
    ankle M11.27-
    elbow M11.22-
    foot joint M11.27-
    hand joint M11.24-
    hip M11.25-
    knee M11.26-
    multiple site M11.29
    shoulder M11.21-
    vertebrae M11.28
    wrist M11.23-
  vertebrae M11.28
  wrist M11.23-
Chondrodermatitis nodularis helicis or
    anthelicis —*see* Perichondritis, ear
Chondrodysplasia Q78.9
  with hemangioma Q78.4
  calcificans congenita Q77.3
  fetalis Q77.4
  metaphyseal (Jansen's) (McKusick's)
      (Schmid's) Q78.8 ◀▥
  punctata Q77.3
Chondrodystrophy, chondrodystrophia
      (familial) (fetalis) (hypoplastic) Q78.9
  calcificans congenita Q77.3
  myotonic (congenital) G71.13
  punctata Q77.3
Chondroectodermal dysplasia Q77.6
Chondrogenesis imperfecta Q77.4
Chondrolysis M94.35-
Chondroma —*see also* Neoplasm, cartilage,
      benign
  juxtacortical —*see* Neoplasm, bone, benign
  periosteal —*see* Neoplasm, bone, benign
Chondromalacia (systemic) M94.20
  acromioclavicular joint M94.21-
  ankle M94.27-
  elbow M94.22-
  foot joint M94.27-
  glenohumeral joint M94.21-
  hand joint M94.24-
  hip M94.25-
  knee M94.26-
    patella M22.4-
  multiple sites M94.29
  patella M22.4-
  rib M94.28
  sacroiliac joint M94.259
  shoulder M94.21-
  sternoclavicular joint M94.21-
  vertebral joint M94.28
  wrist M94.23-
Chondromatosis —*see also* Neoplasm, cartilage,
      uncertain behavior
  internal Q78.4
Chondromyxosarcoma —*see* Neoplasm,
      cartilage, malignant
Chondro-osteodysplasia (Morquio-Brailsford
      type) E76.219
Chondro-osteodystrophy E76.29
Chondro-osteoma —*see* Neoplasm, bone, benign
Chondropathia tuberosa M94.0
Chondrosarcoma —*see* Neoplasm, cartilage,
      malignant
  juxtacortical —*see* Neoplasm, bone, malignant
  mesenchymal —*see* Neoplasm, connective
      tissue, malignant
  myxoid —*see* Neoplasm, cartilage, malignant
Chordee (nonvenereal) N48.89
  congenital Q54.4
  gonococcal A54.09

Chorditis (fibrinous) (nodosa) (tuberosa) J38.2
Chordoma —see Neoplasm, vertebral (column),
   malignant
Chorea (chronic) (gravis) (posthemiplegic)
   (senile) (spasmodic) G25.5
  with
    heart involvement I02.0
     active or acute (conditions in I01-) I02.0
     rheumatic I02.9
      with valvular disorder I02.0
     rheumatic heart disease (chronic) (inactive)
      (quiescent) — code to rheumatic heart
      condition involved
  drug-induced G25.4
  habit F95.8
  hereditary G10
  Huntington's G10
  hysterical F44.4
  minor I02.9
   with heart involvement I02.0
  progressive G25.5
   hereditary G10
  rheumatic (chronic) I02.9
   with heart involvement I02.0
  Sydenham's I02.9
   with heart involvement —see Chorea, with
    rheumatic heart disease
  nonrheumatic G25.5
Choreoathetosis (paroxysmal) G25.5
Chorioadenoma (destruens) D39.2
Chorioamnionitis O41.12-
Chorioangioma D26.7
Choriocarcinoma —see Neoplasm, malignant,
   by site
  combined with
   embryonal carcinoma —see Neoplasm,
    malignant, by site
   other germ cell elements —see Neoplasm,
    malignant, by site
   teratoma —see Neoplasm, malignant, by
    site
  specified site —see Neoplasm, malignant, by
   site
  unspecified site
   female C58
   male C62.90
Chorioencephalitis (acute) (lymphocytic)
   (serous) A87.2
Chorioepithelioma —see Choriocarcinoma
Choriomeningitis (acute) (lymphocytic)
   (serous) A87.2
Chorionepithelioma —see Choriocarcinoma
Chorioretinitis —see also Inflammation,
   chorioretinal
  disseminated —see also Inflammation,
   chorioretinal, disseminated
   in neurosyphilis A52.19
  Egyptian B76.9 [D63.8]
  focal —see also Inflammation, chorioretinal,
   focal
  histoplasmic B39.9 [H32]
  in (due to)
   histoplasmosis B39.9 [H32]
   syphilis (secondary) A51.43
    late A52.71
   toxoplasmosis (acquired) B58.01
    congenital (active) P37.1 [H32]
   tuberculosis A18.53
  juxtapapillary, juxtapapillaris —see
   Inflammation, chorioretinal, focal,
   juxtapapillary
  leprous A30.9 [H32]
  miner's B76.9 [D63.8]
  progressive myopia (degeneration) H44.2-
  syphilitic (secondary) A51.43
   congenital (early) A50.01 [H32]
    late A50.32
   late A52.71
  tuberculous A18.53
Chorioretinopathy, central serous H35.71-
Choroid —see condition

Choroideremia H31.21
Choroiditis —see Chorioretinitis
Choroidopathy —see Disorder, choroid
Choroidoretinitis —see Chorioretinitis
Choroidoretinopathy, central serous —see
   Chorioretinopathy, central serous
Christian-Weber disease M35.6
Christmas disease D67
Chromaffinoma —see also Neoplasm, benign,
   by site
  malignant —see Neoplasm, malignant, by site
Chromatopsia —see Deficiency, color vision
Chromhidrosis, chromidrosis L75.1
Chromoblastomycosis —see Chromomycosis
Chromoconversion R82.91
Chromomycosis B43.9
  brain abscess B43.1
  cerebral B43.1
  cutaneous B43.0
  skin B43.0
  specified NEC B43.8
  subcutaneous abscess or cyst B43.2
Chromophytosis B36.0
Chromosome —see condition by chromosome
   involved
  D (1) —see condition, chromosome 13
  E (3) —see condition, chromosome 18
  G —see condition, chromosome 21
Chromotrichomycosis B36.8
Chronic —see condition
  fracture —see Fracture, pathological
Churg-Strauss syndrome M30.1
Chyle cyst, mesentery I89.8
Chylocele (nonfilarial) I89.8
  filarial —see also Infestation, filarial B74.9
   [N51]
  tunica vaginalis N50.89 ◀▥
   filarial —see also Infestation, filarial B74.9
    [N51]
Chylomicronemia (fasting) (with
   hyperprebetalipoproteinemia) E78.3
Chylopericardium I31.3
  acute I30.9
Chylothorax (nonfilarial) I89.8
  filarial —see also Infestation, filarial B74.9
   [J91.8]
Chylous —see condition
Chyluria (nonfilarial) R82.0
  due to
   bilharziasis B65.0
   Brugia (malayi) B74.1
    timori B74.2
   schistosomiasis (bilharziasis) B65.0
   Wuchereria (bancrofti) B74.0
  filarial —see Infestation, filarial
Cicatricial (deformity) —see Cicatrix
Cicatrix (adherent) (contracted) (painful)
   (vicious) —see also Scar L90.5
  adenoid (and tonsil) J35.8
  alveolar process M26.79
  anus K62.89
  auricle —see Disorder, pinna, specified type
   NEC
  bile duct (common) (hepatic) K83.8
  bladder N32.89
  bone —see Disorder, bone, specified type
   NEC
  brain G93.89
  cervix (postoperative) (postpartal) N88.1
  common duct K83.8
  cornea H17.9
   tuberculous A18.59
  duodenum (bulb), obstructive K31.5
  esophagus K22.2
  eyelid —see Disorder, eyelid function
  hypopharynx J39.2
  lacrimal passages —see Obstruction, lacrimal
  larynx J38.7
  lung J98.4
  middle ear —see subcategory H74.8
  mouth K13.79

Cicatrix (Continued)
  muscle M62.89
   with contracture —see Contraction, muscle
    NEC
  nasopharynx J39.2
  palate (soft) K13.79
  penis N48.89
  pharynx J39.2
  prostate N42.89
  rectum K62.89
  retina —see Scar, chorioretinal
  semilunar cartilage —see Derangement,
   meniscus
  seminal vesicle N50.89 ◀▥
  skin L90.5
   infected L08.89
   postinfective L90.5
   tuberculous B90.8
  specified site NEC L90.5
  throat J39.2
  tongue K14.8
  tonsil (and adenoid) J35.8
  trachea J39.8
  tuberculous NEC B90.9
  urethra N36.8
  uterus N85.8
  vagina N89.8
   postoperative N99.2
  vocal cord J38.3
  wrist, constricting (annular) L90.5
CIDP (chronic inflammatory demyelinating
   polyneuropathy) G61.81
CIN —see Neoplasia, intraepithelial, cervix
CINCA (chronic infantile neurological, cutaneous
   and articular syndrome) M04.2 ◀
Cinchonism —see Deafness, ototoxic
  correct substance properly administered —see
   Table of Drugs and Chemicals, by drug,
   adverse effect
  overdose or wrong substance given or
   taken —see Table of Drugs and
   Chemicals, by drug, poisoning
Circle of Willis —see condition
Circular —see condition
Circulating anticoagulants —see also - Disorder,
   hemorrhagic D68.318
  due to drugs —see also - Disorder,
   hemorrhagic D68.32
  following childbirth O72.3
Circulation
  collateral, any site I99.8
  defective (lower extremity) I99.8
   congenital Q28.9
  embryonic Q28.9
  failure (peripheral) R57.9
   newborn P29.89
  fetal, persistent P29.3
  heart, incomplete Q28.9
Circulatory system —see condition
Circulus senilis (cornea) —see Degeneration,
   cornea, senile
Circumcision (in absence of medical indication)
   (ritual) (routine) Z41.2
Circumscribed —see condition
Circumvallate placenta O43.11-
Cirrhosis, cirrhotic (hepatic) (liver)
   K74.60
  alcoholic K70.30
   with ascites K70.31
  atrophic —see Cirrhosis, liver
  Baumgarten-Cruveilhier K74.69
  biliary (cholangiolitic) (cholangitic)
   (hypertrophic) (obstructive)
   (pericholangiolitic) K74.5
   due to
    Clonorchiasis B66.1
    flukes B66.3
   primary K74.3
   secondary K74.4
  cardiac (of liver) K76.1
  Charcot's K74.3

◀ New   ◀▥ Revised   ~~deleted~~ Deleted

Cirrhosis, cirrhotic (Continued)
cholangiolitic, cholangitic, cholostatic
(primary) K74.3
congestive K76.1
Cruveilhier-Baumgarten K74.69
cryptogenic (liver) K74.69
due to
hepatolenticular degeneration E83.01
Wilson's disease E83.01
xanthomatosis E78.2
fatty K76.0
alcoholic K70.0
Hanot's (hypertrophic) K74.3
hepatic —see Cirrhosis, liver
hypertrophic K74.3
Indian childhood K74.69
kidney —see Sclerosis, renal
Laennec's K70.30
with ascites K70.31
alcoholic K70.30
with ascites K70.31
nonalcoholic K74.69
liver K74.60
alcoholic K70.30
with ascites K70.31
fatty K70.0
congenital P78.81
syphilitic A52.74
lung (chronic) J84.10
macronodular K74.69
alcoholic K70.30
with ascites K70.31
micronodular K74.69
alcoholic K70.30
with ascites K70.31
mixed type K74.69
monolobular K74.3
nephritis —see Sclerosis, renal
nutritional K74.69
alcoholic K70.30
with ascites K70.31
obstructive —see Cirrhosis, biliary
ovarian N83.8
pancreas (duct) K86.89 ◄▥
pigmentary E83.110
portal K74.69
alcoholic K70.30
with ascites K70.31
postnecrotic K74.69
alcoholic K70.30
with ascites K70.31
pulmonary J84.10
renal —see Sclerosis, renal
spleen D73.2
stasis K76.1
Todd's K74.3
unilobar K74.3
xanthomatous (biliary) K74.5
due to xanthomatosis (familial) (metabolic)
(primary) E78.2
Cistern, subarachnoid R93.0
Citrullinemia E72.23
Citrullinuria E72.23
Civatte's disease or poikiloderma L57.3
Clam digger's itch B65.3
Clammy skin R23.1
Clap —see Gonorrhea
Clarke-Hadfield syndrome (pancreatic
infantilism) K86.89 ◄▥
Clark's paralysis G80.9
Clastothrix L67.8
Claude Bernard-Horner syndrome G90.2
traumatic —see Injury, nerve, cervical
sympathetic
Claude's disease or syndrome G46.3
Claudicatio venosa intermittens I87.8
~~Claudication, intermittent I73.9~~
~~cerebral (artery) G45.9~~
~~spinal cord (arteriosclerotic) G95.19~~
~~syphilitic A52.09~~
~~venous (axillary) I87.8~~

Claudication (intermittent) I73.9 ◄
cerebral (artery) G45.9 ◄
spinal cord (arteriosclerotic) G95.19 ◄
syphilitic A52.09
venous (axillary) I87.8 ◄
Claustrophobia F40.240
Clavus (infected) L84
Clawfoot (congenital) Q66.89
acquired —see Deformity, limb, clawfoot
Clawhand (acquired) —see also Deformity, limb,
clawhand
congenital Q68.1
Clawtoe (congenital) Q66.89
acquired —see Deformity, toe, specified
NEC
Clay eating —see Pica
Cleansing of artificial opening —see Attention
to, artificial, opening
Cleft (congenital) —see also Imperfect, closure
alveolar process M26.79
branchial (cyst) (persistent) Q18.2
cricoid cartilage, posterior Q31.8
foot Q72.7 ◄
hand Q71.6 ◄
lip (unilateral) Q36.9
with cleft palate Q37.9
hard Q37.1
with soft Q37.5
soft Q37.3
with hard Q37.5
bilateral Q36.0
with cleft palate Q37.8
hard Q37.0
with soft Q37.4
soft Q37.2
with hard Q37.4
median Q36.1
nose Q30.2
palate Q35.9
with cleft lip (unilateral) Q37.9
bilateral Q37.8
hard Q35.1
with
cleft lip (unilateral) Q37.1
bilateral Q37.0
soft Q35.5
with cleft lip (unilateral) Q37.5
bilateral Q37.4
medial Q35.5
soft Q35.3
with
cleft lip (unilateral) Q37.3
bilateral Q37.2
hard Q35.5
with cleft lip (unilateral) Q37.5
bilateral Q37.4
penis Q55.69
scrotum Q55.29
thyroid cartilage Q31.8
uvula Q35.7
Cleidocranial dysostosis Q74.0
Cleptomania F63.2
Clicking hip (newborn) R29.4
Climacteric (female) —see also Menopause
arthritis (any site) NEC —see Arthritis,
specified form NEC
depression (single episode) F32.89 ◄▥
recurrent episode F33.8 ◄
male (symptoms) (syndrome) NEC N50.89 ◄▥
melancholia (single episode) F32.89 ◄
recurrent episode F33.8 ◄
paranoid state F22
polyarthritis NEC —see Arthritis, specified
form NEC
symptoms (female) N95.1
Clinical research investigation (clinical trial)
(control subject) (normal comparison)
(participant) Z00.6
Clitoris —see condition Cloaca (persistent)
Q43.7
Clonorchiasis, clonorchis infection (liver) B66.1

Clonus R25.8
Closed bite M26.29
Clostridium (C.) perfringens, as cause of
disease classified elsewhere B96.7
Closure
congenital, nose Q30.0
cranial sutures, premature Q75.0
defective or imperfect NEC —see Imperfect,
closure
fistula, delayed —see Fistula
foramen ovale, imperfect Q21.1
hymen N89.6
interauricular septum, defective Q21.1
interventricular septum, defective Q21.0
lacrimal duct —see also Stenosis, lacrimal,
duct
congenital Q10.5
nose (congenital) Q30.0
acquired M95.0
of artificial opening —see Attention to,
artificial, opening
primary angle, without glaucoma damage
H40.06-
vagina N89.5
valve —see Endocarditis
vulva N90.5
Clot (blood) —see also Embolism
artery (obstruction) (occlusion) —see
Embolism
bladder N32.89
brain (intradural or extradural) —see
Occlusion, artery, cerebral
circulation I74.9
heart —see also Infarct, myocardium
not resulting in infarction I51.3 ◄▥
vein —see Thrombosis
Clouded state R40.1
epileptic —see Epilepsy, specified NEC
paroxysmal —see Epilepsy, specified NEC
Cloudy antrum, antra J32.0
Clouston's (hidrotic) ectodermal dysplasia
Q82.4
Clubbed nail pachydermoperiostosis M89.40
[L62]
Clubbing of finger (s) (nails) R68.3
Clubfinger R68.3
congenital Q68.1
Clubfoot (congenital) Q66.89
acquired —see Deformity, limb, clubfoot
equinovarus Q66.0
paralytic —see Deformity, limb, clubfoot
Clubhand (congenital) (radial) Q71.4-
acquired —see Deformity, limb, clubhand
Clubnail R68.3
congenital Q84.6
Clump, kidney Q63.1
Clumsiness, clumsy child syndrome F82
Cluttering F98.81
Clutton's joints A50.51 [M12.80]
Coagulation, intravascular (diffuse)
(disseminated) —see also Defibrination
syndrome
complicating abortion —see Abortion, by
type, complicated by, intravascular
coagulation
following ectopic or molar pregnancy O08.1
Coagulopathy —see also Defect, coagulation
consumption D65
intravascular D65
newborn P60
Coalition
calcaneo-scaphoid Q66.89
tarsal Q66.89
Coalminer's
elbow —see Bursitis, elbow, olecranon
lung or pneumoconiosis J60
Coalworker's lung or pneumoconiosis J60
Coarctation
aorta (preductal) (postductal) Q25.1
pulmonary artery Q25.71
Coated tongue K14.3

Coats' disease (exudative retinopathy) —*see*
Retinopathy, exudative
Cocaine-induced ◄
anxiety disorder F14.980 ◄
bipolar and related disorder F14.94 ◄
depressive disorder F14.94 ◄
obsessive-compulsive and related disorder
F14.988 ◄
psychotic disorder F14.959 ◄
sleep disorder F14.982 ◄
sexual dysfunction F14.981 ◄
Cocainism —*see* Disorder, cocaine use ◄▥
Coccidioidomycosis B38.9
cutaneous B38.3
disseminated B38.7
generalized B38.7
meninges B38.4
prostate B38.81
pulmonary B38.2
acute B38.0
chronic B38.1
skin B38.3
specified NEC B38.89
Coccidioidosis —*see* Coccidioidomycosis
Coccidiosis (intestinal) A07.3
Coccydynia, coccygodynia M53.3
Coccyx —*see* condition
Cochin-China diarrhea K90.1
Cockayne's syndrome Q87.1
Cocked up toe —*see* Deformity, toe, specified
NEC
Cock's peculiar tumor L72.3
Codman's tumor —*see* Neoplasm, bone,
benign
Coenurosis B71.8
Coffee-worker's lung J67.8
Cogan's syndrome H16.32-
oculomotor apraxia H51.8
Coitus, painful (female) N94.10 ◄▥
male N53.12
psychogenic F52.6
Cold J00
with influenza, flu, or grippe —*see* Influenza,
with, respiratory manifestations NEC
agglutinin disease or hemoglobinuria
(chronic) D59.1
bronchial —*see* Bronchitis
chest —*see* Bronchitis
common (head) J00
effects of T69.9
specified effect NEC T69.8
excessive, effects of T69.9
specified effect NEC T69.8
exhaustion from T69.8
exposure to T69.9
specified effect NEC T69.8
head J00
injury syndrome (newborn) P80.0
on lung —*see* Bronchitis
rose J30.1
sensitivity, auto-immune D59.1
virus J00
Coldsore B00.1
Colibacillosis A49.8
as the cause of other disease (*see also*
Escherichia coli) B96.20
generalized A41.50
Colic (bilious) (infantile) (intestinal) (recurrent)
(spasmodic) R10.83
abdomen R10.83
psychogenic F45.8
appendix, appendicular K38.8
bile duct —*see* Calculus, bile duct
biliary —*see* Calculus, bile duct
common duct —*see* Calculus, bile duct
cystic duct —*see* Calculus, gallbladder
Devonshire NEC —*see* Poisoning, lead
gallbladder —*see* Calculus, gallbladder
gallstone —*see* Calculus, gallbladder
gallbladder or cystic duct —*see* Calculus,
gallbladder

Colic (*Continued*)
hepatic (duct) —*see* Calculus, bile duct
hysterical F45.8
kidney N23
lead NEC —*see* Poisoning, lead
mucous K58.9
with diarrhea K58.0
psychogenic F54
nephritic N23
painter's NEC —*see* Poisoning, lead
pancreas K86.89 ◄▥
psychogenic F45.8
renal N23
saturnine NEC —*see* Poisoning, lead
ureter N23
urethral N36.8
due to calculus N21.1
uterus NEC N94.89
menstrual —*see* Dysmenorrhea
worm NOS B83.9
Colicystitis —*see* Cystitis
Colitis (acute) (catarrhal) (chronic)
(noninfective) (hemorrhagic) (*see also*
Enteritis) K52.9
allergic K52.29 ◄▥
with ◄
food protein-induced enterocolitis
syndrome K52.21 ◄
proctocolitis K52.82 ◄
amebic (acute) —*see also* Amebiasis A06.0
nondysenteric A06.2
anthrax A22.2
bacillary —*see* Infection, Shigella
balantidial A07.0
Clostridium difficile A04.7
coccidial A07.3
collagenous K52.831 ◄▥
cystica superficialis K52.89
dietary counseling and surveillance (for)
Z71.3
dietetic —*see also* Colitis, allergic K52.29 ◄▥
drug-induced K52.1
due to radiation K52.0
eosinophilic K52.82
food hypersensitivity —*see also* Colitis,
allergic K52.29 ◄▥
giardial A07.1
granulomatous —*see* Enteritis, regional, large
intestine
infectious —*see* Enteritis, infectious
indeterminate, so stated K52.3 ◄
ischemic K55.9
acute (subacute) —*see also* Ischemia,
intestine, acute K55.039 ◄▥
chronic K55.1
due to mesenteric artery insufficiency
K55.1
fulminant (acute) —*see also* Ischemia,
intestine, acute K55.039 ◄▥
left sided K51.50
with
abscess K51.514
complication K51.519
specified NEC K51.518
fistula K51.513
obstruction K51.512
rectal bleeding K51.511
lymphocytic K52.832 ◄▥
membranous
psychogenic F54
microscopic K52.839 ◄▥
specified NEC K52.838 ◄
mucous —*see* Syndrome, irritable, bowel
psychogenic F54
noninfective K52.9
specified NEC K52.89
polyposa —*see* Polyp, colon, inflammatory
protozoal A07.9
pseudomembranous A04.7
pseudomucinous —*see* Syndrome, irritable,
bowel

Colitis (*Continued*)
regional —*see* Enteritis, regional, large
intestine
segmental —*see* Enteritis, regional, large
intestine
septic —*see* Enteritis, infectious
spastic K58.9
with diarrhea K58.0
psychogenic F54
staphylococcal A04.8
foodborne A05.0
subacute ischemic —*see also* Ischemia,
intestine, acute K55.039 ◄▥
thromboulcerative —*see also* Ischemia,
intestine, acute K55.039 ◄▥
toxic NEC K52.1
due to Clostridium difficile A04.7
transmural —*see* Enteritis, regional, large
intestine
trichomonal A07.8
tuberculous (ulcerative) A18.32
ulcerative (chronic) K51.90
with
complication K51.919
abscess K51.914
fistula K51.913
obstruction K51.912
rectal bleeding K51.911
specified complication NEC K51.918
enterocolitis —*see* Enterocolitis, ulcerative
ileocolitis —*see* Ileocolitis, ulcerative
mucosal proctocolitis —*see* Proctocolitis,
mucosal
proctitis —*see* Proctitis, ulcerative
pseudopolyposis —*see* Polyp, colon,
inflammatory
psychogenic F54
rectosigmoiditis —*see* Rectosigmoiditis,
ulcerative
specified type NEC K51.80
with
complication K51.819
abscess K51.814
fistula K51.813
obstruction K51.812
rectal bleeding K51.811
specified complication NEC
K51.818
Collagenosis, collagen disease (nonvascular)
(vascular) M35.9
cardiovascular I42.8
reactive perforating L87.1
specified NEC M35.8
Collapse R55
adrenal E27.2
cardiorespiratory R57.0
cardiovascular R57.0
newborn P29.89
circulatory (peripheral) R57.9
during or after labor and delivery O75.1
following ectopic or molar pregnancy
O08.3
newborn P29.89
during or
after labor and delivery O75.1
resulting from a procedure, not elsewhere
classified T81.10
external ear canal —*see* Stenosis, external ear
canal
general R55
heart —*see* Disease, heart
heat T67.1
hysterical F44.89
labyrinth, membranous (congenital) Q16.5
lung (massive) —*see also* Atelectasis J98.19
pressure due to anesthesia (general) (local)
or other sedation T88.2
during labor and delivery O74.1
in pregnancy O29.02-
postpartum, puerperal O89.09
myocardial —*see* Disease, heart

◄ New ◄▥ Revised ~~deleted~~ Deleted

Collapse (*Continued*)
nervous F48.8
neurocirculatory F45.8
nose M95.0
postoperative T81.10
pulmonary —*see also* Atelectasis J98.19
newborn —*see* Atelectasis
trachea J39.8
tracheobronchial J98.09
valvular —*see* Endocarditis
vascular (peripheral) R57.9
during or after labor and delivery O75.1
following ectopic or molar pregnancy O08.3
newborn P29.89
vertebra M48.50-
cervical region M48.52-
cervicothoracic region M48.53-
in (due to)
metastasis —*see* Collapse, vertebra, in, specified disease NEC
osteoporosis —*see also* Osteoporosis M80.88
cervical region M80.88
cervicothoracic region M80.88
lumbar region M80.88
lumbosacral region M80.88
multiple sites M80.88
occipito-atlanto-axial region M80.88
sacrococcygeal region M80.88
thoracic region M80.88
thoracolumbar region M80.88
specified disease NEC M48.50-
cervical region M48.52-
cervicothoracic region M48.53-
lumbar region M48.56-
lumbosacral region M48.57-
occipito-atlanto-axial region M48.51-
sacrococcygeal region M48.58-
thoracic region M48.54-
thoracolumbar region M48.55-
lumbar region M48.56-
lumbosacral region M48.57-
occipito-atlanto-axial region M48.51-
sacrococcygeal region M48.58-
thoracic region M48.54-
thoracolumbar region M48.55-
Collateral —*see also* condition
circulation (venous) I87.8
dilation, veins I87.8
Colles' fracture S52.53-
Collet (-Sicard) syndrome G52.7
Collier's asthma or lung J60
Collodion baby Q80.2
Colloid nodule (of thyroid) (cystic) E04.1
Coloboma (iris) Q13.0
eyelid Q10.3
fundus Q14.8
lens Q12.2
optic disc (congenital) Q14.2
acquired H47.31-
Coloenteritis —*see* Enteritis
Colon —*see* condition
Colonization
MRSA (Methicillin resistant Staphylococcus aureus) Z22.322
MSSA (Methicillin susceptible Staphylococcus aureus) Z22.321
status —*see* Carrier (suspected) of
Coloptosis K63.4
Color blindness —*see* Deficiency, color vision
Colostomy
attention to Z43.3
fitting or adjustment Z46.89
malfunctioning K94.03
status Z93.3
Colpitis (acute) —*see* Vaginitis
Colpocele N81.5
Colpocystitis —*see* Vaginitis
Colpospasm N94.2
Column, spinal, vertebral —*see* condition

Coma R40.20
with
motor response (none) R40.231
abnormal R40.233
extension R40.232
flexion withdrawal R40.234
motor response (none) (*Continued*)
localizes pain R40.235
obeys commands R40.236
opening of eyes (never) R40.211
in response to
pain R40.212
sound R40.213
spontaneous R40.214
verbal response (none) R40.221
confused conversation R40.224
inappropriate words R40.223
incomprehensible words R40.222
oriented R40.225
eclamptic —*see* Eclampsia
epileptic —*see* Epilepsy
Glasgow, scale score —*see* Glasgow coma scale
hepatic —*see* Failure, hepatic, by type, with coma
hyperglycemic (diabetic) —*see* Diabetes, by type, with hyperosmolarity, with coma ◀▥
hyperosmolar (diabetic) —*see* Diabetes, by type, with hyperosmolarity, with coma ◀▥
hypoglycemic (diabetic) —*see* Diabetes, by type, with hypoglycemia, with coma ◀▥
nondiabetic E15
in diabetes —*see* Diabetes, coma
insulin-induced —*see* Coma, hypoglycemic
myxedematous E03.5
newborn P91.5
persistent vegetative state R40.3
specified NEC, without documented Glasgow coma scale score, or with partial Glasgow coma scale score reported R40.244
Comatose —*see* Coma
Combat fatigue F43.0
Combined —*see* condition
Comedo, comedones (giant) L70.0
Comedocarcinoma —*see also* Neoplasm, breast, malignant
noninfiltrating
breast D05.8-
specified site —*see* Neoplasm, in situ, by site
unspecified site D05.8-
Comedomastitis —*see* Ectasia, mammary duct
Comminuted fracture - code as Fracture, closed
Common
arterial trunk Q20.0
atrioventricular canal Q21.2
atrium Q21.1
cold (head) J00
truncus (arteriosus) Q20.0
variable immunodeficiency —*see* Immunodeficiency, common variable
ventricle Q20.4
Commotio, commotion (current)
brain —*see* Injury, intracranial, concussion
cerebri —*see* Injury, intracranial, concussion
retinae S05.8X-
spinal cord —*see* Injury, spinal cord, by region
spinalis —*see* Injury, spinal cord, by region
Communication
between
base of aorta and pulmonary artery Q21.4
left ventricle and right atrium Q20.5
pericardial sac and pleural sac Q34.8
pulmonary artery and pulmonary vein, congenital Q25.72
congenital between uterus and digestive or urinary tract Q51.7

Compartment syndrome (deep) (posterior) (traumatic) T79.A0
abdomen T79.A3
lower extremity (hip, buttock, thigh, leg, foot, toes) T79.A2
nontraumatic
abdomen M79.A3
lower extremity (hip, buttock, thigh, leg, foot, toes) M79.A2-
specified site NEC M79.A9
upper extremity (shoulder, arm, forearm, wrist, hand, fingers) M79.A1-
specified site NEC T79.A9
upper extremity (shoulder, arm, forearm, wrist, hand, fingers) T79.A1
Compensation
failure —*see* Disease, heart
neurosis, psychoneurosis —*see* Disorder, factitious
Complaint —*see also* Disease
bowel, functional K59.9
psychogenic F45.8
intestine, functional K59.9
psychogenic F45.8
kidney —*see* Disease, renal
miners' J60
Complete —*see* condition
Complex
Addison-Schilder E71.528
cardiorenal —*see* Hypertension, cardiorenal
Costen's M26.69
disseminated mycobacterium avium-intracellulare (DMAC) A31.2
Eisenmenger's (ventricular septal defect) I27.89
hypersexual F52.8
jumped process, spine —*see* Dislocation, vertebra
primary, tuberculous A15.7
Schilder-Addison E71.528
subluxation (vertebral) M99.19
abdomen M99.19
acromioclavicular M99.17
cervical region M99.11
cervicothoracic M99.11
costochondral M99.18
costovertebral M99.18
head region M99.10
hip M99.15
lower extremity M99.16
lumbar region M99.13
lumbosacral M99.13
occipitocervical M99.10
pelvic region M99.15
pubic M99.15
rib cage M99.18
sacral region M99.14
sacrococcygeal M99.14
sacroiliac M99.14
specified NEC M99.19
sternochondral M99.18
sternoclavicular M99.17
thoracic region M99.12
thoracolumbar M99.12
upper extremity M99.17
Taussig-Bing (transposition, aorta and overriding pulmonary artery) Q20.1
Complication (s) (from) (of)
accidental puncture or laceration during a procedure (of) —*see* Complications, intraoperative (intraprocedural), puncture or laceration
amputation stump (surgical) (late) NEC T87.9
dehiscence T87.81
infection or inflammation T87.40
lower limb T87.4-
upper limb T87.4-
necrosis T87.50
lower limb T87.5-
upper limb T87.5-

Complication *(Continued)*
  amputation stump (surgical) (late) (NEC)
      (Continued)
    neuroma T87.30
      lower limb T87.3-
      upper limb T87.3-
    specified type NEC T87.89
  anastomosis (and bypass) —*see also*
      Complications, prosthetic device or
      implant
    intestinal (internal) NEC K91.89
      involving urinary tract N99.89
    urinary tract (involving intestinal tract)
        N99.89
    vascular —*see* Complications,
        cardiovascular device or implant
  anesthesia, anesthetic —*see also* Anesthesia,
      complication T88.59
    brain, postpartum, puerperal O89.2
    cardiac
      in
        labor and delivery O74.2
        pregnancy O29.19-
      postpartum, puerperal O89.1
    central nervous system
      in
        labor and delivery O74.3
        pregnancy O29.29-
      postpartum, puerperal O89.2
    difficult or failed intubation T88.4
      in pregnancy O29.6-
    failed sedation (conscious) (moderate)
        during procedure T88.52
    general, unintended awareness during
        procedure T88.53 ◀
    hyperthermia, malignant T88.3
    hypothermia T88.51
    intubation failure T88.4
    malignant hyperthermia T88.3
    pulmonary
      in
        labor and delivery O74.1
        pregnancy NEC O29.09-
      postpartum, puerperal O89.09
    shock T88.2
    spinal and epidural
      in
        labor and delivery NEC O74.6
          headache O74.5
        pregnancy NEC O29.5X-
      postpartum, puerperal NEC O89.5
        headache O89.4
    unintended awareness under general
        anesthesia during procedure T88.53 ◀
  anti-reflux device —*see* Complications,
      esophageal anti-reflux device
  aortic (bifurcation) graft —*see* Complications,
      graft, vascular
  aortocoronary (bypass) graft —*see*
      Complications, coronary artery (bypass)
      graft
  aortofemoral (bypass) graft —*see*
      Complications, extremity artery
      (bypass) graft
  arteriovenous
    fistula, surgically created T82.9
      embolism T82.818
      fibrosis T82.828
      hemorrhage T82.838
      infection or inflammation T82.7
      mechanical
        breakdown T82.510
        displacement T82.520
        leakage T82.530
        malposition T82.520
        obstruction T82.590
        perforation T82.590
        protrusion T82.590
      pain T82.848
      specified type NEC T82.898
      stenosis T82.858
      thrombosis T82.868

Complication *(Continued)*
  arteriovenous *(Continued)*
    shunt, surgically created T82.9
      embolism T82.818
      fibrosis T82.828
      hemorrhage T82.838
      infection or inflammation T82.7
      mechanical
        breakdown T82.511
        displacement T82.521
        leakage T82.531
        malposition T82.521
        obstruction T82.591
        perforation T82.591
        protrusion T82.591
      pain T82.848
      specified type NEC T82.898
      stenosis T82.858
      thrombosis T82.868
  arthroplasty —*see* Complications, joint
      prosthesis
  artificial
    fertilization or insemination N98.9
      attempted introduction (of)
        embryo in embryo transfer
            N98.3
        ovum following in vitro fertilization
            N98.2
      hyperstimulation of ovaries
          N98.1
      infection N98.0
      specified NEC N98.8
    heart T82.9
      embolism T82.817
      fibrosis T82.827
      hemorrhage T82.837
      infection or inflammation T82.7
      mechanical
        breakdown T82.512
        displacement T82.522
        leakage T82.532
        malposition T82.522
        obstruction T82.592
        perforation T82.592
        protrusion T82.592
      pain T82.847
      specified type NEC T82.897
      stenosis T82.857
      thrombosis T82.867
    opening
      cecostomy —*see* Complications,
          colostomy
      colostomy —*see* Complications,
          colostomy
      cystostomy —*see* Complications,
          cystostomy
      enterostomy —*see* Complications,
          enterostomy
      gastrostomy —*see* Complications,
          gastrostomy
      ileostomy —*see* Complications,
          enterostomy
      jejunostomy —*see* Complications,
          enterostomy
      nephrostomy —*see* Complications,
          stoma, urinary tract
      tracheostomy —*see* Complications,
          tracheostomy
      ureterostomy —*see* Complications,
          stoma, urinary tract
      urethrostomy —*see* Complications,
          stoma, urinary tract
  balloon implant or device
    gastrointestinal T85.9
      embolism T85.818 ◀▥
      fibrosis T85.828 ◀▥
      hemorrhage T85.838 ◀▥
      infection and inflammation T85.79
      pain T85.848 ◀▥
      specified type NEC T85.898 ◀▥
      stenosis T85.858 ◀▥
      thrombosis T85.868 ◀▥

Complication *(Continued)*
  balloon implant or device *(Continued)*
    vascular (counterpulsation) T82.9
      embolism T82.818
      fibrosis T82.828
      hemorrhage T82.838
      infection or inflammation T82.7
      mechanical
        breakdown T82.513
        displacement T82.523
        leakage T82.533
        malposition T82.523
        obstruction T82.593
        perforation T82.593
        protrusion T82.593
      pain T82.848
      specified type NEC T82.898
      stenosis T82.858
      thrombosis T82.868
  bariatric procedure
    gastric band procedure K95.09
      infection K95.01
    specified procedure NEC K95.89
      infection K95.81
  bile duct implant (prosthetic) T85.9
    embolism T85.818 ◀▥
    fibrosis T85.828 ◀▥
    hemorrhage T85.838 ◀▥
    infection and inflammation T85.79
    mechanical
      breakdown T85.510
      displacement T85.520
      malfunction T85.510
      malposition T85.520
      obstruction T85.590
      perforation T85.590
      protrusion T85.590
      specified NEC T85.590
    pain T85.848 ◀▥
    specified type NEC T85.898 ◀▥
    stenosis T85.858 ◀▥
    thrombosis T85.868 ◀▥
  bladder device (auxiliary) —*see*
      Complications, genitourinary, device or
      implant, urinary system
  bleeding (postoperative) —*see* Complication,
      postoperative, hemorrhage
    intraoperative —*see* Complication,
        intraoperative, hemorrhage
  blood vessel graft —*see* Complications, graft,
      vascular
  bone
    device NEC T84.9
      embolism T84.81
      fibrosis T84.82
      hemorrhage T84.83
      infection or inflammation T84.7
      mechanical
        breakdown T84.318
        displacement T84.328
        malposition T84.328
        obstruction T84.398
        perforation T84.398
        protrusion T84.398
      pain T84.84
      specified type NEC T84.89
      stenosis T84.85
      thrombosis T84.86
    graft —*see* Complications, graft, bone
    growth stimulator (electrode) —*see*
        Complications, electronic stimulator
        device, bone
    marrow transplant —*see* Complications,
        transplant, bone, marrow
  brain neurostimulator (electrode) —*see*
      Complications, electronic stimulator
      device, brain
  breast implant (prosthetic) T85.9
    capsular contracture T85.44
    embolism T85.818 ◀▥
    fibrosis T85.828 ◀▥

Complication *(Continued)*
  breast implant (prosthetic) *(Continued)*
    hemorrhage T85.838 ◀▥
    infection and inflammation T85.79
    mechanical
      breakdown T85.41
      displacement T85.42
      leakage T85.43
      malposition T85.42
      obstruction T85.49
      perforation T85.49
      protrusion T85.49
      specified NEC T85.49
    pain T85.848 ◀▥
    specified type NEC T85.898 ◀▥
    stenosis T85.858 ◀▥
    thrombosis T85.868 ◀▥
  bypass —*see also* Complications, prosthetic device or implant
    aortocoronary —*see* Complications, coronary artery (bypass) graft
    arterial —*see also* Complications, graft, vascular
      extremity —*see* Complications, extremity artery (bypass) graft
  cardiac —*see also* Disease, heart
    device, implant or graft T82.9
      embolism T82.817
      fibrosis T82.827
      hemorrhage T82.837
      infection or inflammation T82.7
        valve prosthesis T82.6
      mechanical
        breakdown T82.519
          specified device NEC T82.518
        displacement T82.529
          specified device NEC T82.528
        leakage T82.539
          specified device NEC T82.538
        malposition T82.529
          specified device NEC T82.528
        obstruction T82.599
          specified device NEC T82.598
        perforation T82.599
          specified device NEC T82.598
        protrusion T82.599
          specified device NEC T82.598
      pain T82.847
      specified type NEC T82.897
      stenosis T82.857
      thrombosis T82.867
  cardiovascular device, graft or implant T82.9
    aortic graft —*see* Complications, graft, vascular
    arteriovenous
      fistula, artificial —*see* Complication, arteriovenous, fistula, surgically created
      shunt —*see* Complication, arteriovenous, shunt, surgically created
    artificial heart —*see* Complication, artificial, heart
    balloon (counterpulsation) device —*see* Complication, balloon implant, vascular
    carotid artery graft —*see* Complications, graft, vascular
    coronary bypass graft —*see* Complication, coronary artery (bypass) graft
    dialysis catheter (vascular) —*see* Complication, catheter, dialysis
    electronic T82.9
      electrode T82.9
        embolism T82.817
        fibrosis T82.827
        hemorrhage T82.837
        infection T82.7
        mechanical
          breakdown T82.110
          displacement T82.120

Complication *(Continued)*
  cardiovascular device, graft or implant *(Continued)*
    electronic *(Continued)*
      electrode *(Continued)*
        mechanical *(Continued)*
          leakage T82.190
          obstruction T82.190
          perforation T82.190
          protrusion T82.190
          specified type NEC T82.190
        pain T82.847
        specified NEC T82.897
        stenosis T82.857
        thrombosis T82.867
      embolism T82.817
      fibrosis T82.827
      hemorrhage T82.837
      infection T82.7
      mechanical
        breakdown T82.119
        displacement T82.129
        leakage T82.199
        obstruction T82.199
        perforation T82.199
        protrusion T82.199
        specified type NEC T82.199
      pain T82.847
      pulse generator T82.9
        embolism T82.817
        fibrosis T82.827
        hemorrhage T82.837
        infection T82.7
        mechanical
          breakdown T82.111
          displacement T82.121
          leakage T82.191
          obstruction T82.191
          perforation T82.191
          protrusion T82.191
          specified type NEC T82.191
        pain T82.847
        specified NEC T82.897
        stenosis T82.857
        thrombosis T82.867
      specified condition NEC T82.897
      specified device NEC T82.9
        embolism T82.817
        fibrosis T82.827
        hemorrhage T82.837
        infection T82.7
        mechanical
          breakdown T82.118
          displacement T82.128
          leakage T82.198
          obstruction T82.198
          perforation T82.198
          protrusion T82.198
          specified type NEC T82.198
        pain T82.847
        specified NEC T82.897
        stenosis T82.857
        thrombosis T82.867
      stenosis T82.857
      thrombosis T82.867
    extremity artery graft —*see* Complication, extremity artery (bypass) graft
    femoral artery graft —*see* Complication, extremity artery (bypass) graft
    heart
      transplant —*see* Complication, transplant, heart
      valve —*see* Complication, prosthetic device, heart valve
        graft —*see* Complication, heart, valve, graft
    heart-lung transplant —*see* Complication, transplant, heart, with lung
    infection or inflammation T82.7
    umbrella device —*see* Complication, umbrella device, vascular

Complication *(Continued)*
  cardiovascular device, graft or implant *(Continued)*
    vascular graft (or anastomosis) —*see* Complication, graft, vascular
    carotid artery (bypass) graft —*see* Complications, graft, vascular
    catheter (device) NEC —*see also* Complications, prosthetic device or implant
      cranial infusion ◀
        infection and inflammation T85.735 ◀
        mechanical ◀
          breakdown T85.610 ◀
          displacement T85.620 ◀
          leakage T85.630 ◀
          malfunction T85.690 ◀
          malposition T85.620 ◀
          obstruction T85.690 ◀
          perforation T85.690 ◀
          protrusion T85.690 ◀
          specified NEC T85.690 ◀
      cystostomy T83.9
        embolism T83.81
        fibrosis T83.82
        hemorrhage T83.83
        infection and inflammation T83.510 ◀▥
        mechanical
          breakdown T83.010
          displacement T83.020
          leakage T83.030
          malposition T83.020
          obstruction T83.090
          perforation T83.090
          protrusion T83.090
          specified NEC T83.090
        pain T83.84
        specified type NEC T83.89
        stenosis T83.85
        thrombosis T83.86
      dialysis (vascular) T82.9
        embolism T82.818
        fibrosis T82.828
        hemorrhage T82.838
        infection and inflammation T82.7
        intraperitoneal —*see* Complications, catheter, intraperitoneal
        mechanical
          breakdown T82.41
          displacement T82.42
          leakage T82.43
          malposition T82.42
          obstruction T82.49
          perforation T82.49
          protrusion T82.49
        pain T82.848
        specified type NEC T82.898
        stenosis T82.858
        thrombosis T82.868
      epidural infusion T85.9
        embolism T85.810 ◀▥
        fibrosis T85.820 ◀▥
        hemorrhage T85.830 ◀▥
        infection and inflammation T85.735 ◀▥
        mechanical
          breakdown T85.610
          displacement T85.620
          leakage T85.630
          malfunction T85.610
          malposition T85.620
          obstruction T85.690
          perforation T85.690
          protrusion T85.690
          specified NEC T85.690
        pain T85.840 ◀▥
        specified type NEC T85.890 ◀▥
        stenosis T85.850 ◀▥
        thrombosis T85.860 ◀▥
      intraperitoneal dialysis T85.9
        embolism T85.818 ◀▥
        fibrosis T85.828 ◀▥

Complication *(Continued)*
  catheter NEC *(Continued)*
    intraperitoneal dialysis *(Continued)*
      hemorrhage T85.838 ◄▥
      infection and inflammation T85.71
      mechanical
        breakdown T85.611
        displacement T85.621
        leakage T85.631
        malfunction T85.611
        malposition T85.621
        obstruction T85.691
        perforation T85.691
        protrusion T85.691
        specified NEC T85.691
      pain T85.848 ◄▥
      specified type NEC T85.898 ◄▥
      stenosis T85.858 ◄▥
      thrombosis T85.868 ◄▥
    intrathecal infusion ◄
      infection and inflammation T85.735 ◄
      mechanical ◄
        breakdown T85.610 ◄
        displacement T85.620 ◄
        leakage T85.630 ◄
        malfunction T85.690 ◄
        malposition T85.620 ◄
        obstruction T85.690 ◄
        perforation T85.690 ◄
        protrusion T85.690 ◄
        specified NEC T85.690 ◄
    intravenous infusion T82.9
      embolism T82.818
      fibrosis T82.828
      hemorrhage T82.838
      infection or inflammation T82.7
      mechanical
        breakdown T82.514
        displacement T82.524
        leakage T82.534
        malposition T82.524
        obstruction T82.594
        perforation T82.594
        protrusion T82.594
      pain T82.848
      specified type NEC T82.898
      stenosis T82.858
      thrombosis T82.868
    spinal infusion ◄
      infection and inflammation T85.735 ◄
      mechanical ◄
        breakdown T85.610 ◄
        displacement T85.620 ◄
        leakage T85.630 ◄
        malfunction T85.690 ◄
        malposition T85.620 ◄
        obstruction T85.690 ◄
        perforation T85.690 ◄
        protrusion T85.690 ◄
        specified NEC T85.690 ◄
    subarachnoid infusion ◄
      infection and inflammation T85.735 ◄
      mechanical ◄
        breakdown T85.610 ◄
        displacement T85.620 ◄
        leakage T85.630 ◄
        malfunction T85.690 ◄
        malposition T85.620 ◄
        obstruction T85.690 ◄
        perforation T85.690 ◄
        protrusion T85.690 ◄
        specified NEC T85.690 ◄
    subdural infusion T85.9
      embolism T85.810 ◄▥
      fibrosis T85.820 ◄▥
      hemorrhage T85.830 ◄▥
      infection and inflammation T85.735 ◄▥
      mechanical
        breakdown T85.610
        displacement T85.620
        leakage T85.630

Complication *(Continued)*
  catheter NEC *(Continued)*
    subdural infusion *(Continued)*
      mechanical *(Continued)*
        malfunction T85.610
        malposition T85.620
        obstruction T85.690
        perforation T85.690
        protrusion T85.690
        specified NEC T85.690
      pain T85.840 ◄▥
      specified type NEC T85.890 ◄▥
      stenosis T85.850 ◄▥
      thrombosis T85.860 ◄▥
    ~~urethral, indwelling T83.9~~
      ~~displacement T83.028~~
      ~~embolism T83.81~~
      ~~fibrosis T83.82~~
      ~~hemorrhage T83.83~~
      ~~infection and inflammation T83.51~~
      ~~leakage T83.038~~
      ~~malposition T83.028~~
      ~~mechanical~~
        ~~breakdown T83.018~~
      ~~obstruction (mechanical) T83.098~~
      ~~pain T83.84~~
      ~~perforation T83.098~~
      ~~protrusion T83.098~~
      ~~specified type NEC T83.098~~
      ~~stenosis T83.85~~
      ~~thrombosis T83.86~~
    ~~urinary (indwelling) —see Complications,~~
      ~~catheter, urethral, indwelling~~
    urethral T83.9
      displacement T83.028 ◄
      embolism T83.81 ◄
      fibrosis T83.82 ◄
      hemorrhage T83.83 ◄
      indwelling ◄
        breakdown T83.011 ◄
        displacement T83.021 ◄
        infection and inflammation T83.511 ◄
        leakage T83.031 ◄
        specified complication NEC T83.091 ◄
      infection and inflammation T83.511 ◄
      leakage T83.038 ◄
      malposition T83.028 ◄
      mechanical ◄
        breakdown T83.011 ◄
        obstruction (mechanical) T83.091 ◄
        pain T83.84 ◄
        perforation T83.091 ◄
        protrusion T83.091 ◄
        specified type NEC T83.091 ◄
        stenosis T83.85 ◄
        thrombosis T83.86 ◄
      urinary NEC
        breakdown T83.018 ◄
        displacement T83.028 ◄
        infection and inflammation T83.518 ◄
        leakage T83.038 ◄
        specified complication NEC T83.098 ◄
  cecostomy (stoma) —see Complications,
    colostomy
  cesarean delivery wound NEC O90.89
    disruption O90.0
    hematoma O90.2
    infection (following delivery) O86.0
  chemotherapy (antineoplastic) NEC T88.7
  chin implant (prosthetic) —see Complication,
    prosthetic device or implant, specified
    NEC
  circulatory system I99.8
    intraoperative I97.88
    postprocedural I97.89
      following cardiac surgery I97.19-
        postcardiotomy syndrome I97.0
      hypertension I97.3
      lymphedema after mastectomy I97.2
      postcardiotomy syndrome I97.0
      specified NEC I97.89

Complication *(Continued)*
  colostomy (stoma) K94.00
    hemorrhage K94.01
    infection K94.02
    malfunction K94.03
    mechanical K94.03
    specified complication NEC
      K94.09
  contraceptive device, intrauterine —
    see Complications, intrauterine,
    contraceptive device
  cord (umbilical) —*see* Complications,
    umbilical cord
  corneal graft —*see* Complications, graft,
    cornea
  coronary artery (bypass) graft T82.9
    atherosclerosis —*see* Arteriosclerosis,
      coronary (artery)
    embolism T82.818
    fibrosis T82.828
    hemorrhage T82.838
    infection and inflammation T82.7
    mechanical
      breakdown T82.211
      displacement T82.212
      leakage T82.213
      malposition T82.212
      obstruction T82.218
      perforation T82.218
      protrusion T82.218
      specified NEC T82.218
    pain T82.848
    specified type NEC T82.898 ◄▥
    stenosis T82.858
    thrombosis T82.868
  counterpulsation device (balloon), intra-
    aortic —*see* Complications, balloon
    implant, vascular
  cystostomy (stoma) N99.518
    catheter —*see* Complications, catheter,
      cystostomy
    hemorrhage N99.510
    infection N99.511
    malfunction N99.512
    specified type NEC N99.518
  delivery —*see also* Complications, obstetric
    O75.9
    procedure (instrumental) (manual)
      (surgical) O75.4
    specified NEC O75.89
  dialysis (peritoneal) (renal) —*see also*
    Complications, infusion
    catheter (vascular) —*see* Complication,
      catheter, dialysis
    peritoneal, intraperitoneal —*see*
      Complications, catheter,
      intraperitoneal
  dorsal column (spinal) neurostimulator —*see*
    Complications, electronic stimulator
    device, spinal cord
  drug NEC T88.7
  ear procedure —*see also* Disorder, ear
    intraoperative H95.88-
      hematoma —*see* Complications,
        intraoperative, hematoma (of),
        ear ◄▥
      hemorrhage —*see* Complications,
        intraoperative, hemorrhage (of),
        ear ◄▥
      laceration —*see* Complications,
        intraoperative, puncture or
        laceration..., ear
      seroma —*see* Complications,
        postprocedural, seroma (of),
        mastoid process ◄
      specified NEC H95.88-
    postoperative H95.89-
      external ear canal stenosis H95.81-
      hematoma —*see* Complications,
        postprocedural, hemorrhage
        (hematoma) (of), ear

Complication *(Continued)*
  ear procedure *(Continued)*
    postoperative *(Continued)*
      hemorrhage —*see* Complications,
        postprocedural, hemorrhage
        (hematoma) (of), ear
      postmastoidectomy —*see* Complications,
        postmastoidectomy
      specified NEC H95.89-
  ectopic pregnancy O08.9
    damage to pelvic organs O08.6
    embolism O08.2
    genital infection O08.0
    hemorrhage (delayed) (excessive) O08.1
    metabolic disorder O08.5
    renal failure O08.4
    shock O08.3
    specified type NEC O08.0
    venous complication NEC O08.7
  electronic stimulator device
    bladder (urinary) —*see* Complications,
      electronic stimulator device, urinary
    bone T84.9
      breakdown T84.310
      displacement T84.320
      embolism T84.81
      fibrosis T84.82
      hemorrhage T84.83
      infection or inflammation T84.7
      malfunction T84.310
      malposition T84.320
      mechanical NEC T84.390
      obstruction T84.390
      pain T84.84
      perforation T84.390
      protrusion T84.390
      specified type NEC T84.89
      stenosis T84.85
      thrombosis T84.86
    brain T85.9
      embolism T85.810 ◀▥
      fibrosis T85.820 ◀▥
      hemorrhage T85.830 ◀▥
      infection and inflammation T85.731 ◀▥
      mechanical
        breakdown T85.110
        displacement T85.120
        leakage T85.190
        malposition T85.120
        obstruction T85.190
        perforation T85.190
        protrusion T85.190
        specified NEC T85.190
      pain T85.840 ◀▥
      specified type NEC T85.890 ◀▥
      stenosis T85.850 ◀▥
      thrombosis T85.860 ◀▥
    cardiac (defibrillator) (pacemaker) —*see*
      Complications, cardiovascular device
      or implant, electronic
    generator (brain) (gastric) (peripheral)
      (sacral) (spinal) ◀
      breakdown T85.113 ◀
      displacement T85.123 ◀
      leakage T85.193 ◀
      malposition T85.123 ◀
      obstruction T85.193 ◀
      perforation T85.193 ◀
      protrusion T85.193 ◀
      specified type NEC T85.193 ◀
    muscle T84.9
      breakdown T84.418
      displacement T84.428
      embolism T84.81
      fibrosis T84.82
      hemorrhage T84.83
      infection or inflammation T84.7
      mechanical NEC T84.498
      pain T84.84
      specified type NEC T84.89
      stenosis T84.85
      thrombosis T84.86

Complication *(Continued)*
  electronic stimulator device *(Continued)*
    nervous system T85.9
      brain —*see* Complications, electronic
        stimulator device, brain
      cranial nerve —*see* Complications,
        electronic stimulator device,
        peripheral nerve ◀
      embolism T85.810 ◀▥
      fibrosis T85.820 ◀▥
      gastric nerve —*see* Complications,
        electronic stimulator device,
        peripheral nerve ◀
      hemorrhage T85.830 ◀▥
      infection and inflammation T85.738 ◀▥
      mechanical
        breakdown T85.118
        displacement T85.128
        leakage T85.199
        malposition T85.128
        obstruction T85.199
        perforation T85.199
        protrusion T85.199
        specified NEC T85.199
      pain T85.840 ◀▥
      peripheral nerve —*see* Complications,
        electronic stimulator device,
        peripheral nerve
      sacral nerve —*see* Complications,
        electronic stimulator device,
        peripheral nerve ◀
      specified type NEC T85.890 ◀▥
      spinal cord —*see* Complications,
        electronic stimulator device, spinal
        cord
      stenosis T85.850 ◀▥
      thrombosis T85.860 ◀▥
      vagal nerve —*see* Complications,
        electronic stimulator device,
        peripheral nerve ◀
    peripheral nerve T85.9
      embolism T85.810 ◀▥
      fibrosis T85.820 ◀▥
      hemorrhage T85.830 ◀▥
      infection and inflammation T85.732 ◀▥
      mechanical
        breakdown T85.111
        displacement T85.121
        leakage T85.191
        malposition T85.121
        obstruction T85.191
        perforation T85.191
        protrusion T85.191
        specified NEC T85.191
      pain T85.840 ◀▥
      specified type NEC T85.890 ◀▥
      stenosis T85.850 ◀▥
      thrombosis T85.860 ◀▥
    spinal cord T85.9
      embolism T85.810 ◀▥
      fibrosis T85.820 ◀▥
      hemorrhage T85.830 ◀▥
      infection and inflammation T85.733 ◀▥
      mechanical
        breakdown T85.112
        displacement T85.122
        leakage T85.192
        malposition T85.122
        obstruction T85.192
        perforation T85.192
        protrusion T85.192
        specified NEC T85.192
      pain T85.840 ◀▥
      specified type NEC T85.890 ◀▥
      stenosis T85.850 ◀▥
      thrombosis T85.860 ◀▥
    urinary T83.9
      embolism T83.81
      fibrosis T83.82
      hemorrhage T83.83
      infection and inflammation T83.598 ◀▥

Complication *(Continued)*
  electronic stimulator device *(Continued)*
    urinary *(Continued)*
      mechanical
        breakdown T83.110
        displacement T83.120
        malposition T83.120
        perforation T83.190
        protrusion T83.190
        specified NEC T83.190
      pain T83.84
      specified type NEC T83.89
      stenosis T83.85
      thrombosis T83.86
  electroshock therapy T88.9
    specified NEC T88.8
  endocrine E34.9
    postprocedural
      adrenal hypofunction E89.6
      hypoinsulinemia E89.1
      hypoparathyroidism E89.2
      hypopituitarism E89.3
      hypothyroidism E89.0
      ovarian failure E89.40
        asymptomatic E89.40
        symptomatic E89.41
      specified NEC E89.89
      testicular hypofunction E89.5
  endodontic treatment NEC M27.59
  enterostomy (stoma) K94.10
    hemorrhage K94.11
    infection K94.12
    malfunction K94.13
    mechanical K94.13
    specified complication NEC K94.19
  episiotomy, disruption O90.1
  esophageal anti-reflux device T85.9
    embolism T85.818 ◀▥
    fibrosis T85.828 ◀▥
    hemorrhage T85.838 ◀▥
    infection and inflammation T85.79
    mechanical
      breakdown T85.511
      displacement T85.521
      malfunction T85.511
      malposition T85.521
      obstruction T85.591
      perforation T85.591
      protrusion T85.591
      specified NEC T85.591
    pain T85.848 ◀▥
    specified type NEC T85.898 ◀▥
    stenosis T85.858 ◀▥
    thrombosis T85.868 ◀▥
  esophagostomy K94.30
    hemorrhage K94.31
    infection K94.32
    malfunction K94.33
    mechanical K94.33
    specified complication NEC K94.39
  extracorporeal circulation T80.90
  extremity artery (bypass) graft T82.9
    arteriosclerosis —*see* Arteriosclerosis,
      extremities, bypass graft
    embolism T82.818
    fibrosis T82.828
    hemorrhage T82.838
    infection and inflammation T82.7
    mechanical
      breakdown T82.318
        femoral artery T82.312
      displacement T82.328
        femoral artery T82.322
      leakage T82.338
        femoral artery T82.332
      malposition T82.328
        femoral artery T82.322
      obstruction T82.398
        femoral artery T82.392
      perforation T82.398
        femoral artery T82.392

Complication *(Continued)*
extremity artery (bypass) graft *(Continued)*
  mechanical *(Continued)*
    protrusion T82.398
      femoral artery T82.392
  pain T82.848
  specified type NEC T82.898
  stenosis T82.858
  thrombosis T82.868
eye H57.9
  corneal graft —*see* Complications, graft, cornea
  implant (prosthetic) T85.9
    embolism T85.818 ◄▥
    fibrosis T85.828 ◄▥
    hemorrhage T85.838 ◄▥
    infection and inflammation T85.79
    mechanical
      breakdown T85.318
      displacement T85.328
      leakage T85.398
      malposition T85.328
      obstruction T85.398
      perforation T85.398
      protrusion T85.398
      specified NEC T85.398
    pain T85.848 ◄▥
    specified type NEC T85.898 ◄▥
    stenosis T85.858 ◄▥
    thrombosis T85.868 ◄▥
  intraocular lens —*see* Complications, intraocular lens
  orbital prosthesis —*see* Complications, orbital prosthesis
female genital N94.9
  device, implant or graft NEC —*see* Complications, genitourinary, device or implant, genital tract
femoral artery (bypass) graft —*see* Complication, extremity artery (bypass) graft
fixation device, internal (orthopedic) T84.9
  infection and inflammation T84.60
    arm T84.61-
      humerus T84.61-
      radius T84.61-
      ulna T84.61-
    leg T84.629
      femur T84.62-
      fibula T84.62-
      tibia T84.62-
    specified site NEC T84.69
    spine T84.63
  mechanical
    breakdown
      limb T84.119
        carpal T84.210
        femur T84.11-
        fibula T84.11-
        humerus T84.11-
        metacarpal T84.210
        metatarsal T84.213
        phalanx
          foot T84.213
          hand T84.210
        radius T84.11-
        tarsal T84.213
        tibia T84.11-
        ulna T84.11-
      specified bone NEC T84.218
      spine T84.216
    displacement
      limb T84.129
        carpal T84.220
        femur T84.12-
        fibula T84.12-
        humerus T84.12-
        metacarpal T84.220
        metatarsal T84.223
        phalanx
          foot T84.223
          hand T84.220

Complication *(Continued)*
fixation device, internal *(Continued)*
  mechanical *(Continued)*
    displacement *(Continued)*
      limb *(Continued)*
        radius T84.12-
        tarsal T84.223
        tibia T84.12-
        ulna T84.12-
      specified bone NEC T84.228
      spine T84.226
    malposition —*see* Complications, fixation device, internal, mechanical, displacement
    obstruction —*see* Complications, fixation device, internal, mechanical, specified type NEC
    perforation —*see* Complications, fixation device, internal, mechanical, specified type NEC
    protrusion —*see* Complications, fixation device, internal, mechanical, specified type NEC
    specified type NEC
      limb T84.199
        carpal T84.290
        femur T84.19-
        fibula T84.19-
        humerus T84.19-
        metacarpal T84.290
        metatarsal T84.293
        phalanx
          foot T84.293
          hand T84.290
        radius T84.19-
        tarsal T84.293
        tibia T84.19-
        ulna T84.19-
      specified bone NEC T84.298
      vertebra T84.296
  specified type NEC T84.89
    embolism T84.81
    fibrosis T84.82
    hemorrhage T84.83
    pain T84.84
    specified complication NEC T84.89
    stenosis T84.85
    thrombosis T84.86
following
  acute myocardial infarction NEC I23.8
    aneurysm (false) (of cardiac wall) (of heart wall) (ruptured) I23.3
    angina I23.7
    atrial
      septal defect I23.1
      thrombosis I23.6
    cardiac wall rupture I23.3
    chordae tendinae rupture I23.4
    defect
      septal
        atrial (heart) I23.1
        ventricular (heart) I23.2
    hemopericardium I23.0
    papillary muscle rupture I23.5
    rupture
      cardiac wall I23.3
        with hemopericardium I23.0
      chordae tendineae I23.4
      papillary muscle I23.5
    specified NEC I23.8
    thrombosis
      atrium I23.6
      auricular appendage I23.6
      ventricle (heart) I23.6
    ventricular
      septal defect I23.2
      thrombosis I23.6
  ectopic or molar pregnancy O08.9
    cardiac arrest O08.81
    sepsis O08.82

Complication *(Continued)*
following *(Continued)*
  ectopic or molar pregnancy *(Continued)*
    specified type NEC O08.89
    urinary tract infection O08.83
  termination of pregnancy —*see* Abortion
  gastrointestinal K92.9
    bile duct prosthesis —*see* Complications, bile duct implant
    esophageal anti-reflux device —*see* Complications, esophageal anti-reflux device
    postoperative
      colostomy —*see* Complications, colostomy
      dumping syndrome K91.1
      enterostomy —*see* Complications, enterostomy
      gastrostomy —*see* Complications, gastrostomy
      malabsorption NEC K91.2
      obstruction K91.3
      postcholecystectomy syndrome K91.5
      specified NEC K91.89
      vomiting after GI surgery K91.0
    prosthetic device or implant
      bile duct prosthesis —*see* Complications, bile duct implant
      esophageal anti-reflux device —*see* Complications, esophageal anti-reflux device
      specified type NEC
        embolism T85.818 ◄▥
        fibrosis T85.828 ◄▥
        hemorrhage T85.838 ◄▥
        mechanical
          breakdown T85.518
          displacement T85.528
          malfunction T85.518
          malposition T85.528
          obstruction T85.598
          perforation T85.598
          protrusion T85.598
          specified NEC T85.598
        pain T85.848 ◄▥
        specified complication NEC T85.898 ◄▥
        stenosis T85.858 ◄▥
        thrombosis T85.868 ◄▥
  gastrostomy (stoma) K94.20
    hemorrhage K94.21
    infection K94.22
    malfunction K94.23
    mechanical K94.23
    specified complication NEC K94.29
  genitourinary
    device or implant T83.9
      genital tract T83.9
        infection or inflammation T83.69 ◄▥
        intrauterine contraceptive device —*see* Complications, intrauterine, contraceptive device
        mechanical —*see* Complications, by device, mechanical
        mesh —*see* Complications, mesh
        penile prosthesis —*see* Complications, prosthetic device, penile
        specified type NEC T83.89
          embolism T83.81
          fibrosis T83.82
          hemorrhage T83.83
          pain T83.84
          specified complication NEC T83.89
          stenosis T83.85
          thrombosis T83.86
        vaginal mesh —*see* Complications, mesh
      urinary system T83.9
        cystostomy catheter —*see* Complication, catheter, cystostomy

◄ New   ◄▥ Revised   ~~deleted~~ Deleted

Complication (Continued)
  genitourinary (Continued)
    device or implant (Continued)
      urinary system (Continued)
        electronic stimulator —see
            Complications, electronic
            stimulator device, urinary
        indwelling urethral catheter —see
            Complications, catheter, urethral,
            indwelling
        infection or inflammation T83.598 ◄▥
          ~~indwelling urinary catheter T83.51~~
          indwelling urethral catheter
              T83.511 ◄
        kidney transplant —see Complication,
            transplant, kidney
        organ graft —see Complication, graft,
            urinary organ
        specified type NEC T83.89
          embolism T83.81
          fibrosis T83.82
          hemorrhage T83.83
          mechanical T83.198
            breakdown T83.118
            displacement T83.128
            malfunction T83.118
            malposition T83.128
            obstruction T83.198
            perforation T83.198
            protrusion T83.198
            specified NEC T83.198
          sphincter, implanted T83.191 ◄
          stent (ileal conduit) (nephroureteral)
              T83.193 ◄
          ureteral indwelling T83.192 ◄
          pain T83.84
          specified complication NEC T83.89
          stenosis T83.85
          thrombosis T83.86
        sphincter implant —see
            Complications, implant, urinary
            sphincter
    postprocedural
      pelvic peritoneal adhesions N99.4
      renal failure N99.0
      specified NEC N99.89
      stoma —see Complications, stoma,
          urinary tract
      urethral stricture —see Stricture, urethra,
          postprocedural
      vaginal
        adhesions N99.2
        vault prolapse N99.3
  graft (bypass) (patch) —see also
      Complications, prosthetic device or
      implant
    aorta —see Complications, graft, vascular
    arterial —see Complication, graft, vascular
    bone T86.839
      failure T86.831
      infection T86.832
      mechanical T84.318
        breakdown T84.318
        displacement T84.328
        protrusion T84.398
        specified type NEC T84.398
      rejection T86.830
      specified type NEC T86.838
    carotid artery —see Complications, graft,
        vascular
    cornea T86.849
      failure T86.841
      infection T86.842
      mechanical T85.398
        breakdown T85.318
        displacement T85.328
        protrusion T85.398
        specified type NEC T85.398
      rejection T86.840
      retroprosthetic membrane T85.398
      specified type NEC T86.848

Complication (Continued)
  graft (Continued)
    femoral artery (bypass) —see Complication,
        extremity artery (bypass) graft
    genital organ or tract —see Complications,
        genitourinary, device or implant,
        genital tract
    muscle T84.9
      breakdown T84.410
      displacement T84.420
      embolism T84.81
      fibrosis T84.82
      hemorrhage T84.83
      infection and inflammation T84.7
      mechanical NEC T84.490
      pain T84.84
      specified type NEC T84.89
      stenosis T84.85
      thrombosis T84.86
    nerve —see Complication, prosthetic device
        or implant, specified NEC
    skin —see Complications, prosthetic device
        or implant, skin graft
    tendon T84.9
      breakdown T84.410
      displacement T84.420
      embolism T84.81
      fibrosis T84.82
      hemorrhage T84.83
      infection and inflammation T84.7
      mechanical NEC T84.490
      pain T84.84
      specified type NEC T84.89
      stenosis T84.85
      thrombosis T84.86
    urinary organ T83.9
      embolism T83.81
      fibrosis T83.82
      hemorrhage T83.83
      infection and inflammation
          T83.598 ◄▥
        indwelling urethral catheter
            T83.511 ◄▥
      mechanical
        breakdown T83.21
        displacement T83.22
        erosion T83.24 ◄
        exposure T83.25 ◄
        leakage T83.23
        malposition T83.22
        obstruction T83.29
        perforation T83.29
        protrusion T83.29
        specified NEC T83.29
      pain T83.84
      specified type NEC T83.89
      stenosis T83.85
      thrombosis T83.86
    vascular T82.9
      embolism T82.818
      femoral artery —see Complication,
          extremity artery (bypass) graft
      fibrosis T82.828
      hemorrhage T82.838
      mechanical
        breakdown T82.319
          aorta (bifurcation) T82.310
          carotid artery T82.311
          specified vessel NEC T82.318
        displacement T82.329
          aorta (bifurcation) T82.320
          carotid artery T82.321
          specified vessel NEC T82.328
        leakage T82.339
          aorta (bifurcation) T82.330
          carotid artery T82.331
          specified vessel NEC T82.338
        malposition T82.329
          aorta (bifurcation) T82.320
          carotid artery T82.321
          specified vessel NEC T82.328

Complication (Continued)
  graft (Continued)
    vascular (Continued)
      mechanical (Continued)
        obstruction T82.399
          aorta (bifurcation) T82.390
          carotid artery T82.391
          specified vessel NEC T82.398
        perforation T82.399
          aorta (bifurcation) T82.390
          carotid artery T82.391
          specified vessel NEC T82.398
        protrusion T82.399
          aorta (bifurcation) T82.390
          carotid artery T82.391
          specified vessel NEC T82.398
      pain T82.848
      specified complication NEC
          T82.898
      stenosis T82.858
      thrombosis T82.868
  heart I51.9
    assist device
      infection and inflammation T82.7
    following acute myocardial infarction —
        see Complications, following, acute
        myocardial infarction
    postoperative —see Complications,
        circulatory system
    transplant —see Complication, transplant,
        heart
      and lung (s) —see Complications,
          transplant, heart, with lung
    valve
      graft (biological) T82.9
        embolism T82.817
        fibrosis T82.827
        hemorrhage T82.837
        infection and inflammation
            T82.7
        mechanical T82.228
          breakdown T82.221
          displacement T82.222
          leakage T82.223
          malposition T82.222
          obstruction T82.228
          perforation T82.228
          protrusion T82.228
        pain T82.847
        specified type NEC T82.897
        stenosis T82.857
        thrombosis T82.867
      prosthesis T82.9
        embolism T82.817
        fibrosis T82.827
        hemorrhage T82.837
        infection or inflammation T82.6
        mechanical T82.09
          breakdown T82.01
          displacement T82.02
          leakage T82.03
          malposition T82.02
          obstruction T82.09
          perforation T82.09
          protrusion T82.09
        pain T82.847
        specified type NEC T82.897
          mechanical T82.09
        stenosis T82.857
        thrombosis T82.867
  hematoma
    intraoperative —see Complication,
        intraoperative, hemorrhage
    postprocedural —see Complication,
        postprocedural, hematoma ◄▥
  hemodialysis —see Complications, dialysis
  hemorrhage
    intraoperative —see Complication,
        intraoperative, hemorrhage
    postprocedural —see Complication,
        postprocedural, hemorrhage

Complication *(Continued)*
  ileostomy (stoma) —*see* Complications,
    enterostomy
  immunization (procedure) —*see*
    Complications, vaccination
  implant —*see also* Complications, by site and
    type
    urinary sphincter T83.9
      embolism T83.81
      fibrosis T83.82
      hemorrhage T83.83
      infection and inflammation
        T83.591 ◄
      mechanical
        breakdown T83.111
        displacement T83.121
        leakage T83.191
        malposition T83.121
        obstruction T83.191
        perforation T83.191
        protrusion T83.191
        specified NEC T83.191
      pain T83.84
      specified type NEC T83.89
      stenosis T83.85
      thrombosis T83.86
  infusion (procedure) T80.90
    air embolism T80.0
    blood —*see* Complications, transfusion
    catheter —*see* Complications, catheter
    infection T80.29
    pump —*see* Complications, cardiovascular,
      device or implant
    sepsis T80.29
    serum reaction —*see also* Reaction, serum
      T80.69
      anaphylactic shock —*see also* Shock,
        anaphylactic T80.59
    specified type NEC T80.89
  inhalation therapy NEC T81.81
  injection (procedure) T80.90
    drug reaction —*see* Reaction, drug
    infection T80.29
    sepsis T80.29
    serum (prophylactic) (therapeutic) —*see*
      Complications, vaccination
    specified type NEC T80.89
    vaccine (any) —*see* Complications,
      vaccination
  inoculation (any) —*see* Complications,
    vaccination
  insulin pump
    infection and inflammation T85.72
    mechanical
      breakdown T85.614
      displacement T85.624
      leakage T85.633
      malposition T85.624
      obstruction T85.694
      perforation T85.694
      protrusion T85.694
      specified NEC T85.694
  intestinal pouch NEC K91.858
  intraocular lens (prosthetic) T85.9
    embolism T85.818 ◄
    fibrosis T85.828 ◄
    hemorrhage T85.838 ◄
    infection and inflammation
      T85.79
    mechanical
      breakdown T85.21
      displacement T85.22
      malposition T85.22
      obstruction T85.29
      perforation T85.29
      protrusion T85.29
      specified NEC T85.29
    pain T85.848 ◄
    specified type NEC T85.898 ◄
    stenosis T85.858 ◄
    thrombosis T85.868 ◄

Complication *(Continued)*
  intraoperative (intraprocedural)
    cardiac arrest
      during cardiac surgery I97.710
      during other surgery I97.711
    cardiac functional disturbance NEC
      during cardiac surgery I97.790
      during other surgery I97.791
    hemorrhage (hematoma) (of)
      circulatory system organ or structure
        during cardiac bypass I97.411
        during cardiac catheterization I97.410
        during other circulatory system
          procedure I97.418
        during other procedure I97.42
      digestive system organ
        during procedure on digestive system
          K91.61
        during procedure on other organ
          K91.62
      ear
        during procedure on ear and mastoid
          process H95.21
        during procedure on other organ
          H95.22
      endocrine system organ or structure
        during procedure on endocrine
          system organ or structure E36.01
        during procedure on other organ
          E36.02
      eye and adnexa
        during ophthalmic procedure H59.11-
        during other procedure H59.12-
      genitourinary organ or structure
        during procedure on genitourinary
          organ or structure N99.61
        during procedure on other organ
          N99.62
      mastoid process
        during procedure on ear and mastoid
          process H95.21
        during procedure on other organ
          H95.22
      musculoskeletal structure
        during musculoskeletal surgery
          M96.810
        during non-orthopedic surgery
          M96.811
        during orthopedic surgery M96.810
      nervous system
        during a nervous system procedure
          G97.31
        during other procedure G97.32
      respiratory system
        during other procedure J95.62
        during procedure on respiratory
          system organ or structure J95.61
      skin and subcutaneous tissue
        during a dermatologic procedure
          L76.01
        during a procedure on other organ
          L76.02
      spleen
        during a procedure on other organ
          D78.02
        during a procedure on the spleen
          D78.01
    puncture or laceration (accidental)
      (unintentional) (of)
      brain
        during a nervous system procedure
          G97.48
        during other procedure G97.49
      circulatory system organ or structure
        during circulatory system procedure
          I97.51
        during other procedure I97.52
      digestive system
        during procedure on digestive system
          K91.71
        during procedure on other organ
          K91.72

Complication *(Continued)*
  intraoperative *(Continued)*
    puncture or laceration *(Continued)*
      ear
        during procedure on ear and mastoid
          process H95.31
        during procedure on other organ
          H95.32
      endocrine system organ or structure
        during procedure on endocrine
          system organ or structure E36.11
        during procedure on other organ
          E36.12
      eye and adnexa
        during ophthalmic procedure H59.21-
        during other procedure H59.22-
      genitourinary organ or structure
        during procedure on genitourinary
          organ or structure N99.71
        during procedure on other organ
          N99.72
      mastoid process
        during procedure on ear and mastoid
          process H95.31
        during procedure on other organ
          H95.32
      musculoskeletal structure
        during musculoskeletal surgery
          M96.820
        during non-orthopedic surgery
          M96.821
        during orthopedic surgery M96.820
      nervous system
        during a nervous system procedure
          G97.48
        during other procedure G97.49
      respiratory system
        during other procedure J95.72
        during procedure on respiratory
          system organ or structure J95.71
      skin and subcutaneous tissue
        during a dermatologic procedure
          L76.11
        during a procedure on other organ
          L76.12
      spleen
        during a procedure on other organ
          D78.12
        during a procedure on the spleen
          D78.11
    specified NEC
      circulatory system I97.88
      digestive system K91.81
      ear H95.88
      endocrine system E36.8
      eye and adnexa H59.88
      genitourinary system N99.81
      mastoid process H95.88
      musculoskeletal structure M96.89
      nervous system G97.81
      respiratory system J95.88
      skin and subcutaneous tissue L76.81
      spleen D78.81
  intraperitoneal catheter (dialysis)
    (infusion) —*see* Complications, catheter,
    intraperitoneal
  intrathecal infusion pump ◄
    infection and inflammation T85.738 ◄
    mechanical ◄
      breakdown T85.615 ◄
      displacement T85.625 ◄
      leakage T85.635 ◄
      malfunction T85.695 ◄
      malposition T85.625 ◄
      obstruction T85.695 ◄
      perforation T85.695 ◄
      protrusion T85.695 ◄
      specified NEC T85.695 ◄
  intrauterine
    contraceptive device
      embolism T83.81
      fibrosis T83.82

◄ New   ◄▥ Revised   ~~deleted~~ Deleted

Complication *(Continued)*
intrauterine *(Continued)*
contraceptive device *(Continued)*
hemorrhage T83.83
infection and inflammation T83.69 ◀▥
mechanical
breakdown T83.31
displacement T83.32
malposition T83.32
obstruction T83.39
perforation T83.39
protrusion T83.39
specified NEC T83.39
pain T83.84
specified type NEC T83.89
stenosis T83.85
thrombosis T83.86
procedure (fetal), to newborn P96.5
jejunostomy (stoma) —*see* Complications,
enterostomy
joint prosthesis, internal T84.9
breakage (fracture) T84.01-
dislocation T84.02-
fracture T84.01-
infection or inflammation T84.50
hip T84.5-
knee T84.5-
specified joint NEC T84.59
instability T84.02-
malposition —*see* Complications, joint
prosthesis, mechanical, displacement
mechanical
breakage, broken T84.01-
dislocation T84.02-
fracture T84.01-
instability T84.02-
leakage —*see* Complications, joint
prosthesis, mechanical, specified
NEC
loosening T84.039
hip T84.03-
knee T84.03-
specified joint NEC T84.038
obstruction —*see* Complications, joint
prosthesis, mechanical, specified
NEC
perforation —*see* Complications, joint
prosthesis, mechanical, specified
NEC
periprosthetic
fracture T84.049
hip T84.04-
knee T84.04-
other specified joint T84.048
osteolysis T84.059 ◀
hip T84.05- ◀
knee T84.05- ◀
other specified joint T84.058 ◀
protrusion —*see* Complications, joint
prosthesis, mechanical, specified
NEC
specified complication NEC T84.099
hip T84.09-
knee T84.09-
other specified joint T84.098
subluxation T84.02-
wear of articular bearing surface T84.069
hip T84.06-
knee T84.06-
other specified joint T84.068
specified joint NEC T84.89
embolism T84.81
fibrosis T84.82
hemorrhage T84.83
pain T84.84
specified complication NEC T84.89
stenosis T84.85
thrombosis T84.86
subluxation T84.02-
kidney transplant —*see* Complications,
transplant, kidney

Complication *(Continued)*
labor O75.9
specified NEC O75.89
liver transplant (immune or nonimmune) —
see Complications, transplant, liver
lumbar puncture G97.1
cerebrospinal fluid leak G97.0
headache or reaction G97.1
lung transplant —*see* Complications,
transplant, lung
and heart —*see* Complications, transplant,
lung, with heart
male genital N50.9
device, implant or graft —*see*
Complications, genitourinary, device
or implant, genital tract
postprocedural or postoperative —*see*
Complications, genitourinary,
postprocedural
specified NEC N99.89
mastoid (process) procedure
intraoperative H95.88-
hematoma —*see* Complications,
intraoperative, hemorrhage
(hematoma) (of), mastoid
process
hemorrhage —*see* Complications,
intraoperative, hemorrhage
(hematoma) (of), mastoid
process
laceration —*see* Complications,
intraoperative, puncture or
laceration..., mastoid
process
specified NEC H95.88-
postmastoidectomy —*see* Complications,
postmastoidectomy
postoperative H95.89-
external ear canal stenosis H95.81-
hematoma —*see* Complications...,
postprocedural, hematoma (of),
mastoid process ◀▥
hemorrhage —*see* Complications...,
postprocedural, hemorrhage (of),
mastoid process ◀▥
postmastoidectomy —*see* Complications,
postmastoidectomy
seroma —*see* Complications,
postprocedural, seroma (of),
mastoid process ◀
specified NEC H95.89-
mastoidectomy cavity —*see* Complications,
postmastoidectomy
mechanical —*see* Complications, by site and
type, mechanical
medical procedures (*see also* Complication(s),
intraoperative) T88.9
metabolic E88.9
postoperative E89.89
specified NEC E89.89
molar pregnancy NOS O08.9
damage to pelvic organs O08.6
embolism O08.2
genital infection O08.0
hemorrhage (delayed) (excessive) O08.1
metabolic disorder O08.5
renal failure O08.4
shock O08.3
specified type NEC O08.0
venous complication NEC O08.7
musculoskeletal system —*see also*
Complication, intraoperative
(intraprocedural), by site
device, implant or graft NEC —*see*
Complications, orthopedic, device or
implant
internal fixation (nail) (plate) (rod) —*see*
Complications, fixation device,
internal
joint prosthesis —*see* Complications, joint
prosthesis

Complication *(Continued)*
musculoskeletal system *(Continued)*
postoperative (postprocedural) M96.89
with osteoporosis —*see* Osteoporosis
fracture following insertion of device —
see Fracture, following insertion of
orthopedic implant, joint prosthesis
or bone plate
joint instability after prosthesis removal
M96.89
lordosis M96.4
postlaminectomy syndrome NEC M96.1
kyphosis M96.2 ◀▥
pseudarthrosis M96.0
specified complication NEC M96.89
post radiation M96.89
kyphosis M96.3
scoliosis M96.5
specified complication NEC M96.89
nephrostomy (stoma) —*see* Complications,
stoma, urinary tract, external NEC
nervous system G98.8
central G96.9
device, implant or graft —*see also*
Complication, prosthetic device or
implant, specified NEC
electronic stimulator (electrode (s)) —
see Complications, electronic
stimulator device
specified NEC ◀
infection and inflammation T85.738 ◀
mechanical T85.695 ◀
breakdown T85.615 ◀
displacement T85.625 ◀
leakage T85.635 ◀
malfunction T85.695 ◀
malposition T85.625 ◀
obstruction T85.695 ◀
perforation T85.695 ◀
protrusion T85.695 ◀
specified NEC T85.695 ◀
ventricular shunt —*see* Complications,
ventricular shunt
electronic stimulator (electrode (s)) —*see*
Complications, electronic stimulator
device
postprocedural G97.82
intracranial hypotension G97.2
specified NEC G97.82
spinal fluid leak G97.0
newborn, due to intrauterine (fetal)
procedure P96.5
nonabsorbable (permanent) sutures —*see*
Complication, sutures, permanent
obstetric O75.9
procedure (instrumental) (manual)
(surgical) specified NEC O75.4
specified NEC O75.89
surgical wound NEC O90.89
hematoma O90.2
infection O86.0
ocular lens implant —*see* Complications,
intraocular lens
ophthalmologic
postprocedural bleb —*see* Blebitis
orbital prosthesis T85.9
embolism T85.818 ◀▥
fibrosis T85.828 ◀▥
hemorrhage T85.838 ◀▥
infection and inflammation T85.79
mechanical
breakdown T85.31-
displacement T85.32-
malposition T85.32-
obstruction T85.39-
perforation T85.39-
protrusion T85.39-
specified NEC T85.39-
pain T85.848 ◀▥
specified type NEC T85.898 ◀▥
stenosis T85.858 ◀▥
thrombosis T85.868 ◀▥

Complication (*Continued*)
organ or tissue transplant (partial) (total) —
see Complications, transplant
orthopedic —*see also* Disorder, soft tissue
device or implant T84.9
bone
device or implant —*see* Complication,
bone, device NEC
graft —*see* Complication, graft, bone
breakdown T84.418
displacement T84.428
electronic bone stimulator —*see*
Complications, electronic
stimulator device, bone
embolism T84.81
fibrosis T84.82
fixation device —*see* Complication,
fixation device, internal
hemorrhage T84.83
infection or inflammation T84.7
joint prosthesis —*see* Complication, joint
prosthesis, internal
malfunction T84.418
malposition T84.428
mechanical NEC T84.498
muscle graft —*see* Complications, graft,
muscle
obstruction T84.498
pain T84.84
perforation T84.498
protrusion T84.498
specified complication NEC T84.89
stenosis T84.85
tendon graft —*see* Complications, graft,
tendon
thrombosis T84.86
fracture (following insertion of device) —
see Fracture, following insertion of
orthopedic implant, joint prosthesis
or bone plate
postprocedural M96.89
fracture —*see* Fracture, following
insertion of orthopedic implant,
joint prosthesis or bone plate
postlaminectomy syndrome NEC M96.1
kyphosis M96.3
lordosis M96.4
postradiation
kyphosis M96.2
scoliosis M96.5
pseudarthrosis post-fusion M96.0
specified type NEC M96.89
pacemaker (cardiac) —*see* Complications,
cardiovascular device or implant,
electronic
pancreas transplant —*see* Complications,
transplant, pancreas
penile prosthesis (implant) —*see*
Complications, prosthetic device, penile
perfusion NEC T80.90
perineal repair (obstetrical) NEC O90.89
disruption O90.1
hematoma O90.2
infection (following delivery) O86.0
phototherapy T88.9
specified NEC T88.8
postmastoidectomy NEC H95.19-
cyst, mucosal H95.13-
granulation H95.12-
inflammation, chronic H95.11-
recurrent cholesteatoma H95.0-
postoperative —*see* Complications,
postprocedural
circulatory —*see* Complications, circulatory
system
ear —*see* Complications, ear
endocrine —*see* Complications,
endocrine
eye —*see* Complications, eye
lumbar puncture G97.1
cerebrospinal fluid leak G97.0

Complication (*Continued*)
postoperative (*Continued*)
nervous system (central) (peripheral) —*see*
Complications, nervous system
respiratory system —*see* Complications,
respiratory system
postprocedural —*see also* Complications,
surgical procedure
cardiac arrest
following cardiac surgery I97.120
following other surgery I97.121
cardiac functional disturbance NEC
following cardiac surgery I97.190
following other surgery I97.191
cardiac insufficiency
following cardiac surgery I97.110
following other surgery I97.111
chorioretinal scars following retinal
surgery H59.81-
following cataract surgery
cataract (lens) fragments H59.02-
cystoid macular edema H59.03-
specified NEC H59.09-
vitreous (touch) syndrome H59.01-
heart failure
following cardiac surgery I97.130
following other surgery I97.131
hematoma (of) ◄
circulatory system organ or structure ◄
following cardiac bypass I97.631 ◄
following cardiac catheterization
I97.630 ◄
following other circulatory system
procedure I97.638 ◄
following other procedure I97.621 ◄
digestive system ◄
following procedure on digestive
system K91.870 ◄
following procedure on other organ
K91.871 ◄
ear ◄
following other procedure H95.52 ◄
following procedure on ear and
mastoid process H95.51 ◄
endocrine system ◄
following endocrine system procedure
E89.820 ◄
following other procedure E89.821 ◄
eye and adnexa ◄
following ophthalmic procedure
H59.33-
following other procedure H59.34- ◄
genitourinary organ or structure ◄
following procedure on genitourinary
organ or structure N99.840 ◄
following procedure on other organ
N99.841 ◄
mastoid process ◄
following other procedure H95.52 ◄
following procedure on ear and
mastoid process H95.51 ◄
musculoskeletal structure ◄
following musculoskeletal surgery
M96.840 ◄
following non-orthopedic surgery
M96.841 ◄
following orthopedic surgery
M96.840 ◄
nervous system ◄
following nervous system procedure
G97.61 ◄
following other procedure G97.62 ◄
respiratory system ◄
following other procedure J95.861 ◄
following procedure on respiratory
system organ or structure
J95.860 ◄
skin and subcutaneous tissue ◄
following dermatologic procedure
L76.31 ◄
following procedure on other organ
L76.32 ◄

Complication (*Continued*)
postprocedural (*Continued*)
hematoma (*Continued*)
spleen ◄
following procedure on other organ
D78.32 ◄
following procedure on the spleen
D78.31 ◄
hemorrhage (of) ◄⫻
circulatory system organ or structure
~~following a cardiac bypass I97.611~~
~~following a cardiac catheterization~~
~~I97.610~~
following cardiac bypass I97.611 ◄
following cardiac catheterization
I97.610 ◄
following other circulatory system
procedure I97.618 ◄
following other procedure I97.620 ⫻
digestive system
following procedure on digestive
system K91.840 ◄
following procedure on other organ
K91.841 ◄
ear
following other procedure H95.42 ◄
following procedure on ear and
mastoid process H95.41 ◄
endocrine system
following endocrine system procedure
E89.810 ◄
following other procedure E89.811 ◄
eye and adnexa
following ophthalmic procedure
H59.31-
following other procedure H59.32-
genitourinary organ or structure
following procedure on
genitourinary organ or
structure N99.820 ◄
following procedure on other organ
N99.821 ◄
mastoid process
following other procedure H95.42 ◄
following procedure on ear and
mastoid process H95.41 ◄
musculoskeletal structure
following musculoskeletal surgery
M96.830 ◄
following non-orthopedic surgery
M96.831 ◄
following orthopedic surgery M96.830 ◄
nervous system
~~following a nervous system procedure~~
~~G97.51~~
following nervous system procedure
G97.51 ◄
following other procedure G97.52 ◄
respiratory system
following other procedure J95.831 ◄
following procedure on respiratory
system organ or structure J95.830 ◄
skin and subcutaneous tissue
~~following a dermatologic procedure~~
~~L76.21~~
following dermatologic procedure
L76.21 ◄
following a procedure on other organ
L76.22 ◄
spleen
following procedure on other organ
D78.22 ◄
following procedure on the spleen
D78.21 ◄
seroma (of) ◄
circulatory system organ or structure ◄
following cardiac bypass I97.641 ◄
following cardiac catheterization
I97.640 ◄
following other circulatory system
procedure I97.648 ◄
following other procedure I97.622 ◄

◄ New   ⫻ Revised   ~~deleted~~ Deleted

Complication *(Continued)*
 postprocedural *(Continued)*
  seroma *(Continued)*
   digestive system ◀
    following procedure on digestive
      system K91.872 ◀
    following procedure on other organ
      K91.873 ◀
   ear ◀
    following other procedure H95.54 ◀
    following procedure on ear and
      mastoid process H95.53 ◀
   endocrine system ◀
    following endocrine system procedure
      E89.822 ◀
    following other procedure E89.823 ◀
   eye and adnexa ◀
    following ophthalmic procedure
      H59.35-
    following other procedure H59.36- ◀
   genitourinary organ or structure ◀
    following procedure on genitourinary
      organ or structure N99.842 ◀
    following procedure on other organ
      N99.843 ◀
   mastoid process ◀
    following other procedure H95.54 ◀
    following procedure on ear and
      mastoid process H95.53 ◀
   musculoskeletal structure ◀
    following musculoskeletal surgery
      M96.842 ◀
    following non-orthopedic surgery
      M96.843 ◀
    following orthopedic surgery
      M96.842 ◀
   nervous system ◀
    following nervous system procedure
      G97.63 ◀
    following other procedure G97.64 ◀
   respiratory system ◀
    following other procedure J95.863 ◀
    following procedure on respiratory
      system organ or structure
      J95.862 ◀
   skin and subcutaneous tissue ◀
    following dermatologic procedure
      L76.33 ◀
    following procedure on other organ
      L76.34 ◀
   spleen ◀
    following procedure on other organ
      D78.34 ◀
    following procedure on the spleen
      D78.33 ◀
  specified NEC
   circulatory system I97.89
   digestive K91.89
   ear H95.89
   endocrine E89.89
   eye and adnexa H59.89
   genitourinary N99.89
   mastoid process H95.89
   metabolic E89.89
   musculoskeletal structure M96.89
   nervous system G97.82
   respiratory system J95.89
   skin and subcutaneous tissue L76.82
   spleen D78.89
 pregnancy NEC —*see* Pregnancy,
   complicated by
 prosthetic device or implant T85.9
  bile duct —*see* Complications, bile duct
    implant
  breast —*see* Complications, breast implant
  bulking agent ◀
   ureteral ◀
    erosion T83.714 ◀
    exposure T83.724 ◀
   urethral ◀
    erosion T83.713 ◀
    exposure T83.723 ◀

Complication *(Continued)*
 prosthetic device or implant *(Continued)*
  cardiac and vascular NEC —*see*
    Complications, cardiovascular
    device or implant
  corneal transplant —*see* Complications,
    graft, cornea
  electronic nervous system stimulator —*see*
    Complications, electronic stimulator
    device
  epidural infusion catheter —*see*
    Complications, catheter, epidural
  esophageal anti-reflux device —*see*
    Complications, esophageal anti-reflux
    device
  genital organ or tract —*see* Complications,
    genitourinary, device or implant,
    genital tract
   specified NEC T83.79 ◀
  heart valve —*see* Complications, heart,
    valve, prosthesis
  infection or inflammation T85.79
   intestine transplant T86.892
   liver transplant T86.43
   lung transplant T86.812
   pancreas transplant T86.892
   skin graft T86.822
  intraocular lens —*see* Complications,
    intraocular lens
  intraperitoneal (dialysis) catheter —
    see Complications, catheter,
    intraperitoneal
  joint —*see* Complications, joint prosthesis,
    internal
  mechanical NEC T85.698
   dialysis catheter (vascular) —*see also*
     Complication, catheter, dialysis,
     mechanical
    peritoneal —*see* Complication,
      catheter, intraperitoneal,
      mechanical
   gastrointestinal device T85.598
   ocular device T85.398
   subdural (infusion) catheter T85.690
   suture, permanent T85.692
    that for bone repair —*see*
      Complications, fixation device,
      internal (orthopedic), mechanical
   ventricular shunt
    breakdown T85.01
    displacement T85.02
    leakage T85.03
    malposition T85.02
    obstruction T85.09
    perforation T85.09
    protrusion T85.09
    specified NEC T85.09
  mesh
   erosion (to surrounding organ or tissue)
     T83.717 ◀▥
    urethral (into pelvic floor muscles)
      T83.712 ◀
    vaginal (into pelvic floor muscles)
      T83.711
   exposure (into surrounding organ or
     tissue) T83.727 ◀▥
    urethral (through urethral wall)
      T83.722 ◀
    vaginal (into vagina) (through vaginal
      wall) T83.721
  orbital —*see* Complications, orbital
    prosthesis
  penile T83.9
   embolism T83.81
   fibrosis T83.82
   hemorrhage T83.83
   infection and inflammation T83.61 ◀▥
   mechanical
    breakdown T83.410
    displacement T83.420
    leakage T83.490
    malposition T83.420

Complication *(Continued)*
 prosthetic device or implant *(Continued)*
  penile *(Continued)*
   mechanical *(Continued)*
    obstruction T83.490
    perforation T83.490
    protrusion T83.490
    specified NEC T83.490
   pain T83.84
   specified type NEC T83.89
   stenosis T83.85
   thrombosis T83.86
  prosthetic materials NEC
   erosion (to surrounding organ or tissue)
     T83.718
    ~~vaginal (into pelvic floor muscles)~~
      ~~T83.711~~
   exposure (into surrounding organ or
     tissue) T83.728
    ~~vaginal (into vagina) (through vaginal~~
      ~~wall) T83.721~~
  skin graft T86.829
   artificial skin or decellularized
     allodermis
    embolism T85.818 ◀▥
    fibrosis T85.828 ◀▥
    hemorrhage T85.838 ◀▥
    infection and inflammation T85.79
    mechanical
     breakdown T85.613
     displacement T85.623
     malfunction T85.613
     malposition T85.623
     obstruction T85.693
     perforation T85.693
     protrusion T85.693
     specified NEC T85.693
    pain T85.848 ◀▥
    specified type NEC T85.898 ◀▥
    stenosis T85.858 ◀▥
    thrombosis T85.868 ◀▥
   failure T86.821
   infection T86.822
   rejection T86.820
   specified NEC T86.828
  sling ◀
   urethral (female) (male) ◀
    erosion T83.712 ◀
    exposure T83.722 ◀
  specified NEC T85.9
   embolism T85.818 ◀▥
   fibrosis T85.828 ◀▥
   hemorrhage T85.838 ◀▥
   infection and inflammation T85.79
   mechanical
    breakdown T85.618
    displacement T85.628
    leakage T85.638
    malfunction T85.618
    malposition T85.628
    obstruction T85.698
    perforation T85.698
    protrusion T85.698
    specified NEC T85.698
   pain T85.848 ◀▥
   specified type NEC T85.898 ◀▥
   stenosis T85.858 ◀▥
   thrombosis T85.868 ◀▥
  subdural infusion catheter —*see*
    Complications, catheter, subdural
  sutures —*see* Complications, sutures
  urinary organ or tract NEC —*see*
    Complications, genitourinary, device
    or implant, urinary system
  vascular —*see* Complications,
    cardiovascular device or implant
  ventricular shunt —*see* Complications,
    ventricular shunt (device)
 puerperium —*see* Puerperal
 puncture, spinal G97.1
  cerebrospinal fluid leak G97.0
  headache or reaction G97.1

Complication (*Continued*)
  pyelogram N99.89
  radiation
    kyphosis M96.2
    scoliosis M96.5
  reattached
    extremity (infection) (rejection)
      lower T87.1X-
      upper T87.0X-
    specified body part NEC T87.2
  reconstructed breast
    asymmetry between native and
      reconstructed breast N65.1
    deformity N65.0
    disproportion between native and
      reconstructed breast N65.1
    excess tissue N65.0
    misshappen N65.0
  reimplant NEC —*see also* Complications,
    prosthetic device or implant
    limb (infection) (rejection) —*see*
      Complications, reattached,
      extremity
    organ (partial) (total) —*see* Complications,
      transplant
    prosthetic device NEC —*see* Complications,
      prosthetic device
  renal N28.9
    allograft —*see* Complications, transplant,
      kidney
    dialysis —*see* Complications, dialysis
  respirator
    mechanical J95.850
      specified NEC J95.859
  respiratory system J98.9
    device, implant or graft —*see*
      Complication, prosthetic device or
      implant, specified NEC
    lung transplant —*see* Complications,
      prosthetic device or implant, lung
      transplant
    postoperative J95.89
      air leak J95.812
      Mendelson's syndrome (chemical
        pneumonitis) J95.4
      pneumothorax J95.811
      pulmonary insufficiency (acute) (after
        nonthoracic surgery) J95.2
        chronic J95.3
        following thoracic surgery J95.1
      respiratory failure (acute) J95.821
        acute and chronic J95.822
      specified NEC J95.89
      subglottic stenosis J95.5
      tracheostomy complication —*see*
        Complications, tracheostomy
    therapy T81.89
  sedation during labor and delivery O74.9
    cardiac O74.2
    central nervous system O74.3
    pulmonary NEC O74.1
  shunt —*see also* Complications, prosthetic
    device or implant
    arteriovenous —*see* Complications,
      arteriovenous, shunt
    ventricular (communicating) —*see*
      Complications, ventricular shunt
  skin
    graft T86.829
      failure T86.821
      infection T86.822
      rejection T86.820
      specified type NEC T86.828
  spinal
    anesthesia —*see* Complications, anesthesia,
      spinal
    catheter (epidural) (subdural) —*see*
      Complications, catheter
    puncture or tap G97.1
      cerebrospinal fluid leak G97.0
      headache or reaction G97.1

Complication (*Continued*)
  stent
    bile duct —*see* Complications, bile duct
      prosthesis
    ureteral indwelling ◄
      breakdown T83.112 ◄
      displacement T83.122 ◄
      leakage T83.192 ◄
      malposition T83.122 ◄
      obstruction T83.192 ◄
      perforation T83.192 ◄
      protrusion T83.192 ◄
      specified NEC T83.192 ◄
    urinary (ileal conduit) (nephroureteral)
      T83.193 ◄
      embolism T83.81 ◄
      fibrosis T83.82 ◄
      hemorrhage T83.83 ◄
      infection and inflammation T83.593 ◄
      mechanical ◄
        breakdown T83.113 ◄
        displacement T83.123 ◄
        leakage T83.193 ◄
        malposition T83.123 ◄
        obstruction T83.193 ◄
        perforation T83.193 ◄
        protrusion T83.193 ◄
        specified NEC T83.193 ◄
      pain T83.84 ◄
      specified type NEC T83.89 ◄
      stenosis T83.85 ◄
      thrombosis T83.86 ◄
    vascular ◄
      end stent stenosis —*see* Restenosis,
        stent ◄
      in stent stenosis —*see* Restenosis,
        stent ◄
  stoma
    digestive tract
      colostomy —*see* Complications,
        colostomy
      enterostomy —*see* Complications,
        enterostomy
      esophagostomy —*see* Complications,
        esophagostomy
      gastrostomy —*see* Complications,
        gastrostomy
    urinary tract N99.528 ◄⃫
      continent N99.538 ◄
        hemorrhage N99.530 ◄
        herniation N99.533 ◄
        infection N99.531 ◄
        malfunction N99.532 ◄
        specified type NEC N99.538 ◄
        stenosis N99.534 ◄
      cystostomy —*see* Complications,
        cystostomy
      external NOS N99.528
        ~~hemorrhage N99.520~~
        ~~infection N99.521~~
        ~~malfunction N99.522~~
        ~~specified type NEC N99.528~~
        hemorrhage N99.520 ◄⃫
        herniation N99.523 ◄
      incontinent N99.528 ◄
        hemorrhage N99.520 ◄
        herniation N99.523 ◄
        infection N99.521 ◄
        malfunction N99.522 ◄
        specified type NEC N99.528 ◄
        stenosis N99.524 ◄
      infection N99.521 ◄⃫
      malfunction N99.522 ◄⃫
      specified type NEC N99.528 ◄⃫
      stenosis N99.524 ◄
  stomach banding —*see* Complication (s),
    bariatric procedure
  stomach stapling —*see* Complication (s),
    bariatric procedure
  surgical material, nonabsorbable —*see*
    Complication, suture, permanent

Complication (*Continued*)
  surgical procedure (on) T81.9
    amputation stump (late) —*see*
      Complications, amputation stump
    cardiac —*see* Complications, circulatory
      system
    cholesteatoma, recurrent —*see*
      Complications, postmastoidectomy,
      recurrent cholesteatoma
    circulatory (early) —*see* Complications,
      circulatory system
    digestive system —*see* Complications,
      gastrointestinal
    dumping syndrome (postgastrectomy)
      K91.1
    ear —*see* Complications, ear
    elephantiasis or lymphedema I97.89
      postmastectomy I97.2
    emphysema (surgical) T81.82
    endocrine —*see* Complications, endocrine
    eye —*see* Complications, eye
    fistula (persistent postoperative) T81.83
    foreign body inadvertently left in wound
      (sponge) (suture) (swab) —*see*
      Foreign body, accidentally left during
      a procedure
    gastrointestinal —*see* Complications,
      gastrointestinal
    genitourinary NEC N99.89
    hematoma
      intraoperative —*see* Complication,
        intraoperative, hemorrhage
      postprocedural —*see* Complication,
        postprocedural, hematoma ◄⃫
    hemorrhage
      intraoperative —*see* Complication,
        intraoperative, hemorrhage
      postprocedural —*see* Complication,
        postprocedural, hemorrhage
    hepatic failure K91.82
    hyperglycemia (postpancreatectomy) E89.1
    hypoinsulinemia (postpancreatectomy)
      E89.1
    hypoparathyroidism
      (postparathyroidectomy) E89.2
    hypopituitarism (posthypophysectomy)
      E89.3
    hypothyroidism (post-thyroidectomy)
      E89.0
    intestinal obstruction K91.3
    intracranial hypotension following
      ventricular shunting
      (ventriculostomy) G97.2
    lymphedema I97.89
      postmastectomy I97.2
    malabsorption (postsurgical) NEC K91.2
      osteoporosis —*see* Osteoporosis,
        postsurgical malabsorption
    mastoidectomy cavity NEC —*see*
      Complications, postmastoidectomy
    metabolic E89.89
      specified NEC E89.89
    musculoskeletal —*see* Complications,
      musculoskeletal system
    nervous system (central) (peripheral) —*see*
      Complications, nervous system
    ovarian failure E89.40
      asymptomatic E89.40
      symptomatic E89.41
    peripheral vascular —*see* Complications,
      surgical procedure, vascular
    postcardiotomy syndrome I97.0
    postcholecystectomy syndrome K91.5
    postcommissurotomy syndrome I97.0
    postgastrectomy dumping syndrome K91.1
    postlaminectomy syndrome NEC M96.1
      kyphosis M96.3
    postmastectomy lymphedema syndrome
      I97.2
    postmastoidectomy cholesteatoma —*see*
      Complications, postmastoidectomy,
      recurrent cholesteatoma

◄ New   ◄⃫ Revised   ~~deleted~~ Deleted

Complication (Continued)
  surgical procedure (Continued)
    postvagotomy syndrome K91.1
    postvalvulotomy syndrome I97.0
    pulmonary insufficiency (acute) J95.2
      chronic J95.3
      following thoracic surgery J95.1
    reattached body part —see Complications, reattached
    respiratory —see Complications, respiratory system
    shock (hypovolemic) T81.19
    spleen (postoperative) D78.89
      intraoperative D78.81
    stitch abscess T81.48 ◄▥
    subglottic stenosis (postsurgical) J95.5
    testicular hypofunction E89.5
    transplant —see Complications, organ or tissue transplant
    urinary NEC N99.89
    vaginal vault prolapse (posthysterectomy) N99.3
    vascular (peripheral)
      artery T81.719
        mesenteric T81.710
        renal T81.711
        specified NEC T81.718
      vein T81.72
    wound infection T81.40 ◄▥
  suture, permanent (wire) NEC T85.9
    with repair of bone —see Complications, fixation device, internal
    embolism T85.818 ◄▥
    fibrosis T85.828 ◄▥
    hemorrhage T85.838 ◄▥
    infection and inflammation T85.79
    mechanical
      breakdown T85.612
      displacement T85.622
      malfunction T85.612
      malposition T85.622
      obstruction T85.692
      perforation T85.692
      protrusion T85.692
      specified NEC T85.692
    pain T85.848 ◄▥
    specified type NEC T85.898 ◄▥
    stenosis T85.858 ◄▥
    thrombosis T85.868 ◄▥
  tracheostomy J95.00
    granuloma J95.09
    hemorrhage J95.01
    infection J95.02
    malfunction J95.03
    mechanical J95.03
    obstruction J95.03
    specified type NEC J95.09
    tracheo-esophageal fistula J95.04
  transfusion (blood) (lymphocytes) (plasma) T80.92
    air embolism T80.0
    circulatory overload E87.71
    febrile nonhemolytic transfusion reaction R50.84
    hemochromatosis E83.111
    hemolysis T80.89
    hemolytic reaction (antigen unspecified) T80.919
    incompatibility reaction (antigen unspecified) T80.919
      ABO T80.30
        delayed serologic (DSTR) T80.39
        hemolytic transfusion reaction (HTR) (unspecified time after transfusion) T80.319
          acute (AHTR) (less than 24 hours after transfusion) T80.310
          delayed (DHTR) (24 hours or more after transfusion) T80.311
        specified NEC T80.39

Complication (Continued)
  transfusion (Continued)
    incompatibility reaction (Continued)
      acute (antigen unspecified) T80.910
      delayed (antigen unspecified) T80.911
      delayed serologic (DSTR) T80.89
      Non-ABO (minor antigens (Duffy) (Kell) (Kidd) (Lewis) (M) (N) (P) (S)) T80.A0
        delayed serologic (DSTR) T80.A9
        hemolytic transfusion reaction (HTR) (unspecified time after transfusion) T80.A19
          acute (AHTR) (less than 24 hours after transfusion) T80.A10
          delayed (DHTR) (24 hours or more after transfusion) T80.A11
        specified NEC T80.A9
      Rh (antigens (C) (c) (D) (E) (e)) (factor) T80.40
        delayed serologic (DSTR) T80.49
        hemolytic transfusion reaction (HTR) (unspecified time after transfusion) T80.419
          acute (AHTR) (less than 24 hours after transfusion) T80.410
          delayed (DHTR) (24 hours or more after transfusion) T80.411
        specified NEC T80.49
    infection T80.29
      acute T80.22
    reaction NEC T80.89
    sepsis T80.29
    shock T80.89
  transplant T86.90
    bone T86.839
      failure T86.831
      infection T86.832
      rejection T86.830
      specified type NEC T86.838
    bone marrow T86.00
      failure T86.02
      infection T86.03
      rejection T86.01
      specified type NEC T86.09
    cornea T86.849
      failure T86.841
      infection T86.842
      rejection T86.840
      specified type NEC T86.848
    failure T86.92
    heart T86.20
      with lung T86.30
      cardiac allograft vasculopathy T86.290
        failure T86.32
        infection T86.33
        rejection T86.31
        specified type NEC T86.39
      failure T86.22
      infection T86.23
      rejection T86.21
      specified type NEC T86.298
    infection T86.93
    intestine T86.859
      failure T86.851
      infection T86.852
      rejection T86.850
      specified type NEC T86.858
    kidney T86.10
      failure T86.12
      infection T86.13
      rejection T86.11
      specified type NEC T86.19
    liver T86.40
      failure T86.42
      infection T86.43
      rejection T86.41
      specified type NEC T86.49
    lung T86.819
      with heart T86.30
        failure T86.32
        infection T86.33

Complication (Continued)
  transplant (Continued)
    lung (Continued)
      with heart (Continued)
        rejection T86.31
        specified type NEC T86.39
      failure T86.811
      infection T86.812
      rejection T86.810
      specified type NEC T86.818
    malignant neoplasm C80.2
    pancreas T86.899
      failure T86.891
      infection T86.892
      rejection T86.890
      specified type NEC T86.898
    peripheral blood stem cells T86.5
    post-transplant lymphoproliferative disorder (PTLD) D47.Z1
    rejection T86.91
    skin T86.829
      failure T86.821
      infection T86.822
      rejection T86.820
      specified type NEC T86.828
    specified
      tissue T86.899
        failure T86.891
        infection T86.892
        rejection T86.890
        specified type NEC T86.898
      type NEC T86.99
    stem cell (from peripheral blood) (from umbilical cord) T86.5
    umbilical cord stem cells T86.5
  trauma (early) T79.9
    specified NEC T79.8
  ultrasound therapy NEC T88.9
  umbilical cord NEC
    complicating delivery O69.9
    specified NEC O69.89
  umbrella device, vascular T82.9
    embolism T82.818
    fibrosis T82.828
    hemorrhage T82.838
    infection or inflammation T82.7
    mechanical
      breakdown T82.515
      displacement T82.525
      leakage T82.535
      malposition T82.525
      obstruction T82.595
      perforation T82.595
      protrusion T82.595
    pain T82.848
    specified type NEC T82.898
    stenosis T82.858
    thrombosis T82.868
  urethral catheter —see Complications, catheter, urethral, indwelling
  vaccination T88.1
    anaphylaxis NEC T80.52
    arthropathy —see Arthropathy, postimmunization
    cellulitis T88.0
    encephalitis or encephalomyelitis G04.02
    infection (general) (local) NEC T88.0
    meningitis G03.8
    myelitis G04.02 ◄▥
    protein sickness T80.62
    rash T88.1
    reaction (allergic) T88.1
      serum T80.62
    sepsis T88.0
    serum intoxication, sickness, rash, or other serum reaction NEC T80.62
      anaphylactic shock T80.52
    shock (allergic) (anaphylactic) T80.52
    vaccinia (generalized) (localized) T88.1
  vas deferens device or implant —see Complications, genitourinary, device or implant, genital tract

Complication *(Continued)*
  vascular I99.9
    device or implant T82.9
      embolism T82.818
      fibrosis T82.828
      hemorrhage T82.838
      infection or inflammation T82.7
      mechanical
        breakdown T82.519
          specified device NEC T82.518
        displacement T82.529
          specified device NEC T82.528
        leakage T82.539
          specified device NEC T82.538
        malposition T82.529
          specified device NEC T82.528
        obstruction T82.599
          specified device NEC T82.598
        perforation T82.599
          specified device NEC T82.598
        protrusion T82.599
          specified device NEC T82.598
      pain T82.848
      specified type NEC T82.898
      stenosis T82.858
      thrombosis T82.868
    dialysis catheter —*see* Complication,
      catheter, dialysis
    following infusion, therapeutic injection or
      transfusion T80.1
    graft T82.9
      embolism T82.818
      fibrosis T82.828
      hemorrhage T82.838
      mechanical
        breakdown T82.319
          aorta (bifurcation) T82.310
          carotid artery T82.311
          specified vessel NEC T82.318
        displacement T82.329
          aorta (bifurcation) T82.320
          carotid artery T82.321
          specified vessel NEC T82.328
        leakage T82.339
          aorta (bifurcation) T82.330
          carotid artery T82.331
          specified vessel NEC T82.338
        malposition T82.329
          aorta (bifurcation) T82.320
          carotid artery T82.321
          specified vessel NEC T82.328
        obstruction T82.399
          aorta (bifurcation) T82.390
          carotid artery T82.391
          specified vessel NEC T82.398
        perforation T82.399
          aorta (bifurcation) T82.390
          carotid artery T82.391
          specified vessel NEC T82.398
        protrusion T82.399
          aorta (bifurcation) T82.390
          carotid artery T82.391
          specified vessel NEC T82.398
      pain T82.848
      specified complication NEC T82.898
      stenosis T82.858
      thrombosis T82.868
    postoperative —*see* Complications,
      postoperative, circulatory
    vena cava device (filter) (sieve) (umbrella) —
      see Complications, umbrella device,
      vascular
  ventilation therapy NEC T81.81
  ventilator
    mechanical J95.850
    specified NEC J95.859
  ventricular (communicating) shunt (device)
    T85.9
    embolism T85.810 ◀▥
    fibrosis T85.820 ◀▥
    hemorrhage T85.830 ◀▥

Complication *(Continued)*
  ventricular shunt *(Continued)*
    infection and inflammation T85.730 ◀▥
    mechanical
      breakdown T85.01
      displacement T85.02
      leakage T85.03
      malposition T85.02
      obstruction T85.09
      perforation T85.09
      protrusion T85.09
      specified NEC T85.09
    pain T85.840 ◀▥
    specified type NEC T85.890 ◀▥
    stenosis T85.850 ◀▥
    thrombosis T85.860 ◀▥
  wire suture, permanent (implanted) —*see*
    Complications, suture, permanent
Compressed air disease T70.3
Compression
  with injury - code by Nature of injury
  artery I77.1
    celiac, syndrome I77.4
  brachial plexus G54.0
  brain (stem) G93.5
    due to
      contusion (diffuse) —*see* Injury,
        intracranial, diffuse
      focal —*see* Injury, intracranial, focal
      injury NEC —*see* Injury, intracranial,
        diffuse
      traumatic —*see* Injury, intracranial, diffuse
  bronchus J98.09
  cauda equina G83.4
  celiac (artery) (axis) I77.4
  cerebral —*see* Compression, brain
  cervical plexus G54.2
  cord
    spinal —*see* Compression, spinal
    umbilical —*see* Compression, umbilical
      cord
  cranial nerve G52.9
    eighth —*see* subcategory H93.3
    eleventh G52.8
    fifth G50.8
    first G52.0
    fourth —*see* Strabismus, paralytic, fourth
      nerve
    ninth G52.1
    second —*see* Disorder, nerve, optic
    seventh G52.8
    sixth —*see* Strabismus, paralytic, sixth
      nerve
    tenth G52.2
    third —*see* Strabismus, paralytic, third
      nerve
    twelfth G52.3
  diver's squeeze T70.3
  during birth (newborn) P15.9
  esophagus K22.2
  eustachian tube —*see* Obstruction, eustachian
    tube, cartilaginous
  facies Q67.1
  fracture
    nontraumatic NOS —*see* Collapse,
      vertebra ◀
    pathological —*see* Fracture, pathological ◀
    traumatic —*see* Fracture, traumatic ◀
  heart —*see* Disease, heart
  intestine —*see* Obstruction, intestine
  laryngeal nerve, recurrent G52.2
    with paralysis of vocal cords and larynx
      J38.00
      bilateral J38.02
      unilateral J38.01
  lumbosacral plexus G54.1
  lung J98.4
  lymphatic vessel I89.0
  medulla —*see* Compression, brain
  nerve —*see also* Disorder, nerve G58.9
    arm NEC —*see* Mononeuropathy, upper
      limb

Compression *(Continued)*
  nerve *(Continued)*
    axillary G54.0
    cranial —*see* Compression, cranial nerve
    leg NEC —*see* Mononeuropathy, lower
      limb
    median (in carpal tunnel) —*see* Syndrome,
      carpal tunnel
    optic —*see* Disorder, nerve, optic
    plantar —*see* Lesion, nerve, plantar
    posterior tibial (in tarsal tunnel) —*see*
      Syndrome, tarsal tunnel
    root or plexus NOS (in) G54.9
      intervertebral disc disorder NEC —
        see Disorder, disc, with,
        radiculopathy
        with myelopathy —*see* Disorder, disc,
          with, myelopathy
      neoplastic disease —*see also* Neoplasm
        D49.9 [G55]
      spondylosis —*see* Spondylosis, with
        radiculopathy
    sciatic (acute) —*see* Lesion, nerve, sciatic
    sympathetic G90.8
    traumatic —*see* Injury, nerve
    ulnar —*see* Lesion, nerve, ulnar
    upper extremity NEC —*see*
      Mononeuropathy, upper limb
  spinal (cord) G95.20
    by displacement of intervertebral disc
      NEC —*see also* Disorder, disc, with,
      myelopathy
    nerve root NOS G54.9
      due to displacement of intervertebral
        disc NEC —*see* Disorder, disc, with,
        radiculopathy
        with myelopathy —*see* Disorder, disc,
          with, myelopathy
    specified NEC G95.29
    spondylogenic (cervical) (lumbar,
      lumbosacral) (thoracic) —*see*
      Spondylosis, with myelopathy NEC
    anterior —*see* Syndrome, anterior, spinal
      artery, compression
    traumatic —*see* Injury, spinal cord, by
      region
  subcostal nerve (syndrome) —*see*
    Mononeuropathy, upper limb, specified
    NEC
  sympathetic nerve NEC G90.8
  syndrome T79.5
  trachea J39.8
  ulnar nerve (by scar tissue) —*see* Lesion,
    nerve, ulnar
  umbilical cord
    complicating delivery O69.2
      cord around neck O69.1
      prolapse O69.0
      specified NEC O69.2
  ureter N13.5
  vein I87.1
  vena cava (inferior) (superior) I87.1
Compulsion, compulsive
  gambling F63.0
  neurosis F42.8 ▥
  personality F60.5
  states F42.8 ▥
  swearing F42.8 ◀▥
    in Gilles de la Tourette's syndrome F95.2
  tics and spasms F95.9
Concato's disease (pericardial polyserositis)
  A19.9
  nontubercular I31.1
  pleural —*see* Pleurisy, with effusion
Concavity chest wall M95.4
Concealed penis Q55.69
Concern (normal) **about sick person in family**
  Z63.6
Concrescence (teeth) K00.2
Concretio cordis I31.1
  rheumatic I09.2

◀ New   ◀▥ Revised   ~~deleted~~ Deleted

Concretion —*see also* Calculus
  appendicular K38.1
  canaliculus —*see* Dacryolith
  clitoris N90.89
  conjunctiva H11.12-
  eyelid —*see* Disorder, eyelid, specified type NEC
  lacrimal passages —*see* Dacryolith
  prepuce (male) N47.8
  salivary gland (any) K11.5
  seminal vesicle N50.89 ◀▥
  tonsil J35.8
Concussion (brain) (cerebral) (current) S06.0X9 ◀▥
  with ◀
    loss of consciousness of 30 minutes or less S06.0X1 ◀
    loss of consciousness of unspecified duration S06.0X9 ◀
  blast (air) (hydraulic) (immersion) (underwater)
    abdomen or thorax —*see* Injury, blast, by site
    ear with acoustic nerve injury —*see* Injury, nerve, acoustic, specified type NEC
  cauda equina S34.3
  conus medullaris S34.02
  ocular S05.8X-
  spinal (cord)
    cervical S14.0
    lumbar S34.01
    sacral S34.02
    thoracic S24.0
  syndrome F07.81
  Without loss of consciousness S06.0X0 ◀
Condition —*see* Disease
Conditions arising in the perinatal period —*see* Newborn, affected by
Conduct disorder —*see* Disorder, conduct
Condyloma A63.0
  acuminatum A63.0
  gonorrheal A54.09
  latum A51.31
  syphilitic A51.31
    congenital A50.07
  venereal, syphilitic A51.31
Conflagration —*see also* Burn
  asphyxia (by inhalation of gases, fumes or vapors) —*see also* Table of Drugs and Chemicals T59.9-
Conflict (with) —*see also* Discord
  family Z73.9
  marital Z63.0
    involving divorce or estrangement Z63.5
  parent-child Z62.820
    parent-adopted child Z62.821
    parent-biological child Z62.820
    parent-foster child Z62.822
  social role NEC Z73.5
Confluent —*see* condition
Confusion, confused R41.0
  epileptic F05
  mental state (psychogenic) F44.89
  psychogenic F44.89
  reactive (from emotional stress, psychological trauma) F44.89
Confusional arousals G47.51
Congelation T69.9
Congenital —*see also* condition
  aortic septum Q25.49 ◀▥
  intrinsic factor deficiency D51.0
  malformation —*see* Anomaly
Congestion, congestive
  bladder N32.89
  bowel K63.89
  brain G93.89
  breast N64.59
  bronchial J98.09
  catarrhal J31.0
  chest R09.89
  chill, malarial —*see* Malaria

Congestion, congestive (*Continued*)
  circulatory NEC I99.8
  duodenum K31.89
  eye —*see* Hyperemia, conjunctiva
  facial, due to birth injury P15.4
  general R68.89
  glottis J37.0
  heart —*see* Failure, heart, congestive
  hepatic K76.1
  hypostatic (lung) —*see* Edema, lung
  intestine K63.89
  kidney N28.89
  labyrinth —*see* subcategory H83.8
  larynx J37.0
  liver K76.1
  lung R09.89
    active or acute —*see* Pneumonia
  malaria, malarial —*see* Malaria
  nasal R09.81
  nose R09.81
  orbit, orbital —*see also* Exophthalmos
    inflammatory (chronic) —*see* Inflammation, orbit
  ovary N83.8
  pancreas K86.89 ◀▥
  pelvic, female N94.89
  pleural J94.8
  prostate (active) N42.1
  pulmonary —*see* Congestion, lung
  renal N28.89
  retina H35.81
  seminal vesicle N50.1
  spinal cord G95.19
  spleen (chronic) D73.2
  stomach K31.89
  trachea —*see* Tracheitis
  urethra N36.8
  uterus N85.8
    with subinvolution N85.3
  venous (passive) I87.8
  viscera R68.89
Congestive —*see* Congestion
Conical
  cervix (hypertrophic elongation) N88.4
  cornea —*see* Keratoconus
  teeth K00.2
Conjoined twins Q89.4
Conjugal maladjustment Z63.0
  involving divorce or estrangement Z63.5
Conjunctiva —*see* condition
Conjunctivitis (staphylococcal) (streptococcal) NOS H10.9
  Acanthamoeba B60.12
  acute H10.3-
    atopic H10.1-
    chemical —*see also* Corrosion, cornea H10.21-
    mucopurulent H10.02-
      follicular H10.01-
    pseudomembranous H10.22-
    serous except viral H10.23-
    viral —*see* Conjunctivitis, viral
    toxic H10.21-
  adenoviral (acute) (follicular) B30.1
  allergic (acute) —*see* Conjunctivitis, acute, atopic
    chronic H10.45
    vernal H10.44
  anaphylactic —*see* Conjunctivitis, acute, atopic
  Apollo B30.3
  atopic (acute) —*see* Conjunctivitis, acute, atopic
  Béal's B30.2
  blennorrhagic (gonococcal) (neonatorum) A54.31
  chemical (acute) —*see also* Corrosion, cornea H10.21-
  chlamydial A74.0
    due to trachoma A71.1
    neonatal P39.1

Conjunctivitis (*Continued*)
  chronic (nodosa) (petrificans) (phlyctenular) H10.40-
    allergic H10.45
      vernal H10.44
    follicular H10.43-
    giant papillary H10.41-
    simple H10.42-
    vernal H10.44
  coxsackievirus 24 B30.3
  diphtheritic A36.86
  due to
    dust —*see* Conjunctivitis, acute, atopic
    filariasis B74.9
    mucocutaneous leishmaniasis B55.2
  enterovirus type 70 (hemorrhagic) B30.3
  epidemic (viral) B30.9
    hemorrhagic B30.3
  gonococcal (neonatorum) A54.31
  granular (trachomatous) A71.1
    sequelae (late effect) B94.0
  hemorrhagic (acute) (epidemic) B30.3
  herpes zoster B02.31
  in (due to)
    Acanthamoeba B60.12
    adenovirus (acute) (follicular) B30.1
    Chlamydia A74.0
    coxsackievirus 24 B30.3
    diphtheria A36.86
    enterovirus type 70 (hemorrhagic) B30.3
    filariasis B74.9
    gonococci A54.31
    herpes (simplex) virus B00.53
      zoster B02.31
    infectious disease NEC B99
    meningococci A39.89
    mucocutaneous leishmaniasis B55.2
    rosacea L71.9
    syphilis (late) (A52.71)
    zoster B02.31
  inclusion A74.0
  infantile P39.1
    gonococcal A54.31
  Koch-Weeks' —*see* Conjunctivitis, acute, mucopurulent
  light —*see* Conjunctivitis, acute, atopic
  ligneous —*see* Blepharoconjunctivitis, ligneous
  meningococcal A39.89
  mucopurulent —*see* Conjunctivitis, acute, mucopurulent
  neonatal P39.1
    gonococcal A54.31
  Newcastle B30.8
  of Béal B30.2
  parasitic
    filariasis B74.9
    mucocutaneous leishmaniasis B55.2
  Parinaud's H10.89
  petrificans H10.89
  rosacea L71.9
  specified NEC H10.89
  swimming-pool B30.1
  trachomatous A71.1
    acute A71.0
    sequelae (late effect) B94.0
  traumatic NEC H10.89
  tuberculous A18.59
  tularemic A21.1
  tularensis A21.1
  viral B30.9
    due to
      adenovirus B30.1
      enterovirus B30.3
    specified NEC B30.8
Conjunctivochalasis H11.82-
Connective tissue —*see* condition
Conn's syndrome E26.01
Conradi (-Hunermann) disease Q77.3
Consanguinity Z84.3
  counseling Z71.89

Conscious simulation (of illness) Z76.5
Consecutive —*see* condition
Consolidation lung (base) —*see* Pneumonia, lobar
Constipation (atonic) (neurogenic) (simple) (spastic) K59.00
    chronic K59.09 ◀
        idiopathic K59.04 ◀
    drug-induced K59.03 ◀▥
    functional K59.04 ◀
    outlet dysfunction K59.02
    psychogenic F45.8
    slow transit K59.01
    specified NEC K59.09
Constitutional —*see also* condition
    substandard F60.7
Constitutionally substandard F60.7
Constriction —*see also* Stricture
    auditory canal —*see* Stenosis, external ear canal
    bronchial J98.09
    duodenum K31.5
    esophagus K22.2
    external
        abdomen, abdominal (wall) S30.841
        alveolar process S00.542
        ankle S90.54-
        antecubital space —*see* Constriction, external, forearm
        arm (upper) S40.84-
        auricle —*see* Constriction, external, ear
        axilla —*see* Constriction, external, arm
        back, lower S30.840
        breast S20.14-
        brow S00.84
        buttock S30.840
        calf —*see* Constriction, external, leg
        canthus —*see* Constriction, external, eyelid
        cheek S00.84
            internal S00.542
        chest wall —*see* Constriction, external, thorax
        chin S00.84
        clitoris S30.844
        costal region —*see* Constriction, external, thorax
        digit (s)
            foot —*see* Constriction, external, toe
            hand —*see* Constriction, external, finger
        ear S00.44-
        elbow S50.34-
        epididymis S30.843
        epigastric region S30.841
        esophagus, cervical S10.14
        eyebrow —*see* Constriction, external, eyelid
        eyelid S00.24-
        face S00.84
        finger (s) S60.44-
            index S60.44-
            little S60.44-
            middle S60.44-
            ring S60.44-
        flank S30.841
        foot (except toe (s) alone) S90.84-
            toe —*see* Constriction, external, toe
        forearm S50.84-
            elbow only —*see* Constriction, external, elbow
        forehead S00.84
        genital organs, external
            female S30.846
            male S30.845
        groin S30.841
        gum S00.542
        hand S60.54-
        head S00.94
            ear —*see* Constriction, external, ear
            eyelid —*see* Constriction, external, eyelid
            lip S00.541
            nose S00.34
            oral cavity S00.542

Constriction (*Continued*)
    external (*Continued*)
        head (*Continued*)
            scalp S00.04
            specified site NEC S00.84
        heel —*see* Constriction, external, foot
        hip S70.24-
        inguinal region S30.841
        interscapular region S20.449
        jaw S00.84
        knee S80.24-
        labium (majus) (minus) S30.844
        larynx S10.14
        leg (lower) S80.84-
            knee —*see* Constriction, external, knee
            upper —*see* Constriction, external, thigh
        lip S00.541
        lower back S30.840
        lumbar region S30.840
        malar region S00.84
        mammary —*see* Constriction, external, breast
        mastoid region S00.84
        mouth S00.542
        nail
            finger —*see* Constriction, external, finger
            toe —*see* Constriction, external, toe
        nasal S00.34
        neck S10.94
            specified site NEC S10.84
            throat S10.14
        nose S00.34
        occipital region S00.04
        oral cavity S00.542
        orbital region —*see* Constriction, external, eyelid
        palate S00.542
        palm —*see* Constriction, external, hand
        parietal region S00.04
        pelvis S30.840
        penis S30.842
        perineum
            female S30.844
            male S30.840
        periocular area —*see* Constriction, external, eyelid
        phalanges
            finger —*see* Constriction, external, finger
            toe —*see* Constriction, external, toe
        pharynx S10.14
        pinna —*see* Constriction, external, ear
        popliteal space —*see* Constriction, external, knee
        prepuce S30.842
        pubic region S30.840
        pudendum
            female S30.846
            male S30.845
        sacral region S30.840
        scalp S00.04
        scapular region —*see* Constriction, external, shoulder
        scrotum S30.843
        shin —*see* Constriction, external, leg
        shoulder S40.24-
        sternal region S20.349
        submaxillary region S00.84
        submental region S00.84
        subungual
            finger (s) —*see* Constriction, external, finger
            toe (s) —*see* Constriction, external, toe
        supraclavicular fossa S10.84
        supraorbital S00.84
        temple S00.84
        temporal region S00.84
        testis S30.843
        thigh S70.34-
        thorax, thoracic (wall) S20.94
            back S20.44-
            front S20.34-

Constriction (*Continued*)
    external (*Continued*)
        throat S10.14
        thumb S60.34-
        toe (s) (lesser) S90.44-
            great S90.44-
        tongue S00.542
        trachea S10.14
        tunica vaginalis S30.843
        uvula S00.542
        vagina S30.844
        vulva S30.844
        wrist S60.84-
    gallbladder —*see* Obstruction, gallbladder
    intestine —*see* Obstruction, intestine
    larynx J38.6
        congenital Q31.8
            specified NEC Q31.8
            subglottic Q31.1
    organ or site, congenital NEC —*see* Atresia, by site
    prepuce (acquired) (congenital) N47.1
    pylorus (adult hypertrophic) K31.1
        congenital or infantile Q40.0
        newborn Q40.0
    ring dystocia (uterus) O62.4
    spastic —*see also* Spasm
        ureter N13.5
    ureter N13.5
        with infection N13.6
    urethra —*see* Stricture, urethra
    visual field (peripheral) (functional) —*see* Defect, visual field
Constrictive —*see* condition
Consultation
    without complaint or sickness Z71.9
        feared complaint unfounded Z71.1
        specified reason NEC Z71.89
    medical —*see* Counseling, medical
    religious Z71.81
    specified reason NEC Z71.89
    spiritual Z71.81
Consumption —*see* Tuberculosis
Contact (with) —*see also* Exposure (to)
    acariasis Z20.7
    AIDS virus Z20.6
    air pollution Z77.110
    algae and algae toxins Z77.121
    algae bloom Z77.121
    anthrax Z20.810
    aromatic (hazardous) compounds NEC Z77.028
    aromatic amines Z77.020
    aromatic dyes NOS Z77.028
    arsenic Z77.010
    asbestos Z77.090
    bacterial disease NEC Z20.818
    benzene Z77.021
    blue-green algae bloom Z77.121
    body fluids (potentially hazardous) Z77.21
    brown tide Z77.121
    chemicals (chiefly nonmedicinal) (hazardous) NEC Z77.098
    cholera Z20.09
    chromium compounds Z77.018
    communicable disease Z20.9
        bacterial NEC Z20.818
        specified NEC Z20.89
        viral NEC Z20.828
    cyanobacteria bloom Z77.121
    dyes Z77.098
    Escherichia coli (E. coli) Z20.01
    fiberglass —*see* Table of Drugs and Chemicals, fiberglass
    German measles Z20.4
    gonorrhea Z20.2
    hazardous metals NEC Z77.018
    hazardous substances NEC Z77.29
    hazards in the physical environment NEC Z77.128
    hazards to health NEC Z77.9

◀ New   ◀▥ Revised   ~~deleted~~ Deleted

Contact (Continued)
HIV Z20.6
HTLV-III/LAV Z20.6
human immunodeficiency virus (HIV) Z20.6
infection Z20.9
    specified NEC Z20.89
infestation (parasitic) NEC Z20.7
intestinal infectious disease NEC Z20.09
    Escherichia coli (E. coli) Z20.01
lead Z77.011
meningococcus Z20.811
mold (toxic) Z77.120
nickel dust Z77.018
noise Z77.122
parasitic disease Z20.7
pediculosis Z20.7
pfiesteria piscicida Z77.121
poliomyelitis Z20.89
pollution
    air Z77.110
    environmental NEC Z77.118
    soil Z77.112
    water Z77.111
polycyclic aromatic hydrocarbons Z77.028
rabies Z20.3
radiation, naturally occurring NEC Z77.123
radon Z77.123
red tide (Florida) Z77.121
rubella Z20.4
sexually-transmitted disease Z20.2
smallpox (laboratory) Z20.89
syphilis Z20.2
tuberculosis Z20.1
uranium Z77.012
varicella Z20.820
venereal disease Z20.2
viral disease NEC Z20.828
viral hepatitis Z20.5
water pollution Z77.111
Contamination, food —see Intoxication,
    foodborne
Contraception, contraceptive
advice Z30.09
counseling Z30.09
device (intrauterine) (in situ) Z97.5
    causing menorrhagia T83.83
    checking Z30.431
    complications —see Complications,
        intrauterine, contraceptive device
    in place Z97.5
    initial prescription Z30.014
    reinsertion Z30.433
    removal Z30.432
    replacement Z30.433
emergency (postcoital) Z30.012
initial prescription Z30.019
    barrier Z30.018 ◄
    diaphragm Z30.018 ◄
    injectable Z30.013
    intrauterine device Z30.014
    pills Z30.011
    postcoital (emergency) Z30.012
    specified type NEC Z30.018
    subdermal implantable Z30.017 ◄▥
    transdermal patch hormonal Z30.016 ◄
    vaginal ring hormonal Z30.015 ◄
maintenance Z30.40
    barrier Z30.49 ◄
    diaphragm Z30.49 ◄
    examination Z30.8
    injectable Z30.42
    intrauterine device Z30.431
    pills Z30.41
    specified type NEC Z30.49
    subdermal implantable Z30.46 ◄▥
    transdermal patch hormonal Z30.45 ◄
    vaginal ring hormonal Z30.44 ◄
management Z30.9
    specified NEC Z30.8
postcoital (emergency) Z30.012
prescription Z30.019
    repeat Z30.40

Contraception, contraceptive (Continued)
sterilization Z30.2
surveillance (drug) —see Contraception,
    maintenance
Contraction (s), contracture, contracted
Achilles tendon —see also Short, tendon,
    Achilles
    congenital Q66.89
amputation stump (surgical) (flexion) (late)
    next proximal joint T87.89
anus K59.8
bile duct (common) (hepatic) K83.8
bladder N32.89
    neck or sphincter N32.0
bowel, cecum, colon or intestine, any part —
    see Obstruction, intestine
Braxton Hicks —see False, labor
breast implant, capsular T85.44
bronchial J98.09
burn (old) —see Cicatrix
cervix —see Stricture, cervix
cicatricial —see Cicatrix
conjunctiva, trachomatous, active A71.1
    sequelae (late effect) B94.0
Dupuytren's M72.0
eyelid —see Disorder, eyelid function
fascia (lata) (postural) M72.8
    Dupuytren's M72.0
    palmar M72.0
    plantar M72.2
finger NEC —see also Deformity, finger
    congenital Q68.1
    joint —see Contraction, joint, hand
flaccid —see Contraction, paralytic
gallbladder K82.0
heart valve —see Endocarditis
hip —see Contraction, joint, hip
hourglass
    bladder N32.89
        congenital Q64.79
    gallbladder K82.0
        congenital Q44.1
    stomach K31.89
        congenital Q40.2
        psychogenic F45.8
    uterus (complicating delivery) O62.4
hysterical F44.4
internal os —see Stricture, cervix
joint (abduction) (acquired) (adduction)
        (flexion) (rotation) M24.50
    ankle M24.57-
    congenital NEC Q68.8
        hip Q65.89
    elbow M24.52-
    foot joint M24.57-
    hand joint M24.54-
    hip M24.55-
        congenital Q65.89
    hysterical F44.4
    knee M24.56-
    shoulder M24.51-
    wrist M24.53-
kidney (granular) (secondary) N26.9
    congenital Q63.8
    hydronephritic —see Hydronephrosis
    Page N26.2
    pyelonephritic —see Pyelitis, chronic
    tuberculous A18.11
ligament —see also Disorder, ligament
    congenital Q79.8
muscle (postinfective) (postural) NEC M62.40
    with contracture of joint —see Contraction,
        joint
    ankle M62.47-
    congenital Q79.8
        sternocleidomastoid Q68.0
    extraocular —see Strabismus
    eye (extrinsic) —see Strabismus
    foot M62.47-
    forearm M62.43-
    hand M62.44-

Contraction, contracture, contracted
    (Continued)
muscle (Continued)
    hysterical F44.4
    ischemic (Volkmann's) T79.6
    lower leg M62.46-
    multiple sites M62.49
    pelvic region M62.45-
    posttraumatic —see Strabismus, paralytic
    psychogenic F45.8
        conversion reaction F44.4
    shoulder region M62.41-
    specified site NEC M62.48
    thigh M62.45-
    upper arm M62.42-
neck —see Torticollis
ocular muscle —see Strabismus
organ or site, congenital NEC —see Atresia,
    by site
outlet (pelvis) —see Contraction, pelvis
palmar fascia M72.0
paralytic
    joint —see Contraction, joint
    muscle —see also Contraction, muscle NEC
        ocular —see Strabismus, paralytic
pelvis (acquired) (general) M95.5
    with disproportion (fetopelvic) O33.1
        causing obstructed labor O65.1
        inlet O33.2
        mid-cavity O33.3
        outlet O33.3
plantar fascia M72.2
premature
    atrium I49.1
    auriculoventricular I49.49
    heart I49.49
    junctional I49.2
    supraventricular I49.1
    ventricular I49.3
prostate N42.89
pylorus NEC —see also Pylorospasm
    psychogenic F45.8
rectum, rectal (sphincter) K59.8
ring (Bandl's) (complicating delivery) O62.4
scar —see Cicatrix
spine —see Dorsopathy, deforming
sternocleidomastoid (muscle), congenital
    Q68.0
stomach K31.89
    hourglass K31.89
        congenital Q40.2
        psychogenic F45.8
    psychogenic F45.8
tendon (sheath) M62.40
    with contracture of joint —see Contraction,
        joint
    Achilles —see Short, tendon, Achilles
    ankle M62.47-
        Achilles —see Short, tendon, Achilles
    foot M62.47-
    forearm M62.43-
    hand M62.44-
    lower leg M62.46-
    multiple sites M62.49
    neck M62.48
    pelvic region M62.45-
    shoulder region M62.41-
    specified site NEC M62.48
    thigh M62.45-
    thorax M62.48
    trunk M62.48
    upper arm M62.42-
toe —see Deformity, toe, specified NEC
ureterovesical orifice (postinfectional) N13.5
    with infection N13.6
urethra —see also Stricture, urethra
    orifice N32.0
uterus N85.8
    abnormal NEC O62.9
    clonic (complicating delivery) O62.4
    dyscoordinate (complicating delivery) O62.4

Contraction, contracture, contracted
(Continued)
uterus (Continued)
hourglass (complicating delivery) O62.4
hypertonic O62.4
hypotonic NEC O62.2
inadequate
primary O62.0
secondary O62.1
incoordinate (complicating delivery) O62.4
poor O62.2
tetanic (complicating delivery) O62.4
vagina (outlet) N89.5
vesical N32.89
neck or urethral orifice N32.0
visual field —see Defect, visual field,
generalized
Volkmann's (ischemic) T79.6
Contusion (skin surface intact) T14.8
abdomen, abdominal (muscle) (wall) S30.1
adnexa, eye NEC S05.8X-
adrenal gland S37.812
alveolar process S00.532
ankle S90.0-
antecubital space —see Contusion, forearm
anus S30.3
arm (upper) S40.02-
lower (with elbow) —see Contusion,
forearm
auditory canal —see Contusion, ear
auricle —see Contusion, ear
axilla —see Contusion, arm, upper
back —see also Contusion, thorax, back
lower S30.0
bile duct S36.13
bladder S37.22
bone NEC T14.8
brain (diffuse) —see Injury, intracranial, diffuse
focal —see Injury, intracranial, focal
brainstem S06.38-
breast S20.0-
broad ligament S37.892
brow S00.83
buttock S30.0
canthus, eye S00.1-
cauda equina S34.3
cerebellar, traumatic S06.37-
cerebral S06.33-
left side S06.32-
right side S06.31-
cheek S00.83
internal S00.532
chest (wall) —see Contusion, thorax
chin S00.83
clitoris S30.23
colon —see Injury, intestine, large, contusion
common bile duct S36.13
conjunctiva S05.1-
with foreign body (in conjunctival sac) —
see Foreign body, conjunctival sac
conus medullaris (spine) S34.139
cornea —see Contusion, eyeball
with foreign body —see Foreign body,
cornea
corpus cavernosum S30.21
cortex (brain) (cerebral) —see Injury,
intracranial, diffuse
focal —see Injury, intracranial, focal
costal region —see Contusion, thorax
cystic duct S36.13
diaphragm S27.802
duodenum S36.420
ear S00.43-
elbow S50.0-
with forearm —see Contusion, forearm
epididymis S30.22
epigastric region S30.1
epiglottis S10.0
esophagus (thoracic) S27.812
cervical S10.0
eyeball S05.1-

Contusion (Continued)
eyebrow S00.1-
eyelid (and periocular area) S00.1-
face NEC S00.83
fallopian tube S37.529
bilateral S37.522
unilateral S37.521
femoral triangle S30.1
finger (s) S60.00
with damage to nail (matrix) S60.10
index S60.02-
with damage to nail S60.12-
little S60.05-
with damage to nail S60.15-
middle S60.03-
with damage to nail S60.13-
ring S60.04-
with damage to nail S60.14-
thumb —see Contusion, thumb
flank S30.1
foot (except toe (s) alone) S90.3-
toe —see Contusion, toe
forearm S50.1-
elbow only —see Contusion, elbow
forehead S00.83
gallbladder S36.122
genital organs, external
female S30.202
male S30.201
globe (eye) —see Contusion, eyeball
groin S30.1
gum S00.532
hand S60.22-
finger (s) —see Contusion, finger
wrist —see Contusion, wrist
head S00.93
ear —see Contusion, ear
eyelid —see Contusion, eyelid
lip S00.531
nose S00.33
oral cavity S00.532
scalp S00.03
specified part NEC S00.83
heart —see also Injury, heart S26.91 ◀
heel —see Contusion, foot
hepatic duct S36.13
hip S70.0-
ileum S36.428
iliac region S30.1
inguinal region S30.1
interscapular region S20.229
intra-abdominal organ S36.92
colon —see Injury, intestine, large, contusion
liver S36.112
pancreas —see Contusion, pancreas
rectum S36.62
small intestine —see Injury, intestine, small,
contusion
specified organ NEC S36.892
spleen —see Contusion, spleen
stomach S36.32
iris (eye) —see Contusion, eyeball
jaw S00.83
jejunum S36.428
kidney S37.01-
major (greater than 2 cm) S37.02-
minor (less than 2 cm) S37.01-
knee S80.0-
labium (majus) (minus) S30.23
lacrimal apparatus, gland or sac S05.8X-
larynx S10.0
leg (lower) S80.1-
knee —see Contusion, knee
lens —see Contusion, eyeball
lip S00.531
liver S36.112
lower back S30.0
lumbar region S30.0
lung S27.329
bilateral S27.322
unilateral S27.321

Contusion (Continued)
malar region S00.83
mastoid region S00.83
membrane, brain —see Injury, intracranial,
diffuse
focal —see Injury, intracranial, focal
mesentery S36.892
mesosalpinx S37.892
mouth S00.532
muscle —see Contusion, by site
nail
finger —see Contusion, finger, with
damage to nail
toe —see Contusion, toe, with damage to
nail
nasal S00.33
neck S10.93
specified site NEC S10.83
throat S10.0
nerve —see Injury, nerve
newborn P54.5
nose S00.33
occipital
lobe (brain) —see Injury, intracranial,
diffuse
focal —see Injury, intracranial,
focal
region (scalp) S00.03
orbit (region) (tissues) S05.1-
ovary S37.429
bilateral S37.422
unilateral S37.421
palate S00.532
pancreas S36.229
body S36.221
head S36.220
tail S36.222
parietal
lobe (brain) —see Injury, intracranial,
diffuse
focal —see Injury, intracranial, focal
region (scalp) S00.03
pelvic organ S37.92
adrenal gland S37.812
bladder S37.22
fallopian tube —see Contusion, fallopian
tube
kidney —see Contusion, kidney
ovary —see Contusion, ovary
prostate S37.822
specified organ NEC S37.892
ureter S37.12
urethra S37.32
uterus S37.62
pelvis S30.0
penis S30.21
perineum
female S30.23
male S30.0
periocular area S00.1-
peritoneum S36.81
periurethral tissue —see Contusion,
urethra
pharynx S10.0
pinna —see Contusion, ear
popliteal space —see Contusion, knee
prepuce S30.21
prostate S37.822
pubic region S30.1
pudendum
female S30.202
male S30.201
quadriceps femoris —see Contusion, thigh
rectum S36.62
retroperitoneum S36.892
round ligament S37.892
sacral region S30.0
scalp S00.03
due to birth injury P12.3
scapular region —see Contusion, shoulder
sclera —see Contusion, eyeball

◀ New   ◀|||| Revised   ~~deleted~~ Deleted

Contusion (Continued)
scrotum S30.22
seminal vesicle S37.892
shoulder S40.01-
skin NEC T14.8
small intestine —see Injury, intestine, small, contusion
spermatic cord S30.22
spinal cord —see Injury, spinal cord, by region
cauda equina S34.3
conus medullaris S34.139
spleen S36.029
major S36.021
minor S36.020
sternal region S20.219
stomach S36.32
subconjunctival S05.1-
subcutaneous NEC T14.8
submaxillary region S00.83
submental region S00.83
subperiosteal NEC T14.8
subungual
finger —see Contusion, finger, with damage to nail
toe —see Contusion, toe, with damage to nail
supraclavicular fossa S10.83
supraorbital S00.83
suprarenal gland S37.812
temple (region) S00.83
temporal
lobe (brain) —see Injury, intracranial, diffuse
focal —see Injury, intracranial, focal
region S00.83
testis S30.22
thigh S70.1-
thorax (wall) S20.20
back S20.22-
front S20.21-
throat S10.0
thumb S60.01-
with damage to nail S60.11-
toe (s) (lesser) S90.12-
with damage to nail S90.22-
great S90.11-
with damage to nail S90.21-
specified type NEC S90.221
tongue S00.532
trachea (cervical) S10.0
thoracic S27.52
tunica vaginalis S30.22
tympanum, tympanic membrane —see Contusion, ear
ureter S37.12
urethra S37.32
urinary organ NEC S37.892
uterus S37.62
uvula S00.532
vagina S30.23
vas deferens S37.892
vesical S37.22
vocal cord (s) S10.0
vulva S30.23
wrist S60.21-
Conus (congenital) (any type) Q14.8
cornea —see Keratoconus
medullaris syndrome G95.81
Conversion hysteria, neurosis or reaction F44.9
Converter, tuberculosis (test reaction) R76.11
Conviction (legal), anxiety concerning Z65.0
with imprisonment Z65.1
Convulsions (idiopathic) —see also Seizure(s) R56.9
apoplectiform (cerebral ischemia) I67.82
benign neonatal (familial) —see Epilepsy, generalized, idiopathic
dissociative F44.5
epileptic —see Epilepsy
epileptiform, epileptoid —see Seizure, epileptiform

Convulsions (Continued)
ether (anesthetic) —see Table of Drugs and Chemicals, by drug
febrile R56.00
with status epilepticus G40.901
complex R56.01
with status epilepticus G40.901
simple R56.00
hysterical F44.5
infantile P90
epilepsy —see Epilepsy
jacksonian —see Epilepsy, localization-related, symptomatic, with simple partial seizures
myoclonic G25.3
neonatal, benign (familial) —see Epilepsy, generalized, idiopathic
newborn P90
obstetrical (nephritic) (uremic) —see Eclampsia
paretic A52.17
post traumatic R56.1
psychomotor —see Epilepsy, localization-related, symptomatic, with complex partial seizures
recurrent R56.9
reflex R25.8
scarlatinal A38.8
tetanus, tetanic —see Tetanus
thymic E32.8
Convulsive —see also Convulsions
Cooley's anemia D56.1
Coolie itch B76.9
Cooper's
disease —see Mastopathy, cystic
hernia —see Hernia, abdomen, specified site NEC
Copra itch B88.0
Coprophagy F50.89
Coprophobia F40.298
Coproporphyria, hereditary E80.29
Cor
biloculare Q20.8
bovis, bovinum —see Hypertrophy, cardiac
pulmonale (chronic) I27.81
acute I26.09
triatriatum, triatrium Q24.2
triloculare Q20.8
biatrium Q20.4
biventriculare Q21.1
Corbus' disease (gangrenous balanitis) N48.1
Cord —see also condition
around neck (tightly) (with compression) complicating delivery O69.1
bladder G95.89
tabetic A52.19
Cordis ectopia Q24.8
Corditis (spermatic) N49.1
Corectopia Q13.2
Cori's disease (glycogen storage) E74.03
Corkhandler's disease or lung J67.3
Corkscrew esophagus K22.4
Corkworker's disease or lung J67.3
Corn (infected) L84
Cornea —see also condition
donor Z52.5
plana Q13.4
Cornelia de Lange syndrome Q87.1
Cornu cutaneum L85.8
Cornual gestation or pregnancy O00.80
with intrauterine pregnancy O00.81
Coronary (artery) —see condition
Coronavirus, as cause of disease classified elsewhere B97.29
SARS-associated B97.21
Corpora —see also condition
amylacea, prostate N42.89
cavernosa —see condition
Corpulence —see Obesity
Corpus —see condition
Corrected transposition Q20.5

Corrosion (injury) (acid) (caustic) (chemical) (lime) (external) (internal) T30.4
abdomen, abdominal (muscle) (wall) T21.42
first degree T21.52
second degree T21.62
third degree T21.72
above elbow T22.439
first degree T22.539
left T22.432
first degree T22.532
second degree T22.632
third degree T22.732
right T22.431
first degree T22.531
second degree T22.631
third degree T22.731
second degree T22.639
third degree T22.739
alimentary tract NEC T28.7
ankle T25.419
first degree T25.519
left T25.412
first degree T25.512
second degree T25.612
third degree T25.712
multiple with foot —see Corrosion, lower, limb, multiple, ankle and foot
right T25.411
first degree T25.511
second degree T25.611
third degree T25.711
second degree T25.619
third degree T25.719
anus —see Corrosion, buttock
arm (s) (meaning upper limb (s)) —see Corrosion, upper limb
axilla T22.449
first degree T22.549
left T22.442
first degree T22.542
second degree T22.642
third degree T22.742
right T22.441
first degree T22.541
second degree T22.641
third degree T22.741
second degree T22.649
third degree T22.749
back (lower) T21.44
first degree T21.54
second degree T21.64
third degree T21.74
upper T21.43
first degree T21.53
second degree T21.63
third degree T21.73
blisters - code as Corrosion, second degree, by site
breast (s) —see Corrosion, chest wall
buttock (s) T21.45
first degree T21.55
second degree T21.65
third degree T21.75
calf T24.439
first degree T24.539
left T24.432
first degree T24.532
second degree T24.632
third degree T24.732
right T24.431
first degree T24.531
second degree T24.631
third degree T24.731
second degree T24.639
third degree T24.739
canthus (eye) —see Corrosion, eyelid
cervix T28.8
cheek T20.46
first degree T20.56
second degree T20.66
third degree T20.76

Corrosion *(Continued)*
  chest wall T21.41
    first degree T21.51
    second degree T21.61
    third degree T21.71
  chin T20.43
    first degree T20.53
    second degree T20.63
    third degree T20.73
  colon T28.7
  conjunctiva (and cornea) —*see* Corrosion, cornea
  cornea (and conjunctiva) T26.6-
  deep necrosis of underlying tissue - code as Corrosion, third degree, by site
  dorsum of hand T23.469
    first degree T23.569
    left T23.462
      first degree T23.562
      second degree T23.662
      third degree T23.762
    right T23.461
      first degree T23.561
      second degree T23.661
      third degree T23.761
    second degree T23.669
    third degree T23.769
  ear (auricle) (external) (canal) T20.41
    drum T28.91
    first degree T20.51
    second degree T20.61
    third degree T20.71
  elbow T22.429
    first degree T22.529
    left T22.422
      first degree T22.522
      second degree T22.622
      third degree T22.722
    right T22.421
      first degree T22.521
      second degree T22.621
      third degree T22.721
    second degree T22.629
    third degree T22.729
  entire body —*see* Corrosion, multiple body regions
  epidermal loss - code as Corrosion, second degree, by site
  epiglottis T27.4
  erythema, erythematous - code as Corrosion, first degree, by site
  esophagus T28.6
  extent (percentage of body surface)
    less than 10 percent T32.0
    10-19 percent (0-9 percent third degree) T32.10
      with 10-19 percent third degree T32.11
    20-29 percent (0-9 percent third degree) T32.20
      with
        10-19 percent third degree T32.21
        20-29 percent third degree T32.22
    30-39 percent (0-9 percent third degree) T32.30
      with
        10-19 percent third degree T32.31
        20-29 percent third degree T32.32
        30-39 percent third degree T32.33
    40-49 percent (0-9 percent third degree) T32.40
      with
        10-19 percent third degree T32.41
        20-29 percent third degree T32.42
        30-39 percent third degree T32.43
        40-49 percent third degree T32.44
    50-59 percent (0-9 percent third degree) T32.50
      with
        10-19 percent third degree T32.51
        20-29 percent third degree T32.52

Corrosion *(Continued)*
  extent *(Continued)*
    50-59 percent *(Continued)*
      with *(Continued)*
        30-39 percent third degree T32.53
        40-49 percent third degree T32.54
        50-59 percent third degree T32.55
    60-69 percent (0-9 percent third degree) T32.60
      with
        10-19 percent third degree T32.61
        20-29 percent third degree T32.62
        30-39 percent third degree T32.63
        40-49 percent third degree T32.64
        50-59 percent third degree T32.65
        60-69 percent third degree T32.66
    70-79 percent (0-9 percent third degree) T32.70
      with
        10-19 percent third degree T32.71
        20-29 percent third degree T32.72
        30-39 percent third degree T32.73
        40-49 percent third degree T32.74
        50-59 percent third degree T32.75
        60-69 percent third degree T32.76
        70-79 percent third degree T32.77
    80-89 percent (0-9 percent third degree) T32.80
      with
        10-19 percent third degree T32.81
        20-29 percent third degree T32.82
        30-39 percent third degree T32.83
        40-49 percent third degree T32.84
        50-59 percent third degree T32.85
        60-69 percent third degree T32.86
        70-79 percent third degree T32.87
        80-89 percent third degree T32.88
    90 percent or more (0-9 percent third degree) T32.90
      with
        10-19 percent third degree T32.91
        20-29 percent third degree T32.92
        30-39 percent third degree T32.93
        40-49 percent third degree T32.94
        50-59 percent third degree T32.95
        60-69 percent third degree T32.96
        70-79 percent third degree T32.97
        80-89 percent third degree T32.98
        90-99 percent third degree T32.99
  extremity —*see* Corrosion, limb
  eye (s) and adnexa T26.9-
    with resulting rupture and destruction of eyeball T26.7-
    conjunctival sac —*see* Corrosion, cornea
    cornea —*see* Corrosion, cornea
    lid —*see* Corrosion, eyelid
    periocular area —*see* Corrosion eyelid
    specified site NEC T26.8-
  eyeball —*see* Corrosion, eye
  eyelid (s) T26.5-
  face —*see* Corrosion, head
  finger T23.429
    first degree T23.529
    left T23.422
      first degree T23.522
      second degree T23.622
      third degree T23.722
    multiple sites (without thumb) T23.439
      with thumb T23.449
        first degree T23.549
        left T23.442
          first degree T23.542
          second degree T23.642
          third degree T23.742
        right T23.441
          first degree T23.541
          second degree T23.641
          third degree T23.741
      second degree T23.649
      third degree T23.749

Corrosion *(Continued)*
  finger *(Continued)*
    multiple sites *(Continued)*
      first degree T23.539
      left T23.432
        first degree T23.532
        second degree T23.632
        third degree T23.732
      right T23.431
        first degree T23.531
        second degree T23.631
        third degree T23.731
      second degree T23.639
      third degree T23.739
    right T23.421
      first degree T23.521
      second degree T23.621
      third degree T23.721
    second degree T23.629
    third degree T23.729
  flank —*see* Corrosion, abdomen
  foot T25.429
    first degree T25.529
    left T25.422
      first degree T25.522
      second degree T25.622
      third degree T25.722
    multiple with ankle —*see* Corrosion, lower, limb, multiple, ankle and foot
    right T25.421
      first degree T25.521
      second degree T25.621
      third degree T25.721
    second degree T25.629
    third degree T25.729
  forearm T22.419
    first degree T22.519
    left T22.412
      first degree T22.512
      second degree T22.612
      third degree T22.712
    right T22.411
      first degree T22.511
      second degree T22.611
      third degree T22.711
    second degree T22.619
    third degree T22.719
  forehead T20.46
    first degree T20.56
    second degree T20.66
    third degree T20.76
  fourth degree - code as Corrosion, third degree, by site
  full thickness skin loss - code as Corrosion, third degree, by site
  gastrointestinal tract NEC T28.7
  genital organs
    external
      female T21.47
        first degree T21.57
        second degree T21.67
        third degree T21.77
      male T21.46
        first degree T21.56
        second degree T21.66
        third degree T21.76
    internal T28.8
  groin —*see* Corrosion, abdominal wall
  hand (s) T23.409
    back —*see* Corrosion, dorsum of hand
    finger —*see* Corrosion, finger
    first degree T23.509
    left T23.402
      first degree T23.502
      second degree T23.602
      third degree T23.702
    multiple sites with wrist T23.499
      first degree T23.599
      left T23.492
        first degree T23.592
        second degree T23.692
        third degree T23.792

Corrosion *(Continued)*
  hand (s) *(Continued)*
    multiple sites *(Continued)*
      right T23.491
        first degree T23.591
        second degree T23.691
        third degree T23.791
      second degree T23.699
      third degree T23.799
    palm —*see* Corrosion, palm
    right T23.401
      first degree T23.501
      second degree T23.601
      third degree T23.701
    second degree T23.609
    third degree T23.709
    thumb —*see* Corrosion, thumb
  head (and face) (and neck) T20.40
    cheek —*see* Corrosion, cheek
    chin —*see* Corrosion, chin
    ear —*see* Corrosion, ear
    eye (s) only —*see* Corrosion, eye
    first degree T20.50
    forehead —*see* Corrosion, forehead
    lip —*see* Corrosion, lip
    multiple sites T20.49
      first degree T20.59
      second degree T20.69
      third degree T20.79
    neck —*see* Corrosion, neck
    nose —*see* Corrosion, nose
    scalp —*see* Corrosion, scalp
    second degree T20.60
    third degree T20.70
  hip (s) —*see* Corrosion, lower, limb
  inhalation —*see* Corrosion, respiratory
      tract
  internal organ (s) *(see also* Corrosion, by site)
      T28.90
    alimentary tract T28.7
      esophagus T28.6
    esophagus T28.6
    genitourinary T28.8
    mouth T28.5
    pharynx T28.5
    specified organ NEC T28.99
  interscapular region —*see* Corrosion, back,
      upper
  intestine (large) (small) T28.7
  knee T24.429
    first degree T24.529
    left T24.422
      first degree T24.522
      second degree T24.622
      third degree T24.722
    right T24.421
      first degree T24.521
      second degree T24.621
      third degree T24.721
    second degree T24.629
    third degree T24.729
  labium (majus) (minus) —*see* Corrosion,
      genital organs, external, female
  lacrimal apparatus, duct, gland or sac —*see*
      Corrosion, eye, specified site NEC
  larynx T27.4
    with lung T27.5
  leg (s) (meaning lower limb (s)) —*see*
      Corrosion, lower limb
  limb (s)
    lower —*see* Corrosion, lower, limb
    upper —*see* Corrosion, upper limb
  lip (s) T20.42
    first degree T20.52
    second degree T20.62
    third degree T20.72
  lower
    back —*see* Corrosion, back
    limb T24.409
      ankle —*see* Corrosion, ankle
      calf —*see* Corrosion, calf

Corrosion *(Continued)*
  lower *(Continued)*
    limb *(Continued)*
      first degree T24.509
      foot —*see* Corrosion, foot
      hip —*see* Corrosion, thigh
      knee —*see* Corrosion, knee
      left T24.402
        first degree T24.502
        second degree T24.602
        third degree T24.702
      multiple sites, except ankle and foot
          T24.499
        ankle and foot T25.499
          first degree T25.599
          left T25.492
            first degree T25.592
            second degree T25.692
            third degree T25.792
          right T25.491
            first degree T25.591
            second degree T25.691
            third degree T25.791
          second degree T25.699
          third degree T25.799
        first degree T24.599
        left T24.492
          first degree T24.592
          second degree T24.692
          third degree T24.792
        right T24.491
          first degree T24.591
          second degree T24.691
          third degree T24.791
        second degree T24.699
        third degree T24.799
      right T24.401
        first degree T24.501
        second degree T24.601
        third degree T24.701
      second degree T24.609
      thigh —*see* Corrosion, thigh
      third degree T24.709
  lung (with larynx and trachea)
      T27.5
  mouth T28.5
  neck T20.47
    first degree T20.57
    second degree T20.67
    third degree T20.77
  nose (septum) T20.44
    first degree T20.54
    second degree T20.64
    third degree T20.74
  ocular adnexa —*see* Corrosion, eye
  orbit region —*see* Corrosion, eyelid
  palm T23.459
    first degree T23.559
    left T23.452
      first degree T23.552
      second degree T23.652
      third degree T23.752
    right T23.451
      first degree T23.551
      second degree T23.651
      third degree T23.751
    second degree T23.659
    third degree T23.759
  partial thickness - code as Corrosion,
      unspecified degree, by site
  pelvis —*see* Corrosion, trunk
  penis —*see* Corrosion, genital organs,
      external, male
  perineum
    female —*see* Corrosion, genital organs,
        external, female
    male —*see* Corrosion, genital organs,
        external, male
  periocular area —*see* Corrosion, eyelid
  pharynx T28.5
  rectum T28.7

Corrosion *(Continued)*
  respiratory tract T27.7
    larynx —*see* Corrosion, larynx
    specified part NEC T27.6
    trachea —*see* Corrosion, larynx
  sac, lacrimal —*see* Corrosion, eye,
      specified site NEC
  scalp T20.45
    first degree T20.55
    second degree T20.65
    third degree T20.75
  scapular region T22.469
    first degree T22.569
    left T22.462
      first degree T22.562
      second degree T22.662
      third degree T22.762
    right T22.461
      first degree T22.561
      second degree T22.661
      third degree T22.761
    second degree T22.669
    third degree T22.769
  sclera —*see* Corrosion, eye, specified site
      NEC
  scrotum —*see* Corrosion, genital organs,
      external, male
  shoulder T22.459
    first degree T22.559
    left T22.452
      first degree T22.552
      second degree T22.652
      third degree T22.752
    right T22.451
      first degree T22.551
      second degree T22.651
      third degree T22.751
    second degree T22.659
    third degree T22.759
  stomach T28.7
  temple —*see* Corrosion, head
  testis —*see* Corrosion, genital organs,
      external, male
  thigh T24.419
    first degree T24.519
    left T24.412
      first degree T24.512
      second degree T24.612
      third degree T24.712
    right T24.411
      first degree T24.511
      second degree T24.611
      third degree T24.711
    second degree T24.619
    third degree T24.719
  thorax (external) —*see* Corrosion, trunk
  throat (meaning pharynx) T28.5
  thumb (s) T23.419
    first degree T23.519
    left T23.412
      first degree T23.512
      second degree T23.612
      third degree T23.712
    multiple sites with fingers T23.449
      first degree T23.549
      left T23.442
        first degree T23.542
        second degree T23.642
        third degree T23.742
      right T23.441
        first degree T23.541
        second degree T23.641
        third degree T23.741
      second degree T23.649
      third degree T23.749
    right T23.411
      first degree T23.511
      second degree T23.611
      third degree T23.711
    second degree T23.619
    third degree T23.719

Corrosion *(Continued)*
  toe T25.439
    first degree T25.539
    left T25.432
      first degree T25.532
      second degree T25.632
      third degree T25.732
    right T25.431
      first degree T25.531
      second degree T25.631
      third degree T25.731
    second degree T25.639
    third degree T25.739
  tongue T28.5
  tonsil (s) T28.5
  total body —*see* Corrosion, multiple body
    regions
  trachea T27.4
    with lung T27.5
  trunk T21.40
    abdominal wall —*see* Corrosion,
      abdominal wall
    anus —*see* Corrosion, buttock
    axilla —*see* Corrosion, upper limb
    back —*see* Corrosion, back
    breast —*see* Corrosion, chest wall
    buttock —*see* Corrosion, buttock
    chest wall —*see* Corrosion, chest wall
    first degree T21.50
    flank —*see* Corrosion, abdominal wall
    genital
      female —*see* Corrosion, genital organs,
        external, female
      male —*see* Corrosion, genital organs,
        external, male
    groin —*see* Corrosion, abdominal wall
    interscapular region —*see* Corrosion, back,
      upper
    labia —*see* Corrosion, genital organs,
      external, female
    lower back —*see* Corrosion, back
    penis —*see* Corrosion, genital organs,
      external, male
    perineum
      female —*see* Corrosion, genital organs,
        external, female
      male —*see* Corrosion, genital organs,
        external, male
    scapular region —*see* Corrosion, upper
      limb
    scrotum —*see* Corrosion, genital organs,
      external, male
    second degree T21.60
    shoulder —*see* Corrosion, upper limb
    specified site NEC T21.49
      first degree T21.59
      second degree T21.69
      third degree T21.79
    testes —*see* Corrosion, genital organs,
      external, male
    third degree T21.70
    upper back —*see* Corrosion, back, upper
  vagina T28.8
  vulva —*see* Corrosion, genital organs,
    external, female
  unspecified site with extent of body surface
    involved specified
    less than 10 percent T32.0
    10-19 percent (0-9 percent third degree)
      T32.10
      with 10-19 percent third degree T32.11
    20-29 percent (0-9 percent third degree)
      T32.20
      with
        10-19 percent third degree T32.21
        20-29 percent third degree T32.22
    30-39 percent (0-9 percent third degree)
      T32.30
      with
        10-19 percent third degree T32.31
        20-29 percent third degree T32.32
        30-39 percent third degree T32.33

Corrosion *(Continued)*
  unspecified site with extent of body surface
    involved specified *(Continued)*
    40-49 percent (0-9 percent third degree)
      T32.40
      with
        10-19 percent third degree T32.41
        20-29 percent third degree T32.42
        30-39 percent third degree T32.43
        40-49 percent third degree T32.44
    50-59 percent (0-9 percent third degree)
      T32.50
      with
        10-19 percent third degree T32.51
        20-29 percent third degree T32.52
        30-39 percent third degree T32.53
        40-49 percent third degree T32.54
        50-59 percent third degree T32.55
    60-69 percent (0-9 percent third degree)
      T32.60
      with
        10-19 percent third degree T32.61
        20-29 percent third degree T32.62
        30-39 percent third degree T32.63
        40-49 percent third degree T32.64
        50-59 percent third degree T32.65
        60-69 percent third degree T32.66
    70-79 percent (0-9 percent third degree)
      T32.70
      with
        10-19 percent third degree T32.71
        20-29 percent third degree T32.72
        30-39 percent third degree T32.73
        40-49 percent third degree T32.74
        50-59 percent third degree T32.75
        60-69 percent third degree T32.76
        70-79 percent third degree T32.77
    80-89 percent (0-9 percent third degree)
      T32.80
      with
        10-19 percent third degree T32.81
        20-29 percent third degree T32.82
        30-39 percent third degree T32.83
        40-49 percent third degree T32.84
        50-59 percent third degree T32.85
        60-69 percent third degree T32.86
        70-79 percent third degree T32.87
        80-89 percent third degree T32.88
    90 percent or more (0-9 percent third
      degree) T32.90
      with
        10-19 percent third degree T32.91
        20-29 percent third degree T32.92
        30-39 percent third degree T32.93
        40-49 percent third degree T32.94
        50-59 percent third degree T32.95
        60-69 percent third degree T32.96
        70-79 percent third degree T32.97
        80-89 percent third degree T32.98
        90-99 percent third degree T32.99
  upper limb (axilla) (scapular region) T22.40
    above elbow —*see* Corrosion, above elbow
    axilla —*see* Corrosion, axilla
    elbow —*see* Corrosion, elbow
    first degree T22.50
    forearm —*see* Corrosion, forearm
    hand —*see* Corrosion, hand
    interscapular region —*see* Corrosion, back,
      upper
    multiple sites T22.499
      first degree T22.599
      left T22.492
        first degree T22.592
        second degree T22.692
        third degree T22.792
      right T22.491
        first degree T22.591
        second degree T22.691
        third degree T22.791
      second degree T22.699
      third degree T22.799

Corrosion *(Continued)*
  upper limb (axilla) (scapular region)
    (Continued)
    scapular region —*see* Corrosion, scapular
      region
    second degree T22.60
    shoulder —*see* Corrosion, shoulder
    third degree T22.70
    wrist —*see* Corrosion, hand
  uterus T28.8
  vagina T28.8
  vulva —*see* Corrosion, genital organs,
    external, female
  wrist T23.479
    first degree T23.579
    left T23.472
      first degree T23.572
      second degree T23.672
      third degree T23.772
    multiple sites with hand T23.499
      first degree T23.599
      left T23.492
        first degree T23.592
        second degree T23.692
        third degree T23.792
      right T23.491
        first degree T23.591
        second degree T23.691
        third degree T23.791
      second degree T23.699
      third degree T23.799
    right T23.471
      first degree T23.571
      second degree T23.671
      third degree T23.771
    second degree T23.679
    third degree T23.779
Corrosive burn —*see* Corrosion
Corsican fever —*see* Malaria
Cortical —*see* condition
Cortico-adrenal —*see* condition
Coryza (acute) J00
  with grippe or influenza —*see* Influenza,
    with, respiratory manifestations
    NEC
  syphilitic
    congenital (chronic) A50.05
Costen's syndrome or complex M26.69
Costiveness —*see* Constipation
Costochondritis M94.0
Cot death R99
Cotard's syndrome F22
Cotia virus B08.8
Cotton wool spots (retinal) H35.81
Cotungo's disease —*see* Sciatica
Cough (affected) (chronic) (epidemic) (nervous)
  R05
  with hemorrhage —*see* Hemoptysis
  bronchial R05
    with grippe or influenza —*see* Influenza,
      with, respiratory manifestations
      NEC
  functional F45.8
  hysterical F45.8
  laryngeal, spasmodic R05
  psychogenic F45.8
  smokers' J41.0
  tea taster's B49
Counseling (for) Z71.9
  abuse NEC
    perpetrator Z69.82
    victim Z69.81
  alcohol abuser Z71.41
    family Z71.42
  child abuse
    nonparental
      perpetrator Z69.021
      victim Z69.020
    parental
      perpetrator Z69.011
      victim Z69.010

◀ New   ◀║║║ Revised   ~~deleted~~ Deleted

Counseling *(Continued)*
  consanguinity Z71.89
  contraceptive Z30.09
  dietary Z71.3
  drug abuser Z71.51
    family member Z71.52
  family Z71.89
  fertility preservation (prior to cancer therapy) (prior to removal of gonads) Z31.62
  for non-attending third party Z71.0
    related to sexual behavior or orientation Z70.2
  genetic NEC Z31.5
  gestational carrier Z31.7 ◀
  health (advice) (education) (instruction) —*see* Counseling, medical
  human immunodeficiency virus (HIV) Z71.7
  impotence Z70.1
  insulin pump use Z46.81
  medical (for) Z71.9
    boarding school resident Z59.3
    consanguinity Z71.89
    feared complaint and no disease found Z71.1
    human immunodeficiency virus (HIV) Z71.7
    institutional resident Z59.3
    on behalf of another Z71.0
      related to sexual behavior or orientation Z70.2
    person living alone Z60.2
    specified reason NEC Z71.89
  natural family planning
    procreative Z31.61
    to avoid pregnancy Z30.02
  perpetrator (of)
    abuse NEC Z69.82
    child abuse
      non-parental Z69.021
      parental Z69.011
    rape NEC Z69.82
    spousal abuse Z69.12
  procreative NEC Z31.69
    fertility preservation (prior to cancer therapy) (prior to removal of gonads) Z31.62
    using natural family planning Z31.61
  promiscuity Z70.1
  rape victim Z69.81
  religious Z71.81
  sex, sexual (related to) Z70.9
    attitude (s) Z70.0
    behavior or orientation Z70.1
    combined concerns Z70.3
    non-responsiveness Z70.1
    on behalf of third party Z70.2
    specified reason NEC Z70.8
  specified reason NEC Z71.89
  spiritual Z71.81
  spousal abuse (perpetrator) Z69.12
    victim Z69.11
  substance abuse Z71.89
    alcohol Z71.41
    drug Z71.51
    tobacco Z71.6
  tobacco use Z71.6
  use (of)
    insulin pump Z46.81
  victim (of)
    abuse Z69.81
    child abuse
      by parent Z69.010
      non-parental Z69.020
    rape NEC Z69.81
Coupled rhythm R00.8
Couvelaire syndrome or uterus (complicating delivery) O45.8X-
Cowperitis —*see* Urethritis
Cowper's gland —*see* condition

Cowpox B08.010
  due to vaccination T88.1
Coxa
  magna M91.4-
  plana M91.2-
  valga (acquired) —*see also* Deformity, limb, specified type NEC, thigh
    congenital Q65.81
    sequelae (late effect) of rickets E64.3
  vara (acquired) —*see also* Deformity, limb, specified type NEC, thigh
    congenital Q65.82
    sequelae (late effect) of rickets E64.3
Coxalgia, coxalgic (nontuberculous) —*see also* Pain, joint, hip
  tuberculous A18.02
Coxitis —*see* Monoarthritis, hip
Coxsackie (virus) (infection) B34.1
  as cause of disease classified elsewhere B97.11
  carditis B33.20
  central nervous system NEC A88.8
  endocarditis B33.21
  enteritis A08.39
  meningitis (aseptic) A87.0
  myocarditis B33.22
  pericarditis B33.23
  pharyngitis B08.5
  pleurodynia B33.0
  specific disease NEC B33.8
Crabs, meaning pubic lice B85.3
Crack baby P04.41
Cracked nipple N64.0
  associated with
    lactation O92.13
    pregnancy O92.11-
    puerperium O92.12
Cracked tooth K03.81
Cradle cap L21.0
Craft neurosis F48.8
Cramp (s) R25.2
  abdominal —*see* Pain, abdominal
  bathing T75.1
  colic R10.83
    psychogenic F45.8
  due to immersion T75.1
  fireman T67.2
  heat T67.2
  immersion T75.1
  intestinal —*see* Pain, abdominal
    psychogenic F45.8
  leg, sleep related G47.62
  limb (lower) (upper) NEC R25.2
    sleep related G47.62
  linotypist's F48.8
    organic G25.89
  muscle (limb) (general) R25.2
    due to immersion T75.1
    psychogenic F45.8
  occupational (hand) F48.8
    organic G25.89
  salt-depletion E87.1
  sleep related, leg G47.62
  stoker's T67.2
  swimmer's T75.1
  telegrapher's F48.8
    organic G25.89
  typist's F48.8
    organic G25.89
  uterus N94.89
    menstrual —*see* Dysmenorrhea
  writer's F48.8
    organic G25.89
Cranial —*see* condition
Craniocleidodysostosis Q74.0
Craniofenestria (skull) Q75.8
Craniolacunia (skull) Q75.8
Craniopagus Q89.4
Craniopathy, metabolic M85.2
Craniopharyngeal —*see* condition
Craniopharyngioma D44.4
Craniorachischisis (totalis) Q00.1

Cranioschisis Q75.8
Craniostenosis Q75.0
Craniosynostosis Q75.0
Craniotabes (cause unknown) M83.8
  neonatal P96.3
  rachitic E64.3
  syphilitic A50.56
Cranium —*see* condition
Craw-craw —*see* Onchocerciasis
Creaking joint —*see* Derangement, joint, specified type NEC
Creeping
  eruption B76.9
  palsy or paralysis G12.22
Crenated tongue K14.8
Creotoxism A05.9
Crepitus
  caput Q75.8
  joint —*see* Derangement, joint, specified type NEC
Crescent or conus choroid, congenital Q14.3
CREST syndrome M34.1
Cretin, cretinism (congenital) (endemic) (nongoitrous) (sporadic) E00.9
  pelvis
    with disproportion (fetopelvic) O33.0
      causing obstructed labor O65.0
  type
    hypothyroid E00.1
    mixed E00.2
    myxedematous E00.1
    neurological E00.0
Creutzfeldt-Jakob disease or syndrome (with dementia) A81.00
  familial A81.09
  iatrogenic A81.09
  specified NEC A81.09
  sporadic A81.09
  variant (vCJD) A81.01
Crib death R99
Cribriform hymen Q52.3
Cri-du-chat syndrome Q93.4
Crigler-Najjar disease or syndrome E80.5
Crime, victim of Z65.4
Crimean hemorrhagic fever A98.0
Criminalism F60.2
Crisis
  abdomen R10.0
  acute reaction F43.0
  addisonian E27.2
  adrenal (cortical) E27.2
  celiac K90.0
  Dietl's N13.8
  emotional —*see also* Disorder, adjustment
    acute reaction to stress F43.0
    specific to childhood and adolescence F93.8
  glaucomatocyclitic —*see* Glaucoma, secondary, inflammation
  heart —*see* Failure, heart
  nitritoid I95.2
    correct substance properly administered —*see* Table of Drugs and Chemicals, by drug, adverse effect
    overdose or wrong substance given or taken —*see* Table of Drugs and Chemicals, by drug, poisoning
  oculogyric H51.8
    psychogenic F45.8
  Pel's (tabetic) A52.11
  psychosexual identity F64.2
  renal N28.0
  sickle-cell D57.00
    with
      acute chest syndrome D57.01
      splenic sequestration D57.02
  state (acute reaction) F43.0
  tabetic A52.11
  thyroid —*see* Thyrotoxicosis with thyroid storm
  thyrotoxic —*see* Thyrotoxicosis with thyroid storm

Crocq's disease (acrocyanosis) I73.89
Crohn's disease —see Enteritis, regional
Crooked septum, nasal J34.2
Cross syndrome E70.328
Crossbite (anterior) (posterior) M26.24
Cross-eye —see Strabismus, convergent
   concomitant
Croup, croupous (catarrhal) (infectious)
   (inflammatory) (nondiphtheritic) J05.0
   bronchial J20.9
   diphtheritic A36.2
   false J38.5
   spasmodic J38.5
     diphtheritic A36.2
   stridulous J38.5
     diphtheritic A36.2
Crouzon's disease Q75.1
Crowding, tooth, teeth, fully erupted M26.31
CRST syndrome M34.1
Cruchet's disease A85.8
Cruelty in children —see also Disorder, conduct
Crural ulcer —see Ulcer, lower limb
Crush, crushed, crushing T14.8
   abdomen S38.1
   ankle S97.0-
   arm (upper) (and shoulder) S47.-
   axilla —see Crush, arm
   back, lower S38.1
   buttock S38.1
   cheek S07.0
   chest S28.0
   cranium S07.1
   ear S07.0
   elbow S57.0-
   extremity
     lower
       ankle —see Crush, ankle
       below knee —see Crush, leg
       foot —see Crush, foot
       hip —see Crush, hip
       knee —see Crush, knee
       thigh —see Crush, thigh
       toe —see Crush, toe
     upper
       below elbow S67.9-
       elbow —see Crush, elbow
       finger —see Crush, finger
       forearm —see Crush, forearm
       hand —see Crush, hand
       thumb —see Crush, thumb
       upper arm —see Crush, arm
       wrist —see Crush, wrist
   face S07.0
   finger (s) S67.1-
     with hand (and wrist) —see Crush, hand,
       specified site NEC
     index S67.19-
     little S67.19-
     middle S67.19-
     ring S67.19-
     thumb —see Crush, thumb
   foot S97.8-
     toe —see Crush, toe
   forearm S57.8-
   genitalia, external
     female S38.002
       vagina S38.03
       vulva S38.03
     male S38.001
       penis S38.01
       scrotum S38.02
       testis S38.02
   hand (except fingers alone) S67.2-
     with wrist S67.4-
   head S07.9
     specified NEC S07.8
   heel —see Crush, foot
   hip S77.0-
     with thigh S77.2-
   internal organ (abdomen, chest, or pelvis)
     NEC T14.8

Crush, crushed, crushing (Continued)
   knee S87.0-
   labium (majus) (minus) S38.03
   larynx S17.0
   leg (lower) S87.8-
     knee —see Crush, knee
   lip S07.0
   lower
     back S38.1
     leg —see Crush, leg
   neck S17.9
   nerve —see Injury, nerve
   nose S07.0
   pelvis S38.1
   penis S38.01
   scalp S07.8
   scapular region —see Crush, arm
   scrotum S38.02
   severe, unspecified site T14.8
   shoulder (and upper arm) —see Crush, arm
   skull S07.1
   syndrome (complication of trauma) T79.5
   testis S38.02
   thigh S77.1-
     with hip S77.2-
   throat S17.8
   thumb S67.0-
     with hand (and wrist) —see Crush, hand,
       specified site NEC
   toe (s) S97.10-
     great S97.11-
     lesser S97.12-
   trachea S17.0
   vagina S38.03
   vulva S38.03
   wrist S67.3-
     with hand S67.4-
Crusta lactea L21.0
Crusts R23.4
Crutch paralysis —see Injury, brachial plexus
Cruveilhier-Baumgarten cirrhosis, disease or
   syndrome K74.69
Cruveilhier's atrophy or disease G12.8
Crying (constant) (continuous) (excessive)
   child, adolescent, or adult R45.83
   infant (baby) (newborn) R68.11
Cryofibrinogenemia D89.2
Cryoglobulinemia (essential) (idiopathic)
   (mixed) (primary) (purpura) (secondary)
   (vasculitis) D89.1
   with lung involvement D89.1 [J99]
Cryptitis (anal) (rectal) K62.89
Cryptococcosis, cryptococcus (infection)
   (neoformans) B45.9
   bone B45.3
   cerebral B45.1
   cutaneous B45.2
   disseminated B45.7
   generalized B45.7
   meningitis B45.1
   meningocerebralis B45.1
   osseous B45.3
   pulmonary B45.0
   skin B45.2
   specified NEC B45.8
Cryptopapillitis (anus) K62.89
Cryptophthalmos Q11.2
   syndrome Q87.0
Cryptorchid, cryptorchism, cryptorchidism
   Q53.9
   bilateral Q53.20
     abdominal Q53.21
     perineal Q53.22
   unilateral Q53.10
     abdominal Q53.11
     perineal Q53.12
Cryptosporidiosis A07.2
   hepatobiliary B88.8
   respiratory B88.8
Cryptostromosis J67.6
Crystalluria R82.99

Cubitus
   congenital Q68.8
   valgus (acquired) M21.0-
     congenital Q68.8
     sequelae (late effect) of rickets E64.3
   varus (acquired) M21.1-
     congenital Q68.8
     sequelae (late effect) of rickets E64.3
Cultural deprivation or shock Z60.3
Curling esophagus K22.4
Curling's ulcer —see Ulcer, peptic, acute
Curschmann (-Batten) (-Steinert) disease or
   syndrome G71.11
Curse, Ondine's —see Apnea, sleep
Curvature
   organ or site, congenital NEC —see Distortion
   penis (lateral) Q55.61
   Pott's (spinal) A18.01
   radius, idiopathic, progressive (congenital)
     Q74.0
   spine (acquired) (angular) (idiopathic)
     (incorrect) (postural) —see Dorsopathy,
     deforming
     congenital Q67.5
     due to or associated with
       Charcot-Marie-Tooth disease —see also
         subcategory M49.8 G60.0
       osteitis
         deformans M88.88
         fibrosa cystica —see also subcategory
           M49.8 E21.0
       tuberculosis (Pott's curvature) A18.01
     sequelae (late effect) of rickets E64.3
     tuberculous A18.01
Cushingoid due to steroid therapy E24.2
   correct substance properly administered —see
     Table of Drugs and Chemicals, by drug,
     adverse effect
   overdose or wrong substance given or
     taken —see Table of Drugs and
     Chemicals, by drug, poisoning
Cushing's
   syndrome or disease E24.9
     drug-induced E24.2
     iatrogenic E24.2
     pituitary-dependent E24.0
     specified NEC E24.8
   ulcer —see Ulcer, peptic, acute
Cusp, Carabelli - omit code
Cut (external) —see also Laceration
   muscle —see Injury, muscle
Cutaneous —see also condition
   hemorrhage R23.3
   larva migrans B76.9
Cutis —see also condition
   hyperelastica Q82.8
     acquired L57.4
   laxa (hyperelastica) —see Dermatolysis
   marmorata R23.8
   osteosis L94.2
   pendula —see Dermatolysis
   rhomboidalis nuchae L57.2
   verticis gyrata Q82.8
     acquired L91.8
Cyanosis R23.0
   due to
     patent foramen botalli Q21.1
     persistent foramen ovale Q21.1
   enterogenous D74.8
   paroxysmal digital —see Raynaud's disease
     with gangrene I73.01
   retina, retinal H35.89
Cyanotic heart disease I24.9
   congenital Q24.9
Cycle
   anovulatory N97.0
   menstrual, irregular N92.6
Cyclencephaly Q04.9
Cyclical vomiting (see also Vomiting, cyclical)
   G43.A0
   psychogenic F50.89 ◀▬

Cyclitis —see also Iridocyclitis H20.9
 chronic —see Iridocyclitis, chronic
 Fuchs' heterochromic H20.81-
 granulomatous —see Iridocyclitis, chronic
 lens-induced —see Iridocyclitis,
  lens-induced
 posterior H30.2-
Cycloid personality F34.0
Cyclophoria H50.54
Cyclopia, cyclops Q87.0
Cyclopism Q87.0
Cyclosporiasis A07.4
Cyclothymia F34.0
Cyclothymic personality F34.0
Cyclotropia H50.41-
Cylindroma —see also Neoplasm, malignant,
  by site
 eccrine dermal —see Neoplasm, skin,
  benign
 skin —see Neoplasm, skin, benign
Cylindruria R82.99
Cynanche
 diphtheritic A36.2
 tonsillaris J36
Cynophobia F40.218
Cynorexia R63.2
Cyphosis —see Kyphosis
Cyprus fever —see Brucellosis
Cyst (colloid) (mucous) (simple) (retention)
 adenoid (infected) J35.8
 adrenal gland E27.8
  congenital Q89.1
 air, lung J98.4
 allantoic Q64.4
 alveolar process (jaw bone) M27.40
 amnion, amniotic O41.8X-
 aneurysmal M27.49 ◄
 anterior
  chamber (eye) —see Cyst, iris
  nasopalatine K09.1
 antrum J34.1
 anus K62.89
 apical (tooth) (periodontal) K04.8
 appendix K38.8
 arachnoid, brain (acquired) G93.0
  congenital Q04.6
 arytenoid J38.7
 Baker's M71.2-
  ruptured M66.0
  tuberculous A18.02
 Bartholin's gland N75.0
 bile duct (common) (hepatic) K83.5
 bladder (multiple) (trigone) N32.89
 blue dome (breast) —see Cyst, breast
 bone (local) NEC M85.60
  aneurysmal M85.50
   ankle M85.57-
   foot M85.57-
   forearm M85.53-
   hand M85.54-
   jaw M27.49
   lower leg M85.56-
   multiple site M85.59
   neck M85.58
   rib M85.58
   shoulder M85.51-
   skull M85.58
   specified site NEC M85.58
   thigh M85.55-
   toe M85.57-
   upper arm M85.52-
   vertebra M85.58
  solitary M85.40
   ankle M85.47-
   fibula M85.46-
   foot M85.47-
   hand M85.44-
   humerus M85.42-
   jaw M27.49
   neck M85.48
   pelvis M85.45-

Cyst (Continued)
 bone NEC (Continued)
  solitary (Continued)
   radius M85.43-
   rib M85.48
   shoulder M85.41-
   skull M85.48
   specified site NEC M85.48
   tibia M85.46-
   toe M85.47-
   ulna M85.43-
   vertebra M85.48
  specified type NEC M85.60
   ankle M85.67-
   foot M85.67-
   forearm M85.63-
   hand M85.64-
   jaw M27.40
    developmental (nonodontogenic) K09.1
     odontogenic K09.0
    latent M27.0
   lower leg M85.66-
   multiple site M85.69
   neck M85.68
   rib M85.68
   shoulder M85.61-
   skull M85.68
   specified site NEC M85.68
   thigh M85.65-
   toe M85.67-
   upper arm M85.62-
   vertebra M85.68
 brain (acquired) G93.0
  congenital Q04.6
  hydatid B67.99 [G94]
  third ventricle (colloid), congenital
   Q04.6
 branchial (cleft) Q18.0
 branchiogenic Q18.0
 breast (benign) (blue dome) (pedunculated)
   (solitary) N60.0-
  involution —see Dysplasia, mammary,
   specified type NEC
  sebaceous —see Dysplasia, mammary,
   specified type NEC
 broad ligament (benign) N83.8
 bronchogenic (mediastinal) (sequestration)
   J98.4
  congenital Q33.0
 buccal K09.8
 bulbourethral gland N36.8
 bursa, bursal NEC M71.30
  with rupture —see Rupture, synovium
  ankle M71.37-
  elbow M71.32-
  foot M71.37-
  hand M71.34-
  hip M71.35-
  multiple sites M71.39
  pharyngeal J39.2
  popliteal space —see Cyst, Baker's
  shoulder M71.31-
  specified site NEC M71.38
  wrist M71.33-
 calcifying odontogenic D16.5
  upper jaw (bone) (maxilla) D16.4
 canal of Nuck (female) N94.89
  congenital Q52.4
 canthus —see Cyst, conjunctiva
 carcinomatous —see Neoplasm, malignant,
   by site
 cauda equina G95.89
 cavum septi pellucidi —see Cyst, brain
 celomic (pericardium) Q24.8
 cerebellopontine (angle) —see Cyst, brain
 cerebellum —see Cyst, brain
 cerebral —see Cyst, brain
 cervical lateral Q18.0 ◄▥
 cervix NEC N88.8
  embryonic Q51.6
  nabothian N88.8

Cyst (Continued)
 chiasmal optic NEC —see Disorder, optic,
   chiasm
 chocolate (ovary) N80.1
 choledochus, congenital Q44.4
 chorion O41.8X-
 choroid plexus G93.0
 ciliary body —see Cyst, iris
 clitoris N90.7
 colon K63.89
 common (bile) duct K83.5
 congenital NEC Q89.8
  adrenal gland Q89.1
  epiglottis Q31.8
  esophagus Q39.8
  fallopian tube Q50.4
  kidney Q61.00
   more than one (multiple) Q61.02
    specified as polycystic Q61.3
     adult type Q61.2
     infantile type NEC Q61.19
      collecting duct dilation Q61.11
   solitary Q61.01
  larynx Q31.8
  liver Q44.6
  lung Q33.0
  mediastinum Q34.1
  ovary Q50.1
  oviduct Q50.4
  periurethral (tissue) Q64.79
  prepuce Q55.69
  salivary gland (any) Q38.4
   sublingual Q38.6
   submaxillary gland Q38.6
  thymus (gland) Q89.2
  tongue Q38.3
  ureterovesical orifice Q62.8
  vulva Q52.79
 conjunctiva H11.44-
 cornea H18.89-
 corpora quadrigemina G93.0
 corpus
  albicans N83.29- ◄▥
  luteum (hemorrhagic) (ruptured)
   N83.1- ◄▥
 Cowper's gland (benign) (infected) N36.8
 cranial meninges G93.0
 craniobuccal pouch E23.6
 craniopharyngeal pouch E23.6
 cystic duct K82.8
 Cysticercus —see Cysticercosis
 Dandy-Walker Q03.1
  with spina bifida —see Spina bifida
 dental (root) K04.8
  developmental K09.0
  eruption K09.0
  primordial K09.0
 dentigerous (mandible) (maxilla) K09.0
 dermoid —see Neoplasm, benign, by site
  with malignant transformation C56.-
  implantation
   external area or site (skin) NEC
    L72.0
   iris —see Cyst, iris, implantation
   vagina N89.8
   vulva N90.7
  mouth K09.8
  oral soft tissue K09.8
  sacrococcygeal —see Cyst, pilonidal
 developmental K09.1
  odontogenic K09.0
  oral region (nonodontogenic) K09.1
  ovary, ovarian Q50.1
 dura (cerebral) G93.0
  spinal G96.19
 ear (external) Q18.1
 echinococcal —see Echinococcus
 embryonic
  cervix uteri Q51.6
  fallopian tube Q50.4
  vagina Q51.6

Cyst (Continued)
- endometrium, endometrial (uterus) N85.8
  - ectopic —see Endometriosis
- enterogenous Q43.8
- epidermal, epidermoid (inclusion) (see also Cyst, skin) L72.0
  - mouth K09.8
  - oral soft tissue K09.8
- epididymis N50.3
- epiglottis J38.7
- epiphysis cerebri E34.8
- epithelial (inclusion) L72.0
- epoophoron Q50.5
- eruption K09.0
- esophagus K22.8
- ethmoid sinus J34.1
- external female genital organs NEC N90.7
- eye NEC H57.8
  - congenital Q15.8
- eyelid (sebaceous) H02.829
  - infected —see Hordeolum
  - left H02.826
    - lower H02.825
    - upper H02.824
  - right H02.823
    - lower H02.822
    - upper H02.821
- fallopian tube N83.8
  - congenital Q50.4
- fimbrial (twisted) Q50.4
- fissural (oral region) K09.1
- follicle (graafian) (hemorrhagic) N83.0- ◀▥
  - nabothian N88.8
- follicular (atretic) (hemorrhagic) (ovarian) N83.0- ◀▥
  - dentigerous K09.0
  - odontogenic K09.0
  - skin L72.9
    - specified NEC L72.8
- frontal sinus J34.1
- gallbladder K82.8
- ganglion —see Ganglion
- Gartner's duct Q52.4
- gingiva K09.0
- gland of Moll —see Cyst, eyelid
- globulomaxillary K09.1
- graafian follicle (hemorrhagic) N83.0- ◀▥
- granulosal lutein (hemorrhagic) N83.1- ◀▥
- hemangiomatous D18.00
  - intra-abdominal D18.03
  - intracranial D18.02
  - skin D18.01
  - specified site NEC D18.09
- hemorrhagic M27.49 ◀
- hydatid —see also Echinococcus B67.90
  - brain B67.99 [G94]
  - liver —see also Cyst, liver, hydatid B67.8
  - lung NEC B67.99 [J99]
  - Morgagni
    - female Q50.5
    - male (epididymal) Q55.4
      - testicular Q55.29
  - specified site NEC B67.99
- hymen N89.8
  - embryonic Q52.4
- hypopharynx J39.2
- hypophysis, hypophyseal (duct) (recurrent) E23.6
  - cerebri E23.6
- implantation (dermoid)
  - external area or site (skin) NEC L72.0
  - iris —see Cyst, iris, implantation
  - vagina N89.8
  - vulva N90.7
- incisive canal K09.1
- inclusion (epidermal) (epithelial) (epidermoid) (squamous) L72.0
  - not of skin - code under Cyst, by site
- intestine (large) (small) K63.89
- intracranial —see Cyst, brain
- intraligamentous —see also Disorder, ligament
  - knee —see Derangement, knee

Cyst (Continued)
- intrasellar E23.6
- iris H21.309
  - exudative H21.31-
  - idiopathic H21.30-
  - implantation H21.32-
  - parasitic H21.33-
  - pars plana (primary) H21.34-
    - exudative H21.35-
- jaw (bone) M27.40
  - aneurysmal M27.49
  - developmental (odontogenic) K09.0
  - fissural K09.1
  - hemorrhagic M27.49
  - traumatic M27.49
- joint NEC —see Disorder, joint, specified type NEC
- kidney (acquired) N28.1
  - calyceal —see Hydronephrosis
  - congenital Q61.00
  - more than one (multiple) Q61.02
    - specified as polycystic Q61.3
      - adult type (autosomal dominant) Q61.2
      - infantile type (autosomal recessive) NEC Q61.19
        - collecting duct dilation Q61.11
  - pyelogenic —see Hydronephrosis
  - simple N28.1
  - solitary (single) Q61.01
    - acquired N28.1
- labium (majus) (minus) N90.7
  - sebaceous N90.7
- lacrimal —see also Disorder, lacrimal system, specified NEC
  - gland H04.13-
  - passages or sac —see Disorder, lacrimal system, specified NEC
- larynx J38.7
- lateral periodontal K09.0
- lens H27.8
  - congenital Q12.8
- lip (gland) K13.0
- liver (idiopathic) (simple) K76.89
  - congenital Q44.6
  - hydatid B67.8
    - granulosus B67.0
    - multilocularis B67.5
- lung J98.4
  - congenital Q33.0
  - giant bullous J43.9
- lutein N83.1- ◀▥
- lymphangiomatous D18.1
- lymphoepithelial, oral soft tissue K09.8
- macula —see Degeneration, macula, hole
- malignant —see Neoplasm, malignant, by site
- mammary gland —see Cyst, breast
- mandible M27.40
  - dentigerous K09.0
  - radicular K04.8
- maxilla M27.40
  - dentigerous K09.0
  - radicular K04.8
- medial, face and neck Q18.8
- median
  - anterior maxillary K09.1
  - palatal K09.1
- mediastinum, congenital Q34.1
- meibomian (gland) —see Chalazion
  - infected —see Hordeolum
- membrane, brain G93.0
- meninges (cerebral) G93.0
  - spinal G96.19
- meniscus, knee —see Derangement, knee, meniscus, cystic
- mesentery, mesenteric K66.8
  - chyle I89.8
- mesonephric duct
  - female Q50.5
  - male Q55.4
- milk N64.89

Cyst (Continued)
- Morgagni (hydatid)
  - female Q50.5
  - male (epididymal) Q55.4
    - testicular Q55.29
- mouth K09.8
- Müllerian duct Q50.4
  - appendix testis Q55.29
  - cervix Q51.6
  - fallopian tube Q50.4
  - female Q50.4
  - male Q55.29
  - prostatic utricle Q55.4
  - vagina (embryonal) Q52.4
- multilocular (ovary) D39.10
  - benign —see Neoplasm, benign, by site
- myometrium N85.8
- nabothian (follicle) (ruptured) N88.8
- nasoalveolar K09.1
- nasolabial K09.1
- nasopalatine (anterior) (duct) K09.1
- nasopharynx J39.2
- neoplastic —see Neoplasm, uncertain behavior, by site
  - benign —see Neoplasm, benign, by site
- nervous system NEC G96.8
- neuroenteric (congenital) Q06.8
- nipple —see Cyst, breast
- nose (turbinates) J34.1
  - sinus J34.1
- odontogenic, developmental K09.0
- omentum (lesser) K66.8
  - congenital Q45.8
- ora serrata —see Cyst, retina, ora serrata
- oral
  - region K09.9
    - developmental (nonodontogenic) K09.1
    - specified NEC K09.8
  - soft tissue K09.9
    - specified NEC K09.8
- orbit H05.81-
- ovary, ovarian (twisted) N83.20- ◀▥
  - adherent N83.20- ◀▥
  - chocolate N80.1
  - corpus
    - albicans N83.29- ◀▥
    - luteum (hemorrhagic) N83.1- ◀▥
  - dermoid D27.9
  - developmental Q50.1
  - due to failure of involution NEC N83.20- ◀▥
  - endometrial N80.1
  - follicular (graafian) (hemorrhagic) N83.0- ◀▥
  - hemorrhagic N83.20- ◀▥
  - in pregnancy or childbirth O34.8-
    - with obstructed labor O65.5
  - multilocular D39.10
  - pseudomucinous D27.9
  - retention N83.29- ◀▥
  - serous N83.20- ◀▥
  - specified NEC N83.29- ◀▥
  - theca lutein (hemorrhagic) N83.1- ◀▥
  - tuberculous A18.18
- oviduct N83.8
- palate (median) (fissural) K09.1
- palatine papilla (jaw) K09.1
- pancreas, pancreatic (hemorrhagic) (true) K86.2
  - congenital Q45.2
  - false K86.3
- paralabral
  - hip M24.85-
  - shoulder S43.43-
- paramesonephric duct Q50.4
  - female Q50.4
  - male Q55.29
- paranephric N28.1
- paraphysis, cerebri, congenital Q04.6
- parasitic B89
- parathyroid (gland) E21.4
- paratubal N83.8
- paraurethral duct N36.8
- paroophoron Q50.5

◀ New   ◀▥ Revised   ~~deleted~~ Deleted

Cyst (Continued)
  parotid gland K11.6
  parovarian Q50.5
  pelvis, female N94.89
    in pregnancy or childbirth O34.8-
      causing obstructed labor O65.5
  penis (sebaceous) N48.89
  periapical K04.8
  pericardial (congenital) Q24.8
    acquired (secondary) I31.8
  pericoronal K09.0
  periodontal K04.8
    lateral K09.0
  peripelvic (lymphatic) N28.1
  peritoneum K66.8
    chylous I89.8
  periventricular, acquired, newborn P91.1
  pharynx (wall) J39.2
  pilar L72.11
  pilonidal (infected) (rectum) L05.91
    with abscess L05.01
    malignant C44.59-
  pituitary (duct) (gland) E23.6
  placenta O43.19-
  pleura J94.8
  popliteal —see Cyst, Baker's
  porencephalic Q04.6
    acquired G93.0
  postanal (infected) —see Cyst, pilonidal
  postmastoidectomy cavity (mucosal) —see
      Complications, postmastoidectomy, cyst
  preauricular Q18.1
  prepuce N47.4
    congenital Q55.69
  primordial (jaw) K09.0
  prostate N42.83
  pseudomucinous (ovary) D27.9
  pupillary, miotic H21.27-
  radicular (residual) K04.8
  radiculodental K04.8
  ranular K11.8
  Rathke's pouch E23.6
  rectum (epithelium) (mucous) K62.89
  renal —see Cyst, kidney
  residual (radicular) K04.8
  retention (ovary) N83.29- ◀▥
    salivary gland K11.6
  retina H33.19-
    ora serrata H33.11-
    parasitic H33.12-
  retroperitoneal K68.9
  sacrococcygeal (dermoid) —see Cyst,
      pilonidal
  salivary gland or duct (mucous extravasation
      or retention) K11.6
  Sampson's N80.1
  sclera H15.89
  scrotum L72.9
    sebaceous L72.3
  sebaceous (duct) (gland) L72.3
    breast —see Dysplasia, mammary, specified
        type NEC
    eyelid —see Cyst, eyelid
    genital organ NEC
      female N94.89
      male N50.89 ◀▥
    scrotum L72.3
  semilunar cartilage (knee) (multiple) —see
      Derangement, knee, meniscus, cystic
  seminal vesicle N50.89 ◀▥
  serous (ovary) N83.20- ◀▥
  sinus (accessory) (nasal) J34.1
  Skene's gland N36.8
  skin L72.9
    breast —see Dysplasia, mammary, specified
        type NEC
    epidermal, epidermoid L72.0
    epithelial L72.0
    eyelid —see Cyst, eyelid
    genital organ NEC
      female N90.7
      male N50.89 ◀▥

Cyst (Continued)
  skin (Continued)
    inclusion L72.0
    scrotum L72.9
    sebaceous L72.3
    sweat gland or duct L74.8
  solitary
    bone —see Cyst, bone, solitary
    jaw M27.40
    kidney N28.1
  spermatic cord N50.89 ◀▥
  sphenoid sinus J34.1
  spinal meninges G96.19
  spleen NEC D73.4
    congenital Q89.09
    hydatid —see also Echinococcus B67.99 [D77]
  Stafne's M27.0
  subarachnoid intrasellar R93.0
  subcutaneous, pheomycotic (chromomycotic)
      B43.2
  subdural (cerebral) G93.0
    spinal cord G96.19
  sublingual gland K11.6
  submandibular gland K11.6
  submaxillary gland K11.6
  suburethral N36.8
  suprarenal gland E27.8
  suprasellar —see Cyst, brain
  sweat gland or duct L74.8
  synovial —see also Cyst, bursa
    ruptured —see Rupture, synovium
  tarsal —see Chalazion
  tendon (sheath) —see Disorder, tendon,
      specified type NEC
  testis N44.2
    tunica albuginea N44.1
  theca lutein (ovary) N83.1- ◀▥
  Thornwaldt's J39.2
  thymus (gland) E32.8
  thyroglossal duct (infected) (persistent)
      Q89.2
  thyroid (gland) E04.1
  thyrolingual duct (infected) (persistent)
      Q89.2
  tongue K14.8
  tonsil J35.8
  tooth —see Cyst, dental
  Tornwaldt's J39.2
  trichilemmal (proliferating) L72.12
  trichodermal L72.12
  tubal (fallopian) N83.8
    inflammatory —see Salpingitis, chronic
  tubo-ovarian N83.8
    inflammatory N70.13
  tunica
    albuginea testis N44.1
    vaginalis N50.89 ◀▥
  turbinate (nose) J34.1
  Tyson's gland N48.89
  urachus, congenital Q64.4
  ureter N28.89
  ureterovesical orifice N28.89
  urethra, urethral (gland) N36.8
  uterine ligament N83.8
  uterus (body) (corpus) (recurrent)
      N85.8
    embryonic Q51.818
    cervix Q51.6
  vagina, vaginal (implantation) (inclusion)
      (squamous cell) (wall) N89.8
    embryonic Q52.4
  vallecula, vallecular (epiglottis) J38.7
  vesical (orifice) N32.89
  vitreous body H43.89
  vulva (implantation) (inclusion) N90.7
    congenital Q52.79
    sebaceous gland N90.7
  vulvovaginal gland N90.7
  wolffian
    female Q50.5
    male Q55.4

Cystadenocarcinoma —see Neoplasm,
    malignant, by site
  bile duct C22.1
  endometrioid —see Neoplasm, malignant,
      by site
    specified site —see Neoplasm, malignant,
        by site
    unspecified site
      female C56.9
      male C61
  mucinous
    papillary
      specified site —see Neoplasm,
          malignant, by site
      unspecified site C56.9
    specified site —see Neoplasm, malignant,
        by site
    unspecified site C56.9
  papillary
    mucinous
      specified site —see Neoplasm,
          malignant, by site
      unspecified site C56.9
    pseudomucinous
      specified site —see Neoplasm,
          malignant, by site
      unspecified site C56.9
    serous
      specified site —see Neoplasm,
          malignant, by site
      unspecified site C56.9
    specified site —see Neoplasm, malignant,
        by site
    unspecified site C56.9
  pseudomucinous
    papillary
      specified site —see Neoplasm,
          malignant, by site
      unspecified site C56.9
    specified site —see Neoplasm, malignant,
        by site
    unspecified site C56.9
  serous
    papillary
      specified site —see Neoplasm,
          malignant, by site
      unspecified site C56.9
    specified site —see Neoplasm, malignant,
        by site
    unspecified site C56.9
Cystadenofibroma
  clear cell —see Neoplasm, benign, by site
  endometrioid D27.9
    borderline malignancy D39.1-
    malignant C56.-
  mucinous
    specified site —see Neoplasm, benign, by site
    unspecified site D27.9
  serous
    specified site —see Neoplasm, benign, by site
    unspecified site D27.9
  specified site —see Neoplasm, benign, by site
  unspecified site D27.9
Cystadenoma —see also Neoplasm, benign, by
    site
  bile duct D13.4
  endometrioid —see Neoplasm, benign, by site
    borderline malignancy —see Neoplasm,
        uncertain behavior, by site
  malignant —see Neoplasm, malignant, by site
  mucinous
    borderline malignancy
      ovary C56.-
      specified site NEC —see Neoplasm,
          uncertain behavior, by site
    unspecified site C56.9
    papillary
      borderline malignancy
        ovary C56.-
        specified site NEC —see Neoplasm,
            uncertain behavior, by site
      unspecified site C56.9

Cystadenoma *(Continued)*
  mucinous *(Continued)*
    papillary *(Continued)*
      specified site —*see* Neoplasm, benign, by site
      unspecified site D27.9
    specified site —*see* Neoplasm, benign, by site
    unspecified site D27.9
  papillary
    borderline malignancy
      ovary C56-
      specified site NEC —*see* Neoplasm, uncertain behavior, by site
      unspecified site C56.9
    lymphomatosum
      specified site —*see* Neoplasm, benign, by site
      unspecified site D11.9
    mucinous
      borderline malignancy
        ovary C56.-
        specified site NEC —*see* Neoplasm, uncertain behavior, by site
        unspecified site C56.9
      specified site —*see* Neoplasm, benign, by site
      unspecified site D27.9
    pseudomucinous
      borderline malignancy
        ovary C56.-
        specified site NEC —*see* Neoplasm, uncertain behavior, by site
        unspecified site C56.9
      specified site —*see* Neoplasm, benign, by site
      unspecified site D27.9
    serous
      borderline malignancy
        ovary C56.-
        specified site NEC —*see* Neoplasm, uncertain behavior, by site
        unspecified site C56.9
      specified site —*see* Neoplasm, benign, by site
      unspecified site D27.9
    specified site —*see* Neoplasm, benign, by site
    unspecified site D27.9
  pseudomucinous
    borderline malignancy
      ovary C56.-
      specified site NEC —*see* Neoplasm, uncertain behavior, by site
      unspecified site C56.9
    papillary
      borderline malignancy
        ovary C56.-
        specified site NEC —*see* Neoplasm, uncertain behavior, by site
        unspecified site C56.9
      specified site —*see* Neoplasm, benign, by site
      unspecified site D27.9
    specified site —*see* Neoplasm, benign, by site
    unspecified site D27.9
  serous
    borderline malignancy
      ovary C56.-
      specified site NEC —*see* Neoplasm, uncertain behavior, by site
      unspecified site C56.9
    papillary
      borderline malignancy
        ovary C56.-
        specified site NEC —*see* Neoplasm, uncertain behavior, by site
        unspecified site C56.9
      specified site —*see* Neoplasm, benign, by site
      unspecified site D27.9
    specified site —*see* Neoplasm, benign, by site
    unspecified site D27.9

Cystathionine synthase deficiency E72.11
Cystathioninemia E72.19
Cystathioninuria E72.19
Cystic —*see also* condition
  breast (chronic) —*see* Mastopathy, cystic
  corpora lutea (hemorrhagic) N83.1- ◀
  duct —*see* condition
  eyeball (congenital) Q11.0
  fibrosis —*see* Fibrosis, cystic
  kidney (congenital) Q61.9
    adult type Q61.2
    infantile type NEC Q61.19
      collecting duct dilatation Q61.11
    medullary Q61.5
  liver, congenital Q44.6
  lung disease J98.4
    congenital Q33.0
  mastitis, chronic —*see* Mastopathy, cystic
  medullary, kidney Q61.5
  meniscus —*see* Derangement, knee, meniscus, cystic
  ovary N83.20- ◀
Cysticercosis, cysticerciasis B69.9
  with
    epileptiform fits B69.0
    myositis B69.81
  brain B69.0
  central nervous system B69.0
  cerebral B69.0
  ocular B69.1
  specified NEC B69.89
Cysticercus cellulose infestation —*see* Cysticercosis
Cystinosis (malignant) E72.04
Cystinuria E72.01
Cystitis (exudative) (hemorrhagic) (septic) (suppurative) N30.90
  with
    fibrosis —*see* Cystitis, chronic, interstitial
    hematuria N30.91
    leukoplakia —*see* Cystitis, chronic, interstitial
    malakoplakia —*see* Cystitis, chronic, interstitial
    metaplasia —*see* Cystitis, chronic, interstitial
    prostatitis N41.3
  acute N30.00
    with hematuria N30.01
    of trigone N30.30
      with hematuria N30.31
  allergic —*see* Cystitis, specified type NEC
  amebic A06.81
  bilharzial B65.9 *[N33]*
  blennorrhagic (gonococcal) A54.01
  bullous —*see* Cystitis, specified type NEC
  calculous N21.0
  chlamydial A56.01
  chronic N30.20
    with hematuria N30.21
    interstitial N30.10
      with hematuria N30.11
    of trigone N30.30
      with hematuria N30.31
    specified NEC N30.20
      with hematuria N30.21
  cystic (a) —*see* Cystitis, specified type NEC
  diphtheritic A36.85
  echinococcal
    granulosus B67.39
    multilocularis B67.69
  emphysematous —*see* Cystitis, specified type NEC
  encysted —*see* Cystitis, specified type NEC
  eosinophilic —*see* Cystitis, specified type NEC
  follicular —*see* Cystitis, of trigone
  gangrenous —*see* Cystitis, specified type NEC
  glandularis —*see* Cystitis, specified type NEC

Cystitis *(Continued)*
  gonococcal A54.01
  incrusted —*see* Cystitis, specified type NEC
  interstitial (chronic) —*see* Cystitis, chronic, interstitial
  irradiation N30.40
    with hematuria N30.41
  irritation —*see* Cystitis, specified type NEC
  malignant —*see* Cystitis, specified type NEC
  of trigone N30.30
    with hematuria N30.31
  panmural —*see* Cystitis, chronic, interstitial
  polyposa —*see* Cystitis, specified type NEC
  prostatic N41.3
  puerperal (postpartum) O86.22
  radiation —*see* Cystitis, irradiation
  specified type NEC N30.80
    with hematuria N30.81
  subacute —*see* Cystitis, chronic
  submucous —*see* Cystitis, chronic, interstitial
  syphilitic (late) A52.76
  trichomonal A59.03
  tuberculous A18.12
  ulcerative —*see* Cystitis, chronic, interstitial
Cystocele (-urethrocele)
  female N81.10
    with prolapse of uterus —*see* Prolapse, uterus
    lateral N81.12
    midline N81.11
    paravaginal N81.12
  in pregnancy or childbirth O34.8-
    causing obstructed labor O65.5
  male N32.89
Cystolithiasis N21.0
Cystoma —*see also* Neoplasm, benign, by site
  endometrial, ovary N80.1
  mucinous
    specified site —*see* Neoplasm, benign, by site
    unspecified site D27.9
  serous
    specified site —*see* Neoplasm, benign, by site
    unspecified site D27.9
  simple (ovary) N83.29- ◀
Cystoplegia N31.2
Cystoptosis N32.89
Cystopyelitis —*see* Pyelonephritis
Cystorrhagia N32.89
Cystosarcoma phyllodes D48.6-
  benign D24-
  malignant —*see* Neoplasm, breast, malignant
Cystostomy
  attention to Z43.5
  complication —*see* Complications, cystostomy
  status Z93.50
    appendico-vesicostomy Z93.52
    cutaneous Z93.51
    specified NEC Z93.59
Cystourethritis —*see* Urethritis
Cystourethrocele —*see also* Cystocele
  female N81.10
    with uterine prolapse —*see* Prolapse, uterus
    lateral N81.12
    midline N81.11
    paravaginal N81.12
  male N32.89
Cytomegalic inclusion disease
  congenital P35.1
Cytomegalovirus infection B25.9
Cytomycosis (reticuloendothelial) B39.4
Cytopenia D75.9
  refractory
    with multilineage dysplasia D46.A
      and ring sideroblasts (RCMD RS) D46.B
Czerny's disease (periodic hydrarthrosis of the knee) —*see* Effusion, joint, knee

◀ New   ◀◀ Revised   ~~deleted~~ Deleted

D

Daae (-Finsen) disease (epidemic pleurodynia) B33.0
Dabney's grip B33.0
Da Costa's syndrome F45.8
Dacryoadenitis, dacryadenitis H04.00-
  acute H04.01-
  chronic H04.02-
Dacryocystitis H04.30-
  acute H04.32-
  chronic H04.41-
  neonatal P39.1
  phlegmonous H04.31-
  syphilitic A52.71
    congenital (early) A50.01
  trachomatous, active A71.1
    sequelae (late effect) B94.0
Dacryocystoblenorrhea —see Inflammation, lacrimal, passages, chronic
Dacryocystocele —see Disorder, lacrimal system, changes
Dacryolith, dacryolithiasis H04.51-
Dacryoma —see Disorder, lacrimal system, changes
Dacryopericystitis —see Dacryocystitis
Dacryops H04.11-
Dacryostenosis —see also Stenosis, lacrimal
  congenital Q10.5
Dactylitis
  bone —see Osteomyelitis
  sickle-cell D57.00
    Hb C D57.219
    Hb SS D57.00
    specified NEC D57.819
  skin L08.9
  syphilitic A52.77
  tuberculous A18.03
Dactylolysis spontanea (ainhum) L94.6
Dactylosymphysis Q70.9
  fingers —see Syndactylism, complex, fingers
  toes —see Syndactylism, complex, toes
Damage
  arteriosclerotic —see Arteriosclerosis
  brain (nontraumatic) G93.9
    anoxic, hypoxic G93.1
      resulting from a procedure G97.82
    child NEC G80.9
    due to birth injury P11.2
  cardiorenal (vascular) —see Hypertension, cardiorenal
  cerebral NEC —see Damage, brain
  coccyx, complicating delivery O71.6
  coronary —see Disease, heart, ischemic
  eye, birth injury P15.3
  liver (nontraumatic) K76.9
    alcoholic K70.9
    due to drugs —see Disease, liver, toxic
    toxic —see Disease, liver, toxic
  medication T88.7
  pelvic
    joint or ligament, during delivery O71.6
    organ NEC
      during delivery O71.5
      following ectopic or molar pregnancy O08.6
  renal —see Disease, renal
  subendocardium, subendocardial —see Degeneration, myocardial
  vascular I99.9
Dana-Putnam syndrome (subacute combined sclerosis with pernicious anemia) —see Degeneration, combined
Danbolt (-Cross) syndrome (acrodermatitis enteropathica) E83.2
Dandruff L21.0
Dandy-Walker syndrome Q03.1
  with spina bifida —see Spina bifida
Danlos' syndrome Q79.6
Darier (-White) disease (congenital) Q82.8
  meaning erythema annulare centrifugum L53.1

Darier-Roussy sarcoid D86.3
Darling's disease or histoplasmosis B39.4
Darwin's tubercle Q17.8
Dawson's (inclusion body) encephalitis A81.1
De Beurmann (-Gougerot) disease B42.1
De la Tourette's syndrome F95.2
De Lange's syndrome Q87.1
De Morgan's spots (senile angiomas) I78.1
De Quervain's
  disease (tendon sheath) M65.4
  syndrome E34.51
  thyroiditis (subacute granulomatous thyroiditis) E06.1
De Toni-Fanconi (-Debré) syndrome E72.09
  with cystinosis E72.04
Dead
  fetus, retained (mother) O36.4
    early pregnancy O02.1
  labyrinth —see subcategory H83.2
  ovum, retained O02.0
Deaf nonspeaking NEC H91.3
Deafmutism (acquired) (congenital) NEC H91.3
  hysterical F44.6
  syphilitic, congenital —see also subcategory H94.8 A50.09
Deafness (acquired) (complete) (hereditary) (partial) H91.9-
  with blue sclera and fragility of bone Q78.0
  auditory fatigue —see Deafness, specified type NEC
  aviation T70.0
    nerve injury —see Injury, nerve, acoustic, specified type NEC
  boilermaker's —see subcategory H83.3
  central —see Deafness, sensorineural
  conductive H90.2
    and sensorineural, mixed H90.8
      bilateral H90.6
    and sensorineural ◄
      mixed H90.8 ◄
        bilateral H90.6 ◄
      bilateral H90.0
      unilateral H90.1-
        with restricted hearing on the contralateral side H90.A- ◄
  congenital H90.5
    with blue sclera and fragility of bone Q78.0
  due to toxic agents —see Deafness, ototoxic
  emotional (hysterical) F44.6
  functional (hysterical) F44.6
  high frequency H91.9-
  hysterical F44.6
  low frequency H91.9-
  mental R48.8
  mixed conductive and sensorineural H90.8
    bilateral H90.6
    unilateral H90.7-
  nerve —see Deafness, sensorineural
  neural —see Deafness, sensorineural
  noise-induced —see also subcategory H83.3
    nerve injury —see Injury, nerve, acoustic, specified type NEC
  nonspeaking H91.3
  ototoxic —see subcategory H91.0
  perceptive —see Deafness, sensorineural
  psychogenic (hysterical) F44.6
  sensorineural H90.5
    and conductive, mixed H90.8
      bilateral H90.6
    and conductive ◄
      mixed H90.8 ◄
        bilateral H90.6 ◄
      bilateral H90.3
      unilateral H90.4-
        with restricted hearing on the contralateral side H90.A- ◄
  sensory —see Deafness, sensorineural
  specified type NEC —see subcategory H91.8
  sudden (idiopathic) H91.2-

Deafness (Continued)
  syphilitic A52.15
  transient ischemic H93.01-
  traumatic —see Injury, nerve, acoustic, specified type NEC
  word (developmental) H93.25
Death (cause unknown) (of) (unexplained) (unspecified cause) R99
  brain G93.82
  cardiac (sudden) (with successful resuscitation) — code to underlying disease
    family history of Z82.41
    personal history of Z86.74
  family member (assumed) Z63.4
Debility (chronic) (general) (nervous) R53.81
  congenital or neonatal NOS P96.9
  nervous R53.81
  old age R54
  senile R54
Débove's disease (splenomegaly) R16.1
Decalcification
  bone —see Osteoporosis
  teeth K03.89
Decapsulation, kidney N28.89
Decay
  dental —see Caries, dental
  senile R54
  tooth, teeth —see Caries, dental
Deciduitis (acute)
  following ectopic or molar pregnancy O08.0
Decline (general) —see Debility
  cognitive, age-associated R41.81
Decompensation
  cardiac (acute) (chronic) —see Disease, heart
  cardiovascular —see Disease, cardiovascular
  heart —see Disease, heart
  hepatic —see Failure, hepatic
  myocardial (acute) (chronic) —see Disease, heart
  respiratory J98.8
Decompression sickness T70.3
Decrease (d)
  absolute neutrophile count —see Neutropenia
  blood
    platelets —see Thrombocytopenia
    pressure R03.1
      due to shock following
        injury T79.4
        operation T81.19
  estrogen E28.39
    postablative E89.40
      asymptomatic E89.40
      symptomatic E89.41
  fragility of erythrocytes D58.8
  function
    lipase (pancreatic) K90.3
    ovary in hypopituitarism E23.0
    parenchyma of pancreas K86.89 ◄
    pituitary (gland) (anterior) (lobe) E23.0
      posterior (lobe) E23.0
  functional activity R68.89
  glucose R73.09
  hematocrit R71.0
  hemoglobin R71.0
  leukocytes D72.819
    specified NEC D72.818
  libido R68.82
  lymphocytes D72.810
  platelets D69.6
  respiration, due to shock following injury T79.4
  sexual desire R68.82
  tear secretion NEC —see Syndrome, dry eye
  tolerance
    fat K90.49 ◄
    glucose R73.09
    pancreatic K90.3
    salt and water E87.8
  vision NEC H54.7
  white blood cell count D72.819
    specified NEC D72.818

Decubitus (ulcer) —*see* Ulcer, pressure, by site
   cervix N86
Deepening acetabulum —*see* Derangement,
   joint, specified type NEC, hip
Defect, defective Q89.9
   3-beta-hydroxysteroid dehydrogenase E25.0
   11-hydroxylase E25.0
   21-hydroxylase E25.0
   abdominal wall, congenital Q79.59
   antibody immunodeficiency D80.9
   aorticopulmonary septum Q21.4
   atrial septal (ostium secundum type) Q21.1
     following acute myocardial infarction
       (current complication) I23.1
     ostium primum type Q21.2
   atrioventricular
     canal Q21.2
     septum Q21.2
   auricular septal Q21.1
   bilirubin excretion NEC E80.6
   biosynthesis, androgen (testicular) E29.1
   bulbar septum Q21.0
   catalase E80.3
   cell membrane receptor complex (CR3) D71
   circulation I99.9
     congenital Q28.9
     newborn Q28.9
   coagulation (factor) —*see also* Deficiency,
     factor D68.9
     with
       ectopic pregnancy O08.1
       molar pregnancy O08.1
     acquired D68.4
     antepartum with hemorrhage —*see*
       Hemorrhage, antepartum, with
       coagulation defect
     due to
       liver disease D68.4
       vitamin K deficiency D68.4
     hereditary NEC D68.2
     intrapartum O67.0
     newborn, transient P61.6
     postpartum O72.3
     specified type NEC D68.8
   complement system D84.1
   conduction (heart) I45.9
     bone —*see* Deafness, conductive
   congenital, organ or site not listed —*see*
     Anomaly, by site
   coronary sinus Q21.1
   cushion, endocardial Q21.2
   degradation, glycoprotein E77.1
   dental bridge, crown, fillings —*see* Defect,
     dental restoration
   dental restoration K08.50
     specified NEC K08.59
   dentin (hereditary) K00.5
   Descemet's membrane, congenital Q13.89
   developmental —*see also* Anomaly
     cauda equina Q06.3
   diaphragm
     with elevation, eventration or hernia —*see*
       Hernia, diaphragm
     congenital Q79.1
       with hernia Q79.0
       gross (with hernia) Q79.0
   ectodermal, congenital Q82.9
   Eisenmenger's Q21.8
   enzyme
     catalase E80.3
     peroxidase E80.3
   esophagus, congenital Q39.9
   extensor retinaculum M62.89
   fibrin polymerization D68.2
   filling
     bladder R93.41 ◂▥
     kidney R93.42- ◂▥
     renal pelvis R93.41 ◂
     stomach R93.3
     ureter R93.41 ◂▥
     urinary organs, specified NEC R93.49 ◂

Defect, defective (*Continued*)
   Gerbode Q21.0
   glycoprotein degradation E77.1
   Hageman (factor) D68.2
   hearing —*see* Deafness
   high grade F70
   interatrial septal Q21.1
   interauricular septal Q21.1
   interventricular septal Q21.0
     with dextroposition of aorta, pulmonary
       stenosis and hypertrophy of right
       ventricle Q21.8
     in tetralogy of Fallot Q21.3
   learning (specific) —*see* Disorder, learning
   lymphocyte function antigen-1 (LFA-1) D84.0
   lysosomal enzyme, post-translational
     modification E77.0
   major osseous M89.70
     ankle M89.77-
     carpus M89.74-
     clavicle M89.71-
     femur M89.75-
     fibula M89.76-
     fingers M89.74-
     foot M89.77-
     forearm M89.73-
     hand M89.74-
     humerus M89.72-
     lower leg M89.76-
     metacarpus M89.74-
     metatarsus M89.77-
     multiple sites M89.79
     pelvic region M89.75-
     pelvis M89.75-
     radius M89.73-
     scapula M89.71-
     shoulder region M89.71-
     specified NEC M89.78
     tarsus M89.77-
     thigh M89.75-
     tibia M89.76-
     toes M89.77-
     ulna M89.73-
   mental —*see* Disability, intellectual
   modification, lysosomal enzymes, post-
     translational E77.0
   obstructive, congenital
     renal pelvis Q62.39
     ureter Q62.39
       atresia —*see* Atresia, ureter
       cecoureterocele Q62.32
       megaureter Q62.2
       orthotopic ureterocele Q62.31
   osseous, major M89.70
     ankle M89.77-
     carpus M89.74-
     clavicle M89.71-
     femur M89.75-
     fibula M89.76-
     fingers M89.74-
     foot M89.77-
     forearm M89.73-
     hand M89.74-
     humerus M89.72-
     lower leg M89.76-
     metacarpus M89.74-
     metatarsus M89.77-
     multiple sites M89.9
     pelvic region M89.75-
     pelvis M89.75-
     radius M89.73-
     scapula M89.71-
     shoulder region M89.71-
     specified NEC M89.78
     tarsus M89.77-
     thigh M89.75-
     tibia M89.76-
     toes M89.77-
     ulna M89.73-
   osteochondral NEC —*see also* Deformity
     M95.8-

Defect, defective (*Continued*)
   ostium
     primum Q21.2
     secundum Q21.1
   peroxidase E80.3
   placental blood supply —*see* Insufficiency,
     placental
   platelets, qualitative D69.1
     constitutional D68.0
   postural NEC, spine —*see* Dorsopathy,
     deforming
   reduction
     limb Q73.8
       lower Q72.9-
         absence —*see* Agenesis, leg
         foot —*see* Agenesis, foot
         longitudinal
           femur Q72.4-
           fibula Q72.6-
           tibia Q72.5-
           specified type NEC Q72.89-
         split foot Q72.7-
        specified type NEC Q73.8
       upper Q71.9-
         absence —*see* Agenesis, arm
           forearm —*see* Agenesis, forearm
           hand —*see* Agenesis, hand
         lobster-claw hand Q71.6-
         longitudinal
           radius Q71.4-
           ulna Q71.5-
         specified type NEC Q71.89-
   renal pelvis Q63.8
     obstructive Q62.39
   respiratory system, congenital Q34.9
   restoration, dental K08.50
     specified NEC K08.59
   retinal nerve bundle fibers H35.89
   septal (heart) NOS Q21.9
     acquired (atrial) (auricular) (ventricular)
       (old) I51.0
     atrial Q21.1
       concurrent with acute myocardial
         infarction —*see* Infarct,
         myocardium
       following acute myocardial infarction
         (current complication) I23.1
     ventricular —*see also* Defect, ventricular
       septal Q21.0
   sinus venosus Q21.1
   speech R47.9
     developmental F80.9
     specified NEC R47.89
   Taussig-Bing (aortic transposition and
     overriding pulmonary artery) Q20.1
   teeth, wedge K03.1
   vascular (local) I99.9
     congenital Q27.9
   ventricular septal Q21.0
     concurrent with acute myocardial
       infarction —*see* Infarct, myocardium
     following acute myocardial infarction
       (current complication) I23.2
     in tetralogy of Fallot Q21.3
   vision NEC H54.7
   visual field H53.40
     bilateral
       heteronymous H53.47
       homonymous H53.46-
     generalized contraction H53.48-
     localized
       arcuate H53.43-
       scotoma (central area) H53.41-
         blind spot area H53.42-
       sector H53.43-
       specified type NEC H53.45-
   voice R49.9
     specified NEC R49.8
   wedge, tooth, teeth (abrasion) K03.1
Deferentitis N49.1
   gonorrheal (acute) (chronic) A54.23

◂ New   ◂▥ Revised   ~~deleted~~ Deleted

Defibrination (syndrome) D65
    antepartum —see Hemorrhage, antepartum,
        with coagulation defect, disseminated
        intravascular coagulation
    following ectopic or molar pregnancy O08.1
    intrapartum O67.0
    newborn P60
    postpartum O72.3
Deficiency, deficient
    3-beta hydroxysteroid dehydrogenase E25.0
    11-hydroxylase E25.0
    21-hydroxylase E25.0
    5-alpha reductase (with male
        pseudohermaphroditism) E29.1
    abdominal muscle syndrome Q79.4
    AC globulin (congenital) (hereditary) D68.2
        acquired D68.4
    accelerator globulin (Ac G) (blood) D68.2
    acid phosphatase E83.39
    activating factor (blood) D68.2
    adenosine deaminase (ADA) D81.3
    aldolase (hereditary) E74.19
    alpha-1-antitrypsin E88.01
    amino-acids E72.9
    anemia —see Anemia
    aneurin E51.9
    antibody with
        hyperimmunoglobulinemia D80.6
        near-normal immunoglobins D80.6
    antidiuretic hormone E23.2
    anti-hemophilic
        factor (A) D66
            B D67
            C D68.1
        globulin (AHG) NEC D66
    antithrombin (antithrombin III) D68.59
    ascorbic acid E54
    attention (disorder) (syndrome) F98.8
        with hyperactivity —see Disorder,
            attention-deficit hyperactivity
    autoprothrombin
        I D68.2
        II D67
        C D68.2
    beta-glucuronidase E76.29
    biotin E53.8
    biotin-dependent carboxylase D81.819
    biotinidase D81.810
    brancher enzyme (amylopectinosis) E74.03
    C1 esterase inhibitor (C1-INH) D84.1
    calciferol E55.9
        with
            adult osteomalacia M83.8
            rickets —see Rickets
    calcium (dietary) E58
    calorie, severe E43
        with marasmus E41
            and kwashiorkor E42
    cardiac —see Insufficiency, myocardial
    carnitine E71.40
        due to
            hemodialysis E71.43
            inborn errors of metabolism E71.42
            Valproic acid therapy E71.43
        iatrogenic E71.43
        muscle palmityltransferase E71.314
        primary E71.41
        secondary E71.448
    carotene E50.9
    central nervous system G96.8
    ceruloplasmin (Wilson) E83.01
    choline E53.8
    Christmas factor D67
    chromium E61.4
    clotting (blood) —see also Deficiency,
        coagulation factor D68.9
    clotting factor NEC (hereditary) —see also
        Deficiency, factor D68.2
    coagulation NOS D68.9
        with
            ectopic pregnancy O08.1
            molar pregnancy O08.1

Deficiency, deficient (Continued)
    coagulation NOS (Continued)
        acquired (any) D68.4
        antepartum hemorrhage —see
            Hemorrhage, antepartum, with
            coagulation defect
        clotting factor NEC —see also Deficiency,
            factor D68.2
        due to
            hyperprothrombinemia D68.4
            liver disease D68.4
            vitamin K deficiency D68.4
        newborn, transient P61.6
        postpartum O72.3
        specified NEC D68.8
    cognitive F09
    color vision H53.50
        achromatopsia H53.51
        acquired H53.52
        deuteranomaly H53.53
        protanomaly H53.54
        specified type NEC H53.59
        tritanomaly H53.55
    combined glucocorticoid and
        mineralocorticoid E27.49
    contact factor D68.2
    copper (nutritional) E61.0
    corticoadrenal E27.40
        primary E27.1
    craniofacial axis Q75.0
    cyanocobalamin E53.8
    debrancher enzyme (limit dextrinosis) E74.03
    dehydrogenase
        long chain/very long chain acyl CoA
            E71.310
        medium chain acyl CoA E71.311
        short chain acyl CoA E71.312
    diet E63.9
    dihydropyrimidine dehydrogenase (DPD)
        E88.89
    disaccharidase E73.9
    edema —see Malnutrition, severe
    endocrine E34.9
    energy-supply —see Malnutrition
    enzymes, circulating NEC E88.09
    ergosterol E55.9
        with
            adult osteomalacia M83.8
            rickets —see Rickets
    essential fatty acid (EFA) E63.0
    factor —see also Deficiency, coagulation
        Hageman D68.2
        I (congenital) (hereditary) D68.2
        II (congenital) (hereditary) D68.2
        IX (congenital) (functional) (hereditary)
            (with functional defect) D67
        multiple (congenital) D68.8
            acquired D68.4
        V (congenital) (hereditary) D68.2
        VII (congenital) (hereditary) D68.2
        VIII (congenital) (functional) (hereditary)
            (with functional defect) D66
            with vascular defect D68.0
        X (congenital) (hereditary) D68.2
        XI (congenital) (hereditary) D68.1
        XII (congenital) (hereditary) D68.2
        XIII (congenital) (hereditary) D68.2
    femoral, proximal focal (congenital) —
        see Defect, reduction, lower limb,
        longitudinal, femur
    fibrin-stabilizing factor (congenital)
        (hereditary) D68.2
        acquired D68.4
    fibrinase D68.2
    fibrinogen (congenital) (hereditary) D68.2
        acquired D65
    folate E53.8
    folic acid E53.8
    foreskin N47.3
    fructokinase E74.11
    fructose 1,6-diphosphatase E74.19

Deficiency, deficient (Continued)
    fructose-1-phosphate aldolase E74.19
    galactokinase E74.29
    galactose-1-phosphate uridyl transferase
        E74.29
    gammaglobulin in blood D80.1
        hereditary D80.0
    glass factor D68.2
    glucocorticoid E27.49
        mineralocorticoid E27.49
    glucose-6-phosphatase E74.01
    glucose-6-phosphate dehydrogenase anemia
        D55.0
    glucuronyl transferase E80.5
    glycogen synthetase E74.09
    gonadotropin (isolated) E23.0
    growth hormone (idiopathic) (isolated) E23.0
    Hageman factor D68.2
    hemoglobin D64.9
    hepatophosphorylase E74.09
    homogentisate 1,2-dioxygenase E70.29
    hormone
        anterior pituitary (partial) NEC E23.0
            growth E23.0
        growth (isolated) E23.0
        pituitary E23.0
        testicular E29.1
    hypoxanthine-(guanine)-
        phosphoribosyltransferase (HG-PRT)
        (total HG-PRT) E79.1
    immunity D84.9
        cell-mediated D84.8
            with thrombocytopenia and eczema
                D82.0
        combined D81.9
        humoral D80.9
        IgA (secretory) D80.2
        IgG D80.3
        IgM D80.4
    immuno —see Immunodeficiency
    immunoglobulin, selective
        A (IgA) D80.2
        G (IgG) (subclasses) D80.3
        M (IgM) D80.4
    inositol (B complex) E53.8
    intrinsic
        factor (congenital) D51.0
        sphincter N36.42
            with urethral hypermobility N36.43
    iodine E61.8
        congenital syndrome —see Syndrome,
            iodine-deficiency, congenital
    iron E61.1
        anemia D50.9
    kalium E87.6
    kappa-light chain D80.8
    labile factor (congenital) (hereditary) D68.2
        acquired D68.4
    lacrimal fluid (acquired) —see also Syndrome,
        dry eye
        congenital Q10.6
    lactase
        congenital E73.0
        secondary E73.1
    Laki-Lorand factor D68.2
    lecithin cholesterol acyltransferase E78.6
    lipocaic K86.89
    lipoprotein (familial) (high density) E78.6
    liver phosphorylase E74.09
    lysosomal alpha-1, 4 glucosidase E74.02
    magnesium E61.2
    major histocompatibility complex
        class I D81.6
        class II D81.7
    manganese E61.3
    menadione (vitamin K) E56.1
        newborn P53
    mental (familial) (hereditary) —see Disability,
        intellectual
    methylenetetrahydrofolate reductase
        (MTHFR) E72.12

Deficiency, deficient (Continued)
  mevalonate kinase M04.1 ◄
  mineral NEC E61.8
  mineralocorticoid E27.49
      with glucocorticoid E27.49
  molybdenum (nutritional) E61.5
  moral F60.2
  multiple nutrient elements E61.7
  muscle
      carnitine (palmityltransferase) E71.314
      phosphofructokinase E74.09
  myoadenylate deaminase E79.2
  myocardial —see Insufficiency, myocardial
  myophosphorylase E74.04
  NADH diaphorase or reductase (congenital)
      D74.0
  NADH-methemoglobin reductase
      (congenital) D74.0
  natrium E87.1
  niacin (amide) (-tryptophan) E52
  nicotinamide E52
  nicotinic acid E52
  number of teeth —see Anodontia
  nutrient element E61.9
      multiple E61.7
      specified NEC E61.8
  nutrition, nutritional E63.9
      sequelae —see Sequelae, nutritional
          deficiency
      specified NEC E63.8
  of interleukin 1 receptor antagonist [DIRA]
      M04.8 ◄
  ornithine transcarbamylase E72.4
  ovarian E28.39
  oxygen —see Anoxia
  pantothenic acid E53.8
  parathyroid (gland) E20.9
  perineum (female) N81.89
  phenylalanine hydroxylase E70.1
  phosphoenolpyruvate carboxykinase E74.4
  phosphofructokinase E74.19
  phosphomannomutase E74.8
  phosphomannose isomerase E74.8
  phosphomannosyl mutase E74.8
  phosphorylase kinase, liver E74.09
  pituitary hormone (isolated) E23.0
  plasma thromboplastin
      antecedent (PTA) D68.1
      component (PTC) D67
  platelet NEC D69.1
      constitutional D68.0
  polyglandular E31.8
      autoimmune E31.0
  potassium (K) E87.6
  prepuce N47.3
  proaccelerin (congenital) (hereditary) D68.2
      acquired D68.4
  proconvertin factor (congenital) (hereditary)
      D68.2
      acquired D68.4
  protein —see also Malnutrition E46
      anemia D53.0
      C D68.59
      S D68.59
  prothrombin (congenital) (hereditary) D68.2
      acquired D68.4
  Prower factor D68.2
  pseudocholinesterase E88.09
  PTA (plasma thromboplastin antecedent)
      D68.1
  PTC (plasma thromboplastin component)
      D67
  purine nucleoside phosphorylase (PNP) D81.5
  pyracin (alpha) (beta) E53.1
  pyridoxal E53.1
  pyridoxamine E53.1
  pyridoxine (derivatives) E53.1
  pyruvate
      carboxylase E74.4
      dehydrogenase E74.4
  riboflavin (vitamin B2) E53.0

Deficiency, deficient (Continued)
  salt E87.1
  secretion
      ovary E28.39
      salivary gland (any) K11.7
      urine R34
  selenium (dietary) E59
  serum antitrypsin, familial E88.01
  short stature homeobox gene (SHOX)
      with
          dyschondrosteosis Q78.8
          short stature (idiopathic) E34.3
          Turner's syndrome Q96.9
  sodium (Na) E87.1
  SPCA (factor VII) D68.2
  sphincter, intrinsic N36.42
      with urethral hypermobility N36.43
  stable factor (congenital) (hereditary)
      D68.2
      acquired D68.4
  Stuart-Prower (factor X) D68.2
  sucrase E74.39
  sulfatase E75.29
  sulfite oxidase E72.19
  thiamin, thiaminic (chloride) E51.9
      beriberi (dry) E51.11
      wet E51.12
  thrombokinase D68.2
      newborn P53
  thyroid (gland) —see Hypothyroidism
  tocopherol E56.0
  tooth bud K00.0
  transcobalamine II (anemia) D51.2
  vanadium E61.6
  vascular I99.9
  vasopressin E23.2
  vertical ridge K06.8 ◄
  viosterol —see Deficiency, calciferol
  vitamin (multiple) NOS E56.9
      A E50.9
          with
              Bitot's spot (corneal) E50.1
              follicular keratosis E50.8
              keratomalacia E50.4
              manifestations NEC E50.8
              night blindness E50.5
              scar of cornea, xerophthalmic
                  E50.6
              xeroderma E50.8
              xerophthalmia E50.7
              xerosis
                  conjunctival E50.0
                      and Bitot's spot E50.1
                  cornea E50.2
                      and ulceration E50.3
          sequelae E64.1
      B (complex) NOS E53.9
          with
              beriberi (dry) E51.11
              wet E51.12
              pellagra E52
      B1 NOS E51.9
          beriberi (dry) E51.11
              with circulatory system
                  manifestations E51.11
              wet E51.12
      B12 E53.8
      B2 (riboflavin) E53.0
      B6 E53.1
      C E54
          sequelae E64.2
      D E55.9
          with
              adult osteomalacia M83.8
              rickets —see Rickets
              25-hydroxylase E83.32
      E E56.0
      folic acid E53.8
      G E53.0
      group B E53.9
          specified NEC E53.8

Deficiency, deficient (Continued)
  vitamin (Continued)
      H (biotin) E53.8
      K E56.1
          of newborn P53
      nicotinic E52
      P E56.8
      PP (pellagra-preventing) E52
      specified NEC E56.8
      thiamin E51.9
          beriberi —see Beriberi
  zinc, dietary E60
Deficit —see also Deficiency
  attention and concentration R41.840
      following ◄
          cerebral infarction I69.310 ◄
          cerebrovascular disease I69.910 ◄
              specified disease NEC I69.810 ◄
          nontraumatic ◄
              intracerebral hemorrhage I69.110 ◄
              specified intracranial hemorrhage
                  NEC I69.210 ◄
              subarachnoid hemorrhage I69.010 ◄
  disorder —see Attention, deficit
  cognitive communication R41.841
  cognitive
      communication R41.841 ◄
      emotional ◄
          following ◄
              cerebral infarction I69.315 ◄
              cerebrovascular disease I69.915 ◄
                  specified disease NEC I69.815 ◄
              nontraumatic ◄
                  intracerebral hemorrhage I69.115 ◄
                  specified intracranial hemorrhage
                      NEC I69.215 ◄
                  subarachnoid hemorrhage I69.015 ◄
      following ◄
          cerebral infarction I69.319 ◄
          cerebrovascular disease I69.919 ◄
              specified disease NEC I69.819 ◄
          nontraumatic ◄
              intracerebral hemorrhage I69.119 ◄
              specified intracranial hemorrhage
                  NEC I69.219 ◄
              subarachnoid hemorrhage I69.019 ◄
      social ◄
          following ◄
              cerebral infarction I69.315 ◄
              cerebrovascular disease I69.915 ◄
                  specified disease NEC I69.815 ◄
              nontraumatic ◄
                  intracerebral hemorrhage I69.115 ◄
                  specified intracranial hemorrhage
                      NEC I69.215 ◄
                  subarachnoid hemorrhage I69.015 ◄
  cognitive NEC R41.89
      following
          cerebral infarction I69.318 ◄|||
          cerebrovascular disease I69.918 ◄|||
              specified disease NEC I69.818 ◄|||
          intracerebral hemorrhage I69.11
          nontraumatic intracranial hemorrhage
              NEC I69.21
          nontraumatic ◄
              intracerebral hemorrhage I69.118 ◄
              specified intracranial hemorrhage
                  NEC I69.218 ◄
              subarachnoid hemorrhage I69.018 ◄
              subarachnoid hemorrhage I69.01
  concentration R41.840
  executive function R41.844
      following ◄
          cerebral infarction I69.314 ◄
          cerebrovascular disease I69.914 ◄
              specified disease NEC I69.814 ◄
          nontraumatic ◄
              intracerebral hemorrhage I69.114 ◄
              specified intracranial hemorrhage
                  NEC I69.214 ◄
              subarachnoid hemorrhage I69.014 ◄

◄ New   ◄||| Revised   ~~deleted~~ Deleted

Deficit *(Continued)*
  frontal lobe R41.844
    following ◄
      cerebral infarction I69.314 ◄
      cerebrovascular disease I69.914 ◄
        specified disease NEC I69.814 ◄
      nontraumatic ◄
        intracerebral hemorrhage I69.114 ◄
        specified intracranial hemorrhage
          NEC I69.214 ◄
        subarachnoid hemorrhage I69.014 ◄
  memory ◄
    following ◄
      cerebral infarction I69.311 ◄
      cerebrovascular disease I69.911 ◄
        specified disease NEC I69.811 ◄
      nontraumatic ◄
        intracerebral hemorrhage I69.111 ◄
        specified intracranial hemorrhage
          NEC I69.211 ◄
        subarachnoid hemorrhage
          I69.011 ◄
  neurologic NEC R29.818
    ischemic
      reversible (RIND) I63.9
        prolonged (PRIND) I63.9
  oxygen R09.02
  prolonged reversible ischemic neurologic
    (PRIND) I63.9
  psychomotor R41.843
    following ◄
      cerebral infarction I69.313 ◄
      cerebrovascular disease I69.913 ◄
        specified disease NEC I69.813 ◄
      nontraumatic ◄
        intracerebral hemorrhage I69.113 ◄
        specified intracranial hemorrhage
          NEC I69.213 ◄
        subarachnoid hemorrhage
          I69.013 ◄
  visuospatial R41.842
    following ◄
      cerebral infarction I69.312 ◄
      cerebrovascular disease I69.912 ◄
        specified disease NEC I69.812 ◄
      nontraumatic ◄
        intracerebral hemorrhage I69.112 ◄
        specified intracranial hemorrhage
          NEC I69.212 ◄
        subarachnoid hemorrhage I69.012 ◄
Deflection
  radius —*see* Deformity, limb, specified type
    NEC, forearm
  septum (acquired) (nasal) (nose) J34.2
  spine —*see* Curvature, spine
  turbinate (nose) J34.2
Defluvium
  capillorum —*see* Alopecia
  ciliorum —*see* Madarosis
  unguium L60.8
Deformity Q89.9
  abdomen, congenital Q89.9
  abdominal wall
    acquired M95.8
    congenital Q79.59
  acquired (unspecified site) M95.9
  adrenal gland Q89.1
  alimentary tract, congenital Q45.9
    upper Q40.9
  ankle (joint) (acquired) —*see also* Deformity,
    limb, lower leg
    abduction —*see* Contraction, joint, ankle
    congenital Q68.8
    contraction —*see* Contraction, joint,
      ankle
    specified type NEC —*see* Deformity, limb,
      foot, specified NEC
  anus (acquired) K62.89
    congenital Q43.9
  aorta (arch) (congenital) Q25.40 ◄▥
    acquired I77.89

Deformity *(Continued)*
  aortic
    arch, acquired I77.89
    cusp or valve (congenital) Q23.8
      acquired —*see also* Endocarditis, aortic
        I35.8
  arm (acquired) (upper) —*see also* Deformity,
    limb, upper arm
    congenital Q68.8
    forearm —*see* Deformity, limb, forearm
  artery (congenital) (peripheral) NOS Q27.9
    acquired I77.89
    coronary (acquired) I25.9
      congenital Q24.5
    umbilical Q27.0
  atrial septal Q21.1
  auditory canal (external) (congenital) —*see*
    also Malformation, ear, external
    acquired —*see* Disorder, ear, external,
      specified type NEC
  auricle
    ear (congenital) —*see also* Malformation,
      ear, external
      acquired —*see* Disorder, pinna,
        deformity
  back —*see* Dorsopathy, deforming
  bile duct (common) (congenital) (hepatic)
    Q44.5
    acquired K83.8
  biliary duct or passage (congenital) Q44.5
    acquired K83.8
  bladder (neck) (trigone) (sphincter)
    (acquired) N32.89
    congenital Q64.79
  bone (acquired) NOS M95.9
    congenital Q79.9
    turbinate M95.0
  brain (congenital) Q04.9
    acquired G93.89
    reduction Q04.3
  breast (acquired) N64.89
    congenital Q83.9
    reconstructed N65.0
  bronchus (congenital) Q32.4
    acquired NEC J98.09
  bursa, congenital Q79.9
  canaliculi (lacrimalis) (acquired) —*see also*
    Disorder, lacrimal system, changes
    congenital Q10.6
  canthus, acquired —*see* Disorder, eyelid,
    specified type NEC
  capillary (acquired) I78.8
  cardiovascular system, congenital Q28.9
  caruncle, lacrimal (acquired) —*see also*
    Disorder, lacrimal system, changes
    congenital Q10.6
  cascade, stomach K31.2
  cecum (congenital) Q43.9
    acquired K63.89
  cerebral, acquired G93.89
    congenital Q04.9
  cervix (uterus) (acquired) NEC N88.8
    congenital Q51.9
  cheek (acquired) M95.2
    congenital Q18.9
  chest (acquired) (wall) M95.4
    congenital Q67.8
    sequelae (late effect) of rickets E64.3
  chin (acquired) M95.2
    congenital Q18.9
  choroid (congenital) Q14.3
    acquired H31.8
    plexus Q07.8
      acquired G96.19
  cicatricial —*see* Cicatrix
  cilia, acquired —*see* Disorder, eyelid,
    specified type NEC
  clavicle (acquired) M95.8
    congenital Q68.8
  clitoris (congenital) Q52.6
    acquired N90.89
  clubfoot —*see* Clubfoot

Deformity *(Continued)*
  coccyx (acquired) —*see* subcategory M43.8
  colon (congenital) Q43.9
    acquired K63.89
  concha (ear), congenital —*see also*
    Malformation, ear, external
    acquired —*see* Disorder, pinna, deformity
  cornea (acquired) H18.70
    congenital Q13.4
    descemetocele —*see* Descemetocele
    ectasia —*see* Ectasia, cornea
    specified NEC H18.79-
    staphyloma —*see* Staphyloma, cornea
  coronary artery (acquired) I25.9
    congenital Q24.5
  cranium (acquired) —*see* Deformity, skull
  cricoid cartilage (congenital) Q31.8
    acquired J38.7
  cystic duct (congenital) Q44.5
    acquired K82.8
  Dandy-Walker Q03.1
    with spina bifida —*see* Spina bifida
  diaphragm (congenital) Q79.1
    acquired J98.6
  digestive organ NOS Q45.9
  ductus arteriosus Q25.0
  duodenal bulb K31.89
  duodenum (congenital) Q43.9
    acquired K31.89
  dura —*see* Deformity, meninges
  ear (acquired) —*see also* Disorder, pinna,
    deformity
    congenital (external) Q17.9
      internal Q16.5
      middle Q16.4
        ossicles Q16.3
      ossicles Q16.3
  ectodermal (congenital) NEC Q84.9
  ejaculatory duct (congenital) Q55.4
    acquired N50.89 ◄▥
  elbow (joint) (acquired) —*see also* Deformity,
    limb, upper arm
    congenital Q68.8
    contraction —*see* Contraction, joint, elbow
  endocrine gland NEC Q89.2
  epididymis (congenital) Q55.4
    acquired N50.89 ◄▥
  epiglottis (congenital) Q31.8
    acquired J38.7
  esophagus (congenital) Q39.9
    acquired K22.8
  eustachian tube (congenital) NEC Q17.8
  eye, congenital Q15.9
  eyebrow (congenital) Q18.8
  eyelid (acquired) —*see also* Disorder, eyelid,
    specified type NEC
    congenital Q10.3
  face (acquired) M95.2
    congenital Q18.9
  fallopian tube, acquired N83.8
  femur (acquired) —*see* Deformity, limb,
    specified type NEC, thigh
  fetal
    with fetopelvic disproportion O33.7
    causing obstructed labor O66.3
  finger (acquired) M20.00-
    boutonniere M20.02-
    congenital Q68.1
    flexion contracture —*see* Contraction, joint,
      hand
    mallet finger M20.01-
    specified NEC M20.09-
    swan-neck M20.03-
  flexion (joint) (acquired) —*see also* Deformity,
    limb, flexion M21.20
    congenital NOS Q74.9
      hip Q65.89
  foot (acquired) —*see also* Deformity, limb,
    lower leg
    cavovarus (congenital) Q66.1
    congenital NOS Q66.9
      specified type NEC Q66.89

Deformity (Continued)
  foot (Continued)
    specified type NEC —see Deformity, limb,
      foot, specified NEC
    valgus (congenital) Q66.6
      acquired —see Deformity, valgus, ankle
    varus (congenital) NEC Q66.3
      acquired —see Deformity, varus, ankle
  forearm (acquired) —see also Deformity, limb,
    forearm
    congenital Q68.8
  forehead (acquired) M95.2
    congenital Q75.8
  frontal bone (acquired) M95.2
    congenital Q75.8
  gallbladder (congenital) Q44.1
    acquired K82.8
  gastrointestinal tract (congenital) NOS
    Q45.9
    acquired K63.89
  genitalia, genital organ (s) or system NEC
    female (congenital) Q52.9
      acquired N94.89
      external Q52.70
    male (congenital) Q55.9
      acquired N50.89 ◀▥
  globe (eye) (congenital) Q15.8
    acquired H44.89
  gum, acquired NEC K06.8
  hand (acquired) —see Deformity, limb,
    hand
    congenital Q68.1
  head (acquired) M95.2
    congenital Q75.8
  heart (congenital) Q24.9
    septum Q21.9
      auricular Q21.1
      ventricular Q21.0
    valve (congenital) NEC Q24.8
      acquired —see Endocarditis
  heel (acquired) —see Deformity, foot
  hepatic duct (congenital) Q44.5
    acquired K83.8
  hip (joint) (acquired) —see also Deformity,
    limb, thigh
    congenital Q65.9
    due to (previous) juvenile
      osteochondrosis —see Coxa, plana
    flexion —see Contraction, joint, hip
  hourglass —see Contraction, hourglass
  humerus (acquired) M21.82-
    congenital Q74.0
  hypophyseal (congenital) Q89.2
  ileocecal (coil) (valve) (acquired) K63.89
    congenital Q43.9
  ileum (congenital) Q43.9
    acquired K63.89
  ilium (acquired) M95.5
    congenital Q74.2
  integument (congenital) Q84.9
  intervertebral cartilage or disc (acquired) —
    see Disorder, disc, specified NEC
  intestine (large) (small) (congenital) NOS
    Q43.9
    acquired K63.89
  intrinsic minus or plus (hand) —see
    Deformity, limb, specified type NEC,
    forearm
  iris (acquired) H21.89
    congenital Q13.2
  ischium (acquired) M95.5
    congenital Q74.2
  jaw (acquired) (congenital) M26.9
  joint (acquired) NEC M21.90
    congenital Q68.8
    elbow M21.92-
    hand M21.94-
    hip M21.95-
    knee M21.96-
    shoulder M21.92-
    wrist M21.93-

Deformity (Continued)
  kidney (s) (calyx) (pelvis) (congenital) Q63.9
    acquired N28.89
    artery (congenital) Q27.2
      acquired I77.89
  Klippel-Feil (brevicollis) Q76.1
  knee (acquired) NEC —see also Deformity,
    limb, lower leg
    congenital Q68.2
  labium (majus) (minus) (congenital) Q52.79
    acquired N90.89
  lacrimal passages or duct (congenital) NEC
    Q10.6
    acquired —see Disorder, lacrimal system,
      changes
  larynx (muscle) (congenital) Q31.8
    acquired J38.7
    web (glottic) Q31.0
  leg (upper) (acquired) NEC —see also
    Deformity, limb, thigh
    congenital Q68.8
    lower leg —see Deformity, limb, lower leg
  lens (acquired) H27.8
    congenital Q12.9
  lid (fold) (acquired) —see also Disorder,
    eyelid, specified type NEC
    congenital Q10.3
  ligament (acquired) —see Disorder, ligament
    congenital Q79.9
  limb (acquired) M21.90
    clawfoot M21.53-
    clawhand M21.51-
    clubfoot M21.54-
    clubhand M21.52-
    congenital, except reduction deformity
      Q74.9
    flat foot M21.4-
    flexion M21.20
      ankle M21.27-
      elbow M21.22-
      finger M21.24-
      hip M21.25-
      knee M21.26-
      shoulder M21.21-
      toe M21.27-
      wrist M21.23-
    foot
      claw —see Deformity, limb, clawfoot
      club —see Deformity, limb, clubfoot
      drop M21.37-
      flat —see Deformity, limb, flat foot
      specified NEC M21.6X-
    forearm M21.93-
    hand M21.94-
    lower leg M21.96-
    specified type NEC M21.80
      forearm M21.83-
      lower leg M21.86-
      thigh M21.85-
      upper arm M21.82-
    thigh M21.95-
    unequal length M21.70
      short site is
        femur M21.75-
        fibula M21.76-
        humerus M21.72-
        radius M21.73-
        tibia M21.76-
        ulna M21.73-
    upper arm M21.92-
    valgus —see Deformity, valgus
    varus —see Deformity, varus
    wrist drop M21.33-
  lip (acquired) NEC K13.0
    congenital Q38.0
  liver (congenital) Q44.7
    acquired K76.89
  lumbosacral (congenital) (joint) (region) Q76.49
    acquired —see subcategory M43.8
    kyphosis —see Kyphosis, congenital
    lordosis —see Lordosis, congenital

Deformity (Continued)
  lung (congenital) Q33.9
    acquired J98.4
  lymphatic system, congenital Q89.9
  Madelung's (radius) Q74.0
  mandible (acquired) (congenital) M26.9
  maxilla (acquired) (congenital) M26.9
  meninges or membrane (congenital) Q07.9
    cerebral Q04.8
      acquired G96.19
    spinal cord (congenital) G96.19
      acquired G96.19
  metacarpus (acquired) —see Deformity, limb,
    forearm
    congenital Q74.0
  metatarsus (acquired) —see Deformity,
    foot
    congenital Q66.9
  middle ear (congenital) Q16.4
    ossicles Q16.3
  mitral (leaflets) (valve) I05.8
    parachute Q23.2
    stenosis, congenital Q23.2
  mouth (acquired) K13.79
    congenital Q38.6
  multiple, congenital NEC Q89.7
  muscle (acquired) M62.89
    congenital Q79.9
      sternocleidomastoid Q68.0
  musculoskeletal system (acquired) M95.9
    congenital Q79.9
    specified NEC M95.8
  nail (acquired) L60.8
    congenital Q84.6
  nasal —see Deformity, nose
  neck (acquired) M95.3
    congenital Q18.9
    sternocleidomastoid Q68.0
  nervous system (congenital) Q07.9
  nipple (congenital) Q83.9
    acquired N64.89
  nose (acquired) (cartilage) M95.0
    bone (turbinate) M95.0
    congenital Q30.9
      bent or squashed Q67.4
    saddle M95.0
      syphilitic A50.57
    septum (acquired) J34.2
      congenital Q30.8
    sinus (wall) (congenital) Q30.8
      acquired M95.0
    syphilitic (congenital) A50.57
      late A52.73
  ocular muscle (congenital) Q10.3
    acquired —see Strabismus, mechanical
  opticociliary vessels (congenital) Q13.2
  orbit (eye) (acquired) H05.30
    atrophy —see Atrophy, orbit
    congenital Q10.7
    due to
      bone disease NEC H05.32-
      trauma or surgery H05.33-
    enlargement —see Enlargement, orbit
    exostosis —see Exostosis, orbit
  organ of Corti (congenital) Q16.5
  ovary (congenital) Q50.39
    acquired N83.8
  oviduct, acquired N83.8
  palate (congenital) Q38.5
    acquired M27.8
    cleft (congenital) —see Cleft, palate
  pancreas (congenital) Q45.3
    acquired K86.89 ◀▥
  parathyroid (gland) Q89.2
  parotid (gland) (congenital) Q38.4
    acquired K11.8
  patella (acquired) —see Disorder, patella,
    specified NEC
  pelvis, pelvic (acquired) (bony) M95.5
    with disproportion (fetopelvic) O33.0
      causing obstructed labor O65.0

Deformity *(Continued)*
pelvis, pelvic *(Continued)*
  congenital Q74.2
  rachitic sequelae (late effect) E64.3
penis (glans) (congenital) Q55.69
  acquired N48.89
pericardium (congenital) Q24.8
  acquired —*see* Pericarditis
pharynx (congenital) Q38.8
  acquired J39.2
pinna, acquired —*see also* Disorder, pinna,
  deformity
  congenital Q17.9
pituitary (congenital) Q89.2
posture —*see* Dorsopathy, deforming
prepuce (congenital) Q55.69
  acquired N47.8
prostate (congenital) Q55.4
  acquired N42.89
pupil (congenital) Q13.2
  acquired —*see* Abnormality, pupillary
pylorus (congenital) Q40.3
  acquired K31.89
rachitic (acquired), old or healed E64.3
radius (acquired) —*see also* Deformity, limb,
  forearm
  congenital Q68.8
rectum (congenital) Q43.9
  acquired K62.89
reduction (extremity) (limb), congenital *(see
  also* condition and site) Q73.8
  brain Q04.3
  lower —*see* Defect, reduction, lower limb
  upper —*see* Defect, reduction, upper
    limb
renal —*see* Deformity, kidney
respiratory system (congenital) Q34.9
rib (acquired) M95.4
  congenital Q76.6
    cervical Q76.5
rotation (joint) (acquired) —*see* Deformity,
  limb, specified site NEC
  congenital Q74.9
  hip —*see* Deformity, limb, specified type
    NEC, thigh
    congenital Q65.89
sacroiliac joint (congenital) Q74.2
  acquired —*see* subcategory M43.8
sacrum (acquired) —*see* subcategory
  M43.8
saddle
  back —*see* Lordosis
  nose M95.0
    syphilitic A50.57
salivary gland or duct (congenital) Q38.4
  acquired K11.8
scapula (acquired) M95.8
  congenital Q68.8
scrotum (congenital) —*see also* Malformation,
  testis and scrotum
  acquired N50.89 ◀▥
seminal vesicles (congenital) Q55.4
  acquired N50.89 ◀▥
septum, nasal (acquired) J34.2
shoulder (joint) (acquired) —*see* Deformity,
  limb, upper arm
  congenital Q74.0
  contraction —*see* Contraction, joint,
    shoulder
sigmoid (flexure) (congenital) Q43.9
  acquired K63.89
skin (congenital) Q82.9
skull (acquired) M95.2
  congenital Q75.8
    with
      anencephaly Q00.0
      encephalocele —*see* Encephalocele
      hydrocephalus Q03.9
        with spina bifida —*see* Spina bifida,
          by site, with hydrocephalus
      microcephaly Q02

Deformity *(Continued)*
soft parts, organs or tissues (of pelvis)
  in pregnancy or childbirth NEC O34.8-
    causing obstructed labor O65.5
spermatic cord (congenital) Q55.4
  acquired N50.89 ◀▥
    torsion —*see* Torsion, spermatic cord
spinal —*see* Dorsopathy, deforming
  column (acquired) —*see* Dorsopathy,
    deforming
  congenital Q67.5
  cord (congenital) Q06.9
    acquired G95.89
  nerve root (congenital) Q07.9
spine (acquired) —*see also* Dorsopathy,
  deforming
  congenital Q67.5
  rachitic E64.3
  specified NEC —*see* Dorsopathy,
    deforming, specified NEC
spleen
  acquired D73.89
  congenital Q89.09
Sprengel's (congenital) Q74.0
sternocleidomastoid (muscle), congenital
  Q68.0
sternum (acquired) M95.4
  congenital NEC Q76.7
stomach (congenital) Q40.3
  acquired K31.89
submandibular gland (congenital) Q38.4
submaxillary gland (congenital) Q38.4
  acquired K11.8
talipes —*see* Talipes
testis (congenital) —*see also* Malformation,
  testis and scrotum
  acquired N44.8
    torsion —*see* Torsion, testis
thigh (acquired) —*see also* Deformity, limb,
  thigh
  congenital NEC Q68.8
thorax (acquired) (wall) M95.4
  congenital Q67.8
  sequelae of rickets E64.3
thumb (acquired) —*see also* Deformity, finger
  congenital NEC Q68.1
thymus (tissue) (congenital) Q89.2
thyroid (gland) (congenital) Q89.2
  cartilage Q31.8
    acquired J38.7
tibia (acquired) —*see also* Deformity, limb,
  specified type NEC, lower leg
  congenital NEC Q68.8
  saber (syphilitic) A50.56
toe (acquired) M20.6-
  congenital Q66.9
  hallux rigidus M20.2-
  hallux valgus M20.1-
  hallux varus M20.3-
  hammer toe M20.4-
  specified NEC M20.5X-
tongue (congenital) Q38.3
  acquired K14.8
tooth, teeth K00.2
trachea (rings) (congenital) Q32.1
  acquired J39.8
transverse aortic arch (congenital)
  Q25.49 ◀▥
tricuspid (leaflets) (valve) I07.8
  atresia or stenosis Q22.4
  Ebstein's Q22.5
trunk (acquired) M95.8
  congenital Q89.9
ulna (acquired) —*see also* Deformity, limb,
  forearm
  congenital NEC Q68.8
urachus, congenital Q64.4
ureter (opening) (congenital) Q62.8
  acquired N28.89
urethra (congenital) Q64.79
  acquired N36.8

Deformity *(Continued)*
urinary tract (congenital) Q64.9
  urachus Q64.4
uterus (congenital) Q51.9
  acquired N85.8
uvula (congenital) Q38.5
vagina (acquired) N89.8
  congenital Q52.4
valgus NEC M21.00
  ankle M21.07-
  elbow M21.02-
  hip M21.05-
  knee M21.06-
valve, valvular (congenital) (heart) Q24.8
  acquired —*see* Endocarditis
varus NEC M21.10
  ankle M21.17-
  elbow M21.12-
  hip M21.15
  knee M21.16-
  tibia —*see* Osteochondrosis, juvenile, tibia
vas deferens (congenital) Q55.4
  acquired N50.89 ◀▥
vein (congenital) Q27.9
  great Q26.9
vertebra —*see* Dorsopathy, deforming
vertical talus (congenital) Q66.80
  left foot Q66.82
  right foot Q66.81
vesicourethral orifice (acquired) N32.89
  congenital NEC Q64.79
vessels of optic papilla (congenital) Q14.2
visual field (contraction) —*see* Defect, visual
  field
vitreous body, acquired H43.89
vulva (congenital) Q52.79
  acquired N90.89
wrist (joint) (acquired) —*see also* Deformity,
  limb, forearm
  congenital Q68.8
  contraction —*see* Contraction, joint, wrist
Degeneration, degenerative
adrenal (capsule) (fatty) (gland) (hyaline)
  (infectional) E27.8
amyloid —*see also* Amyloidosis E85.9
anterior cornua, spinal cord G12.29
anterior labral S43.49-
aorta, aortic I70.0
  fatty I77.89
aortic valve (heart) —*see* Endocarditis,
  aortic
arteriovascular —*see* Arteriosclerosis
artery, arterial (atheromatous) (calcareous) —
  see also Arteriosclerosis
  cerebral, amyloid E85.4 [I68.0]
  medial —*see* Arteriosclerosis, extremities
articular cartilage NEC —*see* Derangement,
  joint, articular cartilage, by site
atheromatous —*see* Arteriosclerosis
basal nuclei or ganglia G23.9
  specified NEC G23.8
bone NEC —*see* Disorder, bone, specified
  type NEC
brachial plexus G54.0
brain (cortical) (progressive) G31.9
  alcoholic G31.2
  arteriosclerotic I67.2
  childhood G31.9
    specified NEC G31.89
  cystic G31.89
    congenital Q04.6
  in
    alcoholism G31.2
    beriberi E51.2
    cerebrovascular disease I67.9
    congenital hydrocephalus Q03.9
      with spina bifida —*see also* Spina
        bifida
    Fabry-Anderson disease E75.21
    Gaucher's disease E75.22
    Hunter's syndrome E76.1

Degeneration, degenerative *(Continued)*
  brain *(Continued)*
    in *(Continued)*
      lipidosis
        cerebral E75.4
        generalized E75.6
      mucopolysaccharidosis —*see*
          Mucopolysaccharidosis
      myxedema E03.9 *[G32.89]*
      neoplastic disease —*see also* Neoplasm
          D49.6 *[G32.89]*
      Niemann-Pick disease E75.249 *[G32.89]*
      sphingolipidosis E75.3 *[G32.89]*
      vitamin B12 deficiency E53.8 *[G32.89]*
    senile NEC G31.1
  breast N64.89
  Bruch's membrane —*see* Degeneration,
      choroid
  capillaries (fatty) I78.8
    amyloid E85.8 *[I79.8]*
  cardiac —*see also* Degeneration, myocardial
    valve, valvular —*see* Endocarditis
  cardiorenal —*see* Hypertension, cardiorenal
  cardiovascular —*see also* Disease,
      cardiovascular
    renal —*see* Hypertension, cardiorenal
  cerebellar NOS G31.9
    alcoholic G31.2
    primary (hereditary) (sporadic) G11.9
  cerebral —*see* Degeneration, brain
  cerebrovascular I67.9
    due to hypertension I67.4
  cervical plexus G54.2
  cervix N88.8
    due to radiation (intended effect) N88.8
      adverse effect or misadventure N99.89
  chamber angle H21.21-
  changes, spine or vertebra —*see* Spondylosis
  chorioretinal —*see also* Degeneration, choroid
    hereditary H31.20
  choroid (colloid) (drusen) H31.10-
    atrophy —*see* Atrophy, choroidal
    hereditary —*see* Dystrophy, choroidal,
        hereditary
  ciliary body H21.22-
  cochlear —*see* subcategory H83.8
  combined (spinal cord) (subacute) E53.8
      [G32.0]
    with anemia (pernicious) D51.0 *[G32.0]*
      due to dietary vitamin B12 deficiency
          D51.3 *[G32.0]*
    in (due to)
      vitamin B12 deficiency E53.8 *[G32.0]*
        anemia D51.9 *[G32.0]*
  conjunctiva H11.10
    concretions —*see* Concretion, conjunctiva
    deposits —*see* Deposit, conjunctiva
    pigmentations —*see* Pigmentation,
        conjunctiva
    pinguecula —*see* Pinguecula
    xerosis —*see* Xerosis, conjunctiva
  cornea H18.40
    calcerous H18.43
      band keratopathy H18.42-
    familial, hereditary —*see* Dystrophy, cornea
    hyaline (of old scars) H18.49
    keratomalacia —*see* Keratomalacia
    nodular H18.45-
    peripheral H18.46-
    senile H18.41-
    specified type NEC H18.49
  cortical (cerebellar) (parenchymatous)
      G31.89
    alcoholic G31.2
    diffuse, due to arteriopathy I67.2
  corticobasal G31.85
  cutis L98.8
    amyloid E85.4 *[L99]*
  dental pulp K04.2
  disc disease —*see* Degeneration,
      intervertebral disc NEC

Degeneration, degenerative *(Continued)*
  dorsolateral (spinal cord) —*see* Degeneration,
      combined
  extrapyramidal G25.9
  eye, macular —*see also* Degeneration, macula
    congenital or hereditary —*see* Dystrophy,
        retina
  facet joints —*see* Spondylosis
  fatty
    liver NEC K76.0
      alcoholic K70.0
  grey matter (brain) (Alpers') G31.81
  heart —*see also* Degeneration, myocardial
    amyloid E85.4 *[I43]*
    atheromatous —*see* Disease, heart,
        ischemic, atherosclerotic
    ischemic —*see* Disease, heart, ischemic
  hepatolenticular (Wilson's) E83.01
  hepatorenal K76.7
  hyaline (diffuse) (generalized)
    localized —*see* Degeneration, by site
  infrapatellar fat pad M79.4
  intervertebral disc NOS
    with
      myelopathy —*see* Disorder, disc, with,
          myelopathy
      radiculitis or radiculopathy —*see*
          Disorder, disc, with, radiculopathy
    cervical, cervicothoracic —*see* Disorder,
        disc, cervical, degeneration
      with
        myelopathy —*see* Disorder, disc,
            cervical, with myelopathy
        neuritis, radiculitis or
            radiculopathy —*see* Disorder,
            disc, cervical, with neuritis
    lumbar region M51.36
      with
        myelopathy M51.06
        neuritis, radiculitis, radiculopathy or
            sciatica M51.16
    lumbosacral region M51.37
      with
        neuritis, radiculitis, radiculopathy or
            sciatica M51.17
    sacrococcygeal region M53.3
    thoracic region M51.34
      with
        myelopathy M51.04
        neuritis, radiculitis, radiculopathy
            M51.14
    thoracolumbar region M51.35
      with
        myelopathy M51.05
        neuritis, radiculitis, radiculopathy
            M51.15
  intestine, amyloid E85.4
  iris (pigmentary) H21.23-
  ischemic —*see* Ischemia
  joint disease —*see* Osteoarthritis
  kidney N28.89
    amyloid E85.4 *[N29]*
    cystic, congenital Q61.9
    fatty N28.89
    polycystic Q61.3
      adult type (autosomal dominant)
          Q61.2
      infantile type (autosomal recessive) NEC
          Q61.19
        collecting duct dilatation Q61.11
  Kuhnt-Junius —*see also* Degeneration, macula
      H35.32- ◀▥
  lens —*see* Cataract
  lenticular (familial) (progressive) (Wilson's)
      (with cirrhosis of liver) E83.01
  liver (diffuse) NEC K76.89
    amyloid E85.4 *[K77]*
    cystic K76.89
      congenital Q44.6
    fatty NEC K76.0
      alcoholic K70.0

Degeneration, degenerative *(Continued)*
  liver *(Continued)*
    hypertrophic K76.89
    parenchymatous, acute or subacute
        K72.00
      with coma K72.01
    pigmentary K76.89
    toxic (acute) K71.9
  lung J98.4
  lymph gland I89.8
    hyaline I89.8
  macula, macular (acquired) (age-related)
      (senile) H35.30
    angioid streaks H35.33
    atrophic age-related H35.31- ◀▥
    congenital or hereditary —*see* Dystrophy,
        retina
    cystoid H35.35-
    drusen H35.36-
    dry age-related H35.31- ◀
    exudative H35.32- ◀▥
    hole H35.34-
    nonexudative H35.31- ◀▥
    puckering H35.37-
    toxic H35.38-
    wet age-related H35.32- ◀
  membranous labyrinth, congenital (causing
      impairment of hearing) Q16.5
  meniscus —*see* Derangement, meniscus
  mitral —*see* Insufficiency, mitral
  Mönckeberg's —*see* Arteriosclerosis,
      extremities
  motor centers, senile G31.1
  multi-system G90.3
  mural —*see* Degeneration, myocardial
  muscle (fatty) (fibrous) (hyaline)
      (progressive) M62.89
    heart —*see* Degeneration, myocardial
  myelin, central nervous system G37.9
  myocardial, myocardium (fatty) (hyaline)
      (senile) I51.5
    with rheumatic fever (conditions in I00)
        I09.0
      active, acute or subacute I01.2
        with chorea I02.0
      inactive or quiescent (with chorea) I09.0
    hypertensive —*see* Hypertension, heart
    rheumatic —*see* Degeneration, myocardial,
        with rheumatic fever
    syphilitic A52.06
  nasal sinus (mucosa) J32.9
    frontal J32.1
    maxillary J32.0
  nerve —*see* Disorder, nerve
  nervous system G31.9
    alcoholic G31.2
    amyloid E85.4 *[G99.8]*
    autonomic G90.9
    fatty G31.89
    specified NEC G31.89
  nipple N64.89
  olivopontocerebellar (hereditary) (familial)
      G23.8
  osseous labyrinth —*see* subcategory H83.8
  ovary N83.8
    cystic N83.20- ◀▥
    microcystic N83.20- ◀▥
  pallidal pigmentary (progressive) G23.0
  pancreas K86.89 ◀▥
    tuberculous A18.83
  penis N48.89
  pigmentary (diffuse) (general)
    localized —*see* Degeneration, by site
    pallidal (progressive) G23.0
  pineal gland E34.8
  pituitary (gland) E23.6
  popliteal fat pad M79.4
  posterolateral (spinal cord) —*see*
      Degeneration, combined
  pulmonary valve (heart) I37.8
  pulp (tooth) K04.2

◀ New   ◀▥ Revised   ~~deleted~~ Deleted

Degeneration, degenerative *(Continued)*
  pupillary margin H21.24-
  renal —*see* Degeneration, kidney
  retina H35.9
    hereditary (cerebroretinal) (congenital)
        (juvenile) (macula) (peripheral)
        (pigmentary) —*see* Dystrophy, retina
    Kuhnt-Junius —*see also* Degeneration,
        macula H35.32- ◀▥
    macula (cystic) (exudative) (hole)
        (nonexudative) (pseudohole) (senile)
        (toxic) —*see* Degeneration, macula
    peripheral H35.40
      lattice H35.41-
      microcystoid H35.42-
      paving stone H35.43-
      secondary
        pigmentary H35.45-
        vitreoretinal H35.46-
      senile reticular H35.44-
    pigmentary (primary) —*see also* Dystrophy,
        retina
    secondary —*see* Degeneration, retina,
        peripheral, secondary
    posterior pole —*see* Degeneration, macula
  saccule, congenital (causing impairment of
        hearing) Q16.5
  senile R54
    brain G31.1
    cardiac, heart or myocardium —*see*
        Degeneration, myocardial
    motor centers G31.1
    vascular —*see* Arteriosclerosis
  sinus (cystic) —*see also* Sinusitis
    polypoid J33.1
  skin L98.8
    amyloid E85.4 *[L99]*
    colloid L98.8
  spinal (cord) G31.89
    amyloid E85.4 *[G32.89]*
    combined (subacute) —*see* Degeneration,
        combined
    dorsolateral —*see* Degeneration, combined
    familial NEC G31.89
    fatty G31.89
    funicular —*see* Degeneration, combined
    posterolateral —*see* Degeneration,
        combined
    subacute combined —*see* Degeneration,
        combined
    tuberculous A17.81
  spleen D73.0
    amyloid E85.4 *[D77]*
  stomach K31.89
  striatonigral G23.2
  suprarenal (capsule) (gland) E27.8
  synovial membrane (pulpy) —*see* Disorder,
        synovium, specified type NEC
  tapetoretinal —*see* Dystrophy, retina
  thymus (gland) E32.8
    fatty E32.8
  thyroid (gland) E07.89
  tricuspid (heart) (valve) I07.9
  tuberculous NEC —*see* Tuberculosis
  turbinate J34.89
  uterus (cystic) N85.8
  vascular (senile) —*see* Arteriosclerosis
    hypertensive —*see* Hypertension
  vitreoretinal, secondary —*see* Degeneration,
        retina, peripheral, secondary, vitreoretinal
  vitreous (body) H43.81-
  Wallerian —*see* Disorder, nerve
  Wilson's hepatolenticular E83.01
Deglutition
  paralysis R13.0
    hysterical F44.4
  pneumonia J69.0
Degos' disease I77.89
Dehiscence (of)
  amputation stump T87.81
  cesarean wound O90.0

Dehiscence *(Continued)*
  closure of
    cornea T81.31
    craniotomy T81.32
    fascia (muscular) (superficial) T81.32
    internal organ or tissue T81.32
    laceration (external) (internal) T81.33
    ligament T81.32
    mucosa T81.31
    muscle or muscle flap T81.32
    ribs or rib cage T81.32
    skin and subcutaneous tissue (full-
        thickness) (superficial) T81.31
    skull T81.32
    sternum (sternotomy) T81.32
    tendon T81.32
    traumatic laceration (external) (internal)
        T81.33
  episiotomy O90.1
  operation wound NEC T81.31
    external operation wound (superficial)
        T81.31
    internal operation wound (deep)
        T81.32
  perineal wound (postpartum) O90.1
  traumatic injury wound repair T81.33
  wound T81.30
    traumatic repair T81.33
Dehydration E86.0
  ~~hypertonic E87.0~~
  ~~hypotonic E87.1~~
  newborn P74.1
Déjérine-Roussy syndrome G93.89
Déjérine-Sottas disease or neuropathy
    (hypertrophic) G60.0
Déjérine-Thomas atrophy G23.8
Delay, delayed
  any plane in pelvis
    complicating delivery O66.9
  birth or delivery NOS O63.9
  closure, ductus arteriosus (Botalli) P29.3
  coagulation —*see* Defect, coagulation
  conduction (cardiac) (ventricular) I45.9
  delivery, second twin, triplet, etc O63.2
  development R62.50
    global F88
    intellectual (specific) F81.9
    language F80.9
      due to hearing loss F80.4
    learning F81.9
    pervasive F84.9
    physiological R62.50
      specified stage NEC R62.0
    reading F81.9
    sexual E30.0
    speech F80.9
      due to hearing loss F80.4
    spelling F81.81
  ejaculation F52.32 ◀
  gastric emptying K30
  menarche E30.0
  menstruation (cause unknown) N91.0
  milestone R62.0
  passage of meconium (newborn) P76.0
  primary respiration P28.9
  puberty (constitutional) E30.0
  separation of umbilical cord P96.82
  sexual maturation, female E30.0
  sleep phase syndrome G47.21
  union, fracture —*see* Fracture, by site
  vaccination Z28.9
Deletion (s)
  autosome Q93.9
    identified by fluorescence in situ
        hybridization (FISH) Q93.89
    identified by in situ hybridization (ISH)
        Q93.89
  chromosome
    with complex rearrangements NEC Q93.7
    part of NEC Q93.5
  ◀ seen only at prometaphase Q93.89

Deletion *(Continued)*
  chromosome *(Continued)*
    short arm
      4 Q93.3
      5p Q93.4
      22q11.2 Q93.81
    specified NEC Q93.89
    long arm chromosome 18 or 21 Q93.89
      with complex rearrangements NEC
          Q93.7
    microdeletions NEC Q93.88
Delhi boil or button B55.1
Delinquency (juvenile) (neurotic) F91.8
  group Z72.810
Delinquent immunization status Z28.3
Delirium, delirious (acute or subacute) (not
    alcohol or drug-induced) (with dementia)
    R41.0
  alcoholic (acute) (tremens) (withdrawal)
    F10.921
    with intoxication F10.921
      in
        abuse F10.121
        dependence F10.221
  due to (secondary to)
    alcohol
      intoxication F10.921
        in
          abuse F10.121
          dependence F10.221
      withdrawal F10.231
    amphetamine intoxication F15.921
      in
        abuse F15.121
        dependence F15.221
    anxiolytic
      intoxication F13.921
        in
          abuse F13.121
          dependence F13.221
      withdrawal F13.231
    cannabis intoxication (acute) F12.921
      in
        abuse F12.121
        dependence F12.221
    cocaine intoxication (acute) F14.921
      in
        abuse F14.121
        dependence F14.221
    general medical condition F05
    hallucinogen intoxication F16.921
      in
        abuse F16.121
        dependence F16.221
    hypnotic
      intoxication F13.921
        in
          abuse F13.121
          dependence F13.221
      withdrawal F13.231
    inhalant intoxication (acute) F18.921
      in
        abuse F18.121
        dependence F18.221
    multiple etiologies F05
    opioid intoxication (acute) F11.921
      in
        abuse F11.121
        dependence F11.221
    other (or unknown) substance
        F19.921 ◀
    phencyclidine intoxication (acute)
        F16.921
      in
        abuse F16.121
        dependence F16.221
    psychoactive substance NEC intoxication
        (acute) F19.921
      in
        abuse F19.121
        dependence F19.221

Delirium, delirious (Continued)
  due to (Continued)
    sedative
      intoxication F13.921
        in
          abuse F13.121
          dependence F13.221
      withdrawal F13.231
    unknown etiology F05
  exhaustion F43.0
  hysterical F44.89
  postprocedural (postoperative) F05
  puerperal F05
  thyroid —see Thyrotoxicosis with thyroid
    storm
  traumatic —see Injury, intracranial
  tremens (alcohol-induced) F10.231
    sedative-induced F13.231
Delivery (childbirth) (labor)
  arrested active phase O62.1
  cesarean (for)
    without indication O82
    abnormal
      pelvis (bony) (deformity) (major) NEC
        with disproportion (fetopelvic)
        O33.0
          with obstructed labor O65.0
      presentation or position O32.9
    abruptio placentae —see also Abruptio
      placentae Ø45.9-
    acromion presentation O32.2
    atony, uterus O62.2
    breech presentation O32.1
      incomplete O32.8
    brow presentation O32.3
    cephalopelvic disproportion O33.9
    cerclage O34.3-
    chin presentation O32.3
    cicatrix of cervix O34.4-
    contracted pelvis (general)
      inlet O33.2
      outlet O33.3
    cord presentation or prolapse O69.0
    cystocele O34.8-
    deformity (acquired) (congenital)
      pelvic organs or tissues NEC O34.8-
      pelvis (bony) NEC O33.0
    disproportion NOS O33.9
    eclampsia —see Eclampsia
    face presentation O32.3
    failed
      forceps O66.5
      induction of labor O61.9
        instrumental O61.1
        mechanical O61.1
        medical O61.0
        specified NEC O61.8
        surgical O61.1
      trial of labor NOS O66.40
        following previous cesarean delivery
        O66.41
      vacuum extraction O66.5
      ventouse O66.5
    fetal-maternal hemorrhage O43.01-
    hemorrhage (intrapartum) O67.9
      with coagulation defect O67.0
      specified cause NEC O67.8
    high head at term O32.4
    hydrocephalic fetus O33.6
    incarceration of uterus O34.51-
    incoordinate uterine action O62.4
    increased size, fetus O33.5
    inertia, uterus O62.2
      primary O62.0
      secondary O62.1
    lateroversion, uterus O34.59-
    mal lie O32.9
    malposition
      fetus O32.9
      pelvic organs or tissues NEC O34.8-
      uterus NEC O34.59-

Delivery (Continued)
  cesarean (Continued)
    malpresentation NOS O32.9
    oblique presentation O32.2
    occurring after 37 completed weeks of
      gestation but before 39 completed
      weeks gestation due to (spontaneous)
      onset of labor O75.82
    oversize fetus O33.5
    pelvic tumor NEC O34.8-
    placenta previa O44.0- ◄▦
      complete O44.0-
        with hemorrhage O44.1- ◄
        ~~without hemorrhage O44.0-~~
    placental insufficiency O36.51-
    planned, occurring after 37 completed
      weeks of gestation but before 39
      completed weeks gestation due to
      (spontaneous) onset of labor O75.82
    polyp, cervix O34.4-
      causing obstructed labor O65.5
    poor dilatation, cervix O62.0
    pre-eclampsia O14.94 ◄▦
      mild O14.04 ◄▦
      moderate O14.04 ◄▦
      severe O14.14 ◄▦
        with hemolysis, elevated liver
          enzymes and low platelet count
          (HELLP) O14.24 ◄▦
    previous
      cesarean delivery O34.219 ◄▦
        classical (vertical) scar O34.212 ◄
        low transverse scar O34.211 ◄
      surgery (to)
        cervix O34.4-
        gynecological NEC O34.8-
        rectum O34.7-
        uterus O34.29
        vagina O34.6-
    prolapse
      arm or hand O32.2
      uterus O34.52-
    prolonged labor NOS O63.9
    rectocele O34.8-
    retroversion
      uterus O34.53-
    rigid
      cervix O34.4-
      pelvic floor O34.8-
      perineum O34.7-
      vagina O34.6-
      vulva O34.7-
    sacculation, pregnant uterus O34.59-
    scar (s)
      cervix O34.4-
      cesarean delivery O34.219 ◄▦
        classical (vertical) O34.212 ◄
        low transverse O34.211 ◄
      transmural uterine O34.29 ◄
      uterus O34.29
    Shirodkar suture in situ O34.3-
    shoulder presentation O32.2
    stenosis or stricture, cervix O34.4-
    ~~streptococcus B carrier state O99.824~~
    streptococcus group B (GBS) carrier state
      O99.824 ◄
    transmural uterine scar O34.29 ◄
    transverse presentation or lie O32.2
    tumor, pelvic organs or tissues NEC O34.8-
      cervix O34.4-
    umbilical cord presentation or prolapse
      O69.0
  completely normal case O80
  complicated O75.9
    by
      abnormal, abnormality (of)
        forces of labor O62.9
          specified type NEC O62.8
        glucose O99.814
        uterine contractions NOS O62.9
      abruptio placentae —see also Abruptio
        placentae O45.9-

Delivery (Continued)
  complicated (Continued)
    by (Continued)
      abuse
        physical O9A.32
        psychological O9A.52
        sexual O9A.42
      adherent placenta O72.0
        without hemorrhage O73.0
      alcohol use O99.314
      anemia (pre-existing) O99.02
      anesthetic death O74.8
      annular detachment of cervix O71.3
      atony, uterus O62.2
      attempted vacuum extraction and
        forceps O66.5
      Bandl's ring O62.4
      bariatric surgery status O99.844
      biliary tract disorder O26.62
      bleeding —see Delivery, complicated by,
        hemorrhage
      blood disorder NEC O99.12
      cervical dystocia (hypotonic) O62.2
        primary O62.0
        secondary O62.1
      circulatory system disorder O99.42
      compression of cord (umbilical) NEC
        O69.2
      condition NEC O99.89
      contraction, contracted ring O62.4
      cord (umbilical)
        around neck
          with compression O69.1
          without compression O69.81
        bruising O69.5
        complication O69.9
          specified NEC O69.89
        compression NEC O69.2
        entanglement O69.2
          without compression O69.82
        hematoma O69.5
        presentation O69.0
        prolapse O69.0
        short O69.3
        thrombosis (vessels) O69.5
        vascular lesion O69.5
      Couvelaire uterus O45.8X-
      damage to (injury to) NEC
        perineum O71.82
        periurethral tissue O71.82
        vulva O71.82
      delay following rupture of membranes
        (spontaneous) —see Pregnancy,
        complicated by, premature rupture
        of membranes
      depressed fetal heart tones O76
      diabetes O24.92
        gestational O24.429
          diet controlled O24.420
          insulin controlled O24.424
          oral drug controlled (antidiabetic)
            (hypoglycemic) O24.425 ◄
        pre-existing O24.32
          specified NEC O24.82
          type 1 O24.02
          type 2 O24.12
      diastasis recti (abdominis) O71.89
      dilatation
        bladder O66.8
        cervix incomplete, poor or slow O62.0
      disease NEC O99.89
      disruptio uteri —see Delivery,
        complicated by, rupture, uterus
      drug use O99.324
      dysfunction, uterus NOS O62.9
        hypertonic O62.4
        hypotonic O62.2
          primary O62.0
          secondary O62.1
        incoordinate O62.4
      eclampsia O15.1
      embolism (pulmonary) —see Embolism,
        obstetric

◄ New   ◄▦ Revised   ~~deleted~~ Deleted

Delivery *(Continued)*
  complicated *(Continued)*
    by *(Continued)*
      endocrine, nutritional or metabolic
        disease NEC O99.284
      failed
        attempted vaginal birth after previous
          cesarean delivery O66.41
        induction of labor O61.9
          instrumental O61.1
          mechanical O61.1
          medical O61.0
          specified NEC O61.8
          surgical O61.1
        trial of labor O66.40
      female genital mutilation O65.5
      fetal
        abnormal acid-base balance O68
        acidemia O68
        acidosis O68
        alkalosis O68
        death, early O02.1
        deformity O66.3
        heart rate or rhythm (abnormal) (non-
          reassuring) O76
        hypoxia O77.8
        stress O77.9
          due to drug administration O77.1
          electrocardiographic evidence of
            O77.8
          specified NEC O77.8
          ultrasound evidence of O77.8
      fever during labor O75.2
      gastric banding status O99.844
      gastric bypass status O99.844
      gastrointestinal disease NEC O99.62
      ~~gestational diabetes O24.429~~
        ~~diet controlled O24.420~~
        ~~insulin (and diet) controlled O24.424~~
      gestational ◀
        diabetes O24.429 ◀
          diet controlled O24.420 ◀
          insulin (and diet) controlled
            O24.424 ◀
          oral drug controlled (antidiabetic)
            (hypoglycemic) O24.425 ◀
        edema O12.04 ◀
          with proteinuria O12.24 ◀
        proteinuria O12.14 ◀
      gonorrhea O98.22
      hematoma O71.7
        ischial spine O71.7
        pelvic O71.7
        vagina O71.7
        vulva or perineum O71.7
      hemorrhage (uterine) O67.9
        associated with
          afibrinogenemia O67.0
          coagulation defect O67.0
          hyperfibrinolysis O67.0
          hypofibrinogenemia O67.0
        due to
          low implantation of placenta
            O44.5- ◀
          low-lying placenta O44.5- ◀▦
          placenta previa O44.1-
            marginal O44.3- ◀
            partial O44.3- ◀
          premature separation of placenta
            (normally implanted) *(see also*
            Abruptio placentae) O45.9-
          retained placenta O72.0
          uterine leiomyoma O67.8
        placenta NEC O67.8
        postpartum NEC (atonic) (immediate)
          O72.1
          with retained or trapped placenta
            O72.0
          delayed O72.2
          secondary O72.2
          third stage O72.0

Delivery *(Continued)*
  complicated *(Continued)*
    by *(Continued)*
      hourglass contraction, uterus O62.4
      hypertension, hypertensive (pre-
        existing) *—see* Hypertension,
        complicated by, childbirth (labor)
      hypotension O26.5-
      incomplete dilatation (cervix) O62.0
      incoordinate uterus contractions O62.4
      inertia, uterus O62.2
        during latent phase of labor O62.0
        primary O62.0
        secondary O62.1
      infection (maternal) O98.92
        carrier state NEC O99.834
        gonorrhea O98.22
        human immunodeficiency virus (HIV)
          O98.72
        sexually transmitted NEC O98.32
        specified NEC O98.82
        syphilis O98.12
        tuberculosis O98.02
        viral hepatitis O98.42
        viral NEC O98.52
      injury (to mother) *(see also* Delivery,
        complicated, by, damage to)
        O71.9
        nonobstetric O9A.22
          caused by abuse *—see* Delivery,
            complicated by, abuse
      intrauterine fetal death, early O02.1
      inversion, uterus O71.2
      laceration (perineal) O70.9
        anus (sphincter) O70.4
          with third degree laceration *—see*
            also Delivery, complicated, by,
            laceration, perineum, third
            degree O70.20 ◀▦
            with mucosa O70.3
          without third degree laceration
            O70.4
        bladder (urinary) O71.5
        bowel O71.5
        cervix (uteri) O71.3
        fourchette O70.0
        hymen O70.0
        labia O70.0
        pelvic
          floor O70.1
          organ NEC O71.5
        perineum, perineal O70.9
          first degree O70.0
          fourth degree O70.3
          muscles O70.1
          second degree O70.1
          skin O70.0
          slight O70.0
          third degree O70.20 ◀▦
            with ◀
              both external anal sphincter
                (EAS) and internal anal
                sphincter (IAS) torn (IIIc)
                O70.23 ◀
             less than 50% of external anal
                sphincter (EAS) thickness
                torn (IIIa) O70.21 ◀
             more than 50% external anal
                sphincter (EAS) thickness
                torn (IIIb) O70.22 ◀
            IIIa O70.21 ◀
            IIIb O70.22 ◀
            IIIc O70.23 ◀
        peritoneum (pelvic) O71.5
        rectovaginal (septum) (without
          perineal laceration) O71.4
          with perineum *—see also* Delivery,
            complicated, by, laceration,
            perineum, third degree
            O70.20 ◀▦
          with anal or rectal mucosa O70.3

Delivery *(Continued)*
  complicated *(Continued)*
    by *(Continued)*
      laceration *(Continued)*
        specified NEC O71.89
        sphincter ani *—see* Delivery,
          complicated, by, laceration, anus
          (sphincter)
        urethra O71.5
        uterus O71.81
          before labor O71.81
        vagina, vaginal (deep) (high) (without
          perineal laceration) O71.4
          with perineum O70.0
          muscles, with perineum O70.1
        vulva O70.0
      liver disorder O26.62
      malignancy O9A.12
      malnutrition O25.2
      malposition, malpresentation
        without obstruction O32.9 *—see*
          also Delivery, complicated by,
          obstruction
          breech O32.1
          compound O32.6
          face (brow) (chin) O32.3
          footling O38.8
          high head O32.4
          oblique O32.2
          specified NEC O32.8
          transverse O32.2
          unstable lie O32.0
        placenta O44.0- ◀▦
          ~~without hemorrhage O44.0-~~
          with hemorrhage O44.1- ◀
        uterus or cervix O65.5
      meconium in amniotic fluid O77.0
      mental disorder NEC O99.344
      metrorrhexis *—see* Delivery, complicated
        by, rupture, uterus
      nervous system disorder O99.354
      obesity (pre-existing) O99.214
      obesity surgery status O99.844
      obstetric trauma O71.9
        specified NEC O71.89
      obstructed labor
        due to
          breech (complete) (frank)
            presentation O64.1
            incomplete O64.8
          brow presenation O64.3
          buttock presentation O64.1
          chin presentation O64.2
          compound presentation O64.5
          contracted pelvis O65.1
          deep transverse arrest O64.0
          deformed pelvis O65.0
          dystocia (fetal) O66.9
            due to
              conjoined twins O66.3
              fetal
                abnormality NEC O66.3
                ascites O66.3
                hydrops O66.3
                meningomyelocele O66.3
                sacral teratoma O66.3
                tumor O66.3
             hydrocephalic fetus O66.3
            shoulder O66.0
          face presentation O64.2
          fetopelvic disproportion O65.4
          footling presentation O64.8
          impacted shoulders O66.0
          incomplete rotation of fetal head
            O64.0
          large fetus O66.2
          locked twins O66.1
          malposition O64.9
            specified NEC O64.8
          malpresentation O64.9
            specified NEC O64.8

Delivery *(Continued)*
  complicated *(Continued)*
    by *(Continued)*
      obstructed labor *(Continued)*
        due to *(Continued)*
          multiple fetuses NEC O66.6
          pelvic
            abnormality (maternal) O65.9
              organ O65.5
              specified NEC O65.8
            contraction
              inlet O65.2
              mid-cavity O65.3
              outlet O65.3
          persistent (position)
            occipitoiliac O64.0
            occipitoposterior O64.0
            occipitosacral O64.0
            occipitotransverse O64.0
          prolapsed arm O64.4
          shoulder presentation O64.4
        specified NEC O66.8
      pathological retraction ring, uterus O62.4
      penetration, pregnant uterus by
        instrument O71.1
      perforation —*see* Delivery, complicated
        by, laceration
      placenta, placental
        ablatio —*see also* Abruptio placentae
          O45.9-
        abnormality O43.9-
          specified NEC O43.89-
        abruptio —*see also* Abruptio placentae
          O45.9-
        accreta O43.21-
        adherent (with hemorrhage) O72.0
          without hemorrhage O73.0
         detachment (premature) —*see also*
          Abruptio placentae O45.9-
        disorder O43.9-
          specified NEC O43.89-
        hemorrhage NEC O67.8
        increta O43.22-
        low (implantation) (lying) O44.4- ◄▭
          ~~without hemorrhage O44.0-~~
          with hemorrhage O44.5- ◄
        malformation O43.10-
        malposition O44.0- ◄▭
          without hemorrhage O44.1- ◄▭
        percreta O43.23-
        previa (central) (complete) (lateral)
          (total) O44.0- ◄▭
          ~~without hemorrhage O44.0-~~
          with hemorrhage O44.1- ◄
            marginal O44.2- ◄
              with hemorrhage O44.3- ◄
            partial O44.2- ◄
              with hemorrhage O44.3- ◄
        retained (with hemorrhage) O72.0
          without hemorrhage O73.0
        separation (premature) O45.9-
          specified NEC O45.8X-
        vicious insertion O44.1-
      precipitate labor O62.3
      premature rupture, membranes *(see
        also* Pregnancy, complicated by,
        premature rupture of membranes)
        O42.90
      prolapse
        arm or hand O32.2
        cord (umbilical) O69.0
        foot or leg O32.8
        uterus O34.52-
      prolonged labor O63.9
        first stage O63.0
        second stage O63.1
      protozoal disease (maternal) O98.62
      respiratory disease NEC O99.52
      retained membranes or portions of
        placenta O72.2
        without hemorrhage O73.1
      retarded birth O63.9

Delivery *(Continued)*
  complicated *(Continued)*
    by *(Continued)*
      retention of secundines (with
        hemorrhage) O72.0
        without hemorrhage O73.0
        partial O72.2
          without hemorrhage O73.1
      rupture
        bladder (urinary) O71.5
        cervix O71.3
        pelvic organ NEC O71.5
        urethra O71.5
        uterus (during or after labor) O71.1
          before labor O71.0-
      separation, pubic bone (symphysis
        pubis) O71.6
      shock O75.1
      shoulder presentation O64.4
      skin disorder NEC O99.72
      spasm, cervix O62.4
      stenosis or stricture, cervix O65.5
      ~~streptococcus B carrier state O99.824~~
      streptococcus group B (GBS) carrier state
        O99.824 ◄
      subluxation of symphysis (pubis) O26.72
      syphilis (maternal) O98.12
      tear —*see* Delivery, complicated by,
        laceration
      tetanic uterus O62.4
      trauma (obstetrical) —*see also* Delivery,
        complicated, by, damage to O71.9
        non-obstetric O9A.22
        periurethral O71.82
        specified NEC O71.89
      tuberculosis (maternal) O98.02
      tumor, pelvic organs or tissues NEC
        O65.5
      umbilical cord around neck
        with compression O69.1
        without compression O69.81
      uterine inertia O62.2
        during latent phase of labor O62.0
        primary O62.0
        secondary O62.1
      vasa previa O69.4
      velamentous insertion of cord O43.12-
    specified complication NEC O75.89
  delayed NOS O63.9
    following rupture of membranes
      artificial O75.5
    second twin, triplet, etc. O63.2
  forceps, low following failed vacuum
    extraction O66.5
  missed (at or near term) O36.4
  normal O80
  obstructed —*see* Delivery, complicated by,
    obstruction
  precipitate O62.3
  preterm —*see also* Pregnancy, complicated by,
    preterm labor O60.10
  spontaneous O80
  term pregnancy NOS O80
  uncomplicated O80
  vaginal, following previous cesarean delivery
    O34.219 ◄▭
    classical (vertical) scar O34.212 ◄
    low transverse scar O34.211 ◄
Delusions (paranoid) —*see* Disorder, delusional
Dementia (degenerative (primary)) (old age)
  (persisting) F03.90
  with
    aggressive behavior F03.91
    behavioral disturbance F03.91
    combative behavior F03.91
    Lewy bodies G31.83 *[F02.80]*
      with behavioral disturbance G31.83
        [F02.81]
    Parkinson's disease G20 *[F02.80]*
      with behavioral disturbance G20
        [F02.81]

Dementia *(Continued)*
  with *(Continued)*
    Parkinsonism G31.83 *[F02.80]*
      with behavioral disturbance G31.83
        [F02.81]
    violent behavior F03.91
  alcoholic F10.97
    with dependence F10.27
  Alzheimer's type —*see* Disease, Alzheimer's
  arteriosclerotic —*see* Dementia, vascular
  atypical, Alzheimer's type —*see* Disease,
    Alzheimer's, specified NEC
  congenital —*see* Disability, intellectual
  frontal (lobe) G31.09 *[F02.80]*
    with behavioral disturbance G31.09
      [F02.81]
  frontotemporal G31.09 *[F02.80]*
    with behavioral disturbance G31.09
      [F02.81]
    specified NEC G31.09 *[F02.80]*
      with behavioral disturbance G31.09
        [F02.81]
  in (due to)
    alcohol F10.97
      with dependence F10.27
    Alzheimer's disease —*see* Disease,
      Alzheimer's
    arteriosclerotic brain disease —*see*
      Dementia, vascular
    cerebral lipidoses E75.- *[F02.80]*
      with behavioral disturbance
        E75.- *[F02.81]*
    Creutzfeldt-Jakob disease —*see also*
      Creutzfeldt-Jakob disease or
      syndrome (with dementia) A81.00
    epilepsy G40.- *[F02.80]*
      with behavioral disturbance
        G40.- *[F02.81]*
    hepatolenticular degeneration E83.01
      [F02.80]
      with behavioral disturbance E83.01
        [F02.81]
    human immunodeficiency virus (HIV)
      disease B20 *[F02.80]*
      with behavioral disturbance B20 *[F02.81]*
    Huntington's disease or chorea G10
    hypercalcemia E83.52 *[F02.80]*
      with behavioral disturbance E83.52
        [F02.81]
    hypothyroidism, acquired E03.9 *[F02.80]*
      with behavioral disturbance E03.9
        [F02.81]
    due to iodine deficiency E01.8 *[F02.80]*
      with behavioral disturbance E01.8
        [F02.81]
    inhalants F18.97
      with dependence F18.27
    multiple
      etiologies F03
      sclerosis G35 *[F02.80]*
        with behavioral disturbance G35
          [F02.81]
    neurosyphilis A52.17 *[F02.80]*
      with behavioral disturbance A52.17
        [F02.81]
    juvenile A50.49 *[F02.80]*
      with behavioral disturbance A50.49
        [F02.81]
    niacin deficiency E52 *[F02.80]*
      with behavioral disturbance E52 *[F02.81]*
    paralysis agitans G20 *[F02.80]*
      with behavioral disturbance G20 *[F02.81]*
    Parkinson's disease G20 *[F02.80]*
    pellagra E52 *[F02.80]*
      with behavioral disturbance E52 *[F02.81]*
    Pick's G31.01 *[F02.80]*
      with behavioral disturbance G31.01
        [F02.81]
    polyarteritis nodosa M30.0 *[F02.80]*
      with behavioral disturbance M30.0
        [F02.81]

◄ New   ◄▭ Revised   ~~deleted~~ Deleted

Dementia (Continued)
in (Continued)
psychoactive drug F19.97
with dependence F19.27
inhalants F18.97
with dependence F18.27
sedatives, hypnotics or anxiolytics
F13.97
with dependence F13.27
sedatives, hypnotics or anxiolytics F13.97
with dependence F13.27
systemic lupus erythematosus
M32.- [F02.80]
with behavioral disturbance
M32.- [F02.81]
trypanosomiasis
African B56.9 [F02.80]
with behavioral disturbance B56.9
[F02.81]
unknown etiology F03
vitamin B12 deficiency E53.8 [F02.80]
with behavioral disturbance E53.8
[F02.81]
volatile solvents F18.97
with dependence F18.27
infantile, infantilis F84.3
Lewy body G31.83 [F02.80]
with behavioral disturbance G31.83
[F02.81]
multi-infarct —see Dementia, vascular
paralytica, paralytic (syphilitic) A52.17
[F02.80]
with behavioral disturbance A52.17
[F02.81]
juvenilis A50.45
paretic A52.17
praecox —see Schizophrenia
presenile F03
Alzheimer's type —see Disease,
Alzheimer's, early onset
primary degenerative F03
progressive, syphilitic A52.17
senile F03
with acute confusional state F05
Alzheimer's type —see Disease,
Alzheimer's, late onset
depressed or paranoid type F03
vascular (acute onset) (mixed) (multi-infarct)
(subcortical) F01.50
with behavioral disturbance F01.51
Demineralization, bone —see Osteoporosis
Demodex folliculorum (infestation) B88.0
Demophobia F40.248
Demoralization R45.3
Demyelination, demyelinization
central nervous system G37.9
specified NEC G37.8
corpus callosum (central) G37.1
disseminated, acute G36.9
specified NEC G36.8
global G35
in optic neuritis G36.0
Dengue (classical) (fever) A90
hemorrhagic A91
sandfly A93.1
Dennie-Marfan syphilitic syndrome
A50.45
Dens evaginatus, in dente or invaginatus
K00.2
Dense breasts R92.2
Density
increased, bone (disseminated) (generalized)
(spotted) —see Disorder, bone, density
and structure, specified type NEC
lung (nodular) J98.4
Dental —see also condition
examination Z01.20
with abnormal findings Z01.21
restoration
aesthetically inadequate or displeasing
K08.56

Dental (Continued)
restoration (Continued)
defective K08.50
specified NEC K08.59
failure of marginal integrity K08.51
failure of periodontal anatomical integrity
K08.54
Dentia praecox K00.6
Denticles (pulp) K04.2
Dentigerous cyst K09.0
Dentin
irregular (in pulp) K04.3
opalescent K00.5
secondary (in pulp) K04.3
sensitive K03.89
Dentinogenesis imperfecta K00.5
Dentinoma —see Cyst, calcifying odontogenic
Dentition (syndrome) K00.7
delayed K00.6
difficult K00.7
precocious K00.6
premature K00.6
retarded K00.6
Dependence (on) (syndrome) F19.20
with remission F19.21
alcohol (ethyl) (methyl) (without remission)
F10.20
with
amnestic disorder, persisting F10.26
anxiety disorder F10.280
dementia, persisting F10.27
intoxication F10.229
with delirium F10.221
uncomplicated F10.220
mood disorder F10.24
psychotic disorder F10.259
with
delusions F10.250
hallucinations F10.251
remission F10.21
sexual dysfunction F10.281
sleep disorder F10.282
specified disorder NEC F10.288
withdrawal F10.239
with
delirium F10.231
perceptual disturbance F10.232
uncomplicated F10.230
counseling and surveillance Z71.41
amobarbital —see Dependence, drug,
sedative
amphetamine (s) (type) —see Dependence,
drug, stimulant NEC
amytal (sodium) —see Dependence, drug,
sedative
analgesic NEC F55.8
anesthetic (agent) (gas) (general) (local)
NEC —see Dependence, drug,
psychoactive NEC
anxiolytic NEC —see Dependence, drug,
sedative
barbital (s) —see Dependence, drug, sedative
barbiturate (s) (compounds) (drugs
classifiable to T42) —see Dependence,
drug, sedative
benzedrine —see Dependence, drug,
stimulant NEC
bhang —see Dependence, drug, cannabis
bromide (s) NEC —see Dependence, drug,
sedative
caffeine —see Dependence, drug, stimulant
NEC
cannabis (sativa) (indica) (resin) (derivatives)
(type) —see Dependence, drug, cannabis
chloral (betaine) (hydrate) —see Dependence,
drug, sedative
chlordiazepoxide —see Dependence, drug,
sedative
coca (leaf) (derivatives) —see Dependence,
drug, cocaine
cocaine —see Dependence, drug, cocaine

Dependence (Continued)
codeine —see Dependence, drug, opioid
combinations of drugs F19.20
dagga —see Dependence, drug, cannabis
demerol —see Dependence, drug, opioid
dexamphetamine —see Dependence, drug,
stimulant NEC
dexedrine —see Dependence, drug, stimulant
NEC
dextromethorphan —see Dependence, drug,
opioid
dextromoramide —see Dependence, drug,
opioid
dextro-nor-pseudo-ephedrine —see
Dependence, drug, stimulant NEC
dextrorphan —see Dependence, drug, opioid
diazepam —see Dependence, drug, sedative
dilaudid —see Dependence, drug, opioid
D-lysergic acid diethylamide —see
Dependence, drug, hallucinogen
drug NEC F19.20
with sleep disorder F19.282
cannabis F12.20
with
anxiety disorder F12.280
intoxication F12.229
with
delirium F12.221
perceptual disturbance F12.222
uncomplicated F12.220
other specified disorder F12.288
psychosis F12.259
delusions F12.250
hallucinations F12.251
unspecified disorder F12.29
in remission F12.21
cocaine F14.20
with
anxiety disorder F14.280
intoxication F14.229
with
delirium F14.221
perceptual disturbance F14.222
uncomplicated F14.220
mood disorder F14.24
other specified disorder F14.288
psychosis F14.259
delusions F14.250
hallucinations F14.251
sexual dysfunction F14.281
sleep disorder F14.282
unspecified disorder F14.29
withdrawal F14.23
in remission F14.21
withdrawal symptoms in newborn P96.1
counseling and surveillance Z71.51
hallucinogen F16.20
with
anxiety disorder F16.280
flashbacks F16.283
intoxication F16.229
with delirium F16.221
uncomplicated F16.220
mood disorder F16.24
other specified disorder F16.288
perception disorder, persisting F16.283
psychosis F16.259
delusions F16.250
hallucinations F16.251
unspecified disorder F16.29
in remission F16.21
in remission F19.21
inhalant F18.20
with
anxiety disorder F18.280
dementia, persisting F18.27
intoxication F18.229
with delirium F18.221
uncomplicated F18.220
mood disorder F18.24
other specified disorder F18.288

Dependence (Continued)
  drug NEC (Continued)
    inhalant (Continued)
      with (Continued)
        psychosis F18.259
          delusions F18.250
          hallucinations F18.251
        unspecified disorder F18.29
      in remission F18.21
    nicotine F17.200
      with disorder F17.209
        remission F17.201
        specified disorder NEC F17.208
        withdrawal F17.203
      chewing tobacco F17.220
        with disorder F17.229
          remission F17.221
          specified disorder NEC F17.228
          withdrawal F17.223
      cigarettes F17.210
        with disorder F17.219
          remission F17.211
          specified disorder NEC F17.218
          withdrawal F17.213
      specified product NEC F17.290
        with disorder F17.299
          remission F17.291
          specified disorder NEC F17.298
          withdrawal F17.293
    opioid F11.20
      with
        intoxication F11.229
          with
            delirium F11.221
            perceptual disturbance F11.222
          uncomplicated F11.220
        mood disorder F11.24
        other specified disorder F11.288
        psychosis F11.259
          delusions F11.250
          hallucinations F11.251
        sexual dysfunction F11.281
        sleep disorder F11.282
        unspecified disorder F11.29
        withdrawal F11.23
      in remission F11.21
    psychoactive NEC F19.20
      with
        amnestic disorder F19.26
        anxiety disorder F19.280
        dementia F19.27
        intoxication F19.229
          with
            delirium F19.221
            perceptual disturbance
              F19.222
          uncomplicated F19.220
        mood disorder F19.24
        other specified disorder F19.288
        psychosis F19.259
          delusions F19.250
          hallucinations F19.251
        sexual dysfunction F19.281
        sleep disorder F19.282
        unspecified disorder F19.29
        withdrawal F19.239
          with
            delirium F19.231
            perceptual disturbance
              F19.232
          uncomplicated F19.230
    sedative, hypnotic or anxiolytic F13.20
      with
        amnestic disorder F13.26
        anxiety disorder F13.280
        dementia, persisting F13.27
        intoxication F13.229
          with delirium F13.221
          uncomplicated F13.220
        mood disorder F13.24
        other specified disorder F13.288

Dependence (Continued)
  drug NEC (Continued)
    sedative, hypnotic or anxiolytic (Continued)
      with (Continued)
        psychosis F13.259
          delusions F13.250
          hallucinations F13.251
        sexual dysfunction F13.281
        sleep disorder F13.282
        unspecified disorder F13.29
        withdrawal F13.239
          with
            delirium F13.231
            perceptual disturbance F13.232
          uncomplicated F13.230
      in remission F13.21
    stimulant NEC F15.20
      with
        anxiety disorder F15.280
        intoxication F15.229
          with
            delirium F15.221
            perceptual disturbance F15.222
          uncomplicated F15.220
        mood disorder F15.24
        other specified disorder F15.288
        psychosis F15.259
          delusions F15.250
          hallucinations F15.251
        sexual dysfunction F15.281
        sleep disorder F15.282
        unspecified disorder F15.29
        withdrawal F15.23
      in remission F15.21
    ethyl
      alcohol (without remission) F10.20
        with remission F10.21
      bromide —see Dependence, drug,
        sedative
      carbamate F19.20
      chloride F19.20
      morphine —see Dependence, drug, opioid
    ganja —see Dependence, drug, cannabis
    glue (airplane) (sniffing) —see Dependence,
      drug, inhalant
    glutethimide —see Dependence, drug,
      sedative
    hallucinogenics —see Dependence, drug,
      hallucinogen
    hashish —see Dependence, drug, cannabis
    hemp —see Dependence, drug, cannabis
    heroin (salt) (any) —see Dependence, drug,
      opioid
    hypnotic NEC —see Dependence, drug,
      sedative
    Indian hemp —see Dependence, drug,
      cannabis
    inhalants —see Dependence, drug, inhalant
    khat —see Dependence, drug, stimulant NEC
    laudanum —see Dependence, drug, opioid
    LSD (-25) (derivatives) —see Dependence,
      drug, hallucinogen
    luminal —see Dependence, drug, sedative
    lysergic acid —see Dependence, drug,
      hallucinogen
    maconha —see Dependence, drug, cannabis
    marihuana —see Dependence, drug, cannabis
    meprobamate —see Dependence, drug,
      sedative
    mescaline —see Dependence, drug,
      hallucinogen
    methadone —see Dependence, drug, opioid
    methamphetamine (s) —see Dependence,
      drug, stimulant NEC
    methaqualone —see Dependence, drug,
      sedative
    methyl
      alcohol (without remission) F10.20
        with remission F10.21
      bromide —see Dependence, drug, sedative
      morphine —see Dependence, drug, opioid

Dependence (Continued)
  methyl (Continued)
    phenidate —see Dependence, drug,
      stimulant NEC
    sulfonal —see Dependence, drug, sedative
  morphine (sulfate) (sulfite) (type) —see
    Dependence, drug, opioid
  narcotic (drug) NEC —see Dependence, drug,
    opioid
  nembutal —see Dependence, drug, sedative
  neraval —see Dependence, drug, sedative
  neravan —see Dependence, drug, sedative
  neurobarb —see Dependence, drug, sedative
  nicotine —see Dependence, drug, nicotine
  nitrous oxide F19.20
  nonbarbiturate sedatives and tranquilizers
    with similar effect —see Dependence,
    drug, sedative
  on
    artificial heart (fully implantable)
      (mechanical) Z95.812
    aspirator Z99.0
    care provider (because of) Z74.9
      impaired mobility Z74.09
      need for
        assistance with personal care Z74.1
        continuous supervision Z74.3
      no other household member able to
        render care Z74.2
      specified reason NEC Z74.8
    machine Z99.89
      enabling NEC Z99.89
      specified type NEC Z99.89
    renal dialysis (hemodialysis) (peritoneal)
      Z99.2
    respirator Z99.11
    ventilator Z99.11
    wheelchair Z99.3
  opiate —see Dependence, drug, opioid
  opioids —see Dependence, drug, opioid
  opium (alkaloids) (derivatives) (tincture) —
    see Dependence, drug, opioid
  oxygen (long-term) (supplemental) Z99.81
  paraldehyde —see Dependence, drug,
    sedative
  paregoric —see Dependence, drug, opioid
  PCP (phencyclidine) (or related substance) —
    see Dependence, drug, hallucinogen ◂▦
  pentobarbital —see Dependence, drug,
    sedative
  pentobarbitone (sodium) —see Dependence,
    drug, sedative
  pentothal —see Dependence, drug, sedative
  peyote —see Dependence, drug, hallucinogen
  phencyclidine (PCP) (or related substance) —
    see Dependence, drug, hallucinogen ◂▦
  phenmetrazine —see Dependence, drug,
    stimulant NEC
  phenobarbital —see Dependence, drug,
    sedative
  polysubstance F19.20
  psilocibin, psilocin, psilocyn, psilocyline —see
    Dependence, drug, hallucinogen
  psychostimulant NEC —see Dependence,
    drug, stimulant NEC
  secobarbital —see Dependence, drug, sedative
  seconal —see Dependence, drug, sedative
  sedative NEC —see Dependence, drug,
    sedative
  specified drug NEC —see Dependence, drug
  stimulant NEC —see Dependence, drug,
    stimulant NEC
  substance NEC —see Dependence, drug
  supplemental oxygen Z99.81
  tobacco —see Dependence, drug, nicotine
    counseling and surveillance Z71.6
  tranquilizer NEC —see Dependence, drug,
    sedative
  vitamin B6 E53.1
  volatile solvents —see Dependence, drug,
    inhalant

◀ New   ◂▦ Revised   ~~deleted~~ Deleted

Dependency
  care-provider Z74.9
  passive F60.7
  reactions (persistent) F60.7
Depersonalization (in neurotic state) (neurotic)
  (syndrome) F48.1
Depletion
  extracellular fluid E86.9
  plasma E86.1
  potassium E87.6
    nephropathy N25.89
  salt or sodium E87.1
    causing heat exhaustion or prostration T67.4
    nephropathy N28.9
  volume NOS E86.9
Deployment (current) (military) status Z56.82
  in theater or in support of military war,
    peacekeeping and humanitarian
    operations Z56.82
  personal history of Z91.82
    military war, peacekeeping and
      humanitarian deployment (current or
      past conflict) Z91.82
  returned from Z91.82
Depolarization, premature I49.40
  atrial I49.1
  junctional I49.2
  specified NEC I49.49
  ventricular I49.3
Deposit
  bone in Boeck's sarcoid D86.89
  calcareous, calcium —see Calcification
  cholesterol
    retina H35.89
    vitreous (body) (humor) —see Deposit,
      crystalline
  conjunctiva H11.11-
  cornea H18.00-
    argentous H18.02-
    due to metabolic disorder H18.03-
    Kayser-Fleischer ring H18.04-
    pigmentation —see Pigmentation, cornea
  crystalline, vitreous (body) (humor) H43.2-
  hemosiderin in old scars of cornea —see
    Pigmentation, cornea, stromal
  metallic in lens —see Cataract, specified NEC
  skin R23.8
  tooth, teeth (betel) (black) (green) (materia
    alba) (orange) (tobacco) K03.6
  urate, kidney —see Calculus, kidney
Depraved appetite —see Pica
Depressed
  HDL cholesterol E78.6
Depression (acute) (mental) F32.9
  agitated (single episode) F32.2
  anaclitic —see Disorder, adjustment
  anxiety F41.8
    persistent F34.1
  arches —see also Deformity, limb, flat foot
  atypical (single episode) F32.89 ◀▥▥
    recurrent episode F33.8 ◀
  basal metabolic rate R94.8
  bone marrow D75.89
  central nervous system R09.2
  cerebral R29.818
    newborn P91.4
  cerebrovascular I67.9
  chest wall M95.4
  climacteric (single episode) F32.89 ◀▥▥
    recurrent episode F33.8 ◀
  endogenous (without psychotic symptoms)
    F33.2
    with psychotic symptoms F33.3
  functional activity R68.89
  hysterical F44.89
  involutional (single episode) F32.89 ◀▥▥
    recurrent episode F33.8 ◀
  major F32.9
    with psychotic symptoms F32.3
    recurrent —see Disorder, depressive,
      recurrent

Depression (Continued)
  manic-depressive —see Disorder, depressive,
    recurrent
  masked (single episode) F32.89 ◀▥▥
  medullary G93.89
  menopausal (single episode) F32.89 ◀▥▥
    recurrent episode F33.8 ◀
  metatarsus —see Depression, arches
  monopolar F33.9
  nervous F34.1
  neurotic F34.1
  nose M95.0
  postnatal F53
  postpartum F53
  post-psychotic of schizophrenia F32.89 ◀▥▥
  post-schizophrenic F32.89 ◀▥▥
  psychogenic (reactive) (single episode) F32.9
  psychoneurotic F34.1
  psychotic (single episode) F32.3
    recurrent F33.3
  reactive (psychogenic) (single episode) F32.9
    psychotic (single episode) F32.3
  recurrent —see Disorder, depressive,
    recurrent
  respiratory center G93.89
  seasonal —see Disorder, depressive, recurrent
  senile F03
  severe, single episode F32.2
  situational F43.21
  skull Q67.4
  specified NEC (single episode) F32.89 ◀▥▥
  sternum M95.4
  visual field —see Defect, visual field
  vital (recurrent) (without psychotic
    symptoms) F33.2
    with psychotic symptoms F33.3
    single episode F32.2
Deprivation
  cultural Z60.3
  effects NOS T73.9
    specified NEC T73.8
  emotional NEC Z65.8
    affecting infant or child —see
      Maltreatment, child, psychological
  food T73.0
  protein —see Malnutrition
  sleep Z72.820
  social Z60.4
    affecting infant or child —see
      Maltreatment, child, psychological
  specified NEC T73.8
  vitamins —see Deficiency, vitamin
  water T73.1
Derangement
  ankle (internal) —see Derangement, joint,
    ankle
  cartilage (articular) NEC —see Derangement,
    joint, articular cartilage, by site
    recurrent —see Dislocation, recurrent
  cruciate ligament, anterior, current injury —
    see Sprain, knee, cruciate, anterior
  elbow (internal) —see Derangement, joint,
    elbow
  hip (joint) (internal) (old) —see Derangement,
    joint, hip
  joint (internal) M24.9
    ankylosis —see Ankylosis
    articular cartilage M24.10
      ankle M24.17-
      elbow M24.12-
      foot M24.17-
      hand M24.14-
      hip M24.15-
      knee NEC M23.9-
      loose body —see Loose, body
      shoulder M24.11-
      wrist M24.13-
    contracture —see Contraction, joint
    current injury —see also Dislocation
      knee, meniscus or cartilage —see Tear,
      meniscus

Derangement (Continued)
  joint (Continued)
    dislocation
      pathological —see Dislocation,
        pathological
      recurrent —see Dislocation, recurrent
    knee —see Derangement, knee
    ligament —see Disorder, ligament
    loose body —see Loose, body
    recurrent —see Dislocation, recurrent
    specified type NEC M24.80
      ankle M24.87-
      elbow M24.82-
      foot joint M24.87-
      hand joint M24.84-
      hip M24.85-
      shoulder M24.81-
      wrist M24.83-
    temporomandibular M26.69
  knee (recurrent) M23.9-
    ligament disruption, spontaneous
      M23.60-
      anterior cruciate M23.61-
      capsular M23.67-
      instability, chronic M23.5-
      lateral collateral M23.64-
      medial collateral M23.63-
      posterior cruciate M23.62-
    loose body M23.4-
    meniscus M23.30-
      cystic M23.00-
        lateral M23.002
          anterior horn M23.04-
          posterior horn M23.05-
          specified NEC M23.06-
        medial M23.005
          anterior horn M23.01-
          posterior horn M23.02-
          specified NEC M23.03-
      degenerate —see Derangement, knee,
        meniscus, specified NEC
      detached —see Derangement, knee,
        meniscus, specified NEC
      due to old tear or injury M23.20-
        lateral M23.20-
          anterior horn M23.24-
          posterior horn M23.25-
          specified NEC M23.26-
        medial M23.20-
          anterior horn M23.21-
          posterior horn M23.22-
          specified NEC M23.23-
      retained —see Derangement, knee,
        meniscus, specified NEC
      specified NEC M23.30-
        lateral M23.30-
          anterior horn M23.34-
          posterior horn M23.35-
          specified NEC M23.36-
        medial M23.30-
          anterior horn M23.31-
          posterior horn M23.32-
          specified NEC M23.33-
    old M23.8X-
    specified NEC —see subcategory M23.8
  low back NEC —see Dorsopathy, specified
    NEC
  meniscus —see Derangement, knee,
    meniscus
  mental —see Psychosis
  patella, specified NEC —see Disorder,
    patella, derangement NEC
  semilunar cartilage (knee) —see
    Derangement, knee, meniscus,
    specified NEC
  shoulder (internal) —see Derangement,
    joint, shoulder
Dercum's disease E88.2
Derealization (neurotic) F48.1
Dermal —see condition
Dermaphytid —see Dermatophytosis

Dermatitis (eczematous) L30.9
  ab igne L59.0
  acarine B88.0
  actinic (due to sun) L57.8
    other than from sun L59.8
  allergic —see Dermatitis, contact, allergic
  ambustionis, due to burn or scald —see Burn
  amebic A06.7
  ammonia L22
  arsenical (ingested) L27.8
  artefacta L98.1
    psychogenic F54
  atopic L20.9
    psychogenic F54
    specified NEC L20.89
  autoimmune progesterone L30.8
  berlock, berloque L56.2
  blastomycotic B40.3
  blister beetle L24.89
  bullous, bullosa L13.9
    mucosynechial, atrophic L12.1
    seasonal L30.8
    specified NEC L13.8
  calorica L59.0
    due to burn or scald —see Burn
  caterpillar L24.89
  cercarial B65.3
  combustionis L59.0
    due to burn or scald —see Burn
  congelationis T69.1
  contact (occupational) L25.9
    allergic L23.9
      due to
        adhesives L23.1
        cement L23.5
        chemical products NEC L23.5
        chromium L23.0
        cosmetics L23.2
        dander (cat) (dog) L23.81
        drugs in contact with skin L23.3
        dyes L23.4
        food in contact with skin L23.6
        hair (cat) (dog) L23.81
        insecticide L23.5
        metals L23.0
        nickel L23.0
        plants, non-food L23.7
        plastic L23.5
        rubber L23.5
        specified agent NEC L23.89
    due to
      cement L25.3
      chemical products NEC L25.3
      cosmetics L25.0
      dander (cat) (dog) L23.81
      drugs in contact with skin L25.1
      dyes L25.2
      food in contact with skin L25.4
      hair (cat) (dog) L23.81
      plants, non-food L25.5
      specified agent NEC L25.8
    irritant L24.9
      due to
        cement L24.5 ◄▦
        chemical products NEC L24.5
        cosmetics L24.3
        detergents L24.0
        drugs in contact with skin L24.4
        food in contact with skin L24.6
        oils and greases L24.1
        plants, non-food L24.7
        solvents L24.2
        specified agent NEC L24.89
  contusiformis L52
  diabetic —see E08-E13 with .620
  diaper L22
  diphtheritica A36.3
  dry skin L85.3
  due to
    acetone (contact) (irritant) L24.2
    acids (contact) (irritant) L24.5

Dermatitis (Continued)
  due to (Continued)
    adhesive (s) (allergic) (contact) (plaster)
        L23.1
      irritant L24.5
    alcohol (irritant) (skin contact) (substances in
        category T51) L24.2
      taken internally L27.8
    alkalis (contact) (irritant) L24.5
    arsenic (ingested) L27.8
    carbon disulfide (contact) (irritant) L24.2
    caustics (contact) (irritant) L24.5
    cement (contact) L25.3
    cereal (ingested) L27.2
    chemical (s) NEC L25.3
      taken internally L27.8
    chlorocompounds L24.2
    chromium (contact) (irritant) L24.81
    coffee (ingested) L27.2
    cold weather L30.8
    cosmetics (contact) L25.0
      allergic L23.2
      irritant L24.3
    cyclohexanes L24.2
    dander (cat) (dog) L23.81
    Demodex species B88.0
    Dermanyssus gallinae B88.0
    detergents (contact) (irritant) L24.0
    dichromate L24.81
    drugs and medicaments (generalized)
        (internal use) L27.0
      external —see Dermatitis, due to, drugs,
          in contact with skin
      in contact with skin L25.1
        allergic L23.3
        irritant L24.4
      localized skin eruption L27.1
      specified substance —see Table of Drugs
          and Chemicals
    dyes L25.2
      allergic L23.4
      irritant L24.89
    epidermophytosis —see Dermatophytosis
    esters L24.2
    external irritant NEC L24.9
    fish (ingested) L27.2
    flour (ingested) L27.2
    food (ingested) L27.2
      in contact with skin L25.4
    fruit (ingested) L27.2
    furs (allergic) (contact) L23.81
    glues —see Dermatitis, due to, adhesives
    glycols L24.2
    greases NEC (contact) (irritant) L24.1
    hair (cat) (dog) L23.81
    hot
      objects and materials —see Burn
      weather or places L59.0
    hydrocarbons L24.2
    infrared rays L59.8
    ingestion, ingested substance L27.9
      chemical NEC L27.8
      drugs and medicaments —see
          Dermatitis, due to, drugs
      food L27.2
      specified NEC L27.8
    insecticide in contact with skin L24.5
    internal agent L27.9
      drugs and medicaments (generalized) —
          see Dermatitis, due to, drugs
      food L27.2
    irradiation —see Dermatitis, due to,
        radioactive substance
    ketones L24.2
    lacquer tree (allergic) (contact) L23.7
    light (sun) NEC L57.8
      acute L56.8
      other L59.8
    Liponyssoides sanguineus B88.0
    low temperature L30.8
    meat (ingested) L27.2

Dermatitis (Continued)
  due to (Continued)
    metals, metal salts (contact) (irritant)
        L24.81
    milk (ingested) L27.2
    nickel (contact) (irritant) L24.81
    nylon (contact) (irritant) L24.5
    oils NEC (contact) (irritant) L24.1
    paint solvent (contact) (irritant) L24.2
    petroleum products (contact) (irritant)
        (substances in T52) L24.2
    plants NEC (contact) L25.5
      allergic L23.7
      irritant L24.7
    plasters (adhesive) (any) (allergic) (contact)
        L23.1
      irritant L24.5
    plastic (contact) L25.3
    preservatives (contact) —see Dermatitis,
        due to, chemical, in contact with
        skin
    primrose (allergic) (contact) L23.7
    primula (allergic) (contact) L23.7
    radiation L59.8
      nonionizing (chronic exposure) L57.8
      sun NEC L57.8
        acute L56.8
    radioactive substance L58.9
      acute L58.0
      chronic L58.1
    radium L58.9
      acute L58.0
      chronic L58.1
    ragweed (allergic) (contact) L23.7
    Rhus (allergic) (contact) (diversiloba)
        (radicans) (toxicodendron) (venenata)
        (verniciflua) L23.7
    rubber (contact) L24.5
    Senecio jacobaea (allergic) (contact)
        L23.7
    solvents (contact) (irritant) (substances in
        categories T52) L24.2
    specified agent NEC (contact) L25.8
      allergic L23.89
      irritant L24.89
    sunshine NEC L57.8
      acute L56.8
    tetrachlorethylene (contact) (irritant)
        L24.2
    toluene (contact) (irritant) L24.2
    turpentine (contact) L24.2
    ultraviolet rays (sun NEC) (chronic
        exposure) L57.8
      acute L56.8
    vaccine or vaccination L27.0
      specified substance —see Table of Drugs
          and Chemicals
    varicose veins —see Varix, leg, with,
        inflammation
    X-rays L58.9
      acute L58.0
      chronic L58.1
  dyshydrotic L30.1
  dysmenorrheica N94.6
  escharotica —see Burn
  exfoliative, exfoliativa (generalized) L26
    neonatorum L00
  eyelid —see also Dermatosis, eyelid
    allergic H01.119
      left H01.116
        lower H01.115
        upper H01.114
      right H01.113
        lower H01.112
        upper H01.111
    contact —see Dermatitis, eyelid,
        allergic
    due to
      Demodex species B88.0
      herpes (zoster) B02.39
        simplex B00.59

◄ New   ◄▦ Revised   ~~deleted~~ Deleted

Dermatitis (Continued)
eyelid (Continued)
eczematous H01.139
left H01.136
lower H01.135
upper H01.134
right H01.133
lower H01.132
upper H01.131
facta, factitia, factitial L98.1
psychogenic F54
flexural NEC L20.82
friction L30.4
fungus B36.9
specified type NEC B36.8
gangrenosa, gangrenous infantum L08.0
harvest mite B88.0
heat L59.0
herpesviral, vesicular (ear) (lip) B00.1
herpetiformis (bullous) (erythematous)
(pustular) (vesicular) L13.0
juvenile L12.2
senile L12.0
hiemalis L30.8
hypostatic, hypostatica —see Varix, leg, with,
inflammation
infectious eczematoid L30.3
infective L30.3
irritant —see Dermatitis, contact, irritant
Jacquet's (diaper dermatitis) L22
Leptus B88.0
lichenified NEC L28.0
medicamentosa (generalized) (internal
use) —see Dermatitis, due to drugs
mite B88.0
multiformis L13.0
juvenile L12.2
napkin L22
neurotica L13.0
nummular L30.0
papillaris capillitii L73.0
pellagrous E52
perioral L71.0
photocontact L56.2
polymorpha dolorosa L13.0
pruriginosa L13.0
pruritic NEC L30.8
psychogenic F54
purulent L08.0
pustular
contagious B08.02
subcorneal L13.1
pyococcal L08.0
pyogenica L08.0
repens L40.2
Ritter's (exfoliativa) L00
Schamberg's L81.7
schistosome B65.3
seasonal bullous L30.8
seborrheic L21.9
infantile L21.1
specified NEC L21.8
sensitization NOS L23.9
septic L08.0
solare L57.8
specified NEC L30.8
stasis I87.2
~~with varicose ulcer —see Varix, leg, with~~
~~ulcer, with inflammation~~
with ◀
varicose ulcer —see Varix, leg, with ulcer,
with inflammation ◀
varicose veins —see Varix, leg, with,
inflammation ◀
due to postthrombotic syndrome —see
Syndrome, postthrombotic
suppurative L08.0
traumatic NEC L30.4
trophoneurotica L13.0
ultraviolet (sun) (chronic exposure) L57.8
acute L56.8

Dermatitis (Continued)
varicose —see Varix, leg, with, inflammation
vegetans L10.1
verrucosa B43.0
vesicular, herpesviral B00.1
Dermatoarthritis, lipoid E78.81
Dermatochalasis, eyelid H02.839
left H02.836
lower H02.835
upper H02.834
right H02.833
lower H02.832
upper H02.831
Dermatofibroma (lenticulare) —see Neoplasm,
skin, benign
protuberans —see Neoplasm, skin, uncertain
behavior
Dermatofibrosarcoma (pigmented)
(protuberans) —see Neoplasm, skin,
malignant
Dermatographia L50.3
Dermatolysis (exfoliativa) (congenital)
Q82.8
acquired L57.4
eyelids —see Blepharochalasis
palpebrarum —see Blepharochalasis
senile L57.4
Dermatomegaly NEC Q82.8
Dermatomucosomyositis M33.10
with
myopathy M33.12
respiratory involvement M33.11
specified organ involvement NEC
M33.19
Dermatomycosis B36.9
furfuracea B36.0
specified type NEC B36.8
Dermatomyositis (acute) (chronic) —see also
Dermatopolymyositis
in (due to) neoplastic disease —see also
Neoplasm D49.9 [M36.0]
Dermatoneuritis of children —see Poisoning,
mercury
Dermatophilosis A48.8
Dermatophytid L30.2
Dermatophytide —see Dermatophytosis
Dermatophytosis (epidermophyton) (infection)
(Microsporum) (tinea) (Trichophyton)
B35.9
beard B35.0
body B35.4
capitis B35.0
corporis B35.4
deep-seated B35.8
disseminated B35.8
foot B35.3
granulomatous B35.8
groin B35.6
hand B35.2
nail B35.1
perianal (area) B35.6
scalp B35.0
specified NEC B35.8
Dermatopolymyositis M33.90
with
myopathy M33.92
respiratory involvement M33.91
specified organ involvement NEC
M33.99
in neoplastic disease (see also Neoplasm)
D49.9 [M36.0]
juvenile M33.00
with
myopathy M33.02
respiratory involvement M33.01
specified organ involvement NEC
M33.09
specified NEC M33.10
myopathy M33.12
respiratory involvement M33.11
specified organ involvement NEC M33.19

Dermatopolyneuritis —see Poisoning, mercury
Dermatorrhexis Q79.6
acquired L57.4
Dermatosclerosis —see also Scleroderma
localized L94.0
Dermatosis L98.9
Andrews' L08.89
Bowen's —see Neoplasm, skin, in situ
bullous L13.9
specified NEC L13.8
exfoliativa L26
eyelid (noninfectious)
dermatitis —see Dermatitis, eyelid
discoid lupus erythematosus —see Lupus,
erythematosus, eyelid
xeroderma —see Xeroderma, acquired,
eyelid
factitial L98.1
febrile neutrophilic L98.2
gonococcal A54.89
herpetiformis L13.0
juvenile L12.2
linear IgA L13.8
menstrual NEC L98.8
neutrophilic, febrile L98.2
occupational —see Dermatitis, contact
papulosa nigra L82.1
pigmentary L81.9
progressive L81.7
Schamberg's L81.7
psychogenic F54
purpuric, pigmented L81.7
pustular, subcorneal L13.1
transient acantholytic L11.1
Dermographia, dermographism L50.3
Dermoid (cyst) —see also Neoplasm, benign,
by site
with malignant transformation C56-
due to radiation (nonionizing) L57.8
Dermopathy
infiltrative with thyrotoxicosis —see
Thyrotoxicosis
nephrogenic fibrosing L90.8
Dermophytosis —see Dermatophytosis
Descemetocele H18.73-
Descemet's membrane —see condition
Descending —see condition
Descensus uteri —see Prolapse, uterus
Desert
rheumatism B38.0
sore —see Ulcer, skin
Desertion (newborn) —see Maltreatment
Desmoid (extra-abdominal) (tumor) —see
Neoplasm, connective tissue, uncertain
behavior
abdominal D48.1
Despondency F32.9
Desquamation, skin R23.4
Destruction, destructive —see also Damage
articular facet —see also Derangement, joint,
specified type NEC
knee M23.8X-
vertebra —see Spondylosis
bone —see also Disorder, bone, specified type
NEC
syphilitic A52.77
joint —see also Derangement, joint, specified
type NEC
sacroiliac M53.3
rectal sphincter K62.89
septum (nasal) J34.89
tuberculous NEC —see Tuberculosis
tympanum, tympanic membrane
(nontraumatic) —see Disorder,
tympanic membrane, specified
NEC
vertebral disc —see Degeneration,
intervertebral disc
Destructiveness —see also Disorder, conduct
adjustment reaction —see Disorder,
adjustment

Desultory labor O62.2
Detachment
  cartilage —*see* Sprain
  cervix, annular N88.8
    complicating delivery O71.3
  choroid (old) (postinfectional) (simple)
      (spontaneous) H31.40-
    hemorrhagic H31.41-
    serous H31.42-
  ligament —*see* Sprain
  meniscus (knee) —*see also* Derangement,
      knee, meniscus, specified NEC
    current injury —*see* Tear, meniscus
    due to old tear or injury —*see*
        Derangement, knee, meniscus, due
        to old tear
  retina (without retinal break) (serous) H33.2-
    with retinal:
      break H33.00-
        giant H33.03-
          multiple H33.02-
          single H33.01-
        dialysis H33.04-
    pigment epithelium —*see* Degeneration,
        retina, separation of layers, pigment
        epithelium detachment
    rhegmatogenous —*see* Detachment, retina,
        with retinal, break
    specified NEC H33.8
    total H33.05-
    traction H33.4-
  vitreous (body) H43.81
Detergent asthma J69.8
Deterioration
  epileptic F06.8
  general physical R53.81
  heart, cardiac —*see* Degeneration, myocardial
  mental —*see* Psychosis
  myocardial, myocardium —*see* Degeneration,
      myocardial
  senile (simple) R54
Deuteranomaly (anomalous trichromat) H53.53
Deuteranopia (complete) (incomplete) H53.53
Development
  abnormal, bone Q79.9
  arrested R62.50
    bone —*see* Arrest, development or growth,
        bone
    child R62.50
    due to malnutrition E45
  defective, congenital —*see also* Anomaly, by
      site
    cauda equina Q06.3
    left ventricle Q24.8
      in hypoplastic left heart syndrome
          Q23.4
    valve Q24.8
    pulmonary Q22.3
  delayed (*see also* Delay, development) R62.50
    arithmetical skills F81.2
    language (skills) (expressive) F80.1
    learning skill F81.9
    mixed skills F88
    motor coordination F82
    reading F81.0
    specified learning skill NEC F81.89
    speech F80.9
    spelling F81.81
    written expression F81.81
  imperfect, congenital —*see also* Anomaly, by
      site
    heart Q24.9
    lungs Q33.6
  incomplete
    bronchial tree Q32.4
    organ or site not listed —*see* Hypoplasia,
        by site
    respiratory system Q34.9
    sexual, precocious NEC E30.1
  tardy, mental (*see also* Disability, intellectual)
      F79

Developmental —*see* condition
  ~~testing, child —*see* Examination, child~~
  testing, infant or child —*see* Examination,
      child ◀
Devergie's disease (pityriasis rubra pilaris)
    L44.0
Deviation (in)
  conjugate palsy (eye) (spastic) H51.0
  esophagus (acquired) K22.8
  eye, skew H51.8
  midline (jaw) (teeth) (dental arch) M26.29
    specified site NEC —*see* Malposition
  nasal septum J34.2
    congenital Q67.4
  opening and closing of the mandible M26.53
  organ or site, congenital NEC —*see*
      Malposition, congenital
  septum (nasal) (acquired) J34.2
    congenital Q67.4
  sexual F65.9
    bestiality F65.89
    erotomania F52.8
    exhibitionism F65.2
    fetishism, fetishistic F65.0
      transvestism F65.1
    frotteurism F65.81
    masochism F65.51
    multiple F65.89
    necrophilia F65.89
    nymphomania F52.8
    pederosis F65.4
    pedophilia F65.4
    sadism, sadomasochism F65.52
    satyriasis F52.8
    specified type NEC F65.89
    transvestism F64.1
    voyeurism F65.3
  teeth, midline M26.29
  trachea J39.8
  ureter, congenital Q62.61
Device
  cerebral ventricle (communicating) in situ
      Z98.2
  contraceptive —*see* Contraceptive, device
  drainage, cerebrospinal fluid, in situ Z98.2
Devic's disease G36.0
Devil's
  grip B33.0
  pinches (purpura simplex) D69.2
Devitalized tooth K04.99
Devonshire colic —*see* Poisoning, lead
Dextraposition, aorta Q20.3
  in tetralogy of Fallot Q21.3
Dextrinosis, limit (debrancher enzyme
    deficiency) E74.03
Dextrocardia (true) Q24.0
  with
    complete transposition of viscera Q89.3
    situs inversus Q89.3
Dextrotransposition, aorta Q20.3
d-glycericacidemia E72.59
Dhat syndrome F48.8
Dhobi itch B35.6
Di George's syndrome D82.1
Di Guglielmo's disease C94.0-
Diabetes, diabetic (mellitus) (sugar) E11.9
  with
    amyotrophy E11.44
    arthropathy NEC E11.618
    autonomic (poly)neuropathy E11.43
    cataract E11.36
    Charcot's joints E11.610
    chronic kidney disease E11.22
    circulatory complication NEC E11.59
    complication E11.8
      specified NEC E11.69
    dermatitis E11.620
    foot ulcer E11.621
    gangrene E11.52
    gastroparalysis E11.43 ◀
    gastroparesis E11.43

Diabetes, diabetic (Continued)
  with (Continued)
    glomerulonephrosis, intracapillary E11.21
    glomerulosclerosis, intercapillary E11.21
    hyperglycemia E11.65
    hyperosmolarity E11.00
      with coma E11.01
    hypoglycemia E11.649
      with coma E11.641
    kidney complications NEC E11.29
    Kimmelstiel-Wilson disease E11.21
    loss of protective sensation (LOPS) —*see*
        Diabetes, by type, with neuropathy
    mononeuropathy E11.41
    myasthenia E11.44
    necrobiosis lipoidica E11.620
    nephropathy E11.21
    neuralgia E11.42
    neurologic complication NEC E11.49
    neuropathic arthropathy E11.610
    neuropathy E11.40
    ophthalmic complication NEC E11.39
    oral complication NEC E11.638
    osteomyelitis E11.69 ◀
    periodontal disease E11.630
    peripheral angiopathy E11.51
      with gangrene E11.52
    polyneuropathy E11.42
    renal complication NEC E11.29
    renal tubular degeneration E11.29
    retinopathy E11.319
      with macular edema E11.311
        resolved following treatment
            E11.37 ◀
      nonproliferative E11.329
        with macular edema E11.321
        mild E11.329
          with macular edema E11.321
        moderate E11.339
          with macular edema E11.331
        severe E11.349
          with macular edema E11.341
      proliferative E11.359
        ~~with macular edema E11.351~~
        with ◀
          combined traction retinal
              detachment and
              rhegmatogenous retinal
              detachment E11.354 ◀
          macular edema E11.351 ◀
          stable proliferative diabetic
              retinopathy E11.355 ◀
          traction retinal detachment
              involving the macula
              E11.352 ◀
          traction retinal detachment not
              involving the macula
              E11.353 ◀
    skin complication NEC E11.628
    skin ulcer NEC E11.622
  brittle —*see* Diabetes, type 1 ◀
  bronzed E83.110
  complicating pregnancy —*see* Pregnancy,
      complicated by, diabetes
  dietary counseling and surveillance Z71.3
  due to ◀
    autoimmune process —*see* Diabetes,
        type 1 ◀
    immune mediated pancreatic islet beta-cell
        destruction —*see* Diabetes, type 1 ◀
  due to drug or chemical E09.9
    with
      amyotrophy E09.44
      arthropathy NEC E09.618
      autonomic (poly)neuropathy E09.43
      cataract E09.36
      Charcot's joints E09.610
      chronic kidney disease E09.22
      circulatory complication NEC E09.59
      complication E09.8
        specified NEC E09.69

◀ New   ◀⁞⁞ Revised   ~~deleted~~ Deleted

Diabetes, diabetic *(Continued)*
  due to drug or chemical *(Continued)*
    with *(Continued)*
      dermatitis E09.620
      foot ulcer E09.621
      gangrene E09.52
      gastroparalysis E09.43 ◀
      gastroparesis E09.43
      glomerulonephrosis, intracapillary
        E09.21
      glomerulosclerosis, intercapillary E09.21
      hyperglycemia E09.65
      hyperosmolarity E09.00
        with coma E09.01
      hypoglycemia E09.649
        with coma E09.641
      ketoacidosis E09.10
        with coma E09.11
      kidney complications NEC E09.29
      Kimmelsteil-Wilson disease E09.21
      mononeuropathy E09.41
      myasthenia E09.44
      necrobiosis lipoidica E09.620
      nephropathy E09.21
      neuralgia E09.42
      neurologic complication NEC E09.49
      neuropathic arthropathy E09.610
      neuropathy E09.40
      ophthalmic complication NEC E09.39
      oral complication NEC E09.638
      periodontal disease E09.630
      peripheral angiopathy E09.51
        with gangrene E09.52
      polyneuropathy E09.42
      renal complication NEC E09.29
      renal tubular degeneration E09.29
      retinopathy E09.319
        with macular edema E09.311
          resolved following treatment
            E09.37 ◀
        nonproliferative E09.329
          with macular edema E09.321
          mild E09.329
            with macular edema E09.321
          moderate E09.339
            with macular edema E09.331
          severe E09.349
            with macular edema E09.341
        proliferative E09.359
          ~~with macular edema E09.351~~
          with ◀
            combined traction retinal
              detachment and
              rhegmatogenous retinal
              detachment E09.354 ◀
            macular edema E09.351 ◀
            stable proliferative diabetic
              retinopathy E09.355 ◀
            traction retinal detachment
              involving the macula
              E09.352 ◀
            traction retinal detachment not
              involving the macula
              E09.353 ◀
      skin complication NEC E09.628
      skin ulcer NEC E09.622
  due to underlying condition E08.9
    with
      amyotrophy E08.44
      arthropathy NEC E08.618
      autonomic (poly)neuropathy E08.43
      cataract E08.36
      Charcot's joints E08.610
      chronic kidney disease E08.22
      circulatory complication NEC E08.59
      complication E08.8
        specified NEC E08.69
      dermatitis E08.620
      foot ulcer E08.621
      gangrene E08.52
      gastroparalysis E08.43 ◀

Diabetes, diabetic *(Continued)*
  due to underlying condition *(Continued)*
    with *(Continued)*
      gastroparesis E08.43
      glomerulonephrosis, intracapillary
        E08.21
      glomerulosclerosis, intercapillary E08.21
      hyperglycemia E08.69
      hyperosmolarity E08.00
        with coma E08.01
      hypoglycemia E08.649
        with coma E08.641
      ketoacidosis E08.10
        with coma E08.11
      kidney complications NEC E08.29
      Kimmelsteil-WIlson disease E08.21
      mononeuropathy E08.41
      myasthenia E08.44
      necrobiosis lipoidica E08.620
      nephropathy E08.21
      neuralgia E08.42
      neurologic complication NEC E08.49
      neuropathic arthropathy E08.610
      neuropathy E08.40
      ophthalmic complication NEC
        E08.39
      oral complication NEC E08.638
      periodontal disease E08.630
      peripheral angiopathy E08.51
        with gangrene E08.52
      polyneuropathy E08.42
      renal complication NEC E08.29
      renal tubular degeneration E08.29
      retinopathy E08.319
        with macular edema E08.311
          resolved following treatment
            E08.37 ◀
        nonproliferative E08.329
          with macular edema E08.321
          mild E08.329
            with macular edema E08.321
          moderate E08.339
            with macular edema E08.331
          severe E08.349
            with macular edema E08.341
        proliferative E08.359
          ~~with macular edema E08.351~~
          with ◀
            combined traction retinal
              detachment and
              rhegmatogenous retinal
              detachment E08.354 ◀
            macular edema E08.351 ◀
            stable proliferative diabetic
              retinopathy E08.355 ◀
            traction retinal detachment
              involving the macula
              E08.352 ◀
            traction retinal detachment not
              involving the macula
              E08.353 ◀
      skin complication NEC E08.628
      skin ulcer NEC E08.622
  gestational (in pregnancy) O24.419
    affecting newborn P70.0
    diet-controlled O24.410
    in childbirth O24.429
      diet-controlled O24.420
      insulin (and diet) controlled O24.424
      oral drug controlled (antidiabetic)
        (hypoglycemic) O24.425 ◀
    insulin (and diet) controlled O24.414
    oral drug controlled (antidiabetic)
      (hypoglycemic) O24.415 ◀
    puerperal O24.439
      diet-controlled O24.430
      insulin (and diet) controlled O24.434
      oral drug controlled (antidiabetic)
        (hypoglycemic) O24.435 ◀
  hepatogenous E13.9
  idiopathic —*see* Diabetes, type 1 ◀

Diabetes, diabetic *(Continued)*
  inadequately controlled — code to Diabetes,
    by type, with hyperglycemia
  insipidus E23.2
    nephrogenic N25.1
    pituitary E23.2
    vasopressin resistant N25.1
  insulin dependent — code to type of diabetes
  juvenile-onset —*see* Diabetes, type 1
  ketosis-prone —*see* Diabetes, type 1
  latent R73.03 ◀▥
  neonatal (transient) P70.2
  non-insulin dependent — code to type of
    diabetes
  out of control — code to Diabetes, by type,
    with hyperglycemia
  phosphate E83.39
  poorly controlled — code to Diabetes, by
    type, with hyperglycemia
  postpancreatectomy —*see* Diabetes, specified
    type NEC
  postprocedural —*see* Diabetes, specified type
    NEC
  secondary diabetes mellitus NEC —*see*
    Diabetes, specified type NEC
  specified type NEC E13.9
    with
      amyotrophy E13.44
      arthropathy NEC E13.618
      autonomic (poly)neuropathy E13.43
      cataract E13.36
      Charcot's joints E13.610
      chronic kidney disease E13.22
      circulatory complication NEC E13.59
      complication E13.8
        specified NEC E13.69
      dermatitis E13.620
      foot ulcer E13.621
      gangrene E13.52
      gastroparalysis E13.43 ◀
      gastroparesis E13.43
      glomerulonephrosis, intracapillary
        E13.21
      glomerulosclerosis, intercapillary E13.21
      hyperglycemia E13.65
      hyperosmolarity E13.00
        with coma E13.01
      hypoglycemia E13.649
        with coma E13.641
      ketoacidosis E13.10
        with coma E13.11
      kidney complications NEC E13.29
      Kimmelsteil-Wilson disease E13.21
      mononeuropathy E13.41
      myasthenia E13.44
      necrobiosis lipoidica E13.620
      nephropathy E13.21
      neuralgia E13.42
      neurologic complication NEC E13.49
      neuropathic arthropathy E13.610
      neuropathy E13.40
      ophthalmic complication NEC E13.39
      oral complication NEC E13.638
      periodontal disease E13.630
      peripheral angiopathy E13.51
        with gangrene E13.52
      polyneuropathy E13.42
      renal complication NEC E13.29
      renal tubular degeneration E13.29
      retinopathy E13.319
        with macular edema E13.311
          resolved following treatment
            E13.37 ◀
        nonproliferative E13.329
          with macular edema E13.321
          mild E13.329
            with macular edema E13.321
          moderate E13.339
            with macular edema E13.331
          severe E13.349
            with macular edema E13.341

Diabetes, diabetic *(Continued)*
  specified type NEC *(Continued)*
    with *(Continued)*
      retinopathy *(Continued)*
        proliferative E13.359
         ~~with macular edema E13.351~~
         with ◀
           combined traction retinal
             detachment and
             rhegmatogenous retinal
             detachment E13.354 ◀
           macular edema E13.351 ◀
           stable proliferative diabetic
             retinopathy E13.355 ◀
           traction retinal detachment
             involving the macula
             E13.352 ◀
           traction retinal detachment not
             involving the macula
             E13.353 ◀
      skin complication NEC E13.628
      skin ulcer NEC E13.622
  steroid-induced —*see* Diabetes, due to, drug
    or chemical
  type 1 E10.9
    with
      amyotrophy E10.44
      arthropathy NEC E10.618
      autonomic (poly)neuropathy E10.43
      cataract E10.36
      Charcot's joints E10.610
      chronic kidney disease E10.22
      circulatory complication NEC E10.59
      complication E10.8
        specified NEC E10.69
      dermatitis E10.620
      foot ulcer E10.621
      gangrene E10.52
      gastroparalysis E10.43 ◀
      gastroparesis E10.43
      glomerulonephrosis, intracapillary
        E10.21
      glomerulosclerosis, intercapillary
        E10.21
      hyperglycemia E10.65
      hypoglycemia E10.649
        with coma E10.641
      ketoacidosis E10.10
        with coma E10.11
      kidney complications NEC E10.29
      Kimmelsteil-Wilson disease E10.21
      mononeuropathy E10.41
      myasthenia E10.44
      necrobiosis lipoidica E10.620
      nephropathy E10.21
      neuralgia E10.42
      neurologic complication NEC
        E10.49
      neuropathic arthropathy E10.610
      neuropathy E10.40
      ophthalmic complication NEC
        E10.39
      oral complication NEC E10.638
      periodontal disease E10.630
      peripheral angiopathy E10.51
        with gangrene E10.52
      polyneuropathy E10.42
      renal complication NEC E10.29
      renal tubular degeneration E10.29
      retinopathy E10.319
        with macular edema E10.311
          resolved following treatment
            E10.37 ◀
        nonproliferative E10.329
          with macular edema E10.321
          mild E10.329
            with macular edema E10.321
          moderate E10.339
            with macular edema E10.331
          severe E10.349
            with macular edema E10.341

Diabetes, diabetic *(Continued)*
  type 1 *(Continued)*
    with *(Continued)*
      retinopathy *(Continued)*
        proliferative E10.359
         ~~with macular edema E10.351~~
         with ◀
           combined traction retinal
             detachment and
             rhegmatogenous retinal
             detachment E13.354 ◀
           macular edema E13.351 ◀
           stable proliferative diabetic
             retinopathy E13.355 ◀
           traction retinal detachment
             involving the macula
             E13.352 ◀
           traction retinal detachment not
             involving the macula
             E13.353 ◀
      skin complication NEC E10.628
      skin ulcer NEC E10.622
  type 2 E11.9
    with
      amyotrophy E11.44
      arthropathy NEC E11.618
      autonomic (poly)neuropathy E11.43
      cataract E11.36
      Charcot's joints E11.610
      chronic kidney disease E11.22
      circulatory complication NEC E11.59
      complication E11.8
        specified NEC E11.69
      dermatitis E11.620
      foot ulcer E11.621
      gangrene E11.52
      gastroparalysis E11.43 ◀
      gastroparesis E11.43
      glomerulonephrosis, intracapillary E11.21
      glomerulosclerosis, intercapillary E11.21
      hyperglycemia E11.65
      hyperosmolarity E11.00
        with coma E11.01
      hypoglycemia E11.649
        with coma E11.641
      kidney complications NEC E11.29
      Kimmelsteil-Wilson disease E11.21
      mononeuropathy E11.41
      myasthenia E11.44
      necrobiosis lipoidica E11.620
      nephropathy E11.21
      neuralgia E11.42
      neurologic complication NEC E11.49
      neuropathic arthropathy E11.610
      neuropathy E11.40
      ophthalmic complication NEC E11.39
      oral complication NEC E11.638
      periodontal disease E11.630
      peripheral angiopathy E11.51
        with gangrene E11.52
      polyneuropathy E11.42
      renal complication NEC E11.29
      renal tubular degeneration E11.29
      retinopathy E11.319
        with macular edema E11.311
          resolved following treatment
            E11.37 ◀
        nonproliferative E11.329
          with macular edema E11.321
          mild E11.329
            with macular edema E11.321
          moderate E11.339
            with macular edema E11.331
          severe E11.349
            with macular edema E11.341
        proliferative E11.359
         ~~with macular edema E11.351~~
         with ◀
           combined traction retinal
             detachment and
             rhegmatogenous retinal
             detachment E11.354 ◀

Diabetes, diabetic *(Continued)*
  type 2 *(Continued)*
    with *(Continued)*
      retinopathy *(Continued)*
        proliferative *(Continued)*
         with *(Continued)*
           macular edema E11.351 ◀
           stable proliferative diabetic
             retinopathy E11.355 ◀
           traction retinal detachment
             involving the macula
             E11.352 ◀
           traction retinal detachment not
             involving the macula
             E11.353 ◀
      skin complication NEC E11.628
      skin ulcer NEC E11.622
  uncontrolled ◀
    meaning ◀
      hyperglycemia —*see* Diabetes, by type,
        with, hyperglycemia ◀
      hypoglycemia —*see* Diabetes, by type,
        with, hypoglycemia ◀
Diacyclothrombopathia D69.1
Diagnosis deferred R69
Dialysis (intermittent) (treatment)
  noncompliance (with) Z91.15
  renal (hemodialysis) (peritoneal), status Z99.2
  retina, retinal —*see* Detachment, retina, with
    retinal, dialysis
Diamond-Blackfan anemia (congenital
  hypoplastic) D61.01
Diamond-Gardener syndrome
  (autoerythrocyte sensitization) D69.2
Diaper rash L22
Diaphoresis (excessive) R61
Diaphragm —*see* condition
Diaphragmalgia R07.1
Diaphragmatitis, diaphragmitis J98.6
Diaphysial aclasis Q78.6
Diaphysitis —*see* Osteomyelitis, specified type
  NEC
Diarrhea, diarrheal (disease) (infantile)
  (inflammatory) R19.7
  achlorhydric K31.83
  allergic K52.29 ◀▮▮▮
    due to ◀
      colitis —*see* Colitis, allergic ◀
      enteritis —*see* Enteritis, allergic ◀
  amebic —*see also* Amebiasis A06.0
    with abscess —*see* Abscess, amebic
    acute A06.0
    chronic A06.1
    nondysenteric A06.2
  bacillary —*see* Dysentery, bacillary
  balantidial A07.0
  cachectic NEC K52.89
  Chilomastix A07.8
  choleriformis A00.1
  chronic (noninfectious) K52.9
  coccidial A07.3
  Cochin-China K90.1
    strongyloidiasis B78.0
  Dientamoeba A07.8
  dietetic —*see also* Diarrhea, allergic
    K52.29 ◀▮▮▮
  drug-induced K52.1
  due to
    bacteria A04.9
      specified NEC A04.8
    Campylobacter A04.5
    Capillaria philippinensis B81.1
    Clostridium difficile A04.7
    Clostridium perfringens (C) (F) A04.8
    Cryptosporidium A07.2
    drugs K52.1
    Escherichia coli A04.4
      enteroaggregative A04.4
      enterohemorrhagic A04.3
      enteroinvasive A04.2
      enteropathogenic A04.0

◀ New   ◀▮▮▮ Revised   ~~deleted~~ Deleted

Diarrhea, diarrheal (*Continued*)
  due to (*Continued*)
    Escherichia coli (*Continued*)
      enterotoxigenic A04.1
      specified NEC A04.4
      food hypersensitivity —*see also* Diarrhea,
        allergic K52.29 ◀▥
      Necator americanus B76.1
      S. japonicum B65.2
      specified organism NEC A08.8
        bacterial A04.8
        viral A08.39
      Staphylococcus A04.8
      Trichuris trichiuria B79
      virus —*see* Enteritis, viral
      Yersinia enterocolitica A04.6
  dysenteric A09
  endemic A09
  epidemic A09
  flagellate A07.9
  Flexner's (ulcerative) A03.1
  functional K59.1
    following gastrointestinal surgery K91.89
    psychogenic F45.8
  Giardia lamblia A07.1
  giardial A07.1
  hill K90.1
  infectious A09
  malarial —*see* Malaria
  mite B88.0
  mycotic NEC B49
  neonatal (noninfectious) P78.3
  nervous F45.8
  neurogenic K59.1
  noninfectious K52.9
  postgastrectomy K91.1
  postvagotomy K91.1
  protozoal A07.9
    specified NEC A07.8
  psychogenic F45.8
  specified
    bacterium NEC A04.8
    virus NEC A08.39
  strongyloidiasis B78.0
  toxic K52.1
  trichomonal A07.8
  tropical K90.1
  tuberculous A18.32
  viral —*see* Enteritis, viral
Diastasis
  cranial bones M84.88
    congenital NEC Q75.8
  joint (traumatic) —*see* Dislocation
  muscle M62.00
    ankle M62.07-
    congenital Q79.8
    foot M62.07-
    forearm M62.03-
    hand M62.04-
    lower leg M62.06-
    pelvic region M62.05-
    shoulder region M62.01-
    specified site NEC M62.08
    thigh M62.05-
    upper arm M62.02-
  recti (abdomen)
    complicating delivery O71.89
    congenital Q79.59
Diastema, tooth, teeth, fully erupted M26.32
Diastematomyelia Q06.2
Diataxia, cerebral G80.4
Diathesis
  allergic —*see* History, allergy
  bleeding (familial) D69.9
  cystine (familial) E72.00
  gouty —*see* Gout
  hemorrhagic (familial) D69.9
    newborn NEC P53
  spasmophilic R29.0
Diaz's disease or osteochondrosis (juvenile)
    (talus) —*see* Osteochondrosis, juvenile,
    tarsus

Dibothriocephalus, dibothriocephaliasis
    (latus) (infection) (infestation) B70.0
  larval B70.1
Dicephalus, dicephaly Q89.4
Dichotomy, teeth K00.2
Dichromat, dichromatopsia (congenital) —*see*
  Deficiency, color vision
Dichuchwa A65
Dicroceliasis B66.2
Didelphia, didelphys —*see* Double uterus
Didymytis N45.1
  with orchitis N45.3
Dietary
  inadequacy or deficiency E63.9
  surveillance and counseling Z71.3
Dietl's crisis N13.8
Dieulafoy lesion (hemorrhagic)
  duodenum K31.82
  esophagus K22.8
  intestine (colon) K63.81
  stomach K31.82
Difficult, difficulty (in)
  acculturation Z60.3
  feeding R63.3
    newborn P92.9
      breast P92.5
      specified NEC P92.8
    nonorganic (infant or child) F98.29
  intubation, in anesthesia T88.4
  mechanical, gastroduodenal stoma K91.89
    causing obstruction K91.3
  micturition ◀
    need to immediately re-void R39.191 ◀
    position dependent R39.192 ◀
    specified NEC R39.198 ◀
  reading (developmental) F81.0
    secondary to emotional disorders F93.9
  spelling (specific) F81.81
    with reading disorder F81.89
    due to inadequate teaching Z55.8
  swallowing —*see* Dysphagia
  walking R26.2
  work
    conditions NEC Z56.5
    schedule Z56.3
Diffuse —*see* condition
DiGeorge's syndrome (thymic hypoplasia)
  D82.1
Digestive —*see* condition
Dihydropyrimidine dehydrogenase disease
  (DPD) E88.89
Diktyoma —*see* Neoplasm, malignant, by site
Dilaceration, tooth K00.4
Dilatation
  anus K59.8
    venule —*see* Hemorrhoids
  aorta (focal) (general) —*see* Ectasia, aorta
    with aneurysm —*see* Aneurysm, aorta
    congenital Q25.44 ◀
  artery —*see* Aneurysm
  bladder (sphincter) N32.89
    congenital Q64.79
  blood vessel I99.8
  bronchial J47.9
    with
      exacerbation (acute) J47.1
      lower respiratory infection J47.0
  calyx (due to obstruction) —*see*
    Hydronephrosis
  capillaries I78.8
  cardiac (acute) (chronic) —*see also*
    Hypertrophy, cardiac
    congenital Q24.8
      valve NEC Q24.8
        pulmonary Q22.3
    valve —*see* Endocarditis
  cavum septi pellucidi Q06.8
  cervix (uteri) —*see also* Incompetency,
    cervix
    incomplete, poor, slow complicating
      delivery O62.0

Dilatation (*Continued*)
  colon K59.39 ◀▥
    congenital Q43.1
    psychogenic F45.8
    toxic K59.31 ◀
  common duct (acquired) K83.8
    congenital Q44.5
  cystic duct (acquired) K82.8
    congenital Q44.5
  duct, mammary —*see* Ectasia, mammary duct
  duodenum K59.8
  esophagus K22.8
    congenital Q39.5
    due to achalasia K22.0
  eustachian tube, congenital Q17.8
  gallbladder K82.8
  gastric —*see* Dilatation, stomach
  heart (acute) (chronic) —*see also* Hypertrophy,
    cardiac
    congenital Q24.8
    valve —*see* Endocarditis
  ileum K59.8
    psychogenic F45.8
  jejunum K59.8
    psychogenic F45.8
  kidney (calyx) (collecting structures) (cystic)
    (parenchyma) (pelvis) (idiopathic)
    N28.89
  lacrimal passages or duct —*see* Disorder,
    lacrimal system, changes
  lymphatic vessel I89.0
  mammary duct —*see* Ectasia, mammary duct
  Meckel's diverticulum (congenital) Q43.0
    malignant —*see* Table of Neoplasms, small
      intestine, malignant
  myocardium (acute) (chronic) —*see*
    Hypertrophy, cardiac organ or site,
    congenital NEC —*see* Distortion
  pancreatic duct K86.89 ◀▥
  pericardium —*see* Pericarditis
  pharynx J39.2
  prostate N42.89
  pulmonary
    artery (idiopathic) I28.8
    valve, congenital Q22.3
  pupil H57.04
  rectum K59.39 ◀▥
  saccule, congenital Q16.5
  salivary gland (duct) K11.8
  sphincter ani K62.89
  stomach K31.89
    acute K31.0
    psychogenic F45.8
  submaxillary duct K11.8
  trachea, congenital Q32.1
  ureter (idiopathic) N28.82
    congenital Q62.2
    due to obstruction N13.4
  urethra (acquired) N36.8
  vasomotor I73.9
  vein I86.8
  ventricular, ventricle (acute) (chronic) —*see*
    also Hypertrophy, cardiac
    cerebral, congenital Q04.8
  venule NEC I86.8
  vesical orifice N32.89
Dilated, dilation —*see* Dilatation
Diminished, diminution
  hearing (acuity) —*see* Deafness
  sense or sensation (cold) (heat) (tactile)
    (vibratory) R20.8
  vision NEC H54.7
  vital capacity R94.2
Diminuta taenia B71.0
Dimitri-Sturge-Weber disease Q85.8
Dimple
  ~~parasacral, pilonidal or postanal —see Cyst,~~
    ~~pilonidal~~
  congenital sacral Q82.6 ◀
  parasacral Q82.6 ◀
  pilonidal or postanal —*see* Cyst, pilonidal ◀

Dioctophyme renalis (infection) (infestation) B83.8
Dipetalonemiasis B74.4
Diphallus Q55.69
Diphtheria, diphtheritic (gangrenous) (hemorrhagic) A36.9
  carrier (suspected) Z22.2
  cutaneous A36.3
  faucial A36.0
  infection of wound A36.3
  laryngeal A36.2
  myocarditis A36.81
  nasal, anterior A36.89
  nasopharyngeal A36.1
  neurological complication A36.89
  pharyngeal A36.0
  specified site NEC A36.89
  tonsillar A36.0
Diphyllobothriasis (intestine) B70.0
  larval B70.1
Diplacusis H93.22-
Diplegia (upper limbs) G83.0
  congenital (cerebral) G80.8
  facial G51.0
  lower limbs G82.20
  spastic G80.1
Diplococcus, diplococcal —see condition
Diplopia H53.2
Dipsomania F10.20
  with
    psychosis —see Psychosis, alcoholic
    remission F10.21
Dipylidiasis B71.1
DIRA (deficiency of interleukin 1 receptor antagonist) M04.8 ◀
Direction, teeth, abnormal, fully erupted M26.30
Dirofilariasis B74.8
Dirt-eating child F98.3
Disability, disabilities
  heart —see Disease, heart
  intellectual F79
    with
      autistic features F84.9
    mild (I.Q. 50-69) F70
    moderate (I.Q. 35-49) F71
    profound (I.Q. under 20) F73
    severe (I.Q. 20-34) F72
    specified level NEC F78
  knowledge acquisition F81.9
  learning F81.9
  limiting activities Z73.6
  spelling, specific F81.81
Disappearance of family member Z63.4
Disarticulation —see Amputation
  meaning traumatic amputation —see Amputation, traumatic
Discharge (from)
  abnormal finding in —see Abnormal, specimen
  breast (female) (male) N64.52
  diencephalic autonomic idiopathic —see Epilepsy, specified NEC
  ear —see also Otorrhea
    blood —see Otorrhagia
  excessive urine R35.8
  nipple N64.52
  penile R36.9
  postnasal R09.82
  prison, anxiety concerning Z65.2
  urethral R36.9
    without blood R36.0
    hematospermia R36.1
  vaginal N89.8
Discitis, diskitis M46.40
  cervical region M46.42
  cervicothoracic region M46.43
  lumbar region M46.46
  lumbosacral region M46.47
  multiple sites M46.49
  occipito-atlanto-axial region M46.41

Discitis, diskitis (Continued)
  pyogenic —see Infection, intervertebral disc, pyogenic
  sacrococcygeal region M46.48
  thoracic region M46.44
  thoracolumbar region M46.45
Discoid
  meniscus (congenital) Q68.6
  semilunar cartilage (congenital) —see Derangement, knee, meniscus, specified NEC
Discoloration
  nails L60.8
  teeth (posteruptive) K03.7
    during formation K00.8
Discomfort
  chest R07.89
  visual H53.14-
Discontinuity, ossicles, ear H74.2-
Discord (with)
  boss Z56.4
  classmates Z55.4
  counselor Z64.4
  employer Z56.4
  family Z63.8
  fellow employees Z56.4
  in-laws Z63.1
  landlord Z59.2
  lodgers Z59.2
  neighbors Z59.2
  probation officer Z64.4
  social worker Z64.4
  teachers Z55.4
  workmates Z56.4
Discordant connection
  atrioventricular (congenital) Q20.5
  ventriculoarterial Q20.3
Discrepancy
  centric occlusion maximum intercuspation M26.55
  leg length (acquired) —see Deformity, limb, unequal length
    congenital —see Defect, reduction, lower limb
  uterine size date O26.84-
Discrimination
  ethnic Z60.5
  political Z60.5
  racial Z60.5
  religious Z60.5
  sex Z60.5
Disease, diseased —see also Syndrome
  absorbent system I87.8
  acid-peptic K30
  Acosta's T70.29
  Adams-Stokes (-Morgagni) (syncope with heart block) I45.9
  Addison's anemia (pernicious) D51.0
  adenoids (and tonsils) J35.9
  adrenal (capsule) (cortex) (gland) (medullary) E27.9
    hyperfunction E27.0
    specified NEC E27.8
  ainhum L94.6
  airway
    obstructive, chronic J44.9
      due to
        cotton dust J66.0
        specific organic dusts NEC J66.8
    reactive —see Asthma
  akamushi (scrub typhus) A75.3
  Albers-Schönberg (marble bones) Q78.2
  Albert's —see Tendinitis, Achilles
  alimentary canal K63.9
  alligator-skin Q80.9
    acquired L85.0
  alpha heavy chain C88.3
  alpine T70.29
  altitude T70.20

Disease, diseased (Continued)
  alveolar ridge
    edentulous K06.9
      specified NEC K06.8
  alveoli, teeth K08.9
  Alzheimer's G30.9 [F02.80]
    with behavioral disturbance G30.9 [F02.81]
    early onset G30.0 [F02.80]
      with behavioral disturbance G30.0 [F02.81]
    late onset G30.1 [F02.80]
      with behavioral disturbance G30.1 [F02.81]
    specified NEC G30.8 [F02.80]
      with behavioral disturbance G30.8 [F02.81]
  amyloid —see Amyloidosis
  Andersen's (glycogenosis IV) E74.09
  Andes T70.29
  Andrews' (bacterid) L08.89
  angiospastic I73.9
    cerebral G45.9
    vein I87.8
  anterior
    chamber H21.9
    horn cell G12.29
  antiglomerular basement membrane (anti-GBM) antibody M31.0
    tubulo-interstitial nephritis N12
  antral —see Sinusitis, maxillary
  anus K62.9
    specified NEC K62.89
  aorta (nonsyphilitic) I77.9
    syphilitic NEC A52.02
  aortic (heart) (valve) I35.9
    rheumatic I06.9
  Apollo B30.3
  aponeuroses —see Enthesopathy
  appendix K38.9
    specified NEC K38.8
  aqueous (chamber) H21.9
  Arnold-Chiari —see Arnold-Chiari disease
  arterial I77.9
    occlusive —see Occlusion, by site
      due to stricture or stenosis I77.1
  arteriocardiorenal —see Hypertension, cardiorenal
  arteriolar (generalized) (obliterative) I77.9
  arteriorenal —see Hypertension, kidney
  arteriosclerotic —see also Arteriosclerosis
    cardiovascular —see Disease, heart, ischemic, atherosclerotic
    coronary (artery) —see Disease, heart, ischemic, atherosclerotic
    heart —see Disease, heart, ischemic, atherosclerotic
  artery I77.9
    cerebral I67.9
    coronary I25.10
      with angina pectoris —see Arteriosclerosis, coronary (artery),
  arthropod-borne NOS (viral) A94
    specified type NEC A93.8
  atticoantral, chronic H66.20
    left H66.22
      with right H66.23
    right H66.21
      with left H66.23
  auditory canal —see Disorder, ear, external
  auricle, ear NEC —see Disorder, pinna
  Australian X A83.4
  autoimmune (systemic) NOS M35.9
    hemolytic (cold type) (warm type) D59.1
      drug-induced D59.0
    thyroid E06.3
  aviator's —see Effect, adverse, high altitude
  Ayala's Q78.5
  Ayerza's (pulmonary artery sclerosis with pulmonary hypertension) I27.0

◀ New   ◀║ Revised   ~~deleted~~ Deleted

Disease, diseased *(Continued)*
Babington's (familial hemorrhagic
    telangiectasia) I78.0
bacterial A49.9
    specified NEC A48.8
    zoonotic A28.9
        specified type NEC A28.8
Baelz's (cheilitis glandularis apostematosa)
    K13.0
bagasse J67.1
balloon —*see* Effect, adverse, high altitude
Bang's (brucella abortus) A23.1
Bannister's T78.3
barometer makers' —*see* Poisoning, mercury
Barraquer (-Simons') (progressive
    lipodystrophy) E88.1
Barrett's —*see* Barrett's, esophagus
Bartholin's gland N75.9
basal ganglia G25.9
    degenerative G23.9
        specified NEC G23.8
    specified NEC G25.89
Basedow's (exophthalmic goiter) —*see*
    Hyperthyroidism, with, goiter (diffuse)
Bateman's B08.1
Batten-Steinert G71.11
Battey A31.0
Beard's (neurasthenia) F48.8
Becker
    idiopathic mural endomyocardial I42.3
    myotonia congenita G71.12
Begbie's (exophthalmic goiter) —*see*
    Hyperthyroidism, with, goiter (diffuse)
behavioral, organic F07.9
Beigel's (white piedra) B36.2
Benson's —*see* Deposit, crystalline
Bernard-Soulier (thrombopathy) D69.1
Bernhardt (-Roth) —*see* Mononeuropathy,
    lower limb, meralgia paresthetica
Biermer's (pernicious anemia) D51.0
bile duct (common) (hepatic) K83.9
    with calculus, stones —*see* Calculus, bile
        duct
    specified NEC K83.8
biliary (tract) K83.9
    specified NEC K83.8
Billroth's —*see* Spina bifida
bird fancier's J67.2
black lung J60
bladder N32.9
    in (due to)
        schistosomiasis (bilharziasis) B65.0 [N33]
    specified NEC N32.89
bleeder's D66
blood D75.9
    forming organs D75.9
    vessel I99.9
Bloodgood's —*see* Mastopathy, cystic
Bodechtel-Guttmann (subacute sclerosing
    panencephalitis) A81.1
bone —*see also* Disorder, bone
    aluminum M83.4
    fibrocystic NEC
        jaw M27.49
bone-marrow D75.9
Borna A83.9
Bornholm (epidemic pleurodynia) B33.0
Bouchard's (myopathic dilatation of the
    stomach) K31.0
Bouillaud's (rheumatic heart disease) I01.9
Bourneville (-Brissaud) (tuberous sclerosis)
    Q85.1
Bouveret (-Hoffmann) (paroxysmal
    tachycardia) I47.9
bowel K63.9
    functional K59.9
        psychogenic F45.8
brain G93.9
    arterial, artery I67.9
    arteriosclerotic I67.2
    congenital Q04.9

Disease, diseased *(Continued)*
brain *(Continued)*
    degenerative —*see* Degeneration, brain
    inflammatory —*see* Encephalitis
    organic G93.9
        arteriosclerotic I67.2
    parasitic NEC B71.9 *[G94]*
    senile NEC G31.1
    specified NEC G93.89
breast (*see also* Disorder, breast) N64.9
    cystic (chronic) —*see* Mastopathy, cystic
    fibrocystic —*see* Mastopathy, cystic
    Paget's
        female, unspecified side C50.91-
        male, unspecified side C50.92-
    specified NEC N64.89
Breda's —*see* Yaws
Bretonneau's (diphtheritic malignant angina)
    A36.0
Bright's —*see* Nephritis
    arteriosclerotic —*see* Hypertension, kidney
Brill's (recrudescent typhus) A75.1
Brill-Zinsser (recrudescent typhus) A75.1
Brion-Kayser —*see* Fever, paratyphoid
broad
    beta E78.2
    ligament (noninflammatory) N83.9
        inflammatory —*see* Disease, pelvis,
            inflammatory
        specified NEC N83.8
Brocq-Duhring (dermatitis herpetiformis)
    L13.0
Brocq's
    meaning
        dermatitis herpetiformis L13.0
        prurigo L28.2
bronchopulmonary J98.4
bronchus NEC J98.09
bronze Addison's E27.1
    tuberculous A18.7
budgerigar fancier's J67.2
Buerger's (thromboangiitis obliterans)
    I73.1
bullous L13.9
    chronic of childhood L12.2
    specified NEC L13.8
Bürger-Grütz (essential familial
    hyperlipemia) E78.3
bursa —*see* Bursopathy
caisson T70.3
California —*see* Coccidioidomycosis
capillaries I78.9
    specified NEC I78.8
Carapata A68.0
cardiac —*see* Disease, heart
cardiopulmonary, chronic I27.9
cardiorenal (hepatic) (hypertensive)
    (vascular) —*see* Hypertension,
    cardiorenal
cardiovascular (atherosclerotic) I25.10
    with angina pectoris —*see* Arteriosclerosis,
        coronary (artery),
    congenital Q28.9
    hypertensive —*see* Hypertension, heart
    newborn P29.9
        specified NEC P29.89
    renal (hypertensive) —*see* Hypertension,
        cardiorenal
    syphilitic (asymptomatic) A52.00
cartilage —*see* Disorder, cartilage
Castellani's A69.8
Castleman (unicentric) (multicentric)
    D47.Z2 ◀
    HHV-8-associated —*see also* Herpesvirus,
        human, 8 D47.Z2 ◀
cat-scratch A28.1
Cavare's (familial periodic paralysis) G72.3
cecum K63.9
celiac (adult) (infantile) (with steatorrhea)
    K90.0 ◀▥
cellular tissue L98.9

Disease, diseased *(Continued)*
central core G71.2
cerebellar, cerebellum —*see* Disease, brain
cerebral —*see also* Disease, brain
    degenerative —*see* Degeneration, brain
cerebrospinal G96.9
cerebrovascular I67.9
    acute I67.89
        embolic I63.4-
        thrombotic I63.3-
    arteriosclerotic I67.2
    specified NEC I67.89
cervix (uteri) (noninflammatory) N88.9
    inflammatory —*see* Cervicitis
    specified NEC N88.8
Chabert's A22.9
Chandler's (osteochondritis dissecans, hip) —
    see Osteochondritis, dissecans, hip
Charlouis —*see* Yaws
Chédiak-Steinbrinck (-Higashi) (congenital
    gigantism of peroxidase granules)
    E70.330
chest J98.9
Chiari's (hepatic vein thrombosis) I82.0
Chicago B40.9
Chignon B36.8
chigo, chigoe B88.1
childhood granulomatous D71
Chinese liver fluke B66.1
chlamydial A74.9
    specified NEC A74.89
cholecystic K82.9
choroid H31.9
    specified NEC H31.8
Christmas D67
chronic bullous of childhood L12.2
chylomicron retention E78.3
ciliary body H21.9
    specified NEC H21.89
circulatory (system) NEC I99.8
    newborn P29.9
    syphilitic A52.00
        congenital A50.54
coagulation factor deficiency (congenital) —
    see Defect, coagulation
coccidioidal —*see* Coccidioidomycosis
cold
    agglutinin or hemoglobinuria D59.1
        paroxysmal D59.6
    hemagglutinin (chronic) D59.1
collagen NOS (nonvascular) (vascular) M35.9
    specified NEC M35.8
colon K63.9
    functional K59.9
        congenital Q43.2
    ischemic —*see also* Ischemia, intestine,
        acute K55.039 ◀▥
colonic inflammatory bowel, unclassified
    (IBDU) K52.3 ◀
combined system —*see* Degeneration,
    combined
compressed air T70.3
Concato's (pericardial polyserositis) A19.9
    nontubercular I31.1
    pleural —*see* Pleurisy, with effusion
conjunctiva H11.9
    chlamydial A74.0
    specified NEC H11.89
    viral B30.9
        specified NEC B30.8
connective tissue, systemic (diffuse) M35.9
    in (due to)
        hypogammaglobulinemia D80.1 *[M36.8]*
        ochronosis E70.29 *[M36.8]*
    specified NEC M35.8
Conor and Bruch's (boutonneuse fever) A77.1
Cooper's —*see* Mastopathy, cystic
Cori's (glycogenosis III) E74.03
corkhandler's or corkworker's J67.3
cornea H18.9
    specified NEC H18.89-

Disease, diseased *(Continued)*
coronary (artery) —*see* Disease, heart, ischemic, atherosclerotic
   congenital Q24.5
   ostial, syphilitic (aortic) (mitral) (pulmonary) A52.03
corpus cavernosum N48.9
   specified NEC N48.89
Cotugno's —*see* Sciatica
coxsackie (virus) NEC B34.1
cranial nerve NOS G52.9
Creutzfeldt-Jakob —*see* Creutzfeldt- Jakob disease or syndrome
Crocq's (acrocyanosis) I73.89
Crohn's —*see* Enteritis, regional
Curschmann G71.11
cystic
   breast (chronic) —*see* Mastopathy, cystic
   kidney, congenital Q61.9
   liver, congenital Q44.6
   lung J98.4
     congenital Q33.0
cytomegalic inclusion (generalized) B25.9
   with pneumonia B25.0
   congenital P35.1
cytomegaloviral B25.9
   specified NEC B25.8
Czerny's (periodic hydrarthrosis of the knee) —*see* Effusion, joint, knee
Daae (-Finsen) (epidemic pleurodynia) B33.0
Darling's —*see* Histoplasmosis capsulati
Débove's (splenomegaly) R16.1
deer fly —*see* Tularemia
Degos' I77.8
demyelinating, demyelinizating (nervous system) G37.9
   multiple sclerosis G35
   specified NEC G37.8
dense deposit —*see also* N00-N07 with fourth character .6 N05.6
deposition, hydroxyapatite —*see* Disease, hydroxyapatite deposition
de Quervain's (tendon sheath) M65.4
   thyroid (subacute granulomatous thyroiditis) E06.1
Devergie's (pityriasis rubra pilaris) L44.0
Devic's G36.0
diaphorase deficiency D74.0
diaphragm J98.6
diarrheal, infectious NEC A09
digestive system K92.9
   specified NEC K92.89
disc, degenerative —*see* Degeneration, intervertebral disc
discogenic —*see also* Displacement, intervertebral disc NEC
   with myelopathy —*see* Disorder, disc, with, myelopathy
diverticular —*see* Diverticula
Dubois (thymus) A50.59 *[E35]*
Duchenne-Griesinger G71.0
Duchenne's
   muscular dystrophy G71.0
   pseudohypertrophy, muscles G71.0
ductless glands E34.9
Duhring's (dermatitis herpetiformis) L13.0
duodenum K31.9
   specified NEC K31.89
Dupré's (meningism) R29.1
Dupuytren's (muscle contracture) M72.0
Durand-Nicholas-Favre (climatic bubo) A55
Duroziez's (congenital mitral stenosis) Q23.2
ear —*see* Disorder, ear
Eberth's —*see* Fever, typhoid
Ebola (virus) A98.4
Ebstein's heart Q22.5
Echinococcus —*see* Echinococcus
echovirus NEC B34.1
Eddowes' (brittle bones and blue sclera) Q78.0
edentulous (alveolar) ridge K06.9
   specified NEC K06.8

Disease, diseased *(Continued)*
Edsall's T67.2
Eichstedt's (pityriasis versicolor) B36.0
Ellis-van Creveld (chondroectodermal dysplasia) Q77.6
end stage renal (ESRD) N18.6
   due to hypertension I12.0
endocrine glands or system NEC E34.9
endomyocardial (eosinophilic) I42.3
English (rickets) E55.0
enteroviral, enterovirus NEC B34.1
   central nervous system NEC A88.8
epidemic B99.9
   specified NEC B99.8
epididymis N50.9
Erb (-Landouzy) G71.0
Erdheim-Chester (ECD) E88.89
esophagus K22.9
   functional K22.4
   psychogenic F45.8
   specified NEC K22.8
Eulenburg's (congenital paramyotonia) G71.19
eustachian tube —*see* Disorder, eustachian tube
external
   auditory canal —*see* Disorder, ear, external
   ear —*see* Disorder, ear, external
extrapyramidal G25.9
   specified NEC G25.89
eye H57.9
   anterior chamber H21.9
   inflammatory NEC H57.8
   muscle (external) —*see* Strabismus
   specified NEC H57.8
   syphilitic —*see* Oculopathy, syphilitic
eyeball H44.9
   specified NEC H44.89
eyelid —*see* Disorder, eyelid
   specified NEC —*see* Disorder, eyelid, specified type NEC
eyeworm of Africa B74.3
facial nerve (seventh) G51.9
   newborn (birth injury) P11.3
Fahr (of brain) G23.8
Fahr Volhard (of kidney) I12.-
fallopian tube (noninflammatory) N83.9
   inflammatory —*see* Salpingo-oophoritis
   specified NEC N83.8
familial periodic paralysis G72.3
Fanconi's (congenital pancytopenia) D61.09
fascia NEC —*see also* Disorder, muscle
   inflammatory —*see* Myositis
   specified NEC M62.89
Fauchard's (periodontitis) —*see* Periodontitis
Favre-Durand-Nicolas (climatic bubo) A55
Fede's K14.0
Feer's —*see* Poisoning, mercury
female pelvic inflammatory —*see also* Disease, pelvis, inflammatory N73.9
   syphilitic (secondary) A51.42
   tuberculous A18.17
Fernels' (aortic aneurysm) I71.9
fibrocaseous of lung —*see* Tuberculosis, pulmonary
fibrocystic —*see* Fibrocystic disease
Fiedler's (leptospiral jaundice) A27.0
fifth B08.3
file-cutter's —*see* Poisoning, lead
fish-skin Q80.9
   acquired L85.0
Flajani (-Basedow) (exophthalmic goiter) — *see* Hyperthyroidism, with, goiter (diffuse)
flax-dresser's J66.1
fluke —*see* Infestation, fluke
foot and mouth B08.8
foot process N04.9
Forbes' (glycogenosis III) E74.03
Fordyce-Fox (apocrine miliaria) L75.2
Fordyce's (ectopic sebaceous glands) (mouth) Q38.6

Disease, diseased *(Continued)*
Forestier's (rhizomelic pseudopolyarthritis) M35.3
   meaning ankylosing hyperostosis —*see* Hyperostosis, ankylosing
Fothergill's
   neuralgia —*see* Neuralgia, trigeminal
   scarlatina anginosa A38.9
Fournier (gangrene) N49.3
   female N76.89
fourth B08.8
Fox (-Fordyce) (apocrine miliaria) L75.2
Francis' —*see* Tularemia
Franklin C88.2
Frei's (climatic bubo) A55
Friedreich's
   combined systemic or ataxia G11.1
   myoclonia G25.3
frontal sinus —*see* Sinusitis, frontal
fungus NEC B49
Gaisböck's (polycythemia hypertonica) D75.1
gallbladder K82.9
   calculus —*see* Calculus, gallbladder
   cholecystitis —*see* Cholecystitis
   cholesterolosis K82.4
   fistula —*see* Fistula, gallbladder
   hydrops K82.1
   obstruction —*see* Obstruction, gallbladder
   perforation K82.2
   specified NEC K82.8
gamma heavy chain C88.2
Gamna's (siderotic splenomegaly) D73.2
Gamstorp's (adynamia episodica hereditaria) G72.3
Gandy-Nanta (siderotic splenomegaly) D73.2
ganister J62.8
gastric —*see* Disease, stomach
gastroesophageal reflux (GERD) K21.9
   with esophagitis K21.0
gastrointestinal (tract) K92.9
   amyloid E85.4
   functional K59.9
     psychogenic F45.8
   specified NEC K92.89
Gee (-Herter) (-Heubner) (-Thaysen) (nontropical sprue) K90.0
genital organs
   female N94.9
   male N50.9
Gerhardt's (erythromelalgia) I73.81
Gibert's (pityriasis rosea) L42
Gierke's (glycogenosis I) E74.01
Gilles de la Tourette's (motor-verbal tic) F95.2
gingiva K06.9
   plaque induced K05.00 ◄
   specified NEC K06.8
gland (lymph) I89.9
Glanzmann's (hereditary hemorrhagic thrombasthenia) D69.1
glass-blower's (cataract) —*see* Cataract, specified NEC
   salivary gland hypertrophy K11.1
Glisson's —*see* Rickets
globe H44.9
   specified NEC H44.89
glomerular —*see also* Glomerulonephritis
   with edema —*see* Nephrosis
   acute —*see* Nephritis, acute
   chronic —*see* Nephritis, chronic
   minimal change N05.0
   rapidly progressive N01.9
glycogen storage E74.00
   Andersen's E74.09
   Cori's E74.03
   Forbes' E74.03
   generalized E74.00
   glucose-6-phosphatase deficiency E74.01
   heart E74.02 *[143]*
   hepatorenal E74.09
   Hers' E74.09
   liver and kidney E74.09

◄ New   ⬸ Revised   ~~deleted~~ Deleted

Disease, diseased (Continued)
  glycogen storage (Continued)
    McArdle's E74.04
    muscle phosphofructokinase E74.09
    myocardium E74.02 [I43]
    Pompe's E74.02
    Tauri's E74.09
    type Ø E74.09
    type I E74.Ø1
    type II E74.Ø2
    type III E74.Ø3
    type IV E74.Ø9
    type V E74.Ø4
    type VI-XI E74.Ø9
    Von Gierke's E74.Ø1
  Goldstein's (familial hemorrhagic
      telangiectasia) I78.Ø
  gonococcal NOS A54.9
  graft-versus-host (GVH) D89.813
    acute D89.81Ø
    acute on chronic D89.812
    chronic D89.811
  grainhandler's J67.8
  granulomatous (childhood) (chronic) D71
  Graves' (exophthalmic goiter) —see
      Hyperthyroidism, with, goiter
      (diffuse)
  Griesinger's —see Ancylostomiasis
  Grisel's M43.6
  Gruby's (tinea tonsurans) B35.Ø
  Guillain-Barré G61.Ø
  Guinon's (motor-verbal tic) F95.2
  gum KØ6.9
  gynecological N94.9
  H (Hartnup's) E72.Ø2
  Haff —see Poisoning, mercury
  Hageman (congenital factor XII deficiency)
      D68.2
  hair (color) (shaft) L67.9
    follicles L73.9
      specified NEC L73.8
  Hamman's (spontaneous mediastinal
      emphysema) J98.2
  hand, foot and mouth BØ8.4
  Hansen's —see Leprosy
  Hantavirus, with pulmonary manifestations
      B33.4
    with renal manifestations A98.5
  Harada's H3Ø.81-
  Hartnup (pellagra-cerebellar ataxia-renal
      aminoaciduria) E72.Ø2
  Hart's (pellagra-cerebellar ataxia-renal
      aminoaciduria) E72.Ø2
  Hashimoto's (struma lymphomatosa) EØ6.3
  Hb —see Disease, hemoglobin
  heart (organic) I51.9
    with
      pulmonary edema (acute) —see also
          Failure, ventricular, left I5Ø.1
      rheumatic fever (conditions in IØØ)
          active IØ1.9
            with chorea IØ2.Ø
            specified NEC IØ1.8
          inactive or quiescent (with chorea)
              IØ9.9
            specified NEC IØ9.89
    amyloid E85.4 [I43]
    aortic (valve) I35.9
    arteriosclerotic or sclerotic (senile) —
        see Disease, heart, ischemic,
        atherosclerotic
    artery, arterial —see Disease, heart,
        ischemic, atherosclerotic
    beer drinkers' I42.6
    beriberi (wet) E51.12
    black I27.Ø
    congenital Q24.9
      cyanotic Q24.9
      specified NEC Q24.8
    coronary —see Disease, heart, ischemic
    cryptogenic I51.9

Disease, diseased (Continued)
  heart (Continued)
    fibroid —see Myocarditis
    functional I51.89
      psychogenic F45.8
    glycogen storage E74.02 [I43]
    gonococcal A54.83
    hypertensive —see Hypertension, heart
    hyperthyroid —see also Hyperthyroidism
        EØ5.9Ø [I43]
      with thyroid storm EØ5.91 [I43]
    ischemic (chronic or with a stated duration
        of over 4 weeks) I25.9
      atherosclerotic (of) I25.1Ø
        with angina pectoris —see
            Arteriosclerosis, coronary
            (artery)
        coronary artery bypass graft —see
            Arteriosclerosis, coronary
            (artery),
      cardiomyopathy I25.5
      diagnosed on ECG or other special
          investigation, but currently
          presenting no symptoms I25.6
      silent I25.6
      specified form NEC I25.89
    kyphoscoliotic I27.1
    meningococcal A39.5Ø
      endocarditis A39.51
      myocarditis A39.52
      pericarditis A39.53
    mitral IØ5.9
      specified NEC IØ5.8
    muscular —see Degeneration, myocardial
    psychogenic (functional) F45.8
    pulmonary (chronic) I27.9
      in schistosomiasis B65.9 [I52]
      specified NEC I27.89
    rheumatic (chronic) (inactive) (old)
        (quiescent) (with chorea) IØ9.9
      active or acute IØ1.9
        with chorea (acute) (rheumatic)
            (Sydenham's) IØ2.Ø
      specified NEC IØ9.89
    senile —see Myocarditis
    syphilitic A52.Ø6
      aortic A52.Ø3
        aneurysm A52.Ø1
      congenital A5Ø.54 [I52]
    thyrotoxic —see also Thyrotoxicosis EØ5.9Ø
        [I43]
      with thyroid storm EØ5.91 [I43]
    valve, valvular (obstructive)
        (regurgitant) —see also Endocarditis
      congenital NEC Q24.8
        pulmonary Q22.3
    vascular —see Disease, cardiovascular
  heavy chain NEC C88.2
    alpha C88.3
    gamma C88.2
    mu C88.2
  Hebra's
    pityriasis
      maculata et circinata L42
      rubra pilaris L44.Ø
    prurigo L28.2
  hematopoietic organs D75.9
  hemoglobin or Hb
    abnormal (mixed) NEC D58.2
      with thalassemia D56.9
    AS genotype D57.3
    Bart's D56.Ø
    C (Hb-C) D58.2
      with other abnormal hemoglobin NEC
          D58.2
      elliptocytosis D58.1
      Hb-S D57.2-
      sickle-cell D57.2-
      thalassemia D56.8
    Constant Spring D58.2
    D (Hb-D) D58.2

Disease, diseased (Continued)
  hemoglobin or Hb (Continued)
    E (Hb-E) D58.2
    E-beta thalassemia D56.5
    elliptocytosis D58.1
    H (Hb-H) (thalassemia) D56.Ø
      with other abnormal hemoglobin NEC
          D56.9
      Constant Spring D56.Ø
    I thalassemia D56.9
    M D74.Ø
    S or SS D57.1
    SC D57.2-
    SD D57.8-
    SE D57.8-
    spherocytosis D58.Ø
    unstable, hemolytic D58.2
  hemolytic (newborn) P55.9
    autoimmune (cold type) (warm type) D59.1
    drug-induced D59.Ø
    due to or with
      incompatibility
        ABO (blood group) P55.1
        blood (group) (Duffy) (K(ell)) (Kidd)
            (Lewis) (M) (S) NEC P55.8
        Rh (blood group) (factor) P55.Ø
          Rh negative mother P55.Ø
    specified type NEC P55.8
    unstable hemoglobin D58.2
  hemorrhagic D69.9
    newborn P53
  Henoch (-Schönlein) (purpura nervosa) D69.Ø
  hepatic —see Disease, liver
  hepatobiliary K83.9
    toxic K71.9
  hepatolenticular E83.Ø1
  heredodegenerative NEC
    spinal cord G95.89
  herpesviral, disseminated BØØ.7
  Hers' (glycogenosis VI) E74.Ø9
  Herter (-Gee) (-Heubner) (nontropical sprue)
      K9Ø.Ø
  Heubner-Herter (nontropical sprue) K9Ø.Ø
  high fetal gene or hemoglobin thalassemia
      D56.9
  Hildenbrand's —see Typhus
  hip (joint) M25.9
    congenital Q65.89
    suppurative MØØ.9
    tuberculous A18.Ø2
  His (-Werner) (trench fever) A79.Ø
  Hodgson's I71.2
    ruptured I71.1
  Holla —see Spherocytosis
  hookworm B76.9
    specified NEC B76.8
  host-versus-graft D89.813
    acute D89.81Ø
    acute on chronic D89.812
    chronic D89.811
  human immunodeficiency virus (HIV) B2Ø
  Huntington's G1Ø
  Hutchinson's (cheiropompholyx) —see
      Hutchinson's disease
  hyaline (diffuse) (generalized)
    membrane (lung) (newborn) P22.Ø
      adult J8Ø
  hydatid —see Echinococcus
  hydroxyapatite deposition M11.ØØ
    ankle M11.Ø7-
    elbow M11.Ø2-
    foot joint M11.Ø7-
    hand joint M11.Ø4-
    hip M11.Ø5-
    knee M11.Ø6-
    multiple site M11.Ø9
    shoulder M11.Ø1-
    vertebra M11.Ø8
    wrist M11.Ø3-
  hyperkinetic —see Hyperkinesia
  hypertensive —see Hypertension

Disease, diseased *(Continued)*
  hypophysis E23.7
  Iceland G93.3
  I-cell E77.0
  immune D89.9
  immunoproliferative (malignant) C88.9
    small intestinal C88.3
    specified NEC C88.8
  inclusion B25.9
    salivary gland B25.9
  infectious, infective B99.9
    congenital P37.9
      specified NEC P37.8
      viral P35.9
        specified type NEC P35.8
    specified NEC B99.8
  inflammatory
    penis N48.29
      abscess N48.21
      cellulitis N48.22
    prepuce N47.7
      balanoposthitis N47.6
    tubo-ovarian —*see* Salpingo-oophoritis
  intervertebral disc —*see also* Disorder, disc
    with myelopathy —*see* Disorder, disc, with,
      myelopathy
    cervical, cervicothoracic —*see* Disorder,
      disc, cervical
      with
        myelopathy —*see* Disorder, disc,
          cervical, with myelopathy
        neuritis, radiculitis or
          radiculopathy —*see* Disorder,
          disc, cervical, with neuritis
      specified NEC —*see* Disorder, disc,
        cervical, specified type NEC
    lumbar (with)
      myelopathy M51.06
      neuritis, radiculitis, radiculopathy or
        sciatica M51.16
      specified NEC M51.86
    lumbosacral (with)
      neuritis, radiculitis, radiculopathy or
        sciatica M51.17
      specified NEC M51.87
    specified NEC —*see* Disorder, disc,
      specified NEC
    thoracic (with)
      myelopathy M51.04
      neuritis, radiculitis or radiculopathy
        M51.14
      specified NEC M51.84
    thoracolumbar (with)
      myelopathy M51.05
      neuritis, radiculitis or radiculopathy
        M51.15
      specified NEC M51.85
  intestine K63.9
    functional K59.9
      psychogenic F45.8
      specified NEC K59.8
    organic K63.9
    protozoal A07.9
    specified NEC K63.89
  iris H21.9
    specified NEC H21.89
  iron metabolism or storage E83.10
  island (scrub typhus) A75.3
  itai-itai —*see* Poisoning, cadmium
  Jakob-Creutzfeldt —*see* Creutzfeldt- Jakob
    disease or syndrome
  jaw M27.9
    fibrocystic M27.49
    specified NEC M27.8
  jigger B88.1
  joint —*see also* Disorder, joint
    Charcot's —*see* Arthropathy, neuropathic
      (Charcot)
    degenerative —*see* Osteoarthritis
      multiple M15.9
    spine —*see* Spondylosis

Disease, diseased *(Continued)*
  joint *(Continued)*
    hypertrophic —*see* Osteoarthritis
    sacroiliac M53.3
    specified NEC —*see* Disorder, joint,
      specified type NEC
    spine NEC —*see* Dorsopathy
    suppurative —*see* Arthritis, pyogenic or
      pyemic
  Jourdain's (acute gingivitis) K05.00
    nonplaque induced K05.01
    plaque induced K05.00
  Kaschin-Beck (endemic polyarthritis)
    M12.10
    ankle M12.17-
    elbow M12.12-
    foot joint M12.17-
    hand joint M12.14-
    hip M12.15-
    knee M12.16-
    multiple site M12.19
    shoulder M12.11-
    vertebra M12.18
    wrist M12.13-
  Katayama B65.2
  Kedani (scrub typhus) A75.3
  Keshan E59
  kidney (functional) (pelvis) N28.9
    chronic N18.9
      hypertensive —*see* Hypertension, kidney
      stage 1 N18.1
      stage 2 (mild) N18.2
      stage 3 (moderate) N18.3
      stage 4 (severe) N18.4
      stage 5 N18.5
    complicating pregnancy —*see* Pregnancy,
      complicated by, renal disease
    cystic (congenital) Q61.9
    diabetic - see E08-E13 with .22
    fibrocystic (congenital) Q61.8
    hypertensive —*see* Hypertension, kidney
    in (due to)
      schistosomiasis (bilharziasis) B65.9 *[N29]*
    multicystic Q61.4
    polycystic Q61.3
      adult type Q61.2
      childhood type NEC Q61.19
        collecting duct dilatation Q61.11
  Kimmelstiel (-Wilson) (intercapillary polycystic
    (congenital) glomerulosclerosis) —*see*
    E08-E13 with .21
  Kimura D21.9
    specified site (see Neoplasm, connective
      tissue benign)
  Kinnier Wilson's (hepatolenticular
    degeneration) E83.01
  kissing —*see* Mononucleosis, infectious
  Klebs' —*see also* Glomerulonephritis N05.-
  Klippel-Feil (brevicollis) Q76.1
  Köhler-Pellegrini-Stieda (calcification, knee
    joint) —*see* Bursitis, tibial collateral
  Kok Q89.8
  König's (osteochondritis dissecans) —*see*
    Osteochondritis, dissecans
  Korsakoff's (nonalcoholic) F04
    alcoholic F10.96
      with dependence F10.26
  Kostmann's (infantile genetic
    agranulocytosis) D70.0
  kuru A81.81
  Kyasanur Forest A98.2
  labyrinth, ear —*see* Disorder, ear, inner
  lacrimal system —*see* Disorder, lacrimal
    system
  Lafora's —*see* Epilepsy, generalized,
    idiopathic
  Lancereaux-Mathieu (leptospiral jaundice)
    A27.0
  Landry's G61.0
  Larrey-Weil (leptospiral jaundice) A27.0
  larynx J38.7

Disease, diseased *(Continued)*
  legionnaires' A48.1
    nonpneumonic A48.2
  Lenegre's I44.2
  lens H27.9
    specified NEC H27.8
  Lev's (acquired complete heart block) I44.2
  Lewy body (dementia) G31.83 *[F02.80]*
    with behavioral disturbance G31.83 *[F02.81]*
  Lichtheim's (subacute combined sclerosis
    with pernicious anemia) D51.0
  Lightwood's (renal tubular acidosis) N25.89
  Lignac's (cystinosis) E72.04
  lip K13.0
  lipid-storage E75.6
    specified NEC E75.5
  Lipschütz's N76.6
  liver (chronic) (organic) K76.9
    alcoholic (chronic) K70.9
      acute —*see* Disease, liver, alcoholic,
        hepatitis
      cirrhosis K70.30
        with ascites K70.31
      failure K70.40
        with coma K70.41
      fatty liver K70.0
      fibrosis K70.2
      hepatitis K70.10
        with ascites K70.11
      sclerosis K70.2
    cystic, congenital Q44.6
    drug-induced (idiosyncratic) (toxic)
      (predictable) (unpredictable) —*see*
      Disease, liver, toxic
    end stage K72.90
      due to hepatitis —*see* Hepatitis
    fatty, nonalcoholic (NAFLD) K76.0
      alcoholic K70.0
    fibrocystic (congenital) Q44.6
    fluke
      Chinese B66.1
      oriental B66.1
      sheep B66.3
    glycogen storage E74.09 *[K77]*
    in (due to)
      schistosomiasis (bilharziasis) B65.9 *[K77]*
    inflammatory K75.9
      alcoholic K70.1
      specified NEC K75.89
    polycystic (congenital) Q44.6
    toxic K71.9
      with
        cholestasis K71.0
        cirrhosis (liver) K71.7
        fibrosis (liver) K71.7
        focal nodular hyperplasia K71.8
        hepatic granuloma K71.8
        hepatic necrosis K71.10
          with coma K71.11
        hepatitis NEC K71.6
          acute K71.2
          chronic
            active K71.50
              with ascites K71.51
            lobular K71.4
            persistent K71.3
          lupoid K71.50
            with ascites K71.51
        peliosis hepatis K71.8
        veno-occlusive disease (VOD) of liver
          K71.8
      veno-occlusive K76.5
  Lobo's (keloid blastomycosis) B48.0
  Lobstein's (brittle bones and blue sclera) Q78.0
  Ludwig's (submaxillary cellulitis) K12.2
  lumbosacral region M53.87
  lung J98.4
    black J60
    congenital Q33.9
    cystic J98.4
      congenital Q33.0

◀ New   ◀▦ Revised   ~~deleted~~ Deleted

Disease, diseased (Continued)
  lung (Continued)
    fibroid (chronic) —see Fibrosis, lung
    fluke B66.4
      oriental B66.4
    in
      amyloidosis E85.4 [J99]
      sarcoidosis D86.0
      Sjögren's syndrome M35.02
      systemic
        lupus erythematosus M32.13
        sclerosis M34.81
    interstitial J84.9
      of childhood, specified NEC J84.848
      respiratory bronchiolitis J84.115
      specified NEC J84.89
    obstructive (chronic) J44.9
      with
        acute
          bronchitis J44.0
          exacerbation NEC J44.1
          lower respiratory infection J44.0
        alveolitis, allergic J67.9
        asthma J44.9
        bronchiectasis J47.9
          with
            exacerbation (acute) J47.1
            lower respiratory infection J47.0
        bronchitis J44.9
          with
            exacerbation (acute) J44.1
            lower respiratory infection J44.0
        emphysema J44.9
        hypersensitivity pneumonitis J67.9
      decompensated J44.1
        with
          exacerbation (acute) J44.1
    polycystic J98.4
      congenital Q33.0
    rheumatoid (diffuse) (interstitial) —see
      Rheumatoid, lung
  Lutembacher's (atrial septal defect with
    mitral stenosis) Q21.1
  Lyme A69.20
  lymphatic (gland) (system) (channel) (vessel)
    I89.9
  lymphoproliferative D47.9
    specified NEC D47.Z9
    T-gamma D47.Z9
    X-linked D82.3
  Magitot's M27.2
  malarial —see Malaria
  malignant —see also Neoplasm, malignant,
    by site
  Manson's B65.1
  maple bark J67.6
  maple-syrup-urine E71.0
  Marburg (virus) A98.3
  Marion's (bladder neck obstruction) N32.0
  Marsh's (exophthalmic goiter) —see
    Hyperthyroidism, with, goiter (diffuse)
  mastoid (process) —see Disorder, ear, middle
  Mathieu's (leptospiral jaundice) A27.0
  Maxcy's A75.2
  McArdle (-Schmid-Pearson) (glycogenosis
    V) E74.04
  mediastinum J98.59 ◄▥
  medullary center (idiopathic) (respiratory)
    G93.89
  Meige's (chronic hereditary edema) Q82.0
  meningococcal —see Infection, meningococcal
  mental F99
    organic F09
  mesenchymal M35.9
  mesenteric embolic —see also Ischemia,
    intestine, acute K55.039 ◄▥
  metabolic, metabolism E88.9
    bilirubin E80.7
  metal-polisher's J62.8
  metastatic —see also Neoplasm, secondary, by
    site C79.9

Disease, diseased (Continued)
  microvascular — code to condition
  microvillus
    atrophy Q43.8
    inclusion (MVD) Q43.8
  middle ear —see Disorder, ear, middle
  Mikulicz' (dryness of mouth, absent or
    decreased lacrimation) K11.8
  Milroy's (chronic hereditary edema) Q82.0
  Minamata —see Poisoning, mercury
  minicore G71.2
  Minor's G95.19
  Minot's (hemorrhagic disease, newborn) P53
  Minot-von Willebrand-Jürgens
    (angiohemophilia) D68.0
  Mitchell's (erythromelalgia) I73.81
  mitral (valve) I05.9
    nonrheumatic I34.9
  mixed connective tissue M35.1
  moldy hay J67.0
  Monge's T70.29
  Morgagni-Adams-Stokes (syncope with heart
    block) I45.9
  Morgagni's (syndrome) (hyperostosis
    frontalis interna) M85.2
  Morton's (with metatarsalgia) —see Lesion,
    nerve, plantar
  Morvan's G60.8
  motor neuron (bulbar) (familial) (mixed type)
    (spinal) G12.20
    amyotrophic lateral sclerosis G12.21
    progressive bulbar palsy G12.22
    specified NEC G12.29
  moyamoya I67.5
  mu heavy chain disease C88.2
  multicore G71.2
  muscle —see also Disorder, muscle
    inflammatory —see Myositis
    ocular (external) —see Strabismus
  musculoskeletal system, soft tissue —see also
    Disorder, soft tissue
    specified NEC —see Disorder, soft tissue,
      specified type NEC
  mushroom workers' J67.5
  mycotic B49
  myelodysplastic, not classified C94.6
  myeloproliferative, not classified C94.6
    chronic D47.1
  myocardium, myocardial —see also
    Degeneration, myocardial I51.5
    primary (idiopathic) I42.9
  myoneural G70.9
  Naegeli's D69.1
  nails L60.9
    specified NEC L60.8
  Nairobi (sheep virus) A93.8
  nasal J34.9
  nemaline body G71.2
  nerve —see Disorder, nerve
  nervous system G98.8
    autonomic G90.9
    central G96.9
      specified NEC G96.8
    congenital Q07.9
    parasympathetic G90.9
    specified NEC G98.8
    sympathetic G90.9
    vegetative G90.9
  neuromuscular system G70.9
  Newcastle B30.8
  Nicolas (-Durand)-Favre (climatic bubo)
    A55
  nipple N64.9
    Paget's C50.01-
      female C50.01-
      male C50.02-
  Nishimoto (-Takeuchi) I67.5
  nonarthropod-borne NOS (viral) B34.9
    enterovirus NEC B34.1
  nonautoimmune hemolytic D59.4
    drug-induced D59.2

Disease, diseased (Continued)
  Nonne-Milroy-Meige (chronic hereditary
    edema) Q82.0
  nose J34.9
  nucleus pulposus —see Disorder, disc
  nutritional E63.9
  oast-house-urine E72.19
  ocular
    herpesviral B00.50
    zoster B02.30
  obliterative vascular I77.1
  Ohara's —see Tularemia
  Opitz's (congestive splenomegaly)
    D73.2
  Oppenheim-Urbach (necrobiosis lipoidica
    diabeticorum) —see E08-E13 with .620
  optic nerve NEC —see Disorder, nerve, optic
    orbit —see Disorder, orbit
  Oriental liver fluke B66.1
  Oriental lung fluke B66.4
  Ormond's N13.5
  Oropouche virus A93.0
  Osler-Rendu (familial hemorrhagic
    telangiectasia) I78.0
  osteofibrocystic E21.0
  Otto's M24.7
  outer ear —see Disorder, ear, external
  ovary (noninflammatory) N83.9
    cystic N83.20- ◄▥
    inflammatory —see Salpingo-oophoritis
    polycystic E28.2
    specified NEC N83.8
  Owren's (congenital) —see Defect,
    coagulation
  pancreas K86.9
    cystic K86.2
    fibrocystic E84.9
    specified NEC K86.89 ◄▥
  panvalvular I08.9
    specified NEC I08.8
  parametrium (noninflammatory) N83.9
  parasitic B89
    cerebral NEC B71.9 [G94]
    intestinal NOS B82.9
    mouth B37.0
    skin NOS B88.9
    specified type —see Infestation
    tongue B37.0
  parathyroid (gland) E21.5
    specified NEC E21.4
  Parkinson's G20
  parodontal K05.6
  Parrot's (syphilitic osteochondritis) A50.02
  Parry's (exophthalmic goiter) —see
    Hyperthyroidism, with, goiter (diffuse)
  Parson's (exophthalmic goiter) —see
    Hyperthyroidism, with, goiter (diffuse)
  Paxton's (white piedra) B36.2
  pearl-worker's —see Osteomyelitis, specified
    type NEC
  Pellegrini-Stieda (calcification, knee joint) —
    see Bursitis, tibial collateral
  pelvis, pelvic
    female NOS N94.9
      specified NEC N94.89
    gonococcal (acute) (chronic) A54.24
    inflammatory (female) N73.9
      acute N73.0
      chlamydial A56.11 ◄
      chronic N73.1
      specified NEC N73.8
      syphilitic (secondary) A51.42
        late A52.76
      tuberculous A18.17
    organ, female N94.9
    peritoneum, female NEC N94.89
  penis N48.9
    inflammatory N48.29
      abscess N48.21
      cellulitis N48.22
    specified NEC N48.89

Disease, diseased *(Continued)*
  periapical tissues NOS K04.90
  periodontal K05.6
    specified NEC K05.5
  periosteum —*see* Disorder, bone, specified
      type NEC
  peripheral
    arterial I73.9
    autonomic nervous system G90.9
    nerves —*see* Polyneuropathy
    vascular NOS I73.9
  peritoneum K66.9
    pelvic, female NEC N94.89
    specified NEC K66.8
  persistent mucosal (middle ear) H66.20
    left H66.22
      with right H66.23
    right H66.21
      with left H66.23
  Petit's —*see* Hernia, abdomen, specified site
      NEC
  pharynx J39.2
    specified NEC J39.2
  Phocas' —*see* Mastopathy, cystic
  photochromogenic (acid-fast bacilli)
      (pulmonary) A31.0
    nonpulmonary A31.9
  Pick's G31.01 *[F02.80]*
    with behavioral disturbance G31.01
        [F02.81]
    brain G31.01 *[F02.80]* ◀
      with behavioral disturbance G31.01
          [F02.81] ◀
    of pericardium (pericardial pseudocirrhosis
        of liver) I31.1 ◀
  pigeon fancier's J67.2
  pineal gland E34.8
  pink —*see* Poisoning, mercury
  Pinkus' (lichen nitidus) L44.1
  pinworm B80
  Piry virus A93.8
  pituitary (gland) E23.7
  pituitary-snuff-taker's J67.8
  pleura (cavity) J94.9
    specified NEC J94.8
  pneumatic drill (hammer) T75.21
  Pollitzer's (hidradenitis suppurativa)
      L73.2
  polycystic
    kidney or renal Q61.3
      adult type Q61.2
      childhood type NEC Q61.19
        collecting duct dilatation Q61.11
    liver or hepatic Q44.6
    lung or pulmonary J98.4
      congenital Q33.0
    ovary, ovaries E28.2
    spleen Q89.09
  polyethylene T84.05-
  Pompe's (glycogenosis II) E74.02
  Posadas-Wernicke B38.9
  Potain's (pulmonary edema) —*see* Edema,
      lung
  prepuce N47.8
    inflammatory N47.7
      balanoposthitis N47.6
  Pringle's (tuberous sclerosis) Q85.1
  prion, central nervous system A81.9
    specified NEC A81.89
  prostate N42.9
    specified NEC N42.89
  protozoal B64
    acanthamebiasis —*see* Acanthamebiasis
    African trypanosomiasis —*see* African
        trypanosomiasis
    babesiosis B60.0
    Chagas disease —*see* Chagas disease
    intestine, intestinal A07.9
    leishmaniasis —*see* Leishmaniasis
    malaria —*see* Malaria
    naegleriasis B60.2

Disease, diseased *(Continued)*
  protozoal *(Continued)*
    pneumocystosis B59
    specified organism NEC B60.8
    toxoplasmosis —*see* Toxoplasmosis
  pseudo-Hurler's E77.0
  psychiatric F99
  psychotic —*see* Psychosis
  Puente's (simple glandular cheilitis) K13.0
  puerperal —*see also* Puerperal O90.89
  pulmonary —*see also* Disease, lung
    artery I28.9
    chronic obstructive J44.9
      with
        acute bronchitis J44.0
        exacerbation (acute) J44.1
        lower respiratory infection (acute)
            J44.0
      decompensated J44.1
        with
          exacerbation (acute) J44.1
    heart I27.9
      specified NEC I27.89
    hypertensive (vascular) I27.0
    valve I37.9
      rheumatic I09.89
    pulp (dental) NOS K04.90
  pulseless M31.4
  Putnam's (subacute combined sclerosis with
      pernicious anemia) D51.0
  Pyle (-Cohn) (metaphyseal dysplasia)
      Q78.5 ◀▥
  ragpicker's or ragsorter's A22.1
  Raynaud's —*see* Raynaud's disease
  reactive airway —*see* Asthma
  Reclus' (cystic) —*see* Mastopathy,
      cystic
  rectum K62.9
    specified NEC K62.89
  Refsum's (heredopathia atactica
      polyneuritiformis) G60.1
  renal (functional) (pelvis) —*see also* Disease,
      kidney N28.9
    with
      edema —*see* Nephrosis
      glomerular lesion —*see*
          Glomerulonephritis
        with edema —*see* Nephrosis
      interstitial nephritis N12
    acute N28.9
    chronic —*see also* Disease, kidney, chronic
        N18.9
    cystic, congenital Q61.9
    diabetic —*see* E08-E13 with .22
    end-stage (failure) N18.6
      due to hypertension I12.0
    fibrocystic (congenital) Q61.8
    hypertensive —*see* Hypertension,
        kidney
    lupus M32.14
    phosphate-losing (tubular) N25.0
    polycystic (congenital) Q61.3
      adult type Q61.2
      childhood type NEC Q61.19
        collecting duct dilatation Q61.11
    rapidly progressive N01.9
    subacute N01.9
  Rendu-Osler-Weber (familial hemorrhagic
      telangiectasia) I78.0
  renovascular (arteriosclerotic) —*see*
      Hypertension, kidney
  respiratory (tract) J98.9
    acute or subacute NOS J06.9
      due to
        chemicals, gases, fumes or vapors
            (inhalation) J68.3
        external agent J70.9
          specified NEC J70.8
        radiation J70.0
        smoke inhalation J70.5
    noninfectious J39.8

Disease, diseased *(Continued)*
  respiratory *(Continued)*
    chronic NOS J98.9
      due to
        chemicals, gases, fumes or vapors
            J68.4
        external agent J70.9
          specified NEC J70.8
        radiation J70.1
      newborn P27.9
        specified NEC P27.8
    due to
      chemicals, gases, fumes or vapors J68.9
        acute or subacute NEC J68.3
        chronic J68.4
      external agent J70.9
        specified NEC J70.8
    newborn P28.9
      specified type NEC P28.89
    upper J39.9
      acute or subacute J06.9
      noninfectious NEC J39.8
      specified NEC J39.8
      streptococcal J06.9
  retina, retinal H35.9
    Batten's or Batten-Mayou E75.4 *[H36]*
    specified NEC H35.89
  rheumatoid —*see* Arthritis, rheumatoid
  rickettsial NOS A79.9
    specified type NEC A79.89
  Riga (-Fede) (cachectic aphthae) K14.0
  Riggs' (compound periodontitis) —*see*
      Periodontitis
  Ritter's L00
  Rivalta's (cervicofacial actinomycosis)
      A42.2
  Robles' (onchocerciasis) B73.01
  Roger's (congenital interventricular septal
      defect) Q21.0
  Rosenthal's (factor XI deficiency) D68.1
  Ross River B33.1
  Rossbach's (hyperchlorhydria) K30
  Rotes Quérol —*see* Hyperostosis, ankylosing
  Roth (-Bernhardt) —*see* Mononeuropathy,
      lower limb, meralgia paresthetica
  Runeberg's (progressive pernicious anemia)
      D51.0
  sacroiliac NEC M53.3
  salivary gland or duct K11.9
    inclusion B25.9
    specified NEC K11.8
    virus B25.9
  sandworm B76.9
  Schimmelbusch's —*see* Mastopathy, cystic
  Schmorl's —*see* Schmorl's disease or nodes
  Schönlein (-Henoch) (purpura rheumatica)
      D69.0
  Schottmüller's —*see* Fever, paratyphoid
  Schultz's (agranulocytosis) —*see*
      Agranulocytosis
  Schwalbe-Ziehen-Oppenheim G24.1
  Schwartz-Jampel G71.13
  sclera H15.9
    specified NEC H15.89
  scrofulous (tuberculous) A18.2
  scrotum N50.9
  sebaceous glands L73.9
  semilunar cartilage, cystic —*see also*
      Derangement, knee, meniscus, cystic
  seminal vesicle N50.9
  serum NEC —*see also* Reaction, serum T80.69
  sexually transmitted A64
    anogenital
      herpesviral infection —*see* Herpes,
          anogenital
      warts A63.0
    chancroid A57
    chlamydial infection —*see* Chlamydia
    gonorrhea —*see* Gonorrhea
    granuloma inguinale A58
    specified organism NEC A63.8

◀ New   ◀▥ Revised   ~~deleted~~ Deleted

Disease, diseased *(Continued)*
 sexually transmitted *(Continued)*
  syphilis —*see* Syphilis
  trichomoniasis —*see* Trichomoniasis
 Sézary C84.1-
 shimamushi (scrub typhus) A75.3
 shipyard B30.0
 sickle-cell D57.1
  with crisis (vasoocclusive pain) D57.00
   with
    acute chest syndrome D57.01
    splenic sequestration D57.02
  elliptocytosis D57.8-
  Hb-C D57.20
   with crisis (vasoocclusive pain) D57.219
    with
     acute chest syndrome D57.211
     splenic sequestration D57.212
   without crisis D57.20
  Hb-SD D57.80
   with crisis D57.819
    with
     acute chest syndrome D57.811
     splenic sequestration D57.812
  Hb-SE D57.80
   with crisis D57.819
    with
     acute chest syndrome D57.811
     splenic sequestration D57.812
  specified NEC D57.80
   with crisis D57.819
    with
     acute chest syndrome D57.811
     splenic sequestration D57.812
  spherocytosis D57.80
   with crisis D57.819
    with
     acute chest syndrome D57.811
     splenic sequestration D57.812
  thalassemia D57.40
   with crisis (vasoocclusive pain) D57.419
    with
     acute chest syndrome D57.411
     splenic sequestration D57.412
   without crisis D57.40
 silo-filler's J68.8
  bronchitis J68.0
  pneumonitis J68.0
  pulmonary edema J68.1
 simian B B00.4
 Simons' (progressive lipodystrophy) E88.1
 sin nombre virus B33.4
 sinus —*see* Sinusitis
 Sirkari's B55.0
 sixth B08.20
  due to human herpesvirus 6 B08.21
  due to human herpesvirus 7 B08.22
 skin L98.9
  due to metabolic disorder NEC E88.9
   [L99]
  specified NEC L98.8
 slim (HIV) B20
 small vessel I73.9
 Sneddon-Wilkinson (subcorneal pustular
   dermatosis) L13.1
 South African creeping B88.0
 spinal (cord) G95.9
  congenital Q06.9
  specified NEC G95.89
 spine —*see also* Spondylopathy
  joint —*see* Dorsopathy
  tuberculous A18.01
 spinocerebellar (hereditary) G11.9
  specified NEC G11.8
 spleen D73.9
  amyloid E85.4 [D77]
  organic D73.9
  polycystic Q89.09
  postinfectional D73.89
 sponge-diver's —*see* Toxicity, venom, marine
   animal, sea anemone

Disease, diseased *(Continued)*
 Startle Q89.8
 Steinert's G71.11
 Sticker's (erythema infectiosum) B08.3
 Stieda's (calcification, knee joint) —*see*
   Bursitis, tibial collateral
 Stokes' (exophthalmic goiter) —*see*
   Hyperthyroidism, with, goiter (diffuse)
 Stokes-Adams (syncope with heart block)
   I45.9
 stomach K31.9
  functional, psychogenic F45.8
  specified NEC K31.89
 stonemason's J62.8
 storage
  glycogen —*see* Disease, glycogen storage
  mucopolysaccharide —*see*
    Mucopolysaccharidosis
 striatopallidal system NEC G25.89
 Stuart-Prower (congenital factor X deficiency)
   D68.2
 Stuart's (congenital factor X deficiency) D68.2
 subcutaneous tissue —*see* Disease, skin
 supporting structures of teeth K08.9
  specified NEC K08.89 ◄▬▬
 suprarenal (capsule) (gland) E27.9
  hyperfunction E27.0
  specified NEC E27.8
 sweat glands L74.9
  specified NEC L74.8
 Sweeley-Klionsky E75.21
 Swift (-Feer) —*see* Poisoning, mercury
 swimming-pool granuloma A31.1
 Sylvest's (epidemic pleurodynia) B33.0
 sympathetic nervous system G90.9
 synovium —*see* Disorder, synovium
 syphilitic —*see* Syphilis
 systemic tissue mast cell C96.2
 tanapox (virus) B08.71
 Tangier E78.6
 Tarral-Besnier (pityriasis rubra pilaris) L44.0
 Tauri's E74.09
 tear duct —*see* Disorder, lacrimal system
 tendon, tendinous —*see also* Disorder, tendon
  nodular —*see* Trigger finger
 terminal vessel I73.9
 testis N50.9
 thalassemia Hb-S —*see* Disease, sickle-cell,
   thalassemia
 Thaysen-Gee (nontropical sprue) K90.0
 Thomsen G71.12
 throat J39.2
  septic J02.0
 thromboembolic —*see* Embolism
 thymus (gland) E32.9
  specified NEC E32.8
 thyroid (gland) E07.9
  heart —*see also* Hyperthyroidism E05.90
    [I43]
   with thyroid storm E05.91 [I43]
  specified NEC E07.8
 Tietze's M94.0
 tongue K14.9
  specified NEC K14.89
 tonsils, tonsillar (and adenoids) J35.9
 tooth, teeth K08.9
  hard tissues K03.9
   specified NEC K03.89
  pulp NEC K04.99
  specified NEC K08.89 ◄▬▬
 Tourette's F95.2
 trachea NEC J39.8
 tricuspid I07.9
  nonrheumatic I36.9
 triglyceride-storage E75.5
 trophoblastic —*see* Mole, hydatidiform
 tsutsugamushi A75.3
 tube (fallopian) (noninflammatory) N83.9
  inflammatory —*see* Salpingitis
  specified NEC N83.8
 tuberculous NEC —*see* Tuberculosis

Disease, diseased *(Continued)*
 tubo-ovarian (noninflammatory) N83.9
  inflammatory —*see* Salpingo-oophoritis
  specified NEC N83.8
 tubotympanic, chronic —*see* Otitis, media,
   suppurative, chronic, tubotympanic
 tubulo-interstitial N15.9
  specified NEC N15.8
 tympanum —*see* Disorder, tympanic
   membrane
 Uhl's Q24.8
 Underwood's (sclerema neonatorum) P83.0
 Unverricht (-Lundborg) —*see* Epilepsy,
   generalized, idiopathic
 Urbach-Oppenheim (necrobiosis lipoidica
   diabeticorum) —*see* E08-E13 with .620
 ureter N28.9
  in (due to)
   schistosomiasis (bilharziasis) B65.0 [N29]
 urethra N36.9
  specified NEC N36.8
 urinary (tract) N39.9
  bladder N32.9
   specified NEC N32.89
  specified NEC N39.8
 uterus (noninflammatory) N85.9
  infective —*see* Endometritis
  inflammatory —*see* Endometritis
  specified NEC N85.8
 uveal tract (anterior) H21.9
  posterior H31.9
 vagabond's B85.1
 vagina, vaginal (noninflammatory) N89.9
  inflammatory NEC N76.89
  specified NEC N89.8
 valve, valvular I38
  multiple I08.9
   specified NEC I08.8
 van Creveld-von Gierke (glycogenosis I)
   E74.01
 vas deferens N50.9
 vascular I99.9
  arteriosclerotic —*see* Arteriosclerosis
  ciliary body NEC —*see* Disorder, iris,
    vascular
  hypertensive —*see* Hypertension
  iris NEC —*see* Disorder, iris, vascular
  obliterative I77.1
   peripheral I73.9
  occlusive I99.8
  peripheral (occlusive) I73.9
   in diabetes mellitus —*see* E08-E13 with .51
 vasomotor I73.9
 vasospastic I73.9
 vein I87.9
 venereal —*see also* Disease, sexually
   transmitted A64
  chlamydial NEC A56.8
   anus A56.3
   genitourinary NOS A56.2
   pharynx A56.4
   rectum A56.3
  fifth A55
  sixth A55
  specified nature or type NEC A63.8
 vertebra, vertebral —*see also* Spondylopathy
  disc —*see* Disorder, disc
 vibration —*see* Vibration, adverse effects
 viral, virus —*see also* Disease, by type of virus
   B34.9
  arbovirus NOS A94
  arthropod-borne NOS A94
  congenital P35.9
   specified NEC P35.8
  Hanta (with renal manifestations)
    (Dobrava) (Puumala) (Seoul) A98.5
   with pulmonary manifestations (Andes)
     (Bayou) (Bermejo) (Black Creek
     Canal) (Choclo) (Juquitiba) (Laguna
     negra) (Lechiguanas) (New York)
     (Oran) (Sin nombre) B33.4

Disease, diseased *(Continued)*
  viral, virus *(Continued)*
    Hantaan (Korean hemorrhagic fever) A98.5
    human immunodeficiency (HIV) B20
    Kunjin A83.4
    nonarthropod-borne NOS B34.9
    Powassan A84.8
    Rocio (encephalitis) A83.6
    Sin nombre (Hantavirus) (cardio)-
      pulmonary syndrome B33.4
    Tahyna B33.8
    vesicular stomatitis A93.8
  vitreous H43.9
    specified NEC H43.89
  vocal cord J38.3
  Volkmann's, acquired T79.6
  von Eulenburg's (congenital paramyotonia)
    G71.19
  von Gierke's (glycogenosis I) E74.01
  von Graefe's —*see* Strabismus, paralytic,
    ophthalmoplegia, progressive
  von Willebrand (-Jürgens) (angiohemophilia)
    D68.0
  Vrolik's (osteogenesis imperfecta) Q78.0
  vulva (noninflammatory) N90.9
    inflammatory NEC N76.89
    specified NEC N90.89
  Wallgren's (obstruction of splenic vein with
    collateral circulation) I87.8
  Wassilieff's (leptospiral jaundice) A27.0
  wasting NEC R64
    due to malnutrition E41
  Waterhouse-Friderichsen A39.1
  Wegner's (syphilitic osteochondritis) A50.02
  Weil's (leptospiral jaundice of lung) A27.0
  Weir Mitchell's (erythromelalgia) I73.81
  Werdnig-Hoffmann G12.0
  Wermer's E31.21
  Werner-His (trench fever) A79.0
  Werner-Schultz (neutropenic splenomegaly)
    D73.81
  Wernicke-Posadas B38.9
  whipworm B79
  white blood cells D72.9
    specified NEC D72.89
  white matter R90.82
  white-spot, meaning lichen sclerosus et
    atrophicus L90.0
    penis N48.0
    vulva N90.4
  Wilkie's K55.1
  Wilkinson-Sneddon (subcorneal pustular
    dermatosis) L13.1
  Willis' —*see* Diabetes
  Wilson's (hepatolenticular degeneration)
    E83.01
  woolsorter's A22.1
  yaba monkey tumor B08.72
  yaba pox (virus) B08.72
  Zika virus A92.5 ◀
  zoonotic, bacterial A28.9
    specified type NEC A28.8
Disfigurement (due to scar) L90.5
Disgerminoma —*see* Dysgerminoma
DISH (diffuse idiopathic skeletal
    hyperostosis) —*see* Hyperostosis,
    ankylosing
Disinsertion, retina —*see* Detachment, retina
Dislocatable hip, congenital Q65.6
Dislocation (articular)
  with fracture —*see* Fracture
  acromioclavicular (joint) S43.10-
    with displacement
      100%-200% S43.12-
      more than 200% S43.13-
    inferior S43.14-
    posterior S43.15-
  ankle S93.0-
  astragalus —*see* Dislocation, ankle
  atlantoaxial S13.121
  atlantooccipital S13.111

Dislocation *(Continued)*
  atloidooccipital S13.111
  breast bone S23.29
  capsule, joint code by site under Dislocation
  carpal (bone) —*see* Dislocation, wrist
  carpometacarpal (joint) NEC S63.05-
    thumb S63.04-
  cartilage (joint) - code by site under
    Dislocation
  cervical spine (vertebra) —*see* Dislocation,
    vertebra, cervical
  chronic —*see* Dislocation, recurrent
  clavicle —*see* Dislocation, acromioclavicular
    joint
  coccyx S33.2
  congenital NEC Q68.8
  coracoid —*see* Dislocation, shoulder
  costal cartilage S23.29
  costochondral S23.29
  cricoarytenoid articulation S13.29
  cricothyroid articulation S13.29
  dorsal vertebra —*see* Dislocation, vertebra,
    thoracic
  ear ossicle —*see* Discontinuity, ossicles, ear
  elbow S53.10-
    congenital Q68.8
    pathological —*see* Dislocation, pathological
      NEC, elbow
    radial head alone —*see* Dislocation, radial
      head
    recurrent —*see* Dislocation, recurrent,
      elbow
    traumatic S53.10-
      anterior S53.11-
      lateral S53.14-
      medial S53.13-
      posterior S53.12-
      specified type NEC S53.19-
  eye, nontraumatic —*see* Luxation, globe
  eyeball, nontraumatic —*see* Luxation, globe
  femur
    distal end —*see* Dislocation, knee
    proximal end —*see* Dislocation, hip
  fibula
    distal end —*see* Dislocation, ankle
    proximal end —*see* Dislocation, knee
  finger S63.25-
    index S63.25-
    interphalangeal S63.27-
      distal S63.29-
        index S63.29-
        little S63.29-
        middle S63.29-
        ring S63.29-
      index S63.27-
      little S63.27-
      middle S63.27-
      proximal S63.28-
        index S63.28-
        little S63.28-
        middle S63.28-
        ring S63.28-
      ring S63.27-
    little S63.25-
    metacarpophalangeal S63.26-
      index S63.26-
      little S63.26-
      middle S63.26-
      ring S63.26-
    middle S63.25-
    recurrent —*see* Dislocation, recurrent,
      finger
    ring S63.25-
    thumb —*see* Dislocation, thumb
  foot S93.30-
    recurrent —*see* Dislocation, recurrent,
      foot
    specified site NEC S93.33-
    tarsal joint S93.31-
    tarsometatarsal joint S93.32-
    toe —*see* Dislocation, toe

Dislocation *(Continued)*
  fracture —*see* Fracture
  glenohumeral (joint) —*see* Dislocation,
    shoulder
  glenoid —*see* Dislocation, shoulder
  habitual —*see* Dislocation, recurrent
  hip S73.00-
    anterior S73.03-
      obturator S73.02-
    central S73.04-
    congenital (total) Q65.2
      bilateral Q65.1
      partial Q65.5
        bilateral Q65.4
        unilateral Q65.3-
      unilateral Q65.0-
    developmental M24.85-
    pathological —*see* Dislocation, pathological
      NEC, hip
    posterior S73.01-
    recurrent —*see* Dislocation, recurrent,
      hip
  humerus, proximal end —*see* Dislocation,
    shoulder
  incomplete —*see* Subluxation, by site
  incus —*see* Discontinuity, ossicles, ear
  infracoracoid —*see* Dislocation, shoulder
  innominate (pubic junction) (sacral junction)
    S33.39
    acetabulum —*see* Dislocation, hip
  interphalangeal (joint (s))
    finger S63.279
      distal S63.29-
        index S63.29-
        little S63.29-
        middle S63.29-
        ring S63.29-
      index S63.27-
      little S63.27-
      middle S63.27-
      proximal S63.28-
        index S63.28-
        little S63.28-
        middle S63.28-
        ring S63.28-
      ring S63.27-
    foot or toe —*see* Dislocation, toe
    thumb S63.12-
      distal joint S63.14-
      proximal joint S63.13-
  jaw (cartilage) (meniscus) S03.0- ◀▥
  joint prosthesis —*see* Complications, joint
    prosthesis, mechanical, displacement,
    by site
  knee S83.106
    cap —*see* Dislocation, patella
    congenital Q68.2
    old M23.8X-
    patella —*see* Dislocation, patella
    pathological —*see* Dislocation, pathological
      NEC, knee
    proximal tibia
      anteriorly S83.11-
      laterally S83.14-
      medially S83.13-
      posteriorly S83.12-
    recurrent —*see also* Derangement, knee,
      specified NEC
    specified type NEC S83.19-
  lacrimal gland H04.16-
  lens (complete) H27.10-
    anterior H27.12-
    congenital Q12.1
    ocular implant —*see* Complications,
      intraocular lens
    partial H27.11-
    posterior H27.13-
    traumatic S05.8X-
  ligament code by site under Dislocation
  lumbar (vertebra) —*see* Dislocation, vertebra,
    lumbar

◀ New   ◀▥ Revised   ~~deleted~~ Deleted

Dislocation *(Continued)*
  lumbosacral (vertebra) —*see also* Dislocation,
      vertebra, lumbar
    congenital Q76.49
  mandible S03.0- ◀▥
  meniscus (knee) —*see* Tear, meniscus
    other sites code by site under Dislocation
  metacarpal (bone)
    distal end —*see* Dislocation, finger
    proximal end S63.06-
  metacarpophalangeal (joint)
    finger S63.26-
      index S63.26-
      little S63.26-
      middle S63.26-
      ring S63.26-
      thumb S63.11-
  metatarsal (bone) —*see* Dislocation, foot
  metatarsophalangeal (joint (s)) —*see*
      Dislocation, toe
  midcarpal (joint) S63.03-
  midtarsal (joint) —*see* Dislocation, foot
  neck S13.20
    specified site NEC S13.29
    vertebra —*see* Dislocation, vertebra,
      cervical
  nose (septal cartilage) S03.1
  occipitoatloid S13.111
  old —*see* Derangement, joint, specified type
      NEC
  ossicles, ear —*see* Discontinuity, ossicles, ear
  partial —*see* Subluxation, by site
  patella S83.006
    congenital Q74.1
    lateral S83.01-
    recurrent (nontraumatic) M22.0-
      incomplete M22.1-
    specified type NEC S83.09-
  pathological NEC M24.30
    ankle M24.37-
    elbow M24.32-
    foot joint M24.37-
    hand joint M24.34-
    hip M24.35-
    knee M24.36-
    lumbosacral joint —*see* subcategory M53.2
    pelvic region —*see* Dislocation,
      pathological, hip
    sacroiliac —*see* subcategory M53.2
    shoulder M24.31-
    wrist M24.33-
  pelvis NEC S33.30
    specified NEC S33.39
  phalanx
    finger or hand —*see* Dislocation, finger
    foot or toe —*see* Dislocation, toe
  prosthesis, internal —*see* Complications,
      prosthetic device, by site, mechanical
  radial head S53.006
    anterior S53.01-
    posterior S53.02-
    specified type NEC S53.09-
  radiocarpal (joint) S63.02-
  radiohumeral (joint) —*see* Dislocation, radial
      head
  radioulnar (joint)
    distal S63.01-
    proximal —*see* Dislocation, elbow
  radius
    distal end —*see* Dislocation, wrist
    proximal end —*see* Dislocation, radial head
  recurrent M24.40
    ankle M24.47-
    elbow M24.42-
    finger M24.44-
    foot joint M24.47-
    hand joint M24.44-
    hip M24.45-
    knee M24.46-
      patella —*see* Dislocation, patella,
        recurrent

Dislocation *(Continued)*
  recurrent *(Continued)*
    patella —*see* Dislocation, patella, recurrent
    sacroiliac —*see* subcategory M53.2
    shoulder M24.41-
    toe M24.47-
    vertebra —*see also* subcategory M43.5
      atlantoaxial M43.4
        with myelopathy M43.3
    wrist M24.43-
  rib (cartilage) S23.29
  sacrococcygeal S33.2
  sacroiliac (joint) (ligament) S33.2
    congenital Q74.2
    recurrent —*see* subcategory M53.2
  sacrum S33.2
  scaphoid (bone) (hand) (wrist) —*see*
      Dislocation, wrist
    foot —*see* Dislocation, foot
  scapula —*see* Dislocation, shoulder, girdle,
      scapula
  semilunar cartilage, knee —*see* Tear, meniscus
  septal cartilage (nose) S03.1
  septum (nasal) (old) J34.2
  sesamoid bone code by site under Dislocation
  shoulder (blade) (ligament) (joint) (traumatic)
      S43.006
    acromioclavicular —*see* Dislocation,
      acromioclavicular
    chronic —*see* Dislocation, recurrent,
      shoulder
    congenital Q68.8
    girdle S43.30-
      scapula S43.31-
      specified site NEC S43.39-
    humerus S43.00-
      anterior S43.01-
      inferior S43.03-
      posterior S43.02-
    pathological —*see* Dislocation, pathological
      NEC, shoulder
    recurrent —*see* Dislocation, recurrent,
      shoulder
    specified type NEC S43.08-
  spine
    cervical —*see* Dislocation, vertebra, cervical
    congenital Q76.49
    due to birth trauma P11.5
    lumbar —*see* Dislocation, vertebra, lumbar
    thoracic —*see* Dislocation, vertebra,
      thoracic
  spontaneous —*see* Dislocation, pathological
  sternoclavicular (joint) S43.206
    anterior S43.21-
    posterior S43.22-
  sternum S23.29
  subglenoid —*see* Dislocation, shoulder
  symphysis pubis S33.4
  talus —*see* Dislocation, ankle
  tarsal (bone (s)) (joint (s)) —*see* Dislocation,
      foot
  tarsometatarsal (joint (s)) —*see* Dislocation,
      foot
  temporomandibular (joint) S03.0- ◀▥
  thigh, proximal end —*see* Dislocation, hip
  thorax S23.20
    specified site NEC S23.29
    vertebra —*see* Dislocation, vertebra
  thumb S63.10-
    interphalangeal joint —*see* Dislocation,
      interphalangeal (joint), thumb
    metacarpophalangeal joint —*see*
      Dislocation, metacarpophalangeal
      (joint), thumb
  thyroid cartilage S13.29
  tibia
    distal end —*see* Dislocation, ankle
    proximal end —*see* Dislocation, knee
  tibiofibular (joint)
    distal —*see* Dislocation, ankle
    superior —*see* Dislocation, knee

Dislocation *(Continued)*
  toe (s) S93.106
    great S93.10-
      interphalangeal joint S93.11-
      metatarsophalangeal joint S93.12-
    interphalangeal joint S93.119
    lesser S93.106
      interphalangeal joint S93.11-
      metatarsophalangeal joint S93.12-
    metatarsophalangeal joint S93.12-
  tooth S03.2
  trachea S23.29
  ulna
    distal end S63.07-
    proximal end —*see* Dislocation, elbow
  ulnohumeral (joint) —*see* Dislocation, elbow
  vertebra (articular process) (body)
      (traumatic)
    cervical S13.101
      atlantoaxial joint S13.121
      atlantooccipital joint S13.111
      atloidooccipital joint S13.111
      joint between
        C0 and C1 S13.111
        C1 and C2 S13.121
        C2 and C3 S13.131
        C3 and C4 S13.141
        C4 and C5 S13.151
        C5 and C6 S13.161
        C6 and C7 S13.171
        C7 and T1 S13.181
      occipitoatloid joint S13.111
    congenital Q76.49
    lumbar S33.101
      joint between
        L1 and L2 S33.111
        L2 and L3 S33.121
        L3 and L4 S33.131
        L4 and L5 S33.141
    nontraumatic —*see* Displacement,
      intervertebral disc
    partial —*see* Subluxation, by site
    recurrent NEC —*see* subcategory
      M43.5
    thoracic S23.101
      joint between
        T1 and T2 S23.111
        T2 and T3 S23.121
        T3 and T4 S23.123
        T4 and T5 S23.131
        T5 and T6 S23.133
        T6 and T7 S23.141
        T7 and T8 S23.143
        T8 and T9 S23.151
        T9 and T10 S23.153
        T10 and T11 S23.161
        T11 and T12 S23.163
        T12 and L1 S23.171
  wrist (carpal bone) S63.006
    carpometacarpal joint —*see* Dislocation,
      carpometacarpal (joint)
    distal radioulnar joint —*see* Dislocation,
      radioulnar (joint), distal
    metacarpal bone, proximal —*see*
      Dislocation, metacarpal (bone),
      proximal end
    midcarpal —*see* Dislocation, midcarpal
      (joint)
    radiocarpal joint —*see* Dislocation,
      radiocarpal (joint)
    recurrent —*see* Dislocation, recurrent,
      wrist
    specified site NEC S63.09-
    ulna —*see* Dislocation, ulna, distal end
  xiphoid cartilage S23.29
Disorder (of) —*see also* Disease
  acantholytic L11.9
    specified NEC L11.8
  acute
    psychotic —*see* Psychosis, acute
    stress F43.0

Disorder *(Continued)*
  adjustment (grief) F43.20
    with
      anxiety F43.22
        with depressed mood F43.23
      conduct disturbance F43.24
        with emotional disturbance F43.25
      depressed mood F43.21
        with anxiety F43.23
      other specified symptom F43.29
  adrenal (capsule) (gland) (medullary) E27.9
    specified NEC E27.8
  adrenogenital E25.9
    drug-induced E25.8
    iatrogenic E25.8
    idiopathic E25.8
  adult personality (and behavior) F69
    specified NEC F68.8
  affective (mood) —*see* Disorder, mood
  aggressive, unsocialized F91.1
  alcohol-related F10.99
    with
      amnestic disorder, persisting F10.96
      anxiety disorder F10.980
      dementia, persisting F10.97
      intoxication F10.929
        with delirium F10.921
        uncomplicated F10.920
      mood disorder F10.94
      other specified F10.988
      psychotic disorder F10.959
        with
          delusions F10.950
          hallucinations F10.951
      sexual dysfunction F10.981
      sleep disorder F10.982
  alcohol use ◄
    mild F10.10 ◄
      with ◄
        alcohol-induced ◄
          anxiety disorder F10.180 ◄
          bipolar and related disorder
            F10.14 ◄
          depressive disorder F10.14 ◄
          psychotic disorder F10.159 ◄
          sexual dysfunction F10.181 ◄
          sleep disorder F10.182 ◄
        alcohol intoxication F10.129 ◄
          delirium F10.121 ◄
    moderate or severe F10.20 ◄
      with ◄
        alcohol-induced ◄
          anxiety disorder F10.280 ◄
          bipolar and related disorder
            F10.24 ◄
          depressive disorder F10.24 ◄
          major neurocognitive disorder,
            amnestic-confabulatory type
            F10.26 ◄
          major neurocognitive disorder,
            nonamnestic-confabulatory
            type F10.27 ◄
          mild neurocognitive disorder
            F10.288 ◄
          psychotic disorder F10.259 ◄
          sexual dysfunction F10.281 ◄
          sleep disorder F10.282 ◄
        alcohol intoxication F10.229 ◄
          delirium F10.221 ◄
  allergic —*see* Allergy
  alveolar NEC J84.09
  amino-acid
    cystathioninuria E72.19
    cystinosis E72.04
    cystinuria E72.01
    glycinuria E72.09
    homocystinuria E72.11
    metabolism —*see* Disturbance,
      metabolism, amino-acid
      specified NEC E72.8
    neonatal, transitory P74.8

Disorder *(Continued)*
  amino-acid *(Continued)*
    renal transport NEC E72.09
    transport NEC E72.09
  amnesic, amnestic
    alcohol-induced F10.96
      with dependence F10.26
    due to (secondary to) general medical
      condition F04
    psychoactive NEC-induced F19.96
      with
        abuse F19.16
        dependence F19.26
    sedative, hypnotic or anxiolytic-
      induced F13.96
      with dependence F13.26
  amphetamine-type substance use ◄
    mild F15.10 ◄
    moderate F15.20 ◄
    severe F15.20 ◄
  amphetamine (or other stimulant)
    use ◄
    mild ◄
      with ◄
        amphetamine (or other stimulant)
          -induced ◄
          anxiety disorder F15.180 ◄
          bipolar and related disorder
            F15.14 ◄
          depressive disorder F15.14 ◄
          obsessive-compulsive and related
            disorder F15.188 ◄
          psychotic disorder F15.159 ◄
          sexual dysfunction F15.181 ◄
        amphetamine, cocaine, or other
          stimulant intoxication ◄
          with perceptual disturbances
            F15.122 ◄
          without perceptual disturbances
            F15.129 ◄
          intoxication delirium F15.121 ◄
    moderate or severe ◄
      with ◄
        amphetamine (or other stimulant)
          -induced ◄
          anxiety disorder F15.280 ◄
          obsessive-compulsive and related
            disorder F15.288 ◄
          sexual dysfunction F15.281 ◄
          bipolar and related disorder
            F15.24 ◄
          depressive disorder F15.24 ◄
          psychotic disorder F15.259 ◄
        amphetamine, cocaine, or other
          stimulant intoxication ◄
          with perceptual disturbances
            F15.222 ◄
          without perceptual disturbances
            F15.229 ◄
          intoxication delirium F15.221 ◄
  anaerobic glycolysis with anemia
    D55.2
  anxiety F41.9
    due to (secondary to)
      alcohol F10.980
      amphetamine F15.980
        in
          abuse F15.180
          dependence F15.280
      anxiolytic F13.980
        in
          abuse F13.180
          dependence F13.280
      caffeine F15.980
        in
          abuse F15.180
          dependence F15.280
      cannabis F12.980
        in
          abuse F12.180
          dependence F12.280

Disorder *(Continued)*
  anxiety *(Continued)*
    due to *(Continued)*
      cocaine F14.980
        in
          abuse F14.180
          dependence F14.180
      general medical condition F06.4
      hallucinogen F16.980
        in
          abuse F16.180
          dependence F16.280
      hypnotic F13.980
        in
          abuse F13.180
          dependence F13.280
      inhalant F18.980
        in
          abuse F18.180
          dependence F18.280
      phencyclidine F16.980
        in
          abuse F16.180
          dependence F16.280
      psychoactive substance NEC F19.980
        in
          abuse F19.180
          dependence F19.280
      sedative F13.980
        in
          abuse F13.180
          dependence F13.280
      volatile solvents F18.980
        in
          abuse F18.180
          dependence F18.280
    generalized F41.1
    illness F45.21 ◄
    mixed
      with depression (mild) F41.8
      specified NEC F41.3
    organic F06.4
    phobic F40.9
      of childhood F40.8
    specified NEC F41.8
  aortic valve —*see* Endocarditis, aortic
  aromatic amino-acid metabolism E70.9
    specified NEC E70.8
  arteriole NEC I77.89
  artery NEC I77.89
  articulation —*see* Disorder, joint
  attachment (childhood)
    disinhibited F94.2
    reactive F94.1
  attention-deficit hyperactivity (adolescent)
    (adult) (child) F98.8 ◄▥
    combined type F90.2
    hyperactive type F90.1
    inattentive type F90.0
    specified type NEC F90.8
  attention-deficit without hyperactivity
    (adolescent) (adult) (child) F90.0
  auditory processing (central) H93.25
  autism spectrum F84.0 ◄
  autistic F84.0
  autonomic nervous system G90.9
    specified NEC G90.8
  ~~avoidant, child or adolescent F40.10~~
  avoidant ◄
    child or adolescent F40.10 ◄
    restrictive food intake F50.89 ◄
  balance
    acid-base E87.8
      mixed E87.4
    electrolyte E87.8
    fluid NEC E87.8
  behavioral (disruptive) —*see* Disorder, conduct
  beta-amino-acid metabolism E72.8
  bile acid and cholesterol metabolism E78.70
    Barth syndrome E78.71
    other specified E78.79
    Smith-Lemli-Opitz syndrome E78.72

◄ New   ◄▥ Revised   ~~deleted~~ Deleted

Disorder (Continued)
  bilirubin excretion E80.6
  binge eating F50.81 ◀
  binocular
    movement H51.9
      convergence
        excess H51.12
        insufficiency H51.11
      internuclear ophthalmoplegia —see
        Ophthalmoplegia, internuclear
      palsy of conjugate gaze H51.0
      specified type NEC H51.8
    vision NEC —see Disorder, vision,
        binocular
  bipolar (I) F31.9
    current episode
      depressed F31.9
        with psychotic features F31.5
        without psychotic features
            F31.30
          mild F31.31
          moderate F31.32
          severe (without psychotic features)
              F31.4
            with psychotic features
                F31.5
      hypomanic F31.0
      manic F31.9
        with psychotic features F31.2
        without psychotic features F31.10
          mild F31.11
          moderate F31.12
          severe (without psychotic features)
              F31.13
            with psychotic features F31.2
      mixed F31.60
        mild F31.61
        moderate F31.62
        severe (without psychotic features)
            F31.63
          with psychotic features F31.64
      severe depression (without psychotic
          features) F31.4
        with psychotic features F31.5
    II F31.81
    in remission (currently) F31.70
      in full remission
        most recent episode
          depressed F31.76
          hypomanic F31.72
          manic F31.74
          mixed F31.78
      in partial remission
        most recent episode
          depressed F31.75
          hypomanic F31.71
          manic F31.73
          mixed F31.77
    organic F06.30
    single manic episode F30.9
      mild F30.11
      moderate F30.12
      hhsevere (without psychotic symptoms)
          F30.13
        with psychotic symptoms F30.2
    specified NEC F31.89
  bladder N32.9
    functional NEC N31.9
    in schistosomiasis B65.0 [N33]
    specified NEC N32.89
  bleeding D68.9
  blood D75.9
    in congenital early syphilis A50.09 [D77]
  body dysmorphic F45.22
  bone M89.9
    continuity M84.9
      specified type NEC M84.80
        ankle M84.87-
        fibula M84.86-
        foot M84.87-
        hand M84.84-

Disorder (Continued)
  bone (Continued)
    continuity (Continued)
      specified type (Continued)
        humerus M84.82-
        neck M84.88
        pelvis M84.859
        radius M84.83-
        rib M84.88
        shoulder M84.81-
        skull M84.88
        thigh M84.85-
        tibia M84.86-
        ulna M84.83-
        vertebra M84.88
    density and structure M85.9
      cyst —see also Cyst, bone, specified type
          NEC
        aneurysmal —see Cyst, bone,
            aneurysmal
        solitary —see Cyst, bone, solitary
      diffuse idiopathic skeletal
          hyperostosis —see Hyperostosis,
          ankylosing
      fibrous dysplasia (monostotic) —see
          Dysplasia, fibrous, bone
      fluorosis —see Fluorosis, skeletal
      hyperostosis of skull M85.2
      osteitis condensans —see Osteitis,
          condensans
      specified type NEC M85.8-
        ankle M85.87-
        foot M85.87-
        forearm M85.83-
        hand M85.84-
        lower leg M85.86-
        multiple sites M85.89
        neck M85.88
        rib M85.88
        shoulder M85.81-
        skull M85.88
        thigh M85.85-
        upper arm M85.82-
        vertebra M85.88
    development and growth NEC
        M89.20
      carpus M89.24-
      clavicle M89.21-
      femur M89.25-
      fibula M89.26-
      finger M89.24-
      humerus M89.22-
      ilium M89.259
      ischium M89.259
      metacarpus M89.24-
      metatarsus M89.27-
      multiple sites M89.29
      neck M89.28
      radius M89.23-
      rib M89.28
      scapula M89.21-
      skull M89.28
      tarsus M89.27-
      tibia M89.26-
      toe M89.27-
      ulna M89.23-
      vertebra M89.28
      specified type NEC M89.8X-
    brachial plexus G54.0
    branched-chain amino-acid metabolism
        E71.2
      specified NEC E71.19
    breast N64.9
      agalactia —see Agalactia
      associated with
        lactation O92.70
          specified NEC O92.79
        pregnancy O92.20
          specified NEC O92.29
        puerperium O92.20
          specified NEC O92.29

Disorder (Continued)
  breast (Continued)
    cracked nipple —see Cracked nipple
    galactorrhea —see Galactorrhea
    hypogalactia O92.4
    lactation disorder NEC O92.79
    mastitis —see Mastitis
    nipple infection —see Infection, nipple
    retracted nipple —see Retraction, nipple
    specified type NEC N64.89
  Briquet's F45.0
  bullous, in diseases classified elsewhere
      L14
  caffeine use ◀
    mild ◀
      with ◀
        caffeine-induced ◀
          anxiety disorder F15.180 ◀
          sleep disorder F15.182 ◀
    moderate or severe ◀
      with ◀
        caffeine-induced ◀
          anxiety disorder F15.280 ◀
          sleep disorder F15.282 ◀
  cannabis use
    due to drug abuse —see Abuse, drug,
        cannabis
    due to drug dependence —see
        Dependence, drug, cannabis
    mild F12.10 ◀
      with ◀
        cannabis-induced ◀
          anxiety disorder F12.180 ◀
          psychotic disorder F12.159 ◀
          sleep disorder F12.188 ◀
        cannabis intoxication delirium
            F12.121 ◀
          with perceptual disturbances
              F12.122 ◀
          without perceptual disturbances
              F12.129 ◀
    moderate or severe F12.20 ◀
      with ◀
        cannabis-induced ◀
          anxiety disorder F12.280 ◀
          psychotic disorder F12.259 ◀
          sleep disorder F12.288 ◀
        cannabis intoxication ◀
          with perceptual disturbances
              F12.222 ◀
          without perceptual disturbances
              F12.229 ◀
        delirium F12.221 ◀
  carbohydrate
    absorption, intestinal NEC E74.39
    metabolism (congenital) E74.9
      specified NEC E74.8
  cardiac, functional I51.89
  carnitine metabolism E71.40
  cartilage M94.9
    articular NEC —see Derangement, joint,
        articular cartilage
    chondrocalcinosis —see
        Chondrocalcinosis
    specified type NEC M94.8X-
      articular —see Derangement, joint,
          articular cartilage
    multiple sites M94.8X0
  catatonia (due to known physiological
      condition) (with another mental
      disorder) F06.1 ◀
  catatonic
    due to (secondary to) known physiological
        condition F06.1
    organic F06.1
  central auditory processing H93.25
  cervical
    region NEC M53.82
    root (nerve) NEC G54.2
  character NOS F60.9
  childhood disintegrative NEC F84.3

Disorder *(Continued)*
  cholesterol and bile acid metabolism E78.70
    Barth syndrome E78.71
    other specified E78.79
    Smith-Lemli-Opitz syndrome E78.72
  choroid H31.9
    atrophy —*see* Atrophy, choroid
    degeneration —*see* Degeneration, choroid
    detachment —*see* Detachment, choroid
    dystrophy —*see* Dystrophy, choroid
    hemorrhage —*see* Hemorrhage, choroid
    rupture —*see* Rupture, choroid
    scar —*see* Scar, chorioretinal
    solar retinopathy —*see* Retinopathy,
      solar
    specified type NEC H31.8
  ciliary body —*see* Disorder, iris
    degeneration —*see* Degeneration, ciliary
      body
  coagulation (factor) (*see also* Defect,
    coagulation) D68.9
    newborn, transient P61.6
  cocaine use ◀
    mild F14.10 ◀
      with ◀
        amphetamine, cocaine, or other
          stimulant intoxication ◀
          with perceptual disturbances
            F14.122 ◀
          without perceptual disturbances
            F14.129 ◀
        cocaine-induced ◀
          anxiety disorder F14.180 ◀
          bipolar and related disorder
            F14.14 ◀
          depressive disorder F14.14 ◀
          obsessive-compulsive and related
            disorder F14.188 ◀
          psychotic disorder F14.159 ◀
          sexual dysfunction F14.181 ◀
          sleep disorder F14.182 ◀
        cocaine intoxication delirium
          F14.121 ◀
    moderate or severe F14.20 ◀
      with ◀
        amphetamine, cocaine, or other
          stimulant intoxication ◀
          with perceptual disturbances
            F14.222 ◀
          without perceptual disturbances
            F14.229 ◀
        cocaine-induced ◀
          anxiety disorder F14.280 ◀
          bipolar and related disorder
            F14.24 ◀
          depressive disorder F14.24 ◀
          obsessive-compulsive and related
            disorder F14.288 ◀
          psychotic disorder F14.259 ◀
          sexual dysfunction F14.281 ◀
          sleep disorder F14.282 ◀
        cocaine intoxication delirium
          F14.221 ◀
  coccyx NEC M53.3
  cognitive F09
    due to (secondary to) general medical
      condition F09
    persisting R41.89
      due to
        alcohol F10.97
          with dependence F10.27
        anxiolytics F13.97
          with dependence F13.27
        hypnotics F13.97
          with dependence F13.27
        sedatives F13.97
          with dependence F13.27
        specified substance NEC F19.97
          with
            abuse F19.17
            dependence F19.27

Disorder *(Continued)*
  communication F80.9
    social pragmatic F80.82 ◀
  conduct (childhood) F91.9
    adjustment reaction —*see* Disorder,
      adjustment
    adolescent onset type F91.2
    childhood onset type F91.1
    compulsive F63.9
    confined to family context F91.0
    depressive F91.8
    group type F91.2
    hyperkinetic —*see* Disorder, attention-
      deficit hyperactivity
    oppositional defiance F91.3
    socialized F91.2
    solitary aggressive type F91.1
    specified NEC F91.8
    unsocialized (aggressive) F91.1
  conduction, heart I45.9
  congenital glycosylation (CDG) E74.8
  conjunctiva H11.9
    infection —*see* Conjunctivitis
  connective tissue, localized L94.9
    specified NEC L94.8
  conversion (functional neurological symptom
    disorder) ◀▥
    with ◀
      abnormal movement F44.4 ◀
      anesthesia or sensory loss F44.6 ◀
      attacks or seizures F44.5 ◀
      mixed symptoms F44.7 ◀
      special sensory symptoms F44.6 ◀
      speech symptoms F44.4 ◀
      swallowing symptoms F44.4 ◀
      weakness or paralysis F44.4 ◀
  convulsive (secondary) —*see* Convulsions
  cornea H18.9
    deformity —*see* Deformity, cornea
    degeneration —*see* Degeneration, cornea
    deposits —*see* Deposit, cornea
    due to contact lens H18.82-
      specified as edema —*see* Edema,
        cornea
    edema —*see* Edema, cornea
    keratitis —*see* Keratitis
    keratoconjunctivitis —*see*
      Keratoconjunctivitis
    membrane change —*see* Change, corneal
      membrane
    neovascularization —*see*
      Neovascularization, cornea
    scar —*see* Opacity, cornea
    specified type NEC H18.89-
    ulcer —*see* Ulcer, cornea
  corpus cavernosum N48.9
  cranial nerve —*see* Disorder, nerve, cranial
  cyclothymic F34.0
  defiant oppositional F91.3
  delusional (persistent) (systematized) F22
    induced F24
  depersonalization F48.1
  depressive F32.9
    major F32.9
      with psychotic symptoms F32.3
      in remission (full) F32.5
        partial F32.4
      recurrent F33.9
      single episode F32.9
        mild F32.0
        moderate F32.1
        severe (without psychotic symptoms)
          F32.2
          with psychotic symptoms
            F32.3
    organic F06.31
    persistent F34.1 ◀
    recurrent F33.9
      current episode
        mild F33.0
        moderate F33.1

Disorder *(Continued)*
  depressive *(Continued)*
    recurrent *(Continued)*
      current episode *(Continued)*
        severe (without psychotic symptoms)
          F33.2
          with psychotic symptoms
            F33.3
      in remission F33.40
        full F33.42
        partial F33.41
      specified NEC F33.8
    single episode —*see* Episode, depressive
    specified NEC F32.89 ◀
  developmental F89
    arithmetical skills F81.2
    coordination (motor) F82
    expressive writing F81.81
    language F80.9
      expressive F80.1
      mixed receptive and expressive
        F80.2
      receptive type F80.2
      specified NEC F80.89
    learning F81.9
      arithmetical F81.2
      reading F81.0
    mixed F88
    motor coordination or function F82
    pervasive F84.9
      specified NEC F84.8
    phonological F80.0
    reading F81.0
    scholastic skills —*see also* Disorder,
      learning
      mixed F81.89
    specified NEC F88
    speech F80.9
      articulation F80.0
      specified NEC F80.89
    written expression F81.81
  diaphragm J98.6
  digestive (system) K92.9
    newborn P78.9
      specified NEC P78.89
    postprocedural —*see* Complication,
      gastrointestinal
    psychogenic F45.8
  disc (intervertebral) M51.9
    with
      myelopathy
        cervical region M50.00
        cervicothoracic region M50.03
        high cervical region M50.01
        lumbar region M51.06
        mid-cervical region M50.020 ◀▥
        sacrococcygeal region M53.3
        thoracic region M51.04
        thoracolumbar region M51.05
      radiculopathy
        cervical region M50.10
        cervicothoracic region M50.13
        high cervical region M50.11
        lumbar region M51.16
        lumbosacral region M51.17
        mid-cervical region M50.120 ◀▥
        sacrococcygeal region M53.3
        thoracic region M51.14
        thoracolumbar region M51.15
    cervical M50.90
      with
        myelopathy M50.00
          C2-C3 M50.01
          C3-C4 M50.01
          C4-C5 M50.021 ◀▥
          C5-C6 M50.022 ◀▥
          C6-C7 M50.023 ◀▥
          C7-T1 M50.03
          cervicothoracic region M50.03
          high cervical region M50.01
          mid-cervical region M50.020 ◀▥

◀ New   ◀▥ Revised   ~~deleted~~ Deleted

Disorder *(Continued)*
  disc *(Continued)*
    cervical *(Continued)*
      with *(Continued)*
        neuritis, radiculitis or radiculopathy
          M50.10
          C2-C3 M50.11
          C3-C4 M50.11
          C4-C5 M50.121 ◀▥
          C5-C6 M50.122 ◀▥
          C6-C7 M50.123 ◀▥
          C7-T1 M50.13
          cervicothoracic region M50.13
          high cervical region M50.11
          mid-cervical region M50.120 ◀▥
        C2-C3 M50.91
        C3-C4 M50.91
        C4-C5 M50.921 ◀▥
        C5-C6 M50.922 ◀▥
        C6-C7 M50.923 ◀▥
        C7-T1 M50.93
        cervicothoracic region M50.93
        degeneration M50.30
          C2-C3 M50.31
          C3-C4 M50.31
          C4-C5 M50.321 ◀▥
          C5-C6 M50.322 ◀▥
          C6-C7 M50.323 ◀▥
          C7-T1 M50.33
          cervicothoracic region M50.33
          high cervical region M50.31
          mid-cervical region M50.320 ◀▥
        displacement M50.20
          C2-C3 M50.21
          C3-C4 M50.21
          C4-C5 M50.221 ◀▥
          C5-C6 M50.222 ◀▥
          C6-C7 M50.223 ◀▥
          C7-T1 M50.23
          cervicothoracic region M50.23
          high cervical region M50.21
          mid-cervical region M50.220 ◀▥
        high cervical region M50.91
        mid-cervical region M50.920 ◀▥
        specified type NEC M50.80
          C2-C3 M50.81
          C3-C4 M50.81
          C4-C5 M50.821 ◀▥
          C5-C6 M50.822 ◀▥
          C6-C7 M50.823 ◀▥
          C7-T1 M50.83
          cervicothoracic region M50.83
          high cervical region M50.81
          mid-cervical region M50.820 ◀▥
    specified NEC
      lumbar region M51.86
      lumbosacral region M51.87
      sacrococcygeal region M53.3
      thoracic region M51.84
      thoracolumbar region M51.85
  disinhibited attachment (childhood) F94.2
  disintegrative, childhood NEC F84.3
  disruptive F91.9 ◀
    mood dysregulation F34.81 ◀
    specified NEC F91.8 ◀
  disruptive behavior F91.9 ◀▥
  dissocial personality F60.2
  dissociative F44.9
    affecting
      motor function F44.4
        and sensation F44.7
      sensation F44.6
        and motor function F44.7
    brief reactive F43.0
    due to (secondary to) general medical
      condition F06.8
    mixed F44.7
    organic F06.8
    other specified NEC F44.89
  double heterozygous sickling —*see* Disease,
    sickle-cell

Disorder *(Continued)*
  dream anxiety F51.5
  drug induced hemorrhagic D68.32
  drug related F19.99
    abuse —*see* Abuse, drug
    dependence —*see* Dependence, drug
  dysmorphic body F45.22 ◀▥
  dysthymic F34.1
  ear H93.9-
    bleeding —*see* Otorrhagia
    deafness —*see* Deafness
    degenerative H93.09-
    discharge —*see* Otorrhea
    external H61.9-
      auditory canal stenosis —*see* Stenosis,
        external ear canal
      exostosis —*see* Exostosis, external ear
        canal
      impacted cerumen —*see* Impaction,
        cerumen
      otitis —*see* Otitis, externa
      perichondritis —*see* Perichondritis, ear
      pinna —*see* Disorder, pinna
      specified type NEC H61.89-
        in diseases classified elsewhere
          H62.8X-
    inner H83.9-
      vestibular dysfunction —*see* Disorder,
        vestibular function
    middle H74.9-
      adhesive H74.1-
      ossicle —*see* Abnormal, ear ossicles
      polyp —*see* Polyp, ear (middle)
      specified NEC, in diseases classified
        elsewhere H75.8-
    postprocedural —*see* Complications, ear,
      procedure
    specified NEC, in diseases classified
      elsewhere H94.8-
  eating (adult) (psychogenic) F50.9
    anorexia —*see* Anorexia
    binge F50.81 ◀
    bulimia F50.2
    child F98.29
      pica F98.3
      rumination disorder F98.21
    pica F50.89 ◀▥
      childhood F98.3
  electrolyte (balance) NEC E87.8
    with
      abortion —*see* Abortion by type
        complicated by specified condition
          NEC
      ectopic pregnancy O08.5
      molar pregnancy O08.5
    acidosis (metabolic) (respiratory)
      E87.2
    alkalosis (metabolic) (respiratory)
      E87.3
  elimination, transepidermal L87.9
    specified NEC L87.8
  emotional (persistent) F34.9
    of childhood F93.9
      specified NEC F93.8
  endocrine E34.9
    postprocedural E89.89
    specified NEC E89.89
  erectile (male) (organic) —*see also*
    Dysfunction, sexual, male, erectile
    N52.9
    nonorganic F52.21
  erythematous —*see* Erythema
  esophagus K22.9
    functional K22.4
    psychogenic F45.8
  eustachian tube H69.9-
    infection —*see* Salpingitis, eustachian
    obstruction —*see* Obstruction, eustachian
      tube
    patulous —*see* Patulous, eustachian tube
    specified NEC H69.8-

Disorder *(Continued)*
  extrapyramidal G25.9
    in diseases classified elsewhere —*see*
      category G26
    specified type NEC G25.89
  eye H57.9
    postprocedural —*see* Complication,
      postprocedural, eye
  eyelid H02.9
    cyst —*see* Cyst, eyelid
    degenerative H02.70
      chloasma —*see* Chloasma, eyelid
      madarosis —*see* Madarosis
      specified type NEC H02.79
      vitiligo —*see* Vitiligo, eyelid
      xanthelasma —*see* Xanthelasma
    dermatochalasis —*see* Dermato-chalasis
    edema —*see* Edema, eyelid
    elephantiasis —*see* Elephantiasis, eyelid
    foreign body, retained —*see* Foreign body,
      retained, eyelid
    function H02.59
      abnormal innervation syndrome —*see*
        Syndrome, abnormal innervation
      blepharochalasis —*see* Blepharochalasis
      blepharoclonus —*see* Blepharoclonus
      blepharophimosis —*see*
        Blepharophimosis
      blepharoptosis —*see* Blepharoptosis
      lagophthalmos —*see* Lagophthalmos
      lid retraction —*see* Retraction, lid
    hypertrichosis —*see* Hypertrichosis, eyelid
    specified type NEC H02.89
    vascular H02.879
      left H02.876
        lower H02.875
        upper H02.874
      right H02.873
        lower H02.872
        upper H02.871
  factitious F68.10
    with predominantly
      physical symptoms F68.12
        with psychological symptoms F68.13
      psychological symptoms F68.11
        with physical symptoms F68.13
  factor, coagulation —*see* Defect, coagulation
  fatty acid
    metabolism E71.30
      specified NEC E71.39
    oxidation
      LCAD E71.310
      MCAD E71.311
      SCAD E71.312
      specified deficiency NEC E71.318
  feeding (infant or child) —*see also* Disorder,
    eating R63.3-
  feigned (with obvious motivation) Z76.5
    without obvious motivation —*see* Disorder,
      factitious
  female
    hypoactive sexual desire F52.0
    orgasmic F52.31
    sexual arousal F52.22
  fibroblastic M72.9
    specified NEC M72.8
  fluency
    adult onset F98.5
    childhood onset F80.81
    following
      cerebral infarction I69.323
      cerebrovascular disease I69.923
        specified disease NEC I69.823
      intracerebral hemorrhage I69.123
      nontraumatic intracranial hemorrhage
        NEC I69.223
      subarachnoid hemorrhage I69.023
    in conditions classified elsewhere R47.82
  fluid balance E87.8
  follicular (skin) L73.9
    specified NEC L73.8

Disorder *(Continued)*
  fructose metabolism E74.10
    essential fructosuria E74.11
    fructokinase deficiency E74.11
    fructose-1, 6-diphosphatase deficiency
      E74.19
    hereditary fructose intolerance E74.12
    other specified E74.19
  functional polymorphonuclear neutrophils
    D71
  gallbladder, biliary tract and pancreas in
    diseases classified elsewhere K87
  gamma-glutamyl cycle E72.8
  gastric (functional) K31.9
    motility K30
    psychogenic F45.8
    secretion K30
  gastrointestinal (functional) NOS K92.9
    newborn P78.9
    psychogenic F45.8
  gender-identity or -role F64.9
    childhood F64.2
    effect on relationship F66
    of adolescence or adulthood F64.0 ◀▥
      nontranssexual F64.8 ◀
    specified NEC F64.8
    uncertainty F66
  genito-pelvic pain penetration F52.6 ◀
  genitourinary system
    female N94.9
    male N50.9
    psychogenic F45.8
  globe H44.9
    degenerated condition H44.50
      absolute glaucoma H44.51-
      atrophy H44.52-
      leucocoria H44.53-
    degenerative H44.30
      chalcosis H44.31-
      myopia H44.2-
      siderosis H44.32-
      specified type NEC H44.39-
    endophthalmitis —*see* Endophthalmitis
    foreign body, retained —*see* Foreign body,
      intraocular, old, retained
    hemophthalmos —*see* Hemophthalmos
    hypotony H44.40
      due to
        ocular fistula H44.42-
        specified disorder NEC H44.43-
      flat anterior chamber H44.41-
      primary H44.44-
    luxation —*see* Luxation, globe
    specified type NEC H44.89
  glomerular (in) N05.9
    amyloidosis E85.4 *[N08]*
    cryoglobulinemia D89.1 *[N08]*
    disseminated intravascular coagulation
      D65 *[N08]*
    Fabry's disease E75.21 *[N08]*
    familial lecithin cholesterol acyltransferase
      deficiency E78.6 *[N08]*
    Goodpasture's syndrome M31.0
    hemolytic-uremic syndrome D59.3
    Henoch (-Schönlein) purpura D69.0 *[N08]*
    malariae malaria B52.0
    microscopic polyangiitis M31.7 *[N08]*
    multiple myeloma C90.0- *[N08]*
    mumps B26.83
    schistosomiasis B65.9 *[N08]*
    sepsis NEC A41.- *[N08]*
      streptococcal A40.- *[N08]*
    sickle-cell disorders D57.- *[N08]*
    strongyloidiasis B78.9 *[N08]*
    subacute bacterial endocarditis I33.0 *[N08]*
    syphilis A52.75
    systemic lupus erythematosus M32.14
    thrombotic thrombocytopenic purpura
      M31.1 *[N08]*
    Waldenström macroglobulinemia C88.0
      [N08]
    Wegener's granulomatosis M31.31

Disorder *(Continued)*
  gluconeogenesis E74.4
  glucosaminoglycan metabolism —
    see Disorder, metabolism,
    glucosaminoglycan
  glycine metabolism E72.50
    d-glycericacidemia E72.59
    hyperhydroxyprolinemia E72.59
    hyperoxaluria E72.53
    hyperprolinemia E72.59
    non-ketotic hyperglycinemia E72.51
    oxalosis E72.53
    oxaluria E72.53
    sarcosinemia E72.59
    trimethylaminuria E72.52
  glycoprotein metabolism E77.9
    specified NEC E77.8
  habit (and impulse) F63.9
    involving sexual behavior NEC F65.9
    specified NEC F63.89
  hallucinogen use ◀
    mild F16.10 ◀
      with ◀
        hallucinogen-induced ◀
          anxiety disorder F16.180 ◀
          bipolar and related disorder
            F16.14 ◀
          depressive disorder F16.14 ◀
          psychotic disorder F16.159 ◀
        hallucinogen intoxication delirium
          F16.121 ◀
        other hallucinogen intoxication
          F16.129 ◀
    moderate or severe F16.20 ◀
      with ◀
        hallucinogen-induced ◀
          anxiety disorder F16.280 ◀
          bipolar and related disorder
            F16.24 ◀
          depressive disorder F16.24 ◀
          psychotic disorder F16.259 ◀
        hallucinogen intoxication delirium
          F16.221 ◀
        other hallucinogen intoxication
          F16.229 ◀
  heart action I49.9
  hematological D75.9
    newborn (transient) P61.9
      specified NEC P61.8
  hematopoietic organs D75.9
  hemorrhagic NEC D69.9
    drug-induced D68.32
    due to
      extrinsic circulating anticoagulants
        D68.32
      increase in
        anti-IIa D68.32
        anti-Xa D68.32
      intrinsic
        circulating anticoagulants
          D68.318
        increase in
          antithrombin D68.318
          anti-VIIIa D68.318
          anti-IXa D68.318
          anti-XIa D68.318
    following childbirth O72.3
  hemostasis —*see* Defect, coagulation
  histidine metabolism E70.40
    histidinemia E70.41
    other specified E70.49
  hoarding F42.3 ◀
  hyperkinetic —*see* Disorder, attention-deficit
    hyperactivity
  hyperleucine-isoleucinemia E71.19
  hypervalinemia E71.19
  hypoactive sexual desire F52.0
  hypochondriacal F45.20
    body dysmorphic F45.22
    neurosis F45.21
    other specified F45.29

Disorder *(Continued)*
  identity
    dissociative F44.81
    illness anxiety F45.21 ◀
    of childhood F93.8
  immune mechanism (immunity) D89.9
    specified type NEC D89.89
  impaired renal tubular function
    N25.9
    specified NEC N25.89
  impulse (control) F63.9
  inflammatory
    pelvic, in diseases classified elsewhere —
      see category N74
    penis N48.29
      abscess N48.21
      cellulitis N48.22
  inhalant use ◀
    mild F18.10 ◀
      with ◀
        inhalant-induced ◀
          anxiety disorder F18.180 ◀
          depressive disorder F18.14 ◀
          major neurocognitive disorder
            F18.17 ◀
          mild neurocognitive disorder
            F18.188 ◀
          psychotic disorder F18.159 ◀
        inhalant intoxication F18.129 ◀
        inhalant intoxication delirium
          F18.121 ◀
    moderate or severe F18.20 ◀
      with ◀
        inhalant-induced ◀
          anxiety disorder F18.280 ◀
          depressive disorder F18.24 ◀
          major neurocognitive disorder
            F18.27 ◀
          mild neurocognitive disorder
            F18.288 ◀
          psychotic disorder F18.259 ◀
        inhalant intoxication F18.229 ◀
        inhalant intoxication delirium
          F18.221 ◀
  integument, newborn P83.9
    specified NEC P83.8
  intermittent explosive F63.81
  internal secretion pancreas —*see* Increased,
    secretion, pancreas, endocrine
  intestine, intestinal
    carbohydrate absorption NEC E74.39
      postoperative K91.2
    functional NEC K59.9
      postoperative K91.89
    psychogenic F45.8
    vascular K55.9
      chronic K55.1
      specified NEC K55.8
  intraoperative (intraprocedural) —*see*
    Complications, intraoperative
  involuntary emotional expression (IEED)
    F48.2
  iris H21.9
    adhesions —*see* Adhesions, iris
    atrophy —*see* Atrophy, iris
    chamber angle recession —*see* Recession,
      chamber angle
    cyst —*see* Cyst, iris
    degeneration —*see* Degeneration, iris
    in diseases classified elsewhere H22
    iridodialysis —*see* Iridodialysis
    iridoschisis —*see* Iridoschisis
    miotic pupillary cyst —*see* Cyst, pupillary
    pupillary
      abnormality —*see* Abnormality,
        pupillary
      membrane —*see* Membrane, pupillary
    specified type NEC H21.89
    vascular NEC H21.1X-
  iron metabolism E83.10
    specified NEC E83.19

◀ New   ◀▥ Revised   ~~deleted~~ Deleted

Disorder (Continued)
  isovaleric acidemia E71.110
  jaw, developmental M27.0
    temporomandibular —see also Anomaly,
      dentofacial, temporomandibular joint
      M26.60- ◀▥
  joint M25.9
    derangement —see Derangement, joint
    effusion —see Effusion, joint
    fistula —see Fistula, joint
    hemarthrosis —see Hemarthrosis
    instability —see Instability, joint
    osteophyte —see Osteophyte
    pain —see Pain, joint
    psychogenic F45.8
    specified type NEC M25.80
      ankle M25.87-
      elbow M25.82-
      foot joint M25.87-
      hand joint M25.84-
      hip M25.85-
      knee M25.86-
      shoulder M25.81-
      wrist M25.83-
    stiffness —see Stiffness, joint
  ketone metabolism E71.32
  kidney N28.9
    functional (tubular) N25.9
    in
      schistosomiasis B65.9 [N29]
    tubular function N25.9
      specified NEC N25.89
  lacrimal system H04.9
    changes H04.69
    fistula —see Fistula, lacrimal
    gland H04.19
      atrophy —see Atrophy, lacrimal
        gland
      cyst —see Cyst, lacrimal, gland
      dacryops —see Dacryops
      dislocation —see Dislocation, lacrimal
        gland
      dry eye syndrome —see Syndrome, dry
        eye
      infection —see Dacryoadenitis
      granuloma —see Granuloma, lacrimal
      inflammation —see Inflammation, lacrimal
      obstruction —see Obstruction, lacrimal
      specified NEC H04.89
  lactation NEC O92.79
  language (developmental) F80.9
    expressive F80.1
    mixed receptive and expressive F80.2
    receptive F80.2
  late luteal phase dysphoric N94.89
  learning (specific) F81.9
    acalculia R48.8
    alexia R48.0
    mathematics F81.2
    reading F81.0
    specified NEC F81.89
    spelling F81.81
    written expression F81.81
  lens H27.9
    aphakia —see Aphakia
    cataract —see Cataract
    dislocation —see Dislocation, lens
    specified type NEC H27.8
  ligament M24.20
    ankle M24.27-
    attachment, spine —see Enthesopathy,
      spinal
    elbow M24.22-
    foot joint M24.27-
    hand joint M24.24-
    hip M24.25-
    knee —see Derangement, knee, specified
      NEC
    shoulder M24.21-
    vertebra M24.28
    wrist M24.23-

Disorder (Continued)
  ligamentous attachments —see also
    Enthesopathy
    spine —see Enthesopathy, spinal
  lipid
    metabolism, congenital E78.9
    storage E75.6
      specified NEC E75.5
  lipoprotein
    deficiency (familial) E78.6
    metabolism E78.9
      specified NEC E78.89
  liver K76.9
    malarial B54 [K77]
  low back —see also Dorsopathy, specified
    NEC
  lumbosacral
    plexus G54.1
    root (nerve) NEC G54.4
  lung, interstitial, drug-induced J70.4
    acute J70.2
    chronic J70.3
  lymphoproliferative, post-transplant (PTLD)
    D47.Z1
  lysine and hydroxylysine metabolism E72.3
  major neurocognitive —see Dementia, in (due
    to) ◀
  male
    erectile (organic) —see also Dysfunction,
      sexual, male, erectile N52.9
      nonorganic F52.21
    hypoactive sexual desire F52.0
    orgasmic F52.32
  manic F30.9
    organic F06.33
  mast cell activation —see Activation, mast
    cell ◀
  mastoid —see also Disorder, ear, middle
    postprocedural —see Complications, ear,
      procedure
  meniscus —see Derangement, knee, meniscus
  menopausal N95.9
    specified NEC N95.8
  menstrual N92.6
    psychogenic F45.8
    specified NEC N92.5
  mental (or behavioral) (nonpsychotic) F99
    due to (secondary to)
      amphetamine
        due to drug abuse —see Abuse, drug,
          stimulant
        due to drug dependence —see
          Dependence, drug, stimulant
      brain disease, damage and dysfunction
        F09
      caffeine use
        due to drug abuse —see Abuse, drug,
          stimulant
        due to drug dependence —see
          Dependence, drug, stimulant
      cannabis use
        due to drug abuse —see Abuse, drug,
          cannabis
        due to drug dependence —see
          Dependence, drug, cannabis
      general medical condition F09
      sedative or hypnotic use
        due to drug abuse —see Abuse, drug,
          sedative
        due to drug dependence —see
          Dependence, drug, sedative
      tobacco (nicotine) use —see Dependence,
        drug, nicotine
    following organic brain damage F07.9
      frontal lobe syndrome F07.0
      personality change F07.0
      postconcussional syndrome F07.81
      specified NEC F07.89
    infancy, childhood or adolescence F98.9
    neurotic —see Neurosis
    organic or symptomatic F09

Disorder (Continued)
  mental (Continued)
    presenile, psychotic F03
    problem NEC
    psychoneurotic —see Neurosis
    psychotic —see Psychosis
    puerperal F53
    senile, psychotic NEC F03
  metabolic, amino acid, transitory, newborn
    P74.8
  metabolism NOS E88.9
    amino-acid E72.9
      aromatic E70.9
        albinism —see Albinism
        histidine E70.40
          histidinemia E70.41
          other specified E70.49
        hyperphenylalaninemia E70.1
          classical phenylketonuria E70.0
        other specified E70.8
        tryptophan E70.5
        tyrosine E70.20
          hypertyrosinemia E70.21
          other specified E70.29
      branched chain E71.2
        3-methylglutaconic aciduria E71.111
        hyperleucine-isoleucinemia E71.19
        hypervalinemia E71.19
        isovaleric acidemia E71.110
        maple syrup urine disease E71.0
        methylmalonic acidemia E71.120
        organic aciduria NEC E71.118
        other specified E71.19
        proprionate NEC E71.128
        proprionic acidemia E71.121
      glycine E72.50
        d-glycericacidemia E72.59
        hyperhydroxyprolinemia E72.59
        hyperoxaluria E72.53
        hyperprolinemia E72.59
        non-ketotic hyperglycinemia E72.51
        other specified E72.59
        sarcosinemia E72.59
        trimethylaminuria E72.52
      hydroxylysine E72.3
      lysine E72.3
      ornithine E72.4
      other specified E72.8
        beta-amino acid E72.8
        gamma-glutamyl cycle E72.8
      straight-chain E72.8
      sulfur-bearing E72.10
        homocystinuria E72.11
        methylenetetrahydrofolate reductase
          deficiency E72.12
        other specified E72.19
    bile acid and cholesterol metabolism
      E78.70
    bilirubin E80.7
      specified NEC E80.6
    calcium E83.50
      hypercalcemia E83.52
      hypocalcemia E83.51
      other specified E83.59
    carbohydrate E74.9
      specified NEC E74.8
    cholesterol and bile acid metabolism
      E78.70
    congenital E88.9
    copper E83.00
      specified type NEC E83.09
      Wilson's disease E83.01
    cystinuria E72.01
    fructose E74.10
    galactose E74.20
    glucosaminoglycan E76.9
      mucopolysaccharidosis —see
        Mucopolysaccharidosis
      specified NEC E76.8
    glutamine E72.8
    glycine E72.50

Disorder *(Continued)*
  metabolism *(Continued)*
    glycogen storage (hepatorenal) E74.09
    glycoprotein E77.9
      specified NEC E77.8
    glycosaminoglycan E76.9
      specified NEC E76.8
    in labor and delivery O75.89
    iron E83.10
    isoleucine E71.19
    leucine E71.19
    lipoid E78.9
    lipoprotein E78.9
      specified NEC E78.89
    magnesium E83.40
      hypermagnesemia E83.41
      hypomagnesemia E83.42
      other specified E83.49
    mineral E83.9
      specified NEC E83.89
    mitochondrial E88.40
      MELAS syndrome E88.41
      MERRF syndrome (myoclonic epilepsy
        associated with ragged-red fibers)
        E88.42
      other specified E88.49
    ornithine E72.4
    phosphatases E83.30
    phosphorus E83.30
      acid phosphatase deficiency E83.39
      hypophosphatasia E83.39
      hypophosphatemia E83.39
        familial E83.31
      other specified E83.39
      pseudovitamin D deficiency E83.32
    plasma protein NEC E88.09
    porphyrin —*see* Porphyria
    postprocedural E89.89
      specified NEC E89.89
    purine E79.9
      specified NEC E79.8
    pyrimidine E79.9
      specified NEC E79.8
    pyruvate E74.4
    serine E72.8
    sodium E87.8
    specified NEC E88.89
    threonine E72.8
    valine E71.19
    zinc E83.2
  methylmalonic acidemia E71.120
  micturition NEC —*see also* Difficulty,
    micturition R39.198 ◀▥
    feeling of incomplete emptying R39.14
    hesitancy R39.11
    poor stream R39.12
    psychogenic F45.8
    split stream R39.13
    straining R39.16
    urgency R39.15
  mild neurocognitive G31.84 ◀
  mitochondrial metabolism E88.40
  mitral (valve) —*see* Endocarditis, mitral
  mixed
    anxiety and depressive F41.8
    of scholastic skills (developmental)
      F81.89
    receptive expressive language F80.2
  mood F39
    bipolar —*see* Disorder, bipolar
    depressive —*see* Disorder, depressive
    due to (secondary to)
      alcohol F10.94
      amphetamine F15.94
        in
          abuse F15.14
          dependence F15.24
      anxiolytic F13.94
        in
          abuse F13.14
          dependence F13.24

Disorder *(Continued)*
  mood *(Continued)*
    due to *(Continued)*
      cocaine F14.94
        in
          abuse F14.14
          dependence F14.24
      general medical condition F06.30
      hallucinogen F16.94
        in
          abuse F16.14
          dependence F16.24
      hypnotic F13.94
        in
          abuse F13.14
          dependence F13.24
      inhalant F18.94
        in
          abuse F18.14
          dependence F18.24
      opioid F11.94
        in
          abuse F11.14
          dependence F11.24
      phencyclidine (PCP) F16.94
        in
          abuse F16.14
          dependence F16.24
      physiological condition F06.30
        with
          depressive features F06.31
          major depressive-like episode
            F06.32
          manic features F06.33
          mixed features F06.34
      psychoactive substance NEC F19.94
        in
          abuse F19.14
          dependence F19.24
      sedative F13.94
        in
          abuse F13.14
          dependence F13.24
      volatile solvents F18.94
        in
          abuse F18.14
          dependence F18.24
    manic episode F30.9
      with psychotic symptoms F30.2
      without psychotic symptoms F30.10
        mild F30.11
        moderate F30.12
        severe F30.13
      in remission (full) F30.4
        partial F30.3
      specified type NEC F30.8
    organic F06.30
      right hemisphere F07.89
    persistent F34.9
      cyclothymia F34.0
      dysthymia F34.1
      specified type NEC F34.89 ◀▥
    recurrent F39
    right hemisphere organic F07.89
  movement G25.9
    drug-induced G25.70
      akathisia G25.71
      specified NEC G25.79
    hysterical F44.4
    in diseases classified elsewhere —*see*
      category G26
    periodic limb G47.61
      sleep related G47.61
    sleep related NEC G47.69
    specified NEC G25.89
    stereotyped F98.4
    treatment-induced G25.9
  multiple personality F44.81
  muscle M62.9
    attachment, spine —*see* Enthesopathy,
      spinal

Disorder *(Continued)*
  muscle *(Continued)*
    in trichinellosis —*see* Trichinellosis, with
      muscle disorder
    psychogenic F45.8
    specified type NEC M62.89
    tone, newborn P94.9
      specified NEC P94.8
  muscular
    attachments —*see also* Enthesopathy
      spine —*see* Enthesopathy, spinal
    urethra N36.44
  musculoskeletal system, soft tissue —*see*
    Disorder, soft tissue
    postprocedural M96.89
    psychogenic F45.8
  myoneural G70.9
    due to lead G70.1
    specified NEC G70.89
    toxic G70.1
  myotonic NEC G71.19
  nail, in diseases classified elsewhere L62
  neck region NEC —*see* Dorsopathy, specified
    NEC
  neonatal onset multisystemic inflammatory
    (NOMID) M04.2 ◀
  nerve G58.9
    abducent NEC —*see* Strabismus, paralytic,
      sixth nerve
    accessory G52.8
    acoustic —*see* subcategory H93.3
    auditory —*see* subcategory H93.3
    auriculotemporal G50.8
    axillary G54.0
    cerebral —*see* Disorder, nerve, cranial
    cranial G52.9
      eighth —*see* subcategory H93.3
      eleventh G52.8
      fifth G50.9
      first G52.0
      fourth NEC —*see* Strabismus, paralytic,
        fourth nerve
      multiple G52.7
      ninth G52.1
      second NEC —*see* Disorder, nerve, optic
      seventh NEC G51.8
      sixth NEC —*see* Strabismus, paralytic,
        sixth nerve
      specified NEC G52.8
      tenth G52.2
      third NEC —*see* Strabismus, paralytic,
        third nerve
      twelfth G52.3
    entrapment —*see* Neuropathy, entrapment
    facial G51.9
      specified NEC G51.8
    femoral —*see* Lesion, nerve, femoral
    glossopharyngeal NEC G52.1
    hypoglossal G52.3
    intercostal G58.0
    lateral
      cutaneous of thigh —*see*
        Mononeuropathy, lower limb,
        meralgia paresthetica
      popliteal —*see* Lesion, nerve, popliteal
    lower limb —*see* Mononeuropathy, lower
      limb
    medial popliteal —*see* Lesion, nerve,
      popliteal, medial
    median NEC —*see* Lesion, nerve, median
    multiple G58.7
    oculomotor NEC —*see* Strabismus,
      paralytic, third nerve
    olfactory G52.0
    optic NEC H47.09-
      hemorrhage into sheath —*see*
        Hemorrhage, optic nerve
      ischemic H47.01-
    peroneal —*see* Lesion, nerve, popliteal
    phrenic G58.8
    plantar —*see* Lesion, nerve, plantar

◀ New   ◀▥ Revised   deleted Deleted

Disorder (Continued)
  nerve (Continued)
    pneumogastric G52.2
    posterior tibial —see Syndrome, tarsal
        tunnel
    radial —see Lesion, nerve, radial
    recurrent laryngeal G52.2
    root G54.9
      cervical G54.2
      lumbosacral G54.1
      specified NEC G54.8
      thoracic G54.3
    sciatic NEC —see Lesion, nerve, sciatic
    specified NEC G58.8
      lower limb —see Mononeuropathy,
          lower limb, specified NEC
      upper limb —see Mononeuropathy,
          upper limb, specified NEC
    sympathetic G90.9
    tibial —see Lesion, nerve, popliteal,
        medial
    trigeminal G50.9
      specified NEC G50.8
    trochlear NEC —see Strabismus, paralytic,
        fourth nerve
    ulnar —see Lesion, nerve, ulnar
    upper limb —see Mononeuropathy, upper
        limb
    vagus G52.2
  nervous system G98.8
    autonomic (peripheral) G90.9
      specified NEC G90.8
    central G96.9
      specified NEC G96.8
    parasympathetic G90.9
    specified NEC G98.8
    sympathetic G90.9
    vegetative G90.9
  neurocognitive ◄
    major ◄
      with ◄
        aggressive behavior F01.51 ◄
        combative behavior F01.51 ◄
        violent behavior F01.51 ◄
      due to vascular disease, with behavioral
          disturbance F01.51 ◄
      in (due to) (other diseases classified
          elsewhere) —see also Dementia, in
          (due to) F02.80 ◄
        with ◄
          aggressive behavior F02.81 ◄
          combative behavior F02.81 ◄
          violent behavior F02.81 ◄
        without behavioral disturbance
            F01.50 ◄
    mild G31.84 ◄
  neurodevelopmental F89 ◄
    specified NEC F88 ◄
  neurohypophysis NEC E23.3
  neurological NEC R29.818
  neuromuscular G70.9
    hereditary NEC G71.9
    specified NEC G70.89
    toxic G70.1
  neurotic F48.9
    specified NEC F48.8
  neutrophil, polymorphonuclear D71
  nicotine use —see Dependence, drug,
      nicotine
  nightmare F51.5
  nose J34.9
    specified NEC J34.89
  obsessive-compulsive F42.9 ◄▥
  odontogenesis NOS K00.9
  opioid use
    with
      opioid-induced psychotic disorder
          F11.959
        with
          delusions F11.950
          hallucinations F11.951

Disorder (Continued)
  opioid use (Continued)
    due to drug abuse —see Abuse, drug,
        opioid
    due to drug dependence —see Dependence,
        drug, opioid
    mild F11.10 ◄
      with ◄
        opioid-induced ◄
          anxiety disorder F11.188 ◄
          depressive disorder F11.14 ◄
          sexual dysfunction F11.181 ◄
        opioid intoxication ◄
          with perceptual disturbances
              F11.122 ◄
          delirium F11.121 ◄
          without perceptual disturbances
              F11.129 ◄
    moderate or severe F11.20 ◄
      with ◄
        opioid-induced ◄
          anxiety disorder F11.288 ◄
          anxiety disorder F11.988 ◄
          depressive disorder F11.24 ◄
          depressive disorder F11.94 ◄
          sexual dysfunction F11.281 ◄
          sexual dysfunction F11.981 ◄
        opioid intoxication ◄
          with perceptual disturbances
              F11.222 ◄
          delirium F11.221 ◄
          without perceptual disturbances
              F11.229 ◄
  oppositional defiant F91.3
  optic
    chiasm H47.49
      due to
        inflammatory disorder H47.41
        neoplasm H47.42
        vascular disorder H47.43
    disc H47.39-
      coloboma —see Coloboma, optic disc
      drusen —see Drusen, optic disc
      pseudopapilledema —see
          Pseudopapilledema
    radiations —see Disorder, visual, pathway
    tracts —see Disorder, visual, pathway
  orbit H05.9
    cyst —see Cyst, orbit
    deformity —see Deformity, orbit
    edema —see Edema, orbit
    enophthalmos —see Enophthalmos
    exophthalmos —see Exophthalmos
    hemorrhage —see Hemorrhage, orbit
    inflammation —see Inflammation, orbit
    myopathy —see Myopathy, extraocular
        muscles
    retained foreign body —see Foreign body,
        orbit, old
    specified type NEC H05.89
  organic
    anxiety F06.4
    catatonic F06.1
    delusional F06.2
    dissociative F06.8
    emotionally labile (asthenic) F06.8
    mood (affective) F06.30
    schizophrenia-like F06.2
  orgasmic (female) F52.31
    male F52.32
  ornithine metabolism E72.4
  overanxious F41.1
    of childhood F93.8
  pain
    with related psychological factors F45.42
    exclusively related to psychological factors
        F45.41
    genito-pelvic penetration disorder
        F52.6 ◄
  pancreatic internal secretion E16.9
    specified NEC E16.8

Disorder (Continued)
  panic F41.0
    with agoraphobia F40.01
  papulosquamous L44.9
    in diseases classified elsewhere L45
    specified NEC L44.8
  paranoid F22
    induced F24
    shared F24
  parathyroid (gland) E21.5
    specified NEC E21.4
  parietoalveolar NEC J84.09
  paroxysmal, mixed R56.9
  patella M22.9-
    chondromalacia —see Chondromalacia,
        patella
    derangement NEC M22.3X-
    recurrent
      dislocation —see Dislocation, patella,
          recurrent
      subluxation —see Dislocation, patella,
          recurrent, incomplete
    specified NEC M22.8X-
  patellofemoral M22.2X-
  pentose phosphate pathway with anemia
      D55.1
  perception, due to hallucinogens F16.983
    in
      abuse F16.183
      dependence F16.283
  peripheral nervous system NEC G64
  peroxisomal E71.50
    biogenesis
      neonatal adrenoleukodystrophy E71.511
      specified disorder NEC E71.518
      Zellweger syndrome E71.510
    rhizomelic chondrodysplasia punctata
        E71.540
    specified form NEC E71.548
      group 1 E71.518
      group 2 E71.53
      group 3 E71.542
    X-linked adrenoleukodystrophy
        E71.529
      adolescent E71.521
      adrenomyeloneuropathy E71.522
      childhood E71.520
      specified form NEC E71.528
    Zellweger-like syndrome E71.541
  persistent
    (somatoform) pain F45.41
    affective (mood) F34.9
  personality —see also Personality F60.9
    affective F34.0
    aggressive F60.3
    amoral F60.2
    anankastic F60.5
    antisocial F60.2
    anxious F60.6
    asocial F60.2
    asthenic F60.7
    avoidant F60.6
    borderline F60.3
    change (secondary) due to general medical
        condition F07.0
    compulsive F60.5
    cyclothymic F34.0
    dependent (passive) F60.7
    depressive F34.1
    dissocial F60.2
    emotional instability F60.3
    expansive paranoid F60.0
    explosive F60.3
    following organic brain damage
        F07.9
    histrionic F60.4
    hyperthymic F34.0
    hypothymic F34.1
    hysterical F60.4
    immature F60.89
    inadequate F60.7

Disorder *(Continued)*
  personality *(Continued)*
    labile F60.3
    mixed (nonspecific) F60.89
    moral deficiency F60.2
    narcissistic F60.81
    negativistic F60.89
    obsessional F60.5
    obsessive (-compulsive) F60.5
    organic F07.9
    overconscientious F60.5
    paranoid F60.0
    passive (-dependent) F60.7
    passive-aggressive F60.89
    pathological NEC F60.9
    pseudosocial F60.2
    psychopathic F60.2
    schizoid F60.1
    schizotypal F21
    self-defeating F60.7
    specified NEC F60.89
    type A F60.5
    unstable (emotional) F60.3
  pervasive, developmental F84.9
  phencyclidine use ◀
    mild F16.10 ◀
      with ◀
        phencyclidine-induced ◀
          anxiety disorder F16.180 ◀
          bipolar and related disorder
            F16.14 ◀
          depressive disorder F16.14 ◀
          psychotic disorder F16.159 ◀
        phencyclidine intoxication
          F16.129 ◀
        phencyclidine intoxication delirium
          F16.121 ◀
    moderate or severe F16.20 ◀
      with ◀
        phencyclidine-induced ◀
          anxiety disorder F16.280 ◀
          bipolar and related disorder
            F16.24 ◀
          depressive disorder F16.24 ◀
          psychotic disorder F16.259 ◀
        phencyclidine intoxication F16.229 ◀
        phencyclidine intoxication delirium
          F16.221 ◀
  phobic anxiety, childhood F40.8
  phosphate-losing tubular N25.0
  pigmentation L81.9
    choroid, congenital Q14.3
    diminished melanin formation L81.6
    iron L81.8
    specified NEC L81.8
  pinna (noninfective) H61.10-
    deformity, acquired H61.11-
    hematoma H61.12-
    perichondritis —*see* Perichondritis, ear
    specified type NEC H61.19-
  pituitary gland E23.7
    iatrogenic (postprocedural) E89.3
    specified NEC E23.6
  platelets D69.1
  plexus G54.9
    specified NEC G54.8
  polymorphonuclear neutrophils D71
  porphyrin metabolism —*see* Porphyria
  postconcussional F07.81
  posthallucinogen perception F16.983
    in
      abuse F16.183
      dependence F16.283
  postmenopausal N95.9
    specified NEC N95.8
  postprocedural (postoperative) —*see*
    Complications, postprocedural
  post-transplant lymphoproliferative D47.z1
  post-traumatic stress (PTSD) F43.10
    acute F43.11
    chronic F43.12

Disorder *(Continued)*
  premenstrual dysphoric (PMDD) F32.81 ◁◀
  prepuce N47.8
  propionic acidemia E71.121
  prostate N42.9
    specified NEC N42.89
  psychogenic NOS —*see also* condition F45.9
    anxiety F41.8
    appetite F50.9
    asthenic F48.8
    cardiovascular (system) F45.8
    compulsive F42.8 ◁◀
    cutaneous F54
    depressive F32.9
    digestive (system) F45.8
    dysmenorrheic F45.8
    dyspneic F45.8
    endocrine (system) F54
    eye NEC F45.8
    feeding —*see* Disorder, eating
    functional NEC F45.8
    gastric F45.8
    gastrointestinal (system) F45.8
    genitourinary (system) F45.8
    heart (function) (rhythm) F45.8
    hyperventilatory F45.8
    hypochondriacal —*see* Disorder,
      hypochondriacal
    intestinal F45.8
    joint F45.8
    learning F81.9
    limb F45.8
    lymphatic (system) F45.8
    menstrual F45.8
    micturition F45.8
    monoplegic NEC F44.4
    motor F44.4
    muscle F45.8
    musculoskeletal F45.8
    neurocirculatory F45.8
    obsessive F42.8 ◁◀
    occupational F48.8
    organ or part of body NEC F45.8
    paralytic NEC F44.4
    phobic F40.9
    physical NEC F45.8
    rectal F45.8
    respiratory (system) F45.8
    rheumatic F45.8
    sexual (function) F52.9
    skin (allergic) (eczematous) F54
    sleep F51.9
    specified part of body NEC F45.8
    stomach F45.8
  psychological F99
    associated with
      disease classified elsewhere F54
      sexual
        development F66
        relationship F66
      uncertainty about gender identity
        F64.9 ◁◀
  psychomotor NEC F44.4
    hysterical F44.4
  psychoneurotic —*see also* Neurosis
    mixed NEC F48.8
  psychophysiologic —*see* Disorder,
    somatoform
  psychosexual F65.9
    development F66
    identity of childhood F64.2
  psychosomatic NOS —*see* Disorder,
    somatoform
    multiple F45.0
    undifferentiated F45.1
  psychotic —*see* Psychosis
    transient (acute) F23
  puberty E30.9
    specified NEC E30.8
  pulmonary (valve) —*see* Endocarditis,
    pulmonary

Disorder *(Continued)*
  purine metabolism E79.9
  pyrimidine metabolism E79.9
  pyruvate metabolism E74.4
  reactive attachment (childhood) F94.1
  reading R48.0
    developmental (specific) F81.0
  receptive language F80.2
  receptor, hormonal, peripheral —*see also*
    Syndrome, androgen insensitivity
    E34.50
  recurrent brief depressive F33.8
  reflex R29.2
  refraction H52.7
    aniseikonia H52.32
    anisometropia H52.31
    astigmatism —*see* Astigmatism
    hypermetropia —*see* Hypermetropia
    myopia —*see* Myopia
    presbyopia H52.4
    specified NEC H52.6
  relationship F68.8
    due to sexual orientation F66
  REM sleep behavior G47.52
  renal function, impaired (tubular) N25.9
  resonance R49.9
    specified NEC R49.8
  respiratory function, impaired —*see also*
    Failure, respiration
      postprocedural —*see* Complication,
        postoperative, respiratory system
      psychogenic F45.8
  retina H35.9
    angioid streaks H35.33
    changes in vascular appearance H35.01-
    degeneration —*see* Degeneration, retina
    dystrophy (hereditary) —*see* Dystrophy,
      retina
    edema H35.81
    hemorrhage —*see* Hemorrhage, retina
    ischemia H35.82
    macular degeneration —*see* Degeneration,
      macula
    microaneurysms H35.04-
    microvascular abnormality NEC
      H35.09
    neovascularization —*see*
      Neovascularization, retina
    retinopathy —*see* Retinopathy
    separation of layers H35.70
      central serous chorioretinopathy
        H35.71-
      pigment epithelium detachment (serous)
        H35.72-
        hemorrhagic H35.73-
    specified type NEC H35.89
    telangiectasis —*see* Telangiectasis, retina
    vasculitis —*see* Vasculitis, retina
  retroperitoneal K68.9
  right hemisphere organic affective F07.89
  rumination (infant or child) F98.21
  sacrum, sacrococcygeal NEC M53.3
  schizoaffective F25.9
    bipolar type F25.0
    depressive type F25.1
    manic type F25.0
    mixed type F25.0
    specified NEC F25.8
  schizoid of childhood F84.5
  schizophreniform F20.81
    brief F23
  schizotypal (personality) F21
  secretion, thyrocalcitonin E07.0
  sedative, hypnotic, or anxiolytic use ◀
    mild F13.10 ◀
      with ◀
        sedative, hypnotic, or anxiolytic-
          induced ◀
          anxiety disorder F13.180 ◀
          bipolar and related disorder
            F13.14 ◀

Disorder (Continued)
  sedative, hypnotic, or anxiolytic use
      (Continued)
    mild (Continued)
      with (Continued)
        sedative, hypnotic, or anxiolytic-
            induced (Continued)
          depressive disorder F13.14 ◀
          psychotic disorder F13.159 ◀
          sexual dysfunction F13.181 ◀
        sedative, hypnotic, or anxiolytic
            intoxication F13.129 ◀
        sedative, hypnotic, or anxiolytic
            intoxication delirium F13.121 ◀
    moderate or severe F13.20 ◀
      with ◀
        sedative, hypnotic, or anxiolytic-
            induced ◀
          anxiety disorder F13.280 ◀
          bipolar and related disorder
              F13.24 ◀
          depressive disorder F13.24 ◀
          major neurocognitive disorder
              F13.27 ◀
          mild neurocognitive disorder
              F13.288 ◀
          psychotic disorder F13.259 ◀
          sexual dysfunction F13.281 ◀
        sedative, hypnotic, or anxiolytic
            intoxication F13.229 ◀
        sedative, hypnotic, or anxiolytic
            intoxication delirium F13.221 ◀
  seizure —see also Epilepsy G40.909
    intractable G40.919
      with status epilepticus G40.911
  semantic pragmatic F80.89
    with autism F84.0
  sense of smell R43.1
    psychogenic F45.8
  separation anxiety, of childhood F93.0
  sexual
    arousal, female F52.22
    aversion F52.1
    function, psychogenic F52.9
    maturation F66
    nonorganic F52.9
    preference —see also Deviation, sexual
        F65.9
      fetishistic transvestism F65.1
    relationship F66
  shyness, of childhood and adolescence F40.10
  sibling rivalry F93.8
  sickle-cell (sickling) (homozygous) —see
      Disease, sickle-cell
    heterozygous D57.3
    specified type NEC D57.8-
    trait D57.3
  sinus (nasal) J34.9
    specified NEC J34.89
  skin L98.9
    atrophic L90.9
      specified NEC L90.8
    granulomatous L92.9
      specified NEC L92.8
    hypertrophic L91.9
      specified NEC L91.8
    infiltrative NEC L98.6
    newborn P83.9
      specified NEC P83.8
    picking F42.4 ◀
    psychogenic (allergic) (eczematous) F54
  sleep G47.9
    breathing-related —see Apnea, sleep
    circadian rhythm G47.20
      advance sleep phase type G47.22
      delayed sleep phase type G47.21
      due to
        alcohol
          abuse F10.182
          dependence F10.282
          use F10.982

Disorder (Continued)
  sleep (Continued)
    circadian rhythm (Continued)
      due to (Continued)
        amphetamines
          abuse F15.182
          dependence F15.282
          use F15.982
        caffeine
          abuse F15.182
          dependence F15.282
          use F15.982
        cocaine
          abuse F14.182
          dependence F14.282
          use F14.982
        drug NEC
          abuse F19.182
          dependence F19.282
          use F19.982
        opioid
          abuse F11.182
          dependence F11.282
          use F11.982
        psychoactive substance NEC
          abuse F19.182
          dependence F19.282
          use F19.982
        sedative, hypnotic, or anxiolytic
          abuse F13.182
          dependence F13.282
          use F13.982
        stimulant NEC
          abuse F15.182
          dependence F15.282
          use F15.982
      free running type G47.24
      in conditions classified elsewhere
          G47.27
      irregular sleep wake type
          G47.23
      jet lag type G47.25
      shift work type G47.26
      specified NEC G47.29
    due to
      alcohol
        abuse F10.182
        dependence F10.282
        use F10.982
      amphetamine
        abuse F15.182
        dependence F15.282
        use F15.982
      anxiolytic
        abuse F13.182
        dependence F13.282
        use F13.982
      caffeine
        abuse F15.182
        dependence F15.282
        use F15.982
      cocaine
        abuse F14.182
        dependence F14.282
        use F14.982
      drug NEC
        abuse F19.182
        dependence F19.282
        use F19.982
      hypnotic
        abuse F13.182
        dependence F13.282
        use F13.982
      opioid
        abuse F11.182
        dependence F11.282
        use F11.982
      psychoactive substance NEC
        abuse F19.182
        dependence F19.282
        use F19.982

Disorder (Continued)
  sleep (Continued)
    due to (Continued)
      sedative
        abuse F13.182
        dependence F13.282
        use F13.982
      stimulant NEC
        abuse F15.182
        dependence F15.282
        use F15.982
    emotional F51.9
    excessive somnolence —see Hypersomnia
    hypersomnia type —see Hypersomnia
    initiating or maintaining —see Insomnia
    nightmares F51.5
    nonorganic F51.9
      specified NEC F51.8
    parasomnia type G47.50
    specified NEC G47.8
    terrors F51.4
    walking F51.3
  sleep-wake pattern or schedule —see
      Disorder, sleep, circadian rhythm
  social
    anxiety of childhood F40.10
    functioning in childhood F94.9
      specified NEC F94.8
    pragmatic F80.82 ◀
  soft tissue M79.9
    ankle M79.9
    due to use, overuse and pressure
        M70.90
      ankle M70.97-
      bursitis —see Bursitis
      foot M70.97-
      forearm M70.93-
      hand M70.94-
      lower leg M70.96-
      multiple sites M70.99
      pelvic region M70.95-
      shoulder region M70.91-
      specified site NEC M70.98
      specified type NEC M70.80
        ankle M70.87-
        foot M70.87-
        forearm M70.83-
        hand M70.84-
        lower leg M70.86-
        multiple sites M70.89
        pelvic region M70.85-
        shoulder region M70.81-
        specified site NEC M70.88
        thigh M70.85-
        upper arm M70.82-
      thigh M70.95-
      upper arm M70.92-
    foot M79.9
    forearm M79.9
    hand M79.9
    lower leg M79.9
    multiple sites M79.9
    occupational —see Disorder, soft tissue,
        due to use, overuse and pressure
    pelvic region M79.9
    shoulder region M79.9
    specified type NEC M79.89
    thigh M79.9
    upper arm M79.9
  somatic symptom F45.1 ◀
  somatization F45.0
  somatoform F45.9
    pain (persistent) F45.41
    somatization (multiple) (long-lasting) F45.0
    specified NEC F45.8
    undifferentiated F45.1
  somnolence, excessive —see Hypersomnia
  specific
    arithmetical F81.2
    developmental, of motor F82
    reading F81.0

Disorder *(Continued)*
  specific *(Continued)*
    speech and language F80.9
    spelling F81.81
    written expression F81.81
  speech R47.9
    articulation (functional) (specific) F80.0
    developmental F80.9
    specified NEC R47.89
  speech-sound F80.0 ◀
  spelling (specific) F81.81
  spine —*see also* Dorsopathy
    ligamentous or muscular attachments, peripheral —*see* Enthesopathy, spinal
    specified NEC —*see* Dorsopathy, specified NEC
  stereotyped, habit or movement F98.4
  stimulant use (other) (unspecified) ◀
    mild F15.10 ◀
    moderate or severe F15.20 ◀
  stomach (functional) —*see* Disorder, gastric
  stress F43.9
    acute F43.0 ◀
    post-traumatic F43.10
      acute F43.11
      chronic F43.12
  substance use (other) (unknown) ◀
    mild F19.10 ◀
      with substance-induced ◀
        anxiety disorder F19.180 ◀
        bipolar and related disorder F19.14 ◀
        depressive disorder F19.14 ◀
        major neurocognitive disorder F19.17 ◀
        mild neurocognitive disorder F19.188 ◀
        obsessive-compulsive and related disorder F19.188 ◀
        sexual dysfunction F19.181 ◀
        substance intoxication F19.129 ◀
        substance intoxication delirium F19.121 ◀
    moderate or severe F19.20 ◀
      with substance-induced ◀
        anxiety disorder F19.280 ◀
        bipolar and related disorder F19.24 ◀
        depressive disorder F19.24 ◀
        major neurocognitive disorder F19.27 ◀
        mild neurocognitive disorder F19.288 ◀
        obsessive-compulsive and related disorder F19.288 ◀
        sexual dysfunction F19.281 ◀
        substance intoxication F19.229 ◀
        substance intoxication delirium F19.221 ◀
  sulfur-bearing amino-acid metabolism E72.10
  sweat gland (eccrine) L74.9
    apocrine L75.9
      specified NEC L75.8
    specified NEC L74.8
  synovium M67.90
    acromioclavicular M67.91-
    ankle M67.97-
    elbow M67.92-
    foot M67.97-
    forearm M67.93-
    hand M67.94-
    hip M67.95-
    knee M67.96-
    multiple sites M67.99
    rupture —*see* Rupture, synovium
    shoulder M67.91-
    specified type NEC M67.80
      acromioclavicular M67.81-
      ankle M67.87-
      elbow M67.82-
      foot M67.87-
      hand M67.84-
      hip M67.85-

Disorder *(Continued)*
  synovium *(Continued)*
    specified type *(Continued)*
      knee M67.86-
      multiple sites M67.89
      wrist M67.83-
    synovitis —*see* Synovitis
    upper arm M67.92-
    wrist M67.93-
  temperature regulation, newborn P81.9
    specified NEC P81.8
  temporomandibular joint M26.60- ◀▥
  tendon M67.90
    acromioclavicular M67.91-
    ankle M67.97-
    contracture —*see* Contracture, tendon
    elbow M67.92-
    foot M67.97-
    forearm M67.93-
    hand M67.94-
    hip M67.95-
    knee M67.96-
    multiple sites M67.99
    rupture —*see* Rupture, tendon
    shoulder M67.91-
    specified type NEC M67.80
      acromioclavicular M67.81-
      ankle M67.87-
      elbow M67.82-
      foot M67.87-
      hand M67.84-
      hip M67.85-
      knee M67.86-
      multiple sites M67.89
      trunk M67.88
      wrist M67.83-
    synovitis —*see* Synovitis
    tendinitis —*see* Tendinitis
    tenosynovitis —*see* Tenosynovitis
    trunk M67.98
    upper arm M67.92-
    wrist M67.93-
  thoracic root (nerve) NEC G54.3
  thyrocalcitonin hypersecretion E07.0
  thyroid (gland) E07.9
    function NEC, neonatal, transitory P72.2
    iodine-deficiency related E01.8
    specified NEC E07.89
  tic —*see* Tic
  tobacco use ◀
    mild Z72.0 ◀
    moderate F17.200 ◀
    severe F17.200 ◀
  tooth K08.9
    development K00.9
      specified NEC K00.8
    eruption K00.6
  Tourette's F95.2
  trance and possession F44.89
  trauma and stressor-related F43.9 ◀
    other specified F43.8 ◀
  tricuspid (valve) —*see* Endocarditis, tricuspid
  tryptophan metabolism E70.5
  tubular, phosphate-losing N25.0
  tubulo-interstitial (in)
    brucellosis A23.9 *[N16]*
    cystinosis E72.04
    diphtheria A36.84
    glycogen storage disease E74.00 *[N16]*
    leukemia NEC C95.9- *[N16]*
    lymphoma NEC C85.9- *[N16]*
    mixed cryoglobulinemia D89.1 *[N16]*
    multiple myeloma C90.0- *[N16]*
    Salmonella infection A02.25
    sarcoidosis D86.84
    sepsis A41.9 *[N16]*
      streptococcal A40.9 *[N16]*
    systemic lupus erythematosus M32.15
    toxoplasmosis B58.83
    transplant rejection T86.91 *[N16]*
    Wilson's disease E83.01 *[N16]*

Disorder *(Continued)*
  tubulo-renal function, impaired N25.9
    specified NEC N25.89
  tympanic membrane H73.9-
    atrophy —*see* Atrophy, tympanic membrane
    infection —*see* Myringitis
    perforation —*see* Perforation, tympanum
    specified NEC H73.89-
  unsocialized aggressive F91.1
  urea cycle metabolism E72.20
    argininemia E72.21
    arginosuccinic aciduria E72.22
    citrullinemia E72.23
    ornithine transcarbamylase deficiency E72.4
    other specified E72.29
  ureter (in) N28.9
    schistosomiasis B65.0 *[N29]*
    tuberculosis A18.11
  urethra N36.9
    specified NEC N36.8
  urinary system N39.9
    specified NEC N39.8
  valve, heart
    aortic —*see* Endocarditis, aortic
    mitral —*see* Endocarditis, mitral
    pulmonary —*see* Endocarditis, pulmonary
    rheumatic
      aortic —*see* Endocarditis, aortic, rheumatic
      mitral —*see* Endocarditis, mitral
      pulmonary —*see* Endocarditis, pulmonary, rheumatic
      tricuspid —*see* Endocarditis, tricuspid
    tricuspid —*see* Endocarditis, tricuspid
  vestibular function H81.9-
    specified NEC —*see* subcategory H81.8
    in diseases classified elsewhere H82.-
    vertigo —*see* Vertigo
  vision, binocular H53.30
    abnormal retinal correspondence H53.31
    diplopia H53.2
    fusion with defective stereopsis H53.32
    simultaneous perception H53.33
    suppression H53.34
  visual
    cortex
      blindness H47.619
        left brain H47.612
        right brain H47.611
      due to
        inflammatory disorder H47.629
          left brain H47.622
          right brain H47.621
        neoplasm H47.639
          left brain H47.632
          right brain H47.631
        vascular disorder H47.649
          left brain H47.642
          right brain H47.641
    pathway H47.9
      due to
        inflammatory disorder H47.51-
        neoplasm H47.52-
        vascular disorder H47.53-
    optic chiasm —*see* Disorder, optic, chiasm
  vitreous body H43.9
    crystalline deposits —*see* Deposit, crystalline
    degeneration —*see* Degeneration, vitreous
    hemorrhage —*see* Hemorrhage, vitreous
    opacities —*see* Opacity, vitreous
    prolapse —*see* Prolapse, vitreous
    specified type NEC H43.89
  voice R49.9
    specified type NEC R49.8
  volatile solvent use
    due to drug abuse —*see* Abuse, drug, inhalant
    due to drug dependence —*see* Dependence, drug, inhalant

◀ New   ◀▥ Revised   ~~deleted~~ Deleted

Disorder (Continued)
  white blood cells D72.9
    specified NEC D72.89
  withdrawing, child or adolescent
    F40.10
Disorientation R41.0
Displacement, displaced
  acquired traumatic of bone, cartilage, joint,
    tendon NEC —see Dislocation
  adrenal gland (congenital) Q89.1
  appendix, retrocecal (congenital) Q43.8
  auricle (congenital) Q17.4
  bladder (acquired) N32.89
    congenital Q64.19
  brachial plexus (congenital) Q07.8
  brain stem, caudal (congenital) Q04.8
  canaliculus (lacrimalis), congenital Q10.6
  cardia through esophageal hiatus (congenital)
    Q40.1
  cerebellum, caudal (congenital) Q04.8
  cervix —see Malposition, uterus
  colon (congenital) Q43.3
  device, implant or graft —see also
    Complications, by site and type,
    mechanical T85.628
    arterial graft NEC —see Complication,
      cardiovascular device, mechanical,
      vascular
    breast (implant) T85.42
    catheter NEC T85.628
      dialysis (renal) T82.42
        intraperitoneal T85.621
      infusion NEC T82.524
        spinal (epidural) (subdural)
          T85.620
      urinary ◀▥
        cystostomy T83.020
        Hopkins T83.028 ◀
        ileostomy T83.028 ◀
        indwelling T83.021 ◀
        nephrostomy T83.022 ◀
        specified NEC T83.028 ◀
        urostomy T83.028 ◀
    electronic (electrode) (pulse generator)
      (stimulator) —see Complication,
      electronic stimulator
    fixation, internal (orthopedic) NEC —see
      Complication, fixation device,
      mechanical
    gastrointestinal —see Complications,
      prosthetic device, mechanical,
      gastrointestinal device
    genital NEC T83.428
      intrauterine contraceptive device (string)
        T83.32 ◀▥
      penile prosthesis (cylinder) (implanted)
        (pump) (resevoir) T83.420 ◀▥
      testicular prosthesis T83.421 ◀
    heart NEC —see Complication,
      cardiovascular device, mechanical
    joint prosthesis —see Complications, joint
      prosthesis, mechanical
    ocular —see Complications, prosthetic
      device, mechanical, ocular device
    orthopedic NEC —see Complication,
      orthopedic, device or graft,
      mechanical
    specified NEC T85.628
    urinary NEC T83.128 ◀▥
      graft T83.22
      sphincter, implanted T83.121 ◀
      stent (ileal conduit) (nephroureteral)
        T83.123 ◀
      ureteral indwelling T83.122 ◀
    vascular NEC —see Complication,
      cardiovascular device, mechanical
    ventricular intracranial shunt T85.02
  electronic stimulator
    bone T84.320
    cardiac —see Complications, cardiac
      device, electronic

Displacement, displaced (Continued)
  electronic stimulator (Continued)
    nervous system —see Complication,
      prosthetic device, mechanical,
      electronic nervous system
      stimulator
    urinary —see Complications, electronic
      stimulator, urinary
  esophageal mucosa into cardia of stomach,
    congenital Q39.8
  esophagus (acquired) K22.8
    congenital Q39.8
  eyeball (acquired) (lateral) (old) —see
    Displacement, globe
    congenital Q15.8
    current —see Avulsion, eye
  fallopian tube (acquired) N83.4- ◀▥
    congenital Q50.6
    opening (congenital) Q50.6
  gallbladder (congenital) Q44.1
  gastric mucosa (congenital) Q40.2
  globe (acquired) (old) (lateral) H05.21-
    current —see Avulsion, eye
  heart (congenital) Q24.8
    acquired I51.89
  hymen (upward) (congenital) Q52.4
  intervertebral disc NEC
    with myelopathy —see Disorder, disc, with,
      myelopathy
    cervical, cervicothoracic (with)
      M50.20
      myelopathy —see Disorder, disc,
        cervical, with myelopathy
      neuritis, radiculitis or radiculopathy —
        see Disorder, disc, cervical, with
        neuritis
    due to trauma —see Dislocation, vertebra
    lumbar region M51.26
      with
        neuritis, radiculitis, radiculopathy or
          sciatica M51.16
    lumbosacral region M51.27
      with
        myelopathy M51.07
        neuritis, radiculitis, radiculopathy or
          sciatica M51.17
    sacrococcygeal region M53.3
    thoracic region M51.24
      with
        myelopathy M51.04
        neuritis, radiculitis, radiculopathy
          M51.14
    thoracolumbar region M51.25
      with
        myelopathy M51.05
        neuritis, radiculitis, radiculopathy
          M51.15
  intrauterine device (string) T83.32 ◀▥
  kidney (acquired) N28.83
    congenital Q63.2
  lachrymal, lacrimal apparatus or duct
    (congenital) Q10.6
  lens, congenital Q12.1
  macula (congenital) Q14.1
  Meckel's diverticulum Q43.0
    malignant —see Table of Neoplasms, small
      intestine, malignant
  nail (congenital) Q84.6
    acquired L60.8
  opening of Wharton's duct in mouth Q38.4
  organ or site, congenital NEC —see
    Malposition, congenital
  ovary (acquired) N83.4- ◀▥
    congenital Q50.39
    free in peritoneal cavity (congenital)
      Q50.39
    into hernial sac N83.4- ◀▥
  oviduct (acquired) N83.4- ◀▥
    congenital Q50.6
  parathyroid (gland) E21.4
  parotid gland (congenital) Q38.4

Displacement, displaced (Continued)
  punctum lacrimale (congenital) Q10.6
  sacro-iliac (joint) (congenital) Q74.2
    current injury S33.2
    old —see subcategory M53.2
  salivary gland (any) (congenital) Q38.4
  spleen (congenital) Q89.09
  stomach, congenital Q40.2
  sublingual duct Q38.4
  tongue (downward) (congenital) Q38.3
  tooth, teeth, fully erupted M26.30
    horizontal M26.33
    vertical M26.34
  trachea (congenital) Q32.1
  ureter or ureteric opening or orifice
    (congenital) Q62.62
  uterine opening of oviducts or fallopian tubes
    Q50.6
  uterus, uterine —see Malposition, uterus
  ventricular septum Q21.0
    with rudimentary ventricle Q20.4
Disproportion
  between native and reconstructed breast N65.1
  fiber-type G71.2
Disruptio uteri —see Rupture, uterus
Disruption (of)
  ciliary body NEC H21.89
  closure of
    cornea T81.31
    craniotomy T81.32
    fascia (muscular) (superficial) T81.32
    internal organ or tissue T81.32
    laceration (external) (internal) T81.33
    ligament T81.32
    mucosa T81.31
    muscle or muscle flap T81.32
    ribs or rib cage T81.32
    skin and subcutaneous tissue (full-
      thickness) (superficial) T81.31
    skull T81.32
    sternum (sternotomy) T81.32
    tendon T81.32
    traumatic laceration (external) (internal)
      T81.33
  family Z63.8
    due to
      absence of family member due to
        military deployment Z63.31
      absence of family member NEC Z63.32
      alcoholism and drug addiction in family
        Z63.72
      bereavement Z63.4
      death (assumed) or disappearance of
        family member Z63.4
      divorce or separation Z63.5
      drug addiction in family Z63.72
      return of family member from military
        deployment (current or past
        conflict) Z63.71
      stressful life events NEC Z63.79
  iris NEC H21.89
  ligament (s) —see also Sprain
    knee
      current injury —see Dislocation, knee
      old (chronic) —see Derangement, knee,
        ligament, instability, chronic
      spontaneous NEC —see Derangement,
        knee, disruption ligament
  ossicular chain —see Discontinuity, ossicles, ear
  pelvic ring (stable) S32.810
    unstable S32.811
  traumatic injury wound repair T81.33
  wound T81.30
    episiotomy O90.1
    operation T81.31
      cesarean O90.0
      external operation wound (superficial)
        T81.31
      internal operation wound (deep) T81.32
    perineal (obstetric) O90.1
  traumatic injury repair T81.33

Dissatisfaction with
   employment Z56.9
   school environment Z55.4
Dissecting —see condition
Dissection
   aorta I71.00
      abdominal I71.02
      thoracic I71.01
      thoracoabdominal I71.03
   artery I77.70 ◄▥
      basilar (trunk) I77.75 ◄
      carotid I77.71
      cerebral (nonruptured) I67.0
         ruptured —see Hemorrhage, intracranial,
            subarachnoid
      coronary I25.42
      extremity ◄
         lower I77.77 ◄
         upper I77.76 ◄
      iliac I77.72
      precerebral ◄
         congenital (nonruptured) Q28.1 ◄
         specified site NEC I77.75 ◄
      renal I77.73
      specified NEC I77.79
      vertebral I77.74
   traumatic —see Wound, open, by site
   vascular I99.8
   wound —see Wound, open
Disseminated —see condition
Dissociation
   auriculoventricular or atrioventricular (AV)
      (any degree) (isorhythmic) I45.89
      with heart block I44.2
   interference I45.89
Dissociative reaction, state F44.9
Dissolution, vertebra —see Osteoporosis
Distension, distention
   abdomen R14.0
   bladder N32.89
   cecum K63.89
   colon K63.89
   gallbladder K82.8
   intestine K63.89
   kidney N28.89
   liver K76.89
   seminal vesicle N50.89 ◄▥
   stomach K31.89
      acute K31.0
      psychogenic F45.8
   ureter —see Dilatation, ureter
   uterus N85.8
Distoma hepaticum infestation B66.3
Distomiasis B66.9
   bile passages B66.3
   hemic B65.9
   hepatic B66.3
      due to Clonorchis sinensis B66.1
   intestinal B66.5
   liver B66.3
      due to Clonorchis sinensis B66.1
   lung B66.4
   pulmonary B66.4
Distomolar (fourth molar) K00.1
Disto-occlusion (Division I) (Division II)
   M26.212
Distortion (s) (congenital)
   adrenal (gland) Q89.1
   arm NEC Q68.8
   bile duct or passage Q44.5
   bladder Q64.79
   brain Q04.9
   cervix (uteri) Q51.9
   chest (wall) Q67.8
      bones Q76.8
   clavicle Q74.0
   clitoris Q52.6
   coccyx Q76.49
   common duct Q44.5
   coronary Q24.5
   cystic duct Q44.5

Distortion (Continued)
   ear (auricle) (external) Q17.3
      inner Q16.5
      middle Q16.4
         ossicles Q16.3
   endocrine NEC Q89.2
   eustachian tube Q17.8
   eye (adnexa) Q15.8
   face bone (s) NEC Q75.8
   fallopian tube Q50.6
   femur NEC Q68.8
   fibula NEC Q68.8
   finger (s) Q68.1
   foot Q66.9
   genitalia, genital organ (s)
      female Q52.8
         external Q52.79
         internal NEC Q52.8
   gyri Q04.8
   hand bone (s) Q68.1
   heart (auricle) (ventricle) Q24.8
      valve (cusp) Q24.8
   hepatic duct Q44.5
   humerus NEC Q68.8
   hymen Q52.4
   intrafamilial communications
      Z63.8
   jaw NEC M26.89
   labium (majus) (minus) Q52.79
   leg NEC Q68.8
   lens Q12.8
   liver Q44.7
   lumbar spine Q76.49
      with disproportion O33.8
         causing obstructed labor O65.0
   lumbosacral (joint) (region) Q76.49
      kyphosis —see Kyphosis, congenital
      lordosis —see Lordosis, congenital
   nerve Q07.8
   nose Q30.8
   organ
      of Corti Q16.5
      or site not listed —see Anomaly, by site
         ossicles, ear Q16.3
   oviduct Q50.6
   pancreas Q45.3
   parathyroid (gland) Q89.2
   pituitary (gland) Q89.2
   radius NEC Q68.8
   sacroiliac joint Q74.2
   sacrum Q76.49
   scapula Q74.0
   shoulder girdle Q74.0
   skull bone (s) NEC Q75.8
      with
         anencephalus Q00.0
         encephalocele —see Encephalocele
         hydrocephalus Q03.9
            with spina bifida —see Spina bifida,
               with hydrocephalus
         microcephaly Q02
   spinal cord Q06.8
   spine Q76.49
      kyphosis —see Kyphosis, congenital
      lordosis —see Lordosis, congenital
   spleen Q89.09
   sternum NEC Q76.7
   thorax (wall) Q67.8
      bony Q76.8
   thymus (gland) Q89.2
   thyroid (gland) Q89.2
   tibia NEC Q68.8
   toe (s) Q66.9
   tongue Q38.3
   trachea (cartilage) Q32.1
   ulna NEC Q68.8
   ureter Q62.8
   urethra Q64.79
      causing obstruction Q64.39
   uterus Q51.9
   vagina Q52.4

Distortion (Continued)
   vertebra Q76.49
      kyphosis —see Kyphosis, congenital
      lordosis —see Lordosis, congenital
   visual —see also Disturbance, vision
      shape and size H53.15
   vulva Q52.79
   wrist (bones) (joint) Q68.8
Distress
   abdomen —see Pain, abdominal
   acute respiratory R06.00 ◄▥
      syndrome (adult) (child) J80 ◄
   epigastric R10.13
   fetal P84
      complicating pregnancy —see Stress, fetal
   gastrointestinal (functional) K30
      psychogenic F45.8
   intestinal (functional) NOS K59.9
      psychogenic F45.8
   maternal, during labor and delivery O75.0
   respiratory (adult) (child) R06.00 ◄▥
      adult J80
      child J80
      newborn P22.9
         specified NEC P22.8
      orthopnea R06.01
      psychogenic F45.8
      shortness of breath R06.02
      specified type NEC R06.09
Distribution vessel, atypical Q27.9
   coronary artery Q24.5
   precerebral Q28.1
Distichiasis L68.8
Disturbance (s) —see also Disease
   absorption K90.9
      calcium E58
      carbohydrate K90.49 ◄▥
      fat K90.49 ◄▥
         pancreatic K90.3
      protein K90.49 ◄▥
      starch K90.49 ◄▥
      vitamin —see Deficiency, vitamin
   acid-base equilibrium E87.8
      mixed E87.4
   activity and attention (with hyperkinesis) —
      see Disorder, attention-deficit
      hyperactivity
   amino acid transport E72.00
   assimilation, food K90.9
   auditory nerve, except deafness —see
      subcategory H93.3
   behavior —see Disorder, conduct
   blood clotting (mechanism) —see also Defect,
      coagulation D68.9
   cerebral
      nerve —see Disorder, nerve, cranial
      status, newborn P91.9
         specified NEC P91.8
   circulatory I99.9
   conduct —see also Disorder, conduct F91.9
      adjustment reaction —see Disorder,
         adjustment
      compulsive F63.9
      disruptive F91.9
      hyperkinetic —see Disorder, attention-
         deficit hyperactivity
      socialized F91.2
      specified NEC F91.8
      unsocialized F91.1
   coordination R27.8
   cranial nerve —see Disorder, nerve, cranial
   deep sensibility —see Disturbance,
      sensation
   digestive K30
      psychogenic F45.8
   electrolyte —see also Imbalance, electrolyte
      newborn, transitory P74.4
         hyperammonemia P74.6
         potassium balance P74.3
         sodium balance P74.2
         specified type NEC P74.4

◄ New   ◄▥ Revised   deleted Deleted

Disturbance *(Continued)*
emotions specific to childhood and
adolescence F93.9
with
anxiety and fearfulness NEC F93.8
elective mutism F94.0
oppositional disorder F91.3
sensitivity (withdrawal) F40.10
shyness F40.10
social withdrawal F40.10
involving relationship problems
F93.8
mixed F93.8
specified NEC F93.8
endocrine (gland) E34.9
neonatal, transitory P72.9
specified NEC P72.8
equilibrium R42
fructose metabolism E74.10
gait —*see* Gait
hysterical F44.4
psychogenic F44.4
gastrointestinal (functional) K30
psychogenic F45.8
habit, child F98.9
hearing, except deafness and tinnitus —*see*
Abnormal, auditory perception
heart, functional (conditions in I44-I50)
due to presence of (cardiac) prosthesis
I97.19-
postoperative I97.89
cardiac surgery I97.19-
hormones E34.9
innervation uterus (parasympathetic)
(sympathetic) N85.8
keratinization NEC
gingiva K05.10
nonplaque induced K05.11
plaque induced K05.10
lip K13.0
oral (mucosa) (soft tissue) K13.29
tongue K13.29
learning (specific) —*see* Disorder,
learning
memory —*see* Amnesia
mild, following organic brain damage
F06.8
mental F99
associated with diseases classified
elsewhere F54
metabolism E88.9
with
abortion —*see* Abortion, by type with
other specified complication
ectopic pregnancy O08.5
molar pregnancy O08.5
amino-acid E72.9
aromatic E70.9
branched-chain E71.2
straight-chain E72.8
sulfur-bearing E72.10
ammonia E72.20
arginine E72.21
arginosuccinic acid E72.22
carbohydrate E74.9
cholesterol E78.9
citrulline E72.23
cystathionine E72.19
general E88.9
glutamine E72.8
histidine E70.40
homocystine E72.19
hydroxylysine E72.3
in labor or delivery O75.89
iron E83.10
lipoid E78.9
lysine E72.3
methionine E72.19
neonatal, transitory P74.9
calcium and magnesium P71.9
specified type NEC P71.8

Disturbance *(Continued)*
metabolism *(Continued)*
neonatal, transitory *(Continued)*
carbohydrate metabolism P70.9
specified type NEC P70.8
specified NEC P74.8
ornithine E72.4
phosphate E83.39
sodium NEC E87.8
threonine E72.8
tryptophan E70.5
tyrosine E70.20
urea cycle E72.20
motor R29.2
nervous, functional R45.0
neuromuscular mechanism (eye), due to
syphilis A52.15
nutritional E63.9
nail L60.3
ocular motion H51.9
psychogenic F45.8
oculogyric H51.8
psychogenic F45.8
oculomotor H51.9
psychogenic F45.8
olfactory nerve R43.1
optic nerve NEC —*see* Disorder, nerve, optic
oral epithelium, including tongue NEC
K13.29
perceptual due to
alcohol withdrawal F10.232
amphetamine intoxication F15.922
in
abuse F15.122
dependence F15.222
anxiolytic withdrawal F13.232
cannabis intoxication (acute) F12.922
in
abuse F12.122
dependence F12.222
cocaine intoxication (acute) F14.922
in
abuse F14.122
dependence F14.222
hypnotic withdrawal F13.232
opioid intoxication (acute) F11.922
in
abuse F11.122
dependence F11.222
phencyclidine intoxication (acute)
F16.122 ◀▥
~~in~~
~~abuse F19.122~~
~~dependence F19.222~~
sedative withdrawal F13.232
personality (pattern) (trait) —*see also*
Disorder, personality F60.9
following organic brain damage F07.9
polyglandular E31.9
specified NEC E31.8
potassium balance, newborn P74.3
psychogenic F45.9
psychomotor F44.4
psychophysical visual H53.16
pupillary —*see* Anomaly, pupil, function
reflex R29.2
rhythm, heart I49.9
salivary secretion K11.7
sensation (cold) (heat) (localization) (tactile
discrimination) (texture) (vibratory)
NEC R20.9
hysterical F44.6
skin R20.9
anesthesia R20.0
hyperesthesia R20.3
hypoesthesia R20.1
paresthesia R20.2
specified type NEC R20.8
smell R43.9
and taste (mixed) R43.8
anosmia R43.0

Disturbance *(Continued)*
sensation *(Continued)*
smell *(Continued)*
parosmia R43.1
specified NEC R43.8
taste R43.9
and smell (mixed) R43.8
parageusia R43.2
specified NEC R43.8
sensory —*see* Disturbance, sensation
situational (transient) —*see also* Disorder,
adjustment
acute F43.0
sleep G47.9
nonorganic origin F51.9
smell —*see* Disturbance, sensation,
smell
sociopathic F60.2
sodium balance, newborn P74.2
speech R47.9
developmental F80.9
specified NEC R47.89
stomach (functional) K31.9
sympathetic (nerve) G90.9
taste —*see* Disturbance, sensation,
taste
temperature
regulation, newborn P81.9
specified NEC P81.8
sense R20.8
hysterical F44.6
tooth
eruption K00.6
formation K00.4
structure, hereditary NEC K00.5
touch —*see* Disturbance, sensation
vascular I99.9
arteriosclerotic —*see* Arteriosclerosis
vasomotor I73.9
vasospastic I73.9
vision, visual H53.9
following
cerebral infarction I69.398
cerebrovascular disease I69.998
specified NEC I69.898
intracerebral hemorrhage I69.198
nontraumatic intracranial hemorrhage
NEC I69.298
specified disease NEC I69.898
subarachnoid hemorrhage I69.098
psychophysical H53.16
specified NEC H53.8
subjective H53.10
day blindness H53.11
discomfort H53.14-
distortions of shape and size
H53.15
loss
sudden H53.13-
transient H53.12-
specified type NEC H53.19
voice R49.9
psychogenic F44.4
specified NEC R49.8
Diuresis R35.8
Diver's palsy, paralysis or squeeze T70.3
Diverticulitis (acute) K57.92
bladder —*see* Cystitis
ileum —*see* Diverticulitis, intestine, small
intestine K57.92
with
abscess, perforation or peritonitis
K57.80
with bleeding K57.81
bleeding K57.93
congenital Q43.8
large K57.32
with
abscess, perforation or peritonitis
K57.20
with bleeding K57.21

Diverticulitis (Continued)
  intestine (Continued)
    large (Continued)
      with (Continued)
        bleeding K57.33
        small intestine K57.52
          with
            abscess, perforation or peritonitis
              K57.40
              with bleeding K57.41
            bleeding K57.53
      small K57.12
        with
          abscess, perforation or peritonitis
            K57.00
            with bleeding K57.01
          bleeding K57.13
          large intestine K57.52
            with
              abscess, perforation or peritonitis
                K57.40
                with bleeding K57.41
              bleeding K57.53
Diverticulosis K57.90
  with bleeding K57.91
  large intestine K57.30
    with
      bleeding K57.31
      small intestine K57.50
        with bleeding K57.51
  small intestine K57.10
    with
      bleeding K57.11
      large intestine K57.50
        with bleeding K57.51
Diverticulum, diverticula (multiple) K57.90
  appendix (noninflammatory) K38.2
  bladder (sphincter) N32.3
    congenital Q64.6
  bronchus (congenital) Q32.4
    acquired J98.09
  calyx, calyceal (kidney) N28.89
  cardia (stomach) K31.4
  cecum —see Diverticulosis, intestine, large
    congenital Q43.8
  colon —see Diverticulosis, intestine, large
    congenital Q43.8
  duodenum —see Diverticulosis, intestine,
    small
    congenital Q43.8
  epiphrenic (esophagus) K22.5
  esophagus (congenital) Q39.6
    acquired (epiphrenic) (pulsion) (traction)
      K22.5
  eustachian tube —see Disorder, eustachian
    tube, specified NEC
  fallopian tube N83.8
  gastric K31.4
  heart (congenital) Q24.8
  ileum —see Diverticulosis, intestine, small
  jejunum —see Diverticulosis, intestine, small
  kidney (pelvis) (calyces) N28.89
    with calculus —see Calculus, kidney
  Meckel's (displaced) (hypertrophic) Q43.0
    malignant —see Table of Neoplasms, small
      intestine, malignant
  midthoracic K22.5
  organ or site, congenital NEC —see Distortion
  pericardium (congenital) (cyst) Q24.8
    acquired I31.8
  pharyngoesophageal (congenital) Q39.6
    acquired K22.5
  pharynx (congenital) Q38.7
  rectosigmoid —see Diverticulosis, intestine,
    large
    congenital Q43.8
  rectum —see Diverticulosis, intestine, large
  Rokitansky's K22.5
  seminal vesicle N50.89 ◀━
  sigmoid —see Diverticulosis, intestine, large
    congenital Q43.8

Diverticulum, diverticula (Continued)
  stomach (acquired) K31.4
    congenital Q40.2
  trachea (acquired) J39.8
  ureter (acquired) N28.89
    congenital Q62.8
  ureterovesical orifice N28.89
  urethra (acquired) N36.1
    congenital Q64.79
  ventricle, left (congenital) Q24.8
  vesical N32.3
    congenital Q64.6
  Zenker's (esophagus) K22.5
Division
  cervix uteri (acquired) N88.8
  glans penis Q55.69
  labia minora (congenital) Q52.79
  ligament (partial or complete) (current) —see
    also Sprain
    with open wound —see Wound, open
  muscle (partial or complete) (current) —see
    also Injury, muscle
    with open wound —see Wound, open
  nerve (traumatic) —see Injury, nerve
  spinal cord —see Injury, spinal cord,
    by region
  vein I87.8
Divorce, causing family disruption Z63.5
Dix-Hallpike neurolabyrinthitis —see
  Neuronitis, vestibular
Dizziness R42
  hysterical F44.89
  psychogenic F45.8
DMAC (disseminated mycobacterium avium-
  intracellulare complex) A31.2
DNR (do not resuscitate) Z66
Doan-Wiseman syndrome (primary splenic
  neutropenia) —see Agranulocytosis
Doehle-Heller aortitis A52.02
Dog bite —see Bite
Dohle body panmyelopathic syndrome
  D72.0
Dolichocephaly Q67.2
Dolichocolon Q43.8
Dolichostenomelia —see Syndrome, Marfan's
Donohue's syndrome E34.8
Donor (organ or tissue) Z52.9
  blood (whole) Z52.000
    autologous Z52.010
    specified component (lymphocytes)
      (platelets) NEC Z52.008
      autologous Z52.018
      specified donor NEC Z52.098
    specified donor NEC Z52.090
    stem cells Z52.001
      autologous Z52.011
      specified donor NEC Z52.091
  bone Z52.20
    autologous Z52.21
    marrow Z52.3
    specified type NEC Z52.29
  cornea Z52.5
  egg (Oocyte) Z52.819
    age 35 and over Z52.812
      anonymous recipient Z52.812
      designated recipient Z52.813
    under age 35 Z52.810
      anonymous recipient Z52.810
      designated recipient Z52.811
  kidney Z52.4
  liver Z52.6
  lung Z52.89
  lymphocyte —see Donor, blood, specified
    components NEC
  Oocyte —see Donor, egg
  platelets Z52.008
  potential, examination of Z00.5
  semen Z52.89
  skin Z52.10
    autologous Z52.11
    specified type NEC Z52.19

Donor (Continued)
  specified organ or tissue NEC Z52.89
  sperm Z52.89
Donovanosis A58
Dorsalgia M54.9
  psychogenic F45.41
  specified NEC M54.89
Dorsopathy M53.9
  deforming M43.9
    specified NEC —see subcategory M43.8
  specified NEC M53.80
    cervical region M53.82
    cervicothoracic region M53.83
    lumbar region M53.86
    lumbosacral region M53.87
    occipito-atlanto-axial region M53.81
    sacrococcygeal region M53.88
    thoracic region M53.84
    thoracolumbar region M53.85
Double
  albumin E88.09
  aortic arch Q25.45 ◀━
  auditory canal Q17.8
  auricle (heart) Q20.8
  bladder Q64.79
  cervix Q51.820
    with doubling of uterus (and vagina) Q51.10
      with obstruction Q51.11
  inlet ventricle Q20.4
  kidney with double pelvis (renal) Q63.0
  meatus urinarius Q64.75
  monster Q89.4
  outlet
    left ventricle Q20.2
    right ventricle Q20.1
  pelvis (renal) with double ureter Q62.5
  tongue Q38.3
  ureter (one or both sides) Q62.5
    with double pelvis (renal) Q62.5
  urethra Q64.74
  urinary meatus Q64.75
  uterus Q51.2
    with
      doubling of cervix (and vagina)
        Q51.10
        with obstruction Q51.11
    in pregnancy or childbirth O34.59-
      causing obstructed labor O65.5
  vagina Q52.10
    with doubling of uterus (and cervix)
      Q51.10
      with obstruction Q51.11
  vision H53.2
  vulva Q52.79
Douglas' pouch, cul-de-sac —see condition
Down syndrome Q90.9
  meiotic nondisjunction Q90.0
  mitotic nondisjunction Q90.1
  mosaicism Q90.1
  translocation Q90.2
DPD (dihydropyrimidine dehydrogenase
  deficiency) E88.89
Dracontiasis B72
Dracunculiasis, dracunculosis B72
Dream state, hysterical F44.89
Drepanocytic anemia —see Disease, sickle-cell
Dresbach's syndrome (elliptocytosis) D58.1
Dreschlera (hawaiiensis) (infection) B43.8
Dressler's syndrome I24.1
Drift, ulnar —see Deformity, limb, specified
  type NEC, forearm
Drinking (alcohol)
  excessive, to excess NEC (without
    dependence) F10.10
    habitual (continual) (without remission)
      F10.20
      with remission F10.21
Drip, postnasal (chronic) R09.82
  due to
    allergic rhinitis —see Rhinitis, allergic
    common cold J00

◀ New   ◀━ Revised   ~~deleted~~ Deleted

Drip, postnasal *(Continued)*
  due to *(Continued)*
    gastroesophageal reflux —*see* Reflux,
      gastroesophageal
    nasopharyngitis —*see* Nasopharyngitis
    other known condition — code to
      condition
    sinusitis —*see* Sinusitis
Droop
  facial R29.810
    cerebrovascular disease I69.992
      cerebral infarction I69.392
      intracerebral hemorrhage I69.192
      nontraumatic intracranial hemorrhage
        NEC I69.292
      specified disease NEC I69.892
      subarachnoid hemorrhage I69.092
Drop (in)
  attack NEC R55
  finger —*see* Deformity, finger
  foot —*see* Deformity, limb, foot, drop
  hematocrit (precipitous) R71.0
  hemoglobin R71.0
  toe —*see* Deformity, toe, specified NEC
  wrist —*see* Deformity, limb, wrist drop
Dropped heart beats I45.9
Dropsy, dropsical —*see also* Hydrops
  abdomen R18.8
  brain —*see* Hydrocephalus
  cardiac, heart —*see* Failure, heart, congestive
  gangrenous —*see* Gangrene
  heart —*see* Failure, heart, congestive
  kidney —*see* Nephrosis
  lung —*see* Edema, lung
  newborn due to isoimmunization P56.0
  pericardium —*see* Pericarditis
Drowned, drowning (near) T75.1
Drowsiness R40.0
Drug
  abuse counseling and surveillance Z71.51
  addiction —*see* Dependence
  dependence —*see* Dependence
  habit —*see* Dependence
  harmful use —*see* Abuse, drug
  induced fever R50.2
  overdose —*see* Table of Drugs and Chemicals,
    by drug, poisoning
  poisoning —*see* Table of Drugs and
    Chemicals, by drug, poisoning
  resistant organism infection —*see also*
    Resistant, organism, to, drug Z16.30
  therapy
    long term (current) (prophylactic) —*see*
      Therapy, drug long-term (current)
      (prophylactic)
    short term - omit code
  wrong substance given or taken in error —*see*
    Table of Drugs and Chemicals, by drug,
    poisoning
Drunkenness (without dependence) F10.129
  acute in alcoholism F10.229
  chronic (without remission) F10.20
    with remission F10.21
  pathological (without dependence) F10.129
    with dependence F10.229
  sleep F51.9
Drusen
  macula (degenerative) (retina) —*see*
    Degeneration, macula, drusen
  optic disc H47.32-
Dry, dryness —*see also* condition
  larynx J38.7
  mouth R68.2
    due to dehydration E86.0
  nose J34.89
  socket (teeth) M27.3
  throat J39.2
DSAP L56.5
Duane's syndrome H50.81-
Dubin-Johnson disease or syndrome E80.6
Dubois' disease (thymus gland) A50.59 *[E35]*

Dubowitz' syndrome Q87.1
Duchenne-Aran muscular atrophy G12.21
Duchenne-Griesinger disease G71.0
Duchenne's
  disease or syndrome
    motor neuron disease G12.22
    muscular dystrophy G71.0
  locomotor ataxia (syphilitic) A52.11
  paralysis
    birth injury P14.0
    due to or associated with
      motor neuron disease G12.22
      muscular dystrophy G71.0
Ducrey's chancre A57
Duct, ductus —*see* condition
Duhring's disease (dermatitis herpetiformis)
    L13.0
Dullness, cardiac (decreased) (increased) R01.2
Dumb ague —*see* Malaria
Dumbness —*see* Aphasia
Dumdum fever B55.0
Dumping syndrome (postgastrectomy) K91.1
Duodenitis (nonspecific) (peptic) K29.80
  with bleeding K29.81
Duodenocholangitis —*see* Cholangitis
Duodenum, duodenal —*see* condition
Duplay's bursitis or periarthritis —*see*
    Tendinitis, calcific, shoulder
Duplication, duplex —*see also* Accessory
  alimentary tract Q45.8
  anus Q43.4
  appendix (and cecum) Q43.4
  biliary duct (any) Q44.5
  bladder Q64.79
  cecum (and appendix) Q43.4
  cervix Q51.820
  chromosome NEC
    with complex rearrangements NEC
      Q92.5
    seen only at prometaphase Q92.8
  cystic duct Q44.5
  digestive organs Q45.8
  esophagus Q39.8
  frontonasal process Q75.8
  intestine (large) (small) Q43.4
  kidney Q63.0
  liver Q44.7
  pancreas Q45.3
  penis Q55.69
  respiratory organs NEC Q34.8
  salivary duct Q38.4
  spinal cord (incomplete) Q06.2
  stomach Q40.2
Dupré's disease (meningism) R29.1
Dupuytren's contraction or disease M72.0
Durand-Nicolas-Favre disease A55
Durotomy (inadvertent) (incidental) G97.41
Duroziez's disease (congenital mitral stenosis)
    Q23.2
Dutton's relapsing fever (West African) A68.1
Dwarfism E34.3
  achondroplastic Q77.4
  congenital E34.3
  constitutional E34.3
  hypochondroplastic Q77.4
  hypophyseal E23.0
  infantile E34.3
  Laron-type E34.3
  Lorain (-Levi) type E23.0
  metatropic Q77.8
  nephrotic-glycosuric (with
    hypophosphatemic rickets) E72.09
  nutritional E45
  pancreatic K86.89 ◄▥▥
  pituitary E23.0
  renal N25.0
  thanatophoric Q77.1
Dyke-Young anemia (secondary)
    (symptomatic) D59.1
Dysacusis —*see* Abnormal, auditory
    perception

Dysadrenocortism E27.9
  hyperfunction E27.0
Dysarthria R47.1
  following
    cerebral infarction I69.322
    cerebrovascular disease I69.922
      specified disease NEC I69.822
    intracerebral hemorrhage I69.122
    nontraumatic intracranial hemorrhage
      NEC I69.222
    subarachnoid hemorrhage I69.022
Dysautonomia (familial) G90.1
Dysbarism T70.3
Dysbasia R26.2
  angiosclerotica intermittens I73.9
  hysterical F44.4
  lordotica (progressiva) G24.1
  nonorganic origin F44.4
  psychogenic F44.4
Dysbetalipoproteinemia (familial) E78.2
Dyscalculia R48.8
  developmental F81.2
Dyschezia K59.00
Dyschondroplasia (with hemangiomata)
    Q78.4
Dyschromia (skin) L81.9
Dyscollagenosis M35.9
Dyscranio-pygo-phalangy Q87.0
Dyscrasia
  blood (with) D75.9
    antepartum hemorrhage —*see*
      Hemorrhage, antepartum, with
      coagulation defect
    intrapartum hemorrhage O67.0
    newborn P61.9
      specified type NEC P61.8
    puerperal, postpartum O72.3
  polyglandular, pluriglandular E31.9
Dysendocrinism E34.9
Dysentery, dysenteric (catarrhal) (diarrhea)
    (epidemic) (hemorrhagic) (infectious)
    (sporadic) (tropical) A09
  abscess, liver A06.4
  amebic —*see also* Amebiasis A06.0
    with abscess —*see* Abscess, amebic
    acute A06.0
    chronic A06.1
  arthritis —*see also* category M01 A09
  bacillary —*see also* category M01 A03.9
  bacillary A03.9
    arthritis —*see also* category M01
      A03.9
    Boyd A03.2
    Flexner A03.1
    Schmitz (-Stutzer) A03.0
    Shiga (-Kruse) A03.0
    Shigella A03.9
      boydii A03.2
      dysenteriae A03.0
      flexneri A03.1
      group A A03.0
      group B A03.1
      group C A03.2
      group D A03.3
      sonnei A03.3
      specified type NEC A03.8
    Sonne A03.3
    specified type NEC A03.8
  balantidial A07.0
  Balantidium coli A07.0
  Boyd's A03.2
  candidal B37.82
  Chilomastix A07.8
  Chinese A03.9
  coccidial A07.3
  Dientamoeba (fragilis) A07.8
  Embadomonas A07.8
  Entamoeba, entambic —*see* Dysentery,
    amebic
  Flexner-Boyd A03.2
  Flexner's A03.1

Dysentery, dysenteric (Continued)
  Giardia lamblia A07.1
  Hiss-Russell A03.1
  Lamblia A07.1
  leishmanial B55.0
  malarial —see Malaria
  metazoal B82.0
  monilial B37.82
  protozoal A07.9
  Salmonella A02.0
  schistosomal B65.1
  Schmitz (-Stutzer) A03.0
  Shiga (-Kruse) A03.0
  Shigella NOS —see Dysentery, bacillary
  Sonne A03.3
  strongyloidiasis B78.0
  trichomonal A07.8
  viral —see also Enteritis, viral A08.4
Dysequilibrium R42
Dysesthesia R20.8
  hysterical F44.6
Dysfibrinogenemia (congenital) D68.2
Dysfunction
  adrenal E27.9
    hyperfunction E27.0
  autonomic
    due to alcohol G31.2
    somatoform F45.8
  bladder N31.9
    neurogenic NOS —see Dysfunction,
      bladder, neuromuscular
    neuromuscular NOS N31.9
      atonic (motor) (sensory) N31.2
      autonomous N31.2
      flaccid N31.2
      nonreflex N31.2
      reflex N31.1
      specified NEC N31.8
      uninhibited N31.0
  bleeding, uterus N93.8
  cerebral G93.89
  colon K59.9
    psychogenic F45.8
  colostomy K94.03
  cystic duct K82.8
  cystostomy (stoma) —see Complications,
    cystostomy
  ejaculatory N53.19
    anejaculatory orgasm N53.13
    painful N53.12
    premature F52.4
    retarded N53.11
  endocrine NOS E34.9
  endometrium N85.8
  enterostomy K94.13
  erectile —see Dysfunction, sexual, male,
    erectile ◀
  gallbladder K82.8
  gastrostomy (stoma) K94.23
  gland, glandular NOS E34.9
  heart I51.89
  hemoglobin D75.89
  hepatic K76.89
  hypophysis E23.7
  hypothalamic NEC E23.3
  ileostomy (stoma) K94.13
  jejunostomy (stoma) K94.13
  kidney —see Disease, renal
  labyrinthine —see subcategory H83.2
  left ventricular, following sudden emotional
    stress I51.81
  liver K76.89
  male —see Dysfunction, sexual, male
  orgasmic (female) F52.31
    male F52.32
  ovary E28.9
    specified NEC E28.8
  papillary muscle I51.89
  parathyroid E21.4
  physiological NEC R68.89
    psychogenic F59

Dysfunction (Continued)
  pineal gland E34.8
  pituitary (gland) E23.3
  platelets D69.1
  polyglandular E31.9
    specified NEC E31.8
  psychophysiologic F59
  psychosexual F52.9
    with
      dyspareunia F52.6
      premature ejaculation F52.4
      vaginismus F52.5
  pylorus K31.9
  rectum K59.9
    psychogenic F45.8
  reflex (sympathetic) —see Syndrome, pain,
    complex regional I
  segmental —see Dysfunction, somatic
  senile R54
  sexual (due to) R37
    alcohol F10.981
    amphetamine F15.981
      in
        abuse F15.181
        dependence F15.281
    anxiolytic F13.981
      in
        abuse F13.181
        dependence F13.281
    cocaine F14.981
      in
        abuse F14.181
        dependence F14.281
    excessive sexual drive F52.8
    failure of genital response (male) F52.21
      female F52.22
    female N94.9
      aversion F52.1
      dyspareunia N94.10 ◀
        psychogenic F52.6
      frigidity F52.22
      nymphomania F52.8
      orgasmic F52.31
      psychogenic F52.9
        aversion F52.1
        dyspareunia F52.6
        frigidity F52.22
        nymphomania F52.8
        orgasmic F52.31
        vaginismus F52.5
      vaginismus N94.2
        psychogenic F52.5
    hypnotic F13.981
      in
        abuse F13.181
        dependence F13.281
    inhibited orgasm (female) F52.31
      male F52.32
    lack
      of sexual enjoyment F52.1
      or loss of sexual desire F52.0
    male N53.9
      anejaculatory orgasm N53.13
      ejaculatory N53.19
        painful N53.12
        premature F52.4
        retarded N53.11
      erectile N52.9
        drug induced N52.2
        due to
          disease classified elsewhere N52.1
          drug N52.2
        postoperative (postprocedural) N52.39
          following
            cryotherapy N52.37 ◀
            interstitial seed therapy
              N52.36 ◀
            prostate ablative therapy
              N52.37 ◀
            prostatectomy N52.34
              radical N52.31

Dysfunction (Continued)
  sexual (Continued)
    male (Continued)
      erectile (Continued)
        postoperative (Continued)
          following (Continued)
            radiation therapy N52.35 ◀
            radical cystectomy N52.32
            ultrasound ablative therapy
              N52.37 ◀
            urethral surgery N52.33
        psychogenic F52.9
        specified cause NEC N52.8
        vasculogenic
          arterial insufficiency N52.01
            with corporo-venous occlusive
              N52.03
          corporo-venous occlusive N52.02
            with arterial insufficiency N52.03
      impotence —see Dysfunction, sexual,
        male, erectile
      psychogenic F52.9
        aversion F52.1
        erectile F52.21
        orgasmic F52.32
        premature ejaculation F52.4
        satyriasis F52.8
        specified type NEC F52.8
      specified type NEC N53.8
    nonorganic F52.9
      specified NEC F52.8
    opioid F11.981
      in
        abuse F11.181
        dependence F11.281
    orgasmic dysfunction (female) F52.31
      male F52.32
    premature ejaculation F52.4
    psychoactive substances NEC F19.981
      in
        abuse F19.181
        dependence F19.281
    psychogenic F52.9
    sedative F13.981
      in
        abuse F13.181
        dependence F13.281
    sexual aversion F52.1
    vaginismus (nonorganic) (psychogenic)
      F52.5
  sinoatrial node I49.5
  somatic M99.09
    abdomen M99.09
    acromioclavicular M99.07
    cervical region M99.01
    cervicothoracic M99.01
    costochondral M99.08
    costovertebral M99.08
    head region M99.00
    hip M99.05
    lower extremity M99.06
    lumbar region M99.03
    lumbosacral M99.03
    occipitocervical M99.00
    pelvic region M99.05
    pubic M99.05
    rib cage M99.08
    sacral region M99.04
    sacrococcygeal M99.04
    sacroiliac M99.04
    specified NEC M99.09
    sternochondral M99.08
    sternoclavicular M99.07
    thoracic region M99.02
    thoracolumbar M99.02
    upper extremity M99.07
  somatoform autonomic F45.8
  stomach K31.89
    psychogenic F45.8
  suprarenal E27.9
    hyperfunction E27.0

◀ New   ◀ Revised   deleted Deleted

Dysfunction *(Continued)*
  symbolic R48.9
    specified type NEC R48.8
  temporomandibular (joint) M26.69
    joint-pain syndrome M26.62-◄▥
  testicular (endocrine) E29.9
    specified NEC E29.8
  thymus E32.9
  thyroid E07.9
  ureterostomy (stoma) —*see* Complications,
    stoma, urinary tract
  urethrostomy (stoma) —*see* Complications,
    stoma, urinary tract
  uterus, complicating delivery O62.9
    hypertonic O62.4
    hypotonic O62.2
      primary O62.0
      secondary O62.1
  ventricular I51.9
    with congestive heart failure I50.9-
      left, reversible, following sudden
        emotional stress I51.81
Dysgenesis
  gonadal (due to chromosomal anomaly)
    Q96.9
    pure Q99.1
  renal Q60.5
    bilateral Q60.4
    unilateral Q60.3
  reticular D72.0
  tidal platelet D69.3
Dysgerminoma
  specified site —*see* Neoplasm, malignant,
    by site
  unspecified site
    female C56.9
    male C62.90
Dysgeusia R43.2
Dysgraphia R27.8
Dyshidrosis, dysidrosis L30.1
Dyskaryotic cervical smear R87.619
Dyskeratosis L85.8
  cervix —*see* Dysplasia, cervix
  congenital Q82.8
  uterus NEC N85.8
Dyskinesia G24.9
  biliary (cystic duct or gallbladder) K82.8
  drug induced
    orofacial G24.01
  esophagus K22.4
  hysterical F44.4
  intestinal K59.8
  nonorganic origin F44.4
  orofacial (idiopathic) G24.4
    drug induced G24.01
  psychogenic F44.4
  subacute, drug induced G24.01
  tardive G24.01
    neuroleptic induced G24.01
  trachea J39.8
  tracheobronchial J98.09
Dyslalia (developmental) F80.0
Dyslexia R48.0
  developmental F81.0
Dyslipidemia E78.5
  depressed HDL cholesterol E78.6
  elevated fasting triglycerides E78.1
Dysmaturity —*see also* Light for dates
  pulmonary (newborn) (Wilson-Mikity) P27.0
Dysmenorrhea (essential) (exfoliative) N94.6
  congestive (syndrome) N94.6
  primary N94.4
  psychogenic F45.8
  secondary N94.5
Dysmetabolic syndrome X E88.81
Dysmetria R27.8
Dysmorphism (due to)
  alcohol Q86.0
  exogenous cause NEC Q86.8
  hydantoin Q86.1
  warfarin Q86.2

Dysmorphophobia (nondelusional)
  F45.22
  delusional F22
Dysnomia R47.01
Dysorexia R63.0
  psychogenic F50.89 ◄▥
Dysostosis
  cleidocranial, cleidocranialis Q74.0
  craniofacial Q75.1
  Fairbank's (idiopathic familial generalized
    osteophytosis) Q78.9
  mandibulofacial (incomplete)
    Q75.4
  multiplex E76.01
  oculomandibular Q75.5
Dyspareunia (female) N94.10 ◄▥
  deep N94.12 ◄
  male N53.12
  nonorganic F52.6
  psychogenic F52.6
  secondary N94.19 ◄▥
  specified NEC N94.19 ◄
  superficial (introital) N94.11 ◄
Dyspepsia R10.13
  atonic K30
  functional (allergic) (congenital)
    (gastrointestinal) (occupational) (reflex)
    K30
  intestinal K59.8
  nervous F45.8
  neurotic F45.8
  psychogenic F45.8
Dysphagia R13.10
  cervical R13.19
  following
    cerebral infarction I69.391
    cerebrovascular disease I69.991
      specified NEC I69.891
    intracerebral hemorrhage I69.191
    nontraumatic intracranial hemorrhage
      NEC I69.291
    specified disease NEC I69.891
    subarachnoid hemorrhage I69.091
  functional (hysterical) F45.8
  hysterical F45.8
  nervous (hysterical) F45.8
  neurogenic R13.19
  oral phase R13.11
  oropharyngeal phase R13.12
  pharyneal phase R13.13
  pharyngoesophageal phase R13.14
  psychogenic F45.8
  sideropenic D50.1
  spastica K22.4
  specified NEC R13.19
Dysphagocytosis, congenital D71
Dysphasia R47.02
  developmental
    expressive type F80.1
    receptive type F80.2
  following
    cerebrovascular disease I69.921
      cerebral infarction I69.321
      intracerebral hemorrhage I69.121
    nontraumatic intracranial hemorrhage NEC
      I69.221
      specified disease NEC I69.821
      subarachnoid hemorrhage I69.021
Dysphonia R49.0
  functional F44.4
  hysterical F44.4
  psychogenic F44.4
  spastica J38.3
Dysphoria, postpartal O90.6
Dysphoria ◄
  gender ◄
    in ◄
      adolescence and adulthood F64.0 ◄
      children F64.2 ◄
      postpartal O90.6 ◄
Dyspituitarism E23.3

Dysplasia —*see also* Anomaly
  acetabular, congenital Q65.89
  alveolar capillary, with vein misalignment
    J84.843
  anus (histologically confirmed) (mild)
    (moderate) K62.82
    severe D01.3
  arrhythmogenic right ventricular I42.8
  arterial, fibromuscular I77.3
  asphyxiating thoracic (congenital) Q77.2
  brain Q07.9
  bronchopulmonary, perinatal P27.1
  cervix (uteri) N87.9
    mild N87.0
    moderate N87.1
    severe D06.9
  chondroectodermal Q77.6
  colon D12.6
  craniometaphyseal Q78.58 ◄▥
  dentinal K00.5
  diaphyseal, progressive Q78.3
  dystrophic Q77.5
  ectodermal (anhidrotic) (congenital)
    (hereditary) Q82.4
    hydrotic Q82.8
  epithelial, uterine cervix —*see* Dysplasia,
    cervix
  eye (congenital) Q11.2
  fibrous
    bone NEC (monostotic) M85.00
      ankle M85.07-
      foot M85.07-
      forearm M85.03-
      hand M85.04-
      lower leg M85.06-
      multiple site M85.09
      neck M85.08
      rib M85.08
      shoulder M85.01-
      skull M85.08
      specified site NEC M85.08
      thigh M85.05-
      toe M85.07-
      upper arm M85.02-
      vertebra M85.08
    diaphyseal, progressive Q78.3
    jaw M27.8
    polyostotic Q78.1
  florid osseous —*see also* Cyst, calcifying
    odontogenic
  high grade, focal D12.6
  hip, congenital Q65.89
  joint, congenital Q74.8
  kidney Q61.4
    multicystic Q61.4
  leg Q74.2
  lung, congenital (not associated with short
    gestation) Q33.6
  mammary (gland) (benign) N60.9-
    cyst (solitary) —*see* Cyst, breast
    cystic —*see* Mastopathy, cystic
    duct ectasia —*see* Ectasia, mammary
      duct
    fibroadenosis —*see* Fibroadenosis, breast
    fibrosclerosis —*see* Fibrosclerosis, breast
    specified type NEC N60.8-
  metaphyseal Q78.5 ◄▥
  muscle Q79.8
  oculodentodigital Q87.0
  periapical (cemental) (cemento-osseous) —*see*
    Cyst, calcifying odontogenic
  periosteum —*see* Disorder, bone, specified
    type NEC
  polyostotic fibrous Q78.1
  prostate —*see also* Neoplasia, intraepithelial,
    prostate N42.30 ◄▥
    severe D07.5
    specified NEC N42.39 ◄
  renal Q61.4
    multicystic Q61.4
  retinal, congenital Q14.1

Dysplasia (Continued)
  right ventricular, arrhythmogenic I42.8
  septo-optic Q04.4
  skin L98.8
  spinal cord Q06.1
  spondyloepiphyseal Q77.7
  thymic, with immunodeficiency D82.1
  vagina N89.3
    mild N89.0
    moderate N89.1
    severe NEC D07.2
  vulva N90.3
    mild N90.0
    moderate N90.1
    severe NEC D07.1
Dyspnea (nocturnal) (paroxysmal)
    R06.00
  asthmatic (bronchial) J45.909
    with
      bronchitis J45.909
        with
          exacerbation (acute) J45.901
          status asthmaticus J45.902
        chronic J44.9
      exacerbation (acute) J45.901
      status asthmaticus J45.902
    cardiac —see Failure, ventricular, left
  cardiac —see Failure, ventricular, left
  functional F45.8
  hyperventilation R06.4
  hysterical F45.8
  newborn P28.89
  psychogenic F45.8
  shortness of breath R06.02
  specified type NEC R06.09
Dyspraxia R27.8
  developmental (syndrome) F82
Dysproteinemia E88.09
Dysreflexia, autonomic G90.4
Dysrhythmia
  cardiac I49.9
    newborn
      bradycardia P29.12
      occurring before birth P03.819
        before onset of labor P03.810
        during labor P03.811
      tachycardia P29.11
    postoperative I97.89
  cerebral or cortical —see Epilepsy
Dyssomnia —see Disorder, sleep
Dyssynergia
  biliary K83.8
  bladder sphincter N36.44
  cerebellaris myoclonica (Hunt's ataxia)
    G11.1
Dysthymia F34.1
Dysthyroidism E07.9
Dystocia O66.9
  affecting newborn P03.1
  cervical (hypotonic) O62.2
    affecting newborn P03.6
    primary O62.0
    secondary O62.1
  contraction ring O62.4

Dystocia (Continued)
  fetal O66.9
    abnormality NEC O66.3
    conjoined twins O66.3
    oversize O66.2
  maternal O66.9
  positional O64.9
  shoulder (girdle) O66.0
    causing obstructed labor O66.0
  uterine NEC O62.4
Dystonia G24.9
  deformans progressiva G24.1
  drug induced NEC G24.09
    acute G24.02
    specified NEC G24.09
  familial G24.1
  idiopathic G24.1
    familial G24.1
    nonfamilial G24.2
    orofacial G24.4
  lenticularis G24.8
  musculorum deformans G24.1
  neuroleptic induced (acute) G24.02
  orofacial (idiopathic) G24.4
  oromandibular G24.4
    due to drug G24.01
  specified NEC G24.8
  torsion (familial) (idiopathic) G24.1
    acquired G24.8
    genetic G24.1
    symptomatic (nonfamilial) G24.2
Dystonic movements R25.8
Dystrophy, dystrophia
  adiposogenital E23.6
  Becker's type G71.0
  cervical sympathetic G90.2
  choroid (hereditary) H31.20
    central areolar H31.22
    choroideremia H31.21
    gyrate atrophy H31.23
    specified type NEC H31.29
  cornea (hereditary) H18.50
    endothelial H18.51
    epithelial H18.52
    granular H18.53
    lattice H18.54
    macular H18.55
    specified type NEC H18.59
  Duchenne's type G71.0
  due to malnutrition E45
  Erb's G71.0
  Fuchs' H18.51
  Gower's muscular G71.0
  hair L67.8
  infantile neuraxonal G31.89
  Landouzy-Déjérine G71.0
  Leyden-Möbius G71.0
  muscular G71.0
    benign (Becker type) G71.0
    congenital (hereditary) (progressive)
      (with specific morphological
      abnormalities of the muscle fiber)
      G71.0
      myotonic G71.11

Dystrophy, dystrophia (Continued)
  muscular (Continued)
    distal G71.0
    Duchenne type G71.0
    Emery-Dreifuss G71.0
    Erb type G71.0
    facioscapulohumeral G71.0
    Gower's G71.0
    hereditary (progressive) G71.0
    Landouzy-Déjérine type G71.0
    limb-girdle G71.0
    myotonic G71.11
    progressive (hereditary) G71.0
      Charcot-Marie (-Tooth) type
        G60.0
    pseudohypertrophic (infantile)
      G71.0
    severe (Duchenne type) G71.0
  myocardium, myocardial —see
    Degeneration, myocardial
  nail L60.3
    congenital Q84.6
  nutritional E45
  ocular G71.0
  oculocerebrorenal E72.03
  oculopharyngeal G71.0
  ovarian N83.8
  polyglandular E31.8
  reflex (neuromuscular) (sympathetic) —
    see Syndrome, pain, complex
    regional I
  retinal (hereditary) H35.50
    in
      lipid storage disorders E75.6
        [H36]
      systemic lipidoses E75.6 [H36]
    involving
      pigment epithelium H35.54
      sensory area H35.53
    pigmentary H35.52
    vitreoretinal H35.51
  Salzmann's nodular —see Degeneration,
    cornea, nodular
  scapuloperoneal G71.0
  skin NEC L98.8
  sympathetic (reflex) —see Syndrome, pain,
    complex regional I
    cervical G90.2
  tapetoretinal H35.54
  thoracic, asphyxiating Q77.2
  unguium L60.3
    congenital Q84.6
  vitreoretinal H35.51
  vulva N90.4
  yellow (liver) —see Failure, hepatic
Dysuria R30.0
  psychogenic F45.8

◀ New   ◀⫶ Revised   ~~deleted~~ Deleted

E

Eales' disease H35.06-
Ear —see also condition
  piercing Z41.3
  ~~tropical B36.8~~
  tropical NEC B36.9 [H62.40] ◀
    in ◀
      aspergillosis B44.89 ◀
      candidiasis B37.84 ◀
      moniliasis B37.84 ◀
  wax (impacted) H61.20
    left H61.22
      with right H61.23
    right H61.21
      with left H61.23
Earache —see subcategory H92.0
Early satiety R68.81
Eaton-Lambert syndrome—see Syndrome,
    Lambert-Eaton
Eberth's disease (typhoid fever) A01.00
Ebola virus disease A98.4
Ebstein's anomaly or syndrome (heart) Q22.5
Eccentro-osteochondrodysplasia E76.29
Ecchondroma —see Neoplasm, bone, benign
Ecchondrosis D48.0
Ecchymosis R58
  conjunctiva —see Hemorrhage, conjunctiva
  eye (traumatic) —see Contusion, eyeball
  eyelid (traumatic) —see Contusion, eyelid
  newborn P54.5
  spontaneous R23.3
  traumatic —see Contusion
Echinococciasis —see Echinococcus
Echinococcosis —see Echinococcus
Echinococcus (infection) B67.90
  granulosus B67.4
    bone B67.2
    liver B67.0
    lung B67.1
    multiple sites B67.32
    specified site NEC B67.39
    thyroid B67.31 ◀▥
  liver NOS B67.8
    granulosus B67.0
    multilocularis B67.5
  lung NEC B67.99
    granulosus B67.1
    multilocularis B67.69
  multilocularis B67.7
    liver B67.5
    multiple sites B67.61
    specified site NEC B67.69
  specified site NEC B67.99
    granulosus B67.39
    multilocularis B67.69
  thyroid NEC B67.99
    granulosus B67.31 ◀▥
    multilocularis B67.69 [E35]
Echinorhynchiasis B83.8
Echinostomiasis B66.8
Echolalia R48.8
Echovirus, as cause of disease classified
    elsewhere B97.12
Eclampsia, eclamptic (coma) (convulsions)
    (delirium) (with hypertension) NEC O15.9
  complicating ◀
    labor and delivery O15.1 ◀
    postpartum O15.2 ◀
    pregnancy O15.0- ◀
    puerperium O15.2 ◀
  ~~during labor and delivery O15.1~~
  ~~postpartum O15.2~~
  ~~pregnancy O15.0-~~
  ~~puerperal O15.2~~
Economic circumstances affecting care Z59.9
Economo's disease A85.8
Ectasia, ectasis
  annuloaortic I35.8
  aorta I77.819
    with aneurysm —see Aneurysm, aorta
      abdominal I77.811

Ectasia, ectasis (Continued)
  aorta (Continued)
    thoracic I77.810
    thoracoabdominal I77.812
  breast —see Ectasia, mammary duct
  capillary I78.8
  cornea H18.71-
  gastric antral vascular (GAVE) K31.819
    with hemorrhage K31.811
    without hemorrhage K31.819
  mammary duct N60.4-
  salivary gland (duct) K11.8
  sclera —see Sclerectasia
Ecthyma L08.0
  contagiosum B08.02
  gangrenosum L08.0
  infectiosum B08.02
Ectocardia Q24.8
Ectodermal dysplasia (anhidrotic) Q82.4
Ectodermosis erosiva pluriorificialis
    L51.1
Ectopic, ectopia (congenital)
  abdominal viscera Q45.8
    due to defect in anterior abdominal wall
      Q79.59
  ACTH syndrome E24.3
  adrenal gland Q89.1
  anus Q43.5
  atrial beats I49.1
  beats I49.49
    atrial I49.1
    ventricular I49.3
  bladder Q64.10
  bone and cartilage in lung Q33.5
  brain Q04.8
  breast tissue Q83.8
  cardiac Q24.8
  cerebral Q04.8
  cordis Q24.8
  endometrium —see Endometriosis
  gastric mucosa Q40.2
  gestation —see Pregnancy, by site
  heart Q24.8
  hormone secretion NEC E34.2
  kidney (crossed) (pelvis) Q63.2
  lens, lentis Q12.1
  mole —see Pregnancy, by site
  organ or site NEC —see Malposition,
    congenital
  pancreas Q45.3
  pregnancy —see Pregnancy, ectopic
  pupil —see Abnormality, pupillary
  renal Q63.2
  sebaceous glands of mouth Q38.6
  spleen Q89.09
  testis Q53.00
    bilateral Q53.02
    unilateral Q53.01
  thyroid Q89.2
  tissue in lung Q33.5
  ureter Q62.63
  ventricular beats I49.3
  vesicae Q64.10
Ectromelia Q73.8
  lower limb —see Defect, reduction, limb,
    lower, specified type NEC
  upper limb —see Defect, reduction, limb,
    upper, specified type NEC
Ectropion H02.109
  cervix N86
    with cervicitis N72
  congenital Q10.1
  eyelid (paralytic) H02.109
    cicatricial H02.119
      left H02.116
        lower H02.115
        upper H02.114
      right H02.113
        lower H02.112
        upper H02.111
    congenital Q10.1

Ectropion (Continued)
  eyelid (Continued)
    left H02.106
      lower H02.105
      upper H02.104
    mechanical H02.129
      left H02.126
        lower H02.125
        upper H02.124
      right H02.123
        lower H02.122
        upper H02.121
    right H02.103
      lower H02.102
      upper H02.101
    senile H02.139
      left H02.136
        lower H02.135
        upper H02.134
      right H02.133
        lower H02.132
        upper H02.131
    spastic H02.149
      left H02.146
        lower H02.145
        upper H02.144
      right H02.143
        lower H02.142
        upper H02.141
  iris H21.89
  lip (acquired) K13.0
    congenital Q38.0
  urethra N36.8
  uvea H21.89
Eczema (acute) (chronic) (erythematous)
    (fissum) (rubrum) (squamous) (see also
    Dermatitis) L30.9
  contact —see Dermatitis, contact
  dyshydrotic L30.1
  external ear —see Otitis, externa, acute,
    eczematoid
  flexural L20.82
  herpeticum B00.0
  hypertrophicum L28.0
  hypostatic —see Varix, leg, with,
    inflammation
  impetiginous L01.1
  infantile (due to any substance) L20.83
    intertriginous L21.1
    seborrheic L21.1
  intertriginous NEC L30.4
    infantile L21.1
  intrinsic (allergic) L20.84
  lichenified NEC L28.0
  marginatum (hebrae) B35.6
  pustular L30.3
  stasis I87.2 ◀▥
    with varicose veins —see Varix, leg, with,
      inflammation ◀
  vaccination, vaccinatum T88.1
  varicose —see Varix, leg, with, inflammation
Eczematid L30.2
Eddowes (-Spurway) syndrome Q78.0
Edema, edematous (infectious) (pitting)
    (toxic) R60.9
  with nephritis —see Nephrosis
  allergic T78.3
  amputation stump (surgical) (sequelae
    (late effect)) T87.89
  angioneurotic (allergic) (any site) (with
    urticaria) T78.3
    hereditary D84.1
  angiospastic I73.9
  Berlin's (traumatic) S05.8X-
  brain (cytotoxic) (vasogenic) G93.6
    due to birth injury P11.0
    newborn (anoxia or hypoxia) P52.4
      birth injury P11.0
    traumatic —see Injury, intracranial,
      cerebral edema
  cardiac —see Failure, heart, congestive

Edema, edematous *(Continued)*
cardiovascular —*see* Failure, heart, congestive
cerebral —*see* Edema, brain
cerebrospinal —*see* Edema, brain
cervix (uteri) (acute) N88.8
puerperal, postpartum O90.89
chronic hereditary Q82.0
circumscribed, acute T78.3
hereditary D84.1
conjunctiva H11.42-
cornea H18.2-
idiopathic H18.22-
secondary H18.23-
due to contact lens H18.21-
due to
lymphatic obstruction I89.0
salt retention E87.0
epiglottis —*see* Edema, glottis
essential, acute T78.3
hereditary D84.1
extremities, lower —*see* Edema, legs
eyelid NEC H02.849
left H02.846
lower H02.845
upper H02.844
right H02.843
lower H02.842
upper H02.841
familial, hereditary Q82.0
famine —*see* Malnutrition, severe
generalized R60.1
glottis, glottic, glottidis (obstructive) (passive)
J38.4
allergic T78.3
hereditary D84.1
heart —*see* Failure, heart, congestive
heat T67.7
hereditary Q82.0
inanition —*see* Malnutrition, severe
intracranial G93.6
iris H21.89
joint —*see* Effusion, joint
larynx —*see* Edema, glottis
legs R60.0
due to venous obstruction I87.1
hereditary Q82.0
localized R60.0
due to venous obstruction I87.1
lower limbs —*see* Edema, legs
lung J81.1
with heart condition or failure —*see*
Failure, ventricular, left
acute J81.0
chemical (acute) J68.1
chronic J68.1
chronic J81.1
due to
chemicals, gases, fumes or vapors
(inhalation) J68.1
external agent J70.9
specified NEC J70.8
radiation J70.1
due to
chemicals, fumes or vapors (inhalation)
J68.1
external agent J70.9
specified NEC J70.8
high altitude T70.29
near drowning T75.1
radiation J70.0
meaning failure, left ventricle I50.1
lymphatic I89.0
due to mastectomy I97.2
macula H35.81
cystoid, following cataract surgery —*see*
Complications, postprocedural,
following cataract surgery
diabetic —*see* Diabetes, by type, with,
retinopathy, with macular edema
malignant —*see* Gangrene, gas
Milroy's Q82.0

Edema, edematous *(Continued)*
nasopharynx J39.2
newborn P83.30
hydrops fetalis —*see* Hydrops, fetalis
specified NEC P83.39
nutritional —*see also* Malnutrition, severe
with dyspigmentation, skin and hair E40
optic disc or nerve —*see* Papilledema
orbit H05.22-
pancreas K86.89 ◄▥
papilla, optic —*see* Papilledema
penis N48.89
periodic T78.3
hereditary D84.1
pharynx J39.2
pulmonary —*see* Edema, lung
Quincke's T78.3
hereditary D84.1
renal —*see* Nephrosis
retina H35.81
diabetic —*see* Diabetes, by type, with,
retinopathy, with macular edema
salt E87.0
scrotum N50.89 ◄▥
seminal vesicle N50.89 ◄▥
spermatic cord N50.89 ◄▥
spinal (cord) (vascular) (nontraumatic) G95.19
starvation —*see* Malnutrition, severe
stasis —*see* Hypertension, venous, (chronic)
subglottic —*see* Edema, glottis
supraglottic —*see* Edema, glottis
testis N44.8
tunica vaginalis N50.89 ◄▥
vas deferens N50.89 ◄▥
vulva (acute) N90.89
Edentulism —*see* Absence, teeth, acquired
Edsall's disease T67.2
Educational handicap Z55.9
specified NEC Z55.8
Edward's syndrome —*see* Trisomy, 18
Effect, adverse
abnormal gravitational (G) forces or states
T75.81
abuse —*see* Maltreatment
air pressure T70.9
specified NEC T70.8
altitude (high) —*see* Effect, adverse, high
altitude
anesthesia —*see also* Anesthesia T88.59
in labor and delivery O74.9
~~in pregnancy NEC O29.3~~
local, toxic
in labor and delivery O74.4-
in pregnancy NEC O29.3- ◄
postpartum, puerperal O89.3
postpartum, puerperal O89.9
specified NEC T88.59
in labor and delivery O74.8
postpartum, puerperal O89.8
spinal and epidural T88.59
headache T88.59
in labor and delivery O74.5
postpartum, puerperal O89.4
specified NEC
in labor and delivery O74.6
postpartum, puerperal O89.5
antitoxin —*see* Complications, vaccination
atmospheric pressure T70.9
due to explosion T70.8
high T70.3
low —*see* Effect, adverse, high altitude
specified effect NEC T70.8
biological, correct substance properly
administered —*see* Effect, adverse, drug
blood (derivatives) (serum) (transfusion) —
see Complications, transfusion
chemical substance —*see* Table of Drugs and
Chemicals
cold (temperature) (weather) T69.9
chilblains T69.1
frostbite —*see* Frostbite
specified effect NEC T69.8

Effect, adverse *(Continued)*
drugs and medicaments T88.7
specified drug —*see* Table of Drugs and
Chemicals, by drug, adverse effect
specified effect — code to condition
electric current, electricity (shock) T75.4
burn —*see* Burn
exertion (excessive) T73.3
exposure —*see* Exposure
external cause NEC T75.89
foodstuffs T78.1
allergic reaction —*see* Allergy, food
causing anaphylaxis —*see* Shock,
anaphylactic, due to food
noxious —*see* Poisoning, food, noxious
gases, fumes, or vapors T59.9-
specified agent —*see* Table of Drugs and
Chemicals
glue (airplane) sniffing
due to drug abuse —*see* Abuse, drug,
inhalant
due to drug dependence —*see* Dependence,
drug, inhalant
heat —*see* Heat
high altitude NEC T70.29
anoxia T70.29
on
ears T70.0
sinuses T70.1
polycythemia D75.1
high pressure fluids T70.4
hot weather —*see* Heat
hunger T73.0
immersion, foot —*see* Immersion
immunization —*see* Complications,
vaccination
immunological agents —*see* Complications,
vaccination
infrared (radiation) (rays) NOS T66
dermatitis or eczema L59.8
infusion —*see* Complications, infusion
lack of care of infants —*see* Maltreatment,
child
lightning —*see* Lightning
medical care T88.9
specified NEC T88.8
medicinal substance, correct, properly
administered —*see* Effect, adverse, drug
motion T75.3
noise, on inner ear —*see* subcategory H83.3
overheated places —*see* Heat
psychosocial, of work environment Z56.5
radiation (diagnostic) (infrared) (natural
source) (therapeutic) (ultraviolet)
(X-ray) NOS T66
dermatitis or eczema —*see* Dermatitis, due
to, radiation
fibrosis of lung J70.1
pneumonitis J70.0
pulmonary manifestations
acute J70.0
chronic J70.1
skin L59.9
radioactive substance NOS
dermatitis or eczema —*see* Radiodermatitis
reduced temperature T69.9
immersion foot or hand —*see* Immersion
specified effect NEC T69.8
serum NEC (*see also* Reaction, serum) T80.69
specified NEC T78.8
external cause NEC T75.89
strangulation —*see* Asphyxia, traumatic
submersion T75.1
thirst T73.1
toxic —*see* Toxicity
transfusion —*see* Complications, transfusion
ultraviolet (radiation) (rays) NOS T66
burn —*see* Burn
dermatitis or eczema —*see* Dermatitis, due
to, ultraviolet rays
acute L56.8

◄ New   ◄▥ Revised   ~~deleted~~ Deleted

Effect, adverse (Continued)
vaccine (any) —see Complications, vaccination
vibration —see Vibration, adverse effects
water pressure NEC T70.9
specified NEC T70.8
weightlessness T75.82
whole blood —see Complications, transfusion
work environment Z56.5
Effect (s) (of) (from) —see Effect, adverse NEC
Effects, late —see Sequelae
Effluvium
anagen L65.1
telogen L65.0
Effort syndrome (psychogenic) F45.8
Effusion
amniotic fluid —see Pregnancy, complicated by, prematue rupture of membranes
brain (serous) G93.6
bronchial —see Bronchitis
cerebral G93.6
cerebrospinal —see also Meningitis
vessel G93.6
chest —see Effusion, pleura
chylous, chyliform (pleura) J94.0
intracranial G93.6
joint M25.40
ankle M25.47-
elbow M25.42-
foot joint M25.47-
hand joint M25.44-
hip M25.45-
knee M25.46-
shoulder M25.41-
specified joint NEC M25.48
wrist M25.43-
malignant pleural J91.0
meninges —see Meningitis
pericardium, pericardial (noninflammatory) I31.3
acute —see Pericarditis, acute
peritoneal (chronic) R18.8
pleura, pleurisy, pleuritic, pleuropericardial J90
chylous, chyliform J94.0
due to systemic lupus erythematosis M32.13
influenzal —see Influenza, with, respiratory manifestations NEC
malignant J91.0
newborn P28.89
tuberculous NEC A15.6
primary (progressive) A15.7
spinal —see Meningitis
thorax, thoracic —see Effusion, pleura
Egg shell nails L60.3
congenital Q84.6
Egyptian splenomegaly B65.1
Ehlers-Danlos syndrome Q79.6
Ehrlichiosis A77.40
due to
E. chafeensis A77.41
E. sennetsu A79.81
specified organism NEC A77.49
Eichstedt's disease B36.0
Eisenmenger's
complex or syndrome I27.89
defect Q21.8
Ejaculation
delayed F52.32 ◄
painful N53.12
premature F52.4
retarded N53.11
retrograde N53.14
semen, painful N53.12
psychogenic F52.6
Ekbom's syndrome (restless legs) G25.81
Ekman's syndrome (brittle bones and blue sclera) Q78.0
Elastic skin Q82.8
acquired L57.4

Elastofibroma —see Neoplasm, connective tissue, benign
Elastoma (juvenile) Q82.8
Miescher's L87.2
Elastomyofibrosis I42.4
Elastosis
actinic, solar L57.8
atrophicans (senile) L57.4
perforans serpiginosa L87.2
senilis L57.4
Elbow —see condition
Electric current, electricity, effects (concussion) (fatal) (nonfatal) (shock) T75.4
burn —see Burn
Electric feet syndrome E53.8
Electrocution T75.4
from electroshock gun (taser) T75.4
Electrolyte imbalance E87.8
with
abortion —see Abortion by type, complicated by, electrolyte imbalance
ectopic pregnancy O08.5
molar pregnancy O08.5
Elephantiasis (nonfilarial) I89.0
arabicum —see Infestation, filarial
bancroftian B74.0
congenital (any site) (hereditary) Q82.0
due to
Brugia (malayi) B74.1
timori B74.2
mastectomy I97.2
Wuchereria (bancrofti) B74.0
eyelid H02.859
left H02.856
lower H02.855
upper H02.854
right H02.853
lower H02.852
upper H02.851
filarial, filariensis —see Infestation, filarial
glandular I89.0
graecorum A30.9
lymphangiectatic I89.0
lymphatic vessel I89.0
due to mastectomy I97.2
scrotum (nonfilarial) I89.0
streptococcal I89.0
surgical I97.89
postmastectomy I97.2
telangiectodes I89.0
vulva (nonfilarial) N90.89
Elevated, elevation
antibody titer R76.0
basal metabolic rate R94.8
blood pressure —see also Hypertension
reading (incidental) (isolated) (nonspecific), no diagnosis of hypertension R03.0
blood sugar R73.9
body temperature (of unknown origin) R50.9
C-reactive protein (CRP) R79.82
cancer antigen 125 [CA 125] R97.1
carcinoembryonic antigen [CEA] R97.0
cholesterol E78.00 ◄▥
with high triglycerides E78.2
conjugate, eye H51.0
diaphragm, congenital Q79.1
erythrocyte sedimentation rate R70.0
fasting glucose R73.01
fasting triglycerides E78.1
finding on laboratory examination —see Findings, abnormal, inconclusive, without diagnosis, by type of exam
GFR (glomerular filtration rate) —see Findings, abnormal, inconclusive, without diagnosis, by type of exam
glucose tolerance (oral) R73.02
immunoglobulin level R76.8
indoleacetic acid R82.5
lactic acid dehydrogenase (LDH) level R74.0
leukocytes D72.829
lipoprotein a level E78.8

Elevated, elevation (Continued)
liver function
study R94.5
test R79.89
alkaline phosphatase R74.8
aminotransferase R74.0
bilirubin R17
hepatic enzyme R74.8
lactate dehydrogenase R74.0
lymphocytes D72.820
prostate specific antigen [PSA] R97.20 ◄▥
Rh titer —see Complication (s), transfusion, incompatibility reaction, Rh (factor)
scapula, congenital Q74.0
sedimentation rate R70.0
SGOT R74.0
SGPT R74.0
transaminase level R74.0
triglycerides E78.1
with high cholesterol E78.2
tumor associated antigens [TAA] NEC R97.8
tumor specific antigens [TSA] NEC R97.8
urine level of
17-ketosteroids R82.5
catecholamine R82.5
indoleacetic acid R82.5
steroids R82.5
vanillylmandelic acid (VMA) R82.5
venous pressure I87.8
white blood cell count D72.829
specified NEC D72.828
Elliptocytosis (congenital) (hereditary) D58.1
Hb C (disease) D58.1
hemoglobin disease D58.1
sickle-cell (disease) D57.8-
trait D57.3
Ellison-Zollinger syndrome E16.4
Ellis-van Creveld syndrome (chondroectodermal dysplasia) Q77.6
Elongated, elongation (congenital) —see also Distortion
bone Q79.9
cervix (uteri) Q51.828
acquired N88.4
hypertrophic N88.4
colon Q43.8
common bile duct Q44.5
cystic duct Q44.5
frenulum, penis Q55.69
labia minora (acquired) N90.69 ◄▥
ligamentum patellae Q74.1
petiolus (epiglottidis) Q31.8
tooth, teeth K00.2
uvula Q38.6
Eltor cholera A00.1
Emaciation (due to malnutrition) E41
Embadomoniasis A07.8
Embedded tooth, teeth K01.0
root only K08.3
Embolic —see condition
Embolism (multiple) (paradoxical) I74.9
air (any site) (traumatic) T79.0
following
abortion —see Abortion by type complicated by embolism
ectopic pregnancy O08.2
infusion, therapeutic injection or transfusion T80.0
molar pregnancy O08.2
procedure NEC
artery T81.719
mesenteric T81.710
renal T81.711
specified NEC T81.718
vein T81.72
in pregnancy, childbirth or puerperium —see Embolism, obstetric
amniotic fluid (pulmonary) —see also Embolism, obstetric
following
abortion —see Abortion by type complicated by embolism

Embolism *(Continued)*
  amniotic fluid *(Continued)*
    following *(Continued)*
      ectopic pregnancy O08.2
      molar pregnancy O08.2
  aorta, aortic I74.10
    abdominal I74.09
      saddle I74.01
    bifurcation I74.09
    saddle I74.01
    thoracic I74.11
  artery I74.9
    auditory, internal I65.8
    basilar —*see* Occlusion, artery, basilar
    carotid (common) (internal) —*see*
      Occlusion, artery, carotid
    cerebellar (anterior inferior) (posterior
      inferior) (superior) I66.3
    cerebral —*see* Occlusion, artery, cerebral
    choroidal (anterior) I66.8
    communicating posterior I66.8
    coronary —*see also* Infarct, myocardium
      not resulting in infarction I24.0
    extremity I74.4
      lower I74.3
      upper I74.2
    hypophyseal I66.8
    iliac I74.5
    limb I74.4
      lower I74.3
      upper I74.2
    mesenteric (with gangrene) —*see also*
      Ischemia, intestine, acute K55.09 ◀▥
    ophthalmic —*see* Occlusion, artery, retina
    peripheral I74.4
    pontine I66.8
    precerebral —*see* Occlusion, artery,
      precerebral
    pulmonary —*see* Embolism, pulmonary
    renal N28.0
    retinal —*see* Occlusion, artery, retina
    septic I76
    specified NEC I74.8
    vertebral —*see* Occlusion, artery, vertebral
  basilar (artery) I65.1
  blood clot
    following
      abortion —*see* Abortion by type
        complicated by embolism
      ectopic or molar pregnancy O08.2
    in pregnancy, childbirth or puerperium —
      see Embolism, obstetric
  brain —*see also* Occlusion, artery, cerebral
    following
      abortion —*see* Abortion by type
        complicated by embolism
      ectopic or molar pregnancy O08.2
    puerperal, postpartum, childbirth —*see*
      Embolism, obstetric
  capillary I78.8
  cardiac —*see also* Infarct, myocardium
    not resulting in infarction I51.3 ◀▥
  carotid (artery) (common) (internal) —*see*
    Occlusion, artery, carotid
  cavernous sinus (venous) —*see* Embolism,
    intracranial venous sinus
  cerebral —*see* Occlusion, artery, cerebral
  cholesterol —*see* Atheroembolism
  coronary (artery or vein) (systemic) —*see*
    Occlusion, coronary
  due to device, implant or graft —*see also*
    Complications, by site and type,
      specified NEC
    arterial graft NEC T82.818
    breast (implant) T85.818 ◀▥
    catheter NEC T85.818 ◀▥
      dialysis (renal) T82.818
        intraperitoneal T85.818 ◀▥
      infusion NEC T82.818
        spinal (epidural) (subdural) T85.810 ◀▥
      urinary (indwelling) T83.81

Embolism *(Continued)*
  due to device, implant or graft *(Continued)*
    electronic (electrode) (pulse generator)
      (stimulator)
      bone T84.81
      cardiac T82.817
      nervous system (brain) (peripheral
        nerve) (spinal) T85.810 ◀▥
      urinary T83.81
    fixation, internal (orthopedic) NEC T84.81
    gastrointestinal (bile duct) (esophagus)
      T85.818 ◀▥
    genital NEC T83.81
    heart (graft) (valve) T82.817
    joint prosthesis T84.81
    ocular (corneal graft) (orbital implant)
      T85.818 ◀▥
    orthopedic (bone graft) NEC T86.838
    specified NEC T85.818 ◀▥
    urinary (graft) NEC T83.81
    vascular NEC T82.818
    ventricular intracranial shunt T85.810 ◀▥
  extremities
    lower —*see* Embolism, vein, lower
      extremity
      arterial I74.3
    upper I74.2
  eye H34.9
  fat (cerebral) (pulmonary) (systemic) T79.1
    complicating delivery —*see* Embolism,
      obstetric
    following
      abortion —*see* Abortion by type
        complicated by embolism
      ectopic or molar pregnancy O08.2
  following
    abortion —*see* Abortion by type
      complicated by embolism
    ectopic or molar pregnancy O08.2
    infusion, therapeutic injection or
      transfusion
      air T80.0
  heart (fatty) —*see also* Infarct, myocardium
    not resulting in infarction I51.3 ◀▥
  hepatic (vein) I82.0
  in pregnancy, childbirth or puerperium —*see*
    Embolism, obstetric
  intestine (artery) (vein) (with gangrene) —*see*
    also Ischemia, intestine, acute K55.039 ◀▥
  intracranial —*see also* Occlusion, artery,
    cerebral
    venous sinus (any) G08
      nonpyogenic I67.6
  intraspinal venous sinuses or veins G08
    nonpyogenic G95.19
  kidney (artery) N28.0
  lateral sinus (venous) —*see* Embolism,
    intracranial, venous sinus
  leg —*see* Embolism, vein, lower extremity
    arterial I74.3
  longitudinal sinus (venous) —*see* Embolism,
    intracranial, venous sinus
  lung (massive) —*see* Embolism, pulmonary
  meninges I66.8
  mesenteric (artery) (vein) (with gangrene) —
    see also Ischemia, intestine, acute
      K55.059 ◀▥
  obstetric (in) (pulmonary)
    childbirth O88.22 ◀▥
      air O88.02
      amniotic fluid O88.12
      blood clot O88.22
      fat O88.82
      pyemic O88.32
      septic O88.32
      specified type NEC O88.82
    pregnancy O88.21- ◀▥
      air O88.01-
      amniotic fluid O88.11-
      blood clot O88.21-
      fat O88.81-

Embolism *(Continued)*
  obstetric *(Continued)*
    pregnancy *(Continued)*
      pyemic O88.31-
      septic O88.31-
      specified type NEC O88.81-
    puerperal O88.23 ◀▥
      air O88.03
      amniotic fluid O88.13
      blood clot O88.23
      fat O88.83
      pyemic O88.33
      septic O88.33
      specified type NEC O88.83
  ophthalmic —*see* Occlusion, artery, retina
  penis N48.81
  peripheral artery NOS I74.4
  pituitary E23.6
  popliteal (artery) I74.3
  portal (vein) I81
  postoperative, postprocedural
    artery T81.719
      mesenteric T81.710
      renal T81.711
      specified NEC T81.718
    vein T81.72
  precerebral artery —*see* Occlusion, artery,
    precerebral
  puerperal —*see* Embolism, obstetric
  pulmonary (acute) (artery) (vein) I26.99
    with acute cor pulmonale I26.09
    chronic I27.82
    following
      abortion —*see* Abortion by type
        complicated by embolism
      ectopic or molar pregnancy O08.2
    healed or old Z86.711
    in pregnancy, childbirth or puerperium —
      see Embolism, obstetric
    personal history of Z86.711
    saddle I26.92
      with acute cor pulmonale I26.02
    septic I26.90
      with acute cor pulmonale I26.01
  pyemic (multiple) I76
    following
      abortion —*see* Abortion by type
        complicated by embolism
      ectopic or molar pregnancy O08.2
    Hemophilus influenzae A41.3
    pneumococcal A40.3
      with pneumonia J13
    puerperal, postpartum, childbirth (any
      organism) —*see* Embolism, obstetric
    specified organism NEC A41.89
    staphylococcal A41.2
    streptococcal A40.9
  renal (artery) N28.0
    vein I82.3
  retina, retinal —*see* Occlusion, artery,
    retina
  saddle
    abdominal aorta I74.01
    pulmonary artery I26.92
      with acute cor pulmonale I26.02
  septic (arterial) I76
    complicating abortion —*see* Abortion, by
      type, complicated by, embolism
  sinus —*see* Embolism, intracranial, venous
    sinus
  soap complicating abortion —*see* Abortion,
    by type, complicated by, embolism
  spinal cord G95.19
    pyogenic origin G06.1
  spleen, splenic (artery) I74.8
  upper extremity I74.2
  vein (acute) I82.90
    antecubital I82.61-
      chronic I82.71-
    axillary I82.A1-
      chronic I82.A2-

◀ New   ◀▥ Revised   ~~deleted~~ Deleted

Embolism *(Continued)*
 vein *(Continued)*
  basilic I82.61-
   chronic I82.71-
  brachial I82.62-
   chronic I82.72-
  brachiocephalic (innominate) I82.290
   chronic I82.291
  cephalic I82.61-
   chronic I82.71-
  chronic I82.91
  deep (DVT) I82.40-
   calf I82.4Z-
    chronic I82.5Z-
   lower leg I82.4Z-
    chronic I82.5Z-
   thigh I82.4Y-
    chronic I82.5Y-
   upper leg I82.4Y
    chronic I82.5y--
  femoral I82.41-
   chronic I82.51-
  iliac (iliofemoral) I82.42-
   chronic I82.52-
  innominate I82.290
   chronic I82.291
  internal jugular I82.C1-
   chronic I82.C2-
  lower extremity
   deep I82.40-
    chronic I82.50-
     specified NEC I82.49-
      chronic NEC I82.59-
   distal
    deep I82.4Z-
   proximal
    deep I82.4Y-
     chronic I82.5Y-
   superficial I82.81-
  popliteal I82.43-
   chronic I82.53-
  radial I82.62-
   chronic I82.72-
  renal I82.3
  saphenous (greater) (lesser) I82.81-
  specified NEC I82.890
   chronic NEC I82.891
  subclavian I82.B1-
   chronic I82.B2-
  thoracic NEC I82.290
   chronic I82.291
  tibial I82.44-
   chronic I82.54-
  ulnar I82.62-
   chronic I82.72-
  upper extremity I82.60-
   chronic I82.70-
   deep I82.62-
    chronic I82.72-
   superficial I82.61-
    chronic I82.71-
 vena cava
  inferior (acute) I82.220
   chronic I82.221
  superior (acute) I82.210
   chronic I82.211
 venous sinus G08
 vessels of brain —*see* Occlusion, artery,
   cerebral
Embolus —*see* Embolism
Embryoma —*see also* Neoplasm, uncertain
  behavior, by site
 benign —*see* Neoplasm, benign, by site
 kidney C64.-
 liver C22.0
 malignant —*see also* Neoplasm, malignant,
   by site
  kidney C64.-
  liver C22.0
 testis C62.9-
  descended (scrotal) C62.1-
  undescended C62.0-

Embryoma *(Continued)*
 testis C62.9-
  descended (scrotal) C62.1-
  undescended C62.0-
Embryonic
 circulation Q28.9
 heart Q28.9
 vas deferens Q55.4
Embryopathia NOS Q89.9
Embryotoxon Q13.4
Emesis —*see* Vomiting
Emotional lability R45.86
Emotionality, pathological F60.3
Emotogenic disease —*see* Disorder,
  psychogenic
Emphysema (atrophic) (bullous) (chronic)
  (interlobular) (lung) (obstructive)
  (pulmonary) (senile) (vesicular)
  J43.9
 cellular tissue (traumatic) T79.7
  surgical T81.82
 centrilobular J43.2
 compensatory J98.3
 congenital (interstitial) P25.0
 conjunctiva H11.89
 connective tissue (traumatic) T79.7
  surgical T81.82
 due to chemicals, gases, fumes or vapors
   J68.4
 eyelid (s) —*see* Disorder, eyelid, specified
   type NEC
  surgical T81.82
  traumatic T79.7
 interstitial J98.2
  congenital P25.0
  perinatal period P25.0
 laminated tissue T79.7
  surgical T81.82
 mediastinal J98.2
  newborn P25.2
 orbit, orbital —*see* Disorder, orbit, specified
   type NEC
 panacinar J43.1
 panlobular J43.1
 specified NEC J43.8
 subcutaneous (traumatic) T79.7
  nontraumatic J98.2
  postprocedural T81.82
  surgical T81.82
 surgical T81.82
 thymus (gland) (congenital) E32.8
 traumatic (subcutaneous) T79.7
 unilateral J43.0
Empty nest syndrome Z60.0
Empyema (acute) (chest) (double) (pleura)
  (supradiaphragmatic) (thorax) J86.9
 with fistula J86.0
 accessory sinus (chronic) —*see* Sinusitis
 antrum (chronic) —*see* Sinusitis, maxillary
 brain (any part) —*see* Abscess, brain
 ethmoidal (chronic) (sinus) —*see* Sinusitis,
   ethmoidal
 extradural —*see* Abscess, extradural
 frontal (chronic) (sinus) —*see* Sinusitis,
   frontal
 gallbladder K81.0
 mastoid (process) (acute) —*see* Mastoiditis,
   acute
 maxilla, maxillary M27.2
  sinus (chronic) —*see* Sinusitis,
    maxillary
 nasal sinus (chronic) —*see* Sinusitis
 sinus (accessory) (chronic) (nasal) —*see*
   Sinusitis
 sphenoidal (sinus) (chronic) —*see* Sinusitis,
   sphenoidal
 subarachnoid —*see* Abscess, extradural
 subdural —*see* Abscess, subdural
 tuberculous A15.6
 ureter —*see* Ureteritis
 ventricular —*see* Abscess, brain

En coup de sabre lesion L94.1
Enamel pearls K00.2
Enameloma K00.2
Enanthema, viral B09
Encephalitis (chronic) (hemorrhagic)
  (idiopathic) (nonepidemic) (spurious)
  (subacute) G04.90
 acute —*see also* Encephalitis, viral A86
  disseminated G04.00
   infectious G04.01
   noninfectious G04.81
   postimmunization (postvaccination)
     G04.02
   postinfectious G04.01
  inclusion body A85.8
  necrotizing hemorrhagic G04.30
   postimmunization G04.32
   postinfectious G04.31
   specified NEC G04.39
 arboviral, arbovirus NEC A85.2
 arthropod-borne NEC (viral) A85.2
 Australian A83.4
 California (virus) A83.5
 Central European (tick-borne) A84.1
 Czechoslovakian A84.1
 Dawson's (inclusion body) A81.1
 diffuse sclerosing A81.1
 disseminated, acute G04.00
 due to
  cat scratch disease A28.1
  human immunodeficiency virus (HIV)
    disease B20 *[G05.3]*
  malaria —*see* Malaria
  rickettsiosis —*see* Rickettsiosis
  smallpox inoculation G04.02
  typhus —*see* Typhus
 Eastern equine A83.2
 endemic (viral) A86
 epidemic NEC (viral) A86
 equine (acute) (infectious) (viral) A83.9
  Eastern A83.2
  Venezuelan A92.2
  Western A83.1
 Far Eastern (tick-borne) A84.0
 following vaccination or other immunization
   procedure G04.02
 herpes zoster B02.0
 herpesviral B00.4
  due to herpesvirus 6 B10.01
  due to herpesvirus 7 B10.09
  specified NEC B10.09
 Ilheus (virus) A83.8
 in (due to)
  actinomycosis A42.82
  adenovirus A85.1
  African trypanosomiasis B56.9 *[G05.3]*
  Chagas' disease (chronic) B57.42
  cytomegalovirus B25.8
  enterovirus A85.0
  herpes (simplex) virus B00.4
   due to herpesvirus 6 B10.01
   due to herpesvirus 7 B10.09
   specified NEC B10.09
  infectious disease NEC B99 *[G05.3]*
  influenza —*see* Influenza, with,
    encephalopathy
  listeriosis A32.12
  measles B05.0
  mumps B26.2
  naegleriasis B60.2
  parasitic disease NEC B89 *[G05.3]*
  poliovirus A80.9 *[G05.3]*
  rubella B06.01
  syphilis
   congenital A50.42
   late A52.14
  systemic lupus erythematosus M32.19
  toxoplasmosis (acquired) B58.2
   congenital P37.1
  tuberculosis A17.82
  zoster B02.0

Encephalitis *(Continued)*
  inclusion body A81.1
  infectious (acute) (virus) NEC A86
  Japanese (B type) A83.0
  La Crosse A83.5
  lead —*see* Poisoning, lead
  lethargica (acute) (infectious) A85.8
  louping ill A84.8
  lupus erythematosus, systemic M32.19
  lymphatica A87.2
  Mengo A85.8
  meningococcal A39.81
  Murray Valley A83.4
  otitic NEC H66.40 *[G05.3]*
  parasitic NOS B71.9
  periaxial G37.0
  periaxialis (concentrica) (diffuse) G37.5
  postchickenpox B01.11
  postexanthematous NEC B09
  postimmunization G04.02
  postinfectious NEC G04.01
  postmeasles B05.0
  postvaccinal G04.02
  postvaricella B01.11
  postviral NEC A86
  Powassan A84.8
  Rasmussen G04.81
  Rio Bravo A85.8
  Russian
    autumnal A83.0
    spring-summer (taiga) A84.0
  saturnine —*see* Poisoning, lead
  specified NEC G04.81
  St. Louis A83.3
  subacute sclerosing A81.1
  summer A83.0
  suppurative G04.81
  tick-borne A84.9
  Torula, torular (cryptococcal) B45.1
  toxic NEC G92
  trichinosis B75 *[G05.3]*
  type
    B A83.0
    C A83.3
  van Bogaert's A81.1
  Venezuelan equine A92.2
  Vienna A85.8
  viral, virus A86
    arthropod-borne NEC A85.2
    mosquito-borne A83.9
      Australian X disease A83.4
      California virus A83.5
      Eastern equine A83.2
      Japanese (B type) A83.0
      Murray Valley A83.4
      specified NEC A83.8
      St. Louis A83.3
      type B A83.0
      type C A83.3
      Western equine A83.1
    tick-borne A84.9
      biundulant A84.1
      central European A84.1
      Czechoslovakian A84.1
      diphasic meningoencephalitis A84.1
      Far Eastern A84.0
      Russian spring-summer (taiga) A84.0
      specified NEC A84.8
    specified type NEC A85.8
  Western equine A83.1
Encephalocele Q01.9
  frontal Q01.0
  nasofrontal Q01.1
  occipital Q01.2
  specified NEC Q01.8
Encephalocystocele —*see* Encephalocele
Encephaloduroarteriomyosynangiosis
  (EDAMS) I67.5
Encephalomalacia (brain) (cerebellar)
  (cerebral) —*see* Softening, brain

Encephalomeningitis —*see*
  Meningoencephalitis
Encephalomeningocele —*see* Encephalocele
Encephalomeningomyelitis —*see*
  Meningoencephalitis
Encephalomyelitis —*see also* Encephalitis
  G04.90
  acute disseminated G04.00
    infectious G04.01
    noninfectious G04.81
    postimmunization G04.02
    postinfectious G04.01
  acute necrotizing hemorrhagic G04.30
    postimmunization G04.32
    postinfectious G04.31
    specified NEC G04.39
  benign myalgic G93.3
  equine A83.9
    Eastern A83.2
    Venezuelan A92.2
    Western A83.1
  in diseases classified elsewhere G05.3
  myalgic, benign G93.3
  postchickenpox B01.11
  postinfectious NEC G04.01
  postmeasles B05.0
  postvaccinal G04.02
  postvaricella B01.11
  rubella B06.01
  specified NEC G04.81
  Venezuelan equine A92.2
Encephalomyelocele —*see* Encephalocele
Encephalomyelomeningitis —*see*
  Meningoencephalitis
Encephalomyelopathy G96.9
Encephalomyeloradiculitis (acute) G61.0
Encephalomyeloradiculoneuritis (acute)
  (Guillain-Barré) G61.0
Encephalomyeloradiculopathy G96.9
Encephalopathia hyperbilirubinemica,
  newborn P57.9
  due to isoimmunization (conditions in P55)
    P57.0
Encephalopathy (acute) G93.40
  acute necrotizing hemorrhagic G04.30
    postimmunization G04.32
    postinfectious G04.31
    specified NEC G04.39
  alcoholic G31.2
  anoxic —*see* Damage, brain, anoxic
  arteriosclerotic I67.2
  centrolobar progressive (Schilder) G37.0
  congenital Q07.9
  degenerative, in specified disease NEC
    G32.89
  due to
    drugs (*see also* Table of Drugs and
      Chemicals) G92
  demyelinating callosal G37.1
  hepatic —*see* Failure, hepatic
  hyperbilirubinemic, newborn P57.9
    due to isoimmunization (conditions in P55)
      P57.0
  hypertensive I67.4
  hypoglycemic E16.2
  hypoxic —*see* Damage, brain, anoxic
  hypoxic ischemic P91.60
    mild P91.61
    moderate P91.62
    severe P91.63
  in (due to) (with)
    birth injury P11.1
    hyperinsulinism E16.1 *[G94]*
    influenza —*see* Influenza, with,
      encephalopathy
    lack of vitamin (*see also* Deficiency, vitamin)
      E56.9 *[G32.89]*
    neoplastic disease (*see also* Neoplasm)
      D49.9 *[G13.1]*
    serum (*see also* Reaction, serum) T80.69
    syphilis A52.17

Encephalopathy *(Continued)*
  in *(Continued)*
    trauma (postconcussional) F07.81
      current injury —*see* Injury, intracranial
    vaccination G04.02
  lead —*see* Poisoning, lead
  metabolic G93.41
    drug induced G92
    toxic G92
  myoclonic, early, symptomatic —*see* Epilepsy,
    generalized, specified NEC
  necrotizing, subacute (Leigh) G31.82
  pellagrous E52 *[G32.89]*
  portosystemic —*see* Failure, hepatic
  postcontusional F07.81
    current injury —*see* Injury, intracranial,
      diffuse
  posthypoglycemic (coma) E16.1 *[G94]*
  postradiation G93.89
  saturnine —*see* Poisoning, lead
  septic G93.41
  specified NEC G93.49
  spongioform, subacute (viral) A81.09
  toxic G92
    metabolic G92
  traumatic (postconcussional) F07.81
    current injury —*see* Injury, intracranial
  vitamin B deficiency NEC E53.9 *[G32.89]*
    vitamin B1 E51.2
  Wernicke's E51.2
Encephalorrhagia —*see* Hemorrhage,
  intracranial, intracerebral
Encephalosis, posttraumatic F07.81
Enchondroma —*see also* Neoplasm, bone,
  benign
Enchondromatosis (cartilaginous) (multiple)
  Q78.4
Encopresis R15.9
  functional F98.1
  nonorganic origin F98.1
  psychogenic F98.1
Encounter (with health service) (for) Z76.89
  adjustment and management (of)
    breast implant Z45.81
    implanted device NEC Z45.89
    myringotomy device (stent) (tube)
      Z45.82
  administrative purpose only Z02.9
    examination for
      adoption Z02.82
      armed forces Z02.3
      disability determination Z02.71
      driving license Z02.4
      employment Z02.1
      insurance Z02.6
      medical certificate NEC Z02.79
      paternity testing Z02.81
      residential institution admission Z02.2
      school admission Z02.0
      sports Z02.5
      specified reason NEC Z02.89
  aftercare —*see* Aftercare
  antenatal screening Z36
  assisted reproductive fertility procedure cycle
    Z31.83
  blood typing Z01.83
    Rh typing Z01.83
  breast augmentation or reduction Z41.1
  breast implant exchange (different material)
    (different size) Z45.81
  breast reconstruction following mastectomy
    Z42.1
  check-up —*see* Examination
  chemotherapy for neoplasm Z51.11
  colonoscopy, screening Z12.11
  counseling —*see* Counseling
  delivery, full-term, uncomplicated O80
    cesarean, without indication O82
  desensitization to allergens Z51.6 ◄
  ear piercing Z41.3
  examination —*see* Examination

Encounter (Continued)
  expectant parent (s) (adoptive) pre-birth
      pediatrician visit Z76.81
  fertility preservation procedure (prior to
      cancer therapy) (prior to removal of
      gonads) Z31.84
  fitting (of) —see Fitting (and adjustment) (of)
  genetic
    counseling Z31.5
    testing —see Test, genetic
  hearing conservation and treatment
      Z01.12
  immunotherapy for neoplasm Z51.12
  in vitro fertilization cycle Z31.83
  instruction (in)
    child care (postpartal) (prenatal) Z32.3
    childbirth Z32.2
    natural family planning
      procreative Z31.61
      to avoid pregnancy Z30.02
  insulin pump titration Z46.81
  joint prosthesis insertion following prior
      explantation of joint prosthesis (staged
      procedure)
    hip Z47.32
    knee Z47.33
    shoulder Z47.31
  laboratory (as part of a general medical
      examination) Z00.00
    with abnormal findings Z00.01
  mental health services (for)
    abuse NEC
      perpetrator Z69.82
      victim Z69.81
    child abuse
      nonparental
        perpetrator Z69.021
        victim Z69.020
      parental
        perpetrator Z69.011
        victim Z69.010
    spousal or partner abuse
      perpetrator Z69.12
      victim Z69.11
  observation (for) (ruled out)
    exposure to (suspected)
      anthrax Z03.810
      biological agent NEC Z03.818
  pediatrician visit, by expectant parent (s)
      (adoptive) Z76.81
  plastic and reconstructive surgery following
      medical procedure or healed injury
      NEC Z42.8
  pregnancy
    supervision of —see Pregnancy,
        supervision of
    test Z32.00
      result negative Z32.02
      result positive Z32.01
  procreative management and counseling for
      gestational carrier Z31.7 ◀
  prophylactic measures Z29.9 ◀
    antivenin Z29.12 ◀
    fluoride administration Z29.3 ◀
    immunotherapy for respiratory syncytial
        virus (RSV) Z29.11 ◀
    rabies immune globin Z29.14 ◀
    Rho (D) immune globulin Z29.13 ◀
    specified NEC Z29.8 ◀
  radiation therapy (antineoplastic) Z51.0
  radiological (as part of a general medical
      examination) Z00.00
    with abnormal findings Z00.01
  reconstructive surgery following medical
      procedure or healed injury NEC
      Z42.8
  removal (of) —see also Removal
    artificial
      arm Z44.00-
        complete Z44.01-
        partial Z44.02-

Encounter (Continued)
  removal (Continued)
    artificial (Continued)
      eye Z44.2-
      leg Z44.10-
        complete Z44.11-
        partial Z44.12-
    breast implant Z45.81
      tissue expander (without synchronous
          insertion of permanent implant)
          Z45.81
    device Z46.9
      specified NEC Z46.89
    external
      fixation device — code to fracture with
          seventh character D
      prosthesis, prosthetic device Z44.9
        breast Z44.3-
        specified NEC Z44.8
    implanted device NEC Z45.89
    insulin pump Z46.81
    internal fixation device Z47.2
    myringotomy device (stent) (tube) Z45.82
    nervous system device NEC Z46.2
      brain neuropacemaker Z46.2
      visual substitution device Z46.2
        implanted Z45.31
    non-vascular catheter Z46.82
    orthodontic device Z46.4
    stent
      ureteral Z46.6
    urinary device Z46.6
  repeat cervical smear to confirm findings of
      recent normal smear following initial
      abnormal smear Z01.42
  respirator [ventilator] use during power
      failure (Z99.12)
  Rh typing Z01.83
  screening —see Screening
  specified NEC Z76.89
  sterilization Z30.2
  suspected condition, ruled out
    amniotic cavity and membrane Z03.71
    cervical shortening Z03.75
    fetal anomaly Z03.73
    fetal growth Z03.74
    maternal and fetal conditions NEC Z03.79
    oligohydramnios Z03.71
    placental problem Z03.72
    polyhydramnios Z03.71
  suspected exposure (to), ruled out
    anthrax Z03.810
    biological agents NEC Z03.818
  termination of pregnancy, elective Z33.2
  testing —see Test
  therapeutic drug level monitoring Z51.81
  titration, insulin pump Z46.81
  to determine fetal viability of pregnancy
      O36.80
  training
    insulin pump Z46.81
  X-ray of chest (as part of a general medical
      examination Z00.00)
    with abnormal findings Z00.01
Encystment —see Cyst
Endarteritis (bacterial, subacute) (infective)
      I77.6
  brain I67.7
  cerebral or cerebrospinal I67.7
  deformans —see Arteriosclerosis
  embolic —see Embolism
  obliterans —see also Arteriosclerosis
    pulmonary I28.8
  pulmonary I28.8
  retina —see Vasculitis, retina
  senile —see Arteriosclerosis
  syphilitic A52.09
    brain or cerebral A52.04
    congenital A50.54 [I79.8]
  tuberculous A18.89
Endemic —see condition

Endocarditis (chronic) (marantic) (nonbacterial)
      (thrombotic) (valvular) I38
  with rheumatic fever (conditions in I00)
    active —see Endocarditis, acute, rheumatic
    inactive or quiescent (with chorea) I09.1
  acute or subacute I33.9
    infective I33.0
    rheumatic (aortic) (mitral) (pulmonary)
        (tricuspid) I01.1
      with chorea (acute) (rheumatic)
          (Sydenham's) I02.0
  aortic (heart) (nonrheumatic) (valve) I35.8
    with
      mitral disease I08.0
        with tricuspid (valve) disease I08.3
        active or acute I01.1
          with chorea (acute) (rheumatic)
              (Sydenham's) I02.0
      rheumatic fever (conditions in I00)
        active —see Endocarditis, acute,
            rheumatic
        inactive or quiescent (with chorea)
            I06.9
      tricuspid (valve) disease I08.2
        with mitral (valve) disease I08.3
    acute or subacute I33.9
    arteriosclerotic I35.8
    rheumatic I06.9
      with mitral disease I08.0
        with tricuspid (valve) disease I08.3
        active or acute I01.1
          with chorea (acute) (rheumatic)
              (Sydenham's) I02.0
      active or acute I01.1
        with chorea (acute) (rheumatic)
            (Sydenham's) I02.0
    specified NEC I06.8
    specified cause NEC I35.8
    syphilitic A52.03
  arteriosclerotic I38
  atypical verrucous (Libman-Sacks) M32.11
  bacterial (acute) (any valve) (subacute)
      I33.0
  candidal B37.6
  congenital Q24.8
  constrictive I33.0
  Coxiella burnetii A78 [I39]
  Coxsackie B33.21
  due to
    prosthetic cardiac valve T82.6
    Q fever A78 [I39]
    Serratia marcescens I33.0
    typhoid (fever) A01.02
  gonococcal A54.83
  infectious or infective (acute) (any valve)
      (subacute) I33.0
  lenta (acute) (any valve) (subacute) I33.0
  Libman-Sacks M32.11
  listerial A32.82
  Löffler's I42.3
  malignant (acute) (any valve) (subacute) I33.0
  meningococcal A39.51
  mitral (chronic) (double) (fibroid) (heart)
      (inactive) (valve) (with chorea) I05.9
    with
      aortic (valve) disease I08.0
        with tricuspid (valve) disease I08.3
        active or acute I01.1
          with chorea (acute) (rheumatic)
              (Sydenham's) I02.0
      rheumatic fever (conditions in I00)
        active —see Endocarditis, acute,
            rheumatic
        inactive or quiescent (with chorea)
            I05.9
      tricuspid (valve) disease I08.1
        with aortic (valve) disease I08.3
    active or acute I01.1
      with chorea (acute) (rheumatic)
          (Sydenham's) I02.0
    bacterial I33.0

Endocarditis *(Continued)*
  mitral *(Continued)*
    arteriosclerotic I34.8
    nonrheumatic I34.8
      acute or subacute I33.9
    specified NEC I05.8
  monilial B37.6
  multiple valves I08.9
    specified disorders I08.8
  mycotic (acute) (any valve) (subacute) I33.0
  pneumococcal (acute) (any valve) (subacute)
      I33.0
  pulmonary (chronic) (heart) (valve) I37.8
    with rheumatic fever (conditions in I00)
      active —*see* Endocarditis, acute,
          rheumatic
      inactive or quiescent (with chorea)
          I09.89
        with aortic, mitral or tricuspid disease
            I08.8
    acute or subacute I33.9
      rheumatic I01.1
        with chorea (acute) (rheumatic)
            (Sydenham's) I02.0
    arteriosclerotic I37.8
    congenital Q22.2
    rheumatic (chronic) (inactive) (with chorea)
        I09.89
      active or acute I01.1
        with chorea (acute) (rheumatic)
            (Sydenham's) I02.0
    syphilitic A52.03
  purulent (acute) (any valve) (subacute) I33.0
  Q fever A78 *[I39]*
  rheumatic (chronic) (inactive) (with chorea)
      I09.1
    active or acute (aortic) (mitral)
        (pulmonary) (tricuspid) I01.1
      with chorea (acute) (rheumatic)
          (Sydenham's) I02.0
  rheumatoid —*see* Rheumatoid, carditis
  septic (acute) (any valve) (subacute) I33.0
  streptococcal (acute) (any valve) (subacute)
      I33.0
  subacute —*see* Endocarditis, acute
  suppurative (acute) (any valve) (subacute)
      I33.0
  syphilitic A52.03
  toxic I33.9
  tricuspid (chronic) (heart) (inactive)
      (rheumatic) (valve) (with chorea) I07.9
    with
      aortic (valve) disease I08.2
        mitral (valve) disease I08.3
      mitral (valve) disease I08.1
        aortic (valve) disease I08.3
      rheumatic fever (conditions in I00)
        active —*see* Endocarditis, acute,
            rheumatic
        inactive or quiescent (with chorea)
            I07.8
    active or acute I01.1
      with chorea (acute) (rheumatic)
          (Sydenham's) I02.0
    arteriosclerotic I36.8
    nonrheumatic I36.8
      acute or subacute I33.9
    specified cause, except rheumatic I36.8
  tuberculous —*see* Tuberculosis, endocarditis
  typhoid A01.02
  ulcerative (acute) (any valve) (subacute) I33.0
  vegetative (acute) (any valve) (subacute) I33.0
  verrucous (atypical) (nonbacterial)
      (nonrheumatic) M32.11
Endocardium, endocardial —*see also* condition
  cushion defect Q21.2
Endocervicitis —*see also* Cervicitis
  due to intrauterine (contraceptive) device
      T83.69 ◀▥
  hyperplastic N72
Endocrine —*see* condition

Endocrinopathy, pluriglandular E31.9
Endodontic
  overfill M27.52
  underfill M27.53
Endodontitis K04.01 ◀▥
  irreversible K04.02 ◀
  reversible K04.01 ◀
Endomastoiditis —*see* Mastoiditis
Endometrioma N80.9
Endometriosis N80.9
  appendix N80.5
  bladder N80.8
  bowel N80.5
  broad ligament N80.3
  cervix N80.0
  colon N80.5
  cul-de-sac (Douglas') N80.3
  exocervix N80.0
  fallopian tube N80.2
  female genital organ NEC N80.8
  gallbladder N80.8
  in scar of skin N80.6
  internal N80.0
  intestine N80.5
  lung N80.8
  myometrium N80.0
  ovary N80.1
  parametrium N80.3
  pelvic peritoneum N80.3
  peritoneal (pelvic) N80.3
  rectovaginal septum N80.4
  rectum N80.5
  round ligament N80.3
  skin (scar) N80.6
  specified site NEC N80.8
  stromal D39.0
  umbilicus N80.8
  uterus (internal) N80.0
  vagina N80.4
  vulva N80.8
Endometritis (decidual) (nonspecific) (purulent)
    (senile (atrophic) (suppurative) N71.9
  with ectopic pregnancy O08.0
  acute N71.0
  blenorrhagic (gonococcal) (acute) (chronic)
      A54.24
  cervix, cervical (with erosion or ectropion) —
      see also Cervicitis
    hyperplastic N72
  chlamydial A56.11
  chronic N71.1
  following
    abortion —*see* Abortion by type
        complicated by genital infection
    ectopic or molar pregnancy O08.0
  gonococcal, gonorrheal (acute) (chronic) A54.24
  hyperplastic —*see also* Hyperplasia,
      endometrial N85.00-
    cervix N72
  puerperal, postpartum, childbirth O86.12
  subacute N71.0
  tuberculous A18.17
Endometrium —*see* condition
Endomyocardiopathy, South African I42.3
Endomyocarditis —*see* Endocarditis
Endomyofibrosis I42.3
Endomyometritis —*see* Endometritis
Endopericarditis —*see* Endocarditis
Endoperineuritis —*see* Disorder, nerve
Endophlebitis —*see* Phlebitis
Endophthalmia —*see* Endophthalmitis,
    purulent
Endophthalmitis (acute) (infective) (metastatic)
    (subacute) H44.009
  bleb associated H59.4 —*see also* Bleb,
      inflamed (infected), postprocedural
  gonorrheal A54.39
  in (due to)
    cysticercosis B69.1
    onchocerciasis B73.01
    toxocariasis B83.0

Endophthalmitis *(Continued)*
  panuveitis —*see* Panuveitis
  parasitic H44.12-
  purulent H44.00-
    panophthalmitis —*see* Panophthalmitis
    vitreous abscess H44.02-
  specified NEC H44.19
  sympathetic —*see* Uveitis, sympathetic
Endosalpingioma D28.2
Endosalpingiosis N94.89
Endosteitis —*see* Osteomyelitis
Endothelioma, bone —*see* Neoplasm, bone,
    malignant
Endotheliosis (hemorrhagic infectional) D69.8
Endotoxemia — code to condition
Endotrachelitis —*see* Cervicitis
Engelmann (-Camurati) syndrome Q78.3
English disease —*see* Rickets
Engman's disease L30.3
Engorgement
  breast N64.59
    newborn P83.4
    puerperal, postpartum O92.79
  lung (passive) —*see* Edema, lung
  pulmonary (passive) —*see* Edema, lung
  stomach K31.89
  venous, retina —*see* Occlusion, retina, vein,
      engorgement
Enlargement, enlarged —*see also* Hypertrophy
  adenoids J35.2
    with tonsils J35.3
  alveolar ridge K08.89 ◀▥
    congenital —*see* Anomaly, alveolar
  apertures of diaphragm (congenital)
      Q79.1
  gingival K06.1
  heart, cardiac —*see* Hypertrophy, cardiac
  labium majus, childhood asymmetric
      (CALME) N90.61 ◀
  lacrimal gland, chronic H04.03-
  liver —*see* Hypertrophy, liver
  lymph gland or node R59.9
    generalized R59.1
    localized R59.0
  orbit H05.34-
  organ or site, congenital NEC —*see* Anomaly,
      by site
  parathyroid (gland) E21.0
  pituitary fossa R93.0
  prostate N40.0
    with lower urinary tract symptoms (LUTS)
        N40.1
    without lower urinary tract symptoms
        (LUTS) N40.0
  sella turcica R93.0
  spleen —*see* Splenomegaly
  thymus (gland) (congenital) E32.0
  thyroid (gland) —*see* Goiter
  tongue K14.8
  tonsils J35.1
    with adenoids J35.3
  uterus N85.2
Enophthalmos H05.40-
  due to
    orbital tissue atrophy H05.41-
    trauma or surgery H05.42-
Enostosis M27.8
Entamebic, entamebiasis —*see* Amebiasis
Entanglement
  umbilical cord (s) O69.2
    with compression O69.2
      without compression O69.82
    around neck (with compression) O69.1
      without compression O69.81
    of twins in monoamniotic sac O69.2
Enteralgia —*see* Pain, abdominal
Enteric —*see* condition
Enteritis (acute) (diarrheal) (hemorrhagic)
    (noninfective) K52.9 ◀▥
  adenovirus A08.2
  aertrycke infection A02.0

◀ New   ◀▥ Revised   ~~deleted~~ Deleted

Enteritis (Continued)
  allergic K52.29 ◀▥
    with ◀
      eosinophilic gastritis or gastroenteritis
        K52.81 ◀
      food protein-induced enterocolitis
        syndrome K52.21 ◀
      food protein-induced enteropathy
        K52.22 ◀
  amebic (acute) A06.0
    with abscess —see Abscess, amebic
    chronic A06.1
      with abscess —see Abscess, amebic
      nondysenteric A06.2
    nondysenteric A06.2
  astrovirus A08.32
  bacillary NOS A03.9
  bacterial A04.9
    specified NEC A04.8
  calicivirus A08.31
  candidal B37.82
  Chilomastix A07.8
  choleriformis A00.1
  chronic (noninfectious) K52.9
    ulcerative —see Colitis, ulcerative
  cicatrizing (chronic) —see Enteritis, regional,
    small intestine
  Clostridium
    botulinum (food poisoning) A05.1
    difficile A04.7
  coccidial A07.3
  coxsackie virus A08.39
  dietetic —see also Enteritis, allergic
    K52.29 ◀▥
  drug-induced K52.1
  due to
    astrovirus A08.32
    calicivirus A08.31
    coxsackie virus A08.39
    drugs K52.1
    echovirus A08.39
    enterovirus NEC A08.39
    food hypersensitivity —see also Enteritis,
      allergic K52.29 ◀▥
    infectious organism (bacterial) (viral) —see
      Enteritis, infectious
    torovirus A08.39
    Yersinia enterocolitica A04.6
  echovirus A08.39
  eltor A00.1
  enterovirus NEC A08.39
  eosinophilic K52.81
  epidemic (infectious) A09
  fulminant —see also Ischemia, intestine, acute
    K55.019 ◀▥
  gangrenous —see Enteritis, infectious
  giardial A07.1
  infectious NOS A09
    due to
      adenovirus A08.2
      Aerobacter aerogenes A04.8
      Arizona (bacillus) A02.0
      bacteria NOS A04.9
        specified NEC A04.8
      Campylobacter A04.5
      Clostridium difficile A04.7
      Clostridium perfringens A04.8
      Enterobacter aerogenes A04.8
      enterovirus A08.39
      Escherichia coli A04.4
        enteroaggregative A04.4
        enterohemorrhagic A04.3
        enteroinvasive A04.2
        enteropathogenic A04.0
        enterotoxigenic A04.1
        specified NEC A04.4
      specified
        bacteria NEC A04.8
        virus NEC A08.39
      Staphylococcus A04.8

Enteritis (Continued)
  infectious NOS (Continued)
    due to (Continued)
      virus NEC A08.4
        specified type NEC A08.39
      Yersinia enterocolitica A04.6
    specified organism NEC A08.8
  influenzal —see Influenza, with, digestive
    manifestations
  ischemic K55.9
    acute —see also Ischemia, intestine, acute
      K55.019 ◀▥
    chronic K55.1
  microsporidial A07.8
  mucomembranous, myxomembranous —see
    Syndrome, irritable bowel
  mucous —see Syndrome, irritable bowel
  necroticans A05.2
  necrotizing of newborn —see Enterocolitis,
    necrotizing, in newborn
  neurogenic —see Syndrome, irritable
    bowel
  newborn necrotizing —see Enterocolitis,
    necrotizing, in newborn
  noninfectious K52.9
  norovirus A08.11
  parasitic NEC B82.9
  paratyphoid (fever) —see Fever,
    paratyphoid
  protozoal A07.9
    specified NEC A07.8
  radiation K52.0
  regional (of) K50.90
    with
      complication K50.919
        abscess K50.914
        fistula K50.913
        intestinal obstruction K50.912
        rectal bleeding K50.911
        specified complication NEC
          K50.918
    colon —see Enteritis, regional, large
      intestine
    duodenum —see Enteritis, regional, small
      intestine
    ileum —see Enteritis, regional, small
      intestine
    jejunum —see Enteritis, regional, small
      intestine
    large bowel —see Enteritis, regional, large
      intestine
    large intestine (colon) (rectum) K50.10
      with
        complication K50.119
          abscess K50.114
          fistula K50.113
          intestinal obstruction K50.112
          rectal bleeding K50.111
          small intestine (duodenum) (ileum)
            (jejunum) involvement
            K50.80
          with
            complication K50.819
              abscess K50.814
              fistula K50.813
              intestinal obstruction
                K50.812
              rectal bleeding K50.811
              specified complication NEC
                K50.818
          specified complication NEC
            K50.118
    rectum —see Enteritis, regional, large
      intestine
    small intestine (duodenum) (ileum)
      (jejunum) K50.00
      with
        complication K50.019
          abscess K50.014
          fistula K50.013
          intestinal obstruction K50.012

Enteritis (Continued)
  regional (Continued)
    small intestine (Continued)
      with (Continued)
        complication (Continued)
          large intestine (colon) (rectum)
            involvement K50.80
          with
            complication K50.819
              abscess K50.814
              fistula K50.813
              intestinal obstruction K50.812
              rectal bleeding K50.811
              specified complication NEC
                K50.818
          rectal bleeding K50.011
          specified complication NEC K50.018
  rotaviral A08.0
  Salmonella, salmonellosis (arizonae)
    (cholerae-suis) (enteritidis)
    (typhimurium) A02.0
  segmental —see Enteritis, regional
  septic A09
  Shigella —see Infection, Shigella
  small round structured NEC A08.19
  spasmodic, spastic —see Syndrome, irritable
    bowel
  staphylococcal A04.8
    due to food A05.0
  torovirus A08.39
  toxic NEC K52.1
    due to Clostridium difficile A04.7
  trichomonal A07.8
  tuberculous A18.32
  typhosa A01.00
  ulcerative (chronic) —see Colitis, ulcerative
  viral A08.4
    adenovirus A08.2
    enterovirus A08.39
    Rotavirus A08.0
    small round structured NEC A08.19
    specified NEC A08.39
    virus specified NEC A08.39
Enterobiasis B80
Enterobius vermicularis (infection) (infestation)
  B80
Enterocele —see also Hernia, abdomen
  pelvic, pelvis (acquired) (congenital) N81.5
  vagina, vaginal (acquired) (congenital)
    NEC N81.5
Enterocolitis —see also Enteritis K52.9
  due to Clostridium difficile A04.7
  fulminant ischemic —see also Ischemia,
    intestine, acute K55.059 ◀▥
  granulomatous —see Enteritis, regional
  hemorrhagic (acute) —see also Ischemia,
    intestine, acute K55.059 ◀▥
    chronic K55.1
  infectious NEC A09
  ischemic K55.9
  necrotizing K55.30 ◀▥
    with ◀
      perforation K55.33 ◀
      pneumatosis K55.32 ◀
      and perforation K55.33 ◀
    due to Clostridium difficile A04.7
    in non-newborn K55.30 ◀
      stage 1 (without pneumatosis, without
        perforation) K55.31 ◀
      stage 2 (with pneumatosis, without
        perforation) K55.32 ◀
      stage 3 (with pneumatosis, with
        perforation) K55.33 ◀
    in newborn P77.9
      stage 1 (without pneumatosis, without
        perforation) P77.1
      stage 2 (with pneumatosis, without
        perforation) P77.2
      stage 3 (with pneumatosis, with
        perforation) P77.3
    without pneumatosis or perforation
      K55.31 ◀

Enterocolitis *(Continued)*
  noninfectious K52.9
    newborn —*see* Enterocolitis, necrotizing, in
      newborn
  pseudomembranous (newborn) A04.7
  radiation K52.0
    newborn —*see* Enterocolitis, necrotizing, in
      newborn
  ulcerative (chronic) —*see* Pancolitis,
    ulcerative (chronic)
Enterogastritis —*see* Enteritis
Enteropathy K63.9
  food protein-induced enterocolitis K52.22 ◀
  gluten-sensitive K90.0
    non-celiac K90.41 ◀
  hemorrhagic, terminal —*see also* Ischemia,
    intestine, acute K55.059 ◀
  protein-losing K90.49 ◀
Enteroperitonitis —*see* Peritonitis
Enteroptosis K63.4
Enterorrhagia K92.2
Enterospasm —*see also* Syndrome, irritable,
  bowel
  psychogenic F45.8
Enterostenosis —*see also* Obstruction, intestine
  K56.69
Enterostomy
  complication —*see* Complication,
    enterostomy
  status Z93.4
Enterovirus, as cause of disease classified
  elsewhere B97.10
  coxsackievirus B97.11
  echovirus B97.12
  other specified B97.19
Enthesopathy (peripheral) M77.9
  Achilles tendinitis —*see* Tendinitis,
    Achilles
  ankle and tarsus M77.9
    specified type NEC —*see* Enthesopathy,
      foot, specified type NEC
  anterior tibial syndrome M76.81-
  calcaneal spur —*see* Spur, bone, calcaneal
  elbow region M77.8
    lateral epicondylitis —*see* Epicondylitis,
      lateral
    medial epicondylitis —*see* Epicondylitis,
      medial
  foot NEC M77.9
    metatarsalgia —*see* Metatarsalgia
    specified type NEC M77.5-
  forearm M77.9
  gluteal tendinitis —*see* Tendinitis, gluteal
  hand M77.9
  hip —*see* Enthesopathy, lower limb, specified
    type NEC
  iliac crest spur —*see* Spur, bone, iliac crest
  iliotibial band syndrome —*see* Syndrome,
    iliotibial band
  knee —*see* Enthesopathy, lower limb, lower
    leg, specified type NEC
  lateral epicondylitis —*see* Epicondylitis,
    lateral
  lower limb (excluding foot) M76.9
    Achilles tendinitis —*see* Tendinitis, Achilles
    anterior tibial syndrome M76.81-
    gluteal tendinitis —*see* Tendinitis, gluteal
    iliac crest spur —*see* Spur, bone, iliac crest
    iliotibial band syndrome —*see* Syndrome,
      iliotibial band
    patellar tendinitis —*see* Tendinitis, patellar
    pelvic region —*see* Enthesopathy, lower
      limb, specified type NEC
    peroneal tendinitis —*see* Tendinitis,
      peroneal
    posterior tibial syndrome M76.82-
    psoas tendinitis —*see* Tendinitis, psoas
    shoulder M77.9
    specified type NEC M76.89-
    tibial collateral bursitis —*see* Bursitis, tibial
      collateral

Enthesopathy *(Continued)*
  medial epicondylitis —*see* Epicondylitis,
    medial
  multiple sites M77.9
  patellar tendinitis —*see* Tendinitis, patellar
  pelvis M77.9
  periarthritis of wrist —*see* Periarthritis,
    wrist
  peroneal tendinitis —*see* Tendinitis, peroneal
  posterior tibial syndrome M76.82-
  psoas tendinitis —*see* Tendinitis, psoas
  shoulder region —*see* Lesion, shoulder
  specified site NEC M77.9
  specified type NEC M77.8
  spinal M46.00
    cervical region M46.02
    cervicothoracic region M46.03
    lumbar region M46.06
    lumbosacral region M46.07
    multiple sites M46.09
    occipito-atlanto-axial region M46.01
    sacrococcygeal region M46.08
    thoracic region M46.04
    thoracolumbar region M46.05
  tibial collateral bursitis —*see* Bursitis, tibial
    collateral
  upper arm M77.9
  wrist and carpus NEC M77.8
    calcaneal spur —*see* Spur, bone, calcaneal
    periarthritis of wrist —*see* Periarthritis,
      wrist
Entomophobia F40.218
Entomophthoromycosis B46.8
Entrance, air into vein —*see* Embolism, air
Entrapment, nerve —*see* Neuropathy,
  entrapment
Entropion (eyelid) (paralytic) H02.009
  cicatricial H02.019
    left H02.016
      lower H02.015
      upper H02.014
    right H02.013
      lower H02.012
      upper H02.011
  congenital Q10.2
  left H02.006
    lower H02.005
    upper H02.004
  mechanical H02.029
    left H02.026
      lower H02.025
      upper H02.024
    right H02.023
      lower H02.022
      upper H02.021
  right H02.003
    lower H02.002
    upper H02.001
  senile H02.039
    left H02.036
      lower H02.035
      upper H02.034
    right H02.033
      lower H02.032
      upper H02.031
  spastic H02.049
    left H02.046
      lower H02.045
      upper H02.044
    right H02.043
      lower H02.042
      upper H02.041
Enucleated eye (traumatic, current) S05.7-
Enuresis R32
  functional F98.0
  habit disturbance F98.0
  nocturnal N39.44
    psychogenic F98.0
  nonorganic origin F98.0
  psychogenic F98.0
Eosinopenia —*see* Agranulocytosis

Eosinophilia (allergic) (hereditary) (idiopathic)
  (secondary) D72.1
  with
    angiolymphoid hyperplasia (ALHE)
      D18.01
  infiltrative J82
  Löffler's J82
  peritoneal —*see* Peritonitis, eosinophilic
  pulmonary NEC J82
  tropical (pulmonary) J82
Eosinophilia-myalgia syndrome M35.8
Ependymitis (acute) (cerebral) (chronic)
  (granular) —*see* Encephalomyelitis
Ependymoblastoma
  specified site —*see* Neoplasm, malignant, by
    site
  unspecified site C71.9
Ependymoma (epithelial) (malignant)
  anaplastic
    specified site —*see* Neoplasm, malignant,
      by site
    unspecified site C71.9
  benign
    specified site —*see* Neoplasm, benign, by
      site
    unspecified site D33.2
  myxopapillary D43.2
    specified site —*see* Neoplasm, uncertain
      behavior, by site
    unspecified site D43.2
  papillary D43.2
    specified site —*see* Neoplasm, uncertain
      behavior, by site
    unspecified site D43.2
  specified site —*see* Neoplasm, malignant, by
    site
  unspecified site C71.9
Ependymopathy G93.89
Ephelis, ephelides L81.2
Epiblepharon (congenital) Q10.3
Epicanthus, epicanthic fold (eyelid)
  (congenital) Q10.3
Epicondylitis (elbow)
  lateral M77.1-
  medial M77.0-
Epicystitis —*see* Cystitis
Epidemic —*see* condition
Epidermidalization, cervix —*see* Dysplasia,
  cervix
Epidermis, epidermal —*see* condition
Epidermodysplasia verruciformis B07.8
Epidermolysis
  bullosa (congenital) Q81.9
    acquired L12.30
      drug-induced L12.31
      specified cause NEC L12.35
    dystrophica Q81.2
    letalis Q81.1
    simplex Q81.0
    specified NEC Q81.8
  necroticans combustiformis L51.2
    due to drug —*see* Table of Drugs and
      Chemicals, by drug
Epidermophytid —*see* Dermatophytosis
Epidermophytosis (infected) —*see*
  Dermatophytosis
Epididymis —*see* condition
Epididymitis (acute) (nonvenereal) (recurrent)
  (residual) N45.1
  with orchitis N45.3
  blennorrhagic (gonococcal) A54.23
  caseous (tuberculous) A18.15
  chlamydial A56.19
  filarial —*see also* Infestation, filarial B74.9
    [N51]
  gonococcal A54.23
  syphilitic A52.76
  tuberculous A18.15
Epididymo-orchitis —*see also* Epididymitis
  N45.3
Epidural —*see* condition

◀ New   ◀|||| Revised   ~~deleted~~ Deleted

Epigastrium, epigastric —*see* condition
Epigastrocele —*see* Hernia, ventral
Epiglottis —*see* condition
Epiglottitis, epiglottiditis (acute) J05.10
  with obstruction J05.11
  chronic J37.0
Epignathus Q89.4
Epilepsia partialis continua —*see also*
  Kozhevnikof's epilepsy G40.1-
Epilepsy, epileptic, epilepsia (attack)
  (cerebral) (convulsion) (fit) (seizure)
  G40.909

> Note: the following terms are to be
> considered equivalent to intractable:
> pharmacoresistant (pharmacologically
> resistant), treatment resistant, refractory
> (medically) and poorly controlled

with
  complex partial seizures —*see* Epilepsy,
    localization-related, symptomatic,
    with complex partial seizures
  grand mal seizures on awakening —
    see Epilepsy, generalized, specified
    NEC
  myoclonic absences —*see* Epilepsy,
    generalized, specified NEC
  myoclonic-astatic seizures —*see* Epilepsy,
    generalized, specified NEC
  simple partial seizures —*see* Epilepsy,
    localization-related, symptomatic,
    with simple partial seizures
akinetic —*see* Epilepsy, generalized, specified
  NEC
benign childhood with centrotemporal EEG
  spikes —*see* Epilepsy, localization-
  related, idiopathic
benign myoclonic in infancy G40.80-
Bravais-jacksonian —*see* Epilepsy,
  localization-related, symptomatic,
  with simple partial seizures
childhood
  with occipital EEG paroxysms —*see*
    Epilepsy, localization-related,
    idiopathic
  absence G40.A09
    intractable G40.A19
      with status epilepticus G40.A11
      without status epilepticus G40.A19
    not intractable G40.A09
      with status epilepticus G40.A01
      without status epilepticus
        G40.A09
climacteric —*see* Epilepsy, specified NEC
cysticercosis B69.0
deterioration (mental) F06.8
due to syphilis A52.19
focal —*see* Epilepsy, localization-related,
  symptomatic, with simple partial
  seizures
generalized
  idiopathic G40.309
    intractable G40.319
      with status epilepticus G40.311
      without status epilepticus G40.319
    not intractable G40.309
      with status epilepticus G40.301
      without status epilepticus G40.309
    specified NEC G40.409
    intractable G40.419
      with status epilepticus G40.411
      without status epilepticus G40.419
    not intractable G40.409
      with status epilepticus G40.401
      without status epilepticus G40.409
impulsive petit mal —*see* Epilepsy, juvenile
  myoclonic
intractable G40.919
  with status epilepticus G40.911
  without status epilepticus G40.919

Epilepsy, epileptic, epilepsia (Continued)
  juvenile absence G40.A09
    intractable G40.A19
      with status epilepticus G40.A11
      without status epilepticus G40.A19
    not intractable G40.A09
      with status epilepticus G40.A01
      without status epilepticus G40.A09
  juvenile myoclonic G40.B11
    intractable G40.B19
      with status epilepticus G40.B11
      without status epilepticus G40.B19
    not intractable G40.B09
      with status epilepticus G40.B01
      without status epilepticus G40.B09
  localization-related (focal) (partial)
    idiopathic G40.009
      with seizures of localized onset G40.009
        intractable G40.019
          with status epilepticus G40.011
          without status epilepticus G40.019
        not intractable G40.009
          with status epilepticus G40.001
          without status epilepticus G40.009
    symptomatic
      with complex partial seizures G40.209
        intractable G40.219
          with status epilepticus G40.211
          without status epilepticus G40.219
        not intractable G40.209
          with status epilepticus G40.201
          without status epilepticus
            G40.209
      with simple partial seizures G40.109
        intractable G40.119
          with status epilepticus G40.111
          without status epilepticus
            G40.119
        not intractable G40.109
          with status epilepticus G40.101
          without status epilepticus G40.109
  myoclonus, myoclonic —*see* Epilepsy,
    generalized, specified NEC ◄▥
  progressive —*see* Epilepsy, generalized,
    idiopathic ◄
  not intractable G40.909
    with status epilepticus G40.901
    without status epilepticus G40.909
  on awakening —*see* Epilepsy, generalized,
    specified NEC
  parasitic NOS B71.9 [G94]
  partialis continua —*see also* Kozhevnikof's
    epilepsy G40.1-
  peripheral —*see* Epilepsy, specified NEC
  procursiva —*see* Epilepsy, localization-
    related, symptomatic, with simple
    partial seizures
  progressive (familial) myoclonic —*see*
    Epilepsy, generalized, idiopathic
  reflex —*see* Epilepsy, specified NEC
  related to
    alcohol G40.509
      not intractable G40.509
        with status epilepticus G40.501
        without status epliepticus G40.509
    drugs G40.509
      not intractable G40.509
        with status epilepticus G40.501
        without status epilepticus G40.509
    external causes G40.509
      not intractable G40.509
        with status epilepticus G40.501
        without status epilepticus G40.509
    hormonal changes G40.509
      not intractable G40.509
        with status epilepticus G40.501
        without status epliepticus G40.509
    sleep deprivation G40.509
      not intractable G40.509
        with status epilepticus G40.501
        without status epliepticus G40.509

Epilepsy, epileptic, epilepsia (Continued)
  related to (Continued)
    stress G40.509
      not intractable G40.509
        with status epilepticus G40.501
        without status eplieticus G40.509
    somatomotor —*see* Epilepsy, localization-
      related, symptomatic, with simple
      partial seizures
    somatosensory —*see* Epilepsy, localization-
      related, symptomatic, with simple
      partial seizures
    spasms G40.822
      intractable G40.824
        with status epilepticus G40.823
        without status epilepticus G40.824
      not intractable G40.822
        with status epilepticus G40.821
        without status epilepticus G40.822
    specified NEC G40.802
      intractable G40.804
        with status epilepticus G40.803
        without status epilepticus G40.804
      not intractable G40.802
        with status epilepticus G40.801
        without status epilepticus G40.802
  syndromes
    generalized
      idiopathic G40.309
        intractable G40.319
          with status epilepticus G40.311
          without status epilepticus G40.319
        not intractable G40.309
          with status epilepticus G40.301
          without status epilepticus G40.309
      specified NEC G40.409
        intractable G40.419
          with status epilepticus G40.411
          without status epilepticus G40.419
        not intractable G40.409
          with status epilepticus G40.401
          without status epilepticus G40.409
    localization-related (focal) (partial)
      idiopathic G40.009
        with seizures of localized onset
          G40.009
        intractable G40.019
          with status epilepticus G40.011
          without status epilepticus
            G40.019
        not intractable G40.009
          with status epilepticus G40.001
          without status epilepticus
            G40.009
      symptomatic
        with complex partial seizures
          G40.209
          intractable G40.219
            with status epilepticus G40.211
            without status epilepticus
              G40.219
          not intractable G40.209
            with status epilepticus G40.201
            without status epilepticus G40.209
        with simple partial seizures G40.109
          intractable G40.119
            with status epilepticus G40.111
            without status epilepticus G40.119
          not intractable G40.109
            with status epilepticus G40.101
            without status epilepticus G40.109
    specified NEC G40.802
      intractable G40.804
        with status epilepticus G40.803
        without status epilepticus G40.804
      not intractable G40.802
        with status epilepticus G40.801
        without status epilepticus G40.802
  tonic (-clonic) —*see* Epilepsy, generalized,
    specified NEC
  twilight F05

Epilepsy, epileptic, epilepsia *(Continued)*
  uncinate (gyrus) —*see* Epilepsy, localization-related, symptomatic, with complex partial seizures
  Unverricht (-Lundborg) (familial myoclonic) —*see* Epilepsy, generalized, idiopathic
  visceral —*see* Epilepsy, specified NEC
  visual —*see* Epilepsy, specified NEC
Epiloia Q85.1
Epimenorrhea N92.0
Epipharyngitis —*see* Nasopharyngitis
Epiphora H04.20-
  due to
    excess lacrimation H04.21-
    insufficient drainage H04.22-
Epiphyseal arrest —*see* Arrest, epiphyseal
Epiphyseolysis, epiphysiolysis —*see* Osteochondropathy
Epiphysitis —*see also* Osteochondropathy
  juvenile M92.9
  syphilitic (congenital) A50.02
Epiplocele —*see* Hernia, abdomen
Epiploitis —*see* Peritonitis
Epiplosarcomphalocele —*see* Hernia, umbilicus
Episcleritis (suppurative) H15.10-
  in (due to)
    syphilis A52.71
    tuberculosis A18.51
  nodular H15.12-
  periodica fugax H15.11-
    angioneurotic —*see* Edema, angioneurotic
  syphilitic (late) A52.71
  tuberculous A18.51
Episode
  affective, mixed F39
  depersonalization (in neurotic state) F48.1
  depressive F32.9
    major F32.9
      mild F32.0
      moderate F32.1
      severe (without psychotic symptoms) F32.2
        with psychotic symptoms F32.3
    recurrent F33.9
      brief F33.8
    specified NEC F32.89 ◄▥
  hypomanic F30.8
  manic F30.9
    with
      psychotic symptoms F30.2
      remission (full) F30.4
        partial F30.3
    without psychotic symptoms F30.10
      mild F30.11
      moderate F30.12
      severe (without psychotic symptoms) F30.13
        with psychotic symptoms F30.2
    other specified F30.8
    recurrent F31.89
  psychotic F23
    organic F06.8
  schizophrenic (acute) NEC, brief F23
Epispadias (female) (male) Q64.0
Episplenitis D73.89
Epistaxis (multiple) R04.0
  hereditary I78.0
  vicarious menstruation N94.89
Epithelioma (malignant) —*see also* Neoplasm, malignant, by site
  adenoides cysticum —*see* Neoplasm, skin, benign
  basal cell —*see* Neoplasm, skin, malignant
  benign —*see* Neoplasm, benign, by site
  Bowen's —*see* Neoplasm, skin, in situ
  calcifying, of Malherbe —*see* Neoplasm, skin, benign
  external site —*see* Neoplasm, skin, malignant
  intraepidermal, Jadassohn —*see* Neoplasm, skin, benign
  squamous cell —*see* Neoplasm, malignant, by site

Epitheliomatosis pigmented Q82.1
Epitheliopathy, multifocal placoid pigment H30.14-
Epithelium, epithelial —*see* condition
Epituberculosis (with atelectasis) (allergic) A15.7
Eponychia Q84.6
Epstein's
  nephrosis or syndrome —*see* Nephrosis
  pearl K09.8
Epulis (gingiva) (fibrous) (giant cell) K06.8
Equinia A24.0
Equinovarus (congenital) (talipes) Q66.0
  acquired —*see* Deformity, limb, clubfoot
Equivalent
  convulsive (abdominal) —*see* Epilepsy, specified NEC
  epileptic (psychic) —*see* Epilepsy, localization-related, symptomatic, with complex partial seizures
Erb (-Duchenne) paralysis (birth injury) (newborn) P14.0
Erb's
  disease G71.0
  palsy, paralysis (brachial) (birth) (newborn) P14.0
    spinal (spastic) syphilitic A52.17
  pseudohypertrophic muscular dystrophy G71.0
Erb-Goldflam disease or syndrome G70.00
  with exacerbation (acute) G70.01
  in crisis G70.01
Erdheim's syndrome (acromegalic macrospondylitis) E22.0
Erection, painful (persistent) —*see* Priapism
Ergosterol deficiency (vitamin D) E55.9
  with
    adult osteomalacia M83.8
    rickets —*see* Rickets
Ergotism —*see also* Poisoning, food, noxious, plant
  from ergot used as drug (migraine therapy) —*see* Table of Drugs and Chemicals
Erosio interdigitalis blastomycetica B37.2
Erosion
  artery I77.2
    without rupture I77.89
  bone —*see* Disorder, bone, density and structure, specified NEC
  bronchus J98.09
  cartilage (joint) —*see* Disorder, cartilage, specified type NEC
  cervix (uteri) (acquired) (chronic) (congenital) N86
    with cervicitis N72
  cornea (nontraumatic) —*see* Ulcer, cornea
    recurrent H18.83-
    traumatic —*see* Abrasion, cornea
  dental (idiopathic) (occupational) (due to diet, drugs or vomiting) K03.2
  duodenum, postpyloric —*see* Ulcer, duodenum
  esophagus K22.10
    with bleeding K22.11
  gastric —*see* Ulcer, stomach
  gastrojejunal —*see* Ulcer, gastrojejunal
  implanted mesh —*see* Complications, mesh
  intestine K63.3
  lymphatic vessel I89.8
  pylorus, pyloric (ulcer) —*see* Ulcer, stomach
  spine, aneurysmal A52.09
  stomach —*see* Ulcer, stomach
  subcutaneous device pocket ◄
    nervous system prosthetic device, implant, or graft T85.890 ◄
    other internal prosthetic device, implant, or graft T85.898 ◄
  teeth (idiopathic) (occupational) (due to diet, drugs or vomiting) K03.2
  urethra N36.8
  uterus N85.8

Erotomania F52.8
Error
  metabolism, inborn —*see* Disorder, metabolism
  refractive —*see* Disorder, refraction
Eructation R14.2
  nervous or psychogenic F45.8
Eruption
  creeping B76.9
  drug (generalized) (taken internally) L27.0
    fixed L27.1
    in contact with skin —*see* Dermatitis, due to drugs
    localized L27.1
  Hutchinson, summer L56.4
  Kaposi's varicelliform B00.0
  napkin L22
  polymorphous light (sun) L56.4
  recalcitrant pustular L13.8
  ringed R23.8
  skin (nonspecific) R21
    creeping (meaning hookworm) B76.9
    due to inoculation/vaccination (generalized) —*see also* Dermatitis, due to, vaccine L27.0
      localized L27.1
    erysipeloid A26.0
    feigned L98.1
    Kaposi's varicelliform B00.0
    lichenoid L28.0
    meaning dermatitis —*see* Dermatitis
    toxic NEC L53.0
  tooth, teeth, abnormal (incomplete) (late) (premature) (sequence) K00.6
  vesicular R23.8
Erysipelas (gangrenous) (infantile) (newborn) (phlegmonous) (suppurative) A46
  external ear A46 *[H62.40]*
  puerperal, postpartum O86.89
Erysipeloid A26.9
  cutaneous (Rosenbach's) A26.0
  disseminated A26.8
  sepsis A26.7
  specified NEC A26.8
Erythema, erythematous (infectional) (inflammation) L53.9
  ab igne L59.0
  annulare (centrifugum) (rheumaticum) L53.1
  arthriticum epidemicum A25.1
  brucellum —*see* Brucellosis
  chronic figurate NEC L53.3
  chronicum migrans (Borrelia burgdorferi) A69.20
  diaper L22
  due to
    chemical NEC L53.0
      in contact with skin L24.5
    drug (internal use) —*see* Dermatitis, due to, drugs
  elevatum diutinum L95.1
  endemic E52
  epidemic, arthritic A25.1
  figuratum perstans L53.3
  gluteal L22
  heat - code by site under Burn, first degree
  ichthyosiforme congenitum bullous Q80.3
  in diseases classified elsewhere L54
  induratum (nontuberculous) L52
    tuberculous A18.4
  infectiosum B08.3
  intertrigo L30.4
  iris L51.9
  marginatum L53.2
    in (due to) acute rheumatic fever I00
  medicamentosum —*see* Dermatitis, due to, drugs
  migrans A26.0
    chronicum A69.20
    tongue K14.1

◄ New   ◄▥ Revised   ~~deleted~~ Deleted

Erythema, erythematous *(Continued)*
  multiforme (major) (minor) L51.9
    bullous, bullosum L51.1
    conjunctiva L51.1
    nonbullous L51.0
    pemphigoides L12.0
    specified NEC L51.8
  napkin L22
  neonatorum P83.8
    toxic P83.1
  nodosum L52
    tuberculous A18.4
  palmar L53.8
  pernio T69.1
  rash, newborn P83.8
  scarlatiniform (recurrent) (exfoliative)
    L53.8
  solare L55.0
  specified NEC L53.8
  toxic, toxicum NEC L53.0
    newborn P83.1
  tuberculous (primary) A18.4
Erythematous, erythematosus —*see* condition
Erythermalgia (primary) I73.81
Erythralgia I73.81
Erythrasma L08.1
Erythredema (polyneuropathy) —*see* Poisoning,
  mercury
Erythremia (acute) C94.0-
  chronic D45
  secondary D75.1
Erythroblastopenia —*see also* Aplasia, red cell
  D60.9
  congenital D61.01
Erythroblastophthisis D61.09
Erythroblastosis (fetalis) (newborn) P55.9
  due to
    ABO (antibodies) (incompatibility)
      (isoimmunization) P55.1
    Rh (antibodies) (incompatibility)
      (isoimmunization) P55.0
Erythrocyanosis (crurum) I73.89
Erythrocythemia —*see* Erythremia
Erythrocytosis (megalosplenic) (secondary)
  D75.1
  familial D75.0
  oval, hereditary —*see* Elliptocytosis
  secondary D75.1
  stress D75.1
Erythroderma (secondary) —*see also* Erythema
  L53.9
  bullous ichthyosiform, congenital Q80.3
  desquamativum L21.1
  ichthyosiform, congenital (bullous) Q80.3
  neonatorum P83.8
  psoriaticum L40.8
Erythrodysesthesia, palmar plantar (PPE) L27.1
Erythrogenesis imperfecta D61.09
Erythroleukemia C94.0-
Erythromelalgia I73.81
Erythrophagocytosis D75.89
Erythrophobia F40.298
Erythroplakia, oral epithelium, and tongue
  K13.29
Erythroplasia (Queyrat) D07.4
  specified site —*see* Neoplasm, skin, in situ
  unspecified site D07.4
Escherichia coli (E. coli), as cause of disease
    classified elsewhere B96.20
  non-O157 Shiga toxin-producing (with
    known O group) B96.22
  non-Shiga toxin-producing B96.29
  O157 with confirmation of Shiga toxin when
    H antigen is unknown, or is not H7
    B96.21
  O157:H- (nonmotile) with confirmation of
    Shiga toxin B96.21
  O157:H7 with or without confirmation of
    Shiga toxin-production B96.21
  Shiga toxin-producing (with unspecified O
    group) (STEC) B96.23

Escherichia coli *(Continued)*
  O157 B96.21
  O157:H7 with or without confirmation of
    Shiga toxin-production B96.21
    specified NEC B96.22
  specified NEC B96.29
Esophagismus K22.4
Esophagitis (acute) (alkaline) (chemical)
    (chronic) (infectional) (necrotic) (peptic)
    (postoperative) K20.9
  candidal B37.81
  due to gastrointestinal reflux disease K21.0
  eosinophilic K20.0
  reflux K21.0
  specified NEC K20.8
  tuberculous A18.83
  ulcerative K22.10
    with bleeding K22.11
Esophagocele K22.5
Esophagomalacia K22.8
Esophagospasm K22.4
Esophagostenosis K22.2
Esophagostomiasis B81.8
Esophagotracheal —*see* condition
Esophagus —*see* condition
Esophoria H50.51
  convergence, excess H51.12
  divergence, insufficiency H51.8
Esotropia —*see* Strabismus, convergent
    concomitant
Espundia B55.2
Essential —*see* condition
Esthesioneuroblastoma C30.0
Esthesioneurocytoma C30.0
Esthesioneuroepithelioma C30.0
Esthiomene A55
Estivo-autumnal malaria (fever) B50.9
Estrangement (marital) Z63.5
  parent-child NEC Z62.890
Estriasis —*see* Myiasis
Ethanolism —*see* Alcoholism
Etherism —*see* Dependence, drug, inhalant
Ethmoid, ethmoidal —*see* condition
Ethmoiditis (chronic) (nonpurulent)
    (purulent) —*see also* Sinusitis, ethmoidal
  influenzal —*see* Influenza, with, respiratory
    manifestations NEC
  Woakes' J33.1
Ethylism —*see* Alcoholism
Eulenburg's disease (congenital paramyotonia)
    G71.19
Eumycetoma B47.0
Eunuchoidism E29.1
  hypogonadotropic E23.0
European blastomycosis —*see* Cryptococcosis
Eustachian —*see* condition
Evaluation (for) (of)
  development state
    adolescent Z00.3
    period of
      delayed growth in childhood Z00.70
        with abnormal findings Z00.71
      rapid growth in childhood Z00.2
    puberty Z00.3
  growth and developmental state (period of
    rapid growth) Z00.2
  delayed growth Z00.70
    with abnormal findings Z00.71
  mental health (status) Z00.8
    requested by authority Z04.6
  period of
    delayed growth in childhood Z00.70
      with abnormal findings Z00.71
    rapid growth in childhood Z00.2
  suspected condition —*see* Observation
Evans syndrome D69.41
Event, apparent life threatening in newborn
    and infant (ALTE) R68.13
Eventration —*see also* Hernia, ventral
  colon into chest —*see* Hernia, diaphragm
  diaphragm (congenital) Q79.1

Eversion
  bladder N32.89
  cervix (uteri) N86
    with cervicitis N72
  foot NEC —*see also* Deformity, valgus, ankle
    congenital Q66.6
  punctum lacrimale (postinfectional) (senile)
    H04.52-
  ureter (meatus) N28.89
  urethra (meatus) N36.8
  uterus N81.4
Evidence
  cytologic
    of malignancy on anal smear R85.614
    of malignancy on cervical smear R87.614
    of malignancy on vaginal smear R87.624
Evisceration
  birth injury P15.8
  traumatic NEC
    eye —*see* Enucleated eye
Evulsion —*see* Avulsion
Ewing's sarcoma or tumor —*see* Neoplasm,
    bone, malignant
Examination (for) (following) (general) (of)
    (routine) Z00.00
  with abnormal findings Z00.01
  abuse, physical (alleged), ruled out
    adult Z04.71
    child Z04.72
  adolescent (development state) Z00.3
  alleged rape or sexual assault (victim), ruled
    out
    adult Z04.41
    child Z04.42
  allergy Z01.82
  annual (adult) (periodic) (physical) Z00.00
    with abnormal findings Z00.01
    gynecological Z01.419
      with abnormal findings Z01.411
  antibody response Z01.84
  blood —*see* Examination, laboratory
  blood pressure Z01.30
    with abnormal findings Z01.31
  cancer staging —*see* Neoplasm, malignant,
    by site
  cervical Papanicolaou smear Z12.4
    as part of routine gynecological
      examination Z01.419
      with abnormal findings Z01.411
  child (over 28 days old) Z00.129
    with abnormal findings Z00.121
    under 28 days old —*see* Newborn,
      examination
  clinical research control or normal
    comparison (control) (participant) Z00.6
  contraceptive (drug) maintenance (routine)
    Z30.8
    device (intrauterine) Z30.431
  dental Z01.20
    with abnormal findings Z01.21
  developmental —*see* Examination, child
  donor (potential) Z00.5
  ear Z01.10
    with abnormal findings NEC Z01.118
  eye Z01.00
    with abnormal findings Z01.01
  following
    accident NEC Z04.3
      transport Z04.1
      work Z04.2
    assault, alleged, ruled out
      adult Z04.71
      child Z04.72
    motor vehicle accident Z04.1
    treatment (for) Z09
      combined NEC Z09
        fracture Z09
        malignant neoplasm Z08
      malignant neoplasm Z08
      mental disorder Z09
      specified condition NEC Z09

Examination *(Continued)*
follow-up (routine) (following) Z09
  chemotherapy NEC Z09
    malignant neoplasm Z08
  fracture Z09
  malignant neoplasm Z08
  postpartum Z39.2
  psychotherapy Z09
  radiotherapy NEC Z09
    malignant neoplasm Z08
  surgery NEC Z09
    malignant neoplasm Z08
gynecological Z01.419
  with abnormal findings Z01.411
  for contraceptive maintenance Z30.8
health —*see* Examination, medical
hearing Z01.10
  with abnormal findings NEC Z01.118
  following failed hearing screening Z01.110
immunity status testing Z01.84
laboratory (as part of a general medical
    examination) Z00.00
  with abnormal findings Z00.01
  preprocedural Z01.812
lactating mother Z39.1
medical (adult) (for) (of) Z00.00
  with abnormal findings Z00.01
  administrative purpose only Z02.9
    specified NEC Z02.89
  admission to
    armed forces Z02.3
    old age home Z02.2
    prison Z02.89
    residential institution Z02.2
    school Z02.0
      following illness or medical treatment Z02.0
    summer camp Z02.89
  adoption Z02.82
  blood alcohol or drug level Z02.83
  camp (summer) Z02.89
  clinical research, normal subject (control) (participant) Z00.6
  control subject in clinical research (normal comparison) (participant) Z00.6
  donor (potential) Z00.5
  driving license Z02.4
  general (adult) Z00.00
    with abnormal findings Z00.01
  immigration Z02.89
  insurance purposes Z02.6
  marriage Z02.89
  medicolegal reasons NEC Z04.8
  naturalization Z02.89
  participation in sport Z02.5
  paternity testing Z02.81
  population survey Z00.8
  pre-employment Z02.1
  pre-operative —*see* Examination, pre-procedural
  pre-procedural
    cardiovascular Z01.810
    respiratory Z01.811
    specified NEC Z01.818
  preschool children
    for admission to school Z02.0
  prisoners
    for entrance into prison Z02.89
  recruitment for armed forces Z02.3
  specified NEC Z00.8
  sport competition Z02.5
medicolegal reason NEC Z04.8
newborn —*see* Newborn, examination
pelvic (annual) (periodic) Z01.419
  with abnormal findings Z01.411
period of rapid growth in childhood Z00.2
periodic (adult) (annual) (routine) Z00.00
  with abnormal findings Z00.01
physical (adult) —*see also* Examination, medical Z00.00
  sports Z02.5

Examination *(Continued)*
postpartum
  immediately after delivery Z39.0
  routine follow-up Z39.2
pre-chemotherapy (antineoplastic) Z01.818
prenatal (normal pregnancy) —*see also* Pregnancy, normal Z34.9-
pre-procedural (pre-operative)
  cardiovascular Z01.810
  laboratory Z01.812
  respiratory Z01.811
  specified NEC Z01.818
prior to chemotherapy (antineoplastic) Z01.818
psychiatric NEC Z00.8
  follow-up not needing further care Z09
  requested by authority Z04.6
radiological (as part of a general medical examination) Z00.00
  with abnormal findings Z00.01
repeat cervical smear to confirm findings of recent normal smear following initial abnormal smear Z01.42
skin (hypersensitivity) Z01.82
special —*see also* Examination, by type Z01.89
  specified type NEC Z01.89
specified type or reason NEC Z04.8
teeth Z01.20
  with abnormal findings Z01.21
urine —*see* Examination, laboratory
vision Z01.00
  with abnormal findings Z01.01
Exanthem, exanthema —*see also* Rash
with enteroviral vesicular stomatitis B08.4
Boston A88.0
epidemic with meningitis A88.0 [G02]
subitum B08.20
  due to human herpesvirus 6 B08.21
  due to human herpesvirus 7 B08.22
viral, virus B09
  specified type NEC B08.8
Excess, excessive, excessively
alcohol level in blood R78.0
androgen (ovarian) E28.1
attrition, tooth, teeth K03.0
carotene, carotin (dietary) E67.1
cold, effects of T69.9
  specified effect NEC T69.8
convergence H51.12
crying
  in child, adolescent, or adult R45.83
  in infant R68.11
development, breast N62
divergence H51.8
drinking (alcohol) NEC (without dependence) F10.10
  habitual (continual) (without remission) F10.20
eating R63.2
estrogen E28.0
fat —*see also* Obesity
  in heart —*see* Degeneration, myocardial
  localized E65
foreskin N47.8
gas R14.0
glucagon E16.3
heat —*see* Heat
intermaxillary vertical dimension of fully erupted teeth M26.37
interocclusal distance of fully erupted teeth M26.37
kalium E87.5
large
  colon K59.39 ◀
    congenital Q43.8
  infant P08.0
  organ or site, congenital NEC —*see* Anomaly, by site
long
  organ or site, congenital NEC —*see* Anomaly, by site

Excess, excessive, excessively *(Continued)*
menstruation (with regular cycle) N92.0
  with irregular cycle N92.1
napping Z72.821
natrium E87.0
number of teeth K00.1
nutrient (dietary) NEC R63.2
potassium (K) E87.5
salivation K11.7
secretion —*see also* Hypersecretion
  milk O92.6
  sputum R09.3
  sweat R61
sexual drive F52.8
short
  organ or site, congenital NEC —*see* Anomaly, by site
  umbilical cord in labor or delivery O69.3
~~skin, eyelid (acquired) —see Blepharochalasis~~
~~congenital Q10.3~~
skin L98.7 ◀
  and subcutaneous tissue L98.7 ◀
  eyelid (acquired) —*see* Blepharochalasis ◀
    congenital Q10.3 ◀
sodium (Na) E87.0
spacing of fully erupted teeth M26.32
sputum R09.3
sweating R61
thirst R63.1
  due to deprivation of water T73.1
tuberosity of jaw M26.07
vitamin
  A (dietary) E67.0
    administered as drug (prolonged intake) —*see* Table of Drugs and Chemicals, vitamins, adverse effect
    overdose or wrong substance given or taken —*see* Table of Drugs and Chemicals, vitamins, poisoning
  D (dietary) E67.3
    administered as drug (prolonged intake) —*see* Table of Drugs and Chemicals, vitamins, adverse effect
    overdose or wrong substance given or taken —*see* Table of Drugs and Chemicals, vitamins, poisoning
weight
  gain R63.5
  loss R63.4
Excitability, abnormal, under minor stress (personality disorder) F60.3
Excitation
anomalous atrioventricular I45.6
psychogenic F30.8
reactive (from emotional stress, psychological trauma) F30.8
Excitement
hypomanic F30.8
manic F30.9
mental, reactive (from emotional stress, psychological trauma) F30.8
state, reactive (from emotional stress, psychological trauma) F30.8
Excoriation (traumatic) —*see also* Abrasion
neurotic L98.1
skin picking disorder F42.4 ◀
Exfoliation
due to erythematous conditions according to extent of body surface involved L49.0
  10-19 percent of body surface L49.1
  20-29 percent of body surface L49.2
  30-39 percent of body surface L49.3
  40-49 percent of body surface L49.4
  50-59 percent of body surface L49.5
  60-69 percent of body surface L49.6
  70-79 percent of body surface L49.7
  80-89 percent of body surface L49.8
  90-99 percent of body surface L49.9
  less than 10 percent of body surface L49.0
teeth, due to systemic causes K08.0

◀ New ◀▥ Revised ~~deleted~~ Deleted

Exfoliative —*see* condition
Exhaustion, exhaustive (physical NEC) R53.83
  battle F43.0
  cardiac —*see* Failure, heart
  delirium F43.0
  due to
    cold T69.8
    excessive exertion T73.3
    exposure T73.2
    neurasthenia F48.8
  heart —*see* Failure, heart
  heat —*see also* Heat, exhaustion T67.5
    due to
      salt depletion T67.4
      water depletion T67.3
  maternal, complicating delivery O75.81
  mental F48.8
  myocardium, myocardial —*see* Failure, heart
  nervous F48.8
  old age R54
  psychogenic F48.8
  psychosis F43.0
  senile R54
  vital NEC Z73.0
Exhibitionism F65.2
Exocervicitis —*see* Cervicitis
Exomphalos Q79.2
  meaning hernia —*see* Hernia, umbilicus
Exophoria H50.52
  convergence, insufficiency H51.11
  divergence, excess H51.8
Exophthalmos H05.2-
  congenital Q15.8
  constant NEC H05.24-
  displacement, globe —*see* Displacement,
    globe
  due to thyrotoxicosis (hyperthyroidism) —*see*
    Hyperthyroidism, with, goiter (diffuse)
  dysthyroid —*see* Hyperthyroidism, with,
    goiter (diffuse)
  goiter —*see* Hyperthyroidism, with, goiter
    (diffuse)
  intermittent NEC H05.25-
  malignant —*see* Hyperthyroidism, with,
    goiter (diffuse)
  orbital
    edema —*see* Edema, orbit
    hemorrhage —*see* Hemorrhage, orbit
  pulsating NEC H05.26-
  thyrotoxic, thyrotropic —*see*
    Hyperthyroidism, with, goiter (diffuse)
Exostosis —*see also* Disorder, bone
  cartilaginous —*see* Neoplasm, bone, benign
  congenital (multiple) Q78.6
  external ear canal H61.81-
  gonococcal A54.49
  jaw (bone) M27.8
  multiple, congenital Q78.6
  orbit H05.35-
  osteocartilaginous —*see* Neoplasm, bone,
    benign
  syphilitic A52.77
Exotropia —*see* Strabismus, divergent
  concomitant
Explanation of
  investigation finding Z71.2
  medication Z71.89
Exposure (to) —*see also* Contact, with T75.89
  acariasis Z20.7
  AIDS virus Z20.6
  air pollution Z77.110
  algae and algae toxins Z77.121
  algae bloom Z77.121
  anthrax Z20.810
  aromatic amines Z77.020
  aromatic (hazardous) compounds NEC
    Z77.028
  aromatic dyes NOS Z77.028

Exposure (*Continued*)
  arsenic Z77.010
  asbestos Z77.090
  bacterial disease NEC Z20.818
  benzene Z77.021
  blue-green algae bloom Z77.121
  body fluids (potentially hazardous) Z77.21
  brown tide Z77.121
  chemicals (chiefly nonmedicinal) (hazardous)
    NEC Z77.098
  cholera Z20.09
  chromium compounds Z77.018
  cold, effects of T69.9
    specified effect NEC T69.8
  communicable disease Z20.9
    bacterial NEC Z20.818
    specified NEC Z20.89
    viral NEC Z20.828
  cyanobacteria bloom Z77.121
  disaster Z65.5
  discrimination Z60.5
  dyes Z77.098
  effects of T73.9
  environmental tobacco smoke (acute)
    (chronic) Z77.22
  Escherichia coli (E. coli) Z20.01
  exhaustion due to T73.2
  fiberglass —*see* Table of Drugs and
    Chemicals, fiberglass
  German measles Z20.4
  gonorrhea Z20.2
  hazardous metals NEC Z77.018
  hazardous substances NEC Z77.29
  hazards in the physical environment NEC
    Z77.128
  hazards to health NEC Z77.9
  human immunodeficiency virus (HIV) Z20.6
  human T-lymphotropic virus type-1 (HTLV-1)
    Z20.89
  implanted
    mesh —*see* Complications, mesh
    prosthetic materials NEC —*see*
      Complications, prosthetic materials
      NEC
  infestation (parasitic) NEC Z20.7
  intestinal infectious disease NEC Z20.09
    Escherichia coli (E. coli) Z20.01
  lead Z77.011
  meningococcus Z20.811
  mold (toxic) Z77.120
  nickel dust Z77.018
  noise Z77.122
  occupational
    air contaminants NEC Z57.39
    dust Z57.2
    environmental tobacco smoke Z57.31
    extreme temperature Z57.6
    noise Z57.0
    radiation Z57.1
    risk factors Z57.9
      specified NEC Z57.8
    toxic agents (gases) (liquids) (solids)
      (vapors) in agriculture Z57.4
    toxic agents (gases) (liquids) (solids)
      (vapors) in industry NEC Z57.5
    vibration Z57.7
  parasitic disease NEC Z20.7
  pediculosis Z20.7
  persecution Z60.5
  pfiesteria piscicida Z77.121
  poliomyelitis Z20.89
  pollution
    air Z77.110
    environmental NEC Z77.118
    soil Z77.112
    water Z77.111
  polycyclic aromatic hydrocarbons
    Z77.028

Exposure (*Continued*)
  prenatal (drugs) (toxic chemicals) —*see*
    Newborn, affected by, noxious
    substances transmitted via placenta or
    breast milk ◀▦
  rabies Z20.3
  radiation, naturally occurring NEC Z77.123
  radon Z77.123
  red tide (Florida) Z77.121
  rubella Z20.4
  second hand tobacco smoke (acute) (chronic)
    Z77.22
    in the perinatal period P96.81
  sexually-transmitted disease Z20.2
  smallpox (laboratory) Z20.89
  syphilis Z20.2
  terrorism Z65.4
  torture Z65.4
  tuberculosis Z20.1
  uranium Z77.012
  varicella Z20.820
  venereal disease Z20.2
  viral disease NEC Z20.828
  war Z65.5
  water pollution Z77.111
Exsanguination —*see* Hemorrhage
Exstrophy
  abdominal contents Q45.8
  bladder Q64.10
    cloacal Q64.12
    specified type NEC Q64.19
    supravesical fissure Q64.11
Extensive —*see* condition
Extra —*see also* Accessory
  marker chromosomes (normal individual)
    Q92.61
    in abnormal individual Q92.62
  rib Q76.6
    cervical Q76.5
Extrasystoles (supraventricular) I49.49
  atrial I49.1
  auricular I49.1
  junctional I49.2
  ventricular I49.3
Extrauterine gestation or pregnancy —*see*
  Pregnancy, by site
Extravasation
  blood R58
  chyle into mesentery I89.8
  pelvicalyceal N13.8
  pyelosinus N13.8
  urine (from ureter) R39.0
  vesicant agent
    antineoplastic chemotherapy T80.810
    other agent NEC T80.818
Extremity —*see* condition, limb
Extrophy —*see* Exstrophy
Extroversion
  bladder Q64.19
  uterus N81.4
    complicating delivery O71.2
    postpartal (old) N81.4
Extruded tooth (teeth) M26.34
Extrusion
  breast implant (prosthetic) T85.42
  eye implant (globe) (ball) T85.328
  intervertebral disc —*see* Displacement,
    intervertebral disc
  ocular lens implant (prosthetic) —*see*
    Complications, intraocular lens
  vitreous —*see* Prolapse, vitreous
Exudate
  pleural —*see* Effusion, pleura
  retina H35.89
Exudative —*see* condition
Eye, eyeball, eyelid —*see* condition
Eyestrain —*see* Disturbance, vision, subjective
Eyeworm disease of Africa B74.3

F

Faber's syndrome (achlorhydric anemia) D50.9
Fabry (-Anderson) disease E75.21
Faciocephalalgia, autonomic —see also
    Neuropathy, peripheral, autonomic G90.09
Factor (s)
  psychic, associated with diseases classified
    elsewhere F54
  psychological
    affecting physical conditions F54
    or behavioral
      affecting general medical condition F54
      associated with disorders or diseases
        classified elsewhere F54
Fahr disease (of brain) G23.8
Fahr Volhard disease (of kidney) I12.-
Failure, failed
  abortion —see Abortion, attempted
  aortic (valve) I35.8
    rheumatic I06.8
  attempted abortion —see Abortion, attempted
  biventricular I50.9
  bone marrow —see Anemia, aplastic
  cardiac —see Failure, heart
  cardiorenal (chronic) I50.9
    hypertensive I13.2
  cardiorespiratory (see also Failure, heart)
    R09.2
  cardiovascular (chronic) —see Failure, heart
  cerebrovascular I67.9
  cervical dilatation in labor O62.0
  circulation, circulatory (peripheral) R57.9
    newborn P29.89
  compensation —see Disease, heart
  compliance with medical treatment or
    regimen —see Noncompliance
  congestive —see Failure, heart, congestive
  dental implant (endosseous) M27.69
    due to
      failure of dental prosthesis M27.63
      lack of attached gingiva M27.62
      occlusal trauma (poor prosthetic design)
        M27.62
      parafunctional habits M27.62
      periodontal infection (peri-implantitis)
        M27.62
      poor oral hygiene M27.62
    osseointegration M27.61
      due to
        complications of systemic disease
          M27.61
        poor bone quality M27.61
        iatrogenic M27.61
    post-osseointegration
      biological M27.62
      due to complications of systemic disease
        M27.62
      iatrogenic M27.62
      mechanical M27.63
    pre-integration M27.61
    pre-osseointegration M27.61
    specified NEC M27.69
  descent of head (at term) of pregnancy
    (mother) O32.4
  endosseous dental implant —see Failure,
    dental implant
  engagement of head (term of pregnancy)
    (mother) O32.4
  erection (penile) —see also Dysfunction,
    sexual, male, erectile N52.9
    ~~nonorganic F52.21~~
    nonorganic F52.21 ◄
  examination (s), anxiety concerning Z55.2
  expansion terminal respiratory units
    (newborn) (primary) P28.0
  forceps NOS (with subsequent cesarean
    delivery) O66.5
  gain weight (child over 28 days old) R62.51
    adult R62.7
    newborn P92.6

Failure, failed (Continued)
  genital response (male) F52.21
    female F52.22
  heart (acute) (senile) (sudden) I50.9
    with
      acute pulmonary edema —see Failure,
        ventricular, left
      decompensation —see Failure, heart,
        congestive
      dilatation —see Disease, heart
    arteriosclerotic I70.90
    biventricular I50.9
    combined left-right sided I50.9
    compensated I50.9
    complicating
      anesthesia (general) (local) or other
        sedation
        in labor and delivery O74.2
        in pregnancy O29.12-
        postpartum, puerperal O89.1
      delivery (cesarean) (instrumental) O75.4
    congestive (compensated)
      (decompensated) I50.9
      with rheumatic fever (conditions in I00)
        active I01.8
        inactive or quiescent (with chorea)
          I09.81
      newborn P29.0
      rheumatic (chronic) (inactive) (with
        chorea) I09.81
        active or acute I01.8
        with chorea I02.0
    decompensated I50.9
    degenerative —see Degeneration,
      myocardial
    diastolic (congestive) I50.30
      acute (congestive) I50.31
        and (on) chronic (congestive) I50.33
      chronic (congestive) I50.32
        and (on) acute (congestive) I50.33
      combined with systolic (congestive)
        I50.40
        acute (congestive) I50.41
          and (on) chronic (congestive)
            I50.43
        chronic (congestive) I50.42
          and (on) acute (congestive) I50.43
    due to presence of cardiac prosthesis
      I97.13-
    following cardiac surgery I97.13-
    high output NOS I50.9
    hypertensive —see Hypertension, heart
    left (ventricular) —see Failure, ventricular,
      left
    low output (syndrome) NOS I50.9
    newborn P29.0
    organic —see Disease, heart
    peripartum O90.3
    postprocedural I97.13-
    rheumatic (chronic) (inactive) I09.9
    right (ventricular) (secondary to left
      heart failure) —see Failure, heart,
      congestive
    systolic (congestive) I50.20
      acute (congestive) I50.21
        and (on) chronic (congestive)
          I50.23
      chronic (congestive) I50.22
        and (on) acute (congestive) I50.23
      combined with diastolic (congestive)
        I50.40
        acute (congestive) I50.41
          and (on) chronic (congestive)
            I50.43
        chronic (congestive) I50.42
          and (on) acute (congestive)
            I50.43
    thyrotoxic —see also Thyrotoxicosis
      E05.90 [143]
      with thyroid storm E05.91 [143]
    valvular —see Endocarditis

Failure, failed (Continued)
  hepatic K72.90
    with coma K72.91
    acute or subacute K72.00
      with coma K72.01
      due to drugs K71.10
        with coma K71.11
    alcoholic (acute) (chronic) (subacute)
      K70.40
      with coma K70.41
    chronic K72.10
      with coma K72.11
      due to drugs (acute) (subacute) (chronic)
        K71.10
        with coma K71.11
    due to drugs (acute) (subacute) (chronic)
      K71.10
      with coma K71.11
    postprocedural K91.82
  hepatorenal K76.7
  induction (of labor) O61.9
    abortion —see Abortion, attempted
    by
      oxytocic drugs O61.0
      prostaglandins O61.0
    instrumental O61.1
    mechanical O61.1
    medical O61.0
    specified NEC O61.8
    surgical O61.1
  intubation during anesthesia T88.4
    in pregnancy O29.6-
    labor and delivery O74.7
    postpartum, puerperal O89.6
  involution, thymus (gland) E32.0
  kidney —see also Disease, kidney, chronic N19
    acute —see also Failure, renal, acute N17.9-
    diabetic —see E08-E13 with .22
  lactation (complete) O92.3
    partial O92.4
  Leydig's cell, adult E29.1
  liver —see Failure, hepatic
  menstruation at puberty N91.0
  mitral I05.8
  myocardial, myocardium —see also Failure,
    heart I50.9
    chronic —see also Failure, heart, congestive
      I50.9
    congestive —see also Failure, heart,
      congestive I50.9
  orgasm (female) (psychogenic) F52.31
    male F52.32
  ovarian (primary) E28.39
    iatrogenic E89.40
      asymptomatic E89.40
      symptomatic E89.41
    postprocedural (postablative)
      (postirradiation) (postsurgical)
      E89.40
      asymptomatic E89.40
      symptomatic E89.41
  ovulation causing infertility N97.0
  polyglandular, autoimmune E31.0
  prosthetic joint implant —see Complications,
    joint prosthesis, mechanical,
    breakdown, by site
  renal N19
    with
      tubular necrosis (acute) N17.0
    acute N17.9
      with
        cortical necrosis N17.1
        medullary necrosis N17.2
        tubular necrosis N17.0
      specified NEC N17.8
    chronic N18.9
      hypertensive —see Hypertension,
        kidney
    congenital P96.0
    end stage (chronic) N18.6
      due to hypertension I12.0

◄ New   ◄▥ Revised   ~~deleted~~ Deleted

Failure, failed *(Continued)*
  renal *(Continued)*
    following
      abortion —*see* Abortion by type
        complicated by specified
        condition NEC
      crushing T79.5
      ectopic or molar pregnancy O08.4
      labor and delivery (acute) O90.4
    hypertensive —*see* Hypertension,
      kidney
    postprocedural N99.0
  respiration, respiratory J96.9
    with
      hypercapnia J96.92
      hypoxia J96.91
    acute J96.00
      with
        hypercapnia J96.02
        hypoxia J96.01
    acute and (on) chronic J96.20
      with
        hypercapnia J96.22
        hypoxia J96.21
    center G93.89
    chronic J96.10
      with
        hypercapnia J96.12
        hypoxia J96.11
    newborn P28.5
    postprocedural (acute) J95.821
      acute and chronic J95.822
  rotation
    cecum Q43.3
    colon Q43.3
    intestine Q43.3
    kidney Q63.2
  sedation (conscious) (moderate) during
    procedure T88.52
    history of Z92.83
  segmentation —*see also* Fusion
    fingers —*see* Syndactylism, complex,
      fingers
    vertebra Q76.49
      with scoliosis Q76.3
  seminiferous tubule, adult E29.1
  senile (general) R54
  sexual arousal (male) F52.21
    female F52.22
  testicular endocrine function E29.1
  to thrive (child over 28 days old)
    R62.51
    adult R62.7
    newborn P92.6
  transplant T86.92
    bone T86.831
      marrow T86.02
    cornea T86.841
    heart T86.22
      with lung (s) T86.32
    intestine T86.851
    kidney T86.12
    liver T86.42
    lung (s) T86.811
      with heart T86.32
    pancreas T86.891
    skin (allograft) (autograft) T86.821
    specified organ or tissue NEC T86.891
    stem cell (peripheral blood) (umbilical
      cord) T86.5
  trial of labor (with subsequent cesarean
    delivery) O66.40
    following previous cesarean delivery
      O66.41
  tubal ligation N99.89
  urinary —*see* Disease, kidney, chronic
  vacuum extraction NOS (with subsequent
    cesarean delivery) O66.5
  vasectomy N99.89
  ventouse NOS (with subsequent cesarean
    delivery) O66.5

Failure, failed *(Continued)*
  ventricular —*see also* Failure, heart I50.9
    left I50.1
      with rheumatic fever (conditions in I00)
        active I01.8
          with chorea I02.0
          inactive or quiescent (with chorea)
            I09.81
        rheumatic (chronic) (inactive) (with
          chorea) I09.81
          active or acute I01.8
            with chorea I02.0
    right —*see also* Failure, heart, congestive
      I50.9
  vital centers, newborn P91.8
Fainting (fit) R55
Fallen arches —*see* Deformity, limb, flat foot
Falling, falls (repeated) R29.6
  any organ or part —*see* Prolapse
Fallopian
  insufflation Z31.41
  tube —*see* condition
Fallot's
  pentalogy Q21.8
  tetrad or tetralogy Q21.3
  triad or trilogy Q22.3
False —*see also* condition
  croup J38.5
  joint —*see* Nonunion, fracture
  labor (pains) O47.9
    at or after 37 completed weeks of gestation
      O47.1
    before 37 completed weeks of gestation
      O47.0-
  passage, urethra (prostatic) N36.5
  pregnancy F45.8
Family, familial —*see also* condition
  disruption Z63.8
    involving divorce or separation Z63.5
  Li-Fraumeni (syndrome) Z15.01
  planning advice Z30.09
  problem Z63.9
    specified NEC Z63.8
  retinoblastoma C69.2-
Famine (effects of) T73.0
  edema —*see* Malnutrition, severe
Fanconi (-de Toni)(-Debré) **syndrome** E72.09
  with cystinosis E72.04
Fanconi's anemia (congenital pancytopenia)
  D61.09
Farber's disease or syndrome E75.29
Farcy A24.0
Farmer's
  lung J67.0
  skin L57.8
Farsightedness —*see* Hypermetropia
Fascia —*see* condition
Fasciculation R25.3
Fasciitis M72.9
  diffuse (eosinophilic) M35.4
  infective M72.8
    necrotizing M72.6
  necrotizing M72.6
  nodular M72.4
  perirenal (with ureteral obstruction)
    N13.5
    with infection N13.6
  plantar M72.2
  specified NEC M72.8
  traumatic (old) M72.8
    current - code by site under Sprain
Fascioliasis B66.3
Fasciolopsis, fasciolopsiasis (intestinal)
  B66.5
Fascioscapulohumeral myopathy G71.0
Fast pulse R00.0
Fat
  embolism —*see* Embolism, fat
  excessive —*see also* Obesity
    in heart —*see* Degeneration, myocardial
  in stool R19.5

Fat *(Continued)*
  localized (pad) E65
    heart —*see* Degeneration, myocardial
    knee M79.4
    retropatellar M79.4
  necrosis
    breast N64.1
    mesentery K65.4
    omentum K65.4
  pad E65
    knee M79.4
Fatigue R53.83
  auditory deafness —*see* Deafness
  chronic R53.82
  combat F43.0
  general R53.83
    psychogenic F48.8
  heat (transient) T67.6
  muscle M62.89
  myocardium —*see* Failure, heart
  neoplasm-related R53.0
  nervous, neurosis F48.8
  operational F48.8
  psychogenic (general) F48.8
  senile R54
  voice R49.8
Fatness —*see* Obesity
Fatty —*see also* condition
  apron E65
  degeneration —*see* Degeneration, fatty
  heart (enlarged) —*see* Degeneration,
    myocardial
  liver NEC K76.0
    alcoholic K70.0
    nonalcoholic K76.0
  necrosis —*see* Degeneration, fatty
Fauces —*see* condition
Fauchard's disease (periodontitis) —*see*
  Periodontitis
Faucitis J02.9
Favism (anemia) D55.0
Favus —*see* Dermatophytosis
Fazio-Londe disease or syndrome
  G12.1
Fear complex or reaction F40.9
Fear of —*see* Phobia
Feared complaint unfounded Z71.1
Febris, febrile —*see also* Fever
  flava —*see also* Fever, yellow A95.9
  melitensis A23.0
  pestis —*see* Plague
  recurrens —*see* Fever, relapsing
  rubra A38.9
Fecal
  incontinence R15.9
  smearing R15.1
  soiling R15.1
  urgency R15.2
Fecalith (impaction) K56.41
  appendix K38.1
  congenital P76.8
Fede's disease K14.0
**Feeble rapid pulse due to shock following
  injury** T79.4
Feeble-minded F70
Feeding
  difficulties R63.3
  problem R63.3
    newborn P92.9
      specified NEC P92.8
    nonorganic (adult) —*see* Disorder,
      eating
Feeling (of)
  foreign body in throat R09.89
Feer's disease —*see* Poisoning, mercury
Feet —*see* condition
Feigned illness Z76.5
Feil-Klippel syndrome (brevicollis) Q76.1
Feinmesser's (hidrotic) **ectodermal dysplasia**
  Q82.4
Felinophobia F40.218

Felon —*see also* Cellulitis, digit
  with lymphangitis —*see* Lymphangitis, acute,
    digit
Felty's syndrome M05.00
  ankle M05.07-
  elbow M05.02-
  foot joint M05.07-
  hand joint M05.04-
  hip M05.05-
  knee M05.06-
  multiple site M05.09
  shoulder M05.01-
  vertebra —*see* Spondylitis, ankylosing
  wrist M05.03-
Female genital cutting status —*see* Female
  genital mutilation status (FGM)
Female genital mutilation status (FGM) N90.810
  specified NEC N90.818
  type I (clitorectomy status) N90.811
  type II (clitorectomy with excision of labia
    minora status) N90.812
  type III (infibulation status) N90.813
  type IV N90.818
Femur, femoral —*see* condition
Fenestration, fenestrated —*see also* Imperfect,
  closure
  aortico-pulmonary Q21.4
  cusps, heart valve NEC Q24.8
    pulmonary Q22.3
  pulmonic cusps Q22.3
Fernell's disease (aortic aneurysm) I71.9
Fertile eunuch syndrome E23.0
Fetid
  breath R19.6
  sweat L75.0
Fetishism F65.0
  transvestic F65.1
Fetus, fetal —*see also* condition
  alcohol syndrome (dysmorphic) Q86.0
  compressus O31.0-
  hydantoin syndrome Q86.1
  lung tissue P28.0
  papyraceous O31.0-
Fever (inanition) (of unknown origin)
  (persistent) (with chills) (with rigor) R50.9
  abortus A23.1
  Aden (dengue) A90
  African tick-borne A68.1
  American
    mountain (tick) A93.2
    spotted A77.0
  aphthous B08.8
  arbovirus, arboviral A94
    hemorrhagic A94
    specified NEC A93.8
  Argentinian hemorrhagic A96.0
  Assam B55.0
  Australian Q A78
  Bangkok hemorrhagic A91
  Barmah forest A92.8
  Bartonella A44.0
  bilious, hemoglobinuric B50.8
  blackwater B50.8
  blister B00.1
  Bolivian hemorrhagic A96.1
  Bonvale dam T73.3
  boutonneuse A77.1
  brain —*see* Encephalitis
  Brazilian purpuric A48.4
  breakbone A90
  Bullis A77.0
  Bunyamwera A92.8
  Burdwan B55.0
  Bwamba A92.8
  Cameroon —*see* Malaria
  Canton A75.9
  catarrhal (acute) J00
    chronic J31.0
  cat-scratch A28.1
  Central Asian hemorrhagic A98.0
  cerebral —*see* Encephalitis

Fever (Continued)
  cerebrospinal meningococcal A39.0
  Chagres B50.9
  Chandipura A92.8
  Changuinola A93.1
  Charcot's (biliary) (hepatic) (intermittent) —
    see Calculus, bile duct
  Chikungunya (viral) (hemorrhagic)
    A92.0
  Chitral A93.1
  Colombo —*see* Fever, paratyphoid
  Colorado tick (virus) A93.2
  congestive (remittent) —*see* Malaria
  Congo virus A98.0
  continued malarial B50.9
  Corsican —*see* Malaria
  Crimean-Congo hemorrhagic A98.0
  Cyprus —*see* Brucellosis
  dandy A90
  deer fly —*see* Tularemia
  dengue (virus) A90
    hemorrhagic A91
    sandfly A93.1
  desert B38.0
  drug induced R50.2
  due to
    conditions classified elsewhere
      R50.81
    heat T67.0
  enteric A01.00
  enteroviral exanthematous (Boston
    exanthem) A88.0
  ephemeral (of unknown origin) R50.9
  epidemic hemorrhagic A98.5
  erysipelatous —*see* Erysipelas
  estivo-autumnal (malarial) B50.9
  famine A75.0
  five day A79.0
  following delivery O86.4
  Fort Bragg A27.89
  gastroenteric A01.00
  gastromalarial —*see* Malaria
  Gibraltar —*see* Brucellosis
  glandular —*see* Mononucleosis, infectious
  Guama (viral) A92.8
  Haverhill A25.1
  hay (allergic) J30.1
    with asthma (bronchial) J45.909
      with
        exacerbation (acute) J45.901
        status asthmaticus J45.902
    due to
      allergen other than pollen J30.89
      pollen, any plant or tree J30.1
  heat (effects) T67.0
  hematuric, bilious B50.8
  hemoglobinuric (malarial) (bilious) B50.8
  hemorrhagic (arthropod-borne) NOS A94
    with renal syndrome A98.5
    arenaviral A96.9
      specified NEC A96.8
    Argentinian A96.0
    Bangkok A91
    Bolivian A96.1
    Central Asian A98.0
    Chikungunya A92.0
    Crimean-Congo A98.0
    dengue (virus) A91
    epidemic A98.5
    Junin (virus) A96.0
    Korean A98.5
    Kyasanur forest A98.2
    Machupo (virus) A96.1
    mite-borne A93.8
    mosquito-borne A92.8
    Omsk A98.1
    Philippine A91
    Russian A98.5
    Singapore A91
    Southeast Asia A91
    Thailand A91

Fever (Continued)
  hemorrhagic NOS (Continued)
    tick-borne NEC A93.8
    viral A99
      specified NEC A98.8
  hepatic —*see* Cholecystitis
  herpetic —*see* Herpes
  icterohemorrhagic A27.0
  Indiana A93.8
  infective B99.9
    specified NEC B99.8
  intermittent (bilious) —*see also* Malaria
    of unknown origin R50.9
    pernicious B50.9
  iodide R50.2
  Japanese river A75.3
  jungle —*see also* Malaria
    yellow A95.0
  Junin (virus) hemorrhagic A96.0
  Katayama B65.2
  kedani A75.3
  Kenya (tick) A77.1
  Kew Garden A79.1
  Korean hemorrhagic A98.5
  Lassa A96.2
  Lone Star A77.0
  Machupo (virus) hemorrhagic A96.1
  malaria, malarial —*see* Malaria
  Malta A23.9
  Marseilles A77.1
  marsh —*see* Malaria
  Mayaro (viral) A92.8
  Mediterranean —*see also* Brucellosis A23.9
    familial M04.1 ◀▥
    tick A77.1
  meningeal —*see* Meningitis
  Meuse A79.0
  Mexican A75.2
  mianeh A68.1
  miasmatic —*see* Malaria
  mosquito-borne (viral) A92.9
    hemorrhagic A92.8
  mountain —*see also* Brucellosis
    meaning Rocky Mountain spotted fever
      A77.0
    tick (American) (Colorado) (viral) A93.2
  Mucambo (viral) A92.8
  mud A27.9
  Neapolitan —*see* Brucellosis
  neutropenic D70.9
  newborn P81.9
    environmental P81.0
  Nine-Mile A78
  non-exanthematous tick A93.2
  North Asian tick-borne A77.2
  Omsk hemorrhagic A98.1
  O'nyong-nyong (viral) A92.1
  Oropouche (viral) A93.0
  Oroya A44.0
  paludal —*see* Malaria
  Panama (malarial) B50.9
  Pappataci A93.1
  paratyphoid A01.4
    A A01.1
    B A01.2
    C A01.3
  parrot A70
  periodic (Mediterranean) M04.1 ◀▥
  persistent (of unknown origin) R50.9
  petechial A39.0
  pharyngoconjunctival B30.2
  Philippine hemorrhagic A91
  phlebotomus A93.1
  Piry (virus) A93.8
  Pixuna (viral) A92.8
  Plasmodium ovale B53.0
  polioviral (nonparalytic) A80.4
  Pontiac A48.2
  postimmunization R50.83
  postoperative R50.82
    due to infection T81.40 ◀▥

◀ New   ◀▥ Revised   ~~deleted~~ Deleted

Fever *(Continued)*
posttransfusion R50.84
postvaccination R50.83
presenting with conditions classified
    elsewhere R50.81
pretibial A27.89
puerperal O86.4
Q A78
quadrilateral A78
quartan (malaria) B52.9
Queensland (coastal) (tick) A77.3
quintan A79.0
rabbit —*see* Tularemia
rat-bite A25.9
    due to
        Spirillum A25.0
        Streptobacillus moniliformis A25.1
recurrent —*see* Fever, relapsing
relapsing (Borrelia) A68.9
    Carter's (Asiatic) A68.1
    Dutton's (West African) A68.1
    Koch's A68.9
    louse-borne A68.0
    Novy's
        louse-borne A68.0
        tick-borne A68.1
    Obermeyer's (European) A68.0
    tick-borne A68.1
remittent (bilious) (congestive) (gastric) —*see*
    Malaria
rheumatic (active) (acute) (chronic) (subacute)
    I00
    with central nervous system involvement
        I02.9
    active with heart involvement —*see*
        category I01
    inactive or quiescent with
        cardiac hypertrophy I09.89
        carditis I09.9
        endocarditis I09.1
            aortic (valve) I06.9
                with mitral (valve) disease I08.0
            mitral (valve) I05.9
                with aortic (valve) disease I08.0
            pulmonary (valve) I09.89
            tricuspid (valve) I07.8
        heart disease NEC I09.89
        heart failure (congestive) (conditions in
            I50.9) I09.81
        left ventricular failure (conditions in
            I50.1) I09.81
        myocarditis, myocardial degeneration
            (conditions in I51.4) I09.0
        pancarditis I09.9
        pericarditis I09.2
    Rift Valley (viral) A92.4
    Rocky Mountain spotted A77.0
    rose J30.1
    Ross River B33.1
    Russian hemorrhagic A98.5
    San Joaquin (Valley) B38.0
    sandfly A93.1
    Sao Paulo A77.0
    scarlet A38.9
    seven day (leptospirosis) (autumnal)
        (Japanese) A27.89
        dengue A90
    shin-bone A79.0
    Singapore hemorrhagic A91
    solar A90
    Songo A98.5
    sore B00.1
    South African tick-bite A68.1
    Southeast Asia hemorrhagic A91
    spinal —*see* Meningitis
    spirillary A25.0
    splenic —*see* Anthrax
    spotted A77.9
        American A77.0
        Brazilian A77.0
        cerebrospinal meningitis A39.0

Fever *(Continued)*
    spotted *(Continued)*
        Colombian A77.0
        due to Rickettsia
            australis A77.3
            conorii A77.1
            rickettsii A77.0
            sibirica A77.2
            specified type NEC A77.8
        Ehrlichiosis A77.40
            due to
                E. chafeensis A77.41
                specified organism NEC A77.49
        Rocky Mountain A77.0
    steroid R50.2
    streptobacillary A25.1
    subtertian B50.9
    Sumatran mite A75.3
    sun A90
    swamp A27.9
    swine A02.8
    sylvatic, yellow A95.0
    Tahyna B33.8
    tertian —*see* Malaria, tertian
    Thailand hemorrhagic A91
    thermic T67.0
    three-day A93.1
    tick
        American mountain A93.2
        Colorado A93.2
        Kemerovo A93.8
        Mediterranean A77.1
        mountain A93.2
        nonexanthematous A93.2
        Quaranfil A93.8
    tick-bite NEC A93.8
    tick-borne (hemorrhagic) NEC A93.8
    trench A79.0
    tsutsugamushi A75.3
    typhogastric A01.00
    typhoid (abortive) (hemorrhagic)
        (intermittent) (malignant) A01.00
        complicated by
            arthritis A01.04
            heart involvement A01.02
            meningitis A01.01
            osteomyelitis A01.05
            pneumonia A01.03
            specified NEC A01.09
    typhomalarial —*see* Malaria
    typhus —*see* Typhus (fever)
    undulant —*see* Brucellosis
    unknown origin R50.9
    uveoparotid D86.89
    valley B38.0
    Venezuelan equine A92.2
    vesicular stomatitis A93.8
    viral hemorrhagic —*see* Fever, hemorrhagic,
        by type of virus
    Volhynian A79.0
    Wesselsbron (viral) A92.8
    West
        African B50.8
        Nile (viral) A92.30
            with
                complications NEC A92.39
                cranial nerve disorders A92.32
                encephalitis A92.31
                encephalomyelitis A92.31
                neurologic manifestation NEC
                    A92.32
                optic neuritis A92.32
                polyradiculitis A92.32
    Whitmore's —*see* Melioidosis
    Wolhynian A79.0
    worm B83.9
    yellow A95.9
        jungle A95.0
        sylvatic A95.0
        urban A95.1
    Zika virus A92.5 ◀

Fibrillation
    atrial or auricular (established) I48.91
        chronic I48.2
        paroxysmal I48.0
        permanent I48.2
        persistent I48.1
    cardiac I49.8
    heart I49.8
    muscular M62.89
    ventricular I49.01
Fibrin
    ball or bodies, pleural (sac) J94.1
    chamber, anterior (eye) (gelatinous
        exudate) —*see* Iridocyclitis, acute
Fibrinogenolysis —*see* Fibrinolysis
Fibrinogenopenia D68.8
    acquired D65
    congenital D68.2
Fibrinolysis (hemorrhagic) (acquired) D65
    antepartum hemorrhage —*see* Hemorrhage,
        antepartum, with coagulation defect
    following
        abortion —*see* Abortion by type
            complicated by hemorrhage
        ectopic or molar pregnancy O08.1
    intrapartum O67.0
    newborn, transient P60
    postpartum O72.3
Fibrinopenia (hereditary) D68.2
    acquired D68.4
Fibrinopurulent —*see* condition
Fibrinous —*see* condition
Fibroadenoma
    cellular intracanalicular D24-
    giant D24-
    intracanalicular
        cellular D24-
        giant D24-
        specified site —*see* Neoplasm, benign, by
            site
        unspecified site D24-
    juvenile D24-
    pericanalicular
        specified site —*see* Neoplasm, benign, by
            site
        unspecified site D24-
    phyllodes D24-
    prostate D29.1
    specified site NEC —*see* Neoplasm, benign,
        by site
    unspecified site D24-
Fibroadenosis, breast (chronic) (cystic) (diffuse)
    (periodic) (segmental) N60.2-
Fibroangioma —*see also* Neoplasm, benign, by
    site
    juvenile
        specified site —*see* Neoplasm, benign, by
            site
        unspecified site D10.6
Fibrochondrosarcoma —*see* Neoplasm,
    cartilage, malignant
Fibrocystic
    disease —*see also* Fibrosis, cystic
        breast —*see* Mastopathy, cystic
        jaw M27.49
        kidney (congenital) Q61.8
        liver Q44.6
        pancreas E84.9
    kidney (congenital) Q61.8
Fibrodysplasia ossificans progressiva —*see*
    Myositis, ossificans, progressiva
Fibroelastosis (cordis) (endocardial)
    (endomyocardial) I42.4
Fibroid (tumor) —*see also* Neoplasm, connective
    tissue, benign
    disease, lung (chronic) —*see* Fibrosis, lung
    heart (disease) —*see* Myocarditis
    in pregnancy or childbirth O34.1-
        causing obstructed labor O65.5
    induration, lung (chronic) —*see* Fibrosis, lung
    lung —*see* Fibrosis, lung

Fibroid (Continued)
  pneumonia (chronic) —see Fibrosis, lung
  uterus D25.9
Fibrolipoma —see Lipoma
Fibroliposarcoma —see Neoplasm, connective
    tissue, malignant
Fibroma —see also Neoplasm, connective tissue,
    benign
  ameloblastic —see Cyst, calcifying
    odontogenic
  bone (nonossifying) —see Disorder, bone,
    specified type NEC
    ossifying —see Neoplasm, bone,
      benign
  cementifying —see Neoplasm, bone,
    benign
  chondromyxoid —see Neoplasm, bone,
    benign
  desmoplastic —see Neoplasm, connective
    tissue, uncertain behavior
  durum —see Neoplasm, connective tissue,
    benign
  fascial —see Neoplasm, connective tissue,
    benign
  invasive —see Neoplasm, connective tissue,
    uncertain behavior
  molle —see Lipoma
  myxoid —see Neoplasm, connective tissue,
    benign
  nasopharynx, nasopharyngeal (juvenile)
    D10.6
  nonosteogenic (nonossifying) —see Dysplasia,
    fibrous
  odontogenic (central) —see Cyst, calcifying
    odontogenic
  ossifying —see Neoplasm, bone, benign
  periosteal —see Neoplasm, bone, benign
  soft —see Lipoma
Fibromatosis M72.9
  abdominal —see Neoplasm, connective tissue,
    uncertain behavior
  aggressive —see Neoplasm, connective tissue,
    uncertain behavior
  congenital generalized —see Neoplasm,
    connective tissue, uncertain behavior
  Dupuytren's M72.0
  gingival K06.1
  palmar (fascial) M72.0
  plantar (fascial) M72.2
  pseudosarcomatous (proliferative)
    (subcutaneous) M72.4
  retroperitoneal D48.3
  specified NEC M72.8
Fibromyalgia M79.7
Fibromyoma —see also Neoplasm, connective
    tissue, benign
  uterus (corpus) —see also Leiomyoma, uterus
    in pregnancy or childbirth —see Fibroid, in
      pregnancy or childbirth
    causing obstructed labor O65.5
Fibromyositis M79.7
Fibromyxolipoma D17.9
Fibromyxoma —see Neoplasm, connective
    tissue, benign
Fibromyxosarcoma —see Neoplasm, connective
    tissue, malignant
Fibro-odontoma, ameloblastic —see Cyst,
    calcifying odontogenic
Fibro-osteoma —see Neoplasm, bone, benign
Fibroplasia, retrolental H35.17
Fibropurulent —see condition
Fibrosarcoma —see also Neoplasm, connective
    tissue, malignant
  ameloblastic C41.1
    upper jaw (bone) C41.0
  congenital —see Neoplasm, connective tissue,
    malignant
  fascial —see Neoplasm, connective tissue,
    malignant
  infantile —see Neoplasm, connective tissue,
    malignant

Fibrosarcoma (Continued)
  odontogenic C41.1
    upper jaw (bone) C41.0
  periosteal —see Neoplasm, bone, malignant
Fibrosclerosis
  breast N60.3-
  multifocal M35.5
  penis (corpora cavernosa) N48.6
Fibrosis, fibrotic
  adrenal (gland) E27.8
  amnion O41.8X-
  anal papillae K62.89
  arteriocapillary —see Arteriosclerosis
  bladder N32.89
    interstitial —see Cystitis, chronic,
      interstitial
    localized submucosal —see Cystitis,
      chronic, interstitial
    panmural —see Cystitis, chronic, interstitial
  breast —see Fibrosclerosis, breast
  capillary —see also Arteriosclerosis I70.90
    lung (chronic) —see Fibrosis, lung
  cardiac —see Myocarditis
  cervix N88.8
  chorion O41.8X-
  corpus cavernosum (sclerosing) N48.6
  cystic (of pancreas) E84.9
    with
      distal intestinal obstruction syndrome
        E84.19
      fecal impaction E84.19
      intestinal manifestations NEC E84.19
      pulmonary manifestations E84.0
      specified manifestations NEC E84.8
  due to device, implant or graft —see also
      Complications, by site and type,
      specified NEC T85.828 ◄▥
    arterial graft NEC T82.828
    breast (implant) T85.828 ◄▥
    catheter NEC T85.828 ◄▥
      dialysis (renal) T82.828
        intraperitoneal T85.828 ◄▥
      infusion NEC T82.828
        spinal (epidural) (subdural)
          T85.820 ◄▥
      urinary (indwelling) T83.82
    electronic (electrode) (pulse generator)
        (stimulator)
      bone T84.82
      cardiac T82.827
      nervous system (brain) (peripheral
        nerve) (spinal) T85.820 ◄▥
      urinary T83.82
    fixation, internal (orthopedic) NEC T84.82
    gastrointestinal (bile duct) (esophagus)
      T85.828 ◄▥
    genital NEC T83.82
    heart NEC T82.827
    joint prosthesis T84.82
    ocular (corneal graft) (orbital implant)
      NEC T85.828 ◄▥
    orthopedic NEC T84.82
    specified NEC T85.828 ◄▥
    urinary NEC T83.82
    vascular NEC T82.828
    ventricular intracranial shunt T85.820 ◄▥
  ejaculatory duct N50.89 ◄▥
  endocardium —see Endocarditis
  endomyocardial (tropical) I42.3
  epididymis N50.89 ◄▥
  eye muscle —see Strabismus, mechanical
  heart —see Myocarditis
  hepatic —see Fibrosis, liver
  hepatolienal (portal hypertension) K76.6
  hepatosplenic (portal hypertension) K76.6
  infrapatellar fat pad M79.4
  intrascrotal N50.89 ◄▥
  kidney N26.9
  liver K74.0
    with sclerosis K74.2
    alcoholic K70.2

Fibrosis, fibrotic (Continued)
  lung (atrophic) (chronic) (confluent)
      (massive) (perialveolar) (peribronchial)
      J84.10
    with
      anthracosilicosis J60
      anthracosis J60
      asbestosis J61
      bagassosis J67.1
      bauxite J63.1
      berylliosis J63.2
      byssinosis J66.0
      calcicosis J62.8
      chalicosis J62.8
      dust reticulation J64
      farmer's lung J67.0
      ganister disease J62.8
      graphite J63.3
      pneumoconiosis NOS J64
      siderosis J63.4
      silicosis J62.8
    capillary J84.10
    congenital P27.8
    diffuse (idiopathic) J84.10
      chemicals, gases, fumes or vapors
        (inhalation) J68.4
        interstitial J84.10
          acute J84.114
        talc J62.0
    following radiation J70.1
    idiopathic J84.112
    postinflammatory J84.10
    silicotic J62.8
    tuberculous —see Tuberculosis, pulmonary
  lymphatic gland I89.8
  median bar —see Hyperplasia, prostate
  mediastinum (idiopathic) J98.59 ◄▥
  meninges G96.19
  myocardium, myocardial —see Myocarditis
  ovary N83.8
  oviduct N83.8
  pancreas K86.89 ◄▥
  penis NEC N48.6
  pericardium I31.0
  perineum, in pregnancy or childbirth O34.7-
    causing obstructed labor O65.5
  pleura J94.1
  popliteal fat pad M79.4
  prostate (chronic) —see Hyperplasia, prostate
  pulmonary —see also Fibrosis, lung J84.10
    congenital P27.8
    idiopathic J84.112
  rectal sphincter K62.89
  retroperitoneal, idiopathic (with ureteral
      obstruction) N13.5
    with infection N13.6
  sclerosing mesenteric (idiopathic) K65.4
  scrotum N50.89 ◄▥
  seminal vesicle N50.89 ◄▥
  senile R54
  skin L90.5
  spermatic cord N50.89 ◄▥
  spleen D73.89
    in schistosomiasis (bilharziasis) B65.9
      [D77]
  subepidermal nodular —see Neoplasm, skin,
      benign
  submucous (oral) (tongue) K13.5
  testis N44.8
    chronic, due to syphilis A52.76
  thymus (gland) E32.8
  tongue, submucous K13.5
  tunica vaginalis N50.89 ◄▥
  uterus (non-neoplastic) N85.8
  vagina N89.8
  valve, heart —see Endocarditis
  vas deferens N50.89 ◄▥
  vein I87.8
Fibrositis (periarticular) M79.7
  nodular, chronic (Jaccoud's) (rheumatoid) —
    see Arthropathy, postrheumatic, chronic

◄ New   ◄▥ Revised   ~~deleted~~ Deleted

Fibrothorax J94.1
Fibrotic —*see* Fibrosis
Fibrous —*see* condition
Fibroxanthoma —*see also* Neoplasm, connective tissue, benign
  atypical —*see* Neoplasm, connective tissue, uncertain behavior
  malignant —*see* Neoplasm, connective tissue, malignant
Fibroxanthosarcoma —*see* Neoplasm, connective tissue, malignant
Fiedler's
  disease (icterohemorrhagic leptospirosis) A27.0
  myocarditis (acute) I40.1
Fifth disease B08.3
  venereal A55
Filaria, filarial, filariasis —*see* Infestation, filarial
Filatov's disease —*see* Mononucleosis, infectious
File-cutter's disease —*see* Poisoning, lead
Filling defect
  biliary tract R93.2
  bladder R93.41 ◄▥
  duodenum R93.3
  gallbladder R93.2
  gastrointestinal tract R93.3
  intestine R93.3
  kidney R93.42- ◄▥
  stomach R93.3
  ureter R93.41 ◄▥
  urinary organs, specified NEC R93.49 ◄
Fimbrial cyst Q50.4
Financial problem affecting care NOS Z59.9
  bankruptcy Z59.8
  foreclosure on loan Z59.8
Findings, abnormal, inconclusive, without diagnosis —*see also* Abnormal
  17-ketosteroids, elevated R82.5
  acetonuria R82.4
  alcohol in blood R78.0
  anisocytosis R71.8
  antenatal screening of mother O28.9
    biochemical O28.1
    chromosomal O28.5
    cytological O28.2
    genetic O28.5
    hematological O28.0
    radiological O28.4
    specified NEC O28.8
    ultrasonic O28.3
  antibody titer, elevated R76.0
  anticardiolipin antibody R76.0
  antiphosphatidylglycerol antibody R76.0
  antiphosphatidylinositol antibody R76.0
  antiphosphatidylserine antibody R76.0
  antiphospholipid antibody R76.0
  bacteriuria R82.71 ◄▥
  bicarbonate E87.8
  bile in urine R82.2
  blood sugar R73.09
    high R73.9
    low (transient) E16.2
  body fluid or substance, specified NEC R88.8
  casts, urine R82.99
  catecholamines R82.5
  cells, urine R82.99
  chloride E87.8
  cholesterol E78.9
    high E78.00 ◄▥
      with high triglycerides E78.2
  chyluria R82.0
  cloudy
    dialysis effluent R88.0
    urine R82.90
  creatinine clearance R94.4
  crystals, urine R82.99
  culture
    blood R78.81
    positive —*see* Positive, culture
  echocardiogram R93.1

Findings, abnormal, inconclusive, without diagnosis *(Continued)*
  electrolyte level, urinary R82.99
  function study NEC R94.8
    bladder R94.8
    endocrine NEC R94.7
      thyroid R94.6
    kidney R94.4
    liver R94.5
    pancreas R94.8
    placenta R94.8
    pulmonary R94.2
    spleen R94.8
  gallbladder, nonvisualization R93.2
  glucose (tolerance test) (non-fasting) R73.09
  glycosuria R81
  heart
    shadow R93.1
    sounds R01.2
  hematinuria R82.3
  hematocrit drop (precipitous) R71.0
  hemoglobinuria R82.3
  human papillomavirus (HPV) DNA test positive
    cervix
      high risk R87.810
      low risk R87.820
    vagina
      high risk R87.811
      low risk R87.821
  in blood (of substance not normally found in blood) R78.9
    addictive drug NEC R78.4
    alcohol (excessive level) R78.0
    cocaine R78.2
    hallucinogen R78.3
    heavy metals (abnormal level) R78.79
    lead R78.71
    lithium (abnormal level) R78.89
    opiate drug R78.1
    psychotropic drug R78.5
    specified substance NEC R78.89
    steroid agent R78.6
  indoleacetic acid, elevated R82.5
  ketonuria R82.4
  lactic acid dehydrogenase (LDH) R74.0
  liver function test R79.89
  mammogram NEC R92.8
    calcification (calculus) R92.1
    inconclusive result (due to dense breasts) R92.2
    microcalcification R92.0
  mediastinal shift R93.8
  melanin, urine R82.99
  myoglobinuria R82.1
  neonatal screening P09
  nonvisualization of gallbladder R93.2
  odor of urine NOS R82.90
  Papanicolaou cervix R87.619
    non-atypical endometrial cells R87.618
  pneumoencephalogram R93.0
  poikilocytosis R71.8
  potassium (deficiency) E87.6
    excess E87.5
  PPD R76.11
  radiologic (X-ray) R93.8
    abdomen R93.5
    biliary tract R93.2
    breast R92.8
    gastrointestinal tract R93.3
    genitourinary organs R93.8
    head R93.0
    inconclusive due to excess body fat of patient R93.9
    intrathoracic organs NEC R93.1
    placenta R93.8
    retroperitoneum R93.5
    skin R93.8
    skull R93.0
    subcutaneous tissue R93.8

Findings, abnormal, inconclusive, without diagnosis *(Continued)*
  red blood cell (count) (morphology) (sickling) (volume) R71.8
  scan NEC R94.8
    bladder R94.8
    bone R94.8
    kidney R94.4
    liver R93.2
    lung R94.2
    pancreas R94.8
    placental R94.8
    spleen R94.8
    thyroid R94.6
  sedimentation rate, elevated R70.0
  SGOT R74.0
  SGPT R74.0
  sodium (deficiency) E87.1
    excess E87.0
  specified body fluid NEC R88.8
  stress test R94.39
  thyroid (function) (metabolic rate) (scan) (uptake) R94.6
  transaminase (level) R74.0
  triglycerides E78.9
    high E78.1
      with high cholesterol E78.2
  tuberculin skin test (without active tuberculosis) R76.11
  urine R82.90
    acetone R82.4
    bacteria R82.71 ◄▥
    bile R82.2
    casts or cells R82.99
    chyle R82.0
    culture positive R82.79 ◄▥
    glucose R81
    hemoglobin R82.3
    ketone R82.4
    sugar R81
  vanillylmandelic acid (VMA), elevated R82.5
  vectorcardiogram (VCG) R94.39
  ventriculogram R93.0
  white blood cell (count) (differential) (morphology) D72.9
  xerography R92.8
Finger —*see* condition
Fire, Saint Anthony's —*see* Erysipelas
Fire-setting
  pathological (compulsive) F63.1
Fish hook stomach K31.89
Fishmeal-worker's lung J67.8
Fissure, fissured
  anus, anal K60.2
    acute K60.0
    chronic K60.1
    congenital Q43.8
  ear, lobule, congenital Q17.8
  epiglottis (congenital) Q31.8
  larynx J38.7
    congenital Q31.8
  lip K13.0
    congenital —*see* Cleft, lip
  nipple N64.0
    associated with
      lactation O92.13
      pregnancy O92.11-
      puerperium O92.12
  nose Q30.2
  palate (congenital) —*see* Cleft, palate
  skin R23.4
  spine (congenital) —*see also* Spina bifida
    with hydrocephalus —*see* Spina bifida, by site, with hydrocephalus
  tongue (acquired) K14.5
    congenital Q38.3
Fistula (cutaneous) L98.8
  abdomen (wall) K63.2
    bladder N32.2
    intestine NEC K63.2

Fistula *(Continued)*
  abdomen *(Continued)*
    ureter N28.89
    uterus N82.5
  abdominorectal K63.2
  abdominosigmoidal K63.2
  abdominothoracic J86.0
  abdominouterine N82.5
    congenital Q51.7
  abdominovesical N32.2
  accessory sinuses —*see* Sinusitis
  actinomycotic —*see* Actinomycosis
  alveolar antrum —*see* Sinusitis, maxillary
  alveolar process K04.6
  anorectal K60.5
  antrobuccal —*see* Sinusitis, maxillary
  antrum —*see* Sinusitis, maxillary
  anus, anal (recurrent) (infectional) K60.3
    congenital Q43.6
      with absence, atresia and stenosis Q42.2
    tuberculous A18.32
  aorta-duodenal I77.2
  appendix, appendicular K38.3
  arteriovenous (acquired) (nonruptured) I77.0
    brain I67.1
      congenital Q28.2
        ruptured I60.8
      ruptured I60.8
    cerebral —*see* Fistula, arteriovenous, brain
    congenital (peripheral) —*see also*
      Malformation, arteriovenous
      brain Q28.2
        ruptured I60.8
      coronary Q24.5
      pulmonary Q25.72
    coronary I25.41
      congenital Q24.5
    pulmonary I28.0
      congenital Q25.72
    surgically created (for dialysis) Z99.2
      complication —*see* Complication,
        arteriovenous, fistula, surgically
        created
    traumatic —*see* Injury, blood vessel
  artery I77.2
  aural (mastoid) —*see* Mastoiditis, chronic
  auricle —*see also* Disorder, pinna, specified
    type NEC
    congenital Q18.1
  Bartholin's gland N82.8
  bile duct (common) (hepatic) K83.3
    with calculus, stones —*see* Calculus, bile
      duct
  biliary (tract) —*see* Fistula, bile duct
  bladder (sphincter) NEC —*see also* Fistula,
    vesico- N32.2
    into seminal vesicle N32.2
  bone —*see also* Disorder, bone, specified type
    NEC
    with osteomyelitis, chronic —*see*
      Osteomyelitis, chronic, with draining
      sinus
  brain G93.89
    arteriovenous (acquired) I67.1
      congenital Q28.2
  branchial (cleft) Q18.0
  branchiogenous Q18.0
  breast N61.0 ◀▥
    puerperal, postpartum or gestational, due
      to mastitis (purulent) —*see* Mastitis,
      obstetric, purulent
  bronchial J86.0
  bronchocutaneous, bronchomediastinal,
    bronchopleural,
    bronchopleuromediastinal (infective)
    J86.0
    tuberculous NEC A15.5
  bronchoesophageal J86.0
    congenital Q39.2
      with atresia of esophagus Q39.1
  bronchovisceral J86.0

buccal cavity (infective) K12.2
cecosigmoidal K63.2
cecum K63.2
cerebrospinal (fluid) G96.0
cervical, lateral Q18.1
cervicoaural Q18.1
cervicosigmoidal N82.4
cervicovesical N82.1
cervix N82.8
chest (wall) J86.0
cholecystenteric —*see* Fistula, gallbladder
cholecystocolic —*see* Fistula, gallbladder
cholecystocolonic —*see* Fistula, gallbladder
cholecystoduodenal —*see* Fistula,
  gallbladder
cholecystogastric —*see* Fistula, gallbladder
cholecystointestinal —*see* Fistula,
  gallbladder
choledochoduodenal —*see* Fistula,
  bile duct
cholocolic K82.3
coccyx —*see* Sinus, pilonidal
colon K63.2
colostomy K94.09
common duct —*see* Fistula, bile duct
congenital, site not listed —*see* Anomaly, by
  site
coronary, arteriovenous I25.41
  congenital Q24.5
costal region J86.0
cul-de-sac, Douglas' N82.8
cystic duct —*see also* Fistula, gallbladder
  congenital Q44.5
dental K04.6
diaphragm J86.0
duodenum K31.6
ear (external) (canal) —*see* Disorder, ear,
  external, specified type NEC
enterocolic K63.2
enterocutaneous K63.2
enterouterine N82.4
  congenital Q51.7
enterovaginal N82.4
  congenital Q52.2
  large intestine N82.3
  small intestine N82.2
enterovesical N32.1
epididymis N50.89 ◀▥
  tuberculous A18.15
esophagobronchial J86.0
  congenital Q39.2
    with atresia of esophagus Q39.1
esophagocutaneous K22.8
esophagopleural-cutaneous J86.0
esophagotracheal J86.0
  congenital Q39.2
    with atresia of esophagus Q39.1
esophagus K22.8
  congenital Q39.2
    with atresia of esophagus Q39.1
ethmoid —*see* Sinusitis, ethmoidal
eyeball (cornea) (sclera) —*see* Disorder, globe,
  hypotony
eyelid H01.8
fallopian tube, external N82.5
fecal K63.2
  congenital Q43.6
from periapical abscess K04.6
frontal sinus —*see* Sinusitis, frontal
gallbladder K82.3
  with calculus, cholelithiasis, stones —*see*
    Calculus, gallbladder
gastric K31.6
gastrocolic K31.6
  congenital Q40.2
  tuberculous A18.32
gastroenterocolic K31.6
gastroesophageal K31.6
gastrojejunal K31.6
gastrojejunocolic K31.6

genital tract (female) N82.9
  specified NEC N82.8
  to intestine NEC N82.4
  to skin N82.5
hepatic artery-portal vein, congenital Q26.6
hepatopleural J86.0
hepatopulmonary J86.0
ileorectal or ileosigmoidal K63.2
ileovaginal N82.2
ileovesical N32.1
ileum K63.2
in ano K60.3
  tuberculous A18.32
inner ear (labyrinth) —*see* subcategory H83.1
intestine NEC K63.2
intestinocolonic (abdominal) K63.2
intestinoureteral N28.89
intestinouterine N82.4
intestinovaginal N82.4
  large intestine N82.3
  small intestine N82.2
intestinovesical N32.1
ischiorectal (fossa) K61.3
jejunum K63.2
joint M25.10
  ankle M25.17-
  elbow M25.12-
  foot joint M25.17-
  hand joint M25.14-
  hip M25.15-
  knee M25.16-
  shoulder M25.11-
  specified joint NEC M25.18
  tuberculous —*see* Tuberculosis, joint
  vertebrae M25.18
  wrist M25.13-
kidney N28.89
labium (majus) (minus) N82.8
labyrinth —*see* subcategory H83.1
lacrimal (gland) (sac) H04.61-
lacrimonasal duct —*see* Fistula, lacrimal
laryngotracheal, congenital Q34.8
larynx J38.7
lip K13.0
  congenital Q38.0
lumbar, tuberculous A18.01
lung J86.0
lymphatic I89.8
mammary (gland) N61.0 ◀▥
mastoid (process) (region) —*see* Mastoiditis,
  chronic
maxillary J32.0
medial, face and neck Q18.8
mediastinal J86.0
mediastinobronchial J86.0
mediastinocutaneous J86.0
middle ear —*see* subcategory H74.8
mouth K12.2
nasal J34.89
  sinus —*see* Sinusitis
nasopharynx J39.2
nipple N64.0
nose J34.89
oral (cutaneous) K12.2
  maxillary J32.0
  nasal (with cleft palate) —*see* Cleft, palate
orbit, orbital —*see* Disorder, orbit, specified
  type NEC
oroantral J32.0
oviduct, external N82.5
palate (hard) M27.8
pancreatic K86.89 ◀▥
pancreaticoduodenal K86.89 ◀▥
parotid (gland) K11.4
  region K12.2
penis N48.89
perianal K60.3
pericardium (pleura) (sac) —*see* Pericarditis
pericecal K63.2
perineorectal K60.4
perineosigmoidal K63.2

◀ New   ▥ Revised   ~~deleted~~ Deleted

Fistula (*Continued*)
  perineum, perineal (with urethral
      involvement) NEC N36.Ø
    tuberculous A18.13
    ureter N28.89
  perirectal K6Ø.4
    tuberculous A18.32
  peritoneum K65.9
  pharyngoesophageal J39.2
  pharynx J39.2
    branchial cleft (congenital) Q18.Ø
  pilonidal (infected) (rectum) —*see* Sinus,
      pilonidal
  pleura, pleural, pleurocutaneous,
      pleuroperitoneal J86.Ø
    tuberculous NEC A15.6
  pleuropericardial I31.8
  portal vein-hepatic artery, congenital Q26.6
  postauricular H7Ø.81-
  postoperative, persistent T81.83
    specified site —*see* Fistula, by site
  preauricular (congenital) Q18.1
  prostate N42.89
  pulmonary J86.Ø
    arteriovenous I28.Ø
      congenital Q25.72
    tuberculous —*see* Tuberculosis, pulmonary
  pulmonoperitoneal J86.Ø
  rectolabial N82.4
  rectosigmoid (intercommunicating) K63.2
  rectoureteral N28.89
  rectourethral N36.Ø
    congenital Q64.73
  rectouterine N82.4
    congenital Q51.7
  rectovaginal N82.3
    congenital Q52.2
    tuberculous A18.18
  rectovesical N32.1
    congenital Q64.79
  rectovesicovaginal N82.3
  rectovulval N82.4
    congenital Q52.79
  rectum (to skin) K6Ø.4
    congenital Q43.6
      with absence, atresia and stenosis Q42.Ø
    tuberculous A18.32
  renal N28.89
  retroauricular —*see* Fistula, postauricular
  salivary duct or gland (any) K11.4
    congenital Q38.4
  scrotum (urinary) N5Ø.89 ◀▥
    tuberculous A18.15
  semicircular canals —*see* subcategory H83.1
  sigmoid K63.2
    to bladder N32.1
  sinus —*see* Sinusitis
  skin L98.8
    to genital tract (female) N82.5
  splenocolic D73.89
  stercoral K63.2
  stomach K31.6
  sublingual gland K11.4
  submandibular gland K11.4
  submaxillary (gland) K11.4
    region K12.2
  thoracic J86.Ø
    duct I89.8
  thoracoabdominal J86.Ø
  thoracogastric J86.Ø
  thoracointestinal J86.Ø
  thorax J86.Ø
  thyroglossal duct Q89.2
  thyroid EØ7.89
  trachea, congenital (external) (internal) Q32.1
  tracheoesophageal J86.Ø
    congenital Q39.2
      with atresia of esophagus Q39.1
    following tracheostomy J95.Ø4
  traumatic arteriovenous —*see* Injury, blood
      vessel, by site

Fistula (*Continued*)
  tuberculous - code by site under
      Tuberculosis
  typhoid AØ1.Ø9
  umbilicourinary Q64.8
  urachus, congenital Q64.4
  ureter (persistent) N28.89
  ureteroabdominal N28.89
  ureterorectal N28.89
  ureterosigmoido-abdominal N28.89
  ureterovaginal N82.1
  ureterovesical N32.2
  urethra N36.Ø
    congenital Q64.79
    tuberculous A18.13
  urethroperineal N36.Ø
  urethroperineovesical N32.2
  urethrorectal N36.Ø
    congenital Q64.73
  urethroscrotal N5Ø.89 ◀▥
  urethrovaginal N82.1
  urethrovesical N32.2
  urinary (tract) (persistent) (recurrent)
      N36.Ø
  uteroabdominal N82.5
    congenital Q51.7
  uteroenteric, uterointestinal N82.4
    congenital Q51.7
  uterorectal N82.4
    congenital Q51.7
  uteroureteric N82.1
  uterourethral Q51.7
  uterovaginal N82.8
  uterovesical N82.1
    congenital Q51.7
  uterus N82.8
  vagina (postpartal) (wall) N82.8
  vaginocutaneous (postpartal) N82.5
  vaginointestinal NEC N82.4
    large intestine N82.3
    small intestine N82.2
  vaginoperineal N82.5
  vasocutaneous, congenital Q55.7
  vesical NEC N32.2
  vesicoabdominal N32.2
  vesicocervicovaginal N82.1
  vesicocolic N32.1
  vesicocutaneous N32.2
  vesicoenteric N32.1
  vesicointestinal N32.1
  vesicometrorectal N82.4
  vesicoperineal N32.2
  vesicorectal N32.1
    congenital Q64.79
  vesicosigmoidal N32.1
  vesicosigmoidovaginal N82.3
  vesicoureteral N32.2
  vesicoureterovaginal N82.1
  vesicourethral N32.2
  vesicourethrorectal N32.1
  vesicouterine N82.1
    congenital Q51.7
  vesicovaginal N82.Ø
  vulvorectal N82.4
    congenital Q52.79
Fit R56.9
  epileptic —*see* Epilepsy
  fainting R55
  hysterical F44.5
  newborn P9Ø
Fitting (and adjustment) (of)
  artificial
    arm —*see* Admission, adjustment, artificial,
        arm
    breast Z44.3
    eye Z44.2
    leg —*see* Admission, adjustment, artificial,
        leg
  automatic implantable cardiac defibrillator
      (with synchronous cardiac pacemaker)
      Z45.Ø2

Fitting (*Continued*)
  brain neuropacemaker Z46.2
    implanted Z45.42
  cardiac defibrillator —*see* Fitting (and
      adjustment) (of), automatic implantable
      cardiac defibrillator
  catheter, non-vascular Z46.82
  colostomy belt Z46.89
  contact lenses Z46.Ø
  CRT-D (resynchronization therapy
      defibrillator) Z45.Ø2 ◀
  CRT-P (cardiac resynchronization therapy
      pacemaker) Z45.Ø18 ◀
    pulse generator Z45.Ø1Ø ◀
  cystostomy device Z46.6
  defibrillator, cardiac —*see* Fitting (and
      adjustment) (of), automatic implantable
      cardiac defibrillator
  dentures Z46.3
  device NOS Z46.9
    abdominal Z46.89
    gastrointestinal NEC Z46.59
    implanted NEC Z45.89
    nervous system Z46.2
      implanted —*see* Admission, adjustment,
          device, implanted, nervous
          system
    orthodontic Z46.4
    orthoptic Z46.Ø
    orthotic Z46.89
    prosthetic (external) Z44.9
      breast Z44.3
      dental Z46.3
      eye Z44.2
      specified NEC Z44.8
    specified NEC Z46.89
    substitution
      auditory Z46.2
        implanted —*see* Admission,
            adjustment, device, implanted,
            hearing device
      nervous system Z46.2
        implanted —*see* Admission,
            adjustment, device, implanted,
            nervous system
      visual Z46.2
        implanted Z45.31
    urinary Z46.6
  gastric lap band Z46.51
  gastrointestinal appliance NEC Z46.59
  glasses (reading) Z46.Ø
  hearing aid Z46.1
  ileostomy device Z46.89
  insulin pump Z46.81
  intestinal appliance NEC Z46.89
  myringotomy device (stent) (tube) Z45.82
  neuropacemaker Z46.2
    implanted Z45.42
  non-vascular catheter Z46.82
  orthodontic device Z46.4
  orthopedic device (brace) (cast) (corset)
      (shoes) Z46.89
  pacemaker (cardiac) (cardiac
      resynchronization therapy (CRT-P))
      Z45.Ø18 ◀▥
    nervous system (brain) (peripheral nerve)
        (spinal cord) Z46.2
      implanted Z45.42
    pulse generator Z45.Ø1Ø
  portacath (port-a-cath) Z45.2
  prosthesis (external) Z44.9
    arm —*see* Admission, adjustment, artificial,
        arm
    breast Z44.3
    dental Z46.3
    eye Z44.2
    leg —*see* Admission, adjustment, artificial,
        leg
    specified NEC Z44.8
  spectacles Z46.Ø
  wheelchair Z46.89

Fitzhugh-Curtis syndrome
  due to
    Chlamydia trachomatis A74.81
    Neisseria gonorrhorea (gonococcal
      peritonitis) A54.85
Fitz's syndrome (acute hemorrhagic
  pancreatitis) —see also Pancreatitis, acute
  K85.80 ◀▥
Fixation
  joint —see Ankylosis
  larynx J38.7
  stapes —see Ankylosis, ear ossicles
    deafness —see Deafness, conductive
  uterus (acquired) —see Malposition, uterus
  vocal cord J38.3
Flabby ridge K06.8
Flaccid —see also condition
  palate, congenital Q38.5
Flail
  chest S22.5-
    newborn (birth injury) P13.8
  joint (paralytic) M25.20
    ankle M25.27-
    elbow M25.22-
    foot joint M25.27-
    hand joint M25.24-
    hip M25.25-
    knee M25.26-
    shoulder M25.21-
    specified joint NEC M25.28
    wrist M25.23-
Flajani's disease —see Hyperthyroidism, with,
  goiter (diffuse)
Flap, liver K71.3
Flashbacks (residual to hallucinogen use) F16.283
Flat
  chamber (eye) —see Disorder, globe,
    hypotony, flat anterior chamber
  chest, congenital Q67.8
  foot (acquired) (fixed type) (painful)
    (postural) —see also Deformity, limb,
    flat foot
    congenital (rigid) (spastic) (everted) Q66.5-
    rachitic sequelae (late effect) E64.3
  organ or site, congenital NEC —see Anomaly,
    by site
  pelvis M95.5
    with disproportion (fetopelvic) O33.0
      causing obstructed labor O65.0
    congenital Q74.2
Flatau-Schilder disease G37.0
Flatback syndrome M40.30
  lumbar region M40.36
  lumbosacral region M40.37
  thoracolumbar region M40.35
Flattening
  head, femur M89.8X5
  hip —see Coxa, plana
  lip (congenital) Q18.8
  nose (congenital) Q67.4
    acquired M95.0
Flatulence R14.3
  psychogenic F45.8
Flatus R14.3
  vaginalis N89.8
Flax-dresser's disease J66.1
Flea bite —see Injury, bite, by site, superficial,
  insect
Flecks, glaucomatous (subcapsular) —see
  Cataract, complicated
Fleischer (-Kayser) ring (cornea) H18.04-
Fleshy mole O02.0
Flexibilitas cerea —see Catalepsy
Flexion
  amputation stump (surgical) T87.89
  cervix —see Malposition, uterus
  contracture, joint —see Contraction, joint
  deformity, joint —see also Deformity, limb,
    flexion M21.20
  hip, congenital Q65.89
  uterus —see also Malposition, uterus
    lateral —see Lateroversion, uterus

Flexner-Boyd dysentery A03.2
Flexner's dysentery A03.1
Flexure —see Flexion
Flint murmur (aortic insufficiency) I35.1
Floater, vitreous —see Opacity, vitreous
Floating
  cartilage (joint) —see also Loose, body, joint
    knee —see Derangement, knee, loose body
  gallbladder, congenital Q44.1
  kidney N28.89
    congenital Q63.8
  spleen D73.89
Flooding N92.0
Floor —see condition
Floppy
  baby syndrome (nonspecific) P94.2
  iris syndrome (intraoperative) (IFIS) H21.81
  nonrheumatic mitral valve syndrome I34.1
Flu —see also Influenza
  avian —see also Influenza, due to, identified
    novel influenza A virus J09.X2
  bird —see also Influenza, due to, identified
    novel influenza A virus J09.X2
  intestinal NEC A08.4
  swine (viruses that normally cause infections
    in pigs) —see also Influenza, due to,
    identified novel influenza A virus
    J09.X2
Fluctuating blood pressure I99.8
Fluid
  abdomen R18.8
  chest J94.8
  heart —see Failure, heart, congestive
  joint —see Effusion, joint
  loss (acute) E86.9
    ~~with~~
      ~~hypernatremia E87.0~~
      ~~hyponatremia E87.1~~
  lung —see Edema, lung
  overload E87.70
    specified NEC E87.79
  peritoneal cavity R18.8
  pleural cavity J94.8
  retention R60.9
Flukes NEC —see also Infestation, fluke
  blood NEC —see Schistosomiasis
  liver B66.3
Fluor (vaginalis) N89.8
  trichomonal or due to Trichomonas
    (vaginalis) A59.00
Fluorosis
  dental K00.3
  skeletal M85.10
    ankle M85.17-
    foot M85.17-
    forearm M85.13-
    hand M85.14-
    lower leg M85.16-
    multiple site M85.19
    neck M85.18
    rib M85.18
    shoulder M85.11-
    skull M85.18
    specified site NEC M85.18
    thigh M85.15-
    toe M85.17-
    upper arm M85.12-
    vertebra M85.18
Flush syndrome E34.0
Flushing R23.2
  menopausal N95.1
Flutter
  atrial or auricular I48.92
    atypical I48.4
    type I I48.3
    type II I48.4
    typical I48.3
  heart I49.8
    atrial or auricular I48.92
      atypical I48.4
      type I I48.3

Fistula (Continued)
  heart (Continued)
    atrial or auricular (Continued)
      type II I48.4
      typical I48.3
      ventricular I49.02
    ventricular I49.02
FNHTR (febrile nonhemolytic transfusion
  reaction) R50.84
Fochier's abscess - code by site under Abscess
Focus, Assmann's —see Tuberculosis,
  pulmonary
Fogo selvagem L10.3
Foix-Alajouanine syndrome G95.19
Fold, folds (anomalous) —see also Anomaly,
  by site
  Descemet's membrane —see Change, corneal
    membrane, Descemet's, fold
  epicanthic Q10.3
  heart Q24.8
Folie à deux F24
Follicle
  cervix (nabothian) (ruptured) N88.8
  graafian, ruptured, with hemorrhage
    N83.0- ◀▥
  nabothian N88.8
Follicular —see condition
Folliculitis (superficial) L73.9
  abscedens et suffodiens L66.3
  cyst N83.0- ◀▥
  decalvans L66.2
  deep —see Furuncle, by site
  gonococcal (acute) (chronic) A54.01
  keloid, keloidalis L73.0
  pustular L01.02
  ulerythematosa reticulata L66.4
Folliculome lipidique
  specified site —see Neoplasm, benign,
    by site
  unspecified site
    female D27.9
    male D29.20
Følling's disease E70.0
Follow-up —see Examination, follow-up
Fong's syndrome (hereditary osteo-
  onychodysplasia) Q87.2 ◀▥
Food
  allergy L27.2
  asphyxia (from aspiration or inhalation) —see
    Foreign body, by site
  choked on —see Foreign body, by site
  deprivation T73.0
    specified kind of food NEC E63.8
  intoxication —see Poisoning, food
  lack of T73.0
  poisoning —see Poisoning, food
  rejection NEC —see Disorder, eating
  strangulation or suffocation —see Foreign
    body, by site
  toxemia —see Poisoning, food
Foot —see condition
Foramen ovale (nonclosure) (patent)
  (persistent) Q21.1
Forbes' glycogen storage disease E74.03
Fordyce-Fox disease L75.2
Fordyce's disease (mouth) Q38.6
Forearm —see condition
Foreign body
  with
    laceration —see Laceration, by site, with
      foreign body
    puncture wound —see Puncture, by site,
      with foreign body
  accidentally left following a procedure
    T81.509
    aspiration T81.506
    resulting in
      adhesions T81.516
      obstruction T81.526
      perforation T81.536
      specified complication NEC T81.596

◀ New   ▥ Revised   ~~deleted~~ Deleted

Foreign body *(Continued)*
  accidentally left following a procedure
    (Continued)
    cardiac catheterization T81.505
      resulting in
        acute reaction T81.60
          aseptic peritonitis T81.61
          specified NEC T81.69
        adhesions T81.515
        obstruction T81.525
        perforation T81.535
        specified complication NEC T81.595
      causing
        acute reaction T81.60
          aseptic peritonitis T81.61
          specified complication NEC T81.69
        adhesions T81.519
        aseptic peritonitis T81.61
        obstruction T81.529
        perforation T81.539
        specified complication NEC T81.599
    endoscopy T81.504
      resulting in
        adhesions T81.514
        obstruction T81.524
        perforation T81.534
        specified complication NEC T81.594
    immunization T81.503
      resulting in
        adhesions T81.513
        obstruction T81.523
        perforation T81.533
        specified complication NEC T81.593
    infusion T81.501
      resulting in
        adhesions T81.511
        obstruction T81.521
        perforation T81.531
        specified complication NEC T81.591
    injection T81.503
      resulting in
        adhesions T81.513
        obstruction T81.523
        perforation T81.533
        specified complication NEC T81.593
    kidney dialysis T81.502
      resulting in
        adhesions T81.512
        obstruction T81.522
        perforation T81.532
        specified complication NEC T81.592
    packing removal T81.507
      resulting in
        acute reaction T81.60
          aseptic peritonitis T81.61
          specified NEC T81.69
        adhesions T81.517
        obstruction T81.527
        perforation T81.537
        specified complication NEC T81.597
    puncture T81.506
      resulting in
        adhesions T81.516
        obstruction T81.526
        perforation T81.536
        specified complication NEC T81.596
    specified procedure NEC T81.508
      resulting in
        acute reaction T81.60
          aseptic peritonitis T81.61
          specified NEC T81.69
        adhesions T81.518
        obstruction T81.528
        perforation T81.538
        specified complication NEC
          T81.598
    surgical operation T81.500
      resulting in
        acute reaction T81.60
          aseptic peritonitis T81.61
          specified NEC T81.69

Foreign body *(Continued)*
  accidentally left following a procedure
    (Continued)
    surgical operation *(Continued)*
      resulting in *(Continued)*
        adhesions T81.510
        obstruction T81.520
        perforation T81.530
        specified complication NEC T81.590
    transfusion T81.501
      resulting in
        adhesions T81.511
        obstruction T81.521
        perforation T81.531
        specified complication NEC T81.591
  alimentary tract T18.9
    anus T18.5
    colon T18.4
    esophagus —*see* Foreign body, esophagus
    mouth T18.0
    multiple sites T18.8
    rectosigmoid (junction) T18.5
    rectum T18.5
    small intestine T18.3
    specified site NEC T18.8
    stomach T18.2
  anterior chamber (eye) S05.5-
  auditory canal —*see* Foreign body, entering
    through orifice, ear
  bronchus T17.508
    causing
      asphyxiation T17.500
        food (bone) (seed) T17.520
        gastric contents (vomitus) T17.510
        specified type NEC T17.590
      injury NEC T17.508
        food (bone) (seed) T17.528
        gastric contents (vomitus) T17.518
        specified type NEC T17.598
  canthus —*see* Foreign body, conjunctival sac
  ciliary body (eye) S05.5-
  conjunctival sac T15.1-
  cornea T15.0-
  entering through orifice
    accessory sinus T17.0
    alimentary canal T18.9
      multiple parts T18.8
      specified part NEC T18.8
    alveolar process T18.0
    antrum (Highmore's) T17.0
    anus T18.5
    appendix T18.4
    auditory canal —*see* Foreign body, entering
      through orifice, ear
    auricle —*see* Foreign body, entering
      through orifice, ear
    bladder T19.1
    bronchioles —*see* Foreign body, respiratory
      tract, specified site NEC
    bronchus (main) —*see* Foreign body,
      bronchus
    buccal cavity T18.0
    canthus (inner) —*see* Foreign body,
      conjunctival sac
    cecum T18.4
    cervix (canal) (uteri) T19.3
    colon T18.4
    conjunctival sac —*see* Foreign body,
      conjunctival sac
    cornea —*see* Foreign body, cornea
    digestive organ or tract NOS T18.9
      multiple parts T18.8
      specified part NEC T18.8
    duodenum T18.3
    ear (external) T16.-
    esophagus —*see* Foreign body, esophagus
    eye (external) NOS T15.9-
      conjunctival sac —*see* Foreign body,
        conjunctival sac
      cornea —*see* Foreign body, cornea
      specified part NEC T15.8-

Foreign body *(Continued)*
  entering through orifice *(Continued)*
    eyeball —*see also* Foreign body, entering
      through orifice, eye, specified part
      NEC
      with penetrating wound —*see* Puncture,
        eyeball
    eyelid —*see also* Foreign body, conjunctival
      sac
      with
        laceration —*see* Laceration, eyelid,
          with foreign body
        puncture —*see* Puncture, eyelid, with
          foreign body
        superficial injury —*see* Foreign body,
          superficial, eyelid
    gastrointestinal tract T18.9
      multiple parts T18.8
      specified part NEC T18.8
    genitourinary tract T19.9
      multiple parts T19.8
      specified part NEC T19.8
    globe —*see* Foreign body, entering through
      orifice, eyeball
    gum T18.0
    Highmore's antrum T17.0
    hypopharynx —*see* Foreign body, pharynx
    ileum T18.3
    intestine (small) T18.3
      large T18.4
    lacrimal apparatus (punctum) —*see*
      Foreign body, entering through
      orifice, eye, specified part NEC
    large intestine T18.4
    larynx —*see* Foreign body, larynx
    lung —*see* Foreign body, respiratory tract,
      specified site NEC
    maxillary sinus T17.0
    mouth T18.0
    nasal sinus T17.0
    nasopharynx —*see* Foreign body, pharynx
    nose (passage) T17.1
    nostril T17.1
    oral cavity T18.0
    palate T18.0
    penis T19.4
    pharynx —*see* Foreign body, pharynx
    piriform sinus —*see* Foreign body, pharynx
    rectosigmoid (junction) T18.5
    rectum T18.5
    respiratory tract —*see* Foreign body,
      respiratory tract
    sinus (accessory) (frontal) (maxillary)
      (nasal) T17.0
      piriform —*see* Foreign body, pharynx
    small intestine T18.3
    stomach T18.2
    suffocation by —*see* Foreign body, by site
    tear ducts or glands —*see* Foreign body,
      entering through orifice, eye,
      specified part NEC
    throat —*see* Foreign body, pharynx
    tongue T18.0
    tonsil, tonsillar (fossa) —*see* Foreign body,
      pharynx
    trachea —*see* Foreign body, trachea
    ureter T19.8
    urethra T19.0
    uterus (any part) T19.3
    vagina T19.2
    vulva T19.2
  esophagus T18.108
    causing
      injury NEC T18.108
        food (bone) (seed) T18.128
        gastric contents (vomitus) T18.118
        specified type NEC T18.198
      tracheal compression T18.100
        food (bone) (seed) T18.120
        gastric contents (vomitus) T18.110
        specified type NEC T18.190

Foreign body *(Continued)*
  felling of, in throat R09.89
  fragment —*see* Retained, foreign body
      fragments (type of)
  genitourinary tract T19.9
    bladder T19.1
    multiple parts T19.8
    penis T19.4
    specified site NEC T19.8
    urethra T19.0
    uterus T19.3
      IUD Z97.5
    vagina T19.2
      contraceptive device Z97.5
    vulva T19.2
  granuloma (old) (soft tissue) —*see also*
      Granuloma, foreign body
    skin L92.3
  in
    laceration —*see* Laceration, by site, with
        foreign body
    puncture wound —*see* Puncture, by site,
        with foreign body
    soft tissue (residual) M79.5
  inadvertently left in operation wound —*see*
      Foreign body, accidentally left during a
      procedure
  ingestion, ingested NOS T18.9
  inhalation or inspiration —*see* Foreign body,
      by site
  internal organ, not entering through a natural
      orifice - code as specific injury with
      foreign body
  intraocular S05.5-
    old, retained (nonmagnetic) H44.70-
      anterior chamber H44.71-
      ciliary body H44.72-
      iris H44.72-
      lens H44.73-
      magnetic H44.60-
        anterior chamber H44.61-
        ciliary body H44.62-
        iris H44.62-
        lens H44.63-
        posterior wall H44.64-
        specified site NEC H44.69-
        vitreous body H44.65-
      posterior wall H44.74-
      specified site NEC H44.79-
      vitreous body H44.75-
    iris —*see* Foreign body, intraocular
  lacrimal punctum —*see* Foreign body,
      entering through orifice, eye, specified
      part NEC
  larynx T17.308
    causing
      asphyxiation T17.300
        food (bone) (seed) T17.320
        gastric contents (vomitus) T17.310
        specified type NEC T17.390
      injury NEC T17.308
        food (bone) (seed) T17.328
        gastric contents (vomitus) T17.318
        specified type NEC T17.398
  lens —*see* Foreign body, intraocular
  ocular muscle S05.4-
    old, retained —*see* Foreign body, orbit, old
  old or residual
    soft tissue (residual) M79.5
  operation wound, left accidentally —*see*
      Foreign body, accidentally left during a
      procedure
  orbit S05.4-
    old, retained H05.5-
  pharynx T17.208
    causing
      asphyxiation T17.200
        food (bone) (seed) T17.220
        gastric contents (vomitus)
            T17.210
        specified type NEC T17.290

Foreign body *(Continued)*
  pharynx *(Continued)*
    causing *(Continued)*
      injury NEC T17.208
        food (bone) (seed) T17.228
        gastric contents (vomitus) T17.218
        specified type NEC T17.298
  respiratory tract T17.908
    bronchioles —*see* Foreign body, respiratory
        tract, specified site NEC
    bronchus —*see* Foreign body, bronchus
    causing
      asphyxiation T17.900
        food (bone) (seed) T17.920
        gastric contents (vomitus) T17.910
        specified type NEC T17.990
      injury NEC T17.908
        food (bone) (seed) T17.928
        gastric contents (vomitus) T17.918
        specified type NEC T17.998
    larynx —*see* Foreign body, larynx
    lung —*see* Foreign body, respiratory tract,
        specified site NEC
    multiple parts —*see* Foreign body,
        respiratory tract, specified site NEC
    nasal sinus T17.0
    nasopharynx —*see* Foreign body, pharynx
    nose T17.1
    nostril T17.1
    pharynx —*see* Foreign body, pharynx
    specified site NEC T17.808
      causing
        asphyxiation T17.800
          food (bone) (seed) T17.820
          gastric contents (vomitus) T17.810
          specified type NEC T17.890
        injury NEC T17.808
          food (bone) (seed) T17.828
          gastric contents (vomitus) T17.818
          specified type NEC T17.898
    throat —*see* Foreign body, pharynx
    trachea —*see* Foreign body, trachea
  retained (old) (nonmagnetic) (in)
    anterior chamber (eye) —*see* Foreign body,
        intraocular, old, retained, anterior
        chamber
      magnetic —*see* Foreign body, intraocular,
          old, retained, magnetic, anterior
          chamber
    ciliary body —*see* Foreign body,
        intraocular, old, retained, ciliary body
      magnetic —*see* Foreign body, intraocular,
          old, retained, magnetic, ciliary
          body
    eyelid H02.819
      left H02.816
        lower H02.815
        upper H02.814
      right H02.813
        lower H02.812
        upper H02.811
    fragments —*see* Retained, foreign body
        fragments (type of)
    globe —*see* Foreign body, intraocular, old,
        retained
      magnetic —*see* Foreign body, intraocular,
          old, retained, magnetic
    intraocular —*see* Foreign body, intraocular,
        old, retained
      magnetic —*see* Foreign body, intraocular,
          old, retained, magnetic
    iris —*see* Foreign body, intraocular, old,
        retained, iris
      magnetic —*see* Foreign body, intraocular,
          old, retained, magnetic, iris
    lens —*see* Foreign body, intraocular, old,
        retained, lens
      magnetic —*see* Foreign body, intraocular,
          old, retained, magnetic, lens
    muscle —*see* Foreign body, retained, soft
        tissue

Foreign body *(Continued)*
  retained *(Continued)*
    orbit —*see* Foreign body, orbit, old
    posterior wall of globe —*see* Foreign body,
        intraocular, old, retained, posterior
        wall
      magnetic —*see* Foreign body, intraocular,
          old, retained, magnetic, posterior
          wall
    retrobulbar —*see* Foreign body, orbit, old,
        retrobulbar
    soft tissue M79.5
    vitreous —*see* Foreign body, intraocular,
        old, retained, vitreous body
      magnetic —*see* Foreign body, intraocular,
          old, retained, magnetic, vitreous
          body
  retina S05.5-
  superficial, without open wound
    abdomen, abdominal (wall) S30.851
    alveolar process S00.552
    ankle S90.55-
    antecubital space —*see* Foreign body,
        superficial, forearm
    anus S30.857
    arm (upper) S40.85-
    auditory canal —*see* Foreign body,
        superficial, ear
    auricle —*see* Foreign body, superficial, ear
    axilla —*see* Foreign body, superficial, arm
    back, lower S30.850
    breast S20.15-
    brow S00.85
    buttock S30.850
    calf —*see* Foreign body, superficial, leg
    canthus —*see* Foreign body, superficial,
        eyelid
    cheek S00.85
      internal S00.552
    chest wall —*see* Foreign body, superficial,
        thorax
    chin S00.85
    clitoris S30.854
    costal region —*see* Foreign body,
        superficial, thorax
    digit (s)
      foot —*see* Foreign body, superficial, toe
      hand —*see* Foreign body, superficial,
          finger
    ear S00.45-
    elbow S50.35-
    epididymis S30.853
    epigastric region S30.851
    epiglottis S10.15
    esophagus, cervical S10.15
    eyebrow —*see* Foreign body, superficial,
        eyelid
    eyelid S00.25-
    face S00.85
    finger (s) S60.459
      index S60.45-
      little S60.45-
      middle S60.45-
      ring S60.45-
    flank S30.851
    foot (except toe (s) alone) S90.85-
      toe —*see* Foreign body, superficial, toe
    forearm S50.85-
      elbow only —*see* Foreign body,
          superficial, elbow
    forehead S00.85
    genital organs, external
      female S30.856
      male S30.855
    groin S30.851
    gum S00.552
    hand S60.55-
    head S00.95
      ear —*see* Foreign body, superficial, ear
      eyelid —*see* Foreign body, superficial,
          eyelid

◀ New   ◀▦ Revised   ~~deleted~~ Deleted

Foreign body *(Continued)*
  superficial, without open wound *(Continued)*
    head *(Continued)*
      lip S00.551
      nose S00.35
      oral cavity S00.552
      scalp S00.05
      specified site NEC S00.85
    heel —*see* Foreign body, superficial, foot
    hip S70.25-
    inguinal region S30.851
    interscapular region S20.459
    jaw S00.85
    knee S80.25-
    labium (majus) (minus) S30.854
    larynx S10.15
    leg (lower) S80.85-
      knee —*see* Foreign body, superficial, knee
      upper —*see* Foreign body, superficial, thigh
    lip S00.551
    lower back S30.850
    lumbar region S30.850
    malar region S00.85
    mammary —*see* Foreign body, superficial, breast
    mastoid region S00.85
    mouth S00.552
    nail
      finger —*see* Foreign body, superficial, finger
      toe —*see* Foreign body, superficial, toe
    nape S10.85
    nasal S00.35
    neck S10.95
      specified site NEC S10.85
      throat S10.15
    nose S00.35
    occipital region S00.05
    oral cavity S00.552
    orbital region —*see* Foreign body, superficial, eyelid
    palate S00.552
    palm —*see* Foreign body, superficial, hand
    parietal region S00.05
    pelvis S30.850
    penis S30.852
    perineum
      female S30.854
      male S30.850
    periocular area —*see* Foreign body, superficial, eyelid
    phalanges
      finger —*see* Foreign body, superficial, finger
      toe —*see* Foreign body, superficial, toe
    pharynx S10.15
    pinna —*see* Foreign body, superficial, ear
    popliteal space —*see* Foreign body, superficial, knee
    prepuce S30.852
    pubic region S30.850
    pudendum
      female S30.856
      male S30.855
    sacral region S30.850
    scalp S00.05
    scapular region —*see* Foreign body, superficial, shoulder
    scrotum S30.853
    shin —*see* Foreign body, superficial, leg
    shoulder S40.25-
    sternal region S20.359
    submaxillary region S00.85
    submental region S00.85
    subungual
      finger (s) —*see* Foreign body, superficial, finger
      toe (s) —*see* Foreign body, superficial, toe

Foreign body *(Continued)*
  superficial, without open wound *(Continued)*
    supraclavicular fossa S10.85
    supraorbital S00.85
    temple S00.85
    temporal region S00.85
    testis S30.853
    thigh S70.35-
    thorax, thoracic (wall) S20.95
      back S20.45-
      front S20.35-
    throat S10.15
    thumb S60.35-
    toe (s) (lesser) S90.456
      great S90.45-
    tongue S00.552
    trachea S10.15
    tunica vaginalis S30.853
    tympanum, tympanic membrane —*see* Foreign body, superficial, ear
    uvula S00.552
    vagina S30.854
    vocal cords S10.15
    vulva S30.854
    wrist S60.85-
  swallowed T18.9
  trachea T17.408
    causing
      asphyxiation T17.400
        food (bone) (seed) T17.420
        gastric contents (vomitus) T17.410
        specified type NEC T17.490
      injury NEC T17.408
        food (bone) (seed) T17.428
        gastric contents (vomitus) T17.418
        specified type NEC T17.498
  type of fragment —*see* Retained, foreign body fragments (type of)
  vitreous (humor) S05.5-
Forestier's disease (rhizomelic pseudopolyarthritis) M35.3-
  meaning ankylosing hyperostosis —*see* Hyperostosis, ankylosing
Formation
  hyalin in cornea —*see* Degeneration, cornea
  sequestrum in bone (due to infection) —*see* Osteomyelitis, chronic
  valve
    colon, congenital Q43.8
    ureter (congenital) Q62.39
Formication R20.2
Fort Bragg fever A27.89
Fossa —*see also* condition
  pyriform —*see* condition
Foster-Kennedy syndrome H47.14-
Fothergill's
  disease (trigeminal neuralgia) —*see also* Neuralgia, trigeminal
  scarlatina anginosa A38.9
Foul breath R19.6
Foundling Z76.1
Fournier disease or gangrene N49.3
  female N76.89
Fourth
  cranial nerve —*see* condition
  molar K00.1
Foville's (peduncular) disease or syndrome G46.3
Fox (-Fordyce) disease (apocrine miliaria) L75.2
Fracture, burst —*see* Fracture, traumatic, by site
Fracture, chronic —*see* Fracture, pathological
Fracture, insufficiency —*see* Fracture, pathologic, by site
Fracture, nontraumatic, NEC ◄
  atypical ◄
    femur M84.750- ◄
      complete ◄
        oblique M84.759 ◄
          left side M84.758 ◄
          right side M84.757 ◄

Fracture, nontraumatic *(Continued)*
  atypical *(Continued)*
    femur *(Continued)*
      complete *(Continued)*
        transverse M84.756 ◄
          left side M84.755 ◄
          right side M84.754 ◄
      incomplete M84.753 ◄
        left side M84.752 ◄
        right side M84.751 ◄
Fracture, pathological (pathologic) —*see also* Fracture, traumatic M84.40
  ankle M84.47-
  carpus M84.44-
  clavicle M84.41-
  compression (not due to trauma) —*see also* Collapse, vertebra M48.50- ◄
  dental implant M27.63
  dental restorative material K08.539
    with loss of material K08.531
    without loss of material K08.530
  due to
    neoplastic disease NEC —*see also* Neoplasm M84.50
      ankle M84.57-
      carpus M84.54-
      clavicle M84.51-
      femur M84.55-
      fibula M84.56-
      finger M84.54-
      hip M84.559
      humerus M84.52-
      ilium M84.550
      ischium M84.550
      metacarpus M84.54-
      metatarsus M84.57-
      neck M84.58
      pelvis M84.550
      radius M84.53-
      rib M84.58
      scapula M84.51-
      skull M84.58
      specified site NEC M84.58
      tarsus M84.57-
      tibia M84.56-
      toe M84.57-
      ulna M84.53-
      vertebra M84.58
    osteoporosis M80.00 ◄▥
      disuse —*see* Osteoporosis, specified type NEC, with pathological fracture
      drug-induced —*see* Osteoporosis, drug induced, with pathological fracture
      idiopathic —*see* Osteoporosis, specified type NEC, with pathological fracture
      postmenopausal —*see* Osteoporosis, postmenopausal, with pathological fracture
      postoophorectomy —*see* Osteoporosis, postoophorectomy, with pathological fracture
      postsurgical malabsorption —*see* Osteoporosis, specified type NEC, with pathological fracture
      specified cause NEC —*see* Osteoporosis, specified type NEC, with pathological fracture
    specified disease NEC M84.60
      ankle M84.67-
      carpus M84.64-
      clavicle M84.61-
      femur M84.65-
      fibula M84.66-
      finger M84.64-
      hip M84.65-
      humerus M84.62-
      ilium M84.650
      ischium M84.650
      metacarpus M84.64-
      metatarsus M84.67-

Fracture, pathological (Continued)
  due to (Continued)
    specified disease NEC (Continued)
      neck M84.68
      radius M84.63-
      rib M84.68
      scapula M84.61-
      skull M84.68
      tarsus M84.67-
      tibia M84.66-
      toe M84.67-
      ulna M84.63-
      vertebra M84.68
    femur M84.45-
    fibula M84.46-
    finger M84.44-
    hip M84.459
    humerus M84.42-
    ilium M84.454
    ischium M84.454
    joint prosthesis —see Complications, joint
      prosthesis, mechanical, breakdown, by
      site
    periprosthetic —see Fracture, pathological,
      periprosthetic ◀▥
    metacarpus M84.44-
    metatarsus M84.47-
    neck M84.48
    pelvis M84.454
    periprosthetic M97.9 ◀
      ankle M97.2- ◀
      elbow M97.4- ◀
      finger M97.8 ◀
      hip M97.0- ◀
      knee M97.1- ◀
      other specified joint M97.8 ◀
      shoulder M97.3- ◀
      spinal joint M97.8 ◀
      toe joint M97.8 ◀
      wrist joint M97.8 ◀
    radius M84.43-
    restorative material (dental) K08.539
      with loss of material K08.531
      without loss of material K08.530
    rib M84.48
    scapula M84.41-
    skull M84.48
    tarsus M84.47-
    tibia M84.46-
    toe M84.47-
    ulna M84.43-
    vertebra M84.48
Fracture, traumatic (abduction) (adduction)
  (separation) —see also Fracture,
  pathological T14.8
  acetabulum S32.40-
    column
      anterior (displaced) (iliopubic)
        S32.43-
        nondisplaced S32.436
      posterior (displaced) (ilioischial)
        S32.443
        nondisplaced S32.44-
    dome (displaced) S32.48-
      nondisplaced S32.48
    specified NEC S32.49-
    transverse (displaced) S32.45-
      with associated posterior wall fracture
        (displaced) S32.46-
        nondisplaced S32.46-
      nondisplaced S32.45-
    wall
      anterior (displaced) S32.41-
        nondisplaced S32.41-
      medial (displaced) S32.47-
        nondisplaced S32.47-
      posterior (displaced) S32.42-
        with associated transverse fracture
          (displaced) S32.46-
          nondisplaced S32.46-
        nondisplaced S32.42-

Fracture, traumatic (Continued)
  acromion —see Fracture, scapula, acromial
    process
  ankle S82.899
    bimalleolar (displaced) S82.84-
      nondisplaced S82.84-
    lateral malleolus only (displaced) S82.6-
      nondisplaced S82.6-
    medial malleolus (displaced) S82.5-
      associated with Maisonneuve's
        fracture —see Fracture,
        Maisonneuve's
      nondisplaced S82.5-
    talus —see Fracture, tarsal, talus
    trimalleolar (displaced) S82.85-
      nondisplaced S82.85-
  arm (upper) —see also Fracture, humerus,
    shaft
    humerus —see Fracture, humerus
    radius —see Fracture, radius
    ulna —see Fracture, ulna
  astragalus —see Fracture, tarsal, talus
  atlas —see Fracture, neck, cervical vertebra,
    first
  axis —see Fracture, neck, cervical vertebra,
    second
  back —see Fracture, vertebra
  Barton's —see Barton's fracture
  base of skull —see Fracture, skull, base
  basicervical (basal) (femoral) S72.0
  Bennett's —see Bennett's fracture
  bimalleolar —see Fracture, ankle,
    bimalleolar
  blow-out S02.3- ◀▥
  bone NEC T14.8
    birth injury P13.9
    following insertion of orthopedic implant,
      joint prosthesis or bone plate —see
      Fracture, following insertion of
      orthopedic implant, joint prosthesis
      or bone plate
    in (due to) neoplastic disease NEC —see
      Fracture, pathological, due to,
      neoplastic disease
    pathological (cause unknown) —see
      Fracture, pathological
  breast bone —see Fracture, sternum
  bucket handle (semilunar cartilage) —see
    Tear, meniscus
  burst —see Fracture, traumatic, by site
  calcaneus —see Fracture, tarsal, calcaneus
  carpal bone (s) S62.10-
    capitate (displaced) S62.13-
      nondisplaced S62.13-
    cuneiform —see Fracture, carpal bone,
      triquetrum
    hamate (body) (displaced) S62.143
      hook process (displaced) S62.15-
        nondisplaced S62.15-
      nondisplaced S62.14-
    larger multangular —see Fracture, carpal
      bones, trapezium
    lunate (displaced) S62.12-
      nondisplaced S62.12-
    navicular S62.00-
      distal pole (displaced) S62.01-
        nondisplaced S62.01-
      middle third (displaced) S62.02-
        nondisplaced S62.02-
      proximal third (displaced) S62.03-
        nondisplaced S62.03-
      volar tuberosity —see Fracture, carpal
        bones, navicular, distal pole
    os magnum —see Fracture, carpal bones,
      capitate
    pisiform (displaced) S62.16-
      nondisplaced S62.16-
    semilunar —see Fracture, carpal bones,
      lunate
    smaller multangular —see Fracture, carpal
      bones, trapezoid

Fracture, traumatic (Continued)
  carpal bone (s) (Continued)
    trapezium (displaced) S62.17-
      nondisplaced S62.17-
    trapezoid (displaced) S62.18-
      nondisplaced S62.18-
    triquetrum (displaced) S62.11-
      nondisplaced S62.11-
    unciform —see Fracture, carpal bones,
      hamate
  cervical —see Fracture, vertebra, cervical
  clavicle S42.00-
    acromial end (displaced) S42.03-
      nondisplaced S42.03-
    birth injury P13.4
    lateral end —see Fracture, clavicle, acromial
      end
    shaft (displaced) S42.02-
      nondisplaced S42.02-
    sternal end (anterior) (displaced) S42.01-
      nondisplaced S42.01-
      posterior S42.01-
  coccyx S32.2
  collapsed —see Collapse, vertebra
  collar bone —see Fracture, clavicle
  Colles' —see Colles' fracture
  ~~compression, not due to trauma —see~~
    ~~Collapse, vertebra~~
  coronoid process —see Fracture, ulna, upper
    end, coronoid process
  corpus cavernosum penis S39.840
  costochondral cartilage S23.41
  costochondral, costosternal junction —see
    Fracture, rib
  cranium —see Fracture, skull
  cricoid cartilage S12.8
  cuboid (ankle) —see Fracture, tarsal, cuboid
  cuneiform
    foot —see Fracture, tarsal, cuneiform
    wrist —see Fracture, carpal, triquetrum
  delayed union —see Delay, union, fracture
  dental restorative material K08.539
    with loss of material K08.531
    without loss of material K08.530
  due to
    birth injury —see Birth, injury, fracture
    osteoporosis —see Osteoporosis, with
      fracture
  Dupuytren's —see Fracture, ankle, lateral
    malleolus
  elbow S42.40-
  ethmoid (bone) (sinus) —see Fracture, skull,
    base
  face bone S02.92
  fatigue —see also Fracture, stress
    vertebra M48.40
      cervical region M48.42
      cervicothoracic region M48.43
      lumbar region M48.46
      lumbosacral region M48.47
      occipito-atlanto-axial region M48.41
      sacrococcygeal region M48.48
      thoracic region M48.44
      thoracolumbar region M48.45
  femur, femoral S72.9-
    basicervical (basal) S72.0
    birth injury P13.2
    capital epiphyseal S79.01-
    condyles, epicondyles —see Fracture,
      femur, lower end
    distal end —see Fracture, femur,
      lower end
    epiphysis
      head —see Fracture, femur, upper end,
        epiphysis
      lower —see Fracture, femur, lower end,
        epiphysis
      upper —see Fracture, femur, upper end,
        epiphysis
    following insertion of implant, prosthesis
      or plate M96.66-

◀ New   ◀▥ Revised   ~~deleted~~ Deleted

Fracture, traumatic *(Continued)*
femur, femoral *(Continued)*
  head —*see* Fracture, femur, upper end,
    head
  intertrochanteric —*see* Fracture, femur,
    trochanteric
  intratrochanteric —*see* Fracture, femur,
    trochanteric
  lower end S72.40-
    condyle (displaced) S72.41-
      lateral (displaced) S72.42-
        nondisplaced S72.42-
      medial (displaced) S72.43-
        nondisplaced S72.43-
      nondisplaced S72.41-
    epiphysis (displaced) S72.44-
      nondisplaced S72.44-
    physeal S79.10-
      Salter-Harris
        Type I S79.11-
        Type II S79.12-
        Type III S79.13-
        Type IV S79.14-
        specified NEC S79.19-
    specified NEC S72.49-
    supracondylar (displaced) S72.45-
      with intracondylar extension
        (displaced) S72.46-
        nondisplaced S72.46-
      nondisplaced S72.45-
    torus S72.47-
  neck —*see* Fracture, femur, upper end, neck
  pertrochanteric —*see* Fracture, femur,
    trochanteric
  shaft (lower third) (middle third) (upper
    third) S72.30-
    comminuted (displaced) S72.35-
      nondisplaced S72.35-
    oblique (displaced) S72.33-
      nondisplaced S72.33-
    segmental (displaced) S72.36-
      nondisplaced S72.36-
    specified NEC S72.39-
    spiral (displaced) S72.34-
      nondisplaced S72.34-
    transverse (displaced) S72.32-
      nondisplaced S72.32-
  specified site NEC —*see* subcategory S72.8
  subcapital (displaced) S72.01-
  subtrochanteric (region) (section)
    (displaced) S72.2-
    nondisplaced S72.2-
  transcervical —*see* Fracture, femur, upper
    end, neck
  transtrochanteric —*see* Fracture, femur,
    trochanteric
  trochanteric S72.10-
    apophyseal (displaced) S72.13-
      nondisplaced S72.13-
    greater trochanter (displaced) S72.11-
      nondisplaced S72.11-
    intertrochanteric (displaced) S72.14-
      nondisplaced S72.14-
    lesser trochanter (displaced) S72.12-
      nondisplaced S72.12-
  upper end S72.00-
    apophyseal (displaced) S72.13-
      nondisplaced S72.13-
    cervicotrochanteric —*see* Fracture,
      femur, upper end, neck, base
    epiphysis (displaced) S72.02-
      nondisplaced S72.02-
    head S72.05-
      articular (displaced) S72.06-
        nondisplaced S72.06-
      specified NEC S72.09-
    intertrochanteric (displaced) S72.14-
      nondisplaced S72.14-
    intracapsular S72.01-
    midcervical (displaced) S72.03-
      nondisplaced S72.03-

Fracture, traumatic *(Continued)*
femur, femoral *(Continued)*
  upper end *(Continued)*
    neck S72.00-
      base (displaced) S72.04-
        nondisplaced S72.04-
      specified NEC S72.09-
    pertrochanteric —*see* Fracture, femur,
      upper end, trochanteric
    physeal S79.00-
      Salter-Harris type I S79.01-
      specified NEC S79.09-
    subcapital (displaced) S72.01-
    subtrochanteric (displaced) S72.2-
      nondisplaced S72.2-
    transcervical —*see* Fracture, femur,
      upper end, midcervical
    trochanteric S72.10-
      greater (displaced) S72.11-
        nondisplaced S72.11-
      lesser (displaced) S72.12-
        nondisplaced S72.12-
fibula (shaft) (styloid) S82.40-
  comminuted (displaced) S82.45-
    nondisplaced S82.45-
  following insertion of implant, prosthesis
    or plate M96.67-
  involving ankle or malleolus —*see*
    Fracture, fibula, lateral malleolus
  lateral malleolus (displaced)
    S82.6-
    nondisplaced S82.6-
  lower end
    physeal S89.30-
      Salter-Harris
        Type I S89.31-
        Type II S89.32-
        specified NEC S89.39-
    specified NEC S82.83-
    torus S82.82-
  oblique (displaced) S82.43-
    nondisplaced S82.43-
  segmental (displaced) S82.46-
    nondisplaced S82.46-
  specified NEC S82.49-
  spiral (displaced) S82.44-
    nondisplaced S82.44-
  transverse (displaced) S82.42-
    nondisplaced S82.42-
  upper end
    physeal S89.20-
      Salter-Harris
        Type I S89.21-
        Type II S89.22-
        specified NEC S89.29-
    specified NEC S82.83-
    torus S82.81-
finger (except thumb) S62.60-
  distal phalanx (displaced) S62.63-
    nondisplaced S62.66-
  index S62.60-
    distal phalanx (displaced) S62.63-
      nondisplaced S62.66-
    medial phalanx (displaced) S62.62-
      nondisplaced S62.65-
    proximal phalanx (displaced) S62.61-
      nondisplaced S62.64-
  little S62.60-
    distal phalanx (displaced) S62.63-
      nondisplaced S62.66-
    medial phalanx (displaced) S62.62-
      nondisplaced S62.65-
    proximal phalanx (displaced) S62.61-
      nondisplaced S62.64-
  medial phalanx (displaced) S62.62-
    nondisplaced S62.65-
  middle S62.60-
    distal phalanx (displaced) S62.63-
      nondisplaced S62.66-
    medial phalanx (displaced) S62.62-
      nondisplaced S62.65-

Fracture, traumatic *(Continued)*
finger *(Continued)*
  middle *(Continued)*
    proximal phalanx (displaced) S62.61-
      nondisplaced S62.64-
    proximal phalanx (displaced) S62.61-
      nondisplaced S62.64-
  ring S62.60-
    distal phalanx (displaced) S62.63-
      nondisplaced S62.66-
    medial phalanx (displaced) S62.62-
      nondisplaced S62.65-
    proximal phalanx (displaced) S62.61-
      nondisplaced S62.64-
  thumb —*see* Fracture, thumb
following insertion (intraoperative)
  (postoperative) of orthopedic implant,
  joint prosthesis or bone plate M96.69
  femur M96.66-
  fibula M96.67-
  humerus M96.62-
  pelvis M96.65
  radius M96.63-
  specified bone NEC M96.69
  tibia M96.67-
  ulna M96.63-
foot S92.90-
  astragalus —*see* Fracture, tarsal, talus
  calcaneus —*see* Fracture, tarsal, calcaneus
  cuboid —*see* Fracture, tarsal, cuboid
  cuneiform —*see* Fracture, tarsal, cuneiform
  metatarsal —*see* Fracture, metatarsal
  navicular —*see* Fracture, tarsal, navicular
  sesamoid S92.81- ◀
  specified NEC S92.81- ◀
  talus —*see* Fracture, tarsal, talus
  tarsal —*see* Fracture, tarsal
  toe —*see* Fracture, toe
forearm S52.9-
  radius —*see* Fracture, radius
  ulna —*see* Fracture, ulna
fossa (anterior) (middle) (posterior) S02.19
frontal (bone) (skull) S02.0
  sinus S02.19
glenoid (cavity) (scapula) —*see* Fracture,
  scapula, glenoid cavity
greenstick —*see* Fracture, by site
hallux —*see* Fracture, toe, great
hand S62.9-
  carpal —*see* Fracture, carpal bone
  finger (except thumb) —*see* Fracture, finger
  metacarpal —*see* Fracture, metacarpal
  navicular (scaphoid) (hand) —*see* Fracture,
    carpal bone, navicular
  thumb —*see* Fracture, thumb
healed or old
  with complications - code by Nature of the
    complication
heel bone —*see* Fracture, tarsal, calcaneus
Hill-Sachs S42.29-
hip —*see* Fracture, femur, neck
humerus S42.30-
  anatomical neck —*see* Fracture, humerus,
    upper end
  articular process —*see* Fracture, humerus,
    lower end
  capitellum —*see* Fracture, humerus, lower
    end, condyle, lateral
  distal end —*see* Fracture, humerus, lower
    end
  epiphysis
    lower —*see* Fracture, humerus, lower
      end, physeal
    upper —*see* Fracture, humerus, upper
      end, physeal
  external condyle —*see* Fracture, humerus,
    lower end, condyle, lateral
  following insertion of implant, prosthesis
    or plate M96.62-
  great tuberosity —*see* Fracture, humerus,
    upper end, greater tuberosity

Fracture, traumatic *(Continued)*
  humerus *(Continued)*
    intercondylar —*see* Fracture, humerus, lower end
    internal epicondyle —*see* Fracture, humerus, lower end, epicondyle, medial
    lesser tuberosity —*see* Fracture, humerus, upper end, lesser tuberosity
    lower end S42.40-
      condyle
        lateral (displaced) S42.45-
          nondisplaced S42.45-
        medial (displaced) S42.46-
          nondisplaced S42.46-
      epicondyle
        lateral (displaced) S42.43-
          nondisplaced S42.43-
        medial (displaced) S42.44-
          incarcerated S42.44-
          nondisplaced S42.44-
      physeal S49.10-
        Salter-Harris
          Type I S49.11-
          Type II S49.12-
          Type III S49.13-
          Type IV S49.14-
        specified NEC S49.19-
      specified NEC (displaced) S42.49-
        nondisplaced S42.49-
      supracondylar (simple) (displaced) S42.41-
        with intercondylar fracture —*see* Fracture, humerus, lower end ◄
        comminuted (displaced) S42.42-
          nondisplaced S42.42-
        nondisplaced S42.41-
      torus S42.48-
      transcondylar (displaced) S42.47-
        nondisplaced S42.47-
    proximal end —*see* Fracture, humerus, upper end
    shaft S42.30-
      comminuted (displaced) S42.35-
        nondisplaced S42.35-
      greenstick S42.31-
      oblique (displaced) S42.33-
        nondisplaced S42.33-
      segmental (displaced) S42.36-
        nondisplaced S42.36-
      specified NEC S42.39-
      spiral (displaced) S42.34-
        nondisplaced S42.34-
      transverse (displaced) S42.32-
        nondisplaced S42.32-
    supracondylar —*see* Fracture, humerus, lower end
    surgical neck —*see* Fracture, humerus, upper end, surgical neck
    trochlea —*see* Fracture, humerus, lower end, condyle, medial
    tuberosity —*see* Fracture, humerus, upper end
    upper end S42.20-
      anatomical neck —*see* Fracture, humerus, upper end, specified NEC
      articular head —*see* Fracture, humerus, upper end, specified NEC
      epiphysis —*see* Fracture, humerus, upper end, physeal
      greater tuberosity (displaced) S42.25-
        nondisplaced S42.25-
      lesser tuberosity (displaced) S42.26-
        nondisplaced S42.26-
      physeal S49.00-
        Salter-Harris
          Type I S49.01-
          Type II S49.02-
          Type III S49.03-
          Type IV S49.04-
        specified NEC S49.09-

Fracture, traumatic *(Continued)*
  humerus *(Continued)*
    upper end *(Continued)*
      specified NEC (displaced) S42.29-
        nondisplaced S42.29-
      surgical neck (displaced) S42.21-
        four-part S42.24-
        nondisplaced S42.21-
        three-part S42.23-
        two-part (displaced) S42.22-
          nondisplaced S42.22-
      torus S42.27-
      transepiphyseal —*see* Fracture, humerus, upper end, physeal
  hyoid bone S12.8
  ilium S32.30-
    with disruption of pelvic ring —*see* Disruption, pelvic ring
    avulsion (displaced) S32.31-
      nondisplaced S32.31-
    specified NEC S32.39-
  impaction, impacted - code as Fracture, by site
  innominate bone —*see* Fracture, ilium
  instep —*see* Fracture, foot
  ischium S32.60-
    with disruption of pelvic ring —*see* Disruption, pelvic ring
    avulsion (displaced) S32.61-
      nondisplaced S32.61-
    specified NEC S32.69-
  jaw (bone) (lower) —*see* Fracture, mandible
    upper —*see* Fracture, maxilla
  joint prosthesis —*see* Complications, joint prosthesis, mechanical, breakdown, by site
    periprosthetic —*see* Fracture, traumatic, periprosthetic ◄▥
  knee cap —*see* Fracture, patella
  larynx S12.8
  late effects —*see* Sequelae, fracture
  leg (lower) S82.9-
    ankle —*see* Fracture, ankle
    femur —*see* Fracture, femur
    fibula —*see* Fracture, fibula
    malleolus —*see* Fracture, ankle
    patella —*see* Fracture, patella
    specified site NEC S82.89-
    tibia —*see* Fracture, tibia
  lumbar spine —*see* Fracture, vertebra, lumbar
  lumbosacral spine S32.9
  Maisonneuve's (displaced) S82.86-
    nondisplaced S82.86-
  malar bone —*see also* Fracture, maxilla S02.400
    left side S02.40B ◄
    right side S02.40A ◄
  malleolus —*see* Fracture, ankle
  malunion —*see* Fracture, by site
  mandible (lower jawbone) S02.609
    alveolus S02.67- ◄▥
    angle (of jaw) S02.65- ◄▥
    body, unspecified S02.600-
      left side S02.602 ◄
      right side S02.601 ◄
    condylar process S02.61- ◄▥
    coronoid process S02.63- ◄▥
    ramus, unspecified S02.64- ◄▥
    specified site NEC S02.69
    subcondylar process S02.62- ◄▥
    symphysis S02.66
  manubrium (sterni) S22.21
    dissociation from sternum S22.23
  march —*see* Fracture, traumatic, stress, by site
  maxilla, maxillary (bone) (sinus) (superior) (upper jaw) S02.401
    alveolus S02.42
    inferior —*see* Fracture, mandible
    LeFort I S02.411
    LeFort II S02.412
    LeFort III S02.413

Fracture, traumatic *(Continued)*
  maxilla, maxillary *(Continued)*
    left side S02.40D ◄
    right side S02.40C ◄
  metacarpal S62.309
    base (displaced) S62.319
      nondisplaced S62.349
    fifth S62.30-
      base (displaced) S62.31-
        nondisplaced S62.34-
      neck (displaced) S62.33-
        nondisplaced S62.36-
      shaft (displaced) S62.32-
        nondisplaced S62.35-
      specified NEC S62.398
    first S62.20-
      base NEC (displaced) S62.23-
        nondisplaced S62.23-
      Bennett's —*see* Bennett's fracture
      neck (displaced) S62.25-
        nondisplaced S62.25-
      shaft (displaced) S62.24-
        nondisplaced S62.24-
      specified NEC S62.29-
    fourth S62.30-
      base (displaced) S62.31-
        nondisplaced S62.34-
      neck (displaced) S62.33-
        nondisplaced S62.36-
      shaft (displaced) S62.32-
        nondisplaced S62.35-
      specified NEC S62.39-
    neck (displaced) S62.33-
      nondisplaced S62.36-
    Rolando's —*see* Rolando's fracture
    second S62.30-
      base (displaced) S62.31-
        nondisplaced S62.34-
      neck (displaced) S62.33-
        nondisplaced S62.36-
      shaft (displaced) S62.32-
        nondisplaced S62.35-
      specified NEC S62.39-
    shaft (displaced) S62.32-
      nondisplaced S62.35-
    specified NEC S62.399
    third S62.30-
      base (displaced) S62.31-
        nondisplaced S62.34-
      neck (displaced) S62.33-
        nondisplaced S62.36-
      shaft (displaced) S62.32-
        nondisplaced S62.35-
      specified NEC S62.39-
  metastatic —*see* Fracture, pathological, due to, neoplastic disease —*see also* Neoplasm
  metatarsal bone S92.30-
    fifth (displaced) S92.35-
      nondisplaced S92.35-
    first (displaced) S92.31-
      nondisplaced S92.31-
    fourth (displaced) S92.34-
      nondisplaced S92.34-
    physeal S99.10- ◄
      Salter-Harris ◄
        Type I S99.11- ◄
        Type II S99.12- ◄
        Type III S99.13- ◄
        Type IV S99.14- ◄
      specified NEC S99.19- ◄
    second (displaced) S92.32-
      nondisplaced S92.32-
    third (displaced) S92.33-
      nondisplaced S92.33-
  Monteggia's —*see* Monteggia's fracture
  multiple
    hand (and wrist) NEC —*see* Fracture, by site
    ribs —*see* Fracture, rib, multiple

◄ New   ◄▥ Revised   ~~deleted~~ Deleted

Fracture, traumatic (Continued)
  nasal (bone (s)) S02.2
  navicular (scaphoid) (foot) —see also Fracture,
    tarsal, navicular
    hand —see Fracture, carpal, navicular
  neck S12.9
    cervical vertebra S12.9
      fifth (displaced) S12.400
        nondisplaced S12.401
        specified type NEC (displaced) S12.490
          nondisplaced S12.491
      first (displaced) S12.000
        burst (stable) S12.01
          unstable S12.02
        lateral mass (displaced) S12.040
          nondisplaced S12.041
        nondisplaced S12.001
        posterior arch (displaced) S12.030
          nondisplaced S12.031
        specified type NEC (displaced) S12.090
          nondisplaced S12.091
      fourth (displaced) S12.300
        nondisplaced S12.301
        specified type NEC (displaced) S12.390
          nondisplaced S12.391
      second (displaced) S12.100
        dens (anterior) (displaced) (type II)
          S12.110
          nondisplaced S12.112
          posterior S12.111
          specified type NEC (displaced)
            S12.120
            nondisplaced S12.121
        nondisplaced S12.101
        specified type NEC (displaced)
          S12.190
          nondisplaced S12.191
      seventh (displaced) S12.600
        nondisplaced S12.601
        specified type NEC (displaced)
          S12.690
          ~~displaced S12.691~~
          nondisplaced S12.691 ◀
      sixth (displaced) S12.500
        nondisplaced S12.501
        specified type NEC (displaced)
          S12.590
          ~~displaced S12.591~~
          nondisplaced S12.591 ◀
      third (displaced) S12.200
        nondisplaced S12.201
        specified type NEC (displaced)
          S12.290
          ~~displaced S12.291~~
          nondisplaced S12.291 ◀
  hyoid bone S12.8
  larynx S12.8
  specified site NEC S12.8
  thyroid cartilage S12.8
  trachea S12.8
  neoplastic NEC —see Fracture, pathological,
    due to, neoplastic disease
  neural arch —see Fracture, vertebra
  newborn —see Birth, injury, fracture
  nontraumatic —see Fracture, pathological
  nonunion —see Nonunion, fracture
  nose, nasal (bone) (septum) S02.2
  occiput —see Fracture, skull, base, occiput
  odontoid process —see Fracture, neck,
    cervical vertebra, second
  olecranon (process) (ulna) —see Fracture,
    ulna, upper end, olecranon process
  orbit, orbital (bone) (region) S02.8- ◀▥
    floor (blow-out) S02.3- ◀▥
    roof S02.19
  os
    calcis —see Fracture, tarsal, calcaneus
    magnum —see Fracture, carpal, capitate
    pubis —see Fracture, pubis
  palate S02.8- ◀▥
  parietal bone (skull) S02.0

Fracture, traumatic (Continued)
  patella S82.00-
    comminuted (displaced) S82.04-
      nondisplaced S82.04-
    longitudinal (displaced) S82.02-
      nondisplaced S82.02-
    osteochondral (displaced) S82.01-
      nondisplaced S82.01-
    specified NEC S82.09-
    transverse (displaced) S82.03-
      nondisplaced S82.03-
  pedicle (of vertebral arch) —see Fracture,
    vertebra
  pelvis, pelvic (bone) S32.9
    acetabulum —see Fracture, acetabulum
    circle —see Disruption, pelvic ring
    following insertion of implant, prosthesis
      or plate M96.65
    ilium —see Fracture, ilium
    ischium —see Fracture, ischium
    multiple
      with disruption of pelvic ring (circle) —
        see Disruption, pelvic ring
      without disruption of pelvic ring (circle)
        S32.82
    pubis —see Fracture, pubis
    sacrum —see Fracture, sacrum
    specified site NEC S32.89
  periprosthetic, around internal prosthetic
    joint M97.9 ◀
    ankle M97.2- ◀
    elbow M97.4- ◀
    finger M97.8- ◀
    hip M97.0- ◀
    knee M97.1-- ◀
    shoulder M97.3- ◀
    specified joint NEC M97.8 ◀
    spine M97.8 ◀
    toe M97.8 ◀
    wrist M97.8 ◀
  phalanx
    foot —see Fracture, toe
    hand —see Fracture, finger
  pisiform —see Fracture, carpal, pisiform
  pond —see Fracture, skull
  prosthetic device, internal —see
    Complications, prosthetic device, by
    site, mechanical
  pubis S32.50-
    with disruption of pelvic ring —see
      Disruption, pelvic ring
    specified site NEC S32.59-
    superior rim S32.59-
  radius S52.9-
    distal end —see Fracture, radius,
      lower end
    following insertion of implant, prosthesis
      or plate M96.63-
    head —see Fracture, radius, upper end,
      head
    lower end S52.50-
      Barton's —see Barton's fracture
      Colles' —see Colles' fracture
      extraarticular NEC S52.55-
      intraarticular NEC S52.57-
      physeal S59.20-
        Salter-Harris
          Type I S59.21-
          Type II S59.22-
          Type III S59.23-
          Type IV S59.24-
        specified NEC S59.29-
      Smith's —see Smith's fracture
      specified NEC S52.59-
      styloid process (displaced)
        S52.51-
        nondisplaced S52.51-
      torus S52.52-
    neck —see Fracture, radius, upper end
    proximal end —see Fracture, radius, upper
      end

Fracture, traumatic (Continued)
  radius (Continued)
    shaft S52.30-
      bent bone S52.38-
      comminuted (displaced) S52.35-
        nondisplaced S52.35-
      Galeazzi's —see Galeazzi's fracture
      greenstick S52.31-
      oblique (displaced) S52.33-
        nondisplaced S52.33-
      segmental (displaced) S52.36-
        nondisplaced S52.36-
      specified NEC S52.39-
      spiral (displaced) S52.34-
        nondisplaced S52.34-
      transverse (displaced) S52.32-
        nondisplaced S52.32-
    upper end S52.10-
      head (displaced) S52.12-
        nondisplaced S52.12-
      neck (displaced) S52.13-
        nondisplaced S52.13-
      physeal S59.10-
        Salter-Harris
          Type I S59.11-
          Type II S59.12-
          Type III S59.13-
          Type IV S59.14-
        specified NEC S59.19-
      specified NEC S52.18-
      torus S52.11-
  ramus
    inferior or superior, pubis —see Fracture,
      pubis
    mandible —see Fracture, mandible
  restorative material (dental) K08.539
    with loss of material K08.531
    without loss of material K08.530
  rib S22.3-
    with flail chest —see Flail, chest
    multiple S22.4-
      with flail chest —see Flail, chest
  root, tooth —see Fracture, tooth
  sacrum S32.10
    specified NEC S32.19
    Type
      1 S32.14
      2 S32.15
      3 S32.16
      4 S32.17
    Zone
      I S32.119
        displaced (minimally) S32.111
          severely S32.112
        nondisplaced S32.110
      II S32.129
        displaced (minimally) S32.121
          severely S32.122
        nondisplaced S32.120
      III S32.139
        displaced (minimally) S32.131
          severely S32.132
        nondisplaced S32.130
  scaphoid (hand) —see also Fracture, carpal,
    navicular
    foot —see Fracture, tarsal, navicular
  scapula S42.10-
    acromial process (displaced) S42.12-
      nondisplaced S42.12-
    body (displaced) S42.11-
      nondisplaced S42.11-
    coracoid process (displaced) S42.13-
      nondisplaced S42.13-
    glenoid cavity (displaced) S42.14-
      nondisplaced S42.14-
    neck (displaced) S42.15-
      nondisplaced S42.15-
    specified NEC S42.19-
  semilunar bone, wrist —see Fracture, carpal,
    lunate
  sequelae —see Sequelae, fracture

Fracture, traumatic *(Continued)*
  sesamoid bone
    foot S92.81- ◄
    hand —*see* Fracture, carpal
    other —*see* Fracture, traumatic, by site ◄
    other - code by site under Fracture
  shepherd's —*see* Fracture, tarsal, talus
  shoulder (girdle) S42.9-
    blade —*see* Fracture, scapula
  sinus (ethmoid) (frontal) S02.19
  skull S02.91
    base S02.10- ◄▥
      occiput S02.119
        condyle S02.113
          type I S02.110
            left side S02.11B ◄
            right side S02.11A ◄
          type II S02.111
            left side S02.11D ◄
            right side S02.11C ◄
          type III S02.112
            left side S02.11F ◄
            right side S02.11E ◄
          specified NEC S02.118 ◄
            left side S02.11H ◄
            right side S02.11G ◄
          specified NEC S02.118
      specified NEC S02.19- ◄▥
    birth injury P13.0
    frontal bone S02.0
    parietal bone S02.0
    specified site NEC S02.8
    temporal bone S02.19
    vault S02.0
  Smith's —*see* Smith's fracture
  sphenoid (bone) (sinus) S02.19
  spine —*see* Fracture, vertebra
  spinous process —*see* Fracture, vertebra
  spontaneous (cause unknown) —*see* Fracture,
    pathological
  stave (of thumb) —*see* Fracture, metacarpal,
    first
  sternum S22.20
    with flail chest —*see* Flail, chest
    body S22.22
    manubrium S22.21
    xiphoid (process) S22.24
  stress M84.30
    ankle M84.37-
    carpus M84.34-
    clavicle M84.31-
    femoral neck M84.359
    femur M84.35-
    fibula M84.36-
    finger M84.34-
    hip M84.359
    humerus M84.32-
    ilium M84.350
    ischium M84.350
    metacarpus M84.34-
    metatarsus M84.37-
    neck —*see* Fracture, fatigue, vertebra
    pelvis M84.350
    radius M84.33-
    rib M84.38
    scapula M84.31-
    skull M84.38
    tarsus M84.37-
    tibia M84.36-
    toe M84.37-
    ulna M84.33-
    vertebra —*see* Fracture, fatigue, vertebra
  supracondylar, elbow —*see* Fracture,
    humerus, lower end, supracondylar
  symphysis pubis —*see* Fracture, pubis
  talus (ankle bone) —*see* Fracture, tarsal, talus
  tarsal bone (s) S92.20-
    astragalus —*see* Fracture, tarsal, talus
    calcaneus S92.00-
      anterior process (displaced) S92.02-
        nondisplaced S92.02-

Fracture, traumatic *(Continued)*
  tarsal bone *(Continued)*
    calcaneus *(Continued)*
      body (displaced) S92.01-
        nondisplaced S92.01-
      extraarticular NEC (displaced) S92.05-
        nondisplaced S92.05-
      intraarticular (displaced) S92.06-
        nondisplaced S92.06-
      physeal S99.00- ◄
        Salter-Harris ◄
          Type I S99.01- ◄
          Type II S99.02- ◄
          Type III S99.03- ◄
          Type IV S99.04- ◄
        specified NEC S99.09- ◄
      tuberosity (displaced) S92.04-
        avulsion (displaced) S92.03-
          nondisplaced S92.03-
        nondisplaced S92.04-
    cuboid (displaced) S92.21-
      nondisplaced S92.21-
    cuneiform
      intermediate (displaced) S92.23-
        nondisplaced S92.23-
      lateral (displaced) S92.22-
        nondisplaced S92.22-
      medial (displaced) S92.24-
        nondisplaced S92.24-
    navicular (displaced) S92.25-
      nondisplaced S92.25-
    scaphoid —*see* Fracture, tarsal, navicular
    talus S92.10-
      avulsion (displaced) S92.15-
        nondisplaced S92.15-
      body (displaced) S92.12-
        nondisplaced S92.12-
      dome (displaced) S92.14-
        nondisplaced S92.14-
      head (displaced) S92.12-
        nondisplaced S92.12-
      lateral process (displaced) S92.14-
        nondisplaced S92.14-
      neck (displaced) S92.11-
        nondisplaced S92.11-
      posterior process (displaced) S92.13-
        nondisplaced S92.13-
      specified NEC S92.19-
  temporal bone (styloid) S02.19
  thorax (bony) S22.9
    with flail chest —*see* Flail, chest
    rib S22.3-
      multiple S22.4-
        with flail chest —*see* Flail, chest
    sternum S22.20
      body S22.22
      manubrium S22.21
      xiphoid process S22.24
    vertebra (displaced) S22.009
      burst (stable) S22.001
        unstable S22.002
      eighth S22.069
        burst (stable) S22.061
          unstable S22.062
        specified type NEC S22.068
        wedge compression S22.060
      eleventh S22.089
        burst (stable) S22.081
          unstable S22.082
        specified type NEC S22.088
        wedge compression S22.080
      fifth S22.059
        burst (stable) S22.051
          unstable S22.052
        specified type NEC S22.058
        wedge compression S22.050
      first S22.019
        burst (stable) S22.011
          unstable S22.012
        specified type NEC S22.018
        wedge compression S22.010

Fracture, traumatic *(Continued)*
  thorax *(Continued)*
    vertebra *(Continued)*
      fourth S22.049
        burst (stable) S22.041
          unstable S22.042
        specified type NEC S22.048
        wedge compression S22.040
      ninth S22.079
        burst (stable) S22.071
          unstable S22.072
        specified type NEC S22.078
        wedge compression S22.070
      nondisplaced S22.001
      second S22.029
        burst (stable) S22.021
          unstable S22.022
        specified type NEC S22.028
        wedge compression S22.020
      seventh S22.069
        burst (stable) S22.061
          unstable S22.062
        specified type NEC S22.068
        wedge compression S22.060
      sixth S22.059
        burst (stable) S22.051
          unstable S22.052
        specified type NEC S22.058
        wedge compression S22.050
      specified type NEC S22.008
      tenth S22.079
        burst (stable) S22.071
          unstable S22.072
        specified type NEC S22.078
        wedge compression S22.070
      third S22.039
        burst (stable) S22.031
          unstable S22.032
        specified type NEC S22.038
        wedge compression S22.030
      twelfth S22.089
        burst (stable) S22.081
          unstable S22.082
        specified type NEC S22.088
        wedge compression S22.080
      wedge compression S22.000
  thumb S62.50-
    distal phalanx (displaced) S62.52-
      nondisplaced S62.52-
    proximal phalanx (displaced)
      S62.51-
      nondisplaced S62.51-
  thyroid cartilage S12.8
  tibia (shaft) S82.20-
    comminuted (displaced) S82.25-
      nondisplaced S82.25-
    condyles —*see* Fracture, tibia, upper end
    distal end —*see* Fracture, tibia, lower end
    epiphysis
      lower —*see* Fracture, tibia, lower end
      upper —*see* Fracture, tibia, upper end
    following insertion of implant, prosthesis
      or plate M96.67-
    head (involving knee joint) —*see* Fracture,
      tibia, upper end
    intercondyloid eminence —*see* Fracture,
      tibia, upper end
    involving ankle or malleolus —*see*
      Fracture, ankle, medial malleolus
    lower end S82.30-
      physeal S89.10-
        Salter-Harris
          Type I S89.11-
          Type II S89.12-
          Type III S89.13-
          Type IV S89.14-
        specified NEC S89.19-
      pilon (displaced) S82.87-
        nondisplaced S82.87-
      specified NEC S82.39-
      torus S82.31-

◄ New   ◄▥ Revised   ~~deleted~~ Deleted

Fracture, traumatic *(Continued)*
tibia *(Continued)*
malleolus —*see* Fracture, ankle, medial
malleolus
oblique (displaced) S82.23-
nondisplaced S82.23-
pilon —*see* Fracture, tibia, lower end,
pilon
proximal end —*see* Fracture, tibia, upper
end
segmental (displaced) S82.26-
nondisplaced S82.26-
specified NEC S82.29-
spine —*see* Fracture, upper end, spine
spiral (displaced) S82.24-
nondisplaced S82.24-
transverse (displaced) S82.22-
nondisplaced S82.22-
tuberosity —*see* Fracture, tibia, upper end,
tuberosity
upper end S82.10-
bicondylar (displaced) S82.14-
nondisplaced S82.14-
lateral condyle (displaced) S82.12-
nondisplaced S82.12-
medial condyle (displaced) S82.13-
nondisplaced S82.13-
physeal S89.00-
Salter-Harris
Type I S89.01-
Type II S89.02-
Type III S89.03-
Type IV S89.04-
specified NEC S89.09-
plateau —*see* Fracture, tibia, upper end,
bicondylar
specified NEC S82.19-
spine (displaced) S82.11-
nondisplaced S82.11-
torus S82.16-
tuberosity (displaced) S82.15-
nondisplaced S82.15-
toe S92.91-
great (displaced) S92.40-
distal phalanx (displaced) S92.42-
nondisplaced S92.42-
nondisplaced S92.40-
proximal phalanx (displaced)
S92.41-
nondisplaced S92.41-
specified NEC S92.49-
lesser (displaced) S92.50-
distal phalanx (displaced) S92.53-
nondisplaced S92.53-
medial phalanx (displaced) S92.52-
nondisplaced S92.52-
nondisplaced S92.50-
proximal phalanx (displaced)
S92.51-
nondisplaced S92.51-
specified NEC S92.59-
physeal ◄
phalanx S99.20- ◄
Salter-Harris ◄
Type I S99.21- ◄
Type II S99.22- ◄
Type III S99.23- ◄
Type IV S99.24- ◄
specified NEC S99.29- ◄
tooth (root) S02.5
trachea (cartilage) S12.8
transverse process —*see* Fracture, vertebra
trapezium or trapezoid bone —*see* Fracture,
carpal
trimalleolar —*see* Fracture, ankle, trimalleolar
triquetrum (cuneiform of carpus) —*see*
Fracture, carpal, triquetrum
trochanter —*see* Fracture, femur,
trochanteric
tuberosity (external) —*see* Fracture,
traumatic, by site ◄▥

Fracture, traumatic *(Continued)*
ulna (shaft) S52.20-
bent bone S52.28-
coronoid process —*see* Fracture, ulna,
upper end, coronoid process
distal end —*see* Fracture, ulna, lower end
following insertion of implant, prosthesis
or plate M96.63-
head S52.00-
lower end S52.60-
physeal S59.00-
Salter-Harris
Type I S59.01-
Type II S59.02-
Type III S59.03-
Type IV S59.04-
specified NEC S59.09-
specified NEC S52.69-
styloid process (displaced) S52.61-
nondisplaced S52.61-
torus S52.62-
proximal end —*see* Fracture, ulna, upper
end
shaft S52.20-
comminuted (displaced) S52.25-
nondisplaced S52.25-
greenstick S52.21-
Monteggia's —*see* Monteggia's fracture
oblique (displaced) S52.23-
nondisplaced S52.23-
segmental (displaced) S52.26-
nondisplaced S52.26-
specified NEC S52.29-
spiral (displaced) S52.24-
nondisplaced S52.24-
transverse (displaced) S52.22-
nondisplaced S52.22-
upper end S52.00-
coronoid process (displaced) S52.04-
nondisplaced S52.04-
olecranon process (displaced)
S52.02-
with intraarticular extension
S52.03-
nondisplaced S52.02-
with intraarticular extension
S52.03-
specified NEC S52.09-
torus S52.01-
unciform —*see* Fracture, carpal, hamate
vault of skull S02.0
vertebra, vertebral (arch) (body) (column)
(neural arch) (pedicle) (spinous process)
(transverse process)
atlas —*see* Fracture, neck, cervical vertebra,
first
axis —*see* Fracture, neck, cervical vertebra,
second
cervical (teardrop) S12.9
axis —*see* Fracture, neck, cervical
vertebra, second
first (atlas) —*see* Fracture, neck, cervical
vertebra, first
second (axis) —*see* Fracture, neck,
cervical vertebra, second
chronic M84.48
coccyx S32.2
dorsal —*see* Fracture, thorax, vertebra
lumbar S32.009
burst (stable) S32.001
unstable S32.002
fifth S32.059
burst (stable) S32.051
unstable S32.052
specified type NEC S32.058
wedge compression S32.050
first S32.019
burst (stable) S32.011
unstable S32.012
specified type NEC S32.018
wedge compression S32.010

Fracture, traumatic *(Continued)*
vertebra, vertebral *(Continued)*
lumbar *(Continued)*
fourth S32.049
burst (stable) S32.041
unstable S32.042
specified type NEC S32.048
wedge compression S32.040
second S32.029
burst (stable) S32.021
unstable S32.022
specified type NEC S32.028
wedge compression S32.020
specified type NEC S32.008
third S32.039
burst (stable) S32.031
unstable S32.032
specified type NEC S32.038
wedge compression S32.030
wedge compression S32.000
metastatic —*see* Collapse, vertebra, in,
specified disease NEC —*see also*
Neoplasm
newborn (birth injury) P11.5
sacrum S32.10
specified NEC S32.19
Type
1 S32.14
2 S32.15
3 S32.16
4 S32.17
Zone
I S32.119
displaced (minimally) S32.111
severely S32.112
nondisplaced S32.110
II S32.129
displaced (minimally) S32.121
severely S32.122
nondisplaced S32.120
III S32.139
displaced (minimally) S32.131
severely S32.132
nondisplaced S32.130
thoracic —*see* Fracture, thorax, vertebra
vertex S02.0
vomer (bone) S02.2
wrist S62.10-
carpal —*see* Fracture, carpal bone
navicular (scaphoid) (hand) —*see* Fracture,
carpal, navicular
xiphisternum, xiphoid (process) S22.24
zygoma S02.442
left side S02.40F ◄
right side S02.40E ◄
Fragile, fragility
autosomal site Q95.5
bone, congenital (with blue sclera) Q78.0
capillary (hereditary) D69.8
hair L67.8
nails L60.3
non-sex chromosome site Q95.5
X chromosome Q99.2
Fragilitas
crinium L67.8
ossium (with blue sclerae) (hereditary)
Q78.0
unguium L60.3
congenital Q84.6
Fragments, cataract (lens), **following cataract
surgery** H59.02-
retained foreign body —*see* Retained, foreign
body fragments (type of)
Frailty (frail) R54
mental R41.81
Frambesia, frambesial (tropica) —*see also* Yaws
initial lesion or ulcer A66.0
primary A66.0
Frambeside
gummatous A66.4
of early yaws A66.2

Frambesioma A66.1
Franceschetti-Klein (-Wildervanck) disease or
    syndrome Q75.4
Francis' disease —see Tularemia
Franklin disease C88.2
Frank's essential thrombocytopenia D69.3
Fraser's syndrome Q87.0
Freckle (s) L81.2
    malignant melanoma in —see Melanoma
    melanotic (Hutchinson's) —see Melanoma,
        in situ
    retinal D49.81
Frederickson's hyperlipoproteinemia, type
    I and V E78.3
    IIA E78.00 ◀▥
    IIB and III E78.2
    IV E78.1
Freeman Sheldon syndrome Q87.0
Freezing —see also Effect, adverse, cold T69.9
Freiberg's disease (infraction of metatarsal
        head or osteochondrosis) —see
        Osteochondrosis, juvenile, metatarsus
Frei's disease A55
Fremitus, friction, cardiac R01.2
Frenum, frenulum
    external os Q51.828
    tongue (shortening) (congenital) Q38.1
Frequency micturition (nocturnal) R35.0
    psychogenic F45.8
Frey's syndrome
    auriculotemporal G50.8
    hyperhidrosis L74.52
Friction
    burn —see Burn, by site
    fremitus, cardiac R01.2
    precordial R01.2
    sounds, chest R09.89
Friderichsen-Waterhouse syndrome or disease
        A39.1
Friedländer's B (bacillus) NEC —see also
        condition A49.8
Friedreich's
    ataxia G11.1
    combined systemic disease G11.1
    facial hemihypertrophy Q67.4
    sclerosis (cerebellum) (spinal cord)
        G11.1
Frigidity F52.22
Fröhlich's syndrome E23.6
Frontal —see also condition
    lobe syndrome F07.0
Frostbite (superficial) T33.90
    with
        partial thickness skin loss —see Frostbite
            (superficial), by site
        tissue necrosis T34.90
    abdominal wall T33.3
        with tissue necrosis T34.3
    ankle T33.81-
        with tissue necrosis T34.81-
    arm T33.4-
        with tissue necrosis T34.4-
        finger (s) —see Frostbite, finger
        hand —see Frostbite, hand
        wrist —see Frostbite, wrist
    ear T33.01-
        with tissue necrosis T34.01-
    face T33.09
        with tissue necrosis T34.09
    finger T33.53-
        with tissue necrosis T34.53-
    foot T33.82-
        with tissue necrosis T34.82-
    hand T33.52-
        with tissue necrosis T34.52-
    head T33.09
        with tissue necrosis T34.09
        ear —see Frostbite, ear
        nose —see Frostbite, nose
    hip (and thigh) T33.6-
        with tissue necrosis T34.6-

Frostbite (Continued)
    knee T33.7-
        with tissue necrosis T34.7-
    leg T33.9-
        with tissue necrosis T34.9-
        ankle —see Frostbite, ankle
        foot —see Frostbite, foot
        knee —see Frostbite, knee
        lower T33.7-
            with tissue necrosis T34.7-
        thigh —see Frostbite, hip
        toe —see Frostbite, toe
    limb
        lower T33.99
            with tissue necrosis T34.99
        upper —see Frostbite, arm
    neck T33.1
        with tissue necrosis T34.1
    nose T33.02
        with tissue necrosis T34.02
    pelvis T33.3
        with tissue necrosis T34.3
    specified site NEC T33.99
        with tissue necrosis T34.99
    thigh —see Frostbite, hip
    thorax T33.2
        with tissue necrosis T34.2
    toes T33.83-
        with tissue necrosis T34.83-
    trunk T33.99
        with tissue necrosis T34.99
    wrist T33.51-
        with tissue necrosis T34.51-
Frotteurism F65.81
Frozen —see also Effect, adverse, cold T69.9
    pelvis (female) N94.89
        male K66.8
    shoulder —see Capsulitis, adhesive
Fructokinase deficiency E74.11
Fructose 1,6 diphosphatase deficiency E74.19
Fructosemia (benign) (essential) E74.12
Fructosuria (benign) (essential) E74.11
Fuchs'
    black spot (myopic) H44.2-
    dystrophy (corneal endothelium) H18.51
    heterochromic cyclitis —see Cyclitis, Fuchs'
        heterochromic
Fucosidosis E77.1
Fugue R68.89
    dissociative F44.1
    hysterical (dissociative) F44.1
    postictal in epilepsy —see Epilepsy
    reaction to exceptional stress (transient)
        F43.0
Fulminant, fulminating —see condition
Functional —see also condition
    bleeding (uterus) N93.8
Functioning, intellectual, borderline R41.83
Fundus —see condition
Fungemia NOS B49
Fungus, fungous
    cerebral G93.89
    disease NOS B49
    infection —see Infection, fungus
Funiculitis (acute) (chronic) (endemic) N49.1
    gonococcal (acute) (chronic) A54.23
    tuberculous A18.15
Funnel
    breast (acquired) M95.4
        congenital Q67.6
        sequelae (late effect) of rickets E64.3
    chest (acquired) M95.4
        congenital Q67.6
        sequelae (late effect) of rickets E64.3
    pelvis (acquired) M95.5
        with disproportion (fetopelvic) O33.3
            causing obstructed labor O65.3
        congenital Q74.2
FUO (fever of unknown origin) R50.9
Furfur L21.0
    microsporon B36.0

Furrier's lung J67.8
Furrowed K14.5
    nail (s) (transverse) L60.4
        congenital Q84.6
    tongue K14.5
        congenital Q38.3
Furuncle L02.92
    abdominal wall L02.221
    ankle —see Furuncle, lower limb
    antecubital space —see Furuncle, upper limb
    anus K61.0
    arm —see Furuncle, upper limb
    auditory canal, external —see Abscess, ear,
        external
    auricle (ear) —see Abscess, ear, external
    axilla (region) L02.42-
    back (any part) L02.222
    breast N61.1 ◀▥
    buttock L02.32
    cheek (external) L02.02
    chest wall L02.223
    chin L02.02
    corpus cavernosum N48.21
    ear, external —see Abscess, ear, external
    external auditory canal —see Abscess, ear,
        external
    eyelid —see Abscess, eyelid
    face L02.02
    femoral (region) —see Furuncle, lower
        limb
    finger —see Furuncle, hand
    flank L02.221
    foot L02.62-
    forehead L02.02
    gluteal (region) L02.32
    groin L02.224
    hand L02.52-
    head L02.821
        face L02.02
    hip —see Furuncle, lower limb
    kidney —see Abscess, kidney
    knee —see Furuncle, lower limb
    labium (majus) (minus) N76.4
    lacrimal
        gland —see Dacryoadenitis
        passages (duct) (sac) —see Inflammation,
            lacrimal, passages, acute
    leg (any part) —see Furuncle, lower limb
    lower limb L02.42-
    malignant A22.0
    mouth K12.2
    navel L02.226
    neck L02.12
    nose J34.0
    orbit, orbital —see Abscess, orbit
    palmar (space) —see Furuncle, hand
    partes posteriores L02.32
    pectoral region L02.223
    penis N48.21
    perineum L02.225
    pinna —see Abscess, ear, external
    popliteal —see Furuncle, lower limb
    prepatellar —see Furuncle, lower limb
    scalp L02.821
    seminal vesicle N49.0
    shoulder —see Furuncle, upper limb
    specified site NEC L02.828
    submandibular K12.2
    temple (region) L02.02
    thumb —see Furuncle, hand
    toe —see Furuncle, foot
    trunk L02.229
        abdominal wall L02.221
        back L02.222
        chest wall L02.223
        groin L02.224
        perineum L02.225
        umbilicus L02.226
    umbilicus L02.226
    upper limb L02.42-
    vulva N76.4

◀ New   ◀▥ Revised   ~~deleted~~ Deleted

Furunculosis —*see* Furuncle
Fused —*see* Fusion, fused
Fusion, fused (congenital)
  astragaloscaphoid Q74.2
  atria Q21.1
  auditory canal Q16.1
  auricles, heart Q21.1
  binocular with defective stereopsis H53.32
  bone Q79.8
  cervical spine M43.22
  choanal Q30.0
  commissure, mitral valve Q23.2
  cusps, heart valve NEC Q24.8
    mitral Q23.2
    pulmonary Q22.1
    tricuspid Q22.4
  ear ossicles Q16.3
  fingers Q70.0-
  hymen Q52.3
  joint (acquired) —*see also* Ankylosis
    congenital Q74.8
  kidneys (incomplete) Q63.1
  labium (majus) (minus) Q52.5
  larynx and trachea Q34.8

Fusion, fused *(Continued)*
  limb, congenital Q74.8
    lower Q74.2
    upper Q74.0
  lobes, lung Q33.8
  lumbosacral (acquired) M43.27
    arthrodesis status Z98.1
    congenital Q76.49
    postprocedural status Z98.1
  nares, nose, nasal, nostril (s) Q30.0
  organ or site not listed —*see* Anomaly, by site
  ossicles Q79.9
    auditory Q16.3
  pulmonic cusps Q22.1
  ribs Q76.6
  sacroiliac (joint) (acquired) M43.28
    arthrodesis status Z98.1
    congenital Q74.2
    postprocedural status Z98.1
  spine (acquired) NEC M43.20
    arthrodesis status Z98.1
    cervical region M43.22
    cervicothoracic region M43.23
    congenital Q76.49

Fusion, fused *(Continued)*
  spine *(Continued)*
    lumbar M43.26
    lumbosacral region M43.27
    occipito-atlanto-axial region M43.21
    postoperative status Z98.1
    sacrococcygeal region M43.28
    thoracic region M43.24
    thoracolumbar region M43.25
  sublingual duct with submaxillary duct at
    opening in mouth Q38.4
  testes Q55.1
  toes Q70.2
  tooth, teeth K00.2
  trachea and esophagus Q39.8
  twins Q89.4
  vagina Q52.4
  ventricles, heart Q21.0
  vertebra (arch) —*see* Fusion, spine
  vulva Q52.5
Fusospirillosis (mouth) (tongue) (tonsil)
  A69.1
Fussy baby R68.12

G

Gain in weight (abnormal) (excessive) —see also Weight, gain
Gaisböck's disease (polycythemia hypertonica) D75.1
Gait abnormality R26.9
  ataxic R26.0
  falling R29.6
  hysterical (ataxic) (staggering) F44.4
  paralytic R26.1
  spastic R26.1
  specified type NEC R26.89
  staggering R26.0
  unsteadiness R26.81
  walking difficulty NEC R26.2
Galactocele (breast) N64.89
  puerperal, postpartum O92.79
Galactokinase deficiency E74.29
Galactophoritis N61.0 ◄▥
  gestational, puerperal, postpartum O91.2-
Galactorrhea O92.6
  not associated with childbirth N64.3
Galactosemia (classic) (congenital) E74.21
Galactosuria E74.29
Galacturia R82.0
  schistosomiasis (bilharziasis) B65.0
Galeazzi's fracture S52.37-
Galen's vein —see condition
Galeophobia F40.218
Gall duct —see condition
Gallbladder —see also condition
  acute K81.0
Gallop rhythm R00.8
Gallstone (colic) (cystic duct) (gallbladder) (impacted) (multiple) —see also Calculus, gallbladder
  with
    cholecystitis —see Calculus, gallbladder, with cholecystitis
    bile duct (common) (hepatic) —see Calculus, bile duct
    causing intestinal obstruction K56.3
  specified NEC K80.80
    with obstruction K80.81
Gambling Z72.6
  pathological (compulsive) F63.0
Gammopathy (of undetermined significance [MGUS]) D47.2
  associated with lymphoplasmacytic dyscrasia D47.2
  monoclonal D47.2
  polyclonal D89.0
Gamna's disease (siderotic splenomegaly) D73.1
Gamophobia F40.298
Gampsodactylia (congenital) Q66.7
Gamstorp's disease (adynamia episodica hereditaria) G72.3
Gandy-Nanta disease (siderotic splenomegaly) D73.1
Gang
  membership offenses Z72.810
Gangliocytoma D36.10
Ganglioglioma —see Neoplasm, uncertain behavior, by site
Ganglion (compound) (diffuse) (joint) (tendon (sheath)) M67.40
  ankle M67.47-
  foot M67.47-
  forearm M67.43-
  hand M67.44-
  lower leg M67.46-
  multiple sites M67.49
  of yaws (early) (late) A66.6
  pelvic region M67.45-
  periosteal —see Periostitis
  shoulder region M67.41-
  specified site NEC M67.48
  thigh region M67.45-
  tuberculous A18.09
  upper arm M67.42-
  wrist M67.43-

Ganglioneuroblastoma —see Neoplasm, nerve, malignant
Ganglioneuroma D36.10
  malignant —see Neoplasm, nerve, malignant
Ganglioneuromatosis D36.10
Ganglionitis
  fifth nerve —see Neuralgia, trigeminal
  gasserian (postherpetic) (postzoster) B02.21
  geniculate G51.1
    newborn (birth injury) P11.3
    postherpetic, postzoster B02.21
  herpes zoster B02.21
  postherpetic geniculate B02.21
Gangliosidosis E75.10
  GM1 E75.19
  GM2 E75.00
    other specified E75.09
    Sandhoff disease E75.01
    Tay-Sachs disease E75.02
  GM3 E75.19
  mucolipidosis IV E75.11
Gangosa A66.5
Gangrene, gangrenous (connective tissue) (dropsical) (dry) (moist) (skin) (ulcer) —see also Necrosis I96
  with diabetes (mellitus) —see Diabetes, gangrene
  abdomen (wall) I96
  alveolar M27.3
  appendix K35.80
    with
      perforation or rupture K35.2
      peritoneal abscess K35.3
      peritonitis NEC K35.3
        generalized (with perforation or rupture) K35.2
        localized (with perforation or rupture) K35.3
  arteriosclerotic (general) (senile) —see Arteriosclerosis, extremities, with, gangrene
  auricle I96
  Bacillus welchii A48.0
  bladder (infectious) —see Cystitis, specified type NEC
  bowel, cecum, or colon —see Gangrene, intestine
  Clostridium perfringens or welchii A48.0
  cornea H18.89-
  corpora cavernosa N48.29
    noninfective N48.89
  cutaneous, spreading I96
  decubital —see Ulcer, pressure, by site
  diabetic (any site) —see Diabetes, gangrene
  emphysematous —see Gangrene, gas
  epidemic —see Poisoning, food, noxious, plant
  epididymis (infectional) N45.1
  erysipelas —see Erysipelas
  extremity (lower) (upper) I96
  Fournier N49.3
    female N76.89
  fusospirochetal A69.0
  gallbladder —see Cholecystitis, acute
  gas (bacillus) A48.0
    following
      abortion —see Abortion by type complicated by infection
      ectopic or molar pregnancy O08.0
  glossitis K14.0
  hernia —see Hernia, by site, with gangrene
  intestine, intestinal (hemorrhagic) (massive) —see also Infarct, intestine K55.069 ◄▥
    with
      mesenteric embolism —see also Infarct, intestine K55.069 ◄▥
      obstruction —see Obstruction, intestine
  laryngitis J04.0
  limb (lower) (upper) I96

Gangrene, gangrenous (Continued)
  lung J85.0
    spirochetal A69.8
  lymphangitis I89.1
  Meleney's (synergistic) —see Ulcer, skin
  mesentery —see also Infarct, intestine K55.069 ◄▥
    with
      embolism —see also Infarct, intestine K55.069 ◄▥
      intestinal obstruction —see Obstruction, intestine
  mouth A69.0
  ovary —see Oophoritis
  pancreas —see Pancreatitis, acute ◄▥
  penis N48.29
    noninfective N48.89
  perineum I96
  pharynx —see also Pharyngitis
    Vincent's A69.1
  presenile I73.1
  progressive synergistic —see Ulcer, skin
  pulmonary J85.0
  pulpal (dental) K04.1
  quinsy J36
  Raynaud's (symmetric gangrene) I73.01
  retropharyngeal J39.2
  scrotum N49.3
    noninfective N50.89 ◄▥
  senile (atherosclerotic) —see Arteriosclerosis, extremities, with, gangrene
  spermatic cord N49.1
    noninfective N50.89 ◄▥
  spine I96
  spirochetal NEC A69.8
  spreading cutaneous I96
  stomatitis A69.0
  symmetrical I73.01
  testis (infectional) N45.2
    noninfective N44.8
  throat —see also Pharyngitis
    diphtheritic A36.0
    Vincent's A69.1
  thyroid (gland) E07.89
  tooth (pulp) K04.1
  tuberculous NEC —see Tuberculosis
  tunica vaginalis N49.1
    noninfective N50.89 ◄▥
  umbilicus I96
  uterus —see Endometritis
  uvulitis K12.2
  vas deferens N49.1
    noninfective N50.89 ◄▥
  vulva N76.89
Ganister disease J62.8
Ganser's syndrome (hysterical) F44.89
Gardner-Diamond syndrome (autoerythrocyte sensitization) D69.2
Gargoylism E76.01
Garré's disease, osteitis (sclerosing), osteomyelitis —see Osteomyelitis, specified type NEC
Garrod's pad, knuckle M72.1
Gartner's duct
  cyst Q52.4
  persistent Q50.6
Gas R14.3
  asphyxiation, inhalation, poisoning, suffocation NEC —see Table of Drugs and Chemicals
  excessive R14.0
  gangrene A48.0
    following
      abortion —see Abortion by type complicated by infection
      ectopic or molar pregnancy O08.0
  on stomach R14.0
  pains R14.1
Gastralgia —see also Pain, abdominal
Gastrectasis K31.0
  psychogenic F45.8
Gastric —see condition

◄ New   ◄▥ Revised   ~~deleted~~ Deleted

Gastrinoma
   malignant
      pancreas C25.4
      specified site NEC —*see* Neoplasm,
         malignant, by site
      unspecified site C25.4
   specified site —*see* Neoplasm, uncertain
      behavior
   unspecified site D37.9
Gastritis (simple) K29.70
   with bleeding K29.71
   acute (erosive) K29.00
      with bleeding K29.01
   alcoholic K29.20
      with bleeding K29.21
   allergic K29.60
      with bleeding K29.61
   atrophic (chronic) K29.40
      with bleeding K29.41
   chronic (antral) (fundal) K29.50
      with bleeding K29.51
      atrophic K29.40
         with bleeding K29.41
      superficial K29.30
         with bleeding K29.31
   dietary counseling and surveillance Z71.3
   due to diet deficiency E63.9
   eosinophilic K52.81
   giant hypertrophic K29.60
      with bleeding K29.61
   granulomatous K29.60
      with bleeding K29.61
   hypertrophic (mucosa) K29.60
      with bleeding K29.61
   nervous F54
   spastic K29.60
      with bleeding K29.61
   specified NEC K29.60
      with bleeding K29.61
   superficial chronic K29.30
      with bleeding K29.31
   tuberculous A18.83
   viral NEC A08.4
Gastrocarcinoma —*see* Neoplasm, malignant,
   stomach
Gastrocolic —*see* condition
Gastrodisciasis, gastrodiscoidiasis B66.8
Gastroduodenitis K29.90
   with bleeding K29.91
   virus, viral A08.4
      specified type NEC A08.39
Gastrodynia —*see* Pain, abdominal
Gastroenteritis (acute) (chronic) (noninfectious)
   (*see also* Enteritis) K52.9
   allergic K52.29 ◀▥
   with ◀
      eosinophilic gastritis or gastroenteritis
         K52.81 ◀
      food protein-induced enterocolitis
         syndrome K52.21 ◀
      food protein-induced enteropathy
         K52.22 ◀
   dietetic —*see also* Gastroenteritis, allergic
      K52.29 ◀▥
   drug-induced K52.1
   due to
      Cryptosporidium A07.2
      drugs K52.1
      food poisoning —*see* Intoxication,
         foodborne
      radiation K52.0
   eosinophilic K52.81
   epidemic (infectious) A09
   food hypersensitivity —*see also*
      Gastroenteritis, allergic K52.29 ◀▥
   infectious —*see* Enteritis, infectious
   influenzal —*see* Influenza, with
      gastroenteritis
   noninfectious K52.9
      specified NEC K52.89
   rotaviral A08.0

Gastroenteritis (*Continued*)
   Salmonella A02.0
   toxic K52.1
   viral NEC A08.4
      acute infectious A08.39
         type Norwalk A08.11
      infantile (acute) A08.39
      Norwalk agent A08.11
      rotaviral A08.0
      severe of infants A08.39
      specified type NEC A08.39
Gastroenteropathy —*see also* Gastroenteritis
   K52.9
   acute, due to Norovirus A08.11
   acute, due to Norwalk agent A08.11
   infectious A09
Gastroenteroptosis K63.4
Gastroesophageal laceration-hemorrhage
   syndrome K22.6
Gastrointestinal —*see* condition
Gastrojejunal —*see* condition
Gastrojejunitis —*see also* Enteritis K52.9
Gastrojejunocolic —*see* condition
Gastroliths K31.89
Gastromalacia K31.89
Gastroparalysis K31.84
   diabetic —*see* Diabetes, gastroparalysis
Gastroparesis K31.84
   diabetic —*see* Diabetes, by type, with
      gastroparesis
Gastropathy K31.9
   congestive portal K31.89
   erythematous K29.70
   exudative K90.89
   portal hypertensive K31.89
Gastroptosis K31.89
Gastrorrhagia K92.2
   psychogenic F45.8
Gastroschisis (congenital) Q79.3
Gastrospasm (neurogenic) (reflex) K31.89
   neurotic F45.8
   psychogenic F45.8
Gastrostaxis —*see* Gastritis, with bleeding
Gastrostenosis K31.89
Gastrostomy
   attention to Z43.1
   status Z93.1
Gastrosuccorrhea (continuous) (intermittent)
   K31.89
   neurotic F45.8
   psychogenic F45.8
Gatophobia F40.218
Gaucher's disease or splenomegaly (adult)
   (infantile) E75.22
Gee (-Herter)(-Thaysen) disease (nontropical
   sprue) K90.0
Gélineau's syndrome G47.419
   with cataplexy G47.411
Gemination, tooth, teeth K00.2
Gemistocytoma
   specified site —*see* Neoplasm, malignant, by
      site
   unspecified site C71.9
General, generalized —*see* condition
Genetic
   carrier (status)
      cystic fibrosis Z14.1
      hemophilia A (asymptomatic) Z14.01
         symptomatic Z14.02
      specified NEC Z14.8
   susceptibility to disease NEC Z15.89
      malignant neoplasm Z15.09
         breast Z15.01
         endometrium Z15.04
         ovary Z15.02
         prostate Z15.03
         specified NEC Z15.09
      multiple endocrine neoplasia Z15.81
Genital —*see* condition
Genito-anorectal syndrome A55
Genitourinary system —*see* condition

Genu
   congenital Q74.1
   extrorsum (acquired) —*see also* Deformity,
      varus, knee
      congenital Q74.1
      sequelae (late effect) of rickets E64.3
   introrsum (acquired) —*see also* Deformity,
      valgus, knee
      congenital Q74.1
      sequelae (late effect) of rickets E64.3
   rachitic (old) E64.3
   recurvatum (acquired) —*see also* Deformity,
      limb, specified type NEC, lower leg
      congenital Q68.2
      sequelae (late effect) of rickets E64.3
   valgum (acquired) (knock-knee) M21.06-
      congenital Q74.1
      sequelae (late effect) of rickets E64.3
   varum (acquired) (bowleg) M21.16-
      congenital Q74.1
      sequelae (late effect) of rickets E64.3
Geographic tongue K14.1
Geophagia —*see* Pica
Geotrichosis B48.3
   stomatitis B48.3
Gephyrophobia F40.242
Gerbode defect Q21.0
GERD (gastroesophageal reflux disease) K21.9
Gerhardt's
   disease (erythromelalgia) I73.81
   syndrome (vocal cord paralysis)
      J38.00
      bilateral J38.02
      unilateral J38.01
German measles —*see also* Rubella
   exposure to Z20.4
Germinoblastoma (diffuse) C85.9-
   follicular C82.9-
Germinoma —*see* Neoplasm, malignant, by site
Gerontoxon —*see* Degeneration, cornea, senile
Gerstmann-Sträussler-Scheinker syndrome
   (GSS) A81.82
Gerstmann's syndrome R48.8
   developmental F81.2
Gestation (period) —*see also* Pregnancy
   ectopic —*see* Pregnancy, by site
   multiple O30.9-
      greater than quadruplets —*see* Pregnancy,
         multiple (gestation), specified NEC
      specified NEC —*see* Pregnancy, multiple
         (gestation), specified NEC
Gestational
   mammary abscess O91.11-
   purulent mastitis O91.11-
   subareolar abscess O91.11-
Ghon tubercle, primary infection A15.7
Ghost
   teeth K00.4
   vessels (cornea) H16.41-
Ghoul hand A66.3
Gianotti-Crosti disease L44.4
Giant
   cell
      epulis K06.8
      peripheral granuloma K06.8
   esophagus, congenital Q39.5
   kidney, congenital Q63.3
   urticaria T78.3
      hereditary D84.1
Giardiasis A07.1
Gibert's disease or pityriasis L42
Giddiness R42
   hysterical F44.89
   psychogenic F45.8
Gierke's disease (glycogenosis I) E74.01
Gigantism (cerebral) (hypophyseal) (pituitary)
   E22.0
   constitutional E34.4
Gilbert's disease or syndrome E80.4
Gilchrist's disease B40.9
Gilford-Hutchinson disease E34.8

Gilles de la Tourette's disease or syndrome
    (motor-verbal tic) F95.2
Gingivitis K05.10
    acute (catarrhal) K05.00
        necrotizing A69.1
        nonplaque induced K05.01
        plaque induced K05.00
    chronic (desquamative) (hyperplastic)
        (simple marginal) (pregnancy
        associated) (ulcerative) K05.10 ◀▥
        nonplaque induced K05.11
        plaque induced K05.10
    expulsiva —see Periodontitis
    necrotizing ulcerative (acute) A69.1
    pellagrous E52
        acute necrotizing A69.1
    Vincent's A69.1
Gingivoglossitis K14.0
Gingivopericementitis —see Periodontitis
Gingivosis —see Gingivitis, chronic
Gingivostomatitis K05.10
    herpesviral B00.2
    necrotizing ulcerative (acute) A69.1
Gland, glandular —see condition
Glanders A24.0
Glanzmann (-Naegeli) disease or
    thrombasthenia D69.1
Glasgow coma scale
    total score
        3-8 R40.243
        9-12 R40.242
        13-15 R40.241
Glass-blower's disease (cataract) —see
    Cataract, specified NEC
Glaucoma H40.9
    with
        increased episcleral venous pressure
            H40.81-
        pseudoexfoliation of lens —see Glaucoma,
            open angle, primary, capsular
    absolute H44.51-
    angle-closure (primary) H40.20-
        acute (attack) (crisis) H40.21-
        chronic H40.22-
        intermittent H40.23-
        residual stage H40.24-
    borderline H40.00-
    capsular (with pseudoexfoliation of lens) —
        see Glaucoma, open angle, primary,
        capsular
    childhood Q15.0
    closed angle —see Glaucoma, angle-closure
    congenital Q15.0
    corticosteroid-induced —see Glaucoma,
        secondary, drugs
    hypersecretion H40.82-
    in (due to)
        amyloidosis E85.4 [H42]
        aniridia Q13.1 [H42]
        concussion of globe —see Glaucoma,
            secondary, trauma
        dislocation of lens —see Glaucoma,
            secondary
        disorder of lens NEC —see Glaucoma,
            secondary
        drugs —see Glaucoma, secondary, drugs
        endocrine disease NOS E34.9 [H42]
        eye
            inflammation —see Glaucoma,
                secondary, inflammation
            trauma —see Glaucoma, secondary,
                trauma
        hypermature cataract —see Glaucoma,
            secondary
        iridocyclitis —see Glaucoma, secondary,
            inflammation
        lens disorder —see Glaucoma, secondary,
            Lowe's syndrome E72.03 [H42]
        metabolic disease NOS E88.9 [H42]
        ocular disorders NEC —see Glaucoma,
            secondary

Glaucoma (Continued)
    in (due to) (Continued)
        onchocerciasis B73.02
        pupillary block —see Glaucoma, secondary
        retinal vein occlusion —see Glaucoma,
            secondary
        Rieger's anomaly Q13.81 [H42]
        rubeosis of iris —see Glaucoma, secondary
        tumor of globe —see Glaucoma, secondary
    infantile Q15.0
    low tension —see Glaucoma, open angle,
        primary, low-tension
    malignant H40.83-
    narrow angle —see Glaucoma, angle-closure
    newborn Q15.0
    noncongestive (chronic) —see Glaucoma,
        open angle
    nonobstructive —see Glaucoma, open angle
    obstructive —see also Glaucoma,
        angle-closure
        due to lens changes —see Glaucoma,
            secondary
    open angle H40.10-
        primary H40.11-
            capsular (with pseudoexfoliation of lens)
                H40.14-
            low-tension H40.12-
            pigmentary H40.13-
            residual stage H40.15-
    phacolytic —see Glaucoma, secondary
    pigmentary —see Glaucoma, open angle,
        primary, pigmentary
    postinfectious —see Glaucoma, secondary,
        inflammation
    secondary (to) H40.5-
        drugs H40.6-
        inflammation H40.4-
        trauma H40.3-
    simple (chronic) H40.11- ◀▥
    simplex H40.11- ◀▥
    specified type NEC H40.89
    suspect H40.00-
    syphilitic A52.71
    traumatic —see also Glaucoma, secondary,
        trauma
        newborn (birth injury) P15.3
    tuberculous A18.59
Glaucomatous flecks (subcapsular) —see
    Cataract, complicated
Glazed tongue K14.4
Gleet (gonococcal) A54.01
Glénard's disease K63.4
Glioblastoma (multiforme)
    with sarcomatous component
        specified site —see Neoplasm, malignant,
            by site
        unspecified site C71.9
    giant cell
        specified site —see Neoplasm, malignant,
            by site
        unspecified site C71.9
    specified site —see Neoplasm, malignant, by
        site
    unspecified site C71.9
Glioma (malignant)
    astrocytic
        specified site —see Neoplasm, malignant,
            by site
        unspecified site C71.9
    mixed
        specified site —see Neoplasm, malignant,
            by site
        unspecified site C71.9
    nose Q30.8
    specified site NEC —see Neoplasm,
        malignant, by site
    subependymal D43.2
        specified site —see Neoplasm, uncertain
            behavior, by site
        unspecified site D43.2
    unspecified site C71.9

Gliomatosis cerebri C71.0
Glioneuroma —see Neoplasm, uncertain
    behavior, by site
Gliosarcoma
    specified site —see Neoplasm, malignant, by
        site
    unspecified site C71.9
Gliosis (cerebral) G93.89
    spinal G95.89
Glisson's disease —see Rickets
Globinuria R82.3
Globus (hystericus) F45.8
Glomangioma D18.00
    intra-abdominal D18.03
    intracranial D18.02
    skin D18.01
    specified site NEC D18.09
Glomangiomyoma D18.00
    intra-abdominal D18.03
    intracranial D18.02
    skin D18.01
    specified site NEC D18.09
Glomangiosarcoma —see Neoplasm, connective
    tissue, malignant
Glomerular
    disease in syphilis A52.75
    nephritis —see Glomerulonephritis
Glomerulitis —see Glomerulonephritis
Glomerulonephritis —see also Nephritis N05.9
    with
        edema —see Nephrosis
        minimal change N05.0
        minor glomerular abnormality N05.0
    acute N00.9
    chronic N03.9
    crescentic (diffuse) NEC —see also N00-N07
        with fourth character .7 N05.7
    dense deposit —see also N00-N07 with fourth
        character .6 N05.6
    diffuse
        crescentic —see also N00-N07 with fourth
            character .7 N05.7
        endocapillary proliferative —see also
            N00N07 with fourth character .4
            N05.4
        membranous —see also N00-N07 with
            fourth character .2 N05.2
        mesangial proliferative —see also N00-N07
            with fourth character .3 N05.3
        mesangiocapillary —see also N00-N07 with
            fourth character .5 N05.5
        sclerosing N05.8
    endocapillary proliferative (diffuse) NEC —
        see also N00-N07 with fourth character
        .4 N05.4
    extracapillary NEC —see also N00-N07 with
        fourth character .7 N05.7
    focal (and segmental) —see also N00-N07 with
        fourth character .1 N05.1
    hypocomplementemic —see
        Glomerulonephritis,
        membranoproliferative
    IgA —see Nephropathy, IgA
    immune complex (circulating) NEC
        N05.8
    in (due to)
        amyloidosis E85.4 [N08]
        bilharziasis B65.9 [N08]
        cryoglobulinemia D89.1 [N08]
        defibrination syndrome D65 [N08]
        diabetes mellitus —see Diabetes,
            glomerulosclerosis
        disseminated intravascular coagulation
            D65 [N08]
        Fabry (-Anderson) disease E75.21 [N08]
        Goodpasture's syndrome M31.0
        hemolytic-uremic syndrome D59.3
        Henoch (-Schönlein) purpura D69.0
            [N08]
        lecithin cholesterol acyltransferase
            deficiency E78.6 [N08]

◀ New   ◀▥ Revised   ~~deleted~~ Deleted

Glomerulonephritis *(Continued)*
  in *(Continued)*
    microscopic polyangiitis M31.7 *[N08]*
    multiple myeloma C90.0- *[N08]*
    Plasmodium malariae B52.0
    schistosomiasis B65.9 *[N08]*
    sepsis A41.9- *[N08]*
      streptococcal A40- *[N08]*
    sickle-cell disorders D57.- *[N08]*
    strongyloidiasis B78.9 *[N08]*
    subacute bacterial endocarditis I33.0
      [N08]
    syphilis (late) congenital A50.59 *[N08]*
    systemic lupus erythematosus M32.14
    thrombotic thrombocytopenic purpura
      M31.1 *[N08]*
    typhoid fever A01.09
    Waldenström macroglobulinemia C88.0
      [N08]
    Wegener's granulomatosis M31.31
  latent or quiescent N03.9
  lobular, lobulonodular —*see*
    Glomerulonephritis,
    membranoproliferative
  membranoproliferative (diffuse) (type 1
    or 3) —*see also* N00-N07 with fourth
    character .5 N05.5
    dense deposit (type 2) NEC —*see also*
      N00-N07 with fourth character .6
      N05.6
  membranous (diffuse) NEC —*see also*
    N00-N07 with fourth character .2 N05.2
  mesangial
    IgA/IgG —*see* Nephropathy, IgA
    proliferative (diffuse) NEC —*see also*
      N00-N07 with fourth character .3
      N05.3
  mesangiocapillary (diffuse) NEC —*see also*
    N00-N07 with fourth character .5 N05.5
  necrotic, necrotizing NEC —*see also* N00-N07
    with fourth character .8 N05.8
  nodular —*see* Glomerulonephritis,
    membranoproliferative
  poststreptococcal NEC N05.9
    acute N00.9
    chronic N03.9
    rapidly progressive N01.9
  proliferative NEC —*see also* N00-N07 with
    fourth character .8 N05.8
    diffuse (lupus) M32.14
  rapidly progressive N01.9
  sclerosing, diffuse N05.8
  specified pathology NEC —*see also* N00-N07
    with fourth character .8 N05.8
  subacute N01.9
Glomerulopathy —*see* Glomerulonephritis
Glomerulosclerosis —*see also* Sclerosis, renal
  intercapillary (nodular) (with diabetes) —*see*
    Diabetes, glomerulosclerosis
  intracapillary —*see* Diabetes,
    glomerulosclerosis
Glossagra K14.6
Glossalgia K14.6
Glossitis (chronic superficial) (gangrenous)
  (Moeller's) K14.0
  areata exfoliativa K14.1
  atrophic K14.4
  benign migratory K14.1
  cortical superficial, sclerotic K14.0
  Hunter's D51.0
  interstitial, sclerous K14.0
  median rhomboid K14.2
  pellagrous E52
  superficial, chronic K14.0
Glossocele K14.8
Glossodynia K14.6
  exfoliativa K14.4
Glossoncus K14.8
Glossopathy K14.9
Glossophytia K14.3
Glossoplegia K14.8

Glossoptosis K14.8
Glossopyrosis K14.6
Glossotrichia K14.3
Glossy skin L90.8
Glottis —*see* condition
Glottitis —*see also* Laryngitis J04.0
Glucagonoma
  pancreas
    benign D13.7
    malignant C25.4
    uncertain behavior D37.8
  specified site NEC
    benign —*see* Neoplasm, benign, by site
    malignant —*see* Neoplasm, malignant, by
      site
    uncertain behavior —*see* Neoplasm,
      uncertain behavior, by site
  unspecified site
    benign D13.7
    malignant C25.4
    uncertain behavior D37.8
Glucoglycinuria E72.51
Glucose-galactose malabsorption E74.39
Glue
  ear —*see* Otitis, media, nonsuppurative,
    chronic, mucoid
  sniffing (airplane) —*see* Abuse, drug,
    inhalant
    dependence —*see* Dependence, drug,
      inhalant
Glutaric aciduria E72.3
Glycinemia E72.51
Glycinuria (renal) (with ketosis) E72.09
Glycogen
  infiltration —*see* Disease, glycogen storage
  storage disease —*see* Disease, glycogen
    storage
Glycogenosis (diffuse) (generalized) —*see also*
  Disease, glycogen storage
  cardiac E74.02 *[143]*
  diabetic, secondary —*see* Diabetes,
    glycogenosis, secondary
  pulmonary interstitial J84.842
Glycopenia E16.2
Glycosuria R81
  renal E74.8
Gnathostoma spinigerum (infection)
  (infestation), **gnathostomiasis** (wandering
  swelling) B83.1
Goiter (plunging) (substernal) E04.9
  with
    hyperthyroidism (recurrent) —*see*
      Hyperthyroidism, with, goiter
    thyrotoxicosis —*see* Hyperthyroidism,
      with, goiter
  adenomatous —*see* Goiter, nodular
  cancerous C73
  congenital (nontoxic) E03.0
    diffuse E03.0
    parenchymatous E03.0
    transitory, with normal functioning
      P72.0
  cystic E04.2
    due to iodine-deficiency E01.1
  due to
    enzyme defect in synthesis of thyroid
      hormone E07.1
    iodine-deficiency (endemic) E01.2
  dyshormonogenetic (familial) E07.1
  endemic (iodine-deficiency) E01.2
    diffuse E01.0
    multinodular E01.1
  exophthalmic —*see* Hyperthyroidism, with,
    goiter
  iodine-deficiency (endemic) E01.2
    diffuse E01.0
    multinodular E01.1
    nodular E01.1
  lingual Q89.2
  lymphadenoid E06.3
  malignant C73

Goiter *(Continued)*
  multinodular (cystic) (nontoxic) E04.2
    toxic or with hyperthyroidism E05.20
      with thyroid storm E05.21
  neonatal NEC P72.0
  nodular (nontoxic) (due to) E04.9
    with
      hyperthyroidism E05.20
        with thyroid storm E05.21
      thyrotoxicosis E05.20
        with thyroid storm E05.21
    endemic E01.1
    iodine-deficiency E01.1
    sporadic E04.9
    toxic E05.20
      with thyroid storm E05.21
  nontoxic E04.9
    diffuse (colloid) E04.0
    multinodular E04.2
    simple E04.0
    specified NEC E04.8
    uninodular E04.1
  simple E04.0
  toxic —*see* Hyperthyroidism, with, goiter
  uninodular (nontoxic) E04.1
    toxic or with hyperthyroidism E05.10
      with thyroid storm E05.11
Goiter-deafness syndrome E07.1
Goldberg syndrome Q89.8
Goldberg-Maxwell syndrome E34.51
Goldblatt's hypertension or kidney I70.1
Goldenhar (-Gorlin) **syndrome** Q87.0
Goldflam-Erb disease or syndrome G70.00
  with exacerbation (acute) G70.01
  in crisis G70.01
Goldscheider's disease Q81.8
Goldstein's disease (familial hemorrhagic
  telangiectasia) I78.0
Golfer's elbow —*see* Epicondylitis, medial
Gonadoblastoma
  specified site —*see* Neoplasm, uncertain
    behavior, by site
  unspecified site
    female D39.10
    male D40.10
Gonecystitis —*see* Vesiculitis
Gongylonemiasis B83.8
Goniosynechiae —*see* Adhesions, iris,
  goniosynechiae
Gonococcemia A54.86
Gonococcus, gonococcal (disease) (infection)
  —*see also* condition A54.9
  anus A54.6
  bursa, bursitis A54.49
  conjunctiva, conjunctivitis (neonatorum)
    A54.31
  endocardium A54.83
  eye A54.30
    conjunctivitis A54.31
    iridocyclitis A54.32
    keratitis A54.33
    newborn A54.31
    other specified A54.39
  fallopian tubes (acute) (chronic) A54.24
  genitourinary (organ) (system) (tract) (acute)
    lower A54.00
      with abscess (accessory gland)
        (periurethral) A54.1
    upper —*see also* condition A54.29
  heart A54.83
  iridocyclitis A54.32
  joint A54.42
  lymphatic (gland) (node) A54.89
  meninges, meningitis A54.81
  musculoskeletal A54.40
    arthritis A54.42
    osteomyelitis A54.43
    other specified A54.49
    spondylopathy A54.41
  pelviperitonitis A54.24
  pelvis (acute) (chronic) A54.24

Gonococcus, gonococcal *(Continued)*
  pharynx A54.5
  proctitis A54.6
  pyosalpinx (acute) (chronic) A54.24
  rectum A54.6
  skin A54.89
  specified site NEC A54.89
  tendon sheath A54.49
  throat A54.5
  urethra (acute) (chronic) A54.01
    with abscess (accessory gland)
      (periurethral) A54.1
  vulva (acute) (chronic) A54.02
Gonocytoma
  specified site —*see* Neoplasm, uncertain
    behavior, by site
  unspecified site
    female D39.10
    male D40.10
Gonorrhea (acute) (chronic) A54.9
  Bartholin's gland (acute) (chronic) (purulent)
    A54.02
    with abscess (accessory gland)
      (periurethral) A54.1
  bladder A54.01
  cervix A54.03
  conjunctiva, conjunctivitis (neonatorum)
    A54.31
  contact Z20.2
  Cowper's gland (with abscess) A54.1
  exposure to Z20.2
  fallopian tube (acute) (chronic) A54.24
  kidney (acute) (chronic) A54.21
  lower genitourinary tract A54.00
    with abscess (accessory gland)
      (periurethral) A54.1
  ovary (acute) (chronic) A54.24
  pelvis (acute) (chronic) A54.24
    female pelvic inflammatory disease A54.24
  penis A54.09
  prostate (acute) (chronic) A54.22
  seminal vesicle (acute) (chronic) A54.23
  specified site not listed —*see also* Gonococcus
    A54.89
  spermatic cord (acute) (chronic) A54.23
  urethra A54.01
    with abscess (accessory gland)
      (periurethral) A54.1
  vagina A54.02
  vas deferens (acute) (chronic) A54.23
  vulva A54.02
Goodall's disease A08.19
Goodpasture's syndrome M31.0
Gopalan's syndrome (burning feet) E53.0
Gorlin-Chaudry-Moss syndrome Q87.0
Gottron's papules L94.4
Gougerot's syndrome (trisymptomatic) L81.7
Gougerot-Blum syndrome (pigmented
    purpuric lichenoid dermatitis) L81.7
Gougerot-Carteaud disease or syndrome
    (confluent reticulate papillomatosis) L83
Gouley's syndrome (constrictive pericarditis)
    I31.1
Goundou A66.6
Gout, chronic (*see also* Gout, gouty) M1A.9-
  drug-induced M1A.20
    ankle M1A.27-
    elbow M1A.22-
    foot joint M1A.27-
    hand joint M1A.24-
    hip M1A.25-
    knee M1A.26-
    multiple site M1A.29-
    shoulder M1A.21-
    vertebrae M1A.28
    wrist M1A.23-
  idiopathic M1A.00
    ankle M1A.07-
    elbow M1A.02-
    foot joint M1A.07-
    hand joint M1A.04-

Gout, chronic *(Continued)*
  idiopathic *(Continued)*
    hip M1A.05-
    knee M1A.06-
    multiple site M1A.09
    shoulder M1A.01-
    vertebrae M1A.08
    wrist M1A.03-
  in (due to) renal impairment M1A.30
    ankle M1A.37-
    elbow M1A.32-
    foot joint M1A.37-
    hand joint M1A.34-
    hip M1A.35-
    knee M1A.36-
    multiple site M1A.39
    shoulder M1A.31-
    vertebrae M1A.38
    wrist M1A.33-
  lead-induced M1A.10
    ankle M1A.17-
    elbow M1A.12-
    foot joint M1A.17-
    hand joint M1A.14-
    hip M1A.15-
    knee M1A.16-
    multiple site M1A.19
    shoulder M1A.11-
    vertebrae M1A.18
    wrist M1A.13-
  primary —*see* Gout, chronic, idiopathic
  saturnine —*see* Gout, chronic, lead-induced
  secondary NEC M1A.40
    ankle M1A.47-
    elbow M1A.42-
    foot joint M1A.47-
    hand joint M1A.44-
    hip M1A.45-
    knee M1A.46-
    multiple site M1A.49
    shoulder M1A.41-
    vertebrae M1A.48
    wrist M1A.43-
  syphilitic —*see also* subcategory M14.8-
    A52.77
  tophi M1A.9
Gout, gouty (acute) (attack) (flare) —*see also*
    Gout, chronic M10.9-
  drug-induced M10.20
    ankle M10.27-
    elbow M10.22-
    foot joint M10.27-
    hand joint M10.24-
    hip M10.25-
    knee M10.26-
    multiple site M10.29
    shoulder M10.21-
    vertebrae M10.28
    wrist M10.23-
  idiopathic M10.00
    ankle M10.07-
    elbow M10.02-
    foot joint M10.07-
    hand joint M10.04-
    hip M10.05-
    knee M10.06-
    multiple site M10.09
    shoulder M10.01-
    vertebrae M10.08
    wrist M10.03-
  in (due to) renal impairment M10.30
    ankle M10.37-
    elbow M10.32-
    foot joint M10.37-
    hand joint M10.34-
    hip M10.35-
    knee M10.36-
    multiple site M10.39
    shoulder M10.31-
    vertebrae M10.38
    wrist M10.33-

Gout, gouty *(Continued)*
  lead-induced M10.10
    ankle M10.17-
    elbow M10.12-
    foot joint M10.17-
    hand joint M10.14-
    hip M10.15-
    knee M10.16-
    multiple site M10.19
    shoulder M10.11-
    vertebrae M10.18
    wrist M10.13-
  primary —*see* Gout, idiopathic
  saturnine —*see* Gout, lead-induced
  secondary NEC M10.40
    ankle M10.47-
    elbow M10.42-
    foot joint M10.47-
    hand joint M10.44-
    hip M10.45-
    knee M10.46-
    multiple site M10.49
    shoulder M10.41-
    vertebrae M10.48
    wrist M10.43-
  syphilitic —*see also* subcategory M14.8-
    A52.77
  tophi NEC —*see* Gout, chronic
Gower's
  muscular dystrophy G71.0
  syndrome (vasovagal attack) R55
Gradenigo's syndrome —*see* Otitis, media,
    suppurative, acute
Graefe's disease —*see* Strabismus, paralytic,
    ophthalmoplegia, progressive
Graft-versus-host disease D89.813
  acute D89.810
  acute on chronic D89.812
  chronic D89.811
Grain mite (itch) B88.0
Grainhandler's disease or lung J67.8
Grand mal —*see* Epilepsy, generalized,
    specified NEC
Grand multipara status only (not pregnant)
    Z64.1
  pregnant —*see* Pregnancy, complicated by,
    grand multiparity
Granite worker's lung J62.8
Granular —*see also* condition
  inflammation, pharynx J31.2
  kidney (contracting) —*see* Sclerosis, renal
  liver K74.69
Granulation tissue (abnormal) (excessive) L92.9
  postmastoidectomy cavity —*see*
    Complications, postmastoidectomy,
    granulation
Granulocytopenia (primary) (malignant) —*see*
    Agranulocytosis
Granuloma L92.9
  abdomen K66.8
    from residual foreign body L92.3
    pyogenicum L98.0
  actinic L57.5
  annulare (perforating) L92.0
  apical K04.5
  aural —*see* Otitis, externa, specified NEC
  beryllium (skin) L92.3
  bone
    eosinophilic C96.6
    from residual foreign body —*see*
      Osteomyelitis, specified type NEC
    lung C96.6
  brain (any site) G06.0
    schistosomiasis B65.9 *[G07]*
  canaliculus lacrimalis —*see* Granuloma,
    lacrimal
  candidal (cutaneous) B37.2
  cerebral (any site) G06.0
  coccidioidal (primary) (progressive) B38.7
    lung B38.1
    meninges B38.4

◀ New   ◀··· Revised   ~~deleted~~ Deleted

Granuloma (Continued)
    colon K63.89
    conjunctiva H11.22-
    dental K04.5
    ear, middle —see Cholesteatoma
    eosinophilic C96.6
        bone C96.6
        lung C96.6
        oral mucosa K13.4
        skin L92.2
    eyelid H01.8
    facial (e) L92.2
    foreign body (in soft tissue) NEC M60.20
        ankle M60.27-
        foot M60.27-
        forearm M60.23-
        hand M60.24-
        in operation wound —see Foreign body,
            accidentally left during a procedure
        lower leg M60.26-
        pelvic region M60.25-
        shoulder region M60.21-
        skin L92.3
        specified site NEC M60.28
        subcutaneous tissue L92.3
        thigh M60.25-
        upper arm M60.22-
    gangraenescens M31.2
    genito-inguinale A58
    giant cell (central) (reparative) (jaw) M27.1
        gingiva (peripheral) K06.8
    gland (lymph) I88.8
    hepatic NEC K75.3
        in (due to)
            berylliosis J63.2 [K77]
            sarcoidosis D86.89
    Hodgkin C81.9
    ileum K63.89
    infectious B99.9
        specified NEC B99.8
    inguinale (Donovan) (venereal) A58
    intestine NEC K63.89
    intracranial (any site) G06.0
    intraspinal (any part) G06.1
    iridocyclitis —see Iridocyclitis, chronic
    jaw (bone) (central) M27.1
        reparative giant cell M27.1
    kidney —see also Infection, kidney N15.8
    lacrimal H04.81-
    larynx J38.7
    lethal midline (faciale) (e)) M31.2
    liver NEC —see Granuloma, hepatic
    lung (infectious) —see also Fibrosis, lung
        coccidioidal B38.1
        eosinophilic C96.6
    Majocchi's B35.8
    malignant (facial) (e)) M31.2
    mandible (central) M27.1
    midline (lethal) M31.2
    monilial (cutaneous) B37.2
    nasal sinus —see Sinusitis
    operation wound T81.89
        foreign body —see Foreign body,
            accidentally left during a procedure
        stitch T81.89
        talc —see Foreign body, accidentally left
            during a procedure
    oral mucosa K13.4
    orbit, orbital H05.11-
    paracoccidioidal B41.8
    penis, venereal A58
    periapical K04.5
    peritoneum K66.8
        due to ova of helminths NOS —see also
            Helminthiasis B83.9 [K67]
    postmastoidectomy cavity —see
        Complications, postmastoidectomy,
        recurrent cholesteatoma
    prostate N42.89
    pudendi (ulcerating) A58
    pulp, internal (tooth) K03.3

Granuloma (Continued)
    pyogenic, pyogenicum (of) (skin) L98.0
        gingiva K06.8
        maxillary alveolar ridge K04.5
        oral mucosa K13.4
    rectum K62.89
    reticulohistiocytic D76.3
    rubrum nasi L74.8
    Schistosoma —see Schistosomiasis
    septic (skin) L98.0
    silica (skin) L92.3
    sinus (accessory) (infective) (nasal) —see
        Sinusitis
    skin L92.9
        from residual foreign body L92.3
        pyogenicum L98.0
    spine
        syphilitic (epidural) A52.19
        tuberculous A18.01
    stitch (postoperative) T81.89
    suppurative (skin) L98.0
    swimming pool A31.1
    talc —see also Granuloma, foreign body
        in operation wound —see Foreign body,
            accidentally left during a procedure
    telangiectaticum (skin) L98.0
    tracheostomy J95.09
    trichophyticum B35.8
    tropicum A66.4
    umbilicus L92.9
    urethra N36.8
    uveitis —see Iridocyclitis, chronic
    vagina A58
    venereum A58
    vocal cord J38.3
Granulomatosis L92.9
    lymphoid C83.8-
    miliary (listerial) A32.89
    necrotizing, respiratory M31.30
    progressive septic D71
    specified NEC L92.8
    Wegener's M31.30
        with renal involvement M31.31
Granulomatous tissue (abnormal) (excessive)
    L92.9
Granulosis rubra nasi L74.8
Graphite fibrosis (of lung) J63.3
Graphospasm F48.8
    organic G25.89
Grating scapula M89.8X1
Gravel (urinary) —see Calculus, urinary
Graves' disease —see Hyperthyroidism, with,
    goiter
Gravis —see condition
Grawitz tumor C64.-
Gray syndrome (newborn) P93.0
Grayness, hair (premature) L67.1
    congenital Q84.2
Green sickness D50.8
Greenfield's disease
    meaning
        concentric sclerosis (encephalitis periaxialis
            concentrica) G37.5
        metachromatic leukodystrophy E75.25
Greenstick fracture - code as Fracture, by site
Grey syndrome (newborn) P93.0
Grief F43.21
    prolonged F43.29
    reaction —see also Disorder, adjustment F43.20
Griesinger's disease B76.9
Grinder's lung or pneumoconiosis J62.8
Grinding, teeth
    psychogenic F45.8
    sleep related G47.63
Grip
    Dabney's B33.0
    devil's B33.0
Grippe, grippal —see also Influenza
    Balkan A78
    summer, of Italy A93.1
Grisel's disease M43.6
Groin —see condition

Grooved tongue K14.5
Ground itch B76.9
Grover's disease or syndrome L11.1
Growing pains, children R29.898
Growth (fungoid) (neoplastic) (new) —see also
    Neoplasm
    adenoid (vegetative) J35.8
    benign —see Neoplasm, benign, by site
    malignant —see Neoplasm, malignant, by site
    rapid, childhood Z00.2
    secondary —see Neoplasm, secondary, by site
Gruby's disease B35.0
Gubler-Millard paralysis or syndrome G46.3
Guerin-Stern syndrome Q74.3
Guidance, insufficient anterior (occlusal) M26.54
Guillain-Barré disease or syndrome G61.0
    sequelae G65.0
Guinea worms (infection) (infestation) B72
Guinon's disease (motor-verbal tic) F95.2
Gull's disease E03.4
Gum —see condition
Gumboil K04.7
    with sinus K04.6
Gumma (syphilitic) A52.79
    artery A52.09
        cerebral A52.04
    bone A52.77
        of yaws (late) A66.6
    brain A52.19
    cauda equina A52.19
    central nervous system A52.3
    ciliary body A52.71
    congenital A50.59
    eyelid A52.71
    heart A52.06
    intracranial A52.19
    iris A52.71
    kidney A52.75
    larynx A52.73
    leptomeninges A52.19
    liver A52.74
    meninges A52.19
    myocardium A52.06
    nasopharynx A52.73
    neurosyphilitic A52.3
    nose A52.73
    orbit A52.71
    palate (soft) A52.79
    penis A52.76
    pericardium A52.06
    pharynx A52.73
    pituitary A52.79
    scrofulous (tuberculous) A18.4
    skin A52.79
    specified site NEC A52.79
    spinal cord A52.19
    tongue A52.79
    tonsil A52.73
    trachea A52.73
    tuberculous A18.4
    ulcerative due to yaws A66.4
    ureter A52.75
    yaws A66.4
        bone A66.6
Gunn's syndrome Q07.8
Gunshot wound —see also Wound, open
    fracture - code as Fracture, by site
    internal organs —see Injury, by site
Gynandrism Q56.0
Gynandroblastoma
    specified site —see Neoplasm, uncertain
        behavior, by site
    unspecified site
        female D39.10
        male D40.10
Gynecological examination (periodic) (routine)
    Z01.419
    with abnormal findings Z01.411
Gynecomastia N62
Gynephobia F40.291
Gyrate scalp Q82.8

H

H (Hartnup's) disease E72.02
Haas' disease or osteochondrosis (juvenile)
  (head of humerus) —see Osteochondrosis,
  juvenile, humerus
Habit, habituation
  bad sleep Z72.821
  chorea F95.8
  disturbance, child F98.9
  drug —see Dependence, drug
  irregular sleep Z72.821
  laxative F55.2
  spasm —see Tic
  tic —see Tic
Haemophilus (H.) influenzae, as cause of
  disease classified elsewhere B96.3
Haff disease —see Poisoning, mercury
Hageman's factor defect, deficiency or disease
  D68.2
Haglund's disease or osteochondrosis
  (juvenile) (os tibiale externum) —see
  Osteochondrosis, juvenile, tarsus
Hailey-Hailey disease Q82.8
Hair —see also condition
  plucking F63.3
    in stereotyped movement disorder F98.4
  tourniquet syndrome —see also Constriction,
    external, by site
    finger S60.44-
    penis S30.842
    thumb S60.34-
    toe S90.44-
Hairball in stomach T18.2
Hair-pulling, pathological (compulsive) F63.3
Hairy black tongue K14.3
Half vertebra Q76.49
Halitosis R19.6
Hallerman-Streiff syndrome Q87.0
Hallervorden-Spatz disease G23.0
Hallopeau's acrodermatitis or disease L40.2
Hallucination R44.3
  auditory R44.0
  gustatory R44.2
  olfactory R44.2
  specified NEC R44.2
  tactile R44.2
  visual R44.1
Hallucinosis (chronic) F28
  alcoholic (acute) F10.951
    in
      abuse F10.151
      dependence F10.251
  drug-induced F19.951
    cannabis F12.951
    cocaine F14.951
    hallucinogen F16.151
    in
      abuse F19.151
        cannabis F12.151
        cocaine F14.151
        hallucinogen F16.151
        inhalant F18.151
        opioid F11.151
        sedative, anxiolytic or hypnotic
          F13.151
        stimulant NEC F15.151
      dependence F19.251
        cannabis F12.251
        cocaine F14.251
        hallucinogen F16.251
        inhalant F18.251
        opioid F11.251
        sedative, anxiolytic or hypnotic
          F13.251
        stimulant NEC F15.251
    inhalant F18.951
    opioid F11.951
    sedative, anxiolytic or hypnotic F13.951
    stimulant NEC F15.951
  organic F06.0

Hallux
  deformity (acquired) NEC M20.5X-
  limitus M20.5X-
  malleus (acquired) NEC M20.3-
  rigidus (acquired) M20.2-
    congenital Q74.2
    sequelae (late effect) of rickets E64.3
  valgus (acquired) M20.1-
    congenital Q66.6
  varus (acquired) M20.3-
    congenital Q66.3
Halo, visual H53.19
Hamartoma, hamartoblastoma Q85.9
  epithelial (gingival), odontogenic, central
    or peripheral —see Cyst, calcifying
    odontogenic
Hamartosis Q85.9
Hamman-Rich syndrome J84.114
Hammer toe (acquired) NEC —see also
  Deformity, toe, hammer toe
  congenital Q66.89
  sequelae (late effect) of rickets E64.3
Hand —see condition
Hand-foot syndrome L27.1
Handicap, handicapped
  educational Z55.9
    specified NEC Z55.8
Hand-Schüller-Christian disease or syndrome
  C96.5
Hanging (asphyxia) (strangulation)
  (suffocation) —see Asphyxia, traumatic,
  due to mechanical threat
Hangnail —see also Cellulitis, digit
  with lymphangitis —see Lymphangitis, acute,
    digit
Hangover (alcohol) F10.129
Hanhart's syndrome Q87.0
Hanot-Chauffard (-Troisier) syndrome E83.19
Hanot's cirrhosis or disease K74.3
Hansen's disease —see Leprosy
Hantaan virus disease (Korean hemorrhagic
  fever) A98.5
Hantavirus disease (with renal manifestations)
  (Dobrava) (Puumala) (Seoul) A98.5
  with pulmonary manifestations (Andes)
    (Bayou) (Bermejo) (Black Creek Canal)
    (Choclo) (Juquitiba) (Laguna negra)
    (Lechiguanas) (New York) (Oran) (Sin
    nombre) B33.4
Happy puppet syndrome Q93.5
Harada's disease or syndrome H30.81-
Hardening
  artery —see Arteriosclerosis
  brain G93.89
Harelip (complete) (incomplete) —see Cleft, lip
Harlequin (newborn) Q80.4
Harley's disease D59.6
Harmful use (of)
  alcohol F10.10
  anxiolytics —see Abuse, drug, sedative
  cannabinoids —see Abuse, drug, cannabis
  cocaine —see Abuse, drug, cocaine
  drug —see Abuse, drug
  hallucinogens —see Abuse, drug,
    hallucinogen
  hypnotics —see Abuse, drug, sedative -
    opioids —see Abuse, drug, opioid
  PCP (phencyclidine) —see Abuse, drug,
    hallucinogen
  sedatives —see Abuse, drug, sedative
  stimulants NEC —see Abuse, drug, stimulant
Harris' lines —see Arrest, epiphyseal
Hartnup's disease E72.02
Harvester's lung J67.0
Harvesting ovum for in vitro fertilization
  Z31.83
Hashimoto's disease or thyroiditis E06.3
Hashitoxicosis (transient) E06.3
Hassal-Henle bodies or warts (cornea) H18.49
Haut mal —see Epilepsy, generalized, specified
  NEC

Haverhill fever A25.1
Hay fever —see also Fever, hay J30.1
Hayem-Widal syndrome D59.8
Haygarth's nodes M15.8
Haymaker's lung J67.0
Hb (abnormal)
  Bart's disease D56.0
  disease —see Disease, hemoglobin
  trait —see Trait
Head —see condition
Headache R51
  allergic NEC G44.89
  associated with sexual activity
    G44.82
  chronic daily R51
  cluster G44.009
    chronic G44.029
      intractable G44.021
      not intractable G44.029
    episodic G44.019
      intractable G44.011
      not intractable G44.019
    intractable G44.001
    not intractable G44.009
  cough (primary) G44.83
  daily chronic R51
  drug-induced NEC G44.40
    intractable G44.41
    not intractable G44.40
  exertional (primary) G44.84
  histamine G44.009
    intractable G44.001
    not intractable G44.009
  hypnic G44.81
  lumbar puncture G97.1
  medication overuse G44.40
    intractable G44.41
    not intractable G44.40
  menstrual —see Migraine, menstrual
  migraine (type) —see also Migraine
    G43.909
  nasal septum R51
  neuralgiform, short lasting unilateral, with
    conjunctival injection and tearing
    (SUNCT) G44.059
    intractable G44.051
    not intractable G44.059
  new daily persistent (NDPH) G44.52
  orgasmic G44.82
  periodic syndromes in adults and children
    G43.C0
    with refractory migraine G43.C1
    intractable G43.C1
    not intractable G43.C0
    without refractory migraine G43.C0
  postspinal puncture G97.1
  post-traumatic G44.309
    acute G44.319
      intractable G44.311
      not intractable G44.319
    chronic G44.329
      intractable G44.321
      not intractable G44.329
    intractable G44.301
    not intractable G44.309
  pre-menstrual —see Migraine, menstrual
  preorgasmic G44.82
  primary
    cough G44.83
    exertional G44.84
    stabbing G44.85
    thunderclap G44.53
  rebound G44.40
    intractable G44.41
    not intractable G44.40
  short lasting unilateral neuralgiform, with
    conjunctival injection and tearing
    (SUNCT) G44.059
    intractable G44.051
    not intractable G44.059
  specified syndrome NEC G44.89

◀ New   ◀▦ Revised   ~~deleted~~ Deleted

Headache *(Continued)*
  spinal and epidural anesthesia - induced
    T88.59
    in labor and delivery O74.5
    in pregnancy O29.4-
    postpartum, puerperal O89.4
  spinal fluid loss (from puncture) G97.1
  stabbing (primary) G44.85
  tension (-type) G44.209
    chronic G44.229
      intractable G44.221
      not intractable G44.229
    episodic G44.219
      intractable G44.211
      not intractable G44.219
    intractable G44.201
    not intractable G44.209
  thunderclap (primary) G44.53
  vascular NEC G44.1
Healthy
  infant
    accompanying sick mother Z76.3
    receiving care Z76.2
  person accompanying sick person Z76.3
Hearing examination Z01.10
  with abnormal findings NEC Z01.118
  following failed hearing screening Z01.110
  for hearing conservation and treatment
    Z01.12
Heart —*see* condition
Heart beat
  abnormality R00.9
    specified NEC R00.8
  awareness R00.2
  rapid R00.0
  slow R00.1
Heartburn R12
  psychogenic F45.8
Heat (effects) T67.9
  apoplexy T67.0
  burn —*see also* Burn L55.9
  collapse T67.1
  cramps T67.2
  dermatitis or eczema L59.0
  edema T67.7
  erythema - code by site under Burn, first
    degree
  excessive T67.9
    specified effect NEC T67.8
  exhaustion T67.5
    anhydrotic T67.3
    due to
      salt (and water) depletion T67.4
      water depletion T67.3
        with salt depletion T67.4
  fatigue (transient) T67.6
  fever T67.0
  hyperpyrexia T67.0
  prickly L74.0
  prostration —*see* Heat, exhaustion
  pyrexia T67.0
  rash L74.0
  specified effect NEC T67.8
  stroke T67.0
  sunburn —*see* Sunburn
  syncope T67.1
Heavy-for-dates NEC (infant) (4000g to 4499g)
  P08.1
  exceptionally (4500g or more) P08.0
Hebephrenia, hebephrenic (schizophrenia)
  F20.1
Heberden's disease or nodes (with
  arthropathy) M15.1
Hebra's
  pityriasis L26
  prurigo L28.2
Heel —*see* condition
Heerfordt's disease D86.89
Hegglin's anomaly or syndrome D72.0
Heilmeyer-Schoner disease D45
Heine-Medin disease A80.9

Heinz body anemia, congenital D58.2
Heliophobia F40.228
Heller's disease or syndrome F84.3
HELLP syndrome (hemolysis, elevated liver
  enzymes and low platelet count) O14.2-
  complicating ◄
    childbirth O14.24 ◄
    puerperium O14.25 ◄
Helminthiasis —*see also* Infestation, helminth
  Ancylostoma B76.0
  intestinal B82.0
    mixed types (types classifiable to more
      than one of the titles B65.0-B81.3 and
      B81.8) B81.4
    specified type NEC B81.8
  mixed types (intestinal) (types classifiable to
    more than one of the titles B65.0-B81.3
    and B81.8) B81.4
  Necator (americanus) B76.1
  specified type NEC B83.8
Heloma L84
Hemangioblastoma —*see* Neoplasm,
  connective tissue, uncertain behavior
  malignant —*see* Neoplasm, connective tissue,
    malignant
Hemangioendothelioma —*see also* Neoplasm,
  uncertain behavior, by site
  benign D18.00
    intra-abdominal D18.03
    intracranial D18.02
    skin D18.01
    specified site NEC D18.09
  bone (diffuse) —*see* Neoplasm, bone,
    malignant
  epithelioid —*see also* Neoplasm, uncertain
    behavior, by site
    malignant —*see* Neoplasm, malignant, by
      site
  malignant —*see* Neoplasm, connective tissue,
    malignant
Hemangiofibroma —*see* Neoplasm, benign,
  by site
Hemangiolipoma —*see* Lipoma
Hemangioma D18.00
  arteriovenous D18.00
    intra-abdominal D18.03
    intracranial D18.02
    skin D18.01
    specified site NEC D18.09
  capillary D18.00
    intra-abdominal D18.03
    intracranial D18.02
    skin D18.01
    specified site NEC D18.09
  cavernous D18.00
    intra-abdominal D18.03
    intracranial D18.02
    skin D18.01
    specified site NEC D18.09
  epithelioid D18.00
    intra-abdominal D18.03
    intracranial D18.02
    skin D18.01
    specified site NEC D18.09
  histiocytoid D18.00
    intra-abdominal D18.03
    intracranial D18.02
    skin D18.01
    specified site NEC D18.09
  infantile D18.00
    intra-abdominal D18.03
    intracranial D18.02
    skin D18.01
    specified site NEC D18.09
  intra-abdominal D18.03
  intracranial D18.02
  intramuscular D18.00
    intra-abdominal D18.03
    intracranial D18.02
    skin D18.01
    specified site NEC D18.09

Hemangioma *(Continued)*
  intrathoracic structures D18.09 ◄
  juvenile D18.00
  malignant —*see* Neoplasm, connective tissue,
    malignant
  plexiform D18.00
    intra-abdominal D18.03
    intracranial D18.02
    skin D18.01
    specified site NEC D18.09
  racemose D18.00
    intra-abdominal D18.03
    intracranial D18.02
    skin D18.01
    specified site NEC D18.09
  sclerosing —*see* Neoplasm, skin, benign
  simplex D18.00
    intra-abdominal D18.03
    intracranial D18.02
    skin D18.01
    specified site NEC D18.09
  skin D18.01
  specified site NEC D18.09
  venous D18.00
    intra-abdominal D18.03
    intracranial D18.02
    skin D18.01
    specified site NEC D18.09
  verrucous keratotic D18.00
    intra-abdominal D18.03
    intracranial D18.02
    skin D18.01
    specified site NEC D18.09
Hemangiomatosis (systemic) I78.8
  involving single site —*see* Hemangioma
Hemangiopericytoma —*see also* Neoplasm,
  connective tissue, uncertain behavior
  benign —*see* Neoplasm, connective tissue,
    benign
  malignant —*see* Neoplasm, connective tissue,
    malignant
Hemangiosarcoma —*see* Neoplasm, connective
  tissue, malignant
Hemarthrosis (nontraumatic) M25.00
  ankle M25.07-
  elbow M25.02-
  foot joint M25.07-
  hand joint M25.04-
  hip M25.05-
  in hemophilic arthropathy —*see* Arthropathy,
    hemophilic
  knee M25.06-
  shoulder M25.01-
  specified joint NEC M25.08
  traumatic —*see* Sprain, by site
  vertebrae M25.08
  wrist M25.03-
Hematemesis K92.0
  with ulcer - code by site under Ulcer, with
    hemorrhage K27.4
  newborn, neonatal P54.0
    due to swallowed maternal blood
      P78.2
Hematidrosis L74.8
Hematinuria —*see also* Hemoglobinuria
  malarial B50.8
Hematobilia K83.8
Hematocele
  female NEC N94.89
    with ectopic pregnancy O00.90 ◄▥
      with intrauterine pregnancy O00.91 ◄
    ovary N83.8
  male N50.1
Hematochezia —*see also* Melena K92.1
Hematochyluria —*see also* Infestation, filarial
  schistosomiasis (bilharziasis) B65.0
Hematocolpos (with hematometra or
  hematosalpinx) N89.7
Hematocornea —*see* Pigmentation, cornea,
  stromal
Hematogenous —*see* condition

Hematoma (traumatic) (skin surface intact) —
   see also Contusion
   with
      injury of internal organs —*see* Injury, by site
      open wound —*see* Wound, open
   amputation stump (surgical) (late) T87.89
   aorta, dissecting I71.00
      abdominal I71.02
      thoracic I71.01
      thoracoabdominal I71.03
   aortic intramural —*see* Dissection, aorta
   arterial (complicating trauma) —*see* Injury,
      blood vessel, by site
   auricle —*see* Contusion, ear
      nontraumatic —*see* Disorder, pinna,
         hematoma
   birth injury NEC P15.8
   brain (traumatic)
      with
         cerebral laceration or contusion
            (diffuse) —*see* Injury, intracranial,
               diffuse
            focal —*see* Injury, intracranial, focal
      cerebellar, traumatic S06.37-
      intracerebral, traumatic —*see* Injury,
         intracranial, intracerebral
         hemorrhage
      newborn NEC P52.4
         birth injury P10.1
      nontraumatic —*see* Hemorrhage,
         intracranial
      subarachnoid, arachnoid, traumatic —*see*
         Injury, intracranial, subarachnoid
         hemorrhage
      subdural, traumatic —*see* Injury,
         intracranial, subdural hemorrhage
   breast (nontraumatic) N64.89
   broad ligament (nontraumatic) N83.7
      traumatic S37.892
   cerebellar, traumatic S06.37-
   cerebral —*see* Hematoma, brain
   cerebrum S06.36-
      left S06.35-
      right S06.34-
   cesarean delivery wound O90.2
   complicating delivery (perineal) (pelvic)
      (vagina) (vulva) O71.7
   corpus cavernosum (nontraumatic) N48.89
   epididymis (nontraumatic) N50.1
   epidural (traumatic) —*see* Injury, intracranial,
      epidural hemorrhage
      spinal —*see* Injury, spinal cord, by region
   episiotomy O90.2
   face, birth injury P15.4
   genital organ NEC (nontraumatic)
      female (nonobstetric) N94.89
         traumatic S30.202
      male N50.1
         traumatic S30.201
   internal organs —*see* Injury, by site
   intracerebral, traumatic —*see* Injury,
      intracranial, intracerebral hemorrhage
   intraoperative —*see* Complications,
      intraoperative, hemorrhage
   labia (nontraumatic) (nonobstetric) N90.8
   liver (subcapsular) (nontraumatic) K76.89
      birth injury P15.0
   mediastinum —*see* Injury, intrathoracic
   mesosalpinx (nontraumatic) N83.7
      traumatic S37.898
   muscle - code by site under Contusion
   nontraumatic
      muscle M79.81
      soft tissue M79.81
   obstetrical surgical wound O90.2
   orbit, orbital (nontraumatic) —*see also*
      Hemorrhage, orbit
      traumatic —*see* Contusion, orbit
   pelvis (female) (nontraumatic) (nonobstetric)
      N94.89
      obstetric O71.7
      traumatic —*see* Injury, by site

Hematoma (Continued)
   penis (nontraumatic) N48.89
      birth injury P15.5
   perianal (nontraumatic) K64.5
   perineal S30.23
      complicating delivery O71.7
   perirenal —*see* Injury, kidney
   pinna —*see* Contusion, ear
      nontraumatic —*see* Disorder, pinna,
         hematoma
   placenta O43.89-
   postoperative (postprocedural) —*see*
      Complication, postprocedural,
      hematoma ◀▥
   retroperitoneal (nontraumatic) K66.1
      traumatic S36.892
   scrotum, superficial S30.22
      birth injury P15.5
   seminal vesicle (nontraumatic) N50.1
      traumatic S37.892
   spermatic cord (traumatic) S37.892
      nontraumatic N50.1
   spinal (cord) (meninges) —*see also* Injury,
      spinal cord, by region
      newborn (birth injury) P11.5
   spleen D73.5
      intraoperative —*see* Complications,
         intraoperative, hemorrhage, spleen
      postprocedural (postoperative) —*see*
         Complications, postprocedural,
         hemorrhage, spleen
   sternocleidomastoid, birth injury P15.2
   sternomastoid, birth injury P15.2
   subarachnoid (traumatic) —*see* Injury,
      intracranial, subarachnoid hemorrhage
      newborn (nontraumatic) P52.5
         due to birth injury P10.3
      nontraumatic —*see* Hemorrhage,
         intracranial, subarachnoid
   subdural (traumatic) —*see* Injury, intracranial,
      subdural hemorrhage
      newborn (localized) P52.8
         birth injury P10.0
      nontraumatic —*see* Hemorrhage,
         intracranial, subdural
   superficial, newborn P54.5
   testis (nontraumatic) N50.1
      birth injury P15.5
   tunica vaginalis (nontraumatic) N50.1
   umbilical cord, complicating delivery
      O69.5
   uterine ligament (broad) (nontraumatic)
      N83.7
      traumatic S37.892
   vagina (ruptured) (nontraumatic) N89.8
      complicating delivery O71.7
   vas deferens (nontraumatic) N50.1
      traumatic S37.892
   vitreous —*see* Hemorrhage, vitreous
   vulva (nontraumatic) (nonobstetric) N90.89
      complicating delivery O71.7
      newborn (birth injury) P15.5
Hematometra N85.7
   with hematocolpos N89.7
Hematomyelia (central) G95.19
   newborn (birth injury) P11.5
   traumatic T14.8
Hematomyelitis G04.90
Hematoperitoneum —*see* Hemoperitoneum
Hematophobia F40.230
Hematopneumothorax (*see* Hemothorax)
Hematopoiesis, cyclic D70.4
Hematoporphyria —*see* Porphyria
Hematorachis, hematorrhachis G95.19
   newborn (birth injury) P11.5
Hematosalpinx N83.6
   with
      hematocolpos N89.7
      hematometra N85.7
         with hematocolpos N89.7
   infectional —*see* Salpingitis

Hematospermia R36.1
Hematothorax (*see* Hemothorax)
Hematuria R31.9
   benign (familial) (of childhood) —*see also*
      Hematuria, idiopathic
      essential microscopic R31.1
   due to sulphonamide, sulfonamide —*see* Table
      of Drugs and Chemicals, by drug
   endemic —*see also* Schistosomiasis B65.0
   gross R31.0
   idiopathic N02.9
      with glomerular lesion
         crescentic (diffuse) glomerulonephritis
            N02.7
         dense deposit disease N02.6
         endocapillary proliferative
            glomerulonephritis N02.4
         focal and segmental hyalinosis or
            sclerosis N02.1
         membranoproliferative (diffuse) N02.5
         membranous (diffuse) N02.2
         mesangial proliferative (diffuse) N02.3
         mesangiocapillary (diffuse) N02.5
         minor abnormality N02.0
         proliferative NEC N02.8
         specified pathology NEC N02.8
   intermittent —*see* Hematuria, idiopathic
   malarial B50.8
   microscopic NEC (with symptoms) R31.29 ◀▥
      asymptomatic R31.21 ◀
      benign essential R31.1
   paroxysmal —*see also* Hematuria, idiopathic
      nocturnal D59.5
   persistent —*see* Hematuria, idiopathic
   recurrent —*see* Hematuria, idiopathic
   tropical —*see also* Schistosomiasis B65.0
   tuberculous A18.13
Hemeralopia (day blindness) H53.11
   vitamin A deficiency E50.5
Hemi-akinesia R41.4
Hemianalgesia R20.0
Hemianencephaly Q00.0
Hemianesthesia R20.0
Hemianopia, hemianopsia (heteronymous)
   H53.47
   homonymous H53.46-
   syphilitic A52.71
Hemiathetosis R25.8
Hemiatrophy R68.89
   cerebellar G31.9
   face, facial, progressive (Romberg) G51.8
   tongue K14.8
Hemiballism (us) G25.5
Hemicardia Q24.8
Hemicephalus, hemicephaly Q00.0
Hemichorea G25.5
Hemicolitis, left —*see* Colitis, left sided
Hemicrania
   congenital malformation Q00.0
   continua G44.51
   meaning migraine —*see also* Migraine G43.909
   paroxysmal G44.039
      chronic G44.049
         intractable G44.041
         not intractable G44.049
      episodic G44.039
         intractable G44.031
         not intractable G44.039
      intractable G44.031
      not intractable G44.039
Hemidystrophy —*see* Hemiatrophy
Hemiectromelia Q73.8
Hemihypalgesia R20.8
Hemihypesthesia R20.1
Hemi-inattention R41.4
Hemimelia Q73.8
   lower limb —*see* Defect, reduction, lower
      limb, specified type NEC
   upper limb —*see* Defect, reduction, upper
      limb, specified type NEC
Hemiparalysis —*see* Hemiplegia
Hemiparesis —*see* Hemiplegia

◀ New   ◀▥ Revised   ~~deleted~~ Deleted

Hemiparesthesia R20.2
Hemiparkinsonism G20
Hemiplegia G81.9-
  alternans facialis G83.89
  ascending NEC G81.90
    spinal G95.89
  congenital (cerebral) G80.8
    spastic G80.2
  embolic (current episode) I63.4-
  flaccid G81.0-
  following
    cerebrovascular disease I69.959
      cerebral infarction I69.35-
      intracerebral hemorrhage I69.15-
      nontraumatic intracranial hemorrhage
        NEC I69.25-
      specified disease NEC I69.85-
      stroke NOS I69.35-
      subarachnoid hemorrhage I69.05-
  hysterical F44.4
  newborn NEC P91.8
    birth injury P11.9
  spastic G81.1-
    congenital G80.2
  thrombotic (current episode) I63.3- ◄▥
Hemisection, spinal cord —see Injury, spinal
    cord, by region
Hemispasm (facial) R25.2
Hemisporosis B48.8
Hemitremor R25.1
Hemivertebra Q76.49
  failure of segmentation with scoliosis Q76.3
  fusion with scoliosis Q76.3
Hemochromatosis E83.119
  with refractory anemia D46.1
  due to repeated red blood cell transfusion
    E83.111
  hereditary (primary) E83.110
  primary E83.110
  specified NEC E83.118
Hemoglobin —see also condition
  abnormal (disease) —see Disease, hemoglobin
  AS genotype D57.3
  Constant Spring D58.2
  E-beta thalassemia D56.5
  fetal, hereditary persistence (HPFH) D56.4
  H Constant Spring D56.0
  low NOS D64.9
  S (Hb S), heterozygous D57.3
Hemoglobinemia D59.9
  due to blood transfusion T80.89
  paroxysmal D59.6
    nocturnal D59.5
Hemoglobinopathy (mixed) D58.2
  with thalassemia D56.8
  sickle-cell D57.1
    with thalassemia D57.40
      with crisis (vasoocclusive pain) D57.419
        with
          acute chest syndrome D57.411
          splenic sequestration D57.412
        without crisis D57.40
Hemoglobinuria R82.3
  with anemia, hemolytic, acquired (chronic)
    NEC D59.6
  cold (agglutinin) (paroxysmal) (with
    Raynaud's syndrome) D59.6
  due to exertion or hemolysis NEC D59.6
  intermittent D59.6
  malarial B50.8
  march D59.6
  nocturnal (paroxysmal) D59.5
  paroxysmal (cold) D59.6
    nocturnal D59.5
Hemolymphangioma D18.1
Hemolysis
  intravascular
    with
      abortion —see Abortion, by type,
        complicated by, hemorrhage
      ectopic or molar pregnancy O08.1

Hemolysis (Continued)
  intravascular (Continued)
    with (Continued)
      hemorrhage
        antepartum —see Hemorrhage,
          antepartum, with coagulation
          defect
        intrapartum —see also Hemorrhage,
          complicating, delivery O67.0
        postpartum O72.3
    neonatal (excessive) P58.9
      specified NEC P58.8
Hemolytic —see condition
Hemopericardium I31.2
  following acute myocardial infarction
    (current complication) I23.0
  newborn P54.8
  traumatic —see Injury, heart, with
    hemopericardium
Hemoperitoneum K66.1
  infectional K65.9
  traumatic S36.899
    with open wound —see Wound, open, with
      penetration into peritoneal cavity
Hemophilia (classical) (familial) (hereditary)
    D66
  A D66
  B D67
  C D68.1
  acquired D68.311
  autoimmune D68.311
  calcipriva —see also Defect, coagulation D68.4
  nonfamilial —see also Defect, coagulation
    D68.4
  secondary D68.311
  vascular D68.0
Hemophthalmos H44.81-
Hemopneumothorax —see also Hemothorax
  traumatic S27.2
Hemoptysis R04.2
  newborn P26.9
  tuberculous —see Tuberculosis, pulmonary
Hemorrhage, hemorrhagic (concealed) R58
  abdomen R58
  accidental antepartum —see Hemorrhage,
    antepartum
  acute idiopathic pulmonary, in infants
    R04.81
  adenoid J35.8
  adrenal (capsule) (gland) E27.49
    medulla E27.8
    newborn P54.4
  after delivery —see Hemorrhage, postpartum
  alveolar
    lung, newborn P26.8
    process K08.89 ◄▥
  alveolus K08.89 ◄▥
  amputation stump (surgical) T87.89
  anemia (chronic) D50.0
    acute D62
  antepartum (with) O46.90
    with coagulation defect O46.00-
      afibrinogenemia O46.01-
      disseminated intravascular coagulation
        O46.02-
      hypofibrinogenemia O46.01-
      specified defect NEC O46.09-
    before 20 weeks gestation O20.9
      specified type NEC O20.8
      threatened abortion O20.0
    due to
      abruptio placenta —see also Abruptio
        placentae O45.9-
      leiomyoma, uterus —see Hemorrhage,
        antepartum, specified cause NEC
      placenta previa O44.1-
    specified cause NEC —see subcategory
      O46.8X-
  anus (sphincter) K62.5
  apoplexy (stroke) —see Hemorrhage,
    intracranial, intracerebral

Hemorrhage, hemorrhagic (Continued)
  arachnoid —see Hemorrhage, intracranial,
    subarachnoid
  artery R58
    brain —see Hemorrhage, intracranial,
      intracerebral
  basilar (ganglion) I61.0
  bladder N32.89
  bowel K92.2
    newborn P54.3
  brain (miliary) (nontraumatic) —see
    Hemorrhage, intracranial, intracerebral
    due to
      birth injury P10.1
      syphilis A52.05
    epidural or extradural (traumatic) —
      see Injury, intracranial, epidural
      hemorrhage
    newborn P52.4
      birth injury P10.1
    subarachnoid —see Hemorrhage,
      intracranial, subarachnoid
    subdural —see Hemorrhage, intracranial,
      subdural
  brainstem (nontraumatic) I61.3
    traumatic S06.38-
  breast N64.59
  bronchial tube —see Hemorrhage, lung
  bronchopulmonary —see Hemorrhage, lung
  bronchus —see Hemorrhage, lung
  bulbar I61.5
  capillary I78.8
    primary D69.8
  cecum K92.2
  cerebellar, cerebellum (nontraumatic) I61.4
    newborn P52.6
    traumatic S06.37-
  cerebral, cerebrum —see also Hemorrhage,
    intracranial, intracerebral
    lobe I61.1
    newborn (anoxic) P52.4
      birth injury P10.1
  cerebromeningeal I61.8
  cerebrospinal —see Hemorrhage, intracranial,
    intracerebral
  cervix (uteri) (stump) NEC N88.8
  chamber, anterior (eye) —see Hyphema
  childbirth —see Hemorrhage, complicating,
    delivery
  choroid H31.30-
    expulsive H31.31-
  ciliary body —see Hyphema
  cochlea —see subcategory H83.8
  colon K92.2
  complicating
    abortion —see Abortion, by type,
      complicated by, hemorrhage
    delivery O67.9
      associated with coagulation defect
        (afibrinogenemia) (DIC)
        (hyperfibrinolysis) O67.0
      specified cause NEC O67.8
    surgical procedure —see Hemorrhage,
      intraoperative
  conjunctiva H11.3-
    newborn P54.8
  cord, newborn (stump) P51.9
  corpus luteum (ruptured) cyst N83.1- ◄▥
  cortical (brain) I61.1
  cranial —see Hemorrhage, intracranial
  cutaneous R23.3
    due to autosensitivity, erythrocyte D69.2
    newborn P54.5
  delayed
    following ectopic or molar pregnancy
      O08.1
    postpartum O72.2
  diathesis (familial) D69.9
  disease D69.9
    newborn P53
    specified type NEC D69.8

Hemorrhage, hemorrhagic (Continued)
  due to or associated with
    afibrinogenemia or other coagulation defect
      (conditions in categories D65-D69)
      antepartum —see Hemorrhage,
        antepartum, with coagulation
        defect
      intrapartum O67.0
    dental implant M27.61
    device, implant or graft —see also
      Complications, by site and type,
      specified NEC T85.838 ◄▦
      arterial graft NEC T82.838
      breast T85.838 ◄▦
      catheter NEC T85.838 ◄▦
        dialysis (renal) T82.838
          intraperitoneal T85.838 ◄▦
        infusion NEC T82.838
          spinal (epidural) (subdural)
            T85.830 ◄▦
        urinary (indwelling) T83.83
      electronic (electrode) (pulse generator)
        (stimulator)
        bone T84.83
        cardiac T82.837
        nervous system (brain) (peripheral
          nerve) (spinal) T85.830 ◄▦
        urinary T83.83
      fixation, internal (orthopedic) NEC T84.83
      gastrointestinal (bile duct) (esophagus)
        T85.838 ◄▦
      genital NEC T83.83
      heart NEC T82.837
      joint prosthesis T84.83
      ocular (corneal graft) (orbital implant)
        NEC T85.838 ◄▦
      orthopedic NEC T84.83
        bone graft T86.838
      specified NEC T85.838 ◄▦
      urinary T83.83
      vascular NEC T82.838
      ventricular intracranial shunt T85.838 ◄▦
  duodenum, duodenal K92.2
    ulcer —see Ulcer, duodenum, with
      hemorrhage
  dura mater —see Hemorrhage, intracranial,
    subdural
  endotracheal —see Hemorrhage, lung
  epicranial subaponeurotic (massive), birth
    injury P12.2
  epidural (traumatic) —see also Injury,
    intracranial, epidural hemorrhage
    nontraumatic I62.1
  esophagus K22.8
    varix I85.01
      secondary I85.11
  excessive, following ectopic gestation
    (subsequent episode) O08.1
  extradural (traumatic) —see Injury,
    intracranial, epidural hemorrhage
    birth injury P10.8
    newborn (anoxic) (nontraumatic) P52.8
    nontraumatic I62.1
  eye NEC H57.8
    fundus —see Hemorrhage, retina
    lid —see Disorder, eyelid, specified type
      NEC
  fallopian tube N83.6
  fibrinogenolysis —see Fibrinolysis
  fibrinolytic (acquired) —see Fibrinolysis
  from
    ear (nontraumatic) —see Otorrhagia
    tracheostomy stoma J95.01
  fundus, eye —see Hemorrhage, retina
  funis —see Hemorrhage, umbilicus, cord
  gastric —see Hemorrhage, stomach
  gastroenteric K92.2
    newborn P54.3
  gastrointestinal (tract) K92.2
    newborn P54.3
  genital organ, male N50.1

Hemorrhage, hemorrhagic (Continued)
  genitourinary (tract) NOS R31.9
  gingiva K06.8
  globe (eye) —see Hemophthalmos
  graafian follicle cyst (ruptured) N83.0- ◄▦
  gum K06.8
  heart I51.89
  hypopharyngeal (throat) R04.1
  intermenstrual (regular) N92.3
    irregular N92.1
  internal (organs) NEC R58
    capsule I61.0
    ear —see subcategory H83.8
    newborn P54.8
  intestine K92.2
    newborn P54.3
  intra-abdominal R58
  intra-alveolar (lung), newborn P26.8
  intracerebral (nontraumatic) —see
    Hemorrhage, intracranial,
    intracerebral
  intracranial (nontraumatic) I62.9
    birth injury P10.9
    epidural, nontraumatic I62.1
    extradural, nontraumatic I62.1
    intracerebral (nontraumatic) (in) I61.9
      brain stem I61.3
      cerebellum I61.4
      hemisphere I61.2
        cortical (superficial) I61.1
        subcortical (deep) I61.0
      intraoperative
        during a nervous system procedure
          G97.31
        during other procedure G97.32
      intraventricular I61.5
      multiple localized I61.6
      newborn P52.4
        birth injury P10.1
      postprocedural
        following a nervous system procedure
          G97.51
        following other procedure
          G97.52
      specified NEC I61.8
      superficial I61.1
      traumatic (diffuse) —see Injury,
        intracranial, diffuse
      focal —see Injury, intracranial, focal
    newborn P52.9
      specified NEC P52.8
    subarachnoid (nontraumatic) (from)
      I60.9
      intracranial (cerebral) artery I60.7
        anterior communicating I60.2 ◄▦
        basilar I60.4
        carotid siphon and bifurcation
          I60.0-
        communicating I60.7
          anterior I60.2 ◄▦
          posterior I60.3-
        middle cerebral I60.1-
        posterior communicating I60.3-
        specified artery NEC I60.6
        vertebral I60.5-
      newborn P52.5
        birth injury P10.3
      specified NEC I60.8
      traumatic S06.6X-
    subdural (nontraumatic) I62.00
      acute I62.01
      birth injury P10.0
      chronic I62.03
      newborn (anoxic) (hypoxic) P52.8
        birth injury P10.0
      spinal G95.19
      subacute I62.02
      traumatic —see Injury, intracranial,
        subdural hemorrhage
    traumatic —see Injury, intracranial, focal
      brain injury

Hemorrhage, hemorrhagic (Continued)
  intramedullary NEC G95.19
  intraocular —see Hemophthalmos
  intraoperative, intraprocedural —see
    Complication, hemorrhage (hematoma),
    intraoperative (intraprocedural), by site
  intrapartum —see Hemorrhage, complicating,
    delivery
  intrapelvic
    female N94.89
    male K66.1
  intraperitoneal K66.1
  intrapontine I61.3
  intraprocedural —see Complication,
    hemorrhage (hematoma), intraoperative
    (intraprocedural), by site
  intrauterine N85.7
    complicating delivery —see also Hemorrhage,
      complicating, delivery O67.9
    postpartum —see Hemorrhage, postpartum
  intraventricular I61.5
    newborn (nontraumatic) —see also Newborn,
      affected by, hemorrhage P52.3
      due to birth injury P10.2
      grade
        1 P52.0
        2 P52.1
        3 P52.21
        4 P52.22
  intravesical N32.89
  iris (postinfectional) (postinflammatory)
    (toxic) —see Hyphema
  joint (nontraumatic) —see Hemarthrosis
  kidney N28.89
  knee (joint) (nontraumatic) —see
    Hemarthrosis, knee
  labyrinth —see subcategory H83.8
  lenticular striate artery I61.0
  ligature, vessel —see Hemorrhage,
    postoperative
  liver K76.89
  lung R04.89
    newborn P26.9
      massive P26.1
      specified NEC P26.8
    tuberculous —see Tuberculosis, pulmonary
  massive umbilical, newborn P51.0
  mediastinum —see Hemorrhage, lung
  medulla I61.3
  membrane (brain) I60.8
    spinal cord —see Hemorrhage, spinal cord
  meninges, meningeal (brain) (middle) I60.8
    spinal cord —see Hemorrhage, spinal cord
  mesentery K66.1
  metritis —see Endometritis
  mouth K13.79
  mucous membrane NEC R58
    newborn P54.8
  muscle M62.89
  nail (subungual) L60.8
  nasal turbinate R04.0
    newborn P54.8
  navel, newborn P51.9
  newborn P54.9
    specified NEC P54.8
  nipple N64.59
  nose R04.0
    newborn P54.8
  omentum K66.1
  optic nerve (sheath) H47.02-
  orbit, orbital H05.23-
  ovary NEC N83.8
  oviduct N83.6
  pancreas K86.89 ◄▦
  parathyroid (gland) (spontaneous) E21.4
  parturition —see Hemorrhage, complicating,
    delivery
  penis N48.89
  pericardium, pericarditis I31.2
  peritoneum, peritoneal K66.1
  peritonsillar tissue J35.8
    due to infection J36

Hemorrhage, hemorrhagic (Continued)
petechial R23.3
due to autosensitivity, erythrocyte D69.2
pituitary (gland) E23.6
pleura —see Hemorrhage, lung
polioencephalitis, superior E51.2
polymyositis —see Polymyositis
pons, pontine I61.3
posterior fossa (nontraumatic) I61.8
newborn P52.6
postmenopausal N95.0
postnasal R04.0
postoperative —see Complications,
postprocedural, hemorrhage, by site
postpartum NEC (following delivery of
placenta) O72.1
delayed or secondary O72.2
retained placenta O72.0
third stage O72.0
pregnancy —see Hemorrhage, antepartum
preretinal —see Hemorrhage, retina
prostate N42.1
puerperal —see Hemorrhage, postpartum
delayed or secondary O72.2
pulmonary R04.89
newborn P26.9
massive P26.1
specified NEC P26.8
tuberculous —see Tuberculosis, pulmonary
purpura (primary) D69.3
rectum (sphincter) K62.5
newborn P54.2
recurring, following initial hemorrhage at
time of injury T79.2
renal N28.89
respiratory passage or tract R04.9
specified NEC R04.89
retina, retinal (vessels) H35.6-
diabetic —see Diabetes, retinal, hemorrhage
retroperitoneal R58
scalp R58
scrotum N50.1
secondary (nontraumatic) R58
following initial hemorrhage at time of
injury T79.2
seminal vesicle N50.1
skin R23.3
newborn P54.5
slipped umbilical ligature P51.8
spermatic cord N50.1
spinal (cord) G95.19
newborn (birth injury) P11.5
spleen D73.5
intraoperative —see Complications,
intraoperative, hemorrhage, spleen
postprocedural —see Complications,
postprocedural, hemorrhage, spleen
stomach K92.2
newborn P54.3
ulcer —see Ulcer, stomach, with
hemorrhage
subarachnoid (nontraumatic) —see
Hemorrhage, intracranial, subarachnoid
subconjunctival —see also Hemorrhage,
conjunctiva
birth injury P15.3
subcortical (brain) I61.0
subcutaneous R23.3
subdiaphragmatic R58
subdural (acute) (nontraumatic) —see
Hemorrhage, intracranial, subdural
subependymal
newborn P52.0
with intraventricular extension P52.1
and intracerebral extension P52.22
subgaleal P12.2 ◀▥
subhyaloid —see Hemorrhage, retina
subperiosteal —see Disorder, bone, specified
type NEC
subretinal —see Hemorrhage, retina
subtentorial —see Hemorrhage, intracranial,
subdural

Hemorrhage, hemorrhagic (Continued)
subungual L60.8
suprarenal (capsule) (gland) E27.49
newborn P54.4
tentorium (traumatic) NEC —see
Hemorrhage, brain
newborn (birth injury) P10.4
testis N50.1
third stage (postpartum) O72.0
thorax —see Hemorrhage, lung
throat R04.1
thymus (gland) E32.8
thyroid (cyst) (gland) E07.89
tongue K14.8
tonsil J35.8
trachea —see Hemorrhage, lung
tracheobronchial R04.89
newborn P26.0
traumatic — code to specific injury
cerebellar —see Hemorrhage, brain
intracranial —see Hemorrhage, brain
recurring or secondary (following initial
hemorrhage at time of injury)
T79.2
tuberculous NEC —see also Tuberculosis,
pulmonary A15.0
tunica vaginalis N50.1
ulcer - code by site under Ulcer, with
hemorrhage K27.4
umbilicus, umbilical
cord
after birth, newborn P51.9
complicating delivery O69.5
newborn P51.9
massive P51.0
slipped ligature P51.8
stump P51.9
urethra (idiopathic) N36.8
uterus, uterine (abnormal) N93.9
climacteric N92.4
complicating delivery —see Hemorrhage,
complicating, delivery
dysfunctional or functional N93.8
intermenstrual (regular) N92.3
irregular N92.1
postmenopausal N95.0
postpartum —see Hemorrhage,
postpartum
preclimacteric or premenopausal N92.4
prepubertal N93.8
pubertal N92.2
vagina (abnormal) N93.9
newborn P54.6
vas deferens N50.1
vasa previa O69.4
ventricular I61.5
vesical N32.89
viscera NEC R58
newborn P54.8
vitreous (humor) (intraocular) H43.1-
vulva N90.89

Hemorrhoids (bleeding) (without mention of
degree) K64.9
1st degree (grade/stage I) (without prolapse
outside of anal canal) K64.0
2nd degree (grade/stage II) (that
prolapse with straining but retract
spontaneously) K64.1
3rd degree (grade/stage III) (that prolapse
with straining and require manual
replacement back inside anal canal)
K64.2
4th degree (grade/stage IV) (with prolapsed
tissue that cannot be manually replaced)
K64.3
complicating
pregnancy O22.4
puerperium O87.2
external K64.4
with
thrombosis K64.5

Hemorrhoids (Continued)
internal (without mention of degree) K64.8
prolapsed K64.8
skin tags
anus K64.4
residual K64.4
specified NEC K64.8
strangulated —see also Hemorrhoids, by
degree K64.8
thrombosed —see also Hemorrhoids, by
degree K64.5
ulcerated —see also Hemorrhoids, by degree
K64.8
Hemosalpinx N83.6
with
hematocolpos N89.7
hematometra N85.7
with hematocolpos N89.7
Hemosiderosis (dietary) E83.19
pulmonary, idiopathic E83.1 [J84.03]
transfusion T80.89
Hemothorax (bacterial) (nontuberculous) J94.2
newborn P54.8
traumatic S27.1
with pneumothorax S27.2
tuberculous NEC A15.6
Henoch (-Schönlein) disease or syndrome
(purpura) D69.0
Henpue, henpuye A66.6
Hepar lobatum (syphilitic) A52.74
Hepatalgia K76.89
Hepatitis K75.9
acute B17.9
with coma K72.01
with hepatic failure —see Failure, hepatic
alcoholic —see Hepatitis, alcoholic
infectious B15.9 ◀▥
with hepatic coma B15.0
non-viral K72.0 ◀
viral B17.9
alcoholic (acute) (chronic) K70.10
with ascites K70.11
amebic —see Abscess, liver, amebic
anicteric (viral) —see Hepatitis, viral
antigen-associated (HAA) —see Hepatitis, B
Australia-antigen (positive) —see Hepatitis, B
autoimmune K75.4
B B19.10
with hepatic coma B19.11
acute B16.9
with
delta-agent (coinfection) (without
hepatic coma) B16.1
with hepatic coma B16.0
hepatic coma (without delta-agent
coinfection) B16.2
chronic B18.1
with delta-agent B18.0
bacterial NEC K75.89
C (viral) B19.20
with hepatic coma B19.21
acute B17.10
with hepatic coma B17.11
chronic B18.2
catarrhal (acute) B15.9
with hepatic coma B15.0
cholangiolitic K75.89
cholestatic K75.89
chronic K73.9
active NEC K73.2
lobular NEC K73.1
persistent NEC K73.0
specified NEC K73.8
cytomegaloviral B25.1
due to ethanol (acute) (chronic) —see
Hepatitis, alcoholic
epidemic B15.9
with hepatic coma B15.0
fulminant NEC (viral) —see Hepatitis, viral
granulomatous NEC K75.3
herpesviral B00.81

Hepatitis (Continued)
history of
  B Z86.19
  C Z86.19
homologous serum —see Hepatitis, viral,
  type B
in (due to)
  mumps B26.81
  toxoplasmosis (acquired) B58.1
    congenital (active) P37.1 [K77]
infectious, infective B15.9 ◄▓
  ~~with hepatic coma B15.0~~
  acute (subacute) B17.9 ◄
  chronic B18.9 ◄
inoculation —see Hepatitis, viral, type B
interstitial (chronic) K74.69
lupoid NEC K75.2
malignant NEC (with hepatic failure)
  K72.90
  with coma K72.91
neonatal giant cell P59.29
neonatal (idiopathic) (toxic) P59.29
newborn P59.29
postimmunization —see Hepatitis, viral,
  type B
post-transfusion —see Hepatitis, viral, type B
reactive, nonspecific K75.2
serum —see Hepatitis, viral, type B
specified type NEC
  with hepatic failure —see Failure, hepatic
syphilitic (late) A52.74
  congenital (early) A50.08 [K77]
    late A50.59 [K77]
  secondary A51.45
toxic —see also Disease, liver, toxic K71.6
tuberculous A18.83
viral, virus B19.9
  with hepatic coma B19.0
  acute B17.9
  chronic B18.9
    specified NEC B18.8
    type
      B B18.1
        with delta-agent B18.0
      C B18.2
  congenital P35.3
  coxsackie B33.8 [K77]
  cytomegalic inclusion B25.1
  in remission, any type — code to Hepatitis,
    chronic, by type
  non-A, non-B B17.8
  specified type NEC (with or without coma)
    B17.8
  type
    A B15.9
      with hepatic coma B15.0
    B B19.10
      with hepatic coma B19.11
      acute B16.9
        with
          delta-agent (coinfection) (without
            hepatic coma) B16.1
            with hepatic coma B16.0
          hepatic coma (without delta-
            agent coinfection) B16.2
      chronic B18.1
        with delta-agent B18.0
    C B19.20
      with hepatic coma B19.21
      acute B17.10
        with hepatic coma B17.11
      chronic B18.2
    E B17.2
    non-A, non-B B17.8
Hepatization lung (acute) —see Pneumonia,
  lobar
Hepatoblastoma C22.2
Hepatocarcinoma C22.0
Hepatocholangiocarcinoma C22.0
Hepatocholangioma, benign D13.4
Hepatocholangitis K75.89

Hepatolenticular degeneration E83.01
Hepatoma (malignant) C22.0
benign D13.4
embryonal C22.0
Hepatomegaly —see also Hypertrophy, liver
with splenomegaly R16.2
congenital Q44.7
in mononucleosis
  gammaherpesviral B27.09
  infectious specified NEC B27.89
Hepatoptosis K76.89
**Hepatorenal syndrome following labor and
  delivery** O90.4
Hepatosis K76.89
Hepatosplenomegaly R16.2
hyperlipemic (Bürger-Grütz type) E78.3 [K77]
Hereditary —see condition
Heredodegeneration, macular —see Dystrophy,
  retina
Heredopathia atactica polyneuritiformis G60.1
Heredosyphilis —see Syphilis, congenital
Herlitz' syndrome Q81.1
Hermansky-Pudlak syndrome E70.331
Hermaphrodite, hermaphroditism (true) Q56.0
46,XX with streak gonads Q99.1
46,XX/46,XY Q99.0
46,XY with streak gonads Q99.1
chimera 46,XX/46,XY Q99.0
Hernia, hernial (acquired) (recurrent) K46.9
with
  gangrene —see Hernia, by site, with,
    gangrene
  incarceration —see Hernia, by site, with,
    obstruction
  irreducible —see Hernia, by site, with,
    obstruction
  obstruction —see Hernia, by site, with,
    obstruction
  strangulation —see Hernia, by site, with,
    obstruction
abdomen, abdominal K46.9
  with
    gangrene (and obstruction) K46.1
    obstruction K46.0
  femoral —see Hernia, femoral
  incisional —see Hernia, incisional
  inguinal —see Hernia, inguinal
  specified site NEC K45.8
    with
      gangrene (and obstruction) K45.1
      obstruction K45.0
  umbilical —see Hernia, umbilical
  wall —see Hernia, ventral
appendix —see Hernia, abdomen
bladder (mucosa) (sphincter)
  congenital (female) (male) Q79.51
  female —see Cystocele
  male N32.89
brain, congenital —see Encephalocele
cartilage, vertebra —see Displacement,
  intervertebral disc
cerebral, congenital —see also Encephalocele
  endaural Q01.8
ciliary body (traumatic) S05.2-
colon —see Hernia, abdomen
Cooper's —see Hernia, abdomen, specified
  site NEC
crural —see Hernia, femoral
diaphragm, diaphragmatic K44.9
  with
    gangrene (and obstruction) K44.1
    obstruction K44.0
  congenital Q79.0
direct (inguinal) —see Hernia, inguinal
diverticulum, intestine —see Hernia,
  abdomen
double (inguinal) —see Hernia, inguinal,
  bilateral
due to adhesions (with obstruction) K56.5
epigastric —see also Hernia, ventral K43.9
esophageal hiatus —see Hernia, hiatal

Hernia, hernial (Continued)
external (inguinal) —see Hernia, inguinal
fallopian tube N83.4- ◄▓
fascia M62.89
femoral K41.90
  with
    gangrene (and obstruction) K41.40
      not specified as recurrent K41.40
      recurrent K41.41
    obstruction K41.30
      not specified as recurrent K41.30
      recurrent K41.31
  bilateral K41.20
    with
      gangrene (and obstruction) K41.10
        not specified as recurrent K41.10
        recurrent K41.11
      obstruction K41.00
        not specified as recurrent K41.00
        recurrent K41.01
    not specified as recurrent K41.20
    recurrent K41.21
  not specified as recurrent K41.90
  recurrent K41.91
  unilateral K41.90
    with
      gangrene (and obstruction) K41.40
        not specified as recurrent K41.40
        recurrent K41.41
      obstruction K41.30
        not specified as recurrent K41.30
        recurrent K41.31
    not specified as recurrent K41.90
    recurrent K41.91
foramen magnum G93.5
  congenital Q01.8
funicular (umbilical) —see also Hernia,
  umbilicus
  spermatic (cord) —see Hernia, inguinal
gastrointestinal tract —see Hernia, abdomen
Hesselbach's —see Hernia, femoral, specified
  site NEC
hiatal (esophageal) (sliding) K44.9
  with
    gangrene (and obstruction) K44.1
    obstruction K44.0
  congenital Q40.1
hypogastric —see Hernia, ventral
incarcerated —see also Hernia, by site, with
  obstruction
  with gangrene —see Hernia, by site, with
    gangrene
incisional K43.92
  with
    gangrene (and obstruction) K43.1
    obstruction K43.0
indirect (inguinal) —see Hernia, inguinal
inguinal (direct) (external) (funicular)
  (indirect) (internal) (oblique) (scrotal)
  (sliding) K40.90
  with
    gangrene (and obstruction) K40.40
      not specified as recurrent K40.40
      recurrent K40.41
    obstruction K40.30
      not specified as recurrent K40.30
      recurrent K40.31
  bilateral K40.20
    with
      gangrene (and obstruction)
        K40.10
        not specified as recurrent
          K40.10
        recurrent K40.11
      obstruction K40.00
        not specified as recurrent K40.00
        recurrent K40.01
    not specified as recurrent K40.20
    recurrent K40.21
  not specified as recurrent K40.90
  recurrent K40.91

◄ New   ◄▓ Revised   ~~deleted~~ Deleted

Hernia, hernial (*Continued*)
inguinal (*Continued*)
unilateral K40.90
with
gangrene (and obstruction) K40.40
not specified as recurrent K40.40
recurrent K40.41
obstruction K40.30
not specified as recurrent K40.30
recurrent K40.31
not specified as recurrent K40.90
recurrent K40.91
internal —*see also* Hernia, abdomen
inguinal —*see* Hernia, inguinal
interstitial —*see* Hernia, abdomen
intervertebral cartilage or disc —*see*
Displacement, intervertebral disc
intestine, intestinal —*see* Hernia, by site
intra-abdominal —*see* Hernia, abdomen
iris (traumatic) S05.2-
irreducible —*see also* Hernia, by site, with
obstruction
with gangrene —*see* Hernia, by site, with
gangrene
ischiatic —*see* Hernia, abdomen, specified
site NEC
ischiorectal —*see* Hernia, abdomen, specified
site NEC
lens (traumatic) S05.2-
linea (alba) (semilunaris) —*see* Hernia,
ventral
Littre's —*see* Hernia, abdomen
lumbar —*see* Hernia, abdomen, specified site
NEC
lung (subcutaneous) J98.4
mediastinum J98.59 ◀▥
mesenteric (internal) —*see* Hernia, abdomen
midline —*see* Hernia, ventral
muscle (sheath) M62.89
nucleus pulposus —*see* Displacement,
intervertebral disc
oblique (inguinal) —*see* Hernia, inguinal
obstructive —*see also* Hernia, by site, with
obstruction
with gangrene —*see* Hernia, by site, with
gangrene
obturator —*see* Hernia, abdomen, specified
site NEC
omental —*see* Hernia, abdomen
ovary N83.4- ◀▥
oviduct N83.4- ◀▥
paraesophageal —*see also* Hernia, diaphragm
congenital Q40.1
parastomal K43.5
with
gangrene (and obstruction) K43.4
obstruction K43.3
paraumbilical —*see* Hernia, umbilicus
perineal —*see* Hernia, abdomen, specified
site NEC
Petit's —*see* Hernia, abdomen, specified site
NEC
postoperative —*see* Hernia, incisional
pregnant uterus —*see* Abnormal, uterus in
pregnancy or childbirth
prevesical N32.89
properitoneal —*see* Hernia, abdomen,
specified site NEC
pudendal —*see* Hernia, abdomen, specified
site NEC
rectovaginal N81.6
retroperitoneal —*see* Hernia, abdomen,
specified site NEC
Richter's —*see* Hernia, abdomen, with
obstruction
Rieux's, Riex's —*see* Hernia, abdomen,
specified site NEC
sac condition (adhesion) (dropsy)
(inflammation) (laceration)
(suppuration) - code by site under
Hernia

Hernia, hernial (*Continued*)
sciatic —*see* Hernia, abdomen, specified site
NEC
scrotum, scrotal —*see* Hernia, inguinal
sliding (inguinal) —*see also* Hernia,
inguinal
hiatus —*see* Hernia, hiatal
spigelian —*see* Hernia, ventral
spinal —*see* Spina bifida
strangulated —*see also* Hernia, by site, with
obstruction
with gangrene —*see* Hernia, by site, with
gangrene
subxiphoid —*see* Hernia, ventral
supra-umbilicus —*see* Hernia, ventral
tendon —*see* Disorder, tendon, specified type
NEC
Treitz's (fossa) —*see* Hernia, abdomen,
specified site NEC
tunica vaginalis Q55.29
umbilicus, umbilical K42.9
with
gangrene (and obstruction) K42.1
obstruction K42.0
ureter N28.89
urethra, congenital Q64.79
urinary meatus, congenital Q64.79
uterus N81.4
pregnant —*see* Abnormal, uterus in
pregnancy or childbirth
vaginal (anterior) (wall) —*see* Cystocele
Velpeau's —*see* Hernia, femoral
ventral K43.9
with
gangrene (and obstruction) K43.7
obstruction K43.6
incisional K43.2
with
gangrene (and obstruction) K43.1
obstruction K43.0
recurrent —*see* Hernia, incisional
specified NEC K43.9
with
gangrene (and obstruction) K43.7
obstruction K43.6
vesical
congenital (female) (male) Q79.51
female —*see* Cystocele
male N32.89
vitreous (into wound) S05.2-
into anterior chamber —*see* Prolapse,
vitreous
Herniation —*see also* Hernia
brain (stem) G93.5
cerebral G93.5
mediastinum J98.59 ◀▥
nucleus pulposus —*see* Displacement,
intervertebral disc
Herpangina B08.5
Herpes, herpesvirus, herpetic B00.9
anogenital A60.9
perianal skin A60.1
rectum A60.1
urogenital tract A60.00
cervix A60.03
male genital organ NEC A60.02
penis A60.01
specified site NEC A60.09
vagina A60.04
vulva A60.04
blepharitis (zoster) B02.39
simplex B00.59
circinatus B35.4
bullosus L12.0
conjunctivitis (simplex) B00.53
zoster B02.31
cornea B02.33
encephalitis B00.4
due to herpesvirus 6 B10.01
due to herpesvirus 7 B10.09
specified NEC B10.09

Herpes, herpesvirus, herpetic (*Continued*)
eye (zoster) B02.30
simplex B00.50
eyelid (zoster) B02.39
simplex B00.59
facialis B00.1
febrilis B00.1
geniculate ganglionitis B02.21
genital, genitalis A60.00
female A60.09
male A60.02
gestational, gestationis O26.4-
gingivostomatitis B00.2
human B00.9
1 —*see* Herpes, simplex
2 —*see* Herpes, simplex
3 —*see* Varicella
4 —*see* Mononucleosis, Epstein-Barr (virus)
5 —*see* Disease, cytomegalic inclusion
(generalized)
6
encephalitis B10.01
specified NEC B10.81
7
encephalitis B10.09
specified NEC B10.82
8 B10.89
infection NEC B10.89
Kaposi's sarcoma associated B10.89
iridocyclitis (simplex) B00.51
zoster B02.32
iris (vesicular erythema multiforme) L51.9
iritis (simplex) B00.51
Kaposi's sarcoma associated B10.89
keratitis (simplex) (dendritic) (disciform)
(interstitial) B00.52
zoster (interstitial) B02.33
keratoconjunctivitis (simplex) B00.52
zoster B02.33
labialis B00.1
lip B00.1
meningitis (simplex) B00.3
zoster B02.1
ophthalmicus (zoster) NEC B02.30
simplex B00.50
penis A60.01
perianal skin A60.1
pharyngitis, pharyngotonsillitis B00.2
rectum A60.1
scrotum A60.02
sepsis B00.7
simplex B00.9
complicated NEC B00.89
congenital P35.2
conjunctivitis B00.53
external ear B00.1
eyelid B00.59
hepatitis B00.81
keratitis (interstitial) B00.52
myleitis B00.82
specified complication NEC B00.89
visceral B00.89
stomatitis B00.2
tonsurans B35.0
visceral B00.89
vulva A60.04
whitlow B00.89
zoster —*see also* condition B02.9
auricularis B02.21
complicated NEC B02.8
conjunctivitis B02.31
disseminated B02.7
encephalitis B02.0
eye(lid) B02.39
geniculate ganglionitis B02.21
keratitis (interstitial) B02.33
meningitis B02.1
myelitis B02.24
neuritis, neuralgia B02.29
ophthalmicus NEC B02.30
oticus B02.21

Herpes, herpesvirus, herpetic (Continued)
zoster (Continued)
polyneuropathy B02.23
specified complication NEC B02.8
trigeminal neuralgia B02.22
Herpesvirus (human) —see Herpes
Herpetophobia F40.218
Herrick's anemia —see Disease, sickle-cell
Hers' disease E74.09
Herter-Gee syndrome K90.0
Herxheimer's reaction R68.89
Hesitancy
of micturition R39.11
urinary R39.11
Hesselbach's hernia —see Hernia, femoral,
specified site NEC
Heterochromia (congenital) Q13.2
cataract —see Cataract, complicated
cyclitis (Fuchs) —see Cyclitis, Fuchs'
heterochromic
hair L67.1
iritis —see Cyclitis, Fuchs' heterochromic
retained metallic foreign body
(nonmagnetic) —see Foreign body,
intraocular, old, retained
magnetic —see Foreign body, intraocular,
old, retained, magnetic
uveitis —see Cyclitis, Fuchs' heterochromic
Heterophoria —see Strabismus, heterophoria
Heterophyes, heterophyiasis (small intestine)
B66.8
Heterotopia, heterotopic —see also Malposition,
congenital
cerebralis Q04.8
Heterotropia —see Strabismus
Heubner-Herter disease K90.0
Hexadactylism Q69.9
HGSIL (cytology finding) (high grade
squamous intraepithelial lesion on
cytologic smear) (Pap smear finding)
anus R85.613
cervix R87.613
biopsy (histology) finding — see Neoplasia,
intraepithelial, cervix, grade II or
grade III ◄▥
vagina R87.623
biopsy (histology) finding — see Neoplasia,
intraepithelial, vagina, grade II or
grade III ◄▥
Hibernoma —see Lipoma
Hiccup, hiccough R06.6
epidemic B33.0
psychogenic F45.8
Hidden penis (congenital) Q55.64
acquired N48.83
Hidradenitis (axillaris) (suppurative) L73.2
Hidradenoma (nodular) —see also Neoplasm,
skin, benign
clear cell —see Neoplasm, skin, benign
papillary —see Neoplasm, skin, benign
Hidrocystoma —see Neoplasm, skin, benign
High
altitude effects T70.20
anoxia T70.29
on
ears T70.0
sinuses T70.1
polycythemia D75.1
arch
foot Q66.7
palate, congenital Q38.5
arterial tension —see Hypertension
basal metabolic rate R94.8
blood pressure —see also Hypertension
borderline R03.0
reading (incidental) (isolated)
(nonspecific), without diagnosis of
hypertension R03.0
cholesterol E78.00 ◄▥
with high triglycerides E78.2
diaphragm (congenital) Q79.1

High (Continued)
expressed emotional level within family
Z63.8
head at term O32.4
palate, congenital Q38.5
risk
infant NEC Z76.2
sexual behavior (heterosexual) Z72.51
bisexual Z72.53
homosexual Z72.52
temperature (of unknown origin) R50.9
thoracic rib Q76.6
triglycerides E78.1
with high cholesterol E78.2
Hildenbrand's disease A75.0
Hilum —see condition
Hip —see condition
Hippel's disease Q85.8
Hippophobia F40.218
Hippus H57.09
Hirschsprung's disease or megacolon Q43.1
Hirsutism, hirsuties L68.0
Hirudiniasis
external B88.3
internal B83.4
Hiss-Russell dysentery A03.1
Histidinemia, histidinuria E70.41
Histiocytoma —see also Neoplasm, skin, benign
fibrous —see also Neoplasm, skin, benign
atypical —see Neoplasm, connective tissue,
uncertain behavior
malignant —see Neoplasm, connective
tissue, malignant
Histiocytosis D76.3
acute differentiated progressive C96.0
Langerhans' cell NEC C96.6
multifocal X
multisystemic (disseminated) C96.0
unisystemic C96.5
pulmonary, adult (adult PLCH) J84.82
unifocal (X) C96.6
lipid, lipoid D76.3
essential E75.29
malignant C96.A
mononuclear phagocytes NEC D76.1
Langerhans' cells C96.6
non-Langerhans cell D76.3
polyostotic sclerosing D76.3
sinus, with massive lymphadenopathy
D76.3
syndrome NEC D76.3
X NEC C96.6
acute (progressive) C96.0
chronic C96.6
multifocal C96.5
multisystemic C96.0
unifocal C96.6
Histoplasmosis B39.9
with pneumonia NEC B39.2
African B39.5
American —see Histoplasmosis, capsulati
capsulati B39.4
disseminated B39.3
generalized B39.3
pulmonary B39.2
acute B39.0
chronic B39.1
Darling's B39.4
duboisii B39.5
lung NEC B39.2
History
family (of) —see also History, personal (of)
alcohol abuse Z81.1
allergy NEC Z84.89
anemia Z83.2
arthritis Z82.61
asthma Z82.5
blindness Z82.1
cardiac death (sudden) Z82.41
carrier of genetic disease Z84.81
chromosomal anomaly Z82.79

History (Continued)
family (Continued)
chronic
disabling disease NEC Z82.8
lower respiratory disease Z82.5
colonic polyps Z83.71
congenital malformations and
deformations Z82.79
polycystic kidney Z82.71
consanguinity Z84.3
deafness Z82.2
diabetes mellitus Z83.3
disability NEC Z82.8
disease or disorder (of)
allergic NEC Z84.89
behavioral NEC Z81.8
blood and blood-forming organs Z83.2
cardiovascular NEC Z82.49
chronic disabling NEC Z82.8
digestive Z83.79
ear NEC Z83.52
endocrine NEC Z83.49
eye NEC Z83.518
glaucoma Z83.511
familial hypercholesterolemia Z83.42 ◄
genitourinary NEC Z84.2
glaucoma Z83.511
hematological Z83.2
immune mechanism Z83.2
infectious NEC Z83.1
ischemic heart Z82.49
kidney Z84.1
mental NEC Z81.8
metabolic Z83.49
musculoskeletal NEC Z82.69
neurological NEC Z82.0
nutritional Z83.49
parasitic NEC Z83.1
psychiatric NEC Z81.8
respiratory NEC Z83.6
skin and subcutaneous tissue NEC Z84.0
specified NEC Z84.89
drug abuse NEC Z81.3
epilepsy Z82.0
familial hypercholesterolemia Z83.42 ◄
genetic disease carrier Z84.81
glaucoma Z83.511
hearing loss Z82.2
human immunodeficiency virus (HIV)
infection Z83.0
Huntington's chorea Z82.0
intellectual disability Z81.0
leukemia Z80.6
malignant neoplasm (of) NOS Z80.9
bladder Z80.52
breast Z80.3
bronchus Z80.1
digestive organ Z80.0
gastrointestinal tract Z80.0
genital organ Z80.49
ovary Z80.41
prostate Z80.42
specified organ NEC Z80.49
testis Z80.43
hematopoietic NEC Z80.7
intrathoracic organ NEC Z80.2
kidney Z80.51
lung Z80.1
lymphatic NEC Z80.7
ovary Z80.41
prostate Z80.42
respiratory organ NEC Z80.2
specified site NEC Z80.8
testis Z80.43
trachea Z80.1
urinary organ or tract Z80.59
bladder Z80.52
kidney Z80.51
mental
disorder NEC Z81.8
multiple endocrine neoplasia (MEN)
syndrome Z83.41

◄ New   ◄▥ Revised   deleted Deleted

History *(Continued)*
  family *(Continued)*
    osteoporosis Z82.62
    polycystic kidney Z82.71
    polyps (colon) Z83.71
    psychiatric disorder Z81.8
    psychoactive substance abuse NEC Z81.3
    respiratory condition NEC Z83.6
      asthma and other lower respiratory conditions Z82.5
    self-harmful behavior Z81.8
    SIDS (sudden infant death syndrome) Z84.82 ◄
    skin condition Z84.0
    specified condition NEC Z84.89
    stroke (cerebrovascular) Z82.3
    substance abuse NEC Z81.4
      alcohol Z81.1
      drug NEC Z81.3
      psychoactive NEC Z81.3
      tobacco Z81.2
    ~~sudden cardiac death Z82.41~~
    sudden ◄
      cardiac death Z82.41 ◄
      infant death syndrome (SIDS) Z84.82 ◄
    tobacco abuse Z81.2
    violence, violent behavior Z81.8
    visual loss Z82.1
  personal (of) —*see also* History, family (of)
    abuse
      adult Z91.419
        physical and sexual Z91.410
        psychological Z91.411
      childhood Z62.819
        physical Z62.810
        psychological Z62.811
        sexual Z62.810
    alcohol dependence F10.21
    allergy (to) Z88.9
      analgesic agent NEC Z88.6
      anesthetic Z88.4
      antibiotic agent NEC Z88.1
      anti-infective agent NEC Z88.3
      contrast media Z91.041
      drugs, medicaments and biological substances Z88.9
        specified NEC Z88.8
      food Z91.018
        additives Z91.02
        eggs Z91.012
        milk products Z91.011
        peanuts Z91.010
        seafood Z91.013
        specified food NEC Z91.018
      insect Z91.038
        bee Z91.030
      latex Z91.040
      medicinal agents Z88.9
        specified NEC Z88.8
      narcotic agent NEC Z88.5
      nonmedicinal agents Z91.048
      penicillin Z88.0
      serum Z88.7
      specified NEC Z91.09
      sulfonamides Z88.2
      vaccine Z88.7
    anaphylactic shock Z87.892
    anaphylaxis Z87.892
    behavioral disorders Z86.59
    benign carcinoid tumor Z86.012
    benign neoplasm Z86.018
      brain Z86.011
      carcinoid Z86.012
      colonic polyps Z86.010
    brain injury (traumatic) Z87.820
    breast implant removal Z98.86
    calculi, renal Z87.442
    cancer —*see* History, personal (of), malignant neoplasm (of)
    cardiac arrest (death), successfully resuscitated Z86.74

History *(Continued)*
  personal *(Continued)*
    cerebral infarction without residual deficit Z86.73
    cervical dysplasia Z87.410
    chemotherapy for neoplastic condition Z92.21
    childhood abuse —*see* History, personal (of), abuse
    cleft lip (corrected) Z87.730
    cleft palate (corrected) Z87.730
    collapsed vertebra (healed) Z87.311
      due to osteoporosis Z87.310
    combat and operational stress reaction Z86.51
    congenital malformation (corrected) Z87.798
      circulatory system (corrected) Z87.74
      digestive system (corrected) NEC Z87.738
      ear (corrected) Z87.720
      eye (corrected) Z87.721
      face and neck (corrected) Z87.790
      genitourinary system (corrected) NEC Z87.718
      heart (corrected) Z87.74
      integument (corrected) Z87.76
      limb (s) (corrected) Z87.76
      musculoskeletal system (corrected) Z87.76
      neck (corrected) Z87.790
      nervous system (corrected) NEC Z87.728
      respiratory system (corrected) Z87.75
      sense organs (corrected) NEC Z87.728
      specified NEC Z87.798
    contraception Z92.0
    deployment (military) Z91.82
    diabetic foot ulcer Z86.31
    disease or disorder (of) Z87.898
      blood and blood-forming organs Z86.2
      circulatory system Z86.79
        specified condition NEC Z86.79
      connective tissue NEC Z87.39
      digestive system Z87.19
        colonic polyp Z86.010
        peptic ulcer disease Z87.11
        specified condition NEC Z87.19
      ear Z86.69
      endocrine Z86.39
        diabetic foot ulcer Z86.31
        gestational diabetes Z86.32
        specified type NEC Z86.39
      eye Z86.69
      genital (track) system NEC
        female Z87.42
        male Z87.438
      hematological Z86.2
      Hodgkin Z85.71
      immune mechanism Z86.2
      infectious Z86.19
        malaria Z86.13
        Methicillin resistant Staphylococcus aureus (MRSA) Z86.14
        poliomyelitis Z86.12
        specified NEC Z86.19
        tuberculosis Z86.11
      mental NEC Z86.59
      metabolic Z86.39
        diabetic foot ulcer Z86.31
        gestational diabetes Z86.32
        specified type NEC Z86.39
      musculoskeletal NEC Z87.39
      nervous system Z86.69
      nutritional Z86.39
      parasitic Z86.19
      respiratory system NEC Z87.09
      sense organs Z86.69
      skin Z87.2
      specified site or type NEC Z87.898
      subcutaneous tissue Z87.2

History *(Continued)*
  personal *(Continued)*
    disease or disorder (of) *(Continued)*
      trophoblastic Z87.59
      urinary system NEC Z87.448
    drug dependence —*see* Dependence, drug, by type, in remission
    drug therapy
      antineoplastic chemotherapy Z92.21
      estrogen Z92.23
      immunosuppression Z92.25
      inhaled steroids Z92.240
      monoclonal drug Z92.22
      specified NEC Z92.29
      steroid Z92.241
      systemic steroids Z92.241
    dysplasia
      cervical (mild) (moderate) Z87.410 ◄▥
        severe (grade III) Z86.001 ◄
      prostatic Z87.430
      vaginal Z87.411
      vulvar (mild) (moderate) Z87.412 ◄▥
        severe (grade III) Z86.008 ◄
    embolism (venous) Z86.718
      pulmonary Z86.711
    encephalitis Z86.61
    estrogen therapy Z92.23
    extracorporeal membrane oxygenation (ECMO) Z92.81
    failed conscious sedation Z92.83
    failed moderate sedation Z92.83
    fall, falling Z91.81
    fracture (healed)
      fatigue Z87.312
      fragility Z87.310
      osteoporosis Z87.310
      pathological NEC Z87.311
      stress Z87.312
      traumatic Z87.81
    gestational diabetes Z86.32
    hepatitis
      B Z86.19
      C Z86.19
    Hodgkin disease Z85.71
    hyperthermia, malignant Z88.4
    hypospadias (corrected) Z87.710
    hysterectomy Z90.710
    immunosupression therapy Z92.25
    in situ neoplasm
      breast Z86.000
      cervix uteri Z86.001
      specified NEC Z86.008
    infection NEC Z86.19
      central nervous system Z86.61
      Methicillin resistant Staphylococcus aureus (MRSA) Z86.14
      urinary (tract) Z87.41
    injury NEC Z87.828
    in utero procedure during pregnancy Z98.870
    in utero procedure while a fetus Z98.871
    irradiation Z92.3
    kidney stones Z87.442
    leukemia Z85.6
    lymphoma (non-Hodgkin) Z85.72
    malignant melanoma (skin) Z85.820
    malignant neoplasm (of) Z85.9
      accessory sinuses Z85.22
      anus NEC Z85.048
        carcinoid Z85.040
      bladder Z85.51
      bone Z85.830
      brain Z85.841
      breast Z85.3
      bronchus NEC Z85.118
        carcinoid Z85.110
      carcinoid —*see* History, personal (of), malignant neoplasm, by site, carcinioid
      cervix Z85.41
      colon NEC Z85.038
        carcinoid Z85.030

History *(Continued)*
  personal *(Continued)*
    malignant neoplasm *(Continued)*
      digestive organ Z85.00
        specified NEC Z85.09
      endocrine gland NEC Z85.858
      epididymis Z85.48
      esophagus Z85.01
      eye Z85.840
      gastrointestinal tract —*see* History, malignant neoplasm, digestive organ
      genital organ
        female Z85.40
          specified NEC Z85.44
        male Z85.45
          specified NEC Z85.49
      hematopoietic NEC Z85.79
      intrathoracic organ Z85.20-
      kidney NEC Z85.528
        carcinoid Z85.520
      large intestine NEC Z85.038
        carcinoid Z85.030
      larynx Z85.21
      liver Z85.05
      lung NEC Z85.118
        carcinoid Z85.110
      mediastinum Z85.29
      Merkel cell Z85.821
      middle ear Z85.22
      nasal cavities Z85.22
      nervous system NEC Z85.848
      oral cavity Z85.819
        specified site NEC Z85.818
      ovary Z85.43
      pancreas Z85.07
      pelvis Z85.53
      pharynx Z85.819
        specified site NEC Z85.818
      pleura Z85.29
      prostate Z85.46
      rectosigmoid junction NEC Z85.048
        carcinoid Z85.040
      rectum NEC Z85.048
        carcinoid Z85.040
      respiratory organ Z85.20
      sinuses, accessory Z85.22
      skin NEC Z85.828
        melanoma Z85.820
        Merkel cell Z85.821
      small intestine NEC Z85.068
        carcinoid Z85.060
      soft tissue Z85.831
      specified site NEC Z85.89
      stomach NEC Z85.028
        carcinoid Z85.020
      testis Z85.47
      thymus NEC Z85.238
        carcinoid Z85.230
      thyroid Z85.850
      tongue Z85.810
      trachea Z85.12
      ureter Z85.54
      urinary organ or tract Z85.50
        specified NEC Z85.59
      uterus Z85.42
    maltreatment Z91.89
    medical treatment NEC Z92.89
    melanoma (malignant) (skin) Z85.820
    meningitis Z86.61
    mental disorder Z86.59
    Merkel cell carcinoma (skin) Z85.821
    Methicillin resistant Staphylococcus aureus (MRSA) Z86.14
    military deployment Z91.82
    military war, peacekeeping and humanitarian deployment (current or past conflict) Z91.82
    myocardial infarction (old) I25.2
    neglect (in)
      adult Z91.412
      childhood Z62.812

History *(Continued)*
  personal *(Continued)*
    neoplasm
      benign Z86.018
        brain Z86.011
        colon polyp Z86.010
      in situ
        breast Z86.000
        cervix uteri Z86.001
        specified NEC Z86.008
      malignant —*see* History of, malignant neoplasm
      uncertain behavior Z86.03
    nephrotic syndrome Z87.441
    nicotine dependence Z87.891
    noncompliance with medical treatment or regimen —*see* Noncompliance
    nutritional deficiency Z86.39
    obstetric complications Z87.59
      childbirth Z87.59
      pregnancy Z87.59
      pre-term labor Z87.51
      puerperium Z87.59
    osteoporosis fractures Z87.31
    parasuicide (attempt) Z91.5
    physical trauma NEC Z87.828
      self-harm or suicide attempt Z91.5
    pneumonia (recurrent) Z87.01
    poisoning NEC Z91.89
      self-harm or suicide attempt Z91.5
    poor personal hygiene Z91.89
    preterm labor Z87.51
    procedure during pregnancy Z98.870
    procedure while a fetus Z98.871
    prolonged reversible ischemic neurologic deficit (PRIND) Z86.73
    prostatic dysplasia Z87.430
    psychiatric disorder NEC Z87.89
    psychological
      abuse
        adult Z91.411
        child Z62.811
      trauma, specified NEC Z91.49
    radiation therapy Z92.3
    removal
      implant
        breast Z98.86
    renal calculi Z87.442
    respiratory condition NEC Z87.09
    retained foreign body fully removed Z87.821
    risk factors NEC Z91.89
    self-harm Z91.5
    self-poisoning attempt Z91.5
    sex reassignment Z87.890
    sleep-wake cycle problem Z72.821
    specified NEC Z87.898
    steroid therapy (systemic) Z92.241
      inhaled Z92.240
    stroke without residual deficits Z86.73
    substance abuse NEC F10-F19 with fifth character 1
    sudden cardiac arrest Z86.74
    sudden cardiac death successfully resuscitated Z86.74
    suicide attempt Z91.5
    surgery NEC Z98.890
      with uterine scar Z98.891
      sex reassignment Z87.890
      transplant —*see* Transplant
    thrombophlebitis Z86.72
    thrombosis (venous) Z86.718
      pulmonary Z86.711
    tobacco dependence Z87.891
    transient ischemic attack (TIA) without residual deficits Z86.73
    trauma (physical) NEC Z87.828
      psychological NEC Z91.49
      self-harm Z91.5
    traumatic brain injury Z87.820
    unhealthy sleep-wake cycle Z72.821

History *(Continued)*
  personal *(Continued)*
    unintended awareness under general anesthesia Z92.84
    urinary (recurrent) (tract) infection (s) Z87.440
    urinary calculi Z87.42
    uterine scar from previous surgery Z98.891
    vaginal dysplasia Z87.411
    venous thrombosis or embolism Z86.718
      pulmonary Z86.711
    vulvar dysplasia Z87.412
His-Werner disease A79.0
HIV —*see also* Human, immunodeficiency virus B20
  laboratory evidence (nonconclusive) R75
  nonconclusive test (in infants) R75
  positive, seropositive Z21
Hives (bold) —*see* Urticaria
Hoarseness R49.0
Hobo Z59.0
Hodgkin disease —*see* Lymphoma, Hodgkin
Hodgson's disease I71.2
  ruptured I71.1
Hoffa-Kastert disease E88.89
Hoffa's disease E88.89
Hoffmann-Bouveret syndrome I47.9
Hoffmann's syndrome E03.9 [G73.7]
Hole (round)
  macula H35.34-
  retina (without detachment) —*see* Break, retina, round hole
    with detachment —*see* Detachment, retina, with retinal, break
Holiday relief care Z75.5
Hollenhorst's plaque —*see* Occlusion, artery, retina
Hollow foot (congenital) Q66.7
  acquired —*see* Deformity, limb, foot, specified NEC
Holoprosencephaly Q04.2
Holt-Oram syndrome Q87.2
Homelessness Z59.0
Homesickness —*see* Disorder, adjustment
Homocystinemia, homocystinuria E72.11
Homogentisate 1,2-dioxygenase deficiency E70.29
Homologous serum hepatitis (prophylactic) (therapeutic) —*see* Hepatitis, viral, type B
Honeycomb lung J98.4
  congenital Q33.0
Hooded
  clitoris Q52.6
  penis Q55.69
Hookworm (anemia) (disease) (infection) (infestation) B76.9
  specified NEC B76.8
Hordeolum (eyelid) (externum) (recurrent) H00.019
  internum H00.029
    left H00.026
      lower H00.025
      upper H00.024
    right H00.023
      lower H00.022
      upper H00.021
  left H00.016
    lower H00.015
    upper H00.014
  right H00.013
    lower H00.012
    upper H00.011
Horn
  cutaneous L85.8
  nail L60.2
    congenital Q84.6
Horner (-Claude Bernard) syndrome G90.2
  traumatic —*see* Injury, nerve, cervical sympathetic

New   Revised   ~~deleted~~ Deleted

Horseshoe kidney (congenital) Q63.1
Horton's headache or neuralgia G44.099
 intractable G44.091
 not intractable G44.099
Hospital hopper syndrome —see Disorder,
 factitious
Hospitalism in children —see Disorder,
 adjustment
Hostility R45.5
 towards child Z62.3
Hot flashes
 menopausal N95.1
Hourglass (contracture) —see also Contraction,
 hourglass
 stomach K31.89
  congenital Q40.2
  stricture K31.2
Household, housing circumstance affecting
 care Z59.9
 specified NEC Z59.8
Housemaid's knee —see Bursitis, prepatellar
Hudson (-Stähli) line (cornea) —see
 Pigmentation, cornea, anterior
Human
 bite (open wound) —see also Bite
  intact skin surface —see Bite, superficial
 herpesvirus —see Herpes
 immunodeficiency virus (HIV) disease
  (infection) B20
  asymptomatic status Z21
  contact Z20.6
  counseling Z71.7
  dementia B20 [F02.80]
   with behavioral disturbance B20 [F02.81]
  exposure to Z20.6
  laboratory evidence R75
  type-2 (HIV 2) as cause of disease classified
   elsewhere B97.35
 papillomavirus (HPV)
  DNA test positive
   high risk
    cervix R87.810
    vagina R87.811
   low risk
    cervix R87.820
    vagina R87.821
  screening for Z11.51
 T-cell lymphotropic virus
  type-1 (HTLV-I) infection B33.3
   as cause of disease classified elsewhere
    B97.33
   carrier Z22.6
  type-2 (HTLV-II) as cause of disease
   classified elsewhere B97.34
Humidifier lung or pneumonitis J67.7
Humiliation (experience) in childhood Z62.898
Humpback (acquired) —see Kyphosis
Hunchback (acquired) —see Kyphosis
Hunger T73.0
 air, psychogenic F45.8
Hungry bone syndrome E83.81
Hunner's ulcer —see Cystitis, chronic,
 interstitial
Hunter's
 glossitis D51.0
 syndrome E76.1
Huntington's disease or chorea G10
 with dementia G10 [F02.80]
  with behavioral disturbance G10 [F02.81]
Hunt's
 disease or syndrome (herpetic geniculate
  ganglionitis) B02.21
  dyssynergia cerebellaris myoclonica G11.1
 neuralgia B02.21
Hurler (-Scheie) disease or syndrome E76.02
Hurst's disease G36.1
Hurthle cell
 adenocarcinoma C73
 adenoma D34
 carcinoma C73
 tumor D34

Hutchinson-Boeck disease or syndrome —see
 Sarcoidosis
Hutchinson-Gilford disease or syndrome E34.8
Hutchinson's
 disease, meaning
  angioma serpiginosum L81.7
  pompholyx (cheiropompholyx) L30.1
  prurigo estivalis L56.4
  summer eruption or summer prurigo L56.4
 melanotic freckle —see Melanoma, in situ
  malignant melanoma in —see Melanoma
 teeth or incisors (congenital syphilis) A50.52
 triad (congenital syphilis) A50.53
Hyalin plaque, sclera, senile H15.89
Hyaline membrane (disease) (lung)
 (pulmonary) (newborn) P22.0
Hyalinosis
 cutis (et mucosae) E78.89
 focal and segmental (glomerular) —see also
  N00-N07 with fourth character .1 N05.1
Hyalitis, hyalosis, asteroid —see also Deposit,
 crystalline
 syphilitic (late) A52.71
Hydatid
 cyst or tumor —see Echinococcus
 mole —see Hydatidiform mole
 Morgagni
  female Q50.5
  male (epididymal) Q55.4
  testicular Q55.29
Hydatidiform mole (benign) (complicating
 pregnancy) (delivered) (undelivered)
 O01.9
 classical O01.0
 complete O01.0
 incomplete O01.1
 invasive D39.2
 malignant D39.2
 partial O01.1
Hydatidosis —see Echinococcus
Hydradenitis (axillaris) (suppurative) L73.2
Hydradenoma —see Hidradenoma
Hydramnios O40.-
Hydrancephaly, hydranencephaly Q04.3
 with spina bifida —see Spina bifida, with
  hydrocephalus
Hydrargyrism NEC —see Poisoning, mercury
Hydrarthrosis —see also Effusion, joint
 gonococcal A54.42
 intermittent M12.40
  ankle M12.47-
  elbow M12.42-
  foot joint M12.47-
  hand joint M12.44-
  hip M12.45-
  knee M12.46-
  multiple site M12.49
  shoulder M12.41-
  specified joint NEC M12.48
  wrist M12.43-
 of yaws (early) (late) —see also subcategory
  M14.8- A66.6
 syphilitic (late) A52.77
  congenital A50.55 [M12.80]
Hydremia D64.89
Hydrencephalocele (congenital) —see
 Encephalocele
Hydrencephalomeningocele (congenital) —see
 Encephalocele
Hydroa R23.8
 aestivale L56.4
 vacciniforme L56.4
Hydroadenitis (axillaris) (suppurative) L73.2
Hydrocalycosis —see Hydronephrosis
Hydrocele (spermatic cord) (testis) (tunica
 vaginalis) N43.3
 canal of Nuck N94.89
 communicating N43.2
  congenital P83.5
 congenital P83.5
 encysted N43.0

Hydrocele (Continued)
 female NEC N94.89
 infected N43.1
 newborn P83.5
 round ligament N94.89
 specified NEC N43.2
 spinalis —see Spina bifida
 vulva N90.89
Hydrocephalus (acquired) (external) (internal)
 (malignant) (recurrent) G91.9
 aqueduct Sylvius stricture Q03.0
 causing disproportion O33.6
  with obstructed labor O66.3
 communicating G91.0
 congenital (external) (internal) Q03.9
  with spina bifida Q05.4
   cervical Q05.0
   dorsal Q05.1
   lumbar Q05.2
   lumbosacral Q05.2
   sacral Q05.3
   thoracic Q05.1
   thoracolumbar Q05.1
  specified NEC Q03.8
 due to toxoplasmosis (congenital) P37.1
 foramen Magendie block (acquired) G91.1
  congenital —see also Hydrocephalus,
   congenital Q03.1
 in (due to)
  infectious disease NEC B89 [G91.4]
  neoplastic disease NEC (see also Neoplasm)
   G91.4
  parasitic disease B89 [G91.4]
 newborn Q03.9
  with spina bifida —see Spina bifida, with
   hydrocephalus
 noncommunicating G91.1
 normal pressure G91.2
  secondary G91.0
 obstructive G91.1
 otitic G93.2
 post-traumatic NEC G91.3
 secondary G91.4
  post-traumatic G91.3
 specified NEC G91.8
 syphilitic, congenital A50.49
Hydrocolpos (congenital) N89.8
Hydrocystoma —see Neoplasm, skin, benign
Hydroencephalocele (congenital) —see
 Encephalocele
Hydroencephalomeningocele (congenital) —
 see Encephalocele
Hydrohematopneumothorax —see Hemothorax
Hydromeningitis —see Meningitis
Hydromeningocele (spinal) —see also Spina
 bifida
 cranial —see Encephalocele
Hydrometra N85.8
Hydrometrocolpos N89.8
Hydromicrocephaly Q02
Hydromphalos (since birth) Q45.8
Hydromyelia Q06.4
Hydromyelocele —see Spina bifida
Hydronephrosis (atrophic) (early)
 (functionless) (intermittent) (primary)
 (secondary) NEC N13.30
 with
  infection N13.6
  obstruction (by) (of)
   renal calculus N13.2
    with infection N13.6
   ureteral NEC N13.1
    with infection N13.6
    calculus N13.2
     with infection N13.6
   ureteropelvic junction (congenital) Q62.0
    with infection N13.6
    acquired N13.0 ◀
     with infection N13.6 ◀
   ureteral stricture NEC N13.1
    with infection N13.6

Hydronephrosis NEC *(Continued)*
  congenital Q62.0
    due to acquired occlusion of ureteropelvic
      junction N13.0 ◀
  specified type NEC N13.39
  tuberculous A18.11
Hydropericarditis —*see* Pericarditis
Hydropericardium —*see* Pericarditis
Hydroperitoneum R18.8
Hydrophobia —*see* Rabies
Hydrophthalmos Q15.0
Hydropneumohemothorax —*see* Hemothorax
Hydropneumopericarditis —*see* Pericarditis
Hydropneumopericardium —*see* Pericarditis
Hydropneumothorax J94.8
  traumatic —*see* Injury, intrathoracic, lung
  tuberculous NEC A15.6
Hydrops R60.9
  abdominis R18.8
  articulorum intermittens —*see* Hydrarthrosis,
    intermittent
  cardiac —*see* Failure, heart, congestive
  causing obstructed labor (mother) O66.3
  endolymphatic H81.0-
  fetal —*see* Pregnancy, complicated by,
    hydrops, fetalis
  fetalis P83.2
    due to
      ABO isoimmunization P56.0
      alpha thalassemia D56.0
      hemolytic disease P56.90
        specified NEC P56.99
      isoimmunization (ABO) (Rh) P56.0
      other specified nonhemolytic disease
        NEC P83.2
      Rh incompatibility P56.0
    during pregnancy —*see* Pregnancy,
      complicated by, hydrops, fetalis
  gallbladder K82.1
  joint —*see* Effusion, joint
  labyrinth H81.0
  newborn (idiopathic) P83.2
    due to
      ABO isoimmunization P56.0
      alpha thalassemia D56.0
      hemolytic disease P56.90
        specified NEC P56.99
      isoimmunization (ABO) (Rh) P56.0
      Rh incompatibility P56.0
  nutritional —*see* Malnutrition, severe
  pericardium —*see* Pericarditis
  pleura —*see* Hydrothorax
  spermatic cord —*see* Hydrocele
Hydropyonephrosis N13.6
Hydrorachis Q06.4
Hydrorrhea (nasal) J34.89
  pregnancy —*see* Rupture, membranes,
    premature
Hydrosadenitis (axillaris) (suppurative) L73.2
Hydrosalpinx (fallopian tube) (follicularis)
  N70.11
Hydrothorax (double) (pleura) J94.8
  chylous (nonfilarial) I89.8
    filarial —*see also* Infestation, filarial B74.9
      [J91.8]
  traumatic —*see* Injury, intrathoracic
  tuberculous NEC (non primary) A15.6
Hydroureter —*see also* Hydronephrosis N13.4
  with infection N13.6
  congenital Q62.39
Hydroureteronephrosis —*see* Hydronephrosis
Hydrourethra N36.8
Hydroxykynureninuria E70.8
Hydroxylysinemia E72.3
Hydroxyprolinemia E72.59
Hygiene, sleep
  abuse Z72.821
  inadequate Z72.821
  poor Z72.821
Hygroma (congenital) (cystic) D18.1
  praepatellare, prepatellar —*see* Bursitis,
    prepatellar

Hymen —*see* condition
Hymenolepis, hymenolepiasis (diminuta)
  (infection) (infestation) (nana) B71.0
Hypalgesia R20.8
Hyperacidity (gastric) K31.89
  psychogenic F45.8
Hyperactive, hyperactivity F90.9
  basal cell, uterine cervix —*see* Dysplasia,
    cervix
  bowel sounds R19.12
  cervix epithelial (basal) —*see* Dysplasia,
    cervix
  child F90.9
    attention deficit —*see* Disorder, attention-
      deficit hyperactivity
  detrusor muscle N32.81
  gastrointestinal K31.89
    psychogenic F45.8
  nasal mucous membrane J34.3
  stomach K31.89
  thyroid (gland) —*see* Hyperthyroidism
Hyperacusis H93.23-
Hyperadrenalism E27.5
Hyperadrenocorticism E24.9
  congenital E25.0
  iatrogenic E24.2
    correct substance properly administered —
      see Table of Drugs and Chemicals, by
      drug, adverse effect
    overdose or wrong substance given or
      taken —*see* Table of Drugs and
      Chemicals, by drug, poisoning
  not associated with Cushing's syndrome E27.0
  pituitary-dependent E24.0
Hyperaldosteronism E26.9
  familial (type I) E26.02
  glucocorticoid-remediable E26.02
  primary (due to (bilateral) adrenal
    hyperplasia) E26.09
  primary NEC E26.09
  secondary E26.1
  specified NEC E26.89
Hyperalgesia R20.8
Hyperalimentation R63.2
  carotene, carotin E67.1
  specified NEC E67.8
  vitamin
    A E67.0
    D E67.3
Hyperaminoaciduria
  arginine E72.21
  cystine E72.01
  lysine E72.3
  ornithine E72.4
Hyperammonemia (congenital) E72.20
Hyperazotemia —*see* Uremia
Hyperbetalipoproteinemia (familial) E78.00 ◀▥
  with prebetalipoproteinemia E78.2
Hyperbilirubinemia
  constitutional E80.6
  familial conjugated E80.6
  neonatal (transient) —*see* Jaundice, newborn
Hypercalcemia, hypocalciuric, familial E83.52
Hypercalciuria, idiopathic E83.52
Hypercapnia R06.89
  newborn P84
Hypercarotenemia, hypercarotinemia (dietary)
  E67.1
Hypercementosis K03.4
Hyperchloremia E87.8
Hyperchlorhydria K31.89
  neurotic F45.8
  psychogenic F45.8
Hypercholesterinemia —*see*
  Hypercholesterolemia
Hypercholesterolemia (essential) (primary)
  (pure) E78.00 ◀▥
  with hyperglyceridemia, endogenous E78.2
  dietary counseling and surveillance Z71.3
  familial E78.01 ◀
  hereditary E78.01 ◀

Hyperchylia gastrica, psychogenic F45.8
Hyperchylomicronemia (familial) (primary)
  E78.3
  with hyperbetalipoproteinemia E78.3
Hypercoagulable (state) D68.59
  activated protein C resistance D68.51
  antithrombin (III) deficiency D68.59
  factor V Leiden mutation D68.51
  primary NEC D68.59
  protein C deficiency D68.59
  protein S deficiency D68.59
  prothrombin gene mutation D68.52
  secondary D68.69
  specified NEC D68.69
Hypercoagulation (state) D68.59
Hypercorticalism, pituitary-dependent E24.0
Hypercorticosolism —*see* Cushing's, syndrome
Hypercorticosteronism E24.2
  correct substance properly administered —*see*
    Table of Drugs and Chemicals, by drug,
    adverse effect
  overdose or wrong substance given or
    taken —*see* Table of Drugs and
    Chemicals, by drug, poisoning
Hypercortisonism E24.2
  correct substance properly administered —*see*
    Table of Drugs and Chemicals, by drug,
    adverse effect
  overdose or wrong substance given or
    taken —*see* Table of Drugs and
    Chemicals, by drug, poisoning
Hyperekplexia Q89.8
Hyperelectrolytemia E87.8
Hyperemesis R11.10
  with nausea R11.2
  gravidarum (mild) O21.0
    with
      carbohydrate depletion O21.1
      dehydration O21.1
      electrolyte imbalance O21.1
      metabolic disturbance O21.1
    severe (with metabolic disturbance) O21.1
  projectile R11.12
  psychogenic F45.8
Hyperemia (acute) (passive) R68.89
  anal mucosa K62.89
  bladder N32.89
  cerebral I67.89
  conjunctiva H11.43-
  ear internal, acute —*see* subcategory H83.0
  enteric K59.8
  eye —*see* Hyperemia, conjunctiva
  eyelid (active) (passive) —*see* Disorder,
    eyelid, specified type NEC
  intestine K59.8
  iris —*see* Disorder, iris, vascular
  kidney N28.89
  labyrinth —*see* subcategory H83.0
  liver (active) K76.89
  lung (passive) —*see* Edema, lung
  pulmonary (passive) —*see* Edema, lung
  renal N28.89
  retina H35.89
  stomach K31.89
Hyperesthesia (body surface) R20.3
  larynx (reflex) J38.7
    hysterical F44.89
  pharynx (reflex) J39.2
    hysterical F44.89
Hyperestrogenism (drug-induced) (iatrogenic)
  E28.0
Hyperexplexia Q89.8
Hyperfibrinolysis —*see* Fibrinolysis
Hyperfructosemia E74.19
Hyperfunction
  adrenal cortex, not associated with Cushing's
    syndrome E27.0
    medulla E27.5
      adrenomedullary E27.5
    virilism E25.9
      congenital E25.0

◀ New   ▥ Revised   ~~deleted~~ Deleted

Hyperfunction (Continued)
  ovarian E28.8
  pancreas K86.89 ◄▮▮▮
  parathyroid (gland) E21.3
  pituitary (gland) (anterior) E22.9
    specified NEC E22.8
  polyglandular E31.1
  testicular E29.0
Hypergammaglobulinemia D89.2
  polyclonal D89.0
  Waldenström D89.0
Hypergastrinemia E16.4
Hyperglobulinemia R77.1
Hyperglycemia, hyperglycemic (transient) R73.9
  coma —see Diabetes, by type, with coma
  postpancreatectomy E89.1
Hyperglyceridemia (endogenous) (essential)
    (familial) (hereditary) (pure) E78.1
  mixed E78.3
Hyperglycinemia (non-ketotic) E72.51
Hypergonadism
  ovarian E28.8
  testicular (primary) (infantile) E29.0
Hyperheparinemia D68.32
Hyperhidrosis, hyperidrosis R61
  focal
    primary L74.519
      axilla L74.510
      face L74.511
      palms L74.512
      soles L74.513
    secondary L74.52
  generalized R61
  localized
    primary L74.519
      axilla L74.510
      face L74.511
      palms L74.512
      soles L74.513
    secondary L74.52
  psychogenic F45.8
  secondary R61
    focal L74.52
Hyperhistidinemia E70.41
Hyperhomocysteinemia E72.11
Hyperhydroxyprolinemia E72.59
Hyperinsulinism (functional) E16.1
  with
    coma (hypoglycemic) E15
    encephalopathy E16.1 [G94]
  ectopic E16.1
  therapeutic misadventure (from
      administration of insulin) —see
      subcategory T38.3
Hyperkalemia E87.5
Hyperkeratosis —see also Keratosis L85.9
  cervix N88.0
  due to yaws (early) (late) (palmar or plantar)
      A66.3
  follicularis Q82.8
    penetrans (in cutem) L87.0
  palmoplantaris climacterica L85.1
  pinta A67.1
  senile (with pruritus) L57.0
  universalis congenita Q80.8
  vocal cord J38.3
  vulva N90.4
Hyperkinesia, hyperkinetic (disease) (reaction)
    (syndrome) (childhood) (adolescence) —see
    also Disorder, attention-deficit hyperactivity
  heart I51.89
Hyperleucine-isoleucinemia E71.19
Hyperlipemia, hyperlipidemia E78.5
  combined E78.2
    familial E78.4
  group
    A E78.00 ◄▮▮▮
    B E78.1
    C E78.2
    D E78.3
  mixed E78.2
  specified NEC E78.4

Hyperlipidosis E75.6
  hereditary NEC E75.5
Hyperlipoproteinemia E78.5
  Fredrickson's type
    I E78.3
    IIa E78.00 ◄▮▮▮
    IIb E78.2
    III E78.2
    IV E78.1
    V E78.3
  low-density-lipoprotein-type (LDL) E78.00 ◄▮▮▮
  very-low-density-lipoprotein-type (VLDL)
      E78.1
Hyperlucent lung, unilateral J43.0
Hyperlysinemia E72.3
Hypermagnesemia E83.41
  neonatal P71.8
Hypermenorrhea N92.0
Hypermethioninemia E72.19
Hypermetropia (congenital) H52.0-
Hypermobility, hypermotility
  cecum —see Syndrome, irritable bowel
  coccyx —see subcategory M53.2
  colon —see Syndrome, irritable bowel
    psychogenic F45.8
  ileum K58.9
  intestine —see also Syndrome, irritable bowel
      K58.9
    psychogenic F45.8
  meniscus (knee) —see Derangement, knee,
      meniscus
  scapula —see Instability, joint, shoulder
  stomach K31.89
    psychogenic F45.8
  syndrome M35.7
  urethra N36.41
    with intrinsic sphincter deficiency N36.43
Hypernasality R49.21
Hypernatremia E87.0
Hypernephroma C64.-
Hyperopia —see Hypermetropia
Hyperorexia nervosa F50.2
Hyperornithinemia E72.4
Hyperosmia R43.1
Hyperosmolality E87.0
Hyperostosis (monomelic) —see also Disorder,
    bone, density and structure, specified NEC
  ankylosing (spine) M48.10
    cervical region M48.12
    cervicothoracic region M48.13
    lumbar region M48.16
    lumbosacral region M48.17
    multiple sites M48.19
    occipito-atlanto-axial region M48.11
    sacrococcygeal region M48.18
    thoracic region M48.14
    thoracolumbar region M48.15
  cortical (skull) M85.2
    infantile M89.8X-
  frontal, internal of skull M85.2
  interna frontalis M85.2
  skeletal, diffuse idiopathic —see
      Hyperostosis, ankylosing
  skull M85.2
    congenital Q75.8
  vertebral, ankylosing —see Hyperostosis,
      ankylosing
Hyperovarism E28.8
Hyperoxaluria (primary) E72.53
Hyperparathyroidism E21.3
  primary E21.0
  secondary (renal) N25.81
    non-renal E21.1
  specified NEC E21.2
  tertiary E21.2
Hyperpathia R20.8
Hyperperistalsis R19.2
  psychogenic F45.8
Hyperpermeability, capillary I78.8
Hyperphagia R63.2
Hyperphenylalaninemia NEC E70.1

Hyperphoria (alternating) H50.53
Hyperphosphatemia E83.39
Hyperpiesis, hyperpiesia —see Hypertension
Hyperpigmentation —see also Pigmentation
  melanin NEC L81.4
  postinflammatory L81.0
Hyperpinealism E34.8
Hyperpituitarism E22.9
Hyperplasia, hyperplastic
  adenoids J35.2
  adrenal (capsule) (cortex) (gland) E27.8
    with
      sexual precocity (male) E25.9
        congenital E25.0
      virilism, adrenal E25.9
        congenital E25.0
      virilization (female) E25.9
        congenital E25.0
    congenital E25.0
    salt-losing E25.0
  adrenomedullary E27.5
  angiolymphoid, eosinophilia (ALHE) D18.01
  appendix (lymphoid) K38.0
  artery, fibromuscular I77.3
  bone —see also Hypertrophy, bone
    marrow D75.89
  breast —see also Hypertrophy, breast
    ductal (atypical) N60.9-
  C-cell, thyroid E07.0
  cementation (tooth) (teeth) K03.4
  cervical gland R59.0
  cervix (uteri) (basal cell) (endometrium)
      (polypoid) —see also Dysplasia, cervix
    congenital Q51.828
  clitoris, congenital Q52.6
  denture K06.2
  endocervicitis N72
  endometrium, endometrial (adenomatous)
      (benign) (cystic) (glandular) (glandular-
      cystic) (polypoid) N85.00
    with atypia N85.02
    cervix —see Dysplasia, cervix
    complex (without atypia) N85.01
    simple (without atypia) N85.01
  epithelial L85.9
    focal, oral, including tongue K13.29
    nipple N62
    skin L85.9
    tongue K13.29
    vaginal wall N89.3
  erythroid D75.89
  fibromuscular of artery (carotid) (renal)
      I77.3
  genital
    female NEC N94.89
    male N50.89 ◄▮▮▮
  gingiva K06.1
  glandularis cystica uteri (interstitialis) —see
      also Hyperplasia, endometrial N85.00-
  gum K06.1
  hymen, congenital Q52.4
  irritative, edentulous (alveolar) K06.2
  jaw M26.09
    alveolar M26.79
    lower M26.03
      alveolar M26.72
    upper M26.01
      alveolar M26.71
  kidney (congenital) Q63.3
  labia N90.69 ◄▮▮▮
    epithelial N90.3
  liver (congenital) Q44.7
    nodular, focal K76.89
  lymph gland or node R59.9
  mandible, mandibular M26.03
    alveolar M26.72
    unilateral condylar M27.8
  maxilla, maxillary M26.01
    alveolar M26.71
  myometrium, myometrial N85.2
  neuroendocrine cell, of infancy J84.841

Hyperplasia, hyperplastic *(Continued)*
    nose
        lymphoid J34.89
        polypoid J33.9
    oral mucosa (irritative) K13.6
    organ or site, congenital NEC —*see* Anomaly,
        by site
    ovary N83.8
    palate, papillary (irritative) K13.6
    pancreatic islet cells E16.9
        alpha E16.8
            with excess
                gastrin E16.4
                glucagon E16.3
        beta E16.1
    parathyroid (gland) E21.0
    pharynx (lymphoid) J39.2
    prostate (adenofibromatous) (nodular)
        N40.0
        with lower urinary tract symptoms (LUTS)
            N40.1
        without lower urinary tract symptoms
            (LUTS) N40.0
    renal artery I77.89
    reticulo-endothelial (cell) D75.89
    salivary gland (any) K11.1
    Schimmelbusch's —*see* Mastopathy,
        cystic
    suprarenal capsule (gland) E27.8
    thymus (gland) (persistent) E32.0
    thyroid (gland) —*see* Goiter
    tonsils (faucial) (infective) (lingual)
        (lymphoid) J35.1
        with adenoids J35.3
    unilateral condylar M27.8
    uterus, uterine N85.2
        endometrium (glandular) —*see also*
            Hyperplasia, endometrial
            N85.00-
    vulva N90.69 ◀▥
        epithelial N90.3
Hyperpnea —*see* Hyperventilation
Hyperpotassemia E87.5
Hyperprebetalipoproteinemia (familial)
    E78.1
Hyperprolactinemia E22.1
Hyperprolinemia (type I) (type II) E72.59
Hyperproteinemia E88.09
Hyperprothrombinemia, causing coagulation
    factor deficiency D68.4
Hyperpyrexia R50.9
    heat (effects) T67.0
    malignant, due to anesthetic T88.3
    rheumatic —*see* Fever, rheumatic
    unknown origin R50.9
Hyper-reflexia R29.2
Hypersalivation K11.7
Hypersecretion
    ACTH (not associated with Cushing's
        syndrome) E27.0
        pituitary E24.0
    adrenaline E27.5
    adrenomedullary E27.5
    androgen (testicular) E29.0
        ovarian (drug-induced) (iatrogenic) E28.1
    calcitonin E07.0
    catecholamine E27.5
    corticoadrenal E24.9
    cortisol E24.9
    epinephrine E27.5
    estrogen E28.0
    gastric K31.89
        psychogenic F45.8
    gastrin E16.4
    glucagon E16.3
    hormone (s)
        ACTH (not associated with Cushing's
            syndrome) E27.0
            pituitary E24.0
        antidiuretic E22.2
        growth E22.0

Hypersecretion *(Continued)*
    hormone *(Continued)*
        intestinal NEC E34.1
        ovarian androgen E28.1
        pituitary E22.9
        testicular E29.0
        thyroid stimulating E05.80
            with thyroid storm E05.81
    insulin —*see* Hyperinsulinism
    lacrimal glands —*see* Epiphora
    medulloadrenal E27.5
    milk O92.6
    ovarian androgens E28.1
    salivary gland (any) K11.7
    thyrocalcitonin E07.0
    upper respiratory J39.8
Hypersegmentation, leukocytic, hereditary
    D72.0
Hypersensitive, hypersensitiveness,
    hypersensitivity —*see also* Allergy
    carotid sinus G90.01
    colon —*see* Irritable, colon
    drug T88.7
    gastrointestinal K52.29 ◀▥
        immediate K52.29 ◀
        psychogenic F45.8
    labyrinth —*see* subcategory H83.2
    pain R20.8
    pneumonitis —*see* Pneumonitis,
        allergic
    reaction T78.40
        upper respiratory tract NEC J39.3
Hypersomnia (organic) G47.10
    due to
        alcohol
            abuse F10.182
            dependence F10.282
            use F10.982
        amphetamines
            abuse F15.182
            dependence F15.282
            use F15.982
        caffeine
            abuse F15.182
            dependence F15.282
            use F15.982
        cocaine
            abuse F14.182
            dependence F14.282
            use F14.982
        drug NEC
            abuse F19.182
            dependence F19.282
            use F19.982
        medical condition G47.14
        mental disorder F51.13
        opioid
            abuse F11.182
            dependence F11.282
            use F11.982
        psychoactive substance NEC
            abuse F19.182
            dependence F19.282
            use F19.982
        sedative, hypnotic, or anxiolytic
            abuse F13.182
            dependence F13.282
            use F13.982
        stimulant NEC
            abuse F15.182
            dependence F15.282
            use F15.982
    idiopathic G47.11
        with long sleep time G47.11
        without long sleep time G47.12
    menstrual related G47.13
    nonorganic origin F51.11
        specified NEC F51.19
    not due to a substance or known
        physiological condition F51.11
    specified NEC F51.19

Hypersomnia *(Continued)*
    primary F51.11
    recurrent G47.13
    specified NEC G47.19
Hypersplenia, hypersplenism D73.1
Hyperstimulation, ovaries (associated with
    induced ovulation) N98.1
Hypersusceptibility —*see* Allergy
Hypertelorism (ocular) (orbital) Q75.2
Hypertension, hypertensive (accelerated)
    (benign) (essential) (idiopathic)
    (malignant) (systemic) I10
    with
        heart involvement (conditions in
            I51.4-I51.9 due to hypertension) —*see*
            Hypertension, heart
        kidney involvement —*see* Hypertension,
            kidney
    benign, intracranial G93.2
    borderline R03.0
    cardiorenal (disease) I13.10
        with heart failure I13.0
            with stage 1 through stage 4 chronic
                kidney disease I13.0
            with stage 5 or end stage renal disease
                I13.2
        without heart failure I13.10
            with stage 1 through stage 4 chronic
                kidney disease I13.10
            with stage 5 or end stage renal disease
                I13.11
    cardiovascular
        disease (arteriosclerotic) (sclerotic) —*see*
            Hypertension, heart
        renal (disease) —*see* Hypertension,
            cardiorenal
    chronic venous —*see* Hypertension, venous
        (chronic)
    complicating
        childbirth (labor) O16.4 ◀▥
            ~~with~~
                ~~heart disease O10.12~~
                    ~~with renal disease O10.32~~
                ~~renal disease O10.22~~
                    ~~with heart disease O10.32~~
            ~~essential O10.02~~
            pre-existing O10.92 ◀
                with ◀
                    heart disease O10.12 ◀
                        with renal disease
                            O10.32 ◀
                    pre-eclampsia O11.4 ◀
                    renal disease O10.22 ◀
                        with heart disease
                            O10.32 ◀
                    essential O10.02 ◀
                secondary O10.42
        pregnancy O16.-
            with edema —*see also* Pre-eclampsia
                O14.9-
            gestational (pregnancy induced)
                (without proteinuria) O13.- ◀▥
                with proteinuria O14.9-
                    mild pre-eclampsia O14.0-
                    moderate pre-eclampsia
                        O14.0-
                    severe pre-eclampsia O14.1-
                        with hemolysis, elevated liver
                            enzymes and low platelet
                            count (HELLP) O14.2-
            pre-existing O10.91-
                with
                    heart disease O10.11-
                        with renal disease O10.31-
                    pre-eclampsia —*see* category
                        O11 ◀▥
                    renal disease O10.21-
                        with heart disease O10.31-
                    essential O10.01-
                    secondary O10.41-
            transient O13.- ◀

◀ New   ◀▥ Revised   ~~deleted~~ Deleted

Hypertension, hypertensive *(Continued)*
  complicating *(Continued)*
    puerperium pre-existing O16.5 ◄▐▌
      ~~with~~
        ~~heart disease O10.13~~
          ~~with renal disease O10.33~~
        ~~renal disease O10.23~~
          ~~with heart disease O10.33~~
      ~~essential O10.03~~
      pre-existing ◄
        with ◄
          heart disease O10.13 ◄
            with renal disease O10.33 ◄
          pre-eclampsia O11.5 ◄
          renal disease O10.23 ◄
            with heart disease O10.33 ◄
          essential O10.03 ◄
        pregnancy-induced O13.9
        secondary O10.43
  crisis I16.9 ◄
  due to
    endocrine disorders I15.2
    pheochromocytoma I15.2
    renal disorders NEC I15.1
      arterial I15.0
    renovascular disorders I15.0
    specified disease NEC I15.8
  emergency I16.2 ◄
  encephalopathy I67.4
  gestational (without significant proteinuria)
    (pregnancy-induced) (transient)
    O13.-
    with significant proteinuria —*see*
      Pre-eclampsia
    complicating ◄
      delivery O13.4 ◄
      puerperium O13.5 ◄
  Goldblatt's I70.1
  heart (disease) (conditions in I51.4-I51.9 due
    to hypertension) I11.9
    with
      heart failure (congestive) I11.0
      kidney disease (chronic) —*see*
        Hypertension, cardiorenal
  intracranial (benign) G93.2
  kidney I12.9
    with
      heart disease —*see* Hypertension,
        cardiorenal
      stage 1 through stage 4 chronic kidney
        disease I12.9
      stage 5 chronic kidney disease (CKD)
        or end stage renal disease (ESRD)
        I12.0
  lesser circulation I27.0
  maternal O16.- ◄
  newborn P29.2
    pulmonary (persistent) P29.3
  ocular H40.05-
  pancreatic duct — code to underlying
    condition
    with chronic pancreatitis K86.1
  portal (due to chronic liver disease)
    (idiopathic) K76.6
    gastropathy K31.89
    in (due to) schistosomiasis (bilharziasis)
      B65.9 [K77]
  postoperative I97.3
  psychogenic F45.8
  pulmonary (artery) (secondary) NEC
    I27.2
    with
      cor pulmonale (chronic) I27.2
        acute I26.09
      right heart ventricular strain/failure
        I27.2
        acute I26.09
    of newborn (persistent) P29.3
    primary (idiopathic) I27.0
  renal —*see* Hypertension, kidney
  renovascular I15.0

Hypertension, hypertensive *(Continued)*
  secondary NEC I15.9
    due to
      endocrine disorders I15.2
      pheochromocytoma I15.2
      renal disorders NEC I15.1
        arterial I15.0
      renovascular disorders I15.0
    specified NEC I15.8
  transient, of pregnancy O13.- ◄
  urgency I16.0 ◄
  venous (chronic)
    due to
      deep vein thrombosis —*see* Syndrome,
        postthrombotic
    idiopathic I87.309
      with
        inflammation I87.32-
          with ulcer I87.33-
        specified complication NEC I87.39-
        ulcer I87.31-
          with inflammation I87.33-
      asymptomatic I87.30-
Hypertensive urgency —*see* Hypertension
Hyperthecosis ovary E28.8
Hyperthermia (of unknown origin) —*see also*
    Hyperpyrexia
  malignant, due to anesthesia T88.3
  newborn P81.9
    environmental P81.0
Hyperthyroid (recurrent) —*see*
    Hyperthyroidism
Hyperthyroidism (latent) (pre-adult)
    (recurrent) E05.90
  with
    goiter (diffuse) E05.00
      with thyroid storm E05.01
      nodular (multinodular) E05.20
        with thyroid storm E05.21
        uninodular E05.10
          with thyroid storm E05.11
    storm E05.91
  due to ectopic thyroid tissue E05.30
    with thyroid storm E05.31
  neonatal, transitory P72.1
  specified NEC E05.80
    with thyroid storm E05.81
Hypertony, hypertonia, hypertonicity
  bladder N31.8
  congenital P94.1
  stomach K31.89
    psychogenic F45.8
  uterus, uterine (contractions) (complicating
    delivery) O62.4
Hypertrichosis L68.9
  congenital Q84.2
  eyelid H02.869
    left H02.866
      lower H02.865
      upper H02.864
    right H02.863
      lower H02.862
      upper H02.861
  lanuginosa Q84.2
    acquired L68.1
  localized L68.2
  specified NEC L68.8
Hypertriglyceridemia, essential E78.1
Hypertrophy, hypertrophic
  adenofibromatous, prostate —*see*
    Enlargement, enlarged, prostate
  adenoids (infective) J35.2
    with tonsils J35.3
  adrenal cortex E27.8
  alveolar process or ridge —*see* Anomaly,
    alveolar
  anal papillae K62.89
  artery I77.89
    congenital NEC Q27.8
      digestive system Q27.8
      lower limb Q27.8

Hypertrophy, hypertrophic *(Continued)*
  artery *(Continued)*
    congenital NEC *(Continued)*
      specified site NEC Q27.8
      upper limb Q27.8
  auricular —*see* Hypertrophy, cardiac
  Bartholin's gland N75.8
  bile duct (common) (hepatic) K83.8
  bladder (sphincter) (trigone) N32.89
  bone M89.30
    carpus M89.34-
    clavicle M89.31-
    femur M89.35-
    fibula M89.36-
    finger M89.34-
    humerus M89.32-
    ilium M89.359
    ischium M89.359
    metacarpus M89.34-
    metatarsus M89.37-
    multiple sites M89.39
    neck M89.38
    radius M89.33-
    rib M89.38
    scapula M89.31-
    skull M89.38
    tarsus M89.37-
    tibia M89.36-
    toe M89.37-
    ulna M89.33-
    vertebra M89.38
  brain G93.89
  breast N62
    cystic —*see* Mastopathy, cystic
    newborn P83.4
    pubertal, massive N62
    puerperal, postpartum —*see* Disorder,
      breast, specified type NEC
    senile (parenchymatous) N62
  cardiac (chronic) (idiopathic) I51.7
    with rheumatic fever (conditions in I00)
      active I01.8
      inactive or quiescent (with chorea) I09.89
    congenital NEC Q24.8
    fatty —*see* Degeneration, myocardial
    hypertensive —*see* Hypertension, heart
    rheumatic (with chorea) I09.89
      active or acute I01.8
        with chorea I02.0
    valve —*see* Endocarditis
  cartilage —*see* Disorder, cartilage, specified
    type NEC
  cecum —*see* Megacolon
  cervix (uteri) N88.8
    congenital Q51.828
    elongation N88.4
  clitoris (cirrhotic) N90.89
    congenital Q52.6
  colon —*see also* Megacolon
    congenital Q43.2
  conjunctiva, lymphoid H11.89
  corpora cavernosa N48.89
  cystic duct K82.8
  duodenum K31.89
  endometrium (glandular) —*see also*
    Hyperplasia, endometrial N85.00-
    cervix N88.8
  epididymis N50.89 ◄▐▌
  esophageal hiatus (congenital) Q79.1
    with hernia —*see* Hernia, hiatal
  eyelid —*see* Disorder, eyelid, specified type
    NEC
  fat pad E65
    knee (infrapatellar) (popliteal) (prepatellar)
      (retropatellar) M79.4
  foot (congenital) Q74.2
  frenulum, frenum (tongue) K14.8
    lip K13.0
  gallbladder K82.8
  gastric mucosa K29.60
    with bleeding K29.61

Hypertrophy, hypertrophic *(Continued)*
  gland, glandular R59.9
    generalized R59.1
    localized R59.0
  gum (mucous membrane) K06.1
  heart (idiopathic) —*see also* Hypertrophy,
      cardiac
    valve —*see also* Endocarditis I38
  hemifacial Q67.4
  hepatic —*see* Hypertrophy, liver
  hiatus (esophageal) Q79.1
  hilus gland R59.0
  hymen, congenital Q52.4
  ileum K63.89
  intestine NEC K63.89
  jejunum K63.89
  kidney (compensatory) N28.81
    congenital Q63.3
  labium (majus) (minus) N90.60 ◀⊪
  ligament —*see* Disorder, ligament
  lingual tonsil (infective) J35.1
    with adenoids J35.3
  lip K13.0
    congenital Q18.6
  liver R16.0
    acute K76.89
    cirrhotic —*see* Cirrhosis, liver
    congenital Q44.7
    fatty —*see* Fatty, liver
  lymph, lymphatic gland R59.9
    generalized R59.1
    localized R59.0
    tuberculous —*see* Tuberculosis, lymph
      gland
  mammary gland —*see* Hypertrophy, breast
  Meckel's diverticulum (congenital) Q43.0
    malignant —*see* Table of Neoplasms, small
      intestine, malignant
  median bar —*see* Hyperplasia, prostate
  meibomian gland —*see* Chalazion
  meniscus, knee, congenital Q74.1
  metatarsal head —*see* Hypertrophy, bone,
      metatarsus
  metatarsus —*see* Hypertrophy, bone,
      metatarsus
  mucous membrane
    alveolar ridge K06.2
    gum K06.1
    nose (turbinate) J34.3
  muscle M62.89
  muscular coat, artery I77.89
  myocardium —*see also* Hypertrophy, cardiac
    idiopathic I42.2
  myometrium N85.2
  nail L60.2
    congenital Q84.5
  nasal J34.89
    alae J34.89
    bone J34.89
    cartilage J34.89
    mucous membrane (septum) J34.3
    sinus J34.89
    turbinate J34.3
  nasopharynx, lymphoid (infectional) (tissue)
      (wall) J35.2
  nipple N62
  organ or site, congenital NEC —*see* Anomaly,
      by site - ovary N83.8
  palate (hard) M27.8
    soft K13.79
  pancreas, congenital Q45.3
  parathyroid (gland) E21.0
  parotid gland K11.1
  penis N48.89
  pharyngeal tonsil J35.2
  pharynx J39.2
    lymphoid (infectional) (tissue) (wall)
      J35.2
  pituitary (anterior) (fossa) (gland) E23.6
  prepuce (congenital) N47.8
    female N90.89

Hypertrophy, hypertrophic *(Continued)*
  prostate —*see* Enlargement, enlarged,
      prostate
    congenital Q55.4
  pseudomuscular G71.0
  pylorus (adult) (muscle) (sphincter)
      K31.1
    congenital or infantile Q40.0
  rectal, rectum (sphincter) K62.89
  rhinitis (turbinate) J31.0
  salivary gland (any) K11.1
    congenital Q38.4
  scaphoid (tarsal) —*see* Hypertrophy, bone,
      tarsus
  scar L91.0
  scrotum N50.89 ◀⊪
  seminal vesicle N50.89 ◀⊪
  sigmoid —*see* Megacolon
  skin L91.9
    specified NEC L91.8
  spermatic cord N50.89 ◀⊪
  spleen —*see* Splenomegaly
  spondylitis —*see* Spondylosis
  stomach K31.89
  sublingual gland K11.1
  submandibular gland K11.1
  suprarenal cortex (gland) E27.8
  synovial NEC M67.20
    acromioclavicular M67.21-
    ankle M67.27-
    elbow M67.22-
    foot M67.27-
    hand M67.24-
    hip M67.25-
    knee M67.26-
    multiple sites M67.29
    specified site NEC M67.28
    wrist M67.23-
  tendon —*see* Disorder, tendon, specified type
      NEC
  testis N44.8
    congenital Q55.29
  thymic, thymus (gland) (congenital)
      E32.0
  thyroid (gland) —*see* Goiter
  toe (congenital) Q74.2
    acquired —*see also* Deformity, toe, specified
      NEC
  tongue K14.8
    congenital Q38.2
    papillae (foliate) K14.3
  tonsils (faucial) (infective) (lingual)
      (lymphoid) J35.1
    with adenoids J35.3
  tunica vaginalis N50.89 ◀⊪
  ureter N28.89
  urethra N36.8
  uterus N85.2
    neck (with elongation) N88.4
    puerperal O90.89
  uvula K13.79
  vagina N89.8
  vas deferens N50.89 ◀⊪
  vein I87.8
  ventricle, ventricular (heart) —*see also*
      Hypertrophy, cardiac
    congenital Q24.8
    in tetralogy of Fallot Q21.3
  verumontanum N36.8
  vocal cord J38.3
  vulva N90.60 ◀⊪
    stasis (nonfilarial) N90.69 ◀⊪
Hypertropia H50.2-
Hypertyrosinemia E70.21
Hyperuricemia (asymptomatic)
    E79.0
Hypervalinemia E71.19
Hyperventilation (tetany) R06.4
  hysterical F45.8
  psychogenic F45.8
  syndrome F45.8

Hypervitaminosis (dietary) NEC E67.8
  A E67.0
    administered as drug (prolonged intake) —
      see Table of Drugs and Chemicals,
      vitamins, adverse effect
    overdose or wrong substance given or
      taken —*see* Table of Drugs and
      Chemicals, vitamins, poisoning
  B6 E67.2
  D E67.3
    administered as drug (prolonged intake) —
      see Table of Drugs and Chemicals,
      vitamins, adverse effect
    overdose or wrong substance given or
      taken —*see* Table of Drugs and
      Chemicals, vitamins, poisoning
  K E67.8
    administered as drug (prolonged intake) —
      see Table of Drugs and Chemicals,
      vitamins, adverse effect
    overdose or wrong substance given or
      taken —*see* Table of Drugs and
      Chemicals, vitamins, poisoning
Hypervolemia E87.70
  specified NEC E87.79
Hypesthesia R20.1
  cornea —*see* Anesthesia, cornea
Hyphema H21.0-
  traumatic S05.1-
Hypoacidity, gastric K31.89
  psychogenic F45.8
Hypoadrenalism, hypoadrenia E27.40
  primary E27.1
  tuberculous A18.7
Hypoadrenocorticism E27.40
  pituitary E23.0
  primary E27.1
Hypoalbuminemia E88.09
Hypoaldosteronism E27.40
Hypoalphalipoproteinemia E78.6
Hypobarism T70.29
Hypobaropathy T70.29
Hypobetalipoproteinemia (familial)
    E78.6
Hypocalcemia E83.51
  dietary E58
  neonatal P71.1
    due to cow's milk P71.0
  phosphate-loading (newborn) P71.1
Hypochloremia E87.8
Hypochlorhydria K31.89
  neurotic F45.8
  psychogenic F45.8
Hypochondria, hypochondriac,
    hypochondriasis (reaction) F45.21
  sleep F51.03
Hypochondrogenesis Q77.0
Hypochondroplasia Q77.4
Hypochromasia, blood cells D50.8
Hypodontia —*see* Anodontia
Hypoeosinophilia D72.89
Hypoesthesia R20.1
Hypofibrinogenemia D68.8
  acquired D65
  congenital (hereditary) D68.2
Hypofunction
  adrenocortical E27.40
    drug-induced E27.3
    postprocedural E89.6
    primary E27.1
  adrenomedullary, postprocedural E89.6
  cerebral R29.818
  corticoadrenal NEC E27.40
  intestinal K59.8
  labyrinth —*see* subcategory H83.2
  ovary E28.39
  pituitary (gland) (anterior) E23.0
  testicular E29.1
    postprocedural (postsurgical)
      (postirradiation) (iatrogenic) E89.5
Hypogalactia O92.4

◀ New   ◀⊪ Revised   ~~deleted~~ Deleted

Hypogammaglobulinemia —*see also*
    Agammaglobulinemia D80.1
  hereditary D80.0
  nonfamilial D80.1
  transient, of infancy D80.7
Hypogenitalism (congenital) —*see*
  Hypogonadism
Hypoglossia Q38.3
Hypoglycemia (spontaneous) E16.2
  coma E15
    diabetic —*see* Diabetes, coma
  diabetic —*see* Diabetes, hypoglycemia
  dietary counseling and surveillance Z71.3
  drug-induced E16.0
    with coma (nondiabetic) E15
  due to insulin E16.0
    with coma (nondiabetic) E15
    therapeutic misadventure —*see*
      subcategory T38.3
  functional, nonhyperinsulinemic E16.1
  iatrogenic E16.0
    with coma (nondiabetic) E15
  in infant of diabetic mother P70.1
    gestational diabetes P70.0
  infantile E16.1
  leucine-induced E71.19
  neonatal (transitory) P70.4
    iatrogenic P70.3
  reactive (not drug-induced) E16.1
  transitory neonatal P70.4
Hypogonadism
  female E28.39
  hypogonadotropic E23.0
  male E29.1
  ovarian (primary) E28.39
  pituitary E23.0
  testicular (primary) E29.1
Hypohidrosis, hypoidrosis L74.4
Hypoinsulinemia, postprocedural E89.1
Hypokalemia E87.6
Hypoleukocytosis —*see* Agranulocytosis
Hypolipoproteinemia (alpha) (beta) E78.6
Hypomagnesemia E83.42
  neonatal P71.2
Hypomania, hypomanic reaction F30.8
Hypomenorrhea —*see* Oligomenorrhea
Hypometabolism R63.8
Hypomotility
  gastrointestinal (tract) K31.89
    psychogenic F45.8
  intestine K59.8
    psychogenic F45.8
  stomach K31.89
    psychogenic F45.8
Hyponasality R49.22
Hyponatremia E87.1
Hypo-osmolality E87.1
Hypo-ovarianism, hypo-ovarism E28.39
Hypoparathyroidism E20.9
  familial E20.8
  idiopathic E20.0
  neonatal, transitory P71.4
  postprocedural E89.2
  specified NEC E20.8
Hypoperfusion (in)
  newborn P96.89
Hypopharyngitis —*see* Laryngopharyngitis
Hypophoria H50.53
Hypophosphatemia, hypophosphatasia
  (acquired) (congenital) (renal) E83.39
  familial E83.31
Hypophyseal, hypophysis —*see also* condition
  dwarfism E23.0
  gigantism E22.0
Hypopiesis —*see* Hypotension
Hypopinealism E34.8
Hypopituitarism (juvenile) E23.0
  drug-induced E23.1
  due to
    hypophysectomy E89.3
    radiotherapy E89.3

Hypopituitarism (*Continued*)
  iatrogenic NEC E23.1
  postirradiation E89.3
  postpartum O99.285 ◄▬
  postprocedural E89.3
Hypoplasia, hypoplastic
  adrenal (gland), congenital Q89.1
  alimentary tract, congenital Q45.8
    upper Q40.8
  anus, anal (canal) Q42.3
    with fistula Q42.2
  aorta, aortic Q25.42 ◄▬
    ascending, in hypoplastic left heart
      syndrome Q23.4
    valve Q23.1
      in hypoplastic left heart syndrome
        Q23.4
  areola, congenital Q83.8
  arm (congenital) —*see* Defect, reduction,
    upper limb
  artery (peripheral) Q27.8
    brain (congenital) Q28.3
    coronary Q24.5
    digestive system Q27.8
    lower limb Q27.8
    pulmonary Q25.79
      functional, unilateral J43.0
    retinal (congenital) Q14.1
    specified site NEC Q27.8
    umbilical Q27.0
    upper limb Q27.8
  auditory canal Q17.8
    causing impairment of hearing Q16.9
  biliary duct or passage Q44.5
  bone NOS Q79.9
    face Q75.8
    marrow D61.9
      megakaryocytic D69.49
    skull —*see* Hypoplasia, skull
  brain Q02
    gyri Q04.3
    part of Q04.3
  breast (areola) N64.82
  bronchus Q32.4
  cardiac Q24.8
  carpus —*see* Defect, reduction, upper limb,
    specified type NEC
  cartilage hair Q78.8 ◄▬
  cecum Q42.8
  cementum K00.4
  cephalic Q02
  cerebellum Q04.3
  cervix (uteri), congenital Q51.821
  clavicle (congenital) Q74.0
  coccyx Q76.49
  colon Q42.9
    specified NEC Q42.8
  corpus callosum Q04.0
  cricoid cartilage Q31.2
  digestive organ (s) or tract NEC Q45.8
    upper (congenital) Q40.8
  ear (auricle) (lobe) Q17.2
    middle Q16.4
  enamel of teeth (neonatal) (postnatal)
    (prenatal) K00.4
  endocrine (gland) NEC Q89.2
  endometrium N85.8
  epididymis (congenital) Q55.4
  epiglottis Q31.2
  erythroid, congenital D61.01
  esophagus (congenital) Q39.8
  eustachian tube Q17.8
  eye Q11.2
  eyelid (congenital) Q10.3
  face Q18.8
    bone (s) Q75.8
  femur (congenital) —*see* Defect,
    reduction, lower limb, specified
    type NEC
  fibula (congenital) —*see* Defect, reduction,
    lower limb, specified type NEC

Hypoplasia, hypoplastic (*Continued*)
  finger (congenital) —*see* Defect, reduction,
    upper limb, specified type NEC
  focal dermal Q82.8
  foot —*see* Defect, reduction, lower limb,
    specified type NEC
  gallbladder Q44.0
  genitalia, genital organ (s)
    female, congenital Q52.8
      external Q52.79
      internal NEC Q52.8
    in adiposogenital dystrophy E23.6
  glottis Q31.2
  hair Q84.2
  hand (congenital) —*see* Defect, reduction,
    upper limb, specified type NEC
  heart Q24.8
  humerus (congenital) —*see* Defect, reduction,
    upper limb, specified type NEC
  intestine (small) Q41.9
    large Q42.9
      specified NEC Q42.8
  jaw M26.09
    alveolar M26.79
      lower M26.04
        alveolar M26.74
      upper M26.02
        alveolar M26.73
  kidney (s) Q60.5
    bilateral Q60.4
    unilateral Q60.3
  labium (majus) (minus), congenital Q52.79
  larynx Q31.2
  left heart syndrome Q23.4
  leg (congenital) —*see* Defect, reduction, lower
    limb
  limb Q73.8
    lower (congenital) —*see* Defect, reduction,
      lower limb
    upper (congenital) —*see* Defect, reduction,
      upper limb
  liver Q44.7
  lung (lobe) (not associated with short
    gestation) Q33.6
    associated with immaturity, low birth
      weight, prematurity, or short
      gestation P28.0
  mammary (areola), congenital Q83.8
  mandible, mandibular M26.04
    alveolar M26.74
    unilateral condylar M27.8
  maxillary M26.02
    alveolar M26.73
  medullary D61.9
  megakaryocytic D69.49
  metacarpus —*see* Defect, reduction, upper
    limb, specified type NEC
  metatarsus —*see* Defect, reduction, lower
    limb, specified type NEC
  muscle Q79.8
  nail (s) Q84.6
  nose, nasal Q30.1
  optic nerve H47.03-
  osseous meatus (ear) Q17.8
  ovary, congenital Q50.39
  pancreas Q45.0
  parathyroid (gland) Q89.2
  parotid gland Q38.4
  patella Q74.1
  pelvis, pelvic girdle Q74.2
  penis (congenital) Q55.62
  peripheral vascular system Q27.8
    digestive system Q27.8
    lower limb Q27.8
    specified site NEC Q27.8
    upper limb Q27.8
  pituitary (gland) (congenital) Q89.2
  pulmonary (not associated with short
    gestation) Q33.6
    artery, functional J43.0
    associated with short gestation P28.0

Hypoplasia, hypoplastic *(Continued)*
  radioulnar —*see* Defect, reduction, upper limb, specified type NEC
  radius —*see* Defect, reduction, upper limb
  rectum Q42.1
    with fistula Q42.0
  respiratory system NEC Q34.8
  rib Q76.6
  right heart syndrome Q22.6
  sacrum Q76.49
  scapula Q74.0
  scrotum Q55.1
  shoulder girdle Q74.0
  skin Q82.8
  skull (bone) Q75.8
    with
      anencephaly Q00.0
      encephalocele —*see* Encephalocele
      hydrocephalus Q03.9
        with spina bifida —*see* Spina bifida, by site, with hydrocephalus
      microcephaly Q02
  spinal (cord) (ventral horn cell) Q06.1
  spine Q76.49
  sternum Q76.7
  tarsus —*see* Defect, reduction, lower limb, specified type NEC
  testis Q55.1
  thymic, with immunodeficiency D82.1
  thymus (gland) Q89.2
    with immunodeficiency D82.1
  thyroid (gland) E03.1
    cartilage Q31.2
  tibiofibular (congenital) —*see* Defect, reduction, lower limb, specified type NEC
  toe —*see* Defect, reduction, lower limb, specified type NEC
  tongue Q38.3
  Turner's K00.4
  ulna (congenital) —*see* Defect, reduction, upper limb
  umbilical artery Q27.0
  unilateral condylar M27.8
  ureter Q62.8
  uterus, congenital Q51.811
  vagina Q52.4
  vascular NEC peripheral Q27.8
    brain Q28.3
    digestive system Q27.8
    lower limb Q27.8
    specified site NEC Q27.8
    upper limb Q27.8
  vein (s) (peripheral) Q27.8
    brain Q28.3
    digestive system Q27.8
    great Q26.8
    lower limb Q27.8
    specified site NEC Q27.8
    upper limb Q27.8
  vena cava (inferior) (superior) Q26.8
  vertebra Q76.49
  vulva, congenital Q52.79
  zonule (ciliary) Q12.8

Hypopotassemia E87.6
Hypoproconvertinemia, congenital (hereditary) D68.2
Hypoproteinemia E77.8
Hypoprothrombinemia (congenital) (hereditary) (idiopathic) D68.2
  acquired D68.4
  newborn, transient P61.6
Hypoptyalism K11.7
Hypopyon (eye) (anterior chamber) —*see* Iridocyclitis, acute, hypopyon
Hypopyrexia R68.0
Hyporeflexia R29.2
Hyposecretion
  ACTH E23.0
  antidiuretic hormone E23.2
  ovary E28.39
  salivary gland (any) K11.7
  vasopressin E23.2
Hyposegmentation, leukocytic, hereditary D72.0
Hyposiderinemia D50.9
Hypospadias Q54.9
  balanic Q54.0
  coronal Q54.0
  glandular Q54.0
  penile Q54.1
  penoscrotal Q54.2
  perineal Q54.3
  specified NEC Q54.8
Hypospermatogenesis —*see* Oligospermia
Hyposplenism D73.0
Hypostasis pulmonary, passive —*see* Edema, lung
Hypostatic —*see* condition
Hyposthenuria N28.89
Hypotension (arterial) (constitutional) I95.9
  chronic I95.89
  drug-induced I95.2
  due to (of) hemodialysis I95.3
  iatrogenic I95.89
  idiopathic (permanent) I95.0
  intracranial, following ventricular shunting (ventriculostomy) G97.2
  intra-dialytic I95.3
  maternal, syndrome (following labor and delivery) O26.5-
  neurogenic, orthostatic G90.3
  orthostatic (chronic) I95.1
    due to drugs I95.2
    neurogenic G90.3
  postoperative I95.81
  postural I95.1
  specified NEC I95.89
Hypothermia (accidental) T68
  due to anesthesia, anesthetic T88.51
  low environmental temperature T68
  neonatal P80.9
    environmental (mild) NEC P80.8
    mild P80.8
    severe (chronic) (cold injury syndrome) P80.0
    specified NEC P80.8
  not associated with low environmental temperature R68.0

Hypothyroidism (acquired) E03.9
  congenital (without goiter) E03.1
    with goiter (diffuse) E03.0
  due to
    exogenous substance NEC E03.2
    iodine-deficiency, acquired E01.8
      subclinical E02
    irradiation therapy E89.0
    medicament NEC E03.2
    P-aminosalicylic acid (PAS) E03.2
    phenylbutazone E03.2
    resorcinol E03.2
    sulfonamide E03.2
    surgery E89.0
    thiourea group drugs E03.2
  iatrogenic NEC E03.2
  iodine-deficiency (acquired) E01.8
    congenital —*see* Syndrome, iodine-deficiency, congenital
    subclinical E02
  neonatal, transitory P72.2
  postinfectious E03.3
  postirradiation E89.0
  postprocedural E89.0
  postsurgical E89.0
  specified NEC E03.8
  subclinical, iodine-deficiency related E02
Hypotonia, hypotonicity, hypotony
  bladder N31.2
  congenital (benign) P94.2
  eye —*see* Disorder, globe, hypotony
Hypotrichosis —*see* Alopecia
Hypotropia H50.2-
Hypoventilation R06.89
  congenital central alveolar G47.35
  sleep related
    idiopathic nonobstructive alveolar G47.34
    in conditions classified elsewhere G47.36
Hypovitaminosis —*see* Deficiency, vitamin
Hypovolemia E86.1
  surgical shock T81.19
  traumatic (shock) T79.4
Hypoxemia R09.02
  newborn P84
  sleep related, in conditions classified elsewhere G47.36
Hypoxia —*see also* Anoxia R09.02
  cerebral, during a procedure NEC G97.81
    postprocedural NEC G97.82
  intrauterine P84
  myocardial —*see* Insufficiency, coronary
  newborn P84
  sleep-related G47.34
Hypsarhythmia —*see* Epilepsy, generalized, specified NEC
Hysteralgia, pregnant uterus O26.89-
Hysteria, hysterical (conversion) (dissociative state) F44.9
  anxiety F41.8
  convulsions F44.5
  psychosis, acute F44.9
Hysteroepilepsy F44.5

I

IBDU (colonic inflammatory bowel dissease unclassified) K52.3 ◄
Ichthyoparasitism due to Vandellia cirrhosa B88.8
Ichthyosis (congenital) Q80.9
  acquired L85.0
  fetalis Q80.4
  hystrix Q80.8
  lamellar Q80.2
  lingual K13.29
  palmaris and plantaris Q82.8
  simplex Q80.0
  vera Q80.8
  vulgaris Q80.0
  X-linked Q80.1
Ichthyotoxism —see Poisoning, fish
  bacterial —see Intoxication, foodborne
Icteroanemia, hemolytic (acquired) D59.9
  congenital —see Spherocytosis
Icterus —see also Jaundice
  conjunctiva R17
  gravis, newborn P55.0
  hematogenous (acquired) D59.9
  hemolytic (acquired) D59.9
    congenital —see Spherocytosis
  hemorrhagic (acute) (leptospiral) (spirochetal) A27.0
    newborn P53
  infectious B15.9
    with hepatic coma B15.0
    leptospiral A27.0
    spirochetal A27.0
  neonatorum —see Jaundice, newborn
  newborn P59.9
  spirochetal A27.0
Ictus solaris, solis T67.0
Ideation
  homicidal R45.850
  suicidal R45.851
Identity disorder (child) F64.9
  gender role F64.2
  psychosexual F64.2
Idioglossia F80.0
Idiopathic —see condition
Idiot, idiocy (congenital) F73
  amaurotic (Bielschowsky(-Jansky)) (family) (infantile (late)) (juvenile (late)) (Vogt-Spielmeyer) E75.4
  microcephalic Q02
Id reaction (due to bacteria) L30.2
IgE asthma J45.909
IIAC (idiopathic infantile arterial calcification) Q28.8
Ileitis (chronic) (noninfectious) —see also Enteritis K52.9
  backwash —see Pancolitis, ulcerative (chronic)
  infectious A09
  regional (ulcerative) —see Enteritis, regional, small intestine
  segmental —see Enteritis, regional
  terminal (ulcerative) —see Enteritis, regional, small intestine
Ileocolitis —see also Enteritis K52.9
  infectious A09
  regional —see Enteritis, regional
Ileostomy
  attention to Z43.2
  malfunctioning K94.13
  status Z93.2
    with complication —see Complications, enterostomy
Ileotyphus —see Typhoid
Ileum —see condition
Ileus (bowel) (colon) (inhibitory) (intestine) K56.7
  adynamic K56.0
  due to gallstone (in intestine) K56.3
  duodenal (chronic) K31.5

Ileus (Continued)
  gallstone K56.3
  mechanical NEC K56.69
  meconium P76.0
    in cystic fibrosis E84.11
    meaning meconium plug (without cystic fibrosis) P76.0
  myxedema K59.8
  neurogenic K56.0
    Hirschsprung's disease or megacolon Q43.1
  newborn
    due to meconium P76.0
      in cystic fibrosis E84.11
      meaning meconium plug (without cystic fibrosis) P76.0
    transitory P76.1
  obstructive K56.69
  paralytic K56.0
Iliac —see condition
Iliotibial band syndrome M76.3-
Illiteracy Z55.0
Illness—see also Disease R69
  manic-depressive —see Disorder, bipolar
Imbalance R26.89
  autonomic G90.8
  constituents of food intake E63.1
  electrolyte E87.8
    with
      abortion —see Abortion by type, complicated by, electrolyte imbalance
      molar pregnancy O08.5
    due to hyperemesis gravidarum O21.1
    following ectopic or molar pregnancy O08.5
    neonatal, transitory NEC P74.4
      potassium P74.3
      sodium P74.2
  endocrine E34.9
  eye muscle NOS H50.9
  hormone E34.9
  hysterical F44.4
  labyrinth —see subcategory H83.2
  posture R29.3
  protein-energy —see Malnutrition
  sympathetic G90.8
Imbecile, imbecility (I.Q. 35-49) F71
Imbedding, intrauterine device T83.39
Imbibition, cholesterol (gallbladder) K82.4
Imbrication, teeth, fully erupted M26.30
Imerslund (-Gräsbeck) syndrome D51.1
Immature —see also Immaturity
  birth (less than 37 completed weeks) —see Preterm, newborn
  extremely (less than 28 completed weeks) —see Immaturity, extreme
  personality F60.89
Immaturity (less than 37 completed weeks) —see also Preterm, newborn
  extreme of newborn (less than 28 completed weeks of gestation) (less than 196 completed days of gestation) (unspecified weeks of gestation) P07.20
    gestational age
      23 completed weeks (23 weeks, 0 days through 23 weeks, 6 days) P07.22
      24 completed weeks (24 weeks, 0 days through 24 weeks, 6 days) P07.23
      25 completed weeks (25 weeks, 0 days through 25 weeks, 6 days) P07.24
      26 completed weeks (26 weeks, 0 days through 26 weeks, 6 days) P07.25
      27 completed weeks (27 weeks, 0 days through 27 weeks, 6 days) P07.26
      less than 23 completed weeks P07.21
  fetus or infant light-for-dates —see Light-for-dates
  lung, newborn P28.0
  organ or site NEC —see Hypoplasia
  pulmonary, newborn P28.0
  reaction F60.89
  sexual (female) (male), after puberty E30.0

Immersion T75.1
  foot T69.02-
  hand T69.01-
Immobile, immobility
  complete, due to severe physical disability or frailty R53.2
  intestine K59.8
  syndrome (paraplegic) M62.3
Immune reconstitution (inflammatory) syndrome [IRIS] D89.3
Immunization —see also Vaccination
  ABO —see Incompatibility, ABO
    in newborn P55.1
  complication —see Complications, vaccination
  encounter for Z23
  not done (not carried out) Z28.9
    because (of)
      acute illness of patient Z28.01
      allergy to vaccine (or component) Z28.04
      caregiver refusal Z28.82
      chronic illness of patient Z28.02
      contraindication NEC Z28.09
      group pressure Z28.1
      guardian refusal Z28.82
      immune compromised state of patient Z28.03
      parent refusal Z28.82
      patient's belief Z28.1
      patient had disease being vaccinated against Z28.81
      patient refusal Z28.21
      religious beliefs of patient Z28.1
      specified reason NEC Z28.89
      of patient Z28.29
      unspecified patient reason Z28.20
    Rh factor
      affecting management of pregnancy NEC O36.09-
      anti-D antibody O36.01-
      from transfusion —see Complication (s), transfusion, incompatibility reaction, Rh (factor)
Immunocytoma C83.0-
Immunodeficiency D84.9
  with
    adenosine-deaminase deficiency D81.3
    antibody defects D80.9
      specified type NEC D80.8
    hyperimmunoglobulinemia D80.6
    increased immunoglobulin M (IgM) D80.5
    major defect D82.9
      specified type NEC D82.8
    partial albinism D82.8
    short-limbed stature D82.2
    thrombocytopenia and eczema D82.0
  antibody with
    hyperimmunoglobulinemia D80.6
    near-normal immunoglobulins D80.6
  autosomal recessive, Swiss type D80.0
  combined D81.9
    biotin-dependent carboxylase D81.819
      biotinidase D81.810
      holocarboxylase synthetase D81.818
      specified type NEC D81.818
    severe (SCID) D81.9
      with
        low or normal B-cell numbers D81.2
        low T- and B-cell numbers D81.1
        reticular dysgenesis D81.0
      specified type NEC D81.89
  common variable D83.9
    with
      abnormalities of B-cell numbers and function D83.0
      autoantibodies to B- or T-cells D83.2
      immunoregulatory T-cell disorders D83.1
    specified type NEC D83.8
  following hereditary defective response to Epstein-Barr virus (EBV) D82.3

Immunodeficiency (Continued)
  selective, immunoglobulin
    A (IgA) D80.2
    G (IgG) (subclasses) D80.3
    M (IgM) D80.4
  severe combined (SCID) D81.9
  specified type NEC D84.8
  X-linked, with increased IgM D80.5
Immunotherapy (encounter for)
  antineoplastic Z51.12
Impaction, impacted
  bowel, colon, rectum —see also Impaction,
    fecal K56.49
    by gallstone K56.3
  calculus —see Calculus
  cerumen (ear) (external) H61.2-
  cuspid —see Impaction, tooth
  dental (same or adjacent tooth) K01.1
  fecal, feces K56.41
  fracture —see Fracture, by site
  gallbladder —see Calculus, gallbladder
  gallstone (s) —see Calculus, gallbladder
    bile duct (common) (hepatic) —see
      Calculus, bile duct
    cystic duct —see Calculus, gallbladder
    in intestine, with obstruction (any part)
      K56.3
  intestine (calculous) NEC —see also
    Impaction, fecal K56.49
    gallstone, with ileus K56.3
  intrauterine device (IUD) T83.39
  molar —see Impaction, tooth
  shoulder, causing obstructed labor O66.0
  tooth, teeth K01.1
  turbinate J34.89
Impaired, impairment (function)
  auditory discrimination —see Abnormal,
    auditory perception
  cognitive, mild, so stated G31.84
  dual sensory Z73.82
  fasting glucose R73.01
  glucose tolerance (oral) R73.02
  hearing —see Deafness
  heart —see Disease, heart
  kidney N28.9
    disorder resulting from N25.9
      specified NEC N25.89
  liver K72.90
    with coma K72.91
  mastication K08.89 ◀▥
  mild cognitive, so stated G31.84
  mobility
    ear ossicles —see Ankylosis, ear ossicles
    requiring care provider Z74.09
  myocardium, myocardial —see Insufficiency,
    myocardial
  rectal sphincter R19.8
  renal (acute) (chronic) N28.9
    disorder resulting from N25.9
      specified NEC N25.89
  vision NEC H54.7
    both eyes H54.3
Impediment, speech R47.9
  psychogenic (childhood) F98.8
  slurring R47.81
  specified NEC R47.89
Impending
  coronary syndrome I20.0
  delirium tremens F10.239
  myocardial infarction I20.0
Imperception auditory (acquired) —see also
    Deafness
  congenital H93.25
Imperfect
  aeration, lung (newborn) NEC —see
    Atelectasis
  closure (congenital)
    alimentary tract NEC Q45.8
      lower Q43.8
      upper Q40.8
    atrioventricular ostium Q21.2

Imperfect (Continued)
  closure (Continued)
    atrium (secundum) Q21.1
    branchial cleft or sinus Q18.0
    choroid Q14.3
    cricoid cartilage Q31.8
    cusps, heart valve NEC Q24.8
      pulmonary Q22.3
    ductus
      arteriosus Q25.0
      Botalli Q25.0
    ear drum (causing impairment of hearing)
      Q16.4
    esophagus with communication to
      bronchus or trachea Q39.1
    eyelid Q10.3
    foramen
      botalli Q21.1
      ovale Q21.1
    genitalia, genital organ (s) or system
      female Q52.8
        external Q52.79
        internal NEC Q52.8
      male Q55.8
    glottis Q31.8
    interatrial ostium or septum Q21.1
    interauricular ostium or septum Q21.1
    interventricular ostium or septum Q21.0
    larynx Q31.8
    lip —see Cleft, lip
    nasal septum Q30.3
    nose Q30.2
    omphalomesenteric duct Q43.0
    optic nerve entry Q14.2
    organ or site not listed —see Anomaly, by
      site
    ostium
      interatrial Q21.1
      interauricular Q21.1
      interventricular Q21.0
    palate —see Cleft, palate
    preauricular sinus Q18.1
    retina Q14.1
    roof of orbit Q75.8
    sclera Q13.5
    septum
      aorticopulmonary Q21.4
      atrial (secundum) Q21.1
      between aorta and pulmonary artery
        Q21.4
      heart Q21.9
      interatrial (secundum) Q21.1
      interauricular (secundum) Q21.1
      interventricular Q21.0
        in tetralogy of Fallot Q21.3
      nasal Q30.3
      ventricular Q21.0
        with pulmonary stenosis or atresia,
          dextraposition of aorta, and
          hypertrophy of right ventricle
          Q21.3
        in tetralogy of Fallot Q21.3
    skull Q75.0
      with
        anencephaly Q00.0
        encephalocele —see Encephalocele
        hydrocephalus Q03.9
          with spina bifida —see Spina bifida,
            by site, with hydrocephalus
        microcephaly Q02
    spine (with meningocele) —see Spina
      bifida
    trachea Q32.1
    tympanic membrane (causing impairment
      of hearing) Q16.4
    uterus Q51.818
    vitelline duct Q43.0
  erection —see Dysfunction, sexual, male,
    erectile
  fusion —see Imperfect, closure
  inflation, lung (newborn) —see Atelectasis

Imperfect (Continued)
  posture R29.3
  rotation, intestine Q43.3
  septum, ventricular Q21.0
Imperfectly descended testis —see Cryptorchid
Imperforate (congenital) —see also Atresia
  anus Q42.3
    with fistula Q42.2
  cervix (uteri) Q51.828
  esophagus Q39.0
    with tracheoesophageal fistula Q39.1
  hymen Q52.3
  jejunum Q41.1
  pharynx Q38.8
  rectum Q42.1
    with fistula Q42.0
  urethra Q64.39
  vagina Q52.4
Impervious (congenital) —see also Atresia
  anus Q42.3
    with fistula Q42.2
  bile duct Q44.2
  esophagus Q39.0
    with tracheoesophageal fistula Q39.1
  intestine (small) Q41.9
    large Q42.9
      specified NEC Q42.8
  rectum Q42.1
    with fistula Q42.0
  ureter —see Atresia, ureter
  urethra Q64.39
Impetiginization of dermatoses L01.1
Impetigo (any organism) (any site) (circinate)
    (contagiosa) (simplex) (vulgaris)
    L01.00
  Bockhart's L01.02
  bullous, bullosa L01.03
  external ear L01.00 [H62.40]
  follicularis L01.02
  furfuracea L30.5
  herpetiformis L40.1
    nonobstetrical L40.1
  neonatorum L01.03
  nonbullous L01.01
  specified type NEC L01.09
  ulcerative L01.09
Impingement (on teeth)
  soft tissue
    anterior M26.81
    posterior M26.82
Implant, endometrial N80.9
Implantation
  anomalous —see Anomaly, by site
    ureter Q62.63
  cyst
    external area or site (skin) NEC L72.0
    iris —see Cyst, iris, implantation
    vagina N89.8
    vulva N90.7
  dermoid (cyst) —see Implantation, cyst
Impotence (sexual) N52.9
  counseling Z70.1
  organic origin —see also Dysfunction, sexual,
    male, erectile N52.9
  psychogenic F52.21
Impression, basilar Q75.8
Imprisonment, anxiety concerning Z65.1
Improper care (child) (newborn) —see
    Maltreatment
Improperly tied umbilical cord (causing
    hemorrhage) P51.8
Impulsiveness (impulsive) R45.87
Inability to swallow —see Aphagia
Inaccessible, inaccessibility
  health care NEC Z75.3
    due to
      waiting period Z75.2
        for admission to facility elsewhere
          Z75.1
    other helping agencies Z75.4
Inactive —see condition

◀ New   ◀▥ Revised   ~~deleted~~ Deleted

Inadequate, inadequacy
aesthetics of dental restoration K08.56
biologic, constitutional, functional, or social
  F60.7
development
  child R62.50
  genitalia
    after puberty NEC E30.0
    congenital
      female Q52.8
        external Q52.79
        internal Q52.8
      male Q55.8
  lungs Q33.6
    associated with short gestation P28.0
  organ or site not listed —*see* Anomaly, by
    site
diet (causing nutritional deficiency) E63.9
eating habits Z72.4
environment, household Z59.1
family support Z63.8
food (supply) NEC Z59.4
  hunger effects T73.0
functional F60.7
household care, due to
  family member
    handicapped or ill Z74.2
    on vacation Z75.5
    temporarily away from home Z74.2
  technical defects in home Z59.1
  temporary absence from home of person
    rendering care Z74.2
housing (heating) (space) Z59.1
income (financial) Z59.6
intrafamilial communication Z63.8
material resources Z59.9
mental —*see* Disability, intellectual
parental supervision or control of child Z62.0
personality F60.7
pulmonary
  function R06.89
    newborn P28.5
  ventilation, newborn P28.5
sample of cytologic smear
  anus R85.615
  cervix R87.615
  vagina R87.625
social F60.7
  insurance Z59.7
  skills NEC Z73.4
supervision of child by parent Z62.0
teaching affecting education Z55.8
welfare support Z59.7
Inanition R64
with edema —*see* Malnutrition, severe
due to
  deprivation of food T73.0
  malnutrition —*see* Malnutrition
fever R50.9
Inappropriate
change in quantitative human chorionic
    gonadotropin (hCG) in early pregnancy
    O02.81
diet or eating habits Z72.4
level of quantitative human chorionic
    gonadotropin (hCG) for gestational age
    in early pregnancy O02.81
secretion
  antidiuretic hormone (ADH) (excessive)
    E22.2
  deficiency E23.2
  pituitary (posterior) E22.2
Inattention at or after birth —*see* Neglect
Incarceration, incarcerated
enterocele K46.0
  gangrenous K46.1
epiplocele K46.0
  gangrenous K46.1
exomphalos K42.0 ◄
  gangrenous K42.1 ◄
~~exophthalmos K42.0~~
  ~~gangrenous K42.1~~

Incarceration, incarcerated (*Continued*)
hernia —*see also* Hernia, by site, with
    obstruction
  with gangrene —*see* Hernia, by site, with
    gangrene
iris, in wound —*see* Injury, eye, laceration,
    with prolapse
lens, in wound —*see* Injury, eye, laceration,
    with prolapse
omphalocele K42.0
prison, anxiety concerning Z65.1
rupture —*see* Hernia, by site
sarcoepiplocele K46.0
  gangrenous K46.1
sarcoepiplomphalocele K42.0
  with gangrene K42.1
uterus N85.8
  gravid O34.51-
    causing obstructed labor O65.5
Incised wound
external —*see* Laceration
internal organs —*see* Injury, by site
Incision, incisional
hernia K43.2
  with
    gangrene (and obstruction) K43.1
    obstruction K43.0
surgical, complication —*see* Complications,
    surgical procedure
traumatic
  external —*see* Laceration
  internal organs —*see* Injury, by site
Inclusion
azurophilic leukocytic D72.0
blennorrhea (neonatal) (newborn) P39.1
gallbladder in liver (congenital) Q44.1
Incompatibility
ABO
  affecting management of pregnancy
    O36.11-
    anti-A sensitization O36.11-
    anti-B sensitization O36.19-
    specified NEC O36.19-
  infusion or transfusion reaction —*see*
    Complication (s), transfusion,
    incompatibility reaction, ABO
  newborn P55.1
blood (group) (Duffy) (K(ell)) (Kidd) (Lewis)
    (M) (S) NEC
  affecting management of pregnancy
    O36.11-
    anti-A sensitization O36.11-
    anti-B sensitization O36.19-
  infusion or transfusion reaction T80.89
  newborn P55.8
divorce or estrangement Z63.5
Rh (blood group) (factor) Z31.82
  affecting management of pregnancy NEC
    O36.09-
    anti-D antibody O36.01-
  infusion or transfusion reaction —*see*
    Complication (s), transfusion,
    incompatibility reaction, Rh (factor)
  newborn P55.0
rhesus —*see* Incompatibility, Rh
Incompetency, incompetent, incompetence
annular
  aortic (valve) —*see* Insufficiency, aortic
  mitral (valve) I34.0
  pulmonary valve (heart) I37.1
aortic (valve) —*see* Insufficiency, aortic
cardiac valve —*see* Endocarditis
cervix, cervical (os) N88.3
  in pregnancy O34.3-
chronotropic I45.89
  with
    autonomic dysfunction G90.8
    ischemic heart disease I25.89
    left ventricular dysfunction I51.89
    sinus node dysfunction I49.8
esophagogastric (junction) (sphincter) K22.0

Incompetency, incompetent, incompetence
    (*Continued*)
mitral (valve) —*see* Insufficiency, mitral
pelvic fundus N81.89
pubocervical tissue N81.82
pulmonary valve (heart) I37.1
  congenital Q22.3
rectovaginal tissue N81.83
tricuspid (annular) (valve) —*see* Insufficiency,
    tricuspid
valvular —*see* Endocarditis
  congenital Q24.8
vein, venous (saphenous) (varicose) —*see*
    Varix, leg
Incomplete —*see also* condition
bladder, emptying R33.9
defecation R15.0
expansion lungs (newborn) NEC —*see*
    Atelectasis
rotation, intestine Q43.3
Inconclusive
diagnostic imaging due to excess body fat of
    patient R93.9
findings on diagnostic imaging of breast NEC
    R92.8
mammogram (due to dense breasts) R92.2
Incontinence R32
anal sphincter R15.9
coital N39.491 ◄
feces R15.9
  nonorganic origin F98.1
insensible (urinary) N39.42 ◄
overflow N39.490
postural (urinary) N39.492 ◄
psychogenic F45.8
rectal R15.9
reflex N39.498
stress (female) (male) N39.3
  and urge N39.46
urethral sphincter R32
urge N39.41
  and stress (female) (male) N39.46
urine (urinary) R32
  continuous N39.45
  due to cognitive impairment, or severe
      physical disability or immobility
      R39.81
  functional R39.81 ◄
  insensible N39.42 ◄
  mixed (stress and urge) N39.46
  nocturnal N39.44
  nonorganic origin F98.0
  overflow N39.490
  post dribbling N39.43
  postural N39.492 ◄
  reflex N39.498
  specified NEC N39.498
  stress (female) (male) N39.3
    and urge N39.46
  total N39.498
  unaware N39.42
  urge N39.41
    and stress (female) (male) N39.46
Incontinentia pigmenti Q82.3
Incoordinate, incoordination
esophageal-pharyngeal (newborn) —*see*
    Dysphagia
muscular R27.8
uterus (action) (contractions) (complicating
    delivery) O62.4
Increase, increased
abnormal, in development R63.8
androgens (ovarian) E28.1
anticoagulants (antithrombin) (anti-VIIIa)
    (anti-IXa) (anti-Xa) (anti-XIa) —*see*
    Circulating anticoagulants
cold sense R20.8
estrogen E28.0
function
  adrenal
    cortex —*see* Cushing's, syndrome
    medulla E27.5

Increase, increased (Continued)
  function (Continued)
    pituitary (gland) (anterior) (lobe) E22.9
      posterior E22.2
  heat sense R20.8
  intracranial pressure (benign) G93.2
  permeability, capillaries I78.8
  pressure, intracranial G93.2
  secretion
    gastrin E16.4
    glucagon E16.3
    pancreas, endocrine E16.9
      growth hormone-releasing hormone E16.8
      pancreatic polypeptide E16.8
      somatostatin E16.8
      vasoactive-intestinal polypeptide E16.8
  sphericity, lens Q12.4
  splenic activity D73.1
  venous pressure I87.8
    portal K76.6
Increta placenta O43.22-
Incrustation, cornea, foreign body (lead)
    (zinc) —see Foreign body, cornea
Incyclophoria H50.54
Incyclotropia —see Cyclotropia
Indeterminate sex Q56.4
India rubber skin Q82.8
Indigestion (acid) (bilious) (functional) K30
  catarrhal K31.89
  due to decomposed food NOS A05.9
  nervous F45.8
  psychogenic F45.8
Indirect —see condition
Induratio penis plastica N48.6
Induration, indurated
  brain G93.89
  breast (fibrous) N64.51
    puerperal, postpartum O92.29
  broad ligament N83.8
  chancre
    anus A51.1
    congenital A50.07
    extragenital NEC A51.2
  corpora cavernosa (penis) (plastic) N48.6
  liver (chronic) K76.89
  lung (black) (chronic) (fibroid) —see also
      Fibrosis, lung J84.10
    essential brown J84.03
  penile (plastic) N48.6
  phlebitic —see Phlebitis
  skin R23.4
Inebriety (without dependence) —see Alcohol,
    intoxication
Inefficiency, kidney N28.9
Inelasticity, skin R23.4
Inequality, leg (length) (acquired) —see also
    Deformity, limb, unequal length
  congenital —see Defect, reduction, lower
      limb
  lower leg —see Deformity, limb, unequal
      length
Inertia
  bladder (neurogenic) N31.2
  stomach K31.89
    psychogenic F45.8
  uterus, uterine during labor O62.2
    during latent phase of labor O62.0
    primary O62.0
    secondary O62.1
  vesical (neurogenic) N31.2
Infancy, infantile, infantilism —see also
    condition
  celiac K90.0
  genitalia, genitals (after puberty) E30.0
  Herter's (nontropical sprue) K90.0
  intestinal K90.0
  Lorain E23.0
  pancreatic K86.89 ◀▥
  pelvis M95.5
    with disproportion (fetopelvic) O33.1
      causing obstructed labor O65.1

Infancy, infantile, infantilism (Continued)
  pituitary E23.0
  renal N25.0
  uterus —see Infantile, genitalia
Infant (s) —see also Infancy
  excessive crying R68.11
  irritable child R68.12
  lack of care —see Neglect
  liveborn (singleton) Z38.2
    born in hospital Z38.00
      by cesarean Z38.01
    born outside hospital Z38.1
    multiple NEC Z38.8
      born in hospital Z38.68
        by cesarean Z38.69
      born outside hospital Z38.7
    quadruplet Z38.8
      born in hospital Z38.63
        by cesarean Z38.64
      born outside hospital Z38.7
    quintuplet Z38.8
      born in hospital Z38.65
        by cesarean Z38.66
      born outside hospital Z38.7
    triplet Z38.8
      born in hospital Z38.61
        by cesarean Z38.62
      born outside hospital Z38.7
    twin Z38.5
      born in hospital Z38.30
        by cesarean Z38.31
      born outside hospital Z38.4
  of diabetic mother (syndrome of) P70.1
    gestational diabetes P70.0
Infantile —see also condition
  genitalia, genitals E30.0
  os, uterine E30.0
  penis E30.0
  testis E29.1
  uterus E30.0
Infantilism —see Infancy
Infarct, infarction
  adrenal (capsule) (gland) E27.49
  appendices epiploicae —see also Infarct,
      intestine K55.069 ◀▥
  bowel —see also Infarct, intestine K55.069 ◀▥
  brain (stem) —see Infarct, cerebral
  breast N64.89
  brewer's (kidney) N28.0
  cardiac —see Infarct, myocardium
  cerebellar —see Infarct, cerebral
  cerebral —see also Occlusion, artery cerebral
      or precerebral, with infarction I63.9-
    aborted I63.9
    cortical I63.9
    due to
      cerebral venous thrombosis,
          nonpyogenic I63.6
      embolism
        cerebral arteries I63.4-
        precerebral arteries I63.1-
      occlusion NEC
        cerebral arteries I63.5-
        precerebral arteries I63.2-
      stenosis NEC
        cerebral arteries I63.5-
        precerebral arteries I63.2-
      thrombosis
        cerebral artery I63.3-
        precerebral artery I63.0-
    intraoperative
      during cardiac surgery I97.810
      during other surgery I97.811
    postprocedural
      following cardiac surgery I97.820
      following other surgery I97.821
    specified NEC I63.8
  colon (acute) (agnogenic) (embolic)
      (hemorrhagic) (nonocclusive)
      (nonthrombotic) (occlusive) (segmental)
      (thrombotic) (with gangrene) —see also
      Infarct, intestine K55.049 ◀▥

Infarct, infarction (Continued)
  coronary artery —see Infarct, myocardium
  embolic —see Embolism
  fallopian tube N83.8
  gallbladder K82.8
  heart —see Infarct, myocardium
  hepatic K76.3
  hypophysis (anterior lobe) E23.6
  impending (myocardium) I20.0
  intestine (acute) (agnogenic) (embolic)
      (hemorrhagic) (nonocclusive)
      (nonthrombotic) (occlusive) (thrombotic)
      (with gangrene) K55.069 ◀▥
    diffuse K55.062 ◀
    focal K55.061 ◀
    large K55.049 ◀
      diffuse K55.042 ◀
      focal K55.041 ◀
    small K55.029 ◀
      diffuse K55.022 ◀
      focal K55.021 ◀
  kidney N28.0
  liver K76.3
  lung (embolic) (thrombotic) —see Embolism,
      pulmonary
  lymph node I89.8
  mesentery, mesenteric (embolic) (thrombotic)
      (with gangrene) —see also Infarct,
      intestine K55.069 ◀▥
  muscle (ischemic) M62.20
    ankle M62.27-
    foot M62.27-
    forearm M62.23-
    hand M62.24-
    lower leg M62.26-
    pelvic region M62.25-
    shoulder region M62.21-
    specified site NEC M62.28
    thigh M62.25-
    upper arm M62.22-
  myocardium, myocardial (acute) (with stated
      duration of 4 weeks or less) I21.3
    diagnosed on ECG, but presenting no
        symptoms I25.2
    healed or old I25.2
    intraoperative
      during cardiac surgery I97.790
      during other surgery I97.791
    non-Q wave I21.4
    non-ST elevation (NSTEMI) I21.4
      subsequent I22.2
    nontransmural I21.4
    past (diagnosed on ECG or other
        investigation, but currently
        presenting no symptoms) I25.2
    postprocedural
      following cardiac surgery I97.190
      following other surgery I97.191
    Q wave (see also, Infarct, myocardium, by
        site) I21.3
    ST elevation (STEMI) I21.3
      anterior (anteroapical) (anterolateral)
          (anteroseptal) (Q wave) (wall)
          I21.09
        subsequent I22.0
      inferior (diaphragmatic) (inferolateral)
          (inferoposterior) (wall) NEC I21.19
        subsequent I22.1
      inferoposterior transmural (Q wave)
          I21.11
      involving
        coronary artery of anterior wall NEC
            I21.09
        coronary artery of inferior wall NEC
            I21.19
        diagonal coronary artery I21.02
        left anterior descending coronary
            artery I21.02
        left circumflex coronary artery
            I21.21
        left main coronary artery I21.01

◀ New   ◀▥ Revised   ~~deleted~~ Deleted

Infarct, infarction (Continued)
  myocardium, myocardial (Continued)
    ST elevation (STEMI) (Continued)
      involving (Continued)
        oblique marginal coronary artery I21.21
        right coronary artery I21.11
      lateral (apical-lateral) (basal-lateral)
          (high) I21.29
        subsequent I22.8
      posterior (posterobasal) (posterolateral)
          (posteroseptal) (true) I21.29
        subsequent I22.8
      septal I21.29
        subsequent I22.8
      specified NEC I21.29
        subsequent I22.8
    subsequent I22.9
  subsequent (recurrent) (reinfarction) I22.9
    anterior (anteroapical) (anterolateral)
        (anteroseptal) (wall) I22.0
    diaphragmatic (wall) I22.1
    inferior (diaphragmatic) (inferolateral)
        (inferoposterior) (wall) I22.1
    lateral (apical-lateral) (basal-lateral)
        (high) I22.8
    non-ST elevation (NSTEMI) I22.2
    posterior (posterobasal) (posterolateral)
        (posteroseptal) (true) I22.8
    septal I22.8
    specified NEC I22.8
    ST elevation I22.9
      anterior (anteroapical) (anterolateral)
          (anteroseptal) (wall) I22.0
      inferior (diaphragmatic) (inferolateral)
          (inferoposterior) (wall) I22.1
      specified NEC I22.8
    subendocardial I22.2
    transmural I22.9
      anterior (anteroapical) (anterolateral)
          (anteroseptal) (wall) I22.0
      diaphragmatic (wall) I22.1
      inferior (diaphragmatic) (inferolateral)
          (inferoposterior) (wall) I22.1
      lateral (apical-lateral) (basal-lateral)
          (high) I22.8
      posterior (posterobasal)
          (posterolateral) (posteroseptal)
          (true) I22.8
      specified NEC I22.8
  syphilitic A52.06
  transmural I21.3
    anterior (anteroapical) (anterolateral)
        (anteroseptal) (Q wave) (wall) NEC
        I21.09
    inferior (diaphragmatic) (inferolateral)
        (inferoposterior) (Q wave) (wall)
        NEC I21.19
    inferoposterior (Q wave) I21.11
    lateral (apical-lateral) (basal-lateral)
        (high) NEC I21.29
    posterior (posterobasal) (posterolateral)
        (posteroseptal) (true) NEC I21.29
    septal NEC I21.29
    specified NEC I21.29
  nontransmural I21.4
  omentum —see also Infarct, intestine
      K55.069 ◄▥
  ovary N83.8
  pancreas K86.89 ◄▥
  papillary muscle —see Infarct, myocardium
  parathyroid gland E21.4
  pituitary (gland) E23.6
  placenta O43.81-
  prostate N42.89
  pulmonary (artery) (vein) (hemorrhagic) —
      see Embolism, pulmonary
  renal (embolic) (thrombotic) N28.0
  retina, retinal (artery) —see Occlusion, artery,
      retina
  spinal (cord) (acute) (embolic) (nonembolic)
      G95.11

Infarct, infarction (Continued)
  spleen D73.5
    embolic or thrombotic I74.8
  subendocardial (acute) (nontransmural)
      I21.4
  suprarenal (capsule) (gland) E27.49
  testis N50.1
  thrombotic —see also Thrombosis
    artery, arterial —see Embolism
  thyroid (gland) E07.89
  ventricle (heart) —see Infarct, myocardium
Infecting —see condition
Infection, infected, infective (opportunistic)
    B99.9
  with
    drug resistant organism —see Resistance
        (to), drug —see also specific organism
    lymphangitis —see Lymphangitis
    organ dysfunction (acute) R65.20
      with septic shock R65.21
  abscess (skin) - code by site under Abscess
  Absidia —see Mucormycosis
  Acanthamoeba —see Acanthamebiasis
  Acanthocheilonema (perstans) (streptocerca)
      B74.4
  accessory sinus (chronic) —see Sinusitis
  achorion —see Dermatophytosis
  acromioclavicular M00.9
  Actinobacillus (actinomycetem-comitans)
      A28.8
    mallei A24.0
    muris A25.1
  Actinomadura B47.1
  Actinomyces (israelii) —see also
      Actinomycosis A42.9
  Actinomycetales —see Actinomycosis
  actinomycotic NOS —see Actinomycosis
  adenoid (and tonsil) J03.90
    chronic J35.02
  adenovirus NEC
    as cause of disease classified elsewhere
        B97.0
    unspecified nature or site B34.0
  aerogenes capsulatus A48.0
  aertrycke —see Infection, salmonella
  alimentary canal NOS —see Enteritis,
      infectious
  Allescheria boydii B48.2
  Alternaria B48.8
  alveolus, alveolar (process) K04.7
  Ameba, amebic (histolytica) —see Amebiasis
  amniotic fluid, sac or cavity O41.10-
    chorioamnionitis O41.12-
    placentitis O41.14-
  amputation stump (surgical) —see
      Complication, amputation stump,
      infection
  Ancylostoma (duodenalis) B76.0
  Anisakiasis, Anisakis larvae B81.0
  anthrax —see Anthrax
  antrum (chronic) —see Sinusitis, maxillary
  anus, anal (papillae) (sphincter) K62.89
  arbovirus (arbor virus) A94
    specified type NEC A93.8
  artificial insemination N98.0
  Ascaris lumbricoides —see Ascariasis
  Ascomycetes B47.0
  Aspergillus (flavus) (fumigatus) (terreus) —
      see Aspergillosis
  atypical
    acid-fast (bacilli) —see Mycobacterium,
        atypical
    mycobacteria —see Mycobacterium,
        atypical
    virus A81.9
      specified type NEC A81.89
  auditory meatus (external) —see Otitis,
      externa, infective
  auricle (ear) —see Otitis, externa, infective
  axillary gland (lymph) L04.2

Infection, infected, infective (Continued)
  Bacillus A49.9
    abortus A23.1
    anthracis —see Anthrax
    Ducrey's (any location) A57
    Flexner's A03.1
    Friedländer's NEC A49.8
    gas (gangrene) A48.0
    mallei A24.0
    melitensis A23.0
    paratyphoid, paratyphosus A01.4
      A A01.1
      B A01.2
      C A01.3
    Shiga (-Kruse) A03.0
    suipestifer —see Infection, salmonella
    swimming pool A31.1
    typhosa A01.00
    welchii —see Gangrene, gas
  bacterial NOS A49.9
    as cause of disease classified elsewhere
        B96.89
      Bacteroides fragilis [B. fragilis] B96.6
      Clostridium perfringens [C. perfringens]
          B96.7
      Enterobacter sakazakii B96.89
      Enterococcus B95.2
      Escherichia coli [E. coli] (see also
          Escherichia coli) B96.20
      Helicobacter pylori [H.pylori]
          B96.81
      Hemophilus influenzae [H. influenzae]
          B96.3
      Klebsiella pneumoniae [K. pneumoniae]
          B96.1
      Mycoplasma pneumoniae [M.
          pneumoniae] B96.0
      Proteus (mirabilis) (morganii) B96.4
      Pseudomonas (aeruginosa) (mallei)
          (pseudomallei) B96.5
      Staphylococcus B95.8
        aureus (methicillin susceptible)
            (MSSA) B95.61
          methicillin resistant (MRSA)
              B95.62
        specified NEC B95.7
      Streptococcus B95.5
        group A B95.0
        group B B95.1
        pneumoniae B95.3
        specified NEC B95.4
      Vibrio vulnificus B96.82
    specified NEC A48.8
  Bacterium
    paratyphosum A01.4
      A A01.1
      B A01.2
      C A01.3
    typhosum A01.00
  Bacteroides NEC A49.8
    fragilis, as cause of disease classified
        elsewhere B96.6
  Balantidium coli A07.0
  Bartholin's gland N75.8
  Basidiobolus B46.8
  bile duct (common) (hepatic) —see
      Cholangitis
  bladder —see Cystitis
  Blastomyces, blastomycotic —see also
      Blastomycosis
    brasiliensis —see Paracoccidioidomycosis
    dermatitidis —see Blastomycosis
    European —see Cryptococcosis
    Loboi B48.0
    North American B40.9
    South American —see
        Paracoccidioidomycosis
  bleb, postprocedure —see Blebitis
  bone —see Osteomyelitis
  Bordetella —see Whooping cough
  Borrelia bergdorfi A69.20

Infection, infected, infective *(Continued)*
  brain —*see also* Encephalitis G04.90
    membranes —*see* Meningitis
    septic G06.0
      meninges —*see* Meningitis, bacterial
  branchial cyst Q18.0
  breast —*see* Mastitis
  bronchus —*see* Bronchitis
  Brucella A23.9
    abortus A23.1
    canis A23.3
    melitensis A23.0
    mixed A23.8
    specified NEC A23.8
    suis A23.2
  Brugia (malayi) B74.1
    timori B74.2
  bursa —*see* Bursitis, infective
  buttocks (skin) L08.9
  Campylobacter, intestinal A04.5
    as cause of disease classified elsewhere
        B96.81
  Candida (albicans) (tropicalis) —*see*
        Candidiasis
  candiru B88.8
  Capillaria (intestinal) B81.1
    hepatica B83.8
    philippinensis B81.1
  cartilage —*see* Disorder, cartilage, specified
        type NEC
  catheter-related bloodstream (CRBSI) T80.211
  cat liver fluke B66.0
  cellulitis - code by site under Cellulitis
  central line-associated T80.219
    bloodstream (CLABSI) T80.211
    specified NEC T80.218
  Cephalosporium falciforme B47.0
  cerebrospinal —*see* Meningitis
  cervical gland (lymph) L04.0
  cervix —*see* Cervicitis
  cesarean delivery wound (puerperal) O86.0
  cestodes —*see* Infestation, cestodes
  chest J22
  Chilomastix (intestinal) A07.8
  Chlamydia, chlamydial A74.9
    anus A56.3
    genitourinary tract A56.2
      lower A56.00
        specified NEC A56.19
    lymphogranuloma A55
    pharynx A56.4
    psittaci A70
    rectum A56.3
    sexually transmitted NEC A56.8
  cholera —*see* Cholera
  Cladosporium
    bantianum (brain abscess) B43.1
    carrionii B43.0
    castellanii B36.1
    trichoides (brain abscess) B43.1
    werneckii B36.1
  Clonorchis (sinensis) (liver) B66.1
  Clostridium NEC
    bifermentans A48.0
    botulinum (food poisoning) A05.1
      infant A48.51
      wound A48.52
    difficile
      as cause of disease classified elsewhere
          B96.89
      foodborne (disease) A04.7
      gas gangrene A48.0
      necrotizing enterocolitis A04.7
      sepsis A41.4
    gas-forming NEC A48.0
    histolyticum A48.0
    novyi, causing gas gangrene A48.0
    oedematiens A48.0
    perfringens
      as cause of disease classified elsewhere
          B96.7
      due to food A05.2

Infection, infected, infective *(Continued)*
  Clostridium *(Continued)*
    perfringens *(Continued)*
      foodborne (disease) A05.2
      gas gangrene A48.0
      sepsis A41.4
    septicum, causing gas gangrene A48.0
    sordellii, causing gas gangrene A48.0
    welchii
      as cause of disease classified elsewhere
          B96.7
      foodborne (disease) A05.2
      gas gangrene A48.0
      necrotizing enteritis A05.2
      sepsis A41.4
  Coccidioides (immitis) —*see*
        Coccidioidomycosis
  colon —*see* Enteritis, infectious
  colostomy K94.02
  common duct —*see* Cholangitis
  congenital P39.9
    Candida (albicans) P37.5
    cytomegalovirus P35.1
    hepatitis, viral P35.3
    herpes simplex P35.2
    infectious or parasitic disease P37.9
      specified NEC P37.8
    listeriosis (disseminated) P37.2
    malaria NEC P37.4
      falciparum P37.3
    Plasmodium falciparum P37.3
    poliomyelitis P35.8
    rubella P35.0
    skin P39.4
    toxoplasmosis (acute) (subacute) (chronic)
        P37.1
    tuberculosis P37.0
    urinary (tract) P39.3
    vaccinia P35.8
    virus P35.9
      specified type NEC P35.8
  Conidiobolus B46.8
  coronavirus NEC B34.2
    as cause of disease classified elsewhere
        B97.29
    severe acute respiratory syndrome (SARS
        associated) B97.21
  corpus luteum —*see* Salpingo-oophoritis
  Corynebacterium diphtheriae —*see*
        Diphtheria
  cotia virus B08.8
  Coxiella burnetii A78
  coxsackie —*see* Coxsackie
  Cryptococcus neoformans —*see*
        Cryptococcosis
  Cryptosporidium A07.2
  Cunninghamella —*see* Mucormycosis
  cyst —*see* Cyst
  cystic duct —*see also* Cholecystitis K81.9
  Cysticercus cellulosae —*see* Cysticercosis
  cytomegalovirus, cytomegaloviral B25.9
    congenital P35.1
    maternal, maternal care for (suspected)
        damage to fetus O35.3
    mononucleosis B27.10
      with
        complication NEC B27.19
        meningitis B27.12
        polyneuropathy B27.11
  delta-agent (acute), in hepatitis B carrier
      B17.0
  dental (pulpal origin) K04.7
  Deuteromycetes B47.0
  Dicrocoelium dendriticum B66.2
  Dipetalonema (perstans) (streptocerca) B74.4
  diphtherial —*see* Diphtheria
  Diphyllobothrium (adult) (latum) (pacificum)
      B70.0
    larval B70.1
  Diplogonoporus (grandis) B71.8
  Dipylidium caninum B67.4

Infection, infected, infective *(Continued)*
  Dirofilaria B74.8
  Dracunculus medinensis B72
  Drechslera (hawaiiensis) B43.8
  Ducrey Haemophilus (any location) A57
  due to or resulting from
    artificial insemination N98.0
    central venous catheter T80.219
      bloodstream T80.211
      exit or insertion site T80.212
      localized T80.212
      port or reservoir T80.212
      specified NEC T80.218
      tunnel T80.212
    device, implant or graft —*see also*
        Complications, by site and type,
        infection or inflammation
        T85.79
      arterial graft NEC T82.7
      breast (implant) T85.79
      catheter NEC T85.79
        dialysis (renal) T82.7
          intraperitoneal T85.71
        infusion NEC T82.7
          cranial T85.735 ◀
          intrathecal T85.735 ◀
          spinal (epidural) (subdural)
              T85.735 ◀▥
          subarachnoid T85.735 ◀
        urinary T83.518 ◀▥
          cystostomy T83.510 ◀
          Hopkins T83.518 ◀
          ileostomy T83.518 ◀
          nephrostomy T83.512 ◀
          specified NEC T83.518 ◀
          urethral indwelling T83.511 ◀
          urostomy T83.518 ◀
      electronic (electrode) (pulse generator)
          (stimulator)
        bone T84.7
        cardiac T82.7
        nervous system T85.738 ◀▥
          brain T85.731 ◀
          cranial nerve T85.732 ◀
          gastric nerve T85.732 ◀
          generator pocket T85.734 ◀
          neurostimulator generator
              T85.734 ◀
          peripheral nerve T85.732 ◀
          sacral nerve T85.732 ◀
          spinal cord T85.733 ◀
          vagal nerve T85.732 ◀
        urinary T83.590 ◀▥
      fixation, internal (orthopedic) NEC —*see*
          Complication, fixation device,
          infection
      gastrointestinal (bile duct) (esophagus)
          T85.79
        neurostimulator electrode (lead)
            T85.732 ◀
      genital NEC T83.69 ◀▥
      heart NEC T82.7
        valve (prosthesis) T82.6
          graft T82.7
      joint prosthesis —*see* Complication, joint
          prosthesis, infection
      ocular (corneal graft) (orbital implant)
          NEC T85.79
      orthopedic NEC T84.7
      penile (cylinder) (pump) (resevoir)
          T83.61 ◀
      specified NEC T85.79
      testicular T83.62 ◀
      urinary NEC T83.598 ◀▥
        ileal conduit stent T83.593 ◀
        implanted neurostimulation
            T83.590 ◀
        implanted sphincter T83.591 ◀
        indwelling ureteral stent T83.592 ◀
        nephroureteral stent T83.593 ◀
        specified stent NEC T83.593 ◀

◀ New   ◀▥ Revised   ~~deleted~~ Deleted

Infection, infected, infective (Continued)
due to or resulting from (Continued)
device, implant or graft (Continued)
vascular NEC T82.7
~~ventricular intracranial shunt T85.79~~
ventricular intracranial (communicating)
shunt T85.730 ◀
Hickman catheter T80.219
bloodstream T80.211
localized T80.212
specified NEC T80.218
immunization or vaccination T88.0
infusion, injection or transfusion NEC
T80.29
acute T80.22
injury NEC - code by site under Wound,
open
peripherally inserted central catheter
(PICC) T80.219
bloodstream T80.211
localized T80.212
specified NEC T80.218
portacath (port-a-cath) T80.219
bloodstream T80.211
localized T80.212
specified NEC T80.218
pulmonary artery catheter —see Infection,
due to or resulting from, central
venous catheter ◀
surgery T81.40 ◀⊪
Swan Ganz catheter —see Infection, due to
or resulting from, central venous
catheter ◀
triple lumen catheter T80.219
bloodstream T80.211
localized T80.212
specified NEC T80.218
umbilical venous catheter T80.219
bloodstream T80.211
localized T80.212
specified NEC T80.218
during labor NEC O75.3
ear (middle) —see also Otitis media
external —see Otitis, externa, infective
inner —see subcategory H83.0
Eberthella typhosa A01.00
Echinococcus —see Echinococcus
echovirus
as cause of disease classified elsewhere
B97.12
unspecified nature or site B34.1
endocardium I33.0
endocervix —see Cervicitis
Entamoeba —see Amebiasis
enteric —see Enteritis, infectious
Enterobacter sakazakii B96.89
Enterobius vermicularis B80
enterostomy K94.12
enterovirus B34.1
as cause of disease classified elsewhere
B97.10
coxsackievirus B97.11
echovirus B97.12
specified NEC B97.19
Entomophthora B46.8
Epidermophyton —see Dermatophytosis
epididymis —see Epididymitis
episiotomy (puerperal) O86.0
Erysipelothrix (insidiosa) (rhusiopathiae) —
see Erysipeloid
erythema infectiosum B08.3
Escherichia (E.) coli NEC A49.8
as cause of disease classified elsewhere —
see also Escherichia coli B96.20
congenital P39.8
sepsis P36.4
generalized A41.51
intestinal —see Enteritis, infectious, due to,
Escherichia coli
ethmoidal (chronic) (sinus) —see Sinusitis,
ethmoidal

Infection, infected, infective (Continued)
eustachian tube (ear) —see Salpingitis,
eustachian
external auditory canal (meatus) NEC —see
Otitis, externa, infective
eye (purulent) —see Endophthalmitis,
purulent
eyelid —see Inflammation, eyelid
fallopian tube —see Salpingo-oophoritis
Fasciola (gigantica) (hepatica) (indica)
B66.3
Fasciolopsis (buski) B66.5
filarial —see Infestation, filarial
finger (skin) L08.9
nail L03.01-
fungus B35.1
fish tapeworm B70.0
larval B70.1
flagellate, intestinal A07.9
fluke —see Infestation, fluke
focal
teeth (pulpal origin) K04.7
tonsils J35.01
Fonsecaea (compactum) (pedrosoi) B43.0
food —see Intoxication, foodborne
foot (skin) L08.9
dermatophytic fungus B35.3
Francisella tularensis —see Tularemia
frontal (sinus) (chronic) —see Sinusitis,
frontal
fungus NOS B49
beard B35.0
dermatophytic —see Dermatophytosis
foot B35.3
groin B35.6
hand B35.2
nail B35.1
pathogenic to compromised host only
B48.8
perianal (area) B35.6
scalp B35.0
skin B36.9
foot B35.3
hand B35.2
toenails B35.1
Fusarium B48.8
gallbladder —see Cholecystitis
gas bacillus —see Gangrene, gas
gastrointestinal —see Enteritis, infectious
generalized NEC —see Sepsis
generator pocket, implanted electronic
neurostimulator T85.734 ◀
genital organ or tract
female —see Disease, pelvis,
inflammatory
male N49.9
multiple sites N49.8
specified NEC N49.8
Ghon tubercle, primary A15.7
Giardia lamblia A07.1
gingiva (chronic) K05.10
acute K05.00
nonplaque induced K05.01
plaque induced K05.00
nonplaque induced K05.11
plaque induced K05.10
glanders A24.0
glenosporopsis B48.0
Gnathostoma (spinigerum) B83.1
Gongylonema B83.8
gonococcal —see Gonococcus
gram-negative bacilli NOS A49.9
guinea worm B72
gum (chronic) K05.10
acute K05.00
nonplaque induced K05.01
plaque induced K05.00
nonplaque induced K05.11
plaque induced K05.10
Haemophilus —see Infection, Hemophilus
heart —see Carditis

Infection, infected, infective (Continued)
Helicobacter pylori A04.8
as cause of disease classified elsewhere
B96.81
helminths B83.9
intestinal B82.0
mixed (types classifiable to more than
one of the titles B65.0-B81.3 and
B81.8) B81.4
specified type NEC B81.8
specified type NEC B83.8
Hemophilus
aegyptius, systemic A48.4
ducreyi (any location) A57
generalized A41.3
influenzae NEC A49.2
as cause of disease classified elsewhere
B96.3
herpes (simplex) —see also Herpes
congenital P35.2
disseminated B00.7
zoster B02.9
herpesvirus, herpesviral —see Herpes
Heterophyes (heterophyes) B66.8
hip (joint) NEC M00.9
due to internal joint prosthesis
left T84.52
right T84.51
skin NEC L08.9
Histoplasma —see Histoplasmosis
American B39.4
capsulatum B39.4
hookworm B76.9
human
papilloma virus A63.0
T-cell lymphotropic virus type-1 (HTLV-1)
B33.3
hydrocele N43.0
Hymenolepis B71.0
hypopharynx —see Pharyngitis
inguinal (lymph) glands L04.1
due to soft chancre A57
intervertebral disc, pyogenic M46.30
cervical region M46.32
cervicothoracic region M46.33
lumbar region M46.36
lumbosacral region M46.37
multiple sites M46.39
occipito-atlanto-axial region M46.31
sacrococcygeal region M46.38
thoracic region M46.34
thoracolumbar region M46.35
intestine, intestinal —see Enteritis, infectious
specified NEC A08.8
intra-amniotic affecting newborn NEC P39.2
Isospora belli or hominis A07.3
Japanese B encephalitis A83.0
jaw (bone) (lower) (upper) M27.2
joint NEC M00.9
due to internal joint prosthesis T84.50
kidney (cortex) (hematogenous) N15.9
with calculus N20.0
with hydronephrosis N13.6
following ectopic gestation O08.83
pelvis and ureter (cystic) N28.85
puerperal (postpartum) O86.21
specified NEC N15.8
Klebsiella (K.) pneumoniae NEC A49.8
as cause of disease classified elsewhere B96.1
knee (joint) NEC M00.9
due to internal joint prosthesis
left T84.54
right T84.53
joint M00.9
skin L08.9
Koch's —see Tuberculosis
labia (majora) (minora) (acute) —see Vulvitis
lacrimal
gland —see Dacryoadenitis
passages (duct) (sac) —see Inflammation,
lacrimal, passages

Infection, infected, infective (Continued)
  lancet fluke B66.2
  larynx NEC J38.7
  leg (skin) NOS L08.9
  Legionella pneumophila A48.1
    nonpneumonic A48.2
  Leishmania —see also Leishmaniasis
    aethiopica B55.1
    braziliensis B55.2
    chagasi B55.0
    donovani B55.0
    infantum B55.0
    major B55.1
    mexicana B55.1
    tropica B55.1
  lentivirus, as cause of disease classified
    elsewhere B97.31
  Leptosphaeria senegalensis B47.0
  Leptospira interrogans A27.9
    autumnalis A27.89
    canicola A27.89
    hebdomadis A27.89
    icterohaemorrhagiae A27.0
    pomona A27.89
    specified type NEC A27.89
  leptospirochetal NEC —see Leptospirosis
  Listeria monocytogenes —see also Listeriosis
    congenital P37.2
  Loa loa B74.3
    with conjunctival infestation B74.3
    eyelid B74.3
  Loboa loboi B48.0
  local, skin (staphylococcal) (streptococcal)
    L08.9
    abscess - code by site under Abscess
    cellulitis - code by site under Cellulitis
    specified NEC L08.89
    ulcer —see Ulcer, skin
  Loefflerella mallei A24.0
  lung —see also Pneumonia J18.9
    atypical Mycobacterium A31.0
    spirochetal A69.8
    tuberculous —see Tuberculosis,
      pulmonary
    virus —see Pneumonia, viral
  lymph gland —see also Lymphadenitis,
    acute
    mesenteric I88.0
  lymphoid tissue, base of tongue or posterior
    pharynx, NEC (chronic) J35.03
  Madurella (grisea) (mycetomii) B47.0
  major
    following ectopic or molar pregnancy
      O08.0
    puerperal, postpartum, childbirth O85
  Malassezia furfur B36.0
  Malleomyces
    mallei A24.0
    pseudomallei (whitmori) —see Melioidosis
  mammary gland N61.0 ◀▥
  Mansonella (ozzardi) (perstans) (streptocerca)
    B74.4
  mastoid —see Mastoiditis
  maxilla, maxillary M27.2
    sinus (chronic) —see Sinusitis,
      maxillary
  mediastinum J98.51 ◀▥
  Medina (worm) B72
  meibomian cyst or gland —see Hordeolum
  meninges —see Meningitis, bacterial
  meningococcal —see also condition
    A39.9
    adrenals A39.1
    brain A39.81
    cerebrospinal A39.0
    conjunctiva A39.89
    endocardium A39.51
    heart A39.50
      endocardium A39.51
      myocardium A39.52
      pericardium A39.53

Infection, infected, infective (Continued)
  meningococcal (Continued)
    joint A39.83
    meninges A39.0
    meningococcemia A39.4
      acute A39.2
      chronic A39.3
    myocardium A39.52
    pericardium A39.53
    retrobulbar neuritis A39.82
    specified site NEC A39.89
  mesenteric lymph nodes or glands NEC
    I88.0
  Metagonimus B66.8
  metatarsophalangeal M00.9
  methicillin
    resistant Staphylococcus aureus (MRSA)
      A49.02
    susceptible Staphylococcus aureus (MSSA)
      A49.01
  Microsporum, microsporic —see
    Dermatophytosis
  mixed flora (bacterial) NEC A49.8
  Monilia —see Candidiasis
  Monosporium apiospermum B48.2
  mouth, parasitic B37.0
  Mucor —see Mucormycosis
  muscle NEC —see Myositis, infective
  mycelium NOS B49
  mycetoma B47.9
    actinomycotic NEC B47.1
    mycotic NEC B47.0
  Mycobacterium, mycobacterial —see
    Mycobacterium
  Mycoplasma NEC A49.3
    pneumoniae, as cause of disease classified
      elsewhere B96.0
  mycotic NOS B49
    pathogenic to compromised host only
      B48.8
    skin NOS B36.9
  myocardium NEC I40.0
  nail (chronic)
    with lymphangitis —see Lymphangitis,
      acute, digit
    finger L03.01-
      fungus B35.1
    ingrowing L60.0
    toe L03.03-
      fungus B35.1
  nasal sinus (chronic) —see Sinusitis
  nasopharynx —see Nasopharyngitis
  navel L08.82
  Necator americanus B76.1
  Neisseria —see Gonococcus
  Neotestudina rosatii B47.0
  newborn P39.9
    intra-amniotic NEC P39.2
    skin P39.4
    specified type NEC P39.8
  nipple N61.0 ◀▥
    associated with
      lactation O91.03
      pregnancy O91.01-
      puerperium O91.02
  Nocardia —see Nocardiosis
  obstetrical surgical wound (puerperal)
    O86.0
  Oesophagostomum (apiostomum)
    B81.8
  Oestrus ovis —see Myiasis
  Oidium albicans B37.9
  Onchocerca (volvulus) —see Onchocerciasis -
    oncovirus, as cause of disease classified
    elsewhere B97.32
  operation wound T81.40 ◀▥
  Opisthorchis (felineus) (viverrini) B66.0
  orbit, orbital —see Inflammation, orbit
  orthopoxvirus NEC B08.09
  ovary —see Salpingo-oophoritis
  Oxyuris vermicularis B80

Infection, infected, infective (Continued)
  pancreas (acute) —see Pancreatitis, acute ◀▥
    abscess —see Pancreatitis, acute
    specified NEC —see also Pancreatitis, acute
      K85.80 ◀▥
  papillomavirus, as cause of disease classified
    elsewhere B97.7
  papovavirus NEC B34.4
  Paracoccidioides brasiliensis —see
    Paracoccidioidomycosis
  Paragonimus (westermani) B66.4
  parainfluenza virus B34.8
  parameningococcus NOS A39.9
  parapoxvirus B08.60
    specified NEC B08.69
  parasitic B89
  Parastrongylus
    cantonensis B83.2
    costaricensis B81.3
    paratyphoid A01.4
      Type A A01.1
      Type B A01.2
      Type C A01.3
  paraurethral ducts N34.2
  parotid gland —see Sialoadenitis
  parvovirus NEC B34.3
    as cause of disease classified elsewhere
      B97.6
  Pasteurella NEC A28.0
    multocida A28.0
    pestis —see Plague
    pseudotuberculosis A28.0
    septica (cat bite) (dog bite) A28.0
    tularensis —see Tularemia
  pelvic, female —see Disease, pelvis,
    inflammatory
  Penicillium (marneffei) B48.4
  penis (glans) (retention) NEC N48.29
  periapical K04.5
  peridental, periodontal K05.20
    generalized —see Peridontitis, aggressive,
      generalized ◀▥
    localized —see Peridontitis, aggressive,
      localized ◀▥
  perinatal period P39.9
    specified type NEC P39.8
  perineal repair (puerperal) O86.0
  periorbital —see Inflammation, orbit
  perirectal K62.89
  perirenal —see Infection, kidney
  peritoneal —see Peritonitis
  periureteral N28.89
  Petriellidium boydii B48.2
  pharynx —see also Pharyngitis
    coxsackievirus B08.5
    posterior, lymphoid (chronic) J35.03
  Phialophora
    gougerotii (subcutaneous abscess or cyst)
      B43.2
    jeanselmei (subcutaneous abscess or cyst)
      B43.2
    verrucosa (skin) B43.0
  Piedraia hortae B36.3
  pinta A67.9
    intermediate A67.1
    late A67.2
    mixed A67.3
    primary A67.0
  pinworm B80
  pityrosporum furfur B36.0
  pleuro-pneumonia-like organism (PPLO)
    NEC A49.3
    as cause of disease classified elsewhere
      B96.0
  pneumococcus, pneumococcal NEC A49.1
    as cause of disease classified elsewhere
      B95.3
    generalized (purulent) A40.3
      with pneumonia J13
  Pneumocystis carinii (pneumonia) B59
  Pneumocystis jiroveci (pneumonia) B59

◀ New   ◀▥ Revised   ~~deleted~~ Deleted

Infection, infected, infective (Continued)
  port or reservoir T80.212
  postoperative T81.40 ◀▥
  postoperative wound T81.40 ◀▥
  postprocedural T81.40 ◀▥
    deep incisional surgical site T81.42 ◀
    organ and space surgical site T81.43 ◀
    sepsis T81.49 ◀
    specified surgical site NEC T81.48 ◀
    superficial incisional surgical site T81.41 ◀
  postvaccinal T88.0
  prepuce NEC N47.7
    with penile inflammation N47.6
  prion —see Disease, prion, central nervous
    system
  prostate (capsule) —see Prostatitis
  Proteus (mirabilis) (morganii) (vulgaris) NEC
    A49.8
    as cause of disease classified elsewhere B96.4
  protozoal NEC B64
    intestinal A07.9
      specified NEC A07.8
    specified NEC B60.8
  Pseudoallescheria boydii B48.2
  Pseudomonas NEC A49.8
    as cause of disease classified elsewhere
      B96.5
    mallei A24.0
    pneumonia J15.1
    pseudomallei —see Melioidosis
  puerperal O86.4
    genitourinary tract NEC O86.89
    major or generalized O85
    minor O86.4
    specified NEC O86.89
  pulmonary —see Infection, lung
  purulent —see Abscess
  Pyrenochaeta romeroi B47.0
  Q fever A78
  rectum (sphincter) K62.89
  renal —see also Infection, kidney
    pelvis and ureter (cystic) N28.85
  reovirus, as cause of disease classified
    elsewhere B97.5
  respiratory (tract) NEC J98.8
    acute J22
    chronic J98.8
    influenzal (upper) (acute) —see Influenza,
      with, respiratory manifestations NEC
    lower (acute) J22
      chronic —see Bronchitis, chronic
    rhinovirus J00
    syncytial virus, as cause of disease
      classified elsewhere B97.4
    upper (acute) NOS J06.9
      chronic J39.8
      streptococcal J06.9
      viral NOS J06.9
  resulting from
    presence of internal prosthesis, implant,
      graft —see Complications, by site and
      type, infection
  retortamoniasis A07.8
  retroperitoneal NEC K68.9
  retrovirus B33.3
    as cause of disease classified elsewhere
      B97.30
      human
        immunodeficiency, type 2 (HIV 2)
          B97.35
        T-cell lymphotropic
          type I (HTLV-I) B97.33
          type II (HTLV-II) B97.34
      lentivirus B97.31
      oncovirus B97.32
      specified NEC B97.39
  Rhinosporidium (seeberi) B48.1
  rhinovirus
    as cause of disease classified elsewhere
      B97.89
    unspecified nature or site B34.8

Infection, infected, infective (Continued)
  Rhizopus —see Mucormycosis
  rickettsial NOS A79.9
  roundworm (large) NEC B82.0
    Ascariasis —see also Ascariasis B77.9
  rubella —see Rubella
  Saccharomyces —see Candidiasis
  salivary duct or gland (any) —see
    Sialoadenitis
  Salmonella (aertrycke) (arizonae)
    (callinarum) (cholerae-suis) (enteritidis)
    (suipestifer) (typhimurium)
    A02.9
    with
      (gastro) enteritis A02.0
      sepsis A02.1
      specified manifestation NEC A02.8
    due to food (poisoning) A02.9
    hirschfeldii A01.3
    localized A02.20
      arthritis A02.23
      meningitis A02.21
      osteomyelitis A02.24
      pneumonia A02.22
      pyelonephritis A02.25
      specified NEC A02.29
    paratyphi A01.4
      A A01.1
      B A01.2
      C A01.3
    schottmuelleri A01.2
    typhi, typhosa —see Typhoid
  Sarcocystis A07.8
  scabies B86
  Schistosoma —see Infestation, Schistosoma
  scrotum (acute) NEC N49.2
  seminal vesicle —see Vesiculitis
  septic
    localized, skin —see Abscess
  sheep liver fluke B66.3
  Shigella A03.9
    boydii A03.2
    dysenteriae A03.0
    flexneri A03.1
    group
      A A03.0
      B A03.1
      C A03.2
      D A03.3
    Schmitz (-Stutzer) A03.0
    schmitzii A03.0
    shigae A03.0
    sonnei A03.3
    specified NEC A03.8
  shoulder (joint) NEC M00.9
    due to internal joint prosthesis T84.59
    skin NEC L08.9
  sinus (accessory) (chronic) (nasal) —see also
    Sinusitis
    pilonidal —see Sinus, pilonidal
    skin NEC L08.89
  Skene's duct or gland —see Urethritis
  skin (local) (staphylococcal) (streptococcal)
    L08.9
    abscess - code by site under Abscess
    cellulitis - code by site under Cellulitis
    due to fungus B36.9
      specified type NEC B36.8
    mycotic B36.9
      specified type NEC B36.8
    newborn P39.4
    ulcer —see Ulcer, skin
  slow virus A81.9
    specified NEC A81.89
  Sparganum (mansoni) (proliferum) (baxteri)
    B70.1
  specific —see also Syphilis
    to perinatal period —see Infection,
      congenital
  specified NEC B99.8
  spermatic cord NEC N49.1

Infection, infected, infective (Continued)
  sphenoidal (sinus) —see Sinusitis,
    sphenoidal
  spinal cord NOS —see also Myelitis
    G04.91
    abscess G06.1
    meninges —see Meningitis
    streptococcal G04.89
  Spirillum A25.0
  spirochetal NOS A69.9
    lung A69.8
    specified NEC A69.8
  Spirometra larvae B70.1
  spleen D73.89
  Sporotrichum, Sporothrix (schenckii) —see
    Sporotrichosis
  staphylococcal, unspecified site
    aureus (methicillin susceptible) (MSSA)
      A49.01
      methicillin resistant (MRSA) A49.02
    as cause of disease classified elsewhere
      B95.8
      aureus (methicillin susceptible) (MSSA)
        B95.61
        methicillin resistant (MRSA)
          B95.62
      specified NEC B95.7
    food poisoning A05.0
    generalized (purulent) A41.2
    pneumonia —see Pneumonia,
      staphylococcal
  Stellantchasmus falcatus B66.8
  streptobacillus moniliformis A25.1
  streptococcal NEC A49.1
    as cause of disease classified elsewhere
      B95.5
    B genitourinary complicating
      childbirth O98.82
      pregnancy O98.81-
      puerperium O98.83
    congenital
      sepsis P36.10
        group B P36.0
        specified NEC P36.19
    generalized (purulent) A40.9
  Streptomyces B47.1
  Strongyloides (stercoralis) —see
    Strongyloidiasis
  stump (amputation) (surgical) —see
    Complication, amputation stump,
    infection
  subcutaneous tissue, local L08.9
  suipestifer —see Infection, salmonella
  swimming pool bacillus A31.1
  Taenia —see Infestation, Taenia
  Taeniarhynchus saginatus B68.1
  tapeworm —see Infestation, tapeworm
  tendon (sheath) —see Tenosynovitis, infective
    NEC
  Ternidens diminutus B81.8
  testis —see Orchitis
  threadworm B80
  throat —see Pharyngitis
  thyroglossal duct K14.8
  toe (skin) L08.9
    cellulitis L03.03-
      fungus B35.1
    nail L03.03-
      fungus B35.1
  tongue NEC K14.0
    parasitic B37.0
  tonsil (and adenoid) (faucial) (lingual)
    (pharyngeal) —see Tonsillitis
  tooth, teeth K04.7
    irreversible K04.02 ◀
    periapical K04.7
    peridental, periodontal K05.20
      generalized —see Peridontitis,
        aggressive, generalized ◀▥
      localized —see Peridontitis, aggressive,
        localized ◀▥

Infection, infected, infective (Continued)
  tooth, teeth (Continued)
    pulp K04.01 ◄▥
    reversible K04.01 ◄
    socket M27.3
  TORCH —see Infection, congenital
      without active infection P00.2
  Torula histolytica —see Cryptococcosis
  Toxocara (canis) (cati) (felis) B83.0
  Toxoplasma gondii —see Toxoplasma
  trachea, chronic J42
  trematode NEC —see Infestation, fluke
  trench fever A79.0
  Treponema pallidum —see Syphilis
  Trichinella (spiralis) B75
  Trichomonas A59.9
    cervix A59.09
    intestine A07.8
    prostate A59.02
    specified site NEC A59.8
    urethra A59.03
    urogenitalis A59.00
    vagina A59.01
    vulva A59.01
  Trichophyton, trichophytic —see
      Dermatophytosis
  Trichosporon (beigelii) cutaneum B36.2
  Trichostrongylus B81.2
  Trichuris (trichiura) B79
  Trombicula (irritans) B88.0
  Trypanosoma
    brucei
      gambiense B56.0
      rhodesiense B56.1
    cruzi —see Chagas' disease
  tubal —see Salpingo-oophoritis
  tuberculous NEC —see Tuberculosis
  tubo-ovarian —see Salpingo-oophoritis
  tunica vaginalis N49.1
  tunnel T80.212
  tympanic membrane NEC —see Myringitis
  typhoid (abortive) (ambulant) (bacillus) —see
      Typhoid
  typhus A75.9
    flea-borne A75.2
    mite-borne A75.3
    recrudescent A75.1
    tick-borne A77.9
      African A77.1
      North Asian A77.2
  umbilicus L08.82
  ureter N28.86
  urethra —see Urethritis
  urinary (tract) N39.0
    bladder —see Cystitis
    complicating
      pregnancy O23.4-
        specified type NEC O23.3-
    kidney —see Infection, kidney
    newborn P39.3
    puerperal (postpartum) O86.20
    tuberculous A18.13
    urethra —see Urethritis
  uterus, uterine —see Endometritis
  vaccination T88.0
  vaccinia not from vaccination B08.011
  vagina (acute) —see Vaginitis
  varicella B01.9
  varicose veins —see Varix
  vas deferens NEC N49.1
  vesical —see Cystitis
  Vibrio
    cholerae A00.0
      El Tor A00.1
    parahaemolyticus (food poisoning)
        A05.3
    vulnificus
      as cause of disease classified elsewhere
          B96.82
      foodborne intoxication A05.5
  Vincent's (gum) (mouth) (tonsil) A69.1

Infection, infected, infective (Continued)
  virus, viral NOS B34.9
    adenovirus
      as cause of disease classified elsewhere
          B97.0
      unspecified nature or site B34.0
    arborvirus, arbovirus arthropod-borne A94
    as cause of disease classified elsewhere
        B97.89
      adenovirus B97.0
      coronavirus B97.29
        SARS-associated B97.21
      coxsackievirus B97.11
      echovirus B97.12
      enterovirus B97.10
        coxsackievirus B97.11
        echovirus B97.12
        specified NEC B97.19
      human
        immunodeficiency, type 2 (HIV 2)
            B97.35
        metapneumovirus B97.81
        T-cell lymphotropic,
          type I (HTLV-I) B97.33
          type II (HTLV-II) B97.34
      papillomavirus B97.7
      parvovirus B97.6
      reovirus B97.5
      respiratory syncytial B97.4
      retrovirus B97.30
        human
          immunodeficiency, type 2 (HIV 2)
              B97.35
          T-cell lymphotropic,
            type I (HTLV-I) B97.33
            type II (HTLV-II) B97.34
        lentivirus B97.31
        oncovirus B97.32
        specified NEC B97.39
      specified NEC B97.89
    central nervous system A89
      atypical A81.9
        specified NEC A81.89
      enterovirus NEC A88.8
        meningitis A87.0
      slow virus A81.9
        specified NEC A81.89
      specified NEC A88.8
    chest J98.8
    cotia B08.8
    coxsackie —see also Infection, coxsackie B34.1
      as cause of disease classified elsewhere
          B97.11
    ECHO
      as cause of disease classified elsewhere
          B97.12
      unspecified nature or site B34.1
    encephalitis, tick-borne A84.9
    enterovirus, as cause of disease classified
        elsewhere B97.10
      coxsackievirus B97.11
      echovirus B97.12
      specified NEC B97.19
    exanthem NOS B09
    human metapneumovirus as cause of
        disease classified elsewhere B97.81
    human papilloma as cause of disease
        classified elsewhere B97.7
    intestine —see Enteritis, viral
    respiratory syncytial
      as cause of disease classified elsewhere
          B97.4
      bronchopneumonia J12.1
      common cold syndrome J00
      nasopharyngitis (acute) J00
    rhinovirus
      as cause of disease classified elsewhere
          B97.89
      unspecified nature or site B34.8
    slow A81.9
      specified NEC A81.89

Infection, infected, infective (Continued)
  virus, viral NOS (Continued)
    specified type NEC B33.8
      as cause of disease classified elsewhere
          B97.89
      unspecified nature or site B34.8
    unspecified nature or site B34.9
    West Nile —see Virus, West Nile
    vulva (acute) —see Vulvitis
  West Nile —see Virus, West Nile
  whipworm B79
  worms B83.9
    specified type NEC B83.8
  Wuchereria (bancrofti) B74.0
    malayi B74.1
    yatapoxvirus B08.70
      specified NEC B08.79
  yeast (see also Candidiasis) B37.9
  yellow fever —see Fever, yellow
  Yersinia
    enterocolitica (intestinal) A04.6
    pestis —see Plague
    pseudotuberculosis A28.2
  Zeis' gland —see Hordeolum
  Zika virus A92.5 ◄
  zoonotic bacterial NOS A28.9
  Zopfia senegalensis B47.0
Infective, infectious —see condition
Infertility
  female N97.9
    age-related N97.8
    associated with
      anovulation N97.0
      cervical (mucus) disease or anomaly
          N88.3
      congenital anomaly
        cervix N88.3
        fallopian tube N97.1
        uterus N97.2
        vagina N97.8
      dysmucorrhea N88.3
      fallopian tube disease or anomaly N97.1
      pituitary-hypothalamic origin E23.0
      specified origin NEC N97.8
      Stein-Leventhal syndrome E28.2
      uterine disease or anomaly N97.2
      vaginal disease or anomaly N97.8
    due to
      cervical anomaly N88.3
      fallopian tube anomaly N97.1
      ovarian failure E28.39
      Stein-Leventhal syndrome E28.2
      uterine anomaly N97.2
      vaginal anomaly N97.8
    nonimplantation N97.2
    origin
      cervical N88.3
      tubal (block) (occlusion) (stenosis) N97.1
      uterine N97.2
      vaginal N97.8
  male N46.9
    azoospermia N46.01
      extratesticular cause N46.029
        drug therapy N46.021
        efferent duct obstruction N46.023
        infection N46.022
        radiation N46.024
        specified cause NEC N46.029
        systemic disease N46.025
    oligospermia N46.11
      extratesticular cause N46.129
        drug therapy N46.121
        efferent duct obstruction N46.123
        infection N46.122
        radiation N46.124
        specified cause NEC N46.129
        systemic disease N46.125
    specified type NEC N46.8
Infestation B88.9
  Acanthocheilonema (perstans) (streptocerca)
      B74.4

◄ New　◄▥ Revised　deleted Deleted

Infestation *(Continued)*
  Acariasis B88.0
    demodex folliculorum B88.0
    sarcoptes scabiei B86
    trombiculae B88.0
  Agamofilaria streptocerca B74.4
  Ancylostoma, ankylostoma (braziliense)
      (caninum) (ceylanicum) (duodenale)
      B76.0
    americanum B76.1
    new world B76.1
  Anisakis larvae, anisakiasis B81.0
  arthropod NEC B88.2
  Ascaris lumbricoides —*see* Ascariasis
  Balantidium coli A07.0
  beef tapeworm B68.1
  Bothriocephalus (latus) B70.0
    larval B70.1
  broad tapeworm B70.0
    larval B70.1
  Brugia (malayi) B74.1
    timori B74.2
  candiru B88.8
  Capillaria
    hepatica B83.8
    philippinensis B81.1
  cat liver fluke B66.0
  cestodes B71.9
    diphyllobothrium —*see* Infestation,
        diphyllobothrium
    dipylidiasis B71.1
    hymenolepiasis B71.0
    specified type NEC B71.8
  chigger B88.0
  chigo, chigoe B88.1
  Clonorchis (sinensis) (liver) B66.1
  coccidial A07.3
  crab-lice B85.3
  Cysticercus cellulosae —*see* Cysticercosis
  Demodex (folliculorum) B88.0
  Dermanyssus gallinae B88.0
  Dermatobia (hominis) —*see* Myiasis
  Dibothriocephalus (latus) B70.0
    larval B70.1
  Dicrocoelium dendriticum B66.2
  Diphyllobothrium (adult) (latum) (intestinal)
      (pacificum) B70.0
    larval B70.1
  Diplogonoporus (grandis) B71.8
  Dipylidium caninum B67.4
  Distoma hepaticum B66.3
  dog tapeworm B67.4
  Dracunculus medinensis B72
  dragon worm B72
  dwarf tapeworm B71.0
  Echinococcus —*see* Echinococcus
  Echinostomum ilocanum B66.8
  Entamoeba (histolytica) —*see* Infection,
      Ameba
  Enterobius vermicularis B80
  eyelid
    in (due to)
      leishmaniasis B55.1
      loiasis B74.3
      onchocerciasis B73.09
      phthiriasis B85.3
    parasitic NOS B89
  eyeworm B74.3
  Fasciola (gigantica) (hepatica) (indica) B66.3
  Fasciolopsis (buski) (intestine) B66.5
  filarial B74.9
    bancroftian B74.0
    conjunctiva B74.9
    due to
      Acanthocheilonema (perstans)
          (streptocerca) B74.4
      Brugia (malayi) B74.1
        timori B74.2
      Dracunculus medinensis B72
      guinea worm B72
      loa loa B74.3

Infestation *(Continued)*
  filarial *(Continued)*
    due to *(Continued)*
      Mansonella (ozzardi) (perstans)
          (streptocerca) B74.4
      Onchocerca volvulus B73.00
        eye B73.00
        eyelid B73.09
      Wuchereria (bancrofti) B74.0
    Malayan B74.1
    ozzardi B74.4
    specified type NEC B74.8
  fish tapeworm B70.0
    larval B70.1
  fluke B66.9
    blood NOS —*see* Schistosomiasis
    cat liver B66.0
    intestinal B66.5
    lancet B66.2
    liver (sheep) B66.3
      cat B66.0
      Chinese B66.1
      due to clonorchiasis B66.1
      oriental B66.1
    lung (oriental) B66.4
    sheep liver B66.3
    specified type NEC B66.8
  fly larvae —*see* Myiasis
  Gasterophilus (intestinalis) —*see* Myiasis
  Gastrodiscoides hominis B66.8
  Giardia lamblia A07.1
  Gnathostoma (spinigerum) B83.1
  Gongylonema B83.8
  guinea worm B72
  helminth B83.9
    angiostrongyliasis B83.2
      intestinal B81.3
    gnathostomiasis B83.1
    hirudiniasis, internal B83.4
    intestinal B82.0
      angiostrongyliasis B81.3
      anisakiasis B81.0
      ascariasis —*see* Ascariasis
      capillariasis B81.1
      cysticercosis —*see* Cysticercosis
      diphyllobothriasis —*see* Infestation,
          diphyllobothriasis
      dracunculiasis B72
      echinococcus —*see* Echinococcosis
      enterobiasis B80
      filariasis —*see* Infestation, filarial
      fluke —*see* Infestation, fluke
      hookworm —*see* Infestation, hookworm
      mixed (types classifiable to more than
          one of the titles B65.0-B81.3 and
          B81.8) B81.4
      onchocerciasis —*see* Onchocerciasis
      schistosomiasis —*see* Infestation,
          schistosoma
      specified
        cestode NEC —*see* Infestation, cestode
        type NEC B81.8
      strongyloidiasis —*see* Strongyloidiasis
      taenia —*see* Infestation, taenia
      trichinellosis B75
      trichostrongyliasis B81.2
      trichuriasis B79
      specified type NEC B83.8
    syngamiasis B83.3
    visceral larva migrans B83.0
  Heterophyes (heterophyes) B66.8
  hookworm B76.9
    ancylostomiasis B76.0
    necatoriasis B76.1
    specified type NEC B76.8
  Hymenolepis (diminuta) (nana) B71.0
  intestinal NEC B82.9
  leeches (aquatic) (land) —*see* Hirudiniasis
  Leishmania —*see* Leishmaniasis
  lice, louse —*see* Infestation, Pediculus
  Linguatula B88.8

Infestation *(Continued)*
  Liponyssoides sanguineus B88.0
  Loa loa B74.3
    conjunctival B74.3
    eyelid B74.3
  louse —*see* Infestation, Pediculus
  maggots —*see* Myiasis
  Mansonella (ozzardi) (perstans) (streptocerca)
      B74.4
  Medina (worm) B72
  Metagonimus (yokogawai) B66.8
  microfilaria streptocerca —*see* Onchocerciasis
    eye B73.00
    eyelid B73.09
  mites B88.9
    scabic B86
  Monilia (albicans) —*see* Candidiasis
  mouth B37.0
  Necator americanus B76.1
  nematode NEC (intestinal) B82.0
    Ancylostoma B76.0
    conjunctiva NEC B83.9
    Enterobius vermicularis B80
    Gnathostoma spinigerum B83.1
    physaloptera B80
    specified NEC B81.8
    trichostrongylus B81.2
    trichuris (trichuria) B79
  Oesophagostomum (apiostomum) B81.8
  Oestrus ovis —*see also* Myiasis B87.9
  Onchocerca (volvulus) —*see* Onchocerciasis
  Opisthorchis (felineus) (viverrini) B66.0
  orbit, parasitic NOS B89
  Oxyuris vermicularis B80
  Paragonimus (westermani) B66.4
  parasite, parasitic B89
    eyelid B89
    intestinal NOS B82.9
    mouth B37.0
    skin B88.9
    tongue B37.0
  Parastrongylus
    cantonensis B83.2
    costaricensis B81.3
  Pediculus B85.2
    body B85.1
    capitis (humanus) (any site) B85.0
    corporis (humanus) (any site) B85.1
    head B85.0
    mixed (classifiable to more than one of the
        titles B85.0-B85.3) B85.4
    pubis (any site) B85.3
  Pentastoma B88.8
  Phthirus (pubis) (any site) B85.3
    with any infestation classifiable to
        B85.0-B85.2 B85.4
  pinworm B80
  pork tapeworm (adult) B68.0
  protozoal NEC B64
    intestinal A07.9
      specified NEC A07.8
    specified NEC B60.8
  pubic, louse B85.3
  rat tapeworm B71.0
  red bug B88.0
  roundworm (large) NEC B82.0
    Ascariasis —*see also* Ascariasis B77.9
  sandflea B88.1
  Sarcoptes scabiei B86
  scabies B86
  Schistosoma B65.9
    bovis B65.8
    cercariae B65.3
    haematobium B65.0
    intercalatum B65.8
    japonicum B65.2
    mansoni B65.1
    mattheei B65.8
    mekongi B65.8
    specified type NEC B65.8
    spindale B65.8

Infestation (Continued)
    screw worms —see Myiasis
    skin NOS B88.9
    Sparganum (mansoni) (proliferum) (baxteri)
        B70.1
        larval B70.1
    specified type NEC B88.8
    Spirometra larvae B70.1
    Stellantchasmus falcatus B66.8
    Strongyloides stercoralis —see
        Strongyloidiasis
    Taenia B68.9
        diminuta B71.0
        echinococcus —see Echinococcus
        mediocanellata B68.1
        nana B71.0
        saginata B68.1
        solium (intestinal form) B68.0
            larval form —see Cysticercosis
    Taeniarhynchus saginatus B68.1
    tapeworm B71.9
        beef B68.1
        broad B70.0
            larval B70.1
        dog B67.4
        dwarf B71.0
        fish B70.0
            larval B70.1
        pork B68.0
        rat B71.0
    Ternidens diminutus B81.8
    Tetranychus molestissimus B88.0
    threadworm B80
    tongue B37.0
    Toxocara (canis) (cati) (felis) B83.0
    trematode (s) NEC —see Infestation, fluke
    Trichinella (spiralis) B75
    Trichocephalus B79
    Trichomonas —see Trichomoniasis
    Trichostrongylus B81.2
    Trichuris (trichiura) B79
    Trombicula (irritans) B88.0
    Tunga penetrans B88.1
    Uncinaria americana B76.1
    Vandellia cirrhosa B88.8
    whipworm B79
    worms B83.9
        intestinal B82.0
    Wuchereria (bancrofti) B74.0
Infiltrate, infiltration
    amyloid (generalized) (localized) —see
        Amyloidosis
    calcareous NEC R89.7
        localized —see Degeneration, by site
    calcium salt R89.7
    cardiac
        fatty —see Degeneration, myocardial
        glycogenic E74.02 [I43]
    corneal —see Edema, cornea
    eyelid —see Inflammation, eyelid
    glycogen, glycogenic —see Disease, glycogen
        storage
    heart, cardiac
        fatty —see Degeneration, myocardial
        glycogenic E74.02 [I43]
    inflammatory in vitreous H43.89
    kidney N28.89
    leukemic —see Leukemia
    liver K76.89
        fatty —see Fatty, liver NEC
        glycogen —see also Disease, glycogen
            storage E74.03 [K77]
    lung R91.8
        eosinophilic J82
    lymphatic —see also Leukemia, lymphatic
        C91.9-
        gland I88.9
    muscle, fatty M62.89
    myocardium, myocardial
        fatty —see Degeneration, myocardial
        glycogenic E74.02 [I43]

Infiltrate, infiltration (Continued)
    on chest x-ray R91.8
    pulmonary R91.8
        with eosinophilia J82
    skin (lymphocytic) L98.6
    thymus (gland) (fatty) E32.8
    urine R39.0
    vesicant agent
        antineoplastic chemotherapy T80.810
        other agent NEC T80.818
    vitreous body H43.89
Infirmity R68.89
    senile R54
Inflammation, inflamed, inflammatory (with
    exudation)
    abducent (nerve) —see Strabismus, paralytic,
        sixth nerve
    accessory sinus (chronic) —see Sinusitis
    adrenal (gland) E27.8
    alveoli, teeth M27.3
        scorbutic E54
    anal canal, anus K62.89
    antrum (chronic) —see Sinusitis, maxillary
    appendix —see Appendicitis
    arachnoid —see Meningitis
    areola N61.0 ◄
        puerperal, postpartum or gestational —see
            Infection, nipple
    areolar tissue NOS L08.9
    artery —see Arteritis
    auditory meatus (external) —see Otitis,
        externa
    Bartholin's gland N75.8
    bile duct (common) (hepatic) or passage —see
        Cholangitis
    bladder —see Cystitis
    bone —see Osteomyelitis
    brain —see also Encephalitis
        membrane —see Meningitis
    breast N61.0 ◄
        puerperal, postpartum, gestational —see
            Mastitis, obstetric
    broad ligament —see Disease, pelvis,
        inflammatory
    bronchi —see Bronchitis
    catarrhal J00
    cecum —see Appendicitis
    cerebral —see also Encephalitis
        membrane —see Meningitis
    cerebrospinal
        meningococcal A39.0
    cervix (uteri) —see Cervicitis
    chest J98.8
    chorioretinal H30.9-
        cyclitis —see Cyclitis
        disseminated H30.10-
            generalized H30.13-
            peripheral H30.12-
            posterior pole H30.11-
        epitheliopathy —see Epitheliopathy
        focal H30.00-
            juxtapapillary H30.01-
            macular H30.04-
            paramacular —see Inflammation,
                chorioretinal, focal, macular
            peripheral H30.03-
            posterior pole H30.02-
        specified type NEC H30.89-
    choroid —see Inflammation, chorioretinal
    chronic, postmastoidectomy cavity —see
        Complications, postmastoidectomy,
        inflammation
    colon —see Enteritis
    connective tissue (diffuse) NEC —see
        Disorder, soft tissue, specified type
        NEC
    cornea —see Keratitis
    corpora cavernosa N48.29
    cranial nerve —see Disorder, nerve, cranial
    Douglas' cul-de-sac or pouch (chronic)
        N73.0

Inflammation, inflamed, inflammatory
    (Continued)
    due to device, implant or graft —see also
        Complications, by site and type,
        infection or inflammation
    arterial graft T82.7
    breast (implant) T85.79
    catheter T85.79
        dialysis (renal) T82.7
            intraperitoneal T85.71
        infusion T82.7
            cranial T85.735 ◄
            intrathecal T85.735 ◄
            spinal (epidural) (subdural)
                T85.735 ◄⁗
            subarachnoid T85.735 ◄
        urinary T83.518 ◄⁗
            cystostomy T83.510 ◄
            Hopkins T83.518 ◄
            ileostomy T83.518 ◄
            nephrostomy T83.512 ◄
            specified NEC T83.518 ◄
            urethral indwelling T83.511 ◄
            urostomy T83.518 ◄
    electronic (electrode) (pulse generator)
        (stimulator)
        bone T84.7
        cardiac T82.7
        nervous system T85.738 ◄⁗
            brain T85.731 ◄
            cranial nerve T85.732 ◄
            gastric nerve T85.732 ◄
            neurostimulator generator T85.734 ◄
            peripheral nerve T85.732 ◄
            sacral nerve T85.732 ◄
            spinal cord T85.733 ◄
            vagal nerve T85.732 ◄
        urinary T83.590 ◄⁗
    fixation, internal (orthopedic) NEC —see
        Complication, fixation device,
        infection
    gastrointestinal (bile duct) (esophagus)
        T85.79
    neurostimulator electrode (lead)
        T85.732 ◄
    genital NEC T83.69 ◄⁗
    heart NEC T82.7
        valve (prosthesis) T82.6
            graft T82.7
    joint prosthesis —see Complication, joint
        prosthesis, infection
    ocular (corneal graft) (orbital implant)
        NEC T85.79
    orthopedic NEC T84.7
    penile (cylinder) (pump) (resevoir)
        T83.61 ◄
    specified NEC T85.79
    testicular T83.62 ◄
    urinary NEC T83.598 ◄⁗
        ileal conduit stent T83.593 ◄
        implanted neurostimulation T83.590 ◄
        implanted sphincter T83.591 ◄
        indwelling ureteral stent T83.592 ◄
        nephroureteral stent T83.593 ◄
        specified stent NEC T83.593 ◄
    vascular NEC T82.7
    ~~ventricular intracranial shunt T85.79~~
    ventricular intracranial (communicating)
        shunt T85.730 ◄
    duodenum K29.80
        with bleeding K29.81
    dura mater —see Meningitis
    ear (middle) —see also Otitis, media
        external —see Otitis, externa
        inner —see subcategory H83.0
    epididymis —see Epididymitis
    esophagus K20.9
    ethmoidal (sinus) (chronic) —see Sinusitis,
        ethmoidal
    eustachian tube (catarrhal) —see Salpingitis,
        eustachian

◄ New   ◄⁗ Revised   ~~deleted~~ Deleted

Inflammation, inflamed, inflammatory
(Continued)
  eyelid H01.9
    abscess —*see* Abscess, eyelid
    blepharitis —*see* Blepharitis
    chalazion —*see* Chalazion
    dermatosis (noninfectious) —*see*
      Dermatosis, eyelid
    hordeolum —*see* Hordeolum
    specified NEC H01.8
  fallopian tube —*see* Salpingo-oophoritis
  fascia —*see* Myositis
  follicular, pharynx J31.2
  frontal (sinus) (chronic) —*see* Sinusitis, frontal
  gallbladder —*see* Cholecystitis
  gastric —*see* Gastritis
  gastrointestinal —*see* Enteritis
  genital organ (internal) (diffuse)
    female —*see* Disease, pelvis, inflammatory
    male N49.9
      multiple sites N49.8
      specified NEC N49.8
  gland (lymph) —*see* Lymphadenitis
  glottis —*see* Laryngitis
  granular, pharynx J31.2
  gum K05.10
    nonplaque induced K05.11
    plaque induced K05.10
  heart —*see* Carditis
  hepatic duct —*see* Cholangitis
  ileoanal (internal) pouch K91.850
  ileum —*see also* Enteritis
    regional or terminal —*see* Enteritis, regional
  intestinal pouch K91.850
  intestine (any part) —*see* Enteritis
  jaw (acute) (bone) (chronic) (lower)
    (suppurative) (upper) M27.2
  joint NEC —*see* Arthritis
    sacroiliac M46.1
  kidney —*see* Nephritis
  knee (joint) M13.169
    tuberculous A18.02
  labium (majus) (minus) —*see* Vulvitis
  lacrimal
    gland —*see* Dacryoadenitis
    passages (duct) (sac) —*see also*
      Dacryocystitis
      canaliculitis —*see* Canaliculitis, lacrimal
  larynx —*see* Laryngitis
  leg NOS L08.9
  lip K13.0
  liver (capsule) —*see also* Hepatitis
    chronic K73.9
    suppurative K75.0
  lung (acute) —*see also* Pneumonia
    chronic J98.4
  lymphatic vessel —*see* Lymphangitis
  lymph gland or node —*see* Lymphadenitis
  maxilla, maxillary M27.2
    sinus (chronic) —*see* Sinusitis, maxillary
  membranes of brain or spinal cord —*see*
    Meningitis
  meninges —*see* Meningitis
  mouth K12.1
  muscle —*see* Myositis
  myocardium —*see* Myocarditis
  nasal sinus (chronic) —*see* Sinusitis
  nasopharynx —*see* Nasopharyngitis
  navel L08.82
  nerve NEC —*see* Neuralgia
  nipple N61.0 ◀▥
    puerperal, postpartum or gestational —*see*
      Infection, nipple
  nose —*see* Rhinitis
  oculomotor (nerve) —*see* Strabismus,
    paralytic, third nerve
  optic nerve —*see* Neuritis, optic
  orbit (chronic) H05.10
    acute H05.00
      abscess —*see* Abscess, orbit
      cellulitis —*see* Cellulitis, orbit

Inflammation, inflamed, inflammatory
(Continued)
  orbit (chronic) *(Continued)*
    acute *(Continued)*
      osteomyelitis —*see* Osteomyelitis,
        orbit
      periostitis —*see* Periostitis, orbital
      tenonitis —*see* Tenonitis, eye
    granuloma —*see* Granuloma, orbit
    myositis —*see* Myositis, orbital
  ovary —*see* Salpingo-oophoritis
  oviduct —*see* Salpingo-oophoritis
  pancreas (acute) —*see* Pancreatitis
  parametrium N73.0
  parotid region L08.9
  pelvis, female —*see* Disease, pelvis,
    inflammatory
  penis (corpora cavernosa) N48.29
  perianal K62.89
  pericardium —*see* Pericarditis
  perineum (female) (male) L08.9
  perirectal K62.89
  peritoneum —*see* Peritonitis
  periuterine —*see* Disease, pelvis,
    inflammatory
  perivesical —*see* Cystitis
  petrous bone (acute) (chronic) —*see* Petrositis
  pharynx (acute) —*see* Pharyngitis
  pia mater —*see* Meningitis
  pleura —*see* Pleurisy
  polyp, colon —*see also* Polyp, colon,
    inflammatory K51.40
  prostate —*see also* Prostatitis
    specified type NEC N41.8
  rectosigmoid —*see* Rectosigmoiditis
  rectum —*see also* Proctitis K62.89
  respiratory, upper —*see also* Infection,
    respiratory, upper J06.9
    acute, due to radiation J70.0
    chronic, due to external agent —*see*
      condition, respiratory, chronic, due to
    due to
      chemicals, gases, fumes or vapors
        (inhalation) J68.2
      radiation J70.1
  retina —*see* Chorioretinitis
  retrocecal —*see* Appendicitis
  retroperitoneal —*see* Peritonitis
  salivary duct or gland (any) (suppurative) —
    see Sialoadenitis
  scorbutic, alveoli, teeth E54
  scrotum N49.2
  seminal vesicle —*see* Vesiculitis
  sigmoid —*see* Enteritis
  sinus —*see* Sinusitis
  Skene's duct or gland —*see* Urethritis
  skin L08.9
  sphenoidal (sinus) —*see* Sinusitis, sphenoidal
  spinal
    cord —*see* Encephalitis
    membrane —*see* Meningitis
    nerve —*see* Disorder, nerve
  spine —*see* Spondylopathy, inflammatory
  spleen (capsule) D73.89
  stomach —*see* Gastritis
  subcutaneous tissue L08.9
  suprarenal (gland) E27.8
  synovial —*see* Tenosynovitis
  tendon (sheath) NEC —*see* Tenosynovitis
  testis —*see* Orchitis
  throat (acute) —*see* Pharyngitis
  thymus (gland) E32.8
  thyroid (gland) —*see* Thyroiditis
  tongue K14.0
  tonsil —*see* Tonsillitis
  trachea —*see* Tracheitis
  trochlear (nerve) —*see* Strabismus, paralytic,
    fourth nerve
  tubal —*see* Salpingo-oophoritis
  tuberculous NEC —*see* Tuberculosis

Inflammation, inflamed, inflammatory
(Continued)
  tubo-ovarian —*see* Salpingo-oophoritis
  tunica vaginalis N49.1
  tympanic membrane —*see* Tympanitis
  umbilicus, umbilical L08.82
  uterine ligament —*see* Disease, pelvis,
    inflammatory
  uterus (catarrhal) —*see* Endometritis
  uveal tract (anterior) NOS —*see also*
    Iridocyclitis
    posterior —*see* Chorioretinitis
  vagina —*see* Vaginitis
  vas deferens N49.1
  vein —*see also* Phlebitis
    intracranial or intraspinal (septic) G08
    thrombotic I80.9
      leg —*see* Phlebitis, leg
      lower extremity —*see* Phlebitis, leg
  vocal cord J38.3
  vulva —*see* Vulvitis
  Wharton's duct (suppurative) —*see*
    Sialoadenitis
Inflation, lung, imperfect (newborn) —*see*
  Atelectasis
Influenza (bronchial) (epidemic) (respiratory
  (upper)) (unidentified influenza virus)
  J11.1
  with
    digestive manifestations J11.2
    encephalopathy J11.81
    enteritis J11.2
    gastroenteritis J11.2
    gastrointestinal manifestations J11.2
    laryngitis J11.1
    myocarditis J11.82
    otitis media J11.83
    pharyngitis J11.1
    pneumonia J11.00
      specified type J11.08
    respiratory manifestations NEC J11.1
    specified manifestation NEC J11.89
  A/H5N1 —*see also* Influenza, due to,
    identified novel influenza A virus J09.X2
  avian —*see also* Influenza, due to, identified
    novel influenza A virus J09.X2
  bird —*see also* Influenza, due to, identified
    novel influenza A virus J09.X2
  novel (2009) H1N1 influenza —*see also*
    Influenza, due to, identified influenza
    virus NEC J10.1
  novel influenza A/H1N1 —*see also* Influenza,
    due to, identified influenza virus NEC
    J10.1
  due to
    avian (*see also* Influenza, due to, identified
      novel influenza A virus) J09.X2
    identified influenza virus NEC J10.1
      with
        digestive manifestations J10.2
        encephalopathy J10.81
        enteritis J10.2
        gastroenteritis J10.2
        gastrointestinal manifestations J10.2
        laryngitis J10.1
        myocarditis J10.82
        otitis media J10.83
        pharyngitis J10.1
        pneumonia (unspecified type) J10.00
          with same identified influenza virus
            J10.01
          specified type NEC J10.08
        respiratory manifestations NEC J10.1
        specified manifestation NEC J10.89
    identified novel influenza A virus J09.X2
      with
        digestive manifestations J09.X3
        encephalopathy J09.X9
        enteritis J09.X3
        gastroenteritis J09.X3
        gastrointestinal manifestations J09.X3

Influenza *(Continued)*
  due to *(Continued)*
    identified novel influenza A virus
      (Continued)
      with *(Continued)*
        laryngitis J09.X2
        myocarditis J09.X9
        otitis media J09.X9
        pharyngitis J09.X2
        pneumonia J09.X1
        respiratory manifestations NEC J09.X2
        specified manifestation NEC J09.X9
        upper respiratory symptoms J09.X2
    of other animal origin, not bird or swine *(see also* Influenza, due to, identified novel influenza A virus) J09.X2
    swine (viruses that normally cause infections in pigs) —*see also* Influenza, due to, identified novel influenza A virus J09.X2
Influenza-like disease —*see* Influenza
Influenzal —*see* Influenza
Infraction, Freiberg's (metatarsal head) —*see* Osteochondrosis, juvenile, metatarsus
Infraeruption of tooth (teeth) M26.34
Infusion complication, misadventure, or reaction —*see* Complications, infusion
Ingestion
  chemical —*see* Table of Drugs and Chemicals, by substance, poisoning
  drug or medicament
    correct substance properly administered — *see* Table of Drugs and Chemicals, by drug, adverse effect
    overdose or wrong substance given or taken —*see* Table of Drugs and Chemicals, by drug, poisoning
  foreign body —*see* Foreign body, alimentary tract
  tularemia A21.3
Ingrowing
  hair (beard) L73.1
  nail (finger) (toe) L60.0
Inguinal —*see also* condition
  testicle Q53.9
    bilateral Q53.21
    unilateral Q53.11
Inhalant-induced ◄
  anxiety disorder F18.980 ◄
  depressive disorder F18.94 ◄
  major neurocognitive disorder F18.97 ◄
  mild neurocognitive disorder F18.988 ◄
  psychotic disorder F18.959 ◄
Inhalation
  anthrax A22.1
  flame T27.3
  food or foreign body —*see* Foreign body, by site
  gases, fumes, or vapors NEC T59.9-
    specified agent —*see* Table of Drugs and Chemicals, by substance
  liquid or vomitus —*see* Asphyxia
  meconium (newborn) P24.00
    with
      with respiratory symptoms P24.01
      pneumonia (pneumonitis) P24.01
  mucus —*see* Asphyxia, mucus
  oil or gasoline (causing suffocation) —*see* Foreign body, by site
  smoke J70.5
    due to chemicals, gases, fumes and vapors J68.9
  steam —*see* Toxicity, vapors
  stomach contents or secretions —*see* Foreign body, by site
    due to anesthesia (general) (local) or other sedation T88.59
      in labor and delivery O74.0
      in pregnancy O29.01-
      postpartum, puerperal O89.01

Inhibition, orgasm
  female F52.31
  male F52.32
Inhibitor, systemic lupus erythematosus (presence of) D68.62
Iniencephalus, iniencephaly Q00.2
Injection, traumatic jet (air) (industrial) (water) (paint or dye) T70.4
Injury —*see also* specified injury type T14.90
  abdomen, abdominal S39.91
    blood vessel —*see* Injury, blood vessel, abdomen
    cavity —*see* Injury, intra-abdominal
    contusion S30.1
    internal —*see* Injury, intra-abdominal
    intra-abdominal organ —*see* Injury, intra-abdominal
    nerve —*see* Injury, nerve, abdomen
    open —*see* Wound, open, abdomen
    specified NEC S39.81
    superficial —*see* Injury, superficial, abdomen
  Achilles tendon S86.00-
    laceration S86.02-
    specified type NEC S86.09-
    strain S86.01-
  acoustic, resulting in deafness —*see* Injury, nerve, acoustic
  adrenal (gland) S37.819
    contusion S37.812
    laceration S37.813
    specified type NEC S37.818
  alveolar (process) S09.93
  ankle S99.91-
    contusion —*see* Contusion, ankle
    dislocation —*see* Dislocation, ankle
    fracture —*see* Fracture, ankle
    nerve —*see* Injury, nerve, ankle
    open —*see* Wound, open, ankle
    specified type NEC S99.81-
    sprain —*see* Sprain, ankle
    superficial —*see* Injury, superficial, ankle
  anterior chamber, eye —*see* Injury, eye, specified site NEC
  anus —*see* Injury, abdomen
  aorta (thoracic) S25.00
    abdominal S35.00
      laceration (minor) (superficial) S35.01
        major S35.02
      specified type NEC S35.09
    laceration (minor) (superficial) S25.01
      major S25.02
    specified type NEC S25.09
  arm (upper) S49.9-
    blood vessel —*see* Injury, blood vessel, arm
    contusion —*see* Contusion, arm, upper
    fracture —*see* Fracture, humerus
    lower —*see* Injury, forearm
    muscle —*see* Injury, muscle, shoulder
    nerve —*see* Injury, nerve, arm
    open —*see* Wound, open, arm
    specified type NEC S49.8-
    superficial —*see* Injury, superficial, arm
  artery (complicating trauma) —*see also* Injury, blood vessel, by site
    cerebral or meningeal —*see* Injury, intracranial
  auditory canal (external) (meatus) S09.91
  auricle, auris, ear S09.91
  axilla —*see* Injury, shoulder
  back —*see* Injury, back, lower
  bile duct S36.13
  birth —*see also* Birth, injury P15.9
  bladder (sphincter) S37.20
    at delivery O71.5
    contusion S37.22
    laceration S37.23
    obstetrical trauma O71.5
    specified type NEC S37.29

Injury *(Continued)*
  blast (air) (hydraulic) (immersion) (underwater) NEC T14.8
    acoustic nerve trauma —*see* Injury, nerve, acoustic
    bladder —*see* Injury, bladder
    brain —*see* Concussion
    colon —*see* Injury, intestine, large, blast injury
    ear (primary) S09.31-
      secondary S09.39-
    generalized T70.8
    lung —*see* Injury, intrathoracic, lung, blast injury
    multiple body organs T70.8
    peritoneum S36.81
    rectum S36.61
    retroperitoneum S36.898
    small intestine S36.419
      duodenum S36.410
      specified site NEC S36.418
    specified
      intra-abdominal organ NEC S36.898
      pelvic organ NEC S37.899
  blood vessel NEC T14.8
    abdomen S35.9-
      aorta —*see* Injury, aorta, abdominal
      celiac artery —*see* Injury, blood vessel, celiac artery
      iliac vessel —*see* Injury, blood vessel, iliac
      laceration S35.91
      mesenteric vessel —*see* Injury, mesenteric
      portal vein —*see* Injury, blood vessel, portal vein
      renal vessel —*see* Injury, blood vessel, renal
      specified vessel NEC S35.8X-
      splenic vessel —*see* Injury, blood vessel, splenic
      vena cava —*see* Injury, vena cava, inferior
    ankle —*see* Injury, blood vessel, foot
    aorta (abdominal) (thoracic) —*see* Injury, aorta
    arm (upper) NEC S45.90-
      forearm —*see* Injury, blood vessel, forearm
      laceration S45.91-
      specified
        site NEC S45.80-
          laceration S45.81-
          specified type NEC S45.89-
        type NEC S45.99-
      superficial vein S45.30-
        laceration S45.31-
        specified type NEC S45.39-
    axillary
      artery S45.00-
        laceration S45.01-
        specified type NEC S45.09-
      vein S45.20-
        laceration S45.21-
        specified type NEC S45.29-
    azygos vein —*see* Injury, blood vessel, thoracic, specified site NEC
    brachial
      artery S45.10-
        laceration S45.11-
        specified type NEC S45.19-
      vein S45.20-
        laceration S45.219
        specified type NEC S45.29-
    carotid artery (common) (external) (internal, extracranial) S15.00-
      internal, intracranial S06.8-
      laceration (minor) (superficial) S15.01-
        major S15.02-
      specified type NEC S15.09-

◄ New   ◄|||| Revised   ~~deleted~~ Deleted

Injury *(Continued)*
blood vessel NEC *(Continued)*
celiac artery S35.219
branch S35.299
laceration (minor) (superficial) S35.291
major S35.292
specified NEC S35.298
laceration (minor) (superficial) S35.211
major S35.212
specified type NEC S35.218
cerebral —*see* Injury, intracranial
deep plantar —*see* Injury, blood vessel,
plantar artery
digital (hand) —*see* Injury, blood vessel,
finger
dorsal
artery (foot) S95.00-
laceration S95.01-
specified type NEC S95.09-
vein (foot) S95.20-
laceration S95.21-
specified type NEC S95.29-
due to accidental laceration during
procedure —*see* Laceration, accidental
complicating surgery
extremity —*see* Injury, blood vessel, limb
femoral
artery (common) (superficial) S75.00-
laceration (minor) (superficial)
S75.01-
major S75.02-
specified type NEC S75.09-
vein (hip level) (thigh level) S75.10-
laceration (minor) (superficial) S75.11-
major S75.12-
specified type NEC S75.19-
finger S65.50-
index S65.50-
laceration S65.51-
specified type NEC S65.59-
laceration S65.51-
little S65.50-
laceration S65.51-
specified type NEC S65.59-
middle S65.50-
laceration S65.51-
specified type NEC S65.59-
specified type NEC S65.59-
thumb —*see* Injury, blood vessel, thumb
foot S95.90-
dorsal
artery —*see* Injury, blood vessel,
dorsal, artery
vein —*see* Injury, blood vessel, dorsal,
vein
laceration S95.91-
plantar artery —*see* Injury, blood vessel,
plantar artery
specified
site NEC S95.80-
laceration S95.81-
specified type NEC S95.89-
specified type NEC S95.99-
forearm S55.90-
laceration S55.91-
radial artery —*see* Injury, blood vessel,
radial artery
specified
site NEC S55.80-
laceration S55.81-
specified type NEC S55.89-
type NEC S55.99-
ulnar artery —*see* Injury, blood vessel,
ulnar artery
vein S55.20-
laceration S55.21-
specified type NEC S55.29-
gastric
artery —*see* Injury, mesenteric, artery,
branch
vein —*see* Injury, blood vessel, abdomen

Injury *(Continued)*
blood vessel NEC *(Continued)*
gastroduodenal artery —*see* Injury,
mesenteric, artery, branch
greater saphenous vein (lower leg level)
S85.30-
hip (and thigh) level S75.20-
laceration (minor) (superficial) S75.21-
major S75.22-
specified type NEC S75.29-
laceration S85.31-
specified type NEC S85.39-
hand (level) S65.90-
finger —*see* Injury, blood vessel, finger
laceration S65.91-
palmar arch —*see* Injury, blood vessel,
palmar arch
radial artery —*see* Injury, blood vessel,
radial artery, hand
specified
site NEC S65.80-
laceration S65.81-
specified type NEC S65.89-
type NEC S65.99-
thumb —*see* Injury, blood vessel,
thumb
ulnar artery —*see* Injury, blood vessel,
ulnar artery, hand
head S09.0
intracranial —*see* Injury, intracranial
multiple S09.0
hepatic
artery —*see* Injury, mesenteric, artery
vein —*see* Injury, vena cava, inferior
hip S75.90-
femoral artery —*see* Injury, blood vessel,
femoral, artery
femoral vein —*see* Injury, blood vessel,
femoral, vein
greater saphenous vein —*see* Injury,
blood vessel, greater saphenous,
hip level
laceration S75.91-
specified
site NEC S75.80-
laceration S75.81-
specified type NEC S75.89-
type NEC S75.99-
hypogastric (artery) (vein) —*see* Injury,
blood vessel, iliac
iliac S35.5-
artery S35.51-
specified vessel NEC S35.5-
uterine vessel —*see* Injury, blood vessel,
uterine
vein S35.51-
innominate —*see* Injury, blood vessel,
thoracic, innominate
intercostal (artery) (vein) —*see* Injury,
blood vessel, thoracic, intercostal
jugular vein (external) S15.20-
internal S15.30-
laceration (minor) (superficial) S15.31-
major S15.32-
specified type NEC S15.39-
laceration (minor) (superficial) S15.21-
major S15.22-
specified type NEC S15.29-
leg (level) (lower) S85.90-
greater saphenous —*see* Injury, blood
vessel, greater saphenous
laceration S85.91-
lesser saphenous —*see* Injury, blood
vessel, lesser saphenous
peroneal artery —*see* Injury, blood
vessel, peroneal artery
popliteal
artery —*see* Injury, blood vessel,
popliteal, artery
vein —*see* Injury, blood vessel,
popliteal, vein

Injury *(Continued)*
blood vessel NEC *(Continued)*
leg (level) (lower) *(Continued)*
specified
site NEC S85.80-
laceration S85.81-
specified type NEC S85.89-
type NEC S85.99-
thigh —*see* Injury, blood vessel, hip
tibial artery —*see* Injury, blood vessel,
tibial artery
lesser saphenous vein (lower leg level)
S85.40-
laceration S85.41-
specified type NEC S85.49-
limb
lower —*see* Injury, blood vessel, leg
upper —*see* Injury, blood vessel, arm
lower back —*see* Injury, blood vessel,
abdomen
specified NEC —*see* Injury, blood
vessel, abdomen, specified, site
NEC
mammary (artery) (vein) —*see* Injury,
blood vessel, thoracic, specified site
NEC
mesenteric (inferior) (superior)
artery —*see* Injury, mesenteric, artery
vein —*see* Injury, mesenteric, vein
neck S15.9
specified site NEC S15.8
ovarian (artery) (vein) —*see* subcategory
S35.8
palmar arch (superficial) S65.20-
deep S65.30-
laceration S65.31-
specified type NEC S65.39-
laceration S65.21-
specified type NEC S65.29-
pelvis —*see* Injury, blood vessel, abdomen
specified NEC —*see* Injury, blood vessel,
abdomen, specified, site NEC
peroneal artery S85.20-
laceration S85.21-
specified type NEC S85.29-
plantar artery (deep) (foot) S95.10-
laceration S95.11-
specified type NEC S95.19-
popliteal
artery S85.00-
laceration S85.01-
specified type NEC S85.09-
vein S85.50-
laceration S85.51-
specified type NEC S85.59-
portal vein S35.319
laceration S35.311
specified type NEC S35.318
precerebral —*see* Injury, blood vessel, neck
pulmonary (artery) (vein) —*see* Injury,
blood vessel, thoracic, pulmonary
radial artery (forearm level) S55.10-
hand and wrist (level) S65.10-
laceration S65.11-
specified type NEC S65.19-
laceration S55.11-
specified type NEC S55.19-
renal
artery S35.40-
laceration S35.41-
specified NEC S35.49-
vein S35.40-
laceration S35.41-
specified NEC S35.49-
saphenous vein (greater) (lower leg
level) —*see* Injury, blood vessel,
greater saphenous
hip and thigh level —*see* Injury, blood
vessel, greater saphenous, hip level
lesser —*see* Injury, blood vessel, lesser
saphenous

Injury *(Continued)*
  blood vessel NEC *(Continued)*
    shoulder
      specified NEC —*see* Injury, blood vessel,
        arm, specified site NEC
      superficial vein —*see* Injury, blood
        vessel, arm, superficial vein
    specified NEC T14.8
    splenic
      artery —*see* Injury, blood vessel, celiac
        artery, branch
      vein S35.329
        laceration S35.321
        specified NEC S35.328
    subclavian —*see* Injury, blood vessel,
      thoracic, innominate
    thigh —*see* Injury, blood vessel, hip
    thoracic S25.90
      aorta S25.00
        laceration (minor) (superficial) S25.01
          major S25.02
        specified type NEC S25.09
      azygos vein —*see* Injury, blood vessel,
        thoracic, specified, site NEC
      innominate
        artery S25.10-
          laceration (minor) (superficial)
            S25.11-
              major S25.12-
          specified type NEC S25.19-
        vein S25.30-
          laceration (minor) (superficial)
            S25.31-
              major S25.32-
          specified type NEC S25.39-
      intercostal S25.50-
        laceration S25.51-
        specified type NEC S25.59-
      laceration S25.91
      mammary vessel —*see* Injury, blood
        vessel, thoracic, specified, site NEC
      pulmonary S25.40-
        laceration (minor) (superficial) S25.41-
          major S25.42-
        specified type NEC S25.49-
      specified
        site NEC S25.80-
          laceration S25.81-
          specified type NEC S25.89-
        type NEC S25.99
      subclavian —*see* Injury, blood vessel,
        thoracic, innominate
      vena cava (superior) S25.20
        laceration (minor) (superficial) S25.21
          major S25.22
        specified type NEC S25.29
    thumb S65.40-
      laceration S65.41-
      specified type NEC S65.49-
    tibial artery S85.10-
      anterior S85.13-
        laceration S85.14-
        specified injury NEC S85.15-
      laceration S85.11-
      posterior S85.16-
        laceration S85.17-
        specified injury NEC S85.18-
      specified injury NEC S85.12-
    ulnar artery (forearm level) S55.00-
      hand and wrist (level) S65.00-
        laceration S65.01-
        specified type NEC S65.09-
      laceration S55.01-
      specified type NEC S55.09-
    upper arm (level) —*see* Injury, blood vessel,
      arm
    superficial vein —*see* Injury, blood
      vessel, arm, superficial vein
    uterine S35.5-
      artery S35.53-
      vein S35.53-

Injury *(Continued)*
  blood vessel NEC *(Continued)*
    vena cava —*see* Injury, vena cava
    vertebral artery S15.10-
      laceration (minor) (superficial) S15.11-
        major S15.12-
      specified type NEC S15.19-
    wrist (level) —*see* Injury, blood vessel,
      hand
  brachial plexus S14.3
    newborn P14.3
  brain (traumatic) S06.9-
    diffuse (axonal) S06.2X-
    focal S06.30-
    ~~traumatic —see category S06~~
    brainstem S06.38-
  breast NOS S29.9
  broad ligament —*see* Injury, pelvic organ,
    specified site NEC
  bronchus, bronchi —*see* Injury, intrathoracic,
    bronchus
  brow S09.90
  buttock S39.92
  canthus, eye S05.90
  cardiac plexus —*see* Injury, nerve, thorax,
    sympathetic
  cauda equina S34.3
  cavernous sinus —*see* Injury, intracranial
  cecum —*see* Injury, colon
  celiac ganglion or plexus —*see* Injury, nerve,
    lumbosacral, sympathetic
  cerebellum —*see* Injury, intracranial
  cerebral —*see* Injury, intracranial
  cervix (uteri) —*see* Injury, uterus
  cheek (wall) S09.93
  chest —*see* Injury, thorax
  childbirth (newborn) —*see also* Birth, injury
    maternal NEC O71.9
  chin S09.93
  choroid (eye) —*see* Injury, eye, specified site
    NEC
  clitoris S39.94
  coccyx —*see also* Injury, back, lower
    complicating delivery O71.6
  colon —*see* Injury, intestine, large
  common bile duct —*see* Injury, liver
  conjunctiva (superficial) —*see* Injury, eye,
    conjunctiva
  conus medullaris —*see* Injury, spinal, sacral
  cord
    spermatic (pelvic region) S37.898
      scrotal region S39.848
    spinal —*see* Injury, spinal cord, by region
  cornea —*see* Injury, eye, specified site NEC
    abrasion —*see* Injury, eye, cornea, abrasion
  cortex (cerebral) —*see also* Injury, intracranial
    visual —*see* Injury, nerve, optic
  costal region NEC S29.9
  costochondral NEC S29.9
  cranial
    cavity —*see* Injury, intracranial
    nerve —*see* Injury, nerve, cranial
  crushing —*see* Crush
  cutaneous sensory nerve
  cystic duct —*see* Injury, liver
  deep tissue —*see* Contusion, by site
    meaning pressure ulcer —*see* Ulcer,
      pressure, unstageable, by site
  delivery (newborn) P15.9
    maternal NEC O71.9
  Descemet's membrane —*see* Injury, eyeball,
    penetrating
  diaphragm —*see* Injury, intrathoracic,
    diaphragm
  duodenum —*see* Injury, intestine, small,
    duodenum
  ear (auricle) (external) (canal) S09.91
    abrasion —*see* Abrasion, ear
    bite —*see* Bite, ear
    blister —*see* Blister, ear
    bruise —*see* Contusion, ear

Injury *(Continued)*
  ear *(Continued)*
    contusion —*see* Contusion, ear
    external constriction —*see* Constriction,
      external, ear
    hematoma —*see* Hematoma, ear
    inner —*see* Injury, ear, middle
    laceration —*see* Laceration, ear
    middle S09.30-
      blast —*see* Injury, blast, ear
      specified NEC S09.39-
    puncture —*see* Puncture, ear
    superficial —*see* Injury, superficial, ear
  eighth cranial nerve (acoustic or auditory) —
    see Injury, nerve, acoustic
  elbow S59.90-
    contusion —*see* Contusion, elbow
    dislocation —*see* Dislocation, elbow
    fracture —*see* Fracture, ulna, upper end
    open —*see* Wound, open, elbow
    specified NEC S59.80-
    sprain —*see* Sprain, elbow
    superficial —*see* Injury, superficial, elbow
  eleventh cranial nerve (accessory) —*see*
    Injury, nerve, accessory
  epididymis S39.94
  epigastric region S39.91
  epiglottis NEC S19.89
  esophageal plexus —*see* Injury, nerve, thorax,
    sympathetic
  esophagus (thoracic part) —*see also* Injury,
    intrathoracic, esophagus
    cervical NEC S19.85
  eustachian tube S09.30-
  eye S05.9-
    avulsion S05.7-
    ball —*see* Injury, eyeball
    conjunctiva S05.0-
    cornea
      abrasion S05.0-
      laceration S05.3-
        with prolapse S05.2-
    lacrimal apparatus S05.8X-
    orbit penetration S05.4-
    specified site NEC S05.8X-
  eyeball S05.8X-
    contusion S05.1-
    penetrating S05.6-
      with
        foreign body S05.5-
        prolapse or loss of intraocular tissue
          S05.2-
      without prolapse or loss of intraocular
        tissue S05.3-
    specified type NEC S05.8-
  eyebrow S09.93
  eyelid S09.93
    abrasion —*see* Abrasion, eyelid
    contusion —*see* Contusion, eyelid
    open —*see* Wound, open, eyelid
  face S09.93
  fallopian tube S37.509
    bilateral S37.502
      blast injury S37.512
      contusion S37.522
      laceration S37.532
      specified type NEC S37.592
    blast injury (primary) S37.519
      bilateral S37.512
      secondary —*see* Injury, fallopian tube,
        specified type NEC
      unilateral S37.511
    contusion S37.529
      bilateral S37.522
      unilateral S37.521
    laceration S37.539
      bilateral S37.532
      unilateral S37.531
    specified type NEC S37.599
      bilateral S37.592
      unilateral S37.591

◀ New   ◀ Revised   ~~deleted~~ Deleted

Injury *(Continued)*
  fallopian tube *(Continued)*
    unilateral S37.501
      blast injury S37.511
      contusion S37.521
      laceration S37.531
      specified type NEC S37.591
  fascia —*see* Injury, muscle
  fifth cranial nerve (trigeminal) —*see* Injury,
      nerve, trigeminal
  finger (nail) S69.9-
    blood vessel —*see* Injury, blood vessel,
        finger
    contusion —*see* Contusion, finger
    dislocation —*see* Dislocation, finger
    fracture —*see* Fracture, finger
    muscle —*see* Injury, muscle, finger
    nerve —*see* Injury, nerve, digital, finger
    open —*see* Wound, open, finger
    specified NEC S69.8-
    sprain —*see* Sprain, finger
    superficial —*see* Injury, superficial, finger
  first cranial nerve (olfactory) —*see* Injury,
      nerve, olfactory
  flank —*see* Injury, abdomen
  foot S99.92-
    blood vessel —*see* Injury, blood vessel, foot
    contusion —*see* Contusion, foot
    dislocation —*see* Dislocation, foot
    fracture —*see* Fracture, foot
    muscle —*see* Injury, muscle, foot
    open —*see* Wound, open, foot
    specified type NEC S99.82-
    sprain —*see* Sprain, foot
    superficial —*see* Injury, superficial, foot
  forceps NOS P15.9
  forearm S59.91-
    blood vessel —*see* Injury, blood vessel,
        forearm
    contusion —*see* Contusion, forearm
    fracture —*see* Fracture, forearm
    muscle —*see* Injury, muscle, forearm
    nerve —*see* Injury, nerve, forearm
    open —*see* Wound, open, forearm
    specified NEC S59.81-
    superficial —*see* Injury, superficial,
        forearm
  forehead S09.90
  fourth cranial nerve (trochlear) —*see* Injury,
      nerve, trochlear
  gallbladder S36.129
    contusion S36.122
    laceration S36.123
    specified NEC S36.128
  ganglion
    celiac, coeliac —*see* Injury, nerve,
        lumbosacral, sympathetic
    gasserian —*see* Injury, nerve, trigeminal
    stellate —*see* Injury, nerve, thorax,
        sympathetic
    thoracic sympathetic —*see* Injury, nerve,
        thorax, sympathetic
  gasserian ganglion —*see* Injury, nerve,
      trigeminal
  gastric artery —*see* Injury, blood vessel, celiac
      artery, branch
  gastroduodenal artery —*see* Injury, blood
      vessel, celiac artery, branch
  gastrointestinal tract —*see* Injury,
      intra-abdominal
    with open wound into abdominal cavity —
        see Wound, open, with penetration
        into peritoneal cavity
    colon —*see* Injury, intestine, large
    rectum —*see* Injury, intestine, large, rectum
      with open wound into abdominal cavity
          S36.61
    small intestine —*see* Injury, intestine, small
    specified site NEC —*see* Injury, intra-
        abdominal, specified, site NEC
    stomach —*see* Injury, stomach

Injury *(Continued)*
  genital organ (s)
    external S39.94
      specified NEC S39.848
    internal S37.90
      fallopian tube —*see* Injury, fallopian tube
      ovary —*see* Injury, ovary
      prostate —*see* Injury, prostate
      seminal vesicle —*see* Injury, pelvis,
          organ, specified site NEC
      uterus —*see* Injury, uterus
      vas deferens —*see* Injury, pelvis, organ,
          specified site NEC
    obstetrical trauma O71.9
  gland
    lacrimal laceration —*see* Injury, eye,
        specified site NEC
    salivary S09.93 ◀▥
    thyroid NEC S19.84
  globe (eye) S05.90
    specified NEC S05.8X-
  groin —*see* Injury, abdomen
  gum S09.90
  hand S69.9-
    blood vessel —*see* Injury, blood vessel,
        hand
    contusion —*see* Contusion, hand
    fracture —*see* Fracture, hand
    muscle —*see* Injury, muscle, hand
    nerve —*see* Injury, nerve, hand
    open —*see* Wound, open, hand
    specified NEC S69.8-
    sprain —*see* Sprain, hand
    superficial —*see* Injury, superficial, hand
  head S09.90
    with loss of consciousness S06.9-
    specified NEC S09.8-
  heart S26.90
    with hemopericardium S26.00
      contusion S26.01
      laceration (mild) S26.020
        major S26.022
        moderate S26.021
      specified type NEC S26.09
    without hemopericardium S26.10
      contusion S26.11
      laceration S26.12
      specified type NEC S26.19
    contusion S26.91
    laceration S26.92
    specified type NEC S26.99
  heel —*see* Injury, foot
  hepatic
    artery —*see* Injury, blood vessel, celiac
        artery, branch
    duct —*see* Injury, liver
    vein —*see* Injury, vena cava, inferior
  hip S79.91-
    blood vessel —*see* Injury, blood vessel,
        hip
    contusion —*see* Contusion, hip
    dislocation —*see* Dislocation, hip
    fracture —*see* Fracture, femur, neck
    muscle —*see* Injury, muscle, hip
    nerve —*see* Injury, nerve, hip
    open —*see* Wound, open, hip
    specified NEC S79.81-
    sprain —*see* Sprain, hip
    superficial —*see* Injury, superficial, hip
  hymen S39.94
  hypogastric
    blood vessel —*see* Injury, blood vessel, iliac
    plexus —*see* Injury, nerve, lumbosacral,
        sympathetic
  ileum —*see* Injury, intestine, small
  iliac region S39.91
  instrumental (during surgery) —*see*
      Laceration, accidental complicating
      surgery
    birth injury —*see* Birth, injury
    nonsurgical —*see* Injury, by site

Injury *(Continued)*
  instrumental *(Continued)*
    obstetrical O71.9
      bladder O71.5
      cervix O71.3
      high vaginal O71.4
      perineal NOS O70.9
      urethra O71.5
      uterus O71.5
        with rupture or perforation O71.1
  internal T14.8
    aorta —*see* Injury, aorta
    bladder (sphincter) —*see* Injury, bladder
      with
        ectopic or molar pregnancy O08.6
        following ectopic or molar pregnancy
            O08.6
        obstetrical trauma O71.5
    bronchus, bronchi —*see* Injury,
        intrathoracic, bronchus
    cecum —*see* Injury, intestine, large
    cervix (uteri) —*see also* Injury, uterus
      with ectopic or molar pregnancy O08.6
      following ectopic or molar pregnancy
          O08.6
      obstetrical trauma O71.3
    chest —*see* Injury, intrathoracic
    gastrointestinal tract —*see* Injury,
        intra-abdominal
    heart —*see* Injury, heart
    intestine NEC —*see* Injury, intestine
    intrauterine —*see* Injury, uterus
    mesentery —*see* Injury, intra-abdominal,
        specified, site NEC
    pelvis, pelvic (organ) S37.90
      following ectopic or molar pregnancy
          (subsequent episode) O08.6
      obstetrical trauma NEC O71.5
      rupture or perforation O71.1
      specified NEC S39.83
    rectum —*see* Injury, intestine, large,
        rectum
    stomach —*see* Injury, stomach
    ureter —*see* Injury, ureter
    urethra (sphincter) following ectopic or
        molar pregnancy O08.6
    uterus —*see* Injury, uterus
  interscapular area —*see* Injury, thorax
  intestine
    large S36.509
      ascending (right) S36.500
        blast injury (primary) S36.510
          secondary S36.590
        contusion S36.520
        laceration S36.530
        specified type NEC S36.590
      blast injury (primary) S36.519
        ascending (right) S36.510
        descending (left) S36.512
        rectum S36.61
        sigmoid S36.513
        specified site NEC S36.518
        transverse S36.511
      contusion S36.529
        ascending (right) S36.520
        descending (left) S36.522
        rectum S36.62
        sigmoid S36.523
        specified site NEC S36.528
        transverse S36.521
      descending (left) S36.502
        blast injury (primary) S36.512
          secondary S36.592
        contusion S36.522
        laceration S36.532
        specified type NEC S36.592
      laceration S36.539
        ascending (right) S36.530
        descending (left) S36.532
        rectum S36.63
        sigmoid S36.533

Injury *(Continued)*
  intestine *(Continued)*
    large *(Continued)*
      laceration *(Continued)*
        specified site NEC S36.538
        transverse S36.531
      rectum S36.60
        blast injury (primary) S36.61
          secondary S36.69
        contusion S36.62
        laceration S36.63
        specified type NEC S36.69
      sigmoid S36.503
        blast injury (primary) S36.513
          secondary S36.593
        contusion S36.523
        laceration S36.533
        specified type NEC S36.593
      specified
        site NEC S36.508
          blast injury (primary) S36.518
            secondary S36.598
          contusion S36.528
          laceration S36.538
          specified type NEC S36.598
        type NEC S36.599
          ascending (right) S36.590
          descending (left) S36.592
          rectum S36.69
          sigmoid S36.593
          specified site NEC S36.598
          transverse S36.591
      transverse S36.501
        blast injury (primary) S36.511
          secondary S36.591
        contusion S36.521
        laceration S36.531
        specified type NEC S36.591
    small S36.409
      blast injury (primary) S36.419
        duodenum S36.410
        secondary S36.499
          duodenum S36.490
          specified site NEC S36.498
        specified site NEC S36.418
      contusion S36.429
        duodenum S36.420
        specified site NEC S36.428
      duodenum S36.400
        blast injury (primary) S36.410
          secondary S36.490
        contusion S36.420
        laceration S36.430
        specified NEC S36.490
      laceration S36.439
        duodenum S36.430
        specified site NEC S36.438
      specified
        site NEC S36.408
        type NEC S36.499
          duodenum S36.490
          specified site NEC S36.498
  intra-abdominal S36.90
    adrenal gland —*see* Injury, adrenal gland
    bladder —*see* Injury, bladder
    colon —*see* Injury, intestine, large
    contusion S36.92
    fallopian tube —*see* Injury, fallopian tube
    gallbladder —*see* Injury, gallbladder
    intestine —*see* Injury, intestine
    kidney —*see* Injury, kidney
    laceration S36.93
    liver —*see* Injury, liver
    ovary —*see* Injury, ovary
    pancreas —*see* Injury, pancreas
    pelvic NOS S37.90
    peritoneum —*see* Injury, intra-abdominal,
      specified, site NEC
    prostate —*see* Injury, prostate
    rectum —*see* Injury, intestine, large,
      rectum

Injury *(Continued)*
  intra-abdominal *(Continued)*
    retroperitoneum —*see* Injury, intra-
      abdominal, specified, site NEC
    seminal vesicle —*see* Injury, pelvis, organ,
      specified site NEC
    small intestine —*see* Injury, intestine, small
    specified
      pelvic S37.90
        specified
          site NEC S37.899
            specified type NEC S37.898
          type NEC S37.99
      site NEC S36.899
        contusion S36.892
        laceration S36.893
        specified type NEC S36.898
      type NEC S36.99
    spleen —*see* Injury, spleen
    stomach —*see* Injury, stomach
    ureter —*see* Injury, ureter
    urethra —*see* Injury, urethra
    uterus —*see* Injury, uterus
    vas deferens —*see* Injury, pelvis, organ,
      specified site NEC
  intracranial (traumatic) S06.9-
    cerebellar hemorrhage, traumatic —*see*
      Injury, intracranial, focal
    cerebral edema, traumatic S06.1X-
      diffuse S06.1X-
      focal S06.1X-
    diffuse (axonal) S06.2X-
    epidural hemorrhage (traumatic) S06.4X-
    focal brain injury S06.30-
      contusion —*see* Contusion, cerebral
      laceration —*see* Laceration, cerebral
    intracerebral hemorrhage, traumatic
      S06.36-
      left side S06.35-
      right side S06.34-
    subarachnoid hemorrhage, traumatic
      S06.6X-
    subdural hemorrhage, traumatic S06.5X-
  intraocular —*see* Injury, eyeball, penetrating
  intrathoracic S27.9
    bronchus S27.409
      bilateral S27.402
      blast injury (primary) S27.419
        bilateral S27.412
        secondary —*see* Injury, intrathoracic,
          bronchus, specified type NEC
        unilateral S27.411
      contusion S27.429
        bilateral S27.422
        unilateral S27.421
      laceration S27.439
        bilateral S27.432
        unilateral S27.431
      specified type NEC S27.499
        bilateral S27.492
        unilateral S27.491
      unilateral S27.401
    diaphragm S27.809
      contusion S27.802
      laceration S27.803
      specified type NEC S27.808
    esophagus (thoracic) S27.819
      contusion S27.812
      laceration S27.813
      specified type NEC S27.818
    heart —*see* Injury, heart
    hemopneumothorax S27.2
    hemothorax S27.1
    lung S27.309
      aspiration J69.0
      bilateral S27.302
      blast injury (primary) S27.319
        bilateral S27.312
        secondary —*see* Injury, intrathoracic,
          lung, specified type NEC
        unilateral S27.311

Injury *(Continued)*
  intrathoracic *(Continued)*
    bronchus *(Continued)*
      contusion S27.329
        bilateral S27.322
        unilateral S27.321
      laceration S27.339
        bilateral S27.332
        unilateral S27.331
      specified type NEC S27.399
        bilateral S27.392
        unilateral S27.391
      unilateral S27.301
    pleura S27.60
      laceration S27.63
      specified type NEC S27.69
    pneumothorax S27.0
    specified organ NEC S27.899
      contusion S27.892
      laceration S27.893
      specified type NEC S27.898
    thoracic duct —*see* Injury, intrathoracic,
      specified organ NEC
    thymus gland —*see* Injury, intrathoracic,
      specified organ NEC
    trachea, thoracic S27.50
      blast (primary) S27.51
      contusion S27.52
      laceration S27.53
      specified type NEC S27.59
  iris —*see* Injury, eye, specified site NEC
    penetrating —*see* Injury, eyeball,
      penetrating
  jaw S09.93
  jejunum —*see* Injury, intestine, small
  joint NOS T14.8
    old or residual —*see* Disorder, joint,
      specified type NEC
  kidney S37.00-
    acute (nontraumatic) N17.9
    contusion —*see* Contusion, kidney
    laceration —*see* Laceration, kidney
    specified NEC S37.09-
  knee S89.9-
    contusion —*see* Contusion, knee
    dislocation —*see* Dislocation, knee
    meniscus (lateral) (medial) —*see* Sprain,
      knee, specified site NEC
    old injury or tear —*see* Derangement,
      knee, meniscus, due to old injury
    open —*see* Wound, open, knee
    specified NEC S89.8-
    sprain —*see* Sprain, knee
    superficial —*see* Injury, superficial, knee
  labium (majus) (minus) S39.94
  labyrinth, ear S09.30-
  lacrimal apparatus, duct, gland, or sac —*see*
    Injury, eye, specified site NEC
  larynx NEC S19.81
  leg (lower) S89.9-
    blood vessel —*see* Injury, blood vessel, leg
    contusion —*see* Contusion, leg
    fracture —*see* Fracture, leg
    muscle —*see* Injury, muscle, leg
    nerve —*see* Injury, nerve, leg
    open —*see* Wound, open, leg
    specified NEC S89.8-
    superficial —*see* Injury, superficial, leg
  lens, eye —*see* Injury, eye, specified site NEC
    penetrating —*see* Injury, eyeball, penetrating
  limb NEC T14.8
  lip S09.93
  liver S36.119
    contusion S36.112
    laceration S36.113
      major (stellate) S36.116
      minor S36.114
      moderate S36.115
    specified NEC S36.118
  lower back S39.92
    specified NEC S39.82

◄ New   ⬱ Revised   ~~deleted~~ Deleted

Injury (Continued)
lumbar, lumbosacral (region) S39.92
  plexus —see Injury, lumbosacral plexus
lumbosacral plexus S34.4
lung —see also Injury, intrathoracic, lung
  aspiration J69.0
  transfusion-related (TRALI) J95.84
lymphatic thoracic duct —see Injury,
  intrathoracic, specified organ NEC
malar region S09.93
mastoid region S09.90
maxilla S09.93
mediastinum —see Injury, intrathoracic,
  specified organ NEC
membrane, brain —see Injury, intracranial
meningeal artery —see Injury, intracranial,
  subdural hemorrhage
meninges (cerebral) —see Injury, intracranial
mesenteric
  artery
    branch S35.299
      laceration (minor) (superficial) S35.291
        major S35.292
        specified NEC S35.298
    inferior S35.239
      laceration (minor) (superficial) S35.231
        major S35.232
        specified NEC S35.238
    superior S35.229
      laceration (minor) (superficial) S35.221
        major S35.222
        specified NEC S35.228
    plexus (inferior) (superior) —see Injury,
      nerve, lumbosacral, sympathetic
  vein
    inferior S35.349
      laceration S35.341
      specified NEC S35.348
    superior S35.339
      laceration S35.331
      specified NEC S35.338
mesentery —see Injury, intra-abdominal,
  specified site NEC
mesosalpinx —see Injury, pelvic organ,
  specified site NEC
middle ear S09.30-
midthoracic region NOS S29.9
mouth S09.93
multiple NOS T07
muscle (and fascia) (and tendon)
  abdomen S39.001
    laceration S39.021
    specified type NEC S39.091
    strain S39.011
  abductor
    thumb, forearm level —see Injury,
      muscle, thumb, abductor
  adductor
    thigh S76.20-
      laceration S76.22-
      specified type NEC S76.29-
      strain S76.21-
  ankle —see Injury, muscle, foot
  anterior muscle group, at leg level (lower)
    S86.20-
    laceration S86.22-
    specified type NEC S86.29-
    strain S86.21-
  arm (upper) —see Injury, muscle,
    shoulder
  biceps (parts NEC) S46.20-
    laceration S46.22-
    long head S46.10-
      laceration S46.12-
      specified type NEC S46.19-
      strain S46.11-
    specified type NEC S46.29-
    strain S46.21-
  extensor
    finger (s) (other than thumb) —see Injury,
      muscle, finger by site, extensor

Injury (Continued)
  muscle (Continued)
    extensor (Continued)
      forearm level, specified NEC —see
        Injury, muscle, forearm, extensor
      thumb —see Injury, muscle, thumb,
        extensor
      toe (large) (ankle level) (foot level) —see
        Injury, muscle, toe, extensor
    finger
      extensor (forearm level) S56.40-
        hand level S66.309
          laceration S66.329
          specified type NEC S66.399
          strain S66.319
        laceration S56.429
        specified type NEC S56.499
        strain S56.419
      flexor (forearm level) S56.10-
        hand level S66.109
          laceration S66.129
          specified type NEC S66.199
          strain S66.119
        laceration S56.129
        specified type NEC S56.199
        strain S56.119
      index
        extensor (forearm level)
          hand level S66.308
            laceration S66.32-
            specified type NEC S66.39-
            strain S66.31-
          specified type NEC S56.492-
        flexor (forearm level)
          hand level S66.108
            laceration S66.12-
            specified type NEC
              S66.19-
            strain S66.11-
          specified type NEC S56.19-
          strain S56.11-
        intrinsic S66.50-
          laceration S66.52-
          specified type NEC S66.59-
          strain S66.51-
      intrinsic S66.509
        laceration S66.529
        specified type NEC S66.599
        strain S66.519
      little
        extensor (forearm level)
          hand level S66.30-
            laceration S66.32-
            specified type NEC S66.39-
            strain S66.31-
          laceration S56.42-
          specified type NEC S56.49-
          strain S56.41-
        flexor (forearm level)
          hand level S66.10-
            laceration S66.12-
            specified type NEC S66.19-
            strain S66.11-
          laceration S56.12-
          specified type NEC S56.19-
          strain S56.11-
        intrinsic S66.50-
          laceration S66.52-
          specified type NEC S66.59-
          strain S66.51-
      middle
        extensor (forearm level)
          hand level S66.30-
            laceration S66.32-
            specified type NEC
              S66.39-
            strain S66.31-
          laceration S56.42-
          specified type NEC
           S56.49-
          strain S56.41-

Injury (Continued)
  muscle (Continued)
    finger (Continued)
      middle (Continued)
        flexor (forearm level)
          hand level S66.10-
            laceration S66.12-
            specified type NEC
              S66.19-
            strain S66.11-
          laceration S56.12-
          specified type NEC S56.19-
          strain S56.11-
        intrinsic S66.50-
          laceration S66.52-
          specified type NEC S66.59-
          strain S66.51-
      ring
        extensor (forearm level)
          hand level S66.30-
            laceration S66.32-
            specified type NEC S66.39-
            strain S66.31-
          laceration S56.42-
          specified type NEC S56.49-
          strain S56.41-
        flexor (forearm level)
          hand level S66.10-
            laceration S66.12-
            specified type NEC S66.19-
            strain S66.11-
          laceration S56.12-
          specified type NEC S56.19-
          strain S56.11-
        intrinsic S66.50-
          laceration S66.52-
          specified type NEC S66.59-
          strain S66.51-
    flexor
      finger(s) (other than thumb) — see Injury,
        muscle, finger
      forearm level, specified NEC — see
        Injury, muscle, forearm, flexor
      thumb —see Injury, muscle, thumb,
        flexor
      toe (long) (ankle level) (foot level) —see
        Injury, muscle, toe, flexor
    foot S96.90-
      intrinsic S96.20-
        laceration S96.22-
        specified type NEC S96.29-
        strain S96.21-
      laceration S96.92-
      long extensor, toe —see Injury, muscle,
        toe, extensor
      long flexor, toe —see Injury, muscle, toe,
        flexor
      specified
        site NEC S96.80-
          laceration S96.82-
          specified type NEC
           S96.89-
          strain S96.81-
        type NEC S96.99-
      strain S96.91-
    forearm (level) S56.90-
      extensor S56.50-
        laceration S56.52-
        specified type NEC S56.59-
        strain S56.51-
      flexor S56.20-
        laceration S56.22-
        specified type NEC S56.29-
        strain S56.21-
      laceration S56.92-
      specified S56.99-
        site NEC S56.80-
          laceration S56.82-
          strain S56.81-
        type NEC S56.89-
      strain S56.91-

Injury *(Continued)*
  muscle *(Continued)*
    hand (level) S66.9Ø-
      laceration S66.92-
      specified
        site NEC S66.8Ø-
          laceration S66.82-
          specified type NEC S66.89-
          strain S66.81-
        type NEC S66.99-
      strain S66.91-
    head S09.1Ø
      laceration S09.12
      specified type NEC S09.19
      strain S09.11
    hip NEC S76.ØØ-
      laceration S76.Ø2-
      specified type NEC S76.Ø9-
      strain S76.Ø1-
    intrinsic
      ankle and foot level —*see* Injury, muscle,
        foot, intrinsic
      finger (other than thumb) —*see* Injury,
        muscle, finger by site, intrinsic
      foot (level) —*see* Injury, muscle, foot,
        intrinsic
      thumb —*see* Injury, muscle, thumb,
        intrinsic
    leg (level) (lower) S86.9Ø-
      Achilles tendon —*see* Injury, Achilles
        tendon
      anterior muscle group —*see* Injury,
        muscle, anterior muscle
        group
      laceration S86.92-
      peroneal muscle group —*see* Injury,
        muscle, peroneal muscle group
      posterior muscle group —*see* Injury,
        muscle, posterior muscle group,
        leg level
      specified
        site NEC S86.8Ø-
          laceration S86.82-
          specified type NEC
            S86.89-
          strain S86.81-
        type NEC S86.99-
      strain S86.91-
    long
      extensor toe, at ankle and foot level —*see*
        Injury, muscle, toe, extensor
      flexor, toe, at ankle and foot level —*see*
        Injury, muscle, toe, flexor
      head, biceps —*see* Injury, muscle, biceps,
        long head
    lower back S39.ØØ2
      laceration S39.Ø22
      specified type NEC S39.Ø92
      strain S39.Ø12
    neck (level) S16.9
      laceration S16.2
      specified type NEC S16.8
      strain S16.1
    pelvis S39.ØØ3
      laceration S39.Ø23
      specified type NEC S39.Ø93
      strain S39.Ø13
    peroneal muscle group, at leg level (lower)
      S86.3Ø-
      laceration S86.32-
      specified type NEC S86.39-
      strain S86.31-
    posterior muscle (group)
      leg level (lower) S86.1Ø-
        laceration S86.12-
        specified type NEC S86.19-
        strain S86.11-
      thigh level S76.3Ø-
        laceration S76.32-
        specified type NEC S76.39-
        strain S76.31-

Injury *(Continued)*
  muscle *(Continued)*
    quadriceps (thigh) S76.1Ø-
      laceration S76.12-
      specified type NEC S76.19-
      strain S76.11-
    shoulder S46.9Ø-
      laceration S46.92-
      rotator cuff —*see* Injury, rotator cuff
      specified site NEC S46.8Ø-
        laceration S46.82-
        specified type NEC S46.89-
        strain S46.81-
      specified type NEC S46.99-
      strain S46.91-
    thigh NEC (level) S76.9Ø-
      adductor —*see* Injury, muscle, adductor,
        thigh
      laceration S76.92-
      posterior muscle (group) —*see* Injury,
        muscle, posterior muscle, thigh
        level
      quadriceps —*see* Injury, muscle,
        quadriceps
      specified
        site NEC S76.8Ø-
          laceration S76.82-
          specified type NEC S76.89-
          strain S76.81-
        type NEC S76.99-
      strain S76.91-
    thorax (level) S29.ØØ9
      back wall S29.ØØ2
      front wall S29.ØØ1
      laceration S29.Ø29
        back wall S29.Ø22
        front wall S29.Ø21
      specified type NEC S29.Ø99
        back wall S29.Ø92
        front wall S29.Ø91
      strain S29.Ø19
        back wall S29.Ø12
        front wall S29.Ø11
    thumb
      abductor (forearm level) S56.3Ø-
        laceration S56.32-
        specified type NEC S56.39-
        strain S56.31-
      extensor (forearm level) S56.3Ø-
        hand level S66.2Ø-
          laceration S66.22-
          specified type NEC S66.29-
          strain S66.21-
        laceration S56.32-
        specified type NEC S56.39-
        strain S56.31-
      flexor (forearm level) S56.ØØ-
        hand level S66.ØØ-
          laceration S66.Ø2-
          specified type NEC S66.Ø9-
          strain S66.Ø1-
        laceration S56.Ø2-
        specified type NEC S56.Ø9-
        strain S56.Ø1-
        wrist level —*see* Injury, muscle,
          thumb, flexor, hand level
      intrinsic S66.4Ø-
        laceration S66.42-
        specified type NEC S66.49-
        strain S66.41-
    toe —*see also* Injury, muscle, foot
      extensor, long S96.1Ø-
        laceration S96.12-
        specified type NEC
          S96.19-
        strain S96.11-
      flexor, long S96.ØØ-
        laceration S96.Ø2-
        specified type NEC
          S96.Ø9-
        strain S96.Ø1-

Injury *(Continued)*
  muscle *(Continued)*
    triceps S46.3Ø-
      laceration S46.32-
      specified type NEC S46.39-
      strain S46.31-
    wrist (and hand) level —*see* Injury, muscle,
      hand
  musculocutaneous nerve —*see* Injury, nerve,
    musculocutaneous
  myocardium —*see* Injury, heart
  nape —*see* Injury, neck
  nasal (septum) (sinus) S09.92
  nasopharynx S09.92
  neck S19.9
    specified NEC S19.8Ø
      specified site NEC S19.89
  nerve NEC T14.8
    abdomen S34.9
      peripheral S34.6
      specified site NEC S34.8
    abducens S04.4-
      contusion S04.4-
      laceration S04.4-
      specified type NEC S04.4-
    abducent —*see* Injury, nerve,
      abducens
    accessory S04.7-
      contusion S04.7-
      laceration S04.7-
      specified type NEC S04.7-
    acoustic S04.6-
      contusion S04.6-
      laceration S04.6-
      specified type NEC S04.6-
    ankle S94.9-
      cutaneous sensory S94.3-
      specified site NEC —*see* subcategory S94.8
    anterior crural, femoral —*see* Injury, nerve,
      femoral
    arm (upper) S44.9-
      axillary —*see* Injury, nerve, axillary
      cutaneous —*see* Injury, nerve, cutaneous,
        arm
      median —*see* Injury, nerve, median,
        upper arm
      musculocutaneous —*see* Injury, nerve,
        musculocutaneous
      radial —*see* Injury, nerve, radial, upper
        arm
      specified site NEC —*see* subcategory
        S44.8
      ulnar —*see* Injury, nerve, ulnar, arm
    auditory —*see* Injury, nerve, acoustic
    axillary S44.3-
    brachial plexus —*see* Injury, brachial plexus
    cervical sympathetic S14.5
    cranial S04.9
      contusion S04.9
      eighth (acoustic or auditory) —*see* Injury,
        nerve, acoustic
      eleventh (accessory) —*see* Injury, nerve,
        accessory
      fifth (trigeminal) —*see* Injury, nerve,
        trigeminal
      first (olfactory) —*see* Injury, nerve,
        olfactory
      fourth (trochlear) —*see* Injury, nerve,
        trochlear
      laceration S04.9
      ninth (glossopharyngeal) —*see* Injury,
        nerve, glossopharyngeal
      second (optic) —*see* Injury, nerve, optic
      seventh (facial) —*see* Injury, nerve, facial
      sixth (abducent) —*see* Injury, nerve,
        abducens
      specified
        nerve NEC S04.89-
          contusion S04.89-
          laceration S04.89-
          specified type NEC S04.89-
        type NEC S04.9

◀ New   ◀||| Revised   ~~deleted~~ Deleted

Injury (Continued)
nerve NEC (Continued)
cranial (Continued)
tenth (pneumogastric or vagus) —see Injury, nerve, vagus
third (oculomotor) —see Injury, nerve, oculomotor
twelfth (hypoglossal) —see Injury, nerve, hypoglossal
cutaneous sensory
ankle (level) S94.3-
arm (upper) (level) S44.5-
foot (level) —see Injury, nerve, cutaneous sensory, ankle
forearm (level) S54.3-
hip (level) S74.2-
leg (lower level) S84.2-
shoulder (level) —see Injury, nerve, cutaneous sensory, arm
thigh (level) —see Injury, nerve, cutaneous sensory, hip
deep peroneal —see Injury, nerve, peroneal, foot
digital
finger S64.4-
index S64.49-
little S64.49-
middle S64.49-
ring S64.49-
thumb S64.3-
toe —see Injury, nerve, ankle, specified site NEC
eighth cranial (acoustic or auditory) —see Injury, nerve, acoustic
eleventh cranial (accessory) —see Injury, nerve, accessory
facial S04.5-
contusion S04.5-
laceration S04.5-
newborn P11.3
specified type NEC S04.5-
femoral (hip level) (thigh level) S74.1-
fifth cranial (trigeminal) —see Injury, nerve, trigeminal
finger (digital) —see Injury, nerve, digital, finger
first cranial (olfactory) —see Injury, nerve, olfactory
foot S94.9-
cutaneous sensory S94.3-
deep peroneal S94.2-
lateral plantar S94.0-
medial plantar S94.1-
specified site NEC —see subcategory S94.8
forearm (level) S54.9-
cutaneous sensory —see Injury, nerve, cutaneous sensory, forearm
median —see Injury, nerve, median
radial —see Injury, nerve, radial
specified site NEC —see subcategory S54.8
ulnar —see Injury, nerve, ulnar
fourth cranial (trochlear) —see Injury, nerve, trochlear
glossopharyngeal S04.89-
specified type NEC S04.89-
hand S64.9-
median —see Injury, nerve, median, hand
radial —see Injury, nerve, radial, hand
specified NEC —see subcategory S64.8
ulnar —see Injury, nerve, ulnar, hand
hip (level) S74.9-
cutaneous sensory —see Injury, nerve, cutaneous sensory, hip
femoral —see Injury, nerve, femoral
sciatic —see Injury, nerve, sciatic
specified site NEC —see subcategory S74.8

Injury (Continued)
nerve NEC (Continued)
hypoglossal S04.89-
specified type NEC S04.89-
lateral plantar S94.0-
leg (lower) S84.9-
cutaneous sensory —see Injury, nerve, cutaneous sensory, leg
peroneal —see Injury, nerve, peroneal
specified site NEC —see subcategory S84.8
tibial —see Injury, nerve, tibial
upper —see Injury, nerve, thigh
lower
back —see Injury, nerve, abdomen, specified site NEC
peripheral —see Injury, nerve, abdomen, peripheral
limb —see Injury, nerve, leg
lumbar plexus —see Injury, nerve, lumbosacral, sympathetic
lumbar spinal —see Injury, nerve, spinal, lumbar
lumbosacral
plexus —see Injury, nerve, lumbosacral, sympathetic
sympathetic S34.5
medial plantar S94.1-
median (forearm level) S54.1-
hand (level) S64.1-
upper arm (level) S44.1-
wrist (level) —see Injury, nerve, median, hand
musculocutaneous S44.4-
musculospiral (upper arm level) —see Injury, nerve, radial, upper arm
neck S14.9
peripheral S14.4
specified site NEC S14.8
sympathetic S14.5
ninth cranial (glossopharyngeal) —see Injury, nerve, glossopharyngeal
oculomotor S04.1-
contusion S04.1-
laceration S04.1-
specified type NEC S04.1-
olfactory S04.81-
specified type NEC S04.81-
optic S04.01-
contusion S04.01-
laceration S04.01-
specified type NEC S04.01-
pelvic girdle —see Injury, nerve, hip
pelvis —see Injury, nerve, abdomen, specified site NEC
peripheral —see Injury, nerve, abdomen, peripheral
peripheral NEC T14.8
abdomen —see Injury, nerve, abdomen, peripheral
lower back —see Injury, nerve, abdomen, peripheral
neck —see Injury, nerve, neck, peripheral
pelvis —see Injury, nerve, abdomen, peripheral
specified NEC T14.8
peroneal (lower leg level) S84.1-
foot S94.2-
plexus
brachial —see Injury, brachial plexus
celiac, coeliac —see Injury, nerve, lumbosacral, sympathetic
mesenteric, inferior —see Injury, nerve, lumbosacral, sympathetic
sacral —see Injury, lumbosacral plexus
spinal
brachial —see Injury, brachial plexus
lumbosacral —see Injury, lumbosacral plexus

Injury (Continued)
nerve NEC (Continued)
pneumogastric —see Injury, nerve, vagus
radial (forearm level) S54.2-
hand (level) S64.2-
upper arm (level) S44.2-
wrist (level) —see Injury, nerve, radial, hand
root —see Injury, nerve, spinal, root
sacral plexus —see Injury, lumbosacral plexus
sacral spinal —see Injury, nerve, spinal, sacral
sciatic (hip level) (thigh level) S74.0-
second cranial (optic) —see Injury, nerve, optic
seventh cranial (facial) —see Injury, nerve, facial
shoulder —see Injury, nerve, arm
sixth cranial (abducent) —see Injury, nerve, abducens
spinal
plexus —see Injury, nerve, plexus, spinal
root
cervical S14.2
dorsal S24.2
lumbar S34.21
sacral S34.22
thoracic —see Injury, nerve, spinal, root, dorsal
splanchnic —see Injury, nerve, lumbosacral, sympathetic
sympathetic NEC —see Injury, nerve, lumbosacral, sympathetic
cervical —see Injury, nerve, cervical sympathetic
tenth cranial (pneumogastric or vagus) —see Injury, nerve, vagus
thigh (level) —see Injury, nerve, hip
cutaneous sensory —see Injury, nerve, cutaneous sensory, hip
femoral —see Injury, nerve, femoral
sciatic —see Injury, nerve, sciatic
specified NEC —see Injury, nerve, hip
third cranial (oculomotor) —see Injury, nerve, oculomotor
thorax S24.9
peripheral S24.3
specified site NEC S24.8
sympathetic S24.4
thumb, digital —see Injury, nerve, digital, thumb
tibial (lower leg level) (posterior) S84.0-
toe —see Injury, nerve, ankle
trigeminal S04.3-
contusion S04.3-
laceration S04.3-
specified type NEC S04.3-
trochlear S04.2-
contusion S04.2-
laceration S04.2-
specified type NEC S04.2-
twelfth cranial (hypoglossal) —see Injury, nerve, hypoglossal
ulnar (forearm level) S54.0-
arm (upper) (level) S44.0-
hand (level) S64.0-
wrist (level) —see Injury, nerve, ulnar, hand
vagus S04.89-
specified type NEC S04.89-
wrist (level) —see Injury, nerve, hand
ninth cranial nerve (glossopharyngeal) —see Injury, nerve, glossopharyngeal
nose (septum) S09.92
obstetrical O71.9
specified NEC O71.89
occipital (region) (scalp) S09.90
lobe —see Injury, intracranial
optic chiasm S04.02
optic radiation S04.03-

Injury *(Continued)*
  optic tract and pathways S04.03-
  orbit, orbital (region) —*see* Injury, eye
    penetrating (with foreign body) —*see*
        Injury, eye, orbit, penetrating
    specified NEC —*see* Injury, eye, specified
        site NEC
  ovary, ovarian S37.409
    bilateral S37.402
      contusion S37.422
      laceration S37.432
      specified type NEC S37.492
    blood vessel —*see* Injury, blood vessel,
        ovarian
    contusion S37.429
      bilateral S37.422
      unilateral S37.421
    laceration S37.439
      bilateral S37.432
      unilateral S37.431
    specified type NEC S37.499
      bilateral S37.492
      unilateral S37.491
    unilateral S37.401
      contusion S37.421
      laceration S37.431
      specified type NEC S37.491
  palate (hard) (soft) S09.93
  pancreas S36.209
    body S36.201
      contusion S36.221
      laceration S36.231
        major S36.261
        minor S36.241
        moderate S36.251
      specified type NEC S36.291
    contusion S36.229
    head S36.200
      contusion S36.220
      laceration S36.230
        major S36.260
        minor S36.240
        moderate S36.250
      specified type NEC S36.290
    laceration S36.239
      major S36.269
      minor S36.249
      moderate S36.259
    specified type NEC S36.299
    tail S36.202
      contusion S36.222
      laceration S36.232
        major S36.262
        minor S36.242
        moderate S36.252
      specified type NEC S36.292
  parietal (region) (scalp) S09.90
    lobe —*see* Injury, intracranial
  patellar ligament (tendon) S76.10-
    laceration S76.12-
    specified NEC S76.19-
    strain S76.11-
  pelvis, pelvic (floor) S39.93
    complicating delivery O70.1
    joint or ligament, complicating delivery
        O71.6
    organ S37.90
      with ectopic or molar pregnancy O08.6
      complication of abortion —*see* Abortion
      contusion S37.92
      following ectopic or molar pregnancy
          O08.6
      laceration S37.93
      obstetrical trauma NEC O71.5
      specified
        site NEC S37.899
          contusion S37.892
          laceration S37.893
          specified type NEC S37.898
        type NEC S37.99
    specified NEC S39.83

Injury *(Continued)*
  penis S39.94
  perineum S39.94
  peritoneum S36.81
    laceration S36.893
  periurethral tissue —*see* Injury, urethra
    complicating delivery O71.82
  phalanges
    foot —*see* Injury, foot
    hand —*see* Injury, hand
  pharynx NEC S19.85
  pleura —*see* Injury, intrathoracic, pleura
  plexus
    brachial —*see* Injury, brachial plexus
    cardiac —*see* Injury, nerve, thorax,
        sympathetic
    celiac, coeliac —*see* Injury, nerve,
        lumbosacral, sympathetic
    esophageal —*see* Injury, nerve, thorax,
        sympathetic
    hypogastric —*see* Injury, nerve,
        lumbosacral, sympathetic
    lumbar, lumbosacral —*see* Injury,
        lumbosacral plexus
    mesenteric —*see* Injury, nerve, lumbosacral,
        sympathetic
    pulmonary —*see* Injury, nerve, thorax,
        sympathetic
  postcardiac surgery (syndrome) I97.0
  prepuce S39.94
  prostate S37.829
    contusion S37.822
    laceration S37.823
    specified type NEC S37.828
  pubic region S39.94
  pudendum S39.94
  pulmonary plexus —*see* Injury, nerve, thorax,
      sympathetic
  rectovaginal septum NEC S39.83
  rectum —*see* Injury, intestine, large, rectum
  retina —*see* Injury, eye, specified site NEC
    penetrating —*see* Injury, eyeball,
        penetrating
  retroperitoneal —*see* Injury, intra-abdominal,
      specified site NEC
  rotator cuff (muscle (s)) (tendon (s)) S46.00-
    laceration S46.02-
    specified type NEC S46.09-
    strain S46.01-
  round ligament —*see* Injury, pelvic organ,
      specified site NEC
  sacral plexus —*see* Injury, lumbosacral
      plexus
  salivary duct or gland S09.93
  scalp S09.90
    newborn (birth injury) P12.9
      due to monitoring (electrode) (sampling
          incision) P12.4
      specified NEC P12.89
        caput succedaneum P12.81
  scapular region —*see* Injury, shoulder
  sclera —*see* Injury, eye, specified site NEC
    penetrating —*see* Injury, eyeball,
        penetrating
  scrotum S39.94
  second cranial nerve (optic) —*see* Injury,
      nerve, optic
  seminal vesicle —*see* Injury, pelvic organ,
      specified site NEC
  seventh cranial nerve (facial) —*see* Injury,
      nerve, facial
  shoulder S49.9-
    blood vessel —*see* Injury, blood vessel,
        arm
    contusion —*see* Contusion, shoulder
    dislocation —*see* Dislocation, shoulder
    fracture —*see* Fracture, shoulder
    muscle —*see* Injury, muscle, shoulder
    nerve —*see* Injury, nerve, shoulder
    open —*see* Wound, open, shoulder
    specified type NEC S49.8-

Injury *(Continued)*
  shoulder *(Continued)*
    sprain —*see* Sprain, shoulder girdle
    superficial —*see* Injury, superficial,
        shoulder
  sinus
    cavernous —*see* Injury, intracranial
    nasal S09.92
  sixth cranial nerve (abducent) —*see* Injury,
      nerve, abducens
  skeleton, birth injury P13.9
    specified part NEC P13.8
  skin NEC T14.8
    surface intact —*see* Injury, superficial
  skull NEC S09.90
  specified NEC T14.8
  spermatic cord (pelvic region) S37.898
    scrotal region S39.848
  spinal (cord)
    cervical (neck) S14.109
      anterior cord syndrome S14.139
        C1 level S14.131
        C2 level S14.132
        C3 level S14.133
        C4 level S14.134
        C5 level S14.135
        C6 level S14.136
        C7 level S14.137
        C8 level S14.138
      Brown-Séquard syndrome S14.149
        C1 level S14.141
        C2 level S14.142
        C3 level S14.143
        C4 level S14.144
        C5 level S14.145
        C6 level S14.146
        C7 level S14.147
        C8 level S14.148
      C1 level S14.101
      C2 level S14.102
      C3 level S14.103
      C4 level S14.104
      C5 level S14.105
      C6 level S14.106
      C7 level S14.107
      C8 level S14.108
      central cord syndrome S14.129
        C1 level S14.121
        C2 level S14.122
        C3 level S14.123
        C4 level S14.124
        C5 level S14.125
        C6 level S14.126
        C7 level S14.127
        C8 level S14.128
      complete lesion S14.119
        C1 level S14.111
        C2 level S14.112
        C3 level S14.113
        C4 level S14.114
        C5 level S14.115
        C6 level S14.116
        C7 level S14.117
        C8 level S14.118
      concussion S14.0
      edema S14.0
      incomplete lesion specified NEC S14.159
        C1 level S14.151
        C2 level S14.152
        C3 level S14.153
        C4 level S14.154
        C5 level S14.155
        C6 level S14.156
        C7 level S14.157
        C8 level S14.158
      posterior cord syndrome S14.159
        C1 level S14.151
        C2 level S14.152
        C3 level S14.153
        C4 level S14.154
        C5 level S14.155

◀ New   ◀▦ Revised   ~~deleted~~ Deleted

Injury *(Continued)*
  spinal *(Continued)*
    cervical *(Continued)*
      posterior cord syndrome *(Continued)*
        C6 level S14.156
        C7 level S14.157
        C8 level S14.158
      dorsal —*see* Injury, spinal, thoracic
      lumbar S34.109
        complete lesion S34.119
          L1 level S34.111
          L2 level S34.112
          L3 level S34.113
          L4 level S34.114
          L5 level S34.115
        concussion S34.01
        edema S34.01
        incomplete lesion S34.129
          L1 level S34.121
          L2 level S34.122
          L3 level S34.123
          L4 level S34.124
          L5 level S34.125
        L1 level S34.101
        L2 level S34.102
        L3 level S34.103
        L4 level S34.104
        L5 level S34.105
      nerve root NEC
        cervical —*see* Injury, nerve, spinal, root,
          cervical
        dorsal —*see* Injury, nerve, spinal, root,
          dorsal
        lumbar S34.21
        sacral S34.22
        thoracic —*see* Injury, nerve, spinal, root,
          dorsal
      plexus
        brachial —*see* Injury, brachial plexus
        lumbosacral —*see* Injury, lumbosacral
          plexus
      sacral S34.139
        complete lesion S34.131
        incomplete lesion S34.132
      thoracic S24.109
        anterior cord syndrome S24.139
          T1 level S24.131
          T2-T6 level S24.132
          T7-T10 level S24.133
          T11-T12 level S24.134
        Brown-Séquard syndrome
          S24.149
          T1 level S24.141
          T2-T6 level S24.142
          T7-T10 level S24.143
          T11-T12 level S24.144
        complete lesion S24.119
          T1 level S24.111
          T2-T6 level S24.112
          T7-T10 level S24.113
          T11-T12 level S24.114
        concussion S24.0
        edema S24.0
        incomplete lesion specified NEC
          S24.159
          T1 level S24.151
          T2-T6 level S24.152
          T7-T10 level S24.153
          T11-T12 level S24.154
        posterior cord syndrome
          S24.159
          T1 level S24.151
          T2-T6 level S24.152
          T7-T10 level S24.153
          T11-T12 level S24.154
        T1 level S24.101
        T2-T6 level S24.102
        T7-T10 level S24.103
        T11-T12 level S24.104
    splanchnic nerve —*see* Injury, nerve,
      lumbosacral, sympathetic

Injury *(Continued)*
  spleen S36.00
    contusion S36.029
      major S36.021
      minor S36.020
    laceration S36.039
      major (massive) (stellate) S36.032
      moderate S36.031
      superficial (capsular) (minor) S36.030
    specified type NEC S36.09
  splenic artery —*see* Injury, blood vessel, celiac
    artery, branch
  stellate ganglion —*see* Injury, nerve, thorax,
    sympathetic
  sternal region S29.9
  stomach S36.30
    contusion S36.32
    laceration S36.33
    specified type NEC S36.39
  subconjunctival —*see* Injury, eye, conjunctiva
  subcutaneous NEC T14.8
  submaxillary region S09.93
  submental region S09.93
  subungual
    fingers —*see* Injury, hand
    toes —*see* Injury, foot
  superficial NEC T14.8
    abdomen, abdominal (wall) S30.92
      abrasion S30.811
        bite S30.871
          insect S30.861
        contusion S30.1
        external constriction S30.841
        foreign body S30.851
    abrasion —*see* Abrasion, by site
    adnexa, eye NEC —*see* Injury, eye,
      specified site NEC
    alveolar process —*see* Injury, superficial,
      oral cavity
    ankle S90.91-
      abrasion —*see* Abrasion, ankle
      bite —*see* Bite, ankle
      blister —*see* Blister, ankle
      contusion —*see* Contusion, ankle
      external constriction —*see* Constriction,
        external, ankle
      foreign body —*see* Foreign body,
        superficial, ankle
    anus S30.98
    arm (upper) S40.92-
      abrasion —*see* Abrasion, arm
      bite —*see* Bite, superficial, arm
      blister —*see* Blister, arm (upper)
      contusion —*see* Contusion, arm
      external constriction —*see* Constriction,
        external, arm
      foreign body —*see* Foreign body,
        superficial, arm
    auditory canal (external) (meatus) —*see*
      Injury, superficial, ear
    auricle —*see* Injury, superficial, ear
    axilla —*see* Injury, superficial, arm
    back —*see also* Injury, superficial, thorax,
      back
      lower S30.91
        abrasion S30.810
        contusion S30.0
        external constriction S30.840
        superficial
          bite NEC S30.870
            insect S30.860
          foreign body S30.850
    bite NEC —*see* Bite, superficial NEC, by site
    blister —*see* Blister, by site
    breast S20.10-
      abrasion —*see* Abrasion, breast
      bite —*see* Bite, superficial, breast
      contusion —*see* Contusion, breast
      external constriction —*see* Constriction,
        external, breast
      foreign body —*see* Foreign body,
        superficial, breast

Injury *(Continued)*
  superficial NEC *(Continued)*
    brow —*see* Injury, superficial, head,
      specified NEC
    buttock S30.91
    calf —*see* Injury, superficial, leg
    canthus, eye —*see* Injury, superficial,
      periocular area
    cheek (external) —*see* Injury, superficial,
      head, specified NEC
      internal —*see* Injury, superficial, oral
        cavity
    chest wall —*see* Injury, superficial, thorax
    chin —*see* Injury, superficial, head NEC
    clitoris S30.95
    conjunctiva —*see* Injury, eye, conjunctiva
      with foreign body (in conjunctival
        sac) —*see* Foreign body,
        conjunctival sac
    contusion —*see* Contusion, by site
    costal region —*see* Injury, superficial, thorax
    digit (s)
      hand —*see* Injury, superficial, finger
    ear (auricle) (canal) (external) S00.40-
      abrasion —*see* Abrasion, ear
      bite —*see* Bite, superficial, ear
      contusion —*see* Contusion, ear
      external constriction —*see* Constriction,
        external, ear
      foreign body —*see* Foreign body,
        superficial, ear
    elbow S50.90-
      abrasion —*see* Abrasion, elbow
      bite —*see* Bite, superficial, elbow
      blister —*see* Blister, elbow
      contusion —*see* Contusion, elbow
      external constriction —*see* Constriction,
        external, elbow
      foreign body —*see* Foreign body,
        superficial, elbow
    epididymis S30.94
    epigastric region S30.92
    epiglottis —*see* Injury, superficial, throat
    esophagus
      cervical —*see* Injury, superficial, throat
    external constriction —*see* Constriction,
      external, by site
    extremity NEC T14.8
    eyeball NEC —*see* Injury, eye, specified
      site NEC
    eyebrow —*see* Injury, superficial,
      periocular area
    eyelid S00.20-
      abrasion —*see* Abrasion, eyelid
      bite —*see* Bite, superficial, eyelid
      contusion —*see* Contusion, eyelid
      external constriction —*see* Constriction,
        external, eyelid
      foreign body —*see* Foreign body,
        superficial, eyelid
    face NEC —*see* Injury, superficial, head,
      specified NEC
    finger (s) S60.949
      abrasion —*see* Abrasion, finger
      bite —*see* Bite, superficial, finger
      blister —*see* Blister, finger
      contusion —*see* Contusion, finger
      external constriction —*see* Constriction,
        external, finger
      foreign body —*see* Foreign body,
        superficial, finger
      index S60.94-
      insect bite —*see* Bite, by site, superficial,
        insect
      little S60.94-
      middle S60.94-
      ring S60.94-
    flank S30.92
    foot S90.92-
      abrasion —*see* Abrasion, foot
      bite —*see* Bite, foot

Injury (Continued)
  superficial NEC (Continued)
    foot (Continued)
      blister —see Blister, foot
      contusion —see Contusion, foot
      external constriction —see Constriction, external, foot
      foreign body —see Foreign body, superficial, foot
    forearm S50.91-
      abrasion —see Abrasion, forearm
      bite —see Bite, forearm, superficial
      blister —see Blister, forearm
      contusion —see Contusion, forearm
      elbow only —see Injury, superficial, elbow
      external constriction —see Constriction, external, forearm
      foreign body —see Foreign body, superficial, forearm
    forehead —see Injury, superficial, head NEC
    foreign body —see Foreign body, superficial
    genital organs, external
      female S30.97
      male S30.96
    globe (eye) —see Injury, eye, specified site NEC
    groin S30.92
    gum —see Injury, superficial, oral cavity
    hand S60.92-
      abrasion —see Abrasion, hand
      bite —see Bite, superficial, hand
      contusion —see Contusion, hand
      external constriction —see Constriction, external, hand
      foreign body —see Foreign body, superficial, hand
    head S00.90
      ear —see Injury, superficial, ear
      eyelid —see Injury, superficial, eyelid
      nose S00.30
      oral cavity S00.502
      scalp S00.00
      specified site NEC S00.80
    heel —see Injury, superficial, foot
    hip S70.91-
      abrasion —see Abrasion, hip
      bite —see Bite, superficial, hip
      blister —see Blister, hip
      contusion —see Contusion, hip
      external constriction —see Constriction, external, hip
      foreign body —see Foreign body, superficial, hip
    iliac region —see Injury, superficial, abdomen
    inguinal region —see Injury, superficial, abdomen
    insect bite —see Bite, by site, superficial, insect
    interscapular region —see Injury, superficial, thorax, back
    jaw —see Injury, superficial, head, specified NEC
    knee S80.91-
      abrasion —see Abrasion, knee
      bite —see Bite, superficial, knee
      blister —see Blister, knee
      contusion —see Contusion, knee
      external constriction —see Constriction, external, knee
      foreign body —see Foreign body, superficial, knee
    labium (majus) (minus) S30.95
    lacrimal (apparatus) (gland) (sac) —see Injury, eye, specified site NEC
    larynx —see Injury, superficial, throat
    leg (lower) S80.92-
      abrasion —see Abrasion, leg
      bite —see Bite, superficial, leg

Injury (Continued)
  superficial NEC (Continued)
    leg (Continued)
      contusion —see Contusion, leg
      external constriction —see Constriction, external, leg
      foreign body —see Foreign body, superficial, leg
      knee —see Injury, superficial, knee
    limb NEC T14.8
    lip S00.501
    lower back S30.91
    lumbar region S30.91
    malar region —see Injury, superficial, head, specified NEC
    mammary —see Injury, superficial, breast
    mastoid region —see Injury, superficial, head, specified NEC
    mouth —see Injury, superficial, oral cavity
    muscle NEC T14.8
    nail NEC T14.8
      finger —see Injury, superficial, finger
      toe —see Injury, superficial, toe
    nasal (septum) —see Injury, superficial, nose
    neck S10.90
      specified site NEC S10.80
    nose (septum) S00.30
    occipital region —see Injury, superficial, scalp
    oral cavity S00.502
    orbital region —see Injury, superficial, periocular area
    palate —see Injury, superficial, oral cavity
    palm —see Injury, superficial, hand
    parietal region —see Injury, superficial, scalp
    pelvis S30.91
      girdle —see Injury, superficial, hip
    penis S30.93
    perineum
      female S30.95
      male S30.91
    periocular area S00.20-
      abrasion —see Abrasion, eyelid
      bite —see Bite, superficial, eyelid
      contusion —see Contusion, eyelid
      external constriction —see Constriction, external, eyelid
      foreign body —see Foreign body, superficial, eyelid
    phalanges
      finger —see Injury, superficial, finger
      toe —see Injury, superficial, toe
    pharynx —see Injury, superficial, throat
    pinna —see Injury, superficial, ear
    popliteal space —see Injury, superficial, knee
    prepuce S30.93
    pubic region S30.91
    pudendum
      female S30.97
      male S30.96
    sacral region S30.91
    scalp S00.00
    scapular region —see Injury, superficial, shoulder
    sclera —see Injury, eye, specified site NEC
    scrotum S30.94
    shin —see Injury, superficial, leg
    shoulder S40.91-
      abrasion —see Abrasion, shoulder
      bite —see Bite, superficial, shoulder
      blister —see Blister, shoulder
      contusion —see Contusion, shoulder
      external constriction —see Constriction, external, shoulder
      foreign body —see Foreign body, superficial, shoulder

Injury (Continued)
  superficial NEC (Continued)
    skin NEC T14.8
    sternal region —see Injury, superficial, thorax, front
    subconjunctival —see Injury, eye, specified site NEC
    subcutaneous NEC T14.8
    submaxillary region —see Injury, superficial, head, specified NEC
    submental region —see Injury, superficial, head, specified NEC
    subungual
      finger (s) —see Injury, superficial, finger
      toe (s) —see Injury, superficial, toe
    supraclavicular fossa —see Injury, superficial, neck
    supraorbital —see Injury, superficial, head, specified NEC
    temple —see Injury, superficial, head, specified NEC
    temporal region —see Injury, superficial, head, specified NEC
    testis S30.94
    thigh S70.92-
      abrasion —see Abrasion, thigh
      bite —see Bite, superficial, thigh
      blister —see Blister, thigh
      contusion —see Contusion, thigh
      external constriction —see Constriction, external, thigh
      foreign body —see Foreign body, superficial, thigh
    thorax, thoracic (wall) S20.90
      abrasion —see Abrasion, thorax
      back S20.40-
      bite —see Bite, thorax, superficial
      blister —see Blister, thorax
      contusion —see Contusion, thorax
      external constriction —see Constriction, external, thorax
      foreign body —see Foreign body, superficial, thorax
      front S20.30-
    throat S10.10
      abrasion S10.11
      bite S10.17
        insect S10.16
      blister S10.12
      contusion S10.0
      external constriction S10.14
      foreign body S10.15
    thumb S60.93-
      abrasion —see Abrasion, thumb
      bite —see Bite, superficial, thumb
      blister —see Blister, thumb
      contusion —see Contusion, thumb
      external constriction —see Constriction, external, thumb
      foreign body —see Foreign body, superficial, thumb
      insect bite —see Bite, by site, superficial, insect
      specified type NEC S60.39-
    toe (s) S90.93-
      abrasion —see Abrasion, toe
      bite —see Bite, toe
      blister —see Blister, toe
      contusion —see Contusion, toe
      external constriction —see Constriction, external, toe
      foreign body —see Foreign body, superficial, toe
      great S90.93-
    tongue —see Injury, superficial, oral cavity
    tooth, teeth —see Injury, superficial, oral cavity
    trachea S10.10
    tunica vaginalis S30.94
    tympanum, tympanic membrane —see Injury, superficial, ear

◄ New   ◄||||| Revised   ~~deleted~~ Deleted

Injury (Continued)
  superficial NEC (Continued)
    uvula —see Injury, superficial, oral cavity
    vagina S30.95
    vocal cords —see Injury, superficial, throat
    vulva S30.95
    wrist S60.91-
  supraclavicular region —see Injury, neck
  supraorbital S09.93
  suprarenal gland (multiple) —see Injury,
      adrenal
  surgical complication (external or internal
      site) —see Laceration, accidental
      complicating surgery
  temple S09.90
  temporal region S09.90
  tendon —see also Injury, muscle, by site
    abdomen —see Injury, muscle, abdomen
    Achilles —see Injury, Achilles tendon
    lower back —see Injury, muscle, lower back
    pelvic organs —see Injury, muscle, pelvis
  tenth cranial nerve (pneumogastric or
      vagus) —see Injury, nerve, vagus
  testis S39.94
  thigh S79.92-
    blood vessel —see Injury, blood vessel, hip
    contusion —see Contusion, thigh
    fracture —see Fracture, femur
    muscle —see Injury, muscle, thigh
    nerve —see Injury, nerve, thigh
    open —see Wound, open, thigh
    specified NEC S79.82-
    superficial —see Injury, superficial, thigh
  third cranial nerve (oculomotor) —see Injury,
      nerve, oculomotor
  thorax, thoracic S29.9
    blood vessel —see Injury, blood vessel,
        thorax
    cavity —see Injury, intrathoracic
    dislocation —see Dislocation, thorax
    external (wall) S29.9
      contusion —see Contusion, thorax
      nerve —see Injury, nerve, thorax
      open —see Wound, open, thorax
      specified NEC S29.8
      sprain —see Sprain, thorax
      superficial —see Injury, superficial,
          thorax
    fracture —see Fracture, thorax
    internal —see Injury, intrathoracic
    intrathoracic organ —see Injury,
        intrathoracic
    sympathetic ganglion —see Injury, nerve,
        thorax, sympathetic
  throat —see also Injury, neck S19.9
  thumb S69.9-
    blood vessel —see Injury, blood vessel,
        thumb
    contusion —see Contusion, thumb
    dislocation —see Dislocation, thumb
    fracture —see Fracture, thumb
    muscle —see Injury, muscle, thumb
    nerve —see Injury, nerve, digital, thumb
    open —see Wound, open, thumb
    specified NEC S69.8-
    sprain —see Sprain, thumb
    superficial —see Injury, superficial, thumb
  thymus (gland) —see Injury, intrathoracic,
      specified organ NEC
  thyroid (gland) NEC S19.84
  toe S99.92-
    contusion —see Contusion, toe
    dislocation —see Dislocation, toe
    fracture —see Fracture, toe
    muscle —see Injury, muscle, toe
    open —see Wound, open, toe
    specified type NEC S99.82-
    sprain —see Sprain, toe
    superficial —see Injury, superficial, toe
  tongue S09.93
  tonsil S09.93

Injury (Continued)
  tooth S09.93
  trachea (cervical) NEC S19.82
    thoracic —see Injury, intrathoracic, trachea,
        thoracic
  transfusion-related acute lung (TRALI) J95.84
  tunica vaginalis S39.94
  twelfth cranial nerve (hypoglossal) —see
      Injury, nerve, hypoglossal
  ureter S37.10
    contusion S37.12
    laceration S37.13
    specified type NEC S37.19
  urethra (sphincter) S37.30
    at delivery O71.5
    contusion S37.32
    laceration S37.33
    specified type NEC S37.38
  urinary organ S37.899
    contusion S37.92
    laceration S37.93
    specified
      site NEC S37.899
        contusion S37.892
        laceration S37.893
        specified type NEC S37.898
      type NEC S37.99
  uterus, uterine S37.60
    with ectopic or molar pregnancy O08.6
    blood vessel —see Injury, blood vessel, iliac
    contusion S37.62
    laceration S37.63
      cervix at delivery O71.3
    rupture associated with obstetrics —see
        Rupture, uterus
    specified type NEC S37.69
  uvula S09.93
  vagina S39.93
    abrasion S30.814
    bite S31.45
      insect S30.864
      superficial NEC S30.874
    contusion S30.23
    crush S38.03
    during delivery —see Laceration, vagina,
        during delivery
    external constriction S30.844
    insect bite S30.864
    laceration S31.41
      with foreign body S31.42
    open wound S31.40
    puncture S31.43
      with foreign body S31.44
    superficial S30.95
      foreign body S30.854
  vas deferens —see Injury, pelvic organ,
      specified site NEC
  vascular NEC T14.8
  vein —see Injury, blood vessel
  vena cava (superior) S25.20
    inferior S35.10
      laceration (minor) (superficial) S35.11
        major S35.12
      specified type NEC S35.19
    laceration (minor) (superficial) S25.21
      major S25.22
    specified type NEC S25.29
  vesical (sphincter) —see Injury, bladder
  visual cortex S04.04-
  vitreous (humor) S05.90
    specified NEC S05.8X-
  vocal cord NEC S19.83
  vulva S39.94
    abrasion S30.814
    bite S31.45
      insect S30.864
      superficial NEC S30.874
    contusion S30.23
    crush S38.03
    during delivery —see Laceration,
        perineum, female, during delivery

Injury (Continued)
  vulva (Continued)
    external constriction S30.844
    insect bite S30.864
    laceration S31.41
      with foreign body S31.42
    open wound S31.40
    puncture S31.43
      with foreign body S31.44
    superficial S30.95
      foreign body S30.854
  whiplash (cervical spine) S13.4
  wrist S69.9-
    blood vessel —see Injury, blood vessel,
        hand
    contusion —see Contusion, wrist
    dislocation —see Dislocation, wrist
    fracture —see Fracture, wrist
    muscle —see Injury, muscle, hand
    nerve —see Injury, nerve, hand
    open —see Wound, open, wrist
    specified NEC S69.8-
    sprain —see Sprain, wrist
    superficial —see Injury, superficial, wrist
Inoculation —see also Vaccination
  complication or reaction —see Complications,
      vaccination
Insanity, insane —see also Psychosis
  adolescent —see Schizophrenia
  confusional F28
    acute or subacute F05
  delusional F22
  senile F03
Insect
  bite —see Bite, by site, superficial, insect
  venomous, poisoning NEC (by) —see Venom,
      arthropod
Insensitivity
  adrenocorticotropin hormone (ACTH)
      E27.49
  androgen E34.50
    complete E34.51
    partial E34.52
Insertion
  cord (umbilical) lateral or velamentous
      O43.12-
  intrauterine contraceptive device (encounter
      for) —see Intrauterine contraceptive
      device
Insolation (sunstroke) T67.0
Insomnia (organic) G47.00
  without objective findings F51.02
  adjustment F51.02
  adjustment disorder F51.02
  behavioral, of childhood Z73.819
    combined type Z73.812
    limit setting type Z73.811
    sleep-onset association type Z73.810
  childhood Z73.819
  chronic F51.04
    somatized tension F51.04
  conditioned F51.04
  due to
    alcohol
      abuse F10.182
      dependence F10.282
      use F10.982
    amphetamines
      abuse F15.182
      dependence F15.282
      use F15.982
    anxiety disorder F51.05
    caffeine
      abuse F15.182
      dependence F15.282
      use F15.982
    cocaine
      abuse F14.182
      dependence F14.282
      use F14.982
    depression F51.05

Insomnia *(Continued)*
  due to *(Continued)*
    drug NEC
      abuse F19.182
      dependence F19.282
      use F19.982
    medical condition G47.01
    mental disorder NEC F51.05
    opioid
      abuse F11.182
      dependence F11.282
      use F11.982
    psychoactive substance NEC
      abuse F19.182
      dependence F19.282
      use F19.982
    sedative, hypnotic, or anxiolytic
      abuse F13.182
      dependence F13.282
      use F13.982
    stimulant NEC
      abuse F15.182
      dependence F15.282
      use F15.982
  fatal familial (FFI) A81.83
  idiopathic F51.01
  learned F51.3
  nonorganic origin F51.01
  not due to a substance or known
    physiological condition F51.01
    specified NEC F51.09
  paradoxical F51.03
  primary F51.01
  psychiatric F51.05
  psychophysiologic F51.04
  related to psychopathology F51.05
  short-term F51.02
  specified NEC G47.09
  stress-related F51.02
  transient F51.02
Inspiration
  food or foreign body —*see* Foreign body, by
    site
  mucus —*see* Asphyxia, mucus
Inspissated bile syndrome (newborn)
  P59.1
Instability
  emotional (excessive) F60.3
  joint (post-traumatic) M25.30
    ankle M25.37-
    due to old ligament injury —*see* Disorder,
      ligament
    elbow M25.32-
    flail —*see* Flail, joint
    foot M25.37-
    hand M25.34-
    hip M25.35-
    knee M25.36-
    lumbosacral —*see* subcategory M53.2
    prosthesis —*see* Complications, joint
      prosthesis, mechanical, displacement,
      by site
    sacroiliac —*see* subcategory M53.2
    secondary to
      old ligament injury —*see* Disorder,
        ligament
      removal of joint prosthesis M96.89
    shoulder (region) M25.31-
    spine —*see* subcategory M53.2
    wrist M25.33-
  knee (chronic) M23.5-
  lumbosacral —*see* subcategory M53.2
  nervous F48.8
  personality (emotional) F60.3
  spine —*see* Instability, joint, spine
  vasomotor R55
Institutional syndrome (childhood)
  F94.2
Institutionalization, affecting child
  Z62.22
  disinhibited attachment F94.2

Insufficiency, insufficient
  accommodation, old age H52.4
  adrenal (gland) E27.40
    primary E27.1
  adrenocortical E27.40
    drug-induced E27.3
    iatrogenic E27.3
    primary E27.1
  anatomic crown height K08.89 ◄
  anterior (occlusal) guidance M26.54
  anus K62.89
  aortic (valve) I35.1
    with
      mitral (valve) disease I08.0
        with tricuspid (valve) disease I08.3
      stenosis I35.2
      tricuspid (valve) disease I08.2
        with mitral (valve) disease I08.3
    congenital Q23.1
    rheumatic I06.1
      with
        mitral (valve) disease I08.0
          with tricuspid (valve) disease
            I08.3
        stenosis I06.2
          with mitral (valve) disease I08.0
            with tricuspid (valve) disease
              I08.3
        tricuspid (valve) disease I08.2
          with mitral (valve) disease I08.3
    specified cause NEC I35.1
    syphilitic A52.03
  arterial I77.1
    basilar G45.0
    carotid (hemispheric) G45.1
    cerebral I67.81
    coronary (acute or subacute) I24.8
    mesenteric K55.1
    peripheral I73.9
    precerebral (multiple) (bilateral) G45.2
    vertebral G45.0
  arteriovenous I99.8
  biliary K83.8
  cardiac —*see also* Insufficiency, myocardial
    due to presence of (cardiac) prosthesis
      I97.11-
    postprocedural I97.11-
  cardiorenal, hypertensive I13.2
  cardiovascular —*see* Disease, cardiovascular
  cerebrovascular (acute) I67.81
    with transient focal neurological signs and
      symptoms G45.8
  circulatory NEC I99.8
    newborn P29.89
  clinical crown length K08.89 ◄
  convergence H51.11
  coronary (acute or subacute) I24.8
    chronic or with a stated duration of over 4
      weeks I25.89
  corticoadrenal E27.40
    primary E27.1
  dietary E63.9
  divergence H51.8
  food T73.0
  gastroesophageal K22.8
  gonadal
    ovary E28.39
    testis E29.1
  heart —*see also* Insufficiency, myocardial
    newborn P29.0
    valve —*see* Endocarditis
  hepatic —*see* Failure, hepatic
  idiopathic autonomic G90.09
  interocclusal distance of fully erupted teeth
    (ridge) M26.36
  kidney N28.9
    acute N28.9
    chronic N18.9
  lacrimal (secretion) H04.12-
    passages —*see* Stenosis, lacrimal
  liver —*see* Failure, hepatic

Insufficiency, insufficient *(Continued)*
  lung —*see* Insufficiency, pulmonary
  mental (congenital) —*see* Disability,
    intellectual
  mesenteric K55.1
  mitral (valve) I34.0
    with
      aortic valve disease I08.0
        with tricuspid (valve) disease
          I08.3
      obstruction or stenosis I05.2
        with aortic valve disease I08.0
      tricuspid (valve) disease I08.1
        with aortic (valve) disease I08.3
    congenital Q23.3
    rheumatic I05.1
      with
        aortic valve disease I08.0
          with tricuspid (valve) disease I08.3
        obstruction or stenosis I05.2
          with aortic valve disease I08.0
            with tricuspid (valve) disease
              I08.3
        tricuspid (valve) disease I08.1
          with aortic (valve) disease I08.3
      active or acute I01.1
        with chorea, rheumatic (Sydenham's)
          I02.0
    specified cause, except rheumatic
      I34.0
  muscle —*see also* Disease, muscle
    heart —*see* Insufficiency, myocardial
    ocular NEC H50.9
  myocardial, myocardium (with
    arteriosclerosis) I50.9
    with
      rheumatic fever (conditions in I00)
        I09.0
        active, acute or subacute I01.2
          with chorea I02.0
        inactive or quiescent (with chorea)
          I09.0
    congenital Q24.8
    hypertensive —*see* Hypertension, heart
    newborn P29.0
    rheumatic I09.0
      active, acute, or subacute I01.2
    syphilitic A52.06
  nourishment T73.0
  pancreatic K86.89 ◄▥
    exocrine K86.81 ◄
  parathyroid (gland) E20.9
  peripheral vascular (arterial) I73.9
  pituitary E23.0
  placental (mother) O36.51-
  platelets D69.6
  prenatal care affecting management of
    pregnancy O09.3-
  progressive pluriglandular E31.0
  pulmonary J98.4
    acute, following surgery (nonthoracic)
      J95.2
      thoracic J95.1
    chronic, following surgery J95.3
    following
      shock J98.4
      trauma J98.4
    newborn P28.5
    valve I37.1
      with stenosis I37.2
      congenital Q22.2
      rheumatic I09.89
        with aortic, mitral or tricuspid (valve)
          disease I08.8
  pyloric K31.89
  renal (acute) N28.9
    chronic N18.9
  respiratory R06.89
    newborn P28.5
  rotation —*see* Malrotation
  sleep syndrome F51.12

◄ New   ▥ Revised   ~~deleted~~ Deleted

Insufficiency, insufficient (*Continued*)
  social insurance Z59.7
  suprarenal E27.40
    primary E27.1
  tarso-orbital fascia, congenital Q10.3
  testis E29.1
  thyroid (gland) (acquired) E03.9
    congenital E03.1
  tricuspid (valve) (rheumatic) I07.1
    with
      aortic (valve) disease I08.2
        with mitral (valve) disease I08.3
      mitral (valve) disease I08.1
        with aortic (valve) disease I08.3
      obstruction or stenosis I07.2
        with aortic (valve) disease I08.2
          with mitral (valve) disease
            I08.3
    congenital Q22.8
    nonrheumatic I36.1
      with stenosis I36.2
  urethral sphincter R32
  valve, valvular (heart) —*see* Endocarditis
    congenital Q24.8
  vascular I99.8
    intestine K55.9
      acute —*see also* Ischemia, intestine, acute
        K55.059 ◀▦
      mesenteric K55.1
      peripheral I73.9
      renal —*see* Hypertension, kidney
    velopharyngeal
      acquired K13.79
      congenital Q38.8
  venous (chronic) (peripheral) I87.2
  ventricular —*see* Insufficiency, myocardial
  welfare support Z59.7
Insufflation, fallopian Z31.41
Insular —*see* condition
Insulinoma
  pancreas
    benign D13.7
    malignant C25.4
    uncertain behavior D37.8
  specified site
    benign —*see* Neoplasm, by site, benign
    malignant —*see* Neoplasm, by site,
      malignant
    uncertain behavior —*see* Neoplasm, by site,
      uncertain behavior
  unspecified site
    benign D13.7
    malignant C25.4
    uncertain behavior D37.8
Insuloma —*see* Insulinoma
Interference
  balancing side M26.56
  non-working side M26.56
Intermenstrual —*see* condition
Intermittent —*see* condition
Internal —*see* condition
Interrogation
  cardiac defibrillator (automatic) (implantable)
    Z45.02
  cardiac pacemaker Z45.018
  cardiac (event) (loop) recorder Z45.09
  infusion pump (implanted) (intrathecal)
    Z45.1
  neurostimulator Z46.2
Interruption
  aortic arch Q25.21 ◀
  phase-shift, sleep cycle —*see* Disorder, sleep,
    circadian rhythm
  sleep phase-shift, or 24 hour sleep-wake
    cycle —*see* Disorder, sleep, circadian
    rhythm
Interstitial —*see* condition
Intertrigo L30.4
  labialis K13.0
Intervertebral disc —*see* condition
Intestine, intestinal —*see* condition

Intolerance
  carbohydrate K90.49 ◀▦
  disaccharide, hereditary E73.0
  fat NEC K90.49 ◀▦
    pancreatic K90.3
  food K90.49 ◀▦
    dietary counseling and surveillance Z71.3
  fructose E74.10
    hereditary E74.12
  glucose(-galactose) E74.39
  gluten K90.01 ◀▦
  lactose E73.9
    specified NEC E73.8
  lysine E72.3
  milk NEC K90.49 ◀▦
    lactose E73.9
  protein K90.49 ◀▦
  starch NEC K90.49 ◀▦
  sucrose (-isomaltose) E74.31
Intoxicated NEC (without dependence) —*see*
  Alcohol, intoxication
Intoxication
  acid E87.2
  alcoholic (acute) (without dependence) —*see*
    Alcohol, intoxication
  alimentary canal K52.1
  amphetamine (without dependence) —
    see Abuse, drug, stimulant, with
    intoxication
    with dependence —*see* Dependence, drug,
      stimulant, with intoxication
  anxiolytic (acute) (without dependence) —*see*
    Abuse, drug, sedative, with intoxication
    with dependence —*see* Dependence, drug,
      sedative, with intoxication
  caffeine F15.929 ◀▦
    with dependence —*see* Dependence, drug,
      stimulant, with intoxication
  cannabinoids (acute) (without dependence) —
    see Use, cannabis, with intoxication ◀▦
    ~~with dependence —see Dependence, drug,~~
    ~~cannabis, with intoxication~~
    with ◀
      abuse —*see* Abuse, drug, cannabis, with
        intoxication ◀
      dependence —*see* Dependence, drug,
        cannabis, with intoxication ◀
  chemical —*see* Table of Drugs and Chemicals
    via placenta or breast milk —*see* -
      Absorption, chemical, through
      placenta
  cocaine (acute) (without dependence) —*see*
    Abuse, drug, cocaine, with intoxication
    with dependence —*see* Dependence, drug,
      cocaine, with intoxication
  drug
    acute (without dependence) —*see* Abuse,
      drug, by type with intoxication
    with dependence —*see* Dependence,
      drug, by type with intoxication
    addictive
      via placenta or breast milk —*see*
        Absorption, drug, addictive,
        through placenta
    newborn P93.8
      gray baby syndrome P93.0
    overdose or wrong substance given or
      taken —*see* Table of Drugs and
      Chemicals, by drug, poisoning
  enteric K52.1
  foodborne A05.9
    bacterial A05.9
    classical (Clostridium botulinum) A05.1
    due to
      Bacillus cereus A05.4
      bacterium A05.9
        specified NEC A05.8
      Clostridium
        botulinum A05.1
        perfringens A05.2
        welchii A05.2

Intoxication (*Continued*)
  foodborne (*Continued*)
    due to (*Continued*)
      Salmonella A02.9
        with
          (gastro) enteritis A02.0
          localized infection (s) A02.20
            arthritis A02.23
            meningitis A02.21
            osteomyelitis A02.24
            pneumonia A02.22
            pyelonephritis A02.25
            specified NEC A02.29
          sepsis A02.1
          specified manifestation NEC
            A02.8
      Staphylococcus A05.0
      Vibrio
        parahaemolyticus A05.3
        vulnificus A05.5
    enterotoxin, staphylococcal A05.0
    noxious —*see* Poisoning, food, noxious
  gastrointestinal K52.1
  hallucinogenic (without dependence) —*see*
    Abuse, drug, hallucinogen, with
    intoxication
    with dependence —*see* Dependence, drug,
      hallucinogen, with intoxication
  hypnotic (acute) (without dependence) —*see*
    Abuse, drug, sedative, with intoxication
    with dependence —*see* Dependence, drug,
      sedative, with intoxication
  inhalant (acute) (without dependence) —*see*
    Abuse, drug, inhalant, with intoxication
    with dependence —*see* Dependence, drug,
      inhalant, with intoxication
  meaning
    inebriation —*see* category F10
    poisoning —*see* Table of Drugs and
      Chemicals
  methyl alcohol (acute) (without
    dependence) —*see* Alcohol, intoxication
  opioid (acute) (without dependence) —*see*
    Abuse, drug, opioid, with intoxication
    with dependence —*see* Dependence, drug,
      opioid, with intoxication
  pathologic NEC (without dependence) —*see*
    Alcohol, intoxication
  phencyclidine (without dependence) —*see*
    Abuse, drug, hallucinogen, with
    intoxication ◀▦
    with dependence —*see* Dependence, drug,
      hallucinogen, with intoxication ◀▦
  potassium (K) E87.5
  psychoactive substance NEC (without
    dependence) —*see* Abuse, drug,
    psychoactive NEC, with intoxication
    with dependence —*see* Dependence, drug,
      psychoactive NEC, with intoxication
  sedative (acute) (without dependence) —*see*
    Abuse, drug, sedative, with intoxication
    with dependence —*see* Dependence, drug,
      sedative, with intoxication
  serum —*see also* Reaction, serum T80.69
  uremic —*see* Uremia
  volatile solvents (acute) (without
    dependence) —*see* Abuse, drug, inhalant,
    with intoxication
    with dependence —*see* Dependence, drug,
      inhalant, with intoxication
  water E87.79
Intracranial —*see* condition
Intrahepatic gallbladder Q44.1
Intraligamentous —*see* condition
Intrathoracic —*see also* condition
  kidney Q63.2
Intrauterine contraceptive device
  checking Z30.431
  in situ Z97.5
  insertion Z30.430
    immediately following removal Z30.433

Intrauterine contraceptive device (*Continued*)
  management Z30.431
  reinsertion Z30.433
  removal Z30.432
  replacement Z30.433
  retention in pregnancy O26.3-
Intraventricular —*see* condition
Intrinsic deformity —*see* Deformity
Intubation, difficult or failed T88.4
Intumescence, lens (eye) (cataract) —*see* Cataract
Intussusception (bowel) (colon) (enteric) (ileocecal) (ileocolic) (intestine) (rectum) K56.1
  appendix K38.8
  congenital Q43.8
  ureter (with obstruction) N13.5
Invagination (bowel, colon, intestine or rectum) K56.1
Inversion
  albumin-globulin (A-G) ratio E88.09
  bladder N32.89
  cecum —*see* Intussusception
  cervix N88.8
  chromosome in normal individual Q95.1
  circadian rhythm —*see* Disorder, sleep, circadian rhythm
  nipple N64.59
    congenital Q83.8
    gestational —*see* Retraction, nipple
    puerperal, postpartum —*see* Retraction, nipple
  nyctohemeral rhythm —*see* Disorder, sleep, circadian rhythm
  optic papilla Q14.2
  organ or site, congenital NEC —*see* Anomaly, by site
  sleep rhythm —*see* Disorder, sleep, circadian rhythm
  testis (congenital) Q55.29
  uterus (chronic) (postinfectional) (postpartal, old) N85.5
    postpartum O71.2
  vagina (posthysterectomy) N99.3
  ventricular Q20.5
Investigation —*see also* Examination Z04.9
  clinical research subject (control) (normal comparison) (participant) Z00.6
Involuntary movement, abnormal R25.9
Involution, involutional —*see also* condition
  breast, cystic —*see* Dysplasia, mammary, specified type NEC
  depression (single episode) F32.89 ◄▥
    recurrent episode F33.9
  melancholia (single episode) F32.89 ◄▥
    recurrent episode F33.8 ◄
  ovary, senile —*see* Atrophy, ovary
  thymus failure E32.8
I.Q.
  under 20 F73
  20-34 F72
  35-49 F71
  50-69 F70
IRDS (type I) P22.0
  type II P22.1
Irideremia Q13.1
Iridis rubeosis —*see* Disorder, iris, vascular
Iridochoroiditis (panuveitis) —*see* Panuveitis
Iridocyclitis H20.9-
  acute H20.0-
    hypopyon H20.05-
    primary H20.01-
    recurrent H20.02-
    secondary (noninfectious) H20.04-
      infectious H20.03-
  chronic H20.1-
  due to allergy —*see* Iridocyclitis, acute, secondary
  endogenous —*see* Iridocyclitis, acute, primary
  Fuchs' —*see* Cyclitis, Fuchs' heterochromic
  gonococcal A54.32
  granulomatous —*see* Iridocyclitis, chronic
  herpes, herpetic (simplex) B00.51
    zoster B02.32

Iridocyclitis (*Continued*)
  hypopyon —*see* Iridocyclitis, acute, hypopyon
  in (due to)
    ankylosing spondylitis M45.9
    gonococcal infection A54.32
    herpes (simplex) virus B00.51
      zoster B02.32
    infectious disease NOS B99
    parasitic disease NOS B89 [H22]
    sarcoidosis D86.83
    syphilis A51.43
    tuberculosis A18.54
    zoster B02.32
  lens-induced H20.2-
  nongranulomatous —*see* Iridocyclitis, acute
  recurrent —*see* Iridocyclitis, acute, recurrent
  rheumatic —*see* Iridocyclitis, chronic
  subacute —*see* Iridocyclitis, acute
  sympathetic —*see* Uveitis, sympathetic
  syphilitic (secondary) A51.43
  tuberculous (chronic) A18.54
  Vogt-Koyanagi H20.82-
Iridocyclochoroiditis (panuveitis) —*see* Panuveitis
Iridodialysis H21.53-
Iridodonesis H21.89
Iridoplegia (complete) (partial) (reflex) H57.09
Iridoschisis H21.25-
Iris —*see also* condition
  bombé —*see* Membrane, pupillary
Iritis —*see also* Iridocyclitis
  chronic —*see* Iridocyclitis, chronic
  diabetic —*see* E08-E13 with .39
  due to
    herpes simplex B00.51
    leprosy A30.9 [H22]
  gonococcal A54.32
  gouty —*see also* Gout, by type M10.9 [H22] ◄▥
  granulomatous —*see* Iridocyclitis, chronic
  lens induced —*see* Iridocyclitis, lens-induced
  papulosa (syphilitic) A52.71
  rheumatic —*see* Iridocyclitis, chronic
  syphilitic (secondary) A51.43
    congenital (early) A50.01
    late A52.71
  tuberculous A18.54
Iron —*see* condition
Iron-miner's lung J63.4
Irradiated enamel (tooth, teeth) K03.89
Irradiation effects, adverse T66
Irreducible, irreducibility —*see* condition
Irregular, irregularity
  action, heart I49.9
  alveolar process K08.89 ◄▥
  bleeding N92.6
  breathing R06.89
  contour of cornea (acquired) —*see* Deformity, cornea
    congenital Q13.4
  contour, reconstructed breast N65.0
  dentin (in pulp) K04.3
  eye movements H55.89
    nystagmus —*see* Nystagmus
    saccadic H55.81
  labor O62.2
  menstruation (cause unknown) N92.6
  periods N92.6
  prostate N42.9
  pupil —*see* Abnormality, pupillary
  reconstructed breast N65.0
  respiratory R06.89
  septum (nasal) J34.2
  shape, organ or site, congenital NEC —*see* Distortion
  sleep-wake pattern (rhythm) G47.23
Irritable, irritability R45.4
  bladder N32.89
  bowel (syndrome) K58.9
    ~~with diarrhea K58.0~~
    with ◄
      constipation K58.1 ◄
      diarrhea K58.0 ◄

Irritable, irritability (*Continued*)
  bowel (syndrome) (*Continued*)
    mixed K58.2 ◄
    psychogenic F45.8
    specified NEC K58.8 ◄
  bronchial —*see* Bronchitis
  cerebral, in newborn P91.3
  colon —*see also* Irritable, bowel K58.9 ◄▥
    with diarrhea K58.0
    psychogenic F45.8
  duodenum K59.8
  heart (psychogenic) F45.8
  hip —*see* Derangement, joint, specified type NEC, hip
  ileum K59.8
  infant R68.12
  jejunum K59.8
  rectum K59.8
  stomach K31.89
    psychogenic F45.8
  sympathetic G90.8
  urethra N36.8
Irritation
  anus K62.89
  axillary nerve G54.0
  bladder N32.89
  brachial plexus G54.0
  bronchial —*see* Bronchitis
  cervical plexus G54.2
  cervix —*see* Cervicitis
  choroid, sympathetic —*see* Endophthalmitis
  cranial nerve —*see* Disorder, nerve, cranial
  gastric K31.89
    psychogenic F45.8
  globe, sympathetic —*see* Uveitis, sympathetic
  labyrinth —*see* subcategory H83.2
  lumbosacral plexus G54.1
  meninges (traumatic) —*see* Injury, intracranial
    nontraumatic —*see* Meningismus
  nerve —*see* Disorder, nerve
  nervous R45.0
  penis N48.89
  perineum NEC L29.3
  peripheral autonomic nervous system G90.8
  peritoneum —*see* Peritonitis
  pharynx J39.2
  plantar nerve —*see* Lesion, nerve, plantar
  spinal (cord) (traumatic) —*see also* Injury, spinal cord, by region
    nerve G58.9
      root NEC —*see* Radiculopathy
      nontraumatic —*see* Myelopathy
  stomach K31.89
    psychogenic F45.8
  sympathetic nerve NEC G90.8
  ulnar nerve —*see* Lesion, nerve, ulnar
  vagina N89.8
Ischemia, ischemic I99.8
  bowel (transient)
    acute —*see also* Ischemia, intestine, acute K55.059 ◄▥
    chronic K55.1
    due to mesenteric artery insufficiency K55.1
  brain —*see* Ischemia, cerebral
  cardiac (*see* Disease, heart, ischemic)
  cardiomyopathy I25.5
  cerebral (chronic) (generalized) I67.82
    arteriosclerotic I67.2
    intermittent G45.9
    newborn P91.0
    recurrent focal G45.8
    transient G45.9
  colon chronic (due to mesenteric artery insufficiency) K55.1
  coronary —*see* Disease, heart, ischemic
  demand (coronary) —*see also* Angina I24.8
  heart (chronic or with a stated duration of over 4 weeks) I25.9
    acute or with a stated duration of 4 weeks or less I24.9
    subacute I24.9

◄ New   ◄▥ Revised   ~~deleted~~ Deleted

Ischemia, ischemic *(Continued)*
 infarction, muscle —*see* Infarct, muscle
 intestine (large) (small) (transient) K55.9
  acute K55.059 ◄▥
   diffuse K55.052 ◄
   focal K55.051 ◄
   large K55.039 ◄
    diffuse K55.032 ◄
    focal K55.031 ◄
   small K55.019 ◄
    diffuse K55.012 ◄
    focal K55.011 ◄
  chronic K55.1
  due to mesenteric artery insufficiency
    K55.1
 kidney N28.0
 mesenteric, acute —*see also* Ischemia, intestine,
    acute K55.059 ◄▥
 muscle, traumatic T79.6
 myocardium, myocardial (chronic or with a
    stated duration of over 4 weeks) I25.9
  acute, without myocardial infarction
    I51.3 ◄▥
   silent (asymptomatic) I25.6
   transient of newborn P29.4
 renal N28.0
 retina, retinal —*see* Occlusion, artery, retina
 small bowel
  acute K55.019 ◄▥
   diffuse K55.012 ◄
   focal K55.011 ◄
  chronic K55.1
  due to mesenteric artery insufficiency K55.1
 spinal cord G95.11
 subendocardial —*see* Insufficiency, coronary
 supply (coronary) —*see also* Angina I25.9
  due to vasospasm I20.1
Ischial spine —*see* condition
Ischialgia —*see* Sciatica
Ischiopagus Q89.4
Ischium, ischial —*see* condition
Ischuria R34

Iselin's disease or osteochondrosis —*see*
    Osteochondrosis, juvenile, metatarsus
Islands of
 parotid tissue in
  lymph nodes Q38.6
  neck structures Q38.6
 submaxillary glands in
  fascia Q38.6
  lymph nodes Q38.6
  neck muscles Q38.6
Islet cell tumor, pancreas D13.7
Isoimmunization NEC —*see also* Incompatibility
 affecting management of pregnancy (ABO)
    (with hydrops fetalis) O36.11-
  anti-A sensitization O36.11-
  anti-B sensitization O36.19-
  anti-c sensitization O36.09-
  anti-C sensitization O36.09-
  anti-e sensitization O36.09-
  anti-E sensitization O36.09-
  Rh NEC O36.09-
   anti-D antibody O36.01-
  specified NEC O36.19-
 newborn P55.9
  with
   hydrops fetalis P56.0
   kernicterus P57.0
  ABO (blood groups) P55.1
  Rhesus (Rh) factor P55.0
  specified type NEC P55.8
Isolation, isolated
 dwelling Z59.8
 family Z63.79
 social Z60.4
Isoleucinosis E71.19
Isomerism atrial appendages (with asplenia or
    polysplenia) Q20.6
Isosporiasis, isosporosis A07.3
Isovaleric acidemia E71.110
Issue of
 medical certificate Z02.79
  for disability determination Z02.71

Issue of *(Continued)*
 repeat prescription (appliance) (glasses)
    (medicinal substance, medicament,
    medicine) Z76.0
 contraception —*see* Contraception
Itch, itching —*see also* Pruritus
 baker's L23.6
 barber's B35.0
 bricklayer's L24.5
 cheese B88.0
 clam digger's B65.3
 coolie B76.9
 copra B88.0
 dew B76.9
 dhobi B35.6
 filarial —*see* Infestation, filarial
 grain B88.0
 grocer's B88.0
 ground B76.9
 harvest B88.0
 jock B35.6
 Malabar B35.5
  beard B35.0
  foot B35.3
  scalp B35.0
 meaning scabies B86
 Norwegian B86
 perianal L29.0
 poultrymen's B88.0
 sarcoptic B86
 scabies B86
 scrub B88.0
 straw B88.0
 swimmer's B65.3
 water B76.9
 winter L29.8
Ivemark's syndrome (asplenia with congenital
    heart disease) Q89.01
Ivory bones Q78.2
Ixodiasis NEC B88.8

J

Jaccoud's syndrome —*see* Arthropathy, postrheumatic, chronic
Jackson's
  membrane Q43.3
  paralysis or syndrome G83.89
  veil Q43.3
Jacquet's dermatitis (diaper dermatitis) L22
Jadassohn-Pellizari's disease or anetoderma L90.2
Jadassohn's
  blue nevus —*see* Nevus
  intraepidermal epithelioma —*see* Neoplasm, skin, benign
Jaffe-Lichtenstein (-Uehlinger) syndrome —*see* Dysplasia, fibrous, bone NEC
Jakob-Creutzfeldt disease or syndrome —*see* Creutzfeldt-Jakob disease or syndrome
Jaksch-Luzet disease D64.89
Jamaican
  neuropathy G92
  paraplegic tropical ataxic-spastic syndrome G92
Janet's disease F48.8
Janiceps Q89.4
Jansky-Bielschowsky amaurotic idiocy E75.4
Japanese
  B-type encephalitis A83.0
  river fever A75.3
Jaundice (yellow) R17
  acholuric (familial) (splenomegalic) —*see also* Spherocytosis
    acquired D59.8
  breast-milk (inhibitor) P59.3
  catarrhal (acute) B15.9
    with hepatic coma B15.0
  cholestatic (benign) R17
  due to or associated with
    delayed conjugation P59.8
      associated with (due to) preterm delivery P59.0
    preterm delivery P59.0
  epidemic (catarrhal) B15.9
    with hepatic coma B15.0
    leptospiral A27.0
    spirochetal A27.0
  familial nonhemolytic (congenital) (Gilbert) E80.4
    Crigler-Najjar E80.5
  febrile (acute) B15.9
    with hepatic coma B15.0
    leptospiral A27.0
    spirochetal A27.0
  hematogenous D59.9
  hemolytic (acquired) D59.9
    congenital —*see* Spherocytosis

Jaundice (Continued)
  hemorrhagic (acute) (leptospiral) (spirochetal) A27.0
  infectious (acute) (subacute) B15.9
    with hepatic coma B15.0
    leptospiral A27.0
    spirochetal A27.0
  leptospiral (hemorrhagic) A27.0
  malignant (without coma) K72.90
    with coma K72.91
  neonatal —*see* Jaundice, newborn
  newborn P59.9
    due to or associated with
      ABO
        antibodies P55.1
        incompatibility, maternal/fetal P55.1
        isoimmunization P55.1
      absence or deficiency of enzyme system for bilirubin conjugation (congenital) P59.8
      bleeding P58.1
      breast milk inhibitors to conjugation P59.3
      associated with preterm delivery P59.0
      bruising P58.0
      Crigler-Najjar syndrome E80.5
      delayed conjugation P59.8
        associated with preterm delivery P59.0
      drugs or toxins
        given to newborn P58.42
        transmitted from mother P58.41
      excessive hemolysis P58.9
        due to
          bleeding P58.1
          bruising P58.0
          drugs or toxins
            given to newborn P58.42
            transmitted from mother P58.41
          infection P58.2
          polycythemia P58.3
          swallowed maternal blood P58.5
        specified type NEC P58.8
      galactosemia E74.21
      Gilbert syndrome E80.4
      hemolytic disease P55.9
        ABO isoimmunization P55.1
        Rh isoimmunization P55.0
        specified NEC P55.8
      hepatocellular damage P59.20
        specified NEC P59.29
      hereditary hemolytic anemia P58.8
      hypothyroidism, congenital E03.1
      incompatibility, maternal/fetal NOS P55.9
      infection P58.2

Jaundice (Continued)
  newborn (Continued)
    due to or associated with (Continued)
      inspissated bile syndrome P59.1
      isoimmunization NOS P55.9
      mucoviscidosis E84.9
      polycythemia P58.3
      preterm delivery P59.0
      Rh
        antibodies P55.0
        incompatibility, maternal/fetal P55.0
        isoimmunization P55.0
      specified cause NEC P59.8
      swallowed maternal blood P58.5
    spherocytosis (congenital) D58.0
  nonhemolytic congenital familial (Gilbert) E80.4
  nuclear, newborn —*see also* Kernicterus of newborn P57.9
  obstructive —*see also* Obstruction, bile duct K83.1
  post-immunization —*see* Hepatitis, viral, type, B
  post-transfusion —*see* Hepatitis, viral, type, B
  regurgitation —*see also* Obstruction, bile duct K83.1
  serum (homologous) (prophylactic) (therapeutic) —*see* Hepatitis, viral, type, B
  spirochetal (hemorrhagic) A27.0
  symptomatic R17
    newborn P59.9
Jaw —*see* condition
Jaw-winking phenomenon or syndrome Q07.8
Jealousy
  alcoholic F10.988
  childhood F93.8
  sibling F93.8
Jejunitis —*see* Enteritis
Jejunostomy status Z93.4
Jejunum, jejunal —*see* condition
Jensen's disease —*see* Inflammation, chorioretinal, focal, juxtapapillary
Jerks, myoclonic G25.3
Jervell-Lange-Nielsen syndrome I45.81
Jeune's disease Q77.2
Jigger disease B88.1
Job's syndrome (chronic granulomatous disease) D71
Joint —*see also* condition
  mice —*see* Loose, body, joint
    knee M23.4-
Jordan's anomaly or syndrome D72.0
Joseph-Diamond-Blackfan anemia (congenital hypoplastic) D61.01
Jungle yellow fever A95.0
Jüngling's disease —*see* Sarcoidosis
Juvenile —*see* condition

◀ New ◀▥ Revised ~~deleted~~ Deleted

K

Kahler's disease C90.0-
Kakke E51.11
Kala-azar B55.0
Kallmann's syndrome E23.0
Kanner's syndrome (autism) —see Psychosis, childhood
Kaposi's
  dermatosis (xeroderma pigmentosum) Q82.1
  lichen ruber L44.0
    acuminatus L44.0
  sarcoma
    colon C46.4
    connective tissue C46.1
    gastrointestinal organ C46.4
    lung C46.5-
    lymph node (multiple) C46.3
    palate (hard) (soft) C46.2
    rectum C46.4
    skin (multiple sites) C46.0
    specified site NEC C46.7
    stomach C46.4
    unspecified site C46.9
  varicelliform eruption B00.0
    vaccinia T88.1
Kartagener's syndrome or triad (sinusitis, bronchiectasis, situs inversus) Q89.3
Karyotype
  with abnormality except iso (Xq) Q96.2
  45,X Q96.0
  46,X
    iso (Xq) Q96.1
  46,XX Q98.3
    with streak gonads Q50.32
    hermaphrodite (true) Q99.1
    male Q98.3
  46,XY
    with streak gonads Q56.1
    female Q97.3
    hermaphrodite (true) Q99.1
  47,XXX Q97.0
  47,XXY Q98.0
  47,XYY Q98.5
Kaschin-Beck disease —see Disease, Kaschin-Beck
Katayama's disease or fever B65.2
Kawasaki's syndrome M30.3
Kayser-Fleischer ring (cornea) (pseudosclerosis) H18.04-
Kaznelson's syndrome (congenital hypoplastic anemia) D61.01
Kearns-Sayre syndrome H49.81-
Kedani fever A75.3
Kelis L91.0
Kelly (-Patterson) syndrome (sideropenic dysphagia) D50.1
Keloid, cheloid L91.0
  acne L73.0
  Addison's L94.0
  cornea —see Opacity, cornea
  Hawkin's L91.0
  scar L91.0
Keloma L91.0
Kenya fever A77.1
Keratectasia —see also Ectasia, cornea
  congenital Q13.4
Keratinization of alveolar ridge mucosa
  excessive K13.23
  minimal K13.22
Keratinized residual ridge mucosa
  excessive K13.23
  minimal K13.22
Keratitis (nodular) (nonulcerative) (simple) (zonular) H16.9
  with ulceration (central) (marginal) (perforated) (ring) —see Ulcer, cornea
  actinic —see Photokeratitis
  arborescens (herpes simplex) B00.52
  areolar H16.11-
  bullosa H16.8

Keratitis (Continued)
  deep H16.309
    specified type NEC H16.399
  dendritic (a) (herpes simplex) B00.52
  disciform (is) (herpes simplex) B00.52
    varicella B01.81
  filamentary H16.12-
  gonococcal (congenital or prenatal) A54.33
  herpes, herpetic (simplex) B00.52
    zoster B02.33
  in (due to)
    acanthamebiasis B60.13
    adenovirus B30.0
    exanthema —see also Exanthem B09
    herpes (simplex) virus B00.52
    measles B05.81
    syphilis A50.31
    tuberculosis A18.52
    zoster B02.33
  interstitial (nonsyphilitic) H16.30-
    diffuse H16.32-
    herpes, herpetic (simplex) B00.52
      zoster B02.33
    sclerosing H16.33-
    specified type NEC H16.39-
    syphilitic (congenital) (late) A50.31
    tuberculous A18.52
  macular H16.11-
  nummular H16.11-
  oyster shuckers' H16.8
  parenchymatous —see Keratitis, interstitial
  petrificans H16.8
  postmeasles B05.81
  punctata
    leprosa A30.9 [H16.14-]
    syphilitic (profunda) A50.31
  punctate H16.14-
  purulent H16.8
  rosacea L71.8
  sclerosing H16.33-
  specified type NEC H16.8
  stellate H16.11-
  striate H16.11-
  superficial H16.10-
    with conjunctivitis —see Keratoconjunctivitis
    due to light —see Photokeratitis
  suppurative H16.8
  syphilitic (congenital) (prenatal) A50.31
  trachomatous A71.1
    sequelae B94.0
  tuberculous A18.52
  vesicular H16.8
  xerotic —see also Keratomalacia H16.8
    vitamin A deficiency E50.4
Keratoacanthoma L85.8
Keratocele —see Descemetocele
Keratoconjunctivitis H16.20-
  Acanthamoeba B60.13
  adenoviral B30.0
  epidemic B30.0
  exposure H16.21-
  herpes, herpetic (simplex) B00.52
    zoster B02.33
  in exanthema —see also Exanthem B09
  infectious B30.0
  lagophthalmic —see Keratoconjunctivitis, specified type NEC
  neurotrophic H16.23-
  phlyctenular H16.25-
  postmeasles B05.81
  shipyard B30.0
  sicca (Sjogren's) M35.0-
    not Sjogren's H16.22-
  specified type NEC H16.29-
  tuberculous (phlyctenular) A18.52
  vernal H16.26-
Keratoconus H18.60-
  congenital Q13.4
  stable H18.61-
  unstable H18.62-

Keratocyst (dental) (odontogenic) —see Cyst, calcifying odontogenic
Keratoderma, keratodermia (congenital) (palmaris et plantaris) (symmetrical) Q82.8
  acquired L85.1
    in diseases classified elsewhere L86
  climactericum L85.1
  gonococcal A54.89
  gonorrheal A54.89
  punctata L85.2
  Reiter's —see Reiter's disease
Keratodermatocele —see Descemetocele
Keratoglobus H18.79
  congenital Q15.8
    with glaucoma Q15.0
Keratohemia —see Pigmentation, cornea, stromal
Keratoiritis —see also Iridocyclitis
  syphilitic A50.39
  tuberculous A18.54
Keratoma L57.0
  palmaris and plantaris hereditarium Q82.8
  senile L57.0
Keratomalacia H18.44-
  vitamin A deficiency E50.4
Keratomegaly Q13.4
Keratomycosis B49
  nigrans, nigricans (palmaris) B36.1
Keratopathy H18.9
  band H18.42-
  bullous H18.1-
  bullous (aphakic), following cataract surgery H59.01-
Keratoscleritis, tuberculous A18.52
Keratosis L57.0
  actinic L57.0
  arsenical L85.8
  congenital, specified NEC Q80.8
  female genital NEC N94.89
  follicularis Q82.8
    acquired L11.0
    congenita Q82.8
    et parafollicularis in cutem penetrans L87.0
    spinulosa (decalvans) Q82.8
    vitamin A deficiency E50.8
  gonococcal A54.89
  male genital (external) N50.89 ◀▥
  nigricans L83
  obturans, external ear (canal) —see Cholesteatoma, external ear
  palmaris et plantaris (inherited) (symmetrical) Q82.8
    acquired L85.1
  penile N48.89
  pharynx J39.2
  pilaris, acquired L85.8
  punctata (palmaris et plantaris) L85.2
  scrotal N50.89 ◀▥
  seborrheic L82.1
    inflamed L82.0
  senile L57.0
  solar L57.0
  tonsillaris J35.8
  vagina N89.4
  vegetans Q82.8
  vitamin A deficiency E50.8
  vocal cord J38.3
Kerato-uveitis —see Iridocyclitis
Kerion (celsi) B35.0
Kernicterus of newborn (not due to isoimmunization) P57.9
  due to isoimmunization (conditions in P55.0-P55.9) P57.0
  specified type NEC P57.8
Kerunoparalysis T75.09
Keshan disease E59
Ketoacidosis E87.2
  diabetic —see Diabetes, by type, with ketoacidosis
Ketonuria R82.4

Ketosis NEC E88.89
  diabetic —*see* Diabetes, by type, with
    ketoacidosis
Kew Garden fever A79.1
Kidney —*see* condition
Kienböck's disease —*see also* Osteochondrosis,
  juvenile, hand, carpal lunate
  adult M93.1
Kimmelstiel (-Wilson) disease —*see* Diabetes,
  Kimmelstiel (-Wilson) disease
Kimura disease D21.9
  specified site (see Neoplasm, connective
    tissue benign)
Kink, kinking
  artery I77.1
  hair (acquired) L67.8
  ileum or intestine —*see* Obstruction,
    intestine
  Lane's —*see* Obstruction, intestine
  organ or site, congenital NEC —*see* Anomaly,
    by site
  ureter (pelvic junction) N13.5
    with
      hydronephrosis N13.1
        with infection N13.6
      pyelonephritis (chronic) N11.1
      congenital Q62.39
  vein (s) I87.8
    caval I87.1
    peripheral I87.1
Kinnier Wilson's disease (hepatolenticular
  degeneration) E83.01
Kissing spine M48.20
  cervical region M48.22
  cervicothoracic region M48.23
  lumbar region M48.26
  lumbosacral region M48.27
  occipito-atlanto-axial region M48.21
  thoracic region M48.24
  thoracolumbar region M48.25
Klatskin's tumor C24.0
Klauder's disease A26.8
Klebs' disease —*see also* Glomerulonephritis
  N05.-
Klebsiella (K.) pneumoniae, as cause of
  disease classified elsewhere B96.1
Klein (e)-Levin syndrome G47.13
Kleptomania F63.2
Klinefelter's syndrome Q98.4
  karyotype 47,XXY Q98.0
  male with more than two X chromosomes
    Q98.1
Klippel-Feil deficiency, disease, or syndrome
  (brevicollis) Q76.1
Klippel's disease I67.2
Klippel-Trenaunay (-Weber) syndrome
  Q87.2
Klumpke (-Déjerine) palsy, paralysis (birth)
  (newborn) P14.1
Knee —*see* condition
Knock knee (acquired) M21.06-
  congenital Q74.1

Knot (s)
  intestinal, syndrome (volvulus) K56.2
  surfer S89.8-
  umbilical cord (true) O69.2
Knotting (of)
  hair L67.8
  intestine K56.2
Knuckle pad (Garrod's) M72.1
Koch's
  infection —*see* Tuberculosis
  relapsing fever A68.9
Koch-Weeks' conjunctivitis —*see*
  Conjunctivitis, acute, mucopurulent
Köebner's syndrome Q81.8
Köenig's disease (osteochondritis dissecans) —
  see Osteochondritis, dissecans
Köhler-Pellegrini-Steida disease or syndrome
  (calcification, knee joint) —*see* Bursitis,
  tibial collateral
Köhler's disease
  patellar —*see* Osteochondrosis, juvenile,
    patella
  tarsal navicular —*see* Osteochondrosis,
    juvenile, tarsus
Koilonychia L60.3
  congenital Q84.6
Kojevnikov's, epilepsy —*see* Kozhevnikof's
  epilepsy
Koplik's spots B05.9
Kopp's asthma E32.8
Korsakoff's (Wernicke) disease, psychosis or
  syndrome (alcoholic) F10.96
  with dependence F10.26
  drug-induced
    due to drug abuse —*see* Abuse, drug, by
      type, with amnestic disorder
    due to drug dependence —*see* Dependence,
      drug, by type, with amnestic disorder
  nonalcoholic F04
Korsakov's disease, psychosis or syndrome —
  see Korsakoff's disease
Korsakow's disease, psychosis or syndrome —
  see Korsakoff's disease
Kostmann's disease or syndrome (infantile
  genetic agranulocytosis) —*see*
  Agranulocytosis
Kozhevnikof's epilepsy G40.109
  intractable G40.119
    with status epilepticus G40.111
    without status epilepticus G40.119
  not intractable G40.109
    with status epilepticus G40.101
    without status epilepticus G40.109
Krabbe's
  disease E75.23
  syndrome, congenital muscle hypoplasia
    Q79.8
Kraepelin-Morel disease —*see* Schizophrenia
Kraft-Weber-Dimitri disease Q85.8
Kraurosis
  ani K62.89
  penis N48.0

Kraurosis *(Continued)*
  vagina N89.8
  vulva N90.4
Kreotoxism A05.9
Krukenberg's
  spindle —*see* Pigmentation, cornea, posterior
  tumor C79.6-
Kufs' disease E75.4
Kugelberg-Welander disease G12.1
Kuhnt-Junius degeneration —*see also*
  Degeneration, macula H35.32- ◀▥
Kümmell's disease or spondylitis —*see*
  Spondylopathy, traumatic
Kupffer cell sarcoma C22.3
Kuru A81.81
Kussmaul's
  disease M30.0
  respiration E87.2
    in diabetic acidosis —*see* Diabetes, by type,
      with ketoacidosis
Kwashiorkor E40
  marasmic, marasmus type E42
Kyasanur Forest disease A98.2
Kyphoscoliosis, kyphoscoliotic (acquired) —
  see also Scoliosis M41.9
  congenital Q67.5
  heart (disease) I27.1
  sequelae of rickets E64.3
  tuberculous A18.01
Kyphosis, kyphotic (acquired) M40.209
  cervical region M40.202
  cervicothoracic region M40.203
  congenital Q76.419
    cervical region Q76.412
    cervicothoracic region Q76.413
    occipito-atlanto-axial region Q76.411
    thoracic region Q76.414
    thoracolumbar region Q76.415
  Morquio-Brailsford type (spinal) —*see also*
    subcategory M49.8 E76.219
  postlaminectomy M96.3
  postradiation therapy M96.2
  postural (adolescent) M40.00
    cervicothoracic region M40.03
    thoracic region M40.04
    thoracolumbar region M40.05
  secondary NEC M40.10
    cervical region M40.12
    cervicothoracic region M40.13
    thoracic region M40.14
    thoracolumbar region M40.15
  sequelae of rickets E64.3
  specified type NEC M40.299
    cervical region M40.292
    cervicothoracic region M40.293
    thoracic region M40.294
    thoracolumbar region M40.295
  syphilitic, congenital A50.56
  thoracic region M40.204
  thoracolumbar region M40.205
  tuberculous A18.01
Kyrle disease L87.0

L

Labia, labium —*see* condition
Labile
  blood pressure R09.89
  vasomotor system I73.9
Labioglossal paralysis G12.29
Labium leporinum —*see* Cleft, lip
Labor —*see* Delivery
Labored breathing —*see* Hyperventilation
Labyrinthitis (circumscribed) (destructive)
  (diffuse) (inner ear) (latent) (purulent)
  (suppurative) (*see also* subcategory)
  H83.0
  syphilitic A52.79
Laceration
  with abortion —*see* Abortion, by type,
    complicated by laceration of pelvic
    organs
  abdomen, abdominal
    wall S31.119
      with
        foreign body S31.129
        penetration into peritoneal cavity
          S31.619
          with foreign body S31.629
      epigastric region S31.112
        with
          foreign body S31.122
          penetration into peritoneal cavity
            S31.612
            with foreign body S31.622
      left
        lower quadrant S31.114
          with
            foreign body S31.124
            penetration into peritoneal cavity
              S31.614
              with foreign body S31.624
        upper quadrant S31.111
          with
            foreign body S31.121
            penetration into peritoneal cavity
              S31.611
              with foreign body S31.621
      periumbilic region S31.115
        with
          foreign body S31.125
          penetration into peritoneal cavity
            S31.615
            with foreign body S31.625
      right
        lower quadrant S31.113
          with
            foreign body S31.123
            penetration into peritoneal cavity
              S31.613
              with foreign body S31.623
        upper quadrant S31.110
          with
            foreign body S31.120
            penetration into peritoneal cavity
              S31.610
              with foreign body S31.620
  accidental, complicating surgery —*see*
    Complications, surgical, accidental
    puncture or laceration
  Achilles tendon S86.02-
  adrenal gland S37.813
  alveolar (process) —*see* Laceration, oral cavity
  ankle S91.01-
    with
      foreign body S91.02-
  antecubital space —*see* Laceration, elbow
  anus (sphincter) S31.831
    with
      ectopic or molar pregnancy O08.6
      foreign body S31.832
    complicating delivery —*see* Delivery,
      complicated, by, laceration, anus
      (sphincter)

Laceration *(Continued)*
  anus *(Continued)*
    following ectopic or molar pregnancy
      O08.6
    nontraumatic, nonpuerperal —*see* Fissure,
      anus
  arm (upper) S41.11-
    with foreign body S41.12-
    lower —*see* Laceration, forearm
  auditory canal (external) (meatus) —*see*
    Laceration, ear
  auricle, ear —*see* Laceration, ear
  axilla —*see* Laceration, arm
  back —*see also* Laceration, thorax, back
    lower S31.010
      with
        foreign body S31.020
          with penetration into
            retroperitoneal space S31.021
        penetration into retroperitoneal space
          S31.011
  bile duct S36.13
  bladder S37.23
    with ectopic or molar pregnancy O08.6
    following ectopic or molar pregnancy
      O08.6
    obstetrical trauma O71.5
  blood vessel —*see* Injury, blood vessel
  bowel —*see also* Laceration, intestine
    with ectopic or molar pregnancy O08.6
    complicating abortion —*see* Abortion,
      by type, complicated by, specified
      condition NEC
    following ectopic or molar pregnancy
      O08.6
    obstetrical trauma O71.5
  brain (any part) (cortex) (diffuse)
    (membrane) —*see also* Injury,
    intracranial, diffuse
    during birth P10.8
      with hemorrhage P10.1
    focal —*see* Injury, intracranial, focal brain
      injury
  brainstem S06.38-
  breast S21.01-
    with foreign body S21.02-
  broad ligament S37.893
    with ectopic or molar pregnancy O08.6
    following ectopic or molar pregnancy
      O08.6
    laceration syndrome N83.8
    obstetrical trauma O71.6
    syndrome (laceration) N83.8
  buttock S31.801
    with foreign body S31.802
    left S31.821
      with foreign body S31.822
    right S31.811
      with foreign body S31.812
  calf —*see* Laceration, leg
  canaliculus lacrimalis —*see* Laceration,
    eyelid
  canthus, eye —*see* Laceration, eyelid
  capsule, joint —*see* Sprain
  causing eversion of cervix uteri (old) N86
  central (perineal), complicating delivery
    O70.9
  cerebellum, traumatic S06.37-
  cerebral S06.33-
    during birth P10.8
      with hemorrhage P10.1
    left side S06.32-
    right side S06.31-
  cervix (uteri)
    with ectopic or molar pregnancy O08.6
    following ectopic or molar pregnancy
      O08.6
    nonpuerperal, nontraumatic N88.1
    obstetrical trauma (current) O71.3
    old (postpartal) N88.1
    traumatic S37.63

Laceration *(Continued)*
  cheek (external) S01.41-
    with foreign body S01.42-
    internal —*see* Laceration, oral cavity
  chest wall —*see* Laceration, thorax
  chin —*see* Laceration, head, specified site
    NEC
  chordae tendinae NEC I51.1
    concurrent with acute myocardial
      infarction —*see* Infarct, myocardium
    following acute myocardial infarction
      (current complication) I23.4
  clitoris —*see* Laceration, vulva
  colon —*see* Laceration, intestine, large,
    colon
  common bile duct S36.13
  cortex (cerebral) —*see* Injury, intracranial,
    diffuse
  costal region —*see* Laceration, thorax
  cystic duct S36.13
  diaphragm S27.803
  digit (s)
    foot —*see* Laceration, toe
    hand —*see* Laceration, finger
  duodenum S36.430
  ear (canal) (external) S01.31-
    with foreign body S01.32-
    drum S09.2-
  elbow S51.01-
    with
      foreign body S51.02-
  epididymis —*see* Laceration, testis
  epigastric region —*see* Laceration, abdomen,
    wall, epigastric region
  esophagus K22.8
    traumatic
      cervical S11.21
        with foreign body S11.22
      thoracic S27.813
  eye (ball) S05.3-
    with prolapse or loss of intraocular tissue
      S05.2-
    penetrating S05.6-
  eyebrow —*see* Laceration, eyelid
  eyelid S01.11-
    with foreign body S01.12-
  face NEC —*see* Laceration, head, specified
    site NEC
  fallopian tube S37.539
    bilateral S37.532
    unilateral S37.531
  finger (s) S61.219
    with
      damage to nail S61.319
        with
          foreign body S61.329
      foreign body S61.229
    index S61.218
      with
        damage to nail S61.318
          with
            foreign body S61.328
        foreign body S61.228
    left S61.211
      with
        damage to nail S61.311
          with
            foreign body S61.321
        foreign body S61.221
    right S61.210
      with
        damage to nail S61.310
          with
            foreign body S61.320
        foreign body S61.220
    little S61.218
      with
        damage to nail S61.318
          with
            foreign body S61.328
        foreign body S61.228

Laceration (Continued)
  finger (Continued)
    little (Continued)
      left S61.217
        with
          damage to nail S61.317
            with
              foreign body S61.327
          foreign body S61.227
      right S61.216
        with
          damage to nail S61.316
            with
              foreign body S61.326
          foreign body S61.226
    middle S61.218
      with
        damage to nail S61.318
          with
            foreign body S61.328
        foreign body S61.228
      left S61.213
        with
          damage to nail S61.313
            with
              foreign body S61.323
          foreign body S61.223
      right S61.212
        with
          damage to nail S61.312
            with
              foreign body S61.322
          foreign body S61.222
    ring S61.218
      with
        damage to nail S61.318
          with
            foreign body S61.328
        foreign body S61.228
      left S61.215
        with
          damage to nail S61.315
            with
              foreign body S61.325
          foreign body S61.225
      right S61.214
        with
          damage to nail S61.314
            with
              foreign body S61.324
          foreign body S61.224
  flank S31.119
    with foreign body S31.129
  foot (except toe (s) alone) S91.319
    with foreign body S91.329
    left S91.312
      with foreign body S91.322
    right S91.311
      with foreign body S91.321
    toe —see Laceration, toe
  forearm S51.819
    with
      foreign body S51.829
    elbow only —see Laceration,
      elbow
    left S51.812
      with
        foreign body S51.822
    right S51.811
      with
        foreign body S51.821
  forehead S01.81
    with foreign body S01.82
  fourchette O70.0
    with ectopic or molar pregnancy
      O08.6
    complicating delivery O70.0
    following ectopic or molar pregnancy
      O08.6
  gallbladder S36.123

Laceration (Continued)
  genital organs, external
    female S31.512
      with foreign body S31.522
      vagina —see Laceration, vagina
      vulva —see Laceration, vulva
    male S31.511
      with foreign body S31.521
      penis —see Laceration, penis
      scrotum —see Laceration, scrotum
      testis —see Laceration, testis
  groin —see Laceration, abdomen, wall
  gum —see Laceration, oral cavity
  hand S61.419
    with
      foreign body S61.429
    finger —see Laceration, finger
    left S61.412
      with
        foreign body S61.422
    right S61.411
      with
        foreign body S61.421
    thumb —see Laceration, thumb
  head S01.91
    with foreign body S01.92
    cheek —see Laceration, cheek
    ear —see Laceration, ear
    eyelid —see Laceration, eyelid
    lip —see Laceration, lip
    nose —see Laceration, nose
    oral cavity —see Laceration, oral
      cavity
    scalp S01.01
      with foreign body S01.02
    specified site NEC S01.81
      with foreign body S01.82
    temporomandibular area —see Laceration,
      cheek
  heart —see Injury, heart, laceration
  heel —see Laceration, foot
  hepatic duct S36.13
  hip S71.019
    with foreign body S71.029
    left S71.012
      with foreign body S71.022
    right S71.011
      with foreign body S71.021
  hymen —see Laceration, vagina
  hypochondrium —see Laceration, abdomen,
    wall
  hypogastric region —see Laceration,
    abdomen, wall
  ileum S36.438
  inguinal region —see Laceration, abdomen,
    wall
  instep —see Laceration, foot
  internal organ —see Injury, by site
  interscapular region —see Laceration, thorax,
    back
  intestine
    large
      colon S36.539
        ascending S36.530
        descending S36.532
        sigmoid S36.533
        specified site NEC S36.538
      rectum S36.63
        transverse S36.531
    small S36.439
      duodenum S36.430
      specified site NEC S36.438
  intra-abdominal organ S36.93
    intestine —see Laceration, intestine
    liver —see Laceration, liver
    pancreas —see Laceration, pancreas
    peritoneum S36.81
    specified site NEC S36.893
    spleen —see Laceration, spleen
    stomach —see Laceration, stomach

Laceration (Continued)
  intracranial NEC —see also Injury,
    intracranial, diffuse
    birth injury P10.9
  jaw —see Laceration, head, specified site NEC
  jejunum S36.438
  joint capsule —see Sprain, by site
  kidney S37.03-
    major (greater than 3 cm) (massive)
      (stellate) S37.06-
    minor (less than 1 cm) S37.04-
    moderate (1 to 3 cm) S37.05-
    multiple S37.06-
  knee S81.01-
    with foreign body S81.02-
  labium (majus) (minus) —see Laceration,
    vulva
  lacrimal duct —see Laceration, eyelid
  large intestine —see Laceration, intestine,
    large
  larynx S11.011
    with foreign body S11.012
  leg (lower) S81.819
    with foreign body S81.829
    foot —see Laceration, foot
    knee —see Laceration, knee
    left S81.812
      with foreign body S81.822
    right S81.811
      with foreign body S81.821
    upper —see Laceration, thigh
  ligament —see Sprain
  lip S01.511
    with foreign body S01.521
  liver S36.113
    major (stellate) S36.116
    minor S36.114
    moderate S36.115
  loin —see Laceration, abdomen, wall
  lower back —see Laceration, back, lower
  lumbar region —see Laceration, back, lower
  lung S27.339
    bilateral S27.332
    unilateral S27.331
  malar region —see Laceration, head, specified
    site NEC
  mammary —see Laceration, breast
  mastoid region —see Laceration, head,
    specified site NEC
  meninges —see Injury, intracranial, diffuse
  meniscus —see Tear, meniscus
  mesentery S36.893
  mesosalpinx S37.893
  mouth —see Laceration, oral cavity
  muscle —see Injury, muscle, by site,
    laceration
  nail
    finger —see Laceration, finger, with
      damage to nail
    toe —see Laceration, toe, with damage to nail
  nasal (septum) (sinus) —see Laceration, nose
  nasopharynx —see Laceration, head, specified
    site NEC
  neck S11.91
    with foreign body S11.92
    involving
      cervical esophagus S11.21
        with foreign body S11.22
      larynx —see Laceration, larynx
      pharynx —see Laceration, pharynx
      thyroid gland —see Laceration, thyroid
        gland
      trachea —see Laceration, trachea
    specified site NEC S11.81
      with foreign body S11.82
  nerve —see Injury, nerve
  nose (septum) (sinus) S01.21
    with foreign body S01.22
  ocular NOS S05.3-
    adnexa NOS S01.11-

Laceration (Continued)
  oral cavity S01.512
    with foreign body S01.522
  orbit (eye) —see Wound, open, ocular, orbit
  ovary S37.439
    bilateral S37.432
    unilateral S37.431
  palate —see Laceration, oral cavity
  palm —see Laceration, hand
  pancreas S36.239
    body S36.231
      major S36.261
      minor S36.241
      moderate S36.251
    head S36.230
      major S36.260
      minor S36.240
      moderate S36.250
    major S36.269
    minor S36.249
    moderate S36.259
    tail S36.232
      major S36.262
      minor S36.242
      moderate S36.252
  pelvic S31.010
    with
      foreign body S31.020
        penetration into retroperitoneal cavity S31.021
      penetration into retroperitoneal cavity S31.011
    floor —see also Laceration, back, lower
      with ectopic or molar pregnancy O08.6
      complicating delivery O70.1
      following ectopic or molar pregnancy O08.6
      old (postpartal) N81.89
    organ S37.93
      with ectopic or molar pregnancy O08.6
      adrenal gland S37.813
      bladder S37.23
      fallopian tube —see Laceration, fallopian tube
      following ectopic or molar pregnancy O08.6
      kidney —see Laceration, kidney
      obstetrical trauma O71.5
      ovary —see Laceration, ovary
      prostate S37.823
      specified site NEC S37.893
      ureter S37.13
      urethra S37.33
      uterus S37.63
  penis S31.21
    with foreign body S31.22
  perineum
    female S31.41
      with
        ectopic or molar pregnancy O08.6
        foreign body S31.42
      during delivery O70.9
        first degree O70.0
        fourth degree O70.3
        second degree O70.1
        third degree —see also Delivery, complicated, by, laceration, perineum, third degree O70.20 ◄ⅢⅢ
      old (postpartal) N81.89
      postpartal N81.89
      secondary (postpartal) O90.1
    male S31.119
      with foreign body S31.129
  periocular area (with or without lacrimal passages) —see Laceration, eyelid
  peritoneum S36.893
  periumbilic region —see Laceration, abdomen, wall, periumbilic

Laceration (Continued)
  periurethral tissue —see Laceration, urethra
  phalanges
    finger —see Laceration, finger
    toe —see Laceration, toe
  pharynx S11.21
    with foreign body S11.22
  pinna —see Laceration, ear
  popliteal space —see Laceration, knee
  prepuce —see Laceration, penis
  prostate S37.823
  pubic region S31.119
    with foreign body S31.129
  pudendum —see Laceration, genital organs, external
  rectovaginal septum —see Laceration, vagina
  rectum S36.63
  retroperitoneum S36.893
  round ligament S37.893
  sacral region —see Laceration, back, lower
  sacroiliac region —see Laceration, back, lower
  salivary gland —see Laceration, oral cavity
  scalp S01.01
    with foreign body S01.02
  scapular region —see Laceration, shoulder
  scrotum S31.31
    with foreign body S31.32
  seminal vesicle S37.893
  shin —see Laceration, leg
  shoulder S41.019
    with foreign body S41.029
    left S41.012
      with foreign body S41.022
    right S41.011
      with foreign body S41.021
  small intestine —see Laceration, intestine, small
  spermatic cord —see Laceration, testis
  spinal cord (meninges) —see also Injury, spinal cord, by region
    due to injury at birth P11.5
    newborn (birth injury) P11.5
  spleen S36.039
    major (massive) (stellate) S36.032
    moderate S36.031
    superficial (minor) S36.030
  sternal region —see Laceration, thorax, front
  stomach S36.33
  submaxillary region —see Laceration, head, specified site NEC
  submental region —see Laceration, head, specified site NEC
  subungual
    finger (s) —see Laceration, finger, with damage to nail
    toe (s) —see Laceration, toe, with damage to nail
  suprarenal gland —see Laceration, adrenal gland
  temple, temporal region —see Laceration, head, specified site NEC
  temporomandibular area —see Laceration, cheek
  tendon —see Injury, muscle, by site, laceration
    Achilles S86.02-
  tentorium cerebelli —see Injury, intracranial, diffuse
  testis S31.31
    with foreign body S31.32
  thigh S71.11-
    with foreign body S71.12-
  thorax, thoracic (wall) S21.91
    with foreign body S21.92
      back S21.22-
        with penetration into thoracic cavity S21.42-
      front S21.12-
        with penetration into thoracic cavity S21.32-

Laceration (Continued)
  thorax, thoracic (Continued)
    back S21.21-
      with
        foreign body S21.22-
          with penetration into thoracic cavity S21.42-
        penetration into thoracic cavity S21.41-
    breast —see Laceration, breast
    front S21.11-
      with
        foreign body S21.12-
          with penetration into thoracic cavity S21.32-
        penetration into thoracic cavity S21.31-
  thumb S61.019
    with
      damage to nail S61.119
        with foreign body S61.129
      foreign body S61.029
    left S61.012
      with
        damage to nail S61.112
          with foreign body S61.122
        foreign body S61.022
    right S61.011
      with
        damage to nail S61.111
          with foreign body S61.121
        foreign body S61.021
  thyroid gland S11.11
    with foreign body S11.12
  toe (s) S91.119
    with
      damage to nail S91.219
        with foreign body S91.229
      foreign body S91.129
    great S91.113
      with
        damage to nail S91.213
          with foreign body S91.223
        foreign body S91.123
      left S91.112
        with
          damage to nail S91.212
            with foreign body S91.222
          foreign body S91.122
      right S91.111
        with
          damage to nail S91.211
            with foreign body S91.221
          foreign body S91.121
    lesser S91.116
      with
        damage to nail S91.216
          with foreign body S91.226
        foreign body S91.126
      left S91.115
        with
          damage to nail S91.215
            with foreign body S91.225
          foreign body S91.125
      right S91.114
        with
          damage to nail S91.214
            with foreign body S91.224
          foreign body S91.124
  tongue —see Laceration, oral cavity

Laceration *(Continued)*
  trachea S11.021
    with foreign body S11.022
  tunica vaginalis —*see* Laceration, testis
  tympanum, tympanic membrane —*see*
    Laceration, ear, drum
  umbilical region S31.115
    with foreign body S31.125
  ureter S37.13
  urethra S37.33
    with or following ectopic or molar
      pregnancy O08.6
    obstetrical trauma O71.5
  urinary organ NEC S37.893
  uterus S37.63
    with ectopic or molar pregnancy O08.6
    following ectopic or molar pregnancy
      O08.6
    nonpuerperal, nontraumatic N85.8
    obstetrical trauma NEC O71.81
    old (postpartal) N85.8
  uvula —*see* Laceration, oral cavity
  vagina S31.41
    with
      ectopic or molar pregnancy O08.6
      foreign body S31.42
    during delivery O71.4
      with perineal laceration —*see* Laceration,
        perineum, female, during delivery
    following ectopic or molar pregnancy
      O08.6
    nonpuerperal, nontraumatic N89.8
    old (postpartal) N89.8
  vas deferens S37.893
  vesical —*see* Laceration, bladder
  vocal cords S11.031
    with foreign body S11.032
  vulva S31.41
    with
      ectopic or molar pregnancy O08.6
      foreign body S31.42
    complicating delivery O70.0
    following ectopic or molar pregnancy
      O08.6
    nonpuerperal, nontraumatic N90.89
    old (postpartal) N90.89
  wrist S61.519
    with
      foreign body S61.529
    left S61.512
      with
        foreign body S61.522
    right S61.511
      with
        foreign body S61.521
Lack of
  achievement in school Z55.3
  adequate
    food Z59.4
    intermaxillary vertical dimension of fully
      erupted teeth M26.36
    sleep Z72.820
  appetite *(see* Anorexia) R63.0
  awareness R41.9
  care
    in home Z74.2
    of infant (at or after birth) T76.02
      confirmed T74.02
  cognitive functions R41.9
  coordination R27.9
    ataxia R27.0
    specified type NEC R27.8
  development (physiological) R62.50
    failure to thrive (child over 28 days old)
      R62.51
      adult R62.7
      newborn P92.6
    short stature R62.52
    specified type NEC R62.59
  energy R53.83
  financial resources Z59.6

Lack of *(Continued)*
  food T73.0
  growth R62.52
  heating Z59.1
  housing (permanent) (temporary) Z59.0
    adequate Z59.1
  learning experiences in childhood Z62.898
  leisure time (affecting life-style) Z73.2
  material resources Z59.9
  memory —*see also* Amnesia
    mild, following organic brain damage F06.8
  ovulation N97.0
  parental supervision or control of child Z62.0
  person able to render necessary care Z74.2
  physical exercise Z72.3
  play experience in childhood Z62.898
  posterior occlusal support M26.57
  relaxation (affecting life-style) Z73.2
  sexual
    desire F52.0
    enjoyment F52.1
  shelter Z59.0
  sleep (adequate) Z72.820
  supervision of child by parent Z62.0
  support, posterior occlusal M26.57
  water T73.1
Lacrimal —*see* condition
Lacrimation, abnormal —*see* Epiphora
Lacrimonasal duct —*see* condition
Lactation, lactating (breast) (puerperal,
    postpartum)
  associated
    cracked nipple O92.13
    retracted nipple O92.03
  defective O92.4
  disorder NEC O92.79
  excessive O92.6
  failed (complete) O92.3
    partial O92.4
  mastitis NEC —*see* Mastitis, obstetric
  mother (care and/or examination) Z39.1
  nonpuerperal N64.3
Lacticemia, excessive E87.2
Lacunar skull Q75.8
Laennec's cirrhosis K70.30 ◀▥
  ~~alcoholic K70.30~~
    ~~with ascites K70.31~~
  with ascites K70.31 ◀
  nonalcoholic K74.69 ◀
Lafora's disease —*see* Epilepsy, generalized,
    idiopathic
Lag, lid (nervous) —*see* Retraction, lid
Lagophthalmos (eyelid) (nervous) H02.209
  cicatricial H02.219
    left H02.216
      lower H02.215
      upper H02.214
    right H02.213
      lower H02.212
      upper H02.211
  keratoconjunctivitis —*see* Keratoconjunctivitis
  left H02.206
    lower H02.205
    upper H02.204
  mechanical H02.229
    left H02.226
      lower H02.225
      upper H02.224
    right H02.223
      lower H02.222
      upper H02.221
  paralytic H02.239
    left H02.236
      lower H02.235
      upper H02.234
    right H02.233
      lower H02.232
      upper H02.231
    right H02.203
      lower H02.202
      upper H02.201

Laki-Lorand factor deficiency —*see* Defect,
    coagulation, specified type NEC
Lalling F80.0
Lambert-Eaton syndrome —*see* Syndrome,
    Lambert-Eaton
Lambliasis, lambliosis A07.1
Landau-Kleffner syndrome —*see* Epilepsy,
    specified NEC
Landouzy-Déjérine dystrophy or
    facioscapulohumeral atrophy G71.0
Landouzy's disease (icterohemorrhagic
    leptospirosis) A27.0
Landry-Guillain-Barré, syndrome or paralysis
    G61.0
Landry's disease or paralysis G61.0
Lane's
  band Q43.3
  kink —*see* Obstruction, intestine
  syndrome K90.2
Langdon Down's syndrome —*see* Trisomy, 21
Lapsed immunization schedule status Z28.3
Large
  baby (regardless of gestational age) (4000g to
    4499g) P08.1
  ear, congenital Q17.1
  physiological cup Q14.2
  stature R68.89
Large-for-dates NEC (infant) (4000g to 4499g)
    P08.1
  affecting management of pregnancy O36.6-
  exceptionally (4500g or more) P08.0
Larsen-Johansson disease
    orosteochondrosis —*see* Osteochondrosis,
    juvenile, patella
Larsen's syndrome (flattened facies and
    multiple congenital dislocations) Q74.8
Larva migrans
  cutaneous B76.9
    Ancylostoma B76.0
  visceral B83.0
Laryngeal —*see* condition
Laryngismus (stridulus) J38.5
  congenital P28.89
  diphtheritic A36.2
Laryngitis (acute) (edematous) (fibrinous)
    (infective) (infiltrative) (malignant)
    (membranous) (phlegmonous)
    (pneumococcal) (pseudomembranous)
    (septic) (subglottic) (suppurative)
    (ulcerative) J04.0
  with
    influenza, flu, or grippe —*see* Influenza,
      with, laryngitis
    tracheitis (acute) —*see* Laryngotracheitis
  atrophic J37.0
  catarrhal J37.0
  chronic J37.0
    with tracheitis (chronic) J37.1
  diphtheritic A36.2
  due to external agent —*see* Inflammation,
    respiratory, upper, due to
  Hemophilus influenzae J04.0
  H. influenzae J04.0
  hypertrophic J37.0
  influenzal —*see* Influenza, with, respiratory
    manifestations NEC
  obstructive J05.0
  sicca J37.0
  spasmodic J05.0
    acute J04.0
  streptococcal J04.0
  stridulous J05.0
  syphilitic (late) A52.73
    congenital A50.59 *[J99]*
    early A50.03 *[J99]*
  tuberculous A15.5
  Vincent's A69.1
Laryngocele (congenital) (ventricular) Q31.3
Laryngofissure J38.7
  congenital Q31.8
Laryngomalacia (congenital) Q31.5

◀ New   ◀▥ Revised   ~~deleted~~ Deleted

Laryngopharyngitis (acute) J06.0
  chronic J37.0
  due to external agent —*see* Inflammation,
    respiratory, upper, due to
Laryngoplegia J38.00
  bilateral J38.02
  unilateral J38.01
Laryngoptosis J38.7
Laryngospasm J38.5
Laryngostenosis J38.6
Laryngotracheitis (acute) (Infectional)
  (infective) (viral) J04.2
  atrophic J37.1
  catarrhal J37.1
  chronic J37.1
  diphtheritic A36.2
  due to external agent —*see* Inflammation,
    respiratory, upper, due to
  Hemophilus influenzae J04.2
  hypertrophic J37.1
  influenzal —*see* Influenza, with, respiratory
    manifestations NEC
  pachydermic J38.7
  sicca J37.1
  spasmodic J38.5
    acute J05.0
  streptococcal J04.2
  stridulous J38.5
  syphilitic (late) A52.73
    congenital A50.59 [J99]
      early A50.03 [J99]
  tuberculous A15.5
  Vincent's A69.1
Laryngotracheobronchitis —*see* Bronchitis
Larynx, laryngeal —*see* condition
Lassa fever A96.2
Lassitude —*see* Weakness
Late
  talker R62.0
  walker R62.0
Late effect (s) —*see* Sequelae
Latent —*see* condition
Laterocession —*see* Lateroversion
Lateroflexion —*see* Lateroversion
Lateroversion
  cervix —*see* Lateroversion, uterus
  uterus, uterine (cervix) (postinfectional)
    (postpartal, old) N85.4
    congenital Q51.818
    in pregnancy or childbirth O34.59-
Lathyrism —*see* Poisoning, food, noxious, plant
Launois' syndrome (pituitary gigantism) E22.0
Launois-Bensaude adenolipomatosis E88.89
Laurence-Moon (-Bardet)-Biedl syndrome
  Q87.89
Lax, laxity —*see also* Relaxation
  ligament (ous) —*see also* Disorder, ligament
    familial M35.7
    knee —*see* Derangement, knee
  skin (acquired) L57.4
    congenital Q82.8
Laxative habit F55.2
Lazy leukocyte syndrome D70.8
Lead miner's lung J63.6
Leak, leakage
  air NEC J93.82
    postprocedural J95.812
  amniotic fluid —*see* Rupture, membranes,
    premature
  blood (microscopic), fetal, into maternal
    circulation affecting management of
    pregnancy —*see* Pregnancy, complicated
    by
  cerebrospinal fluid G96.0
    from spinal (lumbar) puncture G97.0
  device, implant or graft —*see also*
    Complications, by site and type,
    mechanical
    arterial graft NEC —*see* Complication,
      cardiovascular device, mechanical,
      vascular

Leak, leakage (*Continued*)
  device, implant or graft (*Continued*)
    breast (implant) T85.43
    catheter NEC T85.638
      dialysis (renal) T82.43
        intraperitoneal T85.631
      infusion NEC T82.534
        spinal (epidural) (subdural) T85.630
      ~~urinary, indwelling T83.038~~
      ~~cystostomy T83.030~~
      urinary T83.038 ◄
        cystostomy T83.030 ◄
        Hopkins T83.038 ◄
        ileostomy T83.038 ◄
        indwelling T83.031 ◄
        nephrostomy T83.032 ◄
        specified NEC T83.038 ◄
        urostomy T83.038 ◄
    gastrointestinal —*see* Complications,
      prosthetic device, mechanical,
      gastrointestinal device
    genital NEC T83.498
      penile prosthesis (cylinder) (implanted)
        (pump) (resevoir) T83.490 ◄▥
      testicular prosthesis T83.491 ◄
    heart NEC —*see* Complication,
      cardiovascular device, mechanical
    joint prosthesis —*see* Complications, joint
      prosthesis, mechanical, specified
      NEC, by site
    ocular NEC —*see* Complications, prosthetic
      device, mechanical, ocular device
    orthopedic NEC —*see* Complication,
      orthopedic, device, mechanical
    persistent air J93.82
    specified NEC T85.638
    urinary NEC —*see also* Complication,
      genitourinary, device, urinary,
      mechanical
      graft T83.23
    vascular NEC —*see* Complication,
      cardiovascular device, mechanical
    ventricular intracranial shunt T85.03
  urine —*see* Incontinence
Leaky heart —*see* Endocarditis
Learning defect (specific) F81.9
Leather bottle stomach C16.9
Leber's
  congenital amaurosis H35.50
  optic atrophy (hereditary) H47.22
Lederer's anemia D59.1
Leeches (external) —*see* Hirudiniasis
Leg —*see* condition
Legg (-Calvé)-Perthes disease, syndrome or
  osteochondrosis M91.1-
Legionellosis A48.1
  nonpneumonic A48.2
Legionnaires'
  disease A48.1
    nonpneumonic A48.2
  pneumonia A48.1
Leigh's disease G31.82
Leiner's disease L21.1
Leiofibromyoma —*see* Leiomyoma
Leiomyoblastoma —*see* Neoplasm, connective
  tissue, benign
Leiomyofibroma —*see also* Neoplasm,
  connective tissue, benign
  uterus (cervix) (corpus) D25.9
Leiomyoma —*see also* Neoplasm, connective
  tissue, benign
  bizarre —*see* Neoplasm, connective tissue,
    benign
  cellular —*see* Neoplasm, connective tissue,
    benign
  epithelioid —*see* Neoplasm, connective
    tissue, benign
  uterus (cervix) (corpus) D25.9
    intramural D25.1
    submucous D25.0
    subserosal D25.2

Leiomyoma (*Continued*)
  vascular —*see* Neoplasm, connective tissue,
    benign
Leiomyoma, leiomyomatosis (intravascular) —
  see Neoplasm, connective tissue, uncertain
  behavior
Leiomyosarcoma —*see also* Neoplasm,
  connective tissue, malignant
  epithelioid —*see* Neoplasm, connective
    tissue, malignant
  myxoid —*see* Neoplasm, connective tissue,
    malignant
Leishmaniasis B55.9
  American (mucocutaneous) B55.2
    cutaneous B55.1
  Asian Desert B55.1
  Brazilian B55.2
  cutaneous (any type) B55.1
  dermal —*see also* Leishmaniasis, cutaneous
    post-kala-azar B55.0
  eyelid B55.1
  infantile B55.0
  Mediterranean B55.0
  mucocutaneous (American) (New World)
    B55.2
  naso-oral B55.2
  nasopharyngeal B55.2
  old world B55.1
  tegumentaria diffusa B55.1
  visceral B55.0
Leishmanoid, dermal —*see also* Leishmaniasis,
  cutaneous
  post-kala-azar B55.0
Lenegre's disease I44.2
Lengthening, leg —*see* Deformity, limb,
  unequal length
Lennert's lymphoma —*see* Lymphoma,
  Lennert's
Lennox-Gastaut syndrome G40.812
  intractable G40.814
    with status epilepticus G40.813
    without status epilepticus G40.814
  not intractable G40.812
    with status epilepticus G40.811
    without status epilepticus G40.812
Lens —*see* condition
Lenticonus (anterior) (posterior) (congenital)
  Q12.8
Lenticular degeneration, progressive E83.01
Lentiglobus (posterior) (congenital) Q12.8
Lentigo (congenital) L81.4
  maligna —*see also* Melanoma, in situ
    melanoma —*see* Melanoma
Lentivirus, as cause of disease classified
  elsewhere B97.31
Leontiasis
  ossium M85.2
  syphilitic (late) A52.78
    congenital A50.59
Lepothrix A48.8
Lepra —*see* Leprosy
Leprechaunism E34.8
Leprosy A30.-
  with muscle disorder A30.9 [M63.80]
    ankle A30.9 [M63.87-]
    foot A30.9 [M63.87-]
    forearm A30.9 [M63.83-]
    hand A30.9 [M63.84-]
    lower leg A30.9 [M63.86-]
    multiple sites A30.9 [M63.89]
    pelvic region A30.9 [M63.85-]
    shoulder region A30.9 [M63.81-]
    specified site NEC A30.9 [M63.88]
    thigh A30.9 [M63.85-]
    upper arm A30.9 [M63.82-]
  anesthetic A30.9
  BB A30.3
  BL A30.4
  borderline (infiltrated) (neuritic) A30.3
    lepromatous A30.4
    tuberculoid A30.2

Leprosy *(Continued)*
  BT A30.2
  dimorphous (infiltrated) (neuritic) A30.3
  I A30.0
  indeterminate (macular) (neuritic) A30.0
  lepromatous (diffuse) (infiltrated) (macular)
    (neuritic) (nodular) A30.5
  LL A30.5
  macular (early) (neuritic) (simple)
    A30.9
  maculoanesthetic A30.9
  mixed A30.3
  neural A30.9
  nodular A30.5
  primary neuritic A30.3
  specified type NEC A30.8
  TT A30.1
  tuberculoid (major) (minor) A30.1
Leptocytosis, hereditary D56.9
Leptomeningitis (chronic) (circumscribed)
    (hemorrhagic) (nonsuppurative) —*see*
    Meningitis
Leptomeningopathy G96.19
Leptospiral —*see* condition
Leptospirochetal —*see* condition
Leptospirosis A27.9
  canicola A27.89
  due to Leptospira interrogans serovar
    icterohaemorrhagiae A27.0
  icterohemorrhagica A27.0
  pomona A27.89
  Weil's disease A27.0
Leptus dermatitis B88.0
Leriche's syndrome (aortic bifurcation
    occlusion) I74.09
Leri's pleonosteosis Q78.8
Leri-Weill syndrome Q77.8
Lermoyez' syndrome —*see* Vertigo, peripheral
    NEC
Lesch-Nyhan syndrome E79.1
Leser-Trélat disease L82.1
  inflamed L82.0
Lesion (s) (nontraumatic)
  abducens nerve —*see* Strabismus, paralytic,
    sixth nerve
  alveolar process K08.9
  angiocentric immunoproliferative D47.Z9
  anorectal K62.9
  aortic (valve) I35.9
  auditory nerve —*see* subcategory H93.3
  basal ganglion G25.9
  bile duct —*see* Disease, bile duct
  biomechanical M99.9
    specified type NEC M99.89
      abdomen M99.89
      acromioclavicular M99.87
      cervical region M99.81
      cervicothoracic M99.81
      costochondral M99.88
      costovertebral M99.88
      head region M99.80
      hip M99.85
      lower extremity M99.86
      lumbar region M99.83
      lumbosacral M99.83
      occipitocervical M99.80
      pelvic region M99.85
      pubic M99.85
      rib cage M99.88
      sacral region M99.84
      sacrococcygeal M99.84
      sacroiliac M99.84
      specified NEC M99.89
      sternochondral M99.88
      sternoclavicular M99.87
      thoracic region M99.82
      thoracolumbar M99.82
      upper extremity M99.87
  bladder N32.9
  bone —*see* Disorder, bone
  brachial plexus G54.0

Lesion *(Continued)*
  brain G93.9
    congenital Q04.9
    vascular I67.9
      degenerative I67.9
      hypertensive I67.4
  buccal cavity K13.79
  calcified —*see* Calcification
  canthus —*see* Disorder, eyelid
  carate —*see* Pinta, lesions
  cardia K31.9 ⬅
  cardiac —*see also* Disease, heart I51.9
    congenital Q24.9
    valvular —*see* Endocarditis
  cauda equina G83.4
  cecum K63.9
  cerebral —*see* Lesion, brain
  cerebrovascular I67.9
    degenerative I67.9
    hypertensive I67.4
  cervical (nerve) root NEC G54.2
  chiasmal —*see* Disorder, optic, chiasm
  chorda tympani G51.8
  coin, lung R91.1
  colon K63.9
  combined periodontic - endodontic K05.5 ◀
  congenital —*see* Anomaly, by site
  conjunctiva H11.9
  conus medullaris —*see* Injury, conus
    medullaris
  coronary artery —*see* Ischemia, heart
  cranial nerve G52.9
    eighth —*see* Disorder, ear
    eleventh G52.9
    fifth G50.9
    first G52.0
    fourth —*see* Strabismus, paralytic, fourth
      nerve
    seventh G51.9
    sixth —*see* Strabismus, paralytic, sixth
      nerve
    tenth G52.2
    twelfth G52.3
  cystic —*see* Cyst
  degenerative —*see* Degeneration
  duodenum K31.9
  edentulous (alveolar) ridge, associated with
    trauma, due to traumatic occlusion
    K06.2
  en coup de sabre L94.1
  eyelid —*see* Disorder, eyelid
  gasserian ganglion G50.8
  gastric K31.9
  gastroduodenal K31.9
  gastrointestinal K63.9
  gingiva, associated with trauma K06.2
  glomerular
    focal and segmental —*see also* N00-N07
      with fourth character .1 N05.1
    minimal change —*see also* N00-N07 with
      fourth character .0 N05.0
  heart (organic) —*see* Disease, heart
  hyperchromic, due to pinta (carate)
    A67.1
  hyperkeratotic —*see* Hyperkeratosis
  hypothalamic E23.7
  ileocecal K63.9
  ileum K63.9
  iliohypogastric nerve G57.8-
  inflammatory —*see* Inflammation
  intestine K63.9
  intracerebral —*see* Lesion, brain
  intrachiasmal (optic) —*see* Disorder, optic,
    chiasm
  intracranial, space-occupying R90.0
  joint —*see* Disorder, joint
    sacroiliac (old) M53.3
  keratotic —*see* Keratosis
  kidney —*see* Disease, renal
  laryngeal nerve (recurrent) G52.2
  lip K13.0

Lesion *(Continued)*
  liver K76.9
  lumbosacral
    plexus G54.1
    root (nerve) NEC G54.4
  lung (coin) R91.1
  maxillary sinus J32.0
  mitral I05.9
  Morel-Lavallée —*see* Hematoma,
    by site
  motor cortex NEC G93.89
  mouth K13.79
  nerve G58.9
    femoral G57.2-
    median G56.1-
      carpal tunnel syndrome —*see* Syndrome,
        carpal tunnel
    plantar G57.6-
    popliteal (lateral) G57.3-
      medial G57.4-
    radial G56.3-
    sciatic G57.0-
    spinal —*see* Injury, nerve, spinal
    ulnar G56.2-
  nervous system, congenital Q07.9
  nonallopathic —*see* Lesion, biomechanical
  nose (internal) J34.89
  obstructive —*see* Obstruction
  obturator nerve G57.8-
  oral mucosa K13.70
  organ or site NEC —*see* Disease, by site
  osteolytic —*see* Osteolysis
  peptic K27.9
  periodontal, due to traumatic occlusion
    K05.5
  pharynx J39.2
  pigment, pigmented (skin) L81.9
  pinta —*see* Pinta, lesions
  polypoid —*see* Polyp
  prechiasmal (optic) —*see* Disorder, optic,
    chiasm
  primary —*see also* Syphilis, primary A51.0
    carate A67.0
    pinta A67.0
    yaws A66.0
  pulmonary J98.4
    valve I37.9
  pylorus K31.9
  rectosigmoid K63.9
  retina, retinal H35.9
  sacroiliac (joint) (old) M53.3
  salivary gland K11.9
    benign lymphoepithelial K11.8
  saphenous nerve G57.8-
  sciatic nerve G57.0-
  secondary —*see* Syphilis, secondary
  shoulder (region) M75.9-
    specified NEC M75.8-
  sigmoid K63.9
  sinus (accessory) (nasal) J34.89
  skin L98.9
    suppurative L08.0
  SLAP S43.43-
  spinal cord G95.9
    congenital Q06.9
  spleen D73.89
  stomach K31.9
  superior glenoid labrum S43.43-
  syphilitic —*see* Syphilis
  tertiary —*see* Syphilis, tertiary
  thoracic root (nerve) NEC G54.3
  tonsillar fossa J35.9
  tooth, teeth K08.9
    white spot
      chewing surface K02.51
      pit and fissure surface K02.51
      smooth surface K02.61
  traumatic —*see* specific type of injury by site
  tricuspid (valve) I07.9
    nonrheumatic I36.9
  trigeminal nerve G50.9

◀ New   ⬅ Revised   ~~deleted~~ Deleted

Lesion *(Continued)*
  ulcerated or ulcerative —*see* Ulcer, skin
  uterus N85.9
  vagus nerve G52.2
  valvular —*see* Endocarditis
  vascular I99.9
    affecting central nervous system I67.9
    following trauma NEC T14.8
    umbilical cord, complicating delivery
      O69.5
  warty —*see* Verruca
  white spot (tooth)
    chewing surface K02.51
    pit and fissure surface K02.51
    smooth surface K02.61
Lethargic —*see* condition
Lethargy R53.83
Letterer-Siwe's disease C96.0
Leukemia, leukemic C95.9-
  acute basophilic C94.8-
  acute bilineal C95.0-
  acute erythroid C94.0-
  acute lymphoblastic C91.0-
  acute megakaryoblastic C94.2-
  acute megakaryocytic C94.2-
  acute mixed lineage C95.0-
  acute monoblastic (monoblastic/monocytic)
    C93.0-
  acute monocytic (monoblastic/monocytic)
    C93.0-
  acute myeloblastic (minimal differentiation)
    (with maturation) C92.0-
  acute myeloid
    with
      11q23-abnormality C92.6-
      dysplasia of remaining hematopoesis
        and/or myelodysplastic disease in
        its history C92.A-
      multilineage dysplasia C92.A-
      variation of MLL-gene C92.6-
    M6 (a)(b) C94.0-
    M7 C94.2-
  acute myelomonocytic C92.5-
  acute promyelocytic C92.4-
  adult T-cell (HTLV-1-associated)
    (acute variant) (chronic variant)
    (lymphomatoid variant) (smouldering
    variant) C91.5-
  aggressive NK-cell C94.8-
  AML (1/ETO) (M0) (M1) (M2) (without a
    FAB classification) C92.0-
  AML M3 C92.4-
  AML M4 (Eo with inv(16) or t(16;16))
    C92.5-
  AML M5 C93.0-
  AML M5a C93.0-
  AML M5b C93.0-
  AML Me with t (15;17) and variants C92.4-
  atypical chronic myeloid, BCR/ABL-negative
    C92.2-
  biphenotypic acute C95.0-
  blast cell C95.0-
  Burkitt-type, mature B-cell C91.A-
  chronic lymphocytic, of B-cell type C91.1-
  chronic monocytic C93.1-
  chronic myelogenous (Philadelphia
    chromosome (Ph1) positive) (t(9;22))
    (q34;q11) (with crisis of blast cells)
    C92.1-
  chronic myeloid, BCR/ABL-positive C92.1-
    atypical, BCR/ABL-negative C92.2-
  chronic myelomonocytic C93.1-
  chronic neutrophilic D47.1
  CMML (-1) (-2) (with eosinophilia) C93.1-
  granulocytic —*see also* Category C92 C92.9-
  hairy-cell C91.4-
  juvenile myelomonocytic C93.3-
  lymphoid C91.9-
    specified NEC C91.Z-
  mast cell C94.3-
  mature B-cell, Burkitt-type C91.A-

Leukemia, leukemic *(Continued)*
  monocytic (subacute) C93.9-
    specified NEC C93.Z-
  myelogenous —*see also* Category C92 C92.9-
  myeloid C92.9-
    specified NEC C92.Z-
  plasma cell C90.1-
  plasmacytic C90.1-
  prolymphocytic
    of B-cell type C91.3-
    of T-cell type C91.6-
  specified NEC C94.8-
  stem cell, of unclear lineage C95.0-
  subacute lymphocytic C91.9-
  T-cell large granular lymphocytic C91.Z-
  unspecified cell type C95.9-
    acute C95.0-
    chronic C95.1-
Leukemoid reaction —*see also* Reaction,
  leukemoid D72.823-
Leukoaraiosis (hypertensive) I67.81
Leukoariosis —*see* Leukoaraiosis
Leukocoria —*see* Disorder, globe, degenerated
  condition, leucocoria
Leukocytopenia D72.819
Leukocytosis D72.829
  eosinophilic D72.1
Leukoderma, leukodermia NEC L81.5
  syphilitic A51.39
    late A52.79
Leukodystrophy E75.29
Leukoedema, oral epithelium K13.29
Leukoencephalitis G04.81
  acute (subacute) hemorrhagic G36.1
    postimmunization or postvaccinal G04.02
  postinfectious G04.01
  subacute sclerosing A81.1
  van Bogaert's (sclerosing) A81.1
Leukoencephalopathy —*see also*
  Encephalopathy G93.49
  Binswanger's I67.3
  heroin vapor G92
  metachromatic E75.25
  multifocal (progressive) A81.2
  postimmunization and postvaccinal G04.02
  progressive multifocal A81.2
  reversible, posterior G93.6
  van Bogaert's (sclerosing) A81.1
  vascular, progressive I67.3
Leukoerythroblastosis D75.9
Leukokeratosis —*see also* Leukoplakia
  mouth K13.21
  nicotina palati K13.24
  oral mucosa K13.21
  tongue K13.21
  vocal cord J38.3
Leukokraurosis vulva (e) N90.4
Leukoma (cornea) —*see also* Opacity, cornea
  adherent H17.0-
  interfering with central vision —*see* Opacity,
    cornea, central
Leukomalacia, cerebral, newborn P91.2
  periventricular P91.2
Leukomelanopathy, hereditary D72.0
Leukonychia (punctata) (striata) L60.8
  congenital Q84.4
Leukopathia unguium L60.8
  congenital Q84.4
Leukopenia D72.819
  basophilic D72.818
  chemotherapy (cancer) induced D70.1
  congenital D70.0
  cyclic D70.0
  drug induced NEC D70.2
    due to cytoreductive cancer chemotherapy
      D70.1
  eosinophilic D72.818
  familial D70.0
  infantile genetic D70.0
  malignant D70.9
  periodic D70.0
  transitory neonatal P61.5

Leukopenic —*see* condition
Leukoplakia
  anus K62.89
  bladder (postinfectional) N32.89
  buccal K13.21
  cervix (uteri) N88.0
  esophagus K22.8
  gingiva K13.21
  hairy (oral mucosa) (tongue) K13.3
  kidney (pelvis) N28.89
  larynx J38.7
  lip K13.21
  mouth K13.21
  oral epithelium, including tongue (mucosa)
    K13.21
  palate K13.21
  pelvis (kidney) N28.89
  penis (infectional) N48.0
  rectum K62.89
  syphilitic (late) A52.79
  tongue K13.21
  ureter (postinfectional) N28.89
  urethra (postinfectional) N36.8
  uterus N85.8
  vagina N89.4
  vocal cord J38.3
  vulva N90.4
Leukorrhea N89.8
  due to Trichomonas (vaginalis)
    A59.00
  trichomonal A59.00
Leukosarcoma C85.9
Levocardia (isolated) Q24.1
  with situs inversus Q89.3
Levotransposition Q20.5
Lev's disease or syndrome (acquired complete
  heart block) I44.2
Levulosuria —*see* Fructosuria
Levurid L30.2
Lewy body (ies) (dementia) (disease)
  G31.83
Leyden-Moebius dystrophy G71.0
Leydig cell
  carcinoma
    specified site —*see* Neoplasm, malignant,
      by site
    unspecified site
      female C56.9-
      male C62.9-
  tumor
    benign
      specified site —*see* Neoplasm, benign,
        by site
      unspecified site
        female D27.-
        male D29.2-
    malignant
      specified site —*see* Neoplasm,
        malignant, by site
      unspecified site
        female C56.-
        male C62.9-
    specified site —*see* Neoplasm, uncertain
      behavior, by site
    unspecified site
      female D39.1-
      male D40.1-
Leydig-Sertoli cell tumor
  specified site —*see* Neoplasm, benign,
    by site
  unspecified site
    female D27.-
    male D29.2-
LGSIL (Low grade squamous intraepithelial
  lesion on cytologic smear of)
  anus R85.612
  cervix R87.612
  vagina R87.622
Liar, pathologic F60.2
Libido
  decreased R68.82

Libman-Sacks disease M32.11
Lice (infestation) B85.2
  body (Pediculus corporis) B85.1
  crab B85.3
  head (Pediculus capitis) B85.0
  mixed (classifiable to more than one of the titles B85.0-B85.3) B85.4
  pubic (Phthirus pubis) B85.3
Lichen L28.0
  albus L90.0
    penis N48.0
    vulva N90.4
  amyloidosis E85.4 [L99]
  atrophicus L90.0
    penis N48.0
    vulva N90.4
  congenital Q82.8
  myxedematosus L98.5
  nitidus L44.1
  pilaris Q82.8
    acquired L85.8
  planopilaris L66.1
  planus (chronicus) L43.9
    annularis L43.8
    bullous L43.1
    follicular L66.1
    hypertrophic L43.0
    moniliformis L44.3
    of Wilson L43.9
    specified NEC L43.8
    subacute (active) L43.3
    tropicus L43.3
  ruber
    acuminatus L44.0
    moniliformis L44.3
    planus L43.9
  sclerosus (et atrophicus) L90.0
    penis N48.0
    vulva N90.4
  scrofulosus (primary) (tuberculous) A18.4
  simplex (chronicus) (circumscriptus) L28.0
  striatus L44.2
  urticatus L28.2
Lichenification L28.0
Lichenoides tuberculosis (primary) A18.4
Lichtheim's disease or syndrome —see Degeneration, combined
Lien migrans D73.89
Ligament —see condition
Light
  for gestational age —see Light for dates
  headedness R42
Light-for-dates (infant) P05.00
  with weight of
    499 grams or less P05.01
    500-749 grams P05.02
    750-999 grams P05.03
    1000-1249 grams P05.04
    1250-1499 grams P05.05
    1500-1749 grams P05.06
    1750-1999 grams P05.07
    2000-2499 grams P05.08
    2500 grams and over P05.09 ◄
  affecting management of pregnancy O36.59-
  and small-for-dates —see Small for dates
  specified NEC P05.09 ◄
Lightning (effects) (stroke) (struck by) T75.00
  burn —see Burn
  foot E53.8
  shock T75.01
  specified effect NEC T75.09
Lightwood-Albright syndrome N25.89
Lightwood's disease or syndrome (renal tubular acidosis) N25.89
Lignac (-de Toni) (-Fanconi) (-Debré) disease or syndrome E72.09
  with cystinosis E72.04
Ligneous thyroiditis E06.5
Likoff's syndrome I20.8
Limb —see condition
Limbic epilepsy personality syndrome F07.0

Limitation, limited
  activities due to disability Z73.6
  cardiac reserve —see Disease, heart
  eye muscle duction, traumatic —see Strabismus, mechanical
  mandibular range of motion M26.52
Lindau (-von Hippel) disease Q85.8
Line (s)
  Beau's L60.4
  Harris' —see Arrest, epiphyseal
  Hudson's (cornea) —see Pigmentation, cornea, anterior
  Stähli's (cornea) —see Pigmentation, cornea, anterior
Linea corneae senilis —see Change, cornea, senile
Lingua
  geographica K14.1
  nigra (villosa) K14.3
  plicata K14.5
  tylosis K13.29
Lingual —see condition
Linguatulosis B88.8
Linitis (gastric) plastica C16.9
Lip —see condition
Lipedema —see Edema
Lipemia —see also Hyperlipidemia
  retina, retinalis E78.3
Lipidosis E75.6
  cerebral (infantile) (juvenile) (late) E75.4
  cerebroretinal E75.4
  cerebroside E75.22
  cholesterol (cerebral) E75.5
  glycolipid E75.21
  hepatosplenomegalic E78.3
  sphingomyelin —see Niemann-Pick disease or syndrome
  sulfatide E75.29
Lipoadenoma —see Neoplasm, benign, by site
Lipoblastoma —see Lipoma
Lipoblastomatosis —see Lipoma
Lipochondrodystrophy E76.01
Lipochrome histiocytosis (familial) D71
Lipodermatosclerosis —see Varix, leg, with, inflammation
  ulcerated —see Varix, leg, with, ulcer, with inflammation by site
Lipodystrophia progressiva E88.1
Lipodystrophy (progressive) E88.1
  insulin E88.1
  intestinal K90.81
  mesenteric K65.4
Lipofibroma —see Lipoma
Lipofuscinosis, neuronal (with ceroidosis) E75.4
Lipogranuloma, sclerosing L92.8
Lipogranulomatosis E78.89
Lipoid —see also condition
  histiocytosis D76.3
    essential E75.29
  nephrosis N04.9
  proteinosis of Urbach E78.89
Lipoidemia —see Hyperlipidemia
Lipoidosis —see Lipidosis
Lipoma D17.9
  fetal D17.9
    fat cell D17.9
  infiltrating D17.9
  intramuscular D17.9
  pleomorphic D17.9
  site classification
    arms (skin) (subcutaneous) D17.2-
    connective tissue D17.30
      intra-abdominal D17.5
      intrathoracic D17.4
      peritoneum D17.79
      retroperitoneum D17.79
      specified site NEC D17.39
      spermatic cord D17.6
    face (skin) (subcutaneous) D17.0
    genitourinary organ NEC D17.72

Lipoma (Continued)
  site classification (Continued)
    head (skin) (subcutaneous) D17.0
    intra-abdominal D17.5
    intrathoracic D17.4
    kidney D17.71
    legs (skin) (subcutaneous) D17.2-
    neck (skin) (subcutaneous) D17.0
    peritoneum D17.79
    retroperitoneum D17.79
    skin D17.30
      specified site NEC D17.39
    specified site NEC D17.79
    spermatic cord D17.6
    subcutaneous D17.30
      specified site NEC D17.39
    trunk (skin) (subcutaneous) D17.1
    unspecified D17.9
  spindle cell D17.9
Lipomatosis E88.2
  dolorosa (Dercum) E88.2
  fetal —see Lipoma
  Launois-Bensaude E88.89
Lipomyoma —see Lipoma
Lipomyxoma —see Lipoma
Lipomyxosarcoma —see Neoplasm, connective tissue, malignant
Lipoprotein metabolism disorder E78.9
Lipoproteinemia E78.5
  broad-beta E78.2
  floating-beta E78.2
  hyper-pre-beta E78.1
Liposarcoma —see also Neoplasm, connective tissue, malignant
  dedifferentiated —see Neoplasm, connective tissue, malignant
  differentiated type —see Neoplasm, connective tissue, malignant
  embryonal —see Neoplasm, connective tissue, malignant
  mixed type —see Neoplasm, connective tissue, malignant
  myxoid —see Neoplasm, connective tissue, malignant
  pleomorphic —see Neoplasm, connective tissue, malignant
  round cell —see Neoplasm, connective tissue, malignant
  well differentiated type —see Neoplasm, connective tissue, malignant
Liposynovitis prepatellaris E88.89
Lipping, cervix N86
Lipschütz disease or ulcer N76.6
Lipuria R82.0
  schistosomiasis (bilharziasis) B65.0
Lisping F80.0
Lissauer's paralysis A52.17
Lissencephalia, lissencephaly Q04.3
Listeriosis, listerellosis A32.9
  congenital (disseminated) P37.2
  cutaneous A32.0
  neonatal, newborn (disseminated) P37.2
  oculoglandular A32.81
  specified NEC A32.89
Lithemia E79.0
Lithiasis —see Calculus
Lithosis J62.8
Lithuria R82.99
Litigation, anxiety concerning Z65.3
Little leaguer's elbow —see Epicondylitis, medial
Little's disease G80.9
Littre's
  gland —see condition
  hernia —see Hernia, abdomen
Littritis —see Urethritis
Livedo (annularis) (racemosa) (reticularis) R23.1
Liver —see condition
Living alone (problems with) Z60.2
  with handicapped person Z74.2

◄ New ◄║ Revised ~~deleted~~ Deleted

Lloyd's syndrome —*see* Adenomatosis, endocrine
Loa loa, loaiasis, loasis B74.3
Lobar —*see* condition
Lobomycosis B48.0
Lobo's disease B48.0
Lobotomy syndrome F07.0
Lobstein (-Ekman) disease or syndrome Q78.0
Lobster-claw hand Q71.6-
Lobulation (congenital) —*see also* Anomaly, by site
  kidney, Q63.1
  liver, abnormal Q44.7
  spleen Q89.09
Lobule, lobular —*see* condition
Local, localized —*see* condition
Locked twins causing obstructed labor O66.1
Locked-in state G83.5
Locking
  joint —*see* Derangement, joint, specified type NEC
    knee —*see* Derangement, knee
Lockjaw —*see* Tetanus
Löffler's
  endocarditis I42.3
  eosinophilia J82
  pneumonia J82
  syndrome (eosinophilic pneumonitis) J82
Loiasis (with conjunctival infestation) (eyelid) B74.3
Lone Star fever A77.0
Long
  labor O63.9
    first stage O63.0
    second stage O63.1
  QT syndrome I45.81
Long-term (current) (prophylactic) drug therapy (use of)
  agents affecting estrogen receptors and estrogen levels NEC Z79.818
  anastrozole (Arimidex) Z79.811
  antibiotics Z79.2
    short-term use - omit code
  anticoagulants Z79.01
  anti-inflammatory, non-steroidal (NSAID) Z79.1
  antiplatelet Z79.02
  antithrombotics Z79.02
  aromatase inhibitors Z79.811
  aspirin Z79.82
  birth control pill or patch Z79.3
  bisphosphonates Z79.83
  contraceptive, oral Z79.3
  drug, specified NEC Z79.899
  estrogen receptor downregulators Z79.818
  Evista Z79.810
  exemestane (Aromasin) Z79.811
  Fareston Z79.810
  fulvestrant (Faslodex) Z79.818
  gonadotropin-releasing hormone (GnRH) agonist Z79.818
  goserelin acetate (Zoladex) Z79.818
  hormone replacement (postmenopausal) Z79.890
  insulin Z79.4
  letrozole (Femara) Z79.811
  leuprolide acetate (leuprorelin) (Lupron) Z79.818
  megestrol acetate (Megace) Z79.818
  methadone for pain management Z79.891
  Nolvadex Z79.810
  non-steroidal anti-inflammatories (NSAID) Z79.1
  opiate analgesic Z79.891
  oral contraceptive Z79.3
  oral ◄
    antidiabetic Z79.84 ◄
    contraceptive Z79.3 ◄
    hypoglycemic Z79.84 ◄
  raloxifene (Evista) Z79.810

Long-term (*Continued*)
  selective estrogen receptor modulators (SERMs) Z79.810
  steroids
    inhaled Z79.51
    systemic Z79.52
  tamoxifen (Nolvadex) Z79.810
  toremifene (Fareston) Z79.810
Longitudinal stripes or grooves, nails L60.8
  congenital Q84.6
Loop
  intestine —*see* Volvulus
  vascular on papilla (optic) Q14.2
Loose —*see also* condition
  body
    joint M24.00
      ankle M24.07-
      elbow M24.02-
      hand M24.04-
      hip M24.05-
      knee M23.4-
      shoulder (region) M24.01-
      specified site NEC M24.08
      toe M24.07-
      vertebra M24.08
      wrist M24.03-
    knee M23.4-
    sheath, tendon —*see* Disorder, tendon, specified type NEC
  cartilage —*see* Loose, body, joint
  skin and subcutaneous tissue (following bariatric surgery weight loss) (following dietary weight loss) L98.7 ◄
  tooth, teeth K08.89 ◄▥
Loosening
  aseptic
    joint prosthesis —*see* Complications, joint prosthesis, mechanical, loosening, by site
  epiphysis —*see* Osteochondropathy
  mechanical
    joint prosthesis —*see* Complications, joint prosthesis, mechanical, loosening, by site
Looser-Milkman (-Debray) syndrome M83.8
Lop ear (deformity) Q17.3
Lorain (-Levi) short stature syndrome E23.0
Lordosis M40.50
  acquired —*see* Lordosis, specified type NEC
  congenital Q76.429
    lumbar region Q76.426
    lumbosacral region Q76.427
    sacral region Q76.428
    sacrococcygeal region Q76.428
    thoracolumbar region Q76.425
  lumbar region M40.56
  lumbosacral region M40.57
  postsurgical M96.4
  postural —*see* Lordosis, specified type NEC
  rachitic (late effect) (sequelae) E64.3
  sequelae of rickets E64.3
  specified type NEC M40.40
    lumbar region M40.46
    lumbosacral region M40.47
    thoracolumbar region M40.45
  thoracolumbar region M40.55
  tuberculous A18.01
Loss (of)
  appetite (*see* Anorexia) R63.0
    hysterical F50.89 ◄▥
    nonorganic origin F50.89 ◄▥
    psychogenic F50.89 ◄▥
  blood —*see* Hemorrhage
  bone —*see* Loss, substance of, bone ◄
  consciousness, transient R55
    traumatic —*see* Injury, intracranial
  control, sphincter, rectum R15.9
    nonorganic origin F98.1
  elasticity, skin R23.4

Loss (*Continued*)
  family (member) in childhood Z62.898
  fluid (acute) E86.9
    with
      hypernatremia E87.0
      hyponatremia E87.1
  function of labyrinth —*see* subcategory H83.2
  hair, nonscarring —*see* Alopecia
  hearing —*see also* Deafness
    central NOS H90.5
    conductive H90.2 ◄
      bilateral H90.0 ◄
      unilateral ◄
        with ◄
          restricted hearing on the contralateral side H90.A1- ◄
          unrestricted hearing on the contralateral side H90.1- ◄
    mixed conductive and sensorineural hearing loss H90.8 ◄
      bilateral H90.6 ◄
      unilateral ◄
        with ◄
          restricted hearing on the contralateral side H90.A3- ◄
          unrestricted hearing on the contralateral side H90.7- ◄
    neural NOS H90.5
    perceptive NOS H90.5
    sensorineural NOS H90.5
      bilateral H90.3 ◄
      unilateral ◄
        with ◄
          restricted hearing on the contralateral side H90.A2- ◄
          unrestricted hearing on the contralateral side H90.4- ◄
    sensory NOS H90.5
  height R29.890
  limb or member, traumatic, current —*see* Amputation, traumatic
  love relationship in childhood Z62.898
  memory —*see also* Amnesia
    mild, following organic brain damage F06.8
  mind —*see* Psychosis
  occlusal vertical dimension of fully erupted teeth M26.37
  organ or part —*see* Absence, by site, acquired
  ossicles, ear (partial) H74.32-
  parent in childhood Z63.4
  pregnancy, recurrent N96
    without current pregnancy N96
    care in current pregnancy O26.2-
  recurrent pregnancy —*see* Loss, pregnancy, recurrent
  self-esteem, in childhood Z62.898
  sense of
    smell —*see* Disturbance, sensation, smell
    taste —*see* Disturbance, sensation, taste
    touch R20.8
  sensory R44.9
    dissociative F44.6
  sexual desire F52.0
  sight (acquired) (complete) (congenital) —*see* Blindness
  substance of
    bone —*see* Disorder, bone, density and structure, specified NEC
      horizontal alveolar K06.3 ◄
    cartilage —*see* Disorder, cartilage, specified type NEC
      auricle (ear) —*see* Disorder, pinna, specified type NEC
    vitreous (humor) H15.89
  tooth, teeth —*see* Absence, teeth, acquired
  vision, visual H54.7
    both eyes H54.3
    one eye H54.60
      left (normal vision on right) H54.62
      right (normal vision on left) H54.61

◄ New   ◄▥ Revised   deleted Deleted

Loss *(Continued)*
　vision, visual *(Continued)*
　　specified as blindness —*see* Blindness
　　subjective
　　　sudden H53.13-
　　　transient H53.12-
　vitreous —*see* Prolapse, vitreous
　voice —*see* Aphonia
　weight (abnormal) (cause unknown) R63.4
Louis-Bar syndrome (ataxia-telangiectasia)
　G11.3
Louping ill (encephalitis) A84.8
Louse, lousiness —*see* Lice
Low
　achiever, school Z55.3
　back syndrome M54.5
　basal metabolic rate R94.8
　birthweight (2499 grams or less) P07.10
　　with weight of
　　　1000-1249 grams P07.14
　　　1250-1499 grams P07.15
　　　1500-1749 grams P07.16
　　　1750-1999 grams P07.17
　　　2000-2499 grams P07.18
　　extreme (999 grams or less) P07.00
　　　with weight of
　　　　499 grams or less P07.01
　　　　500-749 grams P07.02
　　　　750-999 grams P07.03
　　for gestational age —*see* Light for dates
　blood pressure —*see also* Hypotension
　　reading (incidental) (isolated) (nonspecific)
　　　R03.1
　cardiac reserve —*see* Disease, heart
　function —*see also* Hypofunction
　　kidney N28.9
　hematocrit D64.9
　hemoglobin D64.9
　income Z59.6
　level of literacy Z55.0
　lying
　　kidney N28.89
　　organ or site, congenital —*see* Malposition,
　　　congenital
　output syndrome (cardiac) —*see* Failure,
　　heart
　platelets (blood) —*see* Thrombocytopenia
　reserve, kidney N28.89
　salt syndrome E87.1
　self esteem R45.81
　set ears Q17.4
　vision H54.2
　　one eye (other eye normal) H54.50
　　　left (normal vision on right) H54.52
　　　other eye blind —*see* Blindness
　　　right (normal vision on left) H54.51
Low-density-lipoprotein-type (LDL)
　hyperlipoproteinemia E78.00 ◀▥▥▥
Lowe's syndrome E72.03
Lown-Ganong-Levine syndrome I45.6
LSD reaction (acute) (without dependence)
　F16.90
　with dependence F16.20
L-shaped kidney Q63.8
Ludwig's angina or disease K12.2
Lues (venerea), luetic —*see* Syphilis
Luetscher's syndrome (dehydration) E86.0
Lumbago, lumbalgia M54.5
　with sciatica M54.4-
　　due to intervertebral disc disorder
　　　M51.17
　due to displacement, intervertebral disc
　　M51.27
　　with sciatica M51.17
Lumbar —*see* condition
Lumbarization, vertebra, congenital Q76.49
Lumbermen's itch B88.0
Lump —*see* Mass
Lunacy —*see* Psychosis
Lung —*see* condition
Lupoid (miliary) of Boeck D86.3

Lupus
　anticoagulant D68.62
　　with
　　　hemorrhagic disorder D68.312
　　　hypercoagulable state D68.62
　　finding without diagnosis R76.0
　discoid (local) L93.0
　erythematosus (discoid) (local) L93.0
　　disseminated —*see* Lupus, erythematosus,
　　　systemic
　　eyelid H01.129
　　　left H01.126
　　　　lower H01.125
　　　　upper H01.124
　　　right H01.123
　　　　lower H01.122
　　　　upper H01.121
　　profundus L93.2
　　specified NEC L93.2
　　subacute cutaneous L93.1
　　systemic M32.9
　　　with organ or system involvement
　　　　M32.10
　　　　endocarditis M32.11
　　　　lung M32.13
　　　　pericarditis M32.12
　　　　renal (glomerular) M32.14
　　　　　tubulo-interstitial M32.15
　　　　specified organ or system NEC
　　　　　M32.19
　　　drug-induced M32.0
　　　inhibitor (presence of) D68.62
　　　　with
　　　　　hemorrhagic disorder D68.312
　　　　　hypercoagulable state D68.62
　　　　finding without diagnosis R76.0
　　　specified NEC M32.8
　exedens A18.4
　hydralazine M32.0
　　correct substance properly administered —
　　　see Table of Drugs and Chemicals, by
　　　drug, adverse effect
　　overdose or wrong substance given or
　　　taken —*see* Table of Drugs and
　　　Chemicals, by drug, poisoning
　nephritis (chronic) M32.14
　nontuberculous, not disseminated L93.0
　panniculitis L93.2
　pernio (Besnier) D86.3
　systemic —*see* Lupus, erythematosus,
　　systemic
　tuberculous A18.4
　　eyelid A18.4
　vulgaris A18.4
　　eyelid A18.4
Luteinoma D27.-
Lutembacher's disease or syndrome (atrial
　septal defect with mitral stenosis)
　Q21.1
Luteoma D27.-
Lutz (-Splendore-de Almeida) disease —*see*
　Paracoccidioidomycosis
Luxation —*see also* Dislocation
　eyeball (nontraumatic) —*see* Luxation, globe
　　birth injury P15.3
　globe, nontraumatic H44.82-
　lacrimal gland —*see* Dislocation, lacrimal
　　gland
　lens (old) (partial) (spontaneous)
　　congenital Q12.1
　　syphilitic A50.39
Lycanthropy F22
Lyell's syndrome L51.2
　due to drug L51.2
　　correct substance properly administered —
　　　see Table of Drugs and Chemicals, by
　　　drug, adverse effect
　　overdose or wrong substance given or
　　　taken —*see* Table of Drugs and
　　　Chemicals, by drug, poisoning
Lyme disease A69.20

Lymph
　gland or node —*see* condition
　scrotum —*see* Infestation, filarial
Lymphadenitis I88.9
　with ectopic or molar pregnancy O08.0
　acute L04.9
　　axilla L04.2
　　face L04.0
　　head L04.0
　　hip L04.3
　　limb
　　　lower L04.3
　　　upper L04.2
　　neck L04.0
　　shoulder L04.2
　　specified site NEC L04.8
　　trunk L04.1
　anthracosis (occupational) J60
　any site, except mesenteric I88.9
　　chronic I88.1
　　subacute I88.1
　breast
　　gestational —*see* Mastitis, obstetric
　　puerperal, postpartum (nonpurulent)
　　　O91.22
　chancroidal (congenital) A57
　chronic I88.1
　　mesenteric I88.0
　due to
　　Brugia (malayi) B74.1
　　　timori B74.2
　　chlamydial lymphogranuloma A55
　　diphtheria (toxin) A36.89
　　lymphogranuloma venereum A55
　　Wuchereria bancrofti B74.0
　following ectopic or molar pregnancy O08.0
　gonorrheal A54.89
　infective —*see* Lymphadenitis, acute
　mesenteric (acute) (chronic) (nonspecific)
　　(subacute) I88.0
　　due to Salmonella typhi A01.09
　　tuberculous A18.39
　mycobacterial A31.8
　purulent —*see* Lymphadenitis, acute
　pyogenic —*see* Lymphadenitis, acute
　regional, nonbacterial I88.8
　septic —*see* Lymphadenitis, acute
　subacute, unspecified site I88.1
　suppurative —*see* Lymphadenitis, acute
　syphilitic (early) (secondary) A51.49
　　late A52.79
　tuberculous —*see* Tuberculosis, lymph gland
　venereal (chlamydial) A55
Lymphadenoid goiter E06.3
Lymphadenopathy (generalized) R59.1
　angioimmunoblastic, with dysproteinemia
　　(AILD) C86.5
　due to toxoplasmosis (acquired) B58.89
　　congenital (acute) (subacute) (chronic)
　　　P37.1
　localized R59.0
　syphilitic (early) (secondary) A51.49
Lymphadenosis R59.1
Lymphangiectasis I89.0
　conjunctiva H11.89
　postinfectional I89.0
　scrotum I89.0
Lymphangiectatic elephantiasis, nonfilarial
　I89.0
Lymphangioendothelioma D18.1
　malignant —*see* Neoplasm, connective tissue,
　　malignant
Lymphangioleiomyomatosis J84.81
Lymphangioma D18.1
　capillary D18.1
　cavernous D18.1
　cystic D18.1
　malignant —*see* Neoplasm, connective tissue,
　　malignant
Lymphangiomyoma D18.1
Lymphangiomyomatosis J84.81

◀ New　◀▥▥▥ Revised　~~deleted~~ Deleted

Lymphangiosarcoma —*see* Neoplasm, connective tissue, malignant
Lymphangitis I89.1
 with
  abscess - code by site under Abscess
  cellulitis - code by site under Cellulitis
  ectopic or molar pregnancy O08.0
 acute L03.91
  abdominal wall L03.321
  ankle —*see* Lymphangitis, acute, lower limb
  arm —*see* Lymphangitis, acute, upper limb
  auricle (ear) —*see* Lymphangitis, acute, ear
  axilla L03.12-
  back (any part) L03.322
  buttock L03.327
  cervical (meaning neck) L03.222
  cheek (external) L03.212
  chest wall L03.323
  digit
   finger —*see* Lymphangitis, acute, finger
   toe —*see* Lymphangitis, acute, toe
  ear (external) H60.1-
  external auditory canal —*see* Lymphangitis, acute, ear
  eyelid —*see* Abscess, eyelid
  face NEC L03.212
  finger (intrathecal) (periosteal) (subcutaneous) (subcuticular) L03.02-
  foot —*see* Lymphangitis, acute, lower limb
  gluteal (region) L03.327
  groin L03.324
  hand —*see* Lymphangitis, acute, upper limb
  head NEC L03.891
   face (any part, except ear, eye and nose) L03.212
  heel —*see* Lymphangitis, acute, lower limb
  hip —*see* Lymphangitis, acute, lower limb
  jaw (region) L03.212
  knee —*see* Lymphangitis, acute, lower limb
  leg —*see* Lymphangitis, acute, lower limb
  lower limb L03.12-
   toe —*see* Lymphangitis, acute, toe
  navel L03.326
  neck (region) L03.222
  orbit, orbital —*see* Cellulitis, orbit
  pectoral (region) L03.323
  perineal, perineum L03.325
  scalp (any part) L03.891
  shoulder —*see* Lymphangitis, acute, upper limb
  specified site NEC L03.898
  thigh —*see* Lymphangitis, acute, lower limb
  thumb (intrathecal) (periosteal) (subcutaneous) (subcuticular) —*see* Lymphangitis, acute, finger
  toe (intrathecal) (periosteal) (subcutaneous) (subcuticular) L03.04-
  trunk L03.329
   abdominal wall L03.321
   back (any part) L03.322
   buttock L03.327
   chest wall L03.323
   groin L03.324
   perineal, perineum L03.325
   umbilicus L03.326
  umbilicus L03.326
  upper limb L03.12-
   axilla —*see* Lymphangitis, acute, axilla
   finger —*see* Lymphangitis, acute, finger
   thumb —*see* Lymphangitis, acute, finger
  wrist —*see* Lymphangitis, acute, upper limb
 breast
  gestational —*see* Mastitis, obstetric
 chancroidal A57
 chronic (any site) I89.1

Lymphangitis (*Continued*)
 due to
  Brugia (malayi) B74.1
   timori B74.2
  Wuchereria bancrofti B74.0
 following ectopic or molar pregnancy O08.89
 penis
  acute N48.29
  gonococcal (acute) (chronic) A54.09
 puerperal, postpartum, childbirth O86.89
 strumous, tuberculous A18.2
 subacute (any site) I89.1
 tuberculous —*see* Tuberculosis, lymph gland
Lymphatic (vessel) —*see* condition
Lymphatism E32.8
Lymphectasia I89.0
Lymphedema (acquired) —*see also* Elephantiasis
 congenital Q82.0
 hereditary (chronic) (idiopathic) Q82.0
 postmastectomy I97.2
 praecox I89.0
 secondary I89.0
 surgical NEC I97.89
  postmastectomy (syndrome) I97.2
Lymphoblastic —*see* condition
Lymphoblastoma (diffuse) —*see* Lymphoma, lymphoblastic (diffuse)
 giant follicular —*see* Lymphoma, lymphoblastic (diffuse)
 macrofollicular —*see* Lymphoma, lymphoblastic (diffuse)
Lymphocele I89.8
Lymphocytic
 chorioencephalitis (acute) (serous) A87.2
 choriomeningitis (acute) (serous) A87.2
 meningoencephalitis A87.2
Lymphocytoma, benign cutis L98.8
Lymphocytopenia D72.810
Lymphocytosis (symptomatic) D72.820
 infectious (acute) B33.8
Lymphoepithelioma —*see* Neoplasm, malignant, by site
Lymphogranuloma (malignant) —*see also* Lymphoma, Hodgkin
 chlamydial A55
 inguinale A55
 venereum (any site) (chlamydial) (with stricture of rectum) A55
Lymphogranulomatosis (malignant) —*see also* Lymphoma, Hodgkin
 benign (Boeck's sarcoid) (Schaumann's) D86.1
Lymphohistiocytosis, hemophagocytic (familial) D76.1
Lymphoid —*see* condition
Lymphoma (of) (malignant) C85.90
 adult T-cell (HTLV-1-associated) (acute variant) (chronic variant) (lymphomatoid variant) (smouldering variant) C91.5-
 anaplastic large cell
  ALK-negative C84.7-
  ALK-positive C84.6-
  CD30-positive C84.6-
  primary cutaneous C86.6
 angioimmunoblastic T-cell C86.5
 BALT C88.4
 B-cell C85.1-
 B-precursor C83.5-
 blastic NK-cell C86.4
 bronchial-associated lymphoid tissue [BALT-lymphoma] C88.4
 Burkitt (atypical) C83.7-
 Burkitt-like C83.7-
 centrocytic C83.1-
 cutaneous follicle center C82.6-
 cutaneous T-cell C84.A-
 diffuse follicle center C82.5-
 diffuse large cell C83.3-
  anaplastic C83.3-
  B-cell C83.3-

Lymphoma (*Continued*)
 diffuse large cell (*Continued*)
  CD30-positive C83.3-
  centroblastic C83.3-
  immunoblastic C83.3-
  plasmablastic C83.3-
  subtype not specified C83.3-
  T-cell rich C83.3-
 enteropathy-type (associated) (intestinal) T-cell C86.2
 extranodal marginal zone B-cell lymphoma of mucosa-associated lymphoid tissue [MALT-lymphoma] C88.4
 extranodal NK/T-cell, nasal type C86.0
 follicular C82.9-
  grade
   I C82.0-
   II C82.1-
   III C82.2-
   IIIa C82.3-
   IIIb C82.4-
  specified NEC C82.8-
 hepatosplenic T-cell (alpha-beta) (gamma-delta) C86.1
 histiocytic C85.9-
  true C96.A
 Hodgkin C81.9
  classical C81.7-
   lymphocyte-rich C81.4-
   lymphocytic depletion C81.3-
   mixed cellularity C81.2-
   nodular sclerosis C81.1-
   specified NEC C81.7-
  lymphocyte-rich (classical) C81.4- ◀
  lymphocyte depleted (classical) C81.3- ◀
  mixed cellularity (classical) C81.2- ◀
  nodular sclerosis (classical) C81.1- ◀
  specified NEC (classical) C81.7- ◀
  lymphocyte-rich classical C81.4-
  lymphocyte depleted classical C81.3-
  mixed cellularity classical C81.2-
  nodular
   lymphocyte predominant C81.0-
   sclerosis classical C81.1-
   sclerosis (classical) C81.1- ◀
 intravascular large B-cell C83.8-
 Lennert's C84.4-
 lymphoblastic (diffuse) C83.5-
 lymphoblastic B-cell C83.5-
 lymphoblastic T-cell C83.5-
 lymphoepithelioid C84.4-
 lymphoplasmacytic C83.0-
  with IgM-production C88.0
 MALT C88.4
 mantle cell C83.1-
 mature T-cell NEC C84.4-
 mature T/NK-cell C84.9-
  specified NEC C84.Z-
 mediastinal (thymic) large B-cell C85.2-
 Mediterranean C88.3
 mucosa-associated lymphoid tissue [MALT-lymphoma] C88.4
 NK/T cell C84.9-
 nodal marginal zone C83.0-
 non-follicular (diffuse) C83.9-
  specified NEC C83.8-
 non-Hodgkin —*see also* Lymphoma, by type C85.9-
  specified NEC C85.8-
 non-leukemic variant of B-CLL C83.0-
 peripheral T-cell, not classified C84.4-
 primary cutaneous
  anaplastic large cell C86.6
  CD30-positive large T-cell C86.6
 primary effusion B-cell C83.8-
 SALT C88.4
 skin-associated lymphoid tissue [SALT-lymphoma] C88.4

Lymphoma *(Continued)*
    small cell B-cell C83.Ø-
    splenic marginal zone C83.Ø-
    subcutaneous panniculitis-like T-cell
        C86.3
    T-precursor C83.5-
    true histiocytic C96.A
Lymphomatosis *—see* Lymphoma

Lymphopathia venereum, veneris A55
Lymphopenia D72.81Ø
Lymphoplasmacytic leukemia *—see* Leukemia,
    chronic lymphocytic, B-cell type
Lymphoproliferation, X-linked disease
    D82.3
Lymphoreticulosis, benign (of inoculation)
    A28.1

Lymphorrhea I89.8
Lymphosarcoma (diffuse) *—see also* Lymphoma
    C85.9-
Lymphostasis I89.8
Lypemania *—see* Melancholia
Lysine and hydroxylysine metabolism
    disorder E72.3
Lyssa *—see* Rabies

◀ New   ◀▥ Revised   ~~deleted~~ Deleted

M

Macacus ear Q17.3
Maceration, wet feet, tropical (syndrome) T69.02-
MacLeod's syndrome J43.0
Macrocephalia, macrocephaly Q75.3
Macrocheilia, macrochilia (congenital)Q18.6
Macrocolon —see also Megacolon Q43.1
Macrocornea Q15.8
    with glaucoma Q15.0
Macrocytic —see condition
Macrocytosis D75.89
Macrodactylia, macrodactylism (fingers) (thumbs) Q74.0
    toes Q74.2
Macrodontia K00.2
Macrogenia M26.05
Macrogenitosomia (adrenal) (male) (praecox) E25.9
    congenital E25.0
Macroglobulinemia (idiopathic) (primary) C88.0
    monoclonal (essential) D47.2
    Waldenström C88.0
Macroglossia (congenital) Q38.2
    acquired K14.8
Macrognathia, macrognathism (congenital) (mandibular) (maxillary) M26.09
Macrogyria (congenital) Q04.8
Macrohydrocephalus —see Hydrocephalus
Macromastia —see Hypertrophy, breast
Macrophthalmos Q11.3
    in congenital glaucoma Q15.0
Macropsia H53.15
Macrosigmoid K59.39 ◀▥
    congenital Q43.2
Macrospondylitis, acromegalic E22.0
Macrostomia (congenital) Q18.4
Macrotia (external ear) (congenital) Q17.1
Macula
    cornea, corneal —see Opacity, cornea
    degeneration (atrophic) (exudative) (senile) —see also Degeneration, macula
    hereditary —see Dystrophy, retina
Maculae ceruleae — B85.1
Maculopathy, toxic —see Degeneration, macula, toxic
Madarosis (eyelid) H02.729
    left H02.726
        lower H02.725
        upper H02.724
    right H02.723
        lower H02.722
        upper H02.721
Madelung's
    deformity (radius) Q74.0
    disease
        radial deformity Q74.0
        symmetrical lipomas, neck E88.89
Madness —see Psychosis
Madura
    foot B47.9
        actinomycotic B47.1
        mycotic B47.0
Maduromycosis B47.0
Maffucci's syndrome Q78.4
Magnesium metabolism disorder —see Disorder, metabolism, magnesium
Main en griffe (acquired) —see also Deformity, limb, clawhand
    congenital Q74.0
Maintenance (encounter for)
    antineoplastic chemotherapy Z51.11
    antineoplastic radiation therapy Z51.0
    methadone F11.20
Majocchi's
    disease L81.7
    granuloma B35.8
Major —see condition
Malabar itch (any site) B35.5

Malabsorption K90.9
    calcium K90.89
    carbohydrate K90.49 ◀▥
    disaccharide E73.9
    fat K90.49 ◀▥
    galactose E74.20
    glucose(-galactose) E74.39
    intestinal K90.9
        specified NEC K90.89
    isomaltose E74.31
    lactose E73.9
    methionine E72.19
    monosaccharide E74.39
    postgastrectomy K91.2
    postsurgical K91.2
    protein K90.49 ◀▥
    starch K90.49 ◀▥
    sucrose E74.39
    syndrome K90.9
        postsurgical K91.2
Malacia, bone (adult) M83.9
    juvenile —see Rickets
Malacoplakia
    bladder N32.89
    pelvis (kidney) N28.89
    ureter N28.89
    urethra N36.8
Malacosteon, juvenile —see Rickets
Maladaptation —see Maladjustment
Maladie de Roger Q21.0
Maladjustment
    conjugal Z63.0
        involving divorce or estrangement Z63.5
    educational Z55.4
    family Z63.9
    marital Z63.0
        involving divorce or estrangement Z63.5
    occupational NEC Z56.89
    simple, adult —see Disorder, adjustment
    situational —see Disorder, adjustment
    social Z60.9
        due to
            acculturation difficulty Z60.3
            discrimination and persecution (perceived) Z60.5
            exclusion and isolation Z60.4
            life-cycle (phase of life) transition Z60.0
            rejection Z60.4
            specified reason NEC Z60.8
Malaise R53.81
Malakoplakia —see Malacoplakia
Malaria, malarial (fever) B54
    with
        blackwater fever B50.8
            hemoglobinuric (bilious) B50.8
            hemoglobinuria B50.8
    accidentally induced (therapeutically) - code by type under Malaria
    algid B50.9
    cerebral B50.0 [G94]
    clinically diagnosed (without parasitological confirmation) B54
    congenital NEC P37.4
        falciparum P37.3
    congestion, congestive B54
    continued (fever) B50.9
    estivo-autumnal B50.9
    falciparum B50.9
        with complications NEC B50.8
            cerebral B50.0 [G94]
        severe B50.8
    hemorrhagic B54
    malariae B52.9
        with
            complications NEC B52.8
            glomerular disorder B52.0
    malignant (tertian) —see Malaria, falciparum
    mixed infections — code to first listed type in B50-B53
    ovale B53.0
    parasitologically confirmed NEC B53.8

Malaria, malarial (Continued)
    pernicious, acute —see Malaria, falciparum
    Plasmodium (P.)
        falciparum NEC —see Malaria, falciparum
        malariae NEC B52.9
            with Plasmodium
                falciparum (and or vivax) —see Malaria, falciparum
                vivax —see also Malaria, vivax
                    and falciparum —see Malaria, falciparum
        ovale B53.0
            with Plasmodium malariae —see also Malaria, malariae
                and vivax —see also Malaria, vivax
                    and falciparum —see Malaria, falciparum
        simian B53.1
            with Plasmodium malariae —see also Malaria, malariae
                and vivax —see also Malaria, vivax
                    and falciparum —see Malaria, falciparum
        vivax NEC B51.9
            with Plasmodium falciparum —see Malaria, falciparum
    quartan —see Malaria, malariae
    quotidian —see Malaria, falciparum
    recurrent B54
    remittent B54
    specified type NEC (parasitologically confirmed) B53.8
    spleen B54
    subtertian (fever) —see Malaria, falciparum
    tertian (benign) —see also Malaria, vivax
        malignant B50.9
    tropical B50.9
    typhoid B54
    vivax B51.9
        with
            complications NEC B51.8
            ruptured spleen B51.0
Malassez's disease (cystic) N50.89 ◀▥
Malassimilation K90.9
Mal de los pintos —see Pinta
Mal de mer T75.3
Maldescent, testis Q53.9
    bilateral Q53.20
        abdominal Q53.21
        perineal Q53.22
    unilateral Q53.10
        abdominal Q53.11
        perineal Q53.12
Maldevelopment —see also Anomaly
    brain Q07.9
    colon Q43.9
    hip Q74.2
        congenital dislocation Q65.2
            bilateral Q65.1
            unilateral Q65.0-
    mastoid process Q75.8
    middle ear Q16.4
        except ossicles Q16.4
        ossicles Q16.3
    ossicles Q16.3
    spine Q76.49
    toe Q74.2
Male type pelvis Q74.2
    with disproportion (fetopelvic) O33.3
        causing obstructed labor O65.3
Malformation (congenital) —see also Anomaly
    adrenal gland Q89.1
    affecting multiple systems with skeletal changes NEC Q87.5
    alimentary tract Q45.9
        specified type NEC Q45.8
        upper Q40.9
            specified type NEC Q40.8
    aorta Q25.40 ◀▥
        absence Q25.41 ◀
        aneurysm, congenital Q25.43 ◀

Malformation (Continued)
- aorta (Continued)
  - aplasia Q25.41 ◀
  - atresia Q25.29 ◀▥
    - aortic arch Q25.21 ◀
  - coarctation (preductal) (postductal) Q25.1
  - dilatation, congenital Q25.44 ◀
  - hypoplasia Q25.42 ◀
  - patent ductus arteriosus Q25.0
  - specified type NEC Q25.49 ◀▥
  - stenosis Q25.1 ◀▥
    - supravalvular Q25.3 ◀
- aortic valve Q23.9
  - specified NEC Q23.8
- arteriovenous, aneurysmatic (congenital) Q27.30
  - brain Q28.2
  - cerebral Q28.2
  - peripheral Q27.30
    - digestive system Q27.33
    - lower limb Q27.32
    - other specified site Q27.39
    - renal vessel Q27.34
    - upper limb Q27.31
  - precerebral vessels (nonruptured) Q28.0
- auricle
  - ear (congenital) Q17.3
    - acquired H61.119
      - left H61.112
        - with right H61.113
      - right H61.111
        - with left H61.113
- bile duct Q44.5
- bladder Q64.79
  - aplasia Q64.5
  - diverticulum Q64.6
  - exstrophy —see Exstrophy, bladder
  - neck obstruction Q64.31
- bone Q79.9
  - face Q75.9
    - specified type NEC Q75.8
  - skull Q75.9
    - specified type NEC Q75.8
- brain (multiple) Q04.9
  - arteriovenous Q28.2
  - specified type NEC Q04.8
- branchial cleft Q18.2
- breast Q83.9
  - specified type NEC Q83.8
- broad ligament Q50.6
- bronchus Q32.4
- bursa Q79.9
- cardiac
  - chambers Q20.9
    - specified type NEC Q20.8
  - septum Q21.9
    - specified type NEC Q21.8
- cerebral Q04.9
  - vessels Q28.3
- cervix uteri Q51.9
  - specified type NEC Q51.828
- Chiari
  - Type I G93.5
  - Type II Q07.01
- choroid (congenital) Q14.3
  - plexus Q07.8
- circulatory system Q28.9
- cochlea Q16.5
- cornea Q13.4
- coronary vessels Q24.5
- corpus callosum (congenital) Q04.0
- diaphragm Q79.1
- digestive system NEC, specified type NEC Q45.8
- dura Q07.9
  - brain Q04.9
  - spinal Q06.9
- ear Q17.9
  - causing impairment of hearing Q16.9

Malformation (Continued)
- ear (Continued)
  - external Q17.9
    - accessory auricle Q17.0
    - causing impairment of hearing Q16.9
      - absence of
        - auditory canal Q16.1
        - auricle Q16.0
    - macrotia Q17.1
    - microtia Q17.2
    - misplacement Q17.4
    - misshapen NEC Q17.3
    - prominence Q17.5
    - specified type NEC Q17.8
  - inner Q16.5
  - middle Q16.4
    - absence of eustachian tube Q16.2
    - ossicles (fusion) Q16.3
  - ossicles Q16.3
  - specified type NEC Q17.8
- epididymis Q55.4
- esophagus Q39.9
  - specified type NEC Q39.8
- eye Q15.9
  - lid Q10.3
  - specified NEC Q15.8
- fallopian tube Q50.6
- genital organ —see Anomaly, genitalia
- great
  - artery Q25.9
    - aorta —see Malformation, aorta
    - pulmonary artery —see Malformation, pulmonary, artery
    - specified type NEC Q25.8
  - vein Q26.9
    - anomalous
      - portal venous connection Q26.5
      - pulmonary venous connection Q26.4
        - partial Q26.3
        - total Q26.2
    - persistent left superior vena cava Q26.1
    - portal vein-hepatic artery fistula Q26.6
    - specified type NEC Q26.8
    - vena cava stenosis, congenital Q26.0
- gum Q38.6
- hair Q84.2
- heart Q24.9
  - specified type NEC Q24.8
- integument Q84.9
  - specified type NEC Q84.8
- internal ear Q16.5
- intestine Q43.9
  - specified type NEC Q43.8
- iris Q13.2
- joint Q74.9
  - ankle Q74.2
  - lumbosacral Q76.49
  - sacroiliac Q74.2
  - specified type NEC Q74.8
- kidney Q63.9
  - accessory Q63.0
  - giant Q63.3
  - horseshoe Q63.1
  - hydronephrosis Q62.0
  - malposition Q63.2
  - specified type NEC Q63.8
- lacrimal apparatus Q10.6
- lingual Q38.3
- lip Q38.0
- liver Q44.7
- lung Q33.9
- meninges or membrane (congenital) Q07.9
  - cerebral Q04.8
  - spinal (cord) Q06.9
- middle ear Q16.4
  - ossicles Q16.3
- mitral valve Q23.9
  - specified NEC Q23.8
- Mondini's (congenital) (malformation, cochlea) Q16.5

Malformation (Continued)
- mouth (congenital) Q38.6
- multiple types NEC Q89.7
- musculoskeletal system Q79.9
- myocardium Q24.8
- nail Q84.6
- nervous system (central) Q07.9
- nose Q30.9
  - specified type NEC Q30.8
- optic disc Q14.2
- orbit Q10.7
- ovary Q50.39
- palate Q38.5
- parathyroid gland Q89.2
- pelvic organs or tissues NEC
  - in pregnancy or childbirth O34.8-
    - causing obstructed labor O65.5
- penis Q55.69
  - aplasia Q55.5
  - curvature (lateral) Q55.61
  - hypoplasia Q55.62
- pericardium Q24.8
- peripheral vascular system Q27.9
  - specified type NEC Q27.8
- pharynx Q38.8
- precerebral vessels Q28.1
- prostate Q55.4
- pulmonary
  - arteriovenous Q25.72
  - artery Q25.9
    - atresia Q25.5
    - specified type NEC Q25.79
    - stenosis Q25.6
  - valve Q22.3
- renal artery Q27.2
- respiratory system Q34.9
- retina Q14.1
- scrotum —see Malformation, testis and scrotum
- seminal vesicles Q55.4
- sense organs NEC Q07.9
- skin Q82.9
- specified NEC Q89.8
- spinal
  - cord Q06.9
  - nerve root Q07.8
- spine Q76.49
  - kyphosis —see Kyphosis, congenital
  - lordosis —see Lordosis, congenital
- spleen Q89.09
- stomach Q40.3
  - specified type NEC Q40.2
- teeth, tooth K00.9
- tendon Q79.9
- testis and scrotum Q55.20
  - aplasia Q55.0
  - hypoplasia Q55.1
  - polyorchism Q55.21
  - retractile testis Q55.22
  - scrotal transposition Q55.23
  - specified NEC Q55.29
- thorax, bony Q76.9
- throat Q38.8
- thyroid gland Q89.2
- tongue (congenital) Q38.3
  - hypertrophy Q38.2
  - tie Q38.1
- trachea Q32.1
- tricuspid valve Q22.9
  - specified type NEC Q22.8
- umbilical cord NEC (complicating delivery) O69.89
- umbilicus Q89.9
- ureter Q62.8
  - agenesis Q62.4
  - duplication Q62.5
  - malposition —see Malposition, congenital, ureter
  - obstructive defect —see Defect, obstructive, ureter
  - vesico-uretero-renal reflux Q62.7

◀ New   ◀▥ Revised   ~~deleted~~ Deleted

Malformation *(Continued)*
  urethra Q64.79
    aplasia Q64.5
    duplication Q64.74
    posterior valves Q64.2
    prolapse Q64.71
    stricture Q64.32
  urinary system Q64.9
  uterus Q51.9
    specified type NEC Q51.818
  vagina Q52.4
  vascular system, peripheral Q27.9
  vas deferens Q55.4
    atresia Q55.3
  venous —*see* Anomaly, vein (s)
  vulva Q52.70
Malfunction —*see also* Dysfunction
  cardiac electronic device T82.119
    electrode T82.110
    pulse generator T82.111
    specified type NEC T82.118
  catheter device NEC T85.618
    cystostomy T83.010
    dialysis (renal) (vascular) T82.41
      intraperitoneal T85.611
    infusion NEC T82.514
      cranial T85.610 ◀
      epidural T85.610 ◀
      intrathecal T85.610 ◀
      spinal T85.610 ◀▥
      subarachnoid T85.610 ◀
      subdural T85.610 ◀
      ~~urinary, indwelling T83.018~~
    urinary —*see also* Breakdown, device,
      catheter T83.018 ◀
  colostomy K94.03
    valve K94.03
  cystostomy (stoma) N99.512
    catheter T83.010
  enteric stoma K94.13
  enterostomy K94.13
  esophagostomy K94.33
  gastroenteric K31.89
  gastrostomy K94.23
  ileostomy K94.13
    valve K94.13
  intrathecal infusion pump T85.615 ◀
  jejunostomy K94.13
  nervous system device, implant or graft,
    specified NEC T85.615 ◀
  pacemaker —*see* Malfunction, cardiac
    electronic device
  prosthetic device, internal —*see*
    Complications, prosthetic device, by
    site, mechanical
  tracheostomy J95.03
  urinary device NEC —*see* Complication,
    genitourinary, device, urinary,
    mechanical
  valve
    colostomy K94.03
    heart T82.09
    ileostomy K94.13
  vascular graft or shunt NEC —*see*
    Complication, cardiovascular device,
    mechanical, vascular
  ventricular (communicating shunt) T85.01
Malherbe's tumor —*see* Neoplasm, skin, benign
Malibu disease L98.8-
Malignancy —*see also* Neoplasm, malignant,
    by site
  unspecified site (primary) C80.1
Malignant —*see* condition
Malingerer, malingering Z76.5
Mallet finger (acquired) —*see* Deformity, finger,
    mallet finger
  congenital Q74.0
  sequelae of rickets E64.3
Malleus A24.0
Mallory's bodies R89.7
Mallory-Weiss syndrome K22.6

Malnutrition E46
  degree
    first E44.1
    mild (protein) E44.1
    moderate (protein) E44.0
    second E44.0
    severe (protein-energy) E43
      intermediate form E42
        with
          kwashiorkor (and marasmus) E42
          marasmus E41
    third E43
  following gastrointestinal surgery K91.2
  intrauterine
    light-for-dates —*see* Light for dates
    small-for-dates —*see* Small for dates
  lack of care, or neglect (child) (infant) T76.02
    confirmed T74.02
  malignant E40
  protein E46
    calorie E46
      mild E44.1
      moderate E44.0
      severe E43
        intermediate form E42
          with
            kwashiorkor (and marasmus)
              E42
            marasmus E41
    energy E46
      mild E44.1
      moderate E44.0
      severe E43
        intermediate form E42
          with
            kwashiorkor (and marasmus)
              E42
            marasmus E41
  severe (protein-energy) E43
    with
      kwashiorkor (and marasmus) E42
      marasmus E41
Malocclusion (teeth) M26.4
  Angle's M26.219
    class I M26.211
    class II M26.212
    class III M26.213
  due to
    abnormal swallowing M26.59
    mouth breathing M26.59
    tongue, lip or finger habits M26.59
  temporomandibular (joint) M26.69
Malposition
  cervix —*see* Malposition, uterus
  congenital
    adrenal (gland) Q89.1
    alimentary tract Q45.8
      lower Q43.8
      upper Q40.8
    aorta Q25.49 ◀▥
    appendix Q43.8
    arterial trunk Q20.0
    artery (peripheral) Q27.8
      coronary Q24.5
      digestive system Q27.8
      lower limb Q27.8
      pulmonary Q25.79
      specified site NEC Q27.8
      upper limb Q27.8
    auditory canal Q17.8
      causing impairment of hearing Q16.9
    auricle (ear) Q17.4
      causing impairment of hearing Q16.9
    cervical Q18.2
    biliary duct or passage Q44.5
    bladder (mucosa) —*see* Exstrophy,
      bladder
    brachial plexus Q07.8
    brain tissue Q04.8
    breast Q83.8
    bronchus Q32.4

Malposition *(Continued)*
  congenital *(Continued)*
    cecum Q43.8
    clavicle Q74.0
    colon Q43.8
    digestive organ or tract NEC Q45.8
      lower Q43.8
      upper Q40.8
    ear (auricle) (external) Q17.4
      ossicles Q16.3
    endocrine (gland) NEC Q89.2
    epiglottis Q31.8
    eustachian tube Q17.8
    eye Q15.8
    facial features Q18.8
    fallopian tube Q50.6
    finger (s) Q68.1
      supernumerary Q69.0
    foot Q66.9
    gallbladder Q44.1
    gastrointestinal tract Q45.8
    genitalia, genital organ (s) or tract
      female Q52.8
        external Q52.79
        internal NEC Q52.8
      male Q55.8
    glottis Q31.8
    hand Q68.1
    heart Q24.8
      dextrocardia Q24.0
        with complete transposition of viscera
          Q89.3
    hepatic duct Q44.5
    hip (joint) Q65.89
    intestine (large) (small) Q43.8
      with anomalous adhesions, fixation or
        malrotation Q43.3
    joint NEC Q68.8
    kidney Q63.2
    larynx Q31.8
    limb Q68.8
      lower Q68.8
      upper Q68.8
    liver Q44.7
    lung (lobe) Q33.8
    nail (s) Q84.6
    nerve Q07.8
    nervous system NEC Q07.8
    nose, nasal (septum) Q30.8
    organ or site not listed —*see* Anomaly,
      by site
    ovary Q50.39
    pancreas Q45.3
    parathyroid (gland) Q89.2
    patella Q74.1
    peripheral vascular system Q27.8
    pituitary (gland) Q89.2
    respiratory organ or system NEC
      Q34.8
    rib (cage) Q76.6
      supernumerary in cervical region
        Q76.5
    scapula Q74.0
    shoulder Q74.0
    spinal cord Q06.8
    spleen Q89.09
    sternum NEC Q76.7
    stomach Q40.2
    symphysis pubis Q74.2
    thymus (gland) Q89.2
    thyroid (gland) (tissue) Q89.2
      cartilage Q31.8
    toe (s) Q66.9
      supernumerary Q69.2
    tongue Q38.3
    trachea Q32.1
    ureter Q62.60
      deviation Q62.61
      displacement Q62.62
      ectopia Q62.63
      specified type NEC Q62.69

M

Malposition (Continued)
  congenital (Continued)
    uterus Q51.818
    vein (s) (peripheral) Q27.8
      great Q26.8
    vena cava (inferior) (superior) Q26.8
  device, implant or graft —see also
      Complications, by site and type,
      mechanical T85.628
    arterial graft NEC —see Complication,
      cardiovascular device, mechanical,
      vascular
    breast (implant) T85.42
    catheter NEC T85.628
      cystostomy T83.020
      dialysis (renal) T82.42
        intraperitoneal T85.621
      infusion NEC T82.524
        spinal (epidural) (subdural) T85.620
      urinary, indwelling T83.028
      urinary —see also Displacement, device,
        catheter, urinary T83.028 ◄
    electronic (electrode) (pulse generator)
      (stimulator)
      bone T84.320
      cardiac T82.129
        electrode T82.120
        pulse generator T82.121
        specified type NEC T82.128
      nervous system —see Complication,
        prosthetic device, mechanical,
        electronic nervous system
        stimulator
      urinary —see Complication,
        genitourinary, device, urinary,
        mechanical
    fixation, internal (orthopedic) NEC —see
      Complication, fixation device,
      mechanical
    gastrointestinal —see Complications,
      prosthetic device, mechanical,
      gastrointestinal device
    genital NEC T83.428
      intrauterine contraceptive device (string)
        T83.32 ◄║║
      penile prosthesis (cylinder) (implanted)
        (pump) (resevoir) T83.420 ◄║║
      testicular prosthesis T83.421 ◄
    heart NEC —see Complication,
      cardiovascular device, mechanical
    joint prosthesis —see Complication, joint
      prosthesis, mechanical
    ocular NEC —see Complications, prosthetic
      device, mechanical, ocular device
    orthopedic NEC —see Complication,
      orthopedic, device, mechanical
    specified NEC T85.628
    urinary NEC —see also Complication,
      genitourinary, device, urinary,
      mechanical
      graft T83.22
    vascular NEC —see Complication,
      cardiovascular device, mechanical
    ventricular intracranial shunt T85.02
  fetus —see Pregnancy, complicated by
    (management affected by), presentation,
    fetal
  gallbladder K82.8
  gastrointestinal tract, congenital Q45.8
  heart, congenital NEC Q24.8
  joint prosthesis —see Complications, joint
    prosthesis, mechanical, displacement,
    by site
  stomach K31.89
    congenital Q40.2
  tooth, teeth, fully erupted M26.30
  uterus (acute) (acquired) (adherent)
    (asymptomatic) (postinfectional)
    (postpartal, old) N85.4
    anteflexion or anteversion N85.4
      congenital Q51.818

Malposition (Continued)
  uterus (Continued)
    flexion N85.4
      lateral —see Lateroversion, uterus
    inversion N85.5
    lateral (flexion) (version) —see
      Lateroversion, uterus
    in pregnancy or childbirth —see
      subcategory O34.5
    retroflexion or retroversion —see
      Retroversion, uterus
Malposture R29.3
Malrotation
  cecum Q43.3
  colon Q43.3
  intestine Q43.3
  kidney Q63.2
Malta fever —see Brucellosis
Maltreatment
  adult
    abandonment
      confirmed T74.01
      suspected T76.01
    confirmed T74.91
    history of Z91.419
    neglect
      confirmed T74.01
      suspected T76.01
    physical abuse
      confirmed T74.11
      suspected T76.11
    psychological abuse
      confirmed T74.31
      history of Z91.411
      suspected T76.31
    sexual abuse
      confirmed T74.21
      suspected T76.21
    suspected T76.91
  child
    abandonment
      confirmed T74.02
      suspected T76.02
    confirmed T74.92
    history of —see History, personal (of),
      abuse
    neglect
      confirmed T74.02
      history of —see History, personal (of),
        abuse
      suspected T76.02
    physical abuse
      confirmed T74.12
      history of —see History, personal (of),
        abuse
      suspected T76.12
    psychological abuse
      confirmed T74.32
      history of —see History, personal (of),
        abuse
      suspected T76.32
    sexual abuse
      confirmed T74.22
      history of —see History, personal (of),
        abuse
      suspected T76.22
    suspected T76.92
    personal history of Z91.89
Maltworker's lung J67.4
Malunion, fracture —see Fracture, by site
Mammillitis N61.0 ◄║║
  puerperal, postpartum O91.02
Mammitis —see Mastitis
Mammogram (examination) Z12.39
  routine Z12.31
Mammoplasia N62
Management (of)
  bone conduction hearing device (implanted)
    Z45.320
  cardiac pacemaker NEC Z45.018
  cerebrospinal fluid drainage device Z45.41

Management (Continued)
  cochlear device (implanted) Z45.321
  contraceptive Z30.9
    specified NEC Z30.8
  implanted device Z45.9
    specified NEC Z45.89
  infusion pump Z45.1
  procreative Z31.9
    male factor infertility in female Z31.81
    specified NEC Z31.89
  prosthesis (external) —see also Fitting Z44.9
    implanted Z45.9
      specified NEC Z45.89
  renal dialysis catheter Z49.01
  vascular access device Z45.2
Mangled —see specified injury by site
Mania (monopolar) —see also Disorder, mood,
  manic episode
  with psychotic symptoms F30.2
  without psychotic symptoms F30.10
    mild F30.11
    moderate F30.12
    severe F30.13
  Bell's F30.8
  chronic (recurrent) F31.89
  hysterical F44.89
  puerperal F30.8
  recurrent F31.89
Manic-depressive insanity, psychosis, or
  syndrome —see Disorder, bipolar
Mannosidosis E77.1
Mansonelliasis, mansonellosis B74.4
Manson's
  disease B65.1
  schistosomiasis B65.1
Manual —see condition
Maple-bark-stripper's lung (disease) J67.6
Maple-syrup-urine disease E71.0
Marable's syndrome (celiac artery
  compression) I77.4
Marasmus E41
  due to malnutrition E41
  intestinal E41
  nutritional E41
  senile R54
  tuberculous NEC —see Tuberculosis
Marble
  bones Q78.2
  skin R23.8
Marburg virus disease A98.3
March
  fracture —see Fracture, traumatic, stress, by
    site
  hemoglobinuria D59.6
Marchesani (-Weill) syndrome Q87.0
Marchiafava (-Bignami) syndrome or disease
  G37.1
Marchiafava-Micheli syndrome D59.5
Marcus Gunn's syndrome Q07.8
Marfan's syndrome —see Syndrome, Marfan's
Marie-Bamberger disease —see
  Osteoarthropathy, hypertrophic, specified
  NEC
Marie-Charcot-Tooth neuropathic muscular
  atrophy G60.0
Marie's
  cerebellar ataxia (late-onset) G11.2
  disease or syndrome (acromegaly) E22.0
Marie-Strümpell arthritis, disease or
  spondylitis —see Spondylitis, ankylosing
Marion's disease (bladder neck obstruction)
  N32.0
Marital conflict Z63.0
Mark
  port wine Q82.5
  raspberry Q82.5
  strawberry Q82.5
  stretch L90.6
  tattoo L81.8
Marker heterochromatin —see Extra, marker
  chromosomes

Maroteaux-Lamy syndrome (mild) (severe)
E76.29
Marrow (bone)
arrest D61.9
poor function D75.89
Marseilles fever A77.1
Marsh fever —see Malaria
Marshall's (hidrotic) ectodermal dysplasia
Q82.4
Marsh's disease (exophthalmic goiter) E05.00
with storm E05.01
Masculinization (female) with adrenal
hyperplasia E25.9
congenital E25.0
Masculinovoblastoma D27.-
Masochism (sexual) F65.51
Mason's lung J62.8
Mass
abdominal R19.00
epigastric R19.06
generalized R19.07
left lower quadrant R19.04
left upper quadrant R19.02
periumbilic R19.05
right lower quadrant R19.03
right upper quadrant R19.01
specified site NEC R19.09
breast N63
chest R22.2
cystic —see Cyst
ear H93.8-
head R22.0
intra-abdominal (diffuse) (generalized) —see
Mass, abdominal
kidney N28.89
liver R16.0
localized (skin) R22.9
chest R22.2
head R22.0
limb
lower R22.4-
upper R22.3-
neck R22.1
trunk R22.2
lung R91.8
malignant —see Neoplasm, malignant, by site
neck R22.1
pelvic (diffuse) (generalized) —see Mass,
abdominal
specified organ NEC —see Disease, by site
splenic R16.1
substernal thyroid —see Goiter
superficial (localized) R22.9
umbilical (diffuse) (generalized) R19.09
Massive —see condition
Mast cell
disease, systemic tissue D47.0
leukemia C94.3-
sarcoma C96.2
tumor D47.0
malignant C96.2
Mastalgia N64.4
Masters-Allen syndrome N83.8
Mastitis (acute) (diffuse) (nonpuerperal)
(subacute) N61.0 ◀▥
with abscess N61.1 ◀
chronic (cystic) —see Mastopathy, cystic
cystic (Schimmelbusch's type) —see
Mastopathy, cystic
fibrocystic —see Mastopathy, cystic
infective N61.0 ◀▥
newborn P39.0
interstitial, gestational or puerperal —see
Mastitis, obstetric
neonatal (noninfective) P83.4
infective P39.0
obstetric (interstitial) (nonpurulent)
associated with
lactation O91.23
pregnancy O91.21-
puerperium O91.22

Mastitis (Continued)
obstetric (Continued)
purulent
associated with
lactation O91.13
pregnancy O91.11-
puerperium O91.12
periductal —see Ectasia, mammary duct
phlegmonous —see Mastopathy, cystic
plasma cell —see Ectasia, mammary duct
without abscess N61.0 ◀
Mastocytoma D47.0
malignant C96.2
Mastocytosis Q82.2
aggressive systemic C96.2
indolent systemic D47.0
malignant C96.2
systemic, associated with clonal hematopoetic
non-mast-cell disease (SM-AHNMD)
D47.0
Mastodynia N64.4
Mastoid —see condition
Mastoidalgia —see subcategory H92.0
Mastoiditis (coalescent) (hemorrhagic)
(suppurative) H70.9-
acute, subacute H70.00-
complicated NEC H70.09-
subperiosteal H70.01-
chronic (necrotic) (recurrent) H70.1-
in (due to)
infectious disease NEC B99 [H75.0-]
parasitic disease NEC B89 [H75.0-]
tuberculosis A18.03
petrositis —see Petrositis
postauricular fistula —see Fistula,
postauricular
specified NEC H70.89-
tuberculous A18.03
Mastopathy, mastopathia N64.9
chronica cystica —see Mastopathy, cystic
cystic (chronic) (diffuse) N60.1
with epithelial proliferation N60.3-
diffuse cystic —see Mastopathy, cystic
estrogenic, oestrogenica N64.89
ovarian origin N64.89
Mastoplasia, mastoplastia N62
Masturbation (excessive) F98.8
Maternal care (for) —see Pregnancy
(complicated by) (management
affected by)
Matheiu's disease (leptospiral jaundice)
A27.0
Mauclaire's disease or osteochondrosis —
see Osteochondrosis, juvenile, hand,
metacarpal
Maxcy's disease A75.2
Maxilla, maxillary —see condition
May (-Hegglin) anomaly or syndrome
D72.0
McArdle (-Schmid)(-Pearson) disease
(glycogen storage) E74.04
McCune-Albright syndrome Q78.1
McQuarrie's syndrome (idiopathic familial
hypoglycemia) E16.2
Meadow's syndrome Q86.1
Measles (black) (hemorrhagic) (suppressed)
B05.9
with
complications NEC B05.89
encephalitis B05.0
intestinal complications B05.4
keratitis (keratoconjunctivitis) B05.81
meningitis B05.1
otitis media B05.3
pneumonia B05.2
French —see Rubella
German —see Rubella
Liberty —see Rubella
Meatitis, urethral —see Urethritis
Meatus, meatal —see condition
Meat-wrappers' asthma J68.9

Meckel-Gruber syndrome Q61.9
Meckel's diverticulitis, diverticulum
(displaced) (hypertrophic) Q43.0
Meconium
ileus, newborn P76.0
in cystic fibrosis E84.11
meaning meconium plug (without cystic
fibrosis) P76.0
obstruction, newborn P76.0
due to fecaliths P76.0
in mucoviscidosis E84.11
peritonitis P78.0
plug syndrome (newborn) NEC P76.0
Median —see also condition
arcuate ligament syndrome I77.4
bar (prostate) (vesical orifice) —see
Hyperplasia, prostate
rhomboid glossitis K14.2
Mediastinal shift R93.8
Mediastinitis (acute) (chronic)
J98.51 ◀▥
syphilitic A52.73
tuberculous A15.8
Mediastinopericarditis —see also Pericarditis
acute I30.9
adhesive I31.0
chronic I31.8
rheumatic I09.2
Mediastinum, mediastinal —see condition
Medicine poisoning —see Table of Drugs and
Chemicals, by drug, poisoning
Mediterranean
fever —see Brucellosis
familial M04.1 ◀▥
tick A77.1
kala-azar B55.0
leishmaniasis B55.0
tick fever A77.1
Medulla —see condition
Medullary cystic kidney Q61.5
Medullated fibers
optic (nerve) Q14.8
retina Q14.1
Medulloblastoma
desmoplastic C71.6
specified site —see Neoplasm, malignant, by
site
unspecified site C71.6
Medulloepithelioma —see also Neoplasm,
malignant, by site
teratoid —see Neoplasm, malignant, by site
Medullomyoblastoma
specified site —see Neoplasm, malignant, by
site
unspecified site C71.6
Meekeren-Ehlers-Danlos syndrome
Q79.6
Megacolon (acquired) (functional) (not
Hirschsprung's disease) (in) K59.39 ◀▥
Chagas' disease B57.32
congenital, congenitum (aganglionic)
Q43.1
Hirschsprung's (disease) Q43.1
toxic NEC K59.31 ◀▥
due to Clostridium difficile A04.7
Megaesophagus (functional) K22.0
congenital Q39.5
in (due to) Chagas' disease B57.31
Megalencephaly Q04.5
Megalerythema (epidemic) B08.3
Megaloappendix Q43.8
Megalocephalus, megalocephaly NEC Q75.3
Megalocornea Q15.8
with glaucoma Q15.0
Megalocytic anemia D53.1
Megalodactylia (fingers) (thumbs) (congenital)
Q74.0
toes Q74.2
Megaloduodenum Q43.8
Megaloesophagus (functional) K22.0
congenital Q39.5

M

Megalogastria (acquired) K31.89
  congenital Q40.2
Megalophthalmos Q11.3
Megalopsia H53.15
Megalosplenia —see Splenomegaly
Megaloureter N28.82
  congenital Q62.2
Megarectum K62.89
Megasigmoid K59.39 ◀▥
  congenital Q43.2
Megaureter N28.82
  congenital Q62.2
Megavitamin-B6 syndrome E67.2
Megrim —see Migraine
Meibomian
  cyst, infected —see Hordeolum
  gland —see condition
  sty, stye —see Hordeolum
Meibomitis —see Hordeolum
Meige-Milroy disease (chronic hereditary
  edema) Q82.0
Meige's syndrome Q82.0
Melalgia, nutritional E53.8
Melancholia F32.9
  climacteric (single episode) F32.89 ◀▥
    recurrent episode F33.8 ◀▥
  hypochondriac F45.29
  intermittent (single episode) F32.89 ◀▥
    recurrent episode F33.8 ◀▥
  involutional (single episode) F32.89 ◀▥
    recurrent episode F33.8 ◀▥
  menopausal (single episode) F32.89 ◀▥
    recurrent episode F33.8 ◀▥
  puerperal F32.89 ◀▥
  reactive (emotional stress or trauma) F32.3
  recurrent F33.9
  senile F03
  stuporous (single episode) F32.89 ◀▥
    recurrent episode F33.8 ◀▥
Melanemia R79.89
Melanoameloblastoma —see Neoplasm, bone,
  benign
Melanoblastoma —see Melanoma
Melanocarcinoma —see Melanoma
Melanocytoma, eyeball D31.9- ◀▥
Melanocytosis, neurocutaneous Q82.8
Melanoderma, melanodermia L81.4
Melanodontia, infantile K03.89
Melanodontoclasia K03.89
Melanoepithelioma —see Melanoma
Melanoma (malignant) C43.9
  acral lentiginous, malignant —see Melanoma,
    skin, by site
  amelanotic —see Melanoma, skin, by site
  balloon cell —see Melanoma, skin, by site
  benign —see Nevus
  desmoplastic, malignant —see Melanoma,
    skin, by site
  epithelioid cell —see Melanoma, skin, by site
    with spindle cell, mixed —see Melanoma,
      skin, by site
  in
    giant pigmented nevus —see Melanoma,
      skin, by site
    Hutchinson's melanotic freckle —see
      Melanoma, skin, by site
    junctional nevus —see Melanoma, skin,
      by site
    precancerous melanosis —see Melanoma,
      skin, by site
  in situ D03.9
    abdominal wall D03.59
    ala nasi D03.39
    ankle D03.7-
    anus, anal (margin) (skin) D03.51
    arm D03.6-
    auditory canal D03.2-
    auricle (ear) D03.2-
    auricular canal (external) D03.2-
    axilla, axillary fold D03.59
    back D03.59

Melanoma (Continued)
  in situ (Continued)
    breast D03.52
    brow D03.39
    buttock D03.59
    canthus (eye) D03.1-
    cheek (external) D03.39
    chest wall D03.59
    chin D03.39
    choroid D03.8
    conjunctiva D03.8
    ear (external) D03.2-
    external meatus (ear) D03.2-
    eye D03.8
    eyebrow D03.39
    eyelid (lower) (upper) D03.1-
    face D03.30
      specified NEC D03.39
    female genital organ (external) NEC D03.8
    finger D03.6-
    flank D03.59
    foot D03.7-
    forearm D03.6-
    forehead D03.39
    foreskin D03.8
    gluteal region D03.59
    groin D03.59
    hand D03.6-
    heel D03.7-
    helix D03.2-
    hip D03.7-
    interscapular region D03.59
    iris D03.8
    jaw D03.39
    knee D03.7-
    labium (majus) (minus) D03.8
    lacrimal gland D03.8
    leg D03.7-
    lip (lower) (upper) D03.0
    lower limb NEC D03.7-
    male genital organ (external) NEC
      D03.8
    nail D03.9
      finger D03.6-
      toe D03.7-
    neck D03.4
    nose (external) D03.39
    orbit D03.8
    penis D03.8
    perianal skin D03.51
    perineum D03.51
    pinna D03.2-
    popliteal fossa or space D03.7-
    prepuce D03.8
    pudendum D03.8
    retina D03.8
    retrobulbar D03.8
    scalp D03.4
    scrotum D03.8
    shoulder D03.6-
    specified site NEC D03.8
    submammary fold D03.52
    temple D03.39
    thigh D03.7-
    toe D03.7-
    trunk NEC D03.59
    umbilicus D03.59
    upper limb NEC D03.6-
    vulva D03.8
  juvenile —see Nevus
  malignant, of soft parts except skin —see
    Neoplasm, connective tissue, malignant
  metastatic
    breast C79.81
    genital organ C79.82
    specified site NEC C79.89
  neurotropic, malignant —see Melanoma, skin,
    by site
  nodular —see Melanoma, skin, by site
  regressing, malignant —see Melanoma, skin,
    by site

Melanoma (Continued)
  skin C43.9
    abdominal wall C43.59
    ala nasi C43.31
    ankle C43.7-
    anus, anal (skin) C43.51
    arm C43.6-
    auditory canal (external) C43.2-
    auricle (ear) C43.2-
    auricular canal (external) C43.2-
    axilla, axillary fold C43.59
    back C43.59
    breast (female) (male) C43.52
    brow C43.39
    buttock C43.59
    canthus (eye) C43.1-
    cheek (external) C43.39
    chest wall C43.59
    chin C43.39
    ear (external) C43.2-
    elbow C43.6-
    external meatus (ear) C43.2-
    eyebrow C43.39
    eyelid (lower) (upper) C43.1-
    face C43.30
      specified NEC C43.39
    female genital organ (external) NEC
      C51.9
    finger C43.6-
    flank C43.59
    foot C43.7-
    forearm C43.6-
    forehead C43.39
    foreskin C60.0
    glabella C43.39
    gluteal region C43.59
    groin C43.59
    hand C43.6-
    heel C43.7-
    helix C43.2-
    hip C43.7-
    interscapular region C43.59
    jaw (external) C43.39
    knee C43.7-
    labium C51.9
      majus C51.0
      minus C51.1
    leg C43.7-
    lip (lower) (upper) C43.0
    lower limb NEC C43.7-
    male genital organ (external) NEC
      C63.9
    nail
      finger C43.6-
      toe C43.7-
    nasolabial groove C43.39
    nates C43.59
    neck C43.4
    nose (external) C43.31
    overlapping site C43.8
    palpebra C43.1-
    penis C60.9
    perianal skin C43.51
    perineum C43.51
    pinna C43.2-
    popliteal fossa or space C43.7-
    prepuce C60.0
    pudendum C51.9
    scalp C43.4
    scrotum C63.2
    shoulder C43.6-
    skin NEC C43.9
    submammary fold C43.52
    temple C43.39
    thigh C43.7-
    toe C43.7-
    trunk NEC C43.59
    umbilicus C43.59
    upper limb NEC C43.6-
    vulva C51.9
      overlapping sites C51.8

◀ New   ▥ Revised   ~~deleted~~ Deleted

M

Melanoma (Continued)
  spindle cell
    with epithelioid, mixed —see Melanoma,
      skin, by site
    type A C69.4-
    type B C69.4-
  superficial spreading —see Melanoma, skin,
    by site
Melanosarcoma —see also Melanoma
  epithelioid cell —see Melanoma
Melanosis L81.4
  addisonian E27.1
    tuberculous A18.7
  adrenal E27.1
  colon K63.89
  conjunctiva —see Pigmentation, conjunctiva
    congenital Q13.89
  cornea (presenile) (senile) —see also
    Pigmentation, cornea
    congenital Q13.4
  eye NEC H57.8
    congenital Q15.8
  lenticularis progressiva Q82.1
  liver K76.89
  precancerous —see also Melanoma, in situ
    malignant melanoma in —see Melanoma
  Riehl's L81.4
  sclera H15.89
    congenital Q13.89
  suprarenal E27.1
  tar L81.4
  toxic L81.4
Melanuria R82.99
MELAS syndrome E88.41
Melasma L81.1
  adrenal (gland) E27.1
  suprarenal (gland) E27.1
Melena K92.1
  with ulcer - code by site under Ulcer, with
    hemorrhage K27.4
  due to swallowed maternal blood P78.2
  newborn, neonatal P54.1
    due to swallowed maternal blood P78.2
Meleney's
  gangrene (cutaneous) —see Ulcer, skin
  ulcer (chronic undermining) —see Ulcer, skin
Melioidosis A24.9
  acute A24.1
  chronic A24.2
  fulminating A24.1
  pneumonia A24.1
  pulmonary (chronic) A24.2
    acute A24.1
    subacute A24.2
  sepsis A24.1
  specified NEC A24.3
  subacute A24.2
Melitensis, febris A23.0
Melkersson (-Rosenthal) syndrome G51.2
Mellitus, diabetes —see Diabetes
Melorheostosis (bone) —see Disorder, bone,
  density and structure, specified NEC
Meloschisis Q18.4
Melotia Q17.4
Membrana
  capsularis lentis posterior Q13.89
  epipapillaris Q14.2
Membranacea placenta O43.19-
Membranaceous uterus N85.8
Membrane (s), membranous —see also condition
  cyclitic —see Membrane, pupillary
  folds, congenital —see Web
  Jackson's Q43.3
  over face of newborn P28.9
  premature rupture —see Rupture,
    membranes, premature
  pupillary H21.4-
    persistent Q13.89
  retained (with hemorrhage) (complicating
    delivery) O72.2
    without hemorrhage O73.1

Membrane (s), membranous (Continued)
  secondary cataract —see Cataract, secondary
  unruptured (causing asphyxia) —see
    Asphyxia, newborn
  vitreous —see Opacity, vitreous, membranes
    and strands
Membranitis —see Chorioamnionitis
Memory disturbance, lack or loss —see also
  Amnesia
  mild, following organic brain damage F06.8
Menadione deficiency E56.1
Menarche
  delayed E30.0
  precocious E30.1
Mendacity, pathologic F60.2
Mendelson's syndrome (due to anesthesia)
  J95.4
  in labor and delivery O74.0
  in pregnancy O29.01-
  obstetric O74.0
  postpartum, puerperal O89.01
Ménétrier's disease or syndrome K29.60
  with bleeding K29.61
Ménière's disease, syndrome or vertigo H81.0-
Meninges, meningeal —see condition
Meningioma —see also Neoplasm, meninges,
  benign
  angioblastic —see Neoplasm, meninges,
    benign
  angiomatous —see Neoplasm, meninges,
    benign
  endotheliomatous —see Neoplasm, meninges,
    benign
  fibroblastic —see Neoplasm, meninges,
    benign
  fibrous —see Neoplasm, meninges, benign
  hemangioblastic —see Neoplasm, meninges,
    benign
  hemangiopericytic —see Neoplasm,
    meninges, benign
  malignant —see Neoplasm, meninges,
    malignant
  meningiothelial —see Neoplasm, meninges,
    benign
  meningotheliomatous —see Neoplasm,
    meninges, benign
  mixed —see Neoplasm, meninges, benign
  multiple —see Neoplasm, meninges,
    uncertain behavior
  papillary —see Neoplasm, meninges,
    uncertain behavior
  psammomatous —see Neoplasm, meninges,
    benign
  syncytial —see Neoplasm, meninges, benign
  transitional —see Neoplasm, meninges,
    benign
Meningiomatosis (diffuse) —see Neoplasm,
  meninges, uncertain behavior
Meningism —see Meningismus
Meningismus (infectional) (pneumococcal)
  R29.1
  due to serum or vaccine R29.1
  influenzal —see Influenza, with,
    manifestations NEC
Meningitis (basal) (basic) (brain) (cerebral)
  (cervical) (congestive) (diffuse)
  (hemorrhagic) infantile) (membranous)
  (metastatic) (nonspecific) (pontine)
  (progressive) (simple) (spinal) (subacute)
  (sympathetic) (toxic) G03.9
  abacterial G03.0
  actinomycotic A42.81
  adenoviral A87.1
  arbovirus A87.8
  aseptic (acute) G03.0
  bacterial G00.9
    Escherichia coli (E. coli) G00.8
    Friedländer (bacillus) G00.8
    gram-negative G00.9
    H. influenzae G00.0
    Klebsiella G00.8

Meningitis (Continued)
  bacterial (Continued)
    pneumococcal G00.1
    specified organism NEC G00.8
    staphylococcal G00.3
    streptococcal (acute) G00.2
  benign recurrent (Mollaret) G03.2
  candidal B37.5
  caseous (tuberculous) A17.0
  cerebrospinal A39.0
  chronic NEC G03.1
  clear cerebrospinal fluid NEC G03.0
  coxsackievirus A87.0
  cryptococcal B45.1
  diplococcal (gram positive) A39.0
  echovirus A87.0
  enteroviral A87.0
  eosinophilic B83.2
  epidemic NEC A39.0
  Escherichia coli (E. coli) G00.8
  fibrinopurulent G00.9
    specified organism NEC G00.8
  Friedländer (bacillus) G00.8
  gonococcal A54.81
  gram-negative cocci G00.9
  gram-positive cocci G00.9
  Haemophilus (influenzae) G00.0
  H. influenzae G00.0
  in (due to)
    adenovirus A87.1
    African trypanosomiasis B56.9 [G02]
    anthrax A22.8
    bacterial disease NEC A48.8 [G01]
    Chagas' disease (chronic) B57.41
    chickenpox B01.0
    coccidioidomycosis B38.4
    Diplococcus pneumoniae G00.1
    enterovirus A87.0
    herpes (simplex) virus B00.3
      zoster B02.1
    infectious mononucleosis B27.92
    leptospirosis A27.81
    Listeria monocytogenes A32.11
    Lyme disease A69.21
    measles B05.1
    mumps (virus) B26.1
    neurosyphilis (late) A52.13
    parasitic disease NEC B89 [G02]
    poliovirus A80.9 [G02]
    preventive immunization, inoculation or
      vaccination G03.8
    rubella B06.02
    Salmonella infection A02.21
    specified cause NEC G03.8
    Streptococcal pneumoniae G00.1 ◄
    typhoid fever A01.01
    varicella B01.0
    viral disease NEC A87.8
    whooping cough A37.90
    zoster B02.1
  infectious G00.9
  influenzal (H. influenzae) G00.0
  Klebsiella G00.8
  leptospiral (aseptic) A27.81
  lymphocytic (acute) (benign) (serous) A87.2
  meningococcal A39.0
  Mima polymorpha G00.8
  Mollaret (benign recurrent) G03.2
  monilial B37.5
  mycotic NEC B49 [G02]
  Neisseria A39.0
  nonbacterial G03.0
  nonpyogenic NEC G03.0
  ossificans G96.19
  ~~pneumococcal G00.1~~
  pneumococcal streptococcus pneumoniae
    G00.1 ◄
  poliovirus A80.9 [G02]
  postmeasles B05.1
  purulent G00.9
    specified organism NEC G00.8

Meningitis *(Continued)*
  pyogenic G00.9
    specified organism NEC G00.8
  Salmonella (arizonae) (Cholerae-Suis)
    (enteritidis) (typhimurium) A02.21
  septic G00.9
    specified organism NEC G00.8
  serosa circumscripta NEC G03.0
  serous NEC G93.2
  specified organism NEC G00.8
  sporotrichosis B42.81
  staphylococcal G00.3
  sterile G03.0
  Streptococcal (acute) G00.2 ◄▥
    pneumoniae G00.1 ◄
  suppurative G00.9
    specified organism NEC G00.8
  syphilitic (late) (tertiary) A52.13
    acute A51.41
    congenital A50.41
    secondary A51.41
  Torula histolytica (cryptococcal) B45.1
  traumatic (complication of injury)
    T79.8
  tuberculous A17.0
  typhoid A01.01
  viral NEC A87.9
  Yersinia pestis A20.3
Meningocele (spinal) —*see also* Spina bifida
  with hydrocephalus —*see* Spina bifida, by
    site, with hydrocephalus
  acquired (traumatic) G96.19
  cerebral —*see* Encephalocele
Meningocerebritis —*see* Meningoencephalitis
Meningococcemia A39.4
  acute A39.2
  chronic A39.3
Meningococcus, meningococcal —*see also*
    condition A39.9
  adrenalitis, hemorrhagic A39.1
  carrier (suspected) of Z22.31
  meningitis (cerebrospinal) A39.0
Meningoencephalitis —*see also* Encephalitis
    G04.90
  acute NEC —*see also* Encephalitis, viral A86
  bacterial NEC G04.2
  California A83.5
  diphasic A84.1
  eosinophilic B83.2
  epidemic A39.81
  herpesviral, herpetic B00.4
    due to herpesvirus 6 B10.01
    due to herpesvirus 7 B10.09
    specified NEC B10.09
  in (due to)
    blastomycosis NEC B40.81
    diseases classified elsewhere G05.3
    free-living amebae B60.2
    Hemophilus influenzae (H. influenzae)
      G00.0 ◄▥
    herpes B00.4
      due to herpesvirus 6 B10.01
      due to herpesvirus 7 B10.09
      specified NEC B10.09
    H. influenzae G00.0
    Lyme disease A69.22
    mercury —*see* subcategory T56.1
    mumps B26.2
    Naegleria (amebae) (organisms) (fowleri)
      B60.2
    Parastrongylus cantonensis B83.2
    toxoplasmosis (acquired) B58.2
      congenital P37.1
  infectious (acute) (viral) A86
  influenzal (H. influenzae) G00.0 ◄▥
  Listeria monocytogenes A32.12
  lymphocytic (serous) A87.2
  mumps B26.2
  parasitic NEC B89 [G05.3]
  pneumococcal G04.2 ◄▥
  primary amebic B60.2

Meningoencephalitis *(Continued)*
  specific (syphilitic) A52.14
  specified organism NEC G04.81
  staphylococcal G04.2
  streptococcal G04.2
  syphilitic A52.14
  toxic NEC G92
    due to mercury —*see* subcategory T56.1
  tuberculous A17.82
  virus NEC A86
Meningoencephalocele —*see also*
    Encephalocele
  syphilitic A52.19
    congenital A50.49
Meningoencephalomyelitis —*see also*
    Meningoencephalitis
  acute NEC (viral) A86
    disseminated G04.00
      postimmunization or postvaccination
        G04.02
      postinfectious G04.01
  due to
    actinomycosis A42.82
    Torula B45.1
    Toxoplasma or toxoplasmosis (acquired)
      B58.2
      congenital P37.1
  postimmunization or postvaccination G04.02
Meningoencephalomyelopathy G96.9
Meningoencephalopathy G96.9
Meningomyelitis —*see also*
    Meningoencephalitis
  bacterial NEC G04.2
  blastomycotic NEC B40.81
  cryptococcal B45.1
  in diseases classified elsewhere G05.4
  meningococcal A39.81
  syphilitic A52.14
  tuberculous A17.82
Meningomyelocele —*see also* Spina bifida
  syphilitic A52.19
Meningomyeloneuritis —*see*
    Meningoencephalitis
Meningoradiculitis —*see* Meningitis
Meningovascular —*see* condition
Menkes' disease or syndrome E83.09
  meaning maple-syrup-urine disease E71.0
Menometrorrhagia N92.1
Menopause, menopausal (asymptomatic)
    (state) Z78.0
  arthritis (any site) NEC —*see* Arthritis,
    specified form NEC
  bleeding N92.4
  depression (single episode) F32.89 ◄▥
    agitated (single episode) F32.2
      recurrent episode F33.9
    psychotic (single episode) F32.89 ◄▥
      recurrent episode F33.8 ◄▥
    recurrent episode F33.9
    melancholia (single episode) F32.89 ◄▥
      recurrent episode F33.8 ◄▥
  paranoid state F22
  premature E28.319
    asymptomatic E28.319
      postirradiation E89.40
      postsurgical E89.40
    symptomatic E28.310
      postirradiation E89.41
      postsurgical E89.41
  psychosis NEC F28
  symptomatic N95.1
  toxic polyarthritis NEC —*see* Arthritis,
    specified form NEC
Menorrhagia (primary) N92.0
  climacteric N92.4
    menopausal N92.4
  menopausal N92.4
  postclimacteric N95.0
  postmenopausal N95.0
  preclimacteric or premenopausal N92.4
  pubertal (menses retained) N92.2

Menostaxis N92.0
Menses, retention N94.89
Menstrual —*see* Menstruation
Menstruation
  absent —*see* Amenorrhea
  anovulatory N97.0
  cycle, irregular N92.6
  delayed N91.0
  disorder N93.9
    psychogenic F45.8
  during pregnancy O20.8
  excessive (with regular cycle) N92.0
    with irregular cycle N92.1
    at puberty N92.2
  frequent N92.0
  infrequent —*see* Oligomenorrhea
  irregular N92.6
    specified NEC N92.5
  latent N92.5
  membranous N92.5
  painful —*see also* Dysmenorrhea N94.6
    primary N94.4
    psychogenic F45.8
    secondary N94.5
  passage of clots N92.0
  precocious E30.1
  protracted N92.5
  rare —*see* Oligomenorrhea
  retained N94.89
  retrograde N92.5
  scanty —*see* Oligomenorrhea
  suppression N94.89
  vicarious (nasal) N94.89
Mental —*see also* condition
  deficiency —*see* Disability, intellectual
  deterioration —*see* Psychosis
  disorder —*see* Disorder, mental
  exhaustion F48.8
  insufficiency (congenital) —*see* Disability,
    intellectual
  observation without need for further medical
    care Z03.89
  retardation —*see* Disability, intellectual
  subnormality —*see* Disability, intellectual
  upset —*see* Disorder, mental
Meralgia paresthetica G57.1-
Mercurial —*see* condition
Mercurialism —*see* subcategory T56.1
MERRF syndrome (myoclonic epilepsy
    associated with ragged-red fiber)
    E88.42
Merkel cell tumor —*see* Carcinoma,
    Merkel cell
Merocele —*see* Hernia, femoral
Meromelia
  lower limb —*see* Defect, reduction, lower
    limb
    intercalary
      femur —*see* Defect, reduction, lower
        limb, specified type NEC
      tibiofibular (complete) (incomplete) —
        see Defect, reduction, lower
        limb
  upper limb —*see* Defect, reduction, upper
    limb
    intercalary, humeral, radioulnar —*see*
      Agenesis, arm, with hand present
Merzbacher-Pelizaeus disease E75.29
Mesaortitis —*see* Aortitis
Mesarteritis —*see* Arteritis
Mesencephalitis —*see* Encephalitis
Mesenchymoma —*see also* Neoplasm,
    connective tissue, uncertain behavior
  benign —*see* Neoplasm, connective tissue,
    benign
  malignant —*see* Neoplasm, connective tissue,
    malignant
Mesenteritis
  retractile K65.4
  sclerosing K65.4
Mesentery, mesenteric —*see* condition

◄ New   ◄▥ Revised   ~~deleted~~ Deleted

Mesiodens, mesiodentes K00.1
Mesio-occlusion M26.213
Mesocolon —see condition
Mesonephroma (malignant) —see Neoplasm, malignant, by site
  benign —see Neoplasm, benign, by site
Mesophlebitis —see Phlebitis
Mesostromal dysgenesis Q13.89
Mesothelioma (malignant) C45.9
  benign
    mesentery D19.1
    mesocolon D19.1
    omentum D19.1
    peritoneum D19.1
    pleura D19.0
    specified site NEC D19.7
    unspecified site D19.9
  biphasic C45.9
    benign
      mesentery D19.1
      mesocolon D19.1
      omentum D19.1
      peritoneum D19.1
      pleura D19.0
      specified site NEC D19.7
      unspecified site D19.9
  cystic D48.4
  epithelioid C45.9
    benign
      mesentery D19.1
      mesocolon D19.1
      omentum D19.1
      peritoneum D19.1
      pleura D19.0
      specified site NEC D19.7
      unspecified site D19.9
  fibrous C45.9
    benign
      mesentery D19.1
      mesocolon D19.1
      omentum D19.1
      peritoneum D19.1
      pleura D19.0
      specified site NEC D19.7
      unspecified site D19.9
  site classification
    liver C45.7
    lung C45.7
    mediastinum C45.7
    mesentery C45.1
    mesocolon C45.1
    omentum C45.1
    pericardium C45.2
    peritoneum C45.1
    pleura C45.0
      parietal C45.0
    retroperitoneum C45.7
    specified site NEC C45.7
    unspecified C45.9
Metabolic syndrome E88.81
Metagonimiasis B66.8
Metagonimus infestation (intestine) B66.8
Metal
  pigmentation L81.8
  polisher's disease J62.8
Metamorphopsia H53.15
Metaplasia
  apocrine (breast) —see Dysplasia, mammary, specified type NEC
  cervix (squamous) —see Dysplasia, cervix
  endometrium (squamous) (uterus) N85.8
  esophagus K22.7- ◄▥
  kidney (pelvis) (squamous) N28.89
  myelogenous D73.1
  myeloid (agnogenic) (megakaryocytic) D73.1
  spleen D73.1
  squamous cell, bladder N32.89
Metastasis, metastatic
  abscess —see Abscess
  calcification E83.59

Metastasis, metastatic (Continued)
  cancer
    from specified site —see Neoplasm, malignant, by site
    to specified site —see Neoplasm, secondary, by site
    deposits (in) —see Neoplasm, secondary, by site
    disease (see also Neoplasm, secondary, by site) C79.9
    spread (to) —see Neoplasm, secondary, by site
Metastrongyliasis B83.8
Metatarsalgia M77.4-
  anterior G57.6-
  Morton's G57.6-
Metatarsus, metatarsal —see also condition
  adductus, congenital Q66.22 ◄
  valgus (abductus), congenital Q66.6
  varus (congenital) Q66.22 ◄▥
    primus Q66.21 ◄
Methadone use —see Use, opioid ◄▥
Methemoglobinemia D74.9
  acquired (with sulfhemoglobinemia) D74.8
  congenital D74.0
  enzymatic (congenital) D74.0
  Hb M disease D74.0
  hereditary D74.0
  toxic D74.8
Methemoglobinuria —see Hemoglobinuria
Methioninemia E72.19
Methylmalonic acidemia E71.120
Metritis (catarrhal) (hemorrhagic) (septic) (suppurative) —see also Endometritis
  cervical —see Cervicitis
Metropathia hemorrhagica N93.8
Metroperitonitis —see Peritonitis, pelvic, female
Metrorrhagia N92.1
  climacteric N92.4
  menopausal N92.4
  postpartum NEC (atonic) (following delivery of placenta) O72.1
    delayed or secondary O72.2
  preclimacteric or premenopausal N92.4
  psychogenic F45.8
Metrorrhexis —see Rupture, uterus
Metrosalpingitis N70.91
Metrostaxis N93.8
Metrovaginitis —see Endometritis
Meyer-Schwickerath and Weyers syndrome Q87.0
Meynert's amentia (nonalcoholic) F04
  alcoholic F10.96
    with dependence F10.26
Mibelli's disease (porokeratosis) Q82.8
Mice, joint —see Loose, body, joint
  knee M23.4
Micrencephalon, micrencephaly Q02
Microalbuminuria R80.9
Microaneurysm, retinal —see also Disorder, retina, microaneurysms
  diabetic —see E08-E13 with .31
Microangiopathy (peripheral) I73.9
  thrombotic M31.1
Microcalcifications, breast R92.0
Microcephalus, microcephalic, microcephaly Q02
  due to toxoplasmosis (congenital) P37.1
Microcheilia Q18.7
Microcolon (congenital) Q43.8
Microcornea (congenital) Q13.4
Microcytic —see condition D57.40
Microdeletions NEC Q93.88
Microdontia K00.2
Microdrepanocytosis D57.40
  with crisis (vasoocclusive pain) D57.419
    with
      acute chest syndrome D57.411
      splenic sequestration D57.412
Microembolism
  atherothrombotic —see Atheroembolism
  retinal —see Occlusion, artery, retina

Microencephalon Q02
Microfilaria streptocerca infestation —see Onchocerciasis
Microgastria (congenital) Q40.2
Microgenia M26.06
Microgenitalia, congenital
  female Q52.8
  male Q55.8
Microglioma —see Lymphoma, non-Hodgkin, specified NEC
Microglossia (congenital) Q38.3
Micrognathia, micrognathism (congenital) (mandibular) (maxillary) M26.09
Microgyria (congenital) Q04.3
Microinfarct of heart —see Insufficiency, coronary
Microlentia (congenital) Q12.8
Microlithiasis, alveolar, pulmonary J84.02
Micromastia N64.82
Micromyelia (congenital) Q06.8
Micropenis Q55.62
Microphakia (congenital) Q12.8
Microphthalmos, microphthalmia (congenital) Q11.2
  due to toxoplasmosis P37.1
Micropsia H53.15
Microscopic polyangiitis (polyarteritis) M31.7
Microsporidiosis B60.8
  intestinal A07.8
Microsporon furfur infestation B36.0
Microsporosis —see also Dermatophytosis
  nigra B36.1
Microstomia (congenital) Q18.5
Microtia (congenital) (external ear) Q17.2
Microtropia H50.40
Microvillus inclusion disease (MVD) (MVID) Q43.8
Micturition
  disorder NEC —see also Difficulty, micturition R39.198 ◄▥
    psychogenic F45.8
  frequency R35.0
    psychogenic F45.8
  hesitancy R39.11
  incomplete emptying R39.14
  nocturnal R35.1
  painful R30.9
    dysuria R30.0
    psychogenic F45.8
    tenesmus R30.1
  poor stream R39.12
  position dependent R39.192 ◄
  split stream R39.13
  straining R39.16
  urgency R39.15
Mid plane —see condition
Middle
  ear —see condition
  lobe (right) syndrome J98.19
Miescher's elastoma L87.2
Mietens' syndrome Q87.2
Migraine (idiopathic) G43.909
  with refractory migraine G43.919
    with status migrainosus G43.911
    without status migrainosus G43.919
  with aura (acute-onset) (prolonged) (typical) (without headache) G43.109
    with refractory migraine G43.119
      with status migrainosus G43.111
      without status migrainosus G43.119
    intractable G43.119
      with status migrainosus G43.111
      without status migrainosus G43.119
    not intractable G43.109
      with status migrainosus G43.101
      without status migrainosus G43.109
  persistent G43.509
    with cerebral infarction G43.609
      with refractory migraine G43.619
        with status migrainosus G43.611
        without status migrainosus G43.619

M

Migraine *(Continued)*
  with aura *(Continued)*
    persistent *(Continued)*
      with cerebral infarction *(Continued)*
        intractable G43.619
          with status migrainosus G43.611
          without status migrainosus G43.619
        not intractable G43.609
          with status migrainosus G43.601
          without status migrainosus G43.609
        without refractory migraine G43.609
          with status migrainosus G43.601
          without status migrainosus G43.609
      without cerebral infarction G43.509
        with refractory migraine G43.519
          with status migrainosus G43.511
          without status migrainosus G43.519
        intractable G43.519
          with status migrainosus G43.511
          without status migrainosus G43.519
        not intractable G43.509
          with status migrainosus G43.501
          without status migrainosus G43.509
        without refractory migraine G43.509
          with status migrainosus G43.501
          without status migrainosus G43.509
      without mention of refractory migraine G43.109
        with status migrainosus G43.101
        without status migrainosus G43.109
  abdominal G43.D0
    with refractory migraine G43.D1
    intractable G43.D1
    not intractable G43.D0
    without refractory migraine G43.D0
  basilar —*see* Migraine, with aura
  classical —*see* Migraine, with aura
  common —*see* Migraine, without aura
  complicated G43.109
  equivalents —*see* Migraine, with aura
  familiar —*see* Migraine, hemiplegic
  hemiplegic G43.409
    with refractory migraine G43.419
      with status migrainosus G43.411
      without status migrainosus G43.419
    intractable G43.419
      with status migrainosus G43.411
      without status migrainosus G43.419
    not intractable G43.409
      with status migrainosus G43.401
      without status migrainosus G43.409
    without refractory migraine G43.409
      with status migrainosus G43.401
      without status migrainosus G43.409
  intractable G43.919
    with status migrainosus G43.911
    without status migrainosus G43.919
  menstrual G43.829
    with refractory migraine G43.839
      with status migrainosus G43.831
      without status migrainosus G43.839
    intractable G43.839
      with status migrainosus G43.831
      without status migrainosus G43.839
    not intractable G43.829
      with status migrainosus G43.821
      without status migrainosus G43.829
    without refractory migraine G43.829
      with status migrainosus G43.821
      without status migrainosus G43.829
  menstrually related —*see* Migraine, menstrual
  not intractable G43.909
    with status migrainosus G43.901
    without status migrainosus G43.919
  ophthalmoplegic G43.B0
    with refractory migraine G43.B1
    intractable G43.B1
    not intractable G43.B0
      without refractory migraine G43.B0

Migraine *(Continued)*
  persistent aura (with, without) cerebral infarction —*see* Migraine, with aura, persistent
  preceded or accompanied by transient focal neurological phenomena —*see* Migraine, with aura
  pre-menstrual —*see* Migraine, menstrual
  pure menstrual —*see* Migraine, menstrual
  retinal —*see* Migraine, with aura
  specified NEC G43.809
    intractable G43.819
      with status migrainosus G43.811
      without status migrainosus G43.819
    not intractable G43.809
      with status migrainosus G43.801
      without status migrainosus G43.809
  sporadic —*see* Migraine, hemiplegic
  transformed —*see* Migraine, without aura, chronic
  triggered seizures —*see* Migraine, with aura
  without aura G43.009
    with refractory migraine G43.019
      with status migrainosus G43.011
      without status migrainosus G43.019
    chronic G43.709
      with refractory migraine G43.719
        with status migrainosus G43.711
        without status migrainosus G43.719
      intractable
        with status migrainosus G43.711
        without status migrainosus G43.719
      not intractable
        with status migrainosus G43.701
        without status migrainosus G43.709
      without refractory migraine G43.709
        with status migrainosus G43.701
        without status migrainosus G43.709
    intractable
      with status migrainosus G43.011
      without status migrainosus G43.019
    not intractable
      with status migrainosus G43.001
      without status migrainosus G43.009
    without mention of refractory migraine G43.009
      with status migrainosus G43.001
      without status migrainosus G43.009
    without refractory migraine G43.909
      with status migrainosus G43.901
      without status migrainosus G43.919
Migrant, social Z59.0
Migration, anxiety concerning Z60.3
Migratory, migrating —*see also* condition
  person Z59.0
  testis Q55.29
Mikity-Wilson disease or syndrome P27.0
Mikulicz' disease or syndrome K11.8
Miliaria L74.3
  alba L74.1
  apocrine L75.2
  crystallina L74.1
  profunda L74.2
  rubra L74.0
  tropicalis L74.2
Miliary —*see* condition
Milium L72.0
  colloid L57.8
Milk
  crust L21.0
  excessive secretion O92.6
  poisoning —*see* Poisoning, food, noxious
  retention O92.79
  sickness —*see* Poisoning, food, noxious
  spots I31.0
Milk-alkali disease or syndrome E83.52
Milk-leg (deep vessels) (nonpuerperal) —*see* Embolism, vein, lower extremity
  complicating pregnancy O22.3-
  puerperal, postpartum, childbirth O87.1

Milkman's disease or syndrome M83.8
Milky urine —*see* Chyluria
Millard-Gubler (-Foville) paralysis or syndrome G46.3
Millar's asthma J38.5
Miller-Fisher syndrome G61.0
Mills' disease —*see* Hemiplegia
Millstone maker's pneumoconiosis J62.8
Milroy's disease (chronic hereditary edema) Q82.0
Minamata disease T56.1-
Miners' asthma or lung J60
Minkowski-Chauffard syndrome —*see* Spherocytosis
Minor —*see* condition
Minor's disease (hematomyelia) G95.19
Minot's disease (hemorrhagic disease), newborn P53
Minot-von Willebrand-Jurgens disease or syndrome (angiohemophilia) D68.0
Minus (and plus) hand (intrinsic) —*see* Deformity, limb, specified type NEC, forearm
Miosis (pupil) H57.03
Mirizzi's syndrome (hepatic duct stenosis) K83.1
Mirror writing F81.0
Misadventure (of) (prophylactic) (therapeutic) —*see also* Complications T88.9
  administration of insulin (by accident) —*see* subcategory T38.3
  infusion —*see* Complications, infusion
  local applications (of fomentations, plasters, etc.) T88.9
    burn or scald —*see* Burn
    specified NEC T88.8
  medical care (early) (late) T88.9
    adverse effect of drugs or chemicals —*see* Table of Drugs and Chemicals
  medical care (early) (late)
    burn or scald —*see* Burn
    specified NEC T88.8
  specified NEC T88.8
  surgical procedure (early) (late) —*see* Complications, surgical procedure
  transfusion —*see* Complications, transfusion
  vaccination or other immunological procedure —*see* Complications, vaccination
Miscarriage O03.9
Misdirection, aqueous H40.83-
Misperception, sleep state F51.02
Misplaced, misplacement
  ear Q17.4
  kidney (acquired) N28.89
    congenital Q63.2
  organ or site, congenital NEC —*see* Malposition, congenital
Missed
  abortion O02.1
  delivery O36.4
Missing —*see also* Absence
  string of intrauterine contraceptive device T83.32
Misuse of drugs F19.99
Mitchell's disease (erythromelalgia) I73.81
Mite (s) (infestation) B88.9
  diarrhea B88.0
  grain (itch) B88.0
  hair follicle (itch) B88.0
  in sputum B88.0
Mitral —*see* condition
Mittelschmerz N94.0
Mixed —*see* condition
MMN (multifocal motor neuropathy) G61.82
MNGIE (Mitochondrial Neurogastrointestinal Encephalopathy) syndrome E88.49
Mobile, mobility
  cecum Q43.3
  excessive —*see* Hypermobility
  gallbladder, congenital Q44.1

◀ New   ◀▥ Revised   ~~deleted~~ Deleted

Mobile, mobility (Continued)
  kidney N28.89
  organ or site, congenital NEC —see
    Malposition, congenital
Mobitz heart block (atrioventricular) I44.1
Moebius, Möbius
  disease (ophthalmoplegic migraine) —see
    Migraine, ophthalmoplegic
  syndrome Q87.0
    congenital oculofacial paralysis (with other
      anomalies) Q87.0
    ophthalmoplegic migraine —see Migraine,
      ophthalmoplegic
Moeller's glossitis K14.0
Mohr's syndrome (Types I and II) Q87.0
Mola destruens D39.2
Molar pregnancy O02.0
Molarization of premolars K00.2
Molding, head (during birth) - omit code
Mole (pigmented) —see also Nevus
  blood O02.0
  Breus' O02.0
  cancerous —see Melanoma
  carneous O02.0
  destructive D39.2
  fleshy O02.0
  hydatid, hydatidiform (benign) (complicating
      pregnancy) (delivered) (undelivered)
      O01.9
    classical O01.0
    complete O01.0
    incomplete O01.1
    invasive D39.2
    malignant D39.2
    partial O01.1
  intrauterine O02.0
  invasive (hydatidiform) D39.2
  malignant
    meaning
      malignant hydatidiform mole D39.2
      melanoma —see Melanoma
  nonhydatidiform O02.0
  nonpigmented —see Nevus
  pregnancy NEC O02.0
  skin —see Nevus
  tubal O00.10 ◀▥▥
    with intrauterine pregnancy O00.11 ◀
  vesicular —see Mole, hydatidiform
Molimen, molimina (menstrual) N94.3
Molluscum contagiosum (epitheliale) B08.1
Mönckeberg's arteriosclerosis, disease, or
    sclerosis —see Arteriosclerosis, extremities
Mondini's malformation (cochlea) Q16.5
Mondor's disease I80.8
Monge's disease T70.29
Monilethrix (congenital) Q84.1
Moniliasis —see also Candidiasis B37.9
  neonatal P37.5
Monitoring (encounter for)
  therapeutic drug level Z51.81
Monkey malaria B53.1
Monkeypox B04
Monoarthritis M13.10
  ankle M13.17-
  elbow M13.12-
  foot joint M13.17-
  hand joint M13.14-
  hip M13.15-
  knee M13.16-
  shoulder M13.11-
  wrist M13.13-
Monoblastic —see condition
Monochromat (ism), monochromatopsia
    (acquired) (congenital) H53.51
Monocytic —see condition
Monocytopenia D72.818
Monocytosis (symptomatic) D72.821
Monomania —see Psychosis
Mononeuritis G58.9
  cranial nerve —see Disorder, nerve,
    cranial

Mononeuritis (Continued)
  femoral nerve G57.2-
  lateral
    cutaneous nerve of thigh G57.1-
    popliteal nerve G57.3-
  lower limb G57.9-
    specified nerve NEC G57.8-
  medial popliteal nerve G57.4-
  median nerve G56.1-
  multiplex G58.7
  plantar nerve G57.6-
  posterior tibial nerve G57.5-
  radial nerve G56.3-
  sciatic nerve G57.0-
  specified NEC G58.8
  tibial nerve G57.4-
  ulnar nerve G56.2-
  upper limb G56.9-
    specified nerve NEC G56.8-
  vestibular —see subcategory H93.3
Mononeuropathy G58.9
  carpal tunnel syndrome —see Syndrome,
    carpal tunnel
  diabetic NEC —see E08-E13 with .41
  femoral nerve —see Lesion, nerve, femoral
  ilioinguinal nerve G57.8-
  in diseases classified elsewhere —see category
    G59
  intercostal G58.0
  lower limb G57.9-
    causalgia —see Causalgia, lower limb
    femoral nerve —see Lesion, nerve,
      femoral
    meralgia paresthetica G57.1-
    plantar nerve —see Lesion, nerve, plantar
    popliteal nerve —see Lesion, nerve,
      popliteal
    sciatic nerve —see Lesion, nerve, sciatic
    specified NEC G57.8-
    tarsal tunnel syndrome —see Syndrome,
      tarsal tunnel
  median nerve —see Lesion, nerve, median
  multiplex G58.7
  obturator nerve G57.8-
  popliteal nerve —see Lesion, nerve,
    popliteal
  radial nerve —see Lesion, nerve, radial
  saphenous nerve G57.8-
  specified NEC G58.8
  tarsal tunnel syndrome —see Syndrome,
    tarsal tunnel
  tuberculous A17.83
  ulnar nerve —see Lesion, nerve, ulnar
  upper limb G56.9-
    carpal tunnel syndrome —see Syndrome,
      carpal tunnel
    causalgia —see Causalgia
    median nerve —see Lesion, nerve, median
    radial nerve —see Lesion, nerve, radial
    specified site NEC G56.8-
    ulnar nerve —see Lesion, nerve, ulnar
Mononucleosis, infectious B27.90
  with
    complication NEC B27.99
    meningitis B27.92
    polyneuropathy B27.91
  cytomegaloviral B27.10
    with
      complication NEC B27.19
      meningitis B27.12
      polyneuropathy B27.11
  Epstein-Barr (virus) B27.00
    with
      complication NEC B27.09
      meningitis B27.02
      polyneuropathy B27.01
  gammaherpesviral B27.00
    with
      complication NEC B27.09
      meningitis B27.02
      polyneuropathy B27.01

Mononucleosis, infectious (Continued)
  specified NEC B27.80
    with
      complication NEC B27.89
      meningitis B27.82
      polyneuropathy B27.81
Monoplegia G83.3-
  congenital (cerebral) G80.8
    spastic G80.1
  embolic (current episode) I63.4- ◀▥▥
  following
    cerebrovascular disease
      cerebral infarction
        lower limb I69.34-
        upper limb I69.33-
      intracerebral hemorrhage
        lower limb I69.14-
        upper limb I69.13-
        lower limb I69.94-
      nontraumatic intracranial hemorrhage
        NEC
        lower limb I69.24-
        upper limb I69.23-
      specified disease NEC
        lower limb I69.84-
        upper limb I69.83-
      stroke NOS
        lower limb I69.34-
        upper limb I69.33-
      subarachnoid hemorrhage
        lower limb I69.04-
        upper limb I69.03-
        upper limb I69.93-
  hysterical (transient) F44.4
  lower limb G83.1-
  psychogenic (conversion reaction) F44.4
  thrombotic (current episode) I63.3- ◀▥▥
  transient R29.818
  upper limb G83.2-
Monorchism, monorchidism Q55.0
Monosomy —see also Deletion, chromosome
    Q93.9
  specified NEC Q93.89
  whole chromosome
    meiotic nondisjunction Q93.0
    mitotic nondisjunction Q93.1
    mosaicism Q93.1
  X Q96.9
Monster, monstrosity (single) Q89.7
  acephalic Q00.0
  twin Q89.4
Monteggia's fracture (-dislocation) S52.27-
Mooren's ulcer (cornea) —see Ulcer, cornea,
    Mooren's
Moore's syndrome —see Epilepsy, specified
    NEC
Mooser-Neill reaction A75.2
Mooser's bodies A75.2
Morbidity not stated or unknown R69
Morbilli —see Measles
Morbus —see also Disease
  angelicus, anglorum E55.0
  Beigel B36.2
  caducus —see Epilepsy
  celiacus K90.0
  comitialis —see Epilepsy
  cordis —see also Disease, heart I51.9
    valvulorum —see Endocarditis
  coxae senilis M16.9
    tuberculous A18.02
  hemorrhagicus neonatorum P53
  maculosus neonatorum P54.5
Morel (-Stewart)(-Morgagni) syndrome M85.2
Morel-Kraepelin disease —see Schizophrenia
Morel-Moore syndrome M85.2
Morgagni's
  cyst, organ, hydatid, or appendage
    female Q50.5
    male (epididymal) Q55.4
      testicular Q55.29
  syndrome M85.2

M

M

Morgagni-Stewart-Morel syndrome M85.2
Morgagni-Stokes-Adams syndrome I45.9
Morgagni-Turner (-Albright) syndrome Q96.9
Moria F07.0
Moron (I.Q. 50-69) F70
Morphea L94.0
Morphinism (without remission) F11.20
  with remission F11.21
Morphinomania (without remission) F11.20
  with remission F11.21
Morquio (-Ullrich)(-Brailsford) disease or
  syndrome —see Mucopolysaccharidosis
Mortification (dry) (moist) —see Gangrene
Morton's metatarsalgia (neuralgia)(neuroma)
  (syndrome) G57.6
Morvan's disease or syndrome G60.8
Mosaicism, mosaic (autosomal) (chromosomal)
  45,X/46,XX Q96.3
  45,X/other cell lines NEC with abnormal sex
    chromosome Q96.4
  sex chromosome
    female Q97.8
    lines with various numbers of X
      chromosomes Q97.2
    male Q98.7
  XY Q96.3
Moschowitz' disease M31.1
Mother yaw A66.0
Motion sickness (from travel, any vehicle)
  (from roundabouts or swings) T75.3
Mottled, mottling, teeth (enamel) (endemic)
  (nonendemic) K00.3
Mounier-Kuhn syndrome Q32.4
  with bronchiectasis J47.9
    exacerbation (acute) J47.1
    lower respiratory infection J47.0
  acquired J98.09
    with bronchiectasis J47.9
      with
        exacerbation (acute) J47.1
        lower respiratory infection J47.0
Mountain
  sickness T70.29
    with polycythemia , acquired (acute) D75.1
  tick fever A93.2
Mouse, joint —see Loose, body, joint
  knee M23.4-
Mouth —see condition
Movable
  coccyx —see subcategory M53.2
  kidney N28.89
    congenital Q63.8
  spleen D73.89
Movements, dystonic R25.8
Moyamoya disease I67.5
MRSA (Methicillin resistant Staphylococcus
    aureus)
  infection A49.02
    as the cause of diseases classified
      elsewhere B95.62
  sepsis A41.02
MSSA (Methicillin susceptible Staphylococcus
    aureus)
  infection A49.01
    as the cause of diseases classified
      elsewhere B95.61
  sepsis A41.01
Mucha-Habermann disease L41.0
Mucinosis (cutaneous) (focal) (papular)
  (reticular erythematous) (skin) L98.5
  oral K13.79
Mucocele
  appendix K38.8
  buccal cavity K13.79
  gallbladder K82.1
  lacrimal sac, chronic H04.43-
  nasal sinus J34.1
  nose J34.1
  salivary gland (any) K11.6
  sinus (accessory) (nasal) J34.1
  turbinate (bone) (middle) (nasal) J34.1
  uterus N85.8

Mucolipidosis
  I E77.1
  II, III E77.0
  IV E75.11
Mucopolysaccharidosis E76.3
  beta-gluduronidase deficiency E76.29
  cardiopathy E76.3 [I52]
  Hunter's syndrome E76.1
  Hurler's syndrome E76.01
  Hurler-Scheie syndrome E76.02
  Maroteaux-Lamy syndrome E76.29
  Morquio syndrome E76.219
    A E76.210
    B E76.211
    classic E76.210
  Sanfilippo syndrome E76.22
  Scheie's syndrome E76.03
  specified NEC E76.29
  type
    I
      Hurler's syndrome E76.01
      Hurler-Scheie syndrome E76.02
      Scheie's syndrome E76.03
    II E76.1
    III E76.22
    IV E76.219
    IVA E76.210
    IVB E76.211
    VI E76.29
    VII E76.29
Mucormycosis B46.5
  cutaneous B46.3
  disseminated B46.4
  gastrointestinal B46.2
  generalized B46.4
  pulmonary B46.0
  rhinocerebral B46.1
  skin B46.3
  subcutaneous B46.3
Mucositis (ulcerative) K12.30
  due to drugs NEC K12.32
  gastrointestinal K92.81
  mouth (oral) (oropharyngeal) K12.30
    due to antineoplastic therapy K12.31
    due to drugs NEC K12.32
    due to radiation K12.33
    specified NEC K12.39
    viral K12.39
  nasal J34.81
  oral cavity —see Mucositis, mouth
  oral soft tissues —see Mucositis, mouth
  vagina and vulva N76.81
Mucositis necroticans agranulocytica —see
    Agranulocytosis
Mucous —see also condition
  patches (syphilitic) A51.39
    congenital A50.07
Mucoviscidosis E84.9
  with meconium obstruction E84.11
Mucus
  asphyxia or suffocation —see Asphyxia,
    mucus
  in stool R19.5
  plug —see Asphyxia, mucus
Muguet B37.0
Mulberry molars (congenital syphilis)
  A50.52
Müllerian mixed tumor
  specified site —see Neoplasm, malignant, by
    site
  unspecified site C54.9
Multicystic kidney (development) Q61.4
Multiparity (grand) Z64.1
  affecting management of pregnancy, labor
    and delivery (supervision only)
    O09.4-
  requiring contraceptive management —see
    Contraception
Multipartita placenta O43.19-
Multiple, multiplex —see also condition
  digits (congenital) Q69.9

Multiple, multiplex (Continued)
  endocrine neoplasia —see Neoplasia,
    endocrine, multiple [MEN]
  personality F44.81
Mumps B26.9
  arthritis B26.85
  complication NEC B26.89
  encephalitis B26.2
  hepatitis B26.81
  meningitis (aseptic) B26.1
  meningoencephalitis B26.2
  myocarditis B26.82
  oophoritis B26.89
  orchitis B26.0
  pancreatitis B26.3
  polyneuropathy B26.84
Mumu —see also Infestation, filarial B74.9
  [N51]
Münchhausen's syndrome —see Disorder,
  factitious
Münchmeyer's syndrome —see Myositis,
  ossificans, progressiva
Mural —see condition
Murmur (cardiac) (heart) (organic) R01.1
  abdominal R19.15
  aortic (valve) —see Endocarditis, aortic
  benign R01.0
  diastolic —see Endocarditis
  Flint I35.1
  functional R01.0
  Graham Steell I37.1
  innocent R01.0
  mitral (valve) —see Insufficiency, mitral
  nonorganic R01.0
  presystolic, mitral —see Insufficiency, mitral
  pulmonic (valve) I37.8
  systolic R01.1 ◀
  tricuspid (valve) I07.9
  valvular —see Endocarditis
Murri's disease (intermittent hemoglobinuria)
  D59.6
Muscle, muscular —see also condition
  carnitine (palmityltransferase) deficiency
    E71.314
Musculoneuralgia —see Neuralgia
Mushroom-workers' (pickers') disease or lung
  J67.5
Mushrooming hip —see Derangement, joint,
  specified NEC, hip
Mutation (s)
  factor V Leiden D68.51
  surfactant, of lung J84.83
  prothrombin gene D68.52
Mutism —see also Aphasia
  deaf (acquired) (congenital) NEC H91.3
  elective (adjustment reaction) (childhood)
    F94.0
  hysterical F44.4
  selective (childhood) F94.0
MVD (microvillus inclusion disease) Q43.8
MVID (microvillus inclusion disease) Q43.8
Myalgia M79.1
  epidemic (cervical) B33.0
  traumatic NEC T14.8
Myasthenia G70.9
  congenital G70.2
  cordis —see Failure, heart
  developmental G70.2
  gravis G70.00
    with exacerbation (acute) G70.01
    in crisis G70.01
    neonatal, transient P94.0
    pseudoparalytica G70.00
      with exacerbation (acute) G70.01
      in crisis G70.01
  stomach, psychogenic F45.8
  syndrome
    in
      diabetes mellitus —see E08-E13 with .44
      neoplastic disease —see also Neoplasm
        D49.9 [G73.3]

◀ New   ◀▥ Revised   ~~deleted~~ Deleted

Myasthenia *(Continued)*
 syndrome *(Continued)*
  in *(Continued)*
   pernicious anemia D51.0 *[G73.3]*
   thyrotoxicosis E05.90 *[G73.3]*
    with thyroid storm E05.91 *[G73.3]*
Myasthenic M62.81
Mycelium infection B49
Mycetismus —*see* Poisoning, food, noxious, mushroom
Mycetoma B47.9
 actinomycotic B47.1
 bone (mycotic) B47.9 *[M90.80]*
 eumycotic B47.0
 foot B47.9
  actinomycotic B47.1
  mycotic B47.0
 madurae NEC B47.9
  mycotic B47.0
 maduromycotic B47.0
 mycotic B47.0
 nocardial B47.1
Mycobacteriosis —*see* Mycobacterium
Mycobacterium, mycobacterial (infection) A31.9
 anonymous A31.9
 atypical A31.9
  cutaneous A31.1
  pulmonary A31.0
   tuberculous —*see* Tuberculosis, pulmonary
  specified site NEC A31.8
 avium (intracellulare complex) A31.0
 balnei A31.1
 Battey A31.0
 chelonei A31.8
 cutaneous A31.1
 extrapulmonary systemic A31.8
 fortuitum A31.8
 intracellulare (Battey bacillus) A31.0
 kakaferifu A31.8
 kansasii (yellow bacillus) A31.0
 kasongo A31.8
 leprae —*see also* Leprosy A30.9
 luciflavum A31.1
 marinum (M. balnei) A31.1
 nonspecific —*see* Mycobacterium, atypical
 pulmonary (atypical) A31.0
  tuberculous —*see* Tuberculosis, pulmonary
 scrofulaceum A31.8
 simiae A31.8
 systemic, extrapulmonary A31.8
 szulgai A31.8
 terrae A31.8
 triviale A31.8
 tuberculosis (human, bovine) —*see* Tuberculosis
 ulcerans A31.1
 xenopi A31.8
Mycoplasma (M.) pneumoniae, as cause of disease classified elsewhere B96.0
Mycosis, mycotic B49
 cutaneous NEC B36.9
 ear B36.9 ◀▥
  in ◀
   aspergillosis B44.89 ◀
   candidiasis B37.84 ◀
   moniliasis B37.84 ◀
 fungoides (extranodal) (solid organ) C84.0-
 mouth B37.0
 nails B35.1
 opportunistic B48.8
 skin NEC B36.9
 specified NEC B48.8
 stomatitis B37.0
 vagina, vaginitis (candidal) B37.3
Mydriasis (pupil) H57.04
Myelatelia Q06.1
Myelinolysis, pontine, central G37.2

Myelitis (acute) (ascending) (childhood) (chronic) (descending) (diffuse) (disseminated) (idiopathic) (pressure) (progressive) (spinal cord) (subacute) —*see also* Encephalitis G04.91
 herpes simplex B00.82
 herpes zoster B02.24
 in diseases classified elsewhere G05.4
 necrotizing, subacute G37.4
 optic neuritis in G36.0
 postchickenpox B01.12
 postherpetic B02.24
 postimmunization G04.02
 postinfectious NEC G04.89
 postvaccinal G04.02
 specified NEC G04.89
 syphilitic (transverse) A52.14
 toxic G92
 transverse (in demyelinating diseases of central nervous system) G37.3
 tuberculous A17.82
 varicella B01.12
Myeloblastic —*see* condition
Myeloblastoma
 granular cell —*see also* Neoplasm, connective tissue
  malignant —*see* Neoplasm, connective tissue, malignant
 tongue D10.1
Myelocele —*see* Spina bifida
Myelocystocele —*see* Spina bifida
Myelocytic —*see* condition
Myelodysplasia D46.9
 specified NEC D46.Z
 spinal cord (congenital) Q06.1
Myelodysplastic syndrome D46.9
 with
  5q deletion D46.C
  isolated del (5q) chromosomal abnormality C46.C
 specified NEC D46.Z
Myeloencephalitis —*see* Encephalitis
Myelofibrosis D75.81
 with myeloid metaplasia D47.4
 acute C94.4-
 idiopathic (chronic) D47.4
 primary D47.1
 secondary D75.81
  in myeloproliferative disease D47.4
Myelogenous —*see* condition
Myeloid —*see* condition
Myelokathexis D70.9
Myeloleukodystrophy E75.29
Myelolipoma —*see* Lipoma
Myeloma (multiple) C90.0-
 monostotic C90.3
  plasma cell C90.0-
 plasma cell C90.0-
 solitary —*see also* Plasmacytoma, solitary C90.3-
Myelomalacia G95.89
Myelomatosis C90.0-
Myelomeningitis —*see* Meningoencephalitis
Myelomeningocele (spinal cord) —*see* Spina bifida
Myelo-osteo-musculodysplasia hereditaria Q79.8
Myelopathic
 anemia D64.89
 muscle atrophy —*see* Atrophy, muscle, spinal
 pain syndrome G89.0
Myelopathy (spinal cord) G95.9
 drug-induced G95.89
 in (due to)
  degeneration or displacement, intervertebral disc NEC —*see* Disorder, disc, with, myelopathy
  infection —*see* Encephalitis
  intervertebral disc disorder —*see also* Disorder, disc, with, myelopathy
  mercury —*see* subcategory T56.1

Myelopathy *(Continued)*
 in (due to) *(Continued)*
  neoplastic disease —*see also* Neoplasm D49.9 *[G99.2]*
  pernicious anemia D51.0 *[G99.2]*
  spondylosis —*see* Spondylosis, with myelopathy NEC
 necrotic (subacute) (vascular) G95.19
 radiation-induced G95.89
 spondylogenic NEC —*see* Spondylosis, with myelopathy NEC
 toxic G95.89
 transverse, acute G37.3
 vascular G95.19
 vitamin B12 E53.8 *[G32.0]*
Myelophthisis D61.82
Myeloradiculitis G04.91
Myeloradiculodysplasia (spinal) Q06.1
Myelosarcoma C92.3-
Myelosclerosis D75.89
 with myeloid metaplasia D47.4
 disseminated, of nervous system G35
 megakaryocytic D47.4
  with myeloid metaplasia D47.4
Myelosis
 acute C92.0-
 aleukemic C92.9-
 chronic D47.1
 erythremic (acute) C94.0-
 megakaryocytic C94.2-
 nonleukemic D72.828
 subacute C92.9-
Myiasis (cavernous) B87.9
 aural B87.4
 creeping B87.0
 cutaneous B87.0
 dermal B87.0
 ear (external) (middle) B87.4
 eye B87.2
 genitourinary B87.81
 intestinal B87.82
 laryngeal B87.3
 nasopharyngeal B87.3
 ocular B87.2
 orbit B87.2
 skin B87.0
 specified site NEC B87.89
 traumatic B87.1
 wound B87.1
Myoadenoma, prostate —*see* Hyperplasia, prostate
Myoblastoma
 granular cell —*see also* Neoplasm, connective tissue, benign
  malignant —*see* Neoplasm, connective tissue, malignant
 tongue D10.1
Myocardial —*see* condition
Myocardiopathy (congestive) (constrictive) (familial) (hypertrophic nonobstructive) (idiopathic) (infiltrative) (obstructive) (primary) (restrictive) (sporadic) —*see also* Cardiomyopathy I42.9
 alcoholic I42.6
 cobalt-beer I42.6
 glycogen storage E74.02 *[143]*
 hypertrophic obstructive I42.1
 in (due to)
  beriberi E51.12
  cardiac glycogenosis E74.02 *[143]*
  Friedreich's ataxia G11.1 *[143]*
  myotonia atrophica G71.11 *[143]*
  progressive muscular dystrophy G71.0 *[143]*
 obscure (African) I42.8
 secondary I42.9
 thyrotoxic E05.90 *[143]*
  with storm E05.91 *[143]*
 toxic NEC I42.7

Myocarditis (with arteriosclerosis) (chronic)
(fibroid) (interstitial) (old) (progressive)
(senile) I51.4
with
  rheumatic fever (conditions in I00) I09.0
    active —see Myocarditis, acute,
      rheumatic
    inactive or quiescent (with chorea) I09.0
active I40.9
  rheumatic I01.2
    with chorea (acute) (rheumatic)
      (Sydenham's) I02.0
acute or subacute (interstitial) I40.9
  due to
    streptococcus (beta-hemolytic) I01.2
  idiopathic I40.1
  rheumatic I01.2
    with chorea (acute) (rheumatic)
      (Sydenham's) I02.0
  specified NEC I40.8
aseptic of newborn B33.22
bacterial (acute) I40.0
Coxsackie (virus) B33.22
diphtheritic A36.81
eosinophilic I40.1
epidemic of newborn (Coxsackie) B33.22
Fiedler's (acute) (isolated) I40.1
giant cell (acute) (subacute) I40.1
gonococcal A54.83
granulomatous (idiopathic) (isolated)
  (nonspecific) I40.1
hypertensive —see Hypertension, heart
idiopathic (granulomatous) I40.1
in (due to)
  diphtheria A36.81
  epidemic louse-borne typhus A75.0 [I41]
  Lyme disease A69.29
  sarcoidosis D86.85
  scarlet fever A38.1
  toxoplasmosis (acquired) B58.81
  typhoid A01.02
  typhus NEC A75.9 [I41]
infective I40.0
influenzal —see Influenza, with, myocarditis
isolated (acute) I40.1
meningococcal A39.52
mumps B26.82
nonrheumatic, active I40.9
parenchymatous I40.9
pneumococcal I40.0
rheumatic (chronic) (inactive) (with chorea)
  I09.0
  active or acute I01.2
    with chorea (acute) (rheumatic)
      (Sydenham's) I02.0
rheumatoid —see Rheumatoid, carditis
septic I40.0
staphylococcal I40.0
suppurative I40.0
syphilitic (chronic) A52.06
toxic I40.8
  rheumatic —see Myocarditis, acute,
    rheumatic
tuberculous A18.84
typhoid A01.02
valvular —see Endocarditis
virus, viral I40.0
  of newborn (Coxsackie) B33.22
Myocardium, myocardial —see condition
Myocardosis —see Cardiomyopathy
Myoclonus, myoclonic, myoclonia (familial)
  (essential) (multifocal) (simplex) G25.3
drug-induced G25.3
epilepsy —see also Epilepsy, generalized,
  specified NEC G40.4-
  familial (progressive) G25.3
epileptica G40.409
  with status epilepticus G40.401
facial G51.3
familial progressive G25.3
Friedreich's G25.3

Myoclonus, myoclonic, myoclonia (Continued)
jerks G25.3
massive G25.3
palatal G25.3
pharyngeal G25.3
Myocytolysis I51.5
Myodiastasis —see Diastasis, muscle
Myoendocarditis —see Endocarditis
Myoepithelioma —see Neoplasm, benign, by
  site
Myofasciitis (acute) —see Myositis
Myofibroma —see also Neoplasm, connective
  tissue, benign
  uterus (cervix) (corpus) —see Leiomyoma
Myofibromatosis D48.1
  infantile Q89.8
Myofibrosis M62.89
  heart —see Myocarditis
  scapulohumeral —see Lesion, shoulder,
    specified NEC
Myofibrositis M79.7
  scapulohumeral —see Lesion, shoulder,
    specified NEC
Myoglobulinuria, myoglobinuria (primary)
  R82.1
Myokymia, facial G51.4
Myolipoma —see Lipoma
Myoma —see also Neoplasm, connective tissue,
  benign
  malignant —see Neoplasm, connective tissue,
    malignant
  prostate D29.1
  uterus (cervix) (corpus) —see Leiomyoma
Myomalacia M62.89
Myometritis —see Endometritis
Myometrium —see condition
Myonecrosis, clostridial A48.0
Myopathy G72.9
  acute
    necrotizing G72.81
    quadriplegic G72.81
  alcoholic G72.1
  benign congenital G71.2
  central core G71.2
  centronuclear G71.2
  congenital (benign) G71.2
  critical illness G72.81
  distal G71.0
  drug-induced G72.0
  endocrine NEC E34.9 [G73.7]
  extraocular muscles H05.82-
  facioscapulohumeral G71.0
  hereditary G71.9
    specified NEC G71.8
  immune NEC G72.49
  in (due to)
    Addison's disease E27.1 [G73.7]
    alcohol G72.1
    amyloidosis E85.0 [G73.7]
    cretinism E00.9 [G73.7]
    Cushing's syndrome E24.9 [G73.7]
    drugs G72.0
    endocrine disease NEC E34.9 [G73.7]
    giant cell arteritis M31.6 [G73.7]
    glycogen storage disease E74.00 [G73.7]
    hyperadrenocorticism E24.9 [G73.7]
    hyperparathyroidism NEC E21.3 [G73.7]
    hypoparathyroidism E20.9 [G73.7]
    hypopituitarism E23.0 [G73.7]
    hypothyroidism E03.9 [G73.7]
    infectious disease B99 [G73.7]
    lipid storage disease E75.6 [G73.7]
    metabolic disease NEC E88.9 [G73.7]
    myxedema E03.9 [G73.7]
    parasitic disease NEC B89 [G73.7]
    polyarteritis nodosa M30.0 [G73.7]
    rheumatoid arthritis —see Rheumatoid,
      myopathy
    sarcoidosis D86.87
    scleroderma M34.82
    sicca syndrome M35.03

Myopathy (Continued)
  in (due to) (Continued)
    Sjögren's syndrome M35.03
    systemic lupus erythematosus M32.19
    thyrotoxicosis (hyperthyroidism) E05.90
      [G73.7]
      with thyroid storm E05.91 [G73.7]
    toxic agent NEC G72.2
  inflammatory NEC G72.49
  intensive care (ICU) G72.81
  limb-girdle G71.0
  mitochondrial NEC G71.3
  myotubular G71.2
  mytonic, proximal (PROMM) G71.11
  nemaline G71.2
  ocular G71.0
  oculopharyngeal G71.0
  of critical illness G72.81
  primary G71.9
    specified NEC G71.8
  progressive NEC G72.89
  proximal myotonic (PROMM) G71.11
  rod G71.2
  scapulohumeral G71.0
  specified NEC G72.89
  toxic G72.2
Myopericarditis —see also Pericarditis
  chronic rheumatic I09.2
Myopia (axial) (congenital) H52.1-
  degenerative (malignant) H44.2-
  malignant H44.2-
  pernicious H44.2-
  progressive high (degenerative) H44.2-
Myosarcoma —see Neoplasm, connective tissue,
  malignant
Myosis (pupil) H57.03
  stromal (endolymphatic) D39.0
Myositis M60.9
  clostridial A48.0
  due to posture —see Myositis, specified type
    NEC
  epidemic B33.0
  fibrosa or fibrous (chronic), Volkmann's
    T79.6
  foreign body granuloma —see Granuloma,
    foreign body
  in (due to)
    bilharziasis B65.9 [M63.8-]
    cysticercosis B69.81
    leprosy A30.9 [M63.8-]
    mycosis B49 [M63.8-]
    sarcoidosis D86.87
    schistosomiasis B65.9 [M63.8-]
    syphilis
      late A52.78
      secondary A51.49
    toxoplasmosis (acquired) B58.82
    trichinellosis B75 [M63.8-]
    tuberculosis A18.09
  inclusion body [IBM] G72.41
  infective M60.009
    arm M60.002
      left M60.001
      right M60.000
    leg M60.005
      left M60.004
      right M60.003
    lower limb M60.005
      ankle M60.07-
      foot M60.07-
      lower leg M60.06-
      thigh M60.05-
      toe M60.07-
    multiple sites M60.09
    specified site NEC M60.08
    upper limb M60.002
      finger M60.04-
      forearm M60.03-
      hand M60.04-
      shoulder region M60.01-
      upper arm M60.02-

◀ New   ◀⁞⁞ Revised   deleted Deleted

Myositis *(Continued)*
  interstitial M60.10
    ankle M60.17-
    foot M60.17-
    forearm M60.13-
    hand M60.14-
    lower leg M60.16-
    multiple sites M60.19
    shoulder region M60.11-
    specified site NEC M60.18
    thigh M60.15-
    upper arm M60.12-
  mycotic B49 *[M63.8-]*
  ossificans or ossifying (circumscripta) —*see also* Ossification, muscle, specified NEC
    in (due to)
      burns M61.30
        ankle M61.37-
        foot M61.37-
        forearm M61.33-
        hand M61.34-
        lower leg M61.36-
        multiple sites M61.39
        pelvic region M61.35-
        shoulder region M61.31-
        specified site NEC M61.38
        thigh M61.35-
        upper arm M61.32-
      quadriplegia or paraplegia M61.20
        ankle M61.27-
        foot M61.27-
        forearm M61.23-
        hand M61.24-
        lower leg M61.26-
        multiple sites M61.29
        pelvic region M61.25-
        shoulder region M61.21-
        specified site NEC M61.28
        thigh M61.25-
        upper arm M61.22-
    progressiva M61.10
      ankle M61.17-
      finger M61.14-
      foot M61.17-
      forearm M61.13-
      hand M61.14-
      lower leg M61.16-

Myositis *(Continued)*
  ossificans or ossifying *(Continued)*
    progressiva *(Continued)*
      multiple sites M61.19
      pelvic region M61.15-
      shoulder region M61.11-
      specified site NEC M61.18
      thigh M61.15-
      toe M61.17-
      upper arm M61.12-
    traumatica M61.00
      ankle M61.07-
      foot M61.07-
      forearm M61.03-
      hand M61.04-
      lower leg M61.06-
      multiple sites M61.09
      pelvic region M61.05-
      shoulder region M61.01-
      specified site NEC M61.08
      thigh M61.05-
      upper arm M61.02-
  purulent —*see* Myositis, infective
  specified type NEC M60.80
    ankle M60.87-
    foot M60.87-
    forearm M60.83-
    hand M60.84-
    lower leg M60.86-
    multiple sites M60.89
    pelvic region M60.85-
    shoulder region M60.81-
    specified site NEC M60.88
    thigh M60.85-
    upper arm M60.82-
  suppurative —*see* Myositis, infective
  traumatic (old) —*see* Myositis, specified type NEC
Myospasia impulsiva F95.2
Myotonia (acquisita) (intermittens) M62.89
  atrophica G71.11
  chondrodystrophic G71.13
  congenita (acetazolamide responsive) (dominant) (recessive) G71.12
  drug-induced G71.14
  dystrophica G71.11
  fluctuans G71.19

Myotonia *(Continued)*
  levior G71.12
  permanens G71.19
  symptomatic G71.19
Myotonic pupil —*see* Anomaly, pupil, function, tonic pupil
Myriapodiasis B88.2
Myringitis H73.2-
  with otitis media —*see* Otitis, media
  acute H73.00-
    bullous H73.01-
    specified NEC H73.09-
  bullous —*see* Myringitis, acute, bullous
  chronic H73.1-
Mysophobia F40.228
Mytilotoxism —*see* Poisoning, fish
Myxadenitis labialis K13.0
Myxedema (adult) (idiocy) (infantile) (juvenile) —*see also* Hypothyroidism E03.9
  circumscribed E05.90
    with storm E05.91
  coma E03.5
  congenital E00.1
  cutis L98.5
  localized (pretibial) E05.90
    with storm E05.91
  papular L98.5
Myxochondrosarcoma —*see* Neoplasm, cartilage, malignant
Myxofibroma —*see* Neoplasm, connective tissue, benign
  odontogenic —*see* Cyst, calcifying odontogenic
Myxofibrosarcoma —*see* Neoplasm, connective tissue, malignant
Myxolipoma D17.9
Myxoliposarcoma —*see* Neoplasm, connective tissue, malignant
Myxoma —*see also* Neoplasm, connective tissue, benign
  nerve sheath —*see* Neoplasm, nerve, benign
  odontogenic —*see* Cyst, calcifying odontogenic
Myxosarcoma —*see* Neoplasm, connective tissue, malignant

M

N

Naegeli's
   disease Q82.8
   leukemia, monocytic C93.1-
Naegleriasis (with meningoencephalitis)
   B60.2
Naffziger's syndrome G54.0
Naga sore —see Ulcer, skin
Nägele's pelvis M95.5
   with disproportion (fetopelvic) O33.0
      causing obstructed labor O65.0
Nail —see also condition
   biting F98.8
   patella syndrome Q87.2
Nanism, nanosomia —see Dwarfism
Nanophyetiasis B66.8
Nanukayami A27.89
Napkin rash L22
Narcolepsy G47.419
   with cataplexy G47.411
   in conditions classified elsewhere
      G47.429
      with cataplexy G47.421
Narcosis R06.89
Narcotism —see Dependence
NARP (Neuropathy, Ataxia and Retinitis
   pigmentosa) syndrome E88.49
Narrow
   anterior chamber angle H40.03-
   gingival width (of periodontal soft tissue)
      K05.5 ◀
   pelvis —see Contraction, pelvis
Narrowing —see also Stenosis
   artery I77.1
      auditory, internal I65.8
      basilar —see Occlusion, artery, basilar
      carotid —see Occlusion, artery, carotid
      cerebellar —see Occlusion, artery, cerebellar
      cerebral —see Occlusion artery, cerebral
      choroidal —see Occlusion, artery, cerebral,
         specified NEC
      communicating posterior —see Occlusion,
         artery, cerebral, specified NEC
      coronary —see also Disease, heart, ischemic,
         atherosclerotic
         congenital Q24.5
            syphilitic A50.54 [152]
         due to syphilis NEC A52.06
      hypophyseal —see Occlusion, artery,
         cerebral, specified NEC
      pontine —see Occlusion, artery, cerebral,
         specified NEC
      precerebral —see Occlusion, artery,
         precerebral
      vertebral —see Occlusion, artery, vertebral
   auditory canal (external) —see Stenosis,
      external ear canal
   eustachian tube —see Obstruction, eustachian
      tube
   eyelid —see Disorder, eyelid function
   larynx J38.6
   mesenteric artery —see also Ischemia,
      intestine, acute K55.059 ◀▥
   palate M26.89
   palpebral fissure —see Disorder, eyelid
      function
   ureter N13.5
      with infection N13.6
   urethra —see Stricture, urethra
Narrowness, abnormal, eyelid Q10.3
Nasal —see condition
Nasolachrymal, nasolacrimal —see condition
Nasopharyngeal —see also condition
   pituitary gland Q89.2
   torticollis M43.6
Nasopharyngitis (acute) (infective)
   (streptococcal) (subacute) J00
   chronic (suppurative) (ulcerative) J31.1
Nasopharynx, nasopharyngeal —see condition
Natal tooth, teeth K00.6

Nausea (without vomiting) R11.0
   with vomiting R11.2
   gravidarum —see Hyperemesis, gravidarum
   marina T75.3
   navalis T75.3
Navel —see condition
Neapolitan fever —see Brucellosis
Near drowning T75.1
Nearsightedness —see Myopia
Near-syncope R55
Nebula, cornea —see Opacity, cornea
Necator americanus infestation B76.1
Necatoriasis B76.1
Neck —see condition
Necrobiosis R68.89
   lipoidica NEC L92.1
      with diabetes —see E08-E13 with .620
Necrolysis, toxic epidermal L51.2
   due to drug
      correct substance properly administered —
         see Table of Drugs and Chemicals, by
         drug, adverse effect
      overdose or wrong substance given or
         taken —see Table of Drugs and
         Chemicals, by drug, poisoning
Necrophilia F65.89
Necrosis, necrotic (ischemic) —see also
      Gangrene
   adrenal (capsule) (gland) E27.49
   amputation stump (surgical) (late) T87.50
      arm T87.5-
      leg T87.5-
   antrum J32.0
   aorta (hyaline) —see also Aneurysm, aorta
      cystic medial —see Dissection, aorta
   artery I77.5
   bladder (aseptic) (sphincter) N32.89
   bone —see also Osteonecrosis M87.9
      aseptic or avascular —see Osteonecrosis
         idiopathic M87.00
      ethmoid J32.2
      jaw M27.2
      tuberculous —see Tuberculosis, bone
   brain I67.89
   breast (aseptic) (fat) (segmental) N64.1
   bronchus J98.09
   central nervous system NEC I67.89
   cerebellar I67.89
   cerebral I67.89
   colon —see also Infarct, intestine K55.049 ◀▥
   cornea H18.89- ◀▥
   cortical (acute) (renal) N17.1
   cystic medial (aorta) —see Dissection, aorta
   dental pulp K04.1
   esophagus K22.8
   ethmoid (bone) J32.2
   eyelid —see Disorder, eyelid, degenerative
   fat, fatty (generalized) —see also Disorder, soft
      tissue, specified type NEC
      abdominal wall K65.4
      breast (aseptic) (segmental) N64.1
      localized —see Degeneration, by site, fatty
      mesentery K65.4
      omentum K65.4
      pancreas K86.89 ◀▥
      peritoneum K65.4
      skin (subcutaneous), newborn P83.0
      subcutaneous, due to birth injury P15.6
   gallbladder —see Cholecystitis, acute
   heart —see Infarct, myocardium
   hip, aseptic or avascular —see Osteonecrosis,
      by type, femur
   intestine (acute) (hemorrhagic) (massive) —
      see also Infarct, intestine K55.069 ◀▥
   jaw M27.2
   kidney (bilateral) N28.0
      acute N17.9
      cortical (acute) (bilateral) N17.1
         with ectopic or molar pregnancy O08.4
      medullary (bilateral) (in acute renal failure)
         (papillary) N17.2

Necrosis, necrotic (Continued)
   kidney (Continued)
      papillary (bilateral) (in acute renal
         failure) N17.2
      tubular N17.0
         with ectopic or molar pregnancy O08.4
         complicating
            abortion —see Abortion, by type,
               complicated by, tubular necrosis
            ectopic or molar pregnancy O08.4
            pregnancy —see Pregnancy,
               complicated by, diseases of,
               specified type or system NEC
         following ectopic or molar pregnancy
            O08.4
      traumatic T79.5
   larynx J38.7
   liver (with hepatic failure) (cell) —see Failure,
      hepatic
   hemorrhagic, central K76.2
   lung J85.0
   lymphatic gland —see Lymphadenitis, acute
   mammary gland (fat) (segmental) N64.1
   mastoid (chronic) —see Mastoiditis, chronic
   medullary (acute) (renal) N17.2
   mesentery —see also Infarct, intestine
      K55.069 ◀▥
      fat K65.4
   mitral valve —see Insufficiency, mitral
   myocardium, myocardial —see Infarct,
      myocardium
   nose J34.0
   omentum (with mesenteric infarction) —see
      also Infarct, intestine K55.069 ◀▥
      fat K65.4
   orbit, orbital —see Osteomyelitis, orbit
   ossicles, ear —see Abnormal, ear ossicles
   ovary N70.92
   pancreas (aseptic) (duct) (fat) K86.89 ◀▥
      acute (infective) —see Pancreatitis, acute
      infective —see Pancreatitis, acute
   papillary (acute) (renal) N17.2
   perineum N90.89
   peritoneum (with mesenteric infarction) —see
      also Infarct, intestine K55.069 ◀▥
      fat K65.4
   pharynx J02.9
      in granulocytopenia —see Neutropenia
      Vincent's A69.1
   phosphorus —see subcategory T54.2
   pituitary (gland) E23.0 ◀▥
      postpartum O99.285 ◀
      Sheehan O99.285 ◀
   pressure —see Ulcer, pressure, by site
   pulmonary J85.0
   pulp (dental) K04.1
   radiation —see Necrosis, by site
   radium —see Necrosis, by site
   renal —see Necrosis, kidney
   sclera H15.89
   scrotum N50.89 ◀▥
   skin or subcutaneous tissue NEC I96
   spine, spinal (column) —see also
      Osteonecrosis, by type, vertebra
      cord G95.19
   spleen D73.5
   stomach K31.89
   stomatitis (ulcerative) A69.0
   subcutaneous fat, newborn P83.8
   subendocardial (acute) I21.4
      chronic I25.89
   suprarenal (capsule) (gland) E27.49
   testis N50.89 ◀▥
   thymus (gland) E32.8
   tonsil J35.8
   trachea J39.8
   tuberculous NEC —see Tuberculosis
   tubular (acute) (anoxic) (renal) (toxic)
      N17.0
      postprocedural N99.0
   vagina N89.8

◀ New   ◀▥ Revised   ~~deleted~~ Deleted

Necrosis, necrotic *(Continued)*
vertebra —*see also* Osteonecrosis, by type, vertebra
tuberculous A18.01
vulva N90.89
X-ray —*see* Necrosis, by site
Necrospermia —*see* Infertility, male
Need (for)
care provider because (of)
assistance with personal care Z74.1
continuous supervision required Z74.3
impaired mobility Z74.09
no other household member able to render care Z74.2
specified reason NEC Z74.8
immunization —*see* Vaccination
vaccination —*see* Vaccination
Neglect
adult
confirmed T74.01
history of Z91.412
suspected T76.01
child (childhood)
confirmed T74.02
history of Z62.812
suspected T76.02
emotional, in childhood Z62.898
hemispatial R41.4
left-sided R41.4
sensory R41.4
visuospatial R41.4
Neisserian infection NEC —*see* Gonococcus
Nelaton's syndrome G60.8
Nelson's syndrome E24.1
Nematodiasis (intestinal) B82.0
Ancylostoma B76.0
Neonatal —*see also* Newborn
acne L70.4
bradycardia P29.12
screening, abnormal findings on P09
tachycardia P29.11
tooth, teeth K00.6
Neonatorum —*see* condition
Neoplasia
endocrine, multiple (MEN) E31.20
type I E31.21
type IIA E31.22
type IIB E31.23
intraepithelial (histologically confirmed)
anal (AIN) (histologically confirmed) K62.82
grade I K62.82
grade II K62.82
severe D01.3
cervical glandular (histologically confirmed) D06.9
cervix (uteri) (CIN) (histologically confirmed) N87.9
glandular D06.9
grade I N87.0
grade II N87.1
grade III (severe dysplasia) —*see also* Carcinoma, cervix uteri, in situ D06.9
prostate (histologically confirmed) (PIN) N42.31 ◄▥
grade I N42.31 ◄▥
grade II N42.31 ◄▥
grade III (severe dysplasia) D07.5 ◄
severe D07.5
vagina (histologically confirmed) (VAIN) N89.3
grade I N89.0
grade II N89.1
grade III (severe dysplasia) D07.2
vulva (histologically confirmed) (VIN) N90.3
grade I N90.0
grade II N90.1
grade III (severe dysplasia) D07.1

Neoplasm, neoplastic —*see also* Table of Neoplasms
lipomatous, benign —*see* Lipoma
Neovascularization
ciliary body —*see* Disorder, iris, vascular
cornea H16.40-
deep H16.44-
ghost vessels —*see* Ghost, vessels
localized H16.43-
pannus —*see* Pannus
iris —*see* Disorder, iris, vascular
retina H35.05-
Nephralgia N23
Nephritis, nephritic (albuminuric) (azotemic) (congenital) (disseminated) (epithelial) (familial) (focal) (granulomatous) (hemorrhagic) (infantile) (nonsuppurative, excretory) (uremic) N05.9
with
dense deposit disease N05.6
diffuse
crescentic glomerulonephritis N05.7
endocapillary proliferative glomerulonephritis N05.4
membranous glomerulonephritis N05.2
mesangial proliferative glomerulonephritis N05.3
mesangiocapillary glomerulonephritis N05.5
edema —*see* Nephrosis
focal and segmental glomerular lesions N05.1
foot process disease N04.9
glomerular lesion
diffuse sclerosing N05.8
hypocomplementemic —*see* Nephritis, membranoproliferative
IgA —*see* Nephropathy, IgA
lobular, lobulonodular —*see* Nephritis, membranoproliferative
nodular —*see* Nephritis, membranoproliferative
lesion of
glomerulonephritis, proliferative N05.8
renal necrosis N05.9
minor glomerular abnormality N05.0
specified morphological changes NEC N05.8
acute N00.9
with
dense deposit disease N00.6
diffuse
crescentic glomerulonephritis N00.7
endocapillary proliferative glomerulonephritis N00.4
membranous glomerulonephritis N00.2
mesangial proliferative glomerulonephritis N00.3
mesangiocapillary glomerulonephritis N00.5
focal and segmental glomerular lesions N00.1
minor glomerular abnormality N00.0
specified morphological changes NEC N00.8
amyloid E85.4 [N08]
antiglomerular basement membrane (anti-GBM) antibody NEC
in Goodpasture's syndrome M31.0
antitubular basement membrane (tubulo-interstitial) NEC N12
toxic —*see* Nephropathy, toxic
arteriolar —*see* Hypertension, kidney
arteriosclerotic —*see* Hypertension, kidney
ascending —*see* Nephritis, tubulo-interstitial
atrophic N03.9

Nephritis, nephritic *(Continued)*
Balkan (endemic) N15.0
calculous, calculus —*see* Calculus, kidney
cardiac —*see* Hypertension, kidney
cardiovascular —*see* Hypertension, kidney
chronic N03.9
with
dense deposit disease N03.6
diffuse
crescentic glomerulonephritis N03.7
endocapillary proliferative glomerulonephritis N03.4
membranous glomerulonephritis N03.2
mesangial proliferative glomerulonephritis N03.3
mesangiocapillary glomerulonephritis N03.5
focal and segmental glomerular lesions N03.1
minor glomerular abnormality N03.0
specified morphological changes NEC N03.8
arteriosclerotic —*see* Hypertension, kidney
cirrhotic N26.9
complicating pregnancy O26.83-
croupous N00.9
degenerative —*see* Nephrosis
diffuse sclerosing N05.8
due to
diabetes mellitus —*see* E08-E13 with .21
subacute bacterial endocarditis I33.0
systemic lupus erythematosus (chronic) M32.14
typhoid fever A01.09
gonococcal (acute) (chronic) A54.21
hypocomplementemic —*see* Nephritis, membranoproliferative
IgA —*see* Nephropathy, IgA
immune complex (circulating) NEC N05.8
infective —*see* Nephritis, tubulo-interstitial
interstitial —*see* Nephritis, tubulo-interstitial
lead N14.3
membranoproliferative (diffuse) (type 1 or 3) —*see also* N00-N07 with fourth character .5 N05.5
type 2 —*see also* N00-N07 with fourth character .6 N05.6
minimal change N05.0
necrotic, necrotizing NEC —*see also* N00-N07 with fourth character .8 N05.8
nephrotic —*see* Nephrosis
nodular —*see* Nephritis, membranoproliferative
polycystic Q61.3
adult type Q61.2
autosomal
dominant Q61.2
recessive NEC Q61.19
childhood type NEC Q61.19
infantile type NEC Q61.19
poststreptococcal N05.9
acute N00.9
chronic N03.9
rapidly progressive N01.9
proliferative NEC —*see also* N00-N07 with fourth character .8 N05.8
purulent —*see* Nephritis, tubulo-interstitial
rapidly progressive N01.9
with
dense deposit disease N01.6
diffuse
crescentic glomerulonephritis N01.7
endocapillary proliferative glomerulonephritis N01.4

Nephritis, nephritic (Continued)
  rapidly progressive (Continued)
    with (Continued)
      diffuse (Continued)
        membranous glomerulonephritis
          N01.2
        mesangial proliferative
          glomerulonephritis N01.3
        mesangiocapillary glomerulonephritis
          N01.5
        focal and segmental glomerular lesions
          N01.1
        minor glomerular abnormality N01.0
        specified morphological changes NEC
          N01.8
  salt losing or wasting NEC N28.89
  saturnine N14.3
  sclerosing, diffuse N05.8
  septic —see Nephritis, tubulo-interstitial
  specified pathology NEC —see also N00-N07
    with fourth character .8 N05.8
  subacute N01.9
  suppurative —see Nephritis,
    tubulo-interstitial
  syphilitic (late) A52.75
    congenital A50.59 [N08]
    early (secondary) A51.44
  toxic —see Nephropathy, toxic
  tubal, tubular —see Nephritis,
    tubulo-interstitial
  tuberculous A18.11
  tubulo-interstitial (in) N12
    acute (infectious) N10
    chronic (infectious) N11.9
      nonobstructive N11.8
        reflux-associated N11.0
      obstructive N11.1
      specified NEC N11.8
    due to
      brucellosis A23.9 [N16]
      cryoglobulinemia D89.1 [N16]
      glycogen storage disease E74.00
        [N16]
    Sjögren's syndrome M35.04
  vascular —see Hypertension, kidney
  war N00.9
Nephroblastoma (epithelial) (mesenchymal)
  C64-
Nephrocalcinosis E83.59 [N29]
Nephrocystitis, pustular —see Nephritis,
  tubulo-interstitial
Nephrolithiasis (congenital) (pelvis)
  (recurrent) —see also Calculus, kidney
Nephroma C64-
  mesoblastic D41.0-
Nephronephritis —see Nephrosis
Nephronophthisis Q61.5
Nephropathia epidemica A98.5
Nephropathy —see also Nephritis N28.9
  with
    edema —see Nephrosis
    glomerular lesion —see
      Glomerulonephritis
  amyloid, hereditary E85.0
  analgesic N14.0
    with medullary necrosis, acute N17.2
  Balkan (endemic) N15.0
  chemical —see Nephropathy, toxic
  diabetic —see E08-E13 with .21
  drug-induced N14.2
    specified NEC N14.1
  focal and segmental hyalinosis or sclerosis
    N02.1
  heavy metal-induced N14.3
  hereditary NEC N07.9
    with
      dense deposit disease N07.6
      diffuse
        crescentic glomerulonephritis N07.7
        endocapillary proliferative
          glomerulonephritis N07.4

Nephropathy (Continued)
  hereditary NEC (Continued)
    with (Continued)
      diffuse (Continued)
        membranous glomerulonephritis
          N07.2
        mesangial proliferative
          glomerulonephritis N07.3
        mesangiocapillary glomerulonephritis
          N07.5
        focal and segmental glomerular lesions
          N07.1
        minor glomerular abnormality N07.0
        specified morphological changes NEC
          N07.8
  hypercalcemic N25.89
  hypertensive —see Hypertension, kidney
  hypokalemic (vacuolar) N25.89
  IgA N02.8
    with glomerular lesion N02.9
      focal and segmental hyalinosis or
        sclerosis N02.1
      membranoproliferative (diffuse) N02.5
      membranous (diffuse) N02.2
      mesangial proliferative (diffuse) N02.3
      mesangiocapillary (diffuse) N02.5
      proliferative NEC N02.8
      specified pathology NEC N02.8
  lead N14.3
  membranoproliferative (diffuse) N02.5
  membranous (diffuse) N02.2
  mesangial (IgA/IgG) —see Nephropathy, IgA
    proliferative (diffuse) N02.3
  mesangiocapillary (diffuse) N02.5
  obstructive N13.8
  phenacetin N17.2
  phosphate-losing N25.0
  potassium depletion N25.89
  pregnancy-related O26.83-
  proliferative NEC (see also N00-N07 with
    fourth character .8) N05.8
  protein-losing N25.89
  saturnine N14.3
  sickle-cell D57.- [N08]
  toxic NEC N14.4
    due to
      drugs N14.2
        analgesic N14.0
        specified NEC N14.1
      heavy metals N14.3
  vasomotor N17.0
  water-losing N25.89
Nephroptosis N28.83
Nephropyosis —see Abscess, kidney
Nephrorrhagia N28.89
Nephrosclerosis (arteriolar) (arteriosclerotic)
  (chronic) (hyaline) —see also Hypertension,
  kidney
  hyperplastic —see Hypertension, kidney
  senile N26.9
Nephrosis, nephrotic (Epstein's) (syndrome)
  (congenital) N04.9
  with
    foot process disease N04.9
    glomerular lesion N04.1
    hypocomplementemic N04.5
  acute N04.9
  anoxic —see Nephrosis, tubular
  chemical —see Nephrosis, tubular
  cholemic K76.7
  diabetic —see E08-E13 with .21
  Finnish type (congenital) Q89.8
  hemoglobin N10
  hemoglobinuric —see Nephrosis, tubular
  in
    amyloidosis E85.4 [N08]
    diabetes mellitus —see E08-E13 with .21
    epidemic hemorrhagic fever A98.5
    malaria (malariae) B52.0
  ischemic —see Nephrosis, tubular
  lipoid N04.9

Nephrosis, nephrotic (Continued)
  lower nephron —see Nephrosis, tubular
  malarial (malariae) B52.0
  minimal change N04.0
  myoglobin N10
  necrotizing —see Nephrosis, tubular
  osmotic (sucrose) N25.89
  radiation N04.9
  syphilitic (late) A52.75
  toxic —see Nephrosis, tubular
  tubular (acute) N17.0
    postprocedural N99.0
    radiation N04.9
Nephrosonephritis, hemorrhagic (endemic)
  A98.5
Nephrostomy
  attention to Z43.6
  status Z93.6
Nerve —see also condition
  injury —see Injury, nerve, by body site
Nerves R45.0
Nervous —see also condition R45.0
  heart F45.8
  stomach F45.8
  tension R45.0
Nervousness R45.0
Nesidioblastoma
  pancreas D13.7
  specified site NEC —see Neoplasm, benign,
    by site
  unspecified site D13.7
Nettleship's syndrome Q82.2
Neumann's disease or syndrome L10.1
Neuralgia, neuralgic (acute) M79.2
  accessory (nerve) G52.8
  acoustic (nerve) —see subcategory H93.3
  auditory (nerve) —see subcategory H93.3
  ciliary G44.009
    intractable G44.001
    not intractable G44.009
  cranial
    nerve —see also Disorder, nerve, cranial
      fifth or trigeminal —see Neuralgia,
        trigeminal
    postherpetic, postzoster B02.29
  ear —see subcategory H92.0
  facialis vera G51.1
  Fothergill's —see Neuralgia, trigeminal
  glossopharyngeal (nerve) G52.1
  Horton's G44.099
    intractable G44.091
    not intractable G44.099
  Hunt's B02.21
  hypoglossal (nerve) G52.3
  infraorbital —see Neuralgia, trigeminal
  malarial —see Malaria
  migrainous G44.009
    intractable G44.001
    not intractable G44.009
  Morton's G57.6-
  nerve, cranial —see Disorder, nerve,
    cranial
  nose G52.0
  occipital M54.81
  olfactory G52.0
  penis N48.9
  perineum R10.2
  postherpetic NEC B02.29
    trigeminal B02.22
  pubic region R10.2
  scrotum R10.2
  Sluder's G44.89
  specified nerve NEC G58.8
  spermatic cord R10.2
  sphenopalatine (ganglion) G90.09
  trifacial —see Neuralgia, trigeminal
  trigeminal G50.0
    postherpetic, postzoster B02.22
  vagus (nerve) G52.2
  writer's F48.8
    organic G25.89

◀ New   ◀||| Revised   deleted Deleted

Neurapraxia —see Injury, nerve
Neurasthenia F48.8
  cardiac F45.8
  gastric F45.8
  heart F45.8
Neurilemmoma —see also Neoplasm, nerve,
    benign
  acoustic (nerve) D33.3
  malignant —see also Neoplasm, nerve,
    malignant
    acoustic (nerve) C72.4
Neurilemmosarcoma —see Neoplasm, nerve,
  malignant
Neurinoma —see Neoplasm, nerve, benign
Neurinomatosis —see Neoplasm, nerve,
  uncertain behavior
Neuritis (rheumatoid) M79.2
  abducens (nerve) —see Strabismus, paralytic,
    sixth nerve
  accessory (nerve) G52.8
  acoustic (nerve) —see also subcategory H93.3
    in (due to)
      infectious disease NEC B99 [H94.0-]
      parasitic disease NEC B89 [H94.0-]
      syphilitic A52.15
  alcoholic G62.1
    with psychosis —see Psychosis, alcoholic
  amyloid, any site E85.4 [G63]
  auditory (nerve) —see subcategory H93.3
  brachial —see Radiculopathy
    due to displacement, intervertebral disc —
      see Disorder, disc, cervical, with
      neuritis
  cranial nerve
    due to Lyme disease A69.22
    eighth or acoustic or auditory —see
      subcategory H93.3
    eleventh or accessory G52.8
    fifth or trigeminal G51.0
    first or olfactory G52.0
    fourth or trochlear —see Strabismus,
      paralytic, fourth nerve
    second or optic —see Neuritis, optic
    seventh or facial G51.8
      newborn (birth injury) P11.3
    sixth or abducent —see Strabismus,
      paralytic, sixth nerve
    tenth or vagus G52.2
    third or oculomotor —see Strabismus,
      paralytic, third nerve
    twelfth or hypoglossal G52.3
  Déjérine-Sottas G60.0
  diabetic (mononeuropathy) —see E08-E13
    with .41
    polyneuropathy —see E08-E13 with .42
  due to
    beriberi E51.11
    displacement, prolapse or rupture,
      intervertebral disc —see Disorder,
      disc, with, radiculopathy
    herniation, nucleus pulposus M51.9 [G55]
  endemic E51.11
  facial G51.8
    newborn (birth injury) P11.3
  general —see Polyneuropathy
  geniculate ganglion G51.1
    due to herpes (zoster) B02.21
  gouty —see also Gout, by type M10.9 [G63] ◀▥
  hypoglossal (nerve) G52.3
  ilioinguinal (nerve) G57.9-
  infectious (multiple) NEC G61.0
  interstitial hypertrophic progressive G60.0
  lumbar M54.16
  lumbosacral M54.17
  multiple —see also Polyneuropathy
    endemic E51.11
    infective, acute G61.0
  multiplex endemica E51.11
  nerve root —see Radiculopathy
  oculomotor (nerve) —see Strabismus,
    paralytic, third nerve

Neuritis (Continued)
  olfactory nerve G52.0
  optic (nerve) (hereditary) (sympathetic) H46.9
    with demyelination G36.0
    in myelitis G36.0
    nutritional H46.2
    papillitis —see Papillitis, optic
    retrobulbar H46.1-
    specified type NEC H46.8
    toxic H46.3
  peripheral (nerve) G62.9
    multiple —see Polyneuropathy
    single —see Mononeuritis
  pneumogastric (nerve) G52.2
  postherpetic, postzoster B02.29
  progressive hypertrophic interstitial G60.0
  retrobulbar —see also Neuritis, optic,
      retrobulbar
    in (due to)
      late syphilis A52.15
      meningococcal infection A39.82
    meningococcal A39.82
    syphilitic A52.15
  sciatic (nerve) —see also Sciatica
    due to displacement of intervertebral
      disc —see Disorder, disc, with,
      radiculopathy
  serum —see also Reaction, serum T80.69
  shoulder-girdle G54.5
  specified nerve NEC G58.8
  spinal (nerve) root —see Radiculopathy
  syphilitic A52.15
  thenar (median) G56.1-
  thoracic M54.14
  toxic NEC G62.2
  trochlear (nerve) —see Strabismus, paralytic,
    fourth nerve
  vagus (nerve) G52.2
Neuroastrocytoma —see Neoplasm, uncertain
  behavior, by site
Neuroavitaminosis E56.9 [G99.8]
Neuroblastoma
  olfactory C30.0
  specified site —see Neoplasm, malignant, by
    site
  unspecified site C74.90
Neurochorioretinitis —see Chorioretinitis
Neurocirculatory asthenia F45.8
Neurocysticercosis B69.0
Neurocytoma —see Neoplasm, benign, by site
Neurodermatitis (circumscribed)
    (circumscripta) (local) L28.0
  atopic L20.81
  diffuse (Brocq) L20.81
  disseminated L20.81
Neuroencephalomyelopathy, optic G36.0
Neuroepithelioma —see also Neoplasm,
    malignant, by site
  olfactory C30.0
Neurofibroma —see also Neoplasm, nerve,
    benign
  melanotic —see Neoplasm, nerve, benign
  multiple —see Neurofibromatosis
  plexiform —see Neoplasm, nerve, benign
Neurofibromatosis (multiple) (nonmalignant)
    Q85.00
  acoustic Q85.02
  malignant —see Neoplasm, nerve, malignant
  specified NEC Q85.09
  type 1 (von Recklinghausen) Q85.01
  type 2 Q85.02
Neurofibrosarcoma —see Neoplasm, nerve,
  malignant
Neurogenic —see also condition
  bladder (see also Dysfunction, bladder,
      neuromuscular) N31.9
    cauda equina syndrome G83.4
  bowel NEC K59.2
  heart F45.8
Neuroglioma —see Neoplasm, uncertain
  behavior, by site

Neurolabyrinthitis (of Dix and Hallpike) —see
  Neuronitis, vestibular
Neurolathyrism —see Poisoning, food, noxious,
  plant
Neuroleprosy A30.9
Neuroma —see also Neoplasm, nerve, benign
  acoustic (nerve) D33.3
  amputation (stump) (traumatic) (surgical
      complication) (late) T87.3-
    arm T87.3-
    leg T87.3-
  digital (toe) G57.6-
  interdigital G58.8 ◀▥
    lower limb toe G57.8- ◀▥
    upper limb G56.8-
  intermetatarsal G57.8-
  Morton's G57.6-
  nonneoplastic
    arm G56.9-
    leg G57.9-
    lower extremity G57.9-
    upper extremity G56.9-
  optic (nerve) D33.3
  plantar G57.6-
  plexiform —see Neoplasm, nerve,
    benign
  surgical (nonneoplastic)
    arm G56.9-
    leg G57.9-
    lower extremity G57.9-
    upper extremity G56.9-
Neuromyalgia —see Neuralgia
Neuromyasthenia (epidemic) (postinfectious)
    G93.3
Neuromyelitis G36.9
  ascending G61.0
  optica G36.0
Neuromyopathy G70.9
  paraneoplastic D49.9 [G13.0]
Neuromyotonia (Isaacs) G71.19
Neuronevus —see Nevus
Neuronitis G58.9
  ascending (acute) G57.2-
  vestibular H81.2-
Neuroparalytic —see condition
Neuropathy, neuropathic G62.9
  acute motor G62.81
  alcoholic G62.1
    with psychosis —see Psychosis, alcoholic
  arm G56.9-
  autonomic, peripheral —see Neuropathy,
      peripheral, autonomic
  axillary G56.9-
  bladder N31.9
    atonic (motor) (sensory) N31.2
    autonomous N31.2
    flaccid N31.2
    nonreflex N31.2
    reflex N31.1
    uninhibited N31.0
  brachial plexus G54.0
  cervical plexus G54.2
  chronic
    progressive segmentally demyelinating
      G62.89
    relapsing demyelinating G62.89
  Déjérine-Sottas G60.0
  diabetic —see E08-E13 with .40
    mononeuropathy —see E08-E13 with .41
    polyneuropathy —see E08-E13 with .42
  entrapment G58.9
    iliohypogastric nerve G57.8-
    ilioinguinal nerve G57.8-
    lateral cutaneous nerve of thigh
      G57.1-
    median nerve G56.0-
    obturator nerve G57.8-
    peroneal nerve G57.3-
    posterior tibial nerve G57.5-
    saphenous nerve G57.8-
    ulnar nerve G56.2-

Neuropathy, neuropathic (Continued)
- facial nerve G51.9
- hereditary G60.9
  - motor and sensory (types I-IV) G60.0
  - sensory G60.8
  - specified NEC G60.8
- hypertrophic G60.0
  - Charcot-Marie-Tooth G60.0
  - Déjérine-Sottas G60.0
  - interstitial progressive G60.0
  - of infancy G60.0
  - Refsum G60.1
- idiopathic G60.9
  - progressive G60.3
  - specified NEC G60.8
- in association with hereditary ataxia G60.2
- intercostal G58.0
- ischemic —see Disorder, nerve
- Jamaica (ginger) G62.2
- leg NEC G57.9-
- lower extremity G57.9-
- lumbar plexus G54.1
- median nerve G56.1-
- motor and sensory —see also Polyneuropathy
  - hereditary (types I-IV) G60.0
- multifocal motor (MMN) G61.82 ◀
- multiple (acute) (chronic) —see
  - Polyneuropathy
- optic (nerve) —see also Neuritis, optic
  - ischemic H47.01-
- paraneoplastic (sensorial) (Denny Brown)
  - D49.9 [G13.0]
- peripheral (nerve) —see also Polyneuropathy
  - G62.9
  - autonomic G90.9
    - idiopathic G90.09
    - in (due to)
      - amyloidosis E85.4 [G99.0]
      - diabetes mellitus —see E08-E13 with
        - .43
      - endocrine disease NEC E34.9 [G99.0]
      - gout M10.00 [G99.0]
      - hyperthyroidism E05.90 [G99.0]
        - with thyroid storm E05.91 [G99.0]
      - metabolic disease NEC E88.9 [G99.0]
  - idiopathic G60.9
    - progressive G60.3
  - in (due to)
    - antitetanus serum G62.0
    - arsenic G62.2
    - drugs NEC G62.0
    - lead G62.2
    - organophosphate compounds G62.2
    - toxic agent NEC G62.2
- plantar nerves G57.6-
- progressive
  - hypertrophic interstitial G60.0
  - inflammatory G62.81
- radicular NEC —see Radiculopathy
- sacral plexus G54.1
- sciatic G57.0-
- serum G61.1
- toxic NEC G62.2
- trigeminal sensory G50.8
- ulnar nerve G56.2-
- uremic N18.9 [G63]
- vitamin B12 E53.8 [G63]
  - with anemia (pernicious) D51.0 [G63]
  - due to dietary deficiency D51.3 [G63]

Neurophthisis —see also Disorder, nerve
- peripheral, diabetic —see E08-E13 with .42

Neuroretinitis —see Chorioretinitis
Neuroretinopathy, hereditary optic H47.22
Neurosarcoma —see Neoplasm, nerve, malignant
Neurosclerosis —see Disorder, nerve
Neurosis, neurotic F48.9
- anankastic F42.8 ◀▥
- anxiety (state) F41.1
  - panic type F41.0
- asthenic F48.8
- bladder F45.8

Neurosis, neurotic (Continued)
- cardiac (reflex) F45.8
- cardiovascular F45.8
- character F60.9
- colon F45.8
- compensation F68.1
- compulsive, compulsion F42.8 ◀▥
- conversion F44.9
- craft F48.8
- cutaneous F45.8
- depersonalization F48.1
- depressive (reaction) (type) F34.1
- environmental F48.8
- excoriation L98.1
- fatigue F48.8
- functional —see Disorder, somatoform
- gastric F45.8
- gastrointestinal F45.8
- heart F45.8
- hypochondriacal F45.21
- hysterical F44.9
- incoordination F45.8
  - larynx F45.8
  - vocal cord F45.8
- intestine F45.8
- larynx (sensory) F45.8
  - hysterical F44.4
- mixed NEC F48.8
- musculoskeletal F45.8
- obsessional F42.8 ◀▥
- obsessive-compulsive F42.8 ◀▥
- occupational F48.8
- ocular NEC F45.8
- organ —see Disorder, somatoform
- pharynx F45.8
- phobic F40.9
- posttraumatic (situational) F43.10
  - acute F43.11
  - chronic F43.12
- psychasthenic (type) F48.8
- railroad F48.8
- rectum F45.8
- respiratory F45.8
- rumination F45.8
- sexual F65.9
- situational F48.8
- social F40.10
  - generalized F40.11
- specified type NEC F48.8
- state F48.9
  - with depersonalization episode F48.1
- stomach F45.8
- traumatic F43.10
  - acute F43.11
  - chronic F43.12
- vasomotor F45.8
- visceral F45.8
- war F48.8

Neurospongioblastosis diffusa Q85.1
Neurosyphilis (arrested) (early) (gumma) (late)
  (latent) (recurrent) (relapse) A52.3
- with ataxia (cerebellar) (locomotor) (spastic)
  (spinal) A52.19
- aneurysm (cerebral) A52.05
- arachnoid (adhesive) A52.13
- arteritis (any artery) (cerebral) A52.04
- asymptomatic A52.2
- congenital A50.40
- dura (mater) A52.13
- general paresis A52.17
- hemorrhagic A52.05
- juvenile (asymptomatic) (meningeal)
  A50.40
- leptomeninges (aseptic) A52.13
- meningeal, meninges (adhesive) A52.13
- meningitis A52.13
- meningovascular (diffuse) A52.13
- optic atrophy A52.15
- parenchymatous (degenerative) A52.19
- paresis, paretic A52.17
  - juvenile A50.45

Neurosyphilis (Continued)
- remission in (sustained) A52.3
- serological (without symptoms) A52.2
- specified nature or site NEC A52.19
- tabes, tabetic (dorsalis) A52.11
  - juvenile A50.45
- taboparesis A52.17
  - juvenile A50.45
- thrombosis (cerebral) A52.05
- vascular (cerebral) NEC A52.05
Neurothekeoma —see Neoplasm, nerve, benign
Neurotic —see Neurosis
Neurotoxemia —see Toxemia
Neutroclusion M26.211
Neutropenia, neutropenic (chronic) (genetic)
  (idiopathic) (immune) (infantile)
  (malignant) (pernicious) (splenic) D70.9
- congenital (primary) D70.0
- cyclic D70.4
- cytoreductive cancer chemotherapy sequela
  D70.1
- drug-induced D70.2
  - due to cytoreductive cancer chemotherapy
    D70.1
- due to infection D70.3
- fever D70.9
- neonatal, transitory (isoimmune) (maternal
  transfer) P61.5
- periodic D70.4
- secondary (cyclic) (periodic) (splenic) D70.4
  - drug-induced D70.2
    - due to cytoreductive cancer
      chemotherapy D70.1
- toxic D70.8
Neutrophilia, hereditary giant D72.0
Nevocarcinoma —see Melanoma
Nevus D22.9
- achromic —see Neoplasm, skin, benign
- amelanotic —see Neoplasm, skin, benign
- angiomatous D18.00
  - intra-abdominal D18.03
  - intracranial D18.02
  - skin D18.01
  - specified site NEC D18.09
- araneus I78.1
- balloon cell —see Neoplasm, skin, benign
- bathing trunk D48.5
- blue —see Neoplasm, skin, benign
  - cellular —see Neoplasm, skin, benign
  - giant —see Neoplasm, skin, benign
  - Jadassohn's —see Neoplasm, skin, benign
  - malignant —see Melanoma
- capillary D18.00
  - intra-abdominal D18.03
  - intracranial D18.02
  - skin D18.01
  - specified site NEC D18.09
- cavernous D18.00
  - intra-abdominal D18.03
  - intracranial D18.02
  - skin D18.01
  - specified site NEC D18.09
- cellular —see Neoplasm, skin, benign
  - blue —see Neoplasm, skin, benign
- choroid D31.3-
- comedonicus Q82.5
- conjunctiva D31.0-
- dermal —see Neoplasm, skin, benign
  - with epidermal nevus —see Neoplasm,
    skin, benign
- dysplastic —see Neoplasm, skin, benign
- eye D31.9-
- flammeus Q82.5
- hemangiomatous D18.00
  - intra-abdominal D18.03
  - intracranial D18.02
  - skin D18.01
  - specified site NEC D18.09
- iris D31.4-
- lacrimal gland D31.5-
- lymphatic D18.1

◀ New   ◀▥ Revised   ~~deleted~~ Deleted

Nevus (Continued)
  magnocellular
    specified site —*see* Neoplasm, benign, by
      site
    unspecified site D31.40
  malignant —*see* Melanoma
  meaning hemangioma D18.00
    intra-abdominal D18.03
    intracranial D18.02
    skin D18.01
    specified site NEC D18.09
  mouth (mucosa) D10.30
    specified site NEC D10.39
    white sponge Q38.6
  multiplex Q85.1
  non-neoplastic I78.1
  oral mucosa D10.30
    specified site NEC D10.39
    white sponge Q38.6
  orbit D31.6-
  pigmented
    giant —*see also* Neoplasm, skin, uncertain
      behavior D48.5
    malignant melanoma in —*see* Melanoma
  portwine Q82.5
  retina D31.2-
  retrobulbar D31.6-
  sanguineous Q82.5
  senile I78.1
  skin D22.9
    abdominal wall D22.5
    ala nasi D22.39
    ankle D22.7-
    anus, anal D22.5
    arm D22.6-
    auditory canal (external) D22.2-
    auricle (ear) D22.2-
    auricular canal (external) D22.2-
    axilla, axillary fold D22.5
    back D22.5
    breast D22.5
    brow D22.39
    buttock D22.5
    canthus (eye) D22.1-
    cheek (external) D22.39
    chest wall D22.5
    chin D22.39
    ear (external) D22.2-
    external meatus (ear) D22.2-
    eyebrow D22.39
    eyelid (lower) (upper) D22.1-
    face D22.30
      specified NEC D22.39
    female genital organ (external) NEC D28.0
    finger D22.6-
    flank D22.5
    foot D22.7-
    forearm D22.6-
    forehead D22.39
    foreskin D29.0
    genital organ (external) NEC
      female D28.0
      male D29.9
    gluteal region D22.5
    groin D22.5
    hand D22.6-
    heel D22.7-
    helix D22.2-
    hip D22.7-
    interscapular region D22.5
    jaw D22.39
    knee D22.7-
    labium (majus) (minus) D28.0
    leg D22.7-
    lip (lower) (upper) D22.0
    lower limb D22.7-
    male genital organ (external) D29.9
    nail D22.9
      finger D22.6-
      toe D22.7-
    nasolabial groove D22.39
    nates D22.5

Nevus (Continued)
  skin (Continued)
    neck D22.4
    nose (external) D22.39
    palpebra D22.1-
    penis D29.0
    perianal skin D22.5
    perineum D22.5
    pinna D22.2-
    popliteal fossa or space D22.7-
    prepuce D29.0
    pudendum D28.0
    scalp D22.4
    scrotum D29.4
    shoulder D22.6-
    submammary fold D22.5
    temple D22.39
    thigh D22.7-
    toe D22.7-
    trunk NEC D22.5
    umbilicus D22.5
    upper limb D22.6-
    vulva D28.0
  specified site NEC —*see* Neoplasm, benign,
    by site
  spider I78.1
  stellar I78.1
  strawberry Q82.5
  Sutton's —*see* Neoplasm, skin, benign
  unius lateris Q82.5
  Unna's Q82.5
  vascular Q82.5
  verrucous Q82.5

Newborn (infant) (liveborn) (singleton) Z38.2
  abstinence syndrome P96.1
  acne L70.4
  affected by ◀▥
    abnormalities of membranes P02.9
      specified NEC P02.8
    abruptio placenta P02.1
    amino-acid metabolic disorder, transitory
      P74.8
    amniocentesis (while in utero) P00.6
    amnionitis P02.7
    apparent life threatening event (ALTE)
      R68.13
    bleeding (into)
      cerebral cortex P52.22
      germinal matrix P52.0
      ventricles P52.1
    breech delivery P03.0
    cardiac arrest P29.81
    cardiomyopathy I42.8
      congenital I42.4
    cerebral ischemia P91.0
    Cesarean delivery P03.4
    chemotherapy agents P04.1
    chorioamnionitis P02.7
    cocaine (crack) P04.41
    complications of labor and delivery P03.9
      specified NEC P03.89
    compression of umbilical cord NEC P02.5
    contracted pelvis P03.1
    delivery P03.9
      Cesarean P03.4
      forceps P03.2
      vacuum extractor P03.3
    entanglement (knot) in umbilical cord
      P02.5
    environmental chemicals P04.6
    fetal (intrauterine)
      growth retardation P05.9
      malnutrition not light or small for
        gestational age P05.2
    forceps delivery P03.2
    heart rate abnormalities
      bradycardia P29.12
      intrauterine P03.819
        before onset of labor P03.810
        during labor P03.811
      tachycardia P29.11

Newborn (Continued)
  affected by (Continued)
    hemorrhage (antepartum) P02.1
      cerebellar (nontraumatic) P52.6
      intracerebral (nontraumatic) P52.4
      intracranial (nontraumatic) P52.9
        specified NEC P52.8
      intraventricular (nontraumatic) P52.3
        grade 1 P52.0
        grade 2 P52.1
        grade 3 P52.21
        grade 4 P52.22
      posterior fossa (nontraumatic) P52.6
      subarachnoid (nontraumatic) P52.5
      subependymal P52.0
        with intracerebral extension P52.22
        with intraventricular extension P52.1
          with enlargment of ventricles
            P52.21
          without intraventricular extension
            P52.0
    hypoxic ischemic encephalopathy [HIE]
      P91.60
      mild P91.61
      moderate P91.62
      severe P91.63
    induction of labor P03.89
    intestinal perforation P78.0
    intrauterine (fetal) blood loss P50.9
      due to (from)
        cut end of co-twin cord P50.5
        hemorrhage into
          co-twin P50.3
          maternal circulation P50.4
        placenta P50.2
        ruptured cord blood P50.1
        vasa previa P50.0
      specified NEC P50.8
    intrauterine (fetal) hemorrhage P50.9
    intrauterine (in utero) procedure P96.5
    malpresentation (malposition) NEC P03.1
    maternal (complication of) (use of)
      alcohol P04.3
      analgesia (maternal) P04.0
      anesthesia (maternal) P04.0
      blood loss P02.1
      circulatory disease P00.3
      condition P00.9
        specified NEC P00.89
      delivery P03.9
        Cesarean P03.4
        forceps P03.2
        vacuum extractor P03.3
      diabetes mellitus (pre-existing) P70.1
      disorder P00.9
        specified NEC P00.89
      drugs (addictive) (illegal) NEC P04.49
      ectopic pregnancy P01.4
      gestational diabetes P70.0
      hemorrhage P02.1
      hypertensive disorder P00.0
      incompetent cervix P01.0
      infectious disease P00.2
      injury P00.5
      labor and delivery P03.9
      malpresentation before labor P01.7
      maternal death P01.6
      medical procedure P00.7
      medication P04.1
      multiple pregnancy P01.5
      nutritional disorder P00.4
      oligohydramnios P01.2
      parasitic disease P00.2
      periodontal disease P00.81
      placenta previa P02.0
      polyhydramnios P01.3
      precipitate delivery P03.5
      pregnancy P01.9
        specified P01.8
      premature rupture of membranes P01.1
      renal disease P00.1

Newborn *(Continued)*
  affected by *(Continued)*
    maternal *(Continued)*
      respiratory disease P00.3
      surgical procedure P00.6
      urinary tract disease P00.1
      uterine contraction (abnormal) P03.6
    meconium peritonitis P78.0
    medication (legal) (maternal use)
      (prescribed) P04.1
    membrane abnormalities P02.9
      specified NEC P02.8
    membranitis P02.7
    methamphetamine (s) P04.49
    mixed metabolic and respiratory acidosis
      P84
    neonatal abstinence syndrome P96.1
    noxious substances transmitted via
      placenta or breast milk P04.9
      specified NEC P04.8
    nutritional supplements P04.5
    placenta previa P02.0
    placental
      abnormality (functional)
        (morphological) P02.20
        specified NEC P02.29
      dysfunction P02.29
      infarction P02.29
      insufficiency P02.29
      separation NEC P02.1
      transfusion syndromes P02.3
    placentitis P02.7
    precipitate delivery P03.5
    prolapsed cord P02.4
    respiratory arrest P28.81
    slow intrauterine growth P05.9
    tobacco P04.2
    twin to twin transplacental transfusion
      P02.3
    umbilical cord (tightly) around neck P02.5
    umbilical cord condition P02.60
      short cord P02.69
      specified NEC P02.69
    uterine contractions (abnormal) P03.6
    vasa previa P02.69
      from intrauterine blood loss P50.0
  apnea P28.4 ◀▥
    obstructive P28.4
    primary P28.3
    ~~specified P28.4~~
    sleep (central) (obstructive) (primary)
      P28.3 ◀
  born in hospital Z38.00
    by cesarean Z38.01
  born outside hospital Z38.1
  breast buds P96.89
  breast engorgement P83.4
  check-up —*see* Newborn, examination
  convulsion P90
  dehydration P74.1
  examination
    8 to 28 days old Z00.111
    under 8 days old Z00.110
  fever P81.9
    environmentally-induced P81.0
  hyperbilirubinemia P59.9
    of prematurity P59.0
  hypernatremia P74.2
  hyponatremia P74.2
  infection P39.9
    candidal P37.5
    specified NEC P39.8
    urinary tract P39.3
  jaundice P59.9 ◀▥
    due to
      breast milk inhibitor P59.3
      hepatocellular damage P59.20
        specified NEC P59.29
      preterm delivery P59.0
    of prematurity P59.0
    specified NEC P59.8

Newborn *(Continued)*
  late metabolic acidosis P74.0
  mastitis P39.0
    infective P39.0
    noninfective P83.4
  multiple born NEC Z38.8
    born in hospital Z38.68
      by cesarean Z38.69
    born outside hospital Z38.7
  omphalitis P38.9
    with mild hemorrhage P38.1
    without hemorrhage P38.9
  post-term P08.21
  prolonged gestation (over 42 completed
    weeks) P08.22
  quadruplet Z38.8
    born in hospital Z38.63
      by cesarean Z38.64
    born outside hospital Z38.7
  quintuplet Z38.8
    born in hospital Z38.65
      by cesarean Z38.66
    born outside hospital Z38.7
  seizure P90
  sepsis (congenital) P36.9
    due to
      anaerobes NEC P36.5
      Escherichia coli P36.4
      Staphylococcus P36.30
        aureus P36.2
        specified NEC P36.39
      Streptococcus P36.10
        group B P36.0
        specified NEC P36.19
    specified NEC P36.8
  triplet Z38.8
    born in hospital Z38.61
      by cesarean Z38.62
    born outside hospital Z38.7
  twin Z38.5
    born in hospital Z38.30
      by cesarean Z38.31
    born outside hospital Z38.4
  vomiting P92.09
    bilious P92.01
  weight check Z00.111
Newcastle conjunctivitis or disease B30.8
Nezelof's syndrome (pure alymphocytosis)
  D81.4
Niacin (amide) deficiency E52
Nicolas (-Durand)-Favre disease A55
Nicotine —*see* Tobacco
Nicotinic acid deficiency E52
Niemann-Pick disease or syndrome E75.249
  specified NEC E75.248
  type
    A E75.240
    B E75.241
    C E75.242
    D E75.243
Night
  blindness —*see* Blindness, night
  sweats R61
  terrors (child) F51.4
Nightmares (REM sleep type) F51.5
NIHSS (National Institutes of Health Stroke
  Scale) score R29.7- ◀
Nipple —*see* condition
Nisbet's chancre A57
Nishimoto (-Takeuchi) disease I67.5
Nitritoid crisis or reaction —*see* Crisis, nitritoid
Nitrosohemoglobinemia D74.8
Njovera A65
Nocardiosis, nocardiasis A43.9
  cutaneous A43.1
  lung A43.0
  pneumonia A43.0
  pulmonary A43.0
  specified site NEC A43.8
Nocturia R35.1
  psychogenic F45.8

Nocturnal —*see* condition
Nodal rhythm I49.8
Node (s) —*see also* Nodule
  Bouchard's (with arthropathy) M15.2
  Haygarth's M15.8
  Heberden's (with arthropathy) M15.1
  larynx J38.7
  lymph —*see* condition
  milker's B08.03
  Osler's I33.0
  Schmorl's —*see* Schmorl's disease
  singer's J38.2
  teacher's J38.2
  tuberculous —*see* Tuberculosis, lymph
    gland
  vocal cord J38.2
Nodule (s), nodular
  actinomycotic —*see* Actinomycosis
  breast NEC N63
  colloid (cystic), thyroid E04.1
  cutaneous —*see* Swelling, localized
  endometrial (stromal) D26.1
  Haygarth's M15.8
  inflammatory —*see* Inflammation
  juxta-articular
    syphilitic A52.77
    yaws A66.7
  larynx J38.7
  lung, solitary (subsegmental branch of the
    bronchial tree) R91.1
    multiple R91.8
  milker's B08.03
  prostate N40.2
    with lower urinary tract symptoms (LUTS)
      N40.3
    without lower urinary tract symptoms
      (LUTS) N40.2
  pulmonary, solitary (subsegmental branch of
    the bronchial tree) R91.1
  retrocardiac R09.89
  rheumatoid M06.30
    ankle M06.37-
    elbow M06.32-
    foot joint M06.37-
    hand joint M06.34-
    hip M06.35-
    knee M06.36-
    multiple site M06.39
    shoulder M06.31-
    vertebra M06.38
    wrist M06.33-
  scrotum (inflammatory) N49.2
  singer's J38.2
  solitary, lung (subsegmental branch of the
    bronchial tree) R91.1
    multiple R91.8
  subcutaneous —*see* Swelling, localized
  teacher's J38.2
  thyroid (cold) (gland) (nontoxic) E04.1
    with thyrotoxicosis E05.20
      with thyroid storm E05.21
    toxic or with hyperthyroidism E05.20
      with thyroid storm E05.21
  vocal cord J38.2
Noma (gangrenous) (hospital) (infective)
  A69.0
  auricle I96
  mouth A69.0
  pudendi N76.89
  vulvae N76.89
Nomad, nomadism Z59.0
NOMID (neonatal onset multisystemic
  inflammatory disorder) M04.2 ◀
Nonautoimmune hemolytic anemia
  D59.4
  drug-induced D59.2
Nonclosure —*see also* Imperfect, closure
  ductus arteriosus (Botallo's) Q25.0
  foramen
    botalli Q21.1
    ovale Q21.1

Noncompliance Z91.19
    with
        dialysis Z91.15
        dietary regimen Z91.11
        medical treatment Z91.19
        medication regimen NEC Z91.14
            underdosing —see also Table of Drugs
                and Chemicals, categories T36-T50,
                with final character 6 Z91.14
                intentional NEC Z91.128
                    due to financial hardship of patient
                        Z91.120
                unintentional NEC Z91.138
                    due to patient's age related debility
                        Z91.130
        renal dialysis Z91.15
Nondescent (congenital) —see also Malposition,
    congenital
    cecum Q43.3
    colon Q43.3
    testicle Q53.9
        bilateral Q53.20
            abdominal Q53.21
            perineal Q53.22
        unilateral Q53.10
            abdominal Q53.11
            perineal Q53.12
Nondevelopment
    brain Q02
        part of Q04.3
    heart Q24.8
    organ or site, congenital NEC —see
        Hypoplasia
Nonengagement
    head NEC O32.4
        in labor, causing obstructed labor O64.8
Nonexanthematous tick fever A93.2
Nonexpansion, lung (newborn) P28.0
Nonfunctioning
    cystic duct —see also Disease, gallbladder
        K82.8
    gallbladder —see also Disease, gallbladder
        K82.8
    kidney N28.9
    labyrinth —see subcategory H83.2

Non-Hodgkin lymphoma NEC —see
    Lymphoma, non-Hodgkin
Nonimplantation, ovum N97.2
Noninsufflation, fallopian tube N97.1
Non-ketotic hyperglycinemia E72.51
Nonne-Milroy syndrome Q82.0
Nonovulation N97.0
Nonpatent fallopian tube N97.1
Nonpneumatization, lung NEC P28.0
Nonrotation —see Malrotation
Nonsecretion, urine —see Anuria
Nonunion
    fracture —see Fracture, by site
    joint, following fusion or arthrodesis
        M96.0 ◄
    organ or site, congenital NEC —see Imperfect,
        closure
    symphysis pubis, congenital Q74.2
Nonvisualization, gallbladder R93.2
Nonvital, nonvitalized tooth K04.99
Non-working side interference
    M26.56
Noonan's syndrome Q87.1
Normocytic anemia (infectional) due to blood
    loss (chronic) D50.0
    acute D62
Norrie's disease (congenital) Q15.8
North American blastomycosis B40.9
Norwegian itch B86
Nose, nasal —see condition
Nosebleed R04.0
Nose-picking F98.8
Nosomania F45.21
Nosophobia F45.22
Nostalgia F43.20
Notch of iris Q13.2
Notching nose, congenital (tip)
    Q30.2
Nothnagel's
    syndrome —see Strabismus, paralytic, third
        nerve
    vasomotor acroparesthesia I73.89
Novy's relapsing fever A68.9
    louse-borne A68.0
    tick-borne A68.1

Noxious
    foodstuffs, poisoning by —see Poisoning,
        food, noxious, plant
    substances transmitted through placenta or
        breast milk P04.9
Nucleus pulposus —see condition
Numbness R20.0
Nuns' knee —see Bursitis, prepatellar
Nursemaid's elbow S53.03-
Nutcracker esophagus K22.4
Nutmeg liver K76.1
Nutrient element deficiency E61.9
    specified NEC E61.8
Nutrition deficient or insufficient —see also
    Malnutrition E46
    due to
        insufficient food T73.0
        lack of
            care (child) T76.02
                adult T76.01
            food T73.0
Nutritional stunting E45
Nyctalopia (night blindness) —see Blindness,
    night
Nycturia R35.1
    psychogenic F45.8
Nymphomania F52.8
Nystagmus H55.00
    benign paroxysmal —see Vertigo, benign
        paroxysmal
    central positional H81.4-
    congenital H55.01
    dissociated H55.04
    latent H55.02
    miners' H55.09
    positional
        benign paroxysmal H81.4-
        central H81.4-
    specified form NEC H55.09
    visual deprivation H55.03

O

Obermeyer's relapsing fever (European)
A68.0
Obesity E66.9
~~with alveolar hyperventilation E66.2~~
with alveolar hypoventilation E66.2 ◀
adrenal E27.8
complicating
childbirth O99.214
pregnancy O99.21-
puerperium O99.215
constitutional E66.8
dietary counseling and surveillance Z71.3
drug-induced E66.1
due to
drug E66.1
excess calories E66.09
morbid E66.01
severe E66.01
endocrine E66.8
endogenous E66.8
exogenous E66.09 ◀
familial E66.8
glandular E66.8
hypothyroid —see Hypothyroidism
hypoventilation syndrome (OHS)
E66.2 ◀
morbid E66.01
~~with alveolar hypoventilation E66.2~~
with ◀
alveolar hypoventilation E66.2 ◀
obesity hypoventilation syndrome
(OHS) E66.2 ◀
due to excess calories E66.01
nutritional E66.09
pituitary E23.6
severe E66.01
specified type NEC E66.8
Oblique —see condition
Obliteration
appendix (lumen) K38.8
artery I77.1
bile duct (noncalculous) K83.1
common duct (noncalculous) K83.1
cystic duct —see Obstruction, gallbladder
disease, arteriolar I77.1
endometrium N85.8
eye, anterior chamber —see Disorder, globe,
hypotony
fallopian tube N97.1
lymphatic vessel I89.0
due to mastectomy I97.2
organ or site, congenital NEC —see Atresia,
by site
ureter N13.5
with infection N13.6
urethra —see Stricture, urethra
vein I87.8
vestibule (oral) K08.89 ◀▥
Observation (following) (for) (without need for
further medical care) Z04.9
accident NEC Z04.3
at work Z04.2
transport Z04.1
adverse effect of drug Z03.6
alleged rape or sexual assault (victim),
ruled out
adult Z04.41
child Z04.42
criminal assault Z04.8
development state
adolescent Z00.3
period of rapid growth in childhood Z00.2
puberty Z00.3
disease, specified NEC Z03.89
following work accident Z04.2
growth and development state —see
Observation, development state
injuries (accidental) NEC —see also
Observation, accident

Observation (Continued)
newborn (for) ◀▥
suspected condition, related to exposure
from the mother or birth process —
see Newborn, affected by,
maternal ◀
ruled out Z05.9 ◀
cardiac Z05.0 ◀
connective tissue Z05.73 ◀
gastrointestinal Z05.5 ◀
genetic Z05.41 ◀
genitourinary Z05.6 ◀
immunologic Z05.43 ◀
infectious Z05.1 ◀
metabolic Z05.42 ◀
musculoskeletal Z05.72 ◀
neurological Z05.2 ◀
respiratory Z05.3 ◀
skin and subcutaneous tissue
Z05.71 ◀
specified condition NEC
Z05.8 ◀
postpartum
immediately after delivery Z39.0
routine follow-up Z39.2
pregnancy (normal) (without complication)
Z34.9-
high risk O09.9-
suicide attempt, alleged NEC Z03.89
self-poisoning Z03.6
suspected, ruled out —see also Suspected
condition, ruled out
abuse, physical
adult Z04.71
child Z04.72
accident at work Z04.2
adult battering victim Z04.71
child battering victim Z04.72
condition NEC Z03.89
newborn —see also Observation,
newborn (for), suspected condition,
ruled out Z05.9 ◀▥
drug poisoning or adverse effect
Z03.6
exposure (to)
anthrax Z03.810
biological agent NEC Z03.818
inflicted injury NEC Z04.8
suicide attempt, alleged Z03.89
self-poisoning Z03.6
toxic effects from ingested substance (drug)
(poison) Z03.6
toxic effects from ingested substance (drug)
(poison) Z03.6
Obsession, obsessional state F42.8 ◀▥
mixed thoughts and acts F42.2 ◀
Obsessive-compulsive neurosis or reaction
F42.8 ◀▥
Obstetric embolism, septic —see Embolism,
obstetric, septic
Obstetrical trauma (complicating delivery)
O71.9
with or following ectopic or molar pregnancy
O08.6
specified type NEC O71.89
Obstipation —see Constipation
Obstruction, obstructed, obstructive
airway J98.8
with
allergic alveolitis J67.9
asthma J45.909
with
exacerbation (acute) J45.901
status asthmaticus J45.902
bronchiectasis J47.9
with
exacerbation (acute) J47.1
lower respiratory infection
J47.0
bronchitis (chronic) J44.9
emphysema J43.9

Obstruction, obstructed, obstructive
(Continued)
airway (Continued)
chronic J44.9
with
allergic alveolitis —see Pneumonitis,
hypersensitivity
bronchiectasis J47.9
with
exacerbation (acute) J47.1
lower respiratory infection J47.0
due to
foreign body —see Foreign body, by site,
causing asphyxia
inhalation of fumes or vapors J68.9
laryngospasm J38.5
ampulla of Vater K83.1
aortic (heart) (valve) —see Stenosis, aortic
aortoiliac I74.09
aqueduct of Sylvius G91.1
congenital Q03.0
with spina bifida —see Spina bifida, by
site, with hydrocephalus
Arnold-Chiari —see Arnold-Chiari disease
artery (see also Embolism, artery) I74.9
basilar (complete) (partial) —see Occlusion,
artery, basilar
carotid (complete) (partial) —see Occlusion,
artery, carotid
cerebellar —see Occlusion, artery, cerebellar
cerebral (anterior) (middle) (posterior) —
see Occlusion, artery, cerebral
precerebral —see Occlusion, artery,
precerebral
renal N28.0
retinal NEC —see Occlusion, artery, retina
stent —see Restenosis, stent ◀
vertebral (complete) (partial) —see
Occlusion, artery, vertebral
band (intestinal) K56.69
bile duct or passage (common) (hepatic)
(noncalculous) K83.1
with calculus K80.51
congenital (causing jaundice) Q44.3
biliary (duct) (tract) K83.1
gallbladder K82.0
bladder-neck (acquired) N32.0
congenital Q64.31
due to hyperplasia (hypertrophy) of
prostate —see Hyperplasia, prostate
bowel —see Obstruction, intestine
bronchus J98.09
canal, ear —see Stenosis, external ear canal
cardia K22.2
caval veins (inferior) (superior) I87.1
cecum —see Obstruction, intestine
circulatory I99.8
colon —see Obstruction, intestine
common duct (noncalculous) K83.1
coronary (artery) —see Occlusion, coronary
cystic duct —see also Obstruction, gallbladder
with calculus K80.21
device, implant or graft —see also
Complications, by site and type,
mechanical T85.698
arterial graft NEC —see Complication,
cardiovascular device, mechanical,
vascular
catheter NEC T85.628
cystostomy T83.090
dialysis (renal) T82.49
intraperitoneal T85.691
Hopkins T83.098 ◀
ileostomy T83.098 ◀
infusion NEC T82.594
spinal (epidural) (subdural) T85.690
nephrostomy T83.092 ◀
urethral indwelling T83.091 ◀
urinary T83.098 ◀
~~urinary, indwelling T83.098~~
urostomy T83.098 ◀

◀ New ◀▥ Revised ~~deleted~~ Deleted

Obstruction, obstructed, obstructive
(Continued)
device, implant or graft (Continued)
  due to infection T85.79
  gastrointestinal —see Complications,
    prosthetic device, mechanical,
    gastrointestinal device
  genital NEC T83.498
    intrauterine contraceptive device T83.39
    penile prosthesis (cylinder) (implanted)
      (pump) (resevoir) T83.490 ◀▥
    testicular prosthesis T83.491 ◀
  heart NEC —see Complication,
    cardiovascular device, mechanical
  joint prosthesis —see Complications, joint
    prosthesis, mechanical, specified
    NEC, by site
  orthopedic NEC —see Complication,
    orthopedic, device, mechanical
  specified NEC T85.628
  urinary NEC —see also Complication,
    genitourinary, device, urinary,
    mechanical
    graft T83.29
  vascular NEC —see Complication,
    cardiovascular device, mechanical
  ventricular intracranial shunt T85.09
  due to foreign body accidentally left in
    operative wound T81.529
duodenum K31.5
ejaculatory duct N50.89 ◀▥
esophagus K22.2
eustachian tube (complete) (partial) H68.10-
  cartilagenous (extrinsic) H68.13-
    intrinsic H68.12-
  osseous H68.11-
fallopian tube (bilateral) N97.1
fecal K56.41
  with hernia —see Hernia, by site, with
    obstruction
foramen of Monro (congenital) Q03.8
  with spina bifida —see Spina bifida,
    by site, with hydrocephalus
foreign body —see Foreign body
gallbladder K82.0
  with calculus, stones K80.21
  congenital Q44.1
gastric outlet K31.1
gastrointestinal —see Obstruction, intestine
hepatic K76.89
  duct (noncalculous) K83.1
hepatobiliary K83.1
ileum —see Obstruction, intestine
iliofemoral (artery) I74.5
intestine K56.60
  with
    adhesions (intestinal) (peritoneal) K56.5
    adynamic K56.0
    by gallstone K56.3
    congenital (small) Q41.9
      large Q42.9
        specified part NEC Q42.8
    neurogenic K56.0
      Hirschsprung's disease or megacolon
        Q43.1
    newborn P76.9
      due to
        fecaliths P76.8
        inspissated milk P76.2
        meconium (plug) P76.0
          in mucoviscidosis E84.11
        specified NEC P76.8
      postoperative K91.3
      reflex K56.0
      specified NEC K56.69
      volvulus K56.2
intracardiac ball valve prosthesis T82.09
jejunum —see Obstruction, intestine
joint prosthesis —see Complications, joint
    prosthesis, mechanical, specified NEC,
    by site

Obstruction, obstructed, obstructive
(Continued)
kidney (calices) N28.89
labor —see Delivery
lacrimal (passages) (duct)
  by
    dacryolith —see Dacryolith
    stenosis —see Stenosis, lacrimal
  congenital Q10.5
  neonatal H04.53-
lacrimonasal duct —see Obstruction,
  lacrimal
lacteal, with steatorrhea K90.2
laryngitis —see Laryngitis
larynx NEC J38.6
  congenital Q31.8
lung J98.4
  disease, chronic J44.9
lymphatic I89.0
meconium (plug)
  newborn P76.0
    due to fecaliths P76.0
    in mucoviscidosis E84.11
mitral —see Stenosis, mitral
nasal J34.89
nasolacrimal duct —see also Obstruction,
  lacrimal
  congenital Q10.5
nasopharynx J39.2
nose J34.89
organ or site, congenital NEC —see Atresia,
  by site
pancreatic duct K86.89 ◀▥
parotid duct or gland K11.8
pelviureteral junction N13.5
  with hydronephrosis N13.0 ◀
  congenital Q62.39
pharynx J39.2
portal (circulation) (vein) I81
prostate —see also Hyperplasia, prostate
  valve (urinary) N32.0
pulmonary valve (heart) I37.0
pyelonephritis (chronic) N11.1
pylorus
  adult K31.1
  congenital or infantile Q40.0
rectosigmoid —see Obstruction,
  intestine
rectum K62.4
renal N28.89
  outflow N13.8
  pelvis, congenital Q62.39
respiratory J98.8
  chronic J44.9
retinal (vessels) H34.9
salivary duct (any) K11.8
  with calculus K11.5
sigmoid —see Obstruction, intestine
sinus (accessory) (nasal) J34.89
Stensen's duct K11.8
stomach NEC K31.89
  acute K31.0
  congenital Q40.2
  due to pylorospasm K31.3
submandibular duct K11.8
submaxillary gland K11.8
  with calculus K11.5
thoracic duct I89.0
thrombotic —see Thrombosis
trachea J39.8
tracheostomy airway J95.03
tricuspid (valve) —see Stenosis, tricuspid
upper respiratory, congenital Q34.8
ureter (functional) (pelvic junction) NEC
  N13.5
  with
    hydronephrosis N13.1
      with infection N13.6
    pyelonephritis (chronic) N11.1
  congenital Q62.39
  due to calculus —see Calculus, ureter

Obstruction, obstructed, obstructive
(Continued)
urethra NEC N36.8
  congenital Q64.39
urinary (moderate) N13.9
  due to hyperplasia (hypertrophy) of
    prostate —see Hyperplasia, prostate
  organ or tract (lower) N13.9
  prostatic valve N32.0
  specified NEC N13.8
uropathy N13.9
uterus N85.8
vagina N89.5
valvular —see Endocarditis
vein, venous I87.1
  caval (inferior) (superior) I87.1
  thrombotic —see Thrombosis
vena cava (inferior) (superior) I87.1
vesical NEC N32.0
vesicourethral orifice N32.0
  congenital Q64.31
vessel NEC I99.8
  stent —see Restenosis, stent ◀
Obturator —see condition
Occlusal wear, teeth K03.0
Occlusio pupillae —see Membrane, pupillary
Occlusion, occluded
anus K62.4
  congenital Q42.3
    with fistula Q42.2
aortoiliac (chronic) I74.09
aqueduct of Sylvius G91.1
  congenital Q03.0
    with spina bifida —see Spina bifida, by
      site, with hydrocephalus
artery —see also Embolism, artery I74.9
  auditory, internal I65.8
  basilar I65.1
    with
      infarction I63.22
      due to
        embolism I63.12
        thrombosis I63.02
  brain or cerebral I66.9
    with infarction (due to) I63.5- ◀▥
      embolism I63.4- ◀▥
      thrombosis I63.3- ◀▥
  carotid I65.2-
    with
      infarction I63.23-
      due to
        embolism I63.13-
        thrombosis I63.03-
  cerebellar (anterior inferior) (posterior
    inferior) (superior) I66.3
    with infarction I63.54-
      due to
        embolism I63.44-
        thrombosis I63.34-
  cerebral I66.9
    with infarction I63.50
      due to
        embolism I63.40
          specified NEC I63.49
        thrombosis I63.30
          specified NEC I63.39
    anterior I66.1-
      with infarction I63.52-
        due to
          embolism I63.42-
          thrombosis I63.32-
    middle I66.0-
      with infarction I63.51-
        due to
          embolism I63.41-
          thrombosis I63.31-
    posterior I66.2-
      with infarction I63.53-
        due to
          embolism I63.43-
          thrombosis I63.33-

Occlusion, occluded (Continued)
  artery (Continued)
    cerebral (Continued)
      specified NEC I66.8
        with infarction I63.59
          due to
            embolism I63.4- ◀▥
            thrombosis I63.3- ◀▥
      choroidal (anterior) —see Occlusion,
          artery, cerebral, specified NEC
      communicating posterior —see
          Occlusion, artery, precerebral,
          specified NEC
      complete
        coronary I25.82
        extremities I70.92
      coronary (acute) (thrombotic) (without
          myocardial infarction) I24.0
        with myocardial infarction —see
            Infarction, myocardium
        chronic total I25.82
        complete I25.82
        healed or old I25.2
        total (chronic) I25.82
      hypophyseal —see Occlusion, artery,
          precerebral, specified NEC
      iliac I74.5
      lower extremities due to stenosis or
          stricture I77.1
      mesenteric (embolic) (thrombotic) —see also
          Infarct, intestine K55.069 ◀▥
      perforating —see Occlusion, artery,
          cerebral, specified NEC
      peripheral I77.9
        thrombotic or embolic I74.4
      pontine —see Occlusion, artery, cerebral,
          specified NEC
      precerebral I65.9
        with infarction I63.20
          due to
            embolism I63.10
              specified NEC I63.19
            thrombosis I63.00
              specified NEC I63.09
          specified NEC I63.29
        basilar —see Occlusion, artery, basilar
        carotid —see Occlusion, artery, carotid
        puerperal O88.23
        specified NEC I65.8
          with infarction I63.29
            due to
              embolism I63.19
              thrombosis I63.00
        vertebral —see Occlusion, artery,
            vertebral
      renal N28.0
      retinal
        branch H34.23-
        central H34.1-
        partial H34.21-
        transient H34.0-
      spinal —see Occlusion, artery, precerebral,
          vertebral
      total (chronic)
        coronary I25.82
        extremities I70.92
      vertebral I65.0-
        with
          infarction I63.21-
            due to
              embolism I63.11-
              thrombosis I63.01-
  basilar artery —see Occlusion, artery, basilar
  bile duct (common) (hepatic) (noncalculous)
      K83.1
  bowel —see Obstruction, intestine
  carotid (artery) (common) (internal) —see
      Occlusion, artery, carotid
  centric (of teeth) M26.59
    maximum intercuspation discrepancy
        M26.55

Occlusion, occluded (Continued)
  cerebellar (artery) —see Occlusion, artery,
      cerebellar
  cerebral (artery) —see Occlusion, artery,
      cerebral
  cerebrovascular —see also Occlusion, artery,
      cerebral
    with infarction I63.5- ◀▥
  cervical canal —see Stricture, cervix
  cervix (uteri) —see Stricture, cervix
  choanal Q30.0
  choroidal (artery) —see Occlusion, artery,
      precerebral, specified NEC
  colon —see Obstruction, intestine
  communicating posterior artery —see
      Occlusion, artery, precerebral, specified
      NEC
  coronary (artery) (vein) (thrombotic) —see
      also Infarct, myocardium
    chronic total I25.82
    healed or old I25.2
    not resulting in infarction I24.0
    total (chronic) I25.82
  cystic duct —see Obstruction, gallbladder
  embolic —see Embolism
  fallopian tube N97.1
    congenital Q50.6
  gallbladder —see also Obstruction,
      gallbladder
    congenital (causing jaundice) Q44.1
  gingiva, traumatic K06.2
  hymen N89.6
    congenital Q52.3
  hypophyseal (artery) —see Occlusion, artery,
      precerebral, specified NEC
  iliac artery I74.5
  intestine —see Obstruction, intestine
  lacrimal passages —see Obstruction, lacrimal
  lung J98.4
  lymph or lymphatic channel I89.0
  mammary duct N64.89
  mesenteric artery (embolic) (thrombotic) —
      see also Infarct, intestine K55.069 ◀▥
  nose J34.89
    congenital Q30.0
  organ or site, congenital NEC —see Atresia,
      by site
  oviduct N97.1
    congenital Q50.6
  peripheral arteries
    due to stricture or stenosis I77.1
    upper extremity I74.2
  pontine (artery) —see Occlusion, artery,
      precerebral, specified NEC
  posterior lingual, of mandibular teeth M26.29
  precerebral artery —see Occlusion, artery,
      precerebral
  punctum lacrimale —see Obstruction,
      lacrimal
  pupil —see Membrane, pupillary
  pylorus, adult —see also Stricture, pylorus
      K31.1
  renal artery N28.0
  retina, retinal
    artery —see Occlusion, artery, retinal
    vein (central) H34.81-
      engorgement H34.82-
      tributary H34.83-
    vessels H34.9
  spinal artery —see Occlusion, artery,
      precerebral, vertebral
  teeth (mandibular) (posterior lingual) M26.29
  thoracic duct I89.0
  thrombotic —see Thrombosis, artery
  traumatic
    edentulous (alveolar) ridge K06.2
    gingiva K06.2
    periodontal K05.5
  tubal N97.1
  ureter (complete) (partial) N13.5
    congenital Q62.10

Occlusion, occluded (Continued)
  ureteropelvic junction N13.5
    congenital Q62.11
  ureterovesical orifice N13.5
    congenital Q62.12
  urethra —see Stricture, urethra
  uterus N85.8
  vagina N89.5
  vascular NEC I99.8
  vein —see Thrombosis
    retinal —see Occlusion, retinal, vein
  vena cava (inferior) (superior) —see
      Embolism, vena cava
  ventricle (brain) NEC G91.1
  vertebral (artery) —see Occlusion, artery,
      vertebral
  vessel (blood) I99.8
  vulva N90.5
Occult
  blood in feces (stools) R19.5
Occupational
  problems NEC Z56.89
Ochlophobia —see Agoraphobia
Ochronosis (endogenous) E70.29
Ocular muscle —see condition
Oculogyric crisis or disturbance H51.8
  psychogenic F45.8
Oculomotor syndrome H51.9
Oculopathy
  syphilitic NEC A52.71
    congenital
      early A50.01
      late A50.30
    early (secondary) A51.43
    late A52.71
Oddi's sphincter spasm K83.4
Odontalgia K08.89 ◀▥
Odontoameloblastoma —see Cyst, calcifying
    odontogenic
Odontoclasia K03.89
Odontodysplasia, regional K00.4
Odontogenesis imperfecta K00.5
Odontoma (ameloblastic) (complex)
    (compound) (fibroameloblastic) —see Cyst,
    calcifying odontogenic
Odontomyelitis (closed) (open) K04.01 ◀▥
  irreversible K04.02 ◀
  reversible K04.01 ◀
Odontorrhagia K08.89 ◀▥
Odontosarcoma, ameloblastic C41.1
  upper jaw (bone) C41.0
Oestriasis —see Myiasis
Oguchi's disease H53.63
Ohara's disease —see Tularemia
OHS (obesity hypoventilation syndrome)
    E66.2 ◀
Oidiomycosis —see Candidiasis
Oidium albicans infection —see Candidiasis
Old (previous) myocardial infarction
    I25.2
Old age (without mention of debility) R54-
  dementia F03
Olfactory —see condition
Oligemia —see Anemia
Oligoastrocytoma
  specified site —see Neoplasm, malignant,
      by site
  unspecified site C71.9
Oligocythemia D64.9
Oligodendroblastoma
  specified site —see Neoplasm, malignant
  unspecified site C71.9
Oligodendroglioma
  anaplastic type
    specified site —see Neoplasm, malignant,
        by site
    unspecified site C71.9
  specified site —see Neoplasm, malignant,
      by site
  unspecified site C71.9
Oligodontia —see Anodontia

◀ New   ◀▥ Revised   ~~deleted~~ Deleted

Oligoencephalon Q02
Oligohidrosis L74.4
Oligohydramnios O41.0-
Oligohydrosis L74.4
Oligomenorrhea N91.5
   primary N91.3
   secondary N91.4
Oligophrenia —see also Disability, intellectual
   phenylpyruvic E70.0
Oligospermia N46.11
   due to
      drug therapy N46.121
      efferent duct obstruction N46.123
      infection N46.122
      radiation N46.124
      specified cause NEC N46.129
      systemic disease N46.125
Oligotrichia —see Alopecia
Oliguria R34
   with, complicating or following ectopic or
      molar pregnancy O08.4
   postprocedural N99.0
Ollier's disease Q78.4
Omenotocele —see Hernia, abdomen, specified
   site NEC
Omentitis —see Peritonitis
Omentum, omental —see condition
Omphalitis (congenital) (newborn) P38.9
   with mild hemorrhage P38.1
   without hemorrhage P38.9
   not of newborn L08.82
   tetanus A33
Omphalocele Q79.2
Omphalomesenteric duct, persistent
   Q43.0
Omphalorrhagia, newborn P51.9
Omsk hemorrhagic fever A98.1
Onanism (excessive) F98.8
Onchocerciasis, onchocercosis B73.1
   with
      eye disease B73.00
         endophthalmitis B73.01
         eyelid B73.09
         glaucoma B73.02
         specified NEC B73.09
      eye NEC B73.00
      eyelid B73.09
Oncocytoma —see Neoplasm, benign, by site
Oncovirus, as cause of disease classified
   elsewhere B97.32
Ondine's curse —see Apnea, sleep
Oneirophrenia F23
Onychauxis L60.2
   congenital Q84.5
Onychia —see also Cellulitis, digit
   with lymphangitis —see Lymphangitis, acute,
      digit
   candidal B37.2
   dermatophytic B35.1
Onychitis —see also Cellulitis, digit
   with lymphangitis —see Lymphangitis, acute,
      digit
Onychocryptosis L60.0
Onychodystrophy L60.3
   congenital Q84.6
Onychogryphosis, onychogryposis L60.2
Onycholysis L60.1
Onychomadesis L60.8
Onychomalacia L60.3
Onychomycosis (finger) (toe) B35.1
Onycho-osteodysplasia Q87.2 ◀▥
Onychophagia F98.8
Onychophosis L60.8
Onychoptosis L60.8
Onychorrhexis L60.3
   congenital Q84.6
Onychoschizia L60.3
Onyxis (finger) (toe) L60.0
Onyxitis —see also Cellulitis, digit
   with lymphangitis —see Lymphangitis, acute,
      digit

Oophoritis (cystic) (infectional) (interstitial)
   N70.92
   with salpingitis N70.93
   acute N70.02
      with salpingitis N70.03
   chronic N70.12
      with salpingitis N70.13
   complicating abortion —see Abortion, by
      type, complicated by, oophoritis
Oophorocele N83.4- ◀▥
Opacity, opacities
   cornea H17.-
      central H17.1-
      congenital Q13.3
      degenerative —see Degeneration, cornea
      hereditary —see Dystrophy, cornea
      inflammatory —see Keratitis
      minor H17.81-
      peripheral H17.82-
      sequelae of trachoma (healed) B94.0
      specified NEC H17.89
   enamel (teeth) (fluoride) (nonfluoride)
      K00.3
   lens —see Cataract
   snowball —see Deposit, crystalline
   vitreous (humor) NEC H43.39-
      congenital Q14.0
      membranes and strands H43.31-
Opalescent dentin (hereditary) K00.5
Open, opening
   abnormal, organ or site, congenital —see
      Imperfect, closure
   angle with
      borderline
         findings
            high risk H40.02-
            low risk H40.01-
            intraocular pressure H40.00-
         cupping of discs H40.01-
      glaucoma (primary) —see Glaucoma, open
         angle
   bite
      anterior M26.220
      posterior M26.221
   false —see Imperfect, closure
   margin on tooth restoration K08.51
   restoration margins of tooth K08.51
   wound —see Wound, open
Operational fatigue F48.8
Operative —see condition
Operculitis —see Periodontitis
Operculum —see Break, retina
Ophiasis L63.2
Ophthalmia —see also Conjunctivitis H10.9
   actinic rays —see Photokeratitis
   allergic (acute) —see Conjunctivitis, acute,
      atopic
   blennorrhagic (gonococcal) (neonatorum)
      A54.31
   diphtheritic A36.86
   Egyptian A71.1
   electrica —see Photokeratitis
   gonococcal (neonatorum) A54.31
   metastatic —see Endophthalmitis, purulent
   migraine —see Migraine, ophthalmoplegic
   neonatorum, newborn P39.1
      gonococcal A54.31
   nodosa H16.24-
   purulent —see Conjunctivitis, acute,
      mucopurulent
   spring —see Conjunctivitis, acute, atopic
   sympathetic —see Uveitis, sympathetic
Ophthalmitis —see Ophthalmia
Ophthalmocele (congenital) Q15.8
Ophthalmoneuromyelitis G36.0
Ophthalmoplegia —see also Strabismus,
   paralytic
   anterior internuclear —see Ophthalmoplegia,
      internuclear
   ataxia-areflexia G61.0
   diabetic —see E08-E13 with .39

Ophthalmoplegia (Continued)
   exophthalmic E05.00
      with thyroid storm E05.01
   external H49.88-
      progressive H49.4-
         with pigmentary retinopathy —see
            Kearns-Sayre syndrome
      total H49.3-
   internal (complete) (total) H52.51-
   internuclear H51.2-
   migraine —see Migraine, ophthalmoplegic
   Parinaud's H49.88-
   progressive external —see Ophthalmoplegia,
      external, progressive
   supranuclear, progressive G23.1
   total (external) —see Ophthalmoplegia,
      external, total
Opioid (s)
   abuse —see Abuse, drug, opioids
   dependence —see Dependence, drug, opioids
   induced, without use disorder ◀
      anxiety disorder F11.988 ◀
      delirium F11.921 ◀
      depressive disorder F11.94 ◀
      sexual dysfunction F11.981 ◀
      sleep disorder F11.982 ◀
Opisthognathism M26.09
Opisthorchiasis (felineus) (viverrini) B66.0
Opitz' disease D73.2
Opiumism —see Dependence, drug, opioid
Oppenheim's disease G70.2
Oppenheim-Urbach disease (necrobiosis
   lipoidica diabeticorum) —see E08-E13 with
   .620
Optic nerve —see condition
Orbit —see condition
Orchioblastoma C62.9-
Orchitis (gangrenous) (nonspecific) (septic)
   (suppurative) N45.2
   blennorrhagic (gonococcal) (acute) (chronic)
      A54.23
   chlamydial A56.19
   filarial —see also Infestation, filarial B74.9
      [N51]
   gonococcal (acute) (chronic) A54.23
   mumps B26.0
   syphilitic A52.76
   tuberculous A18.15
Orf (virus disease) B08.02
Organic —see also condition
   brain syndrome F09
   heart —see Disease, heart
   mental disorder F09
   psychosis F09
Orgasm
   anejaculatory N53.13
Oriental
   bilharziasis B65.2
   schistosomiasis B65.2
Orifice —see condition
Origin of both great vessels from right
   ventricle Q20.1
Ormond's disease (with ureteral obstruction)
   N13.5
   with infection N13.6
Ornithine metabolism disorder E72.4
Ornithinemia (Type I) (Type II) E72.4
Ornithosis A70
Orotaciduria, oroticaciduria (congenital)
   (hereditary) (pyrimidine deficiency) E79.8
   anemia D53.0
Orthodontics
   adjustment Z46.4
   fitting Z46.4
Orthopnea R06.01
Orthopoxvirus B08.09
   specified NEC B08.09
Os, uterus —see condition
Osgood-Schlatter disease or
   osteochondrosis —see Osteochondrosis,
   juvenile, tibia

Osler (-Weber)-Rendu disease I78.0
Osler's nodes I33.0
Osmidrosis L75.0
Osseous —see condition
Ossification
  artery —see Arteriosclerosis
  auricle (ear) —see Disorder, pinna, specified
    type NEC
  bronchial J98.09
  cardiac —see Degeneration, myocardial
  cartilage (senile) —see Disorder, cartilage,
    specified type NEC
  coronary (artery) —see Disease, heart,
    ischemic, atherosclerotic
  diaphragm J98.6
  ear, middle —see Otosclerosis
  falx cerebri G96.19
  fontanel, premature Q75.0
  heart —see also Degeneration, myocardial
    valve —see Endocarditis
  larynx J38.7
  ligament —see Disorder, tendon, specified
    type NEC
    posterior longitudinal —see
      Spondylopathy, specified NEC
  meninges (cerebral) (spinal) G96.19
  multiple, eccentric centers —see Disorder,
    bone, development or growth
  muscle —see also Calcification, muscle
    due to burns —see Myositis, ossificans, in,
      burns
    paralytic —see Myositis, ossificans, in,
      quadriplegia
    progressive —see Myositis, ossificans,
      progressiva
    specified NEC M61.50
      ankle M61.57-
      foot M61.57-
      forearm M61.53-
      hand M61.54-
      lower leg M61.56-
      multiple sites M61.59
      pelvic region M61.55-
      shoulder region M61.51-
      specified site NEC M61.58
      thigh M61.55-
      upper arm M61.52-
    traumatic —see Myositis, ossificans,
      traumatica
  myocardium, myocardial —see Degeneration,
    myocardial
  penis N48.89
  periarticular —see Disorder, joint, specified
    type NEC
  pinna —see Disorder, pinna, specified type
    NEC
  rider's bone —see Ossification, muscle,
    specified NEC
  sclera H15.89
  subperiosteal, post-traumatic M89.8X-
  tendon —see Disorder, tendon, specified
    type NEC
  trachea J39.8
  tympanic membrane —see Disorder,
    tympanic membrane, specified
    NEC
  vitreous (humor) —see Deposit,
    crystalline
Osteitis —see also Osteomyelitis
  alveolar M27.3
  condensans M85.30
    ankle M85.37-
    foot M85.37-
    forearm M85.33-
    hand M85.34-
    lower leg M85.36-
    multiple site M85.39
    neck M85.38
    rib M85.38
    shoulder M85.31-
    skull M85.38

Osteitis (Continued)
  condensans (Continued)
    specified site NEC M85.38
    thigh M85.35-
    toe M85.37-
    upper arm M85.32-
    vertebra M85.38
  deformans M88.9
    in (due to)
      malignant neoplasm of bone
        C41.9 [M90.60]
      neoplastic disease —see also Neoplasm
        D49.9 [M90.60]
        carpus D49.9 [M90.64-]
        clavicle D49.9 [M90.61-]
        femur D49.9 [M90.65-]
        fibula D49.9 [M90.66-]
        finger D49.9 [M90.64-]
        humerus D49.9 [M90.62-]
        ilium D49.9 [M90.65-]
        ischium D49.9 [M90.65-]
        metacarpus D49.9 [M90.64-]
        metatarsus D49.9 [M90.67-]
        multiple sites D49.9 [M90.69]
        neck D49.9 [M90.68]
        radius D49.9 [M90.63-]
        rib D49.9 [M90.68]
        scapula D49.9 [M90.61-]
        skull D49.9 [M90.68]
        tarsus D49.9 [M90.67-]
        tibia D49.9 [M90.66-]
        toe D49.9 [M90.67-]
        ulna D49.9 [M90.63-]
        vertebra D49.9 [M90.68]
    skull M88.0
    specified NEC —see Paget's disease, bone,
      by site
    vertebra M88.1
  due to yaws A66.6
  fibrosa NEC —see Cyst, bone, by site
    circumscripta —see Dysplasia, fibrous,
      bone NEC
    cystica (generalisata) E21.0
    disseminata Q78.1
    osteoplastica E21.0
  fragilitans Q78.0
  Garr's (sclerosing) —see Osteomyelitis,
    specified type NEC
  jaw (acute) (chronic) (lower) (suppurative)
    (upper) M27.2
  parathyroid E21.0
  petrous bone (acute) (chronic) —see Petrositis
  sclerotic, nonsuppurative —see Osteomyelitis,
    specified type NEC
  tuberculosa A18.09
    cystica D86.89
    multiplex cystoides D86.89
Osteoarthritis M19.90
  ankle M19.07-
  elbow M19.02-
  foot joint M19.07-
  generalized M15.9
    erosive M15.4
    primary M15.0
    specified NEC M15.8
  hand joint M19.04-
    first carpometacarpal joint M18.9-
  hip M16.1-
    bilateral M16.0
    due to hip dysplasia (unilateral)
      M16.3-
      bilateral M16.2
  interphalangeal
    distal (Heberden) M15.1
    proximal (Bouchard) M15.2
  knee M17.9-
    bilateral M17.0
  post-traumatic NEC M19.92
    ankle M19.17-
    elbow M19.12-
    foot joint M19.17-

Osteoarthritis (Continued)
  post-traumatic NEC (Continued)
    hand joint M19.14-
      first carpometacarpal joint M18.3-
        bilateral M18.2
    hip M16.5-
      bilateral M16.4
    knee M17.3-
      bilateral M17.2
    shoulder M19.11-
    wrist M19.13-
  primary M19.91
    ankle M19.07-
    elbow M19.02-
    foot joint M19.07-
    hand joint M19.04-
      first carpometacarpal joint M18.1-
        bilateral M18.0
    hip M16.1-
      bilateral M16.0
    knee M17.1-
      bilateral M17.0
    shoulder M19.01-
    spine —see Spondylosis
    wrist M19.03-
  secondary M19.93
    ankle M19.27-
    elbow M19.22-
    foot joint M19.27-
    hand joint M19.24-
      first carpometacarpal joint M18.5-
        bilateral M18.4
    hip M16.7
      bilateral M16.6
    knee M17.5
      bilateral M17.4
    multiple M15.3
    shoulder M19.21-
    spine —see Spondylosis
    wrist M19.23-
  shoulder M19.01-
  spine —see Spondylosis
  wrist M19.03-
Osteoarthropathy (hypertrophic) M19.90
  ankle —see Osteoarthritis, primary, ankle
  elbow —see Osteoarthritis, primary, elbow
  foot joint —see Osteoarthritis, primary, foot
  hand joint —see Osteoarthritis, primary, hand
    joint
  knee joint —see Osteoarthritis, primary, knee
  multiple site —see Osteoarthritis, primary,
    multiple joint
  pulmonary —see also Osteoarthropathy,
    specified type NEC
    hypertrophic —see Osteoarthropathy,
      hypertrophic, specified type NEC
    secondary —see Osteoarthropathy, specified
      type NEC
  secondary hypertrophic —see
    Osteoarthropathy, specified type NEC
  shoulder —see Osteoarthritis, primary,
    shoulder
  specified joint NEC —see Osteoarthritis,
    primary, specified joint NEC
  specified type NEC M89.40
    carpus M89.44-
    clavicle M89.41-
    femur M89.45-
    fibula M89.46-
    finger M89.44-
    humerus M89.42-
    ilium M89.459
    ischium M89.459
    metacarpus M89.44-
    metatarsus M89.47-
    multiple sites M89.49
    neck M89.48
    radius M89.43-
    rib M89.48
    scapula M89.41-
    skull M89.48

◀ New   ⬰ Revised   ~~deleted~~ Deleted

Osteoarthropathy (*Continued*)
  specified type NEC (*Continued*)
    tarsus M89.47-
    tibia M89.46-
    toe M89.47-
    ulna M89.43-
    vertebra M89.48
  spine —*see* Spondylosis
  wrist —*see* Osteoarthritis, primary, wrist
Osteoarthrosis (degenerative) (hypertrophic)
    (joint) —*see also* Osteoarthritis
  deformans alkaptonurica E70.29 [*M36.8*]
  erosive M15.4
  generalized M15.9
    primary M15.0
  polyarticular M15.9
  spine —*see* Spondylosis
Osteoblastoma —*see* Neoplasm, bone, benign
  aggressive —*see* Neoplasm, bone, uncertain
    behavior
Osteochondroarthrosis deformans
    endemica —*see* Disease, Kaschin-Beck
Osteochondritis —*see also* Osteochondropathy,
    by site
  Brailsford's —*see* Osteochondrosis, juvenile,
    radius
  dissecans M93.20
    ankle M93.27-
    elbow M93.22-
    foot M93.27-
    hand M93.24-
    hip M93.25-
    knee M93.26-
    multiple sites M93.29
    shoulder joint M93.21-
    specified site NEC M93.28
    wrist M93.23-
  juvenile M92.9
    patellar —*see* Osteochondrosis, juvenile,
      patella
  syphilitic (congenital) (early) A50.02
      [*M90.80*]
    ankle A50.02 [*M90.87-*]
    elbow A50.02 [*M90.82-*]
    foot A50.02 [*M90.87-*]
    forearm A50.02 [*M90.83-*]
    hand A50.02 [*M90.84-*]
    hip A50.02 [*M90.85-*]
    knee A50.02 [*M90.86-*]
    multiple sites A50.02 [*M90.89*]
    shoulder joint A50.02 [*M90.81-*]
    specified site NEC A50.02 [*M90.88*]
Osteochondrodysplasia Q78.9
  with defects of growth of tubular bones and
    spine Q77.9
  specified NEC Q77.8
  specified NEC Q78.8
Osteochondrodystrophy E78.9
Osteochondrolysis —*see* Osteochondritis,
    dissecans
Osteochondroma —*see* Neoplasm, bone, benign
Osteochondromatosis D48.0
  syndrome Q78.4
Osteochondromyxosarcoma —*see* Neoplasm,
    bone, malignant
Osteochondropathy M93.90
  ankle M93.97-
  elbow M93.92-
  foot M93.97-
  hand M93.94-
  hip M93.95-
  Kienböck's disease of adults M93.1
  knee M93.96-
  multiple joints M93.99
  osteochondritis dissecans —*see*
    Osteochondritis, dissecans
  osteochondrosis —*see* Osteochondrosis
  shoulder region M93.91-
  slipped upper femoral epiphysis —*see*
    Slipped, epiphysis, upper femoral
  specified joint NEC M93.98

Osteochondropathy (*Continued*)
  specified type NEC M93.80
    ankle M93.87-
    elbow M93.82-
    foot M93.87-
    hand M93.84-
    hip M93.85-
    knee M93.86-
    multiple joints M93.89
    shoulder region M93.81-
    specified joint NEC M93.88
    wrist M93.83-
  syphilitic, congenital
    early A50.02 [*M90.80*]
    late A50.56 [*M90.80*]
  wrist M93.93-
Osteochondrosarcoma —*see* Neoplasm, bone,
    malignant
Osteochondrosis —*see also* Osteochondropathy,
    by site
  acetabulum (juvenile) M91.0
  adult —*see* Osteochondropathy, specified
    type NEC, by site
  astragalus (juvenile) —*see* Osteochondrosis,
    juvenile, tarsus
  Blount's —*see* Osteochondrosis, juvenile, tibia
  Buchanan's M91.0
  Burns' —*see* Osteochondrosis, juvenile, ulna
  calcaneus (juvenile) —*see* Osteochondrosis,
    juvenile, tarsus
  capitular epiphysis (femur) (juvenile) —*see*
    Legg-Calvé-Perthes disease
  carpal (juvenile) (lunate) (scaphoid) —*see*
    Osteochondrosis, juvenile, hand, carpal
    lunate
    adult M93.1
  coxae juvenilis —*see* Legg-Calvé-Perthes
    disease
  deformans juvenilis, coxae —*see* Legg-Calvé-
    Perthes disease
  Diaz's —*see* Osteochondrosis, juvenile,
    tarsus
  dissecans (knee) (shoulder) —*see*
    Osteochondritis, dissecans
  femoral capital epiphysis (juvenile) —*see*
    Legg-Calvé-Perthes disease
  femur (head), juvenile —*see* Legg-Calvé-
    Perthes disease
  fibula (juvenile) —*see* Osteochondrosis,
    juvenile, fibula
  foot NEC (juvenile) M92.8
  Freiberg's —*see* Osteochondrosis, juvenile,
    metatarsus
  Haas' (juvenile) —*see* Osteochondrosis,
    juvenile, humerus
  Haglund's —*see* Osteochondrosis, juvenile,
    tarsus
  hip (juvenile) —*see* Legg-Calvé-Perthes
    disease
  humerus (capitulum) (head) (juvenile) —*see*
    Osteochondrosis, juvenile, humerus
  ilium, iliac crest (juvenile) M91.0
  ischiopubic synchondrosis M91.0
  Iselin's —*see* Osteochondrosis, juvenile,
    metatarsus
  juvenile, juvenilis M92.9
    after congenital dislocation of hip
      reduction —*see* Osteochondrosis,
      juvenile, hip, specified NEC
    arm —*see* Osteochondrosis, juvenile, upper
      limb NEC
    capitular epiphysis (femur) —*see* Legg-
      Calvé-Perthes disease
    clavicle, sternal epiphysis —*see*
      Osteochondrosis, juvenile, upper
      limb NEC
    coxae —*see* Legg-Calvé-Perthes
      disease
    deformans M92.9
    fibula M92.5-
    foot NEC M92.8

Osteochondrosis (*Continued*)
  juvenile, juvenilis (*Continued*)
    hand M92.20
      carpal lunate M92.21-
      metacarpal head M92.22-
      specified site NEC M92.29-
    head of femur —*see* Legg-Calvé-Perthes
      disease
    hip and pelvis M91.9-
      coxa plana —*see* Coxa, plana
      femoral head —*see* Legg-Calvé-Perthes
        disease
      pelvis M91.0
      pseudocoxalgia —*see* Pseudocoxalgia
      specified NEC M91.8-
    humerus M92.0-
    limb
      lower NEC M92.8
      upper NEC —*see* Osteochondrosis,
        juvenile, upper limb NEC
    medial cuneiform bone —*see*
      Osteochondrosis, juvenile, tarsus
    metatarsus M92.7-
    patella M92.4-
    radius M92.1-
    specified site NEC M92.8
    spine M42.00
      cervical region M42.02
      cervicothoracic region M42.03
      lumbar region M42.06
      lumbosacral region M42.07
      multiple sites M42.09
      occipito-atlanto-axial region M42.01
      sacrococcygeal region M42.08
      thoracic region M42.04
      thoracolumbar region M42.05
    tarsus M92.6-
    tibia M92.5-
    ulna M92.1-
    upper limb NEC M92.3-
    vertebra (body) (epiphyseal plates)
      (Calvé's) (Scheuermann's) —*see*
      Osteochondrosis, juvenile, spine
  Kienböck's —*see* Osteochondrosis, juvenile,
    hand, carpal lunate
    adult M93.1
  Köhler's
    patellar —*see* Osteochondrosis, juvenile,
      patella
    tarsal navicular —*see* Osteochondrosis,
      juvenile, tarsus
  Legg-Perthes (-Calvé's) (-Waldenström) —*see*
    Legg-Calvé-Perthes disease
  limb
    lower NEC (juvenile) M92.8
    upper NEC (juvenile) —*see*
      Osteochondrosis, juvenile, upper
      limb NEC
  lunate bone (carpal) (juvenile) —*see also*
    Osteochondrosis, juvenile, hand, carpal
    lunate
    adult M93.1
  Mauclaire's —*see* Osteochondrosis, juvenile,
    hand, metacarpal
  metacarpal (head) (juvenile) —*see*
    Osteochondrosis, juvenile, hand,
    metacarpal
  metatarsus (fifth) (head) (juvenile)
    (second) —*see* Osteochondrosis,
    juvenile, metatarsus
  navicular (juvenile) —*see* Osteochondrosis,
    juvenile, tarsus
  os
    calcis (juvenile) —*see* Osteochondrosis,
      juvenile, tarsus
    tibiale externum (juvenile) —*see*
      Osteochondrosis, juvenile, tarsus
  Osgood-Schlatter —*see* Osteochondrosis,
    juvenile, tibia
  Panner's —*see* Osteochondrosis, juvenile,
    humerus

Osteochondrosis (Continued)
  patellar center (juvenile) (primary)
      (secondary) —see Osteochondrosis,
      juvenile, patella
  pelvis (juvenile) M91.0
  Pierson's M91.0
  radius (head) (juvenile) —see
      Osteochondrosis, juvenile, radius
  Scheuermann's —see Osteochondrosis,
      juvenile, spine
  Sever's —see Osteochondrosis, juvenile,
      tarsus
  Sinding-Larsen —see Osteochondrosis,
      juvenile, patella
  spine M42.9
    adult M42.10
      cervical region M42.12
      cervicothoracic region M42.13
      lumbar region M42.16
      lumbosacral region M42.17
      multiple sites M42.19
      occipito-atlanto-axial region M42.11
      sacrococcygeal region M42.18
      thoracic region M42.14
      thoracolumbar region M42.15
    juvenile —see Osteochondrosis, juvenile,
      spine
  symphysis pubis (juvenile) M91.0
  syphilitic (congenital) A50.02
  talus (juvenile) —see Osteochondrosis,
      juvenile, tarsus
  tarsus (navicular) (juvenile) —see
      Osteochondrosis, juvenile, tarsus
  tibia (proximal) (tubercle) (juvenile) —see
      Osteochondrosis, juvenile, tibia
  tuberculous —see Tuberculosis, bone
  ulna (lower) (juvenile) —see Osteochondrosis,
      juvenile, ulna
  van Neck's M91.0
  vertebral —see Osteochondrosis,
      spine
Osteoclastoma D48.0
  malignant —see Neoplasm, bone,
      malignant
Osteodynia —see Disorder, bone,
    specified type NEC
Osteodystrophy Q78.9
  azotemic N25.0
  congenital Q78.9
  parathyroid, secondary E21.1
  renal N25.0
Osteofibroma —see Neoplasm, bone,
    benign
Osteofibrosarcoma —see Neoplasm,
    bone, malignant
Osteogenesis imperfecta Q78.0
Osteogenic —see condition
Osteolysis M89.50
  carpus M89.54-
  clavicle M89.51-
  femur M89.55-
  fibula M89.56-
  finger M89.54-
  humerus M89.52-
  ilium M89.559
  ischium M89.559
  joint prosthesis (periprosthetic) —see
      Complications, joint prosthesis,
      mechanical, periprosthetic, osteolysis,
      by site
  metacarpus M89.54-
  metatarsus M89.57-
  multiple sites M89.59
  neck M89.58
  periprosthetic —see Complications, joint
      prosthesis, mechanical, periprosthetic,
      osteolysis, by site
  radius M89.53-
  rib M89.58
  scapula M89.51-
  skull M89.58

Osteolysis (Continued)
  tarsus M89.57-
  tibia M89.56-
  toe M89.57-
  ulna M89.53-
  vertebra M89.58
Osteoma —see also Neoplasm, bone, benign
  osteoid —see also Neoplasm, bone, benign
    giant —see Neoplasm, bone, benign
Osteomalacia M83.9
  adult M83.9
    drug-induced NEC M83.5
    due to
      malabsorption (postsurgical) M83.2
      malnutrition M83.3
    specified NEC M83.8
  aluminium-induced M83.4
  infantile —see Rickets
  juvenile —see Rickets
  oncogenic E83.89
  pelvis M83.8
  puerperal M83.0
  senile M83.1
  vitamin-D-resistant in adults E83.31
    [M90.8-]
    carpus E83.31 [M90.84-]
    clavicle E83.31 [M90.81-]
    femur E83.31 [M90.85-]
    fibula E83.31 [M90.86-]
    finger E83.31 [M90.84-]
    humerus E83.31 [M90.82-]
    ilium E83.31 [M90.859]
    ischium E83.31 [M90.859]
    metacarpus E83.31 [M90.84-]
    metatarsus E83.31 [M90.87-]
    multiple sites E83.31 [M90.89]
    neck E83.31 [M90.88]
    radius E83.31 [M90.83-]
    rib E83.31 [M90.88]
    scapula E83.31 [M90.819]
    skull E83.31 [M90.88]
    tarsus E83.31 [M90.879]
    tibia E83.31 [M90.869]
    toe E83.31 [M90.879]
    ulna E83.31 [M90.839]
    vertebra E83.31 [M90.88]
Osteomyelitis (general) (infective)
    (localized) (neonatal) (purulent)
    (septic) (staphylococcal) (streptococcal)
    (suppurative) (with periostitis) M86.9
  acute M86.10
    carpus M86.14-
    clavicle M86.11-
    femur M86.15-
    fibula M86.16-
    finger M86.14-
    hematogenous M86.00
      carpus M86.04-
      clavicle M86.01-
      femur M86.05-
      fibula M86.06-
      finger M86.04-
      humerus M86.02-
      ilium M86.059
      ischium M86.059
      mandible M27.2
      metacarpus M86.04-
      metatarsus M86.07-
      multiple sites M86.09
      neck M86.08
      orbit H05.02-
      petrous bone —see Petrositis
      radius M86.03-
      rib M86.08
      scapula M86.01-
      skull M86.08
      tarsus M86.07-
      tibia M86.06-
      toe M86.07-
      ulna M86.03-
      vertebra —see Osteomyelitis, vertebra

Osteomyelitis (Continued)
  acute (Continued)
    humerus M86.12-
    ilium M86.159
    ischium M86.159
    mandible M27.2
    metacarpus M86.14-
    metatarsus M86.17-
    multiple sites M86.19
    neck M86.18
    orbit H05.02-
    petrous bone —see Petrositis
    radius M86.13-
    rib M86.18
    scapula M86.11-
    skull M86.18
    tarsus M86.17-
    tibia M86.16-
    toe M86.17-
    ulna M86.13-
    vertebra —see Osteomyelitis, vertebra
  chronic (or old) M86.60
    with draining sinus M86.40
      carpus M86.44-
      clavicle M86.41-
      femur M86.45-
      fibula M86.46-
      finger M86.44-
      humerus M86.42-
      ilium M86.459
      ischium M86.459
      mandible M27.2
      metacarpus M86.44-
      metatarsus M86.47-
      multiple sites M86.49
      neck M86.48
      orbit H05.02-
      petrous bone —see Petrositis
      radius M86.43-
      rib M86.48
      scapula M86.41-
      skull M86.48
      tarsus M86.47-
      tibia M86.46-
      toe M86.47-
      ulna M86.43-
      vertebra —see Osteomyelitis,
        vertebra
    carpus M86.64-
    clavicle M86.61-
    femur M86.65-
    fibula M86.66-
    finger M86.64-
    hematogenous NEC M86.50
      carpus M86.54-
      clavicle M86.51-
      femur M86.55-
      fibula M86.56-
      finger M86.54-
      humerus M86.52-
      ilium M86.559
      ischium M86.559
      mandible M27.2
      metacarpus M86.54-
      metatarsus M86.57-
      multifocal M86.30
        carpus M86.34-
        clavicle M86.31-
        femur M86.35-
        fibula M86.36-
        finger M86.34-
        humerus M86.32-
        ilium M86.359
        ischium M86.359
        metacarpus M86.34-
        metatarsus M86.37-
        multiple sites M86.39
        neck M86.38
        radius M86.33-
        rib M86.38
        scapula M86.31-

Osteomyelitis (Continued)
  chronic (Continued)
    hematogenous NEC (Continued)
      multifocal (Continued)
        skull M86.38
        tarsus M86.37-
        tibia M86.36-
        toe M86.37-
        ulna M86.33-
        vertebra —see Osteomyelitis, vertebra
      multiple sites M86.59
      neck M86.58
      orbit H05.02-
      petrous bone —see Petrositis
      radius M86.53-
      rib M86.58
      scapula M86.51-
      skull M86.58
      tarsus M86.57-
      tibia M86.56-
      toe M86.57-
      ulna M86.53-
      vertebra —see Osteomyelitis, vertebra
    humerus M86.62-
    ilium M86.659
    ischium M86.659
    mandible M27.2
    metacarpus M86.64-
    metatarsus M86.67-
    multifocal —see Osteomyelitis, chronic,
        hematogenous, multifocal
    multiple sites M86.69
    neck M86.68
    orbit H05.02-
    petrous bone —see Petrositis
    radius M86.63-
    rib M86.68
    scapula M86.61-
    skull M86.68
    tarsus M86.67-
    tibia M86.66-
    toe M86.67-
    ulna M86.63-
    vertebra —see Osteomyelitis, vertebra
  echinococcal B67.2
  Garr's —see Osteomyelitis, specified type
      NEC
  in diabetes mellitus —see E08-E13 with .69 ◀
  jaw (acute) (chronic) (lower) (neonatal)
      (suppurative) (upper) M27.2
  nonsuppurating —see Osteomyelitis,
      specified type NEC
  orbit H05.02-
  petrous bone —see Petrositis
  Salmonella (arizonae) (cholerae-suis)
      (enteritidis) (typhimurium) A02.24
  sclerosing, nonsuppurative —see
      Osteomyelitis, specified type NEC
  specified type NEC —see also subcategory
      M86.8X-
    mandible M27.2
    orbit H05.02-
    petrous bone —see Petrositis
    vertebra —see Osteomyelitis, vertebra
  subacute M86.20
    carpus M86.24-
    clavicle M86.21-
    femur M86.25-
    fibula M86.26-
    finger M86.24-
    humerus M86.22-
    mandible M27.2
    metacarpus M86.24-
    metatarsus M86.27-
    multiple sites M86.29
    neck M86.28
    orbit H05.02-
    petrous bone —see Petrositis
    radius M86.23-
    rib M86.28
    scapula M86.21-

Osteomyelitis (Continued)
  subacute (Continued)
    skull M86.28
    tarsus M86.27-
    tibia M86.26-
    toe M86.27-
    ulna M86.23-
    vertebra —see Osteomyelitis, vertebra
  syphilitic A52.77
    congenital (early) A50.02 [M90.80]
  tuberculous —see Tuberculosis, bone
  typhoid A01.05
  vertebra M46.20
    cervical region M46.22
    cervicothoracic region M46.23
    lumbar region M46.26
    lumbosacral region M46.27
    occipito-atlanto-axial region
        M46.21
    sacrococcygeal region M46.28
    thoracic region M46.24
    thoracolumbar region M46.25
Osteomyelofibrosis D47.4 ◀▥
Osteomyelosclerosis D75.89
Osteonecrosis M87.9
  due to
    drugs —see Osteonecrosis, secondary, due
        to, drugs
    trauma —see Osteonecrosis, secondary, due
        to, trauma
  idiopathic aseptic M87.00
    ankle M87.07-
    carpus M87.03-
    clavicle M87.01-
    femur M87.05-
    fibula M87.06-
    finger M87.04-
    humerus M87.02-
    ilium M87.050
    ischium M87.050
    metacarpus M87.04-
    metatarsus M87.07-
    multiple sites M87.09
    neck M87.08
    pelvis M87.050
    radius M87.03-
    rib M87.08
    scapula M87.01-
    skull M87.08
    tarsus M87.07-
    tibia M87.06-
    toe M87.07-
    ulna M87.03-
    vertebra M87.08
  secondary NEC M87.30
    carpus M87.33-
    clavicle M87.31-
    due to
      drugs M87.10
        carpus M87.13-
        clavicle M87.11-
        femur M87.15-
        fibula M87.16-
        finger M87.14-
        humerus M87.12-
        ilium M87.159
        ischium M87.159
        jaw M87.180
        lumbosacral M87.17-
        metacarpus M87.14-
        metatarsus M87.17-
        multiple sites M87.19
        neck M87.18
        radius M87.13-
        rib M87.18
        scapula M87.11-
        skull M87.18
        tarsus M87.17-
        tibia M87.16-
        toe M87.17-
        ulna M87.13-
        vertebra M87.18

Osteonecrosis (Continued)
  secondary NEC (Continued)
    due to (Continued)
      hemoglobinopathy NEC D58.2
          [M90.50]
        carpus D58.2 [M90.54-]
        clavicle D58.2 [M90.51-]
        femur D58.2 [M90.55-]
        fibula D58.2 [M90.56-]
        finger D58.2 [M90.54-]
        humerus D58.2 [M90.52-]
        ilium D58.2 [M90.55-]
        ischium D58.2 [M90.55-]
        metacarpus D58.2 [M90.54-]
        metatarsus D58.2 [M90.57-]
        multiple sites D58.2 [M90.58]
        neck D58.2 [M90.58]
        radius D58.2 [M90.53-]
        rib D58.2 [M90.58]
        scapula D58.2 [M90.51-]
        skull D58.2 [M90.58]
        tarsus D58.2 [M90.57-]
        tibia D58.2 [M90.56-]
        toe D58.2 [M90.57-]
        ulna D58.2 [M90.53-]
        vertebra D58.2 [M90.58]
      trauma (previous) M87.20
        carpus M87.23-
        clavicle M87.21-
        femur M87.25-
        fibula M87.26-
        finger M87.24-
        humerus M87.22-
        ilium M87.25-
        ischium M87.25-
        metacarpus M87.24-
        metatarsus M87.27-
        multiple sites M87.29
        neck M87.28
        radius M87.23-
        rib M87.28
        scapula M87.21-
        skull M87.28
        tarsus M87.27-
        tibia M87.26-
        toe M87.27-
        ulna M87.23-
        vertebra M87.28
    femur M87.35-
    fibula M87.36-
    finger M87.34-
    humerus M87.32
    ilium M87.350
    in
      caisson disease T70.3 [M90.50]
        carpus T70.3 [M90.54-]
        clavicle T70.3 [M90.51-]
        femur T70.3 [M90.55-]
        fibula T70.3 [M90.56-]
        finger T70.3 [M90.54-]
        humerus T70.3 [M90.52-]
        ilium T70.3 [M90.55-]
        ischium T70.3 [M90.55-]
        metacarpus T70.3 [M90.54-]
        metatarsus T70.3 [M90.57-]
        multiple sites T70.3 [M90.59]
        neck T70.3 [M90.58]
        radius T70.3 [M90.53-]
        rib T70.3 [M90.58]
        scapula T70.3 [M90.51-]
        skull T70.3 [M90.58]
        tarsus T70.3 [M90.57-]
        tibia T70.3 [M90.56-]
        toe T70.3 [M90.57-]
        ulna T70.3 [M90.53-]
        vertebra T70.3 [M90.58]
    ischium M87.350
    metacarpus M87.34-
    metatarsus M87.37-
    multiple site M87.39
    neck M87.38

Osteonecrosis (Continued)
  secondary NEC (Continued)
    radius M87.33-
    rib M87.38
    scapula M87.319
    skull M87.38
    tarsus M87.379
    tibia M87.366
    toe M87.379
    ulna M87.33-
    vertebra M87.38
  specified type NEC M87.80
    carpus M87.83-
    clavicle M87.81-
    femur M87.85-
    fibula M87.86-
    finger M87.84-
    humerus M87.82-
    ilium M87.85-
    ischium M87.85-
    metacarpus M87.84-
    metatarsus M87.87-
    multiple sites M87.89
    neck M87.88
    radius M87.83-
    rib M87.88-
    scapula M87.81-
    skull M87.88
    tarsus M87.87-
    tibia M87.86-
    toe M87.87-
    ulna M87.83-
    vertebra M87.88
Osteo-onycho-arthro-dysplasia Q87.2 ◀▬▬
Osteo-onychodysplasia, hereditary Q87.2 ◀▬▬
Osteopathia condensans disseminata Q78.8
Osteopathy —see also Osteomyelitis,
    Osteonecrosis, Osteoporosis
  after poliomyelitis M89.60
    carpus M89.64-
    clavicle M89.61-
    femur M89.65-
    fibula M89.66-
    finger M89.64-
    humerus M89.62-
    ilium M89.659
    ischium M89.659
    metacarpus M89.64-
    metatarsus M89.67-
    multiple sites M89.69
    neck M89.68
    radius M89.63-
    rib M89.68
    scapula M89.61-
    skull M89.68
    tarsus M89.67-
    tibia M89.66-
    toe M89.67-
    ulna M89.63-
    vertebra M89.68
  in (due to)
    renal osteodystrophy N25.0
    specified diseases classified elsewhere —
        see subcategory M90.8
Osteopenia M85.8-
  borderline M85.8-
Osteoperiostitis —see Osteomyelitis, specified
    type NEC
Osteopetrosis (familial) Q78.2
Osteophyte M25.70
  ankle M25.77-
  elbow M25.72-
  foot joint M25.77-
  hand joint M25.74-
  hip M25.75-
  knee M25.76-
  shoulder M25.71-
  spine M25.78
  vertebrae M25.78
  wrist M25.73-
Osteopoikilosis Q78.8

Osteoporosis (female) (male) M81.0
  with current pathological fracture M80.00
  age-related M81.0
    with current pathologic fracture M80.00
      carpus M80.04-
      clavicle M80.01-
      fibula M80.06-
      finger M80.04-
      humerus M80.02-
      ilium M80.05-
      ischium M80.05-
      metacarpus M80.04-
      metatarsus M80.07-
      pelvis M80.05-
      radius M80.03-
      scapula M80.01-
      tarsus M80.07-
      tibia M80.06-
      toe M80.07-
      ulna M80.03-
      vertebra M80.08
  disuse M81.8
    with current pathological fracture M80.80
      carpus M80.84-
      clavicle M80.81-
      fibula M80.86-
      finger M80.84-
      humerus M80.82-
      ilium M80.85-
      ischium M80.85-
      metacarpus M80.84-
      metatarsus M80.87-
      pelvis M80.85-
      radius M80.83-
      scapula M80.81-
      tarsus M80.87-
      tibia M80.86-
      toe M80.87-
      ulna M80.83-
      vertebra M80.88
  drug-induced —see Osteoporosis, specified
      type NEC
  idiopathic —see Osteoporosis, specified type
      NEC
  involutional —see Osteoporosis, age-related
  Lequesne M81.6
  localized M81.6
  postmenopausal M81.0
    with pathological fracture M80.00
      carpus M80.04-
      clavicle M80.01-
      fibula M80.06-
      finger M80.04-
      humerus M80.02-
      ilium M80.05-
      ischium M80.05-
      metacarpus M80.04-
      metatarsus M80.07-
      pelvis M80.05-
      radius M80.03-
      scapula M80.01-
      tarsus M80.07-
      tibia M80.06-
      toe M80.07-
      ulna M80.03-
      vertebra M80.08
  postoophorectomy —see Osteoporosis,
      specified type NEC
  postsurgical malabsorption —see
      Osteoporosis, specified type NEC
  post-traumatic —see Osteoporosis, specified
      type NEC
  senile —see Osteoporosis, age-related
  specified type NEC M81.8
    with pathological fracture M80.80
      carpus M80.84-
      clavicle M80.81-
      fibula M80.86-
      finger M80.84-
      humerus M80.82-
      ilium M80.85-

Osteoporosis (Continued)
  specified type NEC (Continued)
    with pathological fracture (Continued)
      ischium M80.85-
      metacarpus M80.84-
      metatarsus M80.87-
      pelvis M80.85-
      radius M80.83-
      scapula M80.81-
      tarsus M80.87-
      tibia M80.86-
      toe M80.87-
      ulna M80.83-
      vertebra M80.88
Osteopsathyrosis (idiopathica) Q78.0
Osteoradionecrosis, jaw (acute) (chronic)
    (lower) (suppurative) (upper)
    M27.2
Osteosarcoma (any form) —see Neoplasm,
    bone, malignant
Osteosclerosis Q78.2
  acquired M85.8-
  congenita Q77.4
  fragilitas (generalisata) Q78.2
  myelofibrosis D75.81
Osteosclerotic anemia D64.89
Osteosis
  cutis L94.2
  renal fibrocystic N25.0
Österreicher-Turner syndrome Q87.2
Ostium
  atrioventriculare commune Q21.2
  primum (arteriosum) (defect) (persistent)
      Q21.2
  secundum (arteriosum) (defect) (patent)
      (persistent) Q21.1
Ostrum-Furst syndrome Q75.8
Otalgia —see subcategory H92.0
Otitis (acute) H66.90
  with effusion —see also Otitis, media,
      nonsuppurative
    purulent —see Otitis, media, suppurative
  adhesive —see subcategory H74.1
  chronic —see also Otitis, media, chronic
    with effusion —see also Otitis, media,
        nonsuppurative, chronic
  externa H60.9-
    abscess —see Abscess, ear, external
    acute (noninfective) H60.50-
      actinic H60.51-
      chemical H60.52-
      contact H60.53-
      eczematoid H60.54-
      infective —see Otitis, externa, infective
      reactive H60.55-
      specified NEC H60.59-
    cellulitis —see Cellulitis, ear
    chronic H60.6-
    diffuse —see Otitis, externa, infective, diffuse
    hemorrhagic —see Otitis, externa, infective,
        hemorrhagic
    in (due to)
      aspergillosis B44.89
      candidiasis B37.84
      erysipelas A46 [H62.40]
      herpes (simplex) virus infection B00.1
          zoster B02.8
      impetigo L01.00 [H62.40]
      infectious disease NEC B99 [H62.4-]
      mycosis NEC B36.9 [H62.40]
      parasitic disease NEC B89 [H62.40]
      viral disease NEC B34.9 [H62.40]
      zoster B02.8
    infective NEC H60.39-
      abscess —see Abscess, ear, external
      cellulitis —see Cellulitis, ear
      diffuse H60.31-
      hemorrhagic H60.32-
      swimmer's ear —see Swimmer's, ear
    malignant H60.2-
    mycotic B36.9 [H62.40]

Otitis (Continued)
  externa (Continued)
    mycotic NEC B36.9 [H62.40] ◄
      in ◄
        aspergillosis B44.89 ◄
        candidiasis B37.84 ◄
        moniliasis B37.84 ◄
    necrotizing —see Otitis, externa, malignant
    Pseudomonas aeruginosa —see Otitis,
        externa, malignant
    reactive —see Otitis, externa, acute, reactive
    specified NEC —see subcategory H60.8
    tropical B36.8
    tropical NEC B36.9 [H62.40] ◄
      in ◄
        aspergillosis B44.89 ◄
        candidiasis B37.84 ◄
        moniliasis B37.84 ◄
  insidiosa —see Otosclerosis
  interna —see subcategory H83.0
  media (hemorrhagic) (staphylococcal)
      (streptococcal) H66.9-
    with effusion (nonpurulent) —see Otitis,
        media, nonsuppurative
    acute, subacute H66.90
      allergic —see Otitis, media,
          nonsuppurative, acute, allergic
      exudative —see Otitis, media,
          suppurative, acute ◄⃟
      mucoid —see Otitis, media,
          nonsuppurative, acute
      necrotizing —see also Otitis, media,
          suppurative, acute
        in
          measles B05.3
          scarlet fever A38.0
      nonsuppurative NEC —see Otitis, media,
          nonsuppurative, acute
      purulent —see Otitis, media,
          suppurative, acute
      sanguinous —see Otitis, media,
          nonsuppurative, acute
      secretory —see Otitis, media,
          nonsuppurative, acute, serous
      seromucinous —see Otitis, media,
          nonsuppurative, acute
      serous —see Otitis, media,
          nonsuppurative, acute, serous
      suppurative —see Otitis, media,
          suppurative, acute
    allergic —see Otitis, media, nonsuppurative
    catarrhal —see Otitis, media,
        nonsuppurative
    chronic H66.90
      with effusion (nonpurulent) —see Otitis,
          media, nonsuppurative, chronic
      allergic —see Otitis, media,
          nonsuppurative, chronic, allergic
      benign suppurative —see Otitis,
          media, suppurative, chronic,
          tubotympanic
      catarrhal —see Otitis, media,
          nonsuppurative, chronic, serous
      exudative —see Otitis, media,
          suppurative, chronic ◄⃟
      mucinous —see Otitis, media,
          nonsuppurative, chronic, mucoid
      mucoid —see Otitis, media,
          nonsuppurative, chronic, mucoid
      nonsuppurative NEC —see Otitis, media,
          nonsuppurative, chronic
      purulent —see Otitis, media,
          suppurative, chronic
      secretory —see Otitis, media,
          nonsuppurative, chronic, mucoid
      seromucinous —see Otitis, media,
          nonsuppurative, chronic
      serous —see Otitis, media,
          nonsuppurative, chronic, serous
      suppurative —see Otitis, media,
          suppurative, chronic

Otitis (Continued)
  media (Continued)
    chronic (Continued)
      transudative —see Otitis, media,
          nonsuppurative, chronic, mucoid
      exudative —see Otitis, media,
          nonsuppurative
    in (due to) (with)
      influenza —see Influenza, with, otitis
          media
      measles B05.3
      scarlet fever A38.0
      tuberculosis A18.6
      viral disease NEC B34.- [H67.-]
    mucoid —see Otitis, media,
        nonsuppurative
    nonsuppurative H65.9-
      acute or subacute NEC H65.19-
        allergic H65.11-
          recurrent H65.11-
        recurrent H65.19-
        secretory —see Otitis, media,
            nonsuppurative, serous
        serous H65.0-
          recurrent H65.0-
      chronic H65.49-
        allergic H65.41-
        mucoid H65.3-
        serous H65.2-
    postmeasles B05.3
    purulent —see Otitis, media, suppurative
    secretory —see Otitis, media,
        nonsuppurative
    seromucinous —see Otitis, media,
        nonsuppurative
    serous —see Otitis, media, nonsuppurative
    suppurative H66.4-
      acute H66.00-
        with rupture of ear drum H66.01-
        recurrent H66.00-
          with rupture of ear drum H66.01-
      chronic —see also subcategory H66.3
        atticoantral H66.2-
        benign —see Otitis, media,
            suppurative, chronic,
            tubotympanic
        tubotympanic H66.1-
      transudative —see Otitis, media,
          nonsuppurative
    tuberculous A18.6
Otocephaly Q18.2
Otolith syndrome —see subcategory H81.8
Otomycosis (diffuse) NEC B36.9 [H62.40]
  in
    aspergillosis B44.89
    candidiasis B37.84
    moniliasis B37.84
Otoporosis —see Otosclerosis
Otorrhagia (nontraumatic) H92.2-
  traumatic - code by Type of injury
Otorrhea H92.1-
  cerebrospinal G96.0
Otosclerosis (general) H80.9-
  cochlear (endosteal) H80.2-
  involving
    otic capsule —see Otosclerosis, cochlear
    oval window
      nonobliterative H80.0-
      obliterative H80.1-
    round window —see Otosclerosis, cochlear
  nonobliterative —see Otosclerosis, involving,
      oval window, nonobliterative
  obliterative —see Otosclerosis, involving, oval
      window, obliterative
  specified NEC H80.8-
Otospongiosis —see Otosclerosis
Otto's disease or pelvis M24.7
Outcome of delivery Z37.9
  multiple births Z37.9
    all liveborn Z37.50
      quadruplets Z37.52
      quintuplets Z37.53

Outcome of delivery (Continued)
  multiple births (Continued)
    all liveborn (Continued)
      sextuplets Z37.54
      specified number NEC Z37.59
      triplets Z37.51
    all stillborn Z37.7
    some liveborn Z37.60
      quadruplets Z37.62
      quintuplets Z37.63
      sextuplets Z37.64
      specified number NEC Z37.69
      triplets Z37.61
    single NEC Z37.9
      liveborn Z37.0
      stillborn Z37.1
    twins NEC Z37.9
      both liveborn Z37.2
      both stillborn Z37.4
      one liveborn, one stillborn Z37.3
Outlet —see condition
Ovalocytosis (congenital) (hereditary) —see
    Elliptocytosis
Ovarian —see Condition
Ovariocele N83.4- ◄⃟
Ovaritis (cystic) —see Oophoritis
Ovary, ovarian —see also condition
  resistant syndrome E28.39
  vein syndrome N13.8
Overactive —see also Hyperfunction
  adrenal cortex NEC E27.0
  bladder N32.81
  hypothalamus E23.3
  thyroid —see Hyperthyroidism
Overactivity R46.3
  child —see Disorder, attention-deficit
      hyperactivity
Overbite (deep) (excessive) (horizontal)
    (vertical) M26.29
Overbreathing —see Hyperventilation
Overconscientious personality F60.5
Overdevelopment —see Hypertrophy
Overdistension —see Distension
Overdose, overdosage (drug) —see Table of
    Drugs and Chemicals, by drug, poisoning
Overeating R63.2
  nonorganic origin F50.89 ◄⃟
  psychogenic F50.89 ◄⃟
Overexertion (effects) (exhaustion) T73.3
Overexposure (effects) T73.9
  exhaustion T73.2
Overfeeding —see Overeating
  newborn P92.4
Overfill, endodontic M27.52
Overgrowth, bone —see Hypertrophy, bone
Overhanging of dental restorative material
    (unrepairable) K08.52
Overheated (places) (effects) —see Heat
Overjet (excessive horizontal) M26.23
Overlaid, overlying (suffocation) —see Asphyxia,
    traumatic, due to mechanical threat
Overlap, excessive horizontal (teeth)
    M26.23
Overl apping toe (acquired) —see also
    Deformity, toe, specified NEC
  congenital (fifth toe) Q66.89
Overload
  circulatory, due to transfusion (blood) (blood
      components) (TACO) E87.71
  fluid E87.70
    due to transfusion (blood) (blood
        components) E87.71
    specified NEC E87.79
  iron, due to repeated red blood cell
      transfusions E83.111
  potassium (K) E87.5
  sodium (Na) E87.0
Overnutrition —see Hyperalimentation
Overproduction —see also Hypersecretion
  ACTH E27.0
  catecholamine E27.5
  growth hormone E22.0

Overprotection, child by parent Z62.1
Overriding
  aorta Q25.49 ◀▥
  finger (acquired) —*see* Deformity, finger
    congenital Q68.1
  toe (acquired) —*see also* Deformity, toe,
    specified NEC
    congenital Q66.89
Overstrained R53.83
  heart —*see* Hypertrophy, cardiac

Overuse, muscle NEC
  M70.8-
Overweight E66.3
Overworked R53.83
Oviduct —*see* condition
Ovotestis Q56.0
Ovulation (cycle)
  failure or lack of N97.0
  pain N94.0
Ovum —*see* condition

Owren's disease or syndrome (parahemophilia)
  D68.2
Ox heart —*see* Hypertrophy, cardiac
Oxalosis E72.53
Oxaluria E72.53
Oxycephaly, oxycephalic Q75.0
  syphilitic, congenital A50.02
Oxyuriasis B80
Oxyuris vermicularis (infestation) B80
Ozena J31.0

P

Pachyderma, pachydermia L85.9
  larynx (verrucosa) J38.7
Pachydermatocele (congenital) Q82.8
Pachydermoperiostosis —*see also*
    Osteoarthropathy, hypertrophic, specified
      type NEC
  clubbed nail M89.40 *[L62]*
Pachygyria Q04.3
Pachymeningitis (adhesive) (basal) (brain)
    (cervical) (chronic) (circumscribed)
    (external) (fibrous) (hemorrhagic)
    (hypertrophic) (internal) (purulent)
    (spinal) (suppurative) —*see* Meningitis
Pachyonychia (congenital) Q84.5
Pacinian tumor —*see* Neoplasm, skin, benign
Pad, knuckle or Garrod's M72.1
Paget-Schroetter syndrome I82.890
Paget's disease
  with infiltrating duct carcinoma —*see*
    Neoplasm, breast, malignant
  bone M88.9
    carpus M88.84-
    clavicle M88.81-
    femur M88.85-
    fibula M88.86-
    finger M88.84-
    humerus M88.82-
    ilium M88.85-
    in neoplastic disease —*see* Osteitis,
      deformans, in neoplastic disease
    ischium M88.85-
    metacarpus M88.84-
    metatarsus M88.87-
    multiple sites M88.89
    neck M88.88
    radius M88.83-
    rib M88.88
    scapula M88.81-
    skull M88.0
    tarsus M88.87-
    tibia M88.86-
    toe M88.87-
    ulna M88.83-
    vertebra M88.88
  breast (female) C50.01-
    male C50.02-
  extramammary —*see also* Neoplasm, skin,
    malignant
    anus C21.0
      margin C44.590
      skin C44.590
  intraductal carcinoma —*see* Neoplasm,
    breast, malignant
  malignant —*see* Neoplasm, skin, malignant
    breast (female) C50.01-
      male C50.02-
    unspecified site (female) C50.01-
      male C50.02-
  mammary —*see* Paget's disease, breast
  nipple —*see* Paget's disease, breast
  osteitis deformans —*see* Paget's disease, bone
Pain(s) —*see also* Painful R52
  abdominal R10.9
    colic R10.83
    generalized R10.84
      with acute abdomen R10.0
    lower R10.30
      left quadrant R10.32
      pelvic or perineal R10.2
      periumbilical R10.33
      right quadrant R10.31
    rebound —*see* Tenderness, abdominal,
      rebound
    severe with abdominal rigidity R10.0
    tenderness —*see* Tenderness, abdominal
    upper R10.10
      epigastric R10.13
      left quadrant R10.12
      right quadrant R10.11

Pain *(Continued)*
  acute R52
    due to trauma G89.11
    neoplasm related G89.3
    postprocedural NEC G89.18
    post-thoracotomy G89.12
    specified by site — code to Pain, by site
  adnexa (uteri) R10.2
  anginoid —*see* Pain, precordial
  anus K62.89
  arm —*see* Pain, limb, upper
  axillary (axilla) M79.62-
  back (postural) M54.9
  bladder R39.89
    associated with micturition —*see*
      Micturition, painful
    chronic R39.82 ◀
  bone —*see* Disorder, bone, specified type
    NEC
  breast N64.4
  broad ligament R10.2
  cancer associated (acute) (chronic) G89.3
  cecum —*see* Pain, abdominal
  cervicobrachial M53.1
  chest (central) R07.9
    anterior wall R07.89
    atypical R07.89
    ischemic I20.9
    musculoskeletal R07.89
    non-cardiac R07.89
    on breathing R07.1
    pleurodynia R07.81
    precordial R07.2
    wall (anterior) R07.89
  chronic G89.29
    associated with significant psychosocial
      dysfunction G89.4
    due to trauma G89.21
    neoplasm related G89.3
    postoperative NEC G89.28
    postprocedural NEC G89.28
    post-thoracotomy G89.22
    specified NEC G89.29
  coccyx M53.3
  colon —*see* Pain, abdominal
  coronary —*see* Angina
  costochondral R07.1
  diaphragm R07.1
  due to cancer G89.3
  due to device, implant or graft —*see also*
      Complications, by site and type,
      specified NEC T85.848 ◀▥
    arterial graft NEC T82.848
    breast (implant) T85.848 ◀▥
    catheter NEC T85.848 ◀▥
      dialysis (renal) T82.848
        intraperitoneal T85.848 ◀▥
      infusion NEC T82.848
        spinal (epidural) (subdural) T85.840 ◀▥
      urinary (indwelling) T83.84
    electronic (electrode) (pulse generator)
      (stimulator)
      bone T84.84
      cardiac T82.847
      nervous system (brain) (peripheral
        nerve) (spinal) T85.840 ◀▥
      urinary T83.84
    fixation, internal (orthopedic) NEC T84.84
    gastrointestinal (bile duct) (esophagus)
      T85.848 ◀▥
    genital NEC T83.84
    heart NEC T82.847
    infusion NEC T85.848 ◀▥
    joint prosthesis T84.84
    ocular (corneal graft) (orbital implant)
      NEC T85.848 ◀▥
    orthopedic NEC T84.84
    specified NEC T85.848 ◀▥
    urinary NEC T83.84
    vascular NEC T82.848
    ventricular intracranial shunt T85.840 ◀▥

Pain *(Continued)*
  due to malignancy (primary) (secondary)
    G89.3
  ear —*see* subcategory H92.0
  epigastric, epigastrium R10.13
  eye —*see* Pain, ocular
  face, facial R51
    atypical G50.1
  female genital organs NEC N94.89
  finger —*see* Pain, limb, upper
  flank —*see* Pain, abdominal
  foot —*see* Pain, limb, lower
  gallbladder K82.9
  gas (intestinal) R14.1
  gastric —*see* Pain, abdominal
  generalized NOS R52
  genital organ
    female N94.89
    male N50.89 ◀▥
  groin —*see* Pain, abdominal, lower
  hand —*see* Pain, limb, upper
  head —*see* Headache
  heart —*see* Pain, precordial
  infra-orbital —*see* Neuralgia, trigeminal
  intercostal R07.82
  intermenstrual N94.0
  jaw R68.84
  joint M25.50
    ankle M25.57-
    elbow M25.52-
    finger M25.54- ◀▥
    foot M25.57-
    hand M25.54- ◀▥
    hip M25.55-
    knee M25.56-
    shoulder M25.51-
    toe M25.57-
    wrist M25.53-
  kidney N23
  laryngeal R07.0
  leg —*see* Pain, limb, lower
  limb M79.609
    lower M79.60-
      foot M79.67-
      lower leg M79.66-
      thigh M79.65-
      toe M79.67-
    upper M79.60-
      axilla M79.62-
      finger M79.64-
      forearm M79.63-
      hand M79.64-
      upper arm M79.62-
  loin M54.5
  low back M54.5
  lumbar region M54.5
  mandibular R68.84
  mastoid —*see* subcategory H92.0
  maxilla R68.84
  menstrual —*see also* Dysmenorrhea N94.6
  metacarpophalangeal (joint) —*see* Pain, joint,
    hand
  metatarsophalangeal (joint) —*see* Pain, joint,
    foot
  mouth K13.79
  muscle —*see* Myalgia
  musculoskeletal —*see also* Pain, by site M79.1
  myofascial M79.1
  nasal J34.89
  nasopharynx J39.2
  neck NEC M54.2
  nerve NEC —*see* Neuralgia
  neuromuscular —*see* Neuralgia
  nose J34.89
  ocular H57.1-
  ophthalmic —*see* Pain, ocular
  orbital region —*see* Pain, ocular
  ovary N94.89
  over heart —*see* Pain, precordial
  ovulation N94.0
  pelvic (female) R10.2

Pain *(Continued)*
 penis N48.89
 pericardial —*see* Pain, precordial
 perineal, perineum R10.2
 pharynx J39.2
 pleura, pleural, pleuritic R07.81
 postoperative NOS G89.18
 postprocedural NOS G89.18
 post-thoracotomy G89.12
 precordial (region) R07.2
 premenstrual N94.3
 psychogenic (persistent) (any site) F45.41
 radicular (spinal) —*see* Radiculopathy
 rectum K62.89
 respiration R07.1
 retrosternal R07.2
 rheumatoid, muscular —*see* Myalgia
 rib R07.81
 root (spinal) —*see* Radiculopathy
 round ligament (stretch) R10.2
 sacroiliac M53.3
 sciatic —*see* Sciatica
 scrotum N50.82 ◄▥
 seminal vesicle N50.89 ◄▥
 shoulder M25.51-
 spermatic cord N50.89 ◄▥
 spinal root —*see* Radiculopathy
 spine M54.9
  cervical M54.2
  low back M54.5
   with sciatica M54.4-
  thoracic M54.6
 stomach —*see* Pain, abdominal
 substernal R07.2
 temporomandibular (joint) M26.62- ◄▥
 testis N50.81- ◄▥
 thoracic spine M54.6
  with radicular and visceral pain
   M54.14
 throat R07.0
 tibia —*see* Pain, limb, lower
 toe —*see* Pain, limb, lower
 tongue K14.6
 tooth K08.89 ◄▥
 trigeminal —*see* Neuralgia, trigeminal
 tumor associated G89.3
 ureter N23
 urinary (organ) (system) N23
 uterus NEC N94.89
 vagina R10.2
 vertebrogenic (syndrome) M54.89
 vesical R39.89
  associated with micturition —*see*
   Micturition, painful
 vulva R10.2
Painful —*see also* Pain
 coitus
  female N94.10 ◄▥
  male N53.12
  psychogenic F52.6
 ejaculation (semen) N53.12
  psychogenic F52.6
 erection —*see* Priapism
 feet syndrome E53.8
 joint replacement (hip) (knee) T84.84
 menstruation —*see* Dysmenorrhea
  psychogenic F45.8
 micturition —*see* Micturition, painful
 respiration R07.1
 scar NEC L90.5
 wire sutures T81.89
Painter's colic —*see* subcategory T56.0
Palate —*see* condition
Palatoplegia K13.79
Palatoschisis —*see* Cleft, palate
Palilalia R48.8
Palliative care Z51.5
Pallor R23.1
 optic disc, temporal —*see* Atrophy, optic
Palmar —*see also* condition
 fascia —*see* condition

Palpable
 cecum K63.89
 kidney N28.89
 ovary N83.8
 prostate N42.9
 spleen —*see* Splenomegaly
Palpitations (heart) R00.2
 psychogenic F45.8
Palsy —*see also* Paralysis G83.9
 atrophic diffuse (progressive) G12.22
 Bell's —*see also* Palsy, facial
  newborn P11.3
 brachial plexus NEC G54.0
  newborn (birth injury) P14.3
 brain —*see* Palsy, cerebral
 bulbar (progressive) (chronic) G12.22
  of childhood (Fazio-Londe) G12.1
  pseudo NEC G12.29
  supranuclear (progressive) G23.1
 cerebral (congenital) G80.9
  ataxic G80.4
  athetoid G80.3
  choreathetoid G80.3
  diplegic G80.8
   spastic G80.1
  dyskinetic G80.3
   athetoid G80.3
   choreathetoid G80.3
   distonic G80.3
  dystonic G80.3
  hemiplegic G80.8
   spastic G80.2
  mixed G80.8
  monoplegic G80.8
   spastic G80.8
  paraplegic G80.8
   spastic G80.1
  quadriplegic G80.8
   spastic G80.0
  spastic G80.1
   diplegic G80.1
   hemiplegic G80.2
   monoplegic G80.1
   quadriplegic G80.0
   specified NEC G80.1
   tetrapelgic G80.0
  specified NEC G80.8
  syphilitic A52.12
   congenital A50.49
  tetraplegic G80.8
   spastic G80.0
 cranial nerve —*see also* Disorder, nerve,
   cranial
  multiple G52.7
   in
    infectious disease B99 *[G53]*
    neoplastic disease —*see also* Neoplasm
     D49.9 *[G53]*
    parasitic disease B89 *[G53]*
    sarcoidosis D86.82
 creeping G12.22
 diver's T70.3
 Erb's P14.0
 facial G51.0
  newborn (birth injury) P11.3
 glossopharyngeal G52.1
 Klumpke (-Déjérine) P14.1
 lead —*see* subcategory T56.0
 median nerve (tardy) G56.1-
 nerve G58.9
  specified NEC G58.8
 peroneal nerve (acute) (tardy) G57.3-
 progressive supranuclear G23.1
 pseudobulbar NEC G12.29
 radial nerve (acute) G56.3-
 seventh nerve —*see also* Palsy, facial
  newborn P11.3
 shaking —*see* Parkinsonism
 spastic (cerebral) (spinal) G80.1
 ulnar nerve (tardy) G56.2-
 wasting G12.29

Paludism —*see* Malaria
Panangiitis M30.0
Panaris, panaritium —*see also* Cellulitis, digit
 with lymphangitis —*see* Lymphangitis, acute,
  digit
Panarteritis nodosa M30.0
 brain or cerebral I67.7
Pancake heart R93.1
 with cor pulmonale (chronic) I27.81
Pancarditis (acute) (chronic) I51.89
 rheumatic I09.89
  active or acute I01.8
Pancoast's syndrome or tumor C34.1-
Pancolitis, ulcerative (chronic) K51.00
 with
  abscess K51.014
  complication K51.019
  fistula K51.013
  obstruction K51.012
  rectal bleeding K51.011
  specified complication NEC K51.018
Pancreas, pancreatic —*see* condition
Pancreatitis (annular) (apoplectic) (calcareous)
  (edematous) (hemorrhagic) (malignant)
  (recurrent) (subacute) (suppurative)
  K85.90 ◄▥
 with necrosis (uninfected) K85.91 ◄
  infected K85.92 ◄
 acute (without necrosis or infection)
  K85.90 ◄▥
  with necrosis (uninfected) K85.91 ◄
   infected K85.92 ◄
  alcohol induced (without necrosis or
   infection) K85.20 ◄▥
   with necrosis (uninfected) K85.21 ◄
    infected K85.22 ◄
  biliary (without necrosis or infection)
   K85.10 ◄▥
   with necrosis (uninfected) K85.11 ◄
    infected K85.12 ◄
  drug induced (without necrosis or
   infection) K85.30 ◄▥
   with necrosis (uninfected) K85.31 ◄
    infected K85.32 ◄
  gallstone (without necrosis or infection)
   K85.10 ◄▥
   with necrosis (uninfected) K85.11 ◄
    infected K85.12 ◄
  idiopathic (without necrosis or infection)
   K85.00 ◄▥
   with necrosis (uninfected) K85.01 ◄
    infected K85.02 ◄
  specified NEC (without necrosis or
   infection) K85.80 ◄▥
   with necrosis (uninfected)
    K85.81 ◄
    infected K85.82 ◄
 chronic (infectious) K86.1
  alcohol-induced K86.0
  recurrent K86.1
  relapsing K86.1
 cystic (chronic) K86.1
 cytomegaloviral B25.2
 fibrous (chronic) K86.1
 gallstone (without necrosis or infection)
  K85.10 ◄▥
  with necrosis (uninfected)
   K85.11 ◄
   infected K85.12 ◄
 gangrenous —*see* Pancreatitis, acute ◄▥
 interstitial (chronic) K86.1
  acute —*see also* Pancreatitis, acute
   K85.80 ◄▥
 mumps B26.3
 recurrent (chronic) K86.1
 relapsing, chronic K86.1
 syphilitic A52.74
Pancreatoblastoma —*see* Neoplasm, pancreas,
  malignant
Pancreolithiasis K86.89 ◄▥
Pancytolysis D75.89

Pancytopenia (acquired) D61.818
  with
    malformations D61.09
    myelodysplastic syndrome —*see*
      Syndrome, myelodysplastic
    antineoplastic chemotherapy induced
      D61.810
  congenital D61.09
  drug-induced NEC D61.811
Panencephalitis, subacute, sclerosing
  A81.1
Panhematopenia D61.9
  congenital D61.09
  constitutional D61.09
  splenic, primary D73.1
Panhemocytopenia D61.9
  congenital D61.09
  constitutional D61.09
Panhypogonadism E29.1
Panhypopituitarism E23.0
  prepubertal E23.0
Panic (attack) (state) F41.0
  reaction to exceptional stress (transient)
    F43.0
Panmyelopathy, familial, constitutional
  D61.09
Panmyelophthisis D61.82
  congenital D61.09
Panmyelosis (acute) (with myelofibrosis)
  C94.4-
Panner's disease —*see* Osteochondrosis,
  juvenile, humerus
Panneuritis endemica E51.11
Panniculitis (nodular) (nonsuppurative) M79.3
  back M54.00
    cervical region M54.02
    cervicothoracic region M54.03
    lumbar region M54.06
    lumbosacral region M54.07
    multiple sites M54.09
    occipito-atlanto-axial region M54.01
    sacrococcygeal region M54.08
    thoracic region M54.04
    thoracolumbar region M54.05
  lupus L93.2
  mesenteric K65.4
  neck M54.02
    cervicothoracic region M54.03
    occipito-atlanto-axial region M54.01
  relapsing M35.6
Panniculus adiposus (abdominal) E65
Pannus (allergic) (cornea) (degenerativus)
    (keratic) H16.42-
  abdominal (symptomatic) E65
  trachomatosus, trachomatous (active) A71.1
Panophthalmitis H44.01-
Pansinusitis (chronic) (hyperplastic)
    (nonpurulent) (purulent) J32.4
  acute J01.40
    recurrent J01.41
  tuberculous A15.8
Panuveitis (sympathetic) H44.11-
Panvalvular disease I08.9
  specified NEC I08.8
PAPA (pyogenic arthritis, pyoderma
    gangrenosum, and acne syndrome)
    M04.8 ◄
Papanicolaou smear, cervix Z12.4
  as part of routine gynecological examination
    Z01.419
    with abnormal findings Z01.411
  for suspected neoplasm Z12.4
  nonspecific abnormal finding R87.619
  routine Z01.419
    with abnormal findings Z01.411
Papilledema (choked disc) H47.10
  associated with
    decreased ocular pressure H47.12
    increased intracranial pressure H47.11
    retinal disorder H47.13
  Foster-Kennedy syndrome H47.14-

Papillitis H46.00
  anus K62.89
  chronic lingual K14.4
  necrotizing, kidney N17.2
  optic H46.0-
  rectum K62.89
  renal, necrotizing N17.2
  tongue K14.0
Papilloma —*see also* Neoplasm, benign,
    by site
  acuminatum (female) (male) (anogenital)
    A63.0
  basal cell L82.1 ◄
    inflamed L82.0 ◄
  benign pinta (primary) A67.0
  bladder (urinary) (transitional cell) D41.4
  choroid plexus (lateral ventricle) (third
      ventricle) D33.0
    anaplastic C71.5
    fourth ventricle D33.1
    malignant C71.5
  renal pelvis (transitional cell) D41.1-
    benign D30.1-
  Schneiderian
    specified site —*see* Neoplasm, benign, by
      site
    unspecified site D14.0
  serous surface
    borderline malignancy
      specified site —*see* Neoplasm, uncertain
        behavior, by site
      unspecified site D39.10
    specified site —*see* Neoplasm, benign, by
      site
    unspecified site D27.9
  transitional (cell)
    bladder (urinary) D41.4
    inverted type —*see* Neoplasm, uncertain
      behavior, by site
    renal pelvis D41.1-
    ureter D41.2-
  ureter (transitional cell) D41.2-
    benign D30.2-
  urothelial —*see* Neoplasm, uncertain
    behavior, by site
  villous —*see* Neoplasm, uncertain behavior,
    by site
    adenocarcinoma in —*see* Neoplasm,
      malignant, by site
    in situ —*see* Neoplasm, in situ
  yaws, plantar or palmar A66.1
Papillomata, multiple, of yaws A66.1
Papillomatosis —*see also* Neoplasm, benign,
    by site
  confluent and reticulated L83
  cystic, breast —*see* Mastopathy, cystic
  ductal, breast —*see* Mastopathy, cystic
  intraductal (diffuse) —*see* Neoplasm, benign,
    by site
  subareolar duct D24-
Papillomavirus, as cause of disease classified
    elsewhere B97.7
Papillon-Léage and Psaume syndrome
  Q87.0
Papule (s) R23.8
  carate (primary) A67.0
  fibrous, of nose D22.39
  Gottron's L94.4
  pinta (primary) A67.0
Papulosis
  lymphomatoid C86.6
  malignant I77.89
Papyraceous fetus O31.0-
Para-albuminemia E88.09
Paracephalus Q89.7
Parachute mitral valve Q23.2
Paracoccidioidomycosis B41.9
  disseminated B41.7
  generalized B41.7
  mucocutaneous-lymphangitic B41.8
  pulmonary B41.0

Paracoccidioidomycosis (*Continued*)
  specified NEC B41.8
  visceral B41.8
Paradentosis K05.4
Paraffinoma T88.8
Paraganglioma D44.7
  adrenal D35.0-
    malignant C74.1-
  aortic body D44.7
    malignant C75.5
  carotid body D44.6
    malignant C75.4
  chromaffin —*see also* Neoplasm, benign, by
    site
    malignant —*see* Neoplasm, malignant, by
      site
  extra-adrenal D44.7
    malignant C75.5
      specified site —*see* Neoplasm,
        malignant, by site
      unspecified site C75.5
    specified site —*see* Neoplasm, uncertain
      behavior, by site
    unspecified site D44.7
  gangliocytic D13.2
    specified site —*see* Neoplasm, benign, by
      site
    unspecified site D13.2
  glomus jugulare D44.7
    malignant C75.5
  jugular D44.7
  malignant C75.5
    specified site —*see* Neoplasm, malignant,
      by site
    unspecified site C75.5
  nonchromaffin D44.7
    malignant C75.5
      specified site —*see* Neoplasm,
        malignant, by site
      unspecified site C75.5
    specified site —*see* Neoplasm, uncertain
      behavior, by site
    unspecified site D44.7
  parasympathetic D44.7
    specified site —*see* Neoplasm, uncertain
      behavior, by site
    unspecified site D44.7
  specified site —*see* Neoplasm, uncertain
    behavior, by site
  sympathetic D44.7
    specified site —*see* Neoplasm, uncertain
      behavior, by site
    unspecified site D44.7
Parageusia R43.2
  psychogenic F45.8
Paragonimiasis B66.4
Paragranuloma, Hodgkin —*see*
  Lymphoma, Hodgkin, classical,
    specified NEC
Parahemophilia —*see also* Defect, coagulation
  D68.2
Parakeratosis R23.4
  variegata L41.0
Paralysis, paralytic (complete) (incomplete)
  G83.9
  with
    syphilis A52.17
  abducens, abducent (nerve) —*see* Strabismus,
    paralytic, sixth nerve
  abductor, lower extremity G57.9-
  accessory nerve G52.8
  accommodation —*see also* Paresis, of
    accommodation
    hysterical F44.89
  acoustic nerve (except Deafness) —*see*
    subcategory H93.3
  agitans —*see also* Parkinsonism G20
    arteriosclerotic G21.4
  alternating (oculomotor) G83.89
  amyotrophic G12.21

Paralysis, paralytic *(Continued)*
  ankle G57.9-
  anus (sphincter) K62.89
  arm —*see* Monoplegia, upper limb
  ascending (spinal), acute G61.0
  association G12.29
  asthenic bulbar G70.00
    with exacerbation (acute) G70.01
    in crisis G70.01
  ataxic (hereditary) G11.9
    general (syphilitic) A52.17
  atrophic G58.9
    infantile, acute —*see* Poliomyelitis, paralytic
    progressive G12.22
    spinal (acute) —*see* Poliomyelitis, paralytic
  axillary G54.0
  Babinski-Nageotte's G83.89
  Bell's G51.0
    newborn P11.3
  Benedikt's G46.3
  birth injury P14.9
    spinal cord P11.5
  bladder (neurogenic) (sphincter)
      N31.2
  bowel, colon or intestine K56.0
  brachial plexus G54.0
    birth injury P14.3
    newborn (birth injury) P14.3
  brain G83.9
    diplegia G83.0
    triplegia G83.89
  bronchial J98.09
  Brown-Séquard G83.81
  bulbar (chronic) (progressive) G12.22
    infantile —*see* Poliomyelitis, paralytic
    poliomyelitic —*see* Poliomyelitis, paralytic
    pseudo G12.29
  bulbospinal G70.00
    with exacerbation (acute) G70.01
    in crisis G70.01
  cardiac —*see also* Failure, heart I50.9
  cerebrocerebellar, diplegic G80.1
  cervical
    plexus G54.2
    sympathetic G90.09
  Céstan-Chenais G46.3
  Charcot-Marie-Tooth type G60.0
  Clark's G80.9
  colon K56.0
  compressed air T70.3
  compression
    arm G56.9-
    leg G57.9-
    lower extremity G57.9-
    upper extremity G56.9-
  congenital (cerebral) —*see* Palsy, cerebral
  conjugate movement (gaze) (of eye) H51.0
    cortical (nuclear) (supranuclear) H51.0
  cordis —*see* Failure, heart
  cranial or cerebral nerve G52.9
  creeping G12.22
  crossed leg G83.89
  crutch —*see* Injury, brachial plexus
  deglutition R13.0
    hysterical F44.4
  dementia A52.17
  descending (spinal) NEC G12.29
  diaphragm (flaccid) J98.6
    due to accidental dissection of phrenic
        nerve during procedure —*see*
        Puncture, accidental complicating
        surgery
  digestive organs NEC K59.8
  diplegic —*see* Diplegia
  divergence (nuclear) H51.8
  diver's T70.3
  Duchenne's
    birth injury P14.0
    due to or associated with
        motor neuron disease G12.22
        muscular dystrophy G71.0

Paralysis, paralytic *(Continued)*
  due to intracranial or spinal birth injury —*see*
      Palsy, cerebral
  embolic (current episode) I63.4- ◀▥
  Erb (-Duchenne) (birth) (newborn) P14.0
  Erb's syphilitic spastic spinal A52.17
  esophagus K22.8
  eye muscle (extrinsic) H49.9
    intrinsic —*see also* Paresis, of
        accommodation
  facial (nerve) G51.0
    birth injury P11.3
    congenital P11.3
    following operation NEC —*see* Puncture,
        accidental complicating surgery
    newborn (birth injury) P11.3
  familial (recurrent) (periodic) G72.3
    spastic G11.4
  fauces J39.2
  finger G56.9-
  gait R26.1
  gastric nerve (nondiabetic) G52.2
  gaze, conjugate H51.0
  general (progressive) (syphilitic) A52.17
    juvenile A50.45
  glottis J38.00
    bilateral J38.02
    unilateral J38.01
  gluteal G54.1
  Gubler (-Millard) G46.3
  hand —*see* Monoplegia, upper limb
  heart —*see* Arrest, cardiac
  hemiplegic —*see* Hemiplegia
  hyperkalemic periodic (familial) G72.3
  hypoglossal (nerve) G52.3
  hypokalemic periodic G72.3
  hysterical F44.4
  ileus K56.0
  infantile —*see also* Poliomyelitis, paralytic
      A80.30
    bulbar —*see* Poliomyelitis, paralytic
    cerebral —*see* Palsy, cerebral
    spastic —*see* Palsy, cerebral, spastic
  infective —*see* Poliomyelitis, paralytic
  inferior nuclear G83.9
  internuclear —*see* Ophthalmoplegia,
      internuclear
  intestine K56.0
  iris H57.09
    due to diphtheria (toxin) A36.89
  ischemic, Volkmann's (complicating trauma)
      T79.6
  Jackson's G83.89
  jake —*see* Poisoning, food, noxious, plant
  Jamaica ginger (jake) G62.2
  juvenile general A50.45
  Klumpke (-Déjérine) (birth) (newborn) P14.1
  labioglossal (laryngeal) (pharyngeal) G12.29
  Landry's G61.0
  laryngeal nerve (recurrent) (superior)
        (unilateral) J38.00
    bilateral J38.02
    unilateral J38.01
  larynx J38.00
    bilateral J38.02
    due to diphtheria (toxin) A36.2
    unilateral J38.01
  lateral G12.21
  lead —*see* subcategory T56.0
  left side —*see* Hemiplegia
  leg G83.1-
    both —*see* Paraplegia
    crossed G83.89
    hysterical F44.4
    psychogenic F44.4
    transient or transitory R29.818
    traumatic NEC —*see* Injury, nerve, leg
  levator palpebrae superioris —*see*
      Blepharoptosis, paralytic
  limb —*see* Monoplegia
  lip K13.0

Paralysis, paralytic *(Continued)*
  Lissauer's A52.17
  lower limb —*see* Monoplegia, lower
      limb
    both —*see* Paraplegia
  lung J98.4
  median nerve G56.1-
  medullary (tegmental) G83.89
  mesencephalic NEC G83.89
    tegmental G83.89
  middle alternating G83.89
  Millard-Gubler-Foville G46.3
  monoplegic —*see* Monoplegia
  motor G83.9
  muscle, muscular NEC G72.89
    due to nerve lesion G58.9
    eye (extrinsic) H49.9
      intrinsic —*see* Paresis, of
          accommodation
      oblique —*see* Strabismus, paralytic,
          fourth nerve
    iris sphincter H21.9
    ischemic (Volkmann's) (complicating
        trauma) T79.6
    progressive G12.21
    pseudohypertrophic G71.0
  musculocutaneous nerve G56.9-
  musculospiral G56.9-
  nerve —*see also* Disorder, nerve
    abducent —*see* Strabismus, paralytic, sixth
        nerve
    accessory G52.8
    auditory (except Deafness) —*see*
        subcategory H93.3
    birth injury P14.9
    cranial or cerebral G52.9
    facial G51.0
      birth injury P11.3
      congenital P11.3
      newborn (birth injury) P11.3
    fourth or trochlear —*see* Strabismus,
        paralytic, fourth nerve
    newborn (birth injury) P14.9
    oculomotor —*see* Strabismus, paralytic,
        third nerve
    phrenic (birth injury) P14.2
    radial G56.3-
    seventh or facial G51.0
      newborn (birth injury) P11.3
    sixth or abducent —*see* Strabismus,
        paralytic, sixth nerve
    syphilitic A52.15
    third or oculomotor —*see* Strabismus,
        paralytic, third nerve
    trigeminal G50.9
    trochlear —*see* Strabismus, paralytic,
        fourth nerve
    ulnar G56.2-
  normokalemic periodic G72.3
  ocular H49.9
    alternating G83.89
  oculofacial, congenital (Moebius) Q87.0
  oculomotor (external bilateral) (nerve) —*see*
      Strabismus, paralytic, third nerve
  palate (soft) K13.79
  paratrigeminal G50.9
  periodic (familial) (hyperkalemic)
      (hypokalemic) (myotonic)
      (normokalemic) (potassium sensitive)
      (secondary) G72.3
  peripheral autonomic nervous system —*see*
      Neuropathy, peripheral, autonomic
  peroneal (nerve) G57.3-
  pharynx J39.2
  phrenic nerve G56.8-
  plantar nerve (s) G57.6-
  pneumogastric nerve G52.2
  poliomyelitis (current) —*see* Poliomyelitis,
      paralytic
  popliteal nerve G57.3-
  postepileptic transitory G83.84

◀ New   ◀▥ Revised   ~~deleted~~ Deleted

Paralysis, paralytic (Continued)
  progressive (atrophic) (bulbar) (spinal)
      G12.22
    general A52.17
    infantile acute —see Poliomyelitis, paralytic
    supranuclear G23.1
  pseudobulbar G12.29
  pseudohypertrophic (muscle) G71.0
  psychogenic F44.4
  quadriceps G57.9-
  quadriplegic —see Tetraplegia
  radial nerve G56.3-
  rectus muscle (eye) H49.9
  recurrent isolated sleep G47.53
  respiratory (muscle) (system) (tract) R06.81
    center NEC G93.89
    congenital P28.89
    newborn P28.89
  right side —see Hemiplegia
  saturnine —see subcategory T56.0
  sciatic nerve G57.0-
  senile G83.9
  shaking —see Parkinsonism
  shoulder G56.9-
  sleep, recurrent isolated G47.53
  spastic G83.9
    cerebral —see Palsy, cerebral, spastic
    congenital (cerebral) —see Palsy, cerebral,
        spastic
    familial G11.4
    hereditary G11.4
    quadriplegic G80.0
    syphilitic (spinal) A52.17
  sphincter, bladder —see Paralysis, bladder
  spinal (cord) G83.9
    accessory nerve G52.8
    acute —see Poliomyelitis, paralytic
    ascending acute G61.0
    atrophic (acute) —see also Poliomyelitis,
        paralytic
      spastic, syphilitic A52.17
    congenital NEC —see Palsy, cerebral
    hereditary G95.89
    infantile —see Poliomyelitis, paralytic
    progressive G12.21
    sequelae NEC G83.89
  sternomastoid G52.8
  stomach K31.84
    diabetic —see Diabetes, by type, with
        gastroparesis
    nerve G52.2
      diabetic —see Diabetes, by type, with
          gastroparesis
  stroke —see Infarct, brain
  subcapsularis G56.8-
  supranuclear (progressive) G23.1
  sympathetic G90.8
    cervical G90.09
    nervous system —see Neuropathy,
        peripheral, autonomic
  syndrome G83.9
    specified NEC G83.89
  syphilitic spastic spinal (Erb's) A52.17
  thigh G57.9-
  throat J39.2
    diphtheritic A36.0
    muscle J39.2
  thrombotic (current episode) I63.3- ◀▥
  thumb G56.9-
  tick —see Toxicity, venom, arthropod,
      specified NEC
  Todd's (postepileptic transitory paralysis)
      G83.84
  toe G57.6-
  tongue K14.8
  transient R29.5
    arm or leg NEC R29.818
    traumatic NEC —see Injury, nerve
  trapezius G52.8
  traumatic, transient NEC —see Injury,
      nerve

Paralysis, paralytic (Continued)
  trembling —see Parkinsonism
  triceps brachii G56.9-
  trigeminal nerve G50.9
  trochlear (nerve) —see Strabismus, paralytic,
      fourth nerve
  ulnar nerve G56.2-
  upper limb —see Monoplegia, upper limb
  uremic N18.9 [G99.8]
  uveoparotitic D86.89
  uvula K13.79
    postdiphtheritic A36.0
  vagus nerve G52.2
  vasomotor NEC G90.8
  velum palati K13.79
  vesical —see Paralysis, bladder
  vestibular nerve (except Vertigo) —see
      subcategory H93.3
  vocal cords J38.00
    bilateral J38.02
    unilateral J38.01
  Volkmann's (complicating trauma)
      T79.6
  wasting G12.29
  Weber's G46.3
  wrist G56.9-
Paramedial urethrovesical orifice
    Q64.79
Paramenia N92.6
Parametritis —see also Disease, pelvis,
    inflammatory N73.2
  acute N73.0
  complicating abortion —see Abortion, by
      type, complicated by, parametritis
Parametrium, parametric —see condition
Paramnesia —see Amnesia
Paramolar K00.1
Paramyloidosis E85.8
Paramyoclonus multiplex G25.3
Paramyotonia (congenita) G71.19
Parangi —see Yaws
Paranoia (querulans) F22
  senile F03
Paranoid
  dementia (senile) F03
    praecox —see Schizophrenia
  personality F60.0
  psychosis (climacteric) (involutional)
      (menopausal) F22
    psychogenic (acute) F23
    senile F03
  reaction (acute) F23
    chronic F22
  schizophrenia F20.0
  state (climacteric) (involutional)
      (menopausal) (simple) F22
    senile F03
  tendencies F60.0
  traits F60.0
  trends F60.0
  type, psychopathic personality F60.0
Paraparesis —see Paraplegia
Paraphasia R47.02
Paraphilia F65.9
Paraphimosis (congenital) N47.2
  chancroidal A57
Paraphrenia, paraphrenic (late) F22
  schizophrenia F20.0
Paraplegia (lower) G82.20
  ataxic —see Degeneration, combined, spinal
      cord
  complete G82.21
  congenital (cerebral) G80.8
    spastic G80.1
  familial spastic G11.4
  functional (hysterical) F44.4
  hereditary, spastic G11.4
  hysterical F44.4
  incomplete G82.22
  Pott's A18.01
  psychogenic F44.4

Paraplegia (Continued)
  spastic
    Erb's spinal, syphilitic A52.17
    hereditary G11.4
    tropical G04.1
  syphilitic (spastic) A52.17
  tropical spastic G04.1
Parapoxvirus B08.60
  specified NEC B08.69
Paraproteinemia D89.2
  benign (familial) D89.2
  monoclonal D47.2
  secondary to malignant disease D47.2
Parapsoriasis L41.9
  en plaques L41.4
  guttata L41.1
  large plaque L41.4
  retiform, retiformis L41.5
  small plaque L41.3
  specified NEC L41.8
  varioliformis (acuta) L41.0
Parasitic —see also condition
  disease NEC B89
  stomatitis B37.0
  sycosis (beard) (scalp) B35.0
  twin Q89.4
Parasitism B89
  intestinal B82.9
  skin B88.9
  specified —see Infestation
Parasitophobia F40.218
Parasomnia G47.50
  due to
    alcohol
      abuse F10.182
      dependence F10.282
      use F10.982
    amphetamines
      abuse F15.182
      dependence F15.282
      use F15.982
    caffeine
      abuse F15.182
      dependence F15.282
      use F15.982
    cocaine
      abuse F14.182
      dependence F14.282
      use F14.982
    drug NEC
      abuse F19.182
      dependence F19.282
      use F19.982
    opioid
      abuse F11.182
      dependence F11.282
      use F11.982
    psychoactive substance NEC
      abuse F19.182
      dependence F19.282
      use F19.982
    sedative, hypnotic, or anxiolytic
      abuse F13.182
      dependence F13.282
      use F13.982
    stimulant NEC
      abuse F15.182
      dependence F15.282
      use F15.982
  in conditions classified elsewhere G47.54
  nonorganic origin F51.8
  organic G47.50
  specified NEC G47.59
Paraspadias Q54.9
Paraspasmus facialis G51.8
Parasuicide (attempt)
  history of (personal) Z91.5
    in family Z81.8
Parathyroid gland —see condition
Parathyroid tetany E20.9
Paratrachoma A74.0

Paratyphilitis —see Appendicitis
Paratyphoid (fever) —see Fever, paratyphoid
Paratyphus —see Fever, paratyphoid
Paraurethral duct Q64.79
    nonorganic origin F51.5
Paraurethritis —see also Urethritis
    gonococcal (acute) (chronic) (with abscess)
        A54.1
Paravaccinia NEC B08.04
Paravaginitis —see Vaginitis
Parencephalitis —see also Encephalitis
    sequelae G09
Parent-child conflict —see Conflict, parent-child
    estrangement NEC Z62.890
Paresis —see also Paralysis
    accommodation —see Paresis, of
        accommodation
    Bernhardt's G57.1-
    bladder (sphincter) —see also Paralysis, bladder
        tabetic A52.17
    bowel, colon or intestine K56.0
    extrinsic muscle, eye H49.9
    general (progressive) (syphilitic) A52.17
        juvenile A50.45
    heart —see Failure, heart
    insane (syphilitic) A52.17
    juvenile (general) A50.45
    of accommodation H52.52-
    peripheral progressive (idiopathic) G60.3
    pseudohypertrophic G71.0
    senile G83.9
    syphilitic (general) A52.17
        congenital A50.45
    vesical NEC N31.2
Paresthesia —see also Disturbance, sensation
    Bernhardt G57.1-
Paretic —see condition
Parinaud's
    conjunctivitis H10.89
    oculoglandular syndrome H10.89
    ophthalmoplegia H49.88
Parkinsonism (idiopathic) (primary) G20
    with neurogenic orthostatic hypotension
        (symptomatic) G90.3
    arteriosclerotic G21.4
    dementia G31.83 [F02.80]
        with behavioral disturbance G31.83
            [F02.81]
    due to
        drugs NEC G21.19
            neuroleptic G21.11
        neuroleptic induced G21.11
    postencephalitic G21.3
    secondary G21.9
        due to
            arteriosclerosis G21.4
            drugs NEC G21.19
                neuroleptic G21.11
            encephalitis G21.3
            external agents NEC G21.2
            syphilis A52.19
        specified NEC G21.8
    syphilitic A52.19
    treatment-induced NEC G21.19
    vascular G21.4
Parkinson's disease, syndrome or tremor —see
    Parkinsonism
Parodontitis —see Periodontitis
Parodontosis K05.4
Paronychia —see also Cellulitis, digit
    with lymphangitis —see Lymphangitis, acute,
        digit
    candidal (chronic) B37.2
    tuberculous (primary) A18.4
Parorexia (psychogenic) F50.89
Parosmia R43.1
    psychogenic F45.8
Parotid gland —see condition
Parotitis, parotiditis (allergic) (nonspecific
    toxic) (purulent) (septic) (suppurative) —
    see also Sialoadenitis

Parotitis, parotiditis (Continued)
    epidemic —see Mumps
    infectious —see Mumps
    postoperative K91.89
    surgical K91.89
Parrot fever A70
Parrot's disease (early congenital syphilitic
    pseudoparalysis) A50.02
Parry-Romberg syndrome G51.8
Parry's disease or syndrome E05.00
    with thyroid storm E05.01
Pars planitis —see Cyclitis
Parsonage (-Aldren)-Turner syndrome G54.5
Parson's disease (exophthalmic goiter) E05.00
    with thyroid storm E05.01
Particolored infant Q82.8
Parturition —see Delivery
Parulis K04.7
    with sinus K04.6
Parvovirus, as cause of disease classified
    elsewhere B97.6
Pasini and Pierini's atrophoderma L90.3
Passage
    false, urethra N36.5
    meconium (newborn) during delivery
        P03.82
    of sounds or bougies —see Attention to,
        artificial, opening
Passive —see condition
    smoking Z77.22
Pasteurella septica A28.0
Pasteurellosis —see Infection, Pasteurella
PAT (paroxysmal atrial tachycardia) I47.1
Patau's syndrome —see Trisomy, 13
Patches
    mucous (syphilitic) A51.39
        congenital A50.07
    smokers' (mouth) K13.24
Patellar —see condition
Patent —see also Imperfect, closure
    canal of Nuck Q52.4
    cervix N88.3
    ductus arteriosus or Botallo's Q25.0
    foramen
        botalli Q21.1
        ovale Q21.1
    interauricular septum Q21.1
    interventricular septum Q21.0
    omphalomesenteric duct Q43.0
    os (uteri) —see Patent, cervix
    ostium secundum Q21.1
    urachus Q64.4
    vitelline duct Q43.0
Paterson (-Brown)(-Kelly) syndrome or web
    D50.1
Pathologic, pathological —see also condition
    asphyxia R09.01
    fire-setting F63.1
    gambling F63.0
    ovum O02.0
    resorption, tooth K03.3
    stealing F63.2
Pathology (of) —see Disease
    periradicular, associated with previous
        endodontic treatment NEC M27.59
Pattern, sleep-wake, irregular G47.23
Patulous —see also Imperfect, closure
    (congenital)
    alimentary tract Q45.8
        lower Q43.8
        upper Q40.8
    eustachian tube H69.0-
Pause, sinoatrial I49.5
Paxton's disease B36.2
Pearl (s)
    enamel K00.2
    Epstein's K09.8
Pearl-worker's disease —see Osteomyelitis,
    specified type NEC
Pectenosis K62.4
Pectoral —see condition

Pectus
    carinatum (congenital) Q67.7
        acquired M95.4
        rachitic sequelae (late effect) E64.3
    excavatum (congenital) Q67.6
        acquired M95.4
        rachitic sequelae (late effect) E64.3
    recurvatum (congenital) Q67.6
Pedatrophia E41
Pederosis F65.4
Pediculosis (infestation) B85.2
    capitis (head-louse) (any site) B85.0
    corporis (body-louse) (any site) B85.1
    eyelid B85.0
    mixed (classifiable to more than one of the
        titles B85.0-B85.3) B85.4
    pubis (pubic louse) (any site) B85.3
    vestimenti B85.1
    vulvae B85.3
Pediculus (infestation) —see Pediculosis
Pedophilia F65.4
Peg-shaped teeth K00.2
Pelade —see Alopecia, areata
Pelger-Huët anomaly or syndrome D72.0
Peliosis (rheumatica) D69.0
    hepatis K76.4
        with toxic liver disease K71.8
Pelizaeus-Merzbacher disease E75.29
Pellagra (alcoholic) (with polyneuropathy) E52
Pellagra-cerebellar-ataxia-renal aminoaciduria
    syndrome E72.02
Pellegrini (-Stieda) disease or syndrome —see
    Bursitis, tibial collateral
Pellizzi's syndrome E34.8
Pel's crisis A52.11
Pelvic —see also condition
    examination (periodic) (routine) Z01.419
        with abnormal findings Z01.411
    kidney, congenital Q63.2
Pelviolithiasis —see Calculus, kidney
Pelviperitonitis —see also Peritonitis, pelvic
    gonococcal A54.24
    puerperal O85
Pelvis —see condition or type
Pemphigoid L12.9
    benign, mucous membrane L12.1
    bullous L12.0
    cicatricial L12.1
    juvenile L12.2
    ocular L12.1
    specified NEC L12.8
Pemphigus L10.9
    benign familial (chronic) Q82.8
    Brazilian L10.3
    circinatus L13.0
    conjunctiva L12.1
    drug-induced L10.5
    erythematosus L10.4
    foliaceous L10.2
    gangrenous —see Gangrene
    neonatorum L01.03
    ocular L12.1
    paraneoplastic L10.81
    specified NEC L10.89
    syphilitic (congenital) A50.06
    vegetans L10.1
    vulgaris L10.0
    wildfire L10.3
Pendred's syndrome E07.1
Pendulous
    abdomen, in pregnancy —see Pregnancy,
        complicated by, abnormal, pelvic organs
        or tissues NEC
    breast N64.89
Penetrating wound —see also Puncture
    with internal injury —see Injury, by site
    eyeball —see Puncture, eyeball
    orbit (with or without foreign body) —see
        Puncture, orbit
    uterus by instrument with or following
        ectopic or molar pregnancy O08.6

◀ New   ◀▮▮ Revised   ~~deleted~~ Deleted

Penicillosis B48.4
Penis —see condition
Penitis N48.29
Pentalogy of Fallot Q21.8
Pentasomy X syndrome Q97.1
Pentosuria (essential) E74.8
Percreta placenta O43.23-
Peregrinating patient —see Disorder, factitious
Perforation, perforated (nontraumatic) (of)
  accidental during procedure (blood vessel)
    (nerve) (organ) —see Complication,
    accidental puncture or laceration
  antrum —see Sinusitis, maxillary
  appendix K35.2
    with localized peritonitis K35.3 ◀
  atrial septum, multiple Q21.1
  attic, ear —see Perforation, tympanum, attic
  bile duct (common) (hepatic) K83.2
    cystic K82.2
  bladder (urinary)
    with or following ectopic or molar
      pregnancy O08.6
    obstetrical trauma O71.5
    traumatic S37.29
    at delivery O71.5
  bowel K63.1
    with or following ectopic or molar
      pregnancy O08.6
    newborn P78.0
    obstetrical trauma O71.5
    traumatic —see Laceration, intestine
  broad ligament N83.8
    with or following ectopic or molar
      pregnancy O08.6
    obstetrical trauma O71.6
  by
    device, implant or graft —see also
      Complications, by site and type,
      mechanical T85.628
      arterial graft NEC —see Complication,
        cardiovascular device, mechanical,
        vascular
      breast (implant) T85.49
      catheter NEC T85.698
        cystostomy T83.090
        dialysis (renal) T82.49
          intraperitoneal T85.691
        infusion NEC T82.594
          spinal (epidural) (subdural) T85.690
        urinary —see also Complications,
          catheter, urinary T83.098 ◀
      electronic (electrode) (pulse generator)
        (stimulator)
        bone T84.390
        cardiac T82.199
          electrode T82.190
          pulse generator T82.191
          specified type NEC T82.198
        nervous system —see Complication,
          prosthetic device, mechanical,
          electronic nervous system
          stimulator
        urinary —see Complication,
          genitourinary, device, urinary,
          mechanical
      fixation, internal (orthopedic) NEC —see
        Complication, fixation device,
        mechanical
      gastrointestinal —see Complications,
        prosthetic device, mechanical,
        gastrointestinal device
      genital NEC T83.498
        intrauterine contraceptive device
          T83.39
        penile prosthesis T83.490
      heart NEC —see Complication,
        cardiovascular device,
        mechanical
      joint prosthesis —see Complications,
        joint prosthesis, mechanical,
        specified NEC, by site

Perforation, perforated (Continued)
  by (Continued)
    urinary (Continued)
      ocular NEC —see Complications,
        prosthetic device, mechanical,
        ocular device
      orthopedic NEC —see Complication,
        orthopedic, device, mechanical
      specified NEC T85.628
      urinary NEC —see also Complication,
        genitourinary, device, urinary,
        mechanical
        graft T83.29
        urinary, indwelling T83.098
      vascular NEC —see Complication,
        cardiovascular device, mechanical
      ventricular intracranial shunt T85.09
    foreign body left accidentally in
      operative wound T81.539
    instrument (any) during a procedure,
      accidental —see Puncture, accidental
      complicating surgery
  cecum K35.2
    with localized peritonitis K35.3 ◀
  cervix (uteri) N88.8
    with or following ectopic or molar
      pregnancy O08.6
    obstetrical trauma O71.3
  colon K63.1
    newborn P78.0
    obstetrical trauma O71.5
    traumatic —see Laceration, intestine, large
  common duct (bile) K83.2
  cornea (due to ulceration) —see Ulcer,
    cornea, perforated
  cystic duct K82.2
  diverticulum (intestine) K57.80
    with bleeding K57.81
    large intestine K57.20
      with
        bleeding K57.21
        small intestine K57.40
          with bleeding K57.41
    small intestine K57.00
      with
        bleeding K57.01
        large intestine K57.40
          with bleeding K57.41
  ear drum —see Perforation, tympanum
  esophagus K22.3
  ethmoidal sinus —see Sinusitis, ethmoidal
  frontal sinus —see Sinusitis, frontal
  gallbladder K82.2
  heart valve —see Endocarditis
  ileum K63.1
    newborn P78.0
    obstetrical trauma O71.5
    traumatic —see Laceration, intestine, small
  instrumental, surgical (accidental) (blood
    vessel) (nerve) (organ) —see Puncture,
    accidental complicating surgery
  intestine NEC K63.1
    with ectopic or molar pregnancy O08.6
    newborn P78.0
    obstetrical trauma O71.5
    traumatic —see Laceration, intestine
    ulcerative NEC K63.1
      newborn P78.0
  jejunum, jejunal K63.1
    obstetrical trauma O71.5
    traumatic —see Laceration, intestine, small
    ulcer —see Ulcer, gastrojejunal, with
      perforation
  joint prosthesis —see Complications, joint
    prosthesis, mechanical, specified NEC,
    by site
  mastoid (antrum) (cell) —see Disorder,
    mastoid, specified NEC
  maxillary sinus —see Sinusitis, maxillary
  membrana tympani —see Perforation,
    tympanum

Perforation, perforated (Continued)
  nasal
    septum J34.89
      congenital Q30.3
      syphilitic A52.73
    sinus J34.89
      congenital Q30.8
      due to sinusitis —see Sinusitis
  palate —see also Cleft, palate Q35.9
    syphilitic A52.79
  palatine vault —see also Cleft, palate, hard
    Q35.1
    syphilitic A52.79
      congenital A50.59
  pars flaccida (ear drum) —see Perforation,
    tympanum, attic
  pelvic
    floor S31.030
      with
        ectopic or molar pregnancy O08.6
        penetration into retroperitoneal space
          S31.031
        retained foreign body S31.040
          with penetration into
            retroperitoneal space S31.041
      following ectopic or molar pregnancy
        O08.6
      obstetrical trauma O70.1
    organ S37.99
      adrenal gland S37.818
      bladder —see Perforation, bladder
      fallopian tube S37.599
        bilateral S37.592
        unilateral S37.591
      kidney S37.09-
      obstetrical trauma O71.5
      ovary S37.499
        bilateral S37.492
        unilateral S37.491
      prostate S37.828
      specified organ NEC S37.898
      ureter —see Perforation, ureter
      urethra —see Perforation, urethra
      uterus —see Perforation, uterus
  perineum —see Laceration, perineum
  pharynx J39.2
  rectum K63.1
    newborn P78.0
    obstetrical trauma O71.5
    traumatic S36.63
  root canal space due to endodontic treatment
    M27.51
  sigmoid K63.1
    newborn P78.0
    obstetrical trauma O71.5
    traumatic S36.533
  sinus (accessory) (chronic) (nasal) J34.89
  sphenoidal sinus —see Sinusitis, sphenoidal
  surgical (accidental) (by instrument) (blood
    vessel) (nerve) (organ) —see Puncture,
    accidental complicating surgery
  traumatic
    external —see Puncture
    eye —see Puncture, eyeball
    internal organ —see Injury, by site
  tympanum, tympanic (membrane) (persistent
    post-traumatic) (postinflammatory)
    H72.9-
    attic H72.1-
      multiple —see Perforation, tympanum,
        multiple
      total —see Perforation, tympanum, total
    central H72.0-
      multiple —see Perforation, tympanum,
        multiple
      total —see Perforation, tympanum, total
    marginal NEC —see subcategory H72.2
    multiple H72.81-
    pars flaccida —see Perforation, tympanum,
      attic
    total H72.82-
    traumatic, current episode S09.2-

Perforation, perforated *(Continued)*
   typhoid, gastrointestinal —*see* Typhoid
   ulcer —*see* Ulcer, by site, with perforation
   ureter N28.89
      traumatic S37.19
   urethra N36.8
      with ectopic or molar pregnancy O08.6
      following ectopic or molar pregnancy O08.6
      obstetrical trauma O71.5
      traumatic S37.39
         at delivery O71.5
   uterus
      with ectopic or molar pregnancy O08.6
      by intrauterine contraceptive device T83.39
      following ectopic or molar pregnancy O08.6
      obstetrical trauma O71.1
      traumatic S37.69
         obstetric O71.1
   uvula K13.79
      syphilitic A52.79
   vagina
      obstetrical trauma O71.4
      other trauma - see Puncture, vagina
Periadenitis mucosa necrotica recurrens K12.0
Periappendicitis (acute) —*see* Appendicitis
Periarteritis nodosa (disseminated) (infectious) (necrotizing) M30.0
Periarthritis (joint) —*see also* Enthesopathy
   Duplay's M75.0-
   gonococcal A54.42
   humeroscapularis —*see* Capsulitis, adhesive
   scapulohumeral —*see* Capsulitis, adhesive
   shoulder —*see* Capsulitis, adhesive
   wrist M77.2-
Periarthrosis (angioneural) —*see* Enthesopathy
Pericapsulitis, adhesive (shoulder) —*see* Capsulitis, adhesive
Pericarditis (with decompensation) (with effusion) I31.9
   with rheumatic fever (conditions in I00)
      active —*see* Pericarditis, rheumatic
      inactive or quiescent I09.2
   acute (hemorrhagic) (nonrheumatic) (Sicca) I30.9
      with chorea (acute) (rheumatic) (Sydenham's) I02.0
      benign I30.8
      nonspecific I30.0
      rheumatic I01.0
         with chorea (acute) (Sydenham's) I02.0
   adhesive or adherent (chronic) (external) (internal) I31.0
      acute —*see* Pericarditis, acute
      rheumatic I09.2
   bacterial (acute) (subacute) (with serous or seropurulent effusion) I30.1
   calcareous I31.1
   cholesterol (chronic) I31.8
      acute I30.9
   chronic (nonrheumatic) I31.9
      rheumatic I09.2
   constrictive (chronic) I31.1
   coxsackie B33.23
   fibrinocaseous (tuberculous) A18.84
   fibrinopurulent I30.1
   fibrinous I30.8
   fibrous I31.0
   gonococcal A54.83
   idiopathic I30.0
   in systemic lupus erythematosus M32.12
   infective I30.1
   meningococcal A39.53
   neoplastic (chronic) I31.8
      acute I30.9
   obliterans, obliterating I31.0
   plastic I31.0
   pneumococcal I30.1

Pericarditis *(Continued)*
   postinfarction I24.1
   purulent I30.1
   rheumatic (active) (acute) (with effusion) (with pneumonia) I01.0
      with chorea (acute) (rheumatic) (Sydenham's) I02.0
      chronic or inactive (with chorea) I09.2
   rheumatoid —*see* Rheumatoid, carditis
   septic I30.1
   serofibrinous I30.8
   staphylococcal I30.1
   streptococcal I30.1
   suppurative I30.1
   syphilitic A52.06
   tuberculous A18.84
   uremic N18.9 *[I32]*
   viral I30.1
Pericardium, pericardial —*see* condition
Pericellulitis —*see* Cellulitis
Pericementitis (chronic) (suppurative) —*see also* Periodontitis
   acute K05.20
      generalized —*see* Peridontitis, aggressive, generalized ◀▥
      localized —*see* Peridontitis, aggressive, localized ◀▥
Perichondritis
   auricle —*see* Perichondritis, ear
   bronchus J98.09
   ear (external) H61.00-
      acute H61.01-
      chronic H61.02-
   external auditory canal —*see* Perichondritis, ear
   larynx J38.7
      syphilitic A52.73
      typhoid A01.09
   nose J34.89
   pinna —*see* Perichondritis, ear
   trachea J39.8
Periclasia K05.4
Pericoronitis —*see* Periodontitis
Pericystitis N30.90
   with hematuria N30.91
Peridiverticulitis (intestine) K57.92
   cecum —*see* Diverticulitis, intestine, large
   colon —*see* Diverticulitis, intestine, large
   duodenum —*see* Diverticulitis, intestine, small
   intestine —*see* Diverticulitis, intestine
   jejunum —*see* Diverticulitis, intestine, small
   rectosigmoid —*see* Diverticulitis, intestine, large
   rectum —*see* Diverticulitis, intestine, large
   sigmoid —*see* Diverticulitis, intestine, large
Periendocarditis —*see* Endocarditis
Periepididymitis N45.1
Perifolliculitis L01.02
   abscedens, caput, scalp L66.3
   capitis, abscedens (et suffodiens) L66.3
   superficial pustular L01.02
Perihepatitis K65.8
Perilabyrinthitis (acute) —*see* subcategory H83.0
Perimeningitis —*see* Meningitis
Perimetritis —*see* Endometritis
Perimetrosalpingitis —*see* Salpingo-oophoritis
Perineocele N81.81
Perinephric, perinephritic —*see* condition
Perinephritis —*see also* Infection, kidney
   purulent —*see* Abscess, kidney
Perineum, perineal —*see* condition
Perineuritis NEC —*see* Neuralgia
Periodic —*see* condition
Periodontitis (chronic) (complex) (compound) (local) (simplex) K05.30
   acute K05.20
      generalized K05.229 ◀▥
         moderate K05.222 ◀
         severe K05.223 ◀
         slight K05.221 ◀

Periodontitis *(Continued)*
   acute *(Continued)*
      localized K05.219 ◀▥
         moderate K05.212 ◀
         severe K05.213 ◀
         slight K05.211 ◀
      apical K04.5
         acute (pulpal origin) K04.4
      generalized K05.329 ◀▥
         moderate K05.322 ◀
         severe K05.323 ◀
         slight K05.321 ◀
      localized K05.319 ◀▥
         moderate K05.312 ◀
         severe K05.313 ◀
         slight K05.311 ◀
Periodontoclasia K05.4
Periodontosis (juvenile) K05.4
Periods —*see also* Menstruation
   heavy N92.0
   irregular N92.6
   shortened intervals (irregular) N92.1
Perionychia —*see also* Cellulitis, digit
   with lymphangitis —*see* Lymphangitis, acute, digit
Perioophoritis —*see* Salpingo-oophoritis
Periorchitis N45.2
Periosteum, periosteal —*see* condition
Periostitis (albuminosa) (circumscribed) (diffuse) (infective) (monomelic) —*see also* Osteomyelitis
   alveolar M27.3
   alveolodental M27.3
   dental M27.3
   gonorrheal A54.43
   jaw (lower) (upper) M27.2
   orbit H05.03-
   syphilitic A52.77
      congenital (early) A50.02 *[M90.80]*
      secondary A51.46
   tuberculous —*see* Tuberculosis, bone
   yaws (hypertrophic) (early) (late) A66.6 *[M90.80]*
Periostosis (hyperplastic) —*see also* Disorder, bone, specified type NEC
   with osteomyelitis —*see* Osteomyelitis, specified type NEC
Peripartum
   cardiomyopathy O90.3
Periphlebitis —*see* Phlebitis
Periproctitis K62.89
Periprostatitis —*see* Prostatitis
Perirectal —*see* condition
Perirenal —*see* condition
Perisalpingitis —*see* Salpingo-oophoritis
Perisplenitis (infectional) D73.89
Peristalsis, visible or reversed R19.2
Peritendinitis —*see* Enthesopathy
Peritoneum, peritoneal —*see* condition
Peritonitis (adhesive) (bacterial) (fibrinous) (hemorrhagic) (idiopathic) (localized) (perforative) (primary) (with adhesions) (with effusion) K65.9
   with or following
      abscess K65.1
      appendicitis K35.3 ◀▥
         with perforation or rupture K35.2
         generalized K35.2
         localized K35.3
      diverticular disease (intestine) K57.80
         with bleeding K57.81
      ectopic or molar pregnancy O08.0
      large intestine K57.20
         with
            bleeding K57.21
            small intestine K57.40
               with bleeding K57.41
      small intestine K57.00
         with
            bleeding K57.01
            large intestine K57.40
               with bleeding K57.41

◀ New   ◀▥ Revised   ~~deleted~~ Deleted

Peritonitis (Continued)
  acute (generalized) K65.0
  aseptic T81.61
  bile, biliary K65.3
  chemical T81.61
  chlamydial A74.81
  chronic proliferative K65.8
  complicating abortion —see Abortion, by
      type, complicated by, pelvic peritonitis
  congenital P78.1
  diaphragmatic K65.0
  diffuse K65.0
  diphtheritic A36.89
  disseminated K65.0
  due to
    bile K65.3
    foreign
      body or object accidentally left during
          a procedure (instrument) (sponge)
          (swab) T81.599
      substance accidentally left during a
          procedure (chemical) (powder)
          (talc) T81.61
    talc T81.61
    urine K65.8
  eosinophilic K65.8
    acute K65.0
  fibrocaseous (tuberculous) A18.31
  fibropurulent K65.0
  following ectopic or molar pregnancy
      O08.0
  general (ized) K65.0
  gonococcal A54.85
  meconium (newborn) P78.0
  neonatal P78.1
    meconium P78.0
  pancreatic K65.0
  paroxysmal, familial E85.0
    benign E85.0
  pelvic
    female N73.5
      acute N73.3
      chronic N73.4
        with adhesions N73.6
    male K65.0
  periodic, familial E85.0
  proliferative, chronic K65.8
  puerperal, postpartum, childbirth O85
  purulent K65.0
  septic K65.0
  specified NEC K65.8
  spontaneous bacterial K65.2
  subdiaphragmatic K65.0
  subphrenic K65.0
  suppurative K65.0
  syphilitic A52.74
    congenital (early) A50.08 [K67]
  talc T81.61
  tuberculous A18.31
  urine K65.8
Peritonsillar —see condition
Peritonsillitis J36
Perityphlitis K37
Periureteritis N28.89
Periurethral —see condition
Periurethritis (gangrenous) —see Urethritis
Periuterine —see condition
Perivaginitis —see Vaginitis
Perivasculitis, retinal H35.06-
Perivasitis (chronic) N49.1
Perivesiculitis (seminal) —see Vesiculitis
Perlèche NEC K13.0
  due to
    candidiasis B37.83
    moniliasis B37.83
    riboflavin deficiency E53.0
    vitamin B2 (riboflavin) deficiency E53.0
Pernicious —see condition
Pernio, perniosis T69.1
Perpetrator (of abuse) —see Index to External
    Causes of Injury, Perpetrator

Persecution
  delusion F22
  social Z60.5
Perseveration (tonic) R48.8
Persistence, persistent (congenital)
  anal membrane Q42.3
    with fistula Q42.2
  arteria stapedia Q16.3
  atrioventricular canal Q21.2
  branchial cleft Q18.0
  bulbus cordis in left ventricle Q21.8
  canal of Cloquet Q14.0
  capsule (opaque) Q12.8
  cilioretinal artery or vein Q14.8
  cloaca Q43.7
  communication —see Fistula, congenital
  convolutions
    aortic arch Q25.46 ◀▥
    fallopian tube Q50.6
    oviduct Q50.6
    uterine tube Q50.6
  double aortic arch Q25.45 ◀▥
  ductus arteriosus (Botalli) Q25.0
  fetal
    circulation P29.3
    form of cervix (uteri) Q51.828
    hemoglobin, hereditary (HPFH) D56.4
  foramen
    Botalli Q21.1
    ovale Q21.1
  Gartner's duct Q52.4
  hemoglobin, fetal (hereditary) (HPFH)
      D56.4
  hyaloid
    artery (generally incomplete) Q14.0
    system Q14.8
  hymen, in pregnancy or childbirth —see
      Pregnancy, complicated by, abnormal,
      vulva
  lanugo Q84.2
  left
    posterior cardinal vein Q26.8
    root with right arch of aorta Q25.49 ◀▥
    superior vena cava Q26.1
  Meckel's diverticulum Q43.0
    malignant —see Table of Neoplasms, small
        intestine, malignant
  mucosal disease (middle ear) —see
      Otitis, media, suppurative, chronic,
      tubotympanic
  nail (s), anomalous Q84.6
  omphalomesenteric duct Q43.0
  organ or site not listed —see Anomaly, by site
  ostium
    atrioventriculare commune Q21.2
    primum Q21.2
    secundum Q21.1
  ovarian rests in fallopian tube Q50.6
  pancreatic tissue in intestinal tract Q43.8
  primary (deciduous)
    teeth K00.6
    vitreous hyperplasia Q14.0
  pupillary membrane Q13.89
  rhesus (Rh)titer —see Complication (s),
      transfusion, incompatibility reaction,
      Rh (factor)
  right aortic arch Q25.47 ◀▥
  sinus
    urogenitalis
      female Q52.8
      male Q55.8
    venosus with imperfect incorporation in
        right auricle Q26.8
  thymus (gland) (hyperplasia) E32.0
  thyroglossal duct Q89.2
  thyrolingual duct Q89.2
  truncus arteriosus or communis Q20.0
  tunica vasculosa lentis Q12.2
  umbilical sinus Q64.4
  urachus Q64.4
  vitelline duct Q43.0

Person (with)
  admitted for clinical research, as a control
      subject (normal comparison)
      (participant) Z00.6
  awaiting admission to adequate facility
      elsewhere Z75.1
  concern (normal) about sick person in family
      Z63.6
  consulting on behalf of another Z71.0
  feigning illness Z76.5
  living (in)
    without
      adequate housing (heating) (space)
          Z59.1
      housing (permanent) (temporary)
          Z59.0
      person able to render necessary care
          Z74.2
      shelter Z59.0
    alone Z60.2
    boarding school Z59.3
    residential institution Z59.3
  on waiting list Z75.1
  sick or handicapped in family Z63.6
Personality (disorder) F60.9
  accentuation of traits (type A pattern) Z73.1
  affective F34.0
  aggressive F60.3
  amoral F60.2
  anacastic, anankastic F60.5
  antisocial F60.2
  anxious F60.6
  asocial F60.2
  asthenic F60.7
  avoidant F60.6
  borderline F60.3
  change due to organic condition (enduring)
      F07.0
  compulsive F60.5
  cycloid F34.0
  cyclothymic F34.0
  dependent F60.7
  depressive F34.1
  dissocial F60.2
  dual F44.81
  eccentric F60.89
  emotionally unstable F60.3
  expansive paranoid F60.0
  explosive F60.3
  fanatic F60.0
  haltlose type F60.89
  histrionic F60.4
  hyperthymic F34.0
  hypothymic F34.1
  hysterical F60.4
  immature F60.89
  inadequate F60.7
  labile (emotional) F60.3
  mixed (nonspecific) F60.89 ◀▥
  morally defective F60.2
  multiple F44.81
  narcissistic F60.81
  obsessional F60.5
  obsessive (-compulsive) F60.5
  organic F07.0
  overconscientious F60.5
  paranoid F60.0
  passive (-dependent) F60.7
  passive-aggressive F60.89
  pathologic F60.9
  pattern defect or disturbance F60.9
  pseudopsychopathic (organic) F07.0
  pseudoretarded (organic) F07.0
  psychoinfantile F60.4
  psychoneurotic NEC F60.89
  psychopathic F60.2
  querulant F60.0
  sadistic F60.89
  schizoid F60.1
  self-defeating F60.7
  sensitive paranoid F60.0

Personality *(Continued)*
  sociopathic (amoral) (antisocial) (asocial)
    (dissocial) F60.2
  specified NEC F60.89
  type A Z73.1
  unstable (emotional) F60.3
Perthes' disease —*see* Legg-Calvé-Perthes
  disease
Pertussis *(see also* Whooping cough) A37.90
Perversion, perverted
  appetite F50.89 ◄▥
    psychogenic F50.89 ◄▥
  function
    pituitary gland E23.2
      posterior lobe E22.2
  sense of smell and taste R43.8
    psychogenic F45.8
  sexual —*see* Deviation, sexual
Pervious, congenital —*see also* Imperfect,
  closure
  ductus arteriosus Q25.0
Pes (congenital) —*see also* Talipes
  acquired —*see also* Deformity, limb, foot,
    specified NEC
    planus —*see* Deformity, limb, flat foot
  adductus Q66.89
  cavus Q66.7
  deformity NEC, acquired —*see* Deformity,
    limb, foot, specified NEC
  planus (acquired) (any degree) —*see also*
    Deformity, limb, flat foot
    rachitic sequelae (late effect) E64.3
  valgus Q66.6
Pest, pestis —*see* Plague
Petechia, petechiae R23.3
  newborn P54.5
Petechial typhus A75.9
Peter's anomaly Q13.4
Petit mal seizure —*see* Epilepsy, generalized,
  specified NEC
Petit's hernia —*see* Hernia, abdomen, specified
  site NEC
Petrellidosis B48.2
Petrositis H70.20-
  acute H70.21-
  chronic H70.22-
Peutz-Jeghers disease or syndrome Q85.8
Peyronie's disease N48.6
PFAPA (periodic fever, aphthous stomatitis,
  pharyngitis, and adenopathy syndrome)
  M04.8 ◄
Pfeiffer's disease —*see* Mononucleosis,
  infectious
Phagedena (dry) (moist) (sloughing) —*see also*
  Gangrene
  geometric L88
  penis N48.29
  tropical —*see* Ulcer, skin
  vulva N76.6
Phagedenic —*see* condition
Phakoma H35.89
Phakomatosis —*see also* specific eponymous
  syndromes Q85.9
  Bourneville's Q85.1
  specified NEC Q85.8
Phantom limb syndrome (without pain)
  G54.7
  with pain G54.6
Pharyngeal pouch syndrome D82.1
Pharyngitis (acute) (catarrhal) (gangrenous)
  (infective) (malignant) (membranous)
  (phlegmonous) (pseudomembranous)
  (simple) (subacute) (suppurative)
  (ulcerative) (viral) J02.9
  with influenza, flu, or grippe —*see* Influenza,
    with, pharyngitis
  aphthous B08.5
  atrophic J31.2
  chlamydial A56.4
  chronic (atrophic) (granular) (hypertrophic)
    J31.2

Pharyngitis *(Continued)*
  coxsackievirus B08.5
  diphtheritic A36.0
  enteroviral vesicular B08.5
  follicular (chronic) J31.2
  fusospirochetal A69.1
  gonococcal A54.5
  granular (chronic) J31.2
  herpesviral B00.2
  hypertrophic J31.2
  infectional, chronic J31.2
  influenzal —*see* Influenza, with, respiratory
    manifestations NEC
  lymphonodular, acute (enteroviral) B08.8
  pneumococcal J02.8
  purulent J02.9
  putrid J02.9
  septic J02.0
  sicca J31.2
  specified organism NEC J02.8
  staphylococcal J02.8
  streptococcal J02.0
  syphilitic, congenital (early) A50.03
  tuberculous A15.8
  vesicular, enteroviral B08.5
  viral NEC J02.8
Pharyngoconjunctivitis, viral B30.2
Pharyngolaryngitis (acute) J06.0
  chronic J37.0
Pharyngoplegia J39.2
Pharyngotonsillitis, herpesviral B00.2
Pharyngotracheitis, chronic J42
Pharynx, pharyngeal —*see* condition
Phencyclidine-induced ◄
  anxiety disorder F16.980 ◄
  bipolar and related disorder F16.94 ◄
  depressive disorder F16.94 ◄
  psychotic disorder F16.959 ◄
Phenomenon
  Arthus' —*see* Arthus' phenomenon
  jaw-winking Q07.8
  lupus erythematosus (LE) cell M32.9
  Raynaud's (secondary) I73.00
    with gangrene I73.01
  vasomotor R55
  vasospastic I73.9
  vasovagal R55
  Wenckebach's I44.1
Phenylketonuria E70.1
  classical E70.0
  maternal E70.1
Pheochromoblastoma
  specified site —*see* Neoplasm, malignant, by
    site
  unspecified site C74.10
Pheochromocytoma
  malignant
    specified site —*see* Neoplasm, malignant,
      by site
    unspecified site C74.10
  specified site —*see* Neoplasm, benign, by site
  unspecified site D35.00
Pheohyphomycosis —*see* Chromomycosis
Pheomycosis —*see* Chromomycosis
Phimosis (congenital) (due to infection) N47.1
  chancroidal A57
Phlebectasia —*see also* Varix
  congenital Q27.4
Phlebitis (infective) (pyemic) (septic)
  (suppurative) I80.9
  antepartum —*see* Thrombophlebitis,
    antepartum
  blue —*see* Phlebitis, leg, deep
  breast, superficial I80.8
  cavernous (venous) sinus —*see* Phlebitis,
    intracranial (venous) sinus
  cerebral (venous) sinus —*see* Phlebitis,
    intracranial (venous) sinus
  chest wall, superficial I80.8
  cranial (venous) sinus —*see* Phlebitis,
    intracranial (venous) sinus

Phlebitis *(Continued)*
  deep (vessels) —*see* Phlebitis, leg, deep
  due to implanted device —*see* Complications,
    by site and type, specified NEC
  during or resulting from a procedure
    T81.72
  femoral vein (superficial) I80.1-
  femoropopliteal vein I80.0-
  gestational —*see* Phlebopathy, gestational
  hepatic veins I80.8
  iliofemoral —*see* Phlebitis, femoral vein
  intracranial (venous) sinus (any) G08
    nonpyogenic I67.6
  intraspinal venous sinuses and veins G08
    nonpyogenic G95.19
  lateral (venous) sinus —*see* Phlebitis,
    intracranial (venous) sinus
  leg I80.3
    antepartum —*see* Thrombophlebitis,
      antepartum
    deep (vessels) NEC I80.20-
      iliac I80.21-
      popliteal vein I80.22-
      specified vessel NEC I80.29-
      tibial vein I80.23-
    femoral vein (superficial) I80.1-
    superficial (vessels) I80.0-
  longitudinal sinus —*see* Phlebitis, intracranial
    (venous) sinus
  lower limb —*see* Phlebitis, leg
  migrans, migrating (superficial) I82.1
  pelvic
    with ectopic or molar pregnancy O08.0
    following ectopic or molar pregnancy
      O08.0
    puerperal, postpartum O87.1
  popliteal vein —*see* Phlebitis, leg, deep,
    popliteal
  portal (vein) K75.1
  postoperative T81.72
  pregnancy —*see* Thrombophlebitis,
    antepartum
  puerperal, postpartum, childbirth O87.0
    deep O87.1
    pelvic O87.1
    superficial O87.0
  retina —*see* Vasculitis, retina
  saphenous (accessory) (great) (long)
    (small) —*see* Phlebitis, leg, superficial
  sinus (meninges) —*see* Phlebitis, intracranial
    (venous) sinus
  specified site NEC I80.8
  syphilitic A52.09
  tibial vein —*see* Phlebitis, leg, deep, tibial
  ulcerative I80.9
    leg —*see* Phlebitis, leg
  umbilicus I80.8
  uterus (septic) —*see* Endometritis
  varicose (leg) (lower limb) —*see* Varix, leg,
    with, inflammation
Phlebofibrosis I87.8
Phleboliths I87.8
Phlebopathy
  gestational O22.9-
  puerperal O87.9
Phlebosclerosis I87.8
Phlebothrombosis —*see also* Thrombosis
  antepartum —*see* Thrombophlebitis,
    antepartum
  pregnancy —*see* Thrombophlebitis,
    antepartum
  puerperal —*see* Thrombophlebitis,
    puerperal
Phlebotomus fever A93.1
Phlegmasia
  alba dolens O87.1
    nonpuerperal —*see* Phlebitis, femoral
      vein
  cerulea dolens —*see* Phlebitis, leg, deep
Phlegmon —*see* Abscess
Phlegmonous —*see* condition

◄ New   ◄▥ Revised   ~~deleted~~ Deleted

Phlyctenulosis (allergic) (keratoconjunctivitis) (nontuberculous) —see also Keratoconjunctivitis
  cornea —see Keratoconjunctivitis
  tuberculous A18.52
Phobia, phobic F40.9
  animal F40.218
    spiders F40.210
  examination F40.298
  reaction F40.9
  simple F40.298
  social F40.10
    generalized F40.11
  specific (isolated) F40.298
    animal F40.218
      spiders F40.210
    blood F40.230
    injection F40.231
    injury F40.233
    men F40.290
    natural environment F40.228
      thunderstorms F40.220
    situational F40.248
      bridges F40.242
      closed in spaces F40.240
      flying F40.243
      heights F40.241
    specified focus NEC F40.298
    transfusion F40.231
    women F40.291
  specified NEC F40.8
    medical care NEC F40.232
  state F40.9
Phocas' disease —see Mastopathy, cystic
Phocomelia Q73.1
  lower limb —see Agenesis, leg, with foot present
  upper limb —see Agenesis, arm, with hand present
Phoria H50.50
Phosphate-losing tubular disorder N25.0
Phosphatemia E83.39
Phosphaturia E83.39
Photodermatitis (sun) L56.8
  chronic L57.8
  due to drug L56.8
  light other than sun L59.8
Photokeratitis H16.13-
Photophobia H53.14-
Photophthalmia —see Photokeratitis
Photopsia H53.19
Photoretinitis —see Retinopathy, solar
Photosensitivity, photosensitization (sun) skin L56.8
  light other than sun L59.8
Phrenitis —see Encephalitis
Phrynoderma (vitamin A deficiency) E50.8
Phthiriasis (pubis) B85.3
  with any infestation classifiable to B85.0-B85.2 B85.4
Phthirus infestation —see Phthiriasis
Phthisis —see also Tuberculosis
  bulbi (infectional) —see Disorder, globe, degenerated condition, atrophy
  eyeball (due to infection) —see Disorder, globe, degenerated condition, atrophy
Phycomycosis —see Zygomycosis
Physalopteriasis B81.8
Physical restraint status Z78.1
Phytobezoar T18.9
  intestine T18.3
  stomach T18.2
Pian —see Yaws
Pianoma A66.1
Pica F50.89 ◀▥
  in adults F50.89 ◀▥
  infant or child F98.3
Picking, nose F98.8
Pick-Niemann disease —see Niemann-Pick disease or syndrome

Pick's
  cerebral atrophy G31.01 [F02.80]
    with behavioral disturbance G31.01 [F02.81]
  disease or syndrome (brain) G31.01 [F02.80]
    with behavioral disturbance G31.01 [F02.81]
    brain G31.01 [F02.80] ◀
      with behavioral disturbance G31.01 [F02.81] ◀
    pericardium (pericardial pseudocirrhosis of liver) I31.1 ◀
  syndrome ◀
    brain G31.01 [F02.80] ◀
      with behavioral disturbance G31.01 [F02.81] ◀
    of heart (pericardial pseudocirrhosis of liver) I31.1 ◀
Pickwickian syndrome E66.2
Piebaldism E70.39
Piedra (beard) (scalp) B36.8
  black B36.3
  white B36.2
Pierre Robin deformity or syndrome Q87.0
Pierson's disease or osteochondrosis M91.0
Pig-bel A05.2
Pigeon
  breast or chest (acquired) M95.4
    congenital Q67.7
    rachitic sequelae (late effect) E64.3
  breeder's disease or lung J67.2
  fancier's disease or lung J67.2
  toe —see Deformity, toe, specified NEC
Pigmentation (abnormal) (anomaly) L81.9
  conjunctiva H11.13-
  cornea (anterior) H18.01-
    posterior H18.05-
    stromal H18.06-
  diminished melanin formation NEC L81.6
  iron L81.8
  lids, congenital Q82.8
  limbus corneae —see Pigmentation, cornea
  metals L81.8
  optic papilla, congenital Q14.2
  retina, congenital (grouped) (nevoid) Q14.1
  scrotum, congenital Q82.8
  tattoo L81.8
Piles —see also Hemorrhoids K64.9
Pili
  annulati or torti (congenital) Q84.1
  incarnati L73.1
Pill roller hand (intrinsic) —see Parkinsonism
Pilomatrixoma —see Neoplasm, skin, benign
  malignant —see Neoplasm, skin, malignant
Pilonidal —see condition
Pimple R23.8
PIN —see Neoplasia, intraepithelial, prostate ◀
Pinched nerve —see Neuropathy, entrapment
Pindborg tumor —see Cyst, calcifying odontogenic
Pineal body or gland —see condition
Pinealoblastoma C75.3
Pinealoma D44.5
  malignant C75.3
Pineoblastoma C75.3
Pineocytoma D44.5
Pinguecula H11.15-
Pingueculitis H10.81-
Pinhole meatus —see also Stricture, urethra N35.9
Pink
  disease —see subcategory T56.1
  eye —see Conjunctivitis, acute, mucopurulent
Pinkus' disease (lichen nitidus) L44.1
Pinpoint
  meatus —see Stricture, urethra
  os (uteri) —see Stricture, cervix
Pins and needles R20.2
Pinta A67.9
  cardiovascular lesions A67.2
  chancre (primary) A67.0

Pinta (Continued)
  erythematous plaques A67.1
  hyperchromic lesions A67.1
  hyperkeratosis A67.1
  lesions A67.9
    cardiovascular A67.2
    hyperchromic A67.1
    intermediate A67.1
    late A67.2
    mixed A67.3
    primary A67.0
    skin (achromic) (cicatricial) (dyschromic) A67.2
      hyperchromic A67.1
      mixed (achromic and hyperchromic) A67.3
  papule (primary) A67.0
  skin lesions (achromic) (cicatricial) (dyschromic) A67.2
    hyperchromic A67.1
    mixed (achromic and hyperchromic) A67.3
  vitiligo A67.2
Pintids A67.1
Pinworm (disease) (infection) (infestation) B80
Piroplasmosis B60.0
Pistol wound —see Gunshot wound
Pitchers' elbow —see Derangement, joint, specified type NEC, elbow
Pithecoid pelvis Q74.2
  with disproportion (fetopelvic) O33.0
    causing obstructed labor O65.0
Pithiatism F48.8
Pitted —see Pitting
Pitting —see also Edema R60.9
  lip R60.0
  nail L60.8
  teeth K00.4
Pituitary gland —see condition
Pituitary-snuff-taker's disease J67.8
Pityriasis (capitis) L21.0
  alba L30.5
  circinata (et maculata) L42
  furfuracea L21.0
  Hebra's L26
  lichenoides L41.0
    chronica L41.1
    et varioliformis (acuta) L41.0
  maculata (et circinata) L30.5
  nigra B36.1
  pilaris, Hebra's L44.0
  rosea L42
  rotunda L44.8
  rubra (Hebra) pilaris L44.0
  simplex L30.5
  specified type NEC L30.5
  streptogenes L30.5
  versicolor (scrotal) B36.0
Placenta, placental —see Pregnancy, complicated by (care of) (management affected by), specified condition
Placentitis O41.14-
Plagiocephaly Q67.3
Plague A20.9
  abortive A20.8
  ambulatory A20.8
  asymptomatic A20.8
  bubonic A20.0
  cellulocutaneous A20.1
  cutaneobubonic A20.1
  lymphatic gland A20.0
  meningitis A20.3
  pharyngeal A20.8
  pneumonic (primary) (secondary) A20.2
  pulmonary, pulmonic A20.2
  septicemic A20.7
  tonsillar A20.8
    septicemic A20.7
Planning, family
  contraception Z30.9
  procreation Z31.69

Plaque (s)
  artery, arterial —see Arteriosclerosis
  calcareous —see Calcification
  coronary, lipid rich I25.83
  epicardial I31.8
  erythematous, of pinta A67.1
  Hollenhorst's —see Occlusion, artery,
    retina
  lipid rich, coronary I25.83
  pleural (without asbestos) J92.9
    with asbestos J92.0
  tongue K13.29
Plasmacytoma C90.3-
  extramedullary C90.2-
  medullary C90.0-
  solitary C90.3-
Plasmacytopenia D72.818
Plasmacytosis D72.822
Plaster ulcer —see Ulcer, pressure, by site
Plateau iris syndrome (post-iridectomy)
    (postprocedural) (without glaucoma)
    H21.82
  with glaucoma H40.22-
Platybasia Q75.8
Platyonychia (congenital) Q84.6
  acquired L60.8
Platypelloid pelvis M95.5
  with disproportion (fetopelvic) O33.0
    causing obstructed labor O65.0
  congenital Q74.2
Platyspondylisis Q76.49
Plaut (-Vincent) disease —see also Vincent's
    A69.1
Plethora R23.2
  newborn P61.1
Pleura, pleural —see condition
Pleuralgia R07.81
Pleurisy (acute) (adhesive) (chronic) (costal)
    (diaphragmatic) (double) (dry) (fibrinous)
    (fibrous) (interlobar) (latent) (plastic)
    (primary) (residual) (sicca) (sterile)
    (subacute) (unresolved) R09.1
  with
    adherent pleura J86.0
    effusion J90
      chylous, chyliform J94.0
      tuberculous (non primary)
        A15.6
        primary (progressive) A15.7
      tuberculosis —see Pleurisy, tuberculous
        (non primary)
  encysted —see Pleurisy, with effusion
  exudative —see Pleurisy, with effusion
  fibrinopurulent, fibropurulent —see
    Pyothorax
  hemorrhagic —see Hemothorax
  pneumococcal J90
  purulent —see Pyothorax
  septic —see Pyothorax
  serofibrinous —see Pleurisy, with effusion
  seropurulent —see Pyothorax
  serous —see Pleurisy, with effusion
  staphylococcal J86.9
  streptococcal J90
  suppurative —see Pyothorax
  traumatic (post) (current) —see Injury,
    intrathoracic, pleura
  tuberculous (with effusion) (non primary)
    A15.6
    primary (progressive) A15.7
Pleuritis sicca —see Pleurisy
Pleurobronchopneumonia —see Pneumonia,
    broncho
Pleurodynia R07.81
  epidemic B33.0
  viral B33.0
Pleuropericarditis —see also Pericarditis
  acute I30.9
Pleuropneumonia (acute) (bilateral) (double)
    (septic) —see also Pneumonia J18.8
  chronic —see Fibrosis, lung

Pleuro-pneumonia-like-organism (PPLO),
    as cause of disease classified elsewhere
    B96.0
Pleurorrhea —see Pleurisy, with effusion
Plexitis, brachial G54.0
Plica
  polonica B85.0
  syndrome, knee M67.5
  tonsil J35.8
Plicated tongue K14.5
Plug
  bronchus NEC J98.09
  meconium (newborn) NEC syndrome P76.0
  mucus —see Asphyxia, mucus
Plumbism —see subcategory T56.0
Plummer's disease E05.20
  with thyroid storm E05.21
Plummer-Vinson syndrome D50.1
Pluricarential syndrome of infancy E40
Plus (and minus) hand (intrinsic) —see
    Deformity, limb, specified type NEC,
    forearm
Pneumathemia —see Air, embolism
Pneumatic hammer (drill) syndrome T75.21
Pneumatocele (lung) J98.4
  intracranial G93.89
  tension J44.9
Pneumatosis
  cystoides intestinalis K63.89
  intestinalis K63.89
  peritonei K66.8
Pneumaturia R39.89
Pneumoblastoma —see Neoplasm, lung,
    malignant
Pneumocephalus G93.89
Pneumococcemia A40.3
Pneumococcus, pneumococcal —see condition
Pneumoconiosis (due to) (inhalation of) J64
  with tuberculosis (any type in A15) J65
  aluminum J63.0
  asbestos J61
  bagasse, bagassosis J67.1
  bauxite J63.1
  beryllium J63.2
  coal miners' (simple) J60
  coalworkers' (simple) J60
  collier's J60
  cotton dust J66.0
  diatomite (diatomaceous earth) J62.8
  dust
    inorganic NEC J63.6
    lime J62.8
    marble J62.8
    organic NEC J66.8
  fumes or vapors (from silo) J68.9
  graphite J63.3
  grinder's J62.8
  kaolin J62.8
  mica J62.8
  millstone maker's J62.8
  mineral fibers NEC J61
  miner's J60
  moldy hay J67.0
  potter's J62.8
  rheumatoid —see Rheumatoid, lung
  sandblaster's J62.8
  silica, silicate NEC J62.8
    with carbon J60
  stonemason's J62.8
  talc (dust) J62.0
Pneumocystis carinii pneumonia B59
Pneumocystis jiroveci (pneumonia) B59
Pneumocystosis (with pneumonia) B59
Pneumohemopericardium I31.2
Pneumohemothorax J94.2
  traumatic S27.2
Pneumohydropericardium —see Pericarditis
Pneumohydrothorax —see Hydrothorax
Pneumomediastinum J98.2
  congenital or perinatal P25.2
Pneumomycosis B49 [J99]

Pneumonia (acute) (double) (migratory)
    (purulent) (septic) (unresolved) J18.9
  with
    influenza —see Influenza, with, pneumonia
    lung abscess J85.1
      due to specified organism —see
        Pneumonia, in (due to)
  adenoviral J12.0
  adynamic J18.2
  alba A50.04
  allergic (eosinophilic) J82
  alveolar —see Pneumonia, lobar
  anaerobes J15.8
  anthrax A22.1
  apex, apical —see Pneumonia, lobar
  Ascaris B77.81
  aspiration J69.0
    due to
      aspiration of microorganisms
        bacterial J15.9
        viral J12.9
      food (regurgitated) J69.0
      gastric secretions J69.0
      milk (regurgitated) J69.0
      oils, essences J69.1
      solids, liquids NEC J69.8
      vomitus J69.0
    newborn P24.81
      amniotic fluid (clear) P24.11
      blood P24.21
      food (regurgitated) P24.31
      liquor (amnii) P24.11
      meconium P24.01
      milk P24.31
      mucus P24.11
      specified NEC P24.81
      stomach contents P24.31
    postprocedural J95.4
  atypical NEC J18.9
  bacillus J15.9
    specified NEC J15.8
  bacterial J15.9
    specified NEC J15.8
  Bacteroides (fragilis) (oralis)
    (melaninogenicus) J15.8
  basal, basic, basilar —see Pneumonia, by type
  bronchiolitis obliterans organized (BOOP)
    J84.89
  broncho-, bronchial (confluent) (croupous)
    (diffuse) (disseminated) (hemorrhagic)
    (involving lobes) (lobar) (terminal) J18.0
  allergic (eosinophilic) J82
  aspiration —see Pneumonia, aspiration
  bacterial J15.9
    specified NEC J15.8
  chronic —see Fibrosis, lung
  diplococcal J13
  Eaton's agent J15.7
  Escherichia coli (E. coli) J15.5
  Friedländer's bacillus J15.0
  Hemophilus influenzae J14
  hypostatic J18.2
  inhalation (see also Pneumonia, aspiration
    due to fumes or vapors (chemical) J68.0
    of oils or essences J69.1
  Klebsiella (pneumoniae) J15.0
  lipid, lipoid J69.1
    endogenous J84.89
  Mycoplasma (pneumoniae) J15.7
  pleuro-pneumonia-like-organisms (PPLO)
    J15.7
  pneumococcal J13
  Proteus J15.6
  Pseudomonas J15.1
  Serratia marcescens J15.6
  specified organism NEC J16.8
  staphylococcal —see Pneumonia,
    staphylococcal
  streptococcal NEC J15.4
    group B J15.3
    pneumoniae J13
  viral, virus —see Pneumonia, viral

◄ New   ◄∥ Revised   ~~deleted~~ Deleted

Pneumonia *(Continued)*
  Butyrivibrio (fibriosolvens) J15.8
  Candida B37.1
  caseous —*see* Tuberculosis, pulmonary
  catarrhal —*see* Pneumonia, broncho
  chlamydial J16.0
    congenital P23.1
  cholesterol J84.89
  cirrhotic (chronic) —*see* Fibrosis, lung
  Clostridium (haemolyticum) (novyi) J15.8
  confluent —*see* Pneumonia, broncho
  congenital (infective) P23.9
    due to
      bacterium NEC P23.6
      Chlamydia P23.1
      Escherichia coli P23.4
      Haemophilus influenzae P23.6
      infective organism NEC P23.8
      Klebsiella pneumoniae P23.6
      Mycoplasma P23.6
      Pseudomonas P23.5
      Staphylococcus P23.2
      Streptococcus (except group B) P23.6
        group B P23.3
      viral agent P23.0
      specified NEC P23.8
  croupous —*see* Pneumonia, lobar
  cryptogenic organizing J84.116
  cytomegalic inclusion B25.0
  cytomegaloviral B25.0
  deglutition —*see* Pneumonia, aspiration
  desquamative interstitial J84.117
  diffuse —*see* Pneumonia, broncho
  diplococcal, diplococcus (broncho-) (lobar)
    J13
  disseminated (focal) —*see* Pneumonia,
    broncho
  Eaton's agent J15.7
  embolic, embolism —*see* Embolism,
    pulmonary
  Enterobacter J15.6
  eosinophilic J82
  Escherichia coli (E. coli) J15.5
  Eubacterium J15.8
  fibrinous —*see* Pneumonia, lobar
  fibroid, fibrous (chronic) —*see* Fibrosis, lung
  Friedländer's bacillus J15.0
  Fusobacterium (nucleatum) J15.8
  gangrenous J85.0
  giant cell (measles) B05.2
  gonococcal A54.84
  gram-negative bacteria NEC J15.6
    anaerobic J15.8
  Hemophilus influenzae (broncho) (lobar) J14
  human metapneumovirus J12.3
  hypostatic (broncho) (lobar) J18.2
  in (due to)
    actinomycosis A42.0
    adenovirus J12.0
    anthrax A22.1
    ascariasis B77.81
    aspergillosis B44.9
    Bacillus anthracis A22.1
    Bacterium anitratum J15.6
    candidiasis B37.1
    chickenpox B01.2
    Chlamydia J16.0
      neonatal P23.1
    coccidioidomycosis B38.2
      acute B38.0
      chronic B38.1
    cytomegalovirus disease B25.0
    Diplococcus (pneumoniae) J13
    Eaton's agent J15.7
    Enterobacter J15.6
    Escherichia coli (E. coli) J15.5
    Friedländer's bacillus J15.0
    fumes and vapors (chemical) (inhalation)
      J68.0
    gonorrhea A54.84
    Hemophilus influenzae (H. influenzae) J14

Pneumonia *(Continued)*
  in *(Continued)*
    Herellea J15.6
    histoplasmosis B39.2
      acute B39.0
      chronic B39.1
    human metapneumovirus J12.3
    Klebsiella (pneumoniae) J15.0
    measles B05.2
    Mycoplasma (pneumoniae) J15.7
    nocardiosis, nocardiasis A43.0
    ornithosis A70
    parainfluenza virus J12.2
    pleuro-pneumonia-like-organism (PPLO)
      J15.7
    pneumococcus J13
    pneumocystosis (Pneumocystis carinii)
      (Pneumocystis jiroveci) B59
    Proteus J15.6
    Pseudomonas NEC J15.1
      pseudomallei A24.1
    psittacosis A70
    Q fever A78
    respiratory syncytial virus J12.1
    rheumatic fever I00 *[J17]*
    rubella B06.81
    Salmonella (infection) A02.22
      typhi A01.03
    schistosomiasis B65.9 *[J17]*
    Serratia marcescens J15.6
    specified
      bacterium NEC J15.8
      organism NEC J16.8
    spirochetal NEC A69.8
    Staphylococcus J15.20
      aureus (methicillin susceptible) (MSSA)
        J15.211
        methicillin resistant (MRSA)
          J15.212
      specified NEC J15.29
    Streptococcus J15.4
      group B J15.3
      pneumoniae J13
      specified NEC J15.4
    toxoplasmosis B58.3
    tularemia A21.2
    typhoid (fever) A01.03
    varicella B01.2
    virus —*see* Pneumonia, viral
    whooping cough A37.91
      due to
        Bordetella parapertussis A37.11
        Bordetella pertussis A37.01
        specified NEC A37.81
    Yersinia pestis A20.2
  inhalation of food or vomit —*see* Pneumonia,
    aspiration
  interstitial J84.9
    chronic J84.111
    desquamative J84.117
    due to
      collagen vascular disease J84.17
      known underlying cause J84.17
    idiopathic NOS J84.111
    in disease classified elsewhere J84.17
    lymphocytic (due to collagen vascular
      disease) (in diseases classified
      elsewhere) J84.17
    lymphoid J84.2
    non-specific J84.89
      due to
        collagen vascular disease J84.17
        known underlying cause J84.17
      idiopathic J84.113
      in diseases classified elsewhere J84.17
    plasma cell B59
    pseudomonas J15.1
    usual J84.112
      due to collagen vascular disease J84.17
      idiopathic J84.112
      in diseases classified elsewhere J84.17

Pneumonia *(Continued)*
  Klebsiella (pneumoniae) J15.0
  lipid, lipoid (exogenous) J69.1
    endogenous J84.89
  lobar (disseminated) (double) (interstitial)
    J18.1
    bacterial J15.9
      specified NEC J15.8
    chronic —*see* Fibrosis, lung
    Escherichia coli (E. coli) J15.5
    Friedländer's bacillus J15.0
    Hemophilus influenzae J14
    hypostatic J18.2
    Klebsiella (pneumoniae) J15.0
    pneumococcal J13
    Proteus J15.6
    Pseudomonas J15.1
    specified organism NEC J16.8
    staphylococcal —*see* Pneumonia,
      staphylococcal
    streptococcal NEC J15.4
    Streptococcus pneumoniae J13
    viral, virus —*see* Pneumonia, viral
  lobular —*see* Pneumonia, broncho
  Löffler's J82
  lymphoid interstitial J84.2
  massive —*see* Pneumonia, lobar
  meconium P24.01
  MRSA (Methicillin resistant Staphylococcus
    aureus) J15.212 ◀
  MSSA (methicillin susceptible Staphylococcus
    aureus) J15.211
  multilobar —*see* Pneumonia, by type
  Mycoplasma (pneumoniae) J15.7
  necrotic J85.0
  neonatal P23.9
    aspiration —*see* Aspiration, by substance,
      with pneumonia
  nitrogen dioxide J68.0 ◀▥
  organizing J84.89
    due to
      collagen vascular disease J84.17
      known underlying cause J84.17
    in diseases classified elsewhere
      J84.17
  orthostatic J18.2
  parainfluenza virus J12.2
  parenchymatous —*see* Fibrosis, lung
  passive J18.2
  patchy —*see* Pneumonia, broncho
  Peptococcus J15.8
  Peptostreptococcus J15.8
  plasma cell (of infants) B59
  pleurolobar —*see* Pneumonia, lobar
  pleuro-pneumonia-like organism (PPLO)
    J15.7
  pneumococcal (broncho) (lobar) J13
  Pneumocystis (carinii) (jiroveci) B59
  postinfectional NEC B99 *[J17]*
  postmeasles B05.2
  Proteus J15.6
  Pseudomonas J15.1
  psittacosis A70
  radiation J70.0
  respiratory syncytial virus J12.1
  resulting from a procedure J95.89
  rheumatic I00 *[J17]*
  Salmonella (arizonae) (cholerae-suis)
    (enteritidis) (typhimurium)
    A02.22
    typhi A01.03
    typhoid fever A01.03
  SARS-associated coronavirus J12.81
  segmented, segmental —*see* Pneumonia,
    broncho-
  Serratia marcescens J15.6
  specified NEC J18.8
    bacterium NEC J15.8
    organism NEC J16.8
    virus NEC J12.89
  spirochetal NEC A69.8

Pneumonia *(Continued)*
  staphylococcal (broncho) (lobar) J15.20
    aureus (methicillin susceptible) (MSSA)
      J15.211
      methicillin resistant (MRSA) J15.212
    specified NEC J15.29
  static, stasis J18.2
  streptococcal NEC (broncho) (lobar) J15.4
    group
      A J15.4
      B J15.3
      specified NEC J15.4
  Streptococcus pneumoniae J13
  syphilitic, congenital (early) A50.04
  traumatic (complication) (early) (secondary)
    T79.8
  tuberculous (any) —*see* Tuberculosis,
    pulmonary
  tularemic A21.2
  varicella B01.2
  Veillonella J15.8
  ventilator associated J95.851
  viral, virus (broncho) (interstitial) (lobar) J12.9
    adenoviral J12.0
    congenital P23.0
    human metapneumovirus J12.3
    parainfluenza J12.2
    respiratory syncytial J12.1
    SARS-associated coronavirus J12.81
    specified NEC J12.89
  white (congenital) A50.04
Pneumonic —*see* condition
Pneumonitis (acute) (primary) —*see also*
    Pneumonia
  air-conditioner J67.7
  allergic (due to) J67.9
    organic dust NEC J67.8
    red cedar dust J67.8
    sequoiosis J67.8
    wood dust J67.8
  aspiration J69.0
    due to
      anesthesia J95.4
        during
          labor and delivery O74.0
          pregnancy O29.01-
          puerperium O89.01
        fumes or gases J68.0
        obstetric O74.0
  chemical (due to gases, fumes or vapors)
    (inhalation) J68.0
    due to anesthesia J95.4
  cholesterol J84.89
  chronic —*see* Fibrosis, lung
  congenital rubella P35.0
  crack (cocaine) J68.0
  due to
    beryllium J68.0
    cadmium J68.0
    crack (cocaine) J68.0
    detergent J69.8
    fluorocarbon-polymer J68.0
    food, vomit (aspiration) J69.0
    fumes or vapors J68.0
    gases, fumes or vapors (inhalation) J68.0
    inhalation
      blood J69.8
      essences J69.1
      food (regurgitated), milk, vomit
        J69.0
      oils, essences J69.1
      saliva J69.0
      solids, liquids NEC J69.8
    manganese J68.0
    nitrogen dioxide J68.0
    oils, essences J69.1
    solids, liquids NEC J69.8
    toxoplasmosis (acquired) B58.3
      congenital P37.1
    vanadium J68.0
  ventilator J95.851

Pneumonitis *(Continued)*
  eosinophilic J82
  hypersensitivity J67.9
    air conditioner lung J67.7
    bagassosis J67.1
    bird fancier's lung J67.2
    farmer's lung J67.0
    maltworker's lung J67.4
    maple bark-stripper's lung J67.6
    mushroom worker's lung J67.5
    specified organic dust NEC J67.8
    suberosis J67.3
  interstitial (chronic) J84.89
    acute J84.114
    lymphoid J84.2
    non-specific J84.89
      idiopathic J84.113
  lymphoid, interstitial J84.2
  meconium P24.01
  postanesthetic J95.4
    correct substance properly administered —
      see Table of Drugs and Chemcials, by
      drug, adverse effect
    in labor and delivery O74.0
    in pregnancy O29.01-
      obstetric O74.0
    overdose or wrong substance given or taken
      (by accident) —*see* Table of Drugs and
      Chemicals, by drug, poisoning
    postpartum, puerperal O89.01
  postoperative J95.4
    obstetric O74.0
  radiation J70.0
  rubella, congenital P35.0
  ventilation (air-conditioning) J67.7
  ventilator associated J95.851
  wood-dust J67.8
Pneumonoconiosis —*see* Pneumoconiosis
Pneumoparotid K11.8
Pneumopathy NEC J98.4
  alveolar J84.09
  due to organic dust NEC J66.8
  parietoalveolar J84.09
Pneumopericarditis —*see also* Pericarditis
  acute I30.9
Pneumopericardium —*see also* Pericarditis
  congenital P25.3
  newborn P25.3
  traumatic (post) —*see* Injury, heart
Pneumophagia (psychogenic) F45.8
Pneumopleurisy, pneumopleuritis —*see also*
    Pneumonia J18.8
Pneumopyopericardium I30.1
Pneumopyothorax —*see* Pyopneumothorax
  with fistula J86.0
Pneumorrhagia —*see also* Hemorrhage, lung
  tuberculous —*see* Tuberculosis, pulmonary
Pneumothorax NOS J93.9
  acute J93.83
  chronic J93.81
  congenital P25.1
  perinatal period P25.1
  postprocedural J95.811
  specified NEC J93.83
  spontaneous NOS J93.83
    newborn P25.1
    primary J93.11
    secondary J93.12
    tension J93.0
  tense valvular, infectional J93.0
  tension (spontaneous) J93.0
  traumatic S27.0
    with hemothorax S27.2
  tuberculous —*see* Tuberculosis, pulmonary
Podagra —*see also* Gout M10.9
Podencephalus Q01.9
Poikilocytosis R71.8
Poikiloderma L81.6
  Civatte's L57.3
  congenital Q82.8
  vasculare atrophicans L94.5

Poikilodermatomyositis M33.10
  with
    myopathy M33.12
    respiratory involvement M33.11
    specified organ involvement NEC M33.19
Pointed ear (congenital) Q17.3
Poison ivy, oak, sumac or other plant
    dermatitis (allergic) (contact) L23.7
Poisoning (acute) —*see also* Table of Drugs and
    Chemicals
  algae and toxins T65.82-
  Bacillus B (aertrycke) (cholerae (suis))
    (paratyphosus) (suipestifer) A02.9
    botulinus A05.1
  bacterial toxins A05.9
  berries, noxious —*see* Poisoning, food,
    noxious, berries
  botulism A05.1
  ciguatera fish T61.0-
  Clostridium botulinum A05.1
  death-cap (Amanita phalloides) (Amanita
    verna) —*see* Poisoning, food, noxious,
    mushrooms
  drug —*see* Table of Drugs and Chemicals, by
    drug, poisoning
  epidemic, fish (noxious) —*see* Poisoning,
    seafood
    bacterial A05.9
  fava bean D55.0
  fish (noxious) T61.9-
    bacterial —*see* Intoxication, foodborne, by
      agent
    ciguatera fish —*see* Poisoning, ciguatera
      fish
    scombroid fish —*see* Poisoning, scombroid
      fish
    specified type NEC T61.77-
  food (acute) (diseased) (infected) (noxious)
    NEC T62.9-
    bacterial —*see* Intoxication, foodborne, by
      agent
    due to
      Bacillus (aertrycke) (choleraesuis)
        (paratyphosus) (suipestifer)
        A02.9
        botulinus A05.1
      Clostridium (perfringens) (Welchii)
        A05.2
      salmonella (aertrycke) (callinarum)
        (choleraesuis) (enteritidis)
        (paratyphi) (suipestifer) A02.9
        with
          gastroenteritis A02.0
          sepsis A02.1
      staphylococcus A05.0
      Vibrio
        parahaemolyticus A05.3
        vulnificus A05.5
    noxious or naturally toxic T62.9-
      berries —*see* subcategory T62.1-
      fish —*see* Poisoning, seafood
      mushrooms —*see* subcategory T62.0X-
      plants NEC —*see* subcategory T62.2X-
      seafood —*see* Poisoning, seafood
      specified NEC —*see* subcategory T62.8X-
    ichthyotoxism —*see* Poisoning, seafood
    kreotoxism, food A05.9
  latex T65.81-
  lead T56.0-
  mushroom —*see* Poisoning, food, noxious,
    mushroom
  mussels —*see also* Poisoning, shellfish
    bacterial —*see* Intoxication, foodborne, by
      agent
  nicotine (tobacco) T65.2-
  noxious foodstuffs —*see* Poisoning, food,
    noxious
  plants, noxious —*see* Poisoning, food,
    noxious, plants NEC
  ptomaine —*see* Poisoning, food
  radiation J70.0

◀ New ⫴⫴⫴ Revised ~~deleted~~ Deleted

Poisoning *(Continued)*
 Salmonella (arizonae) (cholerae-suis)
  (enteritidis) (typhimurium) A02.9
 scombroid fish T61.1-
 seafood (noxious) T61.9-
  bacterial —*see* Intoxication, foodborne, by
   agent
  fish —*see* Poisoning, fish
  shellfish —*see* Poisoning, shellfish
  specified NEC —*see* subcategory T61.8X-
 shellfish (amnesic) (azaspiracid) (diarrheic)
  (neurotoxic) (noxious) (paralytic)
  T61.78-
  bacterial —*see* Intoxication, foodborne, by
   agent
  ciguatera mollusk —*see* Poisoning,
   ciguatera fish
 specified substance NEC T65.891
 Staphylococcus, food A05.0
 tobacco (nicotine) T65.2-
 water E87.79
Poker spine —*see* Spondylitis, ankylosing
Poland syndrome Q79.8
Polioencephalitis (acute) (bulbar) A80.9
 inferior G12.22
 influenzal —*see* Influenza, with,
  encephalopathy
 superior hemorrhagic (acute) (Wernicke's)
  E51.2
 Wernicke's E51.2
Polioencephalomyelitis (acute) (anterior) A80.9
 with beriberi E51.2
Polioencephalopathy, superior hemorrhagic
  E51.2
 with
  beriberi E51.11
  pellagra E52
Poliomeningoencephalitis —*see*
  Meningoencephalitis
Poliomyelitis (acute) (anterior) (epidemic)
  A80.9
 with paralysis (bulbar) —*see* Poliomyelitis,
  paralytic
 abortive A80.4
 ascending (progressive) —*see* Poliomyelitis,
  paralytic
 bulbar (paralytic) —*see* Poliomyelitis,
  paralytic
 congenital P35.8
 nonepidemic A80.9
 nonparalytic A80.4
 paralytic A80.30
  specified NEC A80.39
  vaccine-associated A80.0
  wild virus
   imported A80.1
   indigenous A80.2
 spinal, acute A80.9
Poliosis (eyebrow) (eyelashes) L67.1
 circumscripta, acquired L67.1
Pollakiuria R35.0
 psychogenic F45.8
Pollinosis J30.1
Pollitzer's disease L73.2
Polyadenitis —*see also* Lymphadenitis
 malignant A20.0
Polyalgia M79.89
Polyangiitis M30.0
 microscopic M31.7
 overlap syndrome M30.8
Polyarteritis
 microscopic M31.7
 nodosa M30.0
  with lung involvement M30.1
  juvenile M30.2
  related condition NEC M30.8
Polyarthralgia —*see* Pain, joint
Polyarthritis, polyarthropathy —*see also*
  Arthritis M13.0
 due to or associated with other specified
  conditions —*see* Arthritis

Polyarthritis, polyarthropathy *(Continued)*
 epidemic (Australian) (with exanthema)
  B33.1
 infective —*see* Arthritis, pyogenic or
  pyemic
 inflammatory M06.4
 juvenile (chronic) (seronegative)
  M08.3
 migratory —*see* Fever, rheumatic
 rheumatic, acute —*see* Fever, rheumatic
Polyarthrosis M15.9
 post-traumatic M15.3
 primary M15.0
 specified NEC M15.8
Polycarential syndrome of infancy E40
Polychondritis (atrophic) (chronic) —*see also*
  Disorder, cartilage, specified type
  NEC
 relapsing M94.1
Polycoria Q13.2
Polycystic (disease)
 degeneration, kidney Q61.3
  autosomal dominant (adult type) Q61.2
  autosomal recessive (infantile type) NEC
   Q61.19
 kidney Q61.3
  autosomal
   dominant Q61.2
   recessive NEC Q61.19
  autosomal dominant (adult type) Q61.2
  autosomal recessive (childhood type) NEC
   Q61.19
  infantile type NEC Q61.19
 liver Q44.6
 lung J98.4
  congenital Q33.0
 ovary, ovaries E28.2
 spleen Q89.09
Polycythemia (secondary) D75.1
 acquired D75.1
 benign (familial) D75.0
 due to
  donor twin P61.1
  erythropoietin D75.1
  fall in plasma volume D75.1
  high altitude D75.1
  maternal-fetal transfusion P61.1
  stress D75.1
 emotional D75.1
 erythropoietin D75.1
 familial (benign) D75.0
 Gaisböck's (hypertonica) D75.1
 high altitude D75.1
 hypertonica D75.1
 hypoxemic D75.1
 neonatorum P61.1
 nephrogenous D75.1
 relative D75.1
 secondary D75.1
 spurious D75.1
 stress D75.1
 vera D45
Polycytosis cryptogenica D75.1
Polydactylism, polydactyly Q69.9
 toes Q69.2
Polydipsia R63.1
Polydystrophy, pseudo-Hurler E77.0
Polyembryoma —*see* Neoplasm, malignant,
  by site
Polyglandular
 deficiency E31.0
 dyscrasia E31.9
 dysfunction E31.9
 syndrome E31.8
Polyhydramnios O40.-
Polymastia Q83.1
Polymenorrhea N92.0
Polymyalgia M35.3
 arteritica, giant cell M31.5
 rheumatica M35.3
  with giant cell arteritis M31.5

Polymyositis (acute) (chronic) (hemorrhagic)
  M33.20
 with
  myopathy M33.22
  respiratory involvement M33.21
  skin involvement —*see*
   Dermatopolymyositis
  specified organ involvement NEC M33.29
 ossificans (generalisata) (progressiva) —*see*
  Myositis, ossificans, progressiva
Polyneuritis, polyneuritic —*see also*
  Polyneuropathy
 acute (post-)infective G61.0
 alcoholic G62.1
 cranialis G52.7
 demyelinating, chronic inflammatory (CIDP)
  G61.81
 diabetic —*see* Diabetes, polyneuropathy
 diphtheritic A36.83
 due to lack of vitamin NEC E56.9 *[G63]*
 endemic E51.11
 erythredema —*see* subcategory T56.1
 febrile, acute G61.0
 hereditary ataxic G60.1
 idiopathic, acute G61.0
 infective (acute) G61.0
 inflammatory, chronic demyelinating (CIDP)
  G61.81
 nutritional E63.9 *[G63]*
 postinfective (acute) G61.0
 specified NEC G62.89
Polyneuropathy (peripheral) G62.9
 alcoholic G62.1
 amyloid (Portuguese) E85.1 *[G63]*
 arsenical G62.2
 critical illness G62.81
 demyelinating, chronic inflammatory (CIDP)
  G61.81
 diabetic —*see* Diabetes, polyneuropathy
 drug-induced G62.0
 hereditary G60.9
  specified NEC G60.8
 idiopathic G60.9
  progressive G60.3
 in (due to)
  alcohol G62.1
   sequelae G65.2
  amyloidosis, familial (Portuguese) E85.1
   [G63]
  antitetanus serum G61.1
  arsenic G62.2
   sequelae G65.2
  avitaminosis NEC E56.9 *[G63]*
  beriberi E51.11
  collagen vascular disease NEC M35.9 *[G63]*
  deficiency (of)
   B (-complex) vitamins E53.9 *[G63]*
   vitamin B6 E53.1 *[G63]*
  diabetes —*see* Diabetes, polyneuropathy
  diphtheria A36.83
  drug or medicament G62.0
   correct substance properly
    administered —*see* Table of Drugs
    and Chemicals, by drug, adverse
    effect
   overdose or wrong substance given or
    taken —*see* Table of Drugs and
    Chemicals, by drug, poisoning
  endocrine disease NEC E34.9 *[G63]*
  herpes zoster B02.23
  hypoglycemia E16.2 *[G63]*
  infectious
   disease NEC B99 *[G63]*
   mononucleosis B27.91
  lack of vitamin NEC E56.9 *[G63]*
  lead G62.2
   sequelae G65.2
  leprosy A30.9 *[G63]*
  Lyme disease A69.22
  metabolic disease NEC E88.9 *[G63]*
  microscopic polyangiitis M31.7 *[G63]*

Polyneuropathy *(Continued)*
  in *(Continued)*
    mumps B26.84
    neoplastic disease —*see also* Neoplasm
      D49.9 *[G63]*
    nutritional deficiency NEC E63.9 *[G63]*
    organophosphate compounds G62.2
      sequelae G65.2
    parasitic disease NEC B89 *[G63]*
    pellagra E52 *[G63]*
    polyarteritis nodosa M30.0
    porphyria E80.20 *[G63]*
    radiation G62.82
    rheumatoid arthritis —*see* Rheumatoid,
      polyneuropathy
    sarcoidosis D86.89
    serum G61.1
    syphilis (late) A52.15
      congenital A50.43
    systemic
      connective tissue disorder M35.9
        [G63]
      lupus erythematosus M32.19
    toxic agent NEC G62.2
      sequelae G65.2
    triorthocresyl phosphate G62.2
      sequelae G65.2
    tuberculosis A17.89
    uremia N18.9 *[G63]*
    vitamin B12 deficiency E53.8 *[G63]*
      with anemia (pernicious) D51.0
        [G63]
        due to dietary deficiency D51.3
          [G63]
    zoster B02.23
  inflammatory G61.9
    chronic demyelinating (CIDP) G61.81
    sequelae G65.1
    specified NEC G61.89
  lead G62.2
    sequelae G65.2
  nutritional NEC E63.9 *[G63]*
  postherpetic (zoster) B02.23
  progressive G60.3
  radiation-induced G62.82
  sensory (hereditary) (idiopathic) G60.8
  specified NEC G62.89
  syphilitic (late) A52.15
    congenital A50.43
Polyopia H53.8
Polyorchism, polyorchidism Q55.21
Polyosteoarthritis —*see also* Osteoarthritis,
  generalized M15.9-
  post-traumatic M15.3
  specified NEC M15.8
Polyostotic fibrous dysplasia Q78.1
Polyotia Q17.0
Polyp, polypus
  accessory sinus J33.8
  adenocarcinoma in —*see* Neoplasm,
    malignant, by site
  adenocarcinoma in situ in —*see* Neoplasm, in
    situ, by site
  adenoid tissue J33.0
  adenomatous —*see also* Neoplasm, benign,
    by site
    adenocarcinoma in —*see* Neoplasm,
      malignant, by site
    adenocarcinoma in situ in —*see* Neoplasm,
      in situ, by site
    carcinoma in —*see* Neoplasm, malignant,
      by site
    carcinoma in situ in —*see* Neoplasm, in
      situ, by site
    multiple —*see* Neoplasm, benign
      adenocarcinoma in —*see* Neoplasm,
        malignant, by site
      adenocarcinoma in situ in —*see*
        Neoplasm, in situ, by site
  antrum J33.8
  anus, anal (canal) K62.0

Polyp, polypus *(Continued)*
  Bartholin's gland N84.3
  bladder D41.4
  carcinoma in —*see* Neoplasm, malignant, by
    site
  carcinoma in situ in —*see* Neoplasm, in situ,
    by site
  cecum D12.0
  cervix (uteri) N84.1
    in pregnancy or childbirth —*see* Pregnancy,
      complicated by, abnormal, cervix
    mucous N84.1
    nonneoplastic N84.1
  choanal J33.0
  cholesterol K82.4
  clitoris N84.3
  colon K63.5
    adenomatous D12.6
    ascending D12.2
    cecum D12.0
    descending D12.4
    inflammatory K51.40
      with
        abscess K51.414
        complication K51.419
          specified NEC K51.418
        fistula K51.413
        intestinal obstruction K51.412
        rectal bleeding K51.411
    sigmoid D12.5
    transverse D12.3
  corpus uteri N84.0
  dental K04.01 ◀▥
    irreversible K04.02 ◀
    reversible K04.01 ◀
  duodenum K31.7
  ear (middle) H74.4-
  endometrium N84.0
  ethmoidal (sinus) J33.8
  fallopian tube N84.8
  female genital tract N84.9
    specified NEC N84.8
  frontal (sinus) J33.8
  gallbladder K82.4
  gingiva, gum K06.8
  labia, labium (majus) (minus) N84.3
  larynx (mucous) J38.1
    adenomatous D14.1
  malignant —*see* Neoplasm, malignant, by site
  maxillary (sinus) J33.8
  middle ear —*see* Polyp, ear (middle)
  myometrium N84.0
  nares
    anterior J33.9
    posterior J33.0
  nasal (mucous) J33.9
    cavity J33.0
    septum J33.0
  nasopharyngeal J33.0
  nose (mucous) J33.9
  oviduct N84.8
  pharynx J39.2
  placenta O90.89
  prostate —*see* Enlargement, enlarged,
    prostate
  pudenda, pudendum N84.3
  pulpal (dental) K04.01 ◀▥
    irreversible K04.02 ◀
    reversible K04.01 ◀
  rectum (nonadenomatous) K62.1
    adenomatous —*see* Polyp, adenomatous
  septum (nasal) J33.0
  sinus (accessory) (ethmoidal) (frontal)
    (maxillary) (sphenoidal) J33.8
  sphenoidal (sinus) J33.8
  stomach K31.7
    adenomatous D13.1
  tube, fallopian N84.8
  turbinate, mucous membrane J33.8
  umbilical, newborn P83.6
  ureter N28.89

Polyp, polypus *(Continued)*
  urethra N36.2
  uterus (body) (corpus) (mucous) N84.0
    cervix N84.1
    in pregnancy or childbirth —*see* Pregnancy,
      complicated by, tumor, uterus
  vagina N84.2
  vocal cord (mucous) J38.1
  vulva N84.3
Polyphagia R63.2
Polyploidy Q92.7
Polypoid —*see* condition
Polyposis —*see also* Polyp
  coli (adenomatous) D12.6
    adenocarcinoma in C18.9
    adenocarcinoma in situ in —*see* Neoplasm,
      in situ, by site
    carcinoma in C18.9
  colon (adenomatous) D12.6
  familial D12.6
    adenocarcinoma in situ in —*see* Neoplasm,
      in situ, by site
  intestinal (adenomatous) D12.6
  malignant lymphomatous C83.1
  multiple, adenomatous —*see also* Neoplasm,
    benign D36.9
Polyradiculitis —*see* Polyneuropathy
Polyradiculoneuropathy (acute) (postinfective)
  (segmentally demyelinating) G61.0
Polyserositis
  due to pericarditis I31.1
  pericardial I31.1
  periodic, familial E85.0
  tuberculous A19.9
    acute A19.1
    chronic A19.8
Polysplenia syndrome Q89.09
Polysyndactyly —*see also* Syndactylism,
  syndactyly Q70.4
Polytrichia L68.3
Polyunguia Q84.6
Polyuria R35.8
  nocturnal R35.1
  psychogenic F45.8
Pompe's disease (glycogen storage) E74.02
Pompholyx L30.1
Poncet's disease (tuberculous rheumatism)
  A18.09
Pond fracture —*see* Fracture, skull
Ponos B55.0
Pons, pontine —*see* condition
Poor
  aesthetic of existing restoration of tooth
    K08.56
  contractions, labor O62.2
  gingival margin to tooth restoration K08.51
  personal hygiene R46.0
  prenatal care, affecting management of
    pregnancy —*see* Pregnancy, complicated
    by, insufficient, prenatal care
  sucking reflex (newborn) R29.2
  urinary stream R39.12
  vision NEC H54.7
Poradenitis, nostras inguinalis or venerea A55
Porencephaly (congenital) (developmental)
  (true) Q04.6
  acquired G93.0
  nondevelopmental G93.0
  traumatic (post) F07.89
Porocephaliasis B88.8
Porokeratosis Q82.8
Poroma, eccrine —*see* Neoplasm, skin, benign
Porphyria (South African) E80.20
  acquired E80.20
  acute intermittent (hepatic) (Swedish) E80.21
  cutanea tarda (hereditary) (symptomatic)
    E80.1
  due to drugs E80.20
    correct substance properly administered —
      see Table of Drugs and Chemicals, by
      drug, adverse effect

◀ New   ▥ Revised   ~~deleted~~ Deleted

Porphyria *(Continued)*
  due to drugs *(Continued)*
    overdose or wrong substance given or taken —*see* Table of Drugs and Chemicals, by drug, poisoning
  erythropoietic (congenital) (hereditary) E80.0
    hepatocutaneous type E80.1
  secondary E80.20
  toxic NEC E80.20
  variegata E80.20
Porphyrinuria —*see* Porphyria
Porphyruria —*see* Porphyria
Portal —*see* condition
Port wine nevus, mark, or stain Q82.5
Posadas-Wernicke disease B38.9
Positive
  culture (nonspecific)
    blood R78.81
    bronchial washings R84.5
    cerebrospinal fluid R83.5
    cervix uteri R87.5
    nasal secretions R84.5
    nipple discharge R89.5
    nose R84.5
      staphylococcus (Methicillin susceptible) Z22.321
      Methicillin resistant Z22.322
    peritoneal fluid R85.5
    pleural fluid R84.5
    prostatic secretions R86.5
    saliva R85.5
    seminal fluid R86.5
    sputum R84.5
    synovial fluid R89.5
    throat scrapings R84.5
    urine R82.79 ◀▥
    vagina R87.5
    vulva R87.5
    wound secretions R89.5
  PPD (skin test) R76.11
  serology for syphilis A53.0
    with signs or symptoms - code as Syphilis, by site and stage
    false R76.8
  skin test, tuberculin (without active tuberculosis) R76.11
  test, human immunodeficiency virus (HIV) R75
  VDRL A53.0
    with signs or symptoms - code by site and stage under Syphilis A53.9
  Wassermann reaction A53.0
Postcardiotomy syndrome I97.0
Postcaval ureter Q62.62
Postcholecystectomy syndrome K91.5
Postclimacteric bleeding N95.0
Postcommissurotomy syndrome I97.0
Postconcussional syndrome F07.81
Postcontusional syndrome F07.81
Postcricoid region —*see* condition
Post-dates (40-42 weeks) (pregnancy) (mother) O48.0
  more than 42 weeks gestation O48.1
Postencephalitic syndrome F07.89
Posterior —*see* condition
Posterolateral sclerosis (spinal cord) —*see* Degeneration, combined
Postexanthematous —*see* condition
Postfebrile —*see* condition
Postgastrectomy dumping syndrome K91.1
Posthemiplegic chorea —*see* Monoplegia
Posthemorrhagic anemia (chronic) D50.0
  acute D62
  newborn P61.3
Postherpetic neuralgia (zoster) B02.29
  trigeminal B02.22
Posthitis N47.7
Postimmunization complication or reaction — *see* Complications, vaccination
Postinfectious —*see* condition

Postlaminectomy syndrome NEC M96.1
Postleukotomy syndrome F07.0
Postmastectomy lymphedema (syndrome) I97.2
Postmaturity, postmature (over 42 weeks)
  maternal (over 42 weeks gestation) O48.1
  newborn P08.22
Postmeasles complication NEC —*see also* condition B05.89
Postmenopausal
  endometrium (atrophic) N95.8
    suppurative —*see also* Endometritis N71.9
  osteoporosis —*see* Osteoporosis, postmenopausal
Postnasal drip R09.82
  due to
    allergic rhinitis —*see* Rhinitis, allergic
    common cold J00
    gastroesophageal reflux —*see* Reflux, gastroesophageal
    nasopharyngitis —*see* Nasopharyngitis
    other know condition — code to condition
    sinusitis —*see* Sinusitis
Postnatal —*see* condition
Postoperative (postprocedural) —*see* Complication, postoperative
  pneumothorax, therapeutic Z98.3
  state NEC Z98.890 ◀▥
Postpancreatectomy hyperglycemia E89.1
Postpartum —*see* Puerperal
Postphlebitic syndrome —*see* Syndrome, postthrombotic
Postpolio (myelitic) syndrome G14
Postpoliomyelitic —*see also* condition
  osteopathy —*see* Osteopathy, after poliomyelitis
Postprocedural —*see also* Postoperative
  hypoinsulinemia E89.1
Postschizophrenic depression F32.89 ◀▥
Postsurgery status —*see also* Status (post)
  pneumothorax, therapeutic Z98.3
Post-term (40-42 weeks) (pregnancy) (mother) O48.0
  infant P08.21
  more than 42 weeks gestation (mother) O48.1
Post-traumatic brain syndrome, nonpsychotic F07.81
Post-typhoid abscess A01.09
Postures, hysterical F44.2
Postvaccinal reaction or complication —*see* Complications, vaccination
Postvalvulotomy syndrome I97.0
Potain's
  disease (pulmonary edema) —*see* Edema, lung
  syndrome (gastrectasis with dyspepsia) K31.0
Potter's
  asthma J62.8
  facies Q60.6
  lung J62.8
  syndrome (with renal agenesis) Q60.6
Pott's
  curvature (spinal) A18.01
  disease or paraplegia A18.01
  spinal curvature A18.01
  tumor, puffy —*see* Osteomyelitis, specified type NEC
Pouch
  bronchus Q32.4
  Douglas' —*see* condition
  esophagus, esophageal, congenital Q39.6
    acquired K22.5
  gastric K31.4
  Hartmann's K82.8
  pharynx, pharyngeal (congenital) Q38.7
Pouchitis K91.850
Poultrymen's itch B88.0
Poverty NEC Z59.6
  extreme Z59.5
Poxvirus NEC B08.8
Prader-Willi syndrome Q87.1
Preauricular appendage or tag Q17.0

Prebetalipoproteinemia (acquired) (essential) (familial) (hereditary) (primary) (secondary) E78.1
  with chylomicronemia E78.3
Precipitate labor or delivery O62.3
Preclimacteric bleeding (menorrhagia) N92.4
Precocious
  adrenarche E30.1
  menarche E30.1
  menstruation E30.1
  pubarche E30.1
  puberty E30.1
    central E22.8
  sexual development NEC E30.1
  thelarche E30.8
Precocity, sexual (constitutional) (cryptogenic) (female) (idiopathic) (male) E30.1
  with adrenal hyperplasia E25.9
    congenital E25.0
Precordial pain R07.2
Predeciduous teeth K00.2
Prediabetes, prediabetic R73.03 ◀▥
  complicating
    pregnancy —*see* Pregnancy, complicated by, diseases of, specified type or system NEC
    puerperium O99.89
Predislocation status of hip at birth Q65.6
Pre-eclampsia O14.9-
  with pre-existing hypertension —*see* Hypertension, complicating pregnancy, pre-existing, with, pre-eclampsia
  complicating ◀
    childbirth O14.94 ◀
    puerperium O14.95 ◀
  mild O14.0-
    complicating ◀
      childbirth O14.04 ◀
      puerperium O14.05 ◀
  moderate O14.0-
    complicating ◀
      childbirth O14.04 ◀
      puerperium O14.05 ◀
  severe O14.1-
    with hemolysis, elevated liver enzymes and low platelet count (HELLP) O14.2-
      complicating ◀
        childbirth O14.24 ◀
        puerperium O14.25 ◀
      complicating ◀
        childbirth O14.14 ◀
        puerperium O14.15 ◀
Pre-eruptive color change, teeth, tooth K00.8
Pre-excitation atrioventricular conduction I45.6
Preglaucoma H40.00-
Pregnancy (single) (uterine) —*see also* Delivery and Puerperal

Note: The Tabular must be reviewed for assignment of the appropriate character indicating the trimester of the pregnancy

Note: The Tabular must be reviewed for assignment of appropriate seventh character for multiple gestation codes in Chapter 15

  abdominal (ectopic) O00.00 ◀▥
    with intrauterine pregnancy O00.01 ◀
    with viable fetus O36.7-
  ampullar O00.10 ◀▥
    with intrauterine pregnancy O00.11 ◀
  biochemical O02.81
  broad ligament O00.80 ◀▥
    with intrauterine pregnancy O00.81 ◀
  cervical O00.80 ◀▥
    with intrauterine pregnancy O00.81 ◀
  chemical O02.81
  complicated NOS O26.9-

Pregnancy *(Continued)*
   complicated by (care of) (management
     affected by)
    abnormal, abnormality
     cervix O34.4-
      causing obstructed labor O65.5
     cord (umbilical) O69.9
     findings on antenatal screening of
      mother O28.9
      biochemical O28.1
      chromosomal O28.5
      cytological O28.2
      genetic O28.5
      hematological O28.0
      radiological O28.4
      specified NEC O28.8
      ultrasonic O28.3
     glucose (tolerance) NEC O99.810
     pelvic organs O34.9-
      specified NEC O34.8-
       causing obstructed labor O65.5
     pelvis (bony) (major) NEC O33.0
     perineum O34.7-
     position
      placenta O44.0- ◀▥
      ~~without hemorrhage O44.0-~~
       with hemorrhage O44.1- ◀
      uterus O34.59-
     uterus O34.59-
      causing obstructed labor O65.5
      congenital O34.0-
     vagina O34.6-
      causing obstructed labor O65.5
     vulva O34.7-
      causing obstructed labor O65.5
    abruptio placentae —*see* Abruptio
     placentae
    abscess or cellulitis
     bladder O23.1-
     breast O91.11-
     genital organ or tract O23.9-
    abuse
     physical O9A.31-
     psychological O9A.51-
     sexual O9A.41-
    adverse effect anesthesia O29.9-
     aspiration pneumonitis O29.01-
     cardiac arrest O29.11-
     cardiac complication NEC O29.19-
     cardiac failure O29.12-
     central nervous system complication
      NEC O29.29-
     cerebral anoxia O29.21-
     failed or difficult intubation O29.6-
     inhalation of stomach contents or
      secretions NOS O29.01-
     local, toxic reaction O29.3X
     Mendelson's syndrome O29.01-
     pressure collapse of lung O29.02-
     pulmonary complications NEC O29.09-
     specified NEC O29.8X
     spinal and epidural type NEC O29.5X
      induced headache O29.4-
    albuminuria —*see also* Proteinuria,
     gestational O12.1- ◀▥
    alcohol use O99.31-
    amnionitis O41.12-
    anaphylactoid syndrome of pregnancy
     O88.01-
    anemia (conditions in D50-D64) (pre-
     existing) O99.01-
     complicating the puerperium O99.03
    antepartum hemorrhage O46.9-
     with coagulation defect —*see*
      Hemorrhage, antepartum, with
      coagulation defect
     specified NEC O46.8X-
    appendicitis O99.61-
    atrophy (yellow) (acute) liver (subacute)
     O26.61-
    bariatric surgery status O99.84- ◀▥

Pregnancy *(Continued)*
   complicated by *(Continued)*
    bicornis or bicornuate uterus O34.0- ◀▥
    biliary tract problems O26.61-
    breech presentation O32.1
    cardiovascular diseases (conditions in
     I00-I09, I20-I52, I70-I99) O99.41-
    cerebrovascular disorders (conditions in
     I60-I69) O99.41-
    cervical shortening O26.87-
    cervicitis O23.51-
    chloasma (gravidarum) O26.89-
    cholecystitis O99.61-
    cholestasis (intrahepatic) O26.61-
    chorioamnionitis O41.12-
    circulatory system disorder (conditions in
     I00-I09, I20-I99, O99.41-)
    compound presentation O32.6
    conjoined twins O30.02-
    connective system disorders (conditions in
     M00-M99) O99.89
    contracted pelvis (general) O33.1
     inlet O33.2
     outlet O33.3
    convulsions (eclamptic) (uremic) —*see also*
     Eclampsia O15.9-
    cracked nipple O92.11-
    cystitis O23.1-
    cystocele O34.8-
    death of fetus (near term) O36.4
     early pregnancy O02.1
     of one fetus or more in multiple
      gestation O31.2-
    deciduitis O41.14-
    decreased fetal movement O36.81-
    dental problems O99.61-
    diabetes (mellitus) O24.91-
     gestational (pregnancy induced) —*see*
      Diabetes, gestational
     pre-existing O24.31-
      specified NEC O24.81-
      type 1 O24.01-
      type 2 O24.11-
    digestive system disorders (conditions in
     K00-K93) O99.61-
    diseases of —*see* Pregnancy, complicated
     by, specified body system disease
     biliary tract O26.61-
     blood NEC (conditions in D65-D77)
      O99.11-
     liver O26.61-
     specified NEC O99.89
    disorders of —*see* Pregnancy, complicated
     by, specified body system disorder
     amniotic fluid and membranes O41.9-
      specified NEC O41.8X-
     biliary tract O26.61-
     ear and mastoid process (conditions in
      H60-H95) O99.89
     eye and adnexa (conditions in H00-H59)
      O99.89
     liver O26.61-
     skin (conditions in L00-L99) O99.71-
     specified NEC O99.89
    displacement, uterus NEC O34.59-
     causing obstructed labor O65.5
    disproportion (due to) O33.9
     ~~fetal deformities NEC O33.7~~
     fetal (ascites) (hydrops)
      (meningomyelocele) (sacral
      teratoma) (tumor) deformities NEC
      O33.7 ◀
     generally contracted pelvis O33.1
     hydrocephalic fetus O33.6
     inlet contraction of pelvis O33.2
     mixed maternal and fetal origin O33.4
     specified NEC O33.8
    double uterus O34.0- ◀▥
     causing obstructed labor O65.5
    drug use (conditions in F11-F19)
     O99.32-

Pregnancy *(Continued)*
   complicated by *(Continued)*
    eclampsia, eclamptic (coma) (convulsions)
     (delirium) (nephritis) (uremia) (*see
     also* Eclampsia) O15-
    ectopic pregnancy —*see* Pregnancy, ectopic
    edema O12.0-
     with
      gestational hypertension, mild —*see
       also* Pre-eclampsia O14.0-
      proteinuria O12.2-
    effusion, amniotic fluid —*see* Pregnancy,
     complicated by, premature rupture of
     membranes
    elderly
     multigravida O09.52-
     primigravida O09.51-
    embolism —*see also* Embolism, obstetric,
     pregnancy O88.-
    endocrine diseases NEC O99.28-
    endometritis O86.12
    excessive weight gain O26.0-
    exhaustion O26.81-
     during labor and delivery O75.81
    face presentation O32.3
    failed induction of labor O61.9
    failed or difficult intubation for anesthesia
     O29.6-
     instrumental O61.1
     mechanical O61.1
     medical O61.0
     specified NEC O61.8
     surgical O61.1
    false labor (pains) O47.9
     at or after 37 completed weeks of
      pregnancy O47.1
     before 37 completed weeks of pregnancy
      O47.0-
    fatigue O26.81-
     during labor and delivery O75.81
    fatty metamorphosis of liver O26.61-
    female genital mutilation O34.8- *[N90.81-]*
    fetal (maternal care for)
     abnormality or damage O35.9
      acid-base balance O68
      specified type NEC O35.8
     acidemia O68
     acidosis O68
     alkalosis O68
     anemia and thrombocytopenia O36.82-
     anencephaly O35.0
     chromosomal abnormality (conditions in
      Q90-Q99) O35.1
     conjoined twins O30.02-
     damage from
      amniocentesis O35.7
      biopsy procedures O35.7
      drug addiction O35.5
      hematological investigation O35.7
      intrauterine contraceptive device
       O35.7
      maternal
       alcohol addiction O35.4
       cytomegalovirus infection O35.3
       disease NEC O35.8
       drug addiction O35.5
       listeriosis O35.8
       rubella O35.3
       toxoplasmosis O35.8
       viral infection O35.3
      medical procedure NEC O35.7
      radiation O35.6
     death (near term) O36.4
      early pregnancy O02.1
     decreased movement O36.81-
     disproportion due to deformity (fetal)
      O33.7
     excessive growth (large for dates) O36.6-
     growth retardation O36.59-
      light for dates O36.59-
      small for dates O36.59-

◀ New   ◀▥ Revised   ~~deleted~~ Deleted

Pregnancy *(Continued)*
complicated by *(Continued)*
fetal *(Continued)*
heart rate irregularity (bradycardia) (decelerations) (tachycardia) O76
hereditary disease O35.2
hydrocephalus O35.0
intrauterine death O36.4
poor growth O36.59-
light for dates O36.59-
small for dates O36.59-
problem O36.9-
specified NEC O36.89-
reduction (elective) O31.3-
selective termination O31.3-
spina bifida O35.0
thrombocytopenia O36.82-
fibroid (tumor) (uterus) O34.1-
fissure of nipple O92.11-
gallstones O99.61-
gastric banding status O99.84-
gastric bypass status O99.84-
genital herpes (asymptomatic) (history of) (inactive) O98.51-
genital tract infection O23.9-
glomerular diseases (conditions in N00-N07) O26.83-
with hypertension, pre-existing —*see* Hypertension, complicating, pregnancy, pre-existing, with, renal disease
gonorrhea O98.21-
grand multiparity O09.4
habitual aborter —*see* Pregnancy, complicated by, recurrent pregnancy loss
HELLP syndrome (hemolysis, elevated liver enzymes and low platelet count) O14.2-
hemorrhage
antepartum —*see* Hemorrhage, antepartum
before 20 completed weeks gestation O20.9
specified NEC O20.8
due to premature separation, placenta —*see also* Abruptio placentae O45.9-
early O20.9
specified NEC O20.8
threatened abortion O20.0
hemorrhoids O22.4-
hepatitis (viral) O98.41-
herniation of uterus O34.59-
high
head at term O32.4
risk —*see* Supervision (of) (for), high-risk
history of in utero procedure during previous pregnancy O09.82-
HIV O98.71-
human immunodeficiency virus (HIV) disease O98.71-
hydatidiform mole —*see also* Mole, hydatidiform O01.9-
hydramnios O40.-
hydrocephalic fetus (disproportion) O33.6
hydrops
amnii O40.-
fetalis O36.2-
associated with isoimmunization —*see also* Pregnancy, complicated by, isoimmunization O36.11-
hydrorrhea O42.90
hyperemesis (gravidarum) (mild) —*see also* Hyperemesis, gravidarum O21.0-
hypertension —*see* Hypertension, complicating pregnancy
hypertensive
heart and renal disease, pre-existing —*see* Hypertension, complicating, pregnancy, pre-existing, with, heart disease, with renal disease

Pregnancy *(Continued)*
complicated by *(Continued)*
hypertensive *(Continued)*
heart disease, pre-existing —*see* Hypertension, complicating, pregnancy, pre-existing, with, heart disease
renal disease, pre-existing —*see* Hypertension, complicating, pregnancy, pre-existing, with, renal disease
hypotension O26.5-
immune disorders NEC (conditions in D80-D89) O99.11-
incarceration, uterus O34.51-
incompetent cervix O34.3-
inconclusive fetal viability O36.80
infection (s) O98.91-
amniotic fluid or sac O41.10-
bladder O23.1-
carrier state NEC O99.830
streptococcus B O99.820
genital organ or tract O23.9-
specified NEC O23.59-
genitourinary tract O23.9-
gonorrhea O98.21-
hepatitis (viral) O98.41-
HIV O98.71-
human immunodeficiency virus (HIV) O98.71-
kidney O23.0-
nipple O91.01-
parasitic disease O98.91-
specified NEC O98.81-
protozoal disease O98.61-
sexually transmitted NEC O98.31-
specified type NEC O98.81-
syphilis O98.11-
tuberculosis O98.01-
urethra O23.2-
urinary (tract) O23.4-
specified NEC O23.3-
viral disease O98.51-
injury or poisoning (conditions in S00-T88) O9A.21-
due to abuse
physical O9A.31-
psychological O9A.51-
sexual O9A.41-
insufficient
prenatal care O09.3-
weight gain O26.1-
insulin resistance O26.89
intrauterine fetal death (near term) O36.4
early pregnancy O02.1
multiple gestation (one fetus or more) O31.2-
isoimmunization O36.11-
anti-A sensitization O36.11-
anti-B sensitization O36.19-
Rh O36.09-
anti-D antibody O36.01-
specified NEC O36.19-
laceration of uterus NEC O71.81
malformation
placenta, placental (vessel) O43.10-
specified NEC O43.19-
uterus (congenital) O34.0-
malnutrition (conditions in E40-E46) O25.1-
maternal hypotension syndrome O26.5-
mental disorders (conditions in F01-F09, F20-F99) O99.34-
alcohol use O99.31-
drug use O99.32-
smoking O99.33-
mentum presentation O32.3
metabolic disorders O99.28-
missed
abortion O02.1
delivery O36.4

Pregnancy *(Continued)*
complicated by *(Continued)*
multiple gestations O30.9-
conjoined twins O30.02-
quadruplet —*see* Pregnancy, quadruplet
specified complication NEC O31.8X-
specified number of multiples NEC —*see* Pregnancy, multiple (gestation), specified NEC
triplet —*see* Pregnancy, triplet
twin —*see* Pregnancy, twin
musculoskeletal condition (conditions is M00-M99) O99.89
necrosis, liver (conditions in K72) O26.61-
neoplasm
benign
cervix O34.4-
corpus uteri O34.1-
uterus O34.1-
malignant O9A.11-
nephropathy NEC O26.83-
nervous system condition (conditions in G00-G99) O99.35-
nutritional diseases NEC O99.28-
obesity (pre-existing) O99.21-
obesity surgery status O99.84-
oblique lie or presentation O32.2
older mother —*see* Pregnancy, complicated by, elderly
oligohydramnios O41.0-
with premature rupture of membranes —*see also* Pregnancy, complicated by, premature rupture of membranes O42-
onset (spontaneous) of labor after 37 completed weeks of gestation but before 39 completed weeks gestation, with delivery by (planned) cesarean section O75.82
oophoritis O23.52-
overdose, drug —*see also* Table of Drugs and Chemicals, by drug, poisoning O9A.21-
oversize fetus O33.5
papyraceous fetus O31.0-
pelvic inflammatory disease O99.89
periodontal disease O99.61-
peripheral neuritis O26.82-
peritoneal (pelvic) adhesions O99.89
phlebitis O22.9-
phlebopathy O22.9-
phlebothrombosis (superficial) O22.2-
deep O22.3-
placenta accreta O43.21-
placenta increta O43.22-
placenta percreta O43.23-
placenta previa O44.0- ◀▥
complete O44.0- ◀
with hemorrhage O44.1- ◀
marginal O44.2- ◀
with hemorrhage O44.3- ◀
partial O44.2- ◀
with hemorrhage O44.3- ◀
without hemorrhage O44.0
placental disorder O43.9-
specified NEC O43.89-
placental dysfunction O43.89-
placental infarction O43.81-
placental insufficiency O36.51-
placental transfusion syndromes
fetomaternal O43.01-
fetus to fetus O43.02-
maternofetal O43.01-
placentitis O41.14-
pneumonia O99.51-
poisoning —*see also* Table of Drugs and Chemicals O9A.21-
polyhydramnios O40-
polymorphic eruption of pregnancy O26.86
poor obstetric history NEC O09.29-

Pregnancy *(Continued)*
  complicated by *(Continued)*
    postmaturity (post-term) (40 to 42 weeks) O48.0
      more than 42 completed weeks gestation (prolonged) O48.1
    pre-eclampsia O14.9-
      mild O14.0-
      moderate O14.0-
      severe O14.1-
        with hemolysis, elevated liver enzymes and low platelet count (HELLP) O14.2-
    premature labor —*see* Pregnancy, complicated by, preterm labor
    premature rupture of membranes O42.90
      full-term, unspecified as to length of time between rupture and onset of labor O42.92 ◀
      with onset of labor
        within 24 hours O42.00
          after 37 weeks gestation O42.02
          at or after 37 weeks gestation, onset of labor within 24 hours of rupture O42.02 ◀
          pre-term (before 37 completed weeks of gestation) O42.01-
        after 24 hours O42.10
          after 37 weeks gestation O42.12
          at or after 37 weeks gestation, onset of labor more than 24 hours following rupture O42.12 ◀
          pre-term (before 37 completed weeks of gestation) O42.11-
        after 37 weeks gestation O42.92
        at or after 37 weeks gestation, unspecified as to length of time between rupture and onset of labor O42.92 ◀
        full-term O42.92
        pre-term (before 37 completed weeks of gestation) O42.91-
    premature separation of placenta —*see also* Abruptio placentae O45.9-
    presentation, fetal —*see* Delivery, complicated by, malposition
    preterm delivery O60.10
    preterm labor
      with delivery O60.10
        preterm O60.10
        term O60.20
      second trimester
        with preterm delivery
          second trimester O60.12
          third trimester O60.13
        with term delivery O60.22
        without delivery O60.02
      third trimester
        with term delivery O60.23
        with third trimester preterm delivery O60.14
        without delivery O60.03
      without delivery O60.00
        second trimester O60.02
        third trimester O60.03
    previous history of —*see* Pregnancy, supervision of, high-risk
    prolapse, uterus O34.52-
    proteinuria (gestational) —*see also* Proteinuria, gestational O12.1- ◀≡
      with edema O12.2-
    pruritic urticarial papules and plaques of pregnancy (PUPPP) O26.86
    pruritus (neurogenic) O26.89-
    psychosis or psychoneurosis (puerperal) F53
    ptyalism O26.89-
    PUPPP (pruritic urticarial papules and plaques of pregnancy) O26.86
    pyelitis O23.0-
    recurrent pregnancy loss O26.2-

Pregnancy *(Continued)*
  complicated by *(Continued)*
    renal disease or failure NEC O26.83-
      with secondary hypertension, pre-existing —*see* Hypertension, complicating, pregnancy, pre-existing, secondary
      hypertensive, pre-existing —*see* Hypertension, complicating, pregnancy, pre-existing, with, renal disease
    respiratory condition (conditions in J00-J99) O99.51-
    retained, retention
      dead ovum O02.0
      intrauterine contraceptive device O26.3-
    retroversion, uterus O34.53-
    Rh immunization, incompatibility or sensitization NEC O36.09-
      anti-D antibody O36.01-
    rupture
      amnion (premature) —*see also* Pregnancy, complicated by, premature rupture of membranes O42-
      membranes (premature) —*see also* Pregnancy, complicated by, premature rupture of membranes O42-
      uterus (during labor) O71.1
        before onset of labor O71.0-
    salivation (excessive) O26.89-
    salpingitis O23.52-
    salpingo-oophoritis O23.52-
    sepsis (conditions in A40, A41) O98.81-
    size date discrepancy (uterine) O26.84-
    skin condition (conditions in L00-L99) O99.71-
    smoking (tobacco) O99.33-
    social problem O09.7-
    specified condition NEC O26.89-
    spotting O26.85-
    streptococcus B carrier state O99.820
    streptococcus group B (GBS) carrier state O99.820 ◀
    subluxation of symphysis (pubis) O26.71-
    syphilis (conditions in A50-A53) O98.11-
    threatened
      abortion O20.0
      labor O47.9
        at or after 37 completed weeks of gestation O47.1
        before 37 completed weeks of gestation O47.0-
    thrombophlebitis (superficial) O22.2-
    thrombosis O22.9-
      cerebral venous O22.5-
      cerebrovenous sinus O22.5-
      deep O22.3-
    tobacco use disorder (smoking) O99.33- ◀
    torsion of uterus O34.59-
    toxemia O14.9-
    transverse lie or presentation O32.2
    tuberculosis (conditions in A15-A19) O98.01-
    tumor (benign)
      cervix O34.4-
      malignant O9A.11-
      uterus O34.1-
    unstable lie O32.0
    upper respiratory infection O99.51-
    urethritis O23.2-
    uterine size date discrepancy O26.84-
    vaginitis or vulvitis O23.59-
    varicose veins (lower extremities) O22.0-
      genitals O22.1-
      legs O22.0-
      perineal O22.1-
      vaginal or vulval O22.1-
    venereal disease NEC (conditions in A63.8) O98.31-

Pregnancy *(Continued)*
  complicated by *(Continued)*
    venous disorders O22.9-
      specified NEC O22.8X-
    very young mother —*see* Pregnancy, complicated by, young mother
    viral diseases (conditions in A80-B09, B25-B34) O98.51-
    vomiting O21.9
      due to diseases classified elsewhere O21.8
      hyperemesis gravidarum (mild) —*see also* Hyperemesis, gravidarum O21.0-
      late (occurring after 20 weeks of gestation) O21.2
    young mother
      multigravida O09.62-
      primigravida O09.61-
  concealed O09.3-
  continuing following
    elective fetal reduction of one or more fetus O31.3-
    intrauterine death of one or more fetus O31.2-
    spontaneous abortion of one or more fetus O31.1-
  cornual O00.80 ◀≡
    with intrauterine pregnancy O00.81 ◀
  ectopic (ruptured) O00.90 ◀≡
    with intrauterine pregnancy O00.91 ◀
  abdominal O00.00 ◀≡
    with viable fetus O36.7-
    with ◀
      intrauterine pregnancy O00.01 ◀
      viable fetus O36.7- ◀
  cervical O00.80 ◀≡
    with intrauterine pregnancy O00.81 ◀
  complicated (by) O08.9
    afibrinogenemia O08.1
    cardiac arrest O08.81
    chemical damage of pelvic organ (s) O08.6
    circulatory collapse O08.3
    defibrination syndrome O08.1
    electrolyte imbalance O08.5
    embolism (amniotic fluid) (blood clot) (pulmonary) (septic) O08.2
    endometritis O08.0
    genital tract and pelvic infection O08.0
    hemorrhage (delayed) (excessive) O08.1
    infection
      genital tract or pelvic O08.0
      kidney O08.83
      urinary tract O08.83
    intravascular coagulation O08.1
    laceration of pelvic organ (s) O08.6
    metabolic disorder O08.5
    oliguria O08.4
    oophoritis O08.0
    parametritis O08.0
    pelvic peritonitis O08.0
    perforation of pelvic organ (s) O08.6
    renal failure or shutdown O08.4
    salpingitis or salpingo-oophoritis O08.0
    sepsis O08.82
    shock O08.83
      septic O08.82
    specified condition NEC O08.89
    tubular necrosis (renal) O08.4
    uremia O08.4
    urinary infection O08.83
    venous complication NEC O08.7
      embolism O08.2
  cornual O00.80 ◀≡
    with intrauterine pregnancy O00.81 ◀
  intraligamentous O00.80 ◀≡
    with intrauterine pregnancy O00.81 ◀

◀ New   ◀≡ Revised   ~~deleted~~ Deleted

Pregnancy *(Continued)*
  complicated by *(Continued)*
    mural O00.80 ◄▥
      with intrauterine pregnancy O00.81 ◄
    ovarian O00.20 ◄▥
      with intrauterine pregnancy O00.21 ◄
    specified site NEC O00.80 ◄▥
      with intrauterine pregnancy O00.81 ◄
    tubal (ruptured) O00.10 ◄▥
      with intrauterine pregnancy O00.11 ◄
    examination (normal) Z34.9-
      first Z34.0-
      high-risk —*see* Pregnancy, supervision of, high-risk
      specified Z34.8-
    extrauterine —*see* Pregnancy, ectopic
    fallopian O00.10 ◄▥
      with intrauterine pregnancy O00.11 ◄
    false F45.8
    gestational carrier Z33.3 ◄
    hidden O09.3-
    high-risk —*see* Pregnancy, supervision of, high-risk
    incidental finding Z33.1
    interstitial O00.80 ◄▥
      with intrauterine pregnancy O00.81 ◄
    intraligamentous O00.80 ◄▥
      with intrauterine pregnancy O00.81 ◄
    intramural O00.80 ◄▥
      with intrauterine pregnancy O00.81 ◄
    intraperitoneal O00.00 ◄▥
      with intrauterine pregnancy O00.01 ◄
    isthmian O00.10 ◄▥
      with intrauterine pregnancy O00.11 ◄
    mesometric (mural) O00.80 ◄▥
      with intrauterine pregnancy O00.81 ◄
    molar NEC O02.0
      complicated (by) O08.9
        afibrinogenemia O08.1
        cardiac arrest O08.81
        chemical damage of pelvic organ (s) O08.6
        circulatory collapse O08.3
        defibrination syndrome O08.1
        electrolyte imbalance O08.5
        embolism (amniotic fluid) (blood clot) (pulmonary) (septic) O08.2
        endometritis O08.0
        genital tract and pelvic infection O08.0
        hemorrhage (delayed) (excessive) O08.1
        infection
          genital tract or pelvic O08.0
          kidney O08.83
          urinary tract O08.83
        intravascular coagulation O08.1
        laceration of pelvic organ (s) O08.6
        metabolic disorder O08.5
        oliguria O08.4
        oophoritis O08.0
        parametritis O08.0
        pelvic peritonitis O08.0
        perforation of pelvic organ (s) O08.6
        renal failure or shutdown O08.4
        salpingitis or salpingo-oophoritis O08.0
        sepsis O08.82
        shock O08.3
          septic O08.82
        specified condition NEC O08.89
        tubular necrosis (renal) O08.4
        uremia O08.4
        urinary infection O08.83
        venous complication NEC O08.7
          embolism O08.2
    hydatidiform —*see also* Mole, hydatidiform O01.9-
    multiple (gestation) O30.9-
      greater than quadruplets —*see* Pregnancy, multiple (gestation), specified NEC

Pregnancy *(Continued)*
  multiple (gestation) *(Continued)*
    specified NEC O30.80-
      with
        two or more monoamniotic fetuses O30.82-
        two or more monochorionic fetuses O30.81-
      two or more monoamniotic fetuses O30.82-
      two or more monochorionic fetuses O30.81-
      unable to determine number of placenta and number of amniotic sacs O30.89-
      unspecified number of placenta and unspecified number of amniotic sacs O30.80-
    mural O00.80 ◄▥
      with intrauterine pregnancy O00.81 ◄
    normal (supervision of) Z34.9-
      first Z34.0-
      high-risk —*see* Pregnancy, supervision of, high-risk
      specified Z34.8-
    ovarian O00.20 ◄▥
      with intrauterine pregnancy O00.21 ◄
    postmature (40 to 42 weeks) O48.0
      more than 42 weeks gestation O48.1
    post-term (40 to 42 weeks) O48.0
    prenatal care only Z34.9-
      first Z34.0-
      high-risk —*see* Pregnancy, supervision of, high-risk
      specified Z34.8-
    prolonged (more than 42 weeks gestation) O48.1
    quadruplet O30.20-
      with
        two or more monoamniotic fetuses O30.22-
        two or more monochorionic fetuses O30.21-
      two or more monoamniotic fetuses O30.22-
      two or more monochorionic fetuses O30.21-
      unable to determine number of placenta and number of amniotic sacs O30.29-
      unspecified number of placenta and unspecified number of amniotic sacs O30.20-
    quintuplet —*see* Pregnancy, multiple (gestation), specified NEC
    sextuplet —*see* Pregnancy, multiple (gestation), specified NEC
    supervision of
      concealed pregnancy O09.3-
      elderly mother
        multigravida O09.52-
        primigravida O09.51-
      hidden pregnancy O09.3-
      high-risk O09.9-
        due to (history of)
          ectopic pregnancy O09.1-
          elderly —*see* Pregnancy, supervision, elderly mother
          grand multiparity O09.4
          infertility O09.0-
          insufficient prenatal care O09.3-
          in utero procedure during previous pregnancy O09.82-
          in vitro fertilization O09.81-
          molar pregnancy O09.A- ◄▥
          multiple previous pregnancies O09.4-
          older mother —*see* Pregnancy, supervision of, elderly mother
          poor reproductive or obstetric history NEC O09.29-
          pre-term labor O09.21-
          previous
            neonatal death O09.29-

Pregnancy *(Continued)*
  supervision of *(Continued)*
    high-risk *(Continued)*
      due to *(Continued)*
        social problems O09.7-
        specified NEC O09.89-
        very young mother —*see* Pregnancy, supervision, young mother
      resulting from in vitro fertilization O09.81-
    normal Z34.9-
      first Z34.0-
      specified NEC Z34.8-
    young mother
      multigravida O09.62-
      primigravida O09.61-
  triplet O30.10-
    with
      two or more monoamniotic fetuses O30.12-
      two or more monochorionic fetuses O30.11-
    two or more monoamniotic fetuses O30.12-
    two or more monochorionic fetuses O30.11-
    unable to determine number of placenta and number of amniotic sacs O30.19-
    unspecified number of placenta and unspecified number of amniotic sacs O30.10-
  tubal (with abortion) (with rupture) O00.10 ◄▥
    with intrauterine pregnancy O00.11 ◄
  twin O30.00-
    conjoined O30.02-
    dichorionic/diamniotic (two placenta, two amniotic sacs) O30.04-
    monochorionic/diamniotic (one placenta, two amniotic sacs) O30.03-
    monochorionic/monoamniotic (one placenta, one amniotic sac) O30.01-
    unable to determine number of placenta and number of amniotic sacs O30.09-
    unspecified number of placenta and unspecified number of amniotic sacs O30.00-
  unwanted Z64.0
  weeks of gestation
    8 weeks Z3A.08
    9 weeks Z3A.09
    10 weeks Z3A.10
    11 weeks Z3A.11
    12 weeks Z3A.12
    13 weeks Z3A.13
    14 weeks Z3A.14
    15 weeks Z3A.15
    16 weeks Z3A.16
    17 weeks Z3A.17
    18 weeks Z3A.18
    19 weeks Z3A.19
    20 weeks Z3A.20
    21 weeks Z3A.21
    22 weeks Z3A.22
    23 weeks Z3A.23
    24 weeks Z3A.24
    25 weeks Z3A.25
    26 weeks Z3A.26
    27 weeks Z3A.27
    28 weeks Z3A.28
    29 weeks Z3A.29
    30 weeks Z3A.30
    31 weeks Z3A.31
    32 weeks Z3A.32
    33 weeks Z3A.33
    34 weeks Z3A.34
    35 weeks Z3A.35
    36 weeks Z3A.36
    37 weeks Z3A.37
    38 weeks Z3A.38
    39 weeks Z3A.39
    40 weeks Z3A.40
    41 weeks Z3A.41
    42 weeks Z3A.42

Pregnancy *(Continued)*
  weeks of gestation *(Continued)*
    greater than 42 weeks Z3A.49
    less than 8 weeks Z3A.01
    not specified Z3A.00
Preiser's disease —*see* Osteonecrosis,
  secondary, due to, trauma, metacarpus
Pre-kwashiorkor —*see* Malnutrition, severe
Preleukemia (syndrome) D46.9
Preluxation, hip, congenital Q65.6
Premature —*see also* condition
  adrenarche E27.0
  aging E34.8
  beats I49.40
    atrial I49.1
    auricular I49.1
    supraventricular I49.1
  birth NEC —*see* Preterm, newborn
  closure, foramen ovale Q21.8
  contraction
    atrial I49.1
    atrioventricular I49.49
    auricular I49.1
    auriculoventricular I49.2
    heart (extrasystole) I49.49
    junctional I49.2
    ventricular I49.3
  delivery —*see also* Pregnancy, complicated by,
    preterm labor O60.10
  ejaculation F52.4
  infant NEC —*see* Preterm, newborn
    light-for-dates —*see* Light for dates
  labor —*see* Pregnancy, complicated by,
    preterm labor
  lungs P28.0
  menopause E28.319
    asymptomatic E28.319
    symptomatic E28.310
  newborn
    extreme (less than 28 completed weeks) —
      see Immaturity, extreme
    less than 37 completed weeks —*see*
      Preterm, newborn
  puberty E30.1
  rupture membranes or amnion —*see*
    Pregnancy, complicated by, premature
    rupture of membranes
  senility E34.8
  thelarche E30.8
  ventricular systole I49.3
Prematurity NEC (less than 37 completed
  weeks) —*see* Preterm, newborn
  extreme (less than 28 completed weeks) —*see*
    Immaturity, extreme
Premenstrual
  dysphoric disorder (PMDD) F32.81 ◀▥
  tension (syndrome) N94.3
Premolarization, cuspids K00.2
Prenatal
  care, normal pregnancy —*see* Pregnancy,
    normal
  screening of mother Z36
  teeth K00.6
Preparatory care for subsequent treatment
  NEC
  for dialysis Z49.01
  peritoneal Z49.02
Prepartum —*see* condition
Preponderance, left or right ventricular I51.7
Prepuce —*see* condition
PRES (posterior reversible encephalopathy
  syndrome) I67.83
Presbycardia R54
Presbycusis, presbyacusia H91.1-
Presbyesophagus K22.8
Presbyophrenia F03
Presbyopia H52.4
Prescription of contraceptives (initial) Z30.019
  barrier Z30.018 ◀
  diaphragm Z30.018 ◀
  emergency (postcoital) Z30.012

Prescription of contraceptives *(Continued)*
  implantable subdermal Z30.017 ◀▥
  injectable Z30.013
  intrauterine contraceptive device Z30.014
  pills Z30.011
  postcoital (emergency) Z30.012
  repeat Z30.40
    barrier Z30.49 ◀
    diaphragm Z30.49 ◀
    implantable subdermal Z30.46 ◀▥
    injectable Z30.42
    pills Z30.41
    specified type NEC Z30.49
    transdermal patch hormonal Z30.45 ◀
    vaginal ring hormonal Z30.44 ◀
  specified type NEC Z30.018
    transdermal patch hormonal Z30.016 ◀
    vaginal ring hormonal Z30.015 ◀
Presence (of)
  ankle-joint implant (functional) (prosthesis)
    Z96.66-
  aortocoronary (bypass) graft Z95.1
  arterial-venous shunt (dialysis) Z99.2
  artificial
    eye (globe) Z97.0
    heart (fully implantable) (mechanical)
      Z95.812
      valve Z95.2
    larynx Z96.3
    lens (intraocular) Z96.1
    limb (complete) (partial) Z97.1-
      arm Z97.1-
        bilateral Z97.15
      leg Z97.1-
        bilateral Z97.16
  audiological implant (functional) Z96.29
  bladder implant (functional) Z96.0
  bone
    conduction hearing device Z96.29
    implant (functional) NEC Z96.7
    joint (prosthesis) —*see* Presence, joint
      implant
  cardiac
    defibrillator (functional) (with synchronous
      cardiac pacemaker)Z95.810
    implant or graft Z95.9
      specified type NEC Z95.818
    pacemaker Z95.0
    resynchronization therapy ◀
      defibrillator Z95.810 ◀
      pacemaker Z95.0 ◀
  cerebrospinal fluid drainage device Z98.2
  cochlear implant (functional) Z96.21
  contact lens (es) Z97.3
  coronary artery graft or prosthesis Z95.5
  CRT-D (cardiac resynchronization therapy
    defibrillator) Z95.810 ◀
  CRT-P (cardiac resynchronization therapy
    pacemaker) Z95.0 ◀
  cardioverter-defibrillator (ICD) Z95.810 ◀
  CSF shunt Z98.2
  dental prosthesis device Z97.2
  dentures Z97.2
  device (external) NEC Z97.8
    cardiac NEC Z95.818
    heart assist Z95.811
    implanted (functional) Z96.9
      specified NEC Z96.89
    prosthetic Z97.8
  ear implant Z96.20
    cochlear implant Z96.21
    myringotomy tube Z96.22
    specified type NEC Z96.29
  elbow-joint implant (functional) (prosthesis)
    Z96.62-
  endocrine implant (functional) NEC Z96.49
  eustachian tube stent or device (functional)
    Z96.29
  external hearing-aid or device Z97.4
  finger-joint implant (functional) (prosthetic)
    Z96.69-

Presence *(Continued)*
  functional implant Z96.9
    specified NEC Z96.89
  graft
    cardiac NEC Z95.818
    vascular NEC Z95.828
  hearing-aid or device (external) Z97.4
    implant (bone) (cochlear) (functional)
      Z96.21
  heart assist device Z95.811
  heart valve implant (functional) Z95.2
    prosthetic Z95.2
    specified type NEC Z95.4
    xenogenic Z95.3
  hip-joint implant (functional) (prosthesis)
    Z96.64-
  ICD (cardioverter-defibrillator) Z95.810 ◀
  implanted device (artificial) (functional)
    (prosthetic) Z96.9
    automatic cardiac defibrillator (with
      synchronous cardiac pacemaker)
      Z95.810
    cardiac pacemaker Z95.0
    cochlear Z96.21
    dental Z96.5
    heart Z95.812
    heart valve Z95.2
      prosthetic Z95.2
      specified NEC Z95.4
      xenogenic Z95.3
    insulin pump Z96.41
    intraocular lens Z96.1
    joint Z96.60
      ankle Z96.66-
      elbow Z96.62-
      finger Z96.69-
      hip Z96.64-
      knee Z96.65-
      shoulder Z96.61-
      specified NEC Z96.698
      wrist Z96.63-
    larynx Z96.3
    myringotomy tube Z96.22
    otological Z96.20
      cochlear Z96.21
      eustachian stent Z96.29
      myringotomy Z96.22
      specified NEC Z96.29
      stapes Z96.29
    skin Z96.81
    skull plate Z96.7
    specified NEC Z96.89
    urogenital Z96.0
  insulin pump (functional) Z96.41
  intestinal bypass or anastomosis Z98.0
  intraocular lens (functional) Z96.1
  intrauterine contraceptive device (IUD) Z97.5
  intravascular implant (functional) (prosthetic)
    NEC Z95.9
    coronary artery Z95.5
    defibrillator (with synchronous cardiac
      pacemaker) Z95.810
    peripheral vessel (with angioplasty)
      Z95.820
  joint implant (prosthetic) (any) Z96.60
    ankle —*see* Presence, ankle joint implant
    elbow —*see* Presence, elbow joint implant
    finger —*see* Presence, finger joint implant
    hip —*see* Presence, hip joint implant
    knee —*see* Presence, knee joint implant
    shoulder —*see* Presence, shoulder joint
      implant
    specified joint NEC Z96.698
    wrist —*see* Presence, wrist joint implant
  knee-joint implant (functional) (prosthesis)
    Z96.65-
  laryngeal implant (functional) Z96.3
  mandibular implant (dental) Z96.5
  myringotomy tube (s) Z96.22
  orthopedic-joint implant (prosthetic) (any) —
    see Presence, joint implant

◀ New   ◀▥ Revised   ~~deleted~~ Deleted

Presence *(Continued)*
  otological implant (functional) Z96.29
  shoulder-joint implant (functional)
    (prosthesis) Z96.61-
  skull-plate implant Z96.7
  spectacles Z97.3
  stapes implant (functional) Z96.29
  systemic lupus erythematosus [SLE] inhibitor
    D68.62
  tendon implant (functional) (graft) Z96.7
  tooth root (s) implant Z96.5
  ureteral stent Z96.0
  urethral stent Z96.0
  urogenital implant (functional) Z96.0
  vascular implant or device Z95.9
    access port device Z95.828
    specified type NEC Z95.828
  wrist-joint implant (functional) (prosthesis)
    Z96.63-
Presenile —*see also* condition
  dementia F03
  premature aging E34.8
Presentation, fetal —*see* Delivery, complicated
  by, malposition
Prespondylolisthesis (congenital) Q76.2
Pressure
  area, skin —*see* Ulcer, pressure, by site
  brachial plexus G54.0
  brain G93.5
    injury at birth NEC P11.1
  cerebral —*see* Pressure, brain
  chest R07.89
  cone, tentorial G93.5
  hyposystolic —*see also* Hypotension
    incidental reading, without diagnosis of
      hypotension R03.1
  increased
    intracranial (benign) G93.2
      injury at birth P11.0
    intraocular H40.05-
  lumbosacral plexus G54.1
  mediastinum J98.59 ◄▥
  necrosis (chronic) —*see* Ulcer, pressure,
    by site
  parental, inappropriate (excessive) Z62.6
  sore (chronic) —*see* Ulcer, pressure,
    by site
  spinal cord G95.20
  ulcer (chronic) —*see* Ulcer, pressure,
    by site
  venous, increased I87.8
Pre-syncope R55
Preterm
  delivery (see also Pregnancy, complicated by,
    preterm labor) O60.10
  labor —*see* Pregnancy, complicated by,
    preterm labor
  newborn (infant) P07.30
    gestational age
      28 completed weeks (28 weeks, 0 days
        through 28 weeks, 6 days) P07.31
      29 completed weeks (29 weeks, 0 days
        through 29 weeks, 6 days) P07.32
      30 completed weeks (30 weeks, 0 days
        through 30 weeks, 6 days) P07.33
      31 completed weeks (31 weeks, 0 days
        through 31 weeks, 6 days) P07.34
      32 completed weeks (32 weeks, 0 days
        through 32 weeks, 6 days) P07.35
      33 completed weeks (33 weeks, 0 days
        through 33 weeks, 6 days) P07.36
      34 completed weeks (34 weeks, 0 days
        through 34 weeks, 6 days) P07.37
      35 completed weeks (35 weeks, 0 days
        through 35 weeks, 6 days) P07.38
      36 completed weeks (36 weeks, 0 days
        through 36 weeks, 6 days) P07.39
Previa
  placenta (total) (without hemorrhage)
    O44.0- ◄▥
    ~~without hemorrhage O44.0-~~

Previa *(Continued)*
  placenta *(Continued)*
    with hemorrhage O44.1- ◄
    complete O44.0- ◄
      with hemorrhage O44.1- ◄
    low —*see also* Delivery, complicated, by,
      placenta, low O44.4- ◄
      with hemorrhage O44.5- ◄
    marginal O44.2- ◄
      with hemorrhage O44.3- ◄
    partial O44.2- ◄
      with hemorrhage O44.3- ◄
  vasa O69.4
Priapism N48.30
  due to
    disease classified elsewhere N48.32
    drug N48.33
    specified cause NEC N48.39
    trauma N48.31
Prickling sensation (skin) R20.2
Prickly heat L74.0
Primary —*see* condition
Primigravida
  elderly, affecting management of pregnancy,
    labor and delivery (supervision only) —
    see Pregnancy, complicated by, elderly,
    primigravida
  older, affecting management of pregnancy,
    labor and delivery (supervision only) —
    see Pregnancy, complicated by, elderly,
    primigravida
  very young, affecting management of
    pregnancy, labor and delivery
    (supervision only) —*see* Pregnancy,
    complicated by, young mother,
    primigravida
Primipara
  elderly, affecting management of pregnancy,
    labor and delivery (supervision only) —
    see Pregnancy, complicated by, elderly,
    primigravida
  older, affecting management of pregnancy,
    labor and delivery (supervision only) —
    see Pregnancy, complicated by, elderly,
    primigravida
  very young, affecting management of
    pregnancy, labor and delivery
    (supervision only) —*see* Pregnancy,
    complicated by, young mother,
    primigravida
Primus varus (bilateral) Q66.2
PRIND (Prolonged reversible ischemic
  neurologic deficit) I63.9
Pringle's disease (tuberous sclerosis)Q85.1
Prinzmetal angina I20.1
Prizefighter ear —*see* Cauliflower ear
Problem (with) (related to)
  academic Z55.8
  acculturation Z60.3
  adjustment (to)
    change of job Z56.1
    life-cycle transition Z60.0
    pension Z60.0
    retirement Z60.0
  adopted child Z62.821
  alcoholism in family Z63.72
  atypical parenting situation Z62.9
  bankruptcy Z59.8
  behavioral (adult) F69
    drug seeking Z76.5 ◄▥
  birth of sibling affecting child Z62.898
  care (of)
    provider dependency Z74.9
      specified NEC Z74.8
    sick or handicapped person in family or
      household Z63.6
  child
    abuse (affecting the child) —*see*
      Maltreatment, child
    custody or support proceedings Z65.3
    in care of non-parental family member
      Z62.21

Problem *(Continued)*
  child *(Continued)*
    in foster care Z62.21
    in welfare custody Z62.21
    living in orphanage or group home Z62.22
  child-rearing Z62.9
    specified NEC Z62.898
  communication (developmental) F80.9
  conflict or discord (with)
    boss Z56.4
    classmates Z55.4
    counselor Z64.4
    employer Z56.4
    family Z63.9
      specified NEC Z63.8
    probation officer Z64.4
    social worker Z64.4
    teachers Z55.4
    workmates Z56.4
  conviction in legal proceedings Z65.0
    with imprisonment Z65.1
  counselor Z64.4
  creditors Z59.8
  digestive K92.9
  drug addict in family Z63.72
  ear —*see* Disorder, ear
  economic Z59.9
    affecting care Z59.9
    specified NEC Z59.8
  education Z55.9
    specified NEC Z55.8
  employment Z56.9
    change of job Z56.1
    discord Z56.4
    environment Z56.5
    sexual harassment Z56.81
    specified NEC Z56.89
    stress NEC Z56.6
    stressful schedule Z56.3
    threat of job loss Z56.2
    unemployment Z56.0
  enuresis, child F98.0
  eye H57.9
  failed examinations (school) Z55.2
  falling Z91.81
  family —*see also* Disruption, family Z63.9-
    specified NEC Z63.8
  feeding (elderly) (infant) R63.3
    newborn P92.9
      breast P92.5
      overfeeding P92.4
      slow P92.2
      specified NEC P92.8
      underfeeding P92.3
    nonorganic F50.89 ◄▥
  finance Z59.9
    specified NEC Z59.8
  foreclosure on loan Z59.8
  foster child Z62.822
  frightening experience (s) in childhood
    Z62.898
  genital NEC
    female N94.9
    male N50.9
  health care Z75.9
    specified NEC Z75.8
  hearing —*see* Deafness
  homelessness Z59.0
  housing Z59.9
    inadequate Z59.1
    isolated Z59.8
    specified NEC Z59.8
  identity (of childhood) F93.8
  illegitimate pregnancy (unwanted) Z64.0
  illiteracy Z55.0
  impaired mobility Z74.09
  imprisonment or incarceration Z65.1
  inadequate teaching affecting education
    Z55.8
  inappropriate (excessive) parental pressure
    Z62.6

Problem (Continued)
 influencing health status NEC Z78.9
 in-law Z63.1
 institutionalization, affecting child
  Z62.22
 intrafamilial communication Z63.8
 jealousy, child F93.8
 landlord Z59.2
 language (developmental) F80.9
 learning (developmental) F81.9
 legal Z65.3
  conviction without imprisonment
   Z65.0
  imprisonment Z65.1
  release from prison Z65.2
 life-management Z73.9
  specified NEC Z73.89
 life-style Z72.9
  gambling Z72.6
  high-risk sexual behavior (heterosexual)
   Z72.51
   bisexual Z72.53
   homosexual Z72.52
  inappropriate eating habits Z72.4
  self-damaging behavior NEC Z72.89
  specified NEC Z72.89
  tobacco use Z72.0
 literacy Z55.9
  low level Z55.0
  specified NEC Z55.8
 living alone Z60.2
 lodgers Z59.2
 loss of love relationship in childhood
  Z62.898
 marital Z63.0
  involving
   divorce Z63.5
   estrangement Z63.5
   gender identity F66
 mastication K08.89
 medical
  care, within family Z63.6
  facilities Z75.9
   specified NEC Z75.8
 mental F48.9
 multiparity Z64.1
 negative life events in childhood Z62.9
  altered pattern of family relationships
   Z62.898
  frightening experience Z62.898
  loss of
   love relationship Z62.898
   self-esteem Z62.898
  physical abuse (alleged) —see
   Maltreatment, child
  removal from home Z62.29
  specified event NEC Z62.898
 neighbor Z59.2
 neurological NEC R29.818
 new step-parent affecting child Z62.898
 none (feared complaint unfounded)
  Z71.1
 occupational NEC Z56.89
 parent-child —see Conflict, parent-child
 personal hygiene Z91.89
 personality F69
 phase-of-life transition, adjustment Z60.0
 presence of sick or disabled person in family
  or household Z63.79
  needing care Z63.6
 primary support group (family) Z63.9
  specified NEC Z63.8
 probation officer Z64.4
 psychiatric F99
 psychosexual (development) F66
 psychosocial Z65.9
  specified NEC Z65.8
 relationship Z63.9
  childhood F93.8
 release from prison Z65.2
 removal from home affecting child Z62.29

Problem (Continued)
 seeking and accepting known hazardous and
  harmful
  behavioral or psychological interventions
   Z65.8
  chemical, nutritional or physical
   interventions Z65.8
 sexual function (nonorganic) F52.9
 sight H54.7
 sleep disorder, child F51.9
 smell —see Disturbance, sensation, smell
 social
  environment Z60.9
   specified NEC Z60.8
  exclusion and rejection Z60.4
  worker Z64.4
 speech R47.9
  developmental F80.9
  specified NEC R47.89
 swallowing —see Dysphagia
 taste —see Disturbance, sensation, taste
 tic, child F95.0
 underachievement in school Z55.3
 unemployment Z56.0
  threatened Z56.2
 unwanted pregnancy Z64.0
 upbringing Z62.9
  specified NEC Z62.898
 urinary N39.9
 voice production R47.89
 work schedule (stressful) Z56.3
Procedure (surgical)
 converted ◀
  arthroscopic to open Z53.33 ◀
  laparoscopic to open Z53.31 ◀
  specified procedure NEC to open
   Z53.39 ◀
  thoracoscopic to open Z53.32 ◀
 for purpose other than remedying health
  state Z41.9
  specified NEC Z41.8
 not done Z53.9
  because of
   administrative reasons Z53.8
   contraindication Z53.09
    smoking Z53.01
   patient's decision Z53.20
    for reasons of belief or group pressure
     Z53.1
    left against medical advice (AMA)
     Z53.21
   specified reason NEC Z53.29
  specified reason NEC Z53.8
Procidentia (uteri) N81.3
Proctalgia K62.89
 fugax K59.4
 spasmodic K59.4
Proctitis K62.89
 amebic (acute) A06.0
 chlamydial A56.3
 gonococcal A54.6
 granulomatous —see Enteritis, regional, large
  intestine
 herpetic A60.1
 radiation K62.7
 tuberculous A18.32
 ulcerative (chronic) K51.20
  with
   complication K51.219
    abscess K51.214
    fistula K51.213
    obstruction K51.212
    rectal bleeding K51.211
    specified NEC K51.218
Proctocele
 female (without uterine prolapse) N81.6
  with uterine prolapse N81.2
   complete N81.3
 male K62.3
Proctocolitis, mucosal —see Rectosigmoiditis,
 ulcerative

Proctocolitis ◀
 food-induced eosinophilic K52.82 ◀
 food protein-induced K52.82 ◀
 milk protein-induced K52.82 ◀
 mucosal —see Rectosigmoiditis, ulcerative ◀
Proctoptosis K62.3
Proctorrhagia K62.5
Proctosigmoiditis K63.89
 ulcerative (chronic) —see Rectosigmoiditis,
  ulcerative
Proctospasm K59.4
 psychogenic F45.8
Profichet's disease —see Disorder, soft tissue,
 specified type NEC
Progeria E34.8
Prognathism (mandibular) (maxillary) M26.19
Progonoma (melanotic) —see Neoplasm,
 benign, by site
Progressive —see condition
Prolactinoma
 specified site —see Neoplasm, benign,
  by site
 unspecified site D35.2
Prolapse, prolapsed
 anus, anal (canal) (sphincter) K62.2
 arm or hand O32.2
  causing obstructed labor O64.4
 bladder (mucosa) (sphincter) (acquired)
  congenital Q79.4
  female —see Cystocele
  male N32.89
 breast implant (prosthetic) T85.49
 cecostomy K94.09
 cecum K63.4
 cervix, cervical (hypertrophied) N81.2
  anterior lip, obstructing labor O65.5
  congenital Q51.828
  postpartal, old N81.2
  stump N81.85
 ciliary body (traumatic) —see Laceration,
  eye(ball), with prolapse or loss of
  interocular tissue
 colon (pedunculated) K63.4
 colostomy K94.09
 disc (intervertebral) —see Displacement,
  intervertebral disc
 eye implant (orbital) T85.398
  lens (ocular) —see Complications,
   intraocular lens
 fallopian tube N83.4-
 gastric (mucosa) K31.89
 genital, female N81.9
  specified NEC N81.89
 globe, nontraumatic —see Luxation, globe
 ileostomy bud K94.19
 intervertebral disc —see Displacement,
  intervertebral disc
 intestine (small) K63.4
 iris (traumatic) —see Laceration, eye(ball),
  with prolapse or loss of interocular
  tissue
  nontraumatic H21.89
 kidney N28.83
  congenital Q63.2
 laryngeal muscles or ventricle J38.7
 liver K76.89
 meatus urinarius N36.8
 mitral (valve) I34.1
 ocular lens implant —see Complications,
  intraocular lens
 organ or site, congenital NEC —see
  Malposition, congenital
 ovary N83.4-
 pelvic floor, female N81.89
 perineum, female N81.89
 rectum (mucosa) (sphincter) K62.3
  due to trichuris trichuria B79
 spleen D73.89
 stomach K31.89
 umbilical cord
  complicating delivery O69.0

Prolapse, prolapsed (Continued)
  urachus, congenital Q64.4
  ureter N28.89
    with obstruction N13.5
      with infection N13.6
  ureterovesical orifice N28.89
  urethra (acquired) (infected) (mucosa)
      N36.8
    congenital Q64.71
  urinary meatus N36.8
    congenital Q64.72
  uterovaginal N81.4
    complete N81.3
    incomplete N81.2
  uterus (with prolapse of vagina) N81.4
    complete N81.3
    congenital Q51.818
    first degree N81.2
    in pregnancy or childbirth —see
        Pregnancy, complicated by,
        abnormal, uterus
    incomplete N81.2
    postpartal (old) N81.4
    second degree N81.2
    third degree N81.3
  uveal (traumatic) —see Laceration, eye(ball),
      with prolapse or loss of interocular
      tissue
  vagina (anterior) (wall) —see Cystocele
    with prolapse of uterus N81.4
      complete N81.3
      incomplete N81.2
    posterior wall N81.6
    posthysterectomy N99.3
  vitreous (humor) H43.0-
    in wound —see Laceration, eye(ball), with
        prolapse or loss of interocular tissue
  womb —see Prolapse, uterus
Prolapsus, female N81.9
  specified NEC N81.89
Proliferation (s)
  primary cutaneous CD30-positive large T-cell
      C86.6
  prostate, atypical small acinar N42.32 ◄
Proliferative —see condition
Prolonged, prolongation (of)
  bleeding (time) (idiopathic) R79.1
  coagulation (time) R79.1
  gestation (over 42 completed weeks)
    mother O48.1
    newborn P08.22
  interval I44.0
  labor O63.9
    first stage O63.0
    second stage O63.1
  partial thromboplastin time (PTT) R79.1
  pregnancy (more than 42 weeks gestation)
      O48.1
  prothrombin time R79.1
  QT interval I45.81
  uterine contractions in labor O62.4
Prominence, prominent
  with disproportion (fetopelvic) O33.0
    causing obstructed labor O65.0
  auricle (congenital) (ear) Q17.5
  ischial spine or sacral promontory
  nose (congenital) acquired M95.0
Promiscuity —see High, risk, sexual behavior
Pronation
  ankle —see Deformity, limb, foot, specified
      NEC
  foot —see also Deformity, limb, foot, specified
      NEC
    congenital Q74.2
Prophylactic
  administration of
    antibiotics, long-term Z79.2
      short-term use - omit code
    drug —see also Long-term (current) drug
        therapy (use of) Z79.899-
  medication Z79.899

Prophylactic (Continued)
  organ removal (for neoplasia management)
      Z40.00
    breast Z40.01
    ovary Z40.02
    specified site NEC Z40.09
  surgery Z40.9
    for risk factors related to malignant
        neoplasm —see Prophylactic, organ
        removal
    specified NEC Z40.8
  vaccination Z23
Propionic acidemia E71.121
Proptosis (ocular) —see also Exophthalmos
  thyroid —see Hyperthyroidism, with goiter
Prosection, anxiety concerning Z65.3
Prosopagnosia R48.3
Prostadynia N42.81
Prostate, prostatic —see condition
Prostatism —see Hyperplasia, prostate
Prostatitis (congestive) (suppurative) (with
    cystitis) N41.9
  acute N41.0
  cavitary N41.8
  chronic N41.1
  diverticular N41.8
  due to Trichomonas (vaginalis) A59.02
  fibrous N41.1
  gonococcal (acute) (chronic) A54.22
  granulomatous N41.4
  hypertrophic N41.1
  subacute N41.1
  trichomonal A59.02
  tuberculous A18.14
Prostatocystitis N41.3
Prostatorrhea N42.89
Prostatosis N42.82
Prostration R53.83
  heat —see also Heat, exhaustion
    anhydrotic T67.3
    due to
      salt (and water) depletion T67.4
      water depletion T67.3
  nervous F48.8
  senile R54
Protanomaly (anomalous trichromat) H53.54
Protanopia (complete) (incomplete) H53.54
Protection (against) (from) —see Prophylactic
Protein
  deficiency NEC —see Malnutrition
  malnutrition —see Malnutrition
  sickness —see also Reaction, serum T80.69
Proteinemia R77.9
Proteinosis
  alveolar (pulmonary) J84.01
  lipid or lipoid (of Urbach) E78.89
Proteinuria R80.9
  Bence Jones R80.3
  complicating pregnancy —see Proteinuria,
      gestational
  gestational ◄▥
    with edema O12.2-
    complicating ◄
      childbirth O12.14 ◄
      pregnancy O12.1- ◄
        with edema O12.2- ◄
      puerperium O12.15 ◄
  idiopathic R80.0
  isolated R80.0
    with glomerular lesion N06.9
      dense deposit disease N06.6
      diffuse
        crescentic glomerulonephritis
            N06.7
        endocapillary proliferative
            glomerulonephritis N06.4
        mesangiocapillary glomerulonephritis
            N06.5
        focal and segmental hyalinosis or
            sclerosis N06.1
        membranous (diffuse) N06.2

Proteinuria (Continued)
  isolated (Continued)
    with glomerular lesion (Continued)
      mesangial proliferative (diffuse) N06.3
      minimal change N06.0
      specified pathology NEC N06.8
  orthostatic R80.2
    with glomerular lesion —see Proteinuria,
        isolated, with glomerular lesion
  persistent R80.1
    with glomerular lesion —see Proteinuria,
        isolated, with glomerular lesion
  postural R80.2
    with glomerular lesion —see Proteinuria,
        isolated, with glomerular lesion
  pre-eclamptic —see Pre-eclampsia
  puerperal O12.15 ◄
  specified type NEC R80.8
Proteolysis, pathologic D65
Proteus (mirabilis) (morganii), as cause of
    disease classified elsewhere B96.4
Prothrombin gene mutation D68.52
Protoporphyria, erythropoietic E80.0
Protozoal —see also condition
  disease B64
    specified NEC B60.8
Protrusion, protrusio
  acetabuli M24.7
  acetabulum (into pelvis) M24.7
  device, implant or graft —see also
      Complications, by site and type,
      mechanical T85.698
    arterial graft NEC —see Complication,
        cardiovascular device, mechanical,
        vascular
    breast (implant) T85.49
    catheter NEC T85.698
      cystostomy T83.090
      dialysis (renal) T82.49
        intraperitoneal T85.691
      infusion NEC T82.594
        spinal (epidural) (subdural)
            T85.690
      urinary, indwelling T83.098
      urinary —see also Complications,
          catheter, urinary T83.098 ◄
    electronic (electrode) (pulse generator)
        (stimulator)
      bone T84.390
      nervous system —see Complication,
          prosthetic device, mechanical,
          electronic nervous system
          stimulator
    fixation, internal (orthopedic) NEC —see
        Complication, fixation device,
        mechanical
    gastrointestinal —see Complications,
        prosthetic device, mechanical,
        gastrointestinal device
    genital NEC T83.498
      intrauterine contraceptive device
          T83.39
      penile prosthesis (cylinder) (implanted)
          (pump) (resevoir) T83.490 ◄▥
      testicular prosthesis T83.491 ◄
    heart NEC —see Complication,
        cardiovascular device, mechanical
    joint prosthesis —see Complications, joint
        prosthesis, mechanical, specified
        NEC, by site
    ocular NEC —see Complications, prosthetic
        device, mechanical, ocular device
    orthopedic NEC —see Complication,
        orthopedic, device, mechanical
    specified NEC T85.628
    urinary NEC —see also Complication,
        genitourinary, device, urinary,
        mechanical
      graft T83.29
    vascular NEC —see Complication,
        cardiovascular device, mechanical

Protrusion, protrusio (Continued)
  device, implant or graft (Continued)
    ventricular intracranial shunt T85.09
  intervertebral disc —see Displacement,
      intervertebral disc
  joint prosthesis —see Complications, joint
      prosthesis, mechanical, specified NEC,
      by site
  nucleus pulposus —see Displacement,
      intervertebral disc
Prune belly (syndrome) Q79.4
Prurigo (ferox) (gravis) (Hebrae) (Hebra's)
    (mitis) (simplex) L28.2
  Besnier's L20.0
  estivalis L56.4
  nodularis L28.1
  psychogenic F45.8
Pruritus, pruritic (essential) L29.9
  ani, anus L29.0
    psychogenic F45.8
  anogenital L29.3
    psychogenic F45.8
  due to onchocerca volvulus B73.1
  gravidarum —see Pregnancy, complicated by,
      specified pregnancy-related condition
      NEC
  hiemalis L29.8
  neurogenic (any site) F45.8
  perianal L29.0
  psychogenic (any site) F45.8
  scroti, scrotum L29.1
    psychogenic F45.8
  senile, senilis L29.8
  specified NEC L29.8
    psychogenic F45.8
  Trichomonas A59.9
  vulva, vulvae L29.2
    psychogenic F45.8
Pseudarthrosis, pseudoarthrosis (bone) —see
    Nonunion, fracture
  clavicle, congenital Q74.0
  joint, following fusion or arthrodesis
      M96.0
Pseudoaneurysm —see Aneurysm
Pseudoangina (pectoris) —see Angina
Pseudoangioma I81
Pseudoarteriosus Q28.8
Pseudoarthrosis —see Pseudarthrosis
Pseudobulbar affect (PBA) F48.2
Pseudochromhidrosis L67.8
Pseudocirrhosis, liver, pericardial I31.1
Pseudocowpox B08.03
Pseudocoxalgia M91.3-
Pseudocroup J38.5
Pseudo-Cushing's syndrome, alcohol-induced
    E24.4
Pseudocyesis F45.8
Pseudocyst
  lung J98.4
  pancreas K86.3
  retina —see Cyst, retina
Pseudoelephantiasis neuroarthritica Q82.0
Pseudoexfoliation, capsule (lens) —see
    Cataract, specified NEC
Pseudofolliculitis barbae L73.1
Pseudoglioma H44.89
Pseudohemophilia (Bernuth's) (hereditary)
    (type B) D68.0
  Type A D69.8
  vascular D69.8
Pseudohermaphroditism Q56.3
  adrenal E25.8
  female Q56.2
    with adrenocortical disorder E25.8
    without adrenocortical disorder Q56.2
    adrenal, congenital E25.0
    adrenal (congenital) E25.0 ◄
  male Q56.1
    with
      adrenocortical disorder E25.8
      androgen resistance E34.51

Pseudohermaphroditism (Continued)
  male (Continued)
    with (Continued)
      cleft scrotum Q56.1
      feminizing testis E34.51
      5-alpha-reductase deficiency E29.1
    without gonadal disorder Q56.1
    adrenal E25.8
Pseudo-Hurler's polydystrophy E77.0
Pseudohydrocephalus G93.2
Pseudohypertrophic muscular dystrophy
    (Erb's) G71.0
Pseudohypertrophy, muscle G71.0
Pseudohypoparathyroidism E20.1
Pseudoinsomnia F51.03
Pseudoleukemia, infantile D64.89
Pseudomembranous —see condition
Pseudomeningocele (cerebral) (infective) (post-
    traumatic) G96.19
  postprocedural (spinal) G97.82
Pseudomenses (newborn) P54.6
Pseudomenstruation (newborn) P54.6
Pseudomonas
  aeruginosa, as cause of disease classified
      elsewhere B96.5
  mallei infection A24.0
    as cause of disease classified elsewhere
      B96.5
  pseudomallei, as cause of disease classified
      elsewhere B96.5
Pseudomyotonia G71.19
Pseudomyxoma peritonei C78.6
Pseudoneuritis, optic (nerve) (disc) (papilla),
    congenital Q14.2
Pseudo-obstruction intestine (acute) (chronic)
    (idiopathic) (intermittent secondary)
    (primary) K59.8
Pseudopapilledema H47.33-
  congenital Q14.2
Pseudoparalysis
  arm or leg R29.818
  atonic, congenital P94.2
Pseudopelade L66.0
Pseudophakia Z96.1
Pseudopolyarthritis, rhizomelic M35.3
Pseudopolycythemia D75.1
Pseudopseudohypoparathyroidism
    E20.1
Pseudopterygium H11.81-
Pseudoptosis (eyelid) —see Blepharochalasis
Pseudopuberty, precocious
  female heterosexual E25.8
  male isosexual E25.8
Pseudorickets (renal) N25.0
Pseudorubella B08.20
Pseudoscrema, newborn P83.8
Pseudosclerosis (brain)
  Jakob's —see Creutzfeldt-Jakob disease or
      syndrome
  of Westphal (Strüümpell) E83.01
  spastic —see Creutzfeldt-Jakob disease or
      syndrome
Pseudotetanus —see Convulsions
Pseudotetany R29.0
  hysterical F44.5
Pseudotruncus arteriosus Q25.49 ◄▥▥
Pseudotuberculosis A28.2
  enterocolitis A04.8
  pasteurella (infection) A28.0
Pseudotumor
  cerebri G93.2
  orbital H05.11-
Pseudoxanthoma elasticum Q82.8
Psilosis (sprue) (tropical) K90.1
  nontropical K90.0
Psittacosis A70
Psoitis M60.88
Psoriasis L40.9
  arthropathic L40.50
    arthritis mutilans L40.52
    distal interphalangeal L40.51

Psoriasis (Continued)
  arthropathic (Continued)
    juvenile L40.54
    other specified L40.59
    spondylitis L40.53
  buccal K13.29
  flexural L40.8
  guttate L40.4
  mouth K13.29
  nummular L40.0
  plaque L40.0
  psychogenic F54
  pustular (generalized) L40.1
    palmaris et plantaris L40.3
  specified NEC L40.8
  vulgaris L40.0
Psychasthenia F48.8
Psychiatric disorder or problem F99
Psychogenic —see also condition
  factors associated with physical conditions
      F54
Psychological and behavioral factors affecting
    medical condition F59
Psychoneurosis, psychoneurotic —see also
    Neurosis
  anxiety (state) F41.1
  depersonalization F48.1
  hypochondriacal F45.21
  hysteria F44.9
  neurasthenic F48.8
  personality NEC F60.89
Psychopathy, psychopathic
  affectionless F94.2
  autistic F84.5
  constitution, post-traumatic F07.81
  personality —see Disorder, personality
  sexual —see Deviation, sexual
  state F60.2
Psychosexual identity disorder of childhood
    F64.2
Psychosis, psychotic F29
  acute (transient) F23
    hysterical F44.9
  affective —see Disorder, mood
  alcoholic F10.959
    with
      abuse F10.159
      anxiety disorder F10.980
        with
          abuse F10.180
          dependence F10.280
      delirium tremens F10.231
      delusions F10.950
        with
          abuse F10.150
          dependence F10.250
      dementia F10.97
        with dependence F10.27
      dependence F10.259
      hallucinosis F10.951
        with
          abuse F10.151
          dependence F10.251
      mood disorder F10.94
        with
          abuse F10.14
          dependence F10.24
      paranoia F10.950
        with
          abuse F10.150
          dependence F10.250
      persisting amnesia F10.96
        with dependence F10.26
    amnestic confabulatory F10.96
      with dependence F10.26
    delirium tremens F10.231
    Korsakoff's, Korsakov's, Korsakow's F10.26
    paranoid type F10.950
      with
        abuse F10.150
        dependence F10.250

◄ New   ◄▥▥ Revised   ~~deleted~~ Deleted

Psychosis, psychotic (Continued)
anergastic —see Psychosis, organic
arteriosclerotic (simple type) (uncomplicated)
F01.50
with behavioral disturbance F01.51
childhood F84.0
atypical F84.8
climacteric —see Psychosis, involutional
confusional F29
acute or subacute F05
reactive F23
cycloid F23
depressive —see Disorder, depressive
disintegrative (childhood) F84.3
drug-induced —see F11-F19 with .x59
paranoid and hallucinatory states —see
F11-F19 with .x50 or .x51
due to or associated with
addiction, drug —see F11-F19 with .X59
dependence
alcohol F10.259
drug —see F11-F19 with .x59
epilepsy F06.8
Huntington's chorea F06.8
ischemia, cerebrovascular (generalized)
F06.8
multiple sclerosis F06.8
physical disease F06.8
presenile dementia F03
senile dementia F03
vascular disease (arteriosclerotic) (cerebral)
F01.50
with behavioral disturbance F01.51
epileptic F06.8
episode F23
due to or associated with physical
condition F06.8
exhaustive F43.0
hallucinatory, chronic F28
hypomanic F30.8
hysterical (acute) F44.9
induced F24
infantile F84.0
atypical F84.8
infective (acute) (subacute) F05
involutional F28
depressive —see Disorder, depressive
melancholic —see Disorder, depressive
paranoid (state) F22
Korsakoff's, Korsakov's, Korsakow's
(nonalcoholic) F04
alcoholic F10.96
in dependence F10.26
induced by other psychoactive
substance —see categories F11-F19
with .x5x
mania, manic (single episode) F30.2
recurrent type F31.89
manic-depressive —see Disorder, bipolar ◀▥
menopausal —see Psychosis, involutional
mixed schizophrenic and affective F25.8
multi-infarct (cerebrovascular) F01.50
with behavioral disturbance F01.51
nonorganic F29
specified NEC F28
organic F09
due to or associated with
arteriosclerosis (cerebral) —see
Psychosis, arteriosclerotic
cerebrovascular disease,
arteriosclerotic —see Psychosis,
arteriosclerotic
childbirth —see Psychosis, puerperal
Creutzfeldt-Jakob disease or
syndrome —see Creutzfeldt-Jakob
disease or syndrome
dependence, alcohol F10.259
disease
alcoholic liver F10.259
brain, arteriosclerotic —see Psychosis,
arteriosclerotic

Psychosis, psychotic (Continued)
organic (Continued)
due to or associated with (Continued)
disease (Continued)
cerebrovascular F01.50
with behavioral disturbance
F01.51
Creutzfeldt-Jakob —see Creutzfeldt-
Jakob disease or syndrome
endocrine or metabolic F06.8
acute or subacute F05
liver, alcoholic F10.259
epilepsy transient (acute) F05
infection
brain (intracranial) F06.8
acute or subacute F05
intoxication
alcoholic (acute) F10.259
drug F19 with .X59 F11-
ischemia, cerebrovascular (generalized) —
see Psychosis, arteriosclerotic
puerperium —see Psychosis, puerperal
trauma, brain (birth) (from electric
current) (surgical) F06.8
acute or subacute F05
infective F06.8
acute or subacute F05
post-traumatic F06.8
acute or subacute F05
paranoiac F22
paranoid (climacteric) (involutional)
(menopausal) F22
psychogenic (acute) F23
schizophrenic F20.0
senile F03
postpartum F53
presbyophrenic (type) F03
presenile F03
psychogenic (paranoid) F23
depressive F32.3
puerperal F53
specified type —see Psychosis, by type
reactive (brief) (transient) (emotional stress)
(psychological trauma) F23
depressive F32.3
recurrent F33.3
excitative type F30.8
schizoaffective F25.9
depressive type F25.1
manic type F25.0
schizophrenia, schizophrenic —see
Schizophrenia
schizophrenia-like, in epilepsy F06.2
schizophreniform F20.81
affective type F25.9
brief F23
confusional type F23
depressive type F25.1
manic type F25.0
mixed type F25.0
senile NEC F03
depressed or paranoid type F03
simple deterioration F03
specified type — code to condition
shared F24
situational (reactive) F23
symbiotic (childhood) F84.3
symptomatic F09
Psychosomatic —see Disorder, psychosomatic
Psychosyndrome, organic F07.9
Psychotic episode due to or associated with
physical condition F06.8
Pterygium (eye) H11.00-
amyloid H11.01-
central H11.02-
colli Q18.3
double H11.03-
peripheral
progressive H11.05-
stationary H11.04-
recurrent H11.06-

Ptilosis (eyelid) —see Madarosis
Ptomaine (poisoning) —see Poisoning, food
Ptosis —see also Blepharoptosis
adiposa (false) —see Blepharoptosis
breast N64.81
cecum K63.4
colon K63.4
congenital (eyelid) Q10.0
specified site NEC —see Anomaly, by site
eyelid —see Blepharoptosis
congenital Q10.0
gastric K31.89
intestine K63.4
kidney N28.83
liver K76.89
renal N28.83
splanchnic K63.4
spleen D73.89
stomach K31.89
viscera K63.4
PTP D69.51
Ptyalism (periodic) K11.7
hysterical F45.8
pregnancy —see Pregnancy, complicated by,
specified pregnancy-related condition
NEC
psychogenic F45.8
Ptyalolithiasis K11.5
Pubarche, precocious E30.1
Pubertas praecox E30.1
Puberty (development state) Z00.3
bleeding (excessive) N92.2
delayed E30.0
precocious (constitutional) (cryptogenic)
(idiopathic) E30.1
central E22.8
due to
ovarian hyperfunction E28.1
estrogen E28.0
testicular hyperfunction E29.0
premature E30.1
due to
adrenal cortical hyperfunction E25.8
pineal tumor E34.8
pituitary (anterior) hyperfunction E22.8
Puckering, macula —see Degeneration, macula,
puckering
Pudenda, pudendum —see condition
Puente's disease (simple glandular cheilitis)
K13.0
Puerperal, puerperium (complicated by,
complications)
abnormal glucose (tolerance test) O99.815
abscess
areola O91.02
associated with lactation O91.03
Bartholin's gland O86.19
breast O91.12
associated with lactation O91.13
cervix (uteri) O86.11
genital organ NEC O86.19
kidney O86.21
mammary O91.12
associated with lactation O91.13
nipple O91.02
associated with lactation O91.03
peritoneum O85
subareolar O91.12
associated with lactation O91.13
urinary tract —see Puerperal, infection,
urinary
uterus O86.12
vagina (wall) O86.13
vaginorectal O86.13
vulvovaginal gland O86.13
adnexitis O86.19
afibrinogenemia, or other coagulation defect
O72.3
albuminuria (acute) (subacute) —see
Proteinuria, gestational
alcohol use O99.315

Puerperal, puerperium *(Continued)*
anemia O90.81
  pre-existing (pre-pregnancy) O99.03
anesthetic death O89.8
apoplexy O99.43
bariatric surgery status O99.845
blood disorder NEC O99.13
blood dyscrasia O72.3
cardiomyopathy O90.3
cerebrovascular disorder (conditions in I60-I69) O99.43
cervicitis O86.11
circulatory system disorder O99.43
coagulopathy (any) O72.3
complications O90.9
  specified NEC O90.89
convulsions —*see* Eclampsia
cystitis O86.22
cystopyelitis O86.29
delirium NEC F05
diabetes O24.93
  gestational —*see* Puerperal, gestational diabetes
  pre-existing O24.33
    specified NEC O24.83
    type 1 O24.03
    type 2 O24.13
digestive system disorder O99.63
disease O90.9
  breast NEC O92.29
  cerebrovascular (acute) O99.43
  nonobstetric NEC O99.89
  tubo-ovarian O86.19
  Valsuani's O99.03
disorder O90.9
  biliary tract O26.63
  lactation O92.70
  liver O26.63
  nonobstetric NEC O99.89
disruption
  cesarean wound O90.0
  episiotomy wound O90.1
  perineal laceration wound O90.1
drug use O99.325
eclampsia (with pre-existing hypertension) O15.2
embolism (pulmonary) (blood clot) —*see* Embolism, obstetric, puerperal
endocrine, nutritional or metabolic disease NEC O99.285
endophlebitis —*see* Puerperal, phlebitis
endotrachelitis O86.11
failure
  lactation (complete) O92.3
    partial O92.4
  renal, acute O90.4
fever (of unknown origin) O86.4
  septic O85
fissure, nipple O92.12
  associated with lactation O92.13
fistula
  breast (due to mastitis) O91.12
    associated with lactation O91.13
  nipple O91.02
    associated with lactation O91.03
galactophoritis O91.22
  associated with lactation O91.23
galactorrhea O92.6
gastric banding status O99.845
gastric bypass status O99.845
gastrointestinal disease NEC O99.63
~~gestational diabetes O24.439~~
  ~~diet controlled O24.430~~
  ~~insulin (and diet) controlled O24.434~~
gestational ◄
  diabetes O24.439 ◄
    diet controlled O24.430 ◄
    insulin (and diet) controlled O24.434 ◄
    oral drug controlled (antidiabetic) (hypoglycemic) O24.435 ◄

Puerperal, puerperium *(Continued)*
  gestational *(Continued)*
    edema O12.05 ◄
      with proteinuria O12.25 ◄
    proteinuria O12.15 ◄
  gonorrhea O98.23
  hematoma, subdural O99.43
  hemiplegia, cerebral O99.355-
    due to cerebrovascular disorder O99.43
hemorrhage O72.1
  brain O99.43
  bulbar O99.43
  cerebellar O99.43
  cerebral O99.43
  cortical O99.43
  delayed or secondary O72.2
  extradural O99.43
  internal capsule O99.43
  intracranial O99.43
  intrapontine O99.43
  meningeal O99.43
  pontine O99.43
  retained placenta O72.0
  subarachnoid O99.43
  subcortical O99.43
  subdural O99.43
  third stage O72.0
  uterine, delayed O72.2
  ventricular O99.43
hemorrhoids O87.2
hepatorenal syndrome O90.4
hypertension —*see* Hypertension, complicating, puerperium
hypertrophy, breast O92.29
induration breast (fibrous) O92.29
infection O86.4
  cervix O86.11
  generalized O85
  genital tract NEC O86.19
    obstetric surgical wound O86.0
  kidney (bacillus coli) O86.21
  maternal O98.93
    carrier state NEC O99.835
    gonorrhea O98.23
    human immunodeficiency virus (HIV) O98.73
    protozoal O98.63
    sexually transmitted NEC O98.33
    specified NEC O98.83
    ~~streptococcus B carrier state O99.825~~
    streptococcus group B (GBS) carrier state O99.825 ◄
    syphilis O98.13
    tuberculosis O98.03
    viral hepatitis O98.43
    viral NEC O98.53
  nipple O91.02
    associated with lactation O91.03
  peritoneum O85
  renal O86.21
  specified NEC O86.89
  urinary (asymptomatic) (tract) NEC O86.20
    bladder O86.22
    kidney O86.21
    specified site NEC O86.29
    urethra O86.22
  vagina O86.13
  vein —*see* Puerperal, phlebitis
ischemia, cerebral O99.43
lymphangitis O86.89
  breast O91.22
    associated with lactation O91.23
malignancy O9A.13
malnutrition O25.3
mammillitis O91.02
  associated with lactation O91.03
mammitis O91.22
  associated with lactation O91.23
mania F30.8

Puerperal, puerperium *(Continued)*
mastitis O91.22
  associated with lactation O91.23
  purulent O91.12
    associated with lactation O91.13
melancholia —*see* Disorder, depressive
mental disorder NEC O99.345
metroperitonitis O85
metrorrhagia —*see* Hemorrhage, postpartum
metrosalpingitis O86.19
metrovaginitis O86.13
milk leg O87.1
monoplegia, cerebral O99.43
mood disturbance O90.6
necrosis, liver (acute) (subacute) (conditions in subcategory K72.0) O26.63 ◄
  with renal failure O90.4
nervous system disorder O99.355
neuritis O90.89
obesity (pre-existing prior to pregnancy) O99.215
obesity surgery status O99.845
occlusion, precerebral artery O99.43
paralysis
  bladder (sphincter) O90.89
  cerebral O99.43
paralytic stroke O99.43
parametritis O85
paravaginitis O86.13
pelviperitonitis O85
perimetritis O86.12
perimetrosalpingitis O86.19
perinephritis O86.21
periphlebitis —*see* Puerperal phlebitis
peritoneal infection O85
peritonitis (pelvic) O85
perivaginitis O86.13
phlebitis O87.0
  deep O87.1
  pelvic O87.1
  superficial O87.0
phlebothrombosis, deep O87.1
phlegmasia alba dolens O87.1
placental polyp O90.89
pneumonia, embolic —*see* Embolism, obstetric, puerperal
pre-eclampsia —*see* Pre-eclampsia
psychosis F53
pyelitis O86.21
pyelocystitis O86.29
pyelonephritis O86.21
pyelonephrosis O86.21
pyemia O85
pyocystitis O86.29
pyohemia O85
pyometra O86.12
pyonephritis O86.21
pyosalpingitis O86.19
pyrexia (of unknown origin) O86.4
renal
  disease NEC O90.89
  failure O90.4
respiratory disease NEC O99.53
retention
  decidua —*see* Retention, decidua
  placenta O72.0
  secundines —*see* Retention, secundines
retrated nipple O92.02
salpingo-ovaritis O86.19
salpingoperitonitis O85
secondary perineal tear O90.1
sepsis O85
sepsis (pelvic) O85
septic thrombophlebitis O86.81
skin disorder NEC O99.73
specified condition NEC O99.89
stroke O99.43
subinvolution (uterus) O90.89
subluxation of symphysis (pubis) O26.73

Puerperal, puerperium (Continued)
  suppuration —see Puerperal, abscess
  tetanus A34
  thelitis O91.02
    associated with lactation O91.03
  thrombocytopenia O72.3
  thrombophlebitis (superficial) O87.0
    deep O87.1
    pelvic O87.1
    septic O86.81
  thrombosis (venous) —see Thrombosis,
      puerperal
  thyroiditis O90.5
  toxemia (eclamptic) (pre-eclamptic)
      (with convulsions) O15.2
  trauma, non-obstetric O9A.23
    caused by abuse (physical) (suspected)
        O9A.33
      confirmed O9A.33
      psychological (suspected) O9A.53
        confirmed O9A.53
      sexual (suspected) O9A.43
        confirmed O9A.43
  uremia (due to renal failure)
      O90.4
  urethritis O86.22
  vaginitis O86.13
  varicose veins (legs) O87.4
    vulva or perineum O87.8
  venous O87.9
  vulvitis O86.19
  vulvovaginitis O86.13
  white leg O87.1
Puerperium —see Puerperal
Pulmolithiasis J98.4
Pulmonary —see condition
Pulpitis (acute) (anachoretic) (chronic)
    (hyperplastic) (putrescent) (suppurative)
    (ulcerative) K04.01 ◀▥▥
  irreversible K04.02 ◀▥▥
  reversible K04.01 ◀▥▥
Pulpless tooth K04.99
Pulse
  alternating R00.8
  bigeminal R00.8
  fast R00.0
  feeble, rapid due to shock following injury
      T79.4
  rapid R00.0
  weak R09.89
Pulsus alternans or trigeminus R00.8
Punch drunk F07.81
Punctum lacrimale occlusion —see Obstruction,
    lacrimal
Puncture
  abdomen, abdominal
    wall S31.139
      with
        foreign body S31.149
        penetration into peritoneal cavity
            S31.639
          with foreign body S31.649
      epigastric region S31.132
        with
          foreign body S31.142
          penetration into peritoneal cavity
              S31.632
            with foreign body S31.642
      left
        lower quadrant S31.134
          with
            foreign body S31.144
            penetration into peritoneal cavity
                S31.634
              with foreign body S31.644
        upper quadrant S31.131
          with
            foreign body S31.141
            penetration into peritoneal cavity
                S31.631
              with foreign body S31.641

Puncture (Continued)
  abdomen, abdominal (Continued)
    wall (Continued)
      periumbilic region S31.135
        with
          foreign body S31.145
          penetration into peritoneal cavity
              S31.635
            with foreign body S31.645
      right
        lower quadrant S31.133
          with
            foreign body S31.143
            penetration into peritoneal cavity
                S31.633
              with foreign body S31.643
        upper quadrant S31.130
          with
            foreign body S31.140
            penetration into peritoneal cavity
                S31.630
              with foreign body S31.640
  accidental, complicating surgery —see
      Complication, accidental puncture or
      laceration
  alveolar (process) —see Puncture, oral cavity
  ankle S91.039
    with
      foreign body S91.049
    left S91.032
      with
        foreign body S91.042
    right S91.031
      with
        foreign body S91.041
  anus S31.833
    with foreign body S31.834
  arm (upper) S41.139
    with foreign body S41.149
    left S41.132
      with foreign body S41.142
    lower —see Puncture, forearm
    right S41.131
      with foreign body S41.141
  auditory canal (external) (meatus) —see
      Puncture, ear
  auricle, ear —see Puncture, ear
  axilla —see Puncture, arm
  back —see also Puncture, thorax, back
    lower S31.030
      with
        foreign body S31.040
          with penetration into
              retroperitoneal space S31.041
        penetration into retroperitoneal space
            S31.031
  bladder (traumatic) S37.29
    nontraumatic N32.89
  breast S21.039
    with foreign body S21.049
    left S21.032
      with foreign body S21.042
    right S21.031
      with foreign body S21.041
  buttock S31.803
    with foreign body S31.804
    left S31.823
      with foreign body S31.824
    right S31.813
      with foreign body S31.814
  by
    device, implant or graft —see
        Complications, by site and type,
        mechanical
    foreign body left accidentally in operative
        wound T81.539
    instrument (any) during a procedure,
        accidental —see Puncture, accidental
        complicating surgery
  calf —see Puncture, leg
  canaliculus lacrimalis —see Puncture, eyelid

Puncture (Continued)
  canthus, eye —see Puncture, eyelid
  cervical esophagus S11.23
    with foreign body S11.24
  cheek (external) S01.439
    with foreign body S01.449
    internal —see Puncture, oral cavity
    left S01.432
      with foreign body S01.442
    right S01.431
      with foreign body S01.441
  chest wall —see Puncture, thorax
  chin —see Puncture, head, specified site NEC
  clitoris —see Puncture, vulva
  costal region —see Puncture, thorax
  digit (s)
    foot —see Puncture, toe
    hand —see Puncture, finger
  ear (canal) (external) S01.339
    with foreign body S01.349
    drum S09.2-
    left S01.332
      with foreign body S01.342
    right S01.331
      with foreign body S01.341
  elbow S51.039
    with
      foreign body S51.049
    left S51.032
      with
        foreign body S51.042
    right S51.031
      with
        foreign body S51.041
  epididymis —see Puncture, testis
  epigastric region —see Puncture, abdomen,
      wall, epigastric
  epiglottis S11.83
    with foreign body S11.84
  esophagus
    cervical S11.23
      with foreign body S11.24
    thoracic S27.818
  eyeball S05.6-
    with foreign body S05.5-
  eyebrow —see Puncture, eyelid
  eyelid S01.13-
    with foreign body S01.14-
    left S01.132
      with foreign body S01.142
    right S01.131
      with foreign body S01.141
  face NEC —see Puncture, head, specified site
      NEC
  finger (s) S61.239
    with
      damage to nail S61.339
        with
          foreign body S61.349
      foreign body S61.249
    index S61.238
      with
        damage to nail S61.338
          with
            foreign body S61.348
        foreign body S61.248
      left S61.231
        with
          damage to nail S61.331
            with
              foreign body S61.341
          foreign body S61.241
      right S61.230
        with
          damage to nail S61.330
            with
              foreign body S61.340
          foreign body S61.240
    little S61.238
      with
        damage to nail S61.338

Puncture *(Continued)*
  finger *(Continued)*
    with *(Continued)*
      with *(Continued)*
        damage to nail *(Continued)*
          with
            foreign body S61.348
          foreign body S61.248
      left S61.237
        with
          damage to nail S61.337
            with
              foreign body S61.347
          foreign body S61.247
      right S61.236
        with
          damage to nail S61.336
            with
              foreign body S61.346
          foreign body S61.246
    middle S61.238
      with
        damage to nail S61.338
          with
            foreign body S61.348
        foreign body S61.248
      left S61.233
        with
          damage to nail S61.333
            with
              foreign body S61.343
          foreign body S61.243
      right S61.232
        with
          damage to nail S61.332
            with
              foreign body S61.342
          foreign body S61.242
    ring S61.238
      with
        damage to nail S61.338
          with
            foreign body S61.348
        foreign body S61.248
      left S61.235
        with
          damage to nail S61.335
            with
              foreign body S61.345
          foreign body S61.245
      right S61.234
        with
          damage to nail S61.334
            with
              foreign body S61.344
          foreign body S61.244
  flank S31.139
    with foreign body S31.149
  foot (except toe (s) alone) S91.339
    with foreign body S91.349
    left S91.332
      with foreign body S91.342
    right S91.331
      with foreign body S91.341
    toe —*see* Puncture, toe
  forearm S51.839
    with
      foreign body S51.849
    elbow only —*see* Puncture, elbow
    left S51.832
      with
        foreign body S51.842
    right S51.831
      with
        foreign body S51.841
  forehead —*see* Puncture, head, specified site NEC
  genital organs, external
    female S31.532
      with foreign body S31.542
      vagina —*see* Puncture, vagina
      vulva —*see* Puncture, vulva

Puncture *(Continued)*
  genital organs, external *(Continued)*
    male S31.531
      with foreign body S31.541
      penis —*see* Puncture, penis
      scrotum —*see* Puncture, scrotum
      testis —*see* Puncture, testis
  groin —*see* Puncture, abdomen, wall
  gum —*see* Puncture, oral cavity
  hand S61.439
    with
      foreign body S61.449
    finger —*see* Puncture, finger
    left S61.432
      with
        foreign body S61.442
    right S61.431
      with
        foreign body S61.441
    thumb —*see* Puncture, thumb
  head S01.93
    with foreign body S01.94
    cheek —*see* Puncture, cheek
    ear —*see* Puncture, ear
    eyelid —*see* Puncture, eyelid
    lip —*see* Puncture, oral cavity
    nose —*see* Puncture, nose
    oral cavity —*see* Puncture, oral cavity
    scalp S01.03
      with foreign body S01.04
    specified site NEC S01.83
      with foreign body S01.84
    temporomandibular area —*see* Puncture, cheek
  heart S26.99
    with hemopericardium S26.09
    without hemopericardium S26.19
  heel —*see* Puncture, foot
  hip S71.039
    with foreign body S71.049
    left S71.032
      with foreign body S71.042
    right S71.031
      with foreign body S71.041
  hymen —*see* Puncture, vagina
  hypochondrium —*see* Puncture, abdomen, wall
  hypogastric region —*see* Puncture, abdomen, wall
  inguinal region —*see* Puncture, abdomen, wall
  instep —*see* Puncture, foot
  internal organs —*see* Injury, by site
  interscapular region —*see* Puncture, thorax, back
  intestine
    large
      colon S36.599
        ascending S36.590
        descending S36.592
        sigmoid S36.593
        specified site NEC S36.598
        transverse S36.591
      rectum S36.69
    small S36.499
      duodenum S36.490
      specified site NEC S36.498
  intra-abdominal organ S36.99
    gallbladder S36.128
    intestine —*see* Puncture, intestine
    liver S36.118
    pancreas —*see* Puncture, pancreas
    peritoneum S36.81
    specified site NEC S36.898
    spleen S36.09
    stomach S36.39
  jaw —*see* Puncture, head, specified site NEC
  knee S81.039
    with foreign body S81.049
    left S81.032
      with foreign body S81.042

Puncture *(Continued)*
  knee *(Continued)*
    right S81.031
      with foreign body S81.041
  labium (majus) (minus) —*see* Puncture, vulva
  lacrimal duct —*see* Puncture, eyelid
  larynx S11.013
    with foreign body S11.014
  leg (lower) S81.839
    with foreign body S81.849
    foot —*see* Puncture, foot
    knee —*see* Puncture, knee
    left S81.832
      with foreign body S81.842
    right S81.831
      with foreign body S81.841
    upper —*see* Puncture, thigh
  lip S01.531
    with foreign body S01.541
  loin —*see* Puncture, abdomen, wall
  lower back —*see* Puncture, back, lower
  lumbar region —*see* Puncture, back, lower
  malar region —*see* Puncture, head, specified site NEC
  mammary —*see* Puncture, breast
  mastoid region —*see* Puncture, head, specified site NEC
  mouth —*see* Puncture, oral cavity
  nail
    finger —*see* Puncture, finger, with damage to nail
    toe —*see* Puncture, toe, with damage to nail
  nasal (septum) (sinus) —*see* Puncture, nose
  nasopharynx —*see* Puncture, head, specified site NEC
  neck S11.93
    with foreign body S11.94
    involving
      cervical esophagus —*see* Puncture, cervical esophagus
      larynx —*see* Puncture, larynx
      pharynx —*see* Puncture, pharynx
      thyroid gland —*see* Puncture, thyroid gland
      trachea —*see* Puncture, trachea
    specified site NEC S11.83
      with foreign body S11.84
  nose (septum) (sinus) S01.23
    with foreign body S01.24
  ocular —*see* Puncture, eyeball - oral cavity S01.532
    with foreign body S01.542
  orbit S05.4-
  palate —*see* Puncture, oral cavity
  palm —*see* Puncture, hand
  pancreas S36.299
    body S36.291
    head S36.290
    tail S36.292
  pelvis —*see* Puncture, back, lower
  penis S31.23
    with foreign body S31.24
  perineum
    female S31.43
      with foreign body S31.44
    male S31.139
      with foreign body S31.149
  periocular area (with or without lacrimal passages) —*see* Puncture, eyelid
  phalanges
    finger —*see* Puncture, finger
    toe —*see* Puncture, toe
  pharynx S11.23
    with foreign body S11.24
  pinna —*see* Puncture, ear
  popliteal space —*see* Puncture, knee
  prepuce —*see* Puncture, penis
  pubic region S31.139
    with foreign body S31.149

◀ New   ◀▥ Revised   ~~deleted~~ Deleted

Puncture (Continued)
  pudendum —see Puncture, genital organs,
    external
  rectovaginal septum —see Puncture,
    vagina
  sacral region —see Puncture, back,
    lower
  sacroiliac region —see Puncture, back,
    lower
  salivary gland —see Puncture, oral
    cavity
  scalp S01.03
    with foreign body S01.04
  scapular region —see Puncture,
    shoulder
  scrotum S31.33
    with foreign body S31.34
  shin —see Puncture, leg
  shoulder S41.039
    with foreign body S41.049
    left S41.032
      with foreign body S41.042
    right S41.031
      with foreign body S41.041
  spermatic cord —see Puncture, testis
  sternal region —see Puncture, thorax, front
  submaxillary region —see Puncture, head,
    specified site NEC
  submental region —see Puncture, head,
    specified site NEC
  subungual
    finger (s) —see Puncture, finger, with
      damage to nail
    toe —see Puncture, toe, with damage to
      nail
  supraclavicular fossa —see Puncture, neck,
    specified site NEC
  temple, temporal region —see Puncture, head,
    specified site NEC
  temporomandibular area —see Puncture,
    cheek
  testis S31.33
    with foreign body S31.34
  thigh S71.139
    with foreign body S71.149
    left S71.132
      with foreign body S71.142
    right S71.131
      with foreign body S71.141
  thorax, thoracic (wall) S21.93
    with foreign body S21.94
    back S21.23-
      with
        foreign body S21.24-
          with penetration S21.44
        penetration S21.43
    breast —see Puncture, breast
    front S21.13-
      with
        foreign body S21.14-
          with penetration S21.34
        penetration S21.33
  throat —see Puncture, neck
  thumb S61.039
    with
      damage to nail S61.139
        with
          foreign body S61.149
        foreign body S61.049
    left S61.032
      with
        damage to nail S61.132
          with
            foreign body S61.142
          foreign body S61.042
    right S61.031
      with
        damage to nail S61.131
          with
            foreign body S61.141
        foreign body S61.041

Puncture (Continued)
  thyroid gland S11.13
    with foreign body S11.14
  toe (s) S91.139
    with
      damage to nail S91.239
        with
          foreign body S91.249
      foreign body S91.149
    great S91.133
      with
        damage to nail S91.233
          with
            foreign body S91.243
        foreign body S91.143
      left S91.132
        with
          damage to nail S91.232
            with
              foreign body S91.242
          foreign body S91.142
      right S91.131
        with
          damage to nail S91.231
            with
              foreign body S91.241
          foreign body S91.141
    lesser S91.136
      with
        damage to nail S91.236
          with
            foreign body S91.246
        foreign body S91.146
      left S91.135
        with
          damage to nail S91.235
            with
              foreign body S91.245
          foreign body S91.145
      right S91.134
        with
          damage to nail S91.234
            with
              foreign body S91.244
          foreign body S91.144
  tongue —see Puncture, oral cavity
  trachea S11.023
    with foreign body S11.024
  tunica vaginalis —see Puncture, testis
  tympanum, tympanic membrane
    S09.2-
  umbilical region S31.135
    with foreign body S31.145
  uvula —see Puncture, oral cavity
  vagina S31.43
    with foreign body S31.44
  vocal cords S11.033
    with foreign body S11.034
  vulva S31.43
    with foreign body S31.44
  wrist S61.539
    with
      foreign body S61.549
    left S61.532
      with
        foreign body S61.542
    right S61.531
      with
        foreign body S61.541
PUO (pyrexia of unknown origin) R50.9
Pupillary membrane (persistent) Q13.89
Pupillotonia —see Anomaly, pupil, function,
  tonic pupil
Purpura D69.2
  abdominal D69.0
  allergic D69.0
  anaphylactoid D69.0
  annularis telangiectodes L81.7
  arthritic D69.0
  autoerythrocyte sensitization D69.2
  autoimmune D69.0

Purpura (Continued)
  bacterial D69.0
  Bateman's (senile) D69.2
  capillary fragility (hereditary) (idiopathic)
    D69.8
  cryoglobulinemic D89.1
  Devil's pinches D69.2
  fibrinolytic —see Fibrinolysis
  fulminans, fulminous D65
  gangrenous D65
  hemorrhagic, hemorrhagica D69.3
    not due to thrombocytopenia D69.0
  Henoch (-Schönlein) (allergic) D69.0
  hypergammaglobulinemic (benign)
    (Waldenström's) D89.0
  idiopathic (thrombocytopenic) D69.3
    nonthrombocytopenic D69.0
  immune thrombocytopenic D69.3
  infectious D69.0
  malignant D69.0
  neonatorum P54.5
  nervosa D69.0
  newborn P54.5
  nonthrombocytopenic D69.2
    hemorrhagic D69.0
    idiopathic D69.0
  nonthrombopenic D69.2
  peliosis rheumatica D69.0
  posttransfusion (post-transfusion) (from
    (fresh) whole blood or blood products)
    D69.51
  primary D69.49
  red cell membrane sensitivity D69.2
  rheumatica D69.0
  Schönlein (-Henoch) (allergic) D69.0
  scorbutic E54 [D77]
  senile D69.2
  simplex D69.2
  symptomatica D69.0
  telangiectasia annularis L81.7
  thrombocytopenic D69.49
    congenital D69.42
    hemorrhagic D69.3
    hereditary D69.42
    idiopathic D69.3
    immune D69.3
    neonatal, transitory P61.0
    thrombotic M31.1
  thrombohemolytic —see Fibrinolysis
  thrombolytic —see Fibrinolysis
  thrombopenic D69.49
  thrombotic, thrombocytopenic
    M31.1
  toxic D69.0
  vascular D69.0
  visceral symptoms D69.0
Purpuric spots R23.3
Purulent —see condition
Pus
  in
    stool R19.5
    urine N39.0
  tube (rupture) —see Salpingo-oophoritis
Pustular rash L08.0
Pustule (nonmalignant) L08.9
  malignant A22.0
Pustulosis palmaris et plantaris
  L40.3
Putnam (-Dana) disease or syndrome —see
  Degeneration, combined
Putrescent pulp (dental) K04.1
Pyarthritis, pyarthrosis —see Arthritis,
  pyogenic or pyemic
  tuberculous —see Tuberculosis, joint
Pyelectasis —see Hydronephrosis
Pyelitis (congenital) (uremic) —see also
  Pyelonephritis
  with
    calculus —see category N20
      with hydronephrosis N13.2
    contracted kidney N11.9

Pyelitis *(Continued)*
  acute N10
  chronic N11.9
    with calculus —*see* category N20
      with hydronephrosis N13.2
  cystica N28.84
  puerperal (postpartum) O86.21
  tuberculous A18.11
Pyelocystitis —*see* Pyelonephritis
Pyelonephritis —*see also* Nephritis,
    tubulo-interstitial
  with
    calculus —*see* category N20
      with hydronephrosis N13.2
    contracted kidney N11.9
  acute N10
  calculous —*see* category N20
    with hydronephrosis N13.2
  chronic N11.9
    with calculus —*see* category N20
      with hydronephrosis N13.2
    associated with ureteral obstruction or
      stricture N11.1
    nonobstructive N11.8
      with reflux (vesicoureteral) N11.0
    obstructive N11.1
    specified NEC N11.8
  in (due to)
    brucellosis A23.9 *[N16]*
    cryoglobulinemia (mixed) D89.1 *[N16]*
    cystinosis E72.04
    diphtheria A36.84
    glycogen storage disease E74.09 *[N16]*
    leukemia NEC C95.9- *[N16]*
    lymphoma NEC C85.90 *[N16]*
    multiple myeloma C90.0- *[N16]*
    obstruction N11.1
    Salmonella infection A02.25
    sarcoidosis D86.84
    sepsis A41.9 *[N16]*
    Sjögren's disease M35.04
    toxoplasmosis B58.83
    transplant rejection T86.91 *[N16]*
    Wilson's disease E83.01 *[N16]*
  nonobstructive N12
    with reflux (vesicoureteral) N11.0
    chronic N11.8
  syphilitic A52.75

Pyelonephrosis (obstructive) N11.1
  chronic N11.9
Pyelophlebitis I80.8
Pyeloureteritis cystica N28.85
Pyemia, pyemic (fever) (infection) (purulent) —
    see also Sepsis
  joint —*see* Arthritis, pyogenic or pyemic
  liver K75.1
  pneumococcal A40.3
  portal K75.1
  postvaccinal T88.0
  puerperal, postpartum, childbirth O85
  specified organism NEC A41.89
  tuberculous —*see* Tuberculosis, miliary
Pygopagus Q89.4
Pyknoepilepsy (idiopathic) —*see* Pyknolepsy
Pyknolepsy G40.A09
  intractable G40.A19
    with status epilepticus G40.A11
    without status epilepticus G40.A19
  not intractable G40.A09
    with status epilepticus G40.A01
    without status epilepticus G40.A09
Pylephlebitis K75.1
Pyle's syndrome Q78.5
Pylethrombophlebitis K75.1
Pylethrombosis K75.1
Pyloritis K29.90
  with bleeding K29.91
Pylorospasm (reflex) NEC K31.3
  congenital or infantile Q40.0
  neurotic F45.8
  newborn Q40.0
  psychogenic F45.8
Pylorus, pyloric —*see* condition
Pyoarthrosis —*see* Arthritis, pyogenic or
    pyemic
Pyocele
  mastoid —*see* Mastoiditis, acute
  sinus (accessory) —*see* Sinusitis
  turbinate (bone) J32.9
  urethra —*see also* Urethritis N34.0
Pyocolpos —*see* Vaginitis
Pyocystitis N30.80
  with hematuria N30.81
Pyoderma, pyodermia L08.0
  gangrenosum L88
  newborn P39.4

Pyoderma, pyodermia *(Continued)*
  phagedenic L88
  vegetans L08.81
Pyodermatitis L08.0
  vegetans L08.81
Pyogenic —*see* condition
Pyohydronephrosis N13.6
Pyometra, pyometrium, pyometritis —*see*
    Endometritis
Pyomyositis (tropical) —*see* Myositis,
    infective
Pyonephritis N12
Pyonephrosis N13.6
  tuberculous A18.11
Pyo-oophoritis —*see* Salpingo-oophoritis
Pyo-ovarium —*see* Salpingo-oophoritis
Pyopericarditis, pyopericardium
  I30.1
Pyophlebitis —*see* Phlebitis
Pyopneumopericardium I30.1
Pyopneumothorax (infective) J86.9
  with fistula J86.0
  tuberculous NEC A15.6
Pyosalpinx, pyosalpingitis —*see also*
    Salpingo-oophoritis
Pyothorax J86.9
  with fistula J86.0
  tuberculous NEC A15.6
Pyoureter N28.89
  tuberculous A18.11
Pyramidopallidonigral syndrome
  G20
Pyrexia (of unknown origin) R50.9
  atmospheric T67.0
  during labor NEC O75.2
  heat T67.0
  newborn P81.9
    environmentally-induced P81.0
  persistent R50.9
  puerperal O86.4
Pyroglobulinemia NEC E88.09
Pyromania F63.1
Pyrosis R12
Pyuria (bacterial) N39.0

◀ New   ◀‖‖ Revised   ~~deleted~~ Deleted

Q

Q fever A78
  with pneumonia A78
Quadricuspid aortic valve Q23.8
Quadrilateral fever A78
Quadriparesis —*see* Quadriplegia
  meaning muscle weakness M62.81
Quadriplegia G82.50-
  complete
    C1-C4 level G82.51
    C5-C7 level G82.53
  congenital (cerebral) (spinal) G80.8
    spastic G80.0

Quadriplegia (*Continued*)
  embolic (current episode) I63.4- ◄▥
  functional R53.2
  incomplete
    C1-C4 level G82.52
    C5-C7 level G82.54
  thrombotic (current episode) I63.3- ◄▥
  traumatic — code to injury with seventh
    character S
    current episode —*see* Injury, spinal (cord),
      cervical
Quadruplet, pregnancy —*see* Pregnancy,
  quadruplet
Quarrelsomeness F60.3

Queensland fever A77.3
Quervain's disease M65.4
  thyroid E06.1
Queyrat's erythroplasia D07.4
  penis D07.4
  specified site —*see* Neoplasm, skin,
    in situ
  unspecified site D07.4
Quincke's disease or edema T78.3
  hereditary D84.1
Quinsy (gangrenous) J36
Quintan fever A79.0
Quintuplet, pregnancy —*see* Pregnancy,
  quintuplet

R

Rabbit fever —*see* Tularemia
Rabies A82.9
  contact Z20.3
  exposure to Z20.3
  inoculation reaction —*see* Complications,
    vaccination
  sylvatic A82.0
  urban A82.1
Rachischisis —*see* Spina bifida
Rachitic —*see also* condition
  deformities of spine (late effect) (sequelae)
    E64.3
  pelvis (late effect) (sequelae) E64.3
    with disproportion (fetopelvic) O33.0
      causing obstructed labor O65.0
Rachitis, rachitism (acute) (tarda) —*see also*
    Rickets
  renalis N25.0
  sequelae E64.3
Radial nerve —*see* condition
Radiation
  burn —*see* Burn
  effects NOS T66
  sickness NOS T66
  therapy, encounter for Z51.0
Radiculitis (pressure) (vertebrogenic) —*see*
    Radiculopathy
Radiculomyelitis —*see also* Encephalitis
  toxic, due to
    Clostridium tetani A35
    Corynebacterium diphtheriae A36.82
Radiculopathy M54.10
  cervical region M54.12
  cervicothoracic region M54.13
  due to
    disc disorder
      C3 M50.11
      C4 M50.11
      C5 M50.121 ◀
      C6 M50.122 ◀
      C7 M50.123 ◀
      C8 M50.13
    displacement of intervertebral disc —*see*
      Disorder, disc, with, radiculopathy
  leg M54.1-
  lumbar region M54.16
  lumbosacral region M54.17
  occipito-atlanto-axial region M54.11
  postherpetic B02.29
  sacrococcygeal region M54.18
  syphilitic A52.11
  thoracic region (with visceral pain)
    M54.14
  thoracolumbar region M54.15
Radiodermal burns (acute, chronic, or
    occupational) —*see* Burn
Radiodermatitis L58.9
  acute L58.0
  chronic L58.1
Radiotherapy session Z51.0
RAEB (refractory anemia with excess blasts)
    D46.2- ◀
Rage, meaning rabies —*see* Rabies
Ragpicker's disease A22.1
Ragsorter's disease A22.1
Raillietiniasis B71.8
Railroad neurosis F48.8
Railway spine F48.8
Raised —*see also* Elevated
  antibody titer R76.0
Rake teeth, tooth M26.39
Rales R09.89
Ramifying renal pelvis Q63.8
Ramsay-Hunt disease or syndrome —*see also*
    Hunt's disease B02.21
  meaning dyssynergia cerebellaris myoclonica
    G11.1
Ranula K11.6
  congenital Q38.4

Rape
  adult
    confirmed T74.21
    suspected T76.21
  alleged, observation or examination, ruled out
    adult Z04.41
    child Z04.42
  child
    confirmed T74.22
    suspected T76.22
Rapid
  feeble pulse, due to shock, following injury
    T79.4
  heart (beat) R00.0
    psychogenic F45.8
  second stage (delivery) O62.3
  time-zone change syndrome —*see* Disorder,
    sleep, circadian rhythm, psychogenic
Rarefaction, bone —*see* Disorder, bone, density
    and structure, specified NEC
Rash (toxic) R21
  canker A38.9
  diaper L22
  drug (internal use) L27.0
    contact —*see also* Dermatitis, due to, drugs,
      external L25.1
  following immunization T88.1
  food —*see* Dermatitis, due to, food
  heat L74.0
  napkin (psoriasiform) L22
  nettle —*see* Urticaria
  pustular L08.0
  rose R21
    epidemic B06.9
  scarlet A38.9
  serum —*see also* Reaction, serum T80.69
  wandering tongue K14.1
Rasmussen aneurysm —*see* Tuberculosis,
    pulmonary
Rasmussen encephalitis G04.81
Rat-bite fever A25.9
  due to Streptobacillus moniliformis A25.1
  spirochetal (morsus muris) A25.0
Rathke's pouch tumor D44.3
Raymond (-Céstan) syndrome I65.8
Raynaud's disease, phenomenon or syndrome
    (secondary) I73.00
  with gangrene (symmetric) I73.01
RDS (newborn) (type I) P22.0
  type II P22.1
Reaction —*see also* Disorder
  adaptation —*see* Disorder, adjustment
  adjustment (anxiety) (conduct disorder)
    (depressiveness) (distress) —*see*
      Disorder, adjustment
    with
      mutism, elective (child) (adolescent) F94.0
  adverse
    food (any) (ingested) NEC T78.1
      anaphylactic —*see* Shock, anaphylactic,
        due to food
  anaphylactoid —*see* Shock, anaphylactic
  affective —*see* Disorder, mood
  allergic —*see* Allergy
  anaphylactic —*see* Shock, anaphylactic
  anesthesia —*see* Anesthesia, complication
  antitoxin (prophylactic) (therapeutic) —*see*
      Complications, vaccination
  anxiety F41.1
  Arthus —*see* Arthus' phenomenon
  asthenic F48.8
  combat and operational stress F43.0
  compulsive F42.8 ◀⊪
  conversion F44.9
  crisis, acute F43.0
  deoxyribonuclease (DNA) (DNase)
    hypersensitivity D69.2
  depressive (single episode) F32.9
    affective (single episode) F31.4
      recurrent episode F33.9
    neurotic F34.1
    psychoneurotic F34.1

Reaction (*Continued*)
  depressive (*Continued*)
    psychotic F32.3
    recurrent —*see* Disorder, depressive,
      recurrent
  dissociative F44.9
  drug NEC T88.7
    addictive —*see* Dependence, drug
      transmitted via placenta or breast
        milk —*see* Absorption, drug,
        addictive, through placenta
    allergic —*see* Allergy, drug
    lichenoid L43.2
    newborn P93.8
      gray baby syndrome P93.0
    overdose or poisoning (by accident) —*see*
      Table of Drugs and Chemicals, by
      drug, poisoning
    photoallergic L56.1
    phototoxic L56.0
    withdrawal —*see* Dependence, by drug,
      with, withdrawal
      infant of dependent mother P96.1
      newborn P96.1
    wrong substance given or taken (by
      accident) —*see* Table of Drugs and
      Chemicals, by drug, poisoning
  fear F40.9
    child (abnormal) F93.8
  febrile nonhemolytic transfusion (FNHTR)
    R50.84
  fluid loss, cerebrospinal G97.1
  foreign
    body NEC —*see* Granuloma, foreign body
      in operative wound (inadvertently
        left) —*see* Foreign body,
        accidentally left during a
        procedure
    substance accidentally left during a
      procedure (chemical) (powder) (talc)
      T81.60
      aseptic peritonitis T81.61
      body or object (instrument) (sponge)
        (swab) —*see* Foreign body,
        accidentally left during a
        procedure
      specified reaction NEC T81.69
  grief —*see* Disorder, adjustment
  Herxheimer's R68.89
  hyperkinetic —*see* Hyperkinesia
  hypochondriacal F45.20
  hypoglycemic, due to insulin E16.0
    with coma (diabetic) —*see* Diabetes, coma
      nondiabetic E15
    therapeutic misadventure —*see*
      subcategory T38.3
  hypomanic F30.8
  hysterical F44.9
  immunization —*see* Complications, vaccination
  incompatibility
    ABO blood group (infusion) (transfusion) —
      see Complication (s), transfusion,
      incompatibility reaction, ABO
    delayed serologic T80.39
    minor blood group (Duffy) (E) (K(ell))
      (Kidd) (Lewis) (M) (N) (P) (S) T80.89
    Rh (factor) (infusion) (transfusion) —*see*
      Complication (s), transfusion,
      incompatibility reaction, Rh (factor)
  inflammatory —*see* Infection
  infusion —*see* Complications, infusion
  inoculation (immune serum) —*see*
      Complications, vaccination
  insulin T38.3-
  involutional psychotic —*see* Disorder,
      depressive
  leukemoid D72.823
    basophilic D72.823
    lymphocytic D72.823
    monocytic D72.823
    myelocytic D72.823
    neutrophilic D72.823

◀ New   ⊪ Revised   ~~deleted~~ Deleted

Reaction *(Continued)*
LSD (acute)
due to drug abuse —*see* Abuse, drug, hallucinogen
due to drug dependence —*see* Dependence, drug, hallucinogen
lumbar puncture G97.1
manic-depressive —*see* Disorder, bipolar
neurasthenic F48.8
neurogenic —*see* Neurosis
neurotic F48.9
neurotic-depressive F34.1
nitritoid —*see* Crisis, nitritoid - obsessive-compulsive F42
nonspecific
to
cell mediated immunity measurement of gamma interferon antigen response without active tuberculosis R76.12
QuantiFERON-TB test (QFT) without active tuberculosis R76.12
tuberculin test —*see also* Reaction, tuberculin skin test R76.11
obsessive-compulsive F42.8 ◀▥
organic, acute or subacute —*see* Delirium
paranoid (acute) F23
chronic F22
senile F03
passive dependency F60.7
phobic F40.9
post-traumatic stress, uncomplicated Z73.3
psychogenic F99
psychoneurotic —*see also* Neurosis
compulsive F42.8 ◀▥
depersonalization F48.1
depressive F34.1
hypochondriacal F45.20
neurasthenic F48.8
obsessive F42.8 ◀▥
psychophysiologic —*see* Disorder, somatoform
psychosomatic —*see* Disorder, somatoform
psychotic —*see* Psychosis
scarlet fever toxin —*see* Complications, vaccination
schizophrenic F23
acute (brief) (undifferentiated) F23
latent F21
undifferentiated (acute) (brief) F23
serological for syphilis —*see* Serology for syphilis
serum T80.69
anaphylactic (immediate) —*see also* Shock, anaphylactic T80.59
specified reaction NEC
due to
administration of blood and blood products T80.61
immunization T80.62
serum specified NEC T80.69
vaccination T80.62
situational —*see* Disorder, adjustment
somatization —*see* Disorder, somatoform
spinal puncture G97.1
stress (severe) F43.9
acute (agitation) ("daze") (disorientation) (disturbance of consciousness) (flight reaction) (fugue) F43.0
specified NEC F43.8
surgical procedure —*see* Complications, surgical procedure
tetanus antitoxin —*see* Complications, vaccination
toxic, to local anesthesia T81.59 ◀▥
in labor and delivery O74.4
in pregnancy O29.3X-
postpartum, puerperal O89.3
toxin-antitoxin —*see* Complications, vaccination

Reaction *(Continued)*
transfusion (blood) (bone marrow) (lymphocytes) (allergic) —*see* Complications, transfusion
tuberculin skin test, abnormal R76.11
vaccination (any) —*see* Complications, vaccination
withdrawing, child or adolescent F93.8
Reactive airway disease —*see* Asthma
Reactive depression —*see* Reaction, depressive
Rearrangement
chromosomal
balanced (in) Q95.9
abnormal individual (autosomal) Q95.2
non-sex (autosomal) chromosomes Q95.2
sex/non-sex chromosomes Q95.3
specified NEC Q95.8
Recalcitrant patient —*see* Noncompliance
Recanalization, thrombus —*see* Thrombosis
Recession, receding
chamber angle (eye) H21.55-
chin M26.09
gingival (generalized) (localized) (postinfective) (postoperative) K06.00 ◀▥
Miller Class I K06.01 ◀
Miller Class II K06.02 ◀
Miller Class III K06.03 ◀
Miller Class IV K06.04 ◀
Recklinghausen's disease Q85.01
bones E21.0
Reclus' disease (cystic) —*see* Mastopathy, cystic
Recrudescent typhus (fever) A75.1
Recruitment, auditory H93.21-
Rectalgia K62.89
Rectitis K62.89
Rectocele
female (without uterine prolapse) N81.6
with uterine prolapse N81.4
incomplete N81.2
in pregnancy —*see* Pregnancy, complicated by, abnormal, pelvic organs or tissues NEC
male K62.3
Rectosigmoid junction —*see* condition
Rectosigmoiditis K63.89
ulcerative (chronic) K51.30
with
complication K51.319
abscess K51.314
fistula K51.313
obstruction K51.312
rectal bleeding K51.311
specified NEC K51.318
Rectourethral —*see* condition
Rectovaginal —*see* condition
Rectovesical —*see* condition
Rectum, rectal —*see* condition
Recurrent —*see* condition
pregnancy loss —*see* Loss (of), pregnancy, recurrent
Red bugs B88.0
Red-cedar lung or pneumonitis J67.8
Red tide —*see also* Table of Drugs and Chemicals T65.82-
Reduced
mobility Z74.09
ventilatory or vital capacity R94.2
Redundant, redundancy
anus (congenital) Q43.8
clitoris N90.89
colon (congenital) Q43.8
foreskin (congenital) N47.8
intestine (congenital) Q43.8
labia N90.69 ◀▥
organ or site, congenital NEC —*see* Accessory
panniculus (abdominal) E65
prepuce (congenital) N47.8
pylorus K31.89
rectum (congenital) Q43.8
scrotum N50.89 ◀▥

Redundant, redundancy *(Continued)*
sigmoid (congenital) Q43.8
skin L98.7 ◀▥
~~eyelids — see Blepharochalasis~~
and subcutaneous tissue L98.7 ◀
of face L57.4 ◀
eyelids —*see* Blepharochalasis ◀
stomach K31.89
Reduplication —*see* Duplication
Reflex R29.2
hyperactive gag J39.2
pupillary, abnormal —*see* Anomaly, pupil, function
vasoconstriction I73.9
vasovagal R55
Reflux K21.9
acid K21.9
esophageal K21.9
with esophagitis K21.0
newborn P78.83
gastroesophageal K21.9
with esophagitis K21.0
mitral —*see* Insufficiency, mitral
ureteral —*see* Reflux, vesicoureteral
vesicoureteral (with scarring) N13.70
with
nephropathy N13.729
with hydroureter N13.739
bilateral N13.732
unilateral N13.731
without hydroureter N13.729
bilateral N13.722
unilateral N13.721
bilateral N13.722
unilateral N13.721
pyelonephritis (chronic) N11.0
without nephropathy N13.71
congenital Q62.7
Reforming, artificial openings —*see* Attention to, artificial, opening
Refractive error —*see* Disorder, refraction
Refsum's disease or syndrome G60.1
Refusal of
food, psychogenic F50.89 ◀▥
treatment (because of) Z53.20
left against medical advice (AMA) Z53.21
patient's decision NEC Z53.29
reasons of belief or group pressure Z53.1
Regional —*see* condition
Regurgitation R11.10
aortic (valve) —*see* Insufficiency, aortic
food —*see also* Vomiting
with reswallowing —*see* Rumination
newborn P92.1
gastric contents —*see* Vomiting
heart —*see* Endocarditis
mitral (valve) —*see* Insufficiency, mitral
congenital Q23.3
myocardial —*see* Endocarditis
pulmonary (valve) (heart) I37.1
congenital Q22.2
syphilitic A52.03
tricuspid —*see* Insufficiency, tricuspid
valve, valvular —*see* Endocarditis
congenital Q24.8
vesicoureteral —*see* Reflux, vesicoureteral
Reichmann's disease or syndrome K31.89
Reifenstein syndrome E34.52
~~Reinsertion, contraceptive device Z30.433~~
Reinsertion ◀
implantable subdermal contraceptive Z30.46 ◀
intrauterine contraceptive device Z30.433 ◀
Reiter's disease, syndrome, or urethritis M02.30
ankle M02.37-
elbow M02.32-
foot joint M02.37-
hand joint M02.34-
hip M02.35-
knee M02.36-
multiple site M02.39

Reiter's disease, syndrome, or urethritis
    (Continued)
  shoulder M02.31-
  vertebra M02.38
  wrist M02.33-
Rejection
  food, psychogenic F50.89 ◀▥
  transplant T86.91
    bone T86.830
      marrow T86.01
    cornea T86.840
    heart T86.21
      with lung (s) T86.31
    intestine T86.850
    kidney T86.11
    liver T86.41
    lung (s) T86.810
      with heart T86.31
    organ (immune or nonimmune cause)
        T86.91
    pancreas T86.890
    skin (allograft) (autograft) T86.820
    specified NEC T86.890
    stem cell (peripheral blood) (umbilical
        cord) T86.5
Relapsing fever A68.9
  Carter's (Asiatic) A68.1
  Dutton's (West African) A68.1
  Koch's A68.9
  louse-borne (epidemic) A68.0
  Novy's (American) A68.1
  Obermeyers's (European) A68.0
  Spirillum A68.9
  tick-borne (endemic) A68.1
Relationship
  occlusal
    open anterior M26.220
    open posterior M26.221
Relaxation
  anus (sphincter) K62.89
    psychogenic F45.8
  arch (foot) —see also Deformity, limb, flat
      foot
  back ligaments —see Instability, joint,
      spine
  bladder (sphincter) N31.2
  cardioesophageal K21.9
  cervix —see Incompetency, cervix
  diaphragm J98.6
  joint (capsule) (ligament) (paralytic) —see
      Flail, joint
    congenital NEC Q74.8
  lumbosacral (joint) —see subcategory M53.2
  pelvic floor N81.89
  perineum N81.89
  posture R29.3
  rectum (sphincter) K62.89
  sacroiliac (joint) —see subcategory M53.2
  scrotum N50.89 ◀▥
  urethra (sphincter) N36.44
  vesical N31.2
Release from prison, anxiety concerning
    Z65.2
Remains
  canal of Cloquet Q14.0
  capsule (opaque) Q14.8
Remittent fever (malarial) B54
Remnant
  canal of Cloquet Q14.0
  capsule (opaque) Q14.8
  cervix, cervical stump (acquired)
      (postoperative) N88.8
  cystic duct, postcholecystectomy K91.5
  fingernail L60.8
    congenital Q84.6
  meniscus, knee —see Derangement, knee,
      meniscus, specified NEC
  thyroglossal duct Q89.2
  tonsil J35.8
    infected (chronic) J35.01
  urachus Q64.4

Removal (from) (of)
  artificial
    arm Z44.00-
      complete Z44.01-
      partial Z44.02-
    eye Z44.2-
    leg Z44.10-
      complete Z44.11-
      partial Z44.12-
  breast implant Z45.81
  cardiac pulse generator (battery) (end-of-life)
      Z45.010
  catheter (urinary) (indwelling) Z46.6
    from artificial opening —see Attention to,
        artificial, opening
    non-vascular Z46.82
    vascular NEC Z45.2
  device Z46.9
    contraceptive Z30.432
      implantable subdermal Z30.46 ◀
    implanted NEC Z45.89
    specified NEC Z46.89
  drains Z48.03
  dressing (nonsurgical) Z48.00
    surgical Z48.01
  external
    fixation device — code to fracture with
        seventh character D
    prosthesis, prosthetic device Z44.9
      breast Z44.3-
      specified NEC Z44.8
  home in childhood (to foster home or
      institution) Z62.29
  ileostomy Z43.2
  insulin pump Z46.81
  myringotomy device (stent) (tube) Z45.82
  nervous system device NEC Z46.2
    brain neuropacemaker Z46.2
    visual substitution device Z46.2
      implanted Z45.31
  non-vascular catheter Z46.82
  organ, prophylactic (for neoplasia
      management) —see Prophylactic, organ
      removal
  orthodontic device Z46.4
  staples Z48.02
  stent
    ureteral Z46.6
  suture Z48.02
  urinary device Z46.6
  vascular access device or catheter Z45.2
Ren
  arcuatus Q63.1
  mobile, mobilis N28.89
    congenital Q63.8
  unguliformis Q63.1
Renal —see condition
Rendu-Osler-Weber disease or syndrome
    I78.0
Reninoma D41.0-
Renon-Delille syndrome E23.3
Reovirus, as cause of disease classified
    elsewhere B97.5
Repeated falls NEC R29.6
Replaced chromosome by dicentric ring
    Q93.2
Replacement by artificial or mechanical device
    or prosthesis of
  bladder Z96.0
  blood vessel NEC Z95.828
  bone NEC Z96.7
  cochlea Z96.21
  coronary artery Z95.5
  eustachian tube Z96.29
  eye globe Z97.0
  heart Z95.812
    valve Z95.2
      prosthetic Z95.2
      specified NEC Z95.4
      xenogenic Z95.3
  intestine Z96.89

Replacement by artificial or mechanical device
    or prosthesis of (Continued)
  joint Z96.60
    hip —see Presence, hip joint implant
    knee —see Presence, knee joint implant
    specified site NEC Z96.698
  larynx Z96.3
  lens Z96.1
  limb (s) —see Presence, artificial, limb
  mandible NEC (for tooth root implant (s))
      Z96.5
  organ NEC Z96.89
  peripheral vessel NEC Z95.828
  stapes Z96.29
  teeth Z97.2
  tendon Z96.7
  tissue NEC Z96.89
  tooth root (s) Z96.5
  vessel NEC Z95.828
    coronary (artery) Z95.5
Request for expert evidence Z04.8
Reserve, decreased or low
  cardiac —see Disease, heart
  kidney N28.89
Residual —see also condition
  ovary syndrome N99.83
  state, schizophrenic F20.5
  urine R39.198 ◀▥
Resistance, resistant (to)
  activated protein C D68.51
  complicating pregnancy O26.89
  insulin E88.81
  organism (s)
    to
      drug Z16.30 ◀▥
        aminoglycosides Z16.29
        amoxicillin Z16.11
        ampicillin Z16.11
        antibiotic (s) Z16.20
          multiple Z16.24
          specified NEC Z16.29
        antifungal Z16.32
        antimicrobial (single) Z16.30
          multiple Z16.35
          specified NEC Z16.39
        antimycobacterial (single) Z16.341
          multiple Z16.342
        antimycobacterial (single)
            Z16.341 ◀
          multiple Z16.342 ◀
        antiparasitic Z16.31
        antiviral Z16.33
        beta lactam antibiotics Z16.10
          specified NEC Z16.19
        cephalosporins Z16.19
        extended beta lactamase (ESBL)
            Z16.12
        fluoroquinolones Z16.23
        macrolides Z16.29
        methicillin —see MRSA
        multiple drugs (MDRO)
          antibiotics Z16.24
          antimicrobial Z16.35 ◀
          antimycobacterials
              Z16.342 ◀
        penicillins Z16.11
        quinine (and related compounds)
            Z16.31
        quinolones Z16.23
        sulfonamides Z16.29
        tetracyclines Z16.29
        tuberculostatics (single) Z16.341
          multiple Z16.342
        vancomycin Z16.21
          related antibiotics Z16.22
  thyroid hormone E07.89
Resorption
  dental (roots) K03.3
    alveoli M26.79
  teeth (external) (internal) (pathological)
      (roots) K03.3

◀ New   ◀▥ Revised   ~~deleted~~ Deleted

Respiration
   Cheyne-Stokes R06.3
   decreased due to shock, following injury
      T79.4
   disorder of, psychogenic F45.8
   insufficient, or poor R06.89
      newborn P28.5
   painful R07.1
   sighing, psychogenic F45.8
Respiratory —see also condition
   distress syndrome (newborn) (type I)
      P22.0
      type II P22.1
   syncytial virus, as cause of disease classified
      elsewhere B97.4
Respite care Z75.5
Response (drug)
   photoallergic L56.1
   phototoxic L56.0
Restenosis ◀
   stent ◀
      vascular ◀
         end stent ◀
            adjacent to stent —see
               Arteriosclerosis ◀
            within the stent ◀
               coronary T82.855 ◀
               peripheral T82.856 ◀
            in stent ◀
               coronary vessel T82.855 ◀
               peripheral vessel T82.856 ◀
Restless legs (syndrome) G25.81
Restlessness R45.1
Restoration (of)
   dental
      aesthetically inadequate or displeasing
         K08.56
      defective K08.50
         specified NEC K08.59
      failure of marginal integrity K08.51
      failure of periodontal anatomical intergrity
         K08.54
   organ continuity from previous sterilization
      (tuboplasty) (vasoplasty) Z31.0
      aftercare Z31.42
   tooth (existing)
      contours biologically incompatible with
         oral health K08.54
      open margins K08.51
      overhanging K08.52
      poor aesthetic K08.56
      poor gingival margins K08.51
   unsatisfactory, of tooth K08.50
      specified NEC K08.59
Restorative material (dental)
   allergy to K08.55
   fractured K08.539
      with loss of material K08.531
      without loss of material K08.530
   unrepairable overhanging of K08.52
Restriction of housing space Z59.1
Rests, ovarian, in fallopian tube Q50.6
Restzustand (schizophrenic) F20.5
Retained —see also Retention
   cholelithiasis following cholecystectomy
      K91.86
   foreign body fragments (type of) Z18.9
      acrylics Z18.2
      animal quill (s) or spines Z18.31
      cement Z18.83
      concrete Z18.83
      crystalline Z18.83
      depleted isotope Z18.09
      depleted uranium Z18.01
      diethylhexylphthalates Z18.2
      glass Z18.81
      isocyanate Z18.2
      magnetic metal Z18.11
      metal Z18.10
      nonmagnetic metal Z18.12
      nontherapeutic radioactive Z18.09

Retained (Continued)
   foreign body fragments (Continued)
      organic NEC Z18.39
      plastic Z18.2
      quill (s) (animal) Z18.31
      radioactive (nontherapeutic) NEC
         Z18.09
      specified NEC Z18.89
      spine (s) (animal) Z18.31
      stone Z18.83
      tooth (teeth) Z18.32
      wood Z18.33
   fragments (type of) Z18.9
      acrylics Z18.2
      animal quill (s) or spines Z18.31
      cement Z18.83
      concrete Z18.83
      crystalline Z18.83
      depleted isotope Z18.09
      depleted uranium Z18.01
      diethylhexylphthalates Z18.2
      glass Z18.81
      isocyanate Z18.2
      magnetic metal Z18.11
      metal Z18.10
      nonmagnectic metal Z18.12
      nontherapeutic radioactive Z18.09
      organic NEC Z18.39
      plastic Z18.2
      quill (s) (animal) Z18.31
      radioactive (nontherapeutic) NEC
         Z18.09
      specified NEC Z18.89
      spine (s) (animal) Z18.31
      stone Z18.83
      tooth (teeth) Z18.32
      wood Z18.33
   gallstones, following cholecystectomy K91.86
Retardation
   development, developmental, specific —see
      Disorder, developmental
   endochondral bone growth —see Disorder,
      bone, development or growth
   growth R62.50
      due to malnutrition E45
   mental —see Disability, intellectual
   motor function, specific F82
   physical (child) R62.52
      due to malnutrition E45
   reading (specific) F81.0
   spelling (specific) (without reading disorder)
      F81.81
Retching —see Vomiting
Retention —see also Retained
   bladder —see Retention, urine
   carbon dioxide E87.2
   cholelithiasis following cholecystectomy
      K91.86
   cyst —see Cyst
   dead
      fetus (at or near term) (mother) O36.4
         early fetal death O02.1
      ovum O02.0
   decidua (fragments) (following delivery)
      (with hemorrhage) O72.2
      without hemorrhage O73.1
   deciduous tooth K00.6
   dental root K08.3
   fecal —see Constipation
   fetus
      dead O36.4
      early O02.1
   fluid R60.9
   foreign body —see also Foreign body, retained
      current trauma - code as Foreign body, by
         site or type
   gallstones, following cholecystectomy K91.86
   gastric K31.89
   intrauterine contraceptive device, in
      pregnancy —see Pregnancy, complicated
      by, retention, intrauterine device

Retention (Continued)
   membranes (complicating delivery) (with
      hemorrhage) O72.2
      with abortion —see Abortion, by type
      without hemorrhage O73.1
   meniscus —see Derangement, meniscus
   menses N94.89
   milk (puerperal, postpartum) O92.79
   nitrogen, extrarenal R39.2
   ovary syndrome N99.83
   placenta (total) (with hemorrhage) O72.0
      without hemorrhage O73.0
      portions or fragments (with hemorrhage)
         O72.2
      without hemorrhage O73.1
   products of conception
      early pregnancy (dead fetus) O02.1
      following
         delivery (with hemorrhage) O72.2
         without hemorrhage O73.1
   secundines (following delivery) (with
      hemorrhage) O72.0
      without hemorrhage O73.0
   complicating puerperium (delayed
      hemorrhage) O72.2
      partial O72.2
         without hemorrhage O73.1
   smegma, clitoris N90.89
   urine R33.9
      drug-induced R33.0
      due to hyperplasia (hypertrophy) of
         prostate —see Hyperplasia, prostate
      organic R33.8
         drug-induced R33.0
      psychogenic F45.8
      specified NEC R33.8
   water (in tissues) —see Edema
Reticular erythematous mucinosis L98.5
Reticulation, dust —see Pneumoconiosis
Reticulocytosis R70.1
Reticuloendotheliosis
   acute infantile C96.0
   leukemic C91.4-
   ~~malignant C96.9~~
   nonlipid C96.0
Reticulohistiocytoma (giant-cell) D76.3
Reticuloid, actinic L57.1
Reticulosis (skin)
   acute of infancy C96.0
   hemophagocytic, familial D76.1
   histiocytic medullary C96.A ◀
   lipomelanotic I89.8
   malignant (midline) C86.0
   ~~nonlipid C96.0~~
   polymorphic C86.0
   Sézary —see Sézary disease
Retina, retinal —see also condition
   dark area D49.81
Retinitis —see also Inflammation, chorioretinal
   albuminurica N18.9 [H32]
   diabetic —see Diabetes, retinitis
   disciformis —see Degeneration, macula
   focal —see Inflammation, chorioretinal,
      focal
   gravidarum —see Pregnancy, complicated by,
      specified pregnancy-related condition
      NEC
   juxtapapillaris —see Inflammation,
      chorioretinal, focal, juxtapapillary
   luetic —see Retinitis, syphilitic
   pigmentosa H35.52
   proliferans —see Disorder, globe,
      degenerative, specified type NEC
   proliferating —see Disorder, globe,
      degenerative, specified type NEC
   renal N18.9 [H32]
   syphilitic (early) (secondary) A51.43
      central, recurrent A52.71
      congenital (early) A50.01 [H32]
      late A52.71
   tuberculous A18.53

Retinoblastoma C69.2-
  differentiated C69.2-
  undifferentiated C69.2-
Retinochoroiditis —see also Inflammation,
    chorioretinal
  disseminated —see Inflammation,
      chorioretinal, disseminated
    syphilitic A52.71
  focal —see Inflammation, chorioretinal
  juxtapapillaris —see Inflammation,
      chorioretinal, focal, juxtapapillary
Retinopathy (background) H35.00
  arteriosclerotic I70.8 [H35.0-]
  atherosclerotic I70.8 [H35.0-]
  central serous —see Chorioretinopathy,
      central serous
  Coats H35.02-
  diabetic —see Diabetes, retinopathy
  exudative H35.02-
  hypertensive H35.03-
  in (due to)
    diabetes —see Diabetes, retinopathy
    sickle-cell disorders D57.- [H36]
  of prematurity H35.10-
    stage 0 H35.11-
    stage 1 H35.12-
    stage 2 H35.13-
    stage 3 H35.14-
    stage 4 H35.15-
    stage 5 H35.16-
  pigmentary, congenital —see Dystrophy,
      retina
  proliferative NEC H35.2-
    diabetic —see Diabetes, retinopathy,
        proliferative
    sickle-cell D57.- [H36]
  solar H31.02-
Retinoschisis H33.10-
  congenital Q14.1
  specified type NEC H33.19-
Retortamoniasis A07.8
Retractile testis Q55.22
Retraction
  cervix —see Retroversion, uterus
  drum (membrane) —see Disorder, tympanic
      membrane, specified NEC
  finger —see Deformity, finger
  lid H02.539
    left H02.536
      lower H02.535
      upper H02.534
    right H02.533
      lower H02.532
      upper H02.531
  lung J98.4
  mediastinum J98.59 ◄▥
  nipple N64.53
    associated with
      lactation O92.03
      pregnancy O92.01-
      puerperium O92.02
    congenital Q83.8
  palmar fascia M72.0
  pleura —see Pleurisy
  ring, uterus (Bandl's) (pathological) O62.4
  sternum (congenital) Q76.7
    acquired M95.4
  uterus —see Retroversion, uterus
  valve (heart) —see Endocarditis
Retrobulbar —see condition
Retrocecal —see condition
Retrocession —see Retroversion
Retrodisplacement —see Retroversion
Retroflection, retroflexion —see Retroversion
Retrognathia, retrognathism (mandibular)
    (maxillary) M26.19
Retrograde menstruation N92.5
Retroperineal —see condition
Retroperitoneal —see condition
Retroperitonitis K68.9
Retropharyngeal —see condition

Retroplacental —see condition
Retroposition —see Retroversion
Retroprosthetic membrane T85.398
Retrosternal thyroid (congenital) Q89.2
Retroversion, retroverted
  cervix —see Retroversion, uterus
  female NEC —see Retroversion, uterus
  iris H21.89
  testis (congenital) Q55.29
  uterus (acquired) (acute) (any
      degree) (asymptomatic) (cervix)
      (postinfectional) (postpartal, old) N85.4
    congenital Q51.818
    in pregnancy O34.53-
Retrovirus, as cause of disease classified
    elsewhere B97.30
  human
    immunodeficiency, type 2 (HIV 2) B97.35
    T-cell lymphotropic
      type I (HTLV-I) B97.33
      type II (HTLV-II) B97.34
  lentivirus B97.31
  oncovirus B97.32
  specified NEC B97.39
Retrusion, premaxilla (developmental) M26.09
Rett's disease or syndrome F84.2
Reverse peristalsis R19.2
Reye's syndrome G93.7
Rh (factor)
  hemolytic disease (newborn) P55.0
  incompatibility, immunization or
      sensitization
    affecting management of pregnancy NEC
        O36.09-
      anti-D antibody O36.01-
    newborn P55.0
    transfusion reaction —see Complication (s),
        transfusion, incompatibility reaction,
        Rh (factor)
  negative mother affecting newborn P55.0
  titer elevated —see Complication (s),
      transfusion, incompatibility reaction,
      Rh (factor)
  transfusion reaction —see Complication (s),
      transfusion, incompatibility reaction,
      Rh (factor)
Rhabdomyolysis (idiopathic) NEC M62.82
  traumatic T79.6
Rhabdomyoma —see also Neoplasm, connective
    tissue, benign
  adult —see Neoplasm, connective tissue,
      benign
  fetal —see Neoplasm, connective tissue, benign
  glycogenic —see Neoplasm, connective tissue,
      benign
Rhabdomyosarcoma (any type) —see
    Neoplasm, connective tissue, malignant
Rhabdosarcoma —see Rhabdomyosarcoma
Rhesus (factor) incompatibility —see Rh,
    incompatibility
Rheumatic (acute) (subacute) (chronic)
  adherent pericardium I09.2
  coronary arteritis I01.9
  degeneration, myocardium I09.0
  fever (acute) —see Fever, rheumatic
  heart —see Disease, heart, rheumatic
  myocardial degeneration —see Degeneration,
      myocardium
  myocarditis (chronic) (inactive) (with chorea)
      I09.0
    with chorea (acute) (rheumatic)
        (Sydenham's) I02.0
    active or acute I01.2
  pancarditis, acute I01.8
    with chorea (acute (rheumatic)
        Sydenham's) I02.0
  pericarditis (active) (acute) (with effusion)
      (with pneumonia) I01.0
    with chorea (acute) (rheumatic)
        (Sydenham's) I02.0
    chronic or inactive I09.2

Rheumatic (Continued)
  pneumonia I00 [J17]
  torticollis M43.6
  typhoid fever A01.09
Rheumatism (articular) (neuralgic)
    (nonarticular) M79.0
  gout —see Arthritis, rheumatoid
  intercostal, meaning Tietze's disease M94.0
  palindromic (any site) M12.30
    ankle M12.37-
    elbow M12.32-
    foot joint M12.37-
    hand joint M12.34-
    hip M12.35-
    knee M12.36-
    multiple site M12.39
    shoulder M12.31-
    specified joint NEC M12.38
    vertebrae M12.38
    wrist M12.33-
  sciatic M54.4-
Rheumatoid —see also condition
  arthritis —see also Arthritis, rheumatoid
    with involvement of organs NEC M05.60
      ankle M05.67-
      elbow M05.62-
      foot joint M05.67-
      hand joint M05.64-
      hip M05.65-
      knee M05.66-
      multiple site M05.69
      shoulder M05.61-
      vertebra —see Spondylitis, ankylosing
      wrist M05.63-
    seronegative —see Arthritis, rheumatoid,
        seronegative
    seropositive —see Arthritis, rheumatoid,
        seropositive
  carditis M05.30
    ankle M05.37-
    elbow M05.32-
    foot joint M05.37-
    hand joint M05.34-
    hip M05.35-
    knee M05.36-
    multiple site M05.39
    shoulder M05.31-
    vertebra —see Spondylitis, ankylosing
    wrist M05.33-
  endocarditis —see Rheumatoid, carditis
  lung (disease) M05.10
    ankle M05.17-
    elbow M05.12-
    foot joint M05.17-
    hand joint M05.14-
    hip M05.15-
    knee M05.16-
    multiple site M05.19
    shoulder M05.11-
    vertebra —see Spondylitis, ankylosing
    wrist M05.13-
  myocarditis —see Rheumatoid, carditis
  myopathy M05.40
    ankle M05.47-
    elbow M05.42-
    foot joint M05.47-
    hand joint M05.44-
    hip M05.45-
    knee M05.46-
    multiple site M05.49
    shoulder M05.41-
    vertebra —see Spondylitis, ankylosing
    wrist M05.43-
  pericarditis —see Rheumatoid, carditis
  polyarthritis —see Arthritis, rheumatoid
  polyneuropathy M05.50
    ankle M05.57-
    elbow M05.52-
    foot joint M05.57-
    hand joint M05.54-
    hip M05.55-

Rheumatoid *(Continued)*
  polyneuropathy *(Continued)*
    knee M05.56-
    multiple site M05.59
    shoulder M05.51-
    vertebra —*see* Spondylitis, ankylosing
    wrist M05.53-
  vasculitis M05.20
    ankle M05.27-
    elbow M05.22-
    foot joint M05.27-
    hand joint M05.24-
    hip M05.25-
    knee M05.26-
    multiple site M05.29
    shoulder M05.21-
    vertebra —*see* Spondylitis, ankylosing
    wrist M05.23-
Rhinitis (atrophic) (catarrhal) (chronic)
      (croupous) (fibrinous) (granulomatous)
      (hyperplastic) (hypertrophic)
      (membranous) (obstructive) (purulent)
      (suppurative) (ulcerative) J31.0
  with
    sore throat —*see* Nasopharyngitis
  acute J00
  allergic J30.9
    with asthma J45.909
      with
        exacerbation (acute) J45.901
        status asthmaticus J45.902
      due to
        food J30.5
        pollen J30.1
      nonseasonal J30.89
      perennial J30.89
      seasonal NEC J30.2
      specified NEC J30.89
  infective J00
  pneumococcal J00
  syphilitic A52.73
    congenital A50.05 *[J99]*
  tuberculous A15.8
  vasomotor J30.0
Rhinoantritis (chronic) —*see* Sinusitis,
      maxillary
Rhinodacryolith —*see* Dacryolith
Rhinolith (nasal sinus) J34.89
Rhinomegaly J34.89
Rhinopharyngitis (acute) (subacute) —*see also*
      Nasopharyngitis
  chronic J31.1
  destructive ulcerating A66.5
  mutilans A66.5
Rhinophyma L71.1
Rhinorrhea J34.89
  cerebrospinal (fluid) G96.0
  paroxysmal —*see* Rhinitis, allergic
  spasmodic —*see* Rhinitis, allergic
Rhinosalpingitis —*see* Salpingitis, eustachian
Rhinoscleroma A48.8
Rhinosporidiosis B48.1
Rhinovirus infection NEC B34.8
Rhizomelic chondrodysplasia punctata
      E71.540
Rhythm
  atrioventricular nodal I49.8
  disorder I49.9
    coronary sinus I49.8
    ectopic I49.8
    nodal I49.8
  escape I49.9
  heart, abnormal I49.9
  idioventricular I44.2
  nodal I49.8
  sleep, inversion G47.2-
    nonorganic origin —*see* Disorder, sleep,
      circadian rhythm, psychogenic
Rhytidosis facialis L98.8
Rib —*see also* condition
  cervical Q76.5

Riboflavin deficiency E53.0
Rice bodies —*see also* Loose, body, joint
  knee M23.4-
Richter syndrome —*see* Leukemia, chronic
    lymphocytic, B-cell type
Richter's hernia —*see* Hernia, abdomen, with
    obstruction
Ricinism —*see* Poisoning, food, noxious,
    plant
Rickets (active) (acute) (adolescent) (chest
      wall) (congenital) (current) (infantile)
      (intestinal) E55.0
  adult —*see* Osteomalacia
  celiac K90.0
  hypophosphatemic with nephrotic-glycosuric
    dwarfism E72.09
  inactive E64.3
  kidney N25.0
  renal N25.0
  sequelae, any E64.3
  vitamin-D-resistant E83.31 *[M90.80]*
Rickettsial disease A79.9
  specified type NEC A79.89
Rickettsialpox (Rickettsia akari) A79.1
Rickettsiosis A79.9
  due to
    Ehrlichia sennetsu A79.81
    Rickettsia akari (rickettsialpox) A79.1
  specified type NEC A79.89
  tick-borne A77.9
  vesicular A79.1
Rider's bone —*see* Ossification, muscle,
    specified NEC
Ridge, alveolus —*see also* condition
  flabby K06.8
Ridged ear, congenital Q17.3
Riedel's
  lobe, liver Q44.7
  struma, thyroiditis or disease E06.5
Rieger's anomaly or syndrome Q13.81
Riehl's melanosis L81.4
Rietti-Greppi-Micheli anemia D56.9
Rieux's hernia —*see* Hernia, abdomen, specified
    site NEC
Riga (-Fede) disease K14.0
Riggs' disease —*see* Periodontitis
Right aortic arch Q25.47 ◀
Right middle lobe syndrome J98.11
Rigid, rigidity —*see also* condition
  abdominal R19.30
    with severe abdominal pain R10.0
    epigastric R19.36
    generalized R19.37
    left lower quadrant R19.34
    left upper quadrant R19.32
    periumbilic R19.35
    right lower quadrant R19.33
    right upper quadrant R19.31
  articular, multiple, congenital Q68.8
  cervix (uteri) in pregnancy —*see* Pregnancy,
      complicated by, abnormal, cervix
  hymen (acquired) (congenital) N89.6
  nuchal R29.1
  pelvic floor in pregnancy —*see* Pregnancy,
      complicated by, abnormal, pelvic organs
      or tissues NEC
  perineum or vulva in pregnancy —*see*
      Pregnancy, complicated by, abnormal,
      vulva
  spine —*see* Dorsopathy, specified NEC
  vagina in pregnancy —*see* Pregnancy,
      complicated by, abnormal, vagina
Rigors R68.89
  with fever R50.9
Riley-Day syndrome G90.1
RIND (reversible ischemic neurologic deficit)
      I63.9
Ring (s)
  aorta (vascular) Q25.45 ◀|||
  Bandl's O62.4
  contraction, complicating delivery O62.4

Ring (s) *(Continued)*
  esophageal, lower (muscular) K22.2
  Fleischer's (cornea) H18.04-
  hymenal, tight (acquired) (congenital) N89.6
  Kayser-Fleischer (cornea) H18.04-
  retraction, uterus, pathological O62.4
  Schatzki's (esophagus) (lower) K22.2
    congenital Q39.3
  Soemmerring's —*see* Cataract, secondary
  vascular (congenital) Q25.8
    aorta Q25.45 ◀|||
Ringed hair (congenital) Q84.1
Ringworm B35.9
  beard B35.0
  black dot B35.0
  body B35.4
  Burmese B35.5
  corporeal B35.4
  foot B35.3
  groin B35.6
  hand B35.2
  honeycomb B35.0
  nails B35.1
  perianal (area) B35.6
  scalp B35.0
  specified NEC B35.8
  Tokelau B35.5
Rise, venous pressure I87.8
Rising, PSA following treatment for malignant
      neoplasm of prostate R97.21 ◀
Risk, suicidal
  meaning personal history of attempted
      suicide Z91.5
  meaning suicidal ideation —*see* Ideation,
      suicidal
Ritter's disease L00
Rivalry, sibling Z62.891
Rivalta's disease A42.2
River blindness B73.01
Robert's pelvis Q74.2
  with disproportion (fetopelvic) O33.0
    causing obstructed labor O65.0
Robin (-Pierre) syndrome Q87.0
Robinow-Silvermann-Smith syndrome Q87.1
Robinson's (hidrotic) ectodermal dysplasia or
      syndrome Q82.4
Robles' disease B73.01
Rocky Mountain (spotted) **fever** A77.0
Roetheln —*see* Rubella
Roger's disease Q21.0
Rokitansky-Aschoff sinuses (gallbladder) K82.8
Rolando's fracture (displaced) S62.22-
  nondisplaced S62.22-
Romano-Ward (prolonged QT interval)
      syndrome I45.81
Romberg's disease or syndrome G51.8
Roof, mouth —*see* condition
Rosacea L71.9
  acne L71.9
  keratitis L71.8
  specified NEC L71.8
Rosary, rachitic E55.0
Rose
  cold J30.1
  fever J30.1
  rash R21
    epidemic B06.9
Rosenbach's erysipeloid A26.0
Rosenthal's disease or syndrome D68.1
Roseola B09
  infantum B08.20
    due to human herpesvirus 6 B08.21
    due to human herpesvirus 7 B08.22
Ross River disease or fever B33.1
Rossbach's disease K31.89
  psychogenic F45.8
Rostan's asthma (cardiac) —*see* Failure,
      ventricular, left
Rotation
  anomalous, incomplete or insufficient,
      intestine Q43.3

Rotation *(Continued)*
  cecum (congenital) Q43.3
  colon (congenital) Q43.3
  spine, incomplete or insufficient —*see*
      Dorsopathy, deforming, specified NEC
  tooth, teeth, fully erupted M26.35
  vertebra, incomplete or insufficient —*see*
      Dorsopathy, deforming, specified NEC
Rotes Quérol disease or syndrome —*see*
      Hyperostosis, ankylosing
Roth (-Bernhardt) disease or syndrome —*see*
      Meralgia paraesthetica
Rothmund (-Thomson) syndrome Q82.8
Rotor's disease or syndrome E80.6
Round
  back (with wedging of vertebrae) —*see*
      Kyphosis
  sequelae (late effect) of rickets E64.3
  worms (large) (infestation) NEC B82.0
      Ascariasis —*see also* Ascariasis B77.9
Roussy-Lévy syndrome G60.0
Rubella (German measles) B06.9
  complication NEC B06.09
      neurological B06.00
  congenital P35.0
  contact Z20.4
  exposure to Z20.4
  maternal
      care for (suspected) damage to fetus O35.3
      manifest rubella in infant P35.0
      suspected damage to fetus affecting
          management of pregnancy O35.3
  specified complications NEC B06.89
Rubeola (meaning measles) —*see* Measles
  meaning rubella —*see* Rubella
Rubeosis, iris —*see* Disorder, iris, vascular
Rubinstein-Taybi syndrome Q87.2
Rudimentary (congenital) —*see also* Agenesis
  arm —*see* Defect, reduction, upper limb
  bone Q79.9
  cervix uteri Q51.828
  eye Q11.2
  lobule of ear Q17.3
  patella Q74.1
  respiratory organs in thoracopagus Q89.4
  tracheal bronchus Q32.4
  uterus Q51.818
      in male Q56.1
  vagina Q52.0
Ruled out condition —*see* Observation,
      suspected
Rumination R11.10
  with nausea R11.2
  disorder of infancy F98.21
  neurotic F42.8 ◄▥
  newborn P92.1
  obsessional F42.8 ◄▥
  psychogenic F42.8 ◄▥
Runeberg's disease D51.0
Runny nose R09.89
Rupia (syphilitic) A51.39
  congenital A50.06
  tertiary A52.79
Rupture, ruptured
  abscess (spontaneous) - code by site under
      Abscess
  aneurysm —*see* Aneurysm
  anus (sphincter) —*see* Laceration, anus
  aorta, aortic I71.8
      abdominal I71.3
      arch I71.1
      ascending I71.1
      descending I71.8
          abdominal I71.3
          thoracic I71.1
      syphilitic A52.01
      thoracoabdominal I71.5
      thorax, thoracic I71.1
      transverse I71.1
      traumatic —*see* Injury, aorta, laceration,
          major

Rupture, ruptured *(Continued)*
  aorta, aortic *(Continued)*
      valve or cusp —*see also* Endocarditis, aortic
          I35.8
  appendix (with peritonitis) K35.2
      with localized peritonitis K35.3 ◄
  arteriovenous fistula, brain I60.8
  artery I77.2
      brain —*see* Hemorrhage, intracranial,
          intracerebral
      coronary —*see* Infarct, myocardium
      heart —*see* Infarct, myocardium
      pulmonary I28.8
      traumatic (complication) —*see* Injury,
          blood vessel
  bile duct (common) (hepatic) K83.2
      cystic K82.2
  bladder (sphincter) (nontraumatic)
      (spontaneous) N32.89
      following ectopic or molar pregnancy
          O08.6
      obstetrical trauma O71.5
      traumatic S37.29
  blood vessel —*see also* Hemorrhage
      brain —*see* Hemorrhage, intracranial,
          intracerebral
      heart —*see* Infarct, myocardium
      traumatic (complication) —*see* Injury,
          blood vessel, laceration, major, by site
  bone —*see* Fracture
  bowel (nontraumatic) K63.1
  brain
      aneurysm (congenital) —*see also*
          Hemorrhage, intracranial,
          subarachnoid
      syphilitic A52.05
      hemorrhagic —*see* Hemorrhage,
          intracranial, intracerebral
  capillaries I78.8
  cardiac (auricle) (ventricle) (wall) I23.3
      with hemopericardium I23.0
      infectional I40.9
      traumatic —*see* Injury, heart
  cartilage (articular) (current) —*see also* Sprain
      knee S83.3-
      semilunar —*see* Tear, meniscus
  cecum (with peritonitis) K65.0
      with peritoneal abscess K35.3
      traumatic S36.598
  celiac artery, traumatic —*see* Injury, blood
      vessel, celiac artery, laceration, major
  cerebral aneurysm (congenital) (*see*
      Hemorrhage, intracranial,
      subarachnoid)
  cervix (uteri)
      with ectopic or molar pregnancy O08.6
      following ectopic or molar pregnancy
          O08.6
      obstetrical trauma O71.3
      traumatic S37.69
  chordae tendineae NEC I51.1
      concurrent with acute myocardial
          infarction —*see* Infarct, myocardium
      following acute myocardial infarction
          (current complication) I23.4
  choroid (direct) (indirect) (traumatic) H31.32-
  circle of Willis I60.6
  colon (nontraumatic) K63.1
      traumatic —*see* Injury, intestine, large
  cornea (traumatic) —*see* Injury, eye, laceration
  coronary (artery) (thrombotic) —*see* Infarct,
      myocardium
  corpus luteum (infected) (ovary) N83.1- ◄▥
  cyst —*see* Cyst
  cystic duct K82.2
  Descemet's membrane —*see* Change, corneal
      membrane, Descemet's, rupture
      traumatic —*see* Injury, eye, laceration
  diaphragm, traumatic —*see* Injury,
      intrathoracic, diaphragm
  disc —*see* Rupture, intervertebral disc

Rupture, ruptured *(Continued)*
  diverticulum (intestine) K57.80
      with bleeding K57.81
      bladder N32.3
      large intestine K57.20
          with
              bleeding K57.21
              small intestine K57.40
                  with bleeding K57.41
      small intestine K57.00
          with
              bleeding K57.01
              large intestine K57.40
                  with bleeding K57.41
  duodenal stump K31.89
  ear drum (nontraumatic) —*see also*
      Perforation, tympanum
      traumatic S09.2-
      due to blast injury —*see* Injury, blast, ear
  esophagus K22.3
  eye (without prolapse or loss of intraocular
      tissue) —*see* Injury, eye, laceration
  fallopian tube NEC (nonobstetric)
      (nontraumatic) N83.8
      due to pregnancy O00.10 ◄▥
          with intrauterine pregnancy O00.11 ◄
  fontanel P13.1
  gallbladder K82.2
      traumatic S36.128
  gastric —*see also* Rupture, stomach
      vessel K92.2
  globe (eye) (traumatic) —*see* Injury, eye,
      laceration
  graafian follicle (hematoma) N83.0- ◄▥
  heart —*see* Rupture, cardiac
  hymen (nontraumatic) (nonintentional)
      N89.8
  internal organ, traumatic —*see* Injury,
      by site
  intervertebral disc —*see* Displacement,
      intervertebral disc
      traumatic —*see* Rupture, traumatic,
          intervertebral disc
  intestine NEC (nontraumatic) K63.1
      traumatic —*see* Injury, intestine
  iris —*see also* Abnormality, pupillary
      traumatic —*see* Injury, eye, laceration
  joint capsule, traumatic —*see* Sprain
  kidney (traumatic) S37.06-
      birth injury P15.8
      nontraumatic N28.89
  lacrimal duct (traumatic) —*see* Injury, eye,
      specified site NEC
  lens (cataract) (traumatic) —*see* Cataract,
      traumatic
  ligament, traumatic —*see* Rupture, traumatic,
      ligament, by site
  liver S36.116
      birth injury P15.0
  lymphatic vessel I89.8
  marginal sinus (placental) (with
      hemorrhage) —*see* Hemorrhage,
      antepartum, specified cause NEC
  membrana tympani (nontraumatic) —*see*
      Perforation, tympanum
  membranes (spontaneous)
      artificial
          delayed delivery following O75.5
      delayed delivery following —*see*
          Pregnancy, complicated by,
          premature rupture of membranes
  meningeal artery I60.8
  meniscus (knee) —*see also* Tear, meniscus
      old —*see* Derangement, meniscus
      site other than knee - code as Sprain
  mesenteric artery, traumatic —*see* Injury,
      mesenteric, artery, laceration, major
  mesentery (nontraumatic) K66.8
      traumatic —*see* Injury, intra-abdominal,
          specified, site NEC
  mitral (valve) I34.8

◄ New   ◄▥ Revised   ~~deleted~~ Deleted

Rupture, ruptured *(Continued)*
 muscle (traumatic) —*see also* Strain
  diastasis —*see* Diastasis, muscle
  nontraumatic M62.10
   ankle M62.17-
   foot M62.17-
   forearm M62.13-
   hand M62.14-
   lower leg M62.16-
   pelvic region M62.15-
   shoulder region M62.11-
   specified site NEC M62.18
   thigh M62.15-
   upper arm M62.12-
  traumatic —*see* Strain, by site
 musculotendinous junction NEC,
   nontraumatic —*see* Rupture, tendon,
   spontaneous
 mycotic aneurysm causing cerebral
   hemorrhage —*see* Hemorrhage,
   intracranial, subarachnoid
 myocardium, myocardial —*see* Rupture,
   cardiac
  traumatic —*see* Injury, heart
 nontraumatic, meaning hernia —*see* Hernia
 obstructed —*see* Hernia, by site, obstructed
 operation wound —*see* Disruption, wound,
   operation
 ovary, ovarian N83.8
  corpus luteum cyst N83.1- ◀▥▥
  follicle (graafian) N83.0- ◀▥▥
 oviduct (nonobstetric) (nontraumatic)
   N83.8
  due to pregnancy O00.10 ◀▥▥
   with intrauterine pregnancy
     O00.11 ◀
 pancreas (nontraumatic) K86.89 ◀▥▥
  traumatic S36.299
 papillary muscle NEC I51.2
  following acute myocardial infarction
    (current complication) I23.5
 pelvic
  floor, complicating delivery O70.1
  organ NEC, obstetrical trauma O71.5
 perineum (nonobstetric) (nontraumatic)
   N90.89
  complicating delivery —*see* Delivery,
    complicated, by, laceration, anus
    (sphincter)
 postoperative wound —*see* Disruption,
   wound, operation
 prostate (traumatic) S37.828
 pulmonary
  artery I28.8
  valve (heart) I37.8
  vein I28.8
  vessel I28.8
 pus tube —*see* Salpingitis
 pyosalpinx —*see* Salpingitis
 rectum (nontraumatic) K63.1
  traumatic S36.69
 retina, retinal (traumatic) (without
   detachment) —*see also* Break, retina
  with detachment —*see* Detachment, retina,
    with retinal, break
 rotator cuff (nontraumatic) M75.10-
  complete M75.12-
  incomplete M75.11-
 sclera —*see* Injury, eye, laceration
 sigmoid (nontraumatic) K63.1
  traumatic S36.593
 spinal cord —*see also* Injury, spinal cord, by
   region
  due to injury at birth P11.5
  newborn (birth injury) P11.5
 spleen (traumatic) S36.09
  birth injury P15.1
  congenital (birth injury) P15.1
  due to P. vivax malaria B51.0
  nontraumatic D73.5
  spontaneous D73.5

Rupture, ruptured *(Continued)*
 splenic vein R58
  traumatic —*see* Injury, blood vessel,
    splenic vein
 stomach (nontraumatic) (spontaneous)
   K31.89
  traumatic S36.39
 supraspinatus (complete) (incomplete)
   (nontraumatic) —*see* Tear, rotator
   cuff
 symphysis pubis
  obstetric O71.6
  traumatic S33.4
 synovium (cyst) M66.10
  ankle M66.17-
  elbow M66.12-
  finger M66.14-
  foot M66.17-
  forearm M66.13-
  hand M66.14-
  pelvic region M66.15-
  shoulder region M66.11-
  specified site NEC M66.18
  thigh M66.15-
  toe M66.17-
  upper arm M66.12-
  wrist M66.13-
 tendon (traumatic) —*see* Strain
  nontraumatic (spontaneous) M66.9
   ankle M66.87-
   extensor M66.20
    ankle M66.27-
    foot M66.27-
    forearm M66.23-
    hand M66.24-
    lower leg M66.26-
    multiple sites M66.29
    pelvic region M66.25-
    shoulder region M66.21-
    specified site NEC M66.28
    thigh M66.25-
    upper arm M66.22-
   flexor M66.30
    ankle M66.37-
    foot M66.37-
    forearm M66.33-
    hand M66.34-
    lower leg M66.36-
    multiple sites M66.39
    pelvic region M66.35-
    shoulder region M66.31-
    specified site NEC M66.38
    thigh M66.35-
    upper arm M66.32-
   foot M66.87-
   forearm M66.83-
   hand M66.84-
   lower leg M66.86-
   multiple sites M66.89
   pelvic region M66.85-
   shoulder region M66.81-
   specified
    site NEC M66.88
    tendon M66.80
   thigh M66.85-
   upper arm M66.82-
 thoracic duct I89.8
 tonsil J35.8
 traumatic
  aorta —*see* Injury, aorta, laceration,
    major
  diaphragm —*see* Injury, intrathoracic,
    diaphragm
  external site —*see* Wound, open,
    by site
  eye —*see* Injury, eye, laceration
  internal organ —*see* Injury, by site
  intervertebral disc
   cervical S13.0
   lumbar S33.0
   thoracic S23.0

Rupture, ruptured *(Continued)*
 traumatic *(Continued)*
  kidney S37.06-
  ligament —*see also* Sprain
   ankle —*see* Sprain, ankle
   carpus —*see* Rupture, traumatic,
     ligament, wrist
   collateral (hand) —*see* Rupture,
     traumatic, ligament, finger,
     collateral
   finger (metacarpophalangeal)
     (interphalangeal) S63.40-
    collateral S63.41-
     index S63.41-
     little S63.41-
     middle S63.41-
     ring S63.41-
    index S63.40-
    little S63.40-
    middle S63.40-
    palmar S63.42-
     index S63.42-
     little S63.42-
     middle S63.42-
     ring S63.42-
    ring S63.40-
    specified site NEC S63.499
     index S63.49-
     little S63.49-
     middle S63.49-
     ring S63.49-
    volar plate S63.43-
     index S63.43-
     little S63.43-
     middle S63.43-
     ring S63.43-
   foot —*see* Sprain, foot
   radial collateral S53.2-
   radiocarpal —*see* Rupture, traumatic,
     ligament, wrist, radiocarpal
   ulnar collateral S53.3-
   ulnocarpal —*see* Rupture, traumatic,
     ligament, wrist, ulnocarpal
   wrist S63.30-
    collateral S63.31-
    radiocarpal S63.32-
    specified site NEC S63.39-
    ulnocarpal (palmar) S63.33-
  liver S36.116
  membrana tympani —*see* Rupture, ear
    drum, traumatic
  muscle or tendon —*see* Strain
  myocardium —*see* Injury, heart
  pancreas S36.299
  rectum S36.69
  sigmoid S36.593
  spleen S36.09
  stomach S36.39
  symphysis pubis S33.4
  tympanum, tympanic (membrane) —*see*
    Rupture, ear drum, traumatic
  ureter S37.19
  uterus S37.69
  vagina —*see* Injury, vagina
  vena cava —*see* Injury, vena cava,
    laceration, major
 tricuspid (heart) (valve) I07.8
 tube, tubal (nonobstetric) (nontraumatic)
   N83.8
  abscess —*see* Salpingitis
  due to pregnancy O00.10 ◀▥▥
   with intrauterine pregnancy O00.11 ◀
 tympanum, tympanic (membrane)
   (nontraumatic) —*see also* Perforation,
   tympanic membrane H72.9-
  traumatic —*see* Rupture, ear drum,
    traumatic
 umbilical cord, complicating delivery
   O69.89
 ureter (traumatic) S37.19
  nontraumatic N28.89

Rupture, ruptured (Continued)
  urethra (nontraumatic) N36.8
    with ectopic or molar pregnancy
      O08.6
    following ectopic or molar pregnancy
      O08.6
    obstetrical trauma O71.5
    traumatic S37.39
  uterosacral ligament (nonobstetric)
    (nontraumatic) N83.8
  uterus (traumatic) S37.69
    before labor O71.0-
    during or after labor O71.1

Rupture, ruptured (Continued)
  uterus (Continued)
    nonpuerperal, nontraumatic N85.8
    pregnant (during labor) O71.1
      before labor O71.0-
  vagina —see Injury, vagina
  valve, valvular (heart) —see Endocarditis
  varicose vein —see Varix
  varix —see Varix
  vena cava R58
    traumatic —see Injury, vena cava,
      laceration, major
  vesical (urinary) N32.89

Rupture, ruptured (Continued)
  vessel (blood) R58
    pulmonary I28.8
    traumatic —see Injury, blood vessel
  viscus R19.8
  vulva complicating delivery O70.0
Russell-Silver syndrome Q87.1
Russian spring-summer type encephalitis
  A84.0
Rust's disease (tuberculous cervical spondylitis)
  A18.01
Ruvalcaba-Myhre-Smith syndrome E71.440
Rytand-Lipsitch syndrome I44.2

◀ New   ◀━ Revised   ~~deleted~~ Deleted

S

Saber, sabre shin or tibia (syphilitic) A50.56 [M90.8-]
Sac lacrimal —*see* condition
Saccharomyces infection B37.9
Saccharopinuria E72.3
Saccular —*see* condition
Sacculation
aorta (nonsyphilitic) —*see* Aneurysm, aorta
bladder N32.3
intralaryngeal (congenital) (ventricular) Q31.3
larynx (congenital) (ventricular) Q31.3
organ or site, congenital —*see* Distortion
pregnant uterus —*see* Pregnancy, complicated by, abnormal, uterus
ureter N28.89
urethra N36.1
vesical N32.3
Sachs' amaurotic familial idiocy or disease E75.02
Sachs-Tay disease E75.02
Sacks-Libman disease M32.11
Sacralgia M53.3
Sacralization Q76.49
Sacrodynia M53.3
Sacroiliac joint —*see* condition
Sacroiliitis NEC M46.1
Sacrum —*see* condition
Saddle
back —*see* Lordosis
embolus
abdominal aorta I74.01
pulmonary artery I26.92
with acute cor pulmonale I26.02
injury — code to condition
nose M95.0
due to syphilis A50.57
Sadism (sexual) F65.52
Sadness, postpartal O90.6
Sadomasochism F65.50
Saemisch's ulcer (cornea) —*see* Ulcer, cornea, central
Sagging ◄
skin and subcutaneous tissue (following bariatric surgery weight loss) (following dietary weight loss) L98.7 ◄
Sahib disease B55.0
Sailors' skin L57.8
Saint
Anthony's fire —*see* Erysipelas
triad —*see* Hernia, diaphragm
Vitus' dance —*see* Chorea, Sydenham's
Salaam
attack (s) —*see* Epilepsy, spasms
tic R25.8
Salicylism
abuse F55.8
overdose or wrong substance given —*see* Table of Drugs and Chemicals, by drug, poisoning
Salivary duct or gland —*see* condition
Salivation, excessive K11.7
Salmonella —*see* Infection, Salmonella
Salmonellosis A02.0
Salpingitis (catarrhal) (fallopian tube) (nodular) (pseudofollicular) (purulent) (septic) N70.91
with oophoritis N70.93
acute N70.01
with oophoritis N70.03
chlamydial A56.11
chronic N70.11
with oophoritis N70.13
complicating abortion —*see* Abortion, by type, complicated by, salpingitis
ear —*see* Salpingitis, eustachian
eustachian (tube) H68.00-
acute H68.01-
chronic H68.02-

Salpingitis (Continued)
follicularis N70.11
with oophoritis N70.13
gonococcal (acute) (chronic) A54.24
interstitial, chronic N70.11
with oophoritis N70.13
isthmica nodosa N70.11
with oophoritis N70.13
specific (gonococcal) (acute) (chronic) A54.24
tuberculous (acute) (chronic) A18.17
venereal (gonococcal) (acute) (chronic) A54.24
Salpingocele N83.4- ◄▥
Salpingo-oophoritis (catarrhal) (purulent) (ruptured) (septic) (suppurative) N70.93
acute N70.03
with ectopic or molar pregnancy O08.0
following ectopic or molar pregnancy O08.0
gonococcal A54.24
chronic N70.13
following ectopic or molar pregnancy O08.0
gonococcal (acute) (chronic) A54.24
puerperal O86.19
specific (gonococcal) (acute) (chronic) A54.24
subacute N70.03
tuberculous (acute) (chronic) A18.17
venereal (gonococcal) (acute) (chronic) A54.24
Salpingo-ovaritis —*see* Salpingo-oophoritis
Salpingoperitonitis —*see* Salpingo-oophoritis
Salzmann's nodular dystrophy —*see* Degeneration, cornea, nodular
Sampson's cyst or tumor N80.1
San Joaquin (Valley) **fever** B38.0
Sandblaster's asthma, lung or pneumoconiosis J62.8
Sander's disease (paranoia) F22
Sandfly fever A93.1
Sandhoff's disease E75.01
Sanfilippo (Type B) (Type C) (Type D) **syndrome** E76.22
Sanger-Brown ataxia G11.2
Sao Paulo fever or typhus A77.0
Saponification, mesenteric K65.8
Sarcocele (benign)
syphilitic A52.76
congenital A50.59
Sarcocystosis A07.8
Sarcoepiplocele —*see* Hernia
Sarcoepiplomphalocele Q79.2
Sarcoid —*see also* Sarcoidosis
arthropathy D86.86
Boeck's D86.9
Darier-Roussy D86.3
iridocyclitis D86.83
meningitis D86.81
myocarditis D86.85
myositis D86.87
pyelonephritis D86.84
Spiegler-Fendt L08.89
Sarcoidosis D86.9
with
cranial nerve palsies D86.82
hepatic granuloma D86.89
polyarthritis D86.86
tubulo-interstitial nephropathy D86.84
combined sites NEC D86.89
lung D86.0
and lymph nodes D86.2
lymph nodes D86.1
and lung D86.2
meninges D86.81
skin D86.3
specified type NEC D86.89
Sarcoma (of) —*see also* Neoplasm, connective tissue, malignant
alveolar soft part —*see* Neoplasm, connective tissue, malignant
ameloblastic C41.1
upper jaw (bone) C41.0
botryoid —*see* Neoplasm, connective tissue, malignant

Sarcoma (Continued)
botryoides —*see* Neoplasm, connective tissue, malignant
cerebellar C71.6
circumscribed (arachnoidal) C71.6
circumscribed (arachnoidal) cerebellar C71.6
clear cell —*see also* Neoplasm, connective tissue, malignant
kidney C64.-
dendritic cells (accessory cells) C96.4
embryonal —*see* Neoplasm, connective tissue, malignant
endometrial (stromal) C54.1
isthmus C54.0
epithelioid (cell) —*see* Neoplasm, connective tissue, malignant
Ewing's —*see* Neoplasm, bone, malignant
follicular dendritic cell C96.4
germinoblastic (diffuse) —*see* Lymphoma, diffuse, large cell
follicular —*see* Lymphoma, follicular, specified NEC
giant cell (except of bone) —*see also* Neoplasm, connective tissue, malignant
bone —*see* Neoplasm, bone, malignant
glomoid —*see* Neoplasm, connective tissue, malignant
granulocytic C92.3-
hemangioendothelial —*see* Neoplasm, connective tissue, malignant
hemorrhagic, multiple —*see* Sarcoma, Kaposi's
histiocytic C96.A
Hodgkin —*see* Lymphoma, Hodgkin
immunoblastic (diffuse) —*see* Lymphoma, diffuse large cell
interdigitating dendritic cell C96.4
Kaposi's
colon C46.4
connective tissue C46.1
gastrointestinal organ C46.4
lung C46.5-
lymph node (s) C46.3
palate (hard) (soft) C46.2
rectum C46.4
skin C46.0
specified site NEC C46.7
stomach C46.4
unspecified site C46.9
Kupffer cell C22.3
Langerhans cell C96.4
leptomeningeal —*see* Neoplasm, meninges, malignant
liver NEC C22.4
lymphangioendothelial —*see* Neoplasm, connective tissue, malignant
lymphoblastic —*see* Lymphoma, lymphoblastic (diffuse)
lymphocytic —*see* Lymphoma, small cell B-cell
mast cell C96.2
melanotic —*see* Melanoma
meningeal —*see* Neoplasm, meninges, malignant
meningothelial —*see* Neoplasm, meninges, malignant
mesenchymal —*see also* Neoplasm, connective tissue, malignant
mixed —*see* Neoplasm, connective tissue, malignant
mesothelial —*see* Mesothelioma
monstrocellular
specified site —*see* Neoplasm, malignant, by site
unspecified site C71.9
myeloid C92.3-
neurogenic —*see* Neoplasm, nerve, malignant
odontogenic C41.1
upper jaw (bone) C41.0

Sarcoma *(Continued)*
  osteoblastic —*see* Neoplasm, bone,
      malignant
  osteogenic —*see also* Neoplasm, bone,
      malignant
    juxtacortical —*see* Neoplasm, bone,
        malignant
    periosteal —*see* Neoplasm, bone,
        malignant
  periosteal —*see also* Neoplasm, bone,
      malignant
  osteogenic —*see* Neoplasm, bone,
      malignant
  pleomorphic cell —*see* Neoplasm, connective
      tissue, malignant
  reticulum cell (diffuse) —*see* Lymphoma,
      diffuse large cell
    nodular —*see* Lymphoma, follicular
    pleomorphic cell type —*see* Lymphoma,
        diffuse large cell
  rhabdoid —*see* Neoplasm, malignant, by site
  round cell —*see* Neoplasm, connective tissue,
      malignant
  small cell —*see* Neoplasm, connective tissue,
      malignant
  soft tissue —*see* Neoplasm, connective tissue,
      malignant
  spindle cell —*see* Neoplasm, connective
      tissue, malignant
  stromal (endometrial) C54.1
    isthmus C54.0
  synovial —*see also* Neoplasm, connective
      tissue, malignant
    biphasic —*see* Neoplasm, connective tissue,
        malignant
    epithelioid cell —*see* Neoplasm, connective
        tissue, malignant
    spindle cell —*see* Neoplasm, connective
        tissue, malignant
Sarcomatosis
  meningeal —*see* Neoplasm, meninges,
      malignant
  specified site NEC —*see* Neoplasm,
      connective tissue, malignant
  unspecified site C80.1
Sarcopenia (age-related) M62.84 ◀
Sarcosinemia E72.59
Sarcosporidiosis (intestinal) A07.8
Satiety, early R68.81
Saturnine —*see* condition
Saturnism
  overdose or wrong substance given or
      taken —*see* Table of Drugs and
      Chemicals, by drug, poisoning
Satyriasis F52.8
Sauriasis —*see* Ichthyosis
SBE (subacute bacterial endocarditis) I33.0
Scabies (any site) B86
Scabs R23.4
Scaglietti-Dagnini syndrome E22.0
Scald —*see* Burn
Scalenus anticus (anterior) syndrome G54.0
Scales R23.4
Scaling, skin R23.4
Scalp —*see* condition
Scapegoating affecting child Z62.3
Scaphocephaly Q75.0
Scapulalgia M89.8X1
Scapulohumeral myopathy G71.0
Scar, scarring —*see also* Cicatrix L90.5
  adherent L90.5
  atrophic L90.5
  cervix
    in pregnancy or childbirth —*see* Pregnancy,
        complicated by, abnormal cervix
  cheloid L91.0
  chorioretinal H31.00-
    posterior pole macula H31.01-
    postsurgical H59.81-
    solar retinopathy H31.02-
    specified type NEC H31.09-

Scar, scarring *(Continued)*
  choroid —*see* Scar, chorioretinal
  conjunctiva H11.24-
  cornea H17.9
    xerophthalmic —*see also* Opacity, cornea
        vitamin A deficiency E50.6
  duodenum, obstructive K31.5
  hypertrophic L91.0
  keloid L91.0
  labia N90.89
  lung (base) J98.4
  macula —*see* Scar, chorioretinal, posterior
      pole
  muscle M62.89
  myocardium, myocardial I25.2
  painful L90.5
  posterior pole (eye) —*see* Scar, chorioretinal,
      posterior pole
  retina —*see* Scar, chorioretinal
  trachea J39.8
  transmural uterine, in pregnancy O34.29 ◀
  uterus N85.8
    in pregnancy O34.29
  vagina N89.8
    postoperative N99.2
  vulva N90.89
Scarabiasis B88.2
Scarlatina (anginosa) (maligna) (ulcerosa)
    A38.9
  myocarditis (acute) A38.1
    old —*see* Myocarditis
  otitis media A38.0
Scarlet fever (albuminuria) (angina) A38.9
Schamberg's disease (progressive pigmentary
    dermatosis) L81.7
Schatzki's ring (acquired) (esophagus) (lower)
    K22.2
  congenital Q39.3
Schaufenster krankheit I20.8
Schaumann's
  benign lymphogranulomatosis D86.1
  disease or syndrome —*see* Sarcoidosis
Scheie's syndrome E76.03
Schenck's disease B42.1
Scheuermann's disease or osteochondrosis —
    see Osteochondrosis, juvenile, spine
Schilder (-Flatau) disease G37.0
Schilling-type monocytic leukemia C93.0-
Schimmelbusch's disease, cystic mastitis, or
    hyperplasia —*see* Mastopathy, cystic
Schistosoma infestation —*see* Infestation,
    Schistosoma
Schistosomiasis B65.9
  with muscle disorder B65.9 *[M63.80]*
    ankle B65.9 *[M63.87-]*
    foot B65.9 *[M63.87-]*
    forearm B65.9 *[M63.83-]*
    hand B65.9 *[M63.84-]*
    lower leg B65.9 *[M63.86-]*
    multiple sites B65.9 *[M63.89]*
    pelvic region B65.9 *[M63.85-]*
    shoulder region B65.9 *[M63.81-]*
    specified site NEC B65.9 *[M63.88]*
    thigh B65.9 *[M63.85-]*
    upper arm B65.9 *[M63.82-]*
  Asiatic B65.2
  bladder B65.0
  chestermani B65.8
  colon B65.1
  cutaneous B65.3
  due to
    S. haematobium B65.0
    S. japonicum B65.2
    S. mansoni B65.1
    S. mattheii B65.8
  Eastern B65.2
  genitourinary tract B65.0
  intestinal B65.1
  lung NEC B65.9 *[[99]*
    pneumonia B65.9 *[[17]*
  Manson's (intestinal) B65.1

Schistosomiasis *(Continued)*
  oriental B65.2
  pulmonary NEC B65.9 *[[99]*
    pneumonia B65.9
  Schistosoma
    haematobium B65.0
    japonicum B65.2
    mansoni B65.1
  specified type NEC B65.8
  urinary B65.0
  vesical B65.0
Schizencephaly Q04.6
Schizoaffective psychosis F25.9
Schizodontia K00.2
Schizoid personality F60.1
Schizophrenia, schizophrenic F20.9
  acute (brief) (undifferentiated) F23
  atypical (form) F20.3
  borderline F21
  catalepsy F20.2
  catatonic (type) (excited) (withdrawn) F20.2
  cenesthopathic, cenesthesiopathic F20.89
  childhood type F84.5
  chronic undifferentiated F20.5
  cyclic F25.0
  disorganized (type) F20.1
  flexibilitas cerea F20.2
  hebephrenic (type) F20.1
  incipient F21
  latent F21
  negative type F20.5
  paranoid (type) F20.0
  paraphrenic F20.0
  post-psychotic depression F32.89 ◀║
  prepsychotic F21
  prodromal F21
  pseudoneurotic F21
  pseudopsychopathic F21
  reaction F23
  residual (state) (type) F20.5
  restzustand F20.5
  schizoaffective (type) —*see* Psychosis,
      schizoaffective
  simple (type) F20.89
  simplex F20.89
  specified type NEC F20.89
  stupor F20.2
  syndrome of childhood F84.5
  undifferentiated (type) F20.3
    chronic F20.5
Schizothymia (persistent) F60.1
Schlatter-Osgood disease or
    osteochondrosis —*see* Osteochondrosis,
    juvenile, tibia
Schlatter's tibia —*see* Osteochondrosis,
    juvenile, tibia
Schmidt's syndrome (polyglandular,
    autoimmune) E31.0
Schmincke's carcinoma or tumor —*see*
    Neoplasm, nasopharynx, malignant
Schmitz (-Stutzer) dysentery A03.0
Schmorl's disease or nodes
  lumbar region M51.46
  lumbosacral region M51.47
  sacrococcygeal region M53.3
  thoracic region M51.44
  thoracolumbar region M51.45
Schneiderian
  papilloma —*see* Neoplasm, nasopharynx
      benign
    specified site —*see* Neoplasm, benign, by
        site
    unspecified site D14.0
  specified site —*see* Neoplasm, malignant, by
      site
  unspecified site C30.0
Scholte's syndrome (malignant carcinoid) E34.0
Scholz (-Bielchowsky-Henneberg) disease or
    syndrome E75.25
Schönlein (-Henoch) disease or purpura
    (primary) (rheumatic) D69.0

◀ New   ◀║ Revised   ~~deleted~~ Deleted

Schottmuller's disease A01.4
Schroeder's syndrome (endocrine
  hypertensive) E27.0
Schüller-Christian disease or syndrome C96.5
Schultze's type acroparesthesia, simple I73.89
Schultz's disease or syndrome —*see*
  Agranulocytosis
Schwalbe-Ziehen-Oppenheim disease G24.1
Schwannoma —*see also* Neoplasm, nerve,
  benign
  malignant —*see also* Neoplasm, nerve,
    malignant
    with rhabdomyoblastic differentiation —
      see Neoplasm, nerve, malignant
  melanocytic —*see* Neoplasm, nerve, benign
  pigmented —*see* Neoplasm, nerve, benign
Schwannomatosis Q85.03
Schwartz (-Jampel) syndrome G71.13
Schwartz-Bartter syndrome E22.2
Schweniger-Buzzi anetoderma L90.1
Sciatic —*see* condition
Sciatica (infective)
  with lumbago M54.4-
    due to intervertebral disc disorder —*see*
      Disorder, disc, with, radiculopathy
    due to displacement of intervertebral disc
      (with lumbago) —*see* Disorder, disc,
      with, radiculopathy
  wallet M54.3-
Scimitar syndrome Q26.8
Sclera —*see* condition
Sclerectasia H15.84-
Scleredema
  adultorum —*see* Sclerosis, systemic
  Buschke's —*see* Sclerosis, systemic
  newborn P83.0
Sclerema (adiposum) (edematosum)
  (neonatorum) (newborn) P83.0
  adultorum —*see* Sclerosis, systemic
Scleriasis —*see* Scleroderma
Scleritis H15.00-
  with corneal involvement H15.04-
  anterior H15.01-
  brawny H15.02-
  in (due to) zoster B02.34
  posterior H15.03-
  specified type NEC H15.09-
  syphilitic A52.71
  tuberculous (nodular) A18.51
Sclerochoroiditis H31.8
Scleroconjunctivitis —*see* Scleritis
Sclerocystic ovary syndrome E28.2
Sclerodactyly, sclerodactylia L94.3
Scleroderma, sclerodermia (acrosclerotic)
  (diffuse) (generalized) (progressive)
  (pulmonary) —*see also* Sclerosis, systemic
  M34.9-
  circumscribed L94.0
  linear L94.1
  localized L94.0
  newborn P83.8
  systemic M34.9
Sclerokeratitis H16.8
  tuberculous A18.52
Scleroma nasi A48.8
Scleromalacia (perforans) H15.05-
Scleromyxedema L98.5
Sclérose en plaques G35
Sclerosis, sclerotic
  adrenal (gland) E27.8
  Alzheimer's —*see* Disease, Alzheimer's
  amyotrophic (lateral) G12.21
  aorta, aortic I70.0
    valve —*see* Endocarditis, aortic
  artery, arterial, arteriolar, arteriovascular —
    see Arteriosclerosis
  ascending multiple G35
  brain (generalized) (lobular) G37.9
    artery, arterial I67.2
    diffuse G37.0
    disseminated G35

Sclerosis, sclerotic (*Continued*)
  brain (*Continued*)
    insular G35
    Krabbe's E75.23
    miliary G35
    multiple G35
    presenile (Alzheimer's) —*see* Disease,
      Alzheimer's, early onset
    senile (arteriosclerotic) I67.2
    stem, multiple G35
    tuberous Q85.1
  bulbar, multiple G35
  bundle of His I44.39
  cardiac —*see* Disease, heart, ischemic,
    atherosclerotic
  cardiorenal —*see* Hypertension, cardiorenal
  cardiovascular —*see also* Disease,
    cardiovascular
    renal —*see* Hypertension, cardiorenal
  cerebellar —*see* Sclerosis, brain
  cerebral —*see* Sclerosis, brain
  cerebrospinal (disseminated) (multiple) G35
  cerebrovascular I67.2
  choroid —*see* Degeneration, choroid
  combined (spinal cord) —*see also*
    Degeneration, combined
    multiple G35
  concentric (Balo) G37.5
  cornea —*see* Opacity, cornea
  coronary (artery) I25.10
    with angina pectoris —*see* Arteriosclerosis,
      coronary (artery),
  corpus cavernosum
    female N90.89
    male N48.6
  diffuse (brain) (spinal cord) G37.0
  disseminated G35
  dorsal G35
  dorsolateral (spinal cord) —*see* Degeneration,
    combined
  endometrium N85.5
  extrapyramidal G25.9
  eye, nuclear (senile) —*see* Cataract, senile,
    nuclear
  focal and segmental (glomerular) —*see also*
    N00-N07 with fourth character .1
    N05.1
  Friedreich's (spinal cord) G11.1
  funicular (spermatic cord) N50.89 ◄▦
  general (vascular) —*see* Arteriosclerosis
  gland (lymphatic) I89.8
  hepatic K74.1
    alcoholic K70.2
  hereditary
    cerebellar G11.9
    spinal (Friedreich's ataxia) G11.1
  hippocampal G93.81
  insular G35
  kidney —*see* Sclerosis, renal
  larynx J38.7
  lateral (amyotrophic) (descending) (primary)
    (spinal) G12.21
  lens, senile nuclear —*see* Cataract, senile,
    nuclear
  liver K74.1
    with fibrosis K74.2
      alcoholic K70.2
    alcoholic K70.2
    cardiac K76.1
  lung —*see* Fibrosis, lung
  mastoid —*see* Mastoiditis, chronic
  mesial temporal G93.81
  mitral I05.8
  Mönckeberg's (medial) —*see* Arteriosclerosis,
    extremities
  multiple (brain stem) (cerebral) (generalized)
    (spinal cord) G35
  myocardium, myocardial —*see* Disease, heart,
    ischemic, atherosclerotic
  nuclear (senile), eye —*see* Cataract, senile,
    nuclear

Sclerosis, sclerotic (*Continued*)
  ovary N83.8
  pancreas K86.89 ◄▦
  penis N48.6
  peripheral arteries —*see* Arteriosclerosis,
    extremities
  plaques G35
  pluriglandular E31.8
  polyglandular E31.8
  posterolateral (spinal cord) —*see*
    Degeneration, combined
  presenile (Alzheimer's) —*see* Disease,
    Alzheimer's, early onset
  primary, lateral G12.29
  progressive, systemic M34.0
  pulmonary —*see* Fibrosis, lung
    artery I27.0
    valve (heart) —*see* Endocarditis,
      pulmonary
  renal N26.9
    with
      cystine storage disease E72.09
      hypertensive heart disease (conditions
        in I11) —*see* Hypertension,
        cardiorenal
      arteriolar (hyaline) (hyperplastic) —*see*
        Hypertension, kidney
  retina (senile) (vascular) H35.00
  senile (vascular) —*see* Arteriosclerosis
  spinal (cord) (progressive) G95.89
    ascending G61.0
    combined —*see also* Degeneration,
      combined
      multiple G35
      syphilitic A52.11
    disseminated G35
    dorsolateral —*see* Degeneration, combined
    hereditary (Friedreich's) (mixed form)
      G11.1
    lateral (amyotrophic) G12.21
    multiple G35
    posterior (syphilitic) A52.11
  stomach K31.89
  subendocardial, congenital I42.4
  systemic M34.9
    with
      lung involvement M34.81
      myopathy M34.82
      polyneuropathy M34.83
    drug-induced M34.2
    due to chemicals NEC M34.2
    progressive M34.0
    specified NEC M34.89
  temporal (mesial) G93.81
  tricuspid (heart) (valve) I07.8
  tuberous (brain) Q85.1
  tympanic membrane —*see* Disorder,
    tympanic membrane, specified NEC
  valve, valvular (heart) —*see* Endocarditis
  vascular —*see* Arteriosclerosis
  vein I87.8
Scoliosis (acquired) (postural) M41.9
  adolescent (idiopathic) —*see* Scoliosis,
    idiopathic, adolescent ◄▦
  congenital Q67.5
    due to bony malformation Q76.3
    failure of segmentation (hemivertebra)
      Q76.3
    hemivertebra fusion Q76.3
    postural Q67.5
  idiopathic M41.20
    adolescent M41.129
      cervical region M41.122
      cervicothoracic region M41.123
      lumbar region M41.126
      lumbosacral region M41.127
      thoracic region M41.124
      thoracolumbar region
        M41.125
    cervical region M41.22
    cervicothoracic region M41.23

Scoliosis (Continued)
  idiopathic (Continued)
    infantile M41.00
      cervical region M41.02
      cervicothoracic region M41.03
      lumbar region M41.06
      lumbosacral region M41.07
      sacrococcygeal region M41.08
      thoracic region M41.04
      thoracolumbar region M41.05
    juvenile M41.119
      cervical region M41.112
      cervicothoracic region M41.113
      lumbar region M41.116
      lumbosacral region M41.117
      thoracic region M41.114
      thoracolumbar region M41.115
    lumbar region M41.26
    lumbosacral region M41.27
    thoracic region M41.24
    thoracolumbar region M41.25
  infantile —see Scoliosis, idiopathic,
      infantile ◀
  neuromuscular M41.40
    cervical region M41.42
    cervicothoracic region M41.43
    lumbar region M41.46
    lumbosacral region M41.47
    occipito-atlanto-axial region M41.41
    thoracic region M41.44
    thoracolumbar region M41.45
  paralytic —see Scoliosis, neuromuscular
  postradiation therapy M96.5
  rachitic (late effect or sequelae) E64.3
      [M49.80]
    cervical region E64.3 [M49.82]
    cervicothoracic region E64.3 [M49.83]
    lumbar region E64.3 [M49.86]
    lumbosacral region E64.3 [M49.87]
    multiple sites E64.3 [M49.89]
    occipito-atlanto-axial region E64.3
        [M49.81]
    sacrococcygeal region E64.3 [M49.88]
    thoracic region E64.3 [M49.84]
    thoracolumbar region E64.3 [M49.85]
  sciatic M54.4-
  secondary (to) NEC M41.50
    cerebral palsy, Friedreich's ataxia,
        poliomyelitis, neuromuscular
        disorders —see Scoliosis,
        neuromuscular
    cervical region M41.52
    cervicothoracic region M41.53
    lumbar region M41.56
    lumbosacral region M41.57
    thoracic region M41.54
    thoracolumbar region M41.55
  specified form NEC M41.80
    cervical region M41.82
    cervicothoracic region M41.83
    lumbar region M41.86
    lumbosacral region M41.87
    thoracic region M41.84
    thoracolumbar region M41.85
  thoracogenic M41.30
    thoracic region M41.34
    thoracolumbar region M41.35
  tuberculous A18.01
Scoliotic pelvis
  with disproportion (fetopelvic) O33.0
    causing obstructed labor O65.0
Scorbutus, scorbutic —see also Scurvy
  anemia D53.2
Score, NIHSS (National Institutes of Health
    Stroke Scale) R29.7- ◀
Scotoma (arcuate) (Bjerrum) (central) (ring) —
    see also Defect, visual field, localized,
    scotoma
  scintillating H53.19
Scratch —see Abrasion
Scratchy throat R09.89

Screening (for) Z13.9
  alcoholism Z13.89
  anemia Z13.0
  anomaly, congenital Z13.89
  antenatal, of mother Z36
  arterial hypertension Z13.6
  arthropod-borne viral disease NEC Z11.59
  bacteriuria, asymptomatic Z13.89
  behavioral disorder Z13.89
  brain injury, traumatic Z13.850
  bronchitis, chronic Z13.83
  brucellosis Z11.2
  cardiovascular disorder Z13.6
  cataract Z13.5
  chlamydial diseases Z11.8
  cholera Z11.0
  chromosomal abnormalities (nonprocreative)
      NEC Z13.79
  colonoscopy Z12.11
  congenital
    dislocation of hip Z13.89
    eye disorder Z13.5
    malformation or deformation Z13.89
  contamination NEC Z13.88
  cystic fibrosis Z13.228
  dengue fever Z11.59
  dental disorder Z13.84
  depression Z13.89
  developmental handicap Z13.42 ◀▥
    in early childhood Z13.42 ◀▥
    infant Z13.41 ◀
  diabetes mellitus Z13.1
  diphtheria Z11.2
  disability, intellectual Z13.42 ◀▥
    infant Z13.41 ◀
  disease or disorder Z13.9
    bacterial NEC Z11.2
      intestinal infectious Z11.0
      respiratory tuberculosis Z11.1
    blood or blood-forming organ Z13.0
    cardiovascular Z13.6
    Chagas' Z11.6
    chlamydial Z11.8
    dental Z13.89
    developmental Z13.42 ◀▥
      in child Z13.42 ◀
      infant Z13.41 ◀
    digestive tract NEC Z13.818
      lower GI Z13.811
      upper GI Z13.810
    ear Z13.5
    endocrine Z13.29
    eye Z13.5
    genitourinary Z13.89
    heart Z13.6
    human immunodeficiency virus (HIV)
        infection Z11.4
    immunity Z13.0
    infection
      intestinal Z11.0
        specified NEC Z11.6
    infectious Z11.9
    mental Z13.89
    metabolic Z13.228
    neurological Z13.89
    nutritional Z13.21
      metabolic Z13.228
        lipoid disorders Z13.220
    protozoal Z11.6
      intestinal Z11.0
    respiratory Z13.83
    rheumatic Z13.828
    rickettsial Z11.8
    sexually-transmitted NEC Z11.3
      human immunodeficiency virus (HIV)
          Z11.4
    sickle-cell (trait) Z13.0
    skin Z13.89
    specified NEC Z13.89
    spirochetal Z11.8
    thyroid Z13.29

Screening (Continued)
  disease or disorder (Continued)
    vascular Z13.6
    venereal Z11.3
    viral NEC Z11.59
      human immunodeficiency virus (HIV)
          Z11.4
      intestinal Z11.0
  elevated titer Z13.89
  emphysema Z13.83
  encephalitis, viral (mosquito- or tick-borne)
      Z11.59
  exposure to contaminants (toxic) Z13.88
  fever
    dengue Z11.59
    hemorrhagic Z11.59
    yellow Z11.59
  filariasis Z11.6
  galactosemia Z13.228
  gastrointestinal condition Z13.818
  genetic (nonprocreative)- for procreative
      management —see Testing, genetic, for
      procreative management
    disease carrier status (nonprocreative)
        Z13.71
    specified NEC (nonprocreative) Z13.79
  genitourinary condition Z13.89
  glaucoma Z13.5
  gonorrhea Z11.3
  gout Z13.89
  helminthiasis (intestinal) Z11.6
  hematopoietic malignancy Z12.89
  hemoglobinopathies NEC Z13.0
  hemorrhagic fever Z11.59
  Hodgkin disease Z12.89
  human immunodeficiency virus (HIV)
      Z11.4
  human papillomavirus Z11.51
  hypertension Z13.6
  immunity disorders Z13.0
  infection
    mycotic Z11.8
    parasitic Z11.8
  ingestion of radioactive substance Z13.88
  intellectual disability Z13.42 ◀▥
    infant Z13.41 ◀
  intestinal
    helminthiasis Z11.6
    infectious disease Z11.0
  leishmaniasis Z11.6
  leprosy Z11.2
  leptospirosis Z11.8
  leukemia Z12.89
  lymphoma Z12.89
  malaria Z11.6
  malnutrition Z13.29
    metabolic Z13.228
    nutritional Z13.21
  measles Z11.59
  mental disorder Z13.89
  metabolic errors, inborn Z13.228
  multiphasic Z13.89
  musculoskeletal disorder Z13.828
    osteoporosis Z13.820
  mycoses Z11.8
  myocardial infarction (acute) Z13.6
  neoplasm (malignant) (of) Z12.9
    bladder Z12.6
    blood Z12.89
    breast Z12.39
      routine mammogram Z12.31
    cervix Z12.4
    colon Z12.11
    genitourinary organs NEC Z12.79
      bladder Z12.6
      cervix Z12.4
      ovary Z12.73
      prostate Z12.5
      testis Z12.71
      vagina Z12.72
    hematopoietic system Z12.89

◀ New   ◀▥ Revised   ~~deleted~~ Deleted

Screening *(Continued)*
  neoplasm *(Continued)*
    intestinal tract Z12.10
      colon Z12.11
      rectum Z12.12
      small intestine Z12.13
    lung Z12.2
    lymph (glands) Z12.89
    nervous system Z12.82
    oral cavity Z12.81
    prostate Z12.5
    rectum Z12.12
    respiratory organs Z12.2
    skin Z12.83
    small intestine Z12.13
    specified site NEC Z12.89
    stomach Z12.0
  nephropathy Z13.89
  nervous system disorders NEC Z13.858
  neurological condition Z13.89
  osteoporosis Z13.820
  parasitic infestation Z11.9
    specified NEC Z11.8
  phenylketonuria Z13.228
  plague Z11.2
  poisoning (chemical) (heavy metal)
    Z13.88
  poliomyelitis Z11.59
  postnatal, chromosomal abnormalities
    Z13.89
  prenatal, of mother Z36
  protozoal disease Z11.6
    intestinal Z11.0
  pulmonary tuberculosis Z11.1
  radiation exposure Z13.88
  respiratory condition Z13.83
  respiratory tuberculosis Z11.1
  rheumatoid arthritis Z13.828
  rubella Z11.59
  schistosomiasis Z11.6
  sexually-transmitted disease NEC Z11.3
    human immunodeficiency virus (HIV)
      Z11.4
  sickle-cell disease or trait Z13.0
  skin condition Z13.89
  sleeping sickness Z11.6
  special Z13.9
    specified NEC Z13.89
  syphilis Z11.3
  tetanus Z11.2
  trachoma Z11.8
  traumatic brain injury Z13.850
  trypanosomiasis Z11.6
  tuberculosis, respiratory Z11.1
  venereal disease Z11.3
  viral encephalitis (mosquito- or tick-borne)
    Z11.59
  whooping cough Z11.2
  worms, intestinal Z11.6
  yaws Z11.8
  yellow fever Z11.59
Scrofula, scrofulosis (tuberculosis of cervical
    lymph glands) A18.2
Scrofulide (primary) (tuberculous) A18.4
Scrofuloderma, scrofulodermia (any site)
    (primary) A18.4
Scrofulosus lichen (primary) (tuberculous)
    A18.4
Scrofulous —see condition
Scrotal tongue K14.5
Scrotum —see condition
Scurvy, scorbutic E54
  anemia D53.2
  gum E54
  infantile E54
  rickets E55.0 [M90.80]
Sealpox B08.62
Seasickness T75.3
Seatworm (infection) (infestation) B80
Sebaceous —see also condition
  cyst —see Cyst, sebaceous

Seborrhea, seborrheic L21.9
  capillitii R23.8
  capitis L21.0
  dermatitis L21.9
    infantile L21.1
  eczema L21.9
    infantile L21.1
  sicca L21.0
Seckel's syndrome Q87.1
Seclusion, pupil —see Membrane, pupillary
Second hand tobacco smoke exposure (acute)
    (chronic) Z77.22
  in the perinatal period P96.81
Secondary
  dentin (in pulp) K04.3
  neoplasm, secondaries —see Table of
    Neoplasms, secondary
Secretion
  antidiuretic hormone, inappropriate E22.2
  catecholamine, by pheochromocytoma E27.5
  hormone
    antidiuretic, inappropriate (syndrome)
      E22.2
    by
      carcinoid tumor E34.0
      pheochromocytoma E27.5
    ectopic NEC E34.2
  urinary
    excessive R35.8
    suppression R34
Section
  nerve, traumatic —see Injury, nerve
Sedative, hypnotic, or anxiolytic-induced ◄
  anxiety disorder F13.980 ◄
  bipolar and related disorder F13.94 ◄
  delirium F13.921 ◄
  depressive disorder F13.94 ◄
  major neurocognitive disorder F13.97 ◄
  mild neurocognitive disorder F13.988 ◄
  psychotic disorder F13.959 ◄
  sexual dysfunction F13.981 ◄
  sleep disorder F13.982 ◄
Segmentation, incomplete (congenital) —see
    also Fusion
  bone NEC Q78.8
  lumbosacral (joint) (vertebra) Q76.49
Seitelberger's syndrome (infantile neuraxonal
    dystrophy) G31.89
Seizure(s) —see also Convulsions R56.9
  akinetic —see Epilepsy, generalized, specified
    NEC
  atonic —see Epilepsy, generalized, specified
    NEC
  autonomic (hysterical) F44.5
  convulsive —see Convulsions
  cortical (focal) (motor) —see Epilepsy,
    localization-related, symptomatic, with
    simple partial seizures
  disorder —see also Epilepsy G40.909
  due to stroke —see Sequelae (of), disease,
    cerebrovascular, by type, specified NEC
  epileptic —see Epilepsy
  febrile (simple) R56.00
    with status epilepticus G40.901
    complex (atypical) (complicated) R56.01
      with status epilepticus G40.901
  grand mal G40.409
    intractable G40.419
      with status epilepticus G40.411
      without status epilepticus G40.419
    not intractable G40.409
      with status epilepticus G40.401
      without status epilepticus G40.409
  heart —see Disease, heart
  hysterical F44.5
  intractable G40.919
    with status epilepticus G40.911
  Jacksonian (focal) (motor type) (sensory
    type) —see Epilepsy, localization-
    related, symptomatic, with simple
    partial seizures

Seizure *(Continued)*
  newborn P90
  nonspecific epileptic
    atonic —see Epilepsy, generalized, specified
      NEC
    clonic —see Epilepsy, generalized, specified
      NEC
    myoclonic —see Epilepsy, generalized,
      specified NEC
    tonic —see Epilepsy, generalized, specified
      NEC
    tonic-clonic —see Epilepsy, generalized,
      specified NEC
  partial, developing into secondarily
    generalized seizures
    complex —see Epilepsy, localization-
      related, symptomatic, with complex
      partial seizures
    simple —see Epilepsy, localization-related,
      symptomatic, with simple partial
      seizures
  petit mal G40.409
    intractable G40.419
      with status epilepticus G40.411
      without status epilepticus G40.419
    not intractable G40.409
      with status epilepticus G40.401
      without status epilepticus G40.409
  post traumatic R56.1
  recurrent G40.909
  specified NEC G40.89
  uncinate —see Epilepsy, localization-related,
    symptomatic, with complex partial
    seizures
Selenium deficiency, dietary E59
Self-damaging behavior (life-style) Z72.89
Self-harm (attempted)
  history (personal) Z91.5
  in family Z81.8
Self-mutilation (attempted)
  history (personal) Z91.5
  in family Z81.8
Self-poisoning
  history (personal) Z91.5
  in family Z81.8
  observation following (alleged) attempt Z03.6
Semicoma R40.1
Seminal vesiculitis N49.0
Seminoma C62.9-
  specified site —see Neoplasm, malignant, by
    site
Senear-Usher disease or syndrome L10.4
Senectus R54
Senescence (without mention of psychosis)
    R54
Senile, senility —see also condition R41.81
  with
    acute confusional state F05
    mental changes NOS F03
    psychosis NEC —see Psychosis, senile
  asthenia R54
  cervix (atrophic) N88.8
  debility R54
  endometrium (atrophic) N85.8
  fallopian tube (atrophic) —see Atrophy,
    fallopian tube
  heart (failure) R54
  ovary (atrophic) —see Atrophy, ovary
  premature E34.8
  vagina, vaginitis (atrophic) N95.2
  wart L82.1
Sensation
  burning (skin) R20.8
    tongue K14.6
  loss of R20.8
  prickling (skin) R20.2
  tingling (skin) R20.2
Sense loss
  smell —see Disturbance, sensation, smell
  taste —see Disturbance, sensation, taste
  touch R20.8

Sensibility disturbance (cortical) (deep)
    (vibratory) R20.9
Sensitive, sensitivity —see also Allergy
    carotid sinus G90.01
    child (excessive) F93.8
    cold, autoimmune D59.1
    dentin K03.89
    gluten (non-celiac) K90.41 ◄
    latex Z91.040
    methemoglobin D74.8
    tuberculin, without clinical or radiological
        symptoms R76.11
    visual
        glare H53.71
        impaired contrast H53.72
Sensitiver Beziehungswahn F22
Sensitization, auto-erythrocytic D69.2
Separation
    anxiety, abnormal (of childhood) F93.0
    apophysis, traumatic - code as Fracture, by
        site
    choroid —see Detachment, choroid
    epiphysis, epiphyseal
        nontraumatic —see also
            Osteochondropathy, specified type
            NEC
        upper femoral —see Slipped, epiphysis,
            upper femoral
        traumatic - code as Fracture, by site
    fracture —see Fracture
    infundibulum cardiac from right ventricle by
        a partition Q24.3
    joint (traumatic) (current) - code by site under
        Dislocation
    pubic bone, obstetrical trauma O71.6
    retina, retinal —see Detachment, retina
    symphysis pubis, obstetrical trauma O71.6
    tracheal ring, incomplete, congenital Q32.1
Sepsis (generalized) (unspecified organism)
    A41.9
    with
        organ dysfunction (acute) (multiple) R65.20
            with septic shock R65.21
    actinomycotic A42.7
    adrenal hemorrhage syndrome
        (meningococcal) A39.1
    anaerobic A41.4
    Bacillus anthracis A22.7
    Brucella —see also Brucellosis A23.9
    candidal B37.7
    cryptogenic A41.9
    due to device, implant or graft T85.79
        arterial graft NEC T82.7
        breast (implant) T85.79
        catheter NEC T85.79
            dialysis (renal) T82.7
                intraperitoneal T85.71
            infusion NEC T82.7
                spinal (cranial) (epidural) (intrathecal)
                    (spinal) (subarachnoid)
                    (subdural) T85.735 ◄▥
            urethral indwelling T83.511 ◄
            urinary T83.518 ◄▥
        ectopic or molar pregnancy O08.82
        electronic (electrode) (pulse generator)
            (stimulator)
            bone T84.7
            cardiac T82.7
            nervous system T85.738 ◄▥
                brain T85.731 ◄
                neurostimulator generator T85.734 ◄
                peripheral nerve T85.732 ◄
                spinal cord T85.733 ◄
            urinary T83.590 ◄▥
        fixation, internal (orthopedic) —see
            Complication, fixation device,
            infection
        gastrointestinal (bile duct) (esophagus)
            T85.79
        neurostimulator electrode (lead)
            T85.732 ◄

Sepsis (Continued)
    due to device, implant or graft (Continued)
        genital T83.69 ◄▥
        heart NEC T82.7
            valve (prosthesis) T82.6
                graft T82.7
        joint prosthesis —see Complication, joint
            prosthesis, infection
        ocular (corneal graft) (orbital implant)
            T85.79
        orthopedic NEC T84.7
            fixation device, internal —see
                Complication, fixation device,
                infection
        specified NEC T85.79
        vascular T82.7
        ~~ventricular intracranial shunt T85.79~~
        ventricular intracranial (communicating)
            shunt T85.730 ◄
    during labor O75.3
    Enterococcus A41.81
    Erysipelothrix (rhusiopathiae) (erysipeloid)
        A26.7
    Escherichia coli (E. coli) A41.5
    extraintestinal yersiniosis A28.2
    following
        abortion (subsequent episode) O08.0
            current episode —see Abortion
        ectopic or molar pregnancy O08.82
        immunization T88.0
        infusion, therapeutic injection or
            transfusion NEC T80.29
    gangrenous A41.9
    gonococcal A54.86
    Gram-negative (organism) A41.5
        anaerobic A41.4
    Haemophilus influenzae A41.3
    herpesviral B00.7
    intra-abdominal K65.1
    intraocular —see Endophthalmitis, purulent
    Listeria monocytogenes A32.7
    localized — code to specific localized
        infection
        in operation wound T81.49 ◄▥
        skin —see Abscess
    malleus A24.0
    melioidosis A24.1
    meningeal —see Meningitis
    meningococcal A39.4
        acute A39.2
        chronic A39.3
    MSSA (Methicillin susceptible
        Staphylococcus aureus) A41.01
    newborn P36.9
        due to
            anaerobes NEC P36.5
            Escherichia coli P36.4
            Staphylococcus P36.30
                aureus P36.2
                specified NEC P36.39
            Streptococcus P36.10
                group B P36.0
                specified NEC P36.19
        specified NEC P36.8
    Pasteurella multocida A28.0
    pelvic, puerperal, postpartum, childbirth O85
    pneumococcal A40.3
    postprocedural T81.49 ◄▥
    puerperal, postpartum, childbirth (pelvic)
        O85
    Salmonella (arizonae) (cholerae-suis)
        (enteritidis) (typhimurium) A02.1
    severe R65.20
        with septic shock R65.21
    Shigella (see also Dysentery, bacillary) A03.9
    skin, localized —see Abscess
    specified organism NEC A41.89
    Staphylococcus, staphylococcal A41.2
        aureus (methicillin susceptible) (MSSA)
            A41.01
        methicillin resistant (MRSA) A41.02

Sepsis (Continued)
    Staphylococcus, staphylococcal (Continued)
        coagulase-negative A41.1
        specified NEC A41.1
    Streptococcus, streptococcal A40.9
        agalactiae A40.1
        group
            A A40.0
            B A40.1
            D A41.81
        neonatal P36.10
            group B P36.0
            specified NEC P36.19
        pneumoniae A40.3
        pyogenes A40.0
        specified NEC A40.8
    tracheostomy stoma J95.02
    tularemic A21.7
    umbilical, umbilical cord (newborn) —see
        Sepsis, newborn
    Yersinia pestis A20.7
Septate —see Septum
Septic —see condition
    arm —see Cellulitis, upper limb
        with lymphangitis —see Lymphangitis,
            acute, upper limb
    embolus —see Embolism
    finger —see Cellulitis, digit
        with lymphangitis —see Lymphangitis,
            acute, digit
    foot —see Cellulitis, lower limb
        with lymphangitis —see Lymphangitis,
            acute, lower limb
    gallbladder (acute) K81.0
    hand —see Cellulitis, upper limb
        with lymphangitis —see Lymphangitis,
            acute, upper limb
    joint —see Arthritis, pyogenic or pyemic
    leg —see Cellulitis, lower limb
        with lymphangitis —see Lymphangitis,
            acute, lower limb
    nail —see also Cellulitis, digit
        with lymphangitis —see Lymphangitis,
            acute, digit
    sore —see also Abscess
        throat J02.0
            streptococcal J02.0
    spleen (acute) D73.89
    teeth, tooth (pulpal origin) K04.4
    throat —see Pharyngitis
    thrombus —see Thrombosis
    toe —see Cellulitis, digit
        with lymphangitis —see Lymphangitis,
            acute, digit
    tonsils, chronic J35.01
        with adenoiditis J35.03
    uterus —see Endometritis
Septicemia A41.9
    meaning sepsis —see Sepsis
Septum, septate (congenital) —see also
    Anomaly, by site
    anal Q42.3
        with fistula Q42.2
    aqueduct of Sylvius Q03.0
        with spina bifida —see Spina bifida, by site,
            with hydrocephalus
    uterus (complete) (partial) Q51.2
    vagina Q52.10
        in pregnancy —see Pregnancy, complicated
            by, abnormal vagina
        causing obstructed labor
            O65.5
        longitudinal Q52.129 ◄▥
            microperforate ◄
                left side Q52.124 ◄
                right side Q52.123 ◄
            nonobstruction Q52.120 ◄
            obstructing Q52.129 ◄
                left side Q52.122 ◄
                right side Q52.121 ◄
        transverse Q52.11

◄ New   ◄▥ Revised   ~~deleted~~ Deleted

Sequelae (of) —*see also* condition
  abscess, intracranial or intraspinal (conditions in G06) G09
  amputation — code to injury with seventh character S
  burn and corrosion — code to injury with seventh character S
  calcium deficiency E64.8
  cerebrovascular disease —*see* Sequelae, disease, cerebrovascular
  childbirth O94
  contusion — code to injury with seventh character S
  corrosion —*see* Sequelae, burn and corrosion
  crushing injury — code to injury with seventh character S
  disease
    cerebrovascular I69.90
      alteration of sensation I69.998
      aphasia I69.920
      apraxia I69.990
      ataxia I69.993
      cognitive deficits I69.91
      disturbance of vision I69.998
      dysarthria I69.922
      dysphagia I69.991
      dysphasia I69.921
      facial droop I69.992
      facial weakness I69.992
      fluency disorder I69.923
      hemiplegia I69.95-
      hemorrhage
        intracerebral —*see* Sequelae, hemorrhage, intracerebral
        intracranial, nontraumatic NEC — *see* Sequelae, hemorrhage, intracranial, nontraumatic
        subarachnoid —*see* Sequelae, hemorrhage, subarachnoid
      language deficit I69.928
      monoplegia
        lower limb I69.84-
        upper limb I69.93-
      paralytic syndrome I69.96-
      specified effect NEC I69.998
      specified type NEC I69.80
        alteration of sensation I69.898
        aphasia I69.820
        apraxia I69.890
        ataxia I69.893
        cognitive deficits I69.81
        disturbance of vision I69.898
        dysarthria I69.822
        dysphagia I69.891
        dysphasia I69.821
        facial droop I69.892
        facial weakness I69.892
        fluency disorder I69.823
        hemiplegia I69.85-
        language deficit I69.828
        monoplegia
          lower limb I69.84-
          upper limb I69.83-
        paralytic syndrome I69.86-
        specified effect NEC I69.898
      speech deficit I69.928
        speech deficit I69.828
      stroke NOS —*see* Sequelae, stroke NOS
  dislocation — code to injury with seventh character S
  encephalitis or encephalomyelitis (conditions in G04) G09
    in infectious disease NEC B94.8
    viral B94.1
  external cause — code to injury with seventh character S
  foreign body entering natural orifice — code to injury with seventh character S
  fracture — code to injury with seventh character S

Sequelae (*Continued*)
  frostbite — code to injury with seventh character S
  Hansen's disease B92
  hemorrhage
    intracerebral I69.10
      alteration of sensation I69.198
      aphasia I69.120
      apraxia I69.190
      ataxia I69.193
      cognitive deficits I69.11
      disturbance of vision I69.198
      dysarthria I69.122
      dysphagia I69.191
      dysphasia I69.121
      facial droop I69.192
      facial weakness I69.192
      fluency disorder I69.123
      hemiplegia I69.15-
      language deficit NEC I69.128
      monoplegia
        lower limb I69.14-
        upper limb I69.13-
      paralytic syndrome I69.16-
      specified effect NEC I69.198
      speech deficit NEC I69.128
    intracranial, nontraumatic NEC I69.20
      alteration of sensation I69.298
      aphasia I69.220
      apraxia I69.290
      ataxia I69.293
      cognitive deficits I69.21
      disturbance of vision I69.298
      dysarthria I69.222
      dysphagia I69.291
      dysphasia I69.221
      facial droop I69.292
      facial weakness I69.292
      fluency disorder I69.223
      hemiplegia I69.25-
      language deficit NEC I69.228
      monoplegia
        lower limb I69.24-
        upper limb I69.23-
      paralytic syndrome I69.26-
      specified effect NEC I69.298
      speech deficit NEC I69.228
    subarachnoid I69.00
      alteration of sensation I69.098
      aphasia I69.020
      apraxia I69.090
      ataxia I69.093
      cognitive deficits —*see* subcategory I69.01- ◀
      disturbance of vision I69.098
      dysarthria I69.022
      dysphagia I69.091
      dysphasia I69.021
      facial droop I69.092
      facial weakness I69.092
      fluency disorder I69.023
      hemiplegia I69.05-
      language deficit NEC I69.028
      monoplegia
        lower limb I69.04-
        upper limb I69.03-
      paralytic syndrome I69.06-
      specified effect NEC I69.098
      speech deficit NEC I69.028
  hepatitis, viral B94.2
  hyperalimentation E68
  infarction
    cerebral I69.30
      alteration of sensation I69.398
      aphasia I69.320
      apraxia I69.390
      ataxia I69.393
      cognitive deficits I69.31
      disturbance of vision I69.398
      dysarthria I69.322
      dysphagia I69.391

Sequelae (*Continued*)
  infarction (*Continued*)
    cerebral (*Continued*)
      dysphasia I69.321
      facial droop I69.392
      facial weakness I69.392
      fluency disorder I69.323
      hemiplegia I69.35-
      language deficit NEC I69.328
      monoplegia
        lower limb I69.34-
        upper limb I69.33-
      paralytic syndrome I69.36-
      specified effect NEC I69.398
      speech deficit NEC I69.328
  infection, pyogenic, intracranial or intraspinal G09
  infectious disease B94.9
    specified NEC B94.8
  injury — code to injury with seventh character S
  leprosy B92
  meningitis
    bacterial (conditions in G00) G09
    other or unspecified cause (conditions in G03) G09
  muscle (and tendon) injury — code to injury with seventh character S
  myelitis —*see* Sequelae, encephalitis
  niacin deficiency E64.8
  nutritional deficiency E64.9
    specified NEC E64.8
  obstetrical condition O94
  parasitic disease B94.9
  phlebitis or thrombophlebitis of intracranial or intraspinal venous sinuses and veins (conditions in G08) G09
  poisoning — code to poisoning with seventh character S
    nonmedicinal substance —*see* Sequelae, toxic effect, nonmedicinal substance
  poliomyelitis (acute) B91
  pregnancy O94
  protein-energy malnutrition E64.0
  puerperium O94
  rickets E64.3
  selenium deficiency E64.8
  sprain and strain — code to injury with seventh character S
  stroke NOS I69.30
    alteration in sensation I69.398
    aphasia I69.320
    apraxia I69.390
    ataxia I69.393
    cognitive deficits I69.31
    disturbance of vision I69.398
    dysarthria I69.322
    dysphagia I69.391
    dysphasia I69.321
    facial droop I69.392
    facial weakness I69.392
    hemiplegia I69.35-
    language deficit NEC I69.328
    monoplegia
      lower limb I69.34-
      upper limb I69.33-
    paralytic syndrome I69.36-
    specified effect NEC I69.398
    speech deficit NEC I69.328
  tendon and muscle injury — code to injury with seventh character S
  thiamine deficiency E64.8
  trachoma B94.0
  tuberculosis B90.9
    bones and joints B90.2
    central nervous system B90.0
    genitourinary B90.1
    pulmonary (respiratory) B90.9
    specified organs NEC B90.8

S

Sequelae *(Continued)*
 viral
  encephalitis B94.1
  hepatitis B94.2
 vitamin deficiency NEC E64.8
  A E64.1
  B E64.8
  C E64.2
 wound, open — code to injury with seventh
   character S
Sequestration —*see also* Sequestrum
 disk —*see* Displacement, intervertebral
   disk ◄
 lung, congenital Q33.2
Sequestrum
 bone—*see* Osteomyelitis, chronic
 dental M27.2
 jaw bone M27.2
 orbit —*see* Osteomyelitis, orbit
 sinus (accessory) (nasal) —*see* Sinusitis
Sequoiosis lung or pneumonitis J67.8
Serology for syphilis
 doubtful
  with signs or symptoms - code by site and
    stage under Syphilis
  follow-up of latent syphilis —*see* Syphilis,
    latent
 negative, with signs or symptoms — code by
   site and stage under Syphilis
 positive A53.0
  with signs or symptoms - code by site and
    stage under Syphilis
 reactivated A53.0
Seroma —*see also* Hematoma
 postprocedural —*see* Complication,
   postprocedural, seroma ◄
 traumatic, secondary and recurrent
   T79.2
Seropurulent —*see* condition
Serositis, multiple K65.8
 pericardial I31.1
 peritoneal K65.8
Serous —*see* condition
Sertoli cell
 adenoma
  specified site —*see* Neoplasm, benign, by
    site
  unspecified site
   female D27.9
   male D29.20
 carcinoma
  specified site —*see* Neoplasm, malignant,
    by site
  unspecified site (male) C62.9-
   female C56.9
 tumor
  with lipid storage
   specified site —*see* Neoplasm, benign,
     by site
   unspecified site
    female D27.9
    male D29.20
  specified site —*see* Neoplasm, benign, by
    site
  unspecified site
   female D27.9
   male D29.20
Sertoli-Leydig cell tumor —*see* Neoplasm,
   benign, by site
 specified site —*see* Neoplasm, benign,
   by site
 unspecified site
  female D27.9
  male D29.20
Serum
 allergy, allergic reaction —*see also* Reaction,
   serum T80.69
 shock —*see also* Shock, anaphylactic T80.59
 arthritis —*see also* Reaction, serum T80.69
 complication or reaction NEC —*see also*
   Reaction, serum T80.69

Serum *(Continued)*
 disease NEC —*see also* Reaction, serum
   T80.69
 hepatitis —*see also* Hepatitis, viral, type B
   carrier (suspected) of B18.1 ◄▥
 intoxication —*see also* Reaction, serum T80.69
 neuritis —*see also* Reaction, serum T80.69
 neuropathy G61.1
 poisoning NEC —*see also* Reaction, serum
   T80.69
 rash NEC —*see also* Reaction, serum T80.69
 reaction NEC —*see also* Reaction, serum
   T80.69
 sickness NEC —*see also* Reaction, serum
   T80.69
 urticaria —*see also* Reaction, serum T80.69
Sesamoiditis M25.8-
Sever's disease or osteochondrosis —*see*
   Osteochondrosis, juvenile, tarsus
Severe sepsis R65.20
 with septic shock R65.21
Sex
 chromosome mosaics Q97.8
  lines with various numbers of
    X chromosomes Q97.2
 education Z70.8
 reassignment surgery status Z87.890
Sextuplet pregnancy —*see* Pregnancy,
   sextuplet
Sexual
 function, disorder of (psychogenic) F52.9
 immaturity (female) (male) E30.0
 impotence (psychogenic) organic origin
   NEC —*see* Dysfunction, sexual, male
 precocity (constitutional) (cryptogenic)
   (female) (idiopathic) (male) E30.1
Sexuality, pathologic —*see* Deviation, sexual
Sézary disease C84.1-
Shadow, lung R91.8
Shaking palsy or paralysis —*see* Parkinsonism
Shallowness, acetabulum —*see* Derangement,
   joint, specified type NEC, hip
Shaver's disease J63.1
Sheath (tendon) —*see* condition
Sheathing, retinal vessels H35.01-
Shedding
 nail L60.8
 premature, primary (deciduous) teeth
   K00.6
Sheehan's disease or syndrome E23.0
Shelf, rectal K62.89
Shell teeth K00.5
Shellshock (current) F43.0
 lasting state —*see* Disorder, post-traumatic
   stress
Shield kidney Q63.1
Shift
 auditory threshold (temporary) H93.24-
 mediastinal R93.8
Shifting sleep-work schedule (affecting sleep)
   G47.26
Shiga (-Kruse) dysentery A03.0
Shiga's bacillus A03.0
Shigella (dysentery) —*see* Dysentery, bacillary
Shigellosis A03.9
 Group A A03.0
 Group B A03.1
 Group C A03.2
 Group D A03.3
Shin splints S86.89
Shingles —*see* Herpes, zoster
Shipyard disease or eye B30.0
Shirodkar suture, in pregnancy —*see*
   Pregnancy, complicated by, incompetent
   cervix
Shock R57.9
 with ectopic or molar pregnancy O08.3
 adrenal (cortical) (Addisonian) E27.2
 adverse food reaction (anaphylactic) —*see*
   Shock, anaphylactic, due to food
 allergic —*see* Shock, anaphylactic

Shock *(Continued)*
 anaphylactic T78.2
  chemical —*see* Table of Drugs and
    Chemicals
  due to drug or medicinal substance
   correct substance properly administered
     T88.6
   overdose or wrong substance given or
     taken (by accident) —*see* Table of
     Drugs and Chemicals, by drug,
     poisoning
  due to food (nonpoisonous) T78.00
   additives T78.06
   dairy products T78.07
   eggs T78.08
   fish T78.03
    shellfish T78.02
   fruit T78.04
   milk T78.07
   nuts T78.05
    multiple types T78.05 ◄
    peanuts T78.01
   peanuts T78.01
   seeds T78.05
   specified type NEC T78.09
   vegetable T78.04
  following sting (s) —*see* Venom
  immunization T80.52
  serum T80.59
   blood and blood products T80.51
   immunization T80.52
   specified NEC T80.59
   vaccination T80.52
 anaphylactoid —*see* Shock, anaphylactic
 anesthetic
  correct substance properly administered
    T88.2
  overdose or wrong substance given or
    taken —*see* Table of Drugs and
    Chemicals, by drug, poisoning
  specified anesthetic —*see* Table of
    Drugs and Chemicals, by drug,
    poisoning
 cardiogenic R57.0
 chemical substance —*see* Table of Drugs and
   Chemicals
 complicating ectopic or molar pregnancy O08.3
 culture —*see* Disorder, adjustment
 drug
  due to correct substance properly
    administered T88.6
  overdose or wrong substance given or
    taken (by accident) —*see* Table of
    Drugs and Chemicals, by drug,
    poisoning
 during or after labor and delivery O75.1
 electric T75.4
  (taser) T75.4
 endotoxic R65.21
  postprocedural (resulting from a
    procedure, not elsewhere classified)
    T81.12 ◄▥
 following
  ectopic or molar pregnancy O08.3
  injury (immediate) (delayed) T79.4
  labor and delivery O75.1
 food (anaphylactic) —*see* Shock, anaphylactic,
   due to food
 from electroshock gun (taser) T75.4
 gram-negative R65.21
  postprocedural (resulting from a
    procedure, not elsewhere classified)
    T81.12 ◄▥
 hematologic R57.8
 hemorrhagic
  surgery (intraoperative) (postoperative)
    T81.19
  trauma T79.4
 hypovolemic R57.1
  surgical T81.19
  traumatic T79.4

◄ New   ◄▥ Revised   ~~deleted~~ Deleted

Shock (*Continued*)
  insulin E15
    therapeutic misadventure —*see*
      subcategory T38.3
  kidney N17.Ø
    traumatic (following crushing) T79.5
  lightning T75.Ø1
  liver K72.ØØ ◄
  lung J8Ø
  obstetric O75.1
    with ectopic or molar pregnancy OØ8.3
    following ectopic or molar pregnancy
      OØ8.3
  pleural (surgical) T81.19
    due to trauma T79.4
  postprocedural (postoperative) T81.1Ø
    with ectopic or molar pregnancy OØ8.3
    cardiogenic T81.11
    endotoxic T81.12
    following ectopic or molar pregnancy OØ8.3
    gram-negative T81.12
    hypovolemic T81.19
    septic T81.12
    specified type NEC T81.19
  psychic F43.Ø
  septic (due to severe sepsis) R65.21
  specified NEC R57.8
  surgical T81.1Ø
  taser gun (taser) T75.4
  therapeutic misadventure NEC T81.1Ø
  thyroxin
    overdose or wrong substance given or
      taken —*see* Table of Drugs and
      Chemicals, by drug, poisoning
  toxic, syndrome A48.3
  transfusion —*see* Complications, transfusion
  traumatic (immediate) (delayed) T79.4
Shoemaker's chest M95.4
Short, shortening, shortness
  arm (acquired) —*see also* Deformity, limb,
    unequal length
    congenital Q71.81-
      forearm —*see* Deformity, limb, unequal
        length
  bowel syndrome K91.2
  breath R06.02
  cervical (complicating pregnancy) O26.87-
    non-gravid uterus N88.3
  common bile duct, congenital Q44.5
  cord (umbilical), complicating delivery O69.3
  cystic duct, congenital Q44.5
  esophagus (congenital) Q39.8
  femur (acquired) —*see* Deformity, limb,
    unequal length, femur
    congenital —*see* Defect, reduction, lower
      limb, longitudinal, femur
  frenum, frenulum, linguae (congenital) Q38.1
  hip (acquired) —*see also* Deformity, limb,
    unequal length
    congenital Q65.89
  leg (acquired) —*see also* Deformity, limb,
    unequal length
    congenital Q72.81-
    lower leg —*see also* Deformity, limb,
      unequal length
  limbed stature, with immunodeficiency D82.2
  lower limb (acquired) —*see also* Deformity,
    limb, unequal length
    congenital Q72.81-
  organ or site, congenital NEC —*see* Distortion
  palate, congenital Q38.5
  radius (acquired) —*see also* Deformity, limb,
    unequal length
    congenital —*see* Defect, reduction, upper
      limb, longitudinal, radius
  rib syndrome Q77.2
  stature (child) (hereditary) (idiopathic) NEC
    R62.52
    constitutional E34.3
    due to endocrine disorder E34.3
    Laron-type E34.3

Short, shortening, shortness (*Continued*)
  tendon —*see also* Contraction, tendon
    with contracture of joint —*see* Contraction,
      joint
    Achilles (acquired) M67.Ø-
      congenital Q66.89
    congenital Q79.8
  thigh (acquired) —*see also* Deformity, limb,
    unequal length, femur
    congenital —*see* Defect, reduction, lower
      limb, longitudinal, femur
  tibialis anterior (tendon) —*see* Contraction,
    tendon
  umbilical cord
    complicating delivery O69.3
  upper limb, congenital —*see* Defect,
    reduction, upper limb, specified type
    NEC
  urethra N36.8
  uvula, congenital Q38.5
  vagina (congenital) Q52.4
Shortsightedness —*see* Myopia
Shoshin (acute fulminating beriberi) E51.11
Shoulder —*see* condition
Shovel-shaped incisors KØØ.2
Shower, thromboembolic —*see* Embolism
Shunt
  arterial-venous (dialysis) Z99.2
  arteriovenous, pulmonary (acquired) I28.Ø
    congenital Q25.72
  cerebral ventricle (communicating) in situ
    Z98.2
  surgical, prosthetic, with complications —*see*
    Complications, cardiovascular, device
    or implant Shutdown, renal N28.9
Shutdown, renal N28.9
Shy-Drager syndrome G90.3
Sialadenitis, sialadenosis (any gland) (chronic)
  (periodic) (suppurative) —*see* Sialoadenitis
Sialectasia K11.8
Sialidosis E77.1
Sialitis, silitis (any gland) (chronic)
  (suppurative) —*see* Sialoadenitis
Sialoadenitis (any gland) (periodic)
  (suppurative) K11.2Ø
  acute K11.21
    recurrent K11.22
  chronic K11.23
Sialoadenopathy K11.9
Sialoangitis —*see* Sialoadenitis
Sialodochitis (fibrinosa) —*see* Sialoadenitis
Sialodocholithiasis K11.5
Sialolithiasis K11.5
Sialometaplasia, necrotizing K11.8
Sialorrhea —*see also* Ptyalism
  periodic —*see* Sialoadenitis
Sialosis K11.7
Siamese twin Q89.4
Sibling rivalry Z62.891
Sicard's syndrome G52.7
Sicca syndrome M35.ØØ
  with
    keratoconjunctivitis M35.Ø1
    lung involvement M35.Ø2
    myopathy M35.Ø3
    renal tubulo-interstitial disorders M35.Ø4
    specified organ involvement NEC M35.Ø9
Sick R69
  or handicapped person in family Z63.79
    needing care at home Z63.6
  sinus (syndrome) I49.5
Sick-euthyroid syndrome EØ7.81
Sickle-cell
  anemia —*see* Disease, sickle-cell
  trait D57.3
Sicklemia —*see also* Disease, sickle-cell
  trait D57.3
Sickness
  air (travel) T75.3
  airplane T75.3
  alpine T70.29

Sickness (*Continued*)
  altitude T70.2Ø
  Andes T70.29
  aviator's T70.29
  balloon T70.29
  car T75.3
  compressed air T70.3
  decompression T70.3
  green D50.8
  milk —*see* Poisoning, food, noxious
  motion T75.3
  mountain T70.29
    acute D75.1
  protein —*see also* Reaction, serum T8Ø.69
  radiation T66
  roundabout (motion) T75.3
  sea T75.3
  serum NEC —*see also* Reaction, serum T8Ø.69
  sleeping (African) B56.9
    by Trypanosoma B56.9
      brucei
        gambiense B56.Ø
        rhodesiense B56.1
    East African B56.1
    Gambian B56.Ø
    Rhodesian B56.1
    West African B56.Ø
  swing (motion) T75.3
  train (railway) (travel) T75.3
  travel (any vehicle) T75.3
Sideropenia —*see* Anemia, iron deficiency
Siderosilicosis J62.8
Siderosis (lung) J63.4
  eye (globe) —*see* Disorder, globe,
    degenerative, siderosis
Siemens' syndrome (ectodermal dysplasia) Q82.8
Sighing R06.89
  psychogenic F45.8
Sigmoid —*see also* condition
  flexure —*see* condition
  kidney Q63.1
Sigmoiditis —*see also* Enteritis K52.9
  infectious AØ9
  noninfectious K52.9
Silfverskiöld's syndrome Q78.9
Silicosiderosis J62.8
Silicosis, silicotic (simple) (complicated) J62.8
  with tuberculosis J65
Silicotuberculosis J65
Silo-fillers' disease J68.8
  bronchitis J68.Ø
  pneumonitis J68.Ø
  pulmonary edema J68.1
Silver's syndrome Q87.1
Simian malaria B53.1
Simmonds' cachexia or disease E23.Ø
Simons' disease or syndrome (progressive
  lipodystrophy) E88.1
Simple, simplex —*see* condition
Simulation, conscious (of illness) Z76.5
Simultanagnosia (asimultagnosia) R48.3
Sin Nombre virus disease (Hantavirus)
  (cardio)-pulmonary syndrome) B33.4
Sinding-Larsen disease or osteochondrosis —
  see Osteochondrosis, juvenile, patella
Singapore hemorrhagic fever A91
Singer's node or nodule J38.2
Single
  atrium Q21.2
  coronary artery Q24.5
  umbilical artery Q27.Ø
  ventricle Q20.4
Singultus R06.6
  epidemicus B33.Ø
Sinus —*see also* Fistula
  abdominal K63.89
  arrest I45.5
  arrhythmia I49.8
  bradycardia RØØ.1
  branchial cleft (internal) (external) Q18.Ø
  coccygeal —*see* Sinus, pilonidal

Sinus *(Continued)*
dental K04.6
dermal (congenital) Q06.8
with abscess Q06.8
coccygeal, pilonidal —*see* Sinus, coccygeal
infected, skin NEC L08.89
marginal, ruptured or bleeding —*see* Hemorrhage, antepartum, specified cause NEC
medial, face and neck Q18.8
pause I45.5
pericranii Q01.9
pilonidal (infected) (rectum) L05.92
with abscess L05.02
preauricular Q18.1
rectovaginal N82.3
Rokitansky-Aschoff (gallbladder) K82.8
sacrococcygeal (dermoid) (infected) —*see* Sinus, pilonidal
tachycardia R00.0
paroxysmal I47.1
tarsi syndrome M25.57- ◀▥
testis N50.89 ◀▥
tract (postinfective) —*see* Fistula
urachus Q64.4
Sinusitis (accessory) (chronic) (hyperplastic) (nasal) (nonpurulent) (purulent) J32.9
acute J01.90
ethmoidal J01.20
recurrent J01.21
frontal J01.10
recurrent J01.11
involving more than one sinus, other than pansinusitis J01.80
recurrent J01.81
maxillary J01.00
recurrent J01.01
pansinusitis J01.40
recurrent J01.41
recurrent J01.91
specified NEC J01.80
recurrent J01.81
sphenoidal J01.30
recurrent J01.31
allergic —*see* Rhinitis, allergic
due to high altitude T70.1
ethmoidal J32.2
acute J01.20
recurrent J01.21
frontal J32.1
acute J01.10
recurrent J01.11
influenzal —*see* Influenza, with, respiratory manifestations NEC
involving more than one sinus but not pansinusitis J32.8
acute J01.80
recurrent J01.81
maxillary J32.0
acute J01.00
recurrent J01.01
sphenoidal J32.3
acute J01.30
recurrent J01.31
tuberculous, any sinus A15.8
Sinusitis-bronchiectasis-situs inversus (syndrome) (triad) Q89.3
Sipple's syndrome E31.22
Sirenomelia (syndrome) Q87.2
Siriasis T67.0
Sirkari's disease B55.0
Siti A65
Situation, psychiatric F99
Situational
disturbance (transient) —*see* Disorder, adjustment
acute F43.0
maladjustment —*see* Disorder, adjustment
reaction —*see* Disorder, adjustment
acute F43.0

Situs inversus or transversus (abdominalis) (thoracis) Q89.3
Sixth disease B08.20
due to human herpesvirus 6 B08.21
due to human herpesvirus 7 B08.22
Sjögren-Larsson syndrome Q87.1
Sjögren's syndrome or disease —*see* Sicca syndrome
Skeletal —*see* condition
Skene's gland —*see* condition
Skenitis —*see* Urethritis
Skerljevo A65
Skevas-Zerfus disease —*see* Toxicity, venom, marine animal, sea anemone
Skin —*see also* condition
clammy R23.1
donor —*see* Donor, skin
hidebound M35.9
Slate-dressers' or slate-miners' lung J62.8
Sleep
apnea —*see* Apnea, sleep
deprivation Z72.820
disorder or disturbance G47.9
child F51.9
nonorganic origin F51.9
specified NEC G47.8
disturbance G47.9
nonorganic origin F51.9
drunkenness F51.9
rhythm inversion G47.2-
terrors F51.4
walking F51.3
hysterical F44.89
Sleep hygiene
abuse Z72.821
inadequate Z72.821
poor Z72.821
Sleeping sickness —*see* Sickness, sleeping
Sleeplessness —*see* Insomnia
menopausal N95.11
Sleep-wake schedule disorder G47.20
Slim disease (in HIV infection) B20
Slipped, slipping
epiphysis (traumatic) —*see also* Osteochondropathy, specified type NEC
capital femoral (traumatic)
acute (on chronic) S79.01-
current traumatic - code as Fracture, by site
upper femoral (nontraumatic) M93.00-
acute M93.01-
on chronic M93.03-
chronic M93.02-
intervertebral disc —*see* Displacement, intervertebral disc
ligature, umbilical P51.8
patella —*see* Disorder, patella, derangement NEC
rib M89.8X8
sacroiliac joint —*see* subcategory M53.2
tendon —*see* Disorder, tendon
ulnar nerve, nontraumatic —*see* Lesion, nerve, ulnar
vertebra NEC —*see* Spondylolisthesis
Slocumb's syndrome E27.0
Sloughing (multiple) (phagedena) (skin) —*see also* Gangrene
abscess —*see* Abscess
appendix K38.8
fascia —*see* Disorder, soft tissue, specified type NEC
scrotum N50.89 ◀▥
tendon —*see* Disorder, tendon
transplanted organ —*see* Rejection, transplant
ulcer —*see* Ulcer, skin
Slow
feeding, newborn P92.2
flow syndrome, coronary I20.8
heart(beat) R00.1
Slowing, urinary stream R39.198 ◀▥
Sluder's neuralgia (syndrome) G44.89

Slurred, slurring speech R47.81
Small (ness)
for gestational age —*see* Small for dates
introitus, vagina N89.6
kidney (unknown cause) N27.9
bilateral N27.1
unilateral N27.0
ovary (congenital) Q50.39
pelvis
with disproportion (fetopelvic) O33.1
causing obstructed labor O65.1
uterus N85.8
white kidney N03.9
Small-and-light-for-dates —*see* Small for dates
Small-for-dates (infant) P05.10
with weight of
499 grams or less P05.11
500-749 grams P05.12
750-999 grams P05.13
1000-1249 grams P05.14
1250-1499 grams P05.15
1500-1749 grams P05.16
1750-1999 grams P05.17
2000-2499 grams P05.18
2500 grams and over P05.19 ◀
specified NEC P05.19 ◀
Smallpox B03
Smearing, fecal R15.1
Smith-Lemli-Opitz syndrome E78.72
Smith's fracture S52.54-
Smoker —*see* Dependence, drug, nicotine
Smoker's
bronchitis J41.0
cough J41.0
palate K13.24
throat J31.2
tongue K13.24
Smoking
passive Z77.22
Smothering spells R06.81
Snaggle teeth, tooth M26.39
Snapping
finger —*see* Trigger finger
hip —*see* Derangement, joint, specified type NEC, hip
involving the iliotiblial band M76.3-
knee —*see* Derangement, knee
involving the iliotiblial band M76.3-
Sneddon-Wilkinson disease or syndrome (subcorneal pustular dermatosis) L13.1
Sneezing (intractable) R06.7
Sniffing
cocaine
abuse —*see* Abuse, drug, cocaine
dependence —*see* Dependence, drug, cocaine
gasoline
abuse —*see* Abuse, drug, inhalant
dependence —*see* Dependence, drug, inhalant
glue (airplane)
abuse —*see* Abuse, drug, inhalant
drug dependence —*see* Dependence, drug, inhalant
Sniffles
newborn P28.89
Snoring R06.83
Snow blindness —*see* Photokeratitis
Snuffles (non-syphilitic) R06.5
newborn P28.89
syphilitic (infant) A50.05 *[[99]]*
Social
exclusion Z60.4
due to discrimination or persecution (perceived) Z60.5
migrant Z59.0
acculturation difficulty Z60.3
rejection Z60.4
due to discrimination or persecution Z60.5

◀ New   ◀▥ Revised   ~~deleted~~ Deleted

Social *(Continued)*
  role conflict NEC Z73.5
  skills inadequacy NEC Z73.4
  transplantation Z60.3
Sodoku A25.0
Soemmering's ring —*see* Cataract, secondary
Soft —*see also* condition
  nails L60.3
Softening
  bone —*see* Osteomalacia
  brain (necrotic) (progressive) G93.89
    congenital Q04.8
    embolic I63.4- ◀▥
    hemorrhagic —*see* Hemorrhage,
      intracranial, intracerebral
    occlusive I63.5- ◀▥
    thrombotic I63.3- ◀▥
  cartilage M94.2-
    patella M22.4-
  cerebellar —*see* Softening, brain
  cerebral —*see* Softening, brain
  cerebrospinal —*see* Softening, brain
  myocardial, heart —*see* Degeneration,
    myocardial
  spinal cord G95.89
  stomach K31.89
Soldier's
  heart F45.8
  patches I31.0
Solitary
  cyst, kidney N28.1
  kidney, congenital Q60.0
Solvent abuse —*see* Abuse, drug, inhalant
  dependence —*see* Dependence, drug,
    inhalant
Somatization reaction, somatic reaction —*see*
  Disorder, somatoform
Somnambulism F51.3
  hysterical F44.89
Somnolence R40.0
  nonorganic origin F51.11
Sonne dysentery A03.3
Soor B37.0
Sore
  bed —*see* Ulcer, pressure, by site
  chiclero B55.1
  Delhi B55.1
  desert —*see* Ulcer, skin
  eye H57.1-
  Lahore B55.1
  mouth K13.79
    canker K12.0
  muscle M79.1
  Naga —*see* Ulcer, skin
  of skin —*see* Ulcer, skin - oriental B55.1
  pressure —*see* Ulcer, pressure, by site
  skin L98.9
  soft A57
  throat (acute) —*see also* Pharyngitis
    with influenza, flu, or grippe —*see*
      Influenza, with, respiratory
      manifestations NEC
    chronic J31.2
    coxsackie (virus) B08.5
    diphtheritic A36.0
    herpesviral B00.2
    influenzal —*see* Influenza, with, respiratory
      manifestations NEC
    septic J02.0
    streptococcal (ulcerative) J02.0
    viral NEC J02.8
      coxsackie B08.5
  tropical —*see* Ulcer, skin
  veldt —*see* Ulcer, skin
Soto's syndrome (cerebral gigantism) Q87.3
South African cardiomyopathy syndrome I42.8
Southeast Asian hemorrhagic fever A91
Spacing
  abnormal, tooth, teeth, fully erupted M26.30
  excessive, tooth, fully erupted M26.32
Spade-like hand (congenital) Q68.1

Spading nail L60.8
  congenital Q84.6
Spanish collar N47.1
Sparganosis B70.1
Spasm (s), spastic, spasticity —*see also*
  condition R25.2
  accommodation —*see* Spasm, of
    accommodation
  ampulla of Vater K83.4
  anus, ani (sphincter) (reflex) K59.4
    psychogenic F45.8
  artery I73.9
    cerebral G45.9
  Bell's G51.3
  bladder (sphincter, external or internal) N32.89
    psychogenic F45.8
  bronchus, bronchiole J98.01
  cardia K22.0
  cardiac I20.1
  carpopedal —*see* Tetany
  cerebral (arteries) (vascular) G45.9
  cervix, complicating delivery O62.4
  ciliary body (of accommodation) —*see* Spasm,
    of accommodation
  colon —*see also* Irritable, bowel K58.9 ◀▥
    with diarrhea K58.0
    psychogenic F45.8
  common duct K83.8
  compulsive —*see* Tic
  conjugate H51.8
  coronary (artery) I20.1
  diaphragm (reflex) R06.6
    epidemic B33.0
    psychogenic F45.8
  duodenum K59.8
  epidemic diaphragmatic (transient) B33.0
  esophagus (diffuse) K22.4
    psychogenic F45.8
  facial G51.3
  fallopian tube N83.8
  gastrointestinal (tract) K31.89
    psychogenic F45.8
  glottis J38.5
    hysterical F44.4
    psychogenic F45.8
      conversion reaction F44.4
    reflex through recurrent laryngeal nerve
      J38.5
  habit —*see* Tic
  heart I20.1
  hemifacial (clonic) G51.3
  hourglass —*see* Contraction, hourglass
  hysterical F44.4
  infantile —*see* Epilepsy, spasms
  inferior oblique, eye H51.8
  intestinal —*see also* Syndrome, irritable bowel
    K58.9
    psychogenic F45.8
  larynx, laryngeal J38.5
    hysterical F44.4
    psychogenic F45.8
      conversion reaction F44.4
  levator palpebrae superioris —*see* Disorder,
    eyelid function
  muscle NEC M62.838
    back M62.830
  nerve, trigeminal G51.0
  nervous F45.8
  nodding F98.4
  occupational F48.8
  oculogyric H51.8
    psychogenic F45.8
  of accommodation H52.53-
  ophthalmic artery —*see* Occlusion, artery,
    retina
  perineal, female N94.89
  peroneo-extensor —*see also* Deformity, limb,
    flat foot
  pharynx (reflex) J39.2
    hysterical F45.8
    psychogenic F45.8

Spasm (s), spastic, spasticity *(Continued)*
  psychogenic F45.8
  pylorus NEC K31.3
    adult hypertrophic K31.89
    congenital or infantile Q40.0
    psychogenic F45.8
  rectum (sphincter) K59.4
    psychogenic F45.8
  retinal (artery) —*see* Occlusion, artery, retina
  sigmoid —*see also* Syndrome, irritable bowel
    K58.9
    psychogenic F45.8
  sphincter of Oddi K83.4
  stomach K31.89
    neurotic F45.8
  throat J39.2
    hysterical F45.8
    psychogenic F45.8
  tic F95.9
    chronic F95.1
    transient of childhood F95.0
  tongue K14.8
  torsion (progressive) G24.1
  trigeminal nerve —*see* Neuralgia, trigeminal
  ureter N13.5
  urethra (sphincter) N35.9
  uterus N85.8
    complicating labor O62.4
  vagina N94.2
    psychogenic F52.5
  vascular I73.9
  vasomotor I73.9
  vein NEC I87.8
  viscera —*see* Pain, abdominal
Spasmodic —*see* condition
Spasmophilia —*see* Tetany
Spasmus nutans F98.4
Spastic, spasticity —*see also* Spasm
  child (cerebral) (congenital) (paralysis) G80.1
Speaker's throat R49.8
Specific, specified —*see* condition
Speech
  defect, disorder, disturbance, impediment
    R47.9
    psychogenic, in childhood and adolescence
      F98.8
    slurring R47.81
    specified NEC R47.89
Spencer's disease A08.19
Spens' syndrome (syncope with heart block)
  I45.9
Sperm counts (fertility testing) Z31.41
  postvasectomy Z30.8
  reversal Z31.42
Spermatic cord —*see* condition
Spermatocele N43.40
  congenital Q55.4
  multiple N43.42
  single N43.41
Spermatocystitis N49.0
Spermatocytoma C62.9-
  specified site —*see* Neoplasm, malignant, by
    site
Spermatorrhea N50.89 ◀▥
Sphacelus —*see* Gangrene
Sphenoidal —*see* condition
Sphenoiditis (chronic) —*see* Sinusitis,
  sphenoidal
Sphenopalatine ganglion neuralgia G90.09
Sphericity, increased, lens (congenital)
  Q12.4
Spherocytosis (congenital) (familial)
  (hereditary) D58.0
  hemoglobin disease D58.0
  sickle-cell (disease) D57.8-
Spherophakia Q12.4
Sphincter —*see* condition
Sphincteritis, sphincter of Oddi —*see*
  Cholangitis
Sphingolipidosis E75.3
  specified NEC E75.29

Sphingomyelinosis E75.3
Spicule tooth K00.2
Spider
  bite —see Toxicity, venom, spider
  fingers —see Syndrome, Marfan's
  nevus I78.1
  toes —see Syndrome, Marfan's
  vascular I78.1
Spiegler-Fendt
  benign lymphocytoma L98.8
  sarcoid L08.89
Spielmeyer-Vogt disease E75.4
Spina bifida (aperta) Q05.9
  with hydrocephalus NEC Q05.4
  cervical Q05.5
    with hydrocephalus Q05.0
  dorsal Q05.6
    with hydrocephalus Q05.1
  lumbar Q05.7
    with hydrocephalus Q05.2
  lumbosacral Q05.7
    with hydrocephalus Q05.2
  occulta Q76.0
  sacral Q05.8
    with hydrocephalus Q05.3
  thoracic Q05.6
    with hydrocephalus Q05.1
  thoracolumbar Q05.6
    with hydrocephalus Q05.1
Spindle, Krukenberg's —see Pigmentation,
    cornea, posterior
Spine, spinal —see condition
Spiradenoma (eccrine) —see Neoplasm, skin,
    benign
Spirillosis A25.0
Spirillum
  minus A25.0
  obermeieri infection A68.0
Spirochetal —see condition
Spirochetosis A69.9
  arthritic, arthritica A69.9
  bronchopulmonary A69.8
  icterohemorrhagic A27.0
  lung A69.8
Spirometrosis B70.1
Spitting blood —see Hemoptysis
Splanchnoptosis K63.4
Spleen, splenic —see condition
Splenectasis —see Splenomegaly
Splenitis (interstitial) (malignant) (nonspecific)
    D73.89
  malarial —see also Malaria B54 [D77]
  tuberculous A18.85
Splenocele D73.89
Splenomegaly, splenomegalia (Bengal)
    (cryptogenic) (idiopathic) (tropical) R16.1
  with hepatomegaly R16.2
  cirrhotic D73.2
  congenital Q89.09
  congestive, chronic D73.2
  Egyptian B65.1
  Gaucher's E75.22
  malarial —see also Malaria B54 [D77]
  neutropenic D73.81
  Niemann-Pick —see Niemann-Pick disease or
    syndrome
  siderotic D73.2
  syphilitic A52.79
    congenital (early) A50.08 [D77]
Splenopathy D73.9
Splenoptosis D73.89
Splenosis D73.89
Splinter —see Foreign body, superficial, by site
Split, splitting
  foot Q72.7-
  hand Q71.6 ◄
  heart sounds R01.2
  lip, congenital —see Cleft, lip
  nails L60.3
  urinary stream R39.13
Spondylarthrosis —see Spondylosis

Spondylitis (chronic) —see also Spondylopathy,
    inflammatory
  ankylopoietica —see Spondylitis, ankylosing
  ankylosing (chronic) M45.9
    with lung involvement M45.9 [J99]
    cervical region M45.2
    cervicothoracic region M45.3
    juvenile M08.1
    lumbar region M45.6
    lumbosacral region M45.7
    multiple sites M45.0
    occipito-atlanto-axial region M45.1
    sacrococcygeal region M45.8
    thoracic region M45.4
    thoracolumbar region M45.5
  atrophic (ligamentous) —see Spondylitis,
    ankylosing
  deformans (chronic) —see Spondylosis
  gonococcal A54.41
  gouty —see also Gout, by type, vertebrae
    M10.08 ◄▥
  in (due to)
    brucellosis A23.9 [M49.80]
      cervical region A23.9 [M49.82]
      cervicothoracic region A23.9 [M49.83]
      lumbar region A23.9 [M49.86]
      lumbosacral region A23.9 [M49.87]
      multiple sites A23.9 [M49.89]
      occipito-atlanto-axial region A23.9
        [M49.81]
      sacrococcygeal region A23.9 [M49.88]
      thoracic region A23.9 [M49.84]
      thoracolumbar region A23.9 [M49.85]
    enterobacteria —see also subcategory M49.8
      A04.9
    tuberculosis A18.01
  infectious NEC —see Spondylopathy,
    infective
  juvenile ankylosing (chronic) M08.1
  Kümmell's —see Spondylopathy, traumatic
  Marie-Strümpell —see Spondylitis,
    ankylosing
  muscularis —see Spondylopathy, specified
    NEC
  psoriatic L40.53
  rheumatoid —see Spondylitis, ankylosing
  rhizomelica —see Spondylitis, ankylosing
  sacroiliac NEC M46.1
  senescent, senile —see Spondylosis
  traumatic (chronic) or post-traumatic —see
    Spondylopathy, traumatic
  tuberculous A18.01
  typhosa A01.05
Spondylolisthesis (acquired) (degenerative)
    M43.10
  with disproportion (fetopelvic) O33.0
    causing obstructed labor O65.0
  cervical region M43.12
  cervicothoracic region M43.13
  congenital Q76.2
  lumbar region M43.16
  lumbosacral region M43.17
  multiple sites M43.19
  occipito-atlanto-axial region M43.11
  sacrococcygeal region M43.18
  thoracic region M43.14
  thoracolumbar region M43.15
  traumatic (old) M43.10
    acute
      fifth cervical (displaced) S12.430
        nondisplaced S12.431
        specified type NEC (displaced)
          S12.450
          nondisplaced S12.451
        type III S12.44
      fourth cervical (displaced) S12.330
        nondisplaced S12.331
        specified type NEC (displaced)
          S12.350
          nondisplaced S12.351
        type III S12.34

Spondylolisthesis (Continued)
  traumatic (Continued)
    acute (Continued)
      second cervical (displaced) S12.130
        nondisplaced S12.131
        specified type NEC (displaced)
          S12.150
          nondisplaced S12.151
        type III S12.14
      seventh cervical (displaced) S12.630
        nondisplaced S12.631
        specified type NEC (displaced)
          S12.650
          nondisplaced S12.651
        type III S12.64
      sixth cervical (displaced) S12.530
        nondisplaced S12.531
        specified type NEC (displaced)
          S12.550
          nondisplaced S12.551
        type III S12.54
      third cervical (displaced) S12.230
        nondisplaced S12.231
        specified type NEC (displaced)
          S12.250
          nondisplaced S12.251
        type III S12.24
Spondylolysis (acquired) M43.00
  cervical region M43.02
  cervicothoracic region M43.03
  congenital Q76.2
  lumbar region M43.06
  lumbosacral region M43.07
    with disproportion (fetopelvic) O33.0
      causing obstructed labor O65.8
  multiple sites M43.09
  occipito-atlanto-axial region M43.01
  sacrococcygeal region M43.08
  thoracic region M43.04
  thoracolumbar region M43.05
Spondylopathy M48.9
  infective NEC M46.50
    cervical region M46.52
    cervicothoracic region M46.53
    lumbar region M46.56
    lumbosacral region M46.57
    multiple sites M46.59
    occipito-atlanto-axial region M46.51
    sacrococcygeal region M46.58
    thoracic region M46.54
    thoracolumbar region M46.55
  inflammatory M46.90
    cervical region M46.92
    cervicothoracic region M46.93
    lumbar region M46.96
    lumbosacral region M46.97
    multiple sites M46.99
    occipito-atlanto-axial region M46.91
    sacrococcygeal region M46.98
    specified type NEC M46.80
      cervical region M46.82
      cervicothoracic region M46.83
      lumbar region M46.86
      lumbosacral region M46.87
      multiple sites M46.89
      occipito-atlanto-axial region M46.81
      sacrococcygeal region M46.88
      thoracic region M46.84
      thoracolumbar region M46.85
    thoracic region M46.94
    thoracolumbar region M46.95
  neuropathic, in
    syringomyelia and syringobulbia G95.0
    tabes dorsalis A52.11
  specified NEC —see subcategory M48.8
  traumatic M48.30
    cervical region M48.32
    cervicothoracic region M48.33
    lumbar region M48.36
    lumbosacral region M48.37
    occipito-atlanto-axial region M48.31

◄ New   ◄▥ Revised   ~~deleted~~ Deleted

Spondylopathy (*Continued*)
   traumatic (*Continued*)
      sacrococcygeal region M48.38
      thoracic region M48.34
      thoracolumbar region M48.35
Spondylosis M47.9
   with
      disproportion (fetopelvic) O33.0
         causing obstructed labor O65.0
      myelopathy NEC M47.10
         cervical region M47.12
         cervicothoracic region M47.13
         lumbar region M47.16
         occipito-atlanto-axial region
            M47.11
         thoracic region M47.14
         thoracolumbar region M47.15
      radiculopathy M47.20
         cervical region M47.22
         cervicothoracic region M47.23
         lumbar region M47.26
         lumbosacral region M47.27
         occipito-atlanto-axial region
            M47.21
         sacrococcygeal region M47.28
         thoracic region M47.24
         thoracolumbar region M47.25
   without myelopathy or radiculopathy
      M47.819
      cervical region M47.812
      cervicothoracic region M47.813
      lumbar region M47.816
      lumbosacral region M47.817
      occipito-atlanto-axial region M47.811
      sacrococcygeal region M47.818
      thoracic region M47.814
      thoracolumbar region M47.815
   specified NEC M47.899
      cervical region M47.892
      cervicothoracic region M47.893
      lumbar region M47.896
      lumbosacral region M47.897
      occipito-atlanto-axial region M47.891
      sacrococcygeal region M47.898
      thoracic region M47.894
      thoracolumbar region M47.895
   traumatic —*see* Spondylopathy, traumatic
Sponge
   inadvertently left in operation wound —*see*
      Foreign body, accidentally left during a
      procedure
   kidney (medullary) Q61.5
Sponge-diver's disease —*see* Toxicity, venom,
   marine animal, sea anemone
Spongioblastoma (any type) —*see* Neoplasm,
   malignant, by site
   specified site —*see* Neoplasm, malignant, by
      site
   unspecified site C71.9
Spongioneuroblastoma —*see* Neoplasm,
   malignant, by site
Spontaneous —*see also* condition
   fracture (cause unknown) —*see* Fracture,
      pathological
Spoon nail L60.3
   congenital Q84.6
Sporadic —*see* condition
Sporothrix schenckii infection —*see*
   Sporotrichosis
Sporotrichosis B42.9
   arthritis B42.82
   disseminated B42.7
   generalized B42.7
   lymphocutaneous (fixed) (progressive)
      B42.1
   pulmonary B42.0
   specified NEC B42.89
Spots, spotting (in) (of)
   Bitot's —*see also* Pigmentation, conjunctiva
      in the young child E50.1
      vitamin A deficiency E50.1

Spots, spotting (*Continued*)
   café, au lait L81.3
   Cayenne pepper I78.1
   cotton wool, retina —*see* Occlusion, artery,
      retina
   de Morgan's (senile angiomas) I78.1
   Fuchs' black (myopic) H44.2-
   intermenstrual (regular) N92.0
      irregular N92.1
   Koplik's B05.9
   liver L81.4
   pregnancy O26.85-
   purpuric R23.3
   ruby I78.1
Spotted fever —*see* Fever, spotted N92.3
Sprain (joint) (ligament)
   acromioclavicular joint or ligament S43.5-
   ankle S93.40-
      calcaneofibular ligament S93.41-
      deltoid ligament S93.42-
      internal collateral ligament —*see* Sprain,
         ankle, specified ligament NEC
      specified ligament NEC S93.49-
      talofibular ligament —*see* Sprain, ankle,
         specified ligament NEC
      tibiofibular ligament S93.43-
   anterior longitudinal, cervical S13.4
   atlas, atlanto-axial, atlanto-occipital S13.4
   breast bone —*see* Sprain, sternum
   calcaneofibular —*see* Sprain, ankle
   carpal —*see* Sprain, wrist
   carpometacarpal —*see* Sprain, hand, specified
      site NEC
   cartilage
      costal S23.41
      semilunar (knee) —*see* Sprain, knee,
         specified site NEC
         with current tear —*see* Tear, meniscus
      thyroid region S13.5
      xiphoid —*see* Sprain, sternum
   cervical, cervicodorsal, cervicothoracic
      S13.4
   chondrosternal S23.421
   coracoclavicular S43.8-
   coracohumeral S43.41-
   coronary, knee —*see* Sprain, knee, specified
      site NEC
   costal cartilage S23.41
   cricoarytenoid articulation or ligament S13.5
   cricothyroid articulation S13.5
   cruciate, knee —*see* Sprain, knee, cruciate
   deltoid, ankle —*see* Sprain, ankle
   dorsal (spine) S23.3
   elbow S53.40-
      radial collateral ligament S53.43-
      radiohumeral S53.41-
      rupture
         radial collateral ligament —*see* Rupture,
            traumatic, ligament, radial
            collateral
         ulnar collateral ligament —*see* Rupture,
            traumatic, ligament, ulnar
            collateral
      specified type NEC S53.49-
      ulnar collateral ligament S53.44-
      ulnohumeral S53.42-
   femur, head —*see* Sprain, hip
   fibular collateral, knee —*see* Sprain, knee,
      collateral
   fibulocalcaneal —*see* Sprain, ankle
   finger (s) S63.61-
      index S63.61-
      interphalangeal (joint) S63.63-
         index S63.63-
         little S63.63-
         middle S63.63-
         ring S63.63-
      little S63.61-
      metacarpophalangeal (joint) S63.65-
      middle S63.61-
      ring S63.61-

Sprain (*Continued*)
   finger (s) (*Continued*)
      specified site NEC S63.69-
         index S63.69-
         little S63.69-
         middle S63.69-
         ring S63.69-
   foot S93.60-
      specified ligament NEC S93.69-
      tarsal ligament S93.61-
      tarsometatarsal ligament S93.62-
      toe —*see* Sprain, toe
   hand S63.9-
      finger —*see* Sprain, finger
      specified site NEC —*see* subcategory S63.8
      thumb —*see* Sprain, thumb
   head S03.9
   hip S73.10-
      iliofemoral ligament S73.11-
      ischiocapsular (ligament) S73.12-
      specified NEC S73.19-
   iliofemoral —*see* Sprain, hip
   innominate
      acetabulum —*see* Sprain, hip
      sacral junction S33.6
   internal
      collateral, ankle —*see* Sprain, ankle
      semilunar cartilage —*see* Sprain, knee,
         specified site NEC
   interphalangeal
      finger —*see* Sprain, finger, interphalangeal
         (joint)
      toe —*see* Sprain, toe, interphalangeal joint
   ischiocapsular —*see* Sprain, hip
   ischiofemoral —*see* Sprain, hip
   jaw (articular disc) (cartilage) (meniscus)
      S03.4- ◀▥▥
      old M26.69
   knee S83.9-
      collateral ligament S83.40-
         lateral (fibular) S83.42-
         medial (tibial) S83.41-
      cruciate ligament S83.50-
         anterior S83.51-
         posterior S83.52-
      lateral (fibular) collateral ligament S83.42-
      medial (tibial) collateral ligament S83.41-
      patellar ligament S76.11-
      specified site NEC S83.8X-
      superior tibiofibular joint (ligament) S83.6-
   lateral collateral, knee —*see* Sprain, knee,
      collateral
   lumbar (spine) S33.5
   lumbosacral S33.9
   mandible (articular disc) S03.4- ◀▥▥
      old M26.69
   medial collateral, knee —*see* Sprain, knee,
      collateral
   meniscus
      jaw S03.4- ◀▥▥
         old M26.69
      knee —*see* Sprain, knee, specified site NEC
         with current tear —*see* Tear, meniscus
         old —*see* Derangement, knee,
            meniscus, due to old tear
      mandible S03.4- ◀▥▥
         old M26.69
   metacarpal (distal) (proximal) —*see* Sprain,
      hand, specified site NEC
   metacarpophalangeal —*see* Sprain, finger,
      metacarpophalangeal (joint)
   metatarsophalangeal —*see* Sprain, toe,
      metatarsophalangeal joint
   midcarpal —*see* Sprain, hand, specified site
      NEC
   midtarsal —*see* Sprain, foot, specified site
      NEC
   neck S13.9
      anterior longitudinal cervical ligament
         S13.4
      atlanto-axial joint S13.4

Sprain (Continued)
  neck (Continued)
    atlanto-occipital joint S13.4
    cervical spine S13.4
    cricoarytenoid ligament S13.5
    cricothyroid ligament S13.5
    specified site NEC S13.8
    thyroid region (cartilage) S13.5
  nose S03.8
  orbicular, hip —see Sprain, hip
  patella —see Sprain, knee, specified site NEC
  patellar ligament S76.11-
  pelvis NEC S33.8
  phalanx
    finger —see Sprain, finger
    toe —see Sprain, toe
  pubofemoral —see Sprain, hip
  radiocarpal —see Sprain, wrist
  radiohumeral —see Sprain, elbow
  radius, collateral —see Rupture, traumatic,
      ligament, radial collateral
  rib (cage) S23.41
  rotator cuff (capsule) S43.42-
  sacroiliac (region)
    chronic or old —see subcategory M53.2
    joint S33.6
  scaphoid (hand) —see Sprain, hand, specified
      site NEC
  scapula (r) —see Sprain, shoulder girdle,
      specified site NEC
  semilunar cartilage (knee) —see Sprain, knee,
      specified site NEC
    with current tear —see Tear, meniscus
      old —see Derangement, knee, meniscus,
          due to old tear
  shoulder joint S43.40-
    acromioclavicular joint (ligament) —see
        Sprain, acromioclavicular joint
    blade —see Sprain, shoulder, girdle,
        specified site NEC
    coracoclavicular joint (ligament) —see
        Sprain, coracoclavicular joint
    coracohumeral ligament —see Sprain,
        coracohumeral joint
    girdle S43.9-
      specified site NEC S43.8-
    rotator cuff —see Sprain, rotator cuff
    specified site NEC S43.49-
    sternoclavicular joint (ligament) —see
        Sprain, sternoclavicular joint
  spine
    cervical S13.4
    lumbar S33.5
    thoracic S23.3
  sternoclavicular joint S43.6-
  sternum S23.429
    chondrosternal joint S23.421
    specified site NEC S23.428
    sternoclavicular (joint) (ligament)
        S23.420
  symphysis
    jaw S03.4- ◀▥
      old M26.69
    mandibular S03.4- ◀▥
      old M26.69
  talofibular —see Sprain, ankle
  tarsal —see Sprain, foot, specified site NEC
  tarsometatarsal —see Sprain, foot, specified
      site NEC
  temporomandibular S03.4- ◀▥
    old M26.69
  thorax S23.9
    ribs S23.41
    specified site NEC S23.8
    spine S23.3
    sternum —see Sprain, sternum
  thumb S63.60-
    interphalangeal (joint) S63.62-
    metacarpophalangeal (joint) S63.64-
    specified site NEC S63.68-
  thyroid cartilage or region S13.5

Sprain (Continued)
  tibia (proximal end) —see Sprain, knee,
      specified site NEC
  tibial collateral, knee —see Sprain, knee,
      collateral
  tibiofibular
    distal —see Sprain, ankle
    superior —see Sprain, knee, specified site
        NEC
  toe (s) S93.50-
    great S93.50-
    interphalangeal joint S93.51-
      great S93.51-
      lesser S93.51-
    lesser S93.50-
    metatarsophalangeal joint S93.52-
      great S93.52-
      lesser S93.52-
  ulna, collateral —see Rupture, traumatic,
      ligament, ulnar collateral
  ulnohumeral —see Sprain, elbow
  wrist S63.50-
    carpal S63.51-
    radiocarpal S63.52-
    specified site NEC S63.59-
  xiphoid cartilage —see Sprain, sternum
Sprengel's deformity (congenital) Q74.0
Sprue (tropical) K90.1
  celiac K90.0
  idiopathic K90.49 ◀▥
  meaning thrush B37.0
  nontropical K90.0
Spur, bone —see also Enthesopathy
  calcaneal M77.3-
  iliac crest M76.2-
  nose (septum) J34.89
Spurway's syndrome Q78.0
Sputum
  abnormal (amount) (color) (odor) (purulent)
      R09.3
  blood-stained R04.2
  excessive (cause unknown) R09.3
Squamous —see also condition
  epithelium in
    cervical canal (congenital) Q51.828
    uterine mucosa (congenital) Q51.818
Squashed nose M95.0
  congenital Q67.4
Squeeze, diver's T70.3
Squint —see also Strabismus
  accommodative —see Strabismus, convergent
      concomitant
St. Hubert's disease A82.9
Stab —see also Laceration
  internal organs —see Injury, by site
Stafne's cyst or cavity M27.0
Staggering gait R26.0
  hysterical F44.4
Staghorn calculus —see Calculus, kidney
Ståhli's line (cornea) (pigment) —see
    Pigmentation, cornea, anterior
Stain, staining
  meconium (newborn) P96.83
  port wine Q82.5
  tooth, teeth (hard tissues) (extrinsic) K03.6
    due to
      accretions K03.6
      deposits (betel) (black) (green) (materia
          alba) (orange) (soft) (tobacco) K03.6
      metals (copper) (silver) K03.7
      nicotine K03.6
      pulpal bleeding K03.7
      tobacco K03.6
    intrinsic K00.8
Stammering —see also Disorder, fluency F80.81
Standstill
  auricular I45.5
  cardiac —see Arrest, cardiac
  sinoatrial I45.5
  ventricular —see Arrest, cardiac
Stannosis J63.5

Stanton's disease —see Melioidosis
Staphylitis (acute) (catarrhal) (chronic)
    (gangrenous) (membranous) (suppurative)
    (ulcerative) K12.2
Staphylococcal scalded skin syndrome L00
Staphylococcemia A41.2
Staphylococcus, staphylococcal —see also
    condition
  as cause of disease classified elsewhere
      B95.8
    aureus (methicillin susceptible) (MSSA)
        B95.61
      methicillin resistant (MRSA) B95.62
  specified NEC, as cause of disease classified
      elsewhere B95.7
Staphyloma (sclera)
  cornea H18.72-
  equatorial H15.81-
  localized (anterior) H15.82-
  posticum H15.83-
  ring H15.85-
Stargardt's disease —see Dystrophy, retina
Starvation (inanition) (due to lack of food)
    T73.0
  edema —see Malnutrition, severe
Stasis
  bile (noncalculous) K83.1
  bronchus J98.09
    with infection —see Bronchitis
  cardiac —see Failure, heart, congestive
  cecum K59.8
  colon K59.8
  dermatitis I87.2 ◀▥
    with ◀
      varicose ulcer —see Varix, leg, with ulcer,
          with inflammation ◀
      varicose veins —see Varix, leg, with,
          inflammation ◀
    due to postthrombotic syndrome —see
        Syndrome, postthrombotic ◀
  duodenal K31.5
  eczema —see Varix, leg, with, inflammation
  edema —see Hypertension, venous (chronic),
      idiopathic
  foot T69.0-
  ileocecal coil K59.8
  ileum K59.8
  intestinal K59.8
  jejunum K59.8
  kidney N19
  liver (cirrhotic) K76.1
  lymphatic I89.8
  pneumonia J18.2
  pulmonary —see Edema, lung
  rectal K59.8
  renal N19
    tubular N17.0
  ulcer —see Varix, leg, with, ulcer
    without varicose veins I87.2
  urine —see Retention, urine
  venous I87.8
State (of)
  affective and paranoid, mixed, organic
      psychotic F06.8
  agitated R45.1
    acute reaction to stress F43.0
  anxiety (neurotic) F41.1
  apprehension F41.1
  burn-out Z73.0
  climacteric, female Z78.0
    symptomatic N95.1
  compulsive F42.8 ◀▥
    mixed with obsessional thoughts F42.2 ◀▥
  confusional (psychogenic) F44.89
    acute —see also Delirium
      with
        arteriosclerotic dementia F01.50
          with behavioral disturbance
              F01.51
        senility or dementia F05
  alcoholic F10.231

◀ New   ◀▥ Revised   ~~deleted~~ Deleted

State *(Continued)*
  confusional (psychogenic) *(Continued)*
    epileptic F05
    reactive (from emotional stress, psychological trauma) F44.89
    subacute —*see* Delirium
  convulsive —*see* Convulsions
  crisis F43.0
  depressive F32.9
    neurotic F34.1
  dissociative F44.9
  emotional shock (stress) R45.7
  hypercoagulation —*see* Hypercoagulable
  locked-in G83.5
  menopausal Z78.0
    symptomatic N95.1
  neurotic F48.9
    with depersonalization F48.1
  obsessional F42.8 ◀▥
  oneiroid (schizophrenia-like) F23
  organic
    hallucinatory (nonalcoholic) F06.0
    paranoid (-hallucinatory) F06.2
  panic F41.0
  paranoid F22
    climacteric F22
    involutional F22
    menopausal F22
    organic F06.2
    senile F03
    simple F22
  persistent vegetative R40.3
  phobic F40.9
  postleukotomy F07.0
  ~~pregnant, incidental Z33.1~~
  pregnant ◀
    gestational carrier Z33.3 ◀
    incidental Z33.1 ◀
  psychogenic, twilight F44.89
  psychopathic (constitutional) F60.2
  psychotic, organic —*see also* Psychosis, organic
    mixed paranoid and affective F06.8
    senile or presenile F03
    transient NEC F06.8
      with
        depression F06.31
        hallucinations F06.0
  residual schizophrenic F20.5
  restlessness R45.1
  stress (emotional) R45.7
  tension (mental) F48.9
    specified NEC F48.8
  transient organic psychotic NEC F06.8
    depressive type F06.31
    hallucinatory type F06.0 ◀▥
  twilight
    epileptic F05
    psychogenic F44.89
  vegetative, persistent R40.3
  vital exhaustion Z73.0
  withdrawal —*see* Withdrawal, state
Status (post) —*see also* Presence (of)
  absence, epileptic —*see* Epilepsy, by type, with status epilepticus
  administration of tPA (rtPA) in a different facility within the last 24 hours prior to admission to the current facility Z92.82
  adrenalectomy (unilateral) (bilateral) E89.6
  anastomosis Z98.0
  anginosus I20.9
  angioplasty (peripheral) Z98.62
    with implant Z95.820
    coronary artery Z98.61
      with implant Z95.5
  aortocoronary bypass Z95.1
  arthrodesis Z98.1
  artificial opening (of) Z93.9
    gastrointestinal tract Z93.4
    specified NEC Z93.8

Status *(Continued)*
  artificial opening (of) *(Continued)*
    urinary tract Z93.6
    vagina Z93.8
  asthmaticus —*see* Asthma, by type, with status asthmaticus
  awaiting organ transplant Z76.82
  bariatric surgery Z98.84
  bed confinement Z74.01
  bleb, filtering (vitreous), after glaucoma surgery Z98.83
  breast implant Z98.82
    removal Z98.86
  cataract extraction Z98.4-
  cholecystectomy Z90.49
  clitorectomy N90.811
    with excision of labia minora N90.812
  colectomy (complete) (partial) Z90.49
  colonization —*see* Carrier (suspected) of
  colostomy Z93.3
  convulsivus idiopathicus —*see* Epilepsy, by type, with status epilepticus
  coronary artery angioplasty —*see* Status, angioplasty, coronary artery
  cystectomy (urinary bladder) Z90.6
  cystostomy Z93.50
    appendico-vesicostomy Z93.52
    cutaneous Z93.51
    specified NEC Z93.59
  delinquent immunization Z28.3
  dental Z98.818
    crown Z98.811
    fillings Z98.811
    restoration Z98.811
    sealant Z98.810
    specified NEC Z98.818
  deployment (current) (military) Z56.82
  dialysis (hemodialysis) (peritoneal) Z99.2
  do not resuscitate (DNR) Z66
  donor —*see* Donor
  embedded fragments —*see* Retained, foreign body fragments (type of)
  embedded splinter —*see* Retained, foreign body fragments (type of)
  enterostomy Z93.4
  epileptic, epilepticus —*see also* Epilepsy, by type, with status epilepticus G40.901
  estrogen receptor
    negative Z17.1
    positive Z17.0
  female genital cutting —*see* Female genital mutilation status
  female genital mutilation —*see* Female genital mutilation status
  filtering (vitreous) bleb after glaucoma surgery Z98.83
  gastrectomy (complete) (partial) Z90.3
  gastric banding Z98.84
  gastric bypass for obesity Z98.84
  gastrostomy Z93.1
  human immunodeficiency virus (HIV) infection, asymptomatic Z21
  hysterectomy (complete) (total) Z90.710
    partial (with remaining cervial stump) Z90.711
  ileostomy Z93.2
  implant
    breast Z98.82
  infibulation N90.813
  intestinal bypass Z98.0
  jejunostomy Z93.4
  lapsed immunization schedule Z28.3
  laryngectomy Z90.02
  lymphaticus E32.8
  malignancy ◀
    castrate resistant prostate Z19.2 ◀
    hormone resistant Z19.2 ◀
    hormone sensitive Z19.1 ◀
  marmoratus G80.3
  mastectomy (unilateral) (bilateral) Z90.1-

Status *(Continued)*
  military deployment status (current) Z56.82
    in theater or in support of military war, peacekeeping and humanitarian operations Z56.82
  nephrectomy (unilateral) (bilateral) Z90.5
  nephrostomy Z93.6
  obesity surgery Z98.84
  oophorectomy
    bilateral Z90.722
    unilateral Z90.721
  organ replacement
    by artificial or mechanical device or prosthesis of
      artery Z95.828
      bladder Z96.0
      blood vessel Z95.828
      breast Z97.8
      eye globe Z97.0
      heart Z95.812
        valve Z95.2
      intestine Z97.8
      joint Z96.60
        hip —*see* Presence, hip joint implant
        knee —*see* Presence, knee joint implant
        specified site NEC Z96.698
      kidney Z97.8
      larynx Z96.3
      lens Z96.1
      limbs —*see* Presence, artificial, limb
      liver Z97.8
      lung Z97.8
      pancreas Z97.8
    by organ transplant (heterologous) (homologous) —*see* Transplant
  pacemaker
    brain Z96.89
    cardiac Z95.0
    specified NEC Z96.89
  pancreatectomy Z90.410
    complete Z90.410
    partial Z90.411
    total Z90.410
  pneumonectomy (complete) (partial) Z90.2
  pneumothorax, therapeutic Z98.3
  postcommotio cerebri F07.81
  postoperative (postprocedural) NEC Z98.890 ◀▥
    breast implant Z98.82
    dental Z98.818
      crown Z98.811
      fillings Z98.811
      restoration Z98.811
      sealant Z98.810
      specified NEC Z98.818
    pneumothorax, therapeutic Z98.3
    uterine scar Z98.891 ◀
  postpartum (routine follow-up) Z39.2
    care immediately after delivery Z39.0
  postsurgical (postprocedural) NEC Z98.890 ◀▥
    pneumothorax, therapeutic Z98.3
  pregnancy, incidental Z33.1
  prosthesis coronary angioplasty Z95.5
  pseudophakia Z96.1
  renal dialysis (hemodialysis) (peritoneal) Z99.2
  retained foreign body —*see* Retained, foreign body fragments (type of)
  reversed jejunal transposition (for bypass Z98.0
  salpingo-oophorectomy
    bilateral Z90.722
    unilateral Z90.721
  sex reassignment surgery status Z87.890
  shunt
    arteriovenous (for dialysis) Z99.2
    cerebrospinal fluid Z98.2
    ventricular (communicating) (for drainage) Z98.2

Status (Continued)
  splenectomy Z90.81
  thymicolymphaticus E32.8
  thymicus E32.8
  thymolymphaticus E32.8
  thyroidectomy (hypothyroidism) E89.0
  tooth (teeth) extraction —see also Absence,
      teeth, acquired K08.409
  tPA (rtPA) administration in a different
      facility within the last 24 hours prior to
      admission to current facility Z92.82
  tracheostomy Z93.0
  transplant —see Transplant
    organ removed Z98.85
  tubal ligation Z98.51
  underimmunization Z28.3
  ureterostomy Z93.6
  urethrostomy Z93.6
  vagina, artificial Z93.8
  vasectomy Z98.52
  wheelchair confinement Z99.3
Stealing
  child problem F91.8
    in company with others Z72.810
  pathological (compulsive) F63.2
Steam burn —see Burn
Steatocystoma multiplex L72.2
Steatohepatitis (nonalcoholic) (NASH)
    K75.81
Steatoma L72.3
  eyelid (cystic) —see Dermatosis, eyelid
    infected —see Hordeolum
Steatorrhea (chronic) K90.9
  with lacteal obstruction K90.2
  idiopathic (adult) (infantile) K90.9
  pancreatic K90.3
  primary K90.0
  tropical K90.1
Steatosis E88.89
  heart —see Degeneration, myocardial
  kidney N28.89
  liver NEC K76.0
Steele-Richardson-Olszewski disease or
    syndrome G23.1
Steinbrocker's syndrome G90.8
Steinert's disease G71.11
Stein-Leventhal syndrome E28.2
Stein's syndrome E28.2
STEMI —see also - Infarct, myocardium, ST
    elevation I21.3
Stenocardia I20.8
Stenocephaly Q75.8
Stenosis, stenotic (cicatricial) —see also
    Stricture
  ampulla of Vater K83.1
  anus, anal (canal) (sphincter) K62.4
    and rectum K62.4
    congenital Q42.3
      with fistula Q42.2
  aorta (ascending) (supraventricular)
      (congenital) Q25.1
    arteriosclerotic I70.0
    calcified I70.0
    supravalvular Q25.3
  aortic (valve) I35.0
    with insufficiency I35.2
    congenital Q23.0
    rheumatic I06.0
      with
        incompetency, insufficiency or
            regurgitation I06.2
          with mitral (valve) disease I08.0
            with tricuspid (valve) disease
                I08.3
        mitral (valve) disease I08.0
          with tricuspid (valve) disease
              I08.3
        tricuspid (valve) disease I08.2
          with mitral (valve) disease I08.3
    specified cause NEC I35.0
    syphilitic A52.03

Stenosis, stenotic (Continued)
  aqueduct of Sylvius (congenital) Q03.0
    with spina bifida —see Spina bifida,
        by site, with hydrocephalus
    acquired G91.1
  artery NEC —see also Arteriosclerosis
      I77.1
    celiac I77.4
    cerebral —see Occlusion, artery, cerebral
    extremities —see Arteriosclerosis,
        extremities
    precerebral —see Occlusion, artery,
        precerebral
    pulmonary (congenital) Q25.6
      acquired I28.8
    renal I70.1
    stent
      coronary T82.855
      peripheral T82.856
  bile duct (common) (hepatic) K83.1
    congenital Q44.3
  bladder-neck (acquired) N32.0
    congenital Q64.31
  brain G93.89
  bronchus J98.09
    congenital Q32.3
    syphilitic A52.72
  cardia (stomach) K22.2
    congenital Q39.3
  cardiovascular —see Disease, cardiovascular
  caudal M48.08
  cervix, cervical (canal) N88.2
    congenital Q51.828
    in pregnancy or childbirth —see Pregnancy,
        complicated by, abnormal cervix
  colon —see also Obstruction, intestine
    congenital Q42.9
      specified NEC Q42.8
  colostomy K94.03
  common (bile) duct K83.1
    congenital Q44.3
  coronary (artery) —see Disease, heart,
      ischemic, atherosclerotic
  cystic duct —see Obstruction, gallbladder
  due to presence of device, implant or
      graft —see also Complications, by site
      and type, specified NEC T85.858
    arterial graft NEC T82.858
    breast (implant) T85.858
    catheter T85.858
      dialysis (renal) T82.858
        intraperitoneal T85.858
      infusion NEC T82.858
        spinal (epidural) (subdural)
            T85.850
      urinary (indwelling) T83.85
    fixation, internal (orthopedic) NEC
        T84.85
    gastrointestinal (bile duct) (esophagus)
        T85.858
    genital NEC T83.85
    heart NEC T82.857
    joint prosthesis T84.85
    ocular (corneal graft) (orbital implant)
        NEC T85.858
    orthopedic NEC T84.85
    specified NEC T85.858
    urinary NEC T83.85
    vascular NEC T82.858
    ventricular intracranial shunt T85.850
  duodenum K31.5
    congenital Q41.0
  ejaculatory duct NEC N50.89
  endocervical os —see Stenosis, cervix
  enterostomy K94.13
  esophagus K22.2
    congenital Q39.3
    syphilitic A52.79
      congenital A50.59 [K23]
  eustachian tube —see Obstruction, eustachian
      tube

Stenosis, stenotic (Continued)
  external ear canal (acquired) H61.30-
    congenital Q16.1
    due to
      inflammation H61.32-
      trauma H61.31-
    postprocedural H95.81-
    specified cause NEC H61.39-
  gallbladder —see Obstruction,
      gallbladder
  glottis J38.6
  heart valve (congenital) Q24.8
    aortic Q23.0
    mitral Q23.2
    pulmonary Q22.1
    tricuspid Q22.4
  hepatic duct K83.1
  hymen N89.6
  hypertrophic subaortic (idiopathic) I42.1
  ileum K56.69
    congenital Q41.2
  infundibulum cardia Q24.3
  intervertebral foramina —see also Lesion,
      biomechanical, specified NEC
    connective tissue M99.79
      abdomen M99.79
      cervical region M99.71
      cervicothoracic M99.71
      head region M99.70
      lumbar region M99.73
      lumbosacral M99.73
      occipitocervical M99.70
      sacral region M99.74
      sacrococcygeal M99.74
      sacroiliac M99.74
      specified NEC M99.79
      thoracic region M99.72
      thoracolumbar M99.72
    disc M99.79
      abdomen M99.79
      cervical region M99.71
      cervicothoracic M99.71
      head region M99.70
      lower extremity M99.76
      lumbar region M99.73
      lumbosacral M99.73
      occipitocervical M99.70
      pelvic M99.75
      rib cage M99.78
      sacral region M99.74
      sacrococcygeal M99.74
      sacroiliac M99.74
      specified NEC M99.79
      thoracic region M99.72
      thoracolumbar M99.72
      upper extremity M99.77
    osseous M99.69
      abdomen M99.69
      cervical region M99.61
      cervicothoracic M99.61
      head region M99.60
      lower extremity M99.66
      lumbar region M99.63
      lumbosacral M99.63
      occipitocervical M99.60
      pelvic M99.65
      rib cage M99.68
      sacral region M99.64
      sacrococcygeal M99.64
      sacroiliac M99.64
      specified NEC M99.69
      thoracic region M99.62
      thoracolumbar M99.62
      upper extremity M99.67
    subluxation —see Stenosis, intervertebral
        foramina, osseous
  intestine —see also Obstruction, intestine
    congenital (small) Q41.9
      large Q42.9
        specified NEC Q42.8
      specified NEC Q41.8

◀ New   ◀▥ Revised   ~~deleted~~ Deleted

Stenosis, stenotic (Continued)
  jejunum K56.69
    congenital Q41.1
  lacrimal (passage)
    canaliculi H04.54-
    congenital Q10.5
    duct H04.55-
    punctum H04.56-
    sac H04.57-
  lacrimonasal duct —see Stenosis, lacrimal,
      duct
    congenital Q10.5
  larynx J38.6
    congenital NEC Q31.8
      subglottic Q31.1
    syphilitic A52.73
      congenital A50.59 [J99]
  mitral (chronic) (inactive) (valve) I05.0
    with
      aortic valve disease I08.0
      incompetency, insufficiency or
          regurgitation I05.2
    active or acute I01.1
      with rheumatic or Sydenham's chorea
          I02.0
    congenital Q23.2
    specified cause, except rheumatic I34.2
    syphilitic A52.03
  myocardium, myocardial —see also
      Degeneration, myocardial
    hypertrophic subaortic (idiopathic) I42.1
  nares (anterior) (posterior) J34.89
    congenital Q30.0
  nasal duct —see also Stenosis, lacrimal, duct
    congenital Q10.5
  nasolacrimal duct —see also Stenosis, lacrimal,
      duct
    congenital Q10.5
  neural canal —see also Lesion, biomechanical,
      specified NEC
    connective tissue M99.49
      abdomen M99.49
      cervical region M99.41
      cervicothoracic M99.41
      head region M99.40
      lower extremity M99.46
      lumbar region M99.43
      lumbosacral M99.43
      occipitocervical M99.40
      pelvic M99.45
      rib cage M99.48
      sacral region M99.44
      sacrococcygeal M99.44
      sacroiliac M99.44
      specified NEC M99.49
      thoracic region M99.42
      thoracolumbar M99.42
      upper extremity M99.47
    intervertebral disc M99.59
      abdomen M99.59
      cervical region M99.51
      cervicothoracic M99.51
      head region M99.50
      lower extremity M99.56
      lumbar region M99.53
      lumbosacral M99.53
      occipitocervical M99.50
      pelvic M99.55
      rib cage M99.58
      sacral region M99.54
      sacrococcygeal M99.54
      sacroiliac M99.54
      specified NEC M99.59
      thoracic region M99.52
      thoracolumbar M99.52
      upper extremity M99.57
    osseous M99.39
      abdomen M99.39
      cervical region M99.31
      cervicothoracic M99.31
      head region M99.30

Stenosis, stenotic (Continued)
  neural canal (Continued)
    osseous (Continued)
      lower extremity M99.36
      lumbar region M99.33
      lumbosacral M99.33
      occipitocervical M99.30
      pelvic M99.35
      rib cage M99.38
      sacral region M99.34
      sacrococcygeal M99.34
      sacroiliac M99.34
      specified NEC M99.39
      thoracic region M99.32
      thoracolumbar M99.32
      upper extremity M99.37
    subluxation M99.29
      cervical region M99.21
      cervicothoracic M99.21
      head region M99.20
      lower extremity M99.26
      lumbar region M99.23
      lumbosacral M99.23
      occipitocervical M99.20
      pelvic M99.25
      rib cage M99.28
      sacral region M99.24
      sacrococcygeal M99.24
      sacroiliac M99.24
      specified NEC M99.29
      thoracic region M99.22
      thoracolumbar M99.22
      upper extremity M99.27
  organ or site, congenital NEC —see Atresia,
      by site
  papilla of Vater K83.1
  pulmonary (artery) (congenital) Q25.6
    with ventricular septal defect,
        transposition of aorta, and
        hypertrophy of right ventricle
        Q21.3
    acquired I28.8
    in tetralogy of Fallot Q21.3
    infundibular Q24.3
    subvalvular Q24.3
    supravalvular Q25.6
    valve I37.0
      with insufficiency I37.2
      congenital Q22.1
      rheumatic I09.89
        with aortic, mitral or tricuspid (valve)
            disease I08.8
    vein, acquired I28.8
    vessel NEC I28.8
  pulmonic (congenital) Q22.1
    infundibular Q24.3
    subvalvular Q24.3
  pylorus (hypertrophic) (acquired) K31.1
    adult K31.1
    congenital Q40.0
    infantile Q40.0
  rectum (sphincter) —see Stricture, rectum
  renal artery I70.1
    congenital Q27.1
  salivary duct (any) K11.8
  sphincter of Oddi K83.1
  spinal M48.00
    cervical region M48.02
    cervicothoracic region M48.03
    lumbar region M48.06
    lumbosacral region M48.07
    occipito-atlanto-axial region
        M48.01
    sacrococcygeal region M48.08
    thoracic region M48.04
    thoracolumbar region M48.05
  stent ◄
    vascular ◄
      end stent ◄
        adjacent to stent —see
            Arteriosclerosis ◄

Stenosis, stenotic (Continued)
  stent (Continued)
    vascular (Continued)
      end stent (Continued)
        within the stent ◄
          coronary T82.855 ◄
          peripheral T82.856 ◄
        in stent ◄
          coronary vessel T82.855 ◄
          peripheral vessel T82.856 ◄
  stomach, hourglass K31.2
  subaortic (congenital) Q24.4
    hypertrophic (idiopathic) I42.1
  subglottic J38.6
    congenital Q31.1
    postprocedural J95.5
  trachea J39.8
    congenital Q32.1
    syphilitic A52.73
    tuberculous NEC A15.5
  tracheostomy J95.03
  tricuspid (valve) I07.0
    with
      aortic (valve) disease I08.2
      incompetency, insufficiency or
          regurgitation I07.2
        with aortic (valve) disease I08.2
          with mitral (valve) disease
              I08.3
      mitral (valve) disease I08.1
        with aortic (valve) disease I08.3
    congenital Q22.4
    nonrheumatic I36.0
      with insufficiency I36.2
  tubal N97.1
  ureter —see Atresia, ureter
  ureteropelvic junction, congenital
      Q62.11
  ureterovesical orifice, congenital Q62.12
  urethra (valve) —see also Stricture, urethra
    congenital Q64.32
  urinary meatus, congenital Q64.33
  vagina N89.5
    congenital Q52.4
    in pregnancy —see Pregnancy, complicated
        by, abnormal vagina
      causing obstructed labor O65.5
  valve (cardiac) (heart) —see also Endocarditis
      I38
    congenital Q24.8
      aortic Q23.0
      mitral Q23.2
      pulmonary Q22.1
      tricuspid Q22.4
  vena cava (inferior) (superior) I87.1
    congenital Q26.0
  vesicourethral orifice Q64.31
  vulva N90.5
Stent jail T82.897
Stercolith (impaction) K56.41
  appendix K38.1
Stercoraceous, stercoral ulcer K63.3
  anus or rectum K62.6
Stereotypies NEC F98.4
Sterility —see Infertility
Sterilization —see Encounter (for),
    sterilization
Sternalgia —see Angina
Sternopagus Q89.4
Sternum bifidum Q76.7
Steroid
  effects (adverse) (adrenocortical)
      (iatrogenic)
    cushingoid E24.2
      correct substance properly
          administered —see Table of Drugs
          and Chemicals, by drug, adverse
          effect
      overdose or wrong substance given or
          taken —see Table of Drugs and
          Chemicals, by drug, poisoning

Steroid *(Continued)*
  effects *(Continued)*
    diabetes —*see* category E09
      correct substance properly
        administered —*see* Table of Drugs
        and Chemicals, by drug, adverse
        effect
      overdose or wrong substance given or
        taken —*see* Table of Drugs and
        Chemicals, by drug, poisoning
    fever R50.2
    insufficiency E27.3
      correct substance properly
        administered —*see* Table of Drugs
        and Chemicals, by drug, adverse
        effect
      overdose or wrong substance given or
        taken —*see* Table of Drugs and
        Chemicals, by drug, poisoning
  responder H40.04-
Stevens-Johnson disease or syndrome L51.1
  toxic epidermal necrolysis overlap L51.3
Stewart-Morel syndrome M85.2
Sticker's disease B08.3
Sticky eye —*see* Conjunctivitis, acute,
  mucopurulent
Stieda's disease —*see* Bursitis, tibial collateral
Stiff neck —*see* Torticollis
Stiff-man syndrome G25.82
Stiffness, joint NEC M25.60-
  ankle M25.67-
  ankylosis —*see* Ankylosis, joint
  contracture —*see* Contraction, joint
  elbow M25.62-
  foot M25.67-
  hand M25.64-
  hip M25.65-
  knee M25.66-
  shoulder M25.61-
  wrist M25.63-
Stigmata congenital syphilis A50.59
Stillbirth P95
Still-Felty syndrome —*see* Felty's syndrome
Still's disease or syndrome (juvenile) M08.20
  adult-onset M06.1
  ankle M08.27-
  elbow M08.22-
  foot joint M08.27-
  hand joint M08.24-
  hip M08.25-
  knee M08.26-
  multiple site M08.29
  shoulder M08.21-
  vertebra M08.28
  wrist M08.23-
Stimulation, ovary E28.1
Sting (venomous) (with allergic or anaphylactic
  shock) —*see* Table of Drugs and
  Chemicals, by animal or substance,
  poisoning
Stippled epiphyses Q78.8
Stitch
  abscess T81.48 ◄▥
  burst (in operation wound) —*see* Disruption,
    wound, operation
Stokes-Adams disease or syndrome I45.9
Stokes' disease E05.00
  with thyroid storm E05.01
Stokvis (-Talma) disease D74.8
Stoma malfunction
  colostomy K94.03
  enterostomy K94.13
  gastrostomy K94.23
  ileostomy K94.13
  tracheostomy J95.03
Stomach —*see* condition
Stomatitis (denture) (ulcerative) K12.1
  angular K13.0
    due to dietary or vitamin deficiency E53.0
  aphthous K12.0
  bovine B08.61

Stomatitis *(Continued)*
  candidal B37.0
  catarrhal K12.1
  diphtheritic A36.89
  due to
    dietary deficiency E53.0
    thrush B37.0
    vitamin deficiency
      B group NEC E53.9
      B2 (riboflavin) E53.0
  epidemic B08.8
  epizootic B08.8
  follicular K12.1
  gangrenous A69.0
  Geotrichum B48.3
  herpesviral, herpetic B00.2
  herpetiformis K12.0
  malignant K12.1
  membranous acute K12.1
  monilial B37.0
  mycotic B37.0
  necrotizing ulcerative A69.0
  parasitic B37.0
  septic K12.1
  spirochetal A69.1
  suppurative (acute) K12.2
  ulceromembranous A69.1
  vesicular K12.1
    with exanthem (enteroviral)
      B08.4
    virus disease A93.8
  Vincent's A69.1
Stomatocytosis D58.8
Stomatomycosis B37.0
Stomatorrhagia K13.79
Stone (s) —*see also* Calculus
  bladder (diverticulum) N21.0
  cystine E72.09
  heart syndrome I50.1
  kidney N20.0
  prostate N42.0
  pulpal (dental) K04.2
  renal N20.0
  salivary gland or duct (any) K11.5
  urethra (impacted) N21.1
  urinary (duct) (impacted) (passage)
    N20.9
    bladder (diverticulum) N21.0
    lower tract N21.9
    specified NEC N21.8
  xanthine E79.8 *[N22]*
Stonecutter's lung J62.8
Stonemason's asthma, disease, lung or
  pneumoconiosis J62.8
Stoppage
  heart —*see* Arrest, cardiac
  urine —*see* Retention, urine
Storm, thyroid —*see* Thyrotoxicosis
Strabismus (congenital) (nonparalytic)
  H50.9
  concomitant H50.40
    convergent —*see* Strabismus, convergent
      concomitant
    divergent —*see* Strabismus, divergent
      concomitant
  convergent concomitant H50.00
    accommodative component H50.43
    alternating H50.05
      with
        A pattern H50.06
        specified nonconcomitances NEC
          H50.08
        V pattern H50.07
    monocular H50.01-
      with
        A pattern H50.02-
        specified nonconcomitances NEC
          H50.04-
        V pattern H50.03-
    intermittent H50.31-
      alternating H50.32

Strabismus *(Continued)*
  cyclotropia H50.41 ◄▥
  divergent concomitant H50.10
    alternating H50.15
      with
        A pattern H50.16
        specified noncomitances NEC
          H50.18
        V pattern H50.17
    monocular H50.11-
      with
        A pattern H50.12-
        specified noncomitances NEC
          H50.14-
        V pattern H50.13-
    intermittent H50.33-
      alternating H50.34
  Duane's syndrome H50.81-
  due to adhesions, scars H50.69
  heterophoria H50.50
    alternating H50.55
    cyclophoria H50.54
    esophoria H50.51
    exophoria H50.52
    vertical H50.53
  heterotropia H50.40
    intermittent H50.30
  hypertropia H50.2-
  hypotropia —*see* Hypertropia
  latent H50.50
  mechanical H50.60
    Brown's sheath syndrome H50.61-
    specified type NEC H50.69
  monofixation syndrome H50.42
  paralytic H49.9
    abducens nerve H49.2-
    fourth nerve H49.1-
    Kearns-Sayre syndrome H49.81-
    ophthalmoplegia (external)
      progressive H49.4-
        with pigmentary retinopathy H49.81-
      total H49.3-
    sixth nerve H49.2-
    specified type NEC H49.88-
    third nerve H49.0-
    trochlear nerve H49.1-
  specified type NEC H50.89
  vertical H50.2-
Strain
  back S39.012
  cervical S16.1
  eye NEC —*see* Disturbance, vision, subjective
  heart —*see* Disease, heart
  low back S39.012
  mental NOS Z73.3
    work-related Z56.6
  muscle (tendon) —*see* Injury, muscle, by site,
    strain
  neck S16.1
  physical NOS Z73.3
    work-related Z56.6
  postural —*see also* Disorder, soft tissue, due
    to use
  psychological NEC Z73.3
  tendon —*see* Injury, muscle, by site, strain
Straining, on urination R39.16
Strand, vitreous —*see* Opacity, vitreous,
  membranes and strands
Strangulation, strangulated —*see also*
  Asphyxia, traumatic
  appendix K38.8
  bladder-neck N32.0
  bowel or colon K56.2
  food or foreign body —*see* Foreign body, by
    site
  hemorrhoids —*see* Hemorrhoids, with
    complication
  hernia —*see also* Hernia, by site, with
    obstruction
    with gangrene —*see* Hernia, by site, with
      gangrene

◄ New   ◄▥ Revised   ~~deleted~~ Deleted

Strangulation, strangulated (Continued)
　　intestine (large) (small) K56.2
　　　with hernia —see also Hernia, by site, with
　　　　obstruction
　　　　with gangrene —see Hernia, by site, with
　　　　　gangrene
　　mesentery K56.2
　　mucus —see Asphyxia, mucus
　　omentum K56.2
　　organ or site, congenital NEC —see Atresia,
　　　by site
　　ovary —see Torsion, ovary
　　penis N48.89
　　　foreign body T19.4
　　rupture —see Hernia, by site, with obstruction
　　stomach due to hernia —see also Hernia, by
　　　site, with obstruction
　　　with gangrene —see Hernia, by site, with
　　　　gangrene
　　vesicourethral orifice N32.0
Strangury R30.0
Straw itch B88.0
Strawberry
　　gallbladder K82.4
　　mark Q82.5
　　tongue (red) (white) K14.3
Streak (s)
　　macula, angioid H35.33
　　ovarian Q50.32
Strephosymbolia F81.0
　　secondary to organic lesion R48.8
Streptobacillary fever A25.1
Streptobacillosis A25.1
Streptobacillus moniliformis A25.1
Streptococcus, streptococcal —see also
　　　condition
　　as cause of disease classified elsewhere B95.5
　　group
　　　A, as cause of disease classified elsewhere
　　　　B95.0
　　　B, as cause of disease classified elsewhere
　　　　B95.1
　　　D, as cause of disease classified elsewhere
　　　　B95.2
　　pneumoniae, as cause of disease classified
　　　elsewhere B95.3
　　specified NEC, as cause of disease classified
　　　elsewhere B95.4
Streptomycosis B47.1
Streptotrichosis A48.8
Stress F43.9
　　family —see Disruption, family
　　fetal P84
　　　complicating pregnancy O77.9
　　　due to drug administration O77.1
　　mental NEC Z73.3
　　　work-related Z56.6
　　physical NEC Z73.3
　　　work-related Z56.6
　　polycythemia D75.1
　　reaction —see also Reaction, stress F43.9
　　work schedule Z56.3
Stretching, nerve —see Injury, nerve
Striae albicantes, atrophicae or distensae
　　　(cutis) L90.6
Stricture —see also Stenosis
　　ampulla of Vater K83.1
　　anus (sphincter) K62.4
　　　congenital Q42.3
　　　　with fistula Q42.2
　　　infantile Q42.3
　　　　with fistula Q42.2
　　aorta (ascending) (congenital) Q25.1 ◀▥▥
　　　arteriosclerotic I70.0
　　　calcified I70.0
　　　supravalvular, congenital Q25.3
　　aortic (valve) —see Stenosis, aortic
　　aqueduct of Sylvius (congenital) Q03.0
　　　with spina bifida —see Spina bifida, by site,
　　　　with hydrocephalus
　　　acquired G91.1

Stricture (Continued)
　　artery I77.1
　　　basilar —see Occlusion, artery, basilar
　　　carotid —see Occlusion, artery, carotid
　　　celiac I77.4
　　　congenital (peripheral) Q27.8
　　　　cerebral Q28.3
　　　　coronary Q24.5
　　　　digestive system Q27.8
　　　　lower limb Q27.8
　　　　retinal Q14.1
　　　　specified site NEC Q27.8
　　　　umbilical Q27.0
　　　　upper limb Q27.8
　　　coronary —see Disease, heart, ischemic,
　　　　atherosclerotic
　　　　congenital Q24.5
　　　precerebral —see Occlusion, artery,
　　　　precerebral
　　　pulmonary (congenital) Q25.6
　　　　acquired I28.8
　　　renal I70.1
　　　vertebral —see Occlusion, artery, vertebral
　　auditory canal (external) (congenital)
　　　acquired —see Stenosis, external ear canal
　　bile duct (common) (hepatic) K83.1
　　　congenital Q44.3
　　　postoperative K91.89
　　bladder N32.89
　　　neck N32.0
　　bowel —see Obstruction, intestine
　　brain G93.89
　　bronchus J98.09
　　　congenital Q32.3
　　　syphilitic A52.72
　　cardia (stomach) K22.2
　　　congenital Q39.3
　　cardiac —see also Disease, heart
　　　orifice (stomach) K22.2
　　cecum —see Obstruction, intestine
　　cervix, cervical (canal) N88.2
　　　congenital Q51.828
　　　in pregnancy —see Pregnancy, complicated
　　　　by, abnormal cervix
　　　　causing obstructed labor O65.5
　　colon —see also Obstruction, intestine
　　　congenital Q42.9
　　　　specified NEC Q42.8
　　colostomy K94.03
　　common (bile) duct K83.1
　　coronary (artery) —see Disease, heart,
　　　ischemic, atherosclerotic
　　cystic duct —see Obstruction, gallbladder
　　digestive organs NEC, congenital Q45.8
　　duodenum K31.5
　　　congenital Q41.0
　　ear canal (external) (congenital) Q16.1
　　　acquired —see Stricture, auditory canal,
　　　　acquired
　　ejaculatory duct N50.89 ◀▥▥
　　enterostomy K94.13
　　esophagus K22.2
　　　congenital Q39.3
　　　syphilitic A52.79
　　　　congenital A50.59 [K23]
　　eustachian tube —see also Obstruction,
　　　eustachian tube
　　　congenital Q17.8
　　fallopian tube N97.1
　　　gonococcal A54.24
　　　tuberculous A18.17
　　gallbladder —see Obstruction, gallbladder
　　glottis J38.6
　　heart —see also Disease, heart
　　　valve (see also Endocarditis) I38
　　　　aortic Q23.0
　　　　mitral Q23.4
　　　　pulmonary Q22.1
　　　　tricuspid Q22.4
　　hepatic duct K83.1
　　hourglass, of stomach K31.2

Stricture (Continued)
　　hymen N89.6
　　hypopharynx J39.2
　　ileum K56.69
　　　congenital Q41.2
　　intestine —see also Obstruction, intestine
　　　congenital (small) Q41.9
　　　　large Q42.9
　　　　　specified NEC Q42.8
　　　　specified NEC Q41.8
　　　ischemic K55.1
　　jejunum K56.69
　　　congenital Q41.1
　　lacrimal passages —see also Stenosis, lacrimal
　　　congenital Q10.5
　　larynx J38.6
　　　congenital NEC Q31.8
　　　　subglottic Q31.1
　　　syphilitic A52.73
　　　　congenital A50.59 [J99]
　　meatus
　　　ear (congenital) Q16.1
　　　　acquired —see Stricture, auditory canal,
　　　　　acquired
　　　osseous (ear) (congenital) Q16.1
　　　　acquired —see Stricture, auditory canal,
　　　　　acquired
　　　urinarius —see also Stricture, urethra
　　　　congenital Q64.33
　　mitral (valve) —see Stenosis, mitral
　　myocardium, myocardial I51.5
　　　hypertrophic subaortic (idiopathic)
　　　　I42.1
　　nares (anterior) (posterior) J34.89
　　　congenital Q30.0
　　nasal duct —see also Stenosis, lacrimal, duct
　　　congenital Q10.5
　　nasolacrimal duct —see also Stenosis, lacrimal,
　　　duct
　　　congenital Q10.5
　　nasopharynx J39.2
　　　syphilitic A52.73
　　nose J34.89
　　　congenital Q30.0
　　nostril (anterior) (posterior) J34.89
　　　congenital Q30.0
　　　syphilitic A52.73
　　　　congenital A50.59 [J99]
　　organ or site, congenital NEC —see Atresia,
　　　by site
　　os uteri —see Stricture, cervix
　　osseous meatus (ear) (congenital) Q16.1
　　　acquired —see Stricture, auditory canal,
　　　　acquired
　　oviduct —see Stricture, fallopian tube
　　pelviureteric junction (congenital)
　　　Q62.11
　　　acquired, with hydronephrosis N13.0 ◀
　　penis, by foreign body T19.4
　　pharynx J39.2
　　prostate N42.89
　　pulmonary, pulmonic
　　　artery (congenital) Q25.6
　　　　acquired I28.8
　　　　noncongenital I28.8
　　　infundibulum (congenital) Q24.3
　　　valve I37.0
　　　　congenital Q22.1
　　　vein, acquired I28.8
　　　vessel NEC I28.8
　　punctum lacrimale —see also Stenosis,
　　　lacrimal, punctum
　　　congenital Q10.5
　　pylorus (hypertrophic) K31.1
　　　adult K31.1
　　　congenital Q40.0
　　　infantile Q40.0
　　rectosigmoid K56.69
　　rectum (sphincter) K62.4
　　　congenital Q42.1
　　　　with fistula Q42.0

Stricture *(Continued)*
  rectum (sphincter) *(Continued)*
    due to
      chlamydial lymphogranuloma A55
      irradiation K91.89
      lymphogranuloma venereum A55
      gonococcal A54.6
      inflammatory (chlamydial) A55
      syphilitic A52.74
      tuberculous A18.32
  renal artery I70.1
    congenital Q27.1
  salivary duct or gland (any) K11.8
  sigmoid (flexure) —*see* Obstruction, intestine
  spermatic cord N50.89 ◀▥
  stoma (following) (of)
    colostomy K94.03
    enterostomy K94.13
    gastrostomy K94.23
    ileostomy K94.13
    tracheostomy J95.03
  stomach K31.89
    congenital Q40.2
    hourglass K31.2
  subaortic Q24.4
    hypertrophic (acquired) (idiopathic) I42.1
  subglottic J38.6
  syphilitic NEC A52.79
  trachea J39.8
    congenital Q32.1
    syphilitic A52.73
    tuberculous NEC A15.5
  tracheostomy J95.03
  tricuspid (valve) —*see* Stenosis, tricuspid
  tunica vaginalis N50.89 ◀▥
  ureter (postoperative) N13.5
    with
      hydronephrosis N13.1
        with infection N13.6
      pyelonephritis (chronic) N11.1
    congenital —*see* Atresia, ureter
    tuberculous A18.11
  ureteropelvic junction (congenital) Q62.11
    acquired, with hydronephrosis N13.0 ◀
  ureterovesical orifice N13.5
    with infection N13.6
  urethra (organic) (spasmodic) N35.9
    associated with schistosomiasis B65.0 [N37]
    congenital Q64.39
      valvular (posterior) Q64.2
    due to
      infection —*see* Stricture, urethra,
        postinfective
      trauma —*see* Stricture, urethra,
        post-traumatic
    gonococcal, gonorrheal A54.01
    infective NEC —*see* Stricture, urethra,
      postinfective
    late effect (sequelae) of injury —*see*
      Stricture, urethra, post-traumatic
    postcatheterization —*see* Stricture, urethra,
      postprocedural
    postinfective NEC
      female N35.12
      male N35.119
        anterior urethra N35.114
        bulbous urethra N35.112
        meatal N35.111
        membranous urethra N35.113
    postobstetric N35.021
    postoperative —*see* Stricture, urethra,
      postprocedural
    postprocedural
      female N99.12
      male N99.114
        ~~anterior urethra N99.113~~
        anterior bulbous urethra N99.113 ◀
        bulbous urethra N99.111
        fossa navicularis N99.115 ◀
        meatal N99.110
        membranous urethra N99.112

Stricture *(Continued)*
  urethra (organic) (spasmodic) *(Continued)*
    post-traumatic
      female N35.028
        due to childbirth N35.021
      male N35.014
        anterior urethra N35.013
        bulbous urethra N35.011
        meatal N35.010
        membranous urethra N35.012
    sequela (late effect) of
      childbirth N35.021
      injury —*see* Stricture, urethra,
        post-traumatic
    specified cause NEC N35.8
    syphilitic A52.76
    traumatic —*see* Stricture, urethra,
      post-traumatic
    valvular (posterior), congenital Q64.2
  urinary meatus —*see* Stricture, urethra
  uterus, uterine (synechiae) N85.6
    os (external) (internal) —*see* Stricture,
      cervix
  vagina (outlet) —*see* Stenosis, vagina
  valve (cardiac) (heart) —*see also* Endocarditis
    congenital
      aortic Q23.0
      mitral Q23.2
      pulmonary Q22.1
      tricuspid Q22.4
  vas deferens N50.89 ◀▥
    congenital Q55.4
  vein I87.1
  vena cava (inferior) (superior) NEC I87.1
    congenital Q26.0
  vesicourethral orifice N32.0
    congenital Q64.31
  vulva (acquired) N90.5
Stridor R06.1
  congenital (larynx) P28.89
Stridulous —*see* condition
Stroke (apoplectic) (brain) (embolic) (ischemic)
  (paralytic) (thrombotic) I63.9
  epileptic —*see* Epilepsy
  heat T67.0
  in evolution I63.9
  intraoperative
    during cardiac surgery I97.810
    during other surgery I97.811
  lightning —*see* Lightning
  meaning
    cerebral hemorrhage — code to
      Hemorrhage, intracranial
    cerebral infarction — code to Infarction,
      cerebral
  postprocedural
    following cardiac surgery I97.820
    following other surgery I97.821
  unspecified (NOS) I63.9
Stromatosis, endometrial D39.0
Strongyloidiasis, strongyloidosis B78.9
  cutaneous B78.1
  disseminated B78.7
  intestinal B78.0
Strophulus pruriginosus L28.2
Struck by lightning —*see* Lightning
Struma —*see also* Goiter
  Hashimoto E06.3
  lymphomatosa E06.3
  nodosa (simplex) E04.9
    endemic E01.2
      multinodular E01.1
    multinodular E04.2
      iodine-deficiency related E01.1
    toxic or with hyperthyroidism
      E05.20
      with thyroid storm E05.21
      multinodular E05.20
        with thyroid storm E05.21
      uninodular E05.10
        with thyroid storm E05.11

Struma *(Continued)*
  nodosa (simplex) *(Continued)*
    toxicosa E05.20
      with thyroid storm E05.21
      multinodular E05.20
        with thyroid storm E05.21
      uninodular E05.10
        with thyroid storm E05.11
    uninodular E04.1
  ovarii D27.-
  Riedel's E06.5
Strumipriva cachexia E03.4
Strümpell-Marie spine —*see* Spondylitis,
  ankylosing
Strümpell-Westphal pseudosclerosis E83.01
Stuart deficiency disease (factor X) D68.2
Stuart-Prower factor deficiency (factor X)
  D68.2
Student's elbow —*see* Bursitis, elbow,
  olecranon
Stump —*see* Amputation
Stunting, nutritional E45
Stupor (catatonic) R40.1
  depressive (single episode) F32.89 ◀▥
    recurrent episode F33.8 ◀
  dissociative F44.2
  manic F30.2
  manic-depressive F31.89
  psychogenic (anergic) F44.2
  reaction to exceptional stress (transient)
    F43.0
Sturge (-Weber) (-Dimitri) (-Kalischer) **disease
  or syndrome** Q85.8
Stuttering F80.81
  adult onset F98.5
  childhood onset F80.81
  following cerebrovascular disease —
    see Disorder, fluency, following
    cerebrovascular disease
  in conditions classified elsewhere R47.82
Sty, stye (external) (internal) (meibomian)
  (zeisian) —*see* Hordeolum
Subacidity, gastric K31.89
  psychogenic F45.8
Subacute —*see* condition
Subarachnoid —*see* condition
Subcortical —*see* condition
Subcostal syndrome, nerve compression —*see*
  Mononeuropathy, upper limb, specified
  site NEC
Subcutaneous, subcuticular —*see* condition
Subdural —*see* condition
Subendocardium —*see* condition
Subependymoma
  specified site —*see* Neoplasm, uncertain
    behavior, by site
  unspecified site D43.2
Suberosis J67.3
Subglossitis —*see* Glossitis
Subhemophilia D66
Subinvolution
  breast (postlactational) (postpuerperal)
    N64.89
  puerperal O90.89
  uterus (chronic) (nonpuerperal) N85.3
    puerperal O90.89
Sublingual —*see* condition
Sublinguitis —*see* Sialoadenitis
Subluxatable hip Q65.6
Subluxation —*see also* Dislocation
  acromioclavicular S43.11-
  ankle S93.0-
  atlantoaxial, recurrent M43.4
    with myelopathy M43.3
  carpometacarpal (joint) NEC S63.05-
    thumb S63.04-
  complex, vertebral —*see* Complex,
    subluxation
  congenital —*see also* Malposition, congenital
    hip —*see* Dislocation, hip, congenital,
      partial

◀ New   ◀▥ Revised   ~~deleted~~ Deleted

Subluxation *(Continued)*
congenital *(Continued)*
  joint (excluding hip)
    lower limb Q68.8
    shoulder Q68.8
    upper limb Q68.8
  elbow (traumatic) S53.10-
    anterior S53.11-
    lateral S53.14-
    medial S53.13-
    posterior S53.12-
    specified type NEC S53.19-
  finger S63.20-
    index S63.20-
    interphalangeal S63.22-
      distal S63.24-
        index S63.24-
        little S63.24-
        middle S63.24-
        ring S63.24-
      index S63.22-
      little S63.22-
      middle S63.22-
      proximal S63.23-
        index S63.23-
        little S63.23-
        middle S63.23-
        ring S63.23-
      ring S63.22-
    little S63.20-
    metacarpophalangeal S63.21-
      index S63.21-
      little S63.21-
      middle S63.21-
      ring S63.21-
    middle S63.20-
    ring S63.20-
  foot S93.30-
    specified site NEC S93.33-
    tarsal joint S93.31-
    tarsometatarsal joint S93.32-
    toe —*see* Subluxation, toe
  hip S73.00-
    anterior S73.03-
      obturator S73.02-
    central S73.04-
    posterior S73.01-
  interphalangeal (joint)
    finger S63.22-
      distal joint S63.24-
        index S63.24-
        little S63.24-
        middle S63.24-
        ring S63.24-
      index S63.22-
      little S63.22-
      middle S63.22-
      proximal joint S63.23-
        index S63.23-
        little S63.23-
        middle S63.23-
        ring S63.23-
      ring S63.22-
    thumb S63.12-
      distal joint S63.14-
      proximal joint S63.13-
    toe S93.13-
      great S93.13-
      lesser S93.13-
  joint prosthesis —*see* Complications, joint
    prosthesis, mechanical, displacement,
    by site
  knee S83.10-
    cap —*see* Subluxation, patella
    patella —*see* Subluxation, patella
    proximal tibia
      anteriorly S83.11-
      laterally S83.14-
      medially S83.13-
      posteriorly S83.12-
    specified type NEC S83.19-

Subluxation *(Continued)*
lens —*see* Dislocation, lens, partial
ligament, traumatic —*see* Sprain, by site
metacarpal (bone)
  proximal end S63.06-
metacarpophalangeal (joint)
  finger S63.21-
    index S63.21-
    little S63.21-
    middle S63.21-
    ring S63.21-
  thumb S63.11-
metatarsophalangeal joint S93.14-
  great toe S93.14-
  lesser toe S93.14-
midcarpal (joint) S63.03-
patella S83.00-
  lateral S83.01-
  recurrent (nontraumatic) —*see* Dislocation,
    patella, recurrent, incomplete
  specified type NEC S83.09-
pathological —*see* Dislocation, pathological
radial head S53.00-
  anterior S53.01-
  nursemaid's elbow S53.03-
  posterior S53.02-
  specified type NEC S53.09-
radiocarpal (joint) S63.02-
radioulnar (joint)
  distal S63.01-
  proximal —*see* Subluxation, elbow
shoulder
  congenital Q68.8
  girdle S43.30-
    scapula S43.31-
    specified site NEC S43.39-
  traumatic S43.00-
    anterior S43.01-
    inferior S43.03-
    posterior S43.02-
    specified type NEC S43.08-
sternoclavicular (joint) S43.20-
  anterior S43.21-
  posterior S43.22-
symphysis (pubis)
thumb S63.103
  interphalangeal joint —*see* Subluxation,
    interphalangeal (joint), thumb
  metacarpophalangeal joint —*see*
    Subluxation, metacarpophalangeal
    (joint), thumb
toe (s) S93.10-
  great S93.10-
    interphalangeal joint S93.13-
    metatarsophalangeal joint S93.14-
  interphalangeal joint S93.13-
  lesser S93.10-
    interphalangeal joint S93.13-
    metatarsophalangeal joint S93.14-
  metatarsophalangeal joint S93.149
ulnohumeral joint —*see* Subluxation,
  elbow
vertebral
  recurrent NEC —*see* subcategory
    M43.5
  traumatic
    cervical S13.100
      atlantoaxial joint S13.120
      atlantooccipital joint S13.110
      atloidooccipital joint S13.110
      joint between
        C0 and C1 S13.110
        C1 and C2 S13.120
        C2 and C3 S13.130
        C3 and C4 S13.140
        C4 and C5 S13.150
        C5 and C6 S13.160
        C6 and C7 S13.170
        C7 and T1 S13.180
      occipitoatloid joint
        S13.110

Subluxation *(Continued)*
vertebral *(Continued)*
  traumatic *(Continued)*
    lumbar S33.100
      joint between
        L1 and L2 S33.110
        L2 and L3 S33.120
        L3 and L4 S33.130
        L4 and L5 S33.140
    thoracic S23.100
      joint between
        T1 and T2 S23.110
        T2 and T3 S23.120
        T3 and T4 S23.122
        T4 and T5 S23.130
        T5 and T6 S23.132
        T6 and T7 S23.140
        T7 and T8 S23.142
        T8 and T9 S23.150
        T9 and T10 S23.152
        T10 and T11 S23.160
        T11 and T12 S23.162
        T12 and L1 S23.170
ulna
  distal end S63.07-
  proximal end —*see* Subluxation, elbow
wrist (carpal bone) S63.00-
  carpometacarpal joint —*see* Subluxation,
    carpometacarpal (joint)
  distal radioulnar joint —*see* Subluxation,
    radioulnar (joint), distal
  metacarpal bone, proximal —*see*
    Subluxation, metacarpal (bone),
    proximal end
  midcarpal —*see* Subluxation, midcarpal
    (joint)
  radiocarpal joint —*see* Subluxation,
    radiocarpal (joint)
  recurrent —*see* Dislocation, recurrent, wrist
  specified site NEC S63.09-
  ulna —*see* Subluxation, ulna, distal end
Submaxillary —*see* condition
Submersion (fatal) (nonfatal) T75.1
Submucous —*see* condition
Subnormal, subnormality
  accommodation (old age) H52.4
  mental —*see* Disability, intellectual
  temperature (accidental) T68
Subphrenic —*see* condition
Subscapular nerve —*see* condition
Subseptus uterus Q51.2
Subsiding appendicitis K36
Substance (other psychoactive) -induced ◄
  anxiety disorder F19.980 ◄
  bipolar and related disorder F19.94 ◄
  delirium F19.921 ◄
  depressive disorder F19.94 ◄
  major neurocognitive disorder F19.97 ◄
  mild neurocognitive disorder F19.988 ◄
  obsessive-compulsive and related disorder
    F19.988 ◄
  psychotic disorder F19.959 ◄
  sexual dysfunction F19.981 ◄
  sleep disorder F19.982 ◄
Substernal thyroid E04.9
  congenital Q89.2
Substitution disorder F44.9
Subtentorial —*see* condition
Subthyroidism (acquired) —*see also*
    Hypothyroidism
  congenital E03.1
Succenturiate placenta O43.19-
Sucking thumb, child (excessive) F98.8
Sudamen, sudamina L74.1
Sudanese kala-azar B55.0
Sudden
  hearing loss —*see* Deafness, sudden
  heart failure —*see* Failure, heart
Sudeck's atrophy, disease, or syndrome —*see*
    Algoneurodystrophy
Suffocation —*see* Asphyxia, traumatic

Sugar
  blood
    high (transient) R73.9
    low (transient) E16.2
  in urine R81
Suicide, suicidal (attempted) T14.91
  by poisoning —*see* Table of Drugs and
      Chemicals
  history of (personal) Z91.5
    in family Z81.8
  ideation —*see* Ideation, suicidal
  risk
    meaning personal history of attempted
        suicide Z91.5
    meaning suicidal ideation —*see* Ideation,
        suicidal
  tendencies
    meaning personal history of attempted
        suicide Z91.5
    meaning suicidal ideation —*see* Ideation,
        suicidal
  trauma —*see* nature of injury by site
Suipestifer infection —*see* Infection, salmonella
Sulfhemoglobinemia, sulphemoglobinemia
    (acquired) (with methemoglobinemia)
      D74.8
Sumatran mite fever A75.3
Summer —*see* condition
Sunburn L55.9
  due to ◀
    tanning bed (acute) L56.8 ◀
      chronic L57.8 ◀
    ultraviolet radiation (acute) L56.8 ◀
      chronic L57.8 ◀
  first degree L55.0
  second degree L55.1
  third degree L55.2
SUNCT (short lasting unilateral neuralgiform
      headache with conjunctival injection and
      tearing) G44.059
  intractable G44.051
  not intractable G44.059
Sunken acetabulum —*see* Derangement, joint,
    specified type NEC, hip
Sunstroke T67.0
Superfecundation —*see* Pregnancy,
    multiple
Superfetation —*see* Pregnancy, multiple
Superinvolution (uterus) N85.8
Supernumerary (congenital)
  aortic cusps Q23.8
  auditory ossicles Q16.3
  bone Q79.8
  breast Q83.1
  carpal bones Q74.0
  cusps, heart valve NEC Q24.8
    aortic Q23.8
    mitral Q23.2
    pulmonary Q22.3
  digit (s) Q69.9
  ear (lobule) Q17.0
  fallopian tube Q50.6
  finger Q69.0
  hymen Q52.4
  kidney Q63.0
  lacrimonasal duct Q10.6
  lobule (ear) Q17.0
  mitral cusps Q23.2
  muscle Q79.8
  nipple (s) Q83.3
  organ or site not listed —*see* Accessory
  ossicles, auditory Q16.3
  ovary Q50.31
  oviduct Q50.6
  pulmonary, pulmonic cusps Q22.3
  rib Q76.6
    cervical or first (syndrome) Q76.5
  roots (of teeth) K00.2
  spleen Q89.09
  tarsal bones Q74.2
  teeth K00.1

Supernumerary (Continued)
  testis Q55.29
  thumb Q69.1
  toe Q69.2
  uterus Q51.2
  vagina Q52.1
  vertebra Q76.49
Supervision (of)
  contraceptive —*see* Prescription,
      contraceptives
  dietary (for) Z71.3
    allergy (food) Z71.3
    colitis Z71.3
    diabetes mellitus Z71.3
    food allergy or intolerance Z71.3
    gastritis Z71.3
    hypercholesterolemia Z71.3
    hypoglycemia Z71.3
    intolerance (food) Z71.3
    obesity Z71.3
    specified NEC Z71.3
  healthy infant or child Z76.2
    foundling Z76.1
  high-risk pregnancy —*see* Pregnancy,
      complicated by, high, risk
  lactation Z39.1
  pregnancy —*see* Pregnancy, supervision of
Supplemental teeth K00.1
Suppression
  binocular vision H53.34
  lactation O92.5
  menstruation N94.89
  ovarian secretion E28.39
  renal N28.9
  urine, urinary secretion R34
Suppuration, suppurative —*see also* condition
  accessory sinus (chronic) —*see* Sinusitis
  adrenal gland
  antrum (chronic) —*see* Sinusitis, maxillary
  bladder —*see* Cystitis
  brain G06.0
    sequelae G09
  breast N61.1 ◀▥
    puerperal, postpartum or gestational —*see*
        Mastitis, obstetric, purulent
  dental periosteum M27.3
  ear (middle) —*see also* Otitis, media
    external NEC —*see* Otitis, externa,
        infective
    internal —*see* subcategory H83.0
  ethmoidal (chronic) (sinus) —*see* Sinusitis,
      ethmoidal
  fallopian tube —*see* Salpingo-oophoritis
  frontal (chronic) (sinus) —*see* Sinusitis,
      frontal
  gallbladder (acute) K81.0
  gum K05.20
    generalized —*see* Peridontitis, aggressive,
        generalized ◀▥
    localized —*see* Peridontitis, aggressive,
        localized ◀▥
  intracranial G06.0
  joint —*see* Arthritis, pyogenic or pyemic
  labyrinthine —*see* subcategory H83.0
  lung —*see* Abscess, lung
  mammary gland N61.1 ◀▥
    puerperal, postpartum O91.12
      associated with lactation O91.13
  maxilla, maxillary M27.2
    sinus (chronic) —*see* Sinusitis, maxillary
  muscle —*see* Myositis, infective
  nasal sinus (chronic) —*see* Sinusitis
  pancreas, acute —*see also* Pancreatitis, acute
      K85.80 ◀▥
  parotid gland —*see* Sialoadenitis
  pelvis, pelvic
    female —*see* Disease, pelvis, inflammatory
    male K65.0
  pericranial —*see* Osteomyelitis
  salivary duct or gland (any) —*see*
      Sialoadenitis

Suppuration, suppurative (Continued)
  sinus (accessory) (chronic) (nasal) —*see*
      Sinusitis
  sphenoidal sinus (chronic) —*see* Sinusitis,
      sphenoidal
  thymus (gland) E32.1
  thyroid (gland) E06.0
  tonsil —*see* Tonsillitis
  uterus —*see* Endometritis
Supraeruption of tooth (teeth) M26.34
Supraglottitis J04.30
  with obstruction J04.31
Suprarenal (gland) —*see* condition
Suprascapular nerve —*see* condition
Suprasellar —*see* condition
Surfer's knots or nodules S89.8-
Surgical
  emphysema T81.82
  procedures, complication or misadventure —
      see Complications, surgical procedures
  shock T81.10
Surveillance (of) (for) —*see also* Observation
  alcohol abuse Z71.41
  contraceptive —*see* Prescription,
      contraceptives
  dietary Z71.3
  drug abuse Z71.51
Susceptibility to disease, genetic Z15.89
  malignant neoplasm Z15.09
    breast Z15.01
    endometrium Z15.04
    ovary Z15.02
    prostate Z15.03
    specified NEC Z15.09
  multiple endocrine neoplasia Z15.81
Suspected condition, ruled out —*see also*
    Observation, suspected
  amniotic cavity and membrane Z03.71
  cervical shortening Z03.75
  fetal anomaly Z03.73
  fetal growth Z03.74
  maternal and fetal conditions NEC Z03.79
  newborn —*see also* Observation, newborn,
      suspected condition ruled out Z05.9 ◀
  oligohydramnios Z03.71
  placental problem Z03.72
  polyhydramnios Z03.71
Suspended uterus
  in pregnancy or childbirth —*see* Pregnancy,
      complicated by, abnormal uterus
Sutton's nevus D22.9
Suture
  burst (in operation wound) T81.31
    external operation wound T81.31
    internal operation wound T81.32
  inadvertently left in operation wound —*see*
      Foreign body, accidentally left during a
      procedure
  removal Z48.02
Swab inadvertently left in operation wound —
    see Foreign body, accidentally left during
    a procedure
Swallowed, swallowing
  difficulty —*see* Dysphagia
  foreign body —*see* Foreign body, alimentary
      tract
Swan-neck deformity (finger) —*see* Deformity,
    finger, swan-neck
Swearing, compulsive F42.8 ◀▥
  in Gilles de la Tourette's syndrome F95.2
Sweat, sweats
  fetid L75.0
  night R61
Sweating, excessive R61
Sweeley-Klionsky disease E75.21
Sweet's disease or dermatosis L98.2
Swelling (of) R60.9
  abdomen, abdominal (not referable to any
      particular organ) —*see* Mass,
      abdominal
  ankle —*see* Effusion, joint, ankle

426

Swelling *(Continued)*
  arm M79.89
    forearm M79.89
  breast N63
  Calabar B74.3
  cervical gland R59.0
  chest, localized R22.2
  ear H93.8-
  extremity (lower) (upper) —*see* Disorder, soft
    tissue, specified type NEC
  finger M79.89
  foot M79.89
  glands R59.9
    generalized R59.1
    localized R59.0
  hand M79.89
  head (localized) R22.0
  inflammatory —*see* Inflammation
  intra-abdominal —*see* Mass, abdominal
  joint —*see* Effusion, joint
  leg M79.89
    lower M79.89
  limb —*see* Disorder, soft tissue, specified type
    NEC
  localized (skin) R22.9
    chest R22.2
    head R22.0
    limb
      lower —*see* Mass, localized, limb,
        lower
      upper —*see* Mass, localized, limb,
        upper
    neck R22.1
    trunk R22.2
  neck (localized) R22.1
  pelvic —*see* Mass, abdominal
  scrotum N50.89 ◀‖‖
  splenic —*see* Splenomegaly
  testis N50.89 ◀‖‖
  toe M79.89
  umbilical R19.09
  wandering, due to Gnathostoma
    (spinigerum) B83.1
  white —*see* Tuberculosis, arthritis
Swift (-Feer) disease
  overdose or wrong substance given or
    taken —*see* Table of Drugs and
    Chemicals, by drug, poisoning
Swimmer's
  cramp T75.1
  ear H60.33-
  itch B65.3
Swimming in the head R42
Swollen —*see* Swelling
Swyer syndrome Q99.1
Sycosis L73.8
  barbae (not parasitic) L73.8
  contagiosa (mycotic) B35.0
  lupoides L73.8
  mycotic B35.0
  parasitic B35.0
  vulgaris L73.8
Sydenham's chorea —*see* Chorea, Sydenham's
Sylvatic yellow fever A95.0
Sylvest's disease B33.0
Symblepharon H11.23-
  congenital Q10.3
Symond's syndrome G93.2
Sympathetic —*see* condition
Sympatheticotonia G90.8
Sympathicoblastoma
  specified site —*see* Neoplasm, malignant, by
    site
  unspecified site C74.90
Sympathogonioma —*see* Sympathicoblastoma
Symphalangy (fingers) (toes) Q70.9
Symptoms NEC R68.89
  breast NEC N64.59
  development NEC R63.8
  factitious, self-induced —*see* Disorder,
    factitious

Symptoms NEC *(Continued)*
  genital organs, female R10.2
  involving
    abdomen NEC R19.8
    appearance NEC R46.89
    awareness R41.9
      altered mental status R41.82
      amnesia —*see* Amnesia
      borderline intellectual functioning
        R41.83
      coma —*see* Coma
      disorientation R41.0
      neurologic neglect syndrome R41.4
      senile cognitive decline R41.81
      specified symptom NEC R41.89
    behavior NEC R46.89
    cardiovascular system NEC R09.89
    chest NEC R09.89
    circulatory system NEC R09.89
    cognitive functions R41.9
      altered mental status R41.82
      amnesia —*see* Amnesia
      borderline intellectual functioning
        R41.83
      coma —*see* Coma
      disorientation R41.0
      neurologic neglect syndrome R41.4
      senile cognitive decline R41.81
      specified symptom NEC R41.89
    development NEC R62.50
    digestive system NEC R19.8
    emotional state NEC R45.89
      emotional lability R45.86
    food and fluid intake R63.8
    general perceptions and sensations
      R44.9
      specified NEC R44.8
    musculoskeletal system R29.91
      specified NEC R29.898
    nervous system R29.90
      specified NEC R29.818
    pelvis NEC R19.8
    respiratory system NEC R09.89
    skin and integument R23.9
    urinary system R39.9
  menopausal N95.1
  metabolism NEC R63.8
  neurotic F48.8
  of infancy R68.19
  pelvis NEC, female R10.2
  skin and integument NEC R23.9
  subcutaneous tissue NEC R23.9
Sympus Q74.2
Syncephalus Q89.4
Synchondrosis
  abnormal (congenital) Q78.8
  ischiopubic M91.0
Synchysis (scintillans) (senile) (vitreous body)
  H43.89
Syncope (near) (pre-) R55
  anginosa I20.8
  bradycardia R00.1
  cardiac R55
  carotid sinus G90.01
  due to spinal (lumbar) puncture G97.1
  heart R55
  heat T67.1
  laryngeal R05
  psychogenic F48.8
  tussive R05
  vasoconstriction R55
  vasodepressor R55
  vasomotor R55
  vasovagal R55
Syndactylism, syndactyly Q70.9
  complex (with synostosis)
    fingers Q70.0-
    toes Q70.2-
  simple (without synostosis)
    fingers Q70.1-
    toes Q70.3-

Syndrome —*see also* Disease
  5q minus NOS D46.C
  48,XXXX Q97.1
  49,XXXXX Q97.1
  abdominal
    acute R10.0
    muscle deficiency Q79.4
  abnormal innervation H02.519
    left H02.516
      lower H02.515
      upper H02.514
    right H02.513
      lower H02.512
      upper H02.511
  abstinence, neonatal P96.1
  acid pulmonary aspiration, obstetric O74.0
  acquired immunodeficiency —*see* Human,
    immunodeficiency virus (HIV)
    disease
  acute abdominal R10.0
  acute respiratory distress (adult) (child) J80
    idiopathic J84.114 ◀
  Adair-Dighton Q78.0
  Adams-Stokes (-Morgagni) I45.9
  adiposogenital E23.6
  adrenal
    hemorrhage (meningococcal) A39.1
    meningococcic A39.1
  adrenocortical —*see* Cushing's, syndrome
  adrenogenital E25.9
    congenital, associated with enzyme
      deficiency E25.0
  afferent loop NEC K91.89
  Alagille's Q44.7
  alcohol withdrawal (without convulsions) —
    see Dependence, alcohol, with,
    withdrawal
  Alder's D72.0
  Aldrich (-Wiskott) D82.0
  alien hand R41.4
  Alport Q87.81
  alveolar hypoventilation E66.2
  alveolocapillary block J84.10
  amnesic, amnestic (confabulatory) (due to) —
    see Disorder, amnesic
  amyostatic (Wilson's disease) E83.01
  androgen insensitivity E34.50
    complete E34.51
    partial E34.52
  androgen resistance (*see also* Syndrome,
    androgen insensitivity) E34.50
  Angelman Q93.5
  anginal —*see* Angina
  ankyloglossia superior Q38.1
  anterior
    chest wall R07.89
    cord G83.82
    spinal artery G95.19
      compression M47.019
        cervical region M47.012
        cervicothoracic region M47.013
        lumbar region M47.016
        occipito-atlanto-axial region M47.011
        thoracic region M47.014
        thoracolumbar region M47.015
    tibial M76.81-
  antibody deficiency D80.9
    agammaglobulinemic D80.1
      hereditary D80.0
    congenital D80.0
    hypogammaglobulinemic D80.1
      hereditary D80.0
  anticardiolipin (-antibody) D68.61
  antiphospholipid (-antibody) D68.61
  aortic
    arch M31.4
    bifurcation I74.09
  aortomesenteric duodenum occlusion K31.5
  apical ballooning (transient left ventricular)
    I51.81
  arcuate ligament I77.4

Syndrome (*Continued*)
  argentaffin, argintaffinoma E34.0
  Arnold-Chiari —*see* Arnold-Chiari disease
  Arrillaga-Ayerza I27.0
  arterial tortuosity Q87.82 ◄
  arteriovenous steal T82.898- ◄
  Asherman's N85.6
  aspiration, of newborn —*see* Aspiration, by
      substance, with pneumonia
    meconium P24.01
  ataxia-telangiectasia G11.3
  auriculotemporal G50.8
  autoerythrocyte sensitization (Gardner-
      Diamond) D69.2
  autoimmune lymphoproliferative [ALPS]
    D89.82
  autoimmune polyglandular E31.0
  autoinflammatory M04.9 ◄
    specified type NEC M04.8 ◄
  autosomal —*see* Abnormal, autosomes
  Avellis' G46.8
  Ayerza (-Arrillaga) I27.0
  Babinski-Nageotte G83.89
  Bakwin-Krida Q78.5 ◄▥
  bare lymphocyte D81.6
  Barré-Guillain G61.0
  Barré-Liéou M53.0
  Barrett's —*see* Barrett's, esophagus
  Barsony-Polgar K22.4
  Barsony-Teschendorf K22.4
  Barth E78.71
  Bartter's E26.81
  basal cell nevus Q87.89
  Basedow's E05.00
    with thyroid storm E05.01
  basilar artery G45.0
  Batten-Steinert G71.11
  battered
    baby or child —*see* Maltreatment, child,
      physical abuse
    spouse —*see* Maltreatment, adult, physical
      abuse
  Beals Q87.40
  Beau's I51.5
  Beck's I65.8
  Benedikt's G46.3
  Béquez César (-Steinbrinck-Chédiak-Higashi)
    D70.330
  Bernhardt-Roth —*see* Meralgia paresthetica
  Bernheim's I50.9
  big spleen D73.1
  bilateral polycystic ovarian E28.2
  Bing-Horton's —*see* Horton's headache
  Birt-Hogg-Dube syndrome Q87.89
  Björck (-Thorsen) E34.0
  black
    lung J60
    widow spider bite —*see* Toxicity, venom,
      spider, black widow
  Blackfan-Diamond D61.01
  Blau M04.8 ◄
  blind loop K90.2
    congenital Q43.8
    postsurgical K91.2
  blue sclera Q78.0
  blue toe I75.02-
  Boder-Sedgewick G11.3
  Boerhaave's K22.3
  Borjeson Forssman Lehmann Q89.8
  Bouillaud's I01.9
  Bourneville (-Pringle) Q85.1
  Bouveret (-Hoffman) I47.9
  brachial plexus G54.0
  bradycardia-tachycardia I49.5
  brain (nonpsychotic) F09
    with psychosis, psychotic reaction F09
    acute or subacute —*see* Delirium
    congenital —*see* Disability, intellectual
    organic F09
      post-traumatic (nonpsychotic) F07.81
        psychotic F09

Syndrome (*Continued*)
  brain (nonpsychotic) (*Continued*)
    personality change F07.0
    postcontusional F07.81
    post-traumatic, nonpsychotic F07.81
    psycho-organic F09
    psychotic F06.8
  brain stem stroke G46.3
  Brandt's (acrodermatitis enteropathica) E83.2
  broad ligament laceration N83.8
  Brock's J98.11
  bronze baby P83.8
  Brown-Sequard G83.81
  bubbly lung P27.0
  Buchem's M85.2
  Budd-Chiari I82.0
  bulbar (progressive) G12.22
  Bürger-Grütz E78.3
  Burke's K86.89 ◄▥
  Burnett's (milk-alkali) E83.52
  burning feet E53.9
  Bywaters' T79.5
  Call-Fleming I67.841
  carbohydrate-deficient glycoprotein (CDGS)
    E77.8
  carcinogenic thrombophlebitis I82.1
  carcinoid E34.0
  cardiac asthma I50.1
  cardiacos negros I27.0
  cardiofaciocutaneous Q87.89
  cardiopulmonary-obesity E66.2
  cardiorenal —*see* Hypertension, cardiorenal
  cardiorespiratory distress (idiopathic),
    newborn P22.0
  cardiovascular renal —*see* Hypertension,
    cardiorenal
  carotid
    artery (hemispheric) (internal) G45.1
    body G90.01
    sinus G90.01
  carpal tunnel G56.0-
  Cassidy (-Scholte) E34.0
  cat-cry Q93.4
  cat eye Q92.8
  cauda equina G83.4
  causalgia —*see* Causalgia
  celiac K90.0
    artery compression I77.4
    axis I77.4
  central pain G89.0
  cerebellar
    hereditary G11.9
    stroke G46.4
  cerebellomedullary malformation —*see* Spina
    bifida
  cerebral
    artery
      anterior G46.1
      middle G46.0
      posterior G46.2
    gigantism E22.0
  cervical (root) M53.1
    disc —*see* Disorder, disc, cervical, with
      neuritis
    fusion Q76.1
    posterior, sympathicus M53.0
    rib Q76.5
    sympathetic paralysis G90.2
  cervicobrachial (diffuse) M53.1
  cervicocranial M53.0
  cervicodorsal outlet G54.2
  cervicothoracic outlet G54.0
  Céstan (-Raymond) I65.8
  Charcot's (angina cruris) (intermittent
    claudication) I73.9
  Charcot-Weiss-Baker G90.09
  CHARGE Q89.8
  Chédiak-Higashi (-Steinbrinck) E70.330
  chest wall R07.1
  Chiari's (hepatic vein thrombosis) I82.0
  Chilaiditi's Q43.3

Syndrome (*Continued*)
  child maltreatment —*see* Maltreatment,
    child
  chondrocostal junction M94.0
  chondroectodermal dysplasia Q77.6
  chromosome 4 short arm deletion Q93.3
  chromosome 5 short arm deletion Q93.4
  chronic
    infantile neurological, cutaneous and
      articular (CINCA) M04.2 ◄
    pain G89.4
      personality F68.8
  Clarke-Hadfield K86.89 ◄▥
  Clerambault's automatism G93.89
  Clouston's (hidrotic ectodermal dysplasia)
    Q82.4
  clumsiness, clumsy child F82
  cluster headache G44.009
    intractable G44.001
    not intractable G44.009
  Coffin-Lowry Q89.8
  cold injury (newborn) P80.0
  combined immunity deficiency D81.9
  compartment (deep) (posterior) (traumatic)
    T79.A0
    abdomen T79.A3
    lower extremity (hip, buttock, thigh, leg,
      foot, toes) T79.A2
    nontraumatic
      abdomen M79.A3
      lower extremity (hip, buttock, thigh, leg,
        foot, toes) M79.A2-
      specified site NEC M79.A9
      upper extremity (shoulder, arm, forearm,
        wrist, hand, fingers) M79.A1-
    postprocedural —*see* Syndrome
      compartment, nontraumatic
    specified site NEC T79.A9
    upper extremity (shoulder, arm, forearm,
      wrist, hand, fingers) T79.A1
  complex regional pain —*see* Syndrome, pain,
    complex regional
  compression T79.5
    anterior spinal —*see* Syndrome, anterior,
      spinal artery, compression
    cauda equina G83.4
    celiac artery I77.4
    vertebral artery M47.029
      cervical region M47.022
      occipito-atlanto-axial region M47.021
  concussion F07.81
  congenital
    affecting multiple systems NEC Q87.89
    central alveolar hypoventilation G47.35
    facial diplegia Q87.0
    muscular hypertrophy-cerebral Q87.89
    oculo-auriculovertebral Q87.0
    oculofacial diplegia (Moebius) Q87.0
    rubella (manifest) P35.0
  congestion-fibrosis (pelvic), female N94.89
  congestive dysmenorrhea N94.6
  Conn's E26.01
  connective tissue M35.9
    overlap NEC M35.1
  conus medullaris G95.81
  cord
    anterior G83.82
    posterior G83.83
  coronary
    acute NEC I24.9
    insufficiency or intermediate I20.0
    slow flow I20.8
  Costen's (complex) M26.69
  costochondral junction M94.0
  costoclavicular G54.0
  costovertebral E22.0
  Cowden Q85.8
  craniovertebral M53.0
  Creutzfeldt-Jakob —*see* Creutzfeldt-Jakob
    disease or syndrome
  cri-du-chat Q93.4

◄ New   ◄▥ Revised   ~~deleted~~ Deleted

Syndrome (Continued)
crib death R99
cricopharyngeal —see Dysphagia
croup J05.0
CRPS I —see Syndrome, pain, complex
    regional I
crush T79.5
cubital tunnel —see Lesion, nerve, ulnar
Curschmann (-Batten) (-Steinert) G71.11
Cushing's E24.9
  alcohol-induced E24.4
  drug-induced E24.2
  due to
    alcohol
      drugs E24.2
    ectopic ACTH E24.3
    overproduction of pituitary ACTH E24.0
  overdose or wrong substance given or
    taken —see Table of Drugs and
    Chemicals, by drug, poisoning
  pituitary-dependent E24.0
  specified type NEC E24.8
cryopyrin-associated periodic M04.2 ◄
cryptophthalmos Q87.0
cystic duct stump K91.5
Dana-Putnam D51.0
Danbolt (-Cross) (acrodermatitis
    enteropathica) E83.2
Dandy-Walker Q03.1
  with spina bifida Q07.01
Danlos' Q79.6 ◄⠿
defibrination —see also Fibrinolysis
  with
    antepartum hemorrhage —see
      Hemorrhage, antepartum, with
      coagulation defect
    intrapartum hemorrhage —see
      Hemorrhage, complicating,
      delivery
  newborn P60
  postpartum O72.3
Degos' I77.8
Déjérine-Roussy G89.0
delayed sleep phase G47.21
demyelinating G37.9
dependence —see F10-F19 with fourth
    character .2
depersonalization (-derealization) F48.1
De Quervain E34.51
de Toni-Fanconi (-Debré) E72.09
  with cystinosis E72.04
diabetes mellitus-hypertension-nephrosis —
    see Diabetes, nephrosis
diabetes mellitus in newborn infant P70.2
diabetes-nephrosis —see Diabetes, nephrosis
diabetic amyotrophy —see Diabetes,
    amyotrophy
dialysis associated steal T82.898- ◄
Diamond-Blackfan D61.01
Diamond-Gardener D69.2
DIC (diffuse or disseminated intravascular
    coagulopathy) D65
di George's D82.1
Dighton's Q78.0
disequilibrium E87.8
Döhle body-panmyelopathic D72.0
dorsolateral medullary G46.4
double athetosis G80.3
Down (see also Down syndrome) Q90.9
Dresbach's (elliptocytosis) D58.1
Dressler's (postmyocardial infarction) I24.1
  postcardiotomy I97.0
drug withdrawal, infant of dependent mother
    P96.1
dry eye H04.12-
due to abnormality
  chromosomal Q99.9
    sex
      female phenotype Q97.9
      male phenotype Q98.9
      specified NEC Q99.8

Syndrome (Continued)
dumping (postgastrectomy) K91.1
  nonsurgical K31.89
Dupré's (meningism) R29.1
dysmetabolic X E88.81
dyspraxia, developmental F82
Eagle-Barrett Q79.4
Eaton-Lambert —see Syndrome,
    Lambert-Eaton
Ebstein's Q22.5
ectopic ACTH E24.3
eczema-thrombocytopenia D82.0
Eddowes' Q78.0
effort (psychogenic) F45.8
Ehlers-Danlos Q79.6
Eisenmenger's I27.89
Ekman's Q78.0
electric feet E53.8
Ellis-van Creveld Q77.6
empty nest Z60.0
endocrine-hypertensive E27.0
entrapment —see Neuropathy,
    entrapment
eosinophilia-myalgia M35.8
epileptic —see also Epilepsy, by type
  absence G40.A09
    intractable G40.A19
      with status epilepticus G40.A11
      without status epilepticus G40.A19
    not intractable G40.A09
      with status epilepticus G40.A01
      without status epilepticus G40.A09
Erdheim-Chester (ECD) E88.89
Erdheim's E22.0
erythrocyte fragmentation D59.4
Evans D69.41
exhaustion F48.8
extrapyramidal G25.9
  specified NEC G25.89
eye retraction —see Strabismus
eyelid-malar-mandible Q87.0
Faber's D50.9
facial pain, paroxysmal G50.0
Fallot's Q21.3
familial cold autoinflammatory M04.2 ◄
familial eczema-thrombocytopenia (Wiskott-
    Aldrich) D82.0
Fanconi (-de Toni) (-Debré) E72.09
  with cystinosis E72.04
Fanconi's (anemia) (congenital pancytopenia)
    D61.09
fatigue
  chronic R53.82
  psychogenic F48.8
faulty bowel habit K59.39 ◄⠿
Feil-Klippel (brevicollis) Q76.1
Felty's —see Felty's syndrome
fertile eunuch E23.0
fetal
  alcohol (dysmorphic) Q86.0
  hydantoin Q86.1
Fiedler's I40.1
first arch Q87.0
fish odor E72.8
Fisher's G61.0
Fitzhugh-Curtis
  due to
    Chlamydia trachomatis A74.81
    Neisseria gonorrhorea (gonococcal
      peritonitis) A54.85
Fitz's —see also Pancreatitis, acute K85.80 ◄⠿
Flajani (-Basedow) E05.00
  with thyroid storm E05.01
flatback —see Flatback syndrome
floppy
  baby P94.2
  iris (intraoeprative) (IFIS) H21.81
  mitral valve I34.1
flush E34.0
Foix-Alajouanine G95.19
Fong's Q87.2 ◄⠿

Syndrome (Continued)
food protein-induced enterocolitis K52.21 ◄
foramen magnum G93.5
Foster-Kennedy H47.14-
Foville's (peduncular) G46.3
fragile X Q99.2
Franceschetti Q75.4
Frey's
  auriculotemporal G50.8
  hyperhidrosis L74.52
Friderichsen-Waterhouse A39.1
Froin's G95.89
frontal lobe F07.0
Fukuhara E88.49
functional
  bowel K59.9
  prepubertal castrate E29.1
Gaisböck's D75.1
ganglion (basal ganglia brain) G25.9
  geniculi G51.1
Gardner-Diamond D69.2
gastroesophageal
  junction K22.0
  laceration-hemorrhage K22.6
gastrojejunal loop obstruction K91.89
Gee-Herter-Heubner K90.0
Gelineau's G47.419
  with cataplexy G47.411
genito-anorectal A55
Gerstmann-Sträussler-Scheinker (GSS)
    A81.82
Gianotti-Crosti L44.4
giant platelet (Bernard-Soulier) D69.1
Gilles de la Tourette's F95.2
goiter-deafness E07.1
Goldberg Q89.8
Goldberg-Maxwell E34.51
Good's D83.8
Gopalan' (burning feet) E53.8
Gorlin's Q87.89
Gougerot-Blum L81.7
Gouley's I31.1
Gower's R55
gray or grey (newborn) P93.0
  platelet D69.1
Gubler-Millard G46.3
Guillain-Barré (-Strohl) G61.0
gustatory sweating G50.8
Hadfield-Clarke K86.89 ◄⠿
hair tourniquet —see Constriction, external,
    by site
Hamman's J98.19
hand-foot L27.1
hand-shoulder G90.8
hantavirus (cardio)-pulmonary (HPS) (HCPS)
    B33.4
happy puppet Q93.5
Harada's H30.81-
Hayem-Faber D50.9
headache NEC G44.89
  complicated NEC G44.59
Heberden's I20.8
Hedinger's E34.0
Hegglin's D72.0
HELLP (hemolysis, elevated liver enzymes
    and low platelet count) O14.2-
  complicating ◄
    childbirth O14.24 ◄
      puerperium O14.25 ◄
hemolytic-uremic D59.3
hemophagocytic, infection-associated
    D76.2
Henoch-Schönlein D69.0
hepatic flexure K59.8
hepatopulmonary K76.81
hepatorenal K76.7
  following delivery O90.4
  postoperative or postprocedural K91.83
  postpartum, puerperal O90.4
hepatourologic K76.7
Herter (-Gee) (nontropical sprue) K90.0

Syndrome *(Continued)*
  Heubner-Herter K90.0
  Heyd's K76.7
  Hilger's G90.09
  histamine-like (fish poisoning) —*see*
      Poisoning, fish
  histiocytic D76.3
  histiocytosis NEC D76.3
  HIV infection, acute B20
  Hoffmann-Werdnig G12.0
  Hollander-Simons E88.1
  Hoppe-Goldflam G70.00
      with exacerbation (acute) G70.01
      in crisis G70.01
  Horner's G90.2
  hungry bone E83.81
  hunterian glossitis D51.0
  Hutchinson's triad A50.53
  hyperabduction G54.0
  hyperammonemia-hyperornithinemia-
      homocitrullinemia E72.4
  hypereosinophilic (idiopathic) D72.1
  hyperimmunoglobulin D M04.1 ◀
  hyperimmunoglobulin E (IgE) D82.4
  hyperkalemic E87.5
  hyperkinetic —*see* Hyperkinesia
  hypermobility M35.7
  hypernatremia E87.0
  hyperosmolarity E87.0
  hyperperfusion G97.82
  hypersplenic D73.1
  hypertransfusion, newborn P61.1
  hyperventilation F45.8
  hyperviscosity (of serum)
      polycythemic D75.1
      sclerothymic D58.8
  hypoglycemic (familial) (neonatal) E16.2
  hypokalemic E87.6
  hyponatremic E87.1
  hypopituitarism E23.0
  hypoplastic left-heart Q23.4
  hypopotassemia E87.6
  hyposmolality E87.1
  hypotension, maternal O26.5-
  hypothenar hammer I73.89
  hypoventilation, obesity (OHS) E66.2 ◀
  ICF (intravascular coagulation-fibrinolysis)
      D65
  idiopathic
      cardiorespiratory distress, newborn P22.0
      nephrotic (infantile) N04.9
  iliotibial band M76.3-
  immobility, immobilization (paraplegic) M62.3
  immune reconstitution D89.3
  immune reconstitution inflammatory [IRIS]
      D89.3
  immunity deficiency, combined D81.9
  immunodeficiency
      acquired —*see* Human, immunodeficiency
          virus (HIV) disease
      combined D81.9
  impending coronary I20.0
  impingement, shoulder M75.4-
  inappropriate secretion of antidiuretic
      hormone E22.2
  infant
      gestational diabetes P70.0
      of diabetic mother P70.1
  infantilism (pituitary) E23.0
  inferior vena cava I87.1
  inspissated bile (newborn) P59.1
  institutional (childhood) F94.2
  insufficient sleep F51.12
  intermediate coronary (artery) I20.0
  interspinous ligament —*see* Spondylopathy,
      specified NEC
  intestinal
      carcinoid E34.0
      knot K56.2
  intravascular coagulation-fibrinolysis (ICF)
      D65

Syndrome *(Continued)*
  iodine-deficiency, congenital E00.9
      type
          mixed E00.2
          myxedematous E00.1
          neurological E00.0
  IRDS (idiopathic respiratory distress,
      newborn) P22.0
  irritable
      bowel K58.9
          ~~with diarrhea K58.0~~
          with ◀
              constipation K58.1 ◀
              diarrhea K58.0 ◀
          mixed K58.2 ◀
          psychogenic F45.8
          specified NEC K58.8 ◀
      heart (psychogenic) F45.8
      weakness F48.8
  ~~ischemic bowel (transient) K55.9~~
  ~~chronic K55.1~~
  ~~due to mesenteric artery insufficiency~~
      ~~K55.1~~
  ischemic ◀
      bowel (transient) K55.9 ◀
          chronic K55.1 ◀
          due to mesenteric artery insufficiency
              K55.1 ◀
      steal T82.898 ◀
  IVC (intravascular coagulopathy) D65
  Ivemark's Q89.01
  Jaccoud's —*see* Arthropathy, postrheumatic,
      chronic
  Jackson's G83.89
  Jakob-Creutzfeldt —*see* Creutzfeldt-Jakob
      disease or syndrome
  jaw-winking Q07.8
  Jervell-Lange-Nielsen I45.81
  jet lag G47.25
  Job's D71
  Joseph-Diamond-Blackfan D61.01
  jugular foramen G52.7
  Kabuki Q89.8
  Kanner's (autism) F84.0
  Kartagener's Q89.3
  Kelly's D50.1
  Kimmelstiel-Wilson —*see* Diabetes, specified
      type, with Kimmelstiel-Wilson disease
  Klein (e)-Levine G47.13
  Klippel-Feil (brevicollis) Q76.1
  Köhler-Pellegrini-Steida —*see* Bursitis, tibial
      collateral
  König's K59.8
  Korsakoff (-Wernicke) (nonalcoholic) F04
      alcoholic F10.26
  Kostmann's D70.0
  Krabbe's congenital muscle hypoplasia Q79.8
  labyrinthine —*see* subcategory H83.2
  lacunar NEC G46.7
  Lambert-Eaton G70.80
      in
          neoplastic disease G73.1
          specified disease NEC G70.81
  Landau-Kleffner —*see* Epilepsy, specified
      NEC
  Larsen's Q74.8
  lateral
      cutaneous nerve of thigh G57.1-
      medullary G46.4
  Launois' E22.0
  lazy
      leukocyte D70.8
      posture M62.3
  Lemiere I80.8
  Lennox-Gastaut G40.812
      intractable G40.814
          with status epilepticus G40.813
          without status epilepticus G40.814
      not intractable G40.812
          with status epilepticus G40.811
          without status epilepticus G40.812

Syndrome *(Continued)*
  lenticular, progressive E83.01
  Leopold-Levi's E05.90
  Lev's I44.2
  Li-Fraumeni Z15.01
  Lichtheim's D51.0
  Lightwood's N25.89
  Lignac (de Toni) (-Fanconi) (-Debré) E72.09
      with cystinosis E72.04
  Likoff's I20.8
  limbic epilepsy personality F07.0
  liver-kidney K76.7
  lobotomy F07.0
  Loffler's J82
  long arm 18 or 21 deletion Q93.89
  long QT I45.81
  Louis-Barré G11.3
  low
      atmospheric pressure T70.29
      back M54.5
      output (cardiac) I50.9
  lower radicular, newborn (birth injury) P14.8
  Luetscher's (dehydration) E86.0
  Lupus anticoagulant D68.62
  Lutembacher's Q21.1
  macrophage activation D76.1
      due to infection D76.2
  magnesium-deficiency R29.0
  Majeed M04.8 ◀
  Mal de Debarquement R42
  malabsorption K90.9
      postsurgical K91.2
  malformation, congenital, due to
      alcohol Q86.0
      exogenous cause NEC Q86.8
      hydantoin Q86.1
      warfarin Q86.2
  malignant
      carcinoid E34.0
      neuroleptic G21.0
  Mallory-Weiss K22.6
  mandibulofacial dysostosis Q75.4
  manic-depressive —*see* Disorder, bipolar ◀═
  maple-syrup-urine E71.0
  Marable's I77.4
  Marfan's Q87.40
      with
          cardiovascular manifestations Q87.418
              aortic dilation Q87.410
          ocular manifestations Q87.42
          skeletal manifestations Q87.43
  Marie's (acromegaly) E22.0
  mast cell activation —*see* Activation, mast
      cell ◀
  maternal hypotension —*see* Syndrome,
      hypotension, maternal
  May (-Hegglin) D72.0
  McArdle (-Schmidt) (-Pearson) E74.04
  McQuarrie's E16.2
  meconium plug (newborn) P76.0
  median arcuate ligament I77.4
  Meekeren-Ehlers-Danlos Q79.6
  megavitamin-B6 E67.2
  Meige G24.4
  MELAS E88.41
  Mendelson's O74.0
  MERRF (myoclonic epilepsy associated with
      ragged-red fibers) E88.42
  mesenteric
      artery (superior) K55.1
      vascular insufficiency K55.1
  metabolic E88.81
  metastatic carcinoid E34.0
  micrognathia-glossoptosis Q87.0
  midbrain NEC G93.89
  middle lobe (lung) J98.19
  middle radicular G54.0
  migraine —*see also* Migraine G43.909-
  Mikulicz' K11.8
  milk-alkali E83.52
  Millard-Gubler G46.3

◀ New   ◀═ Revised   ~~deleted~~ Deleted

Syndrome *(Continued)*
  Miller-Dieker Q93.88
  Miller-Fisher G61.0
  Minkowski-Chauffard D58.0
  Mirizzi's K83.1
  MNGIE (Mitochondrial Neurogastrointestinal Encephalopathy) E88.49
  Möbius, ophthalmoplegic migraine —*see* Migraine, ophthalmoplegic
  monofixation H50.42
  Morel-Moore M85.2
  Morel-Morgagni M85.2
  Morgagni (-Morel) (-Stewart) M85.2
  Morgagni-Adams-Stokes I45.9
  Mounier-Kuhn Q32.4
    with bronchiectasis J47.9
      with
        exacerbation (acute) J47.1
        lower respiratory infection J47.0
    acquired J98.09
      with bronchiectasis J47.9
        with
          exacerbation (acute) J47.1
          lower respiratory infection J47.0
  Muckle-Wells M04.2 ◀
  mucocutaneous lymph node (acute febrile) (MCLS) M30.3
  multiple endocrine neoplasia (MEN) —*see* Neoplasia, endocrine, multiple (MEN}
  multiple operations —*see* Disorder, factitious
  myasthenic G70.9
    in
      diabetes mellitus —*see* Diabetes, amyotrophy
      endocrine disease NEC E34.9 *[G73.3]*
      neoplastic disease —*see also* Neoplasm D49.9 *[G73.3]*
      thyrotoxicosis (hyperthyroidism) E05.90 *[G73.3]*
        with thyroid storm E05.91 *[G73.3]*
  myelodysplastic D46.9
    with
      5q deletion D46.C
      isolated del (5q) chromosomal abnormality D46.C
    lesions, low grade D46.20
    specified NEC D46.Z
  myelopathic pain G89.0
  myeloproliferative (chronic) D47.1
  myofascial pain M79.1
  Naffziger's G54.0
  nail patella Q87.2
  NARP (Neuropathy, Ataxia and Retinitis pigmentosa) E88.49
  neonatal abstinence P96.1
  nephritic —*see also* Nephritis
    with edema —*see* Nephrosis
    acute N00.9
    chronic N03.9
    rapidly progressive N01.9
  nephrotic (congenital) —*see also* Nephrosis N04.9
    with
      dense deposit disease N04.6
      diffuse
        crescentic glomerulonephritis N04.7
        endocapillary proliferative glomerulonephritis N04.4
        membranous glomerulonephritis N04.2
        mesangial proliferative glomerulonephritis N04.3
        mesangiocapillary glomerulonephritis N04.5
      focal and segmental glomerular lesions N04.1
      minor glomerular abnormality N04.0
      specified morphological changes NEC N04.8
    diabetic —*see* Diabetes, nephrosis

Syndrome *(Continued)*
  neurologic neglect R41.4
  Nezelof's D81.4
  Nonne-Milroy-Meige Q82.0
  Nothnagel's vasomotor acroparesthesia I73.89
  obesity hypoventilation (OHS) E66.2 ◀
  oculomotor H51.9
  ophthalmoplegia-cerebellar ataxia —*see* Strabismus, paralytic, third nerve
  oral allergy T78.1 ◀
  oral-facial-digital Q87.0
  organic
    affective F06.30
    amnesic (not alcohol- or drug-induced) F04
    brain F09
    depressive F06.31
    hallucinosis F06.0
    personality F07.0
  Ormond's N13.5
  oro-facial-digital Q87.0
  os trigonum Q68.8
  Osler-Weber-Rendu I78.0
  osteoporosis-osteomalacia M83.8
  Osterreicher-Turner Q87.2 ◀⁞⁞
  otolith —*see* subcategory H81.8
  oto-palatal-digital Q87.0
  outlet (thoracic) G54.0
  ovary
    polycystic E28.2
    resistant E28.39
    sclerocystic E28.2
  Owren's D68.2
  Paget-Schroetter I82.890
  pain —*see also* Pain
    complex regional I G90.50
      lower limb G90.52-
        specified site NEC G90.59
      upper limb G90.51-
    complex regional II —*see* Causalgia
  painful
    bruising D69.2
    feet E53.8
    prostate N42.81
  paralysis agitans —*see* Parkinsonism
  paralytic G83.9
    specified NEC G83.89
  Parinaud's H51.0
  parkinsonian —*see* Parkinsonism
  Parkinson's —*see* Parkinsonism
  paroxysmal facial pain G50.0
  Parry's E05.00
    with thyroid storm E05.01
  Parsonage (-Aldren)-Turner G54.5
  patella clunk M25.86-
  Paterson (-Brown) (-Kelly) D50.1
  pectoral girdle I77.89
  pectoralis minor I77.89
  Pelger-Huet D72.0
  pellagra-cerebellar ataxia-renal aminoaciduria E72.02
  pellagroid E52
  Pellegrini-Stieda —*see* Bursitis, tibial collateral
  pelvic congestion-fibrosis, female N94.89
  penta X Q97.1
  peptic ulcer —*see* Ulcer, peptic
  perabduction I77.89
  periodic fever M04.1 ◀
  periodic fever, aphthous stomatitis, pharyngitis, and adenopathy [PFAPA] M04.8 ◀
  periodic headache, in adults and children — *see* Headache, periodic syndromes in adults and children
  periurethral fibrosis N13.5
  phantom limb (without pain) G54.7
    with pain G54.6
  pharyngeal pouch D82.1
  Pick's —*see* Disease, Pick's ◀⁞⁞
  Pickwickian E66.2

Syndrome *(Continued)*
  PIE (pulmonary infiltration with eosinophilia) J82
  pigmentary pallidal degeneration (progressive) G23.0
  pineal E34.8
  pituitary E22.0
  placental transfusion —*see* Pregnancy, complicated by, placental transfusion syndromes
  plantar fascia M72.2
  plateau iris (post-iridectomy) (postprocedural) H21.82
  Plummer-Vinson D50.1
  pluricarential of infancy E40
  plurideficiency E40
  pluriglandular (compensatory) E31.8
    autoimmune E31.0
  pneumatic hammer T75.21
  polyangiitis overlap M30.8
  polycarential of infancy E40
  polyglandular E31.8
    autoimmune E31.0
  polysplenia Q89.09
  pontine NEC G93.89
  popliteal
    artery entrapment I77.89
    web Q87.89
  postcardiac injury
    postcardiotomy I97.0
    postmyocardial infarction I24.1
  postcardiotomy I97.0
  post chemoembolization — code to associated conditions
  postcholecystectomy K91.5
  postcommissurotomy I97.0
  postconcussional F07.81
  postcontusional F07.81
  postencephalitic F07.89
  posterior
    cervical sympathetic M53.0
    cord G83.83
    fossa compression G93.5
    reversible encephalopathy (PRES) I67.83
  postgastrectomy (dumping) K91.1
  postgastric surgery K91.1
  postinfarction I24.1
  postlaminectomy NEC M96.1
  postleukotomy F07.0
  postmastectomy lymphedema I97.2
  postmyocardial infarction I24.1
  postoperative NEC T81.9
    blind loop K90.2
  postpartum panhypopituitary (Sheehan) E23.0
  postpolio (myelitic) G14
  postthrombotic I87.009
    with
      inflammation I87.02-
        with ulcer I87.03-
      specified complication NEC I87.09-
      ulcer I87.01-
        with inflammation I87.03-
    asymptomatic I87.00-
  postvagotomy K91.1
  postvalvulotomy I97.0
  postviral NEC G93.3
    fatigue G93.3
  Potain's K31.0
  potassium intoxication E87.5
  precerebral artery (multiple) (bilateral) G45.2
  preinfarction I20.0
  preleukemic D46.9
  premature senility E34.8
  premenstrual dysphoric F32.89 ◀⁞⁞
  premenstrual tension N94.3
  Prinzmetal-Massumi R07.1
  prune belly Q79.4
  pseudocarpal tunnel (sublimis) —*see* Syndrome, carpal tunnel

Syndrome (Continued)
  pseudoparalytica G70.00
    with exacerbation (acute) G70.01
    in crisis G70.01
  pseudo -Turner's Q87.1
  psycho-organic (nonpsychotic severity) F07.9
    acute or subacute F05
    depressive type F06.31
    hallucinatory type F06.0
    nonpsychotic severity F07.0
    specified NEC F07.89
  pulmonary
    arteriosclerosis I27.0
    dysmaturity (Wilson-Mikity) P27.0
    hypoperfusion (idiopathic) P22.0
    renal (hemorrhagic) (Goodpasture's) M31.0
  pure
    motor lacunar G46.5
    sensory lacunar G46.6
  Putnam-Dana D51.0
  pyogenic arthritis, pyoderma gangrenosum,
    and acne [PAPA] M04.8 ◀
  pyramidopallidonigral G20
  pyriformis —see Lesion, nerve, sciatic
  QT interval prolongation I45.81
  radicular NEC —see Radiculopathy
    upper limbs, newborn (birth injury) P14.3
  rapid time-zone change G47.25
  Rasmussen G04.81
  Raymond (-Céstan) I65.8
  Raynaud's I73.00
    with gangrene I73.01
  RDS (respiratory distress syndrome,
    newborn) P22.0
  reactive airways dysfunction J68.3
  Refsum's G60.1
  Reifenstein E34.52
  renal glomerulohyalinosis-diabetic —see
    Diabetes, nephrosis
  Rendu-Osler-Weber I78.0
  residual ovary N99.83
  resistant ovary E28.39
  respiratory
    distress
      acute J80
        adult J80
        child J80
        idiopathic J84.114 ◀
      newborn (idiopathic) (type I) P22.0
        type II P22.1
  restless legs G25.81
  retinoblastoma (familial) C69.2
  retroperitoneal fibrosis N13.5
  retroviral seroconversion (acute) Z21
  Reye's G93.7
  Richter —see Leukemia, chronic lymphocytic,
    B-cell type
  Ridley's I50.1
  right
    heart, hypoplastic Q22.6
    ventricular obstruction —see Failure, heart,
      congestive
  Romano-Ward (prolonged QT interval) I45.81
  rotator cuff, shoulder —see also Tear, rotator
    cuff M75.10-
  Rotes Quérol —see Hyperostosis, ankylosing
  Roth —see Meralgia paresthetica
  rubella (congenital) P35.0
  Ruvalcaba-Myhre-Smith E71.440
  Rytand-Lipsitch I44.2
  salt
    depletion E87.1
      due to heat NEC T67.8
        causing heat exhaustion or prostration
          T67.4
    low E87.1
  salt-losing N28.89
  Scaglietti-Dagnini E22.0
  scalenus anticus (anterior) G54.0
  scapulocostal —see Mononeuropathy, upper
    limb, specified site NEC

Syndrome (Continued)
  scapuloperoneal G71.0
  schizophrenic, of childhood NEC F84.5
  Schnitzler D47.2
  Scholte's E34.0
  Schroeder's E27.0
  Schüller-Christian C96.5
  Schwachman's —see Syndrome,
    Shwachman's
  Schwartz (-Jampel) G71.13
  Schwartz-Bartter E22.2
  scimitar Q26.8
  sclerocystic ovary E28.2
  Seitelberger's G31.89
  septicemic adrenal hemorrhage A39.1
  seroconversion, retroviral (acute) Z21
  serous meningitis G93.2
  severe acute respiratory (SARS) J12.81
  shaken infant T74.4
  shock (traumatic) T79.4
    kidney N17.0
      following crush injury T79.5
    toxic A48.3
  shock-lung J80
  Shone's — code to specific anomalies
  short
    bowel K91.2
    rib Q77.2
  shoulder-hand —see Algoneurodystrophy
  Shwachman's D70.4
  sicca —see Sicca syndrome
  sick
    cell E87.1
    sinus I49.5
  sick-euthyroid E07.81
  sideropenic D50.1
  Siemens' ectodermal dysplasia Q82.4
  Silfversköld's Q78.9
  Simons' E88.1
  sinus tarsi M25.57- ◀
  sinusitis-bronchiectasis-situs inversus
    Q89.3
  Sipple's E31.22
  sirenomelia Q87.2
  Slocumb's E27.0
  slow flow, coronary I20.8
  Sluder's G44.89
  Smith-Magenis Q93.88
  Sneddon-Wilkinson L13.1
  Sotos' Q87.3 ◀
  South African cardiomyopathy I42.8
  spasmodic
    upward movement, eyes H51.8
    winking F95.8
  Spen's I45.9
  splenic
    agenesis Q89.01
    flexure K59.8
    neutropenia D73.81
  Spurway's Q78.0
  staphylococcal scalded skin L00
  steal ◀
    arteriovenous T82.898- ◀
    ischemic T82.898- ◀
    subclavian G45.8 ◀
  Stein-Leventhal E28.2
  Stein's E28.2
  Stevens-Johnson syndrome L51.1
    toxic epidermal necrolysis overlap L51.3
  Stewart-Morel M85.2
  Stickler Q89.8
  stiff baby Q89.8
  stiff man G25.82
  Still-Felty —see Felty's syndrome
  Stokes (-Adams) I45.9
  stone heart I50.1
  straight back, congenital Q76.49
  subclavian steal G45.8
  subcoracoid-pectoralis minor G54.0
  subcostal nerve compression I77.89
  subphrenic interposition Q43.3

Syndrome (Continued)
  superior
    cerebellar artery I63.8
    mesenteric artery K55.1
    semi-circular canal dehiscence H83.8X-
    vena cava I87.1
  supine hypotensive (maternal) —see
    Syndrome, hypotension, maternal
  suprarenal cortical E27.0
  supraspinatus —see also Tear, rotator cuff
    M75.10-
  Susac G93.49
  swallowed blood P78.2
  sweat retention L74.0
  Swyer Q99.1
  Symond's G93.2
  sympathetic
    cervical paralysis G90.2
    pelvic, female N94.89
  systemic inflammatory response (SIRS), of
    non-infectious origin (without organ
    dysfunction) R65.10
    with acute organ dysfunction R65.11
  tachycardia-bradycardia I49.5
  takotsubo I51.81
  TAR (thrombocytopenia with absent radius)
    Q87.2
  tarsal tunnel G57.5-
  teething K00.7
  tegmental G93.89
  telangiectasic-pigmentation-cataract
    Q82.8
  temporal pyramidal apex —see Otitis,
    media, suppurative, acute
  temporomandibular joint-pain-dysfunction
    M26.62- ◀
  Terry's H44.2-
  testicular feminization —see also Syndrome,
    androgen insensitivity E34.51
  thalamic pain (hyperesthetic) G89.0
  thoracic outlet (compression) G54.0
  Thorson-Björck E34.0
  thrombocytopenia with absent radius (TAR)
    Q87.2
  thyroid-adrenocortical insufficiency E31.0
  tibial
    anterior M76.81-
    posterior M76.82-
  Tietze's M94.0
  time-zone (rapid) G47.25
  Toni-Fanconi E72.09
    with cystinosis E72.04
  Touraine's Q79.8
  tourniquet —see Constriction, external,
    by site
  toxic shock A48.3
  transient left ventricular apical ballooning
    I51.81
  traumatic vasospastic T75.22
  Treacher Collins Q75.4
  triple X, female Q97.0
  trisomy Q92.9
    13 Q91.7
      meiotic nondisjunction Q91.4
      mitotic nondisjunction Q91.5
      mosaicism Q91.5
      translocation Q91.6
    18 Q91.3
      meiotic nondisjunction Q91.0
      mitotic nondisjunction Q91.1
      mosaicism Q91.1
      translocation Q91.2
    20 (q)(p) Q92.8
    21 Q90.9
      meiotic nondisjunction Q90.0
      mitotic nondisjunction Q90.1
      mosaicism Q90.1
      translocation Q90.2
    22 Q92.8
  tropical wet feet T69.0-
  Trousseau's I82.1

◀ New   ◀‖‖ Revised   deleted Deleted

Syndrome (Continued)
  tumor lysis (following antineoplastic chemotherapy) (spontaneous) NEC E88.3
  tumor necrosis factor receptor associated periodic (TRAPS) M04.1 ◀
  Twiddler's (due to)
    automatic implantable defibrillator T82.198
    cardiac pacemaker T82.198
  Unverricht (-Lundborg) —see Epilepsy, generalized, idiopathic
  upward gaze H51.8
  uremia, chronic —see also Disease, kidney, chronic N18.9
  urethral N34.3
  urethro-oculo-articular —see Reiter's disease
  urohepatic K76.7
  vago-hypoglossal G52.7
  van Buchem's M85.2
  van der Hoeve's Q78.0
  vascular NEC in cerebrovascular disease G46.8
  vasoconstriction, reversible cerebrovascular I67.841
  vasomotor I73.9
  vasospastic (traumatic) T75.22
  vasovagal R55
  VATER Q87.2
  velo-cardio-facial Q93.81
  vena cava (inferior) (superior) (obstruction) I87.1
  vertebral
    artery G45.0
      compression —see Syndrome, anterior, spinal artery, compression
    steal G45.0
  vertebro-basilar artery G45.0
  vertebrogenic (pain) M54.89
  vertiginous —see Disorder, vestibular function
  Vinson-Plummer D50.1
  virus B34.9
  visceral larva migrans B83.0
  visual disorientation H53.8
  vitamin B6 deficiency E53.1
  vitreal corneal H59.01-
  vitreous (touch) H59.01-
  Vogt-Koyanagi H20.82-
  Volkmann's T79.6
  von Schroetter's I82.890
  von Willebrand (-Jürgen) D68.0
  Waldenström-Kjellberg D50.1
  Wallenberg's G46.3
  water retention E87.79
  Waterhouse (-Friderichsen) A39.1
  Weber-Gubler G46.3
  Weber-Leyden G46.3
  Weber's G46.3
  Wegener's M31.30
    with
      kidney involvement M31.31
      lung involvement M31.30
        with kidney involvement M31.31
  Weingarten's (tropical eosinophilia) J82
  Weiss-Baker G90.09
  Werdnig-Hoffman G12.0
  Wermer's E31.21
  Werner's E34.8
  Wernicke-Korsakoff (nonalcoholic) F04
    alcoholic F10.26
  West's —see Epilepsy, spasms
  Westphal-Strümpell E83.01
  wet
    feet (maceration) (tropical) T69.0-
    lung, newborn P22.1
  whiplash S13.4
  whistling face Q87.0
  Wilkie's K55.1
  Wilkinson-Sneddon L13.1
  Willebrand (-Jürgens) D68.0

Syndrome (Continued)
  Wilson's (hepatolenticular degeneration) E83.01
  Wiskott-Aldrich D82.0
  withdrawal —see Withdrawal, state
    drug
      infant of dependent mother P96.1
      therapeutic use, newborn P96.2
  Woakes' (ethmoiditis) J33.1
  Wright's (hyperabduction) I77.89
  X I20.9
  XXXX Q97.1
  XXXXX Q97.1
  XXXXY Q98.1
  XXY Q98.0
  yellow nail L60.5
  Zahorsky's B08.5
  Zellweger syndrome E71.510
  Zellweger-like syndrome E71.541
Synechia (anterior) (iris) (posterior) (pupil) — see also Adhesions, iris
  intra-uterine (traumatic) N85.6
Synesthesia R20.8
Syngamiasis, syngamosis B83.3
Synodontia K00.2
Synorchidism, synorchism Q55.1
Synostosis (congenital) Q78.8
  astragalo-scaphoid Q74.2
  radioulnar Q74.0
Synovial sarcoma —see Neoplasm, connective tissue, malignant
Synovioma (malignant) —see also Neoplasm, connective tissue, malignant
  benign —see Neoplasm, connective tissue, benign
Synoviosarcoma —see Neoplasm, connective tissue, malignant
Synovitis —see also Tenosynovitis M65.9 ◀▥
  crepitant
    hand M70.0-
    wrist M70.03-
  gonococcal A54.49
  gouty —see Gout ◀▥
  in (due to)
    crystals M65.8-
    gonorrhea A54.49
    syphilis (late) A52.78
    use, overuse, pressure —see Disorder, soft tissue, due to use
  infective NEC —see Tenosynovitis, infective NEC
  specified NEC —see Tenosynovitis, specified type NEC
  syphilitic A52.78
    congenital (early) A50.02
  toxic —see Synovitis, transient
  transient M67.3-
    ankle M67.37-
    elbow M67.32-
    foot joint M67.37-
    hand joint M67.34-
    hip M67.35-
    knee M67.36-
    multiple site M67.39
    pelvic region M67.35-
    shoulder M67.31-
    specified joint NEC M67.38
    wrist M67.33-
  traumatic, current —see Sprain
  tuberculous —see Tuberculosis, synovitis
  villonodular (pigmented) M12.2-
    ankle M12.27-
    elbow M12.22-
    foot joint M12.27-
    hand joint M12.24-
    hip M12.25-
    knee M12.26-
    multiple site M12.29
    pelvic region M12.25-
    shoulder M12.21-
    specified joint NEC M12.28

Synovitis (Continued)
  villonodular (pigmented) (Continued)
    vertebrae M12.28
    wrist M12.23-
Syphilid A51.39
  congenital A50.06
  newborn A50.06
  tubercular (late) A52.79
Syphilis, syphilitic (acquired) A53.9
  abdomen (late) A52.79
  acoustic nerve A52.15
  adenopathy (secondary) A51.49
  adrenal (gland) (with cortical hypofunction) A52.79
  age under 2 years NOS —see also Syphilis, congenital, early
    acquired A51.9
  alopecia (secondary) A51.32
  anemia (late) A52.79 [D63.8]
  aneurysm (aorta) (ruptured) A52.01
    central nervous system A52.05
    congenital A50.54 [I79.0]
  anus (late) A52.74
    primary A51.1
    secondary A51.39
  aorta (arch) (abdominal) (thoracic) A52.02
    aneurysm A52.01
  aortic (insufficiency) (regurgitation) (stenosis) A52.03
    aneurysm A52.01
  arachnoid (adhesive) (cerebral) (spinal) A52.13
  asymptomatic —see Syphilis, latent
  ataxia (locomotor) A52.11
  atrophoderma maculatum A51.39
  auricular fibrillation A52.06
  bladder (late) A52.76
  bone A52.77
    secondary A51.46
  brain A52.17
  breast (late) A52.79
  bronchus (late) A52.72
  bubo (primary) A51.0
  bulbar palsy A52.19
  bursa (late) A52.78
  cardiac decompensation A52.06
  cardiovascular A52.00
  central nervous system (late) (recurrent) (relapse) (tertiary) A52.3
    with
      ataxia A52.11
      general paralysis A52.17
        juvenile A50.45
      paresis (general) A52.17
        juvenile A50.45
      tabes (dorsalis) A52.11
        juvenile A50.45
      taboparesis A52.17
        juvenile A50.45
    aneurysm A52.05
    congenital A50.40
    juvenile A50.40
    remission in (sustained) A52.3
    serology doubtful, negative, or positive A52.3
    specified nature or site NEC A52.19
    vascular A52.05
  cerebral A52.17
    meningovascular A52.13
    nerves (multiple palsies) A52.15
    sclerosis A52.17
    thrombosis A52.05
  cerebrospinal (tabetic type) A52.12
  cerebrovascular A52.05
  cervix (late) A52.76
  chancre (multiple) A51.0
    extragenital A51.2
    Rollet's A51.0
  Charcot's joint A52.16
  chorioretinitis A51.43
    congenital A50.01
    late A52.71
    prenatal A50.01

Syphilis, syphilitic *(Continued)*
  choroiditis —*see* Syphilitic chorioretinitis
  choroidoretinitis —*see* Syphilitic
      chorioretinitis
  ciliary body (secondary) A51.43
      late A52.71
  colon (late) A52.74
  combined spinal sclerosis A52.11
  condyloma (latum) A51.31
  congenital A50.9
      with
          paresis (general) A50.45
          tabes (dorsalis) A50.45
          taboparesis A50.45
      chorioretinitis, choroiditis A50.01 *[H32]*
      early, or less than 2 years after birth NEC
          A50.2
          with manifestations —*see* Syphilis,
              congenital, early, symptomatic
          latent (without manifestations) A50.1
              negative spinal fluid test A50.1
              serology positive A50.1
          symptomatic A50.09
              cutaneous A50.06
              mucocutaneous A50.07
              oculopathy A50.01
              osteochondropathy A50.02
              pharyngitis A50.03
              pneumonia A50.04
              rhinitis A50.05
              visceral A50.08
      interstitial keratitis A50.31
      juvenile neurosyphilis A50.45
      late, or 2 years or more after birth NEC
          A50.7
          chorioretinitis, choroiditis A50.32
          interstitial keratitis A50.31
          juvenile neurosyphilis A50.45
          latent (without manifestations) A50.6
              negative spinal fluid test A50.6
              serology positive A50.6
          symptomatic or with manifestations
              NEC A50.59
              arthropathy A50.55
              cardiovascular A50.54
              Clutton's joints A50.51
              Hutchinson's teeth A50.52
              Hutchinson's triad A50.53
              osteochondropathy A50.56
              saddle nose A50.57
  conjugal A53.9
      tabes A52.11
  conjunctiva (late) A52.71
  contact Z20.2
  cord bladder A52.19
  cornea, late A52.71
  coronary (artery) (sclerosis) A52.06
  coryza, congenital A50.05
  cranial nerve A52.15
      multiple palsies A52.15
  cutaneous —*see* Syphilis, skin
  dacryocystitis (late) A52.71
  degeneration, spinal cord A52.12
  dementia paralytica A52.17
      juvenilis A50.45
  destruction of bone A52.77
  dilatation, aorta A52.01
  due to blood transfusion A53.9
  dura mater A52.13
  ear A52.79
      inner A52.79
          nerve (eighth) A52.15
          neurorecurrence A52.15
  early A51.9
      cardiovascular A52.00
      central nervous system A52.3
      latent (without manifestations) (less than 2
          years after infection) A51.5
          negative spinal fluid test A51.5
          serological relapse after treatment A51.5
          serology positive A51.5

Syphilis, syphilitic *(Continued)*
  early *(Continued)*
      relapse (treated, untreated) A51.9
      skin A51.39
      symptomatic A51.9
          extragenital chancre A51.2
          primary, except extragenital chancre
              A51.0
          secondary —*see also* Syphilis, secondary
              A51.39
          relapse (treated, untreated) A51.49
      ulcer A51.39
  eighth nerve (neuritis) A52.15
  endemic A65
  endocarditis A52.03
      aortic A52.03
      pulmonary A52.03
  epididymis (late) A52.76
  epiglottis (late) A52.73
  epiphysitis (congenital) (early) A50.02
  episcleritis (late) A52.71
  esophagus A52.79
  eustachian tube A52.73
  exposure to Z20.2
  eye A52.71
  eyelid (late) (with gumma) A52.71
  fallopian tube (late) A52.76
  fracture A52.77
  gallbladder (late) A52.74
  gastric (polyposis) (late) A52.74
  general A53.9
      paralysis A52.17
          juvenile A50.45
  genital (primary) A51.0
  glaucoma A52.71
  gumma NEC A52.79
      cardiovascular system A52.00
      central nervous system A52.3
      congenital A50.59
  heart (block) (decompensation) (disease)
      (failure) A52.06 *[I52]*
      valve NEC A52.03
  hemianesthesia A52.19
  hemianopsia A52.71
  hemiparesis A52.17
  hemiplegia A52.17
  hepatic artery A52.09
  hepatis A52.74
  hepatomegaly, congenital A50.08
  hereditaria tarda —*see* Syphilis, congenital,
      late
  hereditary —*see* Syphilis, congenital
  Hutchinson's teeth A50.52
  hyalitis A52.71
  inactive —*see* Syphilis, latent
  infantum —*see* Syphilis, congenital
  inherited —*see* Syphilis, congenital
  internal ear A52.79
  intestine (late) A52.74
  iris, iritis (secondary) A51.43
      late A52.71
  joint (late) A52.77
  keratitis (congenital) (interstitial) (late) A50.31
  kidney (late) A52.75
  lacrimal passages (late) A52.71
  larynx (late) A52.73
  late A52.9
      cardiovascular A52.00
      central nervous system A52.3
      kidney A52.75
      latent or 2 years or more after infection
          (without manifestations) A52.8
          negative spinal fluid test A52.8
          serology positive A52.8
      paresis A52.17
      specified site NEC A52.79
      symptomatic or with manifestations A52.79
      tabes A52.11
  latent A53.0
      with signs or symptoms - code by site and
          stage under Syphilis

Syphilis, syphilitic *(Continued)*
  latent *(Continued)*
      central nervous system A52.2
      date of infection unspecified A53.0
      early, or less than 2 years after infection
          A51.5
          follow-up of latent syphilis A53.0
              date of infection unspecified A53.0
              late, or 2 years or more after infection
                  A52.8
          late, or 2 years or more after infection
              A52.8
          positive serology (only finding) A53.0
              date of infection unspecified A53.0
              early, or less than 2 years after infection
                  A51.5
              late, or 2 years or more after infection
                  A52.8
  lens (late) A52.71
  leukoderma A51.39
      late A52.79
  lienitis A52.79
  lip A51.39
      chancre (primary) A51.2
      late A52.79
  Lissauer's paralysis A52.17
  liver A52.74
  locomotor ataxia A52.11
  lung A52.72
  lymph gland (early) (secondary) A51.49
      late A52.79
  lymphadenitis (secondary) A51.49
  macular atrophy of skin A51.39
      striated A52.79
  mediastinum (late) A52.73
  meninges (adhesive) (brain) (spinal cord)
      A52.13
  meningitis A52.13
      acute (secondary) A51.41
      congenital A50.41
  meningoencephalitis A52.14
  meningovascular A52.13
      congenital A50.41
  mesarteritis A52.09
      brain A52.04
  middle ear A52.77
  mitral stenosis A52.03
  monoplegia A52.17
  mouth (secondary) A51.39
      late A52.79
  mucocutaneous (secondary) A51.39
      late A52.79
  mucous
      membrane (secondary) A51.39
          late A52.79
      patches A51.39
          congenital A50.07
  mulberry molars A50.52
  muscle A52.78
  myocardium A52.06
  nasal sinus (late) A52.73
  neonatorum —*see* Syphilis, congenital
  nephrotic syndrome (secondary)
      A51.44
  nerve palsy (any cranial nerve) A52.15
      multiple A52.15
  nervous system, central A52.3
  neuritis A52.15
      acoustic A52.15
  neurorecidive of retina A52.19
  neuroretinitis A52.19
  newborn —*see* Syphilis, congenital
  nodular superficial (late) A52.79
  nonvenereal A65
  nose (late) A52.73
      saddle back deformity A50.57
  occlusive arterial disease A52.09
  oculopathy A52.71
  ophthalmic (late) A52.71
  optic nerve (atrophy) (neuritis) (papilla)
      A52.15

◄ New   ◄▦ Revised   ~~deleted~~ Deleted

Syphilis, syphilitic (Continued)
orbit (late) A52.71
organic A53.9
osseous (late) A52.77
osteochondritis (congenital) (early) A50.02
[M90.80]
osteoporosis A52.77
ovary (late) A52.76
oviduct (late) A52.76
palate (late) A52.79
pancreas (late) A52.74
paralysis A52.17
general A52.17
juvenile A50.45
paresis (general) A52.17
juvenile A50.45
paresthesia A52.19
Parkinson's disease or syndrome A52.19
paroxysmal tachycardia A52.06
pemphigus (congenital) A50.06
penis (chancre) A51.0
late A52.76
pericardium A52.06
perichondritis, larynx (late) A52.73
periosteum (late) A52.77
congenital (early) A50.02 [M90.80]
early (secondary) A51.46
peripheral nerve A52.79
petrous bone (late) A52.77
pharynx (late) A52.73
secondary A51.39
pituitary (gland) A52.79
pleura (late) A52.73
pneumonia, white A50.04
pontine lesion A52.17
portal vein A52.09
primary A51.0
anal A51.1
and secondary —see Syphilis, secondary
central nervous system A52.3
extragenital chancre NEC A51.2
fingers A51.2
genital A51.0
lip A51.2
specified site NEC A51.2
tonsils A51.2
prostate (late) A52.76
ptosis (eyelid) A52.71
pulmonary (late) A52.72
artery A52.09
pyelonephritis (late) A52.75
recently acquired, symptomatic A51.9
rectum (late) A52.74
respiratory tract (late) A52.73
retina, late A52.71
retrobulbar neuritis A52.15
salpingitis A52.76
sclera (late) A52.71
sclerosis
cerebral A52.17
coronary A52.06
multiple A52.11
scotoma (central) A52.71
scrotum (late) A52.76

Syphilis, syphilitic (Continued)
secondary (and primary) A51.49
adenopathy A51.49
anus A51.39
bone A51.46
chorioretinitis, choroiditis A51.43
hepatitis A51.45
liver A51.45
lymphadenitis A51.49
meningitis (acute) A51.41
mouth A51.39
mucous membranes A51.39
periosteum, periostitis A51.46
pharynx A51.39
relapse (treated, untreated) A51.49
skin A51.39
specified form NEC A51.49
tonsil A51.39
ulcer A51.39
viscera NEC A51.49
vulva A51.39
seminal vesicle (late) A52.76
seronegative with signs or symptoms - code
by site and stage under Syphilis
seropositive
with signs or symptoms - code by site and
stage under Syphilis
follow-up of latent syphilis —see Syphilis,
latent
only finding —see Syphilis, latent
seventh nerve (paralysis) A52.15
sinus, sinusitis (late) A52.73
skeletal system A52.77
skin (with ulceration) (early) (secondary)
A51.39
late or tertiary A52.79
small intestine A52.74
spastic spinal paralysis A52.17
spermatic cord (late) A52.76
spinal (cord) A52.12
spleen A52.79
splenomegaly A52.79
spondylitis A52.77
staphyloma A52.71
stigmata (congenital) A50.59
stomach A52.74
synovium A52.78
tabes dorsalis (late) A52.11
juvenile A50.45
tabetic type A52.11
juvenile A50.45
taboparesis A52.17
juvenile A50.45
tachycardia A52.06
tendon (late) A52.78
tertiary A52.9
with symptoms NEC A52.79
cardiovascular A52.00
central nervous system A52.3
multiple NEC A52.79
specified site NEC A52.79
testis A52.76
thorax A52.73
throat A52.73

Syphilis, syphilitic (Continued)
thymus (gland) (late) A52.79
thyroid (late) A52.79
tongue (late) A52.79
tonsil (lingual) (late) A52.73
primary A51.2
secondary A51.39
trachea (late) A52.73
tunica vaginalis (late) A52.76
ulcer (any site) (early) (secondary)
A51.39
late A52.79
perforating A52.79
foot A52.11
urethra (late) A52.76
urogenital (late) A52.76
uterus (late) A52.76
uveal tract (secondary) A51.43
late A52.71
uveitis (secondary) A51.43
late A52.71
uvula (late) (perforated) A52.79
vagina A51.0
late A52.76
valvulitis NEC A52.03
vascular A52.00
brain (cerebral) A52.05
ventriculi A52.74
vesicae urinariae (late) A52.76
viscera (abdominal) (late) A52.74
secondary A51.49
vitreous (opacities) (late) A52.71
hemorrhage A52.71
vulva A51.0
late A52.76
secondary A51.39
Syphiloma A52.79
cardiovascular system A52.00
central nervous system A52.3
circulatory system A52.00
congenital A50.59
Syphilophobia F45.29
Syringadenoma —see also Neoplasm, skin,
benign
papillary —see Neoplasm, skin, benign
Syringobulbia G95.0
Syringocystadenoma —see Neoplasm, skin,
benign
papillary —see Neoplasm, skin, benign
Syringoma —see also Neoplasm, skin, benign
chondroid —see Neoplasm, skin, benign
Syringomyelia G95.0
Syringomyelitis —see Encephalitis
Syringomyelocele —see Spina bifida
Syringopontia G95.0
System, systemic —see also condition
disease, combined —see Degeneration,
combined
inflammatory response syndrome (SIRS) of
non-infectious origin (without organ
dysfunction) R65.10
with acute organ dysfunction R65.11
lupus erythematosus M32.9
inhibitor present D68.62

T

Tabacism, tabacosis, tabagism —*see also*
    Poisoning, tobacco
    meaning dependence (without remission)
        F17.200
        with
            disorder F17.299
                remission F17.211
                specified disorder NEC F17.298
                withdrawal F17.203
Tabardillo A75.9
    flea-borne A75.2
    louse-borne A75.0
Tabes, tabetic A52.10
    with
        central nervous system syphilis A52.10
        Charcot's joint A52.16
        cord bladder A52.19
        crisis, viscera (any) A52.19
        paralysis, general A52.17
        paresis (general) A52.17
        perforating ulcer (foot) A52.19
    arthropathy (Charcot) A52.16
    bladder A52.19
    bone A52.11
    cerebrospinal A52.12
    congenital A50.45
    conjugal A52.10
    dorsalis A52.11
        juvenile A50.49
    juvenile A50.49
    latent A52.19
    mesenterica A18.39
    paralysis, insane, general A52.17
    spasmodic A52.17
    syphilis (cerebrospinal) A52.12
Taboparalysis A52.17
Taboparesis (remission) A52.17
    juvenile A50.45
TAC (trigeminal autonomic cephalgia) NEC
        G44.099
    intractable G44.091
    not intractable G44.099
Tache noir S60.22-
Tachyalimentation K91.2
Tachyarrhythmia, tachyrhythmia —*see*
        Tachycardia
Tachycardia R00.0
    atrial (paroxysmal) I47.1
    auricular I47.1
    AV nodal re-entry (re-entrant) I47.1
    junctional (paroxysmal) I47.1
    newborn P29.11
    nodal (paroxysmal) I47.1
    non-paroxysmal AV nodal I45.89
    paroxysmal (sustained) (nonsustained)
        I47.9
        with sinus bradycardia I49.5
        atrial (PAT) I47.1
        atrioventricular (AV) (re-entrant) I47.1
            psychogenic F54
        junctional I47.1
            ectopic I47.1
        nodal I47.1
        psychogenic (atrial) (supraventricular)
            (ventricular) F54
        supraventricular (sustained) I47.1
            psychogenic F54
        ventricular I47.2
            psychogenic F54
    psychogenic F45.8
    sick sinus I49.5
    sinoauricular NOS R00.0
        paroxysmal I47.1
    sinus [sinusal] NOS R00.0
        paroxysmal I47.1
    supraventricular I47.1
    ventricular (paroxysmal) (sustained) I47.2
        psychogenic F54
Tachygastria K31.89

Tachypnea R06.82
    hysterical F45.8
    newborn (idiopathic) (transitory) P22.1
    psychogenic F45.8
    transitory, of newborn P22.1
TACO (transfusion associated circulatory
        overload) E87.71
Taenia (infection) (infestation) B68.9
    diminuta B71.0
    echinococcal infestation B67.90
    mediocanellata B68.1
    nana B71.0
    saginata B68.1
    solium (intestinal form) B68.0
        larval form —*see* Cysticercosis
Taeniasis (intestine) —*see* Taenia
Tag (hypertrophied skin) (infected) L91.8
    adenoid J35.8
    anus K64.4
    hemorrhoidal K64.4
    hymen N89.8
    perineal N90.89
    preauricular Q17.0
    sentinel K64.4
    skin L91.8
        accessory (congenital) Q82.8
        anus K64.4
        congenital Q82.8
        preauricular Q17.0
    tonsil J35.8
    urethra, urethral N36.8
    vulva N90.89
Tahyna fever B33.8
Takahara's disease E80.3
Takayasu's disease or syndrome M31.4
Talcosis (pulmonary) J62.0
Talipes (congenital) Q66.89
    acquired, planus —*see* Deformity, limb, flat
        foot
    asymmetric Q66.89
    calcaneovalgus Q66.4
    calcaneovarus Q66.1
    calcaneus Q66.89
    cavus Q66.7
    equinovalgus Q66.6
    equinovarus Q66.0
    equinus Q66.89
    percavus Q66.7
    planovalgus Q66.6
    planus (acquired) (any degree) —*see also*
        Deformity, limb, flat foot
        congenital Q66.5-
        due to rickets (sequelae) E64.3
    valgus Q66.6
    varus Q66.3
Tall stature, constitutional E34.4
Talma's disease M62.89
Talon noir S90.3-
    hand S60.22-
    heel S90.3-
    toe S90.1-
Tamponade, heart I31.4
Tanapox (virus disease) B08.71
Tangier disease E78.6
Tantrum, child problem F91.8
Tapeworm (infection) (infestation) —*see*
        Infestation, tapeworm
Tapia's syndrome G52.7
TAR (thrombocytopenia with absent radius)
        syndrome Q87.2
Tarral-Besnier disease L44.0
Tarsal tunnel syndrome —*see* Syndrome, tarsal
        tunnel
Tarsalgia —*see* Pain, limb, lower
Tarsitis (eyelid) H01.8
    syphilitic A52.71
    tuberculous A18.4
Tartar (teeth) (dental calculus) K03.6
Tattoo (mark) L81.8
Tauri's disease E74.09
Taurodontism K00.2

Taussig-Bing syndrome Q20.1
Taybi's syndrome Q87.2
Tay-Sachs amaurotic familial idiocy or disease
        E75.02
TBI (traumatic brain injury) S06.9 ◄▥
Teacher's node or nodule J38.2
Tear, torn (traumatic) —*see also* Laceration
    with abortion —*see* Abortion
    annular fibrosis M51.35
    anus, anal (sphincter) S31.831
        complicating delivery
            with third degree perineal laceration —
                see also Delivery, complicated, by,
                laceration, perineum, third degree
                O70.20 ◄▥
                with mucosa O70.3
            without third degree perineal laceration
                O70.4
        nontraumatic (healed) (old) K62.81
    articular cartilage, old —*see* Derangement,
        joint, articular cartilage, by site
    bladder
        with ectopic or molar pregnancy O08.6
        following ectopic or molar pregnancy
            O08.6
        obstetrical O71.5
        traumatic —*see* Injury, bladder
    bowel
        with ectopic or molar pregnancy O08.6
        following ectopic or molar pregnancy
            O08.6
        obstetrical trauma O71.5
    broad ligament
        with ectopic or molar pregnancy O08.6
        following ectopic or molar pregnancy O08.6
        obstetrical trauma O71.6
    bucket handle (knee) (meniscus) —*see* Tear,
        meniscus
    capsule, joint —*see* Sprain
    cartilage —*see also* Sprain
        articular, old —*see* Derangement, joint,
            articular cartilage, by site
    cervix
        with ectopic or molar pregnancy O08.6
        following ectopic or molar pregnancy
            O08.6
        obstetrical trauma (current) O71.3
        old N88.1
        traumatic —*see* Injury, uterus
    dural G97.41
        nontraumatic G96.11
    internal organ —*see* Injury, by site
    knee cartilage
        articular (current) S83.3-
        old —*see* Derangement, knee, meniscus,
            due to old tear
    ligament —*see* Sprain
    meniscus (knee) (current injury) S83.209
        bucket-handle S83.20-
        lateral
            bucket-handle S83.25-
            complex S83.27-
            peripheral S83.26-
            specified type NEC S83.28-
        medial
            bucket-handle S83.21-
            complex S83.23-
            peripheral S83.22-
            specified type NEC S83.24-
        old —*see* Derangement, knee, meniscus,
            due to old tear
        site other than knee - code as Sprain
        specified type NEC S83.20-
    muscle —*see* Strain
    pelvic
        floor, complicating delivery O70.1
        organ NEC, obstetrical trauma O71.5
            with ectopic or molar pregnancy O08.6
            following ectopic or molar pregnancy
                O08.6
    perineal, secondary O90.1

◄ New   ◄▥ Revised   ~~deleted~~ Deleted

Tear, torn *(Continued)*
  periurethral tissue, obstetrical trauma O71.82
    with ectopic or molar pregnancy O08.6
    following ectopic or molar pregnancy O08.6
  rectovaginal septum —*see* Laceration, vagina
  retina, retinal (without detachment)
    (horseshoe) —*see also* Break, retina, horseshoe
    with detachment —*see* Detachment, retina, with retinal, break
  rotator cuff (nontraumatic) M75.10-
    complete M75.12-
    incomplete M75.11-
    traumatic S46.01-
      capsule S43.42-
  semilunar cartilage, knee —*see* Tear, meniscus
  supraspinatus (complete) (incomplete) (nontraumatic) —*see also* Tear, rotator cuff M75.10-
  tendon —*see* Strain
  tentorial, at birth P10.4
  umbilical cord
    complicating delivery O69.89
  urethra
    with ectopic or molar pregnancy O08.6
    following ectopic or molar pregnancy O08.6
    obstetrical trauma O71.5
  uterus —*see* Injury, uterus
  vagina —*see* Laceration, vagina
  vessel, from catheter —*see* Puncture, accidental complicating surgery
  vulva, complicating delivery O70.0
Tear-stone —*see* Dacryolith
Teeth —*see also* condition
  grinding
    psychogenic F45.8
    sleep related G47.63
Teething (syndrome) K00.7
Telangiectasia, telangiectasis (verrucous) I78.1
  ataxic (cerebellar) (Louis-Bar) G11.3
  familial I78.0
  hemorrhagic, hereditary (congenital) (senile) I78.0
  hereditary, hemorrhagic (congenital) (senile) I78.0
  juxtafoveal H35.07-
  macular H35.07-
  parafoveal H35.07-
  retinal (idiopathic) (juxtafoveal) (macular) (parafoveal) H35.07-
  spider I78.1
Telephone scatologia F65.89
Telescoped bowel or intestine K56.1
  congenital Q43.8
Temperature
  body, high (of unknown origin) R50.9
  cold, trauma from T69.9
    newborn P80.0
    specified effect NEC T69.8
Temple —*see* condition
Temporal —*see* condition
Temporomandibular joint pain-dysfunction syndrome M26.62- ◀▥
Temporosphenoidal —*see* condition
Tendency
  bleeding —*see* Defect, coagulation
  suicide
    meaning personal history of attempted suicide Z91.5
    meaning suicidal ideation —*see* Ideation, suicidal
  to fall R29.6
Tenderness, abdominal R10.819
  epigastric R10.816
  generalized R10.817
  left lower quadrant R10.814
  left upper quadrant R10.812
  periumbilic R10.815

Tenderness, abdominal *(Continued)*
  rebound R10.829
    epigastric R10.826
    generalized R10.827
    left lower quadrant R10.824
    left upper quadrant R10.822
    periumbilic R10.825
    right lower quadrant R10.823
    right upper quadrant R10.821
  right lower quadrant R10.813
  right upper quadrant R10.811
Tendinitis, tendonitis —*see also* Enthesopathy
  Achilles M76.6-
  adhesive —*see* Tenosynovitis, specified type NEC
    shoulder —*see* Capsulitis, adhesive
  bicipital M75.2-
  calcific M65.2-
    ankle M65.27-
    foot M65.27-
    forearm M65.23-
    hand M65.24-
    lower leg M65.26-
    multiple sites M65.29
    pelvic region M65.25-
    shoulder M75.3-
    specified site NEC M65.28
    thigh M65.25-
    upper arm M65.22-
  due to use, overuse, pressure —*see also* Disorder, soft tissue, due to use
    specified NEC —*see* Disorder, soft tissue, due to use, specified NEC
  gluteal M76.0-
  patellar M76.5-
  peroneal M76.7-
  psoas M76.1-
  tibial (posterior) M76.82-
    anterior M76.81-
  trochanteric —*see* Bursitis, hip, trochanteric
Tendon —*see* condition
Tendosynovitis —*see* Tenosynovitis
Tenesmus (rectal) R19.8
  vesical R30.1
Tennis elbow —*see* Epicondylitis, lateral
Tenonitis —*see also* Tenosynovitis
  eye (capsule) H05.04-
Tenontosynovitis —*see* Tenosynovitis
Tenontothecitis —*see* Tenosynovitis
Tenophyte —*see* Disorder, synovium, specified type NEC
Tenosynovitis —*see also* Synovitis M65.9
  adhesive —*see* Tenosynovitis, specified type NEC
    shoulder —*see* Capsulitis, adhesive
  bicipital (calcifying) —*see* Tendinitis, bicipital
  gonococcal A54.49
  in (due to)
    crystals M65.8-
    gonorrhea A54.49
    syphilis (late) A52.78
    use, overuse, pressure —*see also* Disorder, soft tissue, due to use
      specified NEC —*see* Disorder, soft tissue, due to use, specified NEC
  infective NEC M65.1-
    ankle M65.17-
    foot M65.17-
    forearm M65.13-
    hand M65.14-
    lower leg M65.16-
    multiple sites M65.19
    pelvic region M65.15-
    shoulder region M65.11-
    specified site NEC M65.18
    thigh M65.15-
    upper arm M65.12-
  radial styloid M65.4
  shoulder region M65.81-
    adhesive —*see* Capsulitis, adhesive

Tenosynovitis *(Continued)*
  specified type NEC M65.88-
    ankle M65.87-
    foot M65.87-
    forearm M65.83-
    hand M65.84-
    lower leg M65.86-
    multiple sites M65.89
    pelvic region M65.85-
    shoulder region M65.81-
    specified site NEC M65.88
    thigh M65.85-
    upper arm M65.82-
  tuberculous —*see* Tuberculosis, tenosynovitis
Tenovaginitis —*see* Tenosynovitis
Tension
  arterial, high —*see also* Hypertension
    without diagnosis of hypertension R03.0
  headache G44.209
    intractable G44.201
    not intractable G44.209
  nervous R45.0
  pneumothorax J93.0
  premenstrual N94.3
  state (mental) F48.9
Tentorium —*see* condition
Teratencephalus Q89.8
Teratism Q89.7
Teratoblastoma (malignant) —*see* Neoplasm, malignant, by site
Teratocarcinoma —*see also* Neoplasm, malignant, by site
  liver C22.7
Teratoma (solid) —*see also* Neoplasm, uncertain behavior, by site
  with embryonal carcinoma, mixed —*see* Neoplasm, malignant, by site
  with malignant transformation —*see* Neoplasm, malignant, by site
  adult (cystic) —*see* Neoplasm, benign, by site
  benign —*see* Neoplasm, benign, by site
  combined with choriocarcinoma —*see* Neoplasm, malignant, by site
  cystic (adult) —*see* Neoplasm, benign, by site
  differentiated —*see* Neoplasm, benign, by site
  embryonal —*see also* Neoplasm, malignant, by site
    liver C22.7
  immature —*see* Neoplasm, malignant, by site
  liver C22.7
    adult, benign, cystic, differentiated type or mature D13.4
  malignant —*see also* Neoplasm, malignant, by site
    anaplastic —*see* Neoplasm, malignant, by site
    intermediate —*see* Neoplasm, malignant, by site
      specified site —*see* Neoplasm, malignant, by site
    unspecified site C62.90
    undifferentiated —*see* Neoplasm, malignant, by site
  mature —*see* Neoplasm, uncertain behavior, by site
    malignant —*see* Neoplasm, by site, malignant, by site
  ovary D27.-
    embryonal, immature or malignant C56-
  solid —*see* Neoplasm, uncertain behavior, by site
  testis C62.9-
    adult, benign, cystic, differentiated type or mature D29.2-
    scrotal C62.1-
    undescended C62.0-
Termination
  anomalous —*see also* Malposition, congenital
    right pulmonary vein Q26.3
  pregnancy, elective Z33.2

Ternidens diminutus infestation B81.8
Ternidensiasis B81.8
Terror (s) night (child) F51.4
Terrorism, victim of Z65.4
Terry's syndrome H44.2-
Tertiary —*see* condition
Test, tests, testing (for)
　adequacy (for dialysis)
　　hemodialysis Z49.31
　　peritoneal Z49.32
　blood pressure Z01.30
　　abnormal reading —*see* Blood, pressure
　blood typing Z01.83
　　Rh typing Z01.83
　blood-alcohol Z04.8
　　positive —*see* Findings, abnormal, in
　　　blood
　blood-drug Z04.8
　　positive —*see* Findings, abnormal, in
　　　blood
　cardiac pulse generator (battery) Z45.010
　fertility Z31.41
　genetic
　　disease carrier status for procreative
　　　management
　　　female Z31.430
　　　male Z31.440
　　male partner of patient with recurrent
　　　pregnancy loss Z31.441
　　procreative management NEC
　　　female Z31.438
　　　male Z31.448
　hearing Z01.10
　　with abnormal findings NEC Z01.118
　HIV (human immunodeficiency virus)
　　nonconclusive (in infants) R75
　　positive Z21
　　seropositive Z21
　immunity status Z01.84
　intelligence NEC Z01.89
　laboratory (as part of a general medical
　　examination) Z00.00
　　with abnormal finding Z00.01
　　for medicolegal reason NEC Z04.8
　male partner of patient with recurrent
　　pregnancy loss Z31.441
　Mantoux (for tuberculosis) Z11.1
　　abnormal result R76.11
　pregnancy, positive first pregnancy —*see*
　　Pregnancy, normal, first
　procreative Z31.49
　　fertility Z31.41
　skin, diagnostic
　　allergy Z01.82
　　　special screening examination —*see*
　　　　Screening, by name of disease
　　Mantoux Z11.1
　　tuberculin Z11.1
　specified NEC Z01.89
　tuberculin Z11.1
　　abnormal result R76.11
　vision Z01.00
　　with abnormal findings Z01.01
　Wassermann Z11.3
　　positive —*see* Serology for syphilis,
　　　positive
Testicle, testicular, testis —*see also* condition
　feminization syndrome —*see also* Syndrome,
　　androgen insensitivity E34.51
　migrans Q55.29
Tetanus, tetanic (cephalic) (convulsions) A35
　with
　　abortion A34
　　ectopic or molar pregnancy O08.0
　　following ectopic or molar pregnancy
　　　O08.0
　　inoculation reaction (due to serum) —*see*
　　　Complications, vaccination
　neonatorum A33
　obstetrical A34
　puerperal, postpartum, childbirth A34

Tetany (due to) R29.0
　alkalosis E87.3
　associated with rickets E55.0
　convulsions R29.0
　　hysterical F44.5
　functional (hysterical) F44.5
　hyperkinetic R29.0
　　hysterical F44.5
　hyperpnea R06.4
　　hysterical F44.5
　　psychogenic F45.8
　hyperventilation —*see also* Hyperventilation
　　R06.4
　　hysterical F44.5
　neonatal (without calcium or magnesium
　　deficiency) P71.3
　parathyroid (gland) E20.9
　parathyroprival E89.2
　post- (para)thyroidectomy E89.2
　postoperative E89.2
　pseudotetany R29.0
　psychogenic (conversion reaction) F44.5
Tetralogy of Fallot Q21.3
Tetraplegia (chronic) —*see also* Quadriplegia
　G82.50-
Thailand hemorrhagic fever A91
Thalassanemia —*see* Thalassemia
Thalassemia (anemia) (disease) D56.9
　with other hemoglobinopathy D56.8
　alpha (major) (severe) (triple gene defect)
　　D56.0
　　minor D56.3
　　silent carrier D56.3
　　trait D56.3
　beta (severe) D56.1
　　homozygous D56.1
　　major D56.1
　　minor D56.3
　　trait D56.3
　delta-beta (homozygous) D56.2
　　minor D56.3
　　trait D56.3
　dominant D56.8
　hemoglobin
　　C D56.8
　　E-beta D56.5
　intermedia D56.1
　major D56.1
　minor D56.3
　mixed D56.8
　sickle-cell —*see* Disease, sickle-cell,
　　thalassemia
　specified type NEC D56.8
　trait D56.3
　variants D56.8
Thanatophoric dwarfism or short stature Q77.1
Thaysen-Gee disease (nontropical sprue) K90.0
Thaysen's disease K90.0
Thecoma D27-
　luteinized D27-
　malignant C56-
Thelarche, premature E30.8
Thelaziasis B83.8
Thelitis N61.0 ◀▥
　puerperal, postpartum or gestational —*see*
　　Infection, nipple
Therapeutic —*see* condition
Therapy
　drug, long-term (current) (prophylactic)
　　agents affecting estrogen receptors and
　　　estrogen levels NEC Z79.818
　　anastrozole (Arimidex) Z79.811
　　antibiotics Z79.2
　　　short-term use - omit code
　　anticoagulants Z79.01
　　anti-inflammatory Z79.1
　　antiplatelet Z79.02
　　antithrombotics Z79.02
　　aromatase inhibitors Z79.811
　　aspirin Z79.82
　　birth control pill or patch Z79.3

Therapy (*Continued*)
　drug, long-term (*Continued*)
　　bisphosphonates Z79.83
　　contraceptive, oral Z79.3
　　drug, specified NEC Z79.899
　　estrogen receptor downregulators
　　　Z79.818
　　Evista Z79.810
　　exemestane (Aromasin) Z79.811
　　Fareston Z79.810
　　fulvestrant (Faslodex) Z79.818
　　gonadotropin-releasing hormone (GnRH)
　　　agonist Z79.818
　　goserelin acetate (Zoladex) Z79.818
　　hormone replacement (postmenopausal)
　　　Z79.890
　　insulin Z79.4
　　letrozole (Femara) Z79.811
　　leuprolide acetate (leuprorelin) (Lupron)
　　　Z79.818
　　megestrol acetate (Megace) Z79.818
　　methadone
　　　for pain management Z79.891
　　　maintenance therapy F11.20
　　Nolvadex Z79.810
　　opiate analgesic Z79.891
　　oral contraceptive Z79.3
　　raloxifene (Evista) Z79.810
　　selective estrogen receptor modulators
　　　(SERMs) Z79.810
　　short term - omit code
　　steroids
　　　inhaled Z79.51
　　　systemic Z79.52
　　tamoxifen (Nolvadex) Z79.810
　　toremifene (Fareston) Z79.810
Thermic —*see* condition
Thermography (abnormal) —*see also* Abnormal,
　　diagnostic imaging R93.8
　breast R92.8
Thermoplegia T67.0
Thesaurismosis, glycogen —*see* Disease,
　　glycogen storage
Thiamin deficiency E51.9
　specified NEC E51.8
Thiaminic deficiency with beriberi E51.11
Thibierge-Weissenbach syndrome —*see*
　　Sclerosis, systemic
Thickening
　bone —*see* Hypertrophy, bone
　breast N64.59
　endometrium R93.8
　epidermal L85.9
　　specified NEC L85.8
　hymen N89.6
　larynx J38.7
　nail L60.2
　　congenital Q84.5
　periosteal —*see* Hypertrophy, bone
　pleura J92.9
　　with asbestos J92.0
　skin R23.4
　subepiglottic J38.7
　tongue K14.8
　valve, heart —*see* Endocarditis
Thigh —*see* condition
Thinning vertebra —*see* Spondylopathy,
　　specified NEC
Thirst, excessive R63.1
　due to deprivation of water T73.1
Thomsen disease G71.12
Thoracic —*see also* condition
　kidney Q63.2
　outlet syndrome G54.0
Thoracogastroschisis (congenital) Q79.8
Thoracopagus Q89.4
Thorax —*see* condition
Thorn's syndrome N28.89
Thorson-Björck syndrome E34.0
Threadworm (infection) (infestation)
　B80

◀ New　⬅▥ Revised　~~deleted~~ Deleted

Threatened
abortion O20.0
  with subsequent abortion O03.9
job loss, anxiety concerning Z56.2
labor (without delivery) O47.9
~~after 37 completed weeks of gestation O47.1~~
  at or after 37 completed weeks of gestation O47.1 ◀
  before 37 completed weeks of gestation O47.0-
loss of job, anxiety concerning Z56.2
miscarriage O20.0
unemployment, anxiety concerning Z56.2
Three-day fever A93.1
Threshers' lung J67.0
Thrix annulata (congenital) Q84.1
Throat —see condition
Thrombasthenia (Glanzmann) (hemorrhagic) (hereditary) D69.1
Thromboangiitis I73.1
obliterans (general) I73.1
  cerebral I67.89
  vessels
    brain I67.89
    spinal cord I67.89
Thromboarteritis —see Arteritis
Thromboasthenia (Glanzmann) (hemorrhagic) (hereditary) D69.1
Thrombocytasthenia (Glanzmann) D69.1
Thrombocythemia (essential) (hemorrhagic) (idiopathic) (primary) D47.3
Thrombocytopathy (dystrophic) (granulopenic) D69.1
Thrombocytopenia, thrombocytopenic D69.6
with absent radius (TAR) Q87.2
congenital D69.42
dilutional D69.59
due to
  drugs D69.59
  extracorporeal circulation of blood D69.59
  (massive)blood transfusion D69.59
  platelet alloimmunization D69.59
essential D69.3
heparin induced (HIT) D75.82
hereditary D69.42
idiopathic D69.3
neonatal, transitory P61.0
  due to
    exchange transfusion P61.0
    idiopathic maternal thrombocytopenia P61.0
    isoimmunization P61.0
primary NEC D69.49
  idiopathic D69.3
puerperal, postpartum O72.3
secondary D69.59
transient neonatal P61.0
Thrombocytosis, essential D47.3
primary D47.3
Thromboembolism —see Embolism
Thrombopathy (Bernard-Soulier) D69.1
constitutional D68.0
Willebrand-Jurgens D68.0
Thrombopenia —see Thrombocytopenia
Thrombophilia D68.59
primary NEC D68.59
secondary NEC D68.69
specified NEC D68.69
Thrombophlebitis I80.9
antepartum O22.2-
  deep O22.3-
  superficial O22.2-
cavernous (venous) sinus G08
  complicating pregnancy O22.5-
  nonpyogenic I67.6
cerebral (sinus) (vein) G08
  nonpyogenic I67.6
  sequelae G09
due to implanted device —see Complications, by site and type, specified NEC

Thrombophlebitis (Continued)
during or resulting from a procedure NEC T81.72
femoral vein (superficial) I80.1-
femoropopliteal vein I80.0-
hepatic (vein) I80.8
idiopathic, recurrent I82.1
iliofemoral I80.1-
intracranial venous sinus (any) G08
  nonpyogenic I67.6
  sequelae G09
intraspinal venous sinuses and veins G08
  nonpyogenic G95.19
lateral (venous) sinus G08
  nonpyogenic I67.6
leg I80.299
  superficial I80.0-
longitudinal (venous) sinus G08
  nonpyogenic I67.6
lower extremity I80.299
migrans, migrating I82.1
pelvic
  with ectopic or molar pregnancy O08.0
  following ectopic or molar pregnancy O08.0
  puerperal O87.1
popliteal vein —see Phlebitis, leg, deep, popliteal
portal (vein) K75.1
postoperative T81.72
pregnancy —see Thrombophlebitis, antepartum
puerperal, postpartum, childbirth O87.0
  deep O87.1
  pelvic O87.1
  septic O86.81
  superficial O87.0
saphenous (greater) (lesser) I80.0-
sinus (intracranial) G08
  nonpyogenic I67.6
specified site NEC I80.8
tibial vein I80.23-
Thrombosis, thrombotic (bland) (multiple) (progressive) (silent) (vessel) I82.90
anal K64.5
antepartum —see Thrombophlebitis, antepartum
aorta, aortic I74.10
  abdominal I74.09
    saddle I74.01
  bifurcation I74.09
  saddle I74.01
  specified site NEC I74.19
  terminal I74.09
  thoracic I74.11
  valve —see Endocarditis, aortic
apoplexy I63.3- ◀▥
artery, arteries (postinfectional) I74.9
  auditory, internal —see Occlusion, artery, precerebral, specified NEC
  basilar —see Occlusion, artery, basilar
  carotid (common) (internal) —see Occlusion, artery, carotid
  cerebellar (anterior inferior) (posterior inferior) (superior) —see Occlusion, artery, cerebellar
  cerebral —see Occlusion, artery, cerebral
  choroidal (anterior) —see Occlusion, artery, cerebral, specified NEC
  communicating, posterior —see Occlusion, artery, cerebral, specified NEC
  coronary —see also Infarct, myocardium
    not resulting in infarction I24.0
  hepatic I74.8
  hypophyseal —see Occlusion, artery, cerebral, specified NEC
  iliac I74.5
  limb I74.4
    lower I74.3
    upper I74.2

Thrombosis, thrombotic (Continued)
artery, arteries (Continued)
  meningeal, anterior or posterior —see Occlusion, artery, cerebral, specified NEC
  mesenteric (with gangrene) —see also Infarct, intestine K55.069 ◀▥
  ophthalmic —see Occlusion, artery, retina
  pontine —see Occlusion, artery, cerebral, specified NEC
  precerebral —see Occlusion, artery, precerebral
  pulmonary (iatrogenic) —see Embolism, pulmonary
  renal N28.0
  retinal —see Occlusion, artery, retina
  spinal, anterior or posterior G95.11
  traumatic NEC T14.8
  vertebral —see Occlusion, artery, vertebral
atrium, auricular —see also Infarct, myocardium
  following acute myocardial infarction (current complication) I23.6
  not resulting in infarction I51.3 ◀▥
basilar (artery) —see Occlusion, artery, basilar
brain (artery) (stem) —see also Occlusion, artery, cerebral
  due to syphilis A52.05
  puerperal O99.43
  sinus —see Thrombosis, intracranial venous sinus
capillary I78.8
cardiac —see also Infarct, myocardium
  not resulting in infarction I51.3 ◀▥
  valve —see Endocarditis
carotid (artery) (common) (internal) —see Occlusion, artery, carotid
cavernous (venous) sinus —see Thrombosis, intracranial venous sinus
cerebellar artery (anterior inferior) (posterior inferior) (superior) I66.3
cerebral (artery) —see Occlusion, artery, cerebral
cerebrovenous sinus —see also Thrombosis, intracranial venous sinus
  puerperium O87.3
chronic I82.91
coronary (artery) (vein) —see also Infarct, myocardium
  not resulting in infarction I24.0
corpus cavernosum N48.89
cortical I66.9
deep —see Embolism, vein, lower extremity
due to device, implant or graft —see also Complications, by site and type, specified NEC T85.868 ◀▥
  arterial graft NEC T82.868
  breast (implant) T85.868 ◀▥
  catheter NEC T85.868 ◀▥
    dialysis (renal) T82.868
      intraperitoneal T85.868 ◀▥
    infusion NEC T82.868
      spinal (epidural) (subdural) T85.860 ◀▥
    urinary (indwelling) T83.86
  electronic (electrode) (pulse generator) (stimulator)
    bone T84.86
    cardiac T82.867
    nervous system (brain) (peripheral nerve) (spinal) T85.860 ◀▥
    urinary T83.86
  fixation, internal (orthopedic) NEC T84.86
  gastrointestinal (bile duct) (esophagus) T85.868 ◀▥
  genital NEC T83.86
  heart T82.867
  joint prosthesis T84.86
  ocular (corneal graft) (orbital implant) NEC T85.868 ◀▥
  orthopedic NEC T84.86

Thrombosis, thrombotic *(Continued)*
  due to device, implant or graft *(Continued)*
    specified NEC T85.868 ◀▥
    urinary NEC T83.86
    vascular NEC T82.868
    ventricular intracranial shunt T85.860 ◀▥
  during the puerperium —*see* Thrombosis, puerperal
  endocardial —*see also* Infarct, myocardium
    not resulting in infarction I51.3 ◀▥
  eye —*see* Occlusion, retina
  genital organ
    female NEC N94.89
      pregnancy —*see* Thrombophlebitis, antepartum
    male N50.1
  gestational —*see* Phlebopathy, gestational
  heart (chamber) —*see also* Infarct, myocardium
    not resulting in infarction I51.3 ◀▥
  hepatic (vein) I82.0
    artery I74.8
  history (of) Z86.718
  intestine (with gangrene) —*see also* Infarct, intestine K55.069 ◀▥
  intracardiac NEC (apical) (atrial) (auricular) (ventricular) (old) I51.3
  intracranial (arterial) I66.9
    venous sinus (any) G08
      nonpyogenic origin I67.6
      puerperium O87.3
  intramural —*see also* Infarct, myocardium
    not resulting in infarction I51.3 ◀▥
  intraspinal venous sinuses and veins G08
    nonpyogenic G95.19
  kidney (artery) N28.0
  lateral (venous) sinus —*see* Thrombosis, intracranial venous sinus
  leg —*see* Thrombosis, vein, lower extremity
    arterial I74.3
  liver (venous) I82.0
    artery I74.8
    portal vein I81
  longitudinal (venous) sinus —*see* Thrombosis, intracranial venous sinus
  lower limb —*see* Thrombosis, vein, lower extremity
  lung (iatrogenic) (postoperative) —*see* Embolism, pulmonary
  meninges (brain) (arterial) I66.8
  mesenteric (artery) (with gangrene) —*see also* Infarct, intestine K55.069 ◀▥
    vein (inferior) (superior) I81
  mitral I34.8
  mural —*see also* Infarct, myocardium
    due to syphilis A52.06
    not resulting in infarction I51.3 ◀▥
  omentum (with gangrene) —*see also* Infarct, intestine K55.069 ◀▥
  ophthalmic —*see* Occlusion, retina
  pampiniform plexus (male) N50.1
  parietal —*see also* Infarct, myocardium
    not resulting in infarction I24.0
  penis, superficial vein N48.81
  perianal venous K64.5
  peripheral arteries I74.4
    upper I74.2
  personal history (of) Z86.718
  portal I81
    due to syphilis A52.09
  precerebral artery —*see* Occlusion, artery, precerebral
  puerperal, postpartum O87.0
    brain (artery) O99.43
      venous (sinus) O87.3
    cardiac O99.43
    cerebral (artery) O99.43
      venous (sinus) O87.3
    superficial O87.0

Thrombosis, thrombotic *(Continued)*
  pulmonary (artery) (iatrogenic) (postoperative) (vein) —*see* Embolism, pulmonary
  renal (artery) N28.0
    vein I82.3
  resulting from presence of device, implant or graft —*see* Complications, by site and type, specified NEC
  retina, retinal —*see* Occlusion, retina
  scrotum N50.1
  seminal vesicle N50.1
  sigmoid (venous) sinus —*see* Thrombosis, intracranial venous sinus
  sinus, intracranial (any) —*see* Thrombosis, intracranial venous sinus
  specified site NEC I82.890
    chronic I82.891
  spermatic cord N50.1
  spinal cord (arterial) G95.11
    due to syphilis A52.09
    pyogenic origin G06.1
  spleen, splenic D73.5
    artery I74.8
  testis N50.1
  traumatic NEC T14.8
  tricuspid I07.8
  tumor —*see* Neoplasm, by site
  tunica vaginalis N50.1
  umbilical cord (vessels), complicating delivery O69.5
  vas deferens N50.1
  vein (acute) I82.90
    antecubital I82.61-
      chronic I82.71-
    axillary I82.A1-
      chronic I82.A2-
    basilic I82.61-
      chronic I82.71-
    brachial I82.62-
      chronic I82.72-
    brachiocephalic (innominate) I82.290
      chronic I82.291
    cerebral, nonpyogenic I67.6
    cephalic I82.61-
      chronic I82.71-
    chronic I82.91
    deep (DVT) I82.40-
      calf I82.4Z-
        chronic I82.5Z-
      lower leg I82.4Z-
        chronic I82.5Z-
      thigh I82.4Y-
        chronic I82.5Y-
      upper leg I82.4Y
        chronic I82.5y-
    femoral I82.41-
      chronic I82.51-
    iliac (iliofemoral) I82.42-
      chronic I82.52-
    innominate I82.290
      chronic I82.291
    internal jugular I82.C1-
      chronic I82.C2-
    lower extremity
      deep I82.40-
        chronic I82.50-
        specified NEC I82.49-
          chronic NEC I82.59-
      distal
        deep I82.4Z-
      proximal
        deep I82.4Y-
          chronic I82.5Y-
      superficial I82.81-
    perianal K64.5
    popliteal I82.43-
      chronic I82.53-
    radial I82.62-
      chronic I82.72-
    renal I82.3

Thrombosis, thrombotic *(Continued)*
  vein *(Continued)*
    saphenous (greater) (lesser) I82.81-
    specified NEC I82.890
      chronic NEC I82.891
    subclavian I82.B1-
      chronic I82.B2-
    thoracic NEC I82.290
      chronic I82.291
    tibial I82.44-
      chronic I82.54-
    ulnar I82.62-
      chronic I82.72-
    upper extremity I82.60-
      chronic I82.70-
      deep I82.62-
        chronic I82.72-
      superficial I82.61-
        chronic I82.71-
  vena cava
    inferior I82.220
      chronic I82.221
    superior I82.210
      chronic I82.211
  venous, perianal K64.5
  ventricle —*see also* Infarct, myocardium
    following acute myocardial infarction (current complication) I23.6
    not resulting in infarction I24.0
Thrombus —*see* Thrombosis
Thrush —*see also* Candidiasis
  newborn P37.5
  oral B37.0
  vaginal B37.3
Thumb —*see also* condition
  sucking (child problem) F98.8
Thymitis E32.8
Thymoma (benign) D15.0
  malignant C37
Thymus, thymic (gland) —*see* condition
Thyrocele —*see* Goiter
Thyroglossal —*see also* condition
  cyst Q89.2
  duct, persistent Q89.2
Thyroid (gland) (body) —*see also* condition
  hormone resistance E07.89
  lingual Q89.2
  nodule (cystic) (nontoxic) (single) E04.1
Thyroiditis E06.9
  acute (nonsuppurative) (pyogenic) (suppurative) E06.0
  autoimmune E06.3
  chronic (nonspecific) (sclerosing) E06.5
    with thyrotoxicosis, transient E06.2
    fibrous E06.5
    lymphadenoid E06.3
    lymphocytic E06.3
    lymphoid E06.3
  de Quervain's E06.1
  drug-induced E06.4
  fibrous (chronic) E06.5
  giant-cell (follicular) E06.1
  granulomatous (de Quervain) (subacute) E06.1
  Hashimoto's (struma lymphomatosa) E06.3
  iatrogenic E06.4
  ligneous E06.5
  lymphocytic (chronic) E06.3
  lymphoid E06.3
  lymphomatous E06.3
  nonsuppurative E06.1
  postpartum, puerperal O90.5
  pseudotuberculous E06.1
  pyogenic E06.0
  radiation E06.4
  Riedel's E06.5
  subacute (granulomatous) E06.1
  suppurative E06.0
  tuberculous A18.81
  viral E06.1
  woody E06.5

◀ New   ◀▥ Revised   ~~deleted~~ Deleted

Thyrolingual duct, persistent Q89.2
Thyromegaly E01.0
Thyrotoxic
   crisis —*see* Thyrotoxicosis
   heart disease or failure —*see also*
         Thyrotoxicosis E05.90 [I43]
      with thyroid storm E05.91 [I43]
   storm —*see* Thyrotoxicosis
Thyrotoxicosis (recurrent) E05.90
   with
      goiter (diffuse) E05.00
         with thyroid storm E05.01
         adenomatous uninodular E05.10
            with thyroid storm E05.11
         multinodular E05.20
            with thyroid storm E05.21
         nodular E05.20
            with thyroid storm E05.21
         uninodular E05.10
            with thyroid storm E05.11
      infiltrative
         dermopathy E05.00
            with thyroid storm E05.01
         ophthalmopathy E05.00
            with thyroid storm E05.01
      single thyroid nodule E05.10
         with thyroid storm E05.11
      thyroid storm E05.91
   due to
      ectopic thyroid nodule or tissue E05.30
         with thyroid storm E05.31
      ingestion of (excessive) thyroid material
         E05.40
         with thyroid storm E05.41
      overproduction of thyroid-stimulating
         hormone E05.80
         with thyroid storm E05.81
      specified cause NEC E05.80
         with thyroid storm E05.81
   factitia E05.40
      with thyroid storm E05.41
   heart E05.90 [I43]
      with thyroid storm E05.91 [I43]
      failure E05.90 [I43]
   neonatal (transient) P72.1
   transient with chronic thyroiditis E06.2
Tibia vara —*see* Osteochondrosis, juvenile, tibia
Tic (disorder) F95.9
   breathing F95.8
   child problem F95.0
   compulsive F95.1
   de la Tourette F95.2
   degenerative (generalized) (localized) G25.69
      facial G25.69
   disorder
      chronic
         motor F95.1
         vocal F95.1
      combined vocal and multiple motor F95.2
      transient F95.0
   douloureux G50.0
      atypical G50.1
      postherpetic, postzoster B02.22
   drug-induced G25.61
   eyelid F95.8
   habit F95.9
      chronic F95.1
      transient of childhood F95.0
   lid, transient of childhood F95.0
   motor-verbal F95.2
   occupational F48.8
   orbicularis F95.8
      transient of childhood F95.0
   organic origin G25.69
   postchoreic G25.69
   provisional F95.0 ◀
   psychogenic, compulsive F95.1
   salaam R25.8
   spasm (motor or vocal) F95.9
      chronic F95.1
      transient of childhood F95.0
   specified NEC F95.8

Tick-borne —*see* condition
Tietze's disease or syndrome M94.0
Tight, tightness
   anus K62.89
   chest R07.89
   fascia (lata) M62.89
   foreskin (congenital) N47.1
   hymen, hymenal ring N89.6
   introitus (acquired) (congenital) N89.6
   rectal sphincter K62.89
   tendon —*see* Short, tendon
   urethral sphincter N35.9
Tilting vertebra —*see* Dorsopathy, deforming,
      specified NEC
Timidity, child F93.8
Tin-miner's lung J63.5
Tinea (intersecta) (tarsi) B35.9
   amiantacea L44.8
   asbestina B35.0
   barbae B35.0
   beard B35.0
   black dot B35.0
   blanca B36.2
   capitis B35.0
   corporis B35.4
   cruris B35.6
   flava B36.0
   foot B35.3
   furfuracea B36.0
   imbricata (Tokelau) B35.5
   kerion B35.0
   manuum B35.2
   microsporic —*see* Dermatophytosis
   nigra B36.1
   nodosa —*see* Piedra
   pedis B35.3
   scalp B35.0
   specified site NEC B35.8
   sycosis B35.0
   tonsurans B35.0
   trichophytic —*see* Dermatophytosis
   unguium B35.1
   versicolor B36.0
Tingling sensation (skin) R20.2
~~Tinnitus (audible) (aurium) (subjective) —see~~
      ~~subcategory H93.1~~
Tinnitus NOS H93.1- ◀
   audible H93.1- ◀
   aurium H93.1- ◀
   pulsatile H93.A- ◀
   subjective H93.1- ◀
Tipped tooth (teeth) M26.33
Tipping
   pelvis M95.5
      with disproportion (fetopelvic) O33.0
         causing obstructed labor O65.0
   tooth (teeth), fully erupted M26.33
Tiredness R53.83
Tissue —*see* condition
Tobacco (nicotine)
   abuse —*see* Tobacco, use ◀
   dependence —*see* Dependence, drug, nicotine
   harmful use Z72.0
   heart —*see* Tobacco, toxic effect
   maternal use, affecting newborn P04.2
   toxic effect —*see* Table of Drugs and
         Chemicals, by substance, poisoning
      chewing tobacco —*see* Table of Drugs
            and Chemicals, by substance,
            poisoning
      cigarettes —*see* Table of Drugs and
            Chemicals, by substance, poisoning
   use Z72.0
      complicating
         childbirth O99.334
         pregnancy O99.33-
         puerperium O99.335
      counseling and surveillance Z71.6
      history Z87.891 ◀
   withdrawal state —*see also* Dependence,
         drug, nicotine F17.203 ◀▥

Tocopherol deficiency E56.0
Todd's
   cirrhosis K74.3
   paralysis (postepileptic) (transitory) G83.84
Toe —*see* condition
Toilet, artificial opening —*see* Attention to,
      artificial, opening
Tokelau (ringworm) B35.5
Tollwut —*see* Rabies
Tommaselli's disease R31.9
   correct substance properly administered —*see*
         Table of Drugs and Chemicals, by drug,
         adverse effect
   overdose or wrong substance given or
         taken —*see* Table of Drugs and
         Chemicals, by drug, poisoning
Tongue —*see also* condition
   tie Q38.1
Tonic pupil —*see* Anomaly, pupil, function,
      tonic pupil
Toni-Fanconi syndrome (cystinosis) E72.09
   with cystinosis E72.04
Tonsil —*see* condition
Tonsillitis (acute) (catarrhal) (croupous)
         (follicular) (gangrenous) (infective)
         (lacunar) (lingual) (malignant)
         (membranous) (parenchymatous)
         (phlegmonous) (pseudomembranous)
         (purulent) (septic) (subacute)
         (suppurative) (toxic) (ulcerative)
         (vesicular) (viral) J03.90
   chronic J35.01
      with adenoiditis J35.03
   diphtheritic A36.0
   hypertrophic J35.01
      with adenoiditis J35.03
   recurrent J03.91
   specified organism NEC J03.80
      recurrent J03.81
   staphylococcal J03.80
      recurrent J03.81
   streptococcal J03.00
      recurrent J03.01
   tuberculous A15.8
   Vincent's A69.1
Tooth, teeth —*see* condition
Toothache K08.89 ◀▥
Topagnosis R20.8
Tophi —*see* Gout, chronic
TORCH infection —*see* Infection, congenital
   without active infection P00.2
Torn —*see* Tear
Tornwaldt's cyst or disease J39.2
Torsion
   accessory tube —*see* Torsion, fallopian tube
   adnexa (female) —*see* Torsion, fallopian tube
   aorta, acquired I77.1
   appendix epididymis N44.04
   appendix testis N44.03
   bile duct (common) (hepatic) K83.8
      congenital Q44.5
   bowel, colon or intestine K56.2
   cervix —*see* Malposition, uterus
   cystic duct K82.8
   dystonia —*see* Dystonia, torsion
   epididymis (appendix) N44.04
   fallopian tube N83.52- ◀▥
      with ovary N83.53
   gallbladder K82.8
      congenital Q44.1
   hydatid of Morgagni
      female N83.52- ◀▥
      male N44.03
   kidney (pedicle) (leading to infarction) N28.0
   Meckel's diverticulum (congenital) Q43.0
      malignant —*see* Table of Neoplasms, small
            intestine, malignant
   mesentery K56.2
   omentum K56.2
   organ or site, congenital NEC —*see* Anomaly,
      by site

Torsion (Continued)
  ovary (pedicle) N83.51- ◀▥
    with fallopian tube N83.53
    congenital Q50.2
  oviduct —see Torsion, fallopian tube
  penis (acquired) N48.82
    congenital Q55.63
  spasm —see Dystonia, torsion
  spermatic cord N44.02
    extravaginal N44.01
    intravaginal N44.02
  spleen D73.5
  testis, testicle N44.00
    appendix N44.03
  tibia —see Deformity, limb, specified type
    NEC, lower leg
  uterus —see Malposition, uterus
Torticollis (intermittent) (spastic) M43.6
  congenital (sternomastoid) Q68.0
  due to birth injury P15.8
  hysterical F44.4
  ocular R29.891
  psychogenic F45.8
    conversion reaction F44.4
  rheumatic M43.6
  rheumatoid M06.88
  spasmodic G24.3
  traumatic, current S13.4
Tortipelvis G24.1
Tortuous
  aortic arch Q25.46 ◀
  artery I77.1
  organ or site, congenital NEC —see Distortion
  retinal vessel, congenital Q14.1
  ureter N13.8
  urethra N36.8
  vein —see Varix
Torture, victim of Z65.4
Torula, torular (histolytica) (infection) —see
    Cryptococcosis
Torulosis —see Cryptococcosis
Torus (mandibularis) (palatinus) M27.0
  fracture —see Fracture, by site, torus
Touraine's syndrome Q79.8
Tourette's syndrome F95.2
Tourniquet syndrome —see Constriction,
    external, by site
Tower skull Q75.0
  with exophthalmos Q87.0
Toxemia R68.89
  bacterial —see Sepsis
  burn —see Burn
  eclamptic (with pre-existing hypertension) —
    see Eclampsia
  erysipelatous —see Erysipelas
  fatigue R68.89
  food —see Poisoning, food
  gastrointestinal K52.1
  intestinal K52.1
  kidney —see Uremia
  malarial —see Malaria
  myocardial —see Myocarditis, toxic
  of pregnancy —see Pre-eclampsia
  pre-eclamptic —see Pre-eclampsia
  small intestine K52.1
  staphylococcal, due to food A05.0
  stasis R68.89
  uremic —see Uremia
  urinary —see Uremia
Toxemica cerebropathia psychica
    (nonalcoholic) F04
  alcoholic —see Alcohol, amnestic disorder
Toxic (poisoning) —see also condition T65.91
  effect —see Table of Drugs and Chemicals, by
    substance, poisoning
  shock syndrome A48.3
  thyroid (gland) —see Thyrotoxicosis
Toxicemia —see Toxemia
Toxicity —see Table of Drugs and Chemicals, by
    substance, poisoning
  fava bean D55.0

Toxic (Continued)
  food, noxious —see Poisoning, food
  from drug or nonmedicinal substance —see
    Table of Drugs and Chemicals, by drug
Toxicosis —see also Toxemia
  capillary, hemorrhagic D69.0
Toxinfection, gastrointestinal K52.1
Toxocariasis B83.0
Toxoplasma, toxoplasmosis (acquired) B58.9
  with
    hepatitis B58.1
    meningoencephalitis B58.2
    ocular involvement B58.00
    other organ involvement B58.89
    pneumonia, pneumonitis B58.3
  congenital (acute) (subacute) (chronic) P37.1
  maternal, manifest toxoplasmosis in infant
    (acute) (subacute) (chronic) P37.1
  tPA (rtPA) administation in a different facility
    within the last 24 hours prior to admission
    to current facility Z92.82
Trabeculation, bladder N32.89
Trachea —see condition
Tracheitis (catarrhal) (infantile) (membranous)
    (plastic) (septal) (suppurative) (viral)
    J04.10
  with
    bronchitis (15 years of age and above) J40
      acute or subacute —see Bronchitis, acute
      chronic J42
      tuberculous NEC A15.5
      under 15 years of age J20.9
    laryngitis (acute) J04.2
      chronic J37.1
      tuberculous NEC A15.5
  acute J04.10
    with obstruction J04.11
  chronic J42
    with
      bronchitis (chronic) J42
      laryngitis (chronic) J37.1
  diphtheritic (membranous) A36.89
  due to external agent —see Inflammation,
    respiratory, upper, due to
  syphilitic A52.73
  tuberculous A15.5
Trachelitis (nonvenereal) —see Cervicitis
Tracheobronchial —see condition
Tracheobronchitis (15 years of age and
    above) —see also Bronchitis
  due to
    Bordetella bronchiseptica A37.80
      with pneumonia A37.81
    Francisella tularensis A21.8
Tracheobronchomegaly Q32.4
  with bronchiectasis J47.9
    with
      exacerbation (acute) J47.1
      lower respiratory infection J47.0
  acquired J98.09
    with bronchiectasis J47.9
      with
        exacerbation (acute) J47.1
        lower respiratory infection J47.0
Tracheobronchopneumonitis —see Pneumonia,
    broncho-
Tracheocele (external) (internal) J39.8
  congenital Q32.1
Tracheomalacia J39.8
  congenital Q32.0
Tracheopharyngitis (acute) J06.9
  chronic J42
  due to external agent —see Inflammation,
    respiratory, upper, due to
Tracheostenosis J39.8
Tracheostomy
  complication —see Complication,
    tracheostomy
  status Z93.0
    attention to Z43.0
    malfunctioning J95.03

Trachoma, trachomatous A71.9
  active (stage) A71.1
  contraction of conjunctiva A71.1
  dubium A71.0
  healed or sequelae B94.0
  initial (stage) A71.0
  pannus A71.1
  Türck's J37.0
Traction, vitreomacular H43.82-
Train sickness T75.3
Trait (s)
  Hb-S D57.3
  hemoglobin
    abnormal NEC D58.2
      with thalassemia D56.3
    C —see Disease, hemoglobin C
    S (Hb-S) D57.3
  Lepore D56.3
  personality, accentuated Z73.1
  sickle-cell D57.3
    with elliptocytosis or spherocytosis D57.3
  type A personality Z73.1
Tramp Z59.0
Trance R41.89
  hysterical F44.89
Transaminasemia R74.0
Transection
  abdomen (partial) S38.3
  aorta (incomplete) —see also Injury, aorta
    complete —see Injury, aorta, laceration,
      major
  carotid artery (incomplete) —see also Injury,
    blood vessel, carotid, laceration
    complete —see Injury, blood vessel, carotid,
      laceration, major
  celiac artery (incomplete) S35.211
    branch (incomplete) S35.291
      complete S35.292
    complete S35.212
  innominate
    artery (incomplete) —see also Injury, blood
      vessel, thoracic, innominate, artery,
      laceration
      complete —see Injury, blood vessel,
        thoracic, innominate, artery,
        laceration, major
    vein (incomplete) —see also Injury, blood
      vessel, thoracic, innominate, vein,
      laceration
      complete —see Injury, blood vessel,
        thoracic, innominate, vein,
        laceration, major
  jugular vein (external) (incomplete) —see
    also Injury, blood vessel, jugular vein,
    laceration
    complete —see Injury, blood vessel, jugular
      vein, laceration, major
    internal (incomplete) —see also Injury,
      blood vessel, jugular vein, internal,
      laceration
      complete —see Injury, blood vessel,
        jugular vein, internal, laceration,
        major
  mesenteric artery (incomplete) —see also
    Injury, mesenteric, artery, laceration
    complete —see Injury, mesenteric artery,
      laceration, major
  pulmonary vessel (incomplete) —see
    also Injury, blood vessel, thoracic,
    pulmonary, laceration
    complete —see Injury, blood vessel,
      thoracic, pulmonary, laceration, major
  subclavian —see Transection, innominate
  vena cava (incomplete) —see also Injury, vena
    cava
    complete —see Injury, vena cava,
      laceration, major
  vertebral artery (incomplete) —see also Injury,
    blood vessel, vertebral, laceration
    complete —see Injury, blood vessel,
      vertebral, laceration, major

◀ New   ◀▥ Revised   ~~deleted~~ Deleted

Transfusion
  associated (red blood cell) hemochromatosis
      E83.111
  blood
    ABO incompatible —see Complication (s),
        transfusion, incompatibility reaction,
        ABO
    minor blood group (Duffy) (E) (K(ell))
        (Kidd) (Lewis) (M) (N) (P) (S)
        T80.89
    reaction or complication —see
        Complications, transfusion
  fetomaternal (mother) —see Pregnancy,
      complicated by, placenta, transfusion
      syndrome
  maternofetal (mother) —see Pregnancy,
      complicated by, placenta, transfusion
      syndrome
  placental (syndrome) (mother) —see
      Pregnancy, complicated by, placenta,
      transfusion syndrome
  reaction (adverse) —see Complications,
      transfusion
  related acute lung injury (TRALI) J95.84
  twin-to-twin —see Pregnancy, complicated by,
      placenta, transfusion syndrome, fetus
      to fetus
Transient (meaning homeless) —see also
      condition Z59.0
Translocation
  balanced autosomal Q95.9
    in normal individual Q95.0
  chromosomes NEC Q99.8
    balanced and insertion in normal
        individual Q95.0
  Down's syndrome Q90.2
  trisomy
    13 Q91.6
    18 Q91.2
    21 Q90.2
Translucency, iris —see Degeneration, iris
Transmission of chemical substances through
      the placenta —see Absorption, chemical,
      through placenta
Transparency, lung, unilateral J43.0
Transplant (ed) (status) Z94.9
  awaiting organ Z76.82
  bone Z94.6
    marrow Z94.81
  candidate Z76.82
  complication —see Complication, transplant
  cornea Z94.7
  heart Z94.1
    and lung (s) Z94.3
    valve Z95.2
      prosthetic Z95.2
      specified NEC Z95.4
      xenogenic Z95.3
  intestine Z94.82
  kidney Z94.0
  liver Z94.4
  lung (s) Z94.2
    and heart Z94.3
  organ (failure) (infection) (rejection)Z94.9
    removal status Z98.85
  pancreas Z94.83
  skin Z94.5
  social Z60.3
  specified organ or tissue NEC Z94.89
  stem cells Z94.84
  tissue Z94.9
Transplants, ovarian, endometrial N80.1
Transposed —see Transposition
Transposition (congenital) —see also
      Malposition, congenital
  abdominal viscera Q89.3
  aorta (dextra) Q20.3
  appendix Q43.8
  colon Q43.8
  corrected Q20.5
  great vessels (complete) (partial) Q20.3

Transposition (Continued)
  heart Q24.0
    with complete transposition of viscera
        Q89.3
  intestine (large) (small) Q43.8
  reversed jejunal (for bypass) (status) Z98.0
  scrotum Q55.23
  stomach Q40.2
    with general transposition of viscera
        Q89.3
  tooth, teeth, fully erupted M26.30
  vessels, great (complete) (partial) Q20.3
  viscera (abdominal) (thoracic) Q89.3
Transsexualism F64.0 ◀▥
Transverse —see also condition
  arrest (deep), in labor O64.0
  lie (mother) O32.2
    causing obstructed labor O64.8
Transvestism, transvestitism (dual-role)
      F64.1
  fetishistic F65.1
Trapped placenta (with hemorrhage) O72.0
  without hemorrhage O73.0
TRAPS (tumor necrosis factor receptor
      associated periodic syndrome) M04.1 ◀
Trauma, traumatism —see also Injury
  acoustic —see subcategory H83.3
  birth —see Birth, injury
  complicating ectopic or molar pregnancy
      O08.6
  during delivery O71.9
  following ectopic or molar pregnancy O08.6
  obstetric O71.9
    specified NEC O71.89
  occlusal ◀
    primary K08.81 ◀
    secondary K08.82 ◀
Traumatic —see also condition
  brain injury S06.9 ◀▥
Treacher Collins syndrome Q75.4
Treitz's hernia —see Hernia, abdomen, specified
      site NEC
Trematode infestation —see Infestation, fluke
Trematodiasis —see Infestation, fluke
Trembling paralysis —see Parkinsonism
Tremor (s) R25.1
  drug induced G25.1
  essential (benign) G25.0
  familial G25.0
  hereditary G25.0
  hysterical F44.4
  intention G25.2
  medication induced postural G25.1
  mercurial —see subcategory T56.1
  Parkinson's —see Parkinsonism
  psychogenic (conversion reaction) F44.4
  senilis R54
  specified type NEC G25.2
Trench
  fever A79.0
  foot —see Immersion, foot
  mouth A69.1
Treponema pallidum infection —see Syphilis
Treponematosis
  due to
    T. pallidum —see Syphilis
    T. pertenue —see Yaws
Triad
  Hutchinson's (congenital syphilis) A50.53
  Kartagener's Q89.3
  Saint's —see Hernia, diaphragm
Trichiasis (eyelid) H02.059
  with entropion —see Entropion
  left H02.056
    lower H02.055
    upper H02.054
  right H02.053
    lower H02.052
    upper H02.051
Trichinella spiralis (infection) (infestation)
      B75

Trichinellosis, trichiniasis, trichinelliasis,
      trichinosis B75
  with muscle disorder B75 [M63.80]
    ankle B75 [M63.87-]
    foot B75 [M63.87-]
    forearm B75 [M63.83-]
    hand B75 [M63.84-]
    lower leg B75 [M63.86-]
    multiple sites B75 [M63.89]
    pelvic region B75 [M63.85-]
    shoulder region B75 [M63.81-]
    specified site NEC B75 [M63.88]
    thigh B75 [M63.85-]
    upper arm B75 [M63.82-]
Trichobezoar T18.9
  intestine T18.3
  stomach T18.2
Trichocephaliasis, trichocephalosis B79
Trichocephalus infestation B79
Trichoclasis L67.8
Trichoepithelioma —see also Neoplasm, skin,
      benign
  malignant —see Neoplasm, skin, malignant
Trichofolliculoma —see Neoplasm, skin,
      benign
Tricholemmoma —see Neoplasm, skin,
      benign
Trichomoniasis A59.9
  bladder A59.03
  cervix A59.09
  intestinal A07.8
  prostate A59.02
  seminal vesicles A59.09
  specified site NEC A59.8
  urethra A59.03
  urogenitalis A59.00
  vagina A59.01
  vulva A59.01
Trichomycosis
  axillaris A48.8
  nodosa, nodularis B36.8
Trichonodosis L67.8
Trichophytid, trichophyton infection —see
      Dermatophytosis
Trichophytobezoar T18.9
  intestine T18.3
  stomach T18.2
Trichophytosis —see Dermatophytosis
Trichoptilosis L67.8
Trichorrhexis (nodosa) (invaginata) L67.0
Trichosis axillaris A48.8
Trichosporosis nodosa B36.2
Trichostasis spinulosa (congenital) Q84.1
Trichostrongyliasis, trichostrongylosis (small
      intestine) B81.2
Trichostrongylus infection B81.2
Trichotillomania F63.3
Trichromat, trichromatopsia, anomalous
      (congenital) H53.55
Trichuriasis B79
Trichuris trichiura (infection) (infestation) (any
      site) B79
Tricuspid (valve) —see condition
Trifid —see also Accessory
  kidney (pelvis) Q63.8
  tongue Q38.3
Trigeminal neuralgia —see Neuralgia,
      trigeminal
Trigeminy R00.8
Trigger finger (acquired) M65.30
  congenital Q74.0
  index finger M65.32-
  little finger M65.35-
  middle finger M65.33-
  ring finger M65.34-
  thumb M65.31-
Trigonitis (bladder) (chronic)
      (pseudomembranous) N30.30
  with hematuria N30.31
Trigonocephaly Q75.0
Trilocular heart —see Cor triloculare

Trimethylaminuria E72.52
Tripartite placenta O43.19-
Triphalangeal thumb Q74.0
Triple —see also Accessory
  kidneys Q63.0
  uteri Q51.818
  X, female Q97.0
Triplegia G83.89
  congenital G80.8
Triplet (newborn) —see also Newborn, triplet
  complicating pregnancy —see Pregnancy,
    triplet
Triplication —see Accessory
Triploidy Q92.7
Trismus R25.2
  neonatorum A33
  newborn A33
Trisomy (syndrome) Q92.9
  13 (partial) Q91.7
    meiotic nondisjunction Q91.4
    mitotic nondisjunction Q91.5
    mosaicism Q91.5
    translocation Q91.6
  18 (partial) Q91.3
    meiotic nondisjunction Q91.0
    mitotic nondisjunction Q91.1
    mosaicism Q91.1
    translocation Q91.2
  20 Q92.8
  21 (partial) Q90.9
    meiotic nondisjunction Q90.0
    mitotic nondisjunction Q90.1
    mosaicism Q90.1
    translocation Q90.2
  22 Q92.8
  autosomes Q92.9
  chromosome specified NEC Q92.8
    partial Q92.2
      due to unbalanced translocation Q92.5
    specified NEC Q92.8
    whole (nonsex chromosome)
      meiotic nondisjunction Q92.0
      mitotic nondisjunction Q92.1
      mosaicism Q92.1
  due to
    dicentrics —see Extra, marker
      chromosomes
    extra rings —see Extra, marker
      chromosomes
    isochromosomes —see Extra, marker
      chromosomes
  specified NEC Q92.8
  whole chromosome Q92.9
    meiotic nondisjunction Q92.0
    mitotic nondisjunction Q92.1
    mosaicism Q92.1
    partial Q92.9
    specified NEC Q92.8
Tritanomaly, tritanopia H53.55
Trombiculosis, trombiculiasis, trombidiosis
  B88.0
Trophedema (congenital) (hereditary) Q82.0
Trophoblastic disease —see also Mole,
  hydatidiform O01.9
Tropholymphedema Q82.0
Trophoneurosis NEC G96.8
  disseminated M34.9
Tropical —see condition
Trouble —see also Disease
  heart —see Disease, heart
  kidney —see Disease, renal
  nervous R45.0
  sinus —see Sinusitis
Trousseau's syndrome (thrombophlebitis
  migrans) I82.1
Truancy, childhood
  from school Z72.810
Truncus
  arteriosus (persistent) Q20.0
  communis Q20.0
Trunk —see condition

Trypanosomiasis
  African B56.9
    by Trypanosoma brucei
      gambiense B56.0
      rhodesiense B56.1
  American —see Chagas' disease
  Brazilian —see Chagas' disease
  by Trypanosoma
    brucei gambiense B56.0
    brucei rhodesiense B56.1
    cruzi —see Chagas' disease
  gambiensis, Gambian B56.0
  rhodesiensis, Rhodesian B56.1
  South American —see Chagas' disease
  where
    African trypanosomiasis is prevalent B56.9
    Chagas' disease is prevalent B57.2
T-shaped incisors K00.2
Tsutsugamushi (disease) (fever) A75.3
Tube, tubal, tubular —see condition
Tubercle —see also Tuberculosis
  brain, solitary A17.81
  Darwin's Q17.8
  Ghon, primary infection A15.7
Tuberculid, tuberculide (indurating,
    subcutaneous) (lichenoid) (miliary)
    (papulonecrotic) (primary) (skin) A18.4
Tuberculoma —see also Tuberculosis
  brain A17.81
  meninges (cerebral) (spinal) A17.1
  spinal cord A17.81
Tuberculosis, tubercular, tuberculous
    (calcification) (calcified) (caseous)
    (chromogenic acid-fast bacilli)
    (degeneration) (fibrocaseous) (fistula)
    (interstitial) (isolated circumscribed
    lesions) (necrosis) (parenchymatous)
    (ulcerative) A15.9
  with pneumoconiosis (any condition in
    J60-J64) J65
  abdomen (lymph gland) A18.39
  abscess (respiratory) A15.9
    bone A18.03
      hip A18.02
      knee A18.02
      sacrum A18.01
      specified site NEC A18.03
      spinal A18.01
      vertebra A18.01
    brain A17.81
    breast A18.89
    Cowper's gland A18.15
    dura (mater) (cerebral) (spinal) A17.81
    epidural (cerebral) (spinal) A17.81
    female pelvis A18.17
    frontal sinus A15.8
    genital organs NEC A18.10
    genitourinary A18.10
    gland (lymphatic) —see Tuberculosis,
      lymph gland
    hip A18.02
    intestine A18.32
    ischiorectal A18.32
    joint NEC A18.02
      hip A18.02
      knee A18.02
      specified NEC A18.02
      vertebral A18.01
    kidney A18.11
    knee A18.02
    latent R76.11
    lumbar (spine) A18.01
    lung —see Tuberculosis, pulmonary
    meninges (cerebral) (spinal) A17.0
    muscle A18.09
    perianal (fistula) A18.32
    perinephritic A18.11
    perirectal A18.32
    rectum A18.32
    retropharyngeal A15.8
    sacrum A18.01

Tuberculosis, tubercular, tuberculous
    (Continued)
  abscess (Continued)
    scrofulous A18.2
    scrotum A18.15
    skin (primary) A18.4
    spinal cord A17.81
    spine or vertebra (column) A18.01
    subdiaphragmatic A18.31
    testis A18.15
    urinary A18.13
    uterus A18.17
  accessory sinus —see Tuberculosis, sinus
  Addison's disease A18.7
  adenitis —see Tuberculosis, lymph gland
  adenoids A15.8
  adenopathy —see Tuberculosis, lymph gland
  adherent pericardium A18.84
  adnexa (uteri) A18.17
  adrenal (capsule) (gland) A18.7
  alimentary canal A18.32
  anemia A18.89
  ankle (joint) (bone) A18.02
  anus A18.32
  apex, apical —see Tuberculosis, pulmonary
  appendicitis, appendix A18.32
  arachnoid A17.0
  artery, arteritis A18.89
    cerebral A18.89
  arthritis (chronic) (synovial) A18.02
    spine or vertebra (column) A18.01
  articular —see Tuberculosis, joint
  ascites A18.31
  asthma —see Tuberculosis, pulmonary
  axilla, axillary (gland) A18.2
  bladder A18.12
  bone A18.03
    hip A18.02
    knee A18.02
    limb NEC A18.03
    sacrum A18.01
    spine or vertebral column A18.01
  bowel (miliary) A18.32
  brain A17.81
  breast A18.89
  broad ligament A18.17
  bronchi, bronchial, bronchus A15.5
    ectasia, ectasis (bronchiectasis) —see
      Tuberculosis, pulmonary
    fistula A15.5
      primary (progressive) A15.7
    gland or node A15.4
      primary (progressive) A15.7
    lymph gland or node A15.4
      primary (progressive) A15.7
  bronchiectasis —see Tuberculosis, pulmonary
  bronchitis A15.5
  bronchopleural A15.6
  bronchopneumonia, bronchopneumonic —see
    Tuberculosis, pulmonary
  bronchorrhagia A15.5
  bronchotracheal A15.5
  bronze disease A18.7
  buccal cavity A18.83
  bulbourethral gland A18.15
  bursa A18.09
  cachexia A15.9
  cardiomyopathy A18.84
  caries —see Tuberculosis, bone
  cartilage A18.02
    intervertebral A18.01
  catarrhal —see Tuberculosis, respiratory
  cecum A18.32
  cellulitis (primary) A18.4
  cerebellum A17.81
  cerebral, cerebrum A17.81
  cerebrospinal A17.81
    meninges A17.0
  cervical (lymph gland or node) A18.2
  cervicitis, cervix (uteri) A18.16
  chest —see Tuberculosis, respiratory

◀ New   ◀||| Revised   ~~deleted~~ Deleted

Tuberculosis, tubercular, tuberculous
(Continued)
chorioretinitis A18.53
choroid, choroiditis A18.53
ciliary body A18.54
colitis A18.32
collier's J65
colliquativa (primary) A18.4
colon A18.32
complex, primary A15.7
congenital P37.0
conjunctiva A18.59
connective tissue (systemic) A18.89
contact Z20.1
cornea (ulcer) A18.52
Cowper's gland A18.15
coxae A18.02
coxalgia A18.02
cul-de-sac of Douglas A18.17
curvature, spine A18.01
cutis (colliquativa) (primary) A18.4
cyst, ovary A18.18
cystitis A18.12
dactylitis A18.03
diarrhea A18.32
diffuse —*see* Tuberculosis, miliary
digestive tract A18.32
disseminated —*see* Tuberculosis, miliary
duodenum A18.32
dura (mater) (cerebral) (spinal) A17.0
    abscess (cerebral) (spinal) A17.81
dysentery A18.32
ear (inner) (middle) A18.6
    bone A18.03
    external (primary) A18.4
    skin (primary) A18.4
elbow A18.02
emphysema —*see* Tuberculosis, pulmonary
empyema A15.6
encephalitis A17.82
endarteritis A18.89
endocarditis A18.84
    aortic A18.84
    mitral A18.84
    pulmonary A18.84
    tricuspid A18.84
endocrine glands NEC A18.82
endometrium A18.17
enteric, enterica, enteritis A18.32
enterocolitis A18.32
epididymis, epididymitis A18.15
epidural abscess (cerebral) (spinal) A17.81
epiglottis A15.5
episcleritis A18.51
erythema (induratum) (nodosum) (primary)
    A18.4
esophagus A18.83
eustachian tube A18.6
exposure (to) Z20.1
exudative —*see* Tuberculosis, pulmonary
eye A18.50
eyelid (primary) (lupus) A18.4
fallopian tube (acute) (chronic) A18.17
fascia A18.09
fauces A15.8
female pelvic inflammatory disease A18.17
finger A18.03
first infection A15.7
gallbladder A18.83
ganglion A18.09
gastritis A18.83
gastrocolic fistula A18.32
gastroenteritis A18.32
gastrointestinal tract A18.32
general, generalized —*see* Tuberculosis,
    miliary
genital organs A18.10
genitourinary A18.10
genu A18.02
glandula suprarenalis A18.7
glandular, general A18.2

Tuberculosis, tubercular, tuberculous
(Continued)
glottis A15.5
grinder's J65
gum A18.83
hand A18.03
heart A18.84
hematogenous —*see* Tuberculosis, miliary
hemoptysis —*see* Tuberculosis, pulmonary
hemorrhage NEC —*see* Tuberculosis,
    pulmonary
hemothorax A15.6
hepatitis A18.83
hilar lymph nodes A15.4
    primary (progressive) A15.7
hip (joint) (disease) (bone) A18.02
hydropneumothorax A15.6
hydrothorax A15.6
hypoadrenalism A18.7
hypopharynx A15.8
ileocecal (hyperplastic) A18.32
ileocolitis A18.32
ileum A18.32
iliac spine (superior) A18.03
immunological findings only A15.7
indurativa (primary) A18.4
infantile A15.7
infection A15.9
    without clinical manifestations A15.7
infraclavicular gland A18.2
inguinal gland A18.2
inguinalis A18.2
intestine (any part) A18.32
iridocyclitis A18.54
iris, iritis A18.54
ischiorectal A18.32
jaw A18.03
jejunum A18.32
joint A18.02
    vertebral A18.01
keratitis (interstitial) A18.52
keratoconjunctivitis A18.52
kidney A18.11
knee (joint) A18.02
kyphosis, kyphoscoliosis A18.01
laryngitis A15.5
larynx A15.5
latent R76.11
leptomeninges, leptomeningitis (cerebral)
    (spinal) A17.0
lichenoides (primary) A18.4
linguae A18.83
lip A18.83
liver A18.83
lordosis A18.01
lung —*see* Tuberculosis, pulmonary
lupus vulgaris A18.4
lymph gland or node (peripheral) A18.2
    abdomen A18.39
    bronchial A15.4
        primary (progressive) A15.7
    cervical A18.2
    hilar A15.4
        primary (progressive) A15.7
    intrathoracic A15.4
        primary (progressive) A15.7
    mediastinal A15.4
        primary (progressive) A15.7
    mesenteric A18.39
    retroperitoneal A18.39
    tracheobronchial A15.4
        primary (progressive) A15.7
lymphadenitis —*see* Tuberculosis, lymph
    gland
lymphangitis —*see* Tuberculosis, lymph
    gland
lymphatic (gland) (vessel) —*see* Tuberculosis,
    lymph gland
mammary gland A18.89
marasmus A15.9
mastoiditis A18.03

Tuberculosis, tubercular, tuberculous
(Continued)
mediastinal lymph gland or node
    A15.4
    primary (progressive) A15.7
mediastinitis A15.8
    primary (progressive) A15.7
mediastinum A15.8
    primary (progressive) A15.7
medulla A17.81
melanosis, Addisonian A18.7
meninges, meningitis (basilar) (cerebral)
    (cerebrospinal) (spinal) A17.0
meningoencephalitis A17.82
mesentery, mesenteric (gland or node)
    A18.39
miliary A19.9
    acute A19.2
        multiple sites A19.1
        single specified site A19.0
    chronic A19.8
    specified NEC A19.8
millstone makers' J65
miner's J65
molder's J65
mouth A18.83
multiple A19.9
    acute A19.1
    chronic A19.8
muscle A18.09
myelitis A17.82
myocardium, myocarditis A18.84
nasal (passage) (sinus) A15.8
nasopharynx A15.8
neck gland A18.2
nephritis A18.11
nerve (mononeuropathy) A17.83
nervous system A17.9
nose (septum) A15.8
ocular A18.50
omentum A18.31
oophoritis (acute) (chronic) A18.17
optic (nerve trunk) (papilla) A18.59
orbit A18.59
orchitis A18.15
organ, specified NEC A18.89
osseous —*see* Tuberculosis, bone
osteitis —*see* Tuberculosis, bone
osteomyelitis —*see* Tuberculosis, bone
otitis media A18.6
ovary, ovaritis (acute) (chronic) A18.17
oviduct (acute) (chronic) A18.17
pachymeningitis A17.0
palate (soft) A18.83
pancreas A18.83
papulonecrotic (a) (primary) A18.4
parathyroid glands A18.82
paronychia (primary) A18.4
parotid gland or region A18.83
pelvis (bony) A18.03
penis A18.15
peribronchitis A15.5
pericardium, pericarditis A18.84
perichondritis, larynx A15.5
periostitis —*see* Tuberculosis, bone
perirectal fistula A18.32
peritoneum NEC A18.31
peritonitis A18.31
pharynx, pharyngitis A15.8
phlyctenulosis (keratoconjunctivitis) A18.52
phthisis NEC —*see* Tuberculosis, pulmonary
pituitary gland A18.82
pleura, pleural, pleurisy, pleuritis (fibrinous)
    (obliterative) (purulent) (simple plastic)
    (with effusion) A15.6
    primary (progressive) A15.7
pneumonia, pneumonic —*see* Tuberculosis,
    pulmonary
pneumothorax (spontaneous) (tense
    valvular) —*see* Tuberculosis, pulmonary
polyneuropathy A17.89

Tuberculosis, tubercular, tuberculous
(Continued)
polyserositis A19.9
acute A19.1
chronic A19.8
potter's J65
prepuce A18.15
primary (complex) A15.7
proctitis A18.32
prostate, prostatitis A18.14
pulmonalis —see Tuberculosis, pulmonary
pulmonary (cavitated) (fibrotic) (infiltrative)
(nodular) A15.0
childhood type or first infection A15.7
primary (complex) A15.7
pyelitis A18.11
pyelonephritis A18.11
pyemia —see Tuberculosis, miliary
pyonephrosis A18.11
pyopneumothorax A15.6
pyothorax A15.6
rectum (fistula) (with abscess) A18.32
reinfection stage —see Tuberculosis,
pulmonary
renal A18.11
renis A18.11
respiratory A15.9
primary A15.7
specified site NEC A15.8
retina, retinitis A18.53
retroperitoneal (lymph gland or node)
A18.39
rheumatism NEC A18.09
rhinitis A15.8
sacroiliac (joint) A18.01
sacrum A18.01
salivary gland A18.83
salpingitis (acute) (chronic) A18.17
sandblaster's J65
sclera A18.51
scoliosis A18.01
scrofulous A18.2
scrotum A18.15
seminal tract or vesicle A18.15
senile A15.9
septic —see Tuberculosis, miliary
shoulder (joint) A18.02
blade A18.03
sigmoid A18.32
sinus (any nasal) A15.8
bone A18.03
epididymis A18.15
skeletal NEC A18.03
skin (any site) (primary) A18.4
small intestine A18.32
soft palate A18.83
spermatic cord A18.15
spine, spinal (column) A18.01
cord A17.81
medulla A17.81
membrane A17.0
meninges A17.0
spleen, splenitis A18.85
spondylitis A18.01
sternoclavicular joint A18.02
stomach A18.83
stonemason's J65
subcutaneous tissue (cellular) (primary)
A18.4
subcutis (primary) A18.4
subdeltoid bursa A18.83
submaxillary (region) A18.83
supraclavicular gland A18.2
suprarenal (capsule) (gland) A18.7
swelling, joint —see also category M01 (see also
Tuberculosis, joint) A18.02
symphysis pubis A18.02
synovitis A18.09
articular A18.02
spine or vertebra A18.01
systemic —see Tuberculosis, miliary

Tuberculosis, tubercular, tuberculous
(Continued)
tarsitis A18.4
tendon (sheath) —see Tuberculosis,
tenosynovitis
tenosynovitis A18.09
spine or vertebra A18.01
testis A18.15
throat A15.8
thymus gland A18.82
thyroid gland A18.81
tongue A18.83
tonsil, tonsillitis A15.8
trachea, tracheal A15.5
lymph gland or node A15.4
primary (progressive) A15.7
tracheobronchial A15.5
lymph gland or node A15.4
primary (progressive) A15.7
tubal (acute) (chronic) A18.17
tunica vaginalis A18.15
ulcer (skin) (primary) A18.4
bowel or intestine A18.32
specified NEC - code under Tuberculosis,
by site
unspecified site A15.9
ureter A18.11
urethra, urethral (gland) A18.13
urinary organ or tract A18.13
uterus A18.17
uveal tract A18.54
uvula A18.83
vagina A18.18
vas deferens A18.15
verruca, verrucosa (cutis) (primary) A18.4
vertebra (column) A18.01
vesiculitis A18.15
vulva A18.18
wrist (joint) A18.02
Tuberculum
Carabelli —see Note at K00.2
occlusal —see Note at K00.2
paramolare K00.2
Tuberosity, enitre maxillary M26.07
Tuberous sclerosis (brain) Q85.1
Tubo-ovarian —see condition
Tuboplasty, after previous sterilization
Z31.0
aftercare Z31.42
Tubotympanitis, catarrhal (chronic) —see Otitis,
media, nonsuppurative, chronic, serous
Tularemia A21.9
with
conjunctivitis A21.1
pneumonia A21.2
abdominal A21.3
bronchopneumonic A21.2
conjunctivitis A21.1
cryptogenic A21.3
enteric A21.3
gastrointestinal A21.3
generalized A21.7
ingestion A21.3
intestinal A21.3
oculoglandular A21.1
ophthalmic A21.1
pneumonia (any), pneumonic A21.2
pulmonary A21.2
sepsis A21.7
specified NEC A21.8
typhoidal A21.7
ulceroglandular A21.0
Tularensis conjunctivitis A21.1
Tumefaction —see also Swelling
liver —see Hypertrophy, liver
Tumor —see also Neoplasm, unspecified
behavior, by site
acinar cell —see Neoplasm, uncertain
behavior, by site
acinic cell —see Neoplasm, uncertain
behavior, by site

Tumor (Continued)
adenocarcinoid —see Neoplasm, malignant,
by site
adenomatoid —see also Neoplasm, benign,
by site
odontogenic —see Cyst, calcifying
odontogenic
adnexal (skin) —see Neoplasm, skin, benign,
by site
adrenal
cortical (benign) D35.0-
malignant C74.0-
rest —see Neoplasm, benign, by site
alpha-cell
malignant
pancreas C25.4
specified site NEC —see Neoplasm,
malignant, by site
unspecified site C25.4
pancreas D13.7
specified site NEC —see Neoplasm, benign,
by site
unspecified site D13.7
aneurysmal —see Aneurysm
aortic body D44.7
malignant C75.5
Askin's —see Neoplasm, connective tissue,
malignant
basal cell —see also Neoplasm, skin, uncertain
behavior D48.5
Bednar —see Neoplasm, skin, malignant
benign (unclassified) —see Neoplasm, benign,
by site
beta-cell
malignant
pancreas C25.4
specified site NEC —see Neoplasm,
malignant, by site
unspecified site C25.4
pancreas D13.7
specified site NEC —see Neoplasm, benign,
by site
unspecified site D13.7
Brenner D27.9
borderline malignancy D39.1-
malignant C56-
proliferating D39.1
bronchial alveolar, intravascular D38.1
Brooke's —see Neoplasm, skin, benign
brown fat —see Lipoma
Burkitt —see Lymphoma, Burkitt
calcifying epithelial odontogenic —see Cyst,
calcifying odontogenic
carcinoid
benign D3A.00
appendix D3A.020
ascending colon D3A.022
bronchus (lung) D3A.090
cecum D3A.021
colon D3A.029
descending colon D3A.024
duodenum D3A.010
foregut NOS D3A.094
hindgut NOS D3A.096
ileum D3A.012
jejunum D3A.011
kidney D3A.093
large intestine D3A.029
lung (bronchus) D3A.090
midgut NOS D3A.095
rectum D3A.026
sigmoid colon D3A.025
small intestine D3A.019
specified NEC D3A.098
stomach D3A.092
thymus D3A.091
transverse colon D3A.023
malignant C7A.00
appendix C7A.020
ascending colon C7A.022
bronchus (lung) C7A.090

◀ New   ◀≣ Revised   ~~deleted~~ Deleted

Tumor *(Continued)*
  carcinoid *(Continued)*
    malignant *(Continued)*
      cecum C7A.021
      colon C7A.029
      descending colon C7A.024
      duodenum C7A.010
      foregut NOS C7A.094
      hindgut NOS C7A.096
      ileum C7A.012
      jejunum C7A.011
      kidney C7A.093
      large intestine C7A.029
      lung (bronchus) C7A.090
      midgut NOS C7A.095
      rectum C7A.026
      sigmoid colon C7A.025
      small intestine C7A.019
      specified NEC C7A.098
      stomach C7A.092
      thymus C7A.091
      transverse colon C7A.023
    mesentary metastasis C7B.04
    secondary C7B.00
      bone C7B.03
      distant lymph nodes C7B.01
      liver C7B.02
      peritoneum C7B.04
      specified NEC C7B.09
  carotid body D44.6
    malignant C75.4
  cells —*see also* Neoplasm, unspecified
      behavior, by site
    benign —*see* Neoplasm, benign,
        by site
    malignant —*see* Neoplasm, malignant,
        by site
    uncertain whether benign or malignant —
        see Neoplasm, uncertain behavior,
        by site
  cervix, in pregnancy or childbirth —*see*
      Pregnancy, complicated by, tumor,
      cervix
  chondromatous giant cell —*see* Neoplasm,
      bone, benign
  chromaffin —*see also* Neoplasm, benign, by
      site
    malignant —*see* Neoplasm, malignant, by
        site
  Cock's peculiar L72.3
  Codman's —*see* Neoplasm, bone, benign
  dentigerous, mixed —*see* Cyst, calcifying
      odontogenic
  dermoid —*see* Neoplasm, benign,
      by site
    with malignant transformation C56-
  desmoid (extra-abdominal) —*see also*
      Neoplasm, connective tissue, uncertain
      behavior
    abdominal —*see* Neoplasm, connective
        tissue, uncertain behavior
  embolus —*see* Neoplasm, secondary,
      by site
  embryonal (mixed) —*see also* Neoplasm,
      uncertain behavior, by site
    liver C22.7
  endodermal sinus
    specified site —*see* Neoplasm, malignant,
        by site
    unspecified site
      female C56.-
      male C62.90
  epithelial
    benign —*see* Neoplasm, benign,
        by site
    malignant —*see* Neoplasm, malignant, by
        site
  Ewing's —*see* Neoplasm, bone, malignant,
      by site
  fatty —*see* Lipoma
  fibroid —*see* Leiomyoma

Tumor *(Continued)*
  G cell
    malignant
      pancreas C25.4
      specified site NEC —*see* Neoplasm,
          malignant, by site
      unspecified site C25.4
    specified site —*see* Neoplasm, uncertain
        behavior, by site
    unspecified site D37.8
  germ cell —*see also* Neoplasm, malignant,
      by site
    mixed —*see* Neoplasm, malignant,
        by site
  ghost cell, odontogenic —*see* Cyst, calcifying
      odontogenic
  giant cell —*see also* Neoplasm, uncertain
      behavior, by site
    bone D48.0
      malignant —*see* Neoplasm, bone,
          malignant
      chondromatous —*see* Neoplasm, bone,
          benign
      malignant —*see* Neoplasm, malignant, by
          site
    soft parts —*see* Neoplasm, connective
        tissue, uncertain behavior
      malignant —*see* Neoplasm, connective
          tissue, malignant
  glomus D18.00
    intra-abdominal D18.03
    intracranial D18.02
    jugulare D44.7
      malignant C75.5
    skin D18.01
    specified site NEC D18.09
  gonadal stromal —*see* Neoplasm, uncertain
      behavior, by site
  granular cell —*see also* Neoplasm, connective
      tissue, benign
    malignant —*see* Neoplasm, connective
        tissue, malignant
  granulosa cell D39.1-
    juvenile D39.1-
    malignant C56-
  granulosa cell-theca cell D39.1-
    malignant C56-
  Grawitz's C64-
  hemorrhoidal —*see* Hemorrhoids
  hilar cell D27-
  hilus cell D27-
  Hurthle cell (benign) D34
    malignant C73
  hydatid —*see* Echinococcus
  hypernephroid —*see also* Neoplasm,
      uncertain behavior, by site
  interstitial cell —*see also* Neoplasm, uncertain
      behavior, by site
    benign —*see* Neoplasm, benign, by site
    malignant —*see* Neoplasm, malignant, by
        site
  intravascular bronchial alveolar D38.1
  islet cell —*see* Neoplasm, benign, by site
    malignant —*see* Neoplasm, malignant, by
        site
      pancreas C25.4
      specified site NEC —*see* Neoplasm,
          malignant, by site
      unspecified site C25.4
    pancreas D13.7
    specified site NEC —*see* Neoplasm, benign,
        by site
    unspecified site D13.7
  juxtaglomerular D41.0-
  Klatskin's C24.0
  Krukenberg's C79.6-
  Leydig cell —*see* Neoplasm, uncertain
      behavior, by site
    benign —*see* Neoplasm, benign, by site
      specified site —*see* Neoplasm, benign,
          by site

Tumor *(Continued)*
  Leydig cell *(Continued)*
    benign *(Continued)*
      unspecified site
        female D27.9
        male D29.20
    malignant —*see* Neoplasm, malignant, by
        site
      specified site —*see* Neoplasm,
          malignant, by site
      unspecified site
        female C56.9
        male C62.90
    specified site —*see* Neoplasm, uncertain
        behavior, by site
    unspecified site
      female D39.10
      male D40.10
  lipid cell, ovary D27-
  lipoid cell, ovary D27-
  malignant —*see also* Neoplasm, malignant, by
      site C80.1
    fusiform cell (type) C80.1
    giant cell (type) C80.1
    localized, plasma cell —*see* Plasmacytoma,
        solitary
    mixed NEC C80.1
    small cell (type) C80.1
    spindle cell (type) C80.1
    unclassified C80.1
  mast cell D47.0
    malignant C96.2
  melanotic, neuroectodermal —*see* Neoplasm,
      benign, by site
  Merkel cell —*see* Carcinoma, Merkel cell
  mesenchymal
    malignant —*see* Neoplasm, connective
        tissue, malignant
    mixed —*see* Neoplasm, connective tissue,
        uncertain behavior
  mesodermal, mixed —*see also* Neoplasm,
      malignant, by site
    liver C22.4
  mesonephric —*see also* Neoplasm, uncertain
      behavior, by site
    malignant —*see* Neoplasm, malignant, by
        site
  metastatic
    from specified site —*see* Neoplasm,
        malignant, by site
    of specified site —*see* Neoplasm,
        malignant, by site
    to specified site —*see* Neoplasm, secondary,
        by site
  mixed NEC —*see also* Neoplasm, benign, by
      site
    malignant —*see* Neoplasm, malignant, by
        site
  mucinous of low malignant potential
    specified site —*see* Neoplasm, malignant,
        by site
    unspecified site C56.9
  mucocarcinoid
    specified site —*see* Neoplasm, malignant,
        by site
    unspecified site C18.1
  mucoepidermoid —*see* Neoplasm, uncertain
      behavior, by site
  Müllerian, mixed
    specified site —*see* Neoplasm, malignant,
        by site
    unspecified site C54.9
  myoepithelial —*see* Neoplasm, benign,
      by site
  neuroectodermal (peripheral) —*see*
      Neoplasm, malignant, by site
    primitive
      specified site —*see* Neoplasm,
          malignant,
          by site
      unspecified site C71.9

Tumor *(Continued)*
  neuroendocrine D3A.8
    malignant poorly differentiated C7A.1
    secondary NEC C7B.8
    specified NEC C7A.8
  neurogenic olfactory C30.0
  nonencapsulated sclerosing C73
  odontogenic (adenomatoid) (benign)
      (calcifying epithelial) (keratocystic)
      (squamous) —*see* Cyst, calcifying
      odontogenic
    malignant C41.1
      upper jaw (bone) C41.0
  ovarian stromal D39.1-
  ovary, in pregnancy —*see* Pregnancy,
      complicated by
  pacinian —*see* Neoplasm, skin, benign
  Pancoast's —*see* Pancoast's syndrome
  papillary —*see also* Papilloma
    cystic D37.9
      mucinous of low malignant potential C56-
        specified site —*see* Neoplasm,
            malignant, by site
        unspecified site C56.9
      serous of low malignant potential
        specified site —*see* Neoplasm,
            malignant, by site
        unspecified site C56.9
  pelvic, in pregnancy or childbirth —*see*
      Pregnancy, complicated by
  phantom F45.8
  phyllodes D48.6-
    benign D24-
    malignant —*see* Neoplasm, breast,
        malignant
  Pindborg —*see* Cyst, calcifying odontogenic
  placental site trophoblastic D39.2
  plasma cell (malignant) (localized) —*see*
      Plasmacytoma, solitary
  polyvesicular vitelline
    specified site —*see* Neoplasm, malignant,
        by site
    unspecified site
      female C56.9
      male C62.90
  Pott's puffy —*see* Osteomyelitis, specified
      NEC
  Rathke's pouch D44.3
  retinal anlage —*see* Neoplasm, benign, by site
  salivary gland type, mixed —*see* Neoplasm,
      salivary gland, benign
    malignant —*see* Neoplasm, salivary gland,
        malignant
  Sampson's N80.1
  Schmincke's —*see* Neoplasm, nasopharynx,
      malignant
  sclerosing stromal D27-
  sebaceous —*see* Cyst, sebaceous
  secondary —*see* Neoplasm, secondary, by site
    carcinoid C7B.00
      bone C7B.03
      distant lymph nodes C7B.01
      liver C7B.02
      peritoneum C7B.04
      specified NEC C7B.09
    neuroendocrine NEC C7B.8
  serous of low malignant potential
    specified site —*see* Neoplasm, malignant,
        by site
    unspecified site C56.9
  Sertoli cell —*see* Neoplasm, benign, by site
    with lipid storage
      specified site —*see* Neoplasm, benign,
          by site
      unspecified site
        female D27.9
        male D29.20
    specified site —*see* Neoplasm, benign, by site
    unspecified site
      female D27.9
      male D29.20

Tumor *(Continued)*
  Sertoli-Leydig cell —*see* Neoplasm, benign,
      by site
    specified site —*see* Neoplasm, benign, by
        site
    unspecified site
      female D27.9
      male D29.20
  sex cord(-stromal) —*see* Neoplasm, uncertain
      behavior, by site
    with annular tubules D39.1-
  skin appendage —*see* Neoplasm, skin,
      benign
  smooth muscle —*see* Neoplasm, connective
      tissue, uncertain behavior
  soft tissue
    benign —*see* Neoplasm, connective tissue,
        benign
    malignant —*see* Neoplasm, connective
        tissue, malignant
  sternomastoid (congenital) Q68.0
  stromal
    endometrial D39.0
    gastric D48.1
      benign D21.4
      malignant C16.9
      uncertain behavior D48.1
    gastrointestinal C49.A- ◀▥
      benign D21.4
      esophagus C49.A1 ◀
      large intestine C49.A4 ◀
      malignant C49.A0 ◀▥
        colon C49.A4 ◀
        duodenum C49.A3 ◀
        esophagus C49.A1 ◀
        ileum C49.A3 ◀
        jejunum C49.A3 ◀
        Meckel diverticulum C49.A3 ◀
        large intestine C49.A4 ◀
        omentum C49.A9 ◀
        peritoneum C49.A9 ◀
        rectum C49.A5 ◀
        small intestine C49.A3 ◀
        specified site NEC C49.A9 ◀
        stomach C49.A2 ◀
      large intestine C49.A4 ◀
      rectum C49.A5 ◀
      small intestine C49.A3 ◀
      specified site NEC C49.A9 ◀
      stomach C49.A2 ◀
      uncertain behavior D48.1
    intestine
      benign D21.4
      malignant ◀▥
        large C49.A4 ◀
        small C49.A3 ◀
      uncertain behavior D48.1
    ovarian D39.1-
    stomach C49.A2 ◀▥
      benign D21.4
      malignant C49.A2 ◀▥
      uncertain behavior D48.1
  sweat gland —*see also* Neoplasm, skin,
      uncertain behavior
    benign —*see* Neoplasm, skin, benign
    malignant —*see* Neoplasm, skin, malignant
  syphilitic, brain A52.17
  testicular D40.10
  testicular stromal D40.1-
  theca cell D27.-
  theca cell-granulosa cell D39.1-
  Triton, malignant —*see* Neoplasm, nerve,
      malignant
  trophoblastic, placental site D39.2
  turban D23.4
  uterus (body), in pregnancy or childbirth —
      see Pregnancy, complicated by, tumor,
      uterus
  vagina, in pregnancy or childbirth —*see*
      Pregnancy, complicated by
  varicose —*see* Varix

Tumor *(Continued)*
  von Recklinghausen's —*see*
      Neurofibromatosis
  vulva or perineum, in pregnancy or
      childbirth —*see* Pregnancy, complicated
      by
    causing obstructed labor O65.5
  Warthin's —*see* Neoplasm, salivary gland,
      benign
  Wilms' C64-
  yolk sac —*see* Neoplasm, malignant, by site
    specified site —*see* Neoplasm, malignant,
        by site
    unspecified site
      female C56.9
      male C62.90
Tumor lysis syndrome (following
    antineoplastic chemotherapy)
    (spontaneous) NEC E88.3
Tumorlet —*see* Neoplasm, uncertain behavior,
    by site
Tungiasis B88.1
Tunica vasculosa lentis Q12.2
Turban tumor D23.4
Türck's trachoma J37.0
Turner-Kieser syndrome Q87.2 ◀▥
Turner-like syndrome Q87.1
Turner's
  hypoplasia (tooth) K00.4
  syndrome Q96.9
    specified NEC Q96.8
  tooth K00.4
Turner-Ullrich syndrome Q96.9
Tussis convulsiva —*see* Whooping cough
Twiddler's syndrome (due to)
  automatic implantable defibrillator T82.198
  cardiac pacemaker T82.198
Twilight state
  epileptic F05
  psychogenic F44.89
Twin (newborn) —*see also* Newborn, twin
  conjoined Q89.4
  pregnancy —*see* Pregnancy, twin, conjoined
Twinning, teeth K00.2
Twist, twisted
  bowel, colon or intestine K56.2
  hair (congenital) Q84.1
  mesentery K56.2
  omentum K56.2
  organ or site, congenital NEC —*see* Anomaly,
      by site
  ovarian pedicle —*see* Torsion, ovary
Twitching R25.3
Tylosis (acquired) L84
  buccalis K13.29
  linguae K13.29
  palmaris et plantaris (congenital) (inherited)
      Q82.8
    acquired L85.1
Tympanism R14.0
Tympanites (abdominal) (intestinal) R14.0
Tympanitis —*see* Myringitis
Tympanosclerosis —*see* subcategory H74.0
Tympanum —*see* condition
Tympany
  abdomen R14.0
  chest R09.89
Type A behavior pattern Z73.1
Typhlitis —*see* Appendicitis
Typhoenteritis —*see* Typhoid
Typhoid (abortive) (ambulant) (any site)
    (clinical) (fever) (hemorrhagic) (infection)
    (intermittent) (malignant) (rheumatic)
    (Widal negative) A01.00
  with pneumonia A01.03
  abdominal A01.09
  arthritis A01.04
  carrier (suspected) of Z22.0
  cholecystitis (current) A01.09
  endocarditis A01.02
  heart involvement A01.02

◀ New   ◀▥ Revised   ~~deleted~~ Deleted

Typhoid (Continued)
  inoculation reaction —see Complications,
    vaccination
  meningitis A01.01
  mesenteric lymph nodes A01.09
  myocarditis A01.02
  osteomyelitis A01.05
  perichondritis, larynx A01.09
  pneumonia A01.03
  specified NEC A01.09
  spine A01.05
  ulcer (perforating) A01.09
Typhomalaria (fever) —see Malaria
Typhomania A01.00
Typhoperitonitis A01.09
Typhus (fever) A75.9
  abdominal, abdominalis —see Typhoid
  African tick A77.1
  amarillic A95.9
  brain A75.9 [G94]

Typhus (Continued)
  cerebral A75.9 [G94]
  classical A75.0
  due to Rickettsia
    prowazekii A75.0
      recrudescent A75.1
    tsutsugamushi A75.3
    typhi A75.2
  endemic (flea-borne) A75.2
  epidemic (louse-borne) A75.0
  exanthematic NEC A75.0
  exanthematicus SAI A75.0
    brillii SAI A75.1
    mexicanus SAI A75.2
    typhus murinus A75.2
  flea-borne A75.2
  India tick A77.1
  Kenya (tick) A77.1
  louse-borne A75.0
  Mexican A75.2

Typhus (Continued)
  mite-borne A75.3
  murine A75.2
  North Asian tick-borne A77.2
  petechial A75.9
  Queensland tick A77.3
  rat A75.2
  recrudescent A75.1
  recurrens —see Fever, relapsing
  Sao Paulo A77.0
  scrub (China) (India) (Malaysia) (New
    Guinea) A75.3
  shop (of Malaysia) A75.2
  Siberian tick A77.2
  tick-borne A77.9
  tropical (mite-borne) A75.3
Tyrosinemia E70.21
  newborn, transitory P74.5
Tyrosinosis E70.21
Tyrosinuria E70.29

U

Uhl's anomaly or disease Q24.8
Ulcer, ulcerated, ulcerating, ulceration, ulcerative
  alveolar process M27.3
  amebic (intestine) A06.1
    skin A06.7
  anastomotic —see Ulcer, gastrojejunal
  anorectal K62.6
  antral —see Ulcer, stomach
  anus (sphincter) (solitary) K62.6
  aorta —see Aneurysm
  aphthous (oral) (recurrent) K12.0
    genital organ (s)
      female N76.6
      male N50.89 ◀▥▥
  artery I77.2
  atrophic —see Ulcer, skin
    decubitus —see Ulcer, pressure, by site
  back L98.429
    with
      bone necrosis L98.424
      exposed fat layer L98.422
      muscle necrosis L98.423
      skin breakdown only L98.421
  Barrett's (esophagus) K22.10
    with bleeding K22.11
  bile duct (common) (hepatic) K83.8
  bladder (solitary) (sphincter) NEC N32.89
    bilharzial B65.9 [N33]
    in schistosomiasis (bilharzial) B65.9 [N33]
    submucosal —see Cystitis, interstitial
    tuberculous A18.12
  bleeding K27.4
  bone —see Osteomyelitis, specified type NEC
  bowel —see Ulcer, intestine
  breast N61.1 ◀▥▥
  bronchus J98.09
  buccal (cavity) (traumatic) K12.1
  Buruli A31.1
  buttock L98.419
    with
      bone necrosis L98.414
      exposed fat layer L98.412
      muscle necrosis L98.413
      skin breakdown only L98.411
  cancerous —see Neoplasm, malignant, by site
  cardia K22.10
    with bleeding K22.11
  cardioesophageal (peptic) K22.10
    with bleeding K22.11
  cecum —see Ulcer, intestine
  cervix (uteri) (decubitus) (trophic) N86
    with cervicitis N72
  chancroidal A57
  chiclero B55.1
  chronic (cause unknown) —see Ulcer, skin
  Cochin-China B55.1
  colon —see Ulcer, intestine
  conjunctiva H10.89
  cornea H16.00-
    with hypopyon H16.03-
    central H16.01-
    dendritic (herpes simplex) B00.52
    marginal H16.04-
    Mooren's H16.05-
    mycotic H16.06-
    perforated H16.07-
    ring H16.02-
    tuberculous (phlyctenular) A18.52
  corpus cavernosum (chronic) N48.5
  crural —see Ulcer, lower limb
  Curling's —see Ulcer, peptic, acute
  Cushing's —see Ulcer, peptic, acute
  cystic duct K82.8
  cystitis (interstitial) —see Cystitis, interstitial
  decubitus —see Ulcer, pressure, by site
  dendritic, cornea (herpes simplex) B00.52
  diabetes, diabetic —see Diabetes, ulcer
  Dieulafoy's K25.0

Ulcer, ulcerated, ulcerating, ulceration, ulcerative (Continued)
  due to
    infection NEC —see Ulcer, skin
    radiation NEC L59.8
    trophic disturbance (any region) —see Ulcer, skin
    X-ray L58.1
  duodenum, duodenal (eroded) (peptic) K26.9
    with
      hemorrhage K26.4
        and perforation K26.6
      perforation K26.5
    acute K26.3
      with
        hemorrhage K26.0
          and perforation K26.2
        perforation K26.1
    chronic K26.7
      with
        hemorrhage K26.4
          and perforation K26.6
        perforation K26.5
  dysenteric A09
  elusive —see Cystitis, interstitial
  endocarditis (acute) (chronic) (subacute) I28.8
  epiglottis J38.7
  esophagus (peptic) K22.10
    with bleeding K22.11
    due to
      aspirin K22.10
        with bleeding K22.11
      gastrointestinal reflux disease K21.0
      ingestion of chemical or medicament K22.10
        with bleeding K22.11
    fungal K22.10
      with bleeding K22.11
    infective K22.10
      with bleeding K22.11
    varicose —see Varix, esophagus
  eyelid (region) H01.8
  fauces J39.2
  Fenwick (-Hunner) (solitary) —see Cystitis, interstitial
  fistulous —see Ulcer, skin
  foot (indolent) (trophic) —see Ulcer, lower limb
  frambesial, initial A66.0
  frenum (tongue) K14.0
  gallbladder or duct K82.8
  gangrenous —see Gangrene
  gastric —see Ulcer, stomach
  gastrocolic —see Ulcer, gastrojejunal
  gastroduodenal —see Ulcer, peptic
  gastroesophageal —see Ulcer, stomach
  gastrointestinal —see Ulcer, gastrojejunal
  gastrojejunal (peptic) K28.9
    with
      hemorrhage K28.4
        and perforation K28.6
      perforation K28.5
    acute K28.3
      with
        hemorrhage K28.0
          and perforation K28.2
        perforation K28.1
    chronic K28.7
      with
        hemorrhage K28.4
          and perforation K28.6
        perforation K28.5
  gastrojejunocolic —see Ulcer, gastrojejunal
  gingiva K06.8
  gingivitis K05.10
    nonplaque induced K05.11
    plaque induced K05.10
  glottis J38.7
  granuloma of pudenda A58
  gum K06.8
  gumma, due to yaws A66.4

Ulcer, ulcerated, ulcerating, ulceration, ulcerative (Continued)
  heel —see Ulcer, lower limb
  hemorrhoid —see also Hemorrhoids, by degree K64.8
  Hunner's —see Cystitis, interstitial
  hypopharynx J39.2
  hypopyon (chronic) (subacute) —see Ulcer, cornea, with hypopyon
  hypostaticum —see Ulcer, varicose
  ileum —see Ulcer, intestine
  intestine, intestinal K63.3
    with perforation K63.1
    amebic A06.1
    duodenal —see Ulcer, duodenum
    granulocytopenic (with hemorrhage) —see Neutropenia
    marginal —see Ulcer, gastrojejunal
    perforating K63.1
      newborn P78.0
    primary, small intestine K63.3
    rectum K62.6
    stercoraceous, stercoral K63.3
    tuberculous A18.32
    typhoid (fever) —see Typhoid
    varicose I86.8
  jejunum, jejunal —see Ulcer, gastrojejunal
  keratitis —see Ulcer, cornea
  knee —see Ulcer, lower limb
  labium (majus) (minus) N76.6
  laryngitis —see Laryngitis
  larynx (aphthous) (contact) J38.7
    diphtheritic A36.2
  leg —see Ulcer, lower limb
  lip K13.0
  Lipschütz's N76.6
  lower limb (atrophic) (chronic) (neurogenic) (perforating) (pyogenic) (trophic) (tropical) L97.909
    with
      bone necrosis L97.904
      exposed fat layer L97.902
      muscle necrosis L97.903
      skin breakdown only L97.901
    ankle L97.309
      with
        bone necrosis L97.304
        exposed fat layer L97.302
        muscle necrosis L97.303
        skin breakdown only L97.301
      left L97.329
        with
          bone necrosis L97.324
          exposed fat layer L97.322
          muscle necrosis L97.323
          skin breakdown only L97.321
      right L97.319
        with
          bone necrosis L97.314
          exposed fat layer L97.312
          muscle necrosis L97.313
          skin breakdown only L97.311
    calf L97.209
      with
        bone necrosis L97.204
        exposed fat layer L97.202
        muscle necrosis L97.203
        skin breakdown only L97.201
      left L97.229
        with
          bone necrosis L97.224
          exposed fat layer L97.222
          muscle necrosis L97.223
          skin breakdown only L97.221
      right L97.219
        with
          bone necrosis L97.214
          exposed fat layer L97.212
          muscle necrosis L97.213
          skin breakdown only L97.211
    decubitus —see Ulcer, pressure, by site

◀ New   ◀▥▥ Revised   ~~deleted~~ Deleted

Ulcer, ulcerated, ulcerating, ulceration, ulcerative (Continued)
lower limb (Continued)
  foot specified NEC L97.509
    with
      bone necrosis L97.504
      exposed fat layer L97.502
      muscle necrosis L97.503
      skin breakdown only L97.501
    left L97.529
      with
        bone necrosis L97.524
        exposed fat layer L97.522
        muscle necrosis L97.523
        skin breakdown only L97.521
    right L97.519
      with
        bone necrosis L97.514
        exposed fat layer L97.512
        muscle necrosis L97.513
        skin breakdown only L97.511
  heel L97.409
    with
      bone necrosis L97.404
      exposed fat layer L97.402
      muscle necrosis L97.403
      skin breakdown only L97.401
    left L97.429
      with
        bone necrosis L97.424
        exposed fat layer L97.422
        muscle necrosis L97.423
        skin breakdown only L97.421
    right L97.419
      with
        bone necrosis L97.414
        exposed fat layer L97.412
        muscle necrosis L97.413
        skin breakdown only L97.411
  left L97.929
    with
      bone necrosis L97.924
      exposed fat layer L97.922
      muscle necrosis L97.923
      skin breakdown only L97.921
  lower leg NOS L97.909
    with
      bone necrosis L97.904
      exposed fat layer L97.902
      muscle necrosis L97.903
      skin breakdown only L97.901
    left L97.929
      with
        bone necrosis L97.924
        exposed fat layer L97.922
        muscle necrosis L97.923
        skin breakdown only L97.921
    right L97.919
      with
        bone necrosis L97.914
        exposed fat layer L97.912
        muscle necrosis L97.913
        skin breakdown only L97.911
  specified site NEC L97.809
    with
      bone necrosis L97.804
      exposed fat layer L97.802
      muscle necrosis L97.803
      skin breakdown only L97.801
    left L97.829
      with
        bone necrosis L97.824
        exposed fat layer L97.822
        muscle necrosis L97.823
        skin breakdown only L97.821
    right L97.819
      with
        bone necrosis L97.814
        exposed fat layer L97.812
        muscle necrosis L97.813
        skin breakdown only L97.811

Ulcer, ulcerated, ulcerating, ulceration, ulcerative (Continued)
lower limb (Continued)
  midfoot L97.409
    with
      bone necrosis L97.404
      exposed fat layer L97.402
      muscle necrosis L97.403
      skin breakdown only L97.401
    left L97.429
      with
        bone necrosis L97.424
        exposed fat layer L97.422
        muscle necrosis L97.423
        skin breakdown only L97.421
    right L97.419
      with
        bone necrosis L97.414
        exposed fat layer L97.412
        muscle necrosis L97.413
        skin breakdown only L97.411
  right L97.919
    with
      bone necrosis L97.914
      exposed fat layer L97.912
      muscle necrosis L97.913
      skin breakdown only L97.911
  thigh L97.109
    with
      bone necrosis L97.104
      exposed fat layer L97.102
      muscle necrosis L97.103
      skin breakdown only L97.101
    left L97.129
      with
        bone necrosis L97.124
        exposed fat layer L97.122
        muscle necrosis L97.123
        skin breakdown only L97.121
    right L97.119
      with
        bone necrosis L97.114
        exposed fat layer L97.112
        muscle necrosis L97.113
        skin breakdown only L97.111
  toe L97.509
    with
      bone necrosis L97.504
      exposed fat layer L97.502
      muscle necrosis L97.503
      skin breakdown only L97.501
    left L97.529
      with
        bone necrosis L97.524
        exposed fat layer L97.522
        muscle necrosis L97.523
        skin breakdown only L97.521
    right L97.519
      with
        bone necrosis L97.514
        exposed fat layer L97.512
        muscle necrosis L97.513
        skin breakdown only L97.511
  leprous A30.1
  syphilitic A52.19
  varicose —see Varix, leg, with, ulcer
luetic —see Ulcer, syphilitic
lung J98.4
  tuberculous —see Tuberculosis, pulmonary
malignant —see Neoplasm, malignant, by site
marginal NEC —see Ulcer, gastrojejunal
meatus (urinarius) N34.2
Meckel's diverticulum Q43.0
  malignant —see Table of Neoplasms, small intestine, malignant
Meleney's (chronic undermining) —see Ulcer, skin
Mooren's (cornea) —see Ulcer, cornea, Mooren's
mycobacterial (skin) A31.1
nasopharynx J39.2

Ulcer, ulcerated, ulcerating, ulceration, ulcerative (Continued)
  neck, uterus N86
  neurogenic NEC —see Ulcer, skin
  nose, nasal (passage) (infective) (septum) J34.0
    skin —see Ulcer, skin
    spirochetal A69.8
    varicose (bleeding) I86.8
  oral mucosa (traumatic) K12.1
  palate (soft) K12.1
  penis (chronic) N48.5
  peptic (site unspecified) K27.9
    with
      hemorrhage K27.4
        and perforation K27.6
      perforation K27.5
    acute K27.3
      with
        hemorrhage K27.0
          and perforation K27.2
        perforation K27.1
    chronic K27.7
      with
        hemorrhage K27.4
          and perforation K27.6
        perforation K27.5
  esophagus K22.10
    with bleeding K22.11
  newborn P78.82
  perforating K27.5
    skin —see Ulcer, skin
  peritonsillar J35.8
  phagedenic (tropical) —see Ulcer, skin
  pharynx J39.2
  phlebitis —see Phlebitis
  plaster —see Ulcer, pressure, by site
  popliteal space —see Ulcer, lower limb
  postpyloric —see Ulcer, duodenum
  prepuce N47.7
  prepyloric —see Ulcer, stomach
  pressure (pressure area) L89.9-
    ankle L89.5-
    back L89.1-
    buttock L89.3-
    coccyx L89.15-
    contiguous site of back, buttock, hip L89.4-
    elbow L89.0-
    face L89.81-
    head L89.81-
    heel L89.6-
    hip L89.2-
    sacral region (tailbone) L89.15-
    specified site NEC L89.89-
    stage 1 (healing) (pre-ulcer skin changes limited to persistent focal edema)
      ankle L89.5-
      back L89.1-
      buttock L89.3-
      coccyx L89.15-
      contiguous site of back, buttock, hip L89.4-
      elbow L89.0-
      face L89.81-
      head L89.81-
      heel L89.6-
      hip L89.2-
      sacral region (tailbone) L89.15-
      specified site NEC L89.89-
    stage 2 (healing) (abrasion, blister, partial thickness skin loss involving epidermis and/or dermis)
      ankle L89.5-
      back L89.1-
      buttock L89.3-
      coccyx L89.15-
      contiguous site of back, buttock, hip L89.4-
      elbow L89.0-
      face L89.81-
      head L89.81-

Ulcer, ulcerated, ulcerating, ulceration, ulcerative *(Continued)*
  pressure *(Continued)*
    stage 2 *(Continued)*
      heel L89.6-
      hip L89.2-
      sacral region (tailbone) L89.15-
      specified site NEC L89.89-
    stage 3 (healing) (full thickness skin loss involving damage or necrosis of subcutaneous tissue)
      ankle L89.5-
      back L89.1-
      buttock L89.3-
      coccyx L89.15-
      contiguous site of back, buttock, hip L89.4-
      elbow L89.0-
      face L89.81-
      head L89.81-
      heel L89.6-
      hip L89.2-
      sacral region (tailbone) L89.15-
      specified site NEC L89.89-
    stage 4 (healing) (necrosis of soft tissues through to underlying muscle, tendon, or bone)
      ankle L89.5-
      back L89.1-
      buttock L89.3-
      coccyx L89.15-
      contiguous site of back, buttock, hip L89.4-
      elbow L89.0-
      face L89.81-
      head L89.81-
      heel L89.6-
      hip L89.2-
      sacral region (tailbone) L89.15-
      specified site NEC L89.89-
    unspecified stage
      ankle L89.5-
      back L89.1-
      buttock L89.3-
      coccyx L89.15-
      contiguous site of back, buttock, hip L89.4-
      elbow L89.0-
      face L89.81-
      head L89.81-
      heel L89.6-
      hip L89.2-
      sacral region (tailbone) L89.15-
      specified site NEC L89.89-
    unstageable
      ankle L89.5-
      back L89.1-
      buttock L89.3-
      coccyx L89.15-
      contiguous site of back, buttock, hip L89.4-
      elbow L89.0-
      face L89.81-
      head L89.81-
      heel L89.6-
      hip L89.2-
      sacral region (tailbone) L89.15-
      specified site NEC L89.89-
  primary of intestine K63.3
    with perforation K63.1
  prostate N41.9
  pyloric —*see* Ulcer, stomach
  rectosigmoid K63.3
    with perforation K63.1
  rectum (sphincter) (solitary) K62.6
    stercoraceous, stercoral K62.6
  retina —*see* Inflammation, chorioretinal
  rodent —*see also* Neoplasm, skin, malignant
  sclera —*see* Scleritis
  scrofulous (tuberculous) A18.2

Ulcer, ulcerated, ulcerating, ulceration, ulcerative *(Continued)*
  scrotum N50.89 ◀
    tuberculous A18.15
    varicose I86.1
  seminal vesicle N50.89 ◀
  sigmoid —*see* Ulcer, intestine
  skin (atrophic) (chronic) (neurogenic) (non-healing) (perforating) (pyogenic) (trophic) (tropical) L98.499
    with gangrene —*see* Gangrene
    amebic A06.7
    back —*see* Ulcer, back
    buttock —*see* Ulcer, buttock
    decubitus —*see* Ulcer, pressure
    lower limb —*see* Ulcer, lower limb
    mycobacterial A31.1
    specified site NEC L98.499
      with
        bone necrosis L98.494
        exposed fat layer L98.492
        muscle necrosis L98.493
        skin breakdown only L98.491
    tuberculous (primary) A18.4
    varicose —*see* Ulcer, varicose
  sloughing —*see* Ulcer, skin
  solitary, anus or rectum (sphincter) K62.6
  sore throat J02.9
    streptococcal J02.0
  spermatic cord N50.89 ◀
  spine (tuberculous) A18.01
  stasis (venous) —*see* Varix, leg, with, ulcer
    without varicose veins I87.2
  stercoraceous, stercoral K63.3
    with perforation K63.1
    anus or rectum K62.6
  stoma, stomal —*see* Ulcer, gastrojejunal
  stomach (eroded) (peptic) (round) K25.9
    with
      hemorrhage K25.4
        and perforation K25.6
      perforation K25.5
    acute K25.3
      with
        hemorrhage K25.0
          and perforation K25.2
        perforation K25.1
    chronic K25.7
      with
        hemorrhage K25.4
          and perforation K25.6
        perforation K25.5
  stomal —*see* Ulcer, gastrojejunal
  stomatitis K12.1
  stress —*see* Ulcer, peptic
  strumous (tuberculous) A18.2
  submucosal, bladder —*see* Cystitis, interstitial
  syphilitic (any site) (early) (secondary) A51.39
    late A52.79
    perforating A52.79
      foot A52.11
  testis N50.89 ◀
  thigh —*see* Ulcer, lower limb
  throat J39.2
    diphtheritic A36.0
  toe —*see* Ulcer, lower limb
  tongue (traumatic) K14.0
  tonsil J35.8
    diphtheritic A36.0
  trachea J39.8
  trophic —*see* Ulcer, skin
  tropical —*see* Ulcer, skin
  tuberculous —*see* Tuberculosis, ulcer
  tunica vaginalis N50.89 ◀
  turbinate J34.89
  typhoid (perforating) —*see* Typhoid

Ulcer, ulcerated, ulcerating, ulceration, ulcerative *(Continued)*
  unspecified site —*see* Ulcer, skin
  urethra (meatus) —*see* Urethritis
  uterus N85.8
    cervix N86
      with cervicitis N72
    neck N86
      with cervicitis N72
  vagina N76.5
    in Behçet's disease M35.2 *[N77.0]*
    pessary N89.8
  valve, heart I33.0
  varicose (lower limb, any part) —*see also* Varix, leg, with, ulcer
    broad ligament I86.2
    esophagus —*see* Varix, esophagus
    inflamed or infected —*see* Varix, leg, with, ulcer, with inflammation
    nasal septum I86.8
    perineum I86.3
    scrotum I86.1
    specified site NEC I86.8
    sublingual I86.0
    vulva I86.3
  vas deferens N50.89 ◀
  vulva (acute) (infectional) N76.6
    in (due to)
      Behçet's disease M35.2 *[N77.0]*
      herpesviral (herpes simplex) infection A60.04
      tuberculosis A18.18
  vulvobuccal, recurring N76.6
  X-ray L58.1
  yaws A66.4
Ulcerosa scarlatina A38.8
Ulcus —*see also* Ulcer
  cutis tuberculosum A18.4
  duodeni —*see* Ulcer, duodenum
  durum (syphilitic) A51.0
    extragenital A51.2
  gastrojejunale —*see* Ulcer, gastrojejunal
  hypostaticum —*see* Ulcer, varicose
  molle (cutis) (skin) A57
  serpens corneae —*see* Ulcer, cornea, central
  ventriculi —*see* Ulcer, stomach
Ulegyria Q04.8
Ulerythema
  ophryogenes, congenital Q84.2
  sycosiforme L73.8
Ullrich(-Bonnevie)(-Turner) syndrome —*see also* Turner's syndrome Q87.1 ◀
Ullrich-Feichtiger syndrome Q87.0
Ulnar —*see* condition
Ulorrhagia, ulorrhea K06.8
Umbilicus, umbilical —*see* condition
Unacceptable
  contours of tooth K08.54
  morphology of tooth K08.54
Unavailability (of)
  bed at medical facility Z75.1
  health service-related agencies Z75.4
  medical facilities (at) Z75.3
    due to
      investigation by social service agency Z75.2
      lack of services at home Z75.0
      remoteness from facility Z75.3
      waiting list Z75.1
    home Z75.0
    outpatient clinic Z75.3
  schooling Z55.1
  social service agencies Z75.4
Uncinaria americana infestation B76.1
Uncinariasis B76.9
Uncongenial work Z56.5
Unconscious (ness) —*see* Coma
Underachievement in school Z55.3
Underdevelopment —*see also* Undeveloped
  nose Q30.1
  sexual E30.0

◀ New   ◀ Revised   ~~deleted~~ Deleted

Underdosing —see also Table of Drugs and
Chemicals, categories T36-T50, with final
character 6 Z91.14
intentional NEC Z91.128
due to financial hardship of patient
Z91.120
unintentional NEC Z91.138
due to patient's age related debility
Z91.130
Underfeeding, newborn P92.3
Underfill, endodontic M27.53
Underimmunization status Z28.3
Undernourishment —see Malnutrition
Undernutrition —see Malnutrition
Under observation —see Observation
Underweight R63.6
for gestational age —see Light for dates
Underwood's disease P83.0
Undescended —see also Malposition, congenital
cecum Q43.3
colon Q43.3
testicle —see Cryptorchid
Undeveloped, undevelopment —see also
Hypoplasia
brain (congenital) Q02
cerebral (congenital) Q02
heart Q24.8
lung Q33.6
testis E29.1
uterus E30.0
Undiagnosed (disease) R69
Undulant fever —see Brucellosis
Unemployment, anxiety concerning Z56.0
threatened Z56.2
Unequal length (acquired) (limb) —see also
Deformity, limb, unequal length
leg —see also Deformity, limb, unequal
length
congenital Q72.9-
Unextracted dental root K08.3
Unguis incarnatus L60.0
Unhappiness R45.2
Unicornate uterus Q51.4
Unilateral —see also condition
development, breast N64.89
organ or site, congenital NEC —see Agenesis,
by site
Unilocular heart Q20.8
Union, abnormal —see also Fusion
larynx and trachea Q34.8
Universal mesentery Q43.3
Unrepairable overhanging of dental
restorative materials K08.52
Unsatisfactory
restoration of tooth K08.50
specified NEC K08.59
sample of cytologic smear
anus R85.615
cervix R87.615
vagina R87.625
surroundings Z59.1
work Z56.5
Unsoundness of mind —see Psychosis
Unstable
back NEC —see Instability, joint, spine
hip (congenital) Q65.6
acquired —see Derangement, joint,
specified type NEC, hip
joint —see Instability, joint
secondary to removal of joint prosthesis
M96.89
lie (mother) O32.0
lumbosacral joint (congenital)
acquired —see subcategory M53.2
sacroiliac —see subcategory M53.2
spine NEC —see Instability, joint, spine
Unsteadiness on feet R26.81
Untruthfulness, child problem F91.8
Unverricht(-Lundborg) disease or epilepsy —
see Epilepsy, generalized, idiopathic
Unwanted pregnancy Z64.0

Upbringing, institutional Z62.22
away from parents NEC Z62.29
in care of non-parental family member Z62.21
in foster care Z62.21
in orphanage or group home Z62.22
in welfare custody Z62.21
Upper respiratory —see condition
Upset
gastric K30
gastrointestinal K30
psychogenic F45.8
intestinal (large) (small) K59.9
psychogenic F45.8
menstruation N93.9
mental F48.9
stomach K30
psychogenic F45.8
Urachus —see also condition
patent or persistent Q64.4
Urbach-Oppenheim disease (necrobiosis
lipoidica diabeticorum) —see E08-E13 with
.620
Urbach's lipoid proteinosis E78.89
Urbach-Wiethe disease E78.89
Urban yellow fever A95.1
Urea
blood, high —see Uremia
cycle metabolism disorder —see Disorder,
urea cycle metabolism
Uremia, uremic N19
with
ectopic or molar pregnancy O08.4
polyneuropathy N18.9 [G63]
chronic —see also Disease, kidney, chronic
N18.9
due to hypertension —see Hypertensive,
kidney
complicating
ectopic or molar pregnancy O08.4
congenital P96.0
extrarenal R39.2
following ectopic or molar pregnancy O08.4
newborn P96.0
prerenal R39.2
Ureter, ureteral —see condition
Ureteralgia N23
Ureterectasis —see Hydroureter
Ureteritis N28.89
cystica N28.86
due to calculus N20.1
with calculus, kidney N20.2
with hydronephrosis N13.2
gonococcal (acute) (chronic) A54.21
nonspecific N28.89
Ureterocele N28.89
congenital (orthotopic) Q62.31
ectopic Q62.32
Ureterolith, ureterolithiasis —see Calculus,
ureter
Ureterostomy
attention to Z43.6
status Z93.6
Urethra, urethral —see condition
Urethralgia R39.89
Urethritis (anterior) (posterior) N34.2
calculous N21.1
candidal B37.41
chlamydial A56.01
diplococcal (gonococcal) A54.01
with abscess (accessory gland)
(periurethral) A54.1
gonococcal A54.01
with abscess (accessory gland)
(periurethral) A54.1
nongonococcal N34.1
Reiter's —see Reiter's disease
nonspecific N34.1
nonvenereal N34.1
postmenopausal N34.2
puerperal O86.22
Reiter's —see Reiter's disease

Urethritis (Continued)
specified NEC N34.2
trichomonal or due to Trichomonas
(vaginalis) A59.03
Urethrocele N81.0
with
cystocele —see Cystocele
prolapse of uterus —see Prolapse, uterus
Urethrolithiasis (with colic or infection) N21.1
Urethrorectal —see condition
Urethrorrhagia N36.8
Urethrorrhea R36.9
Urethrostomy
attention to Z43.6
status Z93.6
Urethrotrigonitis —see Trigonitis
Urethrovaginal —see condition
Urgency
fecal R15.2
hypertensive —see Hypertension
urinary N39.15 ◀▥
Urhidrosis, uridrosis L74.8
Uric acid in blood (increased) E79.0
Uricacidemia (asymptomatic) E79.0
Uricemia (asymptomatic) E79.0
Uricosuria R82.99
Urinary —see condition
Urination
frequent R35.0
painful R30.9
Urine
blood in —see Hematuria
discharge, excessive R35.8
enuresis, nonorganic origin F98.0
extravasation R39.0
frequency R35.0
incontinence R32
nonorganic origin F98.0
intermittent stream R39.198 ◀▥
pus in N39.0
retention or stasis R33.9
organic R33.8
drug-induced R33.0
psychogenic F45.8
secretion
deficient R34
excessive R35.8
frequency R35.0
stream
intermittent R39.198 ◀▥
slowing R39.198 ◀▥
splitting R39.13
weak R39.12
Urinemia —see Uremia
Urinoma, urethra N36.8
Uroarthritis, infectious (Reiter's) —see Reiter's
disease
Urodialysis R34
Urolithiasis —see Calculus, urinary
Uronephrosis —see Hydronephrosis
Uropathy N39.9
obstructive N13.9
specified NEC N13.8
reflux N13.9
specified NEC N13.8
vesicoureteral reflux-associated —see Reflux,
vesicoureteral
Urosepsis — code to condition
Urticaria L50.9
with angioneurotic edema T78.3
hereditary D84.1
allergic L50.0
cholinergic L50.5
chronic L50.8
cold, familial L50.2
contact L50.6
dermatographic L50.3
due to
cold or heat L50.2
drugs L50.0
food L50.0

Urticaria *(Continued)*
 due to *(Continued)*
  inhalants L50.0
  plants L50.6
  serum —*see also* Reaction, serum T80.69
 factitial L50.3
 familial cold M04.2 ◀
 giant T78.3
  hereditary D84.1
 gigantea T78.3
 idiopathic L50.1
 larynx T78.3
  hereditary D84.1
 neonatorum P83.8
 nonallergic L50.1
 papulosa (Hebra) L28.2
 pigmentosa Q82.2
 recurrent periodic L50.8
 serum —*see also* Reaction, serum T80.69
 solar L56.3
 specified type NEC L50.8
 thermal (cold) (heat) L50.2
 vibratory L50.4
 xanthelasmoidea Q82.2
Use (of)
 alcohol Z72.89 ◀▥
  ~~with sleep disorder F10.982~~
  with ◀
   intoxication F10.929 ◀
   sleep disorder F10.982 ◀
  harmful —*see* Abuse, alcohol
 amphetamines —*see* Use, stimulant NEC
 caffeine —*see* Use, stimulant NEC
 cannabis F12.90
  with
   anxiety disorder F12.980
   intoxication F12.929
    with
     delirium F12.921
     perceptual disturbance F12.922
    uncomplicated F12.920
   other specified disorder F12.988
   psychosis F12.959
    delusions F12.950
    hallucinations F12.951
   unspecified disorder F12.99
 cocaine F14.90
  with
   anxiety disorder F14.980
   intoxication F14.929
    with
     delirium F14.921
     perceptual disturbance F14.922
    uncomplicated F14.920
   other specified disorder F14.988
   psychosis F14.959
    delusions F14.950
    hallucinations F14.951
   sexual dysfunction F14.981
   sleep disorder F14.982
   unspecified disorder F14.99
  harmful —*see* Abuse, drug, cocaine
 drug (s) NEC F19.90
  with sleep disorder F19.982
  harmful —*see* Abuse, drug, by type
 hallucinogen NEC F16.90
  with
   anxiety disorder F16.980
   intoxication F16.929
    with
     delirium F16.921
    uncomplicated F16.920
   mood disorder F16.94
   other specified disorder F16.988

Use *(Continued)*
 hallucinogen NEC *(Continued)*
  with *(Continued)*
   perception disorder (flashbacks) F16.983
   psychosis F16.959
    delusions F16.950
    hallucinations F16.951
   unspecified disorder F16.99
  harmful —*see* Abuse, drug, hallucinogen NEC
 inhalants F18.90
  with
   anxiety disorder F18.980
   intoxication F18.929
    with delirium F18.921
    uncomplicated F18.920
   mood disorder F18.94
   other specified disorder F18.988
   persisting dementia F18.97
   psychosis F18.959
    delusions F18.950
    hallucinations F18.951
   unspecified disorder F18.99
  harmful —*see* Abuse, drug, inhalant
 methadone —*see* Use, opioid ◀▥
 nonprescribed drugs F19.90
  harmful —*see* Abuse, non-psychoactive substance
 opioid F11.90
  with
   disorder F11.99
    mood F11.94
    sleep F11.982
    specified type NEC F11.988
   intoxication F11.929
    with
     delirium F11.921
     perceptual disturbance F11.922
    uncomplicated F11.920
   withdrawal F11.93
  harmful —*see* Abuse, drug, opioid
 patent medicines F19.90
  harmful —*see* Abuse, non-psychoactive substance
 psychoactive drug NEC F19.90
  with
   anxiety disorder F19.980
   intoxication F19.929
    with
     delirium F19.921
     perceptual disturbance F19.922
    uncomplicated F19.920
   mood disorder F19.94
   other specified disorder F19.988
   persisting
    amnestic disorder F19.96
    dementia F19.97
   psychosis F19.959
    delusions F19.950
    hallucinations F19.951
   sexual dysfunction F19.981
   sleep disorder F19.982
   unspecified disorder F19.99
   withdrawal F19.939
    with
     delirium F19.931
     perceptual disturbance F19.932
    uncomplicated F19.930
  harmful —*see* Abuse, drug NEC, psychoactive NEC

Use *(Continued)*
 sedative, hypnotic, or anxiolytic F13.90
  with
   anxiety disorder F13.980
   intoxication F13.929
    with
     delirium F13.921
    uncomplicated F13.920
   other specified disorder F13.988
   persisting
    amnestic disorder F13.96
    dementia F13.97
   psychosis F13.959
    delusions F13.950
    hallucinations F13.951
   sexual dysfunction F13.981
   sleep disorder F13.982
   unspecified disorder F13.99
  harmful —*see* Abuse, drug, sedative, hypnotic, or anxiolytic
 stimulant NEC F15.90
  with
   anxiety disorder F15.980
   intoxication F15.929
    with
     delirium F15.921
     perceptual disturbance F15.922
    uncomplicated F15.920
   mood disorder F15.94
   other specified disorder F15.988
   psychosis F15.959
    delusions F15.950
    hallucinations F15.951
   sexual dysfunction F15.981
   sleep disorder F15.982
   unspecified disorder F15.99
   withdrawal F15.93
  harmful —*see* Abuse, drug, stimulant NEC
 tobacco Z72.0
  with dependence —*see* Dependence, drug, nicotine
 volatile solvents —*see also* Use, inhalant F18.90
  harmful —*see* Abuse, drug, inhalant
Usher-Senear disease or syndrome L10.4
Uta B55.1
Uteromegaly N85.2
Uterovaginal —*see* condition
Uterovesical —*see* condition
Uveal —*see* condition
Uveitis (anterior) —*see also* Iridocyclitis
 acute —*see* Iridocyclitis, acute
 chronic —*see* Iridocyclitis, chronic
 due to toxoplasmosis (acquired) B58.09
  congenital P37.1
 granulomatous —*see* Iridocyclitis, chronic
 heterochromic —*see* Cyclitis, Fuchs' heterochromic
 lens-induced —*see* Iridocyclitis, lens-induced
 posterior —*see* Chorioretinitis
 sympathetic H44.13-
 syphilitic (secondary) A51.43
  congenital (early) A50.01
  late A52.71
 tuberculous A18.54
Uveoencephalitis —*see* Inflammation, chorioretinal
Uveokeratitis —*see* Iridocyclitis
Uveoparotitis D86.89
Uvula —*see* condition
Uvulitis (acute) (catarrhal) (chronic) (membranous) (suppurative) (ulcerative) K12.2

◀ New   ◀▥ Revised   ~~deleted~~ Deleted

V

Vaccination (prophylactic)
    complication or reaction —*see* Complications,
        vaccination
    delayed Z28.9
    encounter for Z23
    not done —*see* Immunization, not done,
        because (of)
Vaccinia (generalized) (localized) T88.1
    without vaccination B08.011
    congenital P35.8
Vacuum, in sinus (accessory) (nasal) J34.89
Vagabond, vagabondage Z59.0
Vagabond's disease B85.1
Vagina, vaginal —*see* condition
Vaginalitis (tunica) (testis) N49.1
Vaginismus (reflex) N94.2
    functional F52.5
    nonorganic F52.5
    psychogenic F52.5
    secondary N94.2
Vaginitis (acute) (circumscribed) (diffuse)
        (emphysematous) (nonvenereal)
        (ulcerative) N76.0
    with ectopic or molar pregnancy O08.0
    amebic A06.82
    atrophic, postmenopausal N95.2
    bacterial N76.0
    blennorrhagic (gonococcal) A54.02
    candidal B37.3
    chlamydial A56.02
    chronic N76.1
    due to Trichomonas (vaginalis) A59.01
    following ectopic or molar pregnancy O08.0
    gonococcal A54.02
        with abscess (accessory gland)
            (periurethral) A54.1
    granuloma A58
    in (due to)
        candidiasis B37.3
        herpesviral (herpes simplex) infection
            A60.04
        pinworm infection B80 [N77.1]
    monilial B37.3
    mycotic (candidal) B37.3
    postmenopausal atrophic N95.2
    puerperal (postpartum) O86.13
    senile (atrophic) N95.2
    subacute or chronic N76.1
    syphilitic (early) A51.0
        late A52.76
    trichomonal A59.01
    tuberculous A18.18
Vaginosis —*see* Vaginitis
Vagotonia G52.2
Vagrancy Z59.0
VAIN —*see* Neoplasia, intraepithelial, vagina
Vallecula —*see* condition
Valley fever B38.0
Valsuani's disease —*see* Anemia, obstetric
Valve, valvular (formation) —*see also* condition
    cerebral ventricle (communicating) in situ
        Z98.2
    cervix, internal os Q51.828
    congenital NEC —*see* Atresia, by site
    ureter (pelvic junction) (vesical orifice)
        Q62.39
    urethra (congenital) (posterior) Q64.2
Valvulitis (chronic) —*see* Endocarditis
Valvulopathy —*see* Endocarditis
Van Bogaert's leukoencephalopathy
    (sclerosing) (subacute) A81.1
Van Bogaert-Scherer-Epstein disease or
    syndrome E75.5
Van Buchem's syndrome M85.2
Van Creveld-von Gierke disease E74.01
Van der Hoeve (-de Kleyn) syndrome Q78.0
Van der Woude's syndrome Q38.0
Van Neck's disease or osteochondrosis M91.0
Vanishing lung J44.9

Vapor asphyxia or suffocation T59.9
    specified agent —*see* Table of Drugs and
        Chemicals
Variance, lethal ball, prosthetic heart valve
    T82.09
Variants, thalassemic D56.8
Variations in hair color L67.1
Varicella B01.9
    with
        complications NEC B01.89
        encephalitis B01.11
        encephalomyelitis B01.11
        meningitis B01.0
        myelitis B01.12
        pneumonia B01.2
    congenital P35.8
Varices —*see* Varix
Varicocele (scrotum) (thrombosed) I86.1
    ovary I86.2
    perineum I86.3
    spermatic cord (ulcerated) I86.1
Varicose
    aneurysm (ruptured) I77.0
    dermatitis —*see* Varix, leg, with,
        inflammation
    eczema —*see* Varix, leg, with, inflammation
    phlebitis —*see* Varix, with, inflammation
    tumor —*see* Varix
    ulcer (lower limb, any part) —*see also* Varix,
        leg, with, ulcer
        anus —*see also* Hemorrhoids K64.8
        esophagus —*see* Varix, esophagus
        inflamed or infected —*see* Varix, leg, with
            ulcer, with inflammation
        nasal septum I86.8
        perineum I86.3
        scrotum I86.1
        specified site NEC I86.8
    vein —*see* Varix
    vessel —*see* Varix, leg
Varicosis, varicosities, varicosity —*see* Varix
Variola (major) (minor) B03
Varioloid B03
Varix (lower limb) (ruptured) I83.90
    with
        edema I83.899
        inflammation I83.10
            with ulcer (venous) I83.209
        pain I83.819
        specified complication NEC I83.899
        stasis dermatitis I83.10
            with ulcer (venous) I83.209
        swelling I83.899
        ulcer I83.009
            with inflammation I83.209
    aneurysmal I77.0
    asymptomatic I83.9-
    bladder I86.2
    broad ligament I86.2
    complicating
        childbirth (lower extremity) O87.4
            anus or rectum O87.2
            genital (vagina, vulva or perineum)
                O87.8
        pregnancy (lower extremity) O22.0-
            anus or rectum O22.4-
            genital (vagina, vulva or perineum)
                O22.1-
        puerperium (lower extremity) O87.4
            anus or rectum O87.2
            genital (vagina, vulva, perineum) O87.8
    congenital (any site) Q27.8
    esophagus (idiopathic) (primary) (ulcerated)
        I85.00
        bleeding I85.01
        congenital Q27.8
        in (due to)
            alcoholic liver disease I85.10
                bleeding I85.11
            cirrhosis of liver I85.10
                bleeding I85.11

Varix (*Continued*)
    esophagus (*Continued*)
        in (*Continued*)
            portal hypertension I85.10
                bleeding I85.11
            schistosomiasis I85.10
                bleeding I85.11
            toxic liver disease I85.10
                bleeding I85.11
        secondary I85.10
            bleeding I85.11
    gastric I86.4
    inflamed or infected I83.10
        ulcerated I83.209
    labia (majora) I86.3
    leg (asymptomatic) I83.90
        with
            edema I83.899
            inflammation I83.10
                with ulcer —*see* Varix, leg, with, ulcer,
                    with inflammation by site
            pain I83.819
            specified complication NEC I83.899
            swelling I83.899
            ulcer I83.009
                with inflammation I83.209
            ankle I83.003
                with inflammation I83.203
            calf I83.002
                with inflammation I83.202
            foot NEC I83.005
                with inflammation I83.205
            heel I83.004
                with inflammation I83.204
            lower leg NEC I83.008
                with inflammation I83.208
            midfoot I83.004
                with inflammation I83.204
            thigh I83.001
                with inflammation I83.201
        bilateral (asymptomatic) I83.93
            with
                edema I83.893
                pain I83.813
                specified complication NEC I83.893
                swelling I83.893
                ulcer I83.009
                    with inflammation I83.209
        left (asymptomatic) I83.92
            with
                edema I83.892
                inflammation I83.12
                    with ulcer —*see* Varix, leg, with,
                        ulcer, with inflammation by
                        site
                pain I83.812
                specified complication NEC I83.892
                swelling I83.892
                ulcer I83.029
                    with inflammation I83.229
                ankle I83.023
                    with inflammation I83.223
                calf I83.022
                    with inflammation I83.222
                foot NEC I83.025
                    with inflammation I83.225
                heel I83.024
                    with inflammation I83.224
                lower leg NEC I83.028
                    with inflammation I83.228
                midfoot I83.024
                    with inflammation I83.224
                thigh I83.021
                    with inflammation I83.221
        right (asymptomatic) I83.91
            with
                edema I83.891
                inflammation I83.11
                    with ulcer —*see* Varix, leg, with,
                        ulcer, with inflammation by
                        site

Varix (Continued)
  leg (Continued)
    right (Continued)
      with (Continued)
        pain I83.811
        specified complication NEC I83.891
        swelling I83.891
        ulcer I83.019
          with inflammation I83.219
          ankle I83.013
            with inflammation I83.213
          calf I83.012
            with inflammation I83.212
          foot NEC I83.015
            with inflammation I83.215
          heel I83.014
            with inflammation I83.214
          lower leg NEC I83.018
            with inflammation I83.218
          midfoot I83.014
            with inflammation I83.214
          thigh I83.011
            with inflammation I83.211
  nasal septum I86.8
  orbit I86.8
    congenital Q27.8
  ovary I86.2
  papillary I78.1
  pelvis I86.2
  perineum I86.3
  pharynx I86.8
  placenta O43.89-
  renal papilla I86.8
  retina H35.09
  scrotum (ulcerated) I86.1
  sigmoid colon I86.8
  specified site NEC I86.8
  spinal (cord) (vessels) I86.8
  spleen, splenic (vein) (with phlebolith)
    I86.8
  stomach I86.4
  sublingual I86.0
  ulcerated I83.009
    inflamed or infected I83.209
  uterine ligament I86.2
  vagina I86.8
  vocal cord I86.8
  vulva I86.3
Vas deferens —see condition
Vas deferentitis N49.1
Vasa previa O69.4
  hemorrhage from, affecting newborn
    P50.0
Vascular —see also condition
  loop on optic papilla Q14.2
  spasm I73.9
  spider I78.1
Vascularization, cornea —see
    Neovascularization, cornea
Vasculitis I77.6
  allergic D69.0
  cryoglobulinemic D89.1
  disseminated I77.6
  hypocomplementemic M31.8
  kidney I77.89
  livedoid L95.0
  nodular L95.8
  retina H35.06-
  rheumatic —see Fever, rheumatic
  rheumatoid —see Rheumatoid, vasculitis
  skin (limited to) L95.9
    specified NEC L95.8
Vasculopathy, necrotizing M31.9
  cardiac allograft T86.290
  specified NEC M31.8
Vasitis (nodosa) N49.1
  tuberculous A18.15
Vasodilation I73.9
Vasomotor —see condition
Vasoplasty, after previous sterilization Z31.0
  aftercare Z31.42

Vasospasm (vasoconstriction) I73.9
  cerebral (cerebrovascular) (artery)
    I67.848
    reversible I67.841
  coronary I20.1
  nerve
    arm —see Mononeuropathy, upper limb
    brachial plexus G54.0
    cervical plexus G54.2
    leg —see Mononeuropathy, lower limb
  peripheral NOS I73.9
  retina (artery) —see Occlusion, artery,
    retina
Vasospastic —see condition
Vasovagal attack (paroxysmal) R55
  psychogenic F45.8
VATER syndrome Q87.2
Vater's ampulla —see condition
Vegetation, vegetative
  adenoid (nasal fossa) J35.8
  endocarditis (acute) (any valve) (subacute)
    I33.0
  heart (mycotic) (valve) I33.0
Veil
  Jackson's Q43.3
Vein, venous —see condition
Veldt sore —see Ulcer, skin
Velpeau's hernia —see Hernia, femoral
Venereal
  bubo A55
  disease A64
  granuloma inguinale A58
  lymphogranuloma (Durand-Nicolas-Favre)
    A55
Venofibrosis I87.8
Venom, venomous —see Table of Drugs and
    Chemicals, by animal or substance,
    poisoning
Venous —see condition
Ventilator lung, newborn P27.8
Ventral —see condition
Ventricle, ventricular —see also condition
  escape I49.3
  inversion Q20.5
Ventriculitis (cerebral) —see also Encephalitis
    G04.90
Ventriculostomy status Z98.2
Vernet's syndrome G52.7
Verneuil's disease (syphilitic bursitis) A52.78
Verruca (due to HPV) (filiformis) (simplex)
    (viral) (vulgaris) B07.9
  acuminata A63.0
  necrogenica (primary) (tuberculosa) A18.4
  plana B07.8
  plantaris B07.0
  seborrheica L82.1
    inflamed L82.0
  senile (seborrheic) L82.1
    inflamed L82.0
  tuberculosa (primary) A18.4
  venereal A63.0
Verrucosities —see Verruca
Verruga peruana, peruviana A44.1
Version
  with extraction
  cervix —see Malposition, uterus
  uterus (postinfectional) (postpartal, old) —see
    Malposition, uterus
Vertebra, vertebral —see condition
Vertical talus (congenital) Q66.80
  left foot Q66.82
  right foot Q66.81
Vertigo R42
  auditory —see Vertigo, aural
  aural H81.31-
  benign paroxysmal (positional) H81.1-
  central (origin) H81.4-
  cerebral H81.4-
  Dix and Hallpike (epidemic) —see Neuronitis,
    vestibular
  due to infrasound T75.23

Vertigo (Continued)
  epidemic A88.1
    Dix and Hallpike —see Neuronitis,
      vestibular
    Pedersen's —see Neuronitis, vestibular
    vestibular neuronitis —see Neuronitis,
      vestibular
  hysterical F44.89
  infrasound T75.23
  labyrinthine —see subcategory H81.0
  laryngeal R05
  malignant positional H81.4-
  Ménière's —see subcategory H81.40
  menopausal N95.11
  otogenic —see Vertigo, aural
  paroxysmal positional, benign —see Vertigo,
    benign paroxysmal
  Pedersen's (epidemic) —see Neuronitis,
    vestibular
  peripheral NEC H81.39-
  positional
    benign paroxysmal —see Vertigo, benign
      paroxysmal
    malignant H81.4-
Very-low-density-lipoprotein-type (VLDL)
    hyperlipoproteinemia E78.1
Vesania —see Psychosis
Vesical —see condition
Vesicle
  cutaneous R23.8
  seminal —see condition
  skin R23.8
Vesicocolic —see condition
Vesicoperineal —see condition
Vesicorectal —see condition
Vesicourethrorectal —see condition
Vesicovaginal —see condition
Vesicular —see condition
Vesiculitis (seminal) N49.0
  amebic A06.82
  gonorrheal (acute) (chronic) A54.23
  trichomonal A59.09
  tuberculous A18.15
Vestibulitis (ear) —see also subcategory H83.0
  nose (external) J34.89
  vulvar N94.810
Vestibulopathy, acute peripheral (recurrent) —
    see Neuronitis, vestibular
Vestige, vestigial —see also Persistence
  branchial Q18.0
  structures in vitreous Q14.0
Vibration
  adverse effects T75.20
    pneumatic hammer syndrome T75.21
    specified effect NEC T75.29
    vasospastic syndrome T75.22
    vertigo from infrasound T75.23
  exposure (occupational) Z57.7
  vertigo T75.23
Vibriosis A28.9
Victim (of)
  crime Z65.4
  disaster Z65.5
  terrorism Z65.4
  torture Z65.4
  war Z65.5
Vidal's disease L28.0
Villaret's syndrome G52.7
Villous —see condition
VIN —see Neoplasia, intraepithelial, vulva
Vincent's infection (angina) (gingivitis) A69.1
  stomatitis NEC A69.1
Vinson-Plummer syndrome D50.1
Violence, physical R45.6
Viosterol deficiency —see Deficiency, calciferol
Vipoma —see Neoplasm, malignant, by site
Viremia B34.9
Virilism (adrenal) E25.9
  congenital E25.0
Virilization (female) (suprarenal) E25.9
  congenital E25.0
  isosexual E28.2

◀ New   ◀|||| Revised   ~~deleted~~ Deleted

Virulent bubo A57
Virus, viral —*see also* condition
as cause of disease classified elsewhere B97.89
cytomegalovirus B25.9
human immunodeficiency (HIV) —*see* Human, immunodeficiency virus (HIV) disease
infection —*see* Infection, virus
specified NEC B34.8
~~swine influenza (viruses that normally cause infections in pigs) (see also Influenza, due to, identified novel influenza A virus) J09.X2~~
swine influenza (viruses that normally cause infections in pigs) —*see also* Influenza, due to, identified novel influenza A virus J09.X2 ◀
West Nile (fever) A92.30
with
complications NEC A92.39
cranial nerve disorders A92.32
encephalitis A92.31
encephalomyelitis A92.31
neurologic manifestation NEC A92.32
optic neuritis A92.32
polyradiculitis A92.32
Viscera, visceral —*see* condition
Visceroptosis K63.4
Visible peristalsis R19.2
Vision, visual
binocular, suppression H53.34
blurred, blurring H53.8
hysterical F44.6
defect, defective NEC H54.7
disorientation (syndrome) H53.8
disturbance H53.9
hysterical F44.6
double H53.2
examination Z01.00
with abnormal findings Z01.01
field, limitation (defect) —*see* Defect, visual field
hallucinations R44.1
halos H53.19
loss —*see* Loss, vision
sudden —*see* Disturbance, vision, subjective, loss, sudden
low (both eyes) —*see* Low, vision
perception, simultaneous without fusion H53.33
Vitality, lack or want of R53.83
newborn P96.89
Vitamin deficiency —*see* Deficiency, vitamin
Vitelline duct, persistent Q43.0
Vitiligo L80
eyelid H02.739
left H02.736
lower H02.735
upper H02.734

Vitiligo (*Continued*)
eyelid (*Continued*)
right H02.733
lower H02.732
upper H02.731
pinta A67.2
vulva N90.89
Vitreal corneal syndrome H59.01-
Vitreoretinopathy, proliferative —*see also* Retinopathy, proliferative
with retinal detachment —*see* Detachment, retina, traction
Vitreous —*see also* condition
touch syndrome —*see* Complication, postprocedural, following cataract surgery
Vocal cord —*see* condition
Vogt-Koyanagi syndrome H20.82-
Vogt's disease or syndrome G80.3
Vogt-Spielmeyer amaurotic idiocy or disease E75.4
Voice
change R49.9
specified NEC R49.8
loss —*see* Aphonia
Volhynian fever A79.0
Volkmann's ischemic contracture or paralysis (complicating trauma) T79.6
Volvulus (bowel) (colon) (intestine) K56.2 ◀
with perforation K56.2
congenital Q43.8
duodenum K31.5 ◀
fallopian tube —*see* Torsion, fallopian tube
oviduct —*see* Torsion, fallopian tube
stomach (due to absence of gastrocolic ligament) K31.89
Vomiting R11.10
with nausea R11.2
without nausea R11.11
asphyxia —*see* Foreign body, by site, causing asphyxia, gastric contents
bilious (cause unknown) R11.14
following gastro-intestinal surgery K91.0
in newborn P92.01
blood —*see* Hematemesis
causing asphyxia, choking, or suffocation — *see* Foreign body, by site
cyclical G43.A0
with refractory migraine G43.A1
intractable G43.A1
not intractable G43.A0
psychogenic F50.89 ◀▥
without refractory migraine G43.A0
fecal mater R11.13
following gastrointestinal surgery K91.0
psychogenic F50.89 ◀▥

Vomiting (*Continued*)
functional K31.89
hysterical F50.89 ◀▥
nervous F50.89 ◀▥
neurotic F50.89 ◀▥
newborn NEC P92.09
bilious P92.01
periodic R11.10
psychogenic F50.89 ◀▥
projectile R11.12
psychogenic F50.89 ◀▥
uremic —*see* Uremia
Vomito negro —*see* Fever, yellow
Von Bezold's abscess —*see* Mastoiditis, acute
Von Economo-Cruchet disease A85.8
Von Eulenburg's disease G71.19
Von Gierke's disease E74.01
Von Hippel (-Lindau) disease or syndrome Q85.8
Von Jaksch's anemia or disease D64.89
Von Recklinghausen
disease (neurofibromatosis) Q85.01
bones E21.0
Von Schroetter's syndrome I82.890
Von Willebrand (-Jurgens)(-Minot) disease or syndrome D68.0
Von Zumbusch's disease L40.1
Voyeurism F65.3
Vrolik's disease Q78.0
Vulva —*see* condition
Vulvismus N94.2
Vulvitis (acute) (allergic) (atrophic) (hypertrophic) (intertriginous) (senile) N76.2
with ectopic or molar pregnancy O08.0
adhesive, congenital Q52.79
blennorrhagic (gonococcal) A54.02
candidal B37.3
chlamydial A56.02
due to Haemophilus ducreyi A57
following ectopic or molar pregnancy O08.0
gonococcal A54.02
with abscess (accessory gland) (periurethral) A54.1
herpesviral A60.04
leukoplakic N90.4
monilial B37.3
puerperal (postpartum) O86.19
subacute or chronic N76.3
syphilitic (early) A51.0
late A52.76
trichomonal A59.01
tuberculous A18.18
Vulvodynia N94.819
specified NEC N94.818
Vulvorectal —*see* condition
Vulvovaginitis (acute) —*see* Vaginitis

W

Waiting list, person on Z75.1
- for organ transplant Z76.82
- undergoing social agency investigation Z75.2

Waldenström
- hypergammaglobulinemia D89.0
- syndrome or macroglobulinemia C88.0

Waldenström-Kjellberg syndrome D50.1

Walking
- difficulty R26.2
- - psychogenic F44.4
- sleep F51.3
- - hysterical F44.89

Wall, abdominal —see condition

Wallenberg's disease or syndrome G46.3

Wallgren's disease I87.8

Wandering
- gallbladder, congenital Q44.1
- in diseases classified elsewhere Z91.83
- kidney, congenital Q63.8
- organ or site, congenital NEC —see
    Malposition, congenital, by site
- pacemaker (heart) I49.8
- spleen D73.89

War neurosis F48.8

Wart (due to HPV) (filiform) (infectious) (viral)
    B07.9
- anogenital region (venereal) A63.0
- common B07.8
- external genital organs (venereal) A63.0
- flat B07.8
- Hassal-Henle's (of cornea) H18.49
- Peruvian A44.1
- plantar B07.0
- prosector (tuberculous) A18.4
- seborrheic L82.1
- - inflamed L82.0
- senile (seborrheic) L82.1
- - inflamed L82.0
- tuberculous A18.4
- venereal A63.0

Warthin's tumor —see Neoplasm, salivary
    gland, benign

Wassilieff's disease A27.0

Wasting
- disease R64
- - due to malnutrition E41
- extreme (due to malnutrition) E41
- muscle NEC —see Atrophy, muscle

Water
- clefts (senile cataract) —see Cataract, senile,
    incipient
- deprivation of T73.1
- intoxication E87.79
- itch B76.9
- lack of T73.1
- loading E87.70
- on
- - brain —see Hydrocephalus
- - chest J94.8
- poisoning E87.79

Waterbrash R12

Waterhouse(-Friderichsen) syndrome or
    disease (meningococcal) A39.1

Water-losing nephritis N25.89

Watermelon stomach K31.819
- with hemorrhage K31.811
- without hemorrhage K31.819

Watsoniasis B66.8

Wax in ear —see Impaction, cerumen

Weak, weakening, weakness (generalized)
    R53.1
- arches (acquired) —see also Deformity, limb,
    flat foot
- bladder (sphincter) R32
- facial R29.810
- - following
- - - cerebrovascular disease I69.992
- - - - cerebral infarction I69.392
- - - - intracerebral hemorrhage I69.192

Weak, weakening, weakness (Continued)
- facial (Continued)
- - following (Continued)
- - - cerebrovascular disease (Continued)
- - - - nontraumatic intracranial hemorrhage
        NEC I69.292
- - - - specified disease NEC I69.892
- - - - stroke I69.392
- - - - subarachnoid hemorrhage I69.092
- foot (double) —see Weak, arches
- heart, cardiac —see Failure, heart
- mind F70
- muscle M62.81
- myocardium —see Failure, heart
- newborn P96.89
- pelvic fundus N81.89
- pubocervical tissue N81.82
- rectovaginal tissue N81.83
- senile R54
- urinary stream R39.12
- valvular —see Endocarditis

Wear, worn (with normal or routine use)
- articular bearing surface of internal joint
    prosthesis —see Complications, joint
    prosthesis, mechanical, wear of articular
    bearing surfaces, by site
- device, implant or graft —see Complications,
    by site, mechanical complication
- tooth, teeth (approximal) (hard tissues)
    (interproximal) (occlusal) K03.0

Weather, weathered
- effects of
- - cold T69.9
- - - specified effect NEC T69.8
- - hot —see Heat
- skin L57.8

Weaver's syndrome Q87.3

Web, webbed (congenital)
- duodenal Q43.8
- esophagus Q39.4
- fingers Q70.1
- larynx (glottic) (subglottic) Q31.0
- neck (pterygium colli) Q18.3
- Paterson-Kelly D50.1
- popliteal syndrome Q87.89
- toes Q70.3

Weber-Christian disease M35.6

Weber-Cockayne syndrome (epidermolysis
    bullosa) Q81.8

Weber-Gubler syndrome G46.3

Weber-Leyden syndrome G46.3

Weber-Osler syndrome I78.0

Weber's paralysis or syndrome G46.3

Wedge-shaped or wedging vertebra —see
    Collapse, vertebra NEC

Wegener's granulomatosis or syndrome
    M31.30
- with
- - kidney involvement M31.31
- - lung involvement M31.30
- - - with kidney involvement M31.31

Wegner's disease A50.02

Weight
- 1000-2499 grams at birth (low) —see Low,
    birthweight
- 999 grams or less at birth (extremely low) —
    see Low, birthweight, extreme
- and length below 10th percentile for
    gestational age P05.1- ◀
- below but length above 10th percentile for
    gestational age P05.0- ◀
- gain (abnormal) (excessive) R63.5
- - in pregnancy —see Pregnancy, complicated
    by, excessive weight gain
- - low —see Pregnancy, complicated by,
    insufficient, weight gain
- loss (abnormal) (cause unknown) R63.4

Weightlessness (effect of) T75.82

Weil (l)-Marchesani syndrome Q87.1

Weil's disease A27.0

Weingarten's syndrome J82

Weir Mitchell's disease I73.81

Weiss-Baker syndrome G90.09

Wells' disease L98.3

Wen —see Cyst, sebaceous

Wenckebach's block or phenomenon I44.1

Werdnig-Hoffmann syndrome (muscular
    atrophy) G12.0

Werlhof's disease D69.3

Werner-His disease A79.0

Wermer's disease or syndrome E31.21

Werner's disease or syndrome E34.8

Wernicke-Korsakoff's syndrome or psychosis
    (alcoholic) F10.96
- with dependence F10.26
- drug-induced
- - due to drug abuse —see Abuse, drug, by
        type, with amnestic disorder
- - due to drug dependence —see Dependence,
        drug, by type, with amnestic disorder
- nonalcoholic F04

Wernicke-Posadas disease B38.9

Wernicke's
- developmental aphasia F80.2
- disease or syndrome E51.2
- encephalopathy E51.2
- polioencephalitis, superior E51.2

West African fever B50.8

Westphal-Strümpell syndrome E83.01

West's syndrome —see Epilepsy, spasms

Wet
- feet, tropical (maceration) (syndrome) —see
    Immersion, foot
- lung (syndrome), newborn P22.1

Wharton's duct —see condition

Wheal —see Urticaria

Wheezing R06.2

Whiplash injury S13.4

Whipple's disease —see also subcategory
    M14.8- K90.81

Whipworm (disease) (infection) (infestation)
    B79

Whistling face Q87.0

White —see also condition
- kidney, small N03.9
- leg, puerperal, postpartum, childbirth O87.1
- mouth B37.0
- patches of mouth K13.29
- spot lesions, teeth
- - chewing surface K02.51
- - pit and fissure surface K02.51
- - smooth surface K02.61

Whitehead L70.0

Whitlow —see also Cellulitis, digit
- with lymphangitis —see Lymphangitis, acute,
    digit
- herpesviral B00.89

Whitmore's disease or fever —see Melioidosis

Whooping cough A37.90
- with pneumonia A37.91
- - due to Bordetella
- - - bronchiseptica A37.81
- - - parapertussis A37.11
- - - pertussis A37.01
- - - specified organism NEC A37.81
- due to
- - Bordetella
- - - bronchiseptica A37.80
- - - - with pneumonia A37.81
- - - parapertussis A37.10
- - - - with pneumonia A37.11
- - - pertussis A37.00
- - - - with pneumonia A37.01
- - - specified NEC A37.80
- - - - with pneumonia A37.81

Wichman's asthma J38.5

Wide cranial sutures, newborn P96.3

Widening aorta —see Ectasia, aorta
- with aneurysm —see Aneurysm, aorta

Wilkie's disease or syndrome K55.1

Wilkinson-Sneddon disease or syndrome
    L13.1

◀ New   ◀▥ Revised   ~~deleted~~ Deleted

Willebrand (-Jürgens) thrombopathy D68.0
Willige-Hunt disease or syndrome G23.1
Wilms' tumor C64-
Wilson-Mikity syndrome P27.0
Wilson's
    disease or syndrome E83.01
    hepatolenticular degeneration E83.01
    lichen ruber L43.9
Window —*see also* Imperfect, closure
    aorticopulmonary Q21.4
Winter —*see* condition
Wiskott-Aldrich syndrome D82.0
Withdrawal state —*see also* Dependence, drug
        by type, with withdrawal
    alcohol ◄
        with perceptual disturbances F10.232 ◄
        without perceptual disturbances F10.239 ◄
    caffeine F15.93 ◄
    cannabis F12.288 ◄
    newborn
        correct therapeutic substance properly
            administered P96.2
        infant of dependent mother P96.1
        therapeutic substance, neonatal P96.2
Witts' anemia D50.8
Witzelsucht F07.0
Woakes' ethmoiditis or syndrome J33.1
Wolff-Hirschorn syndrome Q93.3
Wolff-Parkinson-White syndrome I45.6
Wolhynian fever A79.0
Wolman's disease E75.5
Wood lung or pneumonitis J67.8
Woolly, wooly hair (congenital) (nevus) Q84.1
Woolsorter's disease A22.1
Word
    blindness (congenital) (developmental) F81.0
    deafness (congenital) (developmental) H93.25
Worm (s) (infection) (infestation) —*see also*
        Infestation, helminth
    guinea B72
    in intestine NEC B82.0
Worm-eaten soles A66.3
Worn out —*see* Exhaustion
    cardiac
        defibrillator (with synchronous cardiac
            pacemaker) Z45.02
        pacemaker
            battery Z45.010
            lead Z45.018
    device, implant or graft —*see* Complications,
        by site, mechanical
Worried well Z71.1
Worries R45.82
Wound, open
    abdomen, abdominal
        wall S31.109
            with penetration into peritoneal cavity
                S31.609
            bite —*see* Bite, abdomen, wall
            epigastric region S31.102
                with penetration into peritoneal cavity
                    S31.602
                bite —*see* Bite, abdomen, wall,
                    epigastric region
                laceration —*see* Laceration, abdomen,
                    wall, epigastric region
                puncture —*see* Puncture, abdomen,
                    wall, epigastric region
            laceration —*see* Laceration, abdomen,
                wall
            left
                lower quadrant S31.104
                    with penetration into peritoneal
                        cavity S31.604
                    bite —*see* Bite, abdomen, wall, left,
                        lower quadrant
                    laceration —*see* Laceration,
                        abdomen, wall, left, lower
                        quadrant
                    puncture —*see* Puncture, abdomen,
                        wall, left, lower quadrant

Wound, open *(Continued)*
    abdomen, abdominal *(Continued)*
        wall *(Continued)*
            left *(Continued)*
                upper quadrant S31.101
                    with penetration into peritoneal
                        cavity S31.601
                    bite —*see* Bite, abdomen, wall, left,
                        upper quadrant
                    laceration —*see* Laceration,
                        abdomen, wall, left, upper
                        quadrant
                    puncture —*see* Puncture, abdomen,
                        wall, left, upper quadrant
            periumbilic region S31.105
                with penetration into peritoneal cavity
                    S31.605
                bite —*see* Bite, abdomen, wall,
                    periumbilic region
                laceration —*see* Laceration, abdomen,
                    wall, periumbilic region
                puncture —*see* Puncture, abdomen,
                    wall, periumbilic region
            puncture —*see* Puncture, abdomen, wall
            right
                lower quadrant S31.103
                    with penetration into peritoneal
                        cavity S31.603
                    bite —*see* Bite, abdomen, wall, right,
                        lower quadrant
                    laceration —*see* Laceration,
                        abdomen, wall, right, lower
                        quadrant
                    puncture —*see* Puncture, abdomen,
                        wall, right, lower quadrant
                upper quadrant S31.100
                    with penetration into peritoneal
                        cavity S31.600
                    bite —*see* Bite, abdomen, wall, right,
                        upper quadrant
                    laceration —*see* Laceration,
                        abdomen, wall, right, upper
                        quadrant
                    puncture —*see* Puncture, abdomen,
                        wall, right, upper quadrant
    alveolar (process) —*see* Wound, open, oral
        cavity
    ankle S91.00-
        bite —*see* Bite, ankle
        laceration —*see* Laceration, ankle
        puncture —*see* Puncture, ankle
    antecubital space —*see* Wound, open, elbow
    anterior chamber, eye —*see* Wound, open,
        ocular
    anus S31.839
        bite S31.835
        laceration —*see* Laceration, anus
        puncture —*see* Puncture, anus
    arm (upper) S41.10-
        with amputation —*see* Amputation,
            traumatic, arm
        bite —*see* Bite, arm
        forearm —*see* Wound, open, forearm
        laceration —*see* Laceration, arm
        puncture —*see* Puncture, arm
    auditory canal (external) (meatus) —*see*
        Wound, open, ear
    auricle, ear —*see* Wound, open, ear
    axilla —*see* Wound, open, arm
    back —*see also* Wound, open, thorax, back
        lower S31.000
            with penetration into retroperitoneal
                space S31.001
            bite —*see* Bite, back, lower
            laceration —*see* Laceration, back, lower
            puncture —*see* Puncture, back, lower
    bite —*see* Bite
    blood vessel —*see* Injury, blood vessel
    breast S21.00-
        with amputation —*see* Amputation,
            traumatic, breast

Wound, open *(Continued)*
    breast *(Continued)*
        bite —*see* Bite, breast
        laceration —*see* Laceration, breast
        puncture —*see* Puncture, breast
    buttock S31.809
        bite —*see* Bite, buttock
        laceration —*see* Laceration, buttock
        left S31.829
        puncture —*see* Puncture, buttock
        right S31.819
    calf —*see* Wound, open, leg
    canaliculus lacrimalis —*see* Wound, open,
        eyelid
    canthus, eye —*see* Wound, open, eyelid
    cervical esophagus S11.20
        bite S11.25
        laceration —*see* Laceration, esophagus,
            traumatic, cervical
        puncture —*see* Puncture, cervical esophagus
    cheek (external) S01.40-
        bite —*see* Bite, cheek
        internal —*see* Wound, open, oral cavity
        laceration —*see* Laceration, cheek
        puncture —*see* Puncture, cheek
    chest wall —*see* Wound, open, thorax
    chin —*see* Wound, open, head, specified site
        NEC
    choroid —*see* Wound, open, ocular
    ciliary body (eye) —*see* Wound, open, ocular
    clitoris S31.40
        with amputation —*see* Amputation,
            traumatic, clitoris
        bite S31.45
        laceration —*see* Laceration, vulva
        puncture —*see* Puncture, vulva
    conjunctiva —*see* Wound, open, ocular
    cornea —*see* Wound, open, ocular
    costal region —*see* Wound, open, thorax
    Descemet's membrane —*see* Wound, open,
        ocular
    digit (s)
        foot —*see* Wound, open, toe
        hand —*see* Wound, open, finger
    ear (canal) (external) S01.30-
        with amputation —*see* Amputation,
            traumatic, ear
        bite —*see* Bite, ear
        drum S09.2-
        laceration —*see* Laceration, ear
        puncture —*see* Puncture, ear
    elbow S51.00-
        bite —*see* Bite, elbow
        laceration —*see* Laceration, elbow
        puncture —*see* Puncture, elbow
    epididymis —*see* Wound, open, testis
    epigastric region S31.102
        with penetration into peritoneal cavity
            S31.602
        bite —*see* Bite, abdomen, wall, epigastric
            region
        laceration —*see* Laceration, abdomen, wall,
            epigastric region
        puncture —*see* Puncture, abdomen, wall,
            epigastric region
    epiglottis —*see* Wound, open, neck, specified
        site NEC
    esophagus (thoracic) S27.819
        cervical —*see* Wound, open, cervical
            esophagus
        laceration S27.813
        specified type NEC S27.818
    eye —*see* Wound, open, ocular
    eyeball —*see* Wound, open, ocular
    eyebrow —*see* Wound, open, eyelid
    eyelid S01.10-
        bite —*see* Bite, eyelid
        laceration —*see* Laceration, eyelid
        puncture —*see* Puncture, eyelid
    face NEC —*see* Wound, open, head, specified
        site NEC

Wound, open *(Continued)*
finger (s) S61.209
with
amputation —*see* Amputation, traumatic, finger
damage to nail S61.309
bite —*see* Bite, finger
index S61.208
with
damage to nail S61.308
left S61.201
with
damage to nail S61.301
right S61.200
with
damage to nail S61.300
laceration —*see* Laceration, finger
little S61.208
with
damage to nail S61.308
left S61.207
with damage to nail S61.307
right S61.206
with damage to nail S61.306
middle S61.208
with
damage to nail S61.308
left S61.203
with damage to nail S61.303
right S61.202
with damage to nail S61.302
puncture —*see* Puncture, finger
ring S61.208
with
damage to nail S61.308
left S61.205
with damage to nail S61.305
right S61.204
with damage to nail S61.304
flank —*see* Wound, open, abdomen, wall
foot (except toe (s) alone) S91.30-
with amputation —*see* Amputation, traumatic, foot
bite —*see* Bite, foot
laceration —*see* Laceration, foot
puncture —*see* Puncture, foot
toe —*see* Wound, open, toe
forearm S51.80-
with
amputation —*see* Amputation, traumatic, forearm
bite —*see* Bite, forearm
elbow only —*see* Wound, open, elbow
laceration —*see* Laceration, forearm
puncture —*see* Puncture, forearm
forehead —*see* Wound, open, head, specified site NEC
genital organs, external
with amputation —*see* Amputation, traumatic, genital organs
bite —*see* Bite, genital organ
female S31.502
vagina S31.40
vulva S31.40
laceration —*see* Laceration, genital organ
male S31.501
penis S31.20
scrotum S31.30
testes S31.30
puncture —*see* Puncture, genital organ
globe (eye) —*see* Wound, open, ocular
groin —*see* Wound, open, abdomen, wall
gum —*see* Wound, open, oral cavity
hand S61.40-
with
amputation —*see* Amputation, traumatic, hand
bite —*see* Bite, hand
finger (s) —*see* Wound, open, finger
laceration —*see* Laceration, hand

Wound, open *(Continued)*
hand *(Continued)*
puncture —*see* Puncture, hand
thumb —*see* Wound, open, thumb
head S01.90
bite —*see* Bite, head
cheek —*see* Wound, open, cheek
ear —*see* Wound, open, ear
eyelid —*see* Wound, open, eyelid
laceration —*see* Laceration, head
lip —*see* Wound, open, lip
nose S01.20
oral cavity —*see* Wound, open, oral cavity
puncture —*see* Puncture, head
scalp —*see* Wound, open, scalp
specified site NEC S01.80
temporomandibular area —*see* Wound, open, cheek
heel —*see* Wound, open, foot
hip S71.00-
with amputation —*see* Amputation, traumatic, hip
bite —*see* Bite, hip
laceration —*see* Laceration, hip
puncture —*see* Puncture, hip
hymen S31.40
bite —*see* Bite, vulva
laceration —*see* Laceration, vagina
puncture —*see* Puncture, vagina
hypochondrium S31.109
bite —*see* Bite, hypochondrium
laceration —*see* Laceration, hypochondrium
puncture —*see* Puncture, hypochondrium
hypogastric region S31.109
bite —*see* Bite, hypogastric region
laceration —*see* Laceration, hypogastric region
puncture —*see* Puncture, hypogastric region
iliac (region) —*see* Wound, open, inguinal region
inguinal region S31.109
bite —*see* Bite, abdomen, wall, lower quadrant
laceration —*see* Laceration, inguinal region
puncture —*see* Puncture, inguinal region
instep —*see* Wound, open, foot
interscapular region —*see* Wound, open, thorax, back
intraocular —*see* Wound, open, ocular
iris —*see* Wound, open, ocular
jaw —*see* Wound, open, head, specified site NEC
knee S81.00-
bite —*see* Bite, knee
laceration —*see* Laceration, knee
puncture —*see* Puncture, knee
labium (majus) (minus) —*see* Wound, open, vulva
laceration —*see* Laceration, by site
lacrimal duct —*see* Wound, open, eyelid
larynx S11.019
bite —*see* Bite, larynx
laceration —*see* Laceration, larynx
puncture —*see* Puncture, larynx
left
lower quadrant S31.104
with penetration into peritoneal cavity S31.604
bite —*see* Bite, abdomen, wall, left, lower quadrant
laceration —*see* Laceration, abdomen, wall, left, lower quadrant
puncture —*see* Puncture, abdomen, wall, left, lower quadrant
upper quadrant S31.101
with penetration into peritoneal cavity S31.601
bite —*see* Bite, abdomen, wall, left, upper quadrant

Wound, open *(Continued)*
left *(Continued)*
upper quadrant *(Continued)*
laceration —*see* Laceration, abdomen, wall, left, upper quadrant
puncture —*see* Puncture, abdomen, wall, left, upper quadrant
leg (lower) S81.80-
with amputation —*see* Amputation, traumatic, leg
ankle —*see* Wound, open, ankle
bite —*see* Bite, leg
foot —*see* Wound, open, foot
knee —*see* Wound, open, knee
laceration —*see* Laceration, leg
puncture —*see* Puncture, leg
toe —*see* Wound, open, toe
upper —*see* Wound, open, thigh
lip S01.501
bite —*see* Bite, lip
laceration —*see* Laceration, lip
puncture —*see* Puncture, lip
loin S31.109
bite —*see* Bite, abdomen, wall
laceration —*see* Laceration, loin
puncture —*see* Puncture, loin
lower back —*see* Wound, open, back, lower
lumbar region —*see* Wound, open, back, lower
malar region —*see* Wound, open, head, specified site NEC
mammary —*see* Wound, open, breast
mastoid region —*see* Wound, open, head, specified site NEC
mouth —*see* Wound, open, oral cavity
nail
finger —*see* Wound, open, finger, with damage to nail
toe —*see* Wound, open, toe, with damage to nail
nape (neck) —*see* Wound, open, neck
nasal (septum) (sinus) —*see* Wound, open, nose
nasopharynx —*see* Wound, open, head, specified site NEC
neck S11.90
bite —*see* Bite, neck
involving
cervical esophagus S11.20
larynx —*see* Wound, open, larynx
pharynx S11.20
thyroid S11.10
trachea (cervical) S11.029
bite —*see* Bite, trachea
laceration S11.021
with foreign body S11.022
puncture S11.023
with foreign body S11.024
laceration —*see* Laceration, neck
puncture —*see* Puncture, neck
specified site NEC S11.80
specified type NEC S11.89
nose (septum) (sinus) S01.20
with amputation —*see* Amputation, traumatic, nose
bite —*see* Bite, nose
laceration —*see* Laceration, nose
puncture —*see* Puncture, nose
ocular S05.90
avulsion (traumatic enucleation) S05.7-
eyeball S05.6-
with foreign body S05.5-
eyelid —*see* Wound, open, eyelid
laceration and rupture S05.3-
with prolapse or loss of intraocular tissue S05.2-
orbit (penetrating) (with or without foreign body) S05.4-
periocular area —*see* Wound, open, eyelid
specified NEC S05.8X-

◀ New   ◀|||| Revised   ~~deleted~~ Deleted

Wound, open (Continued)
oral cavity S01.502
bite S01.552
laceration —see Laceration, oral cavity
puncture —see Puncture, oral cavity
orbit —see Wound, open, ocular, orbit
palate —see Wound, open, oral cavity
palm —see Wound, open, hand
pelvis, pelvic —see also Wound, open, back,
lower
girdle —see Wound, open, hip
penetrating —see Puncture, by site
penis S31.20
with amputation —see Amputation,
traumatic, penis
bite S31.25
laceration —see Laceration, penis
puncture —see Puncture, penis
perineum
bite —see Bite, perineum
female S31.502
laceration —see Laceration, perineum
male S31.501
puncture —see Puncture, perineum
periocular area (with or without lacrimal
passages) —see Wound, open, eyelid
periumbilic region S31.105
with penetration into peritoneal cavity
S31.605
bite —see Bite, abdomen, wall, periumbilic
region
laceration —see Laceration, abdomen, wall,
periumbilic region
puncture —see Puncture, abdomen, wall,
periumbilic region
phalanges
finger —see Wound, open, finger
toe —see Wound, open, toe
pharynx S11.20
pinna —see Wound, open, ear
popliteal space —see Wound, open, knee
prepuce —see Wound, open, penis
pubic region —see Wound, open, back,
lower
pudendum —see Wound, open, genital
organs, external
puncture wound —see Puncture
rectovaginal septum —see Wound, open,
vagina
right
lower quadrant S31.103
with penetration into peritoneal cavity
S31.603
bite —see Bite, abdomen, wall, right,
lower quadrant
laceration —see Laceration, abdomen,
wall, right, lower quadrant
puncture —see Puncture, abdomen, wall,
right, lower quadrant
upper quadrant S31.100
with penetration into peritoneal cavity
S31.600
bite —see Bite, abdomen, wall, right,
upper quadrant
laceration —see Laceration, abdomen,
wall, right, upper quadrant
puncture —see Puncture, abdomen, wall,
right, upper quadrant
sacral region —see Wound, open, back,
lower
sacroiliac region —see Wound, open, back,
lower
salivary gland —see Wound, open, oral
cavity

Wound, open (Continued)
scalp S01.00
bite S01.05
laceration —see Laceration, scalp
puncture —see Puncture, scalp
scalpel, newborn (birth injury) P15.8
scapular region —see Wound, open, shoulder
sclera —see Wound, open, ocular
scrotum S31.30
with amputation —see Amputation,
traumatic, scrotum
bite S31.35
laceration —see Laceration, scrotum
puncture —see Puncture, scrotum
shin —see Wound, open, leg
shoulder S41.00-
with amputation —see Amputation,
traumatic, arm
bite —see Bite, shoulder
laceration —see Laceration, shoulder
puncture —see Puncture, shoulder
skin NOS T14.8
spermatic cord —see Wound, open, testis
sternal region —see Wound, open, thorax,
front wall
submaxillary region —see Wound, open,
head, specified site NEC
submental region —see Wound, open, head,
specified site NEC
subungual
finger (s) —see Wound, open, finger
toe (s) —see Wound, open, toe
supraclavicular region —see Wound, open,
neck, specified site NEC
temple, temporal region —see Wound, open,
head, specified site NEC
temporomandibular area —see Wound, open,
cheek
testis S31.30
with amputation —see Amputation,
traumatic, testes
bite S31.35
laceration —see Laceration, testis
puncture —see Puncture, testis
thigh S71.10-
with amputation —see Amputation,
traumatic, hip
bite —see Bite, thigh
laceration —see Laceration, thigh
puncture —see Puncture, thigh
thorax, thoracic (wall) S21.90
back S21.20-
with penetration S21.40
bite —see Bite, thorax
breast —see Wound, open, breast
front S21.10-
with penetration S21.30
laceration —see Laceration, thorax
puncture —see Puncture, thorax
throat —see Wound, open, neck
thumb S61.009
with
amputation —see Amputation,
traumatic, thumb
damage to nail S61.109
bite —see Bite, thumb
laceration —see Laceration, thumb
left S61.002
with
damage to nail S61.102
puncture —see Puncture, thumb
right S61.001
with
damage to nail S61.101

Wound, open (Continued)
thyroid (gland) —see Wound, open, neck,
thyroid
toe (s) S91.109
with
amputation —see Amputation,
traumatic, toe
damage to nail S91.209
bite —see Bite, toe
great S91.103
with
damage to nail S91.203
left S91.102
with
damage to nail S91.202
right S91.101
with
damage to nail S91.201
laceration —see Laceration, toe
lesser S91.106
with
damage to nail S91.206
left S91.105
with
damage to nail S91.205
right S91.104
with
damage to nail S91.204
puncture —see Puncture, toe
tongue —see Wound, open, oral cavity
trachea (cervical region) —see Wound, open,
neck, trachea
tunica vaginalis —see Wound, open, testis
tympanum, tympanic membrane S09.2-
laceration —see Laceration, ear, drum
puncture —see Puncture, tympanum
umbilical region —see Wound, open,
abdomen, wall, periumbilic region
uvula —see Wound, open, oral cavity
vagina S31.40
bite S31.45
laceration —see Laceration, vagina
puncture —see Puncture, vagina
vitreous (humor) —see Wound, open,
ocular
vocal cord S11.039
bite —see Bite, vocal cord
laceration S11.031
with foreign body S11.032
puncture S11.033
with foreign body S11.034
vulva S31.40
with amputation —see Amputation,
traumatic, vulva
bite S31.45
laceration —see Laceration, vulva
puncture —see Puncture, vulva
wrist S61.50-
bite —see Bite, wrist
laceration —see Laceration, wrist
puncture —see Puncture, wrist
Wound, superficial —see Injury (see also
specified injury type)
Wright's syndrome G54.0
Wrist —see condition
Wrong drug (by accident) (given in error) —
see Table of Drugs and Chemicals, by
drug, poisoning
Wry neck —see Torticollis
Wuchereria (bancrofti) infestation B74.0
Wuchereriasis B74.0
Wuchernde Struma Langhans C73

W

X

Xanthelasma (eyelid) (palpebrarum) H02.60
  left H02.66
    lower H02.65
    upper H02.64
  right H02.63
    lower H02.62
    upper H02.61
Xanthelasmatosis (essential) E78.2
Xanthinuria, hereditary E79.8
Xanthoastrocytoma
  specified site —see Neoplasm, malignant, by
    site
  unspecified site C71.9
Xanthofibroma —see Neoplasm, connective
    tissue, benign
Xanthogranuloma D76.3
Xanthoma (s), xanthomatosis (primary)
    (familial) (hereditary) E75.5
  with
    hyperlipoproteinemia
      Type I E78.3
      Type III E78.2
      Type IV E78.1
      Type V E78.3
  bone (generalisata) C96.5
  cerebrotendinous E75.5
  cutaneotendinous E75.5

Xanthoma (s), xanthomatosis (Continued)
  disseminatum (skin) E78.2
  eruptive E78.2
  hypercholesterinemic E78.00 ◀▦
  hypercholesterolemic E78.00 ◀▦
  hyperlipidemic E78.5
  joint E75.5
  multiple (skin) E78.2
  tendon (sheath) E75.5
  tuberosum E78.2
  tuberous E78.2
  tubo-eruptive E78.2
  verrucous, oral mucosa K13.4
Xanthosis R23.8
Xenophobia F40.10
Xeroderma —see also Ichthyosis
  acquired L85.0
    eyelid H01.149
      left H01.146
        lower H01.145
        upper H01.144
      right H01.143
        lower H01.142
        upper H01.141
  pigmentosum Q82.1
  vitamin A deficiency E50.8
Xerophthalmia (vitamin A deficiency) E50.7
  unrelated to vitamin A deficiency —see
    Keratoconjunctivitis

Xerosis
  conjunctiva H11.14-
    with Bitot's spots —see also Pigmentation,
      conjunctiva
      vitamin A deficiency E50.1
    vitamin A deficiency E50.0
  cornea H18.89-
    with ulceration —see Ulcer, cornea
      vitamin A deficiency E50.3
    vitamin A deficiency E50.2
  cutis L85.3
  skin L85.3
Xerostomia K11.7
Xiphopagus Q89.4
XO syndrome Q96.9
X-ray (of)
  abnormal findings —see Abnormal,
    diagnostic imaging
  breast (mammogram) (routine) Z12.31
  chest
    routine (as part of a general medical
      examination) Z00.00
    with abnormal findings Z00.01
  routine (as part of a general medical
    examination) Z00.00
    with abnormal findings Z00.01
XXXXY syndrome Q98.1
XXY syndrome Q98.0

X

◀ New   ◀▦ Revised   ~~deleted~~ Deleted

Y

Yaba pox virus disease BØ8.72
Yatapoxvirus BØ8.7Ø
   specified NEC BØ8.79
Yawning RØ6.89
   psychogenic F45.8
Yaws A66.9
   bone lesions A66.6
   butter A66.1
   chancre A66.Ø
   cutaneous, less than five years after infection
      A66.2
   early (cutaneous) (macular) (maculopapular)
      (micropapular) (papular) A66.2
      frambeside A66.2
      skin lesions NEC A66.2
   eyelid A66.2
   ganglion A66.6
   gangosis, gangosa A66.5
   gumma, gummata A66.4
      bone A66.6
   gummatous
      frambeside A66.4
      osteitis A66.6
      periostitis A66.6
   hydrarthrosis —*see also* subcategory
      M14.8- A66.6
   hyperkeratosis (early) (late) A66.3

Yaws *(Continued)*
   initial lesions A66.Ø
   joint lesions —*see also* subcategory
      M14.8- A66.6
   juxta-articular nodules A66.7
   late nodular (ulcerated) A66.4
   latent (without clinical manifestations) (with
      positive serology) A66.8
   mother A66.Ø
   mucosal A66.7
   multiple papillomata A66.1
   nodular, late (ulcerated) A66.4
   osteitis A66.6
   papilloma, plantar or palmar A66.1
   periostitis (hypertrophic) A66.6
   specified NEC A66.7
   ulcers A66.4
   wet crab A66.1
Yeast infection —*see also* Candidiasis B37.9
Yellow
   atrophy (liver) —*see* Failure, hepatic
   fever —*see* Fever, yellow
   jack —*see* Fever, yellow
   jaundice —*see* Jaundice
   nail syndrome L6Ø.5
Yersiniosis —*see also* Infection, Yersinia
   extraintestinal A28.2
   intestinal AØ4.6

Z

Zahorsky's syndrome (herpangina) BØ8.5
Zellweger's syndrome Q87.89
Zenker's diverticulum (esophagus) K22.5
Ziehen-Oppenheim disease G24.1
Zieve's syndrome K7Ø.Ø
Zika NOS A92.5 ◀
Zinc
   deficiency, dietary E6Ø
   metabolism disorder E83.2
Zollinger-Ellison syndrome E16.4
Zona —*see* Herpes, zoster
Zoophobia F4Ø.218
Zoster (herpes) —*see* Herpes, zoster
Zygomycosis B46.9
   specified NEC B46.8
Zymotic —*see* condition

ICD-10-CM
Table of Neoplasms

TABLE OF NEOPLASMS

The list below gives the code numbers for neoplasms by anatomical site. For each site there are six possible code numbers according to whether the neoplasm in question is malignant, benign, in situ, of uncertain behavior, or of unspecified nature. The description of the neoplasm will often indicate which of the six columns is appropriate; e.g., malignant melanoma of skin, benign fibroadenoma of breast, carcinoma in situ of cervix uteri.

Where such descriptors are not present, the remainder of the Index should be consulted where guidance is given to the appropriate column for each morphological (histological) variety listed; e.g., Mesonephroma — *see Neoplasm, malignant*; Embryoma — *see also Neoplasm, uncertain behavior*; Disease, Bowen's — *see Neoplasm, skin, in situ*. However, the guidance in the Index can be overridden if one of the descriptors mentioned above is present; e.g., malignant adenoma of colon is coded to C18.9 and not to D12.6 as the adjective "Malignant" overrides the Index entry 'Adenoma — *see also Neoplasm, benign.*'

Codes listed with a dash -, following the code have a required additional character for laterality. The Tablular must be reviewed for the complete code.

	Malignant Primary	Malignant Secondary	Ca in situ	Benign	Uncertain Behavior	Unspecified Behavior
Neoplasm, neoplastic	C80.1	C79.9	D09.9	D36.9	D48.9	D49.9
abdomen, abdominal	C76.2	C79.8-	D09.8	D36.7	D48.7	D49.89
cavity	C76.2	C79.8-	D09.8	D36.7	D48.7	D49.89
organ	C76.2	C79.8-	D09.8	D36.7	D48.7	D49.89
viscera	C76.2	C79.8-	D09.8	D36.7	D48.7	D49.89
wall — *see also Neoplasm, abdomen, wall, skin*	C44.509	C79.2-	D04.5	D23.5	D48.5	D49.2
connective tissue	C49.4	C79.8-	—	D21.4	D48.1	D49.2
skin	C44.509					
basal cell carcinoma	C44.519	—	—	—	—	—
specified type NEC	C44.599	—	—	—	—	—
squamous cell carcinoma	C44.529	—	—	—	—	—
abdominopelvic	C76.8	C79.8-	—	D36.7	D48.7	D49.89
accessory sinus — *see Neoplasm, sinus*						
acoustic nerve	C72.4-	C79.49	—	D33.3	D43.3	D49.7
adenoid (pharynx) (tissue)	C11.1	C79.89	D00.08	D10.6	D37.05	D49.0
adipose tissue — *see also Neoplasm, connective tissue*	C49.4	C79.89	—	D21.9	D48.1	D49.2
adnexa (uterine)	C57.4	C79.89	D07.39	D28.7	D39.8	D49.59
adrenal	C74.9-	C79.7-	D09.3	D35.0-	D44.1-	D49.7
capsule	C74.9-	C79.7-	D09.3	D35.0-	D44.1-	D49.7
cortex	C74.0-	C79.7-	D09.3	D35.0-	D44.1-	D49.7
gland	C74.9-	C79.7-	D09.3	D35.0-	D44.1-	D49.7
medulla	C74.1-	C79.7-	D09.3	D35.0-	D44.1-	D49.7
ala nasi (external) — *see also Neoplasm, skin, nose*	C44.301	C79.2	D04.39	D23.39	D48.5	D49.2
alimentary canal or tract NEC	C26.9	C78.80	D01.9	D13.9	D37.9	D49.0
alveolar	C03.9	C79.89	D00.03	D10.39	D37.09	D49.0
mucosa	C03.9	C79.89	D00.03	D10.39	D37.09	D49.0
lower	C03.1	C79.89	D00.03	D10.39	D37.09	D49.0
upper	C03.0	C79.89	D00.03	D10.39	D37.09	D49.0
ridge or process	C41.1	C79.51	—	D16.5-	D48.0	D49.2
carcinoma	C03.9	C79.8-	—	—	—	—
lower	C03.1	C79.8-	—	—	—	—
upper	C03.0	C79.8-	—	—	—	—
lower	C41.1	C79.51	—	D16.5-	D48.0	D49.2
mucosa	C03.9	C79.89	D00.03	D10.39	D37.09	D49.0
lower	C03.1	C79.89	D00.03	D10.39	D37.09	D49.0
upper	C03.0	C79.89	D00.03	D10.39	D37.09	D49.0
upper	C41.0	C79.51	—	D16.4-	D48.0	D49.2
sulcus	C06.1	C79.89	D00.02	D10.39	D37.09	D49.0
alveolus	C03.9	C79.89	D00.03	D10.39	D37.09	D49.0
lower	C03.1	C79.89	D00.03	D10.39	D37.09	D49.0
upper	C03.0	C79.89	D00.03	D10.39	D37.09	D49.0
ampulla of Vater	C24.1	C78.89	D01.5	D13.5	D37.6	D49.0
ankle NEC	C76.5-	C79.89	D04.7-	D36.7	D48.7	D49.89
anorectum, anorectal (junction)	C21.8	C78.5	D01.3	D12.9	D37.8	D49.0
antecubital fossa or space	C76.4-	C79.89	D04.6-	D36.7	D48.7	D49.89
antrum (Highmore) (maxillary)	C31.0	C78.39	D02.3	D14.0	D38.5	D49.1
pyloric	C16.3	C78.89	D00.2	D13.1	D37.1	D49.0
tympanicum	C30.1	C78.39	D02.3	D14.0	D38.5	D49.1
anus, anal	C21.0	C78.5	D01.3	D12.9	D37.8	D49.0
canal	C21.1	C78.5	D01.3	D12.9	D37.8	D49.0
cloacogenic zone	C21.2	C78.5	D01.3	D12.9	D37.8	D49.0
margin — *see also Neoplasm, anus, skin*	C44.500	C79.2	D04.5	D23.5	D48.5	D49.2
overlapping lesion with rectosigmoid junction or rectum	C21.8	—	—	—	—	—
skin	C44.500	C79.2	D04.5	D23.5	D48.5	D49.2
basal cell carcinoma	C44.510	—	—	—	—	—
specified type NEC	C44.590	—	—	—	—	—
squamous cell carcinoma	C44.520	—	—	—	—	—
sphincter	C21.1	C78.5	D01.3	D12.9	D37.8	D49.0
aorta (thoracic)	C49.3	C79.89	—	D21.3	D48.1	D49.2
abdominal	C49.4	C79.89	—	D21.4	D48.1	D49.2
aortic body	C75.5	C79.89	—	D35.6	D44.7	D49.7
aponeurosis	C49.9	C79.89	—	D21.9	D48.1	D49.2
palmar	C49.1-	C79.89	—	D21.1-	D48.1	D49.2
plantar	C49.2-	C79.89	—	D21.2-	D48.1	D49.2

◀ New ◀◀ Revised ~~deleted~~ Deleted

TABLE OF NEOPLASMS

TABLE OF NEOPLASMS

	Malignant Primary	Malignant Secondary	Ca in situ	Benign	Uncertain Behavior	Unspecified Behavior
appendix	C18.1	C78.5	D01.0	D12.1	D37.3	D49.0
arachnoid	C70.9	C79.49	—	D32.9	D42.9	D49.7
cerebral	C70.0	C79.32	—	D32.0	D42.0	D49.7
spinal	C70.1	C79.49	—	D32.1	D42.1	D49.7
areola	C50.0-	C79.81	D05.-	D24.-	D48.6-	D49.3
arm NEC	C76.4-	C79.89	D04.6-	D36.7	D48.7	D49.89
artery — *see Neoplasm, connective tissue*						
aryepiglottic fold	C13.1	C79.89	D00.08	D10.7	D37.05	D49.0
hypopharyngeal aspect	C13.1	C79.89	D00.08	D10.7	D37.05	D49.0
laryngeal aspect	C32.1	C78.39	D02.0	D14.1	D38.0	D49.1
marginal zone	C13.1	C79.89	D00.08	D10.7	D37.05	D49.0
arytenoid (cartilage)	C32.3	C78.39	D02.0	D14.1	D38.0	D49.1
fold — *see Neoplasm, aryepiglottic*						
associated with transplanted organ	C80.2	—	—	—	—	—
atlas	C41.2	C79.51	—	D16.6	D48.0	D49.2
atrium, cardiac	C38.0	C79.89	—	D15.1	D48.7	D49.89
auditory						
canal (external) (skin)	C44.20-	C79.2	D04.2-	D23.2-	D48.5	D49.2
internal	C30.1	C78.39	D02.3	D14.0	D38.5	D49.1
nerve	C72.4-	C79.49	—	D33.3	D43.3	D49.7
tube	C30.1	C78.39	D02.3	D14.0	D38.5	D49.1
opening	C11.2	C79.89	D00.08	D10.6	D37.05	D49.0
auricle, ear — *see also Neoplasm, skin, ear*	C44.20-	C79.2	D04.2-	D23.2-	D48.5	D49.2
auricular canal (external) — *see also Neoplasm, skin, ear*	C44.20-	C79.2	D04.2-	D23.2-	D48.5	D49.2
internal	C30.1	C78.39	D02.3	D14.0	D38.5	D49.2
autonomic nerve or nervous system NEC *(see Neoplasm, nerve, peripheral)*						
axilla, axillary	C76.1	C79.89	D09.8	D36.7	D48.7	D49.89
fold — *see also Neoplasm, skin, trunk*	C44.509	C79.2	D04.5	D23.5	D48.5	D49.2
back NEC	C76.8	C79.89	D04.5	D36.7	D48.7	D49.89
Bartholin's gland	C51.0	C79.82	D07.1	D28.0	D39.8	D49.59
basal ganglia	C71.0	C79.31	—	D33.0	D43.0	D49.6
basis pedunculi	C71.7	C79.31	—	D33.1	D43.1	D49.6
bile or biliary (tract)	C24.9	C78.89	D01.5	D13.5	D37.6	D49.0
canaliculi (biliferi) (intrahepatic)	C22.1	C78.7	D01.5	D13.4	D37.6	D49.0
canals, interlobular	C22.1	C78.89	D01.5	D13.4	D37.6	D49.0

	Malignant Primary	Malignant Secondary	Ca in situ	Benign	Uncertain Behavior	Unspecified Behavior
bile or biliary *(Continued)*						
duct or passage (common) (cystic) (extrahepatic)	C24.0	C78.89	D01.5	D13.5	D37.6	D49.0
interlobular	C22.1	C78.89	D01.5	D13.4	D37.6	D49.0
intrahepatic	C22.1	C78.7	D01.5	D13.4	D37.6	D49.0
and extrahepatic	C24.8	C78.89	D01.5	D13.5	D37.6	D49.0
bladder (urinary)	C67.9	C79.11	D09.0	D30.3	D41.4	D49.4
dome	C67.1	C79.11	D09.0	D30.3	D41.4	D49.4
neck	C67.5	C79.11	D09.0	D30.3	D41.4	D49.4
orifice	C67.9	C79.11	D09.0	D30.3	D41.4	D49.4
ureteric	C67.6	C79.11	D09.0	D30.3	D41.4	D49.4
urethral	C67.5	C79.11	D09.0	D30.3	D41.4	D49.4
overlapping lesion	C67.8	—	—	—	—	—
sphincter	C67.8	C79.11	D09.0	D30.3	D41.4	D49.4
trigone	C67.0	C79.11	D09.0	D30.3	D41.4	D49.4
urachus	C67.7	C79.11	D09.0	D30.3	D41.4	D49.4
wall	C67.9	C79.11	D09.0	D30.3	D41.4	D49.4
anterior	C67.3	C79.11	D09.0	D30.3	D41.4	D49.4
lateral	C67.2	C79.11	D09.0	D30.3	D41.4	D49.4
posterior	C67.4	C79.11	D09.0	D30.3	D41.4	D49.4
blood vessel — *see Neoplasm, connective tissue*						
bone (periosteum)	C41.9	C79.51	—	D16.9-	D48.0	D49.2
acetabulum	C41.4	C79.51	—	D16.8-	D48.0	D49.2
ankle	C40.3-	C79.51	—	D16.3-	—	—
arm NEC	C40.0-	C79.51	—	D16.0-	—	—
astragalus	C40.3-	C79.51	—	D16.3-	—	—
atlas	C41.2	C79.51	—	D16.6	D48.0	D49.2
axis	C41.2	C79.51	—	D16.6	D48.0	D49.2
back NEC	C41.2	C79.51	—	D16.6	D48.0	D49.2
calcaneus	C40.3-	C79.51	—	D16.3-	—	—
calvarium	C41.0	C79.51	—	D16.4	D48.0	D49.2
carpus (any)	C40.1-	C79.51	—	D16.1-	—	—
cartilage NEC	C41.9	C79.51	—	D16.9-	D48.0	D49.2
clavicle	C41.3	C79.51	—	D16.7-	D48.0	D49.2
clivus	C41.0	C79.51	—	D16.4	D48.0	D49.2
coccygeal vertebra	C41.4	C79.51	—	D16.8-	D48.0	D49.2
coccyx	C41.4	C79.51	—	D16.8-	D48.0	D49.2
costal cartilage	C41.3	C79.51	—	D16.7-	D48.0	D49.2
costovertebral joint	C41.3	C79.51	—	D16.7-	D48.0	D49.2
cranial	C41.0	C79.51	—	D16.4	D48.0	D49.2
cuboid	C40.3-	C79.51	—	D16.3-	—	—
cuneiform	C41.9	C79.51	—	D16.9-	D48.0	D49.2
elbow	C40.0-	C79.51	—	D16.0-	—	—

◀ New   ◀ Revised   ~~deleted~~ Deleted

bone *(Continued)*	Malignant Primary	Malignant Secondary	Ca in situ	Benign	Uncertain Behavior	Unspecified Behavior
ethmoid (labyrinth)	C41.0	C79.51	—	D16.4-	D48.0	D49.2
face	C41.0	C79.51	—	D16.4-	D48.0	D49.2
femur (any part)	C40.2-	C79.51	—	D16.2-	—	—
fibula (any part)	C40.2-	C79.51	—	D16.2-	—	—
finger (any)	C40.1-	C79.51	—	D16.1-	—	—
foot	C40.3-	C79.51	—	D16.3-	—	—
forearm	C40.0-	C79.51	—	D16.0-	—	—
frontal	C41.0	C79.51	—	D16.4-	D48.0	D49.2
hand	C40.1-	C79.51	—	D16.1-	—	—
heel	C40.3-	C79.51	—	D16.3-	—	—
hip	C41.4	C79.51	—	D16.8-	D48.0	D49.2
humerus (any part)	C40.0-	C79.51	—	D16.0-	—	—
hyoid	C41.0	C79.51	—	D16.4-	D48.0	D49.2
ilium	C41.4	C79.51	—	D16.8-	D48.0	D49.2
innominate	C41.4	C79.51	—	D16.8-	D48.0	D49.2
intervertebral cartilage or disc	C41.2	C79.51	—	D16.6-	D48.0	D49.2
ischium	C41.4	C79.51	—	D16.8-	D48.0	D49.2
jaw (lower)	C41.1	C79.51	—	D16.5-	D48.0	D49.2
knee	C40.2-	C79.51	—	D16.2-	—	—
leg NEC	C40.2-	C79.51	—	D16.2-	—	—
limb NEC	C40.9-	C79.51	—	D16.9-	—	—
lower (long bones)	C40.2-	C79.51	—	D16.2-	—	—
short bones	C40.3-	C79.51	—	D16.3-	—	—
upper (long bones)	C40.0-	C79.51	—	D16.0-	—	—
short bones	C40.1-	C79.51	—	D16.1-	—	—
malar	C41.0	C79.51	—	D16.4-	D48.0	D49.2
mandible	C41.1	C79.51	—	D16.5-	D48.0	D49.2
marrow NEC (any bone)	C96.9	C79.52	—	—	D47.9	D49.89
mastoid	C41.0	C79.51	—	D16.4-	D48.0	D49.2
maxilla, maxillary (superior)	C41.0	C79.51	—	D16.4-	D48.0	D49.2
inferior	C41.1	C79.51	—	D16.5-	D48.0	D49.2
metacarpus (any)	C40.1-	C79.51	—	D16.1-	—	—
metatarsus (any)	C40.3-	C79.51	—	D16.3-	—	—
overlapping sites	C40.8-	—	—	—	—	—
navicular						
ankle	C40.3-	C79.51	—	—	—	—
hand	C40.1-	C79.51	—	—	—	—
nose, nasal	C41.0	C79.51	—	D16.4-	D48.0	D49.2
occipital	C41.0	C79.51	—	D16.4-	D48.0	D49.2
orbit	C41.0	C79.51	—	D16.4-	D48.0	D49.2
parietal	C41.0	C79.51	—	D16.4-	D48.0	D49.2
patella	C40.2-	C79.51	—	—	—	—
pelvic	C41.4	C79.51	—	D16.8	D48.0	D49.2

bone *(Continued)*	Malignant Primary	Malignant Secondary	Ca in situ	Benign	Uncertain Behavior	Unspecified Behavior
phalanges						
foot	C40.3-	C79.51	—	—	—	—
hand	C40.1-	C79.51	—	—	—	—
pubic	C41.4	C79.51	—	D16.8	D48.0	D49.2
radius (any part)	C40.0-	C79.51	—	D16.0-	—	—
rib	C41.3	C79.51	—	D16.7	D48.0	D49.2
sacral vertebra	C41.4	C79.51	—	D16.8	D48.0	D49.2
sacrum	C41.4	C79.51	—	D16.8	D48.0	D49.2
scaphoid						
of ankle	C40.3-	C79.51	—	—	—	—
of hand	C40.1-	C79.51	—	—	—	—
scapula (any part)	C40.0-	C79.51	—	D16.0-	—	—
sella turcica	C41.0	C79.51	—	D16.4-	D48.0	D49.2
shoulder	C40.0-	C79.51	—	D16.0-	—	—
skull	C41.0	C79.51	—	D16.4-	D48.0	D49.2
sphenoid	C41.0	C79.51	—	D16.4-	D48.0	D49.2
spine, spinal (column)	C41.2	C79.51	—	D16.6	D48.0	D49.2
coccyx	C41.4	C79.51	—	D16.8	D48.0	D49.2
sacrum	C41.4	C79.51	—	D16.8	D48.0	D49.2
sternum	C41.3	C79.51	—	D16.7	D48.0	D49.2
tarsus (any)	C40.3-	C79.51	—	—	—	—
temporal	C41.0	C79.51	—	D16.4-	D48.0	D49.2
thumb	C40.1-	C79.51	—	—	—	—
tibia (any part)	C40.2-	C79.51	—	—	—	—
toe (any)	C40.3-	C79.51	—	—	—	—
trapezium	C40.1-	C79.51	—	—	—	—
trapezoid	C40.1-	C79.51	—	—	—	—
turbinate	C41.0	C79.51	—	D16.4-	D48.0	D49.2
ulna (any part)	C40.0-	C79.51	—	D16.0-	—	—
unciform	C40.1-	C79.51	—	—	—	—
vertebra (column)	C41.2	C79.51	—	D16.6	D48.0	D49.2
coccyx	C41.4	C79.51	—	D16.8	D48.0	D49.2
sacrum	C41.4	C79.51	—	D16.8	D48.0	D49.2
vomer	C41.0	C79.51	—	D16.4-	D48.0	D49.2
wrist	C40.1-	C79.51	—	—	—	—
xiphoid process	C41.3	C79.51	—	D16.7	D48.0	D49.2
zygomatic	C41.0	C79.51	—	D16.4-	D48.0	D49.2
book-leaf (mouth)	C06.89	C79.89	D00.00	D10.39	D37.09	D49.0
bowel—*see* Neoplasm, intestine						
brachial plexus	C47.1-	C79.89	—	D36.12	D48.2	D49.2
brain NEC	C71.9	C79.31	—	D33.2	D43.2	D49.6
basal ganglia	C71.0	C79.31	—	D33.0	D43.0	D49.6
cerebellopontine angle	C71.6	C79.31	—	D33.1	D43.1	D49.6

TABLE OF NEOPLASMS

	Malignant Primary	Malignant Secondary	Ca in situ	Benign	Uncertain Behavior	Unspecified Behavior
brain NEC (Continued)						
cerebellum NOS	C71.6	C79.31	—	D33.1	D43.1	D49.6
cerebrum	C71.0	C79.31	—	D33.0	D43.0	D49.6
choroid plexus	C71.7	C79.31	—	D33.1	D43.1	D49.6
corpus callosum	C71.8	C79.31	—	D33.2	D43.2	D49.6
corpus striatum	C71.0	C79.31	—	D33.0	D43.0	D49.6
cortex (cerebral)	C71.0	C79.31	—	D33.0	D43.0	D49.6
frontal lobe	C71.1	C79.31	—	D33.0	D43.0	D49.6
globus pallidus	C71.0	C79.31	—	D33.0	D43.0	D49.6
hippocampus	C71.2	C79.31	—	D33.0	D43.0	D49.6
hypothalamus	C71.0	C79.31	—	D33.0	D43.0	D49.6
internal capsule	C71.0	C79.31	—	D33.0	D43.0	D49.6
medulla oblongata	C71.7	C79.31	—	D33.1	D43.1	D49.6
meninges	C70.0	C79.32	—	D32.0	D42.0	D49.7
midbrain	C71.7	C79.31	—	D33.1	D43.1	D49.6
occipital lobe	C71.4	C79.31	—	D33.0	D43.0	D49.6
overlapping lesion	C71.8	C79.31	—	—	—	—
parietal lobe	C71.3	C79.31	—	D33.0	D43.0	D49.6
peduncle	C71.7	C79.31	—	D33.1	D43.1	D49.6
pons	C71.7	C79.31	—	D33.1	D43.1	D49.6
stem	C71.7	C79.31	—	D33.1	D43.1	D49.6
tapetum	C71.8	C79.31	—	D33.2	D43.2	D49.6
temporal lobe	C71.2	C79.31	—	D33.0	D43.0	D49.6
thalamus	C71.0	C79.31	—	D33.0	D43.0	D49.6
uncus	C71.2	C79.31	—	D33.0	D43.0	D49.6
ventricle (floor)	C71.5	C79.31	—	D33.0	D43.0	D49.6
fourth	C71.7	C79.31	—	D33.1	D43.1	D49.6
branchial (cleft) (cyst) (vestiges)	C10.4	C79.89	D00.08	D10.5	D37.05	D49.0
breast (connective tissue) (glandular tissue) (soft parts)	C50.9-	C79.81	D05.-	D24.-	D48.6-	D49.3
areola	C50.0-	C79.81	D05.-	D24.-	D48.6-	D49.3
axillary tail	C50.6-	C79.81	D05.-	D24.-	D48.6-	D49.3
central portion	C50.1-	C79.81	D05.-	D24.-	D48.6-	D49.3
inner	C50.8-	C79.81	D05.-	D24.-	D48.6-	D49.3
lower	C50.8-	C79.81	D05.-	D24.-	D48.6-	D49.3
lower-inner quadrant	C50.3-	C79.81	D05.-	D24.-	D48.6-	D49.3
lower-outer quadrant	C50.5-	C79.81	D05.-	D24.-	D48.6-	D49.3
mastectomy site (skin) — see also Neoplasm, breast, skin	C44.501	C79.2	—	—	—	—
specified as breast tissue	C50.8-	C79.81	—	—	—	—
midline	C50.8-	C79.81	D05.-	D24.-	D48.6-	D49.3
nipple	C50.0-	C79.81	D05.-	D24.-	D48.6-	D49.3
outer	C50.8-	C79.81	D05.-	D24.-	D48.6-	D49.3
overlapping lesion	C50.8-	—	—	—	—	—

	Malignant Primary	Malignant Secondary	Ca in situ	Benign	Uncertain Behavior	Unspecified Behavior
breast (Continued)						
skin	C44.501	C79.2	D04.5	D23.5	D48.5	D49.2
basal cell carcinoma	C44.511	—	—	—	—	—
specified type NEC	C44.591	—	—	—	—	—
squamous cell carcinoma	C44.521	—	—	—	—	—
tail (axillary)	C50.6-	C79.81	D05.-	D24.-	D48.6-	D49.3
upper	C50.8-	C79.81	D05.-	D24.-	D48.6-	D49.3
upper-inner quadrant	C50.2-	C79.81	D05.-	D24.-	D48.6-	D49.3
upper-outer quadrant	C50.4-	C79.81	D05.-	D24.-	D48.6-	D49.3
broad ligament	C57.1	C79.82	D07.39	D28.2	D39.8	D49.59 ◄▥
bronchiogenic, bronchogenic (lung)	C34.9-	C78.0-	D02.2-	D14.3-	D38.1	D49.1
bronchiole	C34.9-	C78.0-	D02.2-	D14.3-	D38.1	D49.1
bronchus	C34.9-	C78.0-	D02.2-	D14.3-	D38.1	D49.1
carina	C34.0-	C78.0-	D02.2-	D14.3-	D38.1	D49.1
lower lobe of lung	C34.3-	C78.0-	D02.2-	D14.3-	D38.1	D49.1
main	C34.0-	C78.0-	D02.2-	D14.3-	D38.1	D49.1
middle lobe of lung	C34.2	C78.0-	D02.21	D14.31	D38.1	D49.1
overlapping lesion	C34.8-	—	—	—	—	—
upper lobe of lung	C34.1-	C78.0-	D02.2-	D14.3-	D38.1	D49.1
brow	C44.309	C79.2	D04.39	D23.39	D48.5	D49.2
basal cell carcinoma	C44.319	—	—	—	—	—
specified type NEC	C44.399	—	—	—	—	—
squamous cell carcinoma	C44.329	—	—	—	—	—
buccal (cavity)	C06.9	C79.89	D00.00	D10.39	D37.09	D49.0
commissure	C06.0	C79.89	D00.02	D10.39	D37.09	D49.0
groove (lower) (upper)	C06.1	C79.89	D00.02	D10.39	D37.09	D49.0
mucosa	C06.0	C79.89	D00.02	D10.39	D37.09	D49.0
sulcus (lower) (upper)	C06.1	C79.89	D00.02	D10.39	D37.09	D49.0
bulbourethral gland	C68.0	C79.19	D09.19	D30.4	D41.3	D49.59 ◄▥
bursa — see Neoplasm, connective tissue						
buttock NEC	C76.3	C79.89	D04.5	D36.7	D48.7	D49.89
calf	C76.5-	C79.89	D04.7-	D36.7	D48.7	D49.89
calvarium	C41.0	C79.51	—	D16.4-	D48.0	D49.2
calyx, renal	C65.-	C79.0-	D09.19	D30.1-	D41.1-	D49.51- ◄▥
canal						
anal	C21.1	C78.5	D01.3	D12.9	D37.8	D49.0
auditory (external) — see also Neoplasm, skin, ear	C44.20-	C79.2	D04.2-	D23.2-	D48.5	D49.2
auricular (external) — see also Neoplasm, skin, ear	C44.20-	C79.2	D04.2-	D23.2-	D48.5	D49.2
canaliculi, biliary (biliferi) (intrahepatic)	C22.1	C78.7	D01.5	D13.4	D37.6	D49.0

◄ New   ◄▥ Revised   ~~deleted~~ Deleted

	Malignant Primary	Malignant Secondary	Ca in situ	Benign	Uncertain Behavior	Unspecified Behavior
canthus (eye) (inner) (outer)	C44.10-	C79.2	D04.1-	D23.1-	D48.5	D49.2
basal cell carcinoma	C44.11-	—	—	—	—	—
specified type NEC	C44.19-	—	—	—	—	—
squamous cell carcinoma	C44.12-	—	—	—	—	—
capillary — see Neoplasm, connective tissue						
caput coli	C18.0	C78.5	D01.0	D12.0	D37.4	D49.0
carcinoid — see Tumor, carcinoid						
cardia (gastric)	C16.0	C78.89	D00.2	D13.1	D37.1	D49.0
cardiac orifice (stomach)	C16.0	C78.89	D00.2	D13.1	D37.1	D49.0
cardio-esophageal junction	C16.0	C78.89	D00.2	D13.1	D37.1	D49.0
cardio-esophagus	C16.0	C78.89	D00.2	D13.1	D37.1	D49.0
carina (bronchus)	C34.0-	C78.0-	D02.2-	D14.3-	D38.1	D49.1
carotid (artery)	C49.0	C79.89	—	D21.0	D48.1	D49.2
body	C75.4	C79.89	—	D35.5	D44.6	D49.7
carpus (any bone)	C40.1-	C79.51	—	D16.1-	—	—
cartilage (articular) (joint) NEC — see also Neoplasm, bone	C41.9	C79.51	—	D16.9-	D48.0	D49.2
arytenoid	C32.3	C78.39	D02.0	D14.1	D38.0	D49.1
auricular	C49.0	C79.89	—	D21.0	D48.1	D49.2
bronchi	C34.0-	C78.39	—	D14.3-	D38.1	D49.1
costal	C41.3	C79.51	—	D16.7	D48.0	D49.2
cricoid	C32.3	C78.39	D02.0	D14.1	D38.0	D49.1
cuneiform	C32.3	C78.39	D02.0	D14.1	D38.0	D49.1
ear (external)	C49.0	C79.89	—	D21.0	D48.1	D49.2
ensiform	C41.3	C79.51	—	D16.7	D48.0	D49.2
epiglottis	C32.1	C78.39	D02.0	D14.1	D38.0	D49.1
anterior surface	C10.1	C79.89	D00.08	D10.5	D37.05	D49.0
eyelid	C49.0	C79.89	—	D21.0	D48.1	D49.2
intervertebral	C41.2	C79.51	—	D16.6	D48.0	D49.2
larynx, laryngeal	C32.3	C78.39	D02.0	D14.1	D38.0	D49.1
nose, nasal	C30.0	C78.39	D02.3	D14.0	D38.5	D49.1
pinna	C49.0	C79.89	—	D21.0	D48.1	D49.2
rib	C41.3	C79.51	—	D16.7	D48.0	D49.2
semilunar (knee)	C40.2-	C79.51	—	D16.2-	D48.0	D49.2
thyroid	C32.3	C78.39	D02.0	D14.1	D38.0	D49.1
trachea	C33	C78.39	D02.1	D14.2	D38.1	D49.1
cauda equina	C72.1	C79.49	—	D33.4	D43.4	D49.7
cavity						
buccal	C06.9	C79.89	D00.00	D10.30	D37.09	D49.0
nasal	C30.0	C78.39	D02.3	D14.0	D38.5	D49.1
oral	C06.9	C79.89	D00.00	D10.30	D37.09	D49.0
peritoneal	C48.2	C78.6	—	D20.1	D48.4	D49.0
tympanic	C30.1	C78.39	D02.3	D14.0	D38.5	D49.1

	Malignant Primary	Malignant Secondary	Ca in situ	Benign	Uncertain Behavior	Unspecified Behavior
cecum	C18.0	C78.5	D01.0	D12.0	D37.4	D49.0
central nervous system	C72.9	C79.40	—	—	—	—
cerebellopontine (angle)	C71.6	C79.31	—	D33.1	D43.1	D49.6
cerebellum, cerebellar	C71.6	C79.31	—	D33.1	D43.1	D49.6
cerebrum, cerebral (cortex) (hemisphere) (white matter)	C71.0	C79.31	—	D33.0	D43.0	D49.6
meninges	C70.0	C79.32	—	D32.0	D42.0	D49.7
peduncle	C71.7	C79.31	—	D33.1	D43.1	D49.6
ventricle	C71.5	C79.31	—	D33.0	D43.0	D49.6
fourth	C71.7	C79.31	—	D33.1	D43.1	D49.6
cervical region	C76.0	C79.89	D09.8	D36.7	D48.7	D49.89
cervix (cervical) (uteri) (uterus)	C53.9	C79.82	D06.9	D26.0	D39.0	D49.59 ◀
canal	C53.0	C79.82	D06.0	D26.0	D39.0	D49.59 ◀
endocervix (canal) (gland)	C53.0	C79.82	D06.0	D26.0	D39.0	D49.59 ◀
exocervix	C53.1	C79.82	D06.1	D26.0	D39.0	D49.59 ◀
external os	C53.1	C79.82	D06.1	D26.0	D39.0	D49.59 ◀
internal os	C53.0	C79.82	D06.0	D26.0	D39.0	D49.59 ◀
nabothian gland	C53.0	C79.82	D06.0	D26.0	D39.0	D49.59 ◀
overlapping lesion	C53.8	—	—	—	—	—
squamocolumnar junction	C53.8	C79.82	D06.7	D26.0	D39.0	D49.59 ◀
stump	C53.8	C79.82	D06.7	D26.0	D39.0	D49.59 ◀
cheek	C76.0	C79.89	D09.8	D36.7	D48.7	D49.89
external	C44.309	C79.2	D04.39	D23.39	D48.5	D49.2
basal cell carcinoma	C44.319	—	—	—	—	—
specified type NEC	C44.399	—	—	—	—	—
squamous cell carcinoma	C44.329	—	—	—	—	—
inner aspect	C06.0	C79.89	D00.02	D10.39	D37.09	D49.0
internal	C06.0	C79.89	D00.02	D10.39	D37.09	D49.0
mucosa	C06.0	C79.89	D00.02	D10.39	D37.09	D49.0
chest (wall) NEC	C76.1	C79.89	D09.8	D36.7	D48.7	D49.89
chiasma opticum	C72.3-	C79.49	—	D33.3	D43.3	D49.7
chin	C44.309	C79.2	D04.39	D23.39	D48.5	D49.2
basal cell carcinoma	C44.319	—	—	—	—	—
specified type NEC	C44.399	—	—	—	—	—
squamous cell carcinoma	C44.329	—	—	—	—	—
choana	C11.3	C79.89	D00.08	D10.6	D37.05	D49.0
cholangiole	C22.1	C78.89	D01.5	D13.4	D37.6	D49.0
choledochal duct	C24.0	C78.89	D01.5	D13.5	D37.6	D49.0
choroid	C69.3-	C79.49	D09.2-	D31.3-	D48.7	D49.81
plexus	C71.5	C79.31	—	D33.0	D43.0	D49.6
ciliary body	C69.4-	C79.49	D09.2-	D31.4-	D48.7	D49.89
clavicle	C41.3	C79.51	—	D16.7	D48.0	D49.2
clitoris	C51.2	C79.82	D07.1	D28.0	D39.8	D49.59 ◀
clivus	C41.0	C79.51	—	D16.4-	D48.0	D49.2

TABLE OF NEOPLASMS

TABLE OF NEOPLASMS (side margin)

	Malignant Primary	Malignant Secondary	Ca in situ	Benign	Uncertain Behavior	Unspecified Behavior
cloacogenic zone	C21.2	C78.5	D01.3	D12.9	D37.8	D49.0
coccygeal						
body or glomus	C49.5	C79.89	—	D21.5	D48.1	D49.2
vertebra	C41.4	C79.51	—	D16.8	D48.0	D49.2
coccyx	C41.4	C79.51	—	D16.8	D48.0	D49.2
colon — *see also Neoplasm, intestine, large*	C18.9	C78.5	—	—	—	—
with rectum	C19	C78.5	D01.1	D12.7	D37.5	D49.0
column, spinal — *see Neoplasm, spine*						
columnella — *see also Neoplasm, skin, face*	C44.390	C79.2	D04.39	D23.39	D48.5	D49.2
commissure						
labial, lip	C00.6	C79.89	D00.01	D10.39	D37.01	D49.0
laryngeal	C32.0	C78.39	D02.0	D14.1	D38.0	D49.1
common (bile) duct	C24.0	C78.89	D01.5	D13.5	D37.6	D49.0
concha — *see also Neoplasm, skin, ear*	C44.20-	C79.2	D04.2-	D23.2-	D48.5	D49.2
nose	C30.0	C78.39	D02.3	D14.0	D38.5	D49.1
conjunctiva	C69.0-	C79.49	D09.2-	D31.0-	D48.7	D49.89
connective tissue NEC	C49.9	C79.89	—	D21.9	D48.1	D49.2

Note: For neoplasms of connective tissue (blood vessel, bursa, fascia, ligament, muscle, peripheral nerves, sympathetic and parasympathetic nerves and ganglia, synovia, tendon, etc.) or of morphological types that indicate connective tissue, code according to the list under "Neoplasm, connective tissue". For sites that do not appear in this list, code to neoplasm of that site; e.g., fibrosarcoma, pancreas (C25.9)

Note: Morphological types that indicate connective tissue appear in their proper place in the alphabetic index with the instruction "*see Neoplasm, connective tissue ....*"

	Malignant Primary	Malignant Secondary	Ca in situ	Benign	Uncertain Behavior	Unspecified Behavior
abdomen	C49.4	C79.89	—	D21.4	D48.1	D49.2
abdominal wall	C49.4	C79.89	—	D21.4	D48.1	D49.2
ankle	C49.2-	C79.89	—	D21.2-	D48.1	D49.2
antecubital fossa or space	C49.1-	C79.89	—	D21.1-	D48.1	D49.2
arm	C49.1-	C79.89	—	D21.1-	D48.1	D49.2
auricle (ear)	C49.0	C79.89	—	D21.0	D48.1	D49.2
axilla	C49.3	C79.89	—	D21.3	D48.1	D49.2
back	C49.6	C79.89	—	D21.6	D48.1	D49.2
breast — *see Neoplasm, breast*						
buttock	C49.5	C79.89	—	D21.5	D48.1	D49.2
calf	C49.2-	C79.89	—	D21.2-	D48.1	D49.2
cervical region	C49.0	C79.89	—	D21.0	D48.1	D49.2
cheek	C49.0	C79.89	—	D21.0	D48.1	D49.2
chest (wall)	C49.3	C79.89	—	D21.3	D48.1	D49.2
chin	C49.0	C79.89	—	D21.0	D48.1	D49.2

connective tissue NEC *(Continued)*	Malignant Primary	Malignant Secondary	Ca in situ	Benign	Uncertain Behavior	Unspecified Behavior
diaphragm	C49.3	C79.89	—	D21.3	D48.1	D49.2
ear (external)	C49.0	C79.89	—	D21.0	D48.1	D49.2
elbow	C49.1-	C79.89	—	D21.1-	D48.1	D49.2
extrarectal	C49.5	C79.89	—	D21.5	D48.1	D49.2
extremity	C49.9	C79.89	—	D21.9	D48.1	D49.2
lower	C49.2-	C79.89	—	D21.2-	D48.1	D49.2
upper	C49.1-	C79.89	—	D21.1-	D48.1	D49.2
eyelid	C49.0	C79.89	—	D21.0	D48.1	D49.2
face	C49.0	C79.89	—	D21.0	D48.1	D49.2
finger	C49.1-	C79.89	—	D21.1-	D48.1	D49.2
flank	C49.6	C79.89	—	D21.6	D48.1	D49.2
foot	C49.2-	C79.89	—	D21.2-	D48.1	D49.2
forearm	C49.1-	C79.89	—	D21.1-	D48.1	D49.2
forehead	C49.0	C79.89	—	D21.0	D48.1	D49.2
gastric	C49.4	C79.89	—	D21.4	D48.1	D49.2
gastrointestinal	C49.4	C79.89	—	D21.4	D48.1	D49.2
gluteal region	C49.5	C79.89	—	D21.5	D48.1	D49.2
great vessels NEC	C49.3	C79.89	—	D21.3	D48.1	D49.2
groin	C49.5	C79.89	—	D21.5	D48.1	D49.2
hand	C49.1-	C79.89	—	D21.1-	D48.1	D49.2
head	C49.0	C79.89	—	D21.0	D48.1	D49.2
heel	C49.2-	C79.89	—	D21.2-	D48.1	D49.2
hip	C49.2-	C79.89	—	D21.2-	D48.1	D49.2
hypochondrium	C49.4	C79.89	—	D21.4	D48.1	D49.2
iliopsoas muscle	C49.5	C79.89	—	D21.5	D48.1	D49.2
infraclavicular region	C49.3	C79.89	—	D21.3	D48.1	D49.2
inguinal (canal) (region)	C49.5	C79.89	—	D21.5	D48.1	D49.2
intestinal	C49.4	C79.89	—	D21.4	D48.1	D49.2
intrathoracic	C49.3	C79.89	—	D21.3	D48.1	D49.2
ischiorectal fossa	C49.5	C79.89	—	D21.5	D48.1	D49.2
jaw	C03.9	C79.89	D00.03	D10.39	D48.1	D49.0
knee	C49.2-	C79.89	—	D21.2-	D48.1	D49.2
leg	C49.2-	C79.89	—	D21.2-	D48.1	D49.2
limb NEC	C49.9	C79.89	—	D21.9	D48.1	D49.2
lower	C49.2-	C79.89	—	D21.2-	D48.1	D49.2
upper	C49.1-	C79.89	—	D21.1-	D48.1	D49.2
nates	C49.5	C79.89	—	D21.5	D48.1	D49.2
neck	C49.0	C79.89	—	D21.0	D48.1	D49.2
orbit	C69.6-	C79.49	D09.2-	D31.6-	D48.1	D49.89
overlapping lesion	C49.8	—	—	—	—	—
pararectal	C49.5	C79.89	—	D21.5	D48.1	D49.2
para-urethral	C49.5	C79.89	—	D21.5	D48.1	D49.2
paravaginal	C49.5	C79.89	—	D21.5	D48.1	D49.2

◀ New ◀◀◀ Revised ~~deleted~~ Deleted

	Malignant Primary	Malignant Secondary	Ca in situ	Benign	Uncertain Behavior	Unspecified Behavior
connective tissue NEC *(Continued)*						
pelvis (floor)	C49.5	C79.89	—	D21.5	D48.1	D49.2
pelvo-abdominal	C49.8	C79.89	—	D21.6	D48.1	D49.2
perineum	C49.5	C79.89	—	D21.5	D48.1	D49.2
perirectal (tissue)	C49.5	C79.89	—	D21.5	D48.1	D49.2
periurethral (tissue)	C49.5	C79.89	—	D21.5	D48.1	D49.2
popliteal fossa or space	C49.2-	C79.89	—	D21.2-	D48.1	D49.2
presacral	C49.5	C79.89	—	D21.5	D48.1	D49.2
psoas muscle	C49.4	C79.89	—	D21.4	D48.1	D49.2
pterygoid fossa	C49.0	C79.89	—	D21.0	D48.1	D49.2
rectovaginal septum or wall	C49.5	C79.89	—	D21.5	D48.1	D49.2
rectovesical	C49.5	C79.89	—	D21.5	D48.1	D49.2
retroperitoneum	C48.0	C78.6	—	D20.0	D48.3	D49.0
sacrococcygeal region	C49.5	C79.89	—	D21.5	D48.1	D49.2
scalp	C49.0	C79.89	—	D21.0	D48.1	D49.2
scapular region	C49.3	C79.89	—	D21.3	D48.1	D49.2
shoulder	C49.1-	C79.89	—	D21.1-	D48.1	D49.2
skin (dermis) NEC — *see also Neoplasm, skin, by site*	C44.90	C79.2	D04.9	D23.9	D48.5	D49.2
stomach	C49.4	C79.89	—	D21.4	D48.1	D49.2
submental	C49.0	C79.89	—	D21.0	D48.1	D49.2
supraclavicular region	C49.0	C79.89	—	D21.0	D48.1	D49.2
temple	C49.0	C79.89	—	D21.0	D48.1	D49.2
temporal region	C49.0	C79.89	—	D21.0	D48.1	D49.2
thigh	C49.2-	C79.89	—	D21.2-	D48.1	D49.2
thoracic (duct) (wall)	C49.3	C79.89	—	D21.3	D48.1	D49.2
thorax	C49.3	C79.89	—	D21.3	D48.1	D49.2
thumb	C49.1-	C79.89	—	D21.1-	D48.1	D49.2
toe	C49.2-	C79.89	—	D21.2-	D48.1	D49.2
trunk	C49.6	C79.89	—	D21.6	D48.1	D49.2
umbilicus	C49.4	C79.89	—	D21.4	D48.1	D49.2
vesicorectal	C49.5	C79.89	—	D21.5	D48.1	D49.2
wrist	C49.1-	C79.89	—	D21.1-	D48.1	D49.2
conus medullaris	C72.0	C79.49	—	D33.4	D43.4	D49.7
cord (true) (vocal)	C32.0	C78.39	D02.0	D14.1	D38.0	D49.1
false	C32.1	C78.39	D02.0	D14.1	D38.0	D49.1
spermatic	C63.1-	C79.82	D07.69	D29.8	D40.8	D49.59
spinal (cervical) (lumbar) (thoracic)	C72.0	C79.49	—	D33.4	D43.4	D49.7
cornea (limbus)	C69.1-	C79.49	D09.2-	D31.1-	D48.7	D49.89
corpus						
albicans	C56.-	C79.6-	D07.39	D27.-	D39.1-	D49.59
callosum, brain	C71.0	C79.31	—	D33.2	D43.2	D49.6
cavernosum	C60.2	C79.82	D07.4	D29.0	D40.8	D49.59

	Malignant Primary	Malignant Secondary	Ca in situ	Benign	Uncertain Behavior	Unspecified Behavior
corpus *(Continued)*						
gastric	C16.2	C78.89	D00.2	D13.1	D37.1	D49.0
overlapping sites	C54.8	—	—	—	—	—
penis	C60.2	C79.82	D07.4	D29.0	D40.8	D49.59
striatum, cerebrum	C71.0	C79.31	—	D33.0	D43.0	D49.6
uteri	C54.9	C79.82	D07.0	D26.1	D39.0	D49.59
isthmus	C54.0	C79.82	D07.0	D26.1	D39.0	D49.59
cortex						
adrenal	C74.0-	C79.7-	D09.3	D35.0-	D44.1-	D49.7
cerebral	C71.0	C79.31	—	D33.0	D43.0	D49.6
costal cartilage	C41.3	C79.51	—	D16.7	D48.0	D49.2
costovertebral joint	C41.3	C79.51	—	D16.7	D48.0	D49.2
Cowper's gland	C68.0	C79.19	D09.19	D30.4	D41.3	D49.59
cranial (fossa, any)	C71.9	C79.31	—	D33.2	D43.2	D49.6
meninges	C70.0	C79.32	—	D32.0	D42.0	D49.7
nerve	C72.50	C79.49	—	D33.3	D43.3	D49.7
specified NEC	C72.59	C79.49	—	D33.3	D43.3	D49.7
craniobuccal pouch	C75.2	C79.89	D09.3	D35.2	D44.3	D49.7
craniopharyngeal (duct) (pouch)	C75.2	C79.89	D09.3	D35.3	D44.4	D49.7
cricoid	C13.0	C79.89	D00.08	D10.7	D37.05	D49.0
cartilage	C32.3	C78.39	D02.0	D14.1	D38.0	D49.1
cricopharynx	C13.0	C79.89	D00.08	D10.7	D37.05	D49.0
crypt of Morgagni	C21.8	C78.5	D01.3	D12.9	D37.8	D49.0
crystalline lens	C69.4-	C79.49	D09.2-	D31.4-	D48.7	D49.89
cul-de-sac (Douglas')	C48.1	C78.6	—	D20.1	D48.4	D49.0
cuneiform cartilage	C32.3	C78.39	D02.0	D14.1	D38.0	D49.1
cutaneous — *see Neoplasm, skin*						
cutis — *see Neoplasm, skin*						
cystic (bile) duct (common)	C24.0	C78.89	D01.5	D13.5	D37.6	D49.0
dermis — *see Neoplasm, skin*						
diaphragm	C49.3	C79.89	—	D21.3	D48.1	D49.2
digestive organs, system, tube, or tract NEC	C26.9	C78.89	D01.9	D13.9	D37.9	D49.0
disc, intervertebral	C41.2	C79.51	—	D16.6	D48.0	D49.2
disease, generalized	C80.0	—	—	—	—	—
disseminated	C80.0	—	—	—	—	—
Douglas' cul-de-sac or pouch	C48.1	C78.6	—	D20.1	D48.4	D49.0
duodenojejunal junction	C17.8	C78.4	D01.49	D13.39	D37.2	D49.0
duodenum	C17.0	C78.4	D01.49	D13.2	D37.2	D49.0
dura (cranial) (mater)	C70.9	C79.49	—	D32.9	D42.9	D49.7
cerebral	C70.0	C79.32	—	D32.0	D42.0	D49.7
spinal	C70.1	C79.49	—	D32.1	D42.1	D49.7

◀ New ◀ Revised ~~deleted~~ Deleted

TABLE OF NEOPLASMS

	Malignant Primary	Malignant Secondary	Ca in situ	Benign	Uncertain Behavior	Unspecified Behavior
ear (external) — *see also Neoplasm, skin, ear*	C44.20-	C79.2	D04.2-	D23.2-	D48.5	D49.2
auricle or auris — *see also Neoplasm, skin, ear*	C44.20-	C79.2	D04.2-	D23.2-	D48.5	D49.2
canal, external — *see also Neoplasm, skin, ear*	C44.20-	C79.2	D04.2-	D23.2-	D48.5	D49.2
cartilage	C49.0	C79.89	—	D21.0	D48.1	D49.2
external meatus — *see also Neoplasm, skin, ear*	C44.20-	C79.2	D04.2-	D23.2-	D48.5	D49.2
inner	C30.1	C78.39	D02.3	D14.0	D38.5	D49.1
lobule — *see also Neoplasm, skin, ear*	C44.20-	C79.2	D04.2-	D23.2-	D48.5	D49.2
middle	C30.1	C78.39	D02.3	D14.0	D38.5	D49.1
overlapping lesion with accessory sinuses	C31.8	—	—	—	—	—
skin	C44.20-	C79.2	D04.2-	D23.2-	D48.5	D49.2
basal cell carcinoma	C44.21-	—	—	—	—	—
specified type NEC	C44.29-	—	—	—	—	—
squamous cell carcinoma	C44.22-	—	—	—	—	—
earlobe	C44.20-	C79.2	D04.2-	D23.2-	D48.5	D49.2
basal cell carcinoma	C44.21-	—	—	—	—	—
specified type NEC	C44.29-	—	—	—	—	—
squamous cell carcinoma	C44.22-	—	—	—	—	—
ejaculatory duct	C63.7	C79.82	D07.69	D29.8	D40.8	D49.59 ◀
elbow NEC	C76.4-	C79.89	D04.6-	D36.7	D48.7	D49.89
endocardium	C38.0	C79.89	—	D15.1	D48.7	D49.89
endocervix (canal) (gland)	C53.0	C79.82	D06.0	D26.0	D39.0	D49.59 ◀
endocrine gland NEC	C75.9	C79.89	D09.3	D35.9	D44.9	D49.7
pluriglandular	C75.8	C79.89	D09.3	D35.7	D44.9	D49.7
endometrium (gland) (stroma)	C54.1	C79.82	D07.0	D26.1	D39.0	D49.59 ◀
ensiform cartilage	C41.3	C79.51	—	D16.7	D48.0	D49.2
enteric — *see Neoplasm, intestine*						
ependyma (brain)	C71.5	C79.31	—	D33.0	D43.0	D49.6
fourth ventricle	C71.7	C79.31	—	D33.1	D43.1	D49.6
epicardium	C38.0	C79.89	—	D15.1	D48.7	D49.89
epididymis	C63.0-	C79.82	D07.69	D29.3-	D40.8	D49.59 ◀
epidural	C72.9	C79.49	—	D33.9	D43.9	D49.7
epiglottis	C32.1	C78.39	D02.0	D14.1	D38.0	D49.1
anterior aspect or surface	C10.1	C79.89	D00.08	D10.5	D37.05	D49.0
cartilage	C32.3	C78.39	D02.0	D14.1	D38.0	D49.1
free border (margin)	C10.1	C79.89	D00.08	D10.5	D37.05	D49.0
junctional region	C10.8	C79.89	D00.08	D10.5	D37.05	D49.0
posterior (laryngeal) surface	C32.1	C78.39	D02.0	D14.1	D38.0	D49.1
suprahyoid portion	C32.1	C78.39	D02.0	D14.1	D38.0	D49.1

	Malignant Primary	Malignant Secondary	Ca in situ	Benign	Uncertain Behavior	Unspecified Behavior
esophagogastric junction	C16.0	C78.89	D00.2	D13.1	D37.1	D49.0
esophagus	C15.9	C78.89	D00.1	D13.0	D37.8	D49.0
abdominal	C15.5	C78.89	D00.1	D13.0	D37.8	D49.0
cervical	C15.3	C78.89	D00.1	D13.0	D37.8	D49.0
distal (third)	C15.5	C78.89	D00.1	D13.0	D37.8	D49.0
lower (third)	C15.5	C78.89	D00.1	D13.0	D37.8	D49.0
middle (third)	C15.4	C78.89	D00.1	D13.0	D37.8	D49.0
overlapping lesion	C15.8	—	—	—	—	—
proximal (third)	C15.3	C78.89	D00.1	D13.0	D37.8	D49.0
thoracic	C15.4	C78.89	D00.1	D13.0	D37.8	D49.0
upper (third)	C15.3	C78.89	D00.1	D13.0	D37.8	D49.0
ethmoid (sinus)	C31.1	C78.39	D02.3	D14.0	D38.5	D49.1
bone or labyrinth	C41.0	C79.51	—	D16.4-	D48.0	D49.2
eustachian tube	C30.1	C78.39	D02.3	D14.0	D38.5	D49.1
exocervix	C53.1	C79.82	D06.1	D26.0	D39.0	D49.59 ◀
external						
meatus (ear) — *see also Neoplasm, skin, ear*	C44.20-	C79.2	D04.2-	D23.2-	D48.5	D49.2
os, cervix uteri	C53.1	C79.82	D06.1	D26.0	D39.0	D49.59 ◀
extradural	C72.9	C79.49	—	D33.9	D43.9	D49.7
extrahepatic (bile) duct	C24.0	C78.89	D01.5	D13.5	D37.6	D49.0
overlapping lesion with gallbladder	C24.8	—	—	—	—	—
extraocular muscle	C69.6-	C79.49	D09.2-	D31.6-	D48.7	D49.89
extrarectal	C76.3	C79.89	D09.8	D36.7	D48.7	D49.89
extremity	C76.8	C79.89	D04.8	D36.7	D48.7	D49.89
lower	C76.5-	C79.89	D04.7-	D36.7	D48.7	D49.89
upper	C76.4-	C79.89	D04.6-	D36.7	D48.7	D49.89
eye NEC	C69.9-	C79.49	D09.2	D31.9	D48.7	D49.89
overlapping sites	C69.8	—	—	—	—	—
eyeball	C69.9-	C79.49	D09.2-	D31.9-	D48.7	D49.89
eyebrow	C44.309	C79.2	D04.39	D23.39	D48.5	D49.2
basal cell carcinoma	C44.319	—	—	—	—	—
specified type NEC	C44.399	—	—	—	—	—
squamous cell carcinoma	C44.329	—	—	—	—	—
eyelid (lower) (skin) (upper)	C44.10-	—	—	—	—	—
basal cell carcinoma	C44.11-	—	—	—	—	—
cartilage	C49.0	C79.89	—	D21.0	D48.1	D49.2
specified type NEC	C44.19-	—	—	—	—	—
squamous cell carcinoma	C44.12-	—	—	—	—	—
face NEC	C76.0	C79.89	D04.39	D36.7	D48.7	D49.89
fallopian tube (accessory)	C57.0-	C79.82	D07.39	D28.2	D39.8	D49.59 ◀
falx (cerebella) (cerebri)	C70.0	C79.32	—	D32.0	D42.0	D49.7

◀ New ◀ Revised ~~deleted~~ Deleted

	Malignant Primary	Malignant Secondary	Ca in situ	Benign	Uncertain Behavior	Unspecified Behavior
fascia — *see also Neoplasm, connective tissue*						
palmar	C49.1-	C79.89	—	D21.1-	D48.1	D49.2
plantar	C49.2-	C79.89	—	D21.2-	D48.1	D49.2
fatty tissue — *see Neoplasm, connective tissue*						
fauces, faucial NEC	C10.9	C79.89	D00.08	D10.5	D37.05	D49.0
pillars	C09.1	C79.89	D00.08	D10.5	D37.05	D49.0
tonsil	C09.9	C79.89	D00.08	D10.4	D37.05	D49.0
femur (any part)	C40.2-	—	—	D16.2-	—	—
fetal membrane	C58	C79.82	D07.0	D26.7	D39.2	D49.59
fibrous tissue — *see Neoplasm, connective tissue*						
fibula (any part)	C40.2-	C79.51	—	D16.2-	—	—
filum terminale	C72.0	C79.49	—	D33.4	D43.4	D49.7
finger NEC	C76.4-	C79.89	D04.6-	D36.7	D48.7	D49.89
flank NEC	C76.8	C79.89	D04.5	D36.7	D48.7	D49.89
follicle, nabothian	C53.0	C79.82	D06.0	D26.0	D39.0	D49.59
foot NEC	C76.5-	C79.89	D04.7-	D36.7	D48.7	D49.89
forearm NEC	C76.4-	C79.89	D04.6-	D36.7	D48.7	D49.89
forehead (skin)	C44.309	C79.2	D04.39	D23.39	D48.5	D49.2
basal cell carcinoma	C44.319	—	—	—	—	—
specified type NEC	C44.399	—	—	—	—	—
squamous cell carcinoma	C44.329	—	—	—	—	—
foreskin	C60.0	C79.82	D07.4	D29.0	D40.8	D49.59
fornix						
pharyngeal	C11.3	C79.89	D00.08	D10.6	D37.05	D49.0
vagina	C52	C79.82	D07.2	D28.1	D39.8	D49.59
fossa (of)						
anterior (cranial)	C71.9	C79.31	—	D33.2	D43.2	D49.6
cranial	C71.9	C79.31	—	D33.2	D43.2	D49.6
ischiorectal	C76.3	C79.89	D09.8	D36.7	D48.7	D49.89
middle (cranial)	C71.9	C79.31	—	D33.2	D43.2	D49.6
piriform	C12	C79.89	D00.08	D10.7	D37.05	D49.0
pituitary	C75.1	C79.89	D09.3	D35.2	D44.3	D49.7
posterior (cranial)	C71.9	C79.31	—	D33.2	D43.2	D49.6
pterygoid	C49.0	C79.89	—	D21.0	D48.1	D49.2
pyriform	C12	C79.89	D00.08	D10.7	D37.05	D49.0
Rosenmuller	C11.2	C79.89	D00.08	D10.6	D37.05	D49.0
tonsillar	C09.0	C79.89	D00.08	D10.5	D37.05	D49.0
fourchette	C51.9	C79.82	D07.1	D28.0	D39.8	D49.59
frenulum						
labii — *see Neoplasm, lip, internal*						
linguae	C02.2	C79.89	D00.07	D10.1	D37.02	D49.0

	Malignant Primary	Malignant Secondary	Ca in situ	Benign	Uncertain Behavior	Unspecified Behavior
frontal						
bone	C41.0	C79.51	—	D16.4-	D48.0	D49.2
lobe, brain	C71.1	C79.31	—	D33.0	D43.0	D49.6
pole	C71.1	C79.31	—	D33.0	D43.0	D49.6
sinus	C31.2	C78.39	D02.3	D14.0	D38.5	D49.1
fundus						
stomach	C16.1	C78.89	D00.2	D13.1	D37.1	D49.0
uterus	C54.3	C79.82	D07.0	D26.1	D39.0	D49.59
gall duct (extrahepatic)	C24.0	C78.89	D01.5	D13.5	D37.6	D49.0
intrahepatic	C22.1	C78.7	D01.5	D13.4	D37.6	D49.0
gallbladder	C23	C78.89	D01.5	D13.5	D37.6	D49.0
overlapping lesion with extrahepatic bile ducts	C24.8	—	—	—	—	—
ganglia — *see also Neoplasm, nerve, peripheral*	C47.9	C79.89	—	D36.10	D48.2	D49.2
basal	C71.0	C79.31	—	D33.0	D43.0	D49.6
cranial nerve	C72.50	C79.49	—	D33.3	D43.3	D49.7
Gartner's duct	C52	C79.82	D07.2	D28.1	D39.8	D49.59
gastric — *see Neoplasm, stomach*						
gastrocolic	C26.9	C78.89	D01.9	D13.9	D37.9	D49.0
gastroesophageal junction	C16.0	C78.89	D00.2	D13.1	D37.1	D49.0
gastrointestinal (tract) NEC	C26.9	C78.89	D01.9	D13.9	D37.9	D49.0
generalized	C80.0	—	—	—	—	—
genital organ or tract						
female NEC	C57.9	C79.82	D07.30	D28.9	D39.9	D49.59
overlapping lesion	C57.8	—	—	—	—	—
specified site NEC	C57.7	C79.82	D07.39	D28.7	D39.8	D49.59
male NEC	C63.9	C79.82	D07.60	D29.9	D40.9	D49.59
overlapping lesion	C63.8	—	—	—	—	—
specified site NEC	C63.7	C79.82	D07.69	D29.8	D40.8	D49.59
genitourinary tract						
female	C57.9	C79.82	D07.30	D28.9	D39.9	D49.59
male	C63.9	C79.82	D07.60	D29.9	D40.9	D49.59
gingiva (alveolar) (marginal)	C03.9	C79.89	D00.03	D10.39	D37.09	D49.0
lower	C03.1	C79.89	D00.03	D10.39	D37.09	D49.0
mandibular	C03.1	C79.89	D00.03	D10.39	D37.09	D49.0
maxillary	C03.0	C79.89	D00.03	D10.39	D37.09	D49.0
upper	C03.0	C79.89	D00.03	D10.39	D37.09	D49.0
gland, glandular (lymphatic) (system) — *see also Neoplasm, lymph gland*						
endocrine NEC	C75.9	C79.89	D09.3	D35.9	D44.9	D49.7
salivary — *see Neoplasm, salivary gland*						

TABLE OF NEOPLASMS

	Malignant Primary	Malignant Secondary	Ca in situ	Benign	Uncertain Behavior	Unspecified Behavior
glans penis	C60.1	C79.82	D07.4	D29.0	D40.8	D49.59
globus pallidus	C71.0	C79.31	—	D33.0	D43.0	D49.6
glomus						
coccygeal	C49.5	C79.89	—	D21.5	D48.1	D49.2
jugularis	C75.5	C79.89	—	D35.6	D44.7	D49.7
glosso-epiglottic fold(s)	C10.1	C79.89	D00.08	D10.5	D37.05	D49.0
glossopalatine fold	C09.1	C79.89	D00.08	D10.5	D37.05	D49.0
glossopharyngeal sulcus	C09.0	C79.89	D00.08	D10.5	D37.05	D49.0
glottis	C32.0	C78.39	D02.0	D14.1	D38.0	D49.1
gluteal region	C76.3	C79.89	D04.5	D36.7	D48.7	D49.89
great vessels NEC	C49.3	C79.89	—	D21.3	D48.1	D49.2
groin NEC	C76.3	C79.89	D04.5	D36.7	D48.7	D49.89
gum	C03.9	C79.89	D00.03	D10.39	D37.09	D49.0
lower	C03.1	C79.89	D00.03	D10.39	D37.09	D49.0
upper	C03.0	C79.89	D00.03	D10.39	D37.09	D49.0
hand NEC	C76.4-	C79.89	D04.6-	D36.7	D48.7	D49.89
head NEC	C76.0	C79.89	D04.4	D36.7	D48.7	D49.89
heart	C38.0	C79.89	—	D15.1	D48.7	D49.89
heel NEC	C76.5-	C79.89	D04.7-	D36.7	D48.7	D49.89
helix — *see also Neoplasm, skin, ear*	C44.20-	C79.2	D04.2-	D23.2-	D48.5	D49.2
hematopoietic, hemopoietic tissue NEC	C96.9	—	—	—	—	—
specified NEC	C96.Z	—	—	—	—	—
hemisphere, cerebral	C71.0	C79.31	—	D33.0	D43.0	D49.6
hemorrhoidal zone	C21.1	C78.5	D01.3	D12.9	D37.8	D49.0
hepatic — *see also Index to disease, by histology*	C22.9	C78.7	D01.5	D13.4	D37.6	D49.0
duct (bile)	C24.0	C78.89	D01.5	D13.5	D37.6	D49.0
flexure (colon)	C18.3	C78.5	D01.0	D12.3	D37.4	D49.0
primary	C22.8	C78.7	D01.5	D13.4	D37.6	D49.0
hepatobiliary	C24.9	C79.89	D01.5	D13.5	D37.6	D49.0
hepatoblastoma	C22.2	C78.7	D01.5	D13.4	D37.6	D49.0
hepatoma	C22.0	C78.7	D01.5	D13.4	D37.6	D49.0
hilus of lung	C34.0-	C78.0-	D02.2-	D14.3-	D38.1	D49.1
hip NEC	C76.5-	C79.89	D04.7-	D36.7	D48.7	D49.89
hippocampus, brain	C71.2	C79.31	—	D33.0	D43.0	D49.6
humerus (any part)	C40.0-	C79.51	—	D16.0-	—	—
hymen	C52	C79.82	D07.2	D28.1	D39.8	D49.59
hypopharynx, hypopharyngeal NEC	C13.9	C79.89	D00.08	D10.7	D37.05	D49.0
overlapping lesion	C13.8	—	—	—	—	—
postcricoid region	C13.0	C79.89	D00.08	D10.7	D37.05	D49.0
posterior wall	C13.2	C79.89	D00.08	D10.7	D37.05	D49.0
pyriform fossa (sinus)	C12	C79.89	D00.08	D10.7	D37.05	D49.0
hypophysis	C75.1	C79.89	D09.3	D35.2	D44.3	D49.7

	Malignant Primary	Malignant Secondary	Ca in situ	Benign	Uncertain Behavior	Unspecified Behavior
hypothalamus	C71.0	C79.31	—	D33.0	D43.0	D49.6
ileocecum, ileocecal (coil) (junction) (valve)	C18.0	C78.5	D01.0	D12.0	D37.4	D49.0
ileum	C17.2	C78.4	D01.49	D13.39	D37.2	D49.0
ilium	C41.4	C79.51	—	D16.8	D48.0	D49.2
immunoproliferative NEC	C88.9	—	—	—	—	—
infraclavicular (region)	C76.1	C79.89	D04.5	D36.7	D48.7	D49.89
inguinal (region)	C76.3	C79.89	D04.5	D36.7	D48.7	D49.89
insula	C71.0	C79.31	—	D33.0	D43.0	D49.6
insular tissue (pancreas)	C25.4	C78.89	D01.7	D13.7	D37.8	D49.0
brain	C71.0	C79.31	—	D33.0	D43.0	D49.6
interarytenoid fold	C13.1	C79.89	D00.08	D10.7	D37.05	D49.0
hypopharyngeal aspect	C13.1	C79.89	D00.08	D10.7	D37.05	D49.0
laryngeal aspect	C32.1	C78.39	D02.0	D14.1	D38.0	D49.1
marginal zone	C13.1	C79.89	D00.08	D10.7	D37.05	D49.0
interdental papillae	C03.9	C79.89	D00.03	D10.39	D37.09	D49.0
lower	C03.1	C79.89	D00.03	D10.39	D37.09	D49.0
upper	C03.0	C79.89	D00.03	D10.39	D37.09	D49.0
internal						
capsule	C71.0	C79.31	—	D33.0	D43.0	D49.6
os (cervix)	C53.0	C79.82	D06.0	D26.0	D39.0	D49.59
intervertebral cartilage or disc	C41.2	C79.51	—	D16.6	D48.0	D49.2
intestine, intestinal	C26.0	C78.80	D01.40	D13.9	D37.8	D49.0
large	C18.9	C78.5	D01.0	D12.6	D37.4	D49.0
appendix	C18.1	C78.5	D01.0	D12.1	D37.3	D49.0
caput coli	C18.0	C78.5	D01.0	D12.0	D37.4	D49.0
cecum	C18.0	C78.5	D01.0	D12.0	D37.4	D49.0
colon	C18.9	C78.5	D01.0	D12.6	D37.4	D49.0
and rectum	C19	C78.5	D01.1	D12.7	D37.5	D49.0
ascending	C18.2	C78.5	D01.0	D12.2	D37.4	D49.0
caput	C18.0	C78.5	D01.0	D12.0	D37.4	D49.0
descending	C18.6	C78.5	D01.0	D12.4	D37.4	D49.0
distal	C18.6	C78.5	D01.0	D12.4	D37.4	D49.0
left	C18.6	C78.5	D01.0	D12.4	D37.4	D49.0
overlapping lesion	C18.8	—	—	—	—	—
pelvic	C18.7	C78.5	D01.0	D12.5	D37.4	D49.0
right	C18.2	C78.5	D01.0	D12.2	D37.4	D49.0
sigmoid (flexure)	C18.7	C78.5	D01.0	D12.5	D37.4	D49.0
transverse	C18.4	C78.5	D01.0	D12.3	D37.4	D49.0
hepatic flexure	C18.3	C78.5	D01.0	D12.3	D37.4	D49.0
ileocecum, ileocecal (coil) (valve)	C18.0	C78.5	D01.0	D12.0	D37.4	D49.0
overlapping lesion	C18.8	—	—	—	—	—

◄ New   ◄◄ Revised   ~~deleted~~ Deleted

	Malignant Primary	Malignant Secondary	Ca in situ	Benign	Uncertain Behavior	Unspecified Behavior
intestine, intestinal *(Continued)*						
large *(Continued)*						
sigmoid flexure (lower) (upper)	C18.7	C78.5	D01.0	D12.5	D37.4	D49.0
splenic flexure	C18.5	C78.5	D01.0	D12.3	D37.4	D49.0
small	C17.9	C78.4	D01.40	D13.30	D37.2	D49.0
duodenum	C17.0	C78.4	D01.49	D13.2	D37.2	D49.0
ileum	C17.2	C78.4	D01.49	D13.39	D37.2	D49.0
jejunum	C17.1	C78.4	D01.49	D13.39	D37.2	D49.0
overlapping lesion	C17.8	—	—	—	—	—
tract NEC	C26.0	C78.89	D01.40	D13.9	D37.8	D49.0
intra-abdominal	C76.2	C79.89	D09.8	D36.7	D48.7	D49.89
intracranial NEC	C71.9	C79.31	—	D33.2	D43.2	D49.6
intrahepatic (bile) duct	C22.1	C78.7	D01.5	D13.4	D37.6	D49.0
intraocular	C69.9-	C79.49	D09.2-	D31.9-	D48.7	D49.89
intraorbital	C69.6-	C79.49	D09.2-	D31.6-	D48.7	D49.89
intrasellar	C75.1	C79.89	D09.3	D35.2	D44.3	D49.7
intrathoracic (cavity) (organs)	C76.1	C79.89	D09.8	D15.9	D48.7	D49.89
specified NEC	C76.1	C79.89	D09.8	D15.7	—	—
iris	C69.4-	C79.49	D09.2-	D31.4-	D48.7	D49.89
ischiorectal (fossa)	C76.3	C79.89	D09.8	D36.7	D48.7	D49.89
ischium	C41.4	C79.51	—	D16.8	D48.0	D49.2
island of Reil	C71.0	C79.31	—	D33.0	D43.0	D49.6
islands or islets of Langerhans	C25.4	C78.89	D01.7	D13.7	D37.8	D49.0
isthmus uteri	C54.0	C79.82	D07.0	D26.1	D39.0	D49.59
jaw	C76.0	C79.89	D09.8	D36.7	D48.7	D49.89
bone	C41.1	C79.51	—	D16.5-	D48.0	D49.2
lower	C41.1	C79.51	—	D16.5-	—	—
upper	C41.0	C79.51	—	D16.4-	—	—
carcinoma (any type) (lower) (upper)	C76.0	C79.89	—	—	—	—
skin — *see also Neoplasm, skin, face*	C44.309	C79.2	D04.39	D23.39	D48.5	D49.2
soft tissues	C03.9	C79.89	D00.03	D10.39	D37.09	D49.0
lower	C03.1	C79.89	D00.03	D10.39	D37.09	D49.0
upper	C03.0	C79.89	D00.03	D10.39	D37.09	D49.0
jejunum	C17.1	C78.4	D01.49	D13.39	D37.2	D49.0
joint NEC — *see also Neoplasm, bone*	C41.9	C79.51	—	D16.9-	D48.0	D49.2
acromioclavicular	C40.0-	C79.51	—	D16.0-	—	—
bursa or synovial membrane — *see Neoplasm, connective tissue*						
costovertebral	C41.3	C79.51	—	D16.7	D48.0	D49.2
sternocostal	C41.3	C79.51	—	D16.7	D48.0	D49.2
temporomandibular	C41.1	C79.51	—	D16.5-	D48.0	D49.2

	Malignant Primary	Malignant Secondary	Ca in situ	Benign	Uncertain Behavior	Unspecified Behavior
junction						
anorectal	C21.8	C78.5	D01.3	D12.9	D37.8	D49.0
cardioesophageal	C16.0	C78.89	D00.2	D13.1	D37.1	D49.0
esophagogastric	C16.0	C78.89	D00.2	D13.1	D37.1	D49.0
gastroesophageal	C16.0	C78.89	D00.2	D13.1	D37.1	D49.0
hard and soft palate	C05.9	C79.89	D00.00	D10.39	D37.09	D49.0
ileocecal	C18.0	C78.5	D01.0	D12.0	D37.4	D49.0
pelvirectal	C19	C78.5	D01.1	D12.7	D37.5	D49.0
pelviureteric	C65.-	C79.0-	D09.19	D30.1-	D41.1-	D49.59
rectosigmoid	C19	C78.5	D01.1	D12.7	D37.5	D49.0
squamocolumnar, of cervix	C53.8	C79.82	D06.7	D26.0	D39.0	D49.59
Kaposi's sarcoma — *see Kaposi's, sarcoma*						
kidney (parenchymal)	C64.-	C79.0-	D09.19	D30.0-	D41.0-	D49.51-
calyx	C65.-	C79.0-	D09.19	D30.1-	D41.1-	D49.51-
hilus	C65.-	C79.0-	D09.19	D30.1-	D41.1-	D49.51-
pelvis	C65.-	C79.0-	D09.19	D30.1-	D41.1-	D49.51-
knee NEC	C76.5-	C79.89	D04.7-	D36.7	D48.7	D49.89
labia (skin)	C51.9	C79.82	D07.1	D28.0	D39.8	D49.59
majora	C51.0	C79.82	D07.1	D28.0	D39.8	D49.59
minora	C51.1	C79.82	D07.1	D28.0	D39.8	D49.59
labial — *see also Neoplasm, lip*	C00.9	C79.89	D00.01	D10.0	D37.01	D49.0
sulcus (lower) (upper)	C06.1	C79.89	D00.02	D10.39	D37.09	D49.0
labium (skin)	C51.9	C79.82	D07.1	D28.0	D39.8	D49.59
majus	C51.0	C79.82	D07.1	D28.0	D39.8	D49.59
minus	C51.1	C79.82	D07.1	D28.0	D39.8	D49.59
lacrimal						
canaliculi	C69.5-	C79.49	D09.2-	D31.5-	D48.7	D49.89
duct (nasal)	C69.5-	C79.49	D09.2-	D31.5-	D48.7	D49.89
gland	C69.5-	C79.49	D09.2-	D31.5-	D48.7	D49.89
punctum	C69.5-	C79.49	D09.2-	D31.5-	D48.7	D49.89
sac	C69.5-	C79.49	D09.2-	D31.5-	D48.7	D49.89
Langerhans, islands or islets	C25.4	C78.89	D01.7	D13.7	D37.8	D49.0
laryngopharynx	C13.9	C79.89	D00.08	D10.7	D37.05	D49.0
larynx, laryngeal NEC	C32.9	C78.39	D02.0	D14.1	D38.0	D49.1
aryepiglottic fold	C32.1	C78.39	D02.0	D14.1	D38.0	D49.1
cartilage (arytenoid) (cricoid) (cuneiform) (thyroid)	C32.3	C78.39	D02.0	D14.1	D38.0	D49.1
commissure (anterior) (posterior)	C32.0	C78.39	D02.0	D14.1	D38.0	D49.1
extrinsic NEC	C32.1	C78.39	D02.0	D14.1	D38.0	D49.1
meaning hypopharynx	C13.9	C79.89	D00.08	D10.7	D37.05	D49.0
interarytenoid fold	C32.1	C78.39	D02.0	D14.1	D38.0	D49.1
intrinsic	C32.0	C78.39	D02.0	D14.1	D38.0	D49.1

TABLE OF NEOPLASMS

	Malignant Primary	Malignant Secondary	Ca in situ	Benign	Uncertain Behavior	Unspecified Behavior
larynx, laryngeal NEC *(Continued)*						
overlapping lesion	C32.8	—	—	—	—	—
ventricular band	C32.1	C78.39	D02.0	D14.1	D38.0	D49.1
leg NEC	C76.5-	C79.89	D04.7-	D36.7	D48.7	D49.89
lens, crystalline	C69.4-	C79.49	D09.2-	D31.4-	D48.7	D49.89
lid (lower) (upper)	C44.10-	C79.2	D04.1-	D23.1-	D48.5	D49.2
basal cell carcinoma	C44.11-	—	—	—	—	—
specified type NEC	C44.19-	—	—	—	—	—
squamous cell carcinoma	C44.12-	—	—	—	—	—
ligament — *see also Neoplasm, connective tissue*						
broad	C57.1	C79.82	D07.39	D28.2	D39.8	D49.59
Mackenrodt's	C57.7	C79.82	D07.39	D28.7	D39.8	D49.59
non-uterine — *see Neoplasm, connective tissue*						
round	C57.2	C79.82	—	D28.2	D39.8	D49.59
sacro-uterine	C57.3	C79.82	—	D28.2	D39.8	D49.59
uterine	C57.3	C79.82	—	D28.2	D39.8	D49.59
utero-ovarian	C57.7	C79.82	D07.39	D28.2	D39.8	D49.59
uterosacral	C57.3	C79.82	—	D28.2	D39.8	D49.59
limb	C76.8	C79.89	D04.8	D36.7	D48.7	D49.89
lower	C76.5-	C79.89	D04.7-	D36.7	D48.7	D49.89
upper	C76.4-	C79.89	D04.6-	D36.7	D48.7	D49.89
limbus of cornea	C69.1-	C79.49	D09.2-	D31.1-	D48.7	D49.89
lingual NEC — *see also Neoplasm, tongue*	C02.9	C79.89	D00.07	D10.1	D37.02	D49.0
lingula, lung	C34.1-	C78.0-	D02.2-	D14.3-	D38.1	D49.1
lip	C00.9	C79.89	D00.01	D10.0	D37.01	D49.0
buccal aspect — *see Neoplasm, lip, internal*						
commissure	C00.6	C79.89	D00.01	D10.0	D37.01	D49.0
external	C00.2	C79.89	D00.01	D10.0	D37.01	D49.0
lower	C00.1	C79.89	D00.01	D10.0	D37.01	D49.0
upper	C00.0	C79.89	D00.01	D10.0	D37.01	D49.0
frenulum — *see Neoplasm, lip, internal*						
inner aspect — *see Neoplasm, lip, internal*						
internal	C00.5	C79.89	D00.01	D10.0	D37.01	D49.0
lower	C00.4	C79.89	D00.01	D10.0	D37.01	D49.0
upper	C00.3	C79.89	D00.01	D10.0	D37.01	D49.0
lipstick area	C00.2	C79.89	D00.01	D10.0	D37.01	D49.0
lower	C00.1	C79.89	D00.01	D10.0	D37.01	D49.0
upper	C00.0	C79.89	D00.01	D10.0	D37.01	D49.0

	Malignant Primary	Malignant Secondary	Ca in situ	Benign	Uncertain Behavior	Unspecified Behavior
lip *(Continued)*						
lower	C00.1	C79.89	D00.01	D10.0	D37.01	D49.0
internal	C00.4	C79.89	D00.01	D10.0	D37.01	D49.0
mucosa — *see Neoplasm, lip, internal*						
oral aspect — *see Neoplasm, lip, internal*						
overlapping lesion	C00.8	—	—	—	—	—
with oral cavity or pharynx	C14.8	—	—	—	—	—
skin (commissure) (lower) (upper)	C44.00	C79.2	D04.0	D23.0	D48.5	D49.2
basal cell carcinoma	C44.01	—	—	—	—	—
specified type NEC	C44.09	—	—	—	—	—
squamous cell carcinoma	C44.02	—	—	—	—	—
upper	C00.0	C79.89	D00.01	D10.0	D37.01	D49.0
internal	C00.3	C79.89	D00.01	D10.0	D37.01	D49.0
vermilion border	C00.2	C79.89	D00.01	D10.0	D37.01	D49.0
lower	C00.1	C79.89	D00.01	D10.0	D37.01	D49.0
upper	C00.0	C79.89	D00.01	D10.0	D37.01	D49.0
lipomatous — *see Lipoma, by site*						
liver — *see also Index to disease, by histology*	C22.9	C78.7	D01.5	D13.4	D37.6	D49.0
primary	C22.8	C78.7	D01.5	D13.4	D37.6	D49.0
lumbosacral plexus	C47.5	C79.89	—	D36.16	D48.2	D49.2
lung	C34.9-	C78.0-	D02.2-	D14.3-	D38.1	D49.1
azygos lobe	C34.1-	C78.0-	D02.2-	D14.3-	D38.1	D49.1
carina	C34.0-	C78.0-	D02.2-	D14.3-	D38.1	D49.1
hilus	C34.0-	C78.0-	D02.2-	D14.3-	D38.1	D49.1
lingula	C34.1-	C78.0-	D02.2-	D14.3-	D38.1	D49.1
lobe NEC	C34.9-	C78.0-	D02.2-	D14.3-	D38.1	D49.1
lower lobe	C34.3-	C78.0-	D02.2-	D14.3-	D38.1	D49.1
main bronchus	C34.0-	C78.0-	D02.2-	D14.3-	D38.1	D49.1
mesothelioma — *see Mesothelioma*						
middle lobe	C34.2	C78.0-	D02.21	D14.31	D38.1	D49.1
overlapping lesion	C34.8-	—	—	—	—	—
upper lobe	C34.1-	C78.0-	D02.2-	D14.3-	D38.1	D49.1
lymph, lymphatic channel NEC	C49.9	C79.89	—	D21.9	D48.1	D49.2
gland (secondary)	—	C77.9	—	D36.0	D48.7	D49.89
abdominal	—	C77.2	—	D36.0	D48.7	D49.89
aortic	—	C77.2	—	D36.0	D48.7	D49.89
arm	—	C77.3	—	D36.0	D48.7	D49.89
auricular (anterior) (posterior)	—	C77.0	—	D36.0	D48.7	D49.89

◀ New ◀⋯ Revised ~~deleted~~ Deleted

	Malignant Primary	Malignant Secondary	Ca in situ	Benign	Uncertain Behavior	Unspecified Behavior
lymph, lymphatic channel						
NEC *(Continued)*						
gland *(Continued)*						
axilla, axillary	—	C77.3	—	D36.0	D48.7	D49.89
brachial	—	C77.3	—	D36.0	D48.7	D49.89
bronchial	—	C77.1	—	D36.0	D48.7	D49.89
bronchopulmonary	—	C77.1	—	D36.0	D48.7	D49.89
celiac	—	C77.2	—	D36.0	D48.7	D49.89
cervical	—	C77.0	—	D36.0	D48.7	D49.89
cervicofacial	—	C77.0	—	D36.0	D48.7	D49.89
Cloquet	—	C77.4	—	D36.0	D48.7	D49.89
colic	—	C77.2	—	D36.0	D48.7	D49.89
common duct	—	C77.2	—	D36.0	D48.7	D49.89
cubital	—	C77.3	—	D36.0	D48.7	D49.89
diaphragmatic	—	C77.1	—	D36.0	D48.7	D49.89
epigastric, inferior	—	C77.1	—	D36.0	D48.7	D49.89
epitrochlear	—	C77.3	—	D36.0	D48.7	D49.89
esophageal	—	C77.1	—	D36.0	D48.7	D49.89
face	—	C77.0	—	D36.0	D48.7	D49.89
femoral	—	C77.4	—	D36.0	D48.7	D49.89
gastric	—	C77.2	—	D36.0	D48.7	D49.89
groin	—	C77.4	—	D36.0	D48.7	D49.89
head	—	C77.0	—	D36.0	D48.7	D49.89
hepatic	—	C77.2	—	D36.0	D48.7	D49.89
hilar (pulmonary)	—	C77.1	—	D36.0	D48.7	D49.89
splenic	—	C77.2	—	D36.0	D48.7	D49.89
hypogastric	—	C77.5	—	D36.0	D48.7	D49.89
ileocolic	—	C77.2	—	D36.0	D48.7	D49.89
iliac	—	C77.5	—	D36.0	D48.7	D49.89
infraclavicular	—	C77.3	—	D36.0	D48.7	D49.89
inguina, inguinal	—	C77.4	—	D36.0	D48.7	D49.89
innominate	—	C77.1	—	D36.0	D48.7	D49.89
intercostal	—	C77.1	—	D36.0	D48.7	D49.89
intestinal	—	C77.2	—	D36.0	D48.7	D49.89
intrabdominal	—	C77.2	—	D36.0	D48.7	D49.89
intrapelvic	—	C77.5	—	D36.0	D48.7	D49.89
intrathoracic	—	C77.1	—	D36.0	D48.7	D49.89
jugular	—	C77.0	—	D36.0	D48.7	D49.89
leg	—	C77.4	—	D36.0	D48.7	D49.89
limb						
lower	—	C77.4	—	D36.0	D48.7	D49.89
upper	—	C77.3	—	D36.0	D48.7	D49.89
lower limb	—	C77.4	—	D36.0	D48.7	D49.89
lumbar	—	C77.2	—	D36.0	D48.7	D49.89

	Malignant Primary	Malignant Secondary	Ca in situ	Benign	Uncertain Behavior	Unspecified Behavior
lymph, lymphatic channel						
NEC *(Continued)*						
gland *(Continued)*						
mandibular	—	C77.0	—	D36.0	D48.7	D49.89
mediastinal	—	C77.1	—	D36.0	D48.7	D49.89
mesenteric (inferior)						
(superior)	—	C77.2	—	D36.0	D48.7	D49.89
midcolic	—	C77.2	—	D36.0	D48.7	D49.89
multiple sites in categories						
C77.0 - C77.5	—	C77.8	—	D36.0	D48.7	D49.89
neck	—	C77.0	—	D36.0	D48.7	D49.89
obturator	—	C77.5	—	D36.0	D48.7	D49.89
occipital	—	C77.0	—	D36.0	D48.7	D49.89
pancreatic	—	C77.2	—	D36.0	D48.7	D49.89
para-aortic	—	C77.2	—	D36.0	D48.7	D49.89
paracervical	—	C77.5	—	D36.0	D48.7	D49.89
parametrial	—	C77.5	—	D36.0	D48.7	D49.89
parasternal	—	C77.1	—	D36.0	D48.7	D49.89
parotid	—	C77.0	—	D36.0	D48.7	D49.89
pectoral	—	C77.3	—	D36.0	D48.7	D49.89
pelvic	—	C77.5	—	D36.0	D48.7	D49.89
peri-aortic	—	C77.2	—	D36.0	D48.7	D49.89
peripancreatic	—	C77.2	—	D36.0	D48.7	D49.89
popliteal	—	C77.4	—	D36.0	D48.7	D49.89
porta hepatis	—	C77.2	—	D36.0	D48.7	D49.89
portal	—	C77.2	—	D36.0	D48.7	D49.89
preauricular	—	C77.0	—	D36.0	D48.7	D49.89
prelaryngeal	—	C77.0	—	D36.0	D48.7	D49.89
presymphysial	—	C77.5	—	D36.0	D48.7	D49.89
pretracheal	—	C77.0	—	D36.0	D48.7	D49.89
primary (any site) NEC	C96.9	—	—	—	—	—
pulmonary (hiler)	—	C77.1	—	D36.0	D48.7	D49.89
pyloric	—	C77.2	—	D36.0	D48.7	D49.89
retroperitoneal	—	C77.2	—	D36.0	D48.7	D49.89
retropharyngeal	—	C77.0	—	D36.0	D48.7	D49.89
Rosenmuller's	—	C77.4	—	D36.0	D48.7	D49.89
sacral	—	C77.5	—	D36.0	D48.7	D49.89
scalene	—	C77.0	—	D36.0	D48.7	D49.89
site NEC	—	C77.9	—	D36.0	D48.7	D49.89
splenic (hilar)	—	C77.2	—	D36.0	D48.7	D49.89
subclavicular	—	C77.3	—	D36.0	D48.7	D49.89
subinguinal	—	C77.4	—	D36.0	D48.7	D49.89
sublingual	—	C77.0	—	D36.0	D48.7	D49.89
submandibular	—	C77.0	—	D36.0	D48.7	D49.89

◀ New ◀▥ Revised ~~deleted~~ Deleted

TABLE OF NEOPLASMS

	Malignant Primary	Malignant Secondary	Ca in situ	Benign	Uncertain Behavior	Unspecified Behavior
lymph, lymphatic channel NEC (Continued)						
gland (Continued)						
submaxillary	—	C77.0	—	D36.0	D48.7	D49.89
submental	—	C77.0	—	D36.0	D48.7	D49.89
subscapular	—	C77.3	—	D36.0	D48.7	D49.89
supraclavicular	—	C77.0	—	D36.0	D48.7	D49.89
thoracic	—	C77.1	—	D36.0	D48.7	D49.89
tibial	—	C77.4	—	D36.0	D48.7	D49.89
tracheal	—	C77.1	—	D36.0	D48.7	D49.89
tracheobronchial	—	C77.1	—	D36.0	D48.7	D49.89
upper limb	—	C77.3	—	D36.0	D48.7	D49.89
Virchow's	—	C77.0	—	D36.0	D48.7	D49.89
node — see also Neoplasm, lymph gland						
primary NEC	C96.9	—	—	—	—	—
vessel — see also Neoplasm, connective tissue	C49.9	C79.89	—	D21.9	D48.1	D49.2
Mackenrodt's ligament	C57.7	C79.82	D07.39	D28.7	D39.8	D49.59
malar	C41.0	C79.51	—	D16.4-	D48.0	D49.2
region — see Neoplasm, cheek						
mammary gland — see Neoplasm, breast						
mandible	C41.1	C79.51	—	D16.5-	D48.0	D49.2
alveolar						
mucosa (carcinoma)	C03.1	C79.89	D00.03	D10.39	D37.09	D49.0
ridge or process	C41.1	C79.51	—	D16.5-	D48.0	D49.2
marrow (bone) NEC	C96.9	C79.52	—	—	D47.9	D49.89
mastectomy site (skin) — see also Neoplasm, breast, skin	C44.501	C79.2				
specified as breast tissue	C50.8-	C79.81	—	—	—	—
mastoid (air cells) (antrum) (cavity)	C30.1	C78.39	D02.3	D14.0	D38.5	D49.1
bone or process	C41.0	C79.51	—	D16.4-	D48.0	D49.2
maxilla, maxillary (superior)	C41.0	C79.51	—	D16.4-	D48.0	D49.2
alveolar						
mucosa	C03.0	C79.89	D00.03	D10.39	D37.09	D49.0
ridge or process (carcinoma)	C41.0	C79.51	—	D16.4-	D48.0	D49.2
antrum	C31.0	C78.39	D02.3	D14.0	D38.5	D49.1
carcinoma	C03.0	C79.51				
inferior — see Neoplasm, mandible						
sinus	C31.0	C78.39	D02.3	D14.0	D38.5	D49.1
meatus external (ear) — see also Neoplasm, skin, ear	C44.20-	C79.2	D04.2-	D23.2-	D48.5	D49.2
Meckel diverticulum, malignant	C17.3	C78.4	D01.49	D13.39	D37.2	D49.0

	Malignant Primary	Malignant Secondary	Ca in situ	Benign	Uncertain Behavior	Unspecified Behavior
mediastinum, mediastinal	C38.3	C78.1	—	D15.2	D38.3	D49.89
anterior	C38.1	C78.1	—	D15.2	D38.3	D49.89
posterior	C38.2	C78.1	—	D15.2	D38.3	D49.89
medulla						
adrenal	C74.1-	C79.7-	D09.3	D35.0-	D44.1-	D49.7
oblongata	C71.7	C79.31	—	D33.1	D43.1	D49.6
meibomian gland	C44.10-	C79.2	D04.1-	D23.1-	D48.5	D49.2
basal cell carcinoma	C44.11-	—	—	—	—	—
specified type NEC	C44.19-	—	—	—	—	—
squamous cell carcinoma	C44.12-	—	—	—	—	—
melanoma — see Melanoma						
meninges	C70.9	C79.49	—	D32.9	D42.9	D49.7
brain	C70.0	C79.32	—	D32.0	D42.0	D49.7
cerebral	C70.0	C79.32	—	D32.0	D42.0	D49.7
crainial	C70.0	C79.32	—	D32.0	D42.0	D49.7
intracranial	C70.0	C79.32	—	D32.0	D42.0	D49.7
spinal (cord)	C70.1	C79.49	—	D32.1	D42.1	D49.7
meniscus, knee joint (lateral) (medial)	C40.2-	C79.51	—	D16.2-	D48.0	D49.2
Merkel cell — see Carcinoma, Merkel cell						
mesentery, mesenteric	C48.1	C78.6	—	D20.1	D48.4	D49.0
mesoappendix	C48.1	C78.6	—	D20.1	D48.4	D49.0
mesocolon	C48.1	C78.6	—	D20.1	D48.4	D49.0
mesopharynx — see Neoplasm, oropharynx						
mesosalpinx	C57.1	C79.82	D07.39	D28.2	D39.8	D49.59
mesothelial tissue — see Mesothelioma						
mesothelioma — see Mesothelioma						
mesovarium	C57.1	C79.82	D07.39	D28.2	D39.8	D49.59
metacarpus (any bone)	C40.1-	C79.51	—	D16.1-	—	—
metastatic NEC — see also Neoplasm, by site, secondary	—	C79.9	—	—	—	—
metatarsus (any bone)	C40.3-	C79.51	—	D16.3-	—	—
midbrain	C71.7	C79.31	—	D33.1	D43.1	D49.6
milk duct — see Neoplasm, breast						
mons						
pubis	C51.9	C79.82	D07.1	D28.0	D39.8	D49.59
veneris	C51.9	C79.82	D07.1	D28.0	D39.8	D49.59
motor tract	C72.9	C79.49	—	D33.9	D43.9	D49.7
brain	C71.9	C79.31	—	D33.2	D43.2	D49.6
cauda equina	C72.1	C79.49	—	D33.4	D43.4	D49.7
spinal	C72.0	C79.49	—	D33.4	D43.4	D49.7

◀ New ⬅ Revised ~~deleted~~ Deleted

	Malignant Primary	Malignant Secondary	Ca in situ	Benign	Uncertain Behavior	Unspecified Behavior
mouth	C06.9	C79.89	D00.00	D10.30	D37.09	D49.0
book-leaf	C06.89	C79.89	—	—	—	—
floor	C04.9	C79.89	D00.06	D10.2	D37.09	D49.0
anterior portion	C04.0	C79.89	D00.06	D10.2	D37.09	D49.0
lateral portion	C04.1	C79.89	D00.06	D10.2	D37.09	D49.0
overlapping lesion	C04.8	—	—	—	—	—
overlapping NEC	C06.80	—	—	—	—	—
roof	C05.9	C79.89	D00.00	D10.39	D37.09	D49.0
specified part NEC	C06.89	C79.89	D00.00	D10.39	D37.09	D49.0
vestibule	C06.1	C79.89	D00.00	D10.39	D37.09	D49.0
mucosa						
alveolar (ridge or process)	C03.9	C79.89	D00.03	D10.39	D37.09	D49.0
lower	C03.1	C79.89	D00.03	D10.39	D37.09	D49.0
upper	C03.0	C79.89	D00.03	D10.39	D37.09	D49.0
buccal	C06.0	C79.89	D00.02	D10.39	D37.09	D49.0
cheek	C06.0	C79.89	D00.02	D10.39	D37.09	D49.0
lip — *see Neoplasm, lip, internal*						
nasal	C30.0	C78.39	D02.3	D14.0	D38.5	D49.1
oral	C06.0	C79.89	D00.02	D10.39	D37.09	D49.0
Mullerian duct						
female	C57.7	C79.82	D07.39	D28.7	D39.8	D49.59 ◀
male	C63.7	C79.82	D07.69	D29.8	D40.8	D49.59 ◀
muscle — *see also Neoplasm, connective tissue*						
extraocular	C69.6-	C79.49	D09.2-	D31.6-	D48.7	D49.89
myocardium	C38.0	C79.89	—	D15.1	D48.7	D49.89
myometrium	C54.2	C79.82	D07.0	D26.1	D39.0	D49.59 ◀
myopericardium	C38.0	C79.89	—	D15.1	D48.7	D49.89
nabothian gland (follicle)	C53.0	C79.82	D06.0	D26.0	D39.0	D49.59 ◀
nail — *see also Neoplasm, skin, limb*	C44.90	C79.2	D04.9	D23.9	D48.5	D49.2
finger — *see also Neoplasm, skin, limb, upper*	C44.60-	C79.2	D04.6-	D23.6-	D48.5	D49.2
toe — *see also Neoplasm, skin, limb, lower*	C44.70-	C79.2	D04.7-	D23.7-	D48.5	D49.2
nares, naris (anterior) (posterior)	C30.0	C78.39	D02.3	D14.0	D38.5	D49.1
nasal — *see Neoplasm, nose*						
nasolabial groove — *see also Neoplasm, skin, face*	C44.309	C79.2	D04.39	D23.39	D48.5	D49.2
nasolacrimal duct	C69.5-	C79.49	D09.2-	D31.5-	D48.7	D49.89
nasopharynx, nasopharyngeal	C11.9	C79.89	D00.08	D10.6	D37.05	D49.0
floor	C11.3	C79.89	D00.08	D10.6	D37.05	D49.0
overlapping lesion	C11.8	—	—	—	—	—
roof	C11.0	C79.89	D00.08	D10.6	D37.05	D49.0

	Malignant Primary	Malignant Secondary	Ca in situ	Benign	Uncertain Behavior	Unspecified Behavior
nasopharynx, nasopharyngeal *(Continued)*						
wall	C11.9	C79.89	D00.08	D10.6	D37.05	D49.0
anterior	C11.3	C79.89	D00.08	D10.6	D37.05	D49.0
lateral	C11.2	C79.89	D00.08	D10.6	D37.05	D49.0
posterior	C11.1	C79.89	D00.08	D10.6	D37.05	D49.0
superior	C11.0	C79.89	D00.08	D10.6	D37.05	D49.0
nates — *see also Neoplasm, skin, trunk*	C44.509	C79.2	D04.5	D23.5	D48.5	D49.2
neck NEC	C76.0	C79.89	D09.8	D36.7	D48.7	D49.89
skin	C44.40	—	—	—	—	—
basal cell carcinoma	C44.41	—	—	—	—	—
specified type NEC	C44.49	—	—	—	—	—
squamous cell carcinoma	C44.42	—	—	—	—	—
nerve (ganglion)	C47.9	C79.89		D36.10	D48.2	D49.2
abducens	C72.59	C79.49	—	D33.3	D43.3	D49.7
accessory (spinal)	C72.59	C79.49	—	D33.3	D43.3	D49.7
acoustic	C72.4-	C79.49	—	D33.3	D43.3	D49.7
auditory	C72.4-	C79.49	—	D33.3	D43.3	D49.7
autonomic NEC — *see also Neoplasm, nerve, peripheral*	C47.9	C79.89	—	D36.10	D48.2	D49.2
brachial	C47.1-	C79.89	—	D36.12	D48.2	D49.2
cranial	C72.50	C79.49	—	D33.3	D43.3	D49.7
specified NEC	C72.59	C79.49	—	D33.3	D43.3	D49.7
facial	C72.59	C79.49	—	D33.3	D43.3	D49.7
femoral	C47.2-	C79.89	—	D36.13	D48.2	D49.2
ganglion NEC — *see also Neoplasm, nerve, peripheral*	C47.9	C79.89	—	D36.10	D48.2	D49.2
glossopharyngeal	C72.59	C79.49	—	D33.3	D43.3	D49.7
hypoglossal	C72.59	C79.49	—	D33.3	D43.3	D49.7
intercostal	C47.3	C79.89	—	D36.14	D48.2	D49.2
lumbar	C47.6	C79.89	—	D36.17	D48.2	D49.2
median	C47.1-	C79.89	—	D36.12	D48.2	D49.2
obturator	C47.2-	C79.89	—	D36.13	D48.2	D49.2
oculomotor	C72.59	C79.49	—	D33.3	D43.3	D49.7
olfactory	C47.2-	C79.49	—	D33.3	D43.3	D49.7
optic	C72.3-	C79.49	—	D33.3	D43.3	D49.7
parasympathetic NEC	C47.9	C79.89	—	D36.10	D48.2	D49.2
peripheral NEC	C47.9	C79.89	—	D36.10	D48.2	D49.2
abdomen	C47.4	C79.89	—	D36.15	D48.2	D49.2
abdominal wall	C47.4	C79.89	—	D36.15	D48.2	D49.2
ankle	C47.2-	C79.89	—	D36.13	D48.2	D49.2

TABLE OF NEOPLASMS

TABLE OF NEOPLASMS

	Malignant Primary	Malignant Secondary	Ca in situ	Benign	Uncertain Behavior	Unspecified Behavior
nerve *(Continued)*						
peripheral NEC *(Continued)*						
antecubital fossa or space	C47.1-	C79.89	—	D36.12	D48.2	D49.2
arm	C47.1-	C79.89	—	D36.12	D48.2	D49.2
auricle (ear)	C47.0	C79.89	—	D36.11	D48.2	D49.2
axilla	C47.3	C79.89	—	D36.12	D48.2	D49.2
back	C47.6	C79.89	—	D36.17	D48.2	D49.2
buttock	C47.5	C79.89	—	D36.16	D48.2	D49.2
calf	C47.2-	C79.89	—	D36.13	D48.2	D49.2
cervical region	C47.0	C79.89	—	D36.11	D48.2	D49.2
cheek	C47.0	C79.89	—	D36.11	D48.2	D49.2
chest (wall)	C47.3	C79.89	—	D36.14	D48.2	D49.2
chin	C47.0	C79.89	—	D36.11	D48.2	D49.2
ear (external)	C47.0	C79.89	—	D36.11	D48.2	D49.2
elbow	C47.1-	C79.89	—	D36.12	D48.2	D49.2
extrarectal	C47.5	C79.89	—	D36.16	D48.2	D49.2
extremity	C47.9	C79.89	—	D36.10	D48.2	D49.2
lower	C47.2-	C79.89	—	D36.13	D48.2	D49.2
upper	C47.1-	C79.89	—	D36.12	D48.2	D49.2
eyelid	C47.0	C79.89	—	D36.11	D48.2	D49.2
face	C47.0	C79.89	—	D36.11	D48.2	D49.2
finger	C47.1-	C79.89	—	D36.12	D48.2	D49.2
flank	C47.6	C79.89	—	D36.17	D48.2	D49.2
foot	C47.2-	C79.89	—	D36.13	D48.2	D49.2
forearm	C47.1-	C79.89	—	D36.12	D48.2	D49.2
forehead	C47.0	C79.89	—	D36.11	D48.2	D49.2
gluteal region	C47.5	C79.89	—	D36.16	D48.2	D49.2
groin	C47.5	C79.89	—	D36.16	D48.2	D49.2
hand	C47.1-	C79.89	—	D36.12	D48.2	D49.2
head	C47.0	C79.89	—	D36.11	D48.2	D49.2
heel	C47.2-	C79.89	—	D36.13	D48.2	D49.2
hip	C47.2-	C79.89	—	D36.13	D48.2	D49.2
infraclavicular region	C47.3	C79.89	—	D36.14	D48.2	D49.2
inguinal (canal) (region)	C47.5	C79.89	—	D36.16	D48.2	D49.2
intrathoracic	C47.3	C79.89	—	D36.14	D48.2	D49.2
ischiorectal fossa	C47.5	C79.89	—	D36.16	D48.2	D49.2
knee	C47.2-	C79.89	—	D36.13	D48.2	D49.2
leg	C47.2-	C79.89	—	D36.13	D48.2	D49.2
limb NEC	C47.9	C79.89	—	D36.10	D48.2	D49.2
lower	C47.2-	C79.89	—	D36.13	D48.2	D49.2
upper	C47.1-	C79.89	—	D36.12	D48.2	D49.2
nates	C47.5	C79.89	—	D36.16	D48.2	D49.2
neck	C47.0	C79.89	—	D36.11	D48.2	D49.2
orbit	C69.6-	C79.49	—	D31.6-	D48.7	D49.2
nerve *(Continued)*						
peripheral NEC *(Continued)*						
pararectal	C47.5	C79.89	—	D36.16	D48.2	D49.2
paraurethral	C47.5	C79.89	—	D36.16	D48.2	D49.2
paravaginal	C47.5	C79.89	—	D36.16	D48.2	D49.2
pelvis (floor)	C47.5	C79.89	—	D36.16	D48.2	D49.2
pelvoabdominal	C47.8	C79.89	—	D36.17	D48.2	D49.2
perineum	C47.5	C79.89	—	D36.16	D48.2	D49.2
perirectal (tissue)	C47.5	C79.89	—	D36.16	D48.2	D49.2
periurethral (tissue)	C47.5	C79.89	—	D36.16	D48.2	D49.2
popliteal fossa or space	C47.2-	C79.89	—	D36.13	D48.2	D49.2
presacral	C47.5	C79.89	—	D36.16	D48.2	D49.2
pterygoid fossa	C47.0	C79.89	—	D36.11	D48.2	D49.2
rectovaginal septum or wall	C47.5	C79.89	—	D36.16	D48.2	D49.2
rectovesical	C47.5	C79.89	—	D36.16	D48.2	D49.2
sacrococcygeal region	C47.5	C79.89	—	D36.16	D48.2	D49.2
scalp	C47.0	C79.89	—	D36.11	D48.2	D49.2
scapular region	C47.3	C79.89	—	D36.14	D48.2	D49.2
shoulder	C47.1-	C79.89	—	D36.12	D48.2	D49.2
submental	C47.0	C79.89	—	D36.11	D48.2	D49.2
supraclavicular region	C47.0	C79.89	—	D36.11	D48.2	D49.2
temple	C47.0	C79.89	—	D36.11	D48.2	D49.2
temporal region	C47.0	C79.89	—	D36.11	D48.2	D49.2
thigh	C47.2-	C79.89	—	D36.13	D48.2	D49.2
thoracic (duct) (wall)	C47.3	C79.89	—	D36.14	D48.2	D49.2
thorax	C47.3	C79.89	—	D36.14	D48.2	D49.2
thumb	C47.1-	C79.89	—	D36.12	D48.2	D49.2
toe	C47.2-	C79.89	—	D36.13	D48.2	D49.2
trunk	C47.6	C79.89	—	D36.17	D48.2	D49.2
umbilicus	C47.4	C79.89	—	D36.15	D48.2	D49.2
vesicorectal	C47.5	C79.89	—	D36.16	D48.2	D49.2
wrist	C47.1-	C79.89	—	D36.12	D48.2	D49.2
radial	C47.1-	C79.89	—	D36.12	D48.2	D49.2
sacral	C47.5	C79.89	—	D36.16	D48.2	D49.2
sciatic	C47.2-	C79.89	—	D36.13	D48.2	D49.2
spinal NEC	C47.9	C79.89	—	D36.10	D48.2	D49.2
accessory	C72.59	C79.49	—	D33.3	D43.3	D49.7
sympathetic NEC — *see also* Neoplasm, nerve, peripheral	C47.9	C79.89	—	D36.10	D48.2	D49.2
trigeminal	C72.59	C79.49	—	D33.3	D43.3	D49.7
trochlear	C72.59	C79.49	—	D33.3	D43.3	D49.7
ulnar	C47.1-	C79.89	—	D36.12	D48.2	D49.2
vagus	C72.59	C79.49	—	D33.3	D43.3	D49.7

◀ New   ◀‖ Revised   ~~deleted~~ Deleted

	Malignant Primary	Malignant Secondary	Ca in situ	Benign	Uncertain Behavior	Unspecified Behavior
nervous system (central)	C72.9	C79.40	—	D33.9	D43.9	D49.7
autonomic — see Neoplasm, nerve, peripheral						
parasympathetic — see Neoplasm, nerve, peripheral						
specified site NEC	—	C79.49	—	D33.7	D43.8	—
sympathetic — see Neoplasm, nerve, peripheral						
nevus — see Nevus						
nipple	C50.0-	C79.81	D05.-	D24.-	—	—
nose, nasal	C76.0	C79.89	D09.8	D36.7	D48.7	D49.89
ala (external) (nasi) — see also Neoplasm, nose, skin	C44.301	C79.2	D04.39	D23.39	D48.5	D49.2
bone	C41.0	C79.51	—	D16.4-	D48.0	D49.2
cartilage	C30.0	C78.39	D02.3	D14.0	D38.5	D49.1
cavity	C30.0	C78.39	D02.3	D14.0	D38.5	D49.1
choana	C11.3	C79.89	D00.08	D10.6	D37.05	D49.0
external (skin) — see also Neoplasm, nose, skin	C44.301	C79.2	D04.39	D23.39	D48.5	D49.2
fossa	C30.0	C78.39	D02.3	D14.0	D38.5	D49.1
internal	C30.0	C78.39	D02.3	D14.0	D38.5	D49.1
mucosa	C30.0	C78.39	D02.3	D14.0	D38.5	D49.1
septum	C30.0	C78.39	D02.3	D14.0	D38.5	D49.1
posterior margin	C11.3	C79.89	D00.08	D10.6	D37.05	D49.0
sinus — see Neoplasm, sinus						
skin	C44.301	C79.2	D04.39	D23.39	D48.5	D49.2
basal cell carcinoma	C44.311	—	—	—	—	—
specified type NEC	C44.391	—	—	—	—	—
squamous cell carcinoma	C44.321	—	—	—	—	—
turbinate (mucosa)	C30.0	C78.39	D02.3	D14.0	D38.5	D49.1
bone	C41.0	C79.51	—	D16.4-	D48.0	D49.2
vestibule	C30.0	C78.39	D02.3	D14.0	D38.5	D49.1
nostril	C30.0	C78.39	D02.3	D14.0	D38.5	D49.1
nucleus pulposus	C41.2	C79.51	—	D16.6	D48.0	D49.2
occipital						
bone	C41.0	C79.51	—	D16.4-	D48.0	D49.2
lobe or pole, brain	C71.4	C79.31	—	D33.0	D43.0	D49.6
odontogenic — see Neoplasm, jaw bone						
olfactory nerve or bulb	C72.2-	C79.49	—	D33.3	D43.3	D49.7
olive (brain)	C71.7	C79.31	—	D33.1	D43.1	D49.6
omentum	C48.1	C78.6	—	D20.1	D48.4	D49.0
operculum (brain)	C71.0	C79.31	—	D33.0	D43.0	D49.6

	Malignant Primary	Malignant Secondary	Ca in situ	Benign	Uncertain Behavior	Unspecified Behavior
optic nerve, chiasm, or tract	C72.3-	C79.49	—	D33.3	D43.3	D49.7
oral (cavity)	C06.9	C79.89	D00.00	D10.30	D37.09	D49.0
ill-defined	C14.8	C79.89	D00.00	D10.30	D37.09	D49.0
mucosa	C06.0	C79.89	D00.02	D10.39	D37.09	D49.0
orbit	C69.6-	C79.49	D09.2-	D31.6-	D48.7	D49.89
autonomic nerve	C69.6-	C79.49	—	D31.6-	D48.7	D49.2
bone	C41.0	C79.51	—	D16.4-	D48.0	D49.2
eye	C69.6-	C79.49	D09.2-	D31.6-	D48.7	D49.89
peripheral nerves	C69.6-	C79.49	—	D31.6-	D48.7	D49.2
soft parts	C69.6-	C79.49	D09.2-	D31.6-	D48.7	D49.89
organ of Zuckerkandl	C75.5	C79.89	—	D35.6	D44.7	D49.7
oropharynx	C10.9	C79.89	D00.08	D10.5	D37.05	D49.0
branchial cleft (vestige)	C10.4	C79.89	D00.08	D10.5	D37.05	D49.0
junctional region	C10.8	C79.89	D00.08	D10.5	D37.05	D49.0
lateral wall	C10.2	C79.89	D00.08	D10.5	D37.05	D49.0
overlapping lesion	C10.8	—	—	—	—	—
pillars or fauces	C09.1	C79.89	D00.08	D10.5	D37.05	D49.0
posterior wall	C10.3	C79.89	D00.08	D10.5	D37.05	D49.0
vallecula	C10.0	C79.89	D00.08	D10.5	D37.05	D49.0
os						
external	C53.1	C79.82	D06.1	D26.0	D39.0	D49.59
internal	C53.0	C79.82	D06.0	D26.0	D39.0	D49.59
ovary	C56.-	C79.6-	D07.39	D27.-	D39.1-	D49.59
oviduct	C57.0-	C79.82	D07.39	D28.2	D39.8	D49.59
palate	C05.9	C79.89	D00.00	D10.39	D37.09	D49.0
hard	C05.0	C79.89	D00.05	D10.39	D37.09	D49.0
junction of hard and soft palate	C05.9	C79.89	D00.00	D10.39	D37.09	D49.0
overlapping lesions	C05.8	—	—	—	—	—
soft	C05.1	C79.89	D00.04	D10.39	D37.09	D49.0
nasopharyngeal surface	C11.3	C79.89	D00.08	D10.6	D37.05	D49.0
posterior surface	C11.3	C79.89	D00.08	D10.6	D37.05	D49.0
superior surface	C11.3	C79.89	D00.08	D10.6	D37.05	D49.0
palatoglossal arch	C09.1	C79.89	D00.00	D10.5	D37.09	D49.0
palatopharyngeal arch	C09.1	C79.89	D00.00	D10.5	D37.09	D49.0
pallium	C71.0	C79.31	—	D33.0	D43.0	D49.6
palpebra	C44.10-	C79.2	D04.1-	D23.1-	D48.5	D49.2
basal cell carcinoma	C44.11-	—	—	—	—	—
specified type NEC	C44.19-	—	—	—	—	—
squamous cell carcinoma	C44.12-	—	—	—	—	—
pancreas	C25.9	C78.89	D01.7	D13.6	D37.8	D49.0
body	C25.1	C78.89	D01.7	D13.6	D37.8	D49.0
duct (of Santorini) (of Wirsung)	C25.3	C78.89	D01.7	D13.6	D37.8	D49.0
ectopic tissue	C25.7	C78.89	—	D13.6	D37.8	D49.0
head	C25.0	C78.89	D01.7	D13.6	D37.8	D49.0

◀ New ◀ Revised deleted Deleted

TABLE OF NEOPLASMS

	Malignant Primary	Malignant Secondary	Ca in situ	Benign	Uncertain Behavior	Unspecified Behavior
pancreas *(Continued)*						
islet cells	C25.4	C78.89	D01.7	D13.7	D37.8	D49.0
neck	C25.7	C78.89	D01.7	D13.6	D37.8	D49.0
overlapping lesion	C25.8	—	—	—	—	—
tail	C25.2	C78.89	D01.7	D13.6	D37.8	D49.0
para-aortic body	C75.5	C79.89		D35.6	D44.7	D49.7
paraganglion NEC	C75.5	C79.89		D35.6	D44.7	D49.7
parametrium	C57.3	C79.82	—	D28.2	D39.8	D49.59
paranephric	C48.0	C78.6	—	D20.0	D48.3	D49.0
pararectal	C76.3	C79.89		D36.7	D48.7	D49.89
parasagittal (region)	C76.0	C79.89	D09.8	D36.7	D48.7	D49.89
parasellar	C72.9	C79.49	—	D33.9	D43.8	D49.7
parathyroid (gland)	C75.0	C79.89	D09.3	D35.1	D44.2	D49.7
paraurethral	C76.3	C79.89		D36.7	D48.7	D49.89
gland	C68.1	C79.19	D09.19	D30.8	D41.8	D49.59
paravaginal	C76.3	C79.89	—	D36.7	D48.7	D49.89
parenchyma, kidney	C64.-	C79.0-	D09.19	D30.0-	D41.0-	D49.51-
parietal						
bone	C41.0	C79.51	—	D16.4-	D48.0	D49.2
lobe, brain	C71.3	C79.31	—	D33.0	D43.0	D49.6
paroophoron	C57.1	C79.82	D07.39	D28.2	D39.8	D49.59
parotid (duct) (gland)	C07	C79.89	D00.00	D11.0	D37.030	D49.0
parovarium	C57.1	C79.82	D07.39	D28.2	D39.8	D49.59
patella	C40.20	C79.51	—	—	—	—
peduncle, cerebral	C71.7	C79.31	—	D33.1	D43.1	D49.6
pelvirectal junction	C19	C78.5	D01.1	D12.7	D37.5	D49.0
pelvis, pelvic	C76.3	C79.89	D09.8	D36.7	D48.7	D49.89
bone	C41.4	C79.51	—	D16.8	D48.0	D49.2
floor	C76.3	C79.89	D09.8	D36.7	D48.7	D49.89
renal	C65.-	C79.0-	D09.19	D30.1-	D41.1-	D49.51-
viscera	C76.3	C79.89	D09.8	D36.7	D48.7	D49.89
wall	C76.3	C79.89	D09.8	D36.7	D48.7	D49.89
pelvo-abdominal	C76.8	C79.89	D09.8	D36.7	D48.7	D49.89
penis	C60.9	C79.82	D07.4	D29.0	D40.8	D49.59
body	C60.2	C79.82	D07.4	D29.0	D40.8	D49.59
corpus (cavernosum)	C60.2	C79.82	D07.4	D29.0	D40.8	D49.59
glans	C60.1	C79.82	D07.4	D29.0	D40.8	D49.59
overlapping sites	C60.8	—	—	—	—	—
skin NEC	C60.9	C79.82	D07.4	D29.0	D40.8	D49.59
periadrenal (tissue)	C48.0	C78.6	—	D20.0	D48.3	D49.0
perianal (skin) — *see also* Neoplasm, anus, skin	C44.500	C79.2	D04.5	D23.5	D48.5	D49.2
pericardium	C38.0	C79.89	—	D15.1	D48.7	D49.89
perinephric	C48.0	C78.6	—	D20.0	D48.3	D49.0
perineum	C76.3	C79.89	D09.8	D36.7	D48.7	D49.89
periodontal tissue NEC	C03.9	C79.89	D00.03	D10.39	D37.09	D49.0
periosteum — *see Neoplasm, bone*						
peripancreatic	C48.0	C78.6	—	D20.0	D48.3	D49.0
peripheral nerve NEC	C47.9	C79.89	—	D36.10	D48.2	D49.2
perirectal (tissue)	C76.3	C79.89	—	D36.7	D48.7	D49.89
perirenal (tissue)	C48.0	C78.6	—	D20.0	D48.3	D49.0
peritoneum, peritoneal (cavity)	C48.2	C78.6	—	D20.1	D48.4	D49.0
benign mesothelial tissue — *see* Mesothelioma, benign						
overlapping lesion	C48.8	—	—	—	—	—
with digestive organs	C26.9	—	—	—	—	—
parietal	C48.1	C78.6	—	D20.1	D48.4	D49.0
pelvic	C48.1	C78.6	—	D20.1	D48.4	D49.0
specified part NEC	C48.1	C78.6	—	D20.1	D48.4	D49.0
peritonsillar (tissue)	C76.0	C79.89	D09.8	D36.7	D48.7	D49.89
periurethral tissue	C76.3	C79.89	—	D36.7	D48.7	D49.89
phalanges						
foot	C40.3-	C79.51	—	D16.3-	—	—
hand	C40.1-	C79.51	—	D16.1-	—	—
pharynx, pharyngeal	C14.0	C79.89	D00.08	D10.9	D37.05	D49.0
bursa	C11.1	C79.89	D00.08	D10.6	D37.05	D49.0
fornix	C11.3	C79.89	D00.08	D10.6	D37.05	D49.0
recess	C11.2	C79.89	D00.08	D10.6	D37.05	D49.0
region	C14.0	C79.89	D00.08	D10.9	D37.05	D49.0
tonsil	C11.1	C79.89	D00.08	D10.6	D37.05	D49.0
wall (lateral) (posterior)	C14.0	C79.89	D00.08	D10.9	D37.05	D49.0
pia mater	C70.9	C79.40	—	D32.9	D42.9	D49.7
cerebral	C70.0	C79.32	—	D32.0	D42.0	D49.7
cranial	C70.0	C79.32	—	D32.0	D42.0	D49.7
spinal	C70.1	C79.49	—	D32.1	D42.1	D49.7
pillars of fauces	C09.1	C79.89	D00.08	D10.5	D37.05	D49.0
pineal (body) (gland)	C75.3	C79.89	D09.3	D35.4	D44.5	D49.7
pinna (ear) NEC — *see also* Neoplasm, skin, ear	C44.20-	C79.2	D04.2-	D23.2-	D48.5	D49.2
piriform fossa or sinus	C12	C79.89	D00.08	D10.7	D37.05	D49.0
pituitary (body) (fossa) (gland) (lobe)	C75.1	C79.89	D09.3	D35.2	D44.3	D49.7
placenta	C58	C79.82	D07.0	D26.7	D39.2	D49.59
pleura, pleural (cavity)	C38.4	C78.2	—	D19.0	D38.2	D49.1
overlapping lesion with heart or mediastinum	C38.8	—	—	—	—	—
parietal	C38.4	C78.2	—	D19.0	D38.2	D49.1
visceral	C38.4	C78.2	—	D19.0	D38.2	D49.1

◀ New   ◀═ Revised   ~~deleted~~ Deleted

	Malignant Primary	Malignant Secondary	Ca in situ	Benign	Uncertain Behavior	Unspecified Behavior
plexus						
brachial	C47.1-	C79.89	—	D36.12	D48.2	D49.2
cervical	C47.0	C79.89	—	D36.11	D48.2	D49.2
choroid	C71.5	C79.31	—	D33.0	D43.0	D49.6
lumbosacral	C47.5	C79.89	—	D36.16	D48.2	D49.2
sacral	C47.5	C79.89	—	D36.16	D48.2	D49.2
pluriendocrine	C75.8	C79.89	D09.3	D35.7	D44.9	D49.7
pole						
frontal	C71.1	C79.31	—	D33.0	D43.0	D49.6
occipital	C71.4	C79.31	—	D33.0	D43.0	D49.6
pons (varolii)	C71.7	C79.31	—	D33.1	D43.1	D49.6
popliteal fossa or space	C76.5-	C79.89	D04.7-	D36.7	D48.7	D49.89
postcricoid (region)	C13.0	C79.89	D00.08	D10.7	D37.05	D49.0
posterior fossa (cranial)	C71.9	C79.31	—	D33.2	D43.2	D49.6
postnasal space	C11.9	C79.89	D00.08	D10.6	D37.05	D49.0
prepuce	C60.0	C79.82	D07.4	D29.0	D40.8	D49.59 ◄
prepylorus	C16.4	C78.89	D00.2	D13.1	D37.1	D49.0
presacral (region)	C76.3	C79.89	—	D36.7	D48.7	D49.89
prostate (gland)	C61	C79.82	D07.5	D29.1	D40.0	D49.59 ◄
utricle	C68.0	C79.19	D09.19	D30.4	D41.3	D49.59 ◄
pterygoid fossa	C49.0	C79.89	—	D21.0	D48.1	D49.2
pubic bone	C41.4	C79.51	—	D16.8	D48.0	D49.2
pudenda, pudendum (female)	C51.9	C79.82	D07.1	D28.0	D39.8	D49.59 ◄
pulmonary — *see also* Neoplasm, lung	C34.9-	C78.0-	D02.2-	D14.3-	D38.1	D49.1
putamen	C71.0	C79.31	—	D33.0	D43.0	D49.6
pyloric						
antrum	C16.3	C78.89	D00.2	D13.1	D37.1	D49.0
canal	C16.4	C78.89	D00.2	D13.1	D37.1	D49.0
pylorus	C16.4	C78.89	D00.2	D13.1	D37.1	D49.0
pyramid (brain)	C71.7	C79.31	—	D33.1	D43.1	D49.6
pyriform fossa or sinus	C12	C79.89	D00.08	D10.7	D37.05	D49.0
radius (any part)	C40.0-	C79.51	—	D16.0-	—	—
Rathke's pouch	C75.1	C79.89	D09.3	D35.2	D44.3	D49.7
rectosigmoid (junction)	C19	C78.5	D01.1	D12.7	D37.5	D49.0
overlapping lesion with anus or rectum	C21.8	—	—	—	—	—
rectouterine pouch	C48.1	C78.6	—	D20.1	D48.4	D49.0
rectovaginal septum or wall	C76.3	C79.89	D09.8	D36.7	D48.7	D49.89
rectovesical septum	C76.3	C79.89	D09.8	D36.7	D48.7	D49.89
rectum (ampulla)	C20	C78.5	D01.2	D12.8	D37.5	D49.0
and colon	C19	C78.5	D01.1	D12.7	D37.5	D49.0
overlapping lesion with anus or rectosigmoid junction	C21.8	—	—	—	—	—

	Malignant Primary	Malignant Secondary	Ca in situ	Benign	Uncertain Behavior	Unspecified Behavior
renal	C64.-	C79.0-	D09.19	D30.0-	D41.0-	D49.51- ◄
calyx	C65.-	C79.0-	D09.19	D30.1-	D41.1-	D49.51- ◄
hilus	C65.-	C79.0-	D09.19	D30.1-	D41.1-	D49.51- ◄
parenchyma	C64.-	C79.0-	D09.19	D30.0-	D41.0-	D49.51- ◄
pelvis	C65.-	C79.0-	D09.19	D30.1-	D41.1-	D49.51- ◄
respiratory						
organs or system NEC	C39.9	C78.30	D02.4	D14.4	D38.6	D49.1
tract NEC	C39.9	C78.30	D02.4	D14.4	D38.5	D49.1
upper	C39.0	C78.30	D02.4	D14.4	D38.5	D49.1
retina	C69.2-	C79.49	D09.2-	D31.2-	D48.7	D49.81
retrobulbar	C69.6-	C79.49	—	D31.6-	D48.7	D49.89
retrocecal	C48.0	C78.6	—	D20.0	D48.3	D49.0
retromolar (area) (triangle) (trigone)	C06.2	C79.89	D00.00	D10.39	D37.09	D49.0
retro-orbital	C76.0	C79.89	D09.8	D36.7	D48.7	D49.89
retroperitoneal (space) (tissue)	C48.0	C78.6	—	D20.0	D48.3	D49.0
retroperitoneum	C48.0	C78.6	—	D20.0	D48.3	D49.0
retropharyngeal	C14.0	C79.89	D00.08	D10.9	D37.05	D49.0
retrovesical (septum)	C76.3	C79.89	D09.8	D36.7	D48.7	D49.89
rhinencephalon	C71.0	C79.31	—	D33.0	D43.0	D49.6
rib	C41.3	C79.51	—	D16.7	D48.0	D49.2
Rosenmuller's fossa	C11.2	C79.89	D00.08	D10.6	D37.05	D49.0
round ligament	C57.2	C79.82	—	D28.2	D39.8	D49.59 ◄
sacrococcyx, sacrococcygeal	C41.4	C79.51	—	D16.8	D48.0	D49.2
region	C76.3	C79.89	D09.8	D36.7	D48.7	D49.89
sacrouterine ligament	C57.3	C79.82	—	D28.2	D39.8	D49.59 ◄
sacrum, sacral (vertebra)	C41.4	C79.51	—	D16.8	D48.0	D49.2
salivary gland or duct (major)	C08.9	C79.89	D00.00	D11.9	D37.039	D49.0
minor NEC	C06.9	C79.89	D00.00	D10.39	D37.04	D49.0
overlapping lesion	C08.9	—	—	—	—	—
parotid	C07	C79.89	D00.00	D11.0	D37.030	D49.0
pluriglandular	C08.9	C79.89	D00.00	D11.9	D37.039	D49.0
sublingual	C08.1	C79.89	D00.00	D11.7	D37.031	D49.0
submandibular	C08.0	C79.89	D00.00	D11.7	D37.032	D49.0
submaxillary	C08.0	C79.89	D00.00	D11.7	D37.032	D49.0
salpinx (uterine)	C57.0-	C79.82	D07.39	D28.2	D39.8	D49.59 ◄
Santorini's duct	C25.3	C78.89	D01.7	D13.6	D37.8	D49.0
scalp	C44.40	C79.2	D04.4	D23.4	D48.5	D49.2
basal cell carcinoma	C44.41	—	—	—	—	—
specified type NEC	C44.49	—	—	—	—	—
squamous cell carcinoma	C44.42	—	—	—	—	—
scapula (any part)	C40.0-	C79.51	—	D16.0-	—	—
scapular region	C76.1	C79.89	D09.8	D36.7	D48.7	D49.89

◄ New   ◄ Revised   ~~deleted~~ Deleted

TABLE OF NEOPLASMS

	Malignant Primary	Malignant Secondary	Ca in situ	Benign	Uncertain Behavior	Unspecified Behavior
scar NEC — see also Neoplasm, skin, by site	C44.90	C79.2	D04.9	D23.9	D48.5	D49.2
sciatic nerve	C47.2-	C79.89	—	D36.13	D48.2	D49.2
sclera	C69.4-	C79.49	D09.2-	D31.4-	D48.7	D49.89
scrotum (skin)	C63.2	C79.82	D07.61	D29.4	D40.8	D49.59
sebaceous gland — see Neoplasm, skin						
sella turcica	C75.1	C79.89	D09.3	D35.2	D44.3	D49.7
bone	C41.0	C79.51	—	D16.4-	D48.0	D49.2
semilunar cartilage (knee)	C40.2-	C79.51	—	D16.2-	D48.0	D49.2
seminal vesicle	C63.7	C79.82	D07.69	D29.8	D40.8	D49.59
septum						
nasal	C30.0	C78.39	D02.3	D14.0	D38.5	D49.1
posterior margin	C11.3	C79.89	D00.08	D10.6	D37.05	D49.0
rectovaginal	C76.3	C79.89	D09.8	D36.7	D48.7	D49.89
rectovesical	C76.3	C79.89	D09.8	D36.7	D48.7	D49.89
urethrovaginal	C57.9	C79.82	D07.30	D28.9	D39.9	D49.59
vesicovaginal	C57.9	C79.82	D07.30	D28.9	D39.9	D49.59
shoulder NEC	C76.4-	C79.89	D04.6-	D36.7	D48.7	D49.89
sigmoid flexure (lower) (upper)	C18.7	C78.5	D01.0	D12.5	D37.4	D49.0
sinus (accessory)	C31.9	C78.39	D02.3	D14.0	D38.5	D49.1
bone (any)	C41.0	C79.51	—	D16.4-	D48.0	D49.2
ethmoidal	C31.1	C78.39	D02.3	D14.0	D38.5	D49.1
frontal	C31.2	C78.39	D02.3	D14.0	D38.5	D49.1
maxillary	C31.0	C78.39	D02.3	D14.0	D38.5	D49.1
nasal, paranasal NEC	C31.9	C78.39	D02.3	D14.0	D38.5	D49.1
overlapping lesion	C31.8	—	—	—	—	—
pyriform	C12	C79.89	D00.08	D10.7	D37.05	D49.0
sphenoid	C31.3	C78.39	D02.3	D14.0	D38.5	D49.1
skeleton, skeletal NEC	C41.9	C79.51	—	D16.9-	D48.0	D49.2
Skene's gland	C68.1	C79.19	D09.19	D30.8	D41.8	D49.59
skin NOS	C44.90	C79.2	D04.9	D23.9	D48.5	D49.2
abdominal wall	C44.509	C79.2	D04.5	D23.5	D48.5	D49.2
basal cell carcinoma	C44.519	—	—	—	—	—
specified type NEC	C44.599	—	—	—	—	—
squamous cell carcinoma	C44.529	—	—	—	—	—
ala nasi — see also Neoplasm, nose, skin	C44.301	C79.2	D04.39	D23.39	D48.5	D49.2
ankle — see also Neoplasm, skin, limb, lower	C44.70-	C79.2	D04.7-	D23.7-	D48.5	D49.2
antecubital space — see also Neoplasm, skin, limb, upper	C44.60-	C79.2	D04.6-	D23.6-	D48.5	D49.2
skin NOS (Continued)						
anus	C44.500	C79.2	D04.5	D23.5	D48.5	D49.2
basal cell carcinoma	C44.510	—	—	—	—	—
specified type NEC	C44.590	—	—	—	—	—
squamous cell carcinoma	C44.520	—	—	—	—	—
arm — see also Neoplasm, skin, limb, upper	C44.60-	C79.2	D04.6-	D23.6-	D48.5	D49.2
auditory canal (external) — see also Neoplasm, skin, ear	C44.20-	C79.2	D04.2-	D23.2-	D48.5	D49.2
auricle (ear) — see also Neoplasm, skin, ear	C44.20-	C79.2	D04.2-	D23.2-	D48.5	D49.2
auricular canal (external) — see also Neoplasm, skin, ear	C44.20-	C79.2	D04.2-	D23.2-	D48.5	D49.2
axilla, axillary fold — see also Neoplasm, skin, trunk	C44.509	C79.2	D04.5	D23.5	D48.5	D49.2
back — see also Neoplasm, skin, trunk	C44.509	C79.2	D04.5	D23.5	D48.5	D49.2
basal cell carcinoma	C44.91					
breast	C44.501	C79.2	D04.5	D23.5	D48.5	D49.2
basal cell carcinoma	C44.511	—	—	—	—	—
specified type NEC	C44.591	—	—	—	—	—
squamous cell carcinoma	C44.521	—	—	—	—	—
brow — see also Neoplasm, skin, face	C44.309	C79.2	D04.39	D23.39	D48.5	D49.2
buttock — see also Neoplasm, skin, trunk	C44.509	C79.2	D04.5	D23.5	D48.5	D49.2
calf — see also Neoplasm, skin, limb, lower	C44.70-	C79.2	D04.7-	D23.7-	D48.5	D49.2
canthus (eye) (inner) (outer)	C44.10-	C79.2	D04.1-	D23.1-	D48.5	D49.2
basal cell carcinoma	C44.11-	—	—	—	—	—
specified type NEC	C44.19-	—	—	—	—	—
squamous cell carcinoma	C44.12-	—	—	—	—	—
cervical region — see also Neoplasm, skin, neck	C44.40	C79.2	D04.4	D23.4	D48.5	D49.2
cheek (external) — see also Neoplasm, skin, face	C44.309	C79.2	D04.39	D23.39	D48.5	D49.2
chest (wall) — see also Neoplasm, skin, trunk	C44.509	C79.2	D04.5	D23.5	D48.5	D49.2
chin — see also Neoplasm, skin, face	C44.309	C79.2	D04.39	D23.39	D48.5	D49.2
clavicular area — see also Neoplasm, skin, trunk	C44.509	C79.2	D04.5	D23.5	D48.5	D49.2
clitoris	C51.2	C79.82	D07.1	D28.0	D39.8	D49.59
columnella — see also Neoplasm, skin, face	C44.309	C79.2	D04.39	D23.39	D48.5	D49.2

◀ New   ◀▦ Revised   ~~deleted~~ Deleted

	Malignant Primary	Malignant Secondary	Ca in situ	Benign	Uncertain Behavior	Unspecified Behavior
skin NOS *(Continued)*						
concha — *see also Neoplasm, skin, ear*	C44.20-	C79.2	D04.2-	D23.2-	D48.5	D49.2
ear (external)	C44.20-	C79.2	D04.2-	D23.2-	D48.5	D49.2
basal cell carcinoma	C44.21-	—	—	—	—	—
specified type NEC	C44.29-	—	—	—	—	—
squamous cell carcinoma	C44.22-	—	—	—	—	—
elbow — *see also Neoplasm, skin, limb, upper*	C44.60-	C79.2	D04.6-	D23.6-	D48.5	D49.2
eyebrow — *see also Neoplasm, skin, face*	C44.309	C79.2	D04.39	D23.39	D48.5	D49.2
eyelid	C44.10-	C79.2	D04.1-	D23.1-	D48.5	D49.2
basal cell carcinoma	C44.11-	—	—	—	—	—
specified type NEC	C44.19-	—	—	—	—	—
squamous cell carcinoma	C44.12-	—	—	—	—	—
face NOS	C44.300	C79.2	D04.30	D23.30	D48.5	D49.2
basal cell carcinoma	C44.310	—	—	—	—	—
specified type NEC	C44.390	—	—	—	—	—
squamous cell carcinoma	C44.320	—	—	—	—	—
female genital organs (external)	C51.9	C79.82	D07.1	D28.0	D39.8	D49.59 ◄
clitoris	C51.2	C79.82	D07.1	D28.0	D39.8	D49.59 ◄
labium NEC	C51.9	C79.82	D07.1	D28.0	D39.8	D49.59 ◄
majus	C51.0	C79.82	D07.1	D28.0	D39.8	D49.59 ◄
minus	C51.1	C79.82	D07.1	D28.0	D39.8	D49.59 ◄
pudendum	C51.9	C79.82	D07.1	D28.0	D39.8	D49.59 ◄
vulva	C51.9	C79.82	D07.1	D28.0	D39.8	D49.59 ◄
finger — *see also Neoplasm, skin, limb, upper*	C44.60-	C79.2	D04.6-	D23.6-	D48.5	D49.2
flank — *see also Neoplasm, skin, trunk*	C44.509	C79.2	D04.5	D23.5	D48.5	D49.2
foot — *see also Neoplasm, skin, limb, lower*	C44.70-	C79.2	D04.7-	D23.7-	D48.5	D49.2
forearm — *see also Neoplasm, skin, limb, upper*	C44.60-	C79.2	D04.6-	D23.6-	D48.5	D49.2
forehead — *see also Neoplasm, skin, face*	C44.309	C79.2	D04.39	D23.39	D48.5	D49.2
glabella — *see also Neoplasm, skin, face*	C44.309	C79.2	D04.39	D23.39	D48.5	D49.2
gluteal region — *see also Neoplasm, skin, trunk*	C44.509	C79.2	D04.5	D23.5	D48.5	D49.2
groin — *see also Neoplasm, skin, trunk*	C44.509	C79.2	D04.5	D23.5	D48.5	D49.2
hand — *see also Neoplasm, skin, limb, upper*	C44.60-	C79.2	D04.6-	D23.6-	D48.5	D49.2

	Malignant Primary	Malignant Secondary	Ca in situ	Benign	Uncertain Behavior	Unspecified Behavior
skin NOS *(Continued)*						
head NEC — *see also Neoplasm, skin, scalp*	C44.40	C79.2	D04.4	D23.4	D48.5	D49.2
heel — *see also Neoplasm, skin, limb, lower*	C44.70-	C79.2	D04.7-	D23.7-	D48.5	D49.2
helix — *see also Neoplasm, skin, ear*	C44.20-	C79.2	D04.2-	D23.2-	D48.5	D49.2
hip — *see also Neoplasm, skin, limb, lower*	C44.70-	C79.2	D04.7-	D23.7-	D48.5	D49.2
infraclavicular region — *see also Neoplasm, skin, trunk*	C44.509	C79.2	D04.5	D23.5	D48.5	D49.2
inguinal region — *see also Neoplasm, skin, trunk*	C44.509	C79.2	D04.5	D23.5	D48.5	D49.2
jaw — *see also Neoplasm, skin, face*	C44.309	C79.2	D04.39	D23.39	D48.5	D49.2
Kaposi's sarcoma — *see Kaposi's, sarcoma, skin*						
knee — *see also Neoplasm, skin, limb, lower*	C44.70-	C79.2	D04.7-	D23.7-	D48.5	D49.2
labia						
majora	C51.0	C79.82	D07.1	D28.0	D39.8	D49.59 ◄
minora	C51.1	C79.82	D07.1	D28.0	D39.8	D49.59 ◄
leg — *see also Neoplasm, skin, limb, lower*	C44.70-	C79.2	D04.7-	D23.7-	D48.5	D49.2
lid (lower) (upper)	C44.10-	C79.2	D04.1-	D23.1-	D48.5	D49.2
basal cell carcinoma	C44.11-	—	—	—	—	—
specified type NEC	C44.19-	—	—	—	—	—
squamous cell carcinoma	C44.12-	—	—	—	—	—
limb NEC	C44.90	C79.2	D04.9	D23.9	D48.5	D49.2
basal cell carcinoma	C44.91					
lower	C44.70-	C79.2	D04.7-	D23.7-	D48.5	D49.2
basal cell carcinoma	C44.71-	—	—	—	—	—
specified type NEC	C44.79-	—	—	—	—	—
squamous cell carcinoma	C44.72-	—	—	—	—	—
upper	C44.60-	C79.2	D04.6-	D23.6-	D48.5	D49.2
basal cell carcinoma	C44.61-	—	—	—	—	—
specified type NEC	C44.69-	—	—	—	—	—
squamous cell carcinoma	C44.62-	—	—	—	—	—
lip (lower) (upper)	C44.00	C79.2	D04.0	D23.0	D48.5	D49.2
basal cell carcinoma	C44.01	—	—	—	—	—
specified type NEC	C44.09	—	—	—	—	—
squamous cell carcinoma	C44.02	—	—	—	—	—

TABLE OF NEOPLASMS

TABLE OF NEOPLASMS

skin NOS (Continued)

	Malignant Primary	Malignant Secondary	Ca in situ	Benign	Uncertain Behavior	Unspecified Behavior
male genital organs	C63.9	C79.82	D07.60	D29.9	D40.8	D49.59
penis	C60.9	C79.82	D07.4	D29.0	D40.8	D49.59
prepuce	C60.0	C79.82	D07.4	D29.0	D40.8	D49.59
scrotum	C63.2	C79.82	D07.61	D29.4	D40.8	D49.59
mastectomy site (skin) — see also Neoplasm, skin, breast	C44.501	C79.2	—	—	—	—
specified as breast tissue	C50.8-	C79.81	—	—	—	—
meatus, acoustic (external) — see also Neoplasm, skin, ear	C44.20-	C79.2	D04.2-	D23.2-	D48.5	D49.2
melanotic — see Melanoma						
Merkel cell — see Carcinoma, Merkel cell						
nates — see also Neoplasm, skin, trunk	C44.509	C79.2	D04.5	D23.5	D48.5	D49.2
neck	C44.40	C79.2	D04.4	D23.4	D48.5	D49.2
basal cell carcinoma	C44.41	—	—	—	—	—
specified type NEC	C44.49	—	—	—	—	—
squamous cell carcinoma	C44.42	—	—	—	—	—
nevus — see Nevus, skin						
nose (external) — see also Neoplasm, nose, skin	C44.301	C79.2	D04.39	D23.39	D48.5	D49.2
overlapping lesion	C44.80	—	—	—	—	—
basal cell carcinoma	C44.81	—	—	—	—	—
specified type NEC	C44.89	—	—	—	—	—
squamous cell carcinoma	C44.82	—	—	—	—	—
palm — see also Neoplasm, skin, limb, upper	C44.60-	C79.2	D04.6-	D23.6-	D48.5	D49.2
palpebra	C44.10-	C79.2	D04.1-	D23.1-	D48.5	D49.2
basal cell carcinoma	C44.11-	—	—	—	—	—
specified type NEC	C44.19-	—	—	—	—	—
squamous cell carcinoma	C44.12-	—	—	—	—	—
penis NEC	C60.9	C79.82	D07.4	D29.0	D40.8	D49.59
perianal — see also Neoplasm, skin, anus	C44.500	C79.2	D04.5	D23.5	D48.5	D49.2
perineum — see also Neoplasm, skin, anus	C44.500	C79.2	D04.5	D23.5	D48.5	D49.2
pinna — see also Neoplasm, skin, ear	C44.20-	C79.2	D04.2-	D23.2-	D48.5	D49.2
plantar — see also Neoplasm, skin, limb, lower	C44.70-	C79.2	D04.7-	D23.7-	D48.5	D49.2
popliteal fossa or space — see also Neoplasm, skin, limb, lower	C44.70-	C79.2	D04.7-	D23.7-	D48.5	D49.2
prepuce	C60.0	C79.82	D07.4	D29.0	D40.8	D49.59

skin NOS (Continued)

	Malignant Primary	Malignant Secondary	Ca in situ	Benign	Uncertain Behavior	Unspecified Behavior
pubes — see also Neoplasm, skin, trunk	C44.509	C79.2	D04.5	D23.5	D48.5	D49.2
sacrococcygeal region — see also Neoplasm, skin, trunk	C44.509	C79.2	D04.5	D23.5	D48.5	D49.2
scalp	C44.40	C79.2	D04.4	D23.4	D48.5	D49.2
basal cell carcinoma	C44.41	—	—	—	—	—
specified type NEC	C44.49	—	—	—	—	—
squamous cell carcinoma	C44.42	—	—	—	—	—
scapular region — see also Neoplasm, skin, trunk	C44.509	C79.2	D04.5	D23.5	D48.5	D49.2
scrotum	C63.2	C79.82	D07.61	D29.4	D40.8	D49.59
shoulder — see also Neoplasm, skin, limb, upper	C44.60-	C79.2	D04.6-	D23.6-	D48.5	D49.2
sole (foot) — see also Neoplasm, skin, limb, lower	C44.70-	C79.2	D04.7-	D23.7-	D48.5	D49.2
specified sites NEC	C44.80	C79.2	D04.8	D23.9	D48.5	D49.2
basal cell carcinoma	C44.81	—	—	—	—	—
specified type NEC	C44.89	—	—	—	—	—
squamous cell carcinoma	C44.82	—	—	—	—	—
specified type NEC	C44.99	—	—	—	—	—
squamous cell carcinoma	C44.92	—	—	—	—	—
submammary fold — see also Neoplasm, skin, trunk	C44.509	C79.2	D04.5	D23.5	D48.5	D49.2
supraclavicular region — see also Neoplasm, skin, neck	C44.40	C79.2	D04.4	D23.4	D48.5	D49.2
temple — see also Neoplasm, skin, face	C44.309	C79.2	D04.39	D23.39	D48.5	D49.2
thigh — see also Neoplasm, skin, limb, lower	C44.70-	C79.2	D04.7-	D23.7-	D48.5	D49.2
thoracic wall — see also Neoplasm, skin, trunk	C44.509	C79.2	D04.5	D23.5	D48.5	D49.2
thumb — see also Neoplasm, skin, limb, upper	C44.60-	C79.2	D04.6-	D23.6-	D48.5	D49.2
toe — see also Neoplasm, skin, limb, lower	C44.70-	C79.2	D04.7-	D23.7-	D48.5	D49.2
tragus — see also Neoplasm, skin, ear	C44.20-	C79.2	D04.2-	D23.2-	D48.5	D49.2
trunk	C44.509	C79.2	D04.5	D23.5	D48.5	D49.2
basal cell carcinoma	C44.519	—	—	—	—	—
specified type NEC	C44.599	—	—	—	—	—
squamous cell carcinoma	C44.529	—	—	—	—	—
umbilicus — see also Neoplasm, skin, trunk	C44.509	C79.2	D04.5	D23.5	D48.5	D49.2

◀ New ◀▪ Revised ~~deleted~~ Deleted

	Malignant Primary	Malignant Secondary	Ca in situ	Benign	Uncertain Behavior	Unspecified Behavior
skin NOS *(Continued)*						
vulva	C51.9	C79.82	D07.1	D28.0	D39.8	D49.59 ◄
overlapping lesion	C51.8	—				
wrist — *see also Neoplasm, skin, limb, upper*	C44.60-	C79.2	D04.6-	D23.6-	D48.5	D49.2
skull	C41.0	C79.51	—	D16.4-	D48.0	D49.2
soft parts or tissues — *see Neoplasm, connective tissue*						
specified site NEC	C76.8	C79.89	D09.8	D36.7	D48.7	D49.89
spermatic cord	C63.1-	C79.82	D07.69	D29.8	D40.8	D49.59 ◄
sphenoid	C31.3	C78.39	D02.3	D14.0	D38.5	D49.1
bone	C41.0	C79.51	—	D16.4-	D48.0	D49.2
sinus	C31.3	C78.39	D02.3	D14.0	D38.5	D49.1
sphincter						
anal	C21.1	C78.5	D01.3	D12.9	D37.8	D49.0
of Oddi	C24.0	C78.89	D01.5	D13.5	D37.6	D49.0
spine, spinal (column)	C41.2	C79.51	—	D16.6	D48.0	D49.2
bulb	C71.7	C79.31	—	D33.1	D43.1	D49.6
coccyx	C41.4	C79.51	—	D16.8	D48.0	D49.2
cord (cervical) (lumbar) (sacral) (thoracic)	C72.0	C79.49	—	D33.4	D43.4	D49.7
dura mater	C70.1	C79.49	—	D32.1	D42.1	D49.7
lumbosacral	C41.2	C79.51	—	D16.6	D48.0	D49.2
marrow NEC	C96.9	C79.52	—	—	D47.9	D49.89
membrane	C70.1	C79.49	—	D32.1	D42.1	D49.7
meninges	C70.1	C79.49	—	D32.1	D42.1	D49.7
nerve (root)	C47.9	C79.89	—	D36.10	D48.2	D49.2
pia mater	C70.1	C79.49	—	D32.1	D42.1	D49.7
root	C47.9	C79.89	—	D36.10	D48.2	D49.2
sacrum	C41.4	C79.51	—	D16.8	D48.0	D49.2
spleen, splenic NEC	C26.1	C78.89	D01.7	D13.9	D37.8	D49.0
flexure (colon)	C18.5	C78.5	D01.0	D12.3	D37.4	D49.0
stem, brain	C71.7	C79.31	—	D33.1	D43.1	D49.6
Stensen's duct	C07	C79.89	D00.00	D11.0	D37.030	D49.0
sternum	C41.3	C79.51	—	D16.7	D48.0	D49.2
stomach	C16.9	C78.89	D00.2	D13.1	D37.1	D49.0
antrum (pyloric)	C16.3	C78.89	D00.2	D13.1	D37.1	D49.0
body	C16.2	C78.89	D00.2	D13.1	D37.1	D49.0
cardia	C16.0	C78.89	D00.2	D13.1	D37.1	D49.0
cardiac orifice	C16.0	C78.89	D00.2	D13.1	D37.1	D49.0
corpus	C16.2	C78.89	D00.2	D13.1	D37.1	D49.0
fundus	C16.1	C78.89	D00.2	D13.1	D37.1	D49.0
greater curvature NEC	C16.6	C78.89	D00.2	D13.1	D37.1	D49.0
lesser curvature NEC	C16.5	C78.89	D00.2	D13.1	D37.1	D49.0

	Malignant Primary	Malignant Secondary	Ca in situ	Benign	Uncertain Behavior	Unspecified Behavior
stomach *(Continued)*						
overlapping lesion	C16.8	—	—	—	—	—
prepylorus	C16.4	C78.89	D00.2	D13.1	D37.1	D49.0
pylorus	C16.4	C78.89	D00.2	D13.1	D37.1	D49.0
wall NEC	C16.9	C78.89	D00.2	D13.1	D37.1	D49.0
anterior NEC	C16.8	C78.89	D00.2	D13.1	D37.1	D49.0
posterior NEC	C16.8	C78.89	D00.2	D13.1	D37.1	D49.0
stroma, endometrial	C54.1	C79.82	D07.0	D26.1	D39.0	D49.59 ◄
stump, cervical	C53.8	C79.82	D06.7	D26.0	D39.0	D49.59 ◄
subcutaneous (nodule) (tissue) NEC — *see Neoplasm, connective tissue*						
subdural	C70.9	C79.32	—	D32.9	D42.9	D49.7
subglottis, subglottic	C32.2	C78.39	D02.0	D14.1	D38.0	D49.1
sublingual	C04.9	C79.89	D00.06	D10.2	D37.09	D49.0
gland or duct	C08.1	C79.89	D00.00	D11.7	D37.031	D49.0
submandibular gland	C08.0	C79.89	D00.00	D11.7	D37.032	D49.0
submaxillary gland or duct	C08.0	C79.89	D00.00	D11.7	D37.032	D49.0
submental	C76.0	C79.89	D09.8	D36.7	D48.7	D49.89
subpleural	C34.9-	C78.0-	D02.2-	D14.3-	D38.1	D49.1
substernal	C38.1	C78.1	—	D15.2	D38.3	D49.89
sudoriferous, sudoriparous gland, site unspecified	C44.90	C79.2	D04.9	D23.9	D48.5	D49.2
specified site — *see Neoplasm, skin*						
supraclavicular region	C76.0	C79.89	D09.8	D36.7	D48.7	D49.89
supraglottis	C32.1	C78.39	D02.0	D14.1	D38.0	D49.1
suprarenal	C74.9-	C79.7-	D09.3	D35.0-	D44.1-	D49.7
capsule	C74.9-	C79.7-	D09.3	D35.0-	D44.1-	D49.7
cortex	C74.0-	C79.7-	D09.3	D35.0-	D44.1-	D49.7
gland	C74.9-	C79.7-	D09.3	D35.0-	D44.1-	D49.7
medulla	C74.1-	C79.7-	D09.3	D35.0-	D44.1-	D49.7
suprasellar (region)	C71.9	C79.31	—	D33.2	D43.2	D49.6
supratentorial (brain) NEC	C71.0	C79.31	—	D33.0	D43.0	D49.6
sweat gland (apocrine) (eccrine), site unspecified	C44.90	C79.2	D04.9	D23.9	D48.5	D49.2
specified site — *see Neoplasm, skin*						
sympathetic nerve or nervous system NEC	C47.9	C79.89	—	D36.10	D48.2	D49.2
symphysis pubis	C41.4	C79.51	—	D16.8	D48.0	D49.2
synovial membrane — *see Neoplasm, connective tissue*						
tapetum, brain	C71.8	C79.31	—	D33.2	D43.2	D49.6

TABLE OF NEOPLASMS

	Malignant Primary	Malignant Secondary	Ca in situ	Benign	Uncertain Behavior	Unspecified Behavior
tarsus (any bone)	C40.3-	C79.51	—	D16.3-	—	—
temple (skin) — see also Neoplasm, skin, face	C44.309	C79.2	D04.39	D23.39	D48.5	D49.2
temporal						
bone	C41.0	C79.51	—	D16.4-	D48.0	D49.2
lobe or pole	C71.2	C79.31	—	D33.0	D43.0	D49.6
region	C76.0	C79.89	D09.8	D36.7	D48.7	D49.89
skin — see also Neoplasm, skin, face	C44.309	C79.2	D04.39	D23.39	D48.5	D49.2
tendon (sheath) — see Neoplasm, connective tissue						
tentorium (cerebelli)	C70.0	C79.32	—	D32.0	D42.0	D49.7
testis, testes	C62.9-	C79.82	D07.69	D29.2-	D40.1-	D49.59
descended	C62.1-	C79.82	D07.69	D29.2-	D40.1-	D49.59
ectopic	C62.0-	C79.82	D07.69	D29.2-	D40.1-	D49.59
retained	C62.0-	C79.82	D07.69	D29.2-	D40.1-	D49.59
scrotal	C62.1-	C79.82	D07.69	D29.2-	D40.1-	D49.59
undescended	C62.0-	C79.82	D07.69	D29.2-	D40.1-	D49.59
unspecified whether descended or undescended	C62.9-	C79.82	D07.69	D29.2-	D40.1-	D49.59
thalamus	C71.0	C79.31	—	D33.0	D43.0	D49.6
thigh NEC	C76.5-	C79.89	D04.7-	D36.7	D48.7	D49.89
thorax, thoracic (cavity) (organs NEC)	C76.1	C79.89	D09.8	D36.7	D48.7	D49.89
duct	C49.3	C79.89	—	D21.3	D48.1	D49.2
wall NEC	C76.1	C79.89	D09.8	D36.7	D48.7	D49.89
throat	C14.0	C79.89	D00.08	D10.9	D37.05	D49.0
thumb NEC	C76.4-	C79.89	D04.6-	D36.7	D48.7	D49.89
thymus (gland)	C37	C79.89	D09.3	D15.0	D38.4	D49.89
thyroglossal duct	C73	C79.89	D09.3	D34	D44.0	D49.7
thyroid (gland)	C73	C79.89	D09.3	D34	D44.0	D49.7
cartilage	C32.3	C78.39	D02.0	D14.1	D38.0	D49.1
tibia (any part)	C40.2-	C79.51	—	D16.2-	—	—
toe NEC	C76.5-	C79.89	D04.7-	D36.7	D48.7	D49.89
tongue	C02.9	C79.89	D00.07	D10.1	D37.02	D49.0
anterior (two-thirds) NEC	C02.3	C79.89	D00.07	D10.1	D37.02	D49.0
dorsal surface	C02.0	C79.89	D00.07	D10.1	D37.02	D49.0
ventral surface	C02.2	C79.89	D00.07	D10.1	D37.02	D49.0
base (dorsal surface)	C01	C79.89	D00.07	D10.1	D37.02	D49.0
border (lateral)	C02.1	C79.89	D00.07	D10.1	D37.02	D49.0
dorsal surface NEC	C02.0	C79.89	D00.07	D10.1	D37.02	D49.0
fixed part NEC	C01	C79.89	D00.07	D10.1	D37.02	D49.0
foreamen cecum	C02.0	C79.89	D00.07	D10.1	D37.02	D49.0
frenulum linguae	C02.2	C79.89	D00.07	D10.1	D37.02	D49.0

	Malignant Primary	Malignant Secondary	Ca in situ	Benign	Uncertain Behavior	Unspecified Behavior
tongue (Continued)						
junctional zone	C02.8	C79.89	D00.07	D10.1	D37.02	D49.0
margin (lateral)	C02.1	C79.89	D00.07	D10.1	D37.02	D49.0
midline NEC	C02.0	C79.89	D00.07	D10.1	D37.02	D49.0
mobile part NEC	C02.3	C79.89	D00.07	D10.1	D37.02	D49.0
overlapping lesion	C02.8	—	—	—	—	—
posterior (third)	C01	C79.89	D00.07	D10.1	D37.02	D49.0
root	C01	C79.89	D00.07	D10.1	D37.02	D49.0
surface (dorsal)	C02.0	C79.89	D00.07	D10.1	D37.02	D49.0
base	C01	C79.89	D00.07	D10.1	D37.02	D49.0
ventral	C02.2	C79.89	D00.07	D10.1	D37.02	D49.0
tip	C02.1	C79.89	D00.07	D10.1	D37.02	D49.0
tonsil	C02.4	C79.89	D00.07	D10.1	D37.02	D49.0
tonsil	C09.9	C79.89	D00.08	D10.4	D37.05	D49.0
fauces, faucial	C09.9	C79.89	D00.08	D10.4	D37.05	D49.0
lingual	C02.4	C79.89	D00.07	D10.1	D37.02	D49.0
overlapping sites	C09.8	—	—	—	—	—
palatine	C09.9	C79.89	D00.08	D10.4	D37.05	D49.0
pharyngeal	C11.1	C79.89	D00.08	D10.6	D37.05	D49.0
pillar (anterior) (posterior)	C09.1	C79.89	D00.08	D10.5	D37.05	D49.0
tonsillar fossa	C09.0	C79.89	D00.08	D10.5	D37.05	D49.0
tooth socket NEC	C03.9	C79.89	D00.03	D10.39	D37.09	D49.0
trachea (cartilage) (mucosa)	C33	C78.39	D02.1	D14.2	D38.1	D49.1
overlapping lesion with bronchus or lung	C34.8-	—	—	—	—	—
tracheobronchial	C34.8-	C78.39	D02.1	D14.2	D38.1	D49.1
overlapping lesion with lung	C34.8-	—	—	—	—	—
tragus — see also Neoplasm, skin, ear	C44.20-	C79.2	D04.2-	D23.2-	D48.5	D49.2
trunk NEC	C76.8	C79.89	D04.5	D36.7	D48.7	D49.89
tubo-ovarian	C57.8	C79.82	D07.39	D28.7	D39.8	D49.59
tunica vaginalis	C63.7	C79.82	D07.69	D29.8	D40.8	D49.59
turbinate (bone)	C41.0	C79.51	—	D16.4-	D48.0	D49.2
nasal	C30.0	C78.39	D02.3	D14.0	D38.5	D49.1
tympanic cavity	C30.1	C78.39	D02.3	D14.0	D38.5	D49.1
ulna (any part)	C40.0-	C79.51	—	D16.0-	—	—
umbilicus, umbilical — see also Neoplasm, skin, trunk	C44.509	C79.2	D04.5	D23.5	D48.5	D49.2
uncus, brain	C71.2	C79.31	—	D33.0	D43.0	D49.6
unknown site or unspecified	C80.1	C79.9	D09.9	D36.9	D48.9	D49.9
urachus	C67.7	C79.11	D09.0	D30.3	D41.4	D49.4
ureter, ureteral	C66.-	C79.19	D09.19	D30.2-	D41.2-	D49.59
orifice (bladder)	C67.6	C79.11	D09.0	D30.3	D41.4	D49.4
ureter-bladder (junction)	C67.6	C79.11	D09.0	D30.3	D41.4	D49.4

◄ New ◄▦ Revised ~~deleted~~ Deleted

	Malignant Primary	Malignant Secondary	Ca in situ	Benign	Uncertain Behavior	Unspecified Behavior
urethra, urethral (gland)	C68.0	C79.19	D09.19	D30.4	D41.3	D49.59
orifice, internal	C67.5	C79.11	D09.0	D30.3	D41.4	D49.4
urethrovaginal (septum)	C57.9	C79.82	D07.30	D28.9	D39.8	D49.59
urinary organ or system	C68.9	C79.10	D09.10	D30.9	D41.9	D49.59
bladder — see Neoplasm, bladder						
overlapping lesion	C68.8	—	—	—	—	—
specified sites NEC	C68.8	C79.19	D09.19	D30.8	D41.8	D49.59
utero-ovarian	C57.8	C79.82	D07.39	D28.7	D39.8	D49.59
ligament	C57.1	C79.82	D07.39	D28.2	D39.8	D49.59
uterosacral ligament	C57.3	C79.82	—	D28.2	D39.8	D49.59
uterus, uteri, uterine	C55	C79.82	D07.0	D26.9	D39.0	D49.59
adnexa NEC	C57.4	C79.82	D07.39	D28.7	D39.8	D49.59
body	C54.9	C79.82	D07.0	D26.1	D39.0	D49.59
cervix	C53.9	C79.82	D06.9	D26.0	D39.0	D49.59
cornu	C54.9	C79.82	D07.0	D26.1	D39.0	D49.59
corpus	C54.9	C79.82	D07.0	D26.1	D39.0	D49.59
endocervix (canal) (gland)	C53.0	C79.82	D06.0	D26.0	D39.0	D49.59
endometrium	C54.1	C79.82	D07.0	D26.1	D39.0	D49.59
exocervix	C53.1	C79.82	D06.1	D26.0	D39.0	D49.59
external os	C53.1	C79.82	D06.1	D26.0	D39.0	D49.59
fundus	C54.3	C79.82	D07.0	D26.1	D39.0	D49.59
internal os	C53.0	C79.82	D06.0	D26.0	D39.0	D49.59
isthmus	C54.0	C79.82	D07.0	D26.1	D39.0	D49.59
ligament	C57.3	C79.82	—	D28.2	D39.8	D49.59
broad	C57.1	C79.82	D07.39	D28.2	D39.8	D49.59
round	C57.2	C79.82	—	D28.2	D39.8	D49.59
lower segment	C54.0	C79.82	D07.0	D26.1	D39.0	D49.59
myometrium	C54.2	C79.82	D07.0	D26.1	D39.0	D49.59
overlapping sites	C54.8	—	—	—	—	—
squamocolumnar junction	C53.8	C79.82	D06.7	D26.0	D39.0	D49.59
tube	C57.0-	C79.82	D07.39	D28.2	D39.8	D49.59
utricle, prostatic	C68.0	C79.19	D09.19	D30.4	D41.3	D49.59
uveal tract	C69.4-	C79.49	D09.2-	D31.4-	D48.7	D49.89
uvula	C05.2	C79.89	D00.04	D10.39	D37.09	D49.0
vagina, vaginal (fornix) (vault) (wall)	C52	C79.82	D07.2	D28.1	D39.8	D49.59
vaginovesical	C57.9	C79.82	D07.30	D28.9	D39.9	D49.59
septum	C57.9	C79.82	D07.30	D28.9	D39.9	D49.59
vallecula (epiglottis)	C10.0	C79.89	D00.08	D10.5	D37.05	D49.0
vas deferens	C63.1-	C79.82	D07.69	D29.8	D40.8	D49.59
vascular — see Neoplasm, connective tissue						

	Malignant Primary	Malignant Secondary	Ca in situ	Benign	Uncertain Behavior	Unspecified Behavior
Vater's ampulla	C24.1	C78.89	D01.5	D13.5	D37.6	D49.0
vein, venous — see Neoplasm, connective tissue						
vena cava (abdominal) (inferior)	C49.4	C79.89	—	D21.4	D48.1	D49.2
superior	C49.3	C79.89	—	D21.3	D48.1	D49.2
ventricle (cerebral) (floor) (lateral) (third)	C71.5	C79.31	—	D33.0	D43.0	D49.6
cardiac (left) (right)	C38.0	C79.89	—	D15.1	D48.7	D49.89
fourth	C71.7	C79.31	—	D33.1	D43.1	D49.6
ventricular band of larynx	C32.1	C78.39	D02.0	D14.1	D38.0	D49.1
ventriculus — see Neoplasm, stomach						
vermillion border — see Neoplasm, lip						
vermis, cerebellum	C71.6	C79.31	—	D33.1	D43.1	D49.6
vertebra (column)	C41.2	C79.51	—	D16.6	D48.0	D49.2
coccyx	C41.4	C79.51	—	D16.8-	D48.0	D49.2
marrow NEC	C96.9	C79.52	—	D47.9		D49.89
sacrum	C41.4	C79.51	—	D16.8-	D48.0	D49.2
vesical — see Neoplasm, bladder						
vesicle, seminal	C63.7	C79.82	D07.69	D29.8	D40.8	D49.59
vesicocervical tissue	C57.9	C79.82	D07.30	D28.9	D39.9	D49.59
vesicorectal	C76.3	C79.82	D09.8	D36.7	D48.7	D49.89
vesicovaginal	C57.9	C79.82	D07.30	D28.9	D39.9	D49.59
septum	C57.9	C79.82	D07.30	D28.9	D39.8	D49.59
vessel (blood) — see Neoplasm, connective tissue						
vestibular gland, greater	C51.0	C79.82	D07.1	D28.0	D39.8	D49.59
vestibule						
mouth	C06.1	C79.89	D00.00	D10.39	D37.09	D49.0
nose	C30.0	C78.39	D02.3	D14.0	D38.5	D49.1
Virchow's gland	C77.0	C77.0	—	D36.0	D48.7	D49.89
viscera NEC	C76.8	C79.89	D09.8	D36.7	D48.7	D49.89
vocal cords (true)	C32.0	C78.39	D02.0	D14.1	D38.0	D49.1
false	C32.1	C78.39	D02.0	D14.1	D38.0	D49.1
vomer	C41.0	C79.51	—	D16.4-	D48.0	D49.2
vulva	C51.9	C79.82	D07.1	D28.0	D39.8	D49.59
vulvovaginal gland	C51.0	C79.82	D07.1	D28.0	D39.8	D49.59
Waldeyer's ring	C14.2	C79.89	D00.08	D10.9	D37.05	D49.0
Wharton's duct	C08.0	C79.89	D00.00	D11.7	D37.032	D49.0
white matter (central) (cerebral)	C71.0	C79.31	—	D33.0	D43.0	D49.6
windpipe	C33	C78.39	D02.1	D14.2	D38.1	D49.1

TABLE OF NEOPLASMS

	Malignant Primary	Malignant Secondary	Ca in situ	Benign	Uncertain Behavior	Unspecified Behavior
Wirsung's duct	C25.3	C78.89	D01.7	D13.6	D37.8	D49.0
wolffian (body) (duct)						
female	C57.7	C79.82	D07.39	D28.7	D39.8	D49.59
male	C63.7	C79.82	D07.69	D29.8	D40.8	D49.59

	Malignant Primary	Malignant Secondary	Ca in situ	Benign	Uncertain Behavior	Unspecified Behavior
womb — *see Neoplasm, uterus*						
wrist NEC	C76.4-	C79.89	D04.6-	D36.7	D48.7	D49.89
xiphoid process	C41.3	C79.51	—	D16.7	D48.0	D49.2
Zuckerkandl organ	C75.5	C79.89	—	D35.6	D44.7	D49.7

TABLE OF NEOPLASMS

◀ New ◀▦ Revised ~~deleted~~ Deleted

ICD-10-CM
Table of Drugs and Chemicals

Substance	Poisoning, Accidental (Unintentional)	Poisoning, Intentional Self-Harm	Poisoning, Assault	Poisoning, Undetermined	Adverse Effect	Underdosing
#						
1-propanol	T51.3X1	T51.3X2	T51.3X3	T51.3X4	—	—
2-propanol	T51.2X1	T51.2X2	T51.2X3	T51.2X4	—	—
2,4-D (dichlorophen-oxyacetic acid)	T60.3X1	T60.3X2	T60.3X3	T60.3X4	—	—
2,4-toluene diisocyanate	T65.0X1	T65.0X2	T65.0X3	T65.0X4		
2,4,5-T (trichloro-phenoxyacetic acid)	T60.1X1	T60.1X2	T60.1X3	T60.1X4		
14-hydroxydihydro-morphinone	T40.2X1	T40.2X2	T40.2X3	T40.2X4	T40.2X5	T40.2X6
A						
ABOB	T37.5X1	T37.5X2	T37.5X3	T37.5X4	T37.5X5	T37.5X6
Abrine	T62.2X1	T62.2X2	T62.2X3	T62.2X4	—	—
Abrus (seed)	T62.2X1	T62.2X2	T62.2X3	T62.2X4	—	—
Absinthe	T51.0X1	T51.0X2	T51.0X3	T51.0X4	—	—
beverage	T51.0X1	T51.0X2	T51.0X3	T51.0X4	—	—
Acaricide	T60.8X1	T60.8X2	T60.8X3	T60.8X4	—	—
Acebutolol	T44.7X1	T44.7X2	T44.7X3	T44.7X4	T44.7X5	T44.7X6
Acecarbromal	T42.6X1	T42.6X2	T42.6X3	T42.6X4	T42.6X5	T42.6X6
Aceclidine	T44.1X1	T44.1X2	T44.1X3	T44.1X4	T44.1X5	T44.1X6
Acedapsone	T37.0X1	T37.0X2	T37.0X3	T37.0X4	T37.0X5	T37.0X6
Acefylline piperazine	T48.6X1	T48.6X2	T48.6X3	T48.6X4	T48.6X5	T48.6X6
Acemorphan	T40.2X1	T40.2X2	T40.2X3	T40.2X4	T40.2X5	T40.2X6
Acenocoumarin	T45.511	T45.512	T45.513	T45.514	T45.515	T45.516
Acenocoumarol	T45.511	T45.512	T45.513	T45.514	T45.515	T45.516
Acepifylline	T48.6X1	T48.6X2	T48.6X3	T48.6X4	T48.6X5	T48.6X6
Acepromazine	T43.3X1	T43.3X2	T43.3X3	T43.3X4	T43.3X5	T43.3X6
Acesulfamethoxypyridazine	T37.0X1	T37.0X2	T37.0X3	T37.0X4	T37.0X5	T37.0X6
Acetal	T52.8X1	T52.8X2	T52.8X3	T52.8X4	—	—
Acetaldehyde (vapor)	T52.8X1	T52.8X2	T52.8X3	T52.8X4	—	—
liquid	T65.891	T65.892	T65.893	T65.894	—	—
P-Acetamidophenol	T39.1X1	T39.1X2	T39.1X3	T39.1X4	T39.1X5	T39.1X6
Acetaminophen	T39.1X1	T39.1X2	T39.1X3	T39.1X4	T39.1X5	T39.1X6
Acetaminosalol	T39.1X1	T39.1X2	T39.1X3	T39.1X4	T39.1X5	T39.1X6
Acetanilide	T39.1X1	T39.1X2	T39.1X3	T39.1X4	T39.1X5	T39.1X6
Acetarsol	T37.3X1	T37.3X2	T37.3X3	T37.3X4	T37.3X5	T37.3X6
Acetazolamide	T50.2X1	T50.2X2	T50.2X3	T50.2X4	T50.2X5	T50.2X6
Acetiamine	T45.2X1	T45.2X2	T45.2X3	T45.2X4	T45.2X5	T45.2X6
Acetic						
acid	T54.2X1	T54.2X2	T54.2X3	T54.2X4		
with sodium acetate (ointment)	T49.3X1	T49.3X2	T49.3X3	T49.3X4	T49.3X5	T49.3X6

Substance	Poisoning, Accidental (Unintentional)	Poisoning, Intentional Self-Harm	Poisoning, Assault	Poisoning, Undetermined	Adverse Effect	Underdosing
Acetic *(Continued)*						
acid *(Continued)*						
ester (solvent) (vapor)	T52.8X1	T52.8X2	T52.8X3	T52.8X4	—	—
irrigating solution	T50.3X1	T50.3X2	T50.3X3	T50.3X4	T50.3X5	T50.3X6
medicinal (lotion)	T49.2X1	T49.2X2	T49.2X3	T49.2X4	T49.2X5	T49.2X6
anhydride	T65.891	T65.892	T65.893	T65.894		
ether (vapor)	T52.8X1	T52.8X2	T52.8X3	T52.8X4	—	—
Acetohexamide	T38.3X1	T38.3X2	T38.3X3	T38.3X4	T38.3X5	T38.3X6
Acetohydroxamic acid	T50.991	T50.992	T50.993	T50.994	T50.995	T50.996
Acetomenaphthone	T45.7X1	T45.7X2	T45.7X3	T45.7X4	T45.7X5	T45.7X6
Acetomorphine	T40.1X1	T40.1X2	T40.1X3	T40.1X4	—	—
Acetone (oils)	T52.4X1	T52.4X2	T52.4X3	T52.4X4	—	—
chlorinated	T52.4X1	T52.4X2	T52.4X3	T52.4X4	—	—
vapor	T52.4X1	T52.4X2	T52.4X3	T52.4X4	—	—
Acetonitrile	T52.8X1	T52.8X2	T52.8X3	T52.8X4	—	—
Acetophenazine	T43.3X1	T43.3X2	T43.3X3	T43.3X4	T43.3X5	T43.3X6
Acetophenetedin	T39.1X1	T39.1X2	T39.1X3	T39.1X4	T39.1X5	T39.1X6
Acetophenone	T52.4X1	T52.4X2	T52.4X3	T52.4X4	—	—
Acetorphine	T40.2X1	T40.2X2	T40.2X3	T40.2X4	—	—
Acetosulfone (sodium)	T37.1X1	T37.1X2	T37.1X3	T37.1X4	T37.1X5	T37.1X6
Acetrizoate (sodium)	T50.8X1	T50.8X2	T50.8X3	T50.8X4	T50.8X5	T50.8X6
Acetylcarbromal	T42.6X1	T42.6X2	T42.6X3	T42.6X4	T42.6X5	T42.6X6
Acetrizoic acid	T50.8X1	T50.8X2	T50.8X3	T50.8X4	T50.8X5	T50.8X6
Acetyl						
bromide	T53.6X1	T53.6X2	T53.6X3	T53.6X4	—	—
chloride	T53.6X1	T53.6X2	T53.6X3	T53.6X4	—	—
Acetylcholine						
chloride	T44.1X1	T44.1X2	T44.1X3	T44.1X4	T44.1X5	T44.1X6
derivative	T44.1X1	T44.1X2	T44.1X3	T44.1X4	T44.1X5	T44.1X6
Acetylcysteine	T48.4X1	T48.4X2	T48.4X3	T48.4X4	T48.4X5	T48.4X6
Acetyldigitoxin	T46.0X1	T46.0X2	T46.0X3	T46.0X4	T46.0X5	T46.0X6
Acetyldigoxin	T46.0X1	T46.0X2	T46.0X3	T46.0X4	T46.0X5	T46.0X6
Acetyldihydrocodeine	T40.2X1	T40.2X2	T40.2X3	T40.2X4	—	—
Acetyldihydrocodeinone	T40.2X1	T40.2X2	T40.2X3	T40.2X4	—	—
Acetylene (gas)	T59.891	T59.892	T59.893	T59.894	—	—
dichloride	T53.6X1	T53.6X2	T53.6X3	T53.6X4	—	—
incomplete combustion of	T58.11	T58.12	T58.13	T58.14		
industrial	T59.891	T59.892	T59.893	T59.894		
tetrachloride	T53.6X1	T53.6X2	T53.6X3	T53.6X4	—	—
vapor	T53.6X1	T53.6X2	T53.6X3	T53.6X4	—	—
Acetylphenylhydrazine	T39.8X1	T39.8X2	T39.8X3	T39.8X4	T39.8X5	T39.8X6
Acetylpheneturide	T42.6X1	T42.6X2	T42.6X3	T42.6X4	T42.6X5	T42.6X6

◀ New   ◀ Revised   ~~deleted~~ Deleted

Substance	External Cause (T-Code) Poisoning, Accidental (Unintentional)	Poisoning, Intentional Self-Harm	Poisoning, Assault	Poisoning, Undetermined	Adverse Effect	Underdosing
Acetylsalicylic acid (salts)	T39.0X1	T39.0X2	T39.0X3	T39.0X4	T39.0X5	T39.0X6
enteric coated	T39.0X1	T39.0X2	T39.0X3	T39.0X4	T39.0X5	T39.0X6
Acetylsulfamethoxypyridazine	T37.0X1	T37.0X2	T37.0X3	T37.0X4	T37.0X5	T37.0X6
Achromycin	T36.4X1	T36.4X2	T36.4X3	T36.4X4	T36.4X5	T36.4X6
ophthalmic preparation	T49.5X1	T49.5X2	T49.5X3	T49.5X4	T49.5X5	T49.5X6
topical NEC	T49.0X1	T49.0X2	T49.0X3	T49.0X4	T49.0X5	T49.0X6
Aciclovir	T37.5X1	T37.5X2	T37.5X3	T37.5X4	T37.5X5	T37.5X6
Acid (corrosive) NEC	T54.2X1	T54.2X2	T54.2X3	T54.2X4	—	—
Acidifying agent NEC	T50.901	T50.902	T50.903	T50.904	T50.905	T50.906
Acipimox	T46.6X1	T46.6X2	T46.6X3	T46.6X4	T46.6X5	T46.6X6
Acitretin	T50.991	T50.992	T50.993	T50.994	T50.995	T50.996
Aclarubicin	T45.1X1	T45.1X2	T45.1X3	T45.1X4	T45.1X5	T45.1X6
Aclatonium napadisilate	T48.1X1	T48.1X2	T48.1X3	T48.1X4	T48.1X5	T48.1X6
Aconite (wild)	T46.991	T46.992	T46.993	T46.994	T46.995	T46.996
Aconitine	T46.991	T46.992	T46.993	T46.994	T46.995	T46.996
Aconitum ferox	T46.991	T46.992	T46.993	T46.994	T46.995	T46.996
Acridine	T65.6X1	T65.6X2	T65.6X3	T65.6X4	—	—
vapor	T59.891	T59.892	T59.893	T59.894	—	—
Acriflavine	T37.91	T37.92	T37.93	T37.94	T37.95	T37.96
Acriflavinium chloride	T49.0X1	T49.0X2	T49.0X3	T49.0X4	T49.0X5	T49.0X6
Acrinol	T49.0X1	T49.0X2	T49.0X3	T49.0X4	T49.0X5	T49.0X6
Acrisorcin	T49.0X1	T49.0X2	T49.0X3	T49.0X4	T49.0X5	T49.0X6
Acrivastine	T45.0X1	T45.0X2	T45.0X3	T45.0X4	T45.0X5	T45.0X6
Acrolein (gas)	T59.891	T59.892	T59.893	T59.894	—	—
liquid	T54.1X1	T54.1X2	T54.1X3	T54.1X4	—	—
Acrylamide	T65.891	T65.892	T65.893	T65.894	—	—
Acrylic resin	T49.3X1	T49.3X2	T49.3X3	T49.3X4	T49.3X5	T49.3X6
Acrylonitrile	T65.891	T65.892	T65.893	T65.894	—	—
Actaea spicata	T62.2X1	T62.2X2	T62.2X3	T62.2X4	—	—
berry	T62.1X1	T62.1X2	T62.1X3	T62.1X4	—	—
Acterol	T37.3X1	T37.3X2	T37.3X3	T37.3X4	T37.3X5	T37.3X6
ACTH	T38.811	T38.812	T38.813	T38.814	T38.815	T38.816
Actinomycin C	T45.1X1	T45.1X2	T45.1X3	T45.1X4	T45.1X5	T45.1X6
Actinomycin D	T45.1X1	T45.1X2	T45.1X3	T45.1X4	T45.1X5	T45.1X6
Activated charcoal—see also Charcoal, medicinal	T47.6X1	T47.6X2	T47.6X3	T47.6X4	T47.6X5	T47.6X6
Acyclovir	T37.5X1	T37.5X2	T37.5X3	T37.5X4	T37.5X5	T37.5X6
Adenine	T45.2X1	T45.2X2	T45.2X3	T45.2X4	T45.2X5	T45.2X6
arabinoside	T37.5X1	T37.5X2	T37.5X3	T37.5X4	T37.5X5	T37.5X6
Adenosine (phosphate)	T46.2X1	T46.2X2	T46.2X3	T46.2X4	T46.2X5	T46.2X6
ADH	T38.891	T38.892	T38.893	T38.894	T38.895	T38.896
Adhesive NEC	T65.891	T65.892	T65.893	T65.894	—	—

Substance	External Cause (T-Code) Poisoning, Accidental (Unintentional)	Poisoning, Intentional Self-Harm	Poisoning, Assault	Poisoning, Undetermined	Adverse Effect	Underdosing
Adicillin	T36.0X1	T36.0X2	T36.0X3	T36.0X4	T36.0X5	T36.0X6
Adiphenine	T44.3X1	T44.3X2	T44.3X3	T44.3X4	T44.3X5	T44.3X6
Adipiodone	T50.8X1	T50.8X2	T50.8X3	T50.8X4	T50.8X5	T50.8X6
Adjunct, pharmaceutical	T50.901	T50.902	T50.903	T50.904	T50.905	T50.906
Adrenal (extract, cortex or medulla) (glucocorticoids) (hormones) (mineralo corticoids)	T38.0X1	T38.0X2	T38.0X3	T38.0X4	T38.0X5	T38.0X6
ENT agent	T49.6X1	T49.6X2	T49.6X3	T49.6X4	T49.6X5	T49.6X6
ophthalmic preparation	T49.5X1	T49.5X2	T49.5X3	T49.5X4	T49.5X5	T49.5X6
topical NEC	T49.0X1	T49.0X2	T49.0X3	T49.0X4	T49.0X5	T49.0X6
Adrenaline	T44.5X1	T44.5X2	T44.5X3	T44.5X4	T44.5X5	T44.5X6
Adrenalin—see Adrenaline						
Adrenergic NEC	T44.901	T44.902	T44.903	T44.904	T44.905	T44.906
blocking agent NEC	T44.8X1	T44.8X2	T44.8X3	T44.8X4	T44.8X5	T44.8X6
beta, heart	T44.7X1	T44.7X2	T44.7X3	T44.7X4	T44.7X5	T44.7X6
specified NEC	T44.991	T44.992	T44.993	T44.994	T44.995	T44.996
Adrenochrome						
(mono) semicarbazone	T46.991	T46.992	T46.993	T46.994	T46.995	T46.996
derivative	T46.991	T46.992	T46.993	T46.994	T46.995	T46.996
Adrenocorticotrophic hormone	T38.811	T38.812	T38.813	T38.814	T38.815	T38.816
Adrenocorticotrophin	T38.811	T38.812	T38.813	T38.814	T38.815	T38.816
Adriamycin	T45.1X1	T45.1X2	T45.1X3	T45.1X4	T45.1X5	T45.1X6
Aerosol spray NEC	T65.91	T65.92	T65.93	T65.94	—	—
Aerosporin	T36.8X1	T36.8X2	T36.8X3	T36.8X4	T36.8X5	T36.8X6
ENT agent	T49.6X1	T49.6X2	T49.6X3	T49.6X4	T49.6X5	T49.6X6
ophthalmic preparation	T49.5X1	T49.5X2	T49.5X3	T49.5X4	T49.5X5	T49.5X6
topical NEC	T49.0X1	T49.0X2	T49.0X3	T49.0X4	T49.0X5	T49.0X6
Aethusa cynapium	T62.2X1	T62.2X2	T62.2X3	T62.2X4	—	—
Afghanistan black	T40.7X1	T40.7X2	T40.7X3	T40.7X4	T40.7X5	T40.7X6
Aflatoxin	T64.01	T64.02	T64.03	T64.04	—	—
Afloqualone	T42.8X1	T42.8X2	T42.8X3	T42.8X4	T42.8X5	T42.8X6
African boxwood	T62.2X1	T62.2X2	T62.2X3	T62.2X4	—	—
Agar	T47.4X1	T47.4X2	T47.4X3	T47.4X4	T47.4X5	T47.4X6
Agonist						
predominantly						
alpha-adrenoreceptor	T44.4X1	T44.4X2	T44.4X3	T44.4X4	T44.4X5	T44.4X6
beta-adrenoreceptor	T44.5X1	T44.5X2	T44.5X3	T44.5X4	T44.5X5	T44.5X6
Agricultural agent NEC	T65.91	T65.92	T65.93	T65.94	—	—
Agrypnal	T42.3X1	T42.3X2	T42.3X3	T42.3X4	T42.3X5	T42.3X6
AHLG	T50.Z11	T50.Z12	T50.Z13	T50.Z14	T50.Z15	T50.Z16
Air contaminant(s), source/type NOS	T65.91	T65.92	T65.93	T65.94	—	—

◀ New ◀⫶⫶ Revised ~~deleted~~ Deleted

Substance	Poisoning, Accidental (Unintentional)	Poisoning, Intentional Self-Harm	Poisoning, Assault	Poisoning, Undetermined	Adverse Effect	Underdosing
Ajmaline	T46.2X1	T46.2X2	T46.2X3	T46.2X4	T46.2X5	T46.2X6
Akritoin	T37.8X1	T37.8X2	T37.8X3	T37.8X4	T37.8X5	T37.8X6
Akee	T62.1X1	T62.1X2	T62.1X3	T62.1X4	—	—
Akrinol	T49.0X1	T49.0X2	T49.0X3	T49.0X4	T49.0X5	T49.0X6
Alacepril	T46.4X1	T46.4X2	T46.4X3	T46.4X4	T46.4X5	T46.4X6
Alantolactone	T37.4X1	T37.4X2	T37.4X3	T37.4X4	T37.4X5	T37.4X6
Albamycin	T36.8X1	T36.8X2	T36.8X3	T36.8X4	T36.8X5	T36.8X6
Albendazole	T37.4X1	T37.4X2	T37.4X3	T37.4X4	T37.4X5	T37.4X6
Albumin						
bovine	T45.8X1	T45.8X2	T45.8X3	T45.8X4	T45.8X5	T45.8X6
human serum	T45.8X1	T45.8X2	T45.8X3	T45.8X4	T45.8X5	T45.8X6
salt-poor	T45.8X1	T45.8X2	T45.8X3	T45.8X4	T45.8X5	T45.8X6
normal human serum	T45.8X1	T45.8X2	T45.8X3	T45.8X4	T45.8X5	T45.8X6
Albuterol	T48.6X1	T48.6X2	T48.6X3	T48.6X4	T48.6X5	T48.6X6
Albutoin	T42.0X1	T42.0X2	T42.0X3	T42.0X4	T42.0X5	T42.0X6
Alclometasone	T49.0X1	T49.0X2	T49.0X3	T49.0X4	T49.0X5	T49.0X6
Alcohol	T51.91	T51.92	T51.93	T51.94	—	—
absolute	T51.0X1	T51.0X2	T51.0X3	T51.0X4	—	—
beverage	T51.0X1	T51.0X2	T51.0X3	T51.0X4	—	—
allyl	T51.8X1	T51.8X2	T51.8X3	T51.8X4	—	—
amyl	T51.3X1	T51.3X2	T51.3X3	T51.3X4	—	—
antifreeze	T51.1X1	T51.1X2	T51.1X3	T51.1X4	—	—
beverage	T51.0X1	T51.0X2	T51.0X3	T51.0X4	—	—
butyl	T51.3X1	T51.3X2	T51.3X3	T51.3X4	—	—
dehydrated	T51.0X1	T51.0X2	T51.0X3	T51.0X4	—	—
beverage	T51.0X1	T51.0X2	T51.0X3	T51.0X4	—	—
denatured	T51.0X1	T51.0X2	T51.0X3	T51.0X4	—	—
deterrent NEC	T50.6X1	T50.6X2	T50.6X3	T50.6X4	T50.6X5	T50.6X6
diagnostic (gastric function)	T50.8X1	T50.8X2	T50.8X3	T50.8X4	T50.8X5	T50.8X6
ethyl	T51.0X1	T51.0X2	T51.0X3	T51.0X4	—	—
beverage	T51.0X1	T51.0X2	T51.0X3	T51.0X4	—	—
grain	T51.0X1	T51.0X2	T51.0X3	T51.0X4	—	—
beverage	T51.0X1	T51.0X2	T51.0X3	T51.0X4	—	—
industrial	T51.0X1	T51.0X2	T51.0X3	T51.0X4	—	—
isopropyl	T51.2X1	T51.2X2	T51.2X3	T51.2X4	—	—
methyl	T51.1X1	T51.1X2	T51.1X3	T51.1X4	—	—
preparation for consumption	T51.0X1	T51.0X2	T51.0X3	T51.0X4	—	—
propyl	T51.3X1	T51.3X2	T51.3X3	T51.3X4	—	—
secondary	T51.2X1	T51.2X2	T51.2X3	T51.2X4	—	—
radiator	T51.1X1	T51.1X2	T51.1X3	T51.1X4	—	—
rubbing	T51.2X1	T51.2X2	T51.2X3	T51.2X4	—	—
specified type NEC	T51.8X1	T51.8X2	T51.8X3	T51.8X4	—	—

Substance	Poisoning, Accidental (Unintentional)	Poisoning, Intentional Self-Harm	Poisoning, Assault	Poisoning, Undetermined	Adverse Effect	Underdosing
Alcohol *(Continued)*						
surgical	T51.0X1	T51.0X2	T51.0X3	T51.0X4	—	—
vapor (from any type of Alcohol)	T59.891	T59.892	T59.893	T59.894	—	—
wood	T51.1X1	T51.1X2	T51.1X3	T51.1X4	—	—
Alcuronium (chloride)	T48.1X1	T48.1X2	T48.1X3	T48.1X4	T48.1X5	T48.1X6
Aldactone	T50.0X1	T50.0X2	T50.0X3	T50.0X4	T50.0X5	T50.0X6
Aldesulfone sodium	T37.1X1	T37.1X2	T37.1X3	T37.1X4	T37.1X5	T37.1X6
Aldicarb	T60.0X1	T60.0X2	T60.0X3	T60.0X4	—	—
Aldomet	T46.5X1	T46.5X2	T46.5X3	T46.5X4	T46.5X5	T46.5X6
Aldosterone	T50.0X1	T50.0X2	T50.0X3	T50.0X4	T50.0X5	T50.0X6
Aldrin (dust)	T60.1X1	T60.1X2	T60.1X3	T60.1X4	—	—
Aleve — *see Naproxen*						
Alexitol sodium	T47.1X1	T47.1X2	T47.1X3	T47.1X4	T47.1X5	T47.1X6
Alfacalcidol	T45.2X1	T45.2X2	T45.2X3	T45.2X4	T45.2X5	T45.2X6
Alfadolone	T41.1X1	T41.1X2	T41.1X3	T41.1X4	T41.1X5	T41.1X6
Alfaxalone	T41.1X1	T41.1X2	T41.1X3	T41.1X4	T41.1X5	T41.1X6
Alfentanil	T40.4X1	T40.4X2	T40.4X3	T40.4X4	T40.4X5	T40.4X6
Alfuzosin (hydrochloride)	T44.8X1	T44.8X2	T44.8X3	T44.8X4	T44.8X5	T44.8X6
Algae (harmful) (toxin)	T65.821	T65.822	T65.823	T65.824	—	—
Algeldrate	T47.1X1	T47.1X2	T47.1X3	T47.1X4	T47.1X5	T47.1X6
Algin	T47.8X1	T47.8X2	T47.8X3	T47.8X4	T47.8X5	T47.8X6
Alglucerase	T45.3X1	T45.3X2	T45.3X3	T45.3X4	T45.3X5	T45.3X6
Alidase	T45.3X1	T45.3X2	T45.3X3	T45.3X4	T45.3X5	T45.3X6
Alimemazine	T43.3X1	T43.3X2	T43.3X3	T43.3X4	T43.3X5	T43.3X6
Aliphatic thiocyanates	T65.0X1	T65.0X2	T65.0X3	T65.0X4	—	—
Alizapride	T45.0X1	T45.0X2	T45.0X3	T45.0X4	T45.0X5	T45.0X6
Alkali (caustic)	T54.3X1	T54.3X2	T54.3X3	T54.3X4	—	—
Alkalizing agent NEC	T50.901	T50.902	T50.903	T50.904	T50.905	T50.906
Alkaline antiseptic solution (aromatic)	T49.6X1	T49.6X2	T49.6X3	T49.6X4	T49.6X5	T49.6X6
Alkalinizing agents (medicinal)	T50.901	T50.902	T50.903	T50.904	T50.905	T50.906
Alka-seltzer	T39.011	T39.012	T39.013	T39.014	T39.015	T39.016
Alkavervir	T46.5X1	T46.5X2	T46.5X3	T46.5X4	T46.5X5	T46.5X6
Alkonium (bromide)	T49.0X1	T49.0X2	T49.0X3	T49.0X4	T49.0X5	T49.0X6
Alkylating drug NEC	T45.1X1	T45.1X2	T45.1X3	T45.1X4	T45.1X5	T45.1X6
antimyeloproliferative	T45.1X1	T45.1X2	T45.1X3	T45.1X4	T45.1X5	T45.1X6
lymphatic	T45.1X1	T45.1X2	T45.1X3	T45.1X4	T45.1X5	T45.1X6
Alkylisocyanate	T65.0X1	T65.0X2	T65.0X3	T65.0X4	—	—
Allantoin	T49.411	T49.412	T49.413	T49.414	T49.415	T49.416
Allegron	T43.0X1	T43.0X2	T43.0X3	T43.0X4	T43.0X5	T43.0X6
Allethrin	T49.0X1	T49.0X2	T49.0X3	T49.0X4	T49.0X5	T49.0X6
Allobarbital	T42.3X1	T42.3X2	T42.3X3	T42.3X4	T42.3X5	T42.3X6

TABLE OF DRUGS AND CHEMICALS

Substance	Poisoning, Accidental (Unintentional)	Poisoning, Intentional Self-Harm	Poisoning, Assault	Poisoning, Undetermined	Adverse Effect	Underdosing
Allopurinol	T50.4X1	T50.4X2	T50.4X3	T50.4X4	T50.4X5	T50.4X6
Allyl						
alcohol	T51.8X1	T51.8X2	T51.8X3	T51.8X4	—	—
disulfide	T46.6X1	T46.6X2	T46.6X3	T46.6X4	T46.6X5	T46.6X6
Allylestrenol	T38.5X1	T38.5X2	T38.5X3	T38.5X4	T38.5X5	T38.5X6
Allylisopropylacetylurea	T42.6X1	T42.6X2	T42.6X3	T42.6X4	T42.6X5	T42.6X6
Allylisopropylmalonylurea	T42.3X1	T42.3X2	T42.3X3	T42.3X4	T42.3X5	T42.3X6
Allylthiourea	T49.3X1	T49.3X2	T49.3X3	T49.3X4	T49.3X5	T49.3X6
Allyltribromide	T42.6X1	T42.6X2	T42.6X3	T42.6X4	T42.6X5	T42.6X6
Allypropymal	T42.3X1	T42.3X2	T42.3X3	T42.3X4	T42.3X5	T42.3X6
Almagate	T47.1X1	T47.1X2	T47.1X3	T47.1X4	T47.1X5	T47.1X6
Almasilate	T47.1X1	T47.1X2	T47.1X3	T47.1X4	T47.1X5	T47.1X6
Almitrine	T50.7X1	T50.7X2	T50.7X3	T50.7X4	T50.7X5	T50.7X6
Aloes	T47.2X1	T47.2X2	T47.2X3	T47.2X4	T47.2X5	T47.2X6
Aloglutamol	T47.1X1	T47.1X2	T47.1X3	T47.1X4	T47.1X5	T47.1X6
Aloin	T47.2X1	T47.2X2	T47.2X3	T47.2X4	T47.2X5	T47.2X6
Aloxidone	T42.2X1	T42.2X2	T42.2X3	T42.2X4	T42.2X5	T42.2X6
Alpha						
acetyldigoxin	T46.0X1	T46.0X2	T46.0X3	T46.0X4	T46.0X5	T46.0X6
adrenergic blocking drug	T44.6X1	T44.6X2	T44.6X3	T44.6X4	T44.6X5	T44.6X6
amylase	T45.3X1	T45.3X2	T45.3X3	T45.3X4	T45.3X5	T45.3X6
tocoferol (acetate)	T45.2X1	T45.2X2	T45.2X3	T45.2X4	T45.2X5	T45.2X6
tocopherol	T45.2X1	T45.2X2	T45.2X3	T45.2X4	T45.2X5	T45.2X6
Alphadolone	T41.1X1	T41.1X2	T41.1X3	T41.1X4	T41.1X5	T41.1X6
Alphaprodine	T40.4X1	T40.4X2	T40.4X3	T40.4X4	T40.4X5	T40.4X6
Alphaxalone	T41.1X1	T41.1X2	T41.1X3	T41.1X4	T41.1X5	T41.1X6
Alprazolam	T42.4X1	T42.4X2	T42.4X3	T42.4X4	T42.4X5	T42.4X6
Alprenolol	T44.7X1	T44.7X2	T44.7X3	T44.7X4	T44.7X5	T44.7X6
Alprostadil	T46.7X1	T46.7X2	T46.7X3	T46.7X4	T46.7X5	T46.7X6
Alsactide	T38.811	T38.812	T38.813	T38.814	T38.815	T38.816
Alseroxylon	T46.5X1	T46.5X2	T46.5X3	T46.5X4	T46.5X5	T46.5X6
Alteplase	T45.611	T45.612	T45.613	T45.614	T45.615	T45.616
Altizide	T50.2X1	T50.2X2	T50.2X3	T50.2X4	T50.2X5	T50.2X6
Altretamine	T45.1X1	T45.1X2	T45.1X3	T45.1X4	T45.1X5	T45.1X6
Alum (medicinal)	T49.4X1	T49.4X2	T49.4X3	T49.4X4	T49.4X5	T49.4X6
nonmedicinal (ammonium) (potassium)	T56.891	T56.892	T56.893	T56.894	—	—
Aluminium, aluminum						
acetate	T49.2X1	T49.2X2	T49.2X3	T49.2X4	T49.2X5	T49.2X6
solution	T49.0X1	T49.0X2	T49.0X3	T49.0X4	T49.0X5	T49.0X6
aspirin	T39.011	T39.012	T39.013	T39.014	T39.015	T39.016
bis (acetylsalicylate)	T39.011	T39.012	T39.013	T39.014	T39.015	T39.016

Substance	Poisoning, Accidental (Unintentional)	Poisoning, Intentional Self-Harm	Poisoning, Assault	Poisoning, Undetermined	Adverse Effect	Underdosing
Aluminium, aluminum *(Continued)*						
carbonate (gel, basic)	T47.1X1	T47.1X2	T47.1X3	T47.1X4	T47.1X5	T47.1X6
chlorhydroxide-complex	T47.1X1	T47.1X2	T47.1X3	T47.1X4	T47.1X5	T47.1X6
chloride	T49.2X1	T49.2X2	T49.2X3	T49.2X4	T49.2X5	T49.2X6
clofibrate	T46.6X1	T46.6X2	T46.6X3	T46.6X4	T46.6X5	T46.6X6
diacetate	T49.2X1	T49.2X2	T49.2X3	T49.2X4	T49.2X5	T49.2X6
glycinate	T47.1X1	T47.1X2	T47.1X3	T47.1X4	T47.1X5	T47.1X6
hydroxide (gel)	T47.1X1	T47.1X2	T47.1X3	T47.1X4	T47.1X5	T47.1X6
hydroxide-magnesium carb. gel	T47.1X1	T47.1X2	T47.1X3	T47.1X4	T47.1X5	T47.1X6
magnesium silicate	T47.1X1	T47.1X2	T47.1X3	T47.1X4	T47.1X5	T47.1X6
nicotinate	T46.7X1	T46.7X2	T46.7X3	T46.7X4	T46.7X5	T46.7X6
ointment (surgical) (topical)	T49.3X1	T49.3X2	T49.3X3	T49.3X4	T49.3X5	T49.3X6
phosphate	T47.1X1	T47.1X2	T47.1X3	T47.1X4	T47.1X5	T47.1X6
salicylate	T39.091	T39.092	T39.093	T39.094	T39.095	T39.096
silicate	T47.1X1	T47.1X2	T47.1X3	T47.1X4	T47.1X5	T47.1X6
sodium silicate	T47.1X1	T47.1X2	T47.1X3	T47.1X4	T47.1X5	T47.1X6
subacetate	T49.2X1	T49.2X2	T49.2X3	T49.2X4	T49.2X5	T49.2X6
sulfate	T49.0X1	T49.0X2	T49.0X3	T49.0X4	T49.0X5	T49.0X6
tannate	T47.6X1	T47.6X2	T47.6X3	T47.6X4	T47.6X5	T47.6X6
topical NEC	T49.3X1	T49.3X2	T49.3X3	T49.3X4	T49.3X5	T49.3X6
Alurate	T42.3X1	T42.3X2	T42.3X3	T42.3X4	T42.3X5	T42.3X6
Alverine	T44.3X1	T44.3X2	T44.3X3	T44.3X4	T44.3X5	T44.3X6
Alvodine	T40.2X1	T40.2X2	T40.2X3	T40.2X4	T40.2X5	T40.2X6
Amanita phalloides	T62.0X1	T62.0X2	T62.0X3	T62.0X4	—	—
Amanitine	T62.0X1	T62.0X2	T62.0X3	T62.0X4	—	—
Amantadine	T42.8X1	T42.8X2	T42.8X3	T42.8X4	T42.8X5	T42.8X6
Ambazone	T49.6X1	T49.6X2	T49.6X3	T49.6X4	T49.6X5	T49.6X6
Ambenonium (chloride)	T44.0X1	T44.0X2	T44.0X3	T44.0X4	T44.0X5	T44.0X6
Ambroxol	T48.4X1	T48.4X2	T48.4X3	T48.4X4	T48.4X5	T48.4X6
Ambuphylline	T48.6X1	T48.6X2	T48.6X3	T48.6X4	T48.6X5	T48.6X6
Ambutonium bromide	T44.3X1	T44.3X2	T44.3X3	T44.3X4	T44.3X5	T44.3X6
Amcinonide	T49.0X1	T49.0X2	T49.0X3	T49.0X4	T49.0X5	T49.0X6
Amdinocilline	T36.0X1	T36.0X2	T36.0X3	T36.0X4	T36.0X5	T36.0X6
Ametazole	T50.8X1	T50.8X2	T50.8X3	T50.8X4	T50.8X5	T50.8X6
Amethocaine	T41.3X1	T41.3X2	T41.3X3	T41.3X4	T41.3X5	T41.3X6
regional	T41.3X1	T41.3X2	T41.3X3	T41.3X4	T41.3X5	T41.3X6
spinal	T41.3X1	T41.3X2	T41.3X3	T41.3X4	T41.3X5	T41.3X6
Amethopterin	T45.1X1	T45.1X2	T45.1X3	T45.1X4	T45.1X5	T45.1X6
Amezinium metilsulfate	T44.991	T44.992	T44.993	T44.994	T44.995	T44.996
Amfebutamone	T43.291	T43.292	T43.293	T43.294	T43.295	T43.296
Amfepramone	T50.5X1	T50.5X2	T50.5X3	T50.5X4	T50.5X5	T50.5X6

◄ New   ◄ Revised   ~~deleted~~ Deleted

Substance	External Cause (T-Code) Poisoning, Accidental (Unintentional)	Poisoning, Intentional Self-Harm	Poisoning, Assault	Poisoning, Undetermined	Adverse Effect	Underdosing
Amfetamine	T43.621	T43.622	T43.623	T43.624	T43.625	T43.626
Amfetaminil	T43.621	T43.622	T43.623	T43.624	T43.625	T43.626
Amfomycin	T36.8X1	T36.8X2	T36.8X3	T36.8X4	T36.8X5	T36.8X6
Amidefrine mesilate	T48.5X1	T48.5X2	T48.5X3	T48.5X4	T48.5X5	T48.5X6
Amidone	T40.3X1	T40.3X2	T40.3X3	T40.3X4	T40.3X5	T40.3X6
Amidopyrine	T39.2X1	T39.2X2	T39.2X3	T39.2X4	T39.2X5	T39.2X6
Amidotrizoate	T50.8X1	T50.8X2	T50.8X3	T50.8X4	T50.8X5	T50.8X6
Amiflamine	T43.1X1	T43.1X2	T43.1X3	T43.1X4	T43.1X5	T43.1X6
Amikacin	T36.5X1	T36.5X2	T36.5X3	T36.5X4	T36.5X5	T36.5X6
Amikhelline	T46.3X1	T46.3X2	T46.3X3	T46.3X4	T46.3X5	T46.3X6
Amiloride	T50.2X1	T50.2X2	T50.2X3	T50.2X4	T50.2X5	T50.2X6
Aminacrine	T49.0X1	T49.0X2	T49.0X3	T49.0X4	T49.0X5	T49.0X6
Amineptine	T43.011	T43.012	T43.013	T43.014	T43.015	T43.016
Aminitrozole	T37.3X1	T37.3X2	T37.3X3	T37.3X4	T37.3X5	T37.3X6
Aminoacetic acid (derivatives)	T50.3X1	T50.3X2	T50.3X3	T50.3X4	T50.3X5	T50.3X6
Amino acids	T50.3X1	T50.3X2	T50.3X3	T50.3X4	T50.3X5	T50.3X6
Aminoacridine	T49.0X1	T49.0X2	T49.0X3	T49.0X4	T49.0X5	T49.0X6
Aminobenzoic acid (-p)	T49.3X1	T49.3X2	T49.3X3	T49.3X4	T49.3X5	T49.3X6
4-Aminobutyric acid	T43.8X1	T43.8X2	T43.8X3	T43.8X4	T43.8X5	T43.8X6
Aminocaproic acid	T45.621	T45.622	T45.623	T45.624	T45.625	T45.626
Aminofenazone	T39.2X1	T39.2X2	T39.2X3	T39.2X4	T39.2X5	T39.2X6
Aminoethylisothiourium	T45.8X1	T45.8X2	T45.8X3	T45.8X4	T45.8X5	T45.8X6
Aminoglutethimide	T45.1X1	T45.1X2	T45.1X3	T45.1X4	T45.1X5	T45.1X6
Aminohippuric acid	T50.8X1	T50.8X2	T50.8X3	T50.8X4	T50.8X5	T50.8X6
Aminomethylbenzoic acid	T45.691	T45.692	T45.693	T45.694	T45.695	T45.696
Aminometradine	T50.2X1	T50.2X2	T50.2X3	T50.2X4	T50.2X5	T50.2X6
Aminopentamide	T44.3X1	T44.3X2	T44.3X3	T44.3X4	T44.3X5	T44.3X6
Aminophenazone	T39.2X1	T39.2X2	T39.2X3	T39.2X4	T39.2X5	T39.2X6
Aminophenol	T54.0X1	T54.0X2	T54.0X3	T54.0X4	—	—
4-Aminophenol derivatives	T39.1X1	T39.1X2	T39.1X3	T39.1X4	T39.1X5	T39.1X6
Aminophenylpyridone	T43.591	T43.592	T43.593	T43.594	T43.595	T43.596
Aminophylline	T48.6X1	T48.6X2	T48.6X3	T48.6X4	T48.6X5	T48.6X6
Aminopterin sodium	T45.1X1	T45.1X2	T45.1X3	T45.1X4	T45.1X5	T45.1X6
Aminopyrine	T39.2X1	T39.2X2	T39.2X3	T39.2X4	T39.2X5	T39.2X6
8-Aminoquinoline drugs	T37.2X1	T37.2X2	T37.2X3	T37.2X4	T37.2X5	T37.2X6
Aminorex	T50.5X1	T50.5X2	T50.5X3	T50.5X4	T50.5X5	T50.5X6
Aminosalicylic acid	T37.1X1	T37.1X2	T37.1X3	T37.1X4	T37.1X5	T37.1X6
Aminosalylum	T37.1X1	T37.1X2	T37.1X3	T37.1X4	T37.1X5	T37.1X6
Amiodarone	T46.2X1	T46.2X2	T46.2X3	T46.2X4	T46.2X5	T46.2X6
Amiphenazole	T50.7X1	T50.7X2	T50.7X3	T50.7X4	T50.7X5	T50.7X6
Amiquinsin	T46.5X1	T46.5X2	T46.5X3	T46.5X4	T46.5X5	T46.5X6
Amisometradine	T50.2X1	T50.2X2	T50.2X3	T50.2X4	T50.2X5	T50.2X6

Substance	External Cause (T-Code) Poisoning, Accidental (Unintentional)	Poisoning, Intentional Self-Harm	Poisoning, Assault	Poisoning, Undetermined	Adverse Effect	Underdosing
Amisulpride	T43.591	T43.592	T43.593	T43.594	T43.595	T43.596
Amitriptyline	T43.021	T43.022	T43.023	T43.024	T43.025	T43.026
Amitriptylinoxide	T43.021	T43.022	T43.023	T43.024	T43.025	T43.026
Amlexanox	T48.6X1	T48.6X2	T48.6X3	T48.6X4	T48.6X5	T48.6X6
Ammonia (fumes) (gas) (vapor)	T59.891	T59.892	T59.893	T59.894	—	—
aromatic spirit	T48.991	T48.992	T48.993	T48.994	T48.995	T48.996
liquid (household)	T54.3X1	T54.3X2	T54.3X3	T54.3X4	—	—
Ammoniated mercury	T49.0X1	T49.0X2	T49.0X3	T49.0X4	T49.0X5	T49.0X6
Ammonium						
acid tartrate	T49.5X1	T49.5X2	T49.5X3	T49.5X4	T49.5X5	T49.5X6
bromide	T42.6X1	T42.6X2	T42.6X3	T42.6X4	T42.6X5	T42.6X6
carbonate	T54.3X1	T54.3X2	T54.3X3	T54.3X4	—	—
chloride	T50.991	T50.992	T50.993	T50.994	T50.995	T50.996
expectorant	T48.4X1	T48.4X2	T48.4X3	T48.4X4	T48.4X5	T48.4X6
compounds (household) NEC	T54.3X1	T54.3X2	T54.3X3	T54.3X4	—	—
fumes (any usage)	T59.891	T59.892	T59.893	T59.894	—	—
industrial	T54.3X1	T54.3X2	T54.3X3	T54.3X4	—	—
ichthyosulronate	T49.4X1	T49.4X2	T49.4X3	T49.4X4	T49.4X5	T49.4X6
mandelate	T37.91	T37.92	T37.93	T37.94	T37.95	T37.96
sulfamate	T60.3X1	T60.3X2	T60.3X3	T60.3X4	—	—
sulfonate resin	T47.8X1	T47.8X2	T47.8X3	T47.8X4	T47.8X5	T47.8X6
Amobarbital (sodium)	T42.3X1	T42.3X2	T42.3X3	T42.3X4	T42.3X5	T42.3X6
Amodiaquine	T37.2X1	T37.2X2	T37.2X3	T37.2X4	T37.2X5	T37.2X6
Amopyroquin(e)	T37.2X1	T37.2X2	T37.2X3	T37.2X4	T37.2X5	T37.2X6
Amoxapine	T43.011	T43.012	T43.013	T43.014	T43.015	T43.016
Amoxicillin	T36.0X1	T36.0X2	T36.0X3	T36.0X4	T36.0X5	T36.0X6
Amperozide	T43.591	T43.592	T43.593	T43.594	T43.595	T43.596
Amphenidone	T43.591	T43.592	T43.593	T43.594	T43.595	T43.596
Amphetamine NEC	T43.621	T43.622	T43.623	T43.624	T43.625	T43.626
Amphomycin	T36.8X1	T36.8X2	T36.8X3	T36.8X4	T36.8X5	T36.8X6
Amphotalide	T37.4X1	T37.4X2	T37.4X3	T37.4X4	T37.4X5	T37.4X6
Amphotericin B	T36.7X1	T36.7X2	T36.7X3	T36.7X4	T36.7X5	T36.7X6
topical	T49.0X1	T49.0X2	T49.0X3	T49.0X4	T49.0X5	T49.0X6
Ampicillin	T36.0X1	T36.0X2	T36.0X3	T36.0X4	T36.0X5	T36.0X6
Amprotropine	T44.3X1	T44.3X2	T44.3X3	T44.3X4	T44.3X5	T44.3X6
Amsacrine	T45.1X1	T45.1X2	T45.1X3	T45.1X4	T45.1X5	T45.1X6
Amygdaline	T62.2X1	T62.2X2	T62.2X3	T62.2X4	—	—
Amyl						
acetate	T52.8X1	T52.8X2	T52.8X3	T52.8X4	—	—
vapor	T59.891	T59.892	T59.893	T59.894	—	—
alcohol	T51.3X1	T51.3X2	T51.3X3	T51.3X4	—	—
chloride	T53.6X1	T53.6X2	T53.6X3	T53.6X4	—	—

◀ New ◀▥ Revised ~~deleted~~ Deleted

TABLE OF DRUGS AND CHEMICALS

TABLE OF DRUGS AND CHEMICALS

Substance	Poisoning, Accidental (Unintentional)	Poisoning, Intentional Self-Harm	Poisoning, Assault	Poisoning, Undetermined	Adverse Effect	Underdosing
External Cause (T-Code)						
Amyl *(Continued)*						
formate	T52.8X1	T52.8X2	T52.8X3	T52.8X4	—	—
nitrite	T46.3X1	T46.3X2	T46.3X3	T46.3X4	T46.3X5	T46.3X6
propionate	T65.891	T65.892	T65.893	T65.894	—	—
Amylase	T47.5X1	T47.5X2	T47.5X3	T47.5X4	T47.5X5	T47.5X6
Amyleine, regional	T41.3X1	T41.3X2	T41.3X3	T41.3X4	T41.3X5	T41.3X6
Amylene						
dichloride	T53.6X1	T53.6X2	T53.6X3	T53.6X4	—	—
hydrate	T51.3X1	T51.3X2	T51.3X3	T51.3X4	—	—
Amylmetacresol	T49.6X1	T49.6X2	T49.6X3	T49.6X4	T49.6X5	T49.6X6
Amylobarbitone	T42.3X1	T42.3X2	T42.3X3	T42.3X4	T42.3X5	T42.3X6
Amylocaine, regional	T41.3X1	T41.3X2	T41.3X3	T41.3X4	T41.3X5	T41.3X6
infiltration (subcutaneous)	T41.3X1	T41.3X2	T41.3X3	T41.3X4	T41.3X5	T41.3X6
nerve block (peripheral) (plexus)	T41.3X1	T41.3X2	T41.3X3	T41.3X4	T41.3X5	T41.3X6
spinal	T41.3X1	T41.3X2	T41.3X3	T41.3X4	T41.3X5	T41.3X6
topical (surface)	T41.3X1	T41.3X2	T41.3X3	T41.3X4	T41.3X5	T41.3X6
Amylopectin	T47.6X1	T47.6X2	T47.6X3	T47.6X4	T47.6X5	T47.6X6
Amytal (sodium)	T42.3X1	T42.3X2	T42.3X3	T42.3X4	T42.3X5	T42.3X6
Anabolic steroid	T38.7X1	T38.7X2	T38.7X3	T38.7X4	T38.7X5	T38.7X6
Analeptic NEC	T50.7X1	T50.7X2	T50.7X3	T50.7X4	T50.7X5	T50.7X6
Analgesic	T39.91	T39.92	T39.93	T39.94	T39.95	T39.96
anti-inflammatory NEC	T39.91	T39.92	T39.93	T39.94	T39.95	T39.96
propionic acid derivative	T39.311	T39.312	T39.313	T39.314	T39.315	T39.316
antirheumatic NEC	T39.4X1	T39.4X2	T39.4X3	T39.4X4	T39.4X5	T39.4X6
aromatic NEC	T39.1X1	T39.1X2	T39.1X3	T39.1X4	T39.1X5	T39.1X6
narcotic NEC	T40.601	T40.602	T40.603	T40.604	T40.605	T40.606
combination	T40.601	T40.602	T40.603	T40.604	T40.605	T40.606
obstetric	T40.601	T40.602	T40.603	T40.604	T40.605	T40.606
non-narcotic NEC	T39.91	T39.92	T39.93	T39.94	T39.95	T39.96
combination	T39.91	T39.92	T39.93	T39.94	T39.95	T39.96
pyrazole	T39.2X1	T39.2X2	T39.2X3	T39.2X4	T39.2X5	T39.2X6
specified NEC	T39.8X1	T39.8X2	T39.8X3	T39.8X4	T39.8X5	T39.8X6
Analgin	T39.2X1	T39.2X2	T39.2X3	T39.2X4	T39.2X5	T39.2X6
Anamirta cocculus	T62.1X1	T62.1X2	T62.1X3	T62.1X4	—	—
Ancillin	T36.0X1	T36.0X2	T36.0X3	T36.0X4	T36.0X5	T36.0X6
Ancrod	T45.691	T45.692	T45.693	T45.694	T45.695	T45.696
Androgen	T38.7X1	T38.7X2	T38.7X3	T38.7X4	T38.7X5	T38.7X6
Androgen-estrogen mixture	T38.7X1	T38.7X2	T38.7X3	T38.7X4	T38.7X5	T38.7X6
Androstalone	T38.7X1	T38.7X2	T38.7X3	T38.7X4	T38.7X5	T38.7X6
Androstanolone	T38.7X1	T38.7X2	T38.7X3	T38.7X4	T38.7X5	T38.7X6
Androsterone	T38.7X1	T38.7X2	T38.7X3	T38.7X4	T38.7X5	T38.7X6

Substance	Poisoning, Accidental (Unintentional)	Poisoning, Intentional Self-Harm	Poisoning, Assault	Poisoning, Undetermined	Adverse Effect	Underdosing
External Cause (T-Code)						
Anemone pulsatilla	T62.2X1	T62.2X2	T62.2X3	T62.2X4	—	—
Anesthesia						
caudal	T41.3X1	T41.3X2	T41.3X3	T41.3X4	T41.3X5	T41.3X6
endotracheal	T41.0X1	T41.0X2	T41.0X3	T41.0X4	T41.0X5	T41.0X6
epidural	T41.3X1	T41.3X2	T41.3X3	T41.3X4	T41.3X5	T41.3X6
inhalation	T41.0X1	T41.0X2	T41.0X3	T41.0X4	T41.0X5	T41.0X6
local	T41.3X1	T41.3X2	T41.3X3	T41.3X4	T41.3X5	T41.3X6
mucosal	T41.3X1	T41.3X2	T41.3X3	T41.3X4	T41.3X5	T41.3X6
muscle relaxation	T48.1X1	T48.1X2	T48.1X3	T48.1X4	T48.1X5	T48.1X6
nerve blocking	T41.3X1	T41.3X2	T41.3X3	T41.3X4	T41.3X5	T41.3X6
plexus blocking	T41.3X1	T41.3X2	T41.3X3	T41.3X4	T41.3X5	T41.3X6
potentiated	T41.201	T41.202	T41.203	T41.204	T41.205	T41.206
rectal	T41.201	T41.202	T41.203	T41.204	T41.205	T41.206
general	T41.201	T41.202	T41.203	T41.204	T41.205	T41.206
local	T41.3X1	T41.3X2	T41.3X3	T41.3X4	T41.3X5	T41.3X6
regional	T41.3X1	T41.3X2	T41.3X3	T41.3X4	T41.3X5	T41.3X6
surface	T41.3X1	T41.3X2	T41.3X3	T41.3X4	T41.3X5	T41.3X6
Anesthetic NEC—*see also Anesthesia*	T41.41	T41.42	T41.43	T41.44	T41.45	T41.46
with muscle relaxant	T41.201	T41.202	T41.203	T41.204	T41.205	T41.206
general	T41.201	T41.202	T41.203	T41.204	T41.205	T41.206
local	T41.3X1	T41.3X2	T41.3X3	T41.3X4	T41.3X5	T41.3X6
gaseous NEC	T41.0X1	T41.0X2	T41.0X3	T41.0X4	T41.0X5	T41.0X6
general NEC	T41.201	T41.202	T41.203	T41.204	T41.205	T41.206
halogenated hydrocarbon derivatives NEC	T41.0X1	T41.0X2	T41.0X3	T41.0X4	T41.0X5	T41.0X6
infiltration NEC	T41.3X1	T41.3X2	T41.3X3	T41.3X4	T41.3X5	T41.3X6
intravenous NEC	T41.1X1	T41.1X2	T41.1X3	T41.1X4	T41.1X5	T41.1X6
local NEC	T41.3X1	T41.3X2	T41.3X3	T41.3X4	T41.3X5	T41.3X6
rectal	T41.201	T41.202	T41.203	T41.204	T41.205	T41.206
general	T41.201	T41.202	T41.203	T41.204	T41.205	T41.206
local	T41.3X1	T41.3X2	T41.3X3	T41.3X4	T41.3X5	T41.3X6
regional NEC	T41.3X1	T41.3X2	T41.3X3	T41.3X4	T41.3X5	T41.3X6
spinal NEC	T41.3X1	T41.3X2	T41.3X3	T41.3X4	T41.3X5	T41.3X6
thiobarbiturate	T41.1X1	T41.1X2	T41.1X3	T41.1X4	T41.1X5	T41.1X6
topical	T41.3X1	T41.3X2	T41.3X3	T41.3X4	T41.3X5	T41.3X6
Aneurine	T45.2X1	T45.2X2	T45.2X3	T45.2X4	T45.2X5	T45.2X6
Angio-Conray	T50.8X1	T50.8X2	T50.8X3	T50.8X4	T50.8X5	T50.8X6
Angiotensin	T44.5X1	T44.5X2	T44.5X3	T44.5X4	T44.5X5	T44.5X6
Angiotensinamide	T44.991	T44.992	T44.993	T44.994	T44.995	T44.996
Anhydrohydroxy-progesterone	T38.5X1	T38.5X2	T38.5X3	T38.5X4	T38.5X5	T38.5X6
Anhydron	T50.2X1	T50.2X2	T50.2X3	T50.2X4	T50.2X5	T50.2X6
Anileridine	T40.4X1	T40.4X2	T40.4X3	T40.4X4	T40.4X5	T40.4X6

◀ New ⬅ Revised ~~deleted~~ Deleted

Substance	External Cause (T-Code) Poisoning, Accidental (Unintentional)	Poisoning, Intentional Self-Harm	Poisoning, Assault	Poisoning, Undetermined	Adverse Effect	Underdosing
Aniline (dye) (liquid)	T65.3X1	T65.3X2	T65.3X3	T65.3X4	—	—
analgesic	T39.1X1	T39.1X2	T39.1X3	T39.1X4	T39.1X5	T39.1X6
derivatives, therapeutic NEC	T39.1X1	T39.1X2	T39.1X3	T39.1X4	T39.1X5	T39.1X6
vapor	T65.3X1	T65.3X2	T65.3X3	T65.3X4	—	—
Anise oil	T47.5X1	T47.5X2	T47.5X3	T47.5X4	T47.5X5	T47.5X6
Aniscoropine	T44.3X1	T44.3X2	T44.3X3	T44.3X4	T44.3X5	T44.3X6
Anisidine	T65.3X1	T65.3X2	T65.3X3	T65.3X4	—	—
Anisindione	T45.511	T45.512	T45.513	T45.514	T45.515	T45.516
Anisotropine methyl-bromide	T44.3X1	T44.3X2	T44.3X3	T44.3X4	T44.3X5	T44.3X6
Anistreplase	T45.611	T45.612	T45.613	T45.614	T45.615	T45.616
Anorexiant (central)	T50.5X1	T50.5X2	T50.5X3	T50.5X4	T50.5X5	T50.5X6
Anorexic agents	T50.5X1	T50.5X2	T50.5X3	T50.5X4	T50.5X5	T50.5X6
Ansamycin	T36.6X1	T36.6X2	T36.6X3	T36.6X4	T36.6X5	T36.6X6
Ant (bite) (sting)	T63.421	T63.422	T63.423	T63.424	—	—
Antabuse	T50.6X1	T50.6X2	T50.6X3	T50.6X4	T50.6X5	T50.6X6
Ant poison — see Insecticide						
Antacid NEC	T47.1X1	T47.1X2	T47.1X3	T47.1X4	T47.1X5	T47.1X6
Antagonist						
Aldosterone	T50.0X1	T50.0X2	T50.0X3	T50.0X4	T50.0X5	T50.0X6
alpha-adrenoreceptor	T44.6X1	T44.6X2	T44.6X3	T44.6X4	T44.6X5	T44.6X6
anticoagulant	T45.7X1	T45.7X2	T45.7X3	T45.7X4	T45.7X5	T45.7X6
beta-adrenoreceptor	T44.7X1	T44.7X2	T44.7X3	T44.7X4	T44.7X5	T44.7X6
extrapyramidal NEC	T44.3X1	T44.3X2	T44.3X3	T44.3X4	T44.3X5	T44.3X6
folic acid	T45.1X1	T45.1X2	T45.1X3	T45.1X4	T45.1X5	T45.1X6
H2 receptor	T47.0X1	T47.0X2	T47.0X3	T47.0X4	T47.0X5	T47.0X6
heavy metal	T45.8X1	T45.8X2	T45.8X3	T45.8X4	T45.8X5	T45.8X6
narcotic analgesic	T50.7X1	T50.7X2	T50.7X3	T50.7X4	T50.7X5	T50.7X6
opiate	T50.7X1	T50.7X2	T50.7X3	T50.7X4	T50.7X5	T50.7X6
pyrimidine	T45.1X1	T45.1X2	T45.1X3	T45.1X4	T45.1X5	T45.1X6
serotonin	T46.5X1	T46.5X2	T46.5X3	T46.5X4	T46.5X5	T46.5X6
Antazolin(e)	T45.0X1	T45.0X2	T45.0X3	T45.0X4	T45.0X5	T45.0X6
Anterior pituitary hormone NEC	T38.811	T38.812	T38.813	T38.814	T38.815	T38.816
Anthelmintic NEC	T37.4X1	T37.4X2	T37.4X3	T37.4X4	T37.4X5	T37.4X6
Anthiolimine	T37.4X1	T37.4X2	T37.4X3	T37.4X4	T37.4X5	T37.4X6
Anthralin	T49.4X1	T49.4X2	T49.4X3	T49.4X4	T49.4X5	T49.4X6
Anthramycin	T45.1X1	T45.1X2	T45.1X3	T45.1X4	T45.1X5	T45.1X6
Antiadrenergic NEC	T44.8X1	T44.8X2	T44.8X3	T44.8X4	T44.8X5	T44.8X6
Antiallergic NEC	T45.0X1	T45.0X2	T45.0X3	T45.0X4	T45.0X5	T45.0X6
Anti-anemic (drug) (preparation)	T45.8X1	T45.8X2	T45.8X3	T45.8X4	T45.8X5	T45.8X6
Antiandrogen NEC	T38.6X1	T38.6X2	T38.6X3	T38.6X4	T38.6X5	T38.6X6
Antianxiety drug NEC	T43.501	T43.502	T43.503	T43.504	T43.505	T43.506
Antiaris toxicaria	T65.891	T65.892	T65.893	T65.894	—	—

Substance	External Cause (T-Code) Poisoning, Accidental (Unintentional)	Poisoning, Intentional Self-Harm	Poisoning, Assault	Poisoning, Undetermined	Adverse Effect	Underdosing
Antiarteriosclerotic drug	T46.6X1	T46.6X2	T46.6X3	T46.6X4	T46.6X5	T46.6X6
Antiasthmatic drug NEC	T48.6X1	T48.6X2	T48.6X3	T48.6X4	T48.6X5	T48.6X6
Antibiotic NEC	T36.91	T36.92	T36.93	T36.94	T36.95	T36.96
aminoglycoside	T36.5X1	T36.5X2	T36.5X3	T36.5X4	T36.5X5	T36.5X6
anticancer	T45.1X1	T45.1X2	T45.1X3	T45.1X4	T45.1X5	T45.1X6
antifungal	T36.7X1	T36.7X2	T36.7X3	T36.7X4	T36.7X5	T36.7X6
antimycobacterial	T36.5X1	T36.5X2	T36.5X3	T36.5X4	T36.5X5	T36.5X6
antineoplastic	T45.1X1	T45.1X2	T45.1X3	T45.1X4	T45.1X5	T45.1X6
cephalosporin (group)	T36.1X1	T36.1X2	T36.1X3	T36.1X4	T36.1X5	T36.1X6
chloramphenicol (group)	T36.2X1	T36.2X2	T36.2X3	T36.2X4	T36.2X5	T36.2X6
ENT	T49.6X1	T49.6X2	T49.6X3	T49.6X4	T49.6X5	T49.6X6
eye	T49.5X1	T49.5X2	T49.5X3	T49.5X4	T49.5X5	T49.5X6
fungicidal (local)	T49.0X1	T49.0X2	T49.0X3	T49.0X4	T49.0X5	T49.0X6
intestinal	T36.8X1	T36.8X2	T36.8X3	T36.8X4	T36.8X5	T36.8X6
b-lactam NEC	T36.1X1	T36.1X2	T36.1X3	T36.1X4	T36.1X5	T36.1X6
local	T49.0X1	T49.0X2	T49.0X3	T49.0X4	T49.0X5	T49.0X6
macrolides	T36.3X1	T36.3X2	T36.3X3	T36.3X4	T36.3X5	T36.3X6
polypeptide	T36.8X1	T36.8X2	T36.8X3	T36.8X4	T36.8X5	T36.8X6
specified NEC	T36.8X1	T36.8X2	T36.8X3	T36.8X4	T36.8X5	T36.8X6
tetracycline (group)	T36.4X1	T36.4X2	T36.4X3	T36.4X4	T36.4X5	T36.4X6
throat	T49.6X1	T49.6X2	T49.6X3	T49.6X4	T49.6X5	T49.6X6
Anticancer agents NEC	T45.1X1	T45.1X2	T45.1X3	T45.1X4	T45.1X5	T45.1X6
Anticholesterolemic drug NEC	T46.6X1	T46.6X2	T46.6X3	T46.6X4	T46.6X5	T46.6X6
Anticholinergic NEC	T44.3X1	T44.3X2	T44.3X3	T44.3X4	T44.3X5	T44.3X6
Anticholinesterase	T44.0X1	T44.0X2	T44.0X3	T44.0X4	T44.0X5	T44.0X6
organophosphorus	T44.0X1	T44.0X2	T44.0X3	T44.0X4	T44.0X5	T44.0X6
insecticide	T60.0X1	T60.0X2	T60.0X3	T60.0X4	—	—
nerve gas	T59.891	T59.892	T59.893	T59.894	—	—
reversible	T44.0X1	T44.0X2	T44.0X3	T44.0X4	T44.0X5	T44.0X6
ophthalmological	T49.5X1	T49.5X2	T49.5X3	T49.5X4	T49.5X5	T49.5X6
Anticoagulant NEC	T45.511	T45.512	T45.513	T45.514	T45.515	T45.516
Antagonist	T45.7X1	T45.7X2	T45.7X3	T45.7X4	T45.7X5	T45.7X6
Anti-common-cold drug NEC	T48.5X1	T48.5X2	T48.5X3	T48.5X4	T48.5X5	T48.5X6
Anticonvulsant	T42.71	T42.72	T42.73	T42.74	T42.75	T42.76
barbiturate	T42.3X1	T42.3X2	T42.3X3	T42.3X4	T42.3X5	T42.3X6
combination (with barbiturate)	T42.3X1	T42.3X2	T42.3X3	T42.3X4	T42.3X5	T42.3X6
hydantoin	T42.0X1	T42.0X2	T42.0X3	T42.0X4	T42.0X5	T42.0X6
hypnotic NEC	T42.6X1	T42.6X2	T42.6X3	T42.6X4	T42.6X5	T42.6X6
oxazolidinedione	T42.2X1	T42.2X2	T42.2X3	T42.2X4	T42.2X5	T42.2X6
pyrimidinedione	T42.6X1	T42.6X2	T42.6X3	T42.6X4	T42.6X5	T42.6X6
specified NEC	T42.6X1	T42.6X2	T42.6X3	T42.6X4	T42.6X5	T42.6X6
succinimide	T42.2X1	T42.2X2	T42.2X3	T42.2X4	T42.2X5	T42.2X6

◀ New ◀▥ Revised ~~deleted~~ Deleted

Substance	External Cause (T-Code)					
	Poisoning, Accidental (Unintentional)	Poisoning, Intentional Self-Harm	Poisoning, Assault	Poisoning, Undetermined	Adverse Effect	Underdosing
Anti-D immunoglobulin (human)	T50.Z11	T50.Z12	T50.Z13	T50.Z14	T50.Z15	T50.Z16
Antidepressant NEC	T43.201	T43.202	T43.203	T43.204	T43.205	T43.206
monoamine oxidase inhibitor	T43.1X1	T43.1X2	T43.1X3	T43.1X4	T43.1X5	T43.1X6
selective serotonin norepinephrine reuptake inhibitor	T43.211	T43.212	T43.213	T43.214	T43.215	T43.216
selective serotonin reuptake inhibitor	T43.221	T43.222	T43.223	T43.224	T43.225	T43.226
specified NEC	T43.291	T43.292	T43.293	T43.294	T43.295	T43.296
tetracyclic	T43.021	T43.022	T43.023	T43.024	T43.025	T43.026
triazolopyridine	T43.221	T43.222	T43.223	T43.224	T43.225	T43.226
tricyclic	T43.011	T43.012	T43.013	T43.014	T43.015	T43.016
Antidiabetic NEC	T38.3X1	T38.3X2	T38.3X3	T38.3X4	T38.3X5	T38.3X6
biguanide	T38.3X1	T38.3X2	T38.3X3	T38.3X4	T38.3X5	T38.3X6
and sulfonyl combined	T38.3X1	T38.3X2	T38.3X3	T38.3X4	T38.3X5	T38.3X6
combined	T38.3X1	T38.3X2	T38.3X3	T38.3X4	T38.3X5	T38.3X6
sulfonylurea	T38.3X1	T38.3X2	T38.3X3	T38.3X4	T38.3X5	T38.3X6
Antidiarrheal drug NEC	T47.6X1	T47.6X2	T47.6X3	T47.6X4	T47.6X5	T47.6X6
absorbent	T47.6X1	T47.6X2	T47.6X3	T47.6X4	T47.6X5	T47.6X6
Antidiphtheria serum	T50.Z11	T50.Z12	T50.Z13	T50.Z14	T50.Z15	T50.Z16
Antidiuretic hormone	T38.891	T38.892	T38.893	T38.894	T38.895	T38.896
Antidote NEC	T50.6X1	T50.6X2	T50.6X3	T50.6X4	T50.6X5	T50.6X6
heavy metal	T45.8X1	T45.8X2	T45.8X3	T45.8X4	T45.8X5	T45.8X6
Antidysrhythmic NEC	T46.2X1	T46.2X2	T46.2X3	T46.2X4	T46.2X5	T46.2X6
Antiemetic drug	T45.0X1	T45.0X2	T45.0X3	T45.0X4	T45.0X5	T45.0X6
Antiepilepsy agent	T42.71	T42.72	T42.73	T42.74	T42.75	T42.76
combination	T42.5X1	T42.5X2	T42.5X3	T42.5X4	T42.5X5	T42.5X6
mixed	T42.5X1	T42.5X2	T42.5X3	T42.5X4	T42.5X5	T42.5X6
specified, NEC	T42.6X1	T42.6X2	T42.6X3	T42.6X4	T42.6X5	T42.6X6
Antiestrogen NEC	T38.6X1	T38.6X2	T38.6X3	T38.6X4	T38.6X5	T38.6X6
Antifertility pill	T38.4X1	T38.4X2	T38.4X3	T38.4X4	T38.4X5	T38.4X6
Antifibrinolytic drug	T45.621	T45.622	T45.623	T45.624	T45.625	T45.626
Antifilarial drug	T37.4X1	T37.4X2	T37.4X3	T37.4X4	T37.4X5	T37.4X6
Antiflatulent	T47.5X1	T47.5X2	T47.5X3	T47.5X4	T47.5X5	T47.5X6
Antifreeze	T65.91	T65.92	T65.93	T65.94	—	—
alcohol	T51.1X1	T51.1X2	T51.1X3	T51.1X4	—	—
ethylene glycol	T51.8X1	T51.8X2	T51.8X3	T51.8X4	—	—
Antifungal						
antibiotic (systemic)	T36.7X1	T36.7X2	T36.7X3	T36.7X4	T36.7X5	T36.7X6
anti-infective NEC	T37.91	T37.92	T37.93	T37.94	T37.95	T37.96
disinfectant, local	T49.0X1	T49.0X2	T49.0X3	T49.0X4	T49.0X5	T49.0X6
nonmedicinal (spray)	T60.3X1	T60.3X2	T60.3X3	T60.3X4	—	—
topical	T49.0X1	T49.0X2	T49.0X3	T49.0X4	T49.0X5	T49.0X6

Substance	External Cause (T-Code)					
	Poisoning, Accidental (Unintentional)	Poisoning, Intentional Self-Harm	Poisoning, Assault	Poisoning, Undetermined	Adverse Effect	Underdosing
Anti-gastric-secretion drug NEC	T47.1X1	T47.1X2	T47.1X3	T47.1X4	T47.1X5	T47.1X6
Antigonadotrophin NEC	T38.6X1	T38.6X2	T38.6X3	T38.6X4	T38.6X5	T38.6X6
Antihallucinogen	T43.501	T43.502	T43.503	T43.504	T43.505	T43.506
Antihelmintics	T37.4X1	T37.4X2	T37.4X3	T37.4X4	T37.4X5	T37.4X6
Antihemophilic						
factor	T45.8X1	T45.8X2	T45.8X3	T45.8X4	T45.8X5	T45.8X6
fraction	T45.8X1	T45.8X2	T45.8X3	T45.8X4	T45.8X5	T45.8X6
globulin concentrate	T45.7X1	T45.7X2	T45.7X3	T45.7X4	T45.7X5	T45.7X6
human plasma	T45.8X1	T45.8X2	T45.8X3	T45.8X4	T45.8X5	T45.8X6
plasma, dried	T45.7X1	T45.7X2	T45.7X3	T45.7X4	T45.7X5	T45.7X6
Antihemorrhoidal preparation	T49.2X1	T49.2X2	T49.2X3	T49.2X4	T49.2X5	T49.2X6
Antiheparin drug	T45.7X1	T45.7X2	T45.7X3	T45.7X4	T45.7X5	T45.7X6
Antihistamine	T45.0X1	T45.0X2	T45.0X3	T45.0X4	T45.0X5	T45.0X6
Antihookworm drug	T37.4X1	T37.4X2	T37.4X3	T37.4X4	T37.4X5	T37.4X6
Anti-human lymphocytic globulin	T50.Z11	T50.Z12	T50.Z13	T50.Z14	T50.Z15	T50.Z16
Antihyperlipidemic drug	T46.6X1	T46.6X2	T46.6X3	T46.6X4	T46.6X5	T46.6X6
Antihypertensive drug NEC	T46.5X1	T46.5X2	T46.5X3	T46.5X4	T46.5X5	T46.5X6
Anti-infective NEC	T37.91	T37.92	T37.93	T37.94	T37.95	T37.96
anthelmintic	T37.4X1	T37.4X2	T37.4X3	T37.4X4	T37.4X5	T37.4X6
antibiotics	T36.91	T36.92	T36.93	T36.94	T36.95	T36.96
specified NEC	T36.8X1	T36.8X2	T36.8X3	T36.8X4	T36.8X5	T36.8X6
antimalarial	T37.2X1	T37.2X2	T37.2X3	T37.2X4	T37.2X5	T37.2X6
antimycobacterial NEC	T37.1X1	T37.1X2	T37.1X3	T37.1X4	T37.1X5	T37.1X6
antibiotics	T36.5X1	T36.5X2	T36.5X3	T36.5X4	T36.5X5	T36.5X6
antiprotozoal NEC	T37.3X1	T37.3X2	T37.3X3	T37.3X4	T37.3X5	T37.3X6
blood	T37.2X1	T37.2X2	T37.2X3	T37.2X4	T37.2X5	T37.2X6
antiviral	T37.5X1	T37.5X2	T37.5X3	T37.5X4	T37.5X5	T37.5X6
arsenical	T37.8X1	T37.8X2	T37.8X3	T37.8X4	T37.8X5	T37.8X6
bismuth, local	T49.0X1	T49.0X2	T49.0X3	T49.0X4	T49.0X5	T49.0X6
ENT	T49.6X1	T49.6X2	T49.6X3	T49.6X4	T49.6X5	T49.6X6
eye NEC	T49.5X1	T49.5X2	T49.5X3	T49.5X4	T49.5X5	T49.5X6
heavy metals NEC	T37.8X1	T37.8X2	T37.8X3	T37.8X4	T37.8X5	T37.8X6
local NEC	T49.0X1	T49.0X2	T49.0X3	T49.0X4	T49.0X5	T49.0X6
specified NEC	T49.0X1	T49.0X2	T49.0X3	T49.0X4	T49.0X5	T49.0X6
mixed	T37.91	T37.92	T37.93	T37.94	T37.95	T37.96
ophthalmic preparation	T49.5X1	T49.5X2	T49.5X3	T49.5X4	T49.5X5	T49.5X6
topical NEC	T49.0X1	T49.0X2	T49.0X3	T49.0X4	T49.0X5	T49.0X6
Anti-inflammatory drug NEC	T49.0X1	T49.0X2	T49.0X3	T49.0X4	T49.0X5	T49.0X6
local	T49.0X1	T49.0X2	T49.0X3	T49.0X4	T49.0X5	T49.0X6
nonsteroidal NEC	T39.391	T39.392	T39.393	T39.394	T39.395	T39.396
propionic acid derivative	T39.311	T39.312	T39.313	T39.314	T39.315	T39.316
specified NEC	T39.391	T39.392	T39.393	T39.394	T39.395	T39.396

◄ New   ⬅ Revised   ~~deleted~~ Deleted

TABLE OF DRUGS AND CHEMICALS

Substance	Poisoning, Accidental (Unintentional)	Poisoning, Intentional Self-Harm	Poisoning, Assault	Poisoning, Undetermined	Adverse Effect	Underdosing
Antikaluretic	T50.3X1	T50.3X2	T50.3X3	T50.3X4	T50.3X5	T50.3X6
Antiknock (tetraethyl lead)	T56.0X1	T56.0X2	T56.0X3	T56.0X4	—	—
Antilipemic drug NEC	T46.6X1	T46.6X2	T46.6X3	T46.6X4	T46.6X5	T46.6X6
Antimalarial	T37.2X1	T37.2X2	T37.2X3	T37.2X4	T37.2X5	T37.2X6
prophylactic NEC	T37.2X1	T37.2X2	T37.2X3	T37.2X4	T37.2X5	T37.2X6
pyrimidine derivative	T37.2X1	T37.2X2	T37.2X3	T37.2X4	T37.2X5	T37.2X6
Antimetabolite	T45.1X1	T45.1X2	T45.1X3	T45.1X4	T45.1X5	T45.1X6
Antimitotic agent	T45.1X1	T45.1X2	T45.1X3	T45.1X4	T45.1X5	T45.1X6
Antimony (compounds) (vapor) NEC	T56.891	T56.892	T56.893	T56.894	—	—
anti-infectives	T37.8X1	T37.8X2	T37.8X3	T37.8X4	T37.8X5	T37.8X6
dimercaptosuccinate	T37.3X1	T37.3X2	T37.3X3	T37.3X4	T37.3X5	T37.3X6
hydride	T56.891	T56.892	T56.893	T56.894	—	—
pesticide (vapor)	T60.8X1	T60.8X2	T60.8X3	T60.8X4	—	—
potassium (sodium) tartrate	T37.8X1	T37.8X2	T37.8X3	T37.8X4	T37.8X5	T37.8X6
sodium dimercaptosuccinate	T37.3X1	T37.3X2	T37.3X3	T37.3X4	T37.3X5	T37.3X6
tartrated	T37.8X1	T37.8X2	T37.8X3	T37.8X4	T37.8X5	T37.8X6
Antimuscarinic NEC	T44.3X1	T44.3X2	T44.3X3	T44.3X4	T44.3X5	T44.3X6
Antimycobacterial drug NEC	T37.1X1	T37.1X2	T37.1X3	T37.1X4	T37.1X5	T37.1X6
antibiotics	T36.5X1	T36.5X2	T36.5X3	T36.5X4	T36.5X5	T36.5X6
combination	T37.1X1	T37.1X2	T37.1X3	T37.1X4	T37.1X5	T37.1X6
Antinausea drug	T45.0X1	T45.0X2	T45.0X3	T45.0X4	T45.0X5	T45.0X6
Antinematode drug	T37.4X1	T37.4X2	T37.4X3	T37.4X4	T37.4X5	T37.4X6
Antineoplastic NEC	T45.1X1	T45.1X2	T45.1X3	T45.1X4	T45.1X5	T45.1X6
alkaloidal	T45.1X1	T45.1X2	T45.1X3	T45.1X4	T45.1X5	T45.1X6
antibiotics	T45.1X1	T45.1X2	T45.1X3	T45.1X4	T45.1X5	T45.1X6
combination	T45.1X1	T45.1X2	T45.1X3	T45.1X4	T45.1X5	T45.1X6
estrogen	T38.5X1	T38.5X2	T38.5X3	T38.5X4	T38.5X5	T38.5X6
steroid	T38.7X1	T38.7X2	T38.7X3	T38.7X4	T38.7X5	T38.7X6
Antiparasitic drug (systemic)	T37.91	T37.92	T37.93	T37.94	T37.95	T37.96
local	T49.0X1	T49.0X2	T49.0X3	T49.0X4	T49.0X5	T49.0X6
specified NEC	T37.8X1	T37.8X2	T37.8X3	T37.8X4	T37.8X5	T37.8X6
Antiparkinsonism drug NEC	T42.8X1	T42.8X2	T42.8X3	T42.8X4	T42.8X5	T42.8X6
Antiperspirant NEC	T49.2X1	T49.2X2	T49.2X3	T49.2X4	T49.2X5	T49.2X6
Antiphlogistic NEC	T39.4X1	T39.4X2	T39.4X3	T39.4X4	T39.4X5	T39.4X6
Antiplatyhelmintic drug	T37.4X1	T37.4X2	T37.4X3	T37.4X4	T37.4X5	T37.4X6
Antiprotozoal drug NEC	T37.3X1	T37.3X2	T37.3X3	T37.3X4	T37.3X5	T37.3X6
blood	T37.2X1	T37.2X2	T37.2X3	T37.2X4	T37.2X5	T37.2X6
local	T49.0X1	T49.0X2	T49.0X3	T49.0X4	T49.0X5	T49.0X6
Antipruritic drug NEC	T49.1X1	T49.1X2	T49.1X3	T49.1X4	T49.1X5	T49.1X6
Antipsychotic drug	T43.501	T43.502	T43.503	T43.504	T43.505	T43.506
specified NEC	T43.591	T43.592	T43.593	T43.594	T43.595	T43.596

Substance	Poisoning, Accidental (Unintentional)	Poisoning, Intentional Self-Harm	Poisoning, Assault	Poisoning, Undetermined	Adverse Effect	Underdosing
Antipyretic	T39.91	T39.92	T39.93	T39.94	T39.95	T39.96
specified NEC	T39.8X1	T39.8X2	T39.8X3	T39.8X4	T39.8X5	T39.8X6
Antipyrine	T39.2X1	T39.2X2	T39.2X3	T39.2X4	T39.2X5	T39.2X6
Antirabies hyperimmune serum	T50.Z11	T50.Z12	T50.Z13	T50.Z14	T50.Z15	T50.Z16
Antirheumatic NEC	T39.4X1	T39.4X2	T39.4X3	T39.4X4	T39.4X5	T39.4X6
Antirigidity drug NEC	T42.8X1	T42.8X2	T42.8X3	T42.8X4	T42.8X5	T42.8X6
Antischistosomal drug	T37.4X1	T37.4X2	T37.4X3	T37.4X4	T37.4X5	T37.4X6
Antiscorpion sera	T50.Z11	T50.Z12	T50.Z13	T50.Z14	T50.Z15	T50.Z16
Antiseborrheics	T49.4X1	T49.4X2	T49.4X3	T49.4X4	T49.4X5	T49.4X6
Antiseptics (external) (medicinal)	T49.0X1	T49.0X2	T49.0X3	T49.0X4	T49.0X5	T49.0X6
Antistine	T45.0X1	T45.0X2	T45.0X3	T45.0X4	T45.0X5	T45.0X6
Antitapeworm drug	T37.4X1	T37.4X2	T37.4X3	T37.4X4	T37.4X5	T37.4X6
Antitetanus immunoglobulin	T50.Z11	T50.Z12	T50.Z13	T50.Z14	T50.Z15	T50.Z16
Antithyroid drug NEC	T38.2X1	T38.2X2	T38.2X3	T38.2X4	T38.2X5	T38.2X6
Antitoxin	T50.Z11	T50.Z12	T50.Z13	T50.Z14	T50.Z15	T50.Z16
diphtheria	T50.Z11	T50.Z12	T50.Z13	T50.Z14	T50.Z15	T50.Z16
gas gangrene	T50.Z11	T50.Z12	T50.Z13	T50.Z14	T50.Z15	T50.Z16
tetanus	T50.Z11	T50.Z12	T50.Z13	T50.Z14	T50.Z15	T50.Z16
Antitoxin, any	T50.901	T50.902	T50.903	T50.904	T50.905	T50.906
Antitrichomonal drug	T37.3X1	T37.3X2	T37.3X3	T37.3X4	T37.3X5	T37.3X6
Antituberculars	T37.1X1	T37.1X2	T37.1X3	T37.1X4	T37.1X5	T37.1X6
antibiotics	T36.5X1	T36.5X2	T36.5X3	T36.5X4	T36.5X5	T36.5X6
Antitussive NEC	T48.3X1	T48.3X2	T48.3X3	T48.3X4	T48.3X5	T48.3X6
codeine mixture	T40.2X1	T40.2X2	T40.2X3	T40.2X4	T40.2X5	T40.2X6
opiate	T40.2X1	T40.2X2	T40.2X3	T40.2X4	T40.2X5	T40.2X6
Antivaricose drug	T46.8X1	T46.8X2	T46.8X3	T46.8X4	T46.8X5	T46.8X6
Antivenin, antivenom (sera)	T50.Z11	T50.Z12	T50.Z13	T50.Z14	T50.Z15	T50.Z16
crotaline	T50.Z11	T50.Z12	T50.Z13	T50.Z14	T50.Z15	T50.Z16
spider bite	T50.Z11	T50.Z12	T50.Z13	T50.Z14	T50.Z15	T50.Z16
Antivertigo drug	T45.0X1	T45.0X2	T45.0X3	T45.0X4	T45.0X5	T45.0X6
Antiviral drug NEC	T37.5X1	T37.5X2	T37.5X3	T37.5X4	T37.5X5	T37.5X6
eye	T49.5X1	T49.5X2	T49.5X3	T49.5X4	T49.5X5	T49.5X6
Antiwhipworm drug	T37.4X1	T37.4X2	T37.4X3	T37.4X4	T37.4X5	T37.4X6
Ant poisons — see Pesticides						
Antrol — see also by specific chemical substance	T60.91	T60.92	T60.93	T60.94	—	—
fungicide	T60.91	T60.92	T60.93	T60.94	—	—
ANTU (alpha naphthylthiourea)	T60.4X1	T60.4X2	T60.4X3	T60.4X4	—	—
Apalcillin	T36.0X1	T36.0X2	T36.0X3	T36.0X4	T36.0X5	T36.0X6
APC	T48.5X1	T48.5X2	T48.5X3	T48.5X4	T48.5X5	T48.5X6
Aplonidine	T44.4X1	T44.4X2	T44.4X3	T44.4X4	T44.4X5	T44.4X6
Apomorphine	T47.7X1	T47.7X2	T47.7X3	T47.7X4	T47.7X5	T47.7X6

◄ New ◄ Revised ~~deleted~~ Deleted

Substance	External Cause (T-Code)					
	Poisoning, Accidental (Unintentional)	Poisoning, Intentional Self-Harm	Poisoning, Assault	Poisoning, Undetermined	Adverse Effect	Underdosing
Appetite depressants, central	T50.5X1	T50.5X2	T50.5X3	T50.5X4	T50.5X5	T50.5X6
Apraclonidine (hydrochloride)	T44.4X1	T44.4X2	T44.4X3	T44.4X4	T44.4X5	T44.4X6
Apresoline	T46.5X1	T46.5X2	T46.5X3	T46.5X4	T46.5X5	T46.5X6
Aprindine	T46.2X1	T46.2X2	T46.2X3	T46.2X4	T46.2X5	T46.2X6
Aprobarbital	T42.3X1	T42.3X2	T42.3X3	T42.3X4	T42.3X5	T42.3X6
Apronalide	T42.6X1	T42.6X2	T42.6X3	T42.6X4	T42.6X5	T42.6X6
Aprotinin	T45.621	T45.622	T45.623	T45.624	T45.625	T45.626
Aptocaine	T41.3X1	T41.3X2	T41.3X3	T41.3X4	T41.3X5	T41.3X6
Aqua fortis	T54.2X1	T54.2X2	T54.2X3	T54.2X4	—	—
Ara-A	T37.5X1	T37.5X2	T37.5X3	T37.5X4	T37.5X5	T37.5X6
Ara-C	T45.1X1	T45.1X2	T45.1X3	T45.1X4	T45.1X5	T45.1X6
Arachis oil	T49.3X1	T49.3X2	T49.3X3	T49.3X4	T49.3X5	T49.3X6
cathartic	T47.4X1	T47.4X2	T47.4X3	T47.4X4	T47.4X5	T47.4X6
Aralen	T37.2X1	T37.2X2	T37.2X3	T37.2X4	T37.2X5	T37.2X6
Arecoline	T44.1X1	T44.1X2	T44.1X3	T44.1X4	T44.1X5	T44.1X6
Arginine	T50.991	T50.992	T50.993	T50.994	T50.995	T50.996
glutamate	T50.991	T50.992	T50.993	T50.994	T50.995	T50.996
Argyrol	T49.0X1	T49.0X2	T49.0X3	T49.0X4	T49.0X5	T49.0X6
ENT agent	T49.6X1	T49.6X2	T49.6X3	T49.6X4	T49.6X5	T49.6X6
ophthalmic preparation	T49.5X1	T49.5X2	T49.5X3	T49.5X4	T49.5X5	T49.5X6
Aristocort	T38.0X1	T38.0X2	T38.0X3	T38.0X4	T38.0X5	T38.0X6
ENT agent	T49.6X1	T49.6X2	T49.6X3	T49.6X4	T49.6X5	T49.6X6
ophthalmic preparation	T49.5X1	T49.5X2	T49.5X3	T49.5X4	T49.5X5	T49.5X6
topical NEC	T49.0X1	T49.0X2	T49.0X3	T49.0X4	T49.0X5	T49.0X6
Aromatics, corrosive	T54.1X1	T54.1X2	T54.1X3	T54.1X4	—	—
disinfectants	T54.1X1	T54.1X2	T54.1X3	T54.1X4	—	—
Arsenate of lead	T57.0X1	T57.0X2	T57.0X3	T57.0X4	—	—
herbicide	T57.0X1	T57.0X2	T57.0X3	T57.0X4	—	—
Arsenic, arsenicals (compounds) (dust) (vapor) NEC	T57.0X1	T57.0X2	T57.0X3	T57.0X4	—	—
anti-infectives	T37.8X1	T37.8X2	T37.8X3	T37.8X4	T37.8X5	T37.8X6
pesticide (dust) (fumes)	T57.0X1	T57.0X2	T57.0X3	T57.0X4	—	—
Arsine (gas)	T57.0X1	T57.0X2	T57.0X3	T57.0X4	—	—
Arsphenamine (silver)	T37.8X1	T37.8X2	T37.8X3	T37.8X4	T37.8X5	T37.8X6
Arsthinol	T37.3X1	T37.3X2	T37.3X3	T37.3X4	T37.3X5	T37.3X6
Artane	T44.3X1	T44.3X2	T44.3X3	T44.3X4	T44.3X5	T44.3X6
Arthropod (venomous) NEC	T63.481	T63.482	T63.483	T63.484	—	—
Articaine	T41.3X1	T41.3X2	T41.3X3	T41.3X4	T41.3X5	T41.3X6
Asbestos	T57.8X1	T57.8X2	T57.8X3	T57.8X4	—	—
Ascaridole	T37.4X1	T37.4X2	T37.4X3	T37.4X4	T37.4X5	T37.4X6
Ascorbic acid	T45.2X1	T45.2X2	T45.2X3	T45.2X4	T45.2X5	T45.2X6
Asiaticoside	T49.0X1	T49.0X2	T49.0X3	T49.0X4	T49.0X5	T49.0X6

Substance	External Cause (T-Code)					
	Poisoning, Accidental (Unintentional)	Poisoning, Intentional Self-Harm	Poisoning, Assault	Poisoning, Undetermined	Adverse Effect	Underdosing
Asparaginase	T45.1X1	T45.1X2	T45.1X3	T45.1X4	T45.1X5	T45.1X6
Aspidium (oleoresin)	T37.4X1	T37.4X2	T37.4X3	T37.4X4	T37.4X5	T37.4X6
Aspirin (aluminum) (soluble)	T39.011	T39.012	T39.013	T39.014	T39.015	T39.016
Aspoxicillin	T36.0X1	T36.0X2	T36.0X3	T36.0X4	T36.0X5	T36.0X6
Astemizole	T45.0X1	T45.0X2	T45.0X3	T45.0X4	T45.0X5	T45.0X6
Astringent (local)	T49.2X1	T49.2X2	T49.2X3	T49.2X4	T49.2X5	T49.2X6
specified NEC	T49.2X1	T49.2X2	T49.2X3	T49.2X4	T49.2X5	T49.2X6
Astromicin	T36.5X1	T36.5X2	T36.5X3	T36.5X4	T36.5X5	T36.5X6
Ataractic drug NEC	T43.501	T43.502	T43.503	T43.504	T43.505	T43.506
Atenolol	T44.7X1	T44.7X2	T44.7X3	T44.7X4	T44.7X5	T44.7X6
Atonia drug, intestinal	T47.4X1	T47.4X2	T47.4X3	T47.4X4	T47.4X5	T47.4X6
Atophan	T50.4X1	T50.4X2	T50.4X3	T50.4X4	T50.4X5	T50.4X6
Atracurium besilate	T48.1X1	T48.1X2	T48.1X3	T48.1X4	T48.1X5	T48.1X6
Atropine	T44.3X1	T44.3X2	T44.3X3	T44.3X4	T44.3X5	T44.3X6
derivative	T44.3X1	T44.3X2	T44.3X3	T44.3X4	T44.3X5	T44.3X6
methonitrate	T44.3X1	T44.3X2	T44.3X3	T44.3X4	T44.3X5	T44.3X6
Attapulgite	T47.6X1	T47.6X2	T47.6X3	T47.6X4	T47.6X5	T47.6X6
Attenuvax	T50.991	T50.992	T50.993	T50.994	T50.995	T50.996
Auramine	T65.891	T65.892	T65.893	T65.894	—	—
dye	T65.6X1	T65.6X2	T65.6X3	T65.6X4	—	—
fungicide	T60.3X1	T60.3X2	T60.3X3	T60.3X4	—	—
Auranofin	T39.4X1	T39.4X2	T39.4X3	T39.4X4	T39.4X5	T39.4X6
Aurantiin	T46.991	T46.992	T46.993	T46.994	T46.995	T46.996
Aureomycin	T36.4X1	T36.4X2	T36.4X3	T36.4X4	T36.4X5	T36.4X6
ophthalmic preparation	T49.5X1	T49.5X2	T49.5X3	T49.5X4	T49.5X5	T49.5X6
topical NEC	T49.0X1	T49.0X2	T49.0X3	T49.0X4	T49.0X5	T49.0X6
Aurothioglucose	T39.4X1	T39.4X2	T39.4X3	T39.4X4	T39.4X5	T39.4X6
Aurothioglycanide	T39.4X1	T39.4X2	T39.4X3	T39.4X4	T39.4X5	T39.4X6
Aurothiomalate sodium	T39.4X1	T39.4X2	T39.4X3	T39.4X4	T39.4X5	T39.4X6
Aurotioprol	T39.4X1	T39.4X2	T39.4X3	T39.4X4	T39.4X5	T39.4X6
Automobile fuel	T52.0X1	T52.0X2	T52.0X3	T52.0X4	—	—
Autonomic nervous system agent NEC	T44.901	T44.902	T44.903	T44.904	T44.905	T44.906
Avlosulfon	T37.1X1	T37.1X2	T37.1X3	T37.1X4	T37.1X5	T37.1X6
Avomine	T42.6X1	T42.6X2	T42.6X3	T42.6X4	T42.6X5	T42.6X6
Axerophthol	T45.2X1	T45.2X2	T45.2X3	T45.2X4	T45.2X5	T45.2X6
Azacitidine	T45.1X1	T45.1X2	T45.1X3	T45.1X4	T45.1X5	T45.1X6
Azacyclonol	T43.591	T43.592	T43.593	T43.594	T43.595	T43.596
Azadirachta	T60.2X1	T60.2X2	T60.2X3	T60.2X4	—	—
Azanidazole	T37.3X1	T37.3X2	T37.3X3	T37.3X4	T37.3X5	T37.3X6
Azapetine	T46.7X1	T46.7X2	T46.7X3	T46.7X4	T46.7X5	T46.7X6
Azapropazone	T39.2X1	T39.2X2	T39.2X3	T39.2X4	T39.2X5	T39.2X6

◀ New ◀▥ Revised ~~deleted~~ Deleted

Substance	Poisoning, Accidental (Unintentional)	Poisoning, Intentional Self-Harm	Poisoning, Assault	Poisoning, Undetermined	Adverse Effect	Underdosing
Azaribine	T45.1X1	T45.1X2	T45.1X3	T45.1X4	T45.1X5	T45.1X6
Azaserine	T45.1X1	T45.1X2	T45.1X3	T45.1X4	T45.1X5	T45.1X6
Azatadine	T45.0X1	T45.0X2	T45.0X3	T45.0X4	T45.0X5	T45.0X6
Azatepa	T45.1X1	T45.1X2	T45.1X3	T45.1X4	T45.1X5	T45.1X6
Azathioprine	T45.1X1	T45.1X2	T45.1X3	T45.1X4	T45.1X5	T45.1X6
Azelaic acid	T49.0X1	T49.0X2	T49.0X3	T49.0X4	T49.0X5	T49.0X6
Azelastine	T45.0X1	T45.0X2	T45.0X3	T45.0X4	T45.0X5	T45.0X6
Azidocillin	T36.0X1	T36.0X2	T36.0X3	T36.0X4	T36.0X5	T36.0X6
Azidothymidine	T37.5X1	T37.5X2	T37.5X3	T37.5X4	T37.5X5	T37.5X6
Azinphos (ethyl) (methyl)	T60.0X1	T60.0X2	T60.0X3	T60.0X4	—	—
Aziridine (chelating)	T54.1X1	T54.1X2	T54.1X3	T54.1X4	—	—
Azithromycin	T36.3X1	T36.3X2	T36.3X3	T36.3X4	T36.3X5	T36.3X6
Azlocillin	T36.01	T36.02	T36.03	T36.04	T36.05	T36.06
Azobenzene smoke	T65.3X1	T65.3X2	T65.3X3	T65.3X4	—	—
acaricide	T60.8X1	T60.8X2	T60.8X3	T60.8X4	—	—
Azosulfamide	T37.0X1	T37.0X2	T37.0X3	T37.0X4	T37.0X5	T37.0X6
AZT	T37.5X1	T37.5X2	T37.5X3	T37.5X4	T37.5X5	T37.5X6
Aztreonam	T36.1X1	T36.1X2	T36.1X3	T36.1X4	T36.1X5	T36.1X6
Azulfidine	T37.0X1	T37.0X2	T37.0X3	T37.0X4	T37.0X5	T37.0X6
Azuresin	T50.8X1	T50.8X2	T50.8X3	T50.8X4	T50.8X5	T50.8X6
B						
Bacampicillin	T36.0X1	T36.0X2	T36.0X3	T36.0X4	T36.0X5	T36.0X6
Bacillus						
lactobacillus	T47.8X1	T47.8X2	T47.8X3	T47.8X4	T47.8X5	T47.8X6
subtilis	T47.6X1	T47.6X2	T47.6X3	T47.6X4	T47.6X5	T47.6X6
Bacimycin	T49.0X1	T49.0X2	T49.0X3	T49.0X4	T49.0X5	T49.0X6
ophthalmic preparation	T49.5X1	T49.5X2	T49.5X3	T49.5X4	T49.5X5	T49.5X6
Bacitracin zinc	T49.0X1	T49.0X2	T49.0X3	T49.0X4	T49.0X5	T49.0X6
with neomycin	T49.0X1	T49.0X2	T49.0X3	T49.0X4	T49.0X5	T49.0X6
ENT agent	T49.6X1	T49.6X2	T49.6X3	T49.6X4	T49.6X5	T49.6X6
ophthalmic preparation	T49.5X1	T49.5X2	T49.5X3	T49.5X4	T49.5X5	T49.5X6
topical NEC	T49.0X1	T49.0X2	T49.0X3	T49.0X4	T49.0X5	T49.0X6
Baclofen	T42.8X1	T42.8X2	T42.8X3	T42.8X4	T42.8X5	T42.8X6
Baking soda	T50.991	T50.992	T50.993	T50.994	T50.995	T50.996
BAL	T45.8X1	T45.8X2	T45.8X3	T45.8X4	T45.8X5	T45.8X6
Bambuterol	T48.6X1	T48.6X2	T48.6X3	T48.6X4	T48.6X5	T48.6X6
Bamethan (sulfate)	T46.7X1	T46.7X2	T46.7X3	T46.7X4	T46.7X5	T46.7X6
Bamifylline	T48.6X1	T48.6X2	T48.6X3	T48.6X4	T48.6X5	T48.6X6
Bamipine	T45.0X1	T45.0X2	T45.0X3	T45.0X4	T45.0X5	T45.0X6
Baneberry — *see Actaea spicata*						
Banewort — *see Belladonna*						

Substance	Poisoning, Accidental (Unintentional)	Poisoning, Intentional Self-Harm	Poisoning, Assault	Poisoning, Undetermined	Adverse Effect	Underdosing
Barbenyl	T42.3X1	T42.3X2	T42.3X3	T42.3X4	T42.3X5	T42.3X6
Barbexaclone	T42.6X1	T42.6X2	T42.6X3	T42.6X4	T42.6X5	T42.6X6
Barbital	T42.3X1	T42.3X2	T42.3X3	T42.3X4	T42.3X5	T42.3X6
sodium	T42.3X1	T42.3X2	T42.3X3	T42.3X4	T42.3X5	T42.3X6
Barbitone	T42.3X1	T42.3X2	T42.3X3	T42.3X4	T42.3X5	T42.3X6
Barbiturate NEC	T42.3X1	T42.3X2	T42.3X3	T42.3X4	T42.3X5	T42.3X6
with tranquilizer	T42.3X1	T42.3X2	T42.3X3	T42.3X4	T42.3X5	T42.3X6
anesthetic (intravenous)	T41.1X1	T41.1X2	T41.1X3	T41.1X4	T41.1X5	T41.1X6
Barium (carbonate) (chloride) (sulfite)	T57.8X1	T57.8X2	T57.8X3	T57.8X4	—	—
diagnostic agent	T50.8X1	T50.8X2	T50.8X3	T50.8X4	T50.8X5	T50.8X6
pesticide	T60.4X1	T60.4X2	T60.4X3	T60.4X4	—	—
rodenticide	T60.4X1	T60.4X2	T60.4X3	T60.4X4	—	—
sulfate (medicinal)	T50.8X1	T50.8X2	T50.8X3	T50.8X4	T50.8X5	T50.8X6
Barrier cream	T49.3X1	T49.3X2	T49.3X3	T49.3X4	T49.3X5	T49.3X6
Basic fuchsin	T49.0X1	T49.0X2	T49.0X3	T49.0X4	T49.0X5	T49.0X6
Battery acid or fluid	T54.2X1	T54.2X2	T54.2X3	T54.2X4	—	—
Bay rum	T51.8X1	T51.8X2	T51.8X3	T51.8X4	—	—
BCG (vaccine)	T50.A91	T50.A92	T50.A93	T50.A94	T50.A95	T50.A96
BCNU	T45.1X1	T45.1X2	T45.1X3	T45.1X4	T45.1X5	T45.1X6
Bearsfoot	T62.2X1	T62.2X2	T62.2X3	T62.2X4	—	—
Beclamide	T42.6X1	T42.6X2	T42.6X3	T42.6X4	T42.6X5	T42.6X6
Beclomethasone	T44.5X1	T44.5X2	T44.5X3	T44.5X4	T44.5X5	T44.5X6
Bee (sting) (venom)	T63.441	T63.442	T63.443	T63.444	—	—
Befunolol	T49.5X1	T49.5X2	T49.5X3	T49.5X4	T49.5X5	T49.5X6
Bekanamycin	T36.5X1	T36.5X2	T36.5X3	T36.5X4	T36.5X5	T36.5X6
Belladonna — *see also Nightshade*						
alkaloids	T44.3X1	T44.3X2	T44.3X3	T44.3X4	T44.3X5	T44.3X6
extract	T44.3X1	T44.3X2	T44.3X3	T44.3X4	T44.3X5	T44.3X6
herb	T44.3X1	T44.3X2	T44.3X3	T44.3X4	T44.3X5	T44.3X6
Bemegride	T50.7X1	T50.7X2	T50.7X3	T50.7X4	T50.7X5	T50.7X6
Benactyzine	T44.3X1	T44.3X2	T44.3X3	T44.3X4	T44.3X5	T44.3X6
Benadryl	T45.0X1	T45.0X2	T45.0X3	T45.0X4	T45.0X5	T45.0X6
Benaprizine	T44.3X1	T44.3X2	T44.3X3	T44.3X4	T44.3X5	T44.3X6
Benazepril	T46.4X1	T46.4X2	T46.4X3	T46.4X4	T46.4X5	T46.4X6
Bencyclane	T46.7X1	T46.7X2	T46.7X3	T46.7X4	T46.7X5	T46.7X6
Bendazol	T46.3X1	T46.3X2	T46.3X3	T46.3X4	T46.3X5	T46.3X6
Bendrofluazide	T50.2X1	T50.2X2	T50.2X3	T50.2X4	T50.2X5	T50.2X6
Bendroflumethiazide	T50.2X1	T50.2X2	T50.2X3	T50.2X4	T50.2X5	T50.2X6
Benemid	T50.4X1	T50.4X2	T50.4X3	T50.4X4	T50.4X5	T50.4X6
Benethamine penicillin	T36.0X1	T36.0X2	T36.0X3	T36.0X4	T36.0X5	T36.0X6
Benisone	T49.0X1	T49.0X2	T49.0X3	T49.0X4	T49.0X5	T49.0X6

TABLE OF DRUGS AND CHEMICALS

Substance	External Cause (T-Code) Poisoning, Accidental (Unintentional)	Poisoning, Intentional Self-Harm	Poisoning, Assault	Poisoning, Undetermined	Adverse Effect	Underdosing
Benexate	T47.1X1	T47.1X2	T47.1X3	T47.1X4	T47.1X5	T47.1X6
Benfluorex	T46.6X1	T46.6X2	T46.6X3	T46.6X4	T46.6X5	T46.6X6
Benfotiamine	T45.2X1	T45.2X2	T45.2X3	T45.2X4	T45.2X5	T45.2X6
Benomyl	T60.0X1	T60.0X2	T60.0X3	T60.0X4	—	—
Benoquin	T49.8X1	T49.8X2	T49.8X3	T49.8X4	T49.8X5	T49.8X6
Benoxinate	T41.3X1	T41.3X2	T41.3X3	T41.3X4	T41.3X5	T41.3X6
Benperidol	T43.4X1	T43.4X2	T43.4X3	T43.4X4	T43.4X5	T43.4X6
Benproperine	T48.3X1	T48.3X2	T48.3X3	T48.3X4	T48.3X5	T48.3X6
Benserazide	T42.8X1	T42.8X2	T42.8X3	T42.8X4	T42.8X5	T42.8X6
Bentazepam	T42.4X1	T42.4X2	T42.4X3	T42.4X4	T42.4X5	T42.4X6
Bentiromide	T50.8X1	T50.8X2	T50.8X3	T50.8X4	T50.8X5	T50.8X6
Bentonite	T49.3X1	T49.3X2	T49.3X3	T49.3X4	T49.3X5	T49.3X6
Benzalbutyramide	T46.6X1	T46.6X2	T46.6X3	T46.6X4	T46.6X5	T46.6X6
Benzalkonium (chloride)	T49.0X1	T49.0X2	T49.0X3	T49.0X4	T49.0X5	T49.0X6
ophthalmic preparation	T49.5X1	T49.5X2	T49.5X3	T49.5X4	T49.5X5	T49.5X6
Benzamine	T41.3X1	T41.3X2	T41.3X3	T41.3X4	T41.3X5	T41.3X6
lactate	T49.1X1	T49.1X2	T49.1X3	T49.1X4	T49.1X5	T49.1X6
Benzamidosalicylate (calcium)	T37.1X1	T37.1X2	T37.1X3	T37.1X4	T37.1X5	T37.1X6
Benzamphetamine	T50.5X1	T50.5X2	T50.5X3	T50.5X4	T50.5X5	T50.5X6
Benzapril hydrochloride	T46.5X1	T46.5X2	T46.5X3	T46.5X4	T46.5X5	T46.5X6
Benzathine benzylpenicillin	T36.0X1	T36.0X2	T36.0X3	T36.0X4	T36.0X5	T36.0X6
Benzathine penicillin	T36.0X1	T36.0X2	T36.0X3	T36.0X4	T36.0X5	T36.0X6
Benzatropine	T42.8X1	T42.8X2	T42.8X3	T42.8X4	T42.8X5	T42.8X6
Benzbromarone	T50.4X1	T50.4X2	T50.4X3	T50.4X4	T50.4X5	T50.4X6
Benzcarbimine	T45.1X1	T45.1X2	T45.1X3	T45.1X4	T45.1X5	T45.1X6
Benzedrex	T44.991	T44.992	T44.993	T44.994	T44.995	T44.996
Benzedrine (amphetamine)	T43.621	T43.622	T43.623	T43.624	T43.625	T43.626
Benzenamine	T65.3X1	T65.3X2	T65.3X3	T65.3X4	—	—
Benzene	T52.1X1	T52.1X2	T52.1X3	T52.1X4	—	—
homologues (acetyl) (dimethyl) (methyl) (solvent)	T52.2X1	T52.2X2	T52.2X3	T52.2X4	—	—
Benzethonium (chloride)	T49.0X1	T49.0X2	T49.0X3	T49.0X4	T49.0X5	T49.0X6
Benzfetamine	T50.5X1	T50.5X2	T50.5X3	T50.5X4	T50.5X5	T50.5X6
Benzhexol	T44.3X1	T44.3X2	T44.3X3	T44.3X4	T44.3X5	T44.3X6
Benzhydramine (chloride)	T45.0X1	T45.0X2	T45.0X3	T45.0X4	T45.0X5	T45.0X6
Benzidine	T65.891	T65.892	T65.893	T65.894	—	—
Benzilonium bromide	T44.3X1	T44.3X2	T44.3X3	T44.3X4	T44.3X5	T44.3X6
Benzimidazole	T60.3X1	T60.3X2	T60.3X3	T60.3X4	—	—
Benzin(e) — see Ligroin						
Benziodarone	T46.3X1	T46.3X2	T46.3X3	T46.3X4	T46.3X5	T46.3X6
Benznidazole	T37.3X1	T37.3X2	T37.3X3	T37.3X4	T37.3X5	T37.3X6
Benzocaine	T41.3X1	T41.3X2	T41.3X3	T41.3X4	T41.3X5	T41.3X6

Substance	External Cause (T-Code) Poisoning, Accidental (Unintentional)	Poisoning, Intentional Self-Harm	Poisoning, Assault	Poisoning, Undetermined	Adverse Effect	Underdosing
Benzoctamine	T43.0X1	T43.0X2	T43.0X3	T43.0X4	T43.0X5	T43.0X6
Benzodiapin	T42.4X1	T42.4X2	T42.4X3	T42.4X4	T42.4X5	T42.4X6
Benzodiazepine NEC	T42.4X1	T42.4X2	T42.4X3	T42.4X4	T42.4X5	T42.4X6
Benzoic acid	T49.0X1	T49.0X2	T49.0X3	T49.0X4	T49.0X5	T49.0X6
with salicylic acid	T49.0X1	T49.0X2	T49.0X3	T49.0X4	T49.0X5	T49.0X6
Benzoin (tincture)	T48.5X1	T48.5X2	T48.5X3	T48.5X4	T48.5X5	T48.5X6
Benzol (benzene)	T52.1X1	T52.1X2	T52.1X3	T52.1X4	—	—
vapor	T52.0X1	T52.0X2	T52.0X3	T52.0X4	—	—
Benzomorphan	T40.2X1	T40.2X2	T40.2X3	T40.2X4	T40.2X5	T40.2X6
Benzonatate	T48.3X1	T48.3X2	T48.3X3	T48.3X4	T48.3X5	T48.3X6
Benzophenones	T49.3X1	T49.3X2	T49.3X3	T49.3X4	T49.3X5	T49.3X6
Benzopyrone	T46.991	T46.992	T46.993	T46.994	T46.995	T46.996
Benzothiadiazides	T50.2X1	T50.2X2	T50.2X3	T50.2X4	T50.2X5	T50.2X6
Benzoxonium chloride	T49.0X1	T49.0X2	T49.0X3	T49.0X4	T49.0X5	T49.0X6
Benzoyl peroxide	T49.0X1	T49.0X2	T49.0X3	T49.0X4	T49.0X5	T49.0X6
Benzoylpas calcium	T37.1X1	T37.1X2	T37.1X3	T37.1X4	T37.1X5	T37.1X6
Benzperidin	T43.591	T43.592	T43.593	T43.594	T43.595	T43.596
Benzperidol	T43.591	T43.592	T43.593	T43.594	T43.595	T43.596
Benzphetamine	T50.5X1	T50.5X2	T50.5X3	T50.5X4	T50.5X5	T50.5X6
Benzpyrinium bromide	T44.1X1	T44.1X2	T44.1X3	T44.1X4	T44.1X5	T44.1X6
Benzquinamide	T45.0X1	T45.0X2	T45.0X3	T45.0X4	T45.0X5	T45.0X6
Benzthiazide	T50.2X1	T50.2X2	T50.2X3	T50.2X4	T50.2X5	T50.2X6
Benztropine						
anticholinergic	T44.3X1	T44.3X2	T44.3X3	T44.3X4	T44.3X5	T44.3X6
antiparkinson	T42.8X1	T42.8X2	T42.8X3	T42.8X4	T42.8X5	T42.8X6
Benzydamine	T49.0X1	T49.0X2	T49.0X3	T49.0X4	T49.0X5	T49.0X6
Benzyl						
acetate	T52.8X1	T52.8X2	T52.8X3	T52.8X4	—	—
alcohol	T49.0X1	T49.0X2	T49.0X3	T49.0X4	T49.0X5	T49.0X6
benzoate	T49.0X1	T49.0X2	T49.0X3	T49.0X4	T49.0X5	T49.0X6
Benzoic acid	T49.0X1	T49.0X2	T49.0X3	T49.0X4	T49.0X5	T49.0X6
morphine	T40.2X1	T40.2X2	T40.2X3	T40.2X4	—	—
nicotinate	T46.6X1	T46.6X2	T46.6X3	T46.6X4	T46.6X5	T46.6X6
penicillin	T36.0X1	T36.0X2	T36.0X3	T36.0X4	T36.0X5	T36.0X6
Benzylhydrochlorthia-zide	T50.2X1	T50.2X2	T50.2X3	T50.2X4	T50.2X5	T50.2X6
Benzylpenicillin	T36.0X1	T36.0X2	T36.0X3	T36.0X4	T36.0X5	T36.0X6
Benzylthiouracil	T38.2X1	T38.2X2	T38.2X3	T38.2X4	T38.2X5	T38.2X6
Bephenium hydroxy-naphthoate	T37.4X1	T37.4X2	T37.4X3	T37.4X4	T37.4X5	T37.4X6
Bepridil	T46.1X1	T46.1X2	T46.1X3	T46.1X4	T46.1X5	T46.1X6
Bergamot oil	T65.891	T65.892	T65.893	T65.894	—	—
Bergapten	T50.991	T50.992	T50.993	T50.994	T50.995	T50.996
Berries, poisonous	T62.1X1	T62.1X2	T62.1X3	T62.1X4	—	—

◀ New   ◀▥ Revised   ~~deleted~~ Deleted

TABLE OF DRUGS AND CHEMICALS

Substance	Poisoning, Accidental (Unintentional)	Poisoning, Intentional Self-Harm	Poisoning, Assault	Poisoning, Undetermined	Adverse Effect	Underdosing
Beryllium (compounds)	T56.7X1	T56.7X2	T56.7X3	T56.7X4	—	—
b-acetyldigoxin	T46.0X1	T46.0X2	T46.0X3	T46.0X4	T46.0X5	T46.0X6
beta adrenergic blocking agent, heart	T44.7X1	T44.7X2	T44.7X3	T44.7X4	T44.7X5	T44.7X6
b-benzalbutyramide	T46.6X1	T46.6X2	T46.6X3	T46.6X4	T46.6X5	T46.6X6
Betacarotene	T45.2X1	T45.2X2	T45.2X3	T45.2X4	T45.2X5	T45.2X6
b-eucaine	T49.1X1	T49.1X2	T49.1X3	T49.1X4	T49.1X5	T49.1X6
Beta-Chlor	T42.6X1	T42.6X2	T42.6X3	T42.6X4	T42.6X5	T42.6X6
b-galactosidase	T47.5X1	T47.5X2	T47.5X3	T47.5X4	T47.5X5	T47.5X6
Betahistine	T46.7X1	T46.7X2	T46.7X3	T46.7X4	T46.7X5	T46.7X6
Betaine	T47.5X1	T47.5X2	T47.5X3	T47.5X4	T47.5X5	T47.5X6
Betamethasone	T49.0X1	T49.0X2	T49.0X3	T49.0X4	T49.0X5	T49.0X6
topical	T49.0X1	T49.0X2	T49.0X3	T49.0X4	T49.0X5	T49.0X6
Betamicin	T36.8X1	T36.8X2	T36.8X3	T36.8X4	T36.8X5	T36.8X6
Betanidine	T46.5X1	T46.5X2	T46.5X3	T46.5X4	T46.5X5	T46.5X6
b-sitosterol(s)	T46.6X1	T46.6X2	T46.6X3	T46.6X4	T46.6X5	T46.6X6
Betaxolol	T44.7X1	T44.7X2	T44.7X3	T44.7X4	T44.7X5	T44.7X6
Betazole	T50.8X1	T50.8X2	T50.8X3	T50.8X4	T50.8X5	T50.8X6
Bethanechol	T44.1X1	T44.1X2	T44.1X3	T44.1X4	T44.1X5	T44.1X6
chloride	T44.1X1	T44.1X2	T44.1X3	T44.1X4	T44.1X5	T44.1X6
Bethanidine	T46.5X1	T46.5X2	T46.5X3	T46.5X4	T46.5X5	T46.5X6
Betoxycaine	T41.3X1	T41.3X2	T41.3X3	T41.3X4	T41.3X5	T41.3X6
Betula oil	T49.3X1	T49.3X2	T49.3X3	T49.3X4	T49.3X5	T49.3X6
Bevantolol	T44.7X1	T44.7X2	T44.7X3	T44.7X4	T44.7X5	T44.7X6
Bevonium metilsulfate	T44.3X1	T44.3X2	T44.3X3	T44.3X4	T44.3X5	T44.3X6
Bezafibrate	T46.6X1	T46.6X2	T46.6X3	T46.6X4	T46.6X5	T46.6X6
Bezitramide	T40.4X1	T40.4X2	T40.4X3	T40.4X4	T40.4X5	T40.4X6
BHA	T50.991	T50.992	T50.993	T50.994	T50.995	T50.996
Bhang	T40.7X1	T40.7X2	T40.7X3	T40.7X4	T40.7X5	T40.7X6
BHC (medicinal)	T49.0X1	T49.0X2	T49.0X3	T49.0X4	T49.0X5	T49.0X6
nonmedicinal (vapor)	T53.6X1	T53.6X2	T53.6X3	T53.6X4	—	—
Bialamicol	T37.3X1	T37.3X2	T37.3X3	T37.3X4	T37.3X5	T37.3X6
Bibenzonium bromide	T48.3X1	T48.3X2	T48.3X3	T48.3X4	T48.3X5	T48.3X6
Bibrocathol	T49.5X1	T49.5X2	T49.5X3	T49.5X4	T49.5X5	T49.5X6
Bichloride of mercury — see Mercury, chloride						
Bichromates (calcium) (potassium) (sodium) (crystals)	T57.8X1	T57.8X2	T57.8X3	T57.8X4	—	—
fumes	T56.2X1	T56.2X2	T56.2X3	T56.2X4	—	—
Biclotymol	T49.6X1	T49.6X2	T49.6X3	T49.6X4	T49.6X5	T49.6X6
Bicucculine	T50.7X1	T50.7X2	T50.7X3	T50.7X4	T50.7X5	T50.7X6
Bifemelane	T43.291	T43.292	T43.293	T43.294	T43.295	T43.296
Biguanide derivatives, oral	T38.3X1	T38.3X2	T38.3X3	T38.3X4	T38.3X5	T38.3X6

Substance	Poisoning, Accidental (Unintentional)	Poisoning, Intentional Self-Harm	Poisoning, Assault	Poisoning, Undetermined	Adverse Effect	Underdosing
Biligrafin	T50.8X1	T50.8X2	T50.8X3	T50.8X4	T50.8X5	T50.8X6
Bile salts	T47.5X1	T47.5X2	T47.5X3	T47.5X4	T47.5X5	T47.5X6
Bilopaque	T50.8X1	T50.8X2	T50.8X3	T50.8X4	T50.8X5	T50.8X6
Binifibrate	T46.6X1	T46.6X2	T46.6X3	T46.6X4	T46.6X5	T46.6X6
Binitrobenzol	T65.3X1	T65.3X2	T65.3X3	T65.3X4	—	—
Bioflavonoid(s)	T46.991	T46.992	T46.993	T46.994	T46.995	T46.996
Biological substance NEC	T50.901	T50.902	T50.903	T50.904	T50.905	T50.906
Biotin	T45.2X1	T45.2X2	T45.2X3	T45.2X4	T45.2X5	T45.2X6
Biperiden	T44.3X1	T44.3X2	T44.3X3	T44.3X4	T44.3X5	T44.3X6
Bisacodyl	T47.2X1	T47.2X2	T47.2X3	T47.2X4	T47.2X5	T47.2X6
Bisbentiamine	T45.2X1	T45.2X2	T45.2X3	T45.2X4	T45.2X5	T45.2X6
Bisbutiamine	T45.2X1	T45.2X2	T45.2X3	T45.2X4	T45.2X5	T45.2X6
Bisdequalinium (salts) (diacetate)	T49.6X1	T49.6X2	T49.6X3	T49.6X4	T49.6X5	T49.6X6
Bishydroxycoumarin	T45.511	T45.512	T45.513	T45.514	T45.515	T45.516
Bismarsen	T37.8X1	T37.8X2	T37.8X3	T37.8X4	T37.8X5	T37.8X6
Bismuth salts	T47.6X1	T47.6X2	T47.6X3	T47.6X4	T47.6X5	T47.6X6
aluminate	T47.1X1	T47.1X2	T47.1X3	T47.1X4	T47.1X5	T47.1X6
anti-infectives	T37.8X1	T37.8X2	T37.8X3	T37.8X4	T37.8X5	T37.8X6
formic iodide	T49.0X1	T49.0X2	T49.0X3	T49.0X4	T49.0X5	T49.0X6
glycolylarsenate	T49.0X1	T49.0X2	T49.0X3	T49.0X4	T49.0X5	T49.0X6
nonmedicinal (compounds) NEC	T65.91	T65.92	T65.93	T65.94	—	—
subcarbonate	T47.6X1	T47.6X2	T47.6X3	T47.6X4	T47.6X5	T47.6X6
subsalicylate	T37.8X1	T37.8X2	T37.8X3	T37.8X4	T37.8X5	T37.8X6
sulfarsphenamine	T37.8X1	T37.8X2	T37.8X3	T37.8X4	T37.8X5	T37.8X6
Bisoprolol	T44.7X1	T44.7X2	T44.7X3	T44.7X4	T44.7X5	T44.7X6
Bisoxatin	T47.2X1	T47.2X2	T47.2X3	T47.2X4	T47.2X5	T47.2X6
Bisulepin (hydrochloride)	T45.0X1	T45.0X2	T45.0X3	T45.0X4	T45.0X5	T45.0X6
Bithionol	T37.8X1	T37.8X2	T37.8X3	T37.8X4	T37.8X5	T37.8X6
anthelminthic	T37.4X1	T37.4X2	T37.4X3	T37.4X4	T37.4X5	T37.4X6
Bitolterol	T48.6X1	T48.6X2	T48.6X3	T48.6X4	T48.6X5	T48.6X6
Bitoscanate	T37.4X1	T37.4X2	T37.4X3	T37.4X4	T37.4X5	T37.4X6
Bitter almond oil	T62.8X1	T62.8X2	T62.8X3	T62.8X4	—	—
Bittersweet	T62.2X1	T62.2X2	T62.2X3	T62.2X4	—	—
Black						
flag	T60.91	T60.92	T60.93	T60.94	—	—
henbane	T62.2X1	T62.2X2	T62.2X3	T62.2X4	—	—
leaf (40)	T60.91	T60.92	T60.93	T60.94	—	—
widow spider (bite)	T63.311	T63.312	T63.313	T63.314	—	—
antivenin	T50.Z11	T50.Z12	T50.Z13	T50.Z14	T50.Z15	T50.Z16
Blast furnace gas (carbon monoxide from)	T58.8X1	T58.8X2	T58.8X3	T58.8X4	—	—
Bleach	T54.91	T54.92	T54.93	T54.94	—	—

◀ New ◀▥ Revised ~~deleted~~ Deleted

TABLE OF DRUGS AND CHEMICALS

Substance	External Cause (T-Code)					
	Poisoning, Accidental (Unintentional)	Poisoning, Intentional Self-Harm	Poisoning, Assault	Poisoning, Undetermined	Adverse Effect	Underdosing
Bleaching agent (medicinal)	T49.4X1	T49.4X2	T49.4X3	T49.4X4	T49.4X5	T49.4X6
Bleomycin	T45.1X1	T45.1X2	T45.1X3	T45.1X4	T45.1X5	T45.1X6
Blockain	T41.3X1	T41.3X2	T41.3X3	T41.3X4	T41.3X5	T41.3X6
infiltration (subcutaneous)	T41.3X1	T41.3X2	T41.3X3	T41.3X4	T41.3X5	T41.3X6
nerve block (peripheral) (plexus)	T41.3X1	T41.3X2	T41.3X3	T41.3X4	T41.3X5	T41.3X6
topical (surface)	T41.3X1	T41.3X2	T41.3X3	T41.3X4	T41.3X5	T41.3X6
Blockers, calcium channel	T46.1X1	T46.1X2	T46.1X3	T46.1X4	T46.1X5	T46.1X6
Blood (derivatives) (natural) (plasma) (whole)	T45.8X1	T45.8X2	T45.8X3	T45.8X4	T45.8X5	T45.8X6
dried	T45.8X1	T45.8X2	T45.8X3	T45.8X4	T45.8X5	T45.8X6
drug affecting NEC	T45.91	T45.92	T45.93	T45.94	T45.95	T45.96
expander NEC	T45.8X1	T45.8X2	T45.8X3	T45.8X4	T45.8X5	T45.8X6
fraction NEC	T45.8X1	T45.8X2	T45.8X3	T45.8X4	T45.8X5	T45.8X6
substitute (macromolecular)	T45.8X1	T45.8X2	T45.8X3	T45.8X4	T45.8X5	T45.8X6
Blue velvet	T40.2X1	T40.2X2	T40.2X3	T40.2X4	—	—
Bone meal	T62.8X1	T62.8X2	T62.8X3	T62.8X4	—	—
Bonine	T45.0X1	T45.0X2	T45.0X3	T45.0X4	T45.0X5	T45.0X6
Bopindolol	T44.7X1	T44.7X2	T44.7X3	T44.7X4	T44.7X5	T44.7X6
Boracic acid	T49.0X1	T49.0X2	T49.0X3	T49.0X4	T49.0X5	T49.0X6
ENT agent	T49.6X1	T49.6X2	T49.6X3	T49.6X4	T49.6X5	T49.6X6
ophthalmic preparation	T49.5X1	T49.5X2	T49.5X3	T49.5X4	T49.5X5	T49.5X6
Borane complex	T57.8X1	T57.8X2	T57.8X3	T57.8X4	—	—
Borate(s)	T57.8X1	T57.8X2	T57.8X3	T57.8X4	—	—
buffer	T50.991	T50.992	T50.993	T50.994	T50.995	T50.996
cleanser	T54.91	T54.92	T54.93	T54.94	—	—
sodium	T57.8X1	T57.8X2	T57.8X3	T57.8X4	—	—
Borax (cleanser)	T54.91	T54.92	T54.93	T54.94	—	—
Bordeaux mixture	T60.3X1	T60.3X2	T60.3X3	T60.3X4	—	—
Boric acid	T49.0X1	T49.0X2	T49.0X3	T49.0X4	T49.0X5	T49.0X6
ENT agent	T49.6X1	T49.6X2	T49.6X3	T49.6X4	T49.6X5	T49.6X6
ophthalmic preparation	T49.5X1	T49.5X2	T49.5X3	T49.5X4	T49.5X5	T49.5X6
Bornaprine	T44.3X1	T44.3X2	T44.3X3	T44.3X4	T44.3X5	T44.3X6
Boron	T57.8X1	T57.8X2	T57.8X3	T57.8X4	—	—
hydride NEC	T57.8X1	T57.8X2	T57.8X3	T57.8X4	—	—
fumes or gas	T57.8X1	T57.8X2	T57.8X3	T57.8X4	—	—
trifluoride	T59.891	T59.892	T59.893	T59.894	—	—
Botox	T48.291	T48.292	T48.293	T48.294	T48.295	T48.296
Botulinus anti-toxin (type A, B)	T50.Z11	T50.Z12	T50.Z13	T50.Z14	T50.Z15	T50.Z16
Brake fluid vapor	T59.891	T59.892	T59.893	T59.894	—	—
Brallobarbital	T42.3X1	T42.3X2	T42.3X3	T42.3X4	T42.3X5	T42.3X6
Bran (wheat)	T47.4X1	T47.4X2	T47.4X3	T47.4X4	T47.4X5	T47.4X6
Brass (fumes)	T56.891	T56.892	T56.893	T56.894	—	—

Substance	External Cause (T-Code)					
	Poisoning, Accidental (Unintentional)	Poisoning, Intentional Self-Harm	Poisoning, Assault	Poisoning, Undetermined	Adverse Effect	Underdosing
Brasso	T52.0X1	T52.0X2	T52.0X3	T52.0X4	—	—
Bretylium tosilate	T46.2X1	T46.2X2	T46.2X3	T46.2X4	T46.2X5	T46.2X6
Brevital (sodium)	T41.1X1	T41.1X2	T41.1X3	T41.1X4	T41.1X5	T41.1X6
Brinase	T45.3X1	T45.3X2	T45.3X3	T45.3X4	T45.3X5	T45.3X6
British antilewisite	T45.8X1	T45.8X2	T45.8X3	T45.8X4	T45.8X5	T45.8X6
Brodifacoum	T60.4X1	T60.4X2	T60.4X3	T60.4X4	—	—
Bromal (hydrate)	T42.6X1	T42.6X2	T42.6X3	T42.6X4	T42.6X5	T42.6X6
Bromazepam	T42.4X1	T42.4X2	T42.4X3	T42.4X4	T42.4X5	T42.4X6
Bromazine	T45.0X1	T45.0X2	T45.0X3	T45.0X4	T45.0X5	T45.0X6
Brombenzylcyanide	T59.3X1	T59.3X2	T59.3X3	T59.3X4	—	—
Bromelains	T45.3X1	T45.3X2	T45.3X3	T45.3X4	T45.3X5	T45.3X6
Bromethalin	T60.4X1	T60.4X2	T60.4X3	T60.4X4	—	—
Bromhexine	T48.4X1	T48.4X2	T48.4X3	T48.4X4	T48.4X5	T48.4X6
Bromide salts	T42.6X1	T42.6X2	T42.6X3	T42.6X4	T42.6X5	T42.6X6
Bromindione	T45.511	T45.512	T45.513	T45.514	T45.515	T45.516
Bromine						
compounds (medicinal)	T42.6X1	T42.6X2	T42.6X3	T42.6X4	T42.6X5	T42.6X6
sedative	T42.6X1	T42.6X2	T42.6X3	T42.6X4	T42.6X5	T42.6X6
vapor	T59.891	T59.892	T59.893	T59.894	—	—
Bromisovalum	T42.6X1	T42.6X2	T42.6X3	T42.6X4	T42.6X5	T42.6X6
Bromisoval	T42.6X1	T42.6X2	T42.6X3	T42.6X4	T42.6X5	T42.6X6
Bromobenzylcyanide	T59.3X1	T59.3X2	T59.3X3	T59.3X4	—	—
Bromochlorosalicylani-lide	T49.0X1	T49.0X2	T49.0X3	T49.0X4	T49.0X5	T49.0X6
Bromocriptine	T42.8X1	T42.8X2	T42.8X3	T42.8X4	T42.8X5	T42.8X6
Bromodiphenhydramine	T45.0X1	T45.0X2	T45.0X3	T45.0X4	T45.0X5	T45.0X6
Bromoform	T42.6X1	T42.6X2	T42.6X3	T42.6X4	T42.6X5	T42.6X6
Bromophenol blue reagent	T50.991	T50.992	T50.993	T50.994	T50.995	T50.996
Bromopride	T47.8X1	T47.8X2	T47.8X3	T47.8X4	T47.8X5	T47.8X6
Bromosalicylchloranitide	T49.0X1	T49.0X2	T49.0X3	T49.0X4	T49.0X5	T49.0X6
Bromosalicylhydroxamic acid	T37.1X1	T37.1X2	T37.1X3	T37.1X4	T37.1X5	T37.1X6
Bromo-seltzer	T39.1X1	T39.1X2	T39.1X3	T39.1X4	T39.1X5	T39.1X6
Bromoxynil	T60.3X1	T60.3X2	T60.3X3	T60.3X4	—	—
Bromperidol	T43.4X1	T43.4X2	T43.4X3	T43.4X4	T43.4X5	T43.4X6
Brompheniramine	T45.0X1	T45.0X2	T45.0X3	T45.0X4	T45.0X5	T45.0X6
Bromsulfophthalein	T50.8X1	T50.8X2	T50.8X3	T50.8X4	T50.8X5	T50.8X6
Bromural	T42.6X1	T42.6X2	T42.6X3	T42.6X4	T42.6X5	T42.6X6
Bromvaletone	T42.6X1	T42.6X2	T42.6X3	T42.6X4	T42.6X5	T42.6X6
Bronchodilator NEC	T48.6X1	T48.6X2	T48.6X3	T48.6X4	T48.6X5	T48.6X6
Brotizolam	T42.4X1	T42.4X2	T42.4X3	T42.4X4	T42.4X5	T42.4X6
Brovincamine	T46.7X1	T46.7X2	T46.7X3	T46.7X4	T46.7X5	T46.7X6
Brown spider (bite) (venom)	T63.391	T63.392	T63.393	T63.394	—	—

◀ New ◀ Revised ~~deleted~~ Deleted

Substance	Poisoning, Accidental (Unintentional)	Poisoning, Intentional Self-Harm	Poisoning, Assault	Poisoning, Undetermined	Adverse Effect	Underdosing
Brown recluse spider (bite) (venom)	T63.331	T63.332	T63.333	T63.334	—	—
Broxaterol	T48.6X1	T48.6X2	T48.6X3	T48.6X4	T48.6X5	T48.6X6
Broxuridine	T45.1X1	T45.1X2	T45.1X3	T45.1X4	T45.1X5	T45.1X6
Broxyquinoline	T37.8X1	T37.8X2	T37.8X3	T37.8X4	T37.8X5	T37.8X6
Bruceine	T48.291	T48.292	T48.293	T48.294	T48.295	T48.296
Brucia	T62.2X1	T62.2X2	T62.2X3	T62.2X4	—	—
Brucine	T65.1X1	T65.1X2	T65.1X3	T65.1X4	—	—
Brunswick green — see Copper						
Bruten — see Ibuprofen						
Bryonia	T47.2X1	T47.2X2	T47.2X3	T47.2X4	T47.2X5	T47.2X6
Buclizine	T45.0X1	T45.0X2	T45.0X3	T45.0X4	T45.0X5	T45.0X6
Buclosamide	T49.0X1	T49.0X2	T49.0X3	T49.0X4	T49.0X5	T49.0X6
Budesonide	T44.5X1	T44.5X2	T44.5X3	T44.5X4	T44.5X5	T44.5X6
Budralazine	T46.5X1	T46.5X2	T46.5X3	T46.5X4	T46.5X5	T46.5X6
Bufferin	T39.011	T39.012	T39.013	T39.014	T39.015	T39.016
Buflomedil	T46.7X1	T46.7X2	T46.7X3	T46.7X4	T46.7X5	T46.7X6
Buformin	T38.3X1	T38.3X2	T38.3X3	T38.3X4	T38.3X5	T38.3X6
Bufotenine	T40.991	T40.992	T40.993	T40.994	—	—
Bufrolin	T48.6X1	T48.6X2	T48.6X3	T48.6X4	T48.6X5	T48.6X6
Bufylline	T48.6X1	T48.6X2	T48.6X3	T48.6X4	T48.6X5	T48.6X6
Bulk filler	T50.5X1	T50.5X2	T50.5X3	T50.5X4	T50.5X5	T50.5X6
cathartic	T47.4X1	T47.4X2	T47.4X3	T47.4X4	T47.4X5	T47.4X6
Bumetanide	T50.1X1	T50.1X2	T50.1X3	T50.1X4	T50.1X5	T50.1X6
Bunaftine	T46.2X1	T46.2X2	T46.2X3	T46.2X4	T46.2X5	T46.2X6
Bunamiodyl	T50.8X1	T50.8X2	T50.8X3	T50.8X4	T50.8X5	T50.8X6
Bunazosin	T44.6X1	T44.6X2	T44.6X3	T44.6X4	T44.6X5	T44.6X6
Bunitrolol	T44.7X1	T44.7X2	T44.7X3	T44.7X4	T44.7X5	T44.7X6
Buphenine	T46.7X1	T46.7X2	T46.7X3	T46.7X4	T46.7X5	T46.7X6
Bupivacaine	T41.3X1	T41.3X2	T41.3X3	T41.3X4	T41.3X5	T41.3X6
infiltration (subcutaneous)	T41.3X1	T41.3X2	T41.3X3	T41.3X4	T41.3X5	T41.3X6
nerve block (peripheral) (plexus)	T41.3X1	T41.3X2	T41.3X3	T41.3X4	T41.3X5	T41.3X6
spinal	T41.3X1	T41.3X2	T41.3X3	T41.3X4	T41.3X5	T41.3X6
Bupranolol	T44.7X1	T44.7X2	T44.7X3	T44.7X4	T44.7X5	T44.7X6
Buprenorphine	T40.4X1	T40.4X2	T40.4X3	T40.4X4	T40.4X5	T40.4X6
Bupropion	T43.291	T43.292	T43.293	T43.294	T43.295	T43.296
Burimamide	T47.1X1	T47.1X2	T47.1X3	T47.1X4	T47.1X5	T47.1X6
Buserelin	T38.891	T38.892	T38.893	T38.894	T38.895	T38.896
Buspirone	T43.591	T43.592	T43.593	T43.594	T43.595	T43.596
Busulfan, busulphan	T45.1X1	T45.1X2	T45.1X3	T45.1X4	T45.1X5	T45.1X6
Butabarbital (sodium)	T42.3X1	T42.3X2	T42.3X3	T42.3X4	T42.3X5	T42.3X6
Butabarbitone	T42.3X1	T42.3X2	T42.3X3	T42.3X4	T42.3X5	T42.3X6

Substance	Poisoning, Accidental (Unintentional)	Poisoning, Intentional Self-Harm	Poisoning, Assault	Poisoning, Undetermined	Adverse Effect	Underdosing
Butabarpal	T42.3X1	T42.3X2	T42.3X3	T42.3X4	T42.3X5	T42.3X6
Butacaine	T41.3X1	T41.3X2	T41.3X3	T41.3X4	T41.3X5	T41.3X6
Butalamine	T46.7X1	T46.7X2	T46.7X3	T46.7X4	T46.7X5	T46.7X6
Butalbital	T42.3X1	T42.3X2	T42.3X3	T42.3X4	T42.3X5	T42.3X6
Butallylonal	T42.3X1	T42.3X2	T42.3X3	T42.3X4	T42.3X5	T42.3X6
Butamben	T41.3X1	T41.3X2	T41.3X3	T41.3X4	T41.3X5	T41.3X6
Butamirate	T48.3X1	T48.3X2	T48.3X3	T48.3X4	T48.3X5	T48.3X6
Butane (distributed in mobile container)	T59.891	T59.892	T59.893	T59.894	—	—
distributed through pipes	T59.891	T59.892	T59.893	T59.894	—	—
incomplete combustion	T58.11	T58.12	T58.13	T58.14	—	—
Butanilicaine	T41.3X1	T41.3X2	T41.3X3	T41.3X4	T41.3X5	T41.3X6
Butanol	T51.3X1	T51.3X2	T51.3X3	T51.3X4		
Butanone, 2-butanone	T52.4X1	T52.4X2	T52.4X3	T52.4X4	—	—
Butantrone	T49.4X1	T49.4X2	T49.4X3	T49.4X4	T49.4X5	T49.4X6
Butaperazine	T43.3X1	T43.3X2	T43.3X3	T43.3X4	T43.3X5	T43.3X6
Butazolidin	T39.2X1	T39.2X2	T39.2X3	T39.2X4	T39.2X5	T39.2X6
Butetamate	T48.6X1	T48.6X2	T48.6X3	T48.6X4	T48.6X5	T48.6X6
Butethal	T42.3X1	T42.3X2	T42.3X3	T42.3X4	T42.3X5	T42.3X6
Butethamate	T44.3X1	T44.3X2	T44.3X3	T44.3X4	T44.3X5	T44.3X6
Buthalitone (sodium)	T41.1X1	T41.1X2	T41.1X3	T41.1X4	T41.1X5	T41.1X6
Butisol (sodium)	T42.3X1	T42.3X2	T42.3X3	T42.3X4	T42.3X5	T42.3X6
Butizide	T50.2X1	T50.2X2	T50.2X3	T50.2X4	T50.2X5	T50.2X6
Butobarbital	T42.3X1	T42.3X2	T42.3X3	T42.3X4	T42.3X5	T42.3X6
sodium	T42.3X1	T42.3X2	T42.3X3	T42.3X4	T42.3X5	T42.3X6
Butobarbitone	T42.3X1	T42.3X2	T42.3X3	T42.3X4	T42.3X5	T42.3X6
Butoconazole (nitrate)	T49.0X1	T49.0X2	T49.0X3	T49.0X4	T49.0X5	T49.0X6
Butorphanol	T40.4X1	T40.4X2	T40.4X3	T40.4X4	T40.4X5	T40.4X6
Butriptyline	T43.011	T43.012	T43.013	T43.014	T43.015	T43.016
Butropium bromide	T44.3X1	T44.3X2	T44.3X3	T44.3X4	T44.3X5	T44.3X6
Buttercups	T62.2X1	T62.2X2	T62.2X3	T62.2X4	—	—
Butter of antimony — see Antimony						
Butyl						
acetate (secondary)	T52.8X1	T52.8X2	T52.8X3	T52.8X4	—	—
alcohol	T51.3X1	T51.3X2	T51.3X3	T51.3X4		
aminobenzoate	T41.3X1	T41.3X2	T41.3X3	T41.3X4	T41.3X5	T41.3X6
butyrate	T52.8X1	T52.8X2	T52.8X3	T52.8X4	—	—
carbinol	T51.3X1	T51.3X2	T51.3X3	T51.3X4		
carbitol	T52.3X1	T52.3X2	T52.3X3	T52.3X4	—	—
cellosolve	T52.3X1	T52.3X2	T52.3X3	T52.3X4	—	—
chloral (hydrate)	T42.6X1	T42.6X2	T42.6X3	T42.6X4	T42.6X5	T42.6X6
formate	T52.8X1	T52.8X2	T52.8X3	T52.8X4	—	—

Substance	External Cause (T-Code) Poisoning, Accidental (Unintentional)	Poisoning, Intentional Self-Harm	Poisoning, Assault	Poisoning, Undetermined	Adverse Effect	Underdosing
Butyl *(Continued)*						
lactate	T52.8X1	T52.8X2	T52.8X3	T52.8X4	—	—
propionate	T52.8X1	T52.8X2	T52.8X3	T52.8X4	—	—
scopolamine bromide	T44.3X1	T44.3X2	T44.3X3	T44.3X4	T44.3X5	T44.3X6
thiobarbital sodium	T41.1X1	T41.1X2	T41.1X3	T41.1X4	T41.1X5	T41.1X6
Butylated hydroxy-anisole	T50.991	T50.992	T50.993	T50.994	T50.995	T50.996
Butylchloral hydrate	T42.6X1	T42.6X2	T42.6X3	T42.6X4	T42.6X5	T42.6X6
Butyltoluene	T52.2X1	T52.2X2	T52.2X3	T52.2X4	—	—
Butyn	T41.3X1	T41.3X2	T41.3X3	T41.3X4	T41.3X5	T41.3X6
Butyrophenone (-based tranquilizers)	T43.4X1	T43.4X2	T43.4X3	T43.4X4	T43.4X5	T43.4X6
C						
Cabergoline	T42.8X1	T42.8X2	T42.8X3	T42.8X4	T42.8X5	T42.8X6
Cacodyl, cacodylic acid	T57.0X1	T57.0X2	T57.0X3	T57.0X4	—	—
Cactinomycin	T45.1X1	T45.1X2	T45.1X3	T45.1X4	T45.1X5	T45.1X6
Cade oil	T49.4X1	T49.4X2	T49.4X3	T49.4X4	T49.4X5	T49.4X6
Cadexomer iodine	T49.0X1	T49.0X2	T49.0X3	T49.0X4	T49.0X5	T49.0X6
Cadmium (chloride) (fumes) (oxide)	T56.3X1	T56.3X2	T56.3X3	T56.3X4	—	—
sulfide (medicinal) NEC	T49.4X1	T49.4X2	T49.4X3	T49.4X4	T49.4X5	T49.4X6
Cadralazine	T46.5X1	T46.5X2	T46.5X3	T46.5X4	T46.5X5	T46.5X6
Caffeine	T43.611	T43.612	T43.613	T43.614	T43.615	T43.616
Calabar bean	T62.2X1	T62.2X2	T62.2X3	T62.2X4	—	—
Caladium seguinum	T62.2X1	T62.2X2	T62.2X3	T62.2X4	—	—
Calamine (lotion)	T49.3X1	T49.3X2	T49.3X3	T49.3X4	T49.3X5	T49.3X6
Calcifediol	T45.2X1	T45.2X2	T45.2X3	T45.2X4	T45.2X5	T45.2X6
Calciferol	T45.2X1	T45.2X2	T45.2X3	T45.2X4	T45.2X5	T45.2X6
Calcitonin	T50.991	T50.992	T50.993	T50.994	T50.995	T50.996
Calcitriol	T45.2X1	T45.2X2	T45.2X3	T45.2X4	T45.2X5	T45.2X6
Calcium	T50.3X1	T50.3X2	T50.3X3	T50.3X4	T50.3X5	T50.3X6
actylsalicylate	T39.011	T39.012	T39.013	T39.014	T39.015	T39.016
benzamidosalicylate	T37.1X1	T37.1X2	T37.1X3	T37.1X4	T37.1X5	T37.1X6
bromide	T42.6X1	T42.6X2	T42.6X3	T42.6X4	T42.6X5	T42.6X6
bromolactobionate	T42.6X1	T42.6X2	T42.6X3	T42.6X4	T42.6X5	T42.6X6
carbaspirin	T39.011	T39.012	T39.013	T39.014	T39.015	T39.016
carbimide	T50.6X1	T50.6X2	T50.6X3	T50.6X4	T50.6X5	T50.6X6
carbonate	T47.1X1	T47.1X2	T47.1X3	T47.1X4	T47.1X5	T47.1X6
chloride	T50.991	T50.992	T50.993	T50.994	T50.995	T50.996
anhydrous	T50.991	T50.992	T50.993	T50.994	T50.995	T50.996
cyanide	T57.8X1	T57.8X2	T57.8X3	T57.8X4	—	—
dioctyl sulfosuccinate	T47.4X1	T47.4X2	T47.4X3	T47.4X4	T47.4X5	T47.4X6
disodium edathamil	T45.8X1	T45.8X2	T45.8X3	T45.8X4	T45.8X5	T45.8X6

Substance	External Cause (T-Code) Poisoning, Accidental (Unintentional)	Poisoning, Intentional Self-Harm	Poisoning, Assault	Poisoning, Undetermined	Adverse Effect	Underdosing
Calcium *(Continued)*						
disodium edetate	T45.8X1	T45.8X2	T45.8X3	T45.8X4	T45.8X5	T45.8X6
dobesilate	T46.991	T46.992	T46.993	T46.994	T46.995	T46.996
EDTA	T45.8X1	T45.8X2	T45.8X3	T45.8X4	T45.8X5	T45.8X6
ferrous citrate	T45.4X1	T45.4X2	T45.4X3	T45.4X4	T45.4X5	T45.4X6
folinate	T45.8X1	T45.8X2	T45.8X3	T45.8X4	T45.8X5	T45.8X6
glubionate	T50.3X1	T50.3X2	T50.3X3	T50.3X4	T50.3X5	T50.3X6
gluconate	T50.3X1	T50.3X2	T50.3X3	T50.3X4	T50.3X5	T50.3X6
gluconogalactogluconate	T50.3X1	T50.3X2	T50.3X3	T50.3X4	T50.3X5	T50.3X6
hydrate, hydroxide	T54.3X1	T54.3X2	T54.3X3	T54.3X4	—	—
hypochlorite	T54.3X1	T54.3X2	T54.3X3	T54.3X4	—	—
iodide	T48.4X1	T48.4X2	T48.4X3	T48.4X4	T48.4X5	T48.4X6
ipodate	T50.8X1	T50.8X2	T50.8X3	T50.8X4	T50.8X5	T50.8X6
lactate	T50.3X1	T50.3X2	T50.3X3	T50.3X4	T50.3X5	T50.3X6
leucovorin	T45.8X1	T45.8X2	T45.8X3	T45.8X4	T45.8X5	T45.8X6
mandelate	T37.91	T37.92	T37.93	T37.94	T37.95	T37.96
oxide	T54.3X1	T54.3X2	T54.3X3	T54.3X4	—	—
pantothenate	T45.2X1	T45.2X2	T45.2X3	T45.2X4	T45.2X5	T45.2X6
phosphate	T50.3X1	T50.3X2	T50.3X3	T50.3X4	T50.3X5	T50.3X6
salicylate	T39.091	T39.092	T39.093	T39.094	T39.095	T39.096
salts	T50.3X1	T50.3X2	T50.3X3	T50.3X4	T50.3X5	T50.3X6
Calculus-dissolving drug	T50.991	T50.992	T50.993	T50.994	T50.995	T50.996
Calomel	T49.0X1	T49.0X2	T49.0X3	T49.0X4	T49.0X5	T49.0X6
Caloric agent	T50.3X1	T50.3X2	T50.3X3	T50.3X4	T50.3X5	T50.3X6
Calusterone	T38.7X1	T38.7X2	T38.7X3	T38.7X4	T38.7X5	T38.7X6
Camazepam	T42.4X1	T42.4X2	T42.4X3	T42.4X4	T42.4X5	T42.4X6
Camomile	T49.0X1	T49.0X2	T49.0X3	T49.0X4	T49.0X5	T49.0X6
Camoquin	T37.2X1	T37.2X2	T37.2X3	T37.2X4	T37.2X5	T37.2X6
Camphor						
insecticide	T60.2X1	T60.2X2	T60.2X3	T60.2X4	—	—
medicinal	T49.8X1	T49.8X2	T49.8X3	T49.8X4	T49.8X5	T49.8X6
Camylofin	T44.3X1	T44.3X2	T44.3X3	T44.3X4	T44.3X5	T44.3X6
Cancer chemotherapy drug regimen	T45.1X1	T45.1X2	T45.1X3	T45.1X4	T45.1X5	T45.1X6
Candeptin	T49.0X1	T49.0X2	T49.0X3	T49.0X4	T49.0X5	T49.0X6
Candicidin	T49.0X1	T49.0X2	T49.0X3	T49.0X4	T49.0X5	T49.0X6
Cannabinol	T40.7X1	T40.7X2	T40.7X3	T40.7X4	T40.7X5	T40.7X6
Cannabis (derivatives)	T40.7X1	T40.7X2	T40.7X3	T40.7X4	T40.7X5	T40.7X6
Canned heat	T51.1X1	T51.1X2	T51.1X3	T51.1X4	—	—
Canrenoic acid	T50.0X1	T50.0X2	T50.0X3	T50.0X4	T50.0X5	T50.0X6
Canrenone	T50.0X1	T50.0X2	T50.0X3	T50.0X4	T50.0X5	T50.0X6
Cantharides, cantharidin, cantharis	T49.8X1	T49.8X2	T49.8X3	T49.8X4	T49.8X5	T49.8X6

◀ New ◀ Revised ~~deleted~~ Deleted

Substance	Poisoning, Accidental (Unintentional)	Poisoning, Intentional Self-Harm	Poisoning, Assault	Poisoning, Undetermined	Adverse Effect	Underdosing
Canthaxanthin	T50.991	T50.992	T50.993	T50.994	T50.995	T50.996
Capillary-active drug NEC	T46.901	T46.902	T46.903	T46.904	T46.905	T46.906
Capreomycin	T36.8X1	T36.8X2	T36.8X3	T36.8X4	T36.8X5	T36.8X6
Capsicum	T49.4X1	T49.4X2	T49.4X3	T49.4X4	T49.4X5	T49.4X6
Captafol	T60.3X1	T60.3X2	T60.3X3	T60.3X4	—	—
Captan	T60.3X1	T60.3X2	T60.3X3	T60.3X4	—	—
Captodiame, captodiamine	T43.591	T43.592	T43.593	T43.594	T43.595	T43.596
Captopril	T46.4X1	T46.4X2	T46.4X3	T46.4X4	T46.4X5	T46.4X6
Caramiphen	T44.3X1	T44.3X2	T44.3X3	T44.3X4	T44.3X5	T44.3X6
Carazolol	T44.7X1	T44.7X2	T44.7X3	T44.7X4	T44.7X5	T44.7X6
Carbachol	T44.1X1	T44.1X2	T44.1X3	T44.1X4	T44.1X5	T44.1X6
Carbacrylamine (resin)	T50.3X1	T50.3X2	T50.3X3	T50.3X4	T50.3X5	T50.3X6
Carbamate (insecticide)	T60.0X1	T60.0X2	T60.0X3	T60.0X4	—	—
Carbamate (sedative)	T42.6X1	T42.6X2	T42.6X3	T42.6X4	T42.6X5	T42.6X6
herbicide	T60.0X1	T60.0X2	T60.0X3	T60.0X4	—	—
insecticide	T60.0X1	T60.0X2	T60.0X3	T60.0X4	—	—
Carbamazepine	T42.1X1	T42.1X2	T42.1X3	T42.1X4	T42.1X5	T42.1X6
Carbamide	T47.3X1	T47.3X2	T47.3X3	T47.3X4	T47.3X5	T47.3X6
peroxide	T49.0X1	T49.0X2	T49.0X3	T49.0X4	T49.0X5	T49.0X6
topical	T49.8X1	T49.8X2	T49.8X3	T49.8X4	T49.8X5	T49.8X6
Carbamylcholine chloride	T44.1X1	T44.1X2	T44.1X3	T44.1X4	T44.1X5	T44.1X6
Carbaril	T60.0X1	T60.0X2	T60.0X3	T60.0X4	—	—
Carbarsone	T37.3X1	T37.3X2	T37.3X3	T37.3X4	T37.3X5	T37.3X6
Carbaryl	T60.0X1	T60.0X2	T60.0X3	T60.0X4	—	—
Carbaspirin	T39.011	T39.012	T39.013	T39.014	T39.015	T39.016
Carbazochrome (salicylate) (sodium sulfonate)	T49.4X1	T49.4X2	T49.4X3	T49.4X4	T49.4X5	T49.4X6
Carbenicillin	T36.0X1	T36.0X2	T36.0X3	T36.0X4	T36.0X5	T36.0X6
Carbenoxolone	T47.1X1	T47.1X2	T47.1X3	T47.1X4	T47.1X5	T47.1X6
Carbetapentane	T48.3X1	T48.3X2	T48.3X3	T48.3X4	T48.3X5	T48.3X6
Carbethyl salicylate	T39.091	T39.092	T39.093	T39.094	T39.095	T39.096
Carbidopa (with levodopa)	T42.8X1	T42.8X2	T42.8X3	T42.8X4	T42.8X5	T42.8X6
Carbimazole	T38.2X1	T38.2X2	T38.2X3	T38.2X4	T38.2X5	T38.2X6
Carbinol	T51.1X1	T51.1X2	T51.1X3	T51.1X4	—	—
Carbinoxamine	T45.0X1	T45.0X2	T45.0X3	T45.0X4	T45.0X5	T45.0X6
Carbiphene	T39.8X1	T39.8X2	T39.8X3	T39.8X4	T39.8X5	T39.8X6
Carbitol	T52.3X1	T52.3X2	T52.3X3	T52.3X4	—	—
Carbocaine	T41.3X1	T41.3X2	T41.3X3	T41.3X4	T41.3X5	T41.3X6
infiltration (subcutaneous)	T41.3X1	T41.3X2	T41.3X3	T41.3X4	T41.3X5	T41.3X6
nerve block (peripheral) (plexus)	T41.3X1	T41.3X2	T41.3X3	T41.3X4	T41.3X5	T41.3X6
topical (surface)	T41.3X1	T41.3X2	T41.3X3	T41.3X4	T41.3X5	T41.3X6
Carbo medicinalis	T47.6X1	T47.6X2	T47.6X3	T47.6X4	T47.6X5	T47.6X6

Substance	Poisoning, Accidental (Unintentional)	Poisoning, Intentional Self-Harm	Poisoning, Assault	Poisoning, Undetermined	Adverse Effect	Underdosing
Carbomycin	T36.8X1	T36.8X2	T36.8X3	T36.8X4	T36.8X5	T36.8X6
Carbocisteine	T48.4X1	T48.4X2	T48.4X3	T48.4X4	T48.4X5	T48.4X6
Carbocromen	T46.3X1	T46.3X2	T46.3X3	T46.3X4	T46.3X5	T46.3X6
Carbol fuchsin	T49.0X1	T49.0X2	T49.0X3	T49.0X4	T49.0X5	T49.0X6
Carbolic acid — *see also* Phenol	T54.0X1	T54.0X2	T54.0X3	T54.0X4	—	—
Carbolonium (bromide)	T48.1X1	T48.1X2	T48.1X3	T48.1X4	T48.1X5	T48.1X6
Carbon						
bisulfide (liquid)	T65.4X1	T65.4X2	T65.4X3	T65.4X4	—	—
vapor	T65.4X1	T65.4X2	T65.4X3	T65.4X4	—	—
dioxide (gas)	T59.7X1	T59.7X2	T59.7X3	T59.7X4	—	—
medicinal	T41.5X1	T41.5X2	T41.5X3	T41.5X4	T41.5X5	T41.5X6
nonmedicinal	T59.7X1	T59.7X2	T59.7X3	T59.7X4	—	—
snow	T49.4X1	T49.4X2	T49.4X3	T49.4X4	T49.4X5	T49.4X6
disulfide (liquid)	T65.4X1	T65.4X2	T65.4X3	T65.4X4	—	—
vapor	T65.4X1	T65.4X2	T65.4X3	T65.4X4	—	—
monoxide (from incomplete combustion)	T58.91	T58.92	T58.93	T58.94	—	—
blast furnace gas	T58.8X1	T58.8X2	T58.8X3	T58.8X4	—	—
butane (distributed in mobile container)	T58.11	T58.12	T58.13	T58.14	—	—
distributed through pipes	T58.11	T58.12	T58.13	T58.14	—	—
charcoal fumes	T58.2X1	T58.2X2	T58.2X3	T58.2X4	—	—
coal	T58.2X1	T58.2X2	T58.2X3	T58.2X4	—	—
coke (in domestic stoves, fireplaces)	T58.2X1	T58.2X2	T58.2X3	T58.2X4	—	—
gas (piped)	T58.11	T58.12	T58.13	T58.14	—	—
solid (in domestic stoves, fireplaces)	T58.2X1	T58.2X2	T58.2X3	T58.2X4	—	—
exhaust gas (motor) not in transit	T58.01	T58.02	T58.03	T58.04	—	—
combustion engine, any not in watercraft	T58.01	T58.02	T58.03	T58.04	—	—
farm tractor, not in transit	T58.01	T58.02	T58.03	T58.04	—	—
gas engine	T58.01	T58.02	T58.03	T58.04	—	—
motor pump	T58.01	T58.02	T58.03	T58.04	—	—
motor vehicle, not in transit	T58.01	T58.02	T58.03	T58.04	—	—
fuel (in domestic use)	T58.2X1	T58.2X2	T58.2X3	T58.2X4	—	—
gas (piped)	T58.11	T58.12	T58.13	T58.14	—	—
in mobile container	T58.11	T58.12	T58.13	T58.14	—	—
utility	T58.11	T58.12	T58.13	T58.14	—	—
in mobile container	T58.11	T58.12	T58.13	T58.14	—	—
piped (natural)	T58.11	T58.12	T58.13	T58.14	—	—

◀ New   ◀▥ Revised   ~~deleted~~ Deleted

TABLE OF DRUGS AND CHEMICALS

TABLE OF DRUGS AND CHEMICALS

Substance	External Cause (T-Code)					
	Poisoning, Accidental (Unintentional)	Poisoning, Intentional Self-Harm	Poisoning, Assault	Poisoning, Undetermined	Adverse Effect	Underdosing
Carbon *(Continued)*						
monoxide *(Continued)*						
illuminating gas	T58.11	T58.12	T58.13	T58.14	—	—
industrial fuels or gases, any	T58.8X1	T58.8X2	T58.8X3	T58.8X4	—	—
kerosene (in domestic stoves, fireplaces)	T58.2X1	T58.2X2	T58.2X3	T58.2X4	—	—
kiln gas or vapor	T58.8X1	T58.8X2	T58.8X3	T58.8X4	—	—
motor exhaust gas, not in transit	T58.01	T58.02	T58.03	T58.04	—	—
piped gas (manufactured) (natural)	T58.11	T58.12	T58.13	T58.14	—	—
producer gas	T58.8X1	T58.8X2	T58.8X3	T58.8X4	—	—
propane (distributed in mobile container)	T58.11	T58.12	T58.13	T58.14	—	—
distributed through pipes	T58.11	T58.12	T58.13	T58.14	—	—
specified source NEC	T58.8X1	T58.8X2	T58.8X3	T58.8X4	—	—
stove gas	T58.11	T58.12	T58.13	T58.14	—	—
piped	T58.11	T58.12	T58.13	T58.14	—	—
utility gas	T58.11	T58.12	T58.13	T58.14	—	—
piped	T58.11	T58.12	T58.13	T58.14	—	—
water gas	T58.11	T58.12	T58.13	T58.14	—	—
wood (in domestic stoves, fireplaces)	T58.2X1	T58.2X2	T58.2X3	T58.2X4	—	—
tetrachloride (vapor) NEC	T53.0X1	T53.0X2	T53.0X3	T53.0X4	—	—
liquid (cleansing agent) NEC	T53.0X1	T53.0X2	T53.0X3	T53.0X4	—	—
solvent	T53.0X1	T53.0X2	T53.0X3	T53.0X4	—	—
Carbonic acid gas	T59.7X1	T59.7X2	T59.7X3	T59.7X4	—	—
anhydrase inhibitor NEC	T50.2X1	T50.2X2	T50.2X3	T50.2X4	T50.2X5	T50.2X6
Carbophenothion	T60.0X1	T60.0X2	T60.0X3	T60.0X4		
Carboplatin	T45.1X1	T45.1X2	T45.1X3	T45.1X4	T45.1X5	T45.1X6
Carboprost	T48.0X1	T48.0X2	T48.0X3	T48.0X4	T48.0X5	T48.0X6
Carboquone	T45.1X1	T45.1X2	T45.1X3	T45.1X4	T45.1X5	T45.1X6
Carbowax	T49.3X1	T49.3X2	T49.3X3	T49.3X4	T49.3X5	T49.3X6
Carboxymethyl-cellulose	T47.4X1	T47.4X2	T47.4X3	T47.4X4	T47.4X5	T47.4X6
S-Carboxymethyl-cysteine	T48.4X1	T48.4X2	T48.4X3	T48.4X4	T48.4X5	T48.4X6
Carbrital	T42.3X1	T42.3X2	T42.3X3	T42.3X4	T42.3X5	T42.3X6
Carbromal	T42.6X1	T42.6X2	T42.6X3	T42.6X4	T42.6X5	T42.6X6
Carbutamide	T38.3X1	T38.3X2	T38.3X3	T38.3X4	T38.3X5	T38.3X6
Carbuterol	T48.6X1	T48.6X2	T48.6X3	T48.6X4	T48.6X5	T48.6X6
Cardiac						
depressants	T46.2X1	T46.2X2	T46.2X3	T46.2X4	T46.2X5	T46.2X6
rhythm regulator	T46.2X1	T46.2X2	T46.2X3	T46.2X4	T46.2X5	T46.2X6
specified NEC	T46.2X1	T46.2X2	T46.2X3	T46.2X4	T46.2X5	T46.2X6

Substance	External Cause (T-Code)					
	Poisoning, Accidental (Unintentional)	Poisoning, Intentional Self-Harm	Poisoning, Assault	Poisoning, Undetermined	Adverse Effect	Underdosing
Cardiografin	T50.8X1	T50.8X2	T50.8X3	T50.8X4	T50.8X5	T50.8X6
Cardio-green	T50.8X1	T50.8X2	T50.8X3	T50.8X4	T50.8X5	T50.8X6
Cardiotonic (glycoside) NEC	T46.0X1	T46.0X2	T46.0X3	T46.0X4	T46.0X5	T46.0X6
Cardiovascular drug NEC	T46.901	T46.902	T46.903	T46.904	T46.905	T46.906
Cardrase	T50.2X1	T50.2X2	T50.2X3	T50.2X4	T50.2X5	T50.2X6
Carfusin	T49.0X1	T49.0X2	T49.0X3	T49.0X4	T49.0X5	T49.0X6
Carfecillin	T36.0X1	T36.0X2	T36.0X3	T36.0X4	T36.0X5	T36.0X6
Carfenazine	T43.3X1	T43.3X2	T43.3X3	T43.3X4	T43.3X5	T43.3X6
Carindacillin	T36.0X1	T36.0X2	T36.0X3	T36.0X4	T36.0X5	T36.0X6
Carisoprodol	T42.8X1	T42.8X2	T42.8X3	T42.8X4	T42.8X5	T42.8X6
Carmellose	T47.4X1	T47.4X2	T47.4X3	T47.4X4	T47.4X5	T47.4X6
Carminative	T47.5X1	T47.5X2	T47.5X3	T47.5X4	T47.5X5	T47.5X6
Carmofur	T45.1X1	T45.1X2	T45.1X3	T45.1X4	T45.1X5	T45.1X6
Carmustine	T45.1X1	T45.1X2	T45.1X3	T45.1X4	T45.1X5	T45.1X6
Carotene	T45.2X1	T45.2X2	T45.2X3	T45.2X4	T45.2X5	T45.2X6
Carphenazine	T43.3X1	T43.3X2	T43.3X3	T43.3X4	T43.3X5	T43.3X6
Carpipramine	T42.4X1	T42.4X2	T42.4X3	T42.4X4	T42.4X5	T42.4X6
Carprofen	T39.311	T39.312	T39.313	T39.314	T39.315	T39.316
Carpronium chloride	T44.3X1	T44.3X2	T44.3X3	T44.3X4	T44.3X5	T44.3X6
Carrageenan	T47.8X1	T47.8X2	T47.8X3	T47.8X4	T47.8X5	T47.8X6
Carteolol	T44.7X1	T44.7X2	T44.7X3	T44.7X4	T44.7X5	T44.7X6
Carter's Little Pills	T47.2X1	T47.2X2	T47.2X3	T47.2X4	T47.2X5	T47.2X6
Cascara (sagrada)	T47.2X1	T47.2X2	T47.2X3	T47.2X4	T47.2X5	T47.2X6
Cassava	T62.2X1	T62.2X2	T62.2X3	T62.2X4	—	—
Castellani's paint	T49.0X1	T49.0X2	T49.0X3	T49.0X4	T49.0X5	T49.0X6
Castor						
bean	T62.2X1	T62.2X2	T62.2X3	T62.2X4	—	—
oil	T47.2X1	T47.2X2	T47.2X3	T47.2X4	T47.2X5	T47.2X6
Catalase	T45.3X1	T45.3X2	T45.3X3	T45.3X4	T45.3X5	T45.3X6
Caterpillar (sting)	T63.431	T63.432	T63.433	T63.434	—	—
Catha (edulis) (tea)	T43.691	T43.692	T43.693	T43.694	—	—
Cathartic NEC	T47.4X1	T47.4X2	T47.4X3	T47.4X4	T47.4X5	T47.4X6
anthacene derivative	T47.2X1	T47.2X2	T47.2X3	T47.2X4	T47.2X5	T47.2X6
bulk	T47.4X1	T47.4X2	T47.4X3	T47.4X4	T47.4X5	T47.4X6
contact	T47.2X1	T47.2X2	T47.2X3	T47.2X4	T47.2X5	T47.2X6
emollient NEC	T47.4X1	T47.4X2	T47.4X3	T47.4X4	T47.4X5	T47.4X6
irritant NEC	T47.2X1	T47.2X2	T47.2X3	T47.2X4	T47.2X5	T47.2X6
mucilage	T47.4X1	T47.4X2	T47.4X3	T47.4X4	T47.4X5	T47.4X6
saline	T47.3X1	T47.3X2	T47.3X3	T47.3X4	T47.3X5	T47.3X6
vegetable	T47.2X1	T47.2X2	T47.2X3	T47.2X4	T47.2X5	T47.2X6
Cathine	T50.5X1	T50.5X2	T50.5X3	T50.5X4	T50.5X5	T50.5X6
Cathomycin	T36.8X1	T36.8X2	T36.8X3	T36.8X4	T36.8X5	T36.8X6

◀ New ◀ Revised ~~deleted~~ Deleted

Substance	Poisoning, Accidental (Unintentional)	Poisoning, Intentional Self-Harm	Poisoning, Assault	Poisoning, Undetermined	Adverse Effect	Underdosing
Cation exchange resin	T50.3X1	T50.3X2	T50.3X3	T50.3X4	T50.3X5	T50.3X6
Caustic(s) NEC	T54.91	T54.92	T54.93	T54.94	—	—
alkali	T54.3X1	T54.3X2	T54.3X3	T54.3X4	—	—
hydroxide	T54.3X1	T54.3X2	T54.3X3	T54.3X4	—	—
potash	T54.3X1	T54.3X2	T54.3X3	T54.3X4	—	—
soda	T54.3X1	T54.3X2	T54.3X3	T54.3X4	—	—
specified NEC	T54.91	T54.92	T54.93	T54.94	—	—
Ceepryn	T49.0X1	T49.0X2	T49.0X3	T49.0X4	T49.0X5	T49.0X6
ENT agent	T49.6X1	T49.6X2	T49.6X3	T49.6X4	T49.6X5	T49.6X6
lozenges	T49.6X1	T49.6X2	T49.6X3	T49.6X4	T49.6X5	T49.6X6
Cefacetrile	T36.1X1	T36.1X2	T36.1X3	T36.1X4	T36.1X5	T36.1X6
Cefaclor	T36.1X1	T36.1X2	T36.1X3	T36.1X4	T36.1X5	T36.1X6
Cefadroxil	T36.1X1	T36.1X2	T36.1X3	T36.1X4	T36.1X5	T36.1X6
Cefalexin	T36.1X1	T36.1X2	T36.1X3	T36.1X4	T36.1X5	T36.1X6
Cefaloglycin	T36.1X1	T36.1X2	T36.1X3	T36.1X4	T36.1X5	T36.1X6
Cefaloridine	T36.1X1	T36.1X2	T36.1X3	T36.1X4	T36.1X5	T36.1X6
Cefalosporins	T36.1X1	T36.1X2	T36.1X3	T36.1X4	T36.1X5	T36.1X6
Cefalotin	T36.1X1	T36.1X2	T36.1X3	T36.1X4	T36.1X5	T36.1X6
Cefamandole	T36.1X1	T36.1X2	T36.1X3	T36.1X4	T36.1X5	T36.1X6
Cefamycin antibiotic	T36.1X1	T36.1X2	T36.1X3	T36.1X4	T36.1X5	T36.1X6
Cefapirin	T36.1X1	T36.1X2	T36.1X3	T36.1X4	T36.1X5	T36.1X6
Cefatrizine	T36.1X1	T36.1X2	T36.1X3	T36.1X4	T36.1X5	T36.1X6
Cefazedone	T36.1X1	T36.1X2	T36.1X3	T36.1X4	T36.1X5	T36.1X6
Cefazolin	T36.1X1	T36.1X2	T36.1X3	T36.1X4	T36.1X5	T36.1X6
Cefbuperazone	T36.1X1	T36.1X2	T36.1X3	T36.1X4	T36.1X5	T36.1X6
Cefetamet	T36.1X1	T36.1X2	T36.1X3	T36.1X4	T36.1X5	T36.1X6
Cefixime	T36.1X1	T36.1X2	T36.1X3	T36.1X4	T36.1X5	T36.1X6
Cefmenoxime	T36.1X1	T36.1X2	T36.1X3	T36.1X4	T36.1X5	T36.1X6
Cefmetazole	T36.1X1	T36.1X2	T36.1X3	T36.1X4	T36.1X5	T36.1X6
Cefminox	T36.1X1	T36.1X2	T36.1X3	T36.1X4	T36.1X5	T36.1X6
Cefonicid	T36.1X1	T36.1X2	T36.1X3	T36.1X4	T36.1X5	T36.1X6
Cefoperazone	T36.1X1	T36.1X2	T36.1X3	T36.1X4	T36.1X5	T36.1X6
Ceforanide	T36.1X1	T36.1X2	T36.1X3	T36.1X4	T36.1X5	T36.1X6
Cefotaxime	T36.1X1	T36.1X2	T36.1X3	T36.1X4	T36.1X5	T36.1X6
Cefotetan	T36.1X1	T36.1X2	T36.1X3	T36.1X4	T36.1X5	T36.1X6
Cefotiam	T36.1X1	T36.1X2	T36.1X3	T36.1X4	T36.1X5	T36.1X6
Cefoxitin	T36.1X1	T36.1X2	T36.1X3	T36.1X4	T36.1X5	T36.1X6
Cefpimizole	T36.1X1	T36.1X2	T36.1X3	T36.1X4	T36.1X5	T36.1X6
Cefpiramide	T36.1X1	T36.1X2	T36.1X3	T36.1X4	T36.1X5	T36.1X6
Cefradine	T36.1X1	T36.1X2	T36.1X3	T36.1X4	T36.1X5	T36.1X6
Cefroxadine	T36.1X1	T36.1X2	T36.1X3	T36.1X4	T36.1X5	T36.1X6
Cefsulodin	T36.1X1	T36.1X2	T36.1X3	T36.1X4	T36.1X5	T36.1X6

Substance	Poisoning, Accidental (Unintentional)	Poisoning, Intentional Self-Harm	Poisoning, Assault	Poisoning, Undetermined	Adverse Effect	Underdosing
Ceftazidime	T36.1X1	T36.1X2	T36.1X3	T36.1X4	T36.1X5	T36.1X6
Cefteram	T36.1X1	T36.1X2	T36.1X3	T36.1X4	T36.1X5	T36.1X6
Ceftezole	T36.1X1	T36.1X2	T36.1X3	T36.1X4	T36.1X5	T36.1X6
Ceftizoxime	T36.1X1	T36.1X2	T36.1X3	T36.1X4	T36.1X5	T36.1X6
Ceftriaxone	T36.1X1	T36.1X2	T36.1X3	T36.1X4	T36.1X5	T36.1X6
Cefuroxime	T36.1X1	T36.1X2	T36.1X3	T36.1X4	T36.1X5	T36.1X6
Cefuzonam	T36.1X1	T36.1X2	T36.1X3	T36.1X4	T36.1X5	T36.1X6
Celestone	T38.0X1	T38.0X2	T38.0X3	T38.0X4	T38.0X5	T38.0X6
topical	T49.0X1	T49.0X2	T49.0X3	T49.0X4	T49.0X5	T49.0X6
Celiprolol	T44.7X1	T44.7X2	T44.7X3	T44.7X4	T44.7X5	T44.7X6
Cellosolve	T52.91	T52.92	T52.93	T52.94	—	—
Cell stimulants and proliferants	T49.8X1	T49.8X2	T49.8X3	T49.8X4	T49.8X5	T49.8X6
Cellulose						
cathartic	T47.4X1	T47.4X2	T47.4X3	T47.4X4	T47.4X5	T47.4X6
hydroxyethyl	T47.4X1	T47.4X2	T47.4X3	T47.4X4	T47.4X5	T47.4X6
nitrates (topical)	T49.3X1	T49.3X2	T49.3X3	T49.3X4	T49.3X5	T49.3X6
oxidized	T49.4X1	T49.4X2	T49.4X3	T49.4X4	T49.4X5	T49.4X6
Centipede (bite)	T63.411	T63.412	T63.413	T63.414	—	—
Central nervous system						
depressants	T42.71	T42.72	T42.73	T42.74	T42.75	T42.76
anesthetic (general) NEC	T41.201	T41.202	T41.203	T41.204	T41.205	T41.206
gases NEC	T41.0X1	T41.0X2	T41.0X3	T41.0X4	T41.0X5	T41.0X6
intravenous	T41.1X1	T41.1X2	T41.1X3	T41.1X4	T41.1X5	T41.1X6
barbiturates	T42.3X1	T42.3X2	T42.3X3	T42.3X4	T42.3X5	T42.3X6
benzodiazepines	T42.4X1	T42.4X2	T42.4X3	T42.4X4	T42.4X5	T42.4X6
bromides	T42.6X1	T42.6X2	T42.6X3	T42.6X4	T42.6X5	T42.6X6
cannabis sativa	T40.7X1	T40.7X2	T40.7X3	T40.7X4	T40.7X5	T40.7X6
chloral hydrate	T42.6X1	T42.6X2	T42.6X3	T42.6X4	T42.6X5	T42.6X6
ethanol	T51.0X1	T51.0X2	T51.0X3	T51.0X4	—	—
hallucinogenics	T40.901	T40.902	T40.903	T40.904	T40.905	T40.906
hypnotics	T42.71	T42.72	T42.73	T42.74	T42.75	T42.76
specified NEC	T42.6X1	T42.6X2	T42.6X3	T42.6X4	T42.6X5	T42.6X6
muscle relaxants	T42.8X1	T42.8X2	T42.8X3	T42.8X4	T42.8X5	T42.8X6
paraldehyde	T42.6X1	T42.6X2	T42.6X3	T42.6X4	T42.6X5	T42.6X6
sedatives; sedative-hypnotics	T42.71	T42.72	T42.73	T42.74	T42.75	T42.76
mixed NEC	T42.6X1	T42.6X2	T42.6X3	T42.6X4	T42.6X5	T42.6X6
specified NEC	T42.6X1	T42.6X2	T42.6X3	T42.6X4	T42.6X5	T42.6X6
muscle-tone depressants	T42.8X1	T42.8X2	T42.8X3	T42.8X4	T42.8X5	T42.8X6
stimulants	T43.601	T43.602	T43.603	T43.604	T43.605	T43.606
amphetamines	T43.621	T43.622	T43.623	T43.624	T43.625	T43.626
analeptics	T50.7X1	T50.7X2	T50.7X3	T50.7X4	T50.7X5	T50.7X6

◀ New ◀▥ Revised ~~deleted~~ Deleted

TABLE OF DRUGS AND CHEMICALS

TABLE OF DRUGS AND CHEMICALS

Substance	External Cause (T-Code)					
	Poisoning, Accidental (Unintentional)	Poisoning, Intentional Self-Harm	Poisoning, Assault	Poisoning, Undetermined	Adverse Effect	Underdosing
Central nervous system (Continued)						
stimulants (Continued)						
antidepressants	T43.201	T43.202	T43.203	T43.204	T43.205	T43.206
opiate antagonists	T50.7X1	T50.7X2	T50.7X3	T50.7X4	T50.7X5	T50.7X6
specified NEC	T43.691	T43.692	T43.693	T43.694	T43.695	T43.696
Cephalexin	T36.1X1	T36.1X2	T36.1X3	T36.1X4	T36.1X5	T36.1X6
Cephaloglycin	T36.1X1	T36.1X2	T36.1X3	T36.1X4	T36.1X5	T36.1X6
Cephaloridine	T36.1X1	T36.1X2	T36.1X3	T36.1X4	T36.1X5	T36.1X6
Cephalosporins	T36.1X1	T36.1X2	T36.1X3	T36.1X4	T36.1X5	T36.1X6
N (adicillin)	T36.0X1	T36.0X2	T36.0X3	T36.0X4	T36.0X5	T36.0X6
Cephalothin	T36.1X1	T36.1X2	T36.1X3	T36.1X4	T36.1X5	T36.1X6
Cephalotin	T36.1X1	T36.1X2	T36.1X3	T36.1X4	T36.1X5	T36.1X6
Cephradine	T36.1X1	T36.1X2	T36.1X3	T36.1X4	T36.1X5	T36.1X6
Cerbera (odallam)	T62.2X1	T62.2X2	T62.2X3	T62.2X4	—	—
Cerberin	T46.0X1	T46.0X2	T46.0X3	T46.0X4	T46.0X5	T46.0X6
Cerebral stimulants	T43.601	T43.602	T43.603	T43.604	T43.605	T43.606
psychotherapeutic	T43.601	T43.602	T43.603	T43.604	T43.605	T43.606
specified NEC	T43.691	T43.692	T43.693	T43.694	T43.695	T43.696
Cerium oxalate	T45.0X1	T45.0X2	T45.0X3	T45.0X4	T45.0X5	T45.0X6
Cerous oxalate	T45.0X1	T45.0X2	T45.0X3	T45.0X4	T45.0X5	T45.0X6
Ceruletide	T50.8X1	T50.8X2	T50.8X3	T50.8X4	T50.8X5	T50.8X6
Cetalkonium (chloride)	T49.0X1	T49.0X2	T49.0X3	T49.0X4	T49.0X5	T49.0X6
Cethexonium chloride	T49.0X1	T49.0X2	T49.0X3	T49.0X4	T49.0X5	T49.0X6
Cetiedil	T46.7X1	T46.7X2	T46.7X3	T46.7X4	T46.7X5	T46.7X6
Cetirizine	T45.0X1	T45.0X2	T45.0X3	T45.0X4	T45.0X5	T45.0X6
Cetomacrogol	T50.991	T50.992	T50.993	T50.994	T50.995	T50.996
Cetotiamine	T45.2X1	T45.2X2	T45.2X3	T45.2X4	T45.2X5	T45.2X6
Cetoxime	T45.0X1	T45.0X2	T45.0X3	T45.0X4	T45.0X5	T45.0X6
Cetraxate	T47.1X1	T47.1X2	T47.1X3	T47.1X4	T47.1X5	T47.1X6
Cetrimide	T49.0X1	T49.0X2	T49.0X3	T49.0X4	T49.0X5	T49.0X6
Cetrimonium (bromide)	T49.0X1	T49.0X2	T49.0X3	T49.0X4	T49.0X5	T49.0X6
Cetylpyridinium chloride	T49.0X1	T49.0X2	T49.0X3	T49.0X4	T49.0X5	T49.0X6
ENT agent	T49.6X1	T49.6X2	T49.6X3	T49.6X4	T49.6X5	T49.6X6
lozenges	T49.6X1	T49.6X2	T49.6X3	T49.6X4	T49.6X5	T49.6X6
Cevadillasee Sabadilla						
Cevitamic acid	T45.2X1	T45.2X2	T45.2X3	T45.2X4	T45.2X5	T45.2X6
Chalk, precipitated	T47.1X1	T47.1X2	T47.1X3	T47.1X4	T47.1X5	T47.1X6
Chamomile	T49.0X1	T49.0X2	T49.0X3	T49.0X4	T49.0X5	T49.0X6
Ch'an su	T46.0X1	T46.0X2	T46.0X3	T46.0X4	T46.0X5	T46.0X6
Charcoal	T47.6X1	T47.6X2	T47.6X3	T47.6X4	T47.6X5	T47.6X6
activated — see also Charcoal, medicinal	T47.6X1	T47.6X2	T47.6X3	T47.6X4	T47.6X5	T47.6X6

Substance	External Cause (T-Code)					
	Poisoning, Accidental (Unintentional)	Poisoning, Intentional Self-Harm	Poisoning, Assault	Poisoning, Undetermined	Adverse Effect	Underdosing
Charcoal (Continued)						
fumes (Carbon monoxide)	T58.2X1	T58.2X2	T58.2X3	T58.2X4	—	—
industrial	T58.8X1	T58.8X2	T58.8X3	T58.8X4	—	—
medicinal (activated)	T47.6X1	T47.6X2	T47.6X3	T47.6X4	T47.6X5	T47.6X6
antidiarrheal	T47.6X1	T47.6X2	T47.6X3	T47.6X4	T47.6X5	T47.6X6
poison control	T47.8X1	T47.8X2	T47.8X3	T47.8X4	T47.8X5	T47.8X6
specified use other than for diarrhea	T47.8X1	T47.8X2	T47.8X3	T47.8X4	T47.8X5	T47.8X6
topical	T49.8X1	T49.8X2	T49.8X3	T49.8X4	T49.8X5	T49.8X6
Chaulmosulfone	T37.1X1	T37.1X2	T37.1X3	T37.1X4	T37.1X5	T37.1X6
Chelating agent NEC	T50.6X1	T50.6X2	T50.6X3	T50.6X4	T50.6X5	T50.6X6
Chelidonium majus	T62.2X1	T62.2X2	T62.2X3	T62.2X4	—	—
Chemical substance NEC	T65.91	T65.92	T65.93	T65.94	—	—
Chenodeoxycholic acid	T47.5X1	T47.5X2	T47.5X3	T47.5X4	T47.5X5	T47.5X6
Chenodiol	T47.5X1	T47.5X2	T47.5X3	T47.5X4	T47.5X5	T47.5X6
Chenopodium	T37.4X1	T37.4X2	T37.4X3	T37.4X4	T37.4X5	T37.4X6
Cherry laurel	T62.2X1	T62.2X2	T62.2X3	T62.2X4		
Chinidin(e)	T46.2X1	T46.2X2	T46.2X3	T46.2X4	T46.2X5	T46.2X6
Chiniofon	T37.8X1	T37.8X2	T37.8X3	T37.8X4	T37.8X5	T37.8X6
Chlophedianol	T48.3X1	T48.3X2	T48.3X3	T48.3X4	T48.3X5	T48.3X6
Chloral	T42.6X1	T42.6X2	T42.6X3	T42.6X4	T42.6X5	T42.6X6
derivative	T42.6X1	T42.6X2	T42.6X3	T42.6X4	T42.6X5	T42.6X6
hydrate	T42.6X1	T42.6X2	T42.6X3	T42.6X4	T42.6X5	T42.6X6
Chloralamide	T42.6X1	T42.6X2	T42.6X3	T42.6X4	T42.6X5	T42.6X6
Chloralodol	T42.6X1	T42.6X2	T42.6X3	T42.6X4	T42.6X5	T42.6X6
Chloralose	T60.4X1	T60.4X2	T60.4X3	T60.4X4	—	—
Chlorambucil	T45.1X1	T45.1X2	T45.1X3	T45.1X4	T45.1X5	T45.1X6
Chloramine	T57.8X1	T57.8X2	T57.8X3	T57.8X4	—	—
T	T49.0X1	T49.0X2	T49.0X3	T49.0X4	T49.0X5	T49.0X6
topical	T49.0X1	T49.0X2	T49.0X3	T49.0X4	T49.0X5	T49.0X6
Chloramphenicol	T36.2X1	T36.2X2	T36.2X3	T36.2X4	T36.2X5	T36.2X6
ENT agent	T49.6X1	T49.6X2	T49.6X3	T49.6X4	T49.6X5	T49.6X6
ophthalmic preparation	T49.5X1	T49.5X2	T49.5X3	T49.5X4	T49.5X5	T49.5X6
topical NEC	T49.0X1	T49.0X2	T49.0X3	T49.0X4	T49.0X5	T49.0X6
Chlorate (potassium) (sodium) NEC	T60.3X1	T60.3X2	T60.3X3	T60.3X4		
herbicide	T60.3X1	T60.3X2	T60.3X3	T60.3X4	—	—
Chlorazanil	T50.2X1	T50.2X2	T50.2X3	T50.2X4	T50.2X5	T50.2X6
Chlorbenzene, chlorbenzol	T53.7X1	T53.7X2	T53.7X3	T53.7X4		
Chlorbenzoxamine	T44.3X1	T44.3X2	T44.3X3	T44.3X4	T44.3X5	T44.3X6
Chlorbutol	T42.6X1	T42.6X2	T42.6X3	T42.6X4	T42.6X5	T42.6X6
Chlorcyclizine	T45.0X1	T45.0X2	T45.0X3	T45.0X4	T45.0X5	T45.0X6

◀ New   ◀ Revised   deleted Deleted

Substance	Poisoning, Accidental (Unintentional)	Poisoning, Intentional Self-Harm	Poisoning, Assault	Poisoning, Undetermined	Adverse Effect	Underdosing
Chlordan(e) (dust)	T60.1X1	T60.1X2	T60.1X3	T60.1X4	—	—
Chlordantoin	T49.0X1	T49.0X2	T49.0X3	T49.0X4	T49.0X5	T49.0X6
Chlordiazepoxide	T42.4X1	T42.4X2	T42.4X3	T42.4X4	T42.4X5	T42.4X6
Chlordiethyl benzamide	T49.3X1	T49.3X2	T49.3X3	T49.3X4	T49.3X5	T49.3X6
Chloresium	T49.8X1	T49.8X2	T49.8X3	T49.8X4	T49.8X5	T49.8X6
Chlorethiazol	T42.6X1	T42.6X2	T42.6X3	T42.6X4	T42.6X5	T42.6X6
Chlorethyl — *see Ethyl chloride*						
Chloretone	T42.6X1	T42.6X2	T42.6X3	T42.6X4	T42.6X5	T42.6X6
Chlorex	T53.6X1	T53.6X2	T53.6X3	T53.6X4	—	—
insecticide	T60.1X1	T60.1X2	T60.1X3	T60.1X4	—	—
Chlorfenvinphos	T60.0X1	T60.0X2	T60.0X3	T60.0X4	—	—
Chlorhexadol	T42.6X1	T42.6X2	T42.6X3	T42.6X4	T42.6X5	T42.6X6
Chlorhexamide	T45.1X1	T45.1X2	T45.1X3	T45.1X4	T45.1X5	T45.1X6
Chlorhexidine	T49.0X1	T49.0X2	T49.0X3	T49.0X4	T49.0X5	T49.0X6
Chlorhydroxyquinolin	T49.0X1	T49.0X2	T49.0X3	T49.0X4	T49.0X5	T49.0X6
Chloride of lime (bleach)	T54.3X1	T54.3X2	T54.3X3	T54.3X4	—	—
Chlorimipramine	T43.011	T43.012	T43.013	T43.014	T43.015	T43.016
Chlorinated						
camphene	T53.6X1	T53.6X2	T53.6X3	T53.6X4		
diphenyl	T53.7X1	T53.7X2	T53.7X3	T53.7X4		
hydrocarbons NEC	T53.91	T53.92	T53.93	T53.94		
solvents	T53.91	T53.92	T53.93	T53.94		
lime (bleach)	T54.3X1	T54.3X2	T54.3X3	T54.3X4		
and boric acid solution	T49.0X1	T49.0X2	T49.0X3	T49.0X4	T49.0X5	T49.0X6
naphthalene (insecticide)	T60.1X1	T60.1X2	T60.1X3	T60.1X4	—	—
industrial (non-pesticide)	T53.7X1	T53.7X2	T53.7X3	T53.7X4		
pesticide NEC	T60.8X1	T60.8X2	T60.8X3	T60.8X4		
soda — *see also sodium hypochlorite*						
solution	T49.0X1	T49.0X2	T49.0X3	T49.0X4	T49.0X5	T49.0X6
Chlorine (fumes) (gas)	T59.4X1	T59.4X2	T59.4X3	T59.4X4		
bleach	T54.3X1	T54.3X2	T54.3X3	T54.3X4		
compound gas NEC	T59.4X1	T59.4X2	T59.4X3	T59.4X4		
disinfectant	T59.4X1	T59.4X2	T59.4X3	T59.4X4		
releasing agents NEC	T59.4X1	T59.4X2	T59.4X3	T59.4X4		
Chlorisondamine chloride	T46.991	T46.992	T46.993	T46.994	T46.995	T46.996
Chlormadinone	T38.5X1	T38.5X2	T38.5X3	T38.5X4	T38.5X5	T38.5X6
Chlormephos	T60.0X1	T60.0X2	T60.0X3	T60.0X4	—	—
Chlormerodrin	T50.2X1	T50.2X2	T50.2X3	T50.2X4	T50.2X5	T50.2X6
Chlormethiazole	T42.6X1	T42.6X2	T42.6X3	T42.6X4	T42.6X5	T42.6X6
Chlormethine	T45.1X1	T45.1X2	T45.1X3	T45.1X4	T45.1X5	T45.1X6
Chlormethylenecycline	T36.4X1	T36.4X2	T36.4X3	T36.4X4	T36.4X5	T36.4X6

Substance	Poisoning, Accidental (Unintentional)	Poisoning, Intentional Self-Harm	Poisoning, Assault	Poisoning, Undetermined	Adverse Effect	Underdosing
Chlormezanone	T42.6X1	T42.6X2	T42.6X3	T42.6X4	T42.6X5	T42.6X6
Chloroacetic acid	T60.3X1	T60.3X2	T60.3X3	T60.3X4	—	—
Chloroacetone	T59.3X1	T59.3X2	T59.3X3	T59.3X4	—	—
Chloroacetophenone	T59.3X1	T59.3X2	T59.3X3	T59.3X4	—	—
Chloroaniline	T53.7X1	T53.7X2	T53.7X3	T53.7X4	—	—
Chlorobenzene, chlorobenzol	T53.7X1	T53.7X2	T53.7X3	T53.7X4	—	—
Chlorobromomethane (fire extinguisher)	T53.6X1	T53.6X2	T53.6X3	T53.6X4	—	—
Chlorobutanol	T49.0X1	T49.0X2	T49.0X3	T49.0X4	T49.0X5	T49.0X6
Chlorocresol	T49.0X1	T49.0X2	T49.0X3	T49.0X4	T49.0X5	T49.0X6
Chlorodehydro-methyltestosterone	T38.7X1	T38.7X2	T38.7X3	T38.7X4	T38.7X5	T38.7X6
Chlorodinitrobenzene	T53.7X1	T53.7X2	T53.7X3	T53.7X4	—	—
dust or vapor	T53.7X1	T53.7X2	T53.7X3	T53.7X4		
Chlorodiphenyl	T53.7X1	T53.7X2	T53.7X3	T53.7X4	—	—
Chloroethane — *see Ethyl chloride*						
Chloroethylene	T53.6X1	T53.6X2	T53.6X3	T53.6X4	—	—
Chlorofluorocarbons	T53.5X1	T53.5X2	T53.5X3	T53.5X4	—	—
Chloroform (fumes) (vapor)	T53.1X1	T53.1X2	T53.1X3	T53.1X4	—	—
anesthetic	T41.0X1	T41.0X2	T41.0X3	T41.0X4	T41.0X5	T41.0X6
solvent	T53.1X1	T53.1X2	T53.1X3	T53.1X4	—	—
water, concentrated	T41.0X1	T41.0X2	T41.0X3	T41.0X4	T41.0X5	T41.0X6
Chloroguanide	T37.2X1	T37.2X2	T37.2X3	T37.2X4	T37.2X5	T37.2X6
Chloromycetin	T36.2X1	T36.2X2	T36.2X3	T36.2X4	T36.2X5	T36.2X6
ENT agent	T49.6X1	T49.6X2	T49.6X3	T49.6X4	T49.6X5	T49.6X6
ophthalmic preparation	T49.5X1	T49.5X2	T49.5X3	T49.5X4	T49.5X5	T49.5X6
otic solution	T49.6X1	T49.6X2	T49.6X3	T49.6X4	T49.6X5	T49.6X6
topical NEC	T49.0X1	T49.0X2	T49.0X3	T49.0X4	T49.0X5	T49.0X6
Chloronitrobenzene	T53.7X1	T53.7X2	T53.7X3	T53.7X4	—	—
dust or vapor	T53.7X1	T53.7X2	T53.7X3	T53.7X4	—	—
Chlorophacinone	T60.4X1	T60.4X2	T60.4X3	T60.4X4	—	—
Chlorophenol	T53.7X1	T53.7X2	T53.7X3	T53.7X4	—	—
Chlorophenothane	T60.1X1	T60.1X2	T60.1X3	T60.1X4	—	—
Chlorophyll	T50.991	T50.992	T50.993	T50.994	T50.995	T50.996
Chloropicrin (fumes)	T53.6X1	T53.6X2	T53.6X3	T53.6X4	—	—
fumigant	T60.8X1	T60.8X2	T60.8X3	T60.8X4	—	—
fungicide	T60.3X1	T60.3X2	T60.3X3	T60.3X4	—	—
pesticide	T60.8X1	T60.8X2	T60.8X3	T60.8X4	—	—
Chloroprocaine	T41.3X1	T41.3X2	T41.3X3	T41.3X4	T41.3X5	T41.3X6
infiltration (subcutaneous)	T41.3X1	T41.3X2	T41.3X3	T41.3X4	T41.3X5	T41.3X6
nerve block (peripheral) (plexus)	T41.3X1	T41.3X2	T41.3X3	T41.3X4	T41.3X5	T41.3X6
spinal	T41.3X1	T41.3X2	T41.3X3	T41.3X4	T41.3X5	T41.3X6

◀ New   ◀▥ Revised   ~~deleted~~ Deleted

TABLE OF DRUGS AND CHEMICALS

Substance	External Cause (T-Code)					
	Poisoning, Accidental (Unintentional)	Poisoning, Intentional Self-Harm	Poisoning, Assault	Poisoning, Undetermined	Adverse Effect	Underdosing
Chloroptic	T49.5X1	T49.5X2	T49.5X3	T49.5X4	T49.5X5	T49.5X6
Chloropurine	T45.1X1	T45.1X2	T45.1X3	T45.1X4	T45.1X5	T45.1X6
Chloropyramine	T45.0X1	T45.0X2	T45.0X3	T45.0X4	T45.0X5	T45.0X6
Chloropyrifos	T60.0X1	T60.0X2	T60.0X3	T60.0X4	—	—
Chloropyrilene	T45.0X1	T45.0X2	T45.0X3	T45.0X4	T45.0X5	T45.0X6
Chloroquine	T37.2X1	T37.2X2	T37.2X3	T37.2X4	T37.2X5	T37.2X6
Chlorothalonil	T60.3X1	T60.3X2	T60.3X3	T60.3X4	—	—
Chlorothen	T45.0X1	T45.0X2	T45.0X3	T45.0X4	T45.0X5	T45.0X6
Chlorothiazide	T50.2X1	T50.2X2	T50.2X3	T50.2X4	T50.2X5	T50.2X6
Chlorothymol	T49.4X1	T49.4X2	T49.4X3	T49.4X4	T49.4X5	T49.4X6
Chlorotrianisene	T38.5X1	T38.5X2	T38.5X3	T38.5X4	T38.5X5	T38.5X6
Chlorovinyldichloro-arsine, not in war	T57.0X1	T57.0X2	T57.0X3	T57.0X4	—	—
Chloroxine	T49.4X1	T49.4X2	T49.4X3	T49.4X4	T49.4X5	T49.4X6
Chloroxylenol	T49.0X1	T49.0X2	T49.0X3	T49.0X4	T49.0X5	T49.0X6
Chlorphenamine	T45.0X1	T45.0X2	T45.0X3	T45.0X4	T45.0X5	T45.0X6
Chlorphenesin	T42.8X1	T42.8X2	T42.8X3	T42.8X4	T42.8X5	T42.8X6
topical (antifungal)	T49.0X1	T49.0X2	T49.0X3	T49.0X4	T49.0X5	T49.0X6
Chlorpheniramine	T45.0X1	T45.0X2	T45.0X3	T45.0X4	T45.0X5	T45.0X6
Chlorphenoxamine	T45.0X1	T45.0X2	T45.0X3	T45.0X4	T45.0X5	T45.0X6
Chlorphentermine	T50.5X1	T50.5X2	T50.5X3	T50.5X4	T50.5X5	T50.5X6
Chlorprocaine — see Chloroprocaine						
Chlorproguanil	T37.2X1	T37.2X2	T37.2X3	T37.2X4	T37.2X5	T37.2X6
Chlorpromazine	T43.3X1	T43.3X2	T43.3X3	T43.3X4	T43.3X5	T43.3X6
Chlorpropamide	T38.3X1	T38.3X2	T38.3X3	T38.3X4	T38.3X5	T38.3X6
Chlorprothixene	T43.4X1	T43.4X2	T43.4X3	T43.4X4	T43.4X5	T43.4X6
Chlorquinaldol	T49.0X1	T49.0X2	T49.0X3	T49.0X4	T49.0X5	T49.0X6
Chlorquinol	T49.0X1	T49.0X2	T49.0X3	T49.0X4	T49.0X5	T49.0X6
Chlortalidone	T50.2X1	T50.2X2	T50.2X3	T50.2X4	T50.2X5	T50.2X6
Chlortetracycline	T36.4X1	T36.4X2	T36.4X3	T36.4X4	T36.4X5	T36.4X6
Chlorthalidone	T50.2X1	T50.2X2	T50.2X3	T50.2X4	T50.2X5	T50.2X6
Chlorthiophos	T60.0X1	T60.0X2	T60.0X3	T60.0X4	—	—
Chlorotrianisene	T38.5X1	T38.5X2	T38.5X3	T38.5X4	T38.5X5	T38.5X6
Chlor-Trimeton	T45.0X1	T45.0X2	T45.0X3	T45.0X4	T45.0X5	T45.0X6
Chlorthion	T60.0X1	T60.0X2	T60.0X3	T60.0X4	—	—
Chlorzoxazone	T42.8X1	T42.8X2	T42.8X3	T42.8X4	T42.8X5	T42.8X6
Choke damp	T59.7X1	T59.7X2	T59.7X3	T59.7X4	—	—
Cholagogues	T47.5X1	T47.5X2	T47.5X3	T47.5X4	T47.5X5	T47.5X6
Cholebrine	T50.8X1	T50.8X2	T50.8X3	T50.8X4	T50.8X5	T50.8X6
Cholecalciferol	T45.2X1	T45.2X2	T45.2X3	T45.2X4	T45.2X5	T45.2X6
Cholecystokinin	T50.8X1	T50.8X2	T50.8X3	T50.8X4	T50.8X5	T50.8X6
Cholera vaccine	T50.A91	T50.A92	T50.A93	T50.A94	T50.A95	T50.A96

Substance	External Cause (T-Code)					
	Poisoning, Accidental (Unintentional)	Poisoning, Intentional Self-Harm	Poisoning, Assault	Poisoning, Undetermined	Adverse Effect	Underdosing
Choleretic	T47.5X1	T47.5X2	T47.5X3	T47.5X4	T47.5X5	T47.5X6
Cholesterol-lowering agents	T46.6X1	T46.6X2	T46.6X3	T46.6X4	T46.6X5	T46.6X6
Cholestyramine (resin)	T46.6X1	T46.6X2	T46.6X3	T46.6X4	T46.6X5	T46.6X6
Cholic acid	T47.5X1	T47.5X2	T47.5X3	T47.5X4	T47.5X5	T47.5X6
Choline	T48.6X1	T48.6X2	T48.6X3	T48.6X4	T48.6X5	T48.6X6
chloride	T50.991	T50.992	T50.993	T50.994	T50.995	T50.996
dihydrogen citrate	T50.991	T50.992	T50.993	T50.994	T50.995	T50.996
salicylate	T39.091	T39.092	T39.093	T39.094	T39.095	T39.096
theophyllinate	T48.6X1	T48.6X2	T48.6X3	T48.6X4	T48.6X5	T48.6X6
Cholinergic (drug) NEC	T44.1X1	T44.1X2	T44.1X3	T44.1X4	T44.1X5	T44.1X6
muscle tone enhancer	T44.1X1	T44.1X2	T44.1X3	T44.1X4	T44.1X5	T44.1X6
organophosphorus	T44.0X1	T44.0X2	T44.0X3	T44.0X4	T44.0X5	T44.0X6
insecticide	T60.0X1	T60.0X2	T60.0X3	T60.0X4	—	—
nerve gas	T59.891	T59.892	T59.893	T59.894	—	—
trimethyl ammonium propanediol	T44.1X1	T44.1X2	T44.1X3	T44.1X4	T44.1X5	T44.1X6
Cholinesterase reactivator	T50.6X1	T50.6X2	T50.6X3	T50.6X4	T50.6X5	T50.6X6
Cholografin	T50.8X1	T50.8X2	T50.8X3	T50.8X4	T50.8X5	T50.8X6
Chorionic gonadotropin	T38.891	T38.892	T38.893	T38.894	T38.895	T38.896
Chromate	T56.2X1	T56.2X2	T56.2X3	T56.2X4	—	—
dust or mist	T56.2X1	T56.2X2	T56.2X3	T56.2X4	—	—
lead — see also lead	T56.0X1	T56.0X2	T56.0X3	T56.0X4	—	—
paint	T56.0X1	T56.0X2	T56.0X3	T56.0X4	—	—
Chromic						
acid	T56.2X1	T56.2X2	T56.2X3	T56.2X4	—	—
dust or mist	T56.2X1	T56.2X2	T56.2X3	T56.2X4	—	—
phosphate 32P	T45.1X1	T45.1X2	T45.1X3	T45.1X4	T45.1X5	T45.1X6
Chromium	T56.2X1	T56.2X2	T56.2X3	T56.2X4	—	—
compounds — see Chromate						
sesquioxide	T50.8X1	T50.8X2	T50.8X3	T50.8X4	T50.8X5	T50.8X6
Chromomycin A3	T45.1X1	T45.1X2	T45.1X3	T45.1X4	T45.1X5	T45.1X6
Chromonar	T46.3X1	T46.3X2	T46.3X3	T46.3X4	T46.3X5	T46.3X6
Chromyl chloride	T56.2X1	T56.2X2	T56.2X3	T56.2X4	—	—
Chrysarobin	T49.4X1	T49.4X2	T49.4X3	T49.4X4	T49.4X5	T49.4X6
Chrysazin	T47.2X1	T47.2X2	T47.2X3	T47.2X4	T47.2X5	T47.2X6
Chymar	T45.3X1	T45.3X2	T45.3X3	T45.3X4	T45.3X5	T45.3X6
ophthalmic preparation	T49.5X1	T49.5X2	T49.5X3	T49.5X4	T49.5X5	T49.5X6
Chymopapain	T45.3X1	T45.3X2	T45.3X3	T45.3X4	T45.3X5	T45.3X6
Chymotrypsin	T45.3X1	T45.3X2	T45.3X3	T45.3X4	T45.3X5	T45.3X6
ophthalmic preparation	T49.5X1	T49.5X2	T49.5X3	T49.5X4	T49.5X5	T49.5X6
Cianidanol	T50.991	T50.992	T50.993	T50.994	T50.995	T50.996
Cianopramine	T43.011	T43.012	T43.013	T43.014	T43.015	T43.016
Cibenzoline	T46.2X1	T46.2X2	T46.2X3	T46.2X4	T46.2X5	T46.2X6

◀ New ◀|||| Revised ~~deleted~~ Deleted

Substance	Poisoning, Accidental (Unintentional)	Poisoning, Intentional Self-Harm	Poisoning, Assault	Poisoning, Undetermined	Adverse Effect	Underdosing
Ciclacillin	T36.0X1	T36.0X2	T36.0X3	T36.0X4	T36.0X5	T36.0X6
Ciclobarbital — see Hexobarbital						
Ciclonicate	T46.7X1	T46.7X2	T46.7X3	T46.7X4	T46.7X5	T46.7X6
Ciclopirox (olamine)	T49.0X1	T49.0X2	T49.0X3	T49.0X4	T49.0X5	T49.0X6
Ciclosporin	T45.1X1	T45.1X2	T45.1X3	T45.1X4	T45.1X5	T45.1X6
Cicuta maculata or virosa	T62.2X1	T62.2X2	T62.2X3	T62.2X4	—	—
Cicutoxin	T62.2X1	T62.2X2	T62.2X3	T62.2X4	—	—
Cigarette lighter fluid	T52.0X1	T52.0X2	T52.0X3	T52.0X4	—	—
Cigarettes (tobacco)	T65.221	T65.222	T65.223	T65.224		
Ciguatoxin	T61.01	T61.02	T61.03	T61.04	—	—
Cilazapril	T46.4X1	T46.4X2	T46.4X3	T46.4X4	T46.4X5	T46.4X6
Cimetidine	T47.0X1	T47.0X2	T47.0X3	T47.0X4	T47.0X5	T47.0X6
Cimetropium bromide	T44.3X1	T44.3X2	T44.3X3	T44.3X4	T44.3X5	T44.3X6
Cinchocaine	T41.3X1	T41.3X2	T41.3X3	T41.3X4	T41.3X5	T41.3X6
topical (surface)	T41.3X1	T41.3X2	T41.3X3	T41.3X4	T41.3X5	T41.3X6
Cinchona	T37.2X1	T37.2X2	T37.2X3	T37.2X4	T37.2X5	T37.2X6
Cinchonine alkaloids	T37.2X1	T37.2X2	T37.2X3	T37.2X4	T37.2X5	T37.2X6
Cinchophen	T50.4X1	T50.4X2	T50.4X3	T50.4X4	T50.4X5	T50.4X6
Cinepazide	T46.7X1	T46.7X2	T46.7X3	T46.7X4	T46.7X5	T46.7X6
Cinnamedrine	T48.5X1	T48.5X2	T48.5X3	T48.5X4	T48.5X5	T48.5X6
Cinnarizine	T45.0X1	T45.0X2	T45.0X3	T45.0X4	T45.0X5	T45.0X6
Cinoxacin	T37.8X1	T37.8X2	T37.8X3	T37.8X4	T37.8X5	T37.8X6
Ciprofibrate	T46.6X1	T46.6X2	T46.6X3	T46.6X4	T46.6X5	T46.6X6
Ciprofloxacin	T36.8X1	T36.8X2	T36.8X3	T36.8X4	T36.8X5	T36.8X6
Cisapride	T47.8X1	T47.8X2	T47.8X3	T47.8X4	T47.8X5	T47.8X6
Cisplatin	T45.1X1	T45.1X2	T45.1X3	T45.1X4	T45.1X5	T45.1X6
Citalopram	T43.221	T43.222	T43.223	T43.224	T43.225	T43.226
Citanest	T41.3X1	T41.3X2	T41.3X3	T41.3X4	T41.3X5	T41.3X6
infiltration (subcutaneous)	T41.3X1	T41.3X2	T41.3X3	T41.3X4	T41.3X5	T41.3X6
nerve block (peripheral) (plexus)	T41.3X1	T41.3X2	T41.3X3	T41.3X4	T41.3X5	T41.3X6
Citric acid	T47.5X1	T47.5X2	T47.5X3	T47.5X4	T47.5X5	T47.5X6
Citrovorum (factor)	T45.8X1	T45.8X2	T45.8X3	T45.8X4	T45.8X5	T45.8X6
Claviceps purpurea	T62.2X1	T62.2X2	T62.2X3	T62.2X4	—	—
Clavulanic acid	T36.1X1	T36.1X2	T36.1X3	T36.1X4	T36.1X5	T36.1X6
Cleaner, cleansing agent, type not specified	T65.891	T65.892	T65.893	T65.894	—	—
of paint or varnish	T52.91	T52.92	T52.93	T52.94	—	—
specified type NEC	T65.891	T65.892	T65.893	T65.894	—	—
Clebopride	T47.8X1	T47.8X2	T47.8X3	T47.8X4	T47.8X5	T47.8X6
Clefamide	T37.3X1	T37.3X2	T37.3X3	T37.3X4	T37.3X5	T37.3X6
Clemastine	T45.0X1	T45.0X2	T45.0X3	T45.0X4	T45.0X5	T45.0X6
Clematis vitalba	T62.2X1	T62.2X2	T62.2X3	T62.2X4	—	—

Substance	Poisoning, Accidental (Unintentional)	Poisoning, Intentional Self-Harm	Poisoning, Assault	Poisoning, Undetermined	Adverse Effect	Underdosing
Clemizole	T45.0X1	T45.0X2	T45.0X3	T45.0X4	T45.0X5	T45.0X6
penicillin	T36.0X1	T36.0X2	T36.0X3	T36.0X4	T36.0X5	T36.0X6
Clenbuterol	T48.6X1	T48.6X2	T48.6X3	T48.6X4	T48.6X5	T48.6X6
Clidinium bromide	T44.3X1	T44.3X2	T44.3X3	T44.3X4	T44.3X5	T44.3X6
Clindamycin	T36.8X1	T36.8X2	T36.8X3	T36.8X4	T36.8X5	T36.8X6
Clinofibrate	T46.6X1	T46.6X2	T46.6X3	T46.6X4	T46.6X5	T46.6X6
Clioquinol	T37.8X1	T37.8X2	T37.8X3	T37.8X4	T37.8X5	T37.8X6
Cliradon	T40.2X1	T40.2X2	T40.2X3	T40.2X4	—	—
Clobazam	T42.4X1	T42.4X2	T42.4X3	T42.4X4	T42.4X5	T42.4X6
Clobenzorex	T50.5X1	T50.5X2	T50.5X3	T50.5X4	T50.5X5	T50.5X6
Clobetasol	T49.0X1	T49.0X2	T49.0X3	T49.0X4	T49.0X5	T49.0X6
Clobetasone	T49.0X1	T49.0X2	T49.0X3	T49.0X4	T49.0X5	T49.0X6
Clobutinol	T48.3X1	T48.3X2	T48.3X3	T48.3X4	T48.3X5	T48.3X6
Clocapramine	T43.0X1	T43.0X2	T43.0X3	T43.0X4	T43.0X5	T43.0X6
Clocortolone	T38.0X1	T38.0X2	T38.0X3	T38.0X4	T38.0X5	T38.0X6
Clodantoin	T49.0X1	T49.0X2	T49.0X3	T49.0X4	T49.0X5	T49.0X6
Clodronic acid	T50.991	T50.992	T50.993	T50.994	T50.995	T50.996
Clofazimine	T37.1X1	T37.1X2	T37.1X3	T37.1X4	T37.1X5	T37.1X6
Clofedanol	T48.3X1	T48.3X2	T48.3X3	T48.3X4	T48.3X5	T48.3X6
Clofenamide	T50.2X1	T50.2X2	T50.2X3	T50.2X4	T50.2X5	T50.2X6
Clofenotane	T49.0X1	T49.0X2	T49.0X3	T49.0X4	T49.0X5	T49.0X6
Clofezone	T39.2X1	T39.2X2	T39.2X3	T39.2X4	T39.2X5	T39.2X6
Clofibrate	T46.6X1	T46.6X2	T46.6X3	T46.6X4	T46.6X5	T46.6X6
Clofibride	T46.6X1	T46.6X2	T46.6X3	T46.6X4	T46.6X5	T46.6X6
Cloforex	T50.5X1	T50.5X2	T50.5X3	T50.5X4	T50.5X5	T50.5X6
Clomacran	T43.0X1	T43.0X2	T43.0X3	T43.0X4	T43.0X5	T43.0X6
Clomethiazole	T42.6X1	T42.6X2	T42.6X3	T42.6X4	T42.6X5	T42.6X6
Clometocillin	T36.0X1	T36.0X2	T36.0X3	T36.0X4	T36.0X5	T36.0X6
Clomifene	T38.5X1	T38.5X2	T38.5X3	T38.5X4	T38.5X5	T38.5X6
Clomiphene	T38.5X1	T38.5X2	T38.5X3	T38.5X4	T38.5X5	T38.5X6
Clomipramine	T43.011	T43.012	T43.013	T43.014	T43.015	T43.016
Clomocycline	T36.4X1	T36.4X2	T36.4X3	T36.4X4	T36.4X5	T36.4X6
Clonazepam	T42.4X1	T42.4X2	T42.4X3	T42.4X4	T42.4X5	T42.4X6
Clonidine	T46.5X1	T46.5X2	T46.5X3	T46.5X4	T46.5X5	T46.5X6
Clonixin	T39.8X1	T39.8X2	T39.8X3	T39.8X4	T39.8X5	T39.8X6
Clopamide	T50.2X1	T50.2X2	T50.2X3	T50.2X4	T50.2X5	T50.2X6
Clopenthixol	T43.4X1	T43.4X2	T43.4X3	T43.4X4	T43.4X5	T43.4X6
Cloperastine	T48.3X1	T48.3X2	T48.3X3	T48.3X4	T48.3X5	T48.3X6
Clophedianol	T48.3X1	T48.3X2	T48.3X3	T48.3X4	T48.3X5	T48.3X6
Cloponone	T36.2X1	T36.2X2	T36.2X3	T36.2X4	T36.2X5	T36.2X6
Cloprednol	T38.0X1	T38.0X2	T38.0X3	T38.0X4	T38.0X5	T38.0X6
Cloral betaine	T42.6X1	T42.6X2	T42.6X3	T42.6X4	T42.6X5	T42.6X6

TABLE OF DRUGS AND CHEMICALS

Substance	Poisoning, Accidental (Unintentional)	Poisoning, Intentional Self-Harm	Poisoning, Assault	Poisoning, Undetermined	Adverse Effect	Underdosing
Cloramfenicol	T36.2X1	T36.2X2	T36.2X3	T36.2X4	T36.2X5	T36.2X6
Clorazepate (dipotassium)	T42.4X1	T42.4X2	T42.4X3	T42.4X4	T42.4X5	T42.4X6
Clorexolone	T50.2X1	T50.2X2	T50.2X3	T50.2X4	T50.2X5	T50.2X6
Clorox (bleach)	T54.91	T54.92	T54.93	T54.94	—	—
Clorfenamine	T45.0X1	T45.0X2	T45.0X3	T45.0X4	T45.0X5	T45.0X6
Clorgiline	T43.1X1	T43.1X2	T43.1X3	T43.1X4	T43.1X5	T43.1X6
Clorotepine	T44.3X1	T44.3X2	T44.3X3	T44.3X4	T44.3X5	T44.3X6
Clorprenaline	T48.6X1	T48.6X2	T48.6X3	T48.6X4	T48.6X5	T48.6X6
Clortermine	T50.5X1	T50.5X2	T50.5X3	T50.5X4	T50.5X5	T50.5X6
Clotiapine	T43.591	T43.592	T43.593	T43.594	T43.595	T43.596
Clotiazepam	T42.4X1	T42.4X2	T42.4X3	T42.4X4	T42.4X5	T42.4X6
Clotibric acid	T46.6X1	T46.6X2	T46.6X3	T46.6X4	T46.6X5	T46.6X6
Clotrimazole	T49.0X1	T49.0X2	T49.0X3	T49.0X4	T49.0X5	T49.0X6
Cloxacillin	T36.0X1	T36.0X2	T36.0X3	T36.0X4	T36.0X5	T36.0X6
Cloxazolam	T42.4X1	T42.4X2	T42.4X3	T42.4X4	T42.4X5	T42.4X6
Cloxiquine	T49.0X1	T49.0X2	T49.0X3	T49.0X4	T49.0X5	T49.0X6
Clozapine	T42.4X1	T42.4X2	T42.4X3	T42.4X4	T42.4X5	T42.4X6
Coagulant NEC	T45.7X1	T45.7X2	T45.7X3	T45.7X4	T45.7X5	T45.7X6
Coal (carbon monoxide from) — see also Carbon, monoxide, coal	T58.2X1	T58.2X2	T58.2X3	T58.2X4	—	—
oil — see Kerosene						
tar	T49.1X1	T49.1X2	T49.1X3	T49.1X4	T49.1X5	T49.1X6
fumes	T59.891	T59.892	T59.893	T59.894	—	—
medicinal (ointment)	T49.4X1	T49.4X2	T49.4X3	T49.4X4	T49.4X5	T49.4X6
analgesics NEC	T39.2X1	T39.2X2	T39.2X3	T39.2X4	T39.2X5	T39.2X6
naphtha (solvent)	T52.0X1	T52.0X2	T52.0X3	T52.0X4		
Cobalamine	T45.2X1	T45.2X2	T45.2X3	T45.2X4	T45.2X5	T45.2X6
Cobalt (nonmedicinal) (fumes) (industrial)	T56.891	T56.892	T56.893	T56.894		
medicinal (trace) (chloride)	T45.8X1	T45.8X2	T45.8X3	T45.8X4	T45.8X5	T45.8X6
Cobra (venom)	T63.041	T63.042	T63.043	T63.044		
Coca (leaf)	T40.5X1	T40.5X2	T40.5X3	T40.5X4	T40.5X5	T40.5X6
Cocaine	T40.5X1	T40.5X2	T40.5X3	T40.5X4	T40.5X5	T40.5X6
topical anesthetic	T41.3X1	T41.3X2	T41.3X3	T41.3X4	T41.3X5	T41.3X6
Cocarboxylase	T45.3X1	T45.3X2	T45.3X3	T45.3X4	T45.3X5	T45.3X6
Coccidioidin	T50.8X1	T50.8X2	T50.8X3	T50.8X4	T50.8X5	T50.8X6
Cocculus indicus	T62.1X1	T62.1X2	T62.1X3	T62.1X4		
Cochineal	T65.6X1	T65.6X2	T65.6X3	T65.6X4		
medicinal products	T50.991	T50.992	T50.993	T50.994	T50.995	T50.996
Codeine	T40.2X1	T40.2X2	T40.2X3	T40.2X4	T40.2X5	T40.2X6
Cod-liver oil	T45.2X1	T45.2X2	T45.2X3	T45.2X4	T45.2X5	T45.2X6

Substance	Poisoning, Accidental (Unintentional)	Poisoning, Intentional Self-Harm	Poisoning, Assault	Poisoning, Undetermined	Adverse Effect	Underdosing
Coenzyme A	T50.991	T50.992	T50.993	T50.994	T50.995	T50.996
Coffee	T62.8X1	T62.8X2	T62.8X3	T62.8X4	—	—
Cogalactoisomerase	T50.991	T50.992	T50.993	T50.994	T50.995	T50.996
Cogentin	T44.3X1	T44.3X2	T44.3X3	T44.3X4	T44.3X5	T44.3X6
Coke fumes or gas (carbon monoxide)	T58.2X1	T58.2X2	T58.2X3	T58.2X4	—	—
industrial use	T58.8X1	T58.8X2	T58.8X3	T58.8X4	—	—
Colace	T47.4X1	T47.4X2	T47.4X3	T47.4X4	T47.4X5	T47.4X6
Colaspase	T45.1X1	T45.1X2	T45.1X3	T45.1X4	T45.1X5	T45.1X6
Colchicine	T50.4X1	T50.4X2	T50.4X3	T50.4X4	T50.4X5	T50.4X6
Colchicum	T62.2X1	T62.2X2	T62.2X3	T62.2X4	—	—
Cold cream	T49.3X1	T49.3X2	T49.3X3	T49.3X4	T49.3X5	T49.3X6
Colecalciferol	T45.2X1	T45.2X2	T45.2X3	T45.2X4	T45.2X5	T45.2X6
Colestipol	T46.6X1	T46.6X2	T46.6X3	T46.6X4	T46.6X5	T46.6X6
Colestyramine	T46.6X1	T46.6X2	T46.6X3	T46.6X4	T46.6X5	T46.6X6
Colimycin	T36.8X1	T36.8X2	T36.8X3	T36.8X4	T36.8X5	T36.8X6
Colistimethate	T36.8X1	T36.8X2	T36.8X3	T36.8X4	T36.8X5	T36.8X6
Colistin	T36.8X1	T36.8X2	T36.8X3	T36.8X4	T36.8X5	T36.8X6
sulfate (eye preparation)	T49.5X1	T49.5X2	T49.5X3	T49.5X4	T49.5X5	T49.5X6
Collagen	T50.991	T50.992	T50.993	T50.994	T50.995	T50.996
Collagenase	T49.4X1	T49.4X2	T49.4X3	T49.4X4	T49.4X5	T49.4X6
Collodion	T49.3X1	T49.3X2	T49.3X3	T49.3X4	T49.3X5	T49.3X6
Colocynth	T47.2X1	T47.2X2	T47.2X3	T47.2X4	T47.2X5	T47.2X6
Colophony adhesive	T49.3X1	T49.3X2	T49.3X3	T49.3X4	T49.3X5	T49.3X6
Colorant — see also Dye	T50.991	T50.992	T50.993	T50.994	T50.995	T50.996
Coloring matter — see Dye(s)						
Combustion gas (after combustion) — see Carbon, monoxide						
prior to combustion	T59.891	T59.892	T59.893	T59.894	—	—
Compazine	T43.3X1	T43.3X2	T43.3X3	T43.3X4	T43.3X5	T43.3X6
Compound						
42 (warfarin)	T60.4X1	T60.4X2	T60.4X3	T60.4X4	—	—
269 (endrin)	T60.1X1	T60.1X2	T60.1X3	T60.1X4	—	—
497 (dieldrin)	T60.1X1	T60.1X2	T60.1X3	T60.1X4	—	—
1080 (sodium fluoroacetate)	T60.4X1	T60.4X2	T60.4X3	T60.4X4	—	—
3422 (parathion)	T60.0X1	T60.0X2	T60.0X3	T60.0X4	—	—
3911 (phorate)	T60.0X1	T60.0X2	T60.0X3	T60.0X4	—	—
3956 (toxaphene)	T60.1X1	T60.1X2	T60.1X3	T60.1X4	—	—
4049 (malathion)	T60.0X1	T60.0X2	T60.0X3	T60.0X4	—	—
4069 (malathion)	T60.0X1	T60.0X2	T60.0X3	T60.0X4	—	—
4124 (dicapthon)	T60.0X1	T60.0X2	T60.0X3	T60.0X4	—	—

◀ New ◀═ Revised ~~deleted~~ Deleted

TABLE OF DRUGS AND CHEMICALS

Substance	Poisoning, Accidental (Unintentional)	Poisoning, Intentional Self-Harm	Poisoning, Assault	Poisoning, Undetermined	Adverse Effect	Underdosing
Compound (Continued)						
E (cortisone)	T38.0X1	T38.0X2	T38.0X3	T38.0X4	T38.0X5	T38.0X6
F (hydrocortisone)	T38.0X1	T38.0X2	T38.0X3	T38.0X4	T38.0X5	T38.0X6
Congener, anabolic	T38.7X1	T38.7X2	T38.7X3	T38.7X4	T38.7X5	T38.7X6
Congo red	T50.8X1	T50.8X2	T50.8X3	T50.8X4	T50.8X5	T50.8X6
Coniine, conine	T62.2X1	T62.2X2	T62.2X3	T62.2X4	—	—
Conium (maculatum)	T62.2X1	T62.2X2	T62.2X3	T62.2X4	—	—
Conjugated estrogenic substances	T38.5X1	T38.5X2	T38.5X3	T38.5X4	T38.5X5	T38.5X6
Contac	T48.5X1	T48.5X2	T48.5X3	T48.5X4	T48.5X5	T48.5X6
Contact lens solution	T49.5X1	T49.5X2	T49.5X3	T49.5X4	T49.5X5	T49.5X6
Contraceptive (oral)	T38.4X1	T38.4X2	T38.4X3	T38.4X4	T38.4X5	T38.4X6
vaginal	T49.8X1	T49.8X2	T49.8X3	T49.8X4	T49.8X5	T49.8X6
Contrast medium, radiography	T50.8X1	T50.8X2	T50.8X3	T50.8X4	T50.8X5	T50.8X6
Convallaria glycosides	T46.0X1	T46.0X2	T46.0X3	T46.0X4	T46.0X5	T46.0X6
Convallaria majalis	T62.2X1	T62.2X2	T62.2X3	T62.2X4	—	—
berry	T62.1X1	T62.1X2	T62.1X3	T62.1X4	—	—
Copper (dust) (fumes) (nonmedicinal) NEC	T56.4X1	T56.4X2	T56.4X3	T56.4X4		
arsenate, arsenite	T57.0X1	T57.0X2	T57.0X3	T57.0X4		
insecticide	T60.2X1	T60.2X2	T60.2X3	T60.2X4		
emetic	T47.7X1	T47.7X2	T47.7X3	T47.7X4	T47.7X5	T47.7X6
fungicide	T60.3X1	T60.3X2	T60.3X3	T60.3X4	—	—
gluconate	T49.0X1	T49.0X2	T49.0X3	T49.0X4	T49.0X5	T49.0X6
insecticide	T60.2X1	T60.2X2	T60.2X3	T60.2X4		
medicinal (trace)	T45.8X1	T45.8X2	T45.8X3	T45.8X4	T45.8X5	T45.8X6
oleate	T49.0X1	T49.0X2	T49.0X3	T49.0X4	T49.0X5	T49.0X6
sulfate	T56.4X1	T56.4X2	T56.4X3	T56.4X4		
cupric	T56.4X1	T56.4X2	T56.4X3	T56.4X4		
fungicide	T60.3X1	T60.3X2	T60.3X3	T60.3X4	—	—
medicinal						
ear	T49.6X1	T49.6X2	T49.6X3	T49.6X4	T49.6X5	T49.6X6
emetic	T47.7X1	T47.7X2	T47.7X3	T47.7X4	T47.7X5	T47.7X6
eye	T49.5X1	T49.5X2	T49.5X3	T49.5X4	T49.5X5	T49.5X6
cuprous	T56.4X1	T56.4X2	T56.4X3	T56.4X4		
fungicide	T60.3X1	T60.3X2	T60.3X3	T60.3X4	—	—
medicinal						
ear	T49.6X1	T49.6X2	T49.6X3	T49.6X4	T49.6X5	T49.6X6
emetic	T47.7X1	T47.7X2	T47.7X3	T47.7X4	T47.7X5	T47.7X6
eye	T49.5X1	T49.5X2	T49.5X3	T49.5X4	T49.5X5	T49.5X6
Copperhead snake (bite) (venom)	T63.061	T63.062	T63.063	T63.064	—	—
Coral (sting)	T63.691	T63.692	T63.693	T63.694	—	—
snake (bite) (venom)	T63.021	T63.022	T63.023	T63.024	—	—

Substance	Poisoning, Accidental (Unintentional)	Poisoning, Intentional Self-Harm	Poisoning, Assault	Poisoning, Undetermined	Adverse Effect	Underdosing
Corbadrine	T49.6X1	T49.6X2	T49.6X3	T49.6X4	T49.6X5	T49.6X6
Cordran	T49.0X1	T49.0X2	T49.0X3	T49.0X4	T49.0X5	T49.0X6
Cordite	T65.891	T65.892	T65.893	T65.894	—	—
vapor	T59.891	T59.892	T59.893	T59.894	—	—
Corn cures	T49.4X1	T49.4X2	T49.4X3	T49.4X4	T49.4X5	T49.4X6
Cornhusker's lotion	T49.3X1	T49.3X2	T49.3X3	T49.3X4	T49.3X5	T49.3X6
Corn starch	T49.3X1	T49.3X2	T49.3X3	T49.3X4	T49.3X5	T49.3X6
Coronary vasodilator NEC	T46.3X1	T46.3X2	T46.3X3	T46.3X4	T46.3X5	T46.3X6
Corrosive NEC	T54.91	T54.92	T54.93	T54.94	—	—
acid NEC	T54.2X1	T54.2X2	T54.2X3	T54.2X4	—	—
aromatics	T54.1X1	T54.1X2	T54.1X3	T54.1X4	—	—
disinfectant	T54.1X1	T54.1X2	T54.1X3	T54.1X4	—	—
fumes NEC	T54.91	T54.92	T54.93	T54.94	—	—
specified NEC	T54.91	T54.92	T54.93	T54.94	—	—
sublimate	T56.1X1	T56.1X2	T56.1X3	T56.1X4	—	—
Cortate	T38.0X1	T38.0X2	T38.0X3	T38.0X4	T38.0X5	T38.0X6
Cort-Dome	T38.0X1	T38.0X2	T38.0X3	T38.0X4	T38.0X5	T38.0X6
ENT agent	T49.6X1	T49.6X2	T49.6X3	T49.6X4	T49.6X5	T49.6X6
ophthalmic preparation	T49.5X1	T49.5X2	T49.5X3	T49.5X4	T49.5X5	T49.5X6
topical NEC	T49.0X1	T49.0X2	T49.0X3	T49.0X4	T49.0X5	T49.0X6
Cortef	T38.0X1	T38.0X2	T38.0X3	T38.0X4	T38.0X5	T38.0X6
ENT agent	T49.6X1	T49.6X2	T49.6X3	T49.6X4	T49.6X5	T49.6X6
ophthalmic preparation	T49.5X1	T49.5X2	T49.5X3	T49.5X4	T49.5X5	T49.5X6
topical NEC	T49.0X1	T49.0X2	T49.0X3	T49.0X4	T49.0X5	T49.0X6
Corticosteroid	T38.0X1	T38.0X2	T38.0X3	T38.0X4	T38.0X5	T38.0X6
ENT agent	T49.6X1	T49.6X2	T49.6X3	T49.6X4	T49.6X5	T49.6X6
mineral	T50.0X1	T50.0X2	T50.0X3	T50.0X4	T50.0X5	T50.0X6
ophthalmic	T49.5X1	T49.5X2	T49.5X3	T49.5X4	T49.5X5	T49.5X6
topical NEC	T49.0X1	T49.0X2	T49.0X3	T49.0X4	T49.0X5	T49.0X6
Corticotropin	T38.811	T38.812	T38.813	T38.814	T38.815	T38.816
Cortisol	T49.0X1	T49.0X2	T49.0X3	T49.0X4	T49.0X5	T49.0X6
ENT agent	T49.6X1	T49.6X2	T49.6X3	T49.6X4	T49.6X5	T49.6X6
ophthalmic preparation	T49.5X1	T49.5X2	T49.5X3	T49.5X4	T49.5X5	T49.5X6
topical NEC	T49.0X1	T49.0X2	T49.0X3	T49.0X4	T49.0X5	T49.0X6
Cortisone (acetate)	T38.0X1	T38.0X2	T38.0X3	T38.0X4	T38.0X5	T38.0X6
ENT agent	T49.6X1	T49.6X2	T49.6X3	T49.6X4	T49.6X5	T49.6X6
ophthalmic preparation	T49.5X1	T49.5X2	T49.5X3	T49.5X4	T49.5X5	T49.5X6
topical NEC	T49.0X1	T49.0X2	T49.0X3	T49.0X4	T49.0X5	T49.0X6
Cortivazol	T38.0X1	T38.0X2	T38.0X3	T38.0X4	T38.0X5	T38.0X6
Cortogen	T38.0X1	T38.0X2	T38.0X3	T38.0X4	T38.0X5	T38.0X6
ENT agent	T49.6X1	T49.6X2	T49.6X3	T49.6X4	T49.6X5	T49.6X6
ophthalmic preparation	T49.5X1	T49.5X2	T49.5X3	T49.5X4	T49.5X5	T49.5X6

◄ New ◄▬ Revised ~~deleted~~ Deleted

TABLE OF DRUGS AND CHEMICALS

Substance	Poisoning, Accidental (Unintentional)	Poisoning, Intentional Self-Harm	Poisoning, Assault	Poisoning, Undetermined	Adverse Effect	Underdosing
Cortone	T38.0X1	T38.0X2	T38.0X3	T38.0X4	T38.0X5	T38.0X6
ENT agent	T49.6X1	T49.6X2	T49.6X3	T49.6X4	T49.6X5	T49.6X6
ophthalmic preparation	T49.5X1	T49.5X2	T49.5X3	T49.5X4	T49.5X5	T49.5X6
Cortril	T38.0X1	T38.0X2	T38.0X3	T38.0X4	T38.0X5	T38.0X6
ENT agent	T49.6X1	T49.6X2	T49.6X3	T49.6X4	T49.6X5	T49.6X6
ophthalmic preparation	T49.5X1	T49.5X2	T49.5X3	T49.5X4	T49.5X5	T49.5X6
topical NEC	T49.0X1	T49.0X2	T49.0X3	T49.0X4	T49.0X5	T49.0X6
Corynebacterium parvum	T45.1X1	T45.1X2	T45.1X3	T45.1X4	T45.1X5	T45.1X6
Cosmetic preparation	T49.8X1	T49.8X2	T49.8X3	T49.8X4	T49.8X5	T49.8X6
Cosmetics	T49.8X1	T49.8X2	T49.8X3	T49.8X4	T49.8X5	T49.8X6
Cosyntropin	T38.811	T38.812	T38.813	T38.814	T38.815	T38.816
Cotarnine	T45.7X1	T45.7X2	T45.7X3	T45.7X4	T45.7X5	T45.7X6
Co-trimoxazole	T36.8X1	T36.8X2	T36.8X3	T36.8X4	T36.8X5	T36.8X6
Cottonseed oil	T49.3X1	T49.3X2	T49.3X3	T49.3X4	T49.3X5	T49.3X6
Cough mixture (syrup)	T48.4X1	T48.4X2	T48.4X3	T48.4X4	T48.4X5	T48.4X6
containing opiates	T40.2X1	T40.2X2	T40.2X3	T40.2X4	T40.2X5	T40.2X6
expectorants	T48.4X1	T48.4X2	T48.4X3	T48.4X4	T48.4X5	T48.4X6
Coumadin	T45.511	T45.512	T45.513	T45.514	T45.515	T45.516
rodenticide	T60.4X1	T60.4X2	T60.4X3	T60.4X4	—	—
Coumaphos	T60.0X1	T60.0X2	T60.0X3	T60.0X4	—	—
Coumarin	T45.511	T45.512	T45.513	T45.514	T45.515	T45.516
Coumetarol	T45.511	T45.512	T45.513	T45.514	T45.515	T45.516
Cowbane	T62.2X1	T62.2X2	T62.2X3	T62.2X4	—	—
Cozyme	T45.2X1	T45.2X2	T45.2X3	T45.2X4	T45.2X5	T45.2X6
Crack	T40.5X1	T40.5X2	T40.5X3	T40.5X4	—	—
Crataegus extract	T46.0X1	T46.0X2	T46.0X3	T46.0X4	T46.0X5	T46.0X6
Creolin	T54.1X1	T54.1X2	T54.1X3	T54.1X4	—	—
disinfectant	T54.1X1	T54.1X2	T54.1X3	T54.1X4	—	—
Creosol (compound)	T49.0X1	T49.0X2	T49.0X3	T49.0X4	T49.0X5	T49.0X6
Creosote (coal tar) (beechwood)	T49.0X1	T49.0X2	T49.0X3	T49.0X4	T49.0X5	T49.0X6
medicinal (expectorant)	T48.4X1	T48.4X2	T48.4X3	T48.4X4	T48.4X5	T48.4X6
syrup	T48.4X1	T48.4X2	T48.4X3	T48.4X4	T48.4X5	T48.4X6
Cresol(s)	T49.0X1	T49.0X2	T49.0X3	T49.0X4	T49.0X5	T49.0X6
and soap solution	T49.0X1	T49.0X2	T49.0X3	T49.0X4	T49.0X5	T49.0X6
Cresyl acetate	T49.0X1	T49.0X2	T49.0X3	T49.0X4	T49.0X5	T49.0X6
Cresylic acid	T49.0X1	T49.0X2	T49.0X3	T49.0X4	T49.0X5	T49.0X6
Crimidine	T60.4X1	T60.4X2	T60.4X3	T60.4X4	—	—
Croconazole	T37.8X1	T37.8X2	T37.8X3	T37.8X4	T37.8X5	T37.8X6
Cromoglicic acid	T48.6X1	T48.6X2	T48.6X3	T48.6X4	T48.6X5	T48.6X6
Cromolyn	T48.6X1	T48.6X2	T48.6X3	T48.6X4	T48.6X5	T48.6X6
Cromonar	T46.3X1	T46.3X2	T46.3X3	T46.3X4	T46.3X5	T46.3X6

Substance	Poisoning, Accidental (Unintentional)	Poisoning, Intentional Self-Harm	Poisoning, Assault	Poisoning, Undetermined	Adverse Effect	Underdosing
Cropropamide	T39.8X1	T39.8X2	T39.8X3	T39.8X4	T39.8X5	T39.8X6
with crotethamide	T50.7X1	T50.7X2	T50.7X3	T50.7X4	T50.7X5	T50.7X6
Crotamiton	T49.0X1	T49.0X2	T49.0X3	T49.0X4	T49.0X5	T49.0X6
Crotethamide	T39.8X1	T39.8X2	T39.8X3	T39.8X4	T39.8X5	T39.8X6
with cropropamide	T50.7X1	T50.7X2	T50.7X3	T50.7X4	T50.7X5	T50.7X6
Croton (oil)	T47.2X1	T47.2X2	T47.2X3	T47.2X4	T47.2X5	T47.2X6
chloral	T42.6X1	T42.6X2	T42.6X3	T42.6X4	T42.6X5	T42.6X6
Crude oil	T52.0X1	T52.0X2	T52.0X3	T52.0X4	—	—
Cryogenine	T39.8X1	T39.8X2	T39.8X3	T39.8X4	T39.8X5	T39.8X6
Cryolite (vapor)	T60.1X1	T60.1X2	T60.1X3	T60.1X4	—	—
insecticide	T60.1X1	T60.1X2	T60.1X3	T60.1X4	—	—
Cryptenamine (tannates)	T46.5X1	T46.5X2	T46.5X3	T46.5X4	T46.5X5	T46.5X6
Crystal violet	T49.0X1	T49.0X2	T49.0X3	T49.0X4	T49.0X5	T49.0X6
Cuckoopint	T62.2X1	T62.2X2	T62.2X3	T62.2X4	—	—
Cumetharol	T45.511	T45.512	T45.513	T45.514	T45.515	T45.516
Cupric						
acetate	T60.3X1	T60.3X2	T60.3X3	T60.3X4	—	—
acetoarsenite	T57.0X1	T57.0X2	T57.0X3	T57.0X4	—	—
arsenate	T57.0X1	T57.0X2	T57.0X3	T57.0X4	—	—
gluconate	T49.0X1	T49.0X2	T49.0X3	T49.0X4	T49.0X5	T49.0X6
oleate	T49.0X1	T49.0X2	T49.0X3	T49.0X4	T49.0X5	T49.0X6
sulfate	T56.4X1	T56.4X2	T56.4X3	T56.4X4		
Cuprous sulfate — see also Copper sulfate	T56.4X1	T56.4X2	T56.4X3	T56.4X4	—	—
Curare, curarine	T48.1X1	T48.1X2	T48.1X3	T48.1X4	T48.1X5	T48.1X6
Cyamemazine	T43.3X1	T43.3X2	T43.3X3	T43.3X4	T43.3X5	T43.3X6
Cyamopsis tetragono-loba	T46.6X1	T46.6X2	T46.6X3	T46.6X4	T46.6X5	T46.6X6
Cyanacetyl hydrazide	T37.1X1	T37.1X2	T37.1X3	T37.1X4	T37.1X5	T37.1X6
Cyanic acid (gas)	T59.891	T59.892	T59.893	T59.894		
Cyanide(s) (compounds) (potassium) (sodium) NEC	T65.0X1	T65.0X2	T65.0X3	T65.0X4		
dust or gas (inhalation) NEC	T57.3X1	T57.3X2	T57.3X3	T57.3X4	—	—
fumigant	T65.0X1	T65.0X2	T65.0X3	T65.0X4		
hydrogen	T57.3X1	T57.3X2	T57.3X3	T57.3X4		
mercuric — see Mercury						
pesticide (dust) (fumes)	T65.0X1	T65.0X2	T65.0X3	T65.0X4	—	—
Cyanoacrylate adhesive	T49.3X1	T49.3X2	T49.3X3	T49.3X4	T49.3X5	T49.3X6
Cyanocobalamin	T45.8X1	T45.8X2	T45.8X3	T45.8X4	T45.8X5	T45.8X6
Cyanogen (chloride) (gas) NEC	T59.891	T59.892	T59.893	T59.894	—	—
Cyclacillin	T36.0X1	T36.0X2	T36.0X3	T36.0X4	T36.0X5	T36.0X6
Cyclaine	T41.3X1	T41.3X2	T41.3X3	T41.3X4	T41.3X5	T41.3X6
Cyclamate	T50.991	T50.992	T50.993	T50.994	T50.995	T50.996

◀ New ◀ Revised ~~deleted~~ Deleted

Substance	Poisoning, Accidental (Unintentional)	Poisoning, Intentional Self-Harm	Poisoning, Assault	Poisoning, Undetermined	Adverse Effect	Underdosing
Cyclamen europaeum	T62.2X1	T62.2X2	T62.2X3	T62.2X4	—	—
Cyclandelate	T46.7X1	T46.7X2	T46.7X3	T46.7X4	T46.7X5	T46.7X6
Cyclazocine	T50.7X1	T50.7X2	T50.7X3	T50.7X4	T50.7X5	T50.7X6
Cyclizine	T45.0X1	T45.0X2	T45.0X3	T45.0X4	T45.0X5	T45.0X6
Cyclobarbital	T42.3X1	T42.3X2	T42.3X3	T42.3X4	T42.3X5	T42.3X6
Cyclobarbitone	T42.3X1	T42.3X2	T42.3X3	T42.3X4	T42.3X5	T42.3X6
Cyclobenzaprine	T48.1X1	T48.1X2	T48.1X3	T48.1X4	T48.1X5	T48.1X6
Cyclodrine	T44.3X1	T44.3X2	T44.3X3	T44.3X4	T44.3X5	T44.3X6
Cycloguanil embonate	T37.2X1	T37.2X2	T37.2X3	T37.2X4	T37.2X5	T37.2X6
Cycloheptadiene	T43.291	T43.292	T43.293	T43.294	T43.295	T43.296
Cyclohexane	T52.8X1	T52.8X2	T52.8X3	T52.8X4	—	—
Cyclohexanol	T51.8X1	T51.8X2	T51.8X3	T51.8X4	—	—
Cyclohexanone	T52.4X1	T52.4X2	T52.4X3	T52.4X4	—	—
Cycloheximide	T60.3X1	T60.3X2	T60.3X3	T60.3X4	—	—
Cyclohexyl acetate	T52.8X1	T52.8X2	T52.8X3	T52.8X4	—	—
Cycloleucin	T45.1X1	T45.1X2	T45.1X3	T45.1X4	T45.1X5	T45.1X6
Cyclomethycaine	T41.3X1	T41.3X2	T41.3X3	T41.3X4	T41.3X5	T41.3X6
Cyclopentamine	T44.4X1	T44.4X2	T44.4X3	T44.4X4	T44.4X5	T44.4X6
Cyclopenthiazide	T50.2X1	T50.2X2	T50.2X3	T50.2X4	T50.2X5	T50.2X6
Cyclopentolate	T44.3X1	T44.3X2	T44.3X3	T44.3X4	T44.3X5	T44.3X6
Cyclophosphamide	T45.1X1	T45.1X2	T45.1X3	T45.1X4	T45.1X5	T45.1X6
Cycloplegic drug	T49.5X1	T49.5X2	T49.5X3	T49.5X4	T49.5X5	T49.5X6
Cyclopropane	T41.291	T41.292	T41.293	T41.294	T41.295	T41.296
Cyclopyrabital	T39.8X1	T39.8X2	T39.8X3	T39.8X4	T39.8X5	T39.8X6
Cycloserine	T37.1X1	T37.1X2	T37.1X3	T37.1X4	T37.1X5	T37.1X6
Cyclosporin	T45.1X1	T45.1X2	T45.1X3	T45.1X4	T45.1X5	T45.1X6
Cyclothiazide	T50.2X1	T50.2X2	T50.2X3	T50.2X4	T50.2X5	T50.2X6
Cycrimine	T44.3X1	T44.3X2	T44.3X3	T44.3X4	T44.3X5	T44.3X6
Cyhalothrin	T60.1X1	T60.1X2	T60.1X3	T60.1X4	—	—
Cymarin	T46.0X1	T46.0X2	T46.0X3	T46.0X4	T46.0X5	T46.0X6
Cypermethrin	T60.1X1	T60.1X2	T60.1X3	T60.1X4	—	—
Cyphenothrin	T60.2X1	T60.2X2	T60.2X3	T60.2X4	—	—
Cyproheptadine	T45.0X1	T45.0X2	T45.0X3	T45.0X4	T45.0X5	T45.0X6
Cyprolidol	T43.291	T43.292	T43.293	T43.294	T43.295	T43.296
Cyproterone	T38.6X1	T38.6X2	T38.6X3	T38.6X4	T38.6X5	T38.6X6
Cysteamine	T50.6X1	T50.6X2	T50.6X3	T50.6X4	T50.6X5	T50.6X6
Cytarabine	T45.1X1	T45.1X2	T45.1X3	T45.1X4	T45.1X5	T45.1X6
Cytisus						
laburnum	T62.2X1	T62.2X2	T62.2X3	T62.2X4	—	—
scoparius	T62.2X1	T62.2X2	T62.2X3	T62.2X4	—	—
Cytochrome C	T47.5X1	T47.5X2	T47.5X3	T47.5X4	T47.5X5	T47.5X6
Cytomel	T38.1X1	T38.1X2	T38.1X3	T38.1X4	T38.1X5	T38.1X6

Substance	Poisoning, Accidental (Unintentional)	Poisoning, Intentional Self-Harm	Poisoning, Assault	Poisoning, Undetermined	Adverse Effect	Underdosing
Cytosine arabinoside	T45.1X1	T45.1X2	T45.1X3	T45.1X4	T45.1X5	T45.1X6
Cytoxan	T45.1X1	T45.1X2	T45.1X3	T45.1X4	T45.1X5	T45.1X6
Cytozyme	T45.7X1	T45.7X2	T45.7X3	T45.7X4	T45.7X5	T45.7X6
2,4-D	T60.3X1	T60.3X2	T60.3X3	T60.3X4	—	—
D						
Dacarbazine	T45.1X1	T45.1X2	T45.1X3	T45.1X4	T45.1X5	T45.1X6
Dactinomycin	T45.1X1	T45.1X2	T45.1X3	T45.1X4	T45.1X5	T45.1X6
DADPS	T37.1X1	T37.1X2	T37.1X3	T37.1X4	T37.1X5	T37.1X6
Dakin's solution	T49.0X1	T49.0X2	T49.0X3	T49.0X4	T49.0X5	T49.0X6
Dalapon (sodium)	T60.3X1	T60.3X2	T60.3X3	T60.3X4	—	—
Dalmane	T42.4X1	T42.4X2	T42.4X3	T42.4X4	T42.4X5	T42.4X6
Danazol	T38.6X1	T38.6X2	T38.6X3	T38.6X4	T38.6X5	T38.6X6
Danilone	T45.511	T45.512	T45.513	T45.514	T45.515	T45.516
Danthron	T47.2X1	T47.2X2	T47.2X3	T47.2X4	T47.2X5	T47.2X6
Dantrolene	T42.8X1	T42.8X2	T42.8X3	T42.8X4	T42.8X5	T42.8X6
Dantron	T47.2X1	T47.2X2	T47.2X3	T47.2X4	T47.2X5	T47.2X6
Daphne (gnidium) (mezereum)	T62.2X1	T62.2X2	T62.2X3	T62.2X4	—	—
berry	T62.1X1	T62.1X2	T62.1X3	T62.1X4		
Dapsone	T37.1X1	T37.1X2	T37.1X3	T37.1X4	T37.1X5	T37.1X6
Daraprim	T37.2X1	T37.2X2	T37.2X3	T37.2X4	T37.2X5	T37.2X6
Darnel	T62.2X1	T62.2X2	T62.2X3	T62.2X4	—	—
Darvon	T39.8X1	T39.8X2	T39.8X3	T39.8X4	T39.8X5	T39.8X6
Daunomycin	T45.1X1	T45.1X2	T45.1X3	T45.1X4	T45.1X5	T45.1X6
Daunorubicin	T45.1X1	T45.1X2	T45.1X3	T45.1X4	T45.1X5	T45.1X6
DBI	T38.3X1	T38.3X2	T38.3X3	T38.3X4	T38.3X5	T38.3X6
D-Con	T60.91	T60.92	T60.93	T60.94	—	—
insecticide	T60.2X1	T60.2X2	T60.2X3	T60.2X4	—	—
rodenticide	T60.4X1	T60.4X2	T60.4X3	T60.4X4	—	—
DDAVP	T38.891	T38.892	T38.893	T38.894	T38.895	T38.896
DDE (bis(chlorophenyl)-dichloroethylene)	T60.2X1	T60.2X2	T60.2X3	T60.2X4	—	—
DDS	T37.1X1	T37.1X2	T37.1X3	T37.1X4	T37.1X5	T37.1X6
DDT (dust)	T60.1X1	T60.1X2	T60.1X3	T60.1X4	—	—
Deadly nightshade — see also Belladonna	T62.2X1	T62.2X2	T62.2X3	T62.2X4	—	—
berry	T62.1X1	T62.1X2	T62.1X3	T62.1X4		
Deamino-D-arginine vasopressin	T38.891	T38.892	T38.893	T38.894	T38.895	T38.896
Deanol (aceglumate)	T50.991	T50.992	T50.993	T50.994	T50.995	T50.996
Debrisoquine	T46.5X1	T46.5X2	T46.5X3	T46.5X4	T46.5X5	T46.5X6
Decaborane	T57.8X1	T57.8X2	T57.8X3	T57.8X4		
fumes	T59.891	T59.892	T59.893	T59.894		

TABLE OF DRUGS AND CHEMICALS

TABLE OF DRUGS AND CHEMICALS

Substance	External Cause (T-Code)					
	Poisoning, Accidental (Unintentional)	Poisoning, Intentional Self-Harm	Poisoning, Assault	Poisoning, Undetermined	Adverse Effect	Underdosing
Decadron	T38.0X1	T38.0X2	T38.0X3	T38.0X4	T38.0X5	T38.0X6
ENT agent	T49.6X1	T49.6X2	T49.6X3	T49.6X4	T49.6X5	T49.6X6
ophthalmic preparation	T49.5X1	T49.5X2	T49.5X3	T49.5X4	T49.5X5	T49.5X6
topical NEC	T49.0X1	T49.0X2	T49.0X3	T49.0X4	T49.0X5	T49.0X6
Decahydronaphthalene	T52.8X1	T52.8X2	T52.8X3	T52.8X4	—	—
Decalin	T52.8X1	T52.8X2	T52.8X3	T52.8X4	—	—
Decamethonium (bromide)	T48.1X1	T48.1X2	T48.1X3	T48.1X4	T48.1X5	T48.1X6
Decholin	T47.5X1	T47.5X2	T47.5X3	T47.5X4	T47.5X5	T47.5X6
Declomycin	T36.4X1	T36.4X2	T36.4X3	T36.4X4	T36.4X5	T36.4X6
Decongestant, nasal (mucosa)	T48.5X1	T48.5X2	T48.5X3	T48.5X4	T48.5X5	T48.5X6
combination	T48.5X1	T48.5X2	T48.5X3	T48.5X4	T48.5X5	T48.5X6
Deet	T60.8X1	T60.8X2	T60.8X3	T60.8X4	—	—
Deferoxamine	T45.8X1	T45.8X2	T45.8X3	T45.8X4	T45.8X5	T45.8X6
Deflazacort	T38.0X1	T38.0X2	T38.0X3	T38.0X4	T38.0X5	T38.0X6
Deglycyrrhizinized extract of licorice	T48.4X1	T48.4X2	T48.4X3	T48.4X4	T48.4X5	T48.4X6
Dehydrocholic acid	T47.5X1	T47.5X2	T47.5X3	T47.5X4	T47.5X5	T47.5X6
Dehydroemetine	T37.3X1	T37.3X2	T37.3X3	T37.3X4	T37.3X5	T37.3X6
Dekalin	T52.8X1	T52.8X2	T52.8X3	T52.8X4	—	—
Delalutin	T38.5X1	T38.5X2	T38.5X3	T38.5X4	T38.5X5	T38.5X6
Delphinium	T62.2X1	T62.2X2	T62.2X3	T62.2X4	—	—
Deltasone	T38.0X1	T38.0X2	T38.0X3	T38.0X4	T38.0X5	T38.0X6
Deltra	T38.0X1	T38.0X2	T38.0X3	T38.0X4	T38.0X5	T38.0X6
Delvinal	T42.3X1	T42.3X2	T42.3X3	T42.3X4	T42.3X5	T42.3X6
Delorazepam	T42.4X1	T42.4X2	T42.4X3	T42.4X4	T42.4X5	T42.4X6
Deltamethrin	T60.1X1	T60.1X2	T60.1X3	T60.1X4	—	—
Demecarium (bromide)	T49.5X1	T49.5X2	T49.5X3	T49.5X4	T49.5X5	T49.5X6
Demeclocycline	T36.4X1	T36.4X2	T36.4X3	T36.4X4	T36.4X5	T36.4X6
Demecolcine	T45.1X1	T45.1X2	T45.1X3	T45.1X4	T45.1X5	T45.1X6
Demegestone	T38.5X1	T38.5X2	T38.5X3	T38.5X4	T38.5X5	T38.5X6
Demelanizing agents	T49.8X1	T49.8X2	T49.8X3	T49.8X4	T49.8X5	T49.8X6
Demephion -O and -S	T60.0X1	T60.0X2	T60.0X3	T60.0X4	—	—
Demerol	T40.2X1	T40.2X2	T40.2X3	T40.2X4	T40.2X5	T40.2X6
Demethylchlortetracycline	T36.4X1	T36.4X2	T36.4X3	T36.4X4	T36.4X5	T36.4X6
Demethyltetracycline	T36.4X1	T36.4X2	T36.4X3	T36.4X4	T36.4X5	T36.4X6
Demeton -O and -S	T60.0X1	T60.0X2	T60.0X3	T60.0X4	—	—
Demulcent (external)	T49.3X1	T49.3X2	T49.3X3	T49.3X4	T49.3X5	T49.3X6
specified NEC	T49.3X1	T49.3X2	T49.3X3	T49.3X4	T49.3X5	T49.3X6
Demulen	T38.4X1	T38.4X2	T38.4X3	T38.4X4	T38.4X5	T38.4X6
Denatured alcohol	T51.0X1	T51.0X2	T51.0X3	T51.0X4	—	—
Dendrid	T49.5X1	T49.5X2	T49.5X3	T49.5X4	T49.5X5	T49.5X6
Dental drug, topical application NEC	T49.7X1	T49.7X2	T49.7X3	T49.7X4	T49.7X5	T49.7X6

Substance	External Cause (T-Code)					
	Poisoning, Accidental (Unintentional)	Poisoning, Intentional Self-Harm	Poisoning, Assault	Poisoning, Undetermined	Adverse Effect	Underdosing
Dentifrice	T49.7X1	T49.7X2	T49.7X3	T49.7X4	T49.7X5	T49.7X6
Deodorant spray (feminine hygiene)	T49.8X1	T49.8X2	T49.8X3	T49.8X4	T49.8X5	T49.8X6
Deoxycortone	T50.0X1	T50.0X2	T50.0X3	T50.0X4	T50.0X5	T50.0X6
2-Deoxy-5-fluorouridine	T45.1X1	T45.1X2	T45.1X3	T45.1X4	T45.1X5	T45.1X6
5-Deoxy-5-fluorouridine	T45.1X1	T45.1X2	T45.1X3	T45.1X4	T45.1X5	T45.1X6
Deoxyribonuclease (pancreatic)	T45.3X1	T45.3X2	T45.3X3	T45.3X4	T45.3X5	T45.3X6
Depilatory	T49.4X1	T49.4X2	T49.4X3	T49.4X4	T49.4X5	T49.4X6
Deprenalin	T42.8X1	T42.8X2	T42.8X3	T42.8X4	T42.8X5	T42.8X6
Deprenyl	T42.8X1	T42.8X2	T42.8X3	T42.8X4	T42.8X5	T42.8X6
Depressant, appetite	T50.5X1	T50.5X2	T50.5X3	T50.5X4	T50.5X5	T50.5X6
Depressant						
appetite, central	T50.5X1	T50.5X2	T50.5X3	T50.5X4	T50.5X5	T50.5X6
cardiac	T46.2X1	T46.2X2	T46.2X3	T46.2X4	T46.2X5	T46.2X6
central nervous system (anesthetic) — see also Central nervous system, depressants	T42.71	T42.72	T42.73	T42.74	T42.75	T42.76
general anesthetic	T41.201	T41.202	T41.203	T41.204	T41.205	T41.206
muscle tone	T42.8X1	T42.8X2	T42.8X3	T42.8X4	T42.8X5	T42.8X6
muscle tone, central	T42.8X1	T42.8X2	T42.8X3	T42.8X4	T42.8X5	T42.8X6
psychotherapeutic	T43.501	T43.502	T43.503	T43.504	T43.505	T43.506
Deptropine	T45.0X1	T45.0X2	T45.0X3	T45.0X4	T45.0X5	T45.0X6
Dequalinium (chloride)	T49.0X1	T49.0X2	T49.0X3	T49.0X4	T49.0X5	T49.0X6
Derris root	T60.2X1	T60.2X2	T60.2X3	T60.2X4	—	—
Deserpidine	T43.011	T43.012	T43.013	T43.014	T43.015	T43.016
Desferrioxamine	T45.8X1	T45.8X2	T45.8X3	T45.8X4	T45.8X5	T45.8X6
Desipramine	T43.0X1	T43.0X2	T43.0X3	T43.0X4	T43.0X5	T43.0X6
Deslanoside	T46.0X1	T46.0X2	T46.0X3	T46.0X4	T46.0X5	T46.0X6
Desloughing agent	T49.4X1	T49.4X2	T49.4X3	T49.4X4	T49.4X5	T49.4X6
Desmethylimipramine	T43.011	T43.012	T43.013	T43.014	T43.015	T43.016
Desmopressin	T38.891	T38.892	T38.893	T38.894	T38.895	T38.896
Desocodeine	T40.2X1	T40.2X2	T40.2X3	T40.2X4	T40.2X5	T40.2X6
Desogestrel	T38.5X1	T38.5X2	T38.5X3	T38.5X4	T38.5X5	T38.5X6
Desomorphine	T40.2X1	T40.2X2	T40.2X3	T40.2X4	—	—
Desonide	T49.0X1	T49.0X2	T49.0X3	T49.0X4	T49.0X5	T49.0X6
Desoximetasone	T49.0X1	T49.0X2	T49.0X3	T49.0X4	T49.0X5	T49.0X6
Desoxycorticosteroid	T50.0X1	T50.0X2	T50.0X3	T50.0X4	T50.0X5	T50.0X6
Desoxycortone	T50.0X1	T50.0X2	T50.0X3	T50.0X4	T50.0X5	T50.0X6
Desoxyephedrine	T43.621	T43.622	T43.623	T43.624	T43.625	T43.626
Detaxtran	T46.6X1	T46.6X2	T46.6X3	T46.6X4	T46.6X5	T46.6X6
Detergent	T49.2X1	T49.2X2	T49.2X3	T49.2X4	T49.2X5	T49.2X6
external medication	T49.2X1	T49.2X2	T49.2X3	T49.2X4	T49.2X5	T49.2X6
local	T49.2X1	T49.2X2	T49.2X3	T49.2X4	T49.2X5	T49.2X6

◀ New ◀ Revised ~~deleted~~ Deleted

Substance	Poisoning, Accidental (Unintentional)	Poisoning, Intentional Self-Harm	Poisoning, Assault	Poisoning, Undetermined	Adverse Effect	Underdosing
Detergent (*Continued*)						
medicinal	T49.2X1	T49.2X2	T49.2X3	T49.2X4	T49.2X5	T49.2X6
nonmedicinal	T55.1X1	T55.1X2	T55.1X3	T55.1X4	—	—
specified NEC	T55.1X1	T55.1X2	T55.1X3	T55.1X4	T55.1X5	T55.1X6
Deterrent, alcohol	T50.6X1	T50.6X2	T50.6X3	T50.6X4	T50.6X5	T50.6X6
Detoxifying agent	T50.6X1	T50.6X2	T50.6X3	T50.6X4	T50.6X5	T50.6X6
Detrothyronine	T38.1X1	T38.1X2	T38.1X3	T38.1X4	T38.1X5	T38.1X6
Dettol (external medication)	T49.0X1	T49.0X2	T49.0X3	T49.0X4	T49.0X5	T49.0X6
Dexamethasone	T38.0X1	T38.0X2	T38.0X3	T38.0X4	T38.0X5	T38.0X6
ENT agent	T49.6X1	T49.6X2	T49.6X3	T49.6X4	T49.6X5	T49.6X6
ophthalmic preparation	T49.5X1	T49.5X2	T49.5X3	T49.5X4	T49.5X5	T49.5X6
topical NEC	T49.0X1	T49.0X2	T49.0X3	T49.0X4	T49.0X5	T49.0X6
Dexamfetamine	T43.621	T43.622	T43.623	T43.624	T43.625	T43.626
Dexamphetamine	T43.621	T43.622	T43.623	T43.624	T43.625	T43.626
Dexbrompheniramine	T45.0X1	T45.0X2	T45.0X3	T45.0X4	T45.0X5	T45.0X6
Dexchlorpheniramine	T45.0X1	T45.0X2	T45.0X3	T45.0X4	T45.0X5	T45.0X6
Dexedrine	T43.621	T43.622	T43.623	T43.624	T43.625	T43.626
Dexetimide	T44.3X1	T44.3X2	T44.3X3	T44.3X4	T44.3X5	T44.3X6
Dexfenfluramine	T50.5X1	T50.5X2	T50.5X3	T50.5X4	T50.5X5	T50.5X6
Dexpanthenol	T45.2X1	T45.2X2	T45.2X3	T45.2X4	T45.2X5	T45.2X6
Dextran (40) (70) (150)	T45.8X1	T45.8X2	T45.8X3	T45.8X4	T45.8X5	T45.8X6
Dextriferron	T45.4X1	T45.4X2	T45.4X3	T45.4X4	T45.4X5	T45.4X6
Dextroamphetamine	T43.621	T43.622	T43.623	T43.624	T43.625	T43.626
Dextro calcium pantothenate	T45.2X1	T45.2X2	T45.2X3	T45.2X4	T45.2X5	T45.2X6
Dextromethorphan	T48.3X1	T48.3X2	T48.3X3	T48.3X4	T48.3X5	T48.3X6
Dextromoramide	T40.4X1	T40.4X2	T40.4X3	T40.4X4	—	—
topical	T49.8X1	T49.8X2	T49.8X3	T49.8X4	T49.8X5	T49.8X6
Dextro pantothenyl alcohol	T45.2X1	T45.2X2	T45.2X3	T45.2X4	T45.2X5	T45.2X6
Dextropropoxyphene	T40.4X1	T40.4X2	T40.4X3	T40.4X4	T40.4X5	T40.4X6
Dextrorphan	T40.2X1	T40.2X2	T40.2X3	T40.2X4	T40.2X5	T40.2X6
Dextrose	T50.3X1	T50.3X2	T50.3X3	T50.3X4	T50.3X5	T50.3X6
concentrated solution, intravenous	T46.8X1	T46.8X2	T46.8X3	T46.8X4	T46.8X5	T46.8X6
Dextrothyroxin	T38.1X1	T38.1X2	T38.1X3	T38.1X4	T38.1X5	T38.1X6
Dextrothyroxine sodium	T38.1X1	T38.1X2	T38.1X3	T38.1X4	T38.1X5	T38.1X6
DFP	T44.0X1	T44.0X2	T44.0X3	T44.0X4	T44.0X5	T44.0X6
DHE	T37.3X1	T37.3X2	T37.3X3	T37.3X4	T37.3X5	T37.3X6
45	T46.5X1	T46.5X2	T46.5X3	T46.5X4	T46.5X5	T46.5X6
Diabinese	T38.3X1	T38.3X2	T38.3X3	T38.3X4	T38.3X5	T38.3X6
Diacetone alcohol	T52.4X1	T52.4X2	T52.4X3	T52.4X4	—	—
Diacetyl monoxime	T50.991	T50.992	T50.993	T50.994	—	—
Diacetylmorphine	T40.1X1	T40.1X2	T40.1X3	T40.1X4	—	—

Substance	Poisoning, Accidental (Unintentional)	Poisoning, Intentional Self-Harm	Poisoning, Assault	Poisoning, Undetermined	Adverse Effect	Underdosing
Diachylon plaster	T49.4X1	T49.4X2	T49.4X3	T49.4X4	T49.4X5	T49.4X6
Diaethylstilboestrolum	T38.5X1	T38.5X2	T38.5X3	T38.5X4	T38.5X5	T38.5X6
Diagnostic agent NEC	T50.8X1	T50.8X2	T50.8X3	T50.8X4	T50.8X5	T50.8X6
Dial (soap)	T49.2X1	T49.2X2	T49.2X3	T49.2X4	T49.2X5	T49.2X6
sedative	T42.3X1	T42.3X2	T42.3X3	T42.3X4	T42.3X5	T42.3X6
Dialkyl carbonate	T52.91	T52.92	T52.93	T52.94	—	—
Diallylbarbituric acid	T42.3X1	T42.3X2	T42.3X3	T42.3X4	T42.3X5	T42.3X6
Diallymal	T42.3X1	T42.3X2	T42.3X3	T42.3X4	T42.3X5	T42.3X6
Dialysis solution (intraperitoneal)	T50.3X1	T50.3X2	T50.3X3	T50.3X4	T50.3X5	T50.3X6
Diaminodiphenylsulfone	T37.1X1	T37.1X2	T37.1X3	T37.1X4	T37.1X5	T37.1X6
Diamorphine	T40.1X1	T40.1X2	T40.1X3	T40.1X4	—	—
Diamox	T50.2X1	T50.2X2	T50.2X3	T50.2X4	T50.2X5	T50.2X6
Diamthazole	T49.0X1	T49.0X2	T49.0X3	T49.0X4	T49.0X5	T49.0X6
Dianthone	T47.2X1	T47.2X2	T47.2X3	T47.2X4	T47.2X5	T47.2X6
Diaphenylsulfone	T37.0X1	T37.0X2	T37.0X3	T37.0X4	T37.0X5	T37.0X6
Diasone (sodium)	T37.1X1	T37.1X2	T37.1X3	T37.1X4	T37.1X5	T37.1X6
Diastase	T47.5X1	T47.5X2	T47.5X3	T47.5X4	T47.5X5	T47.5X6
Diatrizoate	T50.8X1	T50.8X2	T50.8X3	T50.8X4	T50.8X5	T50.8X6
Diazepam	T42.4X1	T42.4X2	T42.4X3	T42.4X4	T42.4X5	T42.4X6
Diazinon	T60.0X1	T60.0X2	T60.0X3	T60.0X4	—	—
Diazomethane (gas)	T59.891	T59.892	T59.893	T59.894	—	—
Diazoxide	T46.5X1	T46.5X2	T46.5X3	T46.5X4	T46.5X5	T46.5X6
Dibekacin	T36.5X1	T36.5X2	T36.5X3	T36.5X4	T36.5X5	T36.5X6
Dibenamine	T44.6X1	T44.6X2	T44.6X3	T44.6X4	T44.6X5	T44.6X6
Dibenzepin	T43.011	T43.012	T43.013	T43.014	T43.015	T43.016
Dibenzheptropine	T45.0X1	T45.0X2	T45.0X3	T45.0X4	T45.0X5	T45.0X6
Dibenzyline	T44.6X1	T44.6X2	T44.6X3	T44.6X4	T44.6X5	T44.6X6
Diborane (gas)	T59.891	T59.892	T59.893	T59.894	—	—
Dibromochloropropane	T60.8X1	T60.8X2	T60.8X3	T60.8X4	—	—
Dibromodulcitol	T45.1X1	T45.1X2	T45.1X3	T45.1X4	T45.1X5	T45.1X6
Dibromoethane	T53.6X1	T53.6X2	T53.6X3	T53.6X4	—	—
Dibromomannitol	T45.1X1	T45.1X2	T45.1X3	T45.1X4	T45.1X5	T45.1X6
Dibromopropamidine isethionate	T49.0X1	T49.0X2	T49.0X3	T49.0X4	T49.0X5	T49.0X6
Dibrompropamidine	T49.0X1	T49.0X2	T49.0X3	T49.0X4	T49.0X5	T49.0X6
Dibucaine	T41.3X1	T41.3X2	T41.3X3	T41.3X4	T41.3X5	T41.3X6
topical (surface)	T41.3X1	T41.3X2	T41.3X3	T41.3X4	T41.3X5	T41.3X6
Dibunate sodium	T48.3X1	T48.3X2	T48.3X3	T48.3X4	T48.3X5	T48.3X6
Dibutoline sulfate	T44.3X1	T44.3X2	T44.3X3	T44.3X4	T44.3X5	T44.3X6
Dicamba	T60.3X1	T60.3X2	T60.3X3	T60.3X4	—	—
Dicapthon	T60.0X1	T60.0X2	T60.0X3	T60.0X4	—	—
Dichlobenil	T60.3X1	T60.3X2	T60.3X3	T60.3X4	—	—
Dichlone	T60.3X1	T60.3X2	T60.3X3	T60.3X4	—	—

TABLE OF DRUGS AND CHEMICALS

Substance	External Cause (T-Code)					
	Poisoning, Accidental (Unintentional)	Poisoning, Intentional Self-Harm	Poisoning, Assault	Poisoning, Undetermined	Adverse Effect	Underdosing
Dichloralphenozone	T42.6X1	T42.6X2	T42.6X3	T42.6X4	T42.6X5	T42.6X6
Dichlorbenzidine	T65.3X1	T65.3X2	T65.3X3	T65.3X4	—	—
Dichlorhydrin	T52.8X1	T52.8X2	T52.8X3	T52.8X4	—	—
Dichlorhydroxyquinoline	T37.8X1	T37.8X2	T37.8X3	T37.8X4	T37.8X5	T37.8X6
Dichlorobenzene	T53.7X1	T53.7X2	T53.7X3	T53.7X4	—	—
Dichlorobenzyl alcohol	T49.6X1	T49.6X2	T49.6X3	T49.6X4	T49.6X5	T49.6X6
Dichlorodifluoromethane	T53.5X1	T53.5X2	T53.5X3	T53.5X4	—	—
Dichloroethane	T52.8X1	T52.8X2	T52.8X3	T52.8X4	—	—
Sym-Dichloroethyl ether	T53.6X1	T53.6X2	T53.6X3	T53.6X4	—	—
Dichloroethyl sulfide, not in war	T59.891	T59.892	T59.893	T59.894	—	—
Dichloroethylene	T53.6X1	T53.6X2	T53.6X3	T53.6X4	—	—
Dichloroformoxime, not in war	T59.891	T59.892	T59.893	T59.894	—	—
Dichlorohydrin, alpha-dichlorohydrin	T52.8X1	T52.8X2	T52.8X3	T52.8X4	—	—
Dichloromethane (solvent)	T53.4X1	T53.4X2	T53.4X3	T53.4X4	—	—
vapor	T53.4X1	T53.4X2	T53.4X3	T53.4X4	—	—
Dichloronaphthoquinone	T60.3X1	T60.3X2	T60.3X3	T60.3X4	—	—
Dichlorophen	T37.4X1	T37.4X2	T37.4X3	T37.4X4	T37.4X5	T37.4X6
2,4-Dichlorophenoxy-acetic acid	T60.3X1	T60.3X2	T60.3X3	T60.3X4	—	—
Dichloropropene	T60.3X1	T60.3X2	T60.3X3	T60.3X4	—	—
Dichloropropionic acid	T60.3X1	T60.3X2	T60.3X3	T60.3X4	—	—
Dichlorphenamide	T50.2X1	T50.2X2	T50.2X3	T50.2X4	T50.2X5	T50.2X6
Dichlorvos	T60.0X1	T60.0X2	T60.0X3	T60.0X4	—	—
Diclofenac	T39.391	T39.392	T39.393	T39.394	T39.395	T39.396
Diclofenamide	T50.2X1	T50.2X2	T50.2X3	T50.2X4	T50.2X5	T50.2X6
Diclofensine	T43.291	T43.292	T43.293	T43.294	T43.295	T43.296
Diclonixine	T39.8X1	T39.8X2	T39.8X3	T39.8X4	T39.8X5	T39.8X6
Dicloxacillin	T36.0X1	T36.0X2	T36.0X3	T36.0X4	T36.0X5	T36.0X6
Dicophane	T49.0X1	T49.0X2	T49.0X3	T49.0X4	T49.0X5	T49.0X6
Dicoumarol, dicoumarin, dicumarol	T45.511	T45.512	T45.513	T45.514	T45.515	T45.516
Dicrotophos	T60.0X1	T60.0X2	T60.0X3	T60.0X4	—	—
Dicyanogen (gas)	T65.0X1	T65.0X2	T65.0X3	T65.0X4	—	—
Dicyclomine	T44.3X1	T44.3X2	T44.3X3	T44.3X4	T44.3X5	T44.3X6
Dicycloverine	T44.3X1	T44.3X2	T44.3X3	T44.3X4	T44.3X5	T44.3X6
Dideoxycytidine	T37.5X1	T37.5X2	T37.5X3	T37.5X4	T37.5X5	T37.5X6
Dideoxyinosine	T37.5X1	T37.5X2	T37.5X3	T37.5X4	T37.5X5	T37.5X6
Dieldrin (vapor)	T60.1X1	T60.1X2	T60.1X3	T60.1X4	—	—
Diemal	T42.3X1	T42.3X2	T42.3X3	T42.3X4	T42.3X5	T42.3X6
Dienestrol	T38.5X1	T38.5X2	T38.5X3	T38.5X4	T38.5X5	T38.5X6
Dienoestrol	T38.5X1	T38.5X2	T38.5X3	T38.5X4	T38.5X5	T38.5X6
Dietetic drug NEC	T50.901	T50.902	T50.903	T50.904	T50.905	T50.906
Diethazine	T42.8X1	T42.8X2	T42.8X3	T42.8X4	T42.8X5	T42.8X6

Substance	External Cause (T-Code)					
	Poisoning, Accidental (Unintentional)	Poisoning, Intentional Self-Harm	Poisoning, Assault	Poisoning, Undetermined	Adverse Effect	Underdosing
Diethyl						
barbituric acid	T42.3X1	T42.3X2	T42.3X3	T42.3X4	T42.3X5	T42.3X6
carbamazine	T37.4X1	T37.4X2	T37.4X3	T37.4X4	T37.4X5	T37.4X6
carbinol	T51.3X1	T51.3X2	T51.3X3	T51.3X4	—	—
carbonate	T52.8X1	T52.8X2	T52.8X3	T52.8X4	—	—
ether (vapor) — *see also ether*	T41.0X1	T41.0X2	T41.0X3	T41.0X4	T41.0X5	T41.0X6
oxide	T52.8X1	T52.8X2	T52.8X3	T52.8X4	—	—
propion	T50.5X1	T50.5X2	T50.5X3	T50.5X4	T50.5X5	T50.5X6
stilbestrol	T38.5X1	T38.5X2	T38.5X3	T38.5X4	T38.5X5	T38.5X6
toluamide (nonmedicinal)	T60.8X1	T60.8X2	T60.8X3	T60.8X4	—	—
medicinal	T49.3X1	T49.3X2	T49.3X3	T49.3X4	T49.3X5	T49.3X6
Diethylcarbamazine	T37.4X1	T37.4X2	T37.4X3	T37.4X4	T37.4X5	T37.4X6
Diethylene						
dioxide	T52.8X1	T52.8X2	T52.8X3	T52.8X4	—	—
glycol (monoacetate) (monobutyl ether) (monoethyl ether)	T52.3X1	T52.3X2	T52.3X3	T52.3X4	—	—
Diethylhexylphthalate	T65.891	T65.892	T65.893	T65.894	—	—
Diethylpropion	T50.5X1	T50.5X2	T50.5X3	T50.5X4	T50.5X5	T50.5X6
Diethylstilbestrol	T38.5X1	T38.5X2	T38.5X3	T38.5X4	T38.5X5	T38.5X6
Diethylstilboestrol	T38.5X1	T38.5X2	T38.5X3	T38.5X4	T38.5X5	T38.5X6
Diethylsulfone-diethylmethane	T42.6X1	T42.6X2	T42.6X3	T42.6X4	T42.6X5	T42.6X6
Diethyltoluamide	T49.0X1	T49.0X2	T49.0X3	T49.0X4	T49.0X5	T49.0X6
Diethyltryptamine (DET)	T40.991	T40.992	T40.993	T40.994	—	—
Difebarbamate	T42.3X1	T42.3X2	T42.3X3	T42.3X4	T42.3X5	T42.3X6
Difencloxazine	T40.2X1	T40.2X2	T40.2X3	T40.2X4	T40.2X5	T40.2X6
Difenidol	T45.0X1	T45.0X2	T45.0X3	T45.0X4	T45.0X5	T45.0X6
Difenoxin	T47.6X1	T47.6X2	T47.6X3	T47.6X4	T47.6X5	T47.6X6
Difetarsone	T37.3X1	T37.3X2	T37.3X3	T37.3X4	T37.3X5	T37.3X6
Diffusin	T45.3X1	T45.3X2	T45.3X3	T45.3X4	T45.3X5	T45.3X6
Diflorasone	T49.0X1	T49.0X2	T49.0X3	T49.0X4	T49.0X5	T49.0X6
Diflubenzuron	T60.1X1	T60.1X2	T60.1X3	T60.1X4	—	—
Diflos	T44.0X1	T44.0X2	T44.0X3	T44.0X4	T44.0X5	T44.0X6
Diflucortolone	T49.0X1	T49.0X2	T49.0X3	T49.0X4	T49.0X5	T49.0X6
Diflunisal	T39.091	T39.092	T39.093	T39.094	T39.095	T39.096
Difluoromethyldopa	T42.8X1	T42.8X2	T42.8X3	T42.8X4	T42.8X5	T42.8X6
Difluorophate	T44.0X1	T44.0X2	T44.0X3	T44.0X4	T44.0X5	T44.0X6
Digestant NEC	T47.5X1	T47.5X2	T47.5X3	T47.5X4	T47.5X5	T47.5X6
Digitalin(e)	T46.0X1	T46.0X2	T46.0X3	T46.0X4	T46.0X5	T46.0X6
Digitalis (leaf) (glycoside)	T46.0X1	T46.0X2	T46.0X3	T46.0X4	T46.0X5	T46.0X6
lanata	T46.0X1	T46.0X2	T46.0X3	T46.0X4	T46.0X5	T46.0X6
purpurea	T46.0X1	T46.0X2	T46.0X3	T46.0X4	T46.0X5	T46.0X6
Digitoxin	T46.0X1	T46.0X2	T46.0X3	T46.0X4	T46.0X5	T46.0X6

◀ New ⬖ Revised deleted Deleted

Substance	Poisoning, Accidental (Unintentional)	Poisoning, Intentional Self-Harm	Poisoning, Assault	Poisoning, Undetermined	Adverse Effect	Underdosing
Digitoxose	T46.0X1	T46.0X2	T46.0X3	T46.0X4	T46.0X5	T46.0X6
Digoxin	T46.0X1	T46.0X2	T46.0X3	T46.0X4	T46.0X5	T46.0X6
Digoxine	T46.0X1	T46.0X2	T46.0X3	T46.0X4	T46.0X5	T46.0X6
Dihydralazine	T46.5X1	T46.5X2	T46.5X3	T46.5X4	T46.5X5	T46.5X6
Dihydrazine	T46.5X1	T46.5X2	T46.5X3	T46.5X4	T46.5X5	T46.5X6
Dihydrocodeinone	T40.2X1	T40.2X2	T40.2X3	T40.2X4	T40.2X5	T40.2X6
Dihydroergocornine	T46.7X1	T46.7X2	T46.7X3	T46.7X4	T46.7X5	T46.7X6
Dihydroergocristine (mesilate)	T46.7X1	T46.7X2	T46.7X3	T46.7X4	T46.7X5	T46.7X6
Dihydroergokryptine	T46.7X1	T46.7X2	T46.7X3	T46.7X4	T46.7X5	T46.7X6
Dihydroergotamine	T46.5X1	T46.5X2	T46.5X3	T46.5X4	T46.5X5	T46.5X6
Dihydroergotoxine	T46.7X1	T46.7X2	T46.7X3	T46.7X4	T46.7X5	T46.7X6
mesilate	T46.7X1	T46.7X2	T46.7X3	T46.7X4	T46.7X5	T46.7X6
Dihydrohydroxycodein-one	T40.2X1	T40.2X2	T40.2X3	T40.2X4	T40.2X5	T40.2X6
Dihydrohydroxymorphinone	T40.2X1	T40.2X2	T40.2X3	T40.2X4	T40.2X5	T40.2X6
Dihydroisocodeine	T40.2X1	T40.2X2	T40.2X3	T40.2X4	T40.2X5	T40.2X6
Dihydromorphine	T40.2X1	T40.2X2	T40.2X3	T40.2X4	—	—
Dihydromorphinone	T40.2X1	T40.2X2	T40.2X3	T40.2X4	T40.2X5	T40.2X6
Dihydrostreptomycin	T36.5X1	T36.5X2	T36.5X3	T36.5X4	T36.5X5	T36.5X6
Dihydrotachysterol	T45.2X1	T45.2X2	T45.2X3	T45.2X4	T45.2X5	T45.2X6
Dihydroxyaluminum aminoacetate	T47.1X1	T47.1X2	T47.1X3	T47.1X4	T47.1X5	T47.1X6
Dihydroxyaluminum sodium carbonate	T47.1X1	T47.1X2	T47.1X3	T47.1X4	T47.1X5	T47.1X6
Dihydroxyanthraquinone	T47.2X1	T47.2X2	T47.2X3	T47.2X4	T47.2X5	T47.2X6
Dihydroxycodeinone	T40.2X1	T40.2X2	T40.2X3	T40.2X4	T40.2X5	T40.2X6
Dihydroxypropyl theophylline	T50.2X1	T50.2X2	T50.2X3	T50.2X4	T50.2X5	T50.2X6
Diiodohydroxyquin	T37.8X1	T37.8X2	T37.8X3	T37.8X4	T37.8X5	T37.8X6
topical	T49.0X1	T49.0X2	T49.0X3	T49.0X4	T49.0X5	T49.0X6
Diiodohydroxyquinoline	T37.8X1	T37.8X2	T37.8X3	T37.8X4	T37.8X5	T37.8X6
Diiodotyrosine	T38.2X1	T38.2X2	T38.2X3	T38.2X4	T38.2X5	T38.2X6
Diisopromine	T44.3X1	T44.3X2	T44.3X3	T44.3X4	T44.3X5	T44.3X6
Diisopropylamine	T46.3X1	T46.3X2	T46.3X3	T46.3X4	T46.3X5	T46.3X6
Diisopropylfluorophosphonate	T44.0X1	T44.0X2	T44.0X3	T44.0X4	T44.0X5	T44.0X6
Dilantin	T42.0X1	T42.0X2	T42.0X3	T42.0X4	T42.0X5	T42.0X6
Dilaudid	T40.2X1	T40.2X2	T40.2X3	T40.2X4	T40.2X5	T40.2X6
Dilazep	T46.3X1	T46.3X2	T46.3X3	T46.3X4	T46.3X5	T46.3X6
Dill	T47.5X1	T47.5X2	T47.5X3	T47.5X4	T47.5X5	T47.5X6
Diloxanide	T37.3X1	T37.3X2	T37.3X3	T37.3X4	T37.3X5	T37.3X6
Diltiazem	T46.1X1	T46.1X2	T46.1X3	T46.1X4	T46.1X5	T46.1X6
Dimazole	T49.0X1	T49.0X2	T49.0X3	T49.0X4	T49.0X5	T49.0X6
Dimefline	T50.7X1	T50.7X2	T50.7X3	T50.7X4	T50.7X5	T50.7X6
Dimefox	T60.0X1	T60.0X2	T60.0X3	T60.0X4	—	—

Substance	Poisoning, Accidental (Unintentional)	Poisoning, Intentional Self-Harm	Poisoning, Assault	Poisoning, Undetermined	Adverse Effect	Underdosing
Dimemorfan	T48.3X1	T48.3X2	T48.3X3	T48.3X4	T48.3X5	T48.3X6
Dimenhydrinate	T45.0X1	T45.0X2	T45.0X3	T45.0X4	T45.0X5	T45.0X6
Dimercaprol (British anti-lewisite)	T45.8X1	T45.8X2	T45.8X3	T45.8X4	T45.8X5	T45.8X6
Dimercaptopropanol	T45.8X1	T45.8X2	T45.8X3	T45.8X4	T45.8X5	T45.8X6
Dimestrol	T38.5X1	T38.5X2	T38.5X3	T38.5X4	T38.5X5	T38.5X6
Dimetane	T45.0X1	T45.0X2	T45.0X3	T45.0X4	T45.0X5	T45.0X6
Dimethicone	T47.1X1	T47.1X2	T47.1X3	T47.1X4	T47.1X5	T47.1X6
Dimethindene	T45.0X1	T45.0X2	T45.0X3	T45.0X4	T45.0X5	T45.0X6
Dimethisoquin	T49.1X1	T49.1X2	T49.1X3	T49.1X4	T49.1X5	T49.1X6
Dimethisterone	T38.5X1	T38.5X2	T38.5X3	T38.5X4	T38.5X5	T38.5X6
Dimethoate	T60.0X1	T60.0X2	T60.0X3	T60.0X4	—	—
Dimethocaine	T41.3X1	T41.3X2	T41.3X3	T41.3X4	T41.3X5	T41.3X6
Dimethoxanate	T48.3X1	T48.3X2	T48.3X3	T48.3X4	T48.3X5	T48.3X6
Dimethyl						
arsine, arsinic acid	T57.0X1	T57.0X2	T57.0X3	T57.0X4	—	—
carbinol	T51.2X1	T51.2X2	T51.2X3	T51.2X4	—	—
carbonate	T52.8X1	T52.8X2	T52.8X3	T52.8X4	—	—
diguanide	T38.3X1	T38.3X2	T38.3X3	T38.3X4	T38.3X5	T38.3X6
ketone	T52.4X1	T52.4X2	T52.4X3	T52.4X4	—	—
vapor	T52.4X1	T52.4X2	T52.4X3	T52.4X4	—	—
meperidine	T40.2X1	T40.2X2	T40.2X3	T40.2X4	T40.2X5	T40.2X6
parathion	T60.0X1	T60.0X2	T60.0X3	T60.0X4	—	—
phthlate	T49.3X1	T49.3X2	T49.3X3	T49.3X4	T49.3X5	T49.3X6
polysiloxane	T47.8X1	T47.8X2	T47.8X3	T47.8X4	T47.8X5	T47.8X6
sulfate (fumes)	T59.891	T59.892	T59.893	T59.894		
liquid	T65.891	T65.892	T65.893	T65.894		
sulfoxide (nonmedicinal)	T52.8X1	T52.8X2	T52.8X3	T52.8X4	—	—
medicinal	T49.4X1	T49.4X2	T49.4X3	T49.4X4	T49.4X5	T49.4X6
tryptamine	T40.991	T40.992	T40.993	T40.994	—	—
tubocurarine	T48.1X1	T48.1X2	T48.1X3	T48.1X4	T48.1X5	T48.1X6
Dimethylamine sulfate	T49.4X1	T49.4X2	T49.4X3	T49.4X4	T49.4X5	T49.4X6
Dimethylformamide	T52.8X1	T52.8X2	T52.8X3	T52.8X4	—	—
Dimethyltubocurarinium chloride	T48.1X1	T48.1X2	T48.1X3	T48.1X4	T48.1X5	T48.1X6
Dimeticone	T47.1X1	T47.1X2	T47.1X3	T47.1X4	T47.1X5	T47.1X6
Dimetilan	T60.0X1	T60.0X2	T60.0X3	T60.0X4	—	—
Dimetindene	T45.0X1	T45.0X2	T45.0X3	T45.0X4	T45.0X5	T45.0X6
Dimetotiazine	T43.3X1	T43.3X2	T43.3X3	T43.3X4	T43.3X5	T43.3X6
Dimorpholamine	T50.7X1	T50.7X2	T50.7X3	T50.7X4	T50.7X5	T50.7X6
Dimoxyline	T46.3X1	T46.3X2	T46.3X3	T46.3X4	T46.3X5	T46.3X6
Dinitrobenzene	T65.3X1	T65.3X2	T65.3X3	T65.3X4	—	—
vapor	T59.891	T59.892	T59.893	T59.894	—	—

◀ New ◀▏▏▏ Revised ~~deleted~~ Deleted

Substance	External Cause (T-Code) Poisoning, Accidental (Unintentional)	Poisoning, Intentional Self-Harm	Poisoning, Assault	Poisoning, Undetermined	Adverse Effect	Underdosing
Dinitrobenzol	T65.3X1	T65.3X2	T65.3X3	T65.3X4	—	—
vapor	T59.891	T59.892	T59.893	T59.894		
Dinitrobutylphenol	T65.3X1	T65.3X2	T65.3X3	T65.3X4	—	—
Dinitro (-ortho-)cresol (pesticide) (spray)	T65.3X1	T65.3X2	T65.3X3	T65.3X4	—	—
Dinitrocyclohexylphenol	T65.3X1	T65.3X2	T65.3X3	T65.3X4	—	—
Dinitrophenol	T65.3X1	T65.3X2	T65.3X3	T65.3X4		
Dinoprost	T48.0X1	T48.0X2	T48.0X3	T48.0X4	T48.0X5	T48.0X6
Dinoprostone	T48.0X1	T48.0X2	T48.0X3	T48.0X4	T48.0X5	T48.0X6
Dinoseb	T60.3X1	T60.3X2	T60.3X3	T60.3X4		
Dioctyl sulfosuccinate (calcium) (sodium)	T47.4X1	T47.4X2	T47.4X3	T47.4X4	T47.4X5	T47.4X6
Diodone	T50.8X1	T50.8X2	T50.8X3	T50.8X4	T50.8X5	T50.8X6
Diodoquin	T37.8X1	T37.8X2	T37.8X3	T37.8X4	T37.8X5	T37.8X6
Dionin	T40.2X1	T40.2X2	T40.2X3	T40.2X4	T40.2X5	T40.2X6
Diosmin	T46.991	T46.992	T46.993	T46.994	T46.995	T46.996
Dioxane	T52.8X1	T52.8X2	T52.8X3	T52.8X4	—	—
Dioxathion	T60.0X1	T60.0X2	T60.0X3	T60.0X4	—	—
Dioxin	T53.7X1	T53.7X2	T53.7X3	T53.7X4		
Dioxopromethazine	T43.3X1	T43.3X2	T43.3X3	T43.3X4	T43.3X5	T43.3X6
Dioxyline	T46.3X1	T46.3X2	T46.3X3	T46.3X4	T46.3X5	T46.3X6
Dipentene	T52.8X1	T52.8X2	T52.8X3	T52.8X4	—	—
Diperodon	T41.3X1	T41.3X2	T41.3X3	T41.3X4	T41.3X5	T41.3X6
Diphacinone	T60.4X1	T60.4X2	T60.4X3	T60.4X4		—
Diphemanil	T44.3X1	T44.3X2	T44.3X3	T44.3X4	T44.3X5	T44.3X6
metilsulfate	T44.3X1	T44.3X2	T44.3X3	T44.3X4	T44.3X5	T44.3X6
Diphenadione	T45.511	T45.512	T45.513	T45.514	T45.515	T45.516
rodenticide	T60.4X1	T60.4X2	T60.4X3	T60.4X4	—	—
Diphenhydramine	T45.0X1	T45.0X2	T45.0X3	T45.0X4	T45.0X5	T45.0X6
Diphenidol	T45.0X1	T45.0X2	T45.0X3	T45.0X4	T45.0X5	T45.0X6
Diphenoxylate	T47.6X1	T47.6X2	T47.6X3	T47.6X4	T47.6X5	T47.6X6
Diphenylamine	T65.3X1	T65.3X2	T65.3X3	T65.3X4	—	—
Diphenylbutazone	T39.2X1	T39.2X2	T39.2X3	T39.2X4	T39.2X5	T39.2X6
Diphenylchloroarsine, not in war	T57.0X1	T57.0X2	T57.0X3	T57.0X4	—	—
Diphenylhydantoin	T42.0X1	T42.0X2	T42.0X3	T42.0X4	T42.0X5	T42.0X6
Diphenylmethane dye	T52.1X1	T52.1X2	T52.1X3	T52.1X4	—	—
Diphenylpyraline	T45.0X1	T45.0X2	T45.0X3	T45.0X4	T45.0X5	T45.0X6
Diphtheria						
antitoxin	T50.Z11	T50.Z12	T50.Z13	T50.Z14	T50.Z15	T50.Z16
toxoid	T50.A91	T50.A92	T50.A93	T50.A94	T50.A95	T50.A96
with tetanus toxoid	T50.A21	T50.A22	T50.A23	T50.A24	T50.A25	T50.A26
with pertussis component	T50.A11	T50.A12	T50.A13	T50.A14	T50.A15	T50.A16

Substance	External Cause (T-Code) Poisoning, Accidental (Unintentional)	Poisoning, Intentional Self-Harm	Poisoning, Assault	Poisoning, Undetermined	Adverse Effect	Underdosing
Diphtheria (Continued)						
vaccine (combination)	T50.A91	T50.A92	T50.A93	T50.A94	T50.A95	T50.A96
combination						
including pertussis	T50.A11	T50.A12	T50.A13	T50.A14	T50.A15	T50.A16
without pertussis	T50.A21	T50.A22	T50.A23	T50.A24	T50.A25	T50.A26
Diphylline	T50.2X1	T50.2X2	T50.2X3	T50.2X4	T50.2X5	T50.2X6
Dipipanone	T40.4X1	T40.4X2	T40.4X3	T40.4X4	—	—
Dipivefrine	T49.5X1	T49.5X2	T49.5X3	T49.5X4	T49.5X5	T49.5X6
Diplovax	T50.B91	T50.B92	T50.B93	T50.B94	T50.B95	T50.B96
Diprophylline	T50.2X1	T50.2X2	T50.2X3	T50.2X4	T50.2X5	T50.2X6
Dipropyline	T48.291	T48.292	T48.293	T48.294	T48.295	T48.296
Dipyridamole	T46.3X1	T46.3X2	T46.3X3	T46.3X4	T46.3X5	T46.3X6
Dipyrone	T39.2X1	T39.2X2	T39.2X3	T39.2X4	T39.2X5	T39.2X6
Diquat (dibromide)	T60.3X1	T60.3X2	T60.3X3	T60.3X4	—	—
Disinfectant	T65.891	T65.892	T65.893	T65.894	—	—
alkaline	T54.3X1	T54.3X2	T54.3X3	T54.3X4	—	—
aromatic	T54.1X1	T54.1X2	T54.1X3	T54.1X4	—	—
intestinal	T37.8X1	T37.8X2	T37.8X3	T37.8X4	T37.8X5	T37.8X6
Disipal	T42.8X1	T42.8X2	T42.8X3	T42.8X4	T42.8X5	T42.8X6
Disodium edetate	T50.6X1	T50.6X2	T50.6X3	T50.6X4	T50.6X5	T50.6X6
Disoprofol	T41.291	T41.292	T41.293	T41.294	T41.295	T41.296
Disopyramide	T46.2X1	T46.2X2	T46.2X3	T46.2X4	T46.2X5	T46.2X6
Distigmine (bromide)	T44.0X1	T44.0X2	T44.0X3	T44.0X4	T44.0X5	T44.0X6
Disulfamide	T50.2X1	T50.2X2	T50.2X3	T50.2X4	T50.2X5	T50.2X6
Disulfanilamide	T37.0X1	T37.0X2	T37.0X3	T37.0X4	T37.0X5	T37.0X6
Disulfiram	T50.6X1	T50.6X2	T50.6X3	T50.6X4	T50.6X5	T50.6X6
Disulfoton	T60.0X1	T60.0X2	T60.0X3	T60.0X4	—	—
Dithiazanine iodide	T37.4X1	T37.4X2	T37.4X3	T37.4X4	T37.4X5	T37.4X6
Dithiocarbamate	T60.0X1	T60.0X2	T60.0X3	T60.0X4	—	—
Dithranol	T49.4X1	T49.4X2	T49.4X3	T49.4X4	T49.4X5	T49.4X6
Diucardin	T50.2X1	T50.2X2	T50.2X3	T50.2X4	T50.2X5	T50.2X6
Diupres	T50.2X1	T50.2X2	T50.2X3	T50.2X4	T50.2X5	T50.2X6
Diuretic NEC	T50.2X1	T50.2X2	T50.2X3	T50.2X4	T50.2X5	T50.2X6
benzothiadiazine	T50.2X1	T50.2X2	T50.2X3	T50.2X4	T50.2X5	T50.2X6
carbonic acid anhydrase inhibitors	T50.2X1	T50.2X2	T50.2X3	T50.2X4	T50.2X5	T50.2X6
furfuryl NEC	T50.2X1	T50.2X2	T50.2X3	T50.2X4	T50.2X5	T50.2X6
loop (high-ceiling)	T50.1X1	T50.1X2	T50.1X3	T50.1X4	T50.1X5	T50.1X6
mercurial NEC	T50.2X1	T50.2X2	T50.2X3	T50.2X4	T50.2X5	T50.2X6
osmotic	T50.2X1	T50.2X2	T50.2X3	T50.2X4	T50.2X5	T50.2X6
purine NEC	T50.2X1	T50.2X2	T50.2X3	T50.2X4	T50.2X5	T50.2X6
saluretic NEC	T50.2X1	T50.2X2	T50.2X3	T50.2X4	T50.2X5	T50.2X6

◀ New ◀ Revised ~~deleted~~ Deleted

Substance	Poisoning, Accidental (Unintentional)	Poisoning, Intentional Self-Harm	Poisoning, Assault	Poisoning, Undetermined	Adverse Effect	Underdosing
Diuretic NEC *(Continued)*						
sulfonamide	T50.2X1	T50.2X2	T50.2X3	T50.2X4	T50.2X5	T50.2X6
thiazide NEC	T50.2X1	T50.2X2	T50.2X3	T50.2X4	T50.2X5	T50.2X6
xanthine	T50.2X1	T50.2X2	T50.2X3	T50.2X4	T50.2X5	T50.2X6
Diurgin	T50.2X1	T50.2X2	T50.2X3	T50.2X4	T50.2X5	T50.2X6
Diuril	T50.2X1	T50.2X2	T50.2X3	T50.2X4	T50.2X5	T50.2X6
Diuron	T60.3X1	T60.3X2	T60.3X3	T60.3X4	—	—
Divalproex	T42.6X1	T42.6X2	T42.6X3	T42.6X4	T42.6X5	T42.6X6
Divinyl ether	T41.0X1	T41.0X2	T41.0X3	T41.0X4	T41.0X5	T41.0X6
Dixanthogen	T49.0X1	T49.0X2	T49.0X3	T49.0X4	T49.0X5	T49.0X6
Dixyrazine	T43.3X1	T43.3X2	T43.3X3	T43.3X4	T43.3X5	T43.3X6
D-lysergic acid diethylamide	T40.8X1	T40.8X2	T40.8X3	T40.8X4	—	—
DMCT	T36.4X1	T36.4X2	T36.4X3	T36.4X4	T36.4X5	T36.4X6
DMSO — *see Dimethyl sulfoxide*						
DNBP	T60.3X1	T60.3X2	T60.3X3	T60.3X4	—	—
DNOC	T65.3X1	T65.3X2	T65.3X3	T65.3X4	—	—
DOCA	T38.0X1	T38.0X2	T38.0X3	T38.0X4	T38.0X5	T38.0X6
Dobutamine	T44.5X1	T44.5X2	T44.5X3	T44.5X4	T44.5X5	T44.5X6
Docusate sodium	T47.4X1	T47.4X2	T47.4X3	T47.4X4	T47.4X5	T47.4X6
Dodicin	T49.0X1	T49.0X2	T49.0X3	T49.0X4	T49.0X5	T49.0X6
Dofamium chloride	T49.0X1	T49.0X2	T49.0X3	T49.0X4	T49.0X5	T49.0X6
Dolophine	T40.3X1	T40.3X2	T40.3X3	T40.3X4	T40.3X5	T40.3X6
Doloxene	T39.8X1	T39.8X2	T39.8X3	T39.8X4	T39.8X5	T39.8X6
Domestic gas (after combustion) — *see Gas, utility*						
prior to combustion	T59.891	T59.892	T59.893	T59.894	—	—
Domiodol	T48.4X1	T48.4X2	T48.4X3	T48.4X4	T48.4X5	T48.4X6
Domiphen (bromide)	T49.0X1	T49.0X2	T49.0X3	T49.0X4	T49.0X5	T49.0X6
Domperidone	T45.0X1	T45.0X2	T45.0X3	T45.0X4	T45.0X5	T45.0X6
Dopa	T42.8X1	T42.8X2	T42.8X3	T42.8X4	T42.8X5	T42.8X6
Dopamine	T44.991	T44.992	T44.993	T44.994	T44.995	T44.996
Doriden	T42.6X1	T42.6X2	T42.6X3	T42.6X4	T42.6X5	T42.6X6
Dormiral	T42.3X1	T42.3X2	T42.3X3	T42.3X4	T42.3X5	T42.3X6
Dormison	T42.6X1	T42.6X2	T42.6X3	T42.6X4	T42.6X5	T42.6X6
Dornase	T48.4X1	T48.4X2	T48.4X3	T48.4X4	T48.4X5	T48.4X6
Dorsacaine	T41.3X1	T41.3X2	T41.3X3	T41.3X4	T41.3X5	T41.3X6
Dosulepin	T43.011	T43.012	T43.013	T43.014	T43.015	T43.016
Dothiepin	T43.011	T43.012	T43.013	T43.014	T43.015	T43.016
Doxantrazole	T48.6X1	T48.6X2	T48.6X3	T48.6X4	T48.6X5	T48.6X6
Doxapram	T50.7X1	T50.7X2	T50.7X3	T50.7X4	T50.7X5	T50.7X6
Doxazosin	T44.6X1	T44.6X2	T44.6X3	T44.6X4	T44.6X5	T44.6X6
Doxepin	T43.011	T43.012	T43.013	T43.014	T43.015	T43.016

Substance	Poisoning, Accidental (Unintentional)	Poisoning, Intentional Self-Harm	Poisoning, Assault	Poisoning, Undetermined	Adverse Effect	Underdosing
Doxifluridine	T45.1X1	T45.1X2	T45.1X3	T45.1X4	T45.1X5	T45.1X6
Doxorubicin	T45.1X1	T45.1X2	T45.1X3	T45.1X4	T45.1X5	T45.1X6
Doxycycline	T36.4X1	T36.4X2	T36.4X3	T36.4X4	T36.4X5	T36.4X6
Doxylamine	T45.0X1	T45.0X2	T45.0X3	T45.0X4	T45.0X5	T45.0X6
Dramamine	T45.0X1	T45.0X2	T45.0X3	T45.0X4	T45.0X5	T45.0X6
Drano (drain cleaner)	T54.3X1	T54.3X2	T54.3X3	T54.3X4	—	—
Dressing, live pulp	T49.7X1	T49.7X2	T49.7X3	T49.7X4	T49.7X5	T49.7X6
Drocode	T40.2X1	T40.2X2	T40.2X3	T40.2X4	T40.2X5	T40.2X6
Dromoran	T40.2X1	T40.2X2	T40.2X3	T40.2X4	T40.2X5	T40.2X6
Dromostanolone	T38.7X1	T38.7X2	T38.7X3	T38.7X4	T38.7X5	T38.7X6
Dronabinol	T40.7X1	T40.7X2	T40.7X3	T40.7X4	T40.7X5	T40.7X6
Droperidol	T43.591	T43.592	T43.593	T43.594	T43.595	T43.596
Dropropizine	T48.3X1	T48.3X2	T48.3X3	T48.3X4	T48.3X5	T48.3X6
Drostanolone	T38.7X1	T38.7X2	T38.7X3	T38.7X4	T38.7X5	T38.7X6
Drotaverine	T44.3X1	T44.3X2	T44.3X3	T44.3X4	T44.3X5	T44.3X6
Drotrecogin alfa	T45.511	T45.512	T45.513	T45.514	T45.515	T45.516
Drug NEC	T50.901	T50.902	T50.903	T50.904	T50.905	T50.906
specified NEC	T50.991	T50.992	T50.993	T50.994	T50.995	T50.996
DTIC	T45.1X1	T45.1X2	T45.1X3	T45.1X4	T45.1X5	T45.1X6
Duboisine	T44.3X1	T44.3X2	T44.3X3	T44.3X4	T44.3X5	T44.3X6
Dulcolax	T47.2X1	T47.2X2	T47.2X3	T47.2X4	T47.2X5	T47.2X6
Duponol (C) (EP)	T49.2X1	T49.2X2	T49.2X3	T49.2X4	T49.2X5	T49.2X6
Durabolin	T38.7X1	T38.7X2	T38.7X3	T38.7X4	T38.7X5	T38.7X6
Dyclone	T41.3X1	T41.3X2	T41.3X3	T41.3X4	T41.3X5	T41.3X6
Dyclonine	T41.3X1	T41.3X2	T41.3X3	T41.3X4	T41.3X5	T41.3X6
Dydrogesterone	T38.5X1	T38.5X2	T38.5X3	T38.5X4	T38.5X5	T38.5X6
Dye NEC	T65.6X1	T65.6X2	T65.6X3	T65.6X4	—	—
antiseptic	T49.0X1	T49.0X2	T49.0X3	T49.0X4	T49.0X5	T49.0X6
diagnostic agents	T50.8X1	T50.8X2	T50.8X3	T50.8X4	T50.8X5	T50.8X6
pharmaceutical NEC	T50.901	T50.902	T50.903	T50.904	T50.905	T50.906
Dyflos	T44.0X1	T44.0X2	T44.0X3	T44.0X4	T44.0X5	T44.0X6
Dymelor	T38.3X1	T38.3X2	T38.3X3	T38.3X4	T38.3X5	T38.3X6
Dynamite	T65.3X1	T65.3X2	T65.3X3	T65.3X4	—	—
fumes	T59.891	T59.892	T59.893	T59.894	—	—
Dyphylline	T44.3X1	T44.3X2	T44.3X3	T44.3X4	T44.3X5	T44.3X6
E						
Ear drug NEC	T49.6X1	T49.6X2	T49.6X3	T49.6X4	T49.6X5	T49.6X6
Ear preparations	T49.6X1	T49.6X2	T49.6X3	T49.6X4	T49.6X5	T49.6X6
Econazole	T49.0X1	T49.0X2	T49.0X3	T49.0X4	T49.0X5	T49.0X6
Ecothiopate iodide	T49.5X1	T49.5X2	T49.5X3	T49.5X4	T49.5X5	T49.5X6
Echothiophate, echothiopate, ecothiopate	T49.5X1	T49.5X2	T49.5X3	T49.5X4	T49.5X5	T49.5X6

◀ New   ◀▦ Revised   ~~deleted~~ Deleted

TABLE OF DRUGS AND CHEMICALS

Substance	External Cause (T-Code)					
	Poisoning, Accidental (Unintentional)	Poisoning, Intentional Self-Harm	Poisoning, Assault	Poisoning, Undetermined	Adverse Effect	Underdosing
Ecstasy	T43.621	T43.622	T43.623	T43.624	T43.625	T43.626
Ectylurea	T42.6X1	T42.6X2	T42.6X3	T42.6X4	T42.6X5	T42.6X6
Edathamil disodium	T45.8X1	T45.8X2	T45.8X3	T45.8X4	T45.8X5	T45.8X6
Edecrin	T50.1X1	T50.1X2	T50.1X3	T50.1X4	T50.1X5	T50.1X6
Edetate, disodium (calcium)	T45.8X1	T45.8X2	T45.8X3	T45.8X4	T45.8X5	T45.8X6
Edoxudine	T49.5X1	T49.5X2	T49.5X3	T49.5X4	T49.5X5	T49.5X6
Edrophonium	T44.0X1	T44.0X2	T44.0X3	T44.0X4	T44.0X5	T44.0X6
chloride	T44.0X1	T44.0X2	T44.0X3	T44.0X4	T44.0X5	T44.0X6
EDTA	T50.6X1	T50.6X2	T50.6X3	T50.6X4	T50.6X5	T50.6X6
Eflornithine	T37.2X1	T37.2X2	T37.2X3	T37.2X4	T37.2X5	T37.2X6
Efloxate	T46.3X1	T46.3X2	T46.3X3	T46.3X4	T46.3X5	T46.3X6
Elase	T49.8X1	T49.8X2	T49.8X3	T49.8X4	T49.8X5	T49.8X6
Elastase	T47.5X1	T47.5X2	T47.5X3	T47.5X4	T47.5X5	T47.5X6
Elaterium	T47.2X1	T47.2X2	T47.2X3	T47.2X4	T47.2X5	T47.2X6
Elcatonin	T50.991	T50.992	T50.993	T50.994	T50.995	T50.996
Elder	T62.2X1	T62.2X2	T62.2X3	T62.2X4	—	—
berry (unripe)	T62.1X1	T62.1X2	T62.1X3	T62.1X4	—	—
Electrolyte balance drug	T50.3X1	T50.3X2	T50.3X3	T50.3X4	T50.3X5	T50.3X6
Electrolytes NEC	T50.3X1	T50.3X2	T50.3X3	T50.3X4	T50.3X5	T50.3X6
Electrolytic agent NEC	T50.3X1	T50.3X2	T50.3X3	T50.3X4	T50.3X5	T50.3X6
Elemental diet	T50.901	T50.902	T50.903	T50.904	T50.905	T50.906
Elliptinium acetate	T45.1X1	T45.1X2	T45.1X3	T45.1X4	T45.1X5	T45.1X6
Embramine	T45.0X1	T45.0X2	T45.0X3	T45.0X4	T45.0X5	T45.0X6
Emepronium (salts)	T44.3X1	T44.3X2	T44.3X3	T44.3X4	T44.3X5	T44.3X6
bromide	T44.3X1	T44.3X2	T44.3X3	T44.3X4	T44.3X5	T44.3X6
Emetic NEC	T47.7X1	T47.7X2	T47.7X3	T47.7X4	T47.7X5	T47.7X6
Emetine	T37.3X1	T37.3X2	T37.3X3	T37.3X4	T37.3X5	T37.3X6
Emollient NEC	T49.3X1	T49.3X2	T49.3X3	T49.3X4	T49.3X5	T49.3X6
Emorfazone	T39.8X1	T39.8X2	T39.8X3	T39.8X4	T39.8X5	T39.8X6
Emylcamate	T43.591	T43.592	T43.593	T43.594	T43.595	T43.596
Enalapril	T46.4X1	T46.4X2	T46.4X3	T46.4X4	T46.4X5	T46.4X6
Enalaprilat	T46.4X1	T46.4X2	T46.4X3	T46.4X4	T46.4X5	T46.4X6
Encainide	T46.2X1	T46.2X2	T46.2X3	T46.2X4	T46.2X5	T46.2X6
Endocaine	T41.3X1	T41.3X2	T41.3X3	T41.3X4	T41.3X5	T41.3X6
Endosulfan	T60.2X1	T60.2X2	T60.2X3	T60.2X4	—	—
Endothall	T60.3X1	T60.3X2	T60.3X3	T60.3X4	—	—
Endralazine	T46.5X1	T46.5X2	T46.5X3	T46.5X4	T46.5X5	T46.5X6
Endrin	T60.1X1	T60.1X2	T60.1X3	T60.1X4	—	—
Enflurane	T41.0X1	T41.0X2	T41.0X3	T41.0X4	T41.0X5	T41.0X6
Enhexymal	T42.3X1	T42.3X2	T42.3X3	T42.3X4	T42.3X5	T42.3X6
Enocitabine	T45.1X1	T45.1X2	T45.1X3	T45.1X4	T45.1X5	T45.1X6
Enovid	T38.4X1	T38.4X2	T38.4X3	T38.4X4	T38.4X5	T38.4X6

Substance	External Cause (T-Code)					
	Poisoning, Accidental (Unintentional)	Poisoning, Intentional Self-Harm	Poisoning, Assault	Poisoning, Undetermined	Adverse Effect	Underdosing
Enoxacin	T36.8X1	T36.8X2	T36.8X3	T36.8X4	T36.8X5	T36.8X6
Enoxaparin (sodium)	T45.511	T45.512	T45.513	T45.514	T45.515	T45.516
Enpiprazole	T43.591	T43.592	T43.593	T43.594	T43.595	T43.596
Enprofylline	T48.6X1	T48.6X2	T48.6X3	T48.6X4	T48.6X5	T48.6X6
Enprostil	T47.1X1	T47.1X2	T47.1X3	T47.1X4	T47.1X5	T47.1X6
ENT preparations (anti-infectives)	T49.6X1	T49.6X2	T49.6X3	T49.6X4	T49.6X5	T49.6X6
Enviomycin	T36.8X1	T36.8X2	T36.8X3	T36.8X4	T36.8X5	T36.8X6
Enzodase	T45.3X1	T45.3X2	T45.3X3	T45.3X4	T45.3X5	T45.3X6
Enzyme NEC	T45.3X1	T45.3X2	T45.3X3	T45.3X4	T45.3X5	T45.3X6
depolymerizing	T49.8X1	T49.8X2	T49.8X3	T49.8X4	T49.8X5	T49.8X6
fibrolytic	T45.3X1	T45.3X2	T45.3X3	T45.3X4	T45.3X5	T45.3X6
gastric	T47.5X1	T47.5X2	T47.5X3	T47.5X4	T47.5X5	T47.5X6
intestinal	T47.5X1	T47.5X2	T47.5X3	T47.5X4	T47.5X5	T47.5X6
local action	T49.4X1	T49.4X2	T49.4X3	T49.4X4	T49.4X5	T49.4X6
proteolytic	T49.4X1	T49.4X2	T49.4X3	T49.4X4	T49.4X5	T49.4X6
thrombolytic	T45.3X1	T45.3X2	T45.3X3	T45.3X4	T45.3X5	T45.3X6
EPAB	T41.3X1	T41.3X2	T41.3X3	T41.3X4	T41.3X5	T41.3X6
Epanutin	T42.0X1	T42.0X2	T42.0X3	T42.0X4	T42.0X5	T42.0X6
Ephedra	T44.991	T44.992	T44.993	T44.994	T44.995	T44.996
Ephedrine	T44.991	T44.992	T44.993	T44.994	T44.995	T44.996
Epichlorhydrin, epichlorohydrin	T52.8X1	T52.8X2	T52.8X3	T52.8X4	—	—
Epicillin	T36.0X1	T36.0X2	T36.0X3	T36.0X4	T36.0X5	T36.0X6
Epiestriol	T38.5X1	T38.5X2	T38.5X3	T38.5X4	T38.5X5	T38.5X6
Epilim — see Sodium valproate						
Epimestrol	T38.5X1	T38.5X2	T38.5X3	T38.5X4	T38.5X5	T38.5X6
Epinephrine	T44.5X1	T44.5X2	T44.5X3	T44.5X4	T44.5X5	T44.5X6
Epirubicin	T45.1X1	T45.1X2	T45.1X3	T45.1X4	T45.1X5	T45.1X6
Epitiostanol	T38.7X1	T38.7X2	T38.7X3	T38.7X4	T38.7X5	T38.7X6
Epitizide	T50.2X1	T50.2X2	T50.2X3	T50.2X4	T50.2X5	T50.2X6
EPN	T60.0X1	T60.0X2	T60.0X3	T60.0X4	—	—
EPO	T45.8X1	T45.8X2	T45.8X3	T45.8X4	T45.8X5	T45.8X6
Epoetin alpha	T45.8X1	T45.8X2	T45.8X3	T45.8X4	T45.8X5	T45.8X6
Epomediol	T50.991	T50.992	T50.993	T50.994	T50.995	T50.996
Epoprostenol	T45.521	T45.522	T45.523	T45.524	T45.525	T45.526
Epoxy resin	T65.891	T65.892	T65.893	T65.894	—	—
Eprazinone	T48.4X1	T48.4X2	T48.4X3	T48.4X4	T48.4X5	T48.4X6
Epsilon amino-caproic acid	T45.621	T45.622	T45.623	T45.624	T45.625	T45.626
Epsom salt	T47.3X1	T47.3X2	T47.3X3	T47.3X4	T47.3X5	T47.3X6
Eptazocine	T40.4X1	T40.4X2	T40.4X3	T40.4X4	T40.4X5	T40.4X6
Equanil	T43.591	T43.592	T43.593	T43.594	T43.595	T43.596
Equisetum	T62.2X1	T62.2X2	T62.2X3	T62.2X4	—	—
diuretic	T50.2X1	T50.2X2	T50.2X3	T50.2X4	T50.2X5	T50.2X6

◀ New ◀◀◀ Revised ~~deleted~~ Deleted

Substance	Poisoning, Accidental (Unintentional)	Poisoning, Intentional Self-Harm	Poisoning, Assault	Poisoning, Undetermined	Adverse Effect	Underdosing
Ergobasine	T48.0X1	T48.0X2	T48.0X3	T48.0X4	T48.0X5	T48.0X6
Ergocalciferol	T45.2X1	T45.2X2	T45.2X3	T45.2X4	T45.2X5	T45.2X6
Ergoloid mesylates	T46.7X1	T46.7X2	T46.7X3	T46.7X4	T46.7X5	T46.7X6
Ergometrine	T48.0X1	T48.0X2	T48.0X3	T48.0X4	T48.0X5	T48.0X6
Ergonovine	T48.0X1	T48.0X2	T48.0X3	T48.0X4	T48.0X5	T48.0X6
Ergot NEC	T64.81	T64.82	T64.83	T64.84	—	—
derivative	T48.0X1	T48.0X2	T48.0X3	T48.0X4	T48.0X5	T48.0X6
medicinal (alkaloids)	T48.0X1	T48.0X2	T48.0X3	T48.0X4	T48.0X5	T48.0X6
prepared	T48.0X1	T48.0X2	T48.0X3	T48.0X4	T48.0X5	T48.0X6
Ergotamine	T46.5X1	T46.5X2	T46.5X3	T46.5X4	T46.5X5	T46.5X6
Ergotocine	T48.0X1	T48.0X2	T48.0X3	T48.0X4	T48.0X5	T48.0X6
Ergotrate	T48.0X1	T48.0X2	T48.0X3	T48.0X4	T48.0X5	T48.0X6
Eritrityl tetranitrate	T46.3X1	T46.3X2	T46.3X3	T46.3X4	T46.3X5	T46.3X6
Erythrityl tetranitrate	T46.3X1	T46.3X2	T46.3X3	T46.3X4	T46.3X5	T46.3X6
Erythrol tetranitrate	T46.3X1	T46.3X2	T46.3X3	T46.3X4	T46.3X5	T46.3X6
Erythromycin (salts)	T36.3X1	T36.3X2	T36.3X3	T36.3X4	T36.3X5	T36.3X6
ophthalmic preparation	T49.5X1	T49.5X2	T49.5X3	T49.5X4	T49.5X5	T49.5X6
topical NEC	T49.0X1	T49.0X2	T49.0X3	T49.0X4	T49.0X5	T49.0X6
Erythropoietin	T45.8X1	T45.8X2	T45.8X3	T45.8X4	T45.8X5	T45.8X6
human	T45.8X1	T45.8X2	T45.8X3	T45.8X4	T45.8X5	T45.8X6
Escin	T46.991	T46.992	T46.993	T46.994	T46.995	T46.996
Esculin	T45.2X1	T45.2X2	T45.2X3	T45.2X4	T45.2X5	T45.2X6
Esculoside	T45.2X1	T45.2X2	T45.2X3	T45.2X4	T45.2X5	T45.2X6
ESDT (ether-soluble tar distillate)	T49.1X1	T49.1X2	T49.1X3	T49.1X4	T49.1X5	T49.1X6
Eserine	T49.5X1	T49.5X2	T49.5X3	T49.5X4	T49.5X5	T49.5X6
Esflurbiprofen	T39.311	T39.312	T39.313	T39.314	T39.315	T39.316
Eskabarb	T42.3X1	T42.3X2	T42.3X3	T42.3X4	T42.3X5	T42.3X6
Eskalith	T43.8X1	T43.8X2	T43.8X3	T43.8X4	T43.8X5	T43.8X6
Esmolol	T44.7X1	T44.7X2	T44.7X3	T44.7X4	T44.7X5	T44.7X6
Estanozolol	T38.7X1	T38.7X2	T38.7X3	T38.7X4	T38.7X5	T38.7X6
Estazolam	T42.4X1	T42.4X2	T42.4X3	T42.4X4	T42.4X5	T42.4X6
Estradiol	T38.5X1	T38.5X2	T38.5X3	T38.5X4	T38.5X5	T38.5X6
with testosterone	T38.7X1	T38.7X2	T38.7X3	T38.7X4	T38.7X5	T38.7X6
benzoate	T38.5X1	T38.5X2	T38.5X3	T38.5X4	T38.5X5	T38.5X6
Estramustine	T45.1X1	T45.1X2	T45.1X3	T45.1X4	T45.1X5	T45.1X6
Estriol	T38.5X1	T38.5X2	T38.5X3	T38.5X4	T38.5X5	T38.5X6
Estrogen	T38.5X1	T38.5X2	T38.5X3	T38.5X4	T38.5X5	T38.5X6
with progesterone	T38.5X1	T38.5X2	T38.5X3	T38.5X4	T38.5X5	T38.5X6
conjugated	T38.5X1	T38.5X2	T38.5X3	T38.5X4	T38.5X5	T38.5X6
Estrone	T38.5X1	T38.5X2	T38.5X3	T38.5X4	T38.5X5	T38.5X6
Estropipate	T38.5X1	T38.5X2	T38.5X3	T38.5X4	T38.5X5	T38.5X6

Substance	Poisoning, Accidental (Unintentional)	Poisoning, Intentional Self-Harm	Poisoning, Assault	Poisoning, Undetermined	Adverse Effect	Underdosing
Etacrynate sodium	T50.1X1	T50.1X2	T50.1X3	T50.1X4	T50.1X5	T50.1X6
Etacrynic acid	T50.1X1	T50.1X2	T50.1X3	T50.1X4	T50.1X5	T50.1X6
Etafedrine	T48.6X1	T48.6X2	T48.6X3	T48.6X4	T48.6X5	T48.6X6
Etafenone	T46.3X1	T46.3X2	T46.3X3	T46.3X4	T46.3X5	T46.3X6
Etambutol	T37.1X1	T37.1X2	T37.1X3	T37.1X4	T37.1X5	T37.1X6
Etamiphyllin	T48.6X1	T48.6X2	T48.6X3	T48.6X4	T48.6X5	T48.6X6
Etamivan	T50.7X1	T50.7X2	T50.7X3	T50.7X4	T50.7X5	T50.7X6
Etamsylate	T45.7X1	T45.7X2	T45.7X3	T45.7X4	T45.7X5	T45.7X6
Etebenecid	T50.4X1	T50.4X2	T50.4X3	T50.4X4	T50.4X5	T50.4X6
Ethacridine	T49.0X1	T49.0X2	T49.0X3	T49.0X4	T49.0X5	T49.0X6
Ethacrynic acid	T50.1X1	T50.1X2	T50.1X3	T50.1X4	T50.1X5	T50.1X6
Ethadione	T42.2X1	T42.2X2	T42.2X3	T42.2X4	T42.2X5	T42.2X6
Ethambutol	T37.1X1	T37.1X2	T37.1X3	T37.1X4	T37.1X5	T37.1X6
Ethamide	T50.2X1	T50.2X2	T50.2X3	T50.2X4	T50.2X5	T50.2X6
Ethamivan	T50.7X1	T50.7X2	T50.7X3	T50.7X4	T50.7X5	T50.7X6
Ethamsylate	T45.7X1	T45.7X2	T45.7X3	T45.7X4	T45.7X5	T45.7X6
Ethanol	T51.0X1	T51.0X2	T51.0X3	T51.0X4	—	—
beverage	T51.0X1	T51.0X2	T51.0X3	T51.0X4	—	—
Ethanolamine oleate	T46.8X1	T46.8X2	T46.8X3	T46.8X4	T46.8X5	T46.8X6
Ethaverine	T44.3X1	T44.3X2	T44.3X3	T44.3X4	T44.3X5	T44.3X6
Ethchlorvynol	T42.6X1	T42.6X2	T42.6X3	T42.6X4	T42.6X5	T42.6X6
Ethebenecid	T50.4X1	T50.4X2	T50.4X3	T50.4X4	T50.4X5	T50.4X6
Ether (vapor)	T41.0X1	T41.0X2	T41.0X3	T41.0X4	T41.0X5	T41.0X6
anesthetic	T41.0X1	T41.0X2	T41.0X3	T41.0X4	T41.0X5	T41.0X6
divinyl	T41.0X1	T41.0X2	T41.0X3	T41.0X4	T41.0X5	T41.0X6
ethyl (medicinal)	T41.0X1	T41.0X2	T41.0X3	T41.0X4	T41.0X5	T41.0X6
nonmedicinal	T52.8X1	T52.8X2	T52.8X3	T52.8X4	—	—
petroleum — *see Ligroin*						
solvent	T52.8X1	T52.8X2	T52.8X3	T52.8X4	—	—
Ethiazide	T50.2X1	T50.2X2	T50.2X3	T50.2X4	T50.2X5	T50.2X6
Ethidium chloride (vapor)	T59.891	T59.892	T59.893	T59.894	—	—
Ethinamate	T42.6X1	T42.6X2	T42.6X3	T42.6X4	T42.6X5	T42.6X6
Ethinylestradiol, ethinyloestradiol	T38.5X1	T38.5X2	T38.5X3	T38.5X4	T38.5X5	T38.5X6
with						
levonorgestrel	T38.4X1	T38.4X2	T38.4X3	T38.4X4	T38.4X5	T38.4X6
norethisterone	T38.4X1	T38.4X2	T38.4X3	T38.4X4	T38.4X5	T38.4X6
Ethiodized oil (131 I)	T50.8X1	T50.8X2	T50.8X3	T50.8X4	T50.8X5	T50.8X6
Ethion	T60.0X1	T60.0X2	T60.0X3	T60.0X4	—	—
Ethionamide	T37.1X1	T37.1X2	T37.1X3	T37.1X4	T37.1X5	T37.1X6
Ethioniamide	T37.1X1	T37.1X2	T37.1X3	T37.1X4	T37.1X5	T37.1X6
Ethisterone	T38.5X1	T38.5X2	T38.5X3	T38.5X4	T38.5X5	T38.5X6
Ethobral	T42.3X1	T42.3X2	T42.3X3	T42.3X4	T42.3X5	T42.3X6

◀ New   ◀▥ Revised   ~~deleted~~ Deleted

TABLE OF DRUGS AND CHEMICALS

Substance	External Cause (T-Code)					
	Poisoning, Accidental (Unintentional)	Poisoning, Intentional Self-Harm	Poisoning, Assault	Poisoning, Undetermined	Adverse Effect	Underdosing
Ethocaine (infiltration) (topical)	T41.3X1	T41.3X2	T41.3X3	T41.3X4	T41.3X5	T41.3X6
nerve block (peripheral) (plexus)	T41.3X1	T41.3X2	T41.3X3	T41.3X4	T41.3X5	T41.3X6
spinal	T41.3X1	T41.3X2	T41.3X3	T41.3X4	T41.3X5	T41.3X6
Ethoheptazine	T40.4X1	T40.4X2	T40.4X3	T40.4X4	T40.4X5	T40.4X6
Ethopropazine	T44.3X1	T44.3X2	T44.3X3	T44.3X4	T44.3X5	T44.3X6
Ethosuximide	T42.2X1	T42.2X2	T42.2X3	T42.2X4	T42.2X5	T42.2X6
Ethotoin	T42.0X1	T42.0X2	T42.0X3	T42.0X4	T42.0X5	T42.0X6
Ethoxazene	T37.91	T37.92	T37.93	T37.94	T37.95	T37.96
Ethoxazorutoside	T46.991	T46.992	T46.993	T46.994	T46.995	T46.996
2-Ethoxyethanol	T52.3X1	T52.3X2	T52.3X3	T52.3X4	—	—
Ethoxzolamide	T50.2X1	T50.2X2	T50.2X3	T50.2X4	T50.2X5	T50.2X6
Ethyl						
acetate	T52.8X1	T52.8X2	T52.8X3	T52.8X4		
alcohol	T51.0X1	T51.0X2	T51.0X3	T51.0X4	—	—
beverage	T51.0X1	T51.0X2	T51.0X3	T51.0X4	—	—
aldehyde (vapor)	T59.891	T59.892	T59.893	T59.894		
liquid	T52.8X1	T52.8X2	T52.8X3	T52.8X4		
aminobenzoate	T41.3X1	T41.3X2	T41.3X3	T41.3X4	T41.3X5	T41.3X6
aminophenothiazine	T43.3X1	T43.3X2	T43.3X3	T43.3X4	T43.3X5	T43.3X6
benzoate	T52.8X1	T52.8X2	T52.8X3	T52.8X4		
biscoumacetate	T45.511	T45.512	T45.513	T45.514	T45.515	T45.516
bromide (anesthetic)	T41.0X1	T41.0X2	T41.0X3	T41.0X4	T41.0X5	T41.0X6
carbamate	T45.1X1	T45.1X2	T45.1X3	T45.1X4	T45.1X5	T45.1X6
carbinol	T51.3X1	T51.3X2	T51.3X3	T51.3X4	—	—
carbonate	T52.8X1	T52.8X2	T52.8X3	T52.8X4	—	—
chaulmoograte	T37.1X1	T37.1X2	T37.1X3	T37.1X4	T37.1X5	T37.1X6
chloride (anesthetic)	T41.0X1	T41.0X2	T41.0X3	T41.0X4	T41.0X5	T41.0X6
anesthetic (local)	T41.3X1	T41.3X2	T41.3X3	T41.3X4	T41.3X5	T41.3X6
inhaled	T41.0X1	T41.0X2	T41.0X3	T41.0X4	T41.0X5	T41.0X6
local	T49.4X1	T49.4X2	T49.4X3	T49.4X4	T49.4X5	T49.4X6
solvent	T53.6X1	T53.6X2	T53.6X3	T53.6X4	—	—
dibunate	T48.3X1	T48.3X2	T48.3X3	T48.3X4	T48.3X5	T48.3X6
dichloroarsine (vapor)	T57.0X1	T57.0X2	T57.0X3	T57.0X4	—	—
estranol	T38.7X1	T38.7X2	T38.7X3	T38.7X4	T38.7X5	T38.7X6
ether — see also ether	T52.8X1	T52.8X2	T52.8X3	T52.8X4	—	—
formate NEC (solvent)	T52.0X1	T52.0X2	T52.0X3	T52.0X4	—	—
fumarate	T49.4X1	T49.4X2	T49.4X3	T49.4X4	T49.4X5	T49.4X6
hydroxyisobutyrate NEC (solvent)	T52.8X1	T52.8X2	T52.8X3	T52.8X4	—	—
iodoacetate	T59.3X1	T59.3X2	T59.3X3	T59.3X4	—	—
lactate NEC (solvent)	T52.8X1	T52.8X2	T52.8X3	T52.8X4	—	—
loflazepate	T42.4X1	T42.4X2	T42.4X3	T42.4X4	T42.4X5	T42.4X6

Substance	External Cause (T-Code)					
	Poisoning, Accidental (Unintentional)	Poisoning, Intentional Self-Harm	Poisoning, Assault	Poisoning, Undetermined	Adverse Effect	Underdosing
Ethyl (Continued)						
mercuric chloride	T56.1X1	T56.1X2	T56.1X3	T56.1X4	—	—
methylcarbinol	T51.8X1	T51.8X2	T51.8X3	T51.8X4	—	—
morphine	T40.2X1	T40.2X2	T40.2X3	T40.2X4	T40.2X5	T40.2X6
noradrenaline	T48.6X1	T48.6X2	T48.6X3	T48.6X4	T48.6X5	T48.6X6
oxybutyrate NEC (solvent)	T52.8X1	T52.8X2	T52.8X3	T52.8X4		
Ethylene (gas)	T59.891	T59.892	T59.893	T59.894	—	—
anesthetic (general)	T41.0X1	T41.0X2	T41.0X3	T41.0X4	T41.0X5	T41.0X6
chlorohydrin	T52.8X1	T52.8X2	T52.8X3	T52.8X4		
vapor	T53.6X1	T53.6X2	T53.6X3	T53.6X4	—	—
dichloride	T52.8X1	T52.8X2	T52.8X3	T52.8X4		
vapor	T53.6X1	T53.6X2	T53.6X3	T53.6X4	—	—
dinitrate	T52.3X1	T52.3X2	T52.3X3	T52.3X4		
glycol(s)	T52.8X1	T52.8X2	T52.8X3	T52.8X4		
dinitrate	T52.3X1	T52.3X2	T52.3X3	T52.3X4		
monobutyl ether	T52.3X1	T52.3X2	T52.3X3	T52.3X4		
imine	T54.1X1	T54.1X2	T54.1X3	T54.1X4		
oxide (fumigant) (nonmedicinal)	T59.891	T59.892	T59.893	T59.894	—	—
medicinal	T49.0X1	T49.0X2	T49.0X3	T49.0X4	T49.0X5	T49.0X6
Ethylenediamine theophylline	T48.6X1	T48.6X2	T48.6X3	T48.6X4	T48.6X5	T48.6X6
Ethylenediaminetetra-acetic acid	T50.6X1	T50.6X2	T50.6X3	T50.6X4	T50.6X5	T50.6X6
Ethylenedinitrilotetra-acetate	T50.6X1	T50.6X2	T50.6X3	T50.6X4	T50.6X5	T50.6X6
Ethylestrenol	T38.7X1	T38.7X2	T38.7X3	T38.7X4	T38.7X5	T38.7X6
Ethylhydroxycellulose	T47.4X1	T47.4X2	T47.4X3	T47.4X4	T47.4X5	T47.4X6
Ethylidene						
chloride NEC	T53.6X1	T53.6X2	T53.6X3	T53.6X4	—	—
diacetate	T60.3X1	T60.3X2	T60.3X3	T60.3X4		
dicoumarin	T45.511	T45.512	T45.513	T45.514	T45.515	T45.516
dicoumarol	T45.511	T45.512	T45.513	T45.514	T45.515	T45.516
diethyl ether	T52.0X1	T52.0X2	T52.0X3	T52.0X4	—	—
Ethylmorphine	T40.2X1	T40.2X2	T40.2X3	T40.2X4	T40.2X5	T40.2X6
Ethylnorepinephrine	T48.6X1	T48.6X2	T48.6X3	T48.6X4	T48.6X5	T48.6X6
Ethylparachlorophen-oxyisobutyrate	T46.6X1	T46.6X2	T46.6X3	T46.6X4	T46.6X5	T46.6X6
Ethynodiol	T38.4X1	T38.4X2	T38.4X3	T38.4X4	T38.4X5	T38.4X6
with mestranol diacetate	T38.4X1	T38.4X2	T38.4X3	T38.4X4	T38.4X5	T38.4X6
Etidocaine	T41.3X1	T41.3X2	T41.3X3	T41.3X4	T41.3X5	T41.3X6
infiltration (subcutaneous)	T41.3X1	T41.3X2	T41.3X3	T41.3X4	T41.3X5	T41.3X6
nerve (peripheral) (plexus)	T41.3X1	T41.3X2	T41.3X3	T41.3X4	T41.3X5	T41.3X6
Etidronate	T50.991	T50.992	T50.993	T50.994	T50.995	T50.996
Etidronic acid (disodium salt)	T50.991	T50.992	T50.993	T50.994	T50.995	T50.996
Etifoxine	T42.6X1	T42.6X2	T42.6X3	T42.6X4	T42.6X5	T42.6X6

◀ New   ◀◀ Revised   ~~deleted~~ Deleted

Substance	Poisoning, Accidental (Unintentional)	Poisoning, Intentional Self-Harm	Poisoning, Assault	Poisoning, Undetermined	Adverse Effect	Underdosing
Etilefrine	T44.4X1	T44.4X2	T44.4X3	T44.4X4	T44.4X5	T44.4X6
Etilfen	T42.3X1	T42.3X2	T42.3X3	T42.3X4	T42.3X5	T42.3X6
Etinodiol	T38.4X1	T38.4X2	T38.4X3	T38.4X4	T38.4X5	T38.4X6
Etiroxate	T46.6X1	T46.6X2	T46.6X3	T46.6X4	T46.6X5	T46.6X6
Etizolam	T42.4X1	T42.4X2	T42.4X3	T42.4X4	T42.4X5	T42.4X6
Etodolac	T39.391	T39.392	T39.393	T39.394	T39.395	T39.396
Etofamide	T37.3X1	T37.3X2	T37.3X3	T37.3X4	T37.3X5	T37.3X6
Etofibrate	T46.6X1	T46.6X2	T46.6X3	T46.6X4	T46.6X5	T46.6X6
Etofylline	T46.7X1	T46.7X2	T46.7X3	T46.7X4	T46.7X5	T46.7X6
clofibrate	T46.6X1	T46.6X2	T46.6X3	T46.6X4	T46.6X5	T46.6X6
Etoglucid	T45.1X1	T45.1X2	T45.1X3	T45.1X4	T45.1X5	T45.1X6
Etomidate	T41.1X1	T41.1X2	T41.1X3	T41.1X4	T41.1X5	T41.1X6
Etomide	T39.8X1	T39.8X2	T39.8X3	T39.8X4	T39.8X5	T39.8X6
Etomidoline	T44.3X1	T44.3X2	T44.3X3	T44.3X4	T44.3X5	T44.3X6
Etoposide	T45.1X1	T45.1X2	T45.1X3	T45.1X4	T45.1X5	T45.1X6
Etorphine	T40.2X1	T40.2X2	T40.2X3	T40.2X4	T40.2X5	T40.2X6
Etoval	T42.3X1	T42.3X2	T42.3X3	T42.3X4	T42.3X5	T42.3X6
Etozolin	T50.1X1	T50.1X2	T50.1X3	T50.1X4	T50.1X5	T50.1X6
Etretinate	T50.991	T50.992	T50.993	T50.994	T50.995	T50.996
Etryptamine	T43.691	T43.692	T43.693	T43.694	T43.695	T43.696
Etybenzatropine	T44.3X1	T44.3X2	T44.3X3	T44.3X4	T44.3X5	T44.3X6
Etynodiol	T38.4X1	T38.4X2	T38.4X3	T38.4X4	T38.4X5	T38.4X6
Eucaine	T41.3X1	T41.3X2	T41.3X3	T41.3X4	T41.3X5	T41.3X6
Eucalyptus oil	T49.7X1	T49.7X2	T49.7X3	T49.7X4	T49.7X5	T49.7X6
Eucatropine	T49.5X1	T49.5X2	T49.5X3	T49.5X4	T49.5X5	T49.5X6
Eucodal	T40.2X1	T40.2X2	T40.2X3	T40.2X4	T40.2X5	T40.2X6
Euneryl	T42.3X1	T42.3X2	T42.3X3	T42.3X4	T42.3X5	T42.3X6
Euphthalmine	T44.3X1	T44.3X2	T44.3X3	T44.3X4	T44.3X5	T44.3X6
Eurax	T49.0X1	T49.0X2	T49.0X3	T49.0X4	T49.0X5	T49.0X6
Euresol	T49.4X1	T49.4X2	T49.4X3	T49.4X4	T49.4X5	T49.4X6
Euthroid	T38.1X1	T38.1X2	T38.1X3	T38.1X4	T38.1X5	T38.1X6
Evans blue	T50.8X1	T50.8X2	T50.8X3	T50.8X4	T50.8X5	T50.8X6
Evipal	T42.3X1	T42.3X2	T42.3X3	T42.3X4	T42.3X5	T42.3X6
sodium	T41.1X1	T41.1X2	T41.1X3	T41.1X4	T41.1X5	T41.1X6
Evipan	T42.3X1	T42.3X2	T42.3X3	T42.3X4	T42.3X5	T42.3X6
sodium	T41.1X1	T41.1X2	T41.1X3	T41.1X4	T41.1X5	T41.1X6
Exalamide	T49.0X1	T49.0X2	T49.0X3	T49.0X4	T49.0X5	T49.0X6
Exalgin	T39.1X1	T39.1X2	T39.1X3	T39.1X4	T39.1X5	T39.1X6
Excipients, pharmaceutical	T50.901	T50.902	T50.903	T50.904	T50.905	T50.906
Exhaust gas (engine) (motor vehicle)	T58.01	T58.02	T58.03	T58.04	—	—
Ex-Lax (phenolphthalein)	T47.2X1	T47.2X2	T47.2X3	T47.2X4	T47.2X5	T47.2X6
Expectorant NEC	T48.4X1	T48.4X2	T48.4X3	T48.4X4	T48.4X5	T48.4X6

Substance	Poisoning, Accidental (Unintentional)	Poisoning, Intentional Self-Harm	Poisoning, Assault	Poisoning, Undetermined	Adverse Effect	Underdosing
Extended insulin zinc suspension	T38.3X1	T38.3X2	T38.3X3	T38.3X4	T38.3X5	T38.3X6
External medications (skin) (mucous membrane)	T49.91	T49.92	T49.93	T49.94	T49.95	T49.96
dental agent	T49.7X1	T49.7X2	T49.7X3	T49.7X4	T49.7X5	T49.7X6
ENT agent	T49.6X1	T49.6X2	T49.6X3	T49.6X4	T49.6X5	T49.6X6
ophthalmic preparation	T49.5X1	T49.5X2	T49.5X3	T49.5X4	T49.5X5	T49.5X6
specified NEC	T49.8X1	T49.8X2	T49.8X3	T49.8X4	T49.8X5	T49.8X6
Extrapyramidal antagonist NEC	T44.3X1	T44.3X2	T44.3X3	T44.3X4	T44.3X5	T44.3X6
Eye agents (anti-infective)	T49.5X1	T49.5X2	T49.5X3	T49.5X4	T49.5X5	T49.5X6
Eye drug NEC	T49.5X1	T49.5X2	T49.5X3	T49.5X4	T49.5X5	T49.5X6
F						
FAC (fluorouracil + doxorubicin + cyclophosphamide)	T45.1X1	T45.1X2	T45.1X3	T45.1X4	T45.1X5	T45.1X6
Factor						
I (fibrinogen)	T45.8X1	T45.8X2	T45.8X3	T45.8X4	T45.8X5	T45.8X6
III (thromboplastin)	T45.8X1	T45.8X2	T45.8X3	T45.8X4	T45.8X5	T45.8X6
VIII (antihemophilic Factor) (Concentrate)	T45.8X1	T45.8X2	T45.8X3	T45.8X4	T45.8X5	T45.8X6
IX complex	T45.7X1	T45.7X2	T45.7X3	T45.7X4	T45.7X5	T45.7X6
human	T45.8X1	T45.8X2	T45.8X3	T45.8X4	T45.8X5	T45.8X6
Famotidine	T47.0X1	T47.0X2	T47.0X3	T47.0X4	T47.0X5	T47.0X6
Fat suspension, intravenous	T50.991	T50.992	T50.993	T50.994	T50.995	T50.996
Fazadinium bromide	T48.1X1	T48.1X2	T48.1X3	T48.1X4	T48.1X5	T48.1X6
Febarbamate	T42.3X1	T42.3X2	T42.3X3	T42.3X4	T42.3X5	T42.3X6
Fecal softener	T47.4X1	T47.4X2	T47.4X3	T47.4X4	T47.4X5	T47.4X6
Fedrilate	T48.3X1	T48.3X2	T48.3X3	T48.3X4	T48.3X5	T48.3X6
Felodipine	T46.1X1	T46.1X2	T46.1X3	T46.1X4	T46.1X5	T46.1X6
Felypressin	T38.891	T38.892	T38.893	T38.894	T38.895	T38.896
Femoxetine	T43.221	T43.222	T43.223	T43.224	T43.225	T43.226
Fenalcomine	T46.3X1	T46.3X2	T46.3X3	T46.3X4	T46.3X5	T46.3X6
Fenamisal	T37.1X1	T37.1X2	T37.1X3	T37.1X4	T37.1X5	T37.1X6
Fenazone	T39.2X1	T39.2X2	T39.2X3	T39.2X4	T39.2X5	T39.2X6
Fenbendazole	T37.4X1	T37.4X2	T37.4X3	T37.4X4	T37.4X5	T37.4X6
Fenbutrazate	T50.5X1	T50.5X2	T50.5X3	T50.5X4	T50.5X5	T50.5X6
Fencamfamine	T43.691	T43.692	T43.693	T43.694	T43.695	T43.696
Fendiline	T46.1X1	T46.1X2	T46.1X3	T46.1X4	T46.1X5	T46.1X6
Fenetylline	T43.691	T43.692	T43.693	T43.694	T43.695	T43.696
Fenflumizole	T39.391	T39.392	T39.393	T39.394	T39.395	T39.396
Fenfluramine	T50.5X1	T50.5X2	T50.5X3	T50.5X4	T50.5X5	T50.5X6
Fenobarbital	T42.3X1	T42.3X2	T42.3X3	T42.3X4	T42.3X5	T42.3X6
Fenofibrate	T46.6X1	T46.6X2	T46.6X3	T46.6X4	T46.6X5	T46.6X6
Fenoprofen	T39.311	T39.312	T39.313	T39.314	T39.315	T39.316
Fenoterol	T48.6X1	T48.6X2	T48.6X3	T48.6X4	T48.6X5	T48.6X6

TABLE OF DRUGS AND CHEMICALS

Substance	External Cause (T-Code)					
	Poisoning, Accidental (Unintentional)	Poisoning, Intentional Self-Harm	Poisoning, Assault	Poisoning, Undetermined	Adverse Effect	Underdosing
Fenoverine	T44.3X1	T44.3X2	T44.3X3	T44.3X4	T44.3X5	T44.3X6
Fenoxazoline	T48.5X1	T48.5X2	T48.5X3	T48.5X4	T48.5X5	T48.5X6
Fenproporex	T50.5X1	T50.5X2	T50.5X3	T50.5X4	T50.5X5	T50.5X6
Fenquizone	T50.2X1	T50.2X2	T50.2X3	T50.2X4	T50.2X5	T50.2X6
Fentanyl	T40.4X1	T40.4X2	T40.4X3	T40.4X4	T40.4X5	T40.4X6
Fentazin	T43.3X1	T43.3X2	T43.3X3	T43.3X4	T43.3X5	T43.3X6
Fenthion	T60.0X1	T60.0X2	T60.0X3	T60.0X4	—	—
Fenticlor	T49.0X1	T49.0X2	T49.0X3	T49.0X4	T49.0X5	T49.0X6
Fenylbutazone	T39.2X1	T39.2X2	T39.2X3	T39.2X4	T39.2X5	T39.2X6
Feprazone	T39.2X1	T39.2X2	T39.2X3	T39.2X4	T39.2X5	T39.2X6
Fer de lance (bite) (venom)	T63.061	T63.062	T63.063	T63.064	—	—
Ferric — see also Iron						
chloride	T45.4X1	T45.4X2	T45.4X3	T45.4X4	T45.4X5	T45.4X6
citrate	T45.4X1	T45.4X2	T45.4X3	T45.4X4	T45.4X5	T45.4X6
hydroxide						
colloidal	T45.4X1	T45.4X2	T45.4X3	T45.4X4	T45.4X5	T45.4X6
polymaltose	T45.4X1	T45.4X2	T45.4X3	T45.4X4	T45.4X5	T45.4X6
pyrophosphate	T45.4X1	T45.4X2	T45.4X3	T45.4X4	T45.4X5	T45.4X6
Ferritin	T45.4X1	T45.4X2	T45.4X3	T45.4X4	T45.4X5	T45.4X6
Ferrocholinate	T45.4X1	T45.4X2	T45.4X3	T45.4X4	T45.4X5	T45.4X6
Ferrodextrane	T45.4X1	T45.4X2	T45.4X3	T45.4X4	T45.4X5	T45.4X6
Ferropolimaler	T45.4X1	T45.4X2	T45.4X3	T45.4X4	T45.4X5	T45.4X6
Ferrous — see also Iron						
phosphate	T45.4X1	T45.4X2	T45.4X3	T45.4X4	T45.4X5	T45.4X6
salt	T45.4X1	T45.4X2	T45.4X3	T45.4X4	T45.4X5	T45.4X6
with folic acid	T45.4X1	T45.4X2	T45.4X3	T45.4X4	T45.4X5	T45.4X6
Ferrous fumerate, gluconate, lactate, salt NEC, sulfate (medicinal)	T45.4X1	T45.4X2	T45.4X3	T45.4X4	T45.4X5	T45.4X6
Ferrovanadium (fumes)	T59.891	T59.892	T59.893	T59.894	—	—
Ferrum — see Iron						
Fertilizers NEC	T65.891	T65.892	T65.893	T65.894	—	—
with herbicide mixture	T60.3X1	T60.3X2	T60.3X3	T60.3X4	—	—
Fetoxilate	T47.6X1	T47.6X2	T47.6X3	T47.6X4	T47.6X5	T47.6X6
Fiber, dietary	T47.4X1	T47.4X2	T47.4X3	T47.4X4	T47.4X5	T47.4X6
Fibrinogen (human)	T45.8X1	T45.8X2	T45.8X3	T45.8X4	T45.8X5	T45.8X6
Fibrinolysin (human)	T45.691	T45.692	T45.693	T45.694	T45.695	T45.696
Fibrinolysis						
affecting drug	T45.601	T45.602	T45.603	T45.604	T45.605	T45.606
inhibitor NEC	T45.621	T45.622	T45.623	T45.624	T45.625	T45.626
Fibrinolytic drug	T45.611	T45.612	T45.613	T45.614	T45.615	T45.616
Filix mas	T37.4X1	T37.4X2	T37.4X3	T37.4X4	T37.4X5	T37.4X6
Filtering cream	T49.3X1	T49.3X2	T49.3X3	T49.3X4	T49.3X5	T49.3X6

Substance	External Cause (T-Code)					
	Poisoning, Accidental (Unintentional)	Poisoning, Intentional Self-Harm	Poisoning, Assault	Poisoning, Undetermined	Adverse Effect	Underdosing
Fiorinal	T39.011	T39.012	T39.013	T39.014	T39.015	T39.016
Firedamp	T59.891	T59.892	T59.893	T59.894	—	—
Fish, noxious, nonbacterial	T61.91	T61.92	T61.93	T61.94	—	—
ciguatera	T61.01	T61.02	T61.03	T61.04	—	—
scombroid	T61.11	T61.12	T61.13	T61.14	—	—
shell	T61.781	T61.782	T61.783	T61.784	—	—
specified NEC	T61.771	T61.772	T61.773	T61.774	—	—
Flagyl	T37.3X1	T37.3X2	T37.3X3	T37.3X4	T37.3X5	T37.3X6
Flavine adenine dinucleotide	T45.2X1	T45.2X2	T45.2X3	T45.2X4	T45.2X5	T45.2X6
Flavodic acid	T46.991	T46.992	T46.993	T46.994	T46.995	T46.996
Flavoxate	T44.3X1	T44.3X2	T44.3X3	T44.3X4	T44.3X5	T44.3X6
Flaxedil	T48.1X1	T48.1X2	T48.1X3	T48.1X4	T48.1X5	T48.1X6
Flaxseed (medicinal)	T49.3X1	T49.3X2	T49.3X3	T49.3X4	T49.3X5	T49.3X6
Flecainide	T46.2X1	T46.2X2	T46.2X3	T46.2X4	T46.2X5	T46.2X6
Fleroxacin	T36.8X1	T36.8X2	T36.8X3	T36.8X4	T36.8X5	T36.8X6
Floctafenine	T39.8X1	T39.8X2	T39.8X3	T39.8X4	T39.8X5	T39.8X6
Flomax	T44.6X1	T44.6X2	T44.6X3	T44.6X4	T44.6X5	T44.6X6
Flomoxef	T36.1X1	T36.1X2	T36.1X3	T36.1X4	T36.1X5	T36.1X6
Flopropione	T44.3X1	T44.3X2	T44.3X3	T44.3X4	T44.3X5	T44.3X6
Florantyrone	T47.5X1	T47.5X2	T47.5X3	T47.5X4	T47.5X5	T47.5X6
Floraquin	T37.8X1	T37.8X2	T37.8X3	T37.8X4	T37.8X5	T37.8X6
Florinef	T38.0X1	T38.0X2	T38.0X3	T38.0X4	T38.0X5	T38.0X6
ENT agent	T49.6X1	T49.6X2	T49.6X3	T49.6X4	T49.6X5	T49.6X6
ophthalmic preparation	T49.5X1	T49.5X2	T49.5X3	T49.5X4	T49.5X5	T49.5X6
topical NEC	T49.0X1	T49.0X2	T49.0X3	T49.0X4	T49.0X5	T49.0X6
Flowers of sulfur	T49.4X1	T49.4X2	T49.4X3	T49.4X4	T49.4X5	T49.4X6
Floxuridine	T45.1X1	T45.1X2	T45.1X3	T45.1X4	T45.1X5	T45.1X6
Fluanisone	T43.4X1	T43.4X2	T43.4X3	T43.4X4	T43.4X5	T43.4X6
Flubendazole	T37.4X1	T37.4X2	T37.4X3	T37.4X4	T37.4X5	T37.4X6
Fluclorolone acetonide	T49.0X1	T49.0X2	T49.0X3	T49.0X4	T49.0X5	T49.0X6
Flucloxacillin	T36.0X1	T36.0X2	T36.0X3	T36.0X4	T36.0X5	T36.0X6
Fluconazole	T37.8X1	T37.8X2	T37.8X3	T37.8X4	T37.8X5	T37.8X6
Flucytosine	T37.8X1	T37.8X2	T37.8X3	T37.8X4	T37.8X5	T37.8X6
Fludeoxyglucose (18F)	T50.8X1	T50.8X2	T50.8X3	T50.8X4	T50.8X5	T50.8X6
Fludiazepam	T42.4X1	T42.4X2	T42.4X3	T42.4X4	T42.4X5	T42.4X6
Fludrocortisone	T50.0X1	T50.0X2	T50.0X3	T50.0X4	T50.0X5	T50.0X6
ENT agent	T49.6X1	T49.6X2	T49.6X3	T49.6X4	T49.6X5	T49.6X6
ophthalmic preparation	T49.5X1	T49.5X2	T49.5X3	T49.5X4	T49.5X5	T49.5X6
topical NEC	T49.0X1	T49.0X2	T49.0X3	T49.0X4	T49.0X5	T49.0X6
Fludroxycortide	T49.0X1	T49.0X2	T49.0X3	T49.0X4	T49.0X5	T49.0X6
Flufenamic acid	T39.391	T39.392	T39.393	T39.394	T39.395	T39.396
Fluindione	T45.511	T45.512	T45.513	T45.514	T45.515	T45.516

◀ New   ◀▥ Revised   ~~deleted~~ Deleted

Substance	Poisoning, Accidental (Unintentional)	Poisoning, Intentional Self-Harm	Poisoning, Assault	Poisoning, Undetermined	Adverse Effect	Underdosing
Flumequine	T37.8X1	T37.8X2	T37.8X3	T37.8X4	T37.8X5	T37.8X6
Flumethasone	T49.0X1	T49.0X2	T49.0X3	T49.0X4	T49.0X5	T49.0X6
Flumethiazide	T50.2X1	T50.2X2	T50.2X3	T50.2X4	T50.2X5	T50.2X6
Flumidin	T37.5X1	T37.5X2	T37.5X3	T37.5X4	T37.5X5	T37.5X6
Flunarizine	T46.7X1	T46.7X2	T46.7X3	T46.7X4	T46.7X5	T46.7X6
Flunidazole	T37.8X1	T37.8X2	T37.8X3	T37.8X4	T37.8X5	T37.8X6
Flunisolide	T48.6X1	T48.6X2	T48.6X3	T48.6X4	T48.6X5	T48.6X6
Flunitrazepam	T42.4X1	T42.4X2	T42.4X3	T42.4X4	T42.4X5	T42.4X6
Fluocinolone (acetonide)	T49.0X1	T49.0X2	T49.0X3	T49.0X4	T49.0X5	T49.0X6
Fluocinonide	T49.0X1	T49.0X2	T49.0X3	T49.0X4	T49.0X5	T49.0X6
Fluocortin (butyl)	T49.0X1	T49.0X2	T49.0X3	T49.0X4	T49.0X5	T49.0X6
Fluocortolone	T49.0X1	T49.0X2	T49.0X3	T49.0X4	T49.0X5	T49.0X6
Fluohydrocortisone	T38.0X1	T38.0X2	T38.0X3	T38.0X4	T38.0X5	T38.0X6
ENT agent	T49.6X1	T49.6X2	T49.6X3	T49.6X4	T49.6X5	T49.6X6
ophthalmic preparation	T49.5X1	T49.5X2	T49.5X3	T49.5X4	T49.5X5	T49.5X6
topical NEC	T49.0X1	T49.0X2	T49.0X3	T49.0X4	T49.0X5	T49.0X6
Fluonid	T49.0X1	T49.0X2	T49.0X3	T49.0X4	T49.0X5	T49.0X6
Fluopromazine	T43.3X1	T43.3X2	T43.3X3	T43.3X4	T43.3X5	T43.3X6
Fluoroacetate	T60.8X1	T60.8X2	T60.8X3	T60.8X4	—	—
Fluorescein	T50.8X1	T50.8X2	T50.8X3	T50.8X4	T50.8X5	T50.8X6
Fluorhydrocortisone	T50.0X1	T50.0X2	T50.0X3	T50.0X4	T50.0X5	T50.0X6
Fluoride (nonmedicinal) (pesticide) (sodium) NEC	T60.8X1	T60.8X2	T60.8X3	T60.8X4	—	—
hydrogen — *see Hydrofluoric acid*						
medicinal NEC	T50.991	T50.992	T50.993	T50.994	T50.995	T50.996
dental use	T49.7X1	T49.7X2	T49.7X3	T49.7X4	T49.7X5	T49.7X6
not pesticide NEC	T54.91	T54.92	T54.93	T54.94	—	—
stannous	T49.7X1	T49.7X2	T49.7X3	T49.7X4	T49.7X5	T49.7X6
Fluorinated corticosteroids	T38.0X1	T38.0X2	T38.0X3	T38.0X4	T38.0X5	T38.0X6
Fluorine (gas)	T59.5X1	T59.5X2	T59.5X3	T59.5X4	—	—
salt — *see Fluoride(s)*						
Fluoristan	T49.7X1	T49.7X2	T49.7X3	T49.7X4	T49.7X5	T49.7X6
Fluormetholone	T49.0X1	T49.0X2	T49.0X3	T49.0X4	T49.0X5	T49.0X6
Fluoroacetate	T60.8X1	T60.8X2	T60.8X3	T60.8X4	—	—
Fluorocarbon monomer	T53.6X1	T53.6X2	T53.6X3	T53.6X4	—	—
Fluorocytosine	T37.8X1	T37.8X2	T37.8X3	T37.8X4	T37.8X5	T37.8X6
Fluorodeoxyuridine	T45.1X1	T45.1X2	T45.1X3	T45.1X4	T45.1X5	T45.1X6
Fluorometholone	T49.0X1	T49.0X2	T49.0X3	T49.0X4	T49.0X5	T49.0X6
ophthalmic preparation	T49.5X1	T49.5X2	T49.5X3	T49.5X4	T49.5X5	T49.5X6
Fluorophosphate insecticide	T60.0X1	T60.0X2	T60.0X3	T60.0X4	—	—
Fluorosol	T46.3X1	T46.3X2	T46.3X3	T46.3X4	T46.3X5	T46.3X6
Fluorouracil	T45.1X1	T45.1X2	T45.1X3	T45.1X4	T45.1X5	T45.1X6

Substance	Poisoning, Accidental (Unintentional)	Poisoning, Intentional Self-Harm	Poisoning, Assault	Poisoning, Undetermined	Adverse Effect	Underdosing
Fluorphenylalanine	T49.5X1	T49.5X2	T49.5X3	T49.5X4	T49.5X5	T49.5X6
Fluothane	T41.0X1	T41.0X2	T41.0X3	T41.0X4	T41.0X5	T41.0X6
Fluoxetine	T43.221	T43.222	T43.223	T43.224	T43.225	T43.226
Fluoxymesterone	T38.7X1	T38.7X2	T38.7X3	T38.7X4	T38.7X5	T38.7X6
Flupenthixol	T43.4X1	T43.4X2	T43.4X3	T43.4X4	T43.4X5	T43.4X6
Flupentixol	T43.4X1	T43.4X2	T43.4X3	T43.4X4	T43.4X5	T43.4X6
Fluphenazine	T43.3X1	T43.3X2	T43.3X3	T43.3X4	T43.3X5	T43.3X6
Fluprednidene	T49.0X1	T49.0X2	T49.0X3	T49.0X4	T49.0X5	T49.0X6
Fluprednisolone	T38.0X1	T38.0X2	T38.0X3	T38.0X4	T38.0X5	T38.0X6
Fluradoline	T39.8X1	T39.8X2	T39.8X3	T39.8X4	T39.8X5	T39.8X6
Flurandrenolide	T49.0X1	T49.0X2	T49.0X3	T49.0X4	T49.0X5	T49.0X6
Flurandrenolone	T49.0X1	T49.0X2	T49.0X3	T49.0X4	T49.0X5	T49.0X6
Flurazepam	T42.4X1	T42.4X2	T42.4X3	T42.4X4	T42.4X5	T42.4X6
Flurbiprofen	T39.311	T39.312	T39.313	T39.314	T39.315	T39.316
Flurobate	T49.0X1	T49.0X2	T49.0X3	T49.0X4	T49.0X5	T49.0X6
Flurotyl	T43.291	T43.292	T43.293	T43.294	T43.295	T43.296
Fluroxene	T41.0X1	T41.0X2	T41.0X3	T41.0X4	T41.0X5	T41.0X6
Fluspirilene	T43.591	T43.592	T43.593	T43.594	T43.595	T43.596
Flutamide	T38.6X1	T38.6X2	T38.6X3	T38.6X4	T38.6X5	T38.6X6
Flutazolam	T42.4X1	T42.4X2	T42.4X3	T42.4X4	T42.4X5	T42.4X6
Fluticasone propionate	T49.1X1	T49.1X2	T49.1X3	T49.1X4	T49.1X5	T49.1X6
Flutoprazepam	T42.4X1	T42.4X2	T42.4X3	T42.4X4	T42.4X5	T42.4X6
Flutropium bromide	T48.6X1	T48.6X2	T48.6X3	T48.6X4	T48.6X5	T48.6X6
Fluvoxamine	T43.221	T43.222	T43.223	T43.224	T43.225	T43.226
Folacin	T45.8X1	T45.8X2	T45.8X3	T45.8X4	T45.8X5	T45.8X6
Folic acid	T45.8X1	T45.8X2	T45.8X3	T45.8X4	T45.8X5	T45.8X6
with ferrous salt	T45.2X1	T45.2X2	T45.2X3	T45.2X4	T45.2X5	T45.2X6
antagonist	T45.1X1	T45.1X2	T45.1X3	T45.1X4	T45.1X5	T45.1X6
Folinic acid	T45.8X1	T45.8X2	T45.8X3	T45.8X4	T45.8X5	T45.8X6
Folium stramoniae	T48.6X1	T48.6X2	T48.6X3	T48.6X4	T48.6X5	T48.6X6
Follicle-stimulating hormone, human	T38.811	T38.812	T38.813	T38.814	T38.815	T38.816
Folpet	T60.3X1	T60.3X2	T60.3X3	T60.3X4	—	—
Fominoben	T48.3X1	T48.3X2	T48.3X3	T48.3X4	T48.3X5	T48.3X6
Food, foodstuffs, noxious, nonbacterial, NEC	T62.91	T62.92	T62.93	T62.94	—	—
berries	T62.1X1	T62.1X2	T62.1X3	T62.1X4	—	—
fish — *see also Fish*	T61.91	T61.92	T61.93	T61.94	—	—
mushrooms	T62.0X1	T62.0X2	T62.0X3	T62.0X4	—	—
plants	T62.2X1	T62.2X2	T62.2X3	T62.2X4	—	—
seafood	T61.91	T61.92	T61.93	T61.94	—	—
specified NEC	T61.8X1	T61.8X2	T61.8X3	T61.8X4	—	—
seeds	T62.2X1	T62.2X2	T62.2X3	T62.2X4	—	—

◀ New ◀ Revised ~~deleted~~ Deleted

TABLE OF DRUGS AND CHEMICALS

TABLE OF DRUGS AND CHEMICALS

Substance	Poisoning, Accidental (Unintentional)	Poisoning, Intentional Self-Harm	Poisoning, Assault	Poisoning, Undetermined	Adverse Effect	Underdosing
Food, foodstuffs, noxious, nonbacterial, NEC (Continued)						
shellfish	T61.781	T61.782	T61.783	T61.784	—	—
specified NEC	T62.8X1	T62.8X2	T62.8X3	T62.8X4	—	—
Fool's parsley	T62.2X1	T62.2X2	T62.2X3	T62.2X4	—	—
Formaldehyde (solution), gas or vapor	T59.2X1	T59.2X2	T59.2X3	T59.2X4	—	—
fungicide	T60.3X1	T60.3X2	T60.3X3	T60.3X4	—	—
Formalin	T59.2X1	T59.2X2	T59.2X3	T59.2X4	—	—
fungicide	T60.3X1	T60.3X2	T60.3X3	T60.3X4	—	—
vapor	T59.2X1	T59.2X2	T59.2X3	T59.2X4	—	—
Formic acid	T54.2X1	T54.2X2	T54.2X3	T54.2X4	—	—
vapor	T59.891	T59.892	T59.893	T59.894	—	—
Foscarnet sodium	T37.5X1	T37.5X2	T37.5X3	T37.5X4	T37.5X5	T37.5X6
Fosfestrol	T38.5X1	T38.5X2	T38.5X3	T38.5X4	T38.5X5	T38.5X6
Fosfomycin	T36.8X1	T36.8X2	T36.8X3	T36.8X4	T36.8X5	T36.8X6
Fosfonet sodium	T37.5X1	T37.5X2	T37.5X3	T37.5X4	T37.5X5	T37.5X6
Fosinopril	T46.4X1	T46.4X2	T46.4X3	T46.4X4	T46.4X5	T46.4X6
sodium	T46.4X1	T46.4X2	T46.4X3	T46.4X4	T46.4X5	T46.4X6
Fowler's solution	T57.0X1	T57.0X2	T57.0X3	T57.0X4	—	—
Foxglove	T62.2X1	T62.2X2	T62.2X3	T62.2X4	—	—
Framycetin	T36.5X1	T36.5X2	T36.5X3	T36.5X4	T36.5X5	T36.5X6
Frangula	T47.2X1	T47.2X2	T47.2X3	T47.2X4	T47.2X5	T47.2X6
extract	T47.2X1	T47.2X2	T47.2X3	T47.2X4	T47.2X5	T47.2X6
Frei antigen	T50.8X1	T50.8X2	T50.8X3	T50.8X4	T50.8X5	T50.8X6
Freon	T53.5X1	T53.5X2	T53.5X3	T53.5X4	—	—
Fructose	T50.3X1	T50.3X2	T50.3X3	T50.3X4	T50.3X5	T50.3X6
Frusemide	T50.1X1	T50.1X2	T50.1X3	T50.1X4	T50.1X5	T50.1X6
FSH	T38.811	T38.812	T38.813	T38.814	T38.815	T38.816
Ftorafur	T45.1X1	T45.1X2	T45.1X3	T45.1X4	T45.1X5	T45.1X6
Fuel						
automobile	T52.0X1	T52.0X2	T52.0X3	T52.0X4	—	—
exhaust gas, not in transit	T58.01	T58.02	T58.03	T58.04	—	—
vapor NEC	T52.0X1	T52.0X2	T52.0X3	T52.0X4	—	—
gas (domestic use) — see also Carbon, monoxide, fuel, utility	T59.891	T59.892	T59.893	T59.894	—	—
utility	T59.891	T59.892	T59.893	T59.894	—	—
in mobile container	T59.891	T59.892	T59.893	T59.894	—	—
incomplete combustion of — see Carbon, monoxide, fuel, utility						
piped (natural)	T59.891	T59.892	T59.893	T59.894	—	—
industrial, incomplete combustion	T58.8X1	T58.8X2	T58.8X3	T58.8X4	—	—

Substance	Poisoning, Accidental (Unintentional)	Poisoning, Intentional Self-Harm	Poisoning, Assault	Poisoning, Undetermined	Adverse Effect	Underdosing
Fugillin	T36.8X1	T36.8X2	T36.8X3	T36.8X4	T36.8X5	T36.8X6
Fulminate of mercury	T56.1X1	T56.1X2	T56.1X3	T56.1X4	—	—
Fulvicin	T36.7X1	T36.7X2	T36.7X3	T36.7X4	T36.7X5	T36.7X6
Fumadil	T36.8X1	T36.8X2	T36.8X3	T36.8X4	T36.8X5	T36.8X6
Fumagillin	T36.8X1	T36.8X2	T36.8X3	T36.8X4	T36.8X5	T36.8X6
Fumaric acid	T49.4X1	T49.4X2	T49.4X3	T49.4X4	T49.4X5	T49.4X6
Fumes (from)	T59.91	T59.92	T59.93	T59.94	—	—
carbon monoxide — see Carbon, monoxide						
charcoal (domestic use) — see Charcoal, fumes						
chloroform — see Chloroform						
coke (in domestic stoves, fireplaces) — see Coke, fumes						
corrosive NEC	T54.91	T54.92	T54.93	T54.94	—	—
ether — see ether						
freons	T53.5X1	T53.5X2	T53.5X3	T53.5X4	—	—
hydrocarbons	T59.891	T59.892	T59.893	T59.894	—	—
petroleum (liquefied)	T59.891	T59.892	T59.893	T59.894	—	—
distributed through pipes (pure or mixed with air)	T59.891	T59.892	T59.893	T59.894	—	—
lead — see lead						
metal — see Metals, or the specified metal						
nitrogen dioxide	T59.0X1	T59.0X2	T59.0X3	T59.0X4	—	—
pesticides — see Pesticides						
petroleum (liquefied)	T59.891	T59.892	T59.893	T59.894	—	—
distributed through pipes (pure or mixed with air)	T59.891	T59.892	T59.893	T59.894	—	—
polyester	T59.891	T59.892	T59.893	T59.894	—	—
specified source NEC — see also substance specified	T59.891	T59.892	T59.893	T59.894	—	—
sulfur dioxide	T59.1X1	T59.1X2	T59.1X3	T59.1X4	—	—
Fumigant NEC	T60.91	T60.92	T60.93	T60.94	—	—
Fungi, noxious, used as food	T62.0X1	T62.0X2	T62.0X3	T62.0X4	—	—
Fungicide NEC (nonmedicinal)	T60.3X1	T60.3X2	T60.3X3	T60.3X4	—	—
Fungizone	T36.7X1	T36.7X2	T36.7X3	T36.7X4	T36.7X5	T36.7X6
topical	T49.0X1	T49.0X2	T49.0X3	T49.0X4	T49.0X5	T49.0X6
Furacin	T49.0X1	T49.0X2	T49.0X3	T49.0X4	T49.0X5	T49.0X6
Furadantin	T37.91	T37.92	T37.93	T37.94	T37.95	T37.96
Furazolidone	T37.8X1	T37.8X2	T37.8X3	T37.8X4	T37.8X5	T37.8X6
Furazolium chloride	T49.0X1	T49.0X2	T49.0X3	T49.0X4	T49.0X5	T49.0X6
Furfural	T52.8X1	T52.8X2	T52.8X3	T52.8X4	—	—

◀ New ◀▥ Revised ~~deleted~~ Deleted

Substance	Poisoning, Accidental (Unintentional)	Poisoning, Intentional Self-Harm	Poisoning, Assault	Poisoning, Undetermined	Adverse Effect	Underdosing
Furnace (coal burning) (domestic), gas from industrial	T58.2X1	T58.2X2	T58.2X3	T58.2X4	—	—
industrial	T58.8X1	T58.8X2	T58.8X3	T58.8X4	—	—
Furniture polish	T65.891	T65.892	T65.893	T65.894		
Furosemide	T50.1X1	T50.1X2	T50.1X3	T50.1X4	T50.1X5	T50.1X6
Furoxone	T37.91	T37.92	T37.93	T37.94	T37.95	T37.96
Fursultiamine	T45.2X1	T45.2X2	T45.2X3	T45.2X4	T45.2X5	T45.2X6
Fusafungine	T36.8X1	T36.8X2	T36.8X3	T36.8X4	T36.8X5	T36.8X6
Fusel oil (any) (amyl) (butyl) (propyl), vapor	T51.3X1	T51.3X2	T51.3X3	T51.3X4	—	—
Fusidate (ethanolamine) (sodium)	T36.8X1	T36.8X2	T36.8X3	T36.8X4	T36.8X5	T36.8X6
Fusidic acid	T36.8X1	T36.8X2	T36.8X3	T36.8X4	T36.8X5	T36.8X6
Fytic acid, nonasodium	T50.6X1	T50.6X2	T50.6X3	T50.6X4	T50.6X5	T50.6X6
G						
GABA	T43.8X1	T43.8X2	T43.8X3	T43.8X4	T43.8X5	T43.8X6
Gadopentetic acid	T50.8X1	T50.8X2	T50.8X3	T50.8X4	T50.8X5	T50.8X6
Galactose	T50.3X1	T50.3X2	T50.3X3	T50.3X4	T50.3X5	T50.3X6
b-Galactosidase	T47.5X1	T47.5X2	T47.5X3	T47.5X4	T47.5X5	T47.5X6
Galantamine	T44.0X1	T44.0X2	T44.0X3	T44.0X4	T44.0X5	T44.0X6
Gallamine (triethiodide)	T48.1X1	T48.1X2	T48.1X3	T48.1X4	T48.1X5	T48.1X6
Gallium citrate	T50.991	T50.992	T50.993	T50.994	T50.995	T50.996
Gallopamil	T46.1X1	T46.1X2	T46.1X3	T46.1X4	T46.1X5	T46.1X6
Gamboge	T47.2X1	T47.2X2	T47.2X3	T47.2X4	T47.2X5	T47.2X6
Gamimune	T50.Z11	T50.Z12	T50.Z13	T50.Z14	T50.Z15	T50.Z16
Gamma-aminobutyric acid	T43.8X1	T43.8X2	T43.8X3	T43.8X4	T43.8X5	T43.8X6
Gamma-benzene hexachloride (medicinal)	T49.0X1	T49.0X2	T49.0X3	T49.0X4	T49.0X5	T49.0X6
nonmedicinal, vapor	T53.6X1	T53.6X2	T53.6X3	T53.6X4	—	—
Gamma-BHC (medicinal) — see also Gamma-benzene hexachloride	T49.0X1	T49.0X2	T49.0X3	T49.0X4	T49.0X5	T49.0X6
Gamma globulin	T50.Z11	T50.Z12	T50.Z13	T50.Z14	T50.Z15	T50.Z16
Gamulin	T50.Z11	T50.Z12	T50.Z13	T50.Z14	T50.Z15	T50.Z16
Ganciclovir (sodium)	T37.5X1	T37.5X2	T37.5X3	T37.5X4	T37.5X5	T37.5X6
Ganglionic blocking drug NEC	T44.2X1	T44.2X2	T44.2X3	T44.2X4	T44.2X5	T44.2X6
specified NEC	T44.2X1	T44.2X2	T44.2X3	T44.2X4	T44.2X5	T44.2X6
Ganja	T40.7X1	T40.7X2	T40.7X3	T40.7X4	T40.7X5	T40.7X6
Garamycin	T36.5X1	T36.5X2	T36.5X3	T36.5X4	T36.5X5	T36.5X6
ophthalmic preparation	T49.5X1	T49.5X2	T49.5X3	T49.5X4	T49.5X5	T49.5X6
topical NEC	T49.0X1	T49.0X2	T49.0X3	T49.0X4	T49.0X5	T49.0X6
Gardenal	T42.3X1	T42.3X2	T42.3X3	T42.3X4	T42.3X5	T42.3X6
Gardepanyl	T42.3X1	T42.3X2	T42.3X3	T42.3X4	T42.3X5	T42.3X6

Substance	Poisoning, Accidental (Unintentional)	Poisoning, Intentional Self-Harm	Poisoning, Assault	Poisoning, Undetermined	Adverse Effect	Underdosing
Gas	T59.91	T59.92	T59.93	T59.94	—	—
acetylene	T59.891	T59.892	T59.893	T59.894		
incomplete combustion of	T58.11	T58.12	T58.13	T58.14	—	—
air contaminants, source or type not specified	T59.91	T59.92	T59.93	T59.94	—	—
anesthetic	T41.0X1	T41.0X2	T41.0X3	T41.0X4	T41.0X5	T41.0X6
blast furnace	T58.8X1	T58.8X2	T58.8X3	T58.8X4		
butane — see butane						
carbon monoxide — see Carbon, monoxide						
chlorine	T59.4X1	T59.4X2	T59.4X3	T59.4X4		
coal	T58.2X1	T58.2X2	T58.2X3	T58.2X4		
cyanide	T57.3X1	T57.3X2	T57.3X3	T57.3X4		
dicyanogen	T65.0X1	T65.0X2	T65.0X3	T65.0X4		
domestic — see Domestic gas	T57.91	T57.92	T57.93	T57.94		
exhaust	T57.91	T57.92	T57.93	T57.94		
from utility (for cooking, heating, or lighting) (after combustion) — see Carbon, monoxide, fuel, utility						
prior to combustion	T59.891	T59.892	T59.893	T59.894		
from wood or coal-burning stove or fireplace	T57.91	T57.92	T57.93	T57.94		
fuel (domestic use) (after combustion) — see also Carbon, monoxide, fuel	T57.91	T57.92	T57.93	T57.94		
industrial use	T58.8X1	T58.8X2	T58.8X3	T58.8X4		
prior to combustion	T59.891	T59.892	T59.893	T59.894		
utility	T59.891	T59.892	T59.893	T59.894		
in mobile container	T59.891	T59.892	T59.893	T59.894		
incomplete combustion of — see Carbon, monoxide, fuel, utility						
piped (natural)	T59.891	T59.892	T59.893	T59.894		
garage	T58.01	T58.02	T58.03	T58.04		
hydrocarbon NEC	T59.891	T59.892	T59.893	T59.894		
incomplete combustion of — see Carbon, monoxide, fuel, utility						
liquefied — see butane						
piped	T59.891	T59.892	T59.893	T59.894	—	—
hydrocyanic acid	T65.0X1	T65.0X2	T65.0X3	T65.0X4		

TABLE OF DRUGS AND CHEMICALS

Substance	External Cause (T-Code)					
	Poisoning, Accidental (Unintentional)	Poisoning, Intentional Self-Harm	Poisoning, Assault	Poisoning, Undetermined	Adverse Effect	Underdosing
Gas *(Continued)*						
illuminating (after combustion)	T58.11	T58.12	T58.13	T58.14	—	—
prior to combustion	T59.891	T59.892	T59.893	T59.894	—	—
incomplete combustion, any — *see Carbon, monoxide*						
kiln	T58.8X1	T58.8X2	T58.8X3	T58.8X4	—	—
lacrimogenic	T59.3X1	T59.3X2	T59.3X3	T59.3X4	—	—
liquefied petroleum — *see butane*						
marsh	T59.891	T59.892	T59.893	T59.894	—	—
motor exhaust, not in transit	T58.01	T58.02	T58.03	T58.04	—	—
mustard, not in war	T59.891	T59.892	T59.893	T59.894	—	—
natural	T59.891	T59.892	T59.893	T59.894	—	—
nerve, not in war	T59.91	T59.92	T59.93	T59.94	—	—
oil	T52.0X1	T52.0X2	T52.0X3	T52.0X4	—	—
petroleum (liquefied) (distributed in mobile containers)	T59.891	T59.892	T59.893	T59.894	—	—
piped (pure or mixed with air)	T59.891	T59.892	T59.893	T59.894	—	—
piped (manufactured) (natural) NEC	T59.891	T59.892	T59.893	T59.894	—	—
producer	T58.8X1	T58.8X2	T58.8X3	T58.8X4	—	—
propane — *see propane*						
refrigerant (chlorofluoro-carbon)	T53.5X1	T53.5X2	T53.5X3	T53.5X4	—	—
not chlorofluoro-carbon	T59.891	T59.892	T59.893	T59.894	—	—
sewer	T59.91	T59.92	T59.93	T59.94	—	—
specified source NEC	T59.91	T59.92	T59.93	T59.94	—	—
stove (after combustion)	T58.11	T58.12	T58.13	T58.14	—	—
tear	T59.3X1	T59.3X2	T59.3X3	T59.3X4	—	—
therapeutic	T41.5X1	T41.5X2	T41.5X3	T41.5X4	T41.5X5	T41.5X6
utility (for cooking, heating, or lighting) (piped) NEC	T59.891	T59.892	T59.893	T59.894	—	—
in mobile container	T59.891	T59.892	T59.893	T59.894	—	—
incomplete combustion of — *see Carbon, monoxide, fuel, utilty*						
piped (natural)	T59.891	T59.892	T59.893	T59.894	—	—
water	T58.11	T58.12	T58.13	T58.14	—	—
incomplete combustion of — *see Carbon, monoxide, fuel, utility*						

Substance	External Cause (T-Code)					
	Poisoning, Accidental (Unintentional)	Poisoning, Intentional Self-Harm	Poisoning, Assault	Poisoning, Undetermined	Adverse Effect	Underdosing
Gaseous substance — *see Gas*						
Gasoline	T52.0X1	T52.0X2	T52.0X3	T52.0X4	—	—
vapor	T52.0X1	T52.0X2	T52.0X3	T52.0X4	—	—
Gastric enzymes	T47.5X1	T47.5X2	T47.5X3	T47.5X4	T47.5X5	T47.5X6
Gastrografin	T50.8X1	T50.8X2	T50.8X3	T50.8X4	T50.8X5	T50.8X6
Gastrointestinal drug	T47.91	T47.92	T47.93	T47.94	T47.95	T47.96
biological	T47.8X1	T47.8X2	T47.8X3	T47.8X4	T47.8X5	T47.8X6
specified NEC	T47.8X1	T47.8X2	T47.8X3	T47.8X4	T47.8X5	T47.8X6
Gaultheria procumbens	T62.2X1	T62.2X2	T62.2X3	T62.2X4	—	—
Gelatin (intravenous)	T45.8X1	T45.8X2	T45.8X3	T45.8X4	T45.8X5	T45.8X6
absorbable (sponge)	T45.7X1	T45.7X2	T45.7X3	T45.7X4	T45.7X5	T45.7X6
Gefarnate	T44.3X1	T44.3X2	T44.3X3	T44.3X4	T44.3X5	T44.3X6
Gelfilm	T49.8X1	T49.8X2	T49.8X3	T49.8X4	T49.8X5	T49.8X6
Gelfoam	T45.7X1	T45.7X2	T45.7X3	T45.7X4	T45.7X5	T45.7X6
Gelsemine	T50.991	T50.992	T50.993	T50.994	T50.995	T50.996
Gelsemium (sempervirens)	T62.2X1	T62.2X2	T62.2X3	T62.2X4	—	—
Gemeprost	T48.0X1	T48.0X2	T48.0X3	T48.0X4	T48.0X5	T48.0X6
Gemfibrozil	T46.6X1	T46.6X2	T46.6X3	T46.6X4	T46.6X5	T46.6X6
Gemonil	T42.3X1	T42.3X2	T42.3X3	T42.3X4	T42.3X5	T42.3X6
Gentamicin	T36.5X1	T36.5X2	T36.5X3	T36.5X4	T36.5X5	T36.5X6
ophthalmic preparation	T49.5X1	T49.5X2	T49.5X3	T49.5X4	T49.5X5	T49.5X6
topical NEC	T49.0X1	T49.0X2	T49.0X3	T49.0X4	T49.0X5	T49.0X6
Gentian	T47.5X1	T47.5X2	T47.5X3	T47.5X4	T47.5X5	T47.5X6
violet	T49.0X1	T49.0X2	T49.0X3	T49.0X4	T49.0X5	T49.0X6
Gepefrine	T44.4X1	T44.4X2	T44.4X3	T44.4X4	T44.4X5	T44.4X6
Gestonorone caproate	T38.5X1	T38.5X2	T38.5X3	T38.5X4	T38.5X5	T38.5X6
Gexane	T49.0X1	T49.0X2	T49.0X3	T49.0X4	T49.0X5	T49.0X6
Gila monster (venom)	T63.111	T63.112	T63.113	T63.114	—	—
Ginger	T47.5X1	T47.5X2	T47.5X3	T47.5X4	T47.5X5	T47.5X6
Jamaica — *see Jamaica, ginger*						
Gitalin	T46.0X1	T46.0X2	T46.0X3	T46.0X4	T46.0X5	T46.0X6
amorphous	T46.0X1	T46.0X2	T46.0X3	T46.0X4	T46.0X5	T46.0X6
Gitaloxin	T46.0X1	T46.0X2	T46.0X3	T46.0X4	T46.0X5	T46.0X6
Gitoxin	T46.0X1	T46.0X2	T46.0X3	T46.0X4	T46.0X5	T46.0X6
Glafenine	T39.8X1	T39.8X2	T39.8X3	T39.8X4	T39.8X5	T39.8X6
Glandular extract (medicinal) NEC	T50.Z91	T50.Z92	T50.Z93	T50.Z94	T50.Z95	T50.Z96
Glaucarubin	T37.3X1	T37.3X2	T37.3X3	T37.3X4	T37.3X5	T37.3X6
Glibenclamide	T38.3X1	T38.3X2	T38.3X3	T38.3X4	T38.3X5	T38.3X6
Glibornuride	T38.3X1	T38.3X2	T38.3X3	T38.3X4	T38.3X5	T38.3X6
Gliclazide	T38.3X1	T38.3X2	T38.3X3	T38.3X4	T38.3X5	T38.3X6
Glimidine	T38.3X1	T38.3X2	T38.3X3	T38.3X4	T38.3X5	T38.3X6

◄ New   ◄ Revised   ~~deleted~~ Deleted

Substance	Poisoning, Accidental (Unintentional)	Poisoning, Intentional Self-Harm	Poisoning, Assault	Poisoning, Undetermined	Adverse Effect	Underdosing
Glipizide	T38.3X1	T38.3X2	T38.3X3	T38.3X4	T38.3X5	T38.3X6
Gliquidone	T38.3X1	T38.3X2	T38.3X3	T38.3X4	T38.3X5	T38.3X6
Glisolamide	T38.3X1	T38.3X2	T38.3X3	T38.3X4	T38.3X5	T38.3X6
Glisoxepide	T38.3X1	T38.3X2	T38.3X3	T38.3X4	T38.3X5	T38.3X6
Globin zinc insulin	T38.3X1	T38.3X2	T38.3X3	T38.3X4	T38.3X5	T38.3X6
Globulin						
antilymphocytic	T50.Z11	T50.Z12	T50.Z13	T50.Z14	T50.Z15	T50.Z16
antirhesus	T50.Z11	T50.Z12	T50.Z13	T50.Z14	T50.Z15	T50.Z16
antivenin	T50.Z11	T50.Z12	T50.Z13	T50.Z14	T50.Z15	T50.Z16
antiviral	T50.Z11	T50.Z12	T50.Z13	T50.Z14	T50.Z15	T50.Z16
Glucagon	T38.3X1	T38.3X2	T38.3X3	T38.3X4	T38.3X5	T38.3X6
Glucocorticoids	T38.0X1	T38.0X2	T38.0X3	T38.0X4	T38.0X5	T38.0X6
Glucocorticosteroid	T38.0X1	T38.0X2	T38.0X3	T38.0X4	T38.0X5	T38.0X6
Gluconic acid	T50.991	T50.992	T50.993	T50.994	T50.995	T50.996
Glucosamine sulfate	T39.4X1	T39.4X2	T39.4X3	T39.4X4	T39.4X5	T39.4X6
Glucose	T50.3X1	T50.3X2	T50.3X3	T50.3X4	T50.3X5	T50.3X6
with sodium chloride	T50.3X1	T50.3X2	T50.3X3	T50.3X4	T50.3X5	T50.3X6
Glucosulfone sodium	T37.1X1	T37.1X2	T37.1X3	T37.1X4	T37.1X5	T37.1X6
Glucurolactone	T47.8X1	T47.8X2	T47.8X3	T47.8X4	T47.8X5	T47.8X6
Glue NEC	T52.8X1	T52.8X2	T52.8X3	T52.8X4	—	—
Glutamic acid	T47.5X1	T47.5X2	T47.5X3	T47.5X4	T47.5X5	T47.5X6
Glutaral (medicinal)	T49.0X1	T49.0X2	T49.0X3	T49.0X4	T49.0X5	T49.0X6
nonmedicinal	T65.891	T65.892	T65.893	T65.894	—	—
Glutaraldehyde (nonmedicinal)	T65.891	T65.892	T65.893	T65.894	—	—
medicinal	T49.0X1	T49.0X2	T49.0X3	T49.0X4	T49.0X5	T49.0X6
Glutathione	T50.6X1	T50.6X2	T50.6X3	T50.6X4	T50.6X5	T50.6X6
Glutethimide	T42.6X1	T42.6X2	T42.6X3	T42.6X4	T42.6X5	T42.6X6
Glyburide	T38.3X1	T38.3X2	T38.3X3	T38.3X4	T38.3X5	T38.3X6
Glycerin	T47.4X1	T47.4X2	T47.4X3	T47.4X4	T47.4X5	T47.4X6
Glycerol	T47.4X1	T47.4X2	T47.4X3	T47.4X4	T47.4X5	T47.4X6
borax	T49.6X1	T49.6X2	T49.6X3	T49.6X4	T49.6X5	T49.6X6
intravenous	T50.3X1	T50.3X2	T50.3X3	T50.3X4	T50.3X5	T50.3X6
iodinated	T48.4X1	T48.4X2	T48.4X3	T48.4X4	T48.4X5	T48.4X6
Glycerophosphate	T50.991	T50.992	T50.993	T50.994	T50.995	T50.996
Glyceryl						
gualacolate	T48.4X1	T48.4X2	T48.4X3	T48.4X4	T48.4X5	T48.4X6
nitrate	T46.3X1	T46.3X2	T46.3X3	T46.3X4	T46.3X5	T46.3X6
triacetate (topical)	T49.0X1	T49.0X2	T49.0X3	T49.0X4	T49.0X5	T49.0X6
trinitrate	T46.3X1	T46.3X2	T46.3X3	T46.3X4	T46.3X5	T46.3X6
Glycine	T50.3X1	T50.3X2	T50.3X3	T50.3X4	T50.3X5	T50.3X6
Glyclopyramide	T38.3X1	T38.3X2	T38.3X3	T38.3X4	T38.3X5	T38.3X6
Glycobiarsol	T37.3X1	T37.3X2	T37.3X3	T37.3X4	T37.3X5	T37.3X6

Substance	Poisoning, Accidental (Unintentional)	Poisoning, Intentional Self-Harm	Poisoning, Assault	Poisoning, Undetermined	Adverse Effect	Underdosing
Glycols (ether)	T52.3X1	T52.3X2	T52.3X3	T52.3X4	—	—
Glyconiazide	T37.1X1	T37.1X2	T37.1X3	T37.1X4	T37.1X5	T37.1X6
Glycopyrrolate	T44.3X1	T44.3X2	T44.3X3	T44.3X4	T44.3X5	T44.3X6
Glycopyrronium	T44.3X1	T44.3X2	T44.3X3	T44.3X4	T44.3X5	T44.3X6
bromide	T44.3X1	T44.3X2	T44.3X3	T44.3X4	T44.3X5	T44.3X6
Glycoside, cardiac (stimulant)	T46.0X1	T46.0X2	T46.0X3	T46.0X4	T46.0X5	T46.0X6
Glycyclamide	T38.3X1	T38.3X2	T38.3X3	T38.3X4	T38.3X5	T38.3X6
Glycyrrhiza extract	T48.4X1	T48.4X2	T48.4X3	T48.4X4	T48.4X5	T48.4X6
Glycyrrhizic acid	T48.4X1	T48.4X2	T48.4X3	T48.4X4	T48.4X5	T48.4X6
Glycyrrhizinate potassium	T48.4X1	T48.4X2	T48.4X3	T48.4X4	T48.4X5	T48.4X6
Glymidine sodium	T38.3X1	T38.3X2	T38.3X3	T38.3X4	T38.3X5	T38.3X6
Glyphosate	T60.3X1	T60.3X2	T60.3X3	T60.3X4	—	—
Glyphylline	T48.6X1	T48.6X2	T48.6X3	T48.6X4	T48.6X5	T48.6X6
Gold						
colloidal (198Au)	T45.1X1	T45.1X2	T45.1X3	T45.1X4	T45.1X5	T45.1X6
salts	T39.4X1	T39.4X2	T39.4X3	T39.4X4	T39.4X5	T39.4X6
Golden sulfide of antimony	T56.891	T56.892	T56.893	T56.894	—	—
Goldylocks	T62.2X1	T62.2X2	T62.2X3	T62.2X4	—	—
Gonadal tissue extract	T38.901	T38.902	T38.903	T38.904	T38.905	T38.906
female	T38.5X1	T38.5X2	T38.5X3	T38.5X4	T38.5X5	T38.5X6
male	T38.7X1	T38.7X2	T38.7X3	T38.7X4	T38.7X5	T38.7X6
Gonadorelin	T38.891	T38.892	T38.893	T38.894	T38.895	T38.896
Gonadotropin	T38.891	T38.892	T38.893	T38.894	T38.895	T38.896
chorionic	T38.891	T38.892	T38.893	T38.894	T38.895	T38.896
pituitary	T38.811	T38.812	T38.813	T38.814	T38.815	T38.816
Goserelin	T45.1X1	T45.1X2	T45.1X3	T45.1X4	T45.1X5	T45.1X6
Grain alcohol	T51.0X1	T51.0X2	T51.0X3	T51.0X4	—	—
Gramicidin	T49.0X1	T49.0X2	T49.0X3	T49.0X4	T49.0X5	T49.0X6
Granisetron	T45.0X1	T45.0X2	T45.0X3	T45.0X4	T45.0X5	T45.0X6
Gratiola officinalis	T62.2X1	T62.2X2	T62.2X3	T62.2X4	—	—
Grease	T65.891	T65.892	T65.893	T65.894	—	—
Green hellebore	T62.2X1	T62.2X2	T62.2X3	T62.2X4	—	—
Green soap	T49.2X1	T49.2X2	T49.2X3	T49.2X4	T49.2X5	T49.2X6
Grifulvin	T36.7X1	T36.7X2	T36.7X3	T36.7X4	T36.7X5	T36.7X6
Griseofulvin	T36.7X1	T36.7X2	T36.7X3	T36.7X4	T36.7X5	T36.7X6
Growth hormone	T38.811	T38.812	T38.813	T38.814	T38.815	T38.816
Guaiacol derivatives	T48.4X1	T48.4X2	T48.4X3	T48.4X4	T48.4X5	T48.4X6
Guaiac reagent	T50.991	T50.992	T50.993	T50.994	T50.995	T50.996
Guaifenesin	T48.4X1	T48.4X2	T48.4X3	T48.4X4	T48.4X5	T48.4X6
Guaimesal	T48.4X1	T48.4X2	T48.4X3	T48.4X4	T48.4X5	T48.4X6
Guaiphenesin	T48.4X1	T48.4X2	T48.4X3	T48.4X4	T48.4X5	T48.4X6
Guamecycline	T36.4X1	T36.4X2	T36.4X3	T36.4X4	T36.4X5	T36.4X6

◀ New   ◀|||| Revised   ~~deleted~~ Deleted

TABLE OF DRUGS AND CHEMICALS

Substance	External Cause (T-Code)					
	Poisoning, Accidental (Unintentional)	Poisoning, Intentional Self-Harm	Poisoning, Assault	Poisoning, Undetermined	Adverse Effect	Underdosing
Guanabenz	T46.5X1	T46.5X2	T46.5X3	T46.5X4	T46.5X5	T46.5X6
Guanacline	T46.5X1	T46.5X2	T46.5X3	T46.5X4	T46.5X5	T46.5X6
Guanadrel	T46.5X1	T46.5X2	T46.5X3	T46.5X4	T46.5X5	T46.5X6
Guanatol	T37.2X1	T37.2X2	T37.2X3	T37.2X4	T37.2X5	T37.2X6
Guanethidine	T46.5X1	T46.5X2	T46.5X3	T46.5X4	T46.5X5	T46.5X6
Guanfacine	T46.5X1	T46.5X2	T46.5X3	T46.5X4	T46.5X5	T46.5X6
Guano	T65.891	T65.892	T65.893	T65.894	—	—
Guanochlor	T46.5X1	T46.5X2	T46.5X3	T46.5X4	T46.5X5	T46.5X6
Guanoclor	T46.5X1	T46.5X2	T46.5X3	T46.5X4	T46.5X5	T46.5X6
Guanoctine	T46.5X1	T46.5X2	T46.5X3	T46.5X4	T46.5X5	T46.5X6
Guanoxabenz	T46.5X1	T46.5X2	T46.5X3	T46.5X4	T46.5X5	T46.5X6
Guanoxan	T46.5X1	T46.5X2	T46.5X3	T46.5X4	T46.5X5	T46.5X6
Guar gum (medicinal)	T46.6X1	T46.6X2	T46.6X3	T46.6X4	T46.6X5	T46.6X6
H						
Hachimycin	T36.7X1	T36.7X2	T36.7X3	T36.7X4	T36.7X5	T36.7X6
Hair						
dye	T49.4X1	T49.4X2	T49.4X3	T49.4X4	T49.4X5	T49.4X6
preparation NEC	T49.4X1	T49.4X2	T49.4X3	T49.4X4	T49.4X5	T49.4X6
Halazepam	T42.4X1	T42.4X2	T42.4X3	T42.4X4	T42.4X5	T42.4X6
Halcinolone	T49.0X1	T49.0X2	T49.0X3	T49.0X4	T49.0X5	T49.0X6
Halcinonide	T49.0X1	T49.0X2	T49.0X3	T49.0X4	T49.0X5	T49.0X6
Halethazole	T49.0X1	T49.0X2	T49.0X3	T49.0X4	T49.0X5	T49.0X6
Hallucinogen NEC	T40.901	T40.902	T40.903	T40.904	T40.905	T40.906
Halofantrine	T37.2X1	T37.2X2	T37.2X3	T37.2X4	T37.2X5	T37.2X6
Halofenate	T46.6X1	T46.6X2	T46.6X3	T46.6X4	T46.6X5	T46.6X6
Halometasone	T49.0X1	T49.0X2	T49.0X3	T49.0X4	T49.0X5	T49.0X6
Haloperidol	T43.4X1	T43.4X2	T43.4X3	T43.4X4	T43.4X5	T43.4X6
Haloprogin	T49.0X1	T49.0X2	T49.0X3	T49.0X4	T49.0X5	T49.0X6
Halotex	T49.0X1	T49.0X2	T49.0X3	T49.0X4	T49.0X5	T49.0X6
Halothane	T41.0X1	T41.0X2	T41.0X3	T41.0X4	T41.0X5	T41.0X6
Haloxazolam	T42.4X1	T42.4X2	T42.4X3	T42.4X4	T42.4X5	T42.4X6
Halquinols	T49.0X1	T49.0X2	T49.0X3	T49.0X4	T49.0X5	T49.0X6
Hamamelis	T49.2X1	T49.2X2	T49.2X3	T49.2X4	T49.2X5	T49.2X6
Haptendextran	T45.8X1	T45.8X2	T45.8X3	T45.8X4	T45.8X5	T45.8X6
Harmonyl	T46.5X1	T46.5X2	T46.5X3	T46.5X4	T46.5X5	T46.5X6
Hartmann's solution	T50.3X1	T50.3X2	T50.3X3	T50.3X4	T50.3X5	T50.3X6
Hashish	T40.7X1	T40.7X2	T40.7X3	T40.7X4	T40.7X5	T40.7X6
Hawaiian Woodrose seeds	T40.991	T40.992	T40.993	T40.994	—	—
HCB	T60.3X1	T60.3X2	T60.3X3	T60.3X4	—	—
HCH	T53.6X1	T53.6X2	T53.6X3	T53.6X4	—	—
medicinal	T49.0X1	T49.0X2	T49.0X3	T49.0X4	T49.0X5	T49.0X6

Substance	External Cause (T-Code)					
	Poisoning, Accidental (Unintentional)	Poisoning, Intentional Self-Harm	Poisoning, Assault	Poisoning, Undetermined	Adverse Effect	Underdosing
HCN	T57.3X1	T57.3X2	T57.3X3	T57.3X4	—	—
Headache cures, drugs, powders NEC	T50.901	T50.902	T50.903	T50.904	T50.905	T50.906
Heavenly Blue (morning glory)	T40.991	T40.992	T40.993	T40.994	—	—
Heavy metal antidote	T45.8X1	T45.8X2	T45.8X3	T45.8X4	T45.8X5	T45.8X6
Hedaquinium	T49.0X1	T49.0X2	T49.0X3	T49.0X4	T49.0X5	T49.0X6
Hedge hyssop	T62.2X1	T62.2X2	T62.2X3	T62.2X4	—	—
Heet	T49.8X1	T49.8X2	T49.8X3	T49.8X4	T49.8X5	T49.8X6
Helium	T48.991	T48.992	T48.993	T48.994	T48.995	T48.996
Helenin	T37.4X1	T37.4X2	T37.4X3	T37.4X4	T37.4X5	T37.4X6
Hellebore (black) (green) (white)	T62.2X1	T62.2X2	T62.2X3	T62.2X4	—	—
Helium (nonmedicinal) NEC	T59.891	T59.892	T59.893	T59.894	—	—
medicinal	T48.991	T48.992	T48.993	T48.994	T48.995	T48.996
Hematin	T45.8X1	T45.8X2	T45.8X3	T45.8X4	T45.8X5	T45.8X6
Hematinic preparation	T45.8X1	T45.8X2	T45.8X3	T45.8X4	T45.8X5	T45.8X6
Hemlock	T62.2X1	T62.2X2	T62.2X3	T62.2X4	—	—
Hemostatic	T45.621	T45.622	T45.623	T45.624	T45.625	T45.626
drug, systemic	T45.621	T45.622	T45.623	T45.624	T45.625	T45.626
Hemostyptic	T49.4X1	T49.4X2	T49.4X3	T49.4X4	T49.4X5	T49.4X6
Henbane	T62.2X1	T62.2X2	T62.2X3	T62.2X4	—	—
Heparin (sodium)	T45.511	T45.512	T45.513	T45.514	T45.515	T45.516
action reverser	T45.7X1	T45.7X2	T45.7X3	T45.7X4	T45.7X5	T45.7X6
Heparin-fraction	T45.511	T45.512	T45.513	T45.514	T45.515	T45.516
Heparinoid (systemic)	T45.511	T45.512	T45.513	T45.514	T45.515	T45.516
Hepatic secretion stimulant	T47.8X1	T47.8X2	T47.8X3	T47.8X4	T47.8X5	T47.8X6
Hepatitis B						
immune globulin	T50.Z11	T50.Z12	T50.Z13	T50.Z14	T50.Z15	T50.Z16
vaccine	T50.B91	T50.B92	T50.B93	T50.B94	T50.B95	T50.B96
Hepronicate	T46.7X1	T46.7X2	T46.7X3	T46.7X4	T46.7X5	T46.7X6
Heptabarb	T42.3X1	T42.3X2	T42.3X3	T42.3X4	T42.3X5	T42.3X6
Heptabarbitone	T42.3X1	T42.3X2	T42.3X3	T42.3X4	T42.3X5	T42.3X6
Heptabarbital	T42.3X1	T42.3X2	T42.3X3	T42.3X4	T42.3X5	T42.3X6
Heptachlor	T60.1X1	T60.1X2	T60.1X3	T60.1X4	—	—
Heptalgin	T40.2X1	T40.2X2	T40.2X3	T40.2X4	T40.2X5	T40.2X6
Heptaminol	T46.3X1	T46.3X2	T46.3X3	T46.3X4	T46.3X5	T46.3X6
Herbicide NEC	T60.3X1	T60.3X2	T60.3X3	T60.3X4	—	—
Heroin	T40.1X1	T40.1X2	T40.1X3	T40.1X4	—	—
Herplex	T49.5X1	T49.5X2	T49.5X3	T49.5X4	T49.5X5	T49.5X6
HES	T45.8X1	T45.8X2	T45.8X3	T45.8X4	T45.8X5	T45.8X6
Hesperidin	T46.991	T46.992	T46.993	T46.994	T46.995	T46.996
Hetacillin	T36.0X1	T36.0X2	T36.0X3	T36.0X4	T36.0X5	T36.0X6

◀ New   ◀⍾ Revised   ~~deleted~~ Deleted

Substance	External Cause (T-Code)					
	Poisoning, Accidental (Unintentional)	Poisoning, Intentional Self-Harm	Poisoning, Assault	Poisoning, Undetermined	Adverse Effect	Underdosing
Hetastarch	T45.8X1	T45.8X2	T45.8X3	T45.8X4	T45.8X5	T45.8X6
HETP	T60.0X1	T60.0X2	T60.0X3	T60.0X4	—	—
Hexachlorobenzene (vapor)	T60.3X1	T60.3X2	T60.3X3	T60.3X4	—	—
Hexachlorocyclohexane	T53.6X1	T53.6X2	T53.6X3	T53.6X4	—	—
Hexachlorophene	T49.0X1	T49.0X2	T49.0X3	T49.0X4	T49.0X5	T49.0X6
Hexadiline	T46.3X1	T46.3X2	T46.3X3	T46.3X4	T46.3X5	T46.3X6
Hexadimethrine (bromide)	T45.7X1	T45.7X2	T45.7X3	T45.7X4	T45.7X5	T45.7X6
Hexadylamine	T46.3X1	T46.3X2	T46.3X3	T46.3X4	T46.3X5	T46.3X6
Hexaethyl tetraphosphate	T60.0X1	T60.0X2	T60.0X3	T60.0X4	—	—
Hexafluorenium bromide	T48.1X1	T48.1X2	T48.1X3	T48.1X4	T48.1X5	T48.1X6
Hexafluorodiethyl ether	T43.291	T43.292	T43.293	T43.294	T43.295	T43.296
Hexafluronium (bromide)	T48.1X1	T48.1X2	T48.1X3	T48.1X4	T48.1X5	T48.1X6
Hexahydrobenzol	T52.8X1	T52.8X2	T52.8X3	T52.8X4	—	—
Hexahydrocresol(s)	T51.8X1	T51.8X2	T51.8X3	T51.8X4	—	—
arsenide	T57.0X1	T57.0X2	T57.0X3	T57.0X4	—	—
arseniurated	T57.0X1	T57.0X2	T57.0X3	T57.0X4	—	—
cyanide	T57.3X1	T57.3X2	T57.3X3	T57.3X4	—	—
gas	T59.891	T59.892	T59.893	T59.894	—	—
Fluoride (liquid)	T57.8X1	T57.8X2	T57.8X3	T57.8X4	—	—
vapor	T59.891	T59.892	T59.893	T59.894	—	—
phophorated	T60.0X1	T60.0X2	T60.0X3	T60.0X4	—	—
sulfate	T57.8X1	T57.8X2	T57.8X3	T57.8X4	—	—
sulfide (gas)	T59.6X1	T59.6X2	T59.6X3	T59.6X4	—	—
arseniurated	T57.0X1	T57.0X2	T57.0X3	T57.0X4	—	—
sulfurated	T57.8X1	T57.8X2	T57.8X3	T57.8X4	—	—
Hexahydrophenol	T51.8X1	T51.8X2	T51.8X3	T51.8X4	—	—
Hexa-germ	T49.2X1	T49.2X2	T49.2X3	T49.2X4	T49.2X5	T49.2X6
Hexalen	T51.8X1	T51.8X2	T51.8X3	T51.8X4	—	—
Hexamethonium bromide	T44.2X1	T44.2X2	T44.2X3	T44.2X4	T44.2X5	T44.2X6
Hexamethylene	T52.8X1	T52.8X2	T52.8X3	T52.8X4	—	—
Hexamethylmelamine	T45.1X1	T45.1X2	T45.1X3	T45.1X4	T45.1X5	T45.1X6
Hexamidine	T49.0X1	T49.0X2	T49.0X3	T49.0X4	T49.0X5	T49.0X6
Hexamine (mandelate)	T37.8X1	T37.8X2	T37.8X3	T37.8X4	T37.8X5	T37.8X6
Hexanone, 2-hexanone	T52.4X1	T52.4X2	T52.4X3	T52.4X4	—	—
Hexanuorenium	T48.1X1	T48.1X2	T48.1X3	T48.1X4	T48.1X5	T48.1X6
Hexapropymate	T42.6X1	T42.6X2	T42.6X3	T42.6X4	T42.6X5	T42.6X6
Hexasonium iodide	T44.3X1	T44.3X2	T44.3X3	T44.3X4	T44.3X5	T44.3X6
Hexcarbacholine bromide	T48.1X1	T48.1X2	T48.1X3	T48.1X4	T48.1X5	T48.1X6
Hexemal	T42.3X1	T42.3X2	T42.3X3	T42.3X4	T42.3X5	T42.3X6
Hexestrol	T38.5X1	T38.5X2	T38.5X3	T38.5X4	T38.5X5	T38.5X6
Hexethal (sodium)	T42.3X1	T42.3X2	T42.3X3	T42.3X4	T42.3X5	T42.3X6
Hexetidine	T37.8X1	T37.8X2	T37.8X3	T37.8X4	T37.8X5	T37.8X6

Substance	External Cause (T-Code)					
	Poisoning, Accidental (Unintentional)	Poisoning, Intentional Self-Harm	Poisoning, Assault	Poisoning, Undetermined	Adverse Effect	Underdosing
Hexobarbital	T42.3X1	T42.3X2	T42.3X3	T42.3X4	T42.3X5	T42.3X6
rectal	T41.291	T41.292	T41.293	T41.294	T41.295	T41.296
sodium	T41.1X1	T41.1X2	T41.1X3	T41.1X4	T41.1X5	T41.1X6
Hexobendine	T46.3X1	T46.3X2	T46.3X3	T46.3X4	T46.3X5	T46.3X6
Hexocyclium	T44.3X1	T44.3X2	T44.3X3	T44.3X4	T44.3X5	T44.3X6
metilsulfate	T44.3X1	T44.3X2	T44.3X3	T44.3X4	T44.3X5	T44.3X6
Hexoestrol	T38.5X1	T38.5X2	T38.5X3	T38.5X4	T38.5X5	T38.5X6
Hexone	T52.4X1	T52.4X2	T52.4X3	T52.4X4	—	—
Hexoprenaline	T48.6X1	T48.6X2	T48.6X3	T48.6X4	T48.6X5	T48.6X6
Hexylcaine	T41.3X1	T41.3X2	T41.3X3	T41.3X4	T41.3X5	T41.3X6
Hexylresorcinol	T52.2X1	T52.2X2	T52.2X3	T52.2X4	—	—
HGH (human growth hormone)	T38.811	T38.812	T38.813	T38.814	T38.815	T38.816
Hinkle's pills	T47.2X1	T47.2X2	T47.2X3	T47.2X4	T47.2X5	T47.2X6
Histalog	T50.8X1	T50.8X2	T50.8X3	T50.8X4	T50.8X5	T50.8X6
Histamine (phosphate)	T50.8X1	T50.8X2	T50.8X3	T50.8X4	T50.8X5	T50.8X6
Histoplasmin	T50.8X1	T50.8X2	T50.8X3	T50.8X4	T50.8X5	T50.8X6
Holly berries	T62.2X1	T62.2X2	T62.2X3	T62.2X4	—	—
Homatropine	T44.3X1	T44.3X2	T44.3X3	T44.3X4	T44.3X5	T44.3X6
methylbromide	T44.3X1	T44.3X2	T44.3X3	T44.3X4	T44.3X5	T44.3X6
Homochlorcyclizine	T45.0X1	T45.0X2	T45.0X3	T45.0X4	T45.0X5	T45.0X6
Homosalate	T49.3X1	T49.3X2	T49.3X3	T49.3X4	T49.3X5	T49.3X6
Homo-tet	T50.Z11	T50.Z12	T50.Z13	T50.Z14	T50.Z15	T50.Z16
Hormone	T38.801	T38.802	T38.803	T38.804	T38.805	T38.806
adrenal cortical steroids	T38.0X1	T38.0X2	T38.0X3	T38.0X4	T38.0X5	T38.0X6
androgenic	T38.7X1	T38.7X2	T38.7X3	T38.7X4	T38.7X5	T38.7X6
anterior pituitary NEC	T38.811	T38.812	T38.813	T38.814	T38.815	T38.816
antidiabetic agents	T38.3X1	T38.3X2	T38.3X3	T38.3X4	T38.3X5	T38.3X6
antidiuretic	T38.891	T38.892	T38.893	T38.894	T38.895	T38.896
cancer therapy	T45.1X1	T45.1X2	T45.1X3	T45.1X4	T45.1X5	T45.1X6
follicle stimulating	T38.811	T38.812	T38.813	T38.814	T38.815	T38.816
gonadotropic	T38.891	T38.892	T38.893	T38.894	T38.895	T38.896
pituitary	T38.811	T38.812	T38.813	T38.814	T38.815	T38.816
growth	T38.811	T38.812	T38.813	T38.814	T38.815	T38.816
luteinizing	T38.811	T38.812	T38.813	T38.814	T38.815	T38.816
ovarian	T38.5X1	T38.5X2	T38.5X3	T38.5X4	T38.5X5	T38.5X6
oxytocic	T48.0X1	T48.0X2	T48.0X3	T48.0X4	T48.0X5	T48.0X6
parathyroid (derivatives)	T50.991	T50.992	T50.993	T50.994	T50.995	T50.996
pituitary (posterior) NEC	T38.891	T38.892	T38.893	T38.894	T38.895	T38.896
anterior	T38.811	T38.812	T38.813	T38.814	T38.815	T38.816
specified, NEC	T38.891	T38.892	T38.893	T38.894	T38.895	T38.896
thyroid	T38.1X1	T38.1X2	T38.1X3	T38.1X4	T38.1X5	T38.1X6
Hornet (sting)	T63.451	T63.452	T63.453	T63.454	—	—

◀ New ◀▪▪ Revised ~~deleted~~ Deleted

Substance	External Cause (T-Code)					
	Poisoning, Accidental (Unintentional)	Poisoning, Intentional Self-Harm	Poisoning, Assault	Poisoning, Undetermined	Adverse Effect	Underdosing
Horse anti-human lymphocytic serum	T50.Z11	T50.Z12	T50.Z13	T50.Z14	T50.Z15	T50.Z16
Horticulture agent NEC	T65.91	T65.92	T65.93	T65.94	—	—
with pesticide	T60.91	T60.92	T60.93	T60.94	—	—
Human						
albumin	T45.8X1	T45.8X2	T45.8X3	T45.8X4	T45.8X5	T45.8X6
growth hormone (HGH)	T38.811	T38.812	T38.813	T38.814	T38.815	T38.816
immune serum	T50.Z11	T50.Z12	T50.Z13	T50.Z14	T50.Z15	T50.Z16
Hyaluronidase	T45.3X1	T45.3X2	T45.3X3	T45.3X4	T45.3X5	T45.3X6
Hyazyme	T45.3X1	T45.3X2	T45.3X3	T45.3X4	T45.3X5	T45.3X6
Hycodan	T40.2X1	T40.2X2	T40.2X3	T40.2X4	T40.2X5	T40.2X6
Hydantoin derivative NEC	T42.0X1	T42.0X2	T42.0X3	T42.0X4	T42.0X5	T42.0X6
Hydeltra	T38.0X1	T38.0X2	T38.0X3	T38.0X4	T38.0X5	T38.0X6
Hydergine	T44.6X1	T44.6X2	T44.6X3	T44.6X4	T44.6X5	T44.6X6
Hydrabamine penicillin	T36.0X1	T36.0X2	T36.0X3	T36.0X4	T36.0X5	T36.0X6
Hydralazine	T46.5X1	T46.5X2	T46.5X3	T46.5X4	T46.5X5	T46.5X6
Hydrargaphen	T49.0X1	T49.0X2	T49.0X3	T49.0X4	T49.0X5	T49.0X6
Hydrargyri amino-chloridum	T49.0X1	T49.0X2	T49.0X3	T49.0X4	T49.0X5	T49.0X6
Hydrastine	T48.291	T48.292	T48.293	T48.294	T48.295	T48.296
Hydrazine	T54.1X1	T54.1X2	T54.1X3	T54.1X4	—	—
monoamine oxidase inhibitors	T43.1X1	T43.1X2	T43.1X3	T43.1X4	T43.1X5	T43.1X6
Hydrazoic acid, azides	T54.2X1	T54.2X2	T54.2X3	T54.2X4	—	—
Hydriodic acid	T48.4X1	T48.4X2	T48.4X3	T48.4X4	T48.4X5	T48.4X6
Hydrocarbon gas	T59.891	T59.892	T59.893	T59.894	—	—
incomplete combustion of — see Carbon, monoxide, fuel, utility						
liquefied (mobile container)	T59.891	T59.892	T59.893	T59.894	—	—
piped (natural)	T59.891	T59.892	T59.893	T59.894	—	—
Hydrochloric acid (liquid)	T54.2X1	T54.2X2	T54.2X3	T54.2X4	—	—
medicinal (digestant)	T47.5X1	T47.5X2	T47.5X3	T47.5X4	T47.5X5	T47.5X6
vapor	T59.891	T59.892	T59.893	T59.894	—	—
Hydrochlorothiazide	T50.2X1	T50.2X2	T50.2X3	T50.2X4	T50.2X5	T50.2X6
Hydrocodone	T40.2X1	T40.2X2	T40.2X3	T40.2X4	T40.2X5	T40.2X6
Hydrocortisone (derivatives)	T38.0X1	T38.0X2	T38.0X3	T38.0X4	T38.0X5	T38.0X6
aceponate	T49.0X1	T49.0X2	T49.0X3	T49.0X4	T49.0X5	T49.0X6
ENT agent	T49.6X1	T49.6X2	T49.6X3	T49.6X4	T49.6X5	T49.6X6
ophthalmic preparation	T49.5X1	T49.5X2	T49.5X3	T49.5X4	T49.5X5	T49.5X6
topical NEC	T49.0X1	T49.0X2	T49.0X3	T49.0X4	T49.0X5	T49.0X6
Hydrocortone	T38.0X1	T38.0X2	T38.0X3	T38.0X4	T38.0X5	T38.0X6
ENT agent	T49.6X1	T49.6X2	T49.6X3	T49.6X4	T49.6X5	T49.6X6
ophthalmic preparation	T49.5X1	T49.5X2	T49.5X3	T49.5X4	T49.5X5	T49.5X6
topical NEC	T49.0X1	T49.0X2	T49.0X3	T49.0X4	T49.0X5	T49.0X6

Substance	External Cause (T-Code)					
	Poisoning, Accidental (Unintentional)	Poisoning, Intentional Self-Harm	Poisoning, Assault	Poisoning, Undetermined	Adverse Effect	Underdosing
Hydrocyanic acid (liquid)	T57.3X1	T57.3X2	T57.3X3	T57.3X4	—	—
gas	T65.0X1	T65.0X2	T65.0X3	T65.0X4	—	—
Hydroflumethiazide	T50.2X1	T50.2X2	T50.2X3	T50.2X4	T50.2X5	T50.2X6
Hydrofluoric acid (liquid)	T54.2X1	T54.2X2	T54.2X3	T54.2X4	—	—
vapor	T59.891	T59.892	T59.893	T59.894	—	—
Hydrogen	T59.891	T59.892	T59.893	T59.894	—	—
arsenide	T57.0X1	T57.0X2	T57.0X3	T57.0X4	—	—
arseniureted	T57.0X1	T57.0X2	T57.0X3	T57.0X4	—	—
chloride	T57.8X1	T57.8X2	T57.8X3	T57.8X4	—	—
cyanide (salts)	T57.3X1	T57.3X2	T57.3X3	T57.3X4	—	—
gas	T57.3X1	T57.3X2	T57.3X3	T57.3X4	—	—
Fluoride	T59.5X1	T59.5X2	T59.5X3	T59.5X4	—	—
vapor	T59.5X1	T59.5X2	T59.5X3	T59.5X4	—	—
peroxide	T49.0X1	T49.0X2	T49.0X3	T49.0X4	T49.0X5	T49.0X6
phosphureted	T57.1X1	T57.1X2	T57.1X3	T57.1X4	—	—
sulfide	T59.6X1	T59.6X2	T59.6X3	T59.6X4	—	—
arseniureted	T57.0X1	T57.0X2	T57.0X3	T57.0X4	—	—
sulfureted	T59.6X1	T59.6X2	T59.6X3	T59.6X4	—	—
Hydromethylpyridine	T46.7X1	T46.7X2	T46.7X3	T46.7X4	T46.7X5	T46.7X6
Hydromorphinol	T40.2X1	T40.2X2	T40.2X3	T40.2X4	—	—
Hydromorphinone	T40.2X1	T40.2X2	T40.2X3	T40.2X4	T40.2X5	T40.2X6
Hydromorphone	T40.2X1	T40.2X2	T40.2X3	T40.2X4	T40.2X5	T40.2X6
Hydromox	T50.2X1	T50.2X2	T50.2X3	T50.2X4	T50.2X5	T50.2X6
Hydrophilic lotion	T49.3X1	T49.3X2	T49.3X3	T49.3X4	T49.3X5	T49.3X6
Hydroquinidine	T46.2X1	T46.2X2	T46.2X3	T46.2X4	T46.2X5	T46.2X6
Hydroquinone	T52.2X1	T52.2X2	T52.2X3	T52.2X4	—	—
vapor	T59.891	T59.892	T59.893	T59.894	—	—
Hydrosulfuric acid (gas)	T59.6X1	T59.6X2	T59.6X3	T59.6X4	—	—
Hydrotalcite	T47.1X1	T47.1X2	T47.1X3	T47.1X4	T47.1X5	T47.1X6
Hydrous wool fat	T49.3X1	T49.3X2	T49.3X3	T49.3X4	T49.3X5	T49.3X6
Hydroxide, caustic	T54.3X1	T54.3X2	T54.3X3	T54.3X4	—	—
Hydroxocobalamin	T45.8X1	T45.8X2	T45.8X3	T45.8X4	T45.8X5	T45.8X6
Hydroxyamphetamine	T49.5X1	T49.5X2	T49.5X3	T49.5X4	T49.5X5	T49.5X6
Hydroxycarbamide	T45.1X1	T45.1X2	T45.1X3	T45.1X4	T45.1X5	T45.1X6
Hydroxychloroquine	T37.8X1	T37.8X2	T37.8X3	T37.8X4	T37.8X5	T37.8X6
Hydroxydihydrocodeinone	T40.2X1	T40.2X2	T40.2X3	T40.2X4	T40.2X5	T40.2X6
Hydroxyestrone	T38.5X1	T38.5X2	T38.5X3	T38.5X4	T38.5X5	T38.5X6
Hydroxyethyl starch	T45.8X1	T45.8X2	T45.8X3	T45.8X4	T45.8X5	T45.8X6
Hydroxymethylpentanone	T52.4X1	T52.4X2	T52.4X3	T52.4X4	—	—
Hydroxyphenamate	T43.591	T43.592	T43.593	T43.594	T43.595	T43.596
Hydroxyphenylbutazone	T39.2X1	T39.2X2	T39.2X3	T39.2X4	T39.2X5	T39.2X6

◀ New ◀⊨ Revised ~~deleted~~ Deleted

Substance	Poisoning, Accidental (Unintentional)	Poisoning, Intentional Self-Harm	Poisoning, Assault	Poisoning, Undetermined	Adverse Effect	Underdosing
Hydroxyprogesterone	T38.5X1	T38.5X2	T38.5X3	T38.5X4	T38.5X5	T38.5X6
caproate	T38.5X1	T38.5X2	T38.5X3	T38.5X4	T38.5X5	T38.5X6
Hydroxyquinoline (derivatives) NEC	T37.8X1	T37.8X2	T37.8X3	T37.8X4	T37.8X5	T37.8X6
Hydroxystilbamidine	T37.3X1	T37.3X2	T37.3X3	T37.3X4	T37.3X5	T37.3X6
Hydroxytoluene (nonmedicinal)	T54.0X1	T54.0X2	T54.0X3	T54.0X4	—	—
medicinal	T49.0X1	T49.0X2	T49.0X3	T49.0X4	T49.0X5	T49.0X6
Hydroxyurea	T45.1X1	T45.1X2	T45.1X3	T45.1X4	T45.1X5	T45.1X6
Hydroxyzine	T43.591	T43.592	T43.593	T43.594	T43.595	T43.596
Hyoscine	T44.3X1	T44.3X2	T44.3X3	T44.3X4	T44.3X5	T44.3X6
Hyoscyamine	T44.3X1	T44.3X2	T44.3X3	T44.3X4	T44.3X5	T44.3X6
Hyoscyamus	T44.3X1	T44.3X2	T44.3X3	T44.3X4	T44.3X5	T44.3X6
dry extract	T44.3X1	T44.3X2	T44.3X3	T44.3X4	T44.3X5	T44.3X6
Hypaque	T50.8X1	T50.8X2	T50.8X3	T50.8X4	T50.8X5	T50.8X6
Hypertussis	T50.Z11	T50.Z12	T50.Z13	T50.Z14	T50.Z15	T50.Z16
Hypnotic	T42.71	T42.72	T42.73	T42.74	T42.75	T42.76
anticonvulsant	T42.71	T42.72	T42.73	T42.74	T42.75	T42.76
specified NEC	T42.6X1	T42.6X2	T42.6X3	T42.6X4	T42.6X5	T42.6X6
Hypochlorite	T49.0X1	T49.0X2	T49.0X3	T49.0X4	T49.0X5	T49.0X6
Hypophysis, posterior	T38.891	T38.892	T38.893	T38.894	T38.895	T38.896
Hypotensive NEC	T46.5X1	T46.5X2	T46.5X3	T46.5X4	T46.5X5	T46.5X6
Hypromellose	T49.5X1	T49.5X2	T49.5X3	T49.5X4	T49.5X5	T49.5X6
I						
Ibacitabine	T37.5X1	T37.5X2	T37.5X3	T37.5X4	T37.5X5	T37.5X6
Ibopamine	T44.991	T44.992	T44.993	T44.994	T44.995	T44.996
Ibufenac	T39.311	T39.312	T39.313	T39.314	T39.315	T39.316
Ibuprofen	T39.311	T39.312	T39.313	T39.314	T39.315	T39.316
Ibuproxam	T39.311	T39.312	T39.313	T39.314	T39.315	T39.316
Ibuterol	T48.6X1	T48.6X2	T48.6X3	T48.6X4	T48.6X5	T48.6X6
Ichthammol	T49.0X1	T49.0X2	T49.0X3	T49.0X4	T49.0X5	T49.0X6
Ichthyol	T49.4X1	T49.4X2	T49.4X3	T49.4X4	T49.4X5	T49.4X6
Idarubicin	T45.1X1	T45.1X2	T45.1X3	T45.1X4	T45.1X5	T45.1X6
Idrocilamide	T42.8X1	T42.8X2	T42.8X3	T42.8X4	T42.8X5	T42.8X6
Ifenprodil	T46.7X1	T46.7X2	T46.7X3	T46.7X4	T46.7X5	T46.7X6
Ifosfamide	T45.1X1	T45.1X2	T45.1X3	T45.1X4	T45.1X5	T45.1X6
Iletin	T38.3X1	T38.3X2	T38.3X3	T38.3X4	T38.3X5	T38.3X6
Ilex	T62.2X1	T62.2X2	T62.2X3	T62.2X4	—	—
Illuminating gas (after combustion)	T58.11	T58.12	T58.13	T58.14	—	—
prior to combustion	T59.891	T59.892	T59.893	T59.894	—	—
Ilopan	T45.2X1	T45.2X2	T45.2X3	T45.2X4	T45.2X5	T45.2X6
Iloprost	T46.7X1	T46.7X2	T46.7X3	T46.7X4	T46.7X5	T46.7X6

Substance	Poisoning, Accidental (Unintentional)	Poisoning, Intentional Self-Harm	Poisoning, Assault	Poisoning, Undetermined	Adverse Effect	Underdosing
Ilotycin	T36.3X1	T36.3X2	T36.3X3	T36.3X4	T36.3X5	T36.3X6
ophthalmic preparation	T49.5X1	T49.5X2	T49.5X3	T49.5X4	T49.5X5	T49.5X6
topical NEC	T49.0X1	T49.0X2	T49.0X3	T49.0X4	T49.0X5	T49.0X6
Imidazole-4-carboxamide	T45.1X1	T45.1X2	T45.1X3	T45.1X4	T45.1X5	T45.1X6
Imipenem	T36.0X1	T36.0X2	T36.0X3	T36.0X4	T36.0X5	T36.0X6
Imipramine	T43.011	T43.012	T43.013	T43.014	T43.015	T43.016
Iminostilbene	T42.1X1	T42.1X2	T42.1X3	T42.1X4	T42.1X5	T42.1X6
Immu-G	T50.Z11	T50.Z12	T50.Z13	T50.Z14	T50.Z15	T50.Z16
Immuglobin	T50.Z11	T50.Z12	T50.Z13	T50.Z14	T50.Z15	T50.Z16
Immune						
globulin	T50.Z11	T50.Z12	T50.Z13	T50.Z14	T50.Z15	T50.Z16
serum globulin	T50.Z11	T50.Z12	T50.Z13	T50.Z14	T50.Z15	T50.Z16
Immunoglobin human (intravenous) (normal)	T50.Z11	T50.Z12	T50.Z13	T50.Z14	T50.Z15	T50.Z16
unmodified	T50.Z11	T50.Z12	T50.Z13	T50.Z14	T50.Z15	T50.Z16
Immunosuppressive drug	T45.1X1	T45.1X2	T45.1X3	T45.1X4	T45.1X5	T45.1X6
Immu-tetanus	T50.Z11	T50.Z12	T50.Z13	T50.Z14	T50.Z15	T50.Z16
Indalpine	T43.221	T43.222	T43.223	T43.224	T43.225	T43.226
Indanazoline	T48.5X1	T48.5X2	T48.5X3	T48.5X4	T48.5X5	T48.5X6
Indandione (derivatives)	T45.511	T45.512	T45.513	T45.514	T45.515	T45.516
Indapamide	T46.5X1	T46.5X2	T46.5X3	T46.5X4	T46.5X5	T46.5X6
Indendione (derivatives)	T45.511	T45.512	T45.513	T45.514	T45.515	T45.516
Indenolol	T44.7X1	T44.7X2	T44.7X3	T44.7X4	T44.7X5	T44.7X6
Inderal	T44.7X1	T44.7X2	T44.7X3	T44.7X4	T44.7X5	T44.7X6
Indian						
hemp	T40.7X1	T40.7X2	T40.7X3	T40.7X4	T40.7X5	T40.7X6
tobacco	T62.2X1	T62.2X2	T62.2X3	T62.2X4	—	—
Indigo carmine	T50.8X1	T50.8X2	T50.8X3	T50.8X4	T50.8X5	T50.8X6
Indobufen	T45.521	T45.522	T45.523	T45.524	T45.525	T45.526
Indocin	T39.2X1	T39.2X2	T39.2X3	T39.2X4	T39.2X5	T39.2X6
Indocyanine green	T50.8X1	T50.8X2	T50.8X3	T50.8X4	T50.8X5	T50.8X6
Indometacin	T39.391	T39.392	T39.393	T39.394	T39.395	T39.396
Indomethacin	T39.391	T39.392	T39.393	T39.394	T39.395	T39.396
farnesil	T39.4X1	T39.4X2	T39.4X3	T39.4X4	T39.4X5	T39.4X6
Indoramin	T44.6X1	T44.6X2	T44.6X3	T44.6X4	T44.6X5	T44.6X6
Industrial						
alcohol	T51.0X1	T51.0X2	T51.0X3	T51.0X4	—	—
fumes	T59.891	T59.892	T59.893	T59.894	—	—
solvents (fumes) (vapors)	T52.91	T52.92	T52.93	T52.94	—	—
Influenza vaccine	T50.B91	T50.B92	T50.B93	T50.B94	T50.B95	T50.B96
Ingested substance NEC	T65.91	T65.92	T65.93	T65.94	—	—
INH	T37.1X1	T37.1X2	T37.1X3	T37.1X4	T37.1X5	T37.1X6

TABLE OF DRUGS AND CHEMICALS

TABLE OF DRUGS AND CHEMICALS

Substance	External Cause (T-Code)					
	Poisoning, Accidental (Unintentional)	Poisoning, Intentional Self-Harm	Poisoning, Assault	Poisoning, Undetermined	Adverse Effect	Underdosing
Inhalation, gas (noxious) — see Gas						
Inhibitor						
angiotensin-converting enzyme	T46.4X1	T46.4X2	T46.4X3	T46.4X4	T46.4X5	T46.4X6
carbonic anhydrase	T50.2X1	T50.2X2	T50.2X3	T50.2X4	T50.2X5	T50.2X6
fibrinolysis	T45.621	T45.622	T45.623	T45.624	T45.625	T45.626
monoamine oxidase NEC	T43.1X1	T43.1X2	T43.1X3	T43.1X4	T43.1X5	T43.1X6
hydrazine	T43.1X1	T43.1X2	T43.1X3	T43.1X4	T43.1X5	T43.1X6
postsynaptic	T43.8X1	T43.8X2	T43.8X3	T43.8X4	T43.8X5	T43.8X6
prothrombin synthesis	T45.511	T45.512	T45.513	T45.514	T45.515	T45.516
Ink	T65.891	T65.892	T65.893	T65.894	—	—
Inorganic substance NEC	T57.91	T57.92	T57.93	T57.94	—	—
Inosine pranobex	T37.5X1	T37.5X2	T37.5X3	T37.5X4	T37.5X5	T37.5X6
Inositol	T50.991	T50.992	T50.993	T50.994	T50.995	T50.996
nicotinate	T46.7X1	T46.7X2	T46.7X3	T46.7X4	T46.7X5	T46.7X6
Inproquone	T45.1X1	T45.1X2	T45.1X3	T45.1X4	T45.1X5	T45.1X6
Insect (sting), venomous	T63.481	T63.482	T63.483	T63.484	—	—
ant	T63.421	T63.422	T63.423	T63.424	—	—
bee	T63.441	T63.442	T63.443	T63.444	—	—
caterpillar	T63.431	T63.432	T63.433	T63.434	—	—
hornet	T63.451	T63.452	T63.453	T63.454	—	—
wasp	T63.461	T63.462	T63.463	T63.464	—	—
Insecticide NEC	T60.91	T60.92	T60.93	T60.94	—	—
carbamate	T60.0X1	T60.0X2	T60.0X3	T60.0X4	—	—
chlorinated	T60.1X1	T60.1X2	T60.1X3	T60.1X4	—	—
mixed	T60.91	T60.92	T60.93	T60.94	—	—
organochlorine	T60.1X1	T60.1X2	T60.1X3	T60.1X4	—	—
organophosphorus	T60.0X1	T60.0X2	T60.0X3	T60.0X4	—	—
Insular tissue extract	T38.3X1	T38.3X2	T38.3X3	T38.3X4	T38.3X5	T38.3X6
Insulin (amorphous) (globin) (isophane) (Lente) (NPH) (Semilente) (Ultralente)	T38.3X1	T38.3X2	T38.3X3	T38.3X4	T38.3X5	T38.3X6
defalan	T38.3X1	T38.3X2	T38.3X3	T38.3X4	T38.3X5	T38.3X6
human	T38.3X1	T38.3X2	T38.3X3	T38.3X4	T38.3X5	T38.3X6
injection, soluble	T38.3X1	T38.3X2	T38.3X3	T38.3X4	T38.3X5	T38.3X6
biphasic	T38.3X1	T38.3X2	T38.3X3	T38.3X4	T38.3X5	T38.3X6
intermediate acting	T38.3X1	T38.3X2	T38.3X3	T38.3X4	T38.3X5	T38.3X6
protamine zinc	T38.3X1	T38.3X2	T38.3X3	T38.3X4	T38.3X5	T38.3X6
slow acting	T38.3X1	T38.3X2	T38.3X3	T38.3X4	T38.3X5	T38.3X6
zinc						
protamine injection	T38.3X1	T38.3X2	T38.3X3	T38.3X4	T38.3X5	T38.3X6
suspension (amorphous) (crystalline)	T38.3X1	T38.3X2	T38.3X3	T38.3X4	T38.3X5	T38.3X6

Substance	External Cause (T-Code)					
	Poisoning, Accidental (Unintentional)	Poisoning, Intentional Self-Harm	Poisoning, Assault	Poisoning, Undetermined	Adverse Effect	Underdosing
Interferon (alpha) (beta) (gamma)	T37.5X1	T37.5X2	T37.5X3	T37.5X4	T37.5X5	T37.5X6
Intestinal motility control drug	T47.6X1	T47.6X2	T47.6X3	T47.6X4	T47.6X5	T47.6X6
biological	T47.8X1	T47.8X2	T47.8X3	T47.8X4	T47.8X5	T47.8X6
Intranarcon	T41.1X1	T41.1X2	T41.1X3	T41.1X4	T41.1X5	T41.1X6
Intravenous						
amino acids	T50.991	T50.992	T50.993	T50.994	T50.995	T50.996
fat suspension	T50.991	T50.992	T50.993	T50.994	T50.995	T50.996
Inulin	T50.8X1	T50.8X2	T50.8X3	T50.8X4	T50.8X5	T50.8X6
Invert sugar	T50.3X1	T50.3X2	T50.3X3	T50.3X4	T50.3X5	T50.3X6
Inza — see Naproxen						
Iobenzamic acid	T50.8X1	T50.8X2	T50.8X3	T50.8X4	T50.8X5	T50.8X6
Iocarmic acid	T50.8X1	T50.8X2	T50.8X3	T50.8X4	T50.8X5	T50.8X6
Iocetamic acid	T50.8X1	T50.8X2	T50.8X3	T50.8X4	T50.8X5	T50.8X6
Iodamide	T50.8X1	T50.8X2	T50.8X3	T50.8X4	T50.8X5	T50.8X6
Iodide NEC — see also Iodine	T49.0X1	T49.0X2	T49.0X3	T49.0X4	T49.0X5	T49.0X6
mercury (ointment)	T49.0X1	T49.0X2	T49.0X3	T49.0X4	T49.0X5	T49.0X6
methylate	T49.0X1	T49.0X2	T49.0X3	T49.0X4	T49.0X5	T49.0X6
potassium (expectorant) NEC	T48.4X1	T48.4X2	T48.4X3	T48.4X4	T48.4X5	T48.4X6
Iodinated						
contrast medium	T50.8X1	T50.8X2	T50.8X3	T50.8X4	T50.8X5	T50.8X6
glycerol	T48.4X1	T48.4X2	T48.4X3	T48.4X4	T48.4X5	T48.4X6
human serum albumin (131I)	T50.8X1	T50.8X2	T50.8X3	T50.8X4	T50.8X5	T50.8X6
Iodine (antiseptic, external) (tincture) NEC	T49.0X1	T49.0X2	T49.0X3	T49.0X4	T49.0X5	T49.0X6
125 — see also Radiation sickness, and Exposure to radioactivce isotopes	T50.8X1	T50.8X2	T50.8X3	T50.8X4	T50.8X5	T50.8X6
therapeutic	T50.991	T50.992	T50.993	T50.994	T50.995	T50.996
131 — see also Radiation sickness, and Exposure to radioactivce isotopes	T50.8X1	T50.8X2	T50.8X3	T50.8X4	T50.8X5	T50.8X6
therapeutic	T38.2X1	T38.2X2	T38.2X3	T38.2X4	T38.2X5	T38.2X6
diagnostic	T50.8X1	T50.8X2	T50.8X3	T50.8X4	T50.8X5	T50.8X6
for thyroid conditions (antithyroid)	T38.2X1	T38.2X2	T38.2X3	T38.2X4	T38.2X5	T38.2X6
solution	T49.0X1	T49.0X2	T49.0X3	T49.0X4	T49.0X5	T49.0X6
vapor	T59.891	T59.892	T59.893	T59.894	—	—
Iodipamide	T50.8X1	T50.8X2	T50.8X3	T50.8X4	T50.8X5	T50.8X6
Iodized (poppy seed) oil	T50.8X1	T50.8X2	T50.8X3	T50.8X4	T50.8X5	T50.8X6
Iodobismitol	T37.8X1	T37.8X2	T37.8X3	T37.8X4	T37.8X5	T37.8X6
Iodochlorhydroxyquin	T37.8X1	T37.8X2	T37.8X3	T37.8X4	T37.8X5	T37.8X6
topical	T49.0X1	T49.0X2	T49.0X3	T49.0X4	T49.0X5	T49.0X6
Iodochlorhydroxyquino-line	T37.8X1	T37.8X2	T37.8X3	T37.8X4	T37.8X5	T37.8X6
Iodocholesterol (131I)	T50.8X1	T50.8X2	T50.8X3	T50.8X4	T50.8X5	T50.8X6

◀ New ◀◀ Revised ~~deleted~~ Deleted

Substance	Poisoning, Accidental (Unintentional)	Poisoning, Intentional Self-Harm	Poisoning, Assault	Poisoning, Undetermined	Adverse Effect	Underdosing
Iodoform	T49.0X1	T49.0X2	T49.0X3	T49.0X4	T49.0X5	T49.0X6
Iodohippuric acid	T50.8X1	T50.8X2	T50.8X3	T50.8X4	T50.8X5	T50.8X6
Iodopanoic acid	T50.8X1	T50.8X2	T50.8X3	T50.8X4	T50.8X5	T50.8X6
Iodophthalein (sodium)	T50.8X1	T50.8X2	T50.8X3	T50.8X4	T50.8X5	T50.8X6
Iodopyracet	T50.8X1	T50.8X2	T50.8X3	T50.8X4	T50.8X5	T50.8X6
Iodoquinol	T37.8X1	T37.8X2	T37.8X3	T37.8X4	T37.8X5	T37.8X6
Iodoxamic acid	T50.8X1	T50.8X2	T50.8X3	T50.8X4	T50.8X5	T50.8X6
Iofendylate	T50.8X1	T50.8X2	T50.8X3	T50.8X4	T50.8X5	T50.8X6
Ioglycamic acid	T50.8X1	T50.8X2	T50.8X3	T50.8X4	T50.8X5	T50.8X6
Iohexol	T50.8X1	T50.8X2	T50.8X3	T50.8X4	T50.8X5	T50.8X6
Ion exchange resin						
anion	T47.8X1	T47.8X2	T47.8X3	T47.8X4	T47.8X5	T47.8X6
cation	T50.3X1	T50.3X2	T50.3X3	T50.3X4	T50.3X5	T50.3X6
cholestyramine	T46.6X1	T46.6X2	T46.6X3	T46.6X4	T46.6X5	T46.6X6
intestinal	T47.8X1	T47.8X2	T47.8X3	T47.8X4	T47.8X5	T47.8X6
Iopamidol	T50.8X1	T50.8X2	T50.8X3	T50.8X4	T50.8X5	T50.8X6
Iopanoic acid	T50.8X1	T50.8X2	T50.8X3	T50.8X4	T50.8X5	T50.8X6
Iophenoic acid	T50.8X1	T50.8X2	T50.8X3	T50.8X4	T50.8X5	T50.8X6
Iopodate, sodium	T50.8X1	T50.8X2	T50.8X3	T50.8X4	T50.8X5	T50.8X6
Iopodic acid	T50.8X1	T50.8X2	T50.8X3	T50.8X4	T50.8X5	T50.8X6
Iopromide	T50.8X1	T50.8X2	T50.8X3	T50.8X4	T50.8X5	T50.8X6
Iopydol	T50.8X1	T50.8X2	T50.8X3	T50.8X4	T50.8X5	T50.8X6
Iotalamic acid	T50.8X1	T50.8X2	T50.8X3	T50.8X4	T50.8X5	T50.8X6
Iothalamate	T50.8X1	T50.8X2	T50.8X3	T50.8X4	T50.8X5	T50.8X6
Iothiouracil	T38.2X1	T38.2X2	T38.2X3	T38.2X4	T38.2X5	T38.2X6
Iotrol	T50.8X1	T50.8X2	T50.8X3	T50.8X4	T50.8X5	T50.8X6
Iotrolan	T50.8X1	T50.8X2	T50.8X3	T50.8X4	T50.8X5	T50.8X6
Iotroxate	T50.8X1	T50.8X2	T50.8X3	T50.8X4	T50.8X5	T50.8X6
Iotroxic acid	T50.8X1	T50.8X2	T50.8X3	T50.8X4	T50.8X5	T50.8X6
Ioversol	T50.8X1	T50.8X2	T50.8X3	T50.8X4	T50.8X5	T50.8X6
Ioxaglate	T50.8X1	T50.8X2	T50.8X3	T50.8X4	T50.8X5	T50.8X6
Ioxaglic acid	T50.8X1	T50.8X2	T50.8X3	T50.8X4	T50.8X5	T50.8X6
Ioxitalamic acid	T50.8X1	T50.8X2	T50.8X3	T50.8X4	T50.8X5	T50.8X6
Ipecac	T47.7X1	T47.7X2	T47.7X3	T47.7X4	T47.7X5	T47.7X6
Ipecacuanha	T48.4X1	T48.4X2	T48.4X3	T48.4X4	T48.4X5	T48.4X6
Ipodate, calcium	T50.8X1	T50.8X2	T50.8X3	T50.8X4	T50.8X5	T50.8X6
Ipral	T42.3X1	T42.3X2	T42.3X3	T42.3X4	T42.3X5	T42.3X6
Ipratropium (bromide)	T48.6X1	T48.6X2	T48.6X3	T48.6X4	T48.6X5	T48.6X6
Ipriflavone	T46.3X1	T46.3X2	T46.3X3	T46.3X4	T46.3X5	T46.3X6
Iprindole	T43.011	T43.012	T43.013	T43.014	T43.015	T43.016
Iproclozide	T43.1X1	T43.1X2	T43.1X3	T43.1X4	T43.1X5	T43.1X6
Iprofenin	T50.8X1	T50.8X2	T50.8X3	T50.8X4	T50.8X5	T50.8X6

Substance	Poisoning, Accidental (Unintentional)	Poisoning, Intentional Self-Harm	Poisoning, Assault	Poisoning, Undetermined	Adverse Effect	Underdosing
Iproheptine	T49.2X1	T49.2X2	T49.2X3	T49.2X4	T49.2X5	T49.2X6
Iproniazid	T43.1X1	T43.1X2	T43.1X3	T43.1X4	T43.1X5	T43.1X6
Iproplatin	T45.1X1	T45.1X2	T45.1X3	T45.1X4	T45.1X5	T45.1X6
Iproveratril	T46.1X1	T46.1X2	T46.1X3	T46.1X4	T46.1X5	T46.1X6
Iron (compounds) (medicinal) NEC	T45.4X1	T45.4X2	T45.4X3	T45.4X4	T45.4X5	T45.4X6
ammonium	T45.4X1	T45.4X2	T45.4X3	T45.4X4	T45.4X5	T45.4X6
dextran injection	T45.4X1	T45.4X2	T45.4X3	T45.4X4	T45.4X5	T45.4X6
nonmedicinal	T56.891	T56.892	T56.893	T56.894	—	—
salts	T45.4X1	T45.4X2	T45.4X3	T45.4X4	T45.4X5	T45.4X6
sorbitex	T45.4X1	T45.4X2	T45.4X3	T45.4X4	T45.4X5	T45.4X6
sorbitol citric acid complex	T45.4X1	T45.4X2	T45.4X3	T45.4X4	T45.4X5	T45.4X6
Irrigating fluid (vaginal)	T49.8X1	T49.8X2	T49.8X3	T49.8X4	T49.8X5	T49.8X6
eye	T49.5X1	T49.5X2	T49.5X3	T49.5X4	T49.5X5	T49.5X6
Isepamicin	T36.5X1	T36.5X2	T36.5X3	T36.5X4	T36.5X5	T36.5X6
Isoaminile (citrate)	T48.3X1	T48.3X2	T48.3X3	T48.3X4	T48.3X5	T48.3X6
Isoamyl nitrite	T46.3X1	T46.3X2	T46.3X3	T46.3X4	T46.3X5	T46.3X6
Isobenzan	T60.1X1	T60.1X2	T60.1X3	T60.1X4	—	—
Isobutyl acetate	T52.8X1	T52.8X2	T52.8X3	T52.8X4	—	—
Isocarboxazid	T43.1X1	T43.1X2	T43.1X3	T43.1X4	T43.1X5	T43.1X6
Isoconazole	T49.0X1	T49.0X2	T49.0X3	T49.0X4	T49.0X5	T49.0X6
Isocyanate	T65.0X1	T65.0X2	T65.0X3	T65.0X4	—	—
Isoephedrine	T44.991	T44.992	T44.993	T44.994	T44.995	T44.996
Isoetarine	T48.6X1	T48.6X2	T48.6X3	T48.6X4	T48.6X5	T48.6X6
Isoethadione	T42.2X1	T42.2X2	T42.2X3	T42.2X4	T42.2X5	T42.2X6
Isoetharine	T44.5X1	T44.5X2	T44.5X3	T44.5X4	T44.5X5	T44.5X6
Isoflurane	T41.0X1	T41.0X2	T41.0X3	T41.0X4	T41.0X5	T41.0X6
Isoflurophate	T44.0X1	T44.0X2	T44.0X3	T44.0X4	T44.0X5	T44.0X6
Isomaltose, ferric complex	T45.4X1	T45.4X2	T45.4X3	T45.4X4	T45.4X5	T45.4X6
Isometheptene	T44.3X1	T44.3X2	T44.3X3	T44.3X4	T44.3X5	T44.3X6
Isoniazid	T37.1X1	T37.1X2	T37.1X3	T37.1X4	T37.1X5	T37.1X6
with						
rifampicin	T36.6X1	T36.6X2	T36.6X3	T36.6X4	T36.6X5	T36.6X6
thioacetazone	T37.1X1	T37.1X2	T37.1X3	T37.1X4	T37.1X5	T37.1X6
Isonicotinic acid hydrazide	T37.1X1	T37.1X2	T37.1X3	T37.1X4	T37.1X5	T37.1X6
Isonipecaine	T40.4X1	T40.4X2	T40.4X3	T40.4X4	T40.4X5	T40.4X6
Isopentaquine	T37.2X1	T37.2X2	T37.2X3	T37.2X4	T37.2X5	T37.2X6
Isophane insulin	T38.3X1	T38.3X2	T38.3X3	T38.3X4	T38.3X5	T38.3X6
Isophorone	T65.891	T65.892	T65.893	T65.894	—	—
Isophosphamide	T45.1X1	T45.1X2	T45.1X3	T45.1X4	T45.1X5	T45.1X6
Isopregnenone	T38.5X1	T38.5X2	T38.5X3	T38.5X4	T38.5X5	T38.5X6
Isoprenaline	T48.6X1	T48.6X2	T48.6X3	T48.6X4	T48.6X5	T48.6X6
Isopromethazine	T43.3X1	T43.3X2	T43.3X3	T43.3X4	T43.3X5	T43.3X6

◀ New   ◀▥▥ Revised   ~~deleted~~ Deleted

TABLE OF DRUGS AND CHEMICALS

Substance	External Cause (T-Code)					
	Poisoning, Accidental (Unintentional)	Poisoning, Intentional Self-Harm	Poisoning, Assault	Poisoning, Undetermined	Adverse Effect	Underdosing
Isopropamide	T44.3X1	T44.3X2	T44.3X3	T44.3X4	T44.3X5	T44.3X6
iodide	T44.3X1	T44.3X2	T44.3X3	T44.3X4	T44.3X5	T44.3X6
Isopropanol	T51.2X1	T51.2X2	T51.2X3	T51.2X4	—	—
Isopropyl						
acetate	T52.8X1	T52.8X2	T52.8X3	T52.8X4		
alcohol	T51.2X1	T51.2X2	T51.2X3	T51.2X4		
medicinal	T49.4X1	T49.4X2	T49.4X3	T49.4X4	T49.4X5	T49.4X6
ether	T52.8X1	T52.8X2	T52.8X3	T52.8X4	—	—
Isopropylaminophena-zone	T39.2X1	T39.2X2	T39.2X3	T39.2X4	T39.2X5	T39.2X6
Isoproterenol	T48.6X1	T48.6X2	T48.6X3	T48.6X4	T48.6X5	T48.6X6
Isosorbide dinitrate	T46.3X1	T46.3X2	T46.3X3	T46.3X4	T46.3X5	T46.3X6
Isothipendyl	T45.0X1	T45.0X2	T45.0X3	T45.0X4	T45.0X5	T45.0X6
Isotretinoin	T50.991	T50.992	T50.993	T50.994	T50.995	T50.996
Isoxazolyl penicillin	T36.0X1	T36.0X2	T36.0X3	T36.0X4	T36.0X5	T36.0X6
Isoxicam	T39.391	T39.392	T39.393	T39.394	T39.395	T39.396
Isoxsuprine	T46.7X1	T46.7X2	T46.7X3	T46.7X4	T46.7X5	T46.7X6
Ispagula	T47.4X1	T47.4X2	T47.4X3	T47.4X4	T47.4X5	T47.4X6
husk	T47.4X1	T47.4X2	T47.4X3	T47.4X4	T47.4X5	T47.4X6
Isradipine	T46.1X1	T46.1X2	T46.1X3	T46.1X4	T46.1X5	T46.1X6
l-thyroxine sodium	T38.1X1	T38.1X2	T38.1X3	T38.1X4	T38.1X5	T38.1X6
Itraconazole	T37.8X1	T37.8X2	T37.8X3	T37.8X4	T37.8X5	T37.8X6
Itramin tosilate	T46.3X1	T46.3X2	T46.3X3	T46.3X4	T46.3X5	T46.3X6
Ivermectin	T37.4X1	T37.4X2	T37.4X3	T37.4X4	T37.4X5	T37.4X6
Izoniazid	T37.1X1	T37.1X2	T37.1X3	T37.1X4	T37.1X5	T37.1X6
with thioacetazone	T37.1X1	T37.1X2	T37.1X3	T37.1X4	T37.1X5	T37.1X6
J						
Jalap	T47.2X1	T47.2X2	T47.2X3	T47.2X4	T47.2X5	T47.2X6
Jamaica						
dogwood (bark)	T39.8X1	T39.8X2	T39.8X3	T39.8X4	T39.8X5	T39.8X6
ginger	T65.891	T65.892	T65.893	T65.894	—	—
root	T62.2X1	T62.2X2	T62.2X3	T62.2X4	—	—
Jatropha	T62.2X1	T62.2X2	T62.2X3	T62.2X4	—	—
curcas	T62.2X1	T62.2X2	T62.2X3	T62.2X4	—	—
Jectofer	T45.4X1	T45.4X2	T45.4X3	T45.4X4	T45.4X5	T45.4X6
Jellyfish (sting)	T63.621	T63.622	T63.623	T63.624	—	—
Jequirity (bean)	T62.2X1	T62.2X2	T62.2X3	T62.2X4	—	—
Jimson weed (stramonium)	T62.2X1	T62.2X2	T62.2X3	T62.2X4	—	—
seeds	T62.2X1	T62.2X2	T62.2X3	T62.2X4	—	—
Josamycin	T36.3X1	T36.3X2	T36.3X3	T36.3X4	T36.3X5	T36.3X6
Juniper tar	T49.1X1	T49.1X2	T49.1X3	T49.1X4	T49.1X5	T49.1X6

Substance	External Cause (T-Code)					
	Poisoning, Accidental (Unintentional)	Poisoning, Intentional Self-Harm	Poisoning, Assault	Poisoning, Undetermined	Adverse Effect	Underdosing
K						
Kallidinogenase	T46.7X1	T46.7X2	T46.7X3	T46.7X4	T46.7X5	T46.7X6
Kallikrein	T46.7X1	T46.7X2	T46.7X3	T46.7X4	T46.7X5	T46.7X6
Kanamycin	T36.5X1	T36.5X2	T36.5X3	T36.5X4	T36.5X5	T36.5X6
Kantrex	T36.5X1	T36.5X2	T36.5X3	T36.5X4	T36.5X5	T36.5X6
Kaolin	T47.6X1	T47.6X2	T47.6X3	T47.6X4	T47.6X5	T47.6X6
light	T47.6X1	T47.6X2	T47.6X3	T47.6X4	T47.6X5	T47.6X6
Karaya (gum)	T47.4X1	T47.4X2	T47.4X3	T47.4X4	T47.4X5	T47.4X6
Kebuzone	T39.2X1	T39.2X2	T39.2X3	T39.2X4	T39.2X5	T39.2X6
Kelevan	T60.1X1	T60.1X2	T60.1X3	T60.1X4	—	—
Kemithal	T41.1X1	T41.1X2	T41.1X3	T41.1X4	T41.1X5	T41.1X6
Kenacort	T38.0X1	T38.0X2	T38.0X3	T38.0X4	T38.0X5	T38.0X6
Keratolytic drug NEC	T49.4X1	T49.4X2	T49.4X3	T49.4X4	T49.4X5	T49.4X6
anthracene	T49.4X1	T49.4X2	T49.4X3	T49.4X4	T49.4X5	T49.4X6
Keratoplastic NEC	T49.4X1	T49.4X2	T49.4X3	T49.4X4	T49.4X5	T49.4X6
Kerosene, kerosine (fuel) (solvent) NEC	T52.0X1	T52.0X2	T52.0X3	T52.0X4	—	—
insecticide	T52.0X1	T52.0X2	T52.0X3	T52.0X4	—	—
vapor	T52.0X1	T52.0X2	T52.0X3	T52.0X4	—	—
Ketamine	T41.291	T41.292	T41.293	T41.294	T41.295	T41.296
Ketazolam	T42.4X1	T42.4X2	T42.4X3	T42.4X4	T42.4X5	T42.4X6
Ketazon	T39.2X1	T39.2X2	T39.2X3	T39.2X4	T39.2X5	T39.2X6
Ketobemidone	T40.4X1	T40.4X2	T40.4X3	T40.4X4	—	—
Ketoconazole	T49.0X1	T49.0X2	T49.0X3	T49.0X4	T49.0X5	T49.0X6
Ketols	T52.4X1	T52.4X2	T52.4X3	T52.4X4	—	—
Ketone oils	T52.4X1	T52.4X2	T52.4X3	T52.4X4	—	—
Ketoprofen	T39.311	T39.312	T39.313	T39.314	T39.315	T39.316
Ketorolac	T39.8X1	T39.8X2	T39.8X3	T39.8X4	T39.8X5	T39.8X6
Ketotifen	T45.0X1	T45.0X2	T45.0X3	T45.0X4	T45.0X5	T45.0X6
Khat	T43.691	T43.692	T43.693	T43.694	—	—
Khellin	T46.3X1	T46.3X2	T46.3X3	T46.3X4	T46.3X5	T46.3X6
Khelloside	T46.3X1	T46.3X2	T46.3X3	T46.3X4	T46.3X5	T46.3X6
Kiln gas or vapor (carbon monoxide)	T58.8X1	T58.8X2	T58.8X3	T58.8X4	—	—
Kitasamycin	T36.3X1	T36.3X2	T36.3X3	T36.3X4	T36.3X5	T36.3X6
Konsyl	T47.4X1	T47.4X2	T47.4X3	T47.4X4	T47.4X5	T47.4X6
Kosam seed	T62.2X1	T62.2X2	T62.2X3	T62.2X4	—	—
Krait (venom)	T63.091	T63.092	T63.093	T63.094	—	—
Kwell (insecticide)	T60.1X1	T60.1X2	T60.1X3	T60.1X4	—	—
anti-infective (topical)	T49.0X1	T49.0X2	T49.0X3	T49.0X4	T49.0X5	T49.0X6

◀ New ◀▥ Revised ~~deleted~~ Deleted

TABLE OF DRUGS AND CHEMICALS

Substance	Poisoning, Accidental (Unintentional)	Poisoning, Intentional Self-Harm	Poisoning, Assault	Poisoning, Undetermined	Adverse Effect	Underdosing
L						
Labetalol	T44.8X1	T44.8X2	T44.8X3	T44.8X4	T44.8X5	T44.8X6
Laburnum (seeds)	T62.2X1	T62.2X2	T62.2X3	T62.2X4	—	—
leaves	T62.2X1	T62.2X2	T62.2X3	T62.2X4	—	—
Lachesine	T49.5X1	T49.5X2	T49.5X3	T49.5X4	T49.5X5	T49.5X6
Lacidipine	T46.5X1	T46.5X2	T46.5X3	T46.5X4	T46.5X5	T46.5X6
Lacquer	T65.6X1	T65.6X2	T65.6X3	T65.6X4	—	—
Lacrimogenic gas	T59.3X1	T59.3X2	T59.3X3	T59.3X4		
Lactated potassic saline	T50.3X1	T50.3X2	T50.3X3	T50.3X4	T50.3X5	T50.3X6
Lactic acid	T49.8X1	T49.8X2	T49.8X3	T49.8X4	T49.8X5	T49.8X6
Lactobacillus						
acidophilus	T47.6X1	T47.6X2	T47.6X3	T47.6X4	T47.6X5	T47.6X6
compound	T47.6X1	T47.6X2	T47.6X3	T47.6X4	T47.6X5	T47.6X6
bifidus, lyophilized	T47.6X1	T47.6X2	T47.6X3	T47.6X4	T47.6X5	T47.6X6
bulgaricus	T47.6X1	T47.6X2	T47.6X3	T47.6X4	T47.6X5	T47.6X6
sporogenes	T47.6X1	T47.6X2	T47.6X3	T47.6X4	T47.6X5	T47.6X6
Lactoflavin	T45.2X1	T45.2X2	T45.2X3	T45.2X4	T45.2X5	T45.2X6
Lactose (as excipient)	T50.901	T50.902	T50.903	T50.904	T50.905	T50.906
Lactuca (virosa) (extract)	T42.6X1	T42.6X2	T42.6X3	T42.6X4	T42.6X5	T42.6X6
Lactucarium	T42.6X1	T42.6X2	T42.6X3	T42.6X4	T42.6X5	T42.6X6
Lactulose	T47.3X1	T47.3X2	T47.3X3	T47.3X4	T47.3X5	T47.3X6
Laevo — *see Levo-*						
Lanatosides	T46.0X1	T46.0X2	T46.0X3	T46.0X4	T46.0X5	T46.0X6
Lanolin	T49.3X1	T49.3X2	T49.3X3	T49.3X4	T49.3X5	T49.3X6
Largactil	T43.3X1	T43.3X2	T43.3X3	T43.3X4	T43.3X5	T43.3X6
Larkspur	T62.2X1	T62.2X2	T62.2X3	T62.2X4	—	—
Laroxyl	T43.011	T43.012	T43.013	T43.014	T43.015	T43.016
Lassar's paste	T49.4X1	T49.4X2	T49.4X3	T49.4X4	T49.4X5	T49.4X6
Lasix	T50.1X1	T50.1X2	T50.1X3	T50.1X4	T50.1X5	T50.1X6
Latamoxef	T36.1X1	T36.1X2	T36.1X3	T36.1X4	T36.1X5	T36.1X6
Latex	T65.811	T65.812	T65.813	T65.814		
Lathyrus (seed)	T62.2X1	T62.2X2	T62.2X3	T62.2X4	—	—
Laudanum	T40.0X1	T40.0X2	T40.0X3	T40.0X4	T40.0X5	T40.0X6
Laudexium	T48.1X1	T48.1X2	T48.1X3	T48.1X4	T48.1X5	T48.1X6
Laughing gas	T41.0X1	T41.0X2	T41.0X3	T41.0X4	T41.0X5	T41.0X6
Laurel, black or cherry	T62.2X1	T62.2X2	T62.2X3	T62.2X4	—	—
Laurolinium	T49.0X1	T49.0X2	T49.0X3	T49.0X4	T49.0X5	T49.0X6
Lauryl sulfoacetate	T49.2X1	T49.2X2	T49.2X3	T49.2X4	T49.2X5	T49.2X6

Substance	Poisoning, Accidental (Unintentional)	Poisoning, Intentional Self-Harm	Poisoning, Assault	Poisoning, Undetermined	Adverse Effect	Underdosing
Laxative NEC	T47.4X1	T47.4X2	T47.4X3	T47.4X4	T47.4X5	T47.4X6
osmotic	T47.3X1	T47.3X2	T47.3X3	T47.3X4	T47.3X5	T47.3X6
saline	T47.3X1	T47.3X2	T47.3X3	T47.3X4	T47.3X5	T47.3X6
stimulant	T47.2X1	T47.2X2	T47.2X3	T47.2X4	T47.2X5	T47.2X6
L-dopa	T42.8X1	T42.8X2	T42.8X3	T42.8X4	T42.8X5	T42.8X6
Lead (dust) (fumes) (vapor) NEC	T56.0X1	T56.0X2	T56.0X3	T56.0X4	—	—
acetate	T49.2X1	T49.2X2	T49.2X3	T49.2X4	T49.2X5	T49.2X6
alkyl (fuel additive)	T56.0X1	T56.0X2	T56.0X3	T56.0X4	—	—
anti-infectives	T37.8X1	T37.8X2	T37.8X3	T37.8X4	T37.8X5	T37.8X6
antiknock compound (tetraethyl)	T56.0X1	T56.0X2	T56.0X3	T56.0X4	—	—
arsenate, arsenite (dust) (herbicide) (insecticide) (vapor)	T57.0X1	T57.0X2	T57.0X3	T57.0X4	—	—
carbonate	T56.0X1	T56.0X2	T56.0X3	T56.0X4	—	—
paint	T56.0X1	T56.0X2	T56.0X3	T56.0X4	—	—
chromate	T56.0X1	T56.0X2	T56.0X3	T56.0X4	—	—
paint	T56.0X1	T56.0X2	T56.0X3	T56.0X4	—	—
dioxide	T56.0X1	T56.0X2	T56.0X3	T56.0X4	—	—
inorganic	T56.0X1	T56.0X2	T56.0X3	T56.0X4	—	—
iodide	T56.0X1	T56.0X2	T56.0X3	T56.0X4	—	—
pigment (paint)	T56.0X1	T56.0X2	T56.0X3	T56.0X4	—	—
monoxide (dust)	T56.0X1	T56.0X2	T56.0X3	T56.0X4	—	—
paint	T56.0X1	T56.0X2	T56.0X3	T56.0X4	—	—
organic	T56.0X1	T56.0X2	T56.0X3	T56.0X4	—	—
oxide	T56.0X1	T56.0X2	T56.0X3	T56.0X4	—	—
paint	T56.0X1	T56.0X2	T56.0X3	T56.0X4	—	—
paint	T56.0X1	T56.0X2	T56.0X3	T56.0X4	—	—
salts	T56.0X1	T56.0X2	T56.0X3	T56.0X4	—	—
specified compound NEC	T56.0X1	T56.0X2	T56.0X3	T56.0X4	—	—
tetra-ethyl	T56.0X1	T56.0X2	T56.0X3	T56.0X4	—	—
Lebanese red	T40.7X1	T40.7X2	T40.7X3	T40.7X4	T40.7X5	T40.7X6
Lefetamine	T39.8X1	T39.8X2	T39.8X3	T39.8X4	T39.8X5	T39.8X6
Lenperone	T43.4X1	T43.4X2	T43.4X3	T43.4X4	T43.4X5	T43.4X6
Lente lietin (insulin)	T38.3X1	T38.3X2	T38.3X3	T38.3X4	T38.3X5	T38.3X6
Leptazol	T50.7X1	T50.7X2	T50.7X3	T50.7X4	T50.7X5	T50.7X6
Leptophos	T60.0X1	T60.0X2	T60.0X3	T60.0X4	—	—
Leritine	T40.2X1	T40.2X2	T40.2X3	T40.2X4	T40.2X5	T40.2X6
Letosteine	T48.4X1	T48.4X2	T48.4X3	T48.4X4	T48.4X5	T48.4X6
Letter	T38.1X1	T38.1X2	T38.1X3	T38.1X4	T38.1X5	T38.1X6
Lettuce opium	T42.6X1	T42.6X2	T42.6X3	T42.6X4	T42.6X5	T42.6X6
Leucinocaine	T41.3X1	T41.3X2	T41.3X3	T41.3X4	T41.3X5	T41.3X6

◀ New ◀▥ Revised ~~deleted~~ Deleted

Substance	External Cause (T-Code) Poisoning, Accidental (Unintentional)	Poisoning, Intentional Self-Harm	Poisoning, Assault	Poisoning, Undetermined	Adverse Effect	Underdosing
Leucocianidol	T46.991	T46.992	T46.993	T46.994	T46.995	T46.996
Leucovorin (factor)	T45.8X1	T45.8X2	T45.8X3	T45.8X4	T45.8X5	T45.8X6
Leukeran	T45.1X1	T45.1X2	T45.1X3	T45.1X4	T45.1X5	T45.1X6
Leuprolide	T38.891	T38.892	T38.893	T38.894	T38.895	T38.896
Levalbuterol	T48.6X1	T48.6X2	T48.6X3	T48.6X4	T48.6X5	T48.6X6
Levallorphan	T50.7X1	T50.7X2	T50.7X3	T50.7X4	T50.7X5	T50.7X6
Levamisole	T37.4X1	T37.4X2	T37.4X3	T37.4X4	T37.4X5	T37.4X6
Levanil	T42.6X1	T42.6X2	T42.6X3	T42.6X4	T42.6X5	T42.6X6
Levarterenol	T44.4X1	T44.4X2	T44.4X3	T44.4X4	T44.4X5	T44.4X6
Levdropropizine	T48.3X1	T48.3X2	T48.3X3	T48.3X4	T48.3X5	T48.3X6
Levobunolol	T49.5X1	T49.5X2	T49.5X3	T49.5X4	T49.5X5	T49.5X6
Levocabastine (hydrochloride)	T45.0X1	T45.0X2	T45.0X3	T45.0X4	T45.0X5	T45.0X6
Levocarnitine	T50.991	T50.992	T50.993	T50.994	T50.995	T50.996
Levodopa	T42.8X1	T42.8X2	T42.8X3	T42.8X4	T42.8X5	T42.8X6
with carbidopa	T42.8X1	T42.8X2	T42.8X3	T42.8X4	T42.8X5	T42.8X6
Levo-dromoran	T40.2X1	T40.2X2	T40.2X3	T40.2X4	T40.2X5	T40.2X6
Levoglutamide	T50.991	T50.992	T50.993	T50.994	T50.995	T50.996
Levoid	T38.1X1	T38.1X2	T38.1X3	T38.1X4	T38.1X5	T38.1X6
Levo-iso-methadone	T40.3X1	T40.3X2	T40.3X3	T40.3X4	T40.3X5	T40.3X6
Levomepromazine	T43.3X1	T43.3X2	T43.3X3	T43.3X4	T43.3X5	T43.3X6
Levonordefrin	T49.6X1	T49.6X2	T49.6X3	T49.6X4	T49.6X5	T49.6X6
Levonorgestrel	T38.4X1	T38.4X2	T38.4X3	T38.4X4	T38.4X5	T38.4X6
with ethinylestradiol	T38.5X1	T38.5X2	T38.5X3	T38.5X4	T38.5X5	T38.5X6
Levopromazine	T43.3X1	T43.3X2	T43.3X3	T43.3X4	T43.3X5	T43.3X6
Levoprome	T42.6X1	T42.6X2	T42.6X3	T42.6X4	T42.6X5	T42.6X6
Levopropoxyphene	T40.4X1	T40.4X2	T40.4X3	T40.4X4	T40.4X5	T40.4X6
Levopropylhexedrine	T50.5X1	T50.5X2	T50.5X3	T50.5X4	T50.5X5	T50.5X6
Levoproxyphylline	T48.6X1	T48.6X2	T48.6X3	T48.6X4	T48.6X5	T48.6X6
Levorphanol	T40.4X1	T40.4X2	T40.4X3	T40.4X4	T40.4X5	T40.4X6
Levothyroxine	T38.1X1	T38.1X2	T38.1X3	T38.1X4	T38.1X5	T38.1X6
sodium	T38.1X1	T38.1X2	T38.1X3	T38.1X4	T38.1X5	T38.1X6
Levsin	T44.3X1	T44.3X2	T44.3X3	T44.3X4	T44.3X5	T44.3X6
Levulose	T50.3X1	T50.3X2	T50.3X3	T50.3X4	T50.3X5	T50.3X6
Lewisite (gas), not in war	T57.0X1	T57.0X2	T57.0X3	T57.0X4	—	—
Librium	T42.4X1	T42.4X2	T42.4X3	T42.4X4	T42.4X5	T42.4X6
Lidex	T49.0X1	T49.0X2	T49.0X3	T49.0X4	T49.0X5	T49.0X6
Lidocaine	T41.3X1	T41.3X2	T41.3X3	T41.3X4	T41.3X5	T41.3X6
regional	T41.3X1	T41.3X2	T41.3X3	T41.3X4	T41.3X5	T41.3X6
spinal	T41.3X1	T41.3X2	T41.3X3	T41.3X4	T41.3X5	T41.3X6
Lidofenin	T50.8X1	T50.8X2	T50.8X3	T50.8X4	T50.8X5	T50.8X6
Lidoflazine	T46.1X1	T46.1X2	T46.1X3	T46.1X4	T46.1X5	T46.1X6
Lighter fluid	T52.0X1	T52.0X2	T52.0X3	T52.0X4	—	—

Substance	External Cause (T-Code) Poisoning, Accidental (Unintentional)	Poisoning, Intentional Self-Harm	Poisoning, Assault	Poisoning, Undetermined	Adverse Effect	Underdosing
Lignin hemicellulose	T47.6X1	T47.6X2	T47.6X3	T47.6X4	T47.6X5	T47.6X6
Lignocaine	T41.3X1	T41.3X2	T41.3X3	T41.3X4	T41.3X5	T41.3X6
regional	T41.3X1	T41.3X2	T41.3X3	T41.3X4	T41.3X5	T41.3X6
spinal	T41.3X1	T41.3X2	T41.3X3	T41.3X4	T41.3X5	T41.3X6
Ligroin(e) (solvent)	T52.0X1	T52.0X2	T52.0X3	T52.0X4	—	—
vapor	T59.891	T59.892	T59.893	T59.894		
Ligustrum vulgare	T62.2X1	T62.2X2	T62.2X3	T62.2X4		
Lily of the valley	T62.2X1	T62.2X2	T62.2X3	T62.2X4		
Lime (chloride)	T54.3X1	T54.3X2	T54.3X3	T54.3X4		
Limonene	T52.8X1	T52.8X2	T52.8X3	T52.8X4		
Lincomycin	T36.8X1	T36.8X2	T36.8X3	T36.8X4	T36.8X5	T36.8X6
Lindane (insecticide) (nonmedicinal) (vapor)	T53.6X1	T53.6X2	T53.6X3	T53.6X4	—	—
medicinal	T49.0X1	T49.0X2	T49.0X3	T49.0X4	T49.0X5	T49.0X6
Liniments NEC	T49.91	T49.92	T49.93	T49.94	T49.95	T49.96
Linoleic acid	T46.6X1	T46.6X2	T46.6X3	T46.6X4	T46.6X5	T46.6X6
Linolenic acid	T46.6X1	T46.6X2	T46.6X3	T46.6X4	T46.6X5	T46.6X6
Linseed	T47.4X1	T47.4X2	T47.4X3	T47.4X4	T47.4X5	T47.4X6
Liothyronine	T38.1X1	T38.1X2	T38.1X3	T38.1X4	T38.1X5	T38.1X6
Liotrix	T38.1X1	T38.1X2	T38.1X3	T38.1X4	T38.1X5	T38.1X6
Lipancreatin	T47.5X1	T47.5X2	T47.5X3	T47.5X4	T47.5X5	T47.5X6
Lipo-alprostadil	T46.7X1	T46.7X2	T46.7X3	T46.7X4	T46.7X5	T46.7X6
Lipo-Lutin	T38.5X1	T38.5X2	T38.5X3	T38.5X4	T38.5X5	T38.5X6
Lipotropic drug NEC	T50.901	T50.902	T50.903	T50.904	T50.905	T50.906
Liquefied petroleum gases	T59.891	T59.892	T59.893	T59.894	—	—
piped (pure or mixed with air)	T59.891	T59.892	T59.893	T59.894	—	—
Liquid						
paraffin	T47.4X1	T47.4X2	T47.4X3	T47.4X4	T47.4X5	T47.4X6
petrolatum	T47.4X1	T47.4X2	T47.4X3	T47.4X4	T47.4X5	T47.4X6
topical	T49.3X1	T49.3X2	T49.3X3	T49.3X4	T49.3X5	T49.3X6
specified NEC	T65.891	T65.892	T65.893	T65.894		
substance	T65.91	T65.92	T65.93	T65.94		
Liquor creosolis compositus	T65.891	T65.892	T65.893	T65.894		
Liquorice	T48.4X1	T48.4X2	T48.4X3	T48.4X4	T48.4X5	T48.4X6
extract	T47.8X1	T47.8X2	T47.8X3	T47.8X4	T47.8X5	T47.8X6
Lirugen	T50.991	T50.992	T50.993	T50.994	T50.995	T50.996
Lisinopril	T46.4X1	T46.4X2	T46.4X3	T46.4X4	T46.4X5	T46.4X6
Lisuride	T42.8X1	T42.8X2	T42.8X3	T42.8X4	T42.8X5	T42.8X6
Lithane	T43.8X1	T43.8X2	T43.8X3	T43.8X4	T43.8X5	T43.8X6
Lithium	T56.891	T56.892	T56.893	T56.894	—	—
gluconate	T43.591	T43.592	T43.593	T43.594	T43.595	T43.596
salts (carbonate)	T43.591	T43.592	T43.593	T43.594	T43.595	T43.596

◀ New ◀◀ Revised ~~deleted~~ Deleted

Substance	Poisoning, Accidental (Unintentional)	Poisoning, Intentional Self-Harm	Poisoning, Assault	Poisoning, Undetermined	Adverse Effect	Underdosing
Lithonate	T43.8X1	T43.8X2	T43.8X3	T43.8X4	T43.8X5	T43.8X6
Liver						
extract	T45.8X1	T45.8X2	T45.8X3	T45.8X4	T45.8X5	T45.8X6
for parenteral use	T45.8X1	T45.8X2	T45.8X3	T45.8X4	T45.8X5	T45.8X6
fraction 1	T45.8X1	T45.8X2	T45.8X3	T45.8X4	T45.8X5	T45.8X6
hydrolysate	T45.8X1	T45.8X2	T45.8X3	T45.8X4	T45.8X5	T45.8X6
Lizard (bite) (venom)	T63.121	T63.122	T63.123	T63.124	—	—
LMD	T45.8X1	T45.8X2	T45.8X3	T45.8X4	T45.8X5	T45.8X6
Lobelia	T62.2X1	T62.2X2	T62.2X3	T62.2X4	—	—
Lobeline	T50.7X1	T50.7X2	T50.7X3	T50.7X4	T50.7X5	T50.7X6
Local action drug NEC	T49.8X1	T49.8X2	T49.8X3	T49.8X4	T49.8X5	T49.8X6
Locorten	T49.0X1	T49.0X2	T49.0X3	T49.0X4	T49.0X5	T49.0X6
Lofepramine	T43.011	T43.012	T43.013	T43.014	T43.015	T43.016
Lolium temulentum	T62.2X1	T62.2X2	T62.2X3	T62.2X4	—	—
Lomotil	T47.6X1	T47.6X2	T47.6X3	T47.6X4	T47.6X5	T47.6X6
Lomustine	T45.1X1	T45.1X2	T45.1X3	T45.1X4	T45.1X5	T45.1X6
Lonidamine	T45.1X1	T45.1X2	T45.1X3	T45.1X4	T45.1X5	T45.1X6
Loperamide	T47.6X1	T47.6X2	T47.6X3	T47.6X4	T47.6X5	T47.6X6
Loprazolam	T42.4X1	T42.4X2	T42.4X3	T42.4X4	T42.4X5	T42.4X6
Lorajmine	T46.2X1	T46.2X2	T46.2X3	T46.2X4	T46.2X5	T46.2X6
Loratidine	T45.0X1	T45.0X2	T45.0X3	T45.0X4	T45.0X5	T45.0X6
Lorazepam	T42.4X1	T42.4X2	T42.4X3	T42.4X4	T42.4X5	T42.4X6
Lorcainide	T46.2X1	T46.2X2	T46.2X3	T46.2X4	T46.2X5	T46.2X6
Lormetazepam	T42.4X1	T42.4X2	T42.4X3	T42.4X4	T42.4X5	T42.4X6
Lotions NEC	T49.91	T49.92	T49.93	T49.94	T49.95	T49.96
Lotusate	T42.3X1	T42.3X2	T42.3X3	T42.3X4	T42.3X5	T42.3X6
Lovastatin	T46.6X1	T46.6X2	T46.6X3	T46.6X4	T46.6X5	T46.6X6
Loxapine	T43.591	T43.592	T43.593	T43.594	T43.595	T43.596
Lowila	T49.2X1	T49.2X2	T49.2X3	T49.2X4	T49.2X5	T49.2X6
Lozenges (throat)	T49.6X1	T49.6X2	T49.6X3	T49.6X4	T49.6X5	T49.6X6
LSD	T40.8X1	T40.8X2	T40.8X3	T40.8X4	—	—
L-Tryptophan — see amino acid						
Lubricant, eye	T49.5X1	T49.5X2	T49.5X3	T49.5X4	T49.5X5	T49.5X6
Lubricating oil NEC	T52.0X1	T52.0X2	T52.0X3	T52.0X4	—	—
Lucanthone	T37.4X1	T37.4X2	T37.4X3	T37.4X4	T37.4X5	T37.4X6
Luminal	T42.3X1	T42.3X2	T42.3X3	T42.3X4	T42.3X5	T42.3X6
Lung irritant (gas) NEC	T59.91	T59.92	T59.93	T59.94	—	—
Luteinizing hormone	T38.811	T38.812	T38.813	T38.814	T38.815	T38.816
Lutocylol	T38.5X1	T38.5X2	T38.5X3	T38.5X4	T38.5X5	T38.5X6
Lutromone	T38.5X1	T38.5X2	T38.5X3	T38.5X4	T38.5X5	T38.5X6
Lututrin	T48.291	T48.292	T48.293	T48.294	T48.295	T48.296
Lye (Concentrated)	T54.3X1	T54.3X2	T54.3X3	T54.3X4	—	—

Substance	Poisoning, Accidental (Unintentional)	Poisoning, Intentional Self-Harm	Poisoning, Assault	Poisoning, Undetermined	Adverse Effect	Underdosing
Lygranum (skin test)	T50.8X1	T50.8X2	T50.8X3	T50.8X4	T50.8X5	T50.8X6
Lymecycline	T36.4X1	T36.4X2	T36.4X3	T36.4X4	T36.4X5	T36.4X6
Lymphogranuloma venereum antigen	T50.8X1	T50.8X2	T50.8X3	T50.8X4	T50.8X5	T50.8X6
Lynestrenol	T38.4X1	T38.4X2	T38.4X3	T38.4X4	T38.4X5	T38.4X6
Lypressin	T38.891	T38.892	T38.893	T38.894	T38.895	T38.896
Lyovac Sodium Edecrin	T50.1X1	T50.1X2	T50.1X3	T50.1X4	T50.1X5	T50.1X6
Lysergic acid diethylamide	T40.8X1	T40.8X2	T40.8X3	T40.8X4	—	—
Lysergide	T40.8X1	T40.8X2	T40.8X3	T40.8X4	—	—
Lysine vasopressin	T38.891	T38.892	T38.893	T38.894	T38.895	T38.896
Lysol	T54.1X1	T54.1X2	T54.1X3	T54.1X4	—	—
Lysozyme	T49.0X1	T49.0X2	T49.0X3	T49.0X4	T49.0X5	T49.0X6
Lytta (vitatta)	T49.8X1	T49.8X2	T49.8X3	T49.8X4	T49.8X5	T49.8X6

M

Substance	Poisoning, Accidental (Unintentional)	Poisoning, Intentional Self-Harm	Poisoning, Assault	Poisoning, Undetermined	Adverse Effect	Underdosing
Mace	T59.3X1	T59.3X2	T59.3X3	T59.3X4	—	—
Macrogol	T50.991	T50.992	T50.993	T50.994	T50.995	T50.996
Macrolide						
anabolic drug	T38.7X1	T38.7X2	T38.7X3	T38.7X4	T38.7X5	T38.7X6
antibiotic	T36.3X1	T36.3X2	T36.3X3	T36.3X4	T36.3X5	T36.3X6
Mafenide	T49.0X1	T49.0X2	T49.0X3	T49.0X4	T49.0X5	T49.0X6
Magaldrate	T47.1X1	T47.1X2	T47.1X3	T47.1X4	T47.1X5	T47.1X6
Magic mushroom	T40.991	T40.992	T40.993	T40.994	—	—
Magnamycin	T36.8X1	T36.8X2	T36.8X3	T36.8X4	T36.8X5	T36.8X6
Magnesia magma	T47.1X1	T47.1X2	T47.1X3	T47.1X4	T47.1X5	T47.1X6
Magnesium NEC	T56.891	T56.892	T56.893	T56.894	—	—
carbonate	T47.1X1	T47.1X2	T47.1X3	T47.1X4	T47.1X5	T47.1X6
citrate	T47.4X1	T47.4X2	T47.4X3	T47.4X4	T47.4X5	T47.4X6
hydroxide	T47.1X1	T47.1X2	T47.1X3	T47.1X4	T47.1X5	T47.1X6
oxide	T47.1X1	T47.1X2	T47.1X3	T47.1X4	T47.1X5	T47.1X6
peroxide	T49.0X1	T49.0X2	T49.0X3	T49.0X4	T49.0X5	T49.0X6
salicylate	T39.091	T39.092	T39.093	T39.094	T39.095	T39.096
silicofluoride	T50.3X1	T50.3X2	T50.3X3	T50.3X4	T50.3X5	T50.3X6
sulfate	T47.4X1	T47.4X2	T47.4X3	T47.4X4	T47.4X5	T47.4X6
thiosulfate	T45.0X1	T45.0X2	T45.0X3	T45.0X4	T45.0X5	T45.0X6
trisilicate	T47.1X1	T47.1X2	T47.1X3	T47.1X4	T47.1X5	T47.1X6
Malathion (medicinal)	T49.0X1	T49.0X2	T49.0X3	T49.0X4	T49.0X5	T49.0X6
insecticide	T60.0X1	T60.0X2	T60.0X3	T60.0X4	—	—
Male fern extract	T37.4X1	T37.4X2	T37.4X3	T37.4X4	T37.4X5	T37.4X6
M-AMSA	T45.1X1	T45.1X2	T45.1X3	T45.1X4	T45.1X5	T45.1X6
Mandelic acid	T37.8X1	T37.8X2	T37.8X3	T37.8X4	T37.8X5	T37.8X6
Manganese (dioxide) (salts)	T57.2X1	T57.2X2	T57.2X3	T57.2X4	—	—
medicinal	T50.991	T50.992	T50.993	T50.994	T50.995	T50.996

TABLE OF DRUGS AND CHEMICALS

TABLE OF DRUGS AND CHEMICALS

Substance	External Cause (T-Code)					
	Poisoning, Accidental (Unintentional)	Poisoning, Intentional Self-Harm	Poisoning, Assault	Poisoning, Undetermined	Adverse Effect	Underdosing
Mannitol	T47.3X1	T47.3X2	T47.3X3	T47.3X4	T47.3X5	T47.3X6
hexanitrate	T46.3X1	T46.3X2	T46.3X3	T46.3X4	T46.3X5	T46.3X6
Mannomustine	T45.1X1	T45.1X2	T45.1X3	T45.1X4	T45.1X5	T45.1X6
MAO inhibitors	T43.1X1	T43.1X2	T43.1X3	T43.1X4	T43.1X5	T43.1X6
Mapharsen	T37.8X1	T37.8X2	T37.8X3	T37.8X4	T37.8X5	T37.8X6
Maphenide	T49.0X1	T49.0X2	T49.0X3	T49.0X4	T49.0X5	T49.0X6
Maprotiline	T43.021	T43.022	T43.023	T43.024	T43.025	T43.026
Marcaine	T41.3X1	T41.3X2	T41.3X3	T41.3X4	T41.3X5	T41.3X6
infiltration (subcutaneous)	T41.3X1	T41.3X2	T41.3X3	T41.3X4	T41.3X5	T41.3X6
nerve block (peripheral) (plexus)	T41.3X1	T41.3X2	T41.3X3	T41.3X4	T41.3X5	T41.3X6
Marezine	T45.0X1	T45.0X2	T45.0X3	T45.0X4	T45.0X5	T45.0X6
Marihuana	T40.7X1	T40.7X2	T40.7X3	T40.7X4	T40.7X5	T40.7X6
Marijuana	T40.7X1	T40.7X2	T40.7X3	T40.7X4	T40.7X5	T40.7X6
Marine (sting)	T63.691	T63.692	T63.693	T63.694	—	—
animals (sting)	T63.691	T63.692	T63.693	T63.694	—	—
plants (sting)	T63.711	T63.712	T63.713	T63.714	—	—
Marplan	T43.1X1	T43.1X2	T43.1X3	T43.1X4	T43.1X5	T43.1X6
Marsh gas	T59.891	T59.892	T59.893	T59.894	—	—
Marsilid	T43.1X1	T43.1X2	T43.1X3	T43.1X4	T43.1X5	T43.1X6
Matulane	T45.1X1	T45.1X2	T45.1X3	T45.1X4	T45.1X5	T45.1X6
Mazindol	T50.5X1	T50.5X2	T50.5X3	T50.5X4	T50.5X5	T50.5X6
MCPA	T60.3X1	T60.3X2	T60.3X3	T60.3X4	—	—
MDMA	T43.621	T43.622	T43.623	T43.624	T43.625	T43.626
Meadow saffron	T62.2X1	T62.2X2	T62.2X3	T62.2X4	—	—
Measles virus vaccine (attenuated)	T50.B91	T50.B92	T50.B93	T50.B94	T50.B95	T50.B96
Meat, noxious	T62.8X1	T62.8X2	T62.8X3	T62.8X4	—	—
Meballymal	T42.3X1	T42.3X2	T42.3X3	T42.3X4	T42.3X5	T42.3X6
Mebanazine	T43.1X1	T43.1X2	T43.1X3	T43.1X4	T43.1X5	T43.1X6
Mebaral	T42.3X1	T42.3X2	T42.3X3	T42.3X4	T42.3X5	T42.3X6
Mebendazole	T37.4X1	T37.4X2	T37.4X3	T37.4X4	T37.4X5	T37.4X6
Mebeverine	T44.3X1	T44.3X2	T44.3X3	T44.3X4	T44.3X5	T44.3X6
Mebhydrolin	T45.0X1	T45.0X2	T45.0X3	T45.0X4	T45.0X5	T45.0X6
Mebumal	T42.3X1	T42.3X2	T42.3X3	T42.3X4	T42.3X5	T42.3X6
Mebutamate	T43.591	T43.592	T43.593	T43.594	T43.595	T43.596
Mecamylamine	T44.2X1	T44.2X2	T44.2X3	T44.2X4	T44.2X5	T44.2X6
Mechlorethamine	T45.1X1	T45.1X2	T45.1X3	T45.1X4	T45.1X5	T45.1X6
Mecillinam	T36.0X1	T36.0X2	T36.0X3	T36.0X4	T36.0X5	T36.0X6
Meclizine (hydrochloride)	T45.0X1	T45.0X2	T45.0X3	T45.0X4	T45.0X5	T45.0X6
Meclocycline	T36.4X1	T36.4X2	T36.4X3	T36.4X4	T36.4X5	T36.4X6
Meclofenamate	T39.391	T39.392	T39.393	T39.394	T39.395	T39.396
Meclofenamic acid	T39.391	T39.392	T39.393	T39.394	T39.395	T39.396

Substance	External Cause (T-Code)					
	Poisoning, Accidental (Unintentional)	Poisoning, Intentional Self-Harm	Poisoning, Assault	Poisoning, Undetermined	Adverse Effect	Underdosing
Meclofenoxate	T43.691	T43.692	T43.693	T43.694	T43.695	T43.696
Meclozine	T45.0X1	T45.0X2	T45.0X3	T45.0X4	T45.0X5	T45.0X6
Mecobalamin	T45.8X1	T45.8X2	T45.8X3	T45.8X4	T45.8X5	T45.8X6
Mecoprop	T60.3X1	T60.3X2	T60.3X3	T60.3X4	—	—
Mecrilate	T49.3X1	T49.3X2	T49.3X3	T49.3X4	T49.3X5	T49.3X6
Mecysteine	T48.4X1	T48.4X2	T48.4X3	T48.4X4	T48.4X5	T48.4X6
Medazepam	T42.4X1	T42.4X2	T42.4X3	T42.4X4	T42.4X5	T42.4X6
Medicament NEC	T50.901	T50.902	T50.903	T50.904	T50.905	T50.906
Medinal	T42.3X1	T42.3X2	T42.3X3	T42.3X4	T42.3X5	T42.3X6
Medomin	T42.3X1	T42.3X2	T42.3X3	T42.3X4	T42.3X5	T42.3X6
Medrogestone	T38.5X1	T38.5X2	T38.5X3	T38.5X4	T38.5X5	T38.5X6
Medroxalol	T44.8X1	T44.8X2	T44.8X3	T44.8X4	T44.8X5	T44.8X6
Medroxyprogesterone acetate (depot)	T38.5X1	T38.5X2	T38.5X3	T38.5X4	T38.5X5	T38.5X6
Medrysone	T49.0X1	T49.0X2	T49.0X3	T49.0X4	T49.0X5	T49.0X6
Mefenamic acid	T39.391	T39.392	T39.393	T39.394	T39.395	T39.396
Mefenorex	T50.5X1	T50.5X2	T50.5X3	T50.5X4	T50.5X5	T50.5X6
Mefloquine	T37.2X1	T37.2X2	T37.2X3	T37.2X4	T37.2X5	T37.2X6
Mefruside	T50.2X1	T50.2X2	T50.2X3	T50.2X4	T50.2X5	T50.2X6
Megahallucinogen	T40.901	T40.902	T40.903	T40.904	T40.905	T40.906
Megestrol	T38.5X1	T38.5X2	T38.5X3	T38.5X4	T38.5X5	T38.5X6
Meglumine						
antimoniate	T37.8X1	T37.8X2	T37.8X3	T37.8X4	T37.8X5	T37.8X6
diatrizoate	T50.8X1	T50.8X2	T50.8X3	T50.8X4	T50.8X5	T50.8X6
iodipamide	T50.8X1	T50.8X2	T50.8X3	T50.8X4	T50.8X5	T50.8X6
iotroxate	T50.8X1	T50.8X2	T50.8X3	T50.8X4	T50.8X5	T50.8X6
MEK (methyl ethyl ketone)	T52.4X1	T52.4X2	T52.4X3	T52.4X4	—	—
Meladrazine	T44.3X1	T44.3X2	T44.3X3	T44.3X4	T44.3X5	T44.3X6
Meladinin	T49.3X1	T49.3X2	T49.3X3	T49.3X4	T49.3X5	T49.3X6
Melaleuca alternifolia oil	T49.0X1	T49.0X2	T49.0X3	T49.0X4	T49.0X5	T49.0X6
Melanizing agents	T49.3X1	T49.3X2	T49.3X3	T49.3X4	T49.3X5	T49.3X6
Melanocyte-stimulating hormone	T38.891	T38.892	T38.893	T38.894	T38.895	T38.896
Melarsonyl potassium	T37.3X1	T37.3X2	T37.3X3	T37.3X4	T37.3X5	T37.3X6
Melarsoprol	T37.3X1	T37.3X2	T37.3X3	T37.3X4	T37.3X5	T37.3X6
Melia azedarach	T62.2X1	T62.2X2	T62.2X3	T62.2X4	—	—
Melitracen	T43.011	T43.012	T43.013	T43.014	T43.015	T43.016
Mellaril	T43.3X1	T43.3X2	T43.3X3	T43.3X4	T43.3X5	T43.3X6
Meloxine	T49.3X1	T49.3X2	T49.3X3	T49.3X4	T49.3X5	T49.3X6
Melperone	T43.4X1	T43.4X2	T43.4X3	T43.4X4	T43.4X5	T43.4X6
Melphalan	T45.1X1	T45.1X2	T45.1X3	T45.1X4	T45.1X5	T45.1X6
Memantine	T43.8X1	T43.8X2	T43.8X3	T43.8X4	T43.8X5	T43.8X6

◄ New   ◀▥ Revised   deleted Deleted

Substance	Poisoning, Accidental (Unintentional)	Poisoning, Intentional Self-Harm	Poisoning, Assault	Poisoning, Undetermined	Adverse Effect	Underdosing
Menadiol	T45.7X1	T45.7X2	T45.7X3	T45.7X4	T45.7X5	T45.7X6
sodium sulfate	T45.7X1	T45.7X2	T45.7X3	T45.7X4	T45.7X5	T45.7X6
Menadione	T45.7X1	T45.7X2	T45.7X3	T45.7X4	T45.7X5	T45.7X6
sodium bisulfite	T45.7X1	T45.7X2	T45.7X3	T45.7X4	T45.7X5	T45.7X6
Menaphthone	T45.7X1	T45.7X2	T45.7X3	T45.7X4	T45.7X5	T45.7X6
Menaquinone	T45.7X1	T45.7X2	T45.7X3	T45.7X4	T45.7X5	T45.7X6
Menatetrenone	T45.7X1	T45.7X2	T45.7X3	T45.7X4	T45.7X5	T45.7X6
Meningococcal vaccine	T50.A91	T50.A92	T50.A93	T50.A94	T50.A95	T50.A96
Menningovax (-AC) (-C)	T50.A91	T50.A92	T50.A93	T50.A94	T50.A95	T50.A96
Menotropins	T38.811	T38.812	T38.813	T38.814	T38.815	T38.816
Menthol	T48.5X1	T48.5X2	T48.5X3	T48.5X4	T48.5X5	T48.5X6
Mepacrine	T37.2X1	T37.2X2	T37.2X3	T37.2X4	T37.2X5	T37.2X6
Meparfynol	T42.6X1	T42.6X2	T42.6X3	T42.6X4	T42.6X5	T42.6X6
Mepartricin	T36.7X1	T36.7X2	T36.7X3	T36.7X4	T36.7X5	T36.7X6
Mepazine	T43.3X1	T43.3X2	T43.3X3	T43.3X4	T43.3X5	T43.3X6
Mepenzolate	T44.3X1	T44.3X2	T44.3X3	T44.3X4	T44.3X5	T44.3X6
bromide	T44.3X1	T44.3X2	T44.3X3	T44.3X4	T44.3X5	T44.3X6
Meperidine	T40.4X1	T40.4X2	T40.4X3	T40.4X4	T40.4X5	T40.4X6
Mephebarbital	T42.3X1	T42.3X2	T42.3X3	T42.3X4	T42.3X5	T42.3X6
Mephenamin(e)	T42.8X1	T42.8X2	T42.8X3	T42.8X4	T42.8X5	T42.8X6
Mephenesin	T42.8X1	T42.8X2	T42.8X3	T42.8X4	T42.8X5	T42.8X6
Mephenhydramine	T45.0X1	T45.0X2	T45.0X3	T45.0X4	T45.0X5	T45.0X6
Mephenoxalone	T42.8X1	T42.8X2	T42.8X3	T42.8X4	T42.8X5	T42.8X6
Mephentermine	T44.991	T44.992	T44.993	T44.994	T44.995	T44.996
Mephenytoin	T42.0X1	T42.0X2	T42.0X3	T42.0X4	T42.0X5	T42.0X6
with phenobarbital	T42.3X1	T42.3X2	T42.3X3	T42.3X4	T42.3X5	T42.3X6
Mephobarbital	T42.3X1	T42.3X2	T42.3X3	T42.3X4	T42.3X5	T42.3X6
Mephosfolan	T60.0X1	T60.0X2	T60.0X3	T60.0X4	—	—
Mepindolol	T44.7X1	T44.7X2	T44.7X3	T44.7X4	T44.7X5	T44.7X6
Mepiperphenidol	T44.3X1	T44.3X2	T44.3X3	T44.3X4	T44.3X5	T44.3X6
Mepitiostane	T38.7X1	T38.7X2	T38.7X3	T38.7X4	T38.7X5	T38.7X6
Mepivacaine	T41.3X1	T41.3X2	T41.3X3	T41.3X4	T41.3X5	T41.3X6
epidural	T41.3X1	T41.3X2	T41.3X3	T41.3X4	T41.3X5	T41.3X6
Meprednisone	T38.0X1	T38.0X2	T38.0X3	T38.0X4	T38.0X5	T38.0X6
Meprobam	T43.591	T43.592	T43.593	T43.594	T43.595	T43.596
Meprobamate	T43.591	T43.592	T43.593	T43.594	T43.595	T43.596
Meproscillarin	T46.0X1	T46.0X2	T46.0X3	T46.0X4	T46.0X5	T46.0X6
Meprylcaine	T41.3X1	T41.3X2	T41.3X3	T41.3X4	T41.3X5	T41.3X6
Meptazinol	T39.8X1	T39.8X2	T39.8X3	T39.8X4	T39.8X5	T39.8X6
Mepyramine	T45.0X1	T45.0X2	T45.0X3	T45.0X4	T45.0X5	T45.0X6
Mequitazine	T43.3X1	T43.3X2	T43.3X3	T43.3X4	T43.3X5	T43.3X6
Meralluride	T50.2X1	T50.2X2	T50.2X3	T50.2X4	T50.2X5	T50.2X6

Substance	Poisoning, Accidental (Unintentional)	Poisoning, Intentional Self-Harm	Poisoning, Assault	Poisoning, Undetermined	Adverse Effect	Underdosing
Merbaphen	T50.2X1	T50.2X2	T50.2X3	T50.2X4	T50.2X5	T50.2X6
Merbromin	T49.0X1	T49.0X2	T49.0X3	T49.0X4	T49.0X5	T49.0X6
Mercaptobenzothiazole salts	T49.0X1	T49.0X2	T49.0X3	T49.0X4	T49.0X5	T49.0X6
Mercaptomerin	T50.2X1	T50.2X2	T50.2X3	T50.2X4	T50.2X5	T50.2X6
Mercaptopurine	T45.1X1	T45.1X2	T45.1X3	T45.1X4	T45.1X5	T45.1X6
Mercumatilin	T50.2X1	T50.2X2	T50.2X3	T50.2X4	T50.2X5	T50.2X6
Mercuramide	T50.2X1	T50.2X2	T50.2X3	T50.2X4	T50.2X5	T50.2X6
Mercurochrome	T49.0X1	T49.0X2	T49.0X3	T49.0X4	T49.0X5	T49.0X6
Mercurophylline	T50.2X1	T50.2X2	T50.2X3	T50.2X4	T50.2X5	T50.2X6
Mercury, mercurial, mercuric, mercurous (compounds) (cyanide) (fumes) (nonmedicinal) (vapor) NEC	T56.1X1	T56.1X2	T56.1X3	T56.1X4	—	—
ammoniated	T49.0X1	T49.0X2	T49.0X3	T49.0X4	T49.0X5	T49.0X6
anti-infective						
local	T49.0X1	T49.0X2	T49.0X3	T49.0X4	T49.0X5	T49.0X6
systemic	T37.8X1	T37.8X2	T37.8X3	T37.8X4	T37.8X5	T37.8X6
topical	T49.0X1	T49.0X2	T49.0X3	T49.0X4	T49.0X5	T49.0X6
chloride (ammoniated)	T49.0X1	T49.0X2	T49.0X3	T49.0X4	T49.0X5	T49.0X6
fungicide	T56.1X1	T56.1X2	T56.1X3	T56.1X4	—	—
diuretic NEC	T50.2X1	T50.2X2	T50.2X3	T50.2X4	T50.2X5	T50.2X6
fungicide	T56.1X1	T56.1X2	T56.1X3	T56.1X4	—	—
organic (fungicide)	T56.1X1	T56.1X2	T56.1X3	T56.1X4	—	—
oxide, yellow	T49.0X1	T49.0X2	T49.0X3	T49.0X4	T49.0X5	T49.0X6
Mersalyl	T50.2X1	T50.2X2	T50.2X3	T50.2X4	T50.2X5	T50.2X6
Merthiolate	T49.0X1	T49.0X2	T49.0X3	T49.0X4	T49.0X5	T49.0X6
ophthalmic preparation	T49.5X1	T49.5X2	T49.5X3	T49.5X4	T49.5X5	T49.5X6
Meruvax	T50.B91	T50.B92	T50.B93	T50.B94	T50.B95	T50.B96
Mesalazine	T47.8X1	T47.8X2	T47.8X3	T47.8X4	T47.8X5	T47.8X6
Mescal buttons	T40.991	T40.992	T40.993	T40.994	—	—
Mescaline	T40.991	T40.992	T40.993	T40.994	—	—
Mesna	T48.4X1	T48.4X2	T48.4X3	T48.4X4	T48.4X5	T48.4X6
Mesoglycan	T46.6X1	T46.6X2	T46.6X3	T46.6X4	T46.6X5	T46.6X6
Mesoridazine	T43.3X1	T43.3X2	T43.3X3	T43.3X4	T43.3X5	T43.3X6
Mestanolone	T38.7X1	T38.7X2	T38.7X3	T38.7X4	T38.7X5	T38.7X6
Mesterolone	T38.7X1	T38.7X2	T38.7X3	T38.7X4	T38.7X5	T38.7X6
Mestranol	T38.5X1	T38.5X2	T38.5X3	T38.5X4	T38.5X5	T38.5X6
Mesulergine	T42.8X1	T42.8X2	T42.8X3	T42.8X4	T42.8X5	T42.8X6
Mesulfen	T49.0X1	T49.0X2	T49.0X3	T49.0X4	T49.0X5	T49.0X6
Mesuximide	T42.2X1	T42.2X2	T42.2X3	T42.2X4	T42.2X5	T42.2X6
Metabutethamine	T41.3X1	T41.3X2	T41.3X3	T41.3X4	T41.3X5	T41.3X6
Metactesylacetate	T49.0X1	T49.0X2	T49.0X3	T49.0X4	T49.0X5	T49.0X6

TABLE OF DRUGS AND CHEMICALS

Substance	Poisoning, Accidental (Unintentional)	Poisoning, Intentional Self-Harm	Poisoning, Assault	Poisoning, Undetermined	Adverse Effect	Underdosing
Metacycline	T36.4X1	T36.4X2	T36.4X3	T36.4X4	T36.4X5	T36.4X6
Metaldehyde (snail killer) NEC	T60.8X1	T60.8X2	T60.8X3	T60.8X4	—	—
Metals (heavy) (nonmedicinal)	T56.91	T56.92	T56.93	T56.94	—	—
dust, fumes, or vapor NEC	T56.91	T56.92	T56.93	T56.94	—	—
light NEC	T56.91	T56.92	T56.93	T56.94	—	—
dust, fumes, or vapor NEC	T56.91	T56.92	T56.93	T56.94	—	—
specified NEC	T56.891	T56.892	T56.893	T56.894	—	—
thallium	T56.811	T56.812	T56.813	T56.814	—	—
Metamfetamine	T43.621	T43.622	T43.623	T43.624	T43.625	T43.626
Metamizole sodium	T39.2X1	T39.2X2	T39.2X3	T39.2X4	T39.2X5	T39.2X6
Metampicillin	T36.0X1	T36.0X2	T36.0X3	T36.0X4	T36.0X5	T36.0X6
Metamucil	T47.4X1	T47.4X2	T47.4X3	T47.4X4	T47.4X5	T47.4X6
Metaphen	T49.0X1	T49.0X2	T49.0X3	T49.0X4	T49.0X5	T49.0X6
Metandienone	T38.7X1	T38.7X2	T38.7X3	T38.7X4	T38.7X5	T38.7X6
Metandrostenolone	T38.7X1	T38.7X2	T38.7X3	T38.7X4	T38.7X5	T38.7X6
Metaphos	T60.0X1	T60.0X2	T60.0X3	T60.0X4	—	—
Metapramine	T43.011	T43.012	T43.013	T43.014	T43.015	T43.016
Metaproterenol	T48.291	T48.292	T48.293	T48.294	T48.295	T48.296
Metaraminol	T44.4X1	T44.4X2	T44.4X3	T44.4X4	T44.4X5	T44.4X6
Metaxalone	T42.8X1	T42.8X2	T42.8X3	T42.8X4	T42.8X5	T42.8X6
Metenolone	T38.7X1	T38.7X2	T38.7X3	T38.7X4	T38.7X5	T38.7X6
Metergoline	T42.8X1	T42.8X2	T42.8X3	T42.8X4	T42.8X5	T42.8X6
Metescufylline	T46.991	T46.992	T46.993	T46.994	T46.995	T46.996
Metetoin	T42.0X1	T42.0X2	T42.0X3	T42.0X4	T42.0X5	T42.0X6
Metformin	T38.3X1	T38.3X2	T38.3X3	T38.3X4	T38.3X5	T38.3X6
Methacholine	T44.1X1	T44.1X2	T44.1X3	T44.1X4	T44.1X5	T44.1X6
Methacycline	T36.4X1	T36.4X2	T36.4X3	T36.4X4	T36.4X5	T36.4X6
Methadone	T40.3X1	T40.3X2	T40.3X3	T40.3X4	T40.3X5	T40.3X6
Methallenestril	T38.5X1	T38.5X2	T38.5X3	T38.5X4	T38.5X5	T38.5X6
Methallenoestril	T38.5X1	T38.5X2	T38.5X3	T38.5X4	T38.5X5	T38.5X6
Methamphetamine	T43.621	T43.622	T43.623	T43.624	T43.625	T43.626
Methampyrone	T39.2X1	T39.2X2	T39.2X3	T39.2X4	T39.2X5	T39.2X6
Methandienone	T38.7X1	T38.7X2	T38.7X3	T38.7X4	T38.7X5	T38.7X6
Methandriol	T38.7X1	T38.7X2	T38.7X3	T38.7X4	T38.7X5	T38.7X6
Methandrostenolone	T38.7X1	T38.7X2	T38.7X3	T38.7X4	T38.7X5	T38.7X6
Methane	T59.891	T59.892	T59.893	T59.894	—	—
Methanethiol	T59.891	T59.892	T59.893	T59.894	—	—
Methaniazide	T37.1X1	T37.1X2	T37.1X3	T37.1X4	T37.1X5	T37.1X6
Methanol (vapor)	T51.1X1	T51.1X2	T51.1X3	T51.1X4	—	—
Methantheline	T44.3X1	T44.3X2	T44.3X3	T44.3X4	T44.3X5	T44.3X6
Methanthelinium bromide	T44.3X1	T44.3X2	T44.3X3	T44.3X4	T44.3X5	T44.3X6
Methaphenilene	T45.0X1	T45.0X2	T45.0X3	T45.0X4	T45.0X5	T45.0X6

Substance	Poisoning, Accidental (Unintentional)	Poisoning, Intentional Self-Harm	Poisoning, Assault	Poisoning, Undetermined	Adverse Effect	Underdosing
Methapyrilene	T45.0X1	T45.0X2	T45.0X3	T45.0X4	T45.0X5	T45.0X6
Methaqualone (compound)	T42.6X1	T42.6X2	T42.6X3	T42.6X4	T42.6X5	T42.6X6
Metharbital	T42.3X1	T42.3X2	T42.3X3	T42.3X4	T42.3X5	T42.3X6
Methazolamide	T50.2X1	T50.2X2	T50.2X3	T50.2X4	T50.2X5	T50.2X6
Methdilazine	T43.3X1	T43.3X2	T43.3X3	T43.3X4	T43.3X5	T43.3X6
Methedrine	T43.621	T43.622	T43.623	T43.624	T43.625	T43.626
Methenamine (mandelate)	T37.8X1	T37.8X2	T37.8X3	T37.8X4	T37.8X5	T37.8X6
Methenolone	T38.7X1	T38.7X2	T38.7X3	T38.7X4	T38.7X5	T38.7X6
Methergine	T48.0X1	T48.0X2	T48.0X3	T48.0X4	T48.0X5	T48.0X6
Methetoin	T42.0X1	T42.0X2	T42.0X3	T42.0X4	T42.0X5	T42.0X6
Methiacil	T38.2X1	T38.2X2	T38.2X3	T38.2X4	T38.2X5	T38.2X6
Methicillin	T36.0X1	T36.0X2	T36.0X3	T36.0X4	T36.0X5	T36.0X6
Methimazole	T38.2X1	T38.2X2	T38.2X3	T38.2X4	T38.2X5	T38.2X6
Methiodal sodium	T50.8X1	T50.8X2	T50.8X3	T50.8X4	T50.8X5	T50.8X6
Methionine	T50.991	T50.992	T50.993	T50.994	T50.995	T50.996
Methisazone	T37.5X1	T37.5X2	T37.5X3	T37.5X4	T37.5X5	T37.5X6
Methisoprinol	T37.5X1	T37.5X2	T37.5X3	T37.5X4	T37.5X5	T37.5X6
Methitural	T42.3X1	T42.3X2	T42.3X3	T42.3X4	T42.3X5	T42.3X6
Methixene	T44.3X1	T44.3X2	T44.3X3	T44.3X4	T44.3X5	T44.3X6
Methobarbital, methobarbitone	T42.3X1	T42.3X2	T42.3X3	T42.3X4	T42.3X5	T42.3X6
Methocarbamol	T42.8X1	T42.8X2	T42.8X3	T42.8X4	T42.8X5	T42.8X6
skeletal muscle relaxant	T48.1X1	T48.1X2	T48.1X3	T48.1X4	T48.1X5	T48.1X6
Methohexital	T41.1X1	T41.1X2	T41.1X3	T41.1X4	T41.1X5	T41.1X6
Methohexitone	T41.1X1	T41.1X2	T41.1X3	T41.1X4	T41.1X5	T41.1X6
Methoin	T42.0X1	T42.0X2	T42.0X3	T42.0X4	T42.0X5	T42.0X6
Methopholine	T39.8X1	T39.8X2	T39.8X3	T39.8X4	T39.8X5	T39.8X6
Methopromazine	T43.3X1	T43.3X2	T43.3X3	T43.3X4	T43.3X5	T43.3X6
Methorate	T48.3X1	T48.3X2	T48.3X3	T48.3X4	T48.3X5	T48.3X6
Methoserpidine	T46.5X1	T46.5X2	T46.5X3	T46.5X4	T46.5X5	T46.5X6
Methotrexate	T45.1X1	T45.1X2	T45.1X3	T45.1X4	T45.1X5	T45.1X6
Methotrimeprazine	T43.3X1	T43.3X2	T43.3X3	T43.3X4	T43.3X5	T43.3X6
Methoxa-Dome	T49.3X1	T49.3X2	T49.3X3	T49.3X4	T49.3X5	T49.3X6
Methoxamine	T44.4X1	T44.4X2	T44.4X3	T44.4X4	T44.4X5	T44.4X6
Methoxsalen	T50.991	T50.992	T50.993	T50.994	T50.995	T50.996
Methoxyaniline	T65.3X1	T65.3X2	T65.3X3	T65.3X4	—	—
Methoxybenzyl penicillin	T36.0X1	T36.0X2	T36.0X3	T36.0X4	T36.0X5	T36.0X6
Methoxychlor	T53.7X1	T53.7X2	T53.7X3	T53.7X4	—	—
Methoxy-DDT	T53.7X1	T53.7X2	T53.7X3	T53.7X4	—	—
2-Methoxyethanol	T52.3X1	T52.3X2	T52.3X3	T52.3X4	—	—
Methoxyflurane	T41.0X1	T41.0X2	T41.0X3	T41.0X4	T41.0X5	T41.0X6
Methoxyphenamine	T48.6X1	T48.6X2	T48.6X3	T48.6X4	T48.6X5	T48.6X6
Methoxypromazine	T43.3X1	T43.3X2	T43.3X3	T43.3X4	T43.3X5	T43.3X6

◄ New ◄═ Revised ~~deleted~~ Deleted

Substance	Poisoning, Accidental (Unintentional)	Poisoning, Intentional Self-Harm	Poisoning, Assault	Poisoning, Undetermined	Adverse Effect	Underdosing
5-Methoxypsoralen (5-MOP)	T50.991	T50.992	T50.993	T50.994	T50.995	T50.996
8-Methoxypsoralen (8-MOP)	T50.991	T50.992	T50.993	T50.994	T50.995	T50.996
Methscopolamine bromide	T44.3X1	T44.3X2	T44.3X3	T44.3X4	T44.3X5	T44.3X6
Methsuximide	T42.2X1	T42.2X2	T42.2X3	T42.2X4	T42.2X5	T42.2X6
Methyclothiazide	T50.2X1	T50.2X2	T50.2X3	T50.2X4	T50.2X5	T50.2X6
Methyl						
acetate	T52.4X1	T52.4X2	T52.4X3	T52.4X4	—	—
acetone	T52.4X1	T52.4X2	T52.4X3	T52.4X4	—	—
acrylate	T65.891	T65.892	T65.893	T65.894	—	—
alcohol	T51.1X1	T51.1X2	T51.1X3	T51.1X4	—	—
aminophenol	T65.3X1	T65.3X2	T65.3X3	T65.3X4	—	—
amphetamine	T43.621	T43.622	T43.623	T43.624	T43.625	T43.626
androstanolone	T38.7X1	T38.7X2	T38.7X3	T38.7X4	T38.7X5	T38.7X6
atropine	T44.3X1	T44.3X2	T44.3X3	T44.3X4	T44.3X5	T44.3X6
benzene	T52.2X1	T52.2X2	T52.2X3	T52.2X4	—	—
benzoate	T52.8X1	T52.8X2	T52.8X3	T52.8X4	—	—
benzol	T52.2X1	T52.2X2	T52.2X3	T52.2X4	—	—
bromide (gas)	T59.891	T59.892	T59.893	T59.894		
fumigant	T60.8X1	T60.8X2	T60.8X4	T60.8X4		
butanol	T51.3X1	T51.3X2	T51.3X3	T51.3X4	—	—
carbinol	T51.1X1	T51.1X2	T51.1X3	T51.1X4	—	—
carbonate	T52.8X1	T52.8X2	T52.8X3	T52.8X4	—	—
CCNU	T45.1X1	T45.1X2	T45.1X3	T45.1X4	T45.1X5	T45.1X6
cellosolve	T52.91	T52.92	T52.93	T52.94	—	—
cellulose	T47.4X1	T47.4X2	T47.4X3	T47.4X4	T47.4X5	T47.4X6
chloride (gas)	T59.891	T59.892	T59.893	T59.894		
chloroformate	T59.3X1	T59.3X2	T59.3X3	T59.3X4		
cyclohexane	T52.8X1	T52.8X2	T52.8X3	T52.8X4	—	—
cyclohexanol	T51.8X1	T51.8X2	T51.8X3	T51.8X4	—	—
cyclohexanone	T52.8X1	T52.8X2	T52.8X3	T52.8X4	—	—
cyclohexyl acetate	T52.8X1	T52.8X2	T52.8X3	T52.8X4	—	—
demeton	T60.0X1	T60.0X2	T60.0X3	T60.0X4		
dihydromorphinone	T40.2X1	T40.2X2	T40.2X3	T40.2X4	T40.2X5	T40.2X6
ergometrine	T48.0X1	T48.0X2	T48.0X3	T48.0X4	T48.0X5	T48.0X6
ergonovine	T48.0X1	T48.0X2	T48.0X3	T48.0X4	T48.0X5	T48.0X6
ethyl ketone	T52.4X1	T52.4X2	T52.4X3	T52.4X4	—	—
glucamine antimonate	T37.8X1	T37.8X2	T37.8X3	T37.8X4	T37.8X5	T37.8X6
hydrazine	T65.891	T65.892	T65.893	T65.894	—	—
iodide	T65.891	T65.892	T65.893	T65.894	—	—
isobutyl ketone	T52.4X1	T52.4X2	T52.4X3	T52.4X4	—	—
isothiocyanate	T60.3X1	T60.3X2	T60.3X3	T60.3X4	—	—
mercaptan	T59.891	T59.892	T59.893	T59.894		

Substance	Poisoning, Accidental (Unintentional)	Poisoning, Intentional Self-Harm	Poisoning, Assault	Poisoning, Undetermined	Adverse Effect	Underdosing
Methyl *(Continued)*						
morphine NEC	T40.2X1	T40.2X2	T40.2X3	T40.2X4	T40.2X5	T40.2X6
nicotinate	T49.4X1	T49.4X2	T49.4X3	T49.4X4	T49.4X5	T49.4X6
paraben	T49.0X1	T49.0X2	T49.0X3	T49.0X4	T49.0X5	T49.0X6
parafynol	T42.6X1	T42.6X2	T42.6X3	T42.6X4	T42.6X5	T42.6X6
parathion	T60.0X1	T60.0X2	T60.0X3	T60.0X4	—	—
peridol	T43.4X1	T43.4X2	T43.4X3	T43.4X4	T43.4X5	T43.4X6
phenidate	T43.631	T43.632	T43.633	T43.634	T43.635	T43.636
prednisolone	T38.0X1	T38.0X2	T38.0X3	T38.0X4	T38.0X5	T38.0X6
ENT agent	T49.6X1	T49.6X2	T49.6X3	T49.6X4	T49.6X5	T49.6X6
ophthalmic preparation	T49.5X1	T49.5X2	T49.5X3	T49.5X4	T49.5X5	T49.5X6
topical NEC	T49.0X1	T49.0X2	T49.0X3	T49.0X4	T49.0X5	T49.0X6
propylcarbinol	T51.3X1	T51.3X2	T51.3X3	T51.3X4	—	—
rosaniline NEC	T49.0X1	T49.0X2	T49.0X3	T49.0X4	T49.0X5	T49.0X6
salicylate	T49.2X1	T49.2X2	T49.2X3	T49.2X4	T49.2X5	T49.2X6
sulfate (fumes)	T59.891	T59.892	T59.893	T59.894		
liquid	T52.8X1	T52.8X2	T52.8X3	T52.8X4	—	—
sulfonal	T42.6X1	T42.6X2	T42.6X3	T42.6X4	T42.6X5	T42.6X6
testosterone	T38.7X1	T38.7X2	T38.7X3	T38.7X4	T38.7X5	T38.7X6
thiouracil	T38.2X1	T38.2X2	T38.2X3	T38.2X4	T38.2X5	T38.2X6
Methylamphetamine	T43.621	T43.622	T43.623	T43.624	T43.625	T43.626
Methylated spirit	T51.1X1	T51.1X2	T51.1X3	T51.1X4	—	—
Methylatropine nitrate	T44.3X1	T44.3X2	T44.3X3	T44.3X4	T44.3X5	T44.3X6
Methylbenactyzium bromide	T44.3X1	T44.3X2	T44.3X3	T44.3X4	T44.3X5	T44.3X6
Methylbenzethonium chloride	T49.0X1	T49.0X2	T49.0X3	T49.0X4	T49.0X5	T49.0X6
Methylcellulose	T47.4X1	T47.4X2	T47.4X3	T47.4X4	T47.4X5	T47.4X6
laxative	T47.4X1	T47.4X2	T47.4X3	T47.4X4	T47.4X5	T47.4X6
Methylchlorophenoxy-acetic acid	T60.3X1	T60.3X2	T60.3X3	T60.3X4	—	—
Methyldopa	T46.5X1	T46.5X2	T46.5X3	T46.5X4	T46.5X5	T46.5X6
Methyldopate	T46.5X1	T46.5X2	T46.5X3	T46.5X4	T46.5X5	T46.5X6
Methylene						
blue	T50.6X1	T50.6X2	T50.6X3	T50.6X4	T50.6X5	T50.6X6
chloride or dichloride (solvent) NEC	T53.4X1	T53.4X2	T53.4X3	T53.4X4		
Methylenedioxyamphet-amine	T43.621	T43.622	T43.623	T43.624	T43.625	T43.626
Methylenedioxymethamphetamine	T43.621	T43.622	T43.623	T43.624	T43.625	T43.626
Methylergometrine	T48.0X1	T48.0X2	T48.0X3	T48.0X4	T48.0X5	T48.0X6
Methylergonovine	T48.0X1	T48.0X2	T48.0X3	T48.0X4	T48.0X5	T48.0X6
Methylestrenolone	T38.5X1	T38.5X2	T38.5X3	T38.5X4	T38.5X5	T38.5X6
Methylethyl cellulose	T50.991	T50.992	T50.993	T50.994	T50.995	T50.996
Methylhexabital	T42.3X1	T42.3X2	T42.3X3	T42.3X4	T42.3X5	T42.3X6
Methylmorphine	T40.2X1	T40.2X2	T40.2X3	T40.2X4	T40.2X5	T40.2X6

TABLE OF DRUGS AND CHEMICALS

TABLE OF DRUGS AND CHEMICALS

Substance	External Cause (T-Code)					
	Poisoning, Accidental (Unintentional)	Poisoning, Intentional Self-Harm	Poisoning, Assault	Poisoning, Undetermined	Adverse Effect	Underdosing
Methylparaben (ophthalmic)	T49.5X1	T49.5X2	T49.5X3	T49.5X4	T49.5X5	T49.5X6
Methylparafynol	T42.6X1	T42.6X2	T42.6X3	T42.6X4	T42.6X5	T42.6X6
Methylpentynol, methylpenthynol	T42.6X1	T42.6X2	T42.6X3	T42.6X4	T42.6X5	T42.6X6
Methylphenidate	T43.631	T43.632	T43.633	T43.634	T43.635	T43.636
Methylphenobarbital	T42.3X1	T42.3X2	T42.3X3	T42.3X4	T42.3X5	T42.3X6
Methylpolysiloxane	T47.1X1	T47.1X2	T47.1X3	T47.1X4	T47.1X5	T47.1X6
Methylprednisolone — see Methyl, prednisolone						
Methylrosaniline	T49.0X1	T49.0X2	T49.0X3	T49.0X4	T49.0X5	T49.0X6
Methylrosanilinium chloride	T49.0X1	T49.0X2	T49.0X3	T49.0X4	T49.0X5	T49.0X6
Methyltestosterone	T38.7X1	T38.7X2	T38.7X3	T38.7X4	T38.7X5	T38.7X6
Methylthionine chloride	T50.6X1	T50.6X2	T50.6X3	T50.6X4	T50.6X5	T50.6X6
Methylthioninium chloride	T50.6X1	T50.6X2	T50.6X3	T50.6X4	T50.6X5	T50.6X6
Methylthiouracil	T38.2X1	T38.2X2	T38.2X3	T38.2X4	T38.2X5	T38.2X6
Methyprylon	T42.6X1	T42.6X2	T42.6X3	T42.6X4	T42.6X5	T42.6X6
Methysergide	T46.5X1	T46.5X2	T46.5X3	T46.5X4	T46.5X5	T46.5X6
Metiamide	T47.1X1	T47.1X2	T47.1X3	T47.1X4	T47.1X5	T47.1X6
Meticillin	T36.0X1	T36.0X2	T36.0X3	T36.0X4	T36.0X5	T36.0X6
Meticrane	T50.2X1	T50.2X2	T50.2X3	T50.2X4	T50.2X5	T50.2X6
Metildigoxin	T46.0X1	T46.0X2	T46.0X3	T46.0X4	T46.0X5	T46.0X6
Metipranolol	T49.5X1	T49.5X2	T49.5X3	T49.5X4	T49.5X5	T49.5X6
Metirosine	T46.5X1	T46.5X2	T46.5X3	T46.5X4	T46.5X5	T46.5X6
Metisazone	T37.5X1	T37.5X2	T37.5X3	T37.5X4	T37.5X5	T37.5X6
Metixene	T44.3X1	T44.3X2	T44.3X3	T44.3X4	T44.3X5	T44.3X6
Metizoline	T48.5X1	T48.5X2	T48.5X3	T48.5X4	T48.5X5	T48.5X6
Metoclopramide	T45.0X1	T45.0X2	T45.0X3	T45.0X4	T45.0X5	T45.0X6
Metofenazate	T43.3X1	T43.3X2	T43.3X3	T43.3X4	T43.3X5	T43.3X6
Metofoline	T39.8X1	T39.8X2	T39.8X3	T39.8X4	T39.8X5	T39.8X6
Metolazone	T50.2X1	T50.2X2	T50.2X3	T50.2X4	T50.2X5	T50.2X6
Metopon	T40.2X1	T40.2X2	T40.2X3	T40.2X4	T40.2X5	T40.2X6
Metoprine	T45.1X1	T45.1X2	T45.1X3	T45.1X4	T45.1X5	T45.1X6
Metoprolol	T44.7X1	T44.7X2	T44.7X3	T44.7X4	T44.7X5	T44.7X6
Metrifonate	T60.0X1	T60.0X2	T60.0X3	T60.0X4	—	—
Metrizamide	T50.8X1	T50.8X2	T50.8X3	T50.8X4	T50.8X5	T50.8X6
Metrizoic acid	T50.8X1	T50.8X2	T50.8X3	T50.8X4	T50.8X5	T50.8X6
Metronidazole	T37.8X1	T37.8X2	T37.8X3	T37.8X4	T37.8X5	T37.8X6
Metycaine	T41.3X1	T41.3X2	T41.3X3	T41.3X4	T41.3X5	T41.3X6
infiltration (subcutaneous)	T41.3X1	T41.3X2	T41.3X3	T41.3X4	T41.3X5	T41.3X6
nerve block (peripheral) (plexus)	T41.3X1	T41.3X2	T41.3X3	T41.3X4	T41.3X5	T41.3X6
topical (surface)	T41.3X1	T41.3X2	T41.3X3	T41.3X4	T41.3X5	T41.3X6
Metyrapone	T50.8X1	T50.8X2	T50.8X3	T50.8X4	T50.8X5	T50.8X6
Mevinphos	T60.0X1	T60.0X2	T60.0X3	T60.0X4	—	—

Substance	External Cause (T-Code)					
	Poisoning, Accidental (Unintentional)	Poisoning, Intentional Self-Harm	Poisoning, Assault	Poisoning, Undetermined	Adverse Effect	Underdosing
Mexazolam	T42.4X1	T42.4X2	T42.4X3	T42.4X4	T42.4X5	T42.4X6
Mexenone	T49.3X1	T49.3X2	T49.3X3	T49.3X4	T49.3X5	T49.3X6
Mexiletine	T46.2X1	T46.2X2	T46.2X3	T46.2X4	T46.2X5	T46.2X6
Mezereon	T62.2X1	T62.2X2	T62.2X3	T62.2X4	—	—
berries	T62.1X1	T62.1X2	T62.1X3	T62.1X4	—	—
Mezlocillin	T36.0X1	T36.0X2	T36.0X3	T36.0X4	T36.0X5	T36.0X6
Mianserin	T43.021	T43.022	T43.023	T43.024	T43.025	T43.026
Micatin	T49.0X1	T49.0X2	T49.0X3	T49.0X4	T49.0X5	T49.0X6
Miconazole	T49.0X1	T49.0X2	T49.0X3	T49.0X4	T49.0X5	T49.0X6
Micronomicin	T36.5X1	T36.5X2	T36.5X3	T36.5X4	T36.5X5	T36.5X6
Midazolam	T42.4X1	T42.4X2	T42.4X3	T42.4X4	T42.4X5	T42.4X6
Midecamycin	T36.3X1	T36.3X2	T36.3X3	T36.3X4	T36.3X5	T36.3X6
Mifepristone	T38.6X1	T38.6X2	T38.6X3	T38.6X4	T38.6X5	T38.6X6
Milk of magnesia	T47.1X1	T47.1X2	T47.1X3	T47.1X4	T47.1X5	T47.1X6
Millipede (tropical) (venomous)	T63.411	T63.412	T63.413	T63.414	—	—
Miltown	T43.591	T43.592	T43.593	T43.594	T43.595	T43.596
Milverine	T44.3X1	T44.3X2	T44.3X3	T44.3X4	T44.3X5	T44.3X6
Minaprine	T43.291	T43.292	T43.293	T43.294	T43.295	T43.296
Minaxolone	T41.291	T41.292	T41.293	T41.294	T41.295	T41.296
Mineral						
acids	T54.2X1	T54.2X2	T54.2X3	T54.2X4	—	—
oil (laxative) (medicinal)	T47.4X1	T47.4X2	T47.4X3	T47.4X4	T47.4X5	T47.4X6
emulsion	T47.2X1	T47.2X2	T47.2X3	T47.2X4	T47.2X5	T47.2X6
nonmedicinal	T52.0X1	T52.0X2	T52.0X3	T52.0X4	—	—
topical	T49.3X1	T49.3X2	T49.3X3	T49.3X4	T49.3X5	T49.3X6
salt NEC	T50.3X1	T50.3X2	T50.3X3	T50.3X4	T50.3X5	T50.3X6
spirits	T52.0X1	T52.0X2	T52.0X3	T52.0X4	—	—
Mineralocorticosteroid	T50.0X1	T50.0X2	T50.0X3	T50.0X4	T50.0X5	T50.0X6
Minocycline	T36.4X1	T36.4X2	T36.4X3	T36.4X4	T36.4X5	T36.4X6
Minoxidil	T46.7X1	T46.7X2	T46.7X3	T46.7X4	T46.7X5	T46.7X6
Miokamycin	T36.3X1	T36.3X2	T36.3X3	T36.3X4	T36.3X5	T36.3X6
Miotic drug	T49.5X1	T49.5X2	T49.5X3	T49.5X4	T49.5X5	T49.5X6
Mipafox	T60.0X1	T60.0X2	T60.0X3	T60.0X4	—	—
Mirex	T60.1X1	T60.1X2	T60.1X3	T60.1X4	—	—
Mirtazapine	T43.021	T43.022	T43.023	T43.024	T43.025	T43.026
Misonidazole	T37.3X1	T37.3X2	T37.3X3	T37.3X4	T37.3X5	T37.3X6
Misoprostol	T47.1X1	T47.1X2	T47.1X3	T47.1X4	T47.1X5	T47.1X6
Mithramycin	T45.1X1	T45.1X2	T45.1X3	T45.1X4	T45.1X5	T45.1X6
Mitobronitol	T45.1X1	T45.1X2	T45.1X3	T45.1X4	T45.1X5	T45.1X6
Mitoguazone	T45.1X1	T45.1X2	T45.1X3	T45.1X4	T45.1X5	T45.1X6
Mitolactol	T45.1X1	T45.1X2	T45.1X3	T45.1X4	T45.1X5	T45.1X6
Mitomycin	T45.1X1	T45.1X2	T45.1X3	T45.1X4	T45.1X5	T45.1X6

◀ New ◀◀◀ Revised ~~deleted~~ Deleted

Substance	Poisoning, Accidental (Unintentional)	Poisoning, Intentional Self-Harm	Poisoning, Assault	Poisoning, Undetermined	Adverse Effect	Underdosing
Mitopodozide	T45.1X1	T45.1X2	T45.1X3	T45.1X4	T45.1X5	T45.1X6
Mitotane	T45.1X1	T45.1X2	T45.1X3	T45.1X4	T45.1X5	T45.1X6
Mitoxantrone	T45.1X1	T45.1X2	T45.1X3	T45.1X4	T45.1X5	T45.1X6
Mivacurium chloride	T48.1X1	T48.1X2	T48.1X3	T48.1X4	T48.1X5	T48.1X6
Miyari bacteria	T47.6X1	T47.6X2	T47.6X3	T47.6X4	T47.6X5	T47.6X6
Moclobemide	T43.1X1	T43.1X2	T43.1X3	T43.1X4	T43.1X5	T43.1X6
Moderil	T46.5X1	T46.5X2	T46.5X3	T46.5X4	T46.5X5	T46.5X6
Mofebutazone	T39.2X1	T39.2X2	T39.2X3	T39.2X4	T39.2X5	T39.2X6
Mogadon — *see Nitrazepam*						
Molindone	T43.591	T43.592	T43.593	T43.594	T43.595	T43.596
Molsidomine	T46.3X1	T46.3X2	T46.3X3	T46.3X4	T46.3X5	T46.3X6
Mometasone	T49.0X1	T49.0X2	T49.0X3	T49.0X4	T49.0X5	T49.0X6
Monistat	T49.0X1	T49.0X2	T49.0X3	T49.0X4	T49.0X5	T49.0X6
Monkshood	T62.2X1	T62.2X2	T62.2X3	T62.2X4	—	—
Monoamine oxidase inhibitor NEC	T43.1X1	T43.1X2	T43.1X3	T43.1X4	T43.1X5	T43.1X6
hydrazine	T43.1X1	T43.1X2	T43.1X3	T43.1X4	T43.1X5	T43.1X6
Monobenzone	T49.4X1	T49.4X2	T49.4X3	T49.4X4	T49.4X5	T49.4X6
Monochloroacetic acid	T60.3X1	T60.3X2	T60.3X3	T60.3X4	—	—
Monochlorobenzene	T53.7X1	T53.7X2	T53.7X3	T53.7X4	—	—
Monoethanolamine	T46.8X1	T46.8X2	T46.8X3	T46.8X4	T46.8X5	T46.8X6
oleate	T46.8X1	T46.8X2	T46.8X3	T46.8X4	T46.8X5	T46.8X6
Monooctanoin	T50.991	T50.992	T50.993	T50.994	T50.995	T50.996
Monophenylbutazone	T39.2X1	T39.2X2	T39.2X3	T39.2X4	T39.2X5	T39.2X6
Monosodium glutamate	T65.891	T65.892	T65.893	T65.894	—	—
Monosulfiram	T49.0X1	T49.0X2	T49.0X3	T49.0X4	T49.0X5	T49.0X6
Monoxide, carbon — *see Carbon, monoxide*	T57.91	T57.92	T57.93	T57.94	—	—
Monoxidine hydrochloride	T46.1X1	T46.1X2	T46.1X3	T46.1X4	T46.1X5	T46.1X6
Monuron	T60.3X1	T60.3X2	T60.3X3	T60.3X4	—	—
Moperone	T43.4X1	T43.4X2	T43.4X3	T43.4X4	T43.4X5	T43.4X6
Mopidamol	T45.1X1	T45.1X2	T45.1X3	T45.1X4	T45.1X5	T45.1X6
MOPP (mechlorethamine + vincristine + prednisone + procarbazine)	T45.1X1	T45.1X2	T45.1X3	T45.1X4	T45.1X5	T45.1X6
Morfin	T40.2X1	T40.2X2	T40.2X3	T40.2X4	T40.2X5	T40.2X6
Morinamide	T37.1X1	T37.1X2	T37.1X3	T37.1X4	T37.1X5	T37.1X6
Morning glory seeds	T40.991	T40.992	T40.993	T40.994	—	—
Moroxydine	T37.5X1	T37.5X2	T37.5X3	T37.5X4	T37.5X5	T37.5X6
Morphazinamide	T37.1X1	T37.1X2	T37.1X3	T37.1X4	T37.1X5	T37.1X6
Morphine	T40.2X1	T40.2X2	T40.2X3	T40.2X4	T40.2X5	T40.2X6
antagonist	T50.7X1	T50.7X2	T50.7X3	T50.7X4	T50.7X5	T50.7X6
Morpholinylethylmorphine	T40.2X1	T40.2X2	T40.2X3	T40.2X4	—	—
Morsuximide	T42.2X1	T42.2X2	T42.2X3	T42.2X4	T42.2X5	T42.2X6

Substance	Poisoning, Accidental (Unintentional)	Poisoning, Intentional Self-Harm	Poisoning, Assault	Poisoning, Undetermined	Adverse Effect	Underdosing
Mosapramine	T43.591	T43.592	T43.593	T43.594	T43.595	T43.596
Moth balls — *see also Pesticides*	T60.2X1	T60.2X2	T60.2X3	T60.2X4	—	—
naphthalene	T60.2X1	T60.2X2	T60.2X3	T60.2X4	—	—
paradichlorobenzene	T60.1X1	T60.1X2	T60.1X3	T60.1X4	—	—
Motor exhaust gas	T58.01	T58.02	T58.03	T58.04		
Mouthwash (antiseptic) (zinc chloride)	T49.6X1	T49.6X2	T49.6X3	T49.6X4	T49.6X5	T49.6X6
Moxastine	T45.0X1	T45.0X2	T45.0X3	T45.0X4	T45.0X5	T45.0X6
Moxaverine	T44.3X1	T44.3X2	T44.3X3	T44.3X4	T44.3X5	T44.3X6
Moxifensine	T43.291	T43.292	T43.293	T43.294	T43.295	T43.296
Moxisylyte	T46.7X1	T46.7X2	T46.7X3	T46.7X4	T46.7X5	T46.7X6
Mucilage, plant	T47.4X1	T47.4X2	T47.4X3	T47.4X4	T47.4X5	T47.4X6
Mucolytic drug	T48.4X1	T48.4X2	T48.4X3	T48.4X4	T48.4X5	T48.4X6
Mucomyst	T48.4X1	T48.4X2	T48.4X3	T48.4X4	T48.4X5	T48.4X6
Mucous membrane agents (external)	T49.91	T49.92	T49.93	T49.94	T49.95	T49.96
specified NEC	T49.8X1	T49.8X2	T49.8X3	T49.8X4	T49.8X5	T49.8X6
Mumps						
immune globulin (human)	T50.Z11	T50.Z12	T50.Z13	T50.Z14	T50.Z15	T50.Z16
skin test antigen	T50.8X1	T50.8X2	T50.8X3	T50.8X4	T50.8X5	T50.8X6
vaccine	T50.B91	T50.B92	T50.B93	T50.B94	T50.B95	T50.B96
Mumpsvax	T50.B91	T50.B92	T50.B93	T50.B94	T50.B95	T50.B96
Mupirocin	T49.0X1	T49.0X2	T49.0X3	T49.0X4	T49.0X5	T49.0X6
Muriatic acid — *see Hydrochloric acid*						
Muromonab-CD3	T45.1X1	T45.1X2	T45.1X3	T45.1X4	T45.1X5	T45.1X6
Muscle relaxant — *see Relaxant, muscle*						
Muscle-action drug NEC	T48.201	T48.202	T48.203	T48.204	T48.205	T48.206
Muscle affecting agents NEC	T48.201	T48.202	T48.203	T48.204	T48.205	T48.206
oxytocic	T48.0X1	T48.0X2	T48.0X3	T48.0X4	T48.0X5	T48.0X6
relaxants	T48.201	T48.202	T48.203	T48.204	T48.205	T48.206
central nervous system	T42.8X1	T42.8X2	T42.8X3	T42.8X4	T42.8X5	T42.8X6
skeletal	T48.1X1	T48.1X2	T48.1X3	T48.1X4	T48.1X5	T48.1X6
smooth	T44.3X1	T44.3X2	T44.3X3	T44.3X4	T44.3X5	T44.3X6
Muscle-tone depressant, central NEC	T42.8X1	T42.8X2	T42.8X3	T42.8X4	T42.8X5	T42.8X6
specified NEC	T42.8X1	T42.8X2	T42.8X3	T42.8X4	T42.8X5	T42.8X6
Mushroom, noxious	T62.0X1	T62.0X2	T62.0X3	T62.0X4	—	—
Mussel, noxious	T61.781	T61.782	T61.783	T61.784	—	—
Mustard (emetic)	T47.7X1	T47.7X2	T47.7X3	T47.7X4	T47.7X5	T47.7X6
black	T47.7X1	T47.7X2	T47.7X3	T47.7X4	T47.7X5	T47.7X6
gas, not in war	T59.91	T59.92	T59.93	T59.94	—	—
nitrogen	T45.1X1	T45.1X2	T45.1X3	T45.1X4	T45.1X5	T45.1X6

TABLE OF DRUGS AND CHEMICALS

Substance	Poisoning, Accidental (Unintentional)	Poisoning, Intentional Self-Harm	Poisoning, Assault	Poisoning, Undetermined	Adverse Effect	Underdosing
Mustine	T45.1X1	T45.1X2	T45.1X3	T45.1X4	T45.1X5	T45.1X6
M-vac	T45.1X1	T45.1X2	T45.1X3	T45.1X4	T45.1X5	T45.1X6
Mycifradin	T36.5X1	T36.5X2	T36.5X3	T36.5X4	T36.5X5	T36.5X6
topical	T49.0X1	T49.0X2	T49.0X3	T49.0X4	T49.0X5	T49.0X6
Mycitracin	T36.8X1	T36.8X2	T36.8X3	T36.8X4	T36.8X5	T36.8X6
ophthalmic preparation	T49.5X1	T49.5X2	T49.5X3	T49.5X4	T49.5X5	T49.5X6
Mycostatin	T36.7X1	T36.7X2	T36.7X3	T36.7X4	T36.7X5	T36.7X6
topical	T49.0X1	T49.0X2	T49.0X3	T49.0X4	T49.0X5	T49.0X6
Mycotoxins	T64.81	T64.82	T64.83	T64.84	—	—
aflatoxin	T64.01	T64.02	T64.03	T64.04	—	—
specified NEC	T64.81	T64.82	T64.83	T64.84	—	—
Mydriacyl	T44.3X1	T44.3X2	T44.3X3	T44.3X4	T44.3X5	T44.3X6
Mydriatic drug	T49.5X1	T49.5X2	T49.5X3	T49.5X4	T49.5X5	T49.5X6
Myelobromal	T45.1X1	T45.1X2	T45.1X3	T45.1X4	T45.1X5	T45.1X6
Myleran	T45.1X1	T45.1X2	T45.1X3	T45.1X4	T45.1X5	T45.1X6
Myochrysin(e)	T39.2X1	T39.2X2	T39.2X3	T39.2X4	T39.2X5	T39.2X6
Myoneural blocking agents	T48.1X1	T48.1X2	T48.1X3	T48.1X4	T48.1X5	T48.1X6
Myralact	T49.0X1	T49.0X2	T49.0X3	T49.0X4	T49.0X5	T49.0X6
Myristica fragrans	T62.2X1	T62.2X2	T62.2X3	T62.2X4	—	—
Myristicin	T65.891	T65.892	T65.893	T65.894	—	—
Mysoline	T42.3X1	T42.3X2	T42.3X3	T42.3X4	T42.3X5	T42.3X6
N						
Nabilone	T40.7X1	T40.7X2	T40.7X3	T40.7X4	T40.7X5	T40.7X6
Nabumetone	T39.391	T39.392	T39.393	T39.394	T39.395	T39.396
Nadolol	T44.7X1	T44.7X2	T44.7X3	T44.7X4	T44.7X5	T44.7X6
Nafcillin	T36.0X1	T36.0X2	T36.0X3	T36.0X4	T36.0X5	T36.0X6
Nafoxidine	T38.6X1	T38.6X2	T38.6X3	T38.6X4	T38.6X5	T38.6X6
Naftazone	T46.991	T46.992	T46.993	T46.994	T46.995	T46.996
Naftidrofuryl (oxalate)	T46.7X1	T46.7X2	T46.7X3	T46.7X4	T46.7X5	T46.7X6
Naftifine	T49.0X1	T49.0X2	T49.0X3	T49.0X4	T49.0X5	T49.0X6
Nail polish remover	T52.91	T52.92	T52.93	T52.94	—	—
Nalbuphine	T40.4X1	T40.4X2	T40.4X3	T40.4X4	T40.4X5	T40.4X6
Naled	T60.0X1	T60.0X2	T60.0X3	T60.0X4	—	—
Nalidixic acid	T37.8X1	T37.8X2	T37.8X3	T37.8X4	T37.8X5	T37.8X6
Nalorphine	T50.7X1	T50.7X2	T50.7X3	T50.7X4	T50.7X5	T50.7X6
Naloxone	T50.7X1	T50.7X2	T50.7X3	T50.7X4	T50.7X5	T50.7X6
Naltrexone	T50.7X1	T50.7X2	T50.7X3	T50.7X4	T50.7X5	T50.7X6
Namenda	T43.8X1	T43.8X2	T43.8X3	T43.8X4	T43.8X5	T43.8X6
Nandrolone	T38.7X1	T38.7X2	T38.7X3	T38.7X4	T38.7X5	T38.7X6
Naphazoline	T48.5X1	T48.5X2	T48.5X3	T48.5X4	T48.5X5	T48.5X6

Substance	Poisoning, Accidental (Unintentional)	Poisoning, Intentional Self-Harm	Poisoning, Assault	Poisoning, Undetermined	Adverse Effect	Underdosing
Naphtha (painters') (petroleum)	T52.0X1	T52.0X2	T52.0X3	T52.0X4	—	—
solvent	T52.0X1	T52.0X2	T52.0X3	T52.0X4	—	—
vapor	T52.0X1	T52.0X2	T52.0X3	T52.0X4	—	—
Naphthalene (non-chlorinated)	T60.2X1	T60.2X2	T60.2X3	T60.2X4	—	—
chlorinated	T60.1X1	T60.1X2	T60.1X3	T60.1X4	—	—
vapor	T60.1X1	T60.1X2	T60.1X3	T60.1X4	—	—
insecticide or moth repellent	T60.2X1	T60.2X2	T60.2X3	T60.2X4	—	—
chlorinated	T60.1X1	T60.1X2	T60.1X3	T60.1X4	—	—
vapor	T60.2X1	T60.2X2	T60.2X3	T60.2X4	—	—
chlorinated	T60.1X1	T60.1X2	T60.1X3	T60.1X4	—	—
Naphthol	T65.891	T65.892	T65.893	T65.894	—	—
Naphthylamine	T65.891	T65.892	T65.893	T65.894	—	—
Naphthylthiourea (ANTU)	T60.4X1	T60.4X2	T60.4X3	T60.4X4	—	—
Naprosyn — see Naproxen						
Naproxen	T39.311	T39.312	T39.313	T39.314	T39.315	T39.316
Narcotic (drug)	T40.601	T40.602	T40.603	T40.604	T40.605	T40.606
analgesic NEC	T40.601	T40.602	T40.603	T40.604	T40.605	T40.606
antagonist	T50.7X1	T50.7X2	T50.7X3	T50.7X4	T50.7X5	T50.7X6
specified NEC	T40.691	T40.692	T40.693	T40.694	T40.695	T40.696
synthetic	T40.4X1	T40.4X2	T40.4X3	T40.4X4	T40.4X5	T40.4X6
Narcotine	T48.3X1	T48.3X2	T48.3X3	T48.3X4	T48.3X5	T48.3X6
Nardil	T43.1X1	T43.1X2	T43.1X3	T43.1X4	T43.1X5	T43.1X6
Nasal drug NEC	T49.6X1	T49.6X2	T49.6X3	T49.6X4	T49.6X5	T49.6X6
Natamycin	T49.0X1	T49.0X2	T49.0X3	T49.0X4	T49.0X5	T49.0X6
Natrium cyanide — see Cyanide(s)						
Natural gas	T59.891	T59.892	T59.893	T59.894	—	—
incomplete combustion	T57.91	T57.92	T57.93	T57.94	—	—
Natural						
blood (product)	T45.8X1	T45.8X2	T45.8X3	T45.8X4	T45.8X5	T45.8X6
gas (piped)	T59.891	T59.892	T59.893	T59.894	—	—
incomplete combustion	T58.11	T58.12	T58.13	T58.14	—	—
Nealbarbital	T42.3X1	T42.3X2	T42.3X3	T42.3X4	T42.3X5	T42.3X6
Nectadon	T48.3X1	T48.3X2	T48.3X3	T48.3X4	T48.3X5	T48.3X6
Nedocromil	T48.6X1	T48.6X2	T48.6X3	T48.6X4	T48.6X5	T48.6X6
Nefopam	T39.8X1	T39.8X2	T39.8X3	T39.8X4	T39.8X5	T39.8X6
Nematocyst (sting)	T63.691	T63.692	T63.693	T63.694	—	—
Nembutal	T42.3X1	T42.3X2	T42.3X3	T42.3X4	T42.3X5	T42.3X6
Nemonapride	T43.591	T43.592	T43.593	T43.594	T43.595	T43.596
Neoarsphenamine	T37.8X1	T37.8X2	T37.8X3	T37.8X4	T37.8X5	T37.8X6

◀ New   ◀||||| Revised   ~~deleted~~ Deleted

Substance	Poisoning, Accidental (Unintentional)	Poisoning, Intentional Self-Harm	Poisoning, Assault	Poisoning, Undetermined	Adverse Effect	Underdosing
Neocinchophen	T50.4X1	T50.4X2	T50.4X3	T50.4X4	T50.4X5	T50.4X6
Neomycin (derivatives)	T36.5X1	T36.5X2	T36.5X3	T36.5X4	T36.5X5	T36.5X6
with						
bacitracin	T49.0X1	T49.0X2	T49.0X3	T49.0X4	T49.0X5	T49.0X6
neostigmine	T44.0X1	T44.0X2	T44.0X3	T44.0X4	T44.0X5	T44.0X6
ENT agent	T49.6X1	T49.6X2	T49.6X3	T49.6X4	T49.6X5	T49.6X6
ophthalmic preparation	T49.5X1	T49.5X2	T49.5X3	T49.5X4	T49.5X5	T49.5X6
topical NEC	T49.0X1	T49.0X2	T49.0X3	T49.0X4	T49.0X5	T49.0X6
Neonal	T42.3X1	T42.3X2	T42.3X3	T42.3X4	T42.3X5	T42.3X6
Neoprontosil	T37.0X1	T37.0X2	T37.0X3	T37.0X4	T37.0X5	T37.0X6
Neosalvarsan	T37.8X1	T37.8X2	T37.8X3	T37.8X4	T37.8X5	T37.8X6
Neosilversalvarsan	T37.8X1	T37.8X2	T37.8X3	T37.8X4	T37.8X5	T37.8X6
Neosporin	T36.8X1	T36.8X2	T36.8X3	T36.8X4	T36.8X5	T36.8X6
ENT agent	T49.6X1	T49.6X2	T49.6X3	T49.6X4	T49.6X5	T49.6X6
opthalmic preparation	T49.5X1	T49.5X2	T49.5X3	T49.5X4	T49.5X5	T49.5X6
topical NEC	T49.0X1	T49.0X2	T49.0X3	T49.0X4	T49.0X5	T49.0X6
Neostigmine bromide	T44.0X1	T44.0X2	T44.0X3	T44.0X4	T44.0X5	T44.0X6
Neraval	T42.3X1	T42.3X2	T42.3X3	T42.3X4	T42.3X5	T42.3X6
Neravan	T42.3X1	T42.3X2	T42.3X3	T42.3X4	T42.3X5	T42.3X6
Nerium oleander	T62.2X1	T62.2X2	T62.2X3	T62.2X4	—	—
Nerve gas, not in war	T59.91	T59.92	T59.93	T59.94	—	—
Nesacaine	T41.3X1	T41.3X2	T41.3X3	T41.3X4	T41.3X5	T41.3X6
infiltration (subcutaneous)	T41.3X1	T41.3X2	T41.3X3	T41.3X4	T41.3X5	T41.3X6
nerve block (peripheral) (plexus)	T41.3X1	T41.3X2	T41.3X3	T41.3X4	T41.3X5	T41.3X6
Netilmicin	T36.5X1	T36.5X2	T36.5X3	T36.5X4	T36.5X5	T36.5X6
Neurobarb	T42.3X1	T42.3X2	T42.3X3	T42.3X4	T42.3X5	T42.3X6
Neuroleptic drug NEC	T43.501	T43.502	T43.503	T43.504	T43.505	T43.506
Neuromuscular blocking drug	T48.1X1	T48.1X2	T48.1X3	T48.1X4	T48.1X5	T48.1X6
Neutral insulin injection	T38.3X1	T38.3X2	T38.3X3	T38.3X4	T38.3X5	T38.3X6
Neutral spirits	T51.0X1	T51.0X2	T51.0X3	T51.0X4	—	—
beverage	T51.0X1	T51.0X2	T51.0X3	T51.0X4	—	—
Niacin	T46.7X1	T46.7X2	T46.7X3	T46.7X4	T46.7X5	T46.7X6
Niacinamide	T45.2X1	T45.2X2	T45.2X3	T45.2X4	T45.2X5	T45.2X6
Nialamide	T43.1X1	T43.1X2	T43.1X3	T43.1X4	T43.1X5	T43.1X6
Niaprazine	T42.6X1	T42.6X2	T42.6X3	T42.6X4	T42.6X5	T42.6X6
Nicametate	T46.7X1	T46.7X2	T46.7X3	T46.7X4	T46.7X5	T46.7X6
Nicardipine	T46.1X1	T46.1X2	T46.1X3	T46.1X4	T46.1X5	T46.1X6
Nicergoline	T46.7X1	T46.7X2	T46.7X3	T46.7X4	T46.7X5	T46.7X6
Nickel (carbonyl) (tetra-carbonyl) (fumes) (vapor)	T56.891	T56.892	T56.893	T56.894	—	—
Nickelocene	T56.891	T56.892	T56.893	T56.894	—	—
Niclosamide	T37.4X1	T37.4X2	T37.4X3	T37.4X4	T37.4X5	T37.4X6
Nicofuranose	T46.7X1	T46.7X2	T46.7X3	T46.7X4	T46.7X5	T46.7X6
Nicomorphine	T40.2X1	T40.2X2	T40.2X3	T40.2X4	—	—
Nicorandil	T46.3X1	T46.3X2	T46.3X3	T46.3X4	T46.3X5	T46.3X6
Nicotiana (plant)	T62.2X1	T62.2X2	T62.2X3	T62.2X4	—	—
Nicotinamide	T45.2X1	T45.2X2	T45.2X3	T45.2X4	T45.2X5	T45.2X6
Nicotine (insecticide) (spray) (sulfate) NEC	T60.2X1	T60.2X2	T60.2X3	T60.2X4	—	—
from tobacco	T65.291	T65.292	T65.293	T65.294		
cigarettes	T65.221	T65.222	T65.223	T65.224		
not insecticide	T65.291	T65.292	T65.293	T65.294		
Nicotinic acid	T46.7X1	T46.7X2	T46.7X3	T46.7X4	T46.7X5	T46.7X6
Nicotinyl alcohol	T46.7X1	T46.7X2	T46.7X3	T46.7X4	T46.7X5	T46.7X6
Nicoumalone	T45.511	T45.512	T45.513	T45.514	T45.515	T45.516
Nifedipine	T46.1X1	T46.1X2	T46.1X3	T46.1X4	T46.1X5	T46.1X6
Nifenazone	T39.2X1	T39.2X2	T39.2X3	T39.2X4	T39.2X5	T39.2X6
Nifuraldezone	T37.91	T37.92	T37.93	T37.94	T37.95	T37.96
Nifuratel	T37.8X1	T37.8X2	T37.8X3	T37.8X4	T37.8X5	T37.8X6
Nifurtimox	T37.3X1	T37.3X2	T37.3X3	T37.3X4	T37.3X5	T37.3X6
Nifurtoinol	T37.8X1	T37.8X2	T37.8X3	T37.8X4	T37.8X5	T37.8X6
Nightshade, deadly (solanum) — see also Belladonna	T62.2X1	T62.2X2	T62.2X3	T62.2X4		
berry	T62.1X1	T62.1X2	T62.1X3	T62.1X4	—	—
Nikethamide	T50.7X1	T50.7X2	T50.7X3	T50.7X4	T50.7X5	T50.7X6
Nilstat	T36.7X1	T36.7X2	T36.7X3	T36.7X4	T36.7X5	T36.7X6
topical	T49.0X1	T49.0X2	T49.0X3	T49.0X4	T49.0X5	T49.0X6
Nilutamide	T38.6X1	T38.6X2	T38.6X3	T38.6X4	T38.6X5	T38.6X6
Nimesulide	T39.391	T39.392	T39.393	T39.394	T39.395	T39.396
Nimetazepam	T42.4X1	T42.4X2	T42.4X3	T42.4X4	T42.4X5	T42.4X6
Nimodipine	T46.1X1	T46.1X2	T46.1X3	T46.1X4	T46.1X5	T46.1X6
Nimorazole	T37.3X1	T37.3X2	T37.3X3	T37.3X4	T37.3X5	T37.3X6
Nimustine	T45.1X1	T45.1X2	T45.1X3	T45.1X4	T45.1X5	T45.1X6
Niridazole	T37.4X1	T37.4X2	T37.4X3	T37.4X4	T37.4X5	T37.4X6
Nisentil	T40.2X1	T40.2X2	T40.2X3	T40.2X4	T40.2X5	T40.2X6
Nisoldipine	T46.1X1	T46.1X2	T46.1X3	T46.1X4	T46.1X5	T46.1X6
Nitramine	T65.3X1	T65.3X2	T65.3X3	T65.3X4	—	—
Nitrate, organic	T46.3X1	T46.3X2	T46.3X3	T46.3X4	T46.3X5	T46.3X6
Nitrazepam	T42.4X1	T42.4X2	T42.4X3	T42.4X4	T42.4X5	T42.4X6
Nitrefazole	T50.6X1	T50.6X2	T50.6X3	T50.6X4	T50.6X5	T50.6X6
Nitrendipine	T46.1X1	T46.1X2	T46.1X3	T46.1X4	T46.1X5	T46.1X6

TABLE OF DRUGS AND CHEMICALS

Substance	External Cause (T-Code)					
	Poisoning, Accidental (Unintentional)	Poisoning, Intentional Self-Harm	Poisoning, Assault	Poisoning, Undetermined	Adverse Effect	Underdosing
Nitric						
acid (liquid)	T54.2X1	T54.2X2	T54.2X3	T54.2X4	—	—
vapor	T59.891	T59.892	T59.893	T59.894	—	—
oxide (gas)	T59.0X1	T59.0X2	T59.0X3	T59.0X4	—	—
Nitrimidazine	T37.3X1	T37.3X2	T37.3X3	T37.3X4	T37.3X5	T37.3X6
Nitrite, amyl (medicinal) (vapor)	T46.3X1	T46.3X2	T46.3X3	T46.3X4	T46.3X5	T46.3X6
Nitroaniline	T65.3X1	T65.3X2	T65.3X3	T65.3X4	—	—
vapor	T59.891	T59.892	T59.893	T59.894	—	—
Nitrobenzene, nitrobenzol	T65.3X1	T65.3X2	T65.3X3	T65.3X4	—	—
vapor	T65.3X1	T65.3X2	T65.3X3	T65.3X4	—	—
Nitrocellulose	T65.891	T65.892	T65.893	T65.894	—	—
lacquer	T65.891	T65.892	T65.893	T65.894	—	—
Nitrodiphenyl	T65.3X1	T65.3X2	T65.3X3	T65.3X4	—	—
Nitrofural	T49.0X1	T49.0X2	T49.0X3	T49.0X4	T49.0X5	T49.0X6
Nitrofurantoin	T37.8X1	T37.8X2	T37.8X3	T37.8X4	T37.8X5	T37.8X6
Nitrofurazone	T49.0X1	T49.0X2	T49.0X3	T49.0X4	T49.0X5	T49.0X6
Nitrogen	T59.0X1	T59.0X2	T59.0X3	T59.0X4		
mustard	T45.1X1	T45.1X2	T45.1X3	T45.1X4	T45.1X5	T45.1X6
Nitroglycerin, nitro-glycerol (medicinal)	T46.3X1	T46.3X2	T46.3X3	T46.3X4	T46.3X5	T46.3X6
nonmedicinal	T65.5X1	T65.5X2	T65.5X3	T65.5X4	—	—
fumes	T65.5X1	T65.5X2	T65.5X3	T65.5X4	—	—
Nitroglycol	T52.3X1	T52.3X2	T52.3X3	T52.3X4	—	—
Nitrohydrochloric acid	T54.2X1	T54.2X2	T54.2X3	T54.2X4	—	—
Nitromersol	T49.0X1	T49.0X2	T49.0X3	T49.0X4	T49.0X5	T49.0X6
Nitronaphthalene	T65.891	T65.892	T65.893	T65.894	—	—
Nitrophenol	T54.0X1	T54.0X2	T54.0X3	T54.0X4	—	—
Nitropropane	T52.8X1	T52.8X2	T52.8X3	T52.8X4	—	—
Nitroprusside	T46.5X1	T46.5X2	T46.5X3	T46.5X4	T46.5X5	T46.5X6
Nitrosodimethylamine	T65.3X1	T65.3X2	T65.3X3	T65.3X4	—	—
Nitrothiazol	T37.4X1	T37.4X2	T37.4X3	T37.4X4	T37.4X5	T37.4X6
Nitrotoluene, nitrotoluol	T65.3X1	T65.3X2	T65.3X3	T65.3X4	—	—
vapor	T65.3X1	T65.3X2	T65.3X3	T65.3X4	—	—
Nitrous						
acid (liquid)	T54.2X1	T54.2X2	T54.2X3	T54.2X4	—	—
fumes	T59.891	T59.892	T59.893	T59.894	—	—
ether spirit	T46.3X1	T46.3X2	T46.3X3	T46.3X4	T46.3X5	T46.3X6
oxide	T41.0X1	T41.0X2	T41.0X3	T41.0X4	T41.0X5	T41.0X6
Nitroxoline	T37.8X1	T37.8X2	T37.8X3	T37.8X4	T37.8X5	T37.8X6
Nitrozone	T49.0X1	T49.0X2	T49.0X3	T49.0X4	T49.0X5	T49.0X6
Nizatidine	T47.0X1	T47.0X2	T47.0X3	T47.0X4	T47.0X5	T47.0X6

Substance	External Cause (T-Code)					
	Poisoning, Accidental (Unintentional)	Poisoning, Intentional Self-Harm	Poisoning, Assault	Poisoning, Undetermined	Adverse Effect	Underdosing
Nizofenone	T43.8X1	T43.8X2	T43.8X3	T43.8X4	T43.8X5	T43.8X6
Noctec	T42.6X1	T42.6X2	T42.6X3	T42.6X4	T42.6X5	T42.6X6
Noludar	T42.6X1	T42.6X2	T42.6X3	T42.6X4	T42.6X5	T42.6X6
Noptil	T42.3X1	T42.3X2	T42.3X3	T42.3X4	T42.3X5	T42.3X6
Nomegestrol	T38.5X1	T38.5X2	T38.5X3	T38.5X4	T38.5X5	T38.5X6
Nomifensine	T43.291	T43.292	T43.293	T43.294	T43.295	T43.296
Nonoxinol	T49.8X1	T49.8X2	T49.8X3	T49.8X4	T49.8X5	T49.8X6
Nonylphenoxy (polyethoxy-ethanol)	T49.8X1	T49.8X2	T49.8X3	T49.8X4	T49.8X5	T49.8X6
Noptil	T42.3X1	T42.3X2	T42.3X3	T42.3X4	T42.3X5	T42.3X6
Noradrenaline	T44.4X1	T44.4X2	T44.4X3	T44.4X4	T44.4X5	T44.4X6
Noramidopyrine	T39.2X1	T39.2X2	T39.2X3	T39.2X4	T39.2X5	T39.2X6
methanesulfonate sodium	T39.2X1	T39.2X2	T39.2X3	T39.2X4	T39.2X5	T39.2X6
Norbormide	T60.4X1	T60.4X2	T60.4X3	T60.4X4	—	—
Nordazepam	T42.4X1	T42.4X2	T42.4X3	T42.4X4	T42.4X5	T42.4X6
Norepinephrine	T44.4X1	T44.4X2	T44.4X3	T44.4X4	T44.4X5	T44.4X6
Norethandrolone	T38.7X1	T38.7X2	T38.7X3	T38.7X4	T38.7X5	T38.7X6
Norethindrone	T38.4X1	T38.4X2	T38.4X3	T38.4X4	T38.4X5	T38.4X6
Norethisterone (acetate) (enantate)	T38.4X1	T38.4X2	T38.4X3	T38.4X4	T38.4X5	T38.4X6
with ethinylestradiol	T38.5X1	T38.5X2	T38.5X3	T38.5X4	T38.5X5	T38.5X6
Noretynodrel	T38.5X1	T38.5X2	T38.5X3	T38.5X4	T38.5X5	T38.5X6
Norfenefrine	T44.4X1	T44.4X2	T44.4X3	T44.4X4	T44.4X5	T44.4X6
Norfloxacin	T36.8X1	T36.8X2	T36.8X3	T36.8X4	T36.8X5	T36.8X6
Norgestrel	T38.4X1	T38.4X2	T38.4X3	T38.4X4	T38.4X5	T38.4X6
Norgestrienone	T38.4X1	T38.4X2	T38.4X3	T38.4X4	T38.4X5	T38.4X6
Norlestrin	T38.4X1	T38.4X2	T38.4X3	T38.4X4	T38.4X5	T38.4X6
Norlutin	T38.4X1	T38.4X2	T38.4X3	T38.4X4	T38.4X5	T38.4X6
Normal serum albumin (human), salt-poor	T45.8X1	T45.8X2	T45.8X3	T45.8X4	T45.8X5	T45.8X6
Normethandrone	T38.5X1	T38.5X2	T38.5X3	T38.5X4	T38.5X5	T38.5X6
Normison — see Benzodiazepines						
Normorphine	T40.2X1	T40.2X2	T40.2X3	T40.2X4	—	—
Norpseudoephedrine	T50.5X1	T50.5X2	T50.5X3	T50.5X4	T50.5X5	T50.5X6
Nortestosterone (furanpropionate)	T38.7X1	T38.7X2	T38.7X3	T38.7X4	T38.7X5	T38.7X6
Nortriptyline	T43.011	T43.012	T43.013	T43.014	T43.015	T43.016
Noscapine	T48.3X1	T48.3X2	T48.3X3	T48.3X4	T48.3X5	T48.3X6
Nose preparations	T49.6X1	T49.6X2	T49.6X3	T49.6X4	T49.6X5	T49.6X6
Novobiocin	T36.5X1	T36.5X2	T36.5X3	T36.5X4	T36.5X5	T36.5X6
Novocain (infiltration) (topical)	T41.3X1	T41.3X2	T41.3X3	T41.3X4	T41.3X5	T41.3X6
nerve block (peripheral) (plexus)	T41.3X1	T41.3X2	T41.3X3	T41.3X4	T41.3X5	T41.3X6
spinal	T41.3X1	T41.3X2	T41.3X3	T41.3X4	T41.3X5	T41.3X6

◀ New ◀◀◀ Revised ~~deleted~~ Deleted

	External Cause (T-Code)					
Substance	Poisoning, Accidental (Unintentional)	Poisoning, Intentional Self-Harm	Poisoning, Assault	Poisoning, Undetermined	Adverse Effect	Underdosing
Noxious foodstuff	T62.91	T62.92	T62.93	T62.94	—	—
specified NEC	T62.8X1	T62.8X2	T62.8X3	T62.8X4	—	—
Noxiptiline	T43.011	T43.012	T43.013	T43.014	T43.015	T43.016
Noxytiolin	T49.0X1	T49.0X2	T49.0X3	T49.0X4	T49.0X5	T49.0X6
NPH Iletin (insulin)	T38.3X1	T38.3X2	T38.3X3	T38.3X4	T38.3X5	T38.3X6
Numorphan	T40.2X1	T40.2X2	T40.2X3	T40.2X4	T40.2X5	T40.2X6
Nunol	T42.3X1	T42.3X2	T42.3X3	T42.3X4	T42.3X5	T42.3X6
Nupercaine (spinal anesthetic)	T41.3X1	T41.3X2	T41.3X3	T41.3X4	T41.3X5	T41.3X6
topical (surface)	T41.3X1	T41.3X2	T41.3X3	T41.3X4	T41.3X5	T41.3X6
Nutmeg oil (liniment)	T49.3X1	T49.3X2	T49.3X3	T49.3X4	T49.3X5	T49.3X6
Nutritional supplement	T50.901	T50.902	T50.903	T50.904	T50.905	T50.906
Nux vomica	T65.1X1	T65.1X2	T65.1X3	T65.1X4	—	—
Nydrazid	T37.1X1	T37.1X2	T37.1X3	T37.1X4	T37.1X5	T37.1X6
Nylidrin	T46.7X1	T46.7X2	T46.7X3	T46.7X4	T46.7X5	T46.7X6
Nystatin	T36.7X1	T36.7X2	T36.7X3	T36.7X4	T36.7X5	T36.7X6
topical	T49.0X1	T49.0X2	T49.0X3	T49.0X4	T49.0X5	T49.0X6
Nytol	T45.0X1	T45.0X2	T45.0X3	T45.0X4	T45.0X5	T45.0X6
O						
Obidoxime chloride	T50.6X1	T50.6X2	T50.6X3	T50.6X4	T50.6X5	T50.6X6
Octafonium (chloride)	T49.3X1	T49.3X2	T49.3X3	T49.3X4	T49.3X5	T49.3X6
Octamethyl pyrophos-phoramide	T60.0X1	T60.0X2	T60.0X3	T60.0X4	—	—
Octanoin	T50.991	T50.992	T50.993	T50.994	T50.995	T50.996
Octatropine methyl-bromide	T44.3X1	T44.3X2	T44.3X3	T44.3X4	T44.3X5	T44.3X6
Octotiamine	T45.2X1	T45.2X2	T45.2X3	T45.2X4	T45.2X5	T45.2X6
Octoxinol (9)	T49.8X1	T49.8X2	T49.8X3	T49.8X4	T49.8X5	T49.8X6
Octreotide	T38.991	T38.992	T38.993	T38.994	T38.995	T38.996
Octyl nitrite	T46.3X1	T46.3X2	T46.3X3	T46.3X4	T46.3X5	T46.3X6
Oestradiol	T38.5X1	T38.5X2	T38.5X3	T38.5X4	T38.5X5	T38.5X6
Oestriol	T38.5X1	T38.5X2	T38.5X3	T38.5X4	T38.5X5	T38.5X6
Oestrogen	T38.5X1	T38.5X2	T38.5X3	T38.5X4	T38.5X5	T38.5X6
Oestrone	T38.5X1	T38.5X2	T38.5X3	T38.5X4	T38.5X5	T38.5X6
Ofloxacin	T36.8X1	T36.8X2	T36.8X3	T36.8X4	T36.8X5	T36.8X6
Oil (of)	T65.891	T65.892	T65.893	T65.894	—	—
bitter almond	T62.8X1	T62.8X2	T62.8X3	T62.8X4	—	—
cloves	T49.7X1	T49.7X2	T49.7X3	T49.7X4	T49.7X5	T49.7X6
colors	T65.6X1	T65.6X2	T65.6X3	T65.6X4	—	—
fumes	T59.891	T59.892	T59.893	T59.894	—	—
lubricating	T52.0X1	T52.0X2	T52.0X3	T52.0X4	—	—
Niobe	T52.8X1	T52.8X2	T52.8X3	T52.8X4	—	—

	External Cause (T-Code)					
Substance	Poisoning, Accidental (Unintentional)	Poisoning, Intentional Self-Harm	Poisoning, Assault	Poisoning, Undetermined	Adverse Effect	Underdosing
Oil (of) *(Continued)*						
vitriol (liquid)	T54.2X1	T54.2X2	T54.2X3	T54.2X4	—	—
fumes	T54.2X1	T54.2X2	T54.2X3	T54.2X4	—	—
wintergreen (bitter) NEC	T49.3X1	T49.3X2	T49.3X3	T49.3X4	T49.3X5	T49.3X6
Oily preparation (for skin)	T49.3X1	T49.3X2	T49.3X3	T49.3X4	T49.3X5	T49.3X6
Ointment NEC	T49.3X1	T49.3X2	T49.3X3	T49.3X4	T49.3X5	T49.3X6
Olanzapine	T43.591	T43.592	T43.593	T43.594	T43.595	T43.596
Oleander	T62.2X1	T62.2X2	T62.2X3	T62.2X4	—	—
Oleandomycin	T36.3X1	T36.3X2	T36.3X3	T36.3X4	T36.3X5	T36.3X6
Oleandrin	T46.0X1	T46.0X2	T46.0X3	T46.0X4	T46.0X5	T46.0X6
Oleic acid	T46.6X1	T46.6X2	T46.6X3	T46.6X4	T46.6X5	T46.6X6
Oleovitamin A	T45.2X1	T45.2X2	T45.2X3	T45.2X4	T45.2X5	T45.2X6
Oleum ricini	T47.2X1	T47.2X2	T47.2X3	T47.2X4	T47.2X5	T47.2X6
Olive oil (medicinal) NEC	T47.4X1	T47.4X2	T47.4X3	T47.4X4	T47.4X5	T47.4X6
Olivomycin	T45.1X1	T45.1X2	T45.1X3	T45.1X4	T45.1X5	T45.1X6
Olsalazine	T47.8X1	T47.8X2	T47.8X3	T47.8X4	T47.8X5	T47.8X6
Omeprazole	T47.1X1	T47.1X2	T47.1X3	T47.1X4	T47.1X5	T47.1X6
OMPA	T60.0X1	T60.0X2	T60.0X3	T60.0X4	—	—
Ondansetron	T45.0X1	T45.0X2	T45.0X3	T45.0X4	T45.0X5	T45.0X6
Oncovin	T45.1X1	T45.1X2	T45.1X3	T45.1X4	T45.1X5	T45.1X6
Ophthaine	T41.3X1	T41.3X2	T41.3X3	T41.3X4	T41.3X5	T41.3X6
Ophthetic	T41.3X1	T41.3X2	T41.3X3	T41.3X4	T41.3X5	T41.3X6
Opiate NEC	T40.601	T40.602	T40.603	T40.604	T40.605	T40.606
antagonists	T50.7X1	T50.7X2	T50.7X3	T50.7X4	T50.7X5	T50.7X6
Opioid NEC	T40.2X1	T40.2X2	T40.2X3	T40.2X4	T40.2X5	T40.2X6
Opipramol	T43.011	T43.012	T43.013	T43.014	T43.015	T43.016
Opium alkaloids (total)	T40.0X1	T40.0X2	T40.0X3	T40.0X4	T40.0X5	T40.0X6
standardized powdered	T40.0X1	T40.0X2	T40.0X3	T40.0X4	T40.0X5	T40.0X6
tincture (camphorated)	T40.0X1	T40.0X2	T40.0X3	T40.0X4	T40.0X5	T40.0X6
Oracon	T38.4X1	T38.4X2	T38.4X3	T38.4X4	T38.4X5	T38.4X6
Oragrafin	T50.8X1	T50.8X2	T50.8X3	T50.8X4	T50.8X5	T50.8X6
Oral contraceptives	T38.4X1	T38.4X2	T38.4X3	T38.4X4	T38.4X5	T38.4X6
Oral rehydration salts	T50.3X1	T50.3X2	T50.3X3	T50.3X4	T50.3X5	T50.3X6
Orazamide	T50.991	T50.992	T50.993	T50.994	T50.995	T50.996
Orciprenaline	T48.291	T48.292	T48.293	T48.294	T48.295	T48.296
Organidin	T48.4X1	T48.4X2	T48.4X3	T48.4X4	T48.4X5	T48.4X6
Organonitrate NEC	T46.3X1	T46.3X2	T46.3X3	T46.3X4	T46.3X5	T46.3X6
Organophosphates	T60.0X1	T60.0X2	T60.0X3	T60.0X4	—	—
Orimune	T50.B91	T50.B92	T50.B93	T50.B94	T50.B95	T50.B96
Orinase	T38.3X1	T38.3X2	T38.3X3	T38.3X4	T38.3X5	T38.3X6
Ormeloxifene	T38.6X1	T38.6X2	T38.6X3	T38.6X4	T38.6X5	T38.6X6

◄ New   ◀▥ Revised   ~~deleted~~ Deleted

TABLE OF DRUGS AND CHEMICALS

Substance	External Cause (T-Code) Poisoning, Accidental (Unintentional)	Poisoning, Intentional Self-Harm	Poisoning, Assault	Poisoning, Undetermined	Adverse Effect	Underdosing
Ornidazole	T37.3X1	T37.3X2	T37.3X3	T37.3X4	T37.3X5	T37.3X6
Ornithine aspartate	T50.991	T50.992	T50.993	T50.994	T50.995	T50.996
Ornoprostil	T47.1X1	T47.1X2	T47.1X3	T47.1X4	T47.1X5	T47.1X6
Orphenadrine (hydrochloride)	T42.8X1	T42.8X2	T42.8X3	T42.8X4	T42.8X5	T42.8X6
Ortal (sodium)	T42.3X1	T42.3X2	T42.3X3	T42.3X4	T42.3X5	T42.3X6
Orthoboric acid	T49.0X1	T49.0X2	T49.0X3	T49.0X4	T49.0X5	T49.0X6
ENT agent	T49.6X1	T49.6X2	T49.6X3	T49.6X4	T49.6X5	T49.6X6
ophthalmic preparation	T49.5X1	T49.5X2	T49.5X3	T49.5X4	T49.5X5	T49.5X6
Orthocaine	T41.3X1	T41.3X2	T41.3X3	T41.3X4	T41.3X5	T41.3X6
Orthodichlorobenzene	T53.7X1	T53.7X2	T53.7X3	T53.7X4	—	—
Ortho-Novum	T38.4X1	T38.4X2	T38.4X3	T38.4X4	T38.4X5	T38.4X6
Orthotolidine (reagent)	T54.2X1	T54.2X2	T54.2X3	T54.2X4	—	—
Osmic acid (liquid)	T54.2X1	T54.2X2	T54.2X3	T54.2X4	—	—
fumes	T54.2X1	T54.2X2	T54.2X3	T54.2X4	—	—
Osmotic diuretics	T50.2X1	T50.2X2	T50.2X3	T50.2X4	T50.2X5	T50.2X6
Otilonium bromide	T44.3X1	T44.3X2	T44.3X3	T44.3X4	T44.3X5	T44.3X6
Otorhinolaryngological drug NEC	T49.6X1	T49.6X2	T49.6X3	T49.6X4	T49.6X5	T49.6X6
Ouabain(e)	T46.0X1	T46.0X2	T46.0X3	T46.0X4	T46.0X5	T46.0X6
Ovarian						
hormone	T38.5X1	T38.5X2	T38.5X3	T38.5X4	T38.5X5	T38.5X6
stimulant	T38.5X1	T38.5X2	T38.5X3	T38.5X4	T38.5X5	T38.5X6
Ovral	T38.4X1	T38.4X2	T38.4X3	T38.4X4	T38.4X5	T38.4X6
Ovulen	T38.4X1	T38.4X2	T38.4X3	T38.4X4	T38.4X5	T38.4X6
Oxacillin	T36.0X1	T36.0X2	T36.0X3	T36.0X4	T36.0X5	T36.0X6
Oxalic acid	T54.2X1	T54.2X2	T54.2X3	T54.2X4	—	—
ammonium salt	T50.991	T50.992	T50.993	T50.994	T50.995	T50.996
Oxamniquine	T37.4X1	T37.4X2	T37.4X3	T37.4X4	T37.4X5	T37.4X6
Oxanamide	T43.591	T43.592	T43.593	T43.594	T43.595	T43.596
Oxandrolone	T38.7X1	T38.7X2	T38.7X3	T38.7X4	T38.7X5	T38.7X6
Oxantel	T37.4X1	T37.4X2	T37.4X3	T37.4X4	T37.4X5	T37.4X6
Oxapium iodide	T44.3X1	T44.3X2	T44.3X3	T44.3X4	T44.3X5	T44.3X6
Oxaprotiline	T43.021	T43.022	T43.023	T43.024	T43.025	T43.026
Oxaprozin	T39.311	T39.312	T39.313	T39.314	T39.315	T39.316
Oxatomide	T45.0X1	T45.0X2	T45.0X3	T45.0X4	T45.0X5	T45.0X6
Oxazepam	T42.4X1	T42.4X2	T42.4X3	T42.4X4	T42.4X5	T42.4X6
Oxazimedrine	T50.5X1	T50.5X2	T50.5X3	T50.5X4	T50.5X5	T50.5X6
Oxazolam	T42.4X1	T42.4X2	T42.4X3	T42.4X4	T42.4X5	T42.4X6
Oxazolidine derivatives	T42.2X1	T42.2X2	T42.2X3	T42.2X4	T42.2X5	T42.2X6
Oxazolidinedione (derivative)	T42.2X1	T42.2X2	T42.2X3	T42.2X4	T42.2X5	T42.2X6
Ox bile extract	T47.5X1	T47.5X2	T47.5X3	T47.5X4	T47.5X5	T47.5X6
Oxcarbazepine	T42.1X1	T42.1X2	T42.1X3	T42.1X4	T42.1X5	T42.1X6
Oxedrine	T44.4X1	T44.4X2	T44.4X3	T44.4X4	T44.4X5	T44.4X6

Substance	External Cause (T-Code) Poisoning, Accidental (Unintentional)	Poisoning, Intentional Self-Harm	Poisoning, Assault	Poisoning, Undetermined	Adverse Effect	Underdosing
Oxeladin (citrate)	T48.3X1	T48.3X2	T48.3X3	T48.3X4	T48.3X5	T48.3X6
Oxendolone	T38.5X1	T38.5X2	T38.5X3	T38.5X4	T38.5X5	T38.5X6
Oxetacaine	T41.3X1	T41.3X2	T41.3X3	T41.3X4	T41.3X5	T41.3X6
Oxethazine	T41.3X1	T41.3X2	T41.3X3	T41.3X4	T41.3X5	T41.3X6
Oxetorone	T39.8X1	T39.8X2	T39.8X3	T39.8X4	T39.8X5	T39.8X6
Oxiconazole	T49.0X1	T49.0X2	T49.0X3	T49.0X4	T49.0X5	T49.0X6
Oxidizing agent NEC	T54.91	T54.92	T54.93	T54.94	—	—
Oxipurinol	T50.4X1	T50.4X2	T50.4X3	T50.4X4	T50.4X5	T50.4X6
Oxitriptan	T43.291	T43.292	T43.293	T43.294	T43.295	T43.296
Oxitropium bromide	T48.6X1	T48.6X2	T48.6X3	T48.6X4	T48.6X5	T48.6X6
Oxodipine	T46.1X1	T46.1X2	T46.1X3	T46.1X4	T46.1X5	T46.1X6
Oxolamine	T48.3X1	T48.3X2	T48.3X3	T48.3X4	T48.3X5	T48.3X6
Oxolinic acid	T37.8X1	T37.8X2	T37.8X3	T37.8X4	T37.8X5	T37.8X6
Oxomemazine	T43.3X1	T43.3X2	T43.3X3	T43.3X4	T43.3X5	T43.3X6
Oxophenarsine	T37.3X1	T37.3X2	T37.3X3	T37.3X4	T37.3X5	T37.3X6
Oxprenolol	T44.7X1	T44.7X2	T44.7X3	T44.7X4	T44.7X5	T44.7X6
Oxsoralen	T49.3X1	T49.3X2	T49.3X3	T49.3X4	T49.3X5	T49.3X6
Oxtriphylline	T48.6X1	T48.6X2	T48.6X3	T48.6X4	T48.6X5	T48.6X6
Oxybate sodium	T41.291	T41.292	T41.293	T41.294	T41.295	T41.296
Oxybuprocaine	T41.3X1	T41.3X2	T41.3X3	T41.3X4	T41.3X5	T41.3X6
Oxybutynin	T44.3X1	T44.3X2	T44.3X3	T44.3X4	T44.3X5	T44.3X6
Oxychlorosene	T49.0X1	T49.0X2	T49.0X3	T49.0X4	T49.0X5	T49.0X6
Oxycodone	T40.2X1	T40.2X2	T40.2X3	T40.2X4	T40.2X5	T40.2X6
Oxyfedrine	T46.3X1	T46.3X2	T46.3X3	T46.3X4	T46.3X5	T46.3X6
Oxygen	T41.5X1	T41.5X2	T41.5X3	T41.5X4	T41.5X5	T41.5X6
Oxylone	T49.0X1	T49.0X2	T49.0X3	T49.0X4	T49.0X5	T49.0X6
ophthalmic preparation	T49.5X1	T49.5X2	T49.5X3	T49.5X4	T49.5X5	T49.5X6
Oxymesterone	T38.7X1	T38.7X2	T38.7X3	T38.7X4	T38.7X5	T38.7X6
Oxymetazoline	T48.5X1	T48.5X2	T48.5X3	T48.5X4	T48.5X5	T48.5X6
Oxymetholone	T38.7X1	T38.7X2	T38.7X3	T38.7X4	T38.7X5	T38.7X6
Oxymorphone	T40.2X1	T40.2X2	T40.2X3	T40.2X4	T40.2X5	T40.2X6
Oxypertine	T43.591	T43.592	T43.593	T43.594	T43.595	T43.596
Oxyphenbutazone	T39.2X1	T39.2X2	T39.2X3	T39.2X4	T39.2X5	T39.2X6
Oxyphencyclimine	T44.3X1	T44.3X2	T44.3X3	T44.3X4	T44.3X5	T44.3X6
Oxyphenisatine	T47.2X1	T47.2X2	T47.2X3	T47.2X4	T47.2X5	T47.2X6
Oxyphenonium bromide	T44.3X1	T44.3X2	T44.3X3	T44.3X4	T44.3X5	T44.3X6
Oxypolygelatin	T45.8X1	T45.8X2	T45.8X3	T45.8X4	T45.8X5	T45.8X6
Oxyquinoline (derivatives)	T37.8X1	T37.8X2	T37.8X3	T37.8X4	T37.8X5	T37.8X6
Oxytetracycline	T36.4X1	T36.4X2	T36.4X3	T36.4X4	T36.4X5	T36.4X6
Oxytocic drug NEC	T48.0X1	T48.0X2	T48.0X3	T48.0X4	T48.0X5	T48.0X6
Oxytocin (synthetic)	T48.0X1	T48.0X2	T48.0X3	T48.0X4	T48.0X5	T48.0X6
Ozone	T59.891	T59.892	T59.893	T59.894	—	—

◄ New ◄ Revised ~~deleted~~ Deleted

Substance	Poisoning, Accidental (Unintentional)	Poisoning, Intentional Self-Harm	Poisoning, Assault	Poisoning, Undetermined	Adverse Effect	Underdosing
P						
PABA	T49.3X1	T49.3X2	T49.3X3	T49.3X4	T49.3X5	T49.3X6
Packed red cells	T45.8X1	T45.8X2	T45.8X3	T45.8X4	T45.8X5	T45.8X6
Padimate	T49.3X1	T49.3X2	T49.3X3	T49.3X4	T49.3X5	T49.3X6
Paint NEC	T65.6X1	T65.6X2	T65.6X3	T65.6X4	—	—
cleaner	T52.91	T52.92	T52.93	T52.94	—	—
fumes NEC	T59.891	T59.892	T59.893	T59.894	—	—
lead (fumes)	T56.0X1	T56.0X2	T56.0X3	T56.0X4	—	—
solvent NEC	T52.8X1	T52.8X2	T52.8X3	T52.8X4	—	—
stripper	T52.8X1	T52.8X2	T52.8X3	T52.8X4	—	—
Palfium	T40.2X1	T40.2X2	T40.2X3	T40.2X4	—	—
Palm kernel oil	T50.991	T50.992	T50.993	T50.994	T50.995	T50.996
Paludrine	T37.2X1	T37.2X2	T37.2X3	T37.2X4	T37.2X5	T37.2X6
PAM (pralidoxime)	T50.6X1	T50.6X2	T50.6X3	T50.6X4	T50.6X5	T50.6X6
Pamaquine (naphthoute)	T37.2X1	T37.2X2	T37.2X3	T37.2X4	T37.2X5	T37.2X6
Panadol	T39.1X1	T39.1X2	T39.1X3	T39.1X4	T39.1X5	T39.1X6
Pancreatic						
digestive secretion stimulant	T47.8X1	T47.8X2	T47.8X3	T47.8X4	T47.8X5	T47.8X6
dornase	T45.3X1	T45.3X2	T45.3X3	T45.3X4	T45.3X5	T45.3X6
Pancreatin	T47.5X1	T47.5X2	T47.5X3	T47.5X4	T47.5X5	T47.5X6
Pancrelipase	T47.5X1	T47.5X2	T47.5X3	T47.5X4	T47.5X5	T47.5X6
Pancuronium (bromide)	T48.1X1	T48.1X2	T48.1X3	T48.1X4	T48.1X5	T48.1X6
Pangamic acid	T45.2X1	T45.2X2	T45.2X3	T45.2X4	T45.2X5	T45.2X6
Panthenol	T45.2X1	T45.2X2	T45.2X3	T45.2X4	T45.2X5	T45.2X6
topical	T49.8X1	T49.8X2	T49.8X3	T49.8X4	T49.8X5	T49.8X6
Pantopon	T40.0X1	T40.0X2	T40.0X3	T40.0X4	T40.0X5	T40.0X6
Pantothenic acid	T45.2X1	T45.2X2	T45.2X3	T45.2X4	T45.2X5	T45.2X6
Panwarfin	T45.511	T45.512	T45.513	T45.514	T45.515	T45.516
Papain	T47.5X1	T47.5X2	T47.5X3	T47.5X4	T47.5X5	T47.5X6
digestant	T47.5X1	T47.5X2	T47.5X3	T47.5X4	T47.5X5	T47.5X6
Papaveretum	T40.0X1	T40.0X2	T40.0X3	T40.0X4	T40.0X5	T40.0X6
Papaverine	T44.3X1	T44.3X2	T44.3X3	T44.3X4	T44.3X5	T44.3X6
Para-acetamidophenol	T39.1X1	T39.1X2	T39.1X3	T39.1X4	T39.1X5	T39.1X6
Para-aminobenzoic acid	T49.3X1	T49.3X2	T49.3X3	T49.3X4	T49.3X5	T49.3X6
Para-aminophenol derivatives	T39.1X1	T39.1X2	T39.1X3	T39.1X4	T39.1X5	T39.1X6
Para-aminosalicylic acid	T37.1X1	T37.1X2	T37.1X3	T37.1X4	T37.1X5	T37.1X6
Paracetaldehyde	T42.6X1	T42.6X2	T42.6X3	T42.6X4	T42.6X5	T42.6X6
Paracetamol	T39.1X1	T39.1X2	T39.1X3	T39.1X4	T39.1X5	T39.1X6
Parachlorophenol (camphorated)	T49.0X1	T49.0X2	T49.0X3	T49.0X4	T49.0X5	T49.0X6
Paracodin	T40.2X1	T40.2X2	T40.2X3	T40.2X4	T40.2X5	T40.2X6
Paradione	T42.2X1	T42.2X2	T42.2X3	T42.2X4	T42.2X5	T42.2X6

Substance	Poisoning, Accidental (Unintentional)	Poisoning, Intentional Self-Harm	Poisoning, Assault	Poisoning, Undetermined	Adverse Effect	Underdosing
Paraffin(s) (wax)	T52.0X1	T52.0X2	T52.0X3	T52.0X4	—	—
liquid (medicinal)	T47.4X1	T47.4X2	T47.4X3	T47.4X4	T47.4X5	T47.4X6
nonmedicinal	T52.0X1	T52.0X2	T52.0X3	T52.0X4		
Paraformaldehyde	T60.3X1	T60.3X2	T60.3X3	T60.3X4	—	—
Paraldehyde	T42.6X1	T42.6X2	T42.6X3	T42.6X4	T42.6X5	T42.6X6
Paramethadione	T42.2X1	T42.2X2	T42.2X3	T42.2X4	T42.2X5	T42.2X6
Paramethasone	T38.0X1	T38.0X2	T38.0X3	T38.0X4	T38.0X5	T38.0X6
acetate	T49.0X1	T49.0X2	T49.0X3	T49.0X4	T49.0X5	T49.0X6
Paraoxon	T60.0X1	T60.0X2	T60.0X3	T60.0X4	—	—
Paraquat	T60.3X1	T60.3X2	T60.3X3	T60.3X4	—	—
Parasympatholytic NEC	T44.3X1	T44.3X2	T44.3X3	T44.3X4	T44.3X5	T44.3X6
Parasympathomimetic drug NEC	T44.1X1	T44.1X2	T44.1X3	T44.1X4	T44.1X5	T44.1X6
Parathion	T60.0X1	T60.0X2	T60.0X3	T60.0X4	—	—
Parathormone	T50.991	T50.992	T50.993	T50.994	T50.995	T50.996
Parathyroid extract	T50.991	T50.992	T50.993	T50.994	T50.995	T50.996
Paratyphoid vaccine	T50.A91	T50.A92	T50.A93	T50.A94	T50.A95	T50.A96
Paredrine	T44.4X1	T44.4X2	T44.4X3	T44.4X4	T44.4X5	T44.4X6
Paregoric	T40.0X1	T40.0X2	T40.0X3	T40.0X4	T40.0X5	T40.0X6
Pargyline	T46.5X1	T46.5X2	T46.5X3	T46.5X4	T46.5X5	T46.5X6
Paris green	T57.0X1	T57.0X2	T57.0X3	T57.0X4	—	—
insecticide	T57.0X1	T57.0X2	T57.0X3	T57.0X4	—	—
Parnate	T43.1X1	T43.1X2	T43.1X3	T43.1X4	T43.1X5	T43.1X6
Paromomycin	T36.5X1	T36.5X2	T36.5X3	T36.5X4	T36.5X5	T36.5X6
Paroxypropione	T45.1X1	T45.1X2	T45.1X3	T45.1X4	T45.1X5	T45.1X6
Parzone	T40.2X1	T40.2X2	T40.2X3	T40.2X4	T40.2X5	T40.2X6
PAS	T37.1X1	T37.1X2	T37.1X3	T37.1X4	T37.1X5	T37.1X6
Pasiniazid	T37.1X1	T37.1X2	T37.1X3	T37.1X4	T37.1X5	T37.1X6
PBB (polybrominated biphenyls)	T65.891	T65.892	T65.893	T65.894	—	—
PCB	T65.891	T65.892	T65.893	T65.894	—	—
PCP						
meaning pentachlorophenol	T60.1X1	T60.1X2	T60.1X3	T60.1X4		
fungicide	T60.3X1	T60.3X2	T60.3X3	T60.3X4		
herbicide	T60.3X1	T60.3X2	T60.3X3	T60.3X4		
insecticide	T60.1X1	T60.1X2	T60.1X3	T60.1X4		
meaning phencyclidine	T40.991	T40.992	T40.993	T40.994	—	—
Peach kernel oil (emulsion)	T47.4X1	T47.4X2	T47.4X3	T47.4X4	T47.4X5	T47.4X6
Peanut oil (emulsion) NEC	T47.4X1	T47.4X2	T47.4X3	T47.4X4	T47.4X5	T47.4X6
topical	T49.3X1	T49.3X2	T49.3X3	T49.3X4	T49.3X5	T49.3X6
Pearly Gates (morning glory seeds)	T40.991	T40.992	T40.993	T40.994	—	—
Pecazine	T43.3X1	T43.3X2	T43.3X3	T43.3X4	T43.3X5	T43.3X6
Pectin	T47.6X1	T47.6X2	T47.6X3	T47.6X4	T47.6X5	T47.6X6

◄ New ◀▥ Revised ~~deleted~~ Deleted

TABLE OF DRUGS AND CHEMICALS

	External Cause (T-Code)					
Substance	Poisoning, Accidental (Unintentional)	Poisoning, Intentional Self-Harm	Poisoning, Assault	Poisoning, Undetermined	Adverse Effect	Underdosing
Pefloxacin	T37.8X1	T37.8X2	T37.8X3	T37.8X4	T37.8X5	T37.8X6
Pegademase, bovine	T50.Z91	T50.Z92	T50.Z93	T50.Z94	T50.Z95	T50.Z96
Pelletierine tannate	T37.4X1	T37.4X2	T37.4X3	T37.4X4	T37.4X5	T37.4X6
Pemirolast (potassium)	T48.6X1	T48.6X2	T48.6X3	T48.6X4	T48.6X5	T48.6X6
Pemoline	T50.7X1	T50.7X2	T50.7X3	T50.7X4	T50.7X5	T50.7X6
Pempidine	T44.2X1	T44.2X2	T44.2X3	T44.2X4	T44.2X5	T44.2X6
Penamecillin	T36.0X1	T36.0X2	T36.0X3	T36.0X4	T36.0X5	T36.0X6
Penbutolol	T44.7X1	T44.7X2	T44.7X3	T44.7X4	T44.7X5	T44.7X6
Penethamate	T36.0X1	T36.0X2	T36.0X3	T36.0X4	T36.0X5	T36.0X6
Penfluridol	T43.591	T43.592	T43.593	T43.594	T43.595	T43.596
Penflutizide	T50.2X1	T50.2X2	T50.2X3	T50.2X4	T50.2X5	T50.2X6
Pengitoxin	T46.0X1	T46.0X2	T46.0X3	T46.0X4	T46.0X5	T46.0X6
Penicillamine	T50.6X1	T50.6X2	T50.6X3	T50.6X4	T50.6X5	T50.6X6
Penicillin (any)	T36.0X1	T36.0X2	T36.0X3	T36.0X4	T36.0X5	T36.0X6
Penicillinase	T45.3X1	T45.3X2	T45.3X3	T45.3X4	T45.3X5	T45.3X6
Penicilloyl polylysine	T50.8X1	T50.8X2	T50.8X3	T50.8X4	T50.8X5	T50.8X6
Penimepicycline	T36.4X1	T36.4X2	T36.4X3	T36.4X4	T36.4X5	T36.4X6
Pentachloroethane	T53.6X1	T53.6X2	T53.6X3	T53.6X4	—	—
Pentachloronaphthalene	T53.7X1	T53.7X2	T53.7X3	T53.7X4	—	—
Pentachlorophenol (pesticide)	T60.1X1	T60.1X2	T60.1X3	T60.1X4	—	—
fungicide	T60.3X1	T60.3X2	T60.3X3	T60.3X4	—	—
herbicide	T60.3X1	T60.3X2	T60.3X3	T60.3X4	—	—
insecticide	T60.1X1	T60.1X2	T60.1X3	T60.1X4	—	—
Pentaerythritol tetranitrate	T46.3X1	T46.3X2	T46.3X3	T46.3X4	T46.3X5	T46.3X6
Pentaerythritol	T46.3X1	T46.3X2	T46.3X3	T46.3X4	T46.3X5	T46.3X6
chloral	T42.6X1	T42.6X2	T42.6X3	T42.6X4	T42.6X5	T42.6X6
tetranitrate NEC	T46.3X1	T46.3X2	T46.3X3	T46.3X4	T46.3X5	T46.3X6
Pentagastrin	T50.8X1	T50.8X2	T50.8X3	T50.8X4	T50.8X5	T50.8X6
Pentalin	T53.6X1	T53.6X2	T53.6X3	T53.6X4	—	—
Pentamethonium bromide	T44.2X1	T44.2X2	T44.2X3	T44.2X4	T44.2X5	T44.2X6
Pentamidine	T37.3X1	T37.3X2	T37.3X3	T37.3X4	T37.3X5	T37.3X6
Pentanol	T51.3X1	T51.3X2	T51.3X3	T51.3X4	—	—
Pentapyrrolinium (bitartrate)	T44.2X1	T44.2X2	T44.2X3	T44.2X4	T44.2X5	T44.2X6
Pentaquine	T37.2X1	T37.2X2	T37.2X3	T37.2X4	T37.2X5	T37.2X6
Pentazocine	T40.4X1	T40.4X2	T40.4X3	T40.4X4	T40.4X5	T40.4X6
Pentetrazole	T50.7X1	T50.7X2	T50.7X3	T50.7X4	T50.7X5	T50.7X6
Penthienate bromide	T44.3X1	T44.3X2	T44.3X3	T44.3X4	T44.3X5	T44.3X6
Pentifylline	T46.7X1	T46.7X2	T46.7X3	T46.7X4	T46.7X5	T46.7X6
Pentobarbital	T42.3X1	T42.3X2	T42.3X3	T42.3X4	T42.3X5	T42.3X6
sodium	T42.3X1	T42.3X2	T42.3X3	T42.3X4	T42.3X5	T42.3X6
Pentobarbitone	T42.3X1	T42.3X2	T42.3X3	T42.3X4	T42.3X5	T42.3X6
Pentolonium tartrate	T44.2X1	T44.2X2	T44.2X3	T44.2X4	T44.2X5	T44.2X6

	External Cause (T-Code)					
Substance	Poisoning, Accidental (Unintentional)	Poisoning, Intentional Self-Harm	Poisoning, Assault	Poisoning, Undetermined	Adverse Effect	Underdosing
Pentosan polysulfate (sodium)	T39.8X1	T39.8X2	T39.8X3	T39.8X4	T39.8X5	T39.8X6
Pentostatin	T45.1X1	T45.1X2	T45.1X3	T45.1X4	T45.1X5	T45.1X6
Pentothal	T41.1X1	T41.1X2	T41.1X3	T41.1X4	T41.1X5	T41.1X6
Pentoxifylline	T46.7X1	T46.7X2	T46.7X3	T46.7X4	T46.7X5	T46.7X6
Pentoxyverine	T48.3X1	T48.3X2	T48.3X3	T48.3X4	T48.3X5	T48.3X6
Pentrinat	T46.3X1	T46.3X2	T46.3X3	T46.3X4	T46.3X5	T46.3X6
Pentylenetetrazole	T50.7X1	T50.7X2	T50.7X3	T50.7X4	T50.7X5	T50.7X6
Pentylsalicylamide	T37.1X1	T37.1X2	T37.1X3	T37.1X4	T37.1X5	T37.1X6
Pentymal	T42.3X1	T42.3X2	T42.3X3	T42.3X4	T42.3X5	T42.3X6
Peplomycin	T45.1X1	T45.1X2	T45.1X3	T45.1X4	T45.1X5	T45.1X6
Peppermint (oil)	T47.5X1	T47.5X2	T47.5X3	T47.5X4	T47.5X5	T47.5X6
Pepsin	T47.5X1	T47.5X2	T47.5X3	T47.5X4	T47.5X5	T47.5X6
digestant	T47.5X1	T47.5X2	T47.5X3	T47.5X4	T47.5X5	T47.5X6
Pepstatin	T47.1X1	T47.1X2	T47.1X3	T47.1X4	T47.1X5	T47.1X6
Peptavlon	T50.8X1	T50.8X2	T50.8X3	T50.8X4	T50.8X5	T50.8X6
Perazine	T43.3X1	T43.3X2	T43.3X3	T43.3X4	T43.3X5	T43.3X6
Percaine (spinal)	T41.3X1	T41.3X2	T41.3X3	T41.3X4	T41.3X5	T41.3X6
topical (surface)	T41.3X1	T41.3X2	T41.3X3	T41.3X4	T41.3X5	T41.3X6
Perchloroethylene	T53.3X1	T53.3X2	T53.3X3	T53.3X4	—	—
medicinal	T37.4X1	T37.4X2	T37.4X3	T37.4X4	T37.4X5	T37.4X6
vapor	T53.3X1	T53.3X2	T53.3X3	T53.3X4	—	—
Percodan	T40.2X1	T40.2X2	T40.2X3	T40.2X4	T40.2X5	T40.2X6
Percogesic — see also acetaminophen	T45.0X1	T45.0X2	T45.0X3	T45.0X4	T45.0X5	T45.0X6
Percorten	T38.0X1	T38.0X2	T38.0X3	T38.0X4	T38.0X5	T38.0X6
Pergolide	T42.8X1	T42.8X2	T42.8X3	T42.8X4	T42.8X5	T42.8X6
Pergonal	T38.811	T38.812	T38.813	T38.814	T38.815	T38.816
Perhexilene	T46.3X1	T46.3X2	T46.3X3	T46.3X4	T46.3X5	T46.3X6
Perhexiline (maleate)	T46.3X1	T46.3X2	T46.3X3	T46.3X4	T46.3X5	T46.3X6
Periactin	T45.0X1	T45.0X2	T45.0X3	T45.0X4	T45.0X5	T45.0X6
Periciazine	T43.3X1	T43.3X2	T43.3X3	T43.3X4	T43.3X5	T43.3X6
Periclor	T42.6X1	T42.6X2	T42.6X3	T42.6X4	T42.6X5	T42.6X6
Perindopril	T46.4X1	T46.4X2	T46.4X3	T46.4X4	T46.4X5	T46.4X6
Perisoxal	T39.8X1	T39.8X2	T39.8X3	T39.8X4	T39.8X5	T39.8X6
Peritrate	T46.3X1	T46.3X2	T46.3X3	T46.3X4	T46.3X5	T46.3X6
Peritoneal dialysis solution	T50.3X1	T50.3X2	T50.3X3	T50.3X4	T50.3X5	T50.3X6
Perlapine	T42.4X1	T42.4X2	T42.4X3	T42.4X4	T42.4X5	T42.4X6
Permanganate	T65.891	T65.892	T65.893	T65.894	—	—
Permethrin	T60.1X1	T60.1X2	T60.1X3	T60.1X4	—	—
Pernocton	T42.3X1	T42.3X2	T42.3X3	T42.3X4	T42.3X5	T42.3X6
Pernoston	T42.3X1	T42.3X2	T42.3X3	T42.3X4	T42.3X5	T42.3X6
Peronine	T40.2X1	T40.2X2	T40.2X3	T40.2X4	—	—
Perphenazine	T43.3X1	T43.3X2	T43.3X3	T43.3X4	T43.3X5	T43.3X6

◀ New ◀ Revised ~~deleted~~ Deleted

Substance	Poisoning, Accidental (Unintentional)	Poisoning, Intentional Self-Harm	Poisoning, Assault	Poisoning, Undetermined	Adverse Effect	Underdosing
Pertofrane	T43.Ø11	T43.Ø12	T43.Ø13	T43.Ø14	T43.Ø15	T43.Ø16
Pertussis						
immune serum (human)	T5Ø.Z11	T5Ø.Z12	T5Ø.Z13	T5Ø.Z14	T5Ø.Z15	T5Ø.Z16
vaccine (with diphtheria toxoid) (with tetanus toxoid)	T5Ø.A11	T5Ø.A12	T5Ø.A13	T5Ø.A14	T5Ø.A15	T5Ø.A16
Peruvian balsam	T49.ØX1	T49.ØX2	T49.ØX3	T49.ØX4	T49.ØX5	T49.ØX6
Peruvoside	T46.ØX1	T46.ØX2	T46.ØX3	T46.ØX4	T46.ØX5	T46.ØX6
Pesticide (dust) (fumes) (vapor) NEC	T6Ø.91	T6Ø.92	T6Ø.93	T6Ø.94	—	—
arsenic	T57.ØX1	T57.ØX2	T57.ØX3	T57.ØX4	—	—
chlorinated	T6Ø.1X1	T6Ø.1X2	T6Ø.1X3	T6Ø.1X4	—	—
cyanide	T65.ØX1	T65.ØX2	T65.ØX3	T65.ØX4	—	—
kerosene	T52.ØX1	T52.ØX2	T52.ØX3	T52.ØX4	—	—
mixture (of compounds)	T6Ø.91	T6Ø.92	T6Ø.93	T6Ø.94	—	—
naphthalene	T6Ø.2X1	T6Ø.2X2	T6Ø.2X3	T6Ø.2X4	—	—
organochlorine (compounds)	T6Ø.1X1	T6Ø.1X2	T6Ø.1X3	T6Ø.1X4	—	—
petroleum (distillate) (products) NEC	T6Ø.8X1	T6Ø.8X2	T6Ø.8X3	T6Ø.8X4	—	—
specified ingredient NEC	T6Ø.8X1	T6Ø.8X2	T6Ø.8X3	T6Ø.8X4	—	—
strychnine	T65.1X1	T65.1X2	T65.1X3	T65.1X4	—	—
thallium	T6Ø.4X1	T6Ø.4X2	T6Ø.4X3	T6Ø.4X4	—	—
Pethidine	T4Ø.4X1	T4Ø.4X2	T4Ø.4X3	T4Ø.4X4	T4Ø.4X5	T4Ø.4X6
Petrichloral	T42.6X1	T42.6X2	T42.6X3	T42.6X4	T42.6X5	T42.6X6
Petrol	T52.ØX1	T52.ØX2	T52.ØX3	T52.ØX4	—	—
vapor	T52.ØX1	T52.ØX2	T52.ØX3	T52.ØX4	—	—
Petrolatum	T49.3X1	T49.3X2	T49.3X3	T49.3X4	T49.3X5	T49.3X6
hydrophilic	T49.3X1	T49.3X2	T49.3X3	T49.3X4	T49.3X5	T49.3X6
liquid	T47.4X1	T47.4X2	T47.4X3	T47.4X4	T47.4X5	T47.4X6
topical	T49.3X1	T49.3X2	T49.3X3	T49.3X4	T49.3X5	T49.3X6
nonmedicinal	T52.ØX1	T52.ØX2	T52.ØX3	T52.ØX4	—	—
red veterinary	T49.3X1	T49.3X2	T49.3X3	T49.3X4	T49.3X5	T49.3X6
white	T49.3X1	T49.3X2	T49.3X3	T49.3X4	T49.3X5	T49.3X6
Petroleum (products) NEC	T52.ØX1	T52.ØX2	T52.ØX3	T52.ØX4	—	—
benzine(s) — see Ligroin						
ether — see Ligroin						
jelly — see Petrolatum						
naphtha — see Ligroin						
pesticide	T6Ø.8X1	T6Ø.8X2	T6Ø.8X3	T6Ø.8X4	—	—
solids	T52.ØX1	T52.ØX2	T52.ØX3	T52.ØX4	—	—
solvents	T52.ØX1	T52.ØX2	T52.ØX3	T52.ØX4	—	—
vapor	T52.ØX1	T52.ØX2	T52.ØX3	T52.ØX4	—	—
Peyote	T4Ø.991	T4Ø.992	T4Ø.993	T4Ø.994	—	—
Phanodorm, phanodorn	T42.3X1	T42.3X2	T42.3X3	T42.3X4	T42.3X5	T42.3X6

Substance	Poisoning, Accidental (Unintentional)	Poisoning, Intentional Self-Harm	Poisoning, Assault	Poisoning, Undetermined	Adverse Effect	Underdosing
Phanquinone	T37.3X1	T37.3X2	T37.3X3	T37.3X4	T37.3X5	T37.3X6
Phanquone	T37.3X1	T37.3X2	T37.3X3	T37.3X4	T37.3X5	T37.3X6
Pharmaceutical						
adjunct NEC	T5Ø.9Ø1	T5Ø.9Ø2	T5Ø.9Ø3	T5Ø.9Ø4	T5Ø.9Ø5	T5Ø.9Ø6
excipient NEC	T5Ø.9Ø1	T5Ø.9Ø2	T5Ø.9Ø3	T5Ø.9Ø4	T5Ø.9Ø5	T5Ø.9Ø6
sweetener	T5Ø.9Ø1	T5Ø.9Ø2	T5Ø.9Ø3	T5Ø.9Ø4	T5Ø.9Ø5	T5Ø.9Ø6
viscous agent	T5Ø.9Ø1	T5Ø.9Ø2	T5Ø.9Ø3	T5Ø.9Ø4	T5Ø.9Ø5	T5Ø.9Ø6
Phemitone	T42.3X1	T42.3X2	T42.3X3	T42.3X4	T42.3X5	T42.3X6
Phenacaine	T41.3X1	T41.3X2	T41.3X3	T41.3X4	T41.3X5	T41.3X6
Phenacemide	T42.6X1	T42.6X2	T42.6X3	T42.6X4	T42.6X5	T42.6X6
Phenacetin	T39.1X1	T39.1X2	T39.1X3	T39.1X4	T39.1X5	T39.1X6
Phenadoxone	T4Ø.2X1	T4Ø.2X2	T4Ø.2X3	T4Ø.2X4	—	—
Phenaglycodol	T43.591	T43.592	T43.593	T43.594	T43.595	T43.596
Phenantoin	T42.ØX1	T42.ØX2	T42.ØX3	T42.ØX4	T42.ØX5	T42.ØX6
Phenaphthazine reagent	T5Ø.991	T5Ø.992	T5Ø.993	T5Ø.994	T5Ø.995	T5Ø.996
Phenazocine	T4Ø.4X1	T4Ø.4X2	T4Ø.4X3	T4Ø.4X4	T4Ø.4X5	T4Ø.4X6
Phenazone	T39.2X1	T39.2X2	T39.2X3	T39.2X4	T39.2X5	T39.2X6
Phenazopyridine	T39.8X1	T39.8X2	T39.8X3	T39.8X4	T39.8X5	T39.8X6
Phenbenicillin	T36.ØX1	T36.ØX2	T36.ØX3	T36.ØX4	T36.ØX5	T36.ØX6
Phenbutrazate	T5Ø.5X1	T5Ø.5X2	T5Ø.5X3	T5Ø.5X4	T5Ø.5X5	T5Ø.5X6
Phencyclidine	T4Ø.991	T4Ø.992	T4Ø.993	T4Ø.994	T4Ø.995	T4Ø.996
Phendimetrazine	T5Ø.5X1	T5Ø.5X2	T5Ø.5X3	T5Ø.5X4	T5Ø.5X5	T5Ø.5X6
Phenelzine	T43.1X1	T43.1X2	T43.1X3	T43.1X4	T43.1X5	T43.1X6
Phenemal	T42.3X1	T42.3X2	T42.3X3	T42.3X4	T42.3X5	T42.3X6
Phenergan	T42.6X1	T42.6X2	T42.6X3	T42.6X4	T42.6X5	T42.6X6
Pheneticillin	T36.ØX1	T36.ØX2	T36.ØX3	T36.ØX4	T36.ØX5	T36.ØX6
Pheneturide	T42.6X1	T42.6X2	T42.6X3	T42.6X4	T42.6X5	T42.6X6
Phenformin	T38.3X1	T38.3X2	T38.3X3	T38.3X4	T38.3X5	T38.3X6
Phenglutarimide	T44.3X1	T44.3X2	T44.3X3	T44.3X4	T44.3X5	T44.3X6
Phenicarbazide	T39.8X1	T39.8X2	T39.8X3	T39.8X4	T39.8X5	T39.8X6
Phenindamine	T45.ØX1	T45.ØX2	T45.ØX3	T45.ØX4	T45.ØX5	T45.ØX6
Phenindione	T45.511	T45.512	T45.513	T45.514	T45.515	T45.516
Pheniprazine	T43.1X1	T43.1X2	T43.1X3	T43.1X4	T43.1X5	T43.1X6
Pheniramine	T45.ØX1	T45.ØX2	T45.ØX3	T45.ØX4	T45.ØX5	T45.ØX6
Phenisatin	T47.2X1	T47.2X2	T47.2X3	T47.2X4	T47.2X5	T47.2X6
Phenmetrazine	T5Ø.5X1	T5Ø.5X2	T5Ø.5X3	T5Ø.5X4	T5Ø.5X5	T5Ø.5X6
Phenobal	T42.3X1	T42.3X2	T42.3X3	T42.3X4	T42.3X5	T42.3X6
Phenobarbital	T42.3X1	T42.3X2	T42.3X3	T42.3X4	T42.3X5	T42.3X6
with						
mephenytoin	T42.3X1	T42.3X2	T42.3X3	T42.3X4	T42.3X5	T42.3X6
phenytoin	T42.3X1	T42.3X2	T42.3X3	T42.3X4	T42.3X5	T42.3X6
sodium	T42.3X1	T42.3X2	T42.3X3	T42.3X4	T42.3X5	T42.3X6

◀ New   ◀ Revised   ~~deleted~~ Deleted

Substance	External Cause (T-Code) Poisoning, Accidental (Unintentional)	Poisoning, Intentional Self-Harm	Poisoning, Assault	Poisoning, Undetermined	Adverse Effect	Underdosing
Phenobarbitone	T42.3X1	T42.3X2	T42.3X3	T42.3X4	T42.3X5	T42.3X6
Phenobutiodil	T50.8X1	T50.8X2	T50.8X3	T50.8X4	T50.8X5	T50.8X6
Phenoctide	T49.0X1	T49.0X2	T49.0X3	T49.0X4	T49.0X5	T49.0X6
Phenol	T49.0X1	T49.0X2	T49.0X3	T49.0X4	T49.0X5	T49.0X6
disinfectant	T54.0X1	T54.0X2	T54.0X3	T54.0X4	—	—
in oil injection	T46.8X1	T46.8X2	T46.8X3	T46.8X4	T46.8X5	T46.8X6
medicinal	T49.1X1	T49.1X2	T49.1X3	T49.1X4	T49.1X5	T49.1X6
nonmedicinal NEC	T54.0X1	T54.0X2	T54.0X3	T54.0X4	—	—
pesticide	T60.8X1	T60.8X2	T60.8X3	T60.8X4	—	—
red	T50.8X1	T50.8X2	T50.8X3	T50.8X4	T50.8X5	T50.8X6
Phenolic preparation	T49.1X1	T49.1X2	T49.1X3	T49.1X4	T49.1X5	T49.1X6
Phenolphthalein	T47.2X1	T47.2X2	T47.2X3	T47.2X4	T47.2X5	T47.2X6
Phenolsulfonphthalein	T50.8X1	T50.8X2	T50.8X3	T50.8X4	T50.8X5	T50.8X6
Phenomorphan	T40.2X1	T40.2X2	T40.2X3	T40.2X4	—	—
Phenonyl	T42.3X1	T42.3X2	T42.3X3	T42.3X4	T42.3X5	T42.3X6
Phenoperidine	T40.4X1	T40.4X2	T40.4X3	T40.4X4	—	—
Phenopyrazone	T46.991	T46.992	T46.993	T46.994	T46.995	T46.996
Phenoquin	T50.4X1	T50.4X2	T50.4X3	T50.4X4	T50.4X5	T50.4X6
Phenothiazine (psychotropic) NEC	T43.3X1	T43.3X2	T43.3X3	T43.3X4	T43.3X5	T43.3X6
insecticide	T60.2X1	T60.2X2	T60.2X3	T60.2X4	—	—
Phenothrin	T49.0X1	T49.0X2	T49.0X3	T49.0X4	T49.0X5	T49.0X6
Phenoxybenzamine	T46.7X1	T46.7X2	T46.7X3	T46.7X4	T46.7X5	T46.7X6
Phenoxyethanol	T49.0X1	T49.0X2	T49.0X3	T49.0X4	T49.0X5	T49.0X6
Phenoxymethyl penicillin	T36.0X1	T36.0X2	T36.0X3	T36.0X4	T36.0X5	T36.0X6
Phenprobamate	T42.8X1	T42.8X2	T42.8X3	T42.8X4	T42.8X5	T42.8X6
Phenprocoumon	T45.511	T45.512	T45.513	T45.514	T45.515	T45.516
Phensuximide	T42.2X1	T42.2X2	T42.2X3	T42.2X4	T42.2X5	T42.2X6
Phentermine	T50.5X1	T50.5X2	T50.5X3	T50.5X4	T50.5X5	T50.5X6
Phenthicillin	T36.0X1	T36.0X2	T36.0X3	T36.0X4	T36.0X5	T36.0X6
Phentolamine	T46.7X1	T46.7X2	T46.7X3	T46.7X4	T46.7X5	T46.7X6
Phenyl						
butazone	T39.2X1	T39.2X2	T39.2X3	T39.2X4	T39.2X5	T39.2X6
enediamine	T65.3X1	T65.3X2	T65.3X3	T65.3X4	—	—
hydrazine	T65.3X1	T65.3X2	T65.3X3	T65.3X4	—	—
antineoplastic	T45.1X1	T45.1X2	T45.1X3	T45.1X4	T45.1X5	T45.1X6
mercuric compounds — see Mercury						
salicylate	T49.3X1	T49.3X2	T49.3X3	T49.3X4	T49.3X5	T49.3X6
Phenylalanine mustard	T45.1X1	T45.1X2	T45.1X3	T45.1X4	T45.1X5	T45.1X6
Phenylbutazone	T39.2X1	T39.2X2	T39.2X3	T39.2X4	T39.2X5	T39.2X6
Phenylenediamine	T65.3X1	T65.3X2	T65.3X3	T65.3X4	—	—
Phenylephrine	T44.4X1	T44.4X2	T44.4X3	T44.4X4	T44.4X5	T44.4X6

Substance	External Cause (T-Code) Poisoning, Accidental (Unintentional)	Poisoning, Intentional Self-Harm	Poisoning, Assault	Poisoning, Undetermined	Adverse Effect	Underdosing
Phenylethylbiguanide	T38.3X1	T38.3X2	T38.3X3	T38.3X4	T38.3X5	T38.3X6
Phenylmercuric						
acetate	T49.0X1	T49.0X2	T49.0X3	T49.0X4	T49.0X5	T49.0X6
borate	T49.0X1	T49.0X2	T49.0X3	T49.0X4	T49.0X5	T49.0X6
nitrate	T49.0X1	T49.0X2	T49.0X3	T49.0X4	T49.0X5	T49.0X6
Phenylmethylbarbitone	T42.3X1	T42.3X2	T42.3X3	T42.3X4	T42.3X5	T42.3X6
Phenylpropanol	T47.5X1	T47.5X2	T47.5X3	T47.5X4	T47.5X5	T47.5X6
Phenylpropanolamine	T44.991	T44.992	T44.993	T44.994	T44.995	T44.996
Phenylsulfthion	T60.0X1	T60.0X2	T60.0X3	T60.0X4	—	—
Phenyltoloxamine	T45.0X1	T45.0X2	T45.0X3	T45.0X4	T45.0X5	T45.0X6
Phenyramidol, phenyramidon	T39.8X1	T39.8X2	T39.8X3	T39.8X4	T39.8X5	T39.8X6
Phenytoin	T42.0X1	T42.0X2	T42.0X3	T42.0X4	T42.0X5	T42.0X6
with Phenobarbital	T42.3X1	T42.3X2	T42.3X3	T42.3X4	T42.3X5	T42.3X6
pHisoHex	T49.2X1	T49.2X2	T49.2X3	T49.2X4	T49.2X5	T49.2X6
Pholcodine	T48.3X1	T48.3X2	T48.3X3	T48.3X4	T48.3X5	T48.3X6
Pholedrine	T46.991	T46.992	T46.993	T46.994	T46.995	T46.996
Phorate	T60.0X1	T60.0X2	T60.0X3	T60.0X4	—	—
Phosdrin	T60.0X1	T60.0X2	T60.0X3	T60.0X4	—	—
Phosfolan	T60.0X1	T60.0X2	T60.0X3	T60.0X4	—	—
Phosgene (gas)	T59.891	T59.892	T59.893	T59.894	—	—
Phosphamidon	T60.0X1	T60.0X2	T60.0X3	T60.0X4	—	—
Phosphate	T65.891	T65.892	T65.893	T65.894	—	—
laxative	T47.4X1	T47.4X2	T47.4X3	T47.4X4	T47.4X5	T47.4X6
organic	T60.0X1	T60.0X2	T60.0X3	T60.0X4	—	—
solvent	T52.91	T52.92	T52.93	T52.94	—	—
tricresyl	T65.891	T65.892	T65.893	T65.894	—	—
Phosphine	T57.1X1	T57.1X2	T57.1X3	T57.1X4	—	—
fumigant	T57.1X1	T57.1X2	T57.1X3	T57.1X4	—	—
Phospholine	T49.5X1	T49.5X2	T49.5X3	T49.5X4	T49.5X5	T49.5X6
Phosphoric acid	T54.2X1	T54.2X2	T54.2X3	T54.2X4	—	—
Phosphorus (compound) NEC	T57.1X1	T57.1X2	T57.1X3	T57.1X4	—	—
pesticide	T60.0X1	T60.0X2	T60.0X3	T60.0X4	—	—
Phthalates	T65.891	T65.892	T65.893	T65.894	—	—
Phthalic anhydride	T65.891	T65.892	T65.893	T65.894	—	—
Phthalimidoglutarimide	T42.6X1	T42.6X2	T42.6X3	T42.6X4	T42.6X5	T42.6X6
Phthalylsulfathiazole	T37.0X1	T37.0X2	T37.0X3	T37.0X4	T37.0X5	T37.0X6
Phylloquinone	T45.7X1	T45.7X2	T45.7X3	T45.7X4	T45.7X5	T45.7X6
Physeptone	T40.3X1	T40.3X2	T40.3X3	T40.3X4	T40.3X5	T40.3X6
Physostigma venenosum	T62.2X1	T62.2X2	T62.2X3	T62.2X4	—	—
Physostigmine	T49.5X1	T49.5X2	T49.5X3	T49.5X4	T49.5X5	T49.5X6
Phytolacca decandra	T62.2X1	T62.2X2	T62.2X3	T62.2X4	—	—
berries	T62.1X1	T62.1X2	T62.1X3	T62.1X4	—	—

◄ New   ◄ Revised   ~~deleted~~ Deleted

Substance	Poisoning, Accidental (Unintentional)	Poisoning, Intentional Self-Harm	Poisoning, Assault	Poisoning, Undetermined	Adverse Effect	Underdosing
Phytomenadione	T45.7X1	T45.7X2	T45.7X3	T45.7X4	T45.7X5	T45.7X6
Phytonadione	T45.7X1	T45.7X2	T45.7X4	T45.7X4	T45.7X5	T45.7X6
Picoperine	T48.3X1	T48.3X2	T48.3X3	T48.3X4	T48.3X5	T48.3X6
Picosulfate (sodium)	T47.2X1	T47.2X2	T47.2X3	T47.2X4	T47.2X5	T47.2X6
Picric (acid)	T54.2X1	T54.2X2	T54.2X3	T54.2X4	—	—
Picrotoxin	T50.7X1	T50.7X2	T50.7X3	T50.7X4	T50.7X5	T50.7X6
Piketoprofen	T49.0X1	T49.0X2	T49.0X3	T49.0X4	T49.0X5	T49.0X6
Pilocarpine	T44.1X1	T44.1X2	T44.1X3	T44.1X4	T44.1X5	T44.1X6
Pilocarpus (jaborandi) extract	T44.1X1	T44.1X2	T44.1X3	T44.1X4	T44.1X5	T44.1X6
Pilsicainide (hydrochloride)	T46.2X1	T46.2X2	T46.2X3	T46.2X4	T46.2X5	T46.2X6
Pimaricin	T36.7X1	T36.7X2	T36.7X3	T36.7X4	T36.7X5	T36.7X6
Pimeclone	T50.7X1	T50.7X2	T50.7X3	T50.7X4	T50.7X5	T50.7X6
Pimelic ketone	T52.8X1	T52.8X2	T52.8X3	T52.8X4	—	—
Pimethixene	T45.0X1	T45.0X2	T45.0X3	T45.0X4	T45.0X5	T45.0X6
Piminodine	T40.2X1	T40.2X2	T40.2X3	T40.2X4	T40.2X5	T40.2X6
Pimozide	T43.591	T43.592	T43.593	T43.594	T43.595	T43.596
Pinacidil	T46.5X1	T46.5X2	T46.5X3	T46.5X4	T46.5X5	T46.5X6
Pinaverium bromide	T44.3X1	T44.3X2	T44.3X3	T44.3X4	T44.3X5	T44.3X6
Pinazepam	T42.4X1	T42.4X2	T42.4X3	T42.4X4	T42.4X5	T42.4X6
Pindolol	T44.7X1	T44.7X2	T44.7X3	T44.7X4	T44.7X5	T44.7X6
Pindone	T60.4X1	T60.4X2	T60.4X3	T60.4X4	—	—
Pine oil (disinfectant)	T65.891	T65.892	T65.893	T65.894	—	—
Pinkroot	T37.4X1	T37.4X2	T37.4X3	T37.4X4	T37.4X5	T37.4X6
Pipadone	T40.2X1	T40.2X2	T40.2X3	T40.2X4	—	—
Pipamazine	T45.0X1	T45.0X2	T45.0X3	T45.0X4	T45.0X5	T45.0X6
Pipamperone	T43.4X1	T43.4X2	T43.4X3	T43.4X4	T43.4X5	T43.4X6
Pipazetate	T48.3X1	T48.3X2	T48.3X3	T48.3X4	T48.3X5	T48.3X6
Pipemidic acid	T37.8X1	T37.8X2	T37.8X3	T37.8X4	T37.8X5	T37.8X6
Pipenzolate bromide	T44.3X1	T44.3X2	T44.3X3	T44.3X4	T44.3X5	T44.3X6
Piperacetazine	T43.3X1	T43.3X2	T43.3X3	T43.3X4	T43.3X5	T43.3X6
Piperacillin	T36.0X1	T36.0X2	T36.0X3	T36.0X4	T36.0X5	T36.0X6
Piperazine	T37.4X1	T37.4X2	T37.4X3	T37.4X4	T37.4X5	T37.4X6
estrone sulfate	T38.5X1	T38.5X2	T38.5X3	T38.5X4	T38.5X5	T38.5X6
Piper cubeba	T62.2X1	T62.2X2	T62.2X3	T62.2X4	—	—
Piperidione	T48.3X1	T48.3X2	T48.3X3	T48.3X4	—	—
Piperidolate	T44.3X1	T44.3X2	T44.3X3	T44.3X4	T44.3X5	T44.3X6
Piperocaine	T41.3X1	T41.3X2	T41.3X3	T41.3X4	T41.3X5	T41.3X6
infiltration (subcutaneous)	T41.3X1	T41.3X2	T41.3X3	T41.3X4	T41.3X5	T41.3X6
nerve block (peripheral) (plexus)	T41.3X1	T41.3X2	T41.3X3	T41.3X4	T41.3X5	T41.3X6
topical (surface)	T41.3X1	T41.3X2	T41.3X3	T41.3X4	T41.3X5	T41.3X6
Piperonyl butoxide	T60.8X1	T60.8X2	T60.8X3	T60.8X4	—	—
Pipethanate	T44.3X1	T44.3X2	T44.3X3	T44.3X4	T44.3X5	T44.3X6

Substance	Poisoning, Accidental (Unintentional)	Poisoning, Intentional Self-Harm	Poisoning, Assault	Poisoning, Undetermined	Adverse Effect	Underdosing
Pipobroman	T45.1X1	T45.1X2	T45.1X3	T45.1X4	T45.1X5	T45.1X6
Pipofezine	T43.0X1	T43.0X2	T43.0X3	T43.0X4	T43.0X5	T43.0X6
Pipotiazine	T43.3X1	T43.3X2	T43.3X3	T43.3X4	T43.3X5	T43.3X6
Pipoxizine	T45.0X1	T45.0X2	T45.0X3	T45.0X4	T45.0X5	T45.0X6
Pipradrol	T43.691	T43.692	T43.693	T43.694	T43.695	T43.696
Piprinhydrinate	T45.0X1	T45.0X2	T45.0X3	T45.0X4	T45.0X5	T45.0X6
Pirarubicin	T45.1X1	T45.1X2	T45.1X3	T45.1X4	T45.1X5	T45.1X6
Pirazinamide	T37.1X1	T37.1X2	T37.1X3	T37.1X4	T37.1X5	T37.1X6
Pirbuterol	T48.6X1	T48.6X2	T48.6X3	T48.6X4	T48.6X5	T48.6X6
Pirenzepine	T47.1X1	T47.1X2	T47.1X3	T47.1X4	T47.1X5	T47.1X6
Piretanide	T50.1X1	T50.1X2	T50.1X3	T50.1X4	T50.1X5	T50.1X6
Piribedil	T42.8X1	T42.8X2	T42.8X3	T42.8X4	T42.8X5	T42.8X6
Piridoxilate	T46.3X1	T46.3X2	T46.3X3	T46.3X4	T46.3X5	T46.3X6
Piritramide	T40.4X1	T40.4X2	T40.4X3	T40.4X4	—	—
Pirlindole	T43.0X1	T43.0X2	T43.0X3	T43.0X4	T43.0X5	T43.0X6
Piromidic acid	T37.8X1	T37.8X2	T37.8X3	T37.8X4	T37.8X5	T37.8X6
Piroxicam	T39.391	T39.392	T39.393	T39.394	T39.395	T39.396
beta-cyclodextrin complex	T39.8X1	T39.8X2	T39.8X3	T39.8X4	T39.8X5	T39.8X6
Pirozadil	T46.6X1	T46.6X2	T46.6X3	T46.6X4	T46.6X5	T46.6X6
Piscidia (bark) (erythrina)	T39.8X1	T39.8X2	T39.8X3	T39.8X4	T39.8X5	T39.8X6
Pitch	T65.891	T65.892	T65.893	T65.894	—	—
Pitkin's solution	T41.3X1	T41.3X2	T41.3X3	T41.3X4	T41.3X5	T41.3X6
Pitocin	T48.0X1	T48.0X2	T48.0X3	T48.0X4	T48.0X5	T48.0X6
Pitressin (tannate)	T38.891	T38.892	T38.893	T38.894	T38.895	T38.896
Pituitary extracts (posterior)	T38.891	T38.892	T38.893	T38.894	T38.895	T38.896
anterior	T38.811	T38.812	T38.813	T38.814	T38.815	T38.816
Pituitrin	T38.891	T38.892	T38.893	T38.894	T38.895	T38.896
Pivampicillin	T36.0X1	T36.0X2	T36.0X3	T36.0X4	T36.0X5	T36.0X6
Pivmecillinam	T36.0X1	T36.0X2	T36.0X3	T36.0X4	T36.0X5	T36.0X6
Placental hormone	T38.891	T38.892	T38.893	T38.894	T38.895	T38.896
Placidyl	T42.6X1	T42.6X2	T42.6X3	T42.6X4	T42.6X5	T42.6X6
Plague vaccine	T50.A91	T50.A92	T50.A93	T50.A94	T50.A95	T50.A96
Plant						
food or fertilizer NEC	T65.891	T65.892	T65.893	T65.894	—	—
containing herbicide	T60.3X1	T60.3X2	T60.3X3	T60.3X4	—	—
noxious, used as food	T62.2X1	T62.2X2	T62.2X3	T62.2X4	—	—
berries	T62.1X1	T62.1X2	T62.1X3	T62.1X4	—	—
seeds	T62.2X1	T62.2X2	T62.2X3	T62.2X4	—	—
specified type NEC	T62.2X1	T62.2X2	T62.2X3	T62.2X4	—	—
Plasma	T45.8X1	T45.8X2	T45.8X3	T45.8X4	T45.8X5	T45.8X6
expander NEC	T45.8X1	T45.8X2	T45.8X3	T45.8X4	T45.8X5	T45.8X6
protein fraction (human)	T45.8X1	T45.8X2	T45.8X3	T45.8X4	T45.8X5	T45.8X6

◀ New ⬅ Revised ~~deleted~~ Deleted

TABLE OF DRUGS AND CHEMICALS

Substance	External Cause (T-Code)					
	Poisoning, Accidental (Unintentional)	Poisoning, Intentional Self-Harm	Poisoning, Assault	Poisoning, Undetermined	Adverse Effect	Underdosing
Plasmanate	T45.8X1	T45.8X2	T45.8X3	T45.8X4	T45.8X5	T45.8X6
Plasminogen (tissue) activator	T45.611	T45.612	T45.613	T45.614	T45.615	T45.616
Plaster dressing	T49.3X1	T49.3X2	T49.3X3	T49.3X4	T49.3X5	T49.3X6
Plastic dressing	T49.3X1	T49.3X2	T49.3X3	T49.3X4	T49.3X5	T49.3X6
Plegicil	T43.3X1	T43.3X2	T43.3X3	T43.3X4	T43.3X5	T43.3X6
Plicamycin	T45.1X1	T45.1X2	T45.1X3	T45.1X4	T45.1X5	T45.1X6
Podophyllotoxin	T49.8X1	T49.8X2	T49.8X3	T49.8X4	T49.8X5	T49.8X6
Podophyllum (resin)	T49.4X1	T49.4X2	T49.4X3	T49.4X4	T49.4X5	T49.4X6
Poison NEC	T65.91	T65.92	T65.93	T65.94	—	—
Poisonous berries	T62.1X1	T62.1X2	T62.1X3	T62.1X4	—	—
Pokeweed (any part)	T62.2X1	T62.2X2	T62.2X3	T62.2X4	—	—
Poldine metilsulfate	T44.3X1	T44.3X2	T44.3X3	T44.3X4	T44.3X5	T44.3X6
Polidexide (sulfate)	T46.6X1	T46.6X2	T46.6X3	T46.6X4	T46.6X5	T46.6X6
Polidocanol	T46.8X1	T46.8X2	T46.8X3	T46.8X4	T46.8X5	T46.8X6
Poliomyelitis vaccine	T50.B91	T50.B92	T50.B93	T50.B94	T50.B95	T50.B96
Polish (car) (floor) (furniture) (metal) (porcelain) (silver)	T65.891	T65.892	T65.893	T65.894	—	—
abrasive	T65.891	T65.892	T65.893	T65.894	—	—
porcelain	T65.891	T65.892	T65.893	T65.894	—	—
Poloxalkol	T47.4X1	T47.4X2	T47.4X3	T47.4X4	T47.4X5	T47.4X6
Poloxamer	T47.4X1	T47.4X2	T47.4X3	T47.4X4	T47.4X5	T47.4X6
Polyaminostyrene resins	T50.3X1	T50.3X2	T50.3X3	T50.3X4	T50.3X5	T50.3X6
Polycarbophil	T47.4X1	T47.4X2	T47.4X3	T47.4X4	T47.4X5	T47.4X6
Polychlorinated biphenyl	T65.891	T65.892	T65.893	T65.894	—	—
Polycycline	T36.4X1	T36.4X2	T36.4X3	T36.4X4	T36.4X5	T36.4X6
Polyester fumes	T59.891	T59.892	T59.893	T59.894	—	—
Polyester resin hardener	T52.91	T52.92	T52.93	T52.94	—	—
fumes	T59.891	T59.892	T59.893	T59.894	—	—
Polyestradiol phosphate	T38.5X1	T38.5X2	T38.5X3	T38.5X4	T38.5X5	T38.5X6
Polyethanolamine alkyl sulfate	T49.2X1	T49.2X2	T49.2X3	T49.2X4	T49.2X5	T49.2X6
Polyethylene adhesive	T49.3X1	T49.3X2	T49.3X3	T49.3X4	T49.3X5	T49.3X6
Polyferose	T45.4X1	T45.4X2	T45.4X3	T45.4X4	T45.4X5	T45.4X6
Polygeline	T45.8X1	T45.8X2	T45.8X3	T45.8X4	T45.8X5	T45.8X6
Polymyxin	T36.8X1	T36.8X2	T36.8X3	T36.8X4	T36.8X5	T36.8X6
B	T36.8X1	T36.8X2	T36.8X3	T36.8X4	T36.8X5	T36.8X6
ENT agent	T49.6X1	T49.6X2	T49.6X3	T49.6X4	T49.6X5	T49.6X6
ophthalmic preparation	T49.5X1	T49.5X2	T49.5X3	T49.5X4	T49.5X5	T49.5X6
topical NEC	T49.0X1	T49.0X2	T49.0X3	T49.0X4	T49.0X5	T49.0X6
E sulfate (eye preparation)	T49.5X1	T49.5X2	T49.5X3	T49.5X4	T49.5X5	T49.5X6
Polynoxylin	T49.0X1	T49.0X2	T49.0X3	T49.0X4	T49.0X5	T49.0X6
Polyoestradiol phosphate	T38.5X1	T38.5X2	T38.5X3	T38.5X4	T38.5X5	T38.5X6
Polyoxymethyleneurea	T49.0X1	T49.0X2	T49.0X3	T49.0X4	T49.0X5	T49.0X6

Substance	External Cause (T-Code)					
	Poisoning, Accidental (Unintentional)	Poisoning, Intentional Self-Harm	Poisoning, Assault	Poisoning, Undetermined	Adverse Effect	Underdosing
Polysilane	T47.8X1	T47.8X2	T47.8X3	T47.8X4	T47.8X5	T47.8X6
Polytetrafluoroethylene (inhaled)	T59.891	T59.892	T59.893	T59.894	—	—
Polythiazide	T50.2X1	T50.2X2	T50.2X3	T50.2X4	T50.2X5	T50.2X6
Polyvidone	T45.8X1	T45.8X2	T45.8X3	T45.8X4	T45.8X5	T45.8X6
Polyvinylpyrrolidone	T45.8X1	T45.8X2	T45.8X3	T45.8X4	T45.8X5	T45.8X6
Pontocaine (hydrochloride) (infiltration) (topical)	T41.3X1	T41.3X2	T41.3X3	T41.3X4	T41.3X5	T41.3X6
nerve block (peripheral) (plexus)	T41.3X1	T41.3X2	T41.3X3	T41.3X4	T41.3X5	T41.3X6
spinal	T41.3X1	T41.3X2	T41.3X3	T41.3X4	T41.3X5	T41.3X6
Porfiromycin	T45.1X1	T45.1X2	T45.1X3	T45.1X4	T45.1X5	T45.1X6
Posterior pituitary hormone NEC	T38.891	T38.892	T38.893	T38.894	T38.895	T38.896
Pot	T40.7X1	T40.7X2	T40.7X3	T40.7X4	T40.7X5	T40.7X6
Potash (caustic)	T54.3X1	T54.3X2	T54.3X3	T54.3X4	—	—
Potassic saline injection (lactated)	T50.3X1	T50.3X2	T50.3X3	T50.3X4	T50.3X5	T50.3X6
Potassium (salts) NEC	T50.3X1	T50.3X2	T50.3X3	T50.3X4	T50.3X5	T50.3X6
aminobenzoate	T45.8X1	T45.8X2	T45.8X3	T45.8X4	T45.8X5	T45.8X6
aminosalicylate	T37.1X1	T37.1X2	T37.1X3	T37.1X4	T37.1X5	T37.1X6
antimony 'tartrate'	T37.8X1	T37.8X2	T37.8X3	T37.8X4	T37.8X5	T37.8X6
arsenite (solution)	T57.0X1	T57.0X2	T57.0X3	T57.0X4	—	—
bichromate	T56.2X1	T56.2X2	T56.2X3	T56.2X4	—	—
bisulfate	T47.3X1	T47.3X2	T47.3X3	T47.3X4	T47.3X5	T47.3X6
bromide	T42.6X1	T42.6X2	T42.6X3	T42.6X4	T42.6X5	T42.6X6
canrenoate	T50.0X1	T50.0X2	T50.0X3	T50.0X4	T50.0X5	T50.0X6
carbonate	T54.3X1	T54.3X2	T54.3X3	T54.3X4	—	—
chlorate NEC	T65.891	T65.892	T65.893	T65.894	—	—
chloride	T50.3X1	T50.3X2	T50.3X3	T50.3X4	T50.3X5	T50.3X6
citrate	T50.991	T50.992	T50.993	T50.994	T50.995	T50.996
cyanide	T65.0X1	T65.0X2	T65.0X3	T65.0X4	—	—
ferric hexacyanoferrate (medicinal)	T50.6X1	T50.6X2	T50.6X3	T50.6X4	T50.6X5	T50.6X6
nonmedicinal	T65.891	T65.892	T65.893	T65.894	—	—
Fluoride	T57.8X1	T57.8X2	T57.8X3	T57.8X4	—	—
glucaldrate	T47.1X1	T47.1X2	T47.1X3	T47.1X4	T47.1X5	T47.1X6
hydroxide	T54.3X1	T54.3X2	T54.3X3	T54.3X4	—	—
iodate	T49.0X1	T49.0X2	T49.0X3	T49.0X4	T49.0X5	T49.0X6
iodide	T48.4X1	T48.4X2	T48.4X3	T48.4X4	T48.4X5	T48.4X6
nitrate	T57.8X1	T57.8X2	T57.8X3	T57.8X4	—	—
oxalate	T65.891	T65.892	T65.893	T65.894	—	—
perchlorate (nonmedicinal) NEC	T65.891	T65.892	T65.893	T65.894	—	—
antithyroid	T38.2X1	T38.2X2	T38.2X3	T38.2X4	T38.2X5	T38.2X6
medicinal	T38.2X1	T38.2X2	T38.2X3	T38.2X4	T38.2X5	T38.2X6

◀ New　◀▥ Revised　~~deleted~~ Deleted

Substance	Poisoning, Accidental (Unintentional)	Poisoning, Intentional Self-Harm	Poisoning, Assault	Poisoning, Undetermined	Adverse Effect	Underdosing
Permanganate (nonmedicinal)	T65.891	T65.892	T65.893	T65.894	—	—
medicinal	T49.0X1	T49.0X2	T49.0X3	T49.0X4	T49.0X5	T49.0X6
sulfate	T47.2X1	T47.2X2	T47.2X3	T47.2X4	T47.2X5	T47.2X6
Potassium-removing resin	T50.3X1	T50.3X2	T50.3X3	T50.3X4	T50.3X5	T50.3X6
Potassium-retaining drug	T50.3X1	T50.3X2	T50.3X3	T50.3X4	T50.3X5	T50.3X6
Povidone	T45.8X1	T45.8X2	T45.8X3	T45.8X4	T45.8X5	T45.8X6
iodine	T49.0X1	T49.0X2	T49.0X3	T49.0X4	T49.0X5	T49.0X6
Practolol	T44.7X1	T44.7X2	T44.7X3	T44.7X4	T44.7X5	T44.7X6
Prajmalium bitartrate	T46.2X1	T46.2X2	T46.2X3	T46.2X4	T46.2X5	T46.2X6
Pralidoxime (iodide)	T50.6X1	T50.6X2	T50.6X3	T50.6X4	T50.6X5	T50.6X6
chloride	T50.6X1	T50.6X2	T50.6X3	T50.6X4	T50.6X5	T50.6X6
Pramiverine	T44.3X1	T44.3X2	T44.3X3	T44.3X4	T44.3X5	T44.3X6
Pramocaine	T49.1X1	T49.1X2	T49.1X3	T49.1X4	T49.1X5	T49.1X6
Pramoxine	T49.1X1	T49.1X2	T49.1X3	T49.1X4	T49.1X5	T49.1X6
Prasterone	T38.7X1	T38.7X2	T38.7X3	T38.7X4	T38.7X5	T38.7X6
Pravastatin	T46.6X1	T46.6X2	T46.6X3	T46.6X4	T46.6X5	T46.6X6
Prazepam	T42.4X1	T42.4X2	T42.4X3	T42.4X4	T42.4X5	T42.4X6
Praziquantel	T37.4X1	T37.4X2	T37.4X3	T37.4X4	T37.4X5	T37.4X6
Prazitone	T43.291	T43.292	T43.293	T43.294	T43.295	T43.296
Prazosin	T44.6X1	T44.6X2	T44.6X3	T44.6X4	T44.6X5	T44.6X6
Prednicarbate	T49.0X1	T49.0X2	T49.0X3	T49.0X4	T49.0X5	T49.0X6
Prednimustine	T45.1X1	T45.1X2	T45.1X3	T45.1X4	T45.1X5	T45.1X6
Prednisolone	T38.0X1	T38.0X2	T38.0X3	T38.0X4	T38.0X5	T38.0X6
ENT agent	T49.6X1	T49.6X2	T49.6X3	T49.6X4	T49.6X5	T49.6X6
ophthalmic preparation	T49.5X1	T49.5X2	T49.5X3	T49.5X4	T49.5X5	T49.5X6
steaglate	T49.0X1	T49.0X2	T49.0X3	T49.0X4	T49.0X5	T49.0X6
topical NEC	T49.0X1	T49.0X2	T49.0X3	T49.0X4	T49.0X5	T49.0X6
Prednisone	T38.0X1	T38.0X2	T38.0X3	T38.0X4	T38.0X5	T38.0X6
Prednylidene	T38.0X1	T38.0X2	T38.0X3	T38.0X4	T38.0X5	T38.0X6
Pregnandiol	T38.5X1	T38.5X2	T38.5X3	T38.5X4	T38.5X5	T38.5X6
Pregneninolone	T38.5X1	T38.5X2	T38.5X3	T38.5X4	T38.5X5	T38.5X6
Preludin	T43.691	T43.692	T43.693	T43.694	T43.695	T43.696
Premarin	T38.5X1	T38.5X2	T38.5X3	T38.5X4	T38.5X5	T38.5X6
Premedication anesthetic	T41.201	T41.202	T41.203	T41.204	T41.205	T41.206
Prenalterol	T44.5X1	T44.5X2	T44.5X3	T44.5X4	T44.5X5	T44.5X6
Prenoxdiazine	T48.3X1	T48.3X2	T48.3X3	T48.3X4	T48.3X5	T48.3X6
Prenylamine	T46.3X1	T46.3X2	T46.3X3	T46.3X4	T46.3X5	T46.3X6
Preparation, local	T49.4X1	T49.4X2	T49.4X3	T49.4X4	T49.4X5	T49.4X6
Preparation H	T49.8X1	T49.8X2	T49.8X3	T49.8X4	T49.8X5	T49.8X6
Preservative (nonmedicinal)	T65.891	T65.892	T65.893	T65.894	—	—
medicinal	T50.901	T50.902	T50.903	T50.904	T50.905	T50.906
wood	T60.91	T60.92	T60.93	T60.94	—	—

Substance	Poisoning, Accidental (Unintentional)	Poisoning, Intentional Self-Harm	Poisoning, Assault	Poisoning, Undetermined	Adverse Effect	Underdosing
Prethcamide	T50.7X1	T50.7X2	T50.7X3	T50.7X4	T50.7X5	T50.7X6
Pride of China	T62.2X1	T62.2X2	T62.2X3	T62.2X4	—	—
Pridinol	T44.3X1	T44.3X2	T44.3X3	T44.3X4	T44.3X5	T44.3X6
Prifinium bromide	T44.3X1	T44.3X2	T44.3X3	T44.3X4	T44.3X5	T44.3X6
Prilocaine	T41.3X1	T41.3X2	T41.3X3	T41.3X4	T41.3X5	T41.3X6
infiltration (subcutaneous)	T41.3X1	T41.3X2	T41.3X3	T41.3X4	T41.3X5	T41.3X6
nerve block (peripheral) (plexus)	T41.3X1	T41.3X2	T41.3X3	T41.3X4	T41.3X5	T41.3X6
regional	T41.3X1	T41.3X2	T41.3X3	T41.3X4	T41.3X5	T41.3X6
Primaquine	T37.2X1	T37.2X2	T37.2X3	T37.2X4	T37.2X5	T37.2X6
Primidone	T42.6X1	T42.6X2	T42.6X3	T42.6X4	T42.6X5	T42.6X6
Primula (veris)	T62.2X1	T62.2X2	T62.2X3	T62.2X4	—	—
Prinadol	T40.2X1	T40.2X2	T40.2X3	T40.2X4	T40.2X5	T40.2X6
Priscol, Priscoline	T44.6X1	T44.6X2	T44.6X3	T44.6X4	T44.6X5	T44.6X6
Pristinamycin	T36.3X1	T36.3X2	T36.3X3	T36.3X4	T36.3X5	T36.3X6
Privet	T62.2X1	T62.2X2	T62.2X3	T62.2X4	—	—
berries	T62.1X1	T62.1X2	T62.1X3	T62.1X4	—	—
Privine	T44.4X1	T44.4X2	T44.4X3	T44.4X4	T44.4X5	T44.4X6
Pro-Banthine	T44.3X1	T44.3X2	T44.3X3	T44.3X4	T44.3X5	T44.3X6
Probarbital	T42.3X1	T42.3X2	T42.3X3	T42.3X4	T42.3X5	T42.3X6
Probenecid	T50.4X1	T50.4X2	T50.4X3	T50.4X4	T50.4X5	T50.4X6
Probucol	T46.6X1	T46.6X2	T46.6X3	T46.6X4	T46.6X5	T46.6X6
Procainamide	T46.2X1	T46.2X2	T46.2X3	T46.2X4	T46.2X5	T46.2X6
Procaine	T41.3X1	T41.3X2	T41.3X3	T41.3X4	T41.3X5	T41.3X6
benzylpenicillin	T36.0X1	T36.0X2	T36.0X3	T36.0X4	T36.0X5	T36.0X6
nerve block (peripheral) (plexus)	T41.3X1	T41.3X2	T41.3X3	T41.3X4	T41.3X5	T41.3X6
penicillin G	T36.0X1	T36.0X2	T36.0X3	T36.0X4	T36.0X5	T36.0X6
regional	T41.3X1	T41.3X2	T41.3X3	T41.3X4	T41.3X5	T41.3X6
spinal	T41.3X1	T41.3X2	T41.3X3	T41.3X4	T41.3X5	T41.3X6
Procalmidol	T43.591	T43.592	T43.593	T43.594	T43.595	T43.596
Procarbazine	T45.1X1	T45.1X2	T45.1X3	T45.1X4	T45.1X5	T45.1X6
Procaterol	T44.5X1	T44.5X2	T44.5X3	T44.5X4	T44.5X5	T44.5X6
Prochlorperazine	T43.3X1	T43.3X2	T43.3X3	T43.3X4	T43.3X5	T43.3X6
Procyclidine	T44.3X1	T44.3X2	T44.3X3	T44.3X4	T44.3X5	T44.3X6
Producer gas	T58.8X1	T58.8X2	T58.8X3	T58.8X4	—	—
Profadol	T40.4X1	T40.4X2	T40.4X3	T40.4X4	T40.4X5	T40.4X6
Profenamine	T44.3X1	T44.3X2	T44.3X3	T44.3X4	T44.3X5	T44.3X6
Profenil	T44.3X1	T44.3X2	T44.3X3	T44.3X4	T44.3X5	T44.3X6
Proflavine	T49.0X1	T49.0X2	T49.0X3	T49.0X4	T49.0X5	T49.0X6
Progabide	T42.6X1	T42.6X2	T42.6X3	T42.6X4	T42.6X5	T42.6X6
Progestin	T38.5X1	T38.5X2	T38.5X3	T38.5X4	T38.5X5	T38.5X6
oral contraceptive	T38.4X1	T38.4X2	T38.4X3	T38.4X4	T38.4X5	T38.4X6

◀ New　◀║ Revised　~~deleted~~ Deleted

TABLE OF DRUGS AND CHEMICALS

Substance	External Cause (T-Code)					
	Poisoning, Accidental (Unintentional)	Poisoning, Intentional Self-Harm	Poisoning, Assault	Poisoning, Undetermined	Adverse Effect	Underdosing
Progesterone	T38.5X1	T38.5X2	T38.5X3	T38.5X4	T38.5X5	T38.5X6
Progestogen NEC	T38.5X1	T38.5X2	T38.5X3	T38.5X4	T38.5X5	T38.5X6
Progestone	T38.5X1	T38.5X2	T38.5X3	T38.5X4	T38.5X5	T38.5X6
Proglumide	T47.1X1	T47.1X2	T47.1X3	T47.1X4	T47.1X5	T47.1X6
Proguanil	T37.2X1	T37.2X2	T37.2X2	T37.2X4	T37.2X5	T37.2X6
Prolactin	T38.811	T38.812	T38.813	T38.814	T38.815	T38.816
Prolintane	T43.691	T43.692	T43.693	T43.694	T43.695	T43.696
Proloid	T38.1X1	T38.1X2	T38.1X3	T38.1X4	T38.1X5	T38.1X6
Proluton	T38.5X1	T38.5X2	T38.5X3	T38.5X4	T38.5X5	T38.5X6
Promacetin	T37.1X1	T37.1X2	T37.1X3	T37.1X4	T37.1X5	T37.1X6
Promazine	T43.3X1	T43.3X2	T43.3X3	T43.3X4	T43.3X5	T43.3X6
Promedol	T40.2X1	T40.2X2	T40.2X3	T40.2X4	—	—
Promegestone	T38.5X1	T38.5X2	T38.5X3	T38.5X4	T38.5X5	T38.5X6
Promethazine (teoclate)	T43.3X1	T43.3X2	T43.3X3	T43.3X4	T43.3X5	T43.3X6
Promin	T37.1X1	T37.1X2	T37.1X3	T37.1X4	T37.1X5	T37.1X6
Pronase	T45.3X1	T45.3X2	T45.3X3	T45.3X4	T45.3X5	T45.3X6
Pronestyl (hydrochloride)	T46.2X1	T46.2X2	T46.2X3	T46.2X4	T46.2X5	T46.2X6
Pronetalol	T44.7X1	T44.7X2	T44.7X3	T44.7X4	T44.7X5	T44.7X6
Prontosil	T37.0X1	T37.0X2	T37.0X3	T37.0X4	T37.0X5	T37.0X6
Propachlor	T60.3X1	T60.3X2	T60.3X3	T60.3X4	—	—
Propafenone	T46.2X1	T46.2X2	T46.2X3	T46.2X4	T46.2X5	T46.2X6
Propallylonal	T42.3X1	T42.3X2	T42.3X3	T42.3X4	T42.3X5	T42.3X6
Propamidine	T49.0X1	T49.0X2	T49.0X3	T49.0X4	T49.0X5	T49.0X6
Propane (distributed in mobile container)	T59.891	T59.892	T59.893	T59.894	—	—
distributed through pipes	T59.891	T59.892	T59.893	T59.894	—	—
incomplete combustion	T57.11	T57.12	T57.13	T57.14	—	—
Propanidid	T41.291	T41.292	T41.293	T41.294	T41.295	T41.296
Propanil	T60.3X1	T60.3X2	T60.3X3	T60.3X4	—	—
1-Propanol	T51.3X1	T51.3X2	T51.3X3	T51.3X4	—	—
2-Propanol	T51.2X1	T51.2X2	T51.2X3	T51.2X4	—	—
Propantheline	T44.3X1	T44.3X2	T44.3X3	T44.3X4	T44.3X5	T44.3X6
bromide	T44.3X1	T44.3X2	T44.3X3	T44.3X4	T44.3X5	T44.3X6
Proparacaine	T41.3X1	T41.3X2	T41.3X3	T41.3X4	T41.3X5	T41.3X6
Propatylnitrate	T46.3X1	T46.3X2	T46.3X3	T46.3X4	T46.3X5	T46.3X6
Propicillin	T36.0X1	T36.0X2	T36.0X3	T36.0X4	T36.0X5	T36.0X6
Propiolactone	T49.0X1	T49.0X2	T49.0X3	T49.0X4	T49.0X5	T49.0X6
Propiomazine	T45.0X1	T45.0X2	T45.0X3	T45.0X4	T45.0X5	T45.0X6
Propionaldehyde (medicinal)	T42.6X1	T42.6X2	T42.6X3	T42.6X4	T42.6X5	T42.6X6
Propionaldehyde (medicinal) ◄	T42.6X1	T42.6X2	T42.6X3	T42.6X4	T42.6X5	T42.6X6
Propionate (calcium) (sodium)	T49.0X1	T49.0X2	T49.0X3	T49.0X4	T49.0X5	T49.0X6
Propion gel	T49.0X1	T49.0X2	T49.0X3	T49.0X4	T49.0X5	T49.0X6

Substance	External Cause (T-Code)					
	Poisoning, Accidental (Unintentional)	Poisoning, Intentional Self-Harm	Poisoning, Assault	Poisoning, Undetermined	Adverse Effect	Underdosing
Propitocaine	T41.3X1	T41.3X2	T41.3X3	T41.3X4	T41.3X5	T41.3X6
infiltration (subcutaneous)	T41.3X1	T41.3X2	T41.3X3	T41.3X4	T41.3X5	T41.3X6
nerve block (peripheral) (plexus)	T41.3X1	T41.3X2	T41.3X3	T41.3X4	T41.3X5	T41.3X6
Propofol	T41.291	T41.292	T41.293	T41.294	T41.295	T41.296
Propoxur	T60.0X1	T60.0X2	T60.0X3	T60.0X4	—	—
Propoxycaine	T41.3X1	T41.3X2	T41.3X3	T41.3X4	T41.3X5	T41.3X6
infiltration (subcutaneous)	T41.3X1	T41.3X2	T41.3X3	T41.3X4	T41.3X5	T41.3X6
nerve block (peripheral) (plexus)	T41.3X1	T41.3X2	T41.3X3	T41.3X4	T41.3X5	T41.3X6
topical (surface)	T41.3X1	T41.3X2	T41.3X3	T41.3X4	T41.3X5	T41.3X6
Propoxyphene	T40.4X1	T40.4X2	T40.4X3	T40.4X4	T40.4X5	T40.4X6
Propranolol	T44.7X1	T44.7X2	T44.7X3	T44.7X4	T44.7X5	T44.7X6
Propyl						
alcohol	T51.3X1	T51.3X2	T51.3X3	T51.3X4	—	—
carbinol	T51.3X1	T51.3X2	T51.3X3	T51.3X4	—	—
hexadrine	T44.4X1	T44.4X2	T44.4X3	T44.4X4	T44.4X5	T44.4X6
iodone	T50.8X1	T50.8X2	T50.8X3	T50.8X4	T50.8X5	T50.8X6
thiouracil	T38.2X1	T38.2X2	T38.2X3	T38.2X4	T38.2X5	T38.2X6
Propylaminophenothiazine	T43.3X1	T43.3X2	T43.3X3	T43.3X4	T43.3X5	T43.3X6
Propylene	T59.891	T59.892	T59.893	T59.894	—	—
Propylhexedrine	T48.5X1	T48.5X2	T48.5X3	T48.5X4	T48.5X5	T48.5X6
Propyliodone	T50.8X1	T50.8X2	T50.8X3	T50.8X4	T50.8X5	T50.8X6
Propylthiouracil	T38.2X1	T38.2X2	T38.2X3	T38.2X4	T38.2X5	T38.2X6
Propylparaben (ophthalmic)	T49.5X1	T49.5X2	T49.5X3	T49.5X4	T49.5X5	T49.5X6
Propyphenazone	T39.2X1	T39.2X2	T39.2X3	T39.2X4	T39.2X5	T39.2X6
Proquazone	T39.391	T39.392	T39.393	T39.394	T39.395	T39.396
Proscillaridin	T46.0X1	T46.0X2	T46.0X3	T46.0X4	T46.0X5	T46.0X6
Prostacyclin	T45.521	T45.522	T45.523	T45.524	T45.525	T45.526
Prostaglandin (I2)	T45.521	T45.522	T45.523	T45.524	T45.525	T45.526
E1	T46.7X1	T46.7X2	T46.7X3	T46.7X4	T46.7X5	T46.7X6
E2	T48.0X1	T48.0X2	T48.0X3	T48.0X4	T48.0X5	T48.0X6
F2 alpha	T48.0X1	T48.0X2	T48.0X3	T48.0X4	T48.0X5	T48.0X6
Prostigmin	T44.0X1	T44.0X2	T44.0X3	T44.0X4	T44.0X5	T44.0X6
Prosultiamine	T45.2X1	T45.2X2	T45.2X3	T45.2X4	T45.2X5	T45.2X6
Protamine sulfate	T45.7X1	T45.7X2	T45.7X3	T45.7X4	T45.7X5	T45.7X6
zinc insulin	T38.3X1	T38.3X2	T38.3X3	T38.3X4	T38.3X5	T38.3X6
Protease	T47.5X1	T47.5X2	T47.5X3	T47.5X4	T47.5X5	T47.5X6
Protectant, skin NEC	T49.3X1	T49.3X2	T49.3X3	T49.3X4	T49.3X5	T49.3X6
Protein hydrolysate	T50.991	T50.992	T50.993	T50.994	T50.995	T50.996
Prothiaden — see Dothiepin hydrochloride						
Prothionamide	T37.1X1	T37.1X2	T37.1X3	T37.1X4	T37.1X5	T37.1X6

◄ New   ⧏⧏⧏ Revised   ~~deleted~~ Deleted

Substance	Poisoning, Accidental (Unintentional)	Poisoning, Intentional Self-Harm	Poisoning, Assault	Poisoning, Undetermined	Adverse Effect	Underdosing
	External Cause (T-Code)					
Prothipendyl	T43.591	T43.592	T43.593	T43.594	T43.595	T43.596
Prothoate	T60.0X1	T60.0X2	T60.0X3	T60.0X4	—	—
Prothrombin						
activator	T45.7X1	T45.7X2	T45.7X3	T45.7X4	T45.7X5	T45.7X6
synthesis inhibitor	T45.511	T45.512	T45.513	T45.514	T45.515	T45.516
Protionamide	T37.1X1	T37.1X2	T37.1X3	T37.1X4	T37.1X5	T37.1X6
Protirelin	T38.891	T38.892	T38.893	T38.894	T38.895	T38.896
Protokylol	T48.6X1	T48.6X2	T48.6X3	T48.6X4	T48.6X5	T48.6X6
Protopam	T50.6X1	T50.6X2	T50.6X3	T50.6X4	T50.6X5	T50.6X6
Protoveratrine(s) (A) (B)	T46.5X1	T46.5X2	T46.5X3	T46.5X4	T46.5X5	T46.5X6
Protriptyline	T43.011	T43.012	T43.013	T43.014	T43.015	T43.016
Provera	T38.5X1	T38.5X2	T38.5X3	T38.5X4	T38.5X5	T38.5X6
Provitamin A	T45.2X1	T45.2X2	T45.2X3	T45.2X4	T45.2X5	T45.2X6
Proxibarbal	T42.3X1	T42.3X2	T42.3X3	T42.3X4	T42.3X5	T42.3X6
Proxymetacaine	T41.3X1	T41.3X2	T41.3X3	T41.3X4	T41.3X5	T41.3X6
Proxyphylline	T48.6X1	T48.6X2	T48.6X3	T48.6X4	T48.6X5	T48.6X6
Prozac — see Fluoxetine hydrochloride						
Prunus						
laurocerasus	T62.2X1	T62.2X2	T62.2X3	T62.2X4	—	—
virginiana	T62.2X1	T62.2X2	T62.2X3	T62.2X4	—	—
Prussian blue						
commercial	T65.891	T65.892	T65.893	T65.894	—	—
therapeutic	T50.6X1	T50.6X2	T50.6X3	T50.6X4	T50.6X5	T50.6X6
Prussic acid	T65.0X1	T65.0X2	T65.0X3	T65.0X4	—	—
vapor	T57.3X1	T57.3X2	T57.3X3	T57.3X4	—	—
Pseudoephedrine	T44.991	T44.992	T44.993	T44.994	T44.995	T44.996
Psilocin	T40.991	T40.992	T40.993	T40.994	—	—
Psilocybin	T40.991	T40.992	T40.993	T40.994	—	—
Psilocybine	T40.991	T40.992	T40.993	T40.994	—	—
Psoralene (nonmedicinal)	T65.891	T65.892	T65.893	T65.894	—	—
Psoralens (medicinal)	T50.991	T50.992	T50.993	T50.994	T50.995	T50.996
PSP (phenolsulfonphthalein)	T50.8X1	T50.8X2	T50.8X3	T50.8X4	T50.8X5	T50.8X6
Psychodysleptic drug NEC	T40.901	T40.902	T40.903	T40.904	T40.905	T40.906
Psychostimulant	T43.601	T43.602	T43.603	T43.604	T43.605	T43.606
amphetamine	T43.621	T43.622	T43.623	T43.624	T43.625	T43.626
caffeine	T43.611	T43.612	T43.613	T43.614	T43.615	T43.616
methylphenidate	T43.631	T43.632	T43.633	T43.634	T43.635	T43.636
specified NEC	T43.691	T43.692	T43.693	T43.694	T43.695	T43.696
Psychotherapeutic drug NEC	T43.91	T43.92	T43.93	T43.94	T43.95	T43.96
antidepressants — see also Antidepressant	T43.201	T43.202	T43.203	T43.204	T43.205	T43.206

Substance	Poisoning, Accidental (Unintentional)	Poisoning, Intentional Self-Harm	Poisoning, Assault	Poisoning, Undetermined	Adverse Effect	Underdosing
	External Cause (T-Code)					
Psychotherapeutic drug NEC (Continued)						
specified NEC	T43.8X1	T43.8X2	T43.8X3	T43.8X4	T43.8X5	T43.8X6
tranquilizers NEC	T43.501	T43.502	T43.503	T43.504	T43.505	T43.506
Psychotomimetic agents	T40.901	T40.902	T40.903	T40.904	T40.905	T40.906
Psychotropic drug NEC	T43.91	T43.92	T43.93	T43.94	T43.95	T43.96
specified NEC	T43.8X1	T43.8X2	T43.8X3	T43.8X4	T43.8X5	T43.8X6
Psyllium hydrophilic mucilloid	T47.4X1	T47.4X2	T47.4X3	T47.4X4	T47.4X5	T47.4X6
Pteroylglutamic acid	T45.8X1	T45.8X2	T45.8X3	T45.8X4	T45.8X5	T45.8X6
Pteroyltriglutamate	T45.1X1	T45.1X2	T45.1X3	T45.1X4	T45.1X5	T45.1X6
PTFE — see Polytetrafluoroethylene						
Pulp						
devitalizing paste	T49.7X1	T49.7X2	T49.7X3	T49.7X4	T49.7X5	T49.7X6
dressing	T49.7X1	T49.7X2	T49.7X3	T49.7X4	T49.7X5	T49.7X6
Pulsatilla	T62.2X1	T62.2X2	T62.2X3	T62.2X4	—	—
Pumpkin seed extract	T37.4X1	T37.4X2	T37.4X3	T37.4X4	T37.4X5	T37.4X6
Purex (bleach)	T54.91	T54.92	T54.93	T54.94		
Purgative NEC — see also Cathartic	T47.4X1	T47.4X2	T47.4X3	T47.4X4	T47.4X5	T47.4X6
Purine analogue (antineoplastic)	T45.1X1	T45.1X2	T45.1X3	T45.1X4	T45.1X5	T45.1X6
Purine diuretics	T50.2X1	T50.2X2	T50.2X3	T50.2X4	T50.2X5	T50.2X6
Purinethol	T45.1X1	T45.1X2	T45.1X3	T45.1X4	T45.1X5	T45.1X6
PVP	T45.8X1	T45.8X2	T45.8X3	T45.8X4	T45.8X5	T45.8X6
Pyrabital	T39.8X1	T39.8X2	T39.8X3	T39.8X4	T39.8X5	T39.8X6
Pyramidon	T39.2X1	T39.2X2	T39.2X3	T39.2X4	T39.2X5	T39.2X6
Pyrantel	T37.4X1	T37.4X2	T37.4X3	T37.4X4	T37.4X5	T37.4X6
Pyrathiazine	T45.0X1	T45.0X2	T45.0X3	T45.0X4	T45.0X5	T45.0X6
Pyrazinamide	T37.1X1	T37.1X2	T37.1X3	T37.1X4	T37.1X5	T37.1X6
Pyrazinoic acid (amide)	T37.1X1	T37.1X2	T37.1X3	T37.1X4	T37.1X5	T37.1X6
Pyrazole (derivatives)	T39.2X1	T39.2X2	T39.2X3	T39.2X4	T39.2X5	T39.2X6
Pyrazolone analgesic NEC	T39.2X1	T39.2X2	T39.2X3	T39.2X4	T39.2X5	T39.2X6
Pyrethrin, pyrethrum (nonmedicinal)	T60.2X1	T60.2X2	T60.2X3	T60.2X4	—	—
Pyrethrum extract	T49.0X1	T49.0X2	T49.0X3	T49.0X4	T49.0X5	T49.0X6
Pyribenzamine	T45.0X1	T45.0X2	T45.0X3	T45.0X4	T45.0X5	T45.0X6
Pyridine	T52.8X1	T52.8X2	T52.8X3	T52.8X4	—	—
aldoxime methiodide	T50.6X1	T50.6X2	T50.6X3	T50.6X4	T50.6X5	T50.6X6
aldoxime methyl chloride	T50.6X1	T50.6X2	T50.6X3	T50.6X4	T50.6X5	T50.6X6
vapor	T59.891	T59.892	T59.893	T59.894	—	—
Pyridium	T39.8X1	T39.8X2	T39.8X3	T39.8X4	T39.8X5	T39.8X6
Pyridostigmine bromide	T44.0X1	T44.0X2	T44.0X3	T44.0X4	T44.0X5	T44.0X6
Pyridoxal phosphate	T45.2X1	T45.2X2	T45.2X3	T45.2X4	T45.2X5	T45.2X6

◀ New ◀ Revised ~~deleted~~ Deleted

TABLE OF DRUGS AND CHEMICALS

Substance	External Cause (T-Code)					
	Poisoning, Accidental (Unintentional)	Poisoning, Intentional Self-Harm	Poisoning, Assault	Poisoning, Undetermined	Adverse Effect	Underdosing
Pyridoxine	T45.2X1	T45.2X2	T45.2X3	T45.2X4	T45.2X5	T45.2X6
Pyrilamine	T45.0X1	T45.0X2	T45.0X3	T45.0X4	T45.0X5	T45.0X6
Pyrimethamine	T37.2X1	T37.2X2	T37.2X3	T37.2X4	T37.2X5	T37.2X6
with sulfadoxine	T37.2X1	T37.2X2	T37.2X3	T37.2X4	T37.2X5	T37.2X6
Pyrimidine antagonist	T45.1X1	T45.1X2	T45.1X3	T45.1X4	T45.1X5	T45.1X6
Pyriminil	T60.4X1	T60.4X2	T60.4X3	T60.4X4	—	—
Pyrithione zinc	T49.4X1	T49.4X2	T49.4X3	T49.4X4	T49.4X5	T49.4X6
Pyrithyldione	T42.6X1	T42.6X2	T42.6X3	T42.6X4	T42.6X5	T42.6X6
Pyrogallic acid	T49.0X1	T49.0X2	T49.0X3	T49.0X4	T49.0X5	T49.0X6
Pyrogallol	T49.0X1	T49.0X2	T49.0X3	T49.0X4	T49.0X5	T49.0X6
Pyroxylin	T49.3X1	T49.3X2	T49.3X3	T49.3X4	T49.3X5	T49.3X6
Pyrrobutamine	T45.0X1	T45.0X2	T45.0X3	T45.0X4	T45.0X5	T45.0X6
Pyrrolizidine alkaloids	T62.8X1	T62.8X2	T62.8X3	T62.8X4	—	—
Pyrvinium chloride	T37.4X1	T37.4X2	T37.4X3	T37.4X4	T37.4X5	T37.4X6
PZI	T38.3X1	T38.3X2	T38.3X3	T38.3X4	T38.3X5	T38.3X6
Q						
Quaalude	T42.6X1	T42.6X2	T42.6X3	T42.6X4	T42.6X5	T42.6X6
Quarternary ammonium						
anti-infective	T49.0X1	T49.0X2	T49.0X3	T49.0X4	T49.0X5	T49.0X6
ganglion blocking	T44.2X1	T44.2X2	T44.2X3	T44.2X4	T44.2X5	T44.2X6
parasympatholytic	T44.3X1	T44.3X2	T44.3X3	T44.3X4	T44.3X5	T44.3X6
Quazepam	T42.4X1	T42.4X2	T42.4X3	T42.4X4	T42.4X5	T42.4X6
Quicklime	T54.3X1	T54.3X2	T54.3X3	T54.3X4	—	—
Quillaja extract	T48.4X1	T48.4X2	T48.4X3	T48.4X4	T48.4X5	T48.4X6
Quinacrine	T37.2X1	T37.2X2	T37.2X3	T37.2X4	T37.2X5	T37.2X6
Quinaglute	T46.2X1	T46.2X2	T46.2X3	T46.2X4	T46.2X5	T46.2X6
Quinalbarbital	T42.3X1	T42.3X2	T42.3X3	T42.3X4	T42.3X5	T42.3X6
Quinalbarbitone sodium	T42.3X1	T42.3X2	T42.3X3	T42.3X4	T42.3X5	T42.3X6
Quinalphos	T60.0X1	T60.0X2	T60.0X3	T60.0X4	—	—
Quinapril	T46.4X1	T46.4X2	T46.4X3	T46.4X4	T46.4X5	T46.4X6
Quinestradiol	T38.5X1	T38.5X2	T38.5X3	T38.5X4	T38.5X5	T38.5X6
Quinestradol	T38.5X1	T38.5X2	T38.5X3	T38.5X4	T38.5X5	T38.5X6
Quinestrol	T38.5X1	T38.5X2	T38.5X3	T38.5X4	T38.5X5	T38.5X6
Quinethazone	T50.2X1	T50.2X2	T50.2X3	T50.2X4	T50.2X5	T50.2X6
Quingestanol	T38.4X1	T38.4X2	T38.4X3	T38.4X4	T38.4X5	T38.4X6
Quinidine	T46.2X1	T46.2X2	T46.2X3	T46.2X4	T46.2X5	T46.2X6
Quinine	T37.2X1	T37.2X2	T37.2X3	T37.2X4	T37.2X5	T37.2X6
Quiniobine	T37.8X1	T37.8X2	T37.8X3	T37.8X4	T37.8X5	T37.8X6
Quinisocaine	T49.1X1	T49.1X2	T49.1X3	T49.1X4	T49.1X5	T49.1X6
Quinocide	T37.2X1	T37.2X2	T37.2X3	T37.2X4	T37.2X5	T37.2X6
Quinoline (derivatives) NEC	T37.8X1	T37.8X2	T37.8X3	T37.8X4	T37.8X5	T37.8X6

Substance	External Cause (T-Code)					
	Poisoning, Accidental (Unintentional)	Poisoning, Intentional Self-Harm	Poisoning, Assault	Poisoning, Undetermined	Adverse Effect	Underdosing
Quinupramine	T43.011	T43.012	T43.013	T43.014	T43.015	T43.016
Quotane	T41.3X1	T41.3X2	T41.3X3	T41.3X4	T41.3X5	T41.3X6
R						
Rabies						
immune globulin (human)	T50.Z11	T50.Z12	T50.Z13	T50.Z14	T50.Z15	T50.Z16
vaccine	T50.B91	T50.B92	T50.B93	T50.B94	T50.B95	T50.B96
Racemoramide	T40.2X1	T40.2X2	T40.2X3	T40.2X4		
Racemorphan	T40.2X1	T40.2X2	T40.2X3	T40.2X4	T40.2X5	T40.2X6
Racepinefrin	T44.5X1	T44.5X2	T44.5X3	T44.5X4	T44.5X5	T44.5X6
Raclopride	T43.591	T43.592	T43.593	T43.594	T43.595	T43.596
Radiator alcohol	T51.1X1	T51.1X2	T51.1X3	T51.1X4	—	—
Radioactive drug NEC	T50.8X1	T50.8X2	T50.8X3	T50.8X4	T50.8X5	T50.8X6
Radio-opaque (drugs) (materials)	T50.8X1	T50.8X2	T50.8X3	T50.8X4	T50.8X5	T50.8X6
Ramifenazone	T39.2X1	T39.2X2	T39.2X3	T39.2X4	T39.2X5	T39.2X6
Ramipril	T46.4X1	T46.4X2	T46.4X3	T46.4X4	T46.4X5	T46.4X6
Ranitidine	T47.0X1	T47.0X2	T47.0X3	T47.0X4	T47.0X5	T47.0X6
Ranunculus	T62.2X1	T62.2X2	T62.2X3	T62.2X4	—	—
Rat poison NEC	T60.4X1	T60.4X2	T60.4X3	T60.4X4	—	—
Rattlesnake (venom)	T63.011	T63.012	T63.013	T63.014	—	—
Raubasine	T46.7X1	T46.7X2	T46.7X3	T46.7X4	T46.7X5	T46.7X6
Raudixin	T46.5X1	T46.5X2	T46.5X3	T46.5X4	T46.5X5	T46.5X6
Rautensin	T46.5X1	T46.5X2	T46.5X3	T46.5X4	T46.5X5	T46.5X6
Rautina	T46.5X1	T46.5X2	T46.5X3	T46.5X4	T46.5X5	T46.5X6
Rautotal	T46.5X1	T46.5X2	T46.5X3	T46.5X4	T46.5X5	T46.5X6
Rauwiloid	T46.5X1	T46.5X2	T46.5X3	T46.5X4	T46.5X5	T46.5X6
Rauwoldin	T46.5X1	T46.5X2	T46.5X3	T46.5X4	T46.5X5	T46.5X6
Rauwolfia (alkaloids)	T46.5X1	T46.5X2	T46.5X3	T46.5X4	T46.5X5	T46.5X6
Razoxane	T45.1X1	T45.1X2	T45.1X3	T45.1X4	T45.1X5	T45.1X6
Realgar	T57.0X1	T57.0X2	T57.0X3	T57.0X4	—	—
Recombinant (R) — *see specific protein*						
Red blood cells, packed	T45.8X1	T45.8X2	T45.8X3	T45.8X4	T45.8X5	T45.8X6
Red squill (scilliroside)	T60.4X1	T60.4X2	T60.4X3	T60.4X4	—	—
Reducing agent, industrial NEC	T65.891	T65.892	T65.893	T65.894	—	—
Refrigerant gas (chlorofluoro-carbon)	T53.5X1	T53.5X2	T53.5X3	T53.5X4	—	—
not chlorofluoro-carbon	T59.891	T59.892	T59.893	T59.894	—	—
Regroton	T50.2X1	T50.2X2	T50.2X3	T50.2X4	T50.2X5	T50.2X6
Rehydration salts (oral)	T50.3X1	T50.3X2	T50.3X3	T50.3X4	T50.3X5	T50.3X6
Rela	T42.8X1	T42.8X2	T42.8X3	T42.8X4	T42.8X5	T42.8X6

◀ New   ◀|||| Revised   ~~deleted~~ Deleted

Substance	Poisoning, Accidental (Unintentional)	Poisoning, Intentional Self-Harm	Poisoning, Assault	Poisoning, Undetermined	Adverse Effect	Underdosing
Relaxant, muscle						
anesthetic	T48.1X1	T48.1X2	T48.1X3	T48.1X4	T48.1X5	T48.1X6
central nervous system	T42.8X1	T42.8X2	T42.8X3	T42.8X4	T42.8X5	T42.8X6
skeletal NEC	T48.1X1	T48.1X2	T48.1X3	T48.1X4	T48.1X5	T48.1X6
smooth NEC	T44.3X1	T44.3X2	T44.3X3	T44.3X4	T44.3X5	T44.3X6
Remoxipride	T43.591	T43.592	T43.593	T43.594	T43.595	T43.596
Renese	T50.2X1	T50.2X2	T50.2X3	T50.2X4	T50.2X5	T50.2X6
Renografin	T50.8X1	T50.8X2	T50.8X3	T50.8X4	T50.8X5	T50.8X6
Replacement solution	T50.3X1	T50.3X2	T50.3X3	T50.3X4	T50.3X5	T50.3X6
Reproterol	T48.6X1	T48.6X2	T48.6X3	T48.6X4	T48.6X5	T48.6X6
Rescinnamine	T46.5X1	T46.5X2	T46.5X3	T46.5X4	T46.5X5	T46.5X6
Reserpin(e)	T46.5X1	T46.5X2	T46.5X3	T46.5X4	T46.5X5	T46.5X6
Resorcin, resorcinol (nonmedicinal)	T65.891	T65.892	T65.893	T65.894	—	—
medicinal	T49.4X1	T49.4X2	T49.4X3	T49.4X4	T49.4X5	T49.4X6
Respaire	T48.4X1	T48.4X2	T48.4X3	T48.4X4	T48.4X5	T48.4X6
Respiratory drug NEC	T48.901	T48.902	T48.903	T48.904	T48.905	T48.906
antiasthmatic NEC	T48.6X1	T48.6X2	T48.6X3	T48.6X4	T48.6X5	T48.6X6
anti-common-cold NEC	T48.5X1	T48.5X2	T48.5X3	T48.5X4	T48.5X5	T48.5X6
expectorant NEC	T48.4X1	T48.4X2	T48.4X3	T48.4X4	T48.4X5	T48.4X6
stimulant	T48.901	T48.902	T48.903	T48.904	T48.905	T48.906
Retinoic acid	T49.0X1	T49.0X2	T49.0X3	T49.0X4	T49.0X5	T49.0X6
Retinol	T45.2X1	T45.2X2	T45.2X3	T45.2X4	T45.2X5	T45.2X6
Rh (D) immune globulin (human)	T50.Z11	T50.Z12	T50.Z13	T50.Z14	T50.Z15	T50.Z16
Rhodine	T39.011	T39.012	T39.013	T39.014	T39.015	T39.016
RhoGAM	T50.Z11	T50.Z12	T50.Z13	T50.Z14	T50.Z15	T50.Z16
Rhubarb						
dry extract	T47.2X1	T47.2X2	T47.2X3	T47.2X4	T47.2X5	T47.2X6
tincture, compound	T47.2X1	T47.2X2	T47.2X3	T47.2X4	T47.2X5	T47.2X6
Ribavirin	T37.5X1	T37.5X2	T37.5X3	T37.5X4	T37.5X5	T37.5X6
Riboflavin	T45.2X1	T45.2X2	T45.2X3	T45.2X4	T45.2X5	T45.2X6
Ribostamycin	T36.5X1	T36.5X2	T36.5X3	T36.5X4	T36.5X5	T36.5X6
Ricin	T62.2X1	T62.2X2	T62.2X3	T62.2X4	—	—
Ricinus communis	T62.2X1	T62.2X2	T62.2X3	T62.2X4	—	—
Rickettsial vaccine NEC	T50.A91	T50.A92	T50.A93	T50.A94	T50.A95	T50.A96
Rifabutin	T36.6X1	T36.6X2	T36.6X3	T36.6X4	T36.6X5	T36.6X6
Rifamide	T36.6X1	T36.6X2	T36.6X3	T36.6X4	T36.6X5	T36.6X6
Rifampicin	T36.6X1	T36.6X2	T36.6X3	T36.6X4	T36.6X5	T36.6X6
with isoniazid	T37.1X1	T37.1X2	T37.1X3	T37.1X4	T37.1X5	T37.1X6
Rifampin	T36.6X1	T36.6X2	T36.6X3	T36.6X4	T36.6X5	T36.6X6
Rifamycin	T36.6X1	T36.6X2	T36.6X3	T36.6X4	T36.6X5	T36.6X6
Rifaximin	T36.6X1	T36.6X2	T36.6X3	T36.6X4	T36.6X5	T36.6X6

Substance	Poisoning, Accidental (Unintentional)	Poisoning, Intentional Self-Harm	Poisoning, Assault	Poisoning, Undetermined	Adverse Effect	Underdosing
Rimantadine	T37.5X1	T37.5X2	T37.5X3	T37.5X4	T37.5X5	T37.5X6
Rimazolium metilsulfate	T39.8X1	T39.8X2	T39.8X3	T39.8X4	T39.8X5	T39.8X6
Rimifon	T37.1X1	T37.1X2	T37.1X3	T37.1X4	T37.1X5	T37.1X6
Rimiterol	T48.6X1	T48.6X2	T48.6X3	T48.6X4	T48.6X5	T48.6X6
Ringer (lactate) solution	T50.3X1	T50.3X2	T50.3X3	T50.3X4	T50.3X5	T50.3X6
Ristocetin	T36.8X1	T36.8X2	T36.8X3	T36.8X4	T36.8X5	T36.8X6
Ritalin	T43.631	T43.632	T43.633	T43.634	T43.635	T43.636
Ritodrine	T44.5X1	T44.5X2	T44.5X3	T44.5X4	T44.5X5	T44.5X6
Roach killer — see Insecticide						
Rociverine	T44.3X1	T44.3X2	T44.3X3	T44.3X4	T44.3X5	T44.3X6
Rocky Mountain spotted fever vaccine	T50.A91	T50.A92	T50.A93	T50.A94	T50.A95	T50.A96
Rodenticide NEC	T60.4X1	T60.4X2	T60.4X3	T60.4X4	—	—
Rohypnol	T42.4X1	T42.4X2	T42.4X3	T42.4X4	T42.4X5	T42.4X6
Rokitamycin	T36.3X1	T36.3X2	T36.3X3	T36.3X4	T36.3X5	T36.3X6
Rolaids	T47.1X1	T47.1X2	T47.1X3	T47.1X4	T47.1X5	T47.1X6
Rolitetracycline	T36.4X1	T36.4X2	T36.4X3	T36.4X4	T36.4X5	T36.4X6
Romilar	T48.3X1	T48.3X2	T48.3X3	T48.3X4	T48.3X5	T48.3X6
Ronifibrate	T46.6X1	T46.6X2	T46.6X3	T46.6X4	T46.6X5	T46.6X6
Rosaprostol	T47.1X1	T47.1X2	T47.1X3	T47.1X4	T47.1X5	T47.1X6
Rose bengal sodium (1311)	T50.8X1	T50.8X2	T50.8X3	T50.8X4	T50.8X5	T50.8X6
Rose water ointment	T49.3X1	T49.3X2	T49.3X3	T49.3X4	T49.3X5	T49.3X6
Rosoxacin	T37.8X1	T37.8X2	T37.8X3	T37.8X4	T37.8X5	T37.8X6
Rotenone	T60.2X1	T60.2X2	T60.2X3	T60.2X4	—	—
Rotoxamine	T45.0X1	T45.0X2	T45.0X3	T45.0X4	T45.0X5	T45.0X6
Rough-on-rats	T60.4X1	T60.4X2	T60.4X3	T60.4X4	—	—
Roxatidine	T47.0X1	T47.0X2	T47.0X3	T47.0X4	T47.0X5	T47.0X6
Roxithromycin	T36.3X1	T36.3X2	T36.3X3	T36.3X4	T36.3X5	T36.3X6
Rt-PA	T45.611	T45.612	T45.613	T45.614	T45.615	T45.616
Rubbing alcohol	T51.2X1	T51.2X2	T51.2X3	T51.2X4	—	—
Rubefacient	T49.4X1	T49.4X2	T49.4X3	T49.4X4	T49.4X5	T49.4X6
Rubella vaccine	T50.B91	T50.B92	T50.B93	T50.B94	T50.B95	T50.B96
Rubelogen	T50.B91	T50.B92	T50.B93	T50.B94	T50.B95	T50.B96
Rubeovax	T50.991	T50.992	T50.993	T50.994	T50.995	T50.996
Rubidium chloride Rb82	T50.8X1	T50.8X2	T50.8X3	T50.8X4	T50.8X5	T50.8X6
Rubidomycin	T45.1X1	T45.1X2	T45.1X3	T45.1X4	T45.1X5	T45.1X6
Rue	T62.2X1	T62.2X2	T62.2X3	T62.2X4	—	—
Rufocromomycin	T45.1X1	T45.1X2	T45.1X3	T45.1X4	T45.1X5	T45.1X6
Russel's viper venin	T45.7X1	T45.7X2	T45.7X3	T45.7X4	T45.7X5	T45.7X6
Ruta (graveolens)	T62.2X1	T62.2X2	T62.2X3	T62.2X4	—	—
Rutinum	T46.991	T46.992	T46.993	T46.994	T46.995	T46.996
Rutoside	T46.991	T46.992	T46.993	T46.994	T46.995	T46.996

TABLE OF DRUGS AND CHEMICALS

Substance	Poisoning, Accidental (Unintentional)	Poisoning, Intentional Self-Harm	Poisoning, Assault	Poisoning, Undetermined	Adverse Effect	Underdosing
S						
Sabadilla (plant)	T62.2X1	T62.2X2	T62.2X3	T62.2X4	—	—
pesticide	T60.2X1	T60.2X2	T60.2X3	T60.2X4	—	—
Saccharated iron oxide	T45.8X1	T45.8X2	T45.8X3	T45.8X4	T45.8X5	T45.8X6
Saccharin	T50.901	T50.902	T50.903	T50.904	T50.905	T50.906
Saccharomyces boulardii	T47.6X1	T47.6X2	T47.6X3	T47.6X4	T47.6X5	T47.6X6
Safflower oil	T46.6X1	T46.6X2	T46.6X3	T46.6X4	T46.6X5	T46.6X6
Safrazine	T43.1X1	T43.1X2	T43.1X3	T43.1X4	T43.1X5	T43.1X6
Salazosulfapyridine	T37.0X1	T37.0X2	T37.0X3	T37.0X4	T37.0X5	T37.0X6
Salbutamol	T48.6X1	T48.6X2	T48.6X3	T48.6X4	T48.6X5	T48.6X6
Salicylamide	T39.091	T39.092	T39.093	T39.094	T39.095	T39.096
Salicylate NEC	T39.091	T39.092	T39.093	T39.094	T39.095	T39.096
methyl	T49.3X1	T49.3X2	T49.3X3	T49.3X4	T49.3X5	T49.3X6
theobromine calcium	T50.2X1	T50.2X2	T50.2X3	T50.2X4	T50.2X5	T50.2X6
Salicylazosulfapyridine	T37.0X1	T37.0X2	T37.0X3	T37.0X4	T37.0X5	T37.0X6
Salicylhydroxamic acid	T49.0X1	T49.0X2	T49.0X3	T49.0X4	T49.0X5	T49.0X6
Salicylic acid	T49.4X1	T49.4X2	T49.4X3	T49.4X4	T49.4X5	T49.4X6
with benzoic acid	T49.4X1	T49.4X2	T49.4X3	T49.4X4	T49.4X5	T49.4X6
congeners	T39.091	T39.092	T39.093	T39.094	T39.095	T39.096
derivative	T39.091	T39.092	T39.093	T39.094	T39.095	T39.096
salts	T39.091	T39.092	T39.093	T39.094	T39.095	T39.096
Salinazid	T37.1X1	T37.1X2	T37.1X3	T37.1X4	T37.1X5	T37.1X6
Salmeterol	T48.6X1	T48.6X2	T48.6X3	T48.6X4	T48.6X5	T48.6X6
Salol	T49.3X1	T49.3X2	T49.3X3	T49.3X4	T49.3X5	T49.3X6
Salsalate	T39.091	T39.092	T39.093	T39.094	T39.095	T39.096
Salt substitute	T50.901	T50.902	T50.903	T50.904	T50.905	T50.906
Salt-replacing drug	T50.901	T50.902	T50.903	T50.904	T50.905	T50.906
Salt-retaining mineralocorticoid	T50.0X1	T50.0X2	T50.0X3	T50.0X4	T50.0X5	T50.0X6
Saluretic NEC	T50.2X1	T50.2X2	T50.2X3	T50.2X4	T50.2X5	T50.2X6
Saluron	T50.2X1	T50.2X2	T50.2X3	T50.2X4	T50.2X5	T50.2X6
Salvarsan 606 (neosilver) (silver)	T37.8X1	T37.8X2	T37.8X3	T37.8X4	T37.8X5	T37.8X6
Sambucus canadensis	T62.2X1	T62.2X2	T62.2X3	T62.2X4	—	—
berry	T62.1X1	T62.1X2	T62.1X3	T62.1X4	—	—
Sandril	T46.5X1	T46.5X2	T46.5X3	T46.5X4	T46.5X5	T46.5X6
Sanguinaria canadensis	T62.2X1	T62.2X2	T62.2X3	T62.2X4	—	—
Saniflush (cleaner)	T54.2X1	T54.2X2	T54.2X3	T54.2X4	—	—
Santonin	T37.4X1	T37.4X2	T37.4X3	T37.4X4	T37.4X5	T37.4X6
Santyl	T49.8X1	T49.8X2	T49.8X3	T49.8X4	T49.8X5	T49.8X6
Saralasin	T46.5X1	T46.5X2	T46.5X3	T46.5X4	T46.5X5	T46.5X6
Sarcolysin	T45.1X1	T45.1X2	T45.1X3	T45.1X4	T45.1X5	T45.1X6
Sarkomycin	T45.1X1	T45.1X2	T45.1X3	T45.1X4	T45.1X5	T45.1X6
Saroten	T43.011	T43.012	T43.013	T43.014	T43.015	T43.016

Substance	Poisoning, Accidental (Unintentional)	Poisoning, Intentional Self-Harm	Poisoning, Assault	Poisoning, Undetermined	Adverse Effect	Underdosing
Saturnine — *see Lead*						
Savin (oil)	T49.4X1	T49.4X2	T49.4X3	T49.4X4	T49.4X5	T49.4X6
Scammony	T47.2X1	T47.2X2	T47.2X3	T47.2X4	T47.2X5	T47.2X6
Scarlet red	T49.8X1	T49.8X2	T49.8X3	T49.8X4	T49.8X5	T49.8X6
Scheele's green	T57.0X1	T57.0X2	T57.0X3	T57.0X4	—	—
insecticide	T57.0X1	T57.0X2	T57.0X3	T57.0X4	—	—
Schizontozide (blood) (tissue)	T37.2X1	T37.2X2	T37.2X3	T37.2X4	T37.2X5	T37.2X6
Schradan	T60.0X1	T60.0X2	T60.0X3	T60.0X4	—	—
Schweinfurth green	T57.0X1	T57.0X2	T57.0X3	T57.0X4	—	—
insecticide	T57.0X1	T57.0X2	T57.0X3	T57.0X4	—	—
Scilla, rat poison	T60.4X1	T60.4X2	T60.4X3	T60.4X4	—	—
Scillaren	T60.4X1	T60.4X2	T60.4X3	T60.4X4	—	—
Sclerosing agent	T46.8X1	T46.8X2	T46.8X3	T46.8X4	T46.8X5	T46.8X6
Scombrotoxin	T61.11	T61.12	T61.13	T61.14	—	—
Scopolamine	T44.3X1	T44.3X2	T44.3X3	T44.3X4	T44.3X5	T44.3X6
Scopolia extract	T44.3X1	T44.3X2	T44.3X3	T44.3X4	T44.3X5	T44.3X6
Scouring powder	T65.891	T65.892	T65.893	T65.894	—	—
Sea						
anemone (sting)	T63.631	T63.632	T63.633	T63.634	—	—
cucumber (sting)	T63.691	T63.692	T63.693	T63.694	—	—
snake (bite) (venom)	T63.091	T63.092	T63.093	T63.094	—	—
urchin spine (puncture)	T63.691	T63.692	T63.693	T63.694	—	—
Seafood	T61.91	T61.92	T61.93	T61.94	—	—
specified NEC	T61.8X1	T61.8X2	T61.8X3	T61.8X4	—	—
Secbutabarbital	T42.3X1	T42.3X2	T42.3X3	T42.3X4	T42.3X5	T42.3X6
Secbutabarbitone	T42.3X1	T42.3X2	T42.3X3	T42.3X4	T42.3X5	T42.3X6
Secnidazole	T37.3X1	T37.3X2	T37.3X3	T37.3X4	T37.3X5	T37.3X6
Secobarbital	T42.3X1	T42.3X2	T42.3X3	T42.3X4	T42.3X5	T42.3X6
Seconal	T42.3X1	T42.3X2	T42.3X3	T42.3X4	T42.3X5	T42.3X6
Secretin	T50.8X1	T50.8X2	T50.8X3	T50.8X4	T50.8X5	T50.8X6
Sedative NEC	T42.71	T42.72	T42.73	T42.74	T42.75	T42.76
mixed NEC	T42.6X1	T42.6X2	T42.6X3	T42.6X4	T42.6X5	T42.6X6
Sedormid	T42.6X1	T42.6X2	T42.6X3	T42.6X4	T42.6X5	T42.6X6
Seed disinfectant or dressing	T60.8X1	T60.8X2	T60.8X3	T60.8X4	—	—
Seeds (poisonous)	T62.2X1	T62.2X2	T62.2X3	T62.2X4	—	—
Selegiline	T42.8X1	T42.8X2	T42.8X3	T42.8X4	T42.8X5	T42.8X6
Selenium NEC	T56.891	T56.892	T56.893	T56.894	—	—
disulfide or sulfide	T49.4X1	T49.4X2	T49.4X3	T49.4X4	T49.4X5	T49.4X6
fumes	T59.891	T59.892	T59.893	T59.894	—	—
sulfide	T49.4X1	T49.4X2	T49.4X3	T49.4X4	T49.4X5	T49.4X6
Selenomethionine (75Se)	T50.8X1	T50.8X2	T50.8X3	T50.8X4	T50.8X5	T50.8X6
Selsun	T49.4X1	T49.4X2	T49.4X3	T49.4X4	T49.4X5	T49.4X6

◀ New   ◀ Revised   ~~deleted~~ Deleted

Substance	Poisoning, Accidental (Unintentional)	Poisoning, Intentional Self-Harm	Poisoning, Assault	Poisoning, Undetermined	Adverse Effect	Underdosing
Semustine	T45.1X1	T45.1X2	T45.1X3	T45.1X4	T45.1X5	T45.1X6
Senega syrup	T48.4X1	T48.4X2	T48.4X3	T48.4X4	T48.4X5	T48.4X6
Senna	T47.2X1	T47.2X2	T47.2X3	T47.2X4	T47.2X5	T47.2X6
Sennoside A+B	T47.2X1	T47.2X2	T47.2X3	T47.2X4	T47.2X5	T47.2X6
Septisol	T49.2X1	T49.2X2	T49.2X3	T49.2X4	T49.2X5	T49.2X6
Seractide	T38.811	T38.812	T38.813	T38.814	T38.815	T38.816
Serax	T42.4X1	T42.4X2	T42.4X3	T42.4X4	T42.4X5	T42.4X6
Serenesil	T42.6X1	T42.6X2	T42.6X3	T42.6X4	T42.6X5	T42.6X6
Serenium (hydrochloride)	T37.91	T37.92	T37.93	T37.94	T37.95	T37.96
Serepax — see Oxazepam						
Sermorelin	T38.891	T38.892	T38.893	T38.894	T38.895	T38.896
Sernyl	T41.1X1	T41.1X2	T41.1X3	T41.1X4	T41.1X5	T41.1X6
Serotonin	T50.991	T50.992	T50.993	T50.994	T50.995	T50.996
Serpasil	T46.5X1	T46.5X2	T46.5X3	T46.5X4	T46.5X5	T46.5X6
Serrapeptase	T45.3X1	T45.3X2	T45.3X3	T45.3X4	T45.3X5	T45.3X6
Serum						
antibotulinus	T50.Z11	T50.Z12	T50.Z13	T50.Z14	T50.Z15	T50.Z16
anticytotoxic	T50.Z11	T50.Z12	T50.Z13	T50.Z14	T50.Z15	T50.Z16
antidiphtheria	T50.Z11	T50.Z12	T50.Z13	T50.Z14	T50.Z15	T50.Z16
antimeningococcus	T50.Z11	T50.Z12	T50.Z13	T50.Z14	T50.Z15	T50.Z16
anti-Rh	T50.Z11	T50.Z12	T50.Z13	T50.Z14	T50.Z15	T50.Z16
anti-snake-bite	T50.Z11	T50.Z12	T50.Z13	T50.Z14	T50.Z15	T50.Z16
antitetanic	T50.Z11	T50.Z12	T50.Z13	T50.Z14	T50.Z15	T50.Z16
antitoxic	T50.Z11	T50.Z12	T50.Z13	T50.Z14	T50.Z15	T50.Z16
complement (inhibitor)	T45.8X1	T45.8X2	T45.8X3	T45.8X4	T45.8X5	T45.8X6
convalescent	T50.Z11	T50.Z12	T50.Z13	T50.Z14	T50.Z15	T50.Z16
hemolytic complement	T45.8X1	T45.8X2	T45.8X3	T45.8X4	T45.8X5	T45.8X6
immune (human)	T50.Z11	T50.Z12	T50.Z13	T50.Z14	T50.Z15	T50.Z16
protective NEC	T50.Z11	T50.Z12	T50.Z13	T50.Z14	T50.Z15	T50.Z16
Setastine	T45.0X1	T45.0X2	T45.0X3	T45.0X4	T45.0X5	T45.0X6
Setoperone	T43.591	T43.592	T43.593	T43.594	T43.595	T43.596
Sewer gas	T59.91	T59.92	T59.93	T59.94	—	—
Shampoo	T55.0X1	T55.0X2	T55.0X3	T55.0X4	—	—
Shellfish, noxious, nonbacterial	T61.781	T61.782	T61.783	T61.784	—	—
Sildenafil	T46.7X1	T46.7X2	T46.7X3	T46.7X4	T46.7X5	T46.7X6
Silibinin	T50.991	T50.992	T50.993	T50.994	T50.995	T50.996
Silicone NEC	T65.891	T65.892	T65.893	T65.894	—	—
medicinal	T49.3X1	T49.3X2	T49.3X3	T49.3X4	T49.3X5	T49.3X6
Silvadene	T49.0X1	T49.0X2	T49.0X3	T49.0X4	T49.0X5	T49.0X6
Silver	T49.0X1	T49.0X2	T49.0X3	T49.0X4	T49.0X5	T49.0X6
anti-infectives	T49.0X1	T49.0X2	T49.0X3	T49.0X4	T49.0X5	T49.0X6
arsphenamine	T37.8X1	T37.8X2	T37.8X3	T37.8X4	T37.8X5	T37.8X6
Silver (Continued)						
colloidal	T49.0X1	T49.0X2	T49.0X3	T49.0X4	T49.0X5	T49.0X6
nitrate	T49.0X1	T49.0X2	T49.0X3	T49.0X4	T49.0X5	T49.0X6
ophthalmic preparation	T49.5X1	T49.5X2	T49.5X3	T49.5X4	T49.5X5	T49.5X6
toughened (keratolytic)	T49.4X1	T49.4X2	T49.4X3	T49.4X4	T49.4X5	T49.4X6
nonmedicinal (dust)	T56.891	T56.892	T56.893	T56.894	—	—
protein	T49.5X1	T49.5X2	T49.5X3	T49.5X4	T49.5X5	T49.5X6
salvarsan	T37.8X1	T37.8X2	T37.8X3	T37.8X4	T37.8X5	T37.8X6
sulfadiazine	T49.4X1	T49.4X2	T49.4X3	T49.4X4	T49.4X5	T49.4X6
Silymarin	T50.991	T50.992	T50.993	T50.994	T50.995	T50.996
Simaldrate	T47.1X1	T47.1X2	T47.1X3	T47.1X4	T47.1X5	T47.1X6
Simazine	T60.3X1	T60.3X2	T60.3X3	T60.3X4	—	—
Simethicone	T47.1X1	T47.1X2	T47.1X3	T47.1X4	T47.1X5	T47.1X6
Simfibrate	T46.6X1	T46.6X2	T46.6X3	T46.6X4	T46.6X5	T46.6X6
Simvastatin	T46.6X1	T46.6X2	T46.6X3	T46.6X4	T46.6X5	T46.6X6
Sincalide	T50.8X1	T50.8X2	T50.8X3	T50.8X4	T50.8X5	T50.8X6
Sinequan	T43.011	T43.012	T43.013	T43.014	T43.015	T43.016
Singoserp	T46.5X1	T46.5X2	T46.5X3	T46.5X4	T46.5X5	T46.5X6
Sintrom	T45.511	T45.512	T45.513	T45.514	T45.515	T45.516
Sisomicin	T36.5X1	T36.5X2	T36.5X3	T36.5X4	T36.5X5	T36.5X6
Sitosterols	T46.6X1	T46.6X2	T46.6X3	T46.6X4	T46.6X5	T46.6X6
Skeletal muscle relaxants	T48.1X1	T48.1X2	T48.1X3	T48.1X4	T48.1X5	T48.1X6
Skin						
agents (external)	T49.91	T49.92	T49.93	T49.94	T49.95	T49.96
specified NEC	T49.8X1	T49.8X2	T49.8X3	T49.8X4	T49.8X5	T49.8X6
test antigen	T50.8X1	T50.8X2	T50.8X3	T50.8X4	T50.8X5	T50.8X6
Sleep-eze	T45.0X1	T45.0X2	T45.0X3	T45.0X4	T45.0X5	T45.0X6
Sleeping draught, pill	T42.71	T42.72	T42.73	T42.74	T42.75	T42.76
Smallpox vaccine	T50.B11	T50.B12	T50.B13	T50.B14	T50.B15	T50.B16
Smelter fumes NEC	T56.91	T56.92	T56.93	T56.94	—	—
Smog	T59.1X1	T59.1X2	T59.1X3	T59.1X4	—	—
Smoke NEC	T59.811	T59.812	T59.813	T59.814	—	—
Smooth muscle relaxant	T44.3X1	T44.3X2	T44.3X3	T44.3X4	T44.3X5	T44.3X6
Snail killer NEC	T60.8X1	T60.8X2	T60.8X3	T60.8X4	—	—
Snake venom or bite	T63.001	T63.002	T63.003	T63.004		
hemocoagulase	T45.7X1	T45.7X2	T45.7X3	T45.7X4	T45.7X5	T45.7X6
Snuff	T65.211	T65.212	T65.213	T65.214		
Soap (powder) (product)	T55.0X1	T55.0X2	T55.0X3	T55.0X4		
enema	T47.4X1	T47.4X2	T47.4X3	T47.4X4	T47.4X5	T47.4X6
medicinal, soft	T49.2X1	T49.2X2	T49.2X3	T49.2X4	T49.2X5	T49.2X6
superfatted	T49.2X1	T49.2X2	T49.2X3	T49.2X4	T49.2X5	T49.2X6
Sobrerol	T48.4X1	T48.4X2	T48.4X3	T48.4X4	T48.4X5	T48.4X6

◄ New ⬅ Revised ~~deleted~~ Deleted

	External Cause (T-Code)					
Substance	Poisoning, Accidental (Unintentional)	Poisoning, Intentional Self-Harm	Poisoning, Assault	Poisoning, Undetermined	Adverse Effect	Underdosing
Soda (caustic)	T54.3X1	T54.3X2	T54.3X3	T54.3X4	—	—
bicarb	T47.1X1	T47.1X2	T47.1X3	T47.1X4	T47.1X5	T47.1X6
chlorinated — *see Sodium, hypochlorite*						
Sodium						
acetosulfone	T37.1X1	T37.1X2	T37.1X3	T37.1X4	T37.1X5	T37.1X6
acetrizoate	T50.8X1	T50.8X2	T50.8X3	T50.8X4	T50.8X5	T50.8X6
acid phosphate	T50.3X1	T50.3X2	T50.3X3	T50.3X4	T50.3X5	T50.3X6
alginate	T47.8X1	T47.8X2	T47.8X3	T47.8X4	T47.8X5	T47.8X6
amidotrizoate	T50.8X1	T50.8X2	T50.8X3	T50.8X4	T50.8X5	T50.8X6
aminopterin	T45.1X1	T45.1X2	T45.1X3	T45.1X4	T45.1X5	T45.1X6
amylosulfate	T47.8X1	T47.8X2	T47.8X3	T47.8X4	T47.8X5	T47.8X6
amytal	T42.3X1	T42.3X2	T42.3X3	T42.3X4	T42.3X5	T42.3X6
antimony gluconate	T37.3X1	T37.3X2	T37.3X3	T37.3X4	T37.3X5	T37.3X6
arsenate	T57.0X1	T57.0X2	T57.0X3	T57.0X4	—	—
aurothiomalate	T39.4X1	T39.4X2	T39.4X3	T39.4X4	T39.4X5	T39.4X6
aurothiosulfate	T39.4X1	T39.4X2	T39.4X3	T39.4X4	T39.4X5	T39.4X6
barbiturate	T42.3X1	T42.3X2	T42.3X3	T42.3X4	T42.3X5	T42.3X6
basic phosphate	T47.4X1	T47.4X2	T47.4X3	T47.4X4	T47.4X5	T47.4X6
bicarbonate	T47.1X1	T47.1X2	T47.1X3	T47.1X4	T47.1X5	T47.1X6
bichromate	T57.8X1	T57.8X2	T57.8X3	T57.8X4	—	—
biphosphate	T50.3X1	T50.3X2	T50.3X3	T50.3X4	T50.3X5	T50.3X6
bisulfate	T65.891	T65.892	T65.893	T65.894	—	—
borate						
cleanser	T57.8X1	T57.8X2	T57.8X3	T57.8X4	—	—
eye	T49.5X1	T49.5X2	T49.5X3	T49.5X4	T49.5X5	T49.5X6
therapeutic	T49.8X1	T49.8X2	T49.8X3	T49.8X4	T49.8X5	T49.8X6
bromide	T42.6X1	T42.6X2	T42.6X3	T42.6X4	T42.6X5	T42.6X6
cacodylate (nonmedicinal) NEC	T50.8X1	T50.8X2	T50.8X3	T50.8X4	T50.8X5	T50.8X6
anti-infective	T37.8X1	T37.8X2	T37.8X3	T37.8X4	T37.8X5	T37.8X6
herbicide	T60.3X1	T60.3X2	T60.3X3	T60.3X4	—	—
calcium edetate	T45.8X1	T45.8X2	T45.8X3	T45.8X4	T45.8X5	T45.8X6
carbonate NEC	T54.3X1	T54.3X2	T54.3X3	T54.3X4	—	—
chlorate NEC	T65.891	T65.892	T65.893	T65.894	—	—
herbicide	T54.91	T54.92	T54.93	T54.94	—	—
chloride	T50.3X1	T50.3X2	T50.3X3	T50.3X4	T50.3X5	T50.3X6
with glucose	T50.3X1	T50.3X2	T50.3X3	T50.3X4	T50.3X5	T50.3X6
chromate	T65.891	T65.892	T65.893	T65.894	—	—
citrate	T50.991	T50.992	T50.993	T50.994	T50.995	T50.996
cromoglicate	T48.6X1	T48.6X2	T48.6X3	T48.6X4	T48.6X5	T48.6X6
cyanide	T65.0X1	T65.0X2	T65.0X3	T65.0X4	—	—
cyclamate	T50.3X1	T50.3X2	T50.3X3	T50.3X4	T50.3X5	T50.3X6

	External Cause (T-Code)					
Substance	Poisoning, Accidental (Unintentional)	Poisoning, Intentional Self-Harm	Poisoning, Assault	Poisoning, Undetermined	Adverse Effect	Underdosing
Sodium *(Continued)*						
dehydrocholate	T45.8X1	T45.8X2	T45.8X3	T45.8X4	T45.8X5	T45.8X6
diatrizoate	T50.8X1	T50.8X2	T50.8X3	T50.8X4	T50.8X5	T50.8X6
dibunate	T48.4X1	T48.4X2	T48.4X3	T48.4X4	T48.4X5	T48.4X6
dioctyl sulfosuccinate	T47.4X1	T47.4X2	T47.4X3	T47.4X4	T47.4X5	T47.4X6
dipantoyl ferrate	T45.8X1	T45.8X2	T45.8X3	T45.8X4	T45.8X5	T45.8X6
edetate	T45.8X1	T45.8X2	T45.8X3	T45.8X4	T45.8X5	T45.8X6
ethacrynate	T50.1X1	T50.1X2	T50.1X3	T50.1X4	T50.1X5	T50.1X6
feredetate	T45.8X1	T45.8X2	T45.8X3	T45.8X4	T45.8X5	T45.8X6
Fluoride — *see Fluoride*						
fluoroacetate (dust) (pesticide)	T60.4X1	T60.4X2	T60.4X3	T60.4X4	—	—
free salt	T50.3X1	T50.3X2	T50.3X3	T50.3X4	T50.3X5	T50.3X6
fusidate	T36.8X1	T36.8X2	T36.8X3	T36.8X4	T36.8X5	T36.8X6
glucaldrate	T47.1X1	T47.1X2	T47.1X3	T47.1X4	T47.1X5	T47.1X6
glucosulfone	T37.1X1	T37.1X2	T37.1X3	T37.1X4	T37.1X5	T37.1X6
glutamate	T45.8X1	T45.8X2	T45.8X3	T45.8X4	T45.8X5	T45.8X6
hydrogen carbonate	T50.3X1	T50.3X2	T50.3X3	T50.3X4	T50.3X5	T50.3X6
hydroxide	T54.3X1	T54.3X2	T54.3X3	T54.3X4	—	—
hypochlorite (bleach) NEC	T54.3X1	T54.3X2	T54.3X3	T54.3X4	—	—
disinfectant	T54.3X1	T54.3X2	T54.3X3	T54.3X4	—	—
medicinal (anti-infective) (external)	T49.0X1	T49.0X2	T49.0X3	T49.0X4	T49.0X5	T49.0X6
vapor	T54.3X1	T54.3X2	T54.3X3	T54.3X4	—	—
hyposulfite	T49.0X1	T49.0X2	T49.0X3	T49.0X4	T49.0X5	T49.0X6
indigotin disulfonate	T50.8X1	T50.8X2	T50.8X3	T50.8X4	T50.8X5	T50.8X6
iodide	T50.991	T50.992	T50.993	T50.994	T50.995	T50.996
I-131	T50.8X1	T50.8X2	T50.8X3	T50.8X4	T50.8X5	T50.8X6
therapeutic	T38.2X1	T38.2X2	T38.2X3	T38.2X4	T38.2X5	T38.2X6
iodohippurate (131I)	T50.8X1	T50.8X2	T50.8X3	T50.8X4	T50.8X5	T50.8X6
iopodate	T50.8X1	T50.8X2	T50.8X3	T50.8X4	T50.8X5	T50.8X6
iothalamate	T50.8X1	T50.8X2	T50.8X3	T50.8X4	T50.8X5	T50.8X6
iron edetate	T45.4X1	T45.4X2	T45.4X3	T45.4X4	T45.4X5	T45.4X6
lactate (compound solution)	T45.8X1	T45.8X2	T45.8X3	T45.8X4	T45.8X5	T45.8X6
lauryl (sulfate)	T49.2X1	T49.2X2	T49.2X3	T49.2X4	T49.2X5	T49.2X6
(L)-triiodothyronine	T38.1X1	T38.1X2	T38.1X3	T38.1X4	T38.1X5	T38.1X6
magnesium citrate	T50.991	T50.992	T50.993	T50.994	T50.995	T50.996
mersalate	T50.2X1	T50.2X2	T50.2X3	T50.2X4	T50.2X5	T50.2X6
metasilicate	T65.891	T65.892	T65.893	T65.894	—	—
metrizoate	T50.8X1	T50.8X2	T50.8X3	T50.8X4	T50.8X5	T50.8X6
monofluoroacetate (pesticide)	T60.1X1	T60.1X2	T60.1X3	T60.1X4	—	—
morrhuate	T46.8X1	T46.8X2	T46.8X3	T46.8X4	T46.8X5	T46.8X6
nafcillin	T36.0X1	T36.0X2	T36.0X3	T36.0X4	T36.0X5	T36.0X6

◀ New ◀▦ Revised ~~deleted~~ Deleted

Substance	Poisoning, Accidental (Unintentional)	Poisoning, Intentional Self-Harm	Poisoning, Assault	Poisoning, Undetermined	Adverse Effect	Underdosing
Sodium (Continued)						
nitrate (oxidizing agent)	T65.891	T65.892	T65.893	T65.894	—	—
nitrite	T50.6X1	T50.6X2	T50.6X3	T50.6X4	T50.6X5	T50.6X6
nitroferricyanide	T46.5X1	T46.5X2	T46.5X3	T46.5X4	T46.5X5	T46.5X6
nitroprusside	T46.5X1	T46.5X2	T46.5X3	T46.5X4	T46.5X5	T46.5X6
oxalate	T65.891	T65.892	T65.893	T65.894		
oxide/peroxide	T65.891	T65.892	T65.893	T65.894	—	—
oxybate	T41.291	T41.292	T41.293	T41.294	T41.295	T41.296
para-aminohippurate	T50.8X1	T50.8X2	T50.8X3	T50.8X4	T50.8X5	T50.8X6
perborate (nonmedicinal) NEC	T65.891	T65.892	T65.893	T65.894	—	—
medicinal	T49.0X1	T49.0X2	T49.0X3	T49.0X4	T49.0X5	T49.0X6
soap	T55.0X1	T55.0X2	T55.0X3	T55.0X4		
percarbonate — see Sodium, perborate						
pertechnetate Tc99m	T50.8X1	T50.8X2	T50.8X3	T50.8X4	T50.8X5	T50.8X6
phosphate						
cellulose	T45.8X1	T45.8X2	T45.8X3	T45.8X4	T45.8X5	T45.8X6
dibasic	T47.2X1	T47.2X2	T47.2X3	T47.2X4	T47.2X5	T47.2X6
monobasic	T47.2X1	T47.2X2	T47.2X3	T47.2X4	T47.2X5	T47.2X6
phytate	T50.6X1	T50.6X2	T50.6X3	T50.6X4	T50.6X5	T50.6X6
picosulfate	T47.2X1	T47.2X2	T47.2X3	T47.2X4	T47.2X5	T47.2X6
polyhydroxyaluminium monocarbonate	T47.1X1	T47.1X2	T47.1X3	T47.1X4	T47.1X5	T47.1X6
polystyrene sulfonate	T50.3X1	T50.3X2	T50.3X3	T50.3X4	T50.3X5	T50.3X6
propionate	T49.0X1	T49.0X2	T49.0X3	T49.0X4	T49.0X5	T49.0X6
propyl hydroxybenzoate	T50.991	T50.992	T50.993	T50.994	T50.995	T50.996
psylliate	T46.8X1	T46.8X2	T46.8X3	T46.8X4	T46.8X5	T46.8X6
removing resins	T50.3X1	T50.3X2	T50.3X3	T50.3X4	T50.3X5	T50.3X6
salicylate	T39.091	T39.092	T39.093	T39.094	T39.095	T39.096
salt NEC	T50.3X1	T50.3X2	T50.3X3	T50.3X4	T50.3X5	T50.3X6
selenate	T60.2X1	T60.2X2	T60.2X3	T60.2X4	—	—
stibogluconate	T37.3X1	T37.3X2	T37.3X3	T37.3X4	T37.3X5	T37.3X6
sulfate	T47.4X1	T47.4X2	T47.4X3	T47.4X4	T47.4X5	T47.4X6
sulfoxone	T37.1X1	T37.1X2	T37.1X3	T37.1X4	T37.1X5	T37.1X6
tetradecyl sulfate	T46.8X1	T46.8X2	T46.8X3	T46.8X4	T46.8X5	T46.8X6
thiopental	T41.1X1	T41.1X2	T41.1X3	T41.1X4	T41.1X5	T41.1X6
thiosalicylate	T39.091	T39.092	T39.093	T39.094	T39.095	T39.096
thiosulfate	T50.6X1	T50.6X2	T50.6X3	T50.6X4	T50.6X5	T50.6X6
tolbutamide	T38.3X1	T38.3X2	T38.3X3	T38.3X4	T38.3X5	T38.3X6
l-triiodothyronine	T38.1X1	T38.1X2	T38.1X3	T38.1X4	T38.1X5	T38.1X6
tyropanoate	T50.8X1	T50.8X2	T50.8X3	T50.8X4	T50.8X5	T50.8X6
valproate	T42.6X1	T42.6X2	T42.6X3	T42.6X4	T42.6X5	T42.6X6
versenate	T50.6X1	T50.6X2	T50.6X3	T50.6X4	T50.6X5	T50.6X6

Substance	Poisoning, Accidental (Unintentional)	Poisoning, Intentional Self-Harm	Poisoning, Assault	Poisoning, Undetermined	Adverse Effect	Underdosing
Sodium-free salt	T50.901	T50.902	T50.903	T50.904	T50.905	T50.906
Sodium-removing resin	T50.3X1	T50.3X2	T50.3X3	T50.3X4	T50.3X5	T50.3X6
Soft soap	T55.0X1	T55.0X2	T55.0X3	T55.0X4	—	—
Solanine	T62.2X1	T62.2X2	T62.2X3	T62.2X4	—	—
berries	T62.1X1	T62.1X2	T62.1X3	T62.1X4	—	—
Solanum dulcamara	T62.2X1	T62.2X2	T62.2X3	T62.2X4	—	—
berries	T62.1X1	T62.1X2	T62.1X3	T62.1X4	—	—
Solapsone	T37.1X1	T37.1X2	T37.1X3	T37.1X4	T37.1X5	T37.1X6
Solar lotion	T49.3X1	T49.3X2	T49.3X3	T49.3X4	T49.3X5	T49.3X6
Solasulfone	T37.1X1	T37.1X2	T37.1X3	T37.1X4	T37.1X5	T37.1X6
Soldering fluid	T65.891	T65.892	T65.893	T65.894	—	—
Solid substance	T65.91	T65.92	T65.93	T65.94		
specified NEC	T65.891	T65.892	T65.893	T65.894		
Solvent, industrial NEC	T52.91	T52.92	T52.93	T52.94	—	—
naphtha	T52.0X1	T52.0X2	T52.0X3	T52.0X4	—	—
petroleum	T52.0X1	T52.0X2	T52.0X3	T52.0X4	—	—
specified NEC	T52.8X1	T52.8X2	T52.8X3	T52.8X4	—	—
Soma	T42.8X1	T42.8X2	T42.8X3	T42.8X4	T42.8X5	T42.8X6
Somatorelin	T38.891	T38.892	T38.893	T38.894	T38.895	T38.896
Somatostatin	T38.991	T38.992	T38.993	T38.994	T38.995	T38.996
Somatotropin	T38.811	T38.812	T38.813	T38.814	T38.815	T38.816
Somatrem	T38.811	T38.812	T38.813	T38.814	T38.815	T38.816
Somatropin	T38.811	T38.812	T38.813	T38.814	T38.815	T38.816
Sominex	T45.0X1	T45.0X2	T45.0X3	T45.0X4	T45.0X5	T45.0X6
Somnos	T42.6X1	T42.6X2	T42.6X3	T42.6X4	T42.6X5	T42.6X6
Somonal	T42.3X1	T42.3X2	T42.3X3	T42.3X4	T42.3X5	T42.3X6
Soneryl	T42.3X1	T42.3X2	T42.3X3	T42.3X4	T42.3X5	T42.3X6
Soothing syrup	T50.901	T50.902	T50.903	T50.904	T50.905	T50.906
Sopor	T42.6X1	T42.6X2	T42.6X3	T42.6X4	T42.6X5	T42.6X6
Soporific	T42.71	T42.72	T42.73	T42.74	T42.75	T42.76
Soporific drug	T42.71	T42.72	T42.73	T42.74	T42.75	T42.76
specified type NEC	T42.6X1	T42.6X2	T42.6X3	T42.6X4	T42.6X5	T42.6X6
Sorbide nitrate	T46.3X1	T46.3X2	T46.3X3	T46.3X4	T46.3X5	T46.3X6
Sorbitol	T47.4X1	T47.4X2	T47.4X3	T47.4X4	T47.4X5	T47.4X6
Sotalol	T44.7X1	T44.7X2	T44.7X3	T44.7X4	T44.7X5	T44.7X6
Sotradecol	T46.8X1	T46.8X2	T46.8X3	T46.8X4	T46.8X5	T46.8X6
Soysterol	T46.6X1	T46.6X2	T46.6X3	T46.6X4	T46.6X5	T46.6X6
Spacoline	T44.3X1	T44.3X2	T44.3X3	T44.3X4	T44.3X5	T44.3X6
Spanish fly	T49.8X1	T49.8X2	T49.8X3	T49.8X4	T49.8X5	T49.8X6
Sparine	T43.3X1	T43.3X2	T43.3X3	T43.3X4	T43.3X5	T43.3X6
Sparteine	T48.0X1	T48.0X2	T48.0X3	T48.0X4	T48.0X5	T48.0X6

◀ New ◀▥ Revised ~~deleted~~ Deleted

Substance	External Cause (T-Code)					
	Poisoning, Accidental (Unintentional)	Poisoning, Intentional Self-Harm	Poisoning, Assault	Poisoning, Undetermined	Adverse Effect	Underdosing
Spasmolytic						
anticholinergics	T44.3X1	T44.3X2	T44.3X3	T44.3X4	T44.3X5	T44.3X6
autonomic	T44.3X1	T44.3X2	T44.3X3	T44.3X4	T44.3X5	T44.3X6
bronchial NEC	T48.6X1	T48.6X2	T48.6X3	T48.6X4	T48.6X5	T48.6X6
quaternary ammonium	T44.3X1	T44.3X2	T44.3X3	T44.3X4	T44.3X5	T44.3X6
skeletal muscle NEC	T48.1X1	T48.1X2	T48.1X3	T48.1X4	T48.1X5	T48.1X6
Spectinomycin	T36.5X1	T36.5X2	T36.5X3	T36.5X4	T36.5X5	T36.5X6
Speed	T43.621	T43.622	T43.623	T43.624	T43.625	T43.626
Spermicide	T49.8X1	T49.8X2	T49.8X3	T49.8X4	T49.8X5	T49.8X6
Spider (bite) (venom)	T63.391	T63.392	T63.393	T63.394	—	—
antivenin	T50.Z11	T50.Z12	T50.Z13	T50.Z14	T50.Z15	T50.Z16
Spigelia (root)	T37.4X1	T37.4X2	T37.4X3	T37.4X4	T37.4X5	T37.4X6
Spindle inactivator	T50.4X1	T50.4X2	T50.4X3	T50.4X4	T50.4X5	T50.4X6
Spiperone	T43.4X1	T43.4X2	T43.4X3	T43.4X4	T43.4X5	T43.4X6
Spiramycin	T36.3X1	T36.3X2	T36.3X3	T36.3X4	T36.3X5	T36.3X6
Spirapril	T46.4X1	T46.4X2	T46.4X3	T46.4X4	T46.4X5	T46.4X6
Spirilene	T43.591	T43.592	T43.593	T43.594	T43.595	T43.596
Spirit(s) (neutral) NEC	T51.0X1	T51.0X2	T51.0X3	T51.0X4	—	—
beverage	T51.0X1	T51.0X2	T51.0X3	T51.0X4	—	—
industrial	T51.0X1	T51.0X2	T51.0X3	T51.0X4	—	—
mineral	T52.0X1	T52.0X2	T52.0X3	T52.0X4	—	—
of salt — see Hydrochloric acid						
surgical	T51.0X1	T51.0X2	T51.0X3	T51.0X4	—	—
Spironolactone	T50.0X1	T50.0X2	T50.0X3	T50.0X4	T50.0X5	T50.0X6
Spiroperidol	T43.4X1	T43.4X2	T43.4X3	T43.4X4	T43.4X5	T43.4X6
Sponge, absorbable (gelatin)	T45.7X1	T45.7X2	T45.7X3	T45.7X4	T45.7X5	T45.7X6
Sporostacin	T49.0X1	T49.0X2	T49.0X3	T49.0X4	T49.0X5	T49.0X6
Spray (aerosol)	T65.91	T65.92	T65.93	T65.94	—	—
cosmetic	T65.891	T65.892	T65.893	T65.894	—	—
medicinal NEC	T50.901	T50.902	T50.903	T50.904	T50.905	T50.906
pesticides — see Pesticides						
specified content — see specific substance						
Spurge flax	T62.2X1	T62.2X2	T62.2X3	T62.2X4	—	—
Spurges	T62.2X1	T62.2X2	T62.2X3	T62.2X4	—	—
Sputum viscosity-lowering drug	T48.4X1	T48.4X2	T48.4X3	T48.4X4	T48.4X5	T48.4X6
Squill	T46.0X1	T46.0X2	T46.0X3	T46.0X4	T46.0X5	T46.0X6
rat poison	T60.4X1	T60.4X2	T60.4X3	T60.4X4		
Squirting cucumber (cathartic)	T47.2X1	T47.2X2	T47.2X3	T47.2X4	T47.2X5	T47.2X6
Stains	T65.6X1	T65.6X2	T65.6X3	T65.6X4	—	—
Stannous fluoride	T49.7X1	T49.7X2	T49.7X3	T49.7X4	T49.7X5	T49.7X6
Stanolone	T38.7X1	T38.7X2	T38.7X3	T38.7X4	T38.7X5	T38.7X6

Substance	External Cause (T-Code)					
	Poisoning, Accidental (Unintentional)	Poisoning, Intentional Self-Harm	Poisoning, Assault	Poisoning, Undetermined	Adverse Effect	Underdosing
Stanozolol	T38.7X1	T38.7X2	T38.7X3	T38.7X4	T38.7X5	T38.7X6
Staphisagria or stavesacre (pediculicide)	T49.0X1	T49.0X2	T49.0X3	T49.0X4	T49.0X5	T49.0X6
Starch	T50.901	T50.902	T50.903	T50.904	T50.905	T50.906
Stelazine	T43.3X1	T43.3X2	T43.3X3	T43.3X4	T43.3X5	T43.3X6
Stemetil	T43.3X1	T43.3X2	T43.3X3	T43.3X4	T43.3X5	T43.3X6
Stepronin	T48.4X1	T48.4X2	T48.4X3	T48.4X4	T48.4X5	T48.4X6
Sterculia	T47.4X1	T47.4X2	T47.4X3	T47.4X4	T47.4X5	T47.4X6
Sternutator gas	T59.891	T59.892	T59.893	T59.894	—	—
Steroid	T38.0X1	T38.0X2	T38.0X3	T38.0X4	T38.0X5	T38.0X6
anabolic	T38.7X1	T38.7X2	T38.7X3	T38.7X4	T38.7X5	T38.7X6
androgenic	T38.7X1	T38.7X2	T38.7X3	T38.7X4	T38.7X5	T38.7X6
antineoplastic, hormone	T38.7X1	T38.7X2	T38.7X3	T38.7X4	T38.7X5	T38.7X6
estrogen	T38.5X1	T38.5X2	T38.5X3	T38.5X4	T38.5X5	T38.5X6
ENT agent	T49.6X1	T49.6X2	T49.6X3	T49.6X4	T49.6X5	T49.6X6
ophthalmic preparation	T49.5X1	T49.5X2	T49.5X3	T49.5X4	T49.5X5	T49.5X6
topical NEC	T49.0X1	T49.0X2	T49.0X3	T49.0X4	T49.0X5	T49.0X6
Stibine	T56.891	T56.892	T56.893	T56.894	—	—
Stibogluconate	T37.3X1	T37.3X2	T37.3X3	T37.3X4	T37.3X5	T37.3X6
Stibophen	T37.4X1	T37.4X2	T37.4X3	T37.4X4	T37.4X5	T37.4X6
Stilbamidine (isetionate)	T37.3X1	T37.3X2	T37.3X3	T37.3X4	T37.3X5	T37.3X6
Stilbestrol	T38.5X1	T38.5X2	T38.5X3	T38.5X4	T38.5X5	T38.5X6
Stilboestrol	T38.5X1	T38.5X2	T38.5X3	T38.5X4	T38.5X5	T38.5X6
Stimulant						
central nervous system — see also Psychostimulant	T43.601	T43.602	T43.603	T43.604	T43.605	T43.606
analeptics	T50.7X1	T50.7X2	T50.7X3	T50.7X4	T50.7X5	T50.7X6
opiate antagonist	T50.7X1	T50.7X2	T50.7X3	T50.7X4	T50.7X5	T50.7X6
psychotherapeutic NEC — see also Psychotherapeutic drug	T43.601	T43.602	T43.603	T43.604	T43.605	T43.606
specified NEC	T43.691	T43.692	T43.693	T43.694	T43.695	T43.696
respiratory	T48.901	T48.902	T48.903	T48.904	T48.905	T48.906
Stone-dissolving drug	T50.901	T50.902	T50.903	T50.904	T50.905	T50.906
Storage battery (cells) (acid)	T54.2X1	T54.2X2	T54.2X3	T54.2X4	—	—
Stovaine	T41.3X1	T41.3X2	T41.3X3	T41.3X4	T41.3X5	T41.3X6
infiltration (subcutaneous)	T41.3X1	T41.3X2	T41.3X3	T41.3X4	T41.3X5	T41.3X6
nerve block (peripheral) (plexus)	T41.3X1	T41.3X2	T41.3X3	T41.3X4	T41.3X5	T41.3X6
spinal	T41.3X1	T41.3X2	T41.3X3	T41.3X4	T41.3X5	T41.3X6
topical (surface)	T41.3X1	T41.3X2	T41.3X3	T41.3X4	T41.3X5	T41.3X6
Stovarsal	T37.8X1	T37.8X2	T37.8X3	T37.8X4	T37.8X5	T37.8X6
Stove gas — see Gas, stove	T57.91	T57.92	T57.93	T57.94	—	—

◀ New ◀▥ Revised ~~deleted~~ Deleted

Substance	External Cause (T-Code)					
	Poisoning, Accidental (Unintentional)	Poisoning, Intentional Self-Harm	Poisoning, Assault	Poisoning, Undetermined	Adverse Effect	Underdosing
Stoxil	T49.5X1	T49.5X2	T49.5X3	T49.5X4	T49.5X5	T49.5X6
Stramonium	T48.6X1	T48.6X2	T48.6X3	T48.6X4	T48.6X5	T48.6X6
natural state	T62.2X1	T62.2X2	T62.2X3	T62.2X4	—	—
Streptodornase	T45.3X1	T45.3X2	T45.3X3	T45.3X4	T45.3X5	T45.3X6
Streptoduocin	T36.5X1	T36.5X2	T36.5X3	T36.5X4	T36.5X5	T36.5X6
Streptokinase	T45.611	T45.612	T45.613	T45.614	T45.615	T45.616
Streptomycin (derivative)	T36.5X1	T36.5X2	T36.5X3	T36.5X4	T36.5X5	T36.5X6
Streptonivicin	T36.5X1	T36.5X2	T36.5X3	T36.5X4	T36.5X5	T36.5X6
Streptovarycin	T36.5X1	T36.5X2	T36.5X3	T36.5X4	T36.5X5	T36.5X6
Streptozocin	T45.1X1	T45.1X2	T45.1X3	T45.1X4	T45.1X5	T45.1X6
Streptozotocin	T45.1X1	T45.1X2	T45.1X3	T45.1X4	T45.1X5	T45.1X6
Stripper (paint) (solvent)	T52.8X1	T52.8X2	T52.8X3	T52.8X4	—	—
Strobane	T60.1X1	T60.1X2	T60.1X3	T60.1X4	—	—
Strofantina	T46.0X1	T46.0X2	T46.0X3	T46.0X4	T46.0X5	T46.0X6
Strophanthin (g) (k)	T46.0X1	T46.0X2	T46.0X3	T46.0X4	T46.0X5	T46.0X6
Strophanthus	T46.0X1	T46.0X2	T46.0X3	T46.0X4	T46.0X5	T46.0X6
Strophantin	T46.0X1	T46.0X2	T46.0X3	T46.0X4	T46.0X5	T46.0X6
Strophantin-g	T46.0X1	T46.0X2	T46.0X3	T46.0X4	T46.0X5	T46.0X6
Strychnine (nonmedicinal) (pesticide) (salts)	T65.1X1	T65.1X2	T65.1X3	T65.1X4	—	—
medicinal	T48.291	T48.292	T48.293	T48.294	T48.295	T48.296
Strychnos (ignatii) — see Strychnine						
Styramate	T42.8X1	T42.8X2	T42.8X3	T42.8X4	T42.8X5	T42.8X6
Styrene	T65.891	T65.892	T65.893	T65.894	—	—
Succinimide, antiepileptic or anticonvulsant	T42.2X1	T42.2X2	T42.2X3	T42.2X4	T42.2X5	T42.2X6
mercuric — see Mercury						
Succinylcholine	T48.1X1	T48.1X2	T48.1X3	T48.1X4	T48.1X5	T48.1X6
Succinylsulfathiazole	T37.0X1	T37.0X2	T37.0X3	T37.0X4	T37.0X5	T37.0X6
Sucralfate	T47.1X1	T47.1X2	T47.1X3	T47.1X4	T47.1X5	T47.1X6
Sucrose	T50.3X1	T50.3X2	T50.3X3	T50.3X4	T50.3X5	T50.3X6
Sufentanil	T40.4X1	T40.4X2	T40.4X3	T40.4X4	T40.4X5	T40.4X6
Sulbactam	T36.0X1	T36.0X2	T36.0X3	T36.0X4	T36.0X5	T36.0X6
Sulbenicillin	T36.0X1	T36.0X2	T36.0X3	T36.0X4	T36.0X5	T36.0X6
Sulbentine	T49.0X1	T49.0X2	T49.0X3	T49.0X4	T49.0X5	T49.0X6
Sulfacetamide	T49.0X1	T49.0X2	T49.0X3	T49.0X4	T49.0X5	T49.0X6
ophthalmic preparation	T49.5X1	T49.5X2	T49.5X3	T49.5X4	T49.5X5	T49.5X6
Sulfachlorpyridazine	T37.0X1	T37.0X2	T37.0X3	T37.0X4	T37.0X5	T37.0X6
Sulfacitine	T37.0X1	T37.0X2	T37.0X3	T37.0X4	T37.0X5	T37.0X6
Sulfadiasulfone sodium	T37.0X1	T37.0X2	T37.0X3	T37.0X4	T37.0X5	T37.0X6
Sulfadiazine	T37.0X1	T37.0X2	T37.0X3	T37.0X4	T37.0X5	T37.0X6
silver (topical)	T49.0X1	T49.0X2	T49.0X3	T49.0X4	T49.0X5	T49.0X6

Substance	External Cause (T-Code)					
	Poisoning, Accidental (Unintentional)	Poisoning, Intentional Self-Harm	Poisoning, Assault	Poisoning, Undetermined	Adverse Effect	Underdosing
Sulfadimethoxine	T37.0X1	T37.0X2	T37.0X3	T37.0X4	T37.0X5	T37.0X6
Sulfadimidine	T37.0X1	T37.0X2	T37.0X3	T37.0X4	T37.0X5	T37.0X6
Sulfadoxine	T37.0X1	T37.0X2	T37.0X3	T37.0X4	T37.0X5	T37.0X6
with pyrimethamine	T37.2X1	T37.2X2	T37.2X3	T37.2X4	T37.2X5	T37.2X6
Sulfaethidole	T37.0X1	T37.0X2	T37.0X3	T37.0X4	T37.0X5	T37.0X6
Sulfafurazole	T37.0X1	T37.0X2	T37.0X3	T37.0X4	T37.0X5	T37.0X6
Sulfaguanidine	T37.0X1	T37.0X2	T37.0X3	T37.0X4	T37.0X5	T37.0X6
Sulfalene	T37.0X1	T37.0X2	T37.0X3	T37.0X4	T37.0X5	T37.0X6
Sulfaloxate	T37.0X1	T37.0X2	T37.0X3	T37.0X4	T37.0X5	T37.0X6
Sulfaloxic acid	T37.0X1	T37.0X2	T37.0X3	T37.0X4	T37.0X5	T37.0X6
Sulfamazone	T39.2X1	T39.2X2	T39.2X3	T39.2X4	T39.2X5	T39.2X6
Sulfamerazine	T37.0X1	T37.0X2	T37.0X3	T37.0X4	T37.0X5	T37.0X6
Sulfameter	T37.0X1	T37.0X2	T37.0X3	T37.0X4	T37.0X5	T37.0X6
Sulfamethazine	T37.0X1	T37.0X2	T37.0X3	T37.0X4	T37.0X5	T37.0X6
Sulfamethizole	T37.0X1	T37.0X2	T37.0X3	T37.0X4	T37.0X5	T37.0X6
Sulfamethoxazole	T37.0X1	T37.0X2	T37.0X3	T37.0X4	T37.0X5	T37.0X6
with trimethoprim	T36.8X1	T36.8X2	T36.8X3	T36.8X4	T36.8X5	T36.8X6
Sulfamethoxydiazine	T37.0X1	T37.0X2	T37.0X3	T37.0X4	T37.0X5	T37.0X6
Sulfamethoxypyridazine	T37.0X1	T37.0X2	T37.0X3	T37.0X4	T37.0X5	T37.0X6
Sulfamethylthiazole	T37.0X1	T37.0X2	T37.0X3	T37.0X4	T37.0X5	T37.0X6
Sulfametoxydiazine	T37.0X1	T37.0X2	T37.0X3	T37.0X4	T37.0X5	T37.0X6
Sulfamidopyrine	T39.2X1	T39.2X2	T39.2X3	T39.2X4	T39.2X5	T39.2X6
Sulfamonomethoxine	T37.0X1	T37.0X2	T37.0X3	T37.0X4	T37.0X5	T37.0X6
Sulfamoxole	T37.0X1	T37.0X2	T37.0X3	T37.0X4	T37.0X5	T37.0X6
Sulfamylon	T49.0X1	T49.0X2	T49.0X3	T49.0X4	T49.0X5	T49.0X6
Sulfan blue (diagnostic dye)	T50.8X1	T50.8X2	T50.8X3	T50.8X4	T50.8X5	T50.8X6
Sulfanilamide	T37.0X1	T37.0X2	T37.0X3	T37.0X4	—	T37.0X6
Sulfanilylguanidine	T37.0X1	T37.0X2	T37.0X3	T37.0X4	T37.0X5	T37.0X6
Sulfaperin	T37.0X1	T37.0X2	T37.0X3	T37.0X4	T37.0X5	T37.0X6
Sulfaphenazole	T37.0X1	T37.0X2	T37.0X3	T37.0X4	T37.0X5	T37.0X6
Sulfaphenylthiazole	T37.0X1	T37.0X2	T37.0X3	T37.0X4	T37.0X5	T37.0X6
Sulfaproxyline	T37.0X1	T37.0X2	T37.0X3	T37.0X4	T37.0X5	T37.0X6
Sulfapyridine	T37.0X1	T37.0X2	T37.0X3	T37.0X4	T37.0X5	T37.0X6
Sulfapyrimidine	T37.0X1	T37.0X2	T37.0X3	T37.0X4	T37.0X5	T37.0X6
Sulfarsphenamine	T37.8X1	T37.8X2	T37.8X3	T37.8X4	T37.8X5	T37.8X6
Sulfasalazine	T37.0X1	T37.0X2	T37.0X3	T37.0X4	T37.0X5	T37.0X6
Sulfasuxidine	T37.0X1	T37.0X2	T37.0X3	T37.0X4	T37.0X5	T37.0X6
Sulfasymazine	T37.0X1	T37.0X2	T37.0X3	T37.0X4	T37.0X5	T37.0X6
Sulfated amylopectin	T47.8X1	T47.8X2	T47.8X3	T47.8X4	T47.8X5	T47.8X6
Sulfathiazole	T37.0X1	T37.0X2	T37.0X3	T37.0X4	T37.0X5	T37.0X6
Sulfatostearate	T49.2X1	T49.2X2	T49.2X3	T49.2X4	T49.2X5	T49.2X6
Sulfinpyrazone	T50.4X1	T50.4X2	T50.4X3	T50.4X4	T50.4X5	T50.4X6

◀ New   ◀▥ Revised   ~~deleted~~ Deleted

TABLE OF DRUGS AND CHEMICALS

Substance	External Cause (T-Code) Poisoning, Accidental (Unintentional)	Poisoning, Intentional Self-Harm	Poisoning, Assault	Poisoning, Undetermined	Adverse Effect	Underdosing
Sulfiram	T49.0X1	T49.0X2	T49.0X3	T49.0X4	T49.0X5	T49.0X6
Sulfisomidine	T37.0X1	T37.0X2	T37.0X3	T37.0X4	T37.0X5	T37.0X6
Sulfisoxazole	T37.0X1	T37.0X2	T37.0X3	T37.0X4	T37.0X5	T37.0X6
ophthalmic preparation	T49.5X1	T49.5X2	T49.5X3	T49.5X4	T49.5X5	T49.5X6
Sulfobromophthalein (sodium)	T50.8X1	T50.8X2	T50.8X3	T50.8X4	T50.8X5	T50.8X6
Sulfobromphthalein	T50.8X1	T50.8X2	T50.8X3	T50.8X4	T50.8X5	T50.8X6
Sulfogaiacol	T48.4X1	T48.4X2	T48.4X3	T48.4X4	T48.4X5	T48.4X6
Sulfomyxin	T36.8X1	T36.8X2	T36.8X3	T36.8X4	T36.8X5	T36.8X6
Sulfonal	T42.6X1	T42.6X2	T42.6X3	T42.6X4	T42.6X5	T42.6X6
Sulfonamide NEC	T37.0X1	T37.0X2	T37.0X3	T37.0X4	T37.0X5	T37.0X6
eye	T49.5X1	T49.5X2	T49.5X3	T49.5X4	T49.5X5	T49.5X6
Sulfonazide	T37.1X1	T37.1X2	T37.1X3	T37.1X4	T37.1X5	T37.1X6
Sulfones	T37.1X1	T37.1X2	T37.1X3	T37.1X4	T37.1X5	T37.1X6
Sulfonethylmethane	T42.6X1	T42.6X2	T42.6X3	T42.6X4	T42.6X5	T42.6X6
Sulfonmethane	T42.6X1	T42.6X2	T42.6X3	T42.6X4	T42.6X5	T42.6X6
Sulfonphthal, sulfonphthol	T50.8X1	T50.8X2	T50.8X3	T50.8X4	T50.8X5	T50.8X6
Sulfonylurea derivatives, oral	T38.3X1	T38.3X2	T38.3X3	T38.3X4	T38.3X5	T38.3X6
Sulforidazine	T43.3X1	T43.3X2	T43.3X3	T43.3X4	T43.3X5	T43.3X6
Sulfoxone	T37.1X1	T37.1X2	T37.1X3	T37.1X4	T37.1X5	T37.1X6
Sulfur, sulfurated, sulfuric, sulfurous, sulfuryl (compounds NEC) (medicinal)	T49.4X1	T49.4X2	T49.4X3	T49.4X4	T49.4X5	T49.4X6
acid	T54.2X1	T54.2X2	T54.2X3	T54.2X4	—	—
dioxide (gas)	T59.1X1	T59.1X2	T59.1X3	T59.1X4	—	—
ether — see Ether(s)						
hydrogen	T59.6X1	T59.6X2	T59.6X3	T59.6X4	—	—
medicinal (keratolytic) (ointment) NEC	T49.4X1	T49.4X2	T49.4X3	T49.4X4	T49.4X5	T49.4X6
ointment	T49.0X1	T49.0X2	T49.0X3	T49.0X4	T49.0X5	T49.0X6
pesticide (vapor)	T60.91	T60.92	T60.93	T60.94	—	—
vapor NEC	T59.891	T59.892	T59.893	T59.894	—	—
Sulfuric acid	T54.2X1	T54.2X2	T54.2X3	T54.2X4	—	—
Sulglicotide	T47.1X1	T47.1X2	T47.1X3	T47.1X4	T47.1X5	T47.1X6
Sulindac	T39.391	T39.392	T39.393	T39.394	T39.395	T39.396
Sulisatin	T47.2X1	T47.2X2	T47.2X3	T47.2X4	T47.2X5	T47.2X6
Sulisobenzone	T49.3X1	T49.3X2	T49.3X3	T49.3X4	T49.3X5	T49.3X6
Sulkowitch's reagent	T50.8X1	T50.8X2	T50.8X3	T50.8X4	T50.8X5	T50.8X6
Sulmetozine	T44.3X1	T44.3X2	T44.3X3	T44.3X4	T44.3X5	T44.3X6
Suloctidil	T46.7X1	T46.7X2	T46.7X3	T46.7X4	T46.7X5	T46.7X6
Sulph — see also Sulf-						
Sulphadiazine	T37.0X1	T37.0X2	T37.0X3	T37.0X4	T37.0X5	T37.0X6

Substance	External Cause (T-Code) Poisoning, Accidental (Unintentional)	Poisoning, Intentional Self-Harm	Poisoning, Assault	Poisoning, Undetermined	Adverse Effect	Underdosing
Sulphadimethoxine	T37.0X1	T37.0X2	T37.0X3	T37.0X4	T37.0X5	T37.0X6
Sulphadimidine	T37.0X1	T37.0X2	T37.0X3	T37.0X4	T37.0X5	T37.0X6
Sulphadione	T37.1X1	T37.1X2	T37.1X3	T37.1X4	T37.1X5	T37.1X6
Sulphafurazole	T37.0X1	T37.0X2	T37.0X3	T37.0X4	T37.0X5	T37.0X6
Sulphamethizole	T37.0X1	T37.0X2	T37.0X3	T37.0X4	T37.0X5	T37.0X6
Sulphamethoxazole	T37.0X1	T37.0X2	T37.0X3	T37.0X4	T37.0X5	T37.0X6
Sulphan blue	T50.8X1	T50.8X2	T50.8X3	T50.8X4	T50.8X5	T50.8X6
Sulphaphenazole	T37.0X1	T37.0X2	T37.0X3	T37.0X4	T37.0X5	T37.0X6
Sulphapyridine	T37.0X1	T37.0X2	T37.0X3	T37.0X4	T37.0X5	T37.0X6
Sulphasalazine	T37.0X1	T37.0X2	T37.0X3	T37.0X4	T37.0X5	T37.0X6
Sulphinpyrazone	T50.4X1	T50.4X2	T50.4X3	T50.4X4	T50.4X5	T50.4X6
Sulpiride	T43.591	T43.592	T43.593	T43.594	T43.595	T43.596
Sulprostone	T48.0X1	T48.0X2	T48.0X3	T48.0X4	T48.0X5	T48.0X6
Sulpyrine	T39.2X1	T39.2X2	T39.2X3	T39.2X4	T39.2X5	T39.2X6
Sultamicillin	T36.0X1	T36.0X2	T36.0X3	T36.0X4	T36.0X5	T36.0X6
Sulthiame	T42.6X1	T42.6X2	T42.6X3	T42.6X4	T42.6X5	T42.6X6
Sultiame	T42.6X1	T42.6X2	T42.6X3	T42.6X4	T42.6X5	T42.6X6
Sultopride	T43.591	T43.592	T43.593	T43.594	T43.595	T43.596
Sumatriptan	T39.8X1	T39.8X2	T39.8X3	T39.8X4	T39.8X5	T39.8X6
Sunflower seed oil	T46.6X1	T46.6X2	T46.6X3	T46.6X4	T46.6X5	T46.6X6
Superinone	T48.4X1	T48.4X2	T48.4X3	T48.4X4	T48.4X5	T48.4X6
Suprofen	T39.311	T39.312	T39.313	T39.314	T39.315	T39.316
Suramin (sodium)	T37.4X1	T37.4X2	T37.4X3	T37.4X4	T37.4X5	T37.4X6
Surfacaine	T41.3X1	T41.3X2	T41.3X3	T41.3X4	T41.3X5	T41.3X6
Surital	T41.1X1	T41.1X2	T41.1X3	T41.1X4	T41.1X5	T41.1X6
Sutilains	T45.3X1	T45.3X2	T45.3X3	T45.3X4	T45.3X5	T45.3X6
Suxamethonium (chloride)	T48.1X1	T48.1X2	T48.1X3	T48.1X4	T48.1X5	T48.1X6
Suxethonium (chloride)	T48.1X1	T48.1X2	T48.1X3	T48.1X4	T48.1X5	T48.1X6
Suxibuzone	T39.2X1	T39.2X2	T39.2X3	T39.2X4	T39.2X5	T39.2X6
Sweet oil (birch)	T49.3X1	T49.3X2	T49.3X3	T49.3X4	T49.3X5	T49.3X6
Sweet niter spirit	T46.3X1	T46.3X2	T46.3X3	T46.3X4	T46.3X5	T46.3X6
Sweetener	T50.901	T50.902	T50.903	T50.904	T50.905	T50.906
Sym-dichloroethyl ether	T53.6X1	T53.6X2	T53.6X3	T53.6X4	—	—
Sympatholytic NEC	T44.8X1	T44.8X2	T44.8X3	T44.8X4	T44.8X5	T44.8X6
haloalkylamine	T44.8X1	T44.8X2	T44.8X3	T44.8X4	T44.8X5	T44.8X6
Sympathomimetic NEC	T44.901	T44.902	T44.903	T44.904	T44.905	T44.906
anti-common-cold	T48.5X1	T48.5X2	T48.5X3	T48.5X4	T48.5X5	T48.5X6
bronchodilator	T48.6X1	T48.6X2	T48.6X3	T48.6X4	T48.6X5	T48.6X6
specified NEC	T44.991	T44.992	T44.993	T44.994	T44.995	T44.996
Synagis	T50.B91	T50.B92	T50.B93	T50.B94	T50.B95	T50.B96
Synalar	T49.0X1	T49.0X2	T49.0X3	T49.0X4	T49.0X5	T49.0X6
Synthroid	T38.1X1	T38.1X2	T38.1X3	T38.1X4	T38.1X5	T38.1X6

◀ New   ◀||| Revised   ~~deleted~~ Deleted

Substance	Poisoning, Accidental (Unintentional)	Poisoning, Intentional Self-Harm	Poisoning, Assault	Poisoning, Undetermined	Adverse Effect	Underdosing
External Cause (T-Code)						
Syntocinon	T48.0X1	T48.0X2	T48.0X3	T48.0X4	T48.0X5	T48.0X6
Syrosingopine	T46.5X1	T46.5X2	T46.5X3	T46.5X4	T46.5X5	T46.5X6
Systemic drug	T45.91	T45.92	T45.93	T45.94	T45.95	T45.96
specified NEC	T45.8X1	T45.8X2	T45.8X3	T45.8X4	T45.8X5	T45.8X6
2,4,5-T	T60.3X1	T60.3X2	T60.3X3	T60.3X4	—	—
T						
Tablets—see also specified substance	T50.901	T50.902	T50.903	T50.904	T50.905	T50.906
Tace	T38.5X1	T38.5X2	T38.5X3	T38.5X4	T38.5X5	T38.5X6
Tacrine	T44.0X1	T44.0X2	T44.0X3	T44.0X4	T44.0X5	T44.0X6
Tadalafil	T46.7X1	T46.7X2	T46.7X3	T46.7X4	T46.7X5	T46.7X6
Talampicillin	T36.0X1	T36.0X2	T36.0X3	T36.0X4	T36.0X5	T36.0X6
Talbutal	T42.3X1	T42.3X2	T42.3X3	T42.3X4	T42.3X5	T42.3X6
Talc powder	T49.3X1	T49.3X2	T49.3X3	T49.3X4	T49.3X5	T49.3X6
Talcum	T49.3X1	T49.3X2	T49.3X3	T49.3X4	T49.3X5	T49.3X6
Taleranol	T38.6X1	T38.6X2	T38.6X3	T38.6X4	T38.6X5	T38.6X6
Tamoxifen	T38.6X1	T38.6X2	T38.6X3	T38.6X4	T38.6X5	T38.6X6
Tamsulosin	T44.6X1	T44.6X2	T44.6X3	T44.6X4	T44.6X5	T44.6X6
Tandearil, tanderil	T39.2X1	T39.2X2	T39.2X3	T39.2X4	T39.2X5	T39.2X6
Tannic acid	T49.2X1	T49.2X2	T49.2X3	T49.2X4	T49.2X5	T49.2X6
medicinal (astringent)	T49.2X1	T49.2X2	T49.2X3	T49.2X4	T49.2X5	T49.2X6
Tannin—see Tannic acid						
Tansy	T62.2X1	T62.2X2	T62.2X3	T62.2X4	—	—
TAO	T36.3X1	T36.3X2	T36.3X3	T36.3X4	T36.3X5	T36.3X6
Tapazole	T38.2X1	T38.2X2	T38.2X3	T38.2X4	T38.2X5	T38.2X6
Tar NEC	T52.0X1	T52.0X2	T52.0X3	T52.0X4	—	—
camphor	T60.1X1	T60.1X2	T60.1X3	T60.1X4	—	—
distillate	T49.1X1	T49.1X2	T49.1X3	T49.1X4	T49.1X5	T49.1X6
fumes	T59.891	T59.892	T59.893	T59.894	—	—
medicinal	T49.1X1	T49.1X2	T49.1X3	T49.1X4	T49.1X5	T49.1X6
ointment	T49.1X1	T49.1X2	T49.1X3	T49.1X4	T49.1X5	T49.1X6
Taractan	T43.591	T43.592	T43.593	T43.594	T43.595	T43.596
Tarantula (venomous)	T63.321	T63.322	T63.323	T63.324	—	—
Tartar emetic	T37.8X1	T37.8X2	T37.8X3	T37.8X4	T37.8X5	T37.8X6
Tartaric acid	T65.891	T65.892	T65.893	T65.894	—	—
Tartrated antimony (anti-infective)	T37.8X1	T37.8X2	T37.8X3	T37.8X4	T37.8X5	T37.8X6
Tartrate, laxative	T47.4X1	T47.4X2	T47.4X3	T47.4X4	T47.4X5	T47.4X6
Tauromustine	T45.1X1	T45.1X2	T45.1X3	T45.1X4	T45.1X5	T45.1X6
TCA—see Trichloroacetic acid						
TCDD	T53.7X1	T53.7X2	T53.7X3	T53.7X4	—	—
TDI (vapor)	T65.0X1	T65.0X2	T65.0X3	T65.0X4	—	—

Substance	Poisoning, Accidental (Unintentional)	Poisoning, Intentional Self-Harm	Poisoning, Assault	Poisoning, Undetermined	Adverse Effect	Underdosing
External Cause (T-Code)						
Tear						
gas	T59.3X1	T59.3X2	T59.3X3	T59.3X4	—	—
solution	T49.5X1	T49.5X2	T49.5X3	T49.5X4	T49.5X5	T49.5X6
Teclothiazide	T50.2X1	T50.2X2	T50.2X3	T50.2X4	T50.2X5	T50.2X6
Teclozan	T37.3X1	T37.3X2	T37.3X3	T37.3X4	T37.3X5	T37.3X6
Tegafur	T45.1X1	T45.1X2	T45.1X3	T45.1X4	T45.1X5	T45.1X6
Tegretol	T42.1X1	T42.1X2	T42.1X3	T42.1X4	T42.1X5	T42.1X6
Teicoplanin	T36.8X1	T36.8X2	T36.8X3	T36.8X4	T36.8X5	T36.8X6
Telepaque	T50.8X1	T50.8X2	T50.8X3	T50.8X4	T50.8X5	T50.8X6
Tellurium	T56.891	T56.892	T56.893	T56.894	—	—
fumes	T56.891	T56.892	T56.893	T56.894	—	—
TEM	T45.1X1	T45.1X2	T45.1X3	T45.1X4	T45.1X5	T45.1X6
Temazepam	T42.4X1	T42.4X2	T42.4X3	T42.4X4	T42.4X5	T42.4X6
Temocillin	T36.0X1	T36.0X2	T36.0X3	T36.0X4	T36.0X5	T36.0X6
Tenamfetamine	T43.621	T43.622	T43.623	T43.624	T43.625	T43.626
Teniposide	T45.1X1	T45.1X2	T45.1X3	T45.1X4	T45.1X5	T45.1X6
Tenitramine	T46.3X1	T46.3X2	T46.3X3	T46.3X4	T46.3X5	T46.3X6
Tenoglicin	T48.4X1	T48.4X2	T48.4X3	T48.4X4	T48.4X5	T48.4X6
Tenonitrozole	T37.3X1	T37.3X2	T37.3X3	T37.3X4	T37.3X5	T37.3X6
Tenoxicam	T39.391	T39.392	T39.393	T39.394	T39.395	T39.396
TEPA	T45.1X1	T45.1X2	T45.1X3	T45.1X4	T45.1X5	T45.1X6
TEPP	T60.0X1	T60.0X2	T60.0X3	T60.0X4	—	—
Teprotide	T46.5X1	T46.5X2	T46.5X3	T46.5X4	T46.5X5	T46.5X6
Terazosin	T44.6X1	T44.6X2	T44.6X3	T44.6X4	T44.6X5	T44.6X6
Terbufos	T60.0X1	T60.0X2	T60.0X3	T60.0X4	—	—
Terbutaline	T48.6X1	T48.6X2	T48.6X3	T48.6X4	T48.6X5	T48.6X6
Terconazole	T49.0X1	T49.0X2	T49.0X3	T49.0X4	T49.0X5	T49.0X6
Terfenadine	T45.0X1	T45.0X2	T45.0X3	T45.0X4	T45.0X5	T45.0X6
Teriparatide (acetate)	T50.991	T50.992	T50.993	T50.994	T50.995	T50.996
Terizidone	T37.1X1	T37.1X2	T37.1X3	T37.1X4	T37.1X5	T37.1X6
Terlipressin	T38.891	T38.892	T38.893	T38.894	T38.895	T38.896
Terodiline	T46.3X1	T46.3X2	T46.3X3	T46.3X4	T46.3X5	T46.3X6
Teroxalene	T37.4X1	T37.4X2	T37.4X3	T37.4X4	T37.4X5	T37.4X6
Terpin(cis) hydrate	T48.4X1	T48.4X2	T48.4X3	T48.4X4	T48.4X5	T48.4X6
Terramycin	T36.4X1	T36.4X2	T36.4X3	T36.4X4	T36.4X5	T36.4X6
Tertatolol	T44.7X1	T44.7X2	T44.7X3	T44.7X4	T44.7X5	T44.7X6
Tessalon	T48.3X1	T48.3X2	T48.3X3	T48.3X4	T48.3X5	T48.3X6
Testolactone	T38.7X1	T38.7X2	T38.7X3	T38.7X4	T38.7X5	T38.7X6
Testosterone	T38.7X1	T38.7X2	T38.7X3	T38.7X4	T38.7X5	T38.7X6
Tetanus toxoid or vaccine	T50.A91	T50.A92	T50.A93	T50.A94	T50.A95	T50.A96
antitoxin	T50.Z11	T50.Z12	T50.Z13	T50.Z14	T50.Z15	T50.Z16
immune globulin (human)	T50.Z11	T50.Z12	T50.Z13	T50.Z14	T50.Z15	T50.Z16

◀ New ◀▥ Revised ~~deleted~~ Deleted

TABLE OF DRUGS AND CHEMICALS

TABLE OF DRUGS AND CHEMICALS

Substance	External Cause (T-Code)					
	Poisoning, Accidental (Unintentional)	Poisoning, Intentional Self-Harm	Poisoning, Assault	Poisoning, Undetermined	Adverse Effect	Underdosing
Tetanus toxoid or vaccine (Continued)						
toxoid	T50.A91	T50.A92	T50.A93	T50.A94	T50.A95	T50.A96
with diphtheria toxoid	T50.A21	T50.A22	T50.A23	T50.A24	T50.A25	T50.A26
with pertussis	T50.A11	T50.A12	T50.A13	T50.A14	T50.A15	T50.A16
Tetrabenazine	T43.591	T43.592	T43.593	T43.594	T43.595	T43.596
Tetracaine	T41.3X1	T41.3X2	T41.3X3	T41.3X4	T41.3X5	T41.3X6
nerve block (peripheral) (plexus)	T41.3X1	T41.3X2	T41.3X3	T41.3X4	T41.3X5	T41.3X6
regional	T41.3X1	T41.3X2	T41.3X3	T41.3X4	T41.3X5	T41.3X6
spinal	T41.3X1	T41.3X2	T41.3X3	T41.3X4	T41.3X5	T41.3X6
Tetrachlorethylene — see Tetrachloroethylene						
Tetrachlormethiazide	T50.2X1	T50.2X2	T50.2X3	T50.2X4	T50.2X5	T50.2X6
2,3,7,8-Tetrachlorodibenzo-p-dioxin	T53.7X1	T53.7X2	T53.7X3	T53.7X4	—	—
Tetrachloroethane	T53.6X1	T53.6X2	T53.6X3	T53.6X4	—	—
vapor	T53.6X1	T53.6X2	T53.6X3	T53.6X4	—	—
paint or varnish	T53.6X1	T53.6X2	T53.6X3	T53.6X4	—	—
Tetrachloroethylene (liquid)	T53.3X1	T53.3X2	T53.3X3	T53.3X4	—	—
medicinal	T37.4X1	T37.4X2	T37.4X3	T37.4X4	T37.4X5	T37.4X6
vapor	T53.3X1	T53.3X2	T53.3X3	T53.3X4	—	—
Tetrachloromethane — see Carbon tetrachloride						
Tetracosactide	T38.811	T38.812	T38.813	T38.814	T38.815	T38.816
Tetracosactrin	T38.811	T38.812	T38.813	T38.814	T38.815	T38.816
Tetracycline	T36.4X1	T36.4X2	T36.4X3	T36.4X4	T36.4X5	T36.4X6
ophthalmic preparation	T49.5X1	T49.5X2	T49.5X3	T49.5X4	T49.5X5	T49.5X6
topical NEC	T49.0X1	T49.0X2	T49.0X3	T49.0X4	T49.0X5	T49.0X6
Tetradifon	T60.8X1	T60.8X2	T60.8X3	T60.8X4	—	—
Tetradotoxin	T61.771	T61.772	T61.773	T61.774		
Tetraethyl						
lead	T56.0X1	T56.0X2	T56.0X3	T56.0X4	—	—
pyrophosphate	T60.0X1	T60.0X2	T60.0X3	T60.0X4	—	—
Tetraethylammonium chloride	T44.2X1	T44.2X2	T44.2X3	T44.2X4	T44.2X5	T44.2X6
Tetraethylthiuram disulfide	T50.6X1	T50.6X2	T50.6X3	T50.6X4	T50.6X5	T50.6X6
Tetrahydroaminoacridine	T44.0X1	T44.0X2	T44.0X3	T44.0X4	T44.0X5	T44.0X6
Tetrahydrocannabinol	T40.7X1	T40.7X2	T40.7X3	T40.7X4	T40.7X5	T40.7X6
Tetrahydrofuran	T52.8X1	T52.8X2	T52.8X3	T52.8X4	—	—
Tetrahydronaphthalene	T52.8X1	T52.8X2	T52.8X3	T52.8X4	—	—
Tetrahydrozoline	T49.5X1	T49.5X2	T49.5X3	T49.5X4	T49.5X5	T49.5X6
Tetralin	T52.8X1	T52.8X2	T52.8X3	T52.8X4	—	—
Tetramethrin	T60.2X1	T60.2X2	T60.2X3	T60.2X4	—	—
Tetramethylthiuram (disulfide) NEC	T60.3X1	T60.3X2	T60.3X3	T60.3X4	—	—
medicinal	T49.0X1	T49.0X2	T49.0X3	T49.0X4	T49.0X5	T49.0X6
Tetramisole	T37.4X1	T37.4X2	T37.4X3	T37.4X4	T37.4X5	T37.4X6
Tetranicotinoyl fructose	T46.7X1	T46.7X2	T46.7X3	T46.7X4	T46.7X5	T46.7X6
Tetronal	T42.6X1	T42.6X2	T42.6X3	T42.6X4	T42.6X5	T42.6X6
Tetrazepam	T42.4X1	T42.4X2	T42.4X3	T42.4X4	T42.4X5	T42.4X6
Tetryl	T65.3X1	T65.3X2	T65.3X3	T65.3X4	—	—
Tetrylammonium chloride	T44.2X1	T44.2X2	T44.2X3	T44.2X4	T44.2X5	T44.2X6
Tetryzoline	T49.5X1	T49.5X2	T49.5X3	T49.5X4	T49.5X5	T49.5X6
Thalidomide	T45.1X1	T45.1X2	T45.1X3	T45.1X4	T45.1X5	T45.1X6
Thallium (compounds) (dust) NEC	T56.811	T56.812	T56.813	T56.814	—	—
pesticide	T60.4X1	T60.4X2	T60.4X3	T60.4X4	—	—
THC	T40.7X1	T40.7X2	T40.7X3	T40.7X4	T40.7X5	T40.7X6
Thebacon	T48.3X1	T48.3X2	T48.3X3	T48.3X4	T48.3X5	T48.3X6
Thebaine	T40.2X1	T40.2X2	T40.2X3	T40.2X4	T40.2X5	T40.2X6
Thenoic acid	T49.6X1	T49.6X2	T49.6X3	T49.6X4	T49.6X5	T49.6X6
Thenyldiamine	T45.0X1	T45.0X2	T45.0X3	T45.0X4	T45.0X5	T45.0X6
Theobromine (calcium salicylate)	T48.6X1	T48.6X2	T48.6X3	T48.6X4	T48.6X5	T48.6X6
sodium salicylate	T48.6X1	T48.6X2	T48.6X3	T48.6X4	T48.6X5	T48.6X6
Theophyllamine	T48.6X1	T48.6X2	T48.6X3	T48.6X4	T48.6X5	T48.6X6
Theophylline	T48.6X1	T48.6X2	T48.6X3	T48.6X4	T48.6X5	T48.6X6
aminobenzoic acid	T48.6X1	T48.6X2	T48.6X3	T48.6X4	T48.6X5	T48.6X6
ethylenediamine	T48.6X1	T48.6X2	T48.6X3	T48.6X4	T48.6X5	T48.6X6
piperazine p-amino-benzoate	T48.6X1	T48.6X2	T48.6X3	T48.6X4	T48.6X5	T48.6X6
Thiabendazole	T37.4X1	T37.4X2	T37.4X3	T37.4X4	T37.4X5	T37.4X6
Thialbarbital	T41.1X1	T41.1X2	T41.1X3	T41.1X4	T41.1X5	T41.1X6
Thiamazole	T38.2X1	T38.2X2	T38.2X3	T38.2X4	T38.2X5	T38.2X6
Thiambutosine	T37.1X1	T37.1X2	T37.1X3	T37.1X4	T37.1X5	T37.1X6
Thiamine	T45.2X1	T45.2X2	T45.2X3	T45.2X4	T45.2X5	T45.2X6
Thiamphenicol	T36.2X1	T36.2X2	T36.2X3	T36.2X4	T36.2X5	T36.2X6
Thiamylal	T41.1X1	T41.1X2	T41.1X3	T41.1X4	T41.1X5	T41.1X6
sodium	T41.1X1	T41.1X2	T41.1X3	T41.1X4	T41.1X5	T41.1X6
Thiazesim	T43.291	T43.292	T43.293	T43.294	T43.295	T43.296
Thiazides (diuretics)	T50.2X1	T50.2X2	T50.2X3	T50.2X4	T50.2X5	T50.2X6
Thiazinamium metilsulfate	T43.3X1	T43.3X2	T43.3X3	T43.3X4	T43.3X5	T43.3X6
Thiethylperazine	T43.3X1	T43.3X2	T43.3X3	T43.3X4	T43.3X5	T43.3X6
Thimerosal	T49.0X1	T49.0X2	T49.0X3	T49.0X4	T49.0X5	T49.0X6
ophthalmic preparation	T49.5X1	T49.5X2	T49.5X3	T49.5X4	T49.5X5	T49.5X6
Thioacetazone	T37.1X1	T37.1X2	T37.1X3	T37.1X4	T37.1X5	T37.1X6
with isoniazid	T37.1X1	T37.1X2	T37.1X3	T37.1X4	T37.1X5	T37.1X6
Thiobarbital sodium	T41.1X1	T41.1X2	T41.1X3	T41.1X4	T41.1X5	T41.1X6

TABLE OF DRUGS AND CHEMICALS

◀ New ◀ Revised ~~deleted~~ Deleted

Substance	External Cause (T-Code)					
	Poisoning, Accidental (Unintentional)	Poisoning, Intentional Self-Harm	Poisoning, Assault	Poisoning, Undetermined	Adverse Effect	Underdosing
Thiobarbiturate anesthetic	T41.1X1	T41.1X2	T41.1X3	T41.1X4	T41.1X5	T41.1X6
Thiobismol	T37.8X1	T37.8X2	T37.8X3	T37.8X4	T37.8X5	T37.8X6
Thiobutabarbital sodium	T41.1X1	T41.1X2	T41.1X3	T41.1X4	T41.1X5	T41.1X6
Thiocarbamate (insecticide)	T60.0X1	T60.0X2	T60.0X3	T60.0X4	—	—
Thiocarbamide	T38.2X1	T38.2X2	T38.2X3	T38.2X4	T38.2X5	T38.2X6
Thiocarbarsone	T37.8X1	T37.8X2	T37.8X3	T37.8X4	T37.8X5	T37.8X6
Thiocarlide	T37.1X1	T37.1X2	T37.1X3	T37.1X4	T37.1X5	T37.1X6
Thioctamide	T50.991	T50.992	T50.993	T50.994	T50.995	T50.996
Thioctic acid	T50.991	T50.992	T50.993	T50.994	T50.995	T50.996
Thiofos	T60.0X1	T60.0X2	T60.0X3	T60.0X4	—	—
Thioglycolate	T49.4X1	T49.4X2	T49.4X3	T49.4X4	T49.4X5	T49.4X6
Thioglycolic acid	T65.891	T65.892	T65.893	T65.894		
Thioguanine	T45.1X1	T45.1X2	T45.1X3	T45.1X4	T45.1X5	T45.1X6
Thiomercaptomerin	T50.2X1	T50.2X2	T50.2X3	T50.2X4	T50.2X5	T50.2X6
Thiomerin	T50.2X1	T50.2X2	T50.2X3	T50.2X4	T50.2X5	T50.2X6
Thiomersal	T49.0X1	T49.0X2	T49.0X3	T49.0X4	T49.0X5	T49.0X6
Thionazin	T60.0X1	T60.0X2	T60.0X3	T60.0X4	—	—
Thiopental (sodium)	T41.1X1	T41.1X2	T41.1X3	T41.1X4	T41.1X5	T41.1X6
Thiopentone (sodium)	T41.1X1	T41.1X2	T41.1X3	T41.1X4	T41.1X5	T41.1X6
Thiopropazate	T43.3X1	T43.3X2	T43.3X3	T43.3X4	T43.3X5	T43.3X6
Thioproperazine	T43.3X1	T43.3X2	T43.3X3	T43.3X4	T43.3X5	T43.3X6
Thioridazine	T43.3X1	T43.3X2	T43.3X3	T43.3X4	T43.3X5	T43.3X6
Thiosinamine	T49.3X1	T49.3X2	T49.3X3	T49.3X4	T49.3X5	T49.3X6
Thiotepa	T45.1X1	T45.1X2	T45.1X3	T45.1X4	T45.1X5	T45.1X6
Thiothixene	T43.4X1	T43.4X2	T43.4X3	T43.4X4	T43.4X5	T43.4X6
Thiouracil (benzyl) (methyl) (propyl)	T38.2X1	T38.2X2	T38.2X3	T38.2X4	T38.2X5	T38.2X6
Thiourea	T38.2X1	T38.2X2	T38.2X3	T38.2X4	T38.2X5	T38.2X6
Thiphenamil	T44.3X1	T44.3X2	T44.3X3	T44.3X4	T44.3X5	T44.3X6
Thiram	T60.3X1	T60.3X2	T60.3X3	T60.3X4	—	—
medicinal	T49.2X1	T49.2X2	T49.2X3	T49.2X4	T49.2X5	T49.2X6
Thonzylamine (systemic)	T45.0X1	T45.0X2	T45.0X3	T45.0X4	T45.0X5	T45.0X6
mucosal decongestant	T48.5X1	T48.5X2	T48.5X3	T48.5X4	T48.5X5	T48.5X6
Thorazine	T43.3X1	T43.3X2	T43.3X3	T43.3X4	T43.3X5	T43.3X6
Thorium dioxide suspension	T50.8X1	T50.8X2	T50.8X3	T50.8X4	T50.8X5	T50.8X6
Thornapple	T62.2X1	T62.2X2	T62.2X2	T62.2X4	—	—
Throat drug NEC	T49.6X1	T49.6X2	T49.6X3	T49.6X4	T49.6X5	T49.6X6
Thrombin	T45.7X1	T45.7X2	T45.7X3	T45.7X4	T45.7X5	T45.7X6
Thrombolysin	T45.611	T45.612	T45.613	T45.614	T45.615	T45.616
Thromboplastin	T45.7X1	T45.7X2	T45.7X3	T45.7X4	T45.7X5	T45.7X6
Thurfyl nicotinate	T46.7X1	T46.7X2	T46.7X3	T46.7X4	T46.7X5	T46.7X6
Thymol	T49.0X1	T49.0X2	T49.0X3	T49.0X4	T49.0X5	T49.0X6

Substance	External Cause (T-Code)					
	Poisoning, Accidental (Unintentional)	Poisoning, Intentional Self-Harm	Poisoning, Assault	Poisoning, Undetermined	Adverse Effect	Underdosing
Thymopentin	T37.5X1	T37.5X2	T37.5X3	T37.5X4	T37.5X5	T37.5X6
Thymoxamine	T46.7X1	T46.7X2	T46.7X3	T46.7X4	T46.7X5	T46.7X6
Thymus extract	T38.891	T38.892	T38.893	T38.894	T38.895	T38.896
Thyreotrophic hormone	T38.811	T38.812	T38.813	T38.814	T38.815	T38.816
Thyroglobulin	T38.1X1	T38.1X2	T38.1X3	T38.1X4	T38.1X5	T38.1X6
Thyroid (hormone)	T38.1X1	T38.1X2	T38.1X3	T38.1X4	T38.1X5	T38.1X6
Thyrolar	T38.1X1	T38.1X2	T38.1X3	T38.1X4	T38.1X5	T38.1X6
Thyrotrophin	T38.811	T38.812	T38.813	T38.814	T38.815	T38.816
Thyrotropic hormone	T38.811	T38.812	T38.813	T38.814	T38.815	T38.816
Thyroxine	T38.1X1	T38.1X2	T38.1X3	T38.1X4	T38.1X5	T38.1X6
Tiabendazole	T37.4X1	T37.4X2	T37.4X3	T37.4X4	T37.4X5	T37.4X6
Tiamizide	T50.2X1	T50.2X2	T50.2X3	T50.2X4	T50.2X5	T50.2X6
Tianeptine	T43.291	T43.292	T43.293	T43.294	T43.295	T43.296
Tiapamil	T46.1X1	T46.1X2	T46.1X3	T46.1X4	T46.1X5	T46.1X6
Tiapride	T43.591	T43.592	T43.593	T43.594	T43.595	T43.596
Tiaprofenic acid	T39.311	T39.312	T39.313	T39.314	T39.315	T39.316
Tiaramide	T39.8X1	T39.8X2	T39.8X3	T39.8X4	T39.8X5	T39.8X6
Ticarcillin	T36.0X1	T36.0X2	T36.0X3	T36.0X4	T36.0X5	T36.0X6
Ticlatone	T49.0X1	T49.0X2	T49.0X3	T49.0X4	T49.0X5	T49.0X6
Ticlopidine	T45.521	T45.522	T45.523	T45.524	T45.525	T45.526
Ticrynafen	T50.1X1	T50.1X2	T50.1X3	T50.1X4	T50.1X5	T50.1X6
Tidiacic	T50.991	T50.992	T50.993	T50.994	T50.995	T50.996
Tiemonium	T44.3X1	T44.3X2	T44.3X3	T44.3X4	T44.3X5	T44.3X6
iodide	T44.3X1	T44.3X2	T44.3X3	T44.3X4	T44.3X5	T44.3X6
Tienilic acid	T50.1X1	T50.1X2	T50.1X3	T50.1X4	T50.1X5	T50.1X6
Tifenamil	T44.3X1	T44.3X2	T44.3X3	T44.3X4	T44.3X5	T44.3X6
Tigan	T45.0X1	T45.0X2	T45.0X3	T45.0X4	T45.0X5	T45.0X6
Tigloidine	T44.3X1	T44.3X2	T44.3X3	T44.3X4	T44.3X5	T44.3X6
Tilactase	T47.5X1	T47.5X2	T47.5X3	T47.5X4	T47.5X5	T47.5X6
Tiletamine	T41.291	T41.292	T41.293	T41.294	T41.295	T41.296
Tilidine	T40.4X1	T40.4X2	T40.4X3	T40.4X4	—	—
Timepidium bromide	T44.3X1	T44.3X2	T44.3X3	T44.3X4	T44.3X5	T44.3X6
Timiperone	T43.4X1	T43.4X2	T43.4X3	T43.4X4	T43.4X5	T43.4X6
Timolol	T44.7X1	T44.7X2	T44.7X3	T44.7X4	T44.7X5	T44.7X6
Tin (chloride) (dust) (oxide) NEC	T56.6X1	T56.6X2	T56.6X3	T56.6X4	—	—
anti-infectives	T37.8X1	T37.8X2	T37.8X3	T37.8X4	T37.8X5	T37.8X6
Tincture, iodine — see Iodine						
Tindal	T43.3X1	T43.3X2	T43.3X3	T43.3X4	T43.3X5	T43.3X6
Tinidazole	T37.3X1	T37.3X2	T37.3X3	T37.3X4	T37.3X5	T37.3X6
Tinoridine	T39.8X1	T39.8X2	T39.8X3	T39.8X4	T39.8X5	T39.8X6
Tiocarlide	T37.1X1	T37.1X2	T37.1X3	T37.1X4	T37.1X5	T37.1X6
Tioclomarol	T45.511	T45.512	T45.513	T45.514	T45.515	T45.516

TABLE OF DRUGS AND CHEMICALS

TABLE OF DRUGS AND CHEMICALS

Substance	External Cause (T-Code) Poisoning, Accidental (Unintentional)	Poisoning, Intentional Self-Harm	Poisoning, Assault	Poisoning, Undetermined	Adverse Effect	Underdosing
Tioconazole	T49.0X1	T49.0X2	T49.0X3	T49.0X4	T49.0X5	T49.0X6
Tioguanine	T45.1X1	T45.1X2	T45.1X3	T45.1X4	T45.1X5	T45.1X6
Tiopronin	T50.991	T50.992	T50.993	T50.994	T50.995	T50.996
Tiotixene	T43.4X1	T43.4X2	T43.4X3	T43.4X4	T43.4X5	T43.4X6
Tioxolone	T49.4X1	T49.4X2	T49.4X3	T49.4X4	T49.4X5	T49.4X6
Tipepidine	T48.3X1	T48.3X2	T48.3X3	T48.3X4	T48.3X5	T48.3X6
Tiquizium bromide	T44.3X1	T44.3X2	T44.3X3	T44.3X4	T44.3X5	T44.3X6
Tiratricol	T38.1X1	T38.1X2	T38.1X3	T38.1X4	T38.1X5	T38.1X6
Tisopurine	T50.4X1	T50.4X2	T50.4X3	T50.4X4	T50.4X5	T50.4X6
Titanium (compounds) (vapor)	T56.891	T56.892	T56.893	T56.894	—	—
dioxide	T49.3X1	T49.3X2	T49.3X3	T49.3X4	T49.3X5	T49.3X6
ointment	T49.3X1	T49.3X2	T49.3X3	T49.3X4	T49.3X5	T49.3X6
oxide	T49.3X1	T49.3X2	T49.3X3	T49.3X4	T49.3X5	T49.3X6
tetrachloride	T56.891	T56.892	T56.893	T56.894	—	—
Titanocene	T56.891	T56.892	T56.893	T56.894	—	—
Titroid	T38.1X1	T38.1X2	T38.1X3	T38.1X4	T38.1X5	T38.1X6
Tizanidine	T42.8X1	T42.8X2	T42.8X3	T42.8X4	T42.8X5	T42.8X6
TMTD	T60.3X1	T60.3X2	T60.3X3	T60.3X4	—	—
TNT (fumes)	T65.3X1	T65.3X2	T65.3X3	T65.3X4	—	—
Toadstool	T62.0X1	T62.0X2	T62.0X3	T62.0X4	—	—
Tobacco NEC	T65.291	T65.292	T65.293	T65.294	—	—
cigarettes	T65.221	T65.222	T65.223	T65.224	—	—
Indian	T62.2X1	T62.2X2	T62.2X3	T62.2X4	—	—
smoke, second-hand	T65.221	T65.222	T65.223	T65.224	—	—
Tobramycin	T36.5X1	T36.5X2	T36.5X3	T36.5X4	T36.5X5	T36.5X6
Tocainide	T46.2X1	T46.2X2	T46.2X3	T46.2X4	T46.2X5	T46.2X6
Tocoferol	T45.2X1	T45.2X2	T45.2X3	T45.2X4	T45.2X5	T45.2X6
Tocopherol	T45.2X1	T45.2X2	T45.2X3	T45.2X4	T45.2X5	T45.2X6
acetate	T45.2X1	T45.2X2	T45.2X3	T45.2X4	T45.2X5	T45.2X6
Tocosamine	T48.0X1	T48.0X2	T48.0X3	T48.0X4	T48.0X5	T48.0X6
Todralazine	T46.5X1	T46.5X2	T46.5X3	T46.5X4	T46.5X5	T46.5X6
Tofisopam	T42.4X1	T42.4X2	T42.4X3	T42.4X4	T42.4X5	T42.4X6
Tofranil	T43.011	T43.012	T43.013	T43.014	T43.015	T43.016
Toilet deodorizer	T65.891	T65.892	T65.893	T65.894	—	—
Tolamolol	T44.7X1	T44.7X2	T44.7X3	T44.7X4	T44.7X5	T44.7X6
Tolazamide	T38.3X1	T38.3X2	T38.3X3	T38.3X4	T38.3X5	T38.3X6
Tolazoline	T46.7X1	T46.7X2	T46.7X3	T46.7X4	T46.7X5	T46.7X6
Tolbutamide (sodium)	T38.3X1	T38.3X2	T38.3X3	T38.3X4	T38.3X5	T38.3X6
Tolciclate	T49.0X1	T49.0X2	T49.0X3	T49.0X4	T49.0X5	T49.0X6
Tolmetin	T39.391	T39.392	T39.393	T39.394	T39.395	T39.396
Tolnaftate	T49.0X1	T49.0X2	T49.0X3	T49.0X4	T49.0X5	T49.0X6
Tolonidine	T46.5X1	T46.5X2	T46.5X3	T46.5X4	T46.5X5	T46.5X6

Substance	External Cause (T-Code) Poisoning, Accidental (Unintentional)	Poisoning, Intentional Self-Harm	Poisoning, Assault	Poisoning, Undetermined	Adverse Effect	Underdosing
Toloxatone	T42.6X1	T42.6X2	T42.6X3	T42.6X4	T42.6X5	T42.6X6
Tolperisone	T44.3X1	T44.3X2	T44.3X3	T44.3X4	T44.3X5	T44.3X6
Tolserol	T42.8X1	T42.8X2	T42.8X3	T42.8X4	T42.8X5	T42.8X6
Toluene (liquid)	T52.2X1	T52.2X2	T52.2X3	T52.2X4	—	—
diisocyanate	T65.0X1	T65.0X2	T65.0X3	T65.0X4	—	—
Toluidine	T65.891	T65.892	T65.893	T65.894	—	—
vapor	T59.891	T59.892	T59.893	T59.894	—	—
Toluol (liquid)	T52.2X1	T52.2X2	T52.2X3	T52.2X4	—	—
vapor	T52.2X1	T52.2X2	T52.2X3	T52.2X4	—	—
Toluylenediamine	T65.3X1	T65.3X2	T65.3X3	T65.3X4	—	—
Tolylene-2,4-diisocyanate	T65.0X1	T65.0X2	T65.0X3	T65.0X4	—	—
Tonic NEC	T50.901	T50.902	T50.903	T50.904	T50.905	T50.906
Topical action drug NEC	T49.91	T49.92	T49.93	T49.94	T49.95	T49.96
ear, nose or throat	T49.6X1	T49.6X2	T49.6X3	T49.6X4	T49.6X5	T49.6X6
eye	T49.5X1	T49.5X2	T49.5X3	T49.5X4	T49.5X5	T49.5X6
skin	T49.91	T49.92	T49.93	T49.94	T49.95	T49.96
specified NEC	T49.8X1	T49.8X2	T49.8X3	T49.8X4	T49.8X5	T49.8X6
Toquizine	T44.3X1	T44.3X2	T44.3X3	T44.3X4	T44.3X5	T44.3X6
Toremifene	T38.6X1	T38.6X2	T38.6X3	T38.6X4	T38.6X5	T38.6X6
Tosylchloramide sodium	T49.8X1	T49.8X2	T49.8X3	T49.8X4	T49.8X5	T49.8X6
Toxaphene (dust) (spray)	T60.1X1	T60.1X2	T60.1X3	T60.1X4	—	—
Toxin, diphtheria (Schick Test)	T50.8X1	T50.8X2	T50.8X3	T50.8X4	T50.8X5	T50.8X6
Toxoid						
combined	T50.A21	T50.A22	T50.A23	T50.A24	T50.A25	T50.A26
diphtheria	T50.A91	T50.A92	T50.A93	T50.A94	T50.A95	T50.A96
tetanus	T50.A91	T50.A92	T50.A93	T50.A94	T50.A95	T50.A96
Trace element NEC	T45.8X1	T45.8X2	T45.8X3	T45.8X4	T45.8X5	T45.8X6
Tractor fuel NEC	T52.0X1	T52.0X2	T52.0X3	T52.0X4	—	—
Tragacanth	T50.991	T50.992	T50.993	T50.994	T50.995	T50.996
Tramadol	T40.4X1	T40.4X2	T40.4X3	T40.4X4	T40.4X5	T40.4X6
Tramazoline	T48.5X1	T48.5X2	T48.5X3	T48.5X4	T48.5X5	T48.5X6
Tranexamic acid	T45.621	T45.622	T45.623	T45.624	T45.625	T45.626
Tranilast	T45.0X1	T45.0X2	T45.0X3	T45.0X4	T45.0X5	T45.0X6
Tranquilizer NEC	T43.501	T43.502	T43.503	T43.504	T43.505	T43.506
with hypnotic or sedative	T42.6X1	T42.6X2	T42.6X3	T42.6X4	T42.6X5	T42.6X6
benzodiazepine NEC	T42.4X1	T42.4X2	T42.4X3	T42.4X4	T42.4X5	T42.4X6
butyrophenone NEC	T43.4X1	T43.4X2	T43.4X3	T43.4X4	T43.4X5	T43.4X6
carbamate	T43.591	T43.592	T43.593	T43.594	T43.595	T43.596
dimethylamine	T43.3X1	T43.3X2	T43.3X3	T43.3X4	T43.3X5	T43.3X6
ethylamine	T43.3X1	T43.3X2	T43.3X3	T43.3X4	T43.3X5	T43.3X6
hydroxyzine	T43.591	T43.592	T43.593	T43.594	T43.595	T43.596
major NEC	T43.501	T43.502	T43.503	T43.504	T43.505	T43.506

◄ New   ◄▦ Revised   ~~deleted~~ Deleted

Substance	External Cause (T-Code)					
	Poisoning, Accidental (Unintentional)	Poisoning, Intentional Self-Harm	Poisoning, Assault	Poisoning, Undetermined	Adverse Effect	Underdosing
Tranquilizer NEC *(Continued)*						
penothiazine NEC	T43.3X1	T43.3X2	T43.3X3	T43.3X4	T43.3X5	T43.3X6
phenothiazine-based	T43.3X1	T43.3X2	T43.3X3	T43.3X4	T43.3X5	T43.3X6
piperazine NEC	T43.3X1	T43.3X2	T43.3X3	T43.3X4	T43.3X5	T43.3X6
piperidine	T43.3X1	T43.3X2	T43.3X3	T43.3X4	T43.3X5	T43.3X6
propylamine	T43.3X1	T43.3X2	T43.3X3	T43.3X4	T43.3X5	T43.3X6
specified NEC	T43.591	T43.592	T43.593	T43.594	T43.595	T43.596
thioxanthene NEC	T43.591	T43.592	T43.593	T43.594	T43.595	T43.596
Tranxene	T42.4X1	T42.4X2	T42.4X3	T42.4X4	T42.4X5	T42.4X6
Tranylcypromine	T43.1X1	T43.1X2	T43.1X3	T43.1X4	T43.1X5	T43.1X6
Trapidil	T46.3X1	T46.3X2	T46.3X3	T46.3X4	T46.3X5	T46.3X6
Trasentine	T44.3X1	T44.3X2	T44.3X3	T44.3X4	T44.3X5	T44.3X6
Travert	T50.3X1	T50.3X2	T50.3X3	T50.3X4	T50.3X5	T50.3X6
Trazodone	T43.211	T43.212	T43.213	T43.214	T43.215	T43.216
Trecator	T37.1X1	T37.1X2	T37.1X4	T37.1X4	T37.1X5	T37.1X6
Treosulfan	T45.1X1	T45.1X2	T45.1X3	T45.1X4	T45.1X5	T45.1X6
Tretamine	T45.1X1	T45.1X2	T45.1X3	T45.1X4	T45.1X5	T45.1X6
Tretinoin	T49.0X1	T49.0X2	T49.0X3	T49.0X4	T49.0X5	T49.0X6
Tretoquinol	T48.6X1	T48.6X2	T48.6X4	T48.6X4	T48.6X5	T48.6X6
Triacetin	T49.0X1	T49.0X2	T49.0X3	T49.0X4	T49.0X5	T49.0X6
Triacetoxyanthracene	T49.4X1	T49.4X2	T49.4X3	T49.4X4	T49.4X5	T49.4X6
Triacetyloleandomycin	T36.3X1	T36.3X2	T36.3X3	T36.3X4	T36.3X5	T36.3X6
Triamcinolone	T49.0X1	T49.0X2	T49.0X3	T49.0X4	T49.0X5	T49.0X6
ENT agent	T49.6X1	T49.6X2	T49.6X3	T49.6X4	T49.6X5	T49.6X6
hexacetonide	T49.0X1	T49.0X2	T49.0X3	T49.0X4	T49.0X5	T49.0X6
ophthalmic preparation	T49.5X1	T49.5X2	T49.5X3	T49.5X4	T49.5X5	T49.5X6
topical NEC	T49.0X1	T49.0X2	T49.0X3	T49.0X4	T49.0X5	T49.0X6
Triampyzine	T44.3X1	T44.3X2	T44.3X3	T44.3X4	T44.3X5	T44.3X6
Triamterene	T50.2X1	T50.2X2	T50.2X3	T50.2X4	T50.2X5	T50.2X6
Triazine (herbicide)	T60.3X1	T60.3X2	T60.3X3	T60.3X4	—	—
Triaziquone	T45.1X1	T45.1X2	T45.1X3	T45.1X4	T45.1X5	T45.1X6
Triazolam	T42.4X1	T42.4X2	T42.4X3	T42.4X4	T42.4X5	T42.4X6
Triazole (herbicide)	T60.3X1	T60.3X2	T60.3X3	T60.3X4	—	—
Tribenoside	T46.991	T46.992	T46.993	T46.994	T46.995	T46.996
Tribromacetaldehyde	T42.6X1	T42.6X2	T42.6X3	T42.6X4	T42.6X5	T42.6X6
Tribromoethanol, rectal	T41.291	T41.292	T41.293	T41.294	T41.295	T41.296
Tribromomethane	T42.6X1	T42.6X2	T42.6X3	T42.6X4	T42.6X5	T42.6X6
Trichlorethane	T53.2X1	T53.2X2	T53.2X3	T53.2X4	—	—
Trichlorethylene	T53.2X1	T53.2X2	T53.2X3	T53.2X4	—	—
Trichlorfon	T60.0X1	T60.0X2	T60.0X3	T60.0X4	—	—
Trichlormethiazide	T50.2X1	T50.2X2	T50.2X3	T50.2X4	T50.2X5	T50.2X6
Trichlormethine	T45.1X1	T45.1X2	T45.1X3	T45.1X4	T45.1X5	T45.1X6

Substance	External Cause (T-Code)					
	Poisoning, Accidental (Unintentional)	Poisoning, Intentional Self-Harm	Poisoning, Assault	Poisoning, Undetermined	Adverse Effect	Underdosing
Trichloroacetic acid, Trichloracetic acid	T54.2X1	T54.2X2	T54.2X3	T54.2X4	—	—
medicinal	T49.4X1	T49.4X2	T49.4X3	T49.4X4	T49.4X5	T49.4X6
Trichloroethane	T53.2X1	T53.2X2	T53.2X3	T53.2X4	—	—
Trichloroethanol	T42.6X1	T42.6X2	T42.6X3	T42.6X4	T42.6X5	T42.6X6
Trichloroethylene (liquid) (vapor)	T53.2X1	T53.2X2	T53.2X3	T53.2X4	—	—
anesthetic (gas)	T41.0X1	T41.0X2	T41.0X3	T41.0X4	T41.0X5	T41.0X6
vapor NEC	T53.2X1	T53.2X2	T53.2X3	T53.2X4	—	—
Trichloroethyl phosphate	T42.6X1	T42.6X2	T42.6X3	T42.6X4	T42.6X5	T42.6X6
Trichlorofluoromethane NEC	T53.5X1	T53.5X2	T53.5X3	T53.5X4	—	—
Trichloronate	T60.0X1	T60.0X2	T60.0X3	T60.0X4	—	—
2,4,5-Trichlorophen-oxyacetic acid	T60.3X1	T60.3X2	T60.3X3	T60.3X4	—	—
Trichloropropane	T53.6X1	T53.6X2	T53.6X3	T53.6X4	—	—
Trichlorotriethylamine	T45.1X1	T45.1X2	T45.1X3	T45.1X4	T45.1X5	T45.1X6
Trichomonacides NEC	T37.3X1	T37.3X2	T37.3X3	T37.3X4	T37.3X5	T37.3X6
Trichomycin	T36.7X1	T36.7X2	T36.7X3	T36.7X4	T36.7X5	T36.7X6
Triclobisonium chloride	T49.0X1	T49.0X2	T49.0X3	T49.0X4	T49.0X5	T49.0X6
Triclocarban	T49.0X1	T49.0X2	T49.0X3	T49.0X4	T49.0X5	T49.0X6
Triclofos	T42.6X1	T42.6X2	T42.6X3	T42.6X4	T42.6X5	T42.6X6
Triclosan	T49.0X1	T49.0X2	T49.0X3	T49.0X4	T49.0X5	T49.0X6
Tricresyl phosphate	T65.891	T65.892	T65.893	T65.894	—	—
solvent	T52.91	T52.92	T52.93	T52.94	—	—
Tricyclamol chloride	T44.3X1	T44.3X2	T44.3X3	T44.3X4	T44.3X5	T44.3X6
Tridesilon	T49.0X1	T49.0X2	T49.0X3	T49.0X4	T49.0X5	T49.0X6
Tridihexethyl iodide	T44.3X1	T44.3X2	T44.3X3	T44.3X4	T44.3X5	T44.3X6
Tridione	T42.2X1	T42.2X2	T42.2X3	T42.2X4	T42.2X5	T42.2X6
Trientine	T45.8X1	T45.8X2	T45.8X3	T45.8X4	T45.8X5	T45.8X6
Triethanolamine NEC	T54.3X1	T54.3X2	T54.3X3	T54.3X4	—	—
detergent	T54.3X1	T54.3X2	T54.3X3	T54.3X4	—	—
trinitrate (biphosphate)	T46.3X1	T46.3X2	T46.3X3	T46.3X4	T46.3X5	T46.3X6
Triethanomelamine	T45.1X1	T45.1X2	T45.1X3	T45.1X4	T45.1X5	T45.1X6
Triethylenemelamine	T45.1X1	T45.1X2	T45.1X3	T45.1X4	T45.1X5	T45.1X6
Triethylenephosphoramide	T45.1X1	T45.1X2	T45.1X3	T45.1X4	T45.1X5	T45.1X6
Triethylenethiophosphoramide	T45.1X1	T45.1X2	T45.1X3	T45.1X4	T45.1X5	T45.1X6
Trifluoperazine	T43.3X1	T43.3X2	T43.3X3	T43.3X4	T43.3X5	T43.3X6
Trifluoroethyl vinyl ether	T41.0X1	T41.0X2	T41.0X3	T41.0X4	T41.0X5	T41.0X6
Trifluperidol	T43.4X1	T43.4X2	T43.4X3	T43.4X4	T43.4X5	T43.4X6
Triflupromazine	T43.3X1	T43.3X2	T43.3X3	T43.3X4	T43.3X5	T43.3X6
Trifluridine	T37.5X1	T37.5X2	T37.5X3	T37.5X4	T37.5X5	T37.5X6
Triflusal	T45.521	T45.522	T45.523	T45.524	T45.525	T45.526
Trihexyphenidyl	T44.3X1	T44.3X2	T44.3X3	T44.3X4	T44.3X5	T44.3X6
Triiodothyronine	T38.1X1	T38.1X2	T38.1X3	T38.1X4	T38.1X5	T38.1X6

◀ New ◀ Revised ~~deleted~~ Deleted

TABLE OF DRUGS AND CHEMICALS

Substance	External Cause (T-Code)					
	Poisoning, Accidental (Unintentional)	Poisoning, Intentional Self-Harm	Poisoning, Assault	Poisoning, Undetermined	Adverse Effect	Underdosing
Trilene	T41.0X1	T41.0X2	T41.0X3	T41.0X4	T41.0X5	T41.0X6
Trilostane	T38.991	T38.992	T38.993	T38.994	T38.995	T38.996
Trimebutine	T44.3X1	T44.3X2	T44.3X3	T44.3X4	T44.3X5	T44.3X6
Trimecaine	T41.3X1	T41.3X2	T41.3X3	T41.3X4	T41.3X5	T41.3X6
Trimeprazine (tartrate)	T44.3X1	T44.3X2	T44.3X3	T44.3X4	T44.3X5	T44.3X6
Trimetaphan camsilate	T44.2X1	T44.2X2	T44.2X3	T44.2X4	T44.2X5	T44.2X6
Trimetazidine	T46.7X1	T46.7X2	T46.7X3	T46.7X4	T46.7X5	T46.7X6
Trimethadione	T42.2X1	T42.2X2	T42.2X3	T42.2X4	T42.2X5	T42.2X6
Trimethaphan	T44.2X1	T44.2X2	T44.2X3	T44.2X4	T44.2X5	T44.2X6
Trimethidinium	T44.2X1	T44.2X2	T44.2X3	T44.2X4	T44.2X5	T44.2X6
Trimethobenzamide	T45.0X1	T45.0X2	T45.0X3	T45.0X4	T45.0X5	T45.0X6
Trimethoprim	T37.8X1	T37.8X2	T37.8X3	T37.8X4	T37.8X5	T37.8X6
with sulfamethoxazole	T36.8X1	T36.8X2	T36.8X3	T36.8X4	T36.8X5	T36.8X6
Trimethylcarbinol	T51.3X1	T51.3X2	T51.3X3	T51.3X4	—	—
Trimethylpsoralen	T49.3X1	T49.3X2	T49.3X3	T49.3X4	T49.3X5	T49.3X6
Trimeton	T45.0X1	T45.0X2	T45.0X3	T45.0X4	T45.0X5	T45.0X6
Trimetrexate	T45.1X1	T45.1X2	T45.1X3	T45.1X4	T45.1X5	T45.1X6
Trimipramine	T43.011	T43.012	T43.013	T43.014	T43.015	T43.016
Trimustine	T45.1X1	T45.1X2	T45.1X3	T45.1X4	T45.1X5	T45.1X6
Trinitrine	T46.3X1	T46.3X2	T46.3X3	T46.3X4	T46.3X5	T46.3X6
Trinitrobenzol	T65.3X1	T65.3X2	T65.3X3	T65.3X4	—	—
Trinitrophenol	T65.3X1	T65.3X2	T65.3X3	T65.3X4	—	—
Trinitrotoluene (fumes)	T65.3X1	T65.3X2	T65.3X3	T65.3X4	—	—
Trional	T42.6X1	T42.6X2	T42.6X3	T42.6X4	T42.6X5	T42.6X6
Triorthocresyl phosphate	T65.891	T65.892	T65.893	T65.894	—	—
Trioxide of arsenic	T57.0X1	T57.0X2	T57.0X3	T57.0X4		
Trioxysalen	T49.4X1	T49.4X2	T49.4X3	T49.4X4	T49.4X5	T49.4X6
Tripamide	T50.2X1	T50.2X2	T50.2X3	T50.2X4	T50.2X5	T50.2X6
Triparanol	T46.6X1	T46.6X2	T46.6X3	T46.6X4	T46.6X5	T46.6X6
Tripelennamine	T45.0X1	T45.0X2	T45.0X3	T45.0X4	T45.0X5	T45.0X6
Triperiden	T44.3X1	T44.3X2	T44.3X3	T44.3X4	T44.3X5	T44.3X6
Triperidol	T43.4X1	T43.4X2	T43.4X3	T43.4X4	T43.4X5	T43.4X6
Triphenylphosphate	T65.891	T65.892	T65.893	T65.894	—	—
Triple						
bromides	T42.6X1	T42.6X2	T42.6X3	T42.6X4	T42.6X5	T42.6X6
carbonate	T47.1X1	T47.1X2	T47.1X3	T47.1X4	T47.1X5	T47.1X6
vaccine						
DPT	T50.A11	T50.A12	T50.A13	T50.A14	T50.A15	T50.A16
including pertussis	T50.A11	T50.A12	T50.A13	T50.A14	T50.A15	T50.A16
MMR	T50.B91	T50.B92	—	—	—	—
Triprolidine	T45.0X1	T45.0X2	T45.0X3	T45.0X4	T45.0X5	T45.0X6
Trisodium hydrogen edetate	T50.6X1	T50.6X2	T50.6X3	T50.6X4	T50.6X5	T50.6X6

Substance	External Cause (T-Code)					
	Poisoning, Accidental (Unintentional)	Poisoning, Intentional Self-Harm	Poisoning, Assault	Poisoning, Undetermined	Adverse Effect	Underdosing
Trisoralen	T49.3X1	T49.3X2	T49.3X3	T49.3X4	T49.3X5	T49.3X6
Trisulfapyrimidines	T37.0X1	T37.0X2	T37.0X3	T37.0X4	T37.0X5	T37.0X6
Trithiozine	T44.3X1	T44.3X2	T44.3X3	T44.3X4	T44.3X5	T44.3X6
Tritiozine	T44.3X1	T44.3X2	T44.3X3	T44.3X4	T44.3X5	T44.3X6
Tritoqualine	T45.0X1	T45.0X2	T45.0X3	T45.0X4	T45.0X5	T45.0X6
Trofosfamide	T45.1X1	T45.1X2	T45.1X3	T45.1X4	T45.1X5	T45.1X6
Troleandomycin	T36.3X1	T36.3X2	T36.3X3	T36.3X4	T36.3X5	T36.3X6
Trolnitrate (phosphate)	T46.3X1	T46.3X2	T46.3X3	T46.3X4	T46.3X5	T46.3X6
Tromantadine	T37.5X1	T37.5X2	T37.5X3	T37.5X4	T37.5X5	T37.5X6
Trometamol	T50.2X1	T50.2X2	T50.2X3	T50.2X4	T50.2X5	T50.2X6
Tromethamine	T50.2X1	T50.2X2	T50.2X3	T50.2X4	T50.2X5	T50.2X6
Tronothane	T41.3X1	T41.3X2	T41.3X3	T41.3X4	T41.3X5	T41.3X6
Tropacine	T44.3X1	T44.3X2	T44.3X3	T44.3X4	T44.3X5	T44.3X6
Tropatepine	T44.3X1	T44.3X2	T44.3X3	T44.3X4	T44.3X5	T44.3X6
Tropicamide	T44.3X1	T44.3X2	T44.3X3	T44.3X4	T44.3X5	T44.3X6
Trospium chloride	T44.3X1	T44.3X2	T44.3X3	T44.3X4	T44.3X5	T44.3X6
Troxerutin	T46.991	T46.992	T46.993	T46.994	T46.995	T46.996
Troxidone	T42.2X1	T42.2X2	T42.2X3	T42.2X4	T42.2X5	T42.2X6
Tryparsamide	T37.3X1	T37.3X2	T37.3X3	T37.3X4	T37.3X5	T37.3X6
Trypsin	T45.3X1	T45.3X2	T45.3X3	T45.3X4	T45.3X5	T45.3X6
Tryptizol	T43.011	T43.012	T43.013	T43.014	T43.015	T43.016
TSH	T38.811	T38.812	T38.813	T38.814	T38.815	T38.816
Tuaminoheptane	T48.5X1	T48.5X2	T48.5X3	T48.5X4	T48.5X5	T48.5X6
Tuberculin, purified protein derivative (PPD)	T50.8X1	T50.8X2	T50.8X3	T50.8X4	T50.8X5	T50.8X6
Tubocurare	T48.1X1	T48.1X2	T48.1X3	T48.1X4	T48.1X5	T48.1X6
Tubocurarine (chloride)	T48.1X1	T48.1X2	T48.1X3	T48.1X4	T48.1X5	T48.1X6
Tulobuterol	T48.6X1	T48.6X2	T48.6X3	T48.6X4	T48.6X5	T48.6X6
Turpentine (spirits of)	T52.8X1	T52.8X2	T52.8X3	T52.8X4	—	—
vapor	T52.8X1	T52.8X2	T52.8X3	T52.8X4	—	—
Tybamate	T43.591	T43.592	T43.593	T43.594	T43.595	T43.596
Tyloxapol	T48.4X1	T48.4X2	T48.4X3	T48.4X4	T48.4X5	T48.4X6
Tymazoline	T48.5X1	T48.5X2	T48.5X3	T48.5X4	T48.5X5	T48.5X6
Typhoid-paratyphoid vaccine	T50.A91	T50.A92	T50.A93	T50.A94	T50.A95	T50.A96
Typhus vaccine	T50.A91	T50.A92	T50.A93	T50.A94	T50.A95	T50.A96
Tyropanoate	T50.8X1	T50.8X2	T50.8X3	T50.8X4	T50.8X5	T50.8X6
Tyrothricin	T49.6X1	T49.6X2	T49.6X3	T49.6X4	T49.6X5	T49.6X6
ENT agent	T49.6X1	T49.6X2	T49.6X3	T49.6X4	T49.6X5	T49.6X6
ophthalmic preparation	T49.5X1	T49.5X2	T49.5X3	T49.5X4	T49.5X5	T49.5X6
U						
Ufenamate	T39.391	T39.392	T39.393	T39.394	T39.395	T39.396
Ultraviolet light protectant	T49.3X1	T49.3X2	T49.3X3	T49.3X4	T49.3X5	T49.3X6

◀ New   ◀▥ Revised   deleted Deleted

Substance	Poisoning, Accidental (Unintentional)	Poisoning, Intentional Self-Harm	Poisoning, Assault	Poisoning, Undetermined	Adverse Effect	Underdosing
Undecenoic acid	T49.0X1	T49.0X2	T49.0X3	T49.0X4	T49.0X5	T49.0X6
Undecoylium	T49.0X1	T49.0X2	T49.0X3	T49.0X4	T49.0X5	T49.0X6
Undecylenic acid (derivatives)	T49.0X1	T49.0X2	T49.0X3	T49.0X4	T49.0X5	T49.0X6
Unna's boot	T49.3X1	T49.3X2	T49.3X3	T49.3X4	T49.3X5	T49.3X6
Unsaturated fatty acid	T46.6X1	T46.6X2	T46.6X3	T46.6X4	T46.6X5	T46.6X6
Uracil mustard	T45.1X1	T45.1X2	T45.1X3	T45.1X4	T45.1X5	T45.1X6
Uramustine	T45.1X1	T45.1X2	T45.1X3	T45.1X4	T45.1X5	T45.1X6
Urapidil	T46.5X1	T46.5X2	T46.5X3	T46.5X4	T46.5X5	T46.5X6
Urari	T48.1X1	T48.1X2	T48.1X3	T48.1X4	T48.1X5	T48.1X6
Urate oxidase	T50.4X1	T50.4X2	T50.4X3	T50.4X4	T50.4X5	T50.4X6
Urea	T47.3X1	T47.3X2	T47.3X3	T47.3X4	T47.3X5	T47.3X6
peroxide	T49.0X1	T49.0X2	T49.0X3	T49.0X4	T49.0X5	T49.0X6
stibamine	T37.4X1	T37.4X2	T37.4X3	T37.4X4	T37.4X5	T37.4X6
topical	T49.8X1	T49.8X2	T49.8X3	T49.8X4	T49.8X5	T49.8X6
Urethane	T45.1X1	T45.1X2	T45.1X3	T45.1X4	T45.1X5	T45.1X6
Urginea (maritima) (scilla) —*see Squill*						
Uric acid metabolism drug NEC	T50.4X1	T50.4X2	T50.4X3	T50.4X4	T50.4X5	T50.4X6
Uricosuric agent	T50.4X1	T50.4X2	T50.4X3	T50.4X4	T50.4X5	T50.4X6
Urinary anti-infective	T37.8X1	T37.8X2	T37.8X3	T37.8X4	T37.8X5	T37.8X6
Urofollitropin	T38.811	T38.812	T38.813	T38.814	T38.815	T38.816
Urokinase	T45.611	T45.612	T45.613	T45.614	T45.615	T45.616
Urokon	T50.8X1	T50.8X2	T50.8X3	T50.8X4	T50.8X5	T50.8X6
Ursodeoxycholic acid	T50.991	T50.992	T50.993	T50.994	T50.995	T50.996
Ursodiol	T50.991	T50.992	T50.993	T50.994	T50.995	T50.996
Urtica	T62.2X1	T62.2X2	T62.2X3	T62.2X4	—	—
Utility gas —*see Gas, utility*						
V						
Vaccine NEC	T50.Z91	T50.Z92	T50.Z93	T50.Z94	T50.Z95	T50.Z96
antineoplastic	T50.Z91	T50.Z92	T50.Z93	T50.Z94	T50.Z95	T50.Z96
bacterial NEC	T50.A91	T50.A92	T50.A93	T50.A94	T50.A95	T50.A96
with						
other bacterial component	T50.A91	T50.A92	T50.A93	T50.A94	T50.A95	T50.A96
pertussis component	T50.A91	T50.A92	T50.A93	T50.A94	T50.A95	T50.A96
viral-rickettsial component	T50.A91	T50.A92	T50.A93	T50.A94	T50.A95	T50.A96
mixed NEC	T50.A91	T50.A92	T50.A93	T50.A94	T50.A95	T50.A96
BCG	T50.A91	T50.A92	T50.A93	T50.A94	T50.A95	T50.A96
cholera	T50.A91	T50.A92	T50.A93	T50.A94	T50.A95	T50.A96
diphtheria	T50.A91	T50.A92	T50.A93	T50.A94	T50.A95	T50.A96
with tetanus	T50.A21	T50.A22	T50.A23	T50.A24	T50.A25	T50.A26
and pertussis	T50.A11	T50.A12	T50.A13	T50.A14	T50.A15	T50.A16

Substance	Poisoning, Accidental (Unintentional)	Poisoning, Intentional Self-Harm	Poisoning, Assault	Poisoning, Undetermined	Adverse Effect	Underdosing
Vaccine NEC *(Continued)*						
influenza	T50.B91	T50.B92	T50.B93	T50.B94	T50.B95	T50.B96
measles	T50.B91	T50.B92	T50.B93	T50.B94	T50.B95	T50.B96
with mumps and rubella	T50.B91	T50.B92	T50.B93	T50.B94	T50.B95	T50.B96
meningococcal	T50.A91	T50.A92	T50.A93	T50.A94	T50.A95	T50.A96
mumps	T50.B91	T50.B92	T50.B93	T50.B94	T50.B95	T50.B96
paratyphoid	T50.A91	T50.A92	T50.A93	T50.A94	T50.A95	T50.A96
pertussis	T50.A11	T50.A12	T50.A13	T50.A14	T50.A15	T50.A16
with diphtheria	T50.A11	T50.A12	T50.A13	T50.A14	T50.A15	T50.A16
and tetanus	T50.A11	T50.A12	T50.A13	T50.A14	T50.A15	T50.A16
plague	T50.A91	T50.A92	T50.A93	T50.A94	T50.A95	T50.A96
poliomyelitis	T50.B91	T50.B92	T50.B93	T50.B94	T50.B95	T50.B96
poliovirus	T50.B91	T50.B92	T50.B93	T50.B94	T50.B95	T50.B96
rabies	T50.B91	T50.B92	T50.B93	T50.B94	T50.B95	T50.B96
respiratory syncytial virus	T50.B91	T50.B92	T50.B93	T50.B94	T50.B95	T50.B96
rickettsial NEC	T50.A91	T50.A92	T50.A93	T50.A94	T50.A95	T50.A96
with						
bacterial component	T50.A21	T50.A22	T50.A23	T50.A24	T50.A25	T50.A26
Rocky Mountain spotted fever	T50.A91	T50.A92	T50.A93	T50.A94	T50.A95	T50.A96
rubella	T50.B91	T50.B92	T50.B93	T50.B94	T50.B95	T50.B96
sabin oral	T50.B91	T50.B92	T50.B93	T50.B94	T50.B95	T50.B96
smallpox	T50.B11	T50.B12	T50.B13	T50.B14	T50.B15	T50.B16
TAB	T50.A91	T50.A92	T50.A93	T50.A94	T50.A95	T50.A96
tetanus	T50.A91	T50.A92	T50.A93	T50.A94	T50.A95	T50.A96
typhoid	T50.A91	T50.A92	T50.A93	T50.A94	T50.A95	T50.A96
typhus	T50.A91	T50.A92	T50.A93	T50.A94	T50.A95	T50.A96
viral NEC	T50.B91	T50.B92	T50.B93	T50.B94	T50.B95	T50.B96
yellow fever	T50.B91	T50.B92	T50.B93	T50.B94	T50.B95	T50.B96
Vaccinia immune globulin	T50.Z11	T50.Z12	T50.Z13	T50.Z14	T50.Z15	T50.Z16
Vaginal contraceptives	T49.8X1	T49.8X2	T49.8X3	T49.8X4	T49.8X5	T49.8X6
Valerian						
root	T42.6X1	T42.6X2	T42.6X3	T42.6X4	T42.6X5	T42.6X6
tincture	T42.6X1	T42.6X2	T42.6X3	T42.6X4	T42.6X5	T42.6X6
Valethamate bromide	T44.3X1	T44.3X2	T44.3X3	T44.3X4	T44.3X5	T44.3X6
Valisone	T49.0X1	T49.0X2	T49.0X3	T49.0X4	T49.0X5	T49.0X6
Valium	T42.4X1	T42.4X2	T42.4X3	T42.4X4	T42.4X5	T42.4X6
Valmid	T42.6X1	T42.6X2	T42.6X3	T42.6X4	T42.6X5	T42.6X6
Valnoctamide	T42.6X1	T42.6X2	T42.6X3	T42.6X4	T42.6X5	T42.6X6
Valproate (sodium)	T42.6X1	T42.6X2	T42.6X3	T42.6X4	T42.6X5	T42.6X6
Valproic acid	T42.6X1	T42.6X2	T42.6X3	T42.6X4	T42.6X5	T42.6X6
Valpromide	T42.6X1	T42.6X2	T42.6X3	T42.6X4	T42.6X5	T42.6X6
Vanadium	T56.891	T56.892	T56.893	T56.894	—	—

	External Cause (T-Code)					
Substance	Poisoning, Accidental (Unintentional)	Poisoning, Intentional Self-Harm	Poisoning, Assault	Poisoning, Undetermined	Adverse Effect	Underdosing
Vancomycin	T36.8X1	T36.8X2	T36.8X3	T36.8X4	T36.8X5	T36.8X6
Vapor — *see also Gas*	T59.91	T59.92	T59.93	T59.94	—	—
kiln (carbon monoxide)	T58.8X1	T58.8X2	T58.8X3	T58.8X4	—	—
lead — *see lead*						
specified source NEC	T59.891	T59.892	T59.893	T59.894	—	—
Vardenafil	T46.7X1	T46.7X2	T46.7X3	T46.7X4	T46.7X5	T46.7X6
Varicose reduction drug	T46.8X1	T46.8X2	T46.8X3	T46.8X4	T46.8X5	T46.8X6
Varnish	T65.4X1	T65.4X2	T65.4X3	T65.4X4		
cleaner	T52.91	T52.92	T52.93	T52.94	—	—
Vaseline	T49.3X1	T49.3X2	T49.3X3	T49.3X4	T49.3X5	T49.3X6
Vasodilan	T46.7X1	T46.7X2	T46.7X3	T46.7X4	T46.7X5	T46.7X6
Vasodilator						
coronary NEC	T46.3X1	T46.3X2	T46.3X3	T46.3X4	T46.3X5	T46.3X6
peripheral NEC	T46.7X1	T46.7X2	T46.7X3	T46.7X4	T46.7X5	T46.7X6
Vasopressin	T38.891	T38.892	T38.893	T38.894	T38.895	T38.896
Vasopressor drugs	T38.891	T38.892	T38.893	T38.894	T38.895	T38.896
Vecuronium bromide	T48.1X1	T48.1X2	T48.1X3	T48.1X4	T48.1X5	T48.1X6
Vegetable extract, astringent	T49.2X1	T49.2X2	T49.2X3	T49.2X4	T49.2X5	T49.2X6
Venlafaxine	T43.211	T43.212	T43.213	T43.214	T43.215	T43.216
Venom, venomous (bite) (sting)	T63.91	T63.92	T63.93	T63.94	—	—
amphibian NEC	T63.831	T63.832	T63.833	T63.834	—	—
animal NEC	T63.891	T63.892	T63.893	T63.894	—	—
ant	T63.421	T63.422	T63.423	T63.424	—	—
arthropod NEC	T63.481	T63.482	T63.483	T63.484	—	—
bee	T63.441	T63.442	T63.443	T63.444	—	—
centipede	T63.411	T63.412	T63.413	T63.414	—	—
fish	T63.591	T63.592	T63.593	T63.594	—	—
frog	T63.811	T63.812	T63.813	T63.814	—	—
hornet	T63.451	T63.452	T63.453	T63.454	—	—
insect NEC	T63.481	T63.482	T63.483	T63.484	—	—
lizard	T63.121	T63.122	T63.123	T63.124	—	—
marine						
animals	T63.691	T63.692	T63.693	T63.694	—	—
bluebottle	T63.611	T63.612	T63.613	T63.614	—	—
jellyfish NEC	T63.621	T63.622	T63.623	T63.624	—	—
Portugese Man-o-war	T63.611	T63.612	T63.613	T63.614	—	—
sea anemone	T63.631	T63.632	T63.633	T63.634	—	—
specified NEC	T63.691	T63.692	T63.693	T63.694	—	—
fish	T63.591	T63.592	T63.593	T63.594	—	—
plants	T63.711	T63.712	T63.713	T63.714	—	—
sting ray	T63.511	T63.512	T63.513	T63.514		

	External Cause (T-Code)					
Substance	Poisoning, Accidental (Unintentional)	Poisoning, Intentional Self-Harm	Poisoning, Assault	Poisoning, Undetermined	Adverse Effect	Underdosing
Venom, venomous *(Continued)*						
millipede (tropical)	T63.411	T63.412	T63.413	T63.414	—	—
plant NEC	T63.791	T63.792	T63.793	T63.794	—	—
marine	T63.711	T63.712	T63.713	T63.714	—	—
reptile	T63.191	T63.192	T63.193	T63.194	—	—
gila monster	T63.111	T63.112	T63.113	T63.114	—	—
lizard NEC	T63.121	T63.122	T63.123	T63.124	—	—
scorpion	T63.2X1	T63.2X2	T63.2X3	T63.2X4	—	—
snake	T63.001	T63.002	T63.003	T63.004	—	—
African NEC	T63.081	T63.082	T63.083	T63.084	—	—
American (North) (South) NEC	T63.061	T63.062	T63.063	T63.064	—	—
Asian	T63.081	T63.082	T63.083	T63.084	—	—
Australian	T63.071	T63.072	T63.073	T63.074	—	—
cobra	T63.041	T63.042	T63.043	T63.044	—	—
coral snake	T63.021	T63.022	T63.023	T63.024	—	—
rattlesnake	T63.011	T63.012	T63.013	T63.014	—	—
specified NEC	T63.091	T63.092	T63.093	T63.094	—	—
taipan	T63.031	T63.032	T63.033	T63.034	—	—
specified NEC	T63.891	T63.892	T63.893	T63.894	—	—
spider	T63.301	T63.302	T63.303	T63.304	—	—
black widow	T63.311	T63.312	T63.313	T63.314	—	—
brown recluse	T63.331	T63.332	T63.333	T63.334	—	—
specified NEC	T63.391	T63.392	T63.393	T63.394	—	—
tarantula	T63.321	T63.322	T63.323	T63.324	—	—
sting ray	T63.511	T63.512	T63.513	T63.514	—	—
toad	T63.821	T63.822	T63.823	T63.824	—	—
wasp	T63.461	T63.462	T63.463	T63.464	—	—
Venous sclerosing drug NEC	T46.8X1	T46.8X2	T46.8X3	T46.8X4	T46.8X5	T46.8X6
Ventolin — *see Albuterol*						
Verapamil	T46.1X1	T46.1X2	T46.1X3	T46.1X4	T46.1X5	T46.1X6
Veramon	T42.3X1	T42.3X2	T42.3X3	T42.3X4	T42.3X5	T42.3X6
Veratrine	T46.5X1	T46.5X2	T46.5X3	T46.5X4	T46.5X5	T46.5X6
Veratrum						
album	T62.2X1	T62.2X2	T62.2X3	T62.2X4	—	—
alkaloids	T46.5X1	T46.5X2	T46.5X3	T46.5X4	T46.5X5	T46.5X6
viride	T62.2X1	T62.2X2	T62.2X3	T62.2X4	—	—
Verdigris	T60.3X1	T60.3X2	T60.3X3	T60.3X4	—	—
Veronal	T42.3X1	T42.3X2	T42.3X3	T42.3X4	T42.3X5	T42.3X6
Veroxil	T37.4X1	T37.4X2	T37.4X3	T37.4X4	T37.4X5	T37.4X6
Versenate	T50.6X1	T50.6X2	T50.6X3	T50.6X4	T50.6X5	T50.6X6

◀ New ◀▥ Revised ~~deleted~~ Deleted

Substance	Poisoning, Accidental (Unintentional)	Poisoning, Intentional Self-Harm	Poisoning, Assault	Poisoning, Undetermined	Adverse Effect	Underdosing
Versidyne	T39.8X1	T39.8X2	T39.8X3	T39.8X4	T39.8X5	T39.8X6
Vetrabutine	T48.0X1	T48.0X2	T48.0X3	T48.0X4	T48.0X5	T48.0X6
Vidarabine	T37.5X1	T37.5X2	T37.5X3	T37.5X4	T37.5X5	T37.5X6
Vienna						
green	T57.0X1	T57.0X2	T57.0X3	T57.0X4	—	—
insecticide	T60.2X1	T60.2X2	T60.2X3	T60.2X4	—	—
red	T57.0X1	T57.0X2	T57.0X3	T57.0X4	—	—
pharmaceutical dye	T50.991	T50.992	T50.993	T50.994	T50.995	T50.996
Vigabatrin	T42.6X1	T42.6X2	T42.6X3	T42.6X4	T42.6X5	T42.6X6
Viloxazine	T43.291	T43.292	T43.293	T43.294	T43.295	T43.296
Viminol	T39.8X1	T39.8X2	T39.8X3	T39.8X4	T39.8X5	T39.8X6
Vinbarbital, vinbarbitone	T42.3X1	T42.3X2	T42.3X3	T42.3X4	T42.3X5	T42.3X6
Vinblastine	T45.1X1	T45.1X2	T45.1X3	T45.1X4	T45.1X5	T45.1X6
Vinburnine	T46.7X1	T46.7X2	T46.7X3	T46.7X4	T46.7X5	T46.7X6
Vincamine	T45.1X1	T45.1X2	T45.1X3	T45.1X4	T45.1X5	T45.1X6
Vincristine	T45.1X1	T45.1X2	T45.1X3	T45.1X4	T45.1X5	T45.1X6
Vindesine	T45.1X1	T45.1X2	T45.1X3	T45.1X4	T45.1X5	T45.1X6
Vinesthene, vinethene	T41.0X1	T41.0X2	T41.0X3	T41.0X4	T41.0X5	T41.0X6
Vinorelbine tartrate	T45.1X1	T45.1X2	T45.1X3	T45.1X4	T45.1X5	T45.1X6
Vinpocetine	T46.7X1	T46.7X2	T46.7X3	T46.7X4	T46.7X5	T46.7X6
Vinyl						
acetate	T65.891	T65.892	T65.893	T65.894	—	—
bital	T42.3X1	T42.3X2	T42.3X3	T42.3X4	T42.3X5	T42.3X6
bromide	T65.891	T65.892	T65.893	T65.894	—	—
chloride	T59.891	T59.892	T59.893	T59.894	—	—
ether	T41.0X1	T41.0X2	T41.0X3	T41.0X4	T41.0X5	T41.0X6
Vinylbital	T42.3X1	T42.3X2	T42.3X3	T42.3X4	T42.3X5	T42.3X6
Vinylidene chloride	T65.891	T65.892	T65.893	T65.894		
Vioform	T37.8X1	T37.8X2	T37.8X3	T37.8X4	T37.8X5	T37.8X6
topical	T49.0X1	T49.0X2	T49.0X3	T49.0X4	T49.0X5	T49.0X6
Viomycin	T36.8X1	T36.8X2	T36.8X3	T36.8X4	T36.8X5	T36.8X6
Viosterol	T45.2X1	T45.2X2	T45.2X3	T45.2X4	T45.2X5	T45.2X6
Viper (venom)	T63.091	T63.092	T63.093	T63.094	—	—
Viprynium	T37.4X1	T37.4X2	T37.4X3	T37.4X4	T37.4X5	T37.4X6
Viquidil	T46.7X1	T46.7X2	T46.7X3	T46.7X4	T46.7X5	T46.7X6
Viral vaccine NEC	T50.B91	T50.B92	T50.B93	T50.B94	T50.B95	T50.B96
Virginiamycin	T36.8X1	T36.8X2	T36.8X3	T36.8X4	T36.8X5	T36.8X6
Virugon	T37.5X1	T37.5X2	T37.5X3	T37.5X4	T37.5X5	T37.5X6
Viscous agent	T50.901	T50.902	T50.903	T50.904	T50.905	T50.906
Visine	T49.5X1	T49.5X2	T49.5X3	T49.5X4	T49.5X5	T49.5X6
Visnadine	T46.3X1	T46.3X2	T46.3X3	T46.3X4	T46.3X5	T46.3X6

Substance	Poisoning, Accidental (Unintentional)	Poisoning, Intentional Self-Harm	Poisoning, Assault	Poisoning, Undetermined	Adverse Effect	Underdosing
Vitamin NEC	T45.2X1	T45.2X2	T45.2X3	T45.2X4	T45.2X5	T45.2X6
A	T45.2X1	T45.2X2	T45.2X3	T45.2X4	T45.2X5	T45.2X6
B NEC	T45.2X1	T45.2X2	T45.2X3	T45.2X4	T45.2X5	T45.2X6
nicotinic acid	T46.7X1	T46.7X2	T46.7X3	T46.7X4	T46.7X5	T46.7X6
B1	T45.2X1	T45.2X2	T45.2X3	T45.2X4	T45.2X5	T45.2X6
B2	T45.2X1	T45.2X2	T45.2X3	T45.2X4	T45.2X5	T45.2X6
B6	T45.2X1	T45.2X2	T45.2X3	T45.2X4	T45.2X5	T45.2X6
B12	T45.2X1	T45.2X2	T45.2X3	T45.2X4	T45.2X5	T45.2X6
B15	T45.2X1	T45.2X2	T45.2X3	T45.2X4	T45.2X5	T45.2X6
C	T45.2X1	T45.2X2	T45.2X3	T45.2X4	T45.2X5	T45.2X6
D	T45.2X1	T45.2X2	T45.2X3	T45.2X4	T45.2X5	T45.2X6
D2	T45.2X1	T45.2X2	T45.2X3	T45.2X4	T45.2X5	T45.2X6
D3	T45.2X1	T45.2X2	T45.2X3	T45.2X4	T45.2X5	T45.2X6
E	T45.2X1	T45.2X2	T45.2X3	T45.2X4	T45.2X5	T45.2X6
E acetate	T45.2X1	T45.2X2	T45.2X3	T45.2X4	T45.2X5	T45.2X6
hematopoietic	T45.8X1	T45.8X2	T45.8X3	T45.8X4	T45.8X5	T45.8X6
K NEC	T45.7X1	T45.7X2	T45.7X3	T45.7X4	T45.7X5	T45.7X6
K1	T45.7X1	T45.7X2	T45.7X3	T45.7X4	T45.7X5	T45.7X6
K2	T45.7X1	T45.7X2	T45.7X3	T45.7X4	T45.7X5	T45.7X6
PP	T45.2X1	T45.2X2	T45.2X3	T45.2X4	T45.2X5	T45.2X6
ulceroprotectant	T47.1X1	T47.1X2	T47.1X3	T47.1X4	T47.1X5	T47.1X6
Vleminckx's solution	T49.4X1	T49.4X2	T49.4X3	T49.4X4	T49.4X5	T49.4X6
Voltaren — see Diclofenac sodium						
W						
Warfarin	T45.511	T45.512	T45.513	T45.514	T45.515	T45.516
rodenticide	T60.4X1	T60.4X2	T60.4X3	T60.4X4	—	—
sodium	T60.4X1	T60.4X2	T60.4X3	T60.4X4	—	—
Wasp (sting)	T63.461	T63.462	T63.463	T63.464	—	—
Water						
balance drug	T50.3X1	T50.3X2	T50.3X3	T50.3X4	T50.3X5	T50.3X6
distilled	T50.3X1	T50.3X2	T50.3X3	T50.3X4	T50.3X5	T50.3X6
gas — see Gas, water						
incomplete combustion of — see Carbon, monoxide, fuel, utility						
hemlock	T62.2X1	T62.2X2	T62.2X3	T62.2X4	—	—
moccasin (venom)	T63.061	T63.062	T63.063	T63.064	—	—
purified	T50.3X1	T50.3X2	T50.3X3	T50.3X4	T50.3X5	T50.3X6
Wax (paraffin) (petroleum)	T52.0X1	T52.0X2	T52.0X3	T52.0X4	—	—
automobile	T65.891	T65.892	T65.893	T65.894	—	—
floor	T52.0X1	T52.0X2	T52.0X3	T52.0X4	—	—

TABLE OF DRUGS AND CHEMICALS

◀ New ◀▥ Revised ~~deleted~~ Deleted

TABLE OF DRUGS AND CHEMICALS

Substance	Poisoning, Accidental (Unintentional)	Poisoning, Intentional Self-Harm	Poisoning, Assault	Poisoning, Undetermined	Adverse Effect	Underdosing
	External Cause (T-Code)					
Weed killers NEC	T60.3X1	T60.3X2	T60.3X3	T60.3X4	—	—
Welldorm	T42.6X1	T42.6X2	T42.6X3	T42.6X4	T42.6X5	T42.6X6
White						
arsenic	T57.0X1	T57.0X2	T57.0X3	T57.0X4	—	—
hellebore	T62.2X1	T62.2X2	T62.2X3	T62.2X4	—	—
lotion (keratolytic)	T49.4X1	T49.4X2	T49.4X3	T49.4X4	T49.4X5	T49.4X6
spirit	T52.0X1	T52.0X2	T52.0X3	T52.0X4	—	—
Whitewash	T65.891	T65.892	T65.893	T65.894		
Whole blood (human)	T45.8X1	T45.8X2	T45.8X3	T45.8X4	T45.8X5	T45.8X6
Wild						
black cherry	T62.2X1	T62.2X2	T62.2X3	T62.2X4	—	—
poisonous plants NEC	T62.2X1	T62.2X2	T62.2X3	T62.2X4	—	—
Window cleaning fluid	T65.891	T65.892	T65.893	T65.894		
Wintergreen (oil)	T49.3X1	T49.3X2	T49.3X3	T49.3X4	T49.3X5	T49.3X6
Wisterine	T62.2X1	T62.2X2	T62.2X3	T62.2X4	—	—
Witch hazel	T49.2X1	T49.2X2	T49.2X3	T49.2X4	T49.2X5	T49.2X6
Wood alcohol or spirit	T51.1X1	T51.1X2	T51.1X3	T51.1X4	—	—
Wool fat (hydrous)	T49.3X1	T49.3X2	T49.3X3	T49.3X4	T49.3X5	T49.3X6
Woorali	T48.1X1	T48.1X2	T48.1X3	T48.1X4	T48.1X5	T48.1X6
Wormseed, American	T37.4X1	T37.4X2	T37.4X3	T37.4X4	T37.4X5	T37.4X6
X						
Xamoterol	T44.5X1	T44.5X2	T44.5X3	T44.5X4	T44.5X5	T44.5X6
Xanthine diuretics	T50.2X1	T50.2X2	T50.2X3	T50.2X4	T50.2X5	T50.2X6
Xanthinol nicotinate	T46.7X1	T46.7X2	T46.7X3	T46.7X4	T46.7X5	T46.7X6
Xanthotoxin	T49.3X1	T49.3X2	T49.3X3	T49.3X4	T49.3X5	T49.3X6
Xantinol nicotinate	T46.7X1	T46.7X2	T46.7X3	T46.7X4	T46.7X5	T46.7X6
Xantocillin	T36.0X1	T36.0X2	T36.0X3	T36.0X4	T36.0X5	T36.0X6
Xenon (127Xe) (133Xe)	T50.8X1	T50.8X2	T50.8X3	T50.8X4	T50.8X5	T50.8X6
Xenysalate	T49.4X1	T49.4X2	T49.4X3	T49.4X4	T49.4X5	T49.4X6
Xibornol	T37.8X1	T37.8X2	T37.8X3	T37.8X4	T37.8X5	T37.8X6
Xigris	T45.511	T45.512	T45.513	T45.514	T45.515	T45.516
Xipamide	T50.2X1	T50.2X2	T50.2X3	T50.2X4	T50.2X5	T50.2X6
Xylene (vapor)	T52.2X1	T52.2X2	T52.2X3	T52.2X4	—	—
Xylocaine (infiltration) (topical)	T41.3X1	T41.3X2	T41.3X3	T41.3X4	T41.3X5	T41.3X6
nerve block (peripheral) (plexus)	T41.3X1	T41.3X2	T41.3X3	T41.3X4	T41.3X5	T41.3X6
spinal	T41.3X1	T41.3X2	T41.3X3	T41.3X4	T41.3X5	T41.3X6
Xylol (vapor)	T52.2X1	T52.2X2	T52.2X3	T52.2X4	—	—
Xylometazoline	T48.5X1	T48.5X2	T48.5X3	T48.5X4	T48.5X5	T48.5X6

Substance	Poisoning, Accidental (Unintentional)	Poisoning, Intentional Self-Harm	Poisoning, Assault	Poisoning, Undetermined	Adverse Effect	Underdosing
	External Cause (T-Code)					
Y						
Yeast	T45.2X1	T45.2X2	T45.2X3	T45.2X4	T45.2X5	T45.2X6
dried	T45.2X1	T45.2X2	T45.2X3	T45.2X4	T45.2X5	T45.2X6
Yellow						
fever vaccine	T50.B91	T50.B92	T50.B93	T50.B94	T50.B95	T50.B96
jasmine	T62.2X1	T62.2X2	T62.2X3	T62.2X4	—	—
phenolphthalein	T47.2X1	T47.2X2	T47.2X3	T47.2X4	T47.2X5	T47.2X6
Yew	T62.2X1	T62.2X2	T62.2X3	T62.2X4	—	—
Yohimbic acid	T40.991	T40.992	T40.993	T40.994	T40.995	T40.996
Z						
Zactane	T39.8X1	T39.8X2	T39.8X3	T39.8X4	T39.8X5	T39.8X6
Zalcitabine	T37.5X1	T37.5X2	T37.5X3	T37.5X4	T37.5X5	T37.5X6
Zaroxolyn	T50.2X1	T50.2X2	T50.2X3	T50.2X4	T50.2X5	T50.2X6
Zephiran (topical)	T49.0X1	T49.0X2	T49.0X3	T49.0X4	T49.0X5	T49.0X6
ophthalmic preparation	T49.5X1	T49.5X2	T49.5X3	T49.5X4	T49.5X5	T49.5X6
Zeranol	T38.7X1	T38.7X2	T38.7X3	T38.7X4	T38.7X5	T38.7X6
Zerone	T51.1X1	T51.1X2	T51.1X3	T51.1X4	—	—
Zidovudine	T37.5X1	T37.5X2	T37.5X3	T37.5X4	T37.5X5	T37.5X6
Zimeldine	T43.221	T43.222	T43.223	T43.224	T43.225	T43.226
Zinc (compounds) (fumes) (vapor) NEC	T56.5X1	T56.5X2	T56.5X3	T56.5X4	—	—
anti-infectives	T49.0X1	T49.0X2	T49.0X3	T49.0X4	T49.0X5	T49.0X6
antivaricose	T46.8X1	T46.8X2	T46.8X3	T46.8X4	T46.8X5	T46.8X6
bacitracin	T49.0X1	T49.0X2	T49.0X3	T49.0X4	T49.0X5	T49.0X6
chloride (mouthwash)	T49.6X1	T49.6X2	T49.6X3	T49.6X4	T49.6X5	T49.6X6
chromate	T56.5X1	T56.5X2	T56.5X3	T56.5X4	—	—
gelatin	T49.3X1	T49.3X2	T49.3X3	T49.3X4	T49.3X5	T49.3X6
oxide	T49.3X1	T49.3X2	T49.3X3	T49.3X4	T49.3X5	T49.3X6
plaster	T49.3X1	T49.3X2	T49.3X3	T49.3X4	T49.3X5	T49.3X6
peroxide	T49.0X1	T49.0X2	T49.0X3	T49.0X4	T49.0X5	T49.0X6
pesticides	T56.5X1	T56.5X2	T56.5X3	T56.5X4	—	—
phosphide	T60.4X1	T60.4X2	T60.4X3	T60.4X4	—	—
pyrithionate	T49.4X1	T49.4X2	T49.4X3	T49.4X4	T49.4X5	T49.4X6
stearate	T49.3X1	T49.3X2	T49.3X3	T49.3X4	T49.3X5	T49.3X6
sulfate	T49.5X1	T49.5X2	T49.5X3	T49.5X4	T49.5X5	T49.5X6
ENT agent	T49.6X1	T49.6X2	T49.6X3	T49.6X4	T49.6X5	T49.6X6
ophthalmic solution	T49.5X1	T49.5X2	T49.5X3	T49.5X4	T49.5X5	T49.5X6
topical NEC	T49.0X1	T49.0X2	T49.0X3	T49.0X4	T49.0X5	T49.0X6
undecylenate	T49.0X1	T49.0X2	T49.0X3	T49.0X4	T49.0X5	T49.0X6

◀ New   ◀ Revised   ~~deleted~~ Deleted

Substance	Poisoning, Accidental (Unintentional)	Poisoning, Intentional Self-Harm	Poisoning, Assault	Poisoning, Undetermined	Adverse Effect	Underdosing
Zineb	T60.0X1	T60.0X2	T60.0X3	T60.0X4	—	—
Zinostatin	T45.1X1	T45.1X2	T45.1X3	T45.1X4	T45.1X5	T45.1X6
Zipeprol	T48.3X1	T48.3X2	T48.3X3	T48.3X4	T48.3X5	T48.3X6
Zofenopril	T46.4X1	T46.4X2	T46.4X3	T46.4X4	T46.4X5	T46.4X6
Zolpidem	T42.6X1	T42.6X2	T42.6X3	T42.6X4	T42.6X5	T42.6X6
Zomepirac	T39.391	T39.392	T39.393	T39.394	T39.395	T39.396
Zopiclone	T42.6X1	T42.6X2	T42.6X3	T42.6X4	T42.6X5	T42.6X6

Substance	Poisoning, Accidental (Unintentional)	Poisoning, Intentional Self-Harm	Poisoning, Assault	Poisoning, Undetermined	Adverse Effect	Underdosing
Zorubicin	T45.1X1	T45.1X2	T45.1X3	T45.1X4	T45.1X5	T45.1X6
Zotepine	T43.591	T43.592	T43.593	T43.594	T43.595	T43.596
Zovant	T45.511	T45.512	T45.513	T45.514	T45.515	T45.516
Zoxazolamine	T42.8X1	T42.8X2	T42.8X3	T42.8X4	T42.8X5	T42.8X6
Zuclopenthixol	T43.4X1	T43.4X2	T43.4X3	T43.4X4	T43.4X5	T43.4X6
Zygadenus (venenosus)	T62.2X1	T62.2X2	T62.2X3	T62.2X4	—	—
Zyprexa	T43.591	T43.592	T43.593	T43.594	T43.595	T43.596

TABLE OF DRUGS AND CHEMICALS

External Cause
of Injuries Index

A

Abandonment (causing exposure to weather conditions) (with intent to injure or kill) NEC X58

Abuse (adult) (child) (mental) (physical) (sexual) X58

Accident (to) X58

aircraft (in transit) (powered) —*see also* Accident, transport, aircraft

  due to, caused by cataclysm —*see* Forces of nature, by type

animal-drawn vehicle —*see* Accident, transport, animal-drawn vehicle occupant

animal-rider —*see* Accident, transport, animal-rider

automobile —*see* Accident, transport, car occupant

bare foot water skiier V94.4

boat, boating —*see also* Accident, watercraft

  striking swimmer

    powered V94.11

    unpowered V94.12

bus —*see* Accident, transport, bus occupant

cable car, not on rails V98.0

  on rails —*see* Accident, transport, streetcar occupant

car —*see* Accident, transport, car occupant

caused by, due to

  animal NEC W64

  chain hoist W24.0

  cold (excessive) —*see* Exposure, cold

  corrosive liquid, substance —*see* Table of Drugs and Chemicals ◄▥

  cutting or piercing instrument —*see* Contact, with, by type of instrument

  drive belt W24.0

  electric

    current —*see* Exposure, electric current

    motor —*see also* Contact, with, by type of machine W31.3

      current (of) W86.8

  environmental factor NEC X58

  explosive material —*see* Explosion

  fire, flames —*see* Exposure, fire

  firearm missile —*see* Discharge, firearm by type

  heat (excessive) —*see* Heat

  hot —*see* Contact, with, hot

  ignition —*see* Ignition

  lifting device W24.0

  lightning —*see* subcategory T75.0

    causing fire —*see* Exposure, fire

  machine, machinery —*see* Contact, with, by type of machine

  natural factor NEC X58

  pulley (block) W24.0

  radiation —*see* Radiation

  steam X13.1

    inhalation X13.0

    pipe X16

  thunderbolt —*see* subcategory T75.0

    causing fire —*see* Exposure, fire

  transmission device W24.1

coach —*see* Accident, transport, bus occupant

coal car —*see* Accident, transport, industrial vehicle occupant

diving —*see also* Fall, into, water

  with

    drowning or submersion —*see* Drowning

forklift —*see* Accident, transport, industrial vehicle occupant

heavy transport vehicle NOS —*see* Accident, transport, truck occupant

ice yacht V98.2

Accident (*Continued*)

in

  medical, surgical procedure

    as, or due to misadventure —*see* Misadventure

    causing an abnormal reaction or later complication without mention of misadventure —*see also* Complication of or following, by type of procedure Y84.9

land yacht V98.1

late effect of —*see* W00-X58 with 7th character S

logging car —*see* Accident, transport, industrial vehicle occupant

machine, machinery —*see also* Contact, with, by type of machine

  on board watercraft V93.69

    explosion —*see* Explosion, in, watercraft

    fire —*see* Burn, on board watercraft

    powered craft V93.63

      ferry boat V93.61

      fishing boat V93.62

      jetskis V93.63

      liner V93.61

      merchant ship V93.60

      passenger ship V93.61

      sailboat V93.64

mine tram —*see* Accident, transport, industrial vehicle occupant

mobility scooter (motorized) —*see* Accident, transport, pedestrian, conveyance, specified type NEC

motor scooter —*see* Accident, transport, motorcyclist

motor vehicle NOS (traffic) —*see also* Accident, transport V89.2

  nontraffic V89.0

  three-wheeled NOS —*see* Accident, transport, three-wheeled motor vehicle occupant

motorcycle NOS —*see* Accident, transport, motorcyclist

nonmotor vehicle NOS (nontraffic) —*see also* Accident, transport V89.1

  traffic NOS V89.3

nontraffic (victim's mode of transport NOS) V88.9

  collision (between) V88.7

    bus and truck V88.5

    car and:

      bus V88.3

      pickup V88.2

      three-wheeled motor vehicle V88.0

      train V88.6

      truck V88.4

      two-wheeled motor vehicle V88.0

      van V88.2

    specified vehicle NEC and:

      three-wheeled motor vehicle V88.1

      two-wheeled motor vehicle V88.1

  known mode of transport —*see* Accident, transport, by type of vehicle

  noncollision V88.8

on board watercraft V93.89

  powered craft V93.83

    ferry boat V93.81

    fishing boat V93.82

    jetskis V93.83

    liner V93.81

    merchant ship V93.80

    passenger ship V93.81

  unpowered craft V93.88

    canoe V93.85

    inflatable V93.86

      in tow

        recreational V94.31

        specified NEC V94.32

    kayak V93.85

Accident (*Continued*)

on board watercraft (*Continued*)

  unpowered craft (*Continued*)

    sailboat V93.84

    surf-board V93.88

    water skis V93.87

    windsurfer V93.88

parachutist V97.29

  entangled in object V97.21

  injured on landing V97.22

pedal cycle —*see* Accident, transport, pedal cyclist

pedestrian (on foot)

  with

    another pedestrian W51

      with fall W03

        due to ice or snow W00.0

      on pedestrian conveyance NEC V00.09

    roller skater (in-line) V00.01

    skate boarder V00.02

    transport vehicle —*see* Accident, transport

  on pedestrian conveyance —*see* Accident, transport, pedestrian, conveyance

pick-up truck or van —*see* Accident, transport, pickup truck occupant

quarry truck —*see* Accident, transport, industrial vehicle occupant

railway vehicle (any) (in motion) —*see* Accident, transport, railway vehicle occupant

  due to cataclysm —*see* Forces of nature, by type

scooter (non-motorized) —*see* Accident, transport, pedestrian, conveyance, scooter

sequelae of —*see* W00-X58 with 7th character S

skateboard —*see* Accident, transport, pedestrian, conveyance, skateboard

ski (ing) —*see* Accident, transport, pedestrian, conveyance

  lift V98.3

specified cause NEC X58

streetcar —*see* Accident, transport, streetcar occupant

traffic (victim's mode of transport NOS) V87.9

  collision (between) V87.7

    bus and truck V87.5

    car and:

      bus V87.3

      pickup V87.2

      three-wheeled motor vehicle V87.0

      train V87.6

      truck V87.4

      two-wheeled motor vehicle V87.0

      van V87.2

    specified vehicle NEC and:

      three-wheeled motor vehicle V87.1

      two-wheeled motor vehicle V87.1

  known mode of transport —*see* Accident, transport, by type of vehicle

  noncollision V87.8

transport (involving injury to) V99

  18 wheeler —*see* Accident, transport, truck occupant

  agricultural vehicle occupant (nontraffic) V84.9

    driver V84.5

    hanger-on V84.7

    passenger V84.6

    traffic V84.3

      driver V84.0

      hanger-on V84.2

      passenger V84.1

    while boarding or alighting V84.4

Accident (Continued)
  transport (Continued)
    aircraft NEC V97.89
      military NEC V97.818
        with civilian aircraft V97.810
        civilian injured by V97.811
      occupant injured (in)
        nonpowered craft accident
          V96.9
          balloon V96.00
            collision V96.03
            crash V96.01
            explosion V96.05
            fire V96.04
            forced landing V96.02
            specified type NEC V96.09
          glider V96.20
            collision V96.23
            crash V96.21
            explosion V96.25
            fire V96.24
            forced landing V96.22
            specified type NEC V96.29
          hang glider V96.10
            collision V96.13
            crash V96.11
            explosion V96.15
            fire V96.14
            forced landing V96.12
            specified type NEC V96.19
          specified craft NEC V96.8
        powered craft accident V95.9
          fixed wing NEC
            commercial V95.30
              collision V95.33
              crash V95.31
              explosion V95.35
              fire V95.34
              forced landing V95.32
              specified type NEC
                V95.39
            private V95.20
              collision V95.23
              crash V95.21
              explosion V95.25
              fire V95.24
              forced landing V95.22
              specified type NEC
                V95.29
          glider V95.10
            collision V95.13
            crash V95.11
            explosion V95.15
            fire V95.14
            forced landing V95.12
            specified type NEC V95.19
          helicopter V95.00
            collision V95.03
            crash V95.01
            explosion V95.05
            fire V95.04
            forced landing V95.02
            specified type NEC V95.09
          spacecraft V95.40
            collision V95.43
            crash V95.41
            explosion V95.45
            fire V95.44
            forced landing V95.42
            specified type NEC V95.49
          specified craft NEC V95.8
          ultralight V95.10
            collision V95.13
            crash V95.11
            explosion V95.15
            fire V95.14
            forced landing V95.12
            specified type NEC V95.19
        specified accident NEC V97.0
        while boarding or alighting
          V97.1

Accident (Continued)
  transport (Continued)
    aircraft NEC (Continued)
      person (injured by)
        falling from, in or on aircraft V97.0
        machinery on aircraft V97.89
        on ground with aircraft involvement
          V97.39
        rotating propeller V97.32
        struck by object falling from aircraft
          V97.31
        sucked into aircraft jet V97.33
        while boarding or alighting aircraft
          V97.1
    airport (battery-powered) passenger
      vehicle —see Accident, transport,
      industrial vehicle occupant
    all-terrain vehicle occupant (nontraffic)
      V86.99
      driver V86.59
      dune buggy —see Accident, transport,
        dune buggy occupant
      hanger-on V86.79
      passenger V86.69
      snowmobile —see Accident, transport,
        snowmobile occupant
      traffic V86.39
        driver V86.09
        hanger-on V86.29
        passenger V86.19
      while boarding or alighting V86.49
    ambulance occupant (traffic) V86.31
      driver V86.01
      hanger-on V86.21
      nontraffic V86.91
        driver V86.51
        hanger-on V86.71
        passenger V86.61
      passenger V86.11
      while boarding or alighting V86.41
    animal-drawn vehicle occupant (in)
      V80.929
      collision (with)
        animal V80.12
          being ridden V80.711
        animal-drawn vehicle V80.721
        bus V80.42
        car V80.42
        fixed or stationary object V80.82
        military vehicle V80.920
        nonmotor vehicle V80.791
        pedal cycle V80.22
        pedestrian V80.12
        pickup V80.42
        railway train or vehicle V80.62
        specified motor vehicle NEC V80.52
        streetcar V80.731
        truck V80.42
        two-or three-wheeled motor vehicle
          V80.32
        van V80.42
      noncollision V80.02
      specified circumstance NEC V80. 928
    animal-rider V80.919
      collision (with)
        animal V80.11
          being ridden V80.710
        animal-drawn vehicle V80.720
        bus V80.41
        car V80.41
        fixed or stationary object V80.81
        military vehicle V80.910
        nonmotor vehicle V80.790
        pedal cycle V80.21
        pedestrian V80.11
        pickup V80.41
        railway train or vehicle V80.61
        specified motor vehicle NEC
          V80.51
        streetcar V80.730
        truck V80.41

Accident (Continued)
  transport (Continued)
    animal-rider (Continued)
      collision (Continued)
        two- or three-wheeled motor vehicle
          V80.31
        van V80.41
      noncollision V80.018
        specified as horse rider V80.010
      specified circumstance NEC V80.918
    armored car —see Accident, transport,
      truck occupant
    battery-powered truck (baggage) (mail) —
      see Accident, transport, industrial
      vehicle occupant
    bus occupant V79.9
      collision (with)
        animal (traffic) V70.9
          being ridden (traffic) V76.9
            nontraffic V76.3
            while boarding or alighting V76.4
          nontraffic V70.3
          while boarding or alighting V70.4
        animal-drawn vehicle (traffic) V76.9
          nontraffic V76.3
          while boarding or alighting V76.4
        bus (traffic) V74.9
          nontraffic V74.3
          while boarding or alighting V74.4
        car (traffic) V73.9
          nontraffic V73.3
          while boarding or alighting V73.4
        motor vehicle NOS (traffic) V79.60
          nontraffic V79.20
          specified type NEC (traffic) V79.69
            nontraffic V79.29
        pedal cycle (traffic) V71.9
          nontraffic V71.3
          while boarding or alighting V71.4
        pickup truck (traffic) V73.9
          nontraffic V73.3
          while boarding or alighting V73.4
        railway vehicle (traffic) V75.9
          nontraffic V75.3
          while boarding or alighting V75.4
        specified vehicle NEC (traffic) V76.9
          nontraffic V76.3
          while boarding or alighting V76.4
        stationary object (traffic) V77.9
          nontraffic V77.3
          while boarding or alighting V77.4
        streetcar (traffic) V76.9
          nontraffic V76.3
          while boarding or alighting V76.4
        three wheeled motor vehicle (traffic)
          V72.9
          nontraffic V72.3
          while boarding or alighting V72.4
        truck (traffic) V74.9
          nontraffic V74.3
          while boarding or alighting V74.4
        two wheeled motor vehicle (traffic)
          V72.9
          nontraffic V72.3
          while boarding or alighting V72.4
        van (traffic) V73.9
          nontraffic V73.3
          while boarding or alighting V73.4
      driver
        collision (with)
          animal (traffic) V70.5
            being ridden (traffic) V76.5
              nontraffic V76.0
            nontraffic V70.0
          animal-drawn vehicle (traffic)
            V76.5
            nontraffic V76.0
          bus (traffic) V74.5
            nontraffic V74.0
          car (traffic) V73.5
            nontraffic V73.0

Accident *(Continued)*
 transport *(Continued)*
  bus occupant *(Continued)*
   driver *(Continued)*
    collision *(Continued)*
     motor vehicle NOS (traffic) V79.40
      nontraffic V79.00
      specified type NEC (traffic)
       V79.49
       nontraffic V79.09
     pedal cycle (traffic) V71.5
      nontraffic V71.0
     pickup truck (traffic) V73.5
      nontraffic V73.0
     railway vehicle (traffic) V75.5
      nontraffic V75.0
     specified vehicle NEC (traffic)
      V76.5
      nontraffic V76.0
     stationary object (traffic) V77.5
      nontraffic V77.0
     streetcar (traffic) V76.5
      nontraffic V76.0
     three wheeled motor vehicle
      (traffic) V72.5
      nontraffic V72.0
     truck (traffic) V74.5
      nontraffic V74.0
     two wheeled motor vehicle (traffic)
      V72.5
      nontraffic V72.0
     van (traffic) V73.5
      nontraffic V73.0
    noncollision accident (traffic) V78.5
     nontraffic V78.0
   hanger-on
    collision (with)
     animal (traffic) V70.7
      being ridden (traffic) V76.7
       nontraffic V76.2
      nontraffic V70.2
     animal-drawn vehicle (traffic) V76.7
      nontraffic V76.2
     bus (traffic) V74.7
      nontraffic V74.2
     car (traffic) V73.7
      nontraffic V73.2
     pedal cycle (traffic) V71.7
      nontraffic V71.2
     pickup truck (traffic) V73.7
      nontraffic V73.2
     railway vehicle (traffic) V75.7
      nontraffic V75.2
     specified vehicle NEC (traffic) V76.7
      nontraffic V76.2
     stationary object (traffic) V77.7
      nontraffic V77.2
     streetcar (traffic) V76.7
      nontraffic V76.2
     three wheeled motor vehicle
      (traffic) V72.7
      nontraffic V72.2
     truck (traffic) V74.7
      nontraffic V74.2
     two wheeled motor vehicle (traffic)
      V72.7
      nontraffic V72.2
     van (traffic) V73.7
      nontraffic V73.2
    noncollision accident (traffic) V78.7
     nontraffic V78.2
   noncollision accident (traffic) V78.9
    nontraffic V78.3
    while boarding or alighting V78.4
   nontraffic V79.3
   passenger
    collision (with)
     animal (traffic) V70.6
      being ridden (traffic) V76.6
       nontraffic V76.1
      nontraffic V70.1

Accident *(Continued)*
 transport *(Continued)*
  bus occupant *(Continued)*
   passenger *(Continued)*
    collision *(Continued)*
     animal-drawn vehicle (traffic) V76.6
      nontraffic V76.1
     bus (traffic) V74.6
      nontraffic V74.1
     car (traffic) V73.6
      nontraffic V73.1
     motor vehicle NOS (traffic) V79.50
      nontraffic V79.10
      specified type NEC (traffic)
       V79.59
       nontraffic V79.19
     pedal cycle (traffic) V71.6
      nontraffic V71.1
     pickup truck (traffic) V73.6
      nontraffic V73.1
     railway vehicle (traffic) V75.6
      nontraffic V75.1
     specified vehicle NEC (traffic) V76.6
      nontraffic V76.1
     stationary object (traffic) V77.6
      nontraffic V77.1
     streetcar (traffic) V76.6
      nontraffic V76.1
     three wheeled motor vehicle
      (traffic) V72.6
      nontraffic V72.1
     truck (traffic) V74.6
      nontraffic V74.1
     two wheeled motor vehicle (traffic)
      V72.6
      nontraffic V72.1
     van (traffic) V73.6
      nontraffic V73.1
    noncollision accident (traffic) V78.6
     nontraffic V78.1
   specified type NEC V79.88
   military vehicle V79.81
  cable car, not on rails V98.0
   on rails —*see* Accident, transport,
    streetcar occupant
  car occupant V49.9
   ambulance occupant —*see* Accident,
    transport, ambulance occupant
   collision (with)
    animal (traffic) V40.9
     being ridden (traffic) V46.9
      nontraffic V46.3
      while boarding or alighting
       V46.4
     nontraffic V40.3
     while boarding or alighting V40.4
    animal-drawn vehicle (traffic) V46.9
     nontraffic V46.3
     while boarding or alighting V46.4
    bus (traffic) V44.9
     nontraffic V44.3
     while boarding or alighting V44.4
    car (traffic) V43.92
     nontraffic V43.32
     while boarding or alighting V43.42
    motor vehicle NOS (traffic) V49.60
     nontraffic V49.20
     specified type NEC (traffic) V49.69
      nontraffic V49.29
    pedal cycle (traffic) V41.9
     nontraffic V41.3
     while boarding or alighting V41.4
    pickup truck (traffic) V43.93
     nontraffic V43.33
     while boarding or alighting V43.43
    railway vehicle (traffic) V45.9
     nontraffic V45.3
     while boarding or alighting V45.4
    specified vehicle NEC (traffic) V46.9
     nontraffic V46.3
     while boarding or alighting V46.4

Accident *(Continued)*
 transport *(Continued)*
  car occupant *(Continued)*
   collision *(Continued)*
    sport utility vehicle (traffic) V43.91
     nontraffic V43.31
     while boarding or alighting V43.41
    stationary object (traffic) V47.92
     nontraffic V47.32
     while boarding or alighting V47.4
    streetcar (traffic) V46.9
     nontraffic V46.3
     while boarding or alighting V46.4
    three wheeled motor vehicle (traffic)
     V42.9
     nontraffic V42.3
     while boarding or alighting V42.4
    truck (traffic) V44.9
     nontraffic V44.3
     while boarding or alighting V44.4
    two wheeled motor vehicle (traffic)
     V42.9
     nontraffic V42.3
     while boarding or alighting V42.4
    van (traffic) V43.94
     nontraffic V43.34
     while boarding or alighting V43.44
   driver
    collision (with)
     animal (traffic) V40.5
      being ridden (traffic) V46.5
       nontraffic V46.0
      nontraffic V40.0
     animal-drawn vehicle (traffic) V46.5
      nontraffic V46.0
     bus (traffic) V44.5
      nontraffic V44.0
     car (traffic) V43.52
      nontraffic V43.02
     motor vehicle NOS (traffic) V49.40
      nontraffic V49.00
      specified type NEC (traffic)
       V49.49
       nontraffic V49.09
     pedal cycle (traffic) V41.5
      nontraffic V41.0
     pickup truck (traffic) V43.53
      nontraffic V43.03
     railway vehicle (traffic) V45.5
      nontraffic V45.0
     specified vehicle NEC (traffic) V46.5
      nontraffic V46.0
     sport utility vehicle (traffic) V43.51
      nontraffic V43.01
     stationary object (traffic) V47.52
      nontraffic V47.02
     streetcar (traffic) V46.5
      nontraffic V46.0
     three wheeled motor vehicle
      (traffic) V42.5
      nontraffic V42.0
     truck (traffic) V44.5
      nontraffic V44.0
     two wheeled motor vehicle (traffic)
      V42.5
      nontraffic V42.0
     van (traffic) V43.54
      nontraffic V43.04
    noncollision accident (traffic) V48.5
     nontraffic V48.0
   hanger-on
    collision (with)
     animal (traffic) V40.7
      being ridden (traffic) V46.7
       nontraffic V46.2
      nontraffic V40.2
     animal-drawn vehicle (traffic)
      V46.7
      nontraffic V46.2
     bus (traffic) V44.7
      nontraffic V44.2

◀ New ◀⦙⦙⦙ Revised ~~deleted~~ Deleted

Accident (Continued)
  transport (Continued)
    car occupant (Continued)
      hanger-on (Continued)
        collision (Continued)
          car (traffic) V43.72
            nontraffic V43.22
          pedal cycle (traffic) V41.7
            nontraffic V41.2
          pickup truck (traffic) V43.73
            nontraffic V43.23
          railway vehicle (traffic) V45.7
            nontraffic V45.2
          specified vehicle NEC (traffic) V46.7
            nontraffic V46.2
          sport utility vehicle (traffic) V43.71
            nontraffic V43.21
          stationary object (traffic) V47.7
            nontraffic V47.2
          streetcar (traffic) V46.7
            nontraffic V46.2
          three wheeled motor vehicle
              (traffic) V42.7
            nontraffic V42.2
          truck (traffic) V44.7
            nontraffic V44.2
          two wheeled motor vehicle (traffic)
              V42.7
            nontraffic V42.2
          van (traffic) V43.74
            nontraffic V43.24
        noncollision accident (traffic) V48.7
          nontraffic V48.2
      noncollision accident (traffic) V48.9
        nontraffic V48.3
        while boarding or alighting V48.4
      nontraffic V49.3
      passenger
        collision (with)
          animal (traffic) V40.6
            being ridden (traffic) V46.6
              nontraffic V46.1
            nontraffic V40.1
          animal-drawn vehicle (traffic) V46.6
            nontraffic V46.1
          bus (traffic) V44.6
            nontraffic V44.1
          car (traffic) V43.62
            nontraffic V43.12
          motor vehicle NOS (traffic) V49.50
            nontraffic V49.10
            specified type NEC (traffic) V49.59
              nontraffic V49.19
          pedal cycle (traffic) V41.6
            nontraffic V41.1
          pickup truck (traffic) V43.63
            nontraffic V43.13
          railway vehicle (traffic) V45.6
            nontraffic V45.1
          specified vehicle NEC (traffic) V46.6
            nontraffic V46.1
          sport utility vehicle (traffic) V43.61
            nontraffic V43.11
          stationary object (traffic) V47.62
            nontraffic V47.12
          streetcar (traffic) V46.6
            nontraffic V46.1
          three wheeled motor vehicle
              (traffic) V42.6
            nontraffic V42.1
          truck (traffic) V44.6
            nontraffic V44.1
          two wheeled motor vehicle (traffic)
              V42.6
            nontraffic V42.1
          van (traffic) V43.64
            nontraffic V43.14
        noncollision accident (traffic) V48.6
          nontraffic V48.1
      specified type NEC V49.88
        military vehicle V49.81

Accident (Continued)
  transport (Continued)
    coal car —see Accident, transport,
        industrial vehicle occupant
    construction vehicle occupant (nontraffic)
        V85.9
      driver V85.5
      hanger-on V85.7
      passenger V85.6
      traffic V85.3
        driver V85.0
        hanger-on V85.2
        passenger V85.1
      while boarding or alighting V85.4
    dirt bike rider —see Accident, transport,
        all-terrain vehicle occupant
    due to cataclysm —see Forces of nature,
        by type
    dune buggy occupant (nontraffic) V86.93
      driver V86.53
      hanger-on V86.73
      passenger V86.63
      traffic V86.33
        driver V86.03
        hanger-on V86.23
        passenger V86.13
      while boarding or alighting V86.43
    forklift —see Accident, transport, industrial
        vehicle occupant
    go cart —see Accident, transport, all-terrain
        vehicle occupant
    golf cart —see Accident, transport, all-
        terrain vehicle occupant
    heavy transport vehicle occupant —see
        Accident, transport, truck occupant
    ice yacht V98.2
    industrial vehicle occupant (nontraffic)
        V83.9
      driver V83.5
      hanger-on V83.7
      passenger V83.6
      traffic V83.3
        driver V83.0
        hanger-on V83.2
        passenger V83.1
      while boarding or alighting V83.4
    interurban electric car —see Accident,
        transport, streetcar
    land yacht V98.1
    logging car —see Accident, transport,
        industrial vehicle occupant
    military vehicle occupant (traffic) V86.34
      driver V86.04
      hanger-on V86.24
      nontraffic V86.94
        driver V86.54
        hanger-on V86.74
        passenger V86.64
      passenger V86.14
      while boarding or alighting V86.44
    mine tram —see Accident, transport,
        industrial vehicle occupant
    motor vehicle NEC occupant (traffic)
        V89.2 ◄▥▥
      driver V86.09
      hanger-on V86.29
      nontraffic V86.99
        driver V86.59
        hanger-on V86.79
        passenger V86.69
      passenger V86.19
      while boarding or alighting V86.49
    motorcoach —see Accident, transport, bus
        occupant
    motorcyclist V29.9
      collision (with)
        animal (traffic) V20.9
          being ridden (traffic) V26.9
            nontraffic V26.2
            while boarding or alighting V26.3
          nontraffic V20.2
          while boarding or alighting V20.3

Accident (Continued)
  transport (Continued)
    motorcyclist (Continued)
      collision (Continued)
        animal-drawn vehicle (traffic) V26.9
          nontraffic V26.2
          while boarding or alighting V26.3
        bus (traffic) V24.9
          nontraffic V24.2
          while boarding or alighting V24.3
        car (traffic) V23.9
          nontraffic V23.2
          while boarding or alighting V23.3
        motor vehicle NOS (traffic) V29.60
          nontraffic V29.20
          specified type NEC (traffic) V29.69
            nontraffic V29.29
        pedal cycle (traffic) V21.9
          nontraffic V21.2
          while boarding or alighting V21.3
        pickup truck (traffic) V23.9
          nontraffic V23.2
          while boarding or alighting V23.3
        railway vehicle (traffic) V25.9
          nontraffic V25.2
          while boarding or alighting V25.3
        specified vehicle NEC (traffic) V26.9
          nontraffic V26.2
          while boarding or alighting V26.3
        stationary object (traffic) V27.9
          nontraffic V27.2
          while boarding or alighting V27.3
        streetcar (traffic) V26.9
          nontraffic V26.2
          while boarding or alighting V26.3
        three wheeled motor vehicle (traffic)
            V22.9
          nontraffic V22.2
          while boarding or alighting V22.3
        truck (traffic) V24.9
          nontraffic V24.2
          while boarding or alighting V24.3
        two wheeled motor vehicle (traffic)
            V22.9
          nontraffic V22.2
          while boarding or alighting V22.3
        van (traffic) V23.9
          nontraffic V23.2
          while boarding or alighting V23.3
      driver
        collision (with)
          animal (traffic) V20.4
            being ridden (traffic) V26.4
              nontraffic V26.0
            nontraffic V20.0
          animal-drawn vehicle (traffic) V26.4
            nontraffic V26.0
          bus (traffic) V24.4
            nontraffic V24.0
          car (traffic) V23.4
            nontraffic V23.0
          motor vehicle NOS (traffic) V29.40
            nontraffic V29.00
            specified type NEC (traffic)
                V29.49
              nontraffic V29.09
          pedal cycle (traffic) V21.4
            nontraffic V21.0
          pickup truck (traffic) V23.4
            nontraffic V23.0
          railway vehicle (traffic) V25.4
            nontraffic V25.0
          specified vehicle NEC (traffic) V26.4
            nontraffic V26.0
          stationary object (traffic) V27.4
            nontraffic V27.0
          streetcar (traffic) V26.4
            nontraffic V26.0
          three wheeled motor vehicle
              (traffic) V22.4
            nontraffic V22.0

Accident *(Continued)*
  transport *(Continued)*
    motorcyclist *(Continued)*
      driver *(Continued)*
        collision *(Continued)*
          truck (traffic) V24.4
            nontraffic V24.0
          two wheeled motor vehicle (traffic) V22.4
            nontraffic V22.0
          van (traffic) V23.4
            nontraffic V23.0
        noncollision accident (traffic) V28.4
          nontraffic V28.0
      noncollision accident (traffic) V28.9
        nontraffic V28.2
      while boarding or alighting V28.3
      nontraffic V29.3
      passenger
        collision (with)
          animal (traffic) V20.5
            being ridden (traffic) V26.5
              nontraffic V26.1
            nontraffic V20.1
          animal-drawn vehicle (traffic) V26.5
            nontraffic V26.1
          bus (traffic) V24.5
            nontraffic V24.1
          car (traffic) V23.5
            nontraffic V23.1
          motor vehicle NOS (traffic) V29.50
            nontraffic V29.10
            specified type NEC (traffic) V29.59
              nontraffic V29.19
          pedal cycle (traffic) V21.5
            nontraffic V21.1
          pickup truck (traffic) V23.5
            nontraffic V23.1
          railway vehicle (traffic) V25.5
            nontraffic V25.1
          specified vehicle NEC (traffic) V26.5
            nontraffic V26.1
          stationary object (traffic) V27.5
            nontraffic V27.1
          streetcar (traffic) V26.5
            nontraffic V26.1
          three wheeled motor vehicle (traffic) V22.5
            nontraffic V22.1
          truck (traffic) V24.5
            nontraffic V24.1
          two wheeled motor vehicle (traffic) V22.5
            nontraffic V22.1
          van (traffic) V23.5
            nontraffic V23.1
        noncollision accident (traffic) V28.5
          nontraffic V28.1
      specified type NEC V29.88
      military vehicle V29.81
    occupant (of)
      aircraft (powered) V95.9
        fixed wing
          commercial —*see* Accident, transport, aircraft, occupant, powered, fixed wing, commercial
          private —*see* Accident, transport, aircraft, occupant, powered, fixed wing, private
        nonpowered V96.9
        specified NEC V95.8
      airport battery-powered vehicle —*see* Accident, transport, industrial vehicle occupant
      all-terrain vehicle (ATV) —*see* Accident, transport, all-terrain vehicle occupant

Accident *(Continued)*
  transport *(Continued)*
    occupant *(Continued)*
      animal-drawn vehicle —*see* Accident, transport, animal-drawn vehicle occupant
      automobile —*see* Accident, transport, car occupant
      balloon V96.00
      battery-powered vehicle —*see* Accident, transport, industrial vehicle occupant
      bicycle —*see* Accident, transport, pedal cyclist
        motorized —*see* Accident, transport, motorcycle rider
      boat NEC —*see* Accident, transport, watercraft
      bulldozer —*see* Accident, transport, construction vehicle occupant
      bus —*see* Accident, transport, bus occupant
      cable car (on rails) —*see also* Accident, transport, streetcar occupant
        not on rails V98.0
      car —*see also* Accident, transport, car occupant
        cable (on rails) —*see also* Accident, transport, streetcar occupant
          not on rails V98.0
      coach —*see* Accident, transport, bus occupant
      coal-car —*see* Accident, transport, industrial vehicle occupant
      digger —*see* Accident, transport, construction vehicle occupant
      dump truck —*see* Accident, transport, construction vehicle occupant
      earth-leveler —*see* Accident, transport, construction vehicle occupant
      farm machinery (self-propelled) —*see* Accident, transport, agricultural vehicle occupant
      forklift —*see* Accident, transport, industrial vehicle occupant
      glider (unpowered) V96.20
        hang V96.10
        powered (microlight) (ultralight) —*see* Accident, transport, aircraft, occupant, powered, glider
      glider (unpowered) NEC V96.20
      hang-glider V96.10
      harvester —*see* Accident, transport, agricultural vehicle occupant
      heavy (transport) vehicle —*see* Accident, transport, truck occupant
      helicopter —*see* Accident, transport, aircraft, occupant, helicopter
      ice-yacht V98.2
      kite (carrying person) V96.8
      land-yacht V98.1
      logging car —*see* Accident, transport, industrial vehicle occupant
      mechanical shovel —*see* Accident, transport, construction vehicle occupant
      microlight —*see* Accident, transport, aircraft, occupant, powered, glider
      minibus —*see* Accident, transport, pickup truck occupant ◄▪▪▪
      minivan —*see* Accident, transport, pickup truck occupant ◄▪▪▪
      moped —*see* Accident, transport, motorcycle
      motor scooter —*see* Accident, transport, motorcycle
      motorcycle (with sidecar) —*see* Accident, transport, motorcycle
      pedal cycle —*see also* Accident, transport, pedal cyclist
      pick-up (truck) —*see* Accident, transport, pickup truck occupant

Accident *(Continued)*
  transport *(Continued)*
    occupant *(Continued)*
      railway (train) (vehicle) (subterranean) (elevated) —*see* Accident, transport, railway vehicle occupant
      rickshaw —*see* Accident, transport, pedal cycle
        pedal driven —*see* Accident, transport, pedal cyclist
      road-roller —*see* Accident, transport, construction vehicle occupant
      ship NOS V94.9
      ski-lift (chair) (gondola) V98.3
      snowmobile —*see* Accident, transport, snowmobile occupant
      spacecraft, spaceship —*see* Accident, transport, aircraft, occupant, spacecraft
      sport utility vehicle —*see* Accident, transport, pickup truck occupant ◄▪▪▪
      streetcar (interurban) (operating on public street or highway) —*see* Accident, transport, streetcar occupant
      SUV —*see* Accident, transport, pickup truck occupant ◄▪▪▪
      téléférique V98.0
      three-wheeled vehicle (motorized) —*see also* Accident, transport, three-wheeled motor vehicle occupant
        nonmotorized —*see* Accident, transport, pedal cycle
      tractor (farm) (and trailer) —*see* Accident, transport, agricultural vehicle occupant
      train —*see* Accident, transport, railway vehicle occupant
      tram —*see* Accident, transport, streetcar occupant
        in mine or quarry —*see* Accident, transport, industrial vehicle occupant
      tricycle —*see* Accident, transport, pedal cycle
        motorized —*see* Accident, transport, three-wheeled motor vehicle
      trolley —*see* Accident, transport, streetcar occupant
        in mine or quarry —*see* Accident, transport, industrial vehicle occupant
      tub, in mine or quarry —*see* Accident, transport, industrial vehicle occupant
      ultralight —*see* Accident, transport, aircraft, occupant, powered, glider
      van —*see* Accident, transport, van occupant
      vehicle NEC V89.9
        heavy transport —*see* Accident, transport, truck occupant
        motor (traffic) NEC V89.2
          nontraffic NEC V89.0
      watercraft NOS V94.9
        causing drowning —*see* Drowning, resulting from accident to boat ◄
    parachutist V97.29
      after accident to aircraft —*see* Accident, transport, aircraft
      entangled in object V97.21
      injured on landing V97.22
    pedal cyclist V19.9
      collision (with)
        animal (traffic) V10.9
          being ridden (traffic) V16.9
            nontraffic V16.2
            while boarding or alighting V16.3
          nontraffic V10.2
          while boarding or alighting V10.3

◄ New   ◄▪▪▪ Revised   ~~deleted~~ Deleted

Accident *(Continued)*
  transport *(Continued)*
    pedal cyclist *(Continued)*
      collision *(Continued)*
        animal-drawn vehicle (traffic) V16.9
          nontraffic V16.2
          while boarding or alighting V16.3
        bus (traffic) V14.9
          nontraffic V14.2
          while boarding or alighting V14.3
        car (traffic) V13.9
          nontraffic V13.2
          while boarding or alighting V13.3
        motor vehicle NOS (traffic) V19.60
          nontraffic V19.20
          specified type NEC (traffic) V19.69
            nontraffic V19.29
        pedal cycle (traffic) V11.9
          nontraffic V11.2
          while boarding or alighting V11.3
        pickup truck (traffic) V13.9
          nontraffic V13.2
          while boarding or alighting V13.3
        railway vehicle (traffic) V15.9
          nontraffic V15.2
          while boarding or alighting V15.3
        specified vehicle NEC (traffic) V16.9
          nontraffic V16.2
          while boarding or alighting V16.3
        stationary object (traffic) V17.9
          nontraffic V17.2
          while boarding or alighting V17.3
        streetcar (traffic) V16.9
          nontraffic V16.2
          while boarding or alighting V16.3
        three wheeled motor vehicle (traffic)
            V12.9
          nontraffic V12.2
          while boarding or alighting V12.3
        truck (traffic) V14.9
          nontraffic V14.2
          while boarding or alighting V14.3
        two wheeled motor vehicle (traffic)
            V12.9
          nontraffic V12.2
          while boarding or alighting V12.3
        van (traffic) V13.9
          nontraffic V13.2
          while boarding or alighting V13.3
      driver
        collision (with)
          animal (traffic) V10.4
            being ridden (traffic) V16.4
              nontraffic V16.0
            nontraffic V10.0
          animal-drawn vehicle (traffic) V16.4
            nontraffic V16.0
          bus (traffic) V14.4
            nontraffic V14.0
          car (traffic) V13.4
            nontraffic V13.0
          motor vehicle NOS (traffic) V19.40
            nontraffic V19.00
            specified type NEC (traffic)
                V19.49
              nontraffic V19.09
          pedal cycle (traffic) V11.4
            nontraffic V11.0
          pickup truck (traffic) V13.4
            nontraffic V13.0
          railway vehicle (traffic) V15.4
            nontraffic V15.0
          specified vehicle NEC (traffic) V16.4
            nontraffic V16.0
          stationary object (traffic) V17.4
            nontraffic V17.0
          streetcar (traffic) V16.4
            nontraffic V16.0
          three wheeled motor vehicle
              (traffic) V12.4
            nontraffic V12.0

Accident *(Continued)*
  transport *(Continued)*
    pedal cyclist *(Continued)*
      driver *(Continued)*
        collision *(Continued)*
          truck (traffic) V14.4
            nontraffic V14.0
          two wheeled motor vehicle (traffic)
              V12.4
            nontraffic V12.0
          van (traffic) V13.4
            nontraffic V13.0
        noncollision accident (traffic) V18.4
          nontraffic V18.0
      noncollision accident (traffic) V18.9
        nontraffic V18.2
        while boarding or alighting V18.3
      nontraffic V19.3
      passenger
        collision (with)
          animal (traffic) V10.5
            being ridden (traffic) V16.5
              nontraffic V16.1
            nontraffic V10.1
          animal-drawn vehicle (traffic) V16.5
            nontraffic V16.1
          bus (traffic) V14.5
            nontraffic V14.1
          car (traffic) V13.5
            nontraffic V13.1
          motor vehicle NOS (traffic) V19.50
            nontraffic V19.10
            specified type NEC (traffic)
                V19.59
              nontraffic V19.19
          pedal cycle (traffic) V11.5
            nontraffic V11.1
          pickup truck (traffic) V13.5
            nontraffic V13.1
          railway vehicle (traffic) V15.5
            nontraffic V15.1
          specified vehicle NEC (traffic) V16.5
            nontraffic V16.1
          stationary object (traffic) V17.5
            nontraffic V17.1
          streetcar (traffic) V16.5
            nontraffic V16.1
          three wheeled motor vehicle
              (traffic) V12.5
            nontraffic V12.1
          truck (traffic) V14.5
            nontraffic V14.1
          two wheeled motor vehicle (traffic)
              V12.5
            nontraffic V12.1
          van (traffic) V13.5
            nontraffic V13.1
        noncollision accident (traffic) V18.5
          nontraffic V18.1
      specified type NEC V19.88
      military vehicle V19.81
    pedestrian
      conveyance (occupant) V09.9
        babystroller V00.828
          collision (with) V09.9
            animal being ridden or animal
                drawn vehicle V06.99
              nontraffic V06.09
              traffic V06.19
            bus or heavy transport V04.99
              nontraffic V04.09
              traffic V04.19
            car V03.99
              nontraffic V03.09
              traffic V03.19
            pedal cycle V01.99
              nontraffic V01.09
              traffic V01.19
            pick-up truck or van V03.99
              nontraffic V03.09
              traffic V03.19

Accident *(Continued)*
  transport *(Continued)*
    pedestrian *(Continued)*
      conveyance *(Continued)*
        babystroller *(Continued)*
          collision *(Continued)*
            railway (train) (vehicle) V05.99
              nontraffic V05.09
              traffic V05.19
            stationary object V00.822
            streetcar V06.99
              nontraffic V06.09
              traffic V06.19
            two- or three-wheeled motor
                vehicle V02.99
              nontraffic V02.09
              traffic V02.19
            vehicle V09.9
              animal-drawn V06.99
                nontraffic V06.09
                traffic V06.19
              motor
                nontraffic V09.00
                traffic V09.20
          fall V00.821
          nontraffic V09.1
            involving motor vehicle NEC
                V09.00
          traffic V09.3
            involving motor vehicle NEC
                V09.20
        flat-bottomed NEC V00.388
          collision (with) V09.9
            animal being ridden or animal
                drawn vehicle V06.99
              nontraffic V06.09
              traffic V06.19
            bus or heavy transport V04.99
              nontraffic V04.09
              traffic V04.19
            car V03.99
              nontraffic V03.09
              traffic V03.19
            pedal cycle V01.99
              nontraffic V01.09
              traffic V01.19
            pick-up truck or van V03.99
              nontraffic V03.09
              traffic V03.19
            railway (train) (vehicle) V05.99
              nontraffic V05.09
              traffic V05.19
            stationary object V00.382
            streetcar V06.99
              nontraffic V06.09
              traffic V06.19
            two-or three-wheeled motor
                vehicle V02.99
              nontraffic V02.09
              traffic V02.19
            vehicle V09.9
              animal-drawn V06.99
                nontraffic V06.09
                traffic V06.19
              motor
                nontraffic V09.00
                traffic V09.20
          fall V00.381
          nontraffic V09.1
            involving motor vehicle NEC
                V09.00
          snow
            board —*see* Accident, transport,
                pedestrian, conveyance,
                snow board
            ski —*see* Accident, transport,
                pedestrian, conveyance, skis
                (snow)
          traffic V09.3
            involving motor vehicle NEC
                V09.20

Accident *(Continued)*
  transport *(Continued)*
    pedestrian *(Continued)*
      conveyance *(Continued)*
        gliding type NEC V00.288
          collision (with) V09.9
            animal being ridden or animal
                drawn vehicle V06.99
              nontraffic V06.09
              traffic V06.19
            bus or heavy transport
                V04.99
              nontraffic V04.09
              traffic V04.19
            car V03.99
              nontraffic V03.09
              traffic V03.19
            pedal cycle V01.99
              nontraffic V01.09
              traffic V01.19
            pick-up truck or van V03.99
              nontraffic V03.09
              traffic V03.19
            railway (train) (vehicle) V05.99
              nontraffic V05.09
              traffic V05.19
            stationary object V00.282
            streetcar V06.99
              nontraffic V06.09
              traffic V06.19
            two- or three-wheeled motor
                vehicle V02.99
              nontraffic V02.09
              traffic V02.19
            vehicle V09.9
              animal-drawn V06.99
                nontraffic V06.09
                traffic V06.19
              motor
                nontraffic V09.00
                traffic V09.20
          fall V00.281
          heelies —*see* Accident, transport,
              pedestrian, conveyance,
              heelies
          ice skate —*see* Accident, transport,
              pedestrian, conveyance, ice
              skate
          nontraffic V09.1
            involving motor vehicle NEC
                V09.00
          sled —*see* Accident, transport,
              pedestrian, conveyance, sled
          traffic V09.3
            involving motor vehicle NEC
                V09.20
              wheelies —*see* Accident,
                  transport, pedestrian,
                  conveyance, heelies
        heelies V00.158
          colliding with stationary object
              V00.152
          fall V00.151
        ice skates V00.218
          collision (with) V09.9
            animal being ridden or animal
                drawn vehicle V06.99
              nontraffic V06.09
              traffic V06.19
            bus or heavy transport V04.99
              nontraffic V04.09
              traffic V04.19
            car V03.99
              nontraffic V03.09
              traffic V03.19
            pedal cycle V01.99
              nontraffic V01.09
              traffic V01.19
            pick-up truck or van V03.99
              nontraffic V03.09
              traffic V03.19

Accident *(Continued)*
  transport *(Continued)*
    pedestrian *(Continued)*
      conveyance *(Continued)*
        ice skates *(Continued)*
          collision *(Continued)*
            railway (train) (vehicle)
                V05.99
              nontraffic V05.09
              traffic V05.19
            stationary object V00.212
            streetcar V06.99
              nontraffic V06.09
              traffic V06.19
            two- or three-wheeled motor
                vehicle V02.99
              nontraffic V02.09
              traffic V02.19
            vehicle V09.9
              animal-drawn V06.99
                nontraffic V06.09
                traffic V06.19
              motor
                nontraffic V09.00
                traffic V09.20
          fall V00.211
          nontraffic V09.1
            involving motor vehicle NEC
                V09.00
          traffic V09.3
            involving motor vehicle NEC
                V09.20
        motorized mobility scooter
            V00.838
          collision with stationary object
              V00.832
          fall from V00.831
        nontraffic V09.1
          involving motor vehicle
              V09.00
            military V09.01
            specified type NEC V09.09
        roller skates (non in-line) V00.128
          collision (with) V09.9
            animal being ridden or animal
                drawn vehicle V06.91
              nontraffic V06.01
              traffic V06.11
            bus or heavy transport
                V04.91
              nontraffic V04.01
              traffic V04.11
            car V03.91
              nontraffic V03.01
              traffic V03.11
            pedal cycle V01.91
              nontraffic V01.01
              traffic V01.11
            pick-up truck or van V03.91
              nontraffic V03.01
              traffic V03.11
            railway (train) (vehicle)
                V05.91
              nontraffic V05.01
              traffic V05.11
            stationary object V00.122
            streetcar V06.91
              nontraffic V06.01
              traffic V06.11
            two- or three-wheeled motor
                vehicle V02.91
              nontraffic V02.01
              traffic V02.11
            vehicle V09.9
              animal-drawn V06.91
                nontraffic V06.01
                traffic V06.11
              motor
                nontraffic V09.00
                traffic V09.20
          fall V00.121

Accident *(Continued)*
  transport *(Continued)*
    pedestrian *(Continued)*
      conveyance *(Continued)*
        roller skates *(Continued)*
          in-line V00.118
            collision —*see also* Accident,
                transport, pedestrian,
                conveyance occupant, roller
                skates, collision
              with stationary object
                  V00.112
            fall V00.111
            nontraffic V09.1
              involving motor vehicle NEC
                  V09.00
            traffic V09.3
              involving motor vehicle NEC
                  V09.20
        rolling shoes V00.158
          colliding with stationary object
              V00.152
          fall V00.151
        rolling type NEC V00.188
          collision (with) V09.9
            animal being ridden or animal
                drawn vehicle V06.99
              nontraffic V06.09
              traffic V06.19
            bus or heavy transport V04.99
              nontraffic V04.09
              traffic V04.19
            car V03.99
              nontraffic V03.09
              traffic V03.19
            pedal cycle V01.99
              nontraffic V01.09
              traffic V01.19
            pick-up truck or van V03.99
              nontraffic V03.09
              traffic V03.19
            railway (train) (vehicle)
                V05.99
              nontraffic V05.09
              traffic V05.19
            stationary object V00.182
            streetcar V06.99
              nontraffic V06.09
              traffic V06.19
            two- or three-wheeled motor
                vehicle V02.99
              nontraffic V02.09
              traffic V02.19
            vehicle V09.9
              animal-drawn V06.99
                nontraffic V06.09
                traffic V06.19
              motor
                nontraffic V09.00
                traffic V09.20
          fall V00.181
          in-line roller skate —*see* Accident,
              transport, pedestrian,
              conveyance, roller skate,
              in-line
          nontraffic V09.1
            involving motor vehicle NEC
                V09.00
          roller skate —*see* Accident,
              transport, pedestrian,
              conveyance, roller skate
          scooter (non-motorized) —
              see Accident, transport,
              pedestrian, conveyance,
              scooter
          skateboard —*see* Accident,
              transport, pedestrian,
              conveyance, skateboard
          traffic V09.3
            involving motor vehicle NEC
                V09.20

◀ New   ◀▥ Revised   ~~deleted~~ Deleted

Accident (Continued)
  transport (Continued)
    pedestrian (Continued)
      conveyance (Continued)
        scooter (non-motorized) V00.148
          collision (with) V09.9
            animal being ridden or animal
              drawn vehicle V06.99
              nontraffic V06.09
              traffic V06.19
            bus or heavy transport
              V04.99
              nontraffic V04.09
              traffic V04.19
            car V03.99
              nontraffic V03.09
              traffic V03.19
            pedal cycle V01.99
              nontraffic V01.09
              traffic V01.19
            pick-up truck or van V03.99
              nontraffic V03.09
              traffic V03.19
            railway (train) (vehicle)
              V05.99
              nontraffic V05.09
              traffic V05.19
            stationary object V00.142
            streetcar V06.99
              nontraffic V06.09
              traffic V06.19
            two- or three-wheeled motor
              vehicle V02.99
              nontraffic V02.09
              traffic V02.19
            vehicle V09.9
              animal-drawn V06.99
                nontraffic V06.09
                traffic V06.19
              motor
                nontraffic V09.00
                traffic V09.20
          fall V00.141
          nontraffic V09.1
            involving motor vehicle NEC
              V09.00
          traffic V09.3
            involving motor vehicle NEC
              V09.20
        skate board V00.138
          collision (with) V09.9
            animal being ridden or
              animal drawn vehicle
              V06.92
              nontraffic V06.02
              traffic V06.12
            bus or heavy transport
              V04.92
              nontraffic V04.02
              traffic V04.12
            car V03.92
              nontraffic V03.02
              traffic V03.12
            pedal cycle V01.92
              nontraffic V01.02
              traffic V01.12
            pick-up truck or van V03.92
              nontraffic V03.02
              traffic V03.12
            railway (train) (vehicle)
              V05.92
              nontraffic V05.02
              traffic V05.12
            stationary object V00.132
            streetcar V06.92
              nontraffic V06.02
              traffic V06.12
            two- or three-wheeled motor
              vehicle V02.92
              nontraffic V02.02
              traffic V02.12

Accident (Continued)
  transport (Continued)
    pedestrian (Continued)
      conveyance (Continued)
        skate board (Continued)
          collision (Continued)
            vehicle V09.9
              animal-drawn V06.92
                nontraffic V06.02
                traffic V06.12
              motor
                nontraffic V09.00
                traffic V09.20
          fall V00.131
          nontraffic V09.1
            involving motor vehicle NEC
              V09.00
          traffic V09.3
            involving motor vehicle NEC
              V09.20
        skis (snow) V00.328
          collision (with) V09.9
            animal being ridden or animal
              drawn vehicle V06.99
              nontraffic V06.09
              traffic V06.19
            bus or heavy transport V04.99
              nontraffic V04.09
              traffic V04.19
            car V03.99
              nontraffic V03.09
              traffic V03.19
            pedal cycle V01.99
              nontraffic V01.09
              traffic V01.19
            pick-up truck or van V03.99
              nontraffic V03.09
              traffic V03.19
            railway (train) (vehicle) V05.99
              nontraffic V05.09
              traffic V05.19
            stationary object V00.322
            streetcar V06.99
              nontraffic V06.09
              traffic V06.19
            two- or three-wheeled motor
              vehicle V02.99
              nontraffic V02.09
              traffic V02.19
            vehicle V09.9
              animal-drawn V06.99
                nontraffic V06.09
                traffic V06.19
              motor
                nontraffic V09.00
                traffic V09.20
          fall V00.321
          nontraffic V09.1
            involving motor vehicle NEC
              V09.00
          traffic V09.3
            involving motor vehicle NEC
              V09.20
        sled V00.228
          collision (with) V09.9
            animal being ridden or animal
              drawn vehicle V06.99
              nontraffic V06.09
              traffic V06.19
            bus or heavy transport V04.99
              nontraffic V04.09
              traffic V04.19
            car V03.99
              nontraffic V03.09
              traffic V03.19
            pedal cycle V01.99
              nontraffic V01.09
              traffic V01.19
            pick-up truck or van V03.99
              nontraffic V03.09
              traffic V03.19

Accident (Continued)
  transport (Continued)
    pedestrian (Continued)
      conveyance (Continued)
        sled (Continued)
          collision (Continued)
            railway (train) (vehicle)
              V05.99
              nontraffic V05.09
              traffic V05.19
            stationary object V00.222
            streetcar V06.99
              nontraffic V06.09
              traffic V06.19
            two- or three-wheeled motor
              vehicle V02.99
              nontraffic V02.09
              traffic V02.19
            vehicle V09.9
              animal-drawn V06.99
                nontraffic V06.09
                traffic V06.19
              motor
                nontraffic V09.00
                traffic V09.20
          fall V00.221
          nontraffic V09.1
            involving motor vehicle NEC
              V09.00
          traffic V09.3
            involving motor vehicle NEC
              V09.20
        snow board V00.318
          collision (with) V09.9
            animal being ridden or animal
              drawn vehicle V06.99
              nontraffic V06.09
              traffic V06.19
            bus or heavy transport V04.99
              nontraffic V04.09
              traffic V04.19
            car V03.99
              nontraffic V03.09
              traffic V03.19
            pedal cycle V01.99
              nontraffic V01.09
              traffic V01.19
            pick-up truck or van V03.99
              nontraffic V03.09
              traffic V03.19
            railway (train) (vehicle) V05.99
              nontraffic V05.09
              traffic V05.19
            stationary object V00.312
            streetcar V06.99
              nontraffic V06.09
              traffic V06.19
            two- or three-wheeled motor
              vehicle V02.99
              nontraffic V02.09
              traffic V02.19
            vehicle V09.9
              animal-drawn V06.99
                nontraffic V06.09
                traffic V06.19
              motor
                nontraffic V09.00
                traffic V09.20
          fall V00.311
          nontraffic V09.1
            involving motor vehicle NEC
              V09.00
          traffic V09.3
            involving motor vehicle NEC
              V09.20
        specified type NEC V00.898
          collision (with) V09.9
            animal being ridden or animal
              drawn vehicle V06.99
              nontraffic V06.09
              traffic V06.19

Accident (Continued)
  transport (Continued)
    pedestrian (Continued)
      conveyance (Continued)
        specified type NEC (Continued)
          collision (Continued)
            bus or heavy transport
              V04.99
              nontraffic V04.09
              traffic V04.19
            car V03.99
              nontraffic V03.09
              traffic V03.19
            pedal cycle V01.99
              nontraffic V01.09
              traffic V01.19
            pick-up truck or van V03.99
              nontraffic V03.09
              traffic V03.19
            railway (train) (vehicle)
              V05.99
              nontraffic V05.09
              traffic V05.19
            stationary object V00.892
            streetcar V06.99
              nontraffic V06.09
              traffic V06.19
            two- or three-wheeled motor
              vehicle V02.99
              nontraffic V02.09
              traffic V02.19
            vehicle V09.9
              animal-drawn V06.99
                nontraffic V06.09
                traffic V06.19
              motor
                nontraffic V09.00
                traffic V09.20
          fall V00.891
          nontraffic V09.1
            involving motor vehicle NEC
              V09.00
          traffic V09.3
            involving motor vehicle NEC
              V09.20
        traffic V09.3
         involving motor vehicle V09.20
          military V09.21
          specified type NEC V09.29
      wheelchair (powered) V00.818
        collision (with) V09.9
          animal being ridden or
            animal drawn vehicle
            V06.99
            nontraffic V06.09
            traffic V06.19
          bus or heavy transport
            V04.99
            nontraffic V04.09
            traffic V04.19
          car V03.99
            nontraffic V03.09
            traffic V03.19
          pedal cycle V01.99
            nontraffic V01.09
            traffic V01.19
          pick-up truck or van V03.99
            nontraffic V03.09
            traffic V03.19
          railway (train) (vehicle)
            V05.99
            nontraffic V05.09
            traffic V05.19
          stationary object V00.812
          streetcar V06.99
            nontraffic V06.09
            traffic V06.19
          two- or three-wheeled motor
            vehicle V02.99
            nontraffic V02.09
            traffic V02.19

Accident (Continued)
  transport (Continued)
    pedestrian (Continued)
      conveyance (Continued)
        wheelchair (Continued)
          collision (Continued)
            vehicle V09.9
              animal-drawn V06.99
                nontraffic V06.09
                traffic V06.19
              motor
                nontraffic V09.00
                traffic V09.20
          fall V00.811
          nontraffic V09.1
            involving motor vehicle NEC
              V09.00
          traffic V09.3
            involving motor vehicle NEC
              V09.20
        wheeled shoe V00.158
          colliding with stationary object
            V00.152
          fall V00.151
    on foot —see also Accident, pedestrian
      collision (with)
        animal being ridden or animal
          drawn vehicle V06.90
          nontraffic V06.00
          traffic V06.10
        bus or heavy transport V04.90
          nontraffic V04.00
          traffic V04.10
        car V03.90
          nontraffic V03.00
          traffic V03.10
        pedal cycle V01.90
          nontraffic V01.00
          traffic V01.10
        pick-up truck or van V03.90
          nontraffic V03.00
          traffic V03.10
        railway (train) (vehicle) V05.90
          nontraffic V05.00
          traffic V05.10
        streetcar V06.90
          nontraffic V06.00
          traffic V06.10
        two- or three-wheeled motor
          vehicle V02.90
          nontraffic V02.00
          traffic V02.10
        vehicle V09.9
          animal-drawn V06.90
           nontraffic V06.00
           traffic V06.10
          motor
           nontraffic V09.00
           traffic V09.20
      nontraffic V09.1
        involving motor vehicle V09.00
          military V09.01
          specified type NEC V09.09
      traffic V09.3
        involving motor vehicle V09.20
          military V09.21
          specified type NEC V09.29
    person NEC (unknown way or
      transportation) V99
      collision (between)
        bus (with)
          heavy transport vehicle (traffic)
           V87.5
          nontraffic V88.5
        car (with)
          nontraffic V88.5
          bus (traffic) V87.3
           nontraffic V88.3
          heavy transport vehicle (traffic)
           V87.4
          nontraffic V88.4

Accident (Continued)
  transport (Continued)
    person NEC (Continued)
      collision (Continued)
        car (Continued)
          pick-up truck or van (traffic) V87.2
           nontraffic V88.2
          train or railway vehicle (traffic)
           V87.6
           nontraffic V88.6
          two- or three-wheeled motor
           vehicle (traffic) V87.0
           nontraffic V88.0
        motor vehicle (traffic) NEC V87.7
          nontraffic V88.7
        two- or three-wheeled vehicle (with)
          (traffic)
          motor vehicle NEC V87.1
           nontraffic V88.1
        nonmotor vehicle (collision)
          (noncollision) (traffic) V87.9
          nontraffic V88.9
      pickup truck occupant V59.9
        collision (with)
          animal (traffic) V50.9
           being ridden (traffic) V56.9
            nontraffic V56.3
             while boarding or alighting V56.4
           nontraffic V50.3
            while boarding or alighting V50.4
          animal-drawn vehicle (traffic) V56.9
           nontraffic V56.3
           while boarding or alighting V56.4
          bus (traffic) V54.9
           nontraffic V54.3
           while boarding or alighting V54.4
          car (traffic) V53.9
           nontraffic V53.3
           while boarding or alighting V53.4
          motor vehicle NOS (traffic) V59.60
           nontraffic V59.20
           specified type NEC (traffic) V59.69
            nontraffic V59.29
          pedal cycle (traffic) V51.9
           nontraffic V51.3
           while boarding or alighting V51.4
          pickup truck (traffic) V53.9
           nontraffic V53.3
           while boarding or alighting V53.4
          railway vehicle (traffic) V55.9
           nontraffic V55.3
           while boarding or alighting V55.4
          specified vehicle NEC (traffic) V56.9
           nontraffic V56.3
           while boarding or alighting V56.4
          stationary object (traffic) V57.9
           nontraffic V57.3
           while boarding or alighting V57.4
          streetcar (traffic) V56.9
           nontraffic V56.3
           while boarding or alighting V56.4
          three wheeled motor vehicle (traffic)
           V52.9
           nontraffic V52.3
           while boarding or alighting V52.4
          truck (traffic) V54.9
           nontraffic V54.3
           while boarding or alighting V54.4
          two wheeled motor vehicle (traffic)
           V52.9
           nontraffic V52.3
           while boarding or alighting V52.4
          van (traffic) V53.9
           nontraffic V53.3
           while boarding or alighting V53.4
        driver
          collision (with)
           animal (traffic) V50.5
            being ridden (traffic) V56.5
             nontraffic V56.0
            nontraffic V50.0

◀ New   ◀▪▪▪ Revised   deleted Deleted

Accident *(Continued)*
  transport *(Continued)*
    pickup truck occupant *(Continued)*
      driver *(Continued)*
        collision *(Continued)*
          animal-drawn vehicle (traffic) V56.5
            nontraffic V56.0
          bus (traffic) V54.5
            nontraffic V54.0
          car (traffic) V53.5
            nontraffic V53.0
          motor vehicle NOS (traffic) V59.40
            nontraffic V59.00
            specified type NEC (traffic) V59.49
              nontraffic V59.09
          pedal cycle (traffic) V51.5
            nontraffic V51.0
          pickup truck (traffic) V53.5
            nontraffic V53.0
          railway vehicle (traffic) V55.5
            nontraffic V55.0
          specified vehicle NEC (traffic) V56.5
            nontraffic V56.0
          stationary object (traffic) V57.5
            nontraffic V57.0
          streetcar (traffic) V56.5
            nontraffic V56.0
          three wheeled motor vehicle (traffic) V52.5
            nontraffic V52.0
          truck (traffic) V54.5
            nontraffic V54.0
          two wheeled motor vehicle (traffic) V52.5
            nontraffic V52.0
          van (traffic) V53.5
            nontraffic V53.0
        noncollision accident (traffic) V58.5
          nontraffic V58.0
      hanger-on
        collision (with)
          animal (traffic) V50.7
            being ridden (traffic) V56.7
              nontraffic V56.2
            nontraffic V50.2
          animal-drawn vehicle (traffic) V56.7
            nontraffic V56.2
          bus (traffic) V54.7
            nontraffic V54.2
          car (traffic) V53.7
            nontraffic V53.2
          pedal cycle (traffic) V51.7
            nontraffic V51.2
          pickup truck (traffic) V53.7
            nontraffic V53.2
          railway vehicle (traffic) V55.7
            nontraffic V55.2
          specified vehicle NEC (traffic) V56.7
            nontraffic V56.2
          stationary object (traffic) V57.7
            nontraffic V57.2
          streetcar (traffic) V56.7
            nontraffic V56.2
          three wheeled motor vehicle (traffic) V52.7
            nontraffic V52.2
          truck (traffic) V54.7
            nontraffic V54.2
          two wheeled motor vehicle (traffic) V52.7
            nontraffic V52.2
          van (traffic) V53.7
            nontraffic V53.2
        noncollision accident (traffic) V58.7
          nontraffic V58.2
        noncollision accident (traffic) V58.9
         nontraffic V58.3
        while boarding or alighting V58.4
        nontraffic V59.3

Accident *(Continued)*
  transport *(Continued)*
    pickup truck occupant *(Continued)*
      passenger
        collision (with)
          animal (traffic) V50.6
            being ridden (traffic) V56.6
              nontraffic V56.1
            nontraffic V50.1
          animal-drawn vehicle (traffic) V56.6
            nontraffic V56.1
          bus (traffic) V54.6
            nontraffic V54.1
          car (traffic) V53.6
            nontraffic V53.1
          motor vehicle NOS (traffic) V59.50
            nontraffic V59.10
            specified type NEC (traffic) V59.59
             nontraffic V59.19
          pedal cycle (traffic) V51.6
            nontraffic V51.1
          pickup truck (traffic) V53.6
            nontraffic V53.1
          railway vehicle (traffic) V55.6
            nontraffic V55.1
          specified vehicle NEC (traffic) V56.6
            nontraffic V56.1
          stationary object (traffic) V57.6
            nontraffic V57.1
          streetcar (traffic) V56.6
            nontraffic V56.1
          three wheeled motor vehicle (traffic) V52.6
            nontraffic V52.1
          truck (traffic) V54.6
            nontraffic V54.1
          two wheeled motor vehicle (traffic) V52.6
            nontraffic V52.1
          van (traffic) V53.6
            nontraffic V53.1
        noncollision accident (traffic) V58.6
         nontraffic V58.1
      specified type NEC V59.88
        military vehicle V59.81
      quarry truck —*see* Accident, transport, industrial vehicle occupant
      race car —*see* Accident, transport, motor vehicle NEC occupant
    railway vehicle occupant V81.9
      collision (with) V81.3
        motor vehicle (non-military) (traffic) V81.1
        military V81.83
        nontraffic V81.0
        rolling stock V81.2
        specified object NEC V81.3
      during derailment V81.7
        with antecedent collision —*see* Accident, transport, railway vehicle occupant, collision ◀
      explosion V81.81
      fall (in railway vehicle) V81.5
        during derailment V81.7
          with antecedent collision —*see* Accident, transport, railway vehicle occupant, collision ◀
        from railway vehicle V81.6
          during derailment V81.7
            with antecedent collision —*see* Accident, transport, railway vehicle occupant, collision ◀
        while boarding or alighting V81.81
      fire V81.81
      object falling onto train V81.82
      specified type NEC V81.89
      while boarding or alighting V81.4
    ski lift V98.3

Accident *(Continued)*
  transport *(Continued)*
    snowmobile occupant (nontraffic) V86.92
      driver V86.52
      hanger-on V86.72
      passenger V86.62
      traffic V86.32
        driver V86.02
        hanger-on V86.22
        passenger V86.12
      while boarding or alighting V86.42
    specified NEC V98.8
    sport utility vehicle occupant —*see also* Accident, transport, pickup truck occupant ◀▥
      ~~collision (with)~~
        ~~stationary object (traffic) V47.91~~
        ~~nontraffic V47.31~~
      ~~driver~~
        ~~collision (with)~~
          ~~stationary object (traffic) V47.51~~
          ~~nontraffic V47.01~~
      ~~passenger~~
        ~~collision (with)~~
          ~~stationary object (traffic) V47.61~~
          ~~nontraffic V47.11~~
    streetcar occupant V82.9
      collision (with) V82.3
        motor vehicle (traffic) V82.1
        nontraffic V82.0
        rolling stock V82.2
      during derailment V82.7
        with antecedent collision —*see* Accident, transport, streetcar occupant, collision ◀
      fall (in streetcar) V82.5
        during derailment V82.7
          with antecedent collision —*see* Accident, transport, streetcar occupant, collision ◀
        from streetcar V82.6
          during derailment V82.7
            with antecedent collision —*see* Accident, transport, streetcar occupant, collision ◀
        while boarding or alighting V82.4
      while boarding or alighting V82.4
      specified type NEC V82.8
      while boarding or alighting V82.4
    three-wheeled motor vehicle occupant V39.9
      collision (with)
        animal (traffic) V30.9
          being ridden (traffic) V36.9
            nontraffic V36.3
              while boarding or alighting V36.4
          nontraffic V30.3
            while boarding or alighting V30.4
        animal-drawn vehicle (traffic) V36.9
          nontraffic V36.3
            while boarding or alighting V36.4
        bus (traffic) V34.9
          nontraffic V34.3
            while boarding or alighting V34.4
        car (traffic) V33.9
          nontraffic V33.3
            while boarding or alighting V33.4
        motor vehicle NOS (traffic) V39.60
          nontraffic V39.20
            specified type NEC (traffic) V39.69
             nontraffic V39.29
        pedal cycle (traffic) V31.9
          nontraffic V31.3
            while boarding or alighting V31.4
        pickup truck (traffic) V33.9
          nontraffic V33.3
            while boarding or alighting V33.4
        railway vehicle (traffic) V35.9
          nontraffic V35.3
            while boarding or alighting V35.4

Accident *(Continued)*
  transport *(Continued)*
    three-wheeled motor vehicle occupant
      (Continued)
      collision *(Continued)*
        specified vehicle NEC (traffic) V36.9
          nontraffic V36.3
          while boarding or alighting V36.4
        stationary object (traffic) V37.9
          nontraffic V37.3
          while boarding or alighting V37.4
        streetcar (traffic) V36.9
          nontraffic V36.3
          while boarding or alighting V36.4
        three wheeled motor vehicle (traffic)
          V32.9
          nontraffic V32.3
          while boarding or alighting V32.4
        truck (traffic) V34.9
          nontraffic V34.3
          while boarding or alighting V34.4
        two wheeled motor vehicle (traffic)
          V32.9
          nontraffic V32.3
          while boarding or alighting V32.4
        van (traffic) V33.9
          nontraffic V33.3
          while boarding or alighting V33.4
      driver
        collision (with)
          animal (traffic) V30.5
            being ridden (traffic) V36.5
              nontraffic V36.0
            nontraffic V30.0
          animal-drawn vehicle (traffic) V36.5
            nontraffic V36.0
          bus (traffic) V34.5
            nontraffic V34.0
          car (traffic) V33.5
            nontraffic V33.0
          motor vehicle NOS (traffic) V39.40
            nontraffic V39.00
            specified type NEC (traffic)
              V39.49
              nontraffic V39.09
          pedal cycle (traffic) V31.5
            nontraffic V31.0
          pickup truck (traffic) V33.5
            nontraffic V33.0
          railway vehicle (traffic) V35.5
            nontraffic V35.0
          specified vehicle NEC (traffic) V36.5
            nontraffic V36.0
          stationary object (traffic) V37.5
            nontraffic V37.0
          streetcar (traffic) V36.5
            nontraffic V36.0
          three wheeled motor vehicle
            (traffic) V32.5
            nontraffic V32.0
          truck (traffic) V34.5
            nontraffic V34.0
          two wheeled motor vehicle (traffic)
            V32.5
            nontraffic V32.0
          van (traffic) V33.5
            nontraffic V33.0
        noncollision accident (traffic) V38.5
          nontraffic V38.0
      hanger-on
        collision (with)
          animal (traffic) V30.7
            being ridden (traffic) V36.7
              nontraffic V36.2
            nontraffic V30.2
          animal-drawn vehicle (traffic) V36.7
            nontraffic V36.2
          bus (traffic) V34.7
            nontraffic V34.2
          car (traffic) V33.7
            nontraffic V33.2

Accident *(Continued)*
  transport *(Continued)*
    three-wheeled motor vehicle occupant
      (Continued)
      hanger-on *(Continued)*
        collision *(Continued)*
          pedal cycle (traffic) V31.7
            nontraffic V31.2
          pickup truck (traffic) V33.7
            nontraffic V33.2
          railway vehicle (traffic) V35.7
            nontraffic V35.2
          specified vehicle NEC (traffic) V36.7
            nontraffic V36.2
          stationary object (traffic) V37.7
            nontraffic V37.2
          streetcar (traffic) V36.7
            nontraffic V36.2
          three wheeled motor vehicle
            (traffic) V32.7
            nontraffic V32.2
          truck (traffic) V34.7
            nontraffic V34.2
          two wheeled motor vehicle (traffic)
            V32.7
            nontraffic V32.2
          van (traffic) V33.7
            nontraffic V33.2
        noncollision accident (traffic) V38.7
          nontraffic V38.2
      noncollision accident (traffic) V38.9
        nontraffic V38.3
        while boarding or alighting V38.4
      nontraffic V39.3
      passenger
        collision (with)
          animal (traffic) V30.6
            being ridden (traffic) V36.6
              nontraffic V36.1
            nontraffic V30.1
          animal-drawn vehicle (traffic) V36.6
            nontraffic V36.1
          bus (traffic) V34.6
            nontraffic V34.1
          car (traffic) V33.6
            nontraffic V33.1
          motor vehicle NOS (traffic) V39.50
            nontraffic V39.10
            specified type NEC (traffic)
              V39.59
              nontraffic V39.19
          pedal cycle (traffic) V31.6
            nontraffic V31.1
          pickup truck (traffic) V33.6
            nontraffic V33.1
          railway vehicle (traffic) V35.6
            nontraffic V35.1
          specified vehicle NEC (traffic)
            V36.6
            nontraffic V36.1
          stationary object (traffic) V37.6
            nontraffic V37.1
          streetcar (traffic) V36.6
            nontraffic V36.1
          three wheeled motor vehicle
            (traffic) V32.6
            nontraffic V32.1
          truck (traffic) V34.6
            nontraffic V34.1
          two wheeled motor vehicle (traffic)
            V32.6
            nontraffic V32.1
          van (traffic) V33.6
            nontraffic V33.1
        noncollision accident (traffic) V38.6
          nontraffic V38.1
      specified type NEC V39.89
        military vehicle V39.81
      tractor (farm) (and trailer) —*see* Accident,
        transport, agricultural vehicle
        occupant

Accident *(Continued)*
  transport *(Continued)*
    tram —*see* Accident, transport, streetcar
      in mine or quarry —*see* Accident,
      transport, industrial vehicle
      occupant
    trolley —*see* Accident, transport, streetcar
      in mine or quarry —*see* Accident,
      transport, industrial vehicle
      occupant
    truck (heavy) occupant V69.9
      collision (with)
        animal (traffic) V60.9
          being ridden (traffic) V66.9
            nontraffic V66.3
            while boarding or alighting V66.4
          nontraffic V60.3
          while boarding or alighting V60.4
        animal-drawn vehicle (traffic) V66.9
          nontraffic V66.3
          while boarding or alighting V66.4
        bus (traffic) V64.9
          nontraffic V64.3
          while boarding or alighting V64.4
        car (traffic) V63.9
          nontraffic V63.3
          while boarding or alighting V63.4
        motor vehicle NOS (traffic) V69.60
          nontraffic V69.20
          specified type NEC (traffic) V69.69
            nontraffic V69.29
        pedal cycle (traffic) V61.9
          nontraffic V61.3
          while boarding or alighting V61.4
        pickup truck (traffic) V63.9
          nontraffic V63.3
          while boarding or alighting V63.4
        railway vehicle (traffic) V65.9
          nontraffic V65.3
          while boarding or alighting V65.4
        specified vehicle NEC (traffic) V66.9
          nontraffic V66.3
          while boarding or alighting V66.4
        stationary object (traffic) V67.9
          nontraffic V67.3
          while boarding or alighting V67.4
        streetcar (traffic) V66.9
          nontraffic V66.3
          while boarding or alighting V66.4
        three wheeled motor vehicle (traffic)
          V62.9
          nontraffic V62.3
          while boarding or alighting V62.4
        truck (traffic) V64.9
          nontraffic V64.3
          while boarding or alighting V64.4
        two wheeled motor vehicle (traffic)
          V62.9
          nontraffic V62.3
          while boarding or alighting V62.4
        van (traffic) V63.9
          nontraffic V63.3
          while boarding or alighting V63.4
      driver
        collision (with)
          animal (traffic) V60.5
            being ridden (traffic) V66.5
              nontraffic V66.0
            nontraffic V60.0
          animal-drawn vehicle (traffic)
            V66.5
            nontraffic V66.0
          bus (traffic) V64.5
            nontraffic V64.0
          car (traffic) V63.5
            nontraffic V63.0
          motor vehicle NOS (traffic) V69.40
            nontraffic V69.00
            specified type NEC (traffic)
              V69.49
              nontraffic V69.09

◀ New   ◀▥ Revised   ~~deleted~~ Deleted

Accident *(Continued)*
  transport *(Continued)*
    truck occupant *(Continued)*
      driver *(Continued)*
        collision *(Continued)*
          pedal cycle (traffic) V61.5
            nontraffic V61.0
          pickup truck (traffic) V63.5
            nontraffic V63.0
          railway vehicle (traffic) V65.5
            nontraffic V65.0
          specified vehicle NEC (traffic) V66.5
            nontraffic V66.0
          stationary object (traffic) V67.5
            nontraffic V67.0
          streetcar (traffic) V66.5
            nontraffic V66.0
          three wheeled motor vehicle
            (traffic) V62.5
            nontraffic V62.0
          truck (traffic) V64.5
            nontraffic V64.0
          two wheeled motor vehicle (traffic)
            V62.5
            nontraffic V62.0
          van (traffic) V63.5
            nontraffic V63.0
        noncollision accident (traffic) V68.5
          nontraffic V68.0
      dump —*see* Accident, transport,
        construction vehicle occupant
      hanger-on
        collision (with)
          animal (traffic) V60.7
            being ridden (traffic) V66.7
              nontraffic V66.2
            nontraffic V60.2
          animal-drawn vehicle (traffic) V66.7
            nontraffic V66.2
          bus (traffic) V64.7
            nontraffic V64.2
          car (traffic) V63.7
            nontraffic V63.2
          pedal cycle (traffic) V61.7
            nontraffic V61.2
          pickup truck (traffic) V63.7
            nontraffic V63.2
          railway vehicle (traffic) V65.7
            nontraffic V65.2
          specified vehicle NEC (traffic) V66.7
            nontraffic V66.2
          stationary object (traffic) V67.7
            nontraffic V67.2
          streetcar (traffic) V66.7
            nontraffic V66.2
          three wheeled motor vehicle
            (traffic) V62.7
            nontraffic V62.2
          truck (traffic) V64.7
            nontraffic V64.2
          two wheeled motor vehicle (traffic)
            V62.7
            nontraffic V62.2
          van (traffic) V63.7
            nontraffic V63.2
        noncollision accident (traffic) V68.7
          nontraffic V68.2
      noncollision accident (traffic) V68.9
        nontraffic V68.3
        while boarding or alighting V68.4
      nontraffic V69.3
      passenger
        collision (with)
          animal (traffic) V60.6
            being ridden (traffic) V66.6
              nontraffic V66.1
            nontraffic V60.1
          animal-drawn vehicle (traffic) V66.6
            nontraffic V66.1
          bus (traffic) V64.6
            nontraffic V64.1

Accident *(Continued)*
  transport *(Continued)*
    truck occupant *(Continued)*
      passenger *(Continued)*
        collision *(Continued)*
          car (traffic) V63.6
            nontraffic V63.1
          motor vehicle NOS (traffic) V69.50
            nontraffic V69.10
            specified type NEC (traffic)
              V69.59
              nontraffic V69.19
          pedal cycle (traffic) V61.6
            nontraffic V61.1
          pickup truck (traffic) V63.6
            nontraffic V63.1
          railway vehicle (traffic) V65.6
            nontraffic V65.1
          specified vehicle NEC (traffic)
            V66.6
            nontraffic V66.1
          stationary object (traffic) V67.6
            nontraffic V67.1
          streetcar (traffic) V66.6
            nontraffic V66.1
          three wheeled motor vehicle
            (traffic) V62.6
            nontraffic V62.1
          truck (traffic) V64.6
            nontraffic V64.1
          two wheeled motor vehicle (traffic)
            V62.6
            nontraffic V62.1
          van (traffic) V63.6
            nontraffic V63.1
        noncollision accident (traffic) V68.6
          nontraffic V68.1
      pickup —*see* Accident, transport, pickup
        truck occupant
      specified type NEC V69.88
      military vehicle V69.81
    van occupant V59.9
      collision (with)
        animal (traffic) V50.9
          being ridden (traffic) V56.9
            nontraffic V56.3
            while boarding or alighting
              V56.4
          nontraffic V50.3
          while boarding or alighting V50.4
        animal-drawn vehicle (traffic) V56.9
          nontraffic V56.3
          while boarding or alighting V56.4
        bus (traffic) V54.9
          nontraffic V54.3
          while boarding or alighting V54.4
        car (traffic) V53.9
          nontraffic V53.3
          while boarding or alighting V53.4
        motor vehicle NOS (traffic) V59.60
          nontraffic V59.20
          specified type NEC (traffic) V59.69
            nontraffic V59.29
        pedal cycle (traffic) V51.9
          nontraffic V51.3
          while boarding or alighting V51.4
        pickup truck (traffic) V53.9
          nontraffic V53.3
          while boarding or alighting V53.4
        railway vehicle (traffic) V55.9
          nontraffic V55.3
          while boarding or alighting V55.4
        specified vehicle NEC (traffic) V56.9
          nontraffic V56.3
          while boarding or alighting V56.4
        stationary object (traffic) V57.9
          nontraffic V57.3
          while boarding or alighting V57.4
        streetcar (traffic) V56.9
          nontraffic V56.3
          while boarding or alighting V56.4

Accident *(Continued)*
  transport *(Continued)*
    van occupant *(Continued)*
      collision *(Continued)*
        three wheeled motor vehicle (traffic)
          V52.9
          nontraffic V52.3
          while boarding or alighting V52.4
        truck (traffic) V54.9
          nontraffic V54.3
          while boarding or alighting V54.4
        two wheeled motor vehicle (traffic)
          V52.9
          nontraffic V52.3
          while boarding or alighting V52.4
        van (traffic) V53.9
          nontraffic V53.3
          while boarding or alighting V53.4
      driver
        collision (with)
          animal (traffic) V50.5
            being ridden (traffic) V56.5
              nontraffic V56.0
            nontraffic V50.0
          animal-drawn vehicle (traffic) V56.5
            nontraffic V56.0
          bus (traffic) V54.5
            nontraffic V54.0
          car (traffic) V53.5
            nontraffic V53.0
          motor vehicle NOS (traffic) V59.40
            nontraffic V59.00
            specified type NEC (traffic)
              V59.49
              nontraffic V59.09
          pedal cycle (traffic) V51.5
            nontraffic V51.0
          pickup truck (traffic) V53.5
            nontraffic V53.0
          railway vehicle (traffic) V55.5
            nontraffic V55.0
          specified vehicle NEC (traffic) V56.5
            nontraffic V56.0
          stationary object (traffic) V57.5
            nontraffic V57.0
          streetcar (traffic) V56.5
            nontraffic V56.0
          three wheeled motor vehicle
            (traffic) V52.5
            nontraffic V52.0
          truck (traffic) V54.5
            nontraffic V54.0
          two wheeled motor vehicle (traffic)
            V52.5
            nontraffic V52.0
          van (traffic) V53.5
            nontraffic V53.0
        noncollision accident (traffic) V58.5
          nontraffic V58.0
      hanger-on
        collision (with)
          animal (traffic) V50.7
            being ridden (traffic) V56.7
              nontraffic V56.2
            nontraffic V50.2
          animal-drawn vehicle (traffic) V56.7
            nontraffic V56.2
          bus (traffic) V54.7
            nontraffic V54.2
          car (traffic) V53.7
            nontraffic V53.2
          pedal cycle (traffic) V51.7
            nontraffic V51.2
          pickup truck (traffic) V53.7
            nontraffic V53.2
          railway vehicle (traffic) V55.7
            nontraffic V55.2
          specified vehicle NEC (traffic) V56.7
            nontraffic V56.2
          stationary object (traffic) V57.7
            nontraffic V57.2

Accident *(Continued)*
  transport *(Continued)*
    van occupant *(Continued)*
      hanger-on *(Continued)*
        collision *(Continued)*
          streetcar (traffic) V56.7
            nontraffic V56.2
          three wheeled motor vehicle
            (traffic) V52.7
            nontraffic V52.2
          truck (traffic) V54.7
            nontraffic V54.2
          two wheeled motor vehicle (traffic)
            V52.7
            nontraffic V52.2
          van (traffic) V53.7
            nontraffic V53.2
        noncollision accident (traffic) V58.7
          nontraffic V58.2
      noncollision accident (traffic) V58.9
        nontraffic V58.3
        while boarding or alighting V58.4
      nontraffic V59.3
      passenger
        collision (with)
          animal (traffic) V50.6
            being ridden (traffic) V56.6
              nontraffic V56.1
            nontraffic V50.1
          animal-drawn vehicle (traffic) V56.6
            nontraffic V56.1
          bus (traffic) V54.6
            nontraffic V54.1
          car (traffic) V53.6
            nontraffic V53.1
          motor vehicle NOS (traffic) V59.50
            nontraffic V59.10
            specified type NEC (traffic) V59.59
              nontraffic V59.19
          pedal cycle (traffic) V51.6
            nontraffic V51.1
          pickup truck (traffic) V53.6
            nontraffic V53.1
          railway vehicle (traffic) V55.6
            nontraffic V55.1
          specified vehicle NEC (traffic) V56.6
            nontraffic V56.1
          stationary object (traffic) V57.6
            nontraffic V57.1
          streetcar (traffic) V56.6
            nontraffic V56.1
          three wheeled motor vehicle
            (traffic) V52.6
            nontraffic V52.1
          truck (traffic) V54.6
            nontraffic V54.1
          two wheeled motor vehicle (traffic)
            V52.6
            nontraffic V52.1
          van (traffic) V53.6
            nontraffic V53.1
        noncollision accident (traffic) V58.6
          nontraffic V58.1
        specified type NEC V59.88
        military vehicle V59.81
    watercraft occupant —*see* Accident,
      watercraft
   vehicle NEC V89.9
    animal-drawn NEC —*see* Accident,
      transport, animal-drawn vehicle
      occupant
    special
      agricultural —*see* Accident, transport,
        agricultural vehicle occupant
      construction —*see* Accident, transport,
        construction vehicle occupant
      industrial —*see* Accident, transport,
        industrial vehicle occupant
      three-wheeled NEC (motorized) —*see*
        Accident, transport, three-wheeled
        motor vehicle occupant

Accident *(Continued)*
  watercraft V94.9
    causing
      drowning —*see* Drowning, due to,
        accident to, watercraft ◄
      injury NEC V91.89
        crushed between craft and object
          V91.19
        powered craft V91.13
          ferry boat V91.11
          fishing boat V91.12
          jetskis V91.13
          liner V91.11
          merchant ship V91.10
          passenger ship V91.11
        unpowered craft V91.18
          canoe V91.15
          inflatable V91.16
          kayak V91.15
          sailboat V91.14
          surf-board V91.18
          windsurfer V91.18
      fall on board V91.29
        powered craft V91.23
          ferry boat V91.21
          fishing boat V91.22
          jetskis V91.23
          liner V91.21
          merchant ship V91.20
          passenger ship V91.21
        unpowered craft
          canoe V91.25
          inflatable V91.26
          kayak V91.25
          sailboat V91.24
      fire on board causing burn V91.09
        powered craft V91.03
          ferry boat V91.01
          fishing boat V91.02
          jetskis V91.03
          liner V91.01
          merchant ship V91.00
          passenger ship V91.01
        unpowered craft V91.08
          canoe V91.05
          inflatable V91.06
          kayak V91.05
          sailboat V91.04
          surf-board V91.08
          water skis V91.07
          windsurfer V91.08
      hit by falling object V91.39
        powered craft V91.33
          ferry boat V91.31
          fishing boat V91.32
          jetskis V91.33
          liner V91.31
          merchant ship V91.30
          passenger ship V91.31
        unpowered craft V91.38
          canoe V91.35
          inflatable V91.36
          kayak V91.35
          sailboat V91.34
          surf-board V91.38
          water skis V91.37
          windsurfer V91.38
      specified type NEC V91.89
        powered craft V91.83
          ferry boat V91.81
          fishing boat V91.82
          jetskis V91.83
          liner V91.81
          merchant ship V91.80
          passenger ship V91.81
        unpowered craft V91.88
          canoe V91.85
          inflatable V91.86
          kayak V91.85
          sailboat V91.84
          surf-board V91.88

Accident *(Continued)*
  watercraft *(Continued)*
    causing *(Continued)*
      injury NEC *(Continued)*
        specified type NEC *(Continued)*
          unpowered craft *(Continued)*
            water skis V91.87
            windsurfer V91.88
      due to, caused by cataclysm —*see* Forces of
        nature, by type
      military NEC V94.818
        with civilian watercraft V94.810
        civilian in water injured by V94.811
      nonpowered, struck by
        nonpowered vessel V94.22
        powered vessel V94.21
      specified type NEC V94.89
      striking swimmer
        powered V94.11
        unpowered V94.12
Acid throwing (assault) Y08.89
Activity (involving) (of victim at time of event)
  Y93.9
  aerobic and step exercise (class) Y93.A3
  alpine skiing Y93.23
  animal care NEC Y93.K9
  arts and handcrafts NEC Y93.D9
  athletics NEC Y93.79
  athletics played as a team or group NEC
    Y93.69
  athletics played individually NEC Y93.59
  baking Y93.G3
  ballet Y93.41
  barbells Y93.B3
  BASE (Building, Antenna, Span, Earth)
    jumping Y93.33
  baseball Y93.64
  basketball Y93.67
  bathing (personal) Y93.E1
  beach volleyball Y93.68
  bike riding Y93.55
  blackout game Y93.85 ◄
  boogie boarding Y93.18
  bowling Y93.54
  boxing Y93.71
  brass instrument playing Y93.J4
  building construction Y93.H3
  bungee jumping Y93.34
  calisthenics Y93.A2
  canoeing (in calm and turbulent water) Y93.16
  capture the flag Y93.6A
  cardiorespiratory exercise NEC Y93.A9
  caregiving (providing) NEC Y93.F9
    bathing Y93.F1
    lifting Y93.F2
  cellular
    communication device Y93.C2
    telephone Y93.C2
  challenge course Y93.A5
  cheerleading Y93.45
  choking game Y93.85 ◄
  circuit training Y93.A4
  cleaning
    floor Y93.E5
  climbing NEC Y93.39
    mountain Y93.31
    rock Y93.31
    wall Y93.31
  clothing care and maintenance NEC Y93.E9
  combatives Y93.75
  computer
    keyboarding Y93.C1
    technology NEC Y93.C9
  confidence course Y93.A5
  construction (building) Y93.H3
  cooking and baking Y93.G3
  cool down exercises Y93.A2
  cricket Y93.69
  crocheting Y93.D1
  cross country skiing Y93.24
  dancing (all types) Y93.41

◄ New   ◄▥ Revised   ~~deleted~~ Deleted

Activity *(Continued)*
- digging
  - dirt Y93.H1
- dirt digging Y93.H1
- dishwashing Y93.G1
- diving (platform) (springboard) Y93.12
  - underwater Y93.15
- dodge ball Y93.6A
- downhill skiing Y93.23
- drum playing Y93.J2
- dumbbells Y93.B3
- electronic
  - devices NEC Y93.C9
    - hand held interactive Y93.C2
  - game playing (using) (with)
    - interactive device Y93.C2
    - keyboard or other stationary device Y93.C1
- elliptical machine Y93.A1
- exercise (s)
  - machines ((primarily) for)
    - cardiorespiratory conditioning Y93.A1
    - muscle strengthening Y93.B1
  - muscle strengthening (non-machine) NEC Y93.B9
- external motion NEC Y93.I9
  - rollercoaster Y93.I1
- fainting game Y93.85 ◄
- field hockey Y93.65
- figure skating (pairs) (singles) Y93.21
- flag football Y93.62
- floor mopping and cleaning Y93.E5
- food preparation and clean up Y93.G1
- football (American) NOS Y93.61
  - flag Y93.62
  - tackle Y93.61
  - touch Y93.62
- four square Y93.6A
- free weights Y93.B3
- frisbee (ultimate) Y93.74
- furniture
  - building Y93.D3
  - finishing Y93.D3
  - repair Y93.D3
- game playing (electronic)
  - using interactive device Y93.C2
  - using keyboard or other stationary device Y93.C1
- gardening Y93.H2
- golf Y93.53
- grass drills Y93.A6
- grilling and smoking food Y93.G2
- grooming and shearing an animal Y93.K3
- guerilla drills Y93.A6
- gymnastics (rhythmic) Y93.43
- hand held interactive electronic device Y93.C2
- handball Y93.73
- handcrafts NEC Y93.D9
- hang gliding Y93.35
- hiking (on level or elevated terrain) Y93.Ø1
- hockey (ice) Y93.22
  - field Y93.65
- horseback riding Y93.52
- household (interior) maintenance NEC Y93. E9
- ice NEC Y93.29
  - dancing Y93.21
  - hockey Y93.22
  - skating Y93.21
- inline roller skating Y93.51
- ironing Y93.E4
- judo Y93.75
- jumping (off) NEC Y93.39
  - BASE (Building, Antenna, Span, Earth) Y93.33
  - bungee Y93.34
  - jacks Y93.A2
  - rope Y93.56
- jumping jacks Y93.A2
- jumping rope Y93.56
- karate Y93.75

Activity *(Continued)*
- kayaking (in calm and turbulent water) Y93.16
- keyboarding (computer) Y93.C1
- kickball Y93.6A
- knitting Y93.D1
- lacrosse Y93.65
- land maintenance NEC Y93.H9
- landscaping Y93.H2
- laundry Y93.E2
- machines (exercise)
  - primarily for cardiorespiratory conditioning Y93.A1
  - primarily for muscle strengthening Y93.B1
- maintenance
  - exterior building NEC Y93.H9
  - household (interior) NEC Y93.E9
  - land Y93.H9
  - property Y93.H9
- marching (on level or elevated terrain) Y93.Ø1
- martial arts Y93.75
- microwave oven Y93.G3
- milking an animal Y93.K2
- mopping (floor) Y93.E5
- mountain climbing Y93.31
- muscle strengthening
  - exercises (non-machine) NEC Y93.B9
  - machines Y93.B1
- musical keyboard (electronic) playing Y93.J1
- nordic skiing Y93.24
- obstacle course Y93.A5
- oven (microwave) Y93.G3
- packing up and unpacking in moving to a new residence Y93.E6
- parasailing Y93.19
- pass out game Y93.85 ◄
- percussion instrument playing NEC Y93.J2
- personal
  - bathing and showering Y93.E1
  - hygiene NEC Y93.E8
  - showering Y93.E1
- physical games generally associated with school recess, summer camp and children Y93.6A
- physical training NEC Y93.A9
- piano playing Y93.J1
- pilates Y93.B4
- platform diving Y93.12
- playing musical instrument
  - brass instrument Y93.J4
  - drum Y93.J2
  - musical keyboard (electronic) Y93.J1
  - percussion instrument NEC Y93.J2
  - piano Y93.J1
  - string instrument Y93.J3
  - winds instrument Y93.J4
- property maintenance
  - exterior NEC Y93.H9
  - interior NEC Y93.E9
- pruning (garden and lawn) Y93.H2
- pull-ups Y93.B2
- push-ups Y93.B2
- racquetball Y93.73
- rafting (in calm and turbulent water) Y93.16
- raking (leaves) Y93.H1
- rappelling Y93.32
- refereeing a sports activity Y93.81
- residential relocation Y93.E6
- rhythmic gymnastics Y93.43
- rhythmic movement NEC Y93.49
- riding
  - horseback Y93.52
  - rollercoaster Y93.I1
- rock climbing Y93.31
- roller skating (inline) Y93.51
- rollercoaster riding Y93.I1
- rough housing and horseplay Y93.83
- rowing (in calm and turbulent water) Y93.16
- rugby Y93.63
- SCUBA diving Y93.15
- sewing Y93.D2

Activity *(Continued)*
- shoveling Y93.H1
  - dirt Y93.H1
  - snow Y93.H1
- showering (personal) Y93.E1
- sit-ups Y93.B2
- skateboarding Y93.51
- skating (ice) Y93.21
  - roller Y93.51
- skiing (alpine) (downhill) Y93.23
  - cross country Y93.24
  - nordic Y93.24
  - water Y93.17
- sledding (snow) Y93.23
- sleeping (sleep) Y93.84
- smoking and grilling food Y93.G2
- snorkeling Y93.15
- snow NEC Y93.29
  - boarding Y93.23
  - shoveling Y93.H1
  - sledding Y93.23
  - tubing Y93.23
- soccer Y93.66
- softball Y93.64
- specified NEC Y93.89
- spectator at an event Y93.82
- sports NEC Y93.79
  - sports played as a team or group NEC Y93.69
  - sports played individually NEC Y93.59
- springboard diving Y93.12
- squash Y93.73
- stationary bike Y93.A1
- step (stepping) exercise (class) Y93.A3
- stepper machine Y93.A1
- stove Y93.G3
- string instrument playing Y93.J3
- surfing Y93.18
  - wind Y93.18
- swimming Y93.11
- tackle football Y93.61
- tap dancing Y93.41
- tennis Y93.73
- tobogganing Y93.23
- touch football Y93.62
- track and field events (non-running) Y93.57
  - running Y93.Ø2
- trampoline Y93.44
- treadmill Y93.A1
- trimming shrubs Y93.H2
- tubing (in calm and turbulent water) Y93.16
  - snow Y93.23
- ultimate frisbee Y93.74
- underwater diving Y93.15
- unpacking in moving to a new residence Y93.E6
- use of stove, oven and microwave oven Y93. G3
- vacuuming Y93.E3
- volleyball (beach) (court) Y93.68
- wake boarding Y93.17
- walking (on level or elevated terrain) Y93.Ø1
  - an animal Y93.K1
- walking an animal Y93.K1
- wall climbing Y93.31
- warm up and cool down exercises Y93.A2
- water NEC Y93.19
  - aerobics Y93.14
  - craft NEC Y93.19
  - exercise Y93.14
  - polo Y93.13
  - skiing Y93.17
  - sliding Y93.18
  - survival training and testing Y93.19
- weeding (garden and lawn) Y93.H2
- wind instrument playing Y93.J4
- windsurfing Y93.18
- wrestling Y93.72
- yoga Y93.42

Adverse effect of drugs —*see* Table of Drugs and Chemicals

A

Aerosinusitis —*see* Air, pressure
After-effect, late —*see* Sequelae
Air
  blast in war operations —*see* War operations,
    air blast
  pressure
    change, rapid
      during
        ascent W94.29
          while (in) (surfacing from)
            aircraft W94.23
            deep water diving W94.21
            underground W94.22
        descent W94.39
          in
            aircraft W94.31
            water W94.32
    high, prolonged W94.0
    low, prolonged W94.12
      due to residence or long visit at high
        altitude W94.11
Alpine sickness W94.11
Altitude sickness W94.11
Anaphylactic shock, anaphylaxis —*see* Table of
  Drugs and Chemicals ◄░░
Andes disease W94.11
Arachnidism, arachnoidism X58
Arson (with intent to injure or kill) X97
Asphyxia, asphyxiation
  by
    food (bone) (seed) —*see* categories T17
      and T18
    gas —*see also* Table of Drugs and
      Chemicals ◄░░
      legal
        execution —*see* Legal, intervention,
          gas
        intervention —*see* Legal, intervention,
          gas
  from
    fire —*see also* Exposure, fire
      in war operations —*see* War operations,
        fire
    ignition —*see* Ignition
    vomitus T17.81
  in war operations —*see* War operations,
    restriction of airway
Aspiration
  food (any type) (into respiratory tract) (with
    asphyxia, obstruction respiratory tract,
    suffocation) —*see* categories T17 and T18
  foreign body —*see* Foreign body, aspiration
  vomitus (with asphyxia, obstruction
    respiratory tract, suffocation) T17.81
Assassination (attempt) —*see* Assault
Assault (homicidal) (by) (in) Y09
  arson X97
  bite (of human being) Y04.1
  bodily force Y04.8
    bite Y04.1
    bumping into Y04.2
    sexual —*see* subcategories T74.0, T76.0
    unarmed fight Y04.0

Assault *(Continued)*
  bomb X96.9
    antipersonnel X96.0
    fertilizer X96.3
    gasoline X96.1
    letter X96.2
    petrol X96.1
    pipe X96.3
    specified NEC X96.8
  brawl (hand) (fists) (foot) (unarmed) Y04.0
  burning, burns (by fire) NEC X97
    acid Y08.89
    caustic, corrosive substance Y08.89
    chemical from swallowing caustic,
      corrosive substance —*see* Table of
      Drugs and Chemicals ◄░░
    cigarette(s) X97
    hot object X98.9
      fluid NEC X98.2
      household appliance X98.3
      specified NEC X98.8
      steam X98.0
      tap water X98.1
      vapors X98.0
    scalding —*see* Assault, burning
    steam X98.0
    vitriol Y08.89
  caustic, corrosive substance (gas) Y08.89
  crashing of
    aircraft Y08.81
    motor vehicle Y03.8
      pushed in front of Y02.0
      run over Y03.0
      specified NEC Y03.8
  cutting or piercing instrument X99.9
    dagger X99.2
    glass X99.0
    knife X99.1
    specified NEC X99.8
    sword X99.2
  dagger X99.2
  drowning (in) X92.9
    bathtub X92.0
    natural water X92.3
    specified NEC X92.8
    swimming pool X92.1
      following fall X92.2
  dynamite X96.8
  explosive (s) (material) X96.9
  fight (hand) (fists) (foot) (unarmed) Y04.0
    with weapon —*see* Assault, by type of
      weapon
  fire X97
  firearm X95.9
    airgun X95.01
    handgun X93
    hunting rifle X94.1
    larger X94.9
      specified NEC X94.8
    machine gun X94.2
    shotgun X94.0
    specified NEC X95.8

Assault *(Continued)*
  from high place Y01
  gunshot (wound) NEC —*see* Assault, firearm,
    by type
  incendiary device X97
  injury Y09
    to child due to criminal abortion attempt
      NEC Y08.89
  knife X99.1
  late effect of —*see* X92-Y08 with 7th character
    S
  placing before moving object NEC Y02.8
    motor vehicle Y02.0
  poisoning —*see* categories T36-T65 with 7th
    character S
  puncture, any part of body —*see* Assault,
    cutting or piercing instrument
  pushing
    before moving object NEC Y02.8
      motor vehicle Y02.0
      subway train Y02.1
      train Y02.1
  rape T74.2-
  scalding —*see* Assault, burning
  sequelae of —*see* X92-Y08 with 7th character
    S
  sexual (by bodily force) T74.2-
  shooting —*see* Assault, firearm
  specified means NEC Y08.89
  stab, any part of body —*see* Assault, cutting
    or piercing instrument
  steam X98.0
  striking against
    other person Y04.2
    sports equipment Y08.09
      baseball bat Y08.02
      hockey stick Y08.01
  struck by
    sports equipment Y08.09
      baseball bat Y08.02
      hockey stick Y08.01
  submersion —*see* Assault, drowning
  violence Y09
  weapon Y09
    blunt Y00
    cutting or piercing —*see* Assault, cutting or
      piercing instrument
    firearm —*see* Assault, firearm
  wound Y09
    cutting —*see* Assault, cutting or piercing
      instrument
    gunshot —*see* Assault, firearm
    knife X99.1
    piercing —*see* Assault, cutting or piercing
      instrument
    puncture —*see* Assault, cutting or piercing
      instrument
    stab —*see* Assault, cutting or piercing
      instrument
Attack by mammals NEC W55.89
Avalanche —*see* Landslide ◄
Aviator's disease —*see* Air, pressure

◄ New   ◄░░ Revised   ~~deleted~~ Deleted

B

Barotitis, barodontalgia, barosinusitis, barotrauma (otitic) (sinus) —see Air, pressure
Battered (baby) (child) (person) (syndrome) X58
Bayonet wound W26.1
  in
    legal intervention —see Legal, intervention, sharp object, bayonet
    war operations —see War operations, combat
  stated as undetermined whether accidental or intentional Y28.8
  suicide (attempt) X78.2
Bean in nose —see categories T17 and T18
Bed set on fire NEC —see Exposure, fire, uncontrolled, building, bed
Beheading (by guillotine)
  homicide X99.9
  legal execution —see Legal, intervention
Bending, injury in (prolonged) (static) X50.1 ◀▥▥
Bends —see Air, pressure, change
Bite, bitten by
  alligator W58.01
  arthropod (nonvenomous) NEC W57
  bull W55.21
  cat W55.01
  cow W55.21
  crocodile W58.11
  dog W54.0
  goat W55.31
  hoof stock NEC W55.31
  horse W55.11
  human being (accidentally) W50.3
    with intent to injure or kill Y04.1
    as, or caused by a crowd or human stampede (with fall) W52
    assault Y04.1
    homicide (attempt) Y04.1
    in
      fight Y04.1
  insect (nonvenomous) W57
  lizard (nonvenomous) W59.01
  mammal NEC W55.81
    marine W56.31 ◀
  marine animal (nonvenomous) W56.81
  millipede W57
  moray eel W56.51
  mouse W53.01
  person (s) (accidentally) W50.3
    with intent to injure or kill Y04.1
    as, or caused by a crowd or human stampede (with fall) W52
    assault Y04.1
    homicide (attempt) Y04.1
    in
      fight Y04.1
  pig W55.41
  raccoon W55.51
  rat W53.11
  reptile W59.81
    lizard W59.01
    snake W59.11
    turtle W59.21
      terrestrial W59.81
  rodent W53.81
    mouse W53.01
    rat W53.11
    specified NEC W53.81
    squirrel W53.21
  shark W56.41
  sheep W55.31
  snake (nonvenomous) W59.11
  spider (nonvenomous) W57
  squirrel W53.21
Blast (air) in war operations —see War operations, blast
Blizzard X37.2

Blood alcohol level Y90.9
  20-39mg/100ml Y90.1
  40-59mg/100ml Y90.2
  60-79mg/100ml Y90.3
  80-99mg/100ml Y90.4
  100-119mg/100ml Y90.5
  120-199mg/100ml Y90.6
  200-239mg/100ml Y90.7
  less than 20mg/100ml Y90.0
  presence in blood, level not specified Y90.9
Blow X58
  by law-enforcing agent, police (on duty) —see Legal, intervention, manhandling
    blunt object —see Legal, intervention, blunt object
Blowing up —see Explosion
Brawl (hand) (fists) (foot) Y04.0
Breakage (accidental) (part of)
  ladder (causing fall) W11
  scaffolding (causing fall) W12
Broken
  glass, contact with —see Contact, with, glass
  power line (causing electric shock) W85
Bumping against, into (accidentally)
  object NEC W22.8
    with fall —see Fall, due to, bumping against, object
    caused by crowd or human stampede (with fall) W52
    sports equipment W21.9
  person (s) W51
    with fall W03
      due to ice or snow W00.0
    assault Y04.2
    caused by, a crowd or human stampede (with fall) W52
    homicide (attempt) Y04.2
  sports equipment W21.9
Burn, burned, burning (accidental) (by) (from) (on)
  acid NEC —see Table of Drugs and Chemicals ◀▥▥
  bed linen —see Exposure, fire, uncontrolled, in building, bed
  blowtorch X08.8
    with ignition of clothing NEC X06.2
      nightwear X05
  bonfire, campfire (controlled) —see also Exposure, fire, controlled, not in building
    uncontrolled —see Exposure, fire, uncontrolled, not in building
  candle X08.8
    with ignition of clothing NEC X06.2
      nightwear X05
  caustic liquid, substance (external) (internal) NEC —see Table of Drugs and Chemicals ◀▥▥
  chemical (external) (internal) —see also Table of Drugs and Chemicals ◀▥▥
    in war operations —see War operations, fire
  cigar (s) or cigarette (s) X08.8
    with ignition of clothing NEC X06.2
      nightwear X05
  clothes, clothing NEC (from controlled fire) X06.2
    with conflagration —see Exposure, fire, uncontrolled, building
    not in building or structure —see Exposure, fire, uncontrolled, not in building
  cooker (hot) X15.8
    stated as undetermined whether accidental or intentional Y27.3
    suicide (attempt) X77.3
  electric blanket X16
  engine (hot) X17
  fire, flames —see Exposure, fire
  flare, Very pistol —see Discharge, firearm NEC

Burn, burned, burning (Continued)
  heat
    from appliance (electrical) (household) X15.8
      cooker X15.8
      hotplate X15.2
      kettle X15.8
      light bulb X15.8
      saucepan X15.3
      skillet X15.3
      stated as undetermined whether accidental or intentional Y27.3
      stove X15.0
      suicide (attempt) X77.3
      toaster X15.1
    in local application or packing during medical or surgical procedure Y63.5
  heating
    appliance, radiator or pipe X16
  homicide (attempt) —see Assault, burning
  hot
    air X14.1
    cooker X15.8
    drink X10.0
    engine X17
    fat X10.2
    fluid NEC X12
    food X10.1
    gases X14.1
    heating appliance X16
    household appliance NEC X15.8
    kettle X15.8
    liquid NEC X12
    machinery X17
    metal (molten) (liquid) NEC X18
    object (not producing fire or flames) NEC X19
    oil (cooking) X10.2
    pipe (s) X16
    radiator X16
    saucepan (glass) (metal) X15.3
    stove (kitchen) X15.0
    substance NEC X19
      caustic or corrosive NEC —see Table of Drugs and Chemicals ◀▥▥
    toaster X15.1
    tool X17
    vapor X13.1
    water (tap) —see Contact, with, hot, tap water
  hotplate X15.2
    suicide (attempt) X77.3
  ignition —see Ignition
  in war operations —see War operations, fire
  inflicted by other person X97
    by hot objects, hot vapor, and steam —see Assault, burning, hot object
  internal, from swallowed caustic, corrosive liquid, substance —see Table of Drugs and Chemicals ◀▥▥
  iron (hot) X15.8
    stated as undetermined whether accidental or intentional Y27.3
    suicide (attempt) X77.3
  kettle (hot) X15.8
    stated as undetermined whether accidental or intentional Y27.3
    suicide (attempt) X77.3
  lamp (flame) X08.8
    with ignition of clothing NEC X06.2
      nightwear X05
  lighter (cigar) (cigarette) X08.8
    with ignition of clothing NEC X06.2
      nightwear X05
  lightning —see subcategory T75.0
    causing fire —see Exposure, fire
  liquid (boiling) (hot) NEC X12
    stated as undetermined whether accidental or intentional Y27.2
    suicide (attempt) X77.2

Burn, burned, burning (*Continued*)
 local application of externally applied
  substance in medical or surgical care
  Y63.5
 machinery (hot) X17
 matches X08.8
  with ignition of clothing NEC X06.2
   nightwear X05
 mattress —*see* Exposure, fire, uncontrolled,
  building, bed
 medicament, externally applied Y63.5
 metal (hot) (liquid) (molten) NEC X18
 nightwear (nightclothes, nightdress, gown,
  pajamas, robe) X05
 object (hot) NEC X19
 on board watercraft
  due to
   accident to watercraft V91.09
    powered craft V91.03
     ferry boat V91.01
     fishing boat V91.02
     jetskis V91.03
     liner V91.01
     merchant ship V91.00
     passenger ship V91.01
    unpowered craft V91.08
     canoe V91.05
     inflatable V91.06
     kayak V91.05
     sailboat V91.04
     surf-board V91.08
     water skis V91.07
     windsurfer V91.08
   fire on board V93.09
    ferry boat V93.01
    fishing boat V93.02
    jetskis V93.03
    liner V93.01
    merchant ship V93.00
    passenger ship V93.01
    powered craft NEC V93.03
    sailboat V93.04

Burn, burned, burning (*Continued*)
 on board watercraft (*Continued*)
  due to (*Continued*)
   specified heat source NEC on board
    V93.19
    ferry boat V93.11
    fishing boat V93.12
    jetskis V93.13
    liner V93.11
    merchant ship V93.10
    passenger ship V93.11
    powered craft NEC V93.13
    sailboat V93.14
 pipe (hot) X16
  smoking X08.8
   with ignition of clothing NEC X06.2
    nightwear X05
 powder —*see* Powder burn
 radiator (hot) X16
 saucepan (hot) (glass) (metal) X15.3
  stated as undetermined whether
   accidental or intentional
   Y27.3
  suicide (attempt) X77.3
 self-inflicted X76
  stated as undetermined whether
   accidental or intentional
   Y26
 stated as undetermined whether
  accidental or intentional Y27.0
 steam X13.1
  pipe X16
  stated as undetermined whether
   accidental or intentional
   Y27.8
  stated as undetermined whether
   accidental or intentional Y27.0
  suicide (attempt) X77.0
 stove (hot) (kitchen) X15.0
  stated as undetermined whether
   accidental or intentional Y27.3
  suicide (attempt) X77.3

Burn, burned, burning (*Continued*)
 substance (hot) NEC X19
  boiling X12
   stated as undetermined whether
    accidental or intentional Y27.2
   suicide (attempt) X77.2
  molten (metal) X18
 suicide (attempt) NEC X76
  hot
   household appliance X77.3
   object X77.9
 stated as undetermined whether accidental or
  intentional Y27.0
 therapeutic misadventure
  heat in local application or packing during
   medical or surgical procedure Y63.5
  overdose of radiation Y63.2
 toaster (hot) X15.1
  stated as undetermined whether accidental
   or intentional Y27.3
  suicide (attempt) X77.3
 tool (hot) X17
 torch, welding X08.8
  with ignition of clothing NEC X06.2
   nightwear X05
 trash fire (controlled) —*see* Exposure, fire,
  controlled, not in building
  uncontrolled —*see* Exposure, fire,
   uncontrolled, not in building
 vapor (hot) X13.1
  stated as undetermined whether accidental
   or intentional Y27.0
  suicide (attempt) X77.0
 Very pistol —*see* Discharge, firearm NEC
Butted by animal W55.82
 bull W55.22
 cow W55.22
 goat W55.32
 horse W55.12
 pig W55.42
 sheep W55.32

◀ New ◀▥▥ Revised ~~deleted~~ Deleted

C

Caisson disease —*see* Air, pressure, change
Campfire (exposure to) (controlled) —*see also* Exposure, fire, controlled, not in building
  uncontrolled —*see* Exposure, fire, uncontrolled, not in building
Capital punishment (any means) —*see* Legal, intervention
Car sickness T75.3
Casualty (not due to war) NEC X58
  war —*see* War operations
Cat
  bite W55.01
  scratch W55.03
Cataclysm, cataclysmic (any injury) NEC —*see* Forces of nature
Catching fire —*see* Exposure, fire
Caught
  between
    folding object W23.0
    objects (moving) (stationary and moving) W23.0
      and machinery —*see* Contact, with, by type of machine
      stationary W23.1
    sliding door and door frame W23.0
  by, in
    machinery (moving parts of) —*see* Contact, with, by type of machine
    washing-machine wringer W23.0
    under packing crate (due to losing grip) W23.1
Cave-in caused by cataclysmic earth surface movement or eruption —*see* Landslide
Change(s) in air pressure —*see* Air, pressure, change
Choked, choking (on) (any object except food or vomitus)
  food (bone) (seed) —*see* categories T17 and T18
  vomitus T17.81-
Civil insurrection —*see* War operations
Cloudburst (any injury) X37.8
Cold, exposure to (accidental) (excessive) (extreme) (natural) (place) NEC —*see* Exposure, cold
Collapse
  building W20.1
    burning (uncontrolled fire) X00.2
  dam or man-made structure (causing earth movement) X36.0
  machinery —*see* Contact, with, by type of machine
  structure W20.1
    burning (uncontrolled fire) X00.2
Collision (accidental) NEC —*see also* Accident, transport V89.9
  pedestrian W51
    with fall W03
      due to ice or snow W00.0
      involving pedestrian conveyance —*see* Accident, transport, pedestrian, conveyance
    and
      crowd or human stampede (with fall) W52
      object W22.8
        with fall —*see* Fall, due to, bumping against, object
  person (s) —*see* Collision, pedestrian
  transport vehicle NEC V89.9
    and
      avalanche, fallen or not moving —*see* Accident, transport
      falling or moving —*see* Landslide ◀
      landslide, fallen or not moving —*see* Accident, transport
      falling or moving —*see* Landslide

Collision NEC *(Continued)*
  transport vehicle NEC *(Continued)*
    due to cataclysm —*see* Forces of nature, by type
    intentional, purposeful suicide (attempt) —*see* Suicide, collision
Combustion, spontaneous —*see* Ignition
Complication (delayed) of or following
  (medical or surgical procedure) Y84.9
  with misadventure —*see* Misadventure
  amputation of limb (s) Y83.5
  anastomosis (arteriovenous) (blood vessel) (gastrojejunal) (tendon) (natural or artificial material) Y83.2
  aspiration (of fluid) Y84.4
    tissue Y84.8
  biopsy Y84.8
  blood
    sampling Y84.7
    transfusion
      procedure Y84.8
  bypass Y83.2
  catheterization (urinary) Y84.6
    cardiac Y84.0
  colostomy Y83.3
  cystostomy Y83.3
  dialysis (kidney) Y84.1
  drug —*see* Table of Drugs and Chemicals ◀▥
  due to misadventure —*see* Misadventure
  duodenostomy Y83.3
  electroshock therapy Y84.3
  external stoma, creation of Y83.3
  formation of external stoma Y83.3
  gastrostomy Y83.3
  graft Y83.2
  hypothermia (medically-induced) Y84.8
  implant, implantation (of)
    artificial
      internal device (cardiac pacemaker) (electrodes in brain) (heart valve prosthesis) (orthopedic) Y83.1
      material or tissue (for anastomosis or bypass) Y83.2
        with creation of external stoma Y83.3
    natural tissues (for anastomosis or bypass) Y83.2
      with creation of external stoma Y83.3
  infusion
    procedure Y84.8
  injection —*see* Table of Drugs and Chemicals ◀▥
    procedure Y84.8
  insertion of gastric or duodenal sound Y84.5
  insulin-shock therapy Y84.3
  paracentesis (abdominal) (thoracic) (aspirative) Y84.4
  procedures other than surgical operation —*see* Complication of or following, by type of procedure
  radiological procedure or therapy Y84.2
  removal of organ (partial) (total) NEC Y83.6
  sampling
    blood Y84.7
    fluid NEC Y84.4
    tissue Y84.8
  shock therapy Y84.3
  surgical operation NEC —*see also* Complication of or following, by type of operation Y83.9
    reconstructive NEC Y83.4
      with
        anastomosis, bypass or graft Y83.2
        formation of external stoma Y83.3
    specified NEC Y83.8
  transfusion —*see also* Table of Drugs and Chemicals ◀▥
    procedure Y84.8
  transplant, transplantation (heart) (kidney) (liver) (whole organ, any) Y83.0
    partial organ Y83.4
  ureterostomy Y83.3

Complication of or following *(Continued)*
  vaccination —*see also* Table of Drugs and Chemicals ◀▥
    procedure Y84.8
Compression
  divers' squeeze —*see* Air, pressure, change
  trachea by
    food (lodged in esophagus) —*see* categories T17 and T18
    vomitus (lodged in esophagus) T17.81-
Conflagration —*see* Exposure, fire, uncontrolled
Constriction (external)
  hair W49.01
  jewelry W49.04
  ring W49.04
  rubber band W49.03
  specified item NEC W49.09
  string W49.02
  thread W49.02
Contact (accidental)
  with
    abrasive wheel (metalworking) W31.1
    alligator W58.09
      bite W58.01
      crushing W58.03
      strike W58.02
    amphibian W62.9
      frog W62.0
      toad W62.1
    animal (nonvenomous) NEC W64
      marine W56.89
        bite W56.81
        dolphin —*see* Contact, with, dolphin
        fish NEC —*see* Contact, with, fish
        mammal —*see* Contact, with, mammal, marine
        orca —*see* Contact, with, orca
        sea lion —*see* Contact, with, sea lion
        shark —*see* Contact, with, shark
        strike W56.82
    animate mechanical force NEC W64
    arrow W21.89
      not thrown, projected or falling W45.8
    arthropods (nonvenomous) W57
    axe W27.0
    band-saw (industrial) W31.2
    bayonet —*see* Bayonet wound
    bee (s) X58
    bench-saw (industrial) W31.2
    bird W61.99
      bite W61.91
      chicken —*see* Contact, with, chicken
      duck —*see* Contact, with, duck
      goose —*see* Contact, with, goose
      macaw —*see* Contact, with, macaw
      parrot —*see* Contact, with, parrot
      psittacine —*see* Contact, with, psittacine
      strike W61.92
      turkey —*see* Contact, with, turkey
    blender W29.0
    boiling water X12
      stated as undetermined whether accidental or intentional Y27.2
      suicide (attempt) X77.2
    bore, earth-drilling or mining (land) (seabed) W31.0
    buffalo —*see* Contact, with, hoof stock NEC
    bull W55.29
      bite W55.21
      gored W55.22
      strike W55.22
    bumper cars W31.81
    camel —*see* Contact, with, hoof stock NEC
    can
      lid W26.8 ◀▥
      opener W27.4
        powered W29.0
    cat W55.09
      bite W55.01
      scratch W55.03
    caterpillar (venomous) X58

Contact *(Continued)*
  with *(Continued)*
    centipede (venomous) X58
    chain
      hoist W24.0
        agricultural operations W30.89
      saw W29.3
    chicken W61.39
      peck W61.33
      strike W61.32
    chisel W27.0
    circular saw W31.2
    cobra X58
    combine (harvester) W30.0
    conveyer belt W24.1
    cooker (hot) X15.8
      stated as undetermined whether
        accidental or intentional Y27.3
      suicide (attempt) X77.3
    coral X58
    cotton gin W31.82
    cow W55.29
      bite W55.21
      strike W55.22
    crane W24.0
      agricultural operations W30.89
    crocodile W58.19
      bite W58.11
      crushing W58.13
      strike W58.12
    dagger W26.1
      stated as undetermined whether
        accidental or intentional Y28.2
      suicide (attempt) X78.2
    dairy equipment W31.82
    dart W21.89
      not thrown, projected or falling W45.8
    deer —*see* Contact, with, hoof stock
      NEC
    derrick W24.0
      agricultural operations W30.89
        hay W30.2
    dog W54.8
      bite W54.0
      strike W54.1
    dolphin W56.09
      bite W56.01
      strike W56.02
    donkey —*see* Contact, with, hoof stock
      NEC
    drill (powered) W29.8
      earth (land) (seabed) W31.0
      nonpowered W27.8
    drive belt W24.0
      agricultural operations W30.89
    dry ice —*see* Exposure, cold, man-made
    dryer (clothes) (powered) (spin) W29.2
    duck W61.69
      bite W61.61
      strike W61.62
    earth(-)
      drilling machine (industrial) W31.0
      scraping machine in stationary use
        W31.83
    edge of stiff paper W26.2 ◄▥▥
    electric
      beater W29.0
      blanket X16
      fan W29.2
        commercial W31.82
      knife W29.1
      mixer W29.0
    elevator (building) W24.0
      agricultural operations W30.89
        grain W30.3
    engine (s), hot NEC X17
    excavating machine W31.0
    farm machine W30.9
    feces —*see* Contact, with, by type of
      animal
    fer de lance X58

Contact *(Continued)*
  with *(Continued)*
    fish W56.59
      bite W56.51
      shark —*see* Contact, with, shark
      strike W56.52
    flying horses W31.81
    forging (metalworking) machine
      W31.1
    fork W27.4
    forklift (truck) W24.0
      agricultural operations W30.89
    frog W62.0
    garden
      cultivator (powered) W29.3
        riding W30.89
      fork W27.1
    gas turbine W31.3
    Gila monster X58
    giraffe —*see* Contact, with, hoof stock
      NEC
    glass (sharp) (broken) W25
      with subsequent fall W18.02
      assault X99.0
      due to fall —*see* Fall, by type
      stated as undetermined whether
        accidental or intentional Y28. 0
      suicide (attempt) X78.0
    goat W55.39
      bite W55.31
      strike W55.32
    goose W61.59
      bite W61.51
      strike W61.52
    hand
      saw W27.0
      tool (not powered) NEC W27.8
        powered W29.8
    harvester W30.0
    hay-derrick W30.2
    heat NEC X19
      from appliance (electrical)
        (household) —*see* Contact, with,
        hot, household appliance
      heating appliance X16
    heating
      appliance (hot) X16
      pad (electric) X16
    hedge-trimmer (powered) W29.3
    hoe W27.1
    hoist (chain) (shaft) NEC W24.0
      agricultural W30.89
    hoof stock NEC W55.39
      bite W55.31
      strike W55.32
    hornet (s) X58
    horse W55.19
      bite W55.11
      strike W55.12
    hot
      air X14.1
        inhalation X14.0
      cooker X15.8
      drinks X10.0
      engine X17
      fats X10.2
      fluids NEC X12
        assault X98.2
        suicide (attempt) X77.2
        undetermined whether accidental or
          intentional Y27.2
      food X10.1
      gases X14.1
        inhalation X14.0
      heating appliance X16
      household appliance X15.8
        assault X98.3
        cooker X15.8
        hotplate X15.2
        kettle X15.8
        light bulb X15.8

Contact *(Continued)*
  with *(Continued)*
    hot *(Continued)*
      household appliance *(Continued)*
        object NEC X19
          assault X98.8
          stated as undetermined whether
            accidental or intentional Y27.9
          suicide (attempt) X77.8
        saucepan X15.3
        skillet X15.3
        stated as undetermined whether
          accidental or intentional Y27.3
        stove X15.0
        suicide (attempt) X77.3
        toaster X15.1
      kettle X15.8
      light bulb X15.8
      liquid NEC —*see also* Burn X12 ◄▥▥
        drinks X10.0
        stated as undetermined whether
          accidental or intentional Y27.2
        suicide (attempt) X77.2
        tap water X11.8
          stated as undetermined whether
            accidental or intentional Y27.1
          suicide (attempt) X77.1
      machinery X17
      metal (molten) (liquid) NEC X18
      object (not producing fire or flames)
        NEC X19
      oil (cooking) X10.2
      pipe X16
      plate X15.2
      radiator X16
      saucepan (glass) (metal) X15.3
      skillet X15.3
      stove (kitchen) X15.0
      substance NEC X19
      tap-water X11.8
        assault X98.1
        heated on stove X12
          stated as undetermined whether
            accidental or intentional Y27.2
          suicide (attempt) X77.2
        in bathtub X11.0
        running X11.1
        stated as undetermined whether
          accidental or intentional Y27.1
        suicide (attempt) X77.1
      toaster X15.1
      tool X17
      vapors X13.1
        inhalation X13.0
      water (tap) X11.8
        boiling X12
          stated as undetermined whether
            accidental or intentional Y27.2
          suicide (attempt) X77.2
        heated on stove X12
          stated as undetermined whether
            accidental or intentional Y27.2
          suicide (attempt) X77.2
        in bathtub X11.0
        running X11.1
        stated as undetermined whether
          accidental or intentional Y27.1
        suicide (attempt) X77.1
    hotplate X15.2
    ice-pick W27.4
    insect (nonvenomous) NEC W57
    kettle (hot) X15.8
    knife W26.0
      assault X99.1
      electric W29.1
      stated as undetermined whether
        accidental or intentional Y28.1
      suicide (attempt) X78.1
    lathe (metalworking) W31.1
      turnings W45.8
      woodworking W31.2

◄ New   ◄▥▥ Revised   ~~deleted~~ Deleted

Contact *(Continued)*
  with *(Continued)*
    lawnmower (powered) (ridden) W28
      causing electrocution W86.8
        suicide (attempt) X83.1
      unpowered W27.1
    lift, lifting (devices) W24.0
      agricultural operations W30.89
      shaft W24.0
    liquefied gas —*see* Exposure, cold, man-made
    liquid air, hydrogen, nitrogen —*see* Exposure, cold, man-made
    lizard (nonvenomous) W59.09
      bite W59.01
      strike W59.02
    llama —*see* Contact, with, hoof stock NEC
    macaw W61.19
      bite W61.11
      strike W61.12
    machine, machinery W31.9
      abrasive wheel W31.1
      agricultural including animal-powered W30.9
        combine harvester W30.0
        grain storage elevator W30.3
        hay derrick W30.2
        power take-off device W30.1
        reaper W30.0
        specified NEC W30.89
        thresher W30.0
        transport vehicle, stationary W30.81
      band saw W31.2
      bench saw W31.2
      circular saw W31.2
      commercial NEC W31.82
      drilling, metal (industrial) W31.1
      earth-drilling W31.0
      earthmoving or scraping W31.89
      excavating W31.89
      forging machine W31.1
      gas turbine W31.3
      hot X17
      internal combustion engine W31.3
      land drill W31.0
      lathe W31.1
      lifting (devices) W24.0
      metal drill W31.1
      metalworking (industrial) W31.1
      milling, metal W31.1
      mining W31.0
      molding W31.2
      overhead plane W31.2
      power press, metal W31.1
      prime mover W31.3
      printing W31.89
      radial saw W31.2
      recreational W31.81
      roller-coaster W31.81
      rolling mill, metal W31.1
      sander W31.2
      seabed drill W31.0
      shaft
        hoist W31.0
        lift W31.0
      specified NEC W31.89
      spinning W31.89
      steam engine W31.3
      transmission W24.1
      undercutter W31.0
      water driven turbine W31.3
      weaving W31.89
      woodworking or forming (industrial) W31.2
    mammal (feces) (urine) W55.89
      bull —*see* Contact, with, bull
      cat —*see* Contact, with, cat
      cow —*see* Contact, with, cow
      goat —*see* Contact, with, goat
      hoof stock —*see* Contact, with, hoof stock

Contact *(Continued)*
  with *(Continued)*
    mammal *(Continued)*
      horse —*see* Contact, with, horse
      marine W56.39
        dolphin —*see* Contact, with, dolphin
        orca —*see* Contact, with, orca
        sea lion —*see* Contact, with, sea lion
        specified NEC W56.39
          bite W56.31
          strike W56.32
      pig —*see* Contact, with, pig
      raccoon —*see* Contact, with, raccoon
      rodent —*see* Contact, with, rodent
      sheep —*see* Contact, with, sheep
      specified NEC W55.89
        bite W55.81
        strike W55.82
    marine
      animal W56.89
        bite W56.81
        dolphin —*see* Contact, with, dolphin
        fish NEC —*see* Contact, with, fish
        mammal —*see* Contact, with, mammal, marine
        orca —*see* Contact, with, orca
        sea lion —*see* Contact, with, sea lion
        shark —*see* Contact, with, shark
        strike W56.82
    meat
      grinder (domestic) W29.0
        industrial W31.82
        nonpowered W27.4
      slicer (domestic) W29.0
        industrial W31.82
    merry go round W31.81
    metal, (hot) (liquid) (molten) NEC X18
    millipede W57
    nail W45.0
      gun W29.4
    needle (sewing) W27.3
      hypodermic W46.0
        contaminated W46.1
    object (blunt) NEC
      hot NEC X19
      legal intervention —*see* Legal, intervention, blunt object
      sharp NEC W45.8
        inflicted by other person NEC W45.8
          stated as
            intentional homicide (attempt) —*see* Assault, cutting or piercing instrument
        legal intervention —*see* Legal, intervention, sharp object
        self-inflicted X78.9
    orca W56.29
      bite W56.21
      strike W56.22
    overhead plane W31.2
    paper (as sharp object) W26.2 ◀▥
    paper-cutter W27.5
    parrot W61.09
      bite W61.01
      strike W61.02
    pig W55.49
      bite W55.41
      strike W55.42
    pipe, hot X16
    pitchfork W27.1
    plane (metal) (wood) W27.0
      overhead W31.2
    plant thorns, spines, sharp leaves or other mechanisms W60
    powered
      garden cultivator W29.3
      household appliance, implement, or machine W29.8
      saw (industrial) W31.2
        hand W29.8
    printing machine W31.89

Contact *(Continued)*
  with *(Continued)*
    psittacine bird W61.29
      bite W61.21
      macaw —*see* Contact, with, macaw ◀▥
      parrot —*see* Contact, with, parrot
      strike W61.22
    pulley (block) (transmission) W24.0
      agricultural operations W30.89
    raccoon W55.59
      bite W55.51
      strike W55.52
    radial-saw (industrial) W31.2
    radiator (hot) X16
    rake W27.1
    rattlesnake X58
    reaper W30.0
    reptile W59.89
      lizard —*see* Contact, with, lizard
      snake —*see* Contact, with, snake
      specified NEC W59.89
        bite W59.81
        crushing W59.83
        strike W59.82
      turtle —*see* Contact, with, turtle
    rivet gun (powered) W29.4
    road scraper —*see* Accident, transport, construction vehicle
    rodent (feces) (urine) W53.89
      bite W53.81
      mouse W53.09
        bite W53.01
      rat W53.19
        bite W53.11
      specified NEC W53.89
        bite W53.81
      squirrel W53.29
        bite W53.21
    roller coaster W31.81
    rope NEC W24.0
      agricultural operations W30.89
    saliva —*see* Contact, with, by type of animal
    sander W29.8
      industrial W31.2
    saucepan (hot) (glass) (metal) X15.3
    saw W27.0
      band (industrial) W31.2
      bench (industrial) W31.2
      chain W29.3
      hand W27.0
    sawing machine, metal W31.1
    scissors W27.2
    scorpion X58
    screwdriver W27.0
      powered W29.8
    sea
      anemone, cucumber or urchin (spine) X58
      lion W56.19
        bite W56.11
        strike W56.12
    serpent —*see* Contact, with, snake, by type
    sewing-machine (electric) (powered) W29.2
      not powered W27.8
    shaft (hoist) (lift) (transmission) NEC W24.0
      agricultural W30.89
    shark W56.49
      bite W56.41
      strike W56.42
    sharp object(s) W26.9 ◀
      specified NEC W26.8 ◀
    shears (hand) W27.2
      powered (industrial) W31.1
        domestic W29.2
    sheep W55.39
      bite W55.31
      strike W55.32
    shovel W27.8
      steam —*see* Accident, transport, construction vehicle

◀ New   ◀▥ Revised   ~~deleted~~ Deleted

Contact *(Continued)*
  with *(Continued)*
    snake (nonvenomous) W59.19
      bite W59.11
      crushing W59.13
      strike W59.12
    spade W27.1
    spider (venomous) X58
    spin-drier W29.2
    spinning machine W31.89
    splinter W45.8
    sports equipment W21.9
    staple gun (powered) W29.8
    steam X13.1
      engine W31.3
      inhalation X13.0
      pipe X16
      shovel W31.89
    stove (hot) (kitchen) X15.0
    substance, hot NEC X19
      molten (metal) X18
    sword W26.1
      assault X99.2
      stated as undetermined whether
        accidental or intentional
        Y28.2
      suicide (attempt) X78.2
    tarantula X58
    thresher W30.0 ◀▥▥
    tin can lid W26.8 ◀▥▥
    toad W62.1
    toaster (hot) X15.1
    tool W27.8
      hand (not powered) W27.8
        auger W27.0
        axe W27.0
        can opener W27.4
        chisel W27.0
        fork W27.4
        garden W27.1
        handsaw W27.0
        hoe W27.1
        ice-pick W27.4
        kitchen utensil W27.4
        manual
          lawn mower W27.1
          sewing machine W27.8
        meat grinder W27.4
        needle (sewing) W27.3
          hypodermic W46.0
            contaminated W46.1
        paper cutter W27.5
        pitchfork W27.1
        rake W27.1
        scissors W27.2
        screwdriver W27.0
        specified NEC W27.8
        workbench W27.0
      hot X17
      powered W29.8
        blender W29.0
          commercial W31.82
        can opener W29.0
          commercial W31.82
        chainsaw W29.3
        clothes dryer W29.2
          commercial W31.82
        dishwasher W29.2
          commercial W31.82
        edger W29.3
        electric fan W29.2
          commercial W31.82
        electric knife W29.1
        food processor W29.0
          commercial W31.82
        garbage disposal W29.0
          commercial W31.82

Contact *(Continued)*
  with *(Continued)*
    tool *(Continued)*
      powered *(Continued)*
        garden tool W29.3
        hedge trimmer W29.3
        ice maker W29.0
          commercial W31.82
        kitchen appliance W29.0
          commercial W31.82
        lawn mower W28
        meat grinder W29.0
          commercial W31.82
        mixer W29.0
          commercial W31.82
        rototiller W29.3
        sewing machine W29.2
          commercial W31.82
        washing machine W29.2
          commercial W31.82
      transmission device (belt, cable, chain,
        gear, pinion, shaft) W24.1
        agricultural operations W30.89
      turbine (gas) (water-driven) W31.3
      turkey W61.49
        peck W61.43
        strike W61.42
      turtle (nonvenomous) W59.29
        bite W59.21
        strike W59.22
        terrestrial W59.89
          bite W59.81
          crushing W59.83
          strike W59.82
      under-cutter W31.0
      urine —*see* Contact, with, by type of animal
      vehicle
        agricultural use (transport) —*see*
          Accident, transport, agricultural
          vehicle
          not on public highway W30.81
        industrial use (transport) —*see*
          Accident, transport, industrial
          vehicle
          not on public highway W31.83
        off-road use (transport) —*see* Accident,
          transport, all-terrain or off-road
          vehicle
          not on public highway W31.83
        special construction use (transport) —*see*
          Accident, transport, construction
          vehicle
          not on public highway W31.83
      venomous
        animal X58
        arthropods X58
        lizard X58
        marine animal NEC X58
        marine plant NEC X58
        millipedes (tropical) X58
        plant (s) X58
        snake X58
        spider X58
        viper X58
      washing-machine (powered) W29.2
      wasp X58
      weaving-machine W31.89
      winch W24.0
        agricultural operations W30.89
      wire NEC W24.0
        agricultural operations W30.89
      wood slivers W45.8
      yellow jacket X58
      zebra —*see* Contact, with, hoof stock NEC
    pressure X50.9 ◀
    stress X50.9 ◀
Coup de soleil X32

Crash
  aircraft (in transit) (powered) V95.9
    balloon V96.01
    fixed wing NEC (private) V95.21
      commercial V95.31
    glider V96.21
      hang V96.11
      powered V95.11
    helicopter V95.01
    in war operations —*see* War operations,
      destruction of aircraft
    microlight V95.11
    nonpowered V96.9
      specified NEC V96.8
    powered NEC V95.8
    stated as
      homicide (attempt) Y08.81
      suicide (attempt) X83.0
    ultralight V95.11
  spacecraft V95.41
  transport vehicle NEC —*see also* Accident,
    transport V89.9
    homicide (attempt) Y03.8
    motor NEC (traffic) V89.2
      homicide (attempt) Y03.8
    suicide (attempt) —*see* Suicide, collision
Cruelty (mental) (physical) (sexual) X58
Crushed (accidentally) X58
  between objects (moving) (stationary and
    moving) W23.0
    stationary W23.1
  by
    alligator W58.03
    avalanche NEC —*see* Landslide ◀
    cave-in W20.0
      caused by cataclysmic earth surface
        movement —*see* Landslide ◀
    crocodile W58.13
    crowd or human stampede W52
    falling
      aircraft V97.39
        in war operations —*see* War
          operations, destruction of aircraft
      earth, material W20.0
        caused by cataclysmic earth surface
          movement —*see* Landslide
      object NEC W20.8
    landslide NEC —*see* Landslide ◀
    lizard (nonvenomous) W59.09
    machinery —*see* Contact, with, by type of
      machine
    reptile NEC W59.89
    snake (nonvenomous) W59.13
  in
    machinery —*see* Contact, with, by type of
      machine
Cut, cutting (any part of body) (accidental) —
  see also Contact, with, by object or machine
  during medical or surgical treatment as
    misadventure —*see* Index to Diseases
    and Injuries, Complications ◀▥▥
  homicide (attempt) —*see* Assault, cutting or
    piercing instrument
  inflicted by other person —*see* Assault,
    cutting or piercing instrument
  legal
    execution —*see* Legal, intervention
    intervention —*see* Legal, intervention,
      sharp object
  machine NEC —*see also* Contact, with, by
    type of machine W31.9
  self-inflicted —*see* Suicide, cutting or piercing
    instrument
  suicide (attempt) —*see* Suicide, cutting or
    piercing instrument
Cyclone (any injury) X37.1

◀ New   ◀▥▥ Revised   ~~deleted~~ Deleted

D

Decapitation (accidental circumstances)
NEC X58
homicide X99.9
legal execution —*see* Legal, intervention
Dehydration from lack of water X58
Deprivation X58
Derailment (accidental)
railway (rolling stock) (train) (vehicle)
(without antecedent collision) V81.7
with antecedent collision —*see* Accident,
transport, railway vehicle occupant
streetcar (without antecedent collision)
V82.7
with antecedent collision —*see* Accident,
transport, streetcar occupant
Descent
parachute (voluntary) (without accident to
aircraft) V97.29
due to accident to aircraft —*see* Accident,
transport, aircraft
Desertion X58
Destitution X58
Disability, late effect or sequela of injury —*see*
Sequelae
Discharge (accidental)
airgun W34.010
assault X95.01
homicide (attempt) X95.01
stated as undetermined whether accidental
or intentional Y24.0
suicide (attempt) X74.01
BB gun —*see* Discharge, airgun
firearm (accidental) W34.00
assault X95.9
handgun (pistol) (revolver) W32.0
assault X93
homicide (attempt) X93
legal intervention —*see* Legal,
intervention, firearm, handgun
stated as undetermined whether
accidental or intentional Y22
suicide (attempt) X72
homicide (attempt) X95.9
hunting rifle W33.02
assault X94.1
homicide (attempt) X94.1
legal intervention
injuring
bystander Y35.032
law enforcement personnel
Y35.031
suspect Y35.033
stated as undetermined whether
accidental or intentional Y23.1
suicide (attempt) X73.1
larger W33.00
assault X94.9
homicide (attempt) X94.9
hunting rifle —*see* Discharge, firearm,
hunting rifle
legal intervention —*see* Legal,
intervention, firearm by type of
firearm
machine gun —*see* Discharge, firearm,
machine gun
shotgun —*see* Discharge, firearm,
shotgun
specified NEC W33.09
assault X94.8
homicide (attempt) X94.8
legal intervention
injuring
bystander Y35.092
law enforcement personnel
Y35.091
suspect Y35.093
stated as undetermined whether
accidental or intentional Y23.8
suicide (attempt) X73.8

Discharge *(Continued)*
firearm *(Continued)*
larger *(Continued)*
stated as undetermined whether
accidental or intentional Y23.9
suicide (attempt) X73.9
legal intervention
injuring
bystander Y35.002
law enforcement personnel Y35.001
suspect Y35.03
using rubber bullet
injuring
bystander Y35.042
law enforcement personnel
Y35.041
suspect Y35.043
machine gun W33.03
assault X94.2
homicide (attempt) X94.2
legal intervention —*see* Legal,
intervention, firearm, machine gun
stated as undetermined whether
accidental or intentional Y23.3
suicide (attempt) X73.2
pellet gun —*see* Discharge, airgun
shotgun W33.01
assault X94.0
homicide (attempt) X94.0
legal intervention —*see* Legal,
intervention, firearm, specified NEC
stated as undetermined whether
accidental or intentional Y23.0
suicide (attempt) X73.0
specified NEC W34.09
assault X95.8
homicide (attempt) X95.8
legal intervention —*see* Legal,
intervention, firearm, specified NEC
stated as undetermined whether
accidental or intentional Y24.8
suicide (attempt) X74.8
stated as undetermined whether accidental
or intentional Y24.9
suicide (attempt) X74.9
Very pistol W34.09
assault X95.8
homicide (attempt) X95.8
stated as undetermined whether
accidental or intentional Y24.8
suicide (attempt) X74.8
firework (s) W39
stated as undetermined whether accidental
or intentional Y25
gas-operated gun NEC W34.018
airgun —*see* Discharge, airgun
assault X95.09
homicide (attempt) X95.09
paintball gun —*see* Discharge, paintball
gun
stated as undetermined whether accidental
or intentional Y24.8
suicide (attempt) X74.09
gun NEC —*see also* Discharge, firearm NEC
air —*see* Discharge, airgun
BB —*see* Discharge, airgun
for single hand use —*see* Discharge,
firearm, handgun
hand —*see* Discharge, firearm, handgun
machine —*see* Discharge, firearm, machine
gun
other specified —*see* Discharge, firearm
NEC
paintball —*see* Discharge, paintball gun
pellet —*see* Discharge, airgun
handgun —*see* Discharge, firearm, handgun
machine gun —*see* Discharge, firearm,
machine gun
paintball gun W34.011
assault X95.02
homicide (attempt) X95.02

Discharge *(Continued)*
paintball gun *(Continued)*
stated as undetermined whether accidental
or intentional Y24.8
suicide (attempt) X74.02
pistol —*see* Discharge, firearm, handgun
flare —*see* Discharge, firearm, Very pistol
pellet —*see* Discharge, airgun
Very —*see* Discharge, firearm, Very pistol
revolver —*see* Discharge, firearm, handgun
rifle (hunting) —*see* Discharge, firearm,
hunting rifle
shotgun —*see* Discharge, firearm, shotgun
spring-operated gun NEC W34.018
assault X95.09
homicide (attempt) X95.09
stated as undetermined whether accidental
or intentional Y24.8
suicide (attempt) X74.09
Disease
Andes W94.11
aviator's —*see* Air, pressure
range W94.11
Diver's disease, palsy, paralysis, squeeze —*see*
Air, pressure
Diving (into water) —*see* Accident, diving
Dog bite W54.0
Dragged by transport vehicle NEC —*see also*
Accident, transport V09.9
Drinking poison (accidental) —*see* Table of
Drugs and Chemicals ◀▥
Dropped (accidentally) while being carried or
supported by other person W04
Drowning (accidental) W74
assault X92.9
due to
accident (to)
machinery —*see* Contact, with, by type
of machine
watercraft V90.89
burning V90.29
powered V90.23
fishing boat V90.22
jetskis V90.23
merchant ship V90.20
passenger ship V90.21
unpowered V90.28
canoe V90.25
inflatable V90.26
kayak V90.25
sailboat V90.24
water skis V90.27
crushed V90.39
powered V90.33
fishing boat V90.32
jetskis V90.33
merchant ship V90.30
passenger ship V90.31
unpowered V90.38
canoe V90.35
inflatable V90.36
kayak V90.35
sailboat V90.34
water skis V90.37
overturning V90.09
powered V90.03
fishing boat V90.02
jetskis V90.03
merchant ship V90.00
passenger ship V90.01
unpowered V90.08
canoe V90.05
inflatable V90.06
kayak V90.05
sailboat V90.04
sinking V90.19
powered V90.13
fishing boat V90.12
jetskis V90.13
merchant ship V90.10
passenger ship V90.11

Drowning *(Continued)*
  due to *(Continued)*
    accident *(Continued)*
      watercraft *(Continued)*
        sinking *(Continued)*
          unpowered V90.18
            canoe V90.15
            inflatable V90.16
            kayak V90.15
            sailboat V90.14
          specified type NEC V90.89
            powered V90.83
              fishing boat V90.82
              jetskis V90.83
              merchant ship V90.80
              passenger ship V90.81
            unpowered V90.88
              canoe V90.85
              inflatable V90.86
              kayak V90.85
              sailboat V90.84
              water skis V90.87
    avalanche —*see* Landslide ◄
    cataclysmic
      earth surface movement NEC —*see*
        Forces of nature, earth movement ◄
      storm —*see* Forces of nature, cataclysmic
        storm ◄
    cloudburst X37.8
    cyclone X37.1
    fall overboard (from) V92.09
      powered craft V92.03
        ferry boat V92.01
        fishing boat V92.02
        jetskis V92.03
        liner V92.01
        merchant ship V92.00
        passenger ship V92.01
      resulting from
        accident to watercraft —*see* Drowning,
          due to, accident to, watercraft
        being washed overboard (from)
          V92.29
          powered craft V92.23
            ferry boat V92.21
             fishing boat V92.22
             jetskis V92.23
             liner V92.21
             merchant ship V92.20
             passenger ship V92.21
          unpowered craft V92.28
            canoe V92.25
            inflatable V92.26
            kayak V92.25
            sailboat V92.24
            surf-board V92.28
            water skis V92.27
            windsurfer V92.28
        motion of watercraft V92.19
          powered craft V92.13
            ferry boat V92.11
            fishing boat V92.12
            jetskis V92.13
            liner V92.11
            merchant ship V92.10
            passenger ship V92.11
          unpowered craft
            canoe V92.15
            inflatable V92.16
            kayak V92.15
            sailboat V92.14
      unpowered craft V92.08
        canoe V92.05
        inflatable V92.06
        kayak V92.05

Drowning *(Continued)*
  due to *(Continued)*
    fall overboard *(Continued)*
      unpowered craft *(Continued)*
        sailboat V92.04
        surf-board V92.08
        water skis V92.07
        windsurfer V92.08
    hurricane X37.0
    jumping into water from watercraft
      (involved in accident) —*see also*
      Drowning, due to, accident to,
      watercraft
      without accident to or on watercraft
      W16.711
    tidal wave NEC —*see* Forces of nature,
      tidal wave ◄
    torrential rain X37.8
  following
    fall
      into
        bathtub W16.211
        bucket W16.221
        fountain —*see* Drowning, following,
          fall, into, water, specified NEC
        quarry —*see* Drowning, following,
          fall, into, water, specified NEC
        reservoir —*see* Drowning, following,
          fall, into, water, specified NEC
        swimming-pool W16.011
          stated as undetermined whether
            accidental or intentional
            Y21.3
          striking
            bottom W16.021
            wall W16.031
          suicide (attempt) X71.2
        water NOS W16.41
          natural (lake) (open sea) (river)
            (stream) (pond) W16.111
            striking
              bottom W16.121
              side W16.131
          specified NEC W16.311
            striking
              bottom W16.321
              wall W16.331
      overboard NEC —*see* Drowning, due to,
        fall overboard
    jump or dive
      from boat W16.711
        striking bottom W16.721
      into
        fountain —*see* Drowning, following,
          jump or dive, into, water,
          specified NEC
        quarry —*see* Drowning, following,
          jump or dive, into, water,
          specified NEC
        reservoir —*see* Drowning, following,
          jump or dive, into, water,
          specified NEC
        swimming-pool W16.511
          striking
            bottom W16.521
            wall W16.531
          suicide (attempt) X71.2
        water NOS W16.91
          natural (lake) (open sea) (river)
            (stream) (pond) W16.611
          specified NEC W16.811
           striking
            bottom W16.821
            wall W16.831
          striking bottom W16.621

Drowning *(Continued)*
  homicide (attempt) X92.9
  in
    bathtub (accidental) W65
      assault X92.0
      following fall W16.211
        stated as undetermined whether
          accidental or intentional
          Y21.1
      stated as undetermined whether
        accidental or intentional Y21.0
      suicide (attempt) X71.0
    lake —*see* Drowning, in, natural water
    natural water (lake) (open sea) (river)
      (stream) (pond) W69
      assault X92.3
      following
        dive or jump W16.611
          striking bottom W16.621
        fall W16.111
          striking
            bottom W16.121
            side W16.131
      stated as undetermined whether
        accidental or intentional Y21.4
      suicide (attempt) X71.3
    quarry —*see* Drowning, in, specified place
      NEC
    quenching tank —*see* Drowning, in,
      specified place NEC
    reservoir —*see* Drowning, in, specified
      place NEC
    river —*see* Drowning, in, natural water
    sea —*see* Drowning, in, natural water
    specified place NEC W73
      assault X92.8
      following
        dive or jump W16.811
          striking
            bottom W16.821
            wall W16.831
        fall W16.311
          striking
            bottom W16.321
            wall W16.331
      stated as undetermined whether
        accidental or intentional Y21.8
      suicide (attempt) X71.8
    stream —*see* Drowning, in, natural water
    swimming-pool W67
      assault X92.1
      following fall X92.2
      following
        dive or jump W16.511
          striking
            bottom W16.521
            wall W16.531
        fall W16.011
          striking
            bottom W16.021
            wall W16.031
      stated as undetermined whether
        accidental or intentional Y21.2
        following fall Y21.3
      suicide (attempt) X71.1
        following fall X71.2
    war operations —*see* War operations,
      restriction of airway
  resulting from accident to watercraft —*see*
    Drowning, due to, accident, watercraft
  self-inflicted X71.9
  stated as undetermined whether accidental or
    intentional Y21.9
  suicide (attempt) X71.9

◄ New   ◀▮▮ Revised   ~~deleted~~ Deleted

E

Earth (surface) movement NEC —*see* Forces of nature, earth movement ◀▦

Earth falling (on) W20.0
  caused by cataclysmic earth surface movement or eruption —*see* Landslide ◀

Earthquake (any injury) X34

Effect (s) (adverse) of
  air pressure (any) —*see* Air, pressure
  cold, excessive (exposure to) —*see* Exposure, cold
  heat (excessive) —*see* Heat
  hot place (weather) —*see* Heat ◀▦
  insolation X30
  late —*see* Sequelae
  motion —*see* Motion
  nuclear explosion or weapon in war operations —*see* War operations, nuclear weapon
  radiation —*see* Radiation
  travel —*see* Travel

Electric shock (accidental) (by) (in) —*see* Exposure, electric current

Electrocution (accidental) —*see* Exposure, electric current

Endotracheal tube wrongly placed during anesthetic procedure Y65.3

Entanglement
  in
    bed linen, causing suffocation —*see* category T71
    wheel of pedal cycle V19.88

Entry of foreign body or material —*see* Foreign body

Environmental pollution related condition — *see* Z57

Execution, legal (any method) —*see* Legal, intervention

Exhaustion
  cold —*see* Exposure, cold
  due to excessive exertion —*see also* Overexertion X50.9 ◀▦
  heat —*see* Heat

Explosion (accidental) (of) (with secondary fire) W40.9
  acetylene W40.1
  aerosol can W36.1
  air tank (compressed) (in machinery) W36.2
  aircraft (in transit) (powered) NEC V95.9
    balloon V96.05
    fixed wing NEC (private) V95.25
      commercial V95.35
    glider V96.25
      hang V96.15
      powered V95.15
    helicopter V95.05
    in war operations —*see* War operations, destruction of aircraft
    microlight V95.15
    nonpowered V96.9
      specified NEC V96.8
    powered NEC V95.8
    stated as
      homicide (attempt) Y03.8
      suicide (attempt) X83.0
    ultralight V95.15
  anesthetic gas in operating room W40.1
  antipersonnel bomb W40.8
    assault X96.0
    homicide (attempt) X96.0
    suicide (attempt) X75
  assault X96.9
  bicycle tire W37.0
  blasting (cap) (materials) W40.0
  boiler (machinery), not on transport vehicle W35
    on watercraft —*see* Explosion, in, watercraft
  butane W40.1
  caused by other person X96.9
  coal gas W40.1

Explosion (*Continued*)
  detonator W40.0
  dump (munitions) W40.8
  dynamite W40.0
    in
      assault X96.8
      homicide (attempt) X96.8
      legal intervention
        injuring
          bystander Y35.112
          law enforcement personnel Y35.111
          suspect Y35.113
      suicide (attempt) X75
  explosive (material) W40.9
    gas W40.1
    in blasting operation W40.0
    specified NEC W40.8
      in
        assault X96.8
        homicide (attempt) X96.8
        legal intervention
          injuring
            bystander Y35.192
            law enforcement personnel Y35.191
            suspect Y35.193
        suicide (attempt) X75
  factory (munitions) W40.8
  fertilizer bomb W40.8
    assault X96.3
    homicide (attempt) X96.3
    suicide (attempt) X75
  fire-damp W40.1
  firearm (parts) NEC W34.19
    airgun W34.110
    BB gun W34.110
    gas, air or spring-operated gun NEC W34.118
    handgun W32.1
    hunting rifle W33.12
    larger firearm W33.10
      specified NEC W33.19
    machine gun W33.13
    paintball gun W34.111
    pellet gun W34.110
    shotgun W33.11
    Very pistol [flare] W34.19
  fireworks W39
  gas (coal) (explosive) W40.1
    cylinder W36.9
      aerosol can W36.1
      air tank W36.2
      pressurized W36.3
      specified NEC W36.8
  gasoline (fumes) (tank) not in moving motor vehicle W40.1
    bomb W40.8
      assault X96.1
      homicide (attempt) X96.1
      suicide (attempt) X75
    in motor vehicle —*see* Accident, transport, by type of vehicle
  grain store W40.8
  grenade W40.8
    in
      assault X96.8
      homicide (attempt) X96.8
      legal intervention
        injuring
          bystander Y35.192
          law enforcement personnel Y35.191
          suspect Y35.193
      suicide (attempt) X75
  handgun (parts) —*see* Explosion, firearm, handgun (parts)
  homicide (attempt) X96.9
    antipersonnel bomb —*see* Explosion, antipersonnel bomb
    fertilizer bomb —*see* Explosion, fertilizer bomb

Explosion (*Continued*)
  homicide (*Continued*)
    gasoline bomb —*see* Explosion, gasoline bomb
    letter bomb —*see* Explosion, letter bomb
    pipe bomb —*see* Explosion, pipe bomb
    specified NEC X96.8
  hose, pressurized W37.8
  hot water heater, tank (in machinery) W35
    on watercraft —*see* Explosion, in, watercraft
  in, on
    dump W40.8
    factory W40.8
    mine (of explosive gases) NEC W40.1
    watercraft V93.59
      powered craft V93.53
        ferry boat V93.51
        fishing boat V93.52
        jetskis V93.53
        liner V93.51
        merchant ship V93.50
        passenger ship V93.51
        sailboat V93.54
  letter bomb W40.8
    assault X96.2
    homicide (attempt) X96.2
    suicide (attempt) X75
  machinery —*see also* Contact, with, by type of machine
    on board watercraft —*see* Explosion, in, watercraft
    pressure vessel —*see* Explosion, by type of vessel
  methane W40.1
  mine W40.1
  missile NEC W40.8
  mortar bomb W40.8
    in
      assault X96.8
      homicide (attempt) X96.8
      legal intervention
        injuring
          bystander Y35.192
          law enforcement personnel Y35.191
          suspect Y35.193
      suicide (attempt) X75
  munitions (dump) (factory) W40.8
  pipe, pressurized W37.8
    bomb W40.8
      assault X96.4
      homicide (attempt) X96.4
      suicide (attempt) X75
  pressure, pressurized
    cooker W38
    gas tank (in machinery) W36.3
    hose W37.8
    pipe W37.8
    specified device NEC W38
    tire W37.8
      bicycle W37.0
    vessel (in machinery) W38
  propane W40.1
  self-inflicted X75
  shell (artillery) NEC W40.8
    during war operations —*see* War operations, explosion
    in
      legal intervention
        injuring
          bystander Y35.122
          law enforcement personnel Y35.121
          suspect Y35.123
    war —*see* War operations, explosion
  spacecraft V95.45
  stated as undetermined whether accidental or intentional Y25
  steam or water lines (in machinery) W37.8
  stove W40.9
  suicide (attempt) X75

Explosion (Continued)
tire, pressurized W37.8
  bicycle W37.Ø
undetermined whether accidental or
    intentional Y25
vehicle tire NEC W37.8
  bicycle W37.Ø
war operations —see War operations,
    explosion
Exposure (to) X58
air pressure change —see Air, pressure
cold (accidental) (excessive) (extreme)
    (natural) (place) X31
  assault YØ8.89
  due to
    man-made conditions W93.8
      dry ice (contact) W93.Ø1
        inhalation W93.Ø2
      liquid air (contact) (hydrogen)
          (nitrogen) W93.11
        inhalation W93.12
      refrigeration unit (deep freeze)
          W93.2
    suicide (attempt) X83.2
    weather (conditions) X31
  homicide (attempt) YØ8.89
  self-inflicted X83.2
due to abandonment or neglect X58
electric current W86.8
  appliance (faulty) W86.8
    domestic W86.Ø
  caused by other person YØ8.89
  conductor (faulty) W86.1
  control apparatus (faulty) W86.1
  electric power generating plant,
      distribution station W86.1
  electroshock gun —see Exposure, electric
      current, taser
  high-voltage cable W85
  homicide (attempt) YØ8.89
  legal execution —see Legal, intervention,
      specified means NEC
  lightning —see subcategory T75.Ø
  live rail W86.8
  misadventure in medical or surgical
      procedure in electroshock therapy
      Y63.4
  motor (electric) (faulty) W86.8
    domestic W86.Ø
  self-inflicted X83.1
  specified NEC W86.8
    domestic W86.Ø
  stun gun —see Exposure, electric current,
      taser
  suicide (attempt) X83.1
  taser W86.8
    assault YØ8.89
    legal intervention —see category Y35
    self-harm (intentional) X83.8
    undetermined intent Y33
  third rail W86.8
  transformer (faulty) W86.1
  transmission lines W85
environmental tobacco smoke X58
excessive
  cold —see Exposure, cold
  heat (natural) NEC X3Ø
    man-made W92
factor (s) NOS X58
  environmental NEC X58
    man-made NEC W99
    natural NEC —see Forces of nature ◀
  specified NEC X58
fire, flames (accidental) XØ8.8
  assault X97
  campfire —see Exposure, fire, controlled,
      not in building
  controlled (in)
    with ignition (of) clothing —see also
        Ignition, clothes XØ6.2
      nightwear XØ5

Exposure (Continued)
fire, flames (Continued)
  controlled (Continued)
    bonfire —see Exposure, fire, controlled,
        not in building
    brazier (in building or structure) —see
        also Exposure, fire, controlled,
        building
    not in building or structure —see
        Exposure, fire, controlled, not in
        building
    building or structure XØ2.Ø
      with
        fall from building XØ2.3
        from building XØ2.5
        injury due to building collapse
            XØ2.2
        smoke inhalation XØ2.1
      hit by object from building XØ2.4
      specified mode of injury NEC XØ2.8
    fireplace, furnace or stove —see
        Exposure, fire, controlled, building
    not in building or structure XØ3.Ø
      with
        fall XØ3.3
        smoke inhalation XØ3.1
      hit by object XØ3.4
      specified mode of injury NEC XØ3.8
    trash —see Exposure, fire, controlled, not
        in building
  fireplace —see Exposure, fire, controlled,
      building
  fittings or furniture (in building or
      structure) (uncontrolled) —see
      Exposure, fire, uncontrolled, building
  forest (uncontrolled) —see Exposure, fire,
      uncontrolled, not in building
  grass (uncontrolled) —see Exposure, fire,
      uncontrolled, not in building
  hay (uncontrolled) —see Exposure, fire,
      uncontrolled, not in building
  homicide (attempt) X97
  ignition of highly flammable material XØ4
  in, of, on, starting in
    machinery —see Contact, with, by type
        of machine
    motor vehicle (in motion) —see also
        Accident, transport, occupant by
        type of vehicle V87.8
      with collision —see Collision
    railway rolling stock, train, vehicle
        V81.81
      with collision —see Accident,
          transport, railway vehicle
          occupant
    street car (in motion) V82.8
      with collision —see Accident,
          transport, streetcar occupant
    transport vehicle NEC —see also
        Accident, transport
      with collision —see Collision
    war operations —see also War operations,
        fire
      from nuclear explosion —see War
          operations, nuclear weapons
    watercraft (in transit) (not in transit)
        V91.Ø9
      localized —see Burn, on board
          watercraft, due to, fire on board
      powered craft V91.Ø3
        ferry boat V91.Ø1
        fishing boat V91.Ø2
        jet skis V91.Ø3
        liner V91.Ø1
        merchant ship V91.ØØ
        passenger ship V91.Ø1
      unpowered craft V91.Ø8
        canoe V91.Ø5
        inflatable V91.Ø6
        kayak V91.Ø5
        sailboat V91.Ø4

Exposure (Continued)
fire, flames (Continued)
  in, of, on, starting in (Continued)
    watercraft (Continued)
      unpowered craft (Continued)
        surf-board V91.Ø8
        waterskis V91.Ø7
        windsurfer V91.Ø8
    lumber (uncontrolled) —see Exposure, fire,
        uncontrolled, not in building
    mine (uncontrolled) —see Exposure, fire,
        uncontrolled, not in building
    prairie (uncontrolled) —see Exposure, fire,
        uncontrolled, not in building
  resulting from
    explosion —see Explosion
    lightning XØ8.8
  self-inflicted X76
  specified NEC XØ8.8
  started by other person X97
  stated as undetermined whether accidental
      or intentional Y26
  stove —see Exposure, fire, controlled,
      building
  suicide (attempt) X76
  tunnel (uncontrolled) —see Exposure, fire,
      uncontrolled, not in building
  uncontrolled
    in building or structure XØØ.Ø
      with
        fall from building XØØ.3
        injury due to building collapse
            XØØ.2
        jump from building XØØ.5
        smoke inhalation XØØ.1
      bed XØ8.ØØ
        due to
          cigarette XØ8.Ø1
          specified material NEC XØ8.Ø9
      furniture NEC XØ8.2Ø
        due to
          cigarette XØ8.21
          specified material NEC XØ8.29
      hit by object from building XØØ.4
      sofa XØ8.1Ø
        due to
          cigarette XØ8.11
          specified material NEC
              XØ8.19
      specified mode of injury NEC
          XØØ.8
    not in building or structure (any)
        XØ1.Ø
      with
        fall XØ1.3
        smoke inhalation XØ1.1
      hit by object XØ1.4
      specified mode of injury NEC
          XØ1.8
  undetermined whether accidental or
      intentional Y26
forces of nature NEC —see Forces of nature ◀
G-forces (abnormal) W49.9
gravitational forces (abnormal) W49.9
heat (natural) NEC —see Heat
high-pressure jet (hydraulic) (pneumatic)
    W49.9
hydraulic jet W49.9
inanimate mechanical force W49.9
jet, high-pressure (hydraulic) (pneumatic)
    W49.9
lightning —see subcategory T75.Ø
  causing fire —see Exposure, fire
mechanical forces NEC W49.9
  animate NEC W64
  inanimate NEC W49.9
noise W42.9
  supersonic W42.Ø
noxious substance —see Table of Drugs and
    Chemicals ◀▥▥
pneumatic jet W49.9

◀ New   ◀▥▥ Revised   ~~deleted~~ Deleted

Exposure (Continued)
  prolonged in deep-freeze unit or refrigerator
    W93.2
  radiation —see Radiation
  smoke —see also Exposure, fire
    tobacco, second hand Z77.22
  specified factors NEC X58
  sunlight X32
    man-made (sun lamp) W89.8
      tanning bed W89.1
  supersonic waves W42.0
  transmission line (s), electric W85
  vibration W49.9

Exposure (Continued)
  waves
    infrasound W49.9
    sound W42.9
    supersonic W42.0
  weather NEC —see Forces of nature ◀
External cause status Y99.9
  child assisting in compensated work for
    family Y99.8
  civilian activity done for financial or other
    compensation Y99.0
  civilian activity done for income or pay
    Y99.0

External cause status (Continued)
  family member assisting in compensated
    work for other family member Y99.8
  hobby not done for income Y99.8
  leisure activity Y99.8
  military activity Y99.1
  off-duty activity of military personnel Y99.8
  recreation or sport not for income or while a
    student Y99.8
  specified NEC Y99.8
  student activity Y99.8
  volunteer activity Y99.2

F

Factors, supplemental
  alcohol
    blood level
      less than 20mg/100ml Y90.0
      presence in blood, level not specified
        Y90.9
      20-39mg/100ml Y90.1
      40-59mg/100ml Y90.2
      60-79mg/100ml Y90.3
      80-99mg/100ml Y90.4
      100-119mg/100ml Y90.5
      120-199mg/100ml Y90.6
      200-239mg/100ml Y90.7
      240mg/100ml or more Y90.8
    presence in blood, but level not specified
      Y90.9
  environmental-pollution-related condition —
    see Z57
  nosocomial condition Y95
  work-related condition Y99.0
Failure
  in suture or ligature during surgical
    procedure Y65.2
  mechanical, of instrument or apparatus
    (any) (during any medical or surgical
    procedure) Y65.8
  sterile precautions (during medical and
    surgical care) —*see* Misadventure,
    failure, sterile precautions, by type of
    procedure
  to
    introduce tube or instrument Y65.4
    endotracheal tube during anesthesia Y65.3
    make curve (transport vehicle) NEC —*see*
      Accident, transport
    remove tube or instrument Y65.4
Fall, falling (accidental) W19
  building W20.1
    burning (uncontrolled fire) X00.3
  down
    embankment W17.81
    escalator W10.0
    hill W17.81
    ladder W11
    ramp W10.2
    stairs, steps W10.9
  due to
    bumping against
      object W18.00
        sharp glass W18.02
        specified NEC W18.09
        sports equipment W18.01
      person W03
        due to ice or snow W00.0
        on pedestrian conveyance —*see*
          Accident, transport, pedestrian,
          conveyance
    collision with another person W03
      due to ice or snow W00.0
      involving pedestrian conveyance —*see*
        Accident, transport, pedestrian,
        conveyance
    grocery cart tipping over W17.82
    ice or snow W00.9
      from one level to another W00.2
        on stairs or steps W00.1
      involving pedestrian conveyance —*see*
        Accident, transport, pedestrian,
        conveyance
      on same level W00.0
    slipping (on moving sidewalk) W01.0
      with subsequent striking against object
        W01.10
        furniture W01.190
        sharp object W01.119
          glass W01.110
          power tool or machine W01.111
          specified NEC W01.118
        specified NEC W01.198

Fall, falling *(Continued)*
  due to *(Continued)*
    striking against
      object W18.00
        sharp glass W18.02
        specified NEC W18.09
        sports equipment W18.01
      person W03
        due to ice or snow W00.0
        on pedestrian conveyance —*see*
          Accident, transport, pedestrian,
          conveyance
  earth (with asphyxia or suffocation (by
    pressure)) —*see* Earth, falling
  from, off, out of
    aircraft NEC (with accident to aircraft
      NEC) V97.0
      while boarding or alighting V97.1
    balcony W13.0
    bed W06
    boat, ship, watercraft NEC (with
      drowning or submersion) —
      see Drowning, due to, fall
      overboard
      with hitting bottom or object V94.0
    bridge W13.1
    building W13.9
      burning (uncontrolled fire) X00.3
    cavity W17.2
    chair W07
    cherry picker W17.89
    cliff W15
    dock W17.4
    embankment W17.81
    escalator W10.0
    flagpole W13.8
    furniture NEC W08
    grocery cart W17.82
    haystack W17.89
    high place NEC W17.89
      stated as undetermined whether
        accidental or intentional Y30
    hole W17.2
    incline W10.2
    ladder W11
    lifting device W17.89
    machine, machinery —*see also* Contact,
      with, by type of machine
      not in operation W17.89
    manhole W17.1
    mobile elevated work platform [MEWP]
      W17.89
    motorized mobility scooter W05.2
    one level to another NEC W17.89
      intentional, purposeful, suicide
        (attempt) X80
      stated as undetermined whether
        accidental or intentional Y30
    pit W17.2
    playground equipment W09.8
      jungle gym W09.2
      slide W09.0
      swing W09.1
    quarry W17.89
    railing W13.9
    ramp W10.2
    roof W13.2
    scaffolding W12
    scooter (nonmotorized) W05.1
      motorized mobility W05.2
    sky lift W17.89
    stairs, steps W10.9
      curb W10.1
      due to ice or snow W00.1
      escalator W10.0
      incline W10.2
      ramp W10.2
      sidewalk curb W10.1
      specified NEC W10.8
    stepladder W11
    storm drain W17.1

Fall, falling *(Continued)*
  from, off, out of *(Continued)*
    streetcar NEC V82.6
      with antecedent collision —*see*
        Accident, transport, streetcar
        occupant
      while boarding or alighting V82.4
    structure NEC W13.8
      burning (uncontrolled fire) X00.3
    table W08
    toilet W18.11
      with subsequent striking against object
        W18.12
    train NEC V81.6
      during derailment (without antecedent
        collision) V81.7
      with antecedent collision —*see*
        Accident, transport, railway
        vehicle occupant
      while boarding or alighting V81.4
    transport vehicle after collision —*see*
      Accident, transport, by type of
      vehicle, collision
    tree W14
    vehicle (in motion) NEC —*see also*
      Accident, transport V89.9
      motor NEC —*see also* Accident,
        transport, occupant, by type of
        vehicle V87.8
      stationary W17.89
      while boarding or alighting —*see*
        Accident, transport, by type of
        vehicle, while boarding or
        alighting ◄
    viaduct W13.8
    wall W13.8
    watercraft —*see also* Drowning, due to, fall
      overboard
      with hitting bottom or object V94.0
    well W17.0
    wheelchair, non-moving W05.0
      powered —*see* Accident, transport,
        pedestrian, conveyance occupant,
        specified type NEC
    window W13.4
  in, on
    aircraft NEC V97.0
      with accident to aircraft V97.0
      while boarding or alighting
        V97.1
    bathtub (empty) W18.2
      filled W16.212
        causing drowning W16.211
    escalator W10.0
    incline W10.2
    ladder W11
    machine, machinery —*see* Contact, with,
      by type of machine
    object, edged, pointed or sharp (with
      cut) —*see* Fall, by type
    playground equipment W09.8
      jungle gym W09.2
      slide W09.0
      swing W09.1
    ramp W10.2
    scaffolding W12
    shower W18.2
      causing drowning W16.211
    staircase, stairs, steps W10.9
      curb W10.1
      due to ice or snow W00.1
      escalator W10.0
      incline W10.2
      specified NEC W10.8
    streetcar (without antecedent collision)
      V82.5
      with antecedent collision —*see*
        Accident, transport, streetcar
        occupant
      while boarding or alighting
        V82.4

◀ New   ◀▦ Revised   ~~deleted~~ Deleted

Fall, falling (Continued)
in, on (Continued)
train (without antecedent collision) V81.5
with antecedent collision —see Accident, transport, railway vehicle occupant
during derailment (without antecedent collision) V81.7
with antecedent collision —see Accident, transport, railway vehicle occupant
while boarding or alighting V81.4
transport vehicle after collision —see Accident, transport, by type of vehicle, collision
watercraft V93.39
due to
accident to craft V91.29
powered craft V91.23
ferry boat V91.21
fishing boat V91.22
jetskis V91.23
liner V91.21
merchant ship V91.20
passenger ship V91.21
unpowered craft
canoe V91.25
inflatable V91.26
kayak V91.25
sailboat V91.24
powered craft V93.33
ferry boat V93.31
fishing boat V93.32
jetskis V93.33
liner V93.31
merchant ship V93.30
passenger ship V93.31
unpowered craft V93.38
canoe V93.35
inflatable V93.36
kayak V93.35
sailboat V93.34
surf-board V93.38
windsurfer V93.38
into
cavity W17.2
dock W17.4
fire —see Exposure, fire, by type
haystack W17.89
hole W17.2
lake —see Fall, into, water
manhole W17.1
moving part of machinery —see Contact, with, by type of machine
ocean —see Fall, into, water
opening in surface NEC W17.89
pit W17.2
pond —see Fall, into, water
quarry W17.89
river —see Fall, into, water
shaft W17.89
storm drain W17.1
stream —see Fall, into, water
swimming pool —see also Fall, into, water, in, swimming pool
empty W17.3
tank W17.89
water W16.42
causing drowning W16.41
from watercraft —see Drowning, due to, fall overboard
hitting diving board W21.4
in
bathtub W16.212
causing drowning W16.211
bucket W16.222
causing drowning W16.221
natural body of water W16.112
causing drowning W16.111
striking
bottom W16.122
causing drowning W16.121

Fall, falling (Continued)
into (Continued)
water (Continued)
in (Continued)
natural body of water (Continued)
striking (Continued)
side W16.132
causing drowning W16.131
specified water NEC W16.312
causing drowning W16.311
striking
bottom W16.322
causing drowning W16.321
wall W16.332
causing drowning W16.331
swimming pool W16.012
causing drowning W16.011
striking
bottom W16.022
causing drowning W16.021
wall W16.032
causing drowning W16.031
utility bucket W16.222
causing drowning W16.221
well W17.0
involving
bed W06
chair W07
furniture NEC W08
glass —see Fall, by type
playground equipment W09.8
jungle gym W09.2
slide W09.0
swing W09.1
roller blades —see Accident, transport, pedestrian, conveyance
skateboard (s) —see Accident, transport, pedestrian, conveyance
skates (ice) (in line) (roller) —see Accident, transport, pedestrian, conveyance
skis —see Accident, transport, pedestrian, conveyance
table W08
wheelchair, non-moving W05.0
powered —see Accident, transport, pedestrian, conveyance, specified type NEC
object —see Struck by, object, falling
off
toilet W18.11
with subsequent striking against object W18.12
on same level W18.30
due to
specified NEC W18.39
stepping on an object W18.31
out of
bed W06
building NEC W13.8
chair W07
furniture NEC W08
wheelchair, non-moving W05.0
powered —see Accident, transport, pedestrian, conveyance, specified type NEC
window W13.4
over
animal W01.0
cliff W15
embankment W17.81
small object W01.0
rock W20.8
same level W18.30
from
being crushed, pushed, or stepped on by a crowd or human stampede W52
collision, pushing, shoving, by or with other person W03
slipping, stumbling, tripping W01.0

Fall, falling (Continued)
same level (Continued)
involving ice or snow W00.0
involving skates (ice) (roller), skateboard, skis —see Accident, transport, pedestrian, conveyance
snowslide (avalanche) —see Landslide ◄
stone W20.8
structure W20.1
burning (uncontrolled fire) X00.3
through
bridge W13.1
floor W13.3
roof W13.2
wall W13.8
window W13.4
timber W20.8
tree (caused by lightning) W20.8
while being carried or supported by other person (s) W04
Fallen on by
animal (not being ridden) NEC W55.89
Felo-de-se —see Suicide
Fight (hand) (fists) (foot) —see Assault, fight
Fire (accidental) —see Exposure, fire
Firearm discharge —see Discharge, firearm
Fireball effects from nuclear explosion in war operations —see War operations, nuclear weapons
Fireworks (explosion) W39
Flash burns from explosion —see Explosion
Flood (any injury) (caused by) X38
collapse of man-made structure causing earth movement X36.0
tidal wave —see Forces of nature, tidal wave
Food (any type) in
air passages (with asphyxia, obstruction, or suffocation) —see categories T17 and T18
alimentary tract causing asphyxia (due to compression of trachea) —see categories T17 and T18
Forces of nature X39.8
avalanche X36.1
causing transport accident —see Accident, transport, by type of vehicle
blizzard X37.2
cataclysmic storm X37.9
with flood X38
blizzard X37.2
cloudburst X37.8
cyclone X37.1
dust storm X37.3
hurricane X37.0
specified storm NEC X37.8
storm surge X37.0
tornado X37.1
twister X37.1
typhoon X37.0
cloudburst X37.8
cold (natural) X31
cyclone X37.1
dam collapse causing earth movement X36.0
dust storm X37.3
earth movement X36.1
caused by dam or structure collapse X36.0
earthquake X34
earthquake X34
flood (caused by) X38
dam collapse X36.0
tidal wave —see Forces of nature, tidal wave ◄
heat (natural) X30
hurricane X37.0
landslide X36.1
causing transport accident —see Accident, transport, by type of vehicle
lightning —see subcategory T75.0
causing fire —see Exposure, fire
mudslide X36.1
causing transport accident —see Accident, transport, by type of vehicle

Forces of nature (Continued)
  radiation (natural) X39.08
    radon X39.01
  radon X39.01
  specified force NEC X39.8
  storm surge X37.0
  structure collapse causing
    earth movement
      X36.0
  sunlight X32
  tidal wave X37.41
    due to
      earthquake X37.41
      landslide X37.43
      storm X37.42
      volcanic eruption X37.41
  tornado X37.1

Forces of nature (Continued)
  tsunami X37.41
  twister X37.1
  typhoon X37.0
  volcanic eruption X35
Foreign body ◄
  aspiration - see Index to Diseases and
    Injuries, Foreign body, respitory
    tract ◄
  embedded in skin W45 ◄
  entering through skin W45.8 ◄
    can lid W26.2 ◄
    nail W45.0 ◄
    paper W26.2 ◄
    specified NEC 45.8 ◄
    splinter W45.8 ◄

Forest fire (exposure to) —see Exposure, fire,
  uncontrolled, not in building
Found injured X58
  from exposure (to) —see Exposure
  on
    highway, road(way), street V89.9
    railway right of way V81.9
Fracture (circumstances unknown or
  unspecified) X58
  due to specified cause NEC X58
Freezing —see Exposure, cold
Frostbite X31
  due to man-made conditions —see Exposure,
    cold, man-made
Frozen —see Exposure, cold

G

Gored by bull W55.22
Gunshot wound W34.00

H

Hailstones, injured by X39.8
Hanged herself or himself —see Hanging,
  self-inflicted
Hanging (accidental) —see also category T71
  legal execution —see Legal, intervention,
    specified means NEC
Heat (effects of) (excessive) X30
  due to
    man-made conditions W92
      on board watercraft V93.29
        fishing boat V93.22
        merchant ship V93.20
        passenger ship V93.21
        sailboat V93.24
        specified powered craft NEC V93.23
    weather (conditions) X30

Heat (Continued)
  from
    electric heating apparatus causing
      burning X16
    nuclear explosion in war operations —
      see War operations, nuclear
      weapons
    inappropriate in local application or
      packing in medical or surgical
      procedure Y63.5
Hemorrhage
  delayed following medical or surgical
    treatment without mention of
    misadventure —see Index to Diseases
    and Injuries, Complication(s) ◄▥
  during medical or surgical treatment as
    misadventure —see Index to Diseases
    and Injuries, Complication(s) ◄▥

High
  altitude (effects) —see Air, pressure, low
  level of radioactivity, effects —see Radiation
  pressure (effects) —see Air, pressure, high
  temperature, effects —see Heat
Hit, hitting (accidental) by —see Struck by
Hitting against —see Striking against
Homicide (attempt) (justifiable) —see Assault
Hot
  place, effects —see also Heat
  weather, effects X30
House fire (uncontrolled) —see Exposure, fire,
  uncontrolled, building
Humidity, causing problem X39.8
Hunger X58
Hurricane (any injury) X37.0
Hypobarism, hypobaropathy —see Air,
  pressure, low

◄ New   ◄▥ Revised   ~~deleted~~ Deleted

F, G, & H

I

Ictus
caloris —*see also* Heat
solaris X30
Ignition (accidental) —*see also* Exposure, fire
X08.8
anesthetic gas in operating room W40.1
apparel X06.2
from highly flammable material X04
nightwear X05
bed linen (sheets) (spreads) (pillows)
(mattress) —*see* Exposure, fire,
uncontrolled, building, bed
benzine X04
clothes, clothing NEC (from controlled fire)
X06.2
from
highly flammable material X04
ether X04
in operating room W40.1
explosive material —*see* Explosion
gasoline X04
jewelry (plastic) (any) X06.0
kerosene X04
material
explosive —*see* Explosion
highly flammable with secondary
explosion X04
nightwear X05
paraffin X04
petrol X04
Immersion (accidental) —*see also* Drowning
hand or foot due to cold (excessive) X31
Implantation of quills of porcupine
W55.89
Inanition (from) (hunger) X58
thirst X58.8
Inappropriate operation performed
correct operation on wrong side or body
part (wrong side) (wrong site)
Y65.53
operation intended for another patient done
on wrong patient Y65.52
wrong operation performed on correct
patient Y65.51
Inattention after, at birth (homicidal intent)
(infanticidal intent) X58
Incident, adverse
device
anesthesiology Y70.8
accessory Y70.2
diagnostic Y70.0
miscellaneous Y70.8
monitoring Y70.0
prosthetic Y70.2
rehabilitative Y70.1
surgical Y70.3
therapeutic Y70.1
cardiovascular Y71.8
accessory Y71.2
diagnostic Y71.0
miscellaneous Y71.8
monitoring Y71.0
prosthetic Y71.2
rehabilitative Y71.1
surgical Y71.3
therapeutic Y71.1
gastroenterology Y73.8
accessory Y73.2
diagnostic Y73.0
miscellaneous Y73.8
monitoring Y73.0
prosthetic Y73.2
rehabilitative Y73.1
surgical Y73.3
therapeutic Y73.1
general
hospital Y74.8
accessory Y74.2
diagnostic Y74.0

Incident, adverse *(Continued)*
device *(Continued)*
general *(Continued)*
hospital *(Continued)*
miscellaneous Y74.8
monitoring Y74.0
prosthetic Y74.2
rehabilitative Y74.1
surgical Y74.3
therapeutic Y74.1
surgical Y81.8
accessory Y81.2
diagnostic Y81.0
miscellaneous Y81.8
monitoring Y81.0
prosthetic Y81.2
rehabilitative Y81.1
surgical Y81.3
therapeutic Y81.1
gynecological Y76.8
accessory Y76.2
diagnostic Y76.0
miscellaneous Y76.8
monitoring Y76.0
prosthetic Y76.2
rehabilitative Y76.1
surgical Y76.3
therapeutic Y76.1
medical Y82.9
specified type NEC Y82.8
neurological Y75.8
accessory Y75.2
diagnostic Y75.0
miscellaneous Y75.8
monitoring Y75.0
prosthetic Y75.2
rehabilitative Y75.1
surgical Y75.3
therapeutic Y75.1
obstetrical Y76.8
accessory Y76.2
diagnostic Y76.0
miscellaneous Y76.8
monitoring Y76.0
prosthetic Y76.2
rehabilitative Y76.1
surgical Y76.3
therapeutic Y76.1
ophthalmic Y77.8
accessory Y77.2
diagnostic Y77.0
miscellaneous Y77.8
monitoring Y77.0
prosthetic Y77.2
rehabilitative Y77.1
surgical Y77.3
therapeutic Y77.1
orthopedic Y79.8
accessory Y79.2
diagnostic Y79.0
miscellaneous Y79.8
monitoring Y79.0
prosthetic Y79.2
rehabilitative Y79.1
surgical Y79.3
therapeutic Y79.1
otorhinolaryngological Y72.8
accessory Y72.2
diagnostic Y72.0
miscellaneous Y72.8
monitoring Y72.0
prosthetic Y72.2
rehabilitative Y72.1
surgical Y72.3
therapeutic Y72.1
personal use Y74.8
accessory Y74.2
diagnostic Y74.0
miscellaneous Y74.8
monitoring Y74.0
prosthetic Y74.2

Incident, adverse *(Continued)*
device *(Continued)*
personal use *(Continued)*
rehabilitative Y74.1
surgical Y74.3
therapeutic Y74.1
physical medicine Y80.8
accessory Y80.2
diagnostic Y80.0
miscellaneous Y80.8
monitoring Y80.0
prosthetic Y80.2
rehabilitative Y80.1
surgical Y80.3
therapeutic Y80.1
plastic surgical Y81.8
accessory Y81.2
diagnostic Y81.0
miscellaneous Y81.8
monitoring Y81.0
prosthetic Y81.2
rehabilitative Y81.1
surgical Y81.3
therapeutic Y81.1
radiological Y78.8
accessory Y78.2
diagnostic Y78.0
miscellaneous Y78.8
monitoring Y78.0
prosthetic Y78.2
rehabilitative Y78.1
surgical Y78.3
therapeutic Y78.1
urology Y73.8
accessory Y73.2
diagnostic Y73.0
miscellaneous Y73.8
monitoring Y73.0
prosthetic Y73.2
rehabilitative Y73.1
surgical Y73.3
therapeutic Y73.1
Incineration (accidental) —*see* Exposure, fire
Infanticide —*see* Assault
Infrasound waves (causing injury) W49.9
Ingestion
foreign body (causing injury) (with
obstruction) —*see* Foreign body,
alimentary canal
poisonous
plant (s) X58
substance NEC —*see* Table of Drugs and
Chemicals ◀▥
Inhalation
excessively cold substance, man-made —*see*
Exposure, cold, man-made
food (any type) (into respiratory tract) (with
asphyxia, obstruction respiratory tract,
suffocation) —*see* categories T17 and T18
foreign body —*see* Foreign body, aspiration
gastric contents (with asphyxia, obstruction
respiratory passage, suffocation) T17.81-
hot air or gases X14.0
liquid air, hydrogen, nitrogen W93.12
suicide (attempt) X83.2
steam X13.0
assault X98.0
stated as undetermined whether accidental
or intentional Y27.0
suicide (attempt) X77.0
toxic gas —*see* Table of Drugs and
Chemicals ◀▥
vomitus (with asphyxia, obstruction
respiratory passage, suffocation)T17.81-
Injury, injured (accidental(ly)) **NOS** X58
by, caused by, from
assault —*see* Assault
law-enforcing agent, police, in course
of legal intervention —*see* Legal
intervention
suicide (attempt) X83.8

Injury, injured NOS *(Continued)*
  due to, in
    civil insurrection —*see* War
      operations
    fight —*see also* Assault, fight
      Y04.0
    war operations —*see* War
      operations
  homicide —*see also* Assault Y09
  inflicted (by)
    in course of arrest (attempted), suppression
      of disturbance, maintenance of order,
      by law-enforcing agents —*see* Legal
      intervention

Injury, injured NOS *(Continued)*
  inflicted *(Continued)*
    other person
      stated as
        accidental X58
        intentional, homicide (attempt) —*see*
          Assault
        undetermined whether accidental or
          intentional Y33
    purposely (inflicted) by other person (s) —*see*
      Assault
    self-inflicted X83.8
      stated as accidental X58
    specified cause NEC X58

Injury, injured NOS *(Continued)*
  undetermined whether accidental or
    intentional Y33
Insolation, effects X30
Insufficient nourishment X58
Interruption of respiration (by)
  food (lodged in esophagus) —*see* categories
    T17 and T18
  vomitus (lodged in esophagus) T17.81-
Intervention, legal —*see* Legal intervention
Intoxication
  drug —*see* Table of Drugs and Chemicals ◄▥
  poison —*see* Table of Drugs and
    Chemicals ◄▥

J

Jammed (accidentally)
  between objects (moving) (stationary and
    moving) W23.0
    stationary W23.1
Jumped, jumping
  before moving object NEC X81.8
    motor vehicle X81.0
    subway train X81.1
    train X81.1
    undetermined whether accidental or
      intentional Y31
  from
    boat (into water) voluntarily,
      without accident (to or on boat)
      W16.712
      with
        accident to or on boat —*see* Accident,
          watercraft
        drowning or submersion W16.711
          suicide (attempt) X71.3

Jumped, jumping *(Continued)*
  from *(Continued)*
    boat voluntarily, without accident
      (Continued)
      striking bottom W16.722
        causing drowning W16.721
    building —*see also* Jumped, from,
      high place W13.9
      burning (uncontrolled fire)
        X00.5
    high place NEC W17.89
      suicide (attempt) X80
      undetermined whether accidental or
        intentional Y30
    structure —*see also* Jumped, from, high
      place W13.9
      burning (uncontrolled fire)
        X00.5
  into water W16.92
    causing drowning W16.91
    from, off watercraft —*see* Jumped, from,
      boat

Jumped, jumping *(Continued)*
  into water *(Continued)*
    in
      natural body W16.612
        causing drowning W16.611
        striking bottom W16.622
          causing drowning W16.621
      specified place NEC W16.812
        causing drowning W16.811
        striking
          bottom W16.822
            causing drowning W16.821
          wall W16.832
            causing drowning W16.831
      swimming pool W16.512
        causing drowning W16.511
        striking
          bottom W16.522
            causing drowning W16.521
          wall W16.532
            causing drowning W16.531
    suicide (attempt) X71.3

K

Kicked by
  animal NEC W55.82
  person (s) (accidentally) W50.1
    with intent to injure or kill Y04.0
    as, or caused by, a crowd or human
      stampede (with fall) W52
    assault Y04.0
    homicide (attempt) Y04.0
    in
      fight Y04.0
      legal intervention
        injuring
          bystander Y35.812
          law enforcement personnel Y35.811
          suspect Y35.813
~~Kicking against~~
~~object W22.8~~
  ~~sports equipment W21.9~~
  ~~stationary W22.09~~
    ~~sports equipment W21.89~~
~~person —see Striking against, person~~
~~sports equipment W21.9~~

Kicking ◄
  against ◄
    object W22.8 ◄
      sports equipment W21.9 ◄
      stationary W22.09 ◄
        sports equipment W21.89 ◄
    person —*see* Striking against, person ◄
    sports equipment W21.9 ◄
  carpet stretcher with knee X50.3 ◄
Killed, killing (accidentally) NOS —*see also*
  Injury X58
  in
    action —*see* War operations
    brawl, fight (hand) (fists) (foot) Y04.0
      by weapon —*see also* Assault
        cutting, piercing —*see* Assault, cutting
          or piercing instrument
        firearm —*see* Discharge, firearm, by
          type, homicide

Killed, killing NOS *(Continued)*
  self
    stated as
      accident NOS X58
      suicide —*see* Suicide
      undetermined whether accidental or
        intentional Y33
Kneeling (prolonged) (static) X50.1 ◄
Knocked down (accidentally) (by) NOS X58
  animal (not being ridden) NEC —*see also*
    Struck by, by type of animal
  crowd or human stampede W52
  person W51
    in brawl, fight Y04.0
  transport vehicle NEC —*see also* Accident,
    transport V09.9

◄ New   ◄▥ Revised   ~~deleted~~ Deleted

L

Laceration NEC —*see* Injury
Lack of
  care (helpless person) (infant) (newborn) X58
  food except as result of abandonment or
    neglect X58
    due to abandonment or neglect X58
  water except as result of transport accident X58
    due to transport accident —*see* Accident,
      transport, by type ◄
  helpless person, infant, newborn X58
Landslide (falling on transport vehicle) X36.1
  caused by collapse of man-made structure
    X36.Ø
Late effect —*see* Sequelae
Legal
  execution (any method) —*see* Legal,
    intervention
  intervention (by)
    baton —*see* Legal, intervention, blunt
      object, baton
    bayonet —*see* Legal, intervention, sharp
      object, bayonet
    blow —*see* Legal, intervention,
      manhandling
    blunt object
      baton
        injuring
          bystander Y35.312
          law enforcement personnel Y35.311
          suspect Y35.313
      injuring
        bystander Y35.3Ø2
        law enforcement personnel Y35.3Ø1
        suspect Y35.3Ø3
      specified NEC
        injuring
          bystander Y35.392
          law enforcement personnel Y35.391
          suspect Y35.393
      stave
        injuring
          bystander Y35.392
          law enforcement personnel Y35.391
          suspect Y35.393
    bomb —*see* Legal, intervention, explosive
    cutting or piercing instrument —*see* Legal,
      intervention, sharp object
    dynamite —*see* Legal, intervention,
      explosive, dynamite
    explosive (s)
      dynamite
        injuring
          bystander Y35.112
          law enforcement personnel Y35.111
          suspect Y35.113
      grenade
        injuring
          bystander Y35.192
          law enforcement personnel Y35.191
          suspect Y35.193
      injuring
        bystander Y35.1Ø2
        law enforcement personnel Y35.1Ø1
        suspect Y35.1Ø3

Legal (*Continued*)
  intervention (*Continued*)
    explosive (*Continued*)
      mortar bomb
        injuring
          bystander Y35.192
          law enforcement personnel
            Y35.191
          suspect Y35.193
      shell
        injuring
          bystander Y35.122
          law enforcement personnel Y35.121
          suspect Y35.123
      specified NEC
        injuring
          bystander Y35.192
          law enforcement personnel Y35.191
          suspect Y35.193
    firearm (s) (discharge)
      handgun
        injuring
          bystander Y35.Ø22
          law enforcement personnel Y35.Ø21
          suspect Y35.Ø23
      injuring
        bystander Y35.ØØ2
        law enforcement personnel Y35.ØØ1
        suspect Y35.ØØ3
      machine gun
        injuring
          bystander Y35.Ø12
          law enforcement personnel Y35.Ø11
          suspect Y35.Ø13
      rifle pellet
        injuring
          bystander Y35.Ø32
          law enforcement personnel Y35.Ø31
          suspect Y35.Ø33
      rubber bullet
        injuring
          bystander Y35.Ø42
          law enforcement personnel Y35.Ø41
          suspect Y35.Ø43
      shotgun —*see* Legal, intervention,
        firearm, specified NEC
      specified NEC
        injuring
          bystander Y35.Ø92
          law enforcement personnel Y35.Ø91
          suspect Y35.Ø93
    gas (asphyxiation) (poisoning)
      injuring
        bystander Y35.2Ø2
        law enforcement personnel Y35.2Ø1
        suspect Y35.2Ø3
      specified NEC
        injuring
          bystander Y35.292
          law enforcement personnel Y35.291
          suspect Y35.293
      tear gas
        injuring
          bystander Y35.212
          law enforcement personnel Y35.211
          suspect Y35.213

Legal (*Continued*)
  intervention (*Continued*)
    grenade —*see* Legal, intervention,
      explosive, grenade
    injuring
      bystander Y35.92
      law enforcement personnel Y35.91
      suspect Y35.93
    late effect (of) —*see* with 7th character S
      Y35
    manhandling
      injuring
        bystander Y35.812
        law enforcement personnel Y35.811
        suspect Y35.813
    sequelae (of) —*see* with 7th character S
      Y35
    sharp objects
      bayonet
        injuring
          bystander Y35.412
          law enforcement personnel
            Y35.411
          suspect Y35.413
      injuring
        bystander Y35.4Ø2
        law enforcement personnel Y35.4Ø1
        suspect Y35.4Ø3
      specified NEC
        injuring
          bystander Y35.492
          law enforcement personnel Y35.491
          suspect Y35.493
    specified means NEC
      injuring
        bystander Y35.892
        law enforcement personnel Y35.891
        suspect Y35.893
    stabbing —*see* Legal, intervention, sharp
      object
    stave —*see* Legal, intervention, blunt
      object, stave
    tear gas —*see* Legal, intervention, gas, tear
      gas
    truncheon —*see* Legal, intervention, blunt
      object, stave
Lifting —*see also* Overexertion ◄
  heavy objects X5Ø.Ø ◄
  weights X5Ø.Ø ◄
Lightning (shock) (stroke) (struck by) —*see*
  subcategory T75.Ø
  causing fire —*see* Exposure, fire
Loss of control (transport vehicle) NEC —*see*
  Accident, transport
Lost at sea NOS —*see* Drowning, due to, fall
  overboard
Low
  pressure (effects) —*see* Air, pressure, low
  temperature (effects) —*see* Exposure, cold
Lying before train, vehicle or other moving
  object X81.8
  subway train X81.1
  train X81.1
  undetermined whether accidental or
    intentional Y31
Lynching —*see* Assault

M

Malfunction (mechanism or component) (of)
　firearm
　　airgun W34.10
　　BB gun W34.110
　　gas, air or spring-operated gun NEC
　　　W34.118
　　handgun W32.1
　　hunting rifle W33.12
　　larger firearm W33.10
　　　specified NEC W33.19
　　machine gun W33.13
　　paintball gun W34.111
　　pellet gun W34.110
　　shotgun W33.11
　　specified NEC W34.19
　　Very pistol [flare] W34.19
　handgun —*see* Malfunction, firearm,
　　handgun
Maltreatment —*see* Perpetrator
Mangled (accidentally) **NOS** X58
Manhandling (in brawl, fight) Y04.0
　legal intervention —*see* Legal, intervention,
　　manhandling
Manslaughter (nonaccidental) —*see* Assault
Mauled by animal NEC W55.89
Medical procedure, complication of
　(delayed or as an abnormal reaction
　　without mention of misadventure) —*see*
　　Complication of or following, by specified
　　type of procedure
　due to or as a result of misadventure —*see*
　　Misadventure
Melting (due to fire) —*see also* Exposure, fire
　apparel NEC X06.3
　clothes, clothing NEC X06.3
　　nightwear X05
　fittings or furniture (burning building)
　　(uncontrolled fire) X00.8
　nightwear X05
　plastic jewelry X06.1
Mental cruelty X58
Military operations (injuries to military and
　civilians occuring during peacetime on
　military property and during routine
　military exercises and operations) (by)
　(from) (involving) Y37.90-
　air blast Y37.20-
　aircraft
　　destruction —*see* Military operations,
　　　destruction of aircraft
　　airway restriction —*see* Military operations,
　　　restriction of airways
　　asphyxiation —*see* Military operations,
　　　restriction of airways
　biological weapons Y37.6X-
　blast Y37.20-
　blast fragments Y37.20-
　blast wave Y37.20-
　blast wind Y37.20-
　bomb Y37.20-
　　dirty Y37.50-
　　gasoline Y37.31-
　　incendiary Y37.31-
　　petrol Y37.31-
　bullet Y37.43-
　　incendiary Y37.32-
　　rubber Y37.41-
　chemical weapons Y37.7X-
　combat
　　hand to hand (unarmed) combat
　　　Y37.44-
　　using blunt or piercing object Y37.45-
　conflagration —*see* Military operations, fire
　conventional warfare NEC Y37.49-
　depth-charge Y37.01-
　destruction of aircraft Y37.10-
　　due to
　　　air to air missile Y37.11-
　　　collision with other aircraft Y37.12-

Military operations (*Continued*)
　destruction of aircraft (*Continued*)
　　due to (*Continued*)
　　　detonation (accidental) of onboard
　　　　munitions and explosives Y37.14-
　　　enemy fire or explosives Y37.11-
　　　explosive placed on aircraft Y37.11-
　　　onboard fire Y37.13-
　　　rocket propelled grenade [RPG] Y37.11-
　　　small arms fire Y37.11-
　　　surface to air missile Y37.11-
　　specified NEC Y37.19-
　detonation (accidental) of
　　onboard marine weapons Y37.05-
　　own munitions or munitions launch device
　　　Y37.24-
　dirty bomb Y37.50-
　explosion (of) Y37.20-
　　aerial bomb Y37.21-
　　bomb NOS —*see also* Military operations,
　　　bomb (s) Y37.20-
　　fragments Y37.20-
　　grenade Y37.29-
　　guided missile Y37.22-
　　improvised explosive device [IED] (person-
　　　borne) (roadside) (vehicle-borne)
　　　Y37.23-
　　land mine Y37.29-
　　marine mine (at sea) (in harbor) Y37.02-
　　marine weapon Y37.00-
　　　specified NEC Y37.09-
　　own munitions or munitions launch device
　　　(accidental) Y37.24-
　　sea-based artillery shell Y37.03-
　　specified NEC Y37.29-
　　torpedo Y37.04-
　fire Y37.30-
　　specified NEC Y37.39-
　firearms
　　discharge Y37.43-
　　pellets Y37.42-
　flamethrower Y37.33-
　fragments (from) (of)
　　improvised explosive device [IED] (person-
　　　borne) (roadside) (vehicle-borne)
　　　Y37.26-
　　munitions Y37.25-
　　specified NEC Y37.29-
　　weapons Y37.27-
　friendly fire Y37.92-
　hand to hand (unarmed) combat Y37.44-
　hot substances —*see* Military operations, fire
　incendiary bullet Y37.32-
　nuclear weapon (effects of) Y37.50-
　　acute radiation exposure Y37.54-
　　blast pressure Y37.51-
　　direct blast Y37.51-
　　direct heat Y37.53-
　　fallout exposure Y37.54-
　　fireball Y37.53-
　　indirect blast (struck or crushed by blast
　　　debris) (being thrown by blast)
　　　Y37.52-
　　ionizing radiation (immediate exposure)
　　　Y37.54-
　　nuclear radiation Y37.54-
　　radiation
　　　ionizing (immediate exposure) Y37.54-
　　　nuclear Y37.54-
　　　thermal Y37.53-
　　secondary effects Y37.54-
　　specified NEC Y37.59-
　　thermal radiation Y37.53-
　restriction of air (airway)
　　intentional Y37.46-
　　unintentional Y37.47-
　rubber bullets Y37.41-
　shrapnel NOS Y37.29-
　suffocation —*see* Military operations,
　　restriction of airways
　unconventional warfare NEC Y37.7X-

Military operations (*Continued*)
　underwater blast NOS Y37.00-
　warfare
　　conventional NEC Y37.49-
　　unconventional NEC Y37.7X-
　weapon of mass destruction [WMD] Y37.91-
　weapons
　　biological weapons Y37.6X-
　　chemical Y37.7X-
　　nuclear (effects of) Y37.50-
　　　acute radiation exposure Y37.54-
　　　blast pressure Y37.51-
　　　direct blast Y37.51-
　　　direct heat Y37.53-
　　　fallout exposure Y37.54-
　　　fireball Y37.53-
　　　~~indirect blast (struck or crushed by blast~~
　　　　~~debris) (being thrown by blast)~~
　　　　~~Y37.52-~~
　　　radiation
　　　　ionizing (immediate exposure) Y37.54-
　　　　nuclear Y37.54-
　　　　thermal Y37.53-
　　　secondary effects Y37.54-
　　　specified NEC Y37.59-
　　of mass destruction [WMD] Y37.91-
**Misadventure (s) to patient (s) during surgical
　or medical care** Y69
　contaminated medical or biological substance
　　(blood, drug, fluid) Y64.9
　　administered (by) NEC Y64.9
　　immunization Y64.1
　　infusion Y64.0
　　injection Y64.1
　　specified means NEC Y64.8
　　transfusion Y64.0
　　vaccination Y64.1
　excessive amount of blood or other fluid
　　during transfusion or infusion Y63.0
　failure
　　in dosage Y63.9
　　　electroshock therapy Y63.4
　　　inappropriate temperature (too hot or
　　　　too cold) in local application and
　　　　packing Y63.5
　　　infusion
　　　　excessive amount of fluid Y63.0
　　　　incorrect dilution of fluid Y63.1
　　　insulin-shock therapy Y63.4
　　　nonadministration of necessary drug or
　　　　biological substance Y63.6 ◀▥
　　　overdose —*see* Table of Drugs and
　　　　Chemicals ◀▥
　　　radiation, in therapy Y63.2
　　　radiation
　　　　overdose Y63.2
　　　specified procedure NEC Y63.8
　　　transfusion
　　　　excessive amount of blood Y63.0
　　mechanical, of instrument or apparatus
　　　(any) (during any procedure) Y65.8
　　sterile precautions (during procedure)
　　　Y62.9
　　aspiration of fluid or tissue (by puncture
　　　or catheterization, except heart)
　　　Y62.6
　　biopsy (except needle aspiration) Y62.8
　　　needle (aspirating) Y62.6
　　blood sampling Y62.6
　　catheterization Y62.6
　　　heart Y62.5
　　dialysis (kidney) Y62.2
　　endoscopic examination Y62.4
　　enema Y62.8
　　immunization Y62.3
　　infusion Y62.1
　　injection Y62.3
　　needle biopsy Y62.6
　　paracentesis (abdominal) (thoracic)
　　　Y62.6
　　perfusion Y62.2

◀ New　◀▥ Revised　~~deleted~~ Deleted

Misadventure (s) to patient (s) during surgical
or medical care *(Continued)*
failure *(Continued)*
sterile precautions *(Continued)*
puncture (lumbar) Y62.6
removal of catheter or packing
Y62.8
specified procedure NEC Y62.8
surgical operation Y62.0
transfusion Y62.1
vaccination Y62.3
suture or ligature during surgical
procedure Y65.2
to introduce or to remove tube or
instrument —*see* Failure, to ◀
hemorrhage —*see* Index to Diseases and
Injuries, Complication(s) ◀▥
inadvertent exposure of patient to radiation
Y63.3
inappropriate
operation performed —*see*
Inappropriate operation
performed
temperature (too hot or too cold) in
local application or packing
Y63.5

infusion —*see also* Misadventure, by type,
infusion Y69
excessive amount of fluid Y63.0
incorrect dilution of fluid Y63.1
wrong fluid Y65.1
mismatched blood in transfusion Y65.0
nonadministration of necessary drug or
biological substance Y63.6 ◀▥
overdose —*see* Table of Drugs and
Chemicals ◀▥
radiation (in therapy) Y63.2
perforation —*see* Index to Diseases and
Injuries, Complication(s) ◀▥
performance of inappropriate operation —*see*
Inappropriate operation performed
puncture —*see* Index to Diseases and Injuries,
Complication(s) ◀▥
specified type NEC Y65.8
failure
suture or ligature during surgical
operation Y65.2
to introduce or to remove tube or
instrument —*see* Failure, to ◀
infusion of wrong fluid Y65.1

specified type NEC *(Continued)*
performance of inappropriate operation —
see Inappropriate operation performed
transfusion of mismatched blood Y65.0
wrong
fluid in infusion Y65.1
placement of endotracheal tube during
anesthetic procedure Y65.3
transfusion —*see* Misadventure, by type,
transfusion
excessive amount of blood Y63.0
mismatched blood Y65.0
wrong
drug given in error —*see* Table of Drugs
and Chemicals ◀▥
fluid in infusion Y65.1
placement of endotracheal tube during
anesthetic procedure Y65.3
Mismatched blood in transfusion Y65.0
Motion sickness T75.3
Mountain sickness W94.11
Mudslide (of cataclysmic nature) —*see*
Landslide
Murder (attempt) —*see* Assault

N

Nail ◀
contact with W45.0 ◀
gun W29.4
embedded in skin W45.0 ◀
~~Nail, contact with W45.0~~
~~gun W29.4~~

Neglect (criminal) (homicidal intent) X58
Noise (causing injury) (pollution) W42.9
supersonic W42.0
Nonadministration (of)
drug or biological substance (necessary)
Y63.6 ◀▥
surgical and medical care Y66
Nosocomial condition Y95

O

Object
falling
from, in, on, hitting
machinery —*see* Contact, with, by type
of machine
set in motion by
accidental explosion or rupture of pressure
vessel W38
firearm —*see* Discharge, firearm, by type
machine (ry) —*see* Contact, with, by type
of machine
Overdose (drug) —*see* Table of Drugs and
Chemicals ◀▥
radiation Y63.2

Overexertion X50.9 ◀▥
from ◀
prolonged static or awkward postures
X50.1 ◀
repetitive movements X50.3 ◀
specified strenuous movements or postures
NEC X50.9 ◀
strenuous movement or load X50.0 ◀
Overexposure (accidental) (to)
cold —*see also* Exposure, cold X31
due to man-made conditions —*see*
Exposure, cold, man-made
heat —*see also* Heat X30
radiation —*see* Radiation
radioactivity W88.0
sun (sunburn) X32

Overexposure *(Continued)*
weather NEC —*see* Forces of nature ◀
wind NEC —*see* Forces of nature ◀
Overheated —*see* Heat
Overturning (accidental)
machinery —*see* Contact, with, by type of
machine
transport vehicle NEC —*see also* Accident,
transport V89.9
watercraft (causing drowning,
submersion) —*see also* Drowning, due to,
accident to, watercraft, overturning
causing injury except drowning or
submersion —*see* Accident, watercraft,
causing, injury NEC ◀

P

Parachute descent (voluntary) (without
accident to aircraft) V97.29
due to accident to aircraft —*see* Accident,
transport, aircraft
Pecked by bird W61.99
Perforation during medical or surgical
treatment as misadventure —*see* Index to
Diseases and Injuries, Complication(s) ◄▥▥
Perpetrator, perpetration, of assault,
maltreatment and neglect (by)
Y07.9
boyfriend Y07.03
brother Y07.410
stepbrother Y07.435
coach Y07.53
cousin
female Y07.491
male Y07.490
daycare provider Y07.519
at-home
adult care Y07.512
childcare Y07.510
care center
adult care Y07.513
childcare Y07.511
family member NEC Y07.499
father Y07.11
adoptive Y07.13
foster Y07.420
stepfather Y07.430
foster father Y07.420
foster mother Y07.421
girl friend Y07.04
healthcare provider Y07.529
mental health Y07.521
specified NEC Y07.528
husband Y07.01
instructor Y07.53
mother Y07.12
adoptive Y07.14
foster Y07.421
stepmother Y07.433
nonfamily member Y07.50
specified NEC Y07.59
nurse Y07.528
occupational therapist Y07.528
partner of parent
female Y07.434
male Y07.432
physical therapist Y07.528
sister Y07.411
speech therapist Y07.528
stepbrother Y07.435
stepfather Y07.430
stepmother Y07.433
stepsister Y07.436
teacher Y07.53
wife Y07.02
Piercing —*see* Contact, with, by type of object
or machine
Pinched
between objects (moving) (stationary and
moving) W23.0
stationary W23.1
Pinned under machine (ry) —*see* Contact, with,
by type of machine
Place of occurrence Y92.9
abandoned house Y92.89
airplane Y92.813
airport Y92.520
ambulatory health services establishment
NEC Y92.538
ambulatory surgery center Y92.530
amusement park Y92.831
apartment (co-op) —*see* Place of occurrence,
residence, apartment
assembly hall Y92.29
bank Y92.510
barn Y92.71
baseball field Y92.320

Place of occurrence (*Continued*)
basketball court Y92.310
beach Y92.832
boarding house —*see* Place of occurrence,
residence, boarding house
boat Y92.814
bowling alley Y92.39
bridge Y92.89
building under construction Y92.61
bus Y92.811
station Y92.521
cafe Y92.511
campsite Y92.833
campus —*see* Place of occurrence, school
canal Y92.89
car Y92.810
casino Y92.59
children's home —*see* Place of occurrence,
residence, institutional, orphanage
church Y92.22
cinema Y92.26
clubhouse Y92.29
coal pit Y92.64
college (community) Y92.214
condominium —*see* Place of occurrence,
residence, apartment
construction area —*see* Place of occurrence,
industrial and construction area
convalescent home —*see* Place of occurrence,
residence, institutional, nursing home
court-house Y92.240
cricket ground Y92.328
cultural building Y92.258
art gallery Y92.250
museum Y92.251
music hall Y92.252
opera house Y92.253
specified NEC Y92.258
theater Y92.254
dancehall Y92.252
day nursery Y92.210
dentist office Y92.531
derelict house Y92.89
desert Y92.820
dock NOS Y92.89
dockyard Y92.62
doctor's office Y92.531
dormitory —*see* Place of occurrence,
residence, institutional, school dormitory
dry dock Y92.62
factory (building) (premises) Y92.63
farm (land under cultivation) (outbuildings)
Y92.79
barn Y92.71
chicken coop Y92.72
field Y92.73
hen house Y92.72
house —*see* Place of occurrence, residence,
house
orchard Y92.74
specified NEC Y92.79
football field Y92.321
forest Y92.821
freeway Y92.411
gallery Y92.250
garage (commercial) Y92.59
boarding house Y92.044
military base Y92.135
mobile home Y92.025
nursing home Y92.124
orphanage Y92.114
private house Y92.015
reform school Y92.155
gas station Y92.524
gasworks Y92.69
golf course Y92.39
gravel pit Y92.64
grocery Y92.512
gymnasium Y92.39
handball court Y92.318
harbor Y92.89

Place of occurrence (*Continued*)
harness racing course Y92.39
healthcare provider office Y92.531
highway (interstate) Y92.411
hill Y92.828
hockey rink Y92.330
home —*see* Place of occurrence, residence
hospice —*see* Place of occurrence, residence,
institutional, nursing home
hospital Y92.239
cafeteria Y92.233
corridor Y92.232
operating room Y92.234
patient
bathroom Y92.231
room Y92.230
specified NEC Y92.238
hotel Y92.59
house —*see also* Place of occurrence, residence
abandoned Y92.89
under construction Y92.61
industrial and construction area (yard)
Y92.69
building under construction Y92.61
dock Y92.62
dry dock Y92.62
factory Y92.63
gasworks Y92.69
mine Y92.64
oil rig Y92.65
pit Y92.64
power station Y92.69
shipyard Y92.62
specified NEC Y92.69
tunnel under construction Y92.69
workshop Y92.69
kindergarten Y92.211
lacrosse field Y92.328
lake Y92.828
library Y92.241
mall Y92.59
market Y92.512
marsh Y92.828
military
base —*see* Place of occurrence, residence,
institutional, military base
training ground Y92.84
mine Y92.64
mosque Y92.22
motel Y92.59
motorway (interstate) Y92.411
mountain Y92.828
movie-house Y92.26
museum Y92.251
music-hall Y92.252
not applicable Y92.9
nuclear power station Y92.69
nursing home —*see* Place of occurrence,
residence, institutional, nursing home
office building Y92.59
offshore installation Y92.65
oil rig Y92.65
old people's home —*see* Place of occurrence,
residence, institutional, specified NEC
opera-house Y92.253
orphanage —*see* Place of occurrence,
residence, institutional, orphanage
outpatient surgery center Y92.530
park (public) Y92.830
amusement Y92.831
parking garage Y92.89
lot Y92.481
pavement Y92.480
physician office Y92.531
polo field Y92.328
pond Y92.828
post office Y92.242
power station Y92.69
prairie Y92.828
prison —*see* Place of occurrence, residence,
institutional, prison

Place of occurrence *(Continued)*
  public
    administration building Y92.248
      city hall Y92.243
      courthouse Y92.240
      library Y92.241
      post office Y92.242
      specified NEC Y92.248
    building NEC Y92.29
    hall Y92.29
    place NOS Y92.89
  race course Y92.39
  radio station Y92.59
  railway line (bridge) Y92.85
  ranch (outbuildings) —*see* Place of
    occurrence, farm
  recreation area Y92.838
    amusement park Y92.831
    beach Y92.832
    campsite Y92.833
    park (public) Y92.830
    seashore Y92.832
    specified NEC Y92.838
  reform school —*see* Place of occurrence,
    residence, institutional, reform school
  religious institution Y92.22
  residence (non-institutional) (private) Y92.009
    apartment Y92.039
      bathroom Y92.031
      bedroom Y92.032
      kitchen Y92.030
      specified NEC Y92.038
    bathroom Y92.002
    bedroom Y92.003
    boarding house Y92.049
      bathroom Y92.041
      bedroom Y92.042
      driveway Y92.043
      garage Y92.044
      garden Y92.046
      kitchen Y92.040
      specified NEC Y92.048
      swimming pool Y92.045
      yard Y92.046
    dining room Y92.001
    garden Y92.007
    home Y92.009
    house, single family Y92.019
      bathroom Y92.012
      bedroom Y92.013
      dining room Y92.011
      driveway Y92.014
      garage Y92.015
      garden Y92.017
      kitchen Y92.010
      specified NEC Y92.018
      swimming pool Y92.016
      yard Y92.017
    institutional Y92.10
      children's home —*see* Place of
        occurrence, residence, institutional,
        orphanage
      hospice —*see* Place of occurrence,
        residence, institutional, nursing
        home
      military base Y92.139
        barracks Y92.133
        garage Y92.135
        garden Y92.137
        kitchen Y92.130
        mess hall Y92.131
        specified NEC Y92.138
        swimming pool Y92.136
        yard Y92.137
      nursing home Y92.129
        bathroom Y92.121
        bedroom Y92.122
        driveway Y92.123
        garage Y92.124
        garden Y92.126
        kitchen Y92.120

Place of occurrence *(Continued)*
  residence *(Continued)*
    institutional *(Continued)*
      nursing home *(Continued)*
        specified NEC Y92.128
        swimming pool Y92.125
        yard Y92.126
      orphanage Y92.119
        bathroom Y92.111
        bedroom Y92.112
        driveway Y92.113
        garage Y92.114
        garden Y92.116
        kitchen Y92.110
        specified NEC Y92.118
        swimming pool Y92.115
        yard Y92.116
      prison Y92.149
        bathroom Y92.142
        cell Y92.143
        courtyard Y92.147
        dining room Y92.141
        kitchen Y92.140
        specified NEC Y92.148
        swimming pool Y92.146
      reform school Y92.159
        bathroom Y92.152
        bedroom Y92.153
        dining room Y92.151
        driveway Y92.154
        garage Y92.155
        garden Y92.157
        kitchen Y92.150
        specified NEC Y92.158
        swimming pool Y92.156
        yard Y92.157
      school dormitory Y92.169
        bathroom Y92.162
        bedroom Y92.163
        dining room Y92.161
        kitchen Y92.160
        specified NEC Y92.168
      specified NEC Y92.199
        bathroom Y92.192
        bedroom Y92.193
        dining room Y92.191
        driveway Y92.194
        garage Y92.195
        garden Y92.197
        kitchen Y92.190
        specified NEC Y92.198
        swimming pool Y92.196
        yard Y92.197
    kitchen Y92.000
    mobile home Y92.029
      bathroom Y92.022
      bedroom Y92.023
      dining room Y92.021
      driveway Y92.024
      garage Y92.025
      garden Y92.027
      kitchen Y92.020
      specified NEC Y92.028
      swimming pool Y92.026
      yard Y92.027
    specified place in residence NEC Y92.008 ◀▥
    specified residence type NEC Y92.099
      bathroom Y92.091
      bedroom Y92.092
      driveway Y92.093
      garage Y92.094
      garden Y92.096
      kitchen Y92.090
      specified NEC Y92.098
      swimming pool Y92.095
      yard Y92.096
    restaurant Y92.511
    riding school Y92.39
    river Y92.828
    road Y92.488
    rodeo ring Y92.39

Place of occurrence *(Continued)*
  rugby field Y92.328
  same day surgery center Y92.530
  sand pit Y92.64
  school (private) (public) (state) Y92.219
    college Y92.214
    daycare center Y92.210
    elementary school Y92.211
    high school Y92.213
    kindergarten Y92.211
    middle school Y92.212
    specified NEC Y92.218
    trace school Y92.215
    university Y92.214
    vocational school Y92.215
  sea (shore) Y92.832
  senior citizen center Y92.29
  service area
    airport Y92.520
    bus station Y92.521
    gas station Y92.524
    highway rest stop Y92.523
    railway station Y92.522
  shipyard Y92.62
  shop (commercial) Y92.513
  sidewalk Y92.480
  silo Y92.79
  skating rink (roller) Y92.331
    ice Y92.330
  slaughter house Y92.86
  soccer field Y92.322
  specified place NEC Y92.89
  sports area Y92.39
    athletic
      court Y92.318
        basketball Y92.310
        specified NEC Y92.318
        squash Y92.311
        tennis Y92.312
      field Y92.328
        baseball Y92.320
        cricket ground Y92.328
        football Y92.321
        hockey Y92.328
        soccer Y92.322
        specified NEC Y92.328
    golf course Y92.39
    gymnasium Y92.39
    riding school Y92.39
    skating rink (roller) Y92.331
      ice Y92.330
    stadium Y92.39
    swimming pool Y92.34
  squash court Y92.311
  stadium Y92.39
  steeplechasing course Y92.39
  store Y92.512
  stream Y92.828
  street and highway Y92.410
    bike path Y92.482
    freeway Y92.411
    highway ramp Y92.415
    interstate highway Y92.411
    local residential or business street
      Y92.414
    motorway Y92.411
    parking lot Y92.481
    parkway Y92.412
    sidewalk Y92.480
    specified NEC Y92.488
    state road Y92.413
  subway car Y92.816
  supermarket Y92.512
  swamp Y92.828
  swimming pool (public) Y92.34
    private (at) Y92.095
      boarding house Y92.045
      military base Y92.136
      mobile home Y92.026
      nursing home Y92.125
      orphanage Y92.115

Place of occurrence *(Continued)*
  swimming pool *(Continued)*
    private *(Continued)*
      prison Y92.146
      reform school Y92.156
      single family residence
        Y92.016
  synagogue Y92.22
  television station Y92.59
  tennis court Y92.312
  theater Y92.254
  trade area Y92.59
    bank Y92.510
    cafe Y92.511
    casino Y92.59
    garage Y92.59
    hotel Y92.59
    market Y92.512
    office building Y92.59
    radio station Y92.59
    restaurant Y92.511
    shop Y92.513
    shopping mall Y92.59
    store Y92.512
    supermarket Y92.512
    television station Y92.59
    warehouse Y92.59
  trailer park, residential —*see* Place of
    occurrence, residence, mobile
    home
  trailer site NOS Y92.89
  train Y92.815
    station Y92.522
  truck Y92.812
  tunnel under construction Y92. 69
  university Y92.214
  urgent (health) care center Y92.532
  vehicle (transport) Y92.818
    airplane Y92.813
    boat Y92.814
    bus Y92.811
    car Y92.810
    specified NEC Y92.818
    subway car Y92.816
    train Y92.815
    truck Y92.812
  warehouse Y92.59
  water reservoir Y92.89
  wilderness area Y92.828
    desert Y92.820
    forest Y92.821
    marsh Y92.828
    mountain Y92.828
    prairie Y92.828
    specified NEC Y92.828
    swamp Y92.828
  workshop Y92.69
  yard, private Y92.096
    boarding house Y92.046
    mobile home Y92.027
    single family house Y92.017

Place of occurrence *(Continued)*
  youth center Y92.29
  zoo (zoological garden) Y92.834
Plumbism —*see* Table of Drugs and Chemicals,
  lead ◄▥
Poisoning (accidental) (by) —*see also* Table of
  Drugs and Chemicals ◄▥
  by plant, thorns, spines, sharp leaves or other
    mechanisms NEC X58
  carbon monoxide
    generated by
      motor vehicle —*see* Accident, transport
      watercraft (in transit) (not in transit)
        V93.89
        ferry boat V93.81
        fishing boat V93.82
        jet skis V93.83
        liner V93.81
        merchant ship V93.80
        passenger ship V93.81
        powered craft NEC V93.83
  caused by injection of poisons into skin by
    plant thorns, spines, sharp leaves X58
    marine or sea plants (venomous) X58
  exhaust gas
    generated by
      motor vehicle —*see* Accident, transport
      watercraft (in transit) (not in transit)
        V93.89
        ferry boat V93.81
        fishing boat V93.82
        jet skis V93.83
        liner V93.81
        merchant ship V93.80
        passenger ship V93.81
        powered craft NEC V93.83
  fumes or smoke due to
    explosion —*see also* Explosion W40.9
    fire —*see* Exposure, fire
    ignition —*see* Ignition
  gas
    in legal intervention —*see* Legal,
      intervention, gas
    legal execution —*see* Legal, intervention,
      gas
  in war operations —*see* War operations
  legal
    execution —*see* Legal, intervention, gas
    intervention
      by gas —*see* Legal, intervention, gas
      other specified means —*see* Legal,
        intervention, specified means
        NEC
Powder burn (by) (from)
  airgun W34.110
  BB gun W34.110
  firearm NEC W34.19
  gas, air or spring-operated gun NEC
    W34.118
  handgun W32.1
  hunting rifle W33.12

Powder burn *(Continued)*
  larger firearm W33.10
    specified NEC W33.19
  machine gun W33.13
  paintball gun W34.111
  pellet gun W34.110
  shotgun W33.11
  Very pistol [flare] W34.19
Premature cessation (of) surgical and medical
  care Y66
Privation (food) (water) X58
Procedure (operation)
  correct, on wrong side or body part (wrong
    side) (wrong site) Y65.53
  intended for another patient done on wrong
    patient Y65.52
  performed on patient not scheduled for
    surgery Y65.52
  performed on wrong patient Y65.52
  wrong, performed on correct patient Y65.51
Prolonged
  sitting in transport vehicle —*see* Travel, by
    type of vehicle
  stay in
    high altitude as cause of anoxia,
      barodontalgia, barotitis or hypoxia
      W94.11
    weightless environment X52
Pulling, excessive —*see also* Overexertion
  X50.9 ◄▥
Puncture, puncturing —*see also* Contact, with,
  by type of object or machine
  by
    plant thorns, spines, sharp leaves or other
      mechanisms NEC W60
  during medical or surgical treatment as
    misadventure —*see* Index to Diseases
    and Injuries, Complication(s) ◄▥
Pushed, pushing (accidental) (injury in) ◄▥
  by other person (s) (accidental) W51
    with fall W03
      due to ice or snow W00.0
    as, or caused by, a crowd or human
      stampede (with fall) W52
    before moving object NEC Y02.8
      motor vehicle Y02.0
      subway train Y02.1
      train Y02.1
    from
      high place NEC
        in accidental circumstances W17.89
        stated as
          intentional, homicide (attempt) Y01
          undetermined whether accidental
            or intentional Y30
      transport vehicle NEC —*see also*
        Accident, transport V89.9
        stated as
          intentional, homicide (attempt)
            Y08.89
    overexertion X50.9 ◄

R

Radiation (exposure to)
arc lamps W89.0
atomic power plant (malfunction) NEC
W88.1
complication of or abnormal reaction to
medical radiotherapy Y84.2
electromagnetic, ionizing W88.0
gamma rays W88.1
in
war operations (from or following
nuclear explosion) —see also War
operations
inadvertent exposure of patient (receiving
test or therapy) Y63.3
infrared (heaters and lamps) W90.1
excessive heat from W92
ionized, ionizing (particles, artificially
accelerated)
radioisotopes W88.1
specified NEC W88.8
x-rays W88.0
isotopes, radioactive —see Radiation,
radioactive isotopes
laser (s) W90.2
in war operations —see War operations
misadventure in medical care Y63.2
light sources (man-made visible and
ultraviolet) W89.9
natural X32
specified NEC W89.8
tanning bed W89.1
welding light W89.0
man-made visible light W89.9
specified NEC W89.8
tanning bed W89.1
welding light W89.0
microwave W90.8
misadventure in medical or surgical
procedure Y63.2

Radiation (Continued)
natural NEC X39.08
radon X39.01
overdose (in medical or surgical procedure)
Y63.2
radar W90.0
radioactive isotopes (any) W88.1
atomic power plant malfunction W88.1
misadventure in medical or surgical
treatment Y63.2
radiofrequency W90.0
radium NEC W88.1
sun X32
ultraviolet (light) (man-made) W89.9
natural X32
specified NEC W89.8
tanning bed W89.1
welding light W89.0
welding arc, torch, or light W89.0
excessive heat from W92
x-rays (hard) (soft) W88.0
Range disease W94.11
Rape (attempted) T74.2-
Rat bite W53.11
Reaching (prolonged) (static) X50.1 ◀
Reaction, abnormal to medical procedure —see
also Complication of or following, by type
of procedure Y84.9
with misadventure —see Misadventure
biologicals —see Table of Drugs and
Chemicals ◀▥
drugs —see Table of Drugs and Chemicals ◀▥
vaccine —see Table of Drugs and
Chemicals ◀▥
Recoil
airgun W34.110
BB gun W34.110
firearm NEC W34.19
gas, air or spring-operated gun NEC W34.118

Recoil (Continued)
handgun W32.1
hunting rifle W33.12
larger firearm W33.10
specified NEC W33.19
machine gun W33.13
paintball gun W34.111
pellet W34.110
shotgun W33.11
Very pistol [flare] W34.19
Reduction in
atmospheric pressure —see Air, pressure,
change
Rock falling on or hitting (accidentally)
(person) W20.8
in cave-in W20.0
Run over (accidentally) (by)
animal (not being ridden) NEC W55.89
machinery —see Contact, with, by specified
type of machine
transport vehicle NEC —see also Accident,
transport V09.9
intentional homicide (attempt) Y03.0
motor NEC V09.20
intentional homicide (attempt) Y03.0
Running
before moving object X81.8
motor vehicle X81.0
Running off, away
animal (being ridden) —see also Accident,
transport V80.918
not being ridden W55.89
animal-drawn vehicle NEC —see also
Accident, transport V80.928
highway, road(way), street
transport vehicle NEC —see also Accident,
transport V89.9
Rupture pressurized devices —see Explosion,
by type of device

S

Saturnism —see Table of Drugs and Chemicals, lead ◀▥

Scald, scalding (accidental) (by) (from) (in) X19
  air (hot) X14.1
  gases (hot) X14.1
  homicide (attempt) —see Assault, burning, hot object
  inflicted by other person
    stated as intentional, homicide (attempt) —see Assault, burning, hot object
  liquid (boiling) (hot) NEC X12
    stated as undetermined whether accidental or intentional Y27.2
    suicide (attempt) X77.2
  local application of externally applied substance in medical or surgical care Y63.5
  metal (molten) (liquid) (hot) NEC X18
  self-inflicted X77.9
  stated as undetermined whether accidental or intentional Y27.8
  steam X13.1
    assault X98.0
    stated as undetermined whether accidental or intentional Y27.0
    suicide (attempt) X77.0
  suicide (attempt) X77.9
  vapor (hot) X13.1
    assault X98.0
    stated as undetermined whether accidental or intentional Y27.0
    suicide (attempt) X77.0

Scratched by
  cat W55.03
  person (s) (accidentally) W50.4
    with intent to injure or kill Y04.0
    as, or caused by, a crowd or human stampede (with fall) W52
    assault Y04.0
    homicide (attempt) Y04.0
    in
      fight Y04.0
      legal intervention
        injuring
          bystander Y35.892
          law enforcement personnel Y35.891
          suspect Y35.893

Seasickness T75.3

Self-harm NEC —see also External cause by type, undetermined whether accidental or intentional
  intentional —see Suicide
  poisoning NEC —see Table of drugs and biologicals, accident

Self-inflicted (injury) NEC —see also External cause by type, undetermined whether accidental or intentional
  intentional —see Suicide
  poisoning NEC —see Table of drugs and biologicals, accident

Sequelae (of)
  accident NEC —see W00-X58 with 7th character S
  assault (homicidal) (any means) —see X92-Y08 with 7th character S
  homicide, attempt (any means) —see X92-Y08 with 7th character S
  injury undetermined whether accidentally or purposely inflicted —see Y21-Y33 with 7th character S
  intentional self-harm (classifiable to X71-X83) —see X71-X83 with 7th character S
  legal intervention (see with 7th character S Y35)
  motor vehicle accident —see V00-V99 with 7th character S
  suicide, attempt (any means) —see X71-X83 with 7th character S

Sequelae (Continued)
  transport accident —see V00-V99 with 7th character S
  war operations —see War operations

Shock
  electric —see Exposure, electric current
  from electric appliance (any) (faulty) W86.8
    domestic W86.0
    suicide (attempt) X83.1

Shooting, shot (accidental (ly)) —see also Discharge, firearm, by type
  herself or himself —see Discharge, firearm by type, self-inflicted
  homicide (attempt) —see Discharge, firearm by type, homicide
  in war operations —see War operations
  inflicted by other person —see Discharge, firearm by type, homicide
    accidental —see Discharge, firearm, by type of firearm
  legal
    execution —see Legal, intervention, firearm
    intervention —see Legal, intervention, firearm
  self-inflicted —see Discharge, firearm by type, suicide
    accidental —see Discharge, firearm, by type of firearm
  suicide (attempt) —see Discharge, firearm by type, suicide

Shoving (accidentally) by other person —see Pushed, by other person ◀▥

Sickness
  alpine W94.11
  motion —see Motion
  mountain W94.11

Sinking (accidental)
  watercraft (causing drowning, submersion) —see also Drowning, due to, accident to, watercraft, sinking
    causing injury except drowning or submersion —see Accident, watercraft, causing, injury NEC ◀

Siriasis X32
Sitting (prolonged) (static) X50.1 ◀
Slashed wrists —see Cut, self-inflicted
Slipping (accidental) (on same level) (with fall) W01.0
  without fall W18.40
    due to
      specified NEC W18.49
      stepping from one level to another W18.43
      stepping into hole or opening W18.42
      stepping on object W18.41
  on
    ice W00.0
      with skates —see Accident, transport, pedestrian, conveyance
    mud W01.0
    oil W01.0
    snow W00.0
      with skis —see Accident, transport, pedestrian, conveyance
    surface (slippery) (wet) NEC W01.0

Sliver, wood, contact with W45.8
Smoldering (due to fire) —see Exposure, fire
Sodomy (attempted) by force T74.2-
Sound waves (causing injury) W42.9
  supersonic W42.0
Splinter, contact with W45.8
Stab, stabbing —see Cut
Standing (prolonged) (static) X50.1 ◀
Starvation X58
Status of external cause Y99.9
  child assisting in compensated work for family Y99.8
  civilian activity done for financial or other compensation Y99.0
  civilian activity done for income or pay Y99.0

Status of external cause (Continued)
  family member assisting in compensated work for other family member Y99.8
  hobby not done for income Y99.8
  leisure activity Y99.8
  military activity Y99.1
  off-duty activity of military personnel Y99.8
  recreation or sport not for income or while a student Y99.8
  specified NEC Y99.8
  student activity Y99.8
  volunteer activity Y99.2

Stepped on
  by
    animal (not being ridden) NEC W55.89
    crowd or human stampede W52
    person W50.0

Stepping on
  object W22.8
    with fall W18.31
      sports equipment W21.9
    stationary W22.09
      sports equipment W21.89
  person W51
    by crowd or human stampede W52
  sports equipment W21.9

Sting
  arthropod, nonvenomous W57
  insect, nonvenomous W57

Storm (cataclysmic) —see Forces of nature, cataclysmic storm ◀▥

Straining, excessive —see also Overexertion X50.9 ◀▥

Strangling —see Strangulation
Strangulation (accidental) —see category T71
Strenuous movements —see also Overexertion X50.9 ◀▥

Striking against
  airbag (automobile) W22.10
    driver side W22.11
    front passenger side W22.12
    specified NEC W22.19
  bottom when
    diving or jumping into water (in) W16.822
      causing drowning W16.821
      from boat W16.722
        causing drowning W16.721
      natural body W16.622
        causing drowning W16.821
      swimming pool W16.522
        causing drowning W16.521
    falling into water (in) W16.322
      causing drowning W16.321
      fountain —see Striking against, bottom when, falling into water, specified NEC
      natural body W16.122
        causing drowning W16.121
      reservoir —see Striking against, bottom when, falling into water, specified NEC
      specified NEC W16.322
        causing drowning W16.321
      swimming pool W16.022
        causing drowning W16.021
  diving board (swimming-pool) W21.4
  object W22.8
    with
      drowning or submersion —see Drowning
      fall —see Fall, due to, bumping against, object
    caused by crowd or human stampede (with fall) W52
    furniture W22.03
    lamppost W22.02
    sports equipment W21.9
    stationary W22.09
      sports equipment W21.89
    wall W22.01

◀ New   ◀▥ Revised   ~~deleted~~ Deleted

Striking against *(Continued)*
  person (s) W51
    with fall W03
      due to ice or snow W00.0
    as, or caused by, a crowd or human
      stampede (with fall) W52
    assault Y04.2
    homicide (attempt) Y04.2
  sports equipment W21.9
  wall (when) W22.01
    diving or jumping into water (in) W16.832
      causing drowning W16.831
      swimming pool W16.532
        causing drowning W16.531
    falling into water (in) W16.332
      causing drowning W16.331
    fountain —*see* Striking against, wall
      when, falling into water, specified
      NEC
    natural body W16.132
      causing drowning W16.131
    reservoir —*see* Striking against, wall
      when, falling into water, specified
      NEC
    specified NEC W16.332
      causing drowning W16.331
    swimming pool W16.032
      causing drowning W16.031
    swimming pool (when) W22.042
      causing drowning W22.041
      diving or jumping into water W16.532
        causing drowning W16.531
      falling into water W16.032
        causing drowning W16.031
Struck (accidentally) by
  airbag (automobile) W22.10
    driver side W22.11
    front passenger side W22.12
    specified NEC W22.19
  alligator W58.02
  animal (not being ridden) NEC W55.89
  avalanche —*see* Landslide ◀
  ball (hit) (thrown) W21.00
    assault Y08.09
    baseball W21.03
    basketball W21.05
    football W21.01
    golf ball W21.04
    football W21.01
    soccer W21.02
    softball W21.07
    specified NEC W21.09
    volleyball W21.06
  bat or racquet
    baseball bat W21.11
      assault Y08.02
    golf club W21.13
      assault Y08.09
    specified NEC W21.19
      assault Y08.09
    tennis racquet W21.12
      assault Y08.09
  bullet —*see also* Discharge, firearm by type
    in war operations —*see* War operations
  crocodile W58.12
  dog W54.1
  flare, Very pistol —*see* Discharge, firearm
    NEC
  hailstones X39.8
  hockey (ice)
    field
      puck W21.221
      stick W21.211
    puck W21.220
    stick W21.210
      assault Y08.01
  landslide —*see* Landslide ◀
  law-enforcement agent (on duty) —*see* Legal,
    intervention, manhandling
    with blunt object —*see* Legal, intervention,
      blunt object

Struck by *(Continued)*
  lightning —*see* subcategory T75.0
    causing fire —*see* Exposure, fire
  machine —*see* Contact, with, by type of
    machine
  mammal NEC W55.89
    marine W56.32
  marine animal W56.82
  missile
    firearm —*see* Discharge, firearm by type
    in war operations —*see* War operations,
      missile
  object W22.8
    blunt W22.8
      assault Y00
      suicide (attempt) X79
      undetermined whether accidental or
        intentional Y29
    falling W20.8
      from, in, on
        building W20.1
          burning (uncontrolled fire) X00.4
        cataclysmic
          earth surface movement NEC —*see*
            Landslide ◀
          storm —*see* Forces of nature,
            cataclysmic storm ◀
        cave-in W20.0
        earthquake X34
        machine (in operation) —*see* Contact,
          with, by type of machine
        structure W20.1
          burning X00.4
        transport vehicle (in motion) —*see*
          Accident, transport, by type of
          vehicle
        watercraft V93.49
          due to
            accident to craft V91.39
            powered craft V91.33
              ferry boat V91.31
              fishing boat V91.32
              jetskis V91.33
              liner V91.31
              merchant ship V91.30
              passenger ship V91.31
            unpowered craft V91.38
              canoe V91.35
              inflatable V91.36
              kayak V91.35
              sailboat V91.34
              surf-board V91.38
              windsurfer V91.38
          powered craft V93.43
           ferry boat V93.41
           fishing boat V93.42
           jetskis V93.43
           liner V93.41
           merchant ship V93.40
           passenger ship V93.41
          unpowered craft V93.48
           sailboat V93.44
           surf-board V93.48
           windsurfer V93.48
    moving NEC W20.8
    projected W20.8
      assault Y00
      in sports W21.9
        assault Y08.09
        ball W21.00
          baseball W21.03
          basketball W21.05
          football W21.01
          golf ball W21.04
          soccer W21.02
          softball W21.07
          specified NEC W21.09
          volleyball W21.06
        bat or racquet
          baseball bat W21.11
           assault Y08.02

Struck by *(Continued)*
  object *(Continued)*
    projected *(Continued)*
      in sports *(Continued)*
        bat or racquet *(Continued)*
          golf club W21.13
           assault Y08.09-
          specified NEC W21.19
           assault Y08.09
          tennis racquet W21.12
           assault Y08.09
        hockey (ice)
          field
           puck W21.221
           stick W21.211
          puck W21.220
          stick W21.210
           assault Y08.01
        specified NEC W21.89
    set in motion by explosion —*see* Explosion
    thrown W20.8
      assault Y00
      in sports W21.9
        assault Y08.09
        ball W21.00
          baseball W21.03
          basketball W21.05
          football W21.01
          golf ball W21.04
          soccer W21.02
          soft ball W21.07
          specified NEC W21.09
          volleyball W21.06
        bat or racquet
          baseball bat W21.11
           assault Y08.02
          golf club W21.13
           assault Y08.09
          specified NEC W21.19
           assault Y08.09
          tennis racquet W21.12
           assault Y08.09
        hockey (ice)
          field
           puck W21.221
           stick W21.211
          puck W21.220
          stick W21.210
           assault Y08.01
        specified NEC W21.89
  other person (s) W50.0
    with
      blunt object W22.8
        intentional, homicide (attempt) Y00
        sports equipment W21.9
        undetermined whether accidental or
          intentional Y29
      fall W03
        due to ice or snow W00.0
      as, or caused by, a crowd or human
        stampede (with fall) W52
      assault Y04.2
      homicide (attempt) Y04.2
      in legal intervention
        injuring
          bystander Y35.812
          law enforcement personnel Y35.811
          suspect Y35.813
      sports equipment W21.9
  police (on duty) —*see* Legal, intervention,
    manhandling
    with blunt object —*see* Legal, intervention,
      blunt object
  sports equipment W21.9
    assault Y08.09
    ball W21.00
      baseball W21.03
      basketball W21.05
      football W21.01
      golf ball W21.04
      soccer W21.02

S

Struck by *(Continued)*
  sports equipment *(Continued)*
    ball *(Continued)*
      soft ball W21.07
      specified NEC W21.09
      volleyball W21.06
    bat or racquet
      baseball bat W21.11
        assault Y08.02
      golf club W21.13
        assault Y08.09
      specified NEC W21.19
      tennis racquet W21.12
        assault Y08.09
    cleats (shoe) W21.31
    foot wear NEC W21.39
    football helmet W21.81
    hockey (ice)
      field
        puck W21.221
        stick W21.211
      puck W21.220
      stick W21.210
        assault Y08.01
    skate blades W21.32
    specified NEC W21.89
      assault Y08.09
  thunderbolt —*see* subcategory
    T75.0
    causing fire —*see* Exposure, fire
  transport vehicle NEC —*see also* Accident,
    transport V09.9
    intentional, homicide (attempt) Y03.0
    motor NEC —*see also* Accident, transport
      V09.20
      homicide Y03.0
  vehicle (transport) NEC —*see* Accident,
    transport, by type of vehicle
    stationary (falling from jack,
      hydraulic lift, ramp)
      W20.8
Stumbling
  without fall W18.40
    due to
      specified NEC W18.49
      stepping from one level to another
        W18.43
      stepping into hole or opening W18.42
      stepping on object W18.41
  over
    animal NEC W01.0
      with fall W18.09
    carpet, rug or (small) object W22.8
      with fall W18.09
    person W51
      with fall W03
        due to ice or snow W00.0

Submersion (accidental) —*see* Drowning
Suffocation (accidental) (by external means) (by
    pressure) (mechanical) —*see also* category
    T71
  due to, by
    avalanche —*see* Landslide
    explosion —*see* Explosion
    fire —*see* Exposure, fire
    food, any type (aspiration) (ingestion)
      (inhalation) —*see* categories T17 and
      T18
    ignition —*see* Ignition
    landslide —*see* Landslide
    machine (ry) —*see* Contact, with, by type
      of machine
    vomitus (aspiration) (inhalation)
      T17.81-
  in
    burning building X00.8
Suicide, suicidal (attempted) (by) X83.8
  blunt object X79
  burning, burns X76
    hot object X77.9
      fluid NEC X77.2
      household appliance X77.3
      specified NEC X77.8
      steam X77.0
      tap water X77.1
      vapors X77.0
  caustic substance —*see* Table of Drugs and
    Chemicals ◄▥
  cold, extreme X83.2
  collision of motor vehicle with
    motor vehicle X82.0
    specified NEC X82.8
    train X82.1
    tree X82.2
  crashing of aircraft X83.0
  cut (any part of body) X78.9
  cutting or piercing instrument X78.9
    dagger X78.2
    glass X78.0
    knife X78.1
    specified NEC X78.8
    sword X78.2
  drowning (in) X71.9
    bathtub X71.0
    natural water X71.3
    specified NEC X71.8
    swimming pool X71.1
      following fall X71.2
  electrocution X83.1
  explosive (s) (material) X75
  fire, flames X76
  firearm X74.9
    airgun X74.01
    handgun X72

Suicide, suicidal *(Continued)*
  firearm *(Continued)*
    hunting rifle X73.1
    larger X73.9
      specified NEC X73.8
    machine gun X73.2
    shotgun X73.0
    specified NEC X74.8
  hanging X83.8
  hot object —*see* Suicide, burning, hot object
  jumping
    before moving object X81.8
      motor vehicle X81.0
      subway train X81.1
      train X81.1
    from high place X80
  late effect of attempt —*see* X71-X83 with 7th
    character S
  lying before moving object, train, vehicle X81.8
  poisoning —*see* Table of Drugs and
    Chemicals ◄▥
  puncture (any part of body) —*see* Suicide,
    cutting or piercing instrument
  scald —*see* Suicide, burning, hot object
  sequelae of attempt —*see* X71-X83 with 7th
    character S
  sharp object (any) —*see* Suicide, cutting or
    piercing instrument
  shooting —*see* Suicide, firearm
  specified means NEC X83.8
  stab (any part of body) —*see* Suicide, cutting
    or piercing instrument
  steam, hot vapors X77.0
  strangulation X83.8
  submersion —*see* Suicide, drowning
  suffocation X83.8
  wound NEC X83.8
Sunstroke X32
Supersonic waves (causing injury) W42.0
Surgical procedure, complication of (delayed
    or as an abnormal reaction without
    mention of misadventure) —*see also*
    Complication of or following, by type of
    procedure
  due to or as a result of misadventure —*see*
    Misadventure
Swallowed, swallowing
  foreign body —*see* Foreign body, alimentary
    canal
  poison —*see* Table of Drugs and Chemicals
  substance
    caustic or corrosive —*see* Table of Drugs
      and Chemicals
    poisonous —*see* Table of Drugs and
      Chemicals

T

Tackle in sport W03
Terrorism (involving) Y38.80
  biological weapons Y38.6X-
  chemical weapons Y38.7X-
  conflagration Y38.3X-
  drowning and submersion Y38.89- ◄
  explosion Y38.2X-
    destruction of aircraft Y38.1X-
    marine weapons Y38.0X-
  fire Y38.3X-
  firearms Y38.4X-
  hot substances Y38.3X- ◄▥
  lasers Y38.89- ◄
  nuclear weapons Y38.5X-
  piercing or stabbing instruments
    Y38.89- ◄
  secondary effects Y38.9X- ◄
  specified method NEC Y38.89- ◄▥
  suicide bomber Y38.81- ◄
Thirst X58
Threat to breathing
  aspiration —see Aspiration
  due to cave-in, falling earth or substance
    NEC —see category T71
Thrown (accidentally)
  against part (any) of or object in transport
    vehicle (in motion) NEC —see also
    Accident, transport

Thrown (Continued)
  from
    high place, homicide (attempt) Y01
    machinery —see Contact, with, by type of
      machine
    transport vehicle NEC —see also Accident,
      transport V89.9
  off —see Thrown, from
Thunderbolt —see subcategory T75.0
  causing fire —see Exposure, fire
Tidal wave (any injury) NEC —see Forces of
  nature, tidal wave ◄▥
Took
  overdose (drug) —see Table of Drugs and
    Chemicals ◄▥
  poison —see Table of Drugs and
    Chemicals ◄▥
Tornado (any injury) X37.1
Torrential rain (any injury) X37.8
Torture X58
Trampled by animal NEC W55.89
Trapped (accidentally)
  between objects (moving) (stationary and
    moving) —see Caught
  by part (any) of
    motorcycle V29.88
    pedal cycle V19.88
    transport vehicle NEC —see also Accident,
      transport V89.9
Travel (effects) (sickness) T75.3

Tree falling on or hitting (accidentally)
  (person) W20.8
Tripping
  without fall W18.40
    due to
      specified NEC W18.49
      stepping from one level to another
        W18.43
      stepping into hole or opening
        W18.42
      stepping on object W18.41
  over
    animal W01.0
      with fall W01.0
    carpet, rug or (small) object W22.8
      with fall W18.09
    person W51
      with fall W03
        due to ice or snow W00.0
Twisted by person (s) (accidentally) W50.2
  with intent to injure or kill Y04.0
  as, or caused by, a crowd or human stampede
    (with fall) W52
  assault Y04.0
  homicide (attempt) Y04.0
  in
    fight Y04.0
    legal intervention —see Legal, intervention,
      manhandling
Twisting (prolonged) (static) X50.1 ◄

U

Underdosing of necessary drugs, medicaments
  or biological substances Y63.6 ◄▥
Undetermined intent (contact)
  (exposure)
  automobile collision Y32
  blunt object Y29
  drowning (submersion) (in) Y21.9
    bathtub Y21.0
      after fall Y21.1
    natural water (lake) (ocean) (pond) (river)
      (stream) Y21.4
    specified place NEC Y21.8
    swimming pool Y21.2
      after fall Y21.3
  explosive material Y25
  fall, jump or push from high place Y30
  falling, lying or running before moving object
    Y31
  fire Y26

Undetermined intent (Continued)
  firearm discharge Y24.9
    airgun (BB) (pellet) Y24.0
    handgun (pistol) (revolver)
      Y22
    hunting rifle Y23.1
    larger Y23.9
      hunting rifle Y23.1
      machine gun Y23.3
      military Y23.2
      shotgun Y23.0
      specified type NEC Y23.8
    machine gun Y23.3
    military Y23.2
    shotgun Y23.0
    specified type NEC Y24.8
    Very pistol Y24.8
  hot object Y27.9
    fluid NEC Y27.2
    household appliance Y27.3
    specified object NEC Y27.8

Undetermined intent (Continued)
  hot object (Continued)
    steam Y27.0
    tap water Y27.1
    vapor Y27.0
  jump, fall or push from high place Y30
  lying, falling or running before moving object
    Y31
  motor vehicle crash Y32
  push, fall or jump from high place Y30
  running, falling or lying before moving object
    Y31
  sharp object Y28.9
    dagger Y28.2
    glass Y28.0
    knife Y28.1
    specified object NEC Y28.8
    sword Y28.2
  smoke Y26
  specified event NEC Y33
Use of hand as hammer X50.3 ◄

V

Vibration (causing injury) W49.9
Victim (of)
  avalanche —see Landslide ◄
  earth movements NEC —see Forces of nature,
    earth movement ◄
  earthquake X34

Victim (Continued)
  flood —see Flood ◄
  landslide —see Landslide ◄
  lightning —see subcategory T75.0
    causing fire —see Exposure, fire
  storm (cataclysmic) NEC —see Forces of
    nature, cataclysmic storm ◄
  volcanic eruption X35

Volcanic eruption (any injury) X35
Vomitus, gastric contents in air passages
  (with asphyxia, obstruction or
    suffocation) T17.81-

T, U, & V

W

Walked into stationary object (any) W22.09
  furniture W22.03
  lamppost W22.02
  wall W22.01
War operations (injuries to military personnel
    and civilians during war, civil insurrection
    and peacekeeping missions) (by) (from)
    (involving) Y36.90-
  after cessation of hostilities Y36.89-
    explosion (of)
      bomb placed during war operations
        Y36.82-
      mine placed during war operations
        Y36.81-
      specified NEC Y36.88-
  air blast Y36.20-
  aircraft
    destruction —see War operations,
      destruction of aircraft
  airway restriction —see War operations,
      restriction of airways
  asphyxiation —see War operations, restriction
      of airways
  biological weapons Y36.6X-
  blast Y36.20-
  blast fragments Y36.20-
  blast wave Y36.20-
  blast wind Y36.20-
  bomb Y36.20-
    dirty Y36.50-
    gasoline Y36.31-
    incendiary Y36.31-
    petrol Y36.31-
  bullet Y36.43-
    incendiary Y36.32-
    rubber Y36.41-
  chemical weapons Y36.7X-
  combat
    hand to hand (unarmed) combat Y36.44-
    using blunt or piercing object Y36.45-
  conflagration —see War operations, fire
  conventional warfare NEC Y36.49-
  depth-charge Y36.01-
  destruction of aircraft Y36.10-
    due to
      air to air missile Y36.11-
      collision with other aircraft Y36.12-
      detonation (accidental) of onboard
        munitions and explosives Y36.14-
      enemy fire or explosives Y36.11-
      explosive placed on aircraft Y36.11-
      onboard fire Y36.13-
      rocket propelled grenade [RPG] Y36.11-
      small arms fire Y36.11-
      surface to air missile Y36.11-
    specified NEC Y36.19-
  detonation (accidental) of
    onboard marine weapons Y36.05-
    own munitions or munitions launch device
      Y36.24-

War operations (Continued)
  dirty bomb Y36.50-
  explosion (of) Y36.20-
    aerial bomb Y36.21-
    after cessation of hostilities
      bomb placed during war operations
        Y36.82-
      mine placed during war operations
        Y36.81-
    bomb NOS —see also War operations,
        bomb (s) Y36.20-
    fragments Y36.20-
    grenade Y36.29-
    guided missile Y36.22-
    improvised explosive device [IED]
        (person-borne) (roadside)
        (vehicle-borne) Y36.23-
    land mine Y36.29-
    marine mine (at sea) (in harbor)
        Y36.02-
    marine weapon Y36.00-
      specified NEC Y36.09-
    own munitions or munitions launch
        device (accidental) Y36.24-
    sea-based artillery shell Y36.03-
    specified NEC Y36.29-
    torpedo Y36.04-
  fire Y36.30-
    specified NEC Y36.39-
  firearms
    discharge Y36.43-
    pellets Y36.42-
  flamethrower Y36.33-
  fragments (from) (of)
    improvised explosive device [IED]
        (person-borne) (roadside)
        (vehicle-borne) Y36.26-
    munitions Y36.25-
    specified NEC Y36.29-
    weapons Y36.27-
  friendly fire Y36.92
  hand to hand (unarmed) combat
      Y36.44-
  hot substances —see War operations,
      fire
  incendiary bullet Y36.32-
  nuclear weapon (effects of) Y36.50-
    acute radiation exposure Y36.54-
    blast pressure Y36.51-
    direct blast Y36.51-
    direct heat Y36.53-
    fallout exposure Y36.54-
    fireball Y36.53-
    indirect blast (struck or crushed by blast
        debris) (being thrown by blast)
        Y36.52-
    ionizing radiation (immediate exposure)
        Y36.54-
    nuclear radiation Y36.54-
    radiation
      ionizing (immediate exposure)
        Y36.54-

War operations (Continued)
  nuclear weapon (Continued)
    radiation (Continued)
      nuclear Y36.54-
      thermal Y36.53-
    secondary effects Y36.54-
    specified NEC Y36.59-
    thermal radiation Y36.53-
  restriction of air (airway)
    intentional Y36.46-
    unintentional Y36.47-
  rubber bullets Y36.41-
  shrapnel NOS Y36.29-
  suffocation —see War operations, restriction
      of airways
  unconventional warfare NEC Y36.7X-
  underwater blast NOS Y36.00-
  warfare
    conventional NEC Y36.49-
    unconventional NEC Y36.7X-
  weapon of mass destruction [WMD] Y36.91
  weapons
    biological weapons Y36.6X-
    chemical Y36.7X-
    nuclear (effects of) Y36.50-
      acute radiation exposure Y36.54-
      blast pressure Y36.51-
      direct blast Y36.51-
      direct heat Y36.53-
      fallout exposure Y36.54-
      fireball Y36.53-
      ~~indirect blast (struck or crushed by blast~~
          ~~debris) (being thrown by blast)~~
          ~~Y36.52-~~
      radiation
        ionizing (immediate exposure) Y36.54-
        nuclear Y36.54-
        thermal Y36.53-
      secondary effects Y36.54-
      specified NEC Y36.59-
  of mass destruction [WMD] Y36.91-
Washed
  away by flood —see Flood
  off road by storm (transport vehicle) —see
      Forces of nature, cataclysmic storm
Weather exposure NEC —see Forces of nature
Weightlessness (causing injury) (effects of) (in
    spacecraft, real or simulated) X52
Work related condition Y99.0
Wound (accidental) NEC —see also Injury X58
  battle —see also War operations Y36.90
  gunshot —see Discharge, firearm by type
Wreck transport vehicle NEC —see also
    Accident, transport V89.9
Wrong
  device implanted into correct surgical site
      Y65.51
  fluid in infusion Y65.1
  patient, procedure performed on Y65.52
  procedure (operation) on correct patient
      Y65.51

ICD-10-CM Tabular List of Diseases and Injuries

CHAPTER 1

CERTAIN INFECTIOUS AND PARASITIC DISEASES (A00-B99)

Chapter-Specific Coding Guidelines

1. **Chapter 1: Certain Infectious and Parasitic Diseases (A00-B99)**

   a. Human Immunodeficiency Virus (HIV) Infections

   1) Code only confirmed cases

   Code only confirmed cases of HIV infection/illness. This is an exception to the hospital inpatient guideline Section II, H.

   In this context, "confirmation" does not require documentation of positive serology or culture for HIV; the provider's diagnostic statement that the patient is HIV positive, or has an HIV-related illness is sufficient.

   2) Selection and sequencing of HIV codes

   (a) Patient admitted for HIV-related condition

   If a patient is admitted for an HIV-related condition, the principal diagnosis should be B20, Human immunodeficiency virus [HIV] disease followed by additional diagnosis codes for all reported HIV-related conditions.

   (b) Patient with HIV disease admitted for unrelated condition

   If a patient with HIV disease is admitted for an unrelated condition (such as a traumatic injury), the code for the unrelated condition (e.g., the nature of injury code) should be the principal diagnosis. Other diagnoses would be B20 followed by additional diagnosis codes for all reported HIV-related conditions.

   (c) Whether the patient is newly diagnosed

   Whether the patient is newly diagnosed or has had previous admissions/encounters for HIV conditions is irrelevant to the sequencing decision.

   (d) Asymptomatic human immunodeficiency virus

   Z21, Asymptomatic human immunodeficiency virus [HIV] infection status, is to be applied when the patient without any documentation of symptoms is listed as being "HIV positive," "known HIV," "HIV test positive," or similar terminology. Do not use this code if the term "AIDS" is used or if the patient is treated for any HIV-related illness or is described as having any condition(s) resulting from his/her HIV positive status; use B20 in these cases.

   (e) Patients with inconclusive HIV serology

   Patients with inconclusive HIV serology, but no definitive diagnosis or manifestations of the illness, may be assigned code R75, Inconclusive laboratory evidence of human immunodeficiency virus [HIV].

   (f) Previously diagnosed HIV-related illness

   Patients with any known prior diagnosis of an HIV-related illness should be coded to B20. Once a patient has developed an HIV-related illness, the patient should always be assigned code B20 on every subsequent admission/encounter. Patients previously diagnosed with any HIV illness (B20) should never be assigned to R75 or Z21, Asymptomatic human immunodeficiency virus [HIV] infection status.

   (g) HIV Infection in Pregnancy, Childbirth and the Puerperium

   During pregnancy, childbirth or the puerperium, a patient admitted (or presenting for a health care encounter) because of an HIV-related illness should receive a principal diagnosis code of O98.7-, Human immunodeficiency [HIV] disease complicating pregnancy, childbirth and the puerperium, followed by B20 and the code(s) for the HIV-related illness(es). Codes from Chapter 15 always take sequencing priority.

   Patients with asymptomatic HIV infection status admitted (or presenting for a health care encounter) during pregnancy, childbirth, or the puerperium should receive codes of O98.7- and Z21.

   (h) Encounters for testing for HIV

   If a patient is being seen to determine his/her HIV status, use code Z11.4, Encounter for screening for human immunodeficiency virus [HIV]. Use additional codes for any associated high risk behavior.

   If a patient with signs or symptoms is being seen for HIV testing, code the signs and symptoms. An additional counseling code Z71.7, Human immunodeficiency virus [HIV] counseling, may be used if counseling is provided during the encounter for the test.

   When a patient returns to be informed of his/her HIV test results and the test result is negative, use code Z71.7, Human immunodeficiency virus [HIV] counseling.

   If the results are positive, see previous guidelines and assign codes as appropriate.

   b. Infectious agents as the cause of diseases classified to other chapters

   Certain infections are classified in chapters other than Chapter 1 and no organism is identified as part of the infection code. In these instances, it is necessary to use an additional code from Chapter 1 to identify the organism. A code from category B95, Streptococcus, Staphylococcus, and Enterococcus as the cause of diseases classified to other chapters, B96, Other bacterial agents as the cause of diseases classified to other chapters, or B97, Viral agents as the cause of diseases classified to other chapters, is to be used as an additional code to identify the organism. An instructional note will be found at the infection code advising that an additional organism code is required.

   c. Infections resistant to antibiotics

   Many bacterial infections are resistant to current antibiotics. It is necessary to identify all infections documented as antibiotic resistant. Assign a code from category Z16, Resistance to antimicrobial drugs, following the infection code only if the infection code does not identify drug resistance.

   d. Sepsis, Severe Sepsis, and Septic Shock

   1) Coding of Sepsis and Severe Sepsis

   (a) Sepsis

   For a diagnosis of sepsis, assign the appropriate code for the underlying systemic infection. If the type of infection or causal organism is not further specified, assign code A41.9, Sepsis, unspecified organism.

   A code from subcategory R65.2, Severe sepsis, should not be assigned unless severe sepsis or an associated acute organ dysfunction is documented.

   (i) Negative or inconclusive blood cultures and sepsis

   Negative or inconclusive blood cultures do not preclude a diagnosis of sepsis in patients with clinical evidence of the condition, however, the provider should be queried.

   (ii) Urosepsis

   The term urosepsis is a nonspecific term. It is not to be considered synonymous with sepsis. It has no default code in the Alphabetic Index. Should a provider use this term, he/she must be queried for clarification.

   (iii) Sepsis with organ dysfunction

   If a patient has sepsis and associated acute organ dysfunction or multiple organ dysfunction (MOD), follow the instructions for coding severe sepsis.

   (iv) Acute organ dysfunction that is not clearly associated with the sepsis

   If a patient has sepsis and an acute organ dysfunction, but the medical record documentation indicates that the acute organ dysfunction is related to a medical condition other than the sepsis, do not assign a code from subcategory R65.2, Severe sepsis. An acute organ dysfunction must be associated with the sepsis in order to assign the severe sepsis code. If the documentation is not clear as to whether an acute organ dysfunction is related to the sepsis or another medical condition, query the provider.

   (b) Severe sepsis

   The coding of severe sepsis requires a minimum of 2 codes: first a code for the underlying systemic infection, followed by a code from subcategory R65.2, Severe sepsis. If the causal organism is not documented, assign code A41.9, Sepsis, unspecified organism, for the infection. Additional code(s) for the associated acute organ dysfunction are also required.

   Due to the complex nature of severe sepsis, some cases may require querying the provider prior to assignment of the codes.

2) Septic shock

(a) Septic shock generally refers to circulatory failure associated with severe sepsis, and therefore, it represents a type of acute organ dysfunction.

For all cases of septic shock, the code for the systemic infection should be sequenced first, followed by code R65.21, Severe sepsis with septic shock or code T81.12, Postprocedural septic shock. Any additional codes for the other acute organ dysfunctions should also be assigned. As noted in the sequencing instructions in the Tabular List, the code for septic shock cannot be assigned as a principal diagnosis.

3) Sequencing of severe sepsis

If severe sepsis is present on admission, and meets the definition of principal diagnosis, the underlying systemic infection should be assigned as principal diagnosis followed by the appropriate code from subcategory R65.2 as required by the sequencing rules in the Tabular List. A code from subcategory R65.2 can never be assigned as a principal diagnosis.

When severe sepsis develops during an encounter (it was not present on admission) the underlying systemic infection and the appropriate code from subcategory R65.2 should be assigned as secondary diagnoses.

Severe sepsis may be present on admission but the diagnosis may not be confirmed until sometime after admission. If the documentation is not clear whether severe sepsis was present on admission, the provider should be queried.

4) Sepsis and severe sepsis with a localized infection

If the reason for admission is both sepsis or severe sepsis and a localized infection, such as pneumonia or cellulitis, a code(s) for the underlying systemic infection should be assigned first and the code for the localized infection should be assigned as a secondary diagnosis. If the patient has severe sepsis, a code from subcategory R65.2 should also be assigned as a secondary diagnosis. If the patient is admitted with a localized infection, such as pneumonia, and sepsis/severe sepsis doesn't develop until after admission, the localized infection should be assigned first, followed by the appropriate sepsis/severe sepsis codes.

5) Sepsis due to a postprocedural infection

(a) Documentation of causal relationship

As with all postprocedural complications, code assignment is based on the provider's documentation of the relationship between the infection and the procedure.

(b) Sepsis due to a postprocedural infection

For such cases, the postprocedural infection code, such as, T80.2, Infections following infusion, transfusion, and therapeutic injection, T81.4, Infection following a procedure, T88.0, Infection following immunization, or O86.0, Infection of obstetric surgical wound, should be coded first, followed by the code for the specific infection. If the patient has severe sepsis the appropriate code from subcategory R65.2 should also be assigned with the additional code(s) for any acute organ dysfunction.

(c) Postprocedural infection and postprocedural septic shock

In cases where a postprocedural infection has occurred and has resulted in severe sepsis the code for the precipitating complication such as code T81.4, Infection following a procedure, or O86.0, Infection of obstetrical surgical wound should be coded first followed by code R65.20, Severe sepsis without septic shock. A Code for the systemic infection should also be assigned.

If a postprocedural infection has resulted in postprocedural septic shock, the code for the precipitating complication such as code T81.4, Infection following a procedure, or O86.0, Infection of obstetrical surgical wound should be coded first followed by code T81.12-, Postprocedural septic shock. A code for the systemic infection should also be assigned.

6) Sepsis and severe sepsis associated with a noninfectious process (condition)

In some cases a noninfectious process (condition), such as trauma, may lead to an infection which can result in sepsis or severe sepsis. If sepsis or severe sepsis is documented as associated with a noninfectious condition, such as a burn or serious injury, and this condition meets the definition for principal diagnosis, the code for the noninfectious condition should be sequenced first, followed by the code for the resulting infection. If severe sepsis is present, a code from subcategory R65.2 should also be assigned with any associated organ dysfunction(s) codes. It is not necessary to assign a code from subcategory R65.1, Systemic inflammatory response syndrome (SIRS) of non-infectious origin, for these cases.

If the infection meets the definition of principal diagnosis it should be sequenced before the non-infectious condition. When both the associated non-infectious condition and the infection meet the definition of principal diagnosis either may be assigned as principal diagnosis.

Only one code from category R65, Symptoms and signs specifically associated with systemic inflammation and infection, should be assigned. Therefore, when a non-infectious condition leads to an infection resulting in severe sepsis, assign the appropriate code from subcategory R65.2, Severe sepsis. Do not additionally assign a code from subcategory R65.1, Systemic inflammatory response syndrome (SIRS) of non-infectious origin.

See Section I.C.18. SIRS due to non-infectious process

7) Sepsis and septic shock complicating abortion, pregnancy, childbirth, and the puerperium

See Section I.C.15. Sepsis and septic shock complicating abortion, pregnancy, childbirth and the puerperium

8) Newborn sepsis

See Section I.C.16. f. Bacterial sepsis of Newborn

e. Methicillin Resistant Staphylococcus aureus (MRSA) Conditions

1) Selection and sequencing of MRSA codes

(a) Combination codes for MRSA infection

When a patient is diagnosed with an infection that is due to methicillin resistant *Staphylococcus aureus* (MRSA), and that infection has a combination code that includes the causal organism (e.g., sepsis, pneumonia) assign the appropriate combination code for the condition (e.g., code A41.02, Sepsis due to Methicillin resistant Staphylococcus aureus or code J15.212, Pneumonia due to Methicillin resistant Staphylococcus aureus). Do not assign code B95.62, Methicillin resistant Staphylococcus aureus infection as the cause of diseases classified elsewhere, as an additional code because the combination code includes the type of infection and the MRSA organism. Do not assign a code from subcategory Z16.11, Resistance to penicillins, as an additional diagnosis.

See Section C.1. for instructions on coding and sequencing of sepsis and severe sepsis.

(b) Other codes for MRSA infection

When there is documentation of a current infection (e.g., wound infection, stitch abscess, urinary tract infection) due to MRSA, and that infection does not have a combination code that includes the causal organism, assign the appropriate code to identify the condition along with code B95.62, Methicillin resistant Staphylococcus aureus infection as the cause of diseases classified elsewhere for the MRSA infection. Do not assign a code from subcategory Z16.11, Resistance to penicillins.

(c) Methicillin susceptible Staphylococcus aureus (MSSA) and MRSA colonization

The condition or state of being colonized or carrying MSSA or MRSA is called colonization or carriage, while an individual person is described as being colonized or being a carrier. Colonization means that MSSA or MSRA is present on or in the body without necessarily causing illness. A positive MRSA colonization test might be documented by the provider as "MRSA screen positive" or "MRSA nasal swab positive".

Assign code Z22.322, Carrier or suspected carrier of Methicillin resistant Staphylococcus aureus, for patients documented as having MRSA colonization. Assign code Z22.321, Carrier or suspected carrier of Methicillin susceptible Staphylococcus aureus, for patient documented as having MSSA colonization. Colonization is not necessarily indicative of a disease process or as the cause of a specific condition the patient may have unless documented as such by the provider.

(d) MRSA colonization and infection

If a patient is documented as having both MRSA colonization and infection during a hospital admission, code Z22.322, Carrier or suspected carrier of Methicillin resistant Staphylococcus aureus, and a code for the MRSA infection may both be assigned.

f. Zika virus infections

1) Code only confirmed cases

Code only a confirmed diagnosis of Zika virus (A92.5, Zika virus disease) as documented by the provider. This is an exception to the hospital inpatient guideline Section II, H.

In this context, "confirmation" does not require documentation of the type of test performed; the physician's diagnostic statement that the condition is confirmed is sufficient. This code should be assigned regardless of the stated mode of transmission.

If the provider documents "suspected", "possible" or "probable" Zika, do not assign code A92.5. Assign a code(s) explaining the reason for encounter (such as fever, rash, or joint pain) or Z20.828, Contact with and (suspected) exposure to other viral communicable diseases.

CHAPTER 1

CERTAIN INFECTIOUS AND PARASITIC DISEASES (A00-B99)

Includes   diseases generally recognized as communicable or transmissible

Use additional code to identify resistance to antimicrobial drugs (Z16.-)

Excludes1   certain localized infections - see body system-related chapters

Excludes2   carrier or suspected carrier of infectious disease (Z22.-)

infectious and parasitic diseases complicating pregnancy, childbirth and the puerperium (O98.-)

infectious and parasitic diseases specific to the perinatal period (P35-P39)

influenza and other acute respiratory infections (J00-J22)

This chapter contains the following blocks:

A00-A09	Intestinal infectious diseases
A15-A19	Tuberculosis
A20-A28	Certain zoonotic bacterial diseases
A30-A49	Other bacterial diseases
A50-A64	Infections with a predominantly sexual mode of transmission
A65-A69	Other spirochetal diseases
A70-A74	Other diseases caused by chlamydiae
A75-A79	Rickettsioses
A80-A89	Viral and prion infections of the central nervous system
A90-A99	Arthropod-borne viral fevers and viral hemorrhagic fevers
B00-B09	Viral infections characterized by skin and mucous membrane lesions
B10	Other human herpesviruses
B15-B19	Viral hepatitis
B20	Human immunodeficiency virus [HIV] disease
B25-B34	Other viral diseases
B35-B49	Mycoses
B50-B64	Protozoal diseases
B65-B83	Helminthiases
B85-B89	Pediculosis, acariasis and other infestations
B90-B94	Sequelae of infectious and parasitic diseases
B95-B97	Bacterial and viral infectious agents
B99	Other infectious diseases

INTESTINAL INFECTIOUS DISEASES (A00-A09)

● **A00** **Cholera**
A serious, often deadly, infectious disease of the small intestine
(Ex:) For category A00 CC codes: A00.0-A00.9

  A00.0 **Cholera due to Vibrio cholerae 01, biovar cholerae**
Classical cholera

  A00.1 **Cholera due to Vibrio cholerae 01, biovar eltor**
Cholera eltor

  A00.9 **Cholera, unspecified**

● **A01** **Typhoid and paratyphoid fevers**
Caused by Salmonella typhi and Salmonella paratyphi A, B, and C bacteria
(Ex:) For category A01 CC codes: A01.00-A01.4

  ● **A01.0** **Typhoid fever**
Infection due to Salmonella typhi

  A01.00 **Typhoid fever, unspecified**

  A01.01 **Typhoid meningitis**

  A01.02 **Typhoid fever with heart involvement**
Typhoid endocarditis
Typhoid myocarditis

  A01.03 **Typhoid pneumonia**

  A01.04 **Typhoid arthritis**

  A01.05 **Typhoid osteomyelitis**

  A01.09 **Typhoid fever with other complications**

  A01.1 **Paratyphoid fever A**

  A01.2 **Paratyphoid fever B**

  A01.3 **Paratyphoid fever C**

  A01.4 **Paratyphoid fever, unspecified**
Infection due to Salmonella paratyphi NOS

● **A02** **Other salmonella infections**
Includes   infection or foodborne intoxication due to any Salmonella species other than S. typhi and S. paratyphi

  A02.0 **Salmonella enteritis**
Salmonellosis
(Ex:) A01.00-A01.09, A01.4-A02.0, A03.9-A05.2, A07.4, A08.0-A09, A48.51-A48.52, K30, K52.1-K52.3, K52.82-K52.9, K58.0-K58.9, K65.0, K65.2, K65.8, K68.12-K68.9, P76.8-P77.9, P78.1, P78.3-P78.89

  A02.1 **Salmonella sepsis**
(Ex:) A02.1, A20.7, A22.7, A26.7, A32.7, A39.2-A39.4, A40.0-A40.1, A40.8-A41.9, A42.7, A48.2-A48.4, A48.8-A49.9, A54.86, B00.7, B37.7, B92, B94.2-B96.89, P36.0-P36.9, P39.2, P39.4-P39.9, R65.10-R65.20, Z16.10-Z16.39

  ● **A02.2** **Localized salmonella infections**

  A02.20 **Localized salmonella infection, unspecified**
Specified in the documentation as localized, but unspecified as to type

  A02.21 **Salmonella meningitis**
Specified as localized in the meninges
(Ex:) A02.21, A17.0-A17.1, A27.81, A39.0, A50.41, A51.41, A52.13, A54.82, A54.84, A54.89-A54.9, A74.81-A74.9, A87.0-A87.9, A96.2, A98.3-A98.4, B26.1, B33.24, B33.4-B33.8, B34.1-B34.2, B34.4-B34.8, B37.5, B38.4, B45.1, B58.2, B92, B94.2-94.9, B97.10, B97.19, B97.29, B97.5-B97.6, B97.81-B97.89, G00.0-G03.9, G04.2, G32.89, G96.8-G96.9, G98.0-G98.8, G99.8

  A02.22 **Salmonella pneumonia**
Specified as localized in the lungs
(Ex:) A02.22, A15.0-A15.6, A15.8-A15.9, A17.9, A18.82, A18.84, A18.89, A20.2, A21.1, A22.1, A31.0, A37.01, A37.11, A37.81, A37.91, A42.0, A43.0, A48.1, B25.0, B39.0-B39.2, B44.0, B58.3, B59, B67.1, J09.X1-J09.X2, J10.00-J10.1, J11.00-J11.1, J12.0-J12.3, J12.89-J18.1, J18.8-J18.9, J22, J60, J62.0-J67.7, J68.0-J70.4, J70.8-J70.9, J98.4, J98.8-J99, R91.1

  A02.23 **Salmonella arthritis**
Specified as localized in the joints
(Ex:) A02.23, A18.02, A18.09, A39.83-A39.84, A54.40, A54.42-A54.43, A54.82, A54.84, A54.89-A54.9, B06.82, M00.00-M02.30, M02.319, M02.329, M02.339, M02.349, M02.359, M02.369, M02.379-M02.9, M05.40-M05.59, M05.70-M06.09, M06.20-M06.39, M06.80-M07.69, M11.00-M11.9, M12.10-M15.0, M15.3-M15.9, M16.2-M16.9, M17.2-M17.9, M18.2-M18.9, M19.111-M19.93, M24.10-M24.176, M25.00, M25.08-M25.18, M25.40-M25.676, M25.80-M25.9, M35.2, M36.1-M36.4, R29.4

  A02.24 **Salmonella osteomyelitis**
Specified as localized in bone
(Ex:) A02.24, A18.03-A18.09, M46.20-M46.39, M86.00-M86.9

  A02.25 **Salmonella pyelonephritis**
Salmonella tubulo-interstitial nephropathy
(Ex:) A02.25-A02.29

  A02.29 **Salmonella with other localized infection**
Specified as localized (because it is still under localized heading) but does not assign into any of the above codes
(Ex:) A02.25-A02.29

Item 1-1   Salmonella is a bacterium that lives in the intestines of fowl and mammals and can spread to humans through improper food preparation and cooking. Salmonellosis is an infection with the bacterium. Symptoms include diarrhea, fever, and abdominal cramps 12 to 72 hours after infection. The illness usually lasts 4 to 7 days, and most persons recover without treatment. The diarrhea may be so severe that the patient needs to be hospitalized. Patients with immunocompromised systems in chronic, ill health are more likely to have the infection invade their bloodstream with life-threatening results. For example, patients with sickle cell disease are more prone to salmonella osteomyelitis than others.

◀ New   ◀◀ Revised   ~~deleted~~ Deleted   Excludes 1   Excludes 2   Includes   Use additional   Code first   Code also   Unspecified

OGCR Official Guidelines   ● Unacceptable Principal Diagnosis   X Assign placeholder X   ● Use Additional Character(s)   ◣ Manifestation Code   **Coding Clinic**

A02.8 Other specified salmonella infections
> *Any specified salmonella infection which does NOT assign into any of the above codes (not specified as localized)*
> (Ex̲) A02.8

A02.9 Salmonella infection, unspecified
> *Unspecified in the documentation as to specific type of salmonella*
> (Ex̲) A02.9

● **A03 Shigellosis**
> *An infectious disease caused by bacteria (Shigella)*

A03.0 Shigellosis due to Shigella dysenteriae
> Group A shigellosis [Shiga-Kruse dysentery]
> (Ex̲) A00.1, A01.00-A01.09, A01.4-A02.0, A03.0, A03.9, A04.9-A05.2, A06.0-A06.2, A06.9, A07.1-A07.9, A08.4-A09, A18.32-A18.39, A18.83, A48.51-A48.52, B37.82, B82.9, J09.X3-J09.X9, J10.2-J10.89, J11.2-J11.89, K30, K31.84, K50.00-K51.919, K52.1-K52.3, K52.82-K55.1, K55.30-K55.33, K55.8-K55.9, K58.0-K58.9, P70.0-P70.4, P70.9-P71.9, P72.1, P72.9-P74.4, P74.9, P76.8-P77.9, P78.1, P78.3-P78.89, P94.0

A03.1 Shigellosis due to Shigella flexneri
> Group B shigellosis

A03.2 Shigellosis due to Shigella boydii
> Group C shigellosis

A03.3 Shigellosis due to Shigella sonnei
> Group D shigellosis

A03.8 Other shigellosis

A03.9 Shigellosis, unspecified
> Bacillary dysentery NOS

● **A04 Other bacterial intestinal infections**
> **Excludes1**   bacterial foodborne intoxications, NEC (A05.-)
> tuberculous enteritis (A18.32)
> (Ex̲) **For category A04 CC codes A04.0-A04.4:** A02.0, A03.9-A05.0, A05.2, A07.4, A08.0-A09, J09.X3-J09.X9, J10.2-J10.89, J11.2-J11.89, K30, K31.84, K52.1-K52.3, K52.82-K52.9, K58.0-K58.9, K65.0, K65.2, K65.8, K68.12-K68.9, P76.8-P77.9, P78.1, P78.3-P78.89 **For category A04 CC codes A04.5-A04.8:** A00.1, A01.00-A01.09, A01.4-A02.0, A03.9, A04.0-A04.8, A04.9-A05.2, A06.0-A06.2, A06.9, A07.1-A09, A18.32-A18.39, A18.83, A48.51-A48.52, B37.82, B82.9, J09.X3-J09.X9, J10.2-J10.89, J11.2-J11.89, K30, K31.84, K50.00-K51.919, K52.1-K52.3, K52.82-K55.1, K55.30-K55.33, K55.8-K55.9, K58.0-K58.9, P70.0-P70.4, P70.9-P71.9, P72.1, P72.9-P74.4, P74.9, P76.8-P77.9, P78.1, P78.3-P78.89, P94.0

A04.0 Enteropathogenic Escherichia coli infection
> *Pertaining to or producing intestinal disease*

A04.1 Enterotoxigenic Escherichia coli infection
> *Producing or containing intestinal toxin*

A04.2 Enteroinvasive Escherichia coli infection
> *Capable of penetrating and spreading through intestinal mucosal epithelium*

A04.3 Enterohemorrhagic Escherichia coli infection
> *Causing bloody diarrhea, resulting from microorganisms*

A04.4 Other intestinal Escherichia coli infections
> Escherichia coli enteritis NOS

A04.5 Campylobacter enteritis
> *Spiral shaped bacterium*

A04.6 Enteritis due to Yersinia enterocolitica
> **Excludes1**   extraintestinal yersiniosis (A28.2)
> *Transmitted by infected food /water and person-to-person contact, affecting intestinal tract*

A04.7 Enterocolitis due to Clostridium difficile
> Foodborne intoxication by Clostridium difficile
> Pseudomembraneous colitis
> *Marked by fibrinous deposit (false membrane) with enmeshed necrotic cells*

A04.8 Other specified bacterial intestinal infections

A04.9 Bacterial intestinal infection, unspecified
> Bacterial enteritis NOS
> (Ex̲) A00.1, A01.00-A01.09, A01.4-A02.0, A03.9-A05.0, A05.2, A06.0-A06.2, A06.9, A07.1-A09, A18.32-A18.39, A18.83, B37.82, B82.9, J09.X3-J09.X9, J10.2-J10.89, J11.2-J11.89, K30, K31.84, K52.1-K52.3, K52.82-K52.9, K58.0-K58.9, K65.0, K65.2, K65.8, K68.12-K68.9, P76.8-P77.9, P78.1, P78.3-P78.89

● **A05 Other bacterial foodborne intoxications, not elsewhere classified**
> **Excludes1**   Clostridium difficile foodborne intoxication and infection (A04.7)
> Escherichia coli infection (A04.0-A04.4)
> listeriosis (A32.-)
> salmonella foodborne intoxication and infection (A02.-)
> toxic effect of noxious foodstuffs (T61-T62)

A05.0 Foodborne staphylococcal intoxication
> (Ex̲) A00.0-A09, A48.51-A48.52

A05.1 Botulism food poisoning
> Botulism NOS
> Classical foodborne intoxication due to Clostridium botulinum
> **Excludes1**   infant botulism (A48.51)
> wound botulism (A48.52)
> (Ex̲) A04.7, A05.0-A05.2, A48.51-A48.52

A05.2 Foodborne Clostridium perfringens [Clostridium welchii] intoxication
> *Type A causes gas gangrene and necrotizing colitis; major cause of food poisoning in humans*
> Enteritis necroticans
> Pig-bel
> (Ex̲) A02.0, A03.9-A05.2, A07.4, A08.0-A09, A48.51-A48.52, J09.X3-J09.X9, J10.2-J10.89, J11.2-J11.89, K30, K31.84, K52.1-K52.3, K52.82-K52.9, K58.0-K58.9, K65.0, K65.2, K65.8, K68.12-K68.9, P76.8-P77.9, P78.1, P78.3-P78.89

A05.3 Foodborne Vibrio parahaemolyticus intoxication
> *Organism that survives only in high salt environment (halophilic), major cause of gastroenteritis due to consumption of raw or improperly cooked fish/seafood*
> (Ex̲) A00.0-A09, A48.51-A48.52

A05.4 Foodborne Bacillus cereus intoxication
> *Spore-forming species commonly found in soil, causes food poisoning from formation of intestinal toxins in contaminated foods*
> (Ex̲) A00.0-A09, A48.51-A48.52

A05.5 Foodborne Vibrio vulnificus intoxication
> *Species that survives in high salt environment (halophilic) with infection by eating raw seafood causes septicemia and cellulitis*
> (Ex̲) A00.0-A09, A48.51-A48.52

A05.8 Other specified bacterial foodborne intoxications
> (Ex̲) A00.0-A09, A48.51-A48.52

A05.9 Bacterial foodborne intoxication, unspecified

CHAPTER 1 (A00-B99)

Figure 1-1   Electron micrograph of escherichia coli (E. coli) expressing P fimbriae. (From Mandell, Bennett, & Dolin: Principles and Practice of Infectious Diseases, ed 7, Churchill Livingstone, An Imprint of Elsevier, 2009)

Item 1-2   *Escherichia coli [E. coli]* is a gram-negative bacterium found in the intestinal tracts of humans and animals and is usually nonpathogenic. Pathogenic strains can cause diarrhea or pyogenic (pus-producing) infections. Can be a threat to food safety.

N Newborn Age: Ø   **P** Pediatric Age: 0–17   **M** Maternity DX: 12–55   **A** Adult Age: 15–124   ♀ Females Only   ♂ Males Only

 Complication\Comorbidity   Major C\C   (Ex̲) CC/MCC Exclusions   Hospital-Acquired Condition

● **A06   Amebiasis**
An intestinal illness caused by the microscopic parasite Entamoeba histolytica

Includes   infection due to Entamoeba histolytica
Excludes1   other protozoal intestinal diseases (A07.-)
Excludes2   acanthamebiasis (B60.1-)
           Naegleriasis (B60.2)

A06.0   Acute amebic dysentery 🔎
Acute amebiasis
Intestinal amebiasis NOS
(Ex:) A06.0-A06.1, A07.4

A06.1   Chronic intestinal amebiasis 🔎
(Ex:) A06.0-A06.1, A07.4

A06.2   Amebic nondysenteric colitis 🔎
Pertaining to single cell microorganism
(Ex:) A02.0, A03.9-A05.0, A05.2, A06.0-A06.2, A06.9, A07.1-A09, B82.9, J09.X3-J09.X9, J10.2-J10.89, J11.2-J11.89, K30, K31.84, K50.00-K51.919, K52.1-K52.3, K52.82-K55.1, K55.30-K55.33, K55.8-K55.9, K58.0-K58.9, P76.8-P77.9, P78.1, P78.3, P78.81-P78.89

A06.3   Ameboma of intestine 🔎
Tumorlike mass produced by localized inflammation often in intestine
Ameboma NOS
(Ex:) A06.0-A06.6, A06.81-A06.89

A06.4   Amebic liver abscess 🔎
Hepatic amebiasis
(Ex:) A06.4, K75.0

A06.5   Amebic lung abscess 🔎
Amebic abscess of lung (and liver)
(Ex:) A06.5, J85.0-J85.2

A06.6   Amebic brain abscess 🔎
Amebic abscess of brain (and liver) (and lung)
(Ex:) A06.6, G06.0

A06.7   Cutaneous amebiasis

● **A06.8   Amebic infection of other sites**

A06.81   Amebic cystitis 🔎
(Ex:) A06.0-A06.6, A06.81-A06.89

A06.82   Other amebic genitourinary infections 🔎
Amebic balanitis
Amebic vesiculitis
Amebic vulvovaginitis
(Ex:) A06.0-A06.6, A06.81-A06.89

A06.89   Other amebic infections 🔎
Amebic appendicitis
Amebic splenic abscess
(Ex:) A06.0-A06.6, A06.81-A06.89

A06.9   Amebiasis, unspecified

● **A07   Other protozoal intestinal diseases**
(Ex:) **For category A07 CC codes unless otherwise indicated:** A02.0, A03.9-A05.0, A05.2, A06.0-A06.2, A06.9, A07.1-A09, B82.9, J09.X3-J09.X9, J10.2-J10.89, J11.2-J11.89, K30, K31.84, K52.1-K52.3, K52.82-K52.9, K58.0-K58.9

A07.0   Balantidiasis
Balantidial dysentery
Infection by protozoa that may cause diarrhea and dysentery, with ulceration of colonic mucous membranes

A07.1   Giardiasis [lambliasis] 🔎
Common infection in small intestine spread by contaminated food, water, or direct person-to-person contact

A07.2   Cryptosporidiosis 🔎
Human infection with protozoa usually seen as self-limited diarrhea in those who work with cattle

A07.3   Isosporiasis 🔎
Human intestinal disease caused by protozoa
Infection due to Isospora belli and Isospora hominis
Intestinal coccidiosis
Isosporosis

A07.4   Cyclosporiasis 🔎
Infection by protozoa with most common species infecting humans being C cayetanensis
(Ex:) A02.0, A03.9-A05.0, A05.2, A06.0-A06.2, A06.9, A07.1-A09, B82.9, J09.X3-J09.X9, J10.2-J10.89, J11.2-J11.89, K30, K31.84, K52.1-K52.3, K52.82-K52.9, K58.0-K58.9, K65.0, K65.2, K65.8, K68.12-K68.9

A07.8   Other specified protozoal intestinal diseases 🔎
Intestinal microsporidiosis
Intestinal trichomoniasis
Sarcocystosis
Sarcosporidiosis

A07.9   Protozoal intestinal disease, unspecified 🔎
Flagellate diarrhea
Protozoal colitis
Protozoal diarrhea
Protozoal dysentery

● **A08   Viral and other specified intestinal infections**
Excludes1   influenza with involvement of gastrointestinal tract (J09.X3, J10.2, J11.2)
(Ex:) **For category A08 CC codes:** A02.0, A03.9-A05.0, A05.2, A06.0-A06.2, A06.9, A07.1-A09, A18.32-A18.39, A18.83, B37.82, B82.9, J09.X3-J09.X9, J10.2-J10.89, J11.2-J11.89, K30, K31.84, K52.1-K52.3, K52.82-K52.9, K58.0-K58.9, K65.0, K65.2, K65.8, K68.12-K68.9, P76.8-P77.9, P78.1, P78.3-P78.89

A08.0   Rotaviral enteritis

● **A08.1   Acute gastroenteropathy due to Norwalk agent and other small round viruses**

A08.11   Acute gastroenteropathy due to Norwalk agent 🔎
Acute gastroenteropathy due to Norovirus
Acute gastroenteropathy due to Norwalk-like agent

A08.19   Acute gastroenteropathy due to other small round viruses 🔎
Acute gastroenteropathy due to small round virus [SRV] NOS

A08.2   Adenoviral enteritis 🔎

● **A08.3   Other viral enteritis**

A08.31   Calicivirus enteritis 🔎

A08.32   Astrovirus enteritis 🔎

A08.39   Other viral enteritis 🔎
Coxsackie virus enteritis
Echovirus enteritis
Enterovirus enteritis NEC
Torovirus enteritis

A08.4   Viral intestinal infection, unspecified
Viral enteritis NOS
Viral gastroenteritis NOS
Viral gastroenteropathy NOS

A08.8   Other specified intestinal infections

A09   Infectious gastroenteritis and colitis, unspecified 🔎
Infectious colitis NOS
Infectious enteritis NOS
Infectious gastroenteritis NOS
Excludes1   colitis NOS (K52.9)
           diarrhea NOS (R19.7)
           enteritis NOS (K52.9)
           gastroenteritis NOS (K52.9)
           noninfective gastroenteritis and colitis, unspecified (K52.9)
(Ex:) A00.0-A09, A48.51-A48.52

◀ New   ◀ Revised   ~~deleted~~ Deleted   Excludes 1   Excludes 2   Includes   Use additional   Code first   Code also   Unspecified

638   OGCR Official Guidelines   ● Unacceptable Principal Diagnosis   X Assign placeholder X   ● Use Additional Character(s)   ▶ Manifestation Code   Coding Clinic

Figure 1-2 Far advanced bilateral pulmonary tuberculosis before and after 8 months of treatment with streptomycin, PAS, and isoniazid. (From Hinshaw HC, Garland LH: Diseases of the Chest, ed 4, Philadelphia, WB Saunders, 1980)

Item 1–3 Tuberculosis is a common and deadly infectious disease caused by the *Mycobacterium tuberculosis* organism. The first tuberculosis infection is called the **primary infection** and most commonly attacks the lungs but can affect the central nervous system, lymphatic system, circulatory system, genitourinary system, bones, joints, and even the skin. A **Ghon** lesion is the **initial lesion.** A **secondary lesion** occurs when the tubercle bacilli are carried to other areas.

Item 1–4 Although it primarily affects the lungs, the bacteria ***Mycobacterium tuberculosis*** can travel from the pulmonary circulation to virtually any organ in the body, much as a cancer metastasizes to a secondary site. If the immune system becomes compromised by age or disease, what would otherwise be a self-limiting primary tuberculosis in the lungs will develop in other organs. These are known as extrapulmonary sites.

TUBERCULOSIS (A15-A19)

Includes	infections due to Mycobacterium tuberculosis and Mycobacterium bovis
Excludes1	congenital tuberculosis (P37.0) nonspecific reaction to test for tuberculosis without active tuberculosis (R76.1-) pneumoconiosis associated with tuberculosis, any type in A15 (J65) positive PPD (R76.11) positive tuberculin skin test without active tuberculosis (R76.11) sequelae of tuberculosis (B90.-) silicotuberculosis (J65)

● **A15   Respiratory tuberculosis**
   Ex: **For category A15 CC codes unless otherwise indicated:** A15.0-A15.9, A17.9, A18.82, A18.84, A18.89-A19.9, A22.1, A31.0, A31.2-A31.9, A37.01, A37.11, A37.81, A37.91, A48.1, A49.3-A49.9, B25.0, B44.0, B90.9, B92, B94.2-B94.9, B96.0, B96.6-B96.89, J09.X1-J09.X2, J10.00-J10.1, J11.00-J11.1, J12.0-J12.3, J12.89-J18.1, J18.8-J18.9, J44.9, J47.0-J70.4, J70.8-J70.9, J98.4, R91.1

   A15.0   Tuberculosis of lung 🔖
      Tuberculous bronchiectasis
         Chronic dilatation of bronchi
      Tuberculous fibrosis of lung
      Tuberculous pneumonia
      Tuberculous pneumothorax

   A15.4   Tuberculosis of intrathoracic lymph nodes 🔖
      Tuberculosis of hilar lymph nodes
      Tuberculosis of mediastinal lymph nodes
      Tuberculosis of tracheobronchial lymph nodes
      | **Excludes1** | tuberculosis specified as primary (A15.7) |

   A15.5   Tuberculosis of larynx, trachea and bronchus 🔖
      Tuberculosis of bronchus
      Tuberculosis of glottis
      Tuberculosis of larynx
      Tuberculosis of trachea

   A15.6   Tuberculous pleurisy 🔖
      Tuberculosis of pleura
      Tuberculous empyema
      | **Excludes1** | primary respiratory tuberculosis (A15.7) |

A15.7   Primary respiratory tuberculosis 🔖
   Ex: A15.0-A17.82, A17.89-A19.9

A15.8   Other respiratory tuberculosis 🔖
   Mediastinal tuberculosis
   Nasopharyngeal tuberculosis
   Tuberculosis of nose
   Tuberculosis of sinus [any nasal]
   Ex: A15.0-A17.82, A17.89, A18.31-A18.39, A18.83, A19.0-A19.9

A15.9   Respiratory tuberculosis unspecified 🔖
   Ex: A15.0-A17.82, A17.89, A18.31-A18.39, A18.83, A19.0-A19.9

● **A17   Tuberculosis of nervous system**
   A17.0   Tuberculous meningitis 🔖
      Tuberculosis of meninges (cerebral) (spinal)
      Tuberculosis leptomeningitis
      | **Excludes1** | tuberculous meningoencephalitis (A17.82) |
      Ex: A02.21, A17.0-A17.1, A17.89-A17.9, A18.82, A18.84, A18.89, A27.81, A31.2-A31.9, A39.0, A49.3-A49.9, A50.41, A51.41, A52.13, A54.82, A54.84, A54.89-A54.9, A87.0-A87.9, B00.3, B02.1, B26.1, B37.5, B38.4, B45.1, B58.2, B90.0, B92, B94.2-B94.9, B96.0, B96.6-B96.89, G00.0-G03.9, G04.2, G32.89, G61.0, G96.8-G96.9, G98.0-G98.8, G99.8

   A17.1   Meningeal tuberculoma 🔖
      Tuberculoma of meninges (cerebral) (spinal)
      | **Excludes2** | tuberculoma of brain and spinal cord (A17.81) |
      Ex: See A17.0

● **A17.8   Other tuberculosis of nervous system**
   A17.81   Tuberculoma of brain and spinal cord 🔖
      Tuberculous abscess of brain and spinal cord
      Ex: A17.81-A17.82, A17.89-A17.9, A18.82, A18.84, A18.89, A31.2-A31.9, A49.3-A49.9, B90.0, B92, B94.2-B94.9, B96.0, B96.6-B96.89

   A17.82   Tuberculous meningoencephalitis 🔖
      Inflammation of brain and meninges; AKA cerebromeningitis and encephalomeningitis
      Tuberculous myelitis
      Ex: See A17.81

   A17.83   Tuberculous neuritis 🔖
      Tuberculous mononeuropathy
      Ex: No exclusions

   A17.89   Other tuberculosis of nervous system 🔖
      Tuberculous polyneuropathy
      Ex: A17.89-A17.9, A18.82, A18.84, A18.89, A31.2-A31.9, A49.3-A49.9, B90.0, B92, B94.2-B94.9, B96.0, B96.6-B96.89

   A17.9   Tuberculosis of nervous system, unspecified 🔖
      Ex: A17.9, A18.82, A18.84, A18.89, A31.2-A31.9, A49.3-A49.9, B92, B94.2-B94.9, B96.0, B96.6-B96.89

● **A18   Tuberculosis of other organs**
   ● **A18.0   Tuberculosis of bones and joints**
      A18.01   Tuberculosis of spine 🔖
         Pott's disease or curvature of spine
         Tuberculous arthritis
         Tuberculous osteomyelitis of spine
         Tuberculous spondylitis
         Ex: A18.01

      A18.02   Tuberculous arthritis of other joints 🔖
         Tuberculosis of hip (joint)
         Tuberculosis of knee (joint)
         Ex: A18.02

      A18.03   Tuberculosis of other bones 🔖
         Tuberculous mastoiditis
         Tuberculous osteomyelitis
         Ex: A18.01, A18.03

      A18.09   Other musculoskeletal tuberculosis 🔖
         Tuberculous myositis
         Tuberculous synovitis
         Tuberculous tenosynovitis
         Ex: A18.01-A18.02, A18.09

N Newborn Age: 0   **P** Pediatric Age: 0–17   **M** Maternity DX: 12–55   **A** Adult Age: 15–124   ♀ Females Only   ♂ Males Only

🔖 Complication\Comorbidity   🔖 Major C\C   Ex: CC/MCC Exclusions   🔖 Hospital-Acquired Condition

639

CHAPTER 1 (A00–B99)

● **A18.1** **Tuberculosis of genitourinary system**

A18.10 **Tuberculosis of genitourinary system, unspecified** 🗝
(Ex:) A17.9, A18.10, A18.82, A18.84, A18.89, A31.2-A31.9, A49.3-A49.9, B90.1, B92, B94.2-B94.9, B96.0, B96.6-B96.89

A18.11 **Tuberculosis of kidney and ureter** 🗝
(Ex:) A17.9, A18.10-A18.13, A18.82, A18.84, A18.89, A31.2-A31.9, A49.3-A49.9, B90.1, B92, B94.2-B94.9, B96.0, B96.6-B96.89

A18.12 **Tuberculosis of bladder** 🗝
(Ex:) See A18.11

A18.13 **Tuberculosis of other urinary organs** 🗝
Tuberculous urethritis
(Ex:) See A18.11

A18.14 **Tuberculosis of prostate** ♂ 🗝   A
(Ex:) A17.9, A18.10, A18.82, A18.84, A18.89, A31.2-A31.9, A49.3-A49.9, B90.1, B92, B94.2-B94.9, B96.0, B96.6-B96.89

A18.15 **Tuberculosis of other male genital organs** ♂ 🗝
(Ex:) See A18.14

A18.16 **Tuberculosis of cervix** ♀ 🗝
(Ex:) A17.9, A18.0, A18.16-A18.18, A18.82, A18.84, A18.89, A31.2-A31.9, A49.3-A49.9, B90.1, B92, B94.2-B94.9, B96.0, B96.6-B96.89

A18.17 **Tuberculous female pelvic inflammatory disease** ♀ 🗝
Tuberculous endometritis
Tuberculous oophoritis and salpingitis
Oophoritis = inflammation of ovary
Salpingitis = inflammation of fallopian tube
(Ex:) See A18.16

A18.18 **Tuberculosis of other female genital organs** ♀ 🗝
Tuberculous ulceration of vulva
(Ex:) See A18.16

A18.2 **Tuberculous peripheral lymphadenopathy** 🗝
Tuberculous adenitis

Excludes2   tuberculosis of bronchial and mediastinal lymph nodes (A15.4)
tuberculosis of mesenteric and retroperitoneal lymph nodes (A18.39)
tuberculous tracheobronchial adenopathy (A15.4)
(Ex:) A17.9, A18.2, A18.82, A18.84, A18.89, A31.2-A31.9, A49.3-A49.9, B92, B94.2-B94.9, B96.0, B96.6-B96.89

● **A18.3** **Tuberculosis of intestines, peritoneum and mesenteric glands**
(Ex:) For category A18.3 CC codes: A17.9, A18.31-A18.39, A18.82-A18.84, A18.89, A31.2-A31.9, A49.3-A49.9, B92, B94.2-B94.9, B96.0, B96.6-B96.89

A18.31 **Tuberculous peritonitis** 🗝
Tuberculous ascites

A18.32 **Tuberculous enteritis** 🗝
Tuberculosis of anus and rectum
Tuberculosis of intestine (large) (small)

A18.39 **Retroperitoneal tuberculosis** 🗝
Tuberculosis of mesenteric glands
Tuberculosis of retroperitoneal (lymph glands)

A18.4 **Tuberculosis of skin and subcutaneous tissue** 🗝
Erythema induratum, tuberculous
Lupus excedens
Lupus vulgaris NOS
Lupus vulgaris of eyelid
Cutaneous tuberculosis characterized by reddish brown plaque on skin surrounded by papules and nodules
Scrofuloderma
Type of cutaneous tuberculosis, with direct extension of tuberculosis into skin from underlying structures; AKA tuberculosis colliquativa
Tuberculosis of external ear

Excludes2   lupus erythematosus (L93.-)
lupus NOS (M32.9)
systemic (M32.-)
(Ex:) A15.0-A17.82, A17.89-A19.9

● **A18.5** **Tuberculosis of eye**

Excludes2   lupus vulgaris of eyelid (A18.4)
(Ex:) For category A18.5 CC codes: A17.9, A18.50-A18.59, A18.82, A18.84, A18.89, A31.2-A31.9, A49.3-A49.9, B92, B94.2-B94.9, B96.0, B96.6-B96.89

A18.50 **Tuberculosis of eye, unspecified** 🗝

A18.51 **Tuberculous episcleritis** 🗝
Inflammation of episclera and adjacent tissues

A18.52 **Tuberculous keratitis** 🗝
Tuberculous interstitial keratitis
Tuberculous keratoconjunctivitis (interstitial) (phlyctenular)
Inflammation of cornea and conjunctiva

A18.53 **Tuberculous chorioretinitis** 🗝
Inflammation of choroid and retina; retinochoroiditis

A18.54 **Tuberculous iridocyclitis** 🗝
Inflammation of iris and ciliary body

A18.59 **Other tuberculosis of eye** 🗝
Tuberculous conjunctivitis

A18.6 **Tuberculosis of (inner) (middle) ear** 🗝
Tuberculous otitis media

Excludes2   tuberculosis of external ear (A18.4)
tuberculous mastoiditis (A18.03)
(Ex:) A17.9, A18.6, A18.82, A18.84, A18.89, A31.2-A31.9, A49.3-A49.9, B92, B94.2-B94.9, B96.0, B96.6-B96.89

A18.7 **Tuberculosis of adrenal glands** 🗝
Tuberculous Addison's disease
(Ex:) A17.9, A18.7, A18.82, A18.84, A18.89, A31.2-A31.9, A49.3-A49.9, B92, B94.2-B94.9, B96.0, B96.6-B96.89

● **A18.8** **Tuberculosis of other specified organs**

A18.81 **Tuberculosis of thyroid gland** 🗝
(Ex:) A17.9, A18.81-A18.82, A18.84, A18.89, A31.2-A31.9, A49.3-A49.9, B92, B94.2-B94.9, B96.0, B96.6-B96.89

A18.82 **Tuberculosis of other endocrine glands** 🗝
Tuberculosis of pituitary gland
Tuberculosis of thymus gland
(Ex:) See A17.9

A18.83 **Tuberculosis of digestive tract organs, not elsewhere classified** 🗝

Excludes1   tuberculosis of intestine (A18.32)
(Ex:) See A18.3

A18.84 **Tuberculosis of heart** 🗝
Tuberculous cardiomyopathy
Tuberculous endocarditis
Tuberculous myocarditis
Tuberculous pericarditis
(Ex:) See A17.9

A18.85 **Tuberculosis of spleen** 🗝
(Ex:) A17.9, A18.82, A18.84-A18.85 A18.89, A31.2-A31.9, A49.3-A49.9, B92, B94.2-B94.9, B96.0, B96.6-B96.89

A18.89 **Tuberculosis of other sites** 🗝
Tuberculosis of muscle
Tuberculous cerebral arteritis
(Ex:) See A17.9

● **A19** **Miliary tuberculosis**

Includes   disseminated tuberculosis
generalized tuberculosis
tuberculous polyserositis
(Ex:) For category A19 CC codes: A17.9, A18.82, A18.84, A18.89, A19.0-A19.9, A31.2-A31.9, A49.3-A49.9, B92, B94.2-B94.9, B96.0, B96.6-B96.89

A19.0 **Acute miliary tuberculosis of a single specified site** 🗝

A19.1 **Acute miliary tuberculosis of multiple sites** 🗝

A19.2 **Acute miliary tuberculosis, unspecified** 🗝

A19.8 **Other miliary tuberculosis** 🗝

A19.9 **Miliary tuberculosis, unspecified** 🗝

◀ New   ◀▪▪ Revised   ~~deleted~~ Deleted   Excludes 1   Excludes 2   Includes   Use additional   Code first   Code also   Unspecified

OGCR Official Guidelines   ● Unacceptable Principal Diagnosis   X Assign placeholder X   🗝 Use Additional Character(s)   ▌Manifestation Code   **Coding Clinic**

Item 1–5 Miliary tuberculosis can be a life-threatening condition. If a tuberculous lesion enters a blood vessel, immense dissemination of tuberculous organisms can occur if the immune system is weak. High-risk populations—children under 4 years of age, the elderly, or the immunocompromised—are particularly prone to this type of infection. The lesions will have a millet seedlike appearance on chest x-ray. Bronchial washings and biopsy may aid in diagnosis.

CERTAIN ZOONOTIC BACTERIAL DISEASES (A20-A28)

● **A20   Plague**
   Infectious disease caused by a Yersinia pestis bacterium, transmitted by a rodent flea bite or handling of infected animal
   Includes   infection due to Yersinia pestis

   A20.0   Bubonic plague 🦠
   (Ex:) A20.0-A20.9

   A20.1   Cellulocutaneous plague 🦠
   Skin and subcutaneous tissue plague
   (Ex:) A20.0-A20.9

   A20.2   Pneumonic plague 🦠
   (Ex:) A20.2, J12.81

   A20.3   Plague meningitis 🦠
   (Ex:) A20.3, A20.8

   A20.7   Septicemic plague 🦠
   (Ex:) A02.1, A20.0-A20.9, A22.7, A26.7, A32.7, A40.0-A40.1, A40.8-A41.9, A42.7, A54.86, B37.7, P36.0-P36.9, P39.2, P39.4-P39.9, R65.10-R65.20

   A20.8   Other forms of plague 🦠
   Abortive plague
   Asymptomatic plague
   Pestis minor
      Systemic bacterial disease
   (Ex:) See A20.3

   A20.9   Plague, unspecified 🦠
   (Ex:) A20.9

● **A21   Tularemia**
   Caused by Francisella tularensis bacterium found in rodents, rabbits, and hares and transmitted to humans by contact with infected animal tissues or by ticks, biting flies, or mosquitoes
   Includes   deer-fly fever
            infection due to Francisella tularensis
            rabbit fever

   A21.0   Ulceroglandular tularemia 🦠
   Most common form of tularemia in humans is painful, swollen, erythematous papule at point of inoculation that ruptures to form shallow ulcer
   (Ex:) A21.0

   A21.1   Oculoglandular tularemia 🦠
   Primary site of entry is conjunctival sac, results in granulomatous corneal lesions
   Ophthalmic tularemia
   (Ex:) A21.1, J12.81

   A21.2   Pulmonary tularemia 🦠
   (Ex:) A22.1, A37.01, A37.11, A37.81, A37.91, A48.1, B25.0, B44.0, J09.X1-J09.X2, J10.00-J10.1, J11.00-J11.1, J15.29, J15.5-J18.0, J18.8-J18.9, J22, J60-J70.4, J70.8-J70.9, J98.4, J98.8-J99, R91.1

   A21.3   Gastrointestinal tularemia 🦠
   Abdominal tularemia
   (Ex:) A21.3

   A21.7   Generalized tularemia 🦠
   (Ex:) A21.0-A21.9

   A21.8   Other forms of tularemia 🦠
   (Ex:) A21.0-A21.9

   A21.9   Tularemia, unspecified 🦠
   (Ex:) A21.0-A21.9

Item 1–6 Brucellosis: An infectious disease caused by the bacterium Brucella. Humans are infected by contact with contaminated animals or animal products. In humans brucellosis symptoms that are similar to the flu include fever, sweats, headaches, back pains, and physical weakness. Severe infections of the central nervous system or lining of the heart may occur. Brucellosis can also cause chronic symptoms that include recurrent fevers, joint pain, and fatigue.

● **A22   Anthrax**
   An acute infectious disease caused by the spore-forming Bacillus anthracis; occurs in humans exposed to infected animals or tissue from infected animals
   Includes   infection due to Bacillus anthracis

   A22.0   Cutaneous anthrax 🦠
   Malignant carbuncle
   Malignant pustule
   (Ex:) A22.0

   A22.1   Pulmonary anthrax 🦠
   Inhalation anthrax
   Ragpicker's disease
   Woolsorter's disease
   (Ex:) A15.0-A15.9, A17.9, A18.82, A18.84, A18.89, A20.2, A21.1-A21.2, A22.1, A31.0, A37.01, A37.11, A37.81, A37.91, A42.0, A43.0, A48.1, B25.0, B39.0-B39.2, B44.0, B58.3, B59, B67.1, J09.X1-J09.X2, J10.00-J10.1, J11.00-J11.1, J12.0-J12.3, J12.81-J18.1, J18.8-J18.9, J22, J44.9, J47.0-J70.4, J70.8-J70.9, J98.4, J98.8-J99, R91.1

   A22.2   Gastrointestinal anthrax 🦠
   (Ex:) A22.2

   A22.7   Anthrax sepsis 🦠
   Infectious bacterial disease
   MCC when PDx is its own MCC
   (Ex:) See A02.1

   A22.8   Other forms of anthrax 🦠
   Anthrax meningitis
   (Ex:) A22.8

   A22.9   Anthrax, unspecified 🦠
   (Ex:) A22.0-A22.9

● **A23   Brucellosis**
   Includes   Malta fever
            Mediterranean fever
            undulant fever

   A23.0   Brucellosis due to Brucella melitensis
   Resulting in flu-like symptoms that may lead to chronic symptoms that include recurrent fevers, joint pain, and fatigue

   A23.1   Brucellosis due to Brucella abortus
   Most common cause of brucellosis in humans; AKA Bang bacillus

   A23.2   Brucellosis due to Brucella suis
   Species found primarily in pigs, rabbits, and reindeer

   A23.3   Brucellosis due to Brucella canis
   Species that causes respiratory tract infection in humans

   A23.8   Other brucellosis 🦠
   (Ex:) A23.0-A23.9

   A23.9   Brucellosis, unspecified 🦠
   (Ex:) A23.0-A23.9

● **A24   Glanders and melioidosis**
   Infection, usually of rodents, which spreads to other animals and humans, caused by Burkholderia pseudomallei through break in skin contaminated with infested soil or water
   (Ex:) **For category A24 CC codes unless otherwise indicated: A24.1-A24.9**

   A24.0   Glanders 🦠
   Infection due to Pseudomonas mallei
   Malleus
   (Ex:) A24.0

   A24.1   Acute and fulminating melioidosis 🦠
   Melioidosis pneumonia
   Melioidosis sepsis

N Newborn Age: 0   **P** Pediatric Age: 0–17   **M** Maternity DX: 12–55   **A** Adult Age: 15–124   ♀ Females Only   ♂ Males Only

🦠 Complication\Comorbidity   🦠 Major C\C   (Ex:) CC/MCC Exclusions   🦠 Hospital-Acquired Condition

641

A24.2   **Subacute and chronic melioidosis** 🔖

A24.3   **Other melioidosis** 🔖

A24.9   **Melioidosis, unspecified** 🔖
     Infection due to Pseudomonas pseudomallei NOS
     Whitmore's disease

● A25   **Rat-bite fevers**
     RBF, infectious disease caused by Streptobacillus moniliformis or
     Spirillum minus.
     (Ex) **For category A25 CC codes:** A25.0-A25.9

     A25.0   **Spirillosis**
         Any disease condition caused by spirilla
         Sodoku

     A25.1   **Streptobacillosis** 🔖
         Acute, febrile human illness caused by bacteria transmitted
         by rats in most cases, passed from rodent to human via
         rodent's urine or mucous secretions; AKA rat fever
         Epidemic arthritic erythema
         Haverhill fever
         Streptobacillary rat-bite fever

     A25.9   **Rat-bite fever, unspecified** 🔖

● A26   **Erysipeloid**
     Infection with Erysipelothrix rhusiopathiae, *occurring often as*
     occupational disease resulting from handling infected fish,
     shellfish, meat, or poultry

     A26.0   **Cutaneous erysipeloid**
         Erythema migrans

     A26.7   **Erysipelothrix sepsis** 🔖
         MCC when PDx is its own MCC
         (Ex) A02.1, A20.7, A22.7, A32.7, A39.2-A39.4, A40.0-A40.1, A40.8-A41.9,
         A42.7, A48.2-A48.4, A48.8-A49.9, A54.86, B00.7, B3.77, B92,
         B94.2-B96.89, R65.10-R65.20, Z16.10-Z16.39

     A26.8   **Other forms of erysipeloid**

     A26.9   **Erysipeloid, unspecified**

● A27   **Leptospirosis**
     Occurs most commonly in the tropics
     (Ex) **For category A27 CC codes unless otherwise indicated:** A27.0-A27.9

     A27.0   **Leptospirosis icterohemorrhagica** 🔖
         Leptospiral or spirochetal jaundice (hemorrhagic)
         Weil's disease

     ● A27.8   **Other forms of leptospirosis**

         A27.81   **Aseptic meningitis in leptospirosis** 🔖
             (Ex) A02.21, A17.0-A17.1, A27.0-A27.9, A39.0, A50.41, A51.41,
             A52.13, A54.82, A54.84, A54.89-A54.9, A74.81-A74.9,
             A87.0-A87.9, A96.2, A98.3-A98.4, B26.1, B33.24, B33.4-B33.8,
             B34.1-B34.2, B34.4-B34.8, B37.5, B38.4, B45.1, B58.2, B92,
             B94.2-B94.9, B97.10, B97.19, B97.29, B97.5-B97.6,
             B97.81-B97.89, G00.0-G03.9, G04.2, G32.89, G61.0,
             G96.8-G96.9, G98.0-G98.8, G99.8

         A27.89   **Other forms of leptospirosis** 🔖

     A27.9   **Leptospirosis, unspecified** 🔖

● A28   **Other zoonotic bacterial diseases, not elsewhere classified**
     (Ex) **For category A28 CC codes unless otherwise indicated:** A26.0, A26.8-A26.9, A28.0,
     A28.2-A28.9, A32.0-A32.12, A32.81-A32.9

     A28.0   **Pasteurellosis** 🔖
         Infection of humans or other animals by species of
         Pasteurella

     A28.1   **Cat-scratch disease** 🔖
         Cat-scratch fever
         (Ex) A28.1, B97.21

     A28.2   **Extraintestinal yersiniosis** 🔖
         Infection from Yersinia enterocolitica; *AKA enteric*
         yersiniosis, intestinal yersiniosis, Yersinia enteritis

         Excludes1   enteritis due to Yersinia enterocolitica
                  (A04.6)
                  plague (A20.-)

     A28.8   **Other specified zoonotic bacterial diseases, not**
         elsewhere classified 🔖

     A28.9   **Zoonotic bacterial disease, unspecified** 🔖

OTHER BACTERIAL DISEASES (A30-A49)

● A30   **Leprosy [Hansen's disease]**
     Chronic infectious disease attacking the skin, peripheral nerves, and
     mucous membranes

     Includes   infection due to Mycobacterium leprae
     Excludes1   sequelae of leprosy (B92)

     A30.0   **Indeterminate leprosy** 🔖
         I leprosy
         (Ex) A30.0

     A30.1   **Tuberculoid leprosy** 🔖
         TT leprosy
         (Ex) A30.1

     A30.2   **Borderline tuberculoid leprosy** 🔖
         BT leprosy
         (Ex) A30.2-A30.4

     A30.3   **Borderline leprosy** 🔖
         BB leprosy
         (Ex) A30.2-A30.4

     A30.4   **Borderline lepromatous leprosy** 🔖
         BL leprosy
         (Ex) A30.2-A30.4

     A30.5   **Lepromatous leprosy** 🔖
         LL leprosy
         (Ex) A30.5

     A30.8   **Other forms of leprosy** 🔖
         (Ex) A30.8

     A30.9   **Leprosy, unspecified** 🔖
         (Ex) A30.9

● A31   **Infection due to other mycobacteria**
     Excludes2   leprosy (A30.-)
                tuberculosis (A15-A19)
     (Ex) **For category A31 CC codes unless otherwise indicated:** A31.0-A31.9

     A31.0   **Pulmonary mycobacterial infection** 🔖
         Infection due to Mycobacterium avium
         Infection due to Mycobacterium intracellulare [Battey
         bacillus]
         Infection due to Mycobacterium kansasii
         (Ex) A15.0-A15.9, A17.9, A18.82, A18.84, A18.89, A22.1, A31.0, A31.2-A31.9,
         A37.01, A37.11, A37.81, A37.91, A48.1, A49.3-A49.9, B25.0, B44.0, B90.0,
         B92, B94.2-B94.9, B96.0, B96.6-B96.89, J09.X1-J09.X2, J10.00-J10.1,
         J11.00-J11.1, J12.0-J12.3, J12.89-J18.1, J18.8-J18.9, J44.9, J47.0-J70.4,
         J70.8-J70.9, J98.4, R91.1

     A31.1   **Cutaneous mycobacterial infection** 🔖
         Buruli ulcer
         Infection due to Mycobacterium marinum
         Infection due to Mycobacterium ulcerans

     A31.2   **Disseminated mycobacterium avium-intracellulare**
         complex (DMAC) 🔖
         MAC sepsis

     A31.8   **Other mycobacterial infections** 🔖

     A31.9   **Mycobacterial infection, unspecified** 🔖
         Atypical mycobacterial infection NOS
         Mycobacteriosis NOS

● A32   **Listeriosis**
     Infection caused by Listeria monocytogenes
     Includes   listerial foodborne infection
     Excludes1   neonatal (disseminated) listeriosis (P37.2)
     (Ex) **For category A32 CC codes unless otherwise indicated:** A26.0, A26.8-A26.9, A28.0,
     A28.2-A28.9, A32.0-A32.12, A32.81-A32.9

     A32.0   **Cutaneous listeriosis** 🔖

     ● A32.1   **Listerial meningitis and meningoencephalitis**

         A32.11   **Listerial meningitis**

         A32.12   **Listerial meningoencephalitis** 🔖

◀ New   ◀ Revised   ~~deleted~~ Deleted   Excludes 1   Excludes 2   Includes   Use additional   Code first   Code also   Unspecified

OGCR Official Guidelines   ● Unacceptable Principal Diagnosis   X Assign placeholder X   ● Use Additional Character(s)   ▶ Manifestation Code   **Coding Clinic**

A32.7　Listerial sepsis
　　MCC when PDx is its own MCC
　　Ex See A26.7

● **A32.8　Other forms of listeriosis**
　A32.81　Oculoglandular listeriosis
　　Primary infection site is conjunctival sac, which if untreated may result in perforation of cornea and optic atrophy
　A32.82　Listerial endocarditis
　　Exudative and proliferative inflammatory condition of endocardium caused by listeria bacteria
　A32.89　Other forms of listeriosis
　　Listerial cerebral arteritis

A32.9　Listeriosis, unspecified

A33　Tetanus neonatorum　　　　　　　　　　　　　　　**N**
　　Neonate = newborn
　　Ex A33, P29.0-P29.2, P29.4, P29.89-P29.9, P94.1-P94.9, P96.0, P96.3-P96.5, P96.82-P96.89

A34　Obstetrical tetanus ♀　　　　　　　　　　　　　**M**
　　Ex A34, O08.0, O08.2-O08.9, O11.4, O11.5, O12.04, O12.05, O12.14, O12.15, O12.24, O12.25, O13.4, O13.5, O14.04, O14.05, O14.14, O14.15, O14.24, O14.25, O14.94, O14.95, O16.4, O16.5, O20.0-O20.9, O25.10-O25.3, O26.10-O26.13, O26.30-O26.43, O26.63-O26.819, O26.841-O26.86, O26.891-O26.93, O29.011-O29.93, O35.7XX0-O35.7XX9, O44.00-O44.13, O44.20-O44.53, O45.8X1-O45.93, O75.4, O75.81, O75.89-O75.9, O80, O90.89, O99.111-O99.285, O99.330-O99.335, O99.350-O99.355, O99.511-O99.73, O99.820-O99.825, O99.840-O9A.53

A35　Other tetanus
　　Tetanus NOS
　　Excludes1　　tetanus neonatorum (A33)
　　　　　　　　　　obstetrical tetanus (A34)
　　Ex A35, B92, B94.2-B94.9

● **A36　Diphtheria**
　　Ex For category A36 CC codes unless otherwise indicated: A36.0-A36.9
　A36.0　Pharyngeal diphtheria
　　Diphtheritic membranous angina
　　Tonsillar diphtheria
　A36.1　Nasopharyngeal diphtheria
　A36.2　Laryngeal diphtheria
　　Diphtheritic laryngotracheitis
　A36.3　Cutaneous diphtheria
　　Excludes2　　erythrasma (L08.1)
　● **A36.8　Other diphtheria**
　　A36.81　Diphtheritic cardiomyopathy
　　　Diphtheritic myocarditis
　　　Ex A36.81, A52.06, B33.20-B33.22, I00, I01.2-I01.9, I09.0, I09.9, I23.0-I23.3, I23.6-I23.8, I40.0-I41, I51.0, I51.4, I87.8-I87.9, I99.8-I99.9
　　A36.82　Diphtheritic radiculomyelitis
　　A36.83　Diphtheritic polyneuritis
　　A36.84　Diphtheritic tubulo-interstitial nephropathy
　　A36.85　Diphtheritic cystitis
　　A36.86　Diphtheritic conjunctivitis
　　A36.89　Other diphtheritic complications
　　　Diphtheritic peritonitis
　A36.9　Diphtheria, unspecified

● **A37　Whooping cough**
　　Pertussis is a highly contagious disease caused by the bacterium Bordetella pertussis and results in a whooping sounding cough.
　　Ex For category A37 CC codes A37.00, A37.10, A37.80, A37.90: A37.00-A37.91
　　For category A37 CC codes A37.01, A37.11, A37.81, A37.91: A15.0-A15.9, A17.9, A18.82, A18.84, A18.89, A21.2, A22.1, A31.0, A37.00-A37.91, A42.0, A43.0, A48.1, B25.0, B39.0-B39.2, B44.0, B58.3, B59, B67.1, J09.X1-J09.X2, J10.00-J10.1, J11.00-J11.1, J12.0-J12.3, J12.89-J18.1, J18.8-J18.9, J22, J44.9, J47.0-J70.4, J70.8-J70.9, J98.4, J98.8-J98.9, Q33.4, R91.1
　● **A37.0　Whooping cough due to Bordetella pertussis**
　　A37.00　Whooping cough due to Bordetella pertussis without pneumonia
　　A37.01　Whooping cough due to Bordetella pertussis with pneumonia
　　　MCC when PDx is its own MCC
　● **A37.1　Whooping cough due to Bordetella parapertussis**
　　A37.10　Whooping cough due to Bordetella parapertussis without pneumonia
　　A37.11　Whooping cough due to Bordetella parapertussis with pneumonia
　　　MCC when PDx is its own MCC
　● **A37.8　Whooping cough due to other Bordetella species**
　　A37.80　Whooping cough due to other Bordetella species without pneumonia
　　A37.81　Whooping cough due to other Bordetella species with pneumonia
　　　MCC when PDx is its own MCC
　● **A37.9　Whooping cough, unspecified species**
　　A37.90　Whooping cough, unspecified species without pneumonia
　　A37.91　Whooping cough, unspecified species with pneumonia
　　　MCC when PDx is its own MCC

● **A38　Scarlet fever**
　　Most commonly caused by the bacteria Streptococcus pneumoniae and Neisseria meningitides
　　Includes　　scarlatina
　　Excludes2　　streptococcal sore throat (J02.0)
　　Ex For category A38 CC codes: A38.0-A38.9, A46, J02.0, J03.00-J03.01
　A38.0　Scarlet fever with otitis media
　A38.1　Scarlet fever with myocarditis
　A38.8　Scarlet fever with other complications
　A38.9　Scarlet fever, uncomplicated
　　Scarlet fever, NOS

● **A39　Meningococcal infection**
　　Most commonly caused by the bacteria Streptococcus pneumoniae and Neisseria meningitides
　A39.0　Meningococcal meningitis
　　Ex A02.21, A17.0-A17.1, A27.81, A39.0, A39.89-A39.9, A49.3-A49.9, A50.41, A51.41, A52.13, A54.82, A54.84, A54.89-A54.9, A87.0-A87.9, B00.3, B02.1, B26.1, B37.5, B38.4, B45.1, B58.2, B92, B94.2-B94.9, B96.0, B96.6-B96.89, G00.0-G03.9, G04.2, G32.89, G61.0, G96.8-G96.9, G98.0-G98.8, G99.8
　A39.1　Waterhouse-Friderichsen syndrome
　　Fulminating complication of meningococcemia
　　Meningococcal hemorrhagic adrenalitis
　　Meningococcic adrenal syndrome
　　Ex A39.1, A39.89-A39.9, A49.3-A49.9, B92, B94.2-B94.9, B96.0, B96.6-B96.89
　A39.2　Acute meningococcemia
　　Ex A02.1, A20.7, A22.7, A26.7, A32.7, A39.2-A39.4, A39.89-A41.9, A42.7, A49.3-A49.9, A54.86, B00.7, B37.7, B92, B94.2-B94.9, B96.0, B96.6-B96.89, R65.10-R65.20
　A39.3　Chronic meningococcemia
　　Ex See A39.2

CHAPTER 1 (A00-B99)

N Newborn Age: 0　　**P** Pediatric Age: 0–17　　**M** Maternity DX: 12–55　　**A** Adult Age: 15–124　　**♀** Females Only　　**♂** Males Only
　　Complication\Comorbidity　　　Major C\C　　Ex CC/MCC Exclusions　　Hospital-Acquired Condition

A39.4   Meningococcemia, unspecified 🔊
      Ex: See A39.2

● **A39.5**   Meningococcal heart disease

    A39.50   Meningococcal carditis, unspecified 🔊
        Ex: A39.50, A39.89-A39.9, A49.3-A49.9, B92, B94.2-B94.9, B96.0, B96.6-B96.89

    A39.51   Meningococcal endocarditis 🔊
        Ex: A39.51, A39.89-A39.9, A49.3-A49.9, B92, B94.2-B94.9, B96.0, B96.6-B96.89

    A39.52   Meningococcal myocarditis 🔊
        Ex: A39.52, A49.3-A49.9, B92, B94.2-B94.9, B96.0, B96.6-B96.89

    A39.53   Meningococcal pericarditis 🔊
        Ex: A39.53, A39.89-A39.9, A49.3-A49.9, B92, B94.2-B94.9, B96.0, B96.6-B96.89

● **A39.8**   Other meningococcal infections

    A39.81   Meningococcal encephalitis 🔊
        Ex: A39.81, A39.89-A39.9, A49.3-A49.9, B92, B94.2-B94.9, B96.0, B96.6-B96.89

    A39.82   Meningococcal retrobulbar neuritis 🔊
        Optic neuritis in portion of optic nerve posterior to eyeball; AKA postocular optic neuritis
        Ex: A39.82, A39.89-A39.9, A49.3-A49.9, B92, B94.2-B94.9, B96.0, B96.6-B96.89

    A39.83   Meningococcal arthritis 🔊
        Ex: A39.83-A39.9, A49.3-A49.9, B92, B94.2-B94.9, B96.0, B96.6-B96.89

    A39.84   Postmeningococcal arthritis 🔊
        Ex: See A39.83

    A39.89   Other meningococcal infections 🔊
        Meningococcal conjunctivitis
        Ex: A39.89-A39.9, A49.3-A49.9, B92, B94.2-B94.9, B96.0, B96.6-B96.89

A39.9   Meningococcal infection, unspecified 🔊
      Meningococcal disease NOS
      Ex: See A39.89

● **A40**   Streptococcal sepsis

    Code first
      postprocedural streptococcal sepsis (T81.4-) ◀▦
      streptococcal sepsis during labor (O75.3)
      streptococcal sepsis following abortion or ectopic or molar pregnancy (O03-O07, O08.0)
      streptococcal sepsis following immunization (T88.0)
      streptococcal sepsis following infusion, transfusion or therapeutic injection (T80.2-)

    Excludes1   neonatal (P36.0-P36.1)
                 puerperal sepsis (O85)
                 sepsis due to Streptococcus, group D (A41.81)

    Ex: **For category A40 CC codes unless otherwise indicated:** A02.1, A20.7, A22.7, A26.7, A32.7, A39.2-A39.4, A40.0-A40.1, A40.8-A41.9, A42.7, A48.2-A48.4, A48.8-A49.9, A54.86, B00.7, B3.77, B92, B94.2-B96.89, R65.10-R65.20, Z16.10-Z16.39

A40.0   Sepsis due to streptococcus, group A 🔊
A40.1   Sepsis due to streptococcus, group B 🔊
A40.3   Sepsis due to Streptococcus pneumoniae 🔊
      Pneumococcal sepsis
      Ex: No exclusions
A40.8   Other streptococcal sepsis 🔊
A40.9   Streptococcal sepsis, unspecified 🔊

● **A41**   Other sepsis

    Code first
      postprocedural sepsis (T81.4-) ◀▦
      sepsis during labor (O75.3)
      sepsis following abortion, ectopic or molar pregnancy (O03-O07, O08.0)
      sepsis following immunization (T88.0)
      sepsis following infusion, transfusion or therapeutic injection (T80.2-)

    Excludes1   bacteremia NOS (R78.81)
                 neonatal (P36.-)
                 puerperal sepsis (O85)
                 ~~sepsis NOS (A41.9)~~
                 streptococcal sepsis (A40.-)

    Excludes2   sepsis (due to) (in) actinomycotic (A42.7)
                 sepsis (due to) (in) anthrax (A22.7)
                 sepsis (due to) (in) candidal (B37.7)
                 sepsis (due to) (in) Erysipelothrix (A26.7)
                 sepsis (due to) (in) extraintestinal yersiniosis (A28.2)
                 sepsis (due to) (in) gonococcal (A54.86)
                 sepsis (due to) (in) herpesviral (B00.7)
                 sepsis (due to) (in) listerial (A32.7)
                 sepsis (due to) (in) melioidosis (A24.1)
                 sepsis (due to) (in) meningococcal (A39.2-A39.4)
                 sepsis (due to) (in) plague (A20.7)
                 sepsis (due to) (in) tularemia (A21.7)
                 toxic shock syndrome (A48.3)

    Ex: **For category A41 CC codes:** A02.1, A20.7, A22.7, A26.7, A32.7, A39.2-A39.4, A40.0-A40.1, A40.8-A41.9, A42.7, A48.2-A48.4, A48.8-A49.9, A54.86, B00.7, B3.77, B92, B94.2-B96.89, R65.10-R65.20, Z16.10-Z16.39

    Coding Clinic: 2016, Q1, P39

● **A41.0**   Sepsis due to Staphylococcus aureus

    A41.01   Sepsis due to Methicillin susceptible Staphylococcus aureus 🔊
        MSSA sepsis
        Staphylococcus aureus sepsis NOS

    A41.02   Sepsis due to Methicillin resistant Staphylococcus aureus 🔊

A41.1   Sepsis due to other specified staphylococcus 🔊
      Coagulase negative staphylococcus sepsis
A41.2   Sepsis due to unspecified staphylococcus 🔊
A41.3   Sepsis due to Hemophilus influenzae 🔊
A41.4   Sepsis due to anaerobes 🔊
    Excludes1   gas gangrene (A48.0)

● **A41.5**   Sepsis due to other Gram-negative organisms

    A41.50   Gram-negative sepsis, unspecified 🔊
        Gram-negative sepsis NOS

    A41.51   Sepsis due to Escherichia coli [E. coli] 🔊

    A41.52   Sepsis due to Pseudomonas 🔊
        Pseudomonas aeroginosa

    A41.53   Sepsis due to Serratia 🔊

    A41.59   Other Gram-negative sepsis 🔊

● **A41.8**   Other specified sepsis

    A41.81   Sepsis due to Enterococcus 🔊

    A41.89   Other specified sepsis 🔊

A41.9   Sepsis, unspecified organism 🔊
      Septicemia NOS

◀ New   ◀▦ Revised   ~~deleted~~ Deleted   Excludes 1   Excludes 2   Includes   Use additional   Code first   Code also   Unspecified

OGCR Official Guidelines   ● Unacceptable Principal Diagnosis   X Assign placeholder X   🔊 Use Additional Character(s)   ▶ Manifestation Code   **Coding Clinic**

● **A42 Actinomycosis**

　　Excludes1   actinomycetoma (B47.1)

　　A42.0 Pulmonary actinomycosis 🦠
　　　　(Ex:) A42.0, A42.81-A43.0, A43.8-A43.9, B47.1, J12.81

　　A42.1 Abdominal actinomycosis 🦠
　　　　(Ex:) A42.1, A42.81-A42.9, A43.8-A43.9, B47.1

　　A42.2 Cervicofacial actinomycosis 🦠
　　　　(Ex:) A42.2, A42.81-A42.9, A43.8-A43.9, B47.1

　　A42.7 Actinomycotic sepsis 🦠
　　　　(Ex:) See A26.7

● 　**A42.8 Other forms of actinomycosis**
　　　　(Ex:) **For category A42.8 CC codes:** A42.0-A42.2, A42.81-A43.9, B47.1-B47.9, L08.1

　　　　A42.81 Actinomycotic meningitis 🦠
　　　　A42.82 Actinomycotic encephalitis 🦠
　　　　A42.89 Other forms of actinomycosis 🦠

　　A42.9 Actinomycosis, unspecified 🦠
　　　　(Ex:) A42.0-A42.2, A42.81-A43.9, B47.1-B47.9, L08.1

● **A43 Nocardiosis**

　　A43.0 Pulmonary nocardiosis 🦠
　　　　(Ex:) See A42.0

　　A43.1 Cutaneous nocardiosis 🦠
　　　　(Ex:) A42.81-A42.9, A43.1-A43.9, B47.1, L08.1

　　A43.8 Other forms of nocardiosis
　　　　(Ex:) See A42.9

　　A43.9 Nocardiosis, unspecified 🦠
　　　　(Ex:) See A42.9

● **A44 Bartonellosis**
　　　　(Ex:) **For category A44 CC codes:** A44.0-A44.9, A68.0-A68.9, A69.20-A69.29, A75.0-A79.9, B55.0-B57.5, B60.0

　　A44.0 Systemic bartonellosis 🦠
　　　　Oroya fever

　　A44.1 Cutaneous and mucocutaneous bartonellosis 🦠
　　　　Verruga peruana

　　A44.8 Other forms of bartonellosis 🦠

　　A44.9 Bartonellosis, unspecified 🦠

A46 Erysipelas

　　Excludes1   postpartum or puerperal erysipelas (O86.89)

● **A48 Other bacterial diseases, not elsewhere classified**

　　Excludes1   actinomycetoma (B47.1)

　　A48.0 Gas gangrene 🦠
　　　　Clostridial cellulitis
　　　　Clostridial myonecrosis
　　　　(Ex:) A48.0, B92, B94.2-B94.9

　　A48.1 Legionnaires' disease 🦠
　　　　(Ex:) A15.0-A15.9, A17.9, A18.82, A18.84, A18.89, A21.2, A22.1, A31.0, A37.01, A37.11, A37.81, A37.91, A42.0, A43.0, A48.1, B25.0, B39.0-B39.2, B44.0, B58.3, B59, B67.1, J09.X1-J09.X2, J10.00-J10.1, J11.00-J11.1, J12.0-J12.3, J12.89-J18.1, J18.8-J18.9, J22, J44.9, J47.0-J70.4, J70.8-J70.9, J98.4, J98.8-J98.9, Q33.4, R91.1

　　A48.2 Nonpneumonic Legionnaires' disease [Pontiac fever]

　　A48.3 Toxic shock syndrome 🦠
　　　　Use additional code to identify the organism (B95, B96)
　　　　Excludes1   endotoxic shock NOS (R57.8)
　　　　　　　sepsis NOS (A41.9)
　　　　(Ex:) A48.3, G89.0-G89.4, R09.89, R29.700-R29.742, R41.0-R41.3, R41.82, R41.9, R44.8-R44.9, R45.83-R45.84, R46.0-R46.89, R52,R57.0-R57.9, R65.21, R68.0-R68.19, R68.81-R68.89, R69

　　A48.4 Brazilian purpuric fever
　　　　Systemic Hemophilus aegyptius infection

Item 1–8 Gas gangrene is a necrotizing subcutaneous infection that will cause tissue death. Patients with poor circulation (e.g., diabetes, peripheral nephropathy) will have low oxygen content in their tissues (hypoxia), which allows the Clostridium bacteria to flourish. Gas gangrene often occurs at the site of a surgical wound or trauma. Onset is sudden and dramatic. Treatment can include debridement, amputation, and/or hyperbaric oxygen treatments.

● 　**A48.5 Other specified botulism**
　　　　Non-foodborne intoxication due to toxins of Clostridium botulinum [C. botulinum]
　　　　Excludes1   food poisoning due to toxins of Clostridium botulinum (A05.1)

　　　　A48.51 Infant botulism 🦠　　　　　　　　P
　　　　　　(Ex:) A04.7, A05.0-A05.2, A48.51-A48.52

　　　　A48.52 Wound botulism 🦠
　　　　　　Non-foodborne botulism NOS
　　　　　　Use additional code for associated wound
　　　　　　(Ex:) A04.7, A05.0-A05.2, A48.51-A48.52

　　A48.8 Other specified bacterial diseases

● **A49 Bacterial infection of unspecified site**

　　Excludes1   bacterial agents as the cause of diseases classified elsewhere (B95-B96)
　　　　　　chlamydial infection NOS (A74.9)
　　　　　　meningococcal infection NOS (A39.9)
　　　　　　rickettsial infection NOS (A79.9)
　　　　　　spirochetal infection NOS (A69.9)

● 　**A49.0 Staphylococcal infection, unspecified site**

　　　　A49.01 Methicillin susceptible Staphylococcus aureus infection, unspecified site
　　　　　　Methicillin susceptible Staphylococcus aureus (MSSA) infection
　　　　　　Staphylococcus aureus infection NOS

　　　　A49.02 Methicillin resistant Staphylococcus aureus infection, unspecified site
　　　　　　Methicillin resistant Staphylococcus aureus (MRSA) infection

　　A49.1 Streptococcal infection, unspecified site

　　A49.2 Hemophilus influenzae infection, unspecified site
　　　　Any of seven bacterium of genus Haemophilus

　　A49.3 Mycoplasma infection, unspecified site
　　　　Bacterium of class Mollicutes, unusual group of bacteria distinguished by absence of cell wall

　　A49.8 Other bacterial infections of unspecified site

　　A49.9 Bacterial infection, unspecified
　　　　Excludes1   bacteremia NOS (R78.81)

INFECTIONS WITH A PREDOMINANTLY SEXUAL MODE OF TRANSMISSION (A50-A64)

　　Excludes1   human immunodeficiency virus [HIV] disease (B20)
　　　　　　nonspecific and nongonococcal urethritis (N34.1)
　　　　　　Reiter's disease (M02.3-)

● **A50 Congenital syphilis**

● 　**A50.0 Early congenital syphilis, symptomatic**
　　　　Any congenital syphilitic condition specified as early or manifest less than two years after birth
　　　　(Ex:) **For category A50.0 CC codes:** A50.01-A51.46, A51.5-A53.9

　　　　A50.01 Early congenital syphilitic oculopathy 🦠

　　　　A50.02 Early congenital syphilitic osteochondropathy 🦠

　　　　A50.03 Early congenital syphilitic pharyngitis 🦠
　　　　　　Early congenital syphilitic laryngitis

　　　　A50.04 Early congenital syphilitic pneumonia 🦠

　　　　A50.05 Early congenital syphilitic rhinitis 🦠

　　　　A50.06 Early cutaneous congenital syphilis 🦠

　　　　A50.07 Early mucocutaneous congenital syphilis 🦠

　　　　A50.08 Early visceral congenital syphilis 🦠

　　　　A50.09 Other early congenital syphilis, symptomatic 🦠

N Newborn Age: 0   **P** Pediatric Age: 0–17   **M** Maternity DX: 12–55   **A** Adult Age: 15–124   ♀ Females Only   ♂ Males Only

🦠 Complication\Comorbidity   🦠 Major C\C   (Ex:) CC/MCC Exclusions   🦠 Hospital-Acquired Condition

CHAPTER 1 (A00-B99)

645

Figure 1-3 Chancre of primary syphilis. (From Mandell, Bennett, & Dolin: Principles and Practice of Infectious Diseases, ed 7, Churchill Livingstone, An Imprint of Elsevier, 2009)

Item 1–9 Syphilis, also known as lues, is the most serious of the venereal diseases caused by *Treponema pallidum*. The **primary** stage is characterized by an ulceration known as **chancre,** which usually appears on the genitals but can also develop on the anus, lips, tonsils, breasts, or fingers. Syphilis is easy to cure in its early stages. A single intramuscular injection of penicillin will usually cure a person who has had syphilis for less than a year.

    The **secondary** stage is characterized by a rash that can affect any area of the body. **Latent** syphilis is divided into **early,** which is diagnosed within two years of infection, and **late,** which is diagnosed two years or more after infection. Additional doses of penicillin or another antibiotic are needed to treat someone who has had syphilis for longer than a year. For those allergic to penicillin, there are other antibiotic treatments. **Congenital** syphilis is also labeled **early** or **late** based on the time of diagnosis.

A50.1   Early congenital syphilis, latent
      Congenital syphilis without clinical manifestations, with positive serological reaction and negative spinal fluid test, less than two years after birth

A50.2   Early congenital syphilis, unspecified
      Congenital syphilis NOS less than two years after birth
      Ex: A50.01-A51.46, A51.5-A54.85, A54.89-A58, A63.8, A64, B92, B94.2-B94.9, M02.30-M02.39, N34.1

● A50.3   Late congenital syphilitic oculopathy
      Excludes1   Hutchinson's triad (A50.53)
      Ex: For category A50.3 CC codes: A50.01-A51.46, A51.5-A53.9

    A50.30   Late congenital syphilitic oculopathy, unspecified
    A50.31   Late congenital syphilitic interstitial keratitis
    A50.32   Late congenital syphilitic chorioretinitis
    A50.39   Other late congenital syphilitic oculopathy

● A50.4   Late congenital neurosyphilis [juvenile neurosyphilis]
      Use additional code to identify any associated mental disorder
      Excludes1   Hutchinson's triad (A50.53)
      Ex: For category A50.4 CC codes unless otherwise indicated: A50.01-A51.46, A51.5-A53.9, A56.00-A56.8, A63.8-A64, B92, B94.2-B94.9, N34.1

    A50.40   Late congenital neurosyphilis, unspecified
      Juvenile neurosyphilis NOS
    A50.41   Late congenital syphilitic meningitis
      Ex: A02.21, A17.0-A17.1, A27.81, A39.0, A50.01-A51.46, A51.5-A53.9, A54.82, A54.84, A54.89-A54.9, A56.00-A56.8, A63.8-A64, A87.0-A87.9, B00.3, B02.1, B26.1, B37.5, B38.4, B45.1, B58.2, B92, B94.2-B94.9, G00.0-G03.9, G04.2, G32.89, G61.0, G96.8-G96.9, G98.0-G98.8, G99.8, N34.1
    A50.42   Late congenital syphilitic encephalitis
    A50.43   Late congenital syphilitic polyneuropathy
    A50.44   Late congenital syphilitic optic nerve atrophy
      Ex: A50.01-A51.46, A51.5-A53.9
    A50.45   Juvenile general paresis
      Dementia paralytica juvenilis
      Juvenile tabetoparetic neurosyphilis
    A50.49   Other late congenital neurosyphilis
      Juvenile tabes dorsalis

● A50.5   Other late congenital syphilis, symptomatic
      Any congenital syphilitic condition specified as late or manifest two years or more after birth
      Ex: For category A50.5 CC codes: A50.01-A51.46, A51.5-A53.9

    A50.51   Clutton's joints
    A50.52   Hutchinson's teeth
    A50.53   Hutchinson's triad
    A50.54   Late congenital cardiovascular syphilis
    A50.55   Late congenital syphilitic arthropathy
    A50.56   Late congenital syphilitic osteochondropathy
    A50.57   Syphilitic saddle nose
    A50.59   Other late congenital syphilis, symptomatic

A50.6   Late congenital syphilis, latent
      Congenital syphilis without clinical manifestations, with positive serological reaction and negative spinal fluid test, two years or more after birth.

A50.7   Late congenital syphilis, unspecified
      Congenital syphilis NOS two years or more after birth.

A50.9   Congenital syphilis, unspecified

● A51   Early syphilis

A51.0   Primary genital syphilis
      Syphilitic chancre NOS

A51.1   Primary anal syphilis

A51.2   Primary syphilis of other sites

● A51.3   Secondary syphilis of skin and mucous membranes

    A51.31   Condyloma latum
      Ex: A50.01-A51.46, A51.5-A53.9
    A51.32   Syphilitic alopecia
      Ex: A50.01-A51.46, A51.5-A54.85, A54.89-A58, A63.8, A64, M02.30-M02.39, N34.1
    A51.39   Other secondary syphilis of skin
      Syphilitic leukoderma
      Syphilitic mucous patch
      Excludes1   late syphilitic leukoderma (A52.79)
      Ex: A50.01-A51.46, A51.5-A53.9

● A51.4   Other secondary syphilis

    A51.41   Secondary syphilitic meningitis
      Ex: A02.21, A17.0-A17.1, A27.81, A39.0, A50.01-A51.46, A51.5-A54.49, A54.5-A54.85, A54.89-A58, A63.8-A64, A74.81-A74.9, A87.0-A87.9, A96.2, A98.3-A98.4, B26.1, B33.24, B33.4-B33.8, B34.1-B34.2, B34.4-B34.8, B37.5, B38.4, B45.1, B58.2, B92, B94.2-B94.9, B97.10, B97.19, B97.29, B97.5-B97.6, B97.81-B97.89, G00.0-G03.9, G04.2, G32.89, G61.0, G96.8-G96.9, G98.0-G98.8, G99.8, M02.30-M02.39, N34.1
    A51.42   Secondary syphilitic female pelvic disease ♀
      Ex: See A50.2
    A51.43   Secondary syphilitic oculopathy
      Secondary syphilitic chorioretinitis
      Secondary syphilitic iridocyclitis, iritis
      Secondary syphilitic uveitis
      Ex: See A50.01-A51.46, A51.5-A53.9
    A51.44   Secondary syphilitic nephritis
      Ex: See A50.2
    A51.45   Secondary syphilitic hepatitis
      Ex: A50.01-A51.46, A51.5-A54.85, A54.89-A58, A63.8, A64, K71.0-K71.9, K73.1-K73.8, K74.0-K74.69, K75.2-K76.0, K76.4-K76.5, K76.89-K76.9, M02.30-M02.39, N34.1

◄ New   ◄■■ Revised   ~~deleted~~ Deleted   Excludes 1   Excludes 2   Includes   Use additional   Code first   Code also   Unspecified

OGCR Official Guidelines   ● Unacceptable Principal Diagnosis   **X** Assign placeholder X   ● Use Additional Character(s)   ▌ Manifestation Code   **Coding Clinic**

A51.46   **Secondary syphilitic osteopathy** 🔖
  (Ex:) A18.09, A50.01-A51.46, A51.5-A54.85, A54.89-A58, A63.8, A64,
  A66.6, M02.30-M02.39,M84.80-M84.9, M85.10-M85.19,
  M85.80-M85.89, M86.30-M86.8X9, M89.20-M89.39,
  M89.50-M89.59, M89.8X0-M89.8X9, M94.1,
  M94.351-M94.8X9, N34.1

A51.49   **Other secondary syphilitic conditions** 🔖
  Secondary syphilitic lymphadenopathy
  Secondary syphilitic myositis

A51.5   **Early syphilis, latent**
  Syphilis (acquired) without clinical manifestations, with
  positive serological reaction and negative spinal
  fluid test, less than two years after infection.

A51.9   **Early syphilis, unspecified**

● A52   **Late syphilis**

  ● A52.0   **Cardiovascular and cerebrovascular syphilis**
    (Ex:) **For category A52.0 CC codes:** A50.01-A51.46, A51.5-A53.9, A56.00-A56.8,
    A63.8-A64, B92, B94.2-B94.9, N34.1

  A52.00   **Cardiovascular syphilis, unspecified** 🔖

  A52.01   **Syphilitic aneurysm of aorta** 🔖

  A52.02   **Syphilitic aortitis** 🔖

  A52.03   **Syphilitic endocarditis** 🔖
    Syphilitic aortic valve incompetence or stenosis
    Syphilitic mitral valve stenosis
    Syphilitic pulmonary valve regurgitation

  A52.04   **Syphilitic cerebral arteritis** 🔖

  A52.05   **Other cerebrovascular syphilis** 🔖
    Syphilitic cerebral aneurysm (ruptured) (non-
    ruptured)
    Syphilitic cerebral thrombosis

  A52.06   **Other syphilitic heart involvement** 🔖
    Syphilitic coronary artery disease
    Syphilitic myocarditis
    Syphilitic pericarditis

  A52.09   **Other cardiovascular syphilis** 🔖

  ● A52.1   **Symptomatic neurosyphilis**
    (Ex:) **For category A52.1 CC codes unless otherwise indicated:** A50.01-A51.46,
    A51.5-A53.9, A56.00-A56.8, A63.8-A64, B92, B94.2-B94.9, N34.1

  A52.10   **Symptomatic neurosyphilis, unspecified** 🔖

  A52.11   **Tabes dorsalis** 🔖
    *Cognitive decline with progressive degeneration of
    posterior columns, roots, and ganglia of spinal
    cord, occur 15-20 years after initial infection
    of syphilis; AKA Duchenne disease*
    Locomotor ataxia (progressive)
    Tabetic neurosyphilis

  A52.12   **Other cerebrospinal syphilis** 🔖

  A52.13   **Late syphilitic meningitis** 🔖
    (Ex:) See A50.41

  A52.14   **Late syphilitic encephalitis** 🔖

  A52.15   **Late syphilitic neuropathy** 🔖
    Late syphilitic acoustic neuritis
    Late syphilitic optic (nerve) atrophy
    Late syphilitic polyneuropathy
    Late syphilitic retrobulbar neuritis

  A52.16   **Charcôt's arthropathy (tabetic)** 🔖
    *Progressive musculoskeletal condition characterized
    by joint dislocation, fractures, and deformities,
    results in progressive destruction of bone and
    soft tissue of weight-bearing joints*

A52.17   **General paresis** 🔖
  *Chronic meningoencephalitis results in loss of
  cortical function, or progressive dementia
  and generalized paralysis, occurring 10-20
  years after initial infection of syphilis; AKA
  Bayle disease, dementia paralytica, paralytic
  dementiaparetic neurosyphilis, syphilitic
  meningoencephalitis*
  Dementia paralytica

A52.19   **Other symptomatic neurosyphilis** 🔖
  Syphilitic parkinsonism

A52.2   **Asymptomatic neurosyphilis** 🔖
  (Ex:) See A52.10

A52.3   **Neurosyphilis, unspecified** 🔖
  Gumma (syphilitic)
  Destructive lesions of syphilis
  Syphilis (late)
  Syphiloma
  (Ex:) See A52.10

● A52.7   **Other symptomatic late syphilis** 🔖
  (Ex:) **For category A52.7 CC codes unless otherwise indicated:** A50.01-A51.46,
  A51.5-A54.85, A54.89-A58, A63.8, A64, M02.30-M02.39, N34.1

  A52.71   **Late syphilitic oculopathy** 🔖
    Late syphilitic chorioretinitis
    Late syphilitic episcleritis
    (Ex:) A18.50-A18.59, A50.001-A51.46, A51.5-A54.85, A54.89-A58,
    A63.8-A64, H15.001-H15.009, H15.091-H15.129,
    M02.30-M02.39, N34.1

  A52.72   **Syphilis of lung and bronchus** 🔖

  A52.73   **Symptomatic late syphilis of other respiratory
    organs** 🔖

  A52.74   **Syphilis of liver and other viscera** 🔖
    Late syphilitic peritonitis

  A52.75   **Syphilis of kidney and ureter** 🔖
    Syphilitic glomerular disease

  A52.76   **Other genitourinary symptomatic late
    syphilis** 🔖
    Late syphilitic female pelvic inflammatory
    disease

  A52.77   **Syphilis of bone and joint** 🔖

  A52.78   **Syphilis of other musculoskeletal tissue** 🔖
    Late syphilitic bursitis
    Syphilis [stage unspecified] of bursa
    Syphilis [stage unspecified] of muscle
    Syphilis [stage unspecified] of synovium
    Syphilis [stage unspecified] of tendon

  A52.79   **Other symptomatic late syphilis** 🔖
    Late syphilitic leukoderma
    Syphilis of adrenal gland
    Syphilis of pituitary gland
    Syphilis of thyroid gland
    Syphilitic splenomegaly
    Excludes1   syphilitic leukoderma
      (secondary) (A51.39)

A52.8   **Late syphilis, latent**
  Syphilis (acquired) without clinical manifestations, with
  positive serological reaction and negative spinal
  fluid test, two years or more after infection

A52.9   **Late syphilis, unspecified**

CHAPTER 1 (A00-B99)

CHAPTER 1 (A00-B99)

● **A53   Other and unspecified syphilis**

  A53.0   Latent syphilis, unspecified as early or late
      Latent syphilis NOS
      Positive serological reaction for syphilis

  A53.9   Syphilis, unspecified
      Infection due to Treponema pallidum NOS
      Syphilis (acquired) NOS

      Excludes1   syphilis NOS under two years of age
                      (A50.2)

● **A54   Gonococcal infection**

  ● **A54.0   Gonococcal infection of lower genitourinary tract
             without periurethral or accessory gland abscess**

      Excludes1   gonococcal infection with genitourinary
                      gland abscess (A54.1)
                      gonococcal infection with periurethral
                      abscess (A54.1)

      Ex: **For category A54.0 CC codes:** A54.00-A54.29, A54.82, A54.84, A54.89,
          A54.9, A56.00-A56.8, A63.8-A64, B92, B94.-B94.9, N34.1

      **A54.00   Gonococcal infection of lower genitourinary
                tract, unspecified**

      **A54.01   Gonococcal cystitis and urethritis,
                unspecified**

      A54.02   Gonococcal vulvovaginitis, unspecified ♀

      A54.03   Gonococcal cervicitis, unspecified ♀

      **A54.09   Other gonococcal infection of lower
                genitourinary tract**

  **A54.1   Gonococcal infection of lower genitourinary tract with
           periurethral and accessory gland abscess**
      Gonococcal Bartholin's gland abscess

  ● **A54.2   Gonococcal pelviperitonitis and other gonococcal
             genitourinary infection**

      Ex: **For category A54.2 CC codes:** A54.00-A54.29, A54.82, A54.84, A54.89,
          A54.9, A56.00-A56.8, A63.8-A64, B92, B94.-B94.9, N34.1

      A54.21   Gonococcal infection of kidney and ureter

      A54.22   Gonococcal prostatitis ♂

      **A54.23   Gonococcal infection of other male genital
                organs ♂**
          Gonococcal epididymitis
          Gonococcal orchitis

      **A54.24   Gonococcal female pelvic inflammatory
                disease ♀**
          Gonococcal pelviperitonitis

          Excludes1   gonococcal peritonitis (A54.85)

      A54.29   Other gonococcal genitourinary infections

  ● **A54.3   Gonococcal infection of eye**

      Ex: **For category A54.3 CC codes:** A50.01-A51.46, A51.5-A54.85, A54.89-A58,
          A63.8, A64, M02.30-M02.39, N34.1

      A54.30   Gonococcal infection of eye, unspecified

      A54.31   Gonococcal conjunctivitis
          *Form of bacterial conjunctivitis contracted by
           newborns during delivery; AKA neonatal
           conjunctivitis*
          Ophthalmia neonatorum due to gonococcus

      A54.32   Gonococcal iridocyclitis
          *Inflammation of iris and of ciliary body due to
           gonococcal infection*

      A54.33   Gonococcal keratitis
          *Inflammation of cornea due to gonococcal infection;
           AKA keratoconjunctivitis, keratopathy*

      A54.39   Other gonococcal eye infection
          Gonococcal endophthalmia

● **A54.4   Gonococcal infection of musculoskeletal system**
      Ex: **For category A54.4 CC codes:** A02.23, A17.9, A18.02, A18.09, A18.82,
          A18.84, A18.89, A39.83-A39.84, A50.01-A51.9, A52.00-A54.89, A54.9-A58,
          A63.8, A64, B06.82, M00.00-M02.9, M05.40-M05.59, M05.70-M06.09,
          M06.20-M06.39, M06.80-M07.69, M11.00-M11.9, M12.10-M15.0,
          M15.3-M15.9, M16.2-M16.9, M17.2-M17.9, M18.2-M18.9, M19.111-M19.93,
          M24.10-M24.176, M25.00, M25.08, M25.10-M25.18, M25.40-M25.676,
          M25.80-M25.9, M35.2, M36.1-M36.4, N34.1, R29.4

  **A54.40   Gonococcal infection of musculoskeletal
            system, unspecified**

  A54.41   Gonococcal spondylopathy
      *Disorder of vertebrae due to gonococcal infection;
       AKA rachiopathy*

  A54.42   Gonococcal arthritis
      Excludes2   gonococcal infection of spine
                      (A54.41)

  A54.43   Gonococcal osteomyelitis
      Excludes2   gonococcal infection of spine
                      (A54.41)

  **A54.49   Gonococcal infection of other musculoskeletal
            tissue**
      Gonococcal bursitis
      Gonococcal myositis
      Gonococcal synovitis
      Gonococcal tenosynovitis

A54.5   Gonococcal pharyngitis

A54.6   Gonococcal infection of anus and rectum

● **A54.8   Other gonococcal infections**

  A54.81   Gonococcal meningitis
      Ex: See A54.41

  A54.82   Gonococcal brain abscess
      Ex: A50.01-A51.46, A51.5-A54.85, A54.89-A58, A63.8, A64,
          M02.30-M02.39, N25.81-N25.89, N34.1

  A54.83   Gonococcal heart infection
      Gonococcal endocarditis
      Gonococcal myocarditis
      Gonococcal pericarditis
      Ex: A01.00-A01.09, A39.51, A50.01-A58, A63.8-A64, A78,
          B33.20-B33.22, B37.6, B40.0-B40.9, I00, I01.1-I02.0,
          I05.0-I05.1, I05.2, I05.8-I08.3, I08.9-I09.1, I09.89-I09.9,
          I23.0-I23.3, I23.6-I23.8, I33.0-I41, I42.4, I51.0, I51.4,
          I87.8-I87.9, I99.8-I99.9, M00.00, M00.08-M00.10,
          M00.18-M00.20, M00.28-M00.80, M00.88-M00.9,
          M02.30-M02.39, N34.1, Q22.2, Q23.8, Q23.9, Q24.8,
          T82.6XX[A]

  A54.84   Gonococcal pneumonia
      Ex: See A54.82

  A54.85   Gonococcal peritonitis
      Excludes1   gonococcal pelviperitonitis
                      (A54.24)
      Ex: A18.31, A34, A50.01-A58, A63.8, A64, K35.2-K35.3, K63.4,
          K63.89-K63.9, K65.1, K65.3, K65.9, K67, K86.81-K86.89,
          K92.89-K92.9, M02.30-M02.39, N34.1, N73.3-N73.4, N73.6,
          O08.0, O08.82, O85, O86.12, O86.81, O86.89, P78.0, R11.13,
          T81.60X[A]-T81.69X[A]

  A54.86   Gonococcal sepsis
      MCC when PDx is its own MCC
      Ex: A02.1, A20.7, A22.7, A26.7, A32.7, A39.2-A39.4, A40.0-A40.1,
          A40.8-A41.9, A42.7, A48.2-A48.4, A48.8-A49.9, A54.86, B00.7,
          B3.77, B92, B94.2-B96.89, R65.10-R65.20, Z16.10-Z16.39

  A54.89   Other gonococcal infections
      Gonococcal keratoderma
      Gonococcal lymphadenitis
      Ex: See A54.82

A54.9   Gonococcal infection, unspecified
      Ex: See A54.82

A55   Chlamydial lymphogranuloma (venereum)
      Climatic or tropical bubo
      Durand-Nicolas-Favre disease
      Esthiomene
      Lymphogranuloma inguinale

Item 1-10 An STD (sexually transmitted disease) caused by **Neisseria
gonorrhoeae** that flourishes in the warm, moist areas of the reproductive
tract. Untreated gonorrhea spreads to other parts of the body, causing
inflammation of the testes or prostate or pelvic inflammatory disease (PID).

◀ New   ◀ᴵᴵᴵ Revised   ~~deleted~~ Deleted   Excludes 1   Excludes 2   Includes   Use additional   Code first   Code also   Unspecified

OGCR Official Guidelines   ● Unacceptable Principal Diagnosis   X Assign placeholder X   ▶ Use Additional Character(s)   ▶ Manifestation Code   **Coding Clinic**

● **A56** **Other sexually transmitted chlamydial diseases**

> **Includes** 　sexually transmitted diseases due to Chlamydia trachomatis
>
> **Excludes1** 　neonatal chlamydial conjunctivitis (P39.1)
> neonatal chlamydial pneumonia (P23.1)
>
> **Excludes2** 　chlamydial lymphogranuloma (A55)
> conditions classified to A74.-

● **A56.0** **Chlamydial infection of lower genitourinary tract**

A56.00 **Chlamydial infection of lower genitourinary tract, unspecified**

A56.01 **Chlamydial cystitis and urethritis**

A56.02 **Chlamydial vulvovaginitis ♀**

A56.09 **Other chlamydial infection of lower genitourinary tract**
Chlamydial cervicitis

● **A56.1** **Chlamydial infection of pelviperitoneum and other genitourinary organs**

A56.11 **Chlamydial female pelvic inflammatory disease ♀**

A56.19 **Other chlamydial genitourinary infection**
Chlamydial epididymitis
Chlamydial orchitis

A56.2 **Chlamydial infection of genitourinary tract, unspecified**

A56.3 **Chlamydial infection of anus and rectum**

A56.4 **Chlamydial infection of pharynx**

A56.8 **Sexually transmitted chlamydial infection of other sites**

A57 **Chancroid**
Ulcus molle
Sexually transmitted infection caused by bacteria, Haemophilus ducreyi

A58 **Granuloma inguinale**
Chronic, progressive, ulcerative granulomatous disease
Donovanosis

● **A59** **Trichomoniasis**

> **Excludes2** 　intestinal trichomoniasis (A07.8)

A common STD caused by a parasite, Trichomonas vaginalis

● **A59.0** **Urogenital trichomoniasis**

A59.00 **Urogenital trichomoniasis, unspecified**
Fluor (vaginalis) due to Trichomonas
Leukorrhea (vaginalis) due to Trichomonas

A59.01 **Trichomonal vulvovaginitis ♀**

A59.02 **Trichomonal prostatitis ♂**

A59.03 **Trichomonal cystitis and urethritis**

A59.09 **Other urogenital trichomoniasis**
Common sexually transmitted disease (STD) caused by single-celled protozoan parasite; AKA trich
Trichomonas cervicitis

A59.8 **Trichomoniasis of other sites**

A59.9 **Trichomoniasis, unspecified**

● **A60** **Anogenital herpesviral [herpes simplex] infections**

● **A60.0** **Herpesviral infection of genitalia and urogenital tract**

A60.00 **Herpesviral infection of urogenital system, unspecified**

A60.01 **Herpesviral infection of penis ♂**

A60.02 **Herpesviral infection of other male genital organs ♂**

A60.03 **Herpesviral cervicitis ♀**

A60.04 **Herpesviral vulvovaginitis ♀**
Herpesviral [herpes simplex] ulceration
Herpesviral [herpes simplex] vaginitis
Herpesviral [herpes simplex] vulvitis

A60.09 **Herpesviral infection of other urogenital tract**

A60.1 **Herpesviral infection of perianal skin and rectum**

A60.9 **Anogenital herpesviral infection, unspecified**

● **A63** **Other predominantly sexually transmitted diseases, not elsewhere classified**

> **Excludes2** 　molluscum contagiosum (B08.1)
> papilloma of cervix (D26.0)

A63.0 **Anogenital (venereal) warts**
Anogenital warts due to (human) papillomavirus [HPV]
Condyloma acuminatum

A63.8 **Other specified predominantly sexually transmitted diseases**

A64 **Unspecified sexually transmitted disease**

OTHER SPIROCHETAL DISEASES (A65-A69)

> **Excludes2** 　leptospirosis (A27.-)
> syphilis (A50-A53)

A65 **Nonvenereal syphilis**
Bejel
Endemic syphilis
Njovera

● **A66** **Yaws**
Endemic, infectious, tropical disease caused by spirochete, spread by direct contact; AKA frambesia, framboesia, frambesia tropica

> **Includes** 　bouba
> frambesia (tropica)
> pian

A66.0 **Initial lesions of yaws**
Chancre of yaws
Frambesia, initial or primary
Initial frambesial ulcer
Mother yaw

A66.1 **Multiple papillomata and wet crab yaws**
Frambesioma
Pianoma
Plantar or palmar papilloma of yaws

A66.2 **Other early skin lesions of yaws**
Cutaneous yaws, less than five years after infection
Early yaws (cutaneous)(macular)(maculopapular)(micropapular)(papular)
Frambeside of early yaws

A66.3 **Hyperkeratosis of yaws**
Hypertrophy of stratum corneum of skin in which there are small, hard, verrucous scales
Ghoul hand
Hyperkeratosis, palmar or plantar (early) (late) due to yaws
Worm-eaten soles

A66.4 **Gummata and ulcers of yaws**
Small, rubbery granuloma with necrotic center and inflamed characteristic of advanced stage of syphilis; AKA syphiloma
Gummatous frambeside
Nodular late yaws (ulcerated)

A66.5 **Gangosa**
Manifestation of yaws that develops in the soft palate and spreads eroding bone, cartilage, and soft tissue
Rhinopharyngitis mutilans

A66.6 **Bone and joint lesions of yaws**
Yaws ganglion
Yaws goundou
Yaws gumma, bone
Yaws gummatous osteitis or periostitis
Yaws hydrarthrosis
Yaws osteitis
Yaws periostitis (hypertrophic)

A66.7 **Other manifestations of yaws**
Juxta-articular nodules of yaws
Mucosal yaws

A66.8 **Latent yaws**
Yaws without clinical manifestations, with positive serology

A66.9 **Yaws, unspecified**

N 　Newborn Age: 0　　P 　Pediatric Age: 0–17　　M 　Maternity DX: 12–55　　A 　Adult Age: 15–124　　♀ Females Only　　♂ Males Only

🔗 Complication\Comorbidity　　🔗 Major C\C　　(Ex:) CC/MCC Exclusions　　🔗 Hospital-Acquired Condition

● A67　Pinta [carate]
　　　　Group of nonvenereal diseases caused by Treponema species
　　A67.0　Primary lesions of pinta
　　　　　Chancre (primary) of pinta
　　　　　Papule (primary) of pinta
　　A67.1　Intermediate lesions of pinta
　　　　　Erythematous plaques of pinta
　　　　　Hyperchromic lesions of pinta
　　　　　Hyperkeratosis of pinta
　　　　　Pintids
　　A67.2　Late lesions of pinta
　　　　　Achromic skin lesions of pinta
　　　　　Cicatricial skin lesions of pinta
　　　　　Dyschromic skin lesions of pinta
　　A67.3　Mixed lesions of pinta
　　　　　Achromic with hyperchromic skin lesions of pinta
　　　　　[carate]
　　A67.9　Pinta, unspecified

● A68　Relapsing fevers
　　　Includes　　recurrent fever
　　　Excludes2　　Lyme disease (A69.2-)
　　　Ⓔⓧ For category A68 CC codes: A44.0-A44.9, A68.0-A68.9, A69.20-A69.29, A75.0-A79.9, B55.0-B57.5, B60.0
　　A68.0　Louse-borne relapsing fever 🔲
　　　　　Relapsing fever due to Borrelia recurrentis
　　A68.1　Tick-borne relapsing fever 🔲
　　　　　Relapsing fever due to any Borrelia species other than
　　　　　Borrelia recurrentis
　　A68.9　Relapsing fever, unspecified 🔲

● A69　Other spirochetal infections
　　A69.0　Necrotizing ulcerative stomatitis
　　　　　Cancrum oris
　　　　　Fusospirochetal gangrene
　　　　　Noma
　　　　　Stomatitis gangrenosa
　　A69.1　Other Vincent's infections 🔲
　　　　　Fusospirochetal pharyngitis
　　　　　Necrotizing ulcerative (acute) gingivitis
　　　　　Necrotizing ulcerative (acute) gingivostomatitis
　　　　　Spirochetal stomatitis
　　　　　Trench mouth
　　　　　Vincent's angina
　　　　　Vincent's gingivitis
　　　　　Ⓔⓧ A69.1
　● A69.2　Lyme disease
　　　　　Erythema chronicum migrans due to Borrelia
　　　　　　burgdorferi
　　　　　Ⓔⓧ For category A69.2 CC codes: See A68
　　　A69.20　Lyme disease, unspecified 🔲
　　　A69.21　Meningitis due to Lyme disease 🔲
　　　A69.22　Other neurologic disorders in Lyme disease 🔲
　　　　　　Cranial neuritis
　　　　　　Meningoencephalitis
　　　　　　Polyneuropathy
　　　A69.23　Arthritis due to Lyme disease 🔲
　　　A69.29　Other conditions associated with Lyme
　　　　　　disease 🔲
　　　　　　Myopericarditis due to Lyme disease
　　A69.8　Other specified spirochetal infections
　　A69.9　Spirochetal infection, unspecified

OTHER DISEASES CAUSED BY CHLAMYDIAE (A70-A74)

　　Excludes1　　sexually transmitted chlamydial diseases
　　　　　　　　(A55-A56)

● A70　Chlamydia psittaci infections 🔲
　　　　Ornithosis
　　　　Parrot fever
　　　　Psittacosis
　　　　Ⓔⓧ A70

● A71　Trachoma
　　　Excludes1　　sequelae of trachoma (B94.0)
　　A71.0　Initial stage of trachoma
　　　　　Trachoma dubium
　　A71.1　Active stage of trachoma
　　　　　Granular conjunctivitis (trachomatous)
　　　　　Trachomatous follicular conjunctivitis
　　　　　Trachomatous pannus
　　A71.9　Trachoma, unspecified

● A74　Other diseases caused by chlamydiae
　　　Excludes1　　neonatal chlamydial conjunctivitis (P39.1)
　　　　　　　　neonatal chlamydial pneumonia (P23.1)
　　　　　　　　Reiter's disease (M02.3-)
　　　　　　　　sexually transmitted chlamydial diseases
　　　　　　　　(A55-A56)
　　　Excludes2　　chlamydial pneumonia (J16.0)
　　A74.0　Chlamydial conjunctivitis
　　　　　Paratrachoma
　● A74.8　Other chlamydial diseases
　　　A74.81　Chlamydial peritonitis
　　　A74.89　Other chlamydial diseases
　　A74.9　Chlamydial infection, unspecified
　　　　　Chlamydiosis NOS

RICKETTSIOSES (A75-A79)

● A75　Typhus fever
　　　Excludes1　　rickettsiosis due to Ehrlichia sennetsu (A79.81)
　　　　Ⓔⓧ For category A75 CC codes unless otherwise indicated: See A68
　　A75.0　Epidemic louse-borne typhus fever due to Rickettsia
　　　　　prowazekii 🔲
　　　　　Organisms transmitted between humans via louse
　　　　　Classical typhus (fever)
　　　　　Epidemic (louse-borne) typhus
　　A75.1　Recrudescent typhus [Brill's disease] 🔲
　　　　　Brill-Zinsser disease
　　A75.2　Typhus fever due to Rickettsia typhi 🔲
　　　　　Murine (flea-borne) typhus
　　A75.3　Typhus fever due to Rickettsia tsutsugamushi 🔲
　　　　　Scrub (mite-borne) typhus
　　　　　Tsutsugamushi fever
　　A75.9　Typhus fever, unspecified 🔲
　　　　　Typhus (fever) NOS
　　　　　Ⓔⓧ A17.82, A44.0-A44.9, A50.42, A52.14, A68.0-A68.9, A69.20-A69.29,
　　　　　A75.0-A79.9, A81.1, A81.82-A81.89, A83.0-A85.8, A87.2, A88.0, A88.8,
　　　　　A92.1-A92.8, A93.0, B00.4, B00.82, B01.11-B01.12, B04, B06.01, B08.09,
　　　　　B08.20-B08.22, B08.60-B08.79, B09, B10.01-B10.09, B26.2, B33.1, B45.0,
　　　　　B45.2-B45.9, B50.9, B55.0-B57.5, B58.2, B60.0, B75, B97.10, B97.21,
　　　　　G04.00-G04.01, G04.31, G04.81-G05.4, G37.0, G37.4-G37.5, J09.X3-J09.
　　　　　X9, J10.2-J10.89, J11.2-J11.89, L44.4, M1A.10X0-M1A.19X1, P35.2-P35.9,
　　　　　P37.0-P37.4, P37.8-P37.9, T56.0X1-T56.0X4[A]

Item 1-12　Rickettsioses are diseases spread from ticks, lice, fleas, or mites to humans.
　　Typhus is spread to humans chiefly by the fleas of rats.
　　Endemic identifies a disease as being present in low numbers of humans at all times, whereas **epidemic** identifies a disease as being present in high numbers of humans at a specific time. Morbidity (death) is higher in epidemic diseases.
　　Brill's disease, also known as **Brill-Zinsser disease,** is spread from human to human by body lice and also from the lice of flying squirrels. **Scrub typhus** is spread in the same ways as Brill's disease.
　　Malaria is spread to humans by mosquitoes.

Item 1-11　Cancrum oris, also known as **noma** or **gangrenous stomatitis,** begins as an ulcer of the gingiva and results in a progressive gangrenous process.

　◀ New　◀━ Revised　d̶e̶l̶e̶t̶e̶d̶ Deleted　Excludes 1　Excludes 2　Includes　Use additional　Code first　Code also　Unspecified
OGCR Official Guidelines　● Unacceptable Principal Diagnosis　X Assign placeholder X　▸ Use Additional Character(s)　▸ Manifestation Code　**Coding Clinic**

● **A77   Spotted fever [tick-borne rickettsioses]**
   (Ex) For category A77 CC codes: See A68

   A77.0   Spotted fever due to Rickettsia rickettsii
      Rocky Mountain spotted fever
      Sao Paulo fever

   A77.1   Spotted fever due to Rickettsia conorii
      African tick typhus
      Boutonneuse fever
      India tick typhus
      Kenya tick typhus
      Marseilles fever
      Mediterranean tick fever

   A77.2   Spotted fever due to Rickettsia siberica
      North Asian tick fever
      Siberian tick typhus

   A77.3   Spotted fever due to Rickettsia australis
      Queensland tick typhus

● **A77.4   Ehrlichiosis**
    Type of tick-borne fever caused by bacteria infection
    Excludes1   Rickettsiosis due to Ehrlichia sennetsu
              (A79.81)

    A77.40   Ehrlichiosis, unspecified
    A77.41   Ehrlichiosis chafeensis [E. chafeensis]
    A77.49   Other ehrlichiosis

   A77.8   Other spotted fevers

   A77.9   Spotted fever, unspecified
      Tick-borne typhus NOS

 A78   Q fever
    Infection due to Coxiella burnetii
    Nine Mile fever
    Quadrilateral fever
    (Ex) See A68

● **A79   Other rickettsioses**
   (Ex) For category A79 CC codes unless otherwise indicated: A77.0-A79.9

   A79.0   Trench fever
      Quintan fever
      Wolhynian fever
      (Ex) See A68

   A79.1   Rickettsialpox due to Rickettsia akari
      Kew Garden fever
      Vesicular rickettsiosis

● **A79.8   Other specified rickettsioses**
    A79.81   Rickettsiosis due to Ehrlichia sennetsu
    A79.89   Other specified rickettsioses

   A79.9   Rickettsiosis, unspecified
      Rickettsial infection NOS

VIRAL AND PRION INFECTIONS OF THE CENTRAL NERVOUS SYSTEM (A80-A89)

    Excludes1   postpolio syndrome (G14)
             sequelae of poliomyelitis (B91)
             sequelae of viral encephalitis (B94.1)

● **A80   Acute poliomyelitis**
   (Ex) For category A80 CC codes: A80.0-A80.39

   A80.0   Acute paralytic poliomyelitis, vaccine-associated
   A80.1   Acute paralytic poliomyelitis, wild virus, imported
   A80.2   Acute paralytic poliomyelitis, wild virus, indigenous
● **A80.3   Acute paralytic poliomyelitis, other and unspecified**
    A80.30   Acute paralytic poliomyelitis, unspecified
    A80.39   Other acute paralytic poliomyelitis

   A80.4   Acute nonparalytic poliomyelitis
   A80.9   Acute poliomyelitis, unspecified

● **A81   Atypical virus infections of central nervous system**
    Includes   diseases of the central nervous system caused by
                prions
   Use additional code to identify:
     dementia with behavioral disturbance (F02.81)
     dementia without behavioral disturbance (F02.80)

● **A81.0   Creutzfeldt-Jakob disease**
    (Ex) For category A81.0 CC codes: A17.82, A50.42, A52.14, A75.9, A79.9,
      A81.00-A81.9, A83.0-A85.8, A87.2, A88.0, A88.8, A92.1-A92.2,
      A92.4-A92.8, A93.0, B00.4, B00.82, B01.11-B01.12, B04, B06.01, B08.09,
      B08.20-B08.22, B08.60-B08.79, B09, B10.01-B10.09, B26.2, B33.1, B45.0,
      B45.2-B45.9, B58.2, B75, B97.10, G04.00-G04.01, G04.31, G04.81-G05.4,
      G37.0, G37.4-G37.5, I67.3, J09.X3-J09.X9, J10.2-J10.89, J11.2-J11.89,
      L44.4, M1A.10X0-M1A.19X1, P35.2-P35.9, P37.0-P37.4, P37.8-P37.9,
      T56.0X1-T56.0X4[A]

    A81.00   Creutzfeldt-Jakob disease, unspecified
       Jakob-Creutzfeldt disease, unspecified

    A81.01   Variant Creutzfeldt-Jakob disease
       vCJD

    A81.09   Other Creutzfeldt-Jakob disease
       CJD
       Familial Creutzfeldt-Jakob disease
       Iatrogenic Creutzfeldt-Jakob disease
       Sporadic Creutzfeldt-Jakob disease
       Subacute spongiform encephalopathy (with
        dementia)

   A81.1   Subacute sclerosing panencephalitis
     Type of viral encephalitis that causes parenchymatous lesions
     in gray and white matter of brain
     Dawson's inclusion body encephalitis
     Van Bogaert's sclerosing leukoencephalopathy
     (Ex) A81.1, B92, B94.2-B94.9

   A81.2   Progressive multifocal leukoencephalopathy
     Group of diseases affecting white matter of brain
     Multifocal leukoencephalopathy NOS
     (Ex) A17.82, A50.42, A52.14, A75.9, A79.9, A81.00-A81.9, A83.0-A85.8, A87.2,
      A88.0, A88.8, A92.1-A92.2, A92.4-A92.8, A93.0, B00.4, B00.82,
      B01.11-B01.12, B04, B06.01, B08.09, B08.20-B08.22, B08.60-B08.79, B09,
      B10.01-B10.09, B26.2, B27.00-B27.99, B33.1, B45.0, B45.2-B45.9, B58.2,
      B75, G04.00-G04.01, G04.31, G04.81-G05.4, G37.0, G37.4-G37.5, I67.3,
      J09.X3-J09.X9, J10.2-J10.89, J11.2-J11.89, L44.4, M1A.10X0-M1A.19X1,
      P35.2-P35.9, P37.0-P37.4, P37.8-P37.9, T56.0X1-T56.0X4[A]

● **A81.8   Other atypical virus infections of central nervous system**
    (Ex) For category A81.8 CC codes unless otherwise indicated:
      A81.00-A81.9, A92.30-A92.39, B97.21, I67.3

    A81.81   Kuru
       (Ex) A81.00-A81.9, I67.3

    A81.82   Gerstmann-Sträussler-Scheinker syndrome
       GSS syndrome

    A81.83   Fatal familial insomnia
       FFI

    A81.89   Other atypical virus infections of central nervous system

   A81.9   Atypical virus infection of central nervous system, unspecified
      Prion diseases of the central nervous system NOS
      (Ex) A81.00-A81.9, I67.3

● **A82   Rabies**
    Viral disease affecting the central nervous system and transmitted
    from infected mammals to man.
    (Ex) For category A82 CC codes: A82.0-A82.9

   A82.0   Sylvatic rabies
   A82.1   Urban rabies
   A82.9   Rabies, unspecified

Item 1-13   Acute Poliomyelitis: Also called infantile paralysis and is caused by the poliovirus, which enters the body orally and infects the intestinal wall and then enters the blood stream and central nervous system, causing muscle weakness and paralysis. This disease has been nearly eradicated with the polio vaccine.

CHAPTER 1 (A00-B99)

N   Newborn Age: 0   **P**   Pediatric Age: 0–17   **M**   Maternity DX: 12–55   **A**   Adult Age: 15–124   ♀   Females Only   ♂   Males Only
 Complication\Comorbidity   Major C\C   (Ex) CC/MCC Exclusions   Hospital-Acquired Condition

651

● **A83**   **Mosquito-borne viral encephalitis**
Inflammation of the brain caused most commonly by Herpes Simplex virus.

> **Includes**   mosquito-borne viral meningoencephalitis
> **Excludes2**   Venezuelan equine encephalitis (A92.2)
>   West Nile fever (A92.3-)
>   West Nile virus (A92.3-)

(Ex.) **For category A83 CC codes:** A17.82, A50.42, A52.14, A75.9, A79.9, A81.1, A81.82-A81.89, A83.0-A85.8, A87.2, A88.0, A88.8, A92.1-A92.8, A93.0, B00.4, B00.82, B01.11-B01.12, B04, B06.01, B08.09, B08.20-B08.22, B08.60-B08.79, B09, B10.01-B10.09, B26.2, B27.00-B27.99, B33.1, B45.0, B45.2-B45.9, B58.2, B75, B97.10-B97.21, G04.00-G04.01, G04.31, G04.81-G04.91, G05.3-G05.4, G37.0, G37.4-G37.5, J09.X3-J09.X9, J10.2-J10.89, J11.2-J11.89, L44.4, M1A.10X0-M1A.19X1, P35.2-P35.9, P37.0-P37.9, T56.0X1-T56.0X4[A]

A83.0   Japanese encephalitis 🦠
A83.1   Western equine encephalitis 🦠
A83.2   Eastern equine encephalitis 🦠
A83.3   St. Louis encephalitis 🦠
A83.4   Australian encephalitis 🦠
        Kunjin virus disease
A83.5   California encephalitis 🦠
        California meningoencephalitis
        La Crosse encephalitis
A83.6   Rocio virus disease 🦠
        Mosquito-borne virus
A83.8   Other mosquito-borne viral encephalitis 🦠
A83.9   Mosquito-borne viral encephalitis, unspecified 🦠

● **A84**   **Tick-borne viral encephalitis**
> **Includes**   tick-borne viral meningoencephalitis

(Ex.) **For category A84 CC codes:** See A83

A84.0   Far Eastern tick-borne encephalitis [Russian spring-summer encephalitis] 🦠
A84.1   Central European tick-borne encephalitis 🦠
A84.8   Other tick-borne viral encephalitis 🦠
        Louping ill
        Powassan virus disease
A84.9   Tick-borne viral encephalitis, unspecified 🦠

● **A85**   **Other viral encephalitis, not elsewhere classified**
> **Includes**   specified viral encephalomyelitis NEC
>   specified viral meningoencephalitis NEC
> **Excludes1**   benign myalgic encephalomyelitis (G93.3)
>   encephalitis due to cytomegalovirus (B25.8)
>   encephalitis due to herpesvirus NEC (B10.0-)
>   encephalitis due to herpesvirus [herpes simplex] (B00.4)
>   encephalitis due to measles virus (B05.0)
>   encephalitis due to mumps virus (B26.2)
>   encephalitis due to poliomyelitis virus (A80.-)
>   encephalitis due to zoster (B02.0)
>   lymphocytic choriomeningitis (A87.2)

(Ex.) **For category A85 CC codes unless otherwise indicated:** A17.82, A50.42, A52.14, A75.9, A79.9, A81.1, A81.82-A81.89, A83.0-A85.8, A87.2, A88.0, A88.8, A92.1-A92.8, A93.0, B00.4, B00.82, B01.11-B01.12, B04, B06.01, B08.09, B08.20-B08.22, B08.60-B08.79, B09, B10.01-B10.09, B26.2, B27.00-B27.99, B33.1, B45.0, B45.2-B45.9, B58.2, B75, B97.10-B97.21, G04.00-G04.01, G04.31, G04.81-G04.91, G05.3-G05.4, G37.0, G37.4-G37.5, H66.40-H66.43, J09.X3-J09.X9, J10.2-J10.89, J11.2-J11.89, L44.4, M1A.10X0-M1A.19X1, M32.0-M32.9, P35.2-P35.9, P37.0-P37.9, T56.0X1-T56.0X4[A]

A85.0   Enteroviral encephalitis 🦠
        Enteroviral encephalomyelitis
A85.1   Adenoviral encephalitis 🦠
        Adenoviral meningoencephalitis
A85.2   Arthropod-borne viral encephalitis, unspecified 🦠
> **Excludes1**   West nile virus with encephalitis (A92.31)
(Ex.) See A83
A85.8   Other specified viral encephalitis 🦠
        Encephalitis lethargica
        Von Economo-Cruchet disease

Item 1-14   **Encephalitis** is an inflammation of the brain most often caused by a virus but may also be caused by a bacteria and most commonly transmitted by a mosquito. **Myelitis** is an inflammation of the spinal cord that may disrupt CNS function. Untreated myelitis may rapidly lead to permanent damage to the spinal cord. **Encephalomyelitis** is a general term for an inflammation of the brain and spinal cord.

● **A86**   **Unspecified viral encephalitis** 🦠
        Viral encephalomyelitis NOS
        Viral meningoencephalitis NOS

(Ex.) A17.82, A50.42, A52.14, A75.9, A79.9, A81.1, A81.82-A81.89, A83.0-A86, A87.2, A88.0, A88.8-A89, A92.1-A92.2, A92.4-A92.8, A93.0, B00.4, B00.82, B01.11-B01.12, B04, B06.01, B08.09, B08.20-B08.22, B08.60-B08.79, B09, B10.01-B10.09, B26.2, B27.00-B27.99, B33.1, B45.0, B45.2-B45.9, B58.2, B75, B97.10, G04.00-G04.01, G04.31, G04.81-G04.91, G05.3-G05.4, G37.0, G37.4-G37.5, H66.40-H66.43, J09.X3-J09.X9, J10.2-J10.89, J11.2-J11.89, L44.4, M1A.10X0-M1A.19X1, M32.0-M32.9, P35.2-P35.9, P37.0-P37.9, T56.0X1-T56.0X4[A]

● **A87**   **Viral meningitis**
> **Excludes1**   meningitis due to herpesvirus [herpes simplex] (B00.3)
>   meningitis due to measles virus (B05.1)
>   meningitis due to mumps virus (B26.1)
>   meningitis due to poliomyelitis virus (A80.-)
>   meningitis due to zoster (B02.1)

(Ex.) **For category A87 CC codes unless otherwise indicated:** A02.21, A17.0-A17.1, A27.81, A39.0, A50.41, A51.41, A52.13, A54.82-A54.84, A54.89-A54.9, A74.81-A74.9, A87.0-A87.9, A96.2, A98.3-A98.4, B26.1, B33.24, B33.4-B33.8, B34.1-B34.8, B37.5, B38.4, B45.1, B58.2, B92, B94.2-B94.9, B97.10, B97.19, B97.29, B97.5-B97.6, B97.81-B97.89, G00.0-G03.9, G04.2, G32.89, G61.0, G96.8-G96.9, G98.0-G98.8, G99.8

A87.0   Enteroviral meningitis 🦠
        Group of common viruses responsible for the majority of viral meningitis
        Coxsackievirus meningitis
        Echovirus meningitis
A87.1   Adenoviral meningitis 🦠
A87.2   Lymphocytic choriomeningitis 🦠
        Lymphocytic meningoencephalitis
(Ex.) A02.21, A17.0-A17.1, A27.81, A39.0, A50.41, A51.41, A52.13, A54.82-A54.84, A54.89-A54.9, A74.81-A74.9, A87.0-A87.9, A92.30-A92.39, A96.2, A98.3-A98.4, B26.1, B33.24, B33.4-B33.8, B34.1-B34.8, B37.5, B38.4, B45.1, B58.2, B92, B94.2-B94.9, B97.10, B97.19, B97.21-B97.29, B97.5-B97.6, B97.81-B97.89, G00.0-G03.9, G04.2, G32.89, G61.0, G96.8-G96.9, G98.0-G98.8, G99.8
A87.8   Other viral meningitis 🦠
A87.9   Viral meningitis, unspecified 🦠

● **A88**   **Other viral infections of central nervous system, not elsewhere classified**
> **Excludes1**   viral encephalitis NOS (A86)
>   viral meningitis NOS (A87.9)

A88.0   Enteroviral exanthematous fever [Boston exanthem] 🦠
        Infectious skin eruption
        (Ex.) See A83
A88.1   Epidemic vertigo
A88.8   Other specified viral infections of central nervous system 🦠
        (Ex.) See A85

● **A89**   **Unspecified viral infection of central nervous system** 🦠
        (Ex.) See A86

ARTHROPOD-BORNE VIRAL FEVERS AND VIRAL HEMORRHAGIC FEVERS (A90-A99)

A90   **Dengue fever [classical dengue]** 🦠
Acute, self-limited disease, characterized by fever, prostration, severe muscle pains, headache, rash, lymphadenopathy, and leukopenia, caused by dengue virus; AKA breakbone, dandy
> **Excludes1**   dengue hemorrhagic fever (A91)
(Ex.) A90

A91   **Dengue hemorrhagic fever** 🦠
Serious follow-up to regular dengue, with symptoms of hemorrhage
(Ex.) A91, A92.0-A94, A98.0-A98.2, A98.8-A99, B33.1

● **A92**   **Other mosquito-borne viral fevers**
> **Excludes1**   Ross River disease (B33.1)

A92.0   Chikungunya virus disease 🦠
        Transmitted by mosquitoes
        Chikungunya (hemorrhagic) fever
        (Ex.) See A91

◀ New   ◀◀ Revised   ~~deleted~~ Deleted   Excludes 1   Excludes 2   Includes   Use additional   Code first   Code also   Unspecified

OGCR Official Guidelines   ● Unacceptable Principal Diagnosis   X Assign placeholder X   ▶ Use Additional Character(s)   ▶ Manifestation Code   **Coding Clinic**

OGCR Section I. C.1.f.

Certain Infectious and Parasitic Diseases (A00–B99)

Zika virus infections

Code only confirmed cases

Code only a confirmed diagnosis of Zika virus (A92.5, Zika virus disease) as documented by the provider. This is an exception to the hospital inpatient guideline Section II, H.

In this context, "confirmation" does not require documentation of the type of test performed; the physician's diagnostic statement that the condition is confirmed is sufficient. This code should be assigned regardless of the stated mode of transmission.

If the provider documents "suspected", "possible" or "probable" Zika, do not assign code A92.5. Assign a code(s) explaining the reason for encounter (such as fever, rash, or joint pain) or Z20.828, Contact with and (suspected) exposure to other viral communicable diseases.

A92.1   **O'nyong-nyong fever** 🦟
Acute, nonfatal febrile disease transmitted by mosquitoes, which clinically resembles dengue and chikungunya
(Ex:) A17.82, A50.42, A52.14, A75.9, A79.9, A81.1, A81.82-A81.89, A83.0-A85.8, A87.2, A88.0, A88.8, A91-A94, A98.0-A98.2, A98.8-A99, B00.4, B00.82, B01.11-B01.12, B04, B06.01, B08.09, B08.20-B08.22, B08.60-B08.79, B09, B10.01-B10.09, B26.2, B27.00-B27.99, B33.1, B45.0, B45.2-B45.9, B58.2, B75, B97.10, B97.21, G04.00-G04.01, G04.31, G04.81-G04.91, G05.3-G05.4, G37.0, G37.4-G37.5, J09.X3-J09.X9, J10.2-J10.89, J11.2-J11.89, L44.4, M1A.10X0-M1A.19X1, P35.2-P35.9, P37.0-P37.9, T56.0X1-T56.0X4[A]

A92.2   **Venezuelan equine fever** 🦟
Venezuelan equine encephalitis
Venezuelan equine encephalomyelitis virus disease
(Ex:) See A92.1

● **A92.3**   **West Nile virus infection**
West Nile fever
(Ex:) **For category A92.3 CC codes:** A17.82, A50.42, A52.14, A75.9, A79.9, A81.1, A81.82-A81.89, A83.0-A85.8, A87.2, A88.0, A88.8, A91, A92.0-A92.2, A92.4-A94, A98.0-A98.2, A98.8-A99, B00.4, B00.82, B01.11-B01.12, B04, B06.01, B08.09, B08.20-B08.22, B08.60-B08.79, B09, B10.01-B10.09, B26.2, B27.00-B27.99, B33.1, B45.0, B45.2-B45.9, B58.2, B75, B97.10, G04.00-G04.01, G04.31, G04.81-G04.91, G05.3-G05.4, G37.0, G37.4-G37.5, J09.X3-J09.X9, J10.2-J10.89, J11.2-J11.89, L44.4, P35.2-P35.9, P37.0-P37.9

    A92.30   **West Nile virus infection, unspecified** 🦟
West Nile fever NOS
West Nile fever without complications
West Nile virus NOS

    A92.31   **West Nile virus infection with encephalitis** 🦟
West Nile encephalitis
West Nile encephalomyelitis

    A92.32   **West Nile virus infection with other neurologic manifestation** 🦟
Use additional code to specify the neurologic manifestation

    A92.39   **West Nile virus infection with other complications** 🦟
Use additional code to specify the other conditions

A92.4   **Rift Valley fever** 🦟
(Ex:) See A92.1

A92.5   **Zika virus disease** 🦟 ◀
Zika virus fever ◀
Zika virus infection ◀
Zika NOS ◀
(Ex:) See A92.1

A92.8   **Other specified mosquito-borne viral fevers** 🦟
(Ex:) See A92.1

A92.9   **Mosquito-borne viral fever, unspecified** 🦟
(Ex:) See A91

● **A93**   **Other arthropod-borne viral fevers, not elsewhere classified**

A93.0   **Oropouche virus disease** 🦟
Tropical viral infection
Oropouche fever
(Ex:) See A92.1

A93.1   **Sandfly fever** 🦟
Pappataci fever
Phlebotomus fever
(Ex:) See A91

A93.2   **Colorado tick fever** 🦟
(Ex:) See A91

A93.8   **Other specified arthropod-borne viral fevers** 🦟
Piry virus disease
Vesicular stomatitis virus disease [Indiana fever]
(Ex:) See A91

A94   **Unspecified arthropod-borne viral fever** 🦟
Arboviral fever NOS
Arbovirus infection NOS
(Ex:) See A91

● **A95**   **Yellow fever**
Acute infectious disease transmitted by mosquitoes
(Ex:) **For category A95 CC codes:** A95.0-A95.9

A95.0   **Sylvatic yellow fever** 🦟
Jungle yellow fever

A95.1   **Urban yellow fever** 🦟

A95.9   **Yellow fever, unspecified** 🦟

● **A96**   **Arenaviral hemorrhagic fever**
Virus that causes various hemorrhagic fevers
(Ex:) **For category A96 CC codes:** A74.81-A74.9, A88.1, A96.0-A96.9, A98.3-A98.5, B25.8-B25.9, B33.24-B34.2, B34.4-B34.8, B97.0-B97.89

A96.0   **Junin hemorrhagic fever** 🦟
Argentinian hemorrhagic fever

A96.1   **Machupo hemorrhagic fever** 🦟
Transmitted by contact with infected rodents
Bolivian hemorrhagic fever

A96.2   **Lassa fever**
Acute type of hemorrhagic fever caused by contact with disease carrying mouse or person

A96.8   **Other arenaviral hemorrhagic fevers** 🦟

A96.9   **Arenaviral hemorrhagic fever, unspecified** 🦟

● **A98**   **Other viral hemorrhagic fevers, not elsewhere classified**
Excludes1   chikungunya hemorrhagic fever (A92.0)
dengue hemorrhagic fever (A91)
(Ex:) **For category A98 CC codes unless otherwise indicated:** See A91

A98.0   **Crimean-Congo hemorrhagic fever** 🦟
Virus transmitted by ticks and contact with blood, secretions, or fluids from infected humans or animals
Central Asian hemorrhagic fever

A98.1   **Omsk hemorrhagic fever** 🦟
Transmitted to humans by bites of infected ticks or contact with infected muskrats

A98.2   **Kyasanur Forest disease** 🦟
Transmitted via infected monkeys, voles, ticks

A98.3   **Marburg virus disease**
Rare, acute, often fatal type of hemorrhagic fever

A98.4   **Ebola virus disease**

A98.5   **Hemorrhagic fever with renal syndrome** 🦟
Epidemic hemorrhagic fever
Korean hemorrhagic fever
Russian hemorrhagic fever
Hantaan virus disease
Hantavirus disease with renal manifestations
Nephropathia epidemica
Songo fever
Excludes1   hantavirus (cardio)-pulmonary syndrome (B33.4)
(Ex:) A17.9, A18.10-A18.11, A18.13, A18.82, A18.84, A18.89, A54.21, A54.29, A54.82, A54.84, A54.89-A54.9, A59.00, A59.8-A59.9, A98.5, B37.41-B37.49, B97.21, E08.21-E08.29, E08.618-E08.638, E08.649-E08.8, E09.21-E09.29, E09.618-E09.638, E09.649-E09.8, E10.21-E10.29, E10.618-E10.638, E10.649, E10.69-E10.8, E11.21-E11.29, E11.618-E11.638, E11.649, E11.69-E11.8, E13.21-E13.29, E13.618-E13.638, E13.649-E13.8, M10.30-M10.39, N00.0-N11.0, N11.8-N13.39, N13.6, N14.0-N17.9, N19, N25.0-N26.1, N26.9-N27.9, N28.1-N29, N36.41-N36.43, N36.8-N36.9, N39.8-N39.9, R31.0-R31.9

A98.8   **Other specified viral hemorrhagic fevers** 🦟

A99   **Unspecified viral hemorrhagic fever** 🦟
(Ex:) See A91

N   Newborn Age: 0   **P**   Pediatric Age: 0–17   **M**   Maternity DX: 12–55   **A**   Adult Age: 15–124   ♀   Females Only   ♂   Males Only

🦟   Complication\Comorbidity   🦟   Major C\C   (Ex:)   CC/MCC Exclusions   🦟   Hospital-Acquired Condition

653

VIRAL INFECTIONS CHARACTERIZED BY SKIN AND MUCOUS MEMBRANE LESIONS (B00-B09)

● **B00   Herpesviral [herpes simplex] infections**

Excludes1   congenital herpesviral infections (P35.2)

Excludes2   anogenital herpesviral infection (A60.-)
gammaherpesviral mononucleosis (B27.0-)
herpangina (B08.5)

B00.0   Eczema herpeticum
Cutaneous eruption caused by herpes simplex virus (HSV) type 1, HSV-2, coxsackievirus A16, or vaccinia virus
Kaposi's varicelliform eruption

B00.1   Herpesviral vesicular dermatitis
Vesicle formation; characteristics include formation of blisters and scabs on feet and legs
Herpes simplex facialis
Herpes simplex labialis
Herpes simplex otitis externa
Vesicular dermatitis of ear
Vesicular dermatitis of lip

B00.2   Herpesviral gingivostomatitis and pharyngotonsillitis 🦠
Inflammation involving both gingivae and oral mucosa
Herpesviral pharyngitis
Inflammation of pharynx and tonsils; AKA tonsillopharyngitis
Ⓔⓧ B00.2

B00.3   Herpesviral meningitis 🦠
Ⓔⓧ A02.21, A17.0-A17.1, A27.81, A39.0, A50.41, A51.41, A52.13, A54.82, A54.84, A54.89-A54.9, A87.0-A87.9, B00.3, B00.82-B00.9, B02.1, B10.81-B10.89, B26.1, B37.5, B38.4, B45.1, B58.2, B92, B94.2-B94.9, G00.0-G03.9, G04.2, G32.89, G61.0, G96.8-G96.9, G98.0-G98.8, G99.8

B00.4   Herpesviral encephalitis 🦠
Herpesviral meningoencephalitis
Simian B disease

Excludes1   herpesviral encephalitis due to herpesvirus 6 and 7 (B10.01, B10.09)
non-simplex herpesviral encephalitis (B10.0-)
Ⓔⓧ B00.4, B00.82-B00.9, B10.01-B10.89, B92, B94.2-B94.9

B00.5   Herpesviral ocular disease 🦠
Ⓔⓧ For category B00.5 CC codes: B00.50-B00.59, B00.89-B00.9, B10.81-B10.89

B00.50   Herpesviral ocular disease, unspecified 🦠

B00.51   Herpesviral iridocyclitis 🦠
Herpesviral iritis
Herpesviral uveitis, anterior

B00.52   Herpesviral keratitis 🦠
Herpesviral keratoconjunctivitis

B00.53   Herpesviral conjunctivitis 🦠

B00.59   Other herpesviral disease of eye 🦠
Herpesviral dermatitis of eyelid

B00.7   Disseminated herpesviral disease 🦠
Herpesviral sepsis
Ⓔⓧ A02.1, A20.7, A22.7, A26.7, A32.7, A39.2-A39.4, A40.0-A41.9, A42.7, A54.86, B00.7, B00.82-B00.9, B10.81-B10.89, B37.7, B92, B94.2-B94.9, R65.10-R65.20

Figure 1-4 Primary herpes simplex in and around the mouth. The infection is usually acquired from siblings or parents and is readily transmitted to other direct contacts. (From Forbes, Jackson: Colour Atlas and Text of Clinical Medicine, International Edition, Mosby, 2002)

Item 1-15   Herpes is a viral disease for which there is no cure. There are two types of the herpes simplex virus: **Type I** causes **cold sores** or **fever blisters,** and **Type II** causes **genital herpes.** The virus can be spread from a sore on the lips to the genitals or from the genitals to the lips.

● **B00.8   Other forms of herpesviral infections**

B00.81   Herpesviral hepatitis 🦠
Ⓔⓧ B00.3, B00.81-B00.9, B10.81-B10.89, B92, B94.2-B94.9

B00.82   Herpes simplex myelitis 🦠
Ⓔⓧ A74.81-A74.9, A96.2, A98.3-A98.4, B00.82-B00.9, B01.12, B02.24, B10.81-B10.89, B33.24, B33.4-B33.8, B34.1-B34.2, B34.4-B34.8, B92, B94.2-B94.9, B97.10, B97.19, B97.29, B97.5-B97.6, B97.81-B97.89, G04.00-G04.01, G04.31, G04.81-G04.89, G05.3-G05.4, G37.3

B00.89   Other herpesviral infection 🦠
Herpesviral whitlow
Ⓔⓧ A74.81-A74.9, A96.2, A98.3-A98.4, B00.82-B00.9, B10.81-B10.89, B33.24, B33.4-B33.8, B34.1-B34.2, B34.4-B34.8, B92, B94.2-B94.9, B97.10, B97.19, B97.29, B97.5-B97.6, B97.81-B97.89

B00.9   Herpesviral infection, unspecified 🦠
Herpes simplex infection NOS

● **B01   Varicella [chickenpox]**
Very contagious disease caused by the varicella zoster virus that results in an itchy outbreak of skin blisters (varicella). The same virus causes shingles (zoster).

B01.0   Varicella meningitis 🦠
Ⓔⓧ A74.81-A74.9, A96.2, A98.3-A98.4, B01.0, B01.12, B01.81-B01.9, B08.04, B33.24, B33.4-B33.8, B34.1-B34.2, B34.4-B34.8, B92, B94.2-B94.9, B97.10, B97.19, B97.29, B97.5-B97.6, B97.81-B97.89

● **B01.1   Varicella encephalitis, myelitis and encephalomyelitis**
Postchickenpox encephalitis, myelitis and encephalomyelitis

B01.11 Varicella encephalitis and encephalomyelitis 🦠
Postchickenpox encephalitis and encephalomyelitis
Ⓔⓧ A74.81-A74.9, A96.2, A98.3-A98.4, B01.0-B01.12, B01.81-B01.9, B08.04, B33.24, B33.4-B33.8, B34.1-B34.2, B34.4-B34.8, B92, B94.2-B94.9, B97.10, B97.19, B97.29, B97.5-B97.6, B97.81-B97.89

B01.12 Varicella myelitis 🦠
Postchickenpox myelitis
Ⓔⓧ A74.81-A74.9, A96.2, A98.3-A98.4, B00.82, B01.0, B01.12, B01.81-B01.9, B02.24, B08.04, B33.24, B33.4-B33.8, B34.1-B34.2, B34.4-B34.8, B92, B94.2-B94.9, B97.10, B97.19, B97.29, B97.5-B97.6, B97.81-B97.89, G04.00-G04.01, G04.31, G04.81-G04.89, G05.3-G05.4, G37.3

B01.2   Varicella pneumonia 🦠
Ⓔⓧ A74.81-A74.9, A96.2, A98.3-A98.4, B01.0, B01.12-B01.9, B08.04, B33.24, B33.4-B33.8, B34.1-B34.2, B34.4-B34.8, B92, B94.2-B94.9, B97.10, B97.19, B97.29, B97.5-B97.6, B97.81-B97.89

● **B01.8   Varicella with other complications**
Ⓔⓧ For category B01.8 CC codes: See B01.0

B01.81   Varicella keratitis 🦠

B01.89   Other varicella complications 🦠

B01.9   Varicella without complication 🦠
Varicella NOS
Ⓔⓧ See B01.0

● **B02   Zoster [herpes zoster]**

Includes   shingles
zona

B02.0   Zoster encephalitis 🦠
Zoster meningoencephalitis
Ⓔⓧ A74.81-A74.9, A96.2, A98.3-A98.4, B00.3, B00.82-B00.9, B02.0-B02.29, B02.7-B02.9, B10.81-B10.89, B33.24, B33.4-B33.8, B34.1-B34.2, B34.4-B34.8, B92, B94.2-B94.9, B97.10, B97.19, B97.29, B97.5-B97.6, B97.81-B97.89

B02.1   Zoster meningitis 🦠
Ⓔⓧ A02.21, A17.0-A17.1, A27.81, A39.0, A50.41, A51.41, A52.13, A54.82, A54.84, A54.89-A54.9, A74.81-A74.9, A87.0-A87.9, A96.2, A98.3-A98.4, B00.3, B00.82-B00.9, B02.0-B02.29, B02.7-B02.9, B10.81-B10.89, B26.1, B33.24, B33.4, B33.8, B34.1-B34.2, B34.4-B34.8, B37.5, B38.4, B45.1, B58.2, B92, B94.2-B94.9, B97.10, B97.19, B97.29, B97.5-B97.6, B97.81-B97.89, G00.0-G03.9, G04.2, G32.89, G61.0, G96.8-G96.9, G98.0-G98.8, G99.8

◀ New   ◀▥ Revised   ~~deleted~~ Deleted   Excludes 1   Excludes 2   Includes   Use additional   Code first   Code also   Unspecified
OGCR Official Guidelines   ● Unacceptable Principal Diagnosis   X Assign placeholder X   ● Use Additional Character(s)   ◼ Manifestation Code   **Coding Clinic**

Item 1-16 Zoster: Also known as *shingles* and is caused by the same virus as chickenpox. After exposure, the virus lies dormant in nerve tissue and is activated by factors including aging, stress, suppression of the immune system, and certain medication. It begins as a unilateral rash that leads to blisters and sores on the skin. It may involve the nerve pathways of the eye, forehead, nose, and eyelids and may be very painful with long-term systemic effects.

● **B02.2   Zoster with other nervous system involvement**
    (Ex) For category B02.2 CC codes unless otherwise indicated: see B02.0

    B02.21   Postherpetic geniculate ganglionitis

    B02.22   Postherpetic trigeminal neuralgia

    B02.23   Postherpetic polyneuropathy

    B02.24   Postherpetic myelitis
        Herpes zoster myelitis
        (Ex) A74.81-A74.9, A96.2, A98.3-A98.4, B00.3, B00.82-B00.9, B01.12, B02.0-B02.29, B02.7-B02.9, B10.81-B10.89, B33.24, B33.4-B33.8, B34.1-B34.2, B34.4-B34.8, B92, B94.2-B94.9, B97.10, B97.19, B97.29, B97.5-B97.6, B97.81-B97.89, G04.00-G04.01, G04.31, G04.81-G04.89, G05.3-G05.4, G37.3

    B02.29   Other postherpetic nervous system involvement
        Postherpetic radiculopathy

● **B02.3   Zoster ocular disease**
    (Ex) For category B02.3 CC codes: B02.30-B02.39

    B02.30   Zoster ocular disease, unspecified

    B02.31   Zoster conjunctivitis

    B02.32   Zoster iridocyclitis

    B02.33   Zoster keratitis
        Herpes zoster keratoconjunctivitis

    B02.34   Zoster scleritis

    B02.39   Other herpes zoster eye disease
        Zoster blepharitis

  B02.7   Disseminated zoster
    (Ex) A60.00-A60.9, A74.81-A74.9, A96.2, A98.3-A98.4, B00.0-B00.2, B00.4-B00.9, B02.0-B02.9, B10.01-B10.89, B33.24, B33.4-B33.8, B34.1-B34.2, B34.4, B34.8, B92, B94.2-B94.9, B97.10, B97.19, B97.29, B97.5-B97.6, B97.81-B97.89

  B02.8   Zoster with other complications
    Herpes zoster otitis externa
    (Ex) See B02.7

  B02.9   Zoster without complications
    Zoster NOS

B03   Smallpox
    Note: In 1980 the 33rd World Health Assembly declared that smallpox had been eradicated. The classification is maintained for surveillance purposes.
    (Ex) B01.0-B01.9, B03, B08.010-B08.04

B04   Monkeypox
    Disease occurring in captive monkeys and other mammals that may be transmitted to humans, clinically similar to smallpox
    (Ex) B04, B08.010-B08.011, B08.09, B08.3, B08.60-B08.79, B09, L44.4

● **B05   Measles**
    Includes   morbilli
    Excludes1   subacute sclerosing panencephalitis (A81.1)

  B05.0   Measles complicated by encephalitis
    Postmeasles encephalitis
    (Ex) A74.81-A74.9, A96.2, A98.3-A98.4, B05.0-B05.1, B05.4, B05.89-B05.9, B33.24, B33.4-B33.8, B34.1-B34.2, B34.4-B34.8, B92, B94.2-B94.9, B97.10, B97.19, B97.29, B97.5-B97.6, B97.81-B97.89

  B05.1   Measles complicated by meningitis
    Postmeasles meningitis
    (Ex) A74.81-A74.9, A96.2, A98.3-A98.4, B05.1, B05.4, B05.89-B05.9, B33.24, B33.4-B33.8, B34.1-B34.2, B34.4-B34.8, B92, B94.2-B94.9, B97.10, B97.19, B97.29, B97.5-B97.6, B97.81-B97.89

  B05.2   Measles complicated by pneumonia
    Postmeasles pneumonia
    (Ex) A74.81-A74.9, A96.2, A98.3-A98.4, B05.1-B05.2, B05.4, B05.89-B05.9, B33.24, B33.4-B33.8, B34.1-B34.2, B34.4-B34.8, B92, B94.2-B94.9, B97.10, B97.19, B97.29, B97.5-B97.6, B97.81-B97.89

  B05.3   Measles complicated by otitis media
    Postmeasles otitis media

  B05.4   Measles with intestinal complications
    (Ex) See B05.1

● **B05.8   Measles with other complications**

    B05.81   Measles keratitis and keratoconjunctivitis
        (Ex) A74.81-A74.9, A96.2, A98.3-A98.4, B05.1, B05.4, B05.81-B05.9, B33.24, B33.4-B33.8, B34.1-B34.2, B34.4-B34.8, B92, B94.2-B94.9, B97.10, B97.19, B97.29, B97.5-B97.6, B97.81-B97.89

    B05.89   Other measles complications
        (Ex) See B05.1

  B05.9   Measles without complication
    Measles NOS

● **B06   Rubella [German measles]**
    Excludes1   congenital rubella (P35.0)

● **B06.0   Rubella with neurological complications**
    (Ex) For category B06.0 CC codes: A74.81-A74.9, A96.2, A98.3-A98.4, B05.1, B05.4, B05.81-B05.9, B06.00-B06.81, B06.89-B06.9, B33.24, B33.4-B33.8, B34.1-B34.2, B34.4-B34.8, B92, B94.2-B94.9, B97.10, B97.19, B97.29, B97.5-B97.6, B97.81-B97.89

    B06.00   Rubella with neurological complication, unspecified

    B06.01   Rubella encephalitis
        Rubella meningoencephalitis

    B06.02   Rubella meningitis

    B06.09   Other neurological complications of rubella

● **B06.8   Rubella with other complications**

    B06.81   Rubella pneumonia
        (Ex) See B06.0

    B06.82   Rubella arthritis
        (Ex) A74.81-A74.9, A96.2, A98.3-A98.4, B05.1, B05.4, B05.81-B05.9, B06.81-B06.82, B06.89-B06.9, B33.24, B33.4-B33.8, B34.1-B34.2, B34.4-B34.8, B92, B94.2-B94.9, B97.10, B97.19, B97.29, B97.5-B97.6, B97.81-B97.89

    B06.89   Other rubella complications
        (Ex) See B06.0

  B06.9   Rubella without complication
    Rubella NOS

Figure 1-5 Photograph of eyelids with marginal blepharitis. (From Mandell, Bennett, & Dolin: Principles and Practice of Infectious Diseases, ed 7, Churchill Livingstone, An Imprint of Elsevier, 2009)

Item 1-17 Blepharitis is a common condition in which the eyelid is swollen and yellow scaling and conjunctivitis develop. Usually the hair on the scalp and brow is involved.

CHAPTER 1 (A00–B99)

N   Newborn Age: 0   **P**   Pediatric Age: 0–17   **M**   Maternity DX: 12–55   **A**   Adult Age: 15–124   ♀ Females Only   ♂ Males Only

 Complication\Comorbidity   Major C\C   (Ex) CC/MCC Exclusions   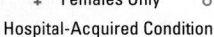 Hospital-Acquired Condition

● **B07** **Viral warts**

> **Includes**   verruca simplex
> verruca vulgaris
> viral warts due to human papillomavirus

> **Excludes2**   anogenital (venereal) warts (A63.0)
> papilloma of bladder (D41.4)
> papilloma of cervix (D26.0)
> papilloma larynx (D14.1)

B07.0 **Plantar wart**
Verruca plantaris

B07.8 **Other viral warts**
Common wart
Flat wart
Verruca plana

B07.9 **Viral wart, unspecified**

● **B08** **Other viral infections characterized by skin and mucous membrane lesions, not elsewhere classified**

> **Excludes1**   vesicular stomatitis virus disease (A93.8)

● **B08.0** **Other orthopoxvirus infections**

> **Excludes2**   monkeypox (B04)

    ● **B08.01** **Cowpox and vaccinia not from vaccine**

         B08.010 **Cowpox**

         B08.011 **Vaccinia not from vaccine**

> **Excludes1**   vaccinia (from vaccination) (generalized) (T88.1)

     B08.02 **Orf virus disease**
Contagious pustular dermatitis
Ecthyma contagiosum

     B08.03 **Pseudocowpox [milker's node]**

     B08.04 **Paravaccinia, unspecified**

     B08.09 **Other orthopoxvirus infections**
Orthopoxvirus infection NOS

B08.1 **Molluscum contagiosum**
Various skin diseases characterized by soft, rounded, cutaneous lesions

● **B08.2** **Exanthema subitum [sixth disease] Roseola infantum**
Acute, short-lived high fever in infants and young children followed by a rash mainly on the trunk, caused by human herpesvirus 6

     B08.20 **Exanthema subitum [sixth disease], unspecified Roseola infantum, unspecified**   P

     B08.21 **Exanthema subitum [sixth disease] due to human herpesvirus 6 Roseola infantum due to human herpesvirus 6**   P
Virus results in sudden rash; infection results in lifelong persistence

     B08.22 **Exanthema subitum [sixth disease] due to human herpesvirus 7 Roseola infantum due to human herpesvirus 7**   P

B08.3 **Erythema infectiosum [fifth disease]** 🔎
Moderately contagious, epidemic disease in children caused by B19 virus; onset of rash that begins as redness of cheeks, later there is rash on trunk and limbs; when this fades, there may be central clearing that leaves lacelike pattern
Ⓔⓧ B08.3, B34.3

B08.4 **Enteroviral vesicular stomatitis with exanthem**
Hand, foot and mouth disease
Check your documentation—this code is HAND, foot, and mouth disease. Code B08.8 is foot and mouth disease.

B08.5 **Enteroviral vesicular pharyngitis**
Herpangina

● **B08.6** **Parapoxvirus infections**

     B08.60 **Parapoxvirus infection, unspecified**

     B08.61 **Bovine stomatitis**

     B08.62 **Sealpox**

     B08.69 **Other parapoxvirus infections**

● **B08.7** **Yatapoxvirus infections**

     B08.70 **Yatapoxvirus infection, unspecified**

     B08.71 **Tanapox virus disease** 🔎
Ⓔⓧ B04, B08.010-B08.011, B08.09, B08.3, B08.60-B08.79, B09, L44.4

     B08.72 **Yaba pox virus disease**
Yaba monkey tumor disease

     B08.79 **Other yatapoxvirus infections**

B08.8 **Other specified viral infections characterized by skin and mucous membrane lesions**
Enteroviral lymphonodular pharyngitis
Foot-and-mouth disease
Check your documentation. Code B08.4 is for HAND, foot, and mouth disease.
Poxvirus NEC

● **B09** **Unspecified viral infection characterized by skin and mucous membrane lesions**
Viral enanthema NOS
Viral exanthema NOS

OTHER HUMAN HERPESVIRUSES (B10)

● **B10** **Other human herpesviruses**

> **Excludes2**   cytomegalovirus (B25.9)
> Epstein-Barr virus (B27.0-)
> herpes NOS (B00.9)
> herpes simplex (B00.-)
> herpes zoster (B02.-)
> human herpesvirus NOS (B00.-)
> human herpesvirus 1 and 2 (B00.-)
> human herpesvirus 3 (B01.-, B02.-)
> human herpesvirus 4 (B27.0-)
> human herpesvirus 5 (B25.-)
> varicella (B01.-)
> zoster (B02.-)

● **B10.0** **Other human herpesvirus encephalitis**

> **Excludes2**   herpes encephalitis NOS (B00.4)
> herpes simplex encephalitis (B00.4)
> human herpesvirus encephalitis (B00.4)
> simian B herpes virus encephalitis (B00.4)
> Ⓔⓧ **For category B10.0 CC codes:** B00.4, B00.82-B00.9, B10.01-B10.89, B92, B94.2-B94.9

     B10.01 **Human herpesvirus 6 encephalitis** 🔎
Sudden rash or roseola

     B10.09 **Other human herpesvirus encephalitis** 🔎
Human herpesvirus 7 encephalitis
Virus closely related to human herpesvirus 6, but not known to cause any disease

● **B10.8** **Other human herpesvirus infection**

     B10.81 **Human herpesvirus 6 infection**
Causative agent of exanthema subitum that results in sudden rash

     B10.82 **Human herpesvirus 7 infection**
Closely related to human herpesvirus 6, but not known cause any disease

     B10.89 **Other human herpesvirus infection**
Human herpesvirus 8 infection
May be the cause of Kaposi sarcoma, a malignant tumor
Kaposi's sarcoma-associated herpesvirus infection

◀ New   ◀▦ Revised   d̶e̶l̶e̶t̶e̶d̶ Deleted   Excludes 1   Excludes 2   Includes   Use additional   Code first   Code also   Unspecified
OGCR Official Guidelines   ● Unacceptable Principal Diagnosis   X Assign placeholder X   ● Use Additional Character(s)   🔎 Manifestation Code   Coding Clinic

Figure 1-6 Hepatitis B viral infection. **A.** Liver parenchyma showing hepatocytes with diffuse granular cytoplasm, so-called ground glass hepatocytes (H&E). **B.** Immunoperoxidase stains from the same case, showing cytoplasmic inclusions of viral particles. (From Kumar: Robbins and Cotran: Pathologic Basis of Disease, ed 8, Saunders, An Imprint of Elsevier, 2009)

Item 1–18   Hepatitis A (HAV) was formerly called epidemic, infectious, short-incubation, or acute catarrhal jaundice hepatitis. The primary transmission mode is the oral–fecal route. **Hepatitis B (HBV)** was formerly called long-incubation period, serum, or homologous serum hepatitis. Transmission modes are through blood from infected persons and from body fluids of infected mother to neonate. **Hepatitis C (HCV),** caused by the hepatitis C virus, is primarily transfusion associated. **Hepatitis D (HDV),** also called delta hepatitis, is caused by the hepatitis D virus in patients formerly or currently infected with hepatitis B. **Hepatitis E (HEV)** is also called enterically transmitted non-A, non-B hepatitis. The primary transmission mode is the oral–fecal route, usually through contaminated water.

VIRAL HEPATITIS (B15-B19)

Excludes1　sequelae of viral hepatitis (B94.2)
Excludes2　cytomegaloviral hepatitis (B25.1)
　　　　　　　herpesviral [herpes simplex] hepatitis (B00.81)

● **B15**　Acute hepatitis A
　　(Ex:) **For category B15 CC codes:** see B15 A74.81-A74.9, A96.2, A98.3-A98.4, B15.0-B19.9, B33.24,
　　B33.4-B33.8, B34.1-B34.2, B34.4-B34.8, B92, B94.2-B94.9, B97.10, B97.19, B97.29,
　　B97.5-B97.6, B97.81-B97.89

　　B15.0　Hepatitis A with hepatic coma 🦠
　　B15.9　Hepatitis A without hepatic coma 🦠
　　　　　　Hepatitis A (acute) (viral) NOS

● **B16**　Acute hepatitis B
　　(Ex:) **For category B16 CC codes:** see B15

　　B16.0　Acute hepatitis B with delta-agent with hepatic coma 🦠
　　B16.1　Acute hepatitis B with delta-agent without hepatic coma 🦠
　　B16.2　Acute hepatitis B without delta-agent with hepatic coma 🦠
　　B16.9　Acute hepatitis B without delta-agent and without hepatic coma 🦠
　　　　　　Hepatitis B (acute) (viral) NOS

● **B17**　Other acute viral hepatitis
　　(Ex:) **For category B17 CC codes:** see B15

　　B17.0　Acute delta-(super) infection of hepatitis B carrier 🦠
● 　**B17.1**　Acute hepatitis C
　　　　B17.10　Acute hepatitis C without hepatic coma 🦠
　　　　　　　　Acute hepatitis C NOS
　　　　B17.11　Acute hepatitis C with hepatic coma 🦠
　　B17.2　Acute hepatitis E 🦠
　　B17.8　Other specified acute viral hepatitis 🦠
　　　　　　Hepatitis non-A non-B (acute) (viral) NEC
　　B17.9　Acute viral hepatitis, **unspecified** 🦠
　　　　　　Acute hepatitis NOS
　　　　　　Acute infectious hepatitis NOS ◀

● **B18**　Chronic viral hepatitis
　　Includes　Carrier of viral hepatitis ◀
　　(Ex:) **For category B18 CC codes:** see B15

　　B18.0　Chronic viral hepatitis B with delta-agent 🦠
　　B18.1　Chronic viral hepatitis B without delta-agent 🦠
　　　　　　Carrier of viral hepatitis B ◀
　　　　　　Chronic (viral) hepatitis B

Figure 1-7　Kaposi's sarcoma. There are large confluent hyperpigmented patch-stage lesions with lymphedema. (From Cohen & Powderly: Infectious Diseases, ed 3, Mosby, An Imprint of Elsevier, 2010)

Item 1–19   AIDS (acquired immune deficiency syndrome) is caused by **HIV** (human immunodeficiency virus). HIV affects certain white blood cells (T-4 lymphocytes) and destroys the ability of the cells to fight infections, making patients susceptible to a host of infectious diseases (e.g., ***Pneumocystis carinii pneumonia (PCP), Kaposi's sarcoma,*** and ***lymphoma).*** ***AIDS-related complex (ARC)*** is an early stage of AIDS in which tests for HIV are positive but the symptoms are mild.

　　B18.2　Chronic viral hepatitis C
　　　　　　Carrier of viral hepatitis C ◀
　　B18.8　Other chronic viral hepatitis 🦠
　　　　　　Carrier of other viral hepatitis ◀
　　B18.9　Chronic viral hepatitis, **unspecified** 🦠
　　　　　　Carrier of unspecified viral hepatitis ◀

● **B19**　Unspecified viral hepatitis
　　(Ex:) **For category B19 CC codes:** see B15

　　B19.0　**Unspecified** viral hepatitis with hepatic coma 🦠
● 　**B19.1**　Unspecified viral hepatitis B
　　　　B19.10　**Unspecified** viral hepatitis B without hepatic coma 🦠
　　　　　　　　Unspecified viral hepatitis B NOS
　　　　B19.11　**Unspecified** viral hepatitis B with hepatic coma 🦠
● 　**B19.2**　Unspecified viral hepatitis C
　　　　B19.20　**Unspecified** viral hepatitis C without hepatic coma 🦠
　　　　　　　　Viral hepatitis C NOS
　　　　B19.21　**Unspecified** viral hepatitis C with hepatic coma 🦠
　　B19.9　**Unspecified** viral hepatitis without hepatic coma 🦠
　　　　　　Viral hepatitis NOS

OGCR　Section I. C.1.a

Certain Infectious and Parasitic Diseases (A00-B99)

a. Human Immunodeficiency Virus (HIV) Infections

1) Code only confirmed cases

Code only confirmed cases of HIV infection illness. This is an exception to the hospital inpatient guideline Section II, H.

In this context, "confirmation" does not require documentation of positive serology or culture for HIV; the provider's diagnostic statement that the patient is HIV positive, or has an HIV-related illness is sufficient.

HUMAN IMMUNODEFICIENCY VIRUS [HIV] DISEASE (B20)

B20　Human immunodeficiency virus [HIV] disease 🦠
　　Includes　acquired immune deficiency syndrome [AIDS]
　　　　　　AIDS-related complex [ARC]
　　　　　　HIV infection, symptomatic

　　Code first Human immunodeficiency virus [HIV] disease complicating pregnancy, childbirth and the puerperium, if applicable (O98.7-)

　　Use additional code(s) to identify all manifestations of HIV infection

　　Excludes1　asymptomatic human immunodeficiency virus [HIV] infection status (Z21)
　　　　　　exposure to HIV virus (Z20.6)
　　　　　　inconclusive serologic evidence of HIV (R75)
　　(Ex:) B20, B92, B94.2-B94.9

N　Newborn Age: 0　　**P**　Pediatric Age: 0–17　　**M**　Maternity DX: 12–55　　**A**　Adult Age: 15–124　　♀ Females Only　　♂ Males Only
🦠 Complication\Comorbidity　　🦠 Major C\C　　(Ex:) CC/MCC Exclusions　　🦠 Hospital-Acquired Condition

657

CHAPTER 1 (A00-B99)

OTHER VIRAL DISEASES (B25-B34)

● **B25** **Cytomegaloviral disease**
AKA: HCMV or Human Herpesvirus 5 (HHV-5)
Excludes1   congenital cytomegalovirus infection (P35.1)
cytomegaloviral mononucleosis (B27.1-)

B25.0 **Cytomegaloviral pneumonitis** 🔊
MCC when PDx is its own MCC
Ⓔ A15.0-A15.9, A17.9, A18.82, A18.84, A18.89, A21.2, A22.1, A31.0, A37.01,
A37.11, A37.81, A37.91, A42.0, A43.0, A48.1, B25.0, B39.0-B39.2, B44.0,
B58.3, B59, B67.1, J09.X1-J09.X2, J10.00-J10.1, J11.00-J11.1, J12.0-J12.3,
J12.89-J18.1, J18.8-J18.9, J22, J44.9, J47.0-J70.4, J70.8-J70.9, J98.4,
J98.8-J98.9, Q33.4, R91.1

B25.1 **Cytomegaloviral hepatitis** 🔊
CC when PDx is its own CC
Ⓔ No exclusions

B25.2 **Cytomegaloviral pancreatitis** 🔊
MCC when PDx is its own MCC
Ⓔ B25.2, K85.00-K86.1, K86.81-K86.9

B25.8 **Other cytomegaloviral diseases** 🔊
Cytomegaloviral encephalitis
Ⓔ A96.0-A96.9, A98.3-A98.5, B25.8-B25.9, B33.24-B34.2, B34.4-B34.8,
B97.0-B97.32, B97.39, B97.5-B97.89

B25.9 **Cytomegaloviral disease, unspecified** 🔊
Ⓔ See B25.8

● **B26** **Mumps**
Includes   epidemic parotitis
infectious parotitis
Acute, contagious, viral disease

B26.0 **Mumps orchitis** ♂ 🔊
Ⓔ A74.81-A74.9, A96.2, A98.3-A98.4, B26.0, B26.82-B26.83, B26.85-B26.9,
B33.24, B33.4-B33.8, B34.1-B34.8, B92, B94.2-B94.9, B97.10, B97.19,
B97.29, B97.5-B97.6, B97.81-B97.89

B26.1 **Mumps meningitis** 🔊
Ⓔ A02.21, A17.0-A17.1, A27.81, A39.0, A50.41, A51.41, A52.13, A54.82,
A54.84, A54.89-A54.9, A74.81-A74.9, A87.0-A87.9, A96.2, A98.3-A98.4,
B00.3, B02.1, B26.1, B26.82-B26.83, B26.85-B26.9, B33.24, B33.4-B33.8,
B34.1-B34.2, B34.4-B34.8, B37.5, B38.4, B45.1, B58.2, B92, B94.2,
B94.8-B94.9, B97.10, B97.19, B97.29, B97.5-B97.6, B97.81-B97.89,
G00.0-G03.9, G04.2, G32.89, G61.0, G96.8-G96.9, G98.0-G98.8, G99.8

B26.2 **Mumps encephalitis** 🔊
Ⓔ A74.81-A74.9, A96.2, A98.3-A98.4, B26.2, B26.82-B26.83, B26.85-B26.9,
B33.24, B33.4, B33.8, B34.1-B34.2, B34.4-B34.8, B92, B94.2, B94.8-B94.9,
B97.10, B97.19, B97.29, B97.5-B97.6, B97.81-B97.89

B26.3 **Mumps pancreatitis** 🔊
Ⓔ A74.81-A74.9, A96.2, A98.3-A98.4, B26.3, B26.82-B26.83, B26.85-B26.9,
B33.24, B33.4, B33.8, B34.1-B34.2, B34.4-B34.8, B92, B94.2, B94.8-B94.9,
B97.10, B97.19, B97.29, B97.5-B97.6, B97.81-B97.89

● **B26.8** **Mumps with other complications** 🔊
Ⓔ For category B26.8 CC codes unless otherwise indicated:
A74.81-A74.9, A96.2, A98.3-A98.4, B26.82-B26.83, B26.85-B26.9, B33.24,
B33.4, B33.8, B34.1-B34.2, B34.4-B34.8, B92, B94.2, B94.8-B94.9, B97.10,
B97.19, B97.29, B97.5-B97.6, B97.81-B97.89

B26.81 **Mumps hepatitis** 🔊
Ⓔ A74.81-A74.9, A96.2, A98.3-A98.4, B26.81-B26.83,
B26.85-B26.9, B33.24, B33.4, B33.8, B34.1-B34.2,
B34.4-B34.8, B92, B94.2, B94.8-B94.9, B97.10, B97.19,
B97.29, B97.5-B97.6, B97.81-B97.89

B26.82 **Mumps myocarditis** 🔊

B26.83 **Mumps nephritis** 🔊

B26.84 **Mumps polyneuropathy** 🔊
Ⓔ A74.81-A74.9, A96.2, A98.3-A98.4, B26.82-B26.9, B33.24,
B33.4, B33.8, B34.1-B34.2, B34.4-B34.8, B92, B94.2,
B94.8-B94.9, B97.10, B97.19, B97.29, B97.5-B97.6,
B97.81-B97.89

B26.85 **Mumps arthritis** 🔊

B26.89 **Other mumps complications** 🔊

B26.9 **Mumps without complication**
Mumps NOS
Mumps parotitis NOS

● **B27** **Infectious mononucleosis**
Includes   glandular fever
monocytic angina
Pfeiffer's disease

● **B27.0** **Gammaherpesviral mononucleosis**
AKA: Pfeiffer's disease, infective mononucleosis
Mononucleosis due to Epstein-Barr virus

B27.00 **Gammaherpesviral mononucleosis without
complication**
Infective mononucleosis

B27.01 **Gammaherpesviral mononucleosis with
polyneuropathy**

B27.02 **Gammaherpesviral mononucleosis with
meningitis**

B27.09 **Gammaherpesviral mononucleosis with other
complications**
Hepatomegaly in gammaherpesviral
mononucleosis

● **B27.1** **Cytomegaloviral mononucleosis**
Infectious disease resembling infectious mononucleosis

B27.10 **Cytomegaloviral mononucleosis without
complications**

B27.11 **Cytomegaloviral mononucleosis with
polyneuropathy**

B27.12 **Cytomegaloviral mononucleosis with
meningitis**

B27.19 **Cytomegaloviral mononucleosis with other
complication**
Hepatomegaly in cytomegaloviral
mononucleosis

● **B27.8** **Other infectious mononucleosis**

B27.80 **Other infectious mononucleosis without
complication**

B27.81 **Other infectious mononucleosis with
polyneuropathy**

B27.82 **Other infectious mononucleosis with
meningitis**

B27.89 **Other infectious mononucleosis with other
complication**
Hepatomegaly in other infectious
mononucleosis

● **B27.9** **Infectious mononucleosis, unspecified**

B27.90 **Infectious mononucleosis, unspecified without
complication**

B27.91 **Infectious mononucleosis, unspecified with
polyneuropathy**

B27.92 **Infectious mononucleosis, unspecified with
meningitis**

B27.99 **Infectious mononucleosis, unspecified with
other complication**
Hepatomegaly in unspecified infectious
mononucleosis

● **B30** **Viral conjunctivitis**
Excludes1   herpesviral [herpes simplex] ocular disease
(B00.5)
ocular zoster (B02.3)

B30.0 **Keratoconjunctivitis due to adenovirus**
Epidemic keratoconjunctivitis
Shipyard eye

B30.1 **Conjunctivitis due to adenovirus**
Acute adenoviral follicular conjunctivitis
Swimming-pool conjunctivitis

B30.2 **Viral pharyngoconjunctivitis**

B30.3 **Acute epidemic hemorrhagic conjunctivitis (enteroviral)**
Conjunctivitis due to coxsackievirus 24
Conjunctivitis due to enterovirus 70
Hemorrhagic conjunctivitis (acute)(epidemic)

B30.8 **Other viral conjunctivitis**
Newcastle conjunctivitis

B30.9 **Viral conjunctivitis, unspecified**

◀ New   ◀▥ Revised   ̶d̶e̶l̶e̶t̶e̶d̶ Deleted   Excludes 1   Excludes 2   Includes   Use additional   Code first   Code also   Unspecified

OGCR Official Guidelines   ● Unacceptable Principal Diagnosis   X Assign placeholder X   ● Use Additional Character(s)   ▶ Manifestation Code   Coding Clinic

● **B33**   **Other viral diseases, not elsewhere classified**

     B33.0   **Epidemic myalgia**
         Acute infectious disease, caused by group A coxsackie viruses or other enteroviruses with symptoms that include sudden pain in chest or upper abdomen with fever
         Bornholm disease

     B33.1   **Ross River disease** 🔗
         Epidemic polyarthritis and exanthema
         Ross River fever
         (Ex:) See A92.1

●   **B33.2**   **Viral carditis**
         Coxsackie (virus) carditis

         B33.20   **Viral carditis, unspecified** 🔗
             (Ex:) A52.06, B33.20-B33.22, I00, I01.2-I01.9, I09.0, I09.9, I23.0-I23.3, I23.6-I23.8, I40.0-I41, I51.0, I51.4, I87.8-I87.9, I99.8-I99.9

         B33.21   **Viral endocarditis** 🔗
             (Ex:) A01.00-A01.09, A39.51, A52.03, A78, B33.21, B37.6, B40.0-B40.9, I00, I01.1, I01.8-I02.0, I05.0-I07.9, I08.1-I08.3, I08.9, I09.1, I09.89-I09.9, I33.0-I39, I42.4, I87.8-I87.9, I99.8-I99.9, Q22.2, Q23.8-Q23.9, Q24.8, T82.6XXA

         B33.22   **Viral myocarditis** 🔗
             (Ex:) See B33.20

         B33.23   **Viral pericarditis** 🔗
             (Ex:) B33.23, I01.0, I09.2, I30.0-I30.9, I31.3-I32, I87.8-I87.9, I99.8-I99.9

         B33.24   **Viral cardiomyopathy**

     B33.3   **Retrovirus infections, not elsewhere classified**
         Retrovirus infection NOS

     B33.4   **Hantavirus (cardio)-pulmonary syndrome [HPS] [HCPS]** 🔗
         Hantavirus disease with pulmonary manifestations
         Sin nombre virus disease

         Use additional code to identify any associated acute kidney failure (N17.9)

         Excludes1   hantavirus disease with renal manifestations (A98.5)
                     hemorrhagic fever with renal manifestations (A98.5)
         (Ex:) A74.81-A74.9, A88.1, A96.0-A96.9, A98.3-A98.5, B19.20-B19.21, B25.8-B25.9, B33.24, B33.3-B34.2, B34.4-B34.8, B97.0-B97.89

     B33.8   **Other specified viral diseases**
         Excludes1   anogenital human papillomavirus infection (A63.0)
                     viral warts due to human papillomavirus infection (B07)

● **B34**   **Viral infection of unspecified site**
     Excludes1   anogenital human papillomavirus infection (A63.0)
             cytomegaloviral disease NOS (B25.9)
             herpesvirus [herpes simplex] infection NOS (B00.9)
             retrovirus infection NOS (B33.3)
             viral agents as the cause of diseases classified elsewhere (B97.-)
             viral warts due to human papillomavirus infection (B07)

     B34.0   **Adenovirus infection, unspecified**

     B34.1   **Enterovirus infection, unspecified**
         Intestinal tract infection
         Coxsackievirus infection NOS
         Echovirus infection NOS

     B34.2   **Coronavirus infection, unspecified**
         Excludes1   pneumonia due to SARS-associated coronavirus (J12.81)

     B34.3   **Parvovirus infection, unspecified** 🔗
         (Ex:) B08.3, B34.3

     B34.4   **Papovavirus infection, unspecified**

     B34.8   **Other viral infections of unspecified site**

     B34.9   **Viral infection, unspecified**
         Viremia NOS

MYCOSES (B35-B49)

     Excludes2   hypersensitivity pneumonitis due to organic dust (J67.-)
                   mycosis fungoides (C84.0-)

● **B35**   **Dermatophytosis**
     AKA tinea or ringworm
     Includes   favus
             infections due to species of Epidermophyton, Micro-sporum and Trichophyton
             tinea, any type except those in B36.-

     B35.0   **Tinea barbae and tinea capitis**
         Beard ringworm
         Kerion
         Scalp ringworm
         Sycosis, mycotic

     B35.1   **Tinea unguium**
         White patches or pits on surface or edges of nails, followed by infection under nail plate
         Dermatophytic onychia
         Dermatophytosis of nail
         Onychomycosis
         Ringworm of nails

     B35.2   **Tinea manuum**
         Tinea of hands
         Dermatophytosis of hand
         Hand ringworm

     B35.3   **Tinea pedis**
         Tinea affecting feet
         Athlete's foot
         Dermatophytosis of foot
         Foot ringworm

     B35.4   **Tinea corporis**
         Infecting skin areas other than hands
         Ringworm of the body

     B35.5   **Tinea imbricata**
         Chronic tropical tinea corporis; AKA Oriental ringworm, tinea inguinalis, tinea cruris
         Tokelau

     B35.6   **Tinea cruris**
         In groin or perineal area, spreading to adjacent regions; AKA jock itch, eczema marginatum, ringworm of groin, or t inguinalis
         Dhobi itch
         Groin ringworm
         Jock itch

     B35.8   **Other dermatophytoses**
         Disseminated dermatophytosis
         Granulomatous dermatophytosis

     B35.9   **Dermatophytosis, unspecified**
         Ringworm NOS

CHAPTER 1 (A00-B99)

● **B36   Other superficial mycoses**

    B36.0   Pityriasis versicolor
          Common, chronic, symptomless disorder that includes
              macular patches of various sizes and shapes; AKA liver
              spots
          Tinea flava
          Tinea versicolor

    B36.1   Tinea nigra
          Minor fungal infection, with dark lesions, usually on skin of
              hands
          Keratomycosis nigricans palmaris
          Microsporosis nigra
          Pityriasis nigra

    B36.2   White piedra
          White to light brown nodules on hair of beard, axilla, or
              groin; AKA trichosporosis
          Tinea blanca

    B36.3   Black piedra
          Characterized by small black or brown nodules on shafts of
              scalp hair

    B36.8   Other specified superficial mycoses

    B36.9   Superficial mycosis, unspecified

● **B37   Candidiasis**

    Includes   candidosis
                moniliasis

    Excludes1   neonatal candidiasis (P37.5)

    B37.0   Candidal stomatitis 🦠
          Oral thrush
          Ⓔⓧ B37.0-B37.9, B48.3, B49, B92, B94.2-B94.9

    B37.1   Pulmonary candidiasis 🦠
          Candidal bronchitis
          Candidal pneumonia
          Ⓔⓧ See B37.0

    B37.2   Candidiasis of skin and nail
          Candidal onychia
          Candidal paronychia
          Excludes2   diaper dermatitis (L22)

    B37.3   Candidiasis of vulva and vagina ♀
          Candidal vulvovaginitis
          Monilial vulvovaginitis
          Vaginal thrush

●   **B37.4   Candidiasis of other urogenital sites**
          Ⓔⓧ For category B37.4 CC codes: B37.1, B37.41-B37.82, B37.84-B37.9,
          N25.81-N25.89

      B37.41   Candidal cystitis and urethritis 🦠🦠

      B37.42   Candidal balanitis ♂
            Male condition only

      B37.49   Other urogenital candidiasis 🦠🦠
            Candidal pyelonephritis

    B37.5   Candidal meningitis 🦠
          Ⓔⓧ A02.21, A17.0-A17.1, A27.81, A39.0, A50.41, A51.41, A52.13, A54.82,
          A54.84, A54.89-A54.9, A87.0-A87.9, B00.3, B02.1, B26.1, B37.0-B38.4,
          B45.1, B48.3, B49, B58.2, B92, B94.2-B94.9, G00.0-G03.9, G04.2, G32.89,
          G61.0, G96.8-G96.9, G98.0, G98.8-G99.8

    B37.6   Candidal endocarditis 🦠
          Ⓔⓧ See B37.0

Figure 1-8   Oral candidiasis (thrush).
(Courtesy of Stephen Raffanti, MD, MPH.)
(From Mandell, Bennett, & Dolin: Principles and
Practice of Infectious Diseases, ed 7, Churchill
Livingstone, An Imprint of Elsevier, 2009)

Item 1–20 Candidiasis, also called oidiomycosis or moniliasis, is a
fungal infection. It most often appears on moist cutaneous areas of the body but
can also be responsible for a variety of systemic infections such as endocarditis,
meningitis, arthritis, and myositis. Antifungal medications cure most yeast
infections.

    B37.7   Candidal sepsis 🦠
          Disseminated candidiasis systemic candidiasis
          MCC when PDx is its own MCC
          Ⓔⓧ A02.1, A20.7, A22.7, A26.7, A32.7, A39.2-A39.4, A40.0-A40.1, A40.8-A41.9,
          A42.7, A48.2-A48.4, A48.8-A49.9, A54.86, B00.7, B37.0-B37.9, B48.3, B49,
          B92, B94.2-B96.89, R65.10-R65.20, Z16.10-Z16.39

●   **B37.8   Candidiasis of other sites**
          Ⓔⓧ For category B37.8 CC codes unless otherwise indicated: B37.0-B37.9,
          B48.3, B49, B92, B94.2-B94.9

      B37.81   Candidal esophagitis 🦠

      B37.82   Candidal enteritis 🦠
            Candidal proctitis

      B37.83   Candidal cheilitis 🦠
            Inflammation affecting lip

      B37.84   Candidal otitis externa 🦠
            Inflammation of external auditory canal

      B37.89   Other sites of candidiasis
            Infection manifested by invasive candidiasis
            Candidal osteomyelitis
            Ⓔⓧ B37.1, B37.5-B37.82, B37.84-B37.9

    B37.9   Candidiasis, unspecified
          Thrush NOS

● **B38   Coccidioidomycosis**
    Fungal disease; AKA coccidioidosis, coccidioidal granuloma, Posadas,
    or Posadas-Wernicke disease

    B38.0   Acute pulmonary coccidioidomycosis 🦠
          Ⓔⓧ B38.0-B38.2, B38.7, B38.89-B38.9, B48.3, B49, B92, B94.2-B94.9

    B38.1   Chronic pulmonary coccidioidomycosis 🦠
          Ⓔⓧ B38.0-B39.9

    B38.2   Pulmonary coccidioidomycosis, unspecified 🦠
          Ⓔⓧ See B38.1

    B38.3   Cutaneous coccidioidomycosis 🦠
          Ⓔⓧ B38.0-B38.9

    B38.4   Coccidioidomycosis meningitis 🦠
          Ⓔⓧ A02.21, A17.0-A17.1, A27.81, A39.0, A50.41, A51.41, A52.13, A54.82,
          A54.84, A54.89-A54.9, A87.0-A87.9, B00.3, B02.1, B26.1, B37.5,
          B38.4-B38.87, B38.89-B38.9, B45.1, B48.3, B49, B58.2, B92, B94.2-B94.9,
          G00.0-G03.9, G04.2, G32.89, G61.0, G96.8-G96.9, G98.0, G98.8-G99.8

    B38.7   Disseminated coccidioidomycosis 🦠
          Generalized coccidioidomycosis
          Ⓔⓧ B38.7, B38.89-B38.9, B48.3, B49, B92, B94.2-B94.9

●   **B38.8   Other forms of coccidioidomycosis**

      B38.81   Prostatic coccidioidomycosis ♂ 🦠
            Ⓔⓧ See B38.3

      B38.89   Other forms of coccidioidomycosis 🦠
            Ⓔⓧ See B38.7

    B38.9   Coccidioidomycosis, unspecified 🦠
          Ⓔⓧ See B38.7

● **B39   Histoplasmosis**
    Infection resulting from inhalation or ingestion of spores; AKA
    Darling disease

    Code first associated AIDS (B20)

    Use additional code for any associated manifestations, such as:
        endocarditis (I39)
        meningitis (G02)
        pericarditis (I32)
        retinitits (H32)

    B39.0   Acute pulmonary histoplasmosis capsulati 🦠
          Ⓔⓧ A22.1, A37.01-A37.11, A37.81, A37.9, A48.1, B25.0, B39.0-B39.4,
          B39.9-B44.0, B48.3, B49, B92, B94.2-B94.9, J09.X1-J09.X2, J10.00-J10.1,
          J11.00-J11.1, J12.0-J12.3, J12.89-J18.1, J18.8-J18.9, J44.9, J47.0-J47.9,
          J60-J70.4, J70.8-J70.9, J98.4, R91.1

    B39.1   Chronic pulmonary histoplasmosis capsulati 🦠
          Ⓔⓧ See B39.0

    B39.2   Pulmonary histoplasmosis capsulati, unspecified 🦠
          Ⓔⓧ See B39.0

    B39.3   Disseminated histoplasmosis capsulati 🦠
          Generalized histoplasmosis capsulati
          Ⓔⓧ B38.0-B39.4

◀ New   ◀ Revised   ~~deleted~~ Deleted   Excludes 1   Excludes 2   Includes   Use additional   Code first   Code also   Unspecified

OGCR Official Guidelines   ● Unacceptable Principal Diagnosis   X Assign placeholder X   ● Use Additional Character(s)   ▶ Manifestation Code   **Coding Clinic**

Item 1–21   Bird and bat droppings that fall into the soil give rise to a fungus that can spread airborne spores. When inhaled into the lungs, these spores divide and multiply into lesions. Histoplasmosis capsulatum takes three forms: primary (lodged in the lungs only), chronic (resembles TB), and disseminated (infection has moved to other organs). This is an opportunistic infection in immunosuppressed patients.

B39.4   **Histoplasmosis capsulati, unspecified**
     American histoplasmosis

B39.5   **Histoplasmosis duboisii**
     African histoplasmosis

B39.9   **Histoplasmosis, unspecified**

● **B40**   **Blastomycosis**
     Rare and potentially fatal infection caused by inhaling fungus found in moist soil in temperate climates.

     Excludes1   Brazilian blastomycosis (B41.-)
         keloidal blastomycosis (B48.0)

     (Ex) **For category B40 CC codes:** B40.0-B40.9, B48.3, B49, B92, B94.2-B94.9

B40.0   **Acute pulmonary blastomycosis** 🪙

B40.1   **Chronic pulmonary blastomycosis** 🪙

B40.2   **Pulmonary blastomycosis, unspecified** 🪙

B40.3   **Cutaneous blastomycosis** 🪙

B40.7   **Disseminated blastomycosis** 🪙
     Generalized blastomycosis

● **B40.8**   **Other forms of blastomycosis**

     B40.81   **Blastomycotic meningoencephalitis** 🪙
         Meningomyelitis due to blastomycosis

     B40.89   **Other forms of blastomycosis** 🪙

B40.9   **Blastomycosis, unspecified** 🪙

● **B41**   **Paracoccidioidomycosis**
     Fungal infection usually chronic that begins in lungs, spreads to mucocutaneous areas which may extend to skin, tonsils, gastrointestinal lymphatics, liver, and spleen; AKA Almeida or Lutz-Splendore-Almeida disease, Brazilian or South American blastomycosis, or paracoccidioidal granuloma

     Includes   Brazilian blastomycosis
         Lutz' disease

     (Ex) **For category B41 CC codes:** B41.0-B41.9, B48.3, B49, B92, B94.2-B94.9

B41.0   **Pulmonary paracoccidioidomycosis** 🪙

B41.7   **Disseminated paracoccidioidomycosis** 🪙
     Generalized paracoccidioidomycosis

B41.8   **Other forms of paracoccidioidomycosis** 🪙

B41.9   **Paracoccidioidomycosis, unspecified** 🪙

● **B42**   **Sporotrichosis**
     Chronic fungal infection with nodular lesions

B42.0   **Pulmonary sporotrichosis**

B42.1   **Lymphocutaneous sporotrichosis**

B42.7   **Disseminated sporotrichosis**
     Generalized sporotrichosis

● **B42.8**   **Other forms of sporotrichosis**

     B42.81   **Cerebral sporotrichosis**
         Meningitis due to sporotrichosis

     B42.82   **Sporotrichosis arthritis**

     B42.89   **Other forms of sporotrichosis**

B42.9   **Sporotrichosis, unspecified**

● **B43**   **Chromomycosis and pheomycotic abscess**
     Chronic fungal infection of skin, initiated at site of puncture affecting lower limb or foot (mossy foot)

B43.0   **Cutaneous chromomycosis**
     Dermatitis verrucosa

B43.1   **Pheomycotic brain abscess**
     Cerebral chromomycosis

B43.2   **Subcutaneous pheomycotic abscess and cyst**

B43.8   **Other forms of chromomycosis**

B43.9   **Chromomycosis, unspecified**

● **B44**   **Aspergillosis**
     Infection marked by inflammatory lesions in skin, ear, orbit, nasal sinuses, lungs, and occasionally bones and meninges

     Includes   aspergilloma

     (Ex) **For category B44 CC codes unless otherwise indicated:** B44.1-B44.7, B44.89-B44.9, B48.3-B48.4, B49, B92, B94.2-B94.9

B44.0   **Invasive pulmonary aspergillosis** 🪙
     MCC when PDx is its own MCC
     (Ex) See B25.0

B44.1   **Other pulmonary aspergillosis** 🪙

B44.2   **Tonsillar aspergillosis** 🪙

B44.7   **Disseminated aspergillosis** 🪙
     Generalized aspergillosis

● **B44.8**   **Other forms of aspergillosis**

     B44.81   **Allergic bronchopulmonary aspergillosis** 🪙
         (Ex) B44.81, J22, J98.8-J98.9

     B44.89   **Other forms of aspergillosis**

B44.9   **Aspergillosis, unspecified** 🪙

● **B45**   **Cryptococcosis**
     Infection in the immunocompromised and fatal if left untreated; AKA torulosis, Buschke, or Busse-Buschke disease

     (Ex) **For category B45 CC codes unless otherwise indicated:** B45.0, B45.2-B45.9, B48.3, B49, B92, B94.2-B94.9

B45.0   **Pulmonary cryptococcosis** 🪙

B45.1   **Cerebral cryptococcosis** 🪙
     Cryptococcal meningitis
     Cryptococcosis meningocerebralis
     MCC when PDx is its own MCC
     (Ex) A02.21, A17.0-A17.1, A27.81, A39.0, A50.41, A51.41, A52.13, A54.82, A54.84, A54.89-A54.9, A87.0-A87.9, B00.3, B02.1, B26.1, B37.5, B38.4, B45.1, B58.2, E08.40-E08.49, E08.618-E08.638, E08.649-E08.8, E09.40-E09.49, E09.618-E09.638, E09.649-E09.8, E10.40-E10.49, E10.618-E10.638, E10.649, E10.69, E10.8, E11.40-E11.49, E11.618-E11.638, E11.649, E11.69-E11.8, E13.40-E13.49, E13.618-E13.638, E13.649-E13.69, E13.8, G00.0-G03.9, G04.2, G32.89, G61.0, G96.8-G96.9, G98.0-G98.8, G99.8

B45.2   **Cutaneous cryptococcosis** 🪙

B45.3   **Osseous cryptococcosis** 🪙

B45.7   **Disseminated cryptococcosis** 🪙
     Generalized cryptococcosis

B45.8   **Other forms of cryptococcosis** 🪙

B45.9   **Cryptococcosis, unspecified** 🪙

● **B46**   **Zygomycosis**
     Fungal infections including subcutaneous lesions and infection of sinuses, brain, or lungs

     (Ex) **For category B46 CC codes:** B46.0-B46.9, B48.3, B49, B92, B94.2-B94.9

B46.0   **Pulmonary mucormycosis** 🪙
     Fungal infection affecting lung

B46.1   **Rhinocerebral mucormycosis** 🪙

B46.2   **Gastrointestinal mucormycosis** 🪙

B46.3   **Cutaneous mucormycosis** 🪙
     Subcutaneous mucormycosis

B46.4   **Disseminated mucormycosis** 🪙
     Generalized mucormycosis

B46.5   **Mucormycosis, unspecified** 🪙

B46.8   **Other zygomycoses** 🪙
     Entomophthoromycosis

B46.9   **Zygomycosis, unspecified** 🪙
     Phycomycosis NOS

N   Newborn Age: 0   **P**   Pediatric Age: 0–17   **M**   Maternity DX: 12–55   **A**   Adult Age: 15–124   ♀   Females Only   ♂   Males Only

🪙   Complication\Comorbidity   🪙   Major C\C   (Ex)   CC/MCC Exclusions   🪙   Hospital-Acquired Condition

● **B47**   **Mycetoma**
Slow progressive, destructive fungal infection of cutaneous and subcutaneous tissues, fascia, and bone, primarily seen in foot (Madura foot) or leg

    B47.0   **Eumycetoma** 🦠
        Madura foot, mycotic Maduromycosis
        (Ex) B47.0, B48.3, B49, B92, B94.2-B94.9

    B47.1   **Actinomycetoma** 🦠
        (Ex) A42.0-A42.2, A42.81-A43.9, B47.1-B47.9, L08.1

    B47.9   **Mycetoma, unspecified**
        Madura foot NOS
        (Ex) A42.81-A42.9, A43.8-A43.9, B47.1-B47.9

● **B48**   **Other mycoses, not elsewhere classified**

    B48.0   **Lobomycosis**
        Infection with symptoms of red, smooth, hard cutaneous nodules resembling keloids
        Keloidal blastomycosis
        Lobo's disease

    B48.1   **Rhinosporidiosis**
        Chronic, localized granulomatous fungal infection, affecting mucocutaneous tissues, usually of nose characterized by polyps, papillomas, and wartlike lesions

    B48.2   **Allescheriasis** 🦠
        Fungal infection
        Infection due to Pseudallescheria boydii
        Excludes1   eumycetoma (B47.0)
        (Ex) B48.2-B48.3, B49, B92, B94.2-B94.9

    B48.3   **Geotrichosis** 🦠
        Fungal infection usually of bronchi, lungs, mouth, or intestinal tract
        Geotrichum stomatitis
        (Ex) B48.3, B49

    B48.4   **Penicillosis** 🦠
        Fungal infection
        (Ex) B44.1-B44.7, B44.89-B44.9, B48.3-B48.4, B49, B92, B94.2-B94.9

    B48.8   **Other specified mycoses** 🦠
        Adiaspiromycosis
        Infection of tissue and organs by Alternaria
        Infection of tissue and organs by Drechslera
        Infection of tissue and organs by Fusarium
        Infection of tissue and organs by saprophytic fungi NEC
        (Ex) B48.3, B48.8-B49, B92, B94.2-B94.9

● **B49**   **Unspecified mycosis** 🦠
      Fungemia NOS
      (Ex) B48.3, B49

PROTOZOAL DISEASES (B50-B64)

    Excludes1   amebiasis (A06.-)
                other protozoal intestinal diseases (A07.-)

● **B50**   **Plasmodium falciparum malaria**
Severe form of malaria that can be fatal
    Includes   mixed infections of Plasmodium falciparum with any other Plasmodium species
    (Ex) For category B50 CC codes: B50.0-B57.5

    B50.0   **Plasmodium falciparum malaria with cerebral complications** 🦠
        Cerebral malaria NOS

    B50.8   **Other severe and complicated Plasmodium falciparum malaria**
        Severe or complicated Plasmodium falciparum malaria NOS

    B50.9   **Plasmodium falciparum malaria, unspecified** 🦠

● **B51**   **Plasmodium vivax malaria**
    Includes   mixed infections of Plasmodium vivax with other Plasmodium species, except Plasmodium falciparum
    Excludes1   plasmodium vivax with Plasmodium falciparum (B50.-)
    (Ex) For category B51 CC codes unless otherwise indicated: B50.0-B57.5

    B51.0   **Plasmodium vivax malaria with rupture of spleen** 🦠
    B51.8   **Plasmodium vivax malaria with other complications** 🦠
    B51.9   **Plasmodium vivax malaria without complication** 🦠
        Plasmodium vivax malaria NOS
        (Ex) A44.0-A44.9, A68.0-A68.9, A69.20-A69.29, B50.0-B57.5, B60.0

● **B52**   **Plasmodium malariae malaria**
Causes fever that recurs at approximately three-day intervals (quartan fever), longer than two-day (tertian) intervals of other malarial parasites
    Includes   mixed infections of Plasmodium malariae with other Plasmodium species, except Plasmodium falciparum and Plasmodium vivax
    Excludes1   plasmodium falciparum (B50.-)
                plasmodium vivax (B51.-)
    (Ex) For category B52 CC codes unless otherwise indicated: B50.0-B57.5

    B52.0   **Plasmodium malariae malaria with nephropathy** 🦠
        CC when PDx is its own CC
        (Ex) A17.9, A18.10-A18.13, A18.82, A18.84, A18.89, A54.21, A54.29, A54.82, A54.84, A54.89-A54.9, A59.00, A59.8-A59.9, B37.41-B37.49, B50.0-B57.5, E08.21-E08.29, E08.618, E08.620-E08.638, E08.649-E08.8, E09.21-E09.29, E09.618-E09.638, E09.649-E09.8, E10.21-E10.29, E10.618-E10.638, E10.649, E10.69-E10.8, E11.21-E11.29, E11.618-E11.638, E11.649, E11.69-E11.8, E13.21-E13.29, E13.618-E13.638, E13.649-E13.8, E88.3, M10.30-M10.39, N00.0-N11.0, N11.8-N13.39, N13.6, N14.0-N19, N25.0-N26.1, N26.9-N27.9, N28.1-N29, N36.41-N36.43, N36.8-N36.9, N39.8-N39.9, R31.0-R31.9

    B52.8   **Plasmodium malariae malaria with other complications** 🦠
    B52.9   **Plasmodium malariae malaria without complication** 🦠
        Plasmodium malariae malaria NOS

● **B53**   **Other specified malaria**
    (Ex) For category B53 CC codes unless otherwise indicated: B50.0-B57.5

    B53.0   **Plasmodium ovale malaria** 🦠
        Least diagnosed type of malaria spread by female mosquitoes of rare species
        Excludes1   plasmodium ovale with Plasmodium falciparum (B50.-)
                      plasmodium ovale with Plasmodium malariae (B52.-)
                      plasmodium ovale with Plasmodium vivax (B51.-)

    B53.1   **Malaria due to simian plasmodia** 🦠
        Malaria-like disease (parasite infection)
        Excludes1   malaria due to simian plasmodia with Plasmodium falciparum (B50.-)
                      malaria due to simian plasmodia with Plasmodium malariae (B52.-)
                      malaria due to simian plasmodia with Plasmodium ovale (B53.0)
                      malaria due to simian plasmodia with Plasmodium vivax (B51.-)

    B53.8   **Other malaria, not elsewhere classified** 🦠

● **B54**   **Unspecified malaria** 🦠
    (Ex) B50.0-B57.5, B97.21

● **B55**   **Leishmaniasis**
Protozoal infection
    (Ex) For category B55 CC codes: A44.0-A44.9, A68.0-A68.9, A69.20-A69.29, A75.0-A79.9, B50.0-B57.5, B60.0

    B55.0   **Visceral leishmaniasis** 🦠
        Kala-azar
        Post-kala-azar dermal leishmaniasis

    B55.1   **Cutaneous leishmaniasis** 🦠
    B55.2   **Mucocutaneous leishmaniasis** 🦠
    B55.9   **Leishmaniasis, unspecified** 🦠

◀ New   ◀▬ Revised   ~~deleted~~ Deleted   Excludes 1   Excludes 2   Includes   Use additional   Code first   Code also   Unspecified

662   OGCR Official Guidelines   ● Unacceptable Principal Diagnosis   X Assign placeholder X   ● Use Additional Character(s)   ▌ Manifestation Code   **Coding Clinic**

● **B56** **African trypanosomiasis**
   Human African trypanosomiasis (HAT) is transmitted by fly bites
   (Ex) **For category B56 CC codes:** A44.0-A44.9, A68.0-A68.9, A69.20-A69.29, A75.0-A79.9, B50.0-B57.5, B60.0

   B56.0 **Gambiense trypanosomiasis** 🔒
      Infection due to Trypanosoma brucei gambiense
      West African sleeping sickness

   B56.1 **Rhodesiense trypanosomiasis** 🔒
      East African sleeping sickness
      Infection due to Trypanosoma brucei rhodesiense

   B56.9 **African trypanosomiasis, unspecified** 🔒
      Sleeping sickness NOS

● **B57** **Chagas' disease**
   Tropical parasitic disease
Includes	American trypanosomiasis
	infection due to Trypanosoma cruzi

   B57.0 **Acute Chagas' disease with heart involvement** 🔒
      Acute Chagas' disease with myocarditis
      (Ex) B57.0, B57.2, B92, B94.2-B94.9

   B57.1 **Acute Chagas' disease without heart involvement** 🔒
      Acute Chagas' disease NOS
      (Ex) See B56

   B57.2 **Chagas' disease (chronic) with heart involvement** 🔒
      American trypanosomiasis NOS
      Chagas' disease (chronic) NOS
      Chagas' disease (chronic) with myocarditis
      Trypanosomiasis NOS
      (Ex) See B57.0

● **B57.3** **Chagas' disease (chronic) with digestive system involvement**
      (Ex) **For category B57.3 CC codes:** A44.0-A44.9, A68.0-A68.9, A69.20-A69.29, A75.0-A79.9, B50.0-B57.5, B60.0

   B57.30 **Chagas' disease with digestive system involvement, unspecified** 🔒

   B57.31 **Megaesophagus in Chagas' disease** 🔒

   B57.32 **Megacolon in Chagas' disease** 🔒

   B57.39 **Other digestive system involvement in Chagas' disease** 🔒

● **B57.4** **Chagas' disease (chronic) with nervous system involvement**
      (Ex) **For category B57.4 CC codes:** A44.0-A44.9, A68.0-A68.9, A69.20-A69.29, A75.0-A79.9, B50.0-B57.5, B60.0

   B57.40 **Chagas' disease with nervous system involvement, unspecified** 🔒

   B57.41 **Meningitis in Chagas' disease** 🔒

   B57.42 **Meningoencephalitis in Chagas' disease** 🔒

   B57.49 **Other nervous system involvement in Chagas' disease** 🔒

   B57.5 **Chagas' disease (chronic) with other organ involvement** 🔒
      (Ex) See B57.4

● **B58** **Toxoplasmosis**
   Infection by protozoon transmitted in cysts in feces of cats
Includes	infection due to Toxoplasma gondii
Excludes1	congenital toxoplasmosis (P37.1)

● **B58.0** **Toxoplasma oculopathy**

   B58.00 **Toxoplasma oculopathy, unspecified** 🔒
      (Ex) B58.00, B58.82-B58.9, B92, B94.2-B94.9

   B58.01 **Toxoplasma chorioretinitis** 🔒
      (Ex) B58.00-B58.01, B58.82-B58.9, B92, B94.2-B94.9

   B58.09 **Other toxoplasma oculopathy** 🔒
      Toxoplasma uveitis
      (Ex) B58.00, B58.09, B58.82-B58.9, B92, B94.2-B94.9

   B58.1 **Toxoplasma hepatitis** 🔒
      (Ex) B58.00, B58.1, B58.82-B58.9, B92, B94.2-B94.9

   B58.2 **Toxoplasma meningoencephalitis** 🔒
      (Ex) B58.00, B58.2, B58.82-B58.9, B92, B94.2-B94.9

Item 1–22 **Toxoplasmosis** is caused by the protozoa **Toxoplasma gondii,** of which the house cat can be a host. Human infection occurs when contact is made with materials containing the pathogen, such as feces, contaminated soil, or ingestion of infected lamb, goat, or pork. Of the infected, very few have symptoms because a healthy person's immune system keeps the parasite from causing illness. When the immune system is compromised, symptoms may occur. Clinical symptoms include flu-like symptoms, but the disease progresses to include the eyes and the brain in babies.

   B58.3 **Pulmonary toxoplasmosis** 🔒
      (Ex) A22.1, A37.01, A37.11, A37.81, A37.91, A48.1, B25.0, B44.0, B58.00, B58.3, B58.82-B58.9, B92, B94.2-B94.9, J09.X1-J09.X2, J10.00-J10.1, J11.00-J11.1, J12.0-J12.3, J12.89-J18.1, J18.8-J18.9, J44.9, J47.0-J70.4, J70.8-J70.9, J98.4, R91.1

● **B58.8** **Toxoplasmosis with other organ involvement**
      (Ex) **For category B58.8 CC codes unless otherwise indicated:** B58.00, B58.82-B58.9, B92, B94.2-B94.9

   B58.81 **Toxoplasma myocarditis** 🔒
      (Ex) B58.00, B58.81-B58.9, B92, B94.2-B94.9

   B58.82 **Toxoplasma myositis** 🔒

   B58.83 **Toxoplasma tubulo-interstitial nephropathy** 🔒
      Toxoplasma pyelonephritis

   B58.89 **Toxoplasmosis with other organ involvement** 🔒

   B58.9 **Toxoplasmosis, unspecified** 🔒
      (Ex) B58.9

● **B59** **Pneumocystosis** 🔒
      Caused by fungus
      Pneumonia due to Pneumocystis carinii
      Pneumonia due to Pneumocystis jiroveci
      (Ex) A22.1, A37.01, A37.11, A37.81, A37.91, A48.1, B25.0, B44.0, B59, B92, B94.2-B94.9, J09.X1-J09.X2, J10.00-J10.1, J11.00-J11.1, J12.0-J12.3, J12.89-J15.20, J15.211-J18.1, J18.8-J18.9, J44.9, J47.0-J70.4, J70.8-J70.9, J98.4, R91.1

● **B60** **Other protozoal diseases, not elsewhere classified**
Excludes1	cryptosporidiosis (A07.2)
	intestinal microsporidiosis (A07.8)
	isosporiasis (A07.3)

   B60.0 **Babesiosis**
      Tickborne disease caused by microscopic organisms
      Piroplasmosis
      (Ex) A44.0-A44.9, A68.0-A68.9, A69.20-A69.29, A75.0-A79.9, B50.0-B57.5, B60.0

● **B60.1** **Acanthamebiasis**
      (Ex) **For category B60.1 CC codes:** B59, B60.10-B60.11, B60.19-B64, B89, B99.8-B99.9, L94.6, M35.2

   B60.10 **Acanthamebiasis, unspecified** 🔒

   B60.11 **Meningoencephalitis due to Acanthamoeba (culbertsoni)**

   B60.12 **Conjunctivitis due to Acanthamoeba**

● **B60.13** **Keratoconjunctivitis due to Acanthamoeba**

   B60.19 **Other acanthamebic disease** 🔒

   B60.2 **Naegleriasis** 🔒
      Infection with microscopic organisms
      Primary amebic meningoencephalitis
      (Ex) B59, B60.10-B60.11, B60.19-B64, B89, B99.8-B99.9, L94.6, M35.2

   B60.8 **Other specified protozoal diseases**
      Microsporidiosis

   B64 **Unspecified protozoal disease**

HELMINTHIASES (B65-B83)
Diseases or infestations caused by parasitic worms

● **B65** **Schistosomiasis [bilharziasis]**
   Infection with flukes (flat parasitic worms)
Includes	snail fever
   (Ex) **For category B64 CC codes:** B65.0-B65.9

   B65.0 **Schistosomiasis due to Schistosoma haematobium [urinary schistosomiasis]** 🔒

   B65.1 **Schistosomiasis due to Schistosoma mansoni [intestinal schistosomiasis]** 🔒

CHAPTER 1 (A00-B99)

B65.2   **Schistosomiasis due to Schistosoma japonicum** 🔖
             Asiatic schistosomiasis

B65.3   **Cercarial dermatitis** 🔖
             Swimmer's itch

B65.8   **Other schistosomiasis** 🔖
             Infection due to Schistosoma intercalatum
             Infection due to Schistosoma mattheei
             Infection due to Schistosoma mekongi

B65.9   **Schistosomiasis, unspecified** 🔖

● **B66**   **Other fluke infections**
             Trematode (parasitic worms)
             (Ex) For category B66 CC codes: B66.0-B66.9

B66.0   **Opisthorchiasis** 🔖
             Infection due to cat liver fluke
             Infection due to Opisthorchis (felineus)(viverrini)

B66.1   **Clonorchiasis** 🔖
             Chinese liver fluke disease
             Infection due to Clonorchis sinensis
             Oriental liver fluke disease

B66.2   **Dicroceliasis** 🔖
             Liver fluke
             Infection due to Dicrocoelium dendriticum
             Lancet fluke infection

B66.3   **Fascioliasis** 🔖
             Infection due to Fasciola gigantica
             Infection due to Fasciola hepatica
             Infection due to Fasciola indica
             Sheep liver fluke disease

B66.4   **Paragonimiasis** 🔖
             Infection due to Paragonimus species
             Lung fluke disease
             Pulmonary distomiasis

B66.5   **Fasciolopsiasis** 🔖
             Largest intestinal fluke in humans
             Infection due to Fasciolopsis buski
             Intestinal distomiasis

B66.8   **Other specified fluke infections** 🔖
             Echinostomiasis
             Heterophyiasis
             Metagonimiasis
             Nanophyetiasis
             Watsoniasis

B66.9   **Fluke infection, unspecified** 🔖

● **B67**   **Echinococcosis**
             Larval forms of tapeworms usually of liver or lungs
             Includes   hydatidosis

B67.0   **Echinococcus granulosus infection of liver** 🔖
             (Ex) B67.0, B67.8-B67.99

B67.1   **Echinococcus granulosus infection of lung** 🔖
             (Ex) B67.1, B67.8-B67.99, J12.81

B67.2   **Echinococcus granulosus infection of bone** 🔖
             (Ex) B67.2, B67.32-B67.39, B67.8-B67.99

● **B67.3** **Echinococcus granulosus infection, other and multiple sites**

B67.31   **Echinococcus granulosus infection, thyroid gland** 🔖
             (Ex) B67.31, B67.8-B67.99

B67.32   **Echinococcus granulosus infection, multiple sites** 🔖
             (Ex) See B67.2

B67.39   **Echinococcus granulosus infection, other sites** 🔖
             (Ex) See B67.2

B67.4   **Echinococcus granulosus infection, unspecified** 🔖
             Dog tapeworm (infection)
             (Ex) B67.4, B67.8-B67.99

B67.5   **Echinococcus multilocularis infection of liver** 🔖
             (Ex) B67.5, B67.8-B67.99

Item 1-23 Echinococcosis: Also known as hydatid disease; is caused by Echinococcus granulosus, E. multilocularis, and E. vogeli tapeworms; and is contracted from infected food. Found in southern South America, the Mediterranean, the Middle East, central Asia, and Africa and uncommon in the United States but has been reported in California, New Mexico, Arizona and Utah. The disease is treated with medication over a long course as it is resistive.

● **B67.6** **Echinococcus multilocularis infection, other and multiple sites**
             (Ex) For category B67.6 CC codes: B67.61-B67.69, B67.8-B67.99

B67.61   **Echinococcus multilocularis infection, multiple sites** 🔖

B67.69   **Echinococcus multilocularis infection, other sites** 🔖

B67.7   **Echinococcus multilocularis infection, unspecified** 🔖
             (Ex) B67.7-B67.99

B67.8   **Echinococcosis, unspecified, of liver** 🔖
             (Ex) B67.8-B67.99

● **B67.9** **Echinococcosis, other and unspecified**
             (Ex) For category B67.9 CC codes: B67.8-B67.99

B67.90   **Echinococcosis, unspecified** 🔖
             Echinococcosis NOS

B67.99   **Other echinococcosis** 🔖

● **B68**   **Taeniasis**
             Intestinal tapeworm (cestode) infection from raw or undercooked meat of infected animal
             Excludes1   cysticercosis (B69.-)

B68.0   **Taenia solium taeniasis** 🔖
             Pork tapeworm (infection)
             (Ex) A00.1, A01.00-A01.09, A01.4-A02.0, A03.9-A05.2, A06.0-A06.2, A06.9, A07.1-A09, A18.32-A18.39, A18.83, A48.51-A48.52, B37.82, B68.0-B71.9, B82.9, J09.X3-J09.X9, J10.2-J10.89, J11.2-J11.89, K30, K31.84, K52.1-K52.3, K52.82-K52.9, K58.0-K58.9, P76.8-P77.9, P78.1, P78.3-P78.89

B68.1   **Taenia saginata taeniasis** 🔖
             Beef tapeworm (infection)
             Infection due to adult tapeworm Taenia saginata
             (Ex) B68.0-B71.9

B68.9   **Taeniasis, unspecified** 🔖
             (Ex) B68.0-B71.9

● **B69**   **Cysticercosis**
             Systemic illness caused by the larvae of pork tapeworm
             Includes   cysticerciasis infection due to larval form of Taenia solium
             (Ex) For category B69 CC codes: B68.0-B71.9

B69.0   **Cysticercosis of central nervous system** 🔖

B69.1   **Cysticercosis of eye** 🔖

● **B69.8** **Cysticercosis of other sites**

B69.81   **Myositis in cysticercosis** 🔖

B69.89   **Cysticercosis of other sites** 🔖

B69.9   **Cysticercosis, unspecified** 🔖

● **B70**   **Diphyllobothriasis and sparganosis**
             Infection with tapeworms seen most often from inadequately cooked fish
             (Ex) For category B70 CC codes: B68.0-B71.9

B70.0   **Diphyllobothriasis** 🔖
             Diphyllobothrium (adult) (latum) (pacificum) infection
             Fish tapeworm (infection)
             Excludes2   larval diphyllobothriasis (B70.1)

B70.1   **Sparganosis** 🔖
             Infection with migrating tapeworm larvae, which invade subcutaneous tissues, causing inflammation and fibrosis that resembles cellulitis
             Infection due to Sparganum (mansoni) (proliferum)
             Infection due to Spirometra larva
             Larval diphyllobothriasis
             Spirometrosis

● **B71**   **Other cestode infections**
     (Ex:) **For category B71 CC codes:** B68.0-B71.9

     B71.0   **Hymenolepiasis** 🔖
         Intestinal infestation with tapeworms
         Dwarf tapeworm infection
         Rat tapeworm (infection)

     B71.1   **Dipylidiasis** 🔖
         Infection with tapeworm common to dogs and cats and seen
         in children having close contact with infected pets

     B71.8   **Other specified cestode infections** 🔖
         Infection by the larval stage of a tapeworm, usually through
         fruit or vegetables
         Coenurosis

     B71.9   **Cestode infection, unspecified**
         Tapeworm (infection) NOS

● **B72**   **Dracunculiasis** 🔖
     Infection with roundworms
     Includes   guinea worm infection
                 infection due to Dracunculus medinensis
     (Ex:) B72-B74.9

● **B73**   **Onchocerciasis**
     Infection with parasitic worm
     Includes   onchocerca volvulus infection
                 onchocercosis
                 river blindness

    ● **B73.0**   **Onchocerciasis with eye disease**
         (Ex:) **For category B73 CC codes:** B72-B74.9

         B73.00   **Onchocerciasis with eye involvement,**
                unspecified 🔖

         B73.01   **Onchocerciasis with endophthalmitis** 🔖

         B73.02   **Onchocerciasis with glaucoma** 🔖

         B73.09   **Onchocerciasis with other eye involvement** 🔖
                Infestation of eyelid due to onchocerciasis

     B73.1   **Onchocerciasis without eye disease** 🔖

● **B74**   **Filariasis**
     Infestation with slender threadlike worms
     Excludes2   onchocerciasis (B73)
                   tropical (pulmonary) eosinophilia NOS (J82)
     (Ex:) **For category B74 CC codes:** B72-B74.9

     B74.0   **Filariasis due to Wuchereria bancrofti** 🔖
         Bancroftian elephantiasis
         Bancroftian filariasis

     B74.1   **Filariasis due to Brugia malayi** 🔖

     B74.2   **Filariasis due to Brugia timori** 🔖

     B74.3   **Loiasis** 🔖
         Infection with round worms growing in subcutaneous
         connective tissue
         Calabar swelling
         Eyeworm disease of Africa
         Loa loa infection

     B74.4   **Mansonelliasis** 🔖
         Infection with filarial parasite
         Infection due to Mansonella ozzardi
         Infection due to Mansonella perstans
         Infection due to Mansonella streptocerca

     B74.8   **Other filariases** 🔖
         Dirofilariasis

     B74.9   **Filariasis, unspecified** 🔖

● **B75**   **Trichinellosis** 🔖
     Infestation with parasitic roundworms ingested in undercooked
     contaminated meat
     Includes   infection due to Trichinella species trichiniasis
     (Ex:) A17.82, A50.42, A52.14, A75.9, A79.9, A81.1, A81.82-A81.89, A83.0-A85.8, A87.2,
         A88.0, A88.8, A92.1-A92.8, A93.0, B00.4, B00.82, B01.11-B01.12, B04, B06.01,
         B08.09, B08.20-B08.22, B08.60-B08.79, B09, B10.01-B10.09, B26.2, B33.1, B45.0,
         B45.2-B45.9, B58.2, B75, B97.10, B97.21, G04.00-G04.01, G04.31, G04.81-G05.4,
         G37.0, G37.4-G37.5, J09.X3-J09.X9, J10.2-J10.89, J11.2-J11.89, L44.4,
         M1A.10X0-M1A.10X1, M1A.1110-M1A.19X1, P35.2-P35.9, P37.0-P37.4, P37.8-P37.9,
         T56.0X1-T56.0X4[A]

● **B76**   **Hookworm diseases**
     Occurs in hot, humid parts of world where larvae are soil borne, enter
     digestive tract through skin of feet/legs or in contaminated food/
     water; AKA ground itch
     Includes   uncinariasis
     (Ex:) **For category B76 CC codes:** B76.0-B76.9

     B76.0   **Ancylostomiasis** 🔖
         Infection due to Ancylostoma species

     B76.1   **Necatoriasis** 🔖
         Infection due to Necator americanus

     B76.8   **Other hookworm diseases** 🔖

     B76.9   **Hookworm disease, unspecified** 🔖
         Cutaneous larva migrans NOS

● **B77**   **Ascariasis**
     Infection by roundworm in small intestine
     Includes   ascaridiasis
                  roundworm infection

     B77.0   **Ascariasis with intestinal complications** 🔖
         (Ex:) B77.0-B78.0, B78.7-B82.0

    ● **B77.8**   **Ascariasis with other complications**

         B77.81   **Ascariasis pneumonia** 🔖
                MCC when PDx is its own MCC
                (Ex:) A15.0-A15.6, A15.8-A15.9, A17.9, A18.82, A18.84, A18.89,
                    A21.2, A22.1, A31.0, A37.01, A37.11, A37.81, A37.91, A42.0,
                    A43.0, A48.1, B25.0, B39.0-B39.2, B44.0, B58.3, B59, B67.1,
                    B77.0-B78.0, B78.7-B82.0, J09.X1-J09.X2, J10.00-J10.1,
                    J11.00-J11.1, J12.0-J12.3, J12.89-J18.1, J18.8-J18.9, J22,
                    J44.9, J47.0-J70.4, J70.8-J70.9, J98.4, J98.8-J99, Q33.4,
                    R91.1

         B77.89   **Ascariasis with other complications** 🔖
                (Ex:) See B77.0

     B77.9   **Ascariasis, unspecified** 🔖
         (Ex:) See B77.0

● **B78**   **Strongyloidiasis**
     Infection with adult female roundworms
     Excludes1   trichostrongyliasis (B81.2)
     (Ex:) **For category B78 CC codes:** B77.0-B78.0, B78.7-B82.0

     B78.0   **Intestinal strongyloidiasis** 🔖

     B78.1   **Cutaneous strongyloidiasis**

     B78.7   **Disseminated strongyloidiasis** 🔖

     B78.9   **Strongyloidiasis, unspecified** 🔖

● **B79**   **Trichuriasis** 🔖
     Intestinal infection with roundworms
     Includes   trichocephaliasis
                  whipworm (disease)(infection)
     (Ex:) See B78

● **B80**   **Enterobiasis** 🔖
     Intestinal infection with pinworms
     Includes   oxyuriasis
                  pinworm infection
                  threadworm infection
     (Ex:) See B78

● **B81**   **Other intestinal helminthiases, not elsewhere classified**
     Diseases or infestations caused by parasitic worms
     Excludes1   angiostrongyliasis due to Parastrongylus
                   cantonensis (B83.2)
     (Ex:) **For category B81 CC codes** B81.0-B81.2: B77.0-B78.0, B78.7-B82.0 **For category**
     B81 CC codes B81.3-B81.8: B77.0-B78.0, B78.7-B83.3, B83.8-B83.9

     B81.0   **Anisakiasis** 🔖
         Roundworm infection via contaminated undercooked infected
         fish or marine mammals
         Infection due to Anisakis larva

     B81.1   **Intestinal capillariasis** 🔖
         Infestation with of parasites (nematodes)
         Capillariasis NOS
         Infection due to Capillaria philippinensis
         Excludes2   hepatic capillariasis (B83.8)

     B81.2   **Trichostrongyliasis** 🔖

N Newborn Age: 0   **P** Pediatric Age: 0–17   **M** Maternity DX: 12–55   **A** Adult Age: 15–124   ♀ Females Only   ♂ Males Only
🔖 Complication\Comorbidity   🔖 Major C\C   (Ex:) CC/MCC Exclusions   🔖 Hospital-Acquired Condition
665

B81.3   Intestinal angiostrongyliasis 🔗
Angiostrongyliasis due to Parastrongylus costaricensis

B81.4   Mixed intestinal helminthiases 🔗
Infection due to intestinal helminths classified to more than one of the categories B65.Ø-B81.3 and B81.8
Mixed helminthiasis NOS

B81.8   Other specified intestinal helminthiases 🔗
Infection due to Oesophagostomum species [esophagostomiasis]
Infection due to Ternidens diminutus [ternidensiasis]

● **B82   Unspecified intestinal parasitism**

B82.Ø   Intestinal helminthiasis, `unspecified` 🔗
Infected with worms
Ⓔ See B81.3

B82.9   Intestinal parasitism, `unspecified`

● **B83   Other helminthiases**
Caused by parasitic worms
> **Excludes1**   capillariasis NOS (B81.1)
> **Excludes2**   intestinal capillariasis (B81.1)

B83.Ø   Visceral larva migrans
Prolonged migration of nematode larvae
Toxocariasis

B83.1   Gnathostomiasis
Infection with nematode occurring from ingested undercooked fish contaminated with larvae; larvae migrate to subcutaneous tissue or deeper tissues, results are abscesses
Wandering swelling

B83.2   Angiostrongyliasis due to Parastrongylus cantonensis
Nematode infection caused by eating contaminated raw snails, slugs, or paratenic hosts such as prawns or crabs; larval worms migrate to central nervous system resulting in eosinophilic meningitis
Eosinophilic meningoencephalitis due to Parastrongylus cantonensis
> **Excludes2**   intestinal angiostrongyliasis (B81.3)

B83.3   Syngamiasis
Infestation with gapeworm from turkey, pheasant, guinea fowl, goose, and wild birds
Syngamosis

B83.4   Internal hirudiniasis
Infestation by leeches
> **Excludes2**   external hirudiniasis (B88.3)

B83.8   Other specified helminthiases
Parasitic worm infestation
Acanthocephaliasis
Gongylonemiasis
Hepatic capillariasis
Metastrongyliasis
Thelaziasis

B83.9   Helminthiasis, `unspecified`
Worms NOS
> **Excludes1**   intestinal helminthiasis NOS (B82.Ø)

PEDICULOSIS, ACARIASIS AND OTHER INFESTATIONS (B85-B89)

● **B85   Pediculosis and phthiriasis**
Infestation of lice

B85.Ø   Pediculosis due to Pediculus humanus capitis
Head-louse infestation

B85.1   Pediculosis due to Pediculus humanus corporis
Body-louse infestation

B85.2   Pediculosis, `unspecified`

B85.3   Phthiriasis
Crab or pubic lice
Infestation by crab-louse
Infestation by Phthirus pubis

B85.4   Mixed pediculosis and phthiriasis
Infestation classifiable to more than one of the categories B85.Ø-B85.3

● **B86   Scabies**
Sarcoptic itch
Contagious dermatitis caused by mites

● **B87   Myiasis**
Infestation by fly maggots
> **Includes**   infestation by larva of flies

B87.Ø   Cutaneous myiasis
Creeping myiasis

B87.1   Wound myiasis
Traumatic myiasis

B87.2   Ocular myiasis

B87.3   Nasopharyngeal myiasis
Laryngeal myiasis

B87.4   Aural myiasis

● **B87.8   Myiasis of other sites**

B87.81   Genitourinary myiasis

B87.82   Intestinal myiasis

B87.89   Myiasis of other sites

B87.9   Myiasis, `unspecified`

● **B88   Other infestations**

B88.Ø   Other acariasis
Acarine dermatitis
Dermatitis due to Demodex species
Dermatitis due to Dermanyssus gallinae
Dermatitis due to Liponyssoides sanguineus
Trombiculosis
> **Excludes2**   scabies (B86)

B88.1   Tungiasis [sandflea infestation]
Inflammatory skin disease caused by infestation of fleas

B88.2   Other arthropod infestations
Scarabiasis

B88.3   External hirudiniasis
Leech infestation NOS
> **Excludes2**   internal hirudiniasis (B83.4)

B88.8   Other specified infestations
Infection of topical fresh water fish parasite
Ichthyoparasitism due to Vandellia cirrhosa
Linguatulosis
Porocephaliasis

B88.9   Infestation, `unspecified`
Infestation (skin) NOS
Infestation by mites NOS
Skin parasites NOS

B89   `Unspecified` parasitic disease

SEQUELAE OF INFECTIOUS AND PARASITIC DISEASES (B9Ø-B94)

Note: Categories B9Ø-B94 are to be used to indicate conditions in categories AØØ-B89 as the cause of sequelae, which are themselves classified elsewhere. The 'sequelae' include conditions specified as such; they also include residuals of diseases classifiable to the above categories if there is evidence that the disease itself is no longer present. Codes from these categories are not to be used for chronic infections. Code chronic current infections to active infectious disease as appropriate.

Code first condition resulting from (sequela) the infectious or parasitic disease

● **B9Ø   Sequelae of tuberculosis**
Condition resulting from tuberculosis

B9Ø.Ø   Sequelae of central nervous system tuberculosis

B9Ø.1   Sequelae of genitourinary tuberculosis

B9Ø.2   Sequelae of tuberculosis of bones and joints

B9Ø.8   Sequelae of tuberculosis of other organs
> **Excludes2**   sequelae of respiratory tuberculosis (B9Ø.9)

B9Ø.9   Sequelae of respiratory and `unspecified` tuberculosis
Sequelae of tuberculosis NOS

◀ New   ◀═ Revised   ~~deleted~~ Deleted   Excludes 1   Excludes 2   Includes   Use additional   Code first   Code also   Unspecified
OGCR Official Guidelines   ● Unacceptable Principal Diagnosis   X Assign placeholder X   ● Use Additional Character(s)   ▶ Manifestation Code   **Coding Clinic**

B91   **Sequelae of poliomyelitis**
    Excludes1   postpolio syndrome (G14)

B92   **Sequelae of leprosy**

● B94   **Sequelae of other and unspecified infectious and parasitic diseases**
    B94.0   **Sequelae of trachoma**
    B94.1   **Sequelae of viral encephalitis**
    B94.2   **Sequelae of viral hepatitis**
    B94.8   **Sequelae of other specified infectious and parasitic diseases**
    B94.9   **Sequelae of unspecified infectious and parasitic disease**

OGCR Section I.C.1.b

> Certain infectious and parasitic diseases
> Infectious agents as the cause of diseases classified to other chapters
> Certain infections are classified in chapters other than Chapter 1 and no organism is identified as part of the infection code. In these instances, it is necessary to use an additional code from Chapter 1 to identify the organism. A code from category B95, Streptococcus, Staphylococcus, and Enterococcus as the cause of diseases classified to other chapters, B96, Other bacterial agents as the cause of diseases classified to other chapters, or B97, Viral agents as the cause of diseases classified to other chapters, is to be used as an additional code to identify the organism. An instructional note will be found at the infection code advising that an additional organism code is required.

BACTERIAL AND VIRAL INFECTIOUS AGENTS (B95-B97)

Note: These categories are provided for use as supplementary or additional codes to identify the infectious agent(s) in diseases classified elsewhere.
Code the disease first, then the bacterium. Do not report codes from B95-B97 for sepsis.

● B95   **Streptococcus, Staphylococcus, and Enterococcus as the cause of diseases classified elsewhere**
    B95.0   **Streptococcus, group A, as the cause of diseases classified elsewhere**
    B95.1   **Streptococcus, group B, as the cause of diseases classified elsewhere**
    B95.2   **Enterococcus as the cause of diseases classified elsewhere**
    B95.3   **Streptococcus pneumoniae as the cause of diseases classified elsewhere**
    B95.4   **Other streptococcus as the cause of diseases classified elsewhere**
    B95.5   **Unspecified streptococcus as the cause of diseases classified elsewhere**
  ● B95.6   **Staphylococcus aureus as the cause of diseases classified elsewhere**
        B95.61   **Methicillin susceptible Staphylococcus aureus infection as the cause of diseases classified elsewhere**
            Methicillin susceptible Staphylococcus aureus (MSSA) infection as the cause of diseases classified elsewhere
            Staphylococcus aureus infection NOS as the cause of diseases classified elsewhere
        B95.62   **Methicillin resistant Staphylococcus aureus infection as the cause of diseases classified elsewhere**
            Methicillin resistant staphylococcus aureus (MRSA) infection as the cause of diseases classified elsewhere
            Coding Clinic: 2016, Q1, P13
    B95.7   **Other staphylococcus as the cause of diseases classified elsewhere**
    B95.8   **Unspecified staphylococcus as the cause of diseases classified elsewhere**

● B96   **Other bacterial agents as the cause of diseases classified elsewhere**
    B96.0   **Mycoplasma pneumoniae [M. pneumoniae] as the cause of diseases classified elsewhere**
        Pleuro-pneumonia-like-organism [PPLO]
    B96.1   **Klebsiella pneumoniae [K. pneumoniae] as the cause of diseases classified elsewhere**
  ● B96.2   **Escherichia coli [E. coli] as the cause of diseases classified elsewhere**
        B96.20   **Unspecified Escherichia coli [E. coli] as the cause of diseases classified elsewhere**
            Escherichia coli [E. coli] NOS
        B96.21   **Shiga toxin-producing Escherichia coli [E. coli] (STEC) O157 as the cause of diseases classified elsewhere**
            E. coli O157:H- (nonmotile) with confirmation of Shiga toxin
            E. coli O157 with confirmation of Shiga toxin when H antigen is unknown, or is not H7
            O157:H7 Escherichia coli [E.coli] with or without confirmation of Shiga toxin-production
            Shiga toxin-producing Escherichia coli [E.coli] O157:H7 with or without confirmation of Shiga toxin-production
            STEC O157:H7 with or without confirmation of Shiga toxin-production
        B96.22   **Other specified Shiga toxin-producing Escherichia coli [E. coli] (STEC) as the cause of diseases classified elsewhere**
            Non-O157 Shiga toxin-producing Escherichia coli [E.coli]
            Non-O157 Shiga toxin-producing Escherichia coli [E.coli] with known O group
        B96.23   **Unspecified Shiga toxin-producing Escherichia coli [E. coli] (STEC) as the cause of diseases classified elsewhere**
            Shiga toxin-producing Escherichia coli [E. coli] with unspecified O group
            STEC NOS
        B96.29   **Other Escherichia coli [E. coli] as the cause of diseases classified elsewhere**
            Non-Shiga toxin-producing E. coli
    B96.3   **Hemophilus influenzae [H. influenzae] as the cause of diseases classified elsewhere**
    B96.4   **Proteus (mirabilis) (morganii) as the cause of diseases classified elsewhere**
    B96.5   **Pseudomonas (aeruginosa) (mallei) (pseudomallei) as the cause of diseases classified elsewhere**
        Coding Clinic: 2015, Q1, P18
    B96.6   **Bacteroides fragilis [B. fragilis] as the cause of diseases classified elsewhere**
    B96.7   **Clostridium perfringens [C. perfringens] as the cause of diseases classified elsewhere**
  ● B96.8   **Other specified bacterial agents as the cause of diseases classified elsewhere**
        B96.81   **Helicobacter pylori [H. pylori] as the cause of diseases classified elsewhere**
        B96.82   **Vibrio vulnificus as the cause of diseases classified elsewhere**
        B96.89   **Other specified bacterial agents as the cause of diseases classified elsewhere**

● B97   **Viral agents as the cause of diseases classified elsewhere**
    B97.0   **Adenovirus as the cause of diseases classified elsewhere**
  ● B97.1   **Enterovirus as the cause of diseases classified elsewhere**
        B97.10   **Unspecified enterovirus as the cause of diseases classified elsewhere**
        B97.11   **Coxsackievirus as the cause of diseases classified elsewhere**
        B97.12   **Echovirus as the cause of diseases classified elsewhere**
        B97.19   **Other enterovirus as the cause of diseases classified elsewhere**

CHAPTER 1 (A00-B99)

N Newborn Age: 0   **P** Pediatric Age: 0–17   **M** Maternity DX: 12–55   **A** Adult Age: 15–124   ♀ Females Only   ♂ Males Only
    Complication\Comorbidity   Major C\C   (Ex) CC/MCC Exclusions   Hospital-Acquired Condition

667

● B97.2 **Coronavirus as the cause of diseases classified elsewhere**

B97.21 **SARS-associated coronavirus as the cause of diseases classified elsewhere** 🔧

> **Excludes1** pneumonia due to SARS-associated coronavirus (J12.81)

> (Ex) A15.0-A15.6, A15.8-A15.9, A17.9, A18.82, A18.84, A18.89, A21.2, A22.1, A31.0, A37.01, A37.11, A37.81, A37.91, A42.0, A43.0, A48.1, B25.0, B34.1-B34.2, B34.4-B34.8, B39.0-B39.2, B44.0, B58.3, B59, B67.1, B97.19-B97.29, B97.5-B97.6, B97.81-B97.89, J09.X1-J09.X2, J10.00-J10.1, J11.00-J11.1, J12.0-J12.3, J12.89-J15.20, J15.211-J18.1, J18.8-J18.9, J22, J44.9, J47.0-J70.4, J70.8-J70.9, J98.4, J98.8-J99, Q33.4, R91.1

B97.29 **Other coronavirus as the cause of diseases classified elsewhere**

● B97.3 **Retrovirus as the cause of diseases classified elsewhere**

> **Excludes1** human immunodeficiency virus [HIV] disease (B20)

B97.30 **Unspecified retrovirus as the cause of diseases classified elsewhere**

B97.31 **Lentivirus as the cause of diseases classified elsewhere**

B97.32 **Oncovirus as the cause of diseases classified elsewhere**

B97.33 **Human T-cell lymphotrophic virus, type I [HTLV-I] as the cause of diseases classified elsewhere** 🔧

> (Ex) A74.81, A74.9, B33.3-B33.4, B34.1-B34.2, B34.4-B34.8, B97.10, B97.19-B97.29, B97.31-B97.39, B97.5-B97.6, B97.81-B97.89

B97.34 **Human T-cell lymphotrophic virus, type II [HTLV-II] as the cause of diseases classified elsewhere** 🔧

> (Ex) A74.81, A74.9, B33.3-B33.4, B34.1-B34.2, B34.4-B34.8, B97.10, B97.19-B97.39, B97.5-B97.6, B97.81, B97.89

Item 1–24 Retrovirus develops by copying its RNA, genetic materials, into the DNA, which then produces new virus particles. It is from the Retroviridae virus family. **Human T-cell lymphotropic virus, Type I (HTLV-I)** is also called human T-cell leukemia virus, Type I, and is a retrovirus thought to cause T-cell leukemia/lymphoma. **Human T-cell lymphotropic virus, Type II (HTLV-II),** is also called human T-cell leukemia virus, Type II, and is a retrovirus associated with hematologic disorders.

HIV-2 is one of the serotypes of HIV and is usually confined to West Africa, whereas HIV-**1** is found worldwide.

B97.35 **Human immunodeficiency virus, type 2 [HIV 2] as the cause of diseases classified elsewhere** 🔧

> (Ex) A74.81, A74.9, B20, B33.3-B33.4, B34.1-B34.2, B34.4, B34.8, B97.10, B97.19-B97.39, B97.5-B97.6, B97.81, B97.89

B97.39 **Other retrovirus as the cause of diseases classified elsewhere**

B97.4 **Respiratory syncytial virus as the cause of diseases classified elsewhere**

B97.5 **Reovirus as the cause of diseases classified elsewhere**

B97.6 **Parvovirus as the cause of diseases classified elsewhere**

B97.7 **Papillomavirus as the cause of diseases classified elsewhere**

● B97.8 **Other viral agents as the cause of diseases classified elsewhere**

B97.81 **Human metapneumovirus as the cause of diseases classified elsewhere**

B97.89 **Other viral agents as the cause of diseases classified elsewhere**

OTHER INFECTIOUS DISEASES (B99)

● B99 **Other and unspecified infectious diseases**

B99.8 **Other infectious disease**

B99.9 **Unspecified infectious disease**

◀ New   ◀▦ Revised   ~~deleted~~ Deleted   Excludes 1   Excludes 2   Includes   Use additional   Code first   Code also   Unspecified

OGCR Official Guidelines   ● Unacceptable Principal Diagnosis   X Assign placeholder X   ● Use Additional Character(s)   ▌ Manifestation Code   **Coding Clinic**

CHAPTER 2

NEOPLASMS (C00-D49)

2. **Chapter 2: Neoplasms (C00-D49)**
General guidelines
Chapter 2 of the ICD-10-CM contains the codes for most benign and all malignant neoplasms. Certain benign neoplasms, such as prostatic adenomas, may be found in the specific body system chapters. To properly code a neoplasm it is necessary to determine from the record if the neoplasm is benign, in-situ, malignant, or of uncertain histologic behavior. If malignant, any secondary (metastatic) sites should also be determined.

Primary malignant neoplasms overlapping site boundaries
A primary malignant neoplasm that overlaps two or more contiguous (next to each other) sites should be classified to the subcategory/code .8 ('overlapping lesion'), unless the combination is specifically indexed elsewhere. For multiple neoplasms of the same site that are not contiguous such as tumors in different quadrants of the same breast, codes for each site should be assigned.

Malignant neoplasm of ectopic tissue
Malignant neoplasms of ectopic tissue are to be coded to the site of origin mentioned, e.g., ectopic pancreatic malignant neoplasms involving the stomach are coded to pancreas, unspecified (C25.9).

The neoplasm table in the Alphabetic Index should be referenced first. However, if the histological term is documented, that term should be referenced first, rather than going immediately to the Neoplasm Table, in order to determine which column in the Neoplasm Table is appropriate. For example, if the documentation indicates "adenoma," refer to the term in the Alphabetic Index to review the entries under this term and the instructional note to "see also neoplasm, by site, benign." The table provides the proper code based on the type of neoplasm and the site. It is important to select the proper column in the table that corresponds to the type of neoplasm. The Tabular List should then be referenced to verify that the correct code has been selected from the table and that a more specific site code does not exist.

See Section I.C.21. Factors influencing health status and contact with health services, Status, for information regarding Z15.0, codes for genetic susceptibility to cancer.

a. **Treatment directed at the malignancy**
If the treatment is directed at the malignancy, designate the malignancy as the principal diagnosis.
The only exception to this guideline is if a patient admission/encounter is solely for the administration of chemotherapy, immunotherapy or radiation therapy, assign the appropriate Z51.— code as the first-listed or principal diagnosis, and the diagnosis or problem for which the service is being performed as a secondary diagnosis.

b. **Treatment of secondary site**
When a patient is admitted because of a primary neoplasm with metastasis and treatment is directed toward the secondary site only, the secondary neoplasm is designated as the principal diagnosis even though the primary malignancy is still present.

c. **Coding and sequencing of complications**
Coding and sequencing of complications associated with the malignancies or with the therapy thereof are subject to the following guidelines:

1) **Anemia associated with malignancy**
When admission/encounter is for management of an anemia associated with the malignancy, and the treatment is only for anemia, the appropriate code for the malignancy is sequenced as the principal or first-listed diagnosis followed by the appropriate code for the anemia (such as code D63.0, Anemia in neoplastic disease).

2) **Anemia associated with chemotherapy, immunotherapy and radiation therapy**
When the admission/encounter is for management of an anemia associated with an adverse effect of the administration of chemotherapy or immunotherapy and the only treatment is for the anemia, the anemia code is sequenced first followed by the appropriate codes for the neoplasm and the adverse effect (T45.1X5, Adverse effect of antineoplastic and immunosuppressive drugs).
When the admission/encounter is for management of an anemia associated with an adverse effect of radiotherapy, the anemia code should be sequenced first, followed by the appropriate neoplasm code and code Y84.2, Radiological procedure and radiotherapy as the cause of abnormal reaction of the patient, or of later complication, without mention of misadventure at the time of the procedure.

3) **Management of dehydration due to the malignancy**
When the admission/encounter is for management of dehydration due to the malignancy and only the dehydration is being treated (intravenous rehydration), the dehydration is sequenced first, followed by the code(s) for the malignancy.

4) **Treatment of a complication resulting from a surgical procedure**
When the admission/encounter is for treatment of a complication resulting from a surgical procedure, designate the complication as the principal or first-listed diagnosis if treatment is directed at resolving the complication.

d. **Primary malignancy previously excised**
When a primary malignancy has been previously excised or eradicated from its site and there is no further treatment directed to that site and there is no evidence of any existing primary malignancy, a code from category Z85, Personal history of malignant neoplasm, should be used to indicate the former site of the malignancy. Any mention of extension, invasion, or metastasis to another site is coded as a secondary malignant neoplasm to that site. The secondary site may be the principal or first-listed with the Z85 code used as a secondary code.

e. **Admissions/Encounters involving chemotherapy, immunotherapy and radiation therapy**

1) **Episode of care involves surgical removal of neoplasm**
When an episode of care involves the surgical removal of a neoplasm, primary or secondary site, followed by adjunct chemotherapy or radiation treatment during the same episode of care, the code for the neoplasm should be assigned as principal or first-listed diagnosis.

2) **Patient admission/encounter solely for administration of chemotherapy, immunotherapy and radiation therapy**
If a patient admission/encounter is solely for the administration of chemotherapy, immunotherapy or radiation therapy assign code Z51.0, Encounter for antineoplastic radiation therapy, or Z51.11, Encounter for antineoplastic chemotherapy, or Z51.12, Encounter for antineoplastic immunotherapy as the first-listed or principal diagnosis. If a patient receives more than one of these therapies during the same admission more than one of these codes may be assigned, in any sequence.
The malignancy for which the therapy is being administered should be assigned as a secondary diagnosis.

3) **Patient admitted for radiation therapy, chemotherapy or immunotherapy and develops complications**
When a patient is admitted for the purpose of radiotherapy, immunotherapy or chemotherapy and develops complications such as uncontrolled nausea and vomiting or dehydration, the principal or first-listed diagnosis is Z51.0, Encounter for antineoplastic radiation therapy, or Z51.11, Encounter for antineoplastic chemotherapy, or Z51.12, Encounter for antineoplastic immunotherapy followed by any codes for the complications.

f. **Admission/encounter to determine extent of malignancy**
When the reason for admission/encounter is to determine the extent of the malignancy, or for a procedure such as paracentesis or thoracentesis, the primary malignancy or appropriate metastatic site is designated as the principal or first-listed diagnosis, even though chemotherapy or radiotherapy is administered.

g. **Symptoms, signs, and abnormal findings listed in Chapter 18 associated with neoplasms**
Symptoms, signs, and ill-defined conditions listed in Chapter 18 characteristic of, or associated with, an existing primary or secondary site malignancy cannot be used to replace the malignancy as principal or first-listed diagnosis, regardless of the number of admissions or encounters for treatment and care of the neoplasm.

See section I.C.21. Factors influencing health status and contact with health services, Encounter for prophylactic organ removal.

h. Admission/encounter for pain control/management
See Section I.C.6. for information on coding admission/encounter for pain control/management.

i. Malignancy in two or more noncontiguous sites
A patient may have more than one malignant tumor in the same organ. These tumors may represent different primaries or metastatic disease, depending on the site. Should the documentation be unclear, the provider should be queried as to the status of each tumor so that the correct codes can be assigned.

j. Disseminated malignant neoplasm, unspecified
Code C80.0, Disseminated malignant neoplasm, unspecified, is for use only in those cases where the patient has advanced metastatic disease and no known primary or secondary sites are specified. It should not be used in place of assigning codes for the primary site and all known secondary sites.

k. Malignant neoplasm without specification of site
Code C80.1, Malignant (primary) neoplasm, unspecified, equates to Cancer, unspecified. This code should only be used when no determination can be made as to the primary site of a malignancy. This code should rarely be used in the inpatient setting.

l. Sequencing of neoplasm codes

1) Encounter for treatment of primary malignancy
If the reason for the encounter is for treatment of a primary malignancy, assign the malignancy as the principal/first-listed diagnosis. The primary site is to be sequenced first, followed by any metastatic sites.

2) Encounter for treatment of secondary malignancy
When an encounter is for a primary malignancy with metastasis and treatment is directed toward the metastatic (secondary) site(s) only, the metastatic site(s) is designated as the principal/first-listed diagnosis. The primary malignancy is coded as an additional code.

3) Malignant neoplasm in a pregnant patient
When a pregnant woman has a malignant neoplasm, a code from subcategory O9A.1-, Malignant neoplasm complicating pregnancy, childbirth, and the puerperium, should be sequenced first, followed by the appropriate code from Chapter 2 to indicate the type of neoplasm.

4) Encounter for complication associated with a neoplasm
When an encounter is for management of a complication associated with a neoplasm, such as dehydration, and the treatment is only for the complication, the complication is coded first, followed by the appropriate code(s) for the neoplasm.

The exception to this guideline is anemia. When the admission/encounter is for management of an anemia associated with the malignancy, and the treatment is only for anemia, the appropriate code for the malignancy is sequenced as the principal or first-listed diagnosis followed by code D63.0, Anemia in neoplastic disease.

5) Complication from surgical procedure for treatment of a neoplasm
When an encounter is for treatment of a complication resulting from a surgical procedure performed for the treatment of the neoplasm, designate the complication as the principal/first-listed diagnosis. See guideline regarding the coding of a current malignancy versus personal history to determine if the code for the neoplasm should also be assigned.

6) Pathologic fracture due to a neoplasm
When an encounter is for a pathological fracture due to a neoplasm, and the focus of treatment is the fracture, a code from subcategory M84.5, Pathological fracture in neoplastic disease, should be sequenced first, followed by the code for the neoplasm.

If the focus of treatment is the neoplasm with an associated pathological fracture, the neoplasm code should be sequenced first, followed by a code from M84.5 for the pathological fracture.

m. Current malignancy versus personal history of malignancy
When a primary malignancy has been excised but further treatment, such as an additional surgery for the malignancy, radiation therapy or chemotherapy is directed to that site, the primary malignancy code should be used until treatment is completed.

When a primary malignancy has been previously excised or eradicated from its site, there is no further treatment (of the malignancy) directed to that site, and there is no evidence of any existing primary malignancy, a code from category Z85, Personal history of malignant neoplasm, should be used to indicate the former site of the malignancy.
See Section I.C.21. Factors influencing health status and contact with health services, History (of)

n. Leukemia, Multiple Myeloma, and Malignant Plasma Cell Neoplasms in remission versus personal history
The categories for leukemia, and category C90, Multiple myeloma and malignant plasma cell neoplasms, have codes indicating whether or not the leukemia has achieved remission. There are also codes Z85.6, Personal history of leukemia, and Z85.79, Personal history of other malignant neoplasms of lymphoid, hematopoietic and related tissues. If the documentation is unclear, as to whether the leukemia has achieved remission, the provider should be queried.
See Section I.C.21. Factors influencing health status and contact with health services, History (of)

o. Aftercare following surgery for neoplasm
See Section I.C.21. Factors influencing health status and contact with health services, Aftercare

p. Follow-up care for completed treatment of a malignancy
See Section I.C.21. Factors influencing health status and contact with health services, Follow-up

q. Prophylactic organ removal for prevention of malignancy
See Section I.C. 21, Factors influencing health status and contact with health services, Prophylactic organ removal

r. Malignant neoplasm associated with transplanted organ
A malignant neoplasm of a transplanted organ should be coded as a transplant complication. Assign first the appropriate code from category T86.-, Complications of transplanted organs and tissue, followed by code C80.2, Malignant neoplasm associated with transplanted organ. Use an additional code for the specific malignancy.

Item 2–1 Neoplasm: Neo = new, plasm = growth, development, formation. This new growth (mass, tumor) can be malignant or benign, which is confirmed by the pathology report. Do not assign a code to a neoplasm until you review the pathology report. Certain CPT codes will specify benign or malignant lesion, so be certain the diagnosis code supports the procedure code.

CHAPTER 2

NEOPLASMS (C00-D49)

This chapter contains the following blocks:

C00-C14	Malignant neoplasms of lip, oral cavity and pharynx
C15-C26	Malignant neoplasms of digestive organs
C30-C39	Malignant neoplasms of respiratory and intrathoracic organs
C40-C41	Malignant neoplasms of bone and articular cartilage
C43-C44	Melanoma and other malignant neoplasms of skin
C45-C49	Malignant neoplasms of mesothelial and soft tissue
C50	Malignant neoplasms of breast
C51-C58	Malignant neoplasms of female genital organs
C60-C63	Malignant neoplasms of male genital organs
C64-C68	Malignant neoplasms of urinary tract
C69-C72	Malignant neoplasms of eye, brain and other parts of central nervous system
C73-C75	Malignant neoplasms of thyroid and other endocrine glands
C7A	Malignant neuroendocrine tumors
C7B	Secondary neuroendocrine tumors
C76-C80	Malignant neoplasms of ill-defined, other secondary and unspecified sites
C81-C96	Malignant neoplasms of lymphoid, hematopoietic and related tissue
D00-D09	In situ neoplasms
D10-D36	Benign neoplasms, except benign neuroendocrine tumors
D3A	Benign neuroendocrine tumors
D37-D48	Neoplasms of uncertain behavior, polycythemia vera and myelodysplastic syndromes
D49	Neoplasms of unspecified behavior

Notes: Functional activity

All neoplasms are classified in this chapter, whether they are functionally active or not. An additional code from Chapter 4 may be used, to identify functional activity associated with any neoplasm.

Morphology [Histology]

Chapter 2 classifies neoplasms primarily by site (topography), with broad groupings for behavior, malignant, in situ, benign, etc. The Table of Neoplasms should be used to identify the correct topography code. In a few cases, such as for malignant melanoma and certain neuroendocrine tumors, the morphology (histologic type) is included in the category and codes.

Primary malignant neoplasms overlapping site boundaries

A primary malignant neoplasm that overlaps two or more contiguous (next to each other) sites should be classified to the subcategory/code .8 ('overlapping lesion'), unless the combination is specifically indexed elsewhere. For multiple neoplasms of the same site that are not contiguous, such as tumors in different quadrants of the same breast, codes for each site should be assigned.

Malignant neoplasm of ectopic tissue

Malignant neoplasms of ectopic tissue are to be coded to the site mentioned, e.g., ectopic pancreatic malignant neoplasms are coded to pancreas, unspecified (C25.9).

MALIGNANT NEOPLASMS (C00-C96)

MALIGNANT NEOPLASMS, STATED OR PRESUMED TO BE PRIMARY (OF SPECIFIED SITES), AND CERTAIN SPECIFIED HISTOLOGIES, EXCEPT NEUROENDOCRINE, AND OF LYMPHOID, HEMATOPOIETIC AND RELATED TISSUE (C00-C75)

MALIGNANT NEOPLASMS OF LIP, ORAL CAVITY AND PHARYNX (C00-C14)

● **C00**   **Malignant neoplasm of lip**

Use additional code to identify:
  alcohol abuse and dependence (F10.-)
  history of tobacco dependence (Z87.891) ◀▥▥
  tobacco dependence (F17.-)
  tobacco use (Z72.0)

Excludes1   malignant melanoma of lip (C43.0)
  Merkel cell carcinoma of lip (C4A.0)
  other and unspecified malignant neoplasm of skin of lip (C44.0-)

C00.0   **Malignant neoplasm of external upper lip**
  Malignant neoplasm of lipstick area of upper lip
  Malignant neoplasm of upper lip NOS
  Malignant neoplasm of vermilion border of upper lip

C00.1   **Malignant neoplasm of external lower lip**
  Malignant neoplasm of lower lip NOS
  Malignant neoplasm of lipstick area of lower lip
  Malignant neoplasm of vermilion border of lower lip

C00.2   **Malignant neoplasm of external lip, unspecified**
  Malignant neoplasm of vermilion border of lip NOS

C00.3   **Malignant neoplasm of upper lip, inner aspect**
  Malignant neoplasm of buccal aspect of upper lip
  Malignant neoplasm of frenulum of upper lip
  Malignant neoplasm of mucosa of upper lip
  Malignant neoplasm of oral aspect of upper lip

C00.4   **Malignant neoplasm of lower lip, inner aspect**
  Malignant neoplasm of buccal aspect of lower lip
  Malignant neoplasm of frenulum of lower lip
  Malignant neoplasm of mucosa of lower lip
  Malignant neoplasm of oral aspect of lower lip

C00.5   **Malignant neoplasm of lip, unspecified, inner aspect**
  Malignant neoplasm of buccal aspect of lip, unspecified
  Malignant neoplasm of frenulum of lip, unspecified
  Malignant neoplasm of mucosa of lip, unspecified
  Malignant neoplasm of oral aspect of lip, unspecified

C00.6   **Malignant neoplasm of commissure of lip, unspecified**
  Commissure: Site of union of corresponding parts

C00.8   **Malignant neoplasm of overlapping sites of lip**

C00.9   **Malignant neoplasm of lip, unspecified**

N Newborn Age: 0   **P** Pediatric Age: 0–17   **M** Maternity DX: 12–55   **A** Adult Age: 15–124   ♀ Females Only   ♂ Males Only

🔹 Complication\Comorbidity   🔹 Major C\C   (Ex) CC/MCC Exclusions   🔹 Hospital-Acquired Condition   **671**

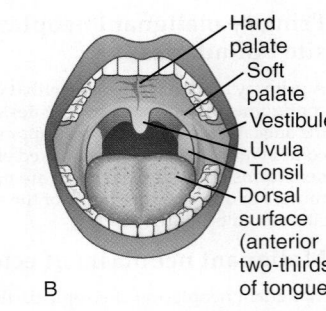

Figure 2-1 Anatomical structures of the mouth and lips. **A.** Transitional or vermilion borders. Lips are connected to the gums by frenulum. **B.** Dorsal surface. **C.** Ventral surface.

CHAPTER 2 (C00-D49)

C01   Malignant neoplasm of base of tongue
   Malignant neoplasm of dorsal surface of base of tongue
   Malignant neoplasm of fixed part of tongue NOS
   Malignant neoplasm of posterior third of tongue

   Use additional code to identify:
      alcohol abuse and dependence (F10.-)
      history of tobacco dependence (Z87.891) ◀▥▥
      tobacco dependence (F17.-)
      tobacco use (Z72.0)

● **C02   Malignant neoplasm of other and unspecified parts of tongue**
   Use additional code to identify:
      alcohol abuse and dependence (F10.-)
      history of tobacco dependence (Z87.891) ◀▥▥
      tobacco dependence (F17.-)
      tobacco use (Z72.0)

   C02.0   Malignant neoplasm of dorsal surface of tongue
      Malignant neoplasm of anterior two-thirds of tongue, dorsal surface

      Excludes2   malignant neoplasm of dorsal surface of base of tongue (C01)

   C02.1   Malignant neoplasm of border of tongue
      Malignant neoplasm of tip of tongue

   C02.2   Malignant neoplasm of ventral surface of tongue
      Malignant neoplasm of anterior two-thirds of tongue, ventral surface
      Malignant neoplasm of frenulum linguae

   C02.3   Malignant neoplasm of anterior two-thirds of tongue, part unspecified
      Malignant neoplasm of middle third of tongue NOS
      Malignant neoplasm of mobile part of tongue NOS

   C02.4   Malignant neoplasm of lingual tonsil
      Lingual tonsil: Aggregation of lymph follicles at root of tongue

      Excludes2   malignant neoplasm of tonsil NOS (C09.9)

   C02.8   Malignant neoplasm of overlapping sites of tongue
      Malignant neoplasm of two or more contiguous sites of tongue

   C02.9   Malignant neoplasm of tongue, unspecified

● **C03   Malignant neoplasm of gum**
   Includes   malignant neoplasm of alveolar (ridge) mucosa
                  malignant neoplasm of gingiva

   Use additional code to identify:
      alcohol abuse and dependence (F10.-)
      history of tobacco dependence (Z87.891) ◀▥▥
      tobacco dependence (F17.-)
      tobacco use (Z72.0)

   Excludes2   malignant odontogenic neoplasms (C41.0-C41.1)

   C03.0   Malignant neoplasm of upper gum
   C03.1   Malignant neoplasm of lower gum
   C03.9   Malignant neoplasm of gum, unspecified

● **C04   Malignant neoplasm of floor of mouth**
   Use additional code to identify:
      alcohol abuse and dependence (F10.-)
      history of tobacco dependence (Z87.891) ◀▥▥
      tobacco dependence (F17.-)
      tobacco use (Z72.0)

   C04.0   Malignant neoplasm of anterior floor of mouth
      Malignant neoplasm of anterior to the premolar-canine junction

   C04.1   Malignant neoplasm of lateral floor of mouth
   C04.8   Malignant neoplasm of overlapping sites of floor of mouth
   C04.9   Malignant neoplasm of floor of mouth, unspecified

● **C05   Malignant neoplasm of palate**
   Use additional code to identify:
      alcohol abuse and dependence (F10.-)
      history of tobacco dependence (Z87.891) ◀▥▥
      tobacco dependence (F17.-)
      tobacco use (Z72.0)

   Excludes1   Kaposi's sarcoma of palate (C46.2)

   C05.0   Malignant neoplasm of hard palate
   C05.1   Malignant neoplasm of soft palate

      Excludes2   malignant neoplasm of nasopharyngeal surface of soft palate (C11.3)

   C05.2   Malignant neoplasm of uvula
   C05.8   Malignant neoplasm of overlapping sites of palate
   C05.9   Malignant neoplasm of palate, unspecified
      Malignant neoplasm of roof of mouth

● **C06   Malignant neoplasm of other and unspecified parts of mouth**
   Use additional code to identify:
      alcohol abuse and dependence (F10.-)
      history of tobacco dependence (Z87.891) ◀▥▥
      tobacco dependence (F17.-)
      tobacco use (Z72.0)

   C06.0   Malignant neoplasm of cheek mucosa
      Malignant neoplasm of buccal mucosa NOS
      Malignant neoplasm of internal cheek

   C06.1   Malignant neoplasm of vestibule of mouth
      Malignant neoplasm of buccal sulcus (upper) (lower)
      Malignant neoplasm of labial sulcus (upper) (lower)

   C06.2   Malignant neoplasm of retromolar area

● **C06.8   Malignant neoplasm of overlapping sites of other and unspecified parts of mouth**

      C06.80   Malignant neoplasm of overlapping sites of unspecified parts of mouth

      C06.89   Malignant neoplasm of overlapping sites of other parts of mouth 'book leaf' neoplasm [ventral surface of tongue and floor of mouth]

   C06.9   Malignant neoplasm of mouth, unspecified
      Malignant neoplasm of minor salivary gland, unspecified site
      Malignant neoplasm of oral cavity NOS

◀ New   ◀▥▥ Revised   ~~deleted~~ Deleted   Excludes 1   Excludes 2   Includes   Use additional   Code first   Code also   Unspecified
OGCR Official Guidelines   ● Unacceptable Principal Diagnosis   X Assign placeholder X   ● Use Additional Character(s)   ▌ Manifestation Code   **Coding Clinic**

Figure 2-2 Major salivary glands.

C07   **Malignant neoplasm of parotid gland**
    Use additional code to identify:
      alcohol abuse and dependence (F10.-)
      exposure to environmental tobacco smoke (Z77.22)
      exposure to tobacco smoke in the perinatal period (P96.81)
      history of tobacco dependence (Z87.891) ◄▥
      occupational exposure to environmental tobacco smoke (Z57.31)
      tobacco dependence (F17.-)
      tobacco use (Z72.0)

C08   **Malignant neoplasm of other and unspecified major salivary glands**
    Includes   malignant neoplasm of salivary ducts
    Use additional code to identify:
      alcohol abuse and dependence (F10.-)
      exposure to environmental tobacco smoke (Z77.22)
      exposure to tobacco smoke in the perinatal period (P96.81)
      history of tobacco dependence (Z87.891) ◄▥
      occupational exposure to environmental tobacco smoke (Z57.31)
      tobacco dependence (F17.-)
      tobacco use (Z72.0)
    Excludes1   malignant neoplasms of specified minor salivary glands which are classified according to their anatomical location
    Excludes2   malignant neoplasms of minor salivary glands NOS (C06.9)
              malignant neoplasm of parotid gland (C07)

C08.0   **Malignant neoplasm of submandibular gland**
      Malignant neoplasm of submaxillary gland

C08.1   **Malignant neoplasm of sublingual gland**

C08.9   **Malignant neoplasm of major salivary gland, unspecified**
      Malignant neoplasm of salivary gland (major) NOS

★ **(See Plate 61 on page 73.)**

C09   **Malignant neoplasm of tonsil**
    Use additional code to identify:
      alcohol abuse and dependence (F10.-)
      exposure to environmental tobacco smoke (Z77.22)
      exposure to tobacco smoke in the perinatal period (P96.81)
      history of tobacco dependence (Z87.891) ◄▥
      occupational exposure to environmental tobacco smoke (Z57.31)
      tobacco dependence (F17.-)
      tobacco use (Z72.0)
    Excludes2   malignant neoplasm of lingual tonsil (C02.4)
              malignant neoplasm of pharyngeal tonsil (C11.1)

C09.0   **Malignant neoplasm of tonsillar fossa**
      Surface of palatine (two masses of lymphatic tissue on sides of throat) tonsils

C09.1   **Malignant neoplasm of tonsillar pillar (anterior) (posterior)**
      Extension from palatine (two masses of lymphatic tissue on sides of throat) tonsils

C09.8   **Malignant neoplasm of overlapping sites of tonsil**

C09.9   **Malignant neoplasm of tonsil, unspecified**
      Malignant neoplasm of tonsil NOS
      Malignant neoplasm of faucial tonsils
      Malignant neoplasm of palatine tonsils

C10   **Malignant neoplasm of oropharynx**
      Area of throat at back of mouth
    Use additional code to identify:
      alcohol abuse and dependence (F10.-)
      exposure to environmental tobacco smoke (Z77.22)
      exposure to tobacco smoke in the perinatal period (P96.81)
      history of tobacco dependence (Z87.891) ◄▥
      occupational exposure to environmental tobacco smoke (Z57.31)
      tobacco dependence (F17.-)
      tobacco use (Z72.0)
    Excludes2   malignant neoplasm of tonsil (C09.-)

C10.0   **Malignant neoplasm of vallecula**
      Vallecula, depression or furrow

C10.1   **Malignant neoplasm of anterior surface of epiglottis**
      Malignant neoplasm of epiglottis, free border [margin]
      Malignant neoplasm of glossoepiglottic fold(s)
      Excludes2   malignant neoplasm of epiglottis (suprahyoid portion) NOS (C32.1)

C10.2   **Malignant neoplasm of lateral wall of oropharynx**

C10.3   **Malignant neoplasm of posterior wall of oropharynx**

C10.4   **Malignant neoplasm of branchial cleft**
      Congenital slitlike openings formed between branchial arches
          pharyngeal groove
      Malignant neoplasm of branchial cyst [site of neoplasm]

C10.8   **Malignant neoplasm of overlapping sites of oropharynx**
      Malignant neoplasm of junctional region of oropharynx

C10.9   **Malignant neoplasm of oropharynx, unspecified**

C11   **Malignant neoplasm of nasopharynx**
    Use additional code to identify:
      exposure to environmental tobacco smoke (Z77.22)
      exposure to tobacco smoke in the perinatal period (P96.81)
      history of tobacco dependence (Z87.891) ◄▥
      occupational exposure to environmental tobacco smoke (Z57.31)
      tobacco dependence (F17.-)
      tobacco use (Z72.0)

C11.0   **Malignant neoplasm of superior wall of nasopharynx**
      Part of pharynx that lies above soft palate
      Malignant neoplasm of roof of nasopharynx

C11.1   **Malignant neoplasm of posterior wall of nasopharynx**
      Malignant neoplasm of adenoid
      Malignant neoplasm of pharyngeal tonsil

C11.2   **Malignant neoplasm of lateral wall of nasopharynx**
      Malignant neoplasm of fossa of Rosenmüller
      Malignant neoplasm of opening of auditory tube
      Malignant neoplasm of pharyngeal recess

C11.3   **Malignant neoplasm of anterior wall of nasopharynx**
      Malignant neoplasm of floor of nasopharynx
      Malignant neoplasm of nasopharyngeal (anterior) (posterior) surface of soft palate
      Malignant neoplasm of posterior margin of nasal choana
      Malignant neoplasm of posterior margin of nasal septum

C11.8   **Malignant neoplasm of overlapping sites of nasopharynx**

C11.9   **Malignant neoplasm of nasopharynx, unspecified**
      Malignant neoplasm of nasopharyngeal wall NOS

C12   **Malignant neoplasm of pyriform sinus**
      Malignant neoplasm of pyriform fossa
    Use additional code to identify:
      exposure to environmental tobacco smoke (Z77.22)
      exposure to tobacco smoke in the perinatal period (P96.81)
      history of tobacco dependence (Z87.891) ◄▥
      occupational exposure to environmental tobacco smoke (Z57.31)
      tobacco dependence (F17.-)
      tobacco use (Z72.0)

CHAPTER 2 (C00-D49)

N   Newborn Age: 0   **P**   Pediatric Age: 0–17   **M**   Maternity DX: 12–55   **A**   Adult Age: 15–124   ♀   Females Only   ♂   Males Only

   Complication\Comorbidity   Major C\C   (Ex)   CC/MCC Exclusions   Hospital-Acquired Condition   **673**

● **C13**   **Malignant neoplasm of hypopharynx**

Use additional code to identify:
exposure to environmental tobacco smoke (Z77.22)
exposure to tobacco smoke in the perinatal period (P96.81)
history of tobacco dependence (Z87.891) ◀▥
occupational exposure to environmental tobacco smoke (Z57.31)
tobacco dependence (F17.-)
tobacco use (Z72.0)

Excludes2   malignant neoplasm of pyriform sinus (C12)

C13.0   **Malignant neoplasm of postcricoid region**
Behind the cricoid cartilage of neck

C13.1   **Malignant neoplasm of aryepiglottic fold, hypopharyngeal aspect**
Arytenoepiglottic fold, triangular opening between side of epiglottis and apex of arytenoid cartilage
Malignant neoplasm of aryepiglottic fold, marginal zone
Malignant neoplasm of aryepiglottic fold NOS
Malignant neoplasm of interarytenoid fold, marginal zone
Malignant neoplasm of interarytenoid fold NOS

Excludes2   malignant neoplasm of aryepiglottic fold or interarytenoid fold, laryngeal aspect (C32.1)

C13.2   **Malignant neoplasm of posterior wall of hypopharynx**

C13.8   **Malignant neoplasm of overlapping sites of hypopharynx**

C13.9   **Malignant neoplasm of hypopharynx, unspecified**
Malignant neoplasm of hypopharyngeal wall NOS

● **C14**   **Malignant neoplasm of other and ill-defined sites in the lip, oral cavity and pharynx**

Use additional code to identify:
alcohol abuse and dependence (F10.-)
exposure to environmental tobacco smoke (Z77.22)
exposure to tobacco smoke in the perinatal period (P96.81)
history of tobacco dependence (Z87.891) ◀▥
occupational exposure to environmental tobacco smoke (Z57.31)
tobacco dependence (F17.-)
tobacco use (Z72.0)

Excludes1   malignant neoplasm of oral cavity NOS (C06.9)

C14.0   **Malignant neoplasm of pharynx, unspecified**

C14.2   **Malignant neoplasm of Waldeyer's ring**

C14.8   **Malignant neoplasm of overlapping sites of lip, oral cavity and pharynx**
Primary malignant neoplasm of two or more contiguous sites of lip, oral cavity and pharynx

Excludes1   'book leaf' neoplasm [ventral surface of tongue and floor of mouth] (C06.89)

MALIGNANT NEOPLASM OF DIGESTIVE ORGANS (C15-C26)

Excludes1   Kaposi's sarcoma of gastrointestinal sites (C46.4)

Excludes2   gastrointestinal stromal tumors (C49.A-) ◀

● **C15**   **Malignant neoplasms of esophagus**

Use additional code to identify:
alcohol abuse and dependence (F10.-)
(Ex) **For category C15 CC codes:** C15.3-C15.9, C26.0, C26.9, C45.7-C45.9, C46.4, C76.8, C7A.00, C7A.098-C7B.00, C7B.1, C80.0-C80.2, D49.0, D49.81-D49.9

C15.3   **Malignant neoplasm of upper third of esophagus** 🔖

C15.4   **Malignant neoplasm of middle third of esophagus** 🔖

C15.5   **Malignant neoplasm of lower third of esophagus** 🔖

Excludes1   malignant neoplasm of cardio-esophageal junction (C16.0)

C15.8   **Malignant neoplasm of overlapping sites of esophagus** 🔖

C15.9   **Malignant neoplasm of esophagus, unspecified** 🔖

● **C16**   **Malignant neoplasm of stomach**

Use additional code to identify:
alcohol abuse and dependence (F10.-)

Excludes2   malignant carcinoid tumor of the stomach (C7A.092)

(Ex) **For category C16 CC codes:** C16.0-C16.9, C26.0, C26.9, C45.7-C45.9, C46.4, C49.A2, C76.8, C7A.00, C7A.092, C7A.094-C7B.00, C7B.1, C80.0-C80.2, D49.0, D49.81-D49.9

C16.0   **Malignant neoplasm of cardia** 🔖
Malignant neoplasm of cardiac orifice
Malignant neoplasm of cardio-esophageal junction
Malignant neoplasm of esophagus and stomach
Malignant neoplasm of gastro-esophageal junction

C16.1   **Malignant neoplasm of fundus of stomach** 🔖

C16.2   **Malignant neoplasm of body of stomach** 🔖

C16.3   **Malignant neoplasm of pyloric antrum** 🔖
Malignant neoplasm of gastric antrum

C16.4   **Malignant neoplasm of pylorus** 🔖
Malignant neoplasm of prepylorus
Malignant neoplasm of pyloric canal

C16.5   **Malignant neoplasm of lesser curvature of stomach, unspecified** 🔖
Malignant neoplasm of lesser curvature of stomach, not classifiable to C16.1-C16.4

C16.6   **Malignant neoplasm of greater curvature of stomach, unspecified** 🔖
Malignant neoplasm of greater curvature of stomach, not classifiable to C16.0-C16.4

C16.8   **Malignant neoplasm of overlapping sites of stomach** 🔖

C16.9   **Malignant neoplasm of stomach, unspecified** 🔖
Gastric cancer NOS

Figure 2-3   The esophagus is the muscular tube that connects the pharynx and the stomach. The 10 inch (25 cm) long esophagus is divided into three parts: **cervical, thoracic,** and **abdominal.**

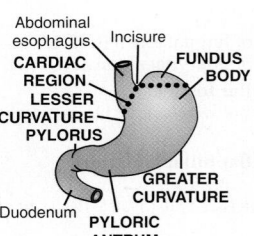

Figure 2-4   Parts of the stomach.

Item 2–2   The esophagus opens into the stomach through the **cardiac orifice,** also called the **cardioesophageal junction.** The **cardia** is adjacent to the cardiac orifice. The stomach widens into the **greater** and **lesser curvatures.** The **pyloric antrum** precedes the **pylorus,** which opens to the duodenum.

◀ New   ◀▥ Revised   ~~deleted~~ Deleted   Excludes 1   Excludes 2   Includes   Use additional   Code first   Code also   Unspecified
OGCR Official Guidelines   ● Unacceptable Principal Diagnosis   X Assign placeholder X   ● Use Additional Character(s)   ▌ Manifestation Code   **Coding Clinic**

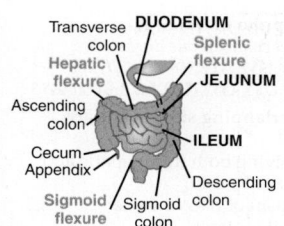

Figure 2-5   Small intestine and colon.

● **C17**   **Malignant neoplasm of small intestine**
> **Excludes1**   malignant carcinoid tumor of the small intestine (C7A.01)

    C17.0   **Malignant neoplasm of duodenum** 🔹
> *First or proximal portion of small intestine, extending from pylorus to jejunum*
> (Ex:) C17.0, C17.8-C17.9, C26.0, C26.9, C45.7-C45.9, C46.4, C76.8, C7A.00-C7A.010, C7A.019, C7A.098-C7B.00, C7B.1, C80.0-C80.2, D49.0, D49.81-D49.9

    C17.1   **Malignant neoplasm of jejunum** 🔹
> *Second section of small intestine, extending from duodenum to ileum*
> (Ex:) C17.1, C17.8-C17.9, C26.0, C26.9, C45.7-C45.9, C46.4, C76.8, C7A.00, C7A.011, C7A.019, C7A.098, C7A.1-C7B.00, C7B.1, C80.0-C80.2, D49.0, D49.81-D49.9

    C17.2   **Malignant neoplasm of ileum** 🔹
> *Distal and longest portion of small intestine, extending from jejunum to cecum*
> **Excludes1**   malignant neoplasm of ileocecal valve (C18.0)
> (Ex:) C17.2, C17.8-C17.9, C26.0, C26.9, C45.7-C45.9, C46.4, C76.8, C7A.00, C7A.012-C7A.019, C7A.098, C7A.1-C7B.00, C7B.1, C80.0-C80.2, D49.0, D49.81-D49.9

    C17.3   **Meckel's diverticulum, malignant** 🔹
> *Appendage of ileum*
> **Excludes1**   Meckel's diverticulum, congenital (Q43.0)
> (Ex:) C17.3-C17.9, C26.0, C26.9, C45.7-C45.9, C46.4, C76.8, C7A.00, C7A.019, C7A.098-C7B.00, C7B.1, C80.0-C80.2, D49.0, D49.81-D49.9

    C17.8   **Malignant neoplasm of overlapping sites of small intestine** 🔹
> (Ex:) C17.8-C17.9, C26.0, C26.9, C45.7-C45.9, C46.4, C76.8, C7A.00, C7A.019, C7A.098, C7A.1-C7B.00, C7B.1, C80.0-C80.2, D49.0, D49.81-D49.9

    C17.9   **Malignant neoplasm of small intestine, unspecified** 🔹
> (Ex:) See C17.8

● **C18**   **Malignant neoplasm of colon**
> **Excludes1**   malignant carcinoid tumors of the colon (C7A.02)

    C18.0   **Malignant neoplasm of cecum** 🔹
> *First section of large intestine*
> Malignant neoplasm of ileocecal valve
> (Ex:) C18.0, C18.8-C18.9, C26.0-C26.9, C45.7-C45.9, C46.4, C76.8, C7A.00, C7A.021, C7A.029, C7A.098-C7B.00, C7B.1, C80.0-C80.2, D49.0, D49.81-D49.9

    C18.1   **Malignant neoplasm of appendix** 🔹
> *Blind ended tube connected to the cecum; AKA vermiform appendix*
> (Ex:) C18.1, C18.8-C18.9, C26.0, C26.9, C45.7-C45.9, C46.4, C76.8, C7A.00, C7A.020, C7A.029, C7A.098, C7A.1-C7B.00, C7B.1, C80.0-C80.2, D49.0, D49.81-D49.9

    C18.2   **Malignant neoplasm of ascending colon** 🔹
> *Ascending colon is between cecum and right colic flexure*
> (Ex:) C18.2, C18.8-C18.9, C26.0, C26.9, C45.7-C45.9, C46.4, C76.8, C7A.00, C7A.022, C7A.029, C7A.098, C7A.1-C7B.00, C7B.1, C80.0-C80.2, D49.0, D49.81-D49.9

    C18.3   **Malignant neoplasm of hepatic flexure** 🔹
> *A flexure is a bending in a structure or organ. Note the three flexures illustrated in Figure 2–5.*
> (Ex:) C18.3, C18.8-C18.9, C26.0, C26.9, C45.7-C45.9, C46.4, C76.8, C7A.00, C7A.029, C7A.098-C7B.00, C7B.1, C80.0-C80.2, D49.0, D49.81-D49.9

    C18.4   **Malignant neoplasm of transverse colon** 🔹
> *Portion of colon that runs transversely across upper part of abdomen, between right and left colic flexures*
> (Ex:) C18.4, C18.8-C18.9, C26.0, C26.9, C45.7-C45.9, C46.4, C76.8, C7A.00, C7A.023, C7A.029, C7A.098, C7A.1-C7B.00, C7B.1, C80.0-C80.2, D49.0, D49.81-D49.9

    C18.5   **Malignant neoplasm of splenic flexure** 🔹
> *Bend at junction of transverse and descending colon*
> (Ex:) C18.5, C18.8-C18.9, C26.0, C26.9, C45.7-C45.9, C46.4, C76.8, C7A.00, C7A.029, C7A.098-C7B.00, C7B.1, C80.0-C80.2, D49.0, D49.81-D49.9

    C18.6   **Malignant neoplasm of descending colon** 🔹
> *Portion between left colic flexure and sigmoid colon at pelvic brim; AKA iliac colon*
> (Ex:) C18.6, C18.8-C18.9, C26.0, C26.9, C45.7-C45.9, C46.4, C76.8, C7A.00, C7A.024, C7A.029, C7A.098-C7B.00, C7B.1, C80.0-C80.2, D49.0, D49.81-D49.9

    C18.7   **Malignant neoplasm of sigmoid colon** 🔹
> *S-shaped part of colon extending from pelvic brim to third segment of sacrum*
> Malignant neoplasm of sigmoid (flexure)
> **Excludes1**   malignant neoplasm of rectosigmoid junction (C19)
> (Ex:) C18.7-C18.9, C26.0, C26.9, C45.7-C45.9, C46.4, C76.8, C7A.00, C7A.025, C7A.029, C7A.098, C7A.1-C7B.00, C7B.1, C80.0-C80.2, D49.0, D49.81-D49.9

    C18.8   **Malignant neoplasm of overlapping sites of colon** 🔹
> (Ex:) C18.8-C18.9, C26.0, C26.9, C45.7-C45.9, C46.4, C76.8, C7A.00, C7A.029, C7A.098, C7A.1-C7B.00, C7B.1, C80.0-C80.2, D49.0, D49.81-D49.9

    C18.9   **Malignant neoplasm of colon, unspecified** 🔹
> Malignant neoplasm of large intestine NOS
> (Ex:) See C18.8

● **C19**   **Malignant neoplasm of rectosigmoid junction** 🔹
> Malignant neoplasm of colon with rectum
> Malignant neoplasm of rectosigmoid (colon)
> **Excludes1**   malignant carcinoid tumors of the colon (C7A.02-)
> (Ex:) C19, C21.2-C21.8, C26.0, C26.9, C45.7-C45.9, C46.4, C76.8, C7A.00, C7A.098, C7A.1-C7B.00, C7B.1, C80.0-C80.2, D49.0, D49.81-D49.9

● **C20**   **Malignant neoplasm of rectum** 🔹
> Malignant neoplasm of rectal ampulla
> **Excludes1**   malignant carcinoid tumor of the rectum (C7A.026)
> (Ex:) C20, C21.2-C21.8, C26.0, C26.9, C45.7-C45.9, C46.4, C76.8, C7A.00, C7A.026, C7A.098, C7A.1-C7B.00, C7B.1, C80.0-C80.2, D49.0, D49.81-D49.9

● **C21**   **Malignant neoplasm of anus and anal canal**
> **Excludes2**   malignant carcinoid tumors of the colon (C7A.02-)
> malignant melanoma of anal margin (C43.51)
> malignant melanoma of anal skin (C43.51)
> malignant melanoma of perianal skin (C43.51)
> other and unspecified malignant neoplasm of anal margin (C44.500, C44.510, C44.520, C44.590)
> other and unspecified malignant neoplasm of anal skin (C44.500, C44.510, C44.520, C44.590)
> other and unspecified malignant neoplasm of perianal skin (C44.500, C44.510, C44.520, C44.590)
> (Ex:) **For category C21 CC codes C21.0-C21.1:** C21.0-C21.8, C26.0, C26.9, C45.7-C45.9, C46.4, C76.8, C7A.00, C7A.098, C7A.1-C7B.00, C7B.1, C80.0-C80.2, D49.0, D49.81-D49.9 **For category C21 CC codes C21.2-C21.8:** C21.2-C21.8, C26.0, C26.9, C45.7-C45.9, C46.4, C76.8, C7A.00, C7A.098, C7A.1-C7B.00, C7B.1, C80.0-C80.2, D49.0, D49.81-D49.9

    C21.0   **Malignant neoplasm of anus, unspecified** 🔹

    C21.1   **Malignant neoplasm of anal canal** 🔹
> *Terminal part of large intestine*
> Malignant neoplasm of anal sphincter

    C21.2   **Malignant neoplasm of cloacogenic zone** 🔹

    C21.8   **Malignant neoplasm of overlapping sites of rectum, anus and anal canal** 🔹
> Malignant neoplasm of anorectal junction
> Malignant neoplasm of anorectum
> Primary malignant neoplasm of two or more contiguous sites of rectum, anus and anal canal

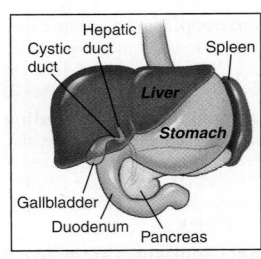

Figure 2-6 Diagram of liver, gallbladder, hepatic duct, pancreas, and spleen. (From Thibodeau and Patton: Anatomy and Physiology, ed 7, Mosby, 2010)

● **C22　Malignant neoplasm of liver and intrahepatic bile ducts**
　　Intrahepatic: Within liver
　　Use additional code to identify:
　　　alcohol abuse and dependence (F10.-)
　　　hepatitis B (B16.-, B18.0-B18.1) hepatitis C (B17.1-, B18.2)
　　　Excludes1　malignant neoplasm of biliary tract NOS (C24.9)
　　　　　secondary malignant neoplasm of liver and
　　　　　intrahepatic bile duct (C78.7)
　　(Ex:) For catgory C22 CC codes: C22.0-C22.9, C26.0, C26.9, C45.7-C45.9, C46.4, C76.8,
　　　　C7A.00, C7A.098, C7A.1-C7B.00, C7B.1, C80.0-C80.2, D49.0, D49.81-D49.9

　C22.0　Liver cell carcinoma 🔖
　　　Hepatocellular carcinoma
　　　Hepatoma
　C22.1　Intrahepatic bile duct carcinoma 🔖
　　　Cholangiocarcinoma
　　　Adenocarcinoma (cancer that originates in glandular tissue)
　　　　arising from epithelium of intrahepatic bile ducts
　　　Excludes1　malignant neoplasm of hepatic duct
　　　　　(C24.0)
　C22.2　Hepatoblastoma 🔖
　　　Malignant intrahepatic tumor
　C22.3　Angiosarcoma of liver 🔖
　　　Kupffer cell sarcoma
　C22.4　Other sarcomas of liver 🔖
　C22.7　Other specified carcinomas of liver 🔖
　C22.8　Malignant neoplasm of liver, primary, unspecified as to type 🔖
　C22.9　Malignant neoplasm of liver, not specified as primary or secondary 🔖

● **C23　Malignant neoplasm of gallbladder** 🔖
　　(Ex:) C23, C24.8-C24.9, C26.0, C26.9, C45.7-C45.9, C46.4, C76.8, C7A.00, C7A.098,
　　　　C7A.1-C7B.00, C7B.1, C8.00-C8.02, D49.0, D49.81-D49.9

● **C24　Malignant neoplasm of other and unspecified parts of biliary tract**
　　　Excludes1　malignant neoplasm of intrahepatic bile duct
　　　　　(C22.1)
　C24.0　Malignant neoplasm of extrahepatic bile duct 🔖
　　　Extrahepatic = outside the liver
　　　Malignant neoplasm of biliary duct or passage NOS
　　　Malignant neoplasm of common bile duct
　　　Malignant neoplasm of cystic duct
　　　Malignant neoplasm of hepatic duct
　　　(Ex:) C24.0, C24.8-C24.9, C26.0, C26.9, C45.7-C45.9, C46.4, C76.8, C7A.00,
　　　　C7A.098-C7B.00, C7B.1, C80.0-C80.2, D49.0, D49.81-D49.9

　C24.1　Malignant neoplasm of ampulla of Vater 🔖
　　　Union of pancreatic duct and common bile duct
　　　(Ex:) C24.1, C24.8-C24.9, C26.0, C26.9, C45.7-C45.9, C46.4, C76.8, C7A.00,
　　　　C7A.098, C7A.1, C7A.8, C7B.00, C7B.1, C80.0-C80.2, D49.0, D49.81-D49.9
　C24.8　Malignant neoplasm of overlapping sites of biliary tract 🔖
　　　Malignant neoplasm involving both intrahepatic and
　　　　extrahepatic bile ducts
　　　Primary malignant neoplasm of two or more
　　　　contiguous sites of biliary tract
　　　(Ex:) C24.8-C24.9, C26.0, C26.9, C45.7-C45.9, C46.4, C76.8, C7A.00, C7A.098-C7A.8,
　　　　C7B.00, C7B.1, C80.0-C80.2, D49.0, D49.81-D49.9
　C24.9　Malignant neoplasm of biliary tract, unspecified 🔖
　　　(Ex:) See C24.8

● **C25　Malignant neoplasm of pancreas**
　　Check documentation for specific site.
　　Code also exocrine pancreatic insufficiency (K86.81) ◀
　　Use additional code to identify:
　　　alcohol abuse and dependence (F10.-)
　　(Ex:) For catgory C25 CC codes: C25.0-C26.0, C26.9, C45.7-C45.9, C46.4, C76.8, C7A.00,
　　　　C7A.098, C7A.1-C7B.00, C7B.1, C8.00-C80.2, D49.0, D49.81-D49.9

　C25.0　Malignant neoplasm of head of pancreas 🔖
　C25.1　Malignant neoplasm of body of pancreas 🔖
　C25.2　Malignant neoplasm of tail of pancreas 🔖
　C25.3　Malignant neoplasm of pancreatic duct 🔖
　C25.4　Malignant neoplasm of endocrine pancreas 🔖
　　　Malignant neoplasm of islets of Langerhans
　　　That part of the pancreas that acts as endocrine gland and
　　　　consists of islets of Langerhans
　　　Use additional code to identify any functional activity.
　C25.7　Malignant neoplasm of other parts of pancreas 🔖
　　　Malignant neoplasm of neck of pancreas
　C25.8　Malignant neoplasm of overlapping sites of pancreas 🔖
　C25.9　Malignant neoplasm of pancreas, unspecified 🔖

● **C26　Malignant neoplasm of other and ill-defined digestive organs**
　　　Excludes1　malignant neoplasm of peritoneum and
　　　　　retroperitoneum (C48.-)
　C26.0　Malignant neoplasm of intestinal tract, part unspecified
　　　Malignant neoplasm of intestine NOS
　C26.1　Malignant neoplasm of spleen
　　　Excludes1　Hodgkin lymphoma (C81.-)
　　　　　non-Hodgkin lymphoma (C82-C85)
　C26.9　Malignant neoplasm of ill-defined sites within the digestive system
　　　Malignant neoplasm of alimentary canal or tract NOS
　　　Malignant neoplasm of gastrointestinal tract NOS
　　　Excludes1　malignant neoplasm of abdominal NOS
　　　　　(C76.2)
　　　　　malignant neoplasm of intra-abdominal
　　　　　NOS (C76.2)

Item 2–3　Islets of Langerhans (endocrine producing cells comprising 1% to 2% of the pancreatic mass) make and secrete hormones that regulate the body's production of insulin, glucagon, and stomach acid. Breakdown of the insulin-producing cells can cause diabetes mellitus. Islet cell tumors can be benign or malignant and include glucagonomas, insulinomas, gastrinomas, and neuroendocrine tumor. The neoplasm table must be consulted for the correct neoplasm code.

◀ New　◀▪▪ Revised　d̶e̶l̶e̶t̶e̶d̶ Deleted　Excludes 1　Excludes 2　Includes　Use additional　Code first　Code also　Unspecified
OGCR Official Guidelines　● Unacceptable Principal Diagnosis　X Assign placeholder X　● Use Additional Character(s)　▸ Manifestation Code　Coding Clinic
676

Figure 2-7 Paranasal sinuses. (From Buck CJ: Step-by-Step Medical Coding, ed 2016, St. Louis, Elsevier, 2016)

Frontal sinus
Sphenoidal sinus
Ethmoidal sinus
Maxillary sinus

MALIGNANT NEOPLASMS OF RESPIRATORY AND INTRATHORACIC ORGANS (C30-C39)

Includes	malignant neoplasm of middle ear
Excludes1	mesothelioma (C45.-)

● **C30   Malignant neoplasm of nasal cavity and middle ear**

C30.0   Malignant neoplasm of nasal cavity
Malignant neoplasm of cartilage of nose
Malignant neoplasm of nasal concha
Malignant neoplasm of internal nose
Malignant neoplasm of septum of nose
Malignant neoplasm of vestibule of nose
Anterior part of nasal cavity

> **Excludes1**   malignant neoplasm of nasal bone (C41.0)
> malignant neoplasm of nose NOS (C76.0)
> malignant neoplasm of olfactory bulb (C72.2-)
> malignant neoplasm of posterior margin of nasal septum and choana (C11.3)
> malignant melanoma of skin of nose (C43.31)
> malignant neoplasm of turbinates (C41.0)
> other and unspecified malignant neoplasm of skin of nose C44.301, C44.311, C44.321, C44.391

C30.1   Malignant neoplasm of middle ear
Malignant neoplasm of antrum tympanicum
Boney cavity or chamber
Malignant neoplasm of auditory tube
Malignant neoplasm of eustachian tube
Malignant neoplasm of inner ear
Malignant neoplasm of mastoid air cells
Malignant neoplasm of tympanic cavity

> **Excludes1**   malignant neoplasm of auricular canal (external) (C43.2-, C44.2-)
> malignant neoplasm of bone of ear (meatus) (C41.0)
> malignant neoplasm of cartilage of ear (C49.0)
> malignant melanoma of skin of (external) ear (C43.2-)
> other and unspecified malignant neoplasm of skin of (external) ear (C44.2-)

● **C31   Malignant neoplasm of accessory sinuses**
Paired sinuses in bones of face

C31.0   Malignant neoplasm of maxillary sinus
Malignant neoplasm of antrum (Highmore) (maxillary)

C31.1   Malignant neoplasm of ethmoidal sinus

C31.2   Malignant neoplasm of frontal sinus

C31.3   Malignant neoplasm of sphenoid sinus

C31.8   Malignant neoplasm of overlapping sites of accessory sinuses

C31.9   Malignant neoplasm of accessory sinus, unspecified

● **C32   Malignant neoplasm of larynx**
Use additional code to identify:
alcohol abuse and dependence (F10.-)
exposure to environmental tobacco smoke (Z77.22)
exposure to tobacco smoke in the perinatal period (P96.81)
history of tobacco dependence (Z87.891) ◄▦
occupational exposure to environmental tobacco smoke (Z57.31)
tobacco dependence (F17.-)
tobacco use (Z72.0)

C32.0   Malignant neoplasm of glottis
Vocal apparatus of larynx, consisting of true vocal cords (plicae vocales) and opening between them (rima glottidis)
Malignant neoplasm of intrinsic larynx
Malignant neoplasm of laryngeal commissure (anterior) (posterior)
Malignant neoplasm of vocal cord (true) NOS
> ***True*** *vocal cords ("lower vocal folds") produce vocalization when air from the lungs passes between them. Check your documentation. Code C32.1 is for malignant neoplasm of the **false** vocal cords.*

C32.1   Malignant neoplasm of supraglottis
Area of pharynx above glottis
Malignant neoplasm of aryepiglottic fold or interarytenoid fold, laryngeal aspect
Malignant neoplasm of epiglottis (suprahyoid portion) NOS
Malignant neoplasm of extrinsic larynx
Malignant neoplasm of false vocal cord
> ***False*** *vocal cords ("upper vocal folds") are not involved in vocalization. Check your documentation. Code C32.0 is for true vocal cords.*
Malignant neoplasm of posterior (laryngeal) surface of epiglottis
Malignant neoplasm of ventricular bands

> **Excludes2**   malignant neoplasm of anterior surface of epiglottis (C10.1)
> malignant neoplasm of aryepiglottic fold or interarytenoid fold, hypopharyngeal aspect (C13.1)
> malignant neoplasm of aryepiglottic fold or interarytenoid fold, marginal zone (C13.1)
> malignant neoplasm of aryepiglottic fold or interarytenoid fold NOS (C13.1)

C32.2   Malignant neoplasm of subglottis
Lowest part of larynx from just below vocal cords down to top of trachea

C32.3   Malignant neoplasm of laryngeal cartilage
Cartilages of larynx, including cricoid, thyroid, and epiglottic, and two each of arytenoid, corniculate, and cuneiform

C32.8   Malignant neoplasm of overlapping sites of larynx

C32.9   Malignant neoplasm of larynx, unspecified

● **C33   Malignant neoplasm of trachea** 🔗
Use additional code to identify:
exposure to environmental tobacco smoke (Z77.22)
exposure to tobacco smoke in the perinatal period (P96.81)
history of tobacco dependence (Z87.891) ◄▦
occupational exposure to environmental tobacco smoke (Z57.31)
tobacco dependence (F17.-)
tobacco use (Z72.0)
(Ex) C33, C34.00-C34.92, C39.9, C45.7-C45.9, C46.50-C46.52, C76.1, C76.8, C78.00-C78.1, C78.30-C78.39, C7A.00, C7A.090, C7A.098-C7B.00, C7B.1, C80.0-C80.2, D49.1, D49.81-D49.9

N Newborn Age: 0   P Pediatric Age: 0-17   M Maternity DX: 12-55   A Adult Age: 15-124   ♀ Females Only   ♂ Males Only
🔗 Complication\Comorbidity   🔗 Major C\C   (Ex) CC/MCC Exclusions   🔗 Hospital-Acquired Condition

677

CHAPTER 2 (C00-D49)

● **C34   Malignant neoplasm of bronchus and lung**

Use additional code to identify:

exposure to environmental tobacco smoke (Z77.22)

exposure to tobacco smoke in the perinatal period (P96.81)

history of tobacco dependence (Z87.891) ◀▥

occupational exposure to environmental tobacco smoke (Z57.31)

tobacco dependence (F17.-)

tobacco use (Z72.0)

Excludes1   Kaposi's sarcoma of lung (C46.5-)

malignant carcinoid tumor of the bronchus and lung (C7A.090)

● **C34.0   Malignant neoplasm of main bronchus**

Malignant neoplasm of carina

Ridgelike structure

Malignant neoplasm of hilus (of lung)

Anatomic depression or pit

Ex: **For catgory C34.0 CC codes:** C34.00-C34.02, C34.80-C34.92, C39.9, C45.7-C45.9, C46.50-C46.52, C76.8, C7A.00, C7A.090, C7A.098, C7A.1-C7B.00, C7B.1, C80.0-C80.2, D49.1, D49.81-D49.9

   C34.00   Malignant neoplasm of unspecified **main bronchus** 🖥

   C34.01   Malignant neoplasm of right main bronchus 🖥

   C34.02   Malignant neoplasm of left main bronchus 🖥

● **C34.1   Malignant neoplasm of upper lobe, bronchus or lung**

Ex: **For catgory C34.1 CC codes:** C34.10-C34.12, C34.80-C34.92, C39.9, C45.7-C45.9, C46.50-C46.52, C76.8, C7A.00, C7A.090, C7A.098-C7B.00, C7B.1, C80.0-C80.2, D49.1, D49.81-D49.9

   C34.10   Malignant neoplasm of unspecified **bronchus or lung** 🖥

   C34.11   Malignant neoplasm of upper lobe, right bronchus or lung 🖥

   C34.12   Malignant neoplasm of upper lobe, left bronchus or lung 🖥

● **C34.2   Malignant neoplasm of middle lobe, bronchus or lung** 🖥

Ex: C34.2, C34.80-C34.92, C39.9, C45.7-C45.9, C46.50-C46.52, C76.8, C7A.00, C7A.090, C7A.098-C7B.00, C7B.1, C80.0-C80.2, D49.1, D49.81-D49.9

● **C34.3   Malignant neoplasm of lower lobe, bronchus or lung**

Ex: **For catgory C34.4 CC codes:** C34.30-C34.92, C39.9, C45.7-C45.9, C46.50-C46.52, C76.8, C7A.00, C7A.090, C7A.098-C7B.00, C7B.1, C80.0-C80.2, D49.1, D49.81-D49.9

   C34.30   Malignant neoplasm of lower lobe, unspecified **bronchus or lung** 🖥

   C34.31   Malignant neoplasm of lower lobe, right bronchus or lung 🖥

   C34.32   Malignant neoplasm of lower lobe, left bronchus or lung 🖥

● **C34.8   Malignant neoplasm of overlapping sites of bronchus and lung**

Ex: **For catgory C34.8 CC codes:** C34.80-C34.92, C39.9, C45.7-C45.9, C46.50-C46.52, C76.8, C7A.00, C7A.090, C7A.098-C7B.00, C7B.1, C80.0-C80.2, D49.1, D49.81-D49.9

   C34.80   Malignant neoplasm of overlapping sites of unspecified **bronchus and lung** 🖥

   C34.81   Malignant neoplasm of overlapping sites of right bronchus and lung 🖥

   C34.82   Malignant neoplasm of overlapping sites of left bronchus and lung 🖥

● **C34.9   Malignant neoplasm of unspecified part of bronchus or lung**

Ex: **For category C34.9 CC codes:** See C34.8

   C34.90   Malignant neoplasm of unspecified **part of unspecified bronchus or lung** 🖥

Lung cancer NOS

   C34.91   Malignant neoplasm of unspecified **part of right bronchus or lung** 🖥

   C34.92   Malignant neoplasm of unspecified **part of left bronchus or lung** 🖥

● **C37   Malignant neoplasm of thymus** 🖥

Excludes1   malignant carcinoid tumor of the thymus (C7A.091)

Ex: C37, C7A.091

● **C38   Malignant neoplasm of heart, mediastinum and pleura**

Excludes1   mesothelioma (C45.-)

Ex: **For catgory C38 CC codes unless otherwise indicated:** C38.1-C38.3, C38.8, C39.9, C45.7-C45.9, C76.8, C7A.00, C7A.098-C7B.00, C7B.1, C80.0-C80.2, D49.1, D49.81-D49.9

   C38.0   Malignant neoplasm of heart 🖥

Malignant neoplasm of pericardium

Excludes1   malignant neoplasm of great vessels (C49.3)

Ex: C38.0, C45.2

   C38.1   Malignant neoplasm of anterior mediastinum 🖥

   C38.2   Malignant neoplasm of posterior mediastinum 🖥

   C38.3   Malignant neoplasm of mediastinum, part unspecified 🖥

   C38.4   Malignant neoplasm of pleura 🖥

Ex: C38.4, C39.9, C45.0, C45.7-C45.9, C76.8, C7A.00, C7A.098, C7A.1-C7B.00, C7B.1, C80.0-C80.2, D49.1, D49.81-D49.9

   C38.8   Malignant neoplasm of overlapping sites of heart, mediastinum and pleura 🖥

Pleura are comprised of serous membrane that lines the thoracic cavity (parietal) and covers the lungs (visceral).

● **C39   Malignant neoplasm of other and ill-defined sites in the respiratory system and intrathoracic organs**

Intrathoracic: within thorax/chest

Use additional code to identify:

exposure to environmental tobacco smoke (Z77.22)

exposure to tobacco smoke in the perinatal period (P96.81)

history of tobacco dependence (Z87.891) ◀▥

occupational exposure to environmental tobacco smoke (Z57.31)

tobacco dependence (F17.-)

tobacco use (Z72.0)

Excludes1   intrathoracic malignant neoplasm NOS (C76.1)

thoracic malignant neoplasm NOS (C76.1)

   C39.0   Malignant neoplasm of upper respiratory tract, part unspecified

   C39.9   Malignant neoplasm of lower respiratory tract, part unspecified

Malignant neoplasm of respiratory tract NOS

MALIGNANT NEOPLASMS OF BONE AND ARTICULAR CARTILAGE (C40-C41)

Includes   malignant neoplasm of cartilage (articular) (joint)

malignant neoplasm of periosteum

Excludes1   malignant neoplasm of bone marrow NOS (C96.9)

malignant neoplasm of synovia (C49.-)

● **C40   Malignant neoplasm of bone and articular cartilage of limbs**

Use additional code to identify major osseous defect, if applicable (M89.7-)

● **C40.0   Malignant neoplasm of scapula and long bones of upper limb**

Ex: **For catgory C40.0 CC codes:** C40.00-C40.02, C40.80-C40.92, C41.9, Z51.0

   C40.00   Malignant neoplasm of scapula and long bones of unspecified **upper limb** 🖥

   C40.01   Malignant neoplasm of scapula and long bones of right upper limb 🖥

   C40.02   Malignant neoplasm of scapula and long bones of left upper limb 🖥

● **C40.1   Malignant neoplasm of short bones of upper limb**

Ex: **For catgory C40.1 CC codes:** C40.10-C40.12, C40.80-C40.92, C41.9, Z51.0

   C40.10   Malignant neoplasm of short bones of unspecified **upper limb** 🖥

   C40.11   Malignant neoplasm of short bones of right upper limb 🖥

   C40.12   Malignant neoplasm of short bones of left upper limb 🖥

◀ New   ◀▥ Revised   ~~deleted~~ Deleted   Excludes 1   Excludes 2   Includes   Use additional   Code first   Code also   Unspecified

OGCR Official Guidelines   ● Unacceptable Principal Diagnosis   X Assign placeholder X   ● Use Additional Character(s)   ▶ Manifestation Code   🖥 Coding Clinic

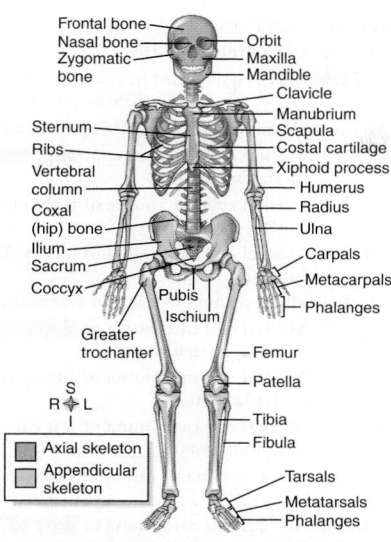

Figure 2-8   Diagram of skeleton of trunk and limbs with bones labeled. (From Thibodeau and Patton: Anatomy and Physiology, ed 7, Mosby, 2010)

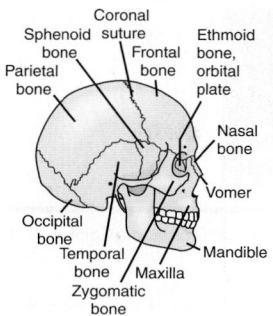

Figure 2-9   Bones of the skull.

● **C40.2**   **Malignant neoplasm of long bones of lower limb**
    (Ex) **For catgory C40.2 CC codes:** C40.20-C40.22, C40.80-C40.92, C41.9, Z51.0

   C40.20   **Malignant neoplasm of long bones of** unspecified **lower limb** 🖐

   C40.21   **Malignant neoplasm of long bones of right lower limb** 🖐

   C40.22   **Malignant neoplasm of long bones of left lower limb** 🖐

● **C40.3**   **Malignant neoplasm of short bones of lower limb**
    (Ex) **For catgory C40.3 CC codes:** C40.30-C40.92, C41.9, Z51.0

   C40.30   **Malignant neoplasm of short bones of** unspecified **lower limb** 🖐

   C40.31   **Malignant neoplasm of short bones of right lower limb** 🖐

   C40.32   **Malignant neoplasm of short bones of left lower limb** 🖐

● **C40.8**   **Malignant neoplasm of overlapping sites of bone and articular cartilage of limb**
    (Ex) **For catgory C40.8 CC codes:** C40.00-C41.9, Z51.0

   C40.80   **Malignant neoplasm of overlapping sites of bone and articular cartilage of** unspecified **limb** 🖐

   C40.81   **Malignant neoplasm of overlapping sites of bone and articular cartilage of right limb** 🖐

   C40.82   **Malignant neoplasm of overlapping sites of bone and articular cartilage of left limb** 🖐

● **C40.9**   **Malignant neoplasm of unspecified bones and articular cartilage of limb**
    (Ex) **For category C40.9 CC codes:** See C40.8

   C40.90   **Malignant neoplasm of** unspecified **bones and articular cartilage of unspecified limb** 🖐

   C40.91   **Malignant neoplasm of** unspecified **bones and articular cartilage of right limb** 🖐

   C40.92   **Malignant neoplasm of** unspecified **bones and articular cartilage of left limb** 🖐

● **C41**   **Malignant neoplasm of bone and articular cartilage of other and unspecified sites**
   Excludes1   malignant neoplasm of bones of limbs (C40.-)
                malignant neoplasm of cartilage of ear (C49.0)
                malignant neoplasm of cartilage of eyelid (C49.0)
                malignant neoplasm of cartilage of larynx (C32.3)
                malignant neoplasm of cartilage of limbs (C40.-)
                malignant neoplasm of cartilage of nose (C30.0)

   C41.0   **Malignant neoplasm of bones of skull and face** 🖐
      Malignant neoplasm of maxilla (superior)
      Malignant neoplasm of orbital bone
     Excludes2   carcinoma, any type except intraosseous or odontogenic of:
                maxillary sinus (C31.0)
                upper jaw (C03.0)
                malignant neoplasm of jaw bone (lower) (C41.1)
      (Ex) C40.80-C41.0, C41.9, Z51.0

   C41.1   **Malignant neoplasm of mandible** 🖐
      Malignant neoplasm of inferior maxilla
      Malignant neoplasm of lower jaw bone
     Excludes2   carcinoma, any type except intraosseous or odontogenic of:
                jaw NOS (C03.9)
                lower (C03.1)
                malignant neoplasm of upper jaw bone (C41.0)
      (Ex) C40.80-C40.92, C41.1, C41.9, Z51.0

   C41.2   **Malignant neoplasm of vertebral column** 🖐
     Excludes1   malignant neoplasm of sacrum and coccyx (C41.4)
      (Ex) C40.80-C40.9, C41.2, C41.9, Z51.0

   C41.3   **Malignant neoplasm of ribs, sternum and clavicle** 🖐
      (Ex) C40.80-C40.92, C41.3, C41.9, Z51.0

   C41.4   **Malignant neoplasm of pelvic bones, sacrum and coccyx** 🖐
      (Ex) C40.80-C40.92, C41.4-C41.9, Z51.0

   C41.9   **Malignant neoplasm of bone and articular cartilage,** unspecified 🖐
      (Ex) See C40.8

MELANOMA AND OTHER MALIGNANT NEOPLASMS OF SKIN (C43-C44)

● **C43**   **Malignant melanoma of skin**
   Excludes1   melanoma in situ (D03.-)
   Excludes2   malignant melanoma of skin of genital organs (C51-C52, C60.-, C63.-)
                Merkel cell carcinoma (C4A.-)
                sites other than skin-code to malignant neoplasm of the site

   C43.0   **Malignant melanoma of lip**
     Excludes1   malignant neoplasm of vermilion border of lip (C00.0-C00.2)

N   Newborn Age: 0   **P**   Pediatric Age: 0–17   **M**   Maternity DX: 12–55   **A**   Adult Age: 15–124   ♀ Females Only   ♂ Males Only
    🖐 Complication\Comorbidity   🖐 Major C\C   (Ex) CC/MCC Exclusions   🖐 Hospital-Acquired Condition

679

CHAPTER 2 (C00-D49)

CHAPTER 2 (C00-D49)

Figure 2-10 Malignant melanoma of skin. (From Goldman: Cecil Textbook of Medicine, ed 22, Saunders, 2004)

Item 2–4 Malignant melanoma is a serious form of skin cancer that affects the melanocytes (pigment-forming cells) and is caused by ultraviolet (UV) rays from the sun that damage skin. It is most commonly seen in the 40- to 60-year-olds with fair skin, blue or green eyes, and red or blond hair who sunburn easily.

Melanoma can spread very rapidly and is the most deadly form of skin cancer. It is less common than other types of skin cancer. The rate of melanoma is increasing and currently is the leading cause of death from skin disease.

- **C43.1 Malignant melanoma of eyelid, including canthus**
  Canthus: Either corner of eye where upper and lower eyelids meet
  - **C43.10 Malignant melanoma of** unspecified **eyelid, including canthus**
  - **C43.11 Malignant melanoma of right eyelid, including canthus**
  - **C43.12 Malignant melanoma of left eyelid, including canthus**
- **C43.2 Malignant melanoma of ear and external auricular canal**
  - **C43.20 Malignant melanoma of** unspecified **ear and external auricular canal**
  - **C43.21 Malignant melanoma of right ear and external auricular canal**
  - **C43.22 Malignant melanoma of left ear and external auricular canal**
- **C43.3 Malignant melanoma of other and unspecified parts of face**
  - **C43.30 Malignant melanoma of** unspecified **part of face**
  - **C43.31 Malignant melanoma of nose**
  - **C43.39 Malignant melanoma of other parts of face**
- **C43.4 Malignant melanoma of scalp and neck**
- **C43.5 Malignant melanoma of trunk**
  > **Excludes2**   malignant neoplasm of anus NOS (C21.0)
  > malignant neoplasm of scrotum (C63.2)
  - **C43.51 Malignant melanoma of anal skin**
    Malignant melanoma of anal margin
    Malignant melanoma of perianal skin
  - **C43.52 Malignant melanoma of skin of breast**
  - **C43.59 Malignant melanoma of other part of trunk**
- **C43.6 Malignant melanoma of upper limb, including shoulder**
  - **C43.60 Malignant melanoma of upper limb, including shoulder,** unspecified **side**
  - **C43.61 Malignant melanoma of right upper limb, including shoulder**
  - **C43.62 Malignant melanoma of left upper limb, including shoulder**
- **C43.7 Malignant melanoma of lower limb, including hip**
  - **C43.70 Malignant melanoma of** unspecified **lower limb, including hip**
  - **C43.71 Malignant melanoma of right lower limb, including hip**
  - **C43.72 Malignant melanoma of left lower limb, including hip**
- **C43.8 Malignant melanoma of overlapping sites of skin**
- **C43.9 Malignant melanoma of skin,** unspecified
  Malignant melanoma of unspecified site of skin
  Melanoma (malignant) NOS

- **C4A Merkel cell carcinoma**
  - **C4A.0 Merkel cell carcinoma of lip**
    > **Excludes1**   malignant neoplasm of vermilion border of lip (C00.0-C00.2)
  - **C4A.1 Merkel cell carcinoma of eyelid, including canthus**
    - **C4A.10 Merkel cell carcinoma of** unspecified **eyelid, including canthus**
    - **C4A.11 Merkel cell carcinoma of right eyelid, including canthus**
    - **C4A.12 Merkel cell carcinoma of left eyelid, including canthus**
  - **C4A.2 Merkel cell carcinoma of ear and external auricular canal**
    - **C4A.20 Merkel cell carcinoma of** unspecified **ear and external auricular canal**
    - **C4A.21 Merkel cell carcinoma of right ear and external auricular canal**
    - **C4A.22 Merkel cell carcinoma of left ear and external auricular canal**
  - **C4A.3 Merkel cell carcinoma of other and unspecified parts of face**
    - **C4A.30 Merkel cell carcinoma of** unspecified **part of face**
    - **C4A.31 Merkel cell carcinoma of nose**
    - **C4A.39 Merkel cell carcinoma of other parts of face**
  - **C4A.4 Merkel cell carcinoma of scalp and neck**
  - **C4A.5 Merkel cell carcinoma of trunk**
    > **Excludes2**   malignant neoplasm of anus NOS (C21.0)
    > malignant neoplasm of scrotum (C63.2)
    - **C4A.51 Merkel cell carcinoma of anal skin**
      Merkel cell carcinoma of anal margin
      Merkel cell carcinoma of perianal skin
    - **C4A.52 Merkel cell carcinoma of skin of breast**
    - **C4A.59 Merkel cell carcinoma of other part of trunk**
  - **C4A.6 Merkel cell carcinoma of upper limb, including shoulder**
    - **C4A.60 Merkel cell carcinoma of** unspecified **upper limb, including shoulder**
    - **C4A.61 Merkel cell carcinoma of right upper limb, including shoulder**
    - **C4A.62 Merkel cell carcinoma of left upper limb, including shoulder**
  - **C4A.7 Merkel cell carcinoma of lower limb, including hip**
    - **C4A.70 Merkel cell carcinoma of** unspecified **lower limb, including hip**
    - **C4A.71 Merkel cell carcinoma of right lower limb, including hip**
    - **C4A.72 Merkel cell carcinoma of left lower limb, including hip**
  - **C4A.8 Merkel cell carcinoma of overlapping sites**
  - **C4A.9 Merkel cell carcinoma,** unspecified
    Merkel cell carcinoma of unspecified site
    Merkel cell carcinoma NOS

- **C44 Other and unspecified malignant neoplasm of skin**
  > **Includes**   malignant neoplasm of sebaceous glands
  > malignant neoplasm of sweat glands
  > **Excludes1**   Kaposi's sarcoma of skin (C46.0)
  > malignant melanoma of skin (C43.-)
  > malignant neoplasm of skin of genital organs (C51-C52, C60.-, C63.2)
  > Merkel cell carcinoma (C4A.-)
  - **C44.0 Other and unspecified malignant neoplasm of skin of lip**
    > **Excludes1**   malignant neoplasm of lip (C00.-)
    - **C44.00 ** Unspecified **malignant neoplasm of skin of lip**
    - **C44.01 Basal cell carcinoma of skin of lip**
    - **C44.02 Squamous cell carcinoma of skin of lip**
    - **C44.09 Other specified malignant neoplasm of skin of lip**

◀ New   ◀▥ Revised   ~~deleted~~ Deleted   Excludes 1   Excludes 2   Includes   Use additional   Code first   Code also   Unspecified

680   **OGCR** Official Guidelines   ● Unacceptable Principal Diagnosis   X Assign placeholder X   ● Use Additional Character(s)   ▲ Manifestation Code   **Coding Clinic**

● **C44.1**   **Other and unspecified malignant neoplasm of skin of eyelid, including canthus**
> **Excludes1**   connective tissue of eyelid (C49.0)

● **C44.10**   Unspecified malignant neoplasm of skin of eyelid, including canthus
    C44.101   Unspecified malignant neoplasm of skin of unspecified eyelid, including canthus
    C44.102   Unspecified malignant neoplasm of skin of right eyelid, including canthus
    C44.109   Unspecified malignant neoplasm of skin of left eyelid, including canthus

● **C44.11**   Basal cell carcinoma of skin of eyelid, including canthus
    C44.111   Basal cell carcinoma of skin of unspecified eyelid, including canthus
    C44.112   Basal cell carcinoma of skin of right eyelid, including canthus
    C44.119   Basal cell carcinoma of skin of left eyelid, including canthus

● **C44.12**   Squamous cell carcinoma of skin of eyelid, including canthus
    C44.121   Squamous cell carcinoma of skin of unspecified eyelid, including canthus
    C44.122   Squamous cell carcinoma of skin of right eyelid, including canthus
    C44.129   Squamous cell carcinoma of skin of left eyelid, including canthus

● **C44.19**   Other specified malignant neoplasm of skin of eyelid, including canthus
    C44.191   Other specified malignant neoplasm of skin of unspecified eyelid, including canthus
    C44.192   Other specified malignant neoplasm of skin of right eyelid, including canthus
    C44.199   Other specified malignant neoplasm of skin of left eyelid, including canthus

● **C44.2**   **Other and unspecified malignant neoplasm of skin of ear and external auricular canal**
> **Excludes1**   connective tissue of ear (C49.0)

● **C44.20**   Unspecified malignant neoplasm of skin of ear and external auricular canal
    C44.201   Unspecified malignant neoplasm of skin of unspecified ear and external auricular canal
    C44.202   Unspecified malignant neoplasm of skin of right ear and external auricular canal
    C44.209   Unspecified malignant neoplasm of skin of left ear and external auricular canal

● **C44.21**   Basal cell carcinoma of skin of ear and external auricular canal
    C44.211   Basal cell carcinoma of skin of unspecified ear and external auricular canal
    C44.212   Basal cell carcinoma of skin of right ear and external auricular canal
    C44.219   Basal cell carcinoma of skin of left ear and external auricular canal

● **C44.22**   Squamous cell carcinoma of skin of ear and external auricular canal
    C44.221   Squamous cell carcinoma of skin of unspecified ear and external auricular canal
    C44.222   Squamous cell carcinoma of skin of right ear and external auricular canal
    C44.229   Squamous cell carcinoma of skin of left ear and external auricular canal

● **C44.29**   Other specified malignant neoplasm of skin of ear and external auricular canal
    C44.291   Other specified malignant neoplasm of skin of unspecified ear and external auricular canal
    C44.292   Other specified malignant neoplasm of skin of right ear and external auricular canal
    C44.299   Other specified malignant neoplasm of skin of left ear and external auricular canal

● **C44.3**   **Other and unspecified malignant neoplasm of skin of other and unspecified parts of face**

● **C44.30**   Unspecified malignant neoplasm of skin of other and unspecified parts of face
    C44.300   Unspecified malignant neoplasm of skin of unspecified part of face
    C44.301   Unspecified malignant neoplasm of skin of nose
    C44.309   Unspecified malignant neoplasm of skin of other parts of face

● **C44.31**   Basal cell carcinoma of skin of other and unspecified parts of face
    C44.310   Basal cell carcinoma of skin of unspecified parts of face
    C44.311   Basal cell carcinoma of skin of nose
    C44.319   Basal cell carcinoma of skin of other parts of face

● **C44.32**   Squamous cell carcinoma of skin of other and unspecified parts of face
    C44.320   Squamous cell carcinoma of skin of unspecified parts of face
    C44.321   Squamous cell carcinoma of skin of nose
    C44.329   Squamous cell carcinoma of skin of other parts of face

● **C44.39**   Other specified malignant neoplasm of skin of other and unspecified parts of face
    C44.390   Other specified malignant neoplasm of skin of unspecified parts of face
    C44.391   Other specified malignant neoplasm of skin of nose
    C44.399   Other specified malignant neoplasm of skin of other parts of face

● **C44.4**   **Other and unspecified malignant neoplasm of skin of scalp and neck**
    C44.40   Unspecified malignant neoplasm of skin of scalp and neck
    C44.41   Basal cell carcinoma of skin of scalp and neck
    C44.42   Squamous cell carcinoma of skin of scalp and neck
    C44.49   Other specified malignant neoplasm of skin of scalp and neck

CHAPTER 2 (C00–D49)

N Newborn Age: 0   **P** Pediatric Age: 0–17   **M** Maternity DX: 12–55   **A** Adult Age: 15–124   ♀ Females Only   ♂ Males Only

Complication\Comorbidity   Major C\C   (Ex) CC/MCC Exclusions   Hospital-Acquired Condition

681

● **C44.5**   **Other and unspecified malignant neoplasm of skin of trunk**

> **Excludes1**   anus NOS (C21.0)
> scrotum (C63.2)

● **C44.50**   **Unspecified malignant neoplasm of skin of trunk**

     C44.500   Unspecified malignant neoplasm of anal skin
> Unspecified malignant neoplasm of anal margin
> Unspecified malignant neoplasm of perianal skin

     C44.501   Unspecified malignant neoplasm of skin of breast

     C44.509   Unspecified malignant neoplasm of skin of other part of trunk

● **C44.51**   **Basal cell carcinoma of skin of trunk**

     C44.510   Basal cell carcinoma of anal skin
> Basal cell carcinoma of anal margin
> Basal cell carcinoma of perianal skin

     C44.511   Basal cell carcinoma of skin of breast

     C44.519   Basal cell carcinoma of skin of other part of trunk

● **C44.52**   **Squamous cell carcinoma of skin of trunk**

     C44.520   Squamous cell carcinoma of anal skin
> Squamous cell carcinoma of anal margin
> Squamous cell carcinoma of perianal skin

     C44.521   Squamous cell carcinoma of skin of breast

     C44.529   Squamous cell carcinoma of skin of other part of trunk

● **C44.59**   **Other specified malignant neoplasm of skin of trunk**

     C44.590   Other specified malignant neoplasm of anal skin
> Other specified malignant neoplasm of anal margin
> Other specified malignant neoplasm of perianal skin

     C44.591   Other specified malignant neoplasm of skin of breast

     C44.599   Other specified malignant neoplasm of skin of other part of trunk

● **C44.6**   **Other and unspecified malignant neoplasm of skin of upper limb, including shoulder**

● **C44.60**   **Unspecified malignant neoplasm of skin of upper limb, including shoulder**

     C44.601   Unspecified malignant neoplasm of skin of unspecified upper limb, including shoulder

     C44.602   Unspecified malignant neoplasm of skin of right upper limb, including shoulder

     C44.609   Unspecified malignant neoplasm of skin of left upper limb, including shoulder

● **C44.61**   **Basal cell carcinoma of skin of upper limb, including shoulder**

     C44.611   Basal cell carcinoma of skin of unspecified upper limb, including shoulder

     C44.612   Basal cell carcinoma of skin of right upper limb, including shoulder

     C44.619   Basal cell carcinoma of skin of left upper limb, including shoulder

● **C44.62**   **Squamous cell carcinoma of skin of upper limb, including shoulder**

     C44.621   Squamous cell carcinoma of skin of unspecified upper limb, including shoulder

     C44.622   Squamous cell carcinoma of skin of right upper limb, including shoulder

     C44.629   Squamous cell carcinoma of skin of left upper limb, including shoulder

● **C44.69**   **Other specified malignant neoplasm of skin of upper limb, including shoulder**

     C44.691   Other specified malignant neoplasm of skin of unspecified upper limb, including shoulder

     C44.692   Other specified malignant neoplasm of skin of right upper limb, including shoulder

     C44.699   Other specified malignant neoplasm of skin of left upper limb, including shoulder

● **C44.7**   **Other and unspecified malignant neoplasm of skin of lower limb, including hip**

● **C44.70**   **Unspecified malignant neoplasm of skin of lower limb, including hip**

     C44.701   Unspecified malignant neoplasm of skin of unspecified lower limb, including hip

     C44.702   Unspecified malignant neoplasm of skin of right lower limb, including hip

     C44.709   Unspecified malignant neoplasm of skin of left lower limb, including hip

● **C44.71**   **Basal cell carcinoma of skin of lower limb, including hip**

     C44.711   Basal cell carcinoma of skin of unspecified lower limb, including hip

     C44.712   Basal cell carcinoma of skin of right lower limb, including hip

     C44.719   Basal cell carcinoma of skin of left lower limb, including hip

● **C44.72**   **Squamous cell carcinoma of skin of lower limb, including hip**

     C44.721   Squamous cell carcinoma of skin of unspecified lower limb, including hip

     C44.722   Squamous cell carcinoma of skin of right lower limb, including hip

     C44.729   Squamous cell carcinoma of skin of left lower limb, including hip

● **C44.79**   **Other specified malignant neoplasm of skin of lower limb, including hip**

     C44.791   Other specified malignant neoplasm of skin of unspecified lower limb, including hip

     C44.792   Other specified malignant neoplasm of skin of right lower limb, including hip

     C44.799   Other specified malignant neoplasm of skin of left lower limb, including hip

● **C44.8**   **Other and unspecified malignant neoplasm of overlapping sites of skin**

     C44.80   Unspecified malignant neoplasm of overlapping sites of skin

     C44.81   Basal cell carcinoma of overlapping sites of skin

     C44.82   Squamous cell carcinoma of overlapping sites of skin

     C44.89   Other specified malignant neoplasm of overlapping sites of skin

◄ New   ◄|||| Revised   ~~deleted~~ Deleted   Excludes 1   Excludes 2   Includes   Use additional   Code first   Code also   Unspecified

OGCR Official Guidelines   ● Unacceptable Principal Diagnosis   **X** Assign placeholder X   ● Use Additional Character(s)   ▶ Manifestation Code   **Coding Clinic**

682

● **C44.9** **Other and unspecified malignant neoplasm of skin, unspecified**

  C44.90 **Unspecified malignant neoplasm of skin, unspecified**
     Malignant neoplasm of unspecified site of skin

  C44.91 **Basal cell carcinoma of skin, unspecified**

  C44.92 **Squamous cell carcinoma of skin, unspecified**

  C44.99 **Other specified malignant neoplasm of skin, unspecified**

MALIGNANT NEOPLASMS OF MESOTHELIAL AND SOFT TISSUE (C45-C49)

● **C45** **Mesothelioma**
  Malignant cells develop in protective lining that covers internal organs (mesothelium) caused by exposure to asbestos

  C45.0 **Mesothelioma of pleura**
     Excludes1 other malignant neoplasm of pleura (C38.4)
     (Ex) C38.4, C39.9, C45.0, C45.7-C45.9, C76.8, C7A.00, C7A.098, C7A.1-C7B.00, C7B.1, C80.0-C80.2, D49.1, D49.81-D49.9

  C45.1 **Mesothelioma of peritoneum**
     Mesothelioma of cul-de-sac
     Mesothelioma of mesentery
     Mesothelioma of mesocolon
     Mesothelioma of omentum
     Mesothelioma of peritoneum (parietal) (pelvic)
     Excludes1 other malignant neoplasm of soft tissue of peritoneum (C48.-)
     (Ex) C45.1, C48.0-C48.8, Z51.0

  C45.2 **Mesothelioma of pericardium**
     Excludes1 other malignant neoplasm of pericardium (C38.0)
     (Ex) C38.0, C45.2

  C45.7 **Mesothelioma of other sites**

  C45.9 **Mesothelioma, unspecified**

● **C46** **Kaposi's sarcoma**
  Code first any human immunodeficiency virus [HIV] disease (B20)

  C46.0 **Kaposi's sarcoma of skin**
     (Ex) C46.0, C46.7-C46.9, Z51.0

  C46.1 **Kaposi's sarcoma of soft tissue**
     Kaposi's sarcoma of blood vessel
     Kaposi's sarcoma of connective tissue
     Kaposi's sarcoma of fascia
     Kaposi's sarcoma of ligament
     Kaposi's sarcoma of lymphatic(s) NEC
     Kaposi's sarcoma of muscle
     Excludes2 Kaposi's sarcoma of lymph glands and nodes (C46.3)
     (Ex) C46.1, C46.7-C46.9, Z51.0

  C46.2 **Kaposi's sarcoma of palate**
     (Ex) C46.2, C46.7-C46.9, Z51.0

  C46.3 **Kaposi's sarcoma of lymph nodes**
     (Ex) C45.7-C45.9, C46.3, C76.8-C77.9, C7A.00, C7A.098-C7B.01, C7B.1, C80.0-C80.2, D49.81-D49.9

  C46.4 **Kaposi's sarcoma of gastrointestinal sites**
     (Ex) C46.4, C46.7-C46.9, Z51.0

Figure 2-11 Kaposi's sarcoma. There are large confluent hyperpigmented patch-stage lesions with lymphedema. (From Cohen & Powderly: Infectious Diseases, ed 3, Mosby, An Imprint of Elsevier, 2010)

Item 2–5 **Kaposi's sarcoma** is a cancer that causes patches of abnormal tissue to grow under the skin; in the lining of the mouth, nose, and throat; or in other organs, often beginning and spreading to other organs. Patients who have had organ transplants or patients with AIDS are at high risk for this malignancy.

● **C46.5** **Kaposi's sarcoma of lung**
     (Ex) For catgory C46.5 CC codes: C34.80-C34.92, C39.9, C45.7-C45.9, C46.50-C46.52, C76.8, C7A.00, C7A.090, C7A.098-C7B.00, C7B.1, C80.0-C80.2, D49.1, D49.81-D49.9

  C46.50 **Kaposi's sarcoma of unspecified lung**

  C46.51 **Kaposi's sarcoma of right lung**

  C46.52 **Kaposi's sarcoma of left lung**

  C46.7 **Kaposi's sarcoma of other sites**
     (Ex) C46.0-C46.9, Z51.0

  C46.9 **Kaposi's sarcoma, unspecified**
     Kaposi's sarcoma of unspecified site
     (Ex) C45.7-C46.9, C51.0-C72.9, C76.0-C79.9, C7A.00, C7A.093, C7A.098-C7B.8, C80.0-C80.2, D00.00-D02.4, D04.0-D09.9, D37.01-D44.9, D48.0-D49.9, Z51.0

● **C47** **Malignant neoplasm of peripheral nerves and autonomic nervous system**
     Includes malignant neoplasm of sympathetic and parasympathetic nerves and ganglia
     Excludes1 Kaposi's sarcoma of soft tissue (C46.1)
     (Ex) For category C47 CC Codes: Z51.0

  C47.0 **Malignant neoplasm of peripheral nerves of head, face and neck**
     Excludes1 malignant neoplasm of peripheral nerves of orbit (C69.6-)

● **C47.1** **Malignant neoplasm of peripheral nerves of upper limb, including shoulder**

  C47.10 **Malignant neoplasm of peripheral nerves of unspecified upper limb, including shoulder**

  C47.11 **Malignant neoplasm of peripheral nerves of right upper limb, including shoulder**

  C47.12 **Malignant neoplasm of peripheral nerves of left upper limb, including shoulder**

● **C47.2** **Malignant neoplasm of peripheral nerves of lower limb, including hip**

  C47.20 **Malignant neoplasm of peripheral nerves of unspecified lower limb, including hip**

  C47.21 **Malignant neoplasm of peripheral nerves of right lower limb, including hip**

  C47.22 **Malignant neoplasm of peripheral nerves of left lower limb, including hip**

  C47.3 **Malignant neoplasm of peripheral nerves of thorax**

  C47.4 **Malignant neoplasm of peripheral nerves of abdomen**

  C47.5 **Malignant neoplasm of peripheral nerves of pelvis**

  C47.6 **Malignant neoplasm of peripheral nerves of trunk, unspecified**
     Malignant neoplasm of peripheral nerves of unspecified part of trunk

  C47.8 **Malignant neoplasm of overlapping sites of peripheral nerves and autonomic nervous system**

  C47.9 **Malignant neoplasm of peripheral nerves and autonomic nervous system, unspecified**
     Malignant neoplasm of unspecified site of peripheral nerves and autonomic nervous system

● **C48** **Malignant neoplasm of retroperitoneum and peritoneum**
     Excludes1 Kaposi's sarcoma of connective tissue (C46.1)
     mesothelioma (C45.-)
     (Ex) For category C48 unless otherwise indicated: C45.1, C48.0-C48.8, Z51.0

  C48.0 **Malignant neoplasm of retroperitoneum**
     Behind/outside of peritoneum
     (Ex) C48.0, Z51.0

  C48.1 **Malignant neoplasm of specified parts of peritoneum**
     Serous membrane lining abdominopelvic walls and covering viscera
     Malignant neoplasm of cul-de-sac
     Malignant neoplasm of mesentery
     Malignant neoplasm of mesocolon
     Malignant neoplasm of omentum
     Malignant neoplasm of parietal peritoneum
     Malignant neoplasm of pelvic peritoneum

  C48.2 **Malignant neoplasm of peritoneum, unspecified**

  C48.8 **Malignant neoplasm of overlapping sites of retroperitoneum and peritoneum**

N Newborn Age: 0   **P** Pediatric Age: 0–17   **M** Maternity DX: 12–55   **A** Adult Age: 15–124   ♀ Females Only   ♂ Males Only

Complication\Comorbidity   Major C\C   (Ex) CC/MCC Exclusions   Hospital-Acquired Condition

683

CHAPTER 2 (C00-D49)

● **C49**   **Malignant neoplasm of other connective and soft tissue**

     Includes   malignant neoplasm of blood vessel
                   malignant neoplasm of bursa
                   malignant neoplasm of cartilage
                   malignant neoplasm of fascia
                   malignant neoplasm of fat
                   malignant neoplasm of ligament, except uterine
                   malignant neoplasm of lymphatic vessel
                   malignant neoplasm of muscle
                   malignant neoplasm of synovia
                   malignant neoplasm of tendon (sheath)

     Excludes1   malignant neoplasm of cartilage (of):
                       articular (C40-C41)
                       larynx (C32.3)
                       nose (C30.0)
                   malignant neoplasm of connective tissue of breast
                       (C50.-)

     Excludes2   Kaposi's sarcoma of soft tissue (C46.1)
                   malignant neoplasm of heart (C38.0)
                   malignant neoplasm of peripheral nerves and
                       autonomic nervous system (C47.-)
                   malignant neoplasm of peritoneum (C48.2)
                   malignant neoplasm of retroperitoneum (C48.0)
                   malignant neoplasm of uterine ligament (C57.3)
                   mesothelioma (C45.-)

     (Ex:) For category C49 unless otherwise indicated: Z51.0

    C49.0   **Malignant neoplasm of connective and soft tissue of head, face and neck** 🔵
        Malignant neoplasm of connective tissue of ear
        Malignant neoplasm of connective tissue of eyelid

        Excludes1   connective tissue of orbit (C69.6-)

● **C49.1**   **Malignant neoplasm of connective and soft tissue of upper limb, including shoulder**

    C49.10   **Malignant neoplasm of connective and soft tissue of unspecified upper limb, including shoulder** 🔵

    C49.11   **Malignant neoplasm of connective and soft tissue of right upper limb, including shoulder** 🔵

    C49.12   **Malignant neoplasm of connective and soft tissue of left upper limb, including shoulder** 🔵

● **C49.2**   **Malignant neoplasm of connective and soft tissue of lower limb, including hip**

    C49.20   **Malignant neoplasm of connective and soft tissue of unspecified lower limb, including hip** 🔵

    C49.21   **Malignant neoplasm of connective and soft tissue of right lower limb, including hip** 🔵

    C49.22   **Malignant neoplasm of connective and soft tissue of left lower limb, including hip** 🔵

    C49.3   **Malignant neoplasm of connective and soft tissue of thorax** 🔵
        Malignant neoplasm of axilla
        Malignant neoplasm of diaphragm
        Malignant neoplasm of great vessels

        Excludes1   malignant neoplasm of breast (C50.-)
                       malignant neoplasm of heart (C38.0)
                       malignant neoplasm of mediastinum
                          (C38.1-C38.3)
                       malignant neoplasm of thymus (C37)

     Coding Clinic: 2015, Q3, P19

    C49.4   **Malignant neoplasm of connective and soft tissue of abdomen** 🔵
        Malignant neoplasm of abdominal wall
        Malignant neoplasm of hypochondrium

    C49.5   **Malignant neoplasm of connective and soft tissue of pelvis** 🔵
        Malignant neoplasm of buttock
        Malignant neoplasm of groin
        Malignant neoplasm of perineum

    C49.6   **Malignant neoplasm of connective and soft tissue of trunk, unspecified** 🔵
        Malignant neoplasm of back NOS

    C49.8   **Malignant neoplasm of overlapping sites of connective and soft tissue** 🔵
        Primary malignant neoplasm of two or more
            contiguous sites of connective and soft tissue

    C49.9   **Malignant neoplasm of connective and soft tissue, unspecified** 🔵

● **C49.A**   **Gastrointestinal stromal tumor** ◀
       (Ex:) For category C49.A CC codes unless otherwise indicated: Z51.0

    C49.A0   **Gastrointestinal stromal tumor, unspecified site** 🔵 ◀

    C49.A1   **Gastrointestinal stromal tumor of esophagus** 🔵 ◀

    C49.A2   **Gastrointestinal stromal tumor of stomach** 🔵 ◀
       (Ex:) D80.0, D80.3-D81.4, D81.6-D81.7, D81.89-D84.0, D84.8-D84.9, D89.3-D89.9

    C49.A3   **Gastrointestinal stromal tumor of small intestine** 🔵 ◀

    C49.A4   **Gastrointestinal stromal tumor of large intestine** 🔵 ◀

    C49.A5   **Gastrointestinal stromal tumor of rectum** 🔵 ◀

    C49.A9   **Gastrointestinal stromal tumor of other sites** 🔵 ◀

MALIGNANT NEOPLASMS OF BREAST (C50)

● **C50**   **Malignant neoplasm of breast**

     Includes   connective tissue of breast
                   Paget's disease of breast
                   Paget's disease of nipple
                   Intraductal carcinoma of breast characterized by eczema-like inflammatory skin changes

     Use additional code to identify estrogen receptor status (Z17.0, Z17.1)

     Excludes1   skin of breast (C44.501, C44.511, C44.521, C44.591)

● **C50.0**   **Malignant neoplasm of nipple and areola**

    ● **C50.01**   **Malignant neoplasm of nipple and areola, female**

       C50.011   **Malignant neoplasm of nipple and areola, right female breast** ♀

       C50.012   **Malignant neoplasm of nipple and areola, left female breast** ♀

       C50.019   **Malignant neoplasm of nipple and areola, unspecified female breast** ♀

    ● **C50.02**   **Malignant neoplasm of nipple and areola, male**

       C50.021   **Malignant neoplasm of nipple and areola, right male breast** ♂

       C50.022   **Malignant neoplasm of nipple and areola, left male breast** ♂

       C50.029   **Malignant neoplasm of nipple and areola, unspecified male breast** ♂

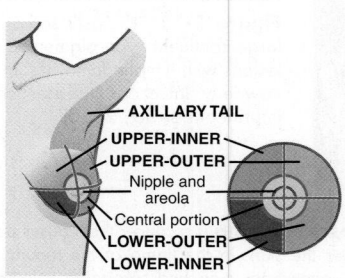

Figure 2-12   Female breast quadrants and axillary tail.

◀ New   ◀▦ Revised   ~~deleted~~ Deleted   Excludes 1   Excludes 2   Includes   Use additional   Code first   Code also   Unspecified
OGCR Official Guidelines   ● Unacceptable Principal Diagnosis   X Assign placeholder X   🔵 Use Additional Character(s)   ▌ Manifestation Code   **Coding Clinic**

- C50.1 Malignant neoplasm of central portion of breast
  - C50.11 Malignant neoplasm of central portion of breast, female
    - C50.111 Malignant neoplasm of central portion of right female breast ♀
    - C50.112 Malignant neoplasm of central portion of left female breast ♀
    - C50.119 Malignant neoplasm of central portion of unspecified female breast ♀
  - C50.12 Malignant neoplasm of central portion of breast, male
    - C50.121 Malignant neoplasm of central portion of right male breast ♂
    - C50.122 Malignant neoplasm of central portion of left male breast ♂
    - C50.129 Malignant neoplasm of central portion of unspecified male breast ♂
- C50.2 Malignant neoplasm of upper-inner quadrant of breast
  - C50.21 Malignant neoplasm of upper-inner quadrant of breast, female
    - C50.211 Malignant neoplasm of upper-inner quadrant of right female breast ♀
    - C50.212 Malignant neoplasm of upper-inner quadrant of left female breast ♀
    - C50.219 Malignant neoplasm of upper-inner quadrant of unspecified female breast ♀
  - C50.22 Malignant neoplasm of upper-inner quadrant of breast, male
    - C50.221 Malignant neoplasm of upper-inner quadrant of right male breast ♂
    - C50.222 Malignant neoplasm of upper-inner quadrant of left male breast ♂
    - C50.229 Malignant neoplasm of upper-inner quadrant of unspecified male breast ♂
- C50.3 Malignant neoplasm of lower-inner quadrant of breast
  - C50.31 Malignant neoplasm of lower-inner quadrant of breast, female
    - C50.311 Malignant neoplasm of lower-inner quadrant of right female breast ♀
    - C50.312 Malignant neoplasm of lower-inner quadrant of left female breast ♀
    - C50.319 Malignant neoplasm of lower-inner quadrant of unspecified female breast ♀
  - C50.32 Malignant neoplasm of lower-inner quadrant of breast, male
    - C50.321 Malignant neoplasm of lower-inner quadrant of right male breast ♂
    - C50.322 Malignant neoplasm of lower-inner quadrant of left male breast ♂
    - C50.329 Malignant neoplasm of lower-inner quadrant of unspecified male breast ♂
- C50.4 Malignant neoplasm of upper-outer quadrant of breast
  - C50.41 Malignant neoplasm of upper-outer quadrant of breast, female
    - C50.411 Malignant neoplasm of upper-outer quadrant of right female breast ♀
    - C50.412 Malignant neoplasm of upper-outer quadrant of left female breast ♀
    - C50.419 Malignant neoplasm of upper-outer quadrant of unspecified female breast ♀
- C50.42 Malignant neoplasm of upper-outer quadrant of breast, male
    - C50.421 Malignant neoplasm of upper-outer quadrant of right male breast ♂
    - C50.422 Malignant neoplasm of upper-outer quadrant of left male breast ♂
    - C50.429 Malignant neoplasm of upper-outer quadrant of unspecified male breast ♂
- C50.5 Malignant neoplasm of lower-outer quadrant of breast
  - C50.51 Malignant neoplasm of lower-outer quadrant of breast, female
    - C50.511 Malignant neoplasm of lower-outer quadrant of right female breast ♀
    - C50.512 Malignant neoplasm of lower-outer quadrant of left female breast ♀
    - C50.519 Malignant neoplasm of lower-outer quadrant of unspecified female breast ♀
  - C50.52 Malignant neoplasm of lower-outer quadrant of breast, male
    - C50.521 Malignant neoplasm of lower-outer quadrant of right male breast ♂
    - C50.522 Malignant neoplasm of lower-outer quadrant of left male breast ♂
    - C50.529 Malignant neoplasm of lower-outer quadrant of unspecified male breast ♂
- C50.6 Malignant neoplasm of axillary tail of breast
  - C50.61 Malignant neoplasm of axillary tail of breast, female
    - C50.611 Malignant neoplasm of axillary tail of right female breast ♀
    - C50.612 Malignant neoplasm of axillary tail of left female breast ♀
    - C50.619 Malignant neoplasm of axillary tail of unspecified female breast ♀
  - C50.62 Malignant neoplasm of axillary tail of breast, male
    - C50.621 Malignant neoplasm of axillary tail of right male breast ♂
    - C50.622 Malignant neoplasm of axillary tail of left male breast ♂
    - C50.629 Malignant neoplasm of axillary tail of unspecified male breast ♂
- C50.8 Malignant neoplasm of overlapping sites of breast
  - C50.81 Malignant neoplasm of overlapping sites of breast, female
    - C50.811 Malignant neoplasm of overlapping sites of right female breast ♀
    - C50.812 Malignant neoplasm of overlapping sites of left female breast ♀
    - C50.819 Malignant neoplasm of overlapping sites of unspecified female breast ♀
  - C50.82 Malignant neoplasm of overlapping sites of breast, male
    - C50.821 Malignant neoplasm of overlapping sites of right male breast ♂
    - C50.822 Malignant neoplasm of overlapping sites of left male breast ♂
    - C50.829 Malignant neoplasm of overlapping sites of unspecified male breast ♂
- C50.9 Malignant neoplasm of breast of unspecified site
  - C50.91 Malignant neoplasm of breast of unspecified site, female
    - C50.911 Malignant neoplasm of unspecified site of right female breast ♀
    - C50.912 Malignant neoplasm of unspecified site of left female breast ♀
    - C50.919 Malignant neoplasm of unspecified site of unspecified female breast ♀

CHAPTER 2 (C00-D49)

● C50.92 **Malignant neoplasm of breast of unspecified site, male**

    C50.921 **Malignant neoplasm of unspecified site of right male breast** ♂

    C50.922 **Malignant neoplasm of unspecified site of left male breast** ♂

    C50.929 **Malignant neoplasm of unspecified site of unspecified male breast** ♂

MALIGNANT NEOPLASMS OF FEMALE GENITAL ORGANS (C51-C58)

Includes   malignant neoplasm of skin of female genital organs

● C51 **Malignant neoplasm of vulva**

    Excludes1   carcinoma in situ of vulva (D07.1)

  C51.0 **Malignant neoplasm of labium majus** ♀
    Outer folds of skin external female genitalia
    Malignant neoplasm of Bartholin's [greater vestibular] gland

  C51.1 **Malignant neoplasm of labium minus** ♀
    Two inner folds surrounding vulva in female genitalia

  C51.2 **Malignant neoplasm of clitoris** ♀

  C51.8 **Malignant neoplasm of overlapping sites of vulva** ♀

  C51.9 **Malignant neoplasm of vulva, unspecified** ♀
    Malignant neoplasm of external female genitalia NOS
    Malignant neoplasm of pudendum

  C52 **Malignant neoplasm of vagina** ♀

    Excludes1   carcinoma in situ of vagina (D07.2)

● C53 **Malignant neoplasm of cervix uteri**

    Excludes1   carcinoma in situ of cervix uteri (D06.-)

  C53.0 **Malignant neoplasm of endocervix** ♀
    Inside the cervix

  C53.1 **Malignant neoplasm of exocervix** ♀
    Outside the cervix

  C53.8 **Malignant neoplasm of overlapping sites of cervix uteri** ♀

  C53.9 **Malignant neoplasm of cervix uteri, unspecified** ♀

● C54 **Malignant neoplasm of corpus uteri**

  C54.0 **Malignant neoplasm of isthmus uteri** ♀
    Constricted part of uterus between cervix and body
    Malignant neoplasm of lower uterine segment

  C54.1 **Malignant neoplasm of endometrium** ♀
    Lining of uterus

  C54.2 **Malignant neoplasm of myometrium** ♀
    Middle layer of uterine wall consisting of smooth muscle supporting stromal and vascular tissue

  C54.3 **Malignant neoplasm of fundus uteri** ♀
    Top rounded portion of uterus

  C54.8 **Malignant neoplasm of overlapping sites of corpus uteri** ♀
    Main body of uterus

  C54.9 **Malignant neoplasm of corpus uteri, unspecified** ♀

● C55 **Malignant neoplasm of uterus, part unspecified** ♀

● C56 **Malignant neoplasm of ovary**

    Use additional code to identify any functional activity

    (Ex) **For category C56 CC Codes:** C45.9, C56.1-C57.4, C76.3, C79.60-C79.62, C7A.00, C7A.098-C7B.00, C7B.1, C80.0-C80.2

  C56.1 **Malignant neoplasm of right ovary** ♀ 🔗

  C56.2 **Malignant neoplasm of left ovary** ♀ 🔗

  C56.9 **Malignant neoplasm of unspecified ovary** ♀ 🔗

● C57 **Malignant neoplasm of other and unspecified female genital organs**

  ● C57.0 **Malignant neoplasm of fallopian tube**
    Malignant neoplasm of oviduct
    Malignant neoplasm of uterine tube

    C57.00 **Malignant neoplasm of unspecified fallopian tube** ♀

    C57.01 **Malignant neoplasm of right fallopian tube** ♀

    C57.02 **Malignant neoplasm of left fallopian tube** ♀

  ● C57.1 **Malignant neoplasm of broad ligament**

    C57.10 **Malignant neoplasm of unspecified broad ligament** ♀

    C57.11 **Malignant neoplasm of right broad ligament** ♀

    C57.12 **Malignant neoplasm of left broad ligament** ♀

  ● C57.2 **Malignant neoplasm of round ligament**

    C57.20 **Malignant neoplasm of unspecified round ligament** ♀

    C57.21 **Malignant neoplasm of right round ligament** ♀

    C57.22 **Malignant neoplasm of left round ligament** ♀

  C57.3 **Malignant neoplasm of parametrium** ♀
    Malignant neoplasm of uterine ligament NOS

  C57.4 **Malignant neoplasm of uterine adnexa, unspecified** ♀

  C57.7 **Malignant neoplasm of other specified female genital organs** ♀
    Malignant neoplasm of wolffian body or duct

  C57.8 **Malignant neoplasm of overlapping sites of female genital organs** ♀
    Primary malignant neoplasm of two or more contiguous sites of the female genital organs whose point of origin cannot be determined
    Primary tubo-ovarian malignant neoplasm whose point of origin cannot be determined
    Primary utero-ovarian malignant neoplasm whose point of origin cannot be determined

  C57.9 **Malignant neoplasm of female genital organ, unspecified** ♀
    Malignant neoplasm of female genitourinary tract NOS

  C58 **Malignant neoplasm of placenta** ♀   M

    Includes   choriocarcinoma NOS
               chorionepithelioma NOS

    Excludes1   chorioadenoma (destruens) (D39.2)
                hydatidiform mole NOS (O01.9)
                invasive hydatidiform mole (D39.2)
                male choriocarcinoma NOS (C62.9-)
                malignant hydatidiform mole (D39.2)

MALIGNANT NEOPLASMS OF MALE GENITAL ORGANS (C60-C63)

Includes   malignant neoplasm of skin of male genital organs

● C60 **Malignant neoplasm of penis**

  C60.0 **Malignant neoplasm of prepuce** ♂
    Malignant neoplasm of foreskin

  C60.1 **Malignant neoplasm of glans penis** ♂

  C60.2 **Malignant neoplasm of body of penis** ♂
    Malignant neoplasm of corpus cavernosum

  C60.8 **Malignant neoplasm of overlapping sites of penis** ♂

  C60.9 **Malignant neoplasm of penis, unspecified** ♂
    Malignant neoplasm of skin of penis NOS

Figure 2-13   Cervix uteri.

Left side margin: CHAPTER 2 (C00-D49)

◀ New   ◀ Revised   ~~deleted~~ Deleted   Excludes 1   Excludes 2   Includes   Use additional   Code first   Code also   Unspecified

OGCR Official Guidelines   ● Unacceptable Principal Diagnosis   X Assign placeholder X   ● Use Additional Character(s)   ▶ Manifestation Code   Coding Clinic

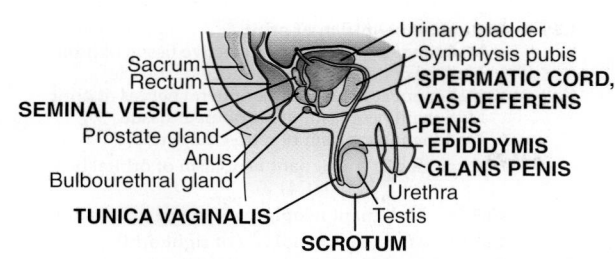

Figure 2-14   Penis and other male genital organs.

C61   **Malignant neoplasm of prostate** ♂
> Use additional code to identify: ◀
> hormone sensitivity status (Z19.1-Z19.2) ◀
> rising PSA following treatment for malignant neoplasm of prostate (R97.21) ◀
> **Excludes1**   malignant neoplasm of seminal vesicle (C63.7)

● C62   **Malignant neoplasm of testis**
> Use additional code to identify any functional activity.

  ● C62.0   **Malignant neoplasm of undescended testis**
> Malignant neoplasm of ectopic testis
> Malignant neoplasm of retained testis

     C62.00   **Malignant neoplasm of unspecified undescended testis** ♂

     C62.01   **Malignant neoplasm of undescended right testis** ♂

     C62.02   **Malignant neoplasm of undescended left testis** ♂

  ● C62.1   **Malignant neoplasm of descended testis**
> Malignant neoplasm of scrotal testis

     C62.10   **Malignant neoplasm of unspecified descended testis, unspecified side** ♂

     C62.11   **Malignant neoplasm of descended right testis** ♂

     C62.12   **Malignant neoplasm of descended left testis** ♂

  ● C62.9   **Malignant neoplasm of testis, unspecified whether descended or undescended**

     C62.90   **Malignant neoplasm of unspecified testis, unspecified whether descended or undescended** ♂
> Malignant neoplasm of testis NOS

     C62.91   **Malignant neoplasm of right testis, unspecified whether descended or undescended** ♂

     C62.92   **Malignant neoplasm of left testis, unspecified whether descended or undescended** ♂

● C63   **Malignant neoplasm of other and unspecified male genital organs**

  ● C63.0   **Malignant neoplasm of epididymis**

     C63.00   **Malignant neoplasm of unspecified epididymis** ♂

     C63.01   **Malignant neoplasm of right epididymis** ♂

     C63.02   **Malignant neoplasm of left epididymis** ♂

  ● C63.1   **Malignant neoplasm of spermatic cord**

     C63.10   **Malignant neoplasm of unspecified spermatic cord** ♂

     C63.11   **Malignant neoplasm of right spermatic cord** ♂

     C63.12   **Malignant neoplasm of left spermatic cord** ♂

   C63.2   **Malignant neoplasm of scrotum** ♂
> Malignant neoplasm of skin of scrotum

   C63.7   **Malignant neoplasm of other specified male genital organs** ♂
> Malignant neoplasm of seminal vesicle
> Malignant neoplasm of tunica vaginalis

   C63.8   **Malignant neoplasm of overlapping sites of male genital organs** ♂
> Primary malignant neoplasm of two or more contiguous sites of male genital organs whose point of origin cannot be determined

C63.9   **Malignant neoplasm of male genital organ, unspecified** ♂
> Malignant neoplasm of male genitourinary tract NOS

MALIGNANT NEOPLASMS OF URINARY TRACT (C64-C68)

● C64   **Malignant neoplasm of kidney, except renal pelvis**
> **Excludes1**   malignant carcinoid tumor of the kidney (C7A.093)
> malignant neoplasm of renal calyces (C65.-)
> malignant neoplasm of renal pelvis (C65.-)
> (Ex) **For category C64 CC Codes:** C45.7-C45.9, C64.1-C65.9, C68.8-C68.9, C76.8, C7A.00, C7A.093, C7A.098-C7B.00, C7B.1, C80.0-C80.2, D49.511-D49.59, D49.81-D49.9

   C64.1   **Malignant neoplasm of right kidney, except renal pelvis** 🅒

   C64.2   **Malignant neoplasm of left kidney, except renal pelvis** 🅒

   C64.9   **Malignant neoplasm of unspecified kidney, except renal pelvis** 🅒

● C65   **Malignant neoplasm of renal pelvis**
> **Includes**   malignant neoplasm of pelviureteric junction
> malignant neoplasm of renal calyces
> (Ex) **For category C65 CC Codes:** See C64

   C65.1   **Malignant neoplasm of right renal pelvis** 🅒

   C65.2   **Malignant neoplasm of left renal pelvis** 🅒

   C65.9   **Malignant neoplasm of unspecified renal pelvis** 🅒

● C66   **Malignant neoplasm of ureter**
> **Excludes1**   malignant neoplasm of ureteric orifice of bladder (C67.6)
> (Ex) **For category C66 CC Codes:** C45.7-C45.9, C66.1-C66.9, C68.8-C68.9, C76.8, C7A.00, C7A.098, C7A.1-C7B.00, C7B.1, C80.0-C80.2, D49.511-D49.59, D49.81-D49.9

   C66.1   **Malignant neoplasm of right ureter** 🅒

   C66.2   **Malignant neoplasm of left ureter** 🅒

   C66.9   **Malignant neoplasm of unspecified ureter** 🅒

● C67   **Malignant neoplasm of bladder**

   C67.0   **Malignant neoplasm of trigone of bladder**
> *Triangular area formed by three openings in the floor of urinary bladder*

   C67.1   **Malignant neoplasm of dome of bladder**
> *Vaulted roof*

   C67.2   **Malignant neoplasm of lateral wall of bladder**
> *Side walls*

   C67.3   **Malignant neoplasm of anterior wall of bladder**
> *Front wall*

   C67.4   **Malignant neoplasm of posterior wall of bladder**
> *Back wall*

   C67.5   **Malignant neoplasm of bladder neck**
> *Joining of bladder and urethra*
> Malignant neoplasm of internal urethral orifice

   C67.6   **Malignant neoplasm of ureteric orifice**
> *Opening from bladder to ureters*

   C67.7   **Malignant neoplasm of urachus**
> *Embryonic canal that connects the urinary bladder with the structure that forms the umbilical cord (allantois)*

   C67.8   **Malignant neoplasm of overlapping sites of bladder**

   C67.9   **Malignant neoplasm of bladder, unspecified**
> **Coding Clinic: 2016, Q1, P19**

● C68   **Malignant neoplasm of other and unspecified urinary organs**
> **Excludes1**   malignant neoplasm of female genitourinary tract NOS (C57.9)
> malignant neoplasm of male genitourinary tract NOS (C63.9)
> (Ex) **For category C68 CC codes C68.0-C68.1:** C68.0-C68.9, C79.82 **For category C68 CC codes C68.8-C68.9:** C6.41-C66.9, C68.0-C68.9, C76.3, C79.00-C79.19, C7A.093

   C68.0   **Malignant neoplasm of urethra** 🅒
> **Excludes1**   malignant neoplasm of urethral orifice of bladder (C67.5)

N   Newborn Age: 0   **P**   Pediatric Age: 0–17   **M**   Maternity DX: 12–55   **A**   Adult Age: 15–124   ♀   Females Only   ♂   Males Only

🅒   Complication\Comorbidity   🅜   Major C\C   (Ex)   CC/MCC Exclusions   🅗   Hospital-Acquired Condition

687

CHAPTER 2 (C00-D49)

CHAPTER 2 (C00-D49)

C68.1 **Malignant neoplasm of paraurethral glands**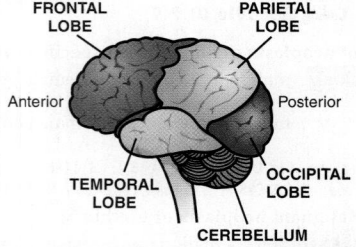
Group of glands of female urethra drained by paraurethral ducts; AKA Skene glands, female prostate

C68.8 **Malignant neoplasm of overlapping sites of urinary organs**
Primary malignant neoplasm of two or more contiguous sites of urinary organs whose point of origin cannot be determined

C68.9 **Malignant neoplasm of urinary organ, unspecified**
Malignant neoplasm of urinary system NOS

MALIGNANT NEOPLASMS OF EYE, BRAIN AND OTHER PARTS OF CENTRAL NERVOUS SYSTEM (C69-C72)

● **C69** **Malignant neoplasm of eye and adnexa**
> **Excludes1** malignant neoplasm of connective tissue of eyelid (C49.0)
> malignant neoplasm of eyelid (skin) (C43.1-, C44.1-)
> malignant neoplasm of optic nerve (C72.3-)

● **C69.0** **Malignant neoplasm of conjunctiva**
    C69.00 **Malignant neoplasm of unspecified conjunctiva**
    C69.01 **Malignant neoplasm of right conjunctiva**
    C69.02 **Malignant neoplasm of left conjunctiva**

● **C69.1** **Malignant neoplasm of cornea**
    C69.10 **Malignant neoplasm of unspecified cornea**
    C69.11 **Malignant neoplasm of right cornea**
    C69.12 **Malignant neoplasm of left cornea**

● **C69.2** **Malignant neoplasm of retina**
> **Excludes1** dark area on retina (D49.81)
> neoplasm of unspecified behavior of retina and choroid (D49.81)
> retinal freckle (D49.81)

    C69.20 **Malignant neoplasm of unspecified retina**
    C69.21 **Malignant neoplasm of right retina**
    C69.22 **Malignant neoplasm of left retina**

● **C69.3** **Malignant neoplasm of choroid**
    C69.30 **Malignant neoplasm of unspecified choroid**
    C69.31 **Malignant neoplasm of right choroid**
    C69.32 **Malignant neoplasm of left choroid**

● **C69.4** **Malignant neoplasm of ciliary body**
    C69.40 **Malignant neoplasm of unspecified ciliary body**
    C69.41 **Malignant neoplasm of right ciliary body**
    C69.42 **Malignant neoplasm of left ciliary body**

● **C69.5** **Malignant neoplasm of lacrimal gland and duct**
Malignant neoplasm of lacrimal sac
Malignant neoplasm of nasolacrimal duct
    C69.50 **Malignant neoplasm of unspecified lacrimal gland and duct**
    C69.51 **Malignant neoplasm of right lacrimal gland and duct**
    C69.52 **Malignant neoplasm of left lacrimal gland and duct**

● **C69.6** **Malignant neoplasm of orbit**
Malignant neoplasm of connective tissue of orbit
Malignant neoplasm of extraocular muscle
Malignant neoplasm of peripheral nerves of orbit
Malignant neoplasm of retrobulbar tissue
Malignant neoplasm of retro-ocular tissue
> **Excludes1** malignant neoplasm of orbital bone (C41.0)

    C69.60 **Malignant neoplasm of unspecified orbit**
    C69.61 **Malignant neoplasm of right orbit**
    C69.62 **Malignant neoplasm of left orbit**

● **C69.8** **Malignant neoplasm of overlapping sites of eye and adnexa**
    C69.80 **Malignant neoplasm of overlapping sites of unspecified eye and adnexa**
    C69.81 **Malignant neoplasm of overlapping sites of right eye and adnexa**
    C69.82 **Malignant neoplasm of overlapping sites of left eye and adnexa**

● **C69.9** **Malignant neoplasm of unspecified site of eye**
Malignant neoplasm of eyeball
    C69.90 **Malignant neoplasm of unspecified site of unspecified eye**
    C69.91 **Malignant neoplasm of unspecified site of right eye**
    C69.92 **Malignant neoplasm of unspecified site of left eye**

● **C70** **Malignant neoplasm of meninges**
    C70.0 **Malignant neoplasm of cerebral meninges**
> (Ex:) C45.7-C45.9, C70.0, C70.9, C72.9, C76.8, C7A.00, C7A.098-C7B.00, C7B.1, C80.0-C80.2, D49.6-D49.9

    C70.1 **Malignant neoplasm of spinal meninges**
> (Ex:) C45.7-C45.9, C70.1, C72.9, C76.8, C7A.00, C7A.098-C7B.00, C7B.1, C80.0-C80.2, D49.6-D49.9

    C70.9 **Malignant neoplasm of meninges, unspecified**
> (Ex:) See C70.0

● **C71** **Malignant neoplasm of brain**
> **Excludes1** malignant neoplasm of cranial nerves (C72.2-C72.5)
> retrobulbar malignant neoplasm (C69.6-)
> (Ex:) For category C71 CC codes: C45.7-C45.9, C70.0, C70.9-C71.9, C72.20-C72.9, C76.8, C7A.00, C7A.098-C7B.00, C7B.1, C80.0-C80.2, D49.6-D49.9

    C71.0 **Malignant neoplasm of cerebrum, except lobes and ventricles**
Malignant neoplasm of supratentorial NOS

    C71.1 **Malignant neoplasm of frontal lobe**
    C71.2 **Malignant neoplasm of temporal lobe**
    C71.3 **Malignant neoplasm of parietal lobe**
    C71.4 **Malignant neoplasm of occipital lobe**
    C71.5 **Malignant neoplasm of cerebral ventricle**
> **Excludes1** malignant neoplasm of fourth cerebral ventricle (C71.7)

    C71.6 **Malignant neoplasm of cerebellum**
    C71.7 **Malignant neoplasm of brain stem**
Malignant neoplasm of fourth cerebral ventricle
Infratentorial malignant neoplasm NOS

    C71.8 **Malignant neoplasm of overlapping sites of brain**
    C71.9 **Malignant neoplasm of brain, unspecified**

● **C72** **Malignant neoplasm of spinal cord, cranial nerves and other parts of central nervous system**
> **Excludes1** malignant neoplasm of meninges (C70.-)
> malignant neoplasm of peripheral nerves and autonomic nervous system (C47.-)
> (Ex:) For category C72 unless otherwise indicated: C45.7-C45.9, C72.20-C72.9, C76.8, C7A.00, C7A.098-C7B.00, C7B.1, C80.0-C80.2, D49.6-D49.9

    C72.0 **Malignant neoplasm of spinal cord**
> (Ex:) C45.7-C45.9, C72.0-C72.1, C72.9, C76.8, C7A.00, C7A.098, C7A.1-C7B.00, C7B.1, C80.0-C80.2, D49.6-D49.9

Figure 2-15 The brain.

FRONTAL LOBE
PARIETAL LOBE
Anterior
Posterior
TEMPORAL LOBE
OCCIPITAL LOBE
CEREBELLUM

◄ New   ◄▦ Revised   ~~deleted~~ Deleted   Excludes 1   Excludes 2   Includes   Use additional   Code first   Code also   Unspecified
OGCR Official Guidelines   ● Unacceptable Principal Diagnosis   X Assign placeholder X   ● Use Additional Character(s)   ▶ Manifestation Code   Coding Clinic

C72.1 **Malignant neoplasm of cauda equina**
Lower end of spinal column
Ⓔ See C72.Ø

● **C72.2** **Malignant neoplasm of olfactory nerve**
Malignant neoplasm of olfactory bulb

C72.2Ø Malignant neoplasm of unspecified olfactory nerve

C72.21 Malignant neoplasm of right olfactory nerve

C72.22 Malignant neoplasm of left olfactory nerve

● **C72.3** **Malignant neoplasm of optic nerve**

C72.3Ø Malignant neoplasm of unspecified optic nerve

C72.31 Malignant neoplasm of right optic nerve

C72.32 Malignant neoplasm of left optic nerve

● **C72.4** **Malignant neoplasm of acoustic nerve**

C72.4Ø Malignant neoplasm of unspecified acoustic nerve

C72.41 Malignant neoplasm of right acoustic nerve

C72.42 Malignant neoplasm of left acoustic nerve

● **C72.5** **Malignant neoplasm of other and unspecified cranial nerves**

C72.5Ø Malignant neoplasm of unspecified cranial nerve
Malignant neoplasm of cranial nerve NOS

C72.59 Malignant neoplasm of other cranial nerves

C72.9 **Malignant neoplasm of central nervous system, unspecified**
Malignant neoplasm of unspecified site of central nervous system
Malignant neoplasm of nervous system NOS
Ⓔ C45.7-C45.9, C7Ø.Ø-C72.9, C76.8, C79.31-C79.49, C7A.ØØ, C7A.Ø98-C7B.ØØ, C7B.1, C8Ø.Ø-C8Ø.2, D49.6-D49.9

MALIGNANT NEOPLASMS OF THYROID AND OTHER ENDOCRINE GLANDS (C73-C75)

C73 **Malignant neoplasm of thyroid gland**
Use additional code to identify any functional activity

● **C74** **Malignant neoplasm of adrenal gland**
Ⓔ For category C74 CC codes: C45.7-C45.9, C74.ØØ-C74.92, C75.9, C76.2, C76.8, C79.7Ø-C79.72, C7A.ØØ, C7A.Ø98-C7B.ØØ, C7B.1, C8Ø.Ø-C8Ø.2

● **C74.Ø** **Malignant neoplasm of cortex of adrenal gland**

C74.ØØ Malignant neoplasm of cortex of unspecified adrenal gland

C74.Ø1 Malignant neoplasm of cortex of right adrenal gland

C74.Ø2 Malignant neoplasm of cortex of left adrenal gland

● **C74.1** **Malignant neoplasm of medulla of adrenal gland**
Pair of glands situated on top of or above each kidney ("suprarenal")

C74.1Ø Malignant neoplasm of medulla of unspecified adrenal gland

C74.11 Malignant neoplasm of medulla of right adrenal gland

C74.12 Malignant neoplasm of medulla of left adrenal gland

● **C74.9** **Malignant neoplasm of unspecified part of adrenal gland**

C74.9Ø Malignant neoplasm of unspecified part of unspecified adrenal gland

C74.91 Malignant neoplasm of unspecified part of right adrenal gland

C74.92 Malignant neoplasm of unspecified part of left adrenal gland

● **C75** **Malignant neoplasm of other endocrine glands and related structures**

Excludes1 malignant carcinoid tumors (C7A.Ø-)
malignant neoplasm of adrenal gland (C74.-)
malignant neoplasm of endocrine pancreas (C25.4)
malignant neoplasm of islets of Langerhans (C25.4)
malignant neoplasm of ovary (C56.-)
malignant neoplasm of testis (C62.-)
malignant neoplasm of thymus (C37)
malignant neoplasm of thyroid gland (C73)
malignant neuroendocrine tumors (C7A.-)

C75.Ø **Malignant neoplasm of parathyroid gland**
Ⓔ C75.Ø, C75.8-C75.9

C75.1 **Malignant neoplasm of pituitary gland**
Ⓔ C75.1-C75.2, Z51.Ø

C75.2 **Malignant neoplasm of craniopharyngeal duct**
Ⓔ See C75.1

C75.3 **Malignant neoplasm of pineal gland**
Ⓔ C75.3, Z51.Ø

C75.4 **Malignant neoplasm of carotid body**
Ⓔ C75.4, C75.8-C75.9

C75.5 **Malignant neoplasm of aortic body and other paraganglia**
Ⓔ C75.4-C75.9

C75.8 **Malignant neoplasm with pluriglandular involvement, unspecified**
Ⓔ C74.ØØ-C75.9

C75.9 **Malignant neoplasm of endocrine gland, unspecified**
Ⓔ See C75.8

MALIGNANT NEUROENDOCRINE TUMORS (C7A)

● **C7A** **Malignant neuroendocrine tumors**
Code also any associated multiple endocrine neoplasia [MEN] syndromes (E31.2-)
Use additional code to identify any associated endocrine syndrome, such as:
carcinoid syndrome (E34.Ø)

Excludes2 malignant pancreatic islet cell tumors (C25.4)
Merkel cell carcinoma (C4A.-)

● **C7A.Ø** **Malignant carcinoid tumors**

C7A.ØØ Malignant carcinoid tumor of unspecified site
Ⓔ C45.7-C45.9, C76.8, C79.89-C79.9, C7A.ØØ-C7B.ØØ, C7B.Ø9-C7B.8, C8Ø.Ø-C8Ø.2, D49.81-D49.9

● **C7A.Ø1** **Malignant carcinoid tumors of the small intestine**

C7A.Ø1Ø Malignant carcinoid tumor of the duodenum
Ⓔ C17.Ø, C17.8-C17.9, C26.Ø, C26.9, C45.7-C45.9, C46.4, C76.8, C7A.ØØ-C7B.ØØ, C7B.1, C8Ø.Ø-C8Ø.2, D49.Ø, D49.81-D49.9

C7A.Ø11 Malignant carcinoid tumor of the jejunum
Ⓔ C17.1, C17.8-C17.9, C26.Ø, C26.9, C45.7-C45.9, C46.4, C76.8, C7A.ØØ-C7B.ØØ, C7B.1, C8Ø.Ø-C8Ø.2, D49.Ø, D49.81-D49.9

C7A.Ø12 Malignant carcinoid tumor of the ileum
Ⓔ C17.2, C17.8-C17.9, C26.Ø, C26.9, C45.7-C45.9, C46.4, C76.8, C7A.ØØ-C7B.ØØ, C7B.1, C8Ø.Ø-C8Ø.2, D49.Ø, D49.81-D49.9

C7A.Ø19 Malignant carcinoid tumor of the small intestine, unspecified portion
Ⓔ C17.8-C17.9, C26.Ø, C26.9, C45.7-C45.9, C46.4, C76.8, C7A.ØØ-C7B.ØØ, C7B.1, C8Ø.Ø-C8Ø.2, D49.Ø, D49.81-D49.9

● **C7A.02**   **Malignant carcinoid tumors of the appendix, large intestine, and rectum**

    C7A.020   **Malignant carcinoid tumor of the appendix** 🐾
       (Ex:) C18.1, C18.8-C18.9, C26.0, C26.9, C45.7-C45.9, C46.4, C76.8, C7A.00-C7B.00, C7B.1, C80.0-C80.2, D49.0, D49.81-D49.9

    C7A.021   **Malignant carcinoid tumor of the cecum** 🐾
       (Ex:) C18.0, C18.8-C18.9, C26.0, C26.9, C45.7-C45.9, C46.4, C76.8, C7A.00-C7B.00, C7B.1, C80.0-C80.2, D49.0, D49.81-D49.9

    C7A.022   **Malignant carcinoid tumor of the ascending colon** 🐾
       (Ex:) C18.2, C18.8-C18.9, C26.0, C26.9, C45.7-C45.9, C46.4, C76.8, C7A.00-C7B.00, C7B.1, C80.0-C80.2, D49.0, D49.81-D49.9

    C7A.023   **Malignant carcinoid tumor of the transverse colon** 🐾
       (Ex:) C18.4, C18.8-C18.9, C26.0, C26.9, C45.7-C45.9, C46.4, C76.8, C7A.00-C7B.00, C7B.1, C80.0-C80.2, D49.0, D49.81-D49.9

    C7A.024   **Malignant carcinoid tumor of the descending colon** 🐾
       (Ex:) C18.6, C18.8-C18.9, C26.0, C26.9, C45.7-C45.9, C46.4, C76.8, C7A.00-C7B.00, C7B.1, C80.0-C80.2, D49.0, D49.81-D49.9

    C7A.025   **Malignant carcinoid tumor of the sigmoid colon** 🐾
       (Ex:) C18.7-C18.9, C26.0, C26.9, C45.7-C45.9, C46.4, C76.8, C7A.00-C7B.00, C7B.1, C80.0-C80.2, D49.0, D49.81-D49.9

    C7A.026   **Malignant carcinoid tumor of the rectum** 🐾
       (Ex:) C20, C21.2-C21.8, C26.0, C26.9, C45.7-C45.9, C46.4, C76.8, C7A.00-C7B.00, C7B.1, C80.0-C80.2, D49.0, D49.81-D49.9

    C7A.029   **Malignant carcinoid tumor of the large intestine, unspecified portion** 🐾
       Malignant carcinoid tumor of the colon NOS
       (Ex:) C18.8-C18.9, C26.0, C26.9, C45.7-C45.9, C46.4, C76.8, C7A.00-C7B.00, C7B.1, C80.0-C80.2, D49.0, D49.81-D49.9

● **C7A.09**   **Malignant carcinoid tumors of other sites**
      (Ex:) For category C7A.09 CC codes unless otherwise indicated: C16.0-C16.9, C26.0, C26.9, C45.7-C45.9, C46.4, C49.A2, C76.8, C7A.00-C7B.00, C7B.1, C80.0-C80.2, D49.0, D49.81-D49.9

    C7A.090   **Malignant carcinoid tumor of the bronchus and lung** 🐾
       (Ex:) C34.80-C34.92, C39.9, C45.7-C45.9, C46.50-C46.52, C76.8, C7A.00-C7B.00, C7B.1, C80.0-C80.2, D49.1, D49.81-D49.9

    C7A.091   **Malignant carcinoid tumor of the thymus** 🐾
       (Ex:) C37, C7A.00-C7A.8

    C7A.092   **Malignant carcinoid tumor of the stomach** 🐾

    C7A.093   **Malignant carcinoid tumor of the kidney** 🐾
       (Ex:) C45.7-C45.9, C64.1-C65.9, C68.8-C68.9, C76.8, C7A.00-C7B.00, C7B.1, C80.0-C80.2, D49.511-D49.59, D49.81-D49.9

    C7A.094   **Malignant carcinoid tumor of the foregut unspecified** 🐾 ◀▥

    C7A.095   **Malignant carcinoid tumor of the midgut unspecified** 🐾 ◀▥

    C7A.096   **Malignant carcinoid tumor of the hindgut unspecified** 🐾 ◀▥

    C7A.098   **Malignant carcinoid tumors of other sites** 🐾
       (Ex:) C45.7-C45.9, C76.8, C79.89-C79.9, C7A.00-C7B.00, C7B.09-C7B.8, C80.0-C80.2, D49.81-D49.9

C7A.1   **Malignant poorly differentiated neuroendocrine tumors** 🐾
    Malignant poorly differentiated neuroendocrine tumor NOS
    Malignant poorly differentiated neuroendocrine carcinoma, any site
    High grade neuroendocrine carcinoma, any site
    (Ex:) See C7A.098

C7A.8   **Other malignant neuroendocrine tumors** 🐾
    Secondary neuroendocrine tumors (C7B)
    (Ex:) See C7A.098

SECONDARY NEUROENDOCRINE TUMORS (C7B)

● **C7B**   **Secondary neuroendocrine tumors**
    Use additional code to identify any functional activity

● **C7B.0**   **Secondary carcinoid tumors**

    C7B.00   **Secondary carcinoid tumors, unspecified site**

    C7B.01   **Secondary carcinoid tumors of distant lymph nodes** 🐾
       (Ex:) C45.7-C45.9, C46.3, C76.8-C77.9, C7A.00, C7A.098-C7B.8, C80.0-C80.2, D49.81-D49.9

    C7B.02   **Secondary carcinoid tumors of liver** 🐾
       (Ex:) C45.7-C45.9, C76.8, C78.7-C78.89, C79.89-C79.9, C7A.00, C7A.098-C7B.8, C80.0-C80.2, D49.81-D49.9

    C7B.03   **Secondary carcinoid tumors of bone** 🐾
       (Ex:) C45.7-C45.9, C76.8, C79.51-C79.52, C79.89-C79.9, C7A.00, C7A.098-C7B.8, C80.0-C80.2, D49.81-D49.9

    C7B.04   **Secondary carcinoid tumors of peritoneum** 🐾
       Mesentary metastasis of carcinoid tumor
       (Ex:) C45.7-C45.9, C76.8, C78.6, C78.80-C78.89, C79.89-C79.9, C7A.00, C7A.098-C7B.8, C80.0-C80.2, D49.81-D49.9

    C7B.09   **Secondary carcinoid tumors of other sites** 🐾
       (Ex:) C45.7-C45.9, C76.8, C79.89-C79.9, C7A.00, C7A.098-C7B.8, C80.0-C80.2, D49.81-D49.9

C7B.1   **Secondary Merkel cell carcinoma**
    Merkel cell carcinoma nodal presentation
    Merkel cell carcinoma visceral metastatic presentation

C7B.8   **Other secondary neuroendocrine tumors** 🐾
    (Ex:) See C7B.09

MALIGNANT NEOPLASMS OF ILL-DEFINED, OTHER SECONDARY AND UNSPECIFIED SITES (C76-C80)

● **C76**   **Malignant neoplasm of other and ill-defined sites**

    Excludes1   malignant neoplasm of female genitourinary tract NOS (C57.9)
       malignant neoplasm of male genitourinary tract NOS (C63.9)
       malignant neoplasm of lymphoid, hematopoietic and related tissue (C81-C96)
       malignant neoplasm of skin (C44.-)
       malignant neoplasm of unspecified site NOS (C80.1)

    C76.0   **Malignant neoplasm of head, face and neck**
      Malignant neoplasm of cheek NOS
      Malignant neoplasm of nose NOS

    C76.1   **Malignant neoplasm of thorax**
      Intrathoracic malignant neoplasm NOS
      Malignant neoplasm of axilla NOS
      Thoracic malignant neoplasm NOS

    C76.2   **Malignant neoplasm of abdomen**

    C76.3   **Malignant neoplasm of pelvis**
      Malignant neoplasm of groin NOS
      Malignant neoplasm of sites overlapping systems within the pelvis
      Rectovaginal (septum) malignant neoplasm
        Between rectum and vagina
      Rectovesical (septum) malignant neoplasm
        Between rectum and urinary bladder; AKA vesicorectal

● **C76.4**   **Malignant neoplasm of upper limb**

    C76.40   **Malignant neoplasm of unspecified upper limb**

    C76.41   **Malignant neoplasm of right upper limb**

    C76.42   **Malignant neoplasm of left upper limb**

◀ New   ◀▥ Revised   ~~deleted~~ Deleted   Excludes 1   Excludes 2   Includes   Use additional   Code first   Code also   Unspecified
OGCR Official Guidelines   ● Unacceptable Principal Diagnosis   X Assign placeholder X   ● Use Additional Character(s)   ▸ Manifestation Code   **Coding Clinic**

● **C76.5** **Malignant neoplasm of lower limb**
   C76.50   Malignant neoplasm of unspecified lower limb
   C76.51   Malignant neoplasm of right lower limb
   C76.52   Malignant neoplasm of left lower limb
C76.8 **Malignant neoplasm of other specified ill-defined sites**
   Malignant neoplasm of overlapping ill-defined sites

● **C77** **Secondary and unspecified malignant neoplasm of lymph nodes**
Excludes1	malignant neoplasm of lymph nodes, specified as primary (C81-C86, C88, C96.-)
	mesentery metastasis of carcinoid tumor (C7B.04)
	secondary carcinoid tumors of distant lymph nodes (C7B.01)

   (Ex) **For category C77 CC codes:** C45.7-C45.9, C46.3, C76.8-C77.9, C7A.00, C7A.098-C7B.01, C7B.1, C80.0-C80.2, D49.81-D49.9

   C77.0 **Secondary and unspecified malignant neoplasm of lymph nodes of head, face and neck** 🅒
      Secondary and unspecified malignant neoplasm of supraclavicular lymph nodes
   C77.1 **Secondary and unspecified malignant neoplasm of intrathoracic lymph nodes** 🅒
   C77.2 **Secondary and unspecified malignant neoplasm of intra-abdominal lymph nodes** 🅒
   C77.3 **Secondary and unspecified malignant neoplasm of axilla and upper limb lymph nodes** 🅒
      Secondary and unspecified malignant neoplasm of pectoral lymph nodes
   C77.4 **Secondary and unspecified malignant neoplasm of inguinal and lower limb lymph nodes** 🅒
   C77.5 **Secondary and unspecified malignant neoplasm of intrapelvic lymph nodes** 🅒
   C77.8 **Secondary and unspecified malignant neoplasm of lymph nodes of multiple regions** 🅒
   C77.9 **Secondary and unspecified malignant neoplasm of lymph node, unspecified** 🅒

● **C78** **Secondary malignant neoplasm of respiratory and digestive organs**
Excludes1	secondary carcinoid tumors of liver (C7B.02)
	secondary carcinoid tumors of peritoneum (C7B.04)

Excludes2	lymph node metastases (C77.0) ◄

   ● **C78.0** **Secondary malignant neoplasm of lung**
      (Ex) **For category C78.0 CC Codes:** C45.7-C45.9, C76.8, C78.00-C78.39, C79.89-C79.9, C7A.00, C7A.098-C7B.00, C7B.09-C7B.8, C80.0-C80.2, D49.81-D49.9

      C78.00   Secondary malignant neoplasm of unspecified lung 🅒
      C78.01   Secondary malignant neoplasm of right lung 🅒
      C78.02   Secondary malignant neoplasm of left lung 🅒
   C78.1 **Secondary malignant neoplasm of mediastinum** 🅒
      Thoracic cavity between pleural cavities
      (Ex) C45.7-C45.9, C76.8, C78.1, C78.30-C78.39, C79.89-C79.9, C7A.00, C7A.098-C7B.00, C7B.09-C7B.8, C80.0-C80.2, D49.81-D49.9
   C78.2 **Secondary malignant neoplasm of pleura** 🅒
      Serous membrane covering lungs and lining thoracic cavity
      (Ex) C45.7-C45.9, C76.8, C78.2-C78.39, C79.89-C79.9, C7A.00, C7A.098-C7B.00, C7B.09-C7B.8, C80.0-C80.2, D49.81-D49.9, J91.0
   ● **C78.3** **Secondary malignant neoplasm of other and unspecified respiratory organs**
      (Ex) **For category C78.3 CC Codes:** C45.7-C45.9, C76.8, C78.00-C78.39, C79.89-C79.9, C7A.00, C7A.098-C7B.00, C7B.09-C7B.8, C80.0-C80.2, D49.81-D49.9

      C78.30   Secondary malignant neoplasm of unspecified respiratory organ 🅒
      C78.39   Secondary malignant neoplasm of other respiratory organs 🅒
   C78.4 **Secondary malignant neoplasm of small intestine** 🅒
      (Ex) C45.7-C45.9, C76.8, C78.4, C78.80-C78.89, C79.89-C79.9, C7A.00, C7A.098-C7B.00, C7B.09-C7B.8, C80.0-C80.2, D49.81-D49.9

C78.5 **Secondary malignant neoplasm of large intestine and rectum** 🅒
   (Ex) C45.7-C45.9, C76.8, C78.5, C78.80-C78.89, C79.89-C79.9, C7A.00, C7A.098-C7B.00, C7B.09-C7B.8, C80.0-C80.2, D49.81-D49.9
C78.6 **Secondary malignant neoplasm of retroperitoneum and peritoneum** 🅒
   (Ex) C45.7-C45.9, C76.8, C78.6, C78.80-C78.89, C79.89-C79.9, C7A.00, C7A.098-C7B.00, C7B.04-C7B.8, C80.0-C80.2, D49.81-D49.9
C78.7 **Secondary malignant neoplasm of liver and intrahepatic bile duct** 🅒
   (Ex) C45.7-C45.9, C76.8, C78.7-C78.89, C79.89-C79.9, C7A.00, C7A.098-C7A.8, C7B.00, C7B.02, C7B.09-C7B.8, C80.0-C80.2, D49.81-D4.99
● **C78.8** **Secondary malignant neoplasm of other and unspecified digestive organs**
   (Ex) **For category C78.8 CC Codes:** C45.7-C45.9, C76.8, C78.4-C78.89, C79.89-C79.9, C7A.00, C7A.098-C7B.00, C7B.02, C7B.04-C7B.8, C80.0-C80.2, D49.81-D49.9

   C78.80   Secondary malignant neoplasm of unspecified digestive organ 🅒
   C78.89   Secondary malignant neoplasm of other digestive organs 🅒
      ► Code also exocrine pancreatic insufficiency (K86.81) ◄

● **C79** **Secondary malignant neoplasm of other and unspecified sites**
Excludes1	secondary carcinoid tumors (C7B.-)
	secondary neuroendocrine tumors (C7B.-)

Excludes2	lymph node metastases (C77.0) ◄

   ● **C79.0** **Secondary malignant neoplasm of kidney and renal pelvis**
      (Ex) **For category C79.0 CC Codes:** C45.7-C45.9, C76.8, C79.00-C79.19, C79.89-C79.9, C7A.00, C7A.098-C7B.00, C7B.09-C7B.8, C80.0-C80.2, D49.81-D49.9

      C79.00   Secondary malignant neoplasm of unspecified kidney and renal pelvis 🅒
      C79.01   Secondary malignant neoplasm of right kidney and renal pelvis 🅒
      C79.02   Secondary malignant neoplasm of left kidney and renal pelvis 🅒
   ● **C79.1** **Secondary malignant neoplasm of bladder and other and unspecified urinary organs**
      (Ex) See C79.0

      C79.10   Secondary malignant neoplasm of unspecified urinary organs 🅒
      C79.11   Secondary malignant neoplasm of bladder 🅒
      C79.19   Secondary malignant neoplasm of other urinary organs 🅒
   C79.2 **Secondary malignant neoplasm of skin** 🅒
Excludes1	secondary Merkel cell carcinoma (C7B.1)
      (Ex) C45.7-C45.9, C76.8, C79.2, C79.89-C79.9, C7A.00, C7A.098-C7B.00, C7B.09-C7B.8, C80.0-C80.2, D49.81-D49.9
   ● **C79.3** **Secondary malignant neoplasm of brain and cerebral meninges**
      C79.31   Secondary malignant neoplasm of brain 🅒
         C45.7-C45.9, C76.8, C79.31, C79.89-C79.9, C7A.00, C7A.098-C7B.00, C7B.09-C7B.8, C80.0-C80.2, D49.81-D49.9
      C79.32   Secondary malignant neoplasm of cerebral meninges 🅒
         (Ex) C45.7-C45.9, C76.8, C79.32-C79.49, C79.89-C79.9, C7A.00, C7A.098-C7B.00, C7B.09-C7B.8, C80.0-C80.2, D49.81-D49.9
   ● **C79.4** **Secondary malignant neoplasm of other and unspecified parts of nervous system**
      (Ex) **For category C79.4 CC codes:** See C79.32

      C79.40   Secondary malignant neoplasm of unspecified part of nervous system 🅒
      C79.49   Secondary malignant neoplasm of other parts of nervous system 🅒

CHAPTER 2 (C00-D49)

Item 2-6 The adrenal glands are a pair of glands situated on top of or above each kidney ("suprarenal") and chiefly responsible for regulating the stress response through the synthesis of corticosteroids and catecholamines, including cortisol and adrenaline.

● **C79.5   Secondary malignant neoplasm of bone and bone marrow**

> Excludes1   secondary carcinoid tumors of bone (C7B.03)

> (Ex) For category C79.5 CC codes: C45.7-C45.9, C76.8, C79.51-C79.52, C79.89-C79.9, C7A.00, C7A.098-C7B.00, C7B.03, C7B.09-C7B.8, C80.0-C80.2, D49.81-D49.9

C79.51   Secondary malignant neoplasm of bone

C79.52   Secondary malignant neoplasm of bone marrow

● **C79.6   Secondary malignant neoplasm of ovary**

> (Ex) For category C79.6 CC codes: C45.7-C45.9, C76.8, C79.60-C79.62, C79.89-C79.9, C7A.00, C7A.098-C7B.00, C7B.09-C7B.8, C80.0-C80.2, D49.81-D49.9

C79.60   Secondary malignant neoplasm of unspecified ovary ♀

C79.61   Secondary malignant neoplasm of right ovary ♀

C79.62   Secondary malignant neoplasm of left ovary ♀

● **C79.7   Secondary malignant neoplasm of adrenal gland**

> (Ex) For category C79.7 CC codes: C45.7-C45.9, C76.8, C79.70-C79.72, C79.89-C79.9, C7A.00, C7A.098-C7B.00, C7B.09-C7B.8, C80.0-C80.2, D49.81-D49.9

C79.70   Secondary malignant neoplasm of unspecified adrenal gland

C79.71   Secondary malignant neoplasm of right adrenal gland

C79.72   Secondary malignant neoplasm of left adrenal gland

● **C79.8   Secondary malignant neoplasm of other specified sites**

C79.81   Secondary malignant neoplasm of breast

> (Ex) C45.7-C45.9, C76.8, C79.81, C79.89-C79.9, C7A.00, C7A.098-C7B.00, C7B.09-C7B.8, C80.0-C80.2, D49.81-D49.9

C79.82   Secondary malignant neoplasm of genital organs

> (Ex) C45.7-C45.9, C76.8, C79.82-C79.9, C7A.00, C7A.098-C7B.00, C7B.09-C7B.8, C80.0-C80.2, D49.81-D49.9

C79.89   Secondary malignant neoplasm of other specified sites

> (Ex) C45.7-C45.9, C76.8, C79.89-C79.9, C7A.00, C7A.098-C7B.00, C7B.09, C7B.1-C7B.8, C80.0-C80.2, D49.81-D49.9

C79.9   Secondary malignant neoplasm of unspecified site
Metastatic cancer NOS
Metastatic disease NOS

> Excludes1   carcinomatosis NOS (C80.0)
> generalized cancer NOS (C80.0)
> malignant (primary) neoplasm of unspecified site (C80.1)

> (Ex) See C79.89

OGCR   Section I.C.2.j and k

Disseminated malignant neoplasm, unspecified

j. Code C80.0, Disseminated malignant neoplasm, unspecified, is for use only in those cases where the patient has advanced metastatic disease and no known primary or secondary sites are specified. It should not be used in place of assigning codes for the primary site and all known secondary sites.

Malignant neoplasm without specification of site

k. Code C80.1, Malignant (primary) neoplasm, unspecified, equates to Cancer, unspecified. This code should only be used when no determination can be made as to the primary site of a malignancy. This code should rarely be used in the inpatient setting.

● C80   **Malignant neoplasm without specification of site**

> Excludes1   malignant carcinoid tumor of unspecified site (C7A.00)
> malignant neoplasm of specified multiple sites- code to each site

C80.0   **Disseminated malignant neoplasm, unspecified**
Carcinomatosis NOS
Generalized cancer, unspecified site (primary) (secondary)
Generalized malignancy, unspecified site (primary) (secondary)

> (Ex) C45.7-C45.9, C76.8, C79.89-C79.9, C7A.00, C7A.098-C7B.00, C7B.09, C7B.1-C7B.8, C80.0-C80.2, D49.81-D49.9

C80.1   **Malignant (primary) neoplasm, unspecified**
Cancer NOS
Cancer unspecified site (primary)
Carcinoma unspecified site (primary)
Malignancy unspecified site (primary)

> Excludes1   secondary malignant neoplasm of unspecified site (C79.9)

● C80.2   **Malignant neoplasm associated with transplanted organ**

> *Code first complication of transplanted organ (T86.-)*
> Use additional code to identify the specific malignancy
> (Ex) See C80.0

★ **(See Plate 315 on page 49.)**

MALIGNANT NEOPLASMS OF LYMPHOID, HEMATOPOIETIC AND RELATED TISSUE (C81-C96)

> Excludes2   Kaposi's sarcoma of lymph nodes (C46.3)
> secondary and unspecified neoplasm of lymph nodes (C77.-)
> secondary neoplasm of bone marrow (C79.52)
> secondary neoplasm of spleen (C78.89)

● C81   **Hodgkin lymphoma**
Form of malignant lymphoma with four types, nodular sclerosis, mixed cellularity, lymphocyte depleted, and lymphocyte predominant

> Excludes1   personal history of Hodgkin lymphoma (Z85.71)

● C81.0   **Nodular lymphocyte predominant Hodgkin lymphoma**
Least aggressive, least common, typically no symptoms
Lymphocytic-histiocytic predominance Hodgkin's disease

C81.00   **Nodular lymphocyte predominant Hodgkin lymphoma, unspecified site**
> (Ex) C81.00-C81.09, C81.40-C81.49, C81.90, C81.98, D49.81-D49.9

C81.01   **Nodular lymphocyte predominant Hodgkin lymphoma, lymph nodes of head, face, and neck**
> (Ex) C81.00-C81.01, C81.08-C81.09, C81.40-C81.41, C81.48-C81.49, C81.90-C81.91, C81.98, D49.81-D49.9

C81.02   **Nodular lymphocyte predominant Hodgkin lymphoma, intrathoracic lymph nodes**
> (Ex) C81.00-C81.02, C81.08-C81.09, C81.40-C81.42, C81.48-C81.49, C81.90-C81.92, C81.98, D49.81-D49.9

C81.03   **Nodular lymphocyte predominant Hodgkin lymphoma, intra-abdominal lymph nodes**
> (Ex) C81.00, C81.03, C81.08-C81.09, C81.40, C81.43, C81.48-C81.49, C81.90, C81.93, C81.98, D49.81-D49.9

C81.04   **Nodular lymphocyte predominant Hodgkin lymphoma, lymph nodes of axilla and upper limb**
> (Ex) C81.00, C81.04, C81.08-C81.09, C81.40, C81.44, C81.48-C81.49, C81.90, C81.94, C81.98, D49.81-D49.9

C81.05   **Nodular lymphocyte predominant Hodgkin lymphoma, lymph nodes of inguinal region and lower limb**
> (Ex) C81.00, C81.05, C81.08-C81.09, C81.40, C81.45, C81.48-C81.49, C81.90, C81.95, C81.98, D49.81-D49.9

C81.06   **Nodular lymphocyte predominant Hodgkin lymphoma, intrapelvic lymph nodes** 🗞
Ex: C81.00, C81.06, C81.08-C81.09, C81.40, C81.46, C81.48-C81.49, C81.90, C81.96, C81.98, D49.81-D49.9

C81.07   **Nodular lymphocyte predominant Hodgkin lymphoma, spleen** 🗞
Ex: C81.00, C81.07-C81.09, C81.40, C81.47-C81.49, C81.90, C81.97-C81.98, D49.81-D49.9

C81.08   **Nodular lymphocyte predominant Hodgkin lymphoma, lymph nodes of multiple sites** 🗞
Ex: See C81.00

C81.09   **Nodular lymphocyte predominant Hodgkin lymphoma, extranodal and solid organ sites** 🗞
Ex: See C81.00

● **C81.1**   **Nodular sclerosis Hodgkin lymphoma** ◀▥
    Nodular sclerosis classical Hodgkin lymphoma ◀
    Moderately aggressive; most common in young adults

C81.10   **Nodular sclerosis Hodgkin lymphoma, unspecified site** 🗞 ◀▥
Ex: C81.10-C81.19, C81.90, C81.98, D49.81-D49.9

C81.11   **Nodular sclerosis Hodgkin lymphoma, lymph nodes of head, face, and neck** 🗞 ◀▥
Ex: C81.10-C81.11, C81.18-C81.19, C81.90-C81.91, C81.98, D49.81-D49.9

C81.12   **Nodular sclerosis Hodgkin lymphoma, intrathoracic lymph nodes** 🗞 ◀▥
Ex: C81.10, C81.12, C81.18-C81.19, C81.90, C81.92, C81.98, D49.81-D49.9

C81.13   **Nodular sclerosis Hodgkin lymphoma, intra-abdominal lymph nodes** 🗞 ◀▥
Ex: C81.10, C81.13, C81.18-C81.19, C81.90, C81.93, C81.98, D49.81-D49.9

C81.14   **Nodular sclerosis Hodgkin lymphoma, lymph nodes of axilla and upper limb** 🗞 ◀▥
Ex: C81.10, C81.14, C81.18-C81.19, C81.90, C81.94, C81.98, D49.81-D49.9

C81.15   **Nodular sclerosis Hodgkin lymphoma, lymph nodes of inguinal region and lower limb** 🗞 ◀▥
Ex: C81.10, C81.15, C81.18-C81.19, C81.90, C81.95, C81.98, D49.81-D49.9

C81.16   **Nodular sclerosis Hodgkin lymphoma, intrapelvic lymph nodes** 🗞 ◀▥
Ex: C81.10, C81.16, C81.18-C81.19, C81.90, C81.96, C81.98, D49.81-D49.9

C81.17   **Nodular sclerosis Hodgkin lymphoma, spleen** 🗞 ◀▥
Ex: C81.10, C81.17-C81.19, C81.90, C81.97-C81.98, D49.81-D49.9

C81.18   **Nodular sclerosis Hodgkin lymphoma, lymph nodes of multiple sites** 🗞 ◀▥
Ex: See C81.10

C81.19   **Nodular sclerosis Hodgkin lymphoma, extranodal and solid organ sites** 🗞 ◀▥
Ex: See C81.10

● **C81.2**   **Mixed cellularity Hodgkin lymphoma** ◀▥
    Mixed cellularity classical Hodgkin lymphoma ◀
    A type of Hodgkin's that is moderately aggressive with mixed cell types

C81.20   **Mixed cellularity Hodgkin lymphoma, unspecified site** 🗞 ◀▥
Ex: C81.20-C81.29, C81.90, C81.98, D49.81-D49.9

C81.21   **Mixed cellularity Hodgkin lymphoma, lymph nodes of head, face, and neck** 🗞 ◀▥
Ex: C81.20-C81.21, C81.28-C81.29, C81.90-C81.91, C81.98, D49.81-D49.9

C81.22   **Mixed cellularity Hodgkin lymphoma, intrathoracic lymph nodes** 🗞 ◀▥
Ex: C81.20, C81.22, C81.28-C81.29, C81.90, C81.92, C81.98, D49.81-D49.9

C81.23   **Mixed cellularity Hodgkin lymphoma, intra-abdominal lymph nodes** 🗞 ◀▥
Ex: C81.20, C81.23, C81.28-C81.29, C81.90, C81.93, C81.98, D49.81-D49.9

C81.24   **Mixed cellularity Hodgkin lymphoma, lymph nodes of axilla and upper limb** 🗞 ◀▥
Ex: C81.20, C81.24, C81.28-C81.29, C81.90, C81.94, C81.98, D49.81-D49.9

C81.25   **Mixed cellularity Hodgkin lymphoma, lymph nodes of inguinal region and lower limb** 🗞 ◀▥
Ex: C81.20, C81.25, C81.28-C81.29, C81.90, C81.95, C81.98, D49.81-D49.9

C81.26   **Mixed cellularity Hodgkin lymphoma, intrapelvic lymph nodes** 🗞 ◀▥
Ex: C81.20, C81.26, C81.28-C81.29, C81.90, C81.96, C81.98, D49.81-D49.9

C81.27   **Mixed cellularity Hodgkin lymphoma, spleen** 🗞 ◀▥
Ex: C81.20, C81.27, C81.28-C81.29, C81.90, C81.97, C81.98, D49.81-D49.9

C81.28   **Mixed cellularity Hodgkin lymphoma, lymph nodes of multiple sites** 🗞 ◀▥
Ex: See C81.20

C81.29   **Mixed cellularity Hodgkin lymphoma, extranodal and solid organ sites** 🗞 ◀▥
Ex: See C81.20

● **C81.3**   **Lymphocyte depleted Hodgkin lymphoma** ◀▥
    Lymphocyte depleted classical Hodgkin lymphoma ◀
    Most aggressive type with poor prognosis

C81.30   **Lymphocyte depleted Hodgkin lymphoma, unspecified site** 🗞 ◀▥
Ex: C81.30-C81.39, C81.90, C81.98, D49.81-D49.9

C81.31   **Lymphocyte depleted Hodgkin lymphoma, lymph nodes of head, face, and neck** 🗞 ◀▥
Ex: C81.30-C81.31, C81.38-C81.39, C81.90-C81.91, C81.98, D49.81-D49.9

C81.32   **Lymphocyte depleted Hodgkin lymphoma, intrathoracic lymph nodes** 🗞 ◀▥
Ex: C81.30, C81.32, C81.38-C81.39, C81.90, C81.92, C81.98, D49.81-D49.9

C81.33   **Lymphocyte depleted Hodgkin lymphoma, intra-abdominal lymph nodes** 🗞 ◀▥
Ex: C81.30, C81.33, C81.38-C81.39, C81.90, C81.93, C81.98, D49.81-D49.9

C81.34   **Lymphocyte depleted Hodgkin lymphoma, lymph nodes of axilla and upper limb** 🗞 ◀▥
Ex: C81.30, C81.34, C81.38-C81.39, C81.90, C81.94, C81.98, D49.81-D49.9

C81.35   **Lymphocyte depleted Hodgkin lymphoma, lymph nodes of inguinal region and lower limb** 🗞 ◀▥
Ex: C81.30, C81.35, C81.38-C81.39, C81.90, C81.95, C81.98, D49.81-D49.9

C81.36   **Lymphocyte depleted Hodgkin lymphoma, intrapelvic lymph nodes** 🗞 ◀▥
Ex: C81.30, C81.36, C81.38-C81.39, C81.90, C81.96, C81.98, D49.81-D49.9

C81.37   **Lymphocyte depleted Hodgkin lymphoma, spleen** 🗞 ◀▥
Ex: C81.30, C81.37, C81.38-C81.39, C81.90, C81.97, C81.98, D49.81-D49.9

C81.38   **Lymphocyte depleted Hodgkin lymphoma, lymph nodes of multiple sites** 🗞 ◀▥
Ex: C81.30-C81.39, C81.98, D49.81-D49.9

C81.39   **Lymphocyte depleted Hodgkin lymphoma, extranodal and solid organ sites** 🗞 ◀▥
Ex: See C81.30

N Newborn Age: 0   **P** Pediatric Age: 0–17   **M** Maternity DX: 12–55   **A** Adult Age: 15–124   ♀ Females Only   ♂ Males Only
🗞 Complication\Comorbidity   🗞 Major C\C   Ex: CC/MCC Exclusions   🗞 Hospital-Acquired Condition
693

CHAPTER 2 (C00-D49)

● **C81.4 Lymphocyte-rich Hodgkin lymphoma** ◄▬
      Lymphocyte-rich classical Hodgkin lymphoma ◄
      Excludes1   nodular lymphocyte predominant
                       Hodgkin lymphoma (C81.0-)

    **C81.40 Lymphocyte-rich Hodgkin
           lymphoma, unspecified site** 🔦 ◄▬
           (Ex) C81.00-C81.09, C81.40-C81.49, C81.90, C81.98, D49.81-D49.9

    **C81.41 Lymphocyte-rich Hodgkin lymphoma, lymph
           nodes of head, face, and neck** 🔦 ◄▬
           (Ex) C81.00-C81.01, C81.08-C81.09, C81.40-C81.41, C81.48-C81.49,
               C81.90-C81.91, C81.98, D49.81-D49.9

    **C81.42 Lymphocyte-rich Hodgkin lymphoma,
           intrathoracic lymph nodes** 🔦 ◄▬
           (Ex) C81.00-C81.02, C81.08-C81.09, C81.40-C81.42, C81.48-C81.49,
               C81.90-C81.92, C81.98, D49.81-D49.9

    **C81.43 Lymphocyte-rich Hodgkin lymphoma, intra-
           abdominal lymph nodes** 🔦 ◄▬
           (Ex) C81.00, C81.03, C81.08-C81.09, C81.40, C81.43, C81.48-C81.49,
               C81.90, C81.93, C81.98, D49.81-D49.9

    **C81.44 Lymphocyte-rich Hodgkin lymphoma, lymph
           nodes of axilla and upper limb** 🔦 ◄▬
           (Ex) C81.00, C81.04, C81.08-C81.09, C81.40, C81.44, C81.48-C81.49,
               C81.90, C81.94, C81.98, D49.81-D49.9

    **C81.45 Lymphocyte-rich Hodgkin lymphoma, lymph
           nodes of inguinal region and lower limb** 🔦 ◄▬
           (Ex) C81.00, C81.05, C81.08-C81.09, C81.40, C81.45, C81.48-C81.49,
               C81.90, C81.95, C81.98, D49.81-D49.9

    **C81.46 Lymphocyte-rich Hodgkin lymphoma,
           intrapelvic lymph nodes** 🔦 ◄▬
           (Ex) C81.00, C81.06, C81.08-C81.09, C81.40, C81.46, C81.48-C81.49,
               C81.90, C81.96, C81.98, D49.81-D49.9

    **C81.47 Lymphocyte-rich Hodgkin lymphoma,
           spleen** 🔦 ◄▬
           (Ex) C81.00, C81.07-C81.09, C81.40, C81.47-C81.49, C81.90,
               C81.97-C81.98, D49.81-D49.9

    **C81.48 Lymphocyte-rich Hodgkin lymphoma, lymph
           nodes of multiple sites** 🔦 ◄▬
           (Ex) See C81.40

    **C81.49 Lymphocyte-rich Hodgkin lymphoma,
           extranodal and solid organ sites** 🔦 ◄▬
           (Ex) See C81.40

● **C81.7 Other Hodgkin lymphoma** ◄▬
      Classical Hodgkin lymphoma NOS
      Other classical Hodgkin lymphoma ◄

    **C81.70 Other Hodgkin lymphoma, unspecified
           site** 🔦 ◄▬
           (Ex) C81.70-C81.79, C81.90, C81.98, D49.81-D49.9

    **C81.71 Other Hodgkin lymphoma, lymph nodes of
           head, face, and neck** 🔦 ◄▬
           (Ex) C81.70-C81.71, C81.78-C81.79, C81.90-C81.91, C81.98,
               D49.81-D49.9

    **C81.72 Other Hodgkin lymphoma, intrathoracic lymph
           nodes** 🔦 ◄▬
           (Ex) C81.70, C81.72, C81.78-C81.79, C81.90, C81.92, C81.98,
               D49.81-D49.9

    **C81.73 Other Hodgkin lymphoma, intra-abdominal
           lymph nodes** 🔦 ◄▬
           (Ex) C81.70, C81.73, C81.78-C81.79, C81.90, C81.93, C81.98,
               D49.81-D49.9

    **C81.74 Other Hodgkin lymphoma, lymph nodes of
           axilla and upper limb** 🔦 ◄▬
           (Ex) C81.70, C81.74, C81.78-C81.79, C81.90, C81.94, C81.98,
               D49.81-D49.9

    **C81.75 Other Hodgkin lymphoma, lymph nodes of
           inguinal region and lower limb** 🔦 ◄▬
           (Ex) C81.70, C81.75, C81.78-C81.79, C81.90, C81.95, C81.98,
               D49.81-D49.9

    **C81.76 Other Hodgkin lymphoma, intrapelvic lymph
           nodes** 🔦 ◄▬
           (Ex) C81.70, C81.76, C81.78-C81.79, C81.90, C81.96, C81.98,
               D49.81-D49.9

    C81.77 Other Hodgkin lymphoma, spleen 🔦 ◄▬
           (Ex) C81.70, C81.77, C81.78-C81.79, C81.90, C81.97, C81.98,
               D49.81-D49.9

    **C81.78 Other Hodgkin lymphoma, lymph nodes of
           multiple sites** 🔦 ◄▬
           (Ex) See C81.70

    **C81.79 Other Hodgkin lymphoma, extranodal and
           solid organ sites** 🔦 ◄▬
           (Ex) See C81.70

● **C81.9 Hodgkin lymphoma, unspecified**

    **C81.90 Hodgkin lymphoma, unspecified, unspecified
           site** 🔦
           (Ex) C81.90-C81.98, D49.81-D49.9

    **C81.91 Hodgkin lymphoma, unspecified, lymph nodes
           of head, face, and neck** 🔦
           (Ex) C81.90-C81.91, C81.98, D49.81-D49.9

    **C81.92 Hodgkin lymphoma, unspecified, intrathoracic
           lymph nodes** 🔦
           (Ex) C81.90, C81.92, C81.98, D49.81-D49.9

    **C81.93 Hodgkin lymphoma, unspecified, intra-
           abdominal lymph nodes** 🔦
           (Ex) C81.90, C81.93, C81.98, D49.81-D49.9

    **C81.94 Hodgkin lymphoma, unspecified, lymph nodes
           of axilla and upper limb** 🔦
           (Ex) C81.90, C81.94, C81.98, D49.81-D49.9

    **C81.95 Hodgkin lymphoma, unspecified, lymph nodes
           of inguinal region and lower limb** 🔦
           (Ex) C81.90, C81.95, C81.98, D49.81-D49.9

    **C81.96 Hodgkin lymphoma, unspecified, intrapelvic
           lymph nodes** 🔦
           (Ex) C81.90, C81.96, C81.98, D49.81-D49.9

    C81.97 Hodgkin lymphoma, unspecified, spleen 🔦
           (Ex) C81.90, C81.97-C81.98, D49.81-D49.9

    **C81.98 Hodgkin lymphoma, unspecified, lymph nodes
           of multiple sites** 🔦
           (Ex) See C81.90

    **C81.99 Hodgkin lymphoma, unspecified, extranodal
           and solid organ sites** 🔦
           (Ex) No exclusions

● **C82 Follicular lymphoma**
      Group of malignant lymphomas
      Includes   follicular lymphoma with or without diffuse
                    areas
      Excludes1   mature T/NK-cell lymphomas (C84.-)
                    personal history of non-Hodgkin lymphoma
                    (Z85.72)

● **C82.0 Follicular lymphoma grade I**

    C82.00 Follicular lymphoma grade I, unspecified site 🔦
           (Ex) C82.00-C82.50, C82.59-C82.99, C83.10, C83.19, C84.40, C84.49,
               C84.60, C84.69-C84.70, C84.79, C84.A0, C84.A9, C84.Z0, C84.
               Z9, C84.90, C84.99-C85.10, C85.19-C85.20, C85.29-C85.80,
               C85.89-C85.90, C85.99, C86.4, C88.4, C96.4, C96.9, C96.Z

    **C82.01 Follicular lymphoma grade I, lymph nodes of
           head, face, and neck** 🔦
           (Ex) C82.00-C82.01, C82.08-C82.11, C82.18-C82.21, C82.28-C82.31,
               C82.38-C82.41, C82.48-C82.49, C82.51, C82.60-C82.61,
               C82.68-C82.81, C82.88-C82.91, C82.98-C82.99, C83.11,
               C84.41, C84.61, C84.71, C84.A1, C84.Z1, C84.91, C85.11,
               C85.21, C85.81, C85.91, C86.0, D49.81-D49.9

    **C82.02 Follicular lymphoma grade I, intrathoracic
           lymph nodes** 🔦
           (Ex) C82.00, C82.02, C82.08-C82.10, C82.12, C82.18-C82.20, C82.22,
               C82.28-C82.30, C82.32, C82.38-C82.40, C82.42,
               C82.48-C82.49, C82.52, C82.60, C82.62, C82.68-C82.80,
               C82.82, C82.88-C82.90, C82.92, C82.98-C82.99, C83.12,
               C84.42, C84.62, C84.72, C84.92, C84.Z2, C85.12,
               C85.22, C85.82, C85.92, D49.81-D49.9

    **C82.03 Follicular lymphoma grade I, intra-abdominal
           lymph nodes** 🔦
           (Ex) C82.00, C82.03, C82.08-C82.10, C82.13, C82.18-C82.20, C12.23,
               C82.28-C82.30, C82.33, C82.38-C82.40, C82.43,
               C82.48-C82.49, C82.53, C82.60, C82.63, C82.68-C82.80,
               C82.83, C82.88-C82.90, C82.93, C82.98-C82.99, C83.13,
               C84.43, C84.63, C84.73, C84.93, C84.A3, C84.Z3, C85.13,
               C85.23, C85.83, C85.93, C86.2, C86.3, D49.81-D49.9

◄ New   ◄▬ Revised   ~~deleted~~ Deleted   Excludes 1   Excludes 2   Includes   Use additional   Code first   Code also   Unspecified

694   OGCR Official Guidelines   ● Unacceptable Principal Diagnosis   X Assign placeholder X   🔦 Use Additional Character(s)   ▶ Manifestation Code   **Coding Clinic**

C82.04   **Follicular lymphoma grade I, lymph nodes of axilla and upper limb** 🔖
    (Ex:) C82.00, C82.04, C82.08-C82.10, C82.14, C82.18-C82.20, C82.24, C82.28-C82.30, C82.34, C82.38-C82.40, C82.44, C82.48-C82.49, C82.54, C82.60, C82.64, C82.68-C82.80, C82.84, C82.88-C82.90, C82.94, C82.98-C82.99, C83.14, C84.44, C84.64, C84.74, C84.94, C84.A4, C84.Z4, C85.14, C85.24, C85.84, C85.94, D49.81-D49.9

C82.05   **Follicular lymphoma grade I, lymph nodes of inguinal region and lower limb** 🔖
    (Ex:) C82.00, C82.05, C82.08-C82.10, C82.15, C82.18-C82.20, C82.25, C82.28-C82.30, C82.35, C82.38-C82.40, C82.45, C82.48-C82.49, C82.55, C82.60, C82.65, C82.68-C82.80, C82.85, C82.88-C82.90, C82.95, C82.98-C82.99, C83.15, C84.45, C84.65, C84.75, C84.95, C84.A5, C84.Z5, C85.15, C85.25, C85.85, C85.95, D49.81-D49.9

C82.06   **Follicular lymphoma grade I, intrapelvic lymph nodes** 🔖
    (Ex:) C82.00, C82.06, C82.08-C82.10, C82.16, C82.18-C82.20, C82.26, C82.28-C82.30, C82.36, C82.38-C82.40, C82.46, C82.48-C82.49, C82.56, C82.60, C82.66, C82.68-C82.80, C82.86, C82.88-C82.90, C82.96, C82.98-C82.99, C83.16, C84.46, C84.66, C84.76, C84.96, C84.A6, C84.Z6, C85.16, C85.26, C85.86, C85.96, D49.81-D49.9

C82.07   **Follicular lymphoma grade I, spleen** 🔖
    (Ex:) C82.00, C82.07, C82.08-C82.10, C82.17-C82.20, C82.27-C82.30, C82.37-C82.40, C82.47-C82.49, C82.57, C82.60, C82.67-C82.80, C82.87-C82.90, C82.97-C82.99, C83.17, C84.47, C84.67, C84.77, C84.97, C84.A7, C84.Z7, C85.17, C85.27, C85.87, C85.97, C86.1, D49.81-D49.9

C82.08   **Follicular lymphoma grade I, lymph nodes of multiple sites** 🔖
    (Ex:) C82.00-C82.49, C82.58, C82.60-C82.99, C83.18, C84.48, C84.68, C84.78, C84.98, C84.A8, C84.Z8, C85.18, C85.28, C85.88, C85.98, D49.81-D49.9

C82.09   **Follicular lymphoma grade I, extranodal and solid organ sites** 🔖
    (Ex:) See C82.00

● **C82.1**   **Follicular lymphoma grade II**

C82.10   **Follicular lymphoma grade II, unspecified site** 🔖
    (Ex:) See C82.00

C82.11   **Follicular lymphoma grade II, lymph nodes of head, face, and neck** 🔖
    (Ex:) See C82.01

C82.12   **Follicular lymphoma grade II, intrathoracic lymph nodes** 🔖
    (Ex:) See C82.02

C82.13   **Follicular lymphoma grade II, intra-abdominal lymph nodes** 🔖
    (Ex:) See C82.03

C82.14   **Follicular lymphoma grade II, lymph nodes of axilla and upper limb** 🔖
    (Ex:) See C82.04

C82.15   **Follicular lymphoma grade II, lymph nodes of inguinal region and lower limb** 🔖
    (Ex:) See C82.05

C82.16   **Follicular lymphoma grade II, intrapelvic lymph nodes** 🔖
    (Ex:) See C82.06

C82.17   **Follicular lymphoma grade II, spleen** 🔖
    (Ex:) See C82.07

C82.18   **Follicular lymphoma grade II, lymph nodes of multiple sites** 🔖
    (Ex:) See C82.08

C82.19   **Follicular lymphoma grade II, extranodal and solid organ sites** 🔖
    (Ex:) See C82.00

● **C82.2**   **Follicular lymphoma grade III, unspecified**

C82.20   **Follicular lymphoma grade III, unspecified, unspecified site** 🔖
    (Ex:) See C82.00

C82.21   **Follicular lymphoma grade III, unspecified, lymph nodes of head, face, and neck** 🔖
    (Ex:) See C82.01

C82.22   **Follicular lymphoma grade III, unspecified, intrathoracic lymph nodes** 🔖
    (Ex:) See C82.02

C82.23   **Follicular lymphoma grade III, unspecified, intra-abdominal lymph nodes** 🔖
    (Ex:) See C82.03

C82.24   **Follicular lymphoma grade III, unspecified, lymph nodes of axilla and upper limb** 🔖
    (Ex:) See C82.04

C82.25   **Follicular lymphoma grade III, unspecified, lymph nodes of inguinal region and lower limb** 🔖
    (Ex:) See C82.05

C82.26   **Follicular lymphoma grade III, unspecified, intrapelvic lymph nodes** 🔖
    (Ex:) See C82.06

C82.27   **Follicular lymphoma grade III, unspecified, spleen** 🔖
    (Ex:) See C82.07

C82.28   **Follicular lymphoma grade III, unspecified, lymph nodes of multiple sites** 🔖
    (Ex:) See C82.08

C82.29   **Follicular lymphoma grade III, unspecified, extranodal and solid organ sites** 🔖
    (Ex:) See C82.00

● **C82.3**   **Follicular lymphoma grade IIIa**

C82.30   **Follicular lymphoma grade IIIa, unspecified site** 🔖
    (Ex:) See C82.00

C82.31   **Follicular lymphoma grade IIIa, lymph nodes of head, face, and neck** 🔖
    (Ex:) See C82.01

C82.32   **Follicular lymphoma grade IIIa, intrathoracic lymph nodes** 🔖
    (Ex:) See C82.02

C82.33   **Follicular lymphoma grade IIIa, intra-abdominal lymph nodes** 🔖
    (Ex:) See C82.03

C82.34   **Follicular lymphoma grade IIIa, lymph nodes of axilla and upper limb** 🔖
    (Ex:) See C82.04

C82.35   **Follicular lymphoma grade IIIa, lymph nodes of inguinal region and lower limb** 🔖
    (Ex:) See C82.05

C82.36   **Follicular lymphoma grade IIIa, intrapelvic lymph nodes** 🔖
    (Ex:) See C82.06

C82.37   **Follicular lymphoma grade IIIa, spleen** 🔖
    (Ex:) See C82.07

C82.38   **Follicular lymphoma grade IIIa, lymph nodes of multiple sites** 🔖
    (Ex:) See C82.08

C82.39   **Follicular lymphoma grade IIIa, extranodal and solid organ sites** 🔖
    (Ex:) See C82.00

● **C82.4**   **Follicular lymphoma grade IIIb**

C82.40   **Follicular lymphoma grade IIIb, unspecified site** 🔖
    (Ex:) See C82.00

C82.41   **Follicular lymphoma grade IIIb, lymph nodes of head, face, and neck** 🔖
    (Ex:) See C82.01

C82.42   **Follicular lymphoma grade IIIb, intrathoracic lymph nodes** 🔖
    (Ex:) See C82.02

N   Newborn Age: 0   **P**   Pediatric Age: 0–17   **M**   Maternity DX: 12–55   **A**   Adult Age: 15–124   ♀   Females Only   ♂   Males Only

🔖   Complication\Comorbidity   🔖   Major C\C   (Ex:)   CC/MCC Exclusions   🔖   Hospital-Acquired Condition

695

C82.43 Follicular lymphoma grade IIIb, intra-abdominal lymph nodes 🔖
Ex: See C82.03

C82.44 Follicular lymphoma grade IIIb, lymph nodes of axilla and upper limb 🔖
Ex: See C82.04

C82.45 Follicular lymphoma grade IIIb, lymph nodes of inguinal region and lower limb 🔖
Ex: See C82.05

C82.46 Follicular lymphoma grade IIIb, intrapelvic lymph nodes 🔖
Ex: See C82.06

C82.47 Follicular lymphoma grade IIIb, spleen 🔖
Ex: See C82.07

C82.48 Follicular lymphoma grade IIIb, lymph nodes of multiple sites 🔖
Ex: See C82.08

C82.49 Follicular lymphoma grade IIIb, extranodal and solid organ sites 🔖
Ex: See C82.00

● **C82.5** Diffuse follicle center lymphoma

C82.50 Diffuse follicle center lymphoma, unspecified site 🔖
Ex: C82.50-C82.59, C83.10-C83.19, C84.40-C84.49, C84.60-C84.79, C84.90-C84.99, C84.A0-C84.Z9, C85.10-C86.4, C88.4, C96.4, C96.9, C96.Z, D49.81-D49.9

C82.51 Diffuse follicle center lymphoma, lymph nodes of head, face, and neck 🔖
Ex: C82.50-C82.51, C82.58-C82.59, C83.10-C83.11, C83.18-C83.19, C84.40-C84.41, C84.48-C84.61, C84.68-C84.71, C84.78-C84.79, C84.90-C84.91, C84.98-C84.99, C84.A0-C84.A1, C84.A8-C84.A9, C84.Z0-C84.Z1, C84.Z8-C84.Z9, C85.10-C85.11, C85.18-C85.21, C85.28-C85.81, C85.88-C85.91, C85.98-C85.99, C86.0, C86.4, C88.4, D49.81-D49.9

C82.52 Diffuse follicle center lymphoma, intrathoracic lymph nodes 🔖
Ex: C82.50, C82.52, C82.58-C82.59, C83.10, C83.12, C83.18-C83.19, C84.40, C84.42, C84.48-C84.60, C84.62, C84.68-C84.70, C84.72, C84.78-C84.79, C84.90, C84.92, C84.98-C84.99, C84.A0, C84.A2, C84.A8-C84.A9, C84.Z0, C84.Z2, C84.Z8-C84.Z9, C85.10, C85.12, C85.18-C85.20, C85.22, C85.28-C85.80, C85.82, C85.88-C85.90, C85.92, C85.98-C85.99, C86.4, C88.4, D49.81-D49.9

C82.53 Diffuse follicle center lymphoma, intra-abdominal lymph nodes 🔖
Ex: C82.50, C82.53, C82.58-C82.59, C83.10, C83.13, C83.18-C83.19, C84.40, C84.43, C84.48-C84.60, C84.63, C84.68-C84.70, C84.73, C84.78-C84.79, C84.90, C84.93, C84.98-C84.99, C84.A0, C84.A3, C84.A8-C84.A9, C84.Z0, C84.Z3, C84.Z8-C84.Z9, C85.10, C85.13, C85.18-C85.20, C85.22, C85.28-C85.80, C85.83, C85.88-C85.90, C85.93, C85.98-C85.99, C86.2-C86.4, C88.4, D49.81-D49.9

C82.54 Diffuse follicle center lymphoma, lymph nodes of axilla and upper limb 🔖
Ex: C82.50, C82.54, C82.58-C82.59, C83.10, C83.14, C83.18-C83.19, C84.40, C84.44, C84.48-C84.60, C84.64, C84.68-C84.70, C84.74, C84.78-C84.79, C84.90, C84.94, C84.98-C84.99, C84.A0, C84.A4, C84.A8-C84.A9, C84.Z0, C84.Z4, C84.Z8-C84.Z9, C85.10, C85.14, C85.18-C85.20, C85.24, C85.28-C85.80, C85.84, C85.88-C85.90, C85.94, C85.98-C85.99, C86.4, C88.4, D49.81-D49.9

C82.55 Diffuse follicle center lymphoma, lymph nodes of inguinal region and lower limb 🔖
Ex: C82.50, C82.55, C82.58-C82.59, C83.10, C83.15, C83.18-C83.19, C84.40, C84.45, C84.48-C84.60, C84.65, C84.68-C84.70, C84.75, C84.78-C84.79, C84.90, C84.95, C84.98-C84.99, C84.A0, C84.A5, C84.A8-C84.A9, C84.Z0, C84.Z5, C84.Z8-C84.Z9, C85.10, C85.15, C85.18-C85.20, C85.25, C85.28-C85.80, C85.85, C85.88-C85.90, C85.95, C85.98-C85.99, C86.4, C88.4, D49.81-D49.9

C82.56 Diffuse follicle center lymphoma, intrapelvic lymph nodes 🔖
Ex: C82.50, C82.56, C82.58-C82.59, C83.10, C83.16, C83.18-C83.19, C84.40, C84.46, C84.48-C84.60, C84.66, C84.68-C84.70, C84.76, C84.78-C84.79, C84.90, C84.96, C84.98-C84.99, C84.A0, C84.A6, C84.A8-C84.A9, C84.Z0, C84.Z6, C84.Z8-C84.Z9, C85.10, C85.16, C85.18-C85.20, C85.26, C85.28-C85.80, C85.86, C85.88-C85.90, C85.96, C85.98-C85.99, C86.4, C88.4, D49.81-D49.9

C82.57 Diffuse follicle center lymphoma, spleen 🔖
Ex: C82.50, C82.57, C82.58-C82.59, C83.10, C83.17, C83.18-C83.19, C84.40, C84.47-C84.49, C84.60, C84.67, C84.68-C84.69, C84.70, C84.77, C84.78-C84.79, C84.90, C84.97-C84.99, C84.A0, C84.A7-C84.A9, C84.Z0, C84.Z7, C84.Z8-C84.Z9, C85.10, C85.17-C85.20, C85.27-C85.29, C85.80, C85.87-C85.90, C85.97-C85.99, C86.1, C86.4, C88.4, D49.81-D49.9

C82.58 Diffuse follicle center lymphoma, lymph nodes of multiple sites 🔖
Ex: C82.50-C82.59, C83.10-C83.19, C84.40-C84.49, C84.60-C84.79, C84.90-C84.99, C84.A0-C84.Z9, C85.10-C86.4, C88.4, D49.81-D49.9

C82.59 Diffuse follicle center lymphoma, extranodal and solid organ sites 🔖
Ex: See C82.50

● **C82.6** Cutaneous follicle center lymphoma

C82.60 Cutaneous follicle center lymphoma, unspecified site 🔖
Ex: See C82.00

C82.61 Cutaneous follicle center lymphoma, lymph nodes of head, face, and neck 🔖
Ex: See C82.01

C82.62 Cutaneous follicle center lymphoma, intrathoracic lymph nodes 🔖
Ex: See C82.02

C82.63 Cutaneous follicle center lymphoma, intra-abdominal lymph nodes 🔖
Ex: See C82.03

C82.64 Cutaneous follicle center lymphoma, lymph nodes of axilla and upper limb 🔖
Ex: See C82.04

C82.65 Cutaneous follicle center lymphoma, lymph nodes of inguinal region and lower limb 🔖
Ex: See C82.05

C82.66 Cutaneous follicle center lymphoma, intrapelvic lymph nodes 🔖
Ex: See C82.06

C82.67 Cutaneous follicle center lymphoma, spleen 🔖
Ex: See C82.07

C82.68 Cutaneous follicle center lymphoma, lymph nodes of multiple sites 🔖
Ex: See C82.08

C82.69 Cutaneous follicle center lymphoma, extranodal and solid organ sites 🔖
Ex: See C82.00

● **C82.8** Other types of follicular lymphoma

C82.80 Other types of follicular lymphoma, unspecified site 🔖
Ex: See C82.00

C82.81 Other types of follicular lymphoma, lymph nodes of head, face, and neck 🔖
Ex: See C82.01

C82.82 Other types of follicular lymphoma, intrathoracic lymph nodes 🔖
Ex: See C82.02

C82.83 Other types of follicular lymphoma, intra-abdominal lymph nodes 🔖
Ex: See C82.03

C82.84 Other types of follicular lymphoma, lymph nodes of axilla and upper limb 🔖
Ex: See C82.04

CHAPTER 2 (C00-D49)

C82.85   Other types of follicular lymphoma, lymph nodes of inguinal region and lower limb 🔗
      (Ex:) See C82.05

C82.86   Other types of follicular lymphoma, intrapelvic lymph nodes 🔗
      (Ex:) See C82.06

C82.87   Other types of follicular lymphoma, spleen 🔗
      (Ex:) See C82.07

C82.88   Other types of follicular lymphoma, lymph nodes of multiple sites 🔗
      (Ex:) See C82.08

C82.89   Other types of follicular lymphoma, extranodal and solid organ sites 🔗
      (Ex:) See C82.00

● **C82.9**   Follicular lymphoma, unspecified

C82.90   Follicular lymphoma, unspecified, unspecified site 🔗
      (Ex:) See C82.00

C82.91   Follicular lymphoma, unspecified, lymph nodes of head, face, and neck 🔗
      (Ex:) See C82.01

C82.92   Follicular lymphoma, unspecified, intrathoracic lymph nodes 🔗
      (Ex:) See C82.02

C82.93   Follicular lymphoma, unspecified, intra-abdominal lymph nodes 🔗
      (Ex:) See C82.03

C82.94   Follicular lymphoma, unspecified, lymph nodes of axilla and upper limb 🔗
      (Ex:) See C82.04

C82.95   Follicular lymphoma, unspecified, lymph nodes of inguinal region and lower limb 🔗
      (Ex:) See C82.05

C82.96   Follicular lymphoma, unspecified, intrapelvic lymph nodes 🔗
      (Ex:) See C82.06

C82.97   Follicular lymphoma, unspecified, spleen 🔗
      (Ex:) See C82.07

C82.98   Follicular lymphoma, unspecified, lymph nodes of multiple sites 🔗
      (Ex:) See C82.08

C82.99   Follicular lymphoma, unspecified, extranodal and solid organ sites 🔗
      (Ex:) See C82.00

● **C83**   Non-follicular lymphoma

    Excludes1   personal history of non-Hodgkin lymphoma (Z85.72)

● **C83.0**   Small cell B-cell lymphoma
    Lymphoplasmacytic lymphoma
    Nodal marginal zone lymphoma
    Non-leukemic variant of B-CLL
    Splenic marginal zone lymphoma

    Excludes1   chronic lymphocytic leukemia (C91.1)
               mature T/NK-cell lymphomas (C84.-)
               Waldenström macroglobulinemia (C88.0)

C83.00   Small cell B-cell lymphoma, unspecified site 🔗
      (Ex:) C83.00-C83.09, C83.80-C83.99, C86.5-C86.6, D49.81-D49.9

C83.01   Small cell B-cell lymphoma, lymph nodes of head, face, and neck 🔗
      (Ex:) C83.00-C83.01, C83.08-C83.09, C83.80-C83.81, C83.88-C83.91, C83.98-C83.99, C86.5-C86.6, D49.81-D49.9

C83.02   Small cell B-cell lymphoma, intrathoracic lymph nodes 🔗
      (Ex:) C83.00, C83.02, C83.08-C83.09, C83.80, C83.82, C83.88-C83.89, C83.90, C83.92, C83.98-C83.99, C86.5-C86.6, D49.81-D49.9

C83.03   Small cell B-cell lymphoma, intra-abdominal lymph nodes 🔗
      (Ex:) C83.00, C83.03, C83.08-C83.09, C83.80, C83.83, C83.88-C83.89, C83.90, C83.93, C83.98-C83.99, C86.5-C86.6, D49.81-D49.9

C83.04   Small cell B-cell lymphoma, lymph nodes of axilla and upper limb 🔗
      (Ex:) C83.00, C83.04, C83.08-C83.09, C83.80, C83.84, C83.88-C83.89, C83.90, C83.94, C83.98-C83.99, C86.5-C86.6, D49.81-D49.9

C83.05   Small cell B-cell lymphoma, lymph nodes of inguinal region and lower limb 🔗
      (Ex:) C83.00, C83.05, C83.08-C83.09, C83.80, C83.85, C83.88-C83.89, C83.90, C83.95, C83.98-C83.99, C86.5-C86.6, D49.81-D49.9

C83.06   Small cell B-cell lymphoma, intrapelvic lymph nodes 🔗
      (Ex:) C83.00, C83.06, C83.08-C83.09, C83.80, C83.86, C83.88-C83.89, C83.90, C83.96, C83.98-C83.99, C86.5-C86.6, D49.81-D49.9

C83.07   Small cell B-cell lymphoma, spleen 🔗
      (Ex:) C83.00, C83.07-C83.09, C83.80, C83.87-C83.89, C83.90, C83.97-C83.99, C86.5-C86.6, D49.81-D49.9

C83.08   Small cell B-cell lymphoma, lymph nodes of multiple sites 🔗
      (Ex:) See C83.00

C83.09   Small cell B-cell lymphoma, extranodal and solid organ sites 🔗
      (Ex:) See C83.00

● **C83.1**   Mantle cell lymphoma
    Centrocytic lymphoma
    Malignant lymphomatous polyposis

C83.10   Mantle cell lymphoma, unspecified site 🔗
      (Ex:) See C82.50

C83.11   Mantle cell lymphoma, lymph nodes of head, face, and neck 🔗
      (Ex:) See C82.51

C83.12   Mantle cell lymphoma, intrathoracic lymph nodes 🔗
      (Ex:) See C82.52

C83.13   Mantle cell lymphoma, intra-abdominal lymph nodes 🔗
      (Ex:) See C82.53

C83.14   Mantle cell lymphoma, lymph nodes of axilla and upper limb 🔗
      (Ex:) See C82.54

C83.15   Mantle cell lymphoma, lymph nodes of inguinal region and lower limb 🔗
      (Ex:) See C82.55

C83.16   Mantle cell lymphoma, intrapelvic lymph nodes 🔗
      (Ex:) See C82.56

C83.17   Mantle cell lymphoma, spleen 🔗
      (Ex:) See C82.57

C83.18   Mantle cell lymphoma, lymph nodes of multiple sites 🔗
      (Ex:) See C82.58

C83.19   Mantle cell lymphoma, extranodal and solid organ sites 🔗
      (Ex:) See C82.50

● **C83.3**   Diffuse large B-cell lymphoma
    Anaplastic diffuse large B-cell lymphoma
    CD30-positive diffuse large B-cell lymphoma
    Centroblastic diffuse large B-cell lymphoma
    Diffuse large B-cell lymphoma, subtype not specified
    Immunoblastic diffuse large B-cell lymphoma
    Plasmablastic diffuse large B-cell lymphoma
    Diffuse large B-cell lymphoma, subtype not specified
    T-cell rich diffuse large B-cell lymphoma

    Excludes1   mediastinal (thymic) large B-cell lymphoma (C85.2-)
               mature T/NK-cell lymphomas (C84.-)

C83.30   Diffuse large B-cell lymphoma, unspecified site 🔗
      (Ex:) C83.30-C83.39, D49.81-D49.9

C83.31   Diffuse large B-cell lymphoma, lymph nodes of head, face, and neck 🔗
      (Ex:) C83.30-C83.31, C83.38-C83.39, D49.81-D49.9

N   Newborn Age: 0   **P**   Pediatric Age: 0–17   **M**   Maternity DX: 12–55   **A**   Adult Age: 15–124   ♀   Females Only   ♂   Males Only

🔗   Complication\Comorbidity   Major C\C   (Ex:)   CC/MCC Exclusions   Hospital-Acquired Condition

697

CHAPTER 2 (C00-D49)

C83.32   Diffuse large B-cell lymphoma, intrathoracic lymph nodes 🔎
Ex: C83.30, C83.32, C83.38-C83.39, D49.81-D49.9

C83.33   Diffuse large B-cell lymphoma, intra-abdominal lymph nodes 🔎
Ex: C83.30, C83.33, C83.38-C83.39, D49.81-D49.9

C83.34   Diffuse large B-cell lymphoma, lymph nodes of axilla and upper limb 🔎
Ex: C83.30, C83.34, C83.38-C83.39, D49.81-D49.9

C83.35   Diffuse large B-cell lymphoma, lymph nodes of inguinal region and lower limb 🔎
Ex: C83.30, C83.35, C83.38-C83.39, D49.81-D49.9

C83.36   Diffuse large B-cell lymphoma, intrapelvic lymph nodes 🔎
Ex: C83.30, C83.36, C83.38-C83.39, D49.81-D49.9

C83.37   Diffuse large B-cell lymphoma, spleen 🔎
Ex: C83.30, C83.37-C83.39, D49.81-D49.9

C83.38   Diffuse large B-cell lymphoma, lymph nodes of multiple sites 🔎
Ex: See C83.30

C83.39   Diffuse large B-cell lymphoma, extranodal and solid organ sites 🔎
Ex: See C83.30

● C83.5   Lymphoblastic (diffuse) lymphoma
Highly malignant type of non-Hodgkin lymphoma with diffuse infiltration
B-precursor lymphoma
Lymphoblastic B-cell lymphoma
Lymphoblastic lymphoma NOS
Lymphoblastic T-cell lymphoma
T-precursor lymphoma

C83.50   Lymphoblastic (diffuse) lymphoma, unspecified site 🔎
Ex: C83.50-C83.59, D49.81-D49.9

C83.51   Lymphoblastic (diffuse) lymphoma, lymph nodes of head, face, and neck 🔎
Ex: C83.50-C83.51, C83.58-C83.59, D49.81-D49.9

C83.52   Lymphoblastic (diffuse) lymphoma, intrathoracic lymph nodes 🔎
Ex: C83.50, C83.52, C83.58-C83.59, D49.81-D49.9

C83.53   Lymphoblastic (diffuse) lymphoma, intra-abdominal lymph nodes 🔎
Ex: C83.50, C83.53, C83.58-C83.59, D49.81-D49.9

C83.54   Lymphoblastic (diffuse) lymphoma, lymph nodes of axilla and upper limb 🔎
Ex: C83.50, C83.54, C83.58-C83.59, D49.81-D49.9

C83.55   Lymphoblastic (diffuse) lymphoma, lymph nodes of inguinal region and lower limb 🔎
Ex: C83.50, C83.55, C83.58-C83.59, D49.81-D49.9

C83.56   Lymphoblastic (diffuse) lymphoma, intrapelvic lymph nodes 🔎
Ex: C83.50, C83.56, C83.58-C83.59, D49.81-D49.9

C83.57   Lymphoblastic (diffuse) lymphoma, spleen 🔎
Ex: C83.50, C83.57-C83.59, D49.81-D49.9

C83.58   Lymphoblastic (diffuse) lymphoma, lymph nodes of multiple sites 🔎
Ex: See C83.50

C83.59   Lymphoblastic (diffuse) lymphoma, extranodal and solid organ sites 🔎
Ex: See C83.50

● C83.7   Burkitt lymphoma
Form of small cell lymphoma
Atypical Burkitt lymphoma
Burkitt-like lymphoma
Excludes1   mature B-cell leukemia Burkitt type (C91.A-)

C83.70   Burkitt lymphoma, unspecified site 🔎
Ex: C83.70-C83.79, D49.81-D49.9

C83.71   Burkitt lymphoma, lymph nodes of head, face, and neck 🔎
Ex: C83.70-C83.71, C83.78-C83.79, D49.81-D49.9

C83.72   Burkitt lymphoma, intrathoracic lymph nodes 🔎
Ex: C83.70, C83.72, C83.78-C83.79, D49.81-D49.9

C83.73   Burkitt lymphoma, intra-abdominal lymph nodes 🔎
Ex: C83.70, C83.73, C83.78-C83.79, D49.81-D49.9

C83.74   Burkitt lymphoma, lymph nodes of axilla and upper limb 🔎
Ex: C83.70, C83.74, C83.78-C83.79, D49.81-D49.9

C83.75   Burkitt lymphoma, lymph nodes of inguinal region and lower limb 🔎
Ex: C83.70, C83.75, C83.78-C83.79, D49.81-D49.9

C83.76   Burkitt lymphoma, intrapelvic lymph nodes 🔎
Ex: C83.70, C83.76, C83.78-C83.79, D49.81-D49.9

C83.77   Burkitt lymphoma, spleen 🔎
Ex: C83.70, C83.77-C83.79, D49.81-D49.9

C83.78   Burkitt lymphoma, lymph nodes of multiple sites 🔎
Ex: See C83.70

C83.79   Burkitt lymphoma, extranodal and solid organ sites 🔎
Ex: See C83.70

● C83.8   Other non-follicular lymphoma
Intravascular large B-cell lymphoma
Lymphoid granulomatosis
Primary effusion B-cell lymphoma
Excludes1   mediastinal (thymic) large B-cell lymphoma (C85.2-)
T-cell rich B-cell lymphoma (C83.3-)

C83.80   Other non-follicular lymphoma, unspecified site 🔎
Ex: See C83.00

C83.81   Other non-follicular lymphoma, lymph nodes of head, face, and neck 🔎
Ex: See C83.01

C83.82   Other non-follicular lymphoma, intrathoracic lymph nodes 🔎
Ex: See C83.02

C83.83   Other non-follicular lymphoma, intra-abdominal lymph nodes 🔎
Ex: See C83.03

C83.84   Other non-follicular lymphoma, lymph nodes of axilla and upper limb 🔎
Ex: See C83.04

C83.85   Other non-follicular lymphoma, lymph nodes of inguinal region and lower limb 🔎
Ex: See C83.05

C83.86   Other non-follicular lymphoma, intrapelvic lymph nodes 🔎
Ex: See C83.06

C83.87   Other non-follicular lymphoma, spleen 🔎
Ex: See C83.07

C83.88   Other non-follicular lymphoma, lymph nodes of multiple sites 🔎
Ex: See C83.00

C83.89   Other non-follicular lymphoma, extranodal and solid organ sites 🔎
Ex: See C83.00

● C83.9   Non-follicular (diffuse) lymphoma, unspecified

C83.90   Non-follicular (diffuse) lymphoma, unspecified, unspecified site 🔎
Ex: See C83.00

C83.91   Non-follicular (diffuse) lymphoma, unspecified, lymph nodes of head, face, and neck 🔎
Ex: See C83.01

C83.92   Non-follicular (diffuse) lymphoma, unspecified, intrathoracic lymph nodes 🔎
Ex: See C83.02

C83.93   Non-follicular (diffuse) lymphoma, unspecified, intra-abdominal lymph nodes 🔎
Ex: See C83.03

C83.94   Non-follicular (diffuse) lymphoma, unspecified, lymph nodes of axilla and upper limb 🔎
Ex: See C83.04

◀ New   ◀⁞⁞ Revised   ~~deleted~~ Deleted   Excludes 1   Excludes 2   Includes   Use additional   Code first   Code also   Unspecified

OGCR Official Guidelines   ● Unacceptable Principal Diagnosis   X Assign placeholder X   ● Use Additional Character(s)   ▶ Manifestation Code   **Coding Clinic**

C83.95   Non-follicular (diffuse) lymphoma, unspecified, lymph nodes of inguinal region and lower limb 🔗
     (Ex:) See C83.05

C83.96   Non-follicular (diffuse) lymphoma, unspecified, intrapelvic lymph nodes 🔗
     (Ex:) See C83.06

C83.97   Non-follicular (diffuse) lymphoma, unspecified, spleen 🔗
     (Ex:) See C83.07

C83.98   Non-follicular (diffuse) lymphoma, unspecified, lymph nodes of multiple sites 🔗
     (Ex:) See C83.00

C83.99   Non-follicular (diffuse) lymphoma, unspecified, extranodal and solid organ sites 🔗
     (Ex:) See C83.00

● **C84**   Mature T/NK-cell lymphomas
     Excludes1   personal history of non-Hodgkin lymphoma (Z85.72)

● **C84.0**   Mycosis fungoides
     Chronic or rapidly progressive form of cutaneous T-cell lymphoma; AKA granuloma fungoides
     Excludes1   peripheral T-cell lymphoma, not classified (C84.4-)

C84.00   Mycosis fungoides, unspecified site 🔗
     (Ex:) C82.50, C82.59, C83.10, C83.19, C84.00-C84.09, C84.40, C84.49, C84.60, C84.69-C84.70, C84.79, C84.90, C84.99, C84.A0, C84.A9-C84.Z0, C84.Z9, C85.10, C85.19-C85.20, C85.29-C85.80, C85.89-C85.90, C85.99, C86.4, C88.4, C96.4, C96.9, C96.Z, D49.81-D49.9

C84.01   Mycosis fungoides, lymph nodes of head, face, and neck 🔗
     (Ex:) C82.51, C83.11, C84.00-C84.01, C84.08-C84.09, C84.41, C84.61, C84.71, C84.91, C84.A1, C84.Z1, C85.11, C85.21, C85.81, C85.91, C86.0, D49.81-D49.9

C84.02   Mycosis fungoides, intrathoracic lymph nodes 🔗
     (Ex:) C82.52, C83.12, C84.00, C84.02, C84.08-C84.09, C84.42, C84.62, C84.72, C84.92, C84.A2, C84.Z2, C85.12, C85.22, C85.82, C85.92, D49.81-D49.9

C84.03   Mycosis fungoides, intra-abdominal lymph nodes 🔗
     (Ex:) C82.53, C83.13, C84.00, C84.03, C84.08-C84.09, C84.43, C84.63, C84.73, C84.93, C84.A3, C84.Z3, C85.13, C85.23, C85.83, C85.93, C86.2-C86.3, D49.81-D49.9

C84.04   Mycosis fungoides, lymph nodes of axilla and upper limb 🔗
     (Ex:) C82.54, C83.14, C84.00, C84.04, C84.08-C84.09, C84.44, C84.64, C84.74, C84.94, C84.A4, C84.Z4, C85.14, C85.24, C85.84, C85.94, D49.81-D49.9

C84.05   Mycosis fungoides, lymph nodes of inguinal region and lower limb 🔗
     (Ex:) C82.55, C83.15, C84.00, C84.05, C84.08-C84.09, C84.45, C84.65, C84.75, C84.95, C84.A5, C84.Z5, C85.15, C85.25, C85.85, C85.95, D49.81-D49.9

C84.06   Mycosis fungoides, intrapelvic lymph nodes 🔗
     (Ex:) C82.56, C83.16, C84.00, C84.06, C84.08-C84.09, C84.46, C84.66, C84.76, C84.96, C84.A6, C84.Z6, C85.16, C85.26, C85.86, C85.96, D49.81-D49.9

C84.07   Mycosis fungoides, spleen 🔗
     (Ex:) C82.57, C83.17, C84.00, C84.07, C84.08-C84.09, C84.47, C84.67, C84.77, C84.97, C84.A7, C84.Z7, C85.17, C85.27, C85.87, C85.97, D49.81-D49.9

C84.08   Mycosis fungoides, lymph nodes of multiple sites 🔗
     (Ex:) C82.58, C83.18, C84.00-C84.09, C84.48, C84.68, C84.78, C84.98, C84.A8, C84.Z8, C85.18, C85.28, C85.88, C85.98, D49.81-D49.9

C84.09   Mycosis fungoides, extranodal and solid organ sites 🔗
     (Ex:) See C84.00

● **C84.1**   Sézary disease
     Type of cutaneous lymphoma affecting T-cells

C84.10   Sézary disease, unspecified site 🔗
     (Ex:) C82.50, C82.59, C83.10, C83.19, C84.10-C84.19, C84.40, C84.49-C84.60, C84.69-C84.70, C84.79, C84.90, C84.99, C84.A0, C84.A9-C84.Z0, C84.Z9, C85.10, C85.19-C85.20, C85.29-C85.80, C85.89-C85.90, C85.99, C86.4, C88.4, C96.4, C96.9, C96.Z, D49.81-D49.9

C84.11   Sézary disease, lymph nodes of head, face, and neck 🔗
     (Ex:) C82.51, C83.11, C84.10-C84.11, C84.18-C84.19, C84.41, C84.61, C84.71, C84.91, C84.A1, C84.Z1, C85.11, C85.21, C85.81, C85.91, C86.0, D49.81-D49.9

C84.12   Sézary disease, intrathoracic lymph nodes 🔗
     (Ex:) C82.52, C83.12, C84.10, C84.12, C84.18-C84.19, C84.42, C84.62, C84.72, C84.92, C84.A2, C84.Z2, C85.12, C85.22, C85.82, C85.92, D49.81-D49.9

C84.13   Sézary disease, intra-abdominal lymph nodes 🔗
     (Ex:) C82.53, C83.13, C84.10, C84.13, C84.18-C84.19, C84.43, C84.73, C84.93, C84.A3, C84.Z3, C85.13, C85.23, C85.83, C85.93, C86.2-C86.3, D49.81-D49.9

C84.14   Sézary disease, lymph nodes of axilla and upper limb 🔗
     (Ex:) C82.54, C83.14, C84.10, C84.14, C84.18-C84.19, C84.44, C84.64, C84.74, C84.94, C84.A4, C84.Z4, C85.14, C85.24, C85.84, C85.94, D49.81-D49.9

C84.15   Sézary disease, lymph nodes of inguinal region and lower limb 🔗
     (Ex:) C82.55, C83.15, C84.10, C84.15, C84.18-C84.19, C84.45, C84.65, C84.75, C84.95, C84.A5, C84.Z5, C85.15, C85.25, C85.85, C85.95, D49.81-D49.9

C84.16   Sézary disease, intrapelvic lymph nodes 🔗
     (Ex:) C82.56, C83.16, C84.10, C84.16, C84.18-C84.19, C84.46, C84.66, C84.76, C84.96, C84.A6, C84.Z6, C85.16, C85.26, C85.86, C85.96, D49.81-D49.9

C84.17   Sézary disease, spleen 🔗
     (Ex:) C82.57, C83.17, C84.10, C84.17-C84.19, C84.47, C84.67, C84.77, C84.97, C84.A7, C84.Z7, C85.17, C85.27, C85.87, C85.97, C86.1, D49.81-D49.9

C84.18   Sézary disease, lymph nodes of multiple sites 🔗
     (Ex:) C82.58, C83.18, C84.10-C84.19, C84.48, C84.68, C84.78, C84.98, C84.A8, C84.Z8, C85.18, C85.28, C85.88, C85.98, D49.81-D49.9

C84.19   Sézary disease, extranodal and solid organ sites 🔗
     (Ex:) See C84.10

● **C84.4**   Peripheral T-cell lymphoma, not classified
     Diverse group of blood carcinomas originating from T-cells, requiring aggressive chemotherapy
     Lennert's lymphoma
     Lymphoepithelioid lymphoma
     Mature T-cell lymphoma, not elsewhere classified

C84.40   Peripheral T-cell lymphoma, not classified, unspecified site 🔗
     (Ex:) See C82.50

C84.41   Peripheral T-cell lymphoma, not classified, lymph nodes of head, face, and neck 🔗
     (Ex:) See C82.51

C84.42   Peripheral T-cell lymphoma, not classified, intrathoracic lymph nodes 🔗
     (Ex:) See C82.52

C84.43   Peripheral T-cell lymphoma, not classified, intra-abdominal lymph nodes 🔗
     (Ex:) See C82.53

C84.44   Peripheral T-cell lymphoma, not classified, lymph nodes of axilla and upper limb 🔗
     (Ex:) See C82.54

CHAPTER 2 (C00-D49)

N   Newborn Age: 0   P   Pediatric Age: 0–17   M   Maternity DX: 12–55   A   Adult Age: 15–124   ♀ Females Only   ♂ Males Only
🔗 Complication\Comorbidity   🔗 Major C\C   (Ex:) CC/MCC Exclusions   🔗 Hospital-Acquired Condition

699

CHAPTER 2 (C00-D49)

C84.45   Peripheral T-cell lymphoma, not classified, lymph nodes of inguinal region and lower limb 🔖
     (Ex:) See C82.55

C84.46   Peripheral T-cell lymphoma, not classified, intrapelvic lymph nodes 🔖
     (Ex:) See C82.56

C84.47   Peripheral T-cell lymphoma, not classified, spleen 🔖
     (Ex:) See C82.57

C84.48   Peripheral T-cell lymphoma, not classified, lymph nodes of multiple sites 🔖
     (Ex:) See C82.58

C84.49   Peripheral T-cell lymphoma, not classified, extranodal and solid organ sites 🔖
     (Ex:) See C82.50

● **C84.6**   Anaplastic large cell lymphoma, ALK-positive
     Anaplastic large cell lymphoma, CD30-positive

C84.60   Anaplastic large cell lymphoma, ALK-positive, unspecified site 🔖
     (Ex:) See C82.50

C84.61   Anaplastic large cell lymphoma, ALK-positive, lymph nodes of head, face, and neck 🔖
     (Ex:) See C82.51

C84.62   Anaplastic large cell lymphoma, ALK-positive, intrathoracic lymph nodes 🔖
     (Ex:) See C82.52

C84.63   Anaplastic large cell lymphoma, ALK-positive, intra-abdominal lymph nodes 🔖
     (Ex:) See C82.53

C84.64   Anaplastic large cell lymphoma, ALK-positive, lymph nodes of axilla and upper limb 🔖
     (Ex:) See C82.54

C84.65   Anaplastic large cell lymphoma, ALK-positive, lymph nodes of inguinal region and lower limb 🔖
     (Ex:) See C82.56

C84.66   Anaplastic large cell lymphoma, ALK-positive, intrapelvic lymph nodes 🔖
     (Ex:) See C82.56

C84.67   Anaplastic large cell lymphoma, ALK-positive, spleen 🔖
     (Ex:) See C82.57

C84.68   Anaplastic large cell lymphoma, ALK-positive, lymph nodes of multiple sites 🔖
     (Ex:) See C82.58

C84.69   Anaplastic large cell lymphoma, ALK-positive, extranodal and solid organ sites 🔖
     (Ex:) See C82.50

● **C84.7**   Anaplastic large cell lymphoma, ALK-negative
     Excludes1   primary cutaneous CD30-positive T-cell proliferations (C86.6-)

C84.70   Anaplastic large cell lymphoma, ALK-negative, unspecified site 🔖
     (Ex:) See C82.50

C84.71   Anaplastic large cell lymphoma, ALK-negative, lymph nodes of head, face, and neck 🔖
     (Ex:) See C82.51

C84.72   Anaplastic large cell lymphoma, ALK-negative, intrathoracic lymph nodes 🔖
     (Ex:) See C82.52

C84.73   Anaplastic large cell lymphoma, ALK-negative, intra-abdominal lymph nodes 🔖
     (Ex:) See C82.53

C84.74   Anaplastic large cell lymphoma, ALK-negative, lymph nodes of axilla and upper limb 🔖
     (Ex:) See C82.54

C84.75   Anaplastic large cell lymphoma, ALK-negative, lymph nodes of inguinal region and lower limb 🔖
     (Ex:) See C82.55

Item 2–7   Lymphosarcoma, also known as malignant lymphoma, is a cancer of the lymph system exhibiting abnormal cells encompassing an entire lymph node creating a diffuse pattern without any definite organization. Diffuse pattern lymphoma has a more unfavorable survival outlook than those with a follicular or nodular pattern. Reticulosarcoma is the most common aggressive form of non-Hodgkin's lymphoma.

C84.76   Anaplastic large cell lymphoma, ALK-negative, intrapelvic lymph nodes 🔖
     (Ex:) See C82.56

C84.77   Anaplastic large cell lymphoma, ALK-negative, spleen 🔖
     (Ex:) See C82.57

C84.78   Anaplastic large cell lymphoma, ALK-negative, lymph nodes of multiple sites 🔖
     (Ex:) See C82.58

C84.79   Anaplastic large cell lymphoma, ALK-negative, extranodal and solid organ sites 🔖
     (Ex:) See C82.50

● **C84.A**   Cutaneous T-cell lymphoma, unspecified

C84.A0   Cutaneous T-cell lymphoma, unspecified, unspecified site 🔖
     (Ex:) See C82.50

C84.A1   Cutaneous T-cell lymphoma, unspecified lymph nodes of head, face, and neck 🔖
     (Ex:) See C82.51

C84.A2   Cutaneous T-cell lymphoma, unspecified, intrathoracic lymph nodes 🔖
     (Ex:) See C82.52

C84.A3   Cutaneous T-cell lymphoma, unspecified, intra-abdominal lymph nodes 🔖
     (Ex:) See C82.53

C84.A4   Cutaneous T-cell lymphoma, unspecified, lymph nodes of axilla and upper limb 🔖
     (Ex:) See C82.54

C84.A5   Cutaneous T-cell lymphoma, unspecified, lymph nodes of inguinal region and lower limb 🔖
     (Ex:) See C82.55

C84.A6   Cutaneous T-cell lymphoma, unspecified, intrapelvic lymph nodes 🔖
     (Ex:) See C82.56

C84.A7   Cutaneous T-cell lymphoma, unspecified, spleen 🔖
     (Ex:) See C82.57

C84.A8   Cutaneous T-cell lymphoma, unspecified, lymph nodes of multiple sites 🔖
     (Ex:) See C82.58

C84.A9   Cutaneous T-cell lymphoma, unspecified, extranodal and solid organ sites 🔖
     (Ex:) See C82.50

● **C84.Z**   Other mature T/NK-cell lymphomas
     Note: If T-cell lineage or involvement is mentioned in conjunction with a specific lymphoma, code to the more specific description.

     Excludes1   angioimmunoblastic T-cell lymphoma (C86.5)
           blastic NK-cell lymphoma (C86.4)
           enteropathy-type T-cell lymphoma (C86.2)
           extranodal NK-cell lymphoma, nasal type (C86.0)
           hepatosplenic T-cell lymphoma (C86.1)
           primary cutaneous CD30-positive T-cell proliferations (C86.6)
           subcutaneous panniculitis-like T-cell lymphoma (C86.3)
           T-cell leukemia (C91.1-)

C84.Z0   Other mature T/NK-cell lymphomas, unspecified site 🔖
     (Ex:) See C82.50

C84.Z1   Other mature T/NK-cell lymphomas, lymph nodes of head, face, and neck 🔖
     (Ex:) See C82.51

◀ New   ◀≡ Revised   ~~deleted~~ Deleted   Excludes 1   Excludes 2   Includes   Use additional   Code first   Code also   Unspecified

OGCR Official Guidelines   ● Unacceptable Principal Diagnosis   X Assign placeholder X   ● Use Additional Character(s)   ▶ Manifestation Code   **Coding Clinic**

C84.Z2   Other mature T/NK-cell lymphomas, intrathoracic lymph nodes 🐾
    (Ex:) See C82.52

C84.Z3   Other mature T/NK-cell lymphomas, intra-abdominal lymph nodes 🐾
    (Ex:) See C82.53

C84.Z4   Other mature T/NK-cell lymphomas, lymph nodes of axilla and upper limb 🐾
    (Ex:) See C82.54

C84.Z5   Other mature T/NK-cell lymphomas, lymph nodes of inguinal region and lower limb 🐾
    (Ex:) See C82.55

C84.Z6   Other mature T/NK-cell lymphomas, intrapelvic lymph nodes 🐾
    (Ex:) See C82.56

C84.Z7   Other mature T/NK-cell lymphomas, spleen 🐾
    (Ex:) See C82.57

C84.Z8   Other mature T/NK-cell lymphomas, lymph nodes of multiple sites 🐾
    (Ex:) See C82.58

C84.Z9   Other mature T/NK-cell lymphomas, extranodal and solid organ sites 🐾
    (Ex:) See C82.50

● **C84.9**   Mature T/NK-cell lymphomas, unspecified
    NK/T cell lymphoma NOS

    Excludes1   mature T-cell lymphoma, not elsewhere classified (C84.4-)

C84.90   Mature T/NK-cell lymphomas, unspecified, unspecified site 🐾
    (Ex:) See C82.50

C84.91   Mature T/NK-cell lymphomas, unspecified, lymph nodes of head, face, and neck 🐾
    (Ex:) See C82.51

C84.92   Mature T/NK-cell lymphomas, unspecified, intrathoracic lymph nodes 🐾
    (Ex:) See C82.52

C84.93   Mature T/NK-cell lymphomas, unspecified, intra-abdominal lymph nodes 🐾
    (Ex:) See C82.53

C84.94   Mature T/NK-cell lymphomas, unspecified, lymph nodes of axilla and upper limb 🐾
    (Ex:) See C82.54

C84.95   Mature T/NK-cell lymphomas, unspecified, lymph nodes of inguinal region and lower limb 🐾
    (Ex:) See C82.55

C84.96   Mature T/NK-cell lymphomas, unspecified, intrapelvic lymph nodes 🐾
    (Ex:) See C82.56

C84.97   Mature T/NK-cell lymphomas, unspecified, spleen 🐾
    (Ex:) See C82.57

C84.98   Mature T/NK-cell lymphomas, unspecified, lymph nodes of multiple sites 🐾
    (Ex:) See C82.58

C84.99   Mature T/NK-cell lymphomas, unspecified, extranodal and solid organ sites 🐾
    (Ex:) See C82.50

● **C85**   Other specified and unspecified types of non-Hodgkin lymphoma

    Excludes1   other specified types of T/NK-cell lymphoma (C86.-)
        personal history of non-Hodgkin lymphoma (Z85.72)

● **C85.1**   Unspecified B-cell lymphoma

    Note: If B-cell lineage or involvement is mentioned in conjunction with a specific lymphoma, code to the more specific description.

C85.10   Unspecified B-cell lymphoma, unspecified site 🐾
    (Ex:) See C82.50

C85.11   Unspecified B-cell lymphoma, lymph nodes of head, face, and neck 🐾
    (Ex:) See C82.51

C85.12   Unspecified B-cell lymphoma, intrathoracic lymph nodes 🐾
    (Ex:) See C82.52

C85.13   Unspecified B-cell lymphoma, intra-abdominal lymph nodes 🐾
    (Ex:) See C82.53

C85.14   Unspecified B-cell lymphoma, lymph nodes of axilla and upper limb 🐾
    (Ex:) See C82.54

C85.15   Unspecified B-cell lymphoma, lymph nodes of inguinal region and lower limb 🐾
    (Ex:) See C82.55

C85.16   Unspecified B-cell lymphoma, intrapelvic lymph nodes 🐾
    (Ex:) See C82.56

C85.17   Unspecified B-cell lymphoma, spleen 🐾
    (Ex:) See C82.57

C85.18   Unspecified B-cell lymphoma, lymph nodes of multiple sites 🐾
    (Ex:) See C82.58

C85.19   Unspecified B-cell lymphoma, extranodal and solid organ sites 🐾
    (Ex:) See C82.50

● **C85.2**   Mediastinal (thymic) large B-cell lymphoma

C85.20   Mediastinal (thymic) large B-cell lymphoma, unspecified site 🐾
    (Ex:) See C82.50

C85.21   Mediastinal (thymic) large B-cell lymphoma, lymph nodes of head, face, and neck 🐾
    (Ex:) See C82.51

C85.22   Mediastinal (thymic) large B-cell lymphoma, intrathoracic lymph nodes 🐾
    (Ex:) See C82.52

C85.23   Mediastinal (thymic) large B-cell lymphoma, intra-abdominal lymph nodes 🐾
    (Ex:) See C82.53

C85.24   Mediastinal (thymic) large B-cell lymphoma, lymph nodes of axilla and upper limb 🐾
    (Ex:) See C82.54

C85.25   Mediastinal (thymic) large B-cell lymphoma, lymph nodes of inguinal region and lower limb 🐾
    (Ex:) See C82.55

C85.26   Mediastinal (thymic) large B-cell lymphoma, intrapelvic lymph nodes 🐾
    (Ex:) See C82.56

C85.27   Mediastinal (thymic) large B-cell lymphoma, spleen 🐾
    (Ex:) See C82.57

C85.28   Mediastinal (thymic) large B-cell lymphoma, lymph nodes of multiple sites 🐾
    (Ex:) See C82.58

C85.29   Mediastinal (thymic) large B-cell lymphoma, extranodal and solid organ sites 🐾
    (Ex:) See C82.50

● **C85.8**   Other specified types of non-Hodgkin lymphoma

C85.80   Other specified types of non-Hodgkin lymphoma, unspecified site 🐾
    (Ex:) See C82.50

C85.81   Other specified types of non-Hodgkin lymphoma, lymph nodes of head, face, and neck 🐾
    (Ex:) See C82.51

C85.82   Other specified types of non-Hodgkin lymphoma, intrathoracic lymph nodes 🐾
    (Ex:) See C82.52

C85.83   Other specified types of non-Hodgkin lymphoma, intra-abdominal lymph nodes 🐾
    (Ex:) See C82.53

CHAPTER 2 (C00-D49)

C85.84   Other specified types of non-Hodgkin lymphoma, lymph nodes of axilla and upper limb 🔗
      (Ex) See C82.54

C85.85   Other specified types of non-Hodgkin lymphoma, lymph nodes of inguinal region and lower limb 🔗
      (Ex) See C82.55

C85.86   Other specified types of non-Hodgkin lymphoma, intrapelvic lymph nodes 🔗
      (Ex) See C82.56

C85.87   Other specified types of non-Hodgkin lymphoma, spleen 🔗
      (Ex) See C82.57

C85.88   Other specified types of non-Hodgkin lymphoma, lymph nodes of multiple sites 🔗
      (Ex) See C82.58

C85.89   Other specified types of non-Hodgkin lymphoma, extranodal and solid organ sites 🔗
      (Ex) See C82.50

● **C85.9**   Non-Hodgkin lymphoma, unspecified
      Lymphoma NOS
      Malignant lymphoma NOS
      Non-Hodgkin lymphoma NOS

C85.90   Non-Hodgkin lymphoma, unspecified, unspecified site 🔗
      (Ex) See C82.50

C85.91   Non-Hodgkin lymphoma, unspecified, lymph nodes of head, face, and neck 🔗
      (Ex) See C82.51

C85.92   Non-Hodgkin lymphoma, unspecified, intrathoracic lymph nodes 🔗
      (Ex) See C82.52

C85.93   Non-Hodgkin lymphoma, unspecified, intra-abdominal lymph nodes 🔗
      (Ex) See C82.53

C85.94   Non-Hodgkin lymphoma, unspecified, lymph nodes of axilla and upper limb 🔗
      (Ex) See C82.54

C85.95   Non-Hodgkin lymphoma, unspecified, lymph nodes of inguinal region and lower limb 🔗
      (Ex) See C82.55

C85.96   Non-Hodgkin lymphoma, unspecified, intrapelvic lymph nodes 🔗
      (Ex) See C82.56

C85.97   Non-Hodgkin lymphoma, unspecified, spleen 🔗
      (Ex) See C82.57

C85.98   Non-Hodgkin lymphoma, unspecified, lymph nodes of multiple sites 🔗
      (Ex) See C82.58

C85.99   Non-Hodgkin lymphoma, unspecified, extranodal and solid organ sites 🔗
      (Ex) See C82.50

● **C86**   Other specified types of T/NK-cell lymphoma
      Excludes1   anaplastic large cell lymphoma, ALK negative (C84.7-)
            anaplastic large cell lymphoma, ALK positive (C84.6-)
            mature T/NK-cell lymphomas (C84.-)
            other specified types of non-Hodgkin lymphoma (C85.8-)

C86.0   Extranodal NK/T-cell lymphoma, nasal type 🔗
      (Ex) See C82.51

C86.1   Hepatosplenic T-cell lymphoma 🔗
      Alpha-beta and gamma delta types
      (Ex) See C82.57

C86.2   Enteropathy-type (intestinal) T-cell lymphoma 🔗
      Enteropathy associated T-cell lymphoma
      (Ex) See C82.53

C86.3   Subcutaneous panniculitis-like T-cell lymphoma 🔗
      (Ex) See C82.53

C86.4   Blastic NK-cell lymphoma 🔗
      (Ex) See C82.50

C86.5   Angioimmunoblastic T-cell lymphoma 🔗
      Angioimmunoblastic lymphadenopathy with dysproteinemia (AILD)
      (Ex) See C83.00

C86.6   Primary cutaneous CD30-positive T-cell proliferations 🔗
      Lymphomatoid papulosis
      Primary cutaneous anaplastic large cell lymphoma
      Primary cutaneous CD30-positive large T-cell lymphoma
      (Ex) See C83.00

● **C88**   Malignant immunoproliferative diseases and certain other B-cell lymphomas
      Diseases involving immune system
      Excludes1   B-cell lymphoma, unspecified (C85.1-)
            personal history of other malignant neoplasms of lymphoid, hematopoietic and related tissues (Z85.79)

C88.0   Waldenström's macroglobulinemia
      Lymphoplasmacytic lymphoma with IgM-production
      Macroglobulinemia (idiopathic) (primary)
      Excludes1   small cell B-cell lymphoma (C83.0)

C88.2   Heavy chain disease 🔗
      Franklin disease
      Gamma heavy chain disease
      Mu heavy chain disease
      (Ex) C88.2-C88.3, C88.8-C90.02, C90.10-C90.12, C90.20-C90.22, C90.30-C90.32, C91.00-C91.02, C91.10-C91.12, C91.30-C91.32, C91.50-C91.52, C91.60-C91.62, C91.90-C91.92, C91.A0-C91.A2, C91.Z0-C91.Z2, C92.00-C92.02, C92.10-C92.12, C92.20-C92.22, C92.30-C92.32, C92.40-C92.42, C92.50-C92.52, C92.60-C92.62, C92.90-C92.92, C92.A0-C92.A2, C92.Z0-C92.Z2, C93.00-C93.02, C93.10-C93.12, C93.30-C93.32, C93.90-C93.92, C93.Z0-C93.Z2, C94.00-C94.02, C94.20-C94.22, C94.30-C94.32, C94.80-C94.82, C95.00-C95.02, C95.10-C95.12, C95.90-C95.92, D49.81-D49.9

C88.3   Immunoproliferative small intestinal disease 🔗
      Alpha heavy chain disease
      Mediterranean lymphoma
      (Ex) See C88.2

C88.4   Extranodal marginal zone B-cell lymphoma of mucosa-associated lymphoid tissue [MALT-lymphoma] 🔗
      Lymphoma of skin-associated lymphoid tissue [SALT-lymphoma]
      Lymphoma of bronchial-associated lymphoid tissue [BALT-lymphoma]
      Excludes1   high malignant (diffuse large B-cell) lymphoma (C83.3-)
      (Ex) See C82.50

C88.8   Other malignant immunoproliferative diseases 🔗
      (Ex) C88.2-C88.3, C88.8-C90.02, C90.10-C90.12, C90.20-C90.22, C90.30-C90.32, C91.00-C91.02, C91.10-C91.12, C91.30-C91.32, C91.40-C91.42, C91.50-C91.52, C91.60-C91.62, C91.90-C91.92, C91.A0-C91.A2, C91.Z0-C91.Z2, C92.00-C92.02, C92.10-C92.12, C92.20-C92.22, C92.30-C92.32, C92.40-C92.42, C92.50-C92.52, C92.60-C92.62, C92.90-C92.92, C92.A0-C92.A2, C92.Z0-C92.Z2, C93.00-C93.02, C93.10-C93.12, C93.30-C93.32, C93.90-C93.92, C93.Z0-C93.Z2, C94.00-C94.02, C94.20-C94.22, C94.30-C94.32, C94.80-C94.82, C95.00-C95.02, C95.10-C95.12, C95.90-C95.92, D45-D46.22, D46.4, D46.9, D46.A-D46.Z, D47.0-D47.1, D47.3, D47.9, D47.Z2, D47.Z9, D48.7-D48.9, D49.81-D49.9

C88.9   Malignant immunoproliferative disease, unspecified 🔗
      Immunoproliferative disease NOS
      (Ex) See C88.2

◀ New   ◀▥ Revised   ~~deleted~~ Deleted   Excludes 1   Excludes 2   Includes   Use additional   Code first   Code also   Unspecified
OGCR Official Guidelines   ● Unacceptable Principal Diagnosis   X Assign placeholder X   ● Use Additional Character(s)   🔗 Manifestation Code   **Coding Clinic**

Item 2–8 Multiple myeloma is a cancer of a plasma cell (a type of white blood cell) and is an incurable but treatable disease. Immunoproliferative neoplasm is a term for diseases (mostly cancers) in which the immune system cells proliferate.

● **C90　Multiple myeloma and malignant plasma cell neoplasms**

　Excludes1　personal history of other malignant neoplasms of lymphoid, hematopoietic and related tissues (Z85.79)

　Ⓔⓧ **For category C90 CC codes:** C88.2-C88.3, C88.8-C90.02, C90.10-C90.12, C90.20-C90.22, C90.30-C90.32, C91.00-C91.02, C91.10-C91.12, C91.30-C91.32, C91.50-C91.52, C91.60-C91.62, C91.90-C91.92, C91.A0-C91.A2, C91.Z0-C91.Z2, C92.00-C92.02, C92.10-C92.12, C92.20-C92.22, C92.30-C92.32, C92.40-C92.42, C92.50-C92.52, C92.60-C92.62, C92.90-C92.92, C92.A0-C92.A2, C92.Z0-C92.Z2, C93.00-C93.02, C93.10-C93.12, C93.30-C93.32, C93.90-C93.92, C93.Z0-C93.Z2, C94.00-C94.02, C94.20-C94.22, C94.30-C94.32, C94.80-C94.82, C95.00-C95.02, C95.10-C95.12, C95.90-C95.92, D49.81-D49.9

● **C90.0　Multiple myeloma**
　　Kahler's disease
　　Medullary plasmacytoma
　　Myelomatosis
　　Plasma cell myeloma

　Excludes1　solitary myeloma (C90.3-)
　　　　　　　solitary plasmacytoma (C90.3-)

　C90.00　Multiple myeloma not having achieved remission 🔖
　　　Multiple myeloma with failed remission
　　　Multiple myeloma NOS

　C90.01　Multiple myeloma in remission 🔖

　C90.02　Multiple myeloma in relapse 🔖

● **C90.1　Plasma cell leukemia**
　　Rare type of acute leukemia
　　Plasmacytic leukemia

　C90.10　Plasma cell leukemia not having achieved remission 🔖
　　　Plasma cell leukemia with failed remission
　　　Plasma cell leukemia NOS

　C90.11　Plasma cell leukemia in remission 🔖

　C90.12　Plasma cell leukemia in relapse 🔖

● **C90.2　Extramedullary plasmacytoma**
　　Malignant monoclonal plasma cell tumor growing in soft tissue; AKA plasma cell dyscrasias

　C90.20　Extramedullary plasmacytoma not having achieved remission 🔖
　　　Extramedullary plasmacytoma with failed remission
　　　Extramedullary plasmacytoma NOS

　C90.21　Extramedullary plasmacytoma in remission 🔖

　C90.22　Extramedullary plasmacytoma in relapse 🔖

● **C90.3　Solitary plasmacytoma**
　　Localized malignant plasma cell tumor NOS
　　Plasmacytoma NOS
　　Solitary myeloma

　C90.30　Solitary plasmacytoma not having achieved remission 🔖
　　　Solitary plasmacytoma with failed remission
　　　Solitary plasmacytoma NOS

　C90.31　Solitary plasmacytoma in remission 🔖

　C90.32　Solitary plasmacytoma in relapse 🔖

● **C91　Lymphoid leukemia**
　Type of leukemia affecting circulating cells of lymphoid origin

　Excludes1　personal history of leukemia (Z85.6)

　Ⓔⓧ **For category C91 CC codes unless otherwise indicated:** C88.2-C88.3, C88.8-C90.02, C90.10-C90.12, C90.20-C90.22, C90.30-C90.32, C91.00-C91.02, C91.10-C91.12, C91.30-C91.32, C91.50-C91.52, C91.60-C91.62, C91.90-C91.92, C91.A0-C91.A2, C91.Z0-C91.Z2, C92.00-C92.02, C92.10-C92.12, C92.20-C92.22, C92.30-C92.32, C92.40-C92.42, C92.50-C92.52, C92.60-C92.62, C92.90-C92.92, C92.A0-C92.A2, C92.Z0-C92.Z2, C93.00-C93.02, C93.10-C93.12, C93.30-C93.32, C93.90-C93.92, C93.Z0-C93.Z2, C94.00-C94.02, C94.20-C94.22, C94.30-C94.32, C94.80-C94.82, C95.00-C95.02, C95.10-C95.12, C95.90-C95.92, D49.81-D49.9

● **C91.0　Acute lymphoblastic leukemia [ALL]**
　　Note:　Code C91.0 should only be used for T-cell and B-cell precursor leukemia

　C91.00　Acute lymphoblastic leukemia not having achieved remission 🔖
　　　Acute lymphoblastic leukemia with failed remission
　　　Acute lymphoblastic leukemia NOS

　C91.01　Acute lymphoblastic leukemia, in remission 🔖

　C91.02　Acute lymphoblastic leukemia, in relapse 🔖

● **C91.1　Chronic lymphocytic leukemia of B-cell type**
　　Lymphoplasmacytic leukemia
　　Richter syndrome

　Excludes1　lymphoplasmacytic lymphoma (C83.0-)

　C91.10　Chronic lymphocytic leukemia of B-cell type not having achieved remission 🔖
　　　Chronic lymphocytic leukemia of B-cell type with failed remission
　　　Chronic lymphocytic leukemia of B-cell type NOS

　C91.11　Chronic lymphocytic leukemia of B-cell type in remission 🔖

　C91.12　Chronic lymphocytic leukemia of B-cell type in relapse 🔖

● **C91.3　Prolymphocytic leukemia of B-cell type**
　　Chronic leukemia with symptoms of large number of circulating lymphocytes

　C91.30　Prolymphocytic leukemia of B-cell type not having achieved remission 🔖
　　　Prolymphocytic leukemia of B-cell type with failed remission
　　　Prolymphocytic leukemia of B-cell type NOS

　C91.31　Prolymphocytic leukemia of B-cell type, in remission 🔖

　C91.32　Prolymphocytic leukemia of B-cell type, in relapse 🔖

● **C91.4　Hairy cell leukemia**
　　Chronic leukemia with splenomegaly and excessive number of abnormal large mononuclear cells covered by hairlike villi
　　Leukemic reticuloendotheliosis

　Ⓔⓧ **For category C91.4 CC codes:** C82.50, C82.59, C83.10, C83.19, C84.40, C84.49-C84.60, C84.69-C84.70, C84.79, C84.90, C84.99, C84.A0, C84.A9-C84.Z0, C84.Z9, C85.10, C85.19-C85.20, C85.29-C85.80, C85.89-C85.90, C85.99, C86.4, C88.4, C91.40-C91.42, C96.4, C96.9, C96.Z, D49.81-D49.9

　C91.40　Hairy cell leukemia not having achieved remission 🔖
　　　Hairy cell leukemia with failed remission
　　　Hairy cell leukemia NOS

　C91.41　Hairy cell leukemia, in remission 🔖

　C91.42　Hairy cell leukemia, in relapse 🔖

Item 2–9 Leukemia is a cancer (acute or chronic) of the blood-forming tissues of the bone marrow. Blood cells all start out as stem cells. They mature and become red cells, white cells, or platelets. There are three main types of leukocytes (white cells that fight infection): monocytes, lymphocytes, and granulocytes. **Acute monocytic leukemia** (AML) affects monocytes. **Acute lymphoid leukemia** (ALL) affects lymphocytes, and **acute myeloid leukemia** (AML) affects cells that typically develop into white blood cells (not lymphocytes), though it may develop in other blood cells.

CHAPTER 2 (C00-D49)

N　Newborn Age: 0　　　**P**　Pediatric Age: 0–17　　　**M**　Maternity DX: 12–55　　　**A**　Adult Age: 15–124　　　♀　Females Only　　　♂　Males Only

🔖　Complication\Comorbidity　　　🔖　Major C\C　　　Ⓔⓧ　CC/MCC Exclusions　　　🔖　Hospital-Acquired Condition

703

● **C91.5** **Adult T-cell lymphoma/leukemia (HTLV-1-associated)**
Acute variant of adult T-cell lymphoma/leukemia (HTLV-1-associated)
Chronic variant of adult T-cell lymphoma/leukemia (HTLV-1-associated)
Lymphomatoid variant of adult T-cell lymphoma/leukemia (HTLV-1-associated)
Smouldering variant of adult T-cell lymphoma/leukemia (HTLV-1-associated)

C91.50 **Adult T-cell lymphoma/leukemia (HTLV-1-associated) not having achieved remission** 🔖 A
Adult T-cell lymphoma/leukemia (HTLV-1-associated) with failed remission
Adult T-cell lymphoma/leukemia (HTLV-1-associated) NOS

C91.51 **Adult T-cell lymphoma/leukemia (HTLV-1-associated), in remission** 🔖 A

C91.52 **Adult T-cell lymphoma/leukemia (HTLV-1-associated), in relapse** 🔖 A

● **C91.6** **Prolymphocytic leukemia of T-cell type**

C91.60 **Prolymphocytic leukemia of T-cell type not having achieved remission** 🔖
Prolymphocytic leukemia of T-cell type with failed remission
Prolymphocytic leukemia of T-cell type NOS

C91.61 **Prolymphocytic leukemia of T-cell type, in remission** 🔖

C91.62 **Prolymphocytic leukemia of T-cell type, in relapse** 🔖

● **C91.A** **Mature B-cell leukemia Burkitt-type**
Excludes1 Burkitt lymphoma (C83.7-)

C91.A0 **Mature B-cell leukemia Burkitt-type not having achieved remission** 🔖
Mature B-cell leukemia Burkitt-type with failed remission
Mature B-cell leukemia Burkitt-type NOS

C91.A1 **Mature B-cell leukemia Burkitt-type, in remission** 🔖

C91.A2 **Mature B-cell leukemia Burkitt-type, in relapse** 🔖

● **C91.Z** **Other lymphoid leukemia**
T-cell large granular lymphocytic leukemia (associated with rheumatoid arthritis)

C91.Z0 **Other lymphoid leukemia not having achieved remission** 🔖
Other lymphoid leukemia with failed remission
Other lymphoid leukemia NOS

C91.Z1 **Other lymphoid leukemia, in remission** 🔖

C91.Z2 **Other lymphoid leukemia, in relapse** 🔖

● **C91.9** **Lymphoid leukemia, unspecified**

C91.90 **Lymphoid leukemia, unspecified not having achieved remission** 🔖
Lymphoid leukemia with failed remission
Lymphoid leukemia NOS

C91.91 **Lymphoid leukemia, unspecified, in remission** 🔖

C91.92 **Lymphoid leukemia, unspecified, in relapse** 🔖

● **C92** **Myeloid leukemia**
Includes granulocytic leukemia
myelogenous leukemia
Excludes1 personal history of leukemia (Z85.6)
(Ex) For category **C92** CC codes: C88.2-C88.3, C88.8-C90.02, C90.10-C90.12, C90.20-C90.22, C90.30-C90.32, C91.00-C91.02, C91.10-C91.12, C91.30-C91.32, C91.50-C91.52, C91.60-C91.62, C91.90-C91.92, C91.A0-C91.A2, C91.Z0-C91.Z2, C92.00-C92.02, C92.10-C92.12, C92.20-C92.22, C92.30-C92.32, C92.40-C92.42, C92.50-C92.52, C92.60-C92.62, C92.90-C92.92, C92.A0-C92.A2, C92.Z0-C92.Z2, C93.00-C93.02, C93.10-C93.12, C93.30-C93.32, C93.90-C93.92, C93.Z0-C93.Z2, C94.00-C94.02, C94.20-C94.22, C94.30-C94.32, C94.80-C94.82, C95.00-C95.02, C95.10-C95.12, C95.90-C95.92, D49.81-D49.9

● **C92.0** **Acute myeloblastic leukemia**
Acute myeloblastic leukemia, minimal differentiation
Acute myeloblastic leukemia (with maturation)
Acute myeloblastic leukemia 1/ETO
Acute myeloblastic leukemia M0
Acute myeloblastic leukemia M1
Acute myeloblastic leukemia M2
Acute myeloblastic leukemia with t(8;21)
Acute myeloblastic leukemia (without a FAB classification) NOS
Refractory anemia with excess blasts in transformation [RAEB T]
Excludes1 acute exacerbation of chronic myeloid leukemia (C92.10)
refractory anemia with excess of blasts not in transformation (D46.2-)

C92.00 **Acute myeloblastic leukemia, not having achieved remission** 🔖
Acute myeloblastic leukemia with failed remission
Acute myeloblastic leukemia NOS

C92.01 **Acute myeloblastic leukemia, in remission** 🔖

C92.02 **Acute myeloblastic leukemia, in relapse** 🔖

● **C92.1** **Chronic myeloid leukemia, BCR/ABL-positive**
Chronic myelogenous leukemia, Philadelphia chromosome (Ph1) positive
Chronic myelogenous leukemia, t(9;22) (q34;q11)
Chronic myelogenous leukemia with crisis of blast cells
Excludes1 atypical chronic myeloid leukemia BCR/ABL-negative (C92.2-)
chronic myelomonocytic leukemia (C93.1-)
chronic myeloproliferative disease (D47.1)

C92.10 **Chronic myeloid leukemia, BCR/ABL-positive, not having achieved remission** 🔖
Chronic myeloid leukemia, BCR/ABL-positive with failed remission
Chronic myeloid leukemia, BCR/ABL-positive NOS

C92.11 **Chronic myeloid leukemia, BCR/ABL-positive, in remission** 🔖

C92.12 **Chronic myeloid leukemia, BCR/ABL-positive, in relapse** 🔖

● **C92.2** **Atypical chronic myeloid leukemia, BCR/ABL-negative**

C92.20 **Atypical chronic myeloid leukemia, BCR/ABL-negative, not having achieved remission** 🔖
Atypical chronic myeloid leukemia, BCR/ABL-negative with failed remission
Atypical chronic myeloid leukemia, BCR/ABL-negative NOS

C92.21 **Atypical chronic myeloid leukemia, BCR/ABL-negative, in remission** 🔖

C92.22 **Atypical chronic myeloid leukemia, BCR/ABL-negative, in relapse** 🔖

◄ New   ◄▥ Revised   d̶e̶l̶e̶t̶e̶d̶ Deleted   Excludes 1   Excludes 2   Includes   Use additional   Code first   Code also   Unspecified
OGCR Official Guidelines   ● Unacceptable Principal Diagnosis   X Assign placeholder X   ● Use Additional Character(s)   ▶ Manifestation Code   Coding Clinic

● **C92.3 Myeloid sarcoma**
A malignant tumor of immature myeloid cells
Chloroma
Granulocytic sarcoma

C92.30 Myeloid sarcoma, not having achieved remission 🔹
Myeloid sarcoma with failed remission
Myeloid sarcoma NOS

C92.31 Myeloid sarcoma, in remission 🔹

C92.32 Myeloid sarcoma, in relapse 🔹

● **C92.4 Acute promyelocytic leukemia**
AML M3
AML Me with t(15;17) and variants

C92.40 Acute promyelocytic leukemia, not having achieved remission 🔹
Acute promyelocytic leukemia with failed remission
Acute promyelocytic leukemia NOS

C92.41 Acute promyelocytic leukemia, in remission 🔹

C92.42 Acute promyelocytic leukemia, in relapse 🔹

● **C92.5 Acute myelomonocytic leukemia**
AML M4
AML M4 Eo with inv(16) or t(16;16)

C92.50 Acute myelomonocytic leukemia, not having achieved remission 🔹
Acute myelomonocytic leukemia with failed remission
Acute myelomonocytic leukemia NOS

C92.51 Acute myelomonocytic leukemia, in remission 🔹

C92.52 Acute myelomonocytic leukemia, in relapse 🔹

● **C92.6 Acute myeloid leukemia with 11q23-abnormality**
Acute myeloid leukemia with variation of MLL-gene

C92.60 Acute myeloid leukemia with 11q23-abnormality not having achieved remission 🔹
Acute myeloid leukemia with 11q23-abnormality with failed remission
Acute myeloid leukemia with 11q23-abnormality NOS

C92.61 Acute myeloid leukemia with 11q23-abnormality in remission 🔹

C92.62 Acute myeloid leukemia with 11q23-abnormality in relapse 🔹

● **C92.A Acute myeloid leukemia with multilineage dysplasia**
Acute myeloid leukemia with dysplasia of remaining hematopoesis and/or myelodysplastic disease in its history

C92.A0 Acute myeloid leukemia with multilineage dysplasia, not having achieved remission 🔹
Acute myeloid leukemia with multilineage dysplasia with failed remission
Acute myeloid leukemia with multilineage dysplasia NOS

C92.A1 Acute myeloid leukemia with multilineage dysplasia, in remission 🔹

C92.A2 Acute myeloid leukemia with multilineage dysplasia, in relapse 🔹

● **C92.Z Other myeloid leukemia**

C92.Z0 Other myeloid leukemia not having achieved remission 🔹
Myeloid leukemia NEC with failed remission
Myeloid leukemia NEC

C92.Z1 Other myeloid leukemia, in remission 🔹

C92.Z2 Other myeloid leukemia, in relapse 🔹

● **C92.9 Myeloid leukemia, unspecified**

C92.90 Myeloid leukemia, unspecified, not having achieved remission 🔹
Myeloid leukemia, unspecified with failed remission
Myeloid leukemia, unspecified NOS

C92.91 Myeloid leukemia, unspecified in remission 🔹

C92.92 Myeloid leukemia, unspecified in relapse 🔹

●● **C93 Monocytic leukemia**

| **Includes** | monocytoid leukemia |
| **Excludes1** | personal history of leukemia (Z85.6) |

Ⓔ For category **C93 CC codes:** C88.2-C88.3, C88.8-C90.02, C90.10-C90.12, C90.20-C90.22, C90.30-C90.32, C91.00-C91.02, C91.10-C91.12, C91.30-C91.32, C91.50-C91.52, C91.60-C91.62, C91.90-C91.92, C91.A0-C91.A2, C91.Z0-C91.Z2, C92.00-C92.02, C92.10-C92.12, C92.20-C92.22, C92.30-C92.32, C92.40-C92.42, C92.50-C92.52, C92.60-C92.62, C92.90-C92.92, C92.A0-C92.A2, C92.Z0-C92.Z2, C93.00-C93.02, C93.10-C93.12, C93.30-C93.32, C93.90-C93.92, C93.Z0-C93.Z2, C94.00-C94.02, C94.20-C94.22, C94.30-C94.32, C94.80-C94.82, C95.00-C95.02, C95.10-C95.12, C95.90-C95.92, D49.81-D49.9

● **C93.0 Acute monoblastic/monocytic leukemia**
AML M5
AML M5a
AML M5b

C93.00 Acute monoblastic/monocytic leukemia, not having achieved remission 🔹
Acute monoblastic/monocytic leukemia with failed remission
Acute monoblastic/monocytic leukemia NOS

C93.01 Acute monoblastic/monocytic leukemia, in remission 🔹

C93.02 Acute monoblastic/monocytic leukemia, in relapse 🔹

● **C93.1 Chronic myelomonocytic leukemia**
Chronic monocytic leukemia
CMML-1
CMML-2
CMML with eosinophilia

C93.10 Chronic myelomonocytic leukemia not having achieved remission 🔹
Chronic myelomonocytic leukemia with failed remission
Chronic myelomonocytic leukemia NOS

C93.11 Chronic myelomonocytic leukemia, in remission 🔹

C93.12 Chronic myelomonocytic leukemia, in relapse 🔹

● **C93.3 Juvenile myelomonocytic leukemia**

C93.30 Juvenile myelomonocytic leukemia, not having achieved remission 🔹   P
Juvenile myelomonocytic leukemia with failed remission
Juvenile myelomonocytic leukemia NOS

C93.31 Juvenile myelomonocytic leukemia, in remission 🔹   P

C93.32 Juvenile myelomonocytic leukemia, in relapse 🔹   P

● **C93.Z Other monocytic leukemia**

C93.Z0 Other monocytic leukemia, not having achieved remission 🔹
Other monocytic leukemia NOS

C93.Z1 Other monocytic leukemia, in remission 🔹

C93.Z2 Other monocytic leukemia, in relapse 🔹

● **C93.9 Monocytic leukemia, unspecified**

C93.90 Monocytic leukemia, unspecified, not having achieved remission 🔹
Monocytic leukemia, unspecified with failed remission
Monocytic leukemia, unspecified NOS

C93.91 Monocytic leukemia, unspecified in remission 🔹

C93.92 Monocytic leukemia, unspecified in relapse 🔹

N Newborn Age: 0   **P** Pediatric Age: 0–17   **M** Maternity DX: 12–55   **A** Adult Age: 15–124   ♀ Females Only   ♂ Males Only

🔹 Complication\Comorbidity   🔹 Major C\C   Ⓔ CC/MCC Exclusions   🔹 Hospital-Acquired Condition

705

● **C94**   **Other leukemias of specified cell type**

> **Excludes1**   leukemic reticuloendotheliosis (C91.4-)
> myelodysplastic syndromes (D46.-)
> personal history of leukemia (Z85.6)
> plasma cell leukemia (C90.1-)

> (Ex) For category **C94** CC codes unless otherwise indicated:C88.2-C88.3, C88.8-C90.02,
> C90.10-C90.12, C90.20-C90.22, C90.30-C90.32, C91.00-C91.02, C91.10-C91.12,
> C91.30-C91.32, C91.50-C91.52, C91.60-C91.62, C91.90-C91.92, C91.A0-C91.A2, C91.
> Z0-C91.Z2, C92.00-C92.02, C92.10-C92.12, C92.20-C92.22, C92.30-C92.32,
> C92.40-C92.42, C92.50-C92.52, C92.60-C92.62, C92.90-C92.92, C92.A0-C92.A2, C92.
> Z0-C92.Z2, C93.00-C93.02, C93.10-C93.12, C93.30-C93.32, C93.90-C93.92, C93.Z0-C93.
> Z2, C94.00-C94.02, C94.20-C94.22, C94.30-C94.32, C94.80-C94.82, C95.00-C95.02,
> C95.10-C95.12, C95.90-C95.92, D49.81-D49.9

● **C94.0**   **Acute erythroid leukemia**
> Acute myeloid leukemia M6(a)(b)
> Erythroleukemia

> **C94.00**   **Acute erythroid leukemia, not having achieved remission** 🔊
> > Acute erythroid leukemia with failed remission
> > Acute erythroid leukemia NOS

> **C94.01**   **Acute erythroid leukemia, in remission** 🔊

> **C94.02**   **Acute erythroid leukemia, in relapse** 🔊

● **C94.2**   **Acute megakaryoblastic leukemia**
> Acute myeloid leukemia M7
> Acute megakaryocytic leukemia

> **C94.20**   **Acute megakaryoblastic leukemia not having achieved remission** 🔊
> > Acute megakaryoblastic leukemia with failed remission ◀▥
> > Acute megakaryoblastic leukemia NOS

> **C94.21**   **Acute megakaryoblastic leukemia, in remission** 🔊

> **C94.22**   **Acute megakaryoblastic leukemia, in relapse** 🔊

● **C94.3**   **Mast cell leukemia**

> **C94.30**   **Mast cell leukemia not having achieved remission** 🔊
> > Mast cell leukemia with failed remission
> > Mast cell leukemia NOS

> **C94.31**   **Mast cell leukemia, in remission** 🔊

> **C94.32**   **Mast cell leukemia, in relapse** 🔊

● **C94.4**   **Acute panmyelosis with myelofibrosis**
> Acute myelofibrosis

> **Excludes1**   myelofibrosis NOS (D75.81)
> > secondary myelofibrosis NOS (D75.81)

> (Ex) For category **C94.4** CC codes: C88.2-C88.3, C88.8-C88.9, C90.10-C90.11,
> C90.20-C90.21, C90.30-C90.31, C91.00-C91.02, C91.10-C91.12,
> C91.30-C91.32, C91.40-C91.42, C91.50-C91.52, C91.60-C91.62,
> C91.90-C91.92, C91.A0-C91.A2, C91.Z0-C91.Z2, C92.00-C92.02,
> C92.10-C92.12, C92.20-C92.22, C92.30-C92.32, C92.40-C92.42,
> C92.50-C92.52, C92.60-C92.62, C92.90-C92.92, C92.A0-C92.A2,
> C92.Z0-C92.Z2, C93.00-C93.02, C93.10-C93.12, C93.30-C93.32,
> C93.90-C93.92, C93.Z0-C93.Z2, C94.00-C94.02, C94.20-C94.22,
> C94.30-C94.32, C94.40-C94.42, C94.6, C94.80-C94.82, C95.00-C95.02,
> C95.10-C95.12, C95.90-C95.92, D45-D46.22, D46.4, D46.9, D46.A-D46.Z,
> D47.0-D47.1, D47.3, D47.9, D47.Z2, D47.Z9, D48.7-D48.9

> **C94.40**   **Acute panmyelosis with myelofibrosis not having achieved remission** 🔊
> > Acute myelofibrosis NOS
> > Acute panmyelosis with myelofibrosis with failed remission
> > Acute panmyelosis NOS

> **C94.41**   **Acute panmyelosis with myelofibrosis, in remission** 🔊

> **C94.42**   **Acute panmyelosis with myelofibrosis, in relapse** 🔊

● **C94.6**   **Myelodysplastic disease, not classified** 🔊
> Myeloproliferative disease, not classified
> (Ex) See C94.4

● **C94.8**   **Other specified leukemias**
> Aggressive NK-cell leukemia
> Acute basophilic leukemia

> **C94.80**   **Other specified leukemias not having achieved remission** 🔊
> > Other specified leukemia with failed remission
> > Other specified leukemias NOS

> **C94.81**   **Other specified leukemias, in remission** 🔊

> **C94.82**   **Other specified leukemias, in relapse** 🔊

● **C95**   **Leukemia of unspecified cell type**

> **Excludes1**   personal history of leukemia (Z85.6)

> (Ex) For category **C95** CC codes: C88.2-C88.3, C88.8-C90.02, C90.10-C90.12,
> C90.20-C90.22, C90.30-C90.32, C91.00-C91.02, C91.10-C91.12, C91.30-C91.32,
> C91.50-C91.52, C91.60-C91.62, C91.90-C91.92, C91.A0-C91.A2, C91.Z0-C91.Z2,
> C92.00-C92.02, C92.10-C92.12, C92.20-C92.22, C92.30-C92.32, C92.40-C92.42,
> C92.50-C92.52, C92.60-C92.62, C92.90-C92.92, C92.A0-C92.A2, C92.Z0-C92.Z2,
> C93.00-C93.02, C93.10-C93.12, C93.30-C93.32, C93.90-C93.92, C93.Z0-C93.Z2,
> C94.00-C94.02, C94.20-C94.22, C94.30-C94.32, C94.80-C94.82, C95.00-C95.02,
> C95.10-C95.12, C95.90-C95.92, D49.81-D49.9

● **C95.0**   **Acute leukemia of unspecified cell type**
> Acute bilineal leukemia
> Acute mixed lineage leukemia
> Biphenotypic acute leukemia
> Stem cell leukemia of unclear lineage

> **Excludes1**   acute exacerbation of unspecified chronic leukemia (C95.10)

> **C95.00**   **Acute leukemia of unspecified cell type not having achieved remission** 🔊
> > Acute leukemia of unspecified cell type with failed remission
> > Acute leukemia NOS

> **C95.01**   **Acute leukemia of unspecified cell type, in remission** 🔊

> **C95.02**   **Acute leukemia of unspecified cell type, in relapse** 🔊

● **C95.1**   **Chronic leukemia of unspecified cell type**

> **C95.10**   **Chronic leukemia of unspecified cell type not having achieved remission** 🔊
> > Chronic leukemia of unspecified cell type with failed remission
> > Chronic leukemia NOS

> **C95.11**   **Chronic leukemia of unspecified cell type, in remission** 🔊

> **C95.12**   **Chronic leukemia of unspecified cell type, in relapse** 🔊

● **C95.9**   **Leukemia, unspecified**

> **C95.90**   **Leukemia, unspecified not having achieved remission** 🔊
> > Leukemia, unspecified with failed remission
> > Leukemia NOS

> **C95.91**   **Leukemia, unspecified, in remission** 🔊

> **C95.92**   **Leukemia, unspecified, in relapse** 🔊

◀ New   ◀▥ Revised   ~~deleted~~ Deleted   Excludes 1   Excludes 2   Includes   Use additional   Code first   Code also   Unspecified

706   OGCR Official Guidelines   ● Unacceptable Principal Diagnosis   X Assign placeholder X   ● Use Additional Character(s)   ▷ Manifestation Code   **Coding Clinic**

● C96 **Other and unspecified malignant neoplasms of lymphoid, hematopoietic and related tissue**

  Excludes1 personal history of other malignant neoplasms of lymphoid, hematopoietic and related tissues (Z85.79)

  C96.0 **Multifocal and multisystemic (disseminated) Langerhans-cell histiocytosis** 🔖
    Histiocytosis X, multisystemic
    Letterer-Siwe disease

    Excludes1 adult pulmonary Langerhans cell histiocytosis (J84.82)
      multifocal and unisystemic Langerhans-cell histiocytosis (C96.5)
      unifocal Langerhans-cell histiocytosis (C96.6)

    (Ex) C82.50, C82.59, C83.10, C83.19, C84.40, C84.49-C84.60, C84.69-C84.70, C84.79, C84.90, C84.99, C84.A0, C84.A9-C84.Z0, C84.Z9, C85.10, C85.19-C85.20, C85.29-C85.80, C85.89-C85.90, C85.99, C86.4, C88.4, C96.0, C96.4, C96.9, C96.Z, D49.81-D49.9

  C96.2 **Malignant mast cell tumor** 🔖
    Aggressive systemic mastocytosis
    Mast cell sarcoma

    Excludes1 indolent mastocytosis (D47.0)
      mast cell leukemia (C94.30)
      mastocytosis (congenital) (cutaneous) (Q82.2)

    (Ex) C82.50, C82.59, C83.10, C83.19, C84.40, C84.49-C84.60, C84.69-C84.70, C84.79, C84.90, C84.99, C84.A0, C84.A9-C84.Z0, C84.Z9, C85.10, C85.19-C85.20, C85.29-C85.80, C85.89-C85.90, C85.99, C86.4, C88.4, C96.2, C96.4, C96.9, C96.Z, D49.81-D49.9

  C96.4 **Sarcoma of dendritic cells (accessory cells)** 🔖
    Follicular dendritic cell sarcoma
    Interdigitating dendritic cell sarcoma
    Langerhans cell sarcoma

    (Ex) C96.4, C96.9, C96.Z, D49.81-D49.9

  C96.5 **Multifocal and unisystemic Langerhans-cell histiocytosis** 🔖
    Hand-Schüller-Christian disease
    Histiocytosis X, multifocal

    Excludes1 multifocal and multisystemic (disseminated) Langerhans-cell histiocytosis (C96.0)
      unifocal Langerhans-cell histiocytosis (C96.6)

    (Ex) E71.310-E71.32, E71.40-E71.548, E80.4-E80.7, E88.40-E88.49, H49.811-H49.819

  C96.6 **Unifocal Langerhans-cell histiocytosis** 🔖
    Eosinophilic granuloma
    Histiocytosis X, unifocal
    Histiocytosis X NOS
    Langerhans-cell histiocytosis NOS

    Excludes1 multifocal and multisysemic (disseminated) Langerhans-cell histiocytosis (C96.0)
      multifocal and unisystemic Langerhans-cell histiocytosis (C96.5)

    (Ex) See C96.5

  C96.A **Histiocytic sarcoma** 🔖
    Malignant histiocytosis

    (Ex) C82.50, C82.59, C83.10, C83.19, C84.40, C84.49-C84.60, C84.69-C84.70, C84.79, C84.90, C84.99, C84.A0, C84.A9-C84.Z0, C84.Z9, C85.10, C85.19-C85.20, C85.29-C85.80, C85.89-C85.90, C85.99, C86.4, C88.4, C96.4, C96.9, C96.A, C96.Z, D49.81-D49.9

  C96.Z **Other specified malignant neoplasms of lymphoid, hematopoietic and related tissue** 🔖
    (Ex) See C96.4

  C96.9 **Malignant neoplasm of lymphoid, hematopoietic and related tissue, unspecified** 🔖
    (Ex) See C96.4

In situ is carcinoma involving cells in localized tissues that has not spread to nearby tissues

IN SITU NEOPLASMS (D00-D09)

  Includes Bowen's disease
    erythroplasia
    grade III intraepithelial neoplasia
    Queyrat's erythroplasia

● D00 **Carcinoma in situ of oral cavity, esophagus and stomach**

  Excludes1 melanoma in situ (D03.-)

  ● D00.0 **Carcinoma in situ of lip, oral cavity and pharynx**
    Use additional code to identify:
    exposure to environmental tobacco smoke (Z77.22)
    exposure to tobacco smoke in the perinatal period (P96.81)
    history of tobacco dependence (Z87.891) ◀▥
    occupational exposure to environmental tobacco smoke (Z57.31)
    tobacco dependence (F17.-)
    tobacco use (Z72.0)

    Excludes1 carcinoma in situ of aryepiglottic fold or interarytenoid fold, laryngeal aspect (D02.0)
      carcinoma in situ of epiglottis NOS (D02.0)
      carcinoma in situ of epiglottis suprahyoid portion (D02.0)
      carcinoma in situ of skin of lip (D03.0, D04.0)

    D00.00 **Carcinoma in situ of oral cavity, unspecified site**
    D00.01 **Carcinoma in situ of labial mucosa and vermilion border**
    D00.02 **Carcinoma in situ of buccal mucosa**
    D00.03 **Carcinoma in situ of gingiva and edentulous alveolar ridge**
    D00.04 **Carcinoma in situ of soft palate**
    D00.05 **Carcinoma in situ of hard palate**
    D00.06 **Carcinoma in situ of floor of mouth**
    D00.07 **Carcinoma in situ of tongue**
    D00.08 **Carcinoma in situ of pharynx**
      Carcinoma in situ of aryepiglottic fold NOS
      Carcinoma in situ of hypopharyngeal aspect of aryepiglottic fold
      Carcinoma in situ of marginal zone of aryepiglottic fold

  D00.1 **Carcinoma in situ of esophagus**
  D00.2 **Carcinoma in situ of stomach**

● D01 **Carcinoma in situ of other and unspecified digestive organs**

  Excludes1 melanoma in situ (D03.-)

  D01.0 **Carcinoma in situ of colon**

    Excludes1 carcinoma in situ of rectosigmoid junction (D01.1)

  D01.1 **Carcinoma in situ of rectosigmoid junction**
  D01.2 **Carcinoma in situ of rectum**
  D01.3 **Carcinoma in situ of anus and anal canal**
    Anal intraepithelial neoplasia III [AIN III] ◀
    Severe dysplasia of anus ◀

    Excludes1 anal intraepithelial neoplasia I and II [AIN I and AIN II] (K62.82) ◀
      carcinoma in situ of anal margin (D04.5)
      carcinoma in situ of anal skin (D04.5)
      carcinoma in situ of perianal skin (D04.5)

  ● D01.4 **Carcinoma in situ of other and unspecified parts of intestine**

    Excludes1 carcinoma in situ of ampulla of Vater (D01.5)

    D01.40 **Carcinoma in situ of unspecified part of intestine**
    D01.49 **Carcinoma in situ of other parts of intestine**

D01.5   **Carcinoma in situ of liver, gallbladder and bile ducts**
     Carcinoma in situ of ampulla of Vater

D01.7   **Carcinoma in situ of other specified digestive organs**
     Carcinoma in situ of pancreas

D01.9   **Carcinoma in situ of digestive organ, unspecified**

● **D02**   **Carcinoma in situ of middle ear and respiratory system**
     Use additional code to identify:
       exposure to environmental tobacco smoke (Z77.22)
       exposure to tobacco smoke in the perinatal period (P96.81)
       history of tobacco dependence (Z87.891) ◄▥
       occupational exposure to environmental tobacco smoke
         (Z57.31)
       tobacco dependence (F17.-)
       tobacco use (Z72.0)
     `Excludes 1`   melanoma in situ (D03.-)

D02.0   **Carcinoma in situ of larynx**
     Carcinoma in situ of aryepiglottic fold or interarytenoid
       fold, laryngeal aspect
     Carcinoma in situ of epiglottis (suprahyoid portion)
     `Excludes 1`   carcinoma in situ of aryepiglottic fold or
                 interarytenoid fold NOS (D00.08)
                 carcinoma in situ of hypopharyngeal
                   aspect (D00.08)
                 carcinoma in situ of marginal zone
                   (D00.08)

D02.1   **Carcinoma in situ of trachea**

● **D02.2**   **Carcinoma in situ of bronchus and lung**
     D02.20   **Carcinoma in situ of unspecified bronchus and
            lung**
     D02.21   **Carcinoma in situ of right bronchus and lung**
     D02.22   **Carcinoma in situ of left bronchus and lung**

D02.3   **Carcinoma in situ of other parts of respiratory system**
     Carcinoma in situ of accessory sinuses
     Carcinoma in situ of middle ear
     Carcinoma in situ of nasal cavities
     `Excludes 1`   carcinoma in situ of ear (external) (skin)
                 (D04.2-)
                 carcinoma in situ of nose NOS (D09.8)
                 carcinoma in situ of skin of nose (D04.3)

D02.4   **Carcinoma in situ of respiratory system, unspecified**

● **D03**   **Melanoma in situ**

D03.0   **Melanoma in situ of lip**

● **D03.1**   **Melanoma in situ of eyelid, including canthus**
     D03.10   **Melanoma in situ of unspecified eyelid,
            including canthus**
     D03.11   **Melanoma in situ of right eyelid, including
            canthus**
     D03.12   **Melanoma in situ of left eyelid, including
            canthus**

● **D03.2**   **Melanoma in situ of ear and external auricular canal**
     D03.20   **Melanoma in situ of unspecified ear and
            external auricular canal**
     D03.21   **Melanoma in situ of right ear and external
            auricular canal**
     D03.22   **Melanoma in situ of left ear and external
            auricular canal**

● **D03.3**   **Melanoma in situ of other and unspecified parts of face**
     D03.30   **Melanoma in situ of unspecified part of face**
     D03.39   **Melanoma in situ of other parts of face**

D03.4   **Melanoma in situ of scalp and neck**

● **D03.5**   **Melanoma in situ of trunk**
     D03.51   **Melanoma in situ of anal skin**
            Melanoma in situ of anal margin
            Melanoma in situ of perianal skin
     D03.52   **Melanoma in situ of breast (skin) (soft tissue)**
     D03.59   **Melanoma in situ of other part of trunk**

● **D03.6**   **Melanoma in situ of upper limb, including shoulder**
     D03.60   **Melanoma in situ of unspecified upper limb,
            including shoulder**

     D03.61   **Melanoma in situ of right upper limb,
            including shoulder**
     D03.62   **Melanoma in situ of left upper limb, including
            shoulder**

● **D03.7**   **Melanoma in situ of lower limb, including hip**
     D03.70   **Melanoma in situ of unspecified lower limb,
            including hip**
     D03.71   **Melanoma in situ of right lower limb, including
            hip**
     D03.72   **Melanoma in situ of left lower limb, including
            hip**

D03.8   **Melanoma in situ of other sites**
     Melanoma in situ of scrotum
     `Excludes 1`   carcinoma in situ of scrotum (D07.61)

D03.9   **Melanoma in situ, unspecified**

● **D04**   **Carcinoma in situ of skin**
     `Excludes 1`   erythroplasia of Queyrat (penis) NOS (D07.4)
                 melanoma in situ (D03.-)

D04.0   **Carcinoma in situ of skin of lip**
     `Excludes 1`   carcinoma in situ of vermilion border of lip
                 (D00.01)

● **D04.1**   **Carcinoma in situ of skin of eyelid, including canthus**
     D04.10   **Carcinoma in situ of skin of unspecified eyelid,
            including canthus**
     D04.11   **Carcinoma in situ of skin of right eyelid,
            including canthus**
     D04.12   **Carcinoma in situ of skin of left eyelid,
            including canthus**

● **D04.2**   **Carcinoma in situ of skin of ear and external auricular
     canal**
     D04.20   **Carcinoma in situ of skin of unspecified ear and
            external auricular canal**
     D04.21   **Carcinoma in situ of skin of right ear and
            external auricular canal**
     D04.22   **Carcinoma in situ of skin of left ear and
            external auricular canal**

● **D04.3**   **Carcinoma in situ of skin of other and unspecified parts
     of face**
     D04.30   **Carcinoma in situ of skin of unspecified part of
            face**
     D04.39   **Carcinoma in situ of skin of other parts of face**

D04.4   **Carcinoma in situ of skin of scalp and neck**

D04.5   **Carcinoma in situ of skin of trunk**
     Carcinoma in situ of anal margin
     Carcinoma in situ of anal skin
     Carcinoma in situ of perianal skin
     Carcinoma in situ of skin of breast
     `Excludes 1`   carcinoma in situ of anus NOS (D01.3)
                 carcinoma in situ of scrotum (D07.61)
                 carcinoma in situ of skin of genital organs
                   (D07.-)

● **D04.6**   **Carcinoma in situ of skin of upper limb, including
     shoulder**
     D04.60   **Carcinoma in situ of skin of unspecified upper
            limb, including shoulder**
     D04.61   **Carcinoma in situ of skin of right upper limb,
            including shoulder**
     D04.62   **Carcinoma in situ of skin of left upper limb,
            including shoulder**

● **D04.7**   **Carcinoma in situ of skin of lower limb, including hip**
     D04.70   **Carcinoma in situ of skin of unspecified lower
            limb, including hip**
     D04.71   **Carcinoma in situ of skin of right lower limb,
            including hip**
     D04.72   **Carcinoma in situ of skin of left lower limb,
            including hip**

D04.8   **Carcinoma in situ of skin of other sites**

D04.9   **Carcinoma in situ of skin, unspecified**

CHAPTER 2 (C00-D49)

● **D05**   **Carcinoma in situ of breast**

> **Excludes1**   carcinoma in situ of skin of breast (D04.5)
> melanoma in situ of breast (skin) (D03.5)
> Paget's disease of breast or nipple (C50.-)

● **D05.0**   **Lobular carcinoma in situ of breast**

    D05.00   **Lobular carcinoma in situ of** unspecified **breast**

    D05.01   **Lobular carcinoma in situ of right breast**

    D05.02   **Lobular carcinoma in situ of left breast**

● **D05.1**   **Intraductal carcinoma in situ of breast**

    D05.10   **Intraductal carcinoma in situ of** unspecified **breast**

    D05.11   **Intraductal carcinoma in situ of right breast**

    D05.12   **Intraductal carcinoma in situ of left breast**

● **D05.8**   **Other specified type of carcinoma in situ of breast**

    D05.80   **Other specified type of carcinoma in situ of** unspecified **breast**

    D05.81   **Other specified type of carcinoma in situ of right breast**

    D05.82   **Other specified type of carcinoma in situ of left breast**

● **D05.9**   **Unspecified type of carcinoma in situ of breast**

    D05.90   Unspecified **type of carcinoma in situ of unspecified breast**

    D05.91   Unspecified **type of carcinoma in situ of right breast**

    D05.92   Unspecified **type of carcinoma in situ of left breast**

● **D06**   **Carcinoma in situ of cervix uteri**

> **Includes**   cervical adenocarcinoma in situ
> cervical intraepithelial glandular neoplasia
> cervical intraepithelial neoplasia III [CIN III]
> severe dysplasia of cervix uteri

> **Excludes1**   cervical intraepithelial neoplasia II [CIN II] (N87.1)
> cytologic evidence of malignancy of cervix without histologic confirmation (R87.614)
> high grade squamous intraepithelial lesion (HGSIL) of cervix (R87.613)
> melanoma in situ of cervix (D03.5)
> moderate cervical dysplasia (N87.1)

   D06.0   **Carcinoma in situ of endocervix** ♀

   D06.1   **Carcinoma in situ of exocervix** ♀

   D06.7   **Carcinoma in situ of other parts of cervix** ♀

   D06.9   **Carcinoma in situ of cervix,** unspecified ♀

● **D07**   **Carcinoma in situ of other and unspecified genital organs**

> **Excludes1**   melanoma in situ of trunk (D03.5)

   D07.0   **Carcinoma in situ of endometrium** ♀

   D07.1   **Carcinoma in situ of vulva** ♀
> Severe dysplasia of vulva
> Vulvar intraepithelial neoplasia III [VIN III]

> **Excludes1**   moderate dysplasia of vulva (N90.1)
> vulvar intraepithelial neoplasia II [VIN II] (N90.1)

   D07.2   **Carcinoma in situ of vagina** ♀
> Severe dysplasia of vagina
> Vaginal intraepithelial neoplasia III [VIN III]

> **Excludes1**   moderate dysplasia of vagina (N89.1)
> vaginal intraepithelial neoplasia II [VIN II] (N89.1)

● **D07.3**   **Carcinoma in situ of other and unspecified female genital organs**

    D07.30   **Carcinoma in situ of** unspecified **female genital organs** ♀

    D07.39   **Carcinoma in situ of other female genital organs** ♀

   D07.4   **Carcinoma in situ of penis** ♂
> Erythroplasia of Queyrat NOS

   D07.5   **Carcinoma in situ of prostate** ♂
> Prostatic intraepithelial neoplasia III (PIN III)
> Severe dysplasia of prostate

> **Excludes1**   dysplasia (mild) (moderate) of prostate (N42.3-) ◀▥
> prostatic intraepithelial neoplasia II [PIN II] (N42.3-) ◀

● **D07.6**   **Carcinoma in situ of other and unspecified male genital organs**

    D07.60   **Carcinoma in situ of** unspecified **male genital organs** ♂

    D07.61   **Carcinoma in situ of scrotum** ♂

    D07.69   **Carcinoma in situ of other male genital organs** ♂

● **D09**   **Carcinoma in situ of other and unspecified sites**

> **Excludes1**   melanoma in situ (D03.-)

   D09.0   **Carcinoma in situ of bladder**

● **D09.1**   **Carcinoma in situ of other and unspecified urinary organs**

    D09.10   **Carcinoma in situ of** unspecified **urinary organ**

    D09.19   **Carcinoma in situ of other urinary organs**

● **D09.2**   **Carcinoma in situ of eye**

> **Excludes1**   carcinoma in situ of skin of eyelid (D04.1-)

    D09.20   **Carcinoma in situ of** unspecified **eye**

    D09.21   **Carcinoma in situ of right eye**

    D09.22   **Carcinoma in situ of left eye**

   D09.3   **Carcinoma in situ of thyroid and other endocrine glands**

> **Excludes1**   carcinoma in situ of endocrine pancreas (D01.7)
> carcinoma in situ of ovary (D07.39)
> carcinoma in situ of testis (D07.69)

   D09.8   **Carcinoma in situ of other specified sites**

   D09.9   **Carcinoma in situ,** unspecified

BENIGN NEOPLASMS, EXCEPT BENIGN NEUROENDOCRINE TUMORS (D10-D36)

● **D10**   **Benign neoplasm of mouth and pharynx**

   D10.0   **Benign neoplasm of lip**
> Benign neoplasm of lip (frenulum) (inner aspect) (mucosa) (vermilion border)

> **Excludes1**   benign neoplasm of skin of lip (D22.0, D23.0)

   D10.1   **Benign neoplasm of tongue**
> Benign neoplasm of lingual tonsil

   D10.2   **Benign neoplasm of floor of mouth**

● **D10.3**   **Benign neoplasm of other and unspecified parts of mouth** ◀▥

    D10.30   **Benign neoplasm of** unspecified **part of mouth**

    D10.39   **Benign neoplasm of other parts of mouth**
> Benign neoplasm of minor salivary gland NOS

> **Excludes1**   benign odontogenic neoplasms (D16.4-D16.5)
> benign neoplasm of mucosa of lip (D10.0)
> benign neoplasm of nasopharyngeal surface of soft palate (D10.6)

   D10.4   **Benign neoplasm of tonsil**
> Benign neoplasm of tonsil (faucial) (palatine)

> **Excludes1**   benign neoplasm of lingual tonsil (D10.1)
> benign neoplasm of pharyngeal tonsil (D10.6)
> benign neoplasm of tonsillar fossa (D10.5)
> benign neoplasm of tonsillar pillars (D10.5)

N Newborn Age: 0   **P** Pediatric Age: 0–17   **M** Maternity DX: 12–55   **A** Adult Age: 15–124   ♀ Females Only   ♂ Males Only

🔹 Complication\Comorbidity   🔹 Major C\C   (Ex) CC/MCC Exclusions   🔹 Hospital-Acquired Condition

709

CHAPTER 2 (C00-D49)

Figure 2-16 The esophagus is the muscular tube that connects the pharynx and the stomach. The 10 inch (25 cm) long esophagus is divided into three parts: **cervical, thoracic,** and **abdominal.**

D10.5   **Benign neoplasm of other parts of oropharynx**
    Division of pharynx lying between soft palate and upper edge of epiglottis
    Benign neoplasm of epiglottis, anterior aspect
    Benign neoplasm of tonsillar fossa
    Benign neoplasm of tonsillar pillars
    Benign neoplasm of vallecula
    Excludes1   benign neoplasm of epiglottis NOS (D14.1)
        benign neoplasm of epiglottis, suprahyoid portion (D14.1)

D10.6   **Benign neoplasm of nasopharynx**
    Segment of pharynx that lies above soft palate
    Benign neoplasm of pharyngeal tonsil
    Benign neoplasm of posterior margin of septum and choanae

D10.7   **Benign neoplasm of hypopharynx**
    Segment of pharynx that lies below upper edge of epiglottis and opens into larynx and esophagus

D10.9   **Benign neoplasm of pharynx, unspecified**

● D11   **Benign neoplasm of major salivary glands**
    Excludes1   benign neoplasms of specified minor salivary glands which are classified according to their anatomical location
        benign neoplasms of minor salivary glands NOS (D10.39)

D11.0   **Benign neoplasm of parotid gland**

D11.7   **Benign neoplasm of other major salivary glands**
    Benign neoplasm of sublingual salivary gland
    Benign neoplasm of submandibular salivary gland

D11.9   **Benign neoplasm of major salivary gland, unspecified**

● D12   **Benign neoplasm of colon, rectum, anus and anal canal**
    Excludes1   benign carcinoid tumors of the large intestine, and rectum (D3A.02-)
    Coding Clinic: 2015, Q2, P14

D12.0   **Benign neoplasm of cecum**
    Benign neoplasm of ileocecal valve

D12.1   **Benign neoplasm of appendix**
    Excludes1   benign carcinoid tumor of the appendix (D3A.020)

D12.2   **Benign neoplasm of ascending colon**

D12.3   **Benign neoplasm of transverse colon**
    Benign neoplasm of hepatic flexure
    Benign neoplasm of splenic flexure
    Flexure is a bending in a structure or organ. Note the three flexures illustrated in Figure 2–17. Hepatic = liver, sigmoid = colon, splenic = spleen.

D12.4   **Benign neoplasm of descending colon**
    Coding Clinic: 2015, Q2, P14

D12.5   **Benign neoplasm of sigmoid colon**

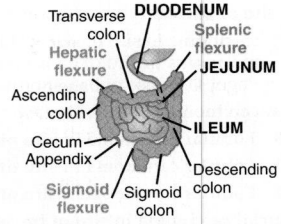

Figure 2-17 Small intestine and colon.

D12.6   **Benign neoplasm of colon, unspecified**
    Adenomatosis of colon
    Benign neoplasm of large intestine NOS
    Polyposis (hereditary) of colon
    Excludes1   inflammatory polyp of colon (K51.4-)
        polyp of colon NOS (K63.5)

D12.7   **Benign neoplasm of rectosigmoid junction**
    Angle where sigmoid colon becomes rectum

D12.8   **Benign neoplasm of rectum**
    Excludes1   benign carcinoid tumor of the rectum (D3A.026)

D12.9   **Benign neoplasm of anus and anal canal**
    Benign neoplasm of anus NOS
    Excludes1   benign neoplasm of anal margin (D22.5, D23.5)
        benign neoplasm of anal skin (D22.5, D23.5)
        benign neoplasm of perianal skin (D22.5, D23.5)

● D13   **Benign neoplasm of other and ill-defined parts of digestive system**
    Excludes1   benign stromal tumors of digestive system (D21.4)

D13.0   **Benign neoplasm of esophagus**

D13.1   **Benign neoplasm of stomach**
    Excludes1   benign carcinoid tumor of the stomach (D3A.092)

D13.2   **Benign neoplasm of duodenum**
    Excludes1   benign carcinoid tumor of the duodenum (D3A.010)

● D13.3   **Benign neoplasm of other and unspecified parts of small intestine**
    Excludes1   benign carcinoid tumors of the small intestine (D3A.01-)
        benign neoplasm of ileocecal valve (D12.0)

D13.30   **Benign neoplasm of unspecified part of small intestine**

D13.39   **Benign neoplasm of other parts of small intestine**

D13.4   **Benign neoplasm of liver**
    Benign neoplasm of intrahepatic bile ducts

D13.5   **Benign neoplasm of extrahepatic bile ducts**
    Extensions of common hepatic bile duct (tube that collects bile from liver)

D13.6   **Benign neoplasm of pancreas**
    Excludes1   benign neoplasm of endocrine pancreas (D13.7)

D13.7   **Benign neoplasm of endocrine pancreas**
    Pancreatic islets: Cells scattered throughout pancreas
    Islet cell tumor
    Benign neoplasm of islets of Langerhans
    Use additional code to identify any functional activity.

D13.9   **Benign neoplasm of ill-defined sites within the digestive system**
    Benign neoplasm of digestive system NOS
    Benign neoplasm of intestine NOS
    Benign neoplasm of spleen

CHAPTER 2 (C00–D49)

● **D14**   **Benign neoplasm of middle ear and respiratory system**

    D14.0   **Benign neoplasm of middle ear, nasal cavity and accessory sinuses**
       Benign neoplasm of cartilage of nose

       Excludes1   benign neoplasm of auricular canal (external) (D22.2-, D23.2-)
                benign neoplasm of bone of ear (D16.4)
                benign neoplasm of bone of nose (D16.4)
                benign neoplasm of cartilage of ear (D21.0)
                benign neoplasm of ear (external) (skin) (D22.2-, D23.2-)
                benign neoplasm of nose NOS (D36.7)
                benign neoplasm of skin of nose (D22.39, D23.39)
                benign neoplasm of olfactory bulb (D33.3)
                benign neoplasm of posterior margin of septum and choanae (D10.6)
                polyp of accessory sinus (J33.8)
                polyp of ear (middle) (H74.4)
                polyp of nasal (cavity) (J33.-)

    D14.1   **Benign neoplasm of larynx**
       Adenomatous polyp of larynx
       Benign neoplasm of epiglottis (suprahyoid portion)
       Horseshoe shaped bone in anterior midline of neck between chin and thyroid cartilage

       Excludes1   benign neoplasm of epiglottis, anterior aspect (D10.5)
                polyp (nonadenomatous) of vocal cord or larynx (J38.1)

    D14.2   **Benign neoplasm of trachea**
●   **D14.3**   **Benign neoplasm of bronchus and lung**
       Excludes1   benign carcinoid tumor of the bronchus and lung (D3A.090)

       D14.30   **Benign neoplasm of unspecified bronchus and lung**
       D14.31   **Benign neoplasm of right bronchus and lung**
       D14.32   **Benign neoplasm of left bronchus and lung**

    D14.4   **Benign neoplasm of respiratory system, unspecified**

● **D15**   **Benign neoplasm of other and unspecified intrathoracic organs**
       Excludes1   benign neoplasm of mesothelial tissue (D19.-)

    D15.0   **Benign neoplasm of thymus**
       Excludes1   benign carcinoid tumor of the thymus (D3A.091)

    D15.1   **Benign neoplasm of heart**
       Excludes1   benign neoplasm of great vessels (D21.3)

    D15.2   **Benign neoplasm of mediastinum**
    D15.7   **Benign neoplasm of other specified intrathoracic organs**
    D15.9   **Benign neoplasm of intrathoracic organ, unspecified**

● **D16**   **Benign neoplasm of bone and articular cartilage**
       Excludes1   benign neoplasm of connective tissue of ear (D21.0)
                benign neoplasm of connective tissue of eyelid (D21.0)
                benign neoplasm of connective tissue of larynx (D14.1)
                benign neoplasm of connective tissue of nose (D14.0)
                benign neoplasm of synovia (D21.-)

●   **D16.0**   **Benign neoplasm of scapula and long bones of upper limb**
       D16.00   **Benign neoplasm of scapula and long bones of unspecified upper limb**
       D16.01   **Benign neoplasm of scapula and long bones of right upper limb**
       D16.02   **Benign neoplasm of scapula and long bones of left upper limb**

● **D16.1**   **Benign neoplasm of short bones of upper limb**
       D16.10   **Benign neoplasm of short bones of unspecified upper limb**
       D16.11   **Benign neoplasm of short bones of right upper limb**
       D16.12   **Benign neoplasm of short bones of left upper limb**

● **D16.2**   **Benign neoplasm of long bones of lower limb**
       D16.20   **Benign neoplasm of long bones of unspecified lower limb**
       D16.21   **Benign neoplasm of long bones of right lower limb**
       D16.22   **Benign neoplasm of long bones of left lower limb**

● **D16.3**   **Benign neoplasm of short bones of lower limb**
       D16.30   **Benign neoplasm of short bones of unspecified lower limb**
       D16.31   **Benign neoplasm of short bones of right lower limb**
       D16.32   **Benign neoplasm of short bones of left lower limb**

    D16.4   **Benign neoplasm of bones of skull and face**
       Benign neoplasm of maxilla (superior)
       Benign neoplasm of orbital bone
       Cavity or socket of skull in which eye and its appendages are located
       Keratocyst of maxilla
       Keratocystic odontogenic tumor of maxilla
       Excludes2   benign neoplasm of lower jaw bone (D16.5) ◄

    D16.5   **Benign neoplasm of lower jaw bone**
       Keratocyst of mandible
       Keratocystic odontogenic tumor of mandible
    D16.6   **Benign neoplasm of vertebral column**
       Excludes1   benign neoplasm of sacrum and coccyx (D16.8)
    D16.7   **Benign neoplasm of ribs, sternum and clavicle**
    D16.8   **Benign neoplasm of pelvic bones, sacrum and coccyx**
    D16.9   **Benign neoplasm of bone and articular cartilage, unspecified**

● **D17**   **Benign lipomatous neoplasm**
       Slow-growing benign tumors (rubbery masses) of mature fat cells enclosed in a thin fibrous capsule

    D17.0   **Benign lipomatous neoplasm of skin and subcutaneous tissue of head, face and neck**
    D17.1   **Benign lipomatous neoplasm of skin and subcutaneous tissue of trunk**
●   **D17.2**   **Benign lipomatous neoplasm of skin and subcutaneous tissue of limb**
       D17.20   **Benign lipomatous neoplasm of skin and subcutaneous tissue of unspecified limb**
       D17.21   **Benign lipomatous neoplasm of skin and subcutaneous tissue of right arm**
       D17.22   **Benign lipomatous neoplasm of skin and subcutaneous tissue of left arm**
       D17.23   **Benign lipomatous neoplasm of skin and subcutaneous tissue of right leg**
       D17.24   **Benign lipomatous neoplasm of skin and subcutaneous tissue of left leg**
●   **D17.3**   **Benign lipomatous neoplasm of skin and subcutaneous tissue of other and unspecified sites**
       D17.30   **Benign lipomatous neoplasm of skin and subcutaneous tissue of unspecified sites**
       D17.39   **Benign lipomatous neoplasm of skin and subcutaneous tissue of other sites**
    D17.4   **Benign lipomatous neoplasm of intrathoracic organs**

CHAPTER 2 (C00-D49)

Figure 2-18   Hemangioma of skin and subcutaneous tissue. (From Yanoff: Ophthalmology, ed 3, Mosby, Inc., 2008)

Item 2–10 **Hemangiomas** are abnormally dense collections of dilated capillaries that occur on the skin or in internal organs. Hemangiomas are both deep and superficial and undergo a rapid growth phase when the size increases rapidly, followed by a rest phase, in which the tumor changes very little, followed by an involutional phase in which the tumor begins to and can disappear altogether. **Lymphangiomas** or cystic hygroma are benign collections of overgrown lymph vessels and, although rare, may occur anywhere but most commonly on the head and neck of children and infants. Visceral organs, lungs, and gastrointestinal tract may also be involved.

D17.5   **Benign lipomatous neoplasm of intra-abdominal organs**

    Excludes1   benign lipomatous neoplasm of peritoneum and retroperitoneum (D17.79)

D17.6   **Benign lipomatous neoplasm of spermatic cord** ♂

● **D17.7**   **Benign lipomatous neoplasm of other sites**

    D17.71   **Benign lipomatous neoplasm of kidney**

    D17.72   **Benign lipomatous neoplasm of other genitourinary organ**

    D17.79   **Benign lipomatous neoplasm of other sites**
                   Benign lipomatous neoplasm of peritoneum
                   Benign lipomatous neoplasm of retroperitoneum

D17.9   **Benign lipomatous neoplasm, unspecified**
      Lipoma NOS

● **D18**   **Hemangioma and lymphangioma, any site**

    Excludes1   benign neoplasm of glomus jugulare (D35.6)
                blue or pigmented nevus (D22.-)
                nevus NOS (D22.-)
                vascular nevus (Q82.5)

● **D18.0**   **Hemangioma**
      Common type of vascular malformation
      Angioma NOS
      Cavernous nevus

    D18.00   **Hemangioma unspecified site**

    D18.01   **Hemangioma of skin and subcutaneous tissue**

    D18.02   **Hemangioma of intracranial structures**

    D18.03   **Hemangioma of intra-abdominal structures**

    D18.09   **Hemangioma of other sites**

  D18.1   **Lymphangioma, any site**

● **D19**   **Benign neoplasm of mesothelial tissue**
    Mesothelial tissue is the membrane lining several body cavities

  D19.0   **Benign neoplasm of mesothelial tissue of pleura**

  D19.1   **Benign neoplasm of mesothelial tissue of peritoneum**

  D19.7   **Benign neoplasm of mesothelial tissue of other sites**

  D19.9   **Benign neoplasm of mesothelial tissue, unspecified**
      Benign mesothelioma NOS

● **D20**   **Benign neoplasm of soft tissue of retroperitoneum and peritoneum**

    Excludes1   benign lipomatous neoplasm of peritoneum and retroperitoneum (D17.79)
                benign neoplasm of mesothelial tissue (D19.-)

  D20.0   **Benign neoplasm of soft tissue of retroperitoneum**

  D20.1   **Benign neoplasm of soft tissue of peritoneum**

● **D21**   **Other benign neoplasms of connective and other soft tissue**

    Includes   benign neoplasm of blood vessel
              benign neoplasm of bursa
              benign neoplasm of cartilage
              benign neoplasm of fascia
              benign neoplasm of fat
              benign neoplasm of ligament, except uterine
              benign neoplasm of lymphatic channel
              benign neoplasm of muscle
              benign neoplasm of synovia
              benign neoplasm of tendon (sheath)
              benign stromal tumors

    Excludes1   benign neoplasm of articular cartilage (D16.-)
              benign neoplasm of cartilage of larynx (D14.1)
              benign neoplasm of cartilage of nose (D14.0)
              benign neoplasm of connective tissue of breast (D24.-)
              benign neoplasm of peripheral nerves and autonomic nervous system (D36.1-)
              benign neoplasm of peritoneum (D20.1)
              benign neoplasm of retroperitoneum (D20.0)
              benign neoplasm of uterine ligament, any (D28.2)
              benign neoplasm of vascular tissue (D18.-)
              hemangioma (D18.0-)
              lipomatous neoplasm (D17.-)
              lymphangioma (D18.1)
              uterine leiomyoma (D25.-)

  D21.0   **Benign neoplasm of connective and other soft tissue of head, face and neck**
      Benign neoplasm of connective tissue of ear
      Benign neoplasm of connective tissue of eyelid

    Excludes1   benign neoplasm of connective tissue of orbit (D31.6-)

● **D21.1**   **Benign neoplasm of connective and other soft tissue of upper limb, including shoulder**

    D21.10   **Benign neoplasm of connective and other soft tissue of unspecified upper limb, including shoulder**

    D21.11   **Benign neoplasm of connective and other soft tissue of right upper limb, including shoulder**

    D21.12   **Benign neoplasm of connective and other soft tissue of left upper limb, including shoulder**

● **D21.2**   **Benign neoplasm of connective and other soft tissue of lower limb, including hip**

    D21.20   **Benign neoplasm of connective and other soft tissue of unspecified lower limb, including hip**

    D21.21   **Benign neoplasm of connective and other soft tissue of right lower limb, including hip**

    D21.22   **Benign neoplasm of connective and other soft tissue of left lower limb, including hip**

  D21.3   **Benign neoplasm of connective and other soft tissue of thorax**
      Benign neoplasm of axilla
      Benign neoplasm of diaphragm
      Benign neoplasm of great vessels

    Excludes1   benign neoplasm of heart (D15.1)
              benign neoplasm of mediastinum (D15.2)
              benign neoplasm of thymus (D15.0)

  D21.4   **Benign neoplasm of connective and other soft tissue of abdomen Benign stromal tumors of abdomen**

  D21.5   **Benign neoplasm of connective and other soft tissue of pelvis**

    Excludes1   benign neoplasm of any uterine ligament (D28.2)
              uterine leiomyoma (D25.-)

  D21.6   **Benign neoplasm of connective and other soft tissue of trunk, unspecified**
      Benign neoplasm of back NOS

  D21.9   **Benign neoplasm of connective and other soft tissue, unspecified**

◀ New   ◀◀ Revised   ~~deleted~~ Deleted   Excludes 1   Excludes 2   Includes   Use additional   Code first   Code also   Unspecified

712   OGCR Official Guidelines   ● Unacceptable Principal Diagnosis   X Assign placeholder X   ● Use Additional Character(s)   ▶ Manifestation Code   **Coding Clinic**

● **D22 Melanocytic nevi**

> **Includes**   atypical nevus
> blue hairy pigmented nevus
> nevus NOS

   D22.0 Melanocytic nevi of lip
      Skin lesions composed of nests of nevus cells with macules/
      papules

● **D22.1 Melanocytic nevi of eyelid, including canthus**
    D22.10   Melanocytic nevi of unspecified eyelid, including canthus
    D22.11   Melanocytic nevi of right eyelid, including canthus
    D22.12   Melanocytic nevi of left eyelid, including canthus

● **D22.2 Melanocytic nevi of ear and external auricular canal**
    D22.20   Melanocytic nevi of unspecified ear and external auricular canal
    D22.21   Melanocytic nevi of right ear and external auricular canal
    D22.22   Melanocytic nevi of left ear and external auricular canal

● **D22.3 Melanocytic nevi of other and unspecified parts of face**
    D22.30   Melanocytic nevi of unspecified part of face
    D22.39   Melanocytic nevi of other parts of face

   D22.4 Melanocytic nevi of scalp and neck

   D22.5 Melanocytic nevi of trunk
      Melanocytic nevi of anal margin
      Melanocytic nevi of anal skin
      Melanocytic nevi of perianal skin
      Melanocytic nevi of skin of breast

● **D22.6 Melanocytic nevi of upper limb, including shoulder**
    D22.60   Melanocytic nevi of unspecified upper limb, including shoulder
    D22.61   Melanocytic nevi of right upper limb, including shoulder
    D22.62   Melanocytic nevi of left upper limb, including shoulder

● **D22.7 Melanocytic nevi of lower limb, including hip**
    D22.70   Melanocytic nevi of unspecified lower limb, including hip
    D22.71   Melanocytic nevi of right lower limb, including hip
    D22.72   Melanocytic nevi of left lower limb, including hip

   D22.9 Melanocytic nevi, unspecified

● **D23 Other benign neoplasms of skin**

> **Includes**   benign neoplasm of hair follicles
> benign neoplasm of sebaceous glands
> benign neoplasm of sweat glands

> **Excludes1**   benign lipomatous neoplasms of skin
> (D17.0-D17.3)
> melanocytic nevi (D22.-)

   D23.0 Other benign neoplasm of skin of lip
> **Excludes1**   benign neoplasm of vermilion border of lip (D10.0)

● **D23.1 Other benign neoplasm of skin of eyelid, including canthus**
    D23.10   Other benign neoplasm of skin unspecified of eyelid, including canthus
    D23.11   Other benign neoplasm of skin of right eyelid, including canthus
    D23.12   Other benign neoplasm of skin of left eyelid, including canthus

● **D23.2 Other benign neoplasm of skin of ear and external auricular canal**
    D23.20   Other benign neoplasm of skin of unspecified ear and external auricular canal
    D23.21   Other benign neoplasm of skin of right ear and external auricular canal
    D23.22   Other benign neoplasm of skin of left ear and external auricular canal

● **D23.3 Other benign neoplasm of skin of other and unspecified parts of face**
    D23.30   Other benign neoplasm of skin of unspecified part of face
    D23.39   Other benign neoplasm of skin of other parts of face

   D23.4 Other benign neoplasm of skin of scalp and neck

   D23.5 Other benign neoplasm of skin of trunk
      Other benign neoplasm of anal margin
      Other benign neoplasm of anal skin
      Other benign neoplasm of perianal skin
      Other benign neoplasm of skin of breast
> **Excludes1**   benign neoplasm of anus NOS (D12.9)

● **D23.6 Other benign neoplasm of skin of upper limb, including shoulder**
    D23.60   Other benign neoplasm of skin of unspecified upper limb, including shoulder
    D23.61   Other benign neoplasm of skin of right upper limb, including shoulder
    D23.62   Other benign neoplasm of skin of left upper limb, including shoulder

● **D23.7 Other benign neoplasm of skin of lower limb, including hip**
    D23.70   Other benign neoplasm of skin of unspecified lower limb, including hip
    D23.71   Other benign neoplasm of skin of right lower limb, including hip
    D23.72   Other benign neoplasm of skin of left lower limb, including hip

   D23.9 Other benign neoplasm of skin, unspecified

● **D24 Benign neoplasm of breast**

> **Includes**   benign neoplasm of connective tissue of breast
> benign neoplasm of soft parts of breast
> fibroadenoma of breast

> **Excludes2**   adenofibrosis of breast (N60.2)
> benign cyst of breast (N60.-)
> benign mammary dysplasia (N60.-)
> benign neoplasm of skin of breast (D22.5, D23.5)
> fibrocystic disease of breast (N60.-)

   D24.1 Benign neoplasm of right breast

   D24.2 Benign neoplasm of left breast

   D24.9 Benign neoplasm of unspecified breast

● **D25 Leiomyoma of uterus**
      Benign tumors or nodules of the uterine wall

> **Includes**   uterine fibroid
> uterine fibromyoma
> uterine myoma

   D25.0 Submucous leiomyoma of uterus ♀

   D25.1 Intramural leiomyoma of uterus ♀
      Interstitial leiomyoma of uterus

   D25.2 Subserosal leiomyoma of uterus ♀
      Subperitoneal leiomyoma of uterus

   D25.9 Leiomyoma of uterus, unspecified ♀

● **D26 Other benign neoplasms of uterus**

   D26.0 Other benign neoplasm of cervix uteri ♀

   D26.1 Other benign neoplasm of corpus uteri ♀

   D26.7 Other benign neoplasm of other parts of uterus ♀

   D26.9 Other benign neoplasm of uterus, unspecified ♀

CHAPTER 2 (C00-D49)

N Newborn Age: 0   **P** Pediatric Age: 0–17   **M** Maternity DX: 12–55   **A** Adult Age: 15–124   ♀ Females Only   ♂ Males Only

Complication\Comorbidity   Major C\C   (Ex) CC/MCC Exclusions   Hospital-Acquired Condition   **713**

Item 2–11 Teratoma: terat = monster, oma = mass, tumor. Alternate terms: dermoid cyst of the ovary, ovarian teratoma. Teratomas are neoplasms and arise from germ cells (ovaries in female and testes in male) and can be benign or malignant. Teratomas have been known to contain hair, nails, and teeth, giving them a bizarre ("monster") appearance.

● **D27   Benign neoplasm of ovary**
　　Use additional code to identify any functional activity.
　　Excludes2   corpus albicans cyst (N83.2-) ◀▥
　　　　　　　 corpus luteum cyst (N83.1-) ◀▥
　　　　　　　 endometrial cyst (N80.1)
　　　　　　　 follicular (atretic) cyst (N83.0-) ◀▥
　　　　　　　 graafian follicle cyst (N83.0-) ◀▥
　　　　　　　 ovarian cyst NEC (N83.2-) ◀▥
　　　　　　　 ovarian retention cyst (N83.2-) ◀▥
　　D27.0   **Benign neoplasm of right ovary** ♀
　　D27.1   **Benign neoplasm of left ovary** ♀
　　D27.9   **Benign neoplasm of** unspecified **ovary** ♀

● **D28   Benign neoplasm of other and unspecified female genital organs**
　　Includes   adenomatous polyp
　　　　　　 benign neoplasm of skin of female genital organs
　　　　　　 benign teratoma
　　Excludes1   epoophoron cyst (Q50.5)
　　　　　　　 fimbrial cyst (Q50.4)
　　　　　　　 Gartner's duct cyst (Q52.4)
　　　　　　　 parovarian cyst (Q50.5)
　　D28.0   **Benign neoplasm of vulva** ♀
　　D28.1   **Benign neoplasm of vagina** ♀
　　D28.2   **Benign neoplasm of uterine tubes and ligaments** ♀
　　　　　　 Benign neoplasm of fallopian tube
　　　　　　 Benign neoplasm of uterine ligament (broad) (round)
　　D28.7   **Benign neoplasm of other specified female genital organs** ♀
　　D28.9   **Benign neoplasm of female genital organ,** unspecified ♀

● **D29   Benign neoplasm of male genital organs**
　　Includes   benign neoplasm of skin of male genital organs
　　D29.0   **Benign neoplasm of penis** ♂
　　D29.1   **Benign neoplasm of prostate** ♂
　　　　　　Excludes1   enlarged prostate (N40.-)
　● D29.2   **Benign neoplasm of testis**
　　　　　　Use additional code to identify any functional activity.
　　　　D29.20   **Benign neoplasm of** unspecified **testis** ♂
　　　　D29.21   **Benign neoplasm of right testis** ♂
　　　　D29.22   **Benign neoplasm of left testis** ♂
　● D29.3   **Benign neoplasm of epididymis**
　　　　D29.30   **Benign neoplasm of** unspecified **epididymis** ♂
　　　　D29.31   **Benign neoplasm of right epididymis** ♂
　　　　D29.32   **Benign neoplasm of left epididymis** ♂
　　D29.4   **Benign neoplasm of scrotum** ♂
　　　　　　 Benign neoplasm of skin of scrotum
　　D29.8   **Benign neoplasm of other specified male genital organs** ♂
　　　　　　 Benign neoplasm of seminal vesicle
　　　　　　 Benign neoplasm of spermatic cord
　　　　　　 Benign neoplasm of tunica vaginalis
　　D29.9   **Benign neoplasm of male genital organ,** unspecified ♂

● **D30   Benign neoplasm of urinary organs**
　● D30.0   **Benign neoplasm of kidney**
　　　　　　Excludes1   benign carcinoid tumor of the kidney (D3A.093)
　　　　　　　　　 benign neoplasm of renal calyces (D30.1-)
　　　　　　　　　 benign neoplasm of renal pelvis (D30.1-)
　　　　D30.00   **Benign neoplasm of** unspecified **kidney**
　　　　D30.01   **Benign neoplasm of right kidney**
　　　　D30.02   **Benign neoplasm of left kidney**
　● D30.1   **Benign neoplasm of renal pelvis**
　　　　D30.10   **Benign neoplasm of** unspecified **renal pelvis**
　　　　D30.11   **Benign neoplasm of right renal pelvis**
　　　　D30.12   **Benign neoplasm of left renal pelvis**
　● D30.2   **Benign neoplasm of ureter**
　　　　　　Excludes1   benign neoplasm of ureteric orifice of bladder (D30.3)
　　　　D30.20   **Benign neoplasm of** unspecified **ureter**
　　　　D30.21   **Benign neoplasm of right ureter**
　　　　D30.22   **Benign neoplasm of left ureter**
　　D30.3   **Benign neoplasm of bladder**
　　　　　　 Benign neoplasm of ureteric orifice of bladder
　　　　　　 Benign neoplasm of urethral orifice of bladder
　　D30.4   **Benign neoplasm of urethra**
　　　　　　Excludes1   benign neoplasm of urethral orifice of bladder (D30.3)
　　D30.8   **Benign neoplasm of other specified urinary organs**
　　　　　　 Benign neoplasm of paraurethral glands
　　D30.9   **Benign neoplasm of urinary organ,** unspecified
　　　　　　 Benign neoplasm of urinary system NOS

● **D31   Benign neoplasm of eye and adnexa**
　　Excludes1   benign neoplasm of connective tissue of eyelid (D21.0)
　　　　　　　 benign neoplasm of optic nerve (D33.3)
　　　　　　　 benign neoplasm of skin of eyelid (D22.1-, D23.1-)
　● D31.0   **Benign neoplasm of conjunctiva**
　　　　D31.00   **Benign neoplasm of** unspecified **conjunctiva**
　　　　D31.01   **Benign neoplasm of right conjunctiva**
　　　　D31.02   **Benign neoplasm of left conjunctiva**
　● D31.1   **Benign neoplasm of cornea**
　　　　D31.10   **Benign neoplasm of** unspecified **cornea**
　　　　D31.11   **Benign neoplasm of right cornea**
　　　　D31.12   **Benign neoplasm of left cornea**
　● D31.2   **Benign neoplasm of retina**
　　　　　　Excludes1   dark area on retina (D49.81)
　　　　　　　　　 hemangioma of retina (D49.81)
　　　　　　　　　 neoplasm of unspecified behavior of retina and choroid (D49.81)
　　　　　　　　　 retinal freckle (D49.81)
　　　　D31.20   **Benign neoplasm of** unspecified **retina**
　　　　D31.21   **Benign neoplasm of right retina**
　　　　D31.22   **Benign neoplasm of left retina**
　● D31.3   **Benign neoplasm of choroid**
　　　　D31.30   **Benign neoplasm of** unspecified **choroid**
　　　　D31.31   **Benign neoplasm of right choroid**
　　　　D31.32   **Benign neoplasm of left choroid**
　● D31.4   **Benign neoplasm of ciliary body**
　　　　D31.40   **Benign neoplasm of** unspecified **ciliary body**
　　　　D31.41   **Benign neoplasm of right ciliary body**
　　　　D31.42   **Benign neoplasm of left ciliary body**

◀ New   ◀▥ Revised   ~~deleted~~ Deleted   Excludes 1   Excludes 2   Includes   Use additional   Code first   Code also   Unspecified

OGCR Official Guidelines   ● Unacceptable Principal Diagnosis   X Assign placeholder X   ● Use Additional Character(s)   ▌ Manifestation Code   **Coding Clinic**

● **D31.5** **Benign neoplasm of lacrimal gland and duct**
Benign neoplasm of lacrimal sac
Benign neoplasm of nasolacrimal duct

D31.50 **Benign neoplasm of unspecified lacrimal gland and duct**

D31.51 **Benign neoplasm of right lacrimal gland and duct**

D31.52 **Benign neoplasm of left lacrimal gland and duct**

● **D31.6** **Benign neoplasm of unspecified site of orbit**
Benign neoplasm of connective tissue of orbit
Benign neoplasm of extraocular muscle
Benign neoplasm of peripheral nerves of orbit
Benign neoplasm of retrobulbar tissue
Benign neoplasm of retro-ocular tissue

Excludes1 benign neoplasm of orbital bone (D16.4)

D31.60 **Benign neoplasm of unspecified site of unspecified orbit**

D31.61 **Benign neoplasm of unspecified site of right orbit**

D31.62 **Benign neoplasm of unspecified site of left orbit**

● **D31.9** **Benign neoplasm of unspecified part of eye**
Benign neoplasm of eyeball

D31.90 **Benign neoplasm of unspecified part of unspecified eye**

D31.91 **Benign neoplasm of unspecified part of right eye**

D31.92 **Benign neoplasm of unspecified part of left eye**

● **D32** **Benign neoplasm of meninges**

D32.0 **Benign neoplasm of cerebral meninges**

D32.1 **Benign neoplasm of spinal meninges**

D32.9 **Benign neoplasm of meninges, unspecified**
Meningioma NOS

● **D33** **Benign neoplasm of brain and other parts of central nervous system**

Excludes1 angioma (D18.0-)
benign neoplasm of meninges (D32.-)
benign neoplasm of peripheral nerves and
autonomic nervous system (D36.1-)
hemangioma (D18.0-)
neurofibromatosis (Q85.0-)
retro-ocular benign neoplasm (D31.6-)

D33.0 **Benign neoplasm of brain, supratentorial**
Benign neoplasm of cerebral ventricle
Benign neoplasm of cerebrum
Benign neoplasm of frontal lobe
Benign neoplasm of occipital lobe
Benign neoplasm of parietal lobe
Benign neoplasm of temporal lobe

Excludes1 benign neoplasm of fourth ventricle
(D33.1)

D33.1 **Benign neoplasm of brain, infratentorial**
Benign neoplasm of brain stem
Benign neoplasm of cerebellum
Benign neoplasm of fourth ventricle

D33.2 **Benign neoplasm of brain, unspecified**

D33.3 **Benign neoplasm of cranial nerves**
Benign neoplasm of olfactory bulb

D33.4 **Benign neoplasm of spinal cord**

D33.7 **Benign neoplasm of other specified parts of central nervous system**

D33.9 **Benign neoplasm of central nervous system, unspecified**
Benign neoplasm of nervous system (central) NOS

D34 **Benign neoplasm of thyroid gland**
Use additional code to identify any functional activity.

● **D35** **Benign neoplasm of other and unspecified endocrine glands**
Use additional code to identify any functional activity.

Excludes1 benign neoplasm of endocrine pancreas (D13.7)
benign neoplasm of ovary (D27.-)
benign neoplasm of testis (D29.2.-)
benign neoplasm of thymus (D15.0)

● **D35.0** **Benign neoplasm of adrenal gland**

D35.00 **Benign neoplasm of unspecified adrenal gland**

D35.01 **Benign neoplasm of right adrenal gland**

D35.02 **Benign neoplasm of left adrenal gland**

D35.1 **Benign neoplasm of parathyroid gland**

D35.2 **Benign neoplasm of pituitary gland**

D35.3 **Benign neoplasm of craniopharyngeal duct**

D35.4 **Benign neoplasm of pineal gland**

D35.5 **Benign neoplasm of carotid body**

D35.6 **Benign neoplasm of aortic body and other paraganglia**
Benign tumor of glomus jugulare

D35.7 **Benign neoplasm of other specified endocrine glands**

D35.9 **Benign neoplasm of endocrine gland, unspecified**
Benign neoplasm of unspecified endocrine gland

● **D36** **Benign neoplasm of other and unspecified sites**

D36.0 **Benign neoplasm of lymph nodes**

Excludes1 lymphangioma (D18.1)

● **D36.1** **Benign neoplasm of peripheral nerves and autonomic nervous system**

Excludes1 benign neoplasm of peripheral nerves of
orbit (D31.6-)
neurofibromatosis (Q85.0-)

D36.10 **Benign neoplasm of peripheral nerves and autonomic nervous system, unspecified**

D36.11 **Benign neoplasm of peripheral nerves and autonomic nervous system of face, head, and neck**

D36.12 **Benign neoplasm of peripheral nerves and autonomic nervous system, upper limb, including shoulder**

D36.13 **Benign neoplasm of peripheral nerves and autonomic nervous system of lower limb, including hip**

D36.14 **Benign neoplasm of peripheral nerves and autonomic nervous system of thorax**

D36.15 **Benign neoplasm of peripheral nerves and autonomic nervous system of abdomen**

D36.16 **Benign neoplasm of peripheral nerves and autonomic nervous system of pelvis**

D36.17 **Benign neoplasm of peripheral nerves and autonomic nervous system of trunk, unspecified**

D36.7 **Benign neoplasm of other specified sites**
Benign neoplasm of nose NOS

D36.9 **Benign neoplasm, unspecified site**

BENIGN NEUROENDOCRINE TUMORS (D3A)

● **D3A** **Benign neuroendocrine tumors**
Code also any associated multiple endocrine neoplasia [MEN]
syndromes (E31.2-)
Use additional code to identify any associated endocrine
syndrome, such as:
carcinoid syndrome (E34.0)

Excludes2 benign pancreatic islet cell tumors (D13.7)

● **D3A.0** **Benign carcinoid tumors**

D3A.00 **Benign carcinoid tumor of unspecified site**
Carcinoid tumor NOS

● **D3A.01   Benign carcinoid tumors of the small intestine**

     D3A.010   Benign carcinoid tumor of the duodenum

     D3A.011   Benign carcinoid tumor of the jejunum

     D3A.012   Benign carcinoid tumor of the ileum

     D3A.019   Benign carcinoid tumor of the small intestine, unspecified portion

● **D3A.02   Benign carcinoid tumors of the appendix, large intestine, and rectum**

     D3A.020   Benign carcinoid tumor of the appendix

     D3A.021   Benign carcinoid tumor of the cecum

     D3A.022   Benign carcinoid tumor of the ascending colon

     D3A.023   Benign carcinoid tumor of the transverse colon

     D3A.024   Benign carcinoid tumor of the descending colon

     D3A.025   Benign carcinoid tumor of the sigmoid colon

     D3A.026   Benign carcinoid tumor of the rectum

     D3A.029   Benign carcinoid tumor of the large intestine, unspecified portion

         Benign carcinoid tumor of the colon NOS

● **D3A.09   Benign carcinoid tumors of other sites**

     D3A.090   Benign carcinoid tumor of the bronchus and lung

     D3A.091   Benign carcinoid tumor of the thymus

     D3A.092   Benign carcinoid tumor of the stomach

     D3A.093   Benign carcinoid tumor of the kidney

     D3A.094   Benign carcinoid tumor of the foregut unspecified ◀▦

     D3A.095   Benign carcinoid tumor of the midgut unspecified ◀▦

     D3A.096   Benign carcinoid tumor of the hindgut unspecified ◀▦

     D3A.098   Benign carcinoid tumors of other sites

D3A.8   Other benign neuroendocrine tumors

     Neuroendocrine tumor NOS

NEOPLASMS OF UNCERTAIN BEHAVIOR, POLYCYTHEMIA VERA AND MYELODYSPLASTIC SYNDROMES (D37-D48)

Note: Categories D37-D44, and D48 classify by site neoplasms of uncertain behavior, i.e., histologic confirmation whether the neoplasm is malignant or benign cannot be made.

     Excludes1   neoplasms of unspecified behavior (D49.-)

● **D37   Neoplasm of uncertain behavior of oral cavity and digestive organs**

     Excludes1   stromal tumors of uncertain behavior of digestive system (D48.1)

● **D37.0   Neoplasm of uncertain behavior of lip, oral cavity and pharynx**

     Excludes1   neoplasm of uncertain behavior of aryepiglottic fold or interarytenoid fold, laryngeal aspect (D38.0)

         neoplasm of uncertain behavior of epiglottis NOS (D38.0)

         neoplasm of uncertain behavior of skin of lip (D48.5)

         neoplasm of uncertain behavior of suprahyoid portion of epiglottis (D38.0)

     D37.01   Neoplasm of uncertain behavior of lip

         Neoplasm of uncertain behavior of vermilion border of lip

     D37.02   Neoplasm of uncertain behavior of tongue

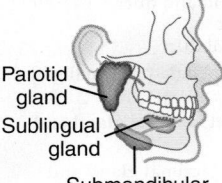

Figure 2-19   Major salivary glands.

Parotid gland

Sublingual gland

Submandibular gland

● **D37.03   Neoplasm of uncertain behavior of the major salivary glands**

     D37.030   Neoplasm of uncertain behavior of the parotid salivary glands

     D37.031   Neoplasm of uncertain behavior of the sublingual salivary glands

     D37.032   Neoplasm of uncertain behavior of the submandibular salivary glands

     D37.039   Neoplasm of uncertain behavior of the major salivary glands, unspecified

     D37.04   Neoplasm of uncertain behavior of the minor salivary glands

         Neoplasm of uncertain behavior of submucosal salivary glands of lip

         Neoplasm of uncertain behavior of submucosal salivary glands of cheek

         Neoplasm of uncertain behavior of submucosal salivary glands of hard palate

         Neoplasm of uncertain behavior of submucosal salivary glands of soft palate

     D37.05   Neoplasm of uncertain behavior of pharynx

         Neoplasm of uncertain behavior of aryepiglottic fold of pharynx NOS

         Neoplasm of uncertain behavior of hypopharyngeal aspect of aryepiglottic fold of pharynx

         Neoplasm of uncertain behavior of marginal zone of aryepiglottic fold of pharynx

     D37.09   Neoplasm of uncertain behavior of other specified sites of the oral cavity

D37.1   Neoplasm of uncertain behavior of stomach

D37.2   Neoplasm of uncertain behavior of small intestine

D37.3   Neoplasm of uncertain behavior of appendix

D37.4   Neoplasm of uncertain behavior of colon

D37.5   Neoplasm of uncertain behavior of rectum

     Neoplasm of uncertain behavior of rectosigmoid junction

     Rectosigmoid junction: Angle where sigmoid colon becomes rectum

D37.6   Neoplasm of uncertain behavior of liver, gallbladder and bile ducts

     Neoplasm of uncertain behavior of ampulla of Vater

     Ampulla of Vater: Enlarged segment of ducts from liver and pancreas at entry point to small intestine

D37.8   Neoplasm of uncertain behavior of other specified digestive organs

     Neoplasm of uncertain behavior of anal canal

     Neoplasm of uncertain behavior of anal sphincter

     Neoplasm of uncertain behavior of anus NOS

     Neoplasm of uncertain behavior of esophagus

     Neoplasm of uncertain behavior of intestine NOS

     Neoplasm of uncertain behavior of pancreas

     Excludes1   neoplasm of uncertain behavior of anal margin (D48.5)

         neoplasm of uncertain behavior of anal skin (D48.5)

         neoplasm of uncertain behavior of perianal skin (D48.5)

D37.9   Neoplasm of uncertain behavior of digestive organ, unspecified

◀ New   ◀▦ Revised   ~~deleted~~ Deleted   Excludes 1   Excludes 2   Includes   Use additional   Code first   Code also   Unspecified

OGCR Official Guidelines   ● Unacceptable Principal Diagnosis   X Assign placeholder X   ● Use Additional Character(s)   ▶ Manifestation Code   **Coding Clinic**

● **D38   Neoplasm of uncertain behavior of middle ear and respiratory and intrathoracic organs**
>   **Excludes1**   neoplasm of uncertain behavior of heart (D48.7)

D38.0   **Neoplasm of uncertain behavior of larynx**
>   Neoplasm of uncertain behavior of aryepiglottic fold or interarytenoid fold, laryngeal aspect
>   Neoplasm of uncertain behavior of epiglottis (suprahyoid portion)
>   **Excludes1**   neoplasm of uncertain behavior of aryepiglottic fold or interarytenoid fold NOS (D37.05)
>   neoplasm of uncertain behavior of hypopharyngeal aspect of aryepiglottic fold (D37.05)
>   neoplasm of uncertain behavior of marginal zone of aryepiglottic fold (D37.05)

D38.1   **Neoplasm of uncertain behavior of trachea, bronchus and lung**

D38.2   **Neoplasm of uncertain behavior of pleura**

D38.3   **Neoplasm of uncertain behavior of mediastinum**

D38.4   **Neoplasm of uncertain behavior of thymus**

D38.5   **Neoplasm of uncertain behavior of other respiratory organs**
>   Neoplasm of uncertain behavior of accessory sinuses
>   Neoplasm of uncertain behavior of cartilage of nose
>   Neoplasm of uncertain behavior of middle ear
>   Neoplasm of uncertain behavior of nasal cavities
>   **Excludes1**   neoplasm of uncertain behavior of ear (external) (skin) (D48.5)
>   neoplasm of uncertain behavior of nose NOS (D48.7)
>   neoplasm of uncertain behavior of skin of nose (D48.5)

D38.6   **Neoplasm of uncertain behavior of respiratory organ, unspecified**

● **D39   Neoplasm of uncertain behavior of female genital organs**

D39.0   **Neoplasm of uncertain behavior of uterus ♀**

● D39.1   **Neoplasm of uncertain behavior of ovary**
>   Use additional code to identify any functional activity.

D39.10   **Neoplasm of uncertain behavior of unspecified ovary ♀**

D39.11   **Neoplasm of uncertain behavior of right ovary ♀**

D39.12   **Neoplasm of uncertain behavior of left ovary ♀**

D39.2   **Neoplasm of uncertain behavior of placenta ♀**   M
>   Chorioadenoma destruens
>   Invasive hydatidiform mole
>   Malignant hydatidiform mole
>   **Excludes1**   hydatidiform mole NOS (O01.9)

D39.8   **Neoplasm of uncertain behavior of other specified female genital organs ♀**
>   Neoplasm of uncertain behavior of skin of female genital organs

D39.9   **Neoplasm of uncertain behavior of female genital organ, unspecified ♀**

● **D40   Neoplasm of uncertain behavior of male genital organs**

D40.0   **Neoplasm of uncertain behavior of prostate ♂**

● D40.1   **Neoplasm of uncertain behavior of testis**

D40.10   **Neoplasm of uncertain behavior of unspecified testis ♂**

D40.11   **Neoplasm of uncertain behavior of right testis ♂**

D40.12   **Neoplasm of uncertain behavior of left testis ♂**

D40.8   **Neoplasm of uncertain behavior of other specified male genital organs ♂**
>   Neoplasm of uncertain behavior of skin of male genital organs

D40.9   **Neoplasm of uncertain behavior of male genital organ, unspecified ♂**

● **D41   Neoplasm of uncertain behavior of urinary organs**

● D41.0   **Neoplasm of uncertain behavior of kidney**
>   **Excludes1**   neoplasm of uncertain behavior of renal pelvis (D41.1-)

D41.00   **Neoplasm of uncertain behavior of unspecified kidney**

D41.01   **Neoplasm of uncertain behavior of right kidney**

D41.02   **Neoplasm of uncertain behavior of left kidney**

● D41.1   **Neoplasm of uncertain behavior of renal pelvis**

D41.10   **Neoplasm of uncertain behavior of unspecified renal pelvis**

D41.11   **Neoplasm of uncertain behavior of right renal pelvis**

D41.12   **Neoplasm of uncertain behavior of left renal pelvis**

● D41.2   **Neoplasm of uncertain behavior of ureter**

D41.20   **Neoplasm of uncertain behavior of unspecified ureter**

D41.21   **Neoplasm of uncertain behavior of right ureter**

D41.22   **Neoplasm of uncertain behavior of left ureter**

D41.3   **Neoplasm of uncertain behavior of urethra**

D41.4   **Neoplasm of uncertain behavior of bladder**

D41.8   **Neoplasm of uncertain behavior of other specified urinary organs**

D41.9   **Neoplasm of uncertain behavior of unspecified urinary organ**

● **D42   Neoplasm of uncertain behavior of meninges**

D42.0   **Neoplasm of uncertain behavior of cerebral meninges**

D42.1   **Neoplasm of uncertain behavior of spinal meninges**

D42.9   **Neoplasm of uncertain behavior of meninges, unspecified**

● **D43   Neoplasm of uncertain behavior of brain and central nervous system**
>   **Excludes1**   neoplasm of uncertain behavior of peripheral nerves and autonomic nervous system (D48.2)

D43.0   **Neoplasm of uncertain behavior of brain, supratentorial**
>   *Superior to tentorium of cerebellum*
>   Neoplasm of uncertain behavior of cerebral ventricle
>   Neoplasm of uncertain behavior of cerebrum
>   Neoplasm of uncertain behavior of frontal lobe
>   Neoplasm of uncertain behavior of occipital lobe
>   Neoplasm of uncertain behavior of parietal lobe
>   Neoplasm of uncertain behavior of temporal lobe
>   **Excludes1**   neoplasm of uncertain behavior of fourth ventricle (D43.1)

D43.1   **Neoplasm of uncertain behavior of brain, infratentorial**
>   *Beneath the tentorium of cerebellum*
>   Neoplasm of uncertain behavior of brain stem
>   Neoplasm of uncertain behavior of cerebellum
>   Neoplasm of uncertain behavior of fourth ventricle

D43.2   **Neoplasm of uncertain behavior of brain, unspecified**

D43.3   **Neoplasm of uncertain behavior of cranial nerves**

D43.4   **Neoplasm of uncertain behavior of spinal cord**

D43.8   **Neoplasm of uncertain behavior of other specified parts of central nervous system**

D43.9   **Neoplasm of uncertain behavior of central nervous system, unspecified**
>   Neoplasm of uncertain behavior of nervous system (central) NOS

CHAPTER 2 (C00-D49)

CHAPTER 2 (C00–D49)

● **D44**   **Neoplasm of uncertain behavior of endocrine glands**

     Excludes1   multiple endocrine adenomatosis (E31.2-)
                   multiple endocrine neoplasia (E31.2-)
                   neoplasm of uncertain behavior of endocrine pancreas (D37.8)
                   neoplasm of uncertain behavior of ovary (D39.1-)
                   neoplasm of uncertain behavior of testis (D40.1-)
                   neoplasm of uncertain behavior of thymus (D38.4)

     D44.0   **Neoplasm of uncertain behavior of thyroid gland**

● **D44.1**   **Neoplasm of uncertain behavior of adrenal gland**

         Use additional code to identify any functional activity.

         D44.10   **Neoplasm of uncertain behavior of unspecified adrenal gland**

         D44.11   **Neoplasm of uncertain behavior of right adrenal gland**

         D44.12   **Neoplasm of uncertain behavior of left adrenal gland**

     D44.2   **Neoplasm of uncertain behavior of parathyroid gland**

     D44.3   **Neoplasm of uncertain behavior of pituitary gland**

         Use additional code to identify any functional activity.

     D44.4   **Neoplasm of uncertain behavior of craniopharyngeal duct**

     D44.5   **Neoplasm of uncertain behavior of pineal gland**

     D44.6   **Neoplasm of uncertain behavior of carotid body**

     D44.7   **Neoplasm of uncertain behavior of aortic body and other paraganglia**

     D44.9   **Neoplasm of uncertain behavior of unspecified endocrine gland**

D45   **Polycythemia vera**

     Excludes1   familial polycythemia (D75.0)
                   secondary polycythemia (D75.1)

     Primary polycythemia. Secondary polycythemia is D75.1. Check your documentation. Polycythemia is caused by too many red blood cells, which increase the thickness of blood (viscosity). This can cause engorgement of the spleen (splenomegaly) with extra RBCs and potential clot formation.

● **D46**   **Myelodysplastic syndromes**

     Use additional code for adverse effect, if applicable, to identify drug (T36-T50 with fifth or sixth character 5)

     Excludes2   drug-induced aplastic anemia (D61.1)

     D46.0   **Refractory anemia without ring sideroblasts, so stated**
         Refractory anemia without sideroblasts, without excess of blasts

     D46.1   **Refractory anemia with ring sideroblasts RARS**

● **D46.2**   **Refractory anemia with excess of blasts [RAEB]** ◀▥
         Form of myelodysplasia with increased immature white blood cells (blasts) in bone marrow

         D46.20   **Refractory anemia with excess of blasts, unspecified RAEB NOS**

         D46.21   **Refractory anemia with excess of blasts 1 RAEB 1**
             Bone marrow disease which results in insufficient RBCs (anemia) in which level of blasts is less than 10%

         D46.22   **Refractory anemia with excess of blasts 2 RAEB 2** ✪
             Bone marrow disease manifested by insufficient numbers of RBCs (anemia) with level of blasts 10-20%
             Ex: See C94.4

     D46.A   **Refractory cytopenia with multilineage dysplasia**

     D46.B   **Refractory cytopenia with multilineage dysplasia and ring sideroblasts**
         RCMD RS

     D46.C   **Myelodysplastic syndrome with isolated del(5q) chromosomal abnormality** ✪
         Myelodysplastic syndrome with 5q deletion
         5q minus syndrome NOS
         Ex: See C94.4

     D46.4   **Refractory anemia, unspecified**

     D46.Z   **Other myelodysplastic syndromes**

         Excludes1   chronic myelomonocytic leukemia (C93.1-)

     D46.9   **Myelodysplastic syndrome, unspecified**
         Myelodysplasia NOS

● **D47**   **Other neoplasms of uncertain behavior of lymphoid, hematopoietic and related tissue**

     D47.0   **Histiocytic and mast cell tumors of uncertain behavior** ✪
         Indolent systemic mastocytosis
         Mast cell tumor NOS
         Mastocytoma NOS

         Excludes1   malignant mast cell tumor (C96.2)
                   mastocytosis (congenital) (cutaneous) (Q82.2)

         Ex: C88.8, C94.40-C94.42, C94.6, D45-D46.22, D46.4, D46.9, D46.A-D46.C, D46.Z, D47.0-D47.1, D47.3, D47.9, D47.Z2, D47.Z9, D75.81, Z51.0

     D47.1   **Chronic myeloproliferative disease** ✪
         Chronic neutrophilic leukemia
         Myeloproliferative disease, unspecified

         Excludes1   atypical chronic myeloid leukemia BCR/ABL-negative (C92.2-)
                   chronic myeloid leukemia BCR/ABL-positive (C92.1-)
                   myelofibrosis NOS (D75.81)
                   myelophthisic anemia (D61.82)
                   myelophthisis (D61.82)
                   secondary myelofibrosis NOS (D75.81)

         Ex: See C94.4

     D47.2   **Monoclonal gammopathy**
         Monoclonal gammopathy of undetermined significance [MGUS]

     D47.3   **Essential (hemorrhagic) thrombocythemia**
         Essential thrombocytosis
         Idiopathic hemorrhagic thrombocythemia

     D47.4   **Osteomyelofibrosis**
         Chronic idiopathic myelofibrosis
         Myelofibrosis (idiopathic) (with myeloid metaplasia)
         Myelosclerosis (megakaryocytic) with myeloid metaplasia
         Secondary myelofibrosis in myeloproliferative disease

         Excludes1   acute myelofibrosis (C94.4-)

● **D47.Z**   **Other specified neoplasms of uncertain behavior of lymphoid, hematopoietic and related tissue**

     ● **D47.Z1**   **Post-transplant lymphoproliferative disorder (PTLD)** ✪

         Code first complications of transplanted organs and tissue (T86.-)
         Ex: D47.Z1, D78.81-D78.89, E89.810-E89.89, H59.011-H59.019, H59.031-H59.099, H59.811-H59.89, H95.811-H95.89, I97.3, M96.89, N98.1-N98.9, T86.850-T86.99

     D47.Z2   **Castleman disease** ✪ ◀

         Code also if applicable human herpesvirus 8 infection (B10.89) ◀

         Excludes2   Kaposi's sarcoma (C46-) ◀
         Ex: See C94.4

     D47.Z9   **Other specified neoplasms of uncertain behavior of lymphoid, hematopoietic and related tissue** ✪
         Histiocytic tumors of uncertain behavior
         Ex: See C94.4

     D47.9   **Neoplasm of uncertain behavior of lymphoid, hematopoietic and related tissue, unspecified** ✪
         Lymphoproliferative disease NOS
         Ex: See C94.4

◀ New   ◀▥ Revised   ~~deleted~~ Deleted   Excludes 1   Excludes 2   Includes   Use additional   Code first   Code also   Unspecified

OGCR Official Guidelines   ● Unacceptable Principal Diagnosis   X Assign placeholder X   ● Use Additional Character(s)   ▶ Manifestation Code   **Coding Clinic**

718

● **D48 Neoplasm of uncertain behavior of other and unspecified sites**

     Excludes1   neurofibromatosis (nonmalignant) (Q85.0-)

     D48.0 Neoplasm of uncertain behavior of bone and articular cartilage

         Excludes1   neoplasm of uncertain behavior of cartilage of ear (D48.1)

                  neoplasm of uncertain behavior of cartilage of larynx (D38.0)

                  neoplasm of uncertain behavior of cartilage of nose (D38.5)

                  neoplasm of uncertain behavior of connective tissue of eyelid (D48.1)

                  neoplasm of uncertain behavior of synovia (D48.1)

     D48.1 Neoplasm of uncertain behavior of connective and other soft tissue

         Neoplasm of uncertain behavior of connective tissue of ear

         Neoplasm of uncertain behavior of connective tissue of eyelid

         Stromal tumors of uncertain behavior of digestive system

         Excludes1   neoplasm of uncertain behavior of articular cartilage (D48.0)

                  neoplasm of uncertain behavior of cartilage of larynx (D38.0)

                  neoplasm of uncertain behavior of cartilage of nose (D38.5)

                  neoplasm of uncertain behavior of connective tissue of breast (D48.6-)

     D48.2 Neoplasm of uncertain behavior of peripheral nerves and autonomic nervous system

         Excludes1   neoplasm of uncertain behavior of peripheral nerves of orbit (D48.7)

     D48.3 Neoplasm of uncertain behavior of retroperitoneum

     D48.4 Neoplasm of uncertain behavior of peritoneum

     D48.5 Neoplasm of uncertain behavior of skin

         Neoplasm of uncertain behavior of anal margin

         Neoplasm of uncertain behavior of anal skin

         Neoplasm of uncertain behavior of perianal skin

         Neoplasm of uncertain behavior of skin of breast

         Excludes1   neoplasm of uncertain behavior of anus NOS (D37.8)

                  neoplasm of uncertain behavior of skin of genital organs (D39.8, D40.8)

                  neoplasm of uncertain behavior of vermilion border of lip (D37.0)

     ● **D48.6 Neoplasm of uncertain behavior of breast**

         Neoplasm of uncertain behavior of connective tissue of breast

         Cystosarcoma phyllodes

         Excludes1   neoplasm of uncertain behavior of skin of breast (D48.5)

         D48.60 Neoplasm of uncertain behavior of unspecified breast

         D48.61 Neoplasm of uncertain behavior of right breast

         D48.62 Neoplasm of uncertain behavior of left breast

     D48.7 Neoplasm of uncertain behavior of other specified sites

         Neoplasm of uncertain behavior of eye

         Neoplasm of uncertain behavior of heart

         Neoplasm of uncertain behavior of peripheral nerves of orbit

         Excludes1   neoplasm of uncertain behavior of connective tissue (D48.1)

                  neoplasm of uncertain behavior of skin of eyelid (D48.5)

     D48.9 Neoplasm of uncertain behavior, unspecified

● **D49 Neoplasms of unspecified behavior**

     Note: Category D49 classifies by site neoplasms of unspecified morphology and behavior. The term 'mass,' unless otherwise stated, is not to be regarded as a neoplastic growth.

     Includes   'growth' NOS

                  neoplasm NOS

                  new growth NOS

                  tumor NOS

     Excludes1   neoplasms of uncertain behavior (D37-D44, D48)

     D49.0 Neoplasm of unspecified behavior of digestive system

         Excludes1   neoplasm of unspecified behavior of margin of anus (D49.2)

                  neoplasm of unspecified behavior of perianal skin (D49.2)

                  neoplasm of unspecified behavior of skin of anus (D49.2)

     D49.1 Neoplasm of unspecified behavior of respiratory system

     D49.2 Neoplasm of unspecified behavior of bone, soft tissue, and skin

         Excludes1   neoplasm of unspecified behavior of anal canal (D49.0)

                  neoplasm of unspecified behavior of anus NOS (D49.0)

                  neoplasm of unspecified behavior of bone marrow (D49.89)

                  neoplasm of unspecified behavior of cartilage of larynx (D49.1)

                  neoplasm of unspecified behavior of cartilage of nose (D49.1)

                  neoplasm of unspecified behavior of connective tissue of breast (D49.3)

                  neoplasm of unspecified behavior of skin of genital organs (D49.59) ◀

                  neoplasm of unspecified behavior of vermilion border of lip (D49.0)

     D49.3 Neoplasm of unspecified behavior of breast

         Excludes1   neoplasm of unspecified behavior of skin of breast (D49.2)

     D49.4 Neoplasm of unspecified behavior of bladder

     ● **D49.5 Neoplasm of unspecified behavior of other genitourinary organs**

         ● **D49.51 Neoplasm of unspecified behavior of kidney** ◀

                 D49.511 Neoplasm of unspecified behavior of right kidney ◀

                 D49.512 Neoplasm of unspecified behavior of left kidney ◀

                 D49.519 Neoplasm of unspecified behavior of unspecified kidney ◀

         D49.59 Neoplasm of unspecified behavior of other genitourinary organ ◀

     D49.6 Neoplasm of unspecified behavior of brain

         Excludes1   neoplasm of unspecified behavior of cerebral meninges (D49.7)

                  neoplasm of unspecified behavior of cranial nerves (D49.7)

     D49.7 Neoplasm of unspecified behavior of endocrine glands and other parts of nervous system

         Excludes1   neoplasm of unspecified behavior of peripheral, sympathetic, and parasympathetic nerves and ganglia (D49.2)

     ● **D49.8 Neoplasm of unspecified behavior of other specified sites**

         Excludes1   neoplasm of unspecified behavior of eyelid (skin) (D49.2)

                  neoplasm of unspecified behavior of eyelid cartilage (D49.2)

                  neoplasm of unspecified behavior of great vessels (D49.2)

                  neoplasm of unspecified behavior of optic nerve (D49.7)

         D49.81 Neoplasm of unspecified behavior of retina and choroid

              Dark area on retina

              Retinal freckle

         D49.89 Neoplasm of unspecified behavior of other specified sites

     D49.9 Neoplasm of unspecified behavior of unspecified site

---

N   Newborn Age: 0   P   Pediatric Age: 0–17   M   Maternity DX: 12–55   A   Adult Age: 15–124   ♀   Females Only   ♂   Males Only

🅒   Complication\Comorbidity   🅜   Major C\C   (Ex)   CC/MCC Exclusions   🅗   Hospital-Acquired Condition

OGCR Chapter-Specific Coding Guidelines

3. Chapter 3: Disease of the blood and blood-forming organs and certain disorders involving the immune mechanism (D50-D89) Reserved for future guideline expansion

CHAPTER 3

DISEASES OF THE BLOOD AND BLOOD-FORMING ORGANS AND CERTAIN DISORDERS INVOLVING THE IMMUNE MECHANISM (D50-D89)

Excludes2   autoimmune disease (systemic) NOS (M35.9)
certain conditions originating in the perinatal period (P00-P96)
complications of pregnancy, childbirth and the puerperium (O00-O9A)
congenital malformations, deformations and chromosomal abnormalities (Q00-Q99)
endocrine, nutritional and metabolic diseases (E00-E88)
human immunodeficiency virus [HIV] disease (B20)
injury, poisoning and certain other consequences of external causes (S00-T88)
neoplasms (C00-D49)
symptoms, signs and abnormal clinical and laboratory findings, not elsewhere classified (R00-R94)

This chapter contains the following blocks:

D50-D53	Nutritional anemias
D55-D59	Hemolytic anemias
D60-D64	Aplastic and other anemias and other bone marrow failure syndromes
D65-D69	Coagulation defects, purpura and other hemorrhagic conditions
D70-D77	Other disorders of blood and blood-forming organs
D78	Intraoperative and postprocedural complications of the spleen
D80-D89	Certain disorders involving the immune mechanism

NUTRITIONAL ANEMIAS (D50-D53)

● **D50** **Iron deficiency anemia**
A disease characterized by a decrease in the number of red cells (hemoglobin) in the blood.

    Includes   asiderotic anemia
hypochromic anemia

  D50.0 **Iron deficiency anemia secondary to blood loss (chronic)**
Posthemorrhagic anemia (chronic)

    Excludes1   acute posthemorrhagic anemia (D62)
congenital anemia from fetal blood loss (P61.3)

  D50.1 **Sideropenic dysphagia**
Web-like growth of membranes in throat that makes swallowing difficult
Kelly-Paterson syndrome
Plummer-Vinson syndrome

  D50.8 **Other iron deficiency anemias**
Iron deficiency anemia due to inadequate dietary iron intake

  D50.9 **Iron deficiency anemia, unspecified**

● **D51** **Vitamin B12 deficiency anemia**

    Excludes1   vitamin B12 deficiency (E53.8)

  D51.0 **Vitamin B12 deficiency anemia due to intrinsic factor deficiency**
Addison anemia
Biermer anemia
Pernicious (congenital) anemia
Congenital intrinsic factor deficiency

  D51.1 **Vitamin B12 deficiency anemia due to selective vitamin B12 malabsorption with proteinuria**
Imerslund (Gräsbeck) syndrome
Megaloblastic hereditary anemia

  D51.2 **Transcobalamin II deficiency**

  D51.3 **Other dietary vitamin B12 deficiency anemia**
Vegan anemia

  D51.8 **Other vitamin B12 deficiency anemias**

  D51.9 **Vitamin B12 deficiency anemia, unspecified**

● **D52** **Folate deficiency anemia**

    Excludes1   folate deficiency without anemia (E53.8)

  D52.0 **Dietary folate deficiency anemia**
Nutritional megaloblastic anemia

  D52.1 **Drug-induced folate deficiency anemia**
Use additional code for adverse effect, if applicable, to identify drug (T36-T50 with fifth or sixth character 5)

  D52.8 **Other folate deficiency anemias**

  D52.9 **Folate deficiency anemia, unspecified**
Folic acid deficiency anemia NOS

● **D53** **Other nutritional anemias**

    Includes   megaloblastic anemia unresponsive to vitamin B12 or folate therapy

  D53.0 **Protein deficiency anemia**
Amino-acid deficiency anemia
Orotaciduric anemia

    Excludes1   Lesch-Nyhan syndrome (E79.1)

  D53.1 **Other megaloblastic anemias, not elsewhere classified**
Megaloblastic anemia NOS

    Excludes1   Di Guglielmo's disease (C94.0)

  D53.2 **Scorbutic anemia**
Anemia resulting from deficiency of ascorbic acid (vitamin C)

    Excludes1   scurvy (E54)

  D53.8 **Other specified nutritional anemias**
Anemia associated with deficiency of copper
Anemia associated with deficiency of molybdenum
Anemia associated with deficiency of zinc

    Excludes1   nutritional deficiencies without anemia, such as:
copper deficiency NOS (E61.0)
molybdenum deficiency NOS (E61.5)
zinc deficiency NOS (E60)

  D53.9 **Nutritional anemia, unspecified**
Simple chronic anemia

    Excludes1   anemia NOS (D64.9)

HEMOLYTIC ANEMIAS (D55-D59)

● **D55** **Anemia due to enzyme disorders**

    Excludes1   drug-induced enzyme deficiency anemia (D59.2)

  D55.0 **Anemia due to glucose-6-phosphate dehydrogenase [G6PD] deficiency**
Favism
G6PD deficiency anemia

  D55.1 **Anemia due to other disorders of glutathione metabolism**
Anemia (due to) enzyme deficiencies, except G6PD, related to the hexose monophosphate [HMP] shunt pathway
Anemia (due to) hemolytic nonspherocytic (hereditary), type I

◀ New   ◀║ Revised   ~~deleted~~ Deleted   Excludes 1   Excludes 2   Includes   Use additional   Code first   Code also   Unspecified
OGCR Official Guidelines   ● Unacceptable Principal Diagnosis   X Assign placeholder X   ● Use Additional Character(s)   ▶ Manifestation Code   **Coding Clinic**

D55.2   Anemia due to disorders of glycolytic enzymes
Hemolytic nonspherocytic (hereditary) anemia, type II
Hexokinase deficiency anemia
Pyruvate kinase [PK] deficiency anemia
Triose-phosphate isomerase deficiency anemia
> **Excludes1**   disorders of glycolysis not associated
> with anemia (E74.8)

D55.3   Anemia due to disorders of nucleotide metabolism

D55.8   Other anemias due to enzyme disorders

D55.9   Anemia due to enzyme disorder, unspecified

● **D56   Thalassemia**
*Hereditary disorders characterized by low production of hemoglobin
or excessive destruction of red blood cells*
> **Excludes1**   sickle-cell thalassemia (D57.4-)

D56.0   Alpha thalassemia
Alpha thalassemia major
Hemoglobin H Constant Spring
Hemoglobin H disease
Hydrops fetalis due to alpha thalassemia
Severe alpha thalassemia
Triple gene defect alpha thalassemia
> Use additional code, if applicable, for hydrops fetalis
> due to alpha thalassemia (P56.99)
> **Excludes1**   alpha thalassemia trait or minor (D56.3)
> asymptomatic alpha thalassemia (D56.3)
> hydrops fetalis due to isoimmunization
> (P56.0)
> hydrops fetalis not due to immune
> hemolysis (P83.2)

D56.1   Beta thalassemia
Beta thalassemia major
Cooley's anemia
Homozygous beta thalassemia
Severe beta thalassemia
Thalassemia intermedia
Thalassemia major
> **Excludes1**   beta thalassemia minor (D56.3)
> beta thalassemia trait (D56.3)
> delta-beta thalassemia (D56.2)
> hemoglobin E-beta thalassemia (D56.5)
> sickle-cell beta thalassemia (D57.4-)

D56.2   Delta-beta thalassemia
Homozygous delta-beta thalassemia
> **Excludes1**   delta-beta thalassemia minor (D56.3)
> delta-beta thalassemia trait (D56.3)

D56.3   Thalassemia minor
*Genetic disorders that have in common defective production
of hemoglobin*
Alpha thalassemia minor
Alpha thalassemia silent carrier
Alpha thalassemia trait
Beta thalassemia minor
Beta thalassemia trait
Delta-beta thalassemia minor
Delta-beta thalassemia trait
Thalassemia trait NOS
> **Excludes1**   alpha thalassemia (D56.0)
> beta thalassemia (D56.1)
> delta-beta thalassemia (D56.2)
> hemoglobin E-beta thalassemia (D56.5)
> sickle-cell trait (D57.3)

D56.4   Hereditary persistence of fetal hemoglobin [HPFH]
Persistent production of hemoglobin

D56.5   Hemoglobin E-beta thalassemia
> **Excludes1**   beta thalassemia (D56.1)
> beta thalassemia minor (D56.3)
> beta thalassemia trait (D56.3)
> delta-beta thalassemia (D56.2)
> delta-beta thalassemia trait (D56.3)
> hemoglobin E disease (D58.2)
> other hemoglobinopathies (D58.2)
> sickle-cell beta thalassemia (D57.4-)

D56.8   Other thalassemias
Dominant thalassemia
Hemoglobin C thalassemia
Mixed thalassemia
Thalassemia with other hemoglobinopathy
> **Excludes1**   hemoglobin C disease (D58.2)
> hemoglobin E disease (D58.2)
> other hemoglobinopathies (D58.2)
> sickle cell anemia (D57.-)
> sickle-cell thalassemia (D57.4)

D56.9   Thalassemia, unspecified
Mediterranean anemia (with other hemoglobinopathy)

● **D57   Sickle-cell disorders**
*Inherited disease in which red blood cells, normally disc-shaped,
become crescent shaped*
> Use additional code for any associated fever (R50.81)
> **Excludes1**   other hemoglobinopathies (D58.-)
> (Ex) **For category D57 CC codes:** D47.4, D50.0-D64.9, D68.312, D68.51-D68.69, D75.81,
> D75.89-D75.9, D77, D89.2

● **D57.0   Hb-SS disease with crisis**
Sickle-cell disease NOS with crisis
Hb-SS disease with vasoocclusive pain

   D57.00   Hb-SS disease with crisis, unspecified 🦠

   D57.01   Hb-SS disease with acute chest syndrome 🦠

   D57.02   Hb-SS disease with splenic sequestration 🦠

**D57.1   Sickle-cell disease without crisis Hb-SS disease without
crisis**
Sickle-cell anemia NOS
Sickle-cell disease NOS
Sickle-cell disorder NOS

● **D57.2   Sickle-cell/Hb-C disease**
Hb-SC disease
Hb-S/Hb-C disease

   D57.20   Sickle-cell/Hb-C disease without crisis

   ● **D57.21   Sickle-cell/Hb-C disease with crisis**

     **D57.211   Sickle-cell/Hb-C disease with acute
chest syndrome** 🦠 🦠
CC when PDX is its own CC

     **D57.212   Sickle-cell/Hb-C disease with splenic
sequestration** 🦠

     **D57.219   Sickle-cell/Hb-C disease with
crisis, unspecified** 🦠
Sickle-cell/Hb-C disease with crisis
NOS

D57.3   Sickle-cell trait
Hb-S trait
Heterozygous hemoglobin S

● **D57.4   Sickle-cell thalassemia**
Sickle-cell beta thalassemia
Thalassemia Hb-S disease

   D57.40   Sickle-cell thalassemia without crisis
Microdrepanocytosis
Sickle-cell thalassemia NOS

   ● **D57.41   Sickle-cell thalassemia with crisis**
*Sickle-cell "crisis" is precipitated when abnormally
crescent-shaped red blood cells form clots and
interrupt blood flow to major organs, causing
severe pain and organ damage.*
Sickle-cell thalassemia with vasoocclusive pain

     **D57.411   Sickle-cell thalassemia with acute
chest syndrome** 🦠 🦠
CC when PDX is its own CC

     **D57.412   Sickle-cell thalassemia with splenic
sequestration** 🦠

     **D57.419   Sickle-cell thalassemia with
crisis, unspecified** 🦠
Sickle-cell thalassemia with crisis
NOS

N   Newborn Age: 0   **P**   Pediatric Age: 0–17   **M**   Maternity DX: 12–55   **A**   Adult Age: 15–124   ♀   Females Only   ♂   Males Only
🦠   Complication\Comorbidity   🦠   Major C\C   (Ex)   CC/MCC Exclusions   🦠   Hospital-Acquired Condition
721

CHAPTER 3 (D50-D89)

● **D57.8   Other sickle-cell disorders**
    Hb-SD disease
    Hb-SE disease

    D57.80   Other sickle-cell disorders without crisis

    ● **D57.81   Other sickle-cell disorders with crisis**

        D57.811   Other sickle-cell disorders with acute chest syndrome 🖋

        D57.812   Other sickle-cell disorders with splenic sequestration 🖋

        D57.819   Other sickle-cell disorders with crisis, unspecified 🖋
            Other sickle-cell disorders with crisis NOS

● **D58   Other hereditary hemolytic anemias**
    Genetic condition in which bone marrow is unable to compensate for premature destruction of red blood cells

    Excludes1   hemolytic anemia of the newborn (P55.-)

    D58.0   Hereditary spherocytosis
        Presence of spherocytes (spherically shaped red blood cells)
        Acholuric (familial) jaundice
        Congenital (spherocytic) hemolytic icterus
        Minkowski-Chauffard syndrome

    D58.1   Hereditary elliptocytosis
        Presence of large numbers of elliptocytes in blood
        Elliptocytosis (congenital)
        Ovalocytosis (congenital) (hereditary)

    D58.2   Other hemoglobinopathies
        Abnormal hemoglobin NOS
        Congenital Heinz body anemia
        Hb-C disease
        Hb-D disease
        Hb-E disease
        Hemoglobinopathy NOS
        Unstable hemoglobin hemolytic disease

        Excludes1   familial polycythemia (D75.0)
                Hb-M disease (D74.0)
                hemoglobin E-beta thalassemia (D56.5)
                hereditary persistence of fetal hemoglobin [HPFH] (D56.4)
                high-altitude polycythemia (D75.1)
                methemoglobinemia (D74.-)
                other hemoglobinopathies with thalassemia (D56.8)

    D58.8   Other specified hereditary hemolytic anemias 🖋
        Stomatocytosis
        (Ex:) D50.0-D64.9, D75.9, P61.2-P61.4

    D58.9   Hereditary hemolytic anemia, unspecified 🖋
        (Ex:) See D58.8

● **D59   Acquired hemolytic anemia**
    (Ex:) **For category D59 CC codes:** D47.4, D50.0-D64.9, D68.312, D68.51-D68.69, D75.81, D75.89-D75.9, D77, D89.2

    D59.0   Drug-induced autoimmune hemolytic anemia 🖋
        Use additional code for adverse effect, if applicable, to identify drug (T36-T50 with fifth or sixth character 5)

    D59.1   Other autoimmune hemolytic anemias 🖋
        Autoimmune hemolytic disease (cold type) (warm type)
        Chronic cold hemagglutinin disease
        Cold agglutinin disease
        Cold agglutinin hemoglobinuria
        Cold type (secondary) (symptomatic) hemolytic anemia
        Warm type (secondary) (symptomatic) hemolytic anemia

        Excludes1   Evans syndrome (D69.41)
                hemolytic disease of newborn (P55.-)
                paroxysmal cold hemoglobinuria (D59.6)

    D59.2   Drug-induced nonautoimmune hemolytic anemia 🖋
        Drug-induced enzyme deficiency anemia

        Use additional code for adverse effect, if applicable, to identify drug (T36-T50 with fifth or sixth character 5)

    D59.3   Hemolytic-uremic syndrome 🖋
        Use additional code to identify associated:
            E. coli infection (B96.2-)
            Pneumococcal pneumonia (J13)
            Shigella dysenteriae (A03.9)

    D59.4   Other nonautoimmune hemolytic anemias 🖋
        Mechanical hemolytic anemia
        Microangiopathic hemolytic anemia
        Toxic hemolytic anemia

    D59.5   Paroxysmal nocturnal hemoglobinuria [Marchiafava-Micheli]
        Excludes1   hemoglobinuria NOS (R82.3)

    D59.6   Hemoglobinuria due to hemolysis from other external causes
        Hemoglobinuria from exertion
        March hemoglobinuria
        Paroxysmal cold hemoglobinuria

        Use additional code (Chapter 20) to identify external cause

        Excludes1   hemoglobinuria NOS (R82.3)

    D59.8   Other acquired hemolytic anemias

    D59.9   Acquired hemolytic anemia, unspecified 🖋
        Idiopathic hemolytic anemia, chronic

APLASTIC AND OTHER ANEMIAS AND OTHER BONE MARROW FAILURE SYNDROMES (D60-D64)

● **D60   Acquired pure red cell aplasia [erythroblastopenia]**
    Deficiency of erythroblasts

    Includes   red cell aplasia (acquired) (adult) (with thymoma)

    Excludes1   congenital red cell aplasia (D61.01)

    (Ex:) **For category D60 CC codes:** D47.4, D50.0-D64.9, D68.312, D68.51-D68.69, D75.81, D75.89-D75.9, D77, D89.2

    D60.0   Chronic acquired pure red cell aplasia 🖋
        Lack of development of blood cell

    D60.1   Transient acquired pure red cell aplasia 🖋

    D60.8   Other acquired pure red cell aplasias 🖋

    D60.9   Acquired pure red cell aplasia, unspecified 🖋

● **D61   Other aplastic anemias and other bone marrow failure syndromes**

    Excludes1   neutropenia (D70.-)

    ● **D61.0   Constitutional aplastic anemia**
        Condition where bone marrow is unable to produce blood cells

        D61.01   Constitutional (pure) red blood cell aplasia 🖋
            Blackfan-Diamond syndrome
            Congenital (pure) red cell aplasia
            Familial hypoplastic anemia
            Primary (pure) red cell aplasia
            Red cell (pure) aplasia of infants
            Excludes1   acquired red cell aplasia (D60.9)
            (Ex:) D50.0-D64.9, D75.9, P61.2-P61.4

        D61.09   Other constitutional aplastic anemia 🖋
            Fanconi's anemia
            Pancytopenia with malformations
            (Ex:) D50.0-D64.9, D69.3-D69.49, D75.9, P61.2-P61.4

    D61.1   Drug-induced aplastic anemia 🖋
        Use additional code for adverse effect, if applicable, to identify drug (T36-T50 with fifth or sixth character 5)
        (Ex:) See D60

    D61.2   Aplastic anemia due to other external agents 🖋
        Code first , if applicable, toxic effects of substances chiefly nonmedicinal as to source (T51-T65)
        (Ex:) See D60

    D61.3   Idiopathic aplastic anemia 🖋
        (Ex:) See D60

◄ New   ◄▦ Revised   ~~deleted~~ Deleted   Excludes 1   Excludes 2   Includes   Use additional   Code first   Code also   Unspecified

722

OGCR Official Guidelines   ● Unacceptable Principal Diagnosis   X Assign placeholder X   ● Use Additional Character(s)   🖋 Manifestation Code   **Coding Clinic**

● **D61.8   Other specified aplastic anemias and other bone marrow failure syndromes**

    (Ex) For category D61.8 CC codes unless otherwise indicated: D60.0-D60.9, D61.1-D64.9, D70.0-D70.9, D72.810-D72.820, D72.823, D72.825-D72.829, D75.9-D76.3, P61.2

   ● **D61.81   Pancytopenia**

      Marked deficiency of all the blood elements: Red blood cells (erythrocytes), white blood cells (leukocytes), and platelets (thrombocytes). Check laboratory results.

      Excludes1   pancytopenia (due to) (with) aplastic anemia (D61.9)

                pancytopenia (due to) (with) bone marrow infiltration (D61.82)

                pancytopenia (due to) (with) congenital (pure) red cell aplasia (D61.01)

                pancytopenia (due to) (with) hairy cell leukemia (C91.4-)

                pancytopenia (due to) (with) human immunodeficiency virus disease (B20.-)

                pancytopenia (due to) (with) leukoerythroblastic anemia (D61.82)

                pancytopenia (due to) (with) myeloproliferative disease (D47.1)

      Excludes2   pancytopenia (due to) (with) myelodysplastic syndromes (D46.-) ◀

    D61.810   Antineoplastic chemotherapy induced pancytopenia 🏥

      Excludes2   aplastic anemia due to antineoplastic chemotherapy (D61.1)

    D61.811   Other drug-induced pancytopenia 🏥

      Excludes2   aplastic anemia due to drugs (D61.1)

    D61.818   Other pancytopenia 🏥

   D61.82   Myelophthisis 🏥

      Leukoerythroblastic anemia

      Myelophthisic anemia

      Panmyelophthisis

      Code also the underlying disorder, such as: malignant neoplasm of breast (C50.-) tuberculosis (A15.-)

      Excludes1   idiopathic myelofibrosis (D47.1)

                myelofibrosis NOS (D75.81)

                myelofibrosis with myeloid metaplasia (D47.4)

                primary myelofibrosis (D47.1)

                secondary myelofibrosis (D75.81)

    D61.89   Other specified aplastic anemias and other bone marrow failure syndromes 🏥

      (Ex) See D60

● **D61.9   Aplastic anemia, unspecified** 🏥

    Hypoplastic anemia NOS

    Medullary hypoplasia

    (Ex) See D60

● **D62   Acute posthemorrhagic anemia** 🏥

   Excludes1   anemia due to chronic blood loss (D50.0)

              blood loss anemia NOS (D50.0)

              congenital anemia from fetal blood loss (P61.3)

    (Ex) D47.4, D50.0-D64.9, D68.312, D68.51-D68.69, D75.81, D75.89-D75.9, D77, D89.2, T79.2XX[A]

● **D63   Anemia in chronic diseases classified elsewhere**

   ▶ **D63.0   Anemia in neoplastic disease**

      Code first neoplasm (C00-D49)

      Excludes1   anemia due to antineoplastic chemotherapy (D64.81)

              aplastic anemia due to antineoplastic chemotherapy (D61.1)

    OGCR Section I.C.2.e.2.

      2) Anemia associated with chemotherapy, immunotherapy and radiation therapy

      When the admission/encounter is for management of an anemia associated with an adverse effect of the administration of chemotherapy or immunotherapy and the only treatment is for the anemia, the anemia code is sequenced first followed by the appropriate codes for the neoplasm and the adverse effect (T45.1X5, Adverse effect of antineoplastic and immunosuppressive drugs).

   ▶ **D63.1   Anemia in chronic kidney disease**

      Erythropoietin resistant anemia (EPO resistant anemia)

      Code first underlying chronic kidney disease (CKD) (N18.-)

   ▶ **D63.8   Anemia in other chronic diseases classified elsewhere**

      Code first underlying disease, such as:

        diphyllobothriasis (B70.0)

        hookworm disease (B76.0-B76.9)

        hypothyroidism (E00.0-E03.9)

        malaria (B50.0-B54)

        symptomatic late syphilis (A52.79)

        tuberculosis (A18.89)

● **D64   Other anemias**

   Excludes1   refractory anemia (D46.-)

              refractory anemia with excess blasts in transformation [RAEB T] (C92.0-)

   D64.0   Hereditary sideroblastic anemia

      Abnormal production RBCs (erythrocytes)

      Sex-linked hypochromic sideroblastic anemia

   ▶ **D64.1   Secondary sideroblastic anemia due to disease**

      Code first underlying disease

   D64.2   Secondary sideroblastic anemia due to drugs and toxins

      Code first poisoning due to drug or toxin, if applicable (T36-T65 with fifth or sixth character 1-4 or 6)

      Use additional code for adverse effect, if applicable, to identify drug (T36-T50 with fifth or sixth character 5)

   D64.3   Other sideroblastic anemias

      Sideroblastic anemia NOS

      Pyridoxine-responsive sideroblastic anemia NEC

   D64.4   Congenital dyserythropoietic anemia

      Any of several rare hereditary anemias, mostly types of macrocytic anemia

      Dyshematopoietic anemia (congenital)

      Excludes1   Blackfan-Diamond syndrome (D61.01)

              Di Guglielmo's disease (C94.0)

● **D64.8   Other specified anemias**

   D64.81   Anemia due to antineoplastic chemotherapy

      Antineoplastic chemotherapy induced anemia

      Excludes1   aplastic anemia due to antineoplastic chemotherapy (D61.1)

      Excludes2   anemia in neoplastic disease (D63.0) ◀

   D64.89   Other specified anemias

      Infantile pseudoleukemia

   D64.9   Anemia, unspecified

CHAPTER 3 (D50-D89)

COAGULATION DEFECTS, PURPURA AND OTHER HEMORRHAGIC CONDITIONS (D65-D69)

D65   Disseminated intravascular coagulation [defibrination syndrome] 🔖

Blood clots form and consume all coagulation proteins and platelets and disrupt normal coagulation, resulting in abnormal bleeding

Afibrinogenemia, acquired
Consumption coagulopathy
Diffuse or disseminated intravascular coagulation [DIC]
Fibrinolytic hemorrhage, acquired
Fibrinolytic purpura
Purpura fulminans

> **Excludes1**   disseminated intravascular coagulation (complicating):
> abortion or ectopic or molar pregnancy (O00-O07, O08.1)
> in newborn (P60)
> pregnancy, childbirth and the puerperium (O45.0, O46.0, O67.0, O72.3)

(Ex) D47.4, D65-D69.9, D75.81-D75.9, D77, D89.2

D66   Hereditary factor VIII deficiency 🔖

Inherited coagulation disorder carried by females but most often affecting males

Classical hemophilia
Deficiency factor VIII (with functional defect)
Hemophilia NOS
Hemophilia A

> **Excludes1**   factor VIII deficiency with vascular defect (D68.0)

(Ex) See D65

D67   Hereditary factor IX deficiency 🔖

Christmas disease
Factor IX deficiency (with functional defect)
Hemophilia B
Plasma thromboplastin component [PTC] deficiency

(Ex) See D65

● **D68   Other coagulation defects**

> **Excludes1**   abnormal coagulation profile (R79.1)
> coagulation defects complicating abortion or ectopic or molar pregnancy (O00-O07, O08.1)
> coagulation defects complicating pregnancy, childbirth and the puerperium (O45.0, O46.0, O67.0, O72.3)

Coding Clinic: 2016, Q1, P14

D68.0   Von Willebrand's disease 🔖

Congenital bleeding disorder

Angiohemophilia
Factor VIII deficiency with vascular defect
Vascular hemophilia

> **Excludes1**   capillary fragility (hereditary) (D69.8)
> factor VIII deficiency NOS (D66)
> factor VIII deficiency with functional defect (D66)

D68.1   Hereditary factor XI deficiency 🔖

Deficiency of blood coagulation resulting in systemic blood-clotting defect

Hemophilia C
Plasma thromboplastin antecedent [PTA] deficiency
Rosenthal's disease

D68.2   Hereditary deficiency of other clotting factors 🔖

Blood clotting disorders caused by hereditary deficiencies of one or more clotting factors

AC globulin deficiency
Congenital afibrinogenemia
Deficiency of factor I [fibrinogen]
Deficiency of factor II [prothrombin]
Deficiency of factor V [labile]
Deficiency of factor VII [stable]
Deficiency of factor X [Stuart-Prower]
Deficiency of factor XII [Hageman]
Deficiency of factor XIII [fibrin stabilizing]
Dysfibrinogenemia (congenital)
Hypoproconvertinemia
Owren's disease
Proaccelerin deficiency

● **D68.3   Hemorrhagic disorder due to circulating anticoagulants**

Blood clotting disorders caused by anticoagulants (warfarin and heparin)

● **D68.31   Hemorrhagic disorder due to intrinsic circulating anticoagulants, antibodies, or inhibitors**

D68.311   Acquired hemophilia 🔖

Autoimmune hemophilia
Autoimmune inhibitors to clotting factors
Secondary hemophilia

(Ex) D47.4, D65-D69.9, D75.82-D75.9, D77, D89.2

D68.312   Antiphospholipid antibody with hemorrhagic disorder 🔖

Lupus anticoagulant (LAC) with hemorrhagic disorder
Systemic lupus erythematosus [SLE] inhibitor with hemorrhagic disorder

> **Excludes1**   antiphospholipid antibody, finding without diagnosis (R76.0)
> antiphospholipid antibody syndrome (D68.61)
> antiphospholipid antibody with hypercoagulable state (D68.61)
> lupus anticoagulant (LAC) finding without diagnosis (R76.0)
> lupus anticoagulant (LAC) with hypercoagulable state (D68.62)
> systemic lupus erythematosus [SLE] inhibitor finding without diagnosis (R76.0)
> systemic lupus erythematosus [SLE] inhibitor with hypercoagulable state (D68.62)

(Ex) D47.4, D68.311-D68.318, D68.51-D68.69, D70.0-D72.9, D73.81, D75.81, D75.89-D77, D89.2

D68.318   Other hemorrhagic disorder due to intrinsic circulating anticoagulants, antibodies, or inhibitors 🔖

Antithromboplastinemia
Antithromboplastinogenemia
Hemorrhagic disorder due to intrinsic increase in antithrombin
Hemorrhagic disorder due to intrinsic increase in anti-VIIIa
Hemorrhagic disorder due to intrinsic increase in anti-IXa
Hemorrhagic disorder due to intrinsic increase in anti-XIa

(Ex) See 68.31

◀ New   ◀▥ Revised   ~~deleted~~ Deleted   Excludes 1   Excludes 2   Includes   Use additional   Code first   Code also   Unspecified

OGCR Official Guidelines   ● Unacceptable Principal Diagnosis   X Assign placeholder X   ● Use Additional Character(s)   ▶ Manifestation Code   **Coding Clinic**

D68.32   Hemorrhagic disorder due to extrinsic circulating anticoagulants 🔗
Drug-induced hemorrhagic disorder
Hemorrhagic disorder due to increase in anti-IIa
Hemorrhagic disorder due to increase in anti-Xa
Hyperheparinemia
Use additional code for adverse effect, if applicable, to identify drug (T45.515, T45.525)
(Ex:) D47.4, D65-D69.9, D75.81-D75.9, D77, D89.2
Coding Clinic: 2016, Q1, P14-15

D68.4   Acquired coagulation factor deficiency 🔗
Deficiency of coagulation factor due to liver disease
Deficiency of coagulation factor due to vitamin K deficiency
Excludes1   vitamin K deficiency of newborn (P53)
(Ex:) See D68.32

● **D68.5   Primary thrombophilia**
AKA idiopathic thrombocytopenia, may be acquired or congenital and is a common cause of coagulation disorders.
Primary hypercoagulable states
Excludes1   antiphospholipid syndrome (D68.61)
lupus anticoagulant (D68.62)
secondary activated protein C resistance (D68.69)
secondary antiphospholipid antibody syndrome (D68.69)
secondary lupus anticoagulant with hypercoagulable state (D68.69)
secondary systemic lupus erythematosus [SLE] inhibitor with hypercoagulable state (D68.69)
systemic lupus erythematosus [SLE] inhibitor finding without diagnosis (R76.0)
systemic lupus erythematosus [SLE] inhibitor with hemorrhagic disorder (D68.312)
thrombotic thrombocytopenic purpura (M31.1)
(Ex:) For category D68.5 CC codes: D47.4, D68.312, D68.51-D68.69, D70.0-D72.9, D73.81, D75.81, D75.89-D77, D89.2

D68.51   Activated protein C resistance 🔗
Factor V Leiden mutation

D68.52   Prothrombin gene mutation 🔗

D68.59   Other primary thrombophilia 🔗
Antithrombin III deficiency
Hypercoagulable state NOS
Primary hypercoagulable state NEC
Primary thrombophilia NEC
Protein C deficiency
Protein S deficiency
Thrombophilia NOS

● **D68.6   Other thrombophilia**
Other hypercoagulable states
Excludes1   diffuse or disseminated intravascular coagulation [DIC] (D65)
heparin induced thrombocytopenia (HIT) (D75.82)
hyperhomocysteinemia (E72.11)
(Ex:) For category D68.6 CC codes: D47.4, D68.312, D68.51-D68.69, D70.0-D72.9, D73.81, D75.81, D75.89-D77, D89.2

D68.61   Antiphospholipid syndrome 🔗
Anticardiolipin syndrome
Antiphospholipid antibody syndrome
Excludes1   anti-phospholipid antibody, finding without diagnosis (R76.0)
anti-phospholipid antibody with hemorrhagic disorder (D68.312)
lupus anticoagulant syndrome (D68.62)

D68.62   Lupus anticoagulant syndrome 🔗
Lupus anticoagulant
Presence of systemic lupus erythematosus [SLE] inhibitor
Excludes1   anticardiolipin syndrome (D68.61)
antiphospholipid syndrome (D68.61)
lupus anticoagulant (LAC) finding without diagnosis (R76.0) ◀
lupus anticoagulant (LAC) with hemorrhagic disorder (D68.312)

D68.69   Other thrombophilia 🔗
Hypercoagulable states NEC
Secondary hypercoagulable state NOS

D68.8   Other specified coagulation defects 🔗
Excludes1   hemorrhagic disease of newborn (P53)
(Ex:) See D68.32

D68.9   Coagulation defect, unspecified 🔗
(Ex:) See D68.32

● **D69   Purpura and other hemorrhagic conditions**
Group of conditions characterized by small hemorrhages in skin, mucous membranes, or serosal surfaces
Excludes1   benign hypergammaglobulinemic purpura (D89.0)
cryoglobulinemic purpura (D89.1)
essential (hemorrhagic) thrombocythemia (D47.3)
hemorrhagic thrombocythemia (D47.3)
purpura fulminans (D65)
thrombotic thrombocytopenic purpura (M31.1)
Waldenström hypergammaglobulinemic purpura (D89.0)

D69.0   Allergic purpura 🔗
Allergic vasculitis
Nonthrombocytopenic hemorrhagic purpura
Nonthrombocytopenic idiopathic purpura
Purpura anaphylactoid
Purpura Henoch(-Schönlein)
Purpura rheumatica
Vascular purpura
Excludes1   thrombocytopenic hemorrhagic purpura (D69.3)
(Ex:) See D68.32

N   Newborn Age: 0   P   Pediatric Age: 0–17   M   Maternity DX: 12–55   A   Adult Age: 15–124   ♀ Females Only   ♂ Males Only
🔗 Complication\Comorbidity   🔗 Major C\C   (Ex:) CC/MCC Exclusions   🔗 Hospital-Acquired Condition

D69.1 **Qualitative platelet defects**
Bernard-Soulier [giant platelet] syndrome
Glanzmann's disease
Grey platelet syndrome
Thromboasthenia (hemorrhagic) (hereditary)
Thrombocytopathy
> **Excludes1**   von Willebrand's disease (D68.0)

D69.2 **Other nonthrombocytopenic purpura**
Purpura NOS
Purpura simplex
Senile purpura

D69.3 **Immune thrombocytopenic purpura** 🔖
Hemorrhagic (thrombocytopenic) purpura
Idiopathic thrombocytopenic purpura
Tidal platelet dysgenesis
(Ex:) See D68.32

● **D69.4** **Other primary thrombocytopenia**
> **Excludes1**   transient neonatal thrombocytopenia (P61.0)
> Wiskott-Aldrich syndrome (D82.0)

     D69.41 **Evans syndrome** 🔖
       Acquired hemolytic anemia and thrombocytopenia
       (Ex:) See D68.32

     D69.42 **Congenital and hereditary thrombocytopenia purpura** 🔖
       Congenital thrombocytopenia
       Hereditary thrombocytopenia
       > **Code first** *congenital or hereditary disorder, such as:*
         thrombocytopenia with absent radius (TAR syndrome) (Q87.2)
       (Ex:) See D68.32

     D69.49 **Other primary thrombocytopenia**
       Megakaryocytic hypoplasia
       Primary thrombocytopenia NOS

● **D69.5** **Secondary thrombocytopenia**
Acquired reduction of number of platelets required for blood clotting
> **Excludes1**   heparin induced thrombocytopenia (HIT) (D75.82)
> transient thrombocytopenia of newborn (P61.0)

     D69.51 **Posttransfusion purpura**
       Posttransfusion purpura from whole blood (fresh) or blood products PTP

     D69.59 **Other secondary thrombocytopenia**

D69.6 **Thrombocytopenia, unspecified**

D69.8 **Other specified hemorrhagic conditions**
Capillary fragility (hereditary)
Vascular pseudohemophilia

D69.9 **Hemorrhagic condition, unspecified**

OTHER DISORDERS OF BLOOD AND BLOOD-FORMING ORGANS (D70-D77)

● **D70** **Neutropenia**
Decrease in number of neutrophils (type of white blood cell)
> **Includes**   agranulocytosis
> decreased absolute neurophile count (ANC)

Use additional code for any associated:
   fever (R50.81)
   mucositis (J34.81, K12.3-, K92.81, N76.81)
> **Excludes1**   neutropenic splenomegaly (D73.81)
> transient neonatal neutropenia (P61.5)

   D70.0 **Congenital agranulocytosis**
       Reduced numbers of neutrophils (type of white blood cell)
       Congenital neutropenia
       Infantile genetic agranulocytosis
       Kostmann's disease

   D70.1 **Agranulocytosis secondary to cancer chemotherapy**
       Decreased numbers of granulocytes (type of white blood cell)
       > **Code also** *underlying neoplasm*
       Use additional code for adverse effect, if applicable, to identify drug (T45.1X5)

   D70.2 **Other drug-induced agranulocytosis**
       Use additional code for adverse effect, if applicable, to identify drug (T36-T50 with fifth or sixth character 5)

   D70.3 **Neutropenia due to infection**

   D70.4 **Cyclic neutropenia**
       Chronic neutropenia (low number of type of white blood cell)
       Cyclic hematopoiesis
       Periodic neutropenia

   D70.8 **Other neutropenia**

   D70.9 **Neutropenia, unspecified**

● **D71** **Functional disorders of polymorphonuclear neutrophils**
Polymorphonuclear: varying shapes of nucleus; AKA PMNs
Cell membrane receptor complex [CR3] defect
Chronic (childhood) granulomatous disease
Congenital dysphagocytosis
Progressive septic granulomatosis

● **D72** **Other disorders of white blood cells**
> **Excludes1**   basophilia (D72.824)
> immunity disorders (D80-D89)
> neutropenia (D70)
> preleukemia (syndrome) (D46.9)

   D72.0 **Genetic anomalies of leukocytes**
       Alder (granulation) (granulocyte) anomaly
       Alder syndrome
       Hereditary leukocytic hypersegmentation
       Hereditary leukocytic hyposegmentation
       Hereditary leukomelanopathy
       May-Hegglin (granulation) (granulocyte) anomaly
       May-Hegglin syndrome
       Pelger-Huët (granulation) (granulocyte) anomaly
       Pelger-Huët syndrome
       > **Excludes1**   Chédiak (-Steinbrinck)-Higashi syndrome (E70.330)

   D72.1 **Eosinophilia**
       Formation and accumulation of high number of white cells in blood/tissue
       Allergic eosinophilia
       Hereditary eosinophilia
       > **Excludes1**   Löffler's syndrome (J82)
       > pulmonary eosinophilia (J82)

●   **D72.8** **Other specified disorders of white blood cells**
       > **Excludes1**   leukemia (C91-C95)

     ● **D72.81** **Decreased white blood cell count**
       > **Excludes1**   neutropenia (D70.-)

       D72.810 **Lymphocytopenia**
         Decreased lymphocytes
         Reduction in number of lympho cytes in blood

       D72.818 **Other decreased white blood cell count**
         Basophilic leukopenia
         Eosinophilic leukopenia
         Monocytopenia
         Other decreased leukocytes
         Plasmacytopenia

       D72.819 **Decreased white blood cell count, unspecified**
         Decreased leukocytes, unspecified
         Leukocytopenia, unspecified
         Leukopenia
         > **Excludes1**   malignant leukopenia (D70.9)

● **D72.82**   **Elevated white blood cell count**
> **Excludes1**   eosinophilia (D72.1)

     D72.820   **Lymphocytosis (symptomatic)**
         Elevated lymphocytes
         Excess of normal lymphocytes

     D72.821   **Monocytosis (symptomatic)**
> **Excludes1**   infectious mononucleosis (B27.-)

     D72.822   **Plasmacytosis**
         Presence of excess plasma cells

     D72.823   **Leukemoid reaction**
         Basophilic leukemoid reaction
         Leukemoid reaction NOS
         Lymphocytic leukemoid reaction
         Monocytic leukemoid reaction
         Myelocytic leukemoid reaction
         Neutrophilic leukemoid reaction

     D72.824   **Basophilia**
         Increase of basophils in blood

     D72.825   **Bandemia**
         Bandemia without diagnosis of specific infection
         Excess number of band cells (immature white blood cells) released by bone marrow
> **Excludes1**   confirmed infection -code to infection
> leukemia (C91.-, C92.-, C93.-, C94.-, C95.-)

     D72.828   **Other elevated white blood cell count**

     D72.829   **Elevated white blood cell count, unspecified**
         Elevated leukocytes, unspecified
         Leukocytosis, unspecified

     D72.89   **Other specified disorders of white blood cells**
         Abnormality of white blood cells NEC

     D72.9   **Disorder of white blood cells, unspecified**
         Abnormal leukocyte differential NOS

● **D73**   **Diseases of spleen**

     D73.0   **Hyposplenism**
         Diminished functioning of spleen
         Atrophy of spleen
> **Excludes1**   asplenia (congenital) (Q89.01)
> postsurgical absence of spleen (Z90.81)

     D73.1   **Hypersplenism**
         Accelerated function of spleen
> **Excludes1**   neutropenic splenomegaly (D73.81)
> primary splenic neutropenia (D73.81)
> splenitis, splenomegaly in late syphilis (A52.79)
> splenitis, splenomegaly in tuberculosis (A18.85)
> splenomegaly NOS (R16.1)
> splenomegaly congenital (Q89.0)

     D73.2   **Chronic congestive splenomegaly**
         Enlargement of spleen

     D73.3   **Abscess of spleen**

     D73.4   **Cyst of spleen**

     D73.5   **Infarction of spleen**
         Splenic rupture, nontraumatic
         Torsion of spleen
> **Excludes1**   rupture of spleen due to Plasmodium vivax malaria (B51.0)
> traumatic rupture of spleen (S36.03-)

     D73.8   **Other diseases of spleen**

     D73.81   **Neutropenic splenomegaly**
         Werner-Schultz disease
         Enlarged spleen responding to inadequate number of neutrophils

     D73.89   **Other diseases of spleen**
         Fibrosis of spleen NOS
         Perisplenitis
         Splenitis NOS

     D73.9   **Disease of spleen, unspecified**

● **D74**   **Methemoglobinemia**
     Excessive methemoglobin (form of hemoglobin)
     (Ex) **For category D74 CC codes:** D56.4, D58.2-D59.2, D59.4-D59.9, D64.4-D64.9, D74.0-D74.9, D75.9

     D74.0   **Congenital methemoglobinemia**
         Congenital NADH-methemoglobin reductase deficiency
         Hemoglobin-M [Hb-M] disease
         Methemoglobinemia, hereditary

     D74.8   **Other methemoglobinemias**
         Acquired methemoglobinemia (with sulfhemoglobinemia)
         Toxic methemoglobinemia

     D74.9   **Methemoglobinemia, unspecified**

● **D75**   **Other and unspecified diseases of blood and blood-forming organs**
> **Excludes2**   acute lymphadenitis (L04.-)
> chronic lymphadenitis (I88.1)
> enlarged lymph nodes (R59.-)
> hypergammaglobulinemia NOS (D89.2)
> lymphadenitis NOS (I88.9)
> mesenteric lymphadenitis (acute) (chronic) (I88.0)

     D75.0   **Familial erythrocytosis**
         Genetic mutation of gene that results in increased circulating RBCs
         Benign polycythemia
         Familial polycythemia
> **Excludes1**   hereditary ovalocytosis (D58.1)

     D75.1   **Secondary polycythemia**
         Increase in total red cell mass
         Acquired polycythemia
         Emotional polycythemia
         Erythrocytosis NOS
         Hypoxemic polycythemia
         Nephrogenous polycythemia
         Polycythemia due to erythropoietin
         Polycythemia due to fall in plasma volume
         Polycythemia due to high altitude
         Polycythemia due to stress
         Polycythemia NOS
         Relative polycythemia
> **Excludes1**   polycythemia neonatorum (P61.1)
> polycythemia vera (D45)

CHAPTER 3 (D50-D89)

● D75.8 **Other specified diseases of blood and blood-forming organs**

▷ D75.81 *Myelofibrosis* 🖉

Replacing bone marrow by fibrous tissue

Myelofibrosis NOS

Secondary myelofibrosis NOS

Code first the underlying disorder, such as:
malignant neoplasm of breast (C50.-)

Use additional code, if applicable, for associated therapy-related myelodysplastic syndrome (D46.-)

Use additional code for adverse effect, if applicable, to identify drug (T45.1X5)

Excludes1   acute myelofibrosis (C94.4-)
idiopathic myelofibrosis (D47.1)
leukoerythroblastic anemia (D61.82)
myelofibrosis with myeloid metaplasia (D47.4)
myelophthisic anemia (D61.82)
myelophthisis (D61.82)
primary myelofibrosis (D47.1)

(Ex) C88.2-C88.3, C88.8-C88.9, C90.10-C90.11, C90.20-C90.21, C90.30-C90.31, C91.00-C91.02, C91.10-C91.12, C91.30-C91.32, C91.40-C91.42, C91.50-C91.52, C91.60-C91.62, C91.90-C91.92, C91.A0-C91.A2, C91.Z0-C91.Z2, C92.00-C92.02, C92.10-C92.12, C92.20-C92.22, C92.30-C92.32, C92.40-C92.42, C92.50-C92.52, C92.60-C92.62, C92.90-C92.92, C92.A0-C92.A2, C92.Z0-C92.Z2, C93.00-C93.02, C93.10-C93.12, C93.30-C93.32, C93.90-C93.92, C93.Z0-C93.Z2, C94.00-C94.02, C94.20-C94.22, C94.30-C94.32, C94.40-C94.42, C94.6, C94.80-C94.82, C95.00-C95.02, C95.10-C95.12, C95.90-C95.92, D45-D46.22, D46.4, D46.9, D46.A-D46.Z, D47.0-D47.1, D47.3, D47.9, D47.Z2, D47.Z9, D48.7-D48.9

D75.82   **Heparin induced thrombocytopenia (HIT)**

D75.89   **Other specified diseases of blood and blood-forming organs**

D75.9   **Disease of blood and blood-forming organs, unspecified**

● D76 **Other specified diseases with participation of lymphoreticular and reticulohistiocytic tissue**

Excludes1   (Abt-) Letterer-Siwe disease (C96.0)
eosinophilic granuloma (C96.6)
Hand-Schüller-Christian disease (C96.5)
histiocytic medullary reticulosis (C96.9) ◀
histiocytic sarcoma (C96.A)
histiocytosis X, multifocal (C96.5)
histiocytosis X, unifocal (C96.6)
Langerhans-cell histiocytosis, multifocal (C96.5)
Langerhans-cell histiocytosis NOS (C96.6)
Langerhans-cell histiocytosis, unifocal (C96.6)
leukemic reticuloendotheliosis (C91.4-) ◀
lipomelanotic reticulosis (I89.8) ◀
malignant histiocytosis (C96.A)
malignant reticulosis (C86.0) ◀
nonlipid reticuloendotheliosis (C96.0) ◀

(Ex) **For category D76 CC codes:** D60.0-D60.9, D61.1-D61.9, D65, D69.3-D70.9, D72.818-D72.819, D75.82, D75.9

D76.1   **Hemophagocytic lymphohistiocytosis** 🖉

Familial hemophagocytic reticulosis

Histiocytoses of mononuclear phagocytes

D76.2   **Hemophagocytic syndrome, infection-associated** 🖉

Use additional code to identify infectious agent or disease.

D76.3   **Other histiocytosis syndromes** 🖉

Reticulohistiocytoma (giant-cell)

Sinus histiocytosis with massive lymphadenopathy

Xanthogranuloma

▷ D77 **Other disorders of blood and blood-forming organs in diseases classified elsewhere**

Code first underlying disease, such as:
amyloidosis (E85.-)
congenital early syphilis (A50.0)
echinococcosis (B67.0-B67.9)
malaria (B50.0-B54)
schistosomiasis [bilharziasis] (B65.0-B65.9)
vitamin C deficiency (E54)

Excludes1   rupture of spleen due to Plasmodium vivax malaria (B51.0)
splenitis, splenomegaly in late syphilis (A52.79)
splenitis, splenomegaly in tuberculosis (A18.85)

INTRAOPERATIVE AND POSTPROCEDURAL COMPLICATIONS OF THE SPLEEN (D78)

● D78 **Intraoperative and postprocedural complications of the spleen**

● D78.0 **Intraoperative hemorrhage and hematoma of the spleen complicating a procedure**

Excludes1   intraoperative hemorrhage and hematoma of the spleen due to accidental puncture or laceration during a procedure (D78.1-)

(Ex) **For category D78.0 CC codes:** D78.01-D78.02, D78.21-D78.89, H95.811-H95.89, I85.01, I85.11, I97.3, K21.9, K22.8, K23-K25.0, K25.2, K25.4, K25.6, K26.0, K26.2, K26.4, K26.6, K27.0, K27.2, K27.4, K27.6, K28.0, K28.2, K28.4, K28.6, K29.01, K29.21, K29.31, K29.41, K29.51, K29.61, K29.71, K29.81, K29.91, K31.811, K55.21, K57.01, K57.11, K57.13, K57.21, K57.31, K57.33, K57.41, K57.51, K57.53, K57.81, K57.91, K57.93, K62.5, K92.0-K92.2, M96.89, N98.1-N98.9, P54.1-P54.3, T81.10X-T81.19X[A], T81.82X[A], T81.89X-T81.9XX[A]

D78.01   **Intraoperative hemorrhage and hematoma of the spleen complicating a procedure on the spleen** 🖉

D78.02   **Intraoperative hemorrhage and hematoma of the spleen complicating other procedure** 🖉

● D78.1 **Accidental puncture and laceration of the spleen during a procedure**

(Ex) **For category D78.1 CC codes:** D78.11-D78.12, D78.81-D78.89, E36.11-E36.8, E89.810-E89.89, G96.11, G97.41-G97.49, H59.011-H59.019, H59.031-H59.099, H59.211-H59.229, H59.811-H59.89, H95.31-H95.32, H95.811-H95.89, I97.3, I97.51-I97.52, J95.71-J95.72, K91.71-K91.72, L76.11-L76.12, L76.81-L76.82, M96.820-M96.821, M96.89, N98.1-N98.9, N99.71-N99.72, T81.82X[A], T81.89X-T81.9XX[A]

D78.11   **Accidental puncture and laceration of the spleen during a procedure on the spleen** 🖉

D78.12   **Accidental puncture and laceration of the spleen during other procedure** 🖉

● D78.2 **Postprocedural hemorrhage of the spleen following a procedure** ◀▥

(Ex) **For category D78.2 CC codes:** See D78.0

D78.21   **Postprocedural hemorrhage of the spleen following a procedure on the spleen** 🖉 ◀▥

D78.22   **Postprocedural hemorrhage of the spleen following other procedure** 🖉 ◀▥

● D78.3 **Postprocedural hematoma and seroma of the spleen following a procedure** ◀

(Ex) **For category D78.3 CC codes:** See D78.0

D78.31   **Postprocedural hematoma of the spleen following a procedure on the spleen** 🖉 ◀

D78.32   **Postprocedural hematoma of the spleen following other procedure** 🖉 ◀

D78.33   **Postprocedural seroma of the spleen following a procedure on the spleen** 🖉 ◀

D78.34   **Postprocedural seroma of the spleen following other procedure** 🖉 ◀

◀ New   ◀▥ Revised   ~~deleted~~ Deleted   Excludes 1   Excludes 2   Includes   Use additional   Code first   Code also   Unspecified

OGCR Official Guidelines   ● Unacceptable Principal Diagnosis   X Assign placeholder X   ● Use Additional Character(s)   ▷ Manifestation Code   **Coding Clinic**

● **D78.8   Other intraoperative and postprocedural complications of the spleen**
     Use additional code, if applicable, to further specify disorder
     ⒺⓍ **For category D78.8 CC codes:** D78.81-D78.89, H95.811-H95.89, I97.3, M96.89, N98.1-N98.9, T81.82X[A], T81.89X-T81.9XX[A]

  D78.81   Other intraoperative complications of the spleen 🔖

  D78.89   Other postprocedural complications of the spleen 🔖

CERTAIN DISORDERS INVOLVING THE IMMUNE MECHANISM (D80-D89)

Includes   defects in the complement system
              immunodeficiency disorders, except human immunodeficiency virus [HIV] disease
              sarcoidosis

Excludes1   autoimmune disease (systemic) NOS (M35.9)
              functional disorders of polymorphonuclear neutrophils (D71)
              human immunodeficiency virus [HIV] disease (B20)

● **D80   Immunodeficiency with predominantly antibody defects**
     ⒺⓍ **For category D80 CC codes unless otherwise indicated:** D80.0, D80.3-D81.4, D81.6-D81.7, D81.89-D84.0, D84.8-D84.9, D89.3-D89.9

  D80.0   Hereditary hypogammaglobulinemia 🔖
          Autosomal recessive agammaglobulinemia (Swiss type)
          X-linked agammaglobulinemia [Bruton] (with growth hormone deficiency)

  D80.1   Nonfamilial hypogammaglobulinemia 🔖
          Abnormally low levels of all classes of immunoglobulins
          Agammaglobulinemia with immunoglobulin-bearing B-lymphocytes
          Common variable agammaglobulinemia [CVAgamma]
          Hypogammaglobulinemia NOS
          ⒺⓍ D80.0-D81.2, D81.4, D81.6-D81.7, D81.89-D84.0, D84.8-D84.9, D89.3-D89.9

  D80.2   Selective deficiency of immunoglobulin A [IgA] 🔖
          ⒺⓍ See D80.1

  D80.3   Selective deficiency of immunoglobulin G [IgG] subclasses 🔖

  D80.4   Selective deficiency of immunoglobulin M [IgM] 🔖

  D80.5   Immunodeficiency with increased immunoglobulin M [IgM] 🔖

  D80.6   Antibody deficiency with near-normal immunoglobulins or with hyperimmunoglobulinemia 🔖
          Abnormally high levels of immunoglobulins in serum

  D80.7   Transient hypogammaglobulinemia of infancy 🔖

  D80.8   Other immunodeficiencies with predominantly antibody defects
          Kappa light chain deficiency

  D80.9   Immunodeficiency with predominantly antibody defects, unspecified 🔖

● **D81   Combined immunodeficiencies**
     Excludes1   autosomal recessive agammaglobulinemia (Swiss type) (D80.0)
     ⒺⓍ **For category D81 CC codes unless otherwise indicated:** See D80

  D81.0   Severe combined immunodeficiency [SCID] with reticular dysgenesis 🔖

  D81.1   Severe combined immunodeficiency [SCID] with low T- and B-cell numbers 🔖

  D81.2   Severe combined immunodeficiency [SCID] with low or normal B-cell numbers 🔖

  D81.3   Adenosine deaminase [ADA] deficiency 🔖
          ⒺⓍ D81.3, D81.5, D81.810, D84.1, E76.01-E76.9, E79.1-E80.29, E80.4-E80.7, E88.81

  D81.4   Nezelof's syndrome 🔖

  D81.5   Purine nucleoside phosphorylase [PNP] deficiency 🔖
          ⒺⓍ See D81.3

  D81.6   Major histocompatibility complex class I deficiency 🔖
          Bare lymphocyte syndrome

  D81.7   Major histocompatibility complex class II deficiency 🔖

● **D81.8   Other combined immunodeficiencies**

  ● **D81.81   Biotin-dependent carboxylase deficiency**
              Multiple carboxylase deficiency
              Excludes1   biotin-dependent carboxylase deficiency due to dietary deficiency of biotin (E53.8)

    D81.810   Biotinidase deficiency

    D81.818   Other biotin-dependent carboxylase deficiency
              Holocarboxylase synthetase deficiency
              Other multiple carboxylase deficiency

    D81.819   Biotin-dependent carboxylase deficiency, unspecified
              Multiple carboxylase deficiency, unspecified

  D81.89   Other combined immunodeficiencies 🔖

  D81.9   Combined immunodeficiency, unspecified 🔖
          Severe combined immunodeficiency disorder [SCID] NOS

● **D82   Immunodeficiency associated with other major defects**
     Excludes1   ataxia telangiectasia [Louis-Bar] (G11.3)

  D82.0   Wiskott-Aldrich syndrome 🔖
          X-linked immunodeficiency
          Immunodeficiency with thrombocytopenia and eczema
          ⒺⓍ See D80

  D82.1   Di George's syndrome 🔖
          Congenital disorder with defective development of third and fourth pharyngeal pouches
          Pharyngeal pouch syndrome
          Thymic alymphoplasia
          Thymic aplasia or hypoplasia with immunodeficiency
          ⒺⓍ See D80

  D82.2   Immunodeficiency with short-limbed stature

  D82.3   Immunodeficiency following hereditary defective response to Epstein-Barr virus
          X-linked lymphoproliferative disease

  D82.4   Hyperimmunoglobulin E [IgE] syndrome
          Suspected genetic defect that produces high levels of antibody immunoglobulin (IgE) that causes skin and lung infections and eczema

  D82.8   Immunodeficiency associated with other specified major defects

  D82.9   Immunodeficiency associated with major defect, unspecified

● **D83   Common variable immunodeficiency**
     ⒺⓍ **For category D83 CC codes:** See D80

  D83.0   Common variable immunodeficiency with predominant abnormalities of B-cell numbers and function 🔖

  D83.1   Common variable immunodeficiency with predominant immunoregulatory T-cell disorders 🔖

  D83.2   Common variable immunodeficiency with autoantibodies to B- or T-cells 🔖

  D83.8   Other common variable immunodeficiencies 🔖

  D83.9   Common variable immunodeficiency, unspecified 🔖

● **D84   Other immunodeficiencies**

  D84.0   Lymphocyte function antigen-1 [LFA-1] defect

  D84.1   Defects in the complement system
          C1 esterase inhibitor [C1-INH] deficiency

  D84.8   Other specified immunodeficiencies 🔖
          ⒺⓍ See D80

  D84.9   Immunodeficiency, unspecified 🔖
          ⒺⓍ See D80

N Newborn Age: 0   **P** Pediatric Age: 0–17   **M** Maternity DX: 12–55   **A** Adult Age: 15–124   ♀ Females Only   ♂ Males Only

 Complication\Comorbidity   Major C\C   ⒺⓍ CC/MCC Exclusions   Hospital-Acquired Condition

Item 3-1 Sarcoidosis: A symptom of an inflammation producing tiny lumps of cells (granulomas) in various organs, most commonly the lungs and lymph nodes, that affect organ function. Cause is unknown occurring primarily in 20- to 40-year-olds, African-American, especially women, and those of Asian, German, Irish, Scandinavian, and Puerto Rican heritage.

● **D86**   **Sarcoidosis**

     D86.0   **Sarcoidosis of lung**

     D86.1   **Sarcoidosis of lymph nodes**

     D86.2   **Sarcoidosis of lung with sarcoidosis of lymph nodes**

     D86.3   **Sarcoidosis of skin**

   ● **D86.8**   **Sarcoidosis of other sites**

         D86.81   **Sarcoid meningitis**

         D86.82   **Multiple cranial nerve palsies in sarcoidosis**

         D86.83   **Sarcoid iridocyclitis**
                Rare large tumor with irregular surface of iris

         D86.84   **Sarcoid pyelonephritis**
                Systemic disease of unknown etiology characterized by chronic granulomatous inflammation with tissue destruction of pelvis kidney
                Tubulo-interstitial nephropathy in sarcoidosis

         D86.85   **Sarcoid myocarditis**

         D86.86   **Sarcoid arthropathy**
                Polyarthritis in sarcoidosis

         D86.87   **Sarcoid myositis**
                Granumloma of muscle

         D86.89   **Sarcoidosis of other sites**
                Hepatic granuloma
                Uveoparotid fever [Heerfordt]

     D86.9   **Sarcoidosis, unspecified**

● **D89**   **Other disorders involving the immune mechanism, not elsewhere classified**

     Excludes1   hyperglobulinemia NOS (R77.1)
                monoclonal gammopathy (of undetermined significance) (D47.2)

     Excludes2   transplant failure and rejection (T86.-)

     D89.0   **Polyclonal hypergammaglobulinemia**
           Benign hypergammaglobulinemic purpura
           Polyclonal gammopathy NOS

     D89.1   **Cryoglobulinemia**
           Cryoglobulin (proteins) in blood that precipitate temperatures below 98.6° F; usually symptomatic of underlying disease
           Cryoglobulinemic purpura
           Cryoglobulinemic vasculitis
           Essential cryoglobulinemia
           Idiopathic cryoglobulinemia
           Mixed cryoglobulinemia
           Primary cryoglobulinemia
           Secondary cryoglobulinemia

     D89.2   **Hypergammaglobulinemia, unspecified**

     D89.3   **Immune reconstitution syndrome**
           Immune reconstitution inflammatory syndrome [IRIS]

           Use additional code for adverse effect, if applicable, to identify drug (T36-T50 with fifth or sixth character 5)

● **D89.4**   **Mast cell activation syndrome and related disorders** ◄

     Excludes1   aggressive systemic mastocytosis (C96.2) ◄
                cutaneous mastocytosis (Q82.2) ◄
                indolent systemic mastocytosis (D47.0) ◄
                malignant mastocytoma (C96.2) ◄
                mast cell leukemia (C94.3-) ◄
                mastocytoma (D47.0) ◄
                systemic mastocytosis associated with a clonal hematologic non-mast cell lineage disease (SM-AHNMD) (D47.0) ◄

     D89.40   **Mast cell activation, unspecified** ◄
           Mast cell activation disorder, unspecified ◄
           Mast cell activation syndrome, NOS ◄

     D89.41   **Monoclonal mast cell activation syndrome** ◄

     D89.42   **Idiopathic mast cell activation syndrome** ◄

     D89.43   **Secondary mast cell activation** ◄
           Secondary mast cell activation syndrome ◄

           Code also underlying etiology, if known ◄

     D89.49   **Other mast cell activation disorder** ◄
           Other mast cell activation syndrome ◄

● **D89.8**   **Other specified disorders involving the immune mechanism, not elsewhere classified**

   ● **D89.81**   **Graft-versus-host disease**

           Code first underlying cause, such as:
           complications of transplanted organs and tissue (T86.-)
           complications of blood transfusion (T80.89)

           Use additional code to identify associated manifestations, such as:
           desquamative dermatitis (L30.8)
           diarrhea (R19.7)
           elevated bilirubin (R17)
           hair loss (L65.9)
           (Ex) **For category D89.81 CC codes:** D78.81-D78.89, D89.810-D89.813, E89.810-E89.89, H59.011-H59.019, H59.031-H59.099, H59.811-H59.89, H95.811-H95.89, I97.3, M96.89, N98.1-N98.9, T86.00-T86.09

     ● **D89.810**   **Acute graft-versus-host disease** ✎

     ● **D89.811**   **Chronic graft-versus-host disease** ✎

     ● **D89.812**   **Acute on chronic graft-versus-host disease** ✎

     ● **D89.813**   **Graft-versus-host disease, unspecified** ✎

     D89.82   **Autoimmune lymphoproliferative syndrome [ALPS]**

     D89.89   **Other specified disorders involving the immune mechanism, not elsewhere classified**

         Excludes1   human immunodeficiency virus disease (B20)

     D89.9   **Disorder involving the immune mechanism, unspecified**
           Immune disease NOS
           Coding Clinic: 2015, Q3, P22

◄ New   ◄▥ Revised   ~~deleted~~ Deleted   Excludes 1   Excludes 2   Includes   Use additional   Code first   Code also   Unspecified

730   OGCR Official Guidelines   ● Unacceptable Principal Diagnosis   X Assign placeholder X   ● Use Additional Character(s)   ◢ Manifestation Code   **Coding Clinic**

CHAPTER 4

ENDOCRINE, NUTRITIONAL AND METABOLIC DISEASES (E00-E89)

OGCR Chapter-Specific Coding Guidelines

4. **Chapter 4: Endocrine, Nutritional, and Metabolic Diseases (E00-E89)**

   a. **Diabetes mellitus**
   The diabetes mellitus codes are combination codes that include the type of diabetes mellitus, the body system affected, and the complications affecting that body system. As many codes within a particular category as are necessary to describe all of the complications of the disease may be used. They should be sequenced based on the reason for a particular encounter. Assign as many codes from categories E08 – E13 as needed to identify all of the associated conditions that the patient has.

   1) **Type of diabetes**
   The age of a patient is not the sole determining factor, though most type 1 diabetics develop the condition before reaching puberty. For this reason type 1 diabetes mellitus is also referred to as juvenile diabetes.

   2) **Type of diabetes mellitus not documented**
   If the type of diabetes mellitus is not documented in the medical record the default is E11.-, Type 2 diabetes mellitus.

   3) **Diabetes mellitus and the use of insulin oral hypoglycemics**
   If the documentation in a medical record does not indicate the type of diabetes but does indicate that the patient uses insulin, code E11, Type 2 diabetes mellitus, should be assigned. Code Z79.4, Long-term (current) use of insulin **or Z79.84, Long term (current) use of oral hypoglycemic drugs**, should also be assigned to indicate that the patient uses insulin **or hypoglycemic drugs**. Code Z79.4 should not be assigned if insulin is given temporarily to bring a type 2 patient's blood sugar under control during an encounter.

   4) **Diabetes mellitus in pregnancy and gestational diabetes**
   See Section I.C.15. Diabetes mellitus in pregnancy.
   See Section I.C.15. Gestational (pregnancy induced) diabetes

   5) **Complications due to insulin pump malfunction**
      (a) **Underdose of insulin due to insulin pump failure**
   An underdose of insulin due to an insulin pump failure should be assigned to a code from subcategory T85.6, Mechanical complication of other specified internal and external prosthetic devices, implants and grafts, that specifies the type of pump malfunction, as the principal or first-listed code, followed by code T38.3X6-, Underdosing of insulin and oral hypoglycemic [antidiabetic] drugs. Additional codes for the type of diabetes mellitus and any associated complications due to the underdosing should also be assigned.

      (b) **Overdose of insulin due to insulin pump failure**
   The principal or first-listed code for an encounter due to an insulin pump malfunction resulting in an overdose of insulin, should also be T85.6-, Mechanical complication of other specified internal and external prosthetic devices, implants and grafts, followed by code T38.3X1-, Poisoning by insulin and oral hypoglycemic [antidiabetic] drugs, accidental (unintentional).

   6) **Secondary diabetes mellitus**
   Codes under categories E08, Diabetes mellitus due to underlying condition, E09, Drug or chemical induced diabetes mellitus and E13, Other specified diabetes mellitus, identify complications/ manifestations associated with secondary diabetes mellitus. Secondary diabetes is always caused by another condition or event (e.g., cystic fibrosis, malignant neoplasm of pancreas, pancreatectomy, adverse effect of drug, or poisoning).

      (a) **Secondary diabetes mellitus and the use of insulin or hypoglycemic drugs**
   For patients who routinely use insulin **or hypoglycemic drugs,** code Z79.4, Long-term (current) use of insulin **or Z79.84, Long term (current) use of oral hypoglycemic drugs**, should also be assigned. Code Z79.4 should not be assigned if insulin is given temporarily to bring a patient's blood sugar under control during an encounter.

      (b) **Assigning and sequencing secondary diabetes codes and its causes**
   The sequencing of the secondary diabetes codes in relationship to codes for the cause of the diabetes is based on the Tabular List instructions for categories E08, E09 and E13.

         (i) **Secondary diabetes mellitus due to pancreatectomy** For postpancreatectomy diabetes mellitus (lack of insulin due to the surgical removal of all or part of the pancreas), assign code E89.1, Postprocedural hypoinsulinemia. Assign a code from category E13 and a code from subcategory Z90.41-, Acquired absence of pancreas, as additional codes.

         (ii) **Secondary diabetes due to drugs** Secondary diabetes may be caused by an adverse effect of correctly administered medications, poisoning or sequela of poisoning.
   See section I.C.19.e for coding of adverse effects and poisoning, and section I.C.20 for external cause code reporting.

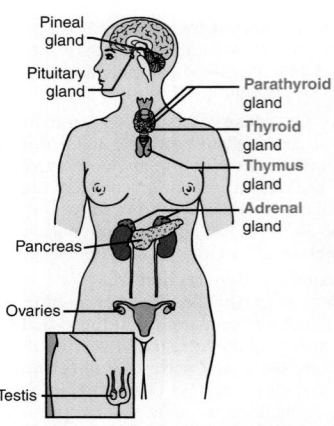

Figure 4-1 The endocrine system. (From Buck CJ: Step-by-Step Medical Coding, ed 2016, St. Louis, Elsevier, 2016)

CHAPTER 4

ENDOCRINE, NUTRITIONAL AND METABOLIC DISEASES (E00-E89)

All neoplasms, whether functionally active or not, are classified in Chapter 2. Appropriate codes in this chapter (i.e., E05.8, E07.0, E16-E31, E34.-) may be used as additional codes to indicate either functional activity by neoplasms and ectopic endocrine tissue or hyperfunction and hypofunction of endocrine glands associated with neoplasms and other conditions classified elsewhere.

Excludes1   transitory endocrine and metabolic disorders specific to newborn (P70-P74)

This chapter contains the following blocks:

E00-E07	Disorders of thyroid gland
E08-E13	Diabetes mellitus
E15-E16	Other disorders of glucose regulation and pancreatic internal secretion
E20-E35	Disorders of other endocrine glands
E36	Intraoperative complications of endocrine system
E40-E46	Malnutrition
E50-E64	Other nutritional deficiencies
E65-E68	Overweight, obesity and other hyperalimentation
E70-E88	Metabolic disorders
E89	Postprocedural endocrine and metabolic complications and disorders, not elsewhere classified

DISORDERS OF THYROID GLAND (E00-E07)

● **E00**   **Congenital iodine-deficiency syndrome**

Use additional code (F70-F79) to identify associated intellectual disabilities.

Excludes1   subclinical iodine-deficiency hypothyroidism (E02)

E00.0   **Congenital iodine-deficiency syndrome, neurological type**
Endemic cretinism, neurological type

E00.1   **Congenital iodine-deficiency syndrome, myxedematous type**
Dry, waxy type of swelling (nonpitting edema) with abnormal deposits of mucin in skin (mucinosis) and other tissues
Endemic hypothyroid cretinism
Endemic cretinism, myxedematous type

E00.2   **Congenital iodine-deficiency syndrome, mixed type**
Endemic cretinism, mixed type

E00.9   **Congenital iodine-deficiency syndrome, unspecified**
Congenital iodine-deficiency hypothyroidism NOS
Endemic cretinism NOS

Figure 4-2   Goiter is an enlargement of the thyroid gland.

Item 4–1   Simple goiter indicates no nodules are present. The most common type of goiter is a **diffuse colloidal,** also called a **nontoxic** or **endemic** goiter.

● **E01**   **Iodine-deficiency related thyroid disorders and allied conditions**

Excludes1   congenital iodine-deficiency syndrome (E00.-)
subclinical iodine-deficiency hypothyroidism (E02)

E01.0   **Iodine-deficiency related diffuse (endemic) goiter**
Thyroid gland is enlarged

E01.1   **Iodine-deficiency related multinodular (endemic) goiter**
Iodine-deficiency related nodular goiter

E01.2   **Iodine-deficiency related (endemic) goiter, unspecified**
Endemic goiter NOS

E01.8   **Other iodine-deficiency related thyroid disorders and allied conditions**
Acquired iodine-deficiency hypothyroidism NOS

E02   **Subclinical iodine-deficiency hypothyroidism**

● **E03**   **Other hypothyroidism**

Excludes1   iodine-deficiency related hypothyroidism (E00-E02)
postprocedural hypothyroidism (E89.0)

E03.0   **Congenital hypothyroidism with diffuse goiter**
Congenital parenchymatous goiter (nontoxic)
Congenital goiter (nontoxic) NOS

Excludes1   transitory congenital goiter with normal function (P72.0)

E03.1   **Congenital hypothyroidism without goiter**
Aplasia of thyroid (with myxedema)
Congenital atrophy of thyroid
Congenital hypothyroidism NOS

E03.2   **Hypothyroidism due to medicaments and other exogenous substances**
Code first poisoning due to drug or toxin, if applicable (T36-T65 with fifth or sixth character 1-4 or 6)
Use additional code for adverse effect, if applicable, to identify drug (T36-T50 with fifth or sixth character 5)

E03.3   **Postinfectious hypothyroidism**

E03.4   **Atrophy of thyroid (acquired)**

Excludes1   congenital atrophy of thyroid (E03.1)

Item 4–2   Hypothyroidism is a condition in which there are insufficient levels of thyroxine. **Cretinism** is congenital hypothyroidism, which can result in mental and physical retardation.

Figure 4-3 Typical appearance of patients with moderately severe primary hypothyroidism or myxedema. (From Larsen: Williams Textbook of Endocrinology, ed 10, Saunders, An Imprint of Elsevier, 2003)

◄ New   ◄ Revised   ~~deleted~~ Deleted   Excludes 1   Excludes 2   Includes   Use additional   Code first   Code also   Unspecified

OGCR Official Guidelines   ● Unacceptable Principal Diagnosis   X Assign placeholder X   ● Use Additional Character(s)   ▶ Manifestation Code   **Coding Clinic**

E03.5   Myxedema coma
Often fatal complication of long-term hypothyroidism
Ⓔ B15.0-B19.9, E03.5, E08.00-E08.59, E09.618-E09.59, E09.618-E10.59,
E10.618-E10.649, E10.69-E11.59, E11.618-E11.649, E11.69-E13.59,
E13.618-E16.2, E89.1, G32.89, G89.0-G89.4, G93.81-G93.9, G96.8-G96.9,
G98.0-G98.8, G99.8, I60.00-I62.9, K72.91, R29.700-R29.742, R40.0-R40.2124,
R40.2210-R40.2224, R40.2310-R40.2324, R40.2340-R40.2344, R40.3-R41.3,
R41.82, R41.9-R42, R45.83-R45.84, R44.8-R44.9, R45.83-R45.84, R46.0-R46.89, R52, R55,
R68.0-R68.83, R68.89-R69, S02.0XX-S02.19X[A,B], S02.91X,
S06.0X1[A], S06.0X9-S06.9X9[A]

E03.8   Other specified hypothyroidism
E03.9   Hypothyroidism, unspecified
Myxedema NOS

● **E04   Other nontoxic goiter**
Excludes1   congenital goiter (NOS) (diffuse)
(parenchymatous) (E03.0)
iodine-deficiency related goiter (E00-E02)

E04.0   Nontoxic diffuse goiter
Thyroid gland is enlarged
Diffuse (colloid) nontoxic goiter
Simple nontoxic goiter

E04.1   Nontoxic single thyroid nodule
Colloid nodule (cystic) (thyroid)
Nontoxic uninodular goiter
Thyroid (cystic) nodule NOS

E04.2   Nontoxic multinodular goiter
Enlarged thyroid gland with multiple nodules
Cystic goiter NOS
Multinodular (cystic) goiter NOS

E04.8   Other specified nontoxic goiter
E04.9   Nontoxic goiter, unspecified
Goiter NOS
Nodular goiter (nontoxic) NOS

● **E05   Thyrotoxicosis [hyperthyroidism]**
Enlarged thyroid gland with multiple nodules
Excludes1   chronic thyroiditis with transient thyrotoxicosis
(E06.2)
neonatal thyrotoxicosis (P72.1)
Ⓔ **For category E05 CC codes:** A17.9, A18.81-A18.82, A18.84, A18.89, E00.0-E03.4,
E03.8-E07.1, E07.89-E07.9, E30.9, E34.1, E34.50-E35, E89.0

● **E05.0   Thyrotoxicosis with diffuse goiter**
Exophthalmic or toxic goiter NOS
Graves' disease
Toxic diffuse goiter

**E05.00   Thyrotoxicosis with diffuse goiter without
thyrotoxic crisis or storm**
**E05.01   Thyrotoxicosis with diffuse goiter with
thyrotoxic crisis or storm**

● **E05.1   Thyrotoxicosis with toxic single thyroid nodule**
Thyrotoxicosis with toxic uninodular goiter

**E05.10   Thyrotoxicosis with toxic single thyroid nodule
without thyrotoxic crisis or storm**
**E05.11   Thyrotoxicosis with toxic single thyroid nodule
with thyrotoxic crisis or storm**

● **E05.2   Thyrotoxicosis with toxic multinodular goiter**
Toxic nodular goiter NOS

**E05.20   Thyrotoxicosis with toxic multinodular goiter
without thyrotoxic crisis or storm**
**E05.21   Thyrotoxicosis with toxic multinodular goiter
with thyrotoxic crisis or storm**

● **E05.3   Thyrotoxicosis from ectopic thyroid tissue**
**E05.30   Thyrotoxicosis from ectopic thyroid tissue
without thyrotoxic crisis or storm**
**E05.31   Thyrotoxicosis from ectopic thyroid tissue with
thyrotoxic crisis or storm**

● **E05.4   Thyrotoxicosis factitia**
**E05.40   Thyrotoxicosis factitia without thyrotoxic crisis
or storm**
**E05.41   Thyrotoxicosis factitia with thyrotoxic crisis or
storm**

● **E05.8   Other thyrotoxicosis**
Overproduction of thyroid-stimulating hormone
**E05.80   Other thyrotoxicosis without thyrotoxic crisis or
storm**
**E05.81   Other thyrotoxicosis with thyrotoxic crisis or
storm**

● **E05.9   Thyrotoxicosis, unspecified**
Hyperthyroidism NOS
**E05.90   Thyrotoxicosis, unspecified without thyrotoxic
crisis or storm**
**E05.91   Thyrotoxicosis, unspecified with thyrotoxic
crisis or storm**

● **E06   Thyroiditis**
*An inflammation of the thyroid gland which results in an inability to
convert iodine into thyroid hormone*
Excludes1   postpartum thyroiditis (O90.5)

E06.0   Acute thyroiditis
Abscess of thyroid
Pyogenic thyroiditis
Suppurative thyroiditis
Use additional code (B95-B97) to identify infectious
agent.
Ⓔ E06.0-E06.9

E06.1   Subacute thyroiditis
*Inflammation of thyroid gland following viral upper
respiratory infection*
de Quervain thyroiditis
Giant-cell thyroiditis
Granulomatous thyroiditis
Nonsuppurative thyroiditis
Viral thyroiditis
Excludes1   autoimmune thyroiditis (E06.3)

E06.2   Chronic thyroiditis with transient thyrotoxicosis
*Chronic inflammation of thyroid gland with intermittent
overproduction of thyroid hormone*
Excludes1   autoimmune thyroiditis (E06.3)

E06.3   Autoimmune thyroiditis
Hashimoto's thyroiditis
Hashitoxicosis (transient)
Lymphadenoid goiter
Lymphocytic thyroiditis
Struma lymphomatosa

E06.4   Drug-induced thyroiditis
Use additional code for adverse effect, if applicable,
to identify drug (T36-T50 with fifth or sixth
character 5)

E06.5   Other chronic thyroiditis
Chronic fibrous thyroiditis
Chronic thyroiditis NOS
Ligneous thyroiditis
Riedel thyroiditis

E06.9   Thyroiditis, unspecified

Figure 4-4   Graves' disease. In Graves'
disease, exophthalmos often looks more
pronounced than it actually is because of the
extreme lid retraction that may occur. This
patient, for instance, had minimal proptosis
of the left eye but marked lid retraction.
(Courtesy Dr. HG Scheie. From Yanoff M, Fine BS: Ocular Pathology, ed 6,
St. Louis, Mosby, 2008)

Item 4–3   Thyrotoxicosis is a condition caused by excessive amounts of the
thyroid hormone thyroxine production or hyperthyroidism. **Graves' disease
is associated with hyperthyroidism** (known as **Basedow's disease**
in Europe).

N Newborn Age: 0   **P** Pediatric Age: 0–17   **M** Maternity DX: 12–55   **A** Adult Age: 15–124   ♀ Females Only   ♂ Males Only
 Complication\Comorbidity   Major C\C   Ⓔ CC/MCC Exclusions   Hospital-Acquired Condition

733

CHAPTER 4 (E00-E90)

- **E07 Other disorders of thyroid**
  - **E07.0 Hypersecretion of calcitonin**
    C-cell hyperplasia of thyroid
    Hypersecretion of thyrocalcitonin
  - **E07.1 Dyshormogenetic goiter**
    Group of several types of goiter resulting from enzyme defects in hormone synthesis
    Familial dyshormogenetic goiter
    Pendred's syndrome
    Excludes1   transitory congenital goiter with normal function (P72.0)
  - **E07.8 Other specified disorders of thyroid**
    - **E07.81 Sick-euthyroid syndrome**
      Euthyroid sick-syndrome
    - **E07.89 Other specified disorders of thyroid**
      Abnormality of thyroid-binding globulin
      Hemorrhage of thyroid
      Infarction of thyroid
  - **E07.9 Disorder of thyroid, unspecified**

OGCR Section I.C.4.a

> **Diabetes mellitus**
>
> The diabetes mellitus codes are combination codes that include the type of diabetes mellitus, body system affected, and the complications affecting that body system. As many codes within a particular category as are necessary to describe all of the complications of the disease may be used. They should be sequenced based on the reason for a particular visit. Assign as many codes from categories E08–E13 as needed to identify all of the associated conditions that the patient has.

DIABETES MELLITUS (E08-E13)

A metabolic disease that results in persistent hyperglycemia.

- **E08 Diabetes mellitus due to underlying condition**
  Code first the underlying condition, such as:
  congenital rubella (P35.0)
  Cushing's syndrome (E24.-)
  cystic fibrosis (E84.-)
  malignant neoplasm (C00-C96)
  malnutrition (E40-E46)
  pancreatitis and other diseases of the pancreas (K85-K86.-)
  Use additional code to identify control using: ◀▥
  insulin (Z79.4) ◀
  oral antidiabetic drugs (Z79.84) ◀
  oral hypoglycemic drugs (Z79.84) ◀
  Excludes1   drug or chemical induced diabetes mellitus (E09.-)
  gestational diabetes (O24.4-)
  neonatal diabetes mellitus (P70.2)
  postpancreatectomy diabetes mellitus (E13.-)
  postprocedural diabetes mellitus (E13.-)
  secondary diabetes mellitus NEC (E13.-)
  type 1 diabetes mellitus (E10.-)
  type 2 diabetes mellitus (E11.-)
  - **E08.0 Diabetes mellitus due to underlying condition with hyperosmolarity**
    (Ex.) For category E08.0 CC codes: E08.00-E08.59, E08.618-E09.59, E09.618-E10.52, E10.59, E10.618-E10.649, E10.69-E11.59, E11.618-E11.649, E11.69-E13.59, E13.618-E16.2, E30.9, E34.1, E34.8-E35, E89.1
    - *E08.00 Diabetes mellitus due to underlying condition with hyperosmolarity without nonketotic hyperglycemic-hyperosmolar coma (NKHHC)* 🌢 🌢
    - *E08.01 Diabetes mellitus due to underlying condition with hyperosmolarity with coma* 🌢 🌢
  - **E08.1 Diabetes mellitus due to underlying condition with ketoacidosis**
    (Ex.) For category E08.1 CC codes: See E08.0
    - *E08.10 Diabetes mellitus due to underlying condition with ketoacidosis without coma* 🌢 🌢
    - *E08.11 Diabetes mellitus due to underlying condition with ketoacidosis with coma* 🌢

- **E08.2 Diabetes mellitus due to underlying condition with kidney complications**
  - *E08.21 Diabetes mellitus due to underlying condition with diabetic nephropathy*
    Diabetes mellitus due to underlying condition with intercapillary glomerulosclerosis
    Diabetes mellitus due to underlying condition with intracapillary glomerulonephrosis
    Diabetes mellitus due to underlying condition with Kimmelstiel-Wilson disease
  - *E08.22 Diabetes mellitus due to underlying condition with diabetic chronic kidney disease*
    Use additional code to identify stage of chronic kidney disease (N18.1-N18.6)
  - *E08.29 Diabetes mellitus due to underlying condition with other diabetic kidney complication*
    Renal tubular degeneration in diabetes mellitus due to underlying condition
- **E08.3 Diabetes mellitus due to underlying condition with ophthalmic complications**
  Changes in blood vessels of retina in which blood vessels swell and leak fluid into retinal surface.
  - **E08.31 Diabetes mellitus due to underlying condition with unspecified diabetic retinopathy**
    - *E08.311 Diabetes mellitus due to underlying condition with unspecified diabetic retinopathy with macular edema*
    - *E08.319 Diabetes mellitus due to underlying condition with unspecified diabetic retinopathy without macular edema*
  - **E08.32 Diabetes mellitus due to underlying condition with mild nonproliferative diabetic retinopathy**
    Diabetes mellitus due to underlying condition with nonproliferative diabetic retinopathy NOS
    One of the following 7th characters is to be assigned to codes in subcategory E08.32 to designate laterality of the disease: ◀

1	right eye ◀
2	left eye ◀
3	bilateral ◀
9	unspecified eye ◀

    - *E08.321 Diabetes mellitus due to underlying condition with mild nonproliferative diabetic retinopathy with macular edema*
    - *E08.329 Diabetes mellitus due to underlying condition with mild nonproliferative diabetic retinopathy without macular edema*
  - **E08.33 Diabetes mellitus due to underlying condition with moderate nonproliferative diabetic retinopathy**
    One of the following 7th characters is to be assigned to codes in subcategory E08.33 to designate laterality of the disease: ◀

1	right eye ◀
2	left eye ◀
3	bilateral ◀
9	unspecified eye ◀

    - *E08.331 Diabetes mellitus due to underlying condition with moderate nonproliferative diabetic retinopathy with macular edema*
    - *E08.339 Diabetes mellitus due to underlying condition with moderate nonproliferative diabetic retinopathy without macular edema*

◀ New   ◀▥ Revised   ~~deleted~~ Deleted   Excludes 1   Excludes 2   Includes   Use additional   Code first   Code also   Unspecified

OGCR Official Guidelines   ● Unacceptable Principal Diagnosis   X Assign placeholder X   ● Use Additional Character(s)   ▶ Manifestation Code   🌢 **Coding Clinic**

● **E08.34** **Diabetes mellitus due to underlying condition with severe nonproliferative diabetic retinopathy**

One of the following 7th characters is to be assigned to codes in subcategory E08.34 to designate laterality of the disease: ◄

1	right eye ◄
2	left eye ◄
3	bilateral ◄
9	unspecified eye ◄

● ▶ **E08.341** *Diabetes mellitus due to underlying condition with severe nonproliferative diabetic retinopathy with macular edema*

● ▶ **E08.349** *Diabetes mellitus due to underlying condition with severe nonproliferative diabetic retinopathy without macular edema*

● **E08.35** **Diabetes mellitus due to underlying condition with proliferative diabetic retinopathy**

One of the following 7th characters is to be assigned to codes in subcategory E08.35 to designate laterality of the disease: ◄

1	right eye ◄
2	left eye ◄
3	bilateral ◄
9	unspecified eye ◄

● ▶ **E08.351** *Diabetes mellitus due to underlying condition with proliferative diabetic retinopathy with macular edema*

● ▶ **E08.352** *Diabetes mellitus due to underlying condition with proliferative diabetic retinopathy with traction retinal detachment involving the macula* 🔗 ◄
(Ex:) G89.0-G89.4, I70.261-I70.269, I96, R29.700-R29.742, R41.0-R41.3, R41.82, R41.9, R44.8, R44.9, R45.83, R45.84, R46.0-R46.89, R52, R68.0-R68.19, R68.81-R68.83, R68.89-R69

● ▶ **E08.353** *Diabetes mellitus due to underlying condition with proliferative diabetic retinopathy with traction retinal detachment not involving the macula* ◄

● ▶ **E08.354** *Diabetes mellitus due to underlying condition with proliferative diabetic retinopathy with combined traction retinal detachment and rhegmatogenous retinal detachment* ◄

● ▶ **E08.355** *Diabetes mellitus due to underlying condition with stable proliferative diabetic retinopathy* ◄

● ▶ **E08.359** *Diabetes mellitus due to underlying condition with proliferative diabetic retinopathy without macular edema* ◄

▶ **E08.36** *Diabetes mellitus due to underlying condition with diabetic cataract*

X ● ▶ **E08.37** *Diabetes mellitus due to underlying condition with diabetic macular edema, resolved following treatment* ◄

One of the following 7th characters is to be assigned to code E08.37 to designate laterality of the disease: ◄

1	right eye ◄
2	left eye ◄
3	bilateral ◄
9	unspecified eye ◄

▶ **E08.39** *Diabetes mellitus due to underlying condition with other diabetic ophthalmic complication*

Use additional code to identify manifestation, such as:
diabetic glaucoma (H40-H42)

● **E08.4** **Diabetes mellitus due to underlying condition with neurological complications**

▶ **E08.40** *Diabetes mellitus due to underlying condition with diabetic neuropathy, unspecified*

▶ **E08.41** *Diabetes mellitus due to underlying condition with diabetic mononeuropathy*

▶ **E08.42** *Diabetes mellitus due to underlying condition with diabetic polyneuropathy*
Diabetes mellitus due to underlying condition with diabetic neuralgia

▶ **E08.43** *Diabetes mellitus due to underlying condition with diabetic autonomic (poly)neuropathy*
Diabetes mellitus due to underlying condition with diabetic gastroparesis

▶ **E08.44** *Diabetes mellitus due to underlying condition with diabetic amyotrophy*

▶ **E08.49** *Diabetes mellitus due to underlying condition with other diabetic neurological complication*

● **E08.5** **Diabetes mellitus due to underlying condition with circulatory complications**

▶ **E08.51** *Diabetes mellitus due to underlying condition with diabetic peripheral angiopathy without gangrene*

▶ **E08.52** *Diabetes mellitus due to underlying condition with diabetic peripheral angiopathy with gangrene* 🔗
Diabetes mellitus due to underlying condition with diabetic gangrene
CC when PDx is its own CC
(Ex:) G89.0-G89.4, I70.261-I70.269, I96, R41.0-R41.3, R41.82, R41.9, R44.8-R44.9, R45.83-R45.84, R46.0-R46.89, R52, R68.0-R68.19, R68.81-R68.83, R68.89-R69

▶ **E08.59** *Diabetes mellitus due to underlying condition with other circulatory complications*

● **E08.6** **Diabetes mellitus due to underlying condition with other specified complications**

● ▶ **E08.61** **Diabetes mellitus due to underlying condition with diabetic arthropathy**

▶ **E08.610** *Diabetes mellitus due to underlying condition with diabetic neuropathic arthropathy*
Diabetes mellitus due to underlying condition with Charcôt's joints

▶ **E08.618** *Diabetes mellitus due to underlying condition with other diabetic arthropathy*

● ▶ **E08.62** **Diabetes mellitus due to underlying condition with skin complications**

▶ **E08.620** *Diabetes mellitus due to underlying condition with diabetic dermatitis*
Diabetes mellitus due to underlying condition with diabetic necrobiosis lipoidica

▶ **E08.621** *Diabetes mellitus due to underlying condition with foot ulcer*
Use additional code to identify site of ulcer (L97.4-, L97.5-)

▶ **E08.622** *Diabetes mellitus due to underlying condition with other skin ulcer*
Use additional code to identify site of ulcer (L97.1-L97.9, L98.41-L98.49)

▶ **E08.628** *Diabetes mellitus due to underlying condition with other skin complications*

● ▶ **E08.63** **Diabetes mellitus due to underlying condition with oral complications**

▶ **E08.630** *Diabetes mellitus due to underlying condition with periodontal disease*

▶ **E08.638** *Diabetes mellitus due to underlying condition with other oral complications*

CHAPTER 4 (E00-E90)

● **E08.64** **Diabetes mellitus due to underlying condition with hypoglycemia**

▸ *E08.641*   *Diabetes mellitus due to underlying condition with hypoglycemia with coma* 🔒
         (Ex) See E08.0

▸ *E08.649*   *Diabetes mellitus due to underlying condition with hypoglycemia without coma*

▸ *E08.65*   *Diabetes mellitus due to underlying condition with hyperglycemia*

▸ *E08.69*   *Diabetes mellitus due to underlying condition with other specified complication*
       Use additional code to identify complication

▸ *E08.8*   *Diabetes mellitus due to underlying condition with unspecified complications*

▸ *E08.9*   *Diabetes mellitus due to underlying condition without complications*

● **E09**   **Drug or chemical induced diabetes mellitus**

     Code first poisoning due to drug or toxin, if applicable (T36-T65 with fifth or sixth character 1-4 or 6)

     Use additional code for adverse effect, if applicable, to identify drug (T36-T50 with fifth or sixth character 5)

     Use additional code to identify control using: ◂▥
       insulin (Z79.4) ◂
       oral antidiabetic drugs (Z79.84) ◂
       oral hypoglycemic drugs (Z79.84) ◂

     Excludes1   diabetes mellitus due to underlying condition (E08.-)
                gestational diabetes (O24.4-)
                neonatal diabetes mellitus (P70.2)
                postpancreatectomy diabetes mellitus (E13.-)
                postprocedural diabetes mellitus (E13.-)
                secondary diabetes mellitus NEC (E13.-)
                type 1 diabetes mellitus (E10.-)
                type 2 diabetes mellitus (E11.-)

● **E09.0**   **Drug or chemical induced diabetes mellitus with hyperosmolarity**
       (Ex) **For category E09.0 CC codes:** See E08.0

     E09.00   **Drug or chemical induced diabetes mellitus with hyperosmolarity without nonketotic hyperglycemic-hyperosmolar coma (NKHHC)** 🔒 🔒

     E09.01   **Drug or chemical induced diabetes mellitus with hyperosmolarity with coma** 🔒 🔒

● **E09.1**   **Drug or chemical induced diabetes mellitus with ketoacidosis**
       (Ex) **For category E09.1 CC codes:** See E08.0

     E09.10   **Drug or chemical induced diabetes mellitus with ketoacidosis without coma** 🔒 🔒

     E09.11   **Drug or chemical induced diabetes mellitus with ketoacidosis with coma** 🔒

● **E09.2**   **Drug or chemical induced diabetes mellitus with kidney complications**

     E09.21   **Drug or chemical induced diabetes mellitus with diabetic nephropathy**
         Drug or chemical induced diabetes mellitus with intercapillary glomerulosclerosis
         Drug or chemical induced diabetes mellitus with intracapillary glomerulonephrosis
         Drug or chemical induced diabetes mellitus with Kimmelstiel-Wilson disease

     E09.22   **Drug or chemical induced diabetes mellitus with diabetic chronic kidney disease**
         Use additional code to identify stage of chronic kidney disease (N18.1-N18.6)

     E09.29   **Drug or chemical induced diabetes mellitus with other diabetic kidney complication**
         Drug or chemical induced diabetes mellitus with renal tubular degeneration

● **E09.3**   **Drug or chemical induced diabetes mellitus with ophthalmic complications**

● **E09.31**   **Drug or chemical induced diabetes mellitus with unspecified diabetic retinopathy**

     E09.311   **Drug or chemical induced diabetes mellitus with unspecified diabetic retinopathy with macular edema**

     E09.319   **Drug or chemical induced diabetes mellitus with unspecified diabetic retinopathy without macular edema**

● **E09.32**   **Drug or chemical induced diabetes mellitus with mild nonproliferative diabetic retinopathy**
       Drug or chemical induced diabetes mellitus with nonproliferative diabetic retinopathy NOS

       One of the following 7th characters is to be assigned to codes in subcategory E09.32 to designate laterality of the disease: ◂

       | | |
       1   right eye ◂
       2   left eye ◂
       3   bilateral ◂
       9   unspecified eye ◂

     ● **E09.321**   **Drug or chemical induced diabetes mellitus with mild nonproliferative diabetic retinopathy with macular edema**

     ● **E09.329**   **Drug or chemical induced diabetes mellitus with mild nonproliferative diabetic retinopathy without macular edema**

● **E09.33**   **Drug or chemical induced diabetes mellitus with moderate nonproliferative diabetic retinopathy**

       One of the following 7th characters is to be assigned to codes in subcategory E09.33 to designate laterality of the disease: ◂

       1   right eye ◂
       2   left eye ◂
       3   bilateral ◂
       9   unspecified eye ◂

     ● **E09.331**   **Drug or chemical induced diabetes mellitus with moderate nonproliferative diabetic retinopathy with macular edema**

     ● **E09.339**   **Drug or chemical induced diabetes mellitus with moderate nonproliferative diabetic retinopathy without macular edema**

● **E09.34**   **Drug or chemical induced diabetes mellitus with severe nonproliferative diabetic retinopathy**

       One of the following 7th characters is to be assigned to codes in subcategory E09.34 to designate laterality of the disease: ◂

       1   right eye ◂
       2   left eye ◂
       3   bilateral ◂
       9   unspecified eye ◂

     ● **E09.341**   **Drug or chemical induced diabetes mellitus with severe nonproliferative diabetic retinopathy with macular edema**

     ● **E09.349**   **Drug or chemical induced diabetes mellitus with severe nonproliferative diabetic retinopathy without macular edema**

◂ New   ◂▥ Revised   ~~deleted~~ Deleted   Excludes 1   Excludes 2   Includes   Use additional   Code first   Code also   Unspecified
OGCR Official Guidelines   ● Unacceptable Principal Diagnosis   X Assign placeholder X   ● Use Additional Character(s)   ▸ Manifestation Code   **Coding Clinic**

● **E09.35**   **Drug or chemical induced diabetes mellitus with proliferative diabetic retinopathy**

One of the following 7th characters is to be assigned to codes in subcategory E09.35 to designate laterality of the disease: ◄

> 1   right eye ◄
> 2   left eye ◄
> 3   bilateral ◄
> 9   unspecified eye ◄

● **E09.351**   Drug or chemical induced diabetes mellitus with proliferative diabetic retinopathy with macular edema

● **E09.352**   Drug or chemical induced diabetes mellitus with proliferative diabetic retinopathy with traction retinal detachment involving the macula ◄

● **E09.353**   Drug or chemical induced diabetes mellitus with proliferative diabetic retinopathy with traction retinal detachment not involving the macula ◄

● **E09.354**   Drug or chemical induced diabetes mellitus with proliferative diabetic retinopathy with combined traction retinal detachment and rhegmatogenous retinal detachment ◄

● **E09.355**   Drug or chemical induced diabetes mellitus with stable proliferative diabetic retinopathy ◄

● **E09.359**   Drug or chemical induced diabetes mellitus with proliferative diabetic retinopathy without macular edema

E09.36   Drug or chemical induced diabetes mellitus with diabetic cataract

X ● **E09.37**   Drug or chemical induced diabetes mellitus with diabetic macular edema, resolved following treatment ◄

One of the following 7th characters is to be assigned to code E09.37 to designate laterality of the disease: ◄

> 1   right eye ◄
> 2   left eye ◄
> 3   bilateral ◄
> 9   unspecified eye ◄

E09.39   Drug or chemical induced diabetes mellitus with other diabetic ophthalmic complication

Use additional code to identify manifestation, such as:
    diabetic glaucoma (H40-H42)

● **E09.4**   **Drug or chemical induced diabetes mellitus with neurological complications**

E09.40   Drug or chemical induced diabetes mellitus with neurological complications with diabetic neuropathy, unspecified

E09.41   Drug or chemical induced diabetes mellitus with neurological complications with diabetic mononeuropathy

E09.42   Drug or chemical induced diabetes mellitus with neurological complications with diabetic polyneuropathy
    Drug or chemical induced diabetes mellitus with diabetic neuralgia

E09.43   Drug or chemical induced diabetes mellitus with neurological complications with diabetic autonomic (poly)neuropathy
    Drug or chemical induced diabetes mellitus with diabetic gastroparesis

E09.44   Drug or chemical induced diabetes mellitus with neurological complications with diabetic amyotrophy

E09.49   Drug or chemical induced diabetes mellitus with neurological complications with other diabetic neurological complication

● **E09.5**   **Drug or chemical induced diabetes mellitus with circulatory complications**

E09.51   Drug or chemical induced diabetes mellitus with diabetic peripheral angiopathy without gangrene

E09.52   Drug or chemical induced diabetes mellitus with diabetic peripheral angiopathy with gangrene 🗍
    Drug or chemical induced diabetes mellitus with diabetic gangrene
    CC when PDx is its own CC
    (Ex:) See E08.52

E09.59   Drug or chemical induced diabetes mellitus with other circulatory complications

● **E09.6**   **Drug or chemical induced diabetes mellitus with other specified complications**

● **E09.61**   Drug or chemical induced diabetes mellitus with diabetic arthropathy

E09.610   Drug or chemical induced diabetes mellitus with diabetic neuropathic arthropathy
    Drug or chemical induced diabetes mellitus with Charcôt's joints
    Progressive degeneration of weight-bearing joint

E09.618   Drug or chemical induced diabetes mellitus with other diabetic arthropathy

● **E09.62**   Drug or chemical induced diabetes mellitus with skin complications

E09.620   Drug or chemical induced diabetes mellitus with diabetic dermatitis
    Drug or chemical induced diabetes mellitus with diabetic necrobiosis lipoidica
    Necrotizing skin condition

E09.621   Drug or chemical induced diabetes mellitus with foot ulcer
    Use additional code to identify site of ulcer (L97.4-, L97.5-)

E09.622   Drug or chemical induced diabetes mellitus with other skin ulcer
    Use additional code to identify site of ulcer (L97.1-L97.9, L98.41-L98.49)

E09.628   Drug or chemical induced diabetes mellitus with other skin complications

● **E09.63**   Drug or chemical induced diabetes mellitus with oral complications

E09.630   Drug or chemical induced diabetes mellitus with periodontal disease

E09.638   Drug or chemical induced diabetes mellitus with other oral complications

● **E09.64**   Drug or chemical induced diabetes mellitus with hypoglycemia

E09.641   Drug or chemical induced diabetes mellitus with hypoglycemia with coma 🗍
    (Ex:) See E08.0

E09.649   Drug or chemical induced diabetes mellitus with hypoglycemia without coma

E09.65   Drug or chemical induced diabetes mellitus with hyperglycemia

E09.69   Drug or chemical induced diabetes mellitus with other specified complication
    Use additional code to identify complication

E09.8   Drug or chemical induced diabetes mellitus with unspecified complications

E09.9   Drug or chemical induced diabetes mellitus without complications

N Newborn Age: 0   **P** Pediatric Age: 0–17   **M** Maternity DX: 12–55   **A** Adult Age: 15–124   ♀ Females Only   ♂ Males Only

🗍 Complication\Comorbidity   🗍 Major C\C   (Ex:) CC/MCC Exclusions   🗍 Hospital-Acquired Condition

737

CHAPTER 4 (E00-E90)

CHAPTER 4 (E00-E90)

● **E10**   **Type 1 diabetes mellitus**

    Includes   brittle diabetes (mellitus)
                      diabetes (mellitus) due to autoimmune process
                      diabetes (mellitus) due to immune mediated
                         pancreatic islet beta-cell destruction
                      idiopathic diabetes (mellitus)
                      juvenile onset diabetes (mellitus)
                      ketosis-prone diabetes (mellitus)

    Excludes1   diabetes mellitus due to underlying condition
                       (E08.-)
                      drug or chemical induced diabetes mellitus (E09.-)
                      gestational diabetes (O24.4-)
                      hyperglycemia NOS (R73.9)
                      neonatal diabetes mellitus (P70.2)
                      postpancreatectomy diabetes mellitus (E13.-)
                      postprocedural diabetes mellitus (E13.-)
                      secondary diabetes mellitus NEC (E13.-)
                      type 2 diabetes mellitus (E11.-)

● **E10.1**   **Type 1 diabetes mellitus with ketoacidosis**
          Acidosis accompanied by accumulation of ketone bodies
          (ketosis) in body tissues and fluids
          Ex: **For category E.10.1 CC codes:** E08.00-E08.59, E08.618-E09.59,
          E09.618-E10.59, E10.618-E10.649, E10.69-E11.59, E11.618-E11.649,
          E11.69-E13.59, E13.618-E16.2, E30.9, E34.1, E34.50-E35, E89.1

    E10.10   **Type 1 diabetes mellitus with ketoacidosis**
               without coma 🚫 🚫
               Coding Clinic: 2013, Q3, P20

    E10.11   **Type 1 diabetes mellitus with ketoacidosis with**
               coma 🚫

● **E10.2**   **Type 1 diabetes mellitus with kidney complications**

    E10.21   **Type 1 diabetes mellitus with diabetic**
               nephropathy
               Type 1 diabetes mellitus with intercapillary
                  glomerulosclerosis
               Type 1 diabetes mellitus with intracapillary
                  glomerulonephrosis
               Type 1 diabetes mellitus with Kimmelstiel-
                  Wilson disease

    E10.22   **Type 1 diabetes mellitus with diabetic chronic**
               kidney disease
               Use additional code to identify stage of chronic
                  kidney disease (N18.1-N18.6)

    E10.29   **Type 1 diabetes mellitus with other diabetic**
               kidney complication
               Type 1 diabetes mellitus with renal tubular
                  degeneration
               Coding Clinic: 2016, Q1, P13

● **E10.3**   **Type 1 diabetes mellitus with ophthalmic complications**

  ● **E10.31**   **Type 1 diabetes mellitus with unspecified**
               diabetic retinopathy

       E10.311   **Type 1 diabetes mellitus**
                   with `unspecified` **diabetic retinopathy**
                   with macular edema

       E10.319   **Type 1 diabetes mellitus**
                   with `unspecified` **diabetic retinopathy**
                   without macular edema

  ● **E10.32**   **Type 1 diabetes mellitus with mild**
               nonproliferative diabetic retinopathy
               Type 1 diabetes mellitus with nonproliferative
                  diabetic retinopathy NOS

               One of the following 7th characters is to be
                  assigned to codes in subcategory E10.32 to
                  designate laterality of the disease: ◄

                1   right eye ◄
                2   left eye ◄
                3   bilateral ◄
                9   unspecified eye ◄

      ● **E10.321**   **Type 1 diabetes mellitus with mild**
                   nonproliferative diabetic retinopathy
                   with macular edema

      ● **E10.329**   **Type 1 diabetes mellitus with mild**
                   nonproliferative diabetic retinopathy
                   without macular edema

● **E10.33**   **Type 1 diabetes mellitus with moderate**
            nonproliferative diabetic retinopathy
          One of the following 7th characters is to be
            assigned to codes in subcategory E10.33 to
            designate laterality of the disease: ◄

         1   right eye ◄
         2   left eye ◄
         3   bilateral ◄
         9   unspecified eye ◄

  ● **E10.331**   **Type 1 diabetes mellitus with**
               moderate nonproliferative diabetic
               retinopathy with macular edema

  ● **E10.339**   **Type 1 diabetes mellitus with**
               moderate nonproliferative diabetic
               retinopathy without macular edema

● **E10.34**   **Type 1 diabetes mellitus with severe**
            nonproliferative diabetic retinopathy
          One of the following 7th characters is to be
            assigned to codes in subcategory E10.34 to
            designate laterality of the disease: ◄

         1   right eye ◄
         2   left eye ◄
         3   bilateral ◄
         9   unspecified eye ◄

  ● **E10.341**   **Type 1 diabetes mellitus with severe**
               nonproliferative diabetic retinopathy
               with macular edema

  ● **E10.349**   **Type 1 diabetes mellitus with severe**
               nonproliferative diabetic retinopathy
               without macular edema

● **E10.35**   **Type 1 diabetes mellitus with proliferative**
            diabetic retinopathy
          One of the following 7th characters is to be
            assigned to codes in subcategory E10.35 to
            designate laterality of the disease: ◄

         1   right eye ◄
         2   left eye ◄
         3   bilateral ◄
         9   unspecified eye ◄

  ● **E10.351**   **Type 1 diabetes mellitus with**
               proliferative diabetic retinopathy
               with macular edema

  ● **E10.352**   **Type 1 diabetes mellitus with**
               proliferative diabetic retinopathy
               with traction retinal detachment
               involving the macula ◄

  ● **E10.353**   **Type 1 diabetes mellitus with**
               proliferative diabetic retinopathy
               with traction retinal detachment not
               involving the macula ◄

  ● **E10.354**   **Type 1 diabetes mellitus with**
               proliferative diabetic retinopathy
               with combined traction retinal
               detachment and rhegmatogenous
               retinal detachment ◄

  ● **E10.355**   **Type 1 diabetes mellitus with stable**
               proliferative diabetic retinopathy ◄

  ● **E10.359**   **Type 1 diabetes mellitus with**
               proliferative diabetic retinopathy
               without macular edema

    E10.36   **Type 1 diabetes mellitus with diabetic cataract**

◄ New   ◄▬ Revised   ~~deleted~~ Deleted   Excludes 1   Excludes 2   Includes   Use additional   Code first   Code also   Unspecified

738   **OGCR** Official Guidelines   ● Unacceptable Principal Diagnosis   X Assign placeholder X   ● Use Additional Character(s)   ▌ Manifestation Code   **Coding Clinic**

X● **E10.37**   **Type 1 diabetes mellitus with diabetic macular edema, resolved following treatment** ◀

One of the following 7th characters is to be assigned to code E10.37 to designate laterality of the disease: ◀

> 1   right eye ◀
> 2   left eye ◀
> 3   bilateral ◀
> 9   unspecified eye ◀

E10.39   **Type 1 diabetes mellitus with other diabetic ophthalmic complication**

Use additional code to identify manifestation, such as:
diabetic glaucoma (H40-H42)

● **E10.4**   **Type 1 diabetes mellitus with neurological complications**

E10.40   **Type 1 diabetes mellitus with diabetic neuropathy, unspecified**

E10.41   **Type 1 diabetes mellitus with diabetic mononeuropathy**

E10.42   **Type 1 diabetes mellitus with diabetic polyneuropathy**

Type 1 diabetes mellitus with diabetic neuralgia

E10.43   **Type 1 diabetes mellitus with diabetic autonomic (poly)neuropathy**

Type 1 diabetes mellitus with diabetic gastroparesis

E10.44   **Type 1 diabetes mellitus with diabetic amyotrophy**

E10.49   **Type 1 diabetes mellitus with other diabetic neurological complication**

● **E10.5**   **Type 1 diabetes mellitus with circulatory complications**

E10.51   **Type 1 diabetes mellitus with diabetic peripheral angiopathy without gangrene**

E10.52   **Type 1 diabetes mellitus with diabetic peripheral angiopathy with gangrene**

Type 1 diabetes mellitus with diabetic gangrene 🦠
CC when PDx is its own CC
(Ex) See E08.52

E10.59   **Type 1 diabetes mellitus with other circulatory complications**

● **E10.6**   **Type 1 diabetes mellitus with other specified complications**

● **E10.61**   **Type 1 diabetes mellitus with diabetic arthropathy**

E10.610   **Type 1 diabetes mellitus with diabetic neuropathic arthropathy**

Type 1 diabetes mellitus with Charcôt's joints

E10.618   **Type 1 diabetes mellitus with other diabetic arthropathy**

● **E10.62**   **Type 1 diabetes mellitus with skin complications**

E10.620   **Type 1 diabetes mellitus with diabetic dermatitis**

Type 1 diabetes mellitus with diabetic necrobiosis lipoidica

E10.621   **Type 1 diabetes mellitus with foot ulcer**

Use additional code to identify site of ulcer (L97.4-, L97.5-)

E10.622   **Type 1 diabetes mellitus with other skin ulcer**

Use additional code to identify site of ulcer (L97.1-L97.9, L98.41-L98.49)

E10.628   **Type 1 diabetes mellitus with other skin complications**

● **E10.63**   **Type 1 diabetes mellitus with oral complications**

E10.630   **Type 1 diabetes mellitus with periodontal disease**

E10.638   **Type 1 diabetes mellitus with other oral complications**

● **E10.64**   **Type 1 diabetes mellitus with hypoglycemia**

E10.641   **Type 1 diabetes mellitus with hypoglycemia with coma** 🦠
(Ex) See E10.1

E10.649   **Type 1 diabetes mellitus with hypoglycemia without coma**
Coding Clinic: 2016, Q1, P13

E10.65   **Type 1 diabetes mellitus with hyperglycemia**
Coding Clinic: 2013, Q3, P20

E10.69   **Type 1 diabetes mellitus with other specified complication**

Use additional code to identify complication
Use this code with E10.65 to report hyperosmolarity in a Type 1 patient

E10.8   **Type 1 diabetes mellitus with unspecified complications**

E10.9   **Type 1 diabetes mellitus without complications**

● **E11**   **Type 2 diabetes mellitus**

Includes   diabetes (mellitus) due to insulin secretory defect
diabetes NOS
insulin resistant diabetes (mellitus)

Use additional code to identify control using: ◀
insulin (Z79.4) ◀
oral antidiabetic drugs (Z79.84) ◀
oral hypoglycemic drugs (Z79.84) ◀

Excludes1   diabetes mellitus due to underlying condition (E08.-)
drug or chemical induced diabetes mellitus (E09.-)
gestational diabetes (O24.4-)
neonatal diabetes mellitus (P70.2)
postpancreatectomy diabetes mellitus (E13.-)
postprocedural diabetes mellitus (E13.-)
secondary diabetes mellitus NEC (E13.-)
type 1 diabetes mellitus (E10.-)

Coding Clinic: 2016, Q2, P10

● **E11.0**   **Type 2 diabetes mellitus with hyperosmolarity**
(Ex) For category E11.0 CC codes: See E08.0

E11.00   **Type 2 diabetes mellitus with hyperosmolarity without nonketotic hyperglycemic-hyperosmolar coma (NKHHC)** 🦠 🦠

E11.01   **Type 2 diabetes mellitus with hyperosmolarity with coma** 🦠 🦠

● **E11.2**   **Type 2 diabetes mellitus with kidney complications**

E11.21   **Type 2 diabetes mellitus with diabetic nephropathy**

Type 2 diabetes mellitus with intercapillary glomerulosclerosis
Type 2 diabetes mellitus with intracapillary glomerulonephrosis
Type 2 diabetes mellitus with Kimmelstiel-Wilson disease

E11.22   **Type 2 diabetes mellitus with diabetic chronic kidney disease**

Use additional code to identify stage of chronic kidney disease (N18.1-N18.6)
Coding Clinic: 2016, Q2, P36, Q1, P13

E11.29   **Type 2 diabetes mellitus with other diabetic kidney complication**

Type 2 diabetes mellitus with renal tubular degeneration

N Newborn Age: Ø   **P** Pediatric Age: Ø–17   **M** Maternity DX: 12–55   **A** Adult Age: 15–124   ♀ Females Only   ♂ Males Only

🦠 Complication\Comorbidity   🦠 Major C\C   (Ex) CC/MCC Exclusions   🦠 Hospital-Acquired Condition

CHAPTER 4 (E00-E90)

739

- E11.3　Type 2 diabetes mellitus with ophthalmic complications
  - E11.31　Type 2 diabetes mellitus with unspecified diabetic retinopathy
    - E11.311　Type 2 diabetes mellitus with `unspecified` diabetic retinopathy with macular edema
    - E11.319　Type 2 diabetes mellitus with `unspecified` diabetic retinopathy without macular edema
      Coding Clinic: 2013, Q3, P20
  - E11.32　Type 2 diabetes mellitus with mild nonproliferative diabetic retinopathy

    Type 2 diabetes mellitus with nonproliferative diabetic retinopathy NOS

    One of the following 7th characters is to be assigned to codes in subcategory E11.32 to designate laterality of the disease: ◀

1	right eye ◀
2	left eye ◀
3	bilateral ◀
9	unspecified eye ◀

    - E11.321　Type 2 diabetes mellitus with mild nonproliferative diabetic retinopathy with macular edema
    - E11.329　Type 2 diabetes mellitus with mild nonproliferative diabetic retinopathy without macular edema
  - E11.33　Type 2 diabetes mellitus with moderate nonproliferative diabetic retinopathy

    One of the following 7th characters is to be assigned to codes in subcategory E11.33 to designate laterality of the disease: ◀

1	right eye ◀
2	left eye ◀
3	bilateral ◀
9	unspecified eye ◀

    - E11.331　Type 2 diabetes mellitus with moderate nonproliferative diabetic retinopathy with macular edema
    - E11.339　Type 2 diabetes mellitus with moderate nonproliferative diabetic retinopathy without macular edema
  - E11.34　Type 2 diabetes mellitus with severe nonproliferative diabetic retinopathy

    One of the following 7th characters is to be assigned to codes in subcategory E11.34 to designate laterality of the disease: ◀

1	right eye ◀
2	left eye ◀
3	bilateral ◀
9	unspecified eye ◀

    - E11.341　Type 2 diabetes mellitus with severe nonproliferative diabetic retinopathy with macular edema
    - E11.349　Type 2 diabetes mellitus with severe nonproliferative diabetic retinopathy without macular edema

- E11.35　Type 2 diabetes mellitus with proliferative diabetic retinopathy

  One of the following 7th characters is to be assigned to codes in subcategory E11.35 to designate laterality of the disease: ◀

1	right eye ◀
2	left eye ◀
3	bilateral ◀
9	unspecified eye ◀

  - E11.351　Type 2 diabetes mellitus with proliferative diabetic retinopathy with macular edema
  - E11.352　Type 2 diabetes mellitus with proliferative diabetic retinopathy with traction retinal detachment involving the macula ◀
  - E11.353　Type 2 diabetes mellitus with proliferative diabetic retinopathy with traction retinal detachment not involving the macula ◀
  - E11.354　Type 2 diabetes mellitus with proliferative diabetic retinopathy with combined traction retinal detachment and rhegmatogenous retinal detachment ◀
  - E11.355　Type 2 diabetes mellitus with stable proliferative diabetic retinopathy ◀
  - E11.359　Type 2 diabetes mellitus with proliferative diabetic retinopathy without macular edema
  - E11.36　Type 2 diabetes mellitus with diabetic cataract
    Coding Clinic: 2016, Q2, P36
  - X ● E11.37　Type 2 diabetes mellitus with diabetic macular edema, resolved following treatment ◀

    One of the following 7th characters is to be assigned to code E11.37 to designate laterality of the disease: ◀

1	right eye ◀
2	left eye ◀
3	bilateral ◀
9	unspecified eye ◀

  - E11.39　Type 2 diabetes mellitus with other diabetic ophthalmic complication

    Use additional code to identify manifestation, such as:
    diabetic glaucoma (H40-H42)

- E11.4　Type 2 diabetes mellitus with neurological complications
  - E11.40　Type 2 diabetes mellitus with diabetic neuropathy, `unspecified`
  - E11.41　Type 2 diabetes mellitus with diabetic mononeuropathy
  - E11.42　Type 2 diabetes mellitus with diabetic polyneuropathy

    Type 2 diabetes mellitus with diabetic neuralgia
    Coding Clinic: 2016, Q1, P13
  - E11.43　Type 2 diabetes mellitus with diabetic autonomic (poly)neuropathy

    Type 2 diabetes mellitus with diabetic gastroparesis
    Coding Clinic: 2016, Q2, P36
  - E11.44　Type 2 diabetes mellitus with diabetic amyotrophy
    Coding Clinic: 2016, Q2, P36
  - E11.49　Type 2 diabetes mellitus with other diabetic neurological complication

◀ New　◀▭ Revised　~~deleted~~ Deleted　Excludes 1　Excludes 2　Includes　Use additional　Code first　Code also　Unspecified
OGCR Official Guidelines　● Unacceptable Principal Diagnosis　X Assign placeholder X　● Use Additional Character(s)　◀ Manifestation Code　Coding Clinic

● **E11.5**   **Type 2 diabetes mellitus with circulatory complications**

     E11.51   **Type 2 diabetes mellitus with diabetic peripheral angiopathy without gangrene**

     E11.52   **Type 2 diabetes mellitus with diabetic peripheral angiopathy with gangrene**
         Type 2 diabetes mellitus with diabetic gangrene 🗌
         CC when PDx is its own CC
         (Ex) See E08.52

     E11.59   **Type 2 diabetes mellitus with other circulatory complications**

● **E11.6**   **Type 2 diabetes mellitus with other specified complications**

   ● **E11.61**   **Type 2 diabetes mellitus with diabetic arthropathy**

     E11.610   **Type 2 diabetes mellitus with diabetic neuropathic arthropathy**
         Type 2 diabetes mellitus with Charcôt's joints
         Coding Clinic: 2016, Q2, P36

     E11.618   **Type 2 diabetes mellitus with other diabetic arthropathy**
         Coding Clinic: 2016, Q2, P36

   ● **E11.62**   **Type 2 diabetes mellitus with skin complications**

     E11.620   **Type 2 diabetes mellitus with diabetic dermatitis**
         Type 2 diabetes mellitus with diabetic necrobiosis lipoidica

     E11.621   **Type 2 diabetes mellitus with foot ulcer**
         Use additional code to identify site of ulcer (L97.4-, L97.5-)
         Coding Clinic: 2016, Q1, P12

     E11.622   **Type 2 diabetes mellitus with other skin ulcer**
         Use additional code to identify site of ulcer (L97.1-L97.9, L98.41-L98.49)

     E11.628   **Type 2 diabetes mellitus with other skin complications**

   ● **E11.63**   **Type 2 diabetes mellitus with oral complications**

     E11.630   **Type 2 diabetes mellitus with periodontal disease**

     E11.638   **Type 2 diabetes mellitus with other oral complications**

   ● **E11.64**   **Type 2 diabetes mellitus with hypoglycemia**

     E11.641   **Type 2 diabetes mellitus with hypoglycemia with coma** 🗌
         (Ex) See E08.0

     E11.649   **Type 2 diabetes mellitus with hypoglycemia without coma**
         Coding Clinic: 2015, Q3, P21

     E11.65   **Type 2 diabetes mellitus with hyperglycemia**
         Coding Clinic: 2013, Q3, P20

     E11.69   **Type 2 diabetes mellitus with other specified complication**
         Use additional code to identify complication
         Use this code with E11.65 to report DKA in a Type 2 patient

   E11.8   **Type 2 diabetes mellitus with unspecified complications**

   E11.9   **Type 2 diabetes mellitus without complications**
     MCE: Questionable admission when principal dx
     Coding Clinic: 2016, Q2, P36

● **E13**   **Other specified diabetes mellitus**

   Includes   diabetes mellitus due to genetic defects of beta-cell function
         diabetes mellitus due to genetic defects in insulin action
         postpancreatectomy diabetes mellitus
         postprocedural diabetes mellitus
         secondary diabetes mellitus NEC

   Use additional code to identify control using: ◄🔲
     insulin (Z79.4) ◄
     oral antidiabetic drugs (Z79.84) ◄
     oral hypoglycemic drugs (Z79.84) ◄

   Excludes1   diabetes (mellitus) due to autoimmune process (E10.-)
         diabetes (mellitus) due to immune mediated pancreatic islet beta-cell destruction (E10.-)
         diabetes mellitus due to underlying condition (E08.-)
         drug or chemical induced diabetes mellitus (E09.-)
         gestational diabetes (O24.4-)
         neonatal diabetes mellitus (P70.2)
         type 1 diabetes mellitus (E10.-) ◄
         type 2 diabetes mellitus (E11.-)

● **E13.0**   **Other specified diabetes mellitus with hyperosmolarity**
     (Ex) For category E13.0 CC codes: See E08.0

     E13.00   **Other specified diabetes mellitus with hyperosmolarity without nonketotic hyperglycemic-hyperosmolar coma (NKHHC)** 🗌 🗌

     E13.01   **Other specified diabetes mellitus with hyperosmolarity with coma** 🗌 🗌

● **E13.1**   **Other specified diabetes mellitus with ketoacidosis**
     (Ex) For category E13.1 CC codes: See E08.0

     E13.10   **Other specified diabetes mellitus with ketoacidosis without coma** 🗌 🗌
         Coding Clinic: 2016, Q2, P10; 2013, Q1, P26

     E13.11   **Other specified diabetes mellitus with ketoacidosis with coma** 🗌

● **E13.2**   **Other specified diabetes mellitus with kidney complications**

     E13.21   **Other specified diabetes mellitus with diabetic nephropathy**
         Other specified diabetes mellitus with intercapillary glomerulosclerosis
         Other specified diabetes mellitus with intracapillary glomerulonephrosis
         Other specified diabetes mellitus with Kimmelstiel-Wilson disease

     E13.22   **Other specified diabetes mellitus with diabetic chronic kidney disease**
         Use additional code to identify stage of chronic kidney disease (N18.1-N18.6)

     E13.29   **Other specified diabetes mellitus with other diabetic kidney complication**
         Other specified diabetes mellitus with renal tubular degeneration

● **E13.3**   **Other specified diabetes mellitus with ophthalmic complications**

   ● **E13.31**   **Other specified diabetes mellitus with unspecified diabetic retinopathy**

     E13.311   **Other specified diabetes mellitus with unspecified diabetic retinopathy with macular edema**

     E13.319   **Other specified diabetes mellitus with unspecified diabetic retinopathy without macular edema**

CHAPTER 4 (E00-E90)

N   Newborn Age: 0   **P**   Pediatric Age: 0–17   **M**   Maternity DX: 12–55   **A**   Adult Age: 15–124   ♀   Females Only   ♂   Males Only

🗌   Complication\Comorbidity   🗌   Major C\C   (Ex)   CC/MCC Exclusions   🗌   Hospital-Acquired Condition

741

● **E13.32**   **Other specified diabetes mellitus with mild nonproliferative diabetic retinopathy**

Other specified diabetes mellitus with nonproliferative diabetic retinopathy NOS

One of the following 7th characters is to be assigned to codes in subcategory E13.32 to designate laterality of the disease: ◄

1	right eye ◄
2	left eye ◄
3	bilateral ◄
9	unspecified eye ◄

● **E13.321**   **Other specified diabetes mellitus with mild nonproliferative diabetic retinopathy with macular edema**

● **E13.329**   **Other specified diabetes mellitus with mild nonproliferative diabetic retinopathy without macular edema**

● **E13.33**   **Other specified diabetes mellitus with moderate nonproliferative diabetic retinopathy**

One of the following 7th characters is to be assigned to codes in subcategory E13.33 to designate laterality of the disease: ◄

1	right eye ◄
2	left eye ◄
3	bilateral ◄
9	unspecified eye ◄

● **E13.331**   **Other specified diabetes mellitus with moderate nonproliferative diabetic retinopathy with macular edema**

● **E13.339**   **Other specified diabetes mellitus with moderate nonproliferative diabetic retinopathy without macular edema**

● **E13.34**   **Other specified diabetes mellitus with severe nonproliferative diabetic retinopathy**

One of the following 7th characters is to be assigned to codes in subcategory E13.34 to designate laterality of the disease: ◄

1	right eye ◄
2	left eye ◄
3	bilateral ◄
9	unspecified eye ◄

● **E13.341**   **Other specified diabetes mellitus with severe nonproliferative diabetic retinopathy with macular edema**

● **E13.349**   **Other specified diabetes mellitus with severe nonproliferative diabetic retinopathy without macular edema**

● **E13.35**   **Other specified diabetes mellitus with proliferative diabetic retinopathy**

One of the following 7th characters is to be assigned to codes in subcategory E13.35 to designate laterality of the disease: ◄

1	right eye ◄
2	left eye ◄
3	bilateral ◄
9	unspecified eye ◄

● **E13.351**   **Other specified diabetes mellitus with proliferative diabetic retinopathy with macular edema**

● **E13.352**   **Other specified diabetes mellitus with proliferative diabetic retinopathy with traction retinal detachment involving the macula ◄**

● **E13.353**   **Other specified diabetes mellitus with proliferative diabetic retinopathy with traction retinal detachment not involving the macula ◄**

● **E13.354**   **Other specified diabetes mellitus with proliferative diabetic retinopathy with combined traction retinal detachment and rhegmatogenous retinal detachment ◄**

● **E13.355**   **Other specified diabetes mellitus with stable proliferative diabetic retinopathy ◄**

● **E13.359**   **Other specified diabetes mellitus with proliferative diabetic retinopathy without macular edema**

E13.36   **Other specified diabetes mellitus with diabetic cataract**

X ● **E13.37**   **Other specified diabetes mellitus with diabetic macular edema, resolved following treatment**

One of the following 7th characters is to be assigned to code E13.37 to designate laterality of the disease: ◄

1	right eye ◄
2	left eye ◄
3	bilateral ◄
9	unspecified eye ◄

E13.39   **Other specified diabetes mellitus with other diabetic ophthalmic complication**

Use additional code to identify manifestation, such as:
diabetic glaucoma (H40-H42)

● **E13.4**   **Other specified diabetes mellitus with neurological complications**

E13.40   **Other specified diabetes mellitus with diabetic neuropathy, unspecified**

E13.41   **Other specified diabetes mellitus with diabetic mononeuropathy**

E13.42   **Other specified diabetes mellitus with diabetic polyneuropathy**

Other specified diabetes mellitus with diabetic neuralgia

E13.43   **Other specified diabetes mellitus with diabetic autonomic (poly)neuropathy**

Other specified diabetes mellitus with diabetic gastroparesis

E13.44   **Other specified diabetes mellitus with diabetic amyotrophy**

E13.49   **Other specified diabetes mellitus with other diabetic neurological complication**

● **E13.5**   **Other specified diabetes mellitus with circulatory complications**

E13.51   **Other specified diabetes mellitus with diabetic peripheral angiopathy without gangrene**

E13.52   **Other specified diabetes mellitus with diabetic peripheral angiopathy with gangrene**

Other specified diabetes mellitus with diabetic gangrene

CC when PDx is its own CC

Ex) See E08.52

E13.59   **Other specified diabetes mellitus with other circulatory complications**

● **E13.6**   **Other specified diabetes mellitus with other specified complications**

● **E13.61**   **Other specified diabetes mellitus with diabetic arthropathy**

E13.610   **Other specified diabetes mellitus with diabetic neuropathic arthropathy**

Other specified diabetes mellitus with Charcôt's joints

E13.618   **Other specified diabetes mellitus with other diabetic arthropathy**

◄ New   ⟸ Revised   ~~deleted~~ Deleted   Excludes 1   Excludes 2   Includes   Use additional   Code first   Code also   Unspecified

OGCR Official Guidelines   ● Unacceptable Principal Diagnosis   X Assign placeholder X   ● Use Additional Character(s)   ▶ Manifestation Code   **Coding Clinic**

CHAPTER 4 (E00-E90)

● **E13.62 Other specified diabetes mellitus with skin complications**

    E13.620 Other specified diabetes mellitus with diabetic dermatitis
        Other specified diabetes mellitus with diabetic necrobiosis lipoidica

    E13.621 Other specified diabetes mellitus with foot ulcer
        Use additional code to identify site of ulcer (L97.4-, L97.5-)

    E13.622 Other specified diabetes mellitus with other skin ulcer
        Use additional code to identify site of ulcer (L97.1-L97.9, L98.41-L98.49)

    E13.628 Other specified diabetes mellitus with other skin complications

● **E13.63 Other specified diabetes mellitus with oral complications**

    E13.630 Other specified diabetes mellitus with periodontal disease

    E13.638 Other specified diabetes mellitus with other oral complications

● **E13.64 Other specified diabetes mellitus with hypoglycemia**

    E13.641 Other specified diabetes mellitus with hypoglycemia with coma
        (Ex) See E08.0

    E13.649 Other specified diabetes mellitus with hypoglycemia without coma

E13.65 Other specified diabetes mellitus with hyperglycemia

E13.69 Other specified diabetes mellitus with other specified complication
    Use additional code to identify complication

E13.8 Other specified diabetes mellitus with unspecified complications

E13.9 Other specified diabetes mellitus without complications
    MCE: Questionable admission when principal dx

OTHER DISORDERS OF GLUCOSE REGULATION AND PANCREATIC INTERNAL SECRETION (E15-E16)

E15 Nondiabetic hypoglycemic coma 🔵 🔵

    Includes drug-induced insulin coma in nondiabetic
    hyperinsulinism with hypoglycemic coma
    hypoglycemic coma NOS

    (Ex) A74.81, A74.9, B33.3-B33.4, B34.1-B34.2, B34.4-B34.8, B97.10, B97.19-B97.29,
    B97.31-B97.39, B97.5-B97.6, B97.81-B97.89, E08.3211-E08.3299, E08.3311-E08.3499,
    E08.3511-E08.3599, E08.37X1-E08.37X9, E09.3211-E09.3319, E09.3391-E09.3399,
    E09.3411-E09.3419, E09.3491-E09.3499, E09.3511-E09.3599, E09.37X1-E09.37X9,
    E10.3211-E10.3599, E10.37X1-E10.37X9, E11.3211-E11.3599, E11.37X1-E11.37X9,
    E13.3211-E13.3599, E13.37X1-E13.37X9

● **E16 Other disorders of pancreatic internal secretion**

E16.0 Drug-induced hypoglycemia without coma

    Excludes1 diabetes with hypoglycemia without coma (E09.692) ◄

    Use additional code for adverse effect, if applicable, to identify drug (T36-T50 with fifth or sixth character 5)

E16.1 Other hypoglycemia
    Functional hyperinsulinism
    Functional nonhyperinsulinemic hypoglycemia
    Hyperinsulinism NOS
    Hyperplasia of pancreatic islet beta cells NOS

    Excludes1 diabetes with hypoglycemia (E08.649, E10.649, E11.649, E13.649) ◄
    hypoglycemia in infant of diabetic mother (P70.1)
    neonatal hypoglycemia (P70.4)

E16.2 Hypoglycemia, unspecified

    Excludes1 diabetes with hypoglycemia (E08.649, E10.649, E11.649, E13.649) ◄

E16.3 Increased secretion of glucagon
    Hyperplasia of pancreatic endocrine cells with glucagon excess

E16.4 Increased secretion of gastrin
    Hypergastrinemia
    Hyperplasia of pancreatic endocrine cells with gastrin excess
    Zollinger-Ellison syndrome

E16.8 Other specified disorders of pancreatic internal secretion
    Increased secretion from endocrine pancreas of growth hormone-releasing hormone
    Increased secretion from endocrine pancreas of pancreatic polypeptide
    Increased secretion from endocrine pancreas of somatostatin
    Increased secretion from endocrine pancreas of vasoactive-intestinal polypeptide

E16.9 Disorder of pancreatic internal secretion, unspecified
    Islet-cell hyperplasia NOS
    Pancreatic endocrine cell hyperplasia NOS

DISORDERS OF OTHER ENDOCRINE GLANDS (E20-E35)

    Excludes1 galactorrhea (N64.3)
    gynecomastia (N62)

● **E20 Hypoparathyroidism**
    Greatly reduced function of parathyroid glands; AKA parathyroid insufficiency

    Excludes1 Di George's syndrome (D82.1)
    postprocedural hypoparathyroidism (E89.2)
    tetany NOS (R29.0)
    transitory neonatal hypoparathyroidism (P71.4)

E20.0 Idiopathic hypoparathyroidism
    Rare condition, unknown cause; short dwarf-like with round face

E20.1 Pseudohypoparathyroidism
    Hereditary condition resembling hypoparathyroidism, but caused by inability to respond to parathyroid hormone

E20.8 Other hypoparathyroidism

E20.9 Hypoparathyroidism, unspecified
    Parathyroid tetany

● **E21 Hyperparathyroidism and other disorders of parathyroid gland**

    Excludes1 adult osteomalacia (M83.-)
    ectopic hyperparathyroidism (E34.2)
    familial hypocalciuric hypercalcemia (E83.52)
    hungry bone syndrome (E83.81)
    infantile and juvenile osteomalacia (E55.0)

E21.0 Primary hyperparathyroidism
    Hyperplasia of parathyroid
    Osteitis fibrosa cystica generalisata [von Recklinghausen's disease of bone]

E21.1 Secondary hyperparathyroidism, not elsewhere classified

    Excludes1 secondary hyperparathyroidism of renal origin (N25.81)

Item 4–4 Hyperparathyroidism is an overactive parathyroid gland that secretes excessive parathormone, causing increased levels of circulating calcium. This results in a loss of calcium in the bone (osteoporosis).
Hypoparathyroidism is an underactive parathyroid gland that results in decreased levels of circulating calcium. The primary manifestation is **tetany,** a continuous muscle spasm.

Figure 4-5 Tetany caused by hypoparathyroidism.

CHAPTER 4 (E00-E90)

N Newborn Age: 0   **P** Pediatric Age: 0–17   **M** Maternity DX: 12–55   **A** Adult Age: 15–124   ♀ Females Only   ♂ Males Only

🔵 Complication\Comorbidity   🔵 Major C\C   (Ex) CC/MCC Exclusions   🔵 Hospital-Acquired Condition

743

Item 4–5 **Hyperadrenalism** is overactivity of the adrenal cortex, which secretes corticosteroid hormones. Excessive glucocorticoid hormone results in hyperglycemia (**Cushing's syndrome**), and excessive aldosterone results in **Conn's syndrome**. **Adrenogenital syndrome** is the result of excessive secretion of androgens, male hormones, which stimulates premature sexual development. **Hypoadrenalism, Addison's disease,** is a condition in which the adrenal glands atrophy.

Figure 4-6 Centripetal and generalized obesity and dorsal kyphosis in a 30-year-old woman with Cushing's disease. (From Larsen: Williams Textbook of Endocrinology, ed 10, Saunders, An Imprint of Elsevier, 2003)

E21.2 **Other hyperparathyroidism**
    Tertiary hyperparathyroidism
    Excludes1 familial hypocalciuric hypercalcemia (E83.52)

E21.3 **Hyperparathyroidism,** unspecified

E21.4 **Other specified disorders of parathyroid gland**

E21.5 **Disorder of parathyroid gland,** unspecified

● **E22** **Hyperfunction of pituitary gland**
    Excludes1 Cushing's syndrome (E24.-)
       Nelson's syndrome (E24.1)
       overproduction of ACTH not associated with Cushing's disease (E27.0)
       overproduction of pituitary ACTH (E24.0)
       overproduction of thyroid-stimulating hormone (E05.8-)
    (Ex) For category E.22 CC codes unless otherwise indicated: E22.1-E22.9

E22.0 **Acromegaly and pituitary gigantism**
    Chronic disease caused by hypersecretion of growth hormone
    Overproduction of growth hormone
    Excludes1 constitutional gigantism (E34.4)
       constitutional tall stature (E34.4)
       increased secretion from endocrine pancreas of growth hormone-releasing hormone (E16.8)

E22.1 **Hyperprolactinemia**
    Increased levels of prolactin
    Use additional code for adverse effect, if applicable, to identify drug (T36-T50 with fifth or sixth character 5)

E22.2 **Syndrome of inappropriate secretion of antidiuretic hormone**
    (Ex) E22.0-E23.7, E24.1, E30.9, E34.1, E34.4, E34.8-E35, E89.3

E22.8 **Other hyperfunction of pituitary gland**
    Central precocious puberty

E22.9 **Hyperfunction of pituitary gland,** unspecified

● **E23** **Hypofunction and other disorders of the pituitary gland**
    Includes the listed conditions whether the disorder is in the pituitary or the hypothalamus
    Excludes1 postprocedural hypopituitarism (E89.3)

E23.0 **Hypopituitarism**
    Fertile eunuch syndrome
    Hypogonadotropic hypogonadism
    Idiopathic growth hormone deficiency
    Isolated deficiency of gonadotropin
    Isolated deficiency of growth hormone
    Isolated deficiency of pituitary hormone
    Kallmann's syndrome
    Lorain-Levi short stature
    Necrosis of pituitary gland (postpartum)
    Panhypopituitarism
    Pituitary cachexia
    Pituitary insufficiency NOS
    Pituitary short stature
    Sheehan's syndrome
    Simmonds' disease
    (Ex) E22.0-E23.7, E24.1, E30.9, E34.1, E34.4-E35, E89.3

E23.1 **Drug-induced hypopituitarism**
    Use additional code for adverse effect, if applicable, to identify drug (T36-T50 with fifth or sixth character 5)

E23.2 **Diabetes insipidus**
    Excludes1 nephrogenic diabetes insipidus (N25.1)
    (Ex) E22.1-E23.7, E24.1, E30.9, E34.1, E34.50-E35, E89.3

E23.3 **Hypothalamic dysfunction, not elsewhere classified**
    Excludes1 Prader-Willi syndrome (Q87.1)
       Russell-Silver syndrome (Q87.1)

E23.6 **Other disorders of pituitary gland**
    Abscess of pituitary
    Adiposogenital dystrophy

E23.7 **Disorder of pituitary gland,** unspecified

● **E24** **Cushing's syndrome**
    Excludes1 congenital adrenal hyperplasia (E25.0)
    (Ex) For category E24 CC codes: E24.0, E24.2-E26.9, E30.9, E34.1, E34.50-E35

E24.0 **Pituitary-dependent Cushing's disease**
    Overproduction of pituitary ACTH
    Pituitary-dependent hypercorticalism

E24.1 **Nelson's syndrome**

E24.2 **Drug-induced Cushing's syndrome**
    Use additional code for adverse effect, if applicable, to identify drug (T36-T50 with fifth or sixth character 5)

E24.3 **Ectopic ACTH syndrome**

E24.4 **Alcohol-induced pseudo-Cushing's syndrome**

E24.8 **Other Cushing's syndrome**

E24.9 **Cushing's syndrome,** unspecified

● **E25** **Adrenogenital disorders**
    Disorder of production of steroid hormone in adrenal gland
    Includes adrenogenital syndromes, virilizing or feminizing, whether acquired or due to adrenal hyperplasia consequent on inborn enzyme defects in hormone synthesis
       female adrenal pseudohermaphroditism
       female heterosexual precocious pseudopuberty
       male isosexual precocious pseudopuberty
       male macrogenitosomia praecox
       male sexual precocity with adrenal hyperplasia
       male virilization (female)
    Excludes1 indeterminate sex and pseudohermaphroditism (Q56)
       chromosomal abnormalities (Q90-Q99)

E25.0 **Congenital adrenogenital disorders associated with enzyme deficiency**
    Congenital adrenal hyperplasia
    21-Hydroxylase deficiency
    Salt-losing congenital adrenal hyperplasia

E25.8 **Other adrenogenital disorders**
    Idiopathic adrenogenital disorder
    Use additional code for adverse effect, if applicable, to identify drug (T36-T50 with fifth or sixth character 5)

E25.9 **Adrenogenital disorder,** unspecified
    Adrenogenital syndrome NOS

◀ New   ◀— Revised   ~~deleted~~ Deleted   Excludes 1   Excludes 2   Includes   Use additional   Code first   Code also   Unspecified

OGCR Official Guidelines   ● Unacceptable Principal Diagnosis   X Assign placeholder X   ▶ Use Additional Character(s)   ▶ Manifestation Code   **Coding Clinic**

● **E26** **Hyperaldosteronism**
Abnormality of electrolyte metabolism caused by excessive secretion of aldosterone

● **E26.0** **Primary hyperaldosteronism**

E26.01 **Conn's syndrome**
Code also adrenal adenoma (D35.0-)

E26.02 **Glucocorticoid-remediable aldosteronism**
Familial aldosteronism type I

E26.09 **Other primary hyperaldosteronism**
Primary aldosteronism due to adrenal hyperplasia (bilateral)

E26.1 **Secondary hyperaldosteronism**

● **E26.8** **Other hyperaldosteronism**

E26.81 **Bartter's syndrome**

E26.89 **Other hyperaldosteronism**

E26.9 **Hyperaldosteronism, unspecified**
Aldosteronism NOS
Hyperaldosteronism NOS

● **E27** **Other disorders of adrenal gland**
Ⓔⓧ **For category E27 CC codes:** A17.9, A18.7, A18.82, A18.84, A18.89, E27.0-E27.9, E30.9, E34.1, E34.50-E35, E89.6

E27.0 **Other adrenocortical overactivity** 🅒
Overproduction of ACTH, not associated with Cushing's disease
Premature adrenarche
Excludes1 Cushing's syndrome (E24.-)

E27.1 **Primary adrenocortical insufficiency** 🅒
Addison's disease
Autoimmune adrenalitis
Excludes1 Addison only phenotype adrenoleukodystrophy (E71.528)
amyloidosis (E85.-)
tuberculous Addison's disease (A18.7)
Waterhouse-Friderichsen syndrome (A39.1)

E27.2 **Addisonian crisis** 🅒
Acute onset of adrenocortical insufficiency
Adrenal crisis
Adrenocortical crisis

E27.3 **Drug-induced adrenocortical insufficiency** 🅒
Use additional code for adverse effect, if applicable, to identify drug (T36-T50 with fifth or sixth character 5)

● **E27.4** **Other and unspecified adrenocortical insufficiency**
Excludes1 adrenoleukodystrophy [Addison-Schilder] (E71.528)
Waterhouse-Friderichsen syndrome (A39.1)

E27.40 **Unspecified adrenocortical insufficiency** 🅒
Adrenocortical insufficiency NOS
Hypoaldosteronism

E27.49 **Other adrenocortical insufficiency** 🅒
Adrenal hemorrhage
Adrenal infarction

E27.5 **Adrenomedullary hyperfunction** 🅒
Adrenomedullary hyperplasia
Catecholamine hypersecretion

E27.8 **Other specified disorders of adrenal gland**
Abnormality of cortisol-binding globulin

E27.9 **Disorder of adrenal gland, unspecified**

● **E28** **Ovarian dysfunction**
Excludes1 isolated gonadotropin deficiency (E23.0)
postprocedural ovarian failure (E89.4-)

E28.0 **Estrogen excess** ♀
Use additional code for adverse effect, if applicable, to identify drug (T36-T50 with fifth or sixth character 5)

E28.1 **Androgen excess** ♀
Hypersecretion of ovarian androgens
Use additional code for adverse effect, if applicable, to identify drug (T36-T50 with fifth or sixth character 5)

E28.2 **Polycystic ovarian syndrome** ♀
Sclerocystic ovary syndrome
Stein-Leventhal syndrome

● **E28.3** **Primary ovarian failure**
Excludes1 pure gonadal dysgenesis (Q99.1)
Turner's syndrome (Q96.-)

● **E28.31** **Premature menopause**

E28.310 **Symptomatic premature menopause** ♀   A
Symptoms such as flushing, sleeplessness, headache, lack of concentration, associated with premature menopause

E28.319 **Asymptomatic premature menopause** ♀   A
Premature menopause NOS

E28.39 **Other primary ovarian failure** ♀
Decreased estrogen
Resistant ovary syndrome

E28.8 **Other ovarian dysfunction** ♀
Ovarian hyperfunction NOS
Excludes1 postprocedural ovarian failure (E89.4-)

E28.9 **Ovarian dysfunction, unspecified** ♀

● **E29** **Testicular dysfunction**
Excludes1 androgen insensitivity syndrome (E34.5-)
azoospermia or oligospermia NOS (N46.0-N46.1)
isolated gonadotropin deficiency (E23.0)
Klinefelter's syndrome (Q98.0-Q98.1, Q98.4) ◀━━

E29.0 **Testicular hyperfunction** ♂
Hypersecretion of testicular hormones

E29.1 **Testicular hypofunction** ♂
Defective biosynthesis of testicular androgen NOS
5-delta-Reductase deficiency (with male pseudohermaphroditism)
Testicular hypogonadism NOS
Use additional code for adverse effect, if applicable, to identify drug (T36-T50 with fifth or sixth character 5)
Excludes1 postprocedural testicular hypofunction (E89.5)

E29.8 **Other testicular dysfunction** ♂

E29.9 **Testicular dysfunction, unspecified** ♂

● **E30** **Disorders of puberty, not elsewhere classified**

E30.0 **Delayed puberty**
Constitutional delay of puberty
Delayed sexual development

E30.1 **Precocious puberty**   P
Sexual maturation at earlier age than normal, or before age 8 in girls and 9 in boys, usually hormonal; AKA sexual precocity or pubertas praecox
Precocious menstruation
Excludes1 Albright (-McCune) (-Sternberg) syndrome (Q78.1)
central precocious puberty (E22.8)
congenital adrenal hyperplasia (E25.0)
female heterosexual precocious pseudopuberty (E25.-)
male isosexual precocious pseudopuberty (E25.-)

E30.8 **Other disorders of puberty**   P
Premature thelarche

E30.9 **Disorder of puberty, unspecified**

CHAPTER 4 (E00-E90)

N Newborn Age: 0   **P** Pediatric Age: 0–17   **M** Maternity DX: 12–55   **A** Adult Age: 15–124   ♀ Females Only   ♂ Males Only
 Complication\Comorbidity   Ⓜ Major C\C   Ⓔⓧ CC/MCC Exclusions   Hospital-Acquired Condition

● E31 **Polyglandular dysfunction**

> **Excludes1** ataxia telangiectasia [Louis-Bar] (G11.3)
> dystrophia myotonica [Steinert] (G71.11)
> pseudohypoparathyroidism (E20.1)

E31.0 **Autoimmune polyglandular failure**
Schmidt's syndrome

E31.1 **Polyglandular hyperfunction**

> **Excludes1** multiple endocrine adenomatosis (E31.2-)
> multiple endocrine neoplasia (E31.2-)

● E31.2 **Multiple endocrine neoplasia [MEN] syndromes**
Adenomatous hyperplasia and malignant tumors in endocrine glands
Multiple endocrine adenomatosis

> Code also any associated malignancies and other conditions associated with the syndromes

E31.20 **Multiple endocrine neoplasia [MEN] syndrome, unspecified**
Multiple endocrine adenomatosis NOS
Multiple endocrine neoplasia [MEN] syndrome NOS

E31.21 **Multiple endocrine neoplasia [MEN] type I**
Wermer's syndrome

E31.22 **Multiple endocrine neoplasia [MEN] type IIA**
Sipple's syndrome

E31.23 **Multiple endocrine neoplasia [MEN] type IIB**

E31.8 **Other polyglandular dysfunction**

E31.9 **Polyglandular dysfunction, unspecified**

● E32 **Diseases of thymus**

> **Excludes1** aplasia or hypoplasia of thymus with immunodeficiency (D82.1)
> myasthenia gravis (G70.0)

E32.0 **Persistent hyperplasia of thymus**
Hypertrophy of thymus

E32.1 **Abscess of thymus** 🔒
(Ex) E30.9, E32.0-E32.9, E34.1, E34.50-E35

E32.8 **Other diseases of thymus**

> **Excludes1** aplasia or hypoplasia with immunodeficiency (D82.1)
> thymoma (D15.0)

E32.9 **Disease of thymus, unspecified**

● E34 **Other endocrine disorders**

> **Excludes1** pseudohypoparathyroidism (E20.1)

E34.0 **Carcinoid syndrome** 🔒
Note: May be used as an additional code to identify functional activity associated with a carcinoid tumor.
(Ex) E30.9, E34.0-E34.2, E34.50-E35

E34.1 **Other hypersecretion of intestinal hormones**

E34.2 **Ectopic hormone secretion, not elsewhere classified**

> **Excludes1** ectopic ACTH syndrome (E24.3)

E34.3 **Short stature due to endocrine disorder**
Constitutional short stature
Laron-type short stature

> **Excludes1** achondroplastic short stature (Q77.4)
> hypochondroplastic short stature (Q77.4)
> nutritional short stature (E45)
> pituitary short stature (E23.0)
> progeria (E34.8)
> renal short stature (N25.0)
> Russell-Silver syndrome (Q87.1)
> short-limbed stature with immunodeficiency (D82.2)
> short stature in specific dysmorphic syndromes - code to syndrome - see Alphabetical Index
> short stature NOS (R62.52)

E34.4 **Constitutional tall stature**
Constitutional gigantism

E34.5 **Androgen insensitivity syndrome**

E34.50 **Androgen insensitivity syndrome, unspecified**
Androgen insensitivity NOS

E34.51 **Complete androgen insensitivity syndrome**
Complete androgen insensitivity
de Quervain syndrome
Goldberg-Maxwell syndrome

E34.52 **Partial androgen insensitivity syndrome**
Partial androgen insensitivity
Reifenstein syndrome

E34.8 **Other specified endocrine disorders**
Pineal gland dysfunction
Progeria

> **Excludes2** pseudohypoparathyroidism (E20.1)

E34.9 **Endocrine disorder, unspecified**
Endocrine disturbance NOS
Hormone disturbance NOS

▶ E35 *Disorders of endocrine glands in diseases classified elsewhere*

> *Code first* underlying disease, such as:
> late congenital syphilis of thymus gland [Dubois disease] (A50.5)

> Use additional code, if applicable, to identify:
> sequelae of tuberculosis of other organs (B90.8)

> **Excludes1** Echinococcus granulosus infection of thyroid gland (B67.3)
> meningococcal hemorrhagic adrenalitis (A39.1)
> syphilis of endocrine gland (A52.79)
> tuberculosis of adrenal gland, except calcification (A18.7)
> tuberculosis of endocrine gland NEC (A18.82)
> tuberculosis of thyroid gland (A18.81)
> Waterhouse-Friderichsen syndrome (A39.1)

INTRAOPERATIVE COMPLICATIONS OF ENDOCRINE SYSTEM (E36)

● E36 **Intraoperative complications of endocrine system**

> **Excludes2** postprocedural endocrine and metabolic complications and disorders, not elsewhere classified (E89.-)

● E36.0 **Intraoperative hemorrhage and hematoma of an endocrine system organ or structure complicating a procedure**

> **Excludes1** intraoperative hemorrhage and hematoma of an endocrine system organ or structure due to accidental puncture or laceration during a procedure (E36.1-)

(Ex) **For category E36.0 CC codes:** E36.01-E36.02, E36.8, E89.810-E89.89, H95.811-H95.89, I85.01, I85.11, I97.3, K21.9, K22.8, K23-K25.0, K25.2, K25.4, K25.6, K26.0, K26.2, K26.4, K26.6, K27.0, K27.2, K27.4, K27.6, K28.0, K28.2, K28.4, K28.6, K29.01, K29.21, K29.31, K29.41, K29.51, K29.61, K29.71, K29.81, K29.91, K31.811, K55.21, K57.01, K57.11, K57.13, K57.21, K57.31, K57.33, K57.41, K57.51, K57.53, K57.81, K57.91, K57.93, K62.5, K92.0-K92.2, M96.89, N98.1-N98.9, P54.1-P54.3, T81.10X-T81.19X[A], T81.82X[A], T81.89X-T81.9XX[A]

E36.01 **Intraoperative hemorrhage and hematoma of an endocrine system organ or structure complicating an endocrine system procedure** 🔒

E36.02 **Intraoperative hemorrhage and hematoma of an endocrine system organ or structure complicating other procedure** 🔒

● E36.1 **Accidental puncture and laceration of an endocrine system organ or structure during a procedure**

(Ex) **For category E36.1 CC codes:** D78.11-D78.12, D78.81-D78.89, E36.11-E36.8, E89.810-E89.89, G96.11, G97.41-G97.49, H59.011-H59.019, H59.031-H59.099, H59.211-H59.229, H59.811-H59.89, H95.31-H95.32, H95.811-H95.89, I97.3, I97.51-I97.52, J95.71-J95.72, K91.71-K91.72, L76.11-L76.12, L76.81-L76.82, M96.820-M96.821, M96.89, N98.1-N98.9, N99.71-N99.72, T81.82X[A], T81.89X-T81.9XX[A]

E36.11 **Accidental puncture and laceration of an endocrine system organ or structure during an endocrine system procedure** 🔒

◀ New ◀ Revised ~~deleted~~ Deleted Excludes 1 Excludes 2 Includes Use additional Code first Code also Unspecified
OGCR Official Guidelines ● Unacceptable Principal Diagnosis X Assign placeholder X ● Use Additional Character(s) ▶ Manifestation Code Coding Clinic

E36.12   **Accidental puncture and laceration of an endocrine system organ or structure during other procedure**

E36.8   **Other intraoperative complications of endocrine system**
Use additional code, if applicable, to further specify disorder

MALNUTRITION (E40-E46)

Excludes1   intestinal malabsorption (K90.-)
sequelae of protein-calorie malnutrition (E64.0)

Excludes2   nutritional anemias (D50-D53)
starvation (T73.0)

E40   **Kwashiorkor**
Malnutrition produced by severe protein deficiency
Severe malnutrition with nutritional edema with dyspigmentation of skin and hair

Excludes1   marasmic kwashiorkor (E42)

Ex: E40-E46, E64.0

E41   **Nutritional marasmus**
Severe malnutrition with marasmus

Excludes1   marasmic kwashiorkor (E42)

Ex: E40-E46, E64.0

E42   **Marasmic kwashiorkor**
Severe protein malnutrition
Intermediate form severe protein-calorie malnutrition
Severe protein-calorie malnutrition with signs of both kwashiorkor and marasmus

Ex: E40-E46, E64.0

E43   **Unspecified severe protein-calorie malnutrition**
Starvation edema

Ex: E40-E46, E64.0

E44   **Protein-calorie malnutrition of moderate and mild degree**
Ex: For category E44 CC codes: E40-E46, E64.0

E44.0   **Moderate protein-calorie malnutrition**

E44.1   **Mild protein-calorie malnutrition**

E45   **Retarded development following protein-calorie malnutrition**
Nutritional short stature
Nutritional stunting
Physical retardation due to malnutrition

Ex: E40-E46, E64.0

E46   **Unspecified protein-calorie malnutrition**
Malnutrition NOS
Protein-calorie imbalance NOS

Excludes1   nutritional deficiency NOS (E63.9)

Ex: E40-E46, E64.0

OTHER NUTRITIONAL DEFICIENCIES (E50-E64)

Excludes2   nutritional anemias (D50-D53)

E50   **Vitamin A deficiency**

Excludes1   sequelae of vitamin A deficiency (E64.1)

E50.0   **Vitamin A deficiency with conjunctival xerosis**

E50.1   **Vitamin A deficiency with Bitot's spot and conjunctival xerosis**
Bitot's spot in the young child

E50.2   **Vitamin A deficiency with corneal xerosis**

E50.3   **Vitamin A deficiency with corneal ulceration and xerosis**

E50.4   **Vitamin A deficiency with keratomalacia**
Eye disorder that results in dry cornea caused by vitamin A deficiency

E50.5   **Vitamin A deficiency with night blindness**

E50.6   **Vitamin A deficiency with xerophthalmic scars of cornea**
Abnormal dryness and thickening of conjunctiva and cornea due to vitamin A deficiency

E50.7   **Other ocular manifestations of vitamin A deficiency**
Xerophthalmia NOS

E50.8   **Other manifestations of vitamin A deficiency**
Follicular keratosis
Xeroderma

E50.9   **Vitamin A deficiency, unspecified**
Hypovitaminosis A NOS

E51   **Thiamine deficiency**

Excludes1   sequelae of thiamine deficiency (E64.8)

E51.1   **Beriberi**
Ex: For category E51.1 CC codes: D81.818-D81.819, E51.11-E53.9, E56.0, E56.8-E63.9, E64.8-E64.9

E51.11   **Dry beriberi**
Thiamine deficiency with nervous system manifestation most often caused by excessive alcohol consumption
Beriberi NOS
Beriberi with polyneuropathy

E51.12   **Wet beriberi**
Thiamine deficiency with cardiovascular manifestation most often caused by excessive alcohol consumption
Beriberi with cardiovascular manifestations
Cardiovascular beriberi
Shoshin disease

E51.2   **Wernicke's encephalopathy**
Acute disease of brain due to thiamine deficiency most often associated with excessive alcohol consumption
Ex: See E51.1

E51.8   **Other manifestations of thiamine deficiency**
Ex: See E51.1

E51.9   **Thiamine deficiency, unspecified**
Ex: See E51.1

CHAPTER 4 (E00-E90)

Item 4–6   Bitot's spots are the result of a buildup of keratin debris found on the superficial surface the conjunctiva; oval, triangular, or irregular in shape; and a sign of vitamin A deficiency and associated with night blindness. The disease may progress to **keratomalacia,** which can result in eventual prolapse of the iris and loss of the lens.

Figure 4-7   Bitot's spot on the conjunctiva.

Figure 4-8   The sharply demarcated, characteristic scaling dermatitis of pellagra. (From Kumar: Robbins and Cotran: Pathologic Basis of Disease, ed 8, Saunders, An Imprint of Elsevier, 2009)

Item 4–7   Pellagra is associated with a deficiency of niacin and its precursor, **tryptophan.** Characteristics of the condition include diarrhea, dermatitis on exposed skin surfaces, dementia, and death. It is prevalent in developing countries where nutrition is inadequate. **Beriberi** is associated with thiamine deficiency.

CHAPTER 4 (E00-E90)

E52   Niacin deficiency [pellagra]
    Niacin (-tryptophan) deficiency
    Nicotinamide deficiency
    Pellagra (alcoholic)
    Excludes1   sequelae of niacin deficiency (E64.8)

● **E53   Deficiency of other B group vitamins**
    Excludes1   sequelae of vitamin B deficiency (E64.8)

    E53.0   Riboflavin deficiency 🔗
        Ariboflavinosis
        Vitamin B2 deficiency
        (Ex) See E51.1

    E53.1   Pyridoxine deficiency
        Vitamin B6 deficiency
        Excludes1   pyridoxine-responsive sideroblastic anemia (D64.3)

    E53.8   Deficiency of other specified B group vitamins
        Biotin deficiency
        Cyanocobalamin deficiency
        Folate deficiency
        Folic acid deficiency
        Pantothenic acid deficiency
        Vitamin B12 deficiency
        Excludes1   folate deficiency anemia (D52.-)
                        vitamin B12 deficiency anemia (D51.-)

    E53.9   Vitamin B deficiency, unspecified

E54   Ascorbic acid deficiency
    Deficiency of vitamin C
    Scurvy
    Excludes1   scorbutic anemia (D53.2)
                 sequelae of vitamin C deficiency (E64.2)

● **E55   Vitamin D deficiency**
    Excludes1   adult osteomalacia (M83.-)
                 osteoporosis (M80.-)
                 sequelae of rickets (E64.3)

    E55.0   Rickets, active 🔗
        Infantile osteomalacia
        Juvenile osteomalacia
        Softening of bone
        Excludes1   celiac rickets (K90.0)
                 Crohn's rickets (K50.-)
                 hereditary vitamin D-dependent rickets (E83.32)
                 inactive rickets (E64.3)
                 renal rickets (N25.0)
                 sequelae of rickets (E64.3)
                 vitamin D-resistant rickets (E83.31)
        (Ex) E55.0-E63.9, E64.3-E64.9, M83.0-M83.9

    E55.9   Vitamin D deficiency, unspecified
        Avitaminosis D

● **E56   Other vitamin deficiencies**
    Excludes1   sequelae of other vitamin deficiencies (E64.8)
    E56.0   Deficiency of vitamin E
    E56.1   Deficiency of vitamin K
        Excludes1   deficiency of coagulation factor due to vitamin K deficiency (D68.4)
                 vitamin K deficiency of newborn (P53)
    E56.8   Deficiency of other vitamins
    E56.9   Vitamin deficiency, unspecified

E58   Dietary calcium deficiency
    Excludes1   disorders of calcium metabolism (E83.5-)
                 sequelae of calcium deficiency (E64.8)

E59   Dietary selenium deficiency
    Keshan disease
    Excludes1   sequelae of selenium deficiency (E64.8)

E60   Dietary zinc deficiency

● **E61   Deficiency of other nutrient elements**
    Use additional code for adverse effect, if applicable, to identify drug (T36-T50 with fifth or sixth character 5)
    Excludes1   disorders of mineral metabolism (E83.-)
                 iodine deficiency related thyroid disorders (E00-E02)
                 sequelae of malnutrition and other nutritional deficiencies (E64.-)
    E61.0   Copper deficiency
    E61.1   Iron deficiency
        Excludes1   iron deficiency anemia (D50.-)
    E61.2   Magnesium deficiency
    E61.3   Manganese deficiency
    E61.4   Chromium deficiency
    E61.5   Molybdenum deficiency
    E61.6   Vanadium deficiency
    E61.7   Deficiency of multiple nutrient elements
    E61.8   Deficiency of other specified nutrient elements
    E61.9   Deficiency of nutrient element, unspecified

● **E63   Other nutritional deficiencies**
    Excludes1   dehydration (E86.0)
                 failure to thrive, adult (R62.7)
                 failure to thrive, child (R62.51)
                 feeding problems in newborn (P92.-)
                 sequelae of malnutrition and other nutritional deficiencies (E64.-)
    E63.0   Essential fatty acid [EFA] deficiency
    E63.1   Imbalance of constituents of food intake
    E63.8   Other specified nutritional deficiencies
    E63.9   Nutritional deficiency, unspecified

● **E64   Sequelae of malnutrition and other nutritional deficiencies**
    Pathological condition resulting from disease, injury, or other trauma
    Note: This category is to be used to indicate conditions in categories E43, E44, E46, E50-E63 as the cause of sequelae, which are themselves classified elsewhere. The 'sequelae' include conditions specified as such; they also include the late effects of diseases classifiable to the above categories if the disease itself is no longer present
    Code first condition resulting from (sequela) of malnutrition and other nutritional deficiencies
    E64.0   Sequelae of protein-calorie malnutrition 🔗
        Excludes2   retarded development following protein-calorie malnutrition (E45)
        (Ex) E40-E46, E64.0
    E64.1   Sequelae of vitamin A deficiency
    E64.2   Sequelae of vitamin C deficiency
    E64.3   Sequelae of rickets
    E64.8   Sequelae of other nutritional deficiencies
    E64.9   Sequelae of unspecified nutritional deficiency

OVERWEIGHT, OBESITY AND OTHER HYPERALIMENTATION (E65-E68)

E65   **Localized adiposity**
       Fat pad

● **E66**   **Overweight and obesity**
       Code first obesity complicating pregnancy, childbirth and the puerperium, if applicable (O99.21-)
       Use additional code to identify body mass index (BMI), if known (Z68.-)

       Excludes1   adiposogenital dystrophy (E23.6)
                      lipomatosis NOS (E88.2)
                      lipomatosis dolorosa [Dercum] (E88.2)
                      Prader-Willi syndrome (Q87.1)

 ● **E66.0**   **Obesity due to excess calories**
       E66.01   **Morbid (severe) obesity due to excess calories** 🖉
                Excludes1   morbid (severe) obesity with alveolar hypoventilation (E66.2)

       E66.09   **Other obesity due to excess calories**
                MCE: Questionable admission when principal dx

      E66.1   **Drug-induced obesity**
            MCE: Questionable admission when principal dx
            Use additional code for adverse effect, if applicable, to identify drug (T36-T50 with fifth or sixth character 5)

      E66.2   **Morbid (severe) obesity with alveolar hypoventilation** 🖉
            Uncommon condition of unknown cause leading to inadequate ventilation in lungs, even though lungs and airways are normal
            Obesity hypoventilation syndrome (OHS) ◄
            Pickwickian syndrome
            (Ex) E66.2, I27.0-I27.81, I27.89-I27.9

      E66.3   **Overweight**
      E66.8   **Other obesity**
            MCE: Questionable admission when principal dx

      E66.9   **Obesity, unspecified**
            Obesity NOS
            MCE: Questionable admission when principal dx

● **E67**   **Other hyperalimentation**
       Ingestion of more than optimal amount of nutrients

       Excludes1   hyperalimentation NOS (R63.2)
                      sequelae of hyperalimentation (E68)

      E67.0   **Hypervitaminosis A**
      E67.1   **Hypercarotinemia**
      E67.2   **Megavitamin-B6 syndrome**
      E67.3   **Hypervitaminosis D**
      E67.8   **Other specified hyperalimentation**

E68   **Sequelae of hyperalimentation**
       Code first condition resulting from (sequela) of hyperalimentation

METABOLIC DISORDERS (E70-E88)

       Excludes1   androgen insensitivity syndrome (E34.5-)
                      congenital adrenal hyperplasia (E25.0)
                      Ehlers-Danlos syndrome (Q79.6)
                      hemolytic anemias attributable to enzyme disorders (D55.-)
                      Marfan's syndrome (Q87.4)
                      5-alpha-reductase deficiency (E29.1)

● **E70**   **Disorders of aromatic amino-acid metabolism**
       (Ex) **For category E70 CC codes:** C88.0, D47.2, D89.0-D89.1, E70.0-E71.30, E72.00-E72.02, E72.04-E74.9, E75.21-E75.249, E75.3, E75.5-E75.6, E77.0-E78.70, E78.79-E78.9, E88.09-E88.2, E88.89

      E70.0   **Classical phenylketonuria** 🖉
            Inherited disorder that increases to harmful levels amino acid phenylalanine

      E70.1   **Other hyperphenylalaninemias** 🖉

 ● **E70.2**   **Disorders of tyrosine metabolism**
       Excludes1   transitory tyrosinemia of newborn (P74.5)

      E70.20   **Disorder of tyrosine metabolism, unspecified** 🖉
           Tyrosine: Nonessential amino acid occurring in most proteins

      E70.21   **Tyrosinemia** 🖉
           Congenital amino acid metabolism
           Hypertyrosinemia

      E70.29   **Other disorders of tyrosine metabolism** 🖉
           Alkaptonuria
           Ochronosis

 ● **E70.3**   **Albinism**
       Congenital condition of reduced or absent pigment in eyes, skin, and hair

      E70.30   **Albinism, unspecified** 🖉
  ● **E70.31**   **Ocular albinism**
       E70.310   **X-linked ocular albinism** 🖉
       E70.311   **Autosomal recessive ocular albinism** 🖉
       E70.318   **Other ocular albinism** 🖉
       E70.319   **Ocular albinism, unspecified** 🖉

  ● **E70.32**   **Oculocutaneous albinism**
       Partial or total lack of melanin pigment in eyes
       Excludes1   Chediak-Higashi syndrome (E70.330)
                      Hermansky-Pudlak syndrome (E70.331)

       E70.320   **Tyrosinase negative oculocutaneous albinism** 🖉
            Albinism I
            Oculocutaneous albinism ty-neg

       E70.321   **Tyrosinase positive oculocutaneous albinism** 🖉
            Albinism II
            Oculocutaneous albinism ty-pos

       E70.328   **Other oculocutaneous albinism** 🖉
            Cross syndrome

       E70.329   **Oculocutaneous albinism, unspecified** 🖉

  ● **E70.33**   **Albinism with hematologic abnormality**
       E70.330   **Chediak-Higashi syndrome** 🖉
       E70.331   **Hermansky-Pudlak syndrome** 🖉
       E70.338   **Other albinism with hematologic abnormality** 🖉
       E70.339   **Albinism with hematologic abnormality, unspecified** 🖉

      E70.39   **Other specified albinism** 🖉
           Piebaldism

 ● **E70.4**   **Disorders of histidine metabolism**
      E70.40   **Disorders of histidine metabolism, unspecified** 🖉
      E70.41   **Histidinemia** 🖉
      E70.49   **Other disorders of histidine metabolism** 🖉

      E70.5   **Disorders of tryptophan metabolism** 🖉
      E70.8   **Other disorders of aromatic amino-acid metabolism** 🖉
      E70.9   **Disorder of aromatic amino-acid metabolism, unspecified** 🖉

CHAPTER 4 (E00-E90)

E71 **Disorders of branched-chain amino-acid metabolism and fatty-acid metabolism**

E71.0 **Maple-syrup-urine disease** 🖉
Due to defect in amino acid catabolism, causing severe ketoacidosis with smell of maple syrup in urine and on body
Ex: See E70

● E71.1 **Other disorders of branched-chain amino-acid metabolism**
Ex: For category E71.1 CC codes: See E70

● E71.11 **Branched-chain organic acidurias**
E71.110 **Isovaleric acidemia** 🖉
E71.111 **3-methylglutaconic aciduria** 🖉
E71.118 **Other branched-chain organic acidurias** 🖉

● E71.12 **Disorders of propionate metabolism**
E71.120 **Methylmalonic acidemia** 🖉
E71.121 **Propionic acidemia** 🖉
E71.128 **Other disorders of propionate metabolism** 🖉

E71.19 **Other disorders of branched-chain amino-acid metabolism**
Hyperleucine-isoleucinemia
Hypervalinemia

E71.2 **Disorder of branched-chain amino-acid metabolism, unspecified** 🖉
Ex: See E70

● E71.3 **Disorders of fatty-acid metabolism**
Excludes1 peroxisomal disorders (E71.5)
Refsum's disease (G60.1)
Schilder's disease (G37.0)
Excludes2 carnitine deficiency due to inborn error of metabolism (E71.42)

E71.30 **Disorder of fatty-acid metabolism, unspecified** 🖉

● E71.31 **Disorders of fatty-acid oxidation**
Ex: For category E71.31 CC codes: C96.5-C96.6, E71.39-E71.548, E80.3, E88.40-E88.49, E88.89, H49.811-H49.819

E71.310 **Long chain/very long chain acyl CoA dehydrogenase deficiency** 🖉
LCAD
VLCAD

E71.311 **Medium chain acyl CoA dehydrogenase deficiency** 🖉
MCAD

E71.312 **Short chain acyl CoA dehydrogenase deficiency** 🖉
SCAD

E71.313 **Glutaric aciduria type II** 🖉
Glutaric aciduria type II A
Glutaric aciduria type II B
Glutaric aciduria type II C
Excludes1 glutaric aciduria (type 1) NOS (E72.3)

E71.314 **Muscle carnitine palmitoyltransferase deficiency** 🖉

E71.318 **Other disorders of fatty-acid oxidation** 🖉

E71.32 **Disorders of ketone metabolism** 🖉
Ex: See E71.31

E71.39 **Other disorders of fatty-acid metabolism** 🖉
Ex: E71.310-E71.32, E71.40-E71.548, E80.4-E80.7, E88.40-E88.49, H49.811-H49.819

● E71.4 **Disorders of carnitine metabolism**
Excludes1 muscle carnitine palmitoyltransferase deficiency (E71.314)

E71.40 **Disorder of carnitine metabolism, unspecified**
E71.41 **Primary carnitine deficiency**
E71.42 **Carnitine deficiency due to inborn errors of metabolism**
Code also associated inborn error or metabolism

E71.43 **Iatrogenic carnitine deficiency**
Iatrogenic: Outcomes from activity of physicians
Carnitine deficiency due to hemodialysis
Carnitine deficiency due to Valproic acid therapy

● E71.44 **Other secondary carnitine deficiency**
E71.440 **Ruvalcaba-Myhre-Smith syndrome**
E71.448 **Other secondary carnitine deficiency**

● E71.5 **Peroxisomal disorders**
Class of conditions which lead to disorders of lipid metabolism
Excludes1 Schilder's disease (G37.0)
Ex: For category E71.5 CC codes: C96.5-C96.6, E71.310-E71.448, E80.3-E80.7, E88.40-E88.49, E88.89, H49.811-H49.819

E71.50 **Peroxisomal disorder, unspecified** 🖉

● E71.51 **Disorders of peroxisome biogenesis**
Group 1 peroxisomal disorders
Excludes1 Refsum's disease (G60.1)
E71.510 **Zellweger syndrome** 🖉
E71.511 **Neonatal adrenoleukodystrophy** 🖉
Excludes1 X-linked adrenoleuko-dystrophy (E71.42-)
E71.518 **Other disorders of peroxisome biogenesis** 🖉

● E71.52 **X-linked adrenoleukodystrophy**
E71.520 **Childhood cerebral X-linked adrenoleukodystrophy** 🖉
E71.521 **Adolescent X-linked adrenoleukodystrophy** 🖉
E71.522 **Adrenomyeloneuropathy** 🖉
E71.528 **Other X-linked adrenoleukodystrophy** 🖉
Addison only phenotype adrenoleukodystrophy
Addison-Schilder adrenoleukodystrophy
E71.529 **X-linked adrenoleukodystrophy, unspecified type** 🖉

E71.53 **Other group 2 peroxisomal disorders** 🖉

● E71.54 **Other peroxisomal disorders**
E71.540 **Rhizomelic chondrodysplasia punctata** 🖉
Rare, severe, inherited disorder with limb shortening, bone and cartilage abnormalities, abnormal facial appearance, severe mental retardation, psychomotor retardation, and cataracts
Excludes1 chondrodysplasia punctata NOS (Q77.3)
E71.541 **Zellweger-like syndrome** 🖉
E71.542 **Other group 3 peroxisomal disorders** 🖉
E71.548 **Other peroxisomal disorders** 🖉

◀ New ⬅ Revised ~~deleted~~ Deleted Excludes 1 Excludes 2 Includes Use additional Code first Code also Unspecified
OGCR Official Guidelines ● Unacceptable Principal Diagnosis X Assign placeholder X ● Use Additional Character(s) 🖉 Manifestation Code **Coding Clinic**

● **E72   Other disorders of amino-acid metabolism**

     Excludes1   disorders of:
                 aromatic amino-acid metabolism (E70.-)
                 branched-chain amino-acid metabolism
                     (E71.0-E71.2)
                 fatty-acid metabolism (E71.3)
                 purine and pyrimidine metabolism (E79.-)
                 gout (M1A.-, M10.-)

     (Ex) For category E72 CC codes unless otherwise noted: See E70

● **E72.0   Disorders of amino-acid transport**

     Excludes1   disorders of tryptophan metabolism
                 (E70.5)

     E72.00   Disorders of amino-acid transport, unspecified 🔖

     E72.01   Cystinuria 🔖
           Hereditary aminoaciduria due to impairment of
           renal transport with predominant symptom of
           urinary cystine calculi

     E72.02   Hartnup's disease 🔖
           Inborn error of metabolism

     E72.03   Lowe's syndrome 🔖
           X-linked disorder with rickets, hydrophthalmia,
           congenital glaucoma, cataracts, mental
           retardation, and renal tubule dysfunction

           Use additional code for associated glaucoma
           (H42)
           (Ex) No exclusion

     E72.04   Cystinosis 🔖
           Genetic disease with excessive depostits of amino
           acid cystine in cells
           Fanconi (-de Toni) (-Debré) syndrome with
           cystinosis

           Excludes1   Fanconi (-de Toni) (-Debré)
                           syndrome without
                           cystinosis (E72.09)

     E72.09   Other disorders of amino-acid transport 🔖
           Fanconi (-de Toni) (-Debré) syndrome,
           unspecified

● **E72.1   Disorders of sulfur-bearing amino-acid metabolism**

     Excludes1   cystinosis (E72.04)
                 cystinuria (E72.01)
                 transcobalamin II deficiency (D51.2)

     E72.10   Disorders of sulfur-bearing amino-acid metabolism, unspecified 🔖

     E72.11   Homocystinuria 🔖
           Cystathionine synthase deficiency

     E72.12   Methylenetetrahydrofolate reductase deficiency 🔖

     E72.19   Other disorders of sulfur-bearing amino-acid metabolism 🔖
           Cystathioninuria
           Methioninemia
           Sulfite oxidase deficiency

● **E72.2   Disorders of urea cycle metabolism**

     Excludes1   disorders of ornithine metabolism (E72.4)

     E72.20   Disorder of urea cycle metabolism, unspecified 🔖
           Hyperammonemia
           Elevated levels of ammonia

           Excludes1   hyperammonemia-
                           hyperornithinemia-
                           homocitrullinemia
                           syndrome E72.4
                           transient hyperammonemia of
                           newborn (P74.6)

     E72.21   Argininemia 🔖
           Disorder in which deficiency of enzyme arginase
           causes build up of arginine and ammonia in
           blood

     E72.22   Arginosuccinic aciduria 🔖
           Gene disorder of urea cycle resulting accumulation
           of ammonia

     E72.23   Citrullinemia 🔖
           Urea cycle disorder that causes ammonia and other
           toxic substances to accumulate in blood

     E72.29   Other disorders of urea cycle metabolism 🔖

● **E72.3   Disorders of lysine and hydroxylysine metabolism** 🔖
       Glutaric aciduria NOS
       Glutaric aciduria (type I)
       Hydroxylysinemia
       Hyperlysinemia

     Excludes1   glutaric aciduria type II (E71.313)
                 Refsum's disease (G60.1)
                 Zellweger syndrome (E71.510)

● **E72.4   Disorders of ornithine metabolism** 🔖
       Hyperammonemia-Hyperornithinemia-
           Homocitrullinemia syndrome
       Ornithinemia (types I, II)
       Ornithine transcarbamylase deficiency

     Excludes1   hereditary choroidal dystrophy (H31.2-)

● **E72.5   Disorders of glycine metabolism**

     E72.50   Disorder of glycine metabolism, unspecified 🔖

     E72.51   Non-ketotic hyperglycinemia 🔖

     E72.52   Trimethylaminuria 🔖

     E72.53   Hyperoxaluria 🔖
           Oxalosis
           Oxaluria

     E72.59   Other disorders of glycine metabolism 🔖
           D-glycericacidemia
           Hyperhydroxyprolinemia
           Hyperprolinemia (types I, II)
           Sarcosinemia

● **E72.8   Other specified disorders of amino-acid metabolism** 🔖
       Disorders of beta-amino-acid metabolism
       Disorders of gamma-glutamyl cycle

● **E72.9   Disorder of amino-acid metabolism, unspecified** 🔖

● **E73   Lactose intolerance**
     Intolerance for lactose, due to inherited deficiency of lactase activity in
     intestinal mucosa

     E73.0   Congenital lactase deficiency

     E73.1   Secondary lactase deficiency

     E73.8   Other lactose intolerance

     E73.9   Lactose intolerance, unspecified

● **E74   Other disorders of carbohydrate metabolism**

     Excludes1   diabetes mellitus (E08-E13)
                 hypoglycemia NOS (E16.2)
                 increased secretion of glucagon (E16.3)
                 mucopolysaccharidosis (E76.0-E76.3)

     (Ex) For category E74 CC codes: See E70

● **E74.0   Glycogen storage disease**

     E74.00   Glycogen storage disease, unspecified 🔖

     E74.01   von Gierke's disease 🔖
           Type I glycogen storage disease

     E74.02   Pompe disease 🔖
           Cardiac glycogenosis
           Type II glycogen storage disease

     E74.03   Cori disease 🔖
           Forbes' disease
           Type III glycogen storage disease

     E74.04   McArdle disease 🔖
           Type V glycogen storage disease

     E74.09   Other glycogen storage disease 🔖
           Andersen disease
           Hers disease
           Tauri disease
           Glycogen storage disease, types 0, IV, VI-XI
           Liver phosphorylase deficiency
           Muscle phosphofructokinase deficiency

CHAPTER 4 (E00-E90)

CHAPTER 4 (E00-E90)

● **E74.1** **Disorders of fructose metabolism**

     Excludes1   muscle phosphofructokinase deficiency (E74.09)

     E74.10 **Disorder of fructose metabolism, unspecified**

     E74.11 **Essential fructosuria**
             Fructokinase deficiency

     E74.12 **Hereditary fructose intolerance**
             Fructosemia

     E74.19 **Other disorders of fructose metabolism**
             Fructose-1, 6-diphosphatase deficiency

● **E74.2** **Disorders of galactose metabolism**

     E74.20 **Disorders of galactose metabolism, unspecified** 🔖

     E74.21 **Galactosemia** 🔖
             Genetic disorders resulting from defective simple sugar (galactose) metabolism

     E74.29 **Other disorders of galactose metabolism** 🔖
             Galactokinase deficiency

● **E74.3** **Other disorders of intestinal carbohydrate absorption**

     Excludes2   lactose intolerance (E73.-)

     E74.31 **Sucrase-isomaltase deficiency**
             Deficiency in metabolism in intestinal mucosa results in malabsorption of sucrose and starch

     E74.39 **Other disorders of intestinal carbohydrate absorption**
             Disorder of intestinal carbohydrate absorption NOS
             Glucose-galactose malabsorption
             Sucrase deficiency

● **E74.4** **Disorders of pyruvate metabolism and gluconeogenesis** 🔖
      Deficiency of phosphoenolpyruvate carboxykinase
      Deficiency of pyruvate carboxylase
      Deficiency of pyruvate dehydrogenase

     Excludes1   disorders of pyruvate metabolism and gluconeogenesis with anemia (D55.-)
                   Leigh's syndrome (G31.82)

● **E74.8** **Other specified disorders of carbohydrate metabolism** 🔖
      Essential pentosuria
      Renal glycosuria

● **E74.9** **Disorder of carbohydrate metabolism, unspecified**

● **E75** **Disorders of sphingolipid metabolism and other lipid storage disorders**

     Excludes1   mucolipidosis, types I-III (E77.0-E77.1)
                   Refsum's disease (G60.1)

● **E75.0** **GM2 gangliosidosis**
      Rare metabolic disorder that causes destruction of nerve cells of brain and spinal cord
     Ⓔˣ **For category E75.0 CC codes:** E75.00-E75.19, E75.4, F84.2, G13.2-G13.8, G30.0-G31.82, G31.84-G31.9, G91.4, G94

     E75.00 **GM2 gangliosidosis, unspecified** 🔖

     E75.01 **Sandhoff disease** 🔖

     E75.02 **Tay-Sachs disease** 🔖

     E75.09 **Other GM2 gangliosidosis** 🔖
             Adult GM2 gangliosidosis
             Juvenile GM2 gangliosidosis

● **E75.1** **Other and unspecified gangliosidosis**
     Ⓔˣ **For category E75.1 CC codes:** See E75.0

     E75.10 **Unspecified gangliosidosis** 🔖
             Gangliosidosis NOS

     E75.11 **Mucolipidosis IV** 🔖
             Disorder with symptoms of psychomotor retardation and severe visual impairment

     E75.19 **Other gangliosidosis** 🔖
             GM1 gangliosidosis
             GM3 gangliosidosis

Item 4–8 **Leukodystrophy** is characterized by degeneration and/or failure of the myelin formation of the central nervous system and sometimes of the peripheral nervous system. The disease is inherited and progressive.

● **E75.2** **Other sphingolipidosis**
      Lysosomal (a particle in a cytoplasm cell that contains digestive enzymes) storage diseases with symptoms of abnormal storage of amino acids

     Excludes1   adrenoleukodystrophy [Addison-Schilder] (E71.528)

     E75.21 **Fabry (-Anderson) disease**

     E75.22 **Gaucher disease**

     E75.23 **Krabbe disease** 🔖
     Ⓔˣ E75.00-E75.19, E75.23, E75.25-E75.29, E75.4, F84.2, G13.2-G13.8, G31.2-G31.82, G32.89, G91.4, G93.81, G93.89-G94, G96.8-G96.9, G98.0-G98.8, G99.8

     ● **E75.24** **Niemann-Pick disease**

         E75.240 **Niemann-Pick disease type A**

         E75.241 **Niemann-Pick disease type B**

         E75.242 **Niemann-Pick disease type C**

         E75.243 **Niemann-Pick disease type D**

         E75.248 **Other Niemann-Pick disease**

         E75.249 **Niemann-Pick disease, unspecified**

     E75.25 **Metachromatic leukodystrophy** 🔖
         Ⓔˣ See E75.23

     E75.29 **Other sphingolipidosis** 🔖
         Farber's syndrome
         Sulfatase deficiency
         Sulfatide lipidosis
         Ⓔˣ See E75.23

● **E75.3** **Sphingolipidosis, unspecified**

● **E75.4** **Neuronal ceroid lipofuscinosis** 🔖
      Batten disease
      Bielschowsky-Jansky disease
      Kufs disease
      Spielmeyer-Vogt disease
     Ⓔˣ See E75.0

● **E75.5** **Other lipid storage disorders**
      Cerebrotendinous cholesterosis [van Bogaert-Scherer-Epstein]
      Wolman's disease

● **E75.6** **Lipid storage disorder, unspecified**

● **E76** **Disorders of glycosaminoglycan metabolism**
     Ⓔˣ **For category E76 CC codes:** D81.3, D81.5, D81.810, D84.1, E76.01-E76.9, E79.1-E80.29, E80.4-E80.7, E85.0, E85.9, E88.81

● **E76.0** **Mucopolysaccharidosis, type I**
      Inborn metabolic disorder of enzymes that break down carbohydrates

     E76.01 **Hurler's syndrome** 🔖

     E76.02 **Hurler-Scheie syndrome** 🔖

     E76.03 **Scheie's syndrome** 🔖

● **E76.1** **Mucopolysaccharidosis, type II** 🔖
      Inborn metabolic disorder of enzymes that break down carbohydrates occurs in 2-4 year old males
      Hunter's syndrome

● **E76.2** **Other mucopolysaccharidoses**

     ● **E76.21** **Morquio mucopolysaccharidoses**

         E76.210 **Morquio A mucopolysaccharidoses** 🔖
             Classic Morquio syndrome
             Morquio syndrome A
             Mucopolysaccharidosis, type IVA

         E76.211 **Morquio B mucopolysaccharidoses** 🔖
             Morquio-like mucopolysaccharidoses
             Morquio-like syndrome
             Morquio syndrome B
             Mucopolysaccharidosis, type IVB

         E76.219 **Morquio mucopolysaccharidoses, unspecified** 🔖
             Morquio syndrome
             Mucopolysaccharidosis, type IV

◀ New   ⬸ Revised   ~~deleted~~ Deleted   Excludes 1   Excludes 2   Includes   Use additional   Code first   Code also   Unspecified

OGCR Official Guidelines   ● Unacceptable Principal Diagnosis   X Assign placeholder X   ● Use Additional Character(s)   🔖 Manifestation Code   **Coding Clinic**

CHAPTER 4 (E00–E90)

E76.22   **Sanfilippo mucopolysaccharidoses**
    Mucopolysaccharidosis, type III (A) (B) (C) (D)
    Sanfilippo A syndrome
    Sanfilippo B syndrome
    Sanfilippo C syndrome
    Sanfilippo D syndrome

E76.29   **Other mucopolysaccharidoses**
    beta-Glucuronidase deficiency
    Maroteaux-Lamy (mild) (severe) syndrome
    Mucopolysaccharidosis, types VI, VII

E76.3   **Mucopolysaccharidosis, unspecified**

E76.8   **Other disorders of glucosaminoglycan metabolism**

E76.9   **Glucosaminoglycan metabolism disorder, unspecified**

E77   **Disorders of glycoprotein metabolism**

E77.0   **Defects in post-translational modification of lysosomal enzymes**
    Mucolipidosis II [I-cell disease]
    Mucolipidosis III [pseudo-Hurler polydystrophy]

E77.1   **Defects in glycoprotein degradation**
    Aspartylglucosaminuria
    Fucosidosis
    Mannosidosis
    Sialidosis [mucolipidosis I]

E77.8   **Other disorders of glycoprotein metabolism**

E77.9   **Disorder of glycoprotein metabolism, unspecified**

E78   **Disorders of lipoprotein metabolism and other lipidemias**
    Excludes1   sphingolipidosis (E75.0-E75.3)

E78.0   **Pure hypercholesterolemia**
    ~~Familial hypercholesterolemia~~
    ~~Hyperlipidemia, Group A~~

E78.00   **Pure hypercholesterolemia, unspecified** ◄
    Fredrickson's hyperlipoproteinemia,
      type IIa ◄
    Hyperbetalipoproteinemia ◄
    Low-density-lipoprotein-type [LDL]
      hyperlipoproteinemia ◄

E78.01   **Familial hypercholesterolemia** ◄

E78.1   **Pure hyperglyceridemia**
    Elevated fasting triglycerides
    Endogenous hyperglyceridemia
    Fredrickson's hyperlipoproteinemia, type IV
    Hyperlipidemia, group B
    Hyperprebetalipoproteinemia
    Very-low-density-lipoprotein-type [VLDL]
      hyperlipoproteinemia

E78.2   **Mixed hyperlipidemia**
    Broad- or floating-betalipoproteinemia
    Combined hyperlipidemia NOS
    Elevated cholesterol with elevated triglycerides NEC
    Fredrickson's hyperlipoproteinemia, type IIb or III
    Hyperbetalipoproteinemia with prebetalipoproteinemia
    Hypercholesteremia with endogenous
      hyperglyceridemia
    Hyperlipidemia, group C
    Tubo-eruptive xanthoma
    Xanthoma tuberosum
    Excludes1   cerebrotendinous cholesterosis [van
        Bogaert-Scherer-Epstein] (E75.5)
        familial combined hyperlipidemia (E78.4)

E78.3   **Hyperchylomicronemia**
    Chylomicron retention disease
    Fredrickson's hyperlipoproteinemia, type I or V
    Hyperlipidemia, group D
    Mixed hyperglyceridemia

E78.4   **Other hyperlipidemia**
    Familial combined hyperlipidemia

E78.5   **Hyperlipidemia, unspecified**

E78.6   **Lipoprotein deficiency**
    Abetalipoproteinemia
    Depressed HDL cholesterol
    High-density lipoprotein deficiency
    Hypoalphalipoproteinemia
    Hypobetalipoproteinemia (familial)
    Lecithin cholesterol acyltransferase deficiency
    Tangier disease

E78.7   **Disorders of bile acid and cholesterol metabolism**
    Excludes1   Niemann-Pick disease type C (E75.242)
    (Ex) For category **E78.7** CC codes: E78.71-E78.72, Q87.1-Q87.89, Q89.8, Q99.2

E78.70   **Disorder of bile acid and cholesterol metabolism, unspecified**

E78.71   **Barth syndrome**

E78.72   **Smith-Lemli-Opitz syndrome**

E78.79   **Other disorders of bile acid and cholesterol metabolism**

E78.8   **Other disorders of lipoprotein metabolism**

E78.81   **Lipoid dermatoarthritis**

E78.89   **Other lipoprotein metabolism disorders**

E78.9   **Disorder of lipoprotein metabolism, unspecified**

E79   **Disorders of purine and pyrimidine metabolism**
    Purines, along with pyrimidines, signal RNA and DNA production
    Excludes1   Ataxia-telangiectasia (Q87.1)
        Bloom's syndrome (Q82.8)
        Cockayne's syndrome (Q87.1)
        calculus of kidney (N20.0)
        combined immunodeficiency disorders (D81.-)
        Fanconi's anemia (D61.09)
        gout (M1A.-, M10.-)
        orotaciduric anemia (D53.0)
        progeria (E34.8)
        Werner's syndrome (E34.8)
        xeroderma pigmentosum (Q82.1)
    (Ex) For category E79 CC codes: D81.3, D81.5, D81.810, D84.1, E76.01-E76.9,
      E79.1-E80.29, E80.4-E80.7, E88.81

E79.0   **Hyperuricemia without signs of inflammatory arthritis and tophaceous disease**
    Asymptomatic hyperuricemia

E79.1   **Lesch-Nyhan syndrome**
    HGPRT deficiency

E79.2   **Myoadenylate deaminase deficiency**

E79.8   **Other disorders of purine and pyrimidine metabolism**
    Hereditary xanthinuria

E79.9   **Disorder of purine and pyrimidine metabolism, unspecified**

E80   **Disorders of porphyrin and bilirubin metabolism**
    Group of chemical compounds in RBC's that combine with iron to form heme
    Includes   defects of catalase and peroxidase
    (Ex) For category E80 CC codes unless otherwise indicated: D81.3, D81.5, D81.810,
      D84.1, E76.01-E76.9, E79.1-E80.29, E80.4-E80.7, E88.81

E80.0   **Hereditary erythropoietic porphyria**
    Congenital erythropoietic porphyria
    Erythropoietic protoporphyria

E80.1   **Porphyria cutanea tarda**

E80.2   **Other and unspecified porphyria**

E80.20   **Unspecified porphyria**
    Porphyria NOS

E80.21   **Acute intermittent (hepatic) porphyria**

E80.29   **Other porphyria**
    Hereditary coproporphyria

E80.3   **Defects of catalase and peroxidase**
    Acatalasia [Takahara]
    (Ex) E71.310-E71.32, E71.40-E71.548, E80.4-E80.7, E88.40-E88.49, H49.811-H49.819

E80.4   **Gilbert syndrome**

E80.5   **Crigler-Najjar syndrome**

E80.6   **Other disorders of bilirubin metabolism**
    Dubin-Johnson syndrome
    Rotor's syndrome

E80.7   **Disorder of bilirubin metabolism, unspecified**

N   Newborn Age: 0   P   Pediatric Age: 0–17   M   Maternity DX: 12–55   A   Adult Age: 15–124   ♀   Females Only   ♂   Males Only
 Complication\Comorbidity   Major C\C   CC/MCC Exclusions   Hospital-Acquired Condition

753

CHAPTER 4 (E00–E90)

● E83   **Disorders of mineral metabolism**
> **Excludes1**   dietary mineral deficiency (E58-E61)
> parathyroid disorders (E20-E21)
> vitamin D deficiency (E55.-)

● E83.0   **Disorders of copper metabolism**

E83.00   **Disorder of copper metabolism, unspecified**

E83.01   **Wilson's disease**
> Code also associated Kayser Fleischer ring (H18.04-)

E83.09   **Other disorders of copper metabolism**
> Menkes' (kinky hair) (steely hair) disease

● E83.1   **Disorders of iron metabolism**
> **Excludes1**   iron deficiency anemia (D50.-)
> sideroblastic anemia (D64.0-D64.3)

E83.10   **Disorder of iron metabolism, unspecified**

● E83.11   **Hemochromatosis**

E83.110   **Hereditary hemochromatosis**
> Bronzed diabetes
> Pigmentary cirrhosis (of liver)
> Primary (hereditary) hemochromatosis

E83.111   **Hemochromatosis due to repeated red blood cell transfusions**
> Iron overload due to repeated red blood cell transfusions
> Transfusion (red blood cell) associated hemochromatosis

E83.118   **Other hemochromatosis**

E83.119   **Hemochromatosis, unspecified**

E83.19   **Other disorders of iron metabolism**
> Use additional code, if applicable, for idiopathic pulmonary hemosiderosis (J84.03)

E83.2   **Disorders of zinc metabolism**
> Acrodermatitis enteropathica

● E83.3   **Disorders of phosphorus metabolism and phosphatases**
> **Excludes1**   adult osteomalacia (M83.-)
> osteoporosis (M80.-)

E83.30   **Disorder of phosphorus metabolism, unspecified**

E83.31   **Familial hypophosphatemia**
> Vitamin D-resistant osteomalacia
> Vitamin D-resistant rickets
> > **Excludes1**   vitamin D-deficiency rickets (E55.0)

E83.32   **Hereditary vitamin D-dependent rickets (type 1) (type 2)**
> 25-hydroxyvitamin D 1-alpha-hydroxylase deficiency
> Pseudovitamin D deficiency
> Vitamin D receptor defect

E83.39   **Other disorders of phosphorus metabolism**
> Acid phosphatase deficiency
> Hypophosphatasia

● E83.4   **Disorders of magnesium metabolism**

E83.40   **Disorders of magnesium metabolism, unspecified**

E83.41   **Hypermagnesemia**

E83.42   **Hypomagnesemia**

E83.49   **Other disorders of magnesium metabolism**

● E83.5   **Disorders of calcium metabolism**
> **Excludes1**   chondrocalcinosis (M11.1-M11.2)
> hungry bone syndrome (E83.81)
> hyperparathyroidism (E21.0-E21.3)

E83.50   **Unspecified disorder of calcium metabolism**

E83.51   **Hypocalcemia**

E83.52   **Hypercalcemia**
> Familial hypocalciuric hypercalcemia

E83.59   **Other disorders of calcium metabolism**
> Idiopathic hypercalciuria

● E83.8   **Other disorders of mineral metabolism**

E83.81   **Hungry bone syndrome**

E83.89   **Other disorders of mineral metabolism**

E83.9   **Disorder of mineral metabolism, unspecified**

● E84   **Cystic fibrosis**
> **Includes**   mucoviscidosis
>
> Code also exocrine pancreatic insufficiency (K86.81) ◄
> Ⓔⓧ For category E84 CC codes: E84.0-E84.9

E84.0   **Cystic fibrosis with pulmonary manifestations** 🔖
> Use additional code to identify any infectious organism present, such as:
> Pseudomonas (B96.5)

● E84.1   **Cystic fibrosis with intestinal manifestations** 🔖

E84.11   **Meconium ileus in cystic fibrosis** 🔖   N
> > **Excludes1**   meconium ileus not due to cystic fibrosis (P76.0)

E84.19   **Cystic fibrosis with other intestinal manifestations** 🔖
> Distal intestinal obstruction syndrome

E84.8   **Cystic fibrosis with other manifestations** 🔖

E84.9   **Cystic fibrosis, unspecified** 🔖

● E85   **Amyloidosis**
> *A disorder resulting from the abnormal deposition of a particular protein (amyloid) into tissues of the body*
>
> **Excludes1**   Alzheimer's disease (G30.0-)
> Ⓔⓧ For category E85CC codes: E85.0-E85.9, E88.81

E85.0   **Non-neuropathic heredofamilial amyloidosis** 🔖
> ~~Familial Mediterranean fever~~
> Hereditary amyloid nephropathy

E85.1   **Neuropathic heredofamilial amyloidosis** 🔖
> Amyloid polyneuropathy (Portuguese)
> **Coding Clinic: 2012, Q4, P100**

E85.2   **Heredofamilial amyloidosis, unspecified** 🔖

E85.3   **Secondary systemic amyloidosis** 🔖
> Hemodialysis-associated amyloidosis

E85.4   **Organ-limited amyloidosis** 🔖
> Localized amyloidosis

E85.8   **Other amyloidosis** 🔖

E85.9   **Amyloidosis, unspecified** 🔖

● E86   **Volume depletion**
> **Excludes1**   dehydration of newborn (P74.1)
> hypovolemic shock NOS (R57.1)
> postprocedural hypovolemic shock (T81.19)
> traumatic hypovolemic shock (T79.4)
>
> Use additional code(s) for any associated disorders of electrolyte and acid-base balance (E87.-) ◄

E86.0   **Dehydration**
> *Excessive loss of body water*

E86.1   **Hypovolemia**
> *Diminished volume of circulating blood*
> Depletion of volume of plasma

E86.9   **Volume depletion, unspecified**

Item 4–9 Circulating fluid volume is regulated by the amount of water and sodium ingested, excreted by the kidneys into the urine, and lost through the gastrointestinal tract, lungs, and skin. To maintain blood volume within a normal range, the kidneys regulate the amount of water and sodium lost into the urine. Too much (**fluid overload**) or too little fluid volume (**volume depletion**) will affect blood pressure. Severe cases of vomiting, diarrhea, bleeding, and burns (fluid loss through exposed burn surface area) can contribute to fluid loss. Internal body environment must maintain a precise balance (homeostasis) between too much fluid and too little fluid. This complex balancing mechanism is critical to good health.

◄ New   ◄◄ Revised   ~~deleted~~ Deleted   Excludes 1   Excludes 2   Includes   Use additional   Code first   Code also   Unspecified

754   **OGCR** Official Guidelines   ● Unacceptable Principal Diagnosis   X Assign placeholder X   ● Use Additional Character(s)   🔖 Manifestation Code   **Coding Clinic**

● **E87** **Other disorders of fluid, electrolyte and acid-base balance**

> Excludes1 diabetes insipidus (E23.2)
> electrolyte imbalance associated with
> hyperemesis gravidarum (O21.1)
> electrolyte imbalance following ectopic or molar
> pregnancy (O08.5)
> familial periodic paralysis (G72.3)
>
> ⒺⓍ **For category E87 CC codes:** E86.0-E87.8

E87.0 **Hyperosmolality and hypernatremia** 🕭
Sodium [Na] excess
Sodium [Na] overload

E87.1 **Hypo-osmolality and hyponatremia** 🕭
Sodium [Na] deficiency

> Excludes1 syndrome of inappropriate secretion of
> antidiuretic hormone (E22.2)

E87.2 **Acidosis** 🕭
Acidosis NOS
Lactic acidosis
Metabolic acidosis
Respiratory acidosis

> Excludes1 diabetic acidosis - see categories E08-E10,
> E13 with ketoacidosis

E87.3 **Alkalosis** 🕭
Alkalosis NOS
Metabolic alkalosis
Respiratory alkalosis

E87.4 **Mixed disorder of acid-base balance** 🕭

E87.5 **Hyperkalemia**
Potassium [K] excess
Potassium [K] overload

E87.6 **Hypokalemia**
Potassium [K] deficiency

● **E87.7** **Fluid overload**

> Excludes1 edema NOS (R60.9)
> fluid retention (R60.9)

E87.70 **Fluid overload, unspecified**

E87.71 **Transfusion associated circulatory overload**
Fluid overload due to transfusion (blood)
(blood components) TACO

E87.79 **Other fluid overload**

E87.8 **Other disorders of electrolyte and fluid balance, not
elsewhere classified**
Electrolyte imbalance NOS
Hyperchloremia
Hypochloremia

● **E88** **Other and unspecified metabolic disorders**

Use additional codes for associated conditions

> Excludes1 histiocytosis X (chronic) (C96.6)

● **E88.0** **Disorders of plasma-protein metabolism, not elsewhere
classified**

> Excludes1 disorder of lipoprotein metabolism (E78.-)
> monoclonal gammopathy (of
> undetermined significance) (D47.2)
> polyclonal hypergammaglobulinemia
> (D89.0)
> Waldenström macroglobulinemia (C88.0)

E88.01 **Alpha-1-antitrypsin deficiency AAT deficiency**

E88.09 **Other disorders of plasma-protein metabolism,
not elsewhere classified**
Bisalbuminemia

E88.1 **Lipodystrophy, not elsewhere classified**
*Defective fat metabolism resulting in absence of subcutaneous
fat*
Lipodystrophy NOS

> Excludes1 Whipple's disease (K90.81)

E88.2 **Lipomatosis, not elsewhere classified**
Abnormal tumorlike accumulations of fat in tissue
Lipomatosis NOS
Lipomatosis (Check) dolorosa [Dercum]

E88.3 **Tumor lysis syndrome** 🕭
Tumor lysis syndrome (spontaneous)
Tumor lysis syndrome following antineoplastic drug
chemotherapy

Use additional code for adverse effect, if applicable, to
identify drug (T45.1X5)

> ⒺⓍ E08.21-E08.29, E09.21-E09.29, E88.3, N00.0-N01.9, N02.8-N02.9,
> N04.7-N05.1, N05.6-N06.1, N06.6-N07.1, N07.6-N08, N14.0-N15.0,
> N15.8-N17.9

● **E88.4** **Mitochondrial metabolism disorders**
Congenital disorder of metabolism

> Excludes1 disorders of pyruvate metabolism (E74.4)
> Kearns-Sayre syndrome (H49.81)
> Leber's disease (H47.22)
> Leigh's encephalopathy (G31.82)
> Mitochondrial myopathy, NEC (G71.3)
> Reye's syndrome (G93.7)
>
> ⒺⓍ **For category E88.4 CC codes:** C96.5-C96.6, E71.310-E71.548, E80.3-E80.7,
> E88.89

E88.40 **Mitochondrial metabolism disorder,
unspecified** 🕭

E88.41 **MELAS syndrome** 🕭
Mitochondrial myopathy, encephalopathy,
lactic acidosis and stroke-like episodes

E88.42 **MERRF syndrome** 🕭
Myoclonic epilepsy associated with ragged-red
fibers

> Code also progressive myoclonic epilepsy
> (G40.3-) ◄━━

E88.49 **Other mitochondrial metabolism disorders** 🕭

● **E88.8** **Other specified metabolic disorders**

E88.81 **Metabolic syndrome**
Dysmetabolic syndrome X

> Use additional codes for associated
> manifestations, such as:
> obesity (E66.-)

E88.89 **Other specified metabolic disorders**
Launois-Bensaude adenolipomatosis

> Excludes1 adult pulmonary Langerhans cell
> histiocytosis (J84.82)

E88.9 **Metabolic disorder, unspecified**

POSTPROCEDURAL ENDOCRINE AND METABOLIC COMPLICATIONS
AND DISORDERS, NOT ELSEWHERE CLASSIFIED (E89)

● **E89** **Postprocedural endocrine and metabolic complications and
disorders, not elsewhere classified**

> Excludes2 intraoperative complications of endocrine system
> organ or structure (E36.0-, E36.1-, E36.8)

E89.0 **Postprocedural hypothyroidism**
Postirradiation hypothyroidism
Postsurgical hypothyroidism

E89.1 **Postprocedural hypoinsulinemia** 🕭
Postpancreatectomy hyperglycemia
Postsurgical hypoinsulinemia

> Use additional code, if applicable, to identify:
> acquired absence of pancreas (Z90.41-)
> diabetes mellitus (postpancreatectomy)
> (postprocedural) (E13.-)
> insulin use (Z79.4)
>
> Excludes1 transient postprocedural hyperglycemia
> (R73.9)
> transient postprocedural hypoglycemia
> (E16.2)
>
> ⒺⓍ E08.00-E08.59, E08.618-E09.59, E09.618-E10.59, E10.618-E10.649,
> E10.69-E11.59, E11.618-E11.649, E11.69-E13.59, E13.618-E16.2, E30.9,
> E34.1, E34.50-E35, E89.1

E89.2 **Postprocedural hypoparathyroidism**
Parathyroprival tetany

E89.3 **Postprocedural hypopituitarism**
Postirradiation hypopituitarism

CHAPTER 4 (E00-E90)

N Newborn Age: 0 P Pediatric Age: 0–17 M Maternity DX: 12–55 A Adult Age: 15–124 ♀ Females Only ♂ Males Only
🕭 Complication\Comorbidity 🕭 Major C\C ⒺⓍ CC/MCC Exclusions 🕭 Hospital-Acquired Condition

755

● **E89.4** **Postprocedural ovarian failure**

    E89.40 **Asymptomatic postprocedural ovarian failure** ♀
        Postprocedural ovarian failure NOS

    E89.41 **Symptomatic postprocedural ovarian failure** ♀
        Symptoms such as flushing, sleeplessness, headache, lack of concentration, associated with postprocedural menopause

E89.5 **Postprocedural testicular hypofunction** ♂

E89.6 **Postprocedural adrenocortical (-medullary) hypofunction** &
    Ex: A17.9, A18.7, A18.82, A18.84, A18.89, E27.0-E27.9, E30.9, E34.1, E34.50-E35, E89.6

● **E89.8** **Other postprocedural endocrine and metabolic complications and disorders**
    Ex: For category E89.8 CC codes: E36.8, E89.810-E89.89, H95.811-H95.89, I97.3, M96.89, N98.1-N98.9, T81.82X[A], T81.89X-T81.9XX[A]

    ● **E89.81** **Postprocedural hemorrhage of an endocrine system organ or structure following a procedure** ◄▥

        E89.810 **Postprocedural hemorrhage of an endocrine system organ or structure following an endocrine system procedure** & ◄▥

        E89.811 **Postprocedural hemorrhage of an endocrine system organ or structure following other procedure** & ◄▥

● **E89.82** **Postprocedural hematoma and seroma of an endocrine system organ or structure** ◄

    E89.820 **Postprocedural hematoma of an endocrine system organ or structure following an endocrine system procedure** & ◄

    E89.821 **Postprocedural hematoma of an endocrine system organ or structure following other procedure** & ◄

    E89.822 **Postprocedural seroma of an endocrine system organ or structure following an endocrine system procedure** & ◄

    E89.823 **Postprocedural seroma of an endocrine system organ or structure following other procedure** & ◄

E89.89 **Other postprocedural endocrine and metabolic complications and disorders** &
    Use additional code, if applicable, to further specify disorder

CHAPTER 5

MENTAL, BEHAVIORAL AND NEURODEVELOPMENTAL DISORDERS (F01-F99)

OGCR Chapter-Specific Coding Guidelines

5. **Chapter 5: Mental, Behavioral and Neurodevelopmental disorders (F01 – F99)**

a. **Pain disorders related to psychological factors**

Assign code F45.41, for pain that is exclusively related to psychological disorders. As indicated by the Excludes 1 note under category G89, a code from category G89 should not be assigned with code F45.41

Code F45.42, Pain disorders with related psychological factors, should be used with a code from category G89, Pain, not elsewhere classified, if there is documentation of a psychological component for a patient with acute or chronic pain.

See Section I.C.6. Pain

c. **Mental and behavioral disorders due to psychoactive substance use**

1) **In Remission**

Selection of codes for "in remission" for categories F10-F19, Mental and behavioral disorders due to psychoactive substance use (categories F10-F19 with -.21) requires the provider's clinical judgment. The appropriate codes for "in remission" are assigned only on the basis of provider documentation (as defined in the Official Guidelines for Coding and Reporting).

2) **Psychoactive Substance Use, Abuse And Dependence**

When the provider documentation refers to use, abuse and dependence of the same substance (e.g. alcohol, opioid, cannabis, etc.), only one code should be assigned to identify the pattern of use based on the following hierarchy:

- If both use and abuse are documented, assign only the code for abuse
- If both abuse and dependence are documented, assign only the code for dependence
- If use, abuse and dependence are all documented, assign only the code for dependence
- If both use and dependence are documented, assign only the code for dependence.

3) **Psychoactive Substance Use**

As with all other diagnoses, the codes for psychoactive substance use (F10.9-, F11.9-, F12.9-, F13.9-, F14.9-, F15.9-, F16.9-) should only be assigned based on provider documentation and when they meet the definition of a reportable diagnosis (see Section III, Reporting Additional Diagnoses). The codes are to be used only when the psychoactive substance use is associated with a mental or behavioral disorder, and such a relationship is documented by the provider.

CHAPTER 5

MENTAL, BEHAVIORAL AND NEURODEVELOPMENTAL DISORDERS (F01-F99)

| **Includes** | disorders of psychological development |
| **Excludes2** | symptoms, signs and abnormal clinical laboratory findings, not elsewhere classified (R00-R99) |

This chapter contains the following blocks:

F01-F09	Mental disorders due to known physiological conditions
F10-F19	Mental and behavioral disorders due to psychoactive substance use
F20-F29	Schizophrenia, schizotypal, delusional, and other non-mood psychotic disorders
F30-F39	Mood [affective] disorders
F40-F48	Anxiety, dissociative, stress-related, somatoform and other nonpsychotic mental disorders
F50-F59	Behavioral syndromes associated with physiological disturbances and physical factors
F60-F69	Disorders of adult personality and behavior
F70-F79	Intellectual disabilities
F80-F89	Pervasive and specific developmental disorders
F90-F98	Behavioral and emotional disorders with onset usually occurring in childhood and adolescence
F99	Unspecified mental disorder

MENTAL DISORDERS DUE TO KNOWN PHYSIOLOGICAL CONDITIONS (F01-F09)

This block comprises a range of mental disorders grouped together on the basis of their having in common a demonstrable etiology in cerebral disease, brain injury, or other insult leading to cerebral dysfunction. The dysfunction may be primary, as in diseases, injuries, and insults that affect the brain directly and selectively; or secondary, as in systemic diseases and disorders that attack the brain only as one of the multiple organs or systems of the body that are involved.

● **F01**   **Vascular dementia**
Vascular dementia as a result of infarction of the brain due to vascular disease, including hypertensive cerebrovascular disease.

     Includes   arteriosclerotic dementia

Code first the underlying physiological condition or sequelae of cerebrovascular disease.

● **F01.5**   **Vascular dementia**

     F01.50   **Vascular dementia without behavioral disturbance**   A
             Major neurocognitive disorder without behavioral disturbance ◄

     F01.51   **Vascular dementia with behavioral disturbance** 🦠   A
             Major neurocognitive disorder due to vascular disease, with behavioral disturbance ◄
             Major neurocognitive disorder with aggressive behavior ◄
             Major neurocognitive disorder with combative behavior ◄
             Major neurocognitive disorder with violent behavior ◄
             Vascular dementia with aggressive behavior
             Vascular dementia with combative behavior
             Vascular dementia with violent behavior
             Use additional code, if applicable, to identify wandering in vascular dementia (Z91.83)
             (Ex) F01.51

CHAPTER 5 (F01-F99)

F02   Dementia in other diseases classified elsewhere

Code first the underlying physiological condition, such as:
Alzheimer's (G30.-)
cerebral lipidosis (E75.4)
Creutzfeldt-Jakob disease (A81.0-)
dementia with Lewy bodies (G31.83)
dementia with Parkinsonism (G31.83) ◀
epilepsy and recurrent seizures (G40.-)
frontotemporal dementia (G31.09)
hepatolenticular degeneration (E83.0)
human immunodeficiency virus [HIV] disease (B20)
Huntington's disease (G10) ◀
hypercalcemia (E83.52)
hypothyroidism, acquired (E00-E03.-)
intoxications (T36-T65)
Jakob-Creutzfeldt disease (A81.0-)
multiple sclerosis (G35)
neurosyphilis (A52.17)
niacin deficiency [pellagra] (E52)
Parkinson's disease (G20)
Pick's disease (G31.01)
polyarteritis nodosa (M30.0)
prion disease (A81.9) ◀
systemic lupus erythematosus (M32.-)
traumatic brain injury (S06.-) ◀
trypanosomiasis (B56.-, B57.-)
vitamin B deficiency (E53.8)

Includes Major neurocognitive disorder in other diseases classified elsewhere ◀

Excludes2 dementia in alcohol and psychoactive substance disorders (F10-F19, with .17, .27, .97)
vascular dementia (F01.5-)

● **F02.8   Dementia in other diseases classified elsewhere**

▶ **F02.80** *Dementia in other diseases classified elsewhere without behavioral disturbance*
Dementia in other diseases classified elsewhere NOS
Major neurocognitive disorder in other diseases classified elsewhere ◀
Coding Clinic: 2016, Q2, P6

▶ **F02.81** *Dementia in other diseases classified elsewhere with behavioral disturbance* 🔗
Dementia in other diseases classified elsewhere with aggressive behavior
Dementia in other diseases classified elsewhere with combative behavior
Dementia in other diseases classified elsewhere with violent behavior
Major neurocognitive disorder in other diseases classified elsewhere with aggressive behavior ◀
Major neurocognitive disorder in other diseases classified elsewhere with combative behavior ◀
Major neurocognitive disorder in other diseases classified elsewhere with violent behavior ◀
Use additional code, if applicable, to identify wandering in dementia in conditions classified elsewhere (Z91.83)
(Ex:) F02.81, F03.91

Item 5-1 Psychosis was a term formerly applied to any mental disorder but is now restricted to disturbances of a great magnitude in which there is a personality disintegration and loss of contact with reality.

● **F03   Unspecified dementia**
Presenile dementia NOS
Presenile psychosis NOS
Primary degenerative dementia NOS
Senile dementia NOS
Senile dementia depressed or paranoid type
Senile psychosis NOS

Excludes1 senility NOS (R41.81)
Excludes2 mild memory disturbance due to known physiological condition (F06.8)
senile dementia with delirium or acute confusional state (F05)

● **F03.9   Unspecified dementia**

F03.90 **Unspecified** dementia without behavioral disturbance   A
Dementia NOS
Coding Clinic: 2012, Q4, P92

F03.91 **Unspecified** dementia with behavioral disturbance 🔗   A
Unspecified dementia with aggressive behavior
Unspecified dementia with combative behavior
Unspecified dementia with violent behavior
Use additional code, if applicable, to identify wandering in unspecified dementia (Z91.83)
(Ex:) F02.81, F03.91

F04   Amnestic disorder due to known physiological condition
Korsakov's psychosis or syndrome, nonalcoholic
Code first the underlying physiological condition

Excludes1 amnesia NOS (R41.3)
anterograde amnesia (R41.1)
dissociative amnesia (F44.0)
retrograde amnesia (R41.2)

Excludes2 alcohol-induced or unspecified Korsakov's syndrome (F10.26, F10.96)
Korsakov's syndrome induced by other psychoactive substances (F13.26, F13.96, F19.16, F19.26, F19.96)

F05   Delirium due to known physiological condition 🔗
Acute or subacute brain syndrome
Acute or subacute confusional state (nonalcoholic)
Acute or subacute infective psychosis
Acute or subacute organic reaction
Acute or subacute psycho-organic syndrome
Delirium of mixed etiology
Delirium superimposed on dementia
Sundowning
Code first the underlying physiological condition
Excludes1 delirium NOS (R41.0)
Excludes2 delirium tremens alcohol-induced or unspecified (F10.231, F10.921)
(Ex:) F05, R45.851

CHAPTER 5 (F01-F99)

758

◀ New   ◀▥ Revised   deleted Deleted   Excludes 1   Excludes 2   Includes   Use additional   Code first   Code also   Unspecified
OGCR Official Guidelines   ● Unacceptable Principal Diagnosis   X Assign placeholder X   ● Use Additional Character(s)   ▶ Manifestation Code   Coding Clinic

● **F06**   **Other mental disorders due to known physiological condition**

> **Includes**   mental disorders due to endocrine disorder
> mental disorders due to exogenous hormone
> mental disorders due to exogenous toxic substance
> mental disorders due to primary cerebral disease
> mental disorders due to somatic illness
> mental disorders due to systemic disease affecting the brain

Code first the underlying physiological condition

> **Excludes1**   unspecified dementia (F03)
> **Excludes2**   delirium due to known physiological condition (F05)
> dementia as classified in F01-F02
> other mental disorders associated with alcohol and other psychoactive substances (F10-F19)

Ⓔˣ **For category F06 CC codes:** F02.80-F02.81, F04-F06.8, F10.10-F11.19, F11.21-F13.19, F13.21-F14.19, F14.21-F15.19, F15.21-F16.19, F16.21-F17.209, F17.213-F17.219, F17.223-F17.229, F17.293-F18.19, F18.21-F19.19, F19.21-F19.99, F53-F55.8, R78

F06.0   **Psychotic disorder with hallucinations due to known physiological condition** 🅒
> Organic hallucinatory state (nonalcoholic)
> **Excludes2**   hallucinations and perceptual disturbance induced by alcohol and other psychoactive substances (F10-F19 with .151, .251, .951)
> schizophrenia (F20.-)

F06.1   **Catatonic disorder due to known physiological condition**
> Catatonia associated with another mental disorder ◄
> Catatonia NOS ◄
> **Excludes1**   catatonic stupor (R40.1)
> stupor NOS (R40.1)
> **Excludes2**   catatonic schizophrenia (F20.2)
> dissociative stupor (F44.2)

F06.2   **Psychotic disorder with delusions due to known physiological condition** 🅒
> Paranoid and paranoid-hallucinatory organic states
> Schizophrenia-like psychosis in epilepsy
> **Excludes2**   alcohol and drug-induced psychotic disorder (F10-F19 with .150, .250, .950)
> brief psychotic disorder (F23)
> delusional disorder (F22)
> schizophrenia (F20.-)

● **F06.3**   **Mood disorder due to known physiological condition**
> **Excludes2**   mood disorders due to alcohol and other psychoactive substances (F10-F19 with .14, .24, .94)
> mood disorders, not due to known physiological condition or unspecified (F30-F39)

F06.30   **Mood disorder due to known physiological condition, unspecified**

F06.31   **Mood disorder due to known physiological condition with depressive features**

F06.32   **Mood disorder due to known physiological condition with major depressive-like episode**

F06.33   **Mood disorder due to known physiological condition with manic features**

F06.34   **Mood disorder due to known physiological condition with mixed features**

F06.4   **Anxiety disorder due to known physiological condition**
> **Excludes2**   anxiety disorders due to alcohol and other psychoactive substances (F10-F19 with .180, .280, .980)
> anxiety disorders, not due to known physiological condition or unspecified (F40.-, F41.-)

F06.8   **Other specified mental disorders due to known physiological condition**
> Epileptic psychosis NOS
> Organic dissociative disorder
> Organic emotionally labile [asthenic] disorder

● **F07**   **Personality and behavioral disorders due to known physiological condition**

Code first the underlying physiological condition

F07.0   **Personality change due to known physiological condition**
> Frontal lobe syndrome
> Limbic epilepsy personality syndrome
> Lobotomy syndrome
> Organic personality disorder
> Organic pseudopsychopathic personality
> Organic pseudoretarded personality
> Postleucotomy syndrome
> *Code first underlying physiological condition*
> **Excludes1**   mild cognitive impairment (G31.84)
> postconcussional syndrome (F07.81)
> postencephalitic syndrome (F07.89)
> signs and symptoms involving emotional state (R45.-)
> **Excludes2**   specific personality disorder (F60.-)

● **F07.8**   **Other personality and behavioral disorders due to known physiological condition**

F07.81   **Postconcussional syndrome**
> Postcontusional syndrome (encephalopathy)
> Post-traumatic brain syndrome, nonpsychotic
> Use additional code to identify associated post-traumatic headache, if applicable (G44.3-)
> **Excludes1**   current concussion (brain) (S06.0-)
> postencephalitic syndrome (F07.89)

F07.89   **Other personality and behavioral disorders due to known physiological condition**
> Postencephalitic syndrome
> *Damage to temporal brain lobes with memory loss and abnormal behavior*
> Right hemispheric organic affective disorder

F07.9   **Unspecified personality and behavioral disorder due to known physiological condition**
> Organic psychosyndrome
> *Due to exposure to organic solvents*

F09   **Unspecified mental disorder due to known physiological condition**
> Mental disorder NOS due to known physiological condition
> Organic brain syndrome NOS
> Organic mental disorder NOS
> Organic psychosis NOS
> Symptomatic psychosis NOS
> *Code first the underlying physiological condition*
> **Excludes1**   psychosis NOS (F29)

MENTAL AND BEHAVIORAL DISORDERS DUE TO PSYCHOACTIVE SUBSTANCE USE (F10-F19)

● **F10**   **Alcohol related disorders**
> Use additional code for blood alcohol level, if applicable (Y90.-)
> Ⓔˣ **For category F10 CC codes:** F02.80-F02.81, F04-F06.8, F10.10-F11.19, F11.21-F13.19, F13.21-F14.19, F14.21-F15.19, F15.21-F16.19, F16.21-F17.209, F17.213-F17.219, F17.223-F17.229, F17.293-F18.19, F18.21-F19.19, F19.21-F19.99, F53-F55.8, R78

● **F10.1**   **Alcohol abuse**
> **Excludes1**   alcohol dependence (F10.2-)
> alcohol use, unspecified (F10.9-)

F10.10   **Alcohol abuse, uncomplicated**
> Alcohol use disorder, mild ◄

● **F10.12**   **Alcohol abuse with intoxication**

F10.120   **Alcohol abuse with intoxication, uncomplicated**

F10.121   **Alcohol abuse with intoxication, delirium** 🅒

F10.129   **Alcohol abuse with intoxication, unspecified**

N Newborn Age: 0   **P** Pediatric Age: 0–17   **M** Maternity DX: 12–55   **A** Adult Age: 15–124   ♀ Females Only   ♂ Males Only

🅒 Complication\Comorbidity   Ⓜ Major C\C   Ⓔˣ CC/MCC Exclusions   Hospital-Acquired Condition

759

CHAPTER 5 (F01-F99)

F10.14　Alcohol abuse with alcohol-induced mood disorder 🦠
　　Alcohol use disorder, mild, with alcohol-induced bipolar or related disorder ◀
　　Alcohol use disorder, mild, with alcohol-induced depressive disorder ◀

● **F10.15　Alcohol abuse with alcohol-induced psychotic disorder**
　　F10.150　Alcohol abuse with alcohol-induced psychotic disorder with delusions
　　F10.151　Alcohol abuse with alcohol-induced psychotic disorder with hallucinations 🦠
　　F10.159　Alcohol abuse with alcohol-induced psychotic disorder, unspecified 🦠

● **F10.18　Alcohol abuse with other alcohol-induced disorders**
　　F10.180　Alcohol abuse with alcohol-induced anxiety disorder 🦠
　　F10.181　Alcohol abuse with alcohol-induced sexual dysfunction 🦠
　　F10.182　Alcohol abuse with alcohol-induced sleep disorder
　　F10.188　Alcohol abuse with other alcohol-induced disorder 🦠

F10.19　Alcohol abuse with unspecified alcohol-induced disorder 🦠

● **F10.2　Alcohol dependence**
　　Excludes1　alcohol abuse (F10.1-)
　　　　　　　　alcohol use, unspecified (F10.9-)
　　Excludes2　toxic effect of alcohol (T51.0-)

F10.20　Alcohol dependence, uncomplicated
　　Alcohol use disorder, moderate ◀
　　Alcohol use disorder, severe ◀

F10.21　Alcohol dependence, in remission

● **F10.22　Alcohol dependence with intoxication**
　　Acute drunkenness (in alcoholism)
　　　Excludes2　alcohol dependence with withdrawal (F10.23-) ◀
　　F10.220　Alcohol dependence with intoxication, uncomplicated
　　F10.221　Alcohol dependence with intoxication delirium 🦠
　　F10.229　Alcohol dependence with intoxication, unspecified

● **F10.23　Alcohol dependence with withdrawal**
　　　Excludes2　alcohol dependence with intoxication (F10.22-) ◀
　　F10.230　Alcohol dependence with withdrawal, uncomplicated 🦠
　　F10.231　Alcohol dependence with withdrawal delirium 🦠
　　F10.232　Alcohol dependence with withdrawal with perceptual disturbance 🦠
　　F10.239　Alcohol dependence with withdrawal, unspecified 🦠
　　　　Coding Clinic: 2015, Q2, P15

F10.24　Alcohol dependence with alcohol-induced mood disorder 🦠
　　Alcohol use disorder, moderate, with alcohol-induced bipolar or related disorder ◀
　　Alcohol use disorder, moderate, with alcohol-induced depressive disorder ◀
　　Alcohol use disorder, severe, with alcohol-induced bipolar or related disorder ◀
　　Alcohol use disorder, severe, with alcohol-induced depressive disorder ◀

● **F10.25　Alcohol dependence with alcohol-induced psychotic disorder**
　　F10.250　Alcohol dependence with alcohol-induced psychotic disorder with delusions
　　F10.251　Alcohol dependence with alcohol-induced psychotic disorder with hallucinations 🦠
　　F10.259　Alcohol dependence with alcohol-induced psychotic disorder, unspecified 🦠

F10.26　Alcohol dependence with alcohol-induced persisting amnestic disorder
　　Alcohol use disorder, moderate, with alcohol-induced major neurocognitive disorder, amnestic-confabulatory type ◀
　　Alcohol use disorder, severe, with alcohol-induced major neurocognitive disorder, amnestic-confabulatory type ◀

F10.27　Alcohol dependence with alcohol-induced persisting dementia 🦠
　　Alcohol use disorder, moderate, with alcohol-induced major neurocognitive disorder, nonamnestic-confabulatory type ◀
　　Alcohol use disorder, severe, with alcohol-induced major neurocognitive disorder, nonamnestic-confabulatory type ◀

● **F10.28　Alcohol dependence with other alcohol-induced disorders**
　　F10.280　Alcohol dependence with alcohol-induced anxiety disorder 🦠
　　F10.281　Alcohol dependence with alcohol-induced sexual dysfunction 🦠
　　F10.282　Alcohol dependence with alcohol-induced sleep disorder
　　F10.288　Alcohol dependence with other alcohol-induced disorder 🦠
　　　　Alcohol use disorder, moderate, with alcohol-induced mild neurocognitive disorder ◀
　　　　Alcohol use disorder, severe, with alcohol-induced mild neurocognitive disorder ◀

F10.29　Alcohol dependence with unspecified alcohol-induced disorder 🦠

● **F10.9　Alcohol use, unspecified**
　　Excludes1　alcohol abuse (F10.1-)
　　　　　　　　alcohol dependence (F10.2-)

● **F10.92　Alcohol use, unspecified with intoxication**
　　F10.920　Alcohol use, unspecified with intoxication, uncomplicated 🦠
　　F10.921　Alcohol use, unspecified with intoxication delirium 🦠
　　F10.929　Alcohol use, unspecified with intoxication, unspecified

F10.94　Alcohol use, unspecified with alcohol-induced mood disorder 🦠
　　Alcohol-induced bipolar or related disorder, without use disorder ◀
　　Alcohol-induced depressive disorder, without use disorder ◀

● **F10.95　Alcohol use, unspecified with alcohol-induced psychotic disorder**
　　F10.950　Alcohol use, unspecified with alcohol-induced psychotic disorder with delusions
　　F10.951　Alcohol use, unspecified with alcohol-induced psychotic disorder with hallucinations 🦠

◀ New　🔙 Revised　~~deleted~~ Deleted　Excludes 1　Excludes 2　Includes　Use additional　Code first　Code also　Unspecified

760

OGCR Official Guidelines　● Unacceptable Principal Diagnosis　X Assign placeholder X　● Use Additional Character(s)　🔺 Manifestation Code　Coding Clinic

F10.959   Alcohol use, unspecified with alcohol-induced psychotic disorder, unspecified 🔗
> Alcohol-induced psychotic disorder without use disorder ◄

F10.96   Alcohol use, unspecified with alcohol-induced persisting amnestic disorder
> Alcohol-induced major neurocognitive disorder, amnestic-confabulatory type, without use disorder ◄

F10.97   Alcohol use, unspecified with alcohol-induced persisting dementia
> Alcohol-induced major neurocognitive disorder, nonamnestic-confabulatory type, without use disorder ◄

● **F10.98**   Alcohol use, unspecified with other alcohol-induced disorders

     F10.980   Alcohol use, unspecified with alcohol-induced anxiety disorder 🔗
> Alcohol-induced anxiety disorder, without use disorder ◄

     F10.981   Alcohol use, unspecified with alcohol-induced sexual dysfunction 🔗
> Alcohol-induced sexual dysfunction, without use disorder ◄

     F10.982   Alcohol use, unspecified with alcohol-induced sleep disorder
> Alcohol-induced sleep disorder, without use disorder ◄

     F10.988   Alcohol use, unspecified with other alcohol-induced disorder 🔗
> Alcohol-induced mild neurocognitive disorder, without use disorder ◄

     F10.99   Alcohol use, unspecified with unspecified alcohol-induced disorder 🔗

● **F11**   Opioid related disorders
> (Ex:) **For category F11 CC codes unless otherwise indicated:** F02.80-F02.81, F04-F06.8, F10.10-F11.19, F11.21-F13.19, F13.21-F14.19, F14.21-F15.19, F15.21-F16.19, F16.21-F17.209, F17.213-F17.219, F17.223-F17.229, F17.293-F18.19, F18.21-F19.19, F19.21-F19.99, F53-F55.8, R78

● **F11.1**   Opioid abuse
> **Excludes1**   opioid dependence (F11.2-)
>   opioid use, unspecified (F11.9-)

     F11.10   Opioid abuse, uncomplicated
> Opioid use disorder, mild ◄

● **F11.12**   Opioid abuse with intoxication

     F11.120   Opioid abuse with intoxication, uncomplicated

     F11.121   Opioid abuse with intoxication delirium 🔗

     F11.122   Opioid abuse with intoxication with perceptual disturbance

     F11.129   Opioid abuse with intoxication, unspecified

     F11.14   Opioid abuse with opioid-induced mood disorder
> Opioid use disorder, mild, with opioid-induced depressive disorder ◄

● **F11.15**   Opioid abuse with opioid-induced psychotic disorder

     F11.150   Opioid abuse with opioid-induced psychotic disorder with delusions 🔗

     F11.151   Opioid abuse with opioid-induced psychotic disorder with hallucinations 🔗

     F11.159   Opioid abuse with opioid-induced psychotic disorder, unspecified

● **F11.18**   Opioid abuse with other opioid-induced disorder

     F11.181   Opioid abuse with opioid-induced sexual dysfunction

     F11.182   Opioid abuse with opioid-induced sleep disorder

     F11.188   Opioid abuse with other opioid-induced disorder

     F11.19   Opioid abuse with unspecified opioid-induced disorder

● **F11.2**   Opioid dependence
> **Excludes1**   opioid abuse (F11.1-)
>   opioid use, unspecified (F11.9-)
>
> **Excludes2**   opioid poisoning (T40.0--T40.2-)

     F11.20   Opioid dependence, uncomplicated 🔗
> Opioid use disorder, moderate ◄
> Opioid use disorder, severe ◄
> (Ex:) No exclusions

     F11.21   Opioid dependence, in remission

● **F11.22**   Opioid dependence with intoxication
> **Excludes1**   opioid dependence with withdrawal (F11.23)

     F11.220   Opioid dependence with intoxication, uncomplicated

     F11.221   Opioid dependence with intoxication delirium 🔗

     F11.222   Opioid dependence with intoxication with perceptual disturbance 🔗
> (Ex:) No exclusions

     F11.229   Opioid dependence with intoxication, unspecified 🔗

     F11.23   Opioid dependence with withdrawal 🔗
> **Excludes1**   opioid dependence with intoxication (F11.22-)

     F11.24   Opioid dependence with opioid-induced mood disorder
> Opioid use disorder, moderate, with opioid-induced depressive disorder ◄

● **F11.25**   Opioid dependence with opioid-induced psychotic disorder

     F11.250   Opioid dependence with opioid-induced psychotic disorder with delusions 🔗

     F11.251   Opioid dependence with opioid-induced psychotic disorder with hallucinations 🔗

     F11.259   Opioid dependence with opioid-induced psychotic disorder, unspecified 🔗
> (Ex:) No exclusions

● **F11.28**   Opioid dependence with other opioid-induced disorder
> (Ex:) **For category F11.28 CC codes:** No exclusions

     F11.281   Opioid dependence with opioid-induced sexual dysfunction 🔗

     F11.282   Opioid dependence with opioid-induced sleep disorder 🔗

     F11.288   Opioid dependence with other opioid-induced disorder 🔗

     F11.29   Opioid dependence with unspecified opioid-induced disorder

● **F11.9**   Opioid use, unspecified
> **Excludes1**   opioid abuse (F11.1-)
>   opioid dependence (F11.2-)

     F11.90   Opioid use, unspecified, uncomplicated

N Newborn Age: 0   **P** Pediatric Age: 0–17   **M** Maternity DX: 12–55   **A** Adult Age: 15–124   ♀ Females Only   ♂ Males Only

🔗 Complication\Comorbidity   🔗 Major C\C   (Ex:) CC/MCC Exclusions   🔗 Hospital-Acquired Condition

● **F11.92** **Opioid use, unspecified with intoxication**
 Excludes1 opioid use, unspecified with withdrawal (F11.93)

  F11.920 **Opioid use, unspecified with intoxication, uncomplicated**

  F11.921 **Opioid use, unspecified with intoxication delirium** 🅒
    Opioid-induced delirium ◀

  F11.922 **Opioid use, unspecified with intoxication with perceptual disturbance**

  F11.929 **Opioid use, unspecified with intoxication, unspecified**

 F11.93 **Opioid use, unspecified with withdrawal** 🅒
  Excludes1 opioid use, unspecified with intoxication (F11.92-)

 F11.94 **Opioid use, unspecified with opioid-induced mood disorder**
   Opioid-induced depressive disorder, without use disorder ◀

● **F11.95** **Opioid use, unspecified with opioid-induced psychotic disorder**

  F11.950 **Opioid use, unspecified with opioid-induced psychotic disorder with delusions** 🅒

  F11.951 **Opioid use, unspecified with opioid-induced psychotic disorder with hallucinations** 🅒

  F11.959 **Opioid use, unspecified with opioid-induced psychotic disorder, unspecified**

● **F11.98** **Opioid use, unspecified with other specified opioid-induced disorder**

  F11.981 **Opioid use, unspecified with opioid-induced sexual dysfunction**
    Opioid-induced sexual dysfunction, without use disorder ◀

  F11.982 **Opioid use, unspecified with opioid-induced sleep disorder**
    Opioid-induced sleep disorder, without use disorder ◀

  F11.988 **Opioid use, unspecified with other opioid-induced disorder**
    Opioid-induced anxiety disorder, without use disorder ◀

 F11.99 **Opioid use, unspecified with unspecified opioid-induced disorder**

● **F12** **Cannabis related disorders**
  Includes marijuana
  Ⓔ **For category F12 CC codes:** F02.80-F02.81, F04-F06.8, F10.10-F11.19, F11.21-F13.19, F13.21-F14.19, F14.21-F15.19, F15.21-F16.19, F16.21-F17.209, F17.213-F17.219, F17.223-F17.229, F17.293-F18.19, F18.21-F19.19, F19.21-F19.99, F53-F55.8, R78

● **F12.1** **Cannabis abuse**
  Excludes1 cannabis dependence (F12.2-)
        cannabis use, unspecified (F12.9-)

  F12.10 **Cannabis abuse, uncomplicated**
    Cannabis use disorder, mild ◀

● **F12.12** **Cannabis abuse with intoxication**

  F12.120 **Cannabis abuse with intoxication, uncomplicated**

  F12.121 **Cannabis abuse with intoxication delirium** 🅒

  F12.122 **Cannabis abuse with intoxication with perceptual disturbance**

  F12.129 **Cannabis abuse with intoxication, unspecified**

● **F12.15** **Cannabis abuse with psychotic disorder**

  F12.150 **Cannabis abuse with psychotic disorder with delusions** 🅒

  F12.151 **Cannabis abuse with psychotic disorder with hallucinations** 🅒

  F12.159 **Cannabis abuse with psychotic disorder, unspecified**

● **F12.18** **Cannabis abuse with other cannabis-induced disorder**

  F12.180 **Cannabis abuse with cannabis-induced anxiety disorder**

  F12.188 **Cannabis abuse with other cannabis-induced disorder**
    Cannabis use disorder, mild, with cannabis-induced sleep disorder ◀

 F12.19 **Cannabis abuse with unspecified cannabis-induced disorder**

● **F12.2** **Cannabis dependence**
  Excludes1 cannabis abuse (F12.1-)
        cannabis use, unspecified (F12.9-)
  Excludes2 cannabis poisoning (T40.7-)

  F12.20 **Cannabis dependence, uncomplicated**
    Cannabis use disorder, moderate ◀
    Cannabis use disorder, severe ◀

  F12.21 **Cannabis dependence, in remission**

● **F12.22** **Cannabis dependence with intoxication**

  F12.220 **Cannabis dependence with intoxication, uncomplicated**

  F12.221 **Cannabis dependence with intoxication delirium** 🅒

  F12.222 **Cannabis dependence with intoxication with perceptual disturbance**

  F12.229 **Cannabis dependence with intoxication, unspecified**

● **F12.25** **Cannabis dependence with psychotic disorder**

  F12.250 **Cannabis dependence with psychotic disorder with delusions** 🅒

  F12.251 **Cannabis dependence with psychotic disorder with hallucinations** 🅒

  F12.259 **Cannabis dependence with psychotic disorder, unspecified**

● **F12.28** **Cannabis dependence with other cannabis-induced disorder**

  F12.280 **Cannabis dependence with cannabis-induced anxiety disorder**

  F12.288 **Cannabis dependence with other cannabis-induced disorder**
    Cannabis use disorder, moderate, with cannabis-induced sleep disorder ◀
    Cannabis use disorder, severe, with cannabis-induced sleep disorder ◀
    Cannabis withdrawal ◀

 F12.29 **Cannabis dependence with unspecified cannabis-induced disorder**

● **F12.9** **Cannabis use, unspecified**
  Excludes1 cannabis abuse (F12.1-)
        cannabis dependence (F12.2-)

  F12.90 **Cannabis use, unspecified, uncomplicated**

● **F12.92** **Cannabis use, unspecified with intoxication**

  F12.920 **Cannabis use, unspecified with intoxication, uncomplicated**

  F12.921 **Cannabis use, unspecified with intoxication delirium** 🅒

◀ New   ◀▥ Revised   ~~deleted~~ Deleted   Excludes 1   Excludes 2   Includes   Use additional   Code first   Code also   Unspecified
OGCR Official Guidelines   ● Unacceptable Principal Diagnosis   X Assign placeholder X   ● Use Additional Character(s)   🅒 Manifestation Code   **Coding Clinic**

F12.922   Cannabis use, unspecified with intoxication with perceptual disturbance

F12.929   Cannabis use, unspecified with intoxication, unspecified

● **F12.95**   Cannabis use, unspecified with psychotic disorder

F12.950   Cannabis use, unspecified with psychotic disorder with delusions 🗪

F12.951   Cannabis use, unspecified with psychotic disorder with hallucinations 🗪

F12.959   Cannabis use, unspecified with psychotic disorder, unspecified
> Cannabis-induced psychotic disorder, without use disorder ◄

● **F12.98**   Cannabis use, unspecified with other cannabis-induced disorder

F12.980   Cannabis use, unspecified with anxiety disorder
> Cannabis-induced anxiety disorder, without use disorder ◄

F12.988   Cannabis use, unspecified with other cannabis-induced disorder
> Cannabis-induced sleep disorder, without use disorder ◄

F12.99   Cannabis use, unspecified with unspecified cannabis-induced disorder

● **F13**   **Sedative, hypnotic, or anxiolytic related disorders**
> (Ex) **For category F13 CC codes unless otherwise indicated:** F02.80-F02.81, F04-F06.8, F10.10-F11.19, F11.21-F13.19, F13.21-F14.19, F14.21-F15.19, F15.21-F16.19, F16.21-F17.209, F17.213-F17.219, F17.223-F17.229, F17.293-F18.19, F18.21-F19.19, F19.21-F19.99, F53-F55.8, R78

● **F13.1**   **Sedative, hypnotic or anxiolytic-related abuse**
> **Excludes1**   sedative, hypnotic or anxiolytic-related dependence (F13.2-)
> sedative, hypnotic, or anxiolytic use, unspecified (F13.9-)

F13.10   Sedative, hypnotic or anxiolytic abuse, uncomplicated
> Sedative, hypnotic, or anxiolytic use disorder, mild ◄

● **F13.12**   Sedative, hypnotic or anxiolytic abuse with intoxication

F13.120   Sedative, hypnotic or anxiolytic abuse with intoxication, uncomplicated

F13.121   Sedative, hypnotic or anxiolytic abuse with intoxication delirium 🗪

F13.129   Sedative, hypnotic or anxiolytic abuse with intoxication, unspecified

F13.14   Sedative, hypnotic or anxiolytic abuse with sedative, hypnotic or anxiolytic-induced mood disorder
> Sedative, hypnotic, or anxiolytic use disorder, mild, with sedative, hypnotic, or anxiolytic-induced bipolar or related disorder ◄
> Sedative, hypnotic, or anxiolytic use disorder, mild, with sedative, hypnotic, or anxiolytic-induced depressive disorder ◄

● **F13.15**   Sedative, hypnotic or anxiolytic abuse with sedative, hypnotic or anxiolytic-induced psychotic disorder

F13.150   Sedative, hypnotic or anxiolytic abuse with sedative, hypnotic or anxiolytic-induced psychotic disorder with delusions 🗪

F13.151   Sedative, hypnotic or anxiolytic abuse with sedative, hypnotic or anxiolytic-induced psychotic disorder with hallucinations 🗪

F13.159   Sedative, hypnotic or anxiolytic abuse with sedative, hypnotic or anxiolytic-induced psychotic disorder, unspecified

● **F13.18**   Sedative, hypnotic or anxiolytic abuse with other sedative, hypnotic or anxiolytic-induced disorders

F13.180   Sedative, hypnotic or anxiolytic abuse with sedative, hypnotic or anxiolytic-induced anxiety disorder

F13.181   Sedative, hypnotic or anxiolytic abuse with sedative, hypnotic or anxiolytic-induced sexual dysfunction

F13.182   Sedative, hypnotic or anxiolytic abuse with sedative, hypnotic or anxiolytic-induced sleep disorder

F13.188   Sedative, hypnotic or anxiolytic abuse with other sedative, hypnotic or anxiolytic-induced disorder

F13.19   Sedative, hypnotic or anxiolytic abuse with unspecified sedative, hypnotic or anxiolytic-induced disorder

● **F13.2**   **Sedative, hypnotic or anxiolytic-related dependence**
> **Excludes1**   sedative, hypnotic or anxiolytic-related abuse (F13.1-)
> sedative, hypnotic, or anxiolytic use, unspecified (F13.9-)
> **Excludes2**   sedative, hypnotic, or anxiolytic poisoning (T42.-)

F13.20   Sedative, hypnotic or anxiolytic dependence, uncomplicated 🗪
> (Ex) No exclusions

F13.21   Sedative, hypnotic or anxiolytic dependence, in remission

● **F13.22**   Sedative, hypnotic or anxiolytic dependence with intoxication
> **Excludes1**   sedative, hypnotic or anxiolytic dependence with withdrawal (F13.23-)

F13.220   Sedative, hypnotic or anxiolytic dependence with intoxication, uncomplicated

F13.221   Sedative, hypnotic or anxiolytic dependence with intoxication delirium 🗪

F13.229   Sedative, hypnotic or anxiolytic dependence with intoxication, unspecified

● **F13.23**   Sedative, hypnotic or anxiolytic dependence with withdrawal
> Sedative, hypnotic, or anxiolytic use disorder, moderate ◄
> Sedative, hypnotic, or anxiolytic use disorder, severe ◄
> **Excludes1**   sedative, hypnotic or anxiolytic dependence with intoxication (F13.22-)

F13.230   Sedative, hypnotic or anxiolytic dependence with withdrawal, uncomplicated 🗪

F13.231   Sedative, hypnotic or anxiolytic dependence with withdrawal delirium 🗪

N Newborn Age: 0   **P** Pediatric Age: 0–17   **M** Maternity DX: 12–55   **A** Adult Age: 15–124   ♀ Females Only   ♂ Males Only

🗪 Complication\Comorbidity   🗪 Major C\C   (Ex) CC/MCC Exclusions   🗪 Hospital-Acquired Condition

763

CHAPTER 5 (F01-F99)

F13.232 **Sedative, hypnotic or anxiolytic dependence with withdrawal with perceptual disturbance** 🔗
> Sedative, hypnotic, or anxiolytic withdrawal with perceptual disturbances ◀

F13.239 **Sedative, hypnotic or anxiolytic dependence with withdrawal, unspecified** 🔗
> Sedative, hypnotic, or anxiolytic withdrawal without perceptual disturbances ◀

F13.24 **Sedative, hypnotic or anxiolytic dependence with sedative, hypnotic or anxiolytic-induced mood disorder**
> Sedative, hypnotic, or anxiolytic use disorder, moderate, with sedative, hypnotic, or anxiolytic-induced bipolar or related disorder ◀
> Sedative, hypnotic, or anxiolytic use disorder, moderate, with sedative, hypnotic, or anxiolytic-induced depressive disorder ◀
> Sedative, hypnotic, or anxiolytic use disorder, severe, with sedative, hypnotic, or anxiolytic-induced bipolar or related disorder ◀
> Sedative, hypnotic, or anxiolytic use disorder, severe, with sedative, hypnotic, or anxiolytic-induced depressive disorder ◀

●F13.25 **Sedative, hypnotic or anxiolytic dependence with sedative, hypnotic or anxiolytic-induced psychotic disorder**

  F13.250 **Sedative, hypnotic or anxiolytic dependence with sedative, hypnotic or anxiolytic-induced psychotic disorder with delusions** 🔗

  F13.251 **Sedative, hypnotic or anxiolytic dependence with sedative, hypnotic or anxiolytic-induced psychotic disorder with hallucinations** 🔗

  F13.259 **Sedative, hypnotic or anxiolytic dependence with sedative, hypnotic or anxiolytic-induced psychotic disorder, unspecified** 🔗
> (Ex:) No exclusions

F13.26 **Sedative, hypnotic or anxiolytic dependence with sedative, hypnotic or anxiolytic-induced persisting amnestic disorder** 🔗
> (Ex:) No exclusions

F13.27 **Sedative, hypnotic or anxiolytic dependence with sedative, hypnotic or anxiolytic-induced persisting dementia** 🔗
> Sedative, hypnotic, or anxiolytic use disorder, moderate, with sedative, hypnotic, or anxiolytic-induced major neurocognitive disorder ◀
> Sedative, hypnotic, or anxiolytic use disorder, severe, with sedative, hypnotic, or anxiolytic-induced major neurocognitive disorder ◀

●F13.28 **Sedative, hypnotic or anxiolytic dependence with other sedative, hypnotic or anxiolytic-induced disorders**
> (Ex:) **For category F13.28 CC codes:** No exclusions

  F13.280 **Sedative, hypnotic or anxiolytic dependence with sedative, hypnotic or anxiolytic-induced anxiety disorder** 🔗

  F13.281 **Sedative, hypnotic or anxiolytic dependence with sedative, hypnotic or anxiolytic-induced sexual dysfunction** 🔗

  F13.282 **Sedative, hypnotic or anxiolytic dependence with sedative, hypnotic or anxiolytic-induced sleep disorder** 🔗

  F13.288 **Sedative, hypnotic or anxiolytic dependence with other sedative, hypnotic or anxiolytic-induced disorder** 🔗
> Sedative, hypnotic, or anxiolytic use disorder, moderate, with sedative, hypnotic, or anxiolytic-induced mild neurocognitive disorder ◀
> Sedative, hypnotic, or anxiolytic use disorder, severe, with sedative, hypnotic, or anxiolytic-induced mild neurocognitive disorder ◀

F13.29 **Sedative, hypnotic or anxiolytic dependence with unspecified sedative, hypnotic or anxiolytic-induced disorder**

●F13.9 **Sedative, hypnotic or anxiolytic-related use, unspecified**
> **Excludes1**   sedative, hypnotic or anxiolytic-related abuse (F13.1-)
> sedative, hypnotic or anxiolytic-related dependence (F13.2-)

F13.90 **Sedative, hypnotic, or anxiolytic use, unspecified, uncomplicated**

●F13.92 **Sedative, hypnotic or anxiolytic use, unspecified with intoxication**
> **Excludes1**   sedative, hypnotic or anxiolytic use, unspecified with withdrawal (F13.93-)

  F13.920 **Sedative, hypnotic or anxiolytic use, unspecified with intoxication, uncomplicated**

  F13.921 **Sedative, hypnotic or anxiolytic use, unspecified with intoxication delirium** 🔗
> Sedative, hypnotic, or anxiolytic-induced delirium ◀

  F13.929 **Sedative, hypnotic or anxiolytic use, unspecified with intoxication, unspecified**

●F13.93 **Sedative, hypnotic or anxiolytic use, unspecified with withdrawal**
> **Excludes1**   sedative, hypnotic or anxiolytic use, unspecified with intoxication (F13.92-)

  F13.930 **Sedative, hypnotic or anxiolytic use, unspecified with withdrawal, uncomplicated** 🔗

  F13.931 **Sedative, hypnotic or anxiolytic use, unspecified with withdrawal delirium** 🔗

  F13.932 **Sedative, hypnotic or anxiolytic use, unspecified with withdrawal with perceptual disturbances** 🔗

  F13.939 **Sedative, hypnotic or anxiolytic use, unspecified with withdrawal, unspecified** 🔗

F13.94 **Sedative, hypnotic or anxiolytic use, unspecified with sedative, hypnotic or anxiolytic-induced mood disorder**
> Sedative, hypnotic, or anxiolytic-induced bipolar or related disorder, without use disorder ◀
> Sedative, hypnotic, or anxiolytic-induced depressive disorder, without use disorder ◀

◀ New   ◀▪ Revised   ~~deleted~~ Deleted   Excludes 1   Excludes 2   Includes   Use additional   Code first   Code also   Unspecified

764

OGCR Official Guidelines   ● Unacceptable Principal Diagnosis   X Assign placeholder X   ● Use Additional Character(s)   ▪ Manifestation Code   **Coding Clinic**

● **F13.95**   **Sedative, hypnotic or anxiolytic use, unspecified with sedative, hypnotic or anxiolytic-induced psychotic disorder**

    F13.950   **Sedative, hypnotic or anxiolytic use, unspecified with sedative, hypnotic or anxiolytic-induced psychotic disorder with delusions** 🦠

    F13.951   **Sedative, hypnotic or anxiolytic use, unspecified with sedative, hypnotic or anxiolytic-induced psychotic disorder with hallucinations** 🦠

    F13.959   **Sedative, hypnotic or anxiolytic use, unspecified with sedative, hypnotic or anxiolytic-induced psychotic disorder, unspecified**
       Sedative, hypnotic, or anxiolytic-induced psychotic disorder, without use disorder ◄

   F13.96   **Sedative, hypnotic or anxiolytic use, unspecified with sedative, hypnotic or anxiolytic-induced persisting amnestic disorder**

   F13.97   **Sedative, hypnotic or anxiolytic use, unspecified with sedative, hypnotic or anxiolytic-induced persisting dementia** 🦠
       Sedative, hypnotic, or anxiolytic-induced major neurocognitive disorder, without use disorder ◄

● **F13.98**   **Sedative, hypnotic or anxiolytic use, unspecified with other sedative, hypnotic or anxiolytic-induced disorders**

    F13.980   **Sedative, hypnotic or anxiolytic use, unspecified with sedative, hypnotic or anxiolytic-induced anxiety disorder**
       Sedative, hypnotic, or anxiolytic-induced anxiety disorder, without use disorder ◄

    F13.981   **Sedative, hypnotic or anxiolytic use, unspecified with sedative, hypnotic or anxiolytic-induced sexual dysfunction**
       Sedative, hypnotic, or anxiolytic-induced sexual dysfunction disorder, without use disorder ◄

    F13.982   **Sedative, hypnotic or anxiolytic use, unspecified with sedative, hypnotic or anxiolytic-induced sleep disorder**
       Sedative, hypnotic, or anxiolytic-induced sleep disorder, without use disorder ◄

    F13.988   **Sedative, hypnotic or anxiolytic use, unspecified with other sedative, hypnotic or anxiolytic-induced disorder**
       Sedative, hypnotic, or anxiolytic-induced mild neurocognitive disorder ◄

   F13.99   **Sedative, hypnotic or anxiolytic use, unspecified with unspecified sedative, hypnotic or anxiolytic-induced disorder**

● **F14**   **Cocaine related disorders**

   Excludes2   other stimulant-related disorders (F15.-)

   (Ex:) **For category F14 CC codes unless otherwise indicated:** F02.80-F02.81, F04-F06.8, F10.10-F11.19, F11.21-F13.19, F13.21-F14.19, F14.21-F15.19, F15.21-F16.19, F16.21-F17.209, F17.213-F17.219, F17.223-F17.229, F17.293-F18.19, F18.21-F19.19, F19.21-F19.99, F53-F55.8, R78

● **F14.1**   **Cocaine abuse**

   Excludes1   cocaine dependence (F14.2-)
          cocaine use, unspecified (F14.9-)

   F14.10   **Cocaine abuse, uncomplicated**
       Cocaine use disorder, mild ◄

● **F14.12**   **Cocaine abuse with intoxication**

    F14.120   **Cocaine abuse with intoxication, uncomplicated**

    F14.121   **Cocaine abuse with intoxication with delirium** 🦠

    F14.122   **Cocaine abuse with intoxication with perceptual disturbance**

    F14.129   **Cocaine abuse with intoxication, unspecified**

   F14.14   **Cocaine abuse with cocaine-induced mood disorder**
       Cocaine use disorder, mild, with cocaine-induced bipolar or related disorder ◄
       Cocaine use disorder, mild, with cocaine-induced depressive disorder ◄

● **F14.15**   **Cocaine abuse with cocaine-induced psychotic disorder**

    F14.150   **Cocaine abuse with cocaine-induced psychotic disorder with delusions** 🦠

    F14.151   **Cocaine abuse with cocaine-induced psychotic disorder with hallucinations** 🦠

    F14.159   **Cocaine abuse with cocaine-induced psychotic disorder, unspecified**

● **F14.18**   **Cocaine abuse with other cocaine-induced disorder**

    F14.180   **Cocaine abuse with cocaine-induced anxiety disorder**

    F14.181   **Cocaine abuse with cocaine-induced sexual dysfunction**

    F14.182   **Cocaine abuse with cocaine-induced sleep disorder**

    F14.188   **Cocaine abuse with other cocaine-induced disorder**
       Cocaine use disorder, mild, with cocaine-induced obsessive-compulsive or related disorder ◄

   F14.19   **Cocaine abuse with unspecified cocaine-induced disorder**

● **F14.2**   **Cocaine dependence**

   Excludes1   cocaine abuse (F14.1-)
          cocaine use, unspecified (F14.9-)

   Excludes2   cocaine poisoning (T40.5-)

   F14.20   **Cocaine dependence, uncomplicated** 🦠
       Cocaine use disorder, moderate ◄
       Cocaine use disorder, severe ◄
       (Ex:) No exclusions

   F14.21   **Cocaine dependence, in remission**

● **F14.22**   **Cocaine dependence with intoxication**

   Excludes1   cocaine dependence with withdrawal (F14.23)

    F14.220   **Cocaine dependence with intoxication, uncomplicated**

    F14.221   **Cocaine dependence with intoxication delirium** 🦠

    F14.222   **Cocaine dependence with intoxication with perceptual disturbance** 🦠
       (Ex:) No exclusions

    F14.229   **Cocaine dependence with intoxication, unspecified** 🦠
       (Ex:) No exclusions

   F14.23   **Cocaine dependence with withdrawal** 🦠

   Excludes1   cocaine dependence with intoxication (F14.22-)

CHAPTER 5 (F01-F99)

F14.24 Cocaine dependence with cocaine-induced mood disorder
Cocaine use disorder, moderate, with cocaine-induced bipolar or related disorder ◄
Cocaine use disorder, moderate, with cocaine-induced depressive disorder ◄
Cocaine use disorder, severe, with cocaine-induced bipolar or related disorder ◄
Cocaine use disorder, severe, with cocaine-induced depressive disorder ◄

● **F14.25 Cocaine dependence with cocaine-induced psychotic disorder**

    F14.250 Cocaine dependence with cocaine-induced psychotic disorder with delusions 🏷

    F14.251 Cocaine dependence with cocaine-induced psychotic disorder with hallucinations 🏷

    F14.259 Cocaine dependence with cocaine-induced psychotic disorder, unspecified 🏷
        (Ex) No exclusions

● **F14.28 Cocaine dependence with other cocaine-induced disorder**
    (Ex) For category F14.28 CC codes: No exclusions

    F14.280 Cocaine dependence with cocaine-induced anxiety disorder 🏷

    F14.281 Cocaine dependence with cocaine-induced sexual dysfunction 🏷

    F14.282 Cocaine dependence with cocaine-induced sleep disorder 🏷

    F14.288 Cocaine dependence with other cocaine-induced disorder 🏷
        Cocaine use disorder, moderate, with cocaine-induced obsessive-compulsive or related disorder ◄
        Cocaine use disorder, severe, with cocaine-induced obsessive-compulsive or related disorder ◄

    F14.29 Cocaine dependence with unspecified cocaine-induced disorder

● **F14.9 Cocaine use, unspecified**
    Excludes1   cocaine abuse (F14.1-)
                 cocaine dependence (F14.2-)

    F14.90 Cocaine use, unspecified, uncomplicated

●   F14.92 Cocaine use, unspecified with intoxication

    F14.920 Cocaine use, unspecified with intoxication, uncomplicated

    F14.921 Cocaine use, unspecified with intoxication delirium 🏷

    F14.922 Cocaine use, unspecified with intoxication with perceptual disturbance

    F14.929 Cocaine use, unspecified with intoxication, unspecified

    F14.94 Cocaine use, unspecified with cocaine-induced mood disorder
        Cocaine-induced bipolar or related disorder, without use disorder ◄
        Cocaine-induced depressive disorder, without use disorder ◄

●   F14.95 Cocaine use, unspecified with cocaine-induced psychotic disorder

    F14.950 Cocaine use, unspecified with cocaine-induced psychotic disorder with delusions 🏷

    F14.951 Cocaine use, unspecified with cocaine-induced psychotic disorder with hallucinations 🏷

    F14.959 Cocaine use, unspecified with cocaine-induced psychotic disorder, unspecified
        Cocaine-induced psychotic disorder, without use disorder ◄

●   F14.98 Cocaine use, unspecified with other specified cocaine-induced disorder

    F14.980 Cocaine use, unspecified with cocaine-induced anxiety disorder
        Cocaine-induced anxiety disorder, without use disorder ◄

    F14.981 Cocaine use, unspecified with cocaine-induced sexual dysfunction
        Cocaine-induced sexual dysfunction, without use disorder ◄

    F14.982 Cocaine use, unspecified with cocaine-induced sleep disorder
        Cocaine-induced sleep disorder, without use disorder ◄

    F14.988 Cocaine use, unspecified with other cocaine-induced disorder
        Cocaine-induced obsessive-compulsive or related disorder ◄

    F14.99 Cocaine use, unspecified with unspecified cocaine-induced disorder

● **F15 Other stimulant related disorders**
    Includes   amphetamine-related disorders
                 caffeine
    Excludes2   cocaine-related disorders (F14.-)
    (Ex) For category F15 CC codes unless otherwise indicated: F02.80-F02.81, F04-F06.8, F10.10-F11.19, F11.21-F13.19, F13.21-F14.19, F14.21-F15.19, F15.21-F16.19, F16.21-F17.209, F17.213-F17.219, F17.223-F17.229, F17.293-F18.19, F18.21-F19.19, F19.21-F19.99, F53-F55.8, R78

● **F15.1 Other stimulant abuse**
    Excludes1   other stimulant dependence (F15.2-)
                 other stimulant use, unspecified (F15.9-)

    F15.10 Other stimulant abuse, uncomplicated
        Amphetamine type substance use disorder, mild ◄
        Other or unspecified stimulant use disorder, mild ◄

●   F15.12 Other stimulant abuse with intoxication

    F15.120 Other stimulant abuse with intoxication, uncomplicated

    F15.121 Other stimulant abuse with intoxication delirium 🏷

    F15.122 Other stimulant abuse with intoxication with perceptual disturbance
        Amphetamine or other stimulant use disorder, mild, with amphetamine or other stimulant intoxication, with perceptual disturbances ◄

    F15.129 Other stimulant abuse with intoxication, unspecified
        Amphetamine or other stimulant use disorder, mild, with amphetamine or other stimulant intoxication, without perceptual disturbances ◄

    F15.14 Other stimulant abuse with stimulant-induced mood disorder
        Amphetamine or other stimulant use disorder, mild, with amphetamine or other stimulant-induced bipolar or related disorder ◄
        Amphetamine or other stimulant use disorder, mild, with amphetamine or other stimulant-induced depressive disorder ◄

◄ New   ◄⃫ Revised   ~~deleted~~ Deleted   Excludes 1   Excludes 2   Includes   Use additional   Code first   Code also   Unspecified
OGCR Official Guidelines   ● Unacceptable Principal Diagnosis   X Assign placeholder X   ● Use Additional Character(s)   ▶ Manifestation Code   **Coding Clinic**

● **F15.15**   **Other stimulant abuse with stimulant-induced psychotic disorder**

     F15.150   **Other stimulant abuse with stimulant-induced psychotic disorder with delusions** ◔

     F15.151   **Other stimulant abuse with stimulant-induced psychotic disorder with hallucinations** ◔

     F15.159   **Other stimulant abuse with stimulant-induced psychotic disorder, unspecified**

● **F15.18**   **Other stimulant abuse with other stimulant-induced disorder**

     F15.180   **Other stimulant abuse with stimulant-induced anxiety disorder**

     F15.181   **Other stimulant abuse with stimulant-induced sexual dysfunction**

     F15.182   **Other stimulant abuse with stimulant-induced sleep disorder**

     F15.188   **Other stimulant abuse with other stimulant-induced disorder**

         Amphetamine or other stimulant use disorder, mild, with amphetamine or other stimulant-induced obsessive-compulsive or related disorder ◄

     F15.19   **Other stimulant abuse with unspecified stimulant-induced disorder**

● **F15.2**   **Other stimulant dependence**

     Excludes1   other stimulant abuse (F15.1-)
                 other stimulant use, unspecified (F15.9-)

     F15.20   **Other stimulant dependence, uncomplicated** ◔

         Amphetamine type substance use disorder, moderate ◄
         Amphetamine type substance use disorder, severe ◄
         Other or unspecified stimulant use disorder, moderate ◄
         Other or unspecified stimulant use disorder, severe ◄
         (Ex) No exclusions

     F15.21   **Other stimulant dependence, in remission**

●   **F15.22**   **Other stimulant dependence with intoxication**

     Excludes1   other stimulant dependence with withdrawal (F15.23)

     F15.220   **Other stimulant dependence with intoxication, uncomplicated**

     F15.221   **Other stimulant dependence with intoxication delirium** ◔

     F15.222   **Other stimulant dependence with intoxication with perceptual disturbance** ◔

         Amphetamine or other stimulant use disorder, moderate, with amphetamine or other stimulant intoxication, with perceptual disturbances ◄
         Amphetamine or other stimulant use disorder, severe, with amphetamine or other stimulant intoxication, with perceptual disturbances ◄
         (Ex) No exclusions

     F15.229   **Other stimulant dependence with intoxication, unspecified**

         Amphetamine or other stimulant use disorder, moderate, with amphetamine or other stimulant intoxication, without perceptual disturbances ◄
         Amphetamine or other stimulant use disorder, severe, with amphetamine or other stimulant intoxication, without perceptual disturbances ◄

     F15.23   **Other stimulant dependence with withdrawal** ◔

         Amphetamine or other stimulant withdrawal ◄

     Excludes1   other stimulant dependence with intoxication (F15.22-)

     F15.24   **Other stimulant dependence with stimulant-induced mood disorder**

         Amphetamine or other stimulant use disorder, moderate, with amphetamine or other stimulant-induced bipolar or related disorder ◄
         Amphetamine or other stimulant use disorder, moderate, with amphetamine or other stimulant-induced depressive disorder ◄
         Amphetamine or other stimulant use disorder, severe, with amphetamine or other stimulant-induced bipolar or related disorder ◄
         Amphetamine or other stimulant use disorder, severe, with amphetamine or other stimulant-induced depressive disorder ◄

● **F15.25**   **Other stimulant dependence with stimulant-induced psychotic disorder**

     F15.250   **Other stimulant dependence with stimulant-induced psychotic disorder with delusions** ◔

     F15.251   **Other stimulant dependence with stimulant-induced psychotic disorder with hallucinations** ◔

     F15.259   **Other stimulant dependence with stimulant-induced psychotic disorder, unspecified** ◔

         (Ex) No exclusions

● **F15.28**   **Other stimulant dependence with other stimulant-induced disorder**

     (Ex) For category F15.28 CC codes: No exclusions

     F15.280   **Other stimulant dependence with stimulant-induced anxiety disorder** ◔

     F15.281   **Other stimulant dependence with stimulant-induced sexual dysfunction** ◔

     F15.282   **Other stimulant dependence with stimulant-induced sleep disorder** ◔

     F15.288   **Other stimulant dependence with other stimulant-induced disorder** ◔

         Amphetamine or other stimulant use disorder, moderate, with amphetamine or other stimulant-induced obsessive-compulsive or related disorder ◄
         Amphetamine or other stimulant use disorder, severe, with amphetamine or other stimulant-induced obsessive-compulsive or related disorder ◄

     F15.29   **Other stimulant dependence with unspecified stimulant-induced disorder**

● **F15.9**   **Other stimulant use, unspecified**

     Excludes1   other stimulant abuse (F15.1-)
                 other stimulant dependence (F15.2-)

     F15.90   **Other stimulant use, unspecified, uncomplicated**

CHAPTER 5 (F01-F99)

● **F15.92   Other stimulant use, unspecified with intoxication**

> **Excludes1**   other stimulant use, unspecified with withdrawal (F15.93)

    F15.920   Other stimulant use, unspecified with intoxication, uncomplicated

    F15.921   Other stimulant use, unspecified with intoxication delirium 🔗
> Amphetamine or other stimulant-induced delirium ◀

    F15.922   Other stimulant use, unspecified with intoxication with perceptual disturbance

    F15.929   Other stimulant use, unspecified with intoxication, unspecified
> Caffeine intoxication ◀

F15.93   Other stimulant use, unspecified with withdrawal 🔗
> Caffeine withdrawal ◀

> **Excludes1**   other stimulant use, unspecified with intoxication (F15.92-)

F15.94   Other stimulant use, unspecified with stimulant-induced mood disorder
> Amphetamine or other stimulant-induced bipolar or related disorder, without use disorder ◀
> Amphetamine or other stimulant-induced depressive disorder, without use disorder ◀

● **F15.95   Other stimulant use, unspecified with stimulant-induced psychotic disorder**

    F15.950   Other stimulant use, unspecified with stimulant-induced psychotic disorder with delusions 🔗

    F15.951   Other stimulant use, unspecified with stimulant-induced psychotic disorder with hallucinations 🔗

    F15.959   Other stimulant use, unspecified with stimulant-induced psychotic disorder, unspecified
> Amphetamine or other stimulant-induced psychotic disorder, without use disorder ◀

● **F15.98   Other stimulant use, unspecified with other stimulant-induced disorder**

    F15.980   Other stimulant use, unspecified with stimulant-induced anxiety disorder
> Amphetamine or other stimulant-induced anxiety disorder, without use disorder ◀
> Caffeine-induced anxiety disorder, without use disorder ◀

    F15.981   Other stimulant use, unspecified with stimulant-induced sexual dysfunction
> Amphetamine or other stimulant-induced sexual dysfunction, without use disorder ◀

    F15.982   Other stimulant use, unspecified with stimulant-induced sleep disorder
> Amphetamine or other stimulant-induced sleep disorder, without use disorder ◀
> Caffeine-induced sleep disorder, without use disorder ◀

    F15.988   Other stimulant use, unspecified with other stimulant-induced disorder
> Amphetamine or other stimulant-induced obsessive-compulsive or related disorder, without use disorder ◀

F15.99   Other stimulant use, unspecified with unspecified stimulant-induced disorder

● **F16   Hallucinogen related disorders**

    Includes   ecstasy
> PCP
> phencyclidine

Ⓔⓧ **For category F16 CC codes unless otherwise indicated:** F02.80-F02.81, F04-F06.8, F10.10-F11.19, F11.21-F13.19, F13.21-F14.19, F14.21-F15.19, F15.21-F16.19, F16.21-F17.209, F17.213-F17.219, F17.223-F17.229, F17.293-F18.19, F18.21-F19.19, F19.21-F19.99, F53-F55.8, R78

● **F16.1   Hallucinogen abuse**

> **Excludes1**   hallucinogen dependence (F16.2-)
> hallucinogen use, unspecified (F16.9-)

    F16.10   Hallucinogen abuse, uncomplicated
> Other hallucinogen use disorder, mild ◀
> Phencyclidine use disorder, mild ◀

● **F16.12   Hallucinogen abuse with intoxication**

    F16.120   Hallucinogen abuse with intoxication, uncomplicated

    F16.121   Hallucinogen abuse with intoxication with delirium 🔗

    F16.122   Hallucinogen abuse with intoxication with perceptual disturbance

    F16.129   Hallucinogen abuse with intoxication, unspecified

F16.14   Hallucinogen abuse with hallucinogen-induced mood disorder
> Other hallucinogen use disorder, mild, with other hallucinogen-induced bipolar or related disorder ◀
> Other hallucinogen use disorder, mild, with other hallucinogen-induced depressive disorder ◀
> Phencyclidine use disorder, mild, with phencyclidine-induced bipolar or related disorder ◀
> Phencyclidine use disorder, mild, with phencyclidine-induced depressive disorder ◀

● **F16.15   Hallucinogen abuse with hallucinogen-induced psychotic disorder**

    F16.150   Hallucinogen abuse with hallucinogen-induced psychotic disorder with delusions 🔗

    F16.151   Hallucinogen abuse with hallucinogen-induced psychotic disorder with hallucinations 🔗

    F16.159   Hallucinogen abuse with hallucinogen-induced psychotic disorder, unspecified

● **F16.18   Hallucinogen abuse with other hallucinogen-induced disorder**

    F16.180   Hallucinogen abuse with hallucinogen-induced anxiety disorder

    F16.183   Hallucinogen abuse with hallucinogen persisting perception disorder (flashbacks)

    F16.188   Hallucinogen abuse with other hallucinogen-induced disorder

F16.19   Hallucinogen abuse with unspecified hallucinogen-induced disorder

● **F16.2   Hallucinogen dependence**

> **Excludes1**   hallucinogen abuse (F16.1-)
> hallucinogen use, unspecified (F16.9-)

    F16.20   Hallucinogen dependence, uncomplicated 🔗
> Other hallucinogen use disorder, moderate ◀
> Other hallucinogen use disorder, severe ◀
> Phencyclidine use disorder, moderate ◀
> Phencyclidine use disorder, severe ◀
> Ⓔⓧ No exclusions

    F16.21   Hallucinogen dependence, in remission

CHAPTER 5 (F01-F99)

◀ New   ◀▥ Revised   ~~deleted~~ Deleted   Excludes 1   Excludes 2   Includes   Use additional   Code first   Code also   Unspecified

OGCR Official Guidelines   ● Unacceptable Principal Diagnosis   X Assign placeholder X   ● Use Additional Character(s)   ▸ Manifestation Code   **Coding Clinic**

● **F16.22**   **Hallucinogen dependence with intoxication**

F16.220   Hallucinogen dependence with intoxication, uncomplicated

F16.221   Hallucinogen dependence with intoxication with delirium 🔗

F16.229   Hallucinogen dependence with intoxication, unspecified

F16.24   **Hallucinogen dependence with hallucinogen-induced mood disorder**

Other hallucinogen use disorder, moderate, with other hallucinogen-induced bipolar or related disorder ◄

Other hallucinogen use disorder, moderate, with other hallucinogen-induced depressive disorder ◄

Other hallucinogen use disorder, severe, with other hallucinogen-induced bipolar or related disorder ◄

Other hallucinogen use disorder, severe, with other hallucinogen-induced depressive disorder ◄

Phencyclidine use disorder, moderate, with phencyclidine-induced bipolar or related disorder ◄

Phencyclidine use disorder, moderate, with phencyclidine-induced depressive disorder ◄

Phencyclidine use disorder, severe, with phencyclidine-induced bipolar or related disorder ◄

Phencyclidine use disorder, severe, with phencyclidine-induced depressive disorder ◄

● **F16.25**   **Hallucinogen dependence with hallucinogen-induced psychotic disorder**

F16.250   Hallucinogen dependence with hallucinogen-induced psychotic disorder with delusions 🔗

F16.251   Hallucinogen dependence with hallucinogen-induced psychotic disorder with hallucinations 🔗

F16.259   Hallucinogen dependence with hallucinogen-induced psychotic disorder, unspecified 🔗

     (Ex:) No exclusions

● **F16.28**   **Hallucinogen dependence with other hallucinogen-induced disorder**

     (Ex:) **For category F16.28 CC codes:** No exclusions

F16.280   Hallucinogen dependence with hallucinogen-induced anxiety disorder 🔗

F16.283   Hallucinogen dependence with hallucinogen persisting perception disorder (flashbacks) 🔗

F16.288   Hallucinogen dependence with other hallucinogen-induced disorder 🔗

F16.29   Hallucinogen dependence with unspecified hallucinogen-induced disorder

● **F16.9**   **Hallucinogen use, unspecified**

     Excludes1   hallucinogen abuse (F16.1-)
                  hallucinogen dependence (F16.2-)

F16.90   Hallucinogen use, unspecified, uncomplicated

● **F16.92**   Hallucinogen use, unspecified with intoxication

F16.920   Hallucinogen use, unspecified with intoxication, uncomplicated

F16.921   Hallucinogen use, unspecified with intoxication with delirium 🔗

Other hallucinogen intoxication delirium ◄

F16.929   Hallucinogen use, unspecified with intoxication, unspecified

● **F16.94**   **Hallucinogen use, unspecified with hallucinogen-induced mood disorder**

Other hallucinogen-induced bipolar or related disorder, without use disorder ◄

Other hallucinogen-induced depressive disorder, without use disorder ◄

Phencyclidine-induced bipolar or related disorder, without use disorder ◄

Phencyclidine-induced depressive disorder, without use disorder ◄

● **F16.95**   **Hallucinogen use, unspecified with hallucinogen-induced psychotic disorder**

F16.950   Hallucinogen use, unspecified with hallucinogen-induced psychotic disorder with delusions 🔗

F16.951   Hallucinogen use, unspecified with hallucinogen-induced psychotic disorder with hallucinations 🔗

F16.959   Hallucinogen use, unspecified with hallucinogen-induced psychotic disorder, unspecified

Other hallucinogen-induced psychotic disorder, without use disorder ◄

Phencyclidine-induced psychotic disorder, without use disorder ◄

● **F16.98**   **Hallucinogen use, unspecified with other specified hallucinogen-induced disorder**

F16.980   Hallucinogen use, unspecified with hallucinogen-induced anxiety disorder

Other hallucinogen-induced anxiety disorder, without use disorder ◄

Phencyclidine-induced anxiety disorder, without use disorder ◄

F16.983   Hallucinogen use, unspecified with hallucinogen persisting perception disorder (flashbacks)

F16.988   Hallucinogen use, unspecified with other hallucinogen-induced disorder

F16.99   Hallucinogen use, unspecified with unspecified hallucinogen-induced disorder

● **F17**   **Nicotine dependence**

     Excludes1   history of tobacco dependence (Z87.891)
                  tobacco use NOS (Z72.0)

     Excludes2   tobacco use (smoking) during pregnancy, childbirth and the puerperium (O99.33-)
                  toxic effect of nicotine (T65.2-)

     (Ex:) **For category F17 CC codes:** F02.80-F02.81, F04-F06.8, F10.10-F11.19, F11.21-F13.19, F13.21-F14.19, F14.21-F15.19, F15.21-F16.19, F16.21-F17.209, F17.213-F17.219, F17.223-F17.229, F17.293-F18.19, F18.21-F19.19, F19.21-F19.99, F53-F55.8, R78

● **F17.2**   **Nicotine dependence**

● **F17.20**   **Nicotine dependence, unspecified**

● **F17.200**   Nicotine dependence, unspecified, uncomplicated

Tobacco use disorder, mild ◄
Tobacco use disorder, moderate ◄
Tobacco use disorder, severe ◄
Coding Clinic: 2016, Q1, P37

● **F17.201**   Nicotine dependence, unspecified, in remission

F17.203   Nicotine dependence unspecified, with withdrawal 🔗

Tobacco withdrawal ◄

F17.208   Nicotine dependence, unspecified, with other nicotine-induced disorders

F17.209   Nicotine dependence, unspecified, with unspecified nicotine-induced disorders

---

N   Newborn Age: Ø   **P**   Pediatric Age: Ø–17   **M**   Maternity DX: 12–55   **A**   Adult Age: 15–124   ♀   Females Only   ♂   Males Only

🔗   Complication\Comorbidity   🔗   Major C\C   (Ex:)   CC/MCC Exclusions   🔗   Hospital-Acquired Condition

CHAPTER 5 (FØ1-F99)

- F17.21   Nicotine dependence, cigarettes
  - F17.210   Nicotine dependence, cigarettes, uncomplicated
  - F17.211   Nicotine dependence, cigarettes, in remission
  - F17.213   Nicotine dependence, cigarettes, with withdrawal 🏷
  - F17.218   Nicotine dependence, cigarettes, with other nicotine-induced disorders
  - F17.219   Nicotine dependence, cigarettes, with unspecified nicotine-induced disorders
- F17.22   Nicotine dependence, chewing tobacco
  - F17.220   Nicotine dependence, chewing tobacco, uncomplicated
  - F17.221   Nicotine dependence, chewing tobacco, in remission
  - F17.223   Nicotine dependence, chewing tobacco, with withdrawal 🏷
  - F17.228   Nicotine dependence, chewing tobacco, with other nicotine-induced disorders
  - F17.229   Nicotine dependence, chewing tobacco, with unspecified nicotine-induced disorders
- F17.29   Nicotine dependence, other tobacco product
  - F17.290   Nicotine dependence, other tobacco product, uncomplicated
  - F17.291   Nicotine dependence, other tobacco product, in remission
  - F17.293   Nicotine dependence, other tobacco product, with withdrawal 🏷
  - F17.298   Nicotine dependence, other tobacco product, with other nicotine-induced disorders
  - F17.299   Nicotine dependence, other tobacco product, with unspecified nicotine-induced disorders

- F18   Inhalant related disorders
  - **Includes**   volatile solvents
  - (Ex): **For category F18 CC codes unless otherwise indicated:** F02.80-F02.81, F04-F06.8, F10.10-F11.19, F11.21-F13.19, F13.21-F14.19, F14.21-F15.19, F15.21-F16.19, F16.21-F17.209, F17.213-F17.219, F17.223-F17.229, F17.293-F18.19, F18.21-F19.19, F19.21-F19.99, F53-F55.8, R78

  - F18.1   Inhalant abuse
    - **Excludes1**   inhalant dependence (F18.2-)
      inhalant use, unspecified (F18.9-)
    - F18.10   Inhalant abuse, uncomplicated
      Inhalant use disorder, mild ◄
    - F18.12   Inhalant abuse with intoxication
      - F18.120   Inhalant abuse with intoxication, uncomplicated
      - F18.121   Inhalant abuse with intoxication delirium 🏷
      - F18.129   Inhalant abuse with intoxication, unspecified
    - F18.14   Inhalant abuse with inhalant-induced mood disorder
      Inhalant use disorder, mild, with inhalant-induced depressive disorder ◄
    - F18.15   Inhalant abuse with inhalant-induced psychotic disorder
      - F18.150   Inhalant abuse with inhalant-induced psychotic disorder with delusions 🏷
      - F18.151   Inhalant abuse with inhalant-induced psychotic disorder with hallucinations 🏷
      - F18.159   Inhalant abuse with inhalant-induced psychotic disorder, unspecified

- F18.17   Inhalant abuse with inhalant-induced dementia 🏷
  Inhalant use disorder, mild, with inhalant-induced major neurocognitive disorder ◄
- F18.18   Inhalant abuse with other inhalant-induced disorders
  - F18.180   Inhalant abuse with inhalant-induced anxiety disorder
  - F18.188   Inhalant abuse with other inhalant-induced disorder
    Inhalant use disorder, mild, with inhalant-induced mild neurocognitive disorder ◄
- F18.19   Inhalant abuse with unspecified inhalant-induced disorder
- F18.2   Inhalant dependence
  - **Excludes1**   inhalant abuse (F18.1-)
    inhalant use, unspecified (F18.9-)
  - F18.20   Inhalant dependence, uncomplicated 🏷
    Inhalant use disorder, moderate ◄
    Inhalant use disorder, severe ◄
    (Ex): No exclusions
  - F18.21   Inhalant dependence, in remission
  - F18.22   Inhalant dependence with intoxication
    - F18.220   Inhalant dependence with intoxication, uncomplicated
    - F18.221   Inhalant dependence with intoxication delirium 🏷
    - F18.229   Inhalant dependence with intoxication, unspecified
  - F18.24   Inhalant dependence with inhalant-induced mood disorder
    Inhalant use disorder, moderate, with inhalant-induced depressive disorder ◄
    Inhalant use disorder, severe, with inhalant-induced depressive disorder ◄
  - F18.25   Inhalant dependence with inhalant-induced psychotic disorder
    - F18.250   Inhalant dependence with inhalant-induced psychotic disorder with delusions 🏷
    - F18.251   Inhalant dependence with inhalant-induced psychotic disorder with hallucinations 🏷
    - F18.259   Inhalant dependence with inhalant-induced psychotic disorder, unspecified 🏷
      (Ex): No exclusions
  - F18.27   Inhalant dependence with inhalant-induced dementia 🏷
    Inhalant use disorder, moderate, with inhalant-induced major neurocognitive disorder ◄
    Inhalant use disorder, severe, with inhalant-induced major neurocognitive disorder ◄
  - F18.28   Inhalant dependence with other inhalant-induced disorders
    (Ex): **For category F18.28 CC codes:** No exclusions
    - F18.280   Inhalant dependence with inhalant-induced anxiety disorder 🏷
    - F18.288   Inhalant dependence with other inhalant-induced disorder 🏷
      Inhalant use disorder, moderate, with inhalant-induced mild neurocognitive disorder ◄
      Inhalant use disorder, severe, with inhalant-induced mild neurocognitive disorder ◄
  - F18.29   Inhalant dependence with unspecified inhalant-induced disorder
- F18.9   Inhalant use, unspecified
  - **Excludes1**   inhalant abuse (F18.1-)
    inhalant dependence (F18.2-)
  - F18.90   Inhalant use, unspecified, uncomplicated

◄ New   ◄⋯ Revised   deleted Deleted   Excludes 1   Excludes 2   Includes   Use additional   Code first   Code also   Unspecified
OGCR Official Guidelines   ● Unacceptable Principal Diagnosis   X Assign placeholder X   ● Use Additional Character(s)   ▶ Manifestation Code   Coding Clinic

CHAPTER 5 (F01-F99)

● **F18.92** Inhalant use, unspecified with intoxication

  F18.920 Inhalant use, unspecified with intoxication, uncomplicated

  F18.921 Inhalant use, unspecified with intoxication with delirium 🔖

  F18.929 Inhalant use, unspecified with intoxication, unspecified

F18.94 Inhalant use, unspecified with inhalant-induced mood disorder
    Inhalant-induced depressive disorder ◄

● **F18.95** Inhalant use, unspecified with inhalant-induced psychotic disorder

  F18.950 Inhalant use, unspecified with inhalant-induced psychotic disorder with delusions 🔖

  F18.951 Inhalant use, unspecified with inhalant-induced psychotic disorder with hallucinations 🔖

  F18.959 Inhalant use, unspecified with inhalant-induced psychotic disorder, unspecified

F18.97 Inhalant use, unspecified with inhalant-induced persisting dementia 🔖
    Inhalant-induced major neurocognitive disorder ◄

● **F18.98** Inhalant use, unspecified with other inhalant-induced disorders

  F18.980 Inhalant use, unspecified with inhalant-induced anxiety disorder

  F18.988 Inhalant use, unspecified with other inhalant-induced disorder
    Inhalant-induced mild neurocognitive disorder ◄

F18.99 Inhalant use, unspecified with unspecified inhalant-induced disorder

● **F19** Other psychoactive substance related disorders

  Includes   polysubstance drug use (indiscriminate drug use)

  Ⓔⓧ **For category F19 CC codes unless otherwise indicated:** F02.80-F02.81, F04-F06.8, F10.10-F11.19, F11.21-F13.19, F13.21-F14.19, F14.21-F15.19, F15.21-F16.19, F16.21-F17.209, F17.213-F17.219, F17.223-F17.229, F17.293-F18.19, F18.21-F19.19, F19.21-F19.99, F53-F55.8, R78

● **F19.1** Other psychoactive substance abuse

  Excludes1   other psychoactive substance dependence (F19.2-)
      other psychoactive substance use, unspecified (F19.9-)

  F19.10 Other psychoactive substance abuse, uncomplicated
    Other (or unknown) substance use disorder, mild ◄

● **F19.12** Other psychoactive substance abuse with intoxication

  F19.120 Other psychoactive substance abuse with intoxication, uncomplicated

  F19.121 Other psychoactive substance abuse with intoxication delirium 🔖

  F19.122 Other psychoactive substance abuse with intoxication with perceptual disturbances

  F19.129 Other psychoactive substance abuse with intoxication, unspecified

F19.14 Other psychoactive substance abuse with psychoactive substance-induced mood disorder
    Other (or unknown) substance use disorder, mild, with other (or unknown) substance-induced bipolar or related disorder ◄
    Other (or unknown) substance use disorder, mild, with other (or unknown) substance-induced depressive disorder ◄

● **F19.15** Other psychoactive substance abuse with psychoactive substance-induced psychotic disorder

  F19.150 Other psychoactive substance abuse with psychoactive substance-induced psychotic disorder with delusions 🔖

  F19.151 Other psychoactive substance abuse with psychoactive substance-induced psychotic disorder with hallucinations 🔖

  F19.159 Other psychoactive substance abuse with psychoactive substance-induced psychotic disorder, unspecified

F19.16 Other psychoactive substance abuse with psychoactive substance-induced persisting amnestic disorder

F19.17 Other psychoactive substance abuse with psychoactive substance-induced persisting dementia 🔖
    Other (or unknown) substance use disorder, mild, with other (or unknown) substance-induced major neurocognitive disorder ◄

● **F19.18** Other psychoactive substance abuse with other psychoactive substance-induced disorders

  F19.180 Other psychoactive substance abuse with psychoactive substance-induced anxiety disorder

  F19.181 Other psychoactive substance abuse with psychoactive substance-induced sexual dysfunction

  F19.182 Other psychoactive substance abuse with psychoactive substance-induced sleep disorder

  F19.188 Other psychoactive substance abuse with other psychoactive substance-induced disorder
    Other (or unknown) substance use disorder, mild, with other (or unknown) substance-induced mild neurocognitive disorder ◄
    Other (or unknown) substance use disorder, mild, with other (or unknown) substance-induced obsessive-compulsive or related disorder ◄

F19.19 Other psychoactive substance abuse with unspecified psychoactive substance-induced disorder

● **F19.2** Other psychoactive substance dependence

  Excludes1   other psychoactive substance abuse (F19.1-)
      other psychoactive substance use, unspecified (F19.9-)

  F19.20 Other psychoactive substance dependence, uncomplicated 🔖
    Other (or unknown) substance use disorder, moderate ◄
    Other (or unknown) substance use disorder, severe ◄
    Ⓔⓧ No exclusions

  F19.21 Other psychoactive substance dependence, in remission

● **F19.22** Other psychoactive substance dependence with intoxication

  Excludes1   other psychoactive substance dependence with withdrawal (F19.23-)

  F19.220 Other psychoactive substance dependence with intoxication, uncomplicated

  F19.221 Other psychoactive substance dependence with intoxication delirium 🔖

N Newborn Age: Ø   **P** Pediatric Age: Ø–17   **M** Maternity DX: 12–55   **A** Adult Age: 15–124   ♀ Females Only   ♂ Males Only

🔖 Complication\Comorbidity   🔖 Major C\C   Ⓔⓧ CC/MCC Exclusions   🔖 Hospital-Acquired Condition

771

F19.222   Other psychoactive substance dependence with intoxication with perceptual disturbance 🔾
      (Ex:) No exclusions

F19.229   Other psychoactive substance dependence with intoxication, unspecified

● **F19.23**   Other psychoactive substance dependence with withdrawal

     Excludes1   other psychoactive substance dependence with intoxication (F19.22-)

F19.230   Other psychoactive substance dependence with withdrawal, uncomplicated 🔾

F19.231   Other psychoactive substance dependence with withdrawal delirium 🔾

F19.232   Other psychoactive substance dependence with withdrawal with perceptual disturbance 🔾

F19.239   Other psychoactive substance dependence with withdrawal, unspecified 🔾

F19.24   Other psychoactive substance dependence with psychoactive substance-induced mood disorder
     Other (or unknown) substance use disorder, moderate, with other (or unknown) substance-induced bipolar or related disorder ◀
     Other (or unknown) substance use disorder, moderate, with other (or unknown) substance-induced depressive disorder ◀
     Other (or unknown) substance use disorder, severe, with other (or unknown) substance-induced bipolar or related disorder ◀
     Other (or unknown) substance use disorder, severe, with other (or unknown) substance-induced depressive disorder ◀

● **F19.25**   Other psychoactive substance dependence with psychoactive substance-induced psychotic disorder

F19.250   Other psychoactive substance dependence with psychoactive substance-induced psychotic disorder with delusions 🔾

F19.251   Other psychoactive substance dependence with psychoactive substance-induced psychotic disorder with hallucinations 🔾

F19.259   Other psychoactive substance dependence with psychoactive substance-induced psychotic disorder, unspecified 🔾
      (Ex:) No exclusions

F19.26   Other psychoactive substance dependence with psychoactive substance-induced persisting amnestic disorder 🔾
      (Ex:) No exclusions

F19.27   Other psychoactive substance dependence with psychoactive substance-induced persisting dementia 🔾
     Other (or unknown) substance use disorder, moderate, with other (or unknown) substance-induced major neurocognitive disorder ◀
     Other (or unknown) substance use disorder, severe, with other (or unknown) substance-induced major neurocognitive disorder ◀

● **F19.28**   Other psychoactive substance dependence with other psychoactive substance-induced disorders
     (Ex:) For category F19.28 CC codes: No exclusions

F19.280   Other psychoactive substance dependence with psychoactive substance-induced anxiety disorder 🔾

F19.281   Other psychoactive substance dependence with psychoactive substance-induced sexual dysfunction 🔾

F19.282   Other psychoactive substance dependence with psychoactive substance-induced sleep disorder 🔾

F19.288   Other psychoactive substance dependence with other psychoactive substance-induced disorder 🔾
     Other (or unknown) substance use disorder, moderate, with other (or unknown) substance-induced mild neurocognitive disorder ◀
     Other (or unknown) substance use disorder, severe, with other (or unknown) substance-induced mild neurocognitive disorder ◀
     Other (or unknown) substance use disorder, moderate, with other (or unknown) substance-induced obsessive-compulsive or related disorder ◀
     Other (or unknown) substance use disorder, severe, with other (or unknown) substance-induced obsessive-compulsive or related disorder ◀

F19.29   Other psychoactive substance dependence with unspecified psychoactive substance-induced disorder

● **F19.9**   Other psychoactive substance use, unspecified
     Excludes1   other psychoactive substance abuse (F19.1-)
                    other psychoactive substance dependence (F19.2-)

F19.90   Other psychoactive substance use, unspecified, uncomplicated

● **F19.92**   Other psychoactive substance use, unspecified with intoxication
     Excludes1   other psychoactive substance use, unspecified with withdrawal (F19.93)

F19.920   Other psychoactive substance use, unspecified with intoxication, uncomplicated

F19.921   Other psychoactive substance use, unspecified with intoxication with delirium 🔾
     Other (or unknown) substance-induced delirium ◀

F19.922   Other psychoactive substance use, unspecified with intoxication with perceptual disturbance

F19.929   Other psychoactive substance use, unspecified with intoxication, unspecified

● **F19.93**   Other psychoactive substance use, unspecified with withdrawal
     Excludes1   other psychoactive substance use, unspecified with intoxication (F19.92-)

F19.930   Other psychoactive substance use, unspecified with withdrawal, uncomplicated 🔾

F19.931   Other psychoactive substance use, unspecified with withdrawal delirium 🔾

◀ New   ◀▥ Revised   ~~deleted~~ Deleted   Excludes 1   Excludes 2   Includes   Use additional   Code first   Code also   Unspecified
OGCR Official Guidelines   ● Unacceptable Principal Diagnosis   X Assign placeholder X   🔾 Use Additional Character(s)   ▶ Manifestation Code   **Coding Clinic**

F19.932   **Other psychoactive substance use, unspecified with withdrawal with perceptual disturbance**

F19.939   **Other psychoactive substance use, unspecified with withdrawal, unspecified**

F19.94   **Other psychoactive substance use, unspecified with psychoactive substance-induced mood disorder**
     Other (or unknown) substance-induced bipolar or related disorder, without use disorder ◄
     Other (or unknown) substance-induced depressive disorder, without use disorder ◄

● **F19.95**   **Other psychoactive substance use, unspecified with psychoactive substance-induced psychotic disorder**

     F19.950   **Other psychoactive substance use, unspecified with psychoactive substance-induced psychotic disorder with delusions**

     F19.951   **Other psychoactive substance use, unspecified with psychoactive substance-induced psychotic disorder with hallucinations**

     F19.959   **Other psychoactive substance use, unspecified with psychoactive substance-induced psychotic disorder, unspecified**
         Other or unknown substance-induced psychotic disorder, without use disorder ◄

F19.96   **Other psychoactive substance use, unspecified with psychoactive substance-induced persisting amnestic disorder**

F19.97   **Other psychoactive substance use, unspecified with psychoactive substance-induced persisting dementia**
     Other (or unknown) substance-induced major neurocognitive disorder, without use disorder ◄

● **F19.98**   **Other psychoactive substance use, unspecified with other psychoactive substance-induced disorders**

     F19.980   **Other psychoactive substance use, unspecified with psychoactive substance-induced anxiety disorder**
         Other (or unknown) substance-induced anxiety disorder, without use disorder ◄

     F19.981   **Other psychoactive substance use, unspecified with psychoactive substance-induced sexual dysfunction**
         Other (or unknown) substance-induced sexual dysfunction, without use disorder ◄

     F19.982   **Other psychoactive substance use, unspecified with psychoactive substance-induced sleep disorder**
         Other (or unknown) substance-induced sleep disorder, without use disorder ◄

     F19.988   **Other psychoactive substance use, unspecified with other psychoactive substance-induced disorder**
         Other (or unknown) substance-induced mild neurocognitive disorder, without use disorder ◄
         Other (or unknown) substance-induced obsessive-compulsive or related disorder, without use disorder ◄

F19.99   **Other psychoactive substance use, unspecified with unspecified psychoactive substance-induced disorder**

SCHIZOPHRENIA, SCHIZOTYPAL, DELUSIONAL, AND OTHER NON-MOOD PSYCHOTIC DISORDERS (F20-F29)

● **F20**   **Schizophrenia**
Personality disorders characterized by multiple mental and behavioral irregularities (may exhibit disorganized thinking, delusions, and auditory hallucinations)

   Excludes1   brief psychotic disorder (F23)
                cyclic schizophrenia (F25.0)
                mood [affective] disorders with psychotic symptoms (F30.2, F31.2, F31.5, F31.64, F32.3, F33.3)
                schizoaffective disorder (F25.-)
                schizophrenic reaction NOS (F23)

   Excludes2   schizophrenic reaction in:
                alcoholism (F10.15-, F10.25-, F10.95-)
                brain disease (F06.2)
                epilepsy (F06.2)
                psychoactive drug use (F11-F19 with .15, .25, .95)
                schizotypal disorder (F21)

(Ex) **For category F20 CC codes:** F07.0-F07.81, F07.9-F09, F20.0-F51.03, F51.12, F51.19, F51.3-F51.9, F52.5, F54, F59-F63.2, F63.81-F63.9, F68.10-F80.4, F80.82-F84.0, F84.3-F99, G44.201-G44.229, H93.25, R45.1-R45.2, R45.5-R45.82, R45.86-R45.87

F20.0   **Paranoid schizophrenia**
     Paraphrenic schizophrenia
   Excludes1   involutional paranoid state (F22)
                paranoia (F22)

F20.1   **Disorganized schizophrenia**
     Hebephrenic schizophrenia
     Hebephrenia

F20.2   **Catatonic schizophrenia**
     Schizophrenic catalepsy
     Schizophrenic catatonia
     Schizophrenic flexibilitas cerea
   Excludes1   catatonic stupor (R40.1)

F20.3   **Undifferentiated schizophrenia**
     Atypical schizophrenia
   Excludes1   acute schizophrenia-like psychotic disorder (F23)
   Excludes2   post-schizophrenic depression (F32.89) ◄▥

F20.5   **Residual schizophrenia**
     Restzustand (schizophrenic)
     Schizophrenic residual state

● **F20.8**   **Other schizophrenia**

     F20.81   **Schizophreniform disorder**
         Schizophreniform psychosis NOS

     F20.89   **Other schizophrenia**
         Cenesthopathic schizophrenia
         Simple schizophrenia

F20.9   **Schizophrenia, unspecified**

F21   **Schizotypal disorder**
Personality disorder characterized by need for social isolation, odd behavior and thinking, and often unconventional beliefs
     Borderline schizophrenia
     Latent schizophrenia
     Latent schizophrenic reaction
     Prepsychotic schizophrenia
     Prodromal schizophrenia
     Pseudoneurotic schizophrenia
     Pseudopsychopathic schizophrenia
     Schizotypal personality disorder
   Excludes2   Asperger's syndrome (F84.5)
                schizoid personality disorder (F60.1)

N Newborn Age: 0   **P** Pediatric Age: 0–17   **M** Maternity DX: 12–55   **A** Adult Age: 15–124   ♀ Females Only   ♂ Males Only
   Complication\Comorbidity   Major C\C   (Ex) CC/MCC Exclusions   Hospital-Acquired Condition

F22   Delusional disorders
    Delusional dysmorphophobia
    Involutional paranoid state
    Paranoia
    Paranoia querulans
    Paranoid psychosis
    Paranoid state
    Paraphrenia (late)
    Sensitiver Beziehungswahn
    Excludes1   mood [affective] disorders with psychotic
                symptoms (F30.2, F31.2, F31.5, F31.64,
                F32.3, F33.3)
                paranoid schizophrenia (F20.0)
    Excludes2   paranoid personality disorder (F60.0)
                paranoid psychosis, psychogenic (F23)
                paranoid reaction (F23)

F23   Brief psychotic disorder 🔍
    Paranoid reaction
    Psychogenic paranoid psychosis
    Excludes2   mood [affective] disorders with psychotic
                symptoms (F30.2, F31.2, F31.5, F31.64,
                F32.3, F33.3)
    (Ex) No exclusions

F24   Shared psychotic disorder
    Folie à deux
    Induced paranoid disorder
    Induced psychotic disorder

● **F25   Schizoaffective disorders**
    *Mental disorder exhibiting major depressive episode, manic episode,
        or mixed episode occurs with symptoms of schizophrenia, and
        mood disorder*
    Excludes1   mood [affective] disorders with psychotic
                symptoms (F30.2, F31.2, F31.5, F31.64, F32.3,
                F33.3)
                schizophrenia (F20.-)
    F25.0   Schizoaffective disorder, bipolar type
            Cyclic schizophrenia
            Schizoaffective disorder, manic type
            Schizoaffective disorder, mixed type
            Schizoaffective psychosis, bipolar type
            Schizophreniform psychosis, manic type
    F25.1   Schizoaffective disorder, depressive type
            Schizoaffective psychosis, depressive type
            Schizophreniform psychosis, depressive type
    F25.8   Other schizoaffective disorders
    F25.9   Schizoaffective disorder, unspecified
            Schizoaffective psychosis NOS

**F28   Other psychotic disorder not due to a substance or known
        physiological condition**
        Chronic hallucinatory psychosis

**F29   Unspecified psychosis not due to a substance or known
        physiological condition**
        Psychosis NOS
    Excludes1   mental disorder NOS (F99)
                unspecified mental disorder due to known
                    physiological condition (F09)

MOOD [AFFECTIVE] DISORDERS (F30-F39)

● **F30   Manic episode**
    Elevated, expansive, or irritable mood
    Includes   bipolar disorder, single manic episode
                mixed affective episode
    Excludes1   bipolar disorder (F31.-)
                major depressive disorder, single episode (F32.-)
                major depressive disorder, recurrent (F33.-)
    (Ex) **For category F30 CC codes unless otherwise indicated:** See F20
    ● **F30.1   Manic episode without psychotic symptoms**
        **F30.10   Manic episode without psychotic
                symptoms, unspecified** 🔍
        **F30.11   Manic episode without psychotic symptoms,
                mild** 🔍

        **F30.12   Manic episode without psychotic symptoms,
                moderate** 🔍
        **F30.13   Manic episode, severe, without psychotic
                symptoms** 🔍
                (Ex) F30.13, F30.2, F31.13-F31.2, F31.4-F31.5, F31.63-F31.64
    F30.2   Manic episode, severe with psychotic symptoms 🔍
            Manic stupor
            Mania with mood-congruent psychotic symptoms
            Mania with mood-incongruent psychotic symptoms
    F30.3   Manic episode in partial remission
    F30.4   Manic episode in full remission
    F30.8   Other manic episodes
            Abnormality of mood resembling mania but less intense
            Hypomania
    F30.9   Manic episode, unspecified 🔍
            Mania NOS

● **F31   Bipolar disorder**
    Mood disorders with history of manic, mixed, or hypomanic episodes
    Includes   manic-depressive illness
                manic-depressive psychosis
                manic-depressive reaction
    Excludes1   bipolar disorder, single manic episode (F30.-)
                major depressive disorder, single episode (F32.-)
                major depressive disorder, recurrent (F33.-)
    Excludes2   cyclothymia (F34.0)
    (Ex) **For category F31 CC codes unless otherwise indicated:** See F20

    F31.0   Bipolar disorder, current episode hypomanic 🔍
    ● **F31.1   Bipolar disorder, current episode manic without
            psychotic features**
        **F31.10   Bipolar disorder, current episode manic without
                psychotic features, unspecified** 🔍
        **F31.11   Bipolar disorder, current episode manic without
                psychotic features, mild** 🔍
        **F31.12   Bipolar disorder, current episode manic without
                psychotic features, moderate** 🔍
        **F31.13   Bipolar disorder, current episode manic without
                psychotic features, severe** 🔍
                (Ex) F31.13-F31.2, F31.63-F31.64
    **F31.2   Bipolar disorder, current episode manic severe with
            psychotic features** 🔍
            Bipolar disorder, current episode manic with mood-
                congruent psychotic symptoms
            Bipolar disorder, current episode manic with mood-
                incongruent psychotic symptoms
    ● **F31.3   Bipolar disorder, current episode depressed, mild or
            moderate severity**
        **F31.30   Bipolar disorder, current episode depressed,
                mild or moderate severity, unspecified** 🔍
        **F31.31   Bipolar disorder, current episode depressed,
                mild** 🔍
        **F31.32   Bipolar disorder, current episode depressed,
                moderate** 🔍
    **F31.4   Bipolar disorder, current episode depressed, severe,
            without psychotic features** 🔍
            (Ex) F31.13-F31.2, F31.4-F31.5, F31.63-F31.64
    **F31.5   Bipolar disorder, current episode depressed, severe, with
            psychotic features** 🔍
            Bipolar disorder, current episode depressed with mood-
                incongruent psychotic symptoms
            Bipolar disorder, current episode depressed with mood-
                congruent psychotic symptoms
    ● **F31.6   Bipolar disorder, current episode mixed**
        **F31.60   Bipolar disorder, current episode
                mixed, unspecified** 🔍
        **F31.61   Bipolar disorder, current episode mixed,
                mild** 🔍
        **F31.62   Bipolar disorder, current episode mixed,
                moderate** 🔍

◀ New   ◀ Revised   ~~deleted~~ Deleted   Excludes 1   Excludes 2   Includes   Use additional   Code first   Code also   Unspecified
OGCR Official Guidelines   ● Unacceptable Principal Diagnosis   **X** Assign placeholder X   ● Use Additional Character(s)   ▶ Manifestation Code   **Coding Clinic**

F31.63 **Bipolar disorder, current episode mixed, severe, without psychotic features**
    (Ex) See F31.4

F31.64 **Bipolar disorder, current episode mixed, severe, with psychotic features**
    Bipolar disorder, current episode mixed with mood-congruent psychotic symptoms
    Bipolar disorder, current episode mixed with mood-incongruent psychotic symptoms

● **F31.7** **Bipolar disorder, currently in remission**

F31.70 **Bipolar disorder, currently in remission, most recent episode unspecified**

F31.71 **Bipolar disorder, in partial remission, most recent episode hypomanic**

F31.72 **Bipolar disorder, in full remission, most recent episode hypomanic**

F31.73 **Bipolar disorder, in partial remission, most recent episode manic**

F31.74 **Bipolar disorder, in full remission, most recent episode manic**

F31.75 **Bipolar disorder, in partial remission, most recent episode depressed**

F31.76 **Bipolar disorder, in full remission, most recent episode depressed**

F31.77 **Bipolar disorder, in partial remission, most recent episode mixed**

F31.78 **Bipolar disorder, in full remission, most recent episode mixed**

● **F31.8** **Other bipolar disorders**

F31.81 **Bipolar II disorder**

F31.89 **Other bipolar disorder**
    Recurrent manic episodes NOS

F31.9 **Bipolar disorder, unspecified**

● **F32** **Major depressive disorder, single episode**

  Includes   single episode of agitated depression
    single episode of depressive reaction
    single episode of major depression
    single episode of psychogenic depression
    single episode of reactive depression
    single episode of vital depression

  Excludes1   bipolar disorder (F31.-)
    manic episode (F30.-)
    recurrent depressive disorder (F33.-)

  Excludes2   adjustment disorder (F43.2)

F32.0 **Major depressive disorder, single episode, mild**
    (Ex) F32.0-F32.3, F33.0-F33.40, F33.9

F32.1 **Major depressive disorder, single episode, moderate**
    (Ex) F32.0-F32.3, F33.0-F33.40, F33.9

F32.2 **Major depressive disorder, single episode, severe without psychotic features**
    (Ex) F32.0-F32.3, F33.0-F33.40, F33.9

F32.3 **Major depressive disorder, single episode, severe with psychotic features**
    Single episode of major depression with mood-congruent psychotic symptoms
    Single episode of major depression with mood-incongruent psychotic symptoms
    Single episode of major depression with psychotic symptoms
    Single episode of psychogenic depressive psychosis
    Single episode of psychotic depression
    Single episode of reactive depressive psychosis
    (Ex) F32.0-F32.3, F33.0-F33.40, F33.9

F32.4 **Major depressive disorder, single episode, in partial remission**

F32.5 **Major depressive disorder, single episode, in full remission**

● **F32.8** **Other depressive episodes**

F32.81 **Premenstrual dysphoric disorder** ♀ ◀
    Excludes1   premenstrual tension syndrome (N94.3) ◀

F32.89 **Other specified depressive episodes** ◀
    Atypical depression ◀
    Post-schizophrenic depression ◀
    Single episode of 'masked' depression NOS ◀

F32.9 **Major depressive disorder, single episode, unspecified**
    Depression NOS
    Depressive disorder NOS
    Major depression NOS

● **F33** **Major depressive disorder, recurrent**

  Includes   recurrent episodes of depressive reaction
    recurrent episodes of endogenous depression
    recurrent episodes of major depression
    recurrent episodes of psychogenic depression
    recurrent episodes of reactive depression
    recurrent episodes of seasonal depressive disorder
    recurrent episodes of vital depression

  Excludes1   bipolar disorder (F31.-)
    manic episode (F30.-)

  (Ex) **For category F33 CC codes unless otherwise indicated:** F32.0-F32.3, F33.0-F33.40, F33.9

F33.0 **Major depressive disorder, recurrent, mild**

F33.1 **Major depressive disorder, recurrent, moderate**

F33.2 **Major depressive disorder, recurrent severe without psychotic features**

F33.3 **Major depressive disorder, recurrent, severe with psychotic symptoms**
    Endogenous depression with psychotic symptoms
    Recurrent severe episodes of major depression with mood-congruent psychotic symptoms
    Recurrent severe episodes of major depression with mood-incongruent psychotic symptoms
    Recurrent severe episodes of major depression with psychotic symptoms
    Recurrent severe episodes of psychogenic depressive psychosis
    Recurrent severe episodes of psychotic depression
    Recurrent severe episodes of reactive depressive psychosis
    (Ex) See F20

● **F33.4** **Major depressive disorder, recurrent, in remission**

F33.40 **Major depressive disorder, recurrent, in remission, unspecified**

F33.41 **Major depressive disorder, recurrent, in partial remission**

F33.42 **Major depressive disorder, recurrent, in full remission**

F33.8 **Other recurrent depressive disorders**
    Recurrent brief depressive episodes
    (Ex) See F20

F33.9 **Major depressive disorder, recurrent, unspecified**
    Monopolar depression NOS

Figure 5-1   PET scan of depressed individual's brain before and after recovery. (From Fortinash KM: Psychiatric Mental Health Nursing, ed 4, St. Louis, Mosby, 2008)

CHAPTER 5 (F01-F99)

N Newborn Age: 0   **P** Pediatric Age: 0–17   **M** Maternity DX: 12–55   **A** Adult Age: 15–124   ♀ Females Only   ♂ Males Only

Complication\Comorbidity   Major C\C   (Ex) CC/MCC Exclusions   Hospital-Acquired Condition   **775**

● **F34**   **Persistent mood [affective] disorders**
(Ex:) **For category F34 CC codes:** F07.0-F07.81, F07.9-F09, F20.0-F51.03, F51.12, F51.19,
F51.3-F51.9, F52.5, F54, F59-F63.2, F63.81-F63.9, F68.10-F80.4, F80.82-F84.0,
F84.3-F99, G44.201-G44.229, H93.25, R45.1-R45.2, R45.5-R45.82, R45.86-R45.87

F34.0   **Cyclothymic disorder**
Affective personality disorder
Cycloid personality
Cyclothymia
Cyclothymic personality

F34.1   **Dysthymic disorder**
Depressive neurosis
Depressive personality disorder
Dysthymia
Neurotic depression
Persistent anxiety depression
Persistent depressive disorder ◄

Excludes2   anxiety depression (mild or not
persistent) (F41.8)

● **F34.8**   **Other persistent mood [affective] disorders**
(Ex:) **For category F34.8 CC codes:** See F20

F34.81   **Disruptive mood dysregulation disorder** 🍂◄

F34.89   **Other specified persistent mood disorders** 🍂◄

F34.9   **Persistent mood [affective] disorder, unspecified** 🍂
(Ex:) See F20

F39   **Unspecified mood [affective] disorder**
Affective psychosis NOS

ANXIETY, DISSOCIATIVE, STRESS-RELATED, SOMATOFORM AND OTHER NONPSYCHOTIC MENTAL DISORDERS (F40-F48)

● **F40**   **Phobic anxiety disorders**
Irrational fear with avoidance of the feared subject, activity, or situation even though the individual knows that the reaction is excessive

● **F40.0**   **Agoraphobia**
Intense, irrational fear of open spaces

F40.00   **Agoraphobia, unspecified**

F40.01   **Agoraphobia with panic disorder**
Panic disorder with agoraphobia

Excludes1   panic disorder without
agoraphobia (F41.0)

F40.02   **Agoraphobia without panic disorder**

● **F40.1**   **Social phobias**
Anthropophobia
Social anxiety disorder of childhood
Social neurosis

F40.10   **Social phobia, unspecified**

F40.11   **Social phobia, generalized**

● **F40.2**   **Specific (isolated) phobias**

Excludes2   dysmorphophobia (nondelusional)
(F45.22)
nosophobia (F45.22)

● **F40.21**   **Animal type phobia**

F40.210   **Arachnophobia**
Fear of spiders

F40.218   **Other animal type phobia**

● **F40.22**   **Natural environment type phobia**

F40.220   **Fear of thunderstorms**

F40.228   **Other natural environment type phobia**

● **F40.23**   **Blood, injection, injury type phobia**

F40.230   **Fear of blood**

F40.231   **Fear of injections and transfusions**

F40.232   **Fear of other medical care**

F40.233   **Fear of injury**

● **F40.24**   **Situational type phobia**

F40.240   **Claustrophobia**
Fear of closed spaces

F40.241   **Acrophobia**
Fear of heights

F40.242   **Fear of bridges**

F40.243   **Fear of flying**

F40.248   **Other situational type phobia**

● **F40.29**   **Other specified phobia**

F40.290   **Androphobia**
Fear of men

F40.291   **Gynephobia**
Fear of women

F40.298   **Other specified phobia**

F40.8   **Other phobic anxiety disorders**
Phobic anxiety disorder of childhood

F40.9   **Phobic anxiety disorder, unspecified**
Phobia NOS
Phobic state NOS

● **F41**   **Other anxiety disorders**

Excludes2   anxiety in:
acute stress reaction (F43.0)
transient adjustment reaction (F43.2)
neurasthenia (F48.8)
psychophysiologic disorders (F45.-)
separation anxiety (F93.0)

F41.0   **Panic disorder [episodic paroxysmal anxiety] without agoraphobia**
Panic attack
Panic state

Excludes1   panic disorder with agoraphobia (F40.01)

F41.1   **Generalized anxiety disorder**
Anxiety neurosis
Anxiety reaction
Anxiety state
Overanxious disorder

Excludes2   neurasthenia (F48.8)

F41.3   **Other mixed anxiety disorders**

F41.8   **Other specified anxiety disorders**
Anxiety depression (mild or not persistent)
Anxiety hysteria
Mixed anxiety and depressive disorder

F41.9   **Anxiety disorder, unspecified**
Anxiety NOS

● **F42**   **Obsessive-compulsive disorder**
Anxiety disorder with recurrent obsessions or compulsions

Excludes2   obsessive-compulsive personality (disorder)
(F60.5)
obsessive-compulsive symptoms occurring in
depression (F32-F33)
obsessive-compulsive symptoms occurring in
schizophrenia (F20.-)

F42.2   **Mixed obsessional thoughts and acts** ◄

F42.3   **Hoarding disorder** ◄

F42.4   **Excoriation (skin-picking) disorder** ◄

Excludes1   factitial dermatitis (L98.1) ◄
other specified behavioral and emotional
disorders with onset usually
occurring in early childhood and
adolescence (F98.8) ◄

F42.8   **Other obsessive-compulsive disorder** ◄
Anancastic neurosis ◄
Obsessive-compulsive neurosis ◄

F42.9   **Obsessive-compulsive disorder, unspecified** ◄

◄ New   ◄ Revised   ~~deleted~~ Deleted   Excludes 1   Excludes 2   Includes   Use additional   Code first   Code also   Unspecified

776   OGCR Official Guidelines   ● Unacceptable Principal Diagnosis   X Assign placeholder X   ● Use Additional Character(s)   ▶ Manifestation Code   **Coding Clinic**

CHAPTER 5 (F01-F99)

● **F43**   **Reaction to severe stress and adjustment disorders**

    F43.0   **Acute stress reaction**
           Acute crisis reaction
           Acute reaction to stress
           Combat and operational stress reaction
           Combat fatigue
           Crisis state
           Psychic shock

   ● **F43.1**   **Post-traumatic stress disorder (PTSD)**
           Traumatic neurosis

       F43.10   **Post-traumatic stress disorder, unspecified**

       F43.11   **Post-traumatic stress disorder, acute**

       F43.12   **Post-traumatic stress disorder, chronic**

   ● **F43.2**   **Adjustment disorders**
           Culture shock
           Grief reaction
           Hospitalism in children

       Excludes2   separation anxiety disorder of childhood (F93.0)

       F43.20   **Adjustment disorder, unspecified**

       F43.21   **Adjustment disorder with depressed mood**

       F43.22   **Adjustment disorder with anxiety**

       F43.23   **Adjustment disorder with mixed anxiety and depressed mood**

       F43.24   **Adjustment disorder with disturbance of conduct**

       F43.25   **Adjustment disorder with mixed disturbance of emotions and conduct**

       F43.29   **Adjustment disorder with other symptoms**

    F43.8   **Other reactions to severe stress**
           Other specified trauma and stressor-related disorder ◄

    F43.9   **Reaction to severe stress, unspecified**
           Trauma and stressor-related disorder, NOS ◄

● **F44**   **Dissociative and conversion disorders**

      Includes   conversion hysteria
                   conversion reaction
                   hysteria
                   hysterical psychosis

      Excludes2   malingering [conscious simulation] (Z76.5)

    F44.0   **Dissociative amnesia**
           Sudden loss of memory for personal information

       Excludes1   amnesia NOS (R41.3)
                   anterograde amnesia (R41.1)
                   dissociative amnesia with dissociative fugue (F44.1) ◄
                   retrograde amnesia (R41.2)

       Excludes2   alcohol-or other psychoactive substance-induced amnestic disorder (F10, F13, F19 with .26, .96)
                   amnestic disorder due to known physiological condition (F04)
                   postictal amnesia in epilepsy (G40.-)

    F44.1   **Dissociative fugue**
           Characterized by episode of sudden, unexpected travel with amnesia for past and partial to total confusion about identity or assumption of new identity
           Dissociative amnesia with dissociative fugue ◄

       Excludes2   postictal fugue in epilepsy (G40.-)

    F44.2   **Dissociative stupor**
           Profound diminution or absence of voluntary movement and responsiveness to external stimuli

       Excludes1   catatonic stupor (R40.1)
                   stupor NOS (R40.1)

       Excludes2   catatonic disorder due to known physiological condition (F06.1)
                   depressive stupor (F32, F33)
                   manic stupor (F30, F31)

    F44.4   **Conversion disorder with motor symptom or deficit**
           Dissociative motor disorders
           Psychogenic aphonia
           Psychogenic dysphonia

    F44.5   **Conversion disorder with seizures or convulsions**
           Dissociative convulsions

    F44.6   **Conversion disorder with sensory symptom or deficit**
           Dissociative anesthesia and sensory loss
           Psychogenic deafness

    F44.7   **Conversion disorder with mixed symptom presentation**

   ● **F44.8**   **Other dissociative and conversion disorders**

       F44.81   **Dissociative identity disorder**
               Multiple personality disorder

       F44.89   **Other dissociative and conversion disorders**
               Ganser's syndrome
               Psychogenic confusion
               Psychogenic twilight state
               Trance and possession disorders

    F44.9   **Dissociative and conversion disorder, unspecified**
           Dissociative disorder NOS

OGCR   Section I.C.5.a

Pain disorders related to psychological factors

Assign code F45.41, for pain that is exclusively psychological. Code F45.41, Pain disorder exclusively related to psychological factors, should be used following the appropriate code from category G89, Pain, not elsewhere classified, if there is documentation of a psychological component for a patient with acute or chronic pain.

See Section I.C.6. Pain

● **F45**   **Somatoform disorders**
           Mental disorders characterized by symptoms suggesting general medical condition

      Excludes2   dissociative and conversion disorders (F44.-)
                   factitious disorders (F68.1-)
                   hair-plucking (F63.3)
                   lalling (F80.0)
                   lisping (F80.0)
                   malingering [conscious simulation] (Z76.5)
                   nail-biting (F98.8)
                   psychological or behavioral factors associated with disorders or diseases classified elsewhere (F54)
                   sexual dysfunction, not due to a substance or known physiological condition (F52.-)
                   thumb-sucking (F98.8)
                   tic disorders (in childhood and adolescence) (F95.-)
                   Tourette's syndrome (F95.2)
                   trichotillomania (F63.3)

    F45.0   **Somatization disorder**
           Briquet's disorder
           Multiple psychosomatic disorder

    F45.1   **Undifferentiated somatoform disorder**
           Somatic symptom disorder ◄
           Undifferentiated psychosomatic disorder

   ● **F45.2**   **Hypochondriacal disorders**
           Persistent, unrealistic preoccupation with possibility of having serious disease

       Excludes2   delusional dysmorphophobia (F22)
                   fixed delusions about bodily functions or shape (F22)

       F45.20   **Hypochondriacal disorder, unspecified**

       F45.21   **Hypochondriasis**
               Hypochondriacal neurosis
               Illness anxiety disorder ◄

       F45.22   **Body dysmorphic disorder**
               Dysmorphophobia (nondelusional)
               Nosophobia

       F45.29   **Other hypochondriacal disorders**

   ● **F45.4**   **Pain disorders related to psychological factors**
       Excludes1   pain NOS (R52)

       F45.41   **Pain disorder exclusively related to psychological factors**
               Somatoform pain disorder (persistent)

       F45.42   **Pain disorder with related psychological factors**
               Code also associated acute or chronic pain (G89.-)

N Newborn Age: 0   **P** Pediatric Age: 0–17   **M** Maternity DX: 12–55   **A** Adult Age: 15–124   ♀ Females Only   ♂ Males Only

Complication\Comorbidity   Major C\C   CC/MCC Exclusions   Hospital-Acquired Condition

777

CHAPTER 5 (F01-F99)

F45.8 **Other somatoform disorders**
Psychogenic dysmenorrhea
Psychogenic dysphagia, including 'globus hystericus'
Psychogenic pruritus
Psychogenic torticollis
Somatoform autonomic dysfunction
Teeth grinding
> **Excludes1** sleep related teeth grinding (G47.63)

F45.9 **Somatoform disorder, unspecified**
Psychosomatic disorder NOS

● **F48** **Other nonpsychotic mental disorders**

F48.1 **Depersonalization-derealization syndrome**

F48.2 **Pseudobulbar affect**
Involuntary emotional expression disorder
Code first underlying cause, if known, such as:
amyotrophic lateral sclerosis (G12.21)
multiple sclerosis (G35)
sequelae of cerebrovascular disease (I69.-)
sequelae of traumatic intracranial injury (S06.-)

F48.8 **Other specified nonpsychotic mental disorders**
Dhat syndrome
Neurasthenia
Occupational neurosis, including writer's cramp
Psychasthenia
Psychasthenic neurosis
Psychogenic syncope

F48.9 **Nonpsychotic mental disorder, unspecified**
Neurosis NOS

BEHAVIORAL SYNDROMES ASSOCIATED WITH PHYSIOLOGICAL DISTURBANCES AND PHYSICAL FACTORS (F50-F59)

● **F50** **Eating disorders**
> **Excludes1** anorexia NOS (R63.0)
> feeding difficulties (R63.3)
> polyphagia (R63.2)
> **Excludes2** feeding disorder in infancy or childhood (F98.2-)

● **F50.0** **Anorexia nervosa**
> **Excludes1** loss of appetite (R63.0)
> psychogenic loss of appetite (F50.89) ◀▥
> (Ex) For category F50.0 CC codes: F45.9, F50.00-F50.9, F59, F98.21-F98.3

F50.00 **Anorexia nervosa, unspecified** 🗨

F50.01 **Anorexia nervosa, restricting type** 🗨

F50.02 **Anorexia nervosa, binge eating/purging type** 🗨
> **Excludes1** bulimia nervosa (F50.2)

F50.2 **Bulimia nervosa** 🗨
Bulimia NOS
Hyperorexia nervosa
> **Excludes1** anorexia nervosa, binge eating/purging
> type (F50.02)
> (Ex) F50.00-F50.9, F98.21-F98.29

● **F50.8** **Other eating disorders**
> **Excludes2** pica of infancy and childhood (F98.3)

F50.81 **Binge eating disorder** ◀

F50.89 **Other specified eating disorder** ◀
Pica in adults ◀
Psychogenic loss of appetite ◀

F50.9 **Eating disorder, unspecified**
Atypical anorexia nervosa
Atypical bulimia nervosa

● **F51** **Sleep disorders not due to a substance or known physiological condition**
> **Excludes2** organic sleep disorders (G47.-)

● **F51.0** **Insomnia not due to a substance or known physiological condition**
> **Excludes2** alcohol related insomnia (F10.182,
> F10.282, F10.982)
> drug-related insomnia (F11.182, F11.282,
> F11.982, F13.182, F13.282, F13.982,
> F14.182, F14.282, F14.982, F15.182,
> F15.282, F15.982, F19.182, F19.282,
> F19.982)
> insomnia NOS (G47.0-)
> insomnia due to known physiological
> condition (G47.0-)
> organic insomnia (G47.0-)
> sleep deprivation (Z72.820)

F51.01 **Primary insomnia**
Idiopathic insomnia

F51.02 **Adjustment insomnia**

F51.03 **Paradoxical insomnia**

F51.04 **Psychophysiologic insomnia**

F51.05 **Insomnia due to other mental disorder**
Code also associated mental disorder

F51.09 **Other insomnia not due to a substance or known physiological condition**

● **F51.1** **Hypersomnia not due to a substance or known physiological condition**
Hypersomnia: Excessive sleeping/sleepiness
> **Excludes2** alcohol related hypersomnia (F10.182,
> F10.282, F10.982)
> drug-related hypersomnia (F11.182,
> F11.282, F11.982, F13.182, F13.282,
> F13.982, F14.182, F14.282, F14.982,
> F15.182, F15.282, F15.982, F19.182,
> F19.282, F19.982)
> hypersomnia NOS (G47.10)
> hypersomnia due to known physiological
> condition (G47.10)
> idiopathic hypersomnia (G47.11, G47.12)
> narcolepsy (G47.4-)

F51.11 **Primary hypersomnia**

F51.12 **Insufficient sleep syndrome**
> **Excludes1** sleep deprivation (Z72.820)

F51.13 **Hypersomnia due to other mental disorder**
Code also associated mental disorder

F51.19 **Other hypersomnia not due to a substance or known physiological condition**

F51.3 **Sleepwalking [somnambulism]**

F51.4 **Sleep terrors [night terrors]**

F51.5 **Nightmare disorder**
Dream anxiety disorder

F51.8 **Other sleep disorders not due to a substance or known physiological condition**

F51.9 **Sleep disorder not due to a substance or known physiological condition, unspecified**
Emotional sleep disorder NOS

● **F52** **Sexual dysfunction not due to a substance or known physiological condition**
> **Excludes2** Dhat syndrome (F48.8)

F52.0 **Hypoactive sexual desire disorder**
Total loss of feeling of sexual pleasure
Lack or loss of sexual desire
Sexual anhedonia ◀
> **Excludes1** decreased libido (R68.82)

F52.1 **Sexual aversion disorder**
Sexual aversion and lack of sexual enjoyment

◀ New   ◀▥ Revised   ~~deleted~~ Deleted   Excludes 1   Excludes 2   Includes   Use additional   Code first   Code also   Unspecified

OGCR Official Guidelines   ● Unacceptable Principal Diagnosis   X Assign placeholder X   ● Use Additional Character(s)   ▮ Manifestation Code   Coding Clinic

● **F52.2**   **Sexual arousal disorders**
Failure of genital response

     F52.21   **Male erectile disorder** ♂
Psychogenic impotence
| **Excludes1** | impotence of organic origin (N52.-) |
| | impotence NOS (N52.-) |

     F52.22   **Female sexual arousal disorder** ♀
~~Frigidity~~

● **F52.3**   **Orgasmic disorder**
Inhibited orgasm
Psychogenic anorgasmy

     F52.31   **Female orgasmic disorder** ♀

     F52.32   **Male orgasmic disorder** ♂
Delayed ejaculation ◀

   F52.4   **Premature ejaculation** ♂

   F52.5   **Vaginismus not due to a substance or known physiological condition** ♀
Psychogenic vaginismus
| **Excludes2** | vaginismus (due to a known physiological condition) (N94.2) |

   F52.6   **Dyspareunia not due to a substance or known physiological condition** ♀
Dyspareunia: Difficult or painful sexual intercourse
Genito-pelvic pain penetration disorder ◀
Psychogenic dyspareunia
| **Excludes2** | dyspareunia (due to a known physiological condition) (N94.1-) ◀ |

   F52.8   **Other sexual dysfunction not due to a substance or known physiological condition**
Excessive sexual drive
Nymphomania
Satyriasis

● **F52.9**   **Unspecified sexual dysfunction not due to a substance or known physiological condition**
Sexual dysfunction NOS

F53   **Puerperal psychosis** ♀   M
Postpartum depression
Acute mental illness with sudden onset following childbirth with symptoms of affective psychosis, disorientation, and confusion are prevalent
Excludes1	mood disorders with psychotic features (F30.2, F31.2, F31.5, F31.64, F32.3, F33.3)
	postpartum dysphoria (O90.6)
	psychosis in schizophrenia, schizotypal, delusional, and other psychotic disorders (F20-F29)

▷ *F54*   *Psychological and behavioral factors associated with disorders or diseases classified elsewhere*
Psychological factors affecting physical conditions
Code first the associated physical disorder, such as:
     asthma (J45.-)
     dermatitis (L23-L25)
     gastric ulcer (K25.-)
     mucous colitis (K58.-)
     ulcerative colitis (K51.-)
     urticaria (L50.-)
| **Excludes2** | tension-type headache (G44.2) |

● **F55**   **Abuse of non-psychoactive substances**
| **Excludes2** | abuse of psychoactive substances (F10-F19) |

   F55.0   **Abuse of antacids**

   F55.1   **Abuse of herbal or folk remedies**

   F55.2   **Abuse of laxatives**

   F55.3   **Abuse of steroids or hormones**

   F55.4   **Abuse of vitamins**

   F55.8   **Abuse of other non-psychoactive substances**

F59   **Unspecified behavioral syndromes associated with physiological disturbances and physical factors**
Psychogenic physiological dysfunction NOS

DISORDERS OF ADULT PERSONALITY AND BEHAVIOR (F60-F69)

● **F60**   **Specific personality disorders**
Long-term patterns of thoughts and behaviors causing serious problems with relationships and work.

   F60.0   **Paranoid personality disorder**
Hostile, devious, and combative response to disappointments
Expansive paranoid personality (disorder)
Fanatic personality (disorder)
Querulant personality (disorder)
Paranoid personality (disorder)
Sensitive paranoid personality (disorder)
Excludes2	paranoia (F22)
	paranoia querulans (F22)
	paranoid psychosis (F22)
	paranoid schizophrenia (F20.0)
	paranoid state (F22)

   F60.1   **Schizoid personality disorder**
Detachment from social relationships with minimal emotional experiences and expressions
Excludes2	Asperger's syndrome (F84.5)
	delusional disorder (F22)
	schizoid disorder of childhood (F84.5)
	schizophrenia (F20.-)
	schizotypal disorder (F21)

   F60.2   **Antisocial personality disorder**
Continuous and chronic antisocial behavior
Amoral personality (disorder)
Asocial personality (disorder)
Dissocial personality disorder
Psychopathic personality (disorder)
Sociopathic personality (disorder)
| **Excludes1** | conduct disorders (F91.-) |
| **Excludes2** | borderline personality disorder (F60.3) |

   F60.3   **Borderline personality disorder**
Instability of mood, self-image or sense of self, and interpersonal relationships
Aggressive personality (disorder)
Emotionally unstable personality disorder
Explosive personality (disorder)
| **Excludes2** | antisocial personality disorder (F60.2) |

   F60.4   **Histrionic personality disorder**
Personality disorder with excessive emotional and attention-seeking behavior
Hysterical personality (disorder)
Psychoinfantile personality (disorder)

   F60.5   **Obsessive-compulsive personality disorder**
Anankastic personality (disorder)
Compulsive personality (disorder)
Obsessional personality (disorder)
| **Excludes2** | obsessive-compulsive disorder (F42-) ◀ |

   F60.6   **Avoidant personality disorder**
Anxious personality disorder

   F60.7   **Dependent personality disorder**
Asthenic personality (disorder)
Inadequate personality (disorder)
Passive personality (disorder)

● **F60.8**   **Other specific personality disorders**

     F60.81   **Narcissistic personality disorder**
Vanity, conceit, egotism or indifference to plight of others

     F60.89   **Other specific personality disorders**
Eccentric personality disorder
'Haltlose' type personality disorder
Immature personality disorder
Passive-aggressive personality disorder
Psychoneurotic personality disorder
Self-defeating personality disorder

   F60.9   **Personality disorder, unspecified**
Character disorder NOS
Character neurosis NOS
Pathological personality NOS

CHAPTER 5 (F01-F99)

CHAPTER 5 (F01–F99)

● **F63   Impulse disorders**
  Excludes2   habitual excessive use of alcohol or psychoactive substances (F10–F19)
  impulse disorders involving sexual behavior (F65.-)

  F63.0   Pathological gambling
    Compulsive gambling
    Excludes1   gambling and betting NOS (Z72.6)
    Excludes2   excessive gambling by manic patients (F30, F31)
    gambling in antisocial personality disorder (F60.2)

  F63.1   Pyromania
    Pathological fire-setting
    Excludes2   fire-setting (by) (in):
      adult with antisocial personality disorder (F60.2)
      alcohol or psychoactive substance intoxication (F10–F19)
      conduct disorders (F91.-)
      mental disorders due to known physiological condition (F01–F09)
      schizophrenia (F20.-)

  F63.2   Kleptomania
    Pathological stealing
    Excludes1   shoplifting as the reason for observation for suspected mental disorder (Z03.8)
    Excludes2   depressive disorder with stealing (F31–F33)
      stealing due to underlying mental condition-code to mental condition
      stealing in mental disorders due to known physiological condition (F01–F09)

  F63.3   Trichotillomania
    Hair plucking
    Excludes2   other stereotyped movement disorder (F98.4)

● **F63.8   Other impulse disorders**
    F63.81   Intermittent explosive disorder
    F63.89   Other impulse disorders

  F63.9   Impulse disorder, unspecified
    Impulse control disorder NOS

● **F64   Gender identity disorders**
  F64.0   Transsexualism ◄
    Gender identity disorder in adolescence and adulthood ◄
    Gender dysphoria in adolescents and adults ◄

  F64.1   Dual role transvestism ◄⟸
    Use additional code to identify sex reassignment status (Z87.890)
    Excludes1   gender identity disorder in childhood (F64.2)
    Excludes2   fetishistic transvestism (F65.1)

  F64.2   Gender identity disorder of childhood   P
    Gender dysphoria in children ◄
    Excludes1   gender identity disorder in adolescence and adulthood (F64.0) ◄⟸
    Excludes2   sexual maturation disorder (F66)

  F64.8   Other gender identity disorders
  F64.9   Gender identity disorder, unspecified
    Gender-role disorder NOS

● **F65   Paraphilias**
  F65.0   Fetishism
    Intense sexual urges and arousing fantasies using inanimate objects

  F65.1   Transvestic fetishism
    Intense sexual urges, arousal, or orgasm associated with fantasized/actual cross-dressing
    Fetishistic transvestism

  F65.2   Exhibitionism

  F65.3   Voyeurism
    Sexual urges or arousal involving real or fantasized observation of unsuspecting people who are naked, disrobing, or engaging in sexual activity

  F65.4   Pedophilia
● **F65.5   Sadomasochism**
    F65.50   Sadomasochism, unspecified
    F65.51   Sexual masochism
    F65.52   Sexual sadism
● **F65.8   Other paraphilias**
    F65.81   Frotteurism
      Sexual arousal or orgasm is achieved by rubbing up against another person (or fantasies of), in crowded place with unsuspecting victim
    F65.89   Other paraphilias
      Necrophilia
  F65.9   Paraphilia, unspecified
    Sexual deviation NOS

  F66   Other sexual disorders
    Sexual maturation disorder
    Sexual relationship disorder

● **F68   Other disorders of adult personality and behavior**
● **F68.1   Factitious disorder**
    Compensation neurosis
    Elaboration of physical symptoms for psychological reasons
    Hospital hopper syndrome
    Münchhausen's syndrome
    Peregrinating patient
    Excludes2   factitial dermatitis (L98.1)
      person feigning illness (with obvious motivation) (Z76.5)
    Ex: For category F68.1 CC codes: See F20
    F68.10   Factitious disorder, unspecified 🔖
    F68.11   Factitious disorder with predominantly psychological signs and symptoms
    F68.12   Factitious disorder with predominantly physical signs and symptoms 🔖
    F68.13   Factitious disorder with combined psychological and physical signs and symptoms
  F68.8   Other specified disorders of adult personality and behavior

  F69   Unspecified disorder of adult personality and behavior   A

INTELLECTUAL DISABILITIES (F70–F79)

  Code first any associated physical or developmental disorders
  Excludes1   borderline intellectual functioning, IQ above 70 to 84 (R41.83)

  F70   Mild intellectual disabilities
    IQ level 50-55 to approximately 70
    Mild mental subnormality

  F71   Moderate intellectual disabilities
    IQ level 35-40 to 50-55
    Moderate mental subnormality

  F72   Severe intellectual disabilities 🔖
    IQ 20-25 to 35-40
    Severe mental subnormality
    Ex: F72-F73

  F73   Profound intellectual disabilities 🔖
    IQ level below 20-25
    Profound mental subnormality
    Ex: F72-F73

◄ New   ⟸ Revised   ~~deleted~~ Deleted   Excludes 1   Excludes 2   Includes   Use additional   Code first   Code also   Unspecified
OGCR Official Guidelines   ● Unacceptable Principal Diagnosis   X Assign placeholder X   ● Use Additional Character(s)   ▶ Manifestation Code   Coding Clinic

F78   Other intellectual disabilities

F79   Unspecified intellectual disabilities
      Mental deficiency NOS
      Mental subnormality NOS

PERVASIVE AND SPECIFIC DEVELOPMENTAL DISORDERS (F80-F89)

● **F80   Specific developmental disorders of speech and language**

  F80.0   Phonological disorder
    Communication disorder of unknown cause, characterized by
      failure to use age-appropriate sounds
    Dyslalia
    Functional speech articulation disorder
    Lalling
    Lisping
    Phonological developmental disorder
    Speech articulation developmental disorder
    Speech-sound disorder ◄

    Excludes1   speech articulation impairment due to
        aphasia NOS (R47.01)
        speech articulation impairment due to
        apraxia (R48.2)

    Excludes2   speech articulation impairment due to
        hearing loss (F80.4)
        speech articulation impairment due to
        intellectual disabilities (F70-F79)
        speech articulation impairment with
        expressive language developmental
        disorder (F80.1)
        speech articulation impairment with
        mixed receptive expressive language
        developmental disorder (F80.2)

  F80.1   Expressive language disorder
    Developmental dysphasia or aphasia, expressive type

    Excludes1   mixed receptive-expressive language
        disorder (F80.2)
        dysphasia and aphasia NOS (R47.-)

    Excludes2   acquired aphasia with epilepsy [Landau-
        Kleffner] (G40.80-)
        intellectual disabilities (F70-F79)
        pervasive developmental disorders
        (F84.-)
        selective mutism (F94.0)

  F80.2   Mixed receptive-expressive language disorder
    Developmental dysphasia or aphasia, receptive type
    Developmental Wernicke's aphasia

    Excludes1   central auditory processing disorder
        (H93.25)
        dysphasia or aphasia NOS (R47.-)
        expressive language disorder (F80.1)
        expressive type dysphasia or aphasia
        (F80.1)
        word deafness (H93.25)

    Excludes2   acquired aphasia with epilepsy [Landau-
        Kleffner] (G40.80-)
        intellectual disabilities (F70-F79)
        pervasive developmental disorders
        (F84.-)
        selective mutism (F94.0)

  F80.4   Speech and language development delay due to hearing loss
    Code also type of hearing loss (H90.-, H91.-)

●   **F80.8   Other developmental disorders of speech or language**

    F80.81   Childhood onset fluency disorder
      Cluttering NOS
      Stuttering NOS

      Excludes1   adult onset fluency disorder
         (F98.5)
         fluency disorder in conditions
          classified elsewhere (R47.82)
         fluency disorder (stuttering)
          following cerebrovascular
          disease (I69. with final
          characters -23)

    F80.82   Social pragmatic communication disorder ◄

      Excludes1   Asperger's syndrome (F84.5) ◄
         autistic disorder (F84.0) ◄

    **F80.89   Other developmental disorders of speech and
        language**

  **F80.9   Developmental disorder of speech and
     language, unspecified**
    Communication disorder NOS
    Language disorder NOS

● **F81   Specific developmental disorders of scholastic skills**

  F81.0   Specific reading disorder
    'Backward reading'
    Developmental dyslexia
    Specific reading retardation

    Excludes1   alexia NOS (R48.0)
        dyslexia NOS (R48.0)

  F81.2   Mathematics disorder
    Developmental acalculia
    Developmental arithmetical disorder
    Developmental Gerstmann's syndrome

    Excludes1   acalculia NOS (R48.8)

    Excludes2   arithmetical difficulties associated with a
        reading disorder (F81.0)
        arithmetical difficulties associated with a
        spelling disorder (F81.81)
        arithmetical difficulties due to inadequate
        teaching (Z55.8)

●   **F81.8   Other developmental disorders of scholastic skills**

    F81.81   Disorder of written expression
      Specific spelling disorder

    **F81.89   Other developmental disorders of scholastic
        skills**

●   **F81.9   Developmental disorder of scholastic skills, unspecified**
    Knowledge acquisition disability NOS
    Learning disability NOS
    Learning disorder NOS

F82   Specific developmental disorder of motor function
    Clumsy child syndrome
    Developmental coordination disorder
    Developmental dyspraxia

    Excludes1   abnormalities of gait and mobility (R26.-)
        lack of coordination (R27.-)

    Excludes2   lack of coordination secondary to intellectual
        disabilities (F70-F79)

● **F84   Pervasive developmental disorders**

    Use additional code to identify any associated medical
      condition and intellectual disabilities.
    (Ex) **For category F84 CC codes unless otherwise indicated:** See F20

  F84.0   Autistic disorder 🔖
    Autism spectrum disorder ◄
    Infantile autism
    Infantile psychosis
    Kanner's syndrome

    Excludes1   Asperger's syndrome (F84.5)

  F84.2   Rett's syndrome 🔖
    Neurodevelopmental disorder

    Excludes1   Asperger's syndrome (F84.5)
        Autistic disorder (F84.0)
        other childhood disintegrative disorder
        (F84.3)
    (Ex) E75.00-E75.19, E75.4, F84.2, G13.2-G13.8, G30.0-G31.82, G31.84-G31.9,
       G91.4, G94

CHAPTER 5 (F01-F99)

CHAPTER 5 (F01-F99)

F84.3   **Other childhood disintegrative disorder** 🗒
Dementia infantilis
At least two years of normal development followed by significant loss of language abilities, social skills, bowel/bladder control, motor skills
Disintegrative psychosis
Heller's syndrome
At least two years of normal development followed by significant loss of language abilities, social skills, bowel/bladder control, motor skills
Symbiotic psychosis
Abnormal relationship to mothering figure, characterized by intense separation anxiety, severe regression, giving up of useful speech, and autism

Use additional code to identify any associated neurological condition.

Excludes1   Asperger's syndrome (F84.5)
Autistic disorder (F84.0)
Rett's syndrome (F84.2)

F84.5   **Asperger's syndrome** 🗒
Developmental disorder
Asperger's disorder
Autistic psychopathy
Schizoid disorder of childhood

F84.8   **Other pervasive developmental disorders** 🗒
Overactive disorder associated with intellectual disabilities and stereotyped movements

F84.9   **Pervasive developmental disorder, unspecified** 🗒
Atypical autism

F88   **Other disorders of psychological development**
Developmental agnosia
Global developmental delay ◀
Other specified neurodevelopmental disorder ◀

F89   **Unspecified disorder of psychological development**
Developmental disorder NOS
Neurodevelopmental disorder NOS ◀

BEHAVIORAL AND EMOTIONAL DISORDERS WITH ONSET USUALLY OCCURRING IN CHILDHOOD AND ADOLESCENCE (F90-F98)

Note: Codes within categories F90-F98 may be used regardless of the age of a patient. These disorders generally have onset within the childhood or adolescent years, but may continue throughout life or not be diagnosed until adulthood.

● **F90**   **Attention-deficit hyperactivity disorders**
Attention deficit disorder with hyperactivity=ADHD

Includes   attention deficit disorder with hyperactivity
attention deficit syndrome with hyperactivity

Excludes2   anxiety disorders (F40.-, F41.-)
mood [affective] disorders (F30-F39)
pervasive developmental disorders (F84.-)
schizophrenia (F20.-)

F90.0   **Attention-deficit hyperactivity disorder, predominantly inattentive type**

F90.1   **Attention-deficit hyperactivity disorder, predominantly hyperactive type**

F90.2   **Attention-deficit hyperactivity disorder, combined type**

F90.8   **Attention-deficit hyperactivity disorder, other type**

F90.9   **Attention-deficit hyperactivity disorder, unspecified type**
Attention-deficit hyperactivity disorder of childhood or adolescence NOS
Attention-deficit hyperactivity disorder NOS

P

● **F91**   **Conduct disorders**
Childhood/adolescence disruptive behavior disorder

Excludes1   antisocial behavior (Z72.81-)
antisocial personality disorder (F60.2)

Excludes2   conduct problems associated with attention-deficit hyperactivity disorder (F90.-)
mood [affective] disorders (F30-F39)
pervasive developmental disorders (F84.-)
schizophrenia (F20.-)

F91.0   **Conduct disorder confined to family context**

F91.1   **Conduct disorder, childhood-onset type**
Unsocialized conduct disorder
Conduct disorder, solitary aggressive type
Unsocialized aggressive disorder

F91.2   **Conduct disorder, adolescent-onset type**
Socialized conduct disorder
Conduct disorder, group type

F91.3   **Oppositional defiant disorder**

F91.8   **Other conduct disorders**
Other specified conduct disorder ◀
Other specified disruptive disorder ◀

F91.9   **Conduct disorder, unspecified**
Behavioral disorder NOS
Conduct disorder NOS
Disruptive behavior disorder NOS
Disruptive disorder NOS ◀

● **F93**   **Emotional disorders with onset specific to childhood**

F93.0   **Separation anxiety disorder of childhood**

Excludes2   mood [affective] disorders (F30-F39)
nonpsychotic mental disorders (F40-F48)
phobic anxiety disorder of childhood (F40.8)
social phobia (F40.1)

F93.8   **Other childhood emotional disorders**
Identity disorder

Excludes2   gender identity disorder of childhood (F64.2)

F93.9   **Childhood emotional disorder, unspecified**

● **F94**   **Disorders of social functioning with onset specific to childhood and adolescence**

F94.0   **Selective mutism**
Elective mutism

Excludes2   pervasive developmental disorders (F84.-)
schizophrenia (F20.-)
specific developmental disorders of speech and language (F80.-)
transient mutism as part of separation anxiety in young children (F93.0)

F94.1   **Reactive attachment disorder of childhood**

Use additional code to identify any associated failure to thrive or growth retardation

Excludes1   disinhibited attachment disorder of childhood (F94.2)
normal variation in pattern of selective attachment

Excludes2   Asperger's syndrome (F84.5)
maltreatment syndromes (T74.-)
sexual or physical abuse in childhood, resulting in psychosocial problems (Z62.81-)

F94.2   **Disinhibited attachment disorder of childhood**
Affectionless psychopathy
Institutional syndrome

Excludes1   reactive attachment disorder of childhood (F94.1)

Excludes2   Asperger's syndrome (F84.5)
attention-deficit hyperactivity disorders (F90.-)
hospitalism in children (F43.2-)

◀ New   ◀▦ Revised   ~~deleted~~ Deleted   Excludes 1   Excludes 2   Includes   Use additional   Code first   Code also   Unspecified
OGCR Official Guidelines   ● Unacceptable Principal Diagnosis   X Assign placeholder X   ● Use Additional Character(s)   ▶ Manifestation Code   **Coding Clinic**

F94.8 **Other childhood disorders of social functioning**

F94.9 **Childhood disorder of social functioning, unspecified**

● F95 **Tic disorder**
Involuntary twitch

F95.0 **Transient tic disorder**
Provisional tic disorder ◀

F95.1 **Chronic motor or vocal tic disorder**

F95.2 **Tourette's disorder**
Combined vocal and multiple motor tic disorder [de la Tourette]
Tourette's syndrome

F95.8 **Other tic disorders**

F95.9 **Tic disorder, unspecified**
Tic NOS

● F98 **Other behavioral and emotional disorders with onset usually occurring in childhood and adolescence**

Excludes2 breath-holding spells (R06.89)
gender identity disorder of childhood (F64.2)
Kleine-Levin syndrome (G47.13)
obsessive-compulsive disorder (F42-) ◀▬▬
sleep disorders not due to a substance or known physiological condition (F51.-)

F98.0 **Enuresis not due to a substance or known physiological condition**
Enuresis: Urinary incontinence
Enuresis (primary) (secondary) of nonorganic origin
Functional enuresis
Psychogenic enuresis
Urinary incontinence of nonorganic origin

Excludes1 enuresis NOS (R32)

F98.1 **Encopresis not due to a substance or known physiological condition**
Encopresis: Fecal incontinence
Functional encopresis
Incontinence of feces of nonorganic origin
Psychogenic encopresis

Use additional code to identify the cause of any coexisting constipation.

Excludes1 encopresis NOS (R15.-)

● F98.2 **Other feeding disorders of infancy and childhood**

Excludes1 feeding difficulties (R63.3)

Excludes2 anorexia nervosa and other eating disorders (F50.-)
feeding problems of newborn (P92.-)
pica of infancy or childhood (F98.3)

F98.21 **Rumination disorder of infancy**

F98.29 **Other feeding disorders of infancy and early childhood**

F98.3 **Pica of infancy and childhood**
Craving and eating substances such as paint, clay, or dirt to replace a nutritional deficit in the body.

F98.4 **Stereotyped movement disorders**
Stereotype/habit disorder

Excludes1 abnormal involuntary movements (R25.-)

Excludes2 compulsions in obsessive-compulsive disorder (F42-) ◀▬▬
hair plucking (F63.3)
movement disorders of organic origin (G20-G25)
nail-biting (F98.8)
nose-picking (F98.8)
stereotypies that are part of a broader psychiatric condition (F01-F95)
thumb-sucking (F98.8)
tic disorders (F95.-)
trichotillomania (F63.3)

F98.5 **Adult onset fluency disorder**

Excludes1 childhood onset fluency disorder (F80.81)
dysphasia (R47.02)
fluency disorder in conditions classified elsewhere (R47.82)
fluency disorder (stuttering) following cerebrovascular disease (I69. with final characters -23)
tic disorders (F95.-)

F98.8 **Other specified behavioral and emotional disorders with onset usually occurring in childhood and adolescence**
Excessive masturbation
Nail-biting
Nose-picking
Thumb-sucking

F98.9 **Unspecified behavioral and emotional disorders with onset usually occurring in childhood and adolescence**

UNSPECIFIED MENTAL DISORDER (F99)

F99 **Mental disorder, not otherwise specified**
Mental illness NOS

Excludes1 unspecified mental disorder due to known physiological condition (F09)

CHAPTER 5 (F01-F99)

Item 5-2 Enuresis: Bed wetting by children at night. Causes can be either psychological or medical (diabetes, urinary tract infections, or abnormalities). **Encopresis:** Overflow incontinence of bowels sometimes resulting from chronic constipation or fecal impaction. Check the documentation for additional diagnoses.

CHAPTER 6

DISEASES OF THE NERVOUS SYSTEM (G00-G99)

OGCR Chapter-Specific Coding Guidelines

6. Chapter 6: Diseases of the Nervous System (G00-G99)

a. Dominant/nondominant side

Codes from category G81, Hemiplegia and hemiparesis, and subcategories, G83.1, Monoplegia of lower limb, G83.2, Monoplegia of upper limb, and G83.3, Monoplegia, unspecified, identify whether the dominant or nondominant side is affected. Should the affected side be documented, but not specified as dominant or nondominant, and the classification system does not indicate a default, code selection is as follows:

- For ambidextrous patients, the default should be dominant.
- If the left side is affected, the default is non-dominant.
- If the right side is affected, the default is dominant.

b. Pain - Category G89

1) General coding information

Codes in category G89, Pain, not elsewhere classified, may be used in conjunction with codes from other categories and chapters to provide more detail about acute or chronic pain and neoplasm-related pain, unless otherwise indicated below.

If the pain is not specified as acute or chronic, post-thoracotomy, postprocedural, or neoplasm-related, do not assign codes from category G89.

A code from category G89 should not be assigned if the underlying (definitive) diagnosis is known, unless the reason for the encounter is pain control/management and not management of the underlying condition.

When an admission or encounter is for a procedure aimed at treating the underlying condition (e.g., spinal fusion, kyphoplasty), a code for the underlying condition (e.g., vertebral fracture, spinal stenosis) should be assigned as the principal diagnosis. No code from category G89 should be assigned.

(a) Category G89 Codes as Principal or First-Listed Diagnosis

Category G89 codes are acceptable as principal diagnosis or the first-listed code:

- When pain control or pain management is the reason for the admission/encounter (e.g., a patient with displaced intervertebral disc, nerve impingement and severe back pain presents for injection of steroid into the spinal canal). The underlying cause of the pain should be reported as an additional diagnosis, if known.
- When a patient is admitted for the insertion of a neurostimulator for pain control, assign the appropriate pain code as the principal or first-listed diagnosis. When an admission or encounter is for a procedure aimed at treating the underlying condition and a neurostimulator is inserted for pain control during the same admission/encounter, a code for the underlying condition should be assigned as the principal diagnosis and the appropriate pain code should be assigned as a secondary diagnosis.

(b) Use of Category G89 Codes in Conjunction with Site Specific Pain Codes

(i) Assigning Category G89 and Site-Specific Pain Codes

Codes from category G89 may be used in conjunction with codes that identify the site of pain (including codes from chapter 18) if the category G89 code provides additional information. For example, if the code describes the site of the pain, but does not fully describe whether the pain is acute or chronic, then both codes should be assigned.

(ii) Sequencing of Category G89 Codes with Site-Specific Pain Codes

The sequencing of category G89 codes with site-specific pain codes (including chapter 18 codes), is dependent on the circumstances of the encounter/admission as follows:

- If the encounter is for pain control or pain management, assign the code from category G89 followed by the code identifying the specific site of pain (e.g., encounter for pain management for acute neck pain from trauma is assigned code G89.11, Acute pain due to trauma, followed by code M54.2, Cervicalgia, to identify the site of pain).
- If the encounter is for any other reason except pain control or pain management, and a related definitive diagnosis has not been established (confirmed) by the provider, assign the code for the specific site of pain first, followed by the appropriate code from category G89.

2) Pain due to devices, implants and grafts

See Section I.C.19. Pain due to medical devices

3) Postoperative Pain

The provider's documentation should be used to guide the coding of postoperative pain, as well as *Section III. Reporting Additional Diagnoses* and *Section IV. Diagnostic Coding and Reporting in the Outpatient Setting.*

The default for post-thoracotomy and other postoperative pain not specified as acute or chronic is the code for the acute form.

Routine or expected postoperative pain immediately after surgery should not be coded.

(a) Postoperative pain not associated with specific postoperative complication

Postoperative pain not associated with a specific postoperative complication is assigned to the appropriate postoperative pain code in category G89.

(b) Postoperative pain associated with specific postoperative complication

Postoperative pain associated with a specific postoperative complication (such as painful wire sutures) is assigned to the appropriate code(s) found in Chapter 19, Injury, poisoning, and certain other consequences of external causes. If appropriate, use additional code(s) from category G89 to identify acute or chronic pain (G89.18 or G89.28).

4) Chronic pain

Chronic pain is classified to subcategory G89.2. There is no time frame defining when pain becomes chronic pain. The provider's documentation should be used to guide use of these codes.

5) Neoplasm Related Pain

Code G89.3 is assigned to pain documented as being related, associated or due to cancer, primary or secondary malignancy, or tumor. This code is assigned regardless of whether the pain is acute or chronic.

This code may be assigned as the principal or first-listed code when the stated reason for the admission/encounter is documented as pain control/pain management. The underlying neoplasm should be reported as an additional diagnosis.

When the reason for the admission/encounter is management of the neoplasm and the pain associated with the neoplasm is also documented, code G89.3 may be assigned as an additional diagnosis. It is not necessary to assign an additional code for the site of the pain.

See Section I.C.2 for instructions on the sequencing of neoplasms for all other stated reasons for the admission/encounter (except for pain control/pain management).

6) Chronic pain syndrome

Central pain syndrome (G89.0) and chronic pain syndrome (G89.4) are different than the term "chronic pain," and therefore codes should only be used when the provider has specifically documented this condition.

See Section I.C.5. Pain disorders related to psychological factors

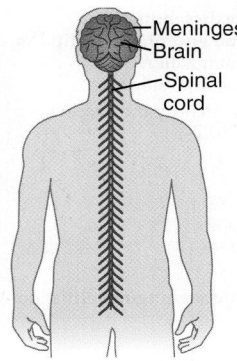

Meninges
Brain
Spinal cord

Figure 6-1 The brain and spinal cord make up the central nervous system.

Item 6-1 The two major classifications of the nervous system are the peripheral nervous system and the central nervous system (CNS). The central nervous system is comprised of the brain and the spinal cord. The peripheral nervous system is comprised of the parasympathetic and sympathetic systems. **Encephalitis** is the swelling of the brain. **Meningitis** is swelling of the covering of the brain, the meninges. Types and causes of brain infections are:

Type	Cause
purulent	bacterial
aseptic/abacterial	viral
chronic meningitis	mycobacterial and fungal

CHAPTER 6

DISEASES OF THE NERVOUS SYSTEM
(G00-G99)

> **Excludes2**   certain conditions originating in the perinatal period (P04-P96)
> certain infectious and parasitic diseases (A00-B99)
> complications of pregnancy, childbirth and the puerperium (O00-O9A)
> congenital malformations, deformations, and chromosomal abnormalities (Q00-Q99)
> endocrine, nutritional and metabolic diseases (E00-E88)
> injury, poisoning and certain other consequences of external causes (S00-T88)
> neoplasms (C00-D49)
> symptoms, signs and abnormal clinical and laboratory findings, not elsewhere classified (R00-R94)

This chapter contains the following blocks:

G00-G09	Inflammatory diseases of the central nervous system
G10-G14	Systemic atrophies primarily affecting the central nervous system
G20-G26	Extrapyramidal and movement disorders
G30-G32	Other degenerative diseases of the nervous system
G35-G37	Demyelinating diseases of the central nervous system
G40-G47	Episodic and paroxysmal disorders
G50-G59	Nerve, nerve root and plexus disorders
G60-G65	Polyneuropathies and other disorders of the peripheral nervous system
G70-G73	Diseases of myoneural junction and muscle
G80-G83	Cerebral palsy and other paralytic syndromes
G89-G99	Other disorders of the nervous system

INFLAMMATORY DISEASES OF THE CENTRAL NERVOUS SYSTEM (G00-G09)

● **G00**   **Bacterial meningitis, not elsewhere classified**
An infection of the cerebrospinal fluid surrounding the spinal cord and brain.

> **Includes**   bacterial arachnoiditis
> bacterial leptomeningitis
> bacterial meningitis
> bacterial pachymeningitis

> **Excludes1**   bacterial:
> meningoencephalitis (G04.2)
> meningomyelitis (G04.2)

Ⓔⓧ **For category G00 CC codes:** 02.21, A17.0-A17.1, A27.81, A39.0, A50.41, A51.41, A52.13, A54.82, A54.84, A54.89-A54.9, A87.0-A87.9, B00.3, B02.1, B26.1, B37.5, B38.4, B45.1, B58.2, E08.40-E08.49, E08.618-E08.638, E08.649-E08.8, E09.40-E09.49, E09.618-E09.638, E09.649-E09.8, E10.40-E10.49, E10.618-E10.638, E10.649, E10.69, E10.8, E11.40-E11.49, E11.618-E11.638, E11.649, E11.69-E11.8, E13.40-E13.49, E13.618-E13.638, E13.649-E13.69, E13.8, G00.0-G03.9, G04.2, G32.89, G61.0, G96.8-G96.9, G98.0-G98.8, G99.8

G00.0   **Hemophilus meningitis** 🔖
Meningitis due to Hemophilus influenzae

G00.1   **Pneumococcal meningitis** 🔖
Meningitis due to Streptococcal pneumoniae ◀

G00.2   **Streptococcal meningitis** 🔖
Use additional code to further identify organism (B95.0-B95.5)

G00.3   **Staphylococcal meningitis** 🔖
Use additional code to further identify organism (B95.61-B95.8)

G00.8   **Other bacterial meningitis** 🔖
Meningitis due to Escherichia coli
Meningitis due to Friedländer bacillus
Meningitis due to Klebsiella
Use additional code to further identify organism (B96.-)

G00.9   **Bacterial meningitis, unspecified** 🔖
Meningitis due to gram-negative bacteria, unspecified
Purulent meningitis NOS
Pyogenic meningitis NOS
Suppurative meningitis NOS

▷ **G01**   *Meningitis in bacterial diseases classified elsewhere* 🔖
Code first underlying disease

> **Excludes1**   meningitis (in):
> gonococcal (A54.81)
> leptospirosis (A27.81)
> listeriosis (A32.11)
> Lyme disease (A69.21)
> meningococcal (A39.0)
> neurosyphilis (A52.13)
> tuberculosis (A17.0)
> meningoencephalitis and meningomyelitis in bacterial diseases classified elsewhere (G05)

Ⓔⓧ See G00

▷ **G02**   *Meningitis in other infectious and parasitic diseases classified elsewhere* 🔖
Code first underlying disease, such as:
African trypanosomiasis (B56.-)
poliovirus infection (A80.-)

> **Excludes1**   candidal meningitis (B37.5)
> coccidioidomycosis meningitis (B38.4)
> cryptococcal meningitis (B45.1)
> herpesviral [herpes simplex] meningitis (B00.3)
> infectious mononucleosis complicated by meningitis (B27.- with fourth character 2)
> measles complicated by meningitis (B05.1)
> meningoencephalitis and meningomyelitis in other infectious and parasitic diseases classified elsewhere (G05)
> mumps meningitis (B26.1)
> rubella meningitis (B06.02)
> varicella [chickenpox] meningitis (B01.0)
> zoster meningitis (B02.1)

Ⓔⓧ A02.21, A17.0-A17.1, A27.81, A39.0, A50.41, A51.41, A52.13, A54.82, A54.84, A54.89-A54.9, A87.0-A87.9, B00.3, B02.1, B26.1, B37.5, B38.4, B45.1, B58.2, G00.0-G03.9, G04.2, G32.89, G61.0, G96.8-G96.9, G98.0-G98.8, G99.8

CHAPTER 6 (G00-G99)

N   Newborn Age: 0   **P**   Pediatric Age: 0-17   **M**   Maternity DX: 12-55   **A**   Adult Age: 15-124   ♀ Females Only   ♂ Males Only

🔖 Complication\Comorbidity   🔖 Major C\C   Ⓔⓧ CC/MCC Exclusions   🔖 Hospital-Acquired Condition

785

● **G03**   **Meningitis due to other and unspecified causes**
   Includes   arachnoiditis NOS
                  leptomeningitis NOS
                  meningitis NOS
                  pachymeningitis NOS
   Excludes1 meningoencephalitis (G04.-)
                  meningomyelitis (G04.-)
   (Ex:) For category G03 CC codes unless otherwise indicated: See G00

   G03.0   **Nonpyogenic meningitis** 🔍
               Aseptic meningitis
               Nonbacterial meningitis

   G03.1   **Chronic meningitis** 🔍

   G03.2   **Benign recurrent meningitis [Mollaret]** 🔍
               (Ex:) A02.21, A17.0-A17.1, A27.81, A39.0, A50.41, A51.41, A52.13,
               A54.82-A54.84, A54.89-A54.9, A74.81-A74.9, A87.0-A87.9, A96.2,
               A98.3-A98.4, B26.1, B33.24, B33.4-B33.8, B34.1-B34.8, B37.5, B38.4,
               B45.1, B58.2, B92, B94.2-B94.9, B97.10, B97.19, B97.29, B97.5-B97.6,
               B97.81-B97.89, G00.0-G03.9, G04.2, G32.89, G61.0, G96.8-G96.9,
               G98.0-G98.8, G99.8

   G03.8   **Meningitis due to other specified causes** 🔍

   G03.9   **Meningitis, unspecified** 🔍
               Arachnoiditis (spinal) NOS

● **G04**   **Encephalitis, myelitis and encephalomyelitis**
   Includes   acute ascending myelitis
                  meningoencephalitis
                  meningomyelitis
   Excludes1 encephalopathy NOS (G93.40)
                  other noninfectious acute disseminated
                  encephalomyelitis (noninfectious ADEM)
                  (G04.81)
   Excludes2 acute transverse myelitis (G37.3-)
                  alcoholic encephalopathy (G31.2)
                  benign myalgic encephalomyelitis (G93.3)
                  multiple sclerosis (G35)
                  subacute necrotizing myelitis (G37.4)
                  toxic encephalitis (G92)
                  toxic encephalopathy (G92)

● **G04.0**   **Acute disseminated encephalitis and encephalomyelitis (ADEM)**
   Excludes1 acute necrotizing hemorrhagic
                  encephalopathy (G04.3-)
   (Ex:) For category G04.0 CC codes unless otherwise indicated: A02.21,
   A17.0-A17.1, A17.82, A27.81, A39.0, A50.41-A50.42, A51.41,
   A52.13-A52.14, A54.82, A54.84, A54.89-A54.9, A81.1, A81.82-A81.89,
   A83.0-A85.8, A87.0-A88.0, A88.8, A92.1-A92.8, A93.0, A96.2, A98.3-A98.4,
   B00.3-B00.4, B00.89-B01.11, B01.81-B02.23, B02.29, B02.7-B02.9, B04,
   B06.01, B08.04-B08.09, B08.20-B08.22, B08.60-B08.79, B09-B10.89,
   B26.1-B26.2, B27.00-B27.99, B33.1, B33.24, B33.4-B33.8, B34.1-B34.2,
   B34.4, B34.8, B37.5, B38.4, B45.1-B58.2, B92, B94.2, B94.8-B94.9, B97.10,
   B97.19-B97.29, B97.5-B97.6, B97.81-B97.89, G00.0-G04.01, G04.2,
   G04.31, G04.81-G05.4, G32.89, G37.0, G37.4-G37.5, G61.0, G96.8-G96.9,
   G98.0-G98.8, G99.8, J09.X3-J09.X9, J10.2-J10.89, J11.2-J11.89, L44.4,
   P35.2-P35.9, P37.0-P37.4, P37.8-P37.9

   G04.00   **Acute disseminated encephalitis and
                encephalomyelitis, unspecified** 🔍

   ▷ **G04.01**   *Postinfectious acute disseminated encephalitis
                  and encephalomyelitis (postinfectious ADEM)* 🔍
                  Excludes1   post chickenpox encephalitis
                                  (B01.1)
                                  post measles encephalitis (B05.0)
                                  post measles myelitis (B05.1)

   G04.02   **Postimmunization acute disseminated
                encephalitis, myelitis and encephalomyelitis** 🔍
                Encephalitis, post immunization
                Encephalomyelitis, post immunization
                Use additional code to identify the vaccine
                (T50.A-, T50.B-, T50.Z-)
                (Ex:) No exclusions

   G04.1   **Tropical spastic paraplegia** 🔍
               (Ex:) G04.1, G11.0-G12.9, G32.0-G37.3, G37.5-G37.9, G80.0-G80.2, G80.4-G80.9,
               G81.00-G83.9, G90.01-G90.09, G90.2, G90.4, G90.50-G90.9, G92,
               G93.40-G93.49, G93.81, G93.89-G95.9, G96.8-G96.9, G98.0-G99.8, I67.83,
               R53.2

   G04.2   **Bacterial meningoencephalitis and meningomyelitis, not
               elsewhere classified** 🔍
               (Ex:) See G00

● **G04.3**   **Acute necrotizing hemorrhagic encephalopathy**
               *Sudden and severe CNS disease with pathology of
               hemorrhages and necrosis of white matter*
   Excludes1   acute disseminated encephalitis and
                   encephalomyelitis (G04.0-)

   G04.30   **Acute necrotizing hemorrhagic
                encephalopathy, unspecified** 🔍
                (Ex:) No exclusions

   G04.31   **Postinfectious acute necrotizing hemorrhagic
                encephalopathy** 🔍
                (Ex:) See G04.0

   G04.32   **Postimmunization acute necrotizing
                hemorrhagic encephalopathy** 🔍
                Use additional code to identify vaccine
                (T50.A-, T50.B-, T50.Z-)
                (Ex:) No exclusions

   G04.39   **Other acute necrotizing hemorrhagic
                encephalopathy** 🔍
                Code also underlying etiology, if applicable
                (Ex:) No exclusions

● **G04.8**   **Other encephalitis, myelitis and encephalomyelitis**
               Code also any associated seizure (G40.-, R56.9)
               (Ex:) For category G04.8 CC codes: See G04.0

   G04.81   **Other encephalitis and encephalomyelitis** 🔍
                Noninfectious acute disseminated
                encephalomyelitis (noninfectious ADEM)

   G04.89   **Other myelitis** 🔍

● **G04.9**   **Encephalitis, myelitis and encephalomyelitis,
               unspecified**
               (Ex:) For category G04.9 CC codes: A17.82, A28.1, A50.42, A52.14, A75.9,
               A79.9, A81.1, A81.82-A81.89, A83.0-A85.8, A87.2, A88.0, A88.8,
               A92.1-A92.8, A93.0, B00.4, B00.82, B01.11-B01.12, B04, B06.01, B08.09,
               B08.20-B08.22, B08.60-B08.79, B09, B10.01-B10.09, B26.2,
               B27.00-B27.99, B33.1, B45.0, B45.2-B45.9, B54, B58.2, B75, B97.10,
               B97.21, G04.00-G04.01, G04.31, G04.81-G05.4, G37.0, G37.4-G37.5,
               H66.40-H66.43, J09.X3-J09.X9, J10.2-J10.89, J11.2-J11.89, L44.4,
               M1A.10X0-M1A.19X1, M32.0-M32.9, P35.2-P35.9, P37.0-P37.9,
               T56.0X1-T56.0X4[A]

   G04.90   **Encephalitis and
                encephalomyelitis, unspecified** 🔍
                Ventriculitis (cerebral) NOS

   G04.91   **Myelitis, unspecified** 🔍

◀ New   ◀ Revised   deleted Deleted   Excludes 1   Excludes 2   Includes   Use additional   Code first   Code also   Unspecified
OGCR Official Guidelines   ● Unacceptable Principal Diagnosis   X Assign placeholder X   ● Use Additional Character(s)   ▷ Manifestation Code   Coding Clinic

CHAPTER 6 (G00-G99)

● **G05 Encephalitis, myelitis and encephalomyelitis in diseases classified elsewhere**

Code first underlying disease, such as:
human immunodeficiency virus [HIV] disease (B20)
poliovirus (A80.-)
suppurative otitis media (H66.01-H66.4)
trichinellosis (B75)

Excludes1   adenoviral encephalitis, myelitis and encephalomyelitis (A85.1)
congenital toxoplasmosis encephalitis, myelitis and encephalomyelitis (P37.1)
cytomegaloviral encephalitis, myelitis and encephalomyelitis (B25.8)
encephalitis, myelitis and encephalomyelitis (in) measles (B05.0)
encephalitis, myelitis and encephalomyelitis (in) systemic lupus erythematosus (M32.19)
enteroviral encephalitis, myelitis and encephalomyelitis (A85.0)
herpesviral [herpes simplex] encephalitis, myelitis and encephalomyelitis (B00.4)
listerial encephalitis, myelitis and encephalomyelitis (A32.12)
meningococcal encephalitis, myelitis and encephalomyelitis (A39.81)
mumps encephalitis, myelitis and encephalomyelitis (B26.2)
postchickenpox encephalitis, myelitis and encephalomyelitis (B01.1-)
rubella encephalitis, myelitis and encephalomyelitis (B06.01)
toxoplasmosis encephalitis, myelitis and encephalomyelitis (B58.2)
zoster encephalitis, myelitis and encephalomyelitis (B02.0)

(Ex:) **For category G05 CC codes:** See G04.0

▶ **G05.3 Encephalitis and encephalomyelitis in diseases classified elsewhere**
Meningoencephalitis in diseases classified elsewhere

▶ **G05.4 Myelitis in diseases classified elsewhere**
Meningomyelitis in diseases classified elsewhere

● **G06 Intracranial and intraspinal abscess and granuloma**
An accumulation of pus in either the brain or spinal cord

Use additional code (B95-B97) to identify infectious agent.

G06.0 Intracranial abscess and granuloma
Brain [any part] abscess (embolic)
Cerebellar abscess (embolic)
Cerebral abscess (embolic)
Intracranial epidural abscess or granuloma
Intracranial extradural abscess or granuloma
Intracranial subdural abscess or granuloma
Otogenic abscess (embolic)

Excludes1   tuberculous intracranial abscess and granuloma (A17.81)

(Ex:) A06.6, A17.81, E08.40-E08.49, E08.618-E08.638, E08.649-E08.8, E09.40-E09.49, E09.618-E09.638, E09.649-E09.8, E10.40-E10.49, E10.618-E10.638, E10.649, E10.69-E10.8, E11.40-E11.49, E11.618-E11.638, E11.649, E11.69-E11.8, E13.40-E13.49, E13.618-E13.638, E13.649-E13.8, G06.0-G08, G93.81, G93.89-G93.9

G06.1 Intraspinal abscess and granuloma
Abscess (embolic) of spinal cord [any part]
Intraspinal epidural abscess or granuloma
Intraspinal extradural abscess or granuloma
Intraspinal subdural abscess or granuloma

Excludes1   tuberculous intraspinal abscess and granuloma (A17.81)

(Ex:) A06.6, A17.81, E08.40-A08.49, E08.618-E08.638, E08.649-E08.8, E09.40-E09.49, E09.618-E09.638, E09.649-E09.8, E10.40-E10.49, E10.618-E10.638, E10.649, E10.69-E10.8, E11.40-E11.49, E11.618-E11.638, E11.649, E11.69-E11.8, E13.40-E13.49, E13.618-E13.638, E13.649-E13.8, G06.1

G06.2 Extradural and subdural abscess, unspecified

(Ex:) A06.6, A17.81, E08.40-E08.49, E08.618-E08.638, E08.649-E08.8, E09.40-E09.49, E09.618-E09.638, E09.649-E09.8, E10.40-E10.49, E10.618-E10.638, E10.649, E10.69-E10.8, E11.40-E11.49, E11.618-E11.638, E11.649, E11.69-E11.8, E13.40-E13.49, E13.618-E13.638, E13.649-E13.8, G06.0-G06.2, G07-G08

▶ **G07 Intracranial and intraspinal abscess and granuloma in diseases classified elsewhere**

Code first underlying disease, such as:
schistosomiasis granuloma of brain (B65.-)

Excludes1   abscess of brain:
amebic (A06.6)
chromomycotic (B43.1)
gonococcal (A54.82)
tuberculous (A17.81)
tuberculoma of meninges (A17.1)

(Ex:) See G06.2

G08 Intracranial and intraspinal phlebitis and thrombophlebitis
Septic embolism of intracranial or intraspinal venous sinuses and veins
Septic endophlebitis of intracranial or intraspinal venous sinuses and veins
Septic phlebitis of intracranial or intraspinal venous sinuses and veins
Septic thrombophlebitis of intracranial or intraspinal venous sinuses and veins
Septic thrombosis of intracranial or intraspinal venous sinuses and veins

Excludes1   intracranial phlebitis and thrombophlebitis complicating:
abortion, ectopic or molar pregnancy (O00-O07, O08.7)
pregnancy, childbirth and the puerperium (O22.5, O87.3)
nonpyogenic intracranial phlebitis and thrombophlebitis (I67.6)

Excludes2   intracranial phlebitis and thrombophlebitis complicating nonpyogenic intraspinal phlebitis and thrombophlebitis (G95.1)

(Ex:) See G06.2

G09 Sequelae of inflammatory diseases of central nervous system
Note: Category G09 is to be used to indicate conditions whose primary classification is to G00-G08 as the cause of sequelae, themselves classifiable elsewhere. The 'sequelae' include conditions specified as residuals.

Code first condition resulting from (sequela) of inflammatory diseases of central nervous system

---

SYSTEMIC ATROPHIES PRIMARILY AFFECTING THE CENTRAL NERVOUS SYSTEM (G10-G14)

G10 Huntington's disease
Genetic disease with degeneration of cells of the nervous system, including brain
Huntington's chorea
Huntington's dementia

(Ex:) G04.1, G20, G21.11-G21.9, G32.89-G37.9, G80.0-G80.2, G80.4-G80.9, G82.20-G83.0, G92, G93.1, G93.40-G93.6, G93.81, G93.89-G93.9, G96.8-G96.9, G98.0-G98.8, G99.8, I67.83, R53.2

Item 6–2 Huntington's chorea is an inherited degenerative disorder of the central nervous system and is characterized by ceaseless, jerky movements and progressive cognitive and behavioral deterioration.

CHAPTER 6 (G00-G99)

 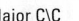

● G11   Hereditary ataxia
Genetic neurological disorder affecting coordination
> **Excludes2**   cerebral palsy (G80.-)
> hereditary and idiopathic neuropathy (G60.-)
> metabolic disorders (E70-E88)

(Ex:) **For category G11 CC codes unless otherwise indicated:** G04.1, G10-G12.9, G21.0, G23.0-G25.79, G25.82-G26, G32.0-G37.9, G80.0-G83.9, G90.01-G90.09, G90.2-G90.9, G92-G93.1, G93.40-G93.49, G93.81, G93.89-G95.9, G96.8-G96.9, G98.0-G99.8, I67.83, R53.2

G11.0   Congenital nonprogressive ataxia 🖉

G11.1   Early-onset cerebellar ataxia 🖉
> Early-onset cerebellar ataxia with essential tremor
> Early-onset cerebellar ataxia with myoclonus [Hunt's ataxia]
> Early-onset cerebellar ataxia with retained tendon reflexes
> Friedreich's ataxia (autosomal recessive)
> X-linked recessive spinocerebellar ataxia

G11.2   Late-onset cerebellar ataxia 🖉   A

G11.3   Cerebellar ataxia with defective DNA repair 🖉
> Ataxia telangiectasia [Louis-Bar]
> > **Excludes2**   Cockayne's syndrome (Q87.1)
> > other disorders of purine and pyrimidine metabolism (E79.-)
> > xeroderma pigmentosum (Q82.1)

G11.4   Hereditary spastic paraplegia 🖉
> (Ex:) G04.1, G10-G12.9, G21.0, G23.0-G25.79, G25.82-G26, G32.0-G37.3, G37.5-G37.9, G80.0-G83.9, G90.01-G90.09, G90.2-G90.9, G92, G93.1, G93.40-G93.49, G93.81, G93.89-G93.9, G95.0-G95.9, G96.12-G96.9, G97.1, G98.0-G99.8, I67.83, R53.2

G11.8   Other hereditary ataxias 🖉

G11.9   Hereditary ataxia, unspecified 🖉
> Hereditary cerebellar ataxia NOS
> Hereditary cerebellar degeneration
> Hereditary cerebellar disease
> Hereditary cerebellar syndrome
> (Ex:) G11.0-G11.9, G32.81

● G12   Spinal muscular atrophy and related syndromes
> (Ex:) **For category G12 CC codes:** E08.40-E08.49, E08.618-E08.638, E08.649-E08.8, E09.40-E09.49, E09.618-E09.638, E09.649-E09.8, E10.40-E10.49, E10.618-E10.638, E10.649, E10.69-E10.8, E11.40-E11.49, E11.618-E11.638, E11.649, E11.69-E11.8, E13.40-E13.49, E13.618-E13.638, E13.649-E13.8, G11.3, G11.8-G12.9, G32, G32.89, G90.01-G90.09, G90.2, G90.4, G90.50-G90.9, G95.0-G95.9, G96.8-G96.9, G98.0-G99.8

G12.0   Infantile spinal muscular atrophy, type I [Werdnig-Hoffman] 🖉

G12.1   Other inherited spinal muscular atrophy 🖉
> Adult form spinal muscular atrophy
> Childhood form, type II spinal muscular atrophy
> Distal spinal muscular atrophy
> Juvenile form, type III spinal muscular atrophy [Kugelberg-Welander]
> Progressive bulbar palsy of childhood [Fazio-Londe]
> Scapuloperoneal form spinal muscular atrophy

● G12.2   Motor neuron disease
> *Progressive disease of motor neurons that carry impulses to muscles to move*

G12.20   Motor neuron disease, unspecified 🖉

G12.21   Amyotrophic lateral sclerosis 🖉   A
> *Lou Gehrig's disease (ALS)*
> Progressive spinal muscle atrophy

G12.22   Progressive bulbar palsy 🖉

G12.29   Other motor neuron disease 🖉
> Familial motor neuron disease
> Primary lateral sclerosis

G12.8   Other spinal muscular atrophies and related syndromes 🖉

G12.9   Spinal muscular atrophy, unspecified 🖉

● G13   Systemic atrophies primarily affecting central nervous system in diseases classified elsewhere

▸ G13.0   *Paraneoplastic neuromyopathy and neuropathy*
> Carcinomatous neuromyopathy
> Sensorial paraneoplastic neuropathy [Denny Brown]
> *Code first underlying neoplasm (C00-D49)*

▸ G13.1   *Other systemic atrophy primarily affecting central nervous system in neoplastic disease*
> Paraneoplastic limbic encephalopathy
> *Code first underlying neoplasm (C00-D49)*

▸ G13.2   *Systemic atrophy primarily affecting the central nervous system in myxedema*
> *Code first underlying disease, such as:*
> hypothyroidism (E03.-)
> myxedematous congenital iodine deficiency (E00.1)

▸ G13.8   *Systemic atrophy primarily affecting central nervous system in other diseases classified elsewhere*
> *Code first underlying disease*

G14   Postpolio syndrome
> **Includes**   Postpolio myelitic syndrome
> **Excludes1**   sequelae of poliomyelitis (B91)

EXTRAPYRAMIDAL AND MOVEMENT DISORDERS (G20-G26)

G20   Parkinson's disease
Progressive disease of the nervous system that affects muscle coordination
> Hemiparkinsonism
> Idiopathic Parkinsonism or Parkinson's disease
> Paralysis agitans
> Parkinsonism or Parkinson's disease NOS
> Primary Parkinsonism or Parkinson's disease
> **Excludes1**   dementia with Parkinsonism (G31.83)

Coding Clinic: 2016, Q2, P7

● G21   Secondary parkinsonism
Symptoms of Parkinson's caused by medicines, illness, or other nervous system disorder
> **Excludes1**   dementia with Parkinsonism (G31.83)
> Huntington's disease (G10)
> Shy-Drager syndrome (G90.3)
> syphilitic Parkinsonism (A52.19)

G21.0   Malignant neuroleptic syndrome 🖉
> Use additional code for adverse effect, if applicable, to identify drug (T43.3X5, T43.4X5, T43.505, T43.595)
> > **Excludes1**   neuroleptic induced parkinsonism (G21.11)
> (Ex:) G10, G21.0, G23.0-G25.79, G25.82-G26, G80.3, G81.00-G81.94, G90.3, G93.2, G93.40-G93.49, I67.83

● G21.1   Other drug-induced secondary parkinsonism
> (Ex:) **For category G21.1 CC codes:** G20, G21.11-G21.9

G21.11   Neuroleptic induced parkinsonism 🖉
> Use additional code for adverse effect, if applicable, to identify drug (T43.3X5, T43.4X5, T43.505, T43.595)
> > **Excludes1**   malignant neuroleptic syndrome (G21.0)

G21.19   Other drug induced secondary parkinsonism 🖉
> Use additional code for adverse effect, if applicable, to identify drug (T36-T50 with fifth or sixth character 5)

G21.2   Secondary parkinsonism due to other external agents 🖉
> *Code first (T51-T65) to identify external agent*

G21.3   Postencephalitic parkinsonism 🖉

G21.4   Vascular parkinsonism

G21.8   Other secondary parkinsonism 🖉

G21.9   Secondary parkinsonism, unspecified 🖉

◀ New   ◀= Revised   ~~deleted~~ Deleted   Excludes 1   Excludes 2   Includes   Use additional   Code first   Code also   Unspecified

788   **OGCR** Official Guidelines   ● Unacceptable Principal Diagnosis   X Assign placeholder X   ● Use Additional Character(s)   ▸ Manifestation Code   **Coding Clinic**

● **G23** **Other degenerative diseases of basal ganglia**
　　　　Excludes2　multi-system degeneration of the autonomic
　　　　　　　　nervous system (G90.3)
　　　(Ex) For category G23 CC codes: G20, G21.11-G21.9, G90.01-G90.09, G93.40-G93.49,
　　　I67.83

　　G23.0 **Hallervorden-Spatz disease** 🕸
　　　　　Pigmentary pallidal degeneration

　　G23.1 **Progressive supranuclear ophthalmoplegia**
　　　　　[Steele-Richardson-Olszewski] 🕸
　　　　　Progressive supranuclear palsy

　　G23.2 **Striatonigral degeneration** 🕸

　　G23.8 **Other specified degenerative diseases of basal ganglia** 🕸
　　　　　Calcification of basal ganglia

　　G23.9 **Degenerative disease of basal ganglia, unspecified** 🕸

● **G24** **Dystonia**
　　　Involuntary movements
　　　Includes　dyskinesia
　　　Excludes2　athetoid cerebral palsy (G80.3)

　● **G24.0** **Drug induced dystonia**
　　　　　Use additional code for adverse effect, if applicable,
　　　　　　to identify drug (T36-T50 with fifth or sixth
　　　　　　character 5)

　　　　G24.01 **Drug induced subacute dyskinesia**
　　　　　　Drug induced blepharospasm
　　　　　　Drug induced orofacial dyskinesia
　　　　　　Neuroleptic induced tardive dyskinesia
　　　　　　Tardive dyskinesia

　　　　G24.02 **Drug induced acute dystonia** 🕸
　　　　　　Acute dystonic reaction to drugs
　　　　　　Neuroleptic induced acute dystonia
　　　　　　(Ex) G20, G21.11-G21.9, G25.70-G25.79, G25.89-G26, G80.3,
　　　　　　　G93.40, G93.41-G93.49, I67.83

　　　　G24.09 **Other drug induced dystonia** 🕸
　　　　　　(Ex) See G24.02

　　G24.1 **Genetic torsion dystonia**
　　　　　Dystonia deformans progressiva
　　　　　Dystonia musculorum deformans
　　　　　Familial torsion dystonia
　　　　　Idiopathic familial dystonia
　　　　　Idiopathic (torsion) dystonia NOS
　　　　　(Schwalbe-) Ziehen-Oppenheim disease

　　G24.2 **Idiopathic nonfamilial dystonia** 🕸
　　　　　(Ex) See G24.02

　　G24.3 **Spasmodic torticollis**
　　　　　Head tilts toward one side and chin is elevated and turned
　　　　　toward opposite side (wry neck)
　　　　　Excludes1　congenital torticollis (Q68.0)
　　　　　　　　hysterical torticollis (F44.4)
　　　　　　　　ocular torticollis (R29.891)
　　　　　　　　psychogenic torticollis (F45.8)
　　　　　　　　torticollis NOS (M43.6)
　　　　　　　　traumatic recurrent torticollis (S13.4)

　　G24.4 **Idiopathic orofacial dystonia**
　　　　　Orofacial dyskinesia
　　　　　Excludes1　drug induced orofacial dyskinesia
　　　　　　　　(G24.01)

　　G24.5 **Blepharospasm**
　　　　　Tonic spasm of orbicularis oculi muscle, producing closure
　　　　　of eyelids
　　　　　Excludes1　drug induced blepharospasm (G24.01)

　　G24.8 **Other dystonia** 🕸
　　　　　Acquired torsion dystonia NOS
　　　　　(Ex) See G24.02

　　G24.9 **Dystonia, unspecified**
　　　　　Dyskinesia NOS

● **G25** **Other extrapyramidal and movement disorders**
　　　Extrapyramidal: Other than pyramidal tracts
　　　Excludes2　sleep related movement disorders (G47.6-)

　　G25.0 **Essential tremor**
　　　　　Familial tremor
　　　　　Excludes1　tremor NOS (R25.1)

　　G25.1 **Drug-induced tremor**
　　　　　Use additional code for adverse effect, if applicable,
　　　　　　to identify drug (T36-T50 with fifth or sixth
　　　　　　character 5)

　　G25.2 **Other specified forms of tremor**
　　　　　Intention tremor

　　G25.3 **Myoclonus**
　　　　　Shocklike contractions muscle(s)
　　　　　Drug-induced myoclonus
　　　　　Palatal myoclonus
　　　　　Use additional code for adverse effect, if applicable,
　　　　　　to identify drug (T36-T50 with fifth or sixth
　　　　　　character 5)
　　　　　Excludes1　facial myokymia (G51.4)
　　　　　　　　myoclonic epilepsy (G40.-)

　　G25.4 **Drug-induced chorea**
　　　　　Use additional code for adverse effect, if applicable,
　　　　　　to identify drug (T36-T50 with fifth or sixth
　　　　　　character 5)

　　G25.5 **Other chorea**
　　　　　Continual, involuntary, jerky, movements
　　　　　Chorea NOS
　　　　　Excludes1　chorea NOS with heart involvement
　　　　　　　　(I02.0)
　　　　　　　　Huntington's chorea (G10)
　　　　　　　　rheumatic chorea (I02.-)
　　　　　　　　Sydenham's chorea (I02.-)

　● **G25.6** **Drug induced tics and other tics of organic origin**
　　　　G25.61 **Drug induced tics**
　　　　　　Use additional code for adverse effect, if
　　　　　　　applicable, to identify drug (T36-T50 with
　　　　　　　fifth or sixth character 5)

　　　　G25.69 **Other tics of organic origin**
　　　　　　Excludes1　habit spasm (F95.9)
　　　　　　　　　tic NOS (F95.9)
　　　　　　　　　Tourette's syndrome (F95.2)

　● **G25.7** **Other and unspecified drug induced movement**
　　　　disorders
　　　　　Use additional code for adverse effect, if applicable,
　　　　　　to identify drug (T36-T50 with fifth or sixth
　　　　　　character 5)

　　　　G25.70 **Drug induced movement disorder, unspecified**

　　　　G25.71 **Drug induced akathisia**
　　　　　　Drug induced acathisia
　　　　　　Neuroleptic induced acute akathisia

　　　　G25.79 **Other drug induced movement disorders**

　● **G25.8** **Other specified extrapyramidal and movement disorders**
　　　　G25.81 **Restless legs syndrome**

　　　　G25.82 **Stiff-man syndrome** 🕸
　　　　　　(Ex) G04.1, G10, G12.22, G20-G21.9, G24.01-G25.79, G25.82-G26,
　　　　　　　G32.89-G37.2, G37.5-G37.9, G80.0-G80.9, G82.20-G83.0, G92,
　　　　　　　G93.1, G93.40-G93.6, G93.81, G93.89-G93.9, G96.8-G96.9,
　　　　　　　G98.0-G98.8, G99.8, I67.83, R53.2

　　　　G25.83 **Benign shuddering attacks**

　　　　G25.89 **Other specified extrapyramidal and movement**
　　　　　　disorders

　　G25.9 **Extrapyramidal and movement disorder, unspecified** 🕸
　　　　　(Ex) See G25.82

▌ **G26** *Extrapyramidal and movement disorders in diseases classified*
　　elsewhere
　　　Code first underlying disease

N Newborn Age: 0　**P** Pediatric Age: 0–17　**M** Maternity DX: 12–55　**A** Adult Age: 15–124　♀ Females Only　♂ Males Only

🕸 Complication\Comorbidity　🕸 Major C\C　(Ex) CC/MCC Exclusions　🕸 Hospital-Acquired Condition

789

CHAPTER 6 (G00-G99)

OTHER DEGENERATIVE DISEASES OF THE NERVOUS SYSTEM (G30-G32)

● **G30   Alzheimer's disease**
Progressive central neurodegenerative disorder

    Includes   Alzheimer's dementia senile and presenile forms

    Use additional code to identify:
      delirium, if applicable (F05)
      dementia with behavioral disturbance (F02.81)
      dementia without behavioral disturbance (F02.80)

    Excludes1   senile degeneration of brain NEC (G31.1)
                      senile dementia NOS (F03)
                      senility NOS (R41.81)

   G30.0   Alzheimer's disease with early onset

   G30.1   Alzheimer's disease with late onset   A

   G30.8   Other Alzheimer's disease

   G30.9   Alzheimer's disease, unspecified
       Coding Clinic: 2016, Q2, P6; 2012, Q4, P95

● **G31   Other degenerative diseases of nervous system, not elsewhere classified**

    Use additional code to identify:
      dementia with behavioral disturbance (F02.81)
      dementia without behavioral disturbance (F02.80)

    Excludes2   Reye's syndrome (G93.7)

 ● **G31.0   Frontotemporal dementia**

    G31.01   Pick's disease
          Primary progressive aphasia
          Progressive isolated aphasia

    G31.09   Other frontotemporal dementia
          Frontal dementia

   G31.1   Senile degeneration of brain, not elsewhere classified

    Excludes1   Alzheimer's disease (G30.-)
                   senility NOS (R41.81)

   G31.2   Degeneration of nervous system due to alcohol
       Alcoholic cerebellar ataxia
       Alcoholic cerebellar degeneration
       Alcoholic cerebral degeneration
       Alcoholic encephalopathy
       Dysfunction of the autonomic nervous system due to alcohol
    Code also associated alcoholism (F10.-)

 ● **G31.8   Other specified degenerative diseases of nervous system**

    G31.81   Alpers' disease 🔖
         Rare neuronal degeneration of cerebral cortex disease of young children
         Grey-matter degeneration
         (Ex:) E75.00-E75.19, E75.4, F84.2, G13.2-G13.8, G30.0-G31.82, G31.84-G31.9, G91.4, G94

    G31.82   Leigh's disease 🔖
         Rare neurometabolic disorder that affects central nervous system
         Subacute necrotizing encephalopathy
         (Ex:) See G31.81

    G31.83   Dementia with Lewy bodies
         Closely allied to Parkinson's Disease
         Dementia with Parkinsonism
         Lewy body dementia
         Lewy body disease

    G31.84   Mild cognitive impairment, so stated

    Excludes1   age related cognitive decline (R41.81)
                   altered mental status (R41.82)
                   cerebral degeneration (G31.9)
                   change in mental status (R41.82)
                   cognitive deficits following (sequelae of) cerebral hemorrhage or infarction (I69.01-, I69.11-, I69.21-, I69.31-, I69.81-, I69.91-) ◀━
                   cognitive impairment due to intracranial or head injury (S06.-)
                   dementia (F01.-, F02.-, F03)
                   mild memory disturbance (F06.8)
                   neurologic neglect syndrome (R41.4)
                   personality change, nonpsychotic (F68.8)

    G31.85   Corticobasal degeneration

    G31.89   Other specified degenerative diseases of nervous system

   G31.9   Degenerative disease of nervous system, unspecified

● **G32   Other degenerative disorders of nervous system in diseases classified elsewhere**

 ▷ **G32.0   *Subacute combined degeneration of spinal cord in diseases classified elsewhere*** 🔖
       Dana-Putnam syndrome
       Sclerosis of spinal cord (combined) (dorsolateral) (posterolateral)

    Code first underlying disease, such as:
      anemia (D51.9)
      dietary (D51.3)
      pernicious (D51.0)
      vitamin B12 deficiency (E53.8)

    Excludes1   syphilitic combined degeneration of spinal cord (A52.11)
      (Ex:) G04.1, G11.3, G11.8-G12.9, G32.0, G32.89-G37.3, G37.5-G37.9, G80.0-G83.9, G90.01-G90.09, G90.2, G90.4-G90.9, G93.1, G93.40-G93.49, G95.0-G96.9, G97.1, G98.0-G99.8, I67.83, R53.2

● **G32.8   Other specified degenerative disorders of nervous system in diseases classified elsewhere**

    Code first underlying disease, such as:
      amyloidosis cerebral degeneration (E85.-)
      cerebral degeneration (due to) hypothyroidism (E00.0-E03.9)
      cerebral degeneration (due to) neoplasm (C00-D49)
      cerebral degeneration (due to) vitamin B deficiency, except thiamine (E52-E53.-)

    Excludes1   superior hemorrhagic polioencephalitis [Wernicke's encephalopathy] (E51.2)

 ▷ **G32.81   *Cerebellar ataxia in diseases classified elsewhere*** 🔖

      Code first underlying disease, such as:
        celiac disease (with gluten ataxia) (K90.0)
        cerebellar ataxia (in) neoplastic disease (paraneoplastic cerebellar degeneration) (C00-D49)
        non-celiac gluten ataxia (M35.9)

      Excludes1   systemic atrophy primarily affecting the central nervous system in alcoholic cerebellar ataxia (G31.2)
                   systemic atrophy primarily affecting the central nervous system in myxedema (G13.2)
       (Ex:) G04.1, G10-G12.9, G21.0, G23.0-G25.79, G25.82-G26, G32.0-G37.9, G80.0-G83.9, G90.01-G90.09, G90.2-G90.9, G92-G93.1, G93.40-G93.49, G93.81, G93.89-G95.9, G96.8-G96.9, G98.0-G99.8, I67.83, R53.2

 ▷ **G32.89   *Other specified degenerative disorders of nervous system in diseases classified elsewhere***
       Degenerative encephalopathy in diseases classified elsewhere

◀ New   ◀━ Revised   ~~deleted~~ Deleted   Excludes 1   Excludes 2   Includes   Use additional   Code first   Code also   Unspecified

OGCR Official Guidelines   ● Unacceptable Principal Diagnosis   X Assign placeholder X   ● Use Additional Character(s)   ▷ Manifestation Code   **Coding Clinic**

CHAPTER 6 (G00-G99)

DEMYELINATING DISEASES OF THE CENTRAL NERVOUS SYSTEM (G35-G37)

G35   Multiple sclerosis
Destruction of central nervous system; four types: relapsing remitting, secondary progressive, primary progressive, and progressive relapsing
Disseminated multiple sclerosis
Generalized multiple sclerosis
Multiple sclerosis NOS
Multiple sclerosis of brain stem
Multiple sclerosis of cord

● **G36   Other acute disseminated demyelination**

> **Excludes1**   postinfectious encephalitis and encephalomyelitis NOS (G04.01)

> (Ex:) **For category G36 CC codes unless otherwise indicated:** G04.1, G10-G12.9, G21.0, G24.01-G25.79, G25.82-G26, G32.0-G37.3, G37.5, G37.8-G37.9, G80.0-G83.9, G90.01-G90.09, G90.2, G90.4-G90.9, G92, G93.40-G93.49, G93.81, G93.89-G95.9, G96.8-G96.9, G98.0-G99.8, I67.83, R53.2

G36.0   Neuromyelitis optica [Devic]
Inflammatory disorder in which immune system attacks optic nerves and spinal cord producing inflammation of optic nerve (optic neuritis) and spinal cord (myelitis)
Demyelination in optic neuritis

> **Excludes1**   optic neuritis NOS (H46)

> (Ex:) G36.0, G93.40-G93.49, I67.83

G36.1   Acute and subacute hemorrhagic leukoencephalitis [Hurst]

G36.8   Other specified acute disseminated demyelination

G36.9   Acute disseminated demyelination, unspecified

● **G37   Other demyelinating diseases of central nervous system**
Destruction of central nervous system

G37.0   Diffuse sclerosis of central nervous system
Periaxial encephalitis
Schilder's disease

> **Excludes1**   X linked adrenoleukodystrophy (E71.52-)

> (Ex:) A92.30-A92.39, B97.21, G93.40-G93.49, I67.83

G37.1   Central demyelination of corpus callosum
> (Ex:) See G36

G37.2   Central pontine myelinolysis
> (Ex:) See G36

G37.3   Acute transverse myelitis in demyelinating disease of central nervous system
Acute transverse myelitis NOS
Acute transverse myelopathy

> **Excludes1**   multiple sclerosis (G35)
> neuromyelitis optica [Devic] (G36.0)

> (Ex:) A02.21, A17.0-A27.81, A39.0, A50.41, A51.41, A52.13, A54.82, A54.84, A54.89-A54.9, A87.0-A87.9, A96.2, A98.3-A98.4, B00.3, B00.89-B00.9, B02.0-B02.29, B02.7-B02.9, B10.81-B10.89, B26.1, B33.24-B33.8, B34.1-B34.2, B34.4-B34.8, B37.5, B38.4, B45.1, B58.2, B92, B94.2-B94.9, B97.10, B97.19, B97.29, B97.5-B97.6, B97.81-B97.89, E08.40-E08.49, E09.40-E09.49, E10.40-E10.49, E11.40-E11.49, E13.40-E13.49, G00.0-G03.9, G04.1-G04.2, G11.3, G11.8-G12.9, G32.0, G32.89-G37.2, G37.5-G37.9, G61.0, G80.0-G80.2, G80.4-G83.9, G90.01-G90.09, G90.2, G90.4-G90.9, G93.1, G93.40-G93.49, G95.0-G95.9, G96.12-G96.9, G97.1, G98.0-G99.8, I67.83, R53.2

G37.4   Subacute necrotizing myelitis of central nervous system
> (Ex:) See G04.9

Item 6–3   Multiple sclerosis (MS) is a nervous system disease affecting the brain and spinal cord by damaging the myelin sheath surrounding and protecting nerve cells. The damage slows down/blocks messages between the brain and body. Symptoms are: visual disturbances, muscle weakness, coordination and balance issues, numbness, prickling, thinking and memory problems. The cause is unknown, though it is thought that it may be an autoimmune disease. It affects women more than men, between 20 and 40 years of age. MS can be mild, but it may cause the loss of ability to write, walk, and speak. There is no cure, but medication may slow or control symptoms.

G37.5   Concentric sclerosis [Baló] of central nervous system
> (Ex:) See G37.0

G37.8   Other specified demyelinating diseases of central nervous system
> (Ex:) See G36

G37.9   Demyelinating disease of central nervous system, unspecified
> (Ex:) See G36

EPISODIC AND PAROXYSMAL DISORDERS (G40-G47)

● **G40   Epilepsy and recurrent seizures**

> **Note:** The following terms are to be considered equivalent to intractable: pharmacoresistant (pharmacologically resistant), treatment resistant, refractory (medically) and poorly controlled

> **Excludes1**   conversion disorder with seizures (F44.5)
> convulsions NOS (R56.9)
> post traumatic seizures (R56.1)
> seizure (convulsive) NOS (R56.9)
> seizure of newborn (P90)

> **Excludes2**   hippocampal sclerosis (G93.81) ◄
> mesial temporal sclerosis (G93.81) ◄
> temporal sclerosis (G93.81) ◄
> Todd's paralysis (G83.84) ◄

● **G40.0   Localization-related (focal) (partial) idiopathic epilepsy and epileptic syndromes with seizures of localized onset**
Benign childhood epilepsy with centrotemporal EEG spikes
Childhood epilepsy with occipital EEG paroxysms

> **Excludes1**   adult onset localization-related epilepsy (G40.1-, G40.2-)

● **G40.00   Localization-related (focal) (partial) idiopathic epilepsy and epileptic syndromes with seizures of localized onset, not intractable**
Localization-related (focal) (partial) idiopathic epilepsy and epileptic syndromes with seizures of localized onset without intractability

G40.001   Localization-related (focal) (partial) idiopathic epilepsy and epileptic syndromes with seizures of localized onset, not intractable, with status epilepticus
> (Ex:) G32.89, G40.001-G40.319, G40.401-G40.919, G40.A01-G40.B19, G93.40-G93.49, G93.9, G96.8-G96.9, G98.0-G98.8, G99.8. I67.83, R56.1

G40.009   Localization-related (focal) (partial) idiopathic epilepsy and epileptic syndromes with seizures of localized onset, not intractable, without status epilepticus
Localization-related (focal) (partial) idiopathic epilepsy and epileptic syndromes with seizures of localized onset NOS
> (Ex:) See G40.001

CHAPTER 6 (G00-G99)

N Newborn Age: 0   **P** Pediatric Age: 0–17   **M** Maternity DX: 12–55   **A** Adult Age: 15–124   ♀ Females Only   ♂ Males Only

   Complication\Comorbidity   Major C\C   (Ex:) CC/MCC Exclusions   Hospital-Acquired Condition

791

● **G40.01** **Localization-related (focal) (partial) idiopathic epilepsy and epileptic syndromes with seizures of localized onset, intractable**

   G40.011 Localization-related (focal) (partial) idiopathic epilepsy and epileptic syndromes with seizures of localized onset, intractable, with status epilepticus 🔗
   (Ex:) E08.40-E08.49, E09.40-E09.49, E10.40-E10.49, E11.40-E11.49, E13.40-E13.49, G32.89, G40.001-G40.319, G40.401-G40.919, G40.A01-G40.A19, G40.B01-G40.B19, G93.81, G93.89-G93.9, G96.8-G96.9, G98.0-G98.8, G99.8, R56.1

   G40.019 Localization-related (focal) (partial) idiopathic epilepsy and epileptic syndromes with seizures of localized onset, intractable, without status epilepticus 🔗
   (Ex:) See G40.011

● **G40.1** **Localization-related (focal) (partial) symptomatic epilepsy and epileptic syndromes with simple partial seizures**
   Attacks without alteration of consciousness
   Epilepsia partialis continua [Kozhevnikof]
   Simple partial seizures developing into secondarily generalized seizures

● **G40.10** **Localization-related (focal) (partial) symptomatic epilepsy and epileptic syndromes with simple partial seizures, not intractable**
   Localization-related (focal) (partial) symptomatic epilepsy and epileptic syndromes with simple partial seizures without intractability

   G40.101 Localization-related (focal) (partial) symptomatic epilepsy and epileptic syndromes with simple partial seizures, not intractable, with status epilepticus 🔗
   (Ex:) See G40.001

   G40.109 Localization-related (focal) (partial) symptomatic epilepsy and epileptic syndromes with simple partial seizures, not intractable, without status epilepticus 🔗
   Localization-related (focal) (partial) symptomatic epilepsy and epileptic syndromes with simple partial seizures NOS
   (Ex:) See G40.001

● **G40.11** **Localization-related (focal) (partial) symptomatic epilepsy and epileptic syndromes with simple partial seizures, intractable**

   G40.111 Localization-related (focal) (partial) symptomatic epilepsy and epileptic syndromes with simple partial seizures, intractable, with status epilepticus 🔗
   (Ex:) See G40.011

   G40.119 Localization-related (focal) (partial) symptomatic epilepsy and epileptic syndromes with simple partial seizures, intractable, without status epilepticus 🔗
   (Ex:) See G40.011

● **G40.2** **Localization-related (focal) (partial) symptomatic epilepsy and epileptic syndromes with complex partial seizures**
   Attacks with alteration of consciousness, often with automatisms
   Complex partial seizures developing into secondarily generalized seizures

● **G40.20** **Localization-related (focal) (partial) symptomatic epilepsy and epileptic syndromes with complex partial seizures, not intractable**
   Localization-related (focal) (partial) symptomatic epilepsy and epileptic syndromes with complex partial seizures without intractability

   G40.201 Localization-related (focal) (partial) symptomatic epilepsy and epileptic syndromes with complex partial seizures, not intractable, with status epilepticus 🔗
   (Ex:) See G40.001

   G40.209 Localization-related (focal) (partial) symptomatic epilepsy and epileptic syndromes with complex partial seizures, not intractable, without status epilepticus 🔗
   Localization-related (focal) (partial) symptomatic epilepsy and epileptic syndromes with complex partial seizures NOS
   (Ex:) See G40.001

● **G40.21** **Localization-related (focal) (partial) symptomatic epilepsy and epileptic syndromes with complex partial seizures, intractable**

   G40.211 Localization-related (focal) (partial) symptomatic epilepsy and epileptic syndromes with complex partial seizures, intractable, with status epilepticus 🔗
   (Ex:) See G40.011

   G40.219 Localization-related (focal) (partial) symptomatic epilepsy and epileptic syndromes with complex partial seizures, intractable, without status epilepticus 🔗
   (Ex:) See G40.011

● **G40.3** **Generalized idiopathic epilepsy and epileptic syndromes**
   Code also MERRF syndrome, if applicable (E88.42)

● **G40.30** **Generalized idiopathic epilepsy and epileptic syndromes, not intractable**
   Generalized idiopathic epilepsy and epileptic syndromes without intractability

   G40.301 Generalized idiopathic epilepsy and epileptic syndromes, not intractable, with status epilepticus 🔗
   (Ex:) E08.40-E08.49, E08.618-E08.638, E08.649-E08.8, E09.40-E09.49, E09.618-E09.638, E09.649-E09.8, E10.40-E10.49, E10.618-E10.638, E10.649, E10.69-E10.8, E11.40-E11.49, E11.618-E11.638, E11.649, E11.69-E11.8, E13.40-E13.49, E13.618-E13.638, E13.649-E13.8, G32.89, G40.001-G40.319, G40.401-G40.419, G40.501-G40.919, G40.A01-G40.B19, G93.81, G93.89-G93.9, G96.8-G96.9, G98.0-G98.8, G99.8, R56.1

   G40.309 Generalized idiopathic epilepsy and epileptic syndromes, not intractable, without status epilepticus
   Generalized idiopathic epilepsy and epileptic syndromes NOS

◀ New   ◀▦ Revised   ~~deleted~~ Deleted   Excludes 1   Excludes 2   Includes   Use additional   Code first   Code also   Unspecified
OGCR Official Guidelines   ● Unacceptable Principal Diagnosis   X Assign placeholder X   ● Use Additional Character(s)   ▶ Manifestation Code   Coding Clinic

● **G40.31** **Generalized idiopathic epilepsy and epileptic syndromes, intractable**

  G40.311 **Generalized idiopathic epilepsy and epileptic syndromes, intractable, with status epilepticus** 🔖
  (Ex:) See G40.301

  G40.319 **Generalized idiopathic epilepsy and epileptic syndromes, intractable, without status epilepticus** 🔖
  (Ex:) See G40.301

● **G40.A** **Absence epileptic syndrome**
  Childhood absence epilepsy [pyknolepsy]
  Juvenile absence epilepsy
  Absence epileptic syndrome, NOS

  ● **G40.A0** **Absence epileptic syndrome, not intractable**

  G40.A01 **Absence epileptic syndrome, not intractable, with status epilepticus**

  G40.A09 **Absence epileptic syndrome, not intractable, without status epilepticus**

  ● **G40.A1** **Absence epileptic syndrome, intractable**

  G40.A11 **Absence epileptic syndrome, intractable, with status epilepticus** 🔖
  (Ex:) See G40.001

  G40.A19 **Absence epileptic syndrome, intractable, without status epilepticus** 🔖
  (Ex:) See G40.001

● **G40.B** **Juvenile myoclonic epilepsy [impulsive petit mal]**
  (Ex:) For category G40.B CC codes: See G40.011

  ● **G40.B0** **Juvenile myoclonic epilepsy, not intractable**

  G40.B01 **Juvenile myoclonic epilepsy, not intractable, with status epilepticus** 🔖

  G40.B09 **Juvenile myoclonic epilepsy, not intractable, without status epilepticus** 🔖

  ● **G40.B1** **Juvenile myoclonic epilepsy, intractable**

  G40.B11 **Juvenile myoclonic epilepsy, intractable, with status epilepticus** 🔖

  G40.B19 **Juvenile myoclonic epilepsy, intractable, without status epilepticus** 🔖

● **G40.4** **Other generalized epilepsy and epileptic syndromes**
  Epilepsy with grand mal seizures on awakening
  Epilepsy with myoclonic absences
  Epilepsy with myoclonic-astatic seizures
  Grand mal seizure NOS
  Nonspecific atonic epileptic seizures
  Nonspecific clonic epileptic seizures
  Nonspecific myoclonic epileptic seizures
  Nonspecific tonic epileptic seizures
  Nonspecific tonic-clonic epileptic seizures
  Symptomatic early myoclonic encephalopathy

  ● **G40.40** **Other generalized epilepsy and epileptic syndromes, not intractable**
  Other generalized epilepsy and epileptic syndromes without intractability
  Other generalized epilepsy and epileptic syndromes NOS

  G40.401 **Other generalized epilepsy and epileptic syndromes, not intractable, with status epilepticus**

  G40.409 **Other generalized epilepsy and epileptic syndromes, not intractable, without status epilepticus**

● **G40.41** **Other generalized epilepsy and epileptic syndromes, intractable**

  G40.411 **Other generalized epilepsy and epileptic syndromes, intractable, with status epilepticus** 🔖
  (Ex:) See G40.011

  G40.419 **Other generalized epilepsy and epileptic syndromes, intractable, without status epilepticus** 🔖
  (Ex:) See G40.011

● **G40.5** **Epileptic seizures related to external causes**
  Epileptic seizures related to alcohol
  Epileptic seizures related to drugs
  Epileptic seizures related to hormonal changes
  Epileptic seizures related to sleep deprivation
  Epileptic seizures related to stress
  Code also, if applicable, associated epilepsy and recurrent seizures (G40.-)
  Use additional code for adverse effect, if applicable, to identify drug (T36-T50 with fifth or sixth character 5)
  (Ex:) For category G40.5 CC codes: See G40.011

  ● **G40.50** **Epileptic seizures related to external causes, not intractable**

  G40.501 **Epileptic seizures related to external causes, not intractable, with status epilepticus** 🔖

  G40.509 **Epileptic seizures related to external causes, not intractable, without status epilepticus** 🔖
  Epileptic seizures related to external causes, NOS

● **G40.8** **Other epilepsy and recurrent seizures**
  Epilepsies and epileptic syndromes undetermined as to whether they are focal or generalized
  Landau-Kleffner syndrome
  (Ex:) For category G40.8 CC codes unless otherwise indicated: See G40.011

  ● **G40.80** **Other epilepsy**

  G40.801 **Other epilepsy, not intractable, with status epilepticus** 🔖
  Other epilepsy without intractability with status epilepticus

  G40.802 **Other epilepsy, not intractable, without status epilepticus** 🔖
  Other epilepsy NOS
  Other epilepsy without intractability without status epilepticus

  G40.803 **Other epilepsy, intractable, with status epilepticus** 🔖

  G40.804 **Other epilepsy, intractable, without status epilepticus** 🔖

  ● **G40.81** **Lennox-Gastaut syndrome**

  G40.811 **Lennox-Gastaut syndrome, not intractable, with status epilepticus** 🔖

  G40.812 **Lennox-Gastaut syndrome, not intractable, without status epilepticus** 🔖

  G40.813 **Lennox-Gastaut syndrome, intractable, with status epilepticus** 🔖

  G40.814 **Lennox-Gastaut syndrome, intractable, without status epilepticus** 🔖

  ● **G40.82** **Epileptic spasms**
  Infantile spasms
  Salaam attacks
  West's syndrome

  G40.821 **Epileptic spasms, not intractable, with status epilepticus** 🔖
  (Ex:) See G40.001

  G40.822 **Epileptic spasms, not intractable, without status epilepticus** 🔖
  (Ex:) See G40.001

CHAPTER 6 (G00-G99)

G40.823 **Epileptic spasms, intractable, with status epilepticus** 🔎

G40.824 **Epileptic spasms, intractable, without status epilepticus** 🔎

G40.89 **Other seizures** 🔎

> **Excludes1**   post traumatic seizures (R56.1)
> recurrent seizures NOS (G40.909)
> seizure NOS (R56.9)

● G40.9 **Epilepsy, unspecified**

  ● G40.90 **Epilepsy, unspecified, not intractable**
  Epilepsy, unspecified, without intractability

    G40.901 **Epilepsy, unspecified, not intractable, with status epilepticus**

    G40.909 **Epilepsy, unspecified, not intractable, without status epilepticus**
    Epilepsy NOS
    Epileptic convulsions NOS
    Epileptic fits NOS
    Epileptic seizures NOS
    Recurrent seizures NOS
    Seizure disorder NOS

  ● G40.91 **Epilepsy, unspecified, intractable**
  Intractable seizure disorder NOS
  > (Ex) **For category G40.91 CC codes:** See G40.011

    G40.911 **Epilepsy, unspecified, intractable, with status epilepticus** 🔎

    G40.919 **Epilepsy, unspecified, intractable, without status epilepticus** 🔎

● G43 **Migraine**

  Note: The following terms are to be considered equivalent to intractable: pharmacoresistant (pharmacologically resistant), treatment resistant, refractory (medically) and poorly controlled

  Use additional code for adverse effect, if applicable, to identify drug (T36-T50 with fifth or sixth character 5)

  > **Excludes1**   headache NOS (R51)
  > lower half migraine (G44.00)

  > **Excludes2**   headache syndromes (G44.-)

  ● G43.0 **Migraine without aura**
  Neurological disorder, generally recurring headaches without early symptom (aura)
  Common migraine
  > **Excludes1**   chronic migraine without aura (G43.7-)

    ● G43.00 **Migraine without aura, not intractable**
    Neurological disorder, generally recurring headaches without early symptom (aura); resistant to cure, relief, or control
    Migraine without aura without mention of refractory migraine

      G43.001 **Migraine without aura, not intractable, with status migrainosus**

      G43.009 **Migraine without aura, not intractable, without status migrainosus**
      Migraine without aura NOS

    ● G43.01 **Migraine without aura, intractable**
    Intractable migraine: Not easily cured or managed; relentless pain from a migraine
    Migraine without aura with refractory migraine

      G43.011 **Migraine without aura, intractable, with status migrainosus**

      G43.019 **Migraine without aura, intractable, without status migrainosus**

Item 6-4   Migraine headache is described as an intense pulsing or throbbing pain in one area of the head. It can be accompanied by extreme sensitivity to light (photophobic) and sound and is three times more common in women than in men. Symptoms include nausea and vomiting. Research indicates migraine headaches are caused by inherited abnormalities in genes that control the activities of certain cell populations in the brain.

  ● G43.1 **Migraine with aura**
  Basilar migraine
  Classical migraine
  Migraine equivalents
  Migraine preceded or accompanied by transient focal neurological phenomena
  Migraine triggered seizures
  Migraine with acute-onset aura
  Migraine with aura without headache (migraine equivalents)
  Migraine with prolonged aura
  Migraine with typical aura
  Retinal migraine
  Code also any associated seizure (G40.-, R56.9)
  > **Excludes1**   persistent migraine aura (G43.5-, G43.6-)

    ● G43.10 **Migraine with aura, not intractable**
    Migraine with aura without mention of refractory migraine

      G43.101 **Migraine with aura, not intractable, with status migrainosus**

      G43.109 **Migraine with aura, not intractable, without status migrainosus**
      Migraine with aura NOS

    ● G43.11 **Migraine with aura, intractable**
    Migraine with aura with refractory migraine

      G43.111 **Migraine with aura, intractable, with status migrainosus**

      G43.119 **Migraine with aura, intractable, without status migrainosus**

  ● G43.4 **Hemiplegic migraine**
  Inherited migraine disorder causing temporary paralysis of one side of body followed by severe headache and nausea
  Familial migraine
  Sporadic migraine

    ● G43.40 **Hemiplegic migraine, not intractable**
    Hemiplegic migraine without refractory migraine

      G43.401 **Hemiplegic migraine, not intractable, with status migrainosus**

      G43.409 **Hemiplegic migraine, not intractable, without status migrainosus**
      Hemiplegic migraine NOS

    ● G43.41 **Hemiplegic migraine, intractable**
    Hemiplegic migraine with refractory migraine

      G43.411 **Hemiplegic migraine, intractable, with status migrainosus**

      G43.419 **Hemiplegic migraine, intractable, without status migrainosus**

  ● G43.5 **Persistent migraine aura without cerebral infarction**

    ● G43.50 **Persistent migraine aura without cerebral infarction, not intractable**
    Persistent migraine aura without cerebral infarction, without refractory migraine

      G43.501 **Persistent migraine aura without cerebral infarction, not intractable, with status migrainosus**

      G43.509 **Persistent migraine aura without cerebral infarction, not intractable, without status migrainosus**
      Persistent migraine aura NOS

CHAPTER 6 (G00-G99)

◀ New   ◀▥ Revised   ~~deleted~~ Deleted | Excludes 1 | | Excludes 2 | | Includes | | Use additional | | Code first | | Code also | | Unspecified |
OGCR Official Guidelines   ● Unacceptable Principal Diagnosis   X Assign placeholder X   ● Use Additional Character(s)   ▶ Manifestation Code   **Coding Clinic**

● **G43.51** **Persistent migraine aura without cerebral infarction, intractable**
Persistent migraine aura without cerebral infarction, with refractory migraine

    G43.511 **Persistent migraine aura without cerebral infarction, intractable, with status migrainosus**

    G43.519 **Persistent migraine aura without cerebral infarction, intractable, without status migrainosus**

● **G43.6** **Persistent migraine aura with cerebral infarction**
Visual, motor, or psychic disturbances, paresthesias, and related neurologic abnormalities accompanying migraine

Code also the type of cerebral infarction (I63.-)

● **G43.6Ø** **Persistent migraine aura with cerebral infarction, not intractable**
Persistent migraine aura with cerebral infarction, without refractory migraine

    (Ex) **For category G43.6 CC codes:** G43.6Ø1-G43.619, I63.ØØ-I66.9

    G43.6Ø1 **Persistent migraine aura with cerebral infarction, not intractable, with status migrainosus** 🔧

    G43.6Ø9 **Persistent migraine aura with cerebral infarction, not intractable, without status migrainosus** 🔧

● **G43.61** **Persistent migraine aura with cerebral infarction, intractable**
Persistent migraine aura with cerebral infarction, with refractory migraine

    G43.611 **Persistent migraine aura with cerebral infarction, intractable, with status migrainosus** 🔧

    G43.619 **Persistent migraine aura with cerebral infarction, intractable, without status migrainosus** 🔧

● **G43.7** **Chronic migraine without aura**
Transformed migraine

Excludes1 migraine without aura (G43.Ø-)

● **G43.7Ø** **Chronic migraine without aura, not intractable**
Chronic migraine without aura, without refractory migraine

    G43.7Ø1 **Chronic migraine without aura, not intractable, with status migrainosus**

    G43.7Ø9 **Chronic migraine without aura, not intractable, without status migrainosus**
Chronic migraine without aura NOS

● **G43.71** **Chronic migraine without aura, intractable**
Chronic migraine without aura, with refractory migraine

    G43.711 **Chronic migraine without aura, intractable, with status migrainosus**

    G43.719 **Chronic migraine without aura, intractable, without status migrainosus**

● **G43.A** **Cyclical vomiting**

    G43.AØ **Cyclical vomiting, not intractable**
Cyclical vomiting, without refractory migraine

    G43.A1 **Cyclical vomiting, intractable**
Cyclical vomiting, with refractory migraine

● **G43.B** **Ophthalmoplegic migraine**

    G43.BØ **Ophthalmoplegic migraine, not intractable**
Ophthalmoplegic migraine, without refractory migraine

    G43.B1 **Ophthalmoplegic migraine, intractable**
Ophthalmoplegic migraine, with refractory migraine

● **G43.C** **Periodic headache syndromes in child or adult**

    G43.CØ **Periodic headache syndromes in child or adult, not intractable**
Periodic headache syndromes in child or adult, without refractory migraine

    G43.C1 **Periodic headache syndromes in child or adult, intractable**
Periodic headache syndromes in child or adult, with refractory migraine

● **G43.D** **Abdominal migraine**

    G43.DØ **Abdominal migraine, not intractable**
Abdominal migraine, without refractory migraine

    G43.D1 **Abdominal migraine, intractable**
Abdominal migraine, with refractory migraine

● **G43.8** **Other migraine**

● **G43.8Ø** **Other migraine, not intractable**
Other migraine, without refractory migraine

    G43.8Ø1 **Other migraine, not intractable, with status migrainosus**

    G43.8Ø9 **Other migraine, not intractable, without status migrainosus**

● **G43.81** **Other migraine, intractable**
Other migraine, with refractory migraine

    G43.811 **Other migraine, intractable, with status migrainosus**

    G43.819 **Other migraine, intractable, without status migrainosus**

● **G43.82** **Menstrual migraine, not intractable**
Menstrual headache, not intractable
Menstrual migraine, without refractory migraine
Menstrually related migraine, not intractable
Pre-menstrual headache, not intractable
Pre-menstrual migraine, not intractable
Pure menstrual migraine, not intractable

Code also associated premenstrual tension syndrome (N94.3)

    G43.821 **Menstrual migraine, not intractable, with status migrainosus** ♀

    G43.829 **Menstrual migraine, not intractable, without status migrainosus** ♀
Menstrual migraine NOS

● **G43.83** **Menstrual migraine, intractable**
Menstrual headache, intractable
Menstrual migraine, with refractory migraine
Menstrually related migraine, intractable
Pre-menstrual headache, intractable
Pre-menstrual migraine, intractable
Pure menstrual migraine, intractable

Code also associated premenstrual tension syndrome (N94.3)

    G43.831 **Menstrual migraine, intractable, with status migrainosus** ♀

    G43.839 **Menstrual migraine, intractable, without status migrainosus** ♀

● **G43.9** **Migraine, unspecified**

● **G43.9Ø** **Migraine, unspecified, not intractable**
Migraine, unspecified, without refractory migraine

    G43.9Ø1 **Migraine, unspecified, not intractable, with status migrainosus**
Status migrainosus NOS

    G43.9Ø9 **Migraine, unspecified, not intractable, without status migrainosus**
Migraine NOS

N Newborn Age: Ø   **P** Pediatric Age: Ø–17   **M** Maternity DX: 12–55   **A** Adult Age: 15–124   ♀ Females Only   ♂ Males Only

🔧 Complication\Comorbidity   🔧 Major C\C   (Ex) CC/MCC Exclusions   🔧 Hospital-Acquired Condition

795

CHAPTER 6 (GØØ-G99)

● **G43.91**   **Migraine, unspecified, intractable**
       Migraine, unspecified, with refractory migraine

     G43.911   **Migraine, unspecified, intractable, with status migrainosus**

     G43.919   **Migraine, unspecified, intractable, without status migrainosus**

● **G44**   **Other headache syndromes**

     Excludes1   headache NOS (R51)

     Excludes2   atypical facial pain (G50.1)
                 headache due to lumbar puncture (G97.1)
                 migraines (G43.-)
                 trigeminal neuralgia (G50.0)

● **G44.0**   **Cluster headaches and other trigeminal autonomic cephalgias (TAC)**

   ● **G44.00**   **Cluster headache syndrome, unspecified**
           Ciliary neuralgia
           Cluster headache NOS
           Histamine cephalgia
           Lower half migraine
           Migrainous neuralgia

     G44.001   **Cluster headache syndrome, unspecified, intractable**

     G44.009   **Cluster headache syndrome, unspecified, not intractable**
                 Cluster headache syndrome NOS

   ● **G44.01**   **Episodic cluster headache**

     G44.011   **Episodic cluster headache, intractable**

     G44.019   **Episodic cluster headache, not intractable**
                 Episodic cluster headache NOS

   ● **G44.02**   **Chronic cluster headache**

     G44.021   **Chronic cluster headache, intractable**

     G44.029   **Chronic cluster headache, not intractable**
                 Chronic cluster headache NOS

   ● **G44.03**   **Episodic paroxysmal hemicrania**
           Paroxysmal hemicrania NOS

     G44.031   **Episodic paroxysmal hemicrania, intractable**

     G44.039   **Episodic paroxysmal hemicrania, not intractable**
                 Episodic paroxysmal hemicrania NOS

   ● **G44.04**   **Chronic paroxysmal hemicrania**
           Unilateral headache

     G44.041   **Chronic paroxysmal hemicrania, intractable**

     G44.049   **Chronic paroxysmal hemicrania, not intractable**
                 Chronic paroxysmal hemicrania NOS

   ● **G44.05**   **Short lasting unilateral neuralgiform headache with conjunctival injection and tearing (SUNCT)**

     G44.051   **Short lasting unilateral neuralgiform headache with conjunctival injection and tearing (SUNCT), intractable**

     G44.059   **Short lasting unilateral neuralgiform headache with conjunctival injection and tearing (SUNCT), not intractable**
                 Short lasting unilateral neuralgiform headache with conjunctival injection and tearing (SUNCT) NOS

   ● **G44.09**   **Other trigeminal autonomic cephalgias (TAC)**
           Cluster headaches

     G44.091   **Other trigeminal autonomic cephalgias (TAC), intractable**

     G44.099   **Other trigeminal autonomic cephalgias (TAC), not intractable**

● **G44.1**   **Vascular headache, not elsewhere classified**

     Excludes2   cluster headache (G44.0)
                 complicated headache syndromes (G44.5-)
                 drug-induced headache (G44.4-)
                 migraine (G43.-)
                 other specified headache syndromes (G44.8-)
                 post-traumatic headache (G44.3-)
                 tension-type headache (G44.2-)

● **G44.2**   **Tension-type headache**

   ● **G44.20**   **Tension-type headache, unspecified**

     G44.201   **Tension-type headache, unspecified, intractable**

     G44.209   **Tension-type headache, unspecified, not intractable**
                 Tension headache NOS

   ● **G44.21**   **Episodic tension-type headache**

     G44.211   **Episodic tension-type headache, intractable**

     G44.219   **Episodic tension-type headache, not intractable**
                 Episodic tension-type headache NOS

   ● **G44.22**   **Chronic tension-type headache**

     G44.221   **Chronic tension-type headache, intractable**

     G44.229   **Chronic tension-type headache, not intractable**
                 Chronic tension-type headache NOS

● **G44.3**   **Post-traumatic headache**

   ● **G44.30**   **Post-traumatic headache, unspecified**

     G44.301   **Post-traumatic headache, unspecified, intractable**

     G44.309   **Post-traumatic headache, unspecified, not intractable**
                 Post-traumatic headache NOS

   ● **G44.31**   **Acute post-traumatic headache**

     G44.311   **Acute post-traumatic headache, intractable**

     G44.319   **Acute post-traumatic headache, not intractable**
                 Acute post-traumatic headache NOS

   ● **G44.32**   **Chronic post-traumatic headache**

     G44.321   **Chronic post-traumatic headache, intractable**

     G44.329   **Chronic post-traumatic headache, not intractable**
                 Chronic post-traumatic headache NOS

● **G44.4**   **Drug-induced headache, not elsewhere classified**
           Medication overuse headache

     Use additional code for adverse effect, if applicable, to identify drug (T36-T50 with fifth or sixth character 5)

     G44.40   **Drug-induced headache, not elsewhere classified, not intractable**

     G44.41   **Drug-induced headache, not elsewhere classified, intractable**

● **G44.5**   **Complicated headache syndromes**

     G44.51   **Hemicrania continua**
           Persistent unilateral headache

     G44.52   **New daily persistent headache (NDPH)**

     G44.53   **Primary thunderclap headache**

     G44.59   **Other complicated headache syndrome**

● **G44.8 Other specified headache syndromes**

G44.81 Hypnic headache
Benign primary headaches

G44.82 Headache associated with sexual activity
Orgasmic headache
Preorgasmic headache

G44.83 Primary cough headache

G44.84 Primary exertional headache

G44.85 Primary stabbing headache

G44.89 Other headache syndrome

● **G45 Transient cerebral ischemic attacks and related syndromes**

Excludes1 neonatal cerebral ischemia (P91.Ø)
transient retinal artery occlusion (H34.Ø-)

(Ex) **For category G45 CC codes:** EØ8.51-EØ8.59, EØ8.618-EØ8.638, EØ8.649-EØ8.8,
EØ9.51-EØ9.59, EØ9.618-EØ9.638, EØ9.649-EØ9.8, E1Ø.51-E1Ø.59, E1Ø.618-E1Ø.638,
E1Ø.649, E1Ø.69-E1Ø.8, E11.51-E11.59, E11.618-E11.638, E11.649, E11.69, E11.8,
E13.51-E13.59, E13.618-E13.638, E13.649-E13.8, G45.Ø-G45.2, G45.8-G46.2,
I63.ØØ-I63.Ø39, I63.Ø9, I63.139, I63.19-I63.239, I63.29, I65.Ø1-I65.9,
I67.841-I67.848, I87.8-I87.9, I99.8-I99.9

G45.Ø Vertebro-basilar artery syndrome 🍏

G45.1 Carotid artery syndrome (hemispheric) 🍏

G45.2 Multiple and bilateral precerebral artery syndromes 🍏

G45.3 Amaurosis fugax 🍏
Transient visual loss in one eye
(Ex) G45.3, H34.ØØ-H34.9

G45.4 Transient global amnesia
Episode of short-term memory loss, nonrecurrent, lasting few hours

Excludes1 amnesia NOS (R41.3)

G45.8 Other transient cerebral ischemic attacks and related syndromes 🍏

G45.9 Transient cerebral ischemic attack, unspecified 🍏
Spasm of cerebral artery
TIA
Transient cerebral ischemia NOS

● **G46 Vascular syndromes of brain in cerebrovascular diseases**

Code first underlying cerebrovascular disease (I6Ø-I69)

G46.Ø Middle cerebral artery syndrome 🍏
(Ex) See G45

G46.1 Anterior cerebral artery syndrome 🍏
(Ex) See G45

G46.2 Posterior cerebral artery syndrome 🍏
(Ex) See G45

G46.3 Brain stem stroke syndrome
Benedikt syndrome
Claude syndrome
Foville syndrome
Millard-Gubler syndrome
Wallenberg syndrome
Weber syndrome

G46.4 Cerebellar stroke syndrome

G46.5 Pure motor lacunar syndrome
Occlusion of single deep penetrating artery

G46.6 Pure sensory lacunar syndrome

G46.7 Other lacunar syndromes

G46.8 Other vascular syndromes of brain in cerebrovascular diseases

● **G47 Sleep disorders**

Excludes2 nightmares (F51.5)
nonorganic sleep disorders (F51.-)
sleep terrors (F51.4)
sleepwalking (F51.3)

● **G47.Ø Insomnia**

Excludes2 alcohol related insomnia (F1Ø.182,
F1Ø.282, F1Ø.982)
drug-related insomnia (F11.182, F11.282,
F11.982, F13.182, F13.282, F13.982,
F14.182, F14.282, F14.982, F15.182,
F15.282, F15.982, F19.182, F19.282,
F19.982)
idiopathic insomnia (F51.Ø1)
insomnia due to a mental disorder (F51.Ø5)
insomnia not due to a substance or known
physiological condition (F51.Ø-)
nonorganic insomnia (F51.Ø-)
primary insomnia (F51.Ø1)
sleep apnea (G47.3-)

G47.ØØ Insomnia, unspecified
Insomnia NOS

G47.Ø1 Insomnia due to medical condition
Code also associated medical condition

G47.Ø9 Other insomnia

● **G47.1 Hypersomnia**

Excludes2 alcohol-related hypersomnia (F1Ø.182,
F1Ø.282, F1Ø.982)
drug-related hypersomnia (F11.182,
F11.282, F11.982, F13.182, F13.282,
F13.982, F14.182, F14.282, F14.982,
F15.182, F15.282, F15.982, F19.182,
F19.282, F19.982)
hypersomnia due to a mental disorder
(F51.13)
hypersomnia not due to a substance
or known physiological condition
(F51.1-)
primary hypersomnia (F51.11)
sleep apnea (G47.3-)

G47.1Ø Hypersomnia, unspecified
Hypersomnia NOS

G47.11 Idiopathic hypersomnia with long sleep time
Idiopathic hypersomnia NOS

G47.12 Idiopathic hypersomnia without long sleep time

G47.13 Recurrent hypersomnia
Kleine-Levin syndrome
Menstrual related hypersomnia

G47.14 Hypersomnia due to medical condition
Code also associated medical condition

G47.19 Other hypersomnia

● **G47.2 Circadian rhythm sleep disorders**
Disorders of the sleep wake schedule
Inversion of nyctohemeral rhythm
Inversion of sleep rhythm

G47.2Ø Circadian rhythm sleep disorder, unspecified type
Sleep wake schedule disorder NOS

G47.21 Circadian rhythm sleep disorder, delayed sleep phase type
Delayed sleep phase syndrome

G47.22 Circadian rhythm sleep disorder, advanced sleep phase type

G47.23 Circadian rhythm sleep disorder, irregular sleep wake type
Irregular sleep-wake pattern

CHAPTER 6 (GØØ-G99)

G47.24   Circadian rhythm sleep disorder, free running type

G47.25   Circadian rhythm sleep disorder, jet lag type

G47.26   Circadian rhythm sleep disorder, shift work type

▶ *G47.27*   *Circadian rhythm sleep disorder in conditions classified elsewhere*
      Code first underlying condition

G47.29   Other circadian rhythm sleep disorder

● G47.3   Sleep apnea
      Characterized by episodes in which breathing stops during sleep
      Code also any associated underlying condition

      Excludes1   apnea NOS (R06.81)
          Cheyne-Stokes breathing (R06.3)
          pickwickian syndrome (E66.2)
          sleep apnea of newborn (P28.3)

G47.30   Sleep apnea, unspecified
      Sleep apnea NOS

G47.31   Primary central sleep apnea

G47.32   High altitude periodic breathing

G47.33   Obstructive sleep apnea (adult) (pediatric)
      Excludes1   obstructive sleep apnea of newborn (P28.3)

G47.34   Idiopathic sleep related nonobstructive alveolar hypoventilation
      Sleep related hypoxia

G47.35   Congenital central alveolar hypoventilation syndrome

▶ *G47.36*   *Sleep related hypoventilation in conditions classified elsewhere*
      Sleep related hypoxemia in conditions classified elsewhere
      Code first underlying condition

▶ *G47.37*   *Central sleep apnea in conditions classified elsewhere*
      Code first underlying condition

G47.39   Other sleep apnea

● G47.4   Narcolepsy and cataplexy
      *Cataplexy is a disorder evidenced by seizures including minor slacking of the facial muscles to complete collapse and often affects people who have **narcolepsy**, a disorder in which there is great difficulty remaining awake during the daytime.*

● G47.41   Narcolepsy

G47.411   Narcolepsy with cataplexy

G47.419   Narcolepsy without cataplexy
      Narcolepsy NOS

G47.42   Narcolepsy in conditions classified elsewhere
      Code first underlying condition

▶ *G47.421*   *Narcolepsy in conditions classified elsewhere with cataplexy*

▶ *G47.429*   *Narcolepsy in conditions classified elsewhere without cataplexy*

● G47.5   Parasomnia
      Excludes1   alcohol induced parasomnia (F10.182, F10.282, F10.982)
          drug induced parasomnia (F11.182, F11.282, F11.982, F13.182, F13.282, F13.982, F14.182, F14.282, F14.982, F15.182, F15.282, F15.982, F19.182, F19.282, F19.982)
          parasomnia not due to a substance or known physiological condition (F51.8)

G47.50   Parasomnia, unspecified
      Parasomnia NOS

G47.51   Confusional arousals

G47.52   REM sleep behavior disorder

G47.53   Recurrent isolated sleep paralysis

▶ *G47.54*   *Parasomnia in conditions classified elsewhere*
      Code first underlying condition

G47.59   Other parasomnia

● G47.6   Sleep related movement disorders
      Excludes2   restless legs syndrome (G25.81)

G47.61   Periodic limb movement disorder
      Periodic limb movement disorder

G47.62   Sleep related leg cramps

G47.63   Sleep related bruxism
      Excludes1   psychogenic bruxism (F45.8)

G47.69   Other sleep related movement disorders

G47.8   Other sleep disorders

G47.9   Sleep disorder, unspecified
      Sleep disorder NOS

★ **(See Plate 118 on page 54.)**

NERVE, NERVE ROOT AND PLEXUS DISORDERS (G50-G59)

      Excludes1   current traumatic nerve, nerve root and plexus disorders - see Injury, nerve by body region
          neuralgia NOS (M79.2)
          neuritis NOS (M79.2)
          peripheral neuritis in pregnancy (O26.82-)
          radiculitis NOS (M54.1-)

● G50   Disorders of trigeminal nerve
      Includes   disorders of 5th cranial nerve

G50.0   Trigeminal neuralgia
      Syndrome of paroxysmal facial pain
      Tic douloureux

G50.1   Atypical facial pain

G50.8   Other disorders of trigeminal nerve

G50.9   Disorder of trigeminal nerve, unspecified

● G51   Facial nerve disorders
      Includes   disorders of 7th cranial nerve

G51.0   Bell's palsy
      Facial palsy

G51.1   Geniculate ganglionitis
      Rare disorder with symptoms of severe pain deep in ear, spreading to ear canal, outer ear, mastoid or eye regions
      Excludes1   postherpetic geniculate ganglionitis (B02.21)

G51.2   Melkersson's syndrome
      Melkersson-Rosenthal syndrome

G51.3   Clonic hemifacial spasm

G51.4   Facial myokymia
      Involuntary facial muscle movement

G51.8   Other disorders of facial nerve

G51.9   Disorder of facial nerve, unspecified

● G52   Disorders of other cranial nerves
      Excludes2   disorders of acoustic [8th] nerve (H93.3)
          disorders of optic [2nd] nerve (H46, H47.0)
          paralytic strabismus due to nerve palsy (H49.0-H49.2)

G52.0   Disorders of olfactory nerve
      Disorders of 1st cranial nerve

G52.1   Disorders of glossopharyngeal nerve
      Disorder of 9th cranial nerve
      Glossopharyngeal neuralgia

G52.2   Disorders of vagus nerve
      Disorders of pneumogastric [10th] nerve

Item 6–5 Trigeminal neuralgia, tic douloureux, is a pain syndrome diagnosed from the patient's history alone. The condition is characterized by pain and a brief facial spasm or tic. Pain is unilateral and follows the sensory distribution of cranial nerve V, typically radiating to the maxillary (V2) or mandibular (V3) area.

Item 6–6   The most common facial nerve disorder is **Bell's Palsy,** which occurs suddenly and results in facial drooping unilaterally. This disorder is the result of a reaction to a virus that causes the facial nerve in the ear to swell resulting in pressure in the bony canal.

◀ New   ◀ Revised   ~~deleted~~ Deleted   Excludes 1   Excludes 2   Includes   Use additional   Code first   Code also   Unspecified

OGCR Official Guidelines   ● Unacceptable Principal Diagnosis   X Assign placeholder X   ● Use Additional Character(s)   ▶ Manifestation Code   **Coding Clinic**

G52.3 Disorders of hypoglossal nerve
Disorders of 12th cranial nerve

G52.7 Disorders of multiple cranial nerves
Polyneuritis cranialis

G52.8 Disorders of other specified cranial nerves

G52.9 Cranial nerve disorder, unspecified

G53 Cranial nerve disorders in diseases classified elsewhere
Code first underlying disease, such as:
neoplasm (C00-D49)

Excludes1   multiple cranial nerve palsy in sarcoidosis
(D86.82)
multiple cranial nerve palsy in syphilis (A52.15)
postherpetic geniculate ganglionitis (B02.21)
postherpetic trigeminal neuralgia (B02.22)

● **G54 Nerve root and plexus disorders**
*Raiculopathy (nerve root disorder) caused by pressure on nerve root,
most common cause is herniation of intervertebral disk. Plexus
disorders (plexopathies) are due to compression or injury.*

Excludes1   current traumatic nerve root and plexus disorders
- see nerve injury by body region
intervertebral disc disorders (M50-M51)
neuralgia or neuritis NOS (M79.2)
neuritis or radiculitis brachial NOS (M54.13)
neuritis or radiculitis lumbar NOS (M54.16)
neuritis or radiculitis lumbosacral NOS (M54.17)
neuritis or radiculitis thoracic NOS (M54.14)
radiculitis NOS (M54.10)
radiculopathy NOS (M54.10)
spondylosis (M47.-)

G54.0 Brachial plexus disorders
Thoracic outlet syndrome

G54.1 Lumbosacral plexus disorders

G54.2 Cervical root disorders, not elsewhere classified

● **G54.3 Thoracic root disorders, not elsewhere classified**

G54.4 Lumbosacral root disorders, not elsewhere classified

G54.5 Neuralgic amyotrophy
Parsonage-Aldren-Turner syndrome
Shoulder-girdle neuritis

Excludes1   neuralgic amyotrophy in diabetes
mellitus (E08-E13 with .44)

G54.6 Phantom limb syndrome with pain
*Sensations (cramping, itching) in a limb that no longer
exists*

G54.7 Phantom limb syndrome without pain
Phantom limb syndrome NOS

G54.8 Other nerve root and plexus disorders

G54.9 Nerve root and plexus disorder, unspecified

*G55 Nerve root and plexus compressions in diseases classified
elsewhere*
Code first underlying disease, such as:
neoplasm (C00-D49)

Excludes1   nerve root compression (due to) (in) ankylosing
spondylitis (M45.-)
nerve root compression (due to) (in)dorsopathies
(M53.-, M54.-)
nerve root compression (due to) (in)intervertebral
disc disorders (M50.1.-, M51.1.-)
nerve root compression (due to) (in)
spondylopathies (M46.-, M48.-)

★**(See Plates 472 and 473 on pages 56 and 57.)**

● **G56 Mononeuropathies of upper limb**
Excludes1   current traumatic nerve disorder - see nerve
injury by body region

● **G56.0 Carpal tunnel syndrome**
**G56.00 Carpal tunnel syndrome, unspecified upper
limb**
G56.01 Carpal tunnel syndrome, right upper limb
G56.02 Carpal tunnel syndrome, left upper limb
**G56.03 Carpal tunnel syndrome, bilateral upper
limbs** ◄

● **G56.1 Other lesions of median nerve**
G56.10 Other lesions of median nerve, unspecified side
**G56.11 Other lesions of median nerve, right upper
limb**
G56.12 Other lesions of median nerve, left upper limb
**G56.13 Other lesions of median nerve, bilateral upper
limbs** ◄

● **G56.2 Lesion of ulnar nerve**
Tardy ulnar nerve palsy
G56.20 Lesion of ulnar nerve, unspecified upper limb
G56.21 Lesion of ulnar nerve, right upper limb
G56.22 Lesion of ulnar nerve, left upper limb
G56.23 Lesion of ulnar nerve, bilateral upper limbs ◄

● **G56.3 Lesion of radial nerve**
G56.30 Lesion of radial nerve, unspecified upper limb
G56.31 Lesion of radial nerve, right upper limb
G56.32 Lesion of radial nerve, left upper limb
G56.33 Lesion of radial nerve, bilateral upper limbs ◄

● **G56.4 Causalgia of upper limb**
Intense burning pain and sensitivity to slight touch
Complex regional pain syndrome II of upper limb
Excludes1   complex regional pain syndrome I of
lower limb (G90.52-)
complex regional pain syndrome I of
upper limb (G90.51-)
complex regional pain syndrome II of
lower limb (G57.7-)
reflex sympathetic dystrophy of lower
limb (G90.52-)
reflex sympathetic dystrophy (G90.51-)
G56.40 Causalgia of unspecified upper limb
G56.41 Causalgia of right upper limb
G56.42 Causalgia of left upper limb
G56.43 Causalgia of bilateral upper limbs ◄

● **G56.8 Other specified mononeuropathies of upper limb**
Disease of a single nerve
Interdigital neuroma of upper limb
**G56.80 Other specified mononeuropathies
of unspecified upper limb**
**G56.81 Other specified mononeuropathies of right
upper limb**
**G56.82 Other specified mononeuropathies of left upper
limb**
**G56.83 Other specified mononeuropathies of bilateral
upper limbs** ◄

● **G56.9 Unspecified mononeuropathy of upper limb**
Disease of a single nerve
**G56.90 Unspecified mononeuropathy of unspecified
upper limb**
**G56.91 Unspecified mononeuropathy of right upper
limb**
**G56.92 Unspecified mononeuropathy of left upper
limb**
**G56.93 Unspecified mononeuropathy of bilateral upper
limbs** ◄

CHAPTER 6 (G00-G99)

N Newborn Age: 0   **P** Pediatric Age: 0–17   **M** Maternity DX: 12–55   **A** Adult Age: 15–124   ♀ Females Only   ♂ Males Only

 Complication\Comorbidity   Major C\C   (Ex) CC/MCC Exclusions   Hospital-Acquired Condition

799

CHAPTER 6 (G00-G99)

● **G57 Mononeuropathies of lower limb**
> Excludes1   current traumatic nerve disorder - see nerve injury by body region

★ **(See Plates 544 and 545 on pages 58 and 59.)**

> ● **G57.0 Lesion of sciatic nerve**
>> Excludes1   sciatica NOS (M54.3-)
>> Excludes2   sciatica attributed to intervertebral disc disorder (M51.1.-)
>> **G57.00 Lesion of sciatic nerve, unspecified lower limb**
>> **G57.01 Lesion of sciatic nerve, right lower limb**
>> **G57.02 Lesion of sciatic nerve, left lower limb**
>> **G57.03 Lesion of sciatic nerve, bilateral lower limbs** ◀

> ● **G57.1 Meralgia paresthetica**
>> *Numbness or pain in outer thigh caused by injury to nerve*
>> Lateral cutaneous nerve of thigh syndrome
>> **G57.10 Meralgia paresthetica, unspecified lower limb**
>> **G57.11 Meralgia paresthetica, right lower limb**
>> **G57.12 Meralgia paresthetica, left lower limb**
>> **G57.13 Meralgia paresthetica, bilateral lower limbs** ◀

> ● **G57.2 Lesion of femoral nerve**
>> **G57.20 Lesion of femoral nerve, unspecified lower limb**
>> **G57.21 Lesion of femoral nerve, right lower limb**
>> **G57.22 Lesion of femoral nerve, left lower limb**
>> **G57.23 Lesion of femoral nerve, bilateral lower limbs** ◀

> ● **G57.3 Lesion of lateral popliteal nerve**
>> Peroneal nerve palsy
>> **G57.30 Lesion of lateral popliteal nerve, unspecified lower limb**
>> **G57.31 Lesion of lateral popliteal nerve, right lower limb**
>> **G57.32 Lesion of lateral popliteal nerve, left lower limb**
>> **G57.33 Lesion of lateral popliteal nerve, bilateral lower limbs** ◀

> ● **G57.4 Lesion of medial popliteal nerve**
>> **G57.40 Lesion of medial popliteal nerve, unspecified lower limb**
>> **G57.41 Lesion of medial popliteal nerve, right lower limb**
>> **G57.42 Lesion of medial popliteal nerve, left lower limb**
>> **G57.43 Lesion of medial popliteal nerve, bilateral lower limbs** ◀

> ● **G57.5 Tarsal tunnel syndrome**
>> **G57.50 Tarsal tunnel syndrome, unspecified lower limb**
>> **G57.51 Tarsal tunnel syndrome, right lower limb**
>> **G57.52 Tarsal tunnel syndrome, left lower limb**
>> **G57.53 Tarsal tunnel syndrome, bilateral lower limbs** ◀

> ● **G57.6 Lesion of plantar nerve**
>> Morton's metatarsalgia
>> **G57.60 Lesion of plantar nerve, unspecified lower limb**
>> **G57.61 Lesion of plantar nerve, right lower limb**
>> **G57.62 Lesion of plantar nerve, left lower limb**
>> **G57.63 Lesion of plantar nerve, bilateral lower limbs** ◀

> ● **G57.7 Causalgia of lower limb**
>> Complex regional pain syndrome II of lower limb
>> Excludes1   complex regional pain syndrome I of lower limb (G90.52-)
>> complex regional pain syndrome I of upper limb (G90.51-)
>> complex regional pain syndrome II of upper limb (G56.4-)
>> reflex sympathetic dystrophy of lower limb (G90.52-)
>> reflex sympathetic dystrophy of upper limb (G90.51-)
>> **G57.70 Causalgia of unspecified lower limb**
>> **G57.71 Causalgia of right lower limb**
>> **G57.72 Causalgia of left lower limb**
>> **G57.73 Causalgia of bilateral lower limbs** ◀

> ● **G57.8 Other specified mononeuropathies of lower limb**
>> Interdigital neuroma of lower limb
>> **G57.80 Other specified mononeuropathies of unspecified lower limb**
>> **G57.81 Other specified mononeuropathies of right lower limb**
>> **G57.82 Other specified mononeuropathies of left lower limb**
>> **G57.83 Other specified mononeuropathies of bilateral lower limbs** ◀

> ● **G57.9 Unspecified mononeuropathy of lower limb**
>> **G57.90 Unspecified mononeuropathy of unspecified lower limb**
>> **G57.91 Unspecified mononeuropathy of right lower limb**
>> **G57.92 Unspecified mononeuropathy of left lower limb**
>> **G57.93 Unspecified mononeuropathy of bilateral lower limbs** ◀

● **G58 Other mononeuropathies**
> **G58.0 Intercostal neuropathy**
> **G58.7 Mononeuritis multiplex**
> **G58.8 Other specified mononeuropathies**
> **G58.9 Mononeuropathy, unspecified**

▌ **G59 *Mononeuropathy in diseases classified elsewhere***
> *Code first underlying disease*
>> Excludes1   diabetic mononeuropathy (E08-E13 with .41)
>> syphilitic nerve paralysis (A52.19)
>> syphilitic neuritis (A52.15)
>> tuberculous mononeuropathy (A17.83)

POLYNEUROPATHIES AND OTHER DISORDERS OF THE PERIPHERAL NERVOUS SYSTEM (G60-G65)

> Excludes1   neuralgia NOS (M79.2)
> neuritis NOS (M79.2)
> peripheral neuritis in pregnancy (O26.82-)
> radiculitis NOS (M54.10)

● **G60 Hereditary and idiopathic neuropathy**
> **G60.0 Hereditary motor and sensory neuropathy**
>> Charcot-Marie-Tooth disease
>> Déjerine-Sottas disease
>> Hereditary motor and sensory neuropathy, types I-IV
>> Hypertrophic neuropathy of infancy
>> Peroneal muscular atrophy (axonal type) (hypertrophic type)
>> Roussy-Lévy syndrome
> **G60.1 Refsum's disease** 🔍
>> *Genetic disorder affecting fatty acid metabolism*
>> Infantile Refsum disease
>> Ⓔⓧ E11.42, G13.0, G13.1, G50.0-G65.2, M34.83
> **G60.2 Neuropathy in association with hereditary ataxia**
> **G60.3 Idiopathic progressive neuropathy**
> **G60.8 Other hereditary and idiopathic neuropathies**
>> Dominantly inherited sensory neuropathy
>> Morvan's disease
>> Nelaton's syndrome
>> Recessively inherited sensory neuropathy
> **G60.9 Hereditary and idiopathic neuropathy, unspecified**

● **G61 Inflammatory polyneuropathy**
> **G61.0 Guillain-Barré syndrome** 🔍
>> *Autoimmune disease affecting peripheral nervous system*
>> Acute (post-)infective polyneuritis
>> Miller Fisher Syndrome
>> Ⓔⓧ A02.21, A17.0-A17.1, A27.81, A39.0, A39.89-A39.9, A49.3-A49.9, A50.41, A51.41, A52.13, A54.82, A54.84, A54.89-A54.9, A87.0-A87.9, B00.3, B02.1, B26.1, B37.5, B38.4, B45.1, B58.2, B92, B94.2-B94.9, B96.0, B96.6-B96.89, G00.0-G03.9, G04.2, G32.89, G61.0, G96.8-G96.9, G98.0-G98.8, G99.8

> **G61.1 Serum neuropathy**
>> Use additional code for adverse effect, if applicable, to identify serum (T50.-)

◀ New   ◀▥ Revised   ~~deleted~~ Deleted   Excludes 1   Excludes 2   Includes   Use additional   Code first   Code also   Unspecified

OGCR Official Guidelines   ● Unacceptable Principal Diagnosis   X Assign placeholder X   ● Use Additional Character(s)   ▌ Manifestation Code   **Coding Clinic**

Item 6–7 The **peripheral nervous system** consists of 31 pairs of spinal nerves, 12 pairs of cranial nerves, and the autonomic nerves, which are divided into the parasympathetic and sympathetic nerves. The cranial nerves are: olfactory (I), optic (II), oculomotor (III), trochlear (IV), trigeminal (V), abducens (VI), facial (VII), vestibulocochlear (VIII), glossopharyngeal (IX), vagus (X), accessory (XI), and hypoglossal (XII).

● **G61.8   Other inflammatory polyneuropathies**

    G61.81   Chronic inflammatory demyelinating polyneuritis 🅒
        Ⓔⓧ G51.0-G54.5, G54.8-G60.9, G61.81-G61.89, G62.81-G62.89, G64

    G61.82   Multifocal motor neuropathy ◀
        MMN ◀

    G61.89   Other inflammatory polyneuropathies

  G61.9   Inflammatory polyneuropathy, unspecified

● **G62   Other and unspecified polyneuropathies**

    G62.0   Drug-induced polyneuropathy
        Use additional code for adverse effect, if applicable, to identify drug (T36-T50 with fifth or sixth character 5)

    G62.1   Alcoholic polyneuropathy
        Malfunction of many peripheral nerves throughout the body

    G62.2   Polyneuropathy due to other toxic agents
        Code first (T51-T65) to identify toxic agent

● **G62.8   Other specified polyneuropathies**

    G62.81   Critical illness polyneuropathy 🅒
        Acute motor neuropathy
        Ⓔⓧ G51.0-G54.5, G54.8-G60.9, G61.81-G61.9, G62.81, G62.89-G62.9, G64

    G62.82   Radiation-induced polyneuropathy
        Use additional external cause code (W88-W90, X39.0-) to identify cause

    G62.89   Other specified polyneuropathies
        Coding Clinic: 2016, Q2, P11

  G62.9   Polyneuropathy, unspecified
    Neuropathy NOS

▷ **G63   Polyneuropathy in diseases classified elsewhere**
    Code first underlying disease, such as:
      amyloidosis (E85.-)
      endocrine disease, except diabetes (E00-E07, E15-E16, E20-E34)
      metabolic diseases (E70-E88)
      neoplasm (C00-D49)
      nutritional deficiency (E40-E64)

    Excludes1   polyneuropathy (in):
      diabetes mellitus (E08-E13 with .42)
      diphtheria (A36.83)
      infectious mononucleosis (B27.0-B27.9 with 1)
      Lyme disease (A69.22)
      mumps (B26.84)
      postherpetic (B02.23)
      rheumatoid arthritis (M05.33)
      scleroderma (M34.83)
      systemic lupus erythematosus (M32.19)

    Coding Clinic: 2012, Q4, P100

  G64   Other disorders of peripheral nervous system
    Disorder of peripheral nervous system NOS

● **G65   Sequelae of inflammatory and toxic polyneuropathies**
    Code first condition resulting from (sequela) of inflammatory and toxic polyneuropathies

    G65.0   Sequelae of Guillain-Barré syndrome

    G65.1   Sequelae of other inflammatory polyneuropathy

    G65.2   Sequelae of toxic polyneuropathy

CHAPTER 6 (G00-G99)

| SYMPATHETIC | PARASYMPATHETIC |

Pupils dilated — — Pupils constricted
Salivation inhibited — — Salivation stimulated
Increased respiration — — Decreased respiration
Bronchial passages dilated — — Bronchial passages constricted
Increased heart rate — — Decreased heart rate
Increased secretion by sweat glands
Hair follicles raised; goose bumps
Secretion of adrenal hormones
Digestion inhibited — — Digestion stimulated
Bladder muscles relaxed (filling) — — Bladder muscles contracted (emptying)

Figure 6-2   Actions of parasympathetic and sympathetic nerves. (From Chabner: The Language of Medicine, ed 9, St. Louis, Saunders, 2011)

N Newborn Age: 0   **P** Pediatric Age: 0–17   **M** Maternity DX: 12–55   **A** Adult Age: 15–124   ♀ Females Only   ♂ Males Only
🅒 Complication\Comorbidity   🅜 Major C\C   Ⓔⓧ CC/MCC Exclusions   🅗 Hospital-Acquired Condition

CHAPTER 6 (G00-G99)

DISEASES OF MYONEURAL JUNCTION AND MUSCLE (G70-G73)

● **G70   Myasthenia gravis and other myoneural disorders**

> **Excludes1**   botulism (A05.1, A48.51-A48.52)
> transient neonatal myasthenia gravis (P94.0)

● **G70.0   Myasthenia gravis**
> *Acquired and results in fatigable muscle weakness*
> *exacerbated by activity and improved with rest*

> **G70.00   Myasthenia gravis without (acute) exacerbation**
> Myasthenia gravis NOS

> **G70.01   Myasthenia gravis with (acute) exacerbation** 🔗
> Myasthenia gravis in crisis
> (Ex) E08.40-E08.49, E08.618-E08.638, E08.649-E08.8,
> E09.40-E09.49, E09.618-E09.638, E09.649-E09.8,
> E10.40-E10.49, E10.618-E10.638, E10.649, E10.69-E10.8,
> E11.40-E11.49, E11.618-E11.638, E11.649, E11.69-E11.8,
> E13.40-E13.49, E13.618-E13.638, E13.649-E13.8, G32.89,
> G70.00-G70.01, G70.80-G70.81, G73.1-G73.3, G96.8-G96.9,
> G98.0-G98.8, G99.8

G70.1   Toxic myoneural disorders
> *Dysfunction at junction of muscle and motor nerve*
> *(myoneural junction)*
> *Code first* (T51-T65) to identify toxic agent

G70.2   Congenital and developmental myasthenia

● **G70.8   Other specified myoneural disorders**

> **G70.80   Lambert-Eaton syndrome, unspecified** 🔗
> Lambert-Eaton syndrome NOS
> (Ex) See G70.01

▷ **G70.81   *Lambert-Eaton syndrome in disease classified elsewhere*** 🔗
> > *Code first* underlying disease
> > **Excludes1**   Lambert-Eaton syndrome in
> > neoplastic disease (G73.1)
> > (Ex) See G70.01

> **G70.89   Other specified myoneural disorders**

G70.9   Myoneural disorder, unspecified

● **G71   Primary disorders of muscles**

> **Excludes2**   arthrogryposis multiplex congenita (Q74.3)
> metabolic disorders (E70-E88)
> myositis (M60.-)

G71.0   Muscular dystrophy 🔗
> Autosomal recessive, childhood type, muscular
> dystrophy resembling Duchenne or Becker
> muscular dystrophy
> Benign [Becker] muscular dystrophy
> Benign scapuloperoneal muscular dystrophy with early
> contractures [Emery-Dreifuss]
> Congenital muscular dystrophy NOS
> Congenital muscular dystrophy with specific
> morphological abnormalities of the muscle fiber
> Distal muscular dystrophy
> Facioscapulohumeral muscular dystrophy
> Limb-girdle muscular dystrophy
> Ocular muscular dystrophy
> Oculopharyngeal muscular dystrophy
> Scapuloperoneal muscular dystrophy
> Severe [Duchenne] muscular dystrophy
> (Ex) E08.40-E08.49, E08.618-E08.638, E08.649-E08.8, E09.40-E09.49,
> E09.618-E09.638, E09.649-E09.8, E10.40-E10.49, E10.618-E10.638,
> E10.649, E10.69-E10.8, E11.40-E11.49, E11.618-E11.638, E11.649,
> E11.69-E11.8, E13.40-E13.49, E13.618-E13.638, E13.649-E13.8, G32.89,
> G71.0, G71.2, G96.8-G96.9, G98.0-G98.8, G99.8

● **G71.1   Myotonic disorders**
> *Inherited disorder that affects muscles tone*

> **G71.11   Myotonic muscular dystrophy**
> Dystrophia myotonica [Steinert]
> Myotonia atrophica
> Myotonic dystrophy
> Proximal myotonic myopathy (PROMM)
> Steinert disease

> **G71.12   Myotonia congenita**
> Acetazolamide responsive myotonia congenita
> Dominant myotonia congenita [Thomsen
> disease]
> Myotonia levior
> Recessive myotonia congenita [Becker disease]

> **G71.13   Myotonic chondrodystrophy**
> Chondrodystrophic myotonia
> Congenital myotonic chondrodystrophy
> Schwartz-Jampel disease

> **G71.14   Drug induced myotonia**
> > Use additional code for adverse effect, if
> > applicable, to identify drug (T36-T50 with
> > fifth or sixth character 5)

> **G71.19   Other specified myotonic disorders**
> Myotonia fluctuans
> Myotonia permanens
> Neuromyotonia [Isaacs]
> Paramyotonia congenita (of von Eulenburg)
> Pseudomyotonia
> Symptomatic myotonia

G71.2   Congenital myopathies 🔗
> Central core disease
> Fiber-type disproportion
> Minicore disease
> Multicore disease
> Myotubular (centronuclear) myopathy
> Nemaline myopathy
> > **Excludes1**   arthrogryposis multiplex congenita
> > (Q74.3)
> > (Ex) See G71.0

G71.3   Mitochondrial myopathy, not elsewhere classified
> *Myopathies associated with increased number of enlarged,*
> *often abnormal, mitochondria in muscle fibers*
> > **Excludes1**   Kearns-Sayre syndrome (H49.81)
> > Leber's disease (H47.21)
> > Leigh's encephalopathy (G31.82)
> > mitochondrial metabolism disorders
> > (E88.4.-)
> > Reye's syndrome (G93.7)

G71.8   Other primary disorders of muscles

G71.9   Primary disorder of muscle, unspecified
> Hereditary myopathy NOS

● **G72   Other and unspecified myopathies**
> **Excludes1**   arthrogryposis multiplex congenita (Q74.3)
> dermatopolymyositis (M33.-)
> ischemic infarction of muscle (M62.2-)
> myositis (M60.-)
> polymyositis (M33.2.-)

G72.0   Drug-induced myopathy 🔗
> > Use additional code for adverse effect, if applicable,
> > to identify drug (T36-T50 with fifth or sixth
> > character 5)
> > (Ex) G32.89, G70.00-G71.0, G71.11-G72.3, G72.81-G73.7, G96.8-G96.9,
> > G98.0-G98.8, G99.8

G72.1   Alcoholic myopathy 🔗
> > Use additional code to identify alcoholism (F10.-)
> > (Ex) See G72.0

G72.2   Myopathy due to other toxic agents 🔗
> *Code first* (T51-T65) to identify toxic agent
> (Ex) See G72.0

Item 6-8   Muscular dystrophies (MD) are a group of rare inherited muscle diseases. Voluntary muscles become progressively weaker. In the late stages of MD, fat and connective tissue replace muscle fibers. In some types of muscular dystrophy, heart muscles, other involuntary muscles, and other organs are affected. **Myopathies** is a general term for neuromuscular diseases in which the muscle fibers dysfunction for any one of many reasons, resulting in muscular weakness.

◀ New   ◀ Revised   ~~deleted~~ Deleted   Excludes 1   Excludes 2   Includes   Use additional   Code first   Code also   Unspecified

OGCR Official Guidelines   ● Unacceptable Principal Diagnosis   X Assign placeholder X   🔗 Use Additional Character(s)   ▷ Manifestation Code   **Coding Clinic**

G72.3   **Periodic paralysis**
Familial periodic paralysis
Hyperkalemic periodic paralysis (familial)
Hypokalemic periodic paralysis (familial)
Myotonic periodic paralysis (familial)
Normokalemic paralysis (familial)
Potassium sensitive periodic paralysis
> **Excludes1**   paramyotonia congenita (of von Eulenburg) (G71.19)

● **G72.4**   **Inflammatory and immune myopathies, not elsewhere classified**

    G72.41   **Inclusion body myositis [IBM]**

    G72.49   **Other inflammatory and immune myopathies, not elsewhere classified**
       Inflammatory myopathy NOS

● **G72.8**   **Other specified myopathies**

    G72.81   **Critical illness myopathy** 🔹
       Acute necrotizing myopathy
       Acute quadriplegic myopathy
       Intensive care (ICU) myopathy
       Myopathy of critical illness
         (Ex:) G70.1-G72.3, G72.81-G73.7

    G72.89   **Other specified myopathies**

   G72.9   **Myopathy, unspecified**

● **G73**   **Disorders of myoneural junction and muscle in diseases classified elsewhere**
     (Ex:) For category G73 CC codes: See G70.01

●▶ **G73.1**   *Lambert-Eaton syndrome in neoplastic disease* 🔹
     Rare autoimmune disorder affecting calcium channels of nerve-muscle (neuromuscular) junction
     Code first underlying neoplasm (C00-D49)
> **Excludes1**   Lambert-Eaton syndrome not associated with neoplasm (G70.80-G70.81)

▶ **G73.3**   *Myasthenic syndromes in other diseases classified elsewhere* 🔹
     Code first underlying disease, such as:
       neoplasm (C00-D49)
       thyrotoxicosis (E05.-)

▶ **G73.7**   *Myopathy in diseases classified elsewhere* 🔹
     Code first underlying disease, such as:
       hyperparathyroidism (E21.0, E21.3)
       hypoparathyroidism (E20.-)
       glycogen storage disease (E74.0)
       lipid storage disorders (E75.-)
> **Excludes1**   myopathy in:
>   rheumatoid arthritis (M05.32)
>   sarcoidosis (D86.87)
>   scleroderma (M34.82)
>   sicca syndrome [Sjögren] (M35.03)
>   systemic lupus erythematosus (M32.19)

CEREBRAL PALSY AND OTHER PARALYTIC SYNDROMES (G80-G83)

● **G80**   **Cerebral palsy**
> **Excludes1**   hereditary spastic paraplegia (G11.4)

   G80.0   **Spastic quadriplegic cerebral palsy** 🔹
     Congenital spastic paralysis (cerebral)
      (Ex:) E08.40-E08.49, E08.618-E08.638, E08.649-E08.8, E09.40-E09.49, E09.618-E09.638, E09.649-E09.8, E10.40-E10.49, E10.618-E10.638, E10.649, E10.69-E10.8, E11.40-E11.49, E11.618-E11.638, E11.649, E11.69-E11.8, E13.40-E13.49, E13.618-E13.638, E13.649-E13.8, G04.1, G32.89, G80.0-G80.2, G80.4-G80.9, G90.1, G93.81, G93.89-G93.9, G96.8-G96.9, G98.0-G98.8, G99.8, Q06.0-Q06.1, Q06.3, Q06.8-Q06.9, Q07.8-Q07.9, R53.2

   G80.1   **Spastic diplegic cerebral palsy** 🔹
     Spastic cerebral palsy NOS
      (Ex:) G80.1, G93.40-G93.49, I67.83

   G80.2   **Spastic hemiplegic cerebral palsy** 🔹
      (Ex:) G80.2, G93.40-G93.49, I67.83

   G80.3   **Athetoid cerebral palsy** 🔹
     Result of damage to cerebellum or basal ganglia responsible for processing neuromuscular signals
     Double athetosis (syndrome)
     Dyskinetic cerebral palsy
     Dystonic cerebral palsy
     Vogt disease
      (Ex:) G20, G21.11-G21.9, G25.70-G25.79, G25.89-G26, G80.0-G80.9, G93.40-G93.49, I67.83

   G80.4   **Ataxic cerebral palsy**
     Poor muscle tone and coordination

   G80.8   **Other cerebral palsy**
     Mixed cerebral palsy syndromes

   G80.9   **Cerebral palsy, unspecified**
     Cerebral palsy NOS

OGCR   **Section I.C.6.a.**
> Dominant/nondominant side
>
> Codes from category G81, Hemiplegia and hemiparesis, and subcategories, G83.1, Monoplegia of lower limb, G83.2, Monoplegia of upper limb, and G83.3, Monoplegia, unspecified, identify whether the dominant and nondominant side is affected. Should the affected side be documented, but not specified as dominant or nondominant, and the classification system does not indicate a default, code selection is as follows:
> - For ambidextrous patients, the default should be dominant.
> - If the left side is affected, the default is non-dominant.
> - If the right side is affected, the default is dominant.

● **G81**   **Hemiplegia and hemiparesis**
   Note: This category is to be used only when hemiplegia (complete)(incomplete) is reported without further specification, or is stated to be old or longstanding but of unspecified cause. The category is also for use in multiple coding to identify these types of hemiplegia resulting from any cause.
> **Excludes1**   congenital cerebral palsy (G80.-)
>   hemiplegia and hemiparesis due to sequela of cerebrovascular disease (I69.05-, I69.15-, I69.25-, I69.35-, I69.85-, I69.95-)
      (Ex:) For category G81 CC codes: G04.1, G11.0-G12.9, G32.0-G37.3, G37.5-G37.9, G80.0-G80.2, G80.4-G80.9, G81.00-G83.9, G90.01-G90.09, G90.2, G90.4, G90.50-G90.9, G92, G93.40-G93.49, G93.81, G93.89-G95.9, G96.8-G96.9, G98.0-G99.8, I67.83, R53.2
     Coding Clinic: 2012, Q4, P106

● **G81.0**   **Flaccid hemiplegia**
     Paralysis of half of body with loss of tone of muscles of paralyzed part and absence of tendon reflexes

    G81.00   **Flaccid hemiplegia affecting unspecified side** 🔹

    G81.01   **Flaccid hemiplegia affecting right dominant side** 🔹

    G81.02   **Flaccid hemiplegia affecting left dominant side** 🔹

    G81.03   **Flaccid hemiplegia affecting right nondominant side** 🔹

    G81.04   **Flaccid hemiplegia affecting left nondominant side** 🔹

Item 6-9   **Hemiplegia** is complete paralysis of one side of the body— arm, leg, and trunk. **Hemiparesis** is a generalized weakness or incomplete paralysis of one side of the body. If most activities (eating, writing) are performed with the right hand, the right is the dominant side, and the left is the nondominant side. **Quadriplegia,** also called tetraplegia, is the complete paralysis of all four limbs. **Quadriparesis** is the incomplete paralysis of all four limbs. Nerve damage in C1–C4 is associated with lower limb paralysis, and C5–C7 damage is associated with upper limb paralysis. **Diplegia** is the paralysis of the upper limbs. **Monoplegia** is the complete paralysis of one limb.

N   Newborn Age: 0   **P**   Pediatric Age: 0–17   **M**   Maternity DX: 12–55   **A**   Adult Age: 15–124   ♀   Females Only   ♂   Males Only

🔹   Complication\Comorbidity   🔹   Major C\C   (Ex:)   CC/MCC Exclusions   🔹   Hospital-Acquired Condition

CHAPTER 6 (G00-G99)

● **G81.1**   **Spastic hemiplegia**
Paralysis of half of body with spasticity of muscles of paralyzed part and increased tendon reflexes

    G81.10   Spastic hemiplegia affecting unspecified side 🖐

    G81.11   Spastic hemiplegia affecting right dominant side 🖐

    G81.12   Spastic hemiplegia affecting left dominant side 🖐

    G81.13   Spastic hemiplegia affecting right nondominant side 🖐

    G81.14   Spastic hemiplegia affecting left nondominant side 🖐

● **G81.9**   **Hemiplegia, unspecified**

    G81.90   Hemiplegia, unspecified affecting unspecified side 🖐

    G81.91   Hemiplegia, unspecified affecting right dominant side 🖐

    G81.92   Hemiplegia, unspecified affecting left dominant side 🖐

    G81.93   Hemiplegia, unspecified affecting right nondominant side 🖐

    G81.94   Hemiplegia, unspecified affecting left nondominant side 🖐
       Coding Clinic: 2015, Q1, P26

● **G82**   **Paraplegia (paraparesis) and quadriplegia (quadriparesis)**
    Note: This category is to be used only when the listed conditions are reported without further specification, or are stated to be old or longstanding but of unspecified cause. The category is also for use in multiple coding to identify these conditions resulting from any cause.

    Excludes1   congenital cerebral palsy (G80.-)
               functional quadriplegia (R53.2)
               hysterical paralysis (F44.4)

● **G82.2**   **Paraplegia**
    Paralysis of both lower limbs NOS
    Paraparesis (lower) NOS
    Paraplegia (lower) NOS
     Ex: For category G82.2 CC codes: See G81

    G82.20   Paraplegia, unspecified 🖐

    G82.21   Paraplegia, complete 🖐

    G82.22   Paraplegia, incomplete 🖐

● **G82.5**   **Quadriplegia**
    Paralysis of all limbs; AKA tetraplegia
     Ex: See G80.0

    G82.50   Quadriplegia, unspecified 🖐

    G82.51   Quadriplegia, C1-C4 complete 🖐

    G82.52   Quadriplegia, C1-C4 incomplete 🖐

    G82.53   Quadriplegia, C5-C7 complete 🖐

    G82.54   Quadriplegia, C5-C7 incomplete 🖐

● **G83**   **Other paralytic syndromes**
    Note: This category is to be used only when the listed conditions are reported without further specification, or are stated to be old or longstanding but of unspecified cause. The category is also for use in multiple coding to identify these conditions resulting from any cause.

    Includes   paralysis (complete) (incomplete), except as in G80-G82

G83.0   **Diplegia of upper limbs** 🖐
    Paralysis affecting limbs on both sides; AKA bilateral paralysis
    Diplegia (upper)
    Paralysis of both upper limbs
     Ex: G32.89, G82.50-G83.0, G83.5-G83.9, G96.8-G96.9, G98.0-G98.8, G99.8, R53.2

● **G83.1**   **Monoplegia of lower limb**
    Paralysis of limb on one side
    Paralysis of lower limb

    Excludes1   monoplegia of lower limbs due to sequela of cerebrovascular disease (I69.04-, I69.14-, I69.24-, I69.34-, I69.84-, I69.94-)
     Coding Clinic: 2012, Q4, P106

    G83.10   Monoplegia of lower limb affecting unspecified side

    G83.11   Monoplegia of lower limb affecting right dominant side

    G83.12   Monoplegia of lower limb affecting left dominant side

    G83.13   Monoplegia of lower limb affecting right nondominant side

    G83.14   Monoplegia of lower limb affecting left nondominant side

● **G83.2**   **Monoplegia of upper limb**
    Paralysis of upper limb

    Excludes1   monoplegia of upper limbs due to sequela of cerebrovascular disease (I69.03-, I69.13-, I69.23-, I69.33-, I69.83-, I69.93-)
     Coding Clinic: 2012, Q4, P106

    G83.20   Monoplegia of upper limb affecting unspecified side

    G83.21   Monoplegia of upper limb affecting right dominant side

    G83.22   Monoplegia of upper limb affecting left dominant side

    G83.23   Monoplegia of upper limb affecting right nondominant side

    G83.24   Monoplegia of upper limb affecting left nondominant side

● **G83.3**   **Monoplegia, unspecified**
     Coding Clinic: 2012, Q4, P106

    G83.30   Monoplegia, unspecified affecting unspecified side

    G83.31   Monoplegia, unspecified affecting right dominant side

    G83.32   Monoplegia, unspecified affecting left dominant side

    G83.33   Monoplegia, unspecified affecting right nondominant side

    G83.34   Monoplegia, unspecified affecting left nondominant side

G83.4   **Cauda equina syndrome** 🖐
    Aching pain due to compression of spinal nerve roots
    Neurogenic bladder due to cauda equina syndrome

    Excludes1   cord bladder NOS (G95.89)
               neurogenic bladder NOS (N31.9)
     Ex: G04.1, G32.89, G82.20-G82.54, G83.10-G83.14, G83.4-G83.9, G96.8-G96.9, G98.0-G98.8, G99.8, R53.2

G83.5   **Locked-in state** 🖐
     Ex: G04.1, G32.89, G80.0-G83.9, G92, G93.40-G93.49, G93.81, G93.89-G93.9, G96.8-G96.9, G98.0-G98.8, G99.8, I67.83, R53.2

● **G83.8**   **Other specified paralytic syndromes**

    Excludes1   paralytic syndromes due to current spinal cord injury-code to spinal cord injury (S14, S24, S34)

    G83.81   Brown-Séquard syndrome

    G83.82   Anterior cord syndrome

    G83.83   Posterior cord syndrome

    G83.84   Todd's paralysis (postepileptic)

    G83.89   Other specified paralytic syndromes

● **G83.9**   **Paralytic syndrome, unspecified**

OTHER DISORDERS OF THE NERVOUS SYSTEM (G89-G99)

● **G89   Pain, not elsewhere classified**

Code also related psychological factors associated with pain (F45.42)

Excludes1   generalized pain NOS (R52)
pain disorders exclusively related to psychological factors (F45.41)
pain NOS (R52)

Excludes2   atypical face pain (G50.1)
headache syndromes (G44.-)
localized pain, unspecified type - code to pain by site, such as:
    abdomen pain (R10.-)
    back pain (M54.9)
    breast pain (N64.4)
    chest pain (R07.1-R07.9)
    ear pain (H92.0-)
    eye pain (H57.1)
    headache (R51)
    joint pain (M25.5-)
    limb pain (M79.6-)
    lumbar region pain (M54.5)
    painful urination (R30.9)
    pelvic and perineal pain (R10.2)
    shoulder pain (M25.51-)
    spine pain (M54.-)
    throat pain (R07.0)
    tongue pain (K14.6)
    tooth pain (K08.8)
renal colic (N23)
migraines (G43.-)
myalgia (M79.1)
pain from prosthetic devices, implants, and grafts (T82.84, T83.84, T84.84, T85.84-) ◄▥
phantom limb syndrome with pain (G54.6)
vulvar vestibulitis (N94.810)
vulvodynia (N94.81-)

G89.0   Central pain syndrome
Neurological condition causing intractable pain resulting from damage to CNS
Déjérine-Roussy syndrome
Myelopathic pain syndrome
Thalamic pain syndrome (hyperesthetic)

● **G89.1   Acute pain, not elsewhere classified**

G89.11   Acute pain due to trauma

G89.12   Acute post-thoracotomy pain
Post-thoracotomy pain NOS

G89.18   Other acute postprocedural pain
Postoperative pain NOS
Postprocedural pain NOS

● **G89.2   Chronic pain, not elsewhere classified**

Excludes1   causalgia, lower limb (G57.7-)
causalgia, upper limb (G56.4-)
central pain syndrome (G89.0)
chronic pain syndrome (G89.4)
complex regional pain syndrome II, lower limb (G57.7-)
complex regional pain syndrome II, upper limb (G56.4-)
neoplasm related chronic pain (G89.3)
reflex sympathetic dystrophy (G90.5-)

G89.21   Chronic pain due to trauma

G89.22   Chronic post-thoracotomy pain

G89.28   Other chronic postprocedural pain
Other chronic postoperative pain

G89.29   Other chronic pain

G89.3   Neoplasm related pain (acute) (chronic)
Cancer associated pain
Pain due to malignancy (primary) (secondary)
Tumor associated pain

G89.4   Chronic pain syndrome
Chronic pain associated with significant psychosocial dysfunction

● **G90   Disorders of autonomic nervous system**

Excludes1   dysfunction of the autonomic nervous system due to alcohol (G31.2)

● **G90.0   Idiopathic peripheral autonomic neuropathy**

G90.01   Carotid sinus syncope
Carotid sinus syndrome

G90.09   Other idiopathic peripheral autonomic neuropathy
Idiopathic peripheral autonomic neuropathy NOS

G90.1   Familial dysautonomia [Riley-Day]
Inherited disorder that affects nerve function

G90.2   Horner's syndrome
Due to damage of the sympathetic nervous system
Bernard(-Horner) syndrome
Cervical sympathetic dystrophy or paralysis

G90.3   Multi-system degeneration of the autonomic nervous system 🖐
Neurogenic orthostatic hypotension [Shy-Drager]
Excludes1   orthostatic hypotension NOS (I95.1)
ⒺⓍ G20, G21.11-G21.9, G90.01-G90.09, G93.40-G93.49, I67.83

G90.4   Autonomic dysreflexia
Syndrome resulting from lesions of spinal cord
Use additional code to identify the cause, such as:
fecal impaction (K56.41)
pressure ulcer (pressure area) (L89.-)
urinary tract infection (N39.0)

● **G90.5   Complex regional pain syndrome I (CRPS I)**
Reflex sympathetic dystrophy
Excludes1   causalgia of lower limb (G57.7-)
causalgia of upper limb (G56.4-)
complex regional pain syndrome II of lower limb (G57.7-)
complex regional pain syndrome II of upper limb (G56.4-)
ⒺⓍ **For category G90.5 CC codes unless otherwise indicated:**
E08.40-E08.49, E09.40-E09.49, E10.40-E10.49, E11.40-E11.49,
E13.40-E13.49, G04.1, G11.3, G11.8-G12.9, G32.0, G32.89-G37.3,
G37.5-G37.9, G80.0-G80.2, G80.4-G83.9, G90.01-G90.09, G90.2,
G90.4-G90.9, G93.1, G93.40-G93.49, G95.0-G95.9, G96.12-G96.9, G97.1,
G98.0-G99.8, I67.83, R53.2

G90.50   Complex regional pain syndrome I, unspecified 🖐
ⒺⓍ G90.50-G90.59

● **G90.51   Complex regional pain syndrome I of upper limb**

G90.511   Complex regional pain syndrome I of right upper limb 🖐

G90.512   Complex regional pain syndrome I of left upper limb 🖐

G90.513   Complex regional pain syndrome I of upper limb, bilateral 🖐

G90.519   Complex regional pain syndrome I of unspecified upper limb 🖐

● **G90.52   Complex regional pain syndrome I of lower limb**

G90.521   Complex regional pain syndrome I of right lower limb 🖐

G90.522   Complex regional pain syndrome I of left lower limb 🖐

G90.523   Complex regional pain syndrome I of lower limb, bilateral 🖐

G90.529   Complex regional pain syndrome I of unspecified lower limb 🖐

G90.59   Complex regional pain syndrome I of other specified site 🖐

G90.8   Other disorders of autonomic nervous system

G90.9   Disorder of the autonomic nervous system, unspecified

CHAPTER 6 (G00-G99)

N   Newborn Age: 0   P   Pediatric Age: 0-17   M   Maternity DX: 12-55   A   Adult Age: 15-124   ♀   Females Only   ♂   Males Only
🖐   Complication\Comorbidity   🖐   Major C\C   ⒺⓍ   CC/MCC Exclusions   🖐   Hospital-Acquired Condition   **805**

● **G91**   **Hydrocephalus**
Dilatation of cerebral ventricles, accompanied by accumulation of cerebrospinal fluid

Includes   acquired hydrocephalus

Excludes1   Arnold-Chiari syndrome with hydrocephalus (Q07.-)
congenital hydrocephalus (Q03.-)
spina bifida with hydrocephalus (Q05.-)

(Ex) **For category G91 CC codes unless otherwise indicated:** E08.40-E08.49, E08.618-E08.638, E08.649-E08.8, E09.40-E09.49, E09.618-E09.638, E09.649-E09.8, E10.40-E10.49, E10.618-E10.638, E10.649, E10.69-E10.8, E11.40-E11.49, E11.618-E11.638, E11.649, E11.69-E11.8, E13.40-E13.49, E13.618-E13.638, E13.649-E13.8, G13.2-G13.8, G31.2, G31.83-G31.9, G91.0-G91.9, G93.81, G93.89-G94, Q03.0-Q03.9, Q04.4-Q04.8, Q05.0-Q05.4, Q05.9-Q06.1, Q06.3, Q06.8-Q06.9, Q07.02-Q07.9

G91.0   **Communicating hydrocephalus** 🔍
Secondary normal pressure hydrocephalus
(Ex) G91.0-G91.3, G91.8-G91.9

G91.1   **Obstructive hydrocephalus** 🔍

G91.2   **(Idiopathic) normal pressure hydrocephalus** 🔍
Normal pressure hydrocephalus NOS
(Ex) G91.0-G91.3, G91.8-G91.9

G91.3   **Post-traumatic hydrocephalus, unspecified** 🔍

▌ **G91.4**   *Hydrocephalus in diseases classified elsewhere*
Code first underlying condition, such as:
congenital syphilis (A50.4-)
neoplasm (C00-D49)

Excludes1   hydrocephalus due to congenital toxoplasmosis (P37.1)

G91.8   **Other hydrocephalus** 🔍

G91.9   **Hydrocephalus, unspecified** 🔍

G92   **Toxic encephalopathy** 🔍
Disorder or disease of brain caused by chemicals
Toxic encephalitis
Toxic metabolic encephalopathy

Code first (T51-T65) to identify toxic agent
(Ex) A17.82, A17.9, A18.82, A18.84, A18.89, A39.81, A50.42, A52.14, A83.0-A85.1, A85.8-A86, A88.8-A89, B00.4, B01.11, B10.01-B10.09, B26.2, B58.2, E08.40-E08.49, E08.618-E08.638, E08.649-E08.8, E09.40-E09.49, E09.618-E09.638, E09.649-E09.8, E10.40-E10.49, E10.618-E10.638, E10.649, E10.69-E10.8, E11.40-E11.49, E11.618-E11.638, E11.649, E11.69-E11.8, E13.40-E13.49, E13.618-E13.638, E13.649-E13.8, G04.00-G04.01, G04.31, G04.81-G05.4, G32.89, G37.3-G37.4, G92, G93.40-G93.49, G93.81, G93.89-G93.9, G96.8-G96.9, G98.0-G98.8, G99.8, I67.83

● **G93**   **Other disorders of brain**
G93.0   **Cerebral cysts**
Arachnoid cyst
Porencephalic cyst, acquired

Excludes1   acquired periventricular cysts of newborn (P91.1)
congenital cerebral cysts (Q04.6)

G93.1   **Anoxic brain damage, not elsewhere classified** 🔍
Permanent brain damage by lack of oxygen perfusion through brain tissues.

Excludes1   cerebral anoxia due to anesthesia during labor and delivery (O74.3)
cerebral anoxia due to anesthesia during the puerperium (O89.2)
neonatal anoxia (P84)

(Ex) E08.40-E08.49, E08.618-E08.638, E08.649-E08.8, E09.40-E09.49, E09.618-E09.638, E09.649-E09.8, E10.40-E10.49, E10.618-E10.638, E10.649, E10.69-E10.8, E11.40-E11.49, E11.618-E11.638, E11.649, E11.69-E11.8, E13.40-E13.49, E13.618-E13.638, E13.649-E13.8, G32.89, G93.1-G93.2, G96.8-G96.9, G98.0-G98.8, G99.8

G93.2   **Benign intracranial hypertension**

Excludes1   hypertensive encephalopathy (I67.4)

G93.3   **Postviral fatigue syndrome**
Benign myalgic encephalomyelitis

Excludes1   chronic fatigue syndrome NOS (R53.82)

● **G93.4**   **Other and unspecified encephalopathy**

Excludes1   alcoholic encephalopathy (G31.2)
encephalopathy in diseases classified elsewhere (G94)
hypertensive encephalopathy (I67.4)
toxic (metabolic) encephalopathy (G92)

G93.40   **Encephalopathy, unspecified** 🔍
(Ex) G21.0, G83.5, G93.41-G93.49, I67.83

G93.41   **Metabolic encephalopathy** 🔍
Septic encephalopathy
(Ex) G21.0, G83.5, G93.40-G93.49, I67.83
Coding Clinic: 2015, Q3, P21

G93.49   **Other encephalopathy** 🔍
Encephalopathy NEC
(Ex) G21.0, G83.5, G93.40-G93.41

G93.5   **Compression of brain** 🔍
Arnold-Chiari type 1 compression of brain
Compression of brain (stem)
Herniation of brain (stem)

Excludes1   diffuse traumatic compression of brain (S06.2-)
focal traumatic compression of brain (S06.3-)

(Ex) G81.90, G93.82

G93.6   **Cerebral edema** 🔍

Excludes1   cerebral edema due to birth injury (P11.0)
traumatic cerebral edema (S06.1-)

(Ex) G93.6, G93.82

G93.7   **Reye's syndrome** 🔍   P
Life-threatening neurological condition, usually follows viral illness
Code first (T39.0-), if salicylates-induced
(Ex) G93.7

● **G93.8**   **Other specified disorders of brain**
G93.81   **Temporal sclerosis**
Hippocampal sclerosis
Mesial temporal sclerosis

G93.82   **Brain death** 🔍
(Ex) B15.0-B19.9, E03.5, E08.00-E08.59, E08.618-E09.59, E09.618-E10.59, E10.618-E10.649, E10.69-E11.59, E11.618-E11.649, E11.69-E13.59, E13.618-E16.2, E89.1, G32.89, G89.0-G89.4, G93.81-G93.9, G96.8-G96.9, G98.0-G98.8, G99.8, I60.00-I62.9, K72.91, R29.700-R29.742, R40.0-R40.2124, R40.2210-R40.2224, R40.2310-R40.2324, R40.2340-R40.2344, R40.3-R41.3, R41.82, R41.9-R42, R44.8-R44.9, R45.83-R45.84, R46.0-R46.89, R52, R55, R68.0-R68.83, R68.89-R69, S02.0XX-S02.19X[A,B], S02.91X[A,B], S06.0X0-S06.0X1[A], S06.0X9-S06.9X9[A]

G93.89   **Other specified disorders of brain**
Postradiation encephalopathy

G93.9   **Disorder of brain, unspecified**

▌ **G94**   *Other disorders of brain in diseases classified elsewhere*
Code first underlying disease

Excludes1   encephalopathy in congenital syphilis (A50.49)
encephalopathy in influenza (J09.X9, J10.81, J11.81)
encephalopathy in syphilis (A52.19)
hydrocephalus in diseases classified elsewhere (G91.4)

● **G95**   **Other and unspecified diseases of spinal cord**

CHAPTER 6 (G00-G99)

Excludes2   myelitis (G04.-)

G95.0   **Syringomyelia and syringobulbia**
Ⓔ G04.1, G11.3, G11.8-G12.9, G32.0, G32.89-G37.3, G37.5-G37.9, G80.0-G80.2, G80.4-G83.9, G90.01-G90.09, G90.2, G90.4-G90.9, G93.40-G93.49, G93.81, G93.89-G93.9, G95.0-G95.9, G96.12-G96.9, G97.1, G98.0-G99.8, I67.83, R53.2

● G95.1   **Vascular myelopathies**
Excludes2   intraspinal phlebitis and thrombophlebitis, except non-pyogenic (G08)
Ⓔ For category G95.1 CC codes: See G90.5

G95.11   **Acute infarction of spinal cord (embolic) (nonembolic)**
Anoxia of spinal cord
Arterial thrombosis of spinal cord

G95.19   **Other vascular myelopathies**
Edema of spinal cord
Hematomyelia
Nonpyogenic intraspinal phlebitis and thrombophlebitis
Subacute necrotic myelopathy

● G95.2   **Other and unspecified cord compression**
Ⓔ For category G95.2 CC codes: E08.40-E08.49, E09.40-E09.49, E10.40-E10.49, E11.40-E11.49, E13.40-E13.49, G04.1, G11.3-G12.9, G32.0, G32.89-G37.9, G80.0-G80.2, G80.4-G83.9, G90.01-G90.09, G90.2, G90.4-G90.9, G93.1, G93.40-G93.49, G95.0-G95.9, G96.12-G96.9, G97.1, G98.0-G99.8, I67.83, R53.2

G95.20   Unspecified **cord compression**
G95.29   **Other cord compression**

● G95.8   **Other specified diseases of spinal cord**
Excludes1   neurogenic bladder NOS (N31.9)
neurogenic bladder due to cauda equina syndrome (G83.4)
neuromuscular dysfunction of bladder without spinal cord lesion (N31.-)
Ⓔ For category G95.8 CC codes: See G90.5

G95.81   **Conus medullaris syndrome**
Damage to gray matter and/or nerve roots in lower end of spinal cord

G95.89   **Other specified diseases of spinal cord**
Cord bladder NOS
Drug-induced myelopathy
Radiation-induced myelopathy
Excludes1   myelopathy NOS (G95.9)

G95.9   **Disease of spinal cord, unspecified**
Myelopathy NOS
Ⓔ See G95.2

● G96   **Other disorders of central nervous system**
G96.0   **Cerebrospinal fluid leak**
Excludes1   cerebrospinal fluid leak from spinal puncture (G97.0)
Ⓔ E08.40-E08.49, E08.618-E08.638, E08.649-E08.8, E09.40-E09.49, E09.618-E09.638, E09.649-E09.8, E10.40-E10.49, E10.618-E10.638, E10.649, E10.69-E10.8, E11.40-E11.49, E11.618-E11.638, E11.649, E11.69-E11.8, E13.40-E13.49, E13.618-E13.638, E13.649-E13.8, G32.89, G96.0, G96.8-G96.9, G98.0-G98.8, G99.8

● G96.1   **Disorders of meninges, not elsewhere classified**
G96.11   **Dural tear**
Excludes1   accidental puncture or laceration of dura during a procedure (G97.41)
Ⓔ D78.11-D78.12, D78.81-D78.89, E36.11-E36.8, E89.810-E89.89, G96.11, G97.41-G97.49, H59.011-H59.019, H59.031-H59.099, H59.211-H59.229, H59.811-H59.89, H95.31-H95.32, H95.811-H95.89, I97.3, I97.51-I97.52, J95.71-J95.72, K91.71-K91.72, L76.11-L76.12, L76.81-L76.82, M96.820-M96.821, M96.89, N98.1-N98.9, N99.71-N99.72, T81.82X[A], T81.89X-T81.9XX[A]

G96.12   **Meningeal adhesions (cerebral) (spinal)**
G96.19   **Other disorders of meninges, not elsewhere classified**

G96.8   **Other specified disorders of central nervous system**
G96.9   **Disorder of central nervous system, unspecified**

● G97   **Intraoperative and postprocedural complications and disorders of nervous system, not elsewhere classified**
Excludes2   intraoperative and postprocedural cerebrovascular infarction (I97.81-, I97.82-)

G97.0   **Cerebrospinal fluid leak from spinal puncture**
Ⓔ D78.81-D78.89, E36.8, E89.810-E89.89, G97.0, G97.2-G97.32, G97.81-G97.82, H59.011-H59.019, H59.031-H59.099, H59.811-H59.89, H95.811-H95.89, I97.3, I97.810-I97.821, L76.81-L76.82, M96.89, N98.1-N98.9, T81.82X[A], T81.89X-T81.9XX[A]

G97.1   **Other reaction to spinal and lumbar puncture**
Headache due to lumbar puncture

G97.2   **Intracranial hypotension following ventricular shunting**
Ⓔ See G97.0

● G97.3   **Intraoperative hemorrhage and hematoma of a nervous system organ or structure complicating a procedure**
Excludes1   intraoperative hemorrhage and hematoma of a nervous system organ or structure due to accidental puncture and laceration during a procedure (G97.4-)
Ⓔ For category G97.3 CC codes: G97.0, G97.2-G97.32, G97.81-G97.82, H95.811-H95.89, I97.3, I97.810-I97.821, M96.89, N98.1-N98.9, T81.82X[A], T81.89X-T81.9XX[A]

G97.31   **Intraoperative hemorrhage and hematoma of a nervous system organ or structure complicating a nervous system procedure**
G97.32   **Intraoperative hemorrhage and hematoma of a nervous system organ or structure complicating other procedure**

● G97.4   **Accidental puncture and laceration of a nervous system organ or structure during a procedure**
Ⓔ For category G97.4 CC codes: See G96.11

G97.41   **Accidental puncture or laceration of dura during a procedure**
Incidental (inadvertent) durotomy

G97.48   **Accidental puncture and laceration of other nervous system organ or structure during a nervous system procedure**

G97.49   **Accidental puncture and laceration of other nervous system organ or structure during other procedure**

● G97.5   **Postprocedural hemorrhage of a nervous system organ or structure following a procedure** ◀▥
Ⓔ For category G97.5 CC codes: G97.51-G97.52, G97.61-G97.64, H95.811-H95.89, I85.01, I85.11, I97.3, K21.9, K22.8, K23-K25.0, K25.2, K25.4, K25.6, K26.0, K26.2, K26.4, K26.6, K27.0, K27.2, K27.4, K27.6, K28.0, K28.2, K28.4, K28.6, K29.01, K29.21, K29.31, K29.41, K29.51, K29.61, K29.71, K29.91, K31.811, K55.21, K57.01, K57.11, K57.13, K57.21, K57.31, K57.33, K57.41, K57.51, K57.53, K57.81, K57.91, K57.93, K62.5, K92.0-K92.2, M96.89, N98.1-N98.9, P54.1-P54.3, T81.10X-T81.19X[A], T81.82X-T81.9XX[A]

G97.51   **Postprocedural hemorrhage of a nervous system organ or structure following a nervous system procedure** ◀▥
G97.52   **Postprocedural hemorrhage of a nervous system organ or structure following other procedure** ◀▥

● G97.6   **Postprocedural hematoma and seroma of a nervous system organ or structure following a procedure** ◀
Ⓔ For category G97.6 CC codes: See G97.5

G97.61   **Postprocedural hematoma of a nervous system organ or structure following a nervous system procedure** ◀
G97.62   **Postprocedural hematoma of a nervous system organ or structure following other procedure** ◀
G97.63   **Postprocedural seroma of a nervous system organ or structure following a nervous system procedure** ◀
G97.64   **Postprocedural seroma of a nervous system organ or structure following other procedure** ◀

CHAPTER 6 (G00-G99)

N   Newborn Age: 0   P   Pediatric Age: 0–17   M   Maternity DX: 12–55   A   Adult Age: 15–124   ♀   Females Only   ♂   Males Only

 Complication\Comorbidity   ◀▥ Major C\C   Ⓔ CC/MCC Exclusions   Hospital-Acquired Condition

● **G97.8 Other intraoperative and postprocedural complications and disorders of nervous system**

Use additional code to further specify disorder

(Ex:) For category G97.8 CC codes: See G97.0

G97.81 Other intraoperative complications of nervous system 🗨

G97.82 Other postprocedural complications and disorders of nervous system 🗨

● **G98 Other disorders of nervous system not elsewhere classified**

Includes   nervous system disorder NOS

G98.0 Neurogenic arthritis, not elsewhere classified

Nonsyphilitic neurogenic arthropathy NEC
Nonsyphilitic neurogenic spondylopathy NEC

Excludes1   spondylopathy (in):
syringomyelia and syringobulbia (G95.0)
tabes dorsalis (A52.11)

G98.8 Other disorders of nervous system

Nervous system disorder NOS

● **G99 Other disorders of nervous system in diseases classified elsewhere**

▌ **G99.0 *Autonomic neuropathy in diseases classified elsewhere*** 🗨

Code first underlying disease, such as:
amyloidosis (E85.-)
gout (M1A.-, M10.-)
hyperthyroidism (E05.-)

Excludes1   diabetic autonomic neuropathy (E08-E13 with .43)

(Ex:) G90.50-G90.59

▌ **G99.2 *Myelopathy in diseases classified elsewhere*** 🗨

Code first underlying disease, such as:
neoplasm (C00-D49)

Excludes1   myelopathy in:
intervertebral disease (M50.0-, M51.0-)
spondylosis (M47.0-, M47.1-)

(Ex:) See G90.5

▌ **G99.8 *Other specified disorders of nervous system in diseases classified elsewhere***

Code first underlying disorder, such as:
amyloidosis (E85.-)
avitaminosis (E56.9)

Excludes1   nervous system involvement in:
cysticercosis (B69.0)
rubella (B06.0-)
syphilis (A52.1-)

◀ New   ◀▬ Revised   ~~deleted~~ Deleted   Excludes 1   Excludes 2   Includes   Use additional   Code first   Code also   Unspecified

OGCR Official Guidelines   ● Unacceptable Principal Diagnosis   X Assign placeholder X   ● Use Additional Character(s)   ▌ Manifestation Code   **Coding Clinic**

CHAPTER 6 (G00-G99)

CHAPTER 7

DISEASES OF THE EYE AND ADNEXA (H00-H59)

OGCR Chapter-Specific Coding Guidelines

> 7. Chapter 7: Diseases of the Eye and Adnexa (H00-H59)
>   a. Glaucoma
>   1) **Assigning Glaucoma Codes**
>   Assign as many codes from category H40, Glaucoma, as needed to identify the type of glaucoma, the affected eye, and the glaucoma stage.
>   2) **Bilateral glaucoma with same type and stage**
>   When a patient has bilateral glaucoma and both eyes are documented as being the same type and stage, and there is a code for bilateral glaucoma, report only the code for the type of glaucoma, bilateral, with the seventh character for the stage.
>   When a patient has bilateral glaucoma and both eyes are documented as being the same type and stage, and the classification does not provide a code for bilateral glaucoma (i.e. subcategories H40.10, H40.11 and H40.20) report only one code for the type of glaucoma with the appropriate seventh character for the stage.
>   3) **Bilateral glaucoma stage with different types or stages**
>   When a patient has bilateral glaucoma and each eye is documented as having a different type or stage, and the classification distinguishes laterality, assign the appropriate code for each eye rather than the code for bilateral glaucoma.
>   When a patient has bilateral glaucoma and each eye is documented as having a different type, and the classification does not distinguish laterality (i.e. subcategories H40.10, H40.11 and H40.20), assign one code for each type of glaucoma with the appropriate seventh character for the stage.
>   When a patient has bilateral glaucoma and each eye is documented as having the same type, but different stage, and the classification does not distinguish laterality (i.e. subcategories H40.10, H40.11 and H40.20), assign a code for the type of glaucoma for each eye with the seventh character for the specific glaucoma stage documented for each eye.
>   4) **Patient admitted with glaucoma and stage evolves during the admission**
>   If a patient is admitted with glaucoma and the stage progresses during the admission, assign the code for highest stage documented.
>   5) **Indeterminate stage glaucoma**
>   Assignment of the seventh character "4" for "indeterminate stage" should be based on the clinical documentation. The seventh character "4" is used for glaucomas whose stage cannot be clinically determined. This seventh character should not be confused with the seventh character "0", unspecified, which should be assigned when there is no documentation regarding the stage of the glaucoma.

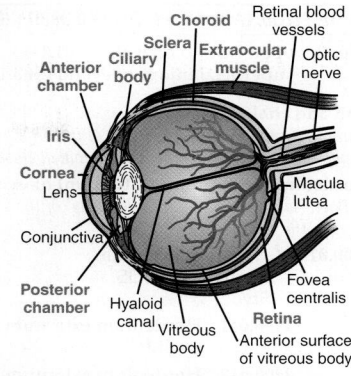

Figure 7-1 Eye and ocular adnexa. (From Buck CJ: Step-by-Step Medical Coding, ed 2016, St. Louis, Elsevier, 2016)

★ **(See Plate 87 on page 63.)**

CHAPTER 7

DISEASES OF THE EYE AND ADNEXA (H00-H59)

Note: Use an external cause code following the code for the eye condition, if applicable, to identify the cause of the eye condition

Excludes2 certain conditions originating in the perinatal period (P04-P96)

certain infectious and parasitic diseases (A00-B99)

complications of pregnancy, childbirth and the puerperium (O00-O9A)

congenital malformations, deformations, and chromosomal abnormalities (Q00-Q99)

diabetes mellitus related eye conditions (E09.3-, E10.3-, E11.3-, E13.3-)

endocrine, nutritional and metabolic diseases (E00-E88)

injury (trauma) of eye and orbit (S05.-)

injury, poisoning and certain other consequences of external causes (S00-T88)

neoplasms (C00-D49)

symptoms, signs and abnormal clinical and laboratory findings, not elsewhere classified (R00-R94)

syphilis related eye disorders (A50.01, A50.3-, A51.43, A52.71)

This chapter contains the following blocks:

H00-H05	Disorders of eyelid, lacrimal system and orbit
H10-H11	Disorders of conjunctiva
H15-H22	Disorders of sclera, cornea, iris and ciliary body
H25-H28	Disorders of lens
H30-H36	Disorders of choroid and retina
H40-H42	Glaucoma
H43-H44	Disorders of vitreous body and globe
H46-H47	Disorders of optic nerve and visual pathways
H49-H52	Disorders of ocular muscles, binocular movement, accommodation and refraction
H53-H54	Visual disturbances and blindness
H55-H57	Other disorders of eye and adnexa
H59	Intraoperative and postprocedural complications and disorders of eye and adnexa, not elsewhere classified

N Newborn Age: 0   **P** Pediatric Age: 0-17   **M** Maternity DX: 12-55   **A** Adult Age: 15-124   ♀ Females Only   ♂ Males Only

🔖 Complication\Comorbidity   🔖 Major C\C   Ⓔⓧ CC/MCC Exclusions   🔖 Hospital-Acquired Condition

809

DISORDERS OF EYELID, LACRIMAL SYSTEM AND ORBIT (H00–H05)

Excludes2   open wound of eyelid (S01.1-)
superficial injury of eyelid (S00.1-, S00.2-)

● **H00**   Hordeolum and chalazion

Hordeolum: inflammatory staphylococcal infection of sebaceous glands of eyelids; AKA stye. Chalazion: eyelid mass

● **H00.0**   Hordeolum (externum) (internum) of eyelid

Bacterial infection (staphylococcus) of the sebaceous gland of the eyelid (stye)

● **H00.01**   Hordeolum externum
Hordeolum NOS
Stye

H00.011   Hordeolum externum right upper eyelid

H00.012   Hordeolum externum right lower eyelid

H00.013   Hordeolum externum right eye, unspecified eyelid

H00.014   Hordeolum externum left upper eyelid

H00.015   Hordeolum externum left lower eyelid

H00.016   Hordeolum externum left eye, unspecified eyelid

H00.019   Hordeolum externum unspecified eye, unspecified eyelid

● **H00.02**   Hordeolum internum
Infection of meibomian gland

H00.021   Hordeolum internum right upper eyelid

H00.022   Hordeolum internum right lower eyelid

H00.023   Hordeolum internum right eye, unspecified eyelid

H00.024   Hordeolum internum left upper eyelid

H00.025   Hordeolum internum left lower eyelid

H00.026   Hordeolum internum left eye, unspecified eyelid

H00.029   Hordeolum internum unspecified eye, unspecified eyelid

● **H00.03**   Abscess of eyelid
Furuncle of eyelid

H00.031   Abscess of right upper eyelid

H00.032   Abscess of right lower eyelid

H00.033   Abscess of eyelid right eye, unspecified eyelid

H00.034   Abscess of left upper eyelid

H00.035   Abscess of left lower eyelid

H00.036   Abscess of eyelid left eye, unspecified eyelid

H00.039   Abscess of eyelid unspecified eye, unspecified eyelid

● **H00.1**   Chalazion

Often caused by accumulation of meibomian gland secretions resulting from a blockage of duct.

Meibomian (gland) cyst

Excludes2   infected meibomian gland (H00.02-)

H00.11   Chalazion right upper eyelid

H00.12   Chalazion right lower eyelid

H00.13   Chalazion right eye, unspecified eyelid

H00.14   Chalazion left upper eyelid

H00.15   Chalazion left lower eyelid

H00.16   Chalazion left eye, unspecified eyelid

H00.19   Chalazion unspecified eye, unspecified eyelid

● **H01**   Other inflammation of eyelid

● **H01.0**   Blepharitis
Inflammation of eyelids

Excludes1   blepharoconjunctivitis (H10.5-)

● **H01.00**   Unspecified blepharitis

H01.001   Unspecified blepharitis right upper eyelid

H01.002   Unspecified blepharitis right lower eyelid

H01.003   Unspecified blepharitis right eye, unspecified eyelid

H01.004   Unspecified blepharitis left upper eyelid

H01.005   Unspecified blepharitis left lower eyelid

H01.006   Unspecified blepharitis left eye, unspecified eyelid

H01.009   Unspecified blepharitis unspecified eye, unspecified eyelid

● **H01.01**   Ulcerative blepharitis

H01.011   Ulcerative blepharitis right upper eyelid

H01.012   Ulcerative blepharitis right lower eyelid

H01.013   Ulcerative blepharitis right eye, unspecified eyelid

H01.014   Ulcerative blepharitis left upper eyelid

H01.015   Ulcerative blepharitis left lower eyelid

H01.016   Ulcerative blepharitis left eye, unspecified eyelid

H01.019   Ulcerative blepharitis unspecified eye, unspecified eyelid

● **H01.02**   Squamous blepharitis

H01.021   Squamous blepharitis right upper eyelid

H01.022   Squamous blepharitis right lower eyelid

H01.023   Squamous blepharitis right eye, unspecified eyelid

H01.024   Squamous blepharitis left upper eyelid

H01.025   Squamous blepharitis left lower eyelid

H01.026   Squamous blepharitis left eye, unspecified eyelid

H01.029   Squamous blepharitis unspecified eye, unspecified eyelid

● **H01.1**   Noninfectious dermatoses of eyelid

● **H01.11**   Allergic dermatitis of eyelid
Contact dermatitis of eyelid

H01.111   Allergic dermatitis of right upper eyelid

H01.112   Allergic dermatitis of right lower eyelid

H01.113   Allergic dermatitis of right eye, unspecified eyelid

H01.114   Allergic dermatitis of left upper eyelid

H01.115   Allergic dermatitis of left lower eyelid

H01.116   Allergic dermatitis of left eye, unspecified eyelid

H01.119   Allergic dermatitis of unspecified eye, unspecified eyelid

◀ New   ◀◀ Revised   ~~deleted~~ Deleted   Excludes 1   Excludes 2   Includes   Use additional   Code first   Code also   Unspecified

OGCR Official Guidelines   ● Unacceptable Principal Diagnosis   X Assign placeholder X   ● Use Additional Character(s)   ▶ Manifestation Code   **Coding Clinic**

● H01.12   Discoid lupus erythematosus of eyelid
     H01.121   Discoid lupus erythematosus of right upper eyelid
     H01.122   Discoid lupus erythematosus of right lower eyelid
     H01.123   Discoid lupus erythematosus of right eye, unspecified eyelid
     H01.124   Discoid lupus erythematosus of left upper eyelid
     H01.125   Discoid lupus erythematosus of left lower eyelid
     H01.126   Discoid lupus erythematosus of left eye, unspecified eyelid
     H01.129   Discoid lupus erythematosus of unspecified eye, unspecified eyelid

● H01.13   Eczematous dermatitis of eyelid
     H01.131   Eczematous dermatitis of right upper eyelid
     H01.132   Eczematous dermatitis of right lower eyelid
     H01.133   Eczematous dermatitis of right eye, unspecified eyelid
     H01.134   Eczematous dermatitis of left upper eyelid
     H01.135   Eczematous dermatitis of left lower eyelid
     H01.136   Eczematous dermatitis of left eye, unspecified eyelid
     H01.139   Eczematous dermatitis of unspecified eye, unspecified eyelid

● H01.14   Xeroderma of eyelid
     Abnormally dry
     H01.141   Xeroderma of right upper eyelid
     H01.142   Xeroderma of right lower eyelid
     H01.143   Xeroderma of right eye, unspecified eyelid
     H01.144   Xeroderma of left upper eyelid
     H01.145   Xeroderma of left lower eyelid
     H01.146   Xeroderma of left eye, unspecified eyelid
     H01.149   Xeroderma of unspecified eye, unspecified eyelid

  H01.8   Other specified inflammations of eyelid

  H01.9   Unspecified inflammation of eyelid
     Inflammation of eyelid NOS

● H02   Other disorders of eyelid
     Turning inward (inversion) of eyelid margin and ingrowing eyelashes
     Excludes1   congenital malformations of eyelid (Q10.0-Q10.3)

● H02.0   Entropion and trichiasis of eyelid
   ● H02.00   Unspecified entropion of eyelid
     H02.001   Unspecified entropion of right upper eyelid
     H02.002   Unspecified entropion of right lower eyelid
     H02.003   Unspecified entropion of right eye, unspecified eyelid
     H02.004   Unspecified entropion of left upper eyelid

     H02.005   Unspecified entropion of left lower eyelid
     H02.006   Unspecified entropion of left eye, unspecified eyelid
     H02.009   Unspecified entropion of unspecified eye, unspecified eyelid

● H02.01   Cicatricial entropion of eyelid
     Scar
     H02.011   Cicatricial entropion of right upper eyelid
     H02.012   Cicatricial entropion of right lower eyelid
     H02.013   Cicatricial entropion of right eye, unspecified eyelid
     H02.014   Cicatricial entropion of left upper eyelid
     H02.015   Cicatricial entropion of left lower eyelid
     H02.016   Cicatricial entropion of left eye, unspecified eyelid
     H02.019   Cicatricial entropion of unspecified eye, unspecified eyelid

● H02.02   Mechanical entropion of eyelid
     Turning inward (inversion) of eyelid margin due to lack of support
     H02.021   Mechanical entropion of right upper eyelid
     H02.022   Mechanical entropion of right lower eyelid
     H02.023   Mechanical entropion of right eye, unspecified eyelid
     H02.024   Mechanical entropion of left upper eyelid
     H02.025   Mechanical entropion of left lower eyelid
     H02.026   Mechanical entropion of left eye, unspecified eyelid
     H02.029   Mechanical entropion of unspecified eye, unspecified eyelid

● H02.03   Senile entropion of eyelid
     Turning inward (inversion) of eyelid margin due to aging
     H02.031   Senile entropion of right upper eyelid   A
     H02.032   Senile entropion of right lower eyelid   A
     H02.033   Senile entropion of right eye, unspecified eyelid   A
     H02.034   Senile entropion of left upper eyelid   A
     H02.035   Senile entropion of left lower eyelid   A
     H02.036   Senile entropion of left eye, unspecified eyelid   A
     H02.039   Senile entropion of unspecified eye, unspecified eyelid   A

● H02.04   Spastic entropion of eyelid
     Turning inward (inversion) of eyelid margin caused by spasm of muscle
     H02.041   Spastic entropion of right upper eyelid
     H02.042   Spastic entropion of right lower eyelid
     H02.043   Spastic entropion of right eye, unspecified eyelid
     H02.044   Spastic entropion of left upper eyelid
     H02.045   Spastic entropion of left lower eyelid
     H02.046   Spastic entropion of left eye, unspecified eyelid
     H02.049   Spastic entropion of unspecified eye, unspecified eyelid

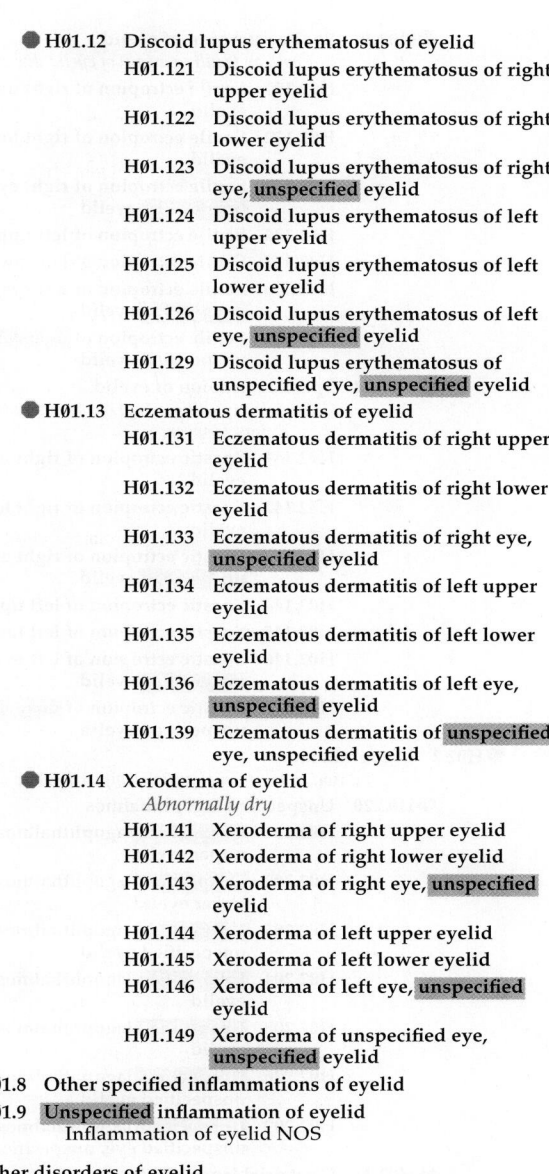

Figure 7-2   Right lower eyelid entropion. Note the inward rotation of the tarsal plate about the horizontal axis and the resultant contact between the mucocutaneous junction and ocular surface. (From Yanoff: Ophthalmology, ed 3, Mosby, Inc., 2008)

CHAPTER 7 (H00-H59)

N   Newborn Age: 0   P   Pediatric Age: 0–17   M   Maternity DX: 12–55   A   Adult Age: 15–124   ♀   Females Only   ♂   Males Only

   🐾   Complication\Comorbidity   🐾   Major C\C   (Ex)   CC/MCC Exclusions   🐾   Hospital-Acquired Condition

● **H02.05**   **Trichiasis without entropian**
Ingrowing hairs of eyelashes

    H02.051   Trichiasis without entropian right upper eyelid

    H02.052   Trichiasis without entropian right lower eyelid

    H02.053   Trichiasis without entropian right eye, unspecified eyelid

    H02.054   Trichiasis without entropian left upper eyelid

    H02.055   Trichiasis without entropian left lower eyelid

    H02.056   Trichiasis without entropian left eye, unspecified eyelid

    H02.059   Trichiasis without entropian unspecified eye, unspecified eyelid

● **H02.1**   **Ectropion of eyelid**
Eversion (pulling away) of eyelid

● **H02.10**   **Unspecified ectropion of eyelid**

    H02.101   Unspecified ectropion of right upper eyelid

    H02.102   Unspecified ectropion of right lower eyelid

    H02.103   Unspecified ectropion of right eye, unspecified eyelid

    H02.104   Unspecified ectropion of left upper eyelid

    H02.105   Unspecified ectropion of left lower eyelid

    H02.106   Unspecified ectropion of left eye, unspecified eyelid

    H02.109   Unspecified ectropion of unspecified eye, unspecified eyelid

● **H02.11**   **Cicatricial ectropion of eyelid**
Pulling of eyelid down and away from eye due to scar or tightening

    H02.111   Cicatricial ectropion of right upper eyelid

    H02.112   Cicatricial ectropion of right lower eyelid

    H02.113   Cicatricial ectropion of right eye, unspecified eyelid

    H02.114   Cicatricial ectropion of left upper eyelid

    H02.115   Cicatricial ectropion of left lower eyelid

    H02.116   Cicatricial ectropion of left eye, unspecified eyelid

    H02.119   Cicatricial ectropion of unspecified eye, unspecified eyelid

● **H02.12**   **Mechanical ectropion of eyelid**
Eversion (pulling away) of eyelid due to lack of support

    H02.121   Mechanical ectropion of right upper eyelid

    H02.122   Mechanical ectropion of right lower eyelid

    H02.123   Mechanical ectropion of right eye, unspecified eyelid

    H02.124   Mechanical ectropion of left upper eyelid

    H02.125   Mechanical ectropion of left lower eyelid

    H02.126   Mechanical ectropion of left eye, unspecified eyelid

    H02.129   Mechanical ectropion of unspecified eye, unspecified eyelid

● **H02.13**   **Senile ectropion of eyelid**
Eversion (pulling away) of eyelid due to age

    H02.131   Senile ectropion of right upper eyelid   A

    H02.132   Senile ectropion of right lower eyelid   A

    H02.133   Senile ectropion of right eye, unspecified eyelid   A

    H02.134   Senile ectropion of left upper eyelid   A

    H02.135   Senile ectropion of left lower eyelid   A

    H02.136   Senile ectropion of left eye, unspecified eyelid   A

    H02.139   Senile ectropion of unspecified eye, unspecified eyelid   A

● **H02.14**   **Spastic ectropion of eyelid**
Eversion (pulling away) of eyelid due to tonic muscle spasm

    H02.141   Spastic ectropion of right upper eyelid

    H02.142   Spastic ectropion of right lower eyelid

    H02.143   Spastic ectropion of right eye, unspecified eyelid

    H02.144   Spastic ectropion of left upper eyelid

    H02.145   Spastic ectropion of left lower eyelid

    H02.146   Spastic ectropion of left eye, unspecified eyelid

    H02.149   Spastic ectropion of unspecified eye, unspecified eyelid

● **H02.2**   **Lagophthalmos**
Condition in which eye cannot completely close

● **H02.20**   **Unspecified lagophthalmos**

    H02.201   Unspecified lagophthalmos right upper eyelid

    H02.202   Unspecified lagophthalmos right lower eyelid

    H02.203   Unspecified lagophthalmos right eye, unspecified eyelid

    H02.204   Unspecified lagophthalmos left upper eyelid

    H02.205   Unspecified lagophthalmos left lower eyelid

    H02.206   Unspecified lagophthalmos left eye, unspecified eyelid

    H02.209   Unspecified lagophthalmos unspecified eye, unspecified eyelid

● **H02.21**   **Cicatricial lagophthalmos**
Upper or lower eyelid does not close due to scar or tightening

    H02.211   Cicatricial lagophthalmos right upper eyelid

    H02.212   Cicatricial lagophthalmos right lower eyelid

    H02.213   Cicatricial lagophthalmos right eye, unspecified eyelid

    H02.214   Cicatricial lagophthalmos left upper eyelid

    H02.215   Cicatricial lagophthalmos left lower eyelid

    H02.216   Cicatricial lagophthalmos left eye, unspecified eyelid

    H02.219   Cicatricial lagophthalmos unspecified eye, unspecified eyelid

◀ New   ◀◀ Revised   ~~deleted~~ Deleted   Excludes 1   Excludes 2   Includes   Use additional   Code first   Code also   Unspecified

812   OGCR Official Guidelines   ● Unacceptable Principal Diagnosis   X Assign placeholder X   ● Use Additional Character(s)   ▶ Manifestation Code   **Coding Clinic**

● **H02.22** **Mechanical lagophthalmos**
    Inability to close lids due to structural disorder
    H02.221 **Mechanical lagophthalmos right upper eyelid**
    H02.222 **Mechanical lagophthalmos right lower eyelid**
    H02.223 **Mechanical lagophthalmos right eye, unspecified eyelid**
    H02.224 **Mechanical lagophthalmos left upper eyelid**
    H02.225 **Mechanical lagophthalmos left lower eyelid**
    H02.226 **Mechanical lagophthalmos left eye, unspecified eyelid**
    H02.229 **Mechanical lagophthalmos unspecified eye, unspecified eyelid**

● **H02.23** **Paralytic lagophthalmos**
    Eyelids do not close due to paralysis
    H02.231 **Paralytic lagophthalmos right upper eyelid**
    H02.232 **Paralytic lagophthalmos right lower eyelid**
    H02.233 **Paralytic lagophthalmos right eye, unspecified eyelid**
    H02.234 **Paralytic lagophthalmos left upper eyelid**
    H02.235 **Paralytic lagophthalmos left lower eyelid**
    H02.236 **Paralytic lagophthalmos left eye, unspecified eyelid**
    H02.239 **Paralytic lagophthalmos unspecified eye, unspecified eyelid**

★ **(See Plate 81, middle, on page 65.)**

● **H02.3** **Blepharochalasis**
    Relaxation of skin of eyelid, due to atrophy of intercellular tissue
    Pseudoptosis
    H02.30 **Blepharochalasis unspecified eye, unspecified eyelid**
    H02.31 **Blepharochalasis right upper eyelid**
    H02.32 **Blepharochalasis right lower eyelid**
    H02.33 **Blepharochalasis right eye, unspecified eyelid**
    H02.34 **Blepharochalasis left upper eyelid**
    H02.35 **Blepharochalasis left lower eyelid**
    H02.36 **Blepharochalasis left eye, unspecified eyelid**

● **H02.4** **Ptosis of eyelid**
    Falling forward, drooping, sagging of eyelid
    ● **H02.40** **Unspecified ptosis of eyelid**
        H02.401 **Unspecified ptosis of right eyelid**
        H02.402 **Unspecified ptosis of left eyelid**
        H02.403 **Unspecified ptosis of bilateral eyelids**
        H02.409 **Unspecified ptosis of unspecified eyelid**
    ● **H02.41** **Mechanical ptosis of eyelid**
        H02.411 **Mechanical ptosis of right eyelid**
        H02.412 **Mechanical ptosis of left eyelid**
        H02.413 **Mechanical ptosis of bilateral eyelids**
        H02.419 **Mechanical ptosis of unspecified eyelid**

● **H02.42** **Myogenic ptosis of eyelid**
    H02.421 **Myogenic ptosis of right eyelid**
    H02.422 **Myogenic ptosis of left eyelid**
    H02.423 **Myogenic ptosis of bilateral eyelids**
    H02.429 **Myogenic ptosis of unspecified eyelid**

● **H02.43** **Paralytic ptosis of eyelid**
    Neurogenic ptosis of eyelid
    H02.431 **Paralytic ptosis of right eyelid**
    H02.432 **Paralytic ptosis of left eyelid**
    H02.433 **Paralytic ptosis of bilateral eyelids**
    H02.439 **Paralytic ptosis unspecified eyelid**

● **H02.5** **Other disorders affecting eyelid function**
    Excludes2 blepharospasm (G24.5)
        organic tic (G25.69)
        psychogenic tic (F95.-)
    ● **H02.51** **Abnormal innervation syndrome**
        H02.511 **Abnormal innervation syndrome right upper eyelid**
        H02.512 **Abnormal innervation syndrome right lower eyelid**
        H02.513 **Abnormal innervation syndrome right eye, unspecified eyelid**
        H02.514 **Abnormal innervation syndrome left upper eyelid**
        H02.515 **Abnormal innervation syndrome left lower eyelid**
        H02.516 **Abnormal innervation syndrome left eye, unspecified eyelid**
        H02.519 **Abnormal innervation syndrome unspecified eye, unspecified eyelid**
    ● **H02.52** **Blepharophimosis**
        Drooping of eyelid with reduced lid size
        Ankyloblepharon
        H02.521 **Blepharophimosis right upper eyelid**
        H02.522 **Blepharophimosis right lower eyelid**
        H02.523 **Blepharophimosis right eye, unspecified eyelid**
        H02.524 **Blepharophimosis left upper eyelid**
        H02.525 **Blepharophimosis left lower eyelid**
        H02.526 **Blepharophimosis left eye, unspecified eyelid**
        H02.529 **Blepharophimosis unspecified eye, unspecified lid**
    ● **H02.53** **Eyelid retraction**
        Eyelid lag
        H02.531 **Eyelid retraction right upper eyelid**
        H02.532 **Eyelid retraction right lower eyelid**
        H02.533 **Eyelid retraction right eye, unspecified eyelid**
        H02.534 **Eyelid retraction left upper eyelid**
        H02.535 **Eyelid retraction left lower eyelid**
        H02.536 **Eyelid retraction left eye, unspecified eyelid**
        H02.539 **Eyelid retraction unspecified eye, unspecified lid**
    H02.59 **Other disorders affecting eyelid function**
        Deficient blink reflex
        Sensory disorders

Figure 7-3 Ptosis of eyelid. (From Yanoff: Ophthalmology, ed 3, Mosby, Inc., 2008)

Item 7-1 Ptosis of eyelid is drooping of the upper eyelid over the pupil when the eyes are fully opened resulting from nerve or muscle damage, which may require surgical correction.

● H02.6   **Xanthelasma of eyelid**
Yellow-to-orange patches or pimples clustered together on eyelid

    H02.60   Xanthelasma of unspecified eye, unspecified eyelid

    H02.61   Xanthelasma of right upper eyelid

    H02.62   Xanthelasma of right lower eyelid

    H02.63   Xanthelasma of right eye, unspecified eyelid

    H02.64   Xanthelasma of left upper eyelid

    H02.65   Xanthelasma of left lower eyelid

    H02.66   Xanthelasma of left eye, unspecified eyelid

● H02.7   **Other and unspecified degenerative disorders of eyelid and periocular area**

    H02.70   Unspecified degenerative disorders of eyelid and periocular area

●   H02.71   **Chloasma of eyelid and periocular area**
Dyspigmentation of eyelid
Hyperpigmentation of eyelid

    H02.711   Chloasma of right upper eyelid and periocular area

    H02.712   Chloasma of right lower eyelid and periocular area

    H02.713   Chloasma of right eye, unspecified eyelid and periocular area

    H02.714   Chloasma of left upper eyelid and periocular area

    H02.715   Chloasma of left lower eyelid and periocular area

    H02.716   Chloasma of left eye, unspecified eyelid and periocular area

    H02.719   Chloasma of unspecified eye, unspecified eyelid and periocular area

●   H02.72   **Madarosis of eyelid and periocular area**
Loss of eyelashes and/or eyebrows
Hypotrichosis of eyelid

    H02.721   Madarosis of right upper eyelid and periocular area

    H02.722   Madarosis of right lower eyelid and periocular area

    H02.723   Madarosis of right eye, unspecified eyelid and periocular area

    H02.724   Madarosis of left upper eyelid and periocular area

    H02.725   Madarosis of left lower eyelid and periocular area

    H02.726   Madarosis of left eye, unspecified eyelid and periocular area

    H02.729   Madarosis of unspecified eye, unspecified eyelid and periocular area

●   H02.73   **Vitiligo of eyelid and periocular area**
Skin pigmentation disease characterized by white patches
Hypopigmentation of eyelid

    H02.731   Vitiligo of right upper eyelid and periocular area

    H02.732   Vitiligo of right lower eyelid and periocular area

    H02.733   Vitiligo of right eye, unspecified eyelid and periocular area

    H02.734   Vitiligo of left upper eyelid and periocular area

    H02.735   Vitiligo of left lower eyelid and periocular area

    H02.736   Vitiligo of left eye, unspecified eyelid and periocular area

    H02.739   Vitiligo of unspecified eye, unspecified eyelid and periocular area

●   H02.79   **Other degenerative disorders of eyelid and periocular area**

● H02.8   **Other specified disorders of eyelid**

●   H02.81   **Retained foreign body in eyelid**
Use additional code to identify the type of retained foreign body (Z18.-)

    Excludes 1   laceration of eyelid with foreign body (S01.12-)
       retained intraocular foreign body (H44.6-, H44.7-)
       superficial foreign body of eyelid and periocular area (S00.25-)

    H02.811   Retained foreign body in right upper eyelid

    H02.812   Retained foreign body in right lower eyelid

    H02.813   Retained foreign body in right eye, unspecified eyelid

    H02.814   Retained foreign body in left upper eyelid

    H02.815   Retained foreign body in left lower eyelid

    H02.816   Retained foreign body in left eye, unspecified eyelid

    H02.819   Retained foreign body in unspecified eye, unspecified eyelid

●   H02.82   **Cysts of eyelid**
Sebaceous cyst of eyelid

    H02.821   Cysts of right upper eyelid

    H02.822   Cysts of right lower eyelid

    H02.823   Cysts of right eye, unspecified eyelid

    H02.824   Cysts of left upper eyelid

    H02.825   Cysts of left lower eyelid

    H02.826   Cysts of left eye, unspecified eyelid

    H02.829   Cysts of unspecified eye, unspecified eyelid

●   H02.83   **Dermatochalasis of eyelid**
Skin is inelastic and hangs loosely in folds

    H02.831   Dermatochalasis of right upper eyelid

    H02.832   Dermatochalasis of right lower eyelid

    H02.833   Dermatochalasis of right eye, unspecified eyelid

    H02.834   Dermatochalasis of left upper eyelid

    H02.835   Dermatochalasis of left lower eyelid

    H02.836   Dermatochalasis of left eye, unspecified eyelid

    H02.839   Dermatochalasis of unspecified eye, unspecified eyelid

●   H02.84   **Edema of eyelid**
Hyperemia of eyelid

    H02.841   Edema of right upper eyelid

    H02.842   Edema of right lower eyelid

    H02.843   Edema of right eye, unspecified eyelid

    H02.844   Edema of left upper eyelid

    H02.845   Edema of left lower eyelid

    H02.846   Edema of left eye, unspecified eyelid

    H02.849   Edema of unspecified eye, unspecified eyelid

●   H02.85   **Elephantiasis of eyelid**
Massive secondary lymphedema with hypertrophy of skin and subcutaneous tissues (pachyderma)

    H02.851   Elephantiasis of right upper eyelid

    H02.852   Elephantiasis of right lower eyelid

    H02.853   Elephantiasis of right eye, unspecified eyelid

    H02.854   Elephantiasis of left upper eyelid

    H02.855   Elephantiasis of left lower eyelid

◀ New   ◀▥ Revised   ~~deleted~~ Deleted   Excludes 1   Excludes 2   Includes   Use additional   Code first   Code also   Unspecified

OGCR Official Guidelines   ● Unacceptable Principal Diagnosis   X Assign placeholder X   ● Use Additional Character(s)   ▸ Manifestation Code   **Coding Clinic**

H02.856   Elephantiasis of left eye, unspecified eyelid

H02.859   Elephantiasis of unspecified eye, unspecified eyelid

● **H02.86**   Hypertrichosis of eyelid
Excessive growth of hair

H02.861   Hypertrichosis of right upper eyelid

H02.862   Hypertrichosis of right lower eyelid

H02.863   Hypertrichosis of right eye, unspecified eyelid

H02.864   Hypertrichosis of left upper eyelid

H02.865   Hypertrichosis of left lower eyelid

H02.866   Hypertrichosis of left eye, unspecified eyelid

H02.869   Hypertrichosis of unspecified eye, unspecified eyelid

● **H02.87**   Vascular anomalies of eyelid

H02.871   Vascular anomalies of right upper eyelid

H02.872   Vascular anomalies of right lower eyelid

H02.873   Vascular anomalies of right eye, unspecified eyelid

H02.874   Vascular anomalies of left upper eyelid

H02.875   Vascular anomalies of left lower eyelid

H02.876   Vascular anomalies of left eye, unspecified eyelid

H02.879   Vascular anomalies of unspecified eye, unspecified eyelid

H02.89   Other specified disorders of eyelid
Hemorrhage of eyelid

H02.9   Unspecified disorder of eyelid
Disorder of eyelid NOS

● **H04**   **Disorders of lacrimal system**
Excludes1   congenital malformations of lacrimal system (Q10.4-Q10.6)

● **H04.0**   Dacryoadenitis
Inflammation of lacrimal gland

● **H04.00**   Unspecified dacryoadenitis

H04.001   Unspecified dacryoadenitis, right lacrimal gland

H04.002   Unspecified dacryoadenitis, left lacrimal gland

H04.003   Unspecified dacryoadenitis, bilateral lacrimal glands

H04.009   Unspecified dacryoadenitis, unspecified lacrimal gland

● **H04.01**   Acute dacryoadenitis

H04.011   Acute dacryoadenitis, right lacrimal gland

H04.012   Acute dacryoadenitis, left lacrimal gland

H04.013   Acute dacryoadenitis, bilateral lacrimal glands

H04.019   Acute dacryoadenitis, unspecified lacrimal gland

Figure 7-4   Lacrimal apparatus. (From Buck CJ: Step-by-Step Medical Coding, 2016, St. Louis, Elsevier, 2016)

★ **(See Plate 82 on page 67.)**

● **H04.02**   Chronic dacryoadenitis

H04.021   Chronic dacryoadenitis, right lacrimal gland

H04.022   Chronic dacryoadenitis, left lacrimal gland

H04.023   Chronic dacryoadenitis, bilateral lacrimal gland

H04.029   Chronic dacryoadenitis, unspecified lacrimal gland

● **H04.03**   Chronic enlargement of lacrimal gland

H04.031   Chronic enlargement of right lacrimal gland

H04.032   Chronic enlargement of left lacrimal gland

H04.033   Chronic enlargement of bilateral lacrimal glands

H04.039   Chronic enlargement of unspecified lacrimal gland

● **H04.1**   Other disorders of lacrimal gland

● **H04.11**   Dacryops
Watery eye or distention of lacrimal duct due to fluid

H04.111   Dacryops of right lacrimal gland

H04.112   Dacryops of left lacrimal gland

H04.113   Dacryops of bilateral lacrimal glands

H04.119   Dacryops of unspecified lacrimal gland

● **H04.12**   Dry eye syndrome
Tear film insufficiency, NOS

H04.121   Dry eye syndrome of right lacrimal gland

H04.122   Dry eye syndrome of left lacrimal gland

H04.123   Dry eye syndrome of bilateral lacrimal glands

H04.129   Dry eye syndrome of unspecified lacrimal gland

● **H04.13**   Lacrimal cyst
Lacrimal cystic degeneration

H04.131   Lacrimal cyst right lacrimal gland

H04.132   Lacrimal cyst left lacrimal gland

H04.133   Lacrimal cyst bilateral lacrimal glands

H04.139   Lacrimal cyst unspecified lacrimal gland

● **H04.14**   Primary lacrimal gland atrophy

H04.141   Primary lacrimal gland atrophy, right lacrimal gland

H04.142   Primary lacrimal gland atrophy, left lacrimal gland

H04.143   Primary lacrimal gland atrophy, bilateral lacrimal glands

H04.149   Primary lacrimal gland atrophy, unspecified lacrimal gland

● **H04.15**   Secondary lacrimal gland atrophy

H04.151   Secondary lacrimal gland atrophy, right lacrimal gland

H04.152   Secondary lacrimal gland atrophy, left lacrimal gland

H04.153   Secondary lacrimal gland atrophy, bilateral lacrimal glands

H04.159   Secondary lacrimal gland atrophy, unspecified lacrimal gland

● **H04.16**   Lacrimal gland dislocation

H04.161   Lacrimal gland dislocation, right lacrimal gland

H04.162   Lacrimal gland dislocation, left lacrimal gland

N Newborn Age: 0   **P** Pediatric Age: 0–17   **M** Maternity DX: 12–55   **A** Adult Age: 15–124   ♀ Females Only   ♂ Males Only

   Complication\Comorbidity   Major C\C   Ⓔ CC/MCC Exclusions   Hospital-Acquired Condition

815

CHAPTER 7 (H00-H59)

H04.163　Lacrimal gland dislocation, bilateral lacrimal glands
H04.169　Lacrimal gland dislocation, unspecified lacrimal gland
H04.19　Other specified disorders of lacrimal gland
● H04.2　Epiphora
Overflow of tears due to stricture of lacrimal passages; AKA lacrimation
　● H04.20　Unspecified epiphora
　　H04.201　Unspecified epiphora, right lacrimal gland
　　H04.202　Unspecified epiphora, left lacrimal gland
　　H04.203　Unspecified epiphora, bilateral lacrimal glands
　　H04.209　Unspecified epiphora, unspecified lacrimal gland
　● H04.21　Epiphora due to excess lacrimation
　　H04.211　Epiphora due to excess lacrimation, right lacrimal gland
　　H04.212　Epiphora due to excess lacrimation, left lacrimal gland
　　H04.213　Epiphora due to excess lacrimation, bilateral lacrimal glands
　　H04.219　Epiphora due to excess lacrimation, unspecified lacrimal gland
　● H04.22　Epiphora due to insufficient drainage
　　H04.221　Epiphora due to insufficient drainage, right lacrimal gland
　　H04.222　Epiphora due to insufficient drainage, left lacrimal gland
　　H04.223　Epiphora due to insufficient drainage, bilateral lacrimal glands
　　H04.229　Epiphora due to insufficient drainage, unspecified lacrimal gland
● H04.3　Acute and unspecified inflammation of lacrimal passages
　　Excludes1　neonatal dacryocystitis (P39.1)
　● H04.30　Unspecified dacryocystitis
　　H04.301　Unspecified dacryocystitis of right lacrimal passage
　　H04.302　Unspecified dacryocystitis of left lacrimal passage
　　H04.303　Unspecified dacryocystitis of bilateral lacrimal passages
　　H04.309　Unspecified dacryocystitis of unspecified lacrimal passage
　● H04.31　Phlegmonous dacryocystitis
Cellulitis of lacrimal sac
　　H04.311　Phlegmonous dacryocystitis of right lacrimal passage
　　H04.312　Phlegmonous dacryocystitis of left lacrimal passage
　　H04.313　Phlegmonous dacryocystitis of bilateral lacrimal passages
　　H04.319　Phlegmonous dacryocystitis of unspecified lacrimal passage
　● H04.32　Acute dacryocystitis
Acute dacryopericystitis
　　H04.321　Acute dacryocystitis of right lacrimal passage
　　H04.322　Acute dacryocystitis of left lacrimal passage
　　H04.323　Acute dacryocystitis of bilateral lacrimal passages
　　H04.329　Acute dacryocystitis of unspecified lacrimal passage

　● H04.33　Acute lacrimal canaliculitis
　　H04.331　Acute lacrimal canaliculitis of right lacrimal passage
　　H04.332　Acute lacrimal canaliculitis of left lacrimal passage
　　H04.333　Acute lacrimal canaliculitis of bilateral lacrimal passages
　　H04.339　Acute lacrimal canaliculitis of unspecified lacrimal passage
● H04.4　Chronic inflammation of lacrimal passages
　● H04.41　Chronic dacryocystitis
Inflammation of lacrimal sac
　　H04.411　Chronic dacryocystitis of right lacrimal passage
　　H04.412　Chronic dacryocystitis of left lacrimal passage
　　H04.413　Chronic dacryocystitis of bilateral lacrimal passages
　　H04.419　Chronic dacryocystitis of unspecified lacrimal passage
　● H04.42　Chronic lacrimal canaliculitis
Inflammation of lacrimal ducts
　　H04.421　Chronic lacrimal canaliculitis of right lacrimal passage
　　H04.422　Chronic lacrimal canaliculitis of left lacrimal passage
　　H04.423　Chronic lacrimal canaliculitis of bilateral lacrimal passages
　　H04.429　Chronic lacrimal canaliculitis of unspecified lacrimal passage
　● H04.43　Chronic lacrimal mucocele
Accumulation of mucous secretion
　　H04.431　Chronic lacrimal mucocele of right lacrimal passage
　　H04.432　Chronic lacrimal mucocele of left lacrimal passage
　　H04.433　Chronic lacrimal mucocele of bilateral lacrimal passages
　　H04.439　Chronic lacrimal mucocele of unspecified lacrimal passage
● H04.5　Stenosis and insufficiency of lacrimal passages
　● H04.51　Dacryolith
Concretion in lacrimal sac/duct; AKA lacrimal calculus
　　H04.511　Dacryolith of right lacrimal passage
　　H04.512　Dacryolith of left lacrimal passage
　　H04.513　Dacryolith of bilateral lacrimal passages
　　H04.519　Dacryolith of unspecified lacrimal passage
　● H04.52　Eversion of lacrimal punctum
Turning out of lacrimal drainage opening
　　H04.521　Eversion of right lacrimal punctum
　　H04.522　Eversion of left lacrimal punctum
　　H04.523　Eversion of bilateral lacrimal punctum
　　H04.529　Eversion of unspecified lacrimal punctum
　● H04.53　Neonatal obstruction of nasolacrimal duct
　　　Excludes1　congenital stenosis and stricture of lacrimal duct (Q10.5)
　　H04.531　Neonatal obstruction of right nasolacrimal duct　　N
　　H04.532　Neonatal obstruction of left nasolacrimal duct　　N
　　H04.533　Neonatal obstruction of bilateral nasolacrimal duct　　N
　　H04.539　Neonatal obstruction of unspecified nasolacrimal duct　　N

CHAPTER 7 (H00-H59)

◀ New　◀▥ Revised　~~deleted~~ Deleted　Excludes 1　Excludes 2　Includes　Use additional　Code first　Code also　Unspecified
OGCR Official Guidelines　● Unacceptable Principal Diagnosis　X Assign placeholder X　● Use Additional Character(s)　▶ Manifestation Code　Coding Clinic

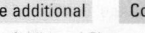

● **H04.54**   Stenosis of lacrimal canaliculi
    H04.541   Stenosis of right lacrimal canaliculi
    H04.542   Stenosis of left lacrimal canaliculi
    H04.543   Stenosis of bilateral lacrimal canaliculi
    H04.549   Stenosis of unspecified lacrimal canaliculi

● **H04.55**   Acquired stenosis of nasolacrimal duct
    H04.551   Acquired stenosis of right nasolacrimal duct
    H04.552   Acquired stenosis of left nasolacrimal duct
    H04.553   Acquired stenosis of bilateral nasolacrimal duct
    H04.559   Acquired stenosis of unspecified nasolacrimal duct

● **H04.56**   Stenosis of lacrimal punctum
    H04.561   Stenosis of right lacrimal punctum
    H04.562   Stenosis of left lacrimal punctum
    H04.563   Stenosis of bilateral lacrimal punctum
    H04.569   Stenosis of unspecified lacrimal punctum

● **H04.57**   Stenosis of lacrimal sac
    H04.571   Stenosis of right lacrimal sac
    H04.572   Stenosis of left lacrimal sac
    H04.573   Stenosis of bilateral lacrimal sac
    H04.579   Stenosis of unspecified lacrimal sac

● **H04.6**   Other changes of lacrimal passages
 ● **H04.61**   Lacrimal fistula
    H04.611   Lacrimal fistula right lacrimal passage
    H04.612   Lacrimal fistula left lacrimal passage
    H04.613   Lacrimal fistula bilateral lacrimal passages
    H04.619   Lacrimal fistula unspecified lacrimal passage
   H04.69   Other changes of lacrimal passages

● **H04.8**   Other disorders of lacrimal system
 ● **H04.81**   Granuloma of lacrimal passages
     Inflammatory response due to infectious or noninfectious agents
    H04.811   Granuloma of right lacrimal passage
    H04.812   Granuloma of left lacrimal passage
    H04.813   Granuloma of bilateral lacrimal passages
    H04.819   Granuloma of unspecified lacrimal passage
   H04.89   Other disorders of lacrimal system
   H04.9   Disorder of lacrimal system, unspecified

● **H05**   **Disorders of orbit**
    Excludes1   congenital malformation of orbit (Q10.7)
 ● **H05.0**   Acute inflammation of orbit
   H05.00   Unspecified acute inflammation of orbit
 ● **H05.01**   Cellulitis of orbit
     Infection of soft tissue of orbit
     Abscess of orbit
     (Ex) **For category H05.01 CC codes:** H05.00-H05.049
    H05.011   Cellulitis of right orbit 🔖
    H05.012   Cellulitis of left orbit 🔖
    H05.013   Cellulitis of bilateral orbits 🔖
    H05.019   Cellulitis of unspecified orbit 🔖

● **H05.02**   Osteomyelitis of orbit
     Infection of boney orbit of eye
     (Ex) **For category H05.02 CC codes:** A02.24, A17.9, A18.03-A18.09, A18.82, A18.84, A18.89, H05.021-H05.029, M46.20-M46.39, M86.00-M86.9
    H05.021   Osteomyelitis of right orbit 🔖
    H05.022   Osteomyelitis of left orbit 🔖
    H05.023   Osteomyelitis of bilateral orbits 🔖
    H05.029   Osteomyelitis of unspecified orbit 🔖

● **H05.03**   Periostitis of orbit
     Inflammation of periosteum (membrane covering bone surface)
     (Ex) **For category H05.03 CC codes:** A02.24, A17.9, A18.03-A18.09, A18.82, A18.84, A18.89, H05.031-H05.039, M46.20-M46.39, M86.00-M86.9
    H05.031   Periostitis of right orbit 🔖
    H05.032   Periostitis of left orbit 🔖
    H05.033   Periostitis of bilateral orbits 🔖
    H05.039   Periostitis of unspecified orbit 🔖

● **H05.04**   Tenonitis of orbit
     Inflammation of tenon capsule (space enclosing fascia of Tenon between eyeball and fat of orbit)
    H05.041   Tenonitis of right orbit
    H05.042   Tenonitis of left orbit
    H05.043   Tenonitis of bilateral orbits
    H05.049   Tenonitis of unspecified orbit

● **H05.1**   Chronic inflammatory disorders of orbit
   H05.10   Unspecified chronic inflammatory disorders of orbit
 ● **H05.11**   Granuloma of orbit
     Pseudotumor (inflammatory) of orbit
    H05.111   Granuloma of right orbit
    H05.112   Granuloma of left orbit
    H05.113   Granuloma of bilateral orbits
    H05.119   Granuloma of unspecified orbit
 ● **H05.12**   Orbital myositis
     Inflammation of extraocular muscles of orbit
    H05.121   Orbital myositis, right orbit
    H05.122   Orbital myositis, left orbit
    H05.123   Orbital myositis, bilateral
    H05.129   Orbital myositis, unspecified orbit

● **H05.2**   Exophthalmic conditions
     Bulging eyes
   H05.20   Unspecified exophthalmos
 ● **H05.21**   Displacement (lateral) of globe
    H05.211   Displacement (lateral) of globe, right eye
    H05.212   Displacement (lateral) of globe, left eye
    H05.213   Displacement (lateral) of globe, bilateral
    H05.219   Displacement (lateral) of globe, unspecified eye
 ● **H05.22**   Edema of orbit
     Orbital congestion
    H05.221   Edema of right orbit
    H05.222   Edema of left orbit
    H05.223   Edema of bilateral orbit
    H05.229   Edema of unspecified orbit
 ● **H05.23**   Hemorrhage of orbit
    H05.231   Hemorrhage of right orbit
    H05.232   Hemorrhage of left orbit
    H05.233   Hemorrhage of bilateral orbit
    H05.239   Hemorrhage of unspecified orbit

CHAPTER 7 (H00-H59)

N   Newborn Age: 0   **P**   Pediatric Age: 0–17   **M**   Maternity DX: 12–55   **A**   Adult Age: 15–124   ♀   Females Only   ♂   Males Only

🔖 Complication\Comorbidity   🔖 Major C\C   (Ex) CC/MCC Exclusions   🔖 Hospital-Acquired Condition

817

Figure 7-5 Exophthalmos. (From Stein: The Ophthalmic Assistant: Fundamentals and Clinical Practice, ed 6, London, Mosby, 1994)

- **H05.24**   Constant exophthalmos
  Constant bulging eyes, often symptom of Graves disease
  - H05.241   Constant exophthalmos, right eye
  - H05.242   Constant exophthalmos, left eye
  - H05.243   Constant exophthalmos, bilateral
  - H05.249   Constant exophthalmos, unspecified eye
- **H05.25**   Intermittent exophthalmos
  Intermittent bulging eye occurring with bending forward or sharp turning of head
  - H05.251   Intermittent exophthalmos, right eye
  - H05.252   Intermittent exophthalmos, left eye
  - H05.253   Intermittent exophthalmos, bilateral
  - H05.259   Intermittent exophthalmos, unspecified eye
- **H05.26**   Pulsating exophthalmos
  Bulging eyes with pulsation and bruit, often due to aneurysm pushing eye forward
  - H05.261   Pulsating exophthalmos, right eye
  - H05.262   Pulsating exophthalmos, left eye
  - H05.263   Pulsating exophthalmos, bilateral
  - H05.269   Pulsating exophthalmos, unspecified eye
- **H05.3**   Deformity of orbit
  | Excludes1 | congenital deformity of orbit (Q10.7) hypertelorism (Q75.2) |
  - H05.30   Unspecified deformity of orbit
  - **H05.31**   Atrophy of orbit
    - H05.311   Atrophy of right orbit
    - H05.312   Atrophy of left orbit
    - H05.313   Atrophy of bilateral orbit
    - H05.319   Atrophy of unspecified orbit
  - **H05.32**   Deformity of orbit due to bone disease
    Code also associated bone disease
    - H05.321   Deformity of right orbit due to bone disease
    - H05.322   Deformity of left orbit due to bone disease
    - H05.323   Deformity of bilateral orbits due to bone disease
    - H05.329   Deformity of unspecified orbit due to bone disease
  - **H05.33**   Deformity of orbit due to trauma or surgery
    - H05.331   Deformity of right orbit due to trauma or surgery
    - H05.332   Deformity of left orbit due to trauma or surgery
    - H05.333   Deformity of bilateral orbits due to trauma or surgery
    - H05.339   Deformity of unspecified orbit due to trauma or surgery

- **H05.34**   Enlargement of orbit
  - H05.341   Enlargement of right orbit
  - H05.342   Enlargement of left orbit
  - H05.343   Enlargement of bilateral orbits
  - H05.349   Enlargement of unspecified orbit
- **H05.35**   Exostosis of orbit
  - H05.351   Exostosis of right orbit
  - H05.352   Exostosis of left orbit
  - H05.353   Exostosis of bilateral orbits
  - H05.359   Exostosis of unspecified orbit
- **H05.4**   Enophthalmos
  Recessed eyeball into orbit
  - **H05.40**   Unspecified enophthalmos
    - H05.401   Unspecified enophthalmos, right eye
    - H05.402   Unspecified enophthalmos, left eye
    - H05.403   Unspecified enophthalmos, bilateral
    - H05.409   Unspecified enophthalmos, unspecified eye
  - **H05.41**   Enophthalmos due to atrophy of orbital tissue
    - H05.411   Enophthalmos due to atrophy of orbital tissue, right eye
    - H05.412   Enophthalmos due to atrophy of orbital tissue, left eye
    - H05.413   Enophthalmos due to atrophy of orbital tissue, bilateral
    - H05.419   Enophthalmos due to atrophy of orbital tissue, unspecified eye
  - **H05.42**   Enophthalmos due to trauma or surgery
    - H05.421   Enophthalmos due to trauma or surgery, right eye
    - H05.422   Enophthalmos due to trauma or surgery, left eye
    - H05.423   Enophthalmos due to trauma or surgery, bilateral
    - H05.429   Enophthalmos due to trauma or surgery, unspecified eye
- **H05.5**   Retained (old) foreign body following penetrating wound of orbit
  Retrobulbar foreign body
  Use additional code to identify the type of retained foreign body (Z18.-)
  | Excludes1 | current penetrating wound of orbit (S05.4-) |
  | Excludes2 | retained foreign body of eyelid (H02.81-) retained intraocular foreign body (H44.6-, H44.7-) |
  - H05.50   Retained (old) foreign body following penetrating wound of unspecified orbit
  - H05.51   Retained (old) foreign body following penetrating wound of right orbit
  - H05.52   Retained (old) foreign body following penetrating wound of left orbit
  - H05.53   Retained (old) foreign body following penetrating wound of bilateral orbits
- **H05.8**   Other disorders of orbit
  - **H05.81**   Cyst of orbit
    Encephalocele of orbit
    - H05.811   Cyst of right orbit
    - H05.812   Cyst of left orbit
    - H05.813   Cyst of bilateral orbits
    - H05.819   Cyst of unspecified orbit

◀ New   ◀ Revised   ~~deleted~~ Deleted   Excludes 1   Excludes 2   Includes   Use additional   Code first   Code also   Unspecified
OGCR Official Guidelines   ● Unacceptable Principal Diagnosis   X Assign placeholder X   ● Use Additional Character(s)   ▌ Manifestation Code   **Coding Clinic**

● H05.82   **Myopathy of extraocular muscles**
Weakness of muscles of eye

    H05.821   **Myopathy of extraocular muscles, right orbit**

    H05.822   **Myopathy of extraocular muscles, left orbit**

    H05.823   **Myopathy of extraocular muscles, bilateral**

    H05.829   **Myopathy of extraocular muscles, unspecified orbit**

   H05.89   **Other disorders of orbit**

H05.9   **Unspecified disorder of orbit**

DISORDERS OF CONJUNCTIVA (H10–H11)

★ **(See Plate 81, upper, on page 66.)**

● H10   **Conjunctivitis**
Inflammation of membrane of the inside of the eyelid or on surface of eye (conjunctiva)

    Excludes1   keratoconjunctivitis (H16.2-)

 ● H10.0   **Mucopurulent conjunctivitis**

  ● H10.01   **Acute follicular conjunctivitis**

    H10.011   **Acute follicular conjunctivitis, right eye**

    H10.012   **Acute follicular conjunctivitis, left eye**

    H10.013   **Acute follicular conjunctivitis, bilateral**

    H10.019   **Acute follicular conjunctivitis, unspecified eye**

  ● H10.02   **Other mucopurulent conjunctivitis**

    H10.021   **Other mucopurulent conjunctivitis, right eye**

    H10.022   **Other mucopurulent conjunctivitis, left eye**

    H10.023   **Other mucopurulent conjunctivitis, bilateral**

    H10.029   **Other mucopurulent conjunctivitis, unspecified eye**

 ● H10.1   **Acute atopic conjunctivitis**
    Acute papillary conjunctivitis

   H10.10   **Acute atopic conjunctivitis, unspecified eye**

   H10.11   **Acute atopic conjunctivitis, right eye**

   H10.12   **Acute atopic conjunctivitis, left eye**

   H10.13   **Acute atopic conjunctivitis, bilateral**

 ● H10.2   **Other acute conjunctivitis**

  ● H10.21   **Acute toxic conjunctivitis**
    Acute chemical conjunctivitis

    Code first (T51-T65) to identify chemical and intent

    Excludes1   burn and corrosion of eye and adnexa (T26.-)

    H10.211   **Acute toxic conjunctivitis, right eye**

    H10.212   **Acute toxic conjunctivitis, left eye**

    H10.213   **Acute toxic conjunctivitis, bilateral**

    H10.219   **Acute toxic conjunctivitis, unspecified eye**

  ● H10.22   **Pseudomembranous conjunctivitis**

    H10.221   **Pseudomembranous conjunctivitis, right eye**

    H10.222   **Pseudomembranous conjunctivitis, left eye**

    H10.223   **Pseudomembranous conjunctivitis, bilateral**

    H10.229   **Pseudomembranous conjunctivitis, unspecified eye**

● H10.23   **Serous conjunctivitis, except viral**

    Excludes1   viral conjunctivitis (B30.-)

    H10.231   **Serous conjunctivitis, except viral, right eye**

    H10.232   **Serous conjunctivitis, except viral, left eye**

    H10.233   **Serous conjunctivitis, except viral, bilateral**

    H10.239   **Serous conjunctivitis, except viral, unspecified eye**

● H10.3   **Unspecified acute conjunctivitis**

    Excludes1   ophthalmia neonatorum NOS (P39.1)

   H10.30   **Unspecified acute conjunctivitis, unspecified eye**

   H10.31   **Unspecified acute conjunctivitis, right eye**

   H10.32   **Unspecified acute conjunctivitis, left eye**

   H10.33   **Unspecified acute conjunctivitis, bilateral**

● H10.4   **Chronic conjunctivitis**

 ● H10.40   **Unspecified chronic conjunctivitis**

    H10.401   **Unspecified chronic conjunctivitis, right eye**

    H10.402   **Unspecified chronic conjunctivitis, left eye**

    H10.403   **Unspecified chronic conjunctivitis, bilateral**

    H10.409   **Unspecified chronic conjunctivitis, unspecified eye**

 ● H10.41   **Chronic giant papillary conjunctivitis**
Inflammation of membrane of the inside of the eyelid or on surface of eye often associated with contact lens wear

    H10.411   **Chronic giant papillary conjunctivitis, right eye**

    H10.412   **Chronic giant papillary conjunctivitis, left eye**

    H10.413   **Chronic giant papillary conjunctivitis, bilateral**

    H10.419   **Chronic giant papillary conjunctivitis, unspecified eye**

 ● H10.42   **Simple chronic conjunctivitis**

    H10.421   **Simple chronic conjunctivitis, right eye**

    H10.422   **Simple chronic conjunctivitis, left eye**

    H10.423   **Simple chronic conjunctivitis, bilateral**

    H10.429   **Simple chronic conjunctivitis, unspecified eye**

 ● H10.43   **Chronic follicular conjunctivitis**
Inflammation of membrane of the inside of the eyelid or on surface of eye due to topical medications or infection

    H10.431   **Chronic follicular conjunctivitis, right eye**

    H10.432   **Chronic follicular conjunctivitis, left eye**

    H10.433   **Chronic follicular conjunctivitis, bilateral**

    H10.439   **Chronic follicular conjunctivitis, unspecified eye**

   H10.44   **Vernal conjunctivitis**
Affecting children, especially boys in which there are flattened papules with thick, gelatinous exudate on conjunctivae on inside of upper lid

    Excludes1   vernal keratoconjunctivitis with limbar and corneal involvement (H16.26-)

   H10.45   **Other chronic allergic conjunctivitis**

N   Newborn Age: 0   **P**   Pediatric Age: 0–17   **M**   Maternity DX: 12–55   **A**   Adult Age: 15–124   ♀   Females Only   ♂   Males Only

   Complication\Comorbidity   Major C\C   (Ex)   CC/MCC Exclusions   Hospital-Acquired Condition   **819**

CHAPTER 7 (H00–H59)

CHAPTER 7 (H00-H59)

- **H10.5 Blepharoconjunctivitis**
  Inflammation of eyelids and conjunctiva
  - **H10.50 Unspecified blepharoconjunctivitis**
    - H10.501 Unspecified blepharoconjunctivitis, right eye
    - H10.502 Unspecified blepharoconjunctivitis, left eye
    - H10.503 Unspecified blepharoconjunctivitis, bilateral
    - H10.509 Unspecified blepharoconjunctivitis, unspecified eye
  - **H10.51 Ligneous conjunctivitis**
    - H10.511 Ligneous conjunctivitis, right eye
    - H10.512 Ligneous conjunctivitis, left eye
    - H10.513 Ligneous conjunctivitis, bilateral
    - H10.519 Ligneous conjunctivitis, unspecified eye
  - **H10.52 Angular blepharoconjunctivitis**
    - H10.521 Angular blepharoconjunctivitis, right eye
    - H10.522 Angular blepharoconjunctivitis, left eye
    - H10.523 Angular blepharoconjunctivitis, bilateral
    - H10.529 Angular blepharoconjunctivitis, unspecified eye
  - **H10.53 Contact blepharoconjunctivitis**
    - H10.531 Contact blepharoconjunctivitis, right eye
    - H10.532 Contact blepharoconjunctivitis, left eye
    - H10.533 Contact blepharoconjunctivitis, bilateral
    - H10.539 Contact blepharoconjunctivitis, unspecified eye
- **H10.8 Other conjunctivitis**
  - **H10.81 Pingueculitis**
    Inflammation of a yellow, raised thickening on the white of the eye associated with chronic dry eyes

    Excludes1   pinguecula (H11.15-)
    - H10.811 Pingueculitis, right eye
    - H10.812 Pingueculitis, left eye
    - H10.813 Pingueculitis, bilateral
    - H10.819 Pingueculitis, unspecified eye
  - H10.89 Other conjunctivitis
  - H10.9 Unspecified conjunctivitis
- **H11 Other disorders of conjunctiva**

  Excludes1   keratoconjunctivitis (H16.2-)
  - **H11.0 Pterygium of eye**

    Excludes1   pseudopterygium (H11.81-)
    - **H11.00 Unspecified pterygium of eye**
      - H11.001 Unspecified pterygium of right eye
      - H11.002 Unspecified pterygium of left eye
      - H11.003 Unspecified pterygium of eye, bilateral
      - H11.009 Unspecified pterygium of unspecified eye
    - **H11.01 Amyloid pterygium**
      - H11.011 Amyloid pterygium of right eye
      - H11.012 Amyloid pterygium of left eye
      - H11.013 Amyloid pterygium of eye, bilateral
      - H11.019 Amyloid pterygium of unspecified eye

Figure 7-6 Double pterygium. Note both nasal and temporal pterygia in a 57-year-old farmer. (From Yanoff: Ophthalmology, ed 3, Mosby, Inc., 2008)

Item 7–2 Pterygium is Greek for batlike. The condition is characterized by a membrane that extends from the limbus to the center of the cornea and resembles a wing.

- **H11.02 Central pterygium of eye**
  - H11.021 Central pterygium of right eye
  - H11.022 Central pterygium of left eye
  - H11.023 Central pterygium of eye, bilateral
  - H11.029 Central pterygium of unspecified eye
- **H11.03 Double pterygium of eye**
  - H11.031 Double pterygium of right eye
  - H11.032 Double pterygium of left eye
  - H11.033 Double pterygium of eye, bilateral
  - H11.039 Double pterygium of unspecified eye
- **H11.04 Peripheral pterygium of eye, stationary**
  - H11.041 Peripheral pterygium, stationary, right eye
  - H11.042 Peripheral pterygium, stationary, left eye
  - H11.043 Peripheral pterygium, stationary, bilateral
  - H11.049 Peripheral pterygium, stationary, unspecified eye
- **H11.05 Peripheral pterygium of eye, progressive**
  - H11.051 Peripheral pterygium, progressive, right eye
  - H11.052 Peripheral pterygium, progressive, left eye
  - H11.053 Peripheral pterygium, progressive, bilateral
  - H11.059 Peripheral pterygium, progressive, unspecified eye
- **H11.06 Recurrent pterygium of eye**
  - H11.061 Recurrent pterygium of right eye
  - H11.062 Recurrent pterygium of left eye
  - H11.063 Recurrent pterygium of eye, bilateral
  - H11.069 Recurrent pterygium of unspecified eye
- **H11.1 Conjunctival degenerations and deposits**

  Excludes2   pseudopterygium (H11.81)
  - H11.10 Unspecified conjunctival degenerations
  - **H11.11 Conjunctival deposits**
    - H11.111 Conjunctival deposits, right eye
    - H11.112 Conjunctival deposits, left eye
    - H11.113 Conjunctival deposits, bilateral
    - H11.119 Conjunctival deposits, unspecified eye
  - **H11.12 Conjunctival concretions**
    White to yellow nodules within or beneath conjunctiva
    - H11.121 Conjunctival concretions, right eye
    - H11.122 Conjunctival concretions, left eye
    - H11.123 Conjunctival concretions, bilateral
    - H11.129 Conjunctival concretions, unspecified eye
  - **H11.13 Conjunctival pigmentations**
    Conjunctival argyrosis [argyria]
    - H11.131 Conjunctival pigmentations, right eye
    - H11.132 Conjunctival pigmentations, left eye
    - H11.133 Conjunctival pigmentations, bilateral
    - H11.139 Conjunctival pigmentations, unspecified eye

● **H11.14**   Conjunctival xerosis, unspecified
> **Excludes1**   xerosis of conjunctiva due to vitamin A deficiency (E50.0, E50.1)

    H11.141   Conjunctival xerosis, unspecified, right eye
    H11.142   Conjunctival xerosis, unspecified, left eye
    H11.143   Conjunctival xerosis, unspecified, bilateral
    H11.149   Conjunctival xerosis, unspecified, unspecified eye

● **H11.15**   Pinguecula
> *Yellowish spot near sclerocorneal junction, usually on nasal side; associated with aging*
> **Excludes1**   pingueculitis (H10.81-)

    H11.151   Pinguecula, right eye
    H11.152   Pinguecula, left eye
    H11.153   Pinguecula, bilateral
    H11.159   Pinguecula, unspecified eye

● **H11.2**   Conjunctival scars
  ● **H11.21**   Conjunctival adhesions and strands (localized)
    H11.211   Conjunctival adhesions and strands (localized), right eye
    H11.212   Conjunctival adhesions and strands (localized), left eye
    H11.213   Conjunctival adhesions and strands (localized), bilateral
    H11.219   Conjunctival adhesions and strands (localized), unspecified eye

  ● **H11.22**   Conjunctival granuloma
    H11.221   Conjunctival granuloma, right eye
    H11.222   Conjunctival granuloma, left eye
    H11.223   Conjunctival granuloma, bilateral
    H11.229   Conjunctival granuloma, unspecified

  ● **H11.23**   Symblepharon
> *Adhesion between tarsal conjunctiva and bulbar conjunctiva*

    H11.231   Symblepharon, right eye
    H11.232   Symblepharon, left eye
    H11.233   Symblepharon, bilateral
    H11.239   Symblepharon, unspecified eye

  ● **H11.24**   Scarring of conjunctiva
    H11.241   Scarring of conjunctiva, right eye
    H11.242   Scarring of conjunctiva, left eye
    H11.243   Scarring of conjunctiva, bilateral
    H11.249   Scarring of conjunctiva, unspecified eye

● **H11.3**   Conjunctival hemorrhage
> Subconjunctival hemorrhage

    H11.30   Conjunctival hemorrhage, unspecified eye
    H11.31   Conjunctival hemorrhage, right eye
    H11.32   Conjunctival hemorrhage, left eye
    H11.33   Conjunctival hemorrhage, bilateral

● **H11.4**   Other conjunctival vascular disorders and cysts
  ● **H11.41**   Vascular abnormalities of conjunctiva
> Conjunctival aneurysm

    H11.411   Vascular abnormalities of conjunctiva, right eye
    H11.412   Vascular abnormalities of conjunctiva, left eye
    H11.413   Vascular abnormalities of conjunctiva, bilateral
    H11.419   Vascular abnormalities of conjunctiva, unspecified eye

● **H11.42**   Conjunctival edema
    H11.421   Conjunctival edema, right eye
    H11.422   Conjunctival edema, left eye
    H11.423   Conjunctival edema, bilateral
    H11.429   Conjunctival edema, unspecified eye

● **H11.43**   Conjunctival hyperemia
    H11.431   Conjunctival hyperemia, right eye
    H11.432   Conjunctival hyperemia, left eye
    H11.433   Conjunctival hyperemia, bilateral
    H11.439   Conjunctival hyperemia, unspecified eye

● **H11.44**   Conjunctival cysts
    H11.441   Conjunctival cysts, right eye
    H11.442   Conjunctival cysts, left eye
    H11.443   Conjunctival cysts, bilateral
    H11.449   Conjunctival cysts, unspecified eye

● **H11.8**   Other specified disorders of conjunctiva
  ● **H11.81**   Pseudopterygium of conjunctiva
> *Conjunctival scar attached to cornea*

    H11.811   Pseudopterygium of conjunctiva, right eye
    H11.812   Pseudopterygium of conjunctiva, left eye
    H11.813   Pseudopterygium of conjunctiva, bilateral
    H11.819   Pseudopterygium of conjunctiva, unspecified eye

  ● **H11.82**   Conjunctivochalasis
> *Conjunctiva bulges over eyelid margin or covers lower punctum*

    H11.821   Conjunctivochalasis, right eye
    H11.822   Conjunctivochalasis, left eye
    H11.823   Conjunctivochalasis, bilateral
    H11.829   Conjunctivochalasis, unspecified eye

    H11.89   Other specified disorders of conjunctiva

   H11.9   Unspecified disorder of conjunctiva

DISORDERS OF SCLERA, CORNEA, IRIS AND CILIARY BODY (H15-H22)

● **H15**   Disorders of sclera
  ● **H15.0**   Scleritis
> *Inflammation of the white (sclera and episclera) of the eye.*

  ● **H15.00**   Unspecified scleritis
    H15.001   Unspecified scleritis, right eye
    H15.002   Unspecified scleritis, left eye
    H15.003   Unspecified scleritis, bilateral
    H15.009   Unspecified scleritis, unspecified eye

  ● **H15.01**   Anterior scleritis
    H15.011   Anterior scleritis, right eye
    H15.012   Anterior scleritis, left eye
    H15.013   Anterior scleritis, bilateral
    H15.019   Anterior scleritis, unspecified eye

  ● **H15.02**   Brawny scleritis
> *Swelling around the cornea that is gelantinous in appearance*

    H15.021   Brawny scleritis, right eye
    H15.022   Brawny scleritis, left eye
    H15.023   Brawny scleritis, bilateral
    H15.029   Brawny scleritis, unspecified eye

  ● **H15.03**   Posterior scleritis
> Sclerotenonitis

    H15.031   Posterior scleritis, right eye
    H15.032   Posterior scleritis, left eye
    H15.033   Posterior scleritis, bilateral
    H15.039   Posterior scleritis, unspecified eye

N Newborn Age: 0   **P** Pediatric Age: 0–17   **M** Maternity DX: 12–55   **A** Adult Age: 15–124   ♀ Females Only   ♂ Males Only
     Complication\Comorbidity   Major C\C   (Ex) CC/MCC Exclusions   Hospital-Acquired Condition

821

CHAPTER 7 (H00–H59)

● H15.04   Scleritis with corneal involvement

    H15.041   Scleritis with corneal involvement, right eye

    H15.042   Scleritis with corneal involvement, left eye

    H15.043   Scleritis with corneal involvement, bilateral

    H15.049   Scleritis with corneal involvement, unspecified eye

● H15.05   Scleromalacia perforans
Necrotic without inflammation; usually associated with rheumatoid arthritis

    H15.051   Scleromalacia perforans, right eye

    H15.052   Scleromalacia perforans, left eye

    H15.053   Scleromalacia perforans, bilateral

    H15.059   Scleromalacia perforans, unspecified eye

● H15.09   Other scleritis
Scleral abscess

    H15.091   Other scleritis, right eye

    H15.092   Other scleritis, left eye

    H15.093   Other scleritis, bilateral

    H15.099   Other scleritis, unspecified eye

● H15.1   Episcleritis
Inflammation of the white (sclera and episclera) of the eye.

● H15.10   Unspecified episcleritis

    H15.101   Unspecified episcleritis, right eye

    H15.102   Unspecified episcleritis, left eye

    H15.103   Unspecified episcleritis, bilateral

    H15.109   Unspecified episcleritis, unspecified eye

● H15.11   Episcleritis periodica fugax
Transient, recurrent inflammation of portion of episclera (connective tissue on the surface of the sclera)

    H15.111   Episcleritis periodica fugax, right eye

    H15.112   Episcleritis periodica fugax, left eye

    H15.113   Episcleritis periodica fugax, bilateral

    H15.119   Episcleritis periodica fugax, unspecified eye

● H15.12   Nodular episcleritis
Characterized by tender, localized, moveable nodule within inflamed area

    H15.121   Nodular episcleritis, right eye

    H15.122   Nodular episcleritis, left eye

    H15.123   Nodular episcleritis, bilateral

    H15.129   Nodular episcleritis, unspecified eye

● H15.8   Other disorders of sclera

    Excludes2   blue sclera (Q13.5)
                 degenerative myopia (H44.2-)

● H15.81   Equatorial staphyloma

    H15.811   Equatorial staphyloma, right eye

    H15.812   Equatorial staphyloma, left eye

    H15.813   Equatorial staphyloma, bilateral

    H15.819   Equatorial staphyloma, unspecified eye

● H15.82   Localized anterior staphyloma

    H15.821   Localized anterior staphyloma, right eye

    H15.822   Localized anterior staphyloma, left eye

    H15.823   Localized anterior staphyloma, bilateral

    H15.829   Localized anterior staphyloma, unspecified eye

● H15.83   Staphyloma posticum

    H15.831   Staphyloma posticum, right eye

    H15.832   Staphyloma posticum, left eye

    H15.833   Staphyloma posticum, bilateral

    H15.839   Staphyloma posticum, unspecified eye

● H15.84   Scleral ectasia

    H15.841   Scleral ectasia, right eye

    H15.842   Scleral ectasia, left eye

    H15.843   Scleral ectasia, bilateral

    H15.849   Scleral ectasia, unspecified eye

● H15.85   Ring staphyloma

    H15.851   Ring staphyloma, right eye

    H15.852   Ring staphyloma, left eye

    H15.853   Ring staphyloma, bilateral

    H15.859   Ring staphyloma, unspecified eye

    H15.89   Other disorders of sclera

  H15.9   Unspecified disorder of sclera

● H16   Keratitis

● H16.0   Corneal ulcer

● H16.00   Unspecified corneal ulcer

    H16.001   Unspecified corneal ulcer, right eye

    H16.002   Unspecified corneal ulcer, left eye

    H16.003   Unspecified corneal ulcer, bilateral

    H16.009   Unspecified corneal ulcer, unspecified eye

● H16.01   Central corneal ulcer

    H16.011   Central corneal ulcer, right eye

    H16.012   Central corneal ulcer, left eye

    H16.013   Central corneal ulcer, bilateral

    H16.019   Central corneal ulcer, unspecified eye

● H16.02   Ring corneal ulcer

    H16.021   Ring corneal ulcer, right eye

    H16.022   Ring corneal ulcer, left eye

    H16.023   Ring corneal ulcer, bilateral

    H16.029   Ring corneal ulcer, unspecified eye

● H16.03   Corneal ulcer with hypopyon

    H16.031   Corneal ulcer with hypopyon, right eye

    H16.032   Corneal ulcer with hypopyon, left eye

    H16.033   Corneal ulcer with hypopyon, bilateral

    H16.039   Corneal ulcer with hypopyon, unspecified eye

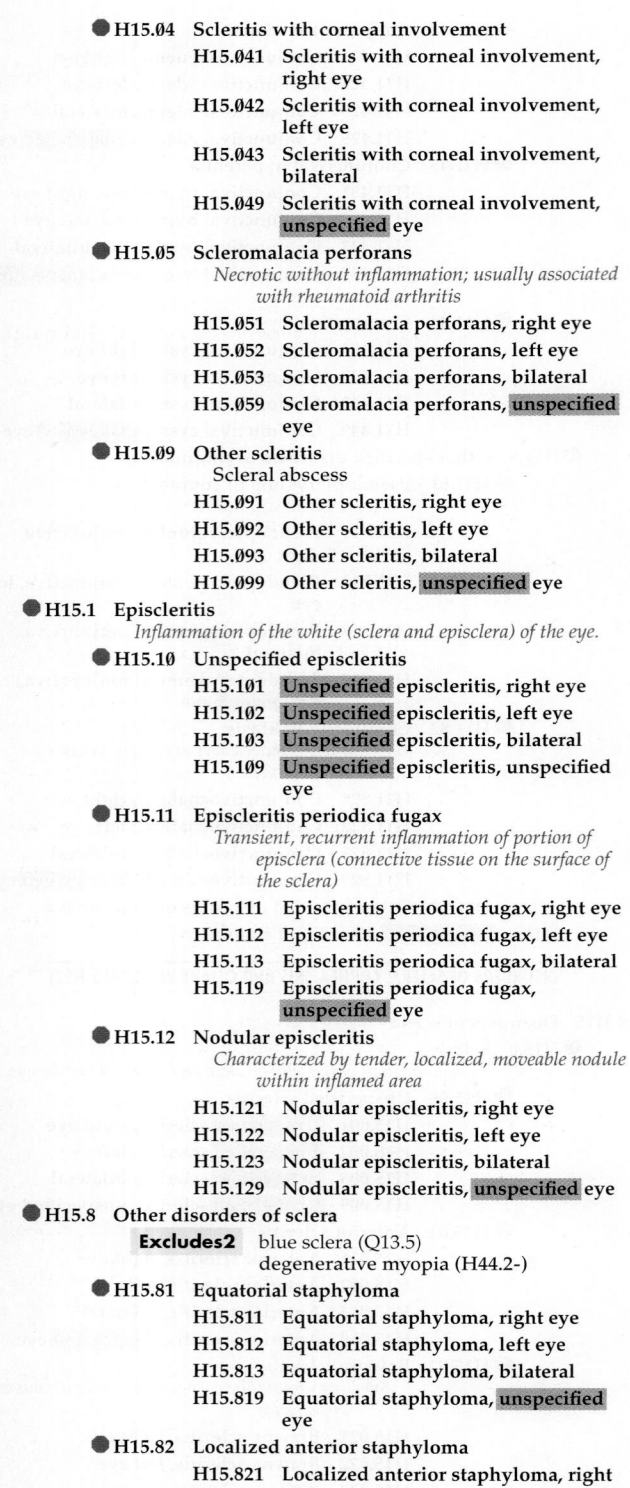

| Marginal (catarrhal) ulcer | Ring ulcer | Central corneal ulcer | Rosacea ulcer | Mooren's (rodent) ulcer |

Figure 7-7   Corneal ulcers: marginal, ring, central corneal, rosacea, and Mooren's.

Item 7–3   An infected ulcer is usually called a **serpiginous** or **hypopyon** ulcer which is a pus sac in the anterior chamber of the eye. **Marginal** ulcers are usually asymptomatic, not primary, and are often superficial and simple. More severe marginal ulcers spread to form a ring ulcer. **Ring** ulcers can extend around the entire corneal periphery. **Central corneal** ulcers develop when there is an abrasion to the epithelium and an infection develops in the eroded area. The **pyocyaneal** ulcer is the most serious corneal infection, which, if left untreated, can lead to loss of the eye.

◀ New   ◀ Revised   ~~deleted~~ Deleted   Excludes 1   Excludes 2   Includes   Use additional   Code first   Code also   Unspecified

OGCR Official Guidelines   ● Unacceptable Principal Diagnosis   X Assign placeholder X   ● Use Additional Character(s)   ▶ Manifestation Code   **Coding Clinic**

● H16.04   Marginal corneal ulcer
     H16.041   Marginal corneal ulcer, right eye
     H16.042   Marginal corneal ulcer, left eye
     H16.043   Marginal corneal ulcer, bilateral
     H16.049   Marginal corneal ulcer, unspecified eye

● H16.05   Mooren's corneal ulcer
     H16.051   Mooren's corneal ulcer, right eye
     H16.052   Mooren's corneal ulcer, left eye
     H16.053   Mooren's corneal ulcer, bilateral
     H16.059   Mooren's corneal ulcer, unspecified eye

● H16.06   Mycotic corneal ulcer
     H16.061   Mycotic corneal ulcer, right eye
     H16.062   Mycotic corneal ulcer, left eye
     H16.063   Mycotic corneal ulcer, bilateral
     H16.069   Mycotic corneal ulcer, unspecified eye

● H16.07   Perforated corneal ulcer
     H16.071   Perforated corneal ulcer, right eye
     H16.072   Perforated corneal ulcer, left eye
     H16.073   Perforated corneal ulcer, bilateral
     H16.079   Perforated corneal ulcer, unspecified eye

● H16.1   Other and unspecified superficial keratitis without conjunctivitis
     ● H16.10   Unspecified superficial keratitis
         H16.101   Unspecified superficial keratitis, right eye
         H16.102   Unspecified superficial keratitis, left eye
         H16.103   Unspecified superficial keratitis, bilateral
         H16.109   Unspecified superficial keratitis, unspecified eye

     ● H16.11   Macular keratitis
         Areolar keratitis
         Nummular keratitis
         Stellate keratitis
         Striate keratitis
         H16.111   Macular keratitis, right eye
         H16.112   Macular keratitis, left eye
         H16.113   Macular keratitis, bilateral
         H16.119   Macular keratitis, unspecified eye

     ● H16.12   Filamentary keratitis
         H16.121   Filamentary keratitis, right eye
         H16.122   Filamentary keratitis, left eye
         H16.123   Filamentary keratitis, bilateral
         H16.129   Filamentary keratitis, unspecified eye

     ● H16.13   Photokeratitis
         Snow blindness
         Welders' keratitis
         H16.131   Photokeratitis, right eye
         H16.132   Photokeratitis, left eye
         H16.133   Photokeratitis, bilateral
         H16.139   Photokeratitis, unspecified eye

     ● H16.14   Punctate keratitis
         H16.141   Punctate keratitis, right eye
         H16.142   Punctate keratitis, left eye
         H16.143   Punctate keratitis, bilateral
         H16.149   Punctate keratitis, unspecified eye

● H16.2   Keratoconjunctivitis
     ● H16.20   Unspecified keratoconjunctivitis
         Superficial keratitis with conjunctivitis NOS
         H16.201   Unspecified keratoconjunctivitis, right eye
         H16.202   Unspecified keratoconjunctivitis, left eye
         H16.203   Unspecified keratoconjunctivitis, bilateral
         H16.209   Unspecified keratoconjunctivitis, unspecified eye

     ● H16.21   Exposure keratoconjunctivitis
         H16.211   Exposure keratoconjunctivitis, right eye
         H16.212   Exposure keratoconjunctivitis, left eye
         H16.213   Exposure keratoconjunctivitis, bilateral
         H16.219   Exposure keratoconjunctivitis, unspecified eye

     ● H16.22   Keratoconjunctivitis sicca, not specified as Sjögren's
         Excludes1   Sjogren's syndrome (M35.01)
         H16.221   Keratoconjunctivitis sicca, not specified as Sjögren's, right eye
         H16.222   Keratoconjunctivitis sicca, not specified as Sjögren's, left eye
         H16.223   Keratoconjunctivitis sicca, not specified as Sjögren's, bilateral
         H16.229   Keratoconjunctivitis sicca, not specified as Sjögren's, unspecified eye

     ● H16.23   Neurotrophic keratoconjunctivitis
         H16.231   Neurotrophic keratoconjunctivitis, right eye
         H16.232   Neurotrophic keratoconjunctivitis, left eye
         H16.233   Neurotrophic keratoconjunctivitis, bilateral
         H16.239   Neurotrophic keratoconjunctivitis, unspecified eye

     ● H16.24   Ophthalmia nodosa
         H16.241   Ophthalmia nodosa, right eye
         H16.242   Ophthalmia nodosa, left eye
         H16.243   Ophthalmia nodosa, bilateral
         H16.249   Ophthalmia nodosa, unspecified eye

     ● H16.25   Phlyctenular keratoconjunctivitis
         H16.251   Phlyctenular keratoconjunctivitis, right eye
         H16.252   Phlyctenular keratoconjunctivitis, left eye
         H16.253   Phlyctenular keratoconjunctivitis, bilateral
         H16.259   Phlyctenular keratoconjunctivitis, unspecified eye

     ● H16.26   Vernal keratoconjunctivitis, with limbar and corneal involvement
         Excludes1   vernal conjunctivitis without limbar and corneal involvement (H10.44)
         H16.261   Vernal keratoconjunctivitis, with limbar and corneal involvement, right eye
         H16.262   Vernal keratoconjunctivitis, with limbar and corneal involvement, left eye

CHAPTER 7 (H00-H59)

     H16.263   Vernal keratoconjunctivitis, with limbar and corneal involvement, bilateral

     H16.269   Vernal keratoconjunctivitis, with limbar and corneal involvement, unspecified eye

● H16.29   Other keratoconjunctivitis

     H16.291   Other keratoconjunctivitis, right eye

     H16.292   Other keratoconjunctivitis, left eye

     H16.293   Other keratoconjunctivitis, bilateral

     H16.299   Other keratoconjunctivitis, unspecified eye

● H16.3   Interstitial and deep keratitis

   ● H16.30   Unspecified interstitial keratitis

     H16.301   Unspecified interstitial keratitis, right eye

     H16.302   Unspecified interstitial keratitis, left eye

     H16.303   Unspecified interstitial keratitis, bilateral

     H16.309   Unspecified interstitial keratitis, unspecified eye

   ● H16.31   Corneal abscess

     H16.311   Corneal abscess, right eye

     H16.312   Corneal abscess, left eye

     H16.313   Corneal abscess, bilateral

     H16.319   Corneal abscess, unspecified eye

   ● H16.32   Diffuse interstitial keratitis
       Cogan's syndrome

     H16.321   Diffuse interstitial keratitis, right eye

     H16.322   Diffuse interstitial keratitis, left eye

     H16.323   Diffuse interstitial keratitis, bilateral

     H16.329   Diffuse interstitial keratitis, unspecified eye

   ● H16.33   Sclerosing keratitis

     H16.331   Sclerosing keratitis, right eye

     H16.332   Sclerosing keratitis, left eye

     H16.333   Sclerosing keratitis, bilateral

     H16.339   Sclerosing keratitis, unspecified eye

   ● H16.39   Other interstitial and deep keratitis

     H16.391   Other interstitial and deep keratitis, right eye

     H16.392   Other interstitial and deep keratitis, left eye

     H16.393   Other interstitial and deep keratitis, bilateral

     H16.399   Other interstitial and deep keratitis, unspecified eye

● H16.4   Corneal neovascularization

   ● H16.40   Unspecified corneal neovascularization

     H16.401   Unspecified corneal neovascularization, right eye

     H16.402   Unspecified corneal neovascularization, left eye

     H16.403   Unspecified corneal neovascularization, bilateral

     H16.409   Unspecified corneal neovascularization, unspecified eye

   ● H16.41   Ghost vessels (corneal)

     H16.411   Ghost vessels (corneal), right eye

     H16.412   Ghost vessels (corneal), left eye

     H16.413   Ghost vessels (corneal), bilateral

     H16.419   Ghost vessels (corneal), unspecified eye

   ● H16.42   Pannus (corneal)

     H16.421   Pannus (corneal), right eye

     H16.422   Pannus (corneal), left eye

     H16.423   Pannus (corneal), bilateral

     H16.429   Pannus (corneal), unspecified eye

   ● H16.43   Localized vascularization of cornea

     H16.431   Localized vascularization of cornea, right eye

     H16.432   Localized vascularization of cornea, left eye

     H16.433   Localized vascularization of cornea, bilateral

     H16.439   Localized vascularization of cornea, unspecified eye

   ● H16.44   Deep vascularization of cornea

     H16.441   Deep vascularization of cornea, right eye

     H16.442   Deep vascularization of cornea, left eye

     H16.443   Deep vascularization of cornea, bilateral

     H16.449   Deep vascularization of cornea, unspecified eye

   ● H16.8   Other keratitis

   ● H16.9   Unspecified keratitis

● H17   Corneal scars and opacities

   ● H17.0   Adherent leukoma

     H17.00   Adherent leukoma, unspecified eye

     H17.01   Adherent leukoma, right eye

     H17.02   Adherent leukoma, left eye

     H17.03   Adherent leukoma, bilateral

   ● H17.1   Central corneal opacity

     H17.10   Central corneal opacity, unspecified eye

     H17.11   Central corneal opacity, right eye

     H17.12   Central corneal opacity, left eye

     H17.13   Central corneal opacity, bilateral

   ● H17.8   Other corneal scars and opacities

   ● H17.81   Minor opacity of cornea
       Corneal nebula

     H17.811   Minor opacity of cornea, right eye

     H17.812   Minor opacity of cornea, left eye

     H17.813   Minor opacity of cornea, bilateral

     H17.819   Minor opacity of cornea, unspecified eye

   ● H17.82   Peripheral opacity of cornea

     H17.821   Peripheral opacity of cornea, right eye

     H17.822   Peripheral opacity of cornea, left eye

     H17.823   Peripheral opacity of cornea, bilateral

     H17.829   Peripheral opacity of cornea, unspecified eye

     H17.89   Other corneal scars and opacities

   ● H17.9   Unspecified corneal scar and opacity

● H18   Other disorders of cornea

   ● H18.0   Corneal pigmentations and deposits

   ● H18.00   Unspecified corneal deposit

     H18.001   Unspecified corneal deposit, right eye

     H18.002   Unspecified corneal deposit, left eye

     H18.003   Unspecified corneal deposit, bilateral

     H18.009   Unspecified corneal deposit, unspecified eye

   ● H18.01   Anterior corneal pigmentations
       Staehli's line

     H18.011   Anterior corneal pigmentations, right eye

     H18.012   Anterior corneal pigmentations, left eye

◀ New   ◀▦ Revised   ~~deleted~~ Deleted   Excludes 1   Excludes 2   Includes   Use additional   Code first   Code also   Unspecified

OGCR Official Guidelines   ● Unacceptable Principal Diagnosis   X Assign placeholder X   ● Use Additional Character(s)   ▶ Manifestation Code   **Coding Clinic**

H18.013   **Anterior corneal pigmentations, bilateral**

H18.019   **Anterior corneal pigmentations, unspecified eye**

● **H18.02**   **Argentous corneal deposits**

H18.021   **Argentous corneal deposits, right eye**

H18.022   **Argentous corneal deposits, left eye**

H18.023   **Argentous corneal deposits, bilateral**

H18.029   **Argentous corneal deposits, unspecified eye**

● **H18.03**   **Corneal deposits in metabolic disorders**

    Code also associated metabolic disorder

H18.031   **Corneal deposits in metabolic disorders, right eye**

H18.032   **Corneal deposits in metabolic disorders, left eye**

H18.033   **Corneal deposits in metabolic disorders, bilateral**

H18.039   **Corneal deposits in metabolic disorders, unspecified eye**

● **H18.04**   **Kayser-Fleischer ring**

    Code also associated Wilson's disease (E83.01)

H18.041   **Kayser-Fleischer ring, right eye**

H18.042   **Kayser-Fleischer ring, left eye**

H18.043   **Kayser-Fleischer ring, bilateral**

H18.049   **Kayser-Fleischer ring, unspecified eye**

● **H18.05**   **Posterior corneal pigmentations**

    Krukenberg's spindle

H18.051   **Posterior corneal pigmentations, right eye**

H18.052   **Posterior corneal pigmentations, left eye**

H18.053   **Posterior corneal pigmentations, bilateral**

H18.059   **Posterior corneal pigmentations, unspecified eye**

● **H18.06**   **Stromal corneal pigmentations**

    Hematocornea

H18.061   **Stromal corneal pigmentations, right eye**

H18.062   **Stromal corneal pigmentations, left eye**

H18.063   **Stromal corneal pigmentations, bilateral**

H18.069   **Stromal corneal pigmentations, unspecified eye**

● **H18.1**   **Bullous keratopathy**

H18.10   **Bullous keratopathy, unspecified eye**

H18.11   **Bullous keratopathy, right eye**

H18.12   **Bullous keratopathy, left eye**

H18.13   **Bullous keratopathy, bilateral**

● **H18.2**   **Other and unspecified corneal edema**

H18.20   **Unspecified corneal edema**

● **H18.21**   **Corneal edema secondary to contact lens**

    Excludes2   other corneal disorders due to contact lens (H18.82-)

H18.211   **Corneal edema secondary to contact lens, right eye**

H18.212   **Corneal edema secondary to contact lens, left eye**

H18.213   **Corneal edema secondary to contact lens, bilateral**

H18.219   **Corneal edema secondary to contact lens, unspecified eye**

● **H18.22**   **Idiopathic corneal edema**

H18.221   **Idiopathic corneal edema, right eye**

H18.222   **Idiopathic corneal edema, left eye**

H18.223   **Idiopathic corneal edema, bilateral**

H18.229   **Idiopathic corneal edema, unspecified eye**

● **H18.23**   **Secondary corneal edema**

H18.231   **Secondary corneal edema, right eye**

H18.232   **Secondary corneal edema, left eye**

H18.233   **Secondary corneal edema, bilateral**

H18.239   **Secondary corneal edema, unspecified eye**

● **H18.3**   **Changes of corneal membranes**

H18.30   **Unspecified corneal membrane change**

● **H18.31**   **Folds and rupture in Bowman's membrane**

H18.311   **Folds and rupture in Bowman's membrane, right eye**

H18.312   **Folds and rupture in Bowman's membrane, left eye**

H18.313   **Folds and rupture in Bowman's membrane, bilateral**

H18.319   **Folds and rupture in Bowman's membrane, unspecified eye**

● **H18.32**   **Folds in Descemet's membrane**

H18.321   **Folds in Descemet's membrane, right eye**

H18.322   **Folds in Descemet's membrane, left eye**

H18.323   **Folds in Descemet's membrane, bilateral**

H18.329   **Folds in Descemet's membrane, unspecified eye**

● **H18.33**   **Rupture in Descemet's membrane**

H18.331   **Rupture in Descemet's membrane, right eye**

H18.332   **Rupture in Descemet's membrane, left eye**

H18.333   **Rupture in Descemet's membrane, bilateral**

H18.339   **Rupture in Descemet's membrane, unspecified eye**

● **H18.4**   **Corneal degeneration**

    Excludes1   Mooren's ulcer (H16.0-)

                recurrent erosion of cornea (H18.83-)

H18.40   **Unspecified corneal degeneration**

● **H18.41**   **Arcus senilis**

    Senile corneal changes

H18.411   **Arcus senilis, right eye**

H18.412   **Arcus senilis, left eye**

H18.413   **Arcus senilis, bilateral**

H18.419   **Arcus senilis, unspecified eye**

● **H18.42**   **Band keratopathy**

H18.421   **Band keratopathy, right eye**

H18.422   **Band keratopathy, left eye**

H18.423   **Band keratopathy, bilateral**

H18.429   **Band keratopathy, unspecified eye**

H18.43   **Other calcerous corneal degeneration**

● **H18.44**   **Keratomalacia**

    Excludes1   keratomalacia due to vitamin A deficiency (E50.4)

H18.441   **Keratomalacia, right eye**

H18.442   **Keratomalacia, left eye**

H18.443   **Keratomalacia, bilateral**

H18.449   **Keratomalacia, unspecified eye**

N Newborn Age: 0   **P** Pediatric Age: 0–17   **M** Maternity DX: 12–55   **A** Adult Age: 15–124   ♀ Females Only   ♂ Males Only

Complication\Comorbidity   Major C\C   (Ex) CC/MCC Exclusions   Hospital-Acquired Condition

825

● H18.45　Nodular corneal degeneration
　　　　H18.451　Nodular corneal degeneration, right eye
　　　　H18.452　Nodular corneal degeneration, left eye
　　　　H18.453　Nodular corneal degeneration, bilateral
　　　　H18.459　Nodular corneal degeneration, unspecified eye
● H18.46　Peripheral corneal degeneration
　　　　H18.461　Peripheral corneal degeneration, right eye
　　　　H18.462　Peripheral corneal degeneration, left eye
　　　　H18.463　Peripheral corneal degeneration, bilateral
　　　　H18.469　Peripheral corneal degeneration, unspecified eye
　　H18.49　Other corneal degeneration
● H18.5　Hereditary corneal dystrophies
　　H18.50　Unspecified hereditary corneal dystrophies
　　H18.51　Endothelial corneal dystrophy
　　　　　　Fuchs' dystrophy
　　H18.52　Epithelial (juvenile) corneal dystrophy
　　H18.53　Granular corneal dystrophy
　　H18.54　Lattice corneal dystrophy
　　H18.55　Macular corneal dystrophy
　　H18.59　Other hereditary corneal dystrophies
● H18.6　Keratoconus
　　H18.60　Keratoconus, unspecified
　　　　H18.601　Keratoconus, unspecified, right eye
　　　　H18.602　Keratoconus, unspecified, left eye
　　　　H18.603　Keratoconus, unspecified, bilateral
　　　　H18.609　Keratoconus, unspecified, unspecified eye
● H18.61　Keratoconus, stable
　　　　H18.611　Keratoconus, stable, right eye
　　　　H18.612　Keratoconus, stable, left eye
　　　　H18.613　Keratoconus, stable, bilateral
　　　　H18.619　Keratoconus, stable, unspecified eye
● H18.62　Keratoconus, unstable
　　　　　　Acute hydrops
　　　　H18.621　Keratoconus, unstable, right eye
　　　　H18.622　Keratoconus, unstable, left eye
　　　　H18.623　Keratoconus, unstable, bilateral
　　　　H18.629　Keratoconus, unstable, unspecified eye

● H18.7　Other and unspecified corneal deformities
　　　Excludes1　congenital malformations of cornea (Q13.3-Q13.4)
　　H18.70　Unspecified corneal deformity
● H18.71　Corneal ectasia
　　　　H18.711　Corneal ectasia, right eye
　　　　H18.712　Corneal ectasia, left eye
　　　　H18.713　Corneal ectasia, bilateral
　　　　H18.719　Corneal ectasia, unspecified eye
● H18.72　Corneal staphyloma
　　　　H18.721　Corneal staphyloma, right eye
　　　　H18.722　Corneal staphyloma, left eye
　　　　H18.723　Corneal staphyloma, bilateral
　　　　H18.729　Corneal staphyloma, unspecified eye
● H18.73　Descemetocele
　　　　H18.731　Descemetocele, right eye
　　　　H18.732　Descemetocele, left eye
　　　　H18.733　Descemetocele, bilateral
　　　　H18.739　Descemetocele, unspecified eye
● H18.79　Other corneal deformities
　　　　H18.791　Other corneal deformities, right eye
　　　　H18.792　Other corneal deformities, left eye
　　　　H18.793　Other corneal deformities, bilateral
　　　　H18.799　Other corneal deformities, unspecified eye
● H18.8　Other specified disorders of cornea
● H18.81　Anesthesia and hypoesthesia of cornea
　　　　H18.811　Anesthesia and hypoesthesia of cornea, right eye
　　　　H18.812　Anesthesia and hypoesthesia of cornea, left eye
　　　　H18.813　Anesthesia and hypoesthesia of cornea, bilateral
　　　　H18.819　Anesthesia and hypoesthesia of cornea, unspecified eye
● H18.82　Corneal disorder due to contact lens
　　　Excludes2　corneal edema due to contact lens (H18.21-)
　　　　H18.821　Corneal disorder due to contact lens, right eye
　　　　H18.822　Corneal disorder due to contact lens, left eye
　　　　H18.823　Corneal disorder due to contact lens, bilateral
　　　　H18.829　Corneal disorder due to contact lens, unspecified eye
● H18.83　Recurrent erosion of cornea
　　　　H18.831　Recurrent erosion of cornea, right eye
　　　　H18.832　Recurrent erosion of cornea, left eye
　　　　H18.833　Recurrent erosion of cornea, bilateral
　　　　H18.839　Recurrent erosion of cornea, unspecified eye
● H18.89　Other specified disorders of cornea
　　　　H18.891　Other specified disorders of cornea, right eye
　　　　H18.892　Other specified disorders of cornea, left eye
　　　　H18.893　Other specified disorders of cornea, bilateral
　　　　H18.899　Other specified disorders of cornea, unspecified eye
● H18.9　Unspecified disorder of cornea

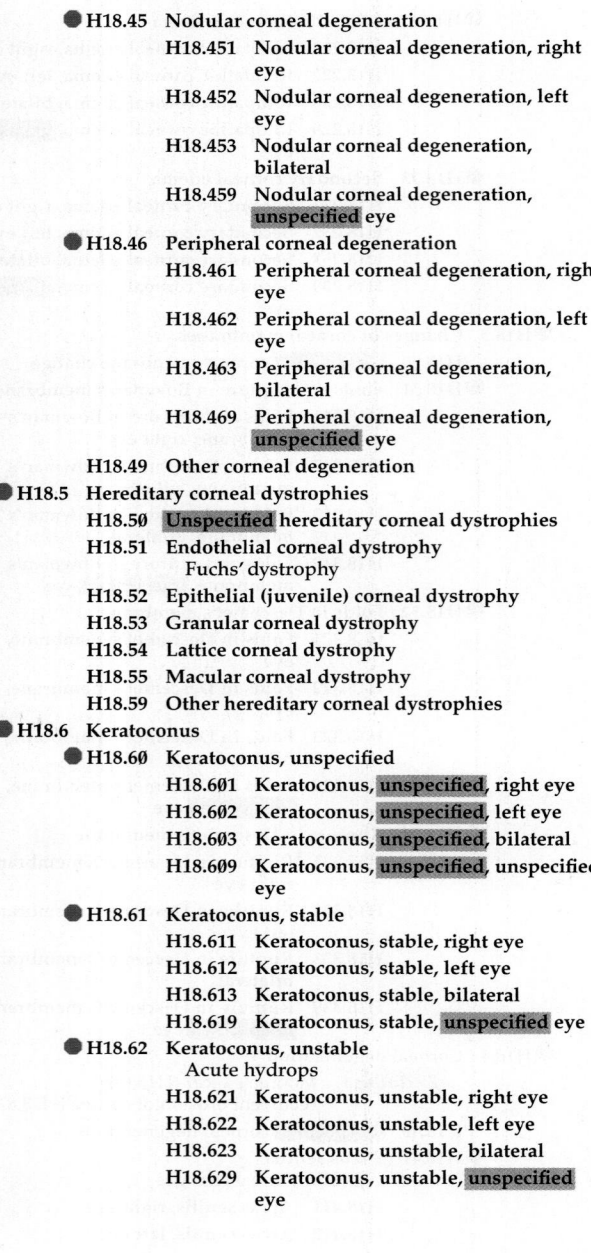

Figure 7-8 Lateral view of the displacement of the cone apex in keratoconus. (From Yanoff: Ophthalmology, ed 3, Mosby, Inc., 2008)

Item 7–4 Keratoconus results in corneal degeneration that begins in childhood, gradually changes the cornea from a round to cone shape, decreasing visual acuity. Treatment includes contact lenses. In severe cases the need for corneal transplant may be the treatment of choice; however, newer technologies may use high frequency radio energy to shrink the edges of the cornea, pulling the central area back to a more normal shape. It can help delay or avoid the need for a corneal transplantation.

◀ New　　◀▥▥ Revised　　~~deleted~~ Deleted　　Excludes 1　　Excludes 2　　Includes　　Use additional　　Code first　　Code also　　Unspecified

OGCR Official Guidelines　　● Unacceptable Principal Diagnosis　　X Assign placeholder X　　● Use Additional Character(s)　　▶ Manifestation Code　　**Coding Clinic**

● **H20   Iridocyclitis**

  ● **H20.0   Acute and subacute iridocyclitis**

      Acute anterior uveitis

      Acute cyclitis

      Acute iritis

      Subacute anterior uveitis

      Subacute cyclitis

      Subacute iritis

      Excludes1   iridocyclitis, iritis, uveitis (due to) (in) diabetes mellitus (E08-E13 with .39)

                   iridocyclitis, iritis, uveitis (due to) (in) diphtheria (A36.89)

                   iridocyclitis, iritis, uveitis (due to) (in) gonococcal (A54.32)

                   iridocyclitis, iritis, uveitis (due to) (in) herpes (simplex) (B00.51)

                   iridocyclitis, iritis, uveitis (due to) (in) herpes zoster (B02.32)

                   iridocyclitis, iritis, uveitis (due to) (in) late congenital syphilis (A50.39)

                   iridocyclitis, iritis, uveitis (due to) (in) late syphilis (A52.71)

                   iridocyclitis, iritis, uveitis (due to) (in) sarcoidosis (D86.83)

                   iridocyclitis, iritis, uveitis (due to) (in) syphilis (A51.43)

                   iridocyclitis, iritis, uveitis (due to) (in) toxoplasmosis (B58.09)

                   iridocyclitis, iritis, uveitis (due to) (in) tuberculosis (A18.54)

      Ex: For category H20 CC codes: A18.54, H20.00-H20.9

      H20.00   Unspecified acute and subacute iridocyclitis

  ● **H20.01**   Primary iridocyclitis

      H20.011   Primary iridocyclitis, right eye

      H20.012   Primary iridocyclitis, left eye

      H20.013   Primary iridocyclitis, bilateral

      H20.019   Primary iridocyclitis, unspecified eye

  ● **H20.02**   Recurrent acute iridocyclitis

      H20.021   Recurrent acute iridocyclitis, right eye

      H20.022   Recurrent acute iridocyclitis, left eye

      H20.023   Recurrent acute iridocyclitis, bilateral

      H20.029   Recurrent acute iridocyclitis, unspecified eye

  ● **H20.03**   Secondary infectious iridocyclitis

      H20.031   Secondary infectious iridocyclitis, right eye

      H20.032   Secondary infectious iridocyclitis, left eye

      H20.033   Secondary infectious iridocyclitis, bilateral

      H20.039   Secondary infectious iridocyclitis, unspecified eye

  ● **H20.04**   Secondary noninfectious iridocyclitis

      H20.041   Secondary noninfectious iridocyclitis, right eye

      H20.042   Secondary noninfectious iridocyclitis, left eye

      H20.043   Secondary noninfectious iridocyclitis, bilateral

      H20.049   Secondary noninfectious iridocyclitis, unspecified eye

  ● **H20.05**   Hypopyon

      H20.051   Hypopyon, right eye

      H20.052   Hypopyon, left eye

      H20.053   Hypopyon, bilateral

      H20.059   Hypopyon, unspecified eye

  ● **H20.1**   Chronic iridocyclitis

      Use additional code for any associated cataract (H26.21-)

      Excludes2   posterior cyclitis (H30.2-)

      H20.10   Chronic iridocyclitis, unspecified eye

      H20.11   Chronic iridocyclitis, right eye

      H20.12   Chronic iridocyclitis, left eye

      H20.13   Chronic iridocyclitis, bilateral

  ● **H20.2**   Lens-induced iridocyclitis

      H20.20   Lens-induced iridocyclitis, unspecified eye

      H20.21   Lens-induced iridocyclitis, right eye

      H20.22   Lens-induced iridocyclitis, left eye

      H20.23   Lens-induced iridocyclitis, bilateral

  ● **H20.8**   Other iridocyclitis

      Excludes2   glaucomatocyclitis crises (H40.4-)

                 posterior cyclitis (H30.2-)

                 sympathetic uveitis (H44.13-)

  ● **H20.81**   Fuchs' heterochromic cyclitis

      H20.811   Fuchs' heterochromic cyclitis, right eye

      H20.812   Fuchs' heterochromic cyclitis, left eye

      H20.813   Fuchs' heterochromic cyclitis, bilateral

      H20.819   Fuchs' heterochromic cyclitis, unspecified eye

  ● **H20.82**   Vogt-Koyanagi syndrome

      H20.821   Vogt-Koyanagi syndrome, right eye

      H20.822   Vogt-Koyanagi syndrome, left eye

      H20.823   Vogt-Koyanagi syndrome, bilateral

      H20.829   Vogt-Koyanagi syndrome, unspecified eye

      H20.9   Unspecified iridocyclitis

      Uveitis NOS

● **H21   Other disorders of iris and ciliary body**

      Excludes2   sympathetic uveitis (H44.1-)

  ● **H21.0**   Hyphema

      Excludes1   traumatic hyphema (S05.1-)

      H21.00   Hyphema, unspecified eye

      H21.01   Hyphema, right eye

      H21.02   Hyphema, left eye

      H21.03   Hyphema, bilateral

  ● **H21.1**   Other vascular disorders of iris and ciliary body

      Neovascularization of iris or ciliary body

      Rubeosis iridis

      Rubeosis of iris

  ● **H21.1X**   Other vascular disorders of iris and ciliary body

      H21.1X1   Other vascular disorders of iris and ciliary body, right eye

      H21.1X2   Other vascular disorders of iris and ciliary body, left eye

      H21.1X3   Other vascular disorders of iris and ciliary body, bilateral

      H21.1X9   Other vascular disorders of iris and ciliary body, unspecified eye

  ● **H21.2**   Degeneration of iris and ciliary body

  ● **H21.21**   Degeneration of chamber angle

      H21.211   Degeneration of chamber angle, right eye

      H21.212   Degeneration of chamber angle, left eye

      H21.213   Degeneration of chamber angle, bilateral

      H21.219   Degeneration of chamber angle, unspecified eye

CHAPTER 7 (H00-H59)

N Newborn Age: Ø   **P** Pediatric Age: Ø–17   **M** Maternity DX: 12–55   **A** Adult Age: 15–124   ♀ Females Only   ♂ Males Only

Complication\Comorbidity   Major C\C   (Ex) CC/MCC Exclusions   Hospital-Acquired Condition

827

● **H21.22 Degeneration of ciliary body**
　　H21.221　Degeneration of ciliary body, right eye
　　H21.222　Degeneration of ciliary body, left eye
　　H21.223　Degeneration of ciliary body, bilateral
　　H21.229　Degeneration of ciliary body, unspecified eye
● **H21.23 Degeneration of iris (pigmentary)**
　　　　Translucency of iris
　　H21.231　Degeneration of iris (pigmentary), right eye
　　H21.232　Degeneration of iris (pigmentary), left eye
　　H21.233　Degeneration of iris (pigmentary), bilateral
　　H21.239　Degeneration of iris (pigmentary), unspecified eye
● **H21.24 Degeneration of pupillary margin**
　　H21.241　Degeneration of pupillary margin, right eye
　　H21.242　Degeneration of pupillary margin, left eye
　　H21.243　Degeneration of pupillary margin, bilateral
　　H21.249　Degeneration of pupillary margin, unspecified eye
● **H21.25 Iridoschisis**
　　H21.251　Iridoschisis, right eye
　　H21.252　Iridoschisis, left eye
　　H21.253　Iridoschisis, bilateral
　　H21.259　Iridoschisis, unspecified eye
● **H21.26 Iris atrophy (essential) (progressive)**
　　H21.261　Iris atrophy (essential) (progressive), right eye
　　H21.262　Iris atrophy (essential) (progressive), left eye
　　H21.263　Iris atrophy (essential) (progressive), bilateral
　　H21.269　Iris atrophy (essential) (progressive), unspecified eye
● **H21.27 Miotic pupillary cyst**
　　H21.271　Miotic pupillary cyst, right eye
　　H21.272　Miotic pupillary cyst, left eye
　　H21.273　Miotic pupillary cyst, bilateral
　　H21.279　Miotic pupillary cyst, unspecified eye
　　H21.29　Other iris atrophy
● **H21.3 Cyst of iris, ciliary body and anterior chamber**
　　Excludes2　miotic pupillary cyst (H21.27-)
● **H21.30　Idiopathic cysts of iris, ciliary body or anterior chamber**
　　　　Cyst of iris, ciliary body or anterior chamber NOS
　　H21.301　Idiopathic cysts of iris, ciliary body or anterior chamber, right eye
　　H21.302　Idiopathic cysts of iris, ciliary body or anterior chamber, left eye
　　H21.303　Idiopathic cysts of iris, ciliary body or anterior chamber, bilateral
　　H21.309　Idiopathic cysts of iris, ciliary body or anterior chamber, unspecified eye
● **H21.31　Exudative cysts of iris or anterior chamber**
　　H21.311　Exudative cysts of iris or anterior chamber, right eye
　　H21.312　Exudative cysts of iris or anterior chamber, left eye
　　H21.313　Exudative cysts of iris or anterior chamber, bilateral
　　H21.319　Exudative cysts of iris or anterior chamber, unspecified eye

● **H21.32　Implantation cysts of iris, ciliary body or anterior chamber**
　　H21.321　Implantation cysts of iris, ciliary body or anterior chamber, right eye
　　H21.322　Implantation cysts of iris, ciliary body or anterior chamber, left eye
　　H21.323　Implantation cysts of iris, ciliary body or anterior chamber, bilateral
　　H21.329　Implantation cysts of iris, ciliary body or anterior chamber, unspecified eye
● **H21.33　Parasitic cyst of iris, ciliary body or anterior chamber**
　　Ex: For category **H21.33** CC codes: H20.051-H20.059, H21.331-H21.339, H33.121-H33.129, H44.001-H44.029, H44.121-H44.129, H44.19
　　H21.331　Parasitic cyst of iris, ciliary body or anterior chamber, right eye 🐾
　　H21.332　Parasitic cyst of iris, ciliary body or anterior chamber, left eye 🐾
　　H21.333　Parasitic cyst of iris, ciliary body or anterior chamber, bilateral 🐾
　　H21.339　Parasitic cyst of iris, ciliary body or anterior chamber, unspecified eye 🐾
● **H21.34　Primary cyst of pars plana**
　　H21.341　Primary cyst of pars plana, right eye
　　H21.342　Primary cyst of pars plana, left eye
　　H21.343　Primary cyst of pars plana, bilateral
　　H21.349　Primary cyst of pars plana, unspecified eye
● **H21.35　Exudative cyst of pars plana**
　　H21.351　Exudative cyst of pars plana, right eye
　　H21.352　Exudative cyst of pars plana, left eye
　　H21.353　Exudative cyst of pars plana, bilateral
　　H21.359　Exudative cyst of pars plana, unspecified eye
● **H21.4　Pupillary membranes**
　　　　Iris bombé
　　　　Pupillary occlusion
　　　　Pupillary seclusion
　　Excludes1　congenital pupillary membranes (Q13.8)
　　H21.40　Pupillary membranes, unspecified eye
　　H21.41　Pupillary membranes, right eye
　　H21.42　Pupillary membranes, left eye
　　H21.43　Pupillary membranes, bilateral
● **H21.5　Other and unspecified adhesions and disruptions of iris and ciliary body**
　　Excludes1　corectopia (Q13.2)
● **H21.50　Unspecified adhesions of iris**
　　　　Synechia (iris) NOS
　　H21.501　Unspecified adhesions of iris, right eye
　　H21.502　Unspecified adhesions of iris, left eye
　　H21.503　Unspecified adhesions of iris, bilateral
　　H21.509　Unspecified adhesions of iris and ciliary body, unspecified eye
● **H21.51　Anterior synechiae (iris)**
　　H21.511　Anterior synechiae (iris), right eye
　　H21.512　Anterior synechiae (iris), left eye
　　H21.513　Anterior synechiae (iris), bilateral
　　H21.519　Anterior synechiae (iris), unspecified eye
● **H21.52　Goniosynechiae**
　　H21.521　Goniosynechiae, right eye
　　H21.522　Goniosynechiae, left eye
　　H21.523　Goniosynechiae, bilateral
　　H21.529　Goniosynechiae, unspecified eye

◀ New　◀|||| Revised　~~deleted~~ Deleted　Excludes 1　Excludes 2　Includes　Use additional　Code first　Code also　Unspecified
OGCR Official Guidelines　● Unacceptable Principal Diagnosis　X Assign placeholder X　● Use Additional Character(s)　▶ Manifestation Code　**Coding Clinic**

● **H21.53 Iridodialysis**
    H21.531 Iridodialysis, right eye
    H21.532 Iridodialysis, left eye
    H21.533 Iridodialysis, bilateral
    H21.539 Iridodialysis, unspecified eye

● **H21.54 Posterior synechiae (iris)**
    H21.541 Posterior synechiae (iris), right eye
    H21.542 Posterior synechiae (iris), left eye
    H21.543 Posterior synechiae (iris), bilateral
    H21.549 Posterior synechiae (iris), unspecified eye

● **H21.55 Recession of chamber angle**
    H21.551 Recession of chamber angle, right eye
    H21.552 Recession of chamber angle, left eye
    H21.553 Recession of chamber angle, bilateral
    H21.559 Recession of chamber angle, unspecified eye

● **H21.56 Pupillary abnormalities**
    Deformed pupil
    Ectopic pupil
    Rupture of sphincter, pupil
    Excludes1   congenital deformity of pupil (Q13.2-)
    H21.561 Pupillary abnormality, right eye
    H21.562 Pupillary abnormality, left eye
    H21.563 Pupillary abnormality, bilateral
    H21.569 Pupillary abnormality, unspecified eye

● **H21.8 Other specified disorders of iris and ciliary body**
    H21.81 Floppy iris syndrome
        Intraoperative floppy iris syndrome (IFIS)
        Use additional code for adverse effect, if applicable, to identify drug (T36-T50 with fifth or sixth character 5)
    H21.82 Plateau iris syndrome (post-iridectomy) (postprocedural)
    H21.89 Other specified disorders of iris and ciliary body
    H21.9 Unspecified disorder of iris and ciliary body

▶ *H22 Disorders of iris and ciliary body in diseases classified elsewhere*
    Code first underlying disease, such as:
        gout (M1A.-, M10.-)
        leprosy (A30.-)
        parasitic disease (B89)

DISORDERS OF LENS (H25-H28)

● **H25 Age-related cataract**
    Senile cataract
    Excludes2   capsular glaucoma with pseudoexfoliation of lens (H40.1-)

● **H25.0 Age-related incipient cataract**
    ● H25.01 Cortical age-related cataract
        H25.011 Cortical age-related cataract, right eye   A
        H25.012 Cortical age-related cataract, left eye   A
        H25.013 Cortical age-related cataract, bilateral   A
        H25.019 Cortical age-related cataract, unspecified eye   A
    ● H25.03 Anterior subcapsular polar age-related cataract
        H25.031 Anterior subcapsular polar age-related cataract, right eye A
        H25.032 Anterior subcapsular polar age-related cataract, left eye   A
        H25.033 Anterior subcapsular polar age-related cataract, bilateral A
        H25.039 Anterior subcapsular polar age-related cataract, unspecified eye A

Figure 7-9   Age-related cataract. Nuclear sclerosis and cortical lens opacities are present. (From Yanoff: Ophthalmology, ed 3, Mosby, Inc., 2008)

Item 7–5   Senile cataracts are linked to the aging process. The most common area for the formation of a cataract is the cortical area of the lens. **Polar cataracts** can be either anterior or posterior. **Anterior polar cataracts** are more common and are small, white, capsular cataracts located on the anterior portion of the lens. **Total cataracts,** also called **complete** or **mature,** cause an opacity of all fibers of the lens. **Hypermature** describes a mature cataract with a swollen, milky cortex that covers the entire lens. **Immature,** also called **incipient,** cataracts have a clear cortex and are only slightly opaque. Treatment for all cataracts is the removal of the lens.

    ● H25.04 Posterior subcapsular polar age-related cataract
        H25.041 Posterior subcapsular polar age-related cataract, right eye   A
        H25.042 Posterior subcapsular polar age-related cataract, left eye   A
        H25.043 Posterior subcapsular polar age-related cataract, bilateral   A
        H25.049 Posterior subcapsular polar age-related cataract, unspecified eye A
    ● H25.09 Other age-related incipient cataract
        Coronary age-related cataract
        Punctate age-related cataract
        Water clefts
        H25.091 Other age-related incipient cataract, right eye   A
        H25.092 Other age-related incipient cataract, left eye   A
        H25.093 Other age-related incipient cataract, bilateral   A
        H25.099 Other age-related incipient cataract, unspecified eye   A

● **H25.1 Age-related nuclear cataract**
    Cataracta brunescens
    Nuclear sclerosis cataract
    H25.10 Age-related nuclear cataract, unspecified eye   A
    H25.11 Age-related nuclear cataract, right eye   A
    H25.12 Age-related nuclear cataract, left eye   A
        Coding Clinic: 2016, Q1, P33
    H25.13 Age-related nuclear cataract, bilateral   A
        Coding Clinic: 2016, Q1, P32

● **H25.2 Age-related cataract, morgagnian type**
    Age-related hypermature cataract
    H25.20 Age-related cataract, morgagnian type, unspecified eye   A
    H25.21 Age-related cataract, morgagnian type, right eye   A
    H25.22 Age-related cataract, morgagnian type, left eye   A
    H25.23 Age-related cataract, morgagnian type, bilateral   A

● **H25.8 Other age-related cataract**
    ● H25.81 Combined forms of age-related cataract
        H25.811 Combined forms of age-related cataract, right eye   A
        H25.812 Combined forms of age-related cataract, left eye   A
        H25.813 Combined forms of age-related cataract, bilateral   A
        H25.819 Combined forms of age-related cataract, unspecified eye   A
    H25.89 Other age-related cataract   A
    H25.9 Unspecified age-related cataract   A

CHAPTER 7 (H00-H59)

● **H26   Other cataract**

    Excludes1   congenital cataract (Q12.0)

   ● **H26.0   Infantile and juvenile cataract**

     ● **H26.00   Unspecified infantile and juvenile cataract**

      H26.001   Unspecified infantile and juvenile cataract, right eye   P

      H26.002   Unspecified infantile and juvenile cataract, left eye   P

      H26.003   Unspecified infantile and juvenile cataract, bilateral   P

      H26.009   Unspecified infantile and juvenile cataract, unspecified eye   P

     ● **H26.01   Infantile and juvenile cortical, lamellar, or zonular cataract**

      H26.011   Infantile and juvenile cortical, lamellar, or zonular cataract, right eye   P

      H26.012   Infantile and juvenile cortical, lamellar, or zonular cataract, left eye   P

      H26.013   Infantile and juvenile cortical, lamellar, or zonular cataract, bilateral   P

      H26.019   Infantile and juvenile cortical, lamellar, or zonular cataract, unspecified eye   P

     ● **H26.03   Infantile and juvenile nuclear cataract**

      H26.031   Infantile and juvenile nuclear cataract, right eye   P

      H26.032   Infantile and juvenile nuclear cataract, left eye   P

      H26.033   Infantile and juvenile nuclear cataract, bilateral   P

      H26.039   Infantile and juvenile nuclear cataract, unspecified eye   P

     ● **H26.04   Anterior subcapsular polar infantile and juvenile cataract**

      H26.041   Anterior subcapsular polar infantile and juvenile cataract, right eye   P

      H26.042   Anterior subcapsular polar infantile and juvenile cataract, left eye   P

      H26.043   Anterior subcapsular polar infantile and juvenile cataract, bilateral   P

      H26.049   Anterior subcapsular polar infantile and juvenile cataract, unspecified eye   P

     ● **H26.05   Posterior subcapsular polar infantile and juvenile cataract**

      H26.051   Posterior subcapsular polar infantile and juvenile cataract, right eye   P

      H26.052   Posterior subcapsular polar infantile and juvenile cataract, left eye   P

      H26.053   Posterior subcapsular polar infantile and juvenile cataract, bilateral   P

      H26.059   Posterior subcapsular polar infantile and juvenile cataract, unspecified eye   P

     ● **H26.06   Combined forms of infantile and juvenile cataract**

      H26.061   Combined forms of infantile and juvenile cataract, right eye   P

      H26.062   Combined forms of infantile and juvenile cataract, left eye   P

      H26.063   Combined forms of infantile and juvenile cataract bilateral   P

      H26.069   Combined forms of infantile and juvenile cataract, unspecified eye   P

     H26.09   Other infantile and juvenile cataract   P

● **H26.1   Traumatic cataract**

    Use additional code (Chapter 20) to identify external cause

   ● **H26.10   Unspecified traumatic cataract**

      H26.101   Unspecified traumatic cataract, right eye

      H26.102   Unspecified traumatic cataract, left eye

      H26.103   Unspecified traumatic cataract, bilateral

      H26.109   Unspecified traumatic cataract, unspecified eye

   ● **H26.11   Localized traumatic opacities**

      H26.111   Localized traumatic opacities, right eye

      H26.112   Localized traumatic opacities, left eye

      H26.113   Localized traumatic opacities, bilateral

      H26.119   Localized traumatic opacities, unspecified eye

   ● **H26.12   Partially resolved traumatic cataract**

      H26.121   Partially resolved traumatic cataract, right eye

      H26.122   Partially resolved traumatic cataract, left eye

      H26.123   Partially resolved traumatic cataract, bilateral

      H26.129   Partially resolved traumatic cataract, unspecified eye

   ● **H26.13   Total traumatic cataract**

      H26.131   Total traumatic cataract, right eye

      H26.132   Total traumatic cataract, left eye

      H26.133   Total traumatic cataract, bilateral

      H26.139   Total traumatic cataract, unspecified eye

● **H26.2   Complicated cataract**

   H26.20   Unspecified complicated cataract

     Cataracta complicata NOS

   ● **H26.21   Cataract with neovascularization**

     Code also associated condition, such as: chronic iridocyclitis (H20.1-)

      H26.211   Cataract with neovascularization, right eye

      H26.212   Cataract with neovascularization, left eye

      H26.213   Cataract with neovascularization, bilateral

      H26.219   Cataract with neovascularization, unspecified eye

   ● **H26.22   Cataract secondary to ocular disorders (degenerative) (inflammatory)**

     Code also associated ocular disorder

      H26.221   Cataract secondary to ocular disorders (degenerative) (inflammatory), right eye

      H26.222   Cataract secondary to ocular disorders (degenerative) (inflammatory), left eye

      H26.223   Cataract secondary to ocular disorders (degenerative) (inflammatory), bilateral

      H26.229   Cataract secondary to ocular disorders (degenerative) (inflammatory), unspecified eye

   ● **H26.23   Glaucomatous flecks (subcapsular)**

     Code first underlying glaucoma (H40-H42)

      H26.231   Glaucomatous flecks (subcapsular), right eye

      H26.232   Glaucomatous flecks (subcapsular), left eye

◀ New   ⇐ Revised   ~~deleted~~ Deleted   Excludes 1   Excludes 2   Includes   Use additional   Code first   Code also   Unspecified
OGCR Official Guidelines   ● Unacceptable Principal Diagnosis   X Assign placeholder X   ● Use Additional Character(s)   ▶ Manifestation Code   **Coding Clinic**

H26.233   Glaucomatous flecks (subcapsular), bilateral

H26.239   Glaucomatous flecks (subcapsular), unspecified eye

● H26.3   **Drug-induced cataract**
Toxic cataract

Use additional code for adverse effect, if applicable, to identify drug (T36-T50 with fifth or sixth character 5)

H26.30   Drug-induced cataract, unspecified eye

H26.31   Drug-induced cataract, right eye

H26.32   Drug-induced cataract, left eye

H26.33   Drug-induced cataract, bilateral

● H26.4   **Secondary cataract**

H26.40   Unspecified secondary cataract

● H26.41   Soemmering's ring

H26.411   Soemmering's ring, right eye

H26.412   Soemmering's ring, left eye

H26.413   Soemmering's ring, bilateral

H26.419   Soemmering's ring, unspecified eye

● H26.49   Other secondary cataract

H26.491   Other secondary cataract, right eye

H26.492   Other secondary cataract, left eye

H26.493   Other secondary cataract, bilateral

H26.499   Other secondary cataract, unspecified eye

H26.8   **Other specified cataract**

H26.9   **Unspecified cataract**

● H27   **Other disorders of lens**

Excludes1   congenital lens malformations (Q12.-)
mechanical complications of intraocular lens implant (T85.2)
pseudophakia (Z96.1)

● H27.0   **Aphakia**
Acquired absence of lens
Acquired aphakia
Aphakia due to trauma

Excludes1   cataract extraction status (Z98.4-)
congenital absence of lens (Q12.3)
congenital aphakia (Q12.3)

H27.00   Aphakia, unspecified eye

H27.01   Aphakia, right eye

H27.02   Aphakia, left eye

H27.03   Aphakia, bilateral

● H27.1   **Dislocation of lens**

H27.10   Unspecified dislocation of lens

● H27.11   Subluxation of lens

H27.111   Subluxation of lens, right eye

H27.112   Subluxation of lens, left eye

H27.113   Subluxation of lens, bilateral

H27.119   Subluxation of lens, unspecified eye

● H27.12   Anterior dislocation of lens

H27.121   Anterior dislocation of lens, right eye

H27.122   Anterior dislocation of lens, left eye

H27.123   Anterior dislocation of lens, bilateral

H27.129   Anterior dislocation of lens, unspecified eye

● H27.13   Posterior dislocation of lens

H27.131   Posterior dislocation of lens, right eye

H27.132   Posterior dislocation of lens, left eye

H27.133   Posterior dislocation of lens, bilateral

H27.139   Posterior dislocation of lens, unspecified eye

H27.8   **Other specified disorders of lens**

H27.9   **Unspecified disorder of lens**

▶ *H28*   *Cataract in diseases classified elsewhere*

Code first underlying disease, such as:
hypoparathyroidism (E20.-)
myotonia (G71.1-)
myxedema (E03.-)
protein-calorie malnutrition (E40-E46)

Excludes1   cataract in diabetes mellitus (E08.36, E09.36, E10.36, E11.36, E13.36)

DISORDERS OF CHOROID AND RETINA (H30-H36)

★ **(See Plate 90 on page 64.)**

● H30   **Chorioretinal inflammation**

● H30.0   **Focal chorioretinal inflammation**
Focal chorioretinitis
Focal choroiditis
Focal retinitis
Focal retinochoroiditis

● H30.00   Unspecified focal chorioretinal inflammation
Focal chorioretinitis NOS
Focal choroiditis NOS
Focal retinitis NOS
Focal retinochoroiditis NOS

H30.001   Unspecified focal chorioretinal inflammation, right eye

H30.002   Unspecified focal chorioretinal inflammation, left eye

H30.003   Unspecified focal chorioretinal inflammation, bilateral

H30.009   Unspecified focal chorioretinal inflammation, unspecified eye

● H30.01   Focal chorioretinal inflammation, juxtapapillary

H30.011   Focal chorioretinal inflammation, juxtapapillary, right eye

H30.012   Focal chorioretinal inflammation, juxtapapillary, left eye

H30.013   Focal chorioretinal inflammation, juxtapapillary, bilateral

H30.019   Focal chorioretinal inflammation, juxtapapillary, unspecified eye

● H30.02   Focal chorioretinal inflammation of posterior pole

H30.021   Focal chorioretinal inflammation of posterior pole, right eye

H30.022   Focal chorioretinal inflammation of posterior pole, left eye

H30.023   Focal chorioretinal inflammation of posterior pole, bilateral

H30.029   Focal chorioretinal inflammation of posterior pole, unspecified eye

● H30.03   Focal chorioretinal inflammation, peripheral

H30.031   Focal chorioretinal inflammation, peripheral, right eye

H30.032   Focal chorioretinal inflammation, peripheral, left eye

H30.033   Focal chorioretinal inflammation, peripheral, bilateral

H30.039   Focal chorioretinal inflammation, peripheral, unspecified eye

● H30.04   Focal chorioretinal inflammation, macular or paramacular

H30.041   Focal chorioretinal inflammation, macular or paramacular, right eye

H30.042   Focal chorioretinal inflammation, macular or paramacular, left eye

H30.043   Focal chorioretinal inflammation, macular or paramacular, bilateral

H30.049   Focal chorioretinal inflammation, macular or paramacular, unspecified eye

CHAPTER 7 (H00–H59)

● **H30.1** **Disseminated chorioretinal inflammation**
Disseminated chorioretinitis
Disseminated choroiditis
Disseminated retinitis
Disseminated retinochoroiditis
   Excludes2   exudative retinopathy (H35.02-)
   Ex: For category H30.1 CC codes: H30.001-H30.93

  ● **H30.10**   **Unspecified disseminated chorioretinal inflammation**
Disseminated chorioretinitis NOS
Disseminated choroiditis NOS
Disseminated retinitis NOS
Disseminated retinochoroiditis NOS

    H30.101   Unspecified disseminated chorioretinal inflammation, right eye

    H30.102   Unspecified disseminated chorioretinal inflammation, left eye

    H30.103   Unspecified disseminated chorioretinal inflammation, bilateral

    H30.109   Unspecified disseminated chorioretinal inflammation, unspecified eye

  ● **H30.11**   **Disseminated chorioretinal inflammation of posterior pole**

    H30.111   Disseminated chorioretinal inflammation of posterior pole, right eye

    H30.112   Disseminated chorioretinal inflammation of posterior pole, left eye

    H30.113   Disseminated chorioretinal inflammation of posterior pole, bilateral

    H30.119   Disseminated chorioretinal inflammation of posterior pole, unspecified eye

  ● **H30.12**   **Disseminated chorioretinal inflammation, peripheral**

    H30.121   Disseminated chorioretinal inflammation, peripheral right eye

    H30.122   Disseminated chorioretinal inflammation, peripheral, left eye

    H30.123   Disseminated chorioretinal inflammation, peripheral, bilateral

    H30.129   Disseminated chorioretinal inflammation, peripheral, unspecified eye

  ● **H30.13**   **Disseminated chorioretinal inflammation, generalized**

    H30.131   Disseminated chorioretinal inflammation, generalized, right eye

    H30.132   Disseminated chorioretinal inflammation, generalized, left eye

    H30.133   Disseminated chorioretinal inflammation, generalized, bilateral

    H30.139   Disseminated chorioretinal inflammation, generalized, unspecified eye

  ● **H30.14**   **Acute posterior multifocal placoid pigment epitheliopathy**

    H30.141   Acute posterior multifocal placoid pigment epitheliopathy, right eye

    H30.142   Acute posterior multifocal placoid pigment epitheliopathy, left eye

    H30.143   Acute posterior multifocal placoid pigment epitheliopathy, bilateral

    H30.149   Acute posterior multifocal placoid pigment epitheliopathy, unspecified eye

● **H30.2**   **Posterior cyclitis**
Pars planitis

    H30.20   Posterior cyclitis, unspecified eye

    H30.21   Posterior cyclitis, right eye

    H30.22   Posterior cyclitis, left eye

    H30.23   Posterior cyclitis, bilateral

● **H30.8**   **Other chorioretinal inflammations**

  ● **H30.81**   **Harada's disease**

    H30.811   Harada's disease, right eye

    H30.812   Harada's disease, left eye

    H30.813   Harada's disease, bilateral

    H30.819   Harada's disease, unspecified eye

  ● **H30.89**   **Other chorioretinal inflammations**
    Ex: For category H30.89 CC codes: H30.001-H30.93

    H30.891   Other chorioretinal inflammations, right eye

    H30.892   Other chorioretinal inflammations, left eye

    H30.893   Other chorioretinal inflammations, bilateral

    H30.899   Other chorioretinal inflammations, unspecified eye

● **H30.9**   **Unspecified chorioretinal inflammation**
Chorioretinitis NOS
Choroiditis NOS
Neuroretinitis NOS
Retinitis NOS
Retinochoroiditis NOS
    Ex: For category H30.9 CC codes: H30.001-H30.93

    H30.90   Unspecified chorioretinal inflammation, unspecified eye

    H30.91   Unspecified chorioretinal inflammation, right eye

    H30.92   Unspecified chorioretinal inflammation, left eye

    H30.93   Unspecified chorioretinal inflammation, bilateral

● **H31**   **Other disorders of choroid**

  ● **H31.0**   **Chorioretinal scars**
    Excludes2   postsurgical chorioretinal scars (H59.81-)

  ● **H31.00**   **Unspecified chorioretinal scars**

    H31.001   Unspecified chorioretinal scars, right eye

    H31.002   Unspecified chorioretinal scars, left eye

    H31.003   Unspecified chorioretinal scars, bilateral

    H31.009   Unspecified chorioretinal scars, unspecified eye

  ● **H31.01**   **Macula scars of posterior pole (postinflammatory) (post-traumatic)**
    Excludes1   postprocedural chorioretinal scar (H59.81-)

    H31.011   Macula scars of posterior pole (postinflammatory) (post-traumatic), right eye

    H31.012   Macula scars of posterior pole (postinflammatory) (post-traumatic), left eye

◀ New   ◀ Revised   deleted Deleted   Excludes 1   Excludes 2   Includes   Use additional   Code first   Code also   Unspecified
OGCR Official Guidelines   ● Unacceptable Principal Diagnosis   X Assign placeholder X   ● Use Additional Character(s)   ▶ Manifestation Code   **Coding Clinic**

H31.013   Macula scars of posterior pole (postinflammatory) (post-traumatic), bilateral

H31.019   Macula scars of posterior pole (postinflammatory) (post-traumatic), unspecified eye

● **H31.02**   Solar retinopathy

H31.021   Solar retinopathy, right eye

H31.022   Solar retinopathy, left eye

H31.023   Solar retinopathy, bilateral

H31.029   Solar retinopathy, unspecified eye

● **H31.09**   Other chorioretinal scars

H31.091   Other chorioretinal scars, right eye

H31.092   Other chorioretinal scars, left eye

H31.093   Other chorioretinal scars, bilateral

H31.099   Other chorioretinal scars, unspecified eye

● **H31.1**   Choroidal degeneration

> **Excludes2**   angioid streaks of macula (H35.33)

● **H31.10**   Unspecified choroidal degeneration
Choroidal sclerosis NOS

H31.101   Choroidal degeneration, unspecified, right eye

H31.102   Choroidal degeneration, unspecified, left eye

H31.103   Choroidal degeneration, unspecified, bilateral

H31.109   Choroidal degeneration, unspecified, unspecified eye

● **H31.11**   Age-related choroidal atrophy

H31.111   Age-related choroidal atrophy, right eye   **A**

H31.112   Age-related choroidal atrophy, left eye   **A**

H31.113   Age-related choroidal atrophy, bilateral   **A**

H31.119   Age-related choroidal atrophy, unspecified eye   **A**

● **H31.12**   Diffuse secondary atrophy of choroid

H31.121   Diffuse secondary atrophy of choroid, right eye

H31.122   Diffuse secondary atrophy of choroid, left eye

H31.123   Diffuse secondary atrophy of choroid, bilateral

H31.129   Diffuse secondary atrophy of choroid, unspecified eye

● **H31.2**   Hereditary choroidal dystrophy

> **Excludes2**   hyperornithinemia (E72.4)
> ornithinemia (E72.4)

H31.20   Hereditary choroidal dystrophy, unspecified

H31.21   Choroideremia

H31.22   Choroidal dystrophy (central areolar) (generalized) (peripapillary)

H31.23   Gyrate atrophy, choroid

H31.29   Other hereditary choroidal dystrophy

● **H31.3**   Choroidal hemorrhage and rupture

● **H31.30**   Unspecified choroidal hemorrhage

H31.301   Unspecified choroidal hemorrhage, right eye

H31.302   Unspecified choroidal hemorrhage, left eye

H31.303   Unspecified choroidal hemorrhage, bilateral

H31.309   Unspecified choroidal hemorrhage, unspecified eye

● **H31.31**   Expulsive choroidal hemorrhage

H31.311   Expulsive choroidal hemorrhage, right eye

H31.312   Expulsive choroidal hemorrhage, left eye

H31.313   Expulsive choroidal hemorrhage, bilateral

H31.319   Expulsive choroidal hemorrhage, unspecified eye

● **H31.32**   Choroidal rupture

> (Ex) **For category H31.32 CC codes:** H31.301-H32

H31.321   Choroidal rupture, right eye 🔗

H31.322   Choroidal rupture, left eye 🔗

H31.323   Choroidal rupture, bilateral 🔗

H31.329   Choroidal rupture, unspecified eye 🔗

● **H31.4**   Choroidal detachment

> (Ex) **For category H31.4 CC codes:** H31.301-H32

● **H31.40**   Unspecified choroidal detachment

H31.401   Unspecified choroidal detachment, right eye 🔗

H31.402   Unspecified choroidal detachment, left eye 🔗

H31.403   Unspecified choroidal detachment, bilateral 🔗

H31.409   Unspecified choroidal detachment, unspecified eye 🔗

● **H31.41**   Hemorrhagic choroidal detachment

H31.411   Hemorrhagic choroidal detachment, right eye 🔗

H31.412   Hemorrhagic choroidal detachment, left eye 🔗

H31.413   Hemorrhagic choroidal detachment, bilateral 🔗

H31.419   Hemorrhagic choroidal detachment, unspecified eye 🔗

● **H31.42**   Serous choroidal detachment

H31.421   Serous choroidal detachment, right eye 🔗

H31.422   Serous choroidal detachment, left eye 🔗

H31.423   Serous choroidal detachment, bilateral 🔗

H31.429   Serous choroidal detachment, unspecified eye 🔗

H31.8   Other specified disorders of choroid

H31.9   Unspecified disorder of choroid

▶ *H32*   *Chorioretinal disorders in diseases classified elsewhere*

> *Code first* underlying disease, such as:
> congenital toxoplasmosis (P37.1)
> histoplasmosis (B39.-)
> leprosy (A30.-)
>
> **Excludes1**   chorioretinitis (in):
>   toxoplasmosis (acquired) (B58.01)
>   tuberculosis (A18.53)

● **H33**   Retinal detachments and breaks

> **Excludes1**   detachment of retinal pigment epithelium (H35.72-, H35.73-)

● **H33.0**   Retinal detachment with retinal break
Rhegmatogenous retinal detachment

> **Excludes1**   serous retinal detachment (without retinal break) (H33.2-)

● **H33.00**   Unspecified retinal detachment with retinal break

H33.001   Unspecified retinal detachment with retinal break, right eye

H33.002   Unspecified retinal detachment with retinal break, left eye

N Newborn Age: 0   **P** Pediatric Age: 0–17   **M** Maternity DX: 12–55   **A** Adult Age: 15–124   ♀ Females Only   ♂ Males Only

🔗 Complication\Comorbidity   Major C\C   (Ex) CC/MCC Exclusions   Hospital-Acquired Condition   **833**

NON-RHEGMATOGENOUS
RETINAL DETACHMENT

— Vitreous
— Retina
— Protein-rich fluid in sub-retinal space
Retinal pigment epithelium

VITREOUS DETACHMENT

— Vitreous
— Posterior hyaloid
Internal limiting membrane

RHEGMATOGENOUS
RETINAL
DETACHMENT

Blood
— Vitreous
— Posterior hyaloid
— Retina
— Retinal tear
— Liquified vitreous
Retinal pigment epithelium

Figure 7-10   Retinal detachment. (From Kumar: Robbins and Cotran: Pathologic Basis of Disease, ed 7, Saunders, 2005)

Item 7–6   Retinal detachments and defects are conditions of the eye in which the retina separates from the underlying tissue. Initial detachment may be localized, requiring rapid treatment (medical emergency) to avoid the entire retina from detaching which leads to vision loss and blindness.

H33.003   Unspecified retinal detachment with retinal break, bilateral

H33.009   Unspecified retinal detachment with retinal break, unspecified eye

● H33.01   Retinal detachment with single break

    H33.011   Retinal detachment with single break, right eye

    H33.012   Retinal detachment with single break, left eye

    H33.013   Retinal detachment with single break, bilateral

    H33.019   Retinal detachment with single break, unspecified eye

● H33.02   Retinal detachment with multiple breaks

    H33.021   Retinal detachment with multiple breaks, right eye

    H33.022   Retinal detachment with multiple breaks, left eye

    H33.023   Retinal detachment with multiple breaks, bilateral

    H33.029   Retinal detachment with multiple breaks, unspecified eye

● H33.03   Retinal detachment with giant retinal tear

    H33.031   Retinal detachment with giant retinal tear, right eye

    H33.032   Retinal detachment with giant retinal tear, left eye

    H33.033   Retinal detachment with giant retinal tear, bilateral

    H33.039   Retinal detachment with giant retinal tear, unspecified eye

● H33.04   Retinal detachment with retinal dialysis

    H33.041   Retinal detachment with retinal dialysis, right eye

    H33.042   Retinal detachment with retinal dialysis, left eye

    H33.043   Retinal detachment with retinal dialysis, bilateral

    H33.049   Retinal detachment with retinal dialysis, unspecified eye

● H33.05   Total retinal detachment

    H33.051   Total retinal detachment, right eye

    H33.052   Total retinal detachment, left eye

    H33.053   Total retinal detachment, bilateral

    H33.059   Total retinal detachment, unspecified eye

● H33.1   Retinoschisis and retinal cysts

    Excludes1   congenital retinoschisis (Q14.1)
       microcystoid degeneration of retina (H35.42-)

● H33.10   Unspecified retinoschisis

    H33.101   Unspecified retinoschisis, right eye

    H33.102   Unspecified retinoschisis, left eye

    H33.103   Unspecified retinoschisis, bilateral

    H33.109   Unspecified retinoschisis, unspecified eye

● H33.11   Cyst of ora serrata

    H33.111   Cyst of ora serrata, right eye

    H33.112   Cyst of ora serrata, left eye

    H33.113   Cyst of ora serrata, bilateral

    H33.119   Cyst of ora serrata, unspecified eye

● H33.12   Parasitic cyst of retina

    (Ex) **For category H33.12 CC codes:** H20.051-H20.059, H21.331-H21.339, H33.121-H33.129, H44.001-H44.029, H44.121-H44.129, H44.19

    H33.121   Parasitic cyst of retina, right eye 🐾

    H33.122   Parasitic cyst of retina, left eye 🐾

    H33.123   Parasitic cyst of retina, bilateral 🐾

    H33.129   Parasitic cyst of retina, unspecified eye 🐾

● H33.19   Other retinoschisis and retinal cysts
    Pseudocyst of retina

    H33.191   Other retinoschisis and retinal cysts, right eye

    H33.192   Other retinoschisis and retinal cysts, left eye

    H33.193   Other retinoschisis and retinal cysts, bilateral

    H33.199   Other retinoschisis and retinal cysts, unspecified eye

● H33.2   Serous retinal detachment
    Retinal detachment NOS
    Retinal detachment without retinal break

    Excludes1   central serous chorioretinopathy (H35.71-)

    (Ex) **For category H33.2 CC codes:** H33.001-H33.119, H33.191-H33.8, H35.70-H35.739

    H33.20   Serous retinal detachment, unspecified eye 🐾

    H33.21   Serous retinal detachment, right eye 🐾

    H33.22   Serous retinal detachment, left eye 🐾

    H33.23   Serous retinal detachment, bilateral 🐾

◀ New   ◀▪▪ Revised   ~~deleted~~ Deleted   Excludes 1   Excludes 2   Includes   Use additional   Code first   Code also   Unspecified

OGCR Official Guidelines   ● Unacceptable Principal Diagnosis   X Assign placeholder X   ● Use Additional Character(s)   ▌ Manifestation Code   **Coding Clinic**

● **H33.3   Retinal breaks without detachment**
　　Excludes1   chorioretinal scars after surgery for
　　　　　　　detachment (H59.81-)
　　　　　　peripheral retinal degeneration without
　　　　　　　break (H35.4-)
　● **H33.30   Unspecified retinal break**
　　　H33.301   Unspecified retinal break, right eye
　　　H33.302   Unspecified retinal break, left eye
　　　H33.303   Unspecified retinal break, bilateral
　　　H33.309   Unspecified retinal break, unspecified
　　　　　　　eye
　● **H33.31   Horseshoe tear of retina without detachment**
　　　Operculum of retina without detachment
　　　H33.311   Horseshoe tear of retina without
　　　　　　　detachment, right eye
　　　H33.312   Horseshoe tear of retina without
　　　　　　　detachment, left eye
　　　H33.313   Horseshoe tear of retina without
　　　　　　　detachment, bilateral
　　　H33.319   Horseshoe tear of retina without
　　　　　　　detachment, unspecified eye
　● **H33.32   Round hole of retina without detachment**
　　　H33.321   Round hole, right eye
　　　H33.322   Round hole, left eye
　　　H33.323   Round hole, bilateral
　　　H33.329   Round hole, unspecified eye
　● **H33.33   Multiple defects of retina without detachment**
　　　H33.331   Multiple defects of retina without
　　　　　　　detachment, right eye
　　　H33.332   Multiple defects of retina without
　　　　　　　detachment, left eye
　　　H33.333   Multiple defects of retina without
　　　　　　　detachment, bilateral
　　　H33.339   Multiple defects of retina without
　　　　　　　detachment, unspecified eye

● **H33.4   Traction detachment of retina**
　　Proliferative vitreo-retinopathy with retinal
　　　detachment
　　(Ex) **For category H33.4 CC codes:** See H33.2
　　H33.40   Traction detachment of retina, unspecified
　　　　　　eye 🦠
　　H33.41   Traction detachment of retina, right eye 🦠
　　H33.42   Traction detachment of retina, left eye 🦠
　　H33.43   Traction detachment of retina, bilateral 🦠
　H33.8   Other retinal detachments 🦠
　　　(Ex) See H33.2

● **H34   Retinal vascular occlusions**
　　Blockage in vessel of the retina
　　Excludes1   amaurosis fugax (G45.3)
　　(Ex) **For category H34 CC codes unless otherwise indicated:** G45.3, H34.00-H34.9
　● **H34.0   Transient retinal artery occlusion**
　　　H34.00   Transient retinal artery occlusion, unspecified
　　　　　　　eye 🦠
　　　H34.01   Transient retinal artery occlusion, right eye 🦠
　　　H34.02   Transient retinal artery occlusion, left eye 🦠
　　　H34.03   Transient retinal artery occlusion, bilateral 🦠
　● **H34.1   Central retinal artery occlusion**
　　　H34.10   Central retinal artery occlusion, unspecified
　　　　　　　eye 🦠
　　　H34.11   Central retinal artery occlusion, right eye 🦠
　　　H34.12   Central retinal artery occlusion, left eye 🦠
　　　H34.13   Central retinal artery occlusion, bilateral 🦠

● **H34.2   Other retinal artery occlusions**
　● **H34.21   Partial retinal artery occlusion**
　　　Hollenhorst's plaque
　　　Retinal microembolism
　　　H34.211   Partial retinal artery occlusion, right
　　　　　　　eye 🦠
　　　H34.212   Partial retinal artery occlusion, left
　　　　　　　eye 🦠
　　　H34.213   Partial retinal artery occlusion,
　　　　　　　bilateral 🦠
　　　H34.219   Partial retinal artery occlusion,
　　　　　　　unspecified eye 🦠
　● **H34.23   Retinal artery branch occlusion**
　　　H34.231   Retinal artery branch occlusion, right
　　　　　　　eye 🦠
　　　H34.232   Retinal artery branch occlusion, left
　　　　　　　eye 🦠
　　　H34.233   Retinal artery branch occlusion,
　　　　　　　bilateral 🦠
　　　H34.239   Retinal artery branch occlusion,
　　　　　　　unspecified eye 🦠
● **H34.8   Other retinal vascular occlusions**
　● **H34.81   Central retinal vein occlusion**
　　　One of the following 7th characters is to
　　　　be assigned to codes in subcategory
　　　　H34.81 to designate the severity of the
　　　　occlusion: ◄

Ø	with macular edema ◄
1	with retinal neovascularization ◄
2	stable ◄
	Old central retinal vein occlusion ◄

　　　(Ex) **For category H34.81 CC codes:** E08.3211-E08.3299,
　　　E08.3511-E08.3599, E08.37X1-E08.37X9, E09.3211-E09.3319,
　　　E09.3411-E09.3419, E09.3511-E09.3599, E09.37X1-E09.37X9,
　　　E10.3211-E10.3599, E10.37X1-E10.37X9, E11.3211-E11.3599,
　　　E11.37X1-E11.37X9, E13.3211-E13.3599, E13.37X1-E13.37X9,
　　　G45.3, H34.00-H34.239, H34.821-H34.9

　　● H34.811   Central retinal vein occlusion, right
　　　　　　　eye 🦠
　　● H34.812   Central retinal vein occlusion, left
　　　　　　　eye 🦠
　　● H34.813   Central retinal vein occlusion,
　　　　　　　bilateral 🦠
　　● H34.819   Central retinal vein occlusion,
　　　　　　　unspecified eye 🦠
　● **H34.82   Venous engorgement**
　　　Incipient retinal vein occlusion
　　　Partial retinal vein occlusion
　　　H34.821   Venous engorgement, right eye
　　　H34.822   Venous engorgement, left eye
　　　H34.823   Venous engorgement, bilateral
　　　H34.829   Venous engorgement, unspecified eye

N   Newborn Age: Ø   **P**   Pediatric Age: Ø-17   **M**   Maternity DX: 12-55   **A**   Adult Age: 15-124   ♀   Females Only   ♂   Males Only

🦠   Complication\Comorbidity   🦠   Major C\C   (Ex)   CC/MCC Exclusions   🦠   Hospital-Acquired Condition   **835**

● **H34.83**   **Tributary (branch) retinal vein occlusion**

> One of the following 7th characters is to be assigned to codes in subcategory H34.83 to designate the severity of the occlusion: ◀

> | | |
> |---|---|
> | 0 | with macular edema ◀ |
> | 1 | with retinal neovascularization ◀ |
> | 2 | stable ◀ |
> | | Old tributary (branch) retinal vein occlusion ◀ |

   ● **H34.831**   Tributary (branch) retinal vein occlusion, right eye

   ● **H34.832**   Tributary (branch) retinal vein occlusion, left eye

   ● **H34.833**   Tributary (branch) retinal vein occlusion, bilateral

   ● **H34.839**   Tributary (branch) retinal vein occlusion, unspecified eye

H34.9   Unspecified retinal vascular occlusion 🔗

● **H35**   **Other retinal disorders**

> **Excludes2**   diabetic retinal disorders (E08.311-E08.359, E09.311-E09.359, E10.311-E10.359, E11.311-E11.359, E13.311-E13.359)

● **H35.0**   **Background retinopathy and retinal vascular changes**

> Code also any associated hypertension (I10.-)

> **OGCR**   Section I. C.9.a.5.

> Hypertensive Retinopathy
>
> Subcategory H35.0, Background retinopathy and retinal vascular changes, should be used with a code from category I10–I15, Hypertensive disease to include the systemic hypertension. The sequencing is based on the reason for the encounter.

   H35.00   Unspecified background retinopathy

  ● **H35.01**   Changes in retinal vascular appearance

> Retinal vascular sheathing

   H35.011   Changes in retinal vascular appearance, right eye

   H35.012   Changes in retinal vascular appearance, left eye

   H35.013   Changes in retinal vascular appearance, bilateral

   H35.019   Changes in retinal vascular appearance, unspecified eye

  ● **H35.02**   Exudative retinopathy

> Coats retinopathy

   H35.021   Exudative retinopathy, right eye

   H35.022   Exudative retinopathy, left eye

   H35.023   Exudative retinopathy, bilateral

   H35.029   Exudative retinopathy, unspecified eye

  ● **H35.03**   Hypertensive retinopathy

   H35.031   Hypertensive retinopathy, right eye

   H35.032   Hypertensive retinopathy, left eye

   H35.033   Hypertensive retinopathy, bilateral

   H35.039   Hypertensive retinopathy, unspecified eye

  ● **H35.04**   Retinal micro-aneurysms, unspecified

   H35.041   Retinal micro-aneurysms, unspecified, right eye

   H35.042   Retinal micro-aneurysms, unspecified, left eye

   H35.043   Retinal micro-aneurysms, unspecified, bilateral

   H35.049   Retinal micro-aneurysms, unspecified, unspecified eye

● **H35.05**   **Retinal neovascularization, unspecified**

   H35.051   Retinal neovascularization, unspecified, right eye

   H35.052   Retinal neovascularization, unspecified, left eye

   H35.053   Retinal neovascularization, unspecified, bilateral

   H35.059   Retinal neovascularization, unspecified, unspecified eye

● **H35.06**   **Retinal vasculitis**

> Eales disease
> Retinal perivasculitis

   H35.061   Retinal vasculitis, right eye

   H35.062   Retinal vasculitis, left eye

   H35.063   Retinal vasculitis, bilateral

   H35.069   Retinal vasculitis, unspecified eye

● **H35.07**   **Retinal telangiectasis**

   H35.071   Retinal telangiectasis, right eye

   H35.072   Retinal telangiectasis, left eye

   H35.073   Retinal telangiectasis, bilateral

   H35.079   Retinal telangiectasis, unspecified eye

H35.09   Other intraretinal microvascular abnormalities

> Retinal varices

H35.1   **Retinopathy of prematurity**

● **H35.10**   Retinopathy of prematurity, unspecified

> Retinopathy of prematurity NOS

   H35.101   Retinopathy of prematurity, unspecified, right eye

   H35.102   Retinopathy of prematurity, unspecified, left eye

   H35.103   Retinopathy of prematurity, unspecified, bilateral

   H35.109   Retinopathy of prematurity, unspecified, unspecified eye

● **H35.11**   Retinopathy of prematurity, stage 0

   H35.111   Retinopathy of prematurity, stage 0, right eye

   H35.112   Retinopathy of prematurity, stage 0, left eye

   H35.113   Retinopathy of prematurity, stage 0, bilateral

   H35.119   Retinopathy of prematurity, stage 0, unspecified eye

● **H35.12**   Retinopathy of prematurity, stage 1

   H35.121   Retinopathy of prematurity, stage 1, right eye

   H35.122   Retinopathy of prematurity, stage 1, left eye

   H35.123   Retinopathy of prematurity, stage 1, bilateral

   H35.129   Retinopathy of prematurity, stage 1, unspecified eye

● **H35.13**   Retinopathy of prematurity, stage 2

   H35.131   Retinopathy of prematurity, stage 2, right eye

   H35.132   Retinopathy of prematurity, stage 2, left eye

   H35.133   Retinopathy of prematurity, stage 2, bilateral

   H35.139   Retinopathy of prematurity, stage 2, unspecified eye

● **H35.14**   **Retinopathy of prematurity, stage 3**

     H35.141   **Retinopathy of prematurity, stage 3, right eye**

     H35.142   **Retinopathy of prematurity, stage 3, left eye**

     H35.143   **Retinopathy of prematurity, stage 3, bilateral**

     H35.149   **Retinopathy of prematurity, stage 3, unspecified eye**

● **H35.15**   **Retinopathy of prematurity, stage 4**

     H35.151   **Retinopathy of prematurity, stage 4, right eye**

     H35.152   **Retinopathy of prematurity, stage 4, left eye**

     H35.153   **Retinopathy of prematurity, stage 4, bilateral**

     H35.159   **Retinopathy of prematurity, stage 4, unspecified eye**

● **H35.16**   **Retinopathy of prematurity, stage 5**

     H35.161   **Retinopathy of prematurity, stage 5, right eye**

     H35.162   **Retinopathy of prematurity, stage 5, left eye**

     H35.163   **Retinopathy of prematurity, stage 5, bilateral**

     H35.169   **Retinopathy of prematurity, stage 5, unspecified eye**

● **H35.17**   **Retrolental fibroplasia**

     H35.171   **Retrolental fibroplasia, right eye**

     H35.172   **Retrolental fibroplasia, left eye**

     H35.173   **Retrolental fibroplasia, bilateral**

     H35.179   **Retrolental fibroplasia, unspecified eye**

● **H35.2**   **Other non-diabetic proliferative retinopathy**
     Proliferative vitreo-retinopathy

     Excludes1   proliferative vitreo-retinopathy with retinal detachment (H33.4-)

     H35.20   **Other non-diabetic proliferative retinopathy, unspecified eye**

     H35.21   **Other non-diabetic proliferative retinopathy, right eye**

     H35.22   **Other non-diabetic proliferative retinopathy, left eye**

     H35.23   **Other non-diabetic proliferative retinopathy, bilateral**

● **H35.3**   **Degeneration of macula and posterior pole**

     H35.30   **Unspecified macular degeneration**   A
     Age-related macular degeneration

● **H35.31**   **Nonexudative age-related macular degeneration**
     Atrophic age-related macular degeneration
     Dry age-related macular degeneration ◄

     One of the following 7th characters is to be assigned to codes in subcategory H35.31 to designate the stage of the disease: ◄

     Ø   stage unspecified ◄
     1   early dry stage ◄
     2   intermediate dry stage ◄
     3   advanced atrophic without subfoveal involvement ◄
        advanced dry stage ◄
     4   advanced atrophic with subfoveal involvement ◄

     ● **H35.311**   **Nonexudative age-related macular degeneration, right eye** ◄   A

     ● **H35.312**   **Nonexudative age-related macular degeneration, left eye** ◄   A

Item 7–7   Macular degeneration is typically age-related, chronic, and is evidenced by deterioration of the macula (the part of the retina that provides for central field vision), resulting in blurred vision or a blind spot in the center of visual field while not affecting peripheral vision.

     ● **H35.313**   **Nonexudative age-related macular degeneration, bilateral** ◄   A

     ● **H35.319**   **Nonexudative age-related macular degeneration, unspecified eye** ◄   A

● **H35.32**   **Exudative age-related macular degeneration**
     Wet age-related macular degeneration ◄

     One of the following 7th characters is to be assigned to codes in subcategory H35.32 to designate the stage of the disease: ◄

     Ø   stage unspecified ◄
     1   with active choroidal neovascularization ◄
     2   with inactive choroidal neovascularization ◄
        with involuted or regressed neovascularization ◄
     3   with inactive scar ◄

     ● **H35.321**   **Exudative age-related macular degeneration, right eye** ◄   A

     ● **H35.322**   **Exudative age-related macular degeneration, left eye** ◄   A

     ● **H35.323**   **Exudative age-related macular degeneration, bilateral** ◄   A

     ● **H35.329**   **Exudative age-related macular degeneration, unspecified eye** ◄   A

     H35.33   **Angioid streaks of macula**

● **H35.34**   **Macular cyst, hole, or pseudohole**

     H35.341   **Macular cyst, hole, or pseudohole, right eye**

     H35.342   **Macular cyst, hole, or pseudohole, left eye**

     H35.343   **Macular cyst, hole, or pseudohole, bilateral**

     H35.349   **Macular cyst, hole, or pseudohole, unspecified eye**

● **H35.35**   **Cystoid macular degeneration**

     Excludes1   cystoid macular edema following cataract surgery (H59.Ø3-)

     H35.351   **Cystoid macular degeneration, right eye**

     H35.352   **Cystoid macular degeneration, left eye**

     H35.353   **Cystoid macular degeneration, bilateral**

     H35.359   **Cystoid macular degeneration, unspecified eye**

● **H35.36**   **Drusen (degenerative) of macula**

     H35.361   **Drusen (degenerative) of macula, right eye**

     H35.362   **Drusen (degenerative) of macula, left eye**

     H35.363   **Drusen (degenerative) of macula, bilateral**

     H35.369   **Drusen (degenerative) of macula, unspecified eye**

CHAPTER 7 (HØØ-H59)

N Newborn Age: Ø   **P** Pediatric Age: Ø–17   **M** Maternity DX: 12–55   **A** Adult Age: 15–124   ♀ Females Only   ♂ Males Only

🔗 Complication\Comorbidity   🔗 Major C\C   (Ex:) CC/MCC Exclusions   🔗 Hospital-Acquired Condition

837

● **H35.37 Puckering of macula**
    H35.371   Puckering of macula, right eye
    H35.372   Puckering of macula, left eye
    H35.373   Puckering of macula, bilateral
    H35.379   Puckering of macula, unspecified eye

● **H35.38 Toxic maculopathy**
> *Code first poisoning due to drug or toxin, if applicable (T36-T65 with fifth or sixth character 1-4 or 6)*
>
> Use additional code for adverse effect, if applicable, to identify drug (T36-T50 with fifth or sixth character 5)

    H35.381   Toxic maculopathy, right eye
    H35.382   Toxic maculopathy, left eye
    H35.383   Toxic maculopathy, bilateral
    H35.389   Toxic maculopathy, unspecified eye

● **H35.4 Peripheral retinal degeneration**
> **Excludes 1**   hereditary retinal degeneration (dystrophy) (H35.5-)
>   peripheral retinal degeneration with retinal break (H33.3-)

    H35.40   Unspecified peripheral retinal degeneration

● **H35.41 Lattice degeneration of retina**
    Palisade degeneration of retina
    H35.411   Lattice degeneration of retina, right eye
    H35.412   Lattice degeneration of retina, left eye
    H35.413   Lattice degeneration of retina, bilateral
    H35.419   Lattice degeneration of retina, unspecified eye

● **H35.42 Microcystoid degeneration of retina**
    H35.421   Microcystoid degeneration of retina, right eye
    H35.422   Microcystoid degeneration of retina, left eye
    H35.423   Microcystoid degeneration of retina, bilateral
    H35.429   Microcystoid degeneration of retina, unspecified eye

● **H35.43 Paving stone degeneration of retina**
    H35.431   Paving stone degeneration of retina, right eye
    H35.432   Paving stone degeneration of retina, left eye
    H35.433   Paving stone degeneration of retina, bilateral
    H35.439   Paving stone degeneration of retina, unspecified eye

● **H35.44 Age-related reticular degeneration of retina**
    H35.441   Age-related reticular degeneration of retina, right eye   A
    H35.442   Age-related reticular degeneration of retina, left eye   A
    H35.443   Age-related reticular degeneration of retina, bilateral   A
    H35.449   Age-related reticular degeneration of retina, unspecified eye   A

● **H35.45 Secondary pigmentary degeneration**
    H35.451   Secondary pigmentary degeneration, right eye
    H35.452   Secondary pigmentary degeneration, left eye
    H35.453   Secondary pigmentary degeneration, bilateral
    H35.459   Secondary pigmentary degeneration, unspecified eye

● **H35.46 Secondary vitreoretinal degeneration**
    H35.461   Secondary vitreoretinal degeneration, right eye
    H35.462   Secondary vitreoretinal degeneration, left eye
    H35.463   Secondary vitreoretinal degeneration, bilateral
    H35.469   Secondary vitreoretinal degeneration, unspecified eye

● **H35.5 Hereditary retinal dystrophy**
> **Excludes 1**   dystrophies primarily involving Bruch's membrane (H31.1-)

    H35.50   Unspecified hereditary retinal dystrophy
    H35.51   Vitreoretinal dystrophy
    H35.52   Pigmentary retinal dystrophy
        Albipunctate retinal dystrophy
        Retinitis pigmentosa
        Tapetoretinal dystrophy
    H35.53   Other dystrophies primarily involving the sensory retina
        Stargardt's disease
    H35.54   Dystrophies primarily involving the retinal pigment epithelium
        Vitelliform retinal dystrophy

● **H35.6 Retinal hemorrhage**
    H35.60   Retinal hemorrhage, unspecified eye
    H35.61   Retinal hemorrhage, right eye
    H35.62   Retinal hemorrhage, left eye
    H35.63   Retinal hemorrhage, bilateral

● **H35.7 Separation of retinal layers**
> **Excludes 1**   retinal detachment (serous) (H33.2-)
>   rhegmatogenous retinal detachment (H33.0-)
>
> ⒺⓍ **For category H35.7 CC codes:** H33.001-H33.119, H33.191-H33.8, H35.70-H35.739

    H35.70   Unspecified separation of retinal layers 🔖

● **H35.71 Central serous chorioretinopathy**
    H35.711   Central serous chorioretinopathy, right eye
    H35.712   Central serous chorioretinopathy, left eye
    H35.713   Central serous chorioretinopathy, bilateral
    H35.719   Central serous chorioretinopathy, unspecified eye

● **H35.72 Serous detachment of retinal pigment epithelium**
    H35.721   Serous detachment of retinal pigment epithelium, right eye 🔖
    H35.722   Serous detachment of retinal pigment epithelium, left eye 🔖
    H35.723   Serous detachment of retinal pigment epithelium, bilateral 🔖
    H35.729   Serous detachment of retinal pigment epithelium, unspecified eye 🔖

● **H35.73 Hemorrhagic detachment of retinal pigment epithelium**

    H35.731 Hemorrhagic detachment of retinal pigment epithelium, right eye 🔗

    H35.732 Hemorrhagic detachment of retinal pigment epithelium, left eye 🔗

    H35.733 Hemorrhagic detachment of retinal pigment epithelium, bilateral 🔗

    H35.739 Hemorrhagic detachment of retinal pigment epithelium, unspecified eye 🔗

● **H35.8 Other specified retinal disorders**

    Excludes2   retinal hemorrhage (H35.6-)

    H35.81 Retinal edema
        Retinal cotton wool spots

    H35.82 Retinal ischemia 🔗
        (Ex) H35.60-H35.63, H35.81-H35.89

    H35.89 Other specified retinal disorders

● **H35.9 Unspecified retinal disorder**

▶ **H36 Retinal disorders in diseases classified elsewhere**

    Code first underlying disease, such as:
        lipid storage disorders (E75.-)
        sickle-cell disorders (D57.-)

    Excludes1   arteriosclerotic retinopathy (H35.0-)
        diabetic retinopathy (E08.3-, E09.3-, E10.3-, E11.3-, E13.3-)

GLAUCOMA (H40-H42)

● **H40 Glaucoma**

    Intraocular pressure (IOP) that is too high results from too much aqueous humor and because of excess production or inadequate drainage, optic nerve damage and vision loss may occur.

    Excludes1   absolute glaucoma (H44.51-)
        congenital glaucoma (Q15.0)
        traumatic glaucoma due to birth injury (P15.3)

● **H40.0 Glaucoma suspect**

  ● **H40.00 Preglaucoma, unspecified**

    H40.001 Preglaucoma, unspecified, right eye

    H40.002 Preglaucoma, unspecified, left eye

    H40.003 Preglaucoma, unspecified, bilateral

    H40.009 Preglaucoma, unspecified, unspecified eye

  ● **H40.01 Open angle with borderline findings, low risk**
    Open angle, low risk

    H40.011 Open angle with borderline findings, low risk, right eye

    H40.012 Open angle with borderline findings, low risk, left eye

    H40.013 Open angle with borderline findings, low risk, bilateral

    H40.019 Open angle with borderline findings, low risk, unspecified eye

  ● **H40.02 Open angle with borderline findings, high risk**
    Open angle, high risk

    H40.021 Open angle with borderline findings, high risk, right eye

    H40.022 Open angle with borderline findings, high risk, left eye

    H40.023 Open angle with borderline findings, high risk, bilateral

    H40.029 Open angle with borderline findings, high risk, unspecified eye

  ● **H40.03 Anatomical narrow angle**
    Primary angle closure suspect

    H40.031 Anatomical narrow angle, right eye

    H40.032 Anatomical narrow angle, left eye

    H40.033 Anatomical narrow angle, bilateral

    H40.039 Anatomical narrow angle, unspecified eye

● **H40.04 Steroid responder**

    H40.041 Steroid responder, right eye

    H40.042 Steroid responder, left eye

    H40.043 Steroid responder, bilateral

    H40.049 Steroid responder, unspecified eye

● **H40.05 Ocular hypertension**

    H40.051 Ocular hypertension, right eye

    H40.052 Ocular hypertension, left eye

    H40.053 Ocular hypertension, bilateral

    H40.059 Ocular hypertension, unspecified eye

● **H40.06 Primary angle closure without glaucoma damage**

    H40.061 Primary angle closure without glaucoma damage, right eye

    H40.062 Primary angle closure without glaucoma damage, left eye

    H40.063 Primary angle closure without glaucoma damage, bilateral

    H40.069 Primary angle closure without glaucoma damage, unspecified eye

● **H40.1 Open-angle glaucoma**

X ● **H40.10 Unspecified open-angle glaucoma**

    One of the following 7th characters is to be assigned to code H40.10 to designate the stage of glaucoma

0	stage unspecified
1	mild stage
2	moderate stage
3	severe stage
4	indeterminate stage

● **H40.11 Primary open-angle glaucoma**
    Chronic simple glaucoma

    One of the following 7th characters is to be assigned to each code in subcategory H40.11 to designate the stage of glaucoma ◀▥

0	stage unspecified
1	mild stage
2	moderate stage
3	severe stage
4	indeterminate stage

  ● **H40.111 Primary open-angle glaucoma, right eye** ◀

  ● **H40.112 Primary open-angle glaucoma, left eye** ◀

  ● **H40.113 Primary open-angle glaucoma, bilateral** ◀

  ● **H40.119 Primary open-angle glaucoma, unspecified eye** ◀

● **H40.12 Low-tension glaucoma**

    One of the following 7th characters is to be assigned to each code in subcategory H40.12 to designate the stage of glaucoma

0	stage unspecified
1	mild stage
2	moderate stage
3	severe stage
4	indeterminate stage

  ●● **H40.121 Low-tension glaucoma, right eye**

  ●● **H40.122 Low-tension glaucoma, left eye**

  ●● **H40.123 Low-tension glaucoma, bilateral**

  ●● **H40.129 Low-tension glaucoma, unspecified eye**

N Newborn Age: 0   **P** Pediatric Age: 0–17   **M** Maternity DX: 12–55   **A** Adult Age: 15–124   ♀ Females Only   ♂ Males Only

🔗 Complication\Comorbidity   Ⓜ Major C\C   (Ex) CC/MCC Exclusions   Hospital-Acquired Condition

839

● H40.13   **Pigmentary glaucoma**

One of the following 7th characters is to be assigned to each code in subcategory H40.13 to designate the stage of glaucoma

0	stage unspecified
1	mild stage
2	moderate stage
3	severe stage
4	indeterminate stage

●● H40.131   **Pigmentary glaucoma, right eye**
●● H40.132   **Pigmentary glaucoma, left eye**
●● H40.133   **Pigmentary glaucoma, bilateral**
●● H40.139   **Pigmentary glaucoma, `unspecified` eye**

● H40.14   **Capsular glaucoma with pseudoexfoliation of lens**

One of the following 7th characters is to be assigned to each code in subcategory H40.14 to designate the stage of glaucoma

0	stage unspecified
1	mild stage
2	moderate stage
3	severe stage
4	indeterminate stage

● H40.141   **Capsular glaucoma with pseudoexfoliation of lens, right eye**
● H40.142   **Capsular glaucoma with pseudoexfoliation of lens, left eye**
● H40.143   **Capsular glaucoma with pseudoexfoliation of lens, bilateral**
● H40.149   **Capsular glaucoma with pseudoexfoliation of lens, `unspecified` eye**

● H40.15   **Residual stage of open-angle glaucoma**

● H40.151   **Residual stage of open-angle glaucoma, right eye**
● H40.152   **Residual stage of open-angle glaucoma, left eye**
● H40.153   **Residual stage of open-angle glaucoma, bilateral**
● H40.159   **Residual stage of open-angle glaucoma, `unspecified` eye**

● H40.2   **Primary angle-closure glaucoma**

`Excludes1`   aqueous misdirection (H40.83-)
           malignant glaucoma (H40.83-)

● H40.20   **`Unspecified` primary angle-closure glaucoma**

One of the following 7th characters is to be assigned to code H40.20 to designate the stage of glaucoma

0	stage unspecified
1	mild stage
2	moderate stage
3	severe stage
4	indeterminate stage

● H40.21   **Acute angle-closure glaucoma**
Acute angle-closure glaucoma attack
Acute angle-closure glaucoma crisis
Ⓔ **For category H40.21 CC codes: H40.211-H40.219**

H40.211   **Acute angle-closure glaucoma, right eye** 🔗
H40.212   **Acute angle-closure glaucoma, left eye** 🔗
H40.213   **Acute angle-closure glaucoma, bilateral** 🔗
H40.219   **Acute angle-closure glaucoma, `unspecified` eye** 🔗

● H40.22   **Chronic angle-closure glaucoma**
Chronic primary angle closure glaucoma

One of the following 7th characters is to be assigned to each code in subcategory H40.22 to designate the stage of glaucoma

0	stage unspecified
1	mild stage
2	moderate stage
3	severe stage
4	indeterminate stage

● H40.221   **Chronic angle-closure glaucoma, right eye**
● H40.222   **Chronic angle-closure glaucoma, left eye**
● H40.223   **Chronic angle-closure glaucoma, bilateral**
● H40.229   **Chronic angle-closure glaucoma, `unspecified` eye**

● H40.23   **Intermittent angle-closure glaucoma**

H40.231   **Intermittent angle-closure glaucoma, right eye**
H40.232   **Intermittent angle-closure glaucoma, left eye**
H40.233   **Intermittent angle-closure glaucoma, bilateral**
H40.239   **Intermittent angle-closure glaucoma, `unspecified` eye**

● H40.24   **Residual stage of angle-closure glaucoma**

H40.241   **Residual stage of angle-closure glaucoma, right eye**
H40.242   **Residual stage of angle-closure glaucoma, left eye**
H40.243   **Residual stage of angle-closure glaucoma, bilateral**
H40.249   **Residual stage of angle-closure glaucoma, `unspecified` eye**

● H40.3   **Glaucoma secondary to eye trauma**
`Code also` underlying condition

One of the following 7th characters is to be assigned to each code in subcategory H40.3 to designate the stage of glaucoma

0	stage unspecified
1	mild stage
2	moderate stage
3	severe stage
4	indeterminate stage

X● H40.30   **Glaucoma secondary to eye trauma, `unspecified` eye**
X● H40.31   **Glaucoma secondary to eye trauma, right eye**
X● H40.32   **Glaucoma secondary to eye trauma, left eye**
X● H40.33   **Glaucoma secondary to eye trauma, bilateral**

CHAPTER 7 (H00-H59)

● **H40.4 Glaucoma secondary to eye inflammation**
    Code also underlying condition
    One of the following 7th characters is to be assigned to
        each code in subcategory H40.4 to designate the
        stage of glaucoma

Ø	stage unspecified
1	mild stage
2	moderate stage
3	severe stage
4	indeterminate stage

X● **H40.40** Glaucoma secondary to eye inflammation,
                unspecified eye
X● **H40.41** Glaucoma secondary to eye inflammation, right
                eye
X● **H40.42** Glaucoma secondary to eye inflammation, left
                eye
X● **H40.43** Glaucoma secondary to eye inflammation,
                bilateral

● **H40.5 Glaucoma secondary to other eye disorders**
    Code also underlying eye disorder
    One of the following 7th characters is to be assigned to
        each code in subcategory H40.5 to designate the
        stage of glaucoma

Ø	stage unspecified
1	mild stage
2	moderate stage
3	severe stage
4	indeterminate stage

X● **H40.50** Glaucoma secondary to other eye disorders,
                unspecified eye
X● **H40.51** Glaucoma secondary to other eye disorders,
                right eye
X● **H40.52** Glaucoma secondary to other eye disorders, left
                eye
X● **H40.53** Glaucoma secondary to other eye disorders,
                bilateral

● **H40.6 Glaucoma secondary to drugs**
    Use additional code for adverse effect, if applicable,
        to identify drug (T36-T50 with fifth or sixth
        character 5)
    One of the following 7th characters is to be assigned to
        each code in subcategory H40.6 to designate the
        stage of glaucoma

Ø	stage unspecified
1	mild stage
2	moderate stage
3	severe stage
4	indeterminate stage

X● **H40.60** Glaucoma secondary to drugs, unspecified eye
X● **H40.61** Glaucoma secondary to drugs, right eye
X● **H40.62** Glaucoma secondary to drugs, left eye
X● **H40.63** Glaucoma secondary to drugs, bilateral

● **H40.8 Other glaucoma**
    ● **H40.81 Glaucoma with increased episcleral venous
                pressure**
        H40.811 Glaucoma with increased episcleral
                    venous pressure, right eye
        H40.812 Glaucoma with increased episcleral
                    venous pressure, left eye
        H40.813 Glaucoma with increased episcleral
                    venous pressure, bilateral
        H40.819 Glaucoma with increased episcleral
                    venous pressure, unspecified eye
    ● **H40.82 Hypersecretion glaucoma**
        H40.821 Hypersecretion glaucoma, right eye
        H40.822 Hypersecretion glaucoma, left eye
        H40.823 Hypersecretion glaucoma, bilateral
        H40.829 Hypersecretion glaucoma, unspecified
                    eye
    ● **H40.83 Aqueous misdirection**
                Malignant glaucoma
        H40.831 Aqueous misdirection, right eye
        H40.832 Aqueous misdirection, left eye
        H40.833 Aqueous misdirection, bilateral
        H40.839 Aqueous misdirection, unspecified
                    eye
    H40.89 Other specified glaucoma
    H40.9 Unspecified glaucoma

▶ **H42 Glaucoma in diseases classified elsewhere**
    Code first underlying condition, such as:
        amyloidosis (E85.-)
        aniridia (Q13.1)
        Lowe's syndrome (E72.Ø3)
        Reiger's anomaly (Q13.81)
        specified metabolic disorder (E7Ø-E88)
    Excludes1 glaucoma (in) onchocerciasis (B73.Ø2) ◀▦
                glaucoma (in) syphilis (A52.71) ◀▦
                glaucoma (in) tuberculous (A18.59) ◀▦
    Excludes2 glaucoma (in) diabetes mellitus (EØ8.39, EØ9.39,
                E1Ø.39, E11.39, E13.39) ◀

DISORDERS OF VITREOUS BODY AND GLOBE (H43-H44)

● **H43 Disorders of vitreous body**
    ● **H43.Ø Vitreous prolapse**
        Excludes1 vitreous syndrome following cataract
                        surgery (H59.Ø-)
                    traumatic vitreous prolapse (SØ5.2-)
        H43.ØØ Vitreous prolapse, unspecified eye
        H43.Ø1 Vitreous prolapse, right eye
        H43.Ø2 Vitreous prolapse, left eye
        H43.Ø3 Vitreous prolapse, bilateral
    ● **H43.1 Vitreous hemorrhage**
        H43.1Ø Vitreous hemorrhage, unspecified eye
        H43.11 Vitreous hemorrhage, right eye
        H43.12 Vitreous hemorrhage, left eye
        H43.13 Vitreous hemorrhage, bilateral
    ● **H43.2 Crystalline deposits in vitreous body**
        H43.2Ø Crystalline deposits in vitreous body,
                    unspecified eye
        H43.21 Crystalline deposits in vitreous body, right eye
        H43.22 Crystalline deposits in vitreous body, left eye
        H43.23 Crystalline deposits in vitreous body, bilateral

CHAPTER 7 (HØØ-H59)

- H43.3 **Other vitreous opacities**
  - H43.31 Vitreous membranes and strands
    - H43.311 Vitreous membranes and strands, right eye
    - H43.312 Vitreous membranes and strands, left eye
    - H43.313 Vitreous membranes and strands, bilateral
    - H43.319 Vitreous membranes and strands, unspecified eye
  - H43.39 Other vitreous opacities
    Vitreous floaters
      Small clumps of cells that float in the vitreous of the eye, appearing as black specks or dots in the field of vision and common in the aging eye.
    - H43.391 Other vitreous opacities, right eye
    - H43.392 Other vitreous opacities, left eye
    - H43.393 Other vitreous opacities, bilateral
    - H43.399 Other vitreous opacities, unspecified eye
- H43.8 **Other disorders of vitreous body**
  - **Excludes1** proliferative vitreo-retinopathy with retinal detachment (H33.4)
  - **Excludes2** vitreous abscess (H44.02-)
  - H43.81 Vitreous degeneration
    Vitreous detachment
    - H43.811 Vitreous degeneration, right eye
    - H43.812 Vitreous degeneration, left eye
    - H43.813 Vitreous degeneration, bilateral
    - H43.819 Vitreous degeneration, unspecified eye
  - H43.82 Vitreomacular adhesion
    Vitreomacular traction
    - H43.821 Vitreomacular adhesion, right eye A
    - H43.822 Vitreomacular adhesion, left eye A
    - H43.823 Vitreomacular adhesion, bilateral A
    - H43.829 Vitreomacular adhesion, unspecified eye A
  - H43.89 Other disorders of vitreous body
- H43.9 Unspecified disorder of vitreous body
- H44 **Disorders of globe**
  - **Includes** disorders affecting multiple structures of eye
  - H44.0 **Purulent endophthalmitis**
    Use additional code to identify organism
    - **Excludes1** bleb associated endophthalmitis (H59.4-)
    - H44.00 Unspecified purulent endophthalmitis
      (Ex:) **For category H44.00 CC codes:** H20.051-H20.059, H21.331-H21.339, H33.121-H33.129, H44.001-H44.029, H44.121-H44.129, H44.19
      - H44.001 Unspecified purulent endophthalmitis, right eye
      - H44.002 Unspecified purulent endophthalmitis, left eye
      - H44.003 Unspecified purulent endophthalmitis, bilateral
      - H44.009 Unspecified purulent endophthalmitis, unspecified eye
    - H44.01 Panophthalmitis (acute)
      (Ex:) **For category H44.01 CC codes:** See H44.00
      - H44.011 Panophthalmitis (acute), right eye
      - H44.012 Panophthalmitis (acute), left eye
      - H44.013 Panophthalmitis (acute), bilateral
      - H44.019 Panophthalmitis (acute), unspecified eye

- H44.02 Vitreous abscess (chronic)
  (Ex:) **For category H44.02 CC codes:** H16.241-H16.249, H21.331-H21.339, H33.121-H33.129, H44.001-H44.19
  - H44.021 Vitreous abscess (chronic), right eye
  - H44.022 Vitreous abscess (chronic), left eye
  - H44.023 Vitreous abscess (chronic), bilateral
  - H44.029 Vitreous abscess (chronic), unspecified eye
- H44.1 **Other endophthalmitis**
  - **Excludes1** bleb associated endophthalmitis (H59.4-)
  - **Excludes2** ophthalmia nodosa (H16.2-)
  - H44.11 Panuveitis
    (Ex:) **For category H44.11 CC codes:** H44.111-H44.119, H44.131-H44.139
    - H44.111 Panuveitis, right eye
    - H44.112 Panuveitis, left eye
    - H44.113 Panuveitis, bilateral
    - H44.119 Panuveitis, unspecified eye
  - H44.12 Parasitic endophthalmitis, unspecified
    (Ex:) **For category H44.12 CC codes:** See H44.00
    - H44.121 Parasitic endophthalmitis, unspecified, right eye
    - H44.122 Parasitic endophthalmitis, unspecified, left eye
    - H44.123 Parasitic endophthalmitis, unspecified, bilateral
    - H44.129 Parasitic endophthalmitis, unspecified, unspecified eye
  - H44.13 Sympathetic uveitis
    (Ex:) **For category H44.13 CC codes:** See H44.11
    - H44.131 Sympathetic uveitis, right eye
    - H44.132 Sympathetic uveitis, left eye
    - H44.133 Sympathetic uveitis, bilateral
    - H44.139 Sympathetic uveitis, unspecified eye
  - H44.19 Other endophthalmitis
    (Ex:) See H44.00
- H44.2 **Degenerative myopia**
  Malignant myopia
  - H44.20 Degenerative myopia, unspecified eye
  - H44.21 Degenerative myopia, right eye
  - H44.22 Degenerative myopia, left eye
  - H44.23 Degenerative myopia, bilateral
- H44.3 **Other and unspecified degenerative disorders of globe**
  - H44.30 Unspecified degenerative disorder of globe
  - H44.31 Chalcosis
    - H44.311 Chalcosis, right eye
    - H44.312 Chalcosis, left eye
    - H44.313 Chalcosis, bilateral
    - H44.319 Chalcosis, unspecified eye
  - H44.32 Siderosis of eye
    - H44.321 Siderosis of eye, right eye
    - H44.322 Siderosis of eye, left eye
    - H44.323 Siderosis of eye, bilateral
    - H44.329 Siderosis of eye, unspecified eye
  - H44.39 Other degenerative disorders of globe
    - H44.391 Other degenerative disorders of globe, right eye
    - H44.392 Other degenerative disorders of globe, left eye
    - H44.393 Other degenerative disorders of globe, bilateral
    - H44.399 Other degenerative disorders of globe, unspecified eye

◀ New   ◀┅ Revised   ~~deleted~~ Deleted   Excludes 1   Excludes 2   Includes   Use additional   Code first   Code also   Unspecified
OGCR Official Guidelines   ● Unacceptable Principal Diagnosis   X Assign placeholder X   ● Use Additional Character(s)   ▶ Manifestation Code   **Coding Clinic**

● **H44.4**   **Hypotony of eye**
     H44.40   Unspecified hypotony of eye
   ● **H44.41**   Flat anterior chamber hypotony of eye
        H44.411   Flat anterior chamber hypotony of right eye
        H44.412   Flat anterior chamber hypotony of left eye
        H44.413   Flat anterior chamber hypotony of eye, bilateral
        H44.419   Flat anterior chamber hypotony of unspecified eye
   ● **H44.42**   Hypotony of eye due to ocular fistula
        H44.421   Hypotony of right eye due to ocular fistula
        H44.422   Hypotony of left eye due to ocular fistula
        H44.423   Hypotony of eye due to ocular fistula, bilateral
        H44.429   Hypotony of unspecified eye due to ocular fistula
   ● **H44.43**   Hypotony of eye due to other ocular disorders
        H44.431   Hypotony of eye due to other ocular disorders, right eye
        H44.432   Hypotony of eye due to other ocular disorders, left eye
        H44.433   Hypotony of eye due to other ocular disorders, bilateral
        H44.439   Hypotony of eye due to other ocular disorders, unspecified eye
   ● **H44.44**   Primary hypotony of eye
        H44.441   Primary hypotony of right eye
        H44.442   Primary hypotony of left eye
        H44.443   Primary hypotony of eye, bilateral
        H44.449   Primary hypotony of unspecified eye
● **H44.5**   **Degenerated conditions of globe**
     H44.50   Unspecified degenerated conditions of globe
   ● **H44.51**   Absolute glaucoma
        H44.511   Absolute glaucoma, right eye
        H44.512   Absolute glaucoma, left eye
        H44.513   Absolute glaucoma, bilateral
        H44.519   Absolute glaucoma, unspecified eye
   ● **H44.52**   Atrophy of globe
              Phthisis bulbi
        H44.521   Atrophy of globe, right eye
        H44.522   Atrophy of globe, left eye
        H44.523   Atrophy of globe, bilateral
        H44.529   Atrophy of globe, unspecified eye
   ● **H44.53**   Leucocoria
        H44.531   Leucocoria, right eye
        H44.532   Leucocoria, left eye
        H44.533   Leucocoria, bilateral
        H44.539   Leucocoria, unspecified eye

● **H44.6**   **Retained (old) intraocular foreign body, magnetic**
       Use additional code to identify magnetic foreign body (Z18.11)

       Excludes1   current intraocular foreign body (S05.-)
       Excludes2   retained foreign body in eyelid (H02.81-)
                     retained (old) foreign body following penetrating wound of orbit (H05.5-)
                     retained (old) intraocular foreign body, nonmagnetic (H44.7-)

   ● **H44.60**   Unspecified retained (old) intraocular foreign body, magnetic
        H44.601   Unspecified retained (old) intraocular foreign body, magnetic, right eye
        H44.602   Unspecified retained (old) intraocular foreign body, magnetic, left eye
        H44.603   Unspecified retained (old) intraocular foreign body, magnetic, bilateral
        H44.609   Unspecified retained (old) intraocular foreign body, magnetic, unspecified eye
   ● **H44.61**   Retained (old) magnetic foreign body in anterior chamber
        H44.611   Retained (old) magnetic foreign body in anterior chamber, right eye
        H44.612   Retained (old) magnetic foreign body in anterior chamber, left eye
        H44.613   Retained (old) magnetic foreign body in anterior chamber, bilateral
        H44.619   Retained (old) magnetic foreign body in anterior chamber, unspecified eye
   ● **H44.62**   Retained (old) magnetic foreign body in iris or ciliary body
        H44.621   Retained (old) magnetic foreign body in iris or ciliary body, right eye
        H44.622   Retained (old) magnetic foreign body in iris or ciliary body, left eye
        H44.623   Retained (old) magnetic foreign body in iris or ciliary body, bilateral
        H44.629   Retained (old) magnetic foreign body in iris or ciliary body, unspecified eye
   ● **H44.63**   Retained (old) magnetic foreign body in lens
        H44.631   Retained (old) magnetic foreign body in lens, right eye
        H44.632   Retained (old) magnetic foreign body in lens, left eye
        H44.633   Retained (old) magnetic foreign body in lens, bilateral
        H44.639   Retained (old) magnetic foreign body in lens, unspecified eye
   ● **H44.64**   Retained (old) magnetic foreign body in posterior wall of globe
        H44.641   Retained (old) magnetic foreign body in posterior wall of globe, right eye
        H44.642   Retained (old) magnetic foreign body in posterior wall of globe, left eye
        H44.643   Retained (old) magnetic foreign body in posterior wall of globe, bilateral
        H44.649   Retained (old) magnetic foreign body in posterior wall of globe, unspecified eye
   ● **H44.65**   Retained (old) magnetic foreign body in vitreous body
        H44.651   Retained (old) magnetic foreign body in vitreous body, right eye
        H44.652   Retained (old) magnetic foreign body in vitreous body, left eye
        H44.653   Retained (old) magnetic foreign body in vitreous body, bilateral
        H44.659   Retained (old) magnetic foreign body in vitreous body, unspecified eye

CHAPTER 7 (H00-H59)

- H44.69   Retained (old) intraocular foreign body, magnetic, in other or multiple sites
  - H44.691   Retained (old) intraocular foreign body, magnetic, in other or multiple sites, right eye
  - H44.692   Retained (old) intraocular foreign body, magnetic, in other or multiple sites, left eye
  - H44.693   Retained (old) intraocular foreign body, magnetic, in other or multiple sites, bilateral
  - H44.699   Retained (old) intraocular foreign body, magnetic, in other or multiple sites, unspecified eye

- H44.7   Retained (old) intraocular foreign body, nonmagnetic

  Use additional code to identify nonmagnetic foreign body (Z18.01-Z18.10, Z18.12, Z18.2-Z18.9)

  Excludes1   current intraocular foreign body (S05.-)

  Excludes2   retained foreign body in eyelid (H02.81-)
  retained (old) foreign body following penetrating wound of orbit (H05.5-)
  retained (old) intraocular foreign body, magnetic (H44.6-)

  - H44.70   Unspecified retained (old) intraocular foreign body, nonmagnetic
    - H44.701   Unspecified retained (old) intraocular foreign body, nonmagnetic, right eye
    - H44.702   Unspecified retained (old) intraocular foreign body, nonmagnetic, left eye
    - H44.703   Unspecified retained (old) intraocular foreign body, nonmagnetic, bilateral
    - H44.709   Unspecified retained (old) intraocular foreign body, nonmagnetic, unspecified eye
      Retained (old) intraocular foreign body NOS
  - H44.71   Retained (nonmagnetic) (old) foreign body in anterior chamber
    - H44.711   Retained (nonmagnetic) (old) foreign body in anterior chamber, right eye
    - H44.712   Retained (nonmagnetic) (old) foreign body in anterior chamber, left eye
    - H44.713   Retained (nonmagnetic) (old) foreign body in anterior chamber, bilateral
    - H44.719   Retained (nonmagnetic) (old) foreign body in anterior chamber, unspecified eye
  - H44.72   Retained (nonmagnetic) (old) foreign body in iris or ciliary body
    - H44.721   Retained (nonmagnetic) (old) foreign body in iris or ciliary body, right eye
    - H44.722   Retained (nonmagnetic) (old) foreign body in iris or ciliary body, left eye
    - H44.723   Retained (nonmagnetic) (old) foreign body in iris or ciliary body, bilateral
    - H44.729   Retained (nonmagnetic) (old) foreign body in iris or ciliary body, unspecified eye
  - H44.73   Retained (nonmagnetic) (old) foreign body in lens
    - H44.731   Retained (nonmagnetic) (old) foreign body in lens, right eye
    - H44.732   Retained (nonmagnetic) (old) foreign body in lens, left eye
    - H44.733   Retained (nonmagnetic) (old) foreign body in lens, bilateral
    - H44.739   Retained (nonmagnetic) (old) foreign body in lens, unspecified eye

- H44.74   Retained (nonmagnetic) (old) foreign body in posterior wall of globe
  - H44.741   Retained (nonmagnetic) (old) foreign body in posterior wall of globe, right eye
  - H44.742   Retained (nonmagnetic) (old) foreign body in posterior wall of globe, left eye
  - H44.743   Retained (nonmagnetic) (old) foreign body in posterior wall of globe, bilateral
  - H44.749   Retained (nonmagnetic) (old) foreign body in posterior wall of globe, unspecified eye
- H44.75   Retained (nonmagnetic) (old) foreign body in vitreous body
  - H44.751   Retained (nonmagnetic) (old) foreign body in vitreous body, right eye
  - H44.752   Retained (nonmagnetic) (old) foreign body in vitreous body, left eye
  - H44.753   Retained (nonmagnetic) (old) foreign body in vitreous body, bilateral
  - H44.759   Retained (nonmagnetic) (old) foreign body in vitreous body, unspecified eye
- H44.79   Retained (old) intraocular foreign body, nonmagnetic, in other or multiple sites
  - H44.791   Retained (old) intraocular foreign body, nonmagnetic, in other or multiple sites, right eye
  - H44.792   Retained (old) intraocular foreign body, nonmagnetic, in other or multiple sites, left eye
  - H44.793   Retained (old) intraocular foreign body, nonmagnetic, in other or multiple sites, bilateral
  - H44.799   Retained (old) intraocular foreign body, nonmagnetic, in other or multiple sites, unspecified eye
- H44.8   Other disorders of globe
  - H44.81   Hemophthalmos
    - H44.811   Hemophthalmos, right eye
    - H44.812   Hemophthalmos, left eye
    - H44.813   Hemophthalmos, bilateral
    - H44.819   Hemophthalmos, unspecified eye
  - H44.82   Luxation of globe
    - H44.821   Luxation of globe, right eye
    - H44.822   Luxation of globe, left eye
    - H44.823   Luxation of globe, bilateral
    - H44.829   Luxation of globe, unspecified eye
  - H44.89   Other disorders of globe
- H44.9   Unspecified disorder of globe

★ **(See Plate 86 on page 55.)**

DISORDERS OF OPTIC NERVE AND VISUAL PATHWAYS (H46-H47)

- H46   Optic neuritis

  Excludes2   ischemic optic neuropathy (H47.01-)
  neuromyelitis optica [Devic] (G36.0)

  (Ex) For category H46 CC codes: H46.00-H46.9

  - H46.0   Optic papillitis
    - H46.00   Optic papillitis, unspecified eye
    - H46.01   Optic papillitis, right eye
    - H46.02   Optic papillitis, left eye
    - H46.03   Optic papillitis, bilateral

◀ New   ◀▥ Revised   ~~deleted~~ Deleted   Excludes 1   Excludes 2   Includes   Use additional   Code first   Code also   Unspecified

OGCR Official Guidelines   ● Unacceptable Principal Diagnosis   X Assign placeholder X   ● Use Additional Character(s)   ▸ Manifestation Code   **Coding Clinic**

● **H46.1**   **Retrobulbar neuritis**
      Retrobulbar neuritis NOS
      Excludes1   syphilitic retrobulbar neuritis (A52.15)
      H46.1Ø   Retrobulbar neuritis, unspecified eye 🝆
      H46.11   Retrobulbar neuritis, right eye 🝆
      H46.12   Retrobulbar neuritis, left eye 🝆
      H46.13   Retrobulbar neuritis, bilateral 🝆
  H46.2   **Nutritional optic neuropathy**
  H46.3   **Toxic optic neuropathy**
      Code first (T51-T65) to identify cause
  H46.8   **Other optic neuritis** 🝆
  H46.9   **Unspecified optic neuritis** 🝆

● **H47**   **Other disorders of optic [2nd] nerve and visual pathways**
 ● **H47.Ø**   **Disorders of optic nerve, not elsewhere classified**
   ● **H47.Ø1**   **Ischemic optic neuropathy**
       H47.Ø11   Ischemic optic neuropathy, right eye
       H47.Ø12   Ischemic optic neuropathy, left eye
       H47.Ø13   Ischemic optic neuropathy, bilateral
       H47.Ø19   Ischemic optic neuropathy, unspecified eye
   ● **H47.Ø2**   **Hemorrhage in optic nerve sheath**
       H47.Ø21   Hemorrhage in optic nerve sheath, right eye
       H47.Ø22   Hemorrhage in optic nerve sheath, left eye
       H47.Ø23   Hemorrhage in optic nerve sheath, bilateral
       H47.Ø29   Hemorrhage in optic nerve sheath, unspecified eye
   ● **H47.Ø3**   **Optic nerve hypoplasia**
       H47.Ø31   Optic nerve hypoplasia, right eye
       H47.Ø32   Optic nerve hypoplasia, left eye
       H47.Ø33   Optic nerve hypoplasia, bilateral
       H47.Ø39   Optic nerve hypoplasia, unspecified eye
   ● **H47.Ø9**   **Other disorders of optic nerve, not elsewhere classified**
       Compression of optic nerve
       H47.Ø91   Other disorders of optic nerve, not elsewhere classified, right eye
       H47.Ø92   Other disorders of optic nerve, not elsewhere classified, left eye
       H47.Ø93   Other disorders of optic nerve, not elsewhere classified, bilateral
       H47.Ø99   Other disorders of optic nerve, not elsewhere classified, unspecified eye
 ● **H47.1**   **Papilledema**
      H47.1Ø   **Unspecified papilledema** 🝆
        ⓔⓧ A17.9, A18.5Ø-A18.59, A18.82, A18.84, A18.89, A39.82,
          EØ8.311-EØ8.39, EØ8.618-EØ8.638, EØ8.649-EØ8.8,
          EØ9.311-EØ9.39, EØ9.618-EØ9.638, EØ9.649-EØ9.8,
          E1Ø.311-E1Ø.39, E1Ø.618-E1Ø.638, E1Ø.649, E1Ø.69-E1Ø.8,
          E11.311-E11.39, E11.618-E11.638, E11.649, E11.69-E11.8,
          E13.311-E13.39, E13.618-E13.638, E13.649-E13.8,
          H47.1Ø-H47.13, H47.231-H47.239, H47.331-H47.339,
          H57.8-H57.9, H59.4Ø-H59.43, Q11.3, Q15.8-Q15.9
      H47.11   **Papilledema associated with increased intracranial pressure** 🝆
        ⓔⓧ See H47.1Ø
      H47.12   **Papilledema associated with decreased ocular pressure**
      H47.13   **Papilledema associated with retinal disorder**
   ● **H47.14**   **Foster-Kennedy syndrome**
       H47.141   Foster-Kennedy syndrome, right eye
       H47.142   Foster-Kennedy syndrome, left eye
       H47.143   Foster-Kennedy syndrome, bilateral
       H47.149   Foster-Kennedy syndrome, unspecified eye

Figure 7-11   Papilledema. (From Behrma: Nelson Textbook of Pediatrics, ed 17, Saunders, 2004)

Item 7–8   Papilledema is swelling of the optic disc caused by increased intracranial pressure. It is most often bilateral and occurs quickly (hours) or over weeks of time. It is a common symptom of a brain tumor. The term should not be used to describe optic disc swelling with underlying infectious, infiltrative, or inflammatory etiologies.

 ● **H47.2**   **Optic atrophy**
      H47.2Ø   **Unspecified optic atrophy**
   ● **H47.21**   **Primary optic atrophy**
       H47.211   Primary optic atrophy, right eye
       H47.212   Primary optic atrophy, left eye
       H47.213   Primary optic atrophy, bilateral
       H47.219   Primary optic atrophy, unspecified eye
      H47.22   **Hereditary optic atrophy**
        Leber's optic atrophy
   ● **H47.23**   **Glaucomatous optic atrophy**
       H47.231   Glaucomatous optic atrophy, right eye
       H47.232   Glaucomatous optic atrophy, left eye
       H47.233   Glaucomatous optic atrophy, bilateral
       H47.239   Glaucomatous optic atrophy, unspecified eye
   ● **H47.29**   **Other optic atrophy**
       Temporal pallor of optic disc
       H47.291   Other optic atrophy, right eye
       H47.292   Other optic atrophy, left eye
       H47.293   Other optic atrophy, bilateral
       H47.299   Other optic atrophy, unspecified eye
 ● **H47.3**   **Other disorders of optic disc**
   ● **H47.31**   **Coloboma of optic disc**
       H47.311   Coloboma of optic disc, right eye
       H47.312   Coloboma of optic disc, left eye
       H47.313   Coloboma of optic disc, bilateral
       H47.319   Coloboma of optic disc, unspecified eye
   ● **H47.32**   **Drusen of optic disc**
       H47.321   Drusen of optic disc, right eye
       H47.322   Drusen of optic disc, left eye
       H47.323   Drusen of optic disc, bilateral
       H47.329   Drusen of optic disc, unspecified eye

N   Newborn Age: Ø   **P**   Pediatric Age: Ø–17   **M**   Maternity DX: 12–55   **A**   Adult Age: 15–124   ♀   Females Only   ♂   Males Only

🝆   Complication\Comorbidity   🝆   Major C\C   ⓔⓧ   CC/MCC Exclusions   🝆   Hospital-Acquired Condition   **845**

● H47.33 Pseudopapilledema of optic disc
   H47.331   Pseudopapilledema of optic disc, right eye
   H47.332   Pseudopapilledema of optic disc, left eye
   H47.333   Pseudopapilledema of optic disc, bilateral
   H47.339   Pseudopapilledema of optic disc, unspecified eye

● H47.39 Other disorders of optic disc
   H47.391   Other disorders of optic disc, right eye
   H47.392   Other disorders of optic disc, left eye
   H47.393   Other disorders of optic disc, bilateral
   H47.399   Other disorders of optic disc, unspecified eye

● H47.4 Disorders of optic chiasm
   Code also underlying condition
   (Ex) For category H47.4 CC codes: H47.41-H47.539
   H47.41   Disorders of optic chiasm in (due to) inflammatory disorders ●
   H47.42   Disorders of optic chiasm in (due to) neoplasm ●
   H47.43   Disorders of optic chiasm in (due to) vascular disorders ●
   H47.49   Disorders of optic chiasm in (due to) other disorders ●

● H47.5 Disorders of other visual pathways
   Disorders of optic tracts, geniculate nuclei and optic radiations
   Code also underlying condition
   (Ex) For category H47.5 CC codes: H47.41-H47.539
   H47.51   Disorders of visual pathways in (due to) inflammatory disorders
      H47.511   Disorders of visual pathways in (due to) inflammatory disorders, right side ●
      H47.512   Disorders of visual pathways in (due to) inflammatory disorders, left side ●
      H47.519   Disorders of visual pathways in (due to) inflammatory disorders, unspecified side ●
   H47.52   Disorders of visual pathways in (due to) neoplasm
      H47.521   Disorders of visual pathways in (due to) neoplasm, right side ●
      H47.522   Disorders of visual pathways in (due to) neoplasm, left side ●
      H47.529   Disorders of visual pathways in (due to) neoplasm, unspecified side ●
   H47.53   Disorders of visual pathways in (due to) vascular disorders
      H47.531   Disorders of visual pathways in (due to) vascular disorders, right side ●
      H47.532   Disorders of visual pathways in (due to) vascular disorders, left side ●
      H47.539   Disorders of visual pathways in (due to) vascular disorders, unspecified side ●

● H47.6 Disorders of visual cortex
   Code also underlying condition
   Excludes1   injury to visual cortex S04.04
   (Ex) For category H47.6 CC codes: H47.611-H47.9
   H47.61   Cortical blindness
      H47.611   Cortical blindness, right side of brain
      H47.612   Cortical blindness, left side of brain
      H47.619   Cortical blindness, unspecified side of brain

● H47.62 Disorders of visual cortex in (due to) inflammatory disorders
   H47.621   Disorders of visual cortex in (due to) inflammatory disorders, right side of brain ●
   H47.622   Disorders of visual cortex in (due to) inflammatory disorders, left side of brain ●
   H47.629   Disorders of visual cortex in (due to) inflammatory disorders, unspecified side of brain ●

● H47.63 Disorders of visual cortex in (due to) neoplasm
   H47.631   Disorders of visual cortex in (due to) neoplasm, right side of brain ●
   H47.632   Disorders of visual cortex in (due to) neoplasm, left side of brain ●
   H47.639   Disorders of visual cortex in (due to) neoplasm, unspecified side of brain ●

● H47.64 Disorders of visual cortex in (due to) vascular disorders
   H47.641   Disorders of visual cortex in (due to) vascular disorders, right side of brain ●
   H47.642   Disorders of visual cortex in (due to) vascular disorders, left side of brain ●
   H47.649   Disorders of visual cortex in (due to) vascular disorders, unspecified side of brain ●

H47.9   Unspecified disorder of visual pathways

DISORDERS OF OCULAR MUSCLES, BINOCULAR MOVEMENT, ACCOMMODATION AND REFRACTION (H49-H52)

Excludes2   nystagmus and other irregular eye movements (H55)

● H49 Paralytic strabismus
   Excludes2   internal ophthalmoplegia (H52.51-)
                internuclear ophthalmoplegia (H51.2-)
                progressive supranuclear ophthalmoplegia (G23.1)
   ● H49.0 Third [oculomotor] nerve palsy
      H49.00   Third [oculomotor] nerve palsy, unspecified eye
      H49.01   Third [oculomotor] nerve palsy, right eye
      H49.02   Third [oculomotor] nerve palsy, left eye
      H49.03   Third [oculomotor] nerve palsy, bilateral
   ● H49.1 Fourth [trochlear] nerve palsy
      H49.10   Fourth [trochlear] nerve palsy, unspecified eye
      H49.11   Fourth [trochlear] nerve palsy, right eye
      H49.12   Fourth [trochlear] nerve palsy, left eye
      H49.13   Fourth [trochlear] nerve palsy, bilateral

Item 7-9 Strabismus or esotropia (crossed eyes) is a condition of the extraocular eye muscles, resulting in an inability of the eyes to focus and also affects depth perception.

A

B

Figure 7-12 A. Image of strabismus. **B.** Exotropia. (**A** from Yanoff: Ophthalmology, ed 3, Mosby, Inc., 2008. **B** from Rakel: Textbook of Family Practice, ed 7, Saunders, 2007)

◀ New   ◀▥ Revised   ~~deleted~~ Deleted   Excludes 1   Excludes 2   Includes   Use additional   Code first   Code also   Unspecified

OGCR Official Guidelines   ● Unacceptable Principal Diagnosis   X Assign placeholder X   ● Use Additional Character(s)   ▶ Manifestation Code   Coding Clinic

- **H49.2** Sixth [abducent] nerve palsy
  - H49.20 Sixth [abducent] nerve palsy, unspecified eye
  - H49.21 Sixth [abducent] nerve palsy, right eye
  - H49.22 Sixth [abducent] nerve palsy, left eye
  - H49.23 Sixth [abducent] nerve palsy, bilateral
- **H49.3** Total (external) ophthalmoplegia
  - H49.30 Total (external) ophthalmoplegia, unspecified eye
  - H49.31 Total (external) ophthalmoplegia, right eye
  - H49.32 Total (external) ophthalmoplegia, left eye
  - H49.33 Total (external) ophthalmoplegia, bilateral
- **H49.4** Progressive external ophthalmoplegia
  - **Excludes1** Kearns-Sayre syndrome (H49.81-)
  - H49.40 Progressive external ophthalmoplegia, unspecified eye
  - H49.41 Progressive external ophthalmoplegia, right eye
  - H49.42 Progressive external ophthalmoplegia, left eye
  - H49.43 Progressive external ophthalmoplegia, bilateral
- **H49.8** Other paralytic strabismus
  - **H49.81** Kearns-Sayre syndrome
    - Progressive external ophthalmoplegia with pigmentary retinopathy
    - Use additional code for other manifestation, such as:
      - heart block (I45.9)
    - (Ex) **For category H49.81 CC codes:** C96.5-C96.6, E71.310-E71.548, E80.3-E80.7, E88.89
    - H49.811 Kearns-Sayre syndrome, right eye 🩸
    - H49.812 Kearns-Sayre syndrome, left eye 🩸
    - H49.813 Kearns-Sayre syndrome, bilateral 🩸
    - H49.819 Kearns-Sayre syndrome, unspecified eye 🩸
  - **H49.88** Other paralytic strabismus
    - External ophthalmoplegia NOS
    - H49.881 Other paralytic strabismus, right eye
    - H49.882 Other paralytic strabismus, left eye
    - H49.883 Other paralytic strabismus, bilateral
    - H49.889 Other paralytic strabismus, unspecified eye
- **H49.9** Unspecified paralytic strabismus
- **H50** **Other strabismus**
  - **H50.0** Esotropia
    - Convergent concomitant strabismus
    - **Excludes1** intermittent esotropia (H50.31-, H50.32)
    - H50.00 Unspecified esotropia
    - **H50.01** Monocular esotropia
      - H50.011 Monocular esotropia, right eye
      - H50.012 Monocular esotropia, left eye
    - **H50.02** Monocular esotropia with A pattern
      - H50.021 Monocular esotropia with A pattern, right eye
      - H50.022 Monocular esotropia with A pattern, left eye
    - **H50.03** Monocular esotropia with V pattern
      - H50.031 Monocular esotropia with V pattern, right eye
      - H50.032 Monocular esotropia with V pattern, left eye

- **H50.04** Monocular esotropia with other noncomitancies
  - H50.041 Monocular esotropia with other noncomitancies, right eye
  - H50.042 Monocular esotropia with other noncomitancies, left eye
- H50.05 Alternating esotropia
- H50.06 Alternating esotropia with A pattern
- H50.07 Alternating esotropia with V pattern
- H50.08 Alternating esotropia with other noncomitancies
- **H50.1** Exotropia
  - *Misalignment in which one eye deviates outward (away from nose) while the other fixates normally*
  - Divergent concomitant strabismus
  - **Excludes1** intermittent exotropia (H50.33-, H50.34)
  - H50.10 Unspecified exotropia
  - **H50.11** Monocular exotropia
    - H50.111 Monocular exotropia, right eye
    - H50.112 Monocular exotropia, left eye
  - **H50.12** Monocular exotropia with A pattern
    - H50.121 Monocular exotropia with A pattern, right eye
    - H50.122 Monocular exotropia with A pattern, left eye
  - **H50.13** Monocular exotropia with V pattern
    - H50.131 Monocular exotropia with V pattern, right eye
    - H50.132 Monocular exotropia with V pattern, left eye
  - **H50.14** Monocular exotropia with other noncomitancies
    - H50.141 Monocular exotropia with other noncomitancies, right eye
    - H50.142 Monocular exotropia with other noncomitancies, left eye
  - H50.15 Alternating exotropia
  - H50.16 Alternating exotropia with A pattern
  - H50.17 Alternating exotropia with V pattern
  - H50.18 Alternating exotropia with other noncomitancies
- **H50.2** Vertical strabismus
  - Hypertropia
  - H50.21 Vertical strabismus, right eye
  - H50.22 Vertical strabismus, left eye
- **H50.3** Intermittent heterotropia
  - *Displacement of an organ or part of an organ from its normal position*
  - H50.30 Unspecified intermittent heterotropia
  - **H50.31** Intermittent monocular esotropia
    - H50.311 Intermittent monocular esotropia, right eye
    - H50.312 Intermittent monocular esotropia, left eye
  - H50.32 Intermittent alternating esotropia
  - **H50.33** Intermittent monocular exotropia
    - H50.331 Intermittent monocular exotropia, right eye
    - H50.332 Intermittent monocular exotropia, left eye
  - H50.34 Intermittent alternating exotropia
- **H50.4** Other and unspecified heterotropia
  - H50.40 Unspecified heterotropia
  - **H50.41** Cyclotropia
    - H50.411 Cyclotropia, right eye
    - H50.412 Cyclotropia, left eye
  - H50.42 Monofixation syndrome
  - H50.43 Accommodative component in esotropia

N Newborn Age: 0   **P** Pediatric Age: 0–17   **M** Maternity DX: 12–55   **A** Adult Age: 15–124   ♀ Females Only   ♂ Males Only

🩸 Complication\Comorbidity   Major C\C   (Ex) CC/MCC Exclusions   Hospital-Acquired Condition

847

● H50.5 **Heterophoria**
One or both eyes wander away from the position where both eyes are looking together in the same direction

 H50.50 **Unspecified** **heterophoria**

 H50.51 **Esophoria**
 Eye deviates inward (toward the nose)

 H50.52 **Exophoria**
 Eye deviates outward (toward the ear)

 H50.53 **Vertical heterophoria**

 H50.54 **Cyclophoria**

 H50.55 **Alternating heterophoria**

● H50.6 **Mechanical strabismus**

 H50.60 **Mechanical strabismus, unspecified**

 ● H50.61 **Brown's sheath syndrome**

 H50.611 **Brown's sheath syndrome, right eye**

 H50.612 **Brown's sheath syndrome, left eye**

 H50.69 **Other mechanical strabismus**
 Strabismus due to adhesions
 Traumatic limitation of duction of eye muscle

● H50.8 **Other specified strabismus**

 ● H50.81 **Duane's syndrome**

 H50.811 **Duane's syndrome, right eye**

 H50.812 **Duane's syndrome, left eye**

 H50.89 **Other specified strabismus**

 H50.9 **Unspecified** **strabismus**

● H51 **Other disorders of binocular movement**

 H51.0 **Palsy (spasm) of conjugate gaze**

 ● H51.1 **Convergence insufficiency and excess**

 H51.11 **Convergence insufficiency**

 H51.12 **Convergence excess**

 ● H51.2 **Internuclear ophthalmoplegia**

 H51.20 **Internuclear ophthalmoplegia, unspecified eye**

 H51.21 **Internuclear ophthalmoplegia, right eye**

 H51.22 **Internuclear ophthalmoplegia, left eye**

 H51.23 **Internuclear ophthalmoplegia, bilateral**

 H51.8 **Other specified disorders of binocular movement**

 H51.9 **Unspecified** **disorder of binocular movement**

● H52 **Disorders of refraction and accommodation**

 ● H52.0 **Hypermetropia**

 H52.00 **Hypermetropia, unspecified eye**

 H52.01 **Hypermetropia, right eye**

 H52.02 **Hypermetropia, left eye**

 H52.03 **Hypermetropia, bilateral**

 ● H52.1 **Myopia**

 Excludes1 degenerative myopia (H44.2-)

 H52.10 **Myopia, unspecified eye**

 H52.11 **Myopia, right eye**

 H52.12 **Myopia, left eye**

 H52.13 **Myopia, bilateral**

● H52.2 **Astigmatism**

 ● H52.20 **Unspecified astigmatism**

 H52.201 **Unspecified** astigmatism, right eye

 H52.202 **Unspecified** astigmatism, left eye

 H52.203 **Unspecified** astigmatism, bilateral

 H52.209 **Unspecified** astigmatism, unspecified eye

 ● H52.21 **Irregular astigmatism**

 H52.211 **Irregular astigmatism, right eye**

 H52.212 **Irregular astigmatism, left eye**

 H52.213 **Irregular astigmatism, bilateral**

 H52.219 **Irregular astigmatism, unspecified eye**

 ● H52.22 **Regular astigmatism**

 H52.221 **Regular astigmatism, right eye**

 H52.222 **Regular astigmatism, left eye**

 H52.223 **Regular astigmatism, bilateral**

 H52.229 **Regular astigmatism, unspecified eye**

● H52.3 **Anisometropia and aniseikonia**

 H52.31 **Anisometropia**

 H52.32 **Aniseikonia**

 H52.4 **Presbyopia**

● H52.5 **Disorders of accommodation**

 ● H52.51 **Internal ophthalmoplegia (complete) (total)**

 H52.511 **Internal ophthalmoplegia (complete) (total), right eye**

 H52.512 **Internal ophthalmoplegia (complete) (total), left eye**

 H52.513 **Internal ophthalmoplegia (complete) (total), bilateral**

 H52.519 **Internal ophthalmoplegia (complete) (total), unspecified eye**

 ● H52.52 **Paresis of accommodation**

 H52.521 **Paresis of accommodation, right eye**

 H52.522 **Paresis of accommodation, left eye**

 H52.523 **Paresis of accommodation, bilateral**

 H52.529 **Paresis of accommodation, unspecified eye**

 ● H52.53 **Spasm of accommodation**

 H52.531 **Spasm of accommodation, right eye**

 H52.532 **Spasm of accommodation, left eye**

 H52.533 **Spasm of accommodation, bilateral**

 H52.539 **Spasm of accommodation, unspecified eye**

 H52.6 **Other disorders of refraction**

 H52.7 **Unspecified** **disorder of refraction**

VISUAL DISTURBANCES AND BLINDNESS (H53-H54)

● H53 **Visual disturbances**

 ● H53.0 **Amblyopia ex anopsia**

 Excludes1 amblyopia due to vitamin A deficiency (E50.5)

 ● H53.00 **Unspecified amblyopia**

 H53.001 **Unspecified** amblyopia, right eye

 H53.002 **Unspecified** amblyopia, left eye

 H53.003 **Unspecified** amblyopia, bilateral

 H53.009 **Unspecified** amblyopia, unspecified eye

 ● H53.01 **Deprivation amblyopia**

 H53.011 **Deprivation amblyopia, right eye**

 H53.012 **Deprivation amblyopia, left eye**

 H53.013 **Deprivation amblyopia, bilateral**

 H53.019 **Deprivation amblyopia, unspecified eye**

Item 7–10 Disorders of refraction: **Hypermetropia,** or farsightedness, means focus at a distance is adequate but not on close objects. **Myopia** is near-sightedness or short-sightedness and means the focus on nearby objects is clear but distant objects appear blurred. **Astigmatism** is warping of the curvature of the cornea so light rays entering do not meet a single focal point, resulting in a distorted image. **Anisometropia** is unequal refractive power in which one eye may be myopic (near-sighted) and the other hyperopic (far-sighted). **Presbyopia** is the loss of focus on near objects, which occurs with age because the lens loses elasticity.

◀ New ◀▥ Revised ~~deleted~~ Deleted | Excludes 1 | Excludes 2 | Includes | Use additional | Code first | Code also | Unspecified

OGCR Official Guidelines ● Unacceptable Principal Diagnosis X Assign placeholder X ● Use Additional Character(s) ▶ Manifestation Code **Coding Clinic**

848

● H53.02   Refractive amblyopia
    H53.021   Refractive amblyopia, right eye
    H53.022   Refractive amblyopia, left eye
    H53.023   Refractive amblyopia, bilateral
    H53.029   Refractive amblyopia, unspecified eye
● H53.03   Strabismic amblyopia
    Excludes1   strabismus (H50.-)
    H53.031   Strabismic amblyopia, right eye
    H53.032   Strabismic amblyopia, left eye
    H53.033   Strabismic amblyopia, bilateral
    H53.039   Strabismic amblyopia, unspecified eye
● H53.04   Amblyopia suspect ◄
    H53.041   Amblyopia suspect, right eye ◄
    H53.042   Amblyopia suspect, left eye ◄
    H53.043   Amblyopia suspect, bilateral ◄
    H53.049   Amblyopia suspect, unspecified eye ◄
● H53.1   Subjective visual disturbances
    Excludes1   subjective visual disturbances due to vitamin A deficiency (E50.5)
                  visual hallucinations (R44.1)
   H53.10   Unspecified subjective visual disturbances
   H53.11   Day blindness
          Hemeralopia
● H53.12   Transient visual loss
          Scintillating scotoma
    Excludes1   amaurosis fugax (G45.3-)
                  transient retinal artery occlusion (H34.0-)
    (Ex) **For category H53.12 CC codes:** H53.10-H53.139, H53.16, R44.1, R48.3
    H53.121   Transient visual loss, right eye ℃
    H53.122   Transient visual loss, left eye ℃
    H53.123   Transient visual loss, bilateral ℃
    H53.129   Transient visual loss, unspecified eye ℃
● H53.13   Sudden visual loss
    (Ex) **For category H53.13 CC codes:** See H53.12
    H53.131   Sudden visual loss, right eye ℃
    H53.132   Sudden visual loss, left eye ℃
    H53.133   Sudden visual loss, bilateral ℃
    H53.139   Sudden visual loss, unspecified eye ℃
● H53.14   Visual discomfort
          Asthenopia
          Photophobia
    H53.141   Visual discomfort, right eye
    H53.142   Visual discomfort, left eye
    H53.143   Visual discomfort, bilateral
    H53.149   Visual discomfort, unspecified
   H53.15   Visual distortions of shape and size
          Metamorphopsia
   H53.16   Psychophysical visual disturbances
   H53.19   Other subjective visual disturbances
          Visual halos
   H53.2   Diplopia
          Double vision
● H53.3   Other and unspecified disorders of binocular vision
   H53.30   Unspecified disorder of binocular vision
   H53.31   Abnormal retinal correspondence
   H53.32   Fusion with defective stereopsis
   H53.33   Simultaneous visual perception without fusion
   H53.34   Suppression of binocular vision

● H53.4   Visual field defects
   H53.40   Unspecified visual field defects
● H53.41   Scotoma involving central area
          Central scotoma
    H53.411   Scotoma involving central area, right eye
    H53.412   Scotoma involving central area, left eye
    H53.413   Scotoma involving central area, bilateral
    H53.419   Scotoma involving central area, unspecified eye
● H53.42   Scotoma of blind spot area
          Enlarged blind spot
    H53.421   Scotoma of blind spot area, right eye
    H53.422   Scotoma of blind spot area, left eye
    H53.423   Scotoma of blind spot area, bilateral
    H53.429   Scotoma of blind spot area, unspecified eye
● H53.43   Sector or arcuate defects
          Arcuate scotoma
          Bjerrum scotoma
    H53.431   Sector or arcuate defects, right eye
    H53.432   Sector or arcuate defects, left eye
    H53.433   Sector or arcuate defects, bilateral
    H53.439   Sector or arcuate defects, unspecified eye
● H53.45   Other localized visual field defect
          Peripheral visual field defect
          Ring scotoma NOS
          Scotoma NOS
    H53.451   Other localized visual field defect, right eye
    H53.452   Other localized visual field defect, left eye
    H53.453   Other localized visual field defect, bilateral
    H53.459   Other localized visual field defect, unspecified eye
● H53.46   Homonymous bilateral field defects
          Homonymous hemianopia
          Homonymous hemianopsia
          Quadrant anopia
          Quadrant anopsia
    H53.461   Homonymous bilateral field defects, right side
    H53.462   Homonymous bilateral field defects, left side
    H53.469   Homonymous bilateral field defects, unspecified side
          Homonymous bilateral field defects NOS
   H53.47   Heteronymous bilateral field defects
          Heteronymous hemianop(s)ia
● H53.48   Generalized contraction of visual field
    H53.481   Generalized contraction of visual field, right eye
    H53.482   Generalized contraction of visual field, left eye
    H53.483   Generalized contraction of visual field, bilateral
    H53.489   Generalized contraction of visual field, unspecified eye

CHAPTER 7 (H00-H59)

N   Newborn Age: 0   P   Pediatric Age: 0–17   M   Maternity DX: 12–55   A   Adult Age: 15–124   ♀   Females Only   ♂   Males Only
℃   Complication\Comorbidity   ℃   Major C\C   (Ex)   CC/MCC Exclusions   ℃   Hospital-Acquired Condition

849

● **H53.5** **Color vision deficiencies**
Color blindness

> **Excludes2**   day blindness (H53.11)

     H53.50 **Unspecified color vision deficiencies**
           Color blindness NOS

     H53.51 **Achromatopsia**

     H53.52 **Acquired color vision deficiency**

     H53.53 **Deuteranomaly**
           Deuteranopia

     H53.54 **Protanomaly**
           Protanopia

     H53.55 **Tritanomaly**
           Tritanopia

     H53.59 **Other color vision deficiencies**

● **H53.6** **Night blindness**

> **Excludes1**   night blindness due to vitamin A deficiency (E50.5)

     H53.60 **Unspecified night blindness**

     H53.61 **Abnormal dark adaptation curve**

     H53.62 **Acquired night blindness**

     H53.63 **Congenital night blindness**

     H53.69 **Other night blindness**

● **H53.7** **Vision sensitivity deficiencies**

     H53.71 **Glare sensitivity**

     H53.72 **Impaired contrast sensitivity**

     H53.8 **Other visual disturbances**

     H53.9 **Unspecified visual disturbance**

● **H54** **Blindness and low vision**

> **Note:** For definition of visual impairment categories see table below.

> *Code first any associated underlying cause of the blindness*

> **Excludes1**   amaurosis fugax (G45.3)

     H54.0 **Blindness, both eyes**
           Visual impairment categories 3, 4, 5 in both eyes.

● **H54.1** **Blindness, one eye, low vision other eye**
           Visual impairment categories 3, 4, 5 in one eye, with categories 1 or 2 in the other eye.

     H54.10 **Blindness, one eye, low vision other eye, unspecified eyes**

     H54.11 **Blindness, right eye, low vision left eye**

     H54.12 **Blindness, left eye, low vision right eye**

     H54.2 **Low vision, both eyes**
           Visual impairment categories 1 or 2 in both eyes.

     H54.3 **Unqualified visual loss, both eyes**
           Visual impairment category 9 in both eyes.

● **H54.4** **Blindness, one eye**
           Visual impairment categories 3, 4, 5 in one eye [normal vision in other eye]

     H54.40 **Blindness, one eye, unspecified eye**

     H54.41 **Blindness, right eye, normal vision left eye**

     H54.42 **Blindness, left eye, normal vision right eye**

● **H54.5** **Low vision, one eye**
           Visual impairment categories 1 or 2 in one eye [normal vision in other eye].

     H54.50 **Low vision, one eye, unspecified eye**

     H54.51 **Low vision, right eye, normal vision left eye**

     H54.52 **Low vision, left eye, normal vision right eye**

● **H54.6** **Unqualified visual loss, one eye**
           Visual impairment category 9 in one eye [normal vision in other eye].

     H54.60 **Unqualified visual loss, one eye, unspecified**

     H54.61 **Unqualified visual loss, right eye, normal vision left eye**

     H54.62 **Unqualified visual loss, left eye, normal vision right eye**

● **H54.7** **Unspecified visual loss**
           Visual impairment category 9 NOS

     H54.8 **Legal blindness, as defined in USA**
           Blindness NOS according to USA definition

> **Excludes1**   legal blindness with specification of impairment level (H54.0-H54.7)

> **Note:** The table below gives a classification of severity of visual impairment recommended by a WHO Study Group on the Prevention of Blindness, Geneva, 6-10 November 1972.

> The term 'low vision' in category H54 comprises categories 1 and 2 of the table, the term 'blindness' categories 3, 4 and 5, and the term 'unqualified visual loss' category 9.

> If the extent of the visual field is taken into account, patients with a field no greater than 10 but greater than 5 around central fixation should be placed in category 3 and patients with a field no greater than 5 around central fixation should be placed in category 4, even if the central acuity is not impaired.

(Document 508 compliance requires all cells in the following table to be filled.)

Category of visual impairment	Visual acuity with best possible correction	
	Maximum less than:	**Minimum equal to or better than:**
—	6/18	6/60
3/10 (0.3)	1/10 (0.1)	—
20/70	20/200	—
—	6/60	3/60
1/10 (0.1)	1/20 (0.05)	—
20/200	20/400	—
—	3/60	1/60 (finger counting at one meter)
1/20 (0.05)	1/50 (0.02)	—
20/400	5/300 (20/1200)	—
—	1/60 (finger counting at one meter)	Light perception
1/50 (0.02)	—	—
5/300	—	—
—	No light perception	—
—	Undetermined or unspecified	—

◀ New   ◀ Revised   ~~deleted~~ Deleted   Excludes 1   Excludes 2   Includes   Use additional   Code first   Code also   Unspecified
OGCR Official Guidelines   ● Unacceptable Principal Diagnosis   X Assign placeholder X   ● Use Additional Character(s)   ▶ Manifestation Code   **Coding Clinic**

OTHER DISORDERS OF EYE AND ADNEXA (H55-H57)

● H55 Nystagmus and other irregular eye movements
 ● H55.0 **Nystagmus**
   Rapid, involuntary movements of the eyes in the horizontal or vertical direction
  H55.00 Unspecified nystagmus
  H55.01 Congenital nystagmus
  H55.02 Latent nystagmus
  H55.03 Visual deprivation nystagmus
  H55.04 Dissociated nystagmus
  H55.09 Other forms of nystagmus
 ● H55.8 Other irregular eye movements
  H55.81 Saccadic eye movements
  H55.89 Other irregular eye movements

● H57 Other disorders of eye and adnexa
 ● H57.0 Anomalies of pupillary function
  H57.00 Unspecified anomaly of pupillary function
  H57.01 Argyll Robertson pupil, atypical
    Excludes1 syphilitic Argyll Robertson pupil (A52.19)
  H57.02 Anisocoria
  H57.03 Miosis
  H57.04 Mydriasis
  ● H57.05 Tonic pupil
   H57.051 Tonic pupil, right eye
   H57.052 Tonic pupil, left eye
   H57.053 Tonic pupil, bilateral
   H57.059 Tonic pupil, unspecified eye
  H57.09 Other anomalies of pupillary function
 ● H57.1 Ocular pain
  H57.10 Ocular pain, unspecified eye
  H57.11 Ocular pain, right eye
  H57.12 Ocular pain, left eye
  H57.13 Ocular pain, bilateral
 ● H57.8 Other specified disorders of eye and adnexa
 ● H57.9 Unspecified disorder of eye and adnexa

INTRAOPERATIVE AND POSTPROCEDURAL COMPLICATIONS AND DISORDERS OF EYE AND ADNEXA, NOT ELSEWHERE CLASSIFIED (H59)

● H59 Intraoperative and postprocedural complications and disorders of eye and adnexa, not elsewhere classified
  Excludes1 mechanical complication of intraocular lens (T85.2)
    mechanical complication of other ocular prosthetic devices, implants and grafts (T85.3)
    pseudophakia (Z96.1)
    secondary cataracts (H26.4-)
 ● H59.0 Disorders of the eye following cataract surgery
   (Ex.) **For category H59.0 CC codes:** H59.011-H59.019, H59.031-H59.099, H59.811-H59.89, H95.811-H95.89, I97.3, M96.89, N98.1-N98.9, T81.82X[A], T81.89X-T81.9XX[A]
  ● H59.01 Keratopathy (bullous aphakic) following cataract surgery
    Vitreal corneal syndrome
    Vitreous (touch) syndrome
   H59.011 Keratopathy (bullous aphakic) following cataract surgery, right eye
   H59.012 Keratopathy (bullous aphakic) following cataract surgery, left eye
   H59.013 Keratopathy (bullous aphakic) following cataract surgery, bilateral
   H59.019 Keratopathy (bullous aphakic) following cataract surgery, unspecified eye

  ● H59.02 Cataract (lens) fragments in eye following cataract surgery
   H59.021 Cataract (lens) fragments in eye following cataract surgery, right eye
   H59.022 Cataract (lens) fragments in eye following cataract surgery, left eye
   H59.023 Cataract (lens) fragments in eye following cataract surgery, bilateral
   H59.029 Cataract (lens) fragments in eye following cataract surgery, unspecified eye
  ● H59.03 Cystoid macular edema following cataract surgery
   H59.031 Cystoid macular edema following cataract surgery, right eye
   H59.032 Cystoid macular edema following cataract surgery, left eye
   H59.033 Cystoid macular edema following cataract surgery, bilateral
   H59.039 Cystoid macular edema following cataract surgery, unspecified eye
  ● H59.09 Other disorders of the eye following cataract surgery
   H59.091 Other disorders of the right eye following cataract surgery
   H59.092 Other disorders of the left eye following cataract surgery
   H59.093 Other disorders of the eye following cataract surgery, bilateral
   H59.099 Other disorders of unspecified eye following cataract surgery
 ● H59.1 Intraoperative hemorrhage and hematoma of eye and adnexa complicating a procedure
  Excludes1 intraoperative hemorrhage and hematoma of eye and adnexa due to accidental puncture or laceration during a procedure (H59.2-)
  (Ex.) **For category H59.1 CC codes:** H59.011-H59.019, H59.031-H59.129, H59.311-H59.329, H59.331-H59.369, H59.811-H59.89, H95.811-H95.89, I85.01, I85.11, I97.3, K21.9, K22.8, K23-K25.0, K25.2, K25.4, K25.6, K26.0, K26.2, K26.4, K26.6, K27.0, K27.2, K27.4, K27.6, K28.0, K28.2, K28.4, K28.6, K29.01, K29.21, K29.31, K29.41, K29.51, K29.61, K29.71, K29.81, K29.91, K31.811, K55.21, K57.01, K57.11, K57.13, K57.21, K57.31, K57.33, K57.41, K57.51, K57.53, K57.81, K57.91, K57.93, K62.5, K92.0-K92.2, M96.89, N98.1-N98.9, P54.1-P54.3, T81.10X-T81.19X[A], T81.82X[A], T81.89X-T81.9XX[A]
  ● H59.11 Intraoperative hemorrhage and hematoma of eye and adnexa complicating an ophthalmic procedure
   H59.111 Intraoperative hemorrhage and hematoma of right eye and adnexa complicating an ophthalmic procedure
   H59.112 Intraoperative hemorrhage and hematoma of left eye and adnexa complicating an ophthalmic procedure
   H59.113 Intraoperative hemorrhage and hematoma of eye and adnexa complicating an ophthalmic procedure, bilateral
   H59.119 Intraoperative hemorrhage and hematoma of unspecified eye and adnexa complicating an ophthalmic procedure

N Newborn Age: 0 **P** Pediatric Age: 0–17 **M** Maternity DX: 12–55 **A** Adult Age: 15–124 ♀ Females Only ♂ Males Only

Complication\Comorbidity Major C\C (Ex.) CC/MCC Exclusions Hospital-Acquired Condition

851

● H59.12 **Intraoperative hemorrhage and hematoma of eye and adnexa complicating other procedure**

   H59.121 **Intraoperative hemorrhage and hematoma of right eye and adnexa complicating other procedure** 🔍

   H59.122 **Intraoperative hemorrhage and hematoma of left eye and adnexa complicating other procedure** 🔍

   H59.123 **Intraoperative hemorrhage and hematoma of eye and adnexa complicating other procedure, bilateral** 🔍

   H59.129 **Intraoperative hemorrhage and hematoma of** unspecified **eye and adnexa complicating other procedure** 🔍

● H59.2 **Accidental puncture and laceration of eye and adnexa during a procedure**

   (Ex) **For category H59.2 CC codes:** D78.11-D78.12, D78.81-D78.89, E36.11-E36.8, E89.810-E89.89, G96.11, G97.41-G97.49, H59.011-H59.019, H59.031-H59.099, H59.211-H59.229, H59.811-H59.89, H95.31-H95.32, H95.811-H95.89, I97.3, I97.51-I97.52, J95.71-J95.72, K91.71-K91.72, L76.11-L76.12, L76.81-L76.82, M96.820-M96.821, M96.89, N98.1-N98.9, N99.71-N99.72, T81.82X[A], T81.89X-T81.9XX[A]

● H59.21 **Accidental puncture and laceration of eye and adnexa during an ophthalmic procedure**

   H59.211 **Accidental puncture and laceration of right eye and adnexa during an ophthalmic procedure** 🔍

   H59.212 **Accidental puncture and laceration of left eye and adnexa during an ophthalmic procedure** 🔍

   H59.213 **Accidental puncture and laceration of eye and adnexa during an ophthalmic procedure, bilateral** 🔍

   H59.219 **Accidental puncture and laceration of** unspecified **eye and adnexa during an ophthalmic procedure** 🔍

● H59.22 **Accidental puncture and laceration of eye and adnexa during other procedure**

   H59.221 **Accidental puncture and laceration of right eye and adnexa during other procedure** 🔍

   H59.222 **Accidental puncture and laceration of left eye and adnexa during other procedure** 🔍

   H59.223 **Accidental puncture and laceration of eye and adnexa during other procedure, bilateral** 🔍

   H59.229 **Accidental puncture and laceration of** unspecified **eye and adnexa during other procedure** 🔍

● H59.3 **Postprocedural hemorrhage, hematoma, and seroma of eye and adnexa following other procedure** ◀▥

   (Ex) **For category H59.3 CC codes:** See H59.1

● H59.31 **Postprocedural hemorrhage of eye and adnexa following an ophthalmic procedure** ◀▥

   H59.311 **Postprocedural hemorrhage of right eye and adnexa following an ophthalmic procedure** 🔍◀▥

   H59.312 **Postprocedural hemorrhage of left eye and adnexa following an ophthalmic procedure** 🔍◀▥

   H59.313 **Postprocedural hemorrhage of eye and adnexa following an ophthalmic procedure, bilateral** 🔍◀▥

   H59.319 **Postprocedural hemorrhage of** unspecified **eye and adnexa following an ophthalmic procedure** 🔍◀▥

● H59.32 **Postprocedural hemorrhage of eye and adnexa following other procedure** ◀▥

   H59.321 **Postprocedural hemorrhage of right eye and adnexa following other procedure** 🔍◀▥

   H59.322 **Postprocedural hemorrhage of left eye and adnexa following other procedure** 🔍◀▥

   H59.323 **Postprocedural hemorrhage of eye and adnexa following other procedure, bilateral** 🔍◀▥

   H59.329 **Postprocedural hemorrhage of** unspecified **eye and adnexa following other procedure** 🔍

● H59.33 **Postprocedural hematoma of eye and adnexa following an ophthalmic procedure** ◀

   H59.331 **Postprocedural hematoma of right eye and adnexa following an ophthalmic procedure** 🔍◀

   H59.332 **Postprocedural hematoma of left eye and adnexa following an ophthalmic procedure** 🔍◀

   H59.333 **Postprocedural hematoma of eye and adnexa following an ophthalmic procedure, bilateral** 🔍◀

   H59.339 **Postprocedural hematoma of** unspecified **eye and adnexa following an ophthalmic procedure** 🔍◀

● H59.34 **Postprocedural hematoma of eye and adnexa following other procedure** ◀

   H59.341 **Postprocedural hematoma of right eye and adnexa following other procedure** 🔍◀

   H59.342 **Postprocedural hematoma of left eye and adnexa following other procedure** 🔍◀

   H59.343 **Postprocedural hematoma of eye and adnexa following other procedure, bilateral** 🔍◀

   H59.349 **Postprocedural hematoma of** unspecified **eye and adnexa following other procedure** 🔍◀

● H59.35 **Postprocedural seroma of eye and adnexa following an ophthalmic procedure** ◀

   H59.351 **Postprocedural seroma of right eye and adnexa following an ophthalmic procedure** 🔍◀

   H59.352 **Postprocedural seroma of left eye and adnexa following an ophthalmic procedure** 🔍◀

   H59.353 **Postprocedural seroma of eye and adnexa following an ophthalmic procedure, bilateral** 🔍◀

   H59.359 **Postprocedural seroma of** unspecified **eye and adnexa following an ophthalmic procedure** 🔍◀

● H59.36 **Postprocedural seroma of eye and adnexa following other procedure** ◀

   H59.361 **Postprocedural seroma of right eye and adnexa following other procedure** 🔍◀

   H59.362 **Postprocedural seroma of left eye and adnexa following other procedure** 🔍◀

   H59.363 **Postprocedural seroma of eye and adnexa following other procedure, bilateral** 🔍◀

   H59.369 **Postprocedural seroma of** unspecified **eye and adnexa following other procedure** 🔍◀

◀ New   ◀▥ Revised   ~~deleted~~ Deleted   Excludes 1   Excludes 2   Includes   Use additional   Code first   Code also   Unspecified

OGCR Official Guidelines   ● Unacceptable Principal Diagnosis   X Assign placeholder X   ● Use Additional Character(s)   ◀ Manifestation Code   **Coding Clinic**

● H59.4 **Inflammation (infection) of postprocedural bleb**
Postprocedural blebitis

   Excludes1 filtering (vitreous) bleb after glaucoma
   surgery status (Z98.83)

   H59.40 **Inflammation (infection) of postprocedural**
   bleb, unspecified

   H59.41 **Inflammation (infection) of postprocedural**
   bleb, stage 1

   H59.42 **Inflammation (infection) of postprocedural**
   bleb, stage 2

   H59.43 **Inflammation (infection) of postprocedural**
   bleb, stage 3
      Bleb endophthalmitis

● H59.8 **Other intraoperative and postprocedural complications**
and disorders of eye and adnexa, not elsewhere classified
   (Ex) **For category H59.8 CC codes:** See H59.0

   ● H59.81 **Chorioretinal scars after surgery for detachment**

      H59.811 **Chorioretinal scars after surgery for**
      detachment, right eye 🗷

      H59.812 **Chorioretinal scars after surgery for**
      detachment, left eye 🗷

      H59.813 **Chorioretinal scars after surgery for**
      detachment, bilateral 🗷

      H59.819 **Chorioretinal scars after surgery for**
      detachment, unspecified eye 🗷

   H59.88 **Other intraoperative complications of eye and**
   adnexa, not elsewhere classified 🗷

   H59.89 **Other postprocedural complications and**
   disorders of eye and adnexa, not elsewhere
   classified 🗷

N Newborn Age: 0   **P** Pediatric Age: 0–17   **M** Maternity DX: 12–55   **A** Adult Age: 15–124   ♀ Females Only   ♂ Males Only

🗷 Complication\Comorbidity   🗷 Major C\C   (Ex) CC/MCC Exclusions   🗷 Hospital-Acquired Condition

853

CHAPTER 8

DISEASES OF THE EAR AND MASTOID PROCESS (H60-H95)

OGCR Chapter-Specific Coding Guidelines

> 8. Chapter 8: Diseases of the Ear and Mastoid Process (H60-H95)
> Reserved for future guideline expansion

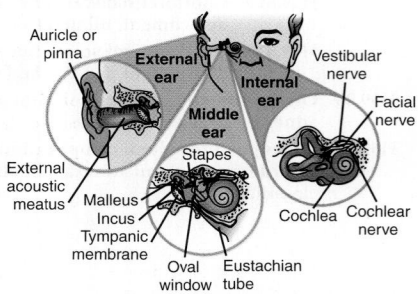

Figure 8-1 Auditory system. (From Buck CJ: Step-by-Step Medical Coding, ed 2016, St. Louis, Elsevier, 2016)

★ **(See Plate 92 on page 68.)**

CHAPTER 8

DISEASES OF THE EAR AND MASTOID PROCESS (H60-H95)

Note: Use an external cause code following the code for the ear condition, if applicable, to identify the cause of the ear condition

> **Excludes2** certain conditions originating in the perinatal period (P04-P96)
> certain infectious and parasitic diseases (A00-B99)
> complications of pregnancy, childbirth and the puerperium (O00-O9A)
> congenital malformations, deformations and chromosomal abnormalities (Q00-Q99)
> endocrine, nutritional and metabolic diseases (E00-E88)
> injury, poisoning and certain other consequences of external causes (S00-T88)
> neoplasms (C00-D49)
> symptoms, signs and abnormal clinical and laboratory findings, not elsewhere classified (R00-R94)

This chapter contains the following blocks:

H60-H62	Diseases of external ear
H65-H75	Diseases of middle ear and mastoid
H80-H83	Diseases of inner ear
H90-H94	Other disorders of ear
H95	Intraoperative and postprocedural complications and disorders of ear and mastoid process, not elsewhere classified

DISEASES OF EXTERNAL EAR (H60-H62)

● **H60**   Otitis externa

● **H60.0**   Abscess of external ear
     Boil of external ear
     Carbuncle of auricle or external auditory canal
     Furuncle of external ear

     H60.00   Abscess of external ear, **unspecified** ear

     H60.01   Abscess of right external ear

     H60.02   Abscess of left external ear

     H60.03   Abscess of external ear, bilateral

● **H60.1**   Cellulitis of external ear
     Cellulitis of auricle
     Cellulitis of external auditory canal

     H60.10   Cellulitis of external ear, **unspecified** ear

     H60.11   Cellulitis of right external ear

     H60.12   Cellulitis of left external ear

     H60.13   Cellulitis of external ear, bilateral

● **H60.2**   Malignant otitis externa
     (Ex) For category H60.2 CC codes: H60.20-H60.23, H70.001-H70.13

     H60.20   Malignant otitis externa, **unspecified** ear

     H60.21   Malignant otitis externa, right ear

     H60.22   Malignant otitis externa, left ear

     H60.23   Malignant otitis externa, bilateral

● **H60.3**   Other infective otitis externa

   ● **H60.31**   Diffuse otitis externa

     H60.311   Diffuse otitis externa, right ear

     H60.312   Diffuse otitis externa, left ear

     H60.313   Diffuse otitis externa, bilateral

     H60.319   Diffuse otitis externa, **unspecified** ear

   ● **H60.32**   Hemorrhagic otitis externa

     H60.321   Hemorrhagic otitis externa, right ear

     H60.322   Hemorrhagic otitis externa, left ear

     H60.323   Hemorrhagic otitis externa, bilateral

     H60.329   Hemorrhagic otitis externa, **unspecified** ear

   ● **H60.33**   Swimmer's ear

     H60.331   Swimmer's ear, right ear

     H60.332   Swimmer's ear, left ear

     H60.333   Swimmer's ear, bilateral

     H60.339   Swimmer's ear, **unspecified** ear

   ● **H60.39**   Other infective otitis externa

     H60.391   Other infective otitis externa, right ear

     H60.392   Other infective otitis externa, left ear

     H60.393   Other infective otitis externa, bilateral

     H60.399   Other infective otitis externa, **unspecified** ear

● **H60.4**   Cholesteatoma of external ear
     Keratosis obturans of external ear (canal)

> **Excludes2** cholesteatoma of middle ear (H71.-)
> recurrent cholesteatoma of postmastoidectomy cavity (H95.0-)

     H60.40   Cholesteatoma of external ear, **unspecified** ear

     H60.41   Cholesteatoma of right external ear

     H60.42   Cholesteatoma of left external ear

     H60.43   Cholesteatoma of external ear, bilateral

● **H60.5**   Acute noninfective otitis externa

   ● **H60.50**   Unspecified acute noninfective otitis externa
     Acute otitis externa NOS

     H60.501   **Unspecified** acute noninfective otitis externa, right ear

     H60.502   **Unspecified** acute noninfective otitis externa, left ear

     H60.503   **Unspecified** acute noninfective otitis externa, bilateral

     H60.509   **Unspecified** acute noninfective otitis externa, unspecified ear

   ● **H60.51**   Acute actinic otitis externa

     H60.511   Acute actinic otitis externa, right ear

     H60.512   Acute actinic otitis externa, left ear

     H60.513   Acute actinic otitis externa, bilateral

     H60.519   Acute actinic otitis externa, **unspecified** ear

◀ New   ◀▥ Revised   ~~deleted~~ Deleted   Excludes 1   Excludes 2   Includes   Use additional   Code first   Code also   Unspecified

OGCR Official Guidelines   ● Unacceptable Principal Diagnosis   X Assign placeholder X   ● Use Additional Character(s)   ▶ Manifestation Code   **Coding Clinic**

● **H60.52 Acute chemical otitis externa**
     H60.521   Acute chemical otitis externa, right ear
     H60.522   Acute chemical otitis externa, left ear
     H60.523   Acute chemical otitis externa, bilateral
     H60.529   Acute chemical otitis externa, unspecified ear

● **H60.53 Acute contact otitis externa**
     H60.531   Acute contact otitis externa, right ear
     H60.532   Acute contact otitis externa, left ear
     H60.533   Acute contact otitis externa, bilateral
     H60.539   Acute contact otitis externa, unspecified ear

● **H60.54 Acute eczematoid otitis externa**
     H60.541   Acute eczematoid otitis externa, right ear
     H60.542   Acute eczematoid otitis externa, left ear
     H60.543   Acute eczematoid otitis externa, bilateral
     H60.549   Acute eczematoid otitis externa, unspecified ear

● **H60.55 Acute reactive otitis externa**
     H60.551   Acute reactive otitis externa, right ear
     H60.552   Acute reactive otitis externa, left ear
     H60.553   Acute reactive otitis externa, bilateral
     H60.559   Acute reactive otitis externa, unspecified ear

● **H60.59 Other noninfective acute otitis externa**
     H60.591   Other noninfective acute otitis externa, right ear
     H60.592   Other noninfective acute otitis externa, left ear
     H60.593   Other noninfective acute otitis externa, bilateral
     H60.599   Other noninfective acute otitis externa, unspecified ear

● **H60.6 Unspecified chronic otitis externa**
     H60.60   Unspecified chronic otitis externa, unspecified ear
     H60.61   Unspecified chronic otitis externa, right ear
     H60.62   Unspecified chronic otitis externa, left ear
     H60.63   Unspecified chronic otitis externa, bilateral

● **H60.8 Other otitis externa**
     ● **H60.8X   Other otitis externa**
         H60.8X1   Other otitis externa, right ear
         H60.8X2   Other otitis externa, left ear
         H60.8X3   Other otitis externa, bilateral
         H60.8X9   Other otitis externa, unspecified ear

● **H60.9 Unspecified otitis externa**
     H60.90   Unspecified otitis externa, unspecified ear
     H60.91   Unspecified otitis externa, right ear
     H60.92   Unspecified otitis externa, left ear
     H60.93   Unspecified otitis externa, bilateral

● **H61 Other disorders of external ear**
     ● **H61.0 Chondritis and perichondritis of external ear**
         Chondrodermatitis nodularis chronica helicis
         Perichondritis of auricle
         Perichondritis of pinna
         ● **H61.00   Unspecified perichondritis of external ear**
             H61.001   Unspecified perichondritis of right external ear
             H61.002   Unspecified perichondritis of left external ear
             H61.003   Unspecified perichondritis of external ear, bilateral
             H61.009   Unspecified perichondritis of external ear, unspecified ear

● **H61.01   Acute perichondritis of external ear**
     H61.011   Acute perichondritis of right external ear
     H61.012   Acute perichondritis of left external ear
     H61.013   Acute perichondritis of external ear, bilateral
     H61.019   Acute perichondritis of external ear, unspecified ear

● **H61.02   Chronic perichondritis of external ear**
     H61.021   Chronic perichondritis of right external ear
     H61.022   Chronic perichondritis of left external ear
     H61.023   Chronic perichondritis of external ear, bilateral
     H61.029   Chronic perichondritis of external ear, unspecified ear

● **H61.03   Chondritis of external ear**
     Chondritis of auricle
     Chondritis of pinna
     H61.031   Chondritis of right external ear
     H61.032   Chondritis of left external ear
         Coding Clinic: 2015, Q1, P18
     H61.033   Chondritis of external ear, bilateral
     H61.039   Chondritis of external ear, unspecified ear

● **H61.1   Noninfective disorders of pinna**
     Excludes2   cauliflower ear (M95.1-)
                 gouty tophi of ear (M1A.-)
     ● **H61.10   Unspecified noninfective disorders of pinna**
         Disorder of pinna NOS
         H61.101   Unspecified noninfective disorders of pinna, right ear
         H61.102   Unspecified noninfective disorders of pinna, left ear
         H61.103   Unspecified noninfective disorders of pinna, bilateral
         H61.109   Unspecified noninfective disorders of pinna, unspecified ear

● **H61.11   Acquired deformity of pinna**
     Acquired deformity of auricle
     Excludes2   cauliflower ear (M95.1-)
     H61.111   Acquired deformity of pinna, right ear
     H61.112   Acquired deformity of pinna, left ear
     H61.113   Acquired deformity of pinna, bilateral
     H61.119   Acquired deformity of pinna, unspecified ear

● **H61.12   Hematoma of pinna**
     Hematoma of auricle
     H61.121   Hematoma of pinna, right ear
     H61.122   Hematoma of pinna, left ear
     H61.123   Hematoma of pinna, bilateral
     H61.129   Hematoma of pinna, unspecified ear

● **H61.19   Other noninfective disorders of pinna**
     H61.191   Noninfective disorders of pinna, right ear
     H61.192   Noninfective disorders of pinna, left ear
     H61.193   Noninfective disorders of pinna, bilateral
     H61.199   Noninfective disorders of pinna, unspecified ear

CHAPTER 8 (H60–H95)

CHAPTER 8 (H60-H95)

● **H61.2   Impacted cerumen**
Wax in ear

    H61.20   Impacted cerumen, unspecified ear
        MCE: Questionable admission when principal dx

    H61.21   Impacted cerumen, right ear
        MCE: Questionable admission when principal dx

    H61.22   Impacted cerumen, left ear
        MCE: Questionable admission when principal dx

    H61.23   Impacted cerumen, bilateral
        MCE: Questionable admission when principal dx

● **H61.3   Acquired stenosis of external ear canal**
Collapse of external ear canal

    Excludes1   postprocedural stenosis of external ear
        canal (H95.81-)

    ● **H61.30   Acquired stenosis of external ear canal,
        unspecified**

        **H61.301   Acquired stenosis of right external ear
            canal, unspecified**

        **H61.302   Acquired stenosis of left external ear
            canal, unspecified**

        **H61.303   Acquired stenosis of external ear
            canal, unspecified, bilateral**

        **H61.309   Acquired stenosis of external ear
            canal, unspecified, unspecified ear**

    ● **H61.31   Acquired stenosis of external ear canal
        secondary to trauma**

        **H61.311   Acquired stenosis of right external ear
            canal secondary to trauma**

        **H61.312   Acquired stenosis of left external ear
            canal secondary to trauma**

        **H61.313   Acquired stenosis of external ear
            canal secondary to trauma, bilateral**

        **H61.319   Acquired stenosis of external
            ear canal secondary to trauma,
            unspecified ear**

    ● **H61.32   Acquired stenosis of external ear canal
        secondary to inflammation and infection**

        **H61.321   Acquired stenosis of right external ear
            canal secondary to inflammation and
            infection**

        **H61.322   Acquired stenosis of left external ear
            canal secondary to inflammation and
            infection**

        **H61.323   Acquired stenosis of external ear
            canal secondary to inflammation and
            infection, bilateral**

        **H61.329   Acquired stenosis of external ear
            canal secondary to inflammation and
            infection, unspecified ear**

    ● **H61.39   Other acquired stenosis of external ear canal**

        **H61.391   Other acquired stenosis of right
            external ear canal**

        **H61.392   Other acquired stenosis of left
            external ear canal**

        **H61.393   Other acquired stenosis of external
            ear canal, bilateral**

        **H61.399   Other acquired stenosis of external
            ear canal, unspecified ear**

● **H61.8   Other specified disorders of external ear**

    ● **H61.81   Exostosis of external canal**

        H61.811   Exostosis of right external canal

        H61.812   Exostosis of left external canal

        H61.813   Exostosis of external canal, bilateral

        **H61.819   Exostosis of external canal,
            unspecified ear**

    ● **H61.89   Other specified disorders of external ear**

        **H61.891   Other specified disorders of right
            external ear**

        **H61.892   Other specified disorders of left
            external ear**

        **H61.893   Other specified disorders of external
            ear, bilateral**

        **H61.899   Other specified disorders of external
            ear, unspecified ear**

● **H61.9   Disorder of external ear, unspecified**

    **H61.90   Disorder of external ear, unspecified,
        unspecified ear**

    H61.91   Disorder of right external ear, unspecified

    H61.92   Disorder of left external ear, unspecified

    H61.93   Disorder of external ear, unspecified, bilateral

● **H62   Disorders of external ear in diseases classified elsewhere**

    ● **H62.4   Otitis externa in other diseases classified elsewhere**

        Code first underlying disease, such as:
            erysipelas (A46)
            impetigo (L01.0)

        Excludes1   otitis externa (in):
            candidiasis (B37.84)
            herpes viral [herpes simplex] (B00.1)
            herpes zoster (B02.8)

        ▌*H62.40   Otitis externa in other diseases classified
            elsewhere, unspecified ear*

        ▌*H62.41   Otitis externa in other diseases classified
            elsewhere, right ear*

        ▌*H62.42   Otitis externa in other diseases classified
            elsewhere, left ear*

        ▌*H62.43   Otitis externa in other diseases classified
            elsewhere, bilateral*

    ● **H62.8   Other disorders of external ear in diseases classified
        elsewhere**

        Code first underlying disease, such as:
            gout (M1A.-, M10.-)

        ● **H62.8X   Other disorders of external ear in diseases
            classified elsewhere**

            ▌*H62.8X1   Other disorders of right external ear in
                diseases classified elsewhere*

            ▌*H62.8X2   Other disorders of left external ear in
                diseases classified elsewhere*

            ▌*H62.8X3   Other disorders of external ear in
                diseases classified elsewhere, bilateral*

            ▌*H62.8X9   Other disorders of external ear
                in diseases classified elsewhere,
                unspecified ear*

DISEASES OF MIDDLE EAR AND MASTOID (H65-H75)

★ **(See Plate 94 on page 69.)**

● **H65   Nonsuppurative otitis media**
*Bacterial or viral infection or inflammation of the middle ear; may result
in fluid accumulation with pain and temporary hearing loss.*

    Includes   nonsuppurative otitis media with myringitis

    Use additional code for any associated perforated tympanic
    membrane (H72.-)

    Use additional code to identify:
    exposure to environmental tobacco smoke (Z77.22)
    exposure to tobacco smoke in the perinatal period (P96.81)
    history of tobacco dependence (Z87.891) ◀▥
    occupational exposure to environmental tobacco smoke
        (Z57.31)
    tobacco dependence (F17.-)
    tobacco use (Z72.0)

    ● **H65.0   Acute serous otitis media**
        Acute and subacute secretory otitis

        H65.00   Acute serous otitis media, unspecified ear

        H65.01   Acute serous otitis media, right ear

        H65.02   Acute serous otitis media, left ear

        H65.03   Acute serous otitis media, bilateral

        H65.04   Acute serous otitis media, recurrent, right ear

        H65.05   Acute serous otitis media, recurrent, left ear

        H65.06   Acute serous otitis media, recurrent, bilateral

        **H65.07   Acute serous otitis media, recurrent,
            unspecified ear**

◀ New   ◀▥ Revised   ~~deleted~~ Deleted   Excludes 1   Excludes 2   Includes   Use additional   Code first   Code also   Unspecified

OGCR Official Guidelines   ● Unacceptable Principal Diagnosis   X Assign placeholder X   ● Use Additional Character(s)   ▌ Manifestation Code   **Coding Clinic**

● **H65.1**   **Other acute nonsuppurative otitis media**
> **Excludes1**   otitic barotrauma (T70.0)
> otitis media (acute) NOS (H66.9)

● **H65.11**   **Acute and subacute allergic otitis media (mucoid) (sanguinous) (serous)**

    H65.111   **Acute and subacute allergic otitis media (mucoid) (sanguinous) (serous), right ear**

    H65.112   **Acute and subacute allergic otitis media (mucoid) (sanguinous) (serous), left ear**

    H65.113   **Acute and subacute allergic otitis media (mucoid) (sanguinous) (serous), bilateral**

    H65.114   **Acute and subacute allergic otitis media (mucoid) (sanguinous) (serous), recurrent, right ear**

    H65.115   **Acute and subacute allergic otitis media (mucoid) (sanguinous) (serous), recurrent, left ear**

    H65.116   **Acute and subacute allergic otitis media (mucoid) (sanguinous) (serous), recurrent, bilateral**

    H65.117   **Acute and subacute allergic otitis media (mucoid) (sanguinous) (serous), recurrent, unspecified ear**

    H65.119   **Acute and subacute allergic otitis media (mucoid) (sanguinous) (serous), unspecified ear**

● **H65.19**   **Other acute nonsuppurative otitis media**
> Acute and subacute mucoid otitis media
> Acute and subacute nonsuppurative otitis media NOS
> Acute and subacute sanguinous otitis media
> Acute and subacute seromucinous otitis media

    H65.191   **Other acute nonsuppurative otitis media, right ear**

    H65.192   **Other acute nonsuppurative otitis media, left ear**

    H65.193   **Other acute nonsuppurative otitis media, bilateral**

    H65.194   **Other acute nonsuppurative otitis media, recurrent, right ear**

    H65.195   **Other acute nonsuppurative otitis media, recurrent, left ear**

    H65.196   **Other acute nonsuppurative otitis media, recurrent, bilateral**

    H65.197   **Other acute nonsuppurative otitis media recurrent, unspecified ear**

    H65.199   **Other acute nonsuppurative otitis media, unspecified ear**

● **H65.2**   **Chronic serous otitis media**
> Chronic tubotympanal catarrh

    H65.20   **Chronic serous otitis media, unspecified ear**

    H65.21   **Chronic serous otitis media, right ear**

    H65.22   **Chronic serous otitis media, left ear**

    H65.23   **Chronic serous otitis media, bilateral**

● **H65.3**   **Chronic mucoid otitis media**
> Chronic mucinous otitis media
> Chronic secretory otitis media
> Chronic transudative otitis media
> Glue ear
> **Excludes1**   adhesive middle ear disease (H74.1)

    H65.30   **Chronic mucoid otitis media, unspecified ear**

    H65.31   **Chronic mucoid otitis media, right ear**

    H65.32   **Chronic mucoid otitis media, left ear**

    H65.33   **Chronic mucoid otitis media, bilateral**

● **H65.4**   **Other chronic nonsuppurative otitis media**

  ● **H65.41**   **Chronic allergic otitis media**

     H65.411   **Chronic allergic otitis media, right ear**

     H65.412   **Chronic allergic otitis media, left ear**

     H65.413   **Chronic allergic otitis media, bilateral**

     H65.419   **Chronic allergic otitis media, unspecified ear**

● **H65.49**   **Other chronic nonsuppurative otitis media**
> Chronic exudative otitis media
> Chronic nonsuppurative otitis media NOS
> Chronic otitis media with effusion (nonpurulent)
> Chronic seromucinous otitis media

    H65.491   **Other chronic nonsuppurative otitis media, right ear**

    H65.492   **Other chronic nonsuppurative otitis media, left ear**

    H65.493   **Other chronic nonsuppurative otitis media, bilateral**

    H65.499   **Other chronic nonsuppurative otitis media, unspecified ear**

● **H65.9**   **Unspecified nonsuppurative otitis media**
> Allergic otitis media NOS
> Catarrhal otitis media NOS
> Exudative otitis media NOS
> Mucoid otitis media NOS
> Otitis media with effusion (nonpurulent) NOS
> Secretory otitis media NOS
> Seromucinous otitis media NOS
> Serous otitis media NOS
> Transudative otitis media NOS

    H65.90   **Unspecified nonsuppurative otitis media, unspecified ear**

    H65.91   **Unspecified nonsuppurative otitis media, right ear**

    H65.92   **Unspecified nonsuppurative otitis media, left ear**

    H65.93   **Unspecified nonsuppurative otitis media, bilateral**

● **H66**   **Suppurative and unspecified otitis media**
> *Suppurative: Discharging pus*
> **Includes**   suppurative and unspecified otitis media with myringitis
> Use additional code to identify:
> exposure to environmental tobacco smoke (Z77.22)
> exposure to tobacco smoke in the perinatal period (P96.81)
> history of tobacco dependence (Z87.891) ◀▥
> occupational exposure to environmental tobacco smoke (Z57.31)
> tobacco dependence (F17.-)
> tobacco use (Z72.0)

  ● **H66.0**   **Acute suppurative otitis media**

    ● **H66.00**   **Acute suppurative otitis media without spontaneous rupture of ear drum**

      H66.001   **Acute suppurative otitis media without spontaneous rupture of ear drum, right ear**
>   **Coding Clinic: 2016, Q1, P34**

      H66.002   **Acute suppurative otitis media without spontaneous rupture of ear drum, left ear**

      H66.003   **Acute suppurative otitis media without spontaneous rupture of ear drum, bilateral**

      H66.004   **Acute suppurative otitis media without spontaneous rupture of ear drum, recurrent, right ear**

      H66.005   **Acute suppurative otitis media without spontaneous rupture of ear drum, recurrent, left ear**

      H66.006   **Acute suppurative otitis media without spontaneous rupture of ear drum, recurrent, bilateral**

      H66.007   **Acute suppurative otitis media without spontaneous rupture of ear drum, recurrent, unspecified ear**

      H66.009   **Acute suppurative otitis media without spontaneous rupture of ear drum, unspecified ear**

N Newborn Age: 0   **P** Pediatric Age: 0–17   **M** Maternity DX: 12–55   **A** Adult Age: 15–124   ♀ Females Only   ♂ Males Only

 Complication\Comorbidity   Major C\C   (Ex) CC/MCC Exclusions   Hospital-Acquired Condition

857

● **H66.01** **Acute suppurative otitis media with spontaneous rupture of ear drum**

    H66.011 Acute suppurative otitis media with spontaneous rupture of ear drum, right ear

    H66.012 Acute suppurative otitis media with spontaneous rupture of ear drum, left ear

    H66.013 Acute suppurative otitis media with spontaneous rupture of ear drum, bilateral

    H66.014 Acute suppurative otitis media with spontaneous rupture of ear drum, recurrent, right ear

    H66.015 Acute suppurative otitis media with spontaneous rupture of ear drum, recurrent, left ear

    H66.016 Acute suppurative otitis media with spontaneous rupture of ear drum, recurrent, bilateral

    H66.017 Acute suppurative otitis media with spontaneous rupture of ear drum, recurrent, unspecified ear

    H66.019 Acute suppurative otitis media with spontaneous rupture of ear drum, unspecified ear

● **H66.1** **Chronic tubotympanic suppurative otitis media**

Benign chronic suppurative otitis media
Chronic tubotympanic disease

Use additional code for any associated perforated tympanic membrane (H72.-)

    H66.10 Chronic tubotympanic suppurative otitis media, unspecified

    H66.11 Chronic tubotympanic suppurative otitis media, right ear

    H66.12 Chronic tubotympanic suppurative otitis media, left ear

    H66.13 Chronic tubotympanic suppurative otitis media, bilateral

● **H66.2** **Chronic atticoantral suppurative otitis media**

Chronic atticoantral disease

Use additional code for any associated perforated tympanic membrane (H72.-)

    H66.20 Chronic atticoantral suppurative otitis media, unspecified ear

    H66.21 Chronic atticoantral suppurative otitis media, right ear

    H66.22 Chronic atticoantral suppurative otitis media, left ear

    H66.23 Chronic atticoantral suppurative otitis media, bilateral

● **H66.3** **Other chronic suppurative otitis media**

Chronic suppurative otitis media NOS

Use additional code for any associated perforated tympanic membrane (H72.-)

Excludes1   tuberculous otitis media (A18.6)

● **H66.3X** **Other chronic suppurative otitis media**

    H66.3X1 Other chronic suppurative otitis media, right ear

    H66.3X2 Other chronic suppurative otitis media, left ear

    H66.3X3 Other chronic suppurative otitis media, bilateral

    H66.3X9 Other chronic suppurative otitis media, unspecified ear

● **H66.4** **Suppurative otitis media, unspecified**

Purulent otitis media NOS

Use additional code for any associated perforated tympanic membrane (H72.-)

    H66.40 Suppurative otitis media, unspecified, unspecified ear

    H66.41 Suppurative otitis media, unspecified, right ear

    H66.42 Suppurative otitis media, unspecified, left ear

    H66.43 Suppurative otitis media, unspecified, bilateral

● **H66.9** **Otitis media, unspecified**

Otitis media NOS
Acute otitis media NOS
Chronic otitis media NOS

Use additional code for any associated perforated tympanic membrane (H72.-)

    H66.90 Otitis media, unspecified, unspecified ear

    H66.91 Otitis media, unspecified, right ear

    H66.92 Otitis media, unspecified, left ear

    H66.93 Otitis media, unspecified, bilateral

● **H67** **Otitis media in diseases classified elsewhere**

Code first underlying disease, such as:
viral disease NEC (B00-B34)

Use additional code for any associated perforated tympanic membrane (H72.-)

Excludes1   otitis media in:
influenza (J09.X9, J10.83, J11.83)
measles (B05.3)
scarlet fever (A38.0)
tuberculosis (A18.6)

▷ *H67.1*   *Otitis media in diseases classified elsewhere, right ear*

▷ *H67.2*   *Otitis media in diseases classified elsewhere, left ear*

▷ *H67.3*   *Otitis media in diseases classified elsewhere, bilateral*

▷ *H67.9*   *Otitis media in diseases classified elsewhere, unspecified ear*

● **H68** **Eustachian salpingitis and obstruction**

● **H68.0** **Eustachian salpingitis**

● **H68.00** **Unspecified Eustachian salpingitis**

    H68.001 Unspecified Eustachian salpingitis, right ear

    H68.002 Unspecified Eustachian salpingitis, left ear

    H68.003 Unspecified Eustachian salpingitis, bilateral

    H68.009 Unspecified Eustachian salpingitis, unspecified ear

● **H68.01** **Acute Eustachian salpingitis**

    H68.011 Acute Eustachian salpingitis, right ear

    H68.012 Acute Eustachian salpingitis, left ear

    H68.013 Acute Eustachian salpingitis, bilateral

    H68.019 Acute Eustachian salpingitis, unspecified ear

● **H68.02** **Chronic Eustachian salpingitis**

    H68.021 Chronic Eustachian salpingitis, right ear

    H68.022 Chronic Eustachian salpingitis, left ear

    H68.023 Chronic Eustachian salpingitis, bilateral

    H68.029 Chronic Eustachian salpingitis, unspecified ear

◀ New   ◀▥ Revised   ~~deleted~~ Deleted   Excludes 1   Excludes 2   Includes   Use additional   Code first   Code also   Unspecified

OGCR Official Guidelines   ● Unacceptable Principal Diagnosis   X Assign placeholder X   ● Use Additional Character(s)   ▷ Manifestation Code   **Coding Clinic**

● **H68.1**   **Obstruction of Eustachian tube**
     Stenosis of Eustachian tube
     Stricture of Eustachian tube
   ● **H68.10**   Unspecified obstruction of Eustachian tube
       H68.101   Unspecified obstruction of Eustachian tube, right ear
       H68.102   Unspecified obstruction of Eustachian tube, left ear
       H68.103   Unspecified obstruction of Eustachian tube, bilateral
       H68.109   Unspecified obstruction of Eustachian tube, unspecified ear
   ● **H68.11**   Osseous obstruction of Eustachian tube
       H68.111   Osseous obstruction of Eustachian tube, right ear
       H68.112   Osseous obstruction of Eustachian tube, left ear
       H68.113   Osseous obstruction of Eustachian tube, bilateral
       H68.119   Osseous obstruction of Eustachian tube, unspecified ear
   ● **H68.12**   Intrinsic cartilagenous obstruction of Eustachian tube
       H68.121   Intrinsic cartilagenous obstruction of Eustachian tube, right ear
       H68.122   Intrinsic cartilagenous obstruction of Eustachian tube, left ear
       H68.123   Intrinsic cartilagenous obstruction of Eustachian tube, bilateral
       H68.129   Intrinsic cartilagenous obstruction of Eustachian tube, unspecified ear
   ● **H68.13**   Extrinsic cartilagenous obstruction of Eustachian tube
       Compression of Eustachian tube
       H68.131   Extrinsic cartilagenous obstruction of Eustachian tube, right ear
       H68.132   Extrinsic cartilagenous obstruction of Eustachian tube, left ear
       H68.133   Extrinsic cartilagenous obstruction of Eustachian tube, bilateral
       H68.139   Extrinsic cartilagenous obstruction of Eustachian tube, unspecified ear

● **H69**   **Other and unspecified disorders of Eustachian tube**
   ● **H69.0**   Patulous Eustachian tube
       H69.00   Patulous Eustachian tube, unspecified ear
       H69.01   Patulous Eustachian tube, right ear
       H69.02   Patulous Eustachian tube, left ear
       H69.03   Patulous Eustachian tube, bilateral
   ● **H69.8**   Other specified disorders of Eustachian tube
       H69.80   Other specified disorders of Eustachian tube, unspecified ear
       H69.81   Other specified disorders of Eustachian tube, right ear
       H69.82   Other specified disorders of Eustachian tube, left ear
       H69.83   Other specified disorders of Eustachian tube, bilateral
   ● **H69.9**   Unspecified Eustachian tube disorder
       H69.90   Unspecified Eustachian tube disorder, unspecified ear
       H69.91   Unspecified Eustachian tube disorder, right ear
       H69.92   Unspecified Eustachian tube disorder, left ear
       H69.93   Unspecified Eustachian tube disorder, bilateral

● **H70**   **Mastoiditis and related conditions**
   ● **H70.0**   **Acute mastoiditis**
     Abscess of mastoid
     Empyema of mastoid
     (Ex) **For category H70.0 CC codes:** A17.9, A18.6, A18.82, A18.84, A18.89, H70.001–H70.213, H70.219–H70.93, H75.00–H75.83, H93.8X1–H93.93, H94.80–H95.199, Q16.1, Q16.9, Q17.3–Q17.9
    ● **H70.00**   Acute mastoiditis without complications
       H70.001   Acute mastoiditis without complications, right ear 🦠
       H70.002   Acute mastoiditis without complications, left ear 🦠
       H70.003   Acute mastoiditis without complications, bilateral 🦠
       H70.009   Acute mastoiditis without complications, unspecified ear 🦠
    ● **H70.01**   Subperiosteal abscess of mastoid
       H70.011   Subperiosteal abscess of mastoid, right ear 🦠
       H70.012   Subperiosteal abscess of mastoid, left ear 🦠
       H70.013   Subperiosteal abscess of mastoid, bilateral 🦠
       H70.019   Subperiosteal abscess of mastoid, unspecified ear 🦠
    ● **H70.09**   Acute mastoiditis with other complications
       H70.091   Acute mastoiditis with other complications, right ear 🦠
       H70.092   Acute mastoiditis with other complications, left ear 🦠
       H70.093   Acute mastoiditis with other complications, bilateral 🦠
       H70.099   Acute mastoiditis with other complications, unspecified ear 🦠
   ● **H70.1**   Chronic mastoiditis
     Caries of mastoid
     Fistula of mastoid
     Excludes1   tuberculous mastoiditis (A18.03)
     H70.10   Chronic mastoiditis, unspecified ear
     H70.11   Chronic mastoiditis, right ear
     H70.12   Chronic mastoiditis, left ear
     H70.13   Chronic mastoiditis, bilateral
   ● **H70.2**   Petrositis
     Inflammation of petrous bone
    ● **H70.20**   Unspecified petrositis
       H70.201   Unspecified petrositis, right ear
       H70.202   Unspecified petrositis, left ear
       H70.203   Unspecified petrositis, bilateral
       H70.209   Unspecified petrositis, unspecified ear
    ● **H70.21**   Acute petrositis
       H70.211   Acute petrositis, right ear
       H70.212   Acute petrositis, left ear
       H70.213   Acute petrositis, bilateral
       H70.219   Acute petrositis, unspecified ear
    ● **H70.22**   Chronic petrositis
       H70.221   Chronic petrositis, right ear
       H70.222   Chronic petrositis, left ear
       H70.223   Chronic petrositis, bilateral
       H70.229   Chronic petrositis, unspecified ear

CHAPTER 8 (H60–H95)

Item 8–1   **Mastoiditis** is an infection of the portion of the temporal bone of the skull that is behind the ear (mastoid process) caused by an untreated otitis media, leading to an infection of the surrounding structures which may include the brain.

N   Newborn Age: 0   P   Pediatric Age: 0–17   M   Maternity DX: 12–55   A   Adult Age: 15–124   ♀   Females Only   ♂   Males Only

🦠   Complication\Comorbidity   🦠   Major C\C   (Ex)   CC/MCC Exclusions   🦠   Hospital-Acquired Condition

CHAPTER 8 (H60-H95)

● **H70.8   Other mastoiditis and related conditions**
    Excludes1   preauricular sinus and cyst (Q18.1)
                      sinus, fistula, and cyst of branchial cleft
                      (Q18.0)

   ● **H70.81   Postauricular fistula**
       H70.811   Postauricular fistula, right ear
       H70.812   Postauricular fistula, left ear
       H70.813   Postauricular fistula, bilateral
       H70.819   Postauricular fistula, unspecified ear

   ● **H70.89   Other mastoiditis and related conditions**
       H70.891   Other mastoiditis and related conditions, right ear
       H70.892   Other mastoiditis and related conditions, left ear
       H70.893   Other mastoiditis and related conditions, bilateral
       H70.899   Other mastoiditis and related conditions, unspecified ear

● **H70.9   Unspecified mastoiditis**
     H70.90   Unspecified mastoiditis, unspecified ear
     H70.91   Unspecified mastoiditis, right ear
     H70.92   Unspecified mastoiditis, left ear
     H70.93   Unspecified mastoiditis, bilateral

● **H71   Cholesteatoma of middle ear**
    Excludes2   cholesteatoma of external ear (H60.4-)
                      recurrent cholesteatoma of postmastoidectomy
                      cavity (H95.0-)

● **H71.0   Cholesteatoma of attic**
     H71.00   Cholesteatoma of attic, unspecified ear
     H71.01   Cholesteatoma of attic, right ear
     H71.02   Cholesteatoma of attic, left ear
     H71.03   Cholesteatoma of attic, bilateral

● **H71.1   Cholesteatoma of tympanum**
     H71.10   Cholesteatoma of tympanum, unspecified ear
     H71.11   Cholesteatoma of tympanum, right ear
     H71.12   Cholesteatoma of tympanum, left ear
     H71.13   Cholesteatoma of tympanum, bilateral

● **H71.2   Cholesteatoma of mastoid**
     H71.20   Cholesteatoma of mastoid, unspecified ear
     H71.21   Cholesteatoma of mastoid, right ear
     H71.22   Cholesteatoma of mastoid, left ear
     H71.23   Cholesteatoma of mastoid, bilateral

● **H71.3   Diffuse cholesteatosis**
     H71.30   Diffuse cholesteatosis, unspecified ear
     H71.31   Diffuse cholesteatosis, right ear
     H71.32   Diffuse cholesteatosis, left ear
     H71.33   Diffuse cholesteatosis, bilateral

● **H71.9   Unspecified cholesteatoma**
     H71.90   Unspecified cholesteatoma, unspecified ear
     H71.91   Unspecified cholesteatoma, right ear
     H71.92   Unspecified cholesteatoma, left ear
     H71.93   Unspecified cholesteatoma, bilateral

★ **(See Plate 93 on page 69.)**

● **H72   Perforation of tympanic membrane**
     Hole or rupture in ear drum
    Includes   persistent post-traumatic perforation of ear drum
                    postinflammatory perforation of ear drum
    Code first any associated otitis media (H65.-, H66.1-, H66.2-,
       H66.3-, H66.4-, H66.9-, H67.-)
    Excludes1   acute suppurative otitis media with rupture of
                      the tympanic membrane (H66.01-)
                      traumatic rupture of ear drum (S09.2-)

● **H72.0   Central perforation of tympanic membrane**
     H72.00   Central perforation of tympanic membrane, unspecified ear
     H72.01   Central perforation of tympanic membrane, right ear
     H72.02   Central perforation of tympanic membrane, left ear
     H72.03   Central perforation of tympanic membrane, bilateral

● **H72.1   Attic perforation of tympanic membrane**
     Perforation of pars flaccida
     H72.10   Attic perforation of tympanic membrane, unspecified ear
     H72.11   Attic perforation of tympanic membrane, right ear
     H72.12   Attic perforation of tympanic membrane, left ear
     H72.13   Attic perforation of tympanic membrane, bilateral

● **H72.2   Other marginal perforations of tympanic membrane**
   ● **H72.2X   Other marginal perforations of tympanic membrane**
       H72.2X1   Other marginal perforations of tympanic membrane, right ear
       H72.2X2   Other marginal perforations of tympanic membrane, left ear
       H72.2X3   Other marginal perforations of tympanic membrane, bilateral
       H72.2X9   Other marginal perforations of tympanic membrane, unspecified ear

● **H72.8   Other perforations of tympanic membrane**
   ● **H72.81   Multiple perforations of tympanic membrane**
       H72.811   Multiple perforations of tympanic membrane, right ear
       H72.812   Multiple perforations of tympanic membrane, left ear
       H72.813   Multiple perforations of tympanic membrane, bilateral
       H72.819   Multiple perforations of tympanic membrane, unspecified ear
   ● **H72.82   Total perforations of tympanic membrane**
       H72.821   Total perforations of tympanic membrane, right ear
       H72.822   Total perforations of tympanic membrane, left ear
       H72.823   Total perforations of tympanic membrane, bilateral
       H72.829   Total perforations of tympanic membrane, unspecified ear

● **H72.9   Unspecified perforation of tympanic membrane**
     H72.90   Unspecified perforation of tympanic membrane, unspecified ear
     H72.91   Unspecified perforation of tympanic membrane, right ear
     H72.92   Unspecified perforation of tympanic membrane, left ear
     H72.93   Unspecified perforation of tympanic membrane, bilateral

◀ New   ◀ Revised   ~~deleted~~ Deleted   Excludes 1   Excludes 2   Includes   Use additional   Code first   Code also   Unspecified
OGCR Official Guidelines   ● Unacceptable Principal Diagnosis   X Assign placeholder X   ● Use Additional Character(s)   ▶ Manifestation Code   **Coding Clinic**

- **H73**   **Other disorders of tympanic membrane**
  - **H73.0**   **Acute myringitis**
    - **Excludes1**   acute myringitis with otitis media (H65, H66)
    - **H73.00**   **Unspecified acute myringitis**
      Acute tympanitis NOS
      - H73.001   Acute myringitis, right ear
      - H73.002   Acute myringitis, left ear
      - H73.003   Acute myringitis, bilateral
      - H73.009   Acute myringitis, unspecified ear
    - **H73.01**   **Bullous myringitis**
      - H73.011   Bullous myringitis, right ear
      - H73.012   Bullous myringitis, left ear
      - H73.013   Bullous myringitis, bilateral
      - H73.019   Bullous myringitis, unspecified ear
    - **H73.09**   **Other acute myringitis**
      - H73.091   Other acute myringitis, right ear
      - H73.092   Other acute myringitis, left ear
      - H73.093   Other acute myringitis, bilateral
      - H73.099   Other acute myringitis, unspecified ear
  - **H73.1**   **Chronic myringitis**
    Chronic tympanitis
    - **Excludes1**   chronic myringitis with otitis media (H65, H66)
    - **H73.10**   Chronic myringitis, unspecified ear
    - **H73.11**   Chronic myringitis, right ear
    - **H73.12**   Chronic myringitis, left ear
    - **H73.13**   Chronic myringitis, bilateral
  - **H73.2**   **Unspecified myringitis**
    - **H73.20**   Unspecified myringitis, unspecified ear
    - **H73.21**   Unspecified myringitis, right ear
    - **H73.22**   Unspecified myringitis, left ear
    - **H73.23**   Unspecified myringitis, bilateral
  - **H73.8**   **Other specified disorders of tympanic membrane**
    - **H73.81**   **Atrophic flaccid tympanic membrane**
      - H73.811   Atrophic flaccid tympanic membrane, right ear
      - H73.812   Atrophic flaccid tympanic membrane, left ear
      - H73.813   Atrophic flaccid tympanic membrane, bilateral
      - H73.819   Atrophic flaccid tympanic membrane, unspecified ear
    - **H73.82**   **Atrophic nonflaccid tympanic membrane**
      - H73.821   Atrophic nonflaccid tympanic membrane, right ear
      - H73.822   Atrophic nonflaccid tympanic membrane, left ear
      - H73.823   Atrophic nonflaccid tympanic membrane, bilateral
      - H73.829   Atrophic nonflaccid tympanic membrane, unspecified ear
    - **H73.89**   **Other specified disorders of tympanic membrane**
      - H73.891   Other specified disorders of tympanic membrane, right ear
      - H73.892   Other specified disorders of tympanic membrane, left ear
      - H73.893   Other specified disorders of tympanic membrane, bilateral
      - H73.899   Other specified disorders of tympanic membrane, unspecified ear

- **H73.9**   **Unspecified disorder of tympanic membrane**
  - **H73.90**   Unspecified disorder of tympanic membrane, unspecified ear
  - **H73.91**   Unspecified disorder of tympanic membrane, right ear
  - **H73.92**   Unspecified disorder of tympanic membrane, left ear
  - **H73.93**   Unspecified disorder of tympanic membrane, bilateral

- **H74**   **Other disorders of middle ear mastoid**
  - **Excludes2**   mastoiditis (H70.-)
  - **H74.0**   **Tympanosclerosis**
    - **H74.01**   Tympanosclerosis, right ear
    - **H74.02**   Tympanosclerosis, left ear
    - **H74.03**   Tympanosclerosis, bilateral
    - **H74.09**   Tympanosclerosis, unspecified ear
  - **H74.1**   **Adhesive middle ear disease**
    Adhesive otitis
    - **Excludes1**   glue ear (H65.3-)
    - **H74.11**   Adhesive right middle ear disease
    - **H74.12**   Adhesive left middle ear disease
    - **H74.13**   Adhesive middle ear disease, bilateral
    - **H74.19**   Adhesive middle ear disease, unspecified ear
  - **H74.2**   **Discontinuity and dislocation of ear ossicles**
    - **H74.20**   Discontinuity and dislocation of ear ossicles, unspecified ear
    - **H74.21**   Discontinuity and dislocation of right ear ossicles
    - **H74.22**   Discontinuity and dislocation of left ear ossicles
    - **H74.23**   Discontinuity and dislocation of ear ossicles, bilateral
  - **H74.3**   **Other acquired abnormalities of ear ossicles**
    - **H74.31**   **Ankylosis of ear ossicles**
      - H74.311   Ankylosis of ear ossicles, right ear
      - H74.312   Ankylosis of ear ossicles, left ear
      - H74.313   Ankylosis of ear ossicles, bilateral
      - H74.319   Ankylosis of ear ossicles, unspecified ear
    - **H74.32**   **Partial loss of ear ossicles**
      - H74.321   Partial loss of ear ossicles, right ear
      - H74.322   Partial loss of ear ossicles, left ear
      - H74.323   Partial loss of ear ossicles, bilateral
      - H74.329   Partial loss of ear ossicles, unspecified ear
    - **H74.39**   **Other acquired abnormalities of ear ossicles**
      - H74.391   Other acquired abnormalities of right ear ossicles
      - H74.392   Other acquired abnormalities of left ear ossicles
      - H74.393   Other acquired abnormalities of ear ossicles, bilateral
      - H74.399   Other acquired abnormalities of ear ossicles, unspecified ear
  - **H74.4**   **Polyp of middle ear**
    - **H74.40**   Polyp of middle ear, unspecified ear
    - **H74.41**   Polyp of right middle ear
    - **H74.42**   Polyp of left middle ear
    - **H74.43**   Polyp of middle ear, bilateral

N   Newborn Age: 0   **P**   Pediatric Age: 0–17   **M**   Maternity DX: 12–55   **A**   Adult Age: 15–124   ♀   Females Only   ♂   Males Only

🅒   Complication\Comorbidity   🅜   Major C\C   ⓔ🆇   CC/MCC Exclusions   🅗   Hospital-Acquired Condition

861

CHAPTER 8 (H60-H95)

● **H74.8** **Other specified disorders of middle ear and mastoid**
  ● **H74.8X** **Other specified disorders of middle ear and mastoid**
    H74.8X1 Other specified disorders of right middle ear and mastoid
    H74.8X2 Other specified disorders of left middle ear and mastoid
    H74.8X3 Other specified disorders of middle ear and mastoid, bilateral
    H74.8X9 Other specified disorders of middle ear and mastoid, unspecified ear
  ● **H74.9** **Unspecified disorder of middle ear and mastoid**
    H74.90 Unspecified disorder of middle ear and mastoid, unspecified ear
    H74.91 Unspecified disorder of right middle ear and mastoid
    H74.92 Unspecified disorder of left middle ear and mastoid
    H74.93 Unspecified disorder of middle ear and mastoid, bilateral

● **H75** **Other disorders of middle ear and mastoid in diseases classified elsewhere**
  Code first underlying disease
  ● **H75.0** **Mastoiditis in infectious and parasitic diseases classified elsewhere**
    Excludes1   mastoiditis (in):
              syphilis (A52.77)
              tuberculosis (A18.03)
    ▶ *H75.00* *Mastoiditis in infectious and parasitic diseases classified elsewhere, unspecified ear*
    ▶ *H75.01* *Mastoiditis in infectious and parasitic diseases classified elsewhere, right ear*
    ▶ *H75.02* *Mastoiditis in infectious and parasitic diseases classified elsewhere, left ear*
    ▶ *H75.03* *Mastoiditis in infectious and parasitic diseases classified elsewhere, bilateral*
  ● **H75.8** **Other specified disorders of middle ear and mastoid in diseases classified elsewhere**
    ▶ *H75.80* *Other specified disorders of middle ear and mastoid in diseases classified elsewhere, unspecified ear*
    ▶ *H75.81* *Other specified disorders of right middle ear and mastoid in diseases classified elsewhere*
    ▶ *H75.82* *Other specified disorders of left middle ear and mastoid in diseases classified elsewhere*
    ▶ *H75.83* *Other specified disorders of middle ear and mastoid in diseases classified elsewhere, bilateral*

DISEASES OF INNER EAR (H80–H83)

★ **(See Plate 95 on page 69.)**

● **H80** **Otosclerosis**
  Inherited middle ear spongelike bone growth causing hearing loss
  Includes   Otospongiosis
  ● **H80.0** **Otosclerosis involving oval window, nonobliterative**
    H80.00 Otosclerosis involving oval window, nonobliterative, unspecified ear
    H80.01 Otosclerosis involving oval window, nonobliterative, right ear
    H80.02 Otosclerosis involving oval window, nonobliterative, left ear
    H80.03 Otosclerosis involving oval window, nonobliterative, bilateral
  ● **H80.1** **Otosclerosis involving oval window, obliterative**
    H80.10 Otosclerosis involving oval window, obliterative, unspecified ear
    H80.11 Otosclerosis involving oval window, obliterative, right ear

● **H80.12** Otosclerosis involving oval window, obliterative, left ear
H80.13 Otosclerosis involving oval window, obliterative, bilateral
  ● **H80.2** **Cochlear otosclerosis**
    Otosclerosis involving otic capsule
    Otosclerosis involving round window
    H80.20 Cochlear otosclerosis, unspecified ear
    H80.21 Cochlear otosclerosis, right ear
    H80.22 Cochlear otosclerosis, left ear
    H80.23 Cochlear otosclerosis, bilateral
  ● **H80.8** **Other otosclerosis**
    H80.80 Other otosclerosis, unspecified ear
    H80.81 Other otosclerosis, right ear
    H80.82 Other otosclerosis, left ear
    H80.83 Other otosclerosis, bilateral
  ● **H80.9** **Unspecified otosclerosis**
    H80.90 Unspecified otosclerosis, unspecified ear
    H80.91 Unspecified otosclerosis, right ear
    H80.92 Unspecified otosclerosis, left ear
    H80.93 Unspecified otosclerosis, bilateral

● **H81** **Disorders of vestibular function**
  Excludes1   epidemic vertigo (A88.1)
              vertigo NOS (R42)
  ● **H81.0** **Ménière's disease**
    Vestibular disorder that produces recurring symptoms including severe and intermittent hearing loss including the feeling of ear pressure or pain
    Labyrinthine hydrops
    Ménière's syndrome or vertigo
    H81.01 Ménière's disease, right ear
    H81.02 Ménière's disease, left ear
    H81.03 Ménière's disease, bilateral
    H81.09 Ménière's disease, unspecified ear
  ● **H81.1** **Benign paroxysmal vertigo**
    H81.10 Benign paroxysmal vertigo, unspecified ear
    H81.11 Benign paroxysmal vertigo, right ear
    H81.12 Benign paroxysmal vertigo, left ear
    H81.13 Benign paroxysmal vertigo, bilateral
  ● **H81.2** **Vestibular neuronitis**
    H81.20 Vestibular neuronitis, unspecified ear
    H81.21 Vestibular neuronitis, right ear
    H81.22 Vestibular neuronitis, left ear
    H81.23 Vestibular neuronitis, bilateral
  ● **H81.3** **Other peripheral vertigo**
    ● **H81.31** **Aural vertigo**
      H81.311 Aural vertigo, right ear
      H81.312 Aural vertigo, left ear
      H81.313 Aural vertigo, bilateral
      H81.319 Aural vertigo, unspecified ear
    ● **H81.39** **Other peripheral vertigo**
      Lermoyez' syndrome
      Otogenic vertigo
      Peripheral vertigo NOS
      H81.391 Other peripheral vertigo, right ear
      H81.392 Other peripheral vertigo, left ear
      H81.393 Other peripheral vertigo, bilateral
      H81.399 Other peripheral vertigo, unspecified ear
  ● **H81.4** **Vertigo of central origin**
    Central positional nystagmus
    H81.41 Vertigo of central origin, right ear
    H81.42 Vertigo of central origin, left ear
    H81.43 Vertigo of central origin, bilateral
    H81.49 Vertigo of central origin, unspecified ear

◀ New   ◀▯ Revised   ~~deleted~~ Deleted   Excludes 1   Excludes 2   Includes   Use additional   Code first   Code also   Unspecified

OGCR Official Guidelines   ● Unacceptable Principal Diagnosis   **X** Assign placeholder X   ● Use Additional Character(s)   ▶ Manifestation Code   **Coding Clinic**

- **H81.8 Other disorders of vestibular function**
  - **H81.8X Other disorders of vestibular function**
    - H81.8X1 Other disorders of vestibular function, right ear
    - H81.8X2 Other disorders of vestibular function, left ear
    - H81.8X3 Other disorders of vestibular function, bilateral
    - H81.8X9 Other disorders of vestibular function, unspecified ear
- **H81.9 Unspecified disorder of vestibular function**
  Vertiginous syndrome NOS
  - H81.90 Unspecified disorder of vestibular function, unspecified ear
  - H81.91 Unspecified disorder of vestibular function, right ear
  - H81.92 Unspecified disorder of vestibular function, left ear
  - H81.93 Unspecified disorder of vestibular function, bilateral
- **H82 Vertiginous syndromes in diseases classified elsewhere**
  Code first underlying disease
  Excludes1 epidemic vertigo (A88.1)
  - *H82.1 Vertiginous syndromes in diseases classified elsewhere, right ear*
  - *H82.2 Vertiginous syndromes in diseases classified elsewhere, left ear*
  - *H82.3 Vertiginous syndromes in diseases classified elsewhere, bilateral*
  - *H82.9 Vertiginous syndromes in diseases classified elsewhere, unspecified ear*
- **H83 Other diseases of inner ear**
  - **H83.0 Labyrinthitis**
    Balance disorder that follows URI or head injury
    - H83.01 Labyrinthitis, right ear
    - H83.02 Labyrinthitis, left ear
    - H83.03 Labyrinthitis, bilateral
    - H83.09 Labyrinthitis, unspecified ear
  - **H83.1 Labyrinthine fistula**
    - H83.11 Labyrinthine fistula, right ear
    - H83.12 Labyrinthine fistula, left ear
    - H83.13 Labyrinthine fistula, bilateral
    - H83.19 Labyrinthine fistula, unspecified ear
  - **H83.2 Labyrinthine dysfunction**
    Labyrinthine hypersensitivity
    Labyrinthine hypofunction
    Labyrinthine loss of function
    - **H83.2X Labyrinthine dysfunction**
      - H83.2X1 Labyrinthine dysfunction, right ear
      - H83.2X2 Labyrinthine dysfunction, left ear
      - H83.2X3 Labyrinthine dysfunction, bilateral
      - H83.2X9 Labyrinthine dysfunction, unspecified ear
  - **H83.3 Noise effects on inner ear**
    Acoustic trauma of inner ear
    Noise-induced hearing loss of inner ear
    - **H83.3X Noise effects on inner ear**
      - H83.3X1 Noise effects on right inner ear
      - H83.3X2 Noise effects on left inner ear
      - H83.3X3 Noise effects on inner ear, bilateral
      - H83.3X9 Noise effects on inner ear, unspecified ear

- **H83.8 Other specified diseases of inner ear**
  - **H83.8X Other specified diseases of inner ear**
    - H83.8X1 Other specified diseases of right inner ear
    - H83.8X2 Other specified diseases of left inner ear
    - H83.8X3 Other specified diseases of inner ear, bilateral
    - H83.8X9 Other specified diseases of inner ear, unspecified ear
- **H83.9 Unspecified disease of inner ear**
  - H83.90 Unspecified disease of inner ear, unspecified ear
  - H83.91 Unspecified disease of right inner ear
  - H83.92 Unspecified disease of left inner ear
  - H83.93 Unspecified disease of inner ear, bilateral

OTHER DISORDERS OF EAR (H90–H94)

- **H90 Conductive and sensorineural hearing loss**
  Excludes1 deaf nonspeaking NEC (H91.3)
  deafness NOS (H91.9-)
  hearing loss NOS (H91.9-)
  noise-induced hearing loss (H83.3-)
  ototoxic hearing loss (H91.0-)
  sudden (idiopathic) hearing loss (H91.2-)
  - H90.0 Conductive hearing loss, bilateral
  - **H90.1 Conductive hearing loss, unilateral with unrestricted hearing on the contralateral side**
    - H90.11 Conductive hearing loss, unilateral, right ear, with unrestricted hearing on the contralateral side
    - H90.12 Conductive hearing loss, unilateral, left ear, with unrestricted hearing on the contralateral side
  - **H90.2 Conductive hearing loss, unspecified**
    Conductive deafness NOS
  - H90.3 Sensorineural hearing loss, bilateral
  - **H90.4 Sensorineural hearing loss, unilateral with unrestricted hearing on the contralateral side**
    - H90.41 Sensorineural hearing loss, unilateral, right ear, with unrestricted hearing on the contralateral side
    - H90.42 Sensorineural hearing loss, unilateral, left ear, with unrestricted hearing on the contralateral side
  - **H90.5 Unspecified sensorineural hearing loss**
    Central hearing loss NOS
    Congenital deafness NOS
    Neural hearing loss NOS
    Perceptive hearing loss NOS
    Sensorineural deafness NOS
    Sensory hearing loss NOS
    Excludes1 abnormal auditory perception (H93.2-)
    psychogenic deafness (F44.6)
  - **H90.6 Mixed conductive and sensorineural hearing loss, bilateral**
    Coding Clinic: 2015, Q2, P7
  - **H90.7 Mixed conductive and sensorineural hearing loss, unilateral with unrestricted hearing on the contralateral side**
    - H90.71 Mixed conductive and sensorineural hearing loss, unilateral, right ear, with unrestricted hearing on the contralateral side
    - H90.72 Mixed conductive and sensorineural hearing loss, unilateral, left ear, with unrestricted hearing on the contralateral side
  - **H90.8 Mixed conductive and sensorineural hearing loss, unspecified**

CHAPTER 8 (H60–H95)

- **H90.A Conductive and sensorineural hearing loss with restricted hearing on the contralateral side** ◀
  - **H90.A1 Conductive hearing loss, unilateral, with restricted hearing on the contralateral side** ◀
    - **H90.A11 Conductive hearing loss, unilateral, right ear with restricted hearing on the contralateral side** ◀
    - **H90.A12 Conductive hearing loss, unilateral, left ear with restricted hearing on the contralateral side** ◀
  - **H90.A2 Sensorineural hearing loss, unilateral, with restricted hearing on the contralateral side** ◀
    - **H90.A21 Sensorineural hearing loss, unilateral, right ear, with restricted hearing on the contralateral side** ◀
    - **H90.A22 Sensorineural hearing loss, unilateral, left ear, with restricted hearing on the contralateral side** ◀
  - **H90.A3 Mixed conductive and sensorineural hearing loss, unilateral with restricted hearing on the contralateral side** ◀
    - **H90.A31 Mixed conductive and sensorineural hearing loss, unilateral, right ear with restricted hearing on the contralateral side** ◀
    - **H90.A32 Mixed conductive and sensorineural hearing loss, unilateral, left ear with restricted hearing on the contralateral side** ◀

- **H91 Other and unspecified hearing loss**
  - **Excludes1**   abnormal auditory perception (H93.2-)
    hearing loss as classified in H90.-
    impacted cerumen (H61.2-)
    noise-induced hearing loss (H83.3-)
    psychogenic deafness (F44.6)
    transient ischemic deafness (H93.01-)
  - **H91.0 Ototoxic hearing loss**
    Code first poisoning due to drug or toxin, if applicable (T36-T65 with fifth or sixth character 1-4 or 6)
    Use additional code for adverse effect, if applicable, to identify drug (T36-T50 with fifth or sixth character 5)
    - **H91.01 Ototoxic hearing loss, right ear**
    - **H91.02 Ototoxic hearing loss, left ear**
    - **H91.03 Ototoxic hearing loss, bilateral**
    - **H91.09 Ototoxic hearing loss, unspecified ear**
  - **H91.1 Presbycusis**
    Presbyacusia
    - **H91.10 Presbycusis, unspecified ear**
    - **H91.11 Presbycusis, right ear**
    - **H91.12 Presbycusis, left ear**
    - **H91.13 Presbycusis, bilateral**
  - **H91.2 Sudden idiopathic hearing loss**
    Sudden hearing loss NOS
    - **H91.20 Sudden idiopathic hearing loss, unspecified ear**
    - **H91.21 Sudden idiopathic hearing loss, right ear**
    - **H91.22 Sudden idiopathic hearing loss, left ear**
    - **H91.23 Sudden idiopathic hearing loss, bilateral**
  - **H91.3 Deaf nonspeaking, not elsewhere classified**
  - **H91.8 Other specified hearing loss**
    - **H91.8X Other specified hearing loss**
      - **H91.8X1 Other specified hearing loss, right ear**
      - **H91.8X2 Other specified hearing loss, left ear**
      - **H91.8X3 Other specified hearing loss, bilateral**
      - **H91.8X9 Other specified hearing loss, unspecified ear**

- **H91.9 Unspecified hearing loss**
  Deafness NOS
  High frequency deafness
  Low frequency deafness
  - **H91.90 Unspecified hearing loss, unspecified ear**
  - **H91.91 Unspecified hearing loss, right ear**
  - **H91.92 Unspecified hearing loss, left ear**
  - **H91.93 Unspecified hearing loss, bilateral**

- **H92 Otalgia and effusion of ear**
  - **H92.0 Otalgia**
    - **H92.01 Otalgia, right ear**
    - **H92.02 Otalgia, left ear**
    - **H92.03 Otalgia, bilateral**
    - **H92.09 Otalgia, unspecified ear**
  - **H92.1 Otorrhea**
    - **Excludes1**   leakage of cerebrospinal fluid through ear (G96.0)
    - **H92.10 Otorrhea, unspecified ear**
    - **H92.11 Otorrhea, right ear**
    - **H92.12 Otorrhea, left ear**
    - **H92.13 Otorrhea, bilateral**
  - **H92.2 Otorrhagia**
    - **Excludes1**   traumatic otorrhagia - code to injury
    - **H92.20 Otorrhagia, unspecified ear**
    - **H92.21 Otorrhagia, right ear**
    - **H92.22 Otorrhagia, left ear**
    - **H92.23 Otorrhagia, bilateral**

- **H93 Other disorders of ear, not elsewhere classified**
  - **H93.0 Degenerative and vascular disorders of ear**
    - **Excludes1**   presbycusis (H91.1)
    - **H93.01 Transient ischemic deafness**
      - **H93.011 Transient ischemic deafness, right ear**
      - **H93.012 Transient ischemic deafness, left ear**
      - **H93.013 Transient ischemic deafness, bilateral**
      - **H93.019 Transient ischemic deafness, unspecified ear**
    - **H93.09 Unspecified degenerative and vascular disorders of ear**
      - **H93.091 Unspecified degenerative and vascular disorders of right ear**
      - **H93.092 Unspecified degenerative and vascular disorders of left ear**
      - **H93.093 Unspecified degenerative and vascular disorders of ear, bilateral**
      - **H93.099 Unspecified degenerative and vascular disorders of unspecified ear**
  - **H93.1 Tinnitus**
    Perception of sound (ringing, buzzing, humming, whistling tunes, or singing)
    - **H93.11 Tinnitus, right ear**
    - **H93.12 Tinnitus, left ear**
    - **H93.13 Tinnitus, bilateral**
    - **H93.19 Tinnitus, unspecified ear**
  - **H93.A Pulsatile tinnitus** ◀
    - **H93.A1 Pulsatile tinnitus, right ear** ◀
    - **H93.A2 Pulsatile tinnitus, left ear** ◀
    - **H93.A3 Pulsatile tinnitus, bilateral** ◀
    - **H93.A9 Pulsatile tinnitus, unspecified ear** ◀
  - **H93.2 Other abnormal auditory perceptions**
    - **Excludes2**   auditory hallucinations (R44.0)
    - **H93.21 Auditory recruitment**
      - **H93.211 Auditory recruitment, right ear**
      - **H93.212 Auditory recruitment, left ear**
      - **H93.213 Auditory recruitment, bilateral**
      - **H93.219 Auditory recruitment, unspecified ear**

◀ New   ◀|||| Revised   ~~deleted~~ Deleted   Excludes 1   Excludes 2   Includes   Use additional   Code first   Code also   Unspecified

864   **OGCR** Official Guidelines   ● Unacceptable Principal Diagnosis   X Assign placeholder X   ● Use Additional Character(s)   ▶ Manifestation Code   **Coding Clinic**

- **H93.22 Diplacusis**
  - H93.221   Diplacusis, right ear
  - H93.222   Diplacusis, left ear
  - H93.223   Diplacusis, bilateral
  - H93.229   Diplacusis, unspecified ear
- **H93.23 Hyperacusis**
  - H93.231   Hyperacusis, right ear
  - H93.232   Hyperacusis, left ear
  - H93.233   Hyperacusis, bilateral
  - H93.239   Hyperacusis, unspecified ear
- **H93.24 Temporary auditory threshold shift**
  - H93.241   Temporary auditory threshold shift, right ear
  - H93.242   Temporary auditory threshold shift, left ear
  - H93.243   Temporary auditory threshold shift, bilateral
  - H93.249   Temporary auditory threshold shift, unspecified ear
- **H93.25 Central auditory processing disorder**
  - Congenital auditory imperception
  - Word deafness
  - **Excludes1**   mixed receptive-expressive language disorder (F80.2)
- **H93.29 Other abnormal auditory perceptions**
  - H93.291   Other abnormal auditory perceptions, right ear
  - H93.292   Other abnormal auditory perceptions, left ear
  - H93.293   Other abnormal auditory perceptions, bilateral
  - H93.299   Other abnormal auditory perceptions, unspecified ear
- **H93.3 Disorders of acoustic nerve**
  - Disorder of 8th cranial nerve
  - **Excludes1**   acoustic neuroma (D33.3)
    - syphilitic acoustic neuritis (A52.15)
  - **H93.3X Disorders of acoustic nerve**
    - H93.3X1   Disorders of right acoustic nerve
    - H93.3X2   Disorders of left acoustic nerve
    - H93.3X3   Disorders of bilateral acoustic nerves
    - H93.3X9   Disorders of unspecified acoustic nerve
- **H93.8 Other specified disorders of ear**
  - **H93.8X Other specified disorders of ear**
    - H93.8X1   Other specified disorders of right ear
    - H93.8X2   Other specified disorders of left ear
    - H93.8X3   Other specified disorders of ear, bilateral
    - H93.8X9   Other specified disorders of ear, unspecified ear
- **H93.9 Unspecified disorder of ear**
  - **H93.90 Unspecified disorder of ear, unspecified ear**
  - **H93.91 Unspecified disorder of right ear**
  - **H93.92 Unspecified disorder of left ear**
  - **H93.93 Unspecified disorder of ear, bilateral**

- **H94 Other disorders of ear in diseases classified elsewhere**
  - **H94.0 Acoustic neuritis in infectious and parasitic diseases classified elsewhere**
    - *Code first* underlying disease, such as:
      - parasitic disease (B65-B89)
    - **Excludes1**   acoustic neuritis (in):
      - herpes zoster (B02.29)
      - syphilis (A52.15)
    - *H94.00   Acoustic neuritis in infectious and parasitic diseases classified elsewhere, unspecified ear*
    - *H94.01   Acoustic neuritis in infectious and parasitic diseases classified elsewhere, right ear*
    - *H94.02   Acoustic neuritis in infectious and parasitic diseases classified elsewhere, left ear*
    - *H94.03   Acoustic neuritis in infectious and parasitic diseases classified elsewhere, bilateral*
  - **H94.8 Other specified disorders of ear in diseases classified elsewhere**
    - *Code first* underlying disease, such as:
      - congenital syphilis (A50.0)
    - **Excludes1**   aural myiasis (B87.4)
      - syphilitic labyrinthitis (A52.79)
    - *H94.80   Other specified disorders of ear in diseases classified elsewhere, unspecified ear*
    - *H94.81   Other specified disorders of right ear in diseases classified elsewhere*
    - *H94.82   Other specified disorders of left ear in diseases classified elsewhere*
    - *H94.83   Other specified disorders of ear in diseases classified elsewhere, bilateral*
- **H95 Intraoperative and postprocedural complications and disorders of ear and mastoid process, not elsewhere classified**
  - **H95.0 Recurrent cholesteatoma of postmastoidectomy cavity**
    - H95.00   Recurrent cholesteatoma of postmastoidectomy cavity, unspecified ear
    - H95.01   Recurrent cholesteatoma of postmastoidectomy cavity, right ear
    - H95.02   Recurrent cholesteatoma of postmastoidectomy cavity, left ear
    - H95.03   Recurrent cholesteatoma of postmastoidectomy cavity, bilateral ears
  - **H95.1 Other disorders of ear and mastoid process following mastoidectomy**
    - **H95.11 Chronic inflammation of postmastoidectomy cavity**
      - H95.111   Chronic inflammation of postmastoidectomy cavity, right ear
      - H95.112   Chronic inflammation of postmastoidectomy cavity, left ear
      - H95.113   Chronic inflammation of postmastoidectomy cavity, bilateral ears
      - H95.119   Chronic inflammation of postmastoidectomy cavity, unspecified ear
    - **H95.12 Granulation of postmastoidectomy cavity**
      - H95.121   Granulation of postmastoidectomy cavity, right ear
      - H95.122   Granulation of postmastoidectomy cavity, left ear
      - H95.123   Granulation of postmastoidectomy cavity, bilateral ears
      - H95.129   Granulation of postmastoidectomy cavity, unspecified ear

CHAPTER 8 (H60–H95)

● **H95.13**   **Mucosal cyst of postmastoidectomy cavity**

    H95.131   Mucosal cyst of postmastoidectomy cavity, right ear

    H95.132   Mucosal cyst of postmastoidectomy cavity, left ear

    H95.133   Mucosal cyst of postmastoidectomy cavity, bilateral ears

    H95.139   Mucosal cyst of postmastoidectomy cavity, unspecified ear

● **H95.19**   **Other disorders following mastoidectomy**

    H95.191   Other disorders following mastoidectomy, right ear

    H95.192   Other disorders following mastoidectomy, left ear

    H95.193   Other disorders following mastoidectomy, bilateral ears

    H95.199   Other disorders following mastoidectomy, unspecified ear

● **H95.2**   **Intraoperative hemorrhage and hematoma of ear and mastoid process complicating a procedure**

    Excludes1   intraoperative hemorrhage and hematoma of ear and mastoid process due to accidental puncture or laceration during a procedure (H95.3-)

    Ex: **For category H95.2 CC codes:** H95.21-H95.22, H95.41-H95.89, I85.01, I85.11, I97.3, K21.9, K22.8, K23-K25.2, K25.4, K25.6, K26.0, K26.2, K26.4, K26.6, K27.0, K27.2, K27.4, K27.6, K28.0, K28.2, K28.4, K28.6, K29.01, K29.21, K29.31, K29.41, K29.51, K29.61, K29.71, K29.81, K29.91, K31.811, K55.21, K57.01, K57.11, K57.13, K57.21, K57.31, K57.33, K57.41, K57.51, K57.53, K57.81, K57.91, K57.93, K62.5, K92.0-K92.2, M96.89, N98.1-N98.9, P54.1-P54.3, T81.10X-T81.19X[A], T81.82X[A], T81.89X-T81.9XX[A]

    H95.21   Intraoperative hemorrhage and hematoma of ear and mastoid process complicating a procedure on the ear and mastoid process

    H95.22   Intraoperative hemorrhage and hematoma of ear and mastoid process complicating other procedure

● **H95.3**   **Accidental puncture and laceration of ear and mastoid process during a procedure**

    Ex: **For category H95.3 CC codes:** D78.11-D78.12, D78.81-D78.89, E36.11-E36.8, E89.810-E89.89, G96.11, G97.41-G97.49, H59.011-H59.019, H59.031-H59.099, H59.211-H59.229, H59.811-H59.89, H95.31-H95.32, H95.811-H95.89, I97.3, I97.51-I97.52, J95.71-J95.72, K91.71-K91.72, L76.11-L76.12, L76.81-L76.82, M96.820-M96.821, M96.89, N98.1-N98.9, N99.71-N99.72, T81.82X[A], T81.89X-T81.9XX[A]

    H95.31   Accidental puncture and laceration of the ear and mastoid process during a procedure on the ear and mastoid process

    H95.32   Accidental puncture and laceration of the ear and mastoid process during other procedure

● **H95.4**   **Postprocedural hemorrhage of ear and mastoid process following a procedure** ◀▥

    Ex: **For category H95.4 CC codes:** See H95.2

    H95.41   Postprocedural hemorrhage of ear and mastoid process following a procedure on the ear and mastoid process ◀▥

    H95.42   Postprocedural hemorrhage of ear and mastoid process following other procedure ◀▥

● **H95.5**   **Postprocedural hematoma and seroma of ear and mastoid process following a procedure** ◀

    Ex: **For category H95.5 CC codes:** See H95.2

    H95.51   Postprocedural hematoma of ear and mastoid process following a procedure on the ear and mastoid process ◀

    H95.52   Postprocedural hematoma of ear and mastoid process following other procedure ◀

    H95.53   Postprocedural seroma of ear and mastoid process following a procedure on the ear and mastoid process ◀

    H95.54   Postprocedural seroma of ear and mastoid process following other procedure ◀

● **H95.8**   **Other intraoperative and postprocedural complications and disorders of the ear and mastoid process, not elsewhere classified**

    Excludes2   postprocedural complications and disorders following mastoidectomy (H95.0-, H95.1-)

    Ex: **For category H95.8 CC codes:** D78.81-D78.89, E36.8, E89.810-E89.89, H59.011-H59.019, H59.031-H59.099, H59.811-H59.89, H95.811-H95.89, I97.3, L76.81-L76.82, M96.89, N98.1-N98.9, T81.82X[A], T81.89X-T81.9XX[A]

    ● **H95.81**   **Postprocedural stenosis of external ear canal**

        H95.811   Postprocedural stenosis of right external ear canal

        H95.812   Postprocedural stenosis of left external ear canal

        H95.813   Postprocedural stenosis of external ear canal, bilateral

        H95.819   Postprocedural stenosis of unspecified external ear canal

    H95.88   Other intraoperative complications and disorders of the ear and mastoid process, not elsewhere classified

        Use additional code, if applicable, to further specify disorder

    H95.89   Other postprocedural complications and disorders of the ear and mastoid process, not elsewhere classified

        Use additional code, if applicable, to further specify disorder

◀ New   ▥ Revised   ~~deleted~~ Deleted   Excludes 1   Excludes 2   Includes   Use additional   Code first   Code also   Unspecified

OGCR Official Guidelines   ● Unacceptable Principal Diagnosis   X Assign placeholder X   ● Use Additional Character(s)   ▷ Manifestation Code   **Coding Clinic**

CHAPTER 9 DISEASES OF THE CIRCULATORY SYSTEM (I00-I99)

OGCR Chapter-Specific Coding Guidelines

9. Chapter 9: Diseases of the Circulatory System (I00-I99)

a. Hypertension

The classification presumes a causal relationship between hypertension and heart involvement and between hypertension and kidney involvement, as the two conditions are linked by the term "with" in the Alphabetic Index. These conditions should be coded as related even in the absence of provider documentation explicitly linking them, unless the documentation clearly states the conditions are unrelated.

For hypertension and conditions not specifically linked by relational terms such as "with," "associated with" or "due to" in the classification, provider documentation must link the conditions in order to code them as related.

1) Hypertension with Heart Disease

Hypertension with heart conditions classified to I50.- or I51.4-I51.9, are assigned to, a code from category I11, Hypertensive heart disease. Use an additional code from category I50, Heart failure, to identify the type of heart failure in those patients with heart failure.

The same heart conditions (I50.-, I51.4-I51.9) with hypertension, are coded separately if the provider has specifically documented a different cause. Sequence according to the circumstances of the admission/encounter.

2) Hypertensive Chronic Kidney Disease

Assign codes from category I12, Hypertensive chronic kidney disease, when both hypertension and a condition classifiable to category N18, Chronic kidney disease (CKD), are present. CKD should not be coded as hypertensive if the physician has specifically documented a different cause.

The appropriate code from category N18 should be used as a secondary code with a code from category I12 to identify the stage of chronic kidney disease.

See Section I.C.14. Chronic kidney disease.

If a patient has hypertensive chronic kidney disease and acute renal failure, an additional code for the acute renal failure is required.

3) Hypertensive Heart and Chronic Kidney Disease

Assign codes from combination category I13, Hypertensive heart and chronic kidney disease, when there is hypertension with both heart and kidney involvement. If heart failure is present, assign an additional code from category I50 to identify the type of heart failure.

The appropriate code from category N18, Chronic kidney disease, should be used as a secondary code with a code from category I13 to identify the stage of chronic kidney disease.

See Section I.C.14. Chronic kidney disease.

The codes in category I13, Hypertensive heart and chronic kidney disease, are combination codes that include hypertension, heart disease and chronic kidney disease. The Includes note at I13 specifies that the conditions included at I11 and I12 are included together in I13. If a patient has hypertension, heart disease and chronic kidney disease then a code from I13 should be used, not individual codes for hypertension, heart disease and chronic kidney disease, or codes from I11 or I12.

For patients with both acute renal failure and chronic kidney disease an additional code for acute renal failure is required.

4) Hypertensive Cerebrovascular Disease

For hypertensive cerebrovascular disease, first assign the appropriate code from categories I60-I69, followed by the appropriate hypertension code.

5) Hypertensive Retinopathy

Subcategory H35.0, Background retinopathy and retinal vascular changes, should be used with a code from category I10 – I15, Hypertensive disease to include the systemic hypertension. The sequencing is based on the reason for the encounter.

6) Hypertension, Secondary

Secondary hypertension is due to an underlying condition. Two codes are required: one to identify the underlying etiology and one from category I15 to identify the hypertension. Sequencing of codes is determined by the reason for admission/encounter.

7) Hypertension, Transient

Assign code R03.0, Elevated blood pressure reading without diagnosis of hypertension, unless patient has an established diagnosis of hypertension. Assign code O13.-, Gestational [pregnancy-induced] hypertension without significant proteinuria, or O14.-, Pre-eclampsia, for transient hypertension of pregnancy.

8) Hypertension, Controlled

This diagnostic statement usually refers to an existing state of hypertension under control by therapy. Assign the appropriate code from categories I10-I15, Hypertensive diseases.

9) Hypertension, Uncontrolled

Uncontrolled hypertension may refer to untreated hypertension or hypertension not responding to current therapeutic regimen. In either case, assign the appropriate code from categories I10-I15, Hypertensive diseases.

10) Hypertensive Crisis

Assign a code from category I16, Hypertensive crisis, for documented hypertensive urgency, hypertensive emergency or unspecified hypertensive crisis. Code also any identified hypertensive disease (I10-I15). The sequencing is based on the reason for the encounter.

b. Atherosclerotic Coronary Artery Disease and Angina

ICD-10-CM has combination codes for atherosclerotic heart disease with angina pectoris. The subcategories for these codes are I25.11, Atherosclerotic heart disease of native coronary artery with angina pectoris and I25.7, Atherosclerosis of coronary artery bypass graft(s) and coronary artery of transplanted heart with angina pectoris.

When using one of these combination codes it is not necessary to use an additional code for angina pectoris. A causal relationship can be assumed in a patient with both atherosclerosis and angina pectoris, unless the documentation indicates the angina is due to something other than the atherosclerosis.

If a patient with coronary artery disease is admitted due to an acute myocardial infarction (AMI), the AMI should be sequenced before the coronary artery disease.

See Section I.C.9. Acute myocardial infarction (AMI)

c. Intraoperative and Postprocedural Cerebrovascular Accident

Medical record documentation should clearly specify the cause-and-effect relationship between the medical intervention and the cerebrovascular accident in order to assign a code for intraoperative or postprocedural cerebrovascular accident.

Proper code assignment depends on whether it was an infarction or hemorrhage and whether it occurred intraoperatively or postoperatively. If it was a cerebral hemorrhage, code assignment depends on the type of procedure performed.

d. Sequelae of Cerebrovascular Disease

1) Category I69, Sequelae of Cerebrovascular disease

Category I69 is used to indicate conditions classifiable to categories I60-I67 as the causes of sequela (neurologic deficits), themselves classified elsewhere. These "late effects" include neurologic deficits that persist after initial onset of conditions classifiable to categories I60-I67. The neurologic deficits caused by cerebrovascular disease may be present from the onset or may arise at any time after the onset of the condition classifiable to categories I60-I67.

Codes from category I69, Sequelae of cerebrovascular disease, that specify hemiplegia, hemiparesis and monoplegia identify whether the dominant or nondominant side is affected. Should the affected side be documented, but not specified as dominant or nondominant, and the classification system does not indicate a default, code selection is as follows:

- For ambidextrous patients, the default should be dominant.
- If the left side is affected, the default is non-dominant.
- If the right side is affected, the default is dominant.

2) Codes from category I69 with codes from I60-I67

Codes from category I69 may be assigned on a health care record with codes from I60-I67, if the patient has a current cerebrovascular disease and deficits from an old cerebrovascular disease.

3) Codes from category I69 and Personal history of transient ischemic attack (TIA) and cerebral infarction (Z86.73)

Codes from category I69 should not be assigned if the patient does not have neurologic deficits.

See Section I.C.21. 4. History (of) for use of personal history codes

e. Acute myocardial infarction (AMI)

1) ST elevation myocardial infarction (STEMI) and non ST elevation myocardial infarction (NSTEMI)

The ICD-10-CM codes for acute myocardial infarction (AMI) identify the site, such as anterolateral wall or true posterior wall. Subcategories I21.0-I21.2 and code I21.3 are used for ST elevation myocardial infarction (STEMI). Code I21.4, Non-ST elevation (NSTEMI) myocardial infarction, is used for non ST elevation myocardial infarction (NSTEMI) and nontransmural MIs.

If NSTEMI evolves to STEMI, assign the STEMI code. If STEMI converts to NSTEMI due to thrombolytic therapy, it is still coded as STEMI.

For encounters occurring while the myocardial infarction is equal to, or less than, four weeks old, including transfers to another acute setting or a postacute setting, and the myocardial infarction **meets the definition for "other diagnoses" (see Section III, Reporting Additional Diagnoses)**, codes from category I21 may continue to be reported. For encounters after the 4 week time frame and the patient is still receiving care related to the myocardial infarction, the appropriate aftercare code should be assigned, rather than a code from category I21. For old or healed myocardial infarctions not requiring further care, code I25.2, Old myocardial infarction, may be assigned.

2) Acute myocardial infarction, unspecified

Code I21.3, ST elevation (STEMI) myocardial infarction of unspecified site, is the default for unspecified acute myocardial infarction. If only STEMI or transmural MI without the site is documented, assign code I21.3.

3) AMI documented as nontransmural or subendocardial but site provided

If an AMI is documented as nontransmural or subendocardial, but the site is provided, it is still coded as a subendocardial AMI.

See Section I.C.21.3 for information on coding status post administration of tPA in a different facility within the last 24 hours.

4) Subsequent acute myocardial infarction

A code from category I22, Subsequent ST elevation (STEMI) and non ST elevation (NSTEMI) myocardial infarction, is to be used when a patient who has suffered an AMI has a new AMI within the 4 week time frame of the initial AMI. A code from category I22 must be used in conjunction with a code from category I21. The sequencing of the I22 and I21 codes depends on the circumstances of the encounter.

Figure 9-1   Cardiovascular valves.

Item 9–1 Rheumatic fever is the inflammation of the valve(s) of the heart, usually the mitral or aortic, which leads to valve damage. Rheumatic heart inflammations are usually **pericarditis** (sac surrounding heart), **endocarditis** (heart cavity), or **myocarditis** (heart muscle).

CHAPTER 9   DISEASES OF THE CIRCULATORY SYSTEM (IØØ-I99)

Excludes2   certain conditions originating in the perinatal period (PØ4-P96)
certain infectious and parasitic diseases (AØØ-B99)
complications of pregnancy, childbirth and the puerperium (OØØ-O9A)
congenital malformations, deformations, and chromosomal abnormalities (QØØ-Q99)
endocrine, nutritional and metabolic diseases (EØØ-E88)
injury, poisoning and certain other consequences of external causes (SØØ-T88)
neoplasms (CØØ-D49)
symptoms, signs and abnormal clinical and laboratory findings, not elsewhere classified (RØØ-R94)
systemic connective tissue disorders (M3Ø-M36)
transient cerebral ischemic attacks and related syndromes (G45.-)

This chapter contains the following blocks:

IØØ-IØ2	Acute rheumatic fever
IØ5-IØ9	Chronic rheumatic heart diseases
I1Ø-I16	Hypertensive diseases ◀
I2Ø-I25	Ischemic heart diseases
I26-I28	Pulmonary heart disease and diseases of pulmonary circulation
I3Ø-I52	Other forms of heart disease
I6Ø-I69	Cerebrovascular diseases
I7Ø-I79	Diseases of arteries, arterioles and capillaries
I8Ø-I89	Diseases of veins, lymphatic vessels and lymph nodes, not elsewhere classified
I95-I99	Other and unspecified disorders of the circulatory system

ACUTE RHEUMATIC FEVER (IØØ-IØ2)

IØØ   **Rheumatic fever without heart involvement**

   Includes   arthritis, rheumatic, acute or subacute
   Excludes1   rheumatic fever with heart involvement (IØ1.Ø-IØ1.9)

● **IØ1**   **Rheumatic fever with heart involvement**

   Excludes1   chronic diseases of rheumatic origin (IØ5-IØ9) unless rheumatic fever is also present or there is evidence of reactivation or activity of the rheumatic process.

IØ1.Ø   **Acute rheumatic pericarditis** 🔖
Any condition in IØØ with pericarditis
Rheumatic pericarditis (acute)

   Excludes1   acute pericarditis not specified as rheumatic (I3Ø.-)
   (Ex:) B33.23, IØ1.Ø, IØ9.2, I3Ø.Ø-I3Ø.9, I31.3-I32, I87.8, I99.8-I99.9

IØ1.1   **Acute rheumatic endocarditis** 🔖
Any condition in IØØ with endocarditis or valvulitis
Acute rheumatic valvulitis
   (Ex:) AØ1.ØØ-AØ1.Ø9, A39.51, A52.Ø3, A78, B33.21, B37.6, IØØ, IØ1.1, IØ1.8-IØ2.Ø, IØ5.Ø-IØ7.9, IØ8.1-IØ8.3, IØ8.9, IØ9.1, IØ9.89-IØ9.9, I33.Ø-I39, I42.4, I87.8-I87.9, I99.8-I99.9, Q22.2, Q23.8-Q23.9, Q24.8, T82.6XX[A]

Item 9–2 Rheumatic chorea, also called Sydenham's, juvenile, minor, simple, or St. Vitus' dance, is a major symptom of rheumatic fever and is characterized by ceaseless, involuntary, jerky, purposeless movements.

I01.2   **Acute rheumatic myocarditis** 🏥
Any condition in I00 with myocarditis
Ⓔⓧ A52.06, B33.20-B33.22, I00, I01.2-I01.9, I09.0, I09.9, I23.0-I23.3, I23.6-I23.8, I40.0-I41, I51.0, I51.4, I87.8, I99.8-I99.9

I01.8   **Other acute rheumatic heart disease** 🏥
Any condition in I00 with other or multiple types of heart involvement
Acute rheumatic pancarditis
Ⓔⓧ I01.0-I09.9, I50.20-I50.43

I01.9   **Acute rheumatic heart disease, unspecified** 🏥
Any condition in I00 with unspecified type of heart involvement
Rheumatic carditis, acute
Rheumatic heart disease, active or acute
Ⓔⓧ I01.0-I09.9

● **I02**   **Rheumatic chorea**
   Includes   Sydenham's chorea
   Excludes1   chorea NOS (G25.5)
             Huntington's chorea (G10)

I02.0   **Rheumatic chorea with heart involvement** 🏥
Chorea NOS with heart involvement
Rheumatic chorea with heart involvement of any type classifiable under I01.-
Ⓔⓧ See I01.8

I02.9   **Rheumatic chorea without heart involvement** 🏥
Rheumatic chorea NOS
Ⓔⓧ See I01.9

CHRONIC RHEUMATIC HEART DISEASES (I05-I09)

● **I05**   **Rheumatic mitral valve diseases**
   Includes   conditions classifiable to both I05.0 and I05.2-I05.9, whether specified as rheumatic or not
   Excludes1   mitral valve disease specified as nonrheumatic (I34.-)
             mitral valve disease with aortic and/or tricuspid valve involvement (I08.-)

I05.0   **Rheumatic mitral stenosis**
Mitral (valve) obstruction (rheumatic)

I05.1   **Rheumatic mitral insufficiency**
Rheumatic mitral incompetence
Rheumatic mitral regurgitation
   Excludes1   mitral insufficiency not specified as rheumatic (I34.0)

I05.2   **Rheumatic mitral stenosis with insufficiency**
Rheumatic mitral stenosis with incompetence or regurgitation

I05.8   **Other rheumatic mitral valve diseases**
Rheumatic mitral (valve) failure

I05.9   **Rheumatic mitral valve disease, unspecified**
Rheumatic mitral (valve) disorder (chronic) NOS

● **I06**   **Rheumatic aortic valve diseases**
   Excludes1   aortic valve disease not specified as rheumatic (I35.-)
             aortic valve disease with mitral and/or tricuspid valve involvement (I08.-)

I06.0   **Rheumatic aortic stenosis**
Rheumatic aortic (valve) obstruction

I06.1   **Rheumatic aortic insufficiency**
Rheumatic aortic incompetence
Rheumatic aortic regurgitation

★ **(See Plate 244 on page 78.)**

Item 9–3 Mitral stenosis is the narrowing of the mitral valve separating the left atrium from the left ventricle. **Mitral insufficiency** is the improper closure of the mitral valve which may lead to enlargement (hypertrophy) of the left atrium.

Item 9–4 Aortic stenosis is the narrowing of the aortic valve located between the left ventricle and the aorta. **Aortic insufficiency** is the improper closure of the aortic valve which may lead to enlargement (hypertrophy) of the left ventricle.

I06.2   **Rheumatic aortic stenosis with insufficiency**
Rheumatic aortic stenosis with incompetence or regurgitation

I06.8   **Other rheumatic aortic valve diseases**

I06.9   **Rheumatic aortic valve disease, unspecified**
Rheumatic aortic (valve) disease NOS

● **I07**   **Rheumatic tricuspid valve diseases**
   Includes   rheumatic tricuspid valve diseases specified as rheumatic or unspecified
   Excludes1   tricuspid valve disease specified as nonrheumatic (I36.-)
             tricuspid valve disease with aortic and/or mitral valve involvement (I08.-)

I07.0   **Rheumatic tricuspid stenosis**
Tricuspid (valve) stenosis (rheumatic)

I07.1   **Rheumatic tricuspid insufficiency**
Tricuspid (valve) insufficiency (rheumatic)

I07.2   **Rheumatic tricuspid stenosis and insufficiency**

I07.8   **Other rheumatic tricuspid valve diseases**

I07.9   **Rheumatic tricuspid valve disease, unspecified**
Rheumatic tricuspid valve disorder NOS

● **I08**   **Multiple valve diseases**
   Includes   multiple valve diseases specified as rheumatic or unspecified
   Excludes1   endocarditis, valve unspecified (I38)
             multiple valve disease specified a nonrheumatic (I34.-, I35.-, I36.-, I37.-, I38.-, Q22.-, Q23.-, Q24.8-)
             rheumatic valve disease NOS (I09.1)

I08.0   **Rheumatic disorders of both mitral and aortic valves**
Involvement of both mitral and aortic valves specified as rheumatic or unspecified

I08.1   **Rheumatic disorders of both mitral and tricuspid valves**

I08.2   **Rheumatic disorders of both aortic and tricuspid valves**

I08.3   **Combined rheumatic disorders of mitral, aortic and tricuspid valves**

I08.8   **Other rheumatic multiple valve diseases**

I08.9   **Rheumatic multiple valve disease, unspecified**

● **I09**   **Other rheumatic heart diseases**

I09.0   **Rheumatic myocarditis** 🏥
   Excludes1   myocarditis not specified as rheumatic (I51.4)
   Ⓔⓧ I00, I01.2-I01.9, I09.0, I09.9, I23.0-I23.3, I23.6-I23.8, I40.0-I41, I51.0, I51.4, I87.8-I87.9, I99.8-I99.9

I09.1   **Rheumatic diseases of endocardium, valve unspecified**
Rheumatic endocarditis (chronic)
Rheumatic valvulitis (chronic)
   Excludes1   endocarditis, valve unspecified (I38)

I09.2   **Chronic rheumatic pericarditis** 🏥
Adherent pericardium, rheumatic
Chronic rheumatic mediastinopericarditis
Chronic rheumatic myopericarditis
   Excludes1   chronic pericarditis not specified as rheumatic (I31.-)
   Ⓔⓧ See I01.0

● **I09.8**   **Other specified rheumatic heart diseases**

I09.81   **Rheumatic heart failure** 🏥
Use additional code to identify type of heart failure (I50.-)
Ⓔⓧ I09.81, I09.9, I11.0, I50.1-I50.9, I87.8-I87.9, I99.8-I99.9

I09.89   **Other specified rheumatic heart diseases**
Rheumatic disease of pulmonary valve

I09.9   **Rheumatic heart disease, unspecified**
Rheumatic carditis
   Excludes1   rheumatoid carditis (M05.31)

N Newborn Age: 0   **P** Pediatric Age: 0–17   **M** Maternity DX: 12–55   **A** Adult Age: 15–124   ♀ Females Only   ♂ Males Only

🏥 Complication\Comorbidity   Major C\C   Ⓔⓧ CC/MCC Exclusions   Hospital-Acquired Condition

869

CHAPTER 9 (I00-I99)

Item 9–5 Hypertension is caused by high arterial blood pressure in the arteries. **Essential, primary,** or **idiopathic** hypertension occurs without identifiable organic cause. **Secondary** hypertension is that which has an organic cause. **Malignant** hypertension is severely elevated blood pressure. **Benign** hypertension is mildly elevated blood pressure.

HYPERTENSIVE DISEASES (I10-I16) ◀▓▓▓

Use additional code to identify:
    exposure to environmental tobacco smoke (Z77.22)
    history of tobacco dependence (Z87.891) ◀▓▓▓
    occupational exposure to environmental tobacco
      smoke (Z57.31)
    tobacco dependence (F17.-)
    tobacco use (Z72.0)

Excludes1 neonatal hypertension (P29.2)
         primary pulmonary hypertension (I27.0)

Excludes2 hypertensive disease complicating pregnancy,
         childbirth and the puerperium (O10-O11,
         O13-O16) ◀

I10   Essential (primary) hypertension

    Includes high blood pressure
         hypertension (arterial) (benign) (essential)
         (malignant) (primary) (systemic)

    Excludes1 hypertensive disease complicating pregnancy,
         childbirth and the puerperium (O10-O11,
         O13-O16)

    Excludes2 essential (primary) hypertension involving
         vessels of brain (I60-I69)
         essential (primary) hypertension involving
         vessels of eye (H35.0-)

    MCE: Questionable admission when principal dx

● I11 Hypertensive heart disease

    Includes any condition in I51.4-I51.9 due to hypertension

    I11.0 Hypertensive heart disease with heart failure
        Hypertensive heart failure

        Use additional code to identify type of heart failure
        (I50.-)

    I11.9 Hypertensive heart disease without heart failure
        Hypertensive heart disease NOS

OGCR Section I.C.9.a.2

Hypertensive Chronic Kidney Disease

Assign codes from category I12, Hypertensive chronic kidney disease, when both hypertension and a condition classifiable to category N18, Chronic kidney disease (CKD), are present. **CKD should not be coded as hypertensive if the physician has specifically documented a different cause.**

The appropriate code from category N18 should be used as a secondary code with a code from category I12 to identify the stage of chronic kidney disease.

See Section I.C.14. Chronic kidney disease.

If a patient has hypertensive chronic kidney disease and acute renal failure, an additional code for the acute renal failure is required.

● I12 Hypertensive chronic kidney disease

    Includes any condition in N18 and N26 - due to
         hypertension
         arteriosclerosis of kidney
         arteriosclerotic nephritis (chronic) (interstitial)
         hypertensive nephropathy
         nephrosclerosis

    Excludes1 hypertension due to kidney disease (I15.0, I15.1)
         renovascular hypertension (I15.0)
         secondary hypertension (I15.-)

    Excludes2 acute kidney failure (N17.-)

    **I12.0 Hypertensive chronic kidney disease with stage 5
        chronic kidney disease or end stage renal disease** 🔖
        Use additional code to identify the stage of chronic
        kidney disease (N18.5, N18.6)
        (Ex:) I10-I16.9, I87.8-I87.9, I99.8-I99.9, N18.6, N26.2

    **I12.9 Hypertensive chronic kidney disease with stage 1
        through stage 4 chronic kidney disease, or unspecified
        chronic kidney disease**
        Hypertensive chronic kidney disease NOS
        Hypertensive renal disease NOS

        Use additional code to identify the stage of chronic
        kidney disease (N18.1-N18.4, N18.9)

OGCR Section I.c.9.a.3

Hypertensive Heart and Chronic Kidney Disease

Assign codes from combination category I13, Hypertensive heart and chronic kidney disease, when **there is hypertension with both heart and kidney involvement.** If heart failure is present, assign an additional code from category I50 to identify the type of heart failure.

The appropriate code from category N18, Chronic kidney disease, should be used as a secondary code with a code from category I13 to identify the stage of chronic kidney disease. *See Section I.C.14. Chronic kidney disease.*

The codes in category I13, Hypertensive heart and chronic kidney disease, are combination codes that include hypertension, heart disease and chronic kidney disease. The Includes note at I13 specifies that the conditions included at I11 and I12 are included together in I13. If a patient has hypertension, heart disease and chronic kidney disease then a code from I13 should be used, not individual codes for hypertension, heart disease and chronic kidney disease, or codes from I11 or I12.

For patients with both acute renal failure and chronic kidney disease an additional code for acute renal failure is required.

● I13 Hypertensive heart and chronic kidney disease

    Includes any condition in I11.- with any condition in I12.-
         cardiorenal disease
         cardiovascular renal disease

    (Ex:) **For category I13 CC codes:** I10-I16.9, I87.8-I87.9, I99.8-I99.9, N26.2

    **I13.0 Hypertensive heart and chronic kidney disease with
        heart failure and stage 1 through stage 4 chronic kidney
        disease, or unspecified chronic kidney disease** 🔖
        Use additional code to identify type of heart failure
        (I50.-)

        Use additional code to identify stage of chronic kidney
        disease (N18.1-N18.4, N18.9)

    **● I13.1 Hypertensive heart and chronic kidney disease without
        heart failure**

        **I13.10 Hypertensive heart and chronic kidney disease
           without heart failure, with stage 1 through
           stage 4 chronic kidney disease, or unspecified
           chronic kidney disease**
           Hypertensive heart disease and hypertensive
           chronic kidney disease NOS

           Use additional code to identify the stage of
           chronic kidney disease (N18.1-N18.4,
           N18.9)

        **I13.11 Hypertensive heart and chronic kidney disease
           without heart failure, with stage 5 chronic
           kidney disease, or end stage renal disease** 🔖
           Use additional code to identify the stage of
           chronic kidney disease (N18.5, N18.6)

    **I13.2 Hypertensive heart and chronic kidney disease with
        heart failure and with stage 5 chronic kidney disease, or
        end stage renal disease** 🔖

        Use additional code to identify type of heart failure (I50.-)

        Use additional code to identify the stage of chronic
        kidney disease (N18.5, N18.6)

◀ New ◀▓▓▓ Revised ~~deleted~~ Deleted Excludes 1 Excludes 2 Includes Use additional Code first Code also Unspecified

OGCR Official Guidelines ● Unacceptable Principal Diagnosis X Assign placeholder X ● Use Additional Character(s) ▶ Manifestation Code **Coding Clinic**

870

OGCR Section I.9.a.6

> Hypertension, Secondary
> Secondary hypertension is due to an underlying condition.
> Two codes are required: one to identify the underlying
> etiology and one from category I15 to identify the
> hypertension. Sequencing of codes is determined by the
> reason for admission/encounter.

● **I15**   **Secondary hypertension**
     Code also underlying condition
     Excludes1   postprocedural hypertension (I97.3)
     Excludes2   secondary hypertension involving vessels of
               brain (I6Ø-I69)
               secondary hypertension involving vessels of eye
               (H35.Ø-)
     I15.Ø   **Renovascular hypertension**
     I15.1   **Hypertension secondary to other renal disorders**
     I15.2   **Hypertension secondary to endocrine disorders**
     I15.8   **Other secondary hypertension**
     I15.9   **Secondary hypertension, unspecified**

● **I16**   **Hypertensive crisis** ◄
     Code also any identified hypertensive disease (I1Ø-I15) ◄
     I16.Ø   **Hypertensive urgency** 🔍 ◄
           (Ex) No exclusions
     I16.1   **Hypertensive emergency** ◄
     I16.9   **Hypertensive crisis, unspecified** 🔍 ◄
           (Ex) No exclusions

ISCHEMIC HEART DISEASES (I2Ø-I25)

Use additional code to identify presence of hypertension
(I1Ø-I16) ◄▥

● **I2Ø**   **Angina pectoris**
     Chest pain/discomfort due to lack of oxygen to the heart muscle.
     Principal symptom of myocardial infarction.
     Use additional code to identify:
       exposure to environmental tobacco smoke (Z77.22)
       history of tobacco dependence (Z87.891) ◄▥
       occupational exposure to environmental tobacco smoke
           (Z57.31)
       tobacco dependence (F17.-)
       tobacco use (Z72.Ø)
     Excludes1   angina pectoris with atherosclerotic heart disease
               of native coronary arteries (I25.1-)
               atherosclerosis of coronary artery bypass graft(s)
               and coronary artery of transplanted heart
               with angina pectoris (I25.7-)
               postinfarction angina (I23.7)
     I2Ø.Ø   **Unstable angina** 🔍
          Accelerated angina
          Crescendo angina
          De novo effort angina
          Intermediate coronary syndrome
          Preinfarction syndrome
          Worsening effort angina
          (Ex) IØ9.81, I11.Ø, I13.Ø, I13.2, I2Ø.Ø-I22.9, I24.Ø, I24.8-I24.9, I25.5-I25.6,
            I25.82-I25.83, I25.89-I25.9, I5Ø.1, I5Ø.9, I87.8-I87.9, I99.8-I99.9, R57.Ø,
            R57.9
     I2Ø.1   **Angina pectoris with documented spasm** 🔍
          Angiospastic angina
          Prinzmetal angina
          Spasm-induced angina
          Variant angina
          (Ex) I2Ø.Ø-I22.9, I24.Ø, I24.8-I24.9, I25.5-I25.6, I25.89-I25.9, I87.8-I87.9,
            I99.8-I99.9

     I2Ø.8   **Other forms of angina pectoris**
          Angina equivalent
          Angina of effort
          Coronary slow flow syndrome
          Stable angina ◄
          Stenocardia
          Use additional code(s) for symptoms associated with
             angina equivalent
     I2Ø.9   **Angina pectoris, unspecified**
          Angina NOS
          Anginal syndrome
          Cardiac angina
          Ischemic chest pain

   I21   **ST elevation (STEMI) and non-ST elevation (NSTEMI)**
      myocardial infarction
     Includes   cardiac infarction
               coronary (artery) embolism
               coronary (artery) occlusion
               coronary (artery) rupture
               coronary (artery) thrombosis
               infarction of heart, myocardium, or ventricle
               myocardial infarction specified as acute or with a
                   stated duration of 4 weeks (28 days) or less
                   from onset
     Use additional code, if applicable, to identify:
       exposure to environmental tobacco smoke (Z77.22)
       history of tobacco dependence (Z87.891) ◄▥
       occupational exposure to environmental tobacco smoke
           (Z57.31)
       status post administration of tPA (rtPA) in a different facility
           within the last 24 hours prior to admission to current
           facility (Z92.82)
       tobacco dependence (F17.-)
       tobacco use (Z72.Ø)
     Excludes2   old myocardial infarction (I25.2)
                postmyocardial infarction syndrome (I24.1)
                subsequent myocardial infarction (I22.-)
     (Ex) **For category I21 CC codes:** I21.Ø1-I22.9, I87.8-I87.9, I99.8-I99.9
     Coding Clinic: 2013, Q1, P25-26; 2012, Q4, P1Ø3

   ● **I21.Ø**   **ST elevation (STEMI) myocardial infarction of anterior**
           wall
           Coding Clinic: 2013, Q1, P26
       I21.Ø1   **ST elevation (STEMI) myocardial infarction**
               involving left main coronary artery 🔍
       I21.Ø2   **ST elevation (STEMI) myocardial infarction**
               involving left anterior descending coronary
               artery 🔍
               ST elevation (STEMI) myocardial infarction
                   involving diagonal coronary artery
               Coding Clinic: 2013, Q1, P26
       I21.Ø9   **ST elevation (STEMI) myocardial infarction**
               involving other coronary artery of anterior
               wall 🔍
               Acute transmural myocardial infarction of
                   anterior wall
               Anteroapical transmural (Q wave) infarction
                   (acute)
               Anterolateral transmural (Q wave) infarction
                   (acute)
               Anteroseptal transmural (Q wave) infarction
                   (acute)
               Transmural (Q wave) infarction (acute) (of)
                   anterior (wall) NOS
               Coding Clinic: 2012, Q4, P1Ø2, 1Ø4

N   Newborn Age: Ø   **P**   Pediatric Age: Ø–17   **M**   Maternity DX: 12–55   **A**   Adult Age: 15–124   ♀   Females Only   ♂   Males Only

🔍   Complication\Comorbidity   🔍   Major C\C   (Ex)   CC/MCC Exclusions   🔍   Hospital-Acquired Condition

871

● **I21.1** **ST elevation (STEMI) myocardial infarction of inferior wall**
Coding Clinic: 2013, Q1, P26

  I21.11 **ST elevation (STEMI) myocardial infarction involving right coronary artery** 🔒
    Inferoposterior transmural (Q wave) infarction (acute)

  I21.19 **ST elevation (STEMI) myocardial infarction involving other coronary artery of inferior wall** 🔒
    Acute transmural myocardial infarction of inferior wall
    Inferolateral transmural (Q wave) infarction (acute)
    Transmural (Q wave) infarction (acute) (of) diaphragmatic wall
    Transmural (Q wave) infarction (acute) (of) inferior (wall) NOS

    Excludes2 ST elevation (STEMI) myocardial infarction involving left circumflex coronary artery (I21.21)

    Coding Clinic: 2012, Q4, P97

● **I21.2** **ST elevation (STEMI) myocardial infarction of other sites**
  Ⓔⓧ For category I21.2 CC codes: I21.01-I22.9, I87.8-I87.9, I99.8-I99.9
  Coding Clinic: 2013, Q1, P26

  I21.21 **ST elevation (STEMI) myocardial infarction involving left circumflex coronary artery** 🔒
    ST elevation (STEMI) myocardial infarction involving oblique marginal coronary artery

  I21.29 **ST elevation (STEMI) myocardial infarction involving other sites** 🔒
    Acute transmural myocardial infarction of other sites
    Apical-lateral transmural (Q wave) infarction (acute)
    Basal-lateral transmural (Q wave) infarction (acute)
    High lateral transmural (Q wave) infarction (acute)
    Lateral (wall) NOS transmural (Q wave) infarction (acute)
    Posterior (true) transmural (Q wave) infarction (acute)
    Posterobasal transmural (Q wave) infarction (acute)
    Posterolateral transmural (Q wave) infarction (acute)
    Posteroseptal transmural (Q wave) infarction (acute)
    Septal transmural (Q wave) infarction (acute) NOS

OGCR Section I.c.9.e.2

Acute myocardial infarction, unspecified
Code I21.3, ST elevation (STEMI) myocardial infarction of unspecified site, is the default for unspecified acute myocardial infarction. If only STEMI or transmural MI without the site is documented, assign I21.3.

I21.3 **ST elevation (STEMI) myocardial infarction of unspecified site** 🔒
  Acute transmural myocardial infarction of unspecified site
  Myocardial infarction (acute) NOS
  Transmural (Q wave) myocardial infarction NOS
  Ⓔⓧ I21.01-I22.9, I87.8-I87.9, I99.8-I99.9
  Coding Clinic: 2013, Q1, P26

I21.4 **Non-ST elevation (NSTEMI) myocardial infarction** 🔒
  Acute subendocardial myocardial infarction
  Non-Q wave myocardial infarction NOS
  Nontransmural myocardial infarction NOS
  Ⓔⓧ I21.01-I22.9, I87.8-I87.9, I99.8-I99.9
  Coding Clinic: 2015, Q2, P16; 2013, Q1, P26

● **I22** **Subsequent ST elevation (STEMI) and non-ST elevation (NSTEMI) myocardial infarction**

  Includes   acute myocardial infarction occurring within four weeks (28 days) of a previous acute myocardial infarction, regardless of site
    cardiac infarction
    coronary (artery) embolism
    coronary (artery) occlusion
    coronary (artery) rupture
    coronary (artery) thrombosis
    infarction of heart, myocardium, or ventricle
    recurrent myocardial infarction
    reinfarction of myocardium
    rupture of heart, myocardium, or ventricle

Use additional code, if applicable, to identify:
  exposure to environmental tobacco smoke (Z77.22)
  history of tobacco dependence (Z87.891) ◀▥
  occupational exposure to environmental tobacco smoke (Z57.31)
  status post administration of tPA (rtPA) in a different facility within the last 24 hours prior to admission to current facility (Z92.82)
  tobacco dependence (F17.-)
  tobacco use (Z72.0)
  Ⓔⓧ For category I22 CC codes: I21.01-I22.9, I87.8-I87.9, I99.8-I99.9
  Coding Clinic: 2013, Q1, P25; 2012, Q4, P103

  I22.0 **Subsequent ST elevation (STEMI) myocardial infarction of anterior wall** 🔒
    Subsequent acute transmural myocardial infarction of anterior wall
    Subsequent transmural (Q wave) infarction (acute)(of) anterior (wall) NOS
    Subsequent anteroapical transmural (Q wave) infarction (acute)
    Subsequent anterolateral transmural (Q wave) infarction (acute)
    Subsequent anteroseptal transmural (Q wave) infarction (acute)

  I22.1 **Subsequent ST elevation (STEMI) myocardial infarction of inferior wall** 🔒
    Subsequent acute transmural myocardial infarction of inferior wall
    Subsequent transmural (Q wave) infarction (acute)(of) diaphragmatic wall
    Subsequent transmural (Q wave) infarction (acute)(of) inferior (wall) NOS
    Subsequent inferolateral transmural (Q wave) infarction (acute)
    Subsequent inferoposterior transmural (Q wave) infarction (acute)
    Coding Clinic: 2012, Q4, P97, 102, 104

  I22.2 **Subsequent non-ST elevation (NSTEMI) myocardial infarction** 🔒
    Subsequent acute subendocardial myocardial infarction
    Subsequent non-Q wave myocardial infarction NOS
    Subsequent nontransmural myocardial infarction NOS

◀ New   ◀▥ Revised   ~~deleted~~ Deleted   Excludes 1   Excludes 2   Includes   Use additional   Code first   Code also   Unspecified
OGCR Official Guidelines   ● Unacceptable Principal Diagnosis   X Assign placeholder X   🔒 Use Additional Character(s)   ▶ Manifestation Code   **Coding Clinic**

I22.8   **Subsequent ST elevation (STEMI) myocardial infarction of other sites** 🩺
     Subsequent acute transmural myocardial infarction of other sites
     Subsequent apical-lateral transmural (Q wave) myocardial infarction (acute)
     Subsequent basal-lateral transmural (Q wave) myocardial infarction (acute)
     Subsequent high lateral transmural (Q wave) myocardial infarction (acute)
     Subsequent transmural (Q wave) myocardial infarction (acute)(of) lateral (wall) NOS
     Subsequent posterior (true) transmural (Q wave) myocardial infarction (acute)
     Subsequent posterobasal transmural (Q wave) myocardial infarction (acute)
     Subsequent posterolateral transmural (Q wave) myocardial infarction (acute)
     Subsequent posteroseptal transmural (Q wave) myocardial infarction (acute)
     Subsequent septal NOS transmural (Q wave) myocardial infarction (acute)

I22.9   **Subsequent ST elevation (STEMI) myocardial infarction of unspecified site** 🩺
     Subsequent acute myocardial infarction of unspecified site
     Subsequent myocardial infarction (acute) NOS

● **I23**   **Certain current complications following ST elevation (STEMI) and non-ST elevation (NSTEMI) myocardial infarction (within the 28 day period)**
     (Ex) **For category I23 CC codes unless otherwise indicated:** E78.71-E78.72, I23.0-I23.8, I40.0-I41, I51.0-I51.2, I51.4, I87.8-I87.9, I97.0-I97.191, I99.8-I99.9, P29.3, Q20.0-Q21.9, Q23.8-Q23.9, Q24.8-Q24.9, Q27.30, Q27.4, Q28.0-Q28.1, Q28.8-Q28.9, Q87.1-Q87.89, Q89.7-Q89.8, Q99.2

I23.0   **Hemopericardium as current complication following acute myocardial infarction** 🩺   A
     Excludes1   hemopericardium not specified as current complication following acute myocardial infarction (I31.2)

I23.1   **Atrial septal defect as current complication following acute myocardial infarction** 🩺   A
     Excludes1   acquired atrial septal defect not specified as current complication following acute myocardial infarction (I51.0)

I23.2   **Ventricular septal defect as current complication following acute myocardial infarction** 🩺   A
     Excludes1   acquired ventricular septal defect not specified as current complication following acute myocardial infarction (I51.0)

I23.3   **Rupture of cardiac wall without hemopericardium as current complication following acute myocardial infarction** 🩺   A

I23.4   **Rupture of chordae tendineae as current complication following acute myocardial infarction** 🩺
     Excludes1   rupture of chordae tendineae not specified as current complication following acute myocardial infarction (I51.1)
     (Ex) I23.0-I23.4, I23.6-I23.8, I51.0-I51.1, I87.8-I87.9, I99.8-I99.9

I23.5   **Rupture of papillary muscle as current complication following acute myocardial infarction** 🩺
     Excludes1   rupture of papillary muscle not specified as current complication following acute myocardial infarction (I51.2)
     (Ex) I23.0-I23.3, I23.5-I23.8, I51.0, I51.2, I87.8-I87.9, I99.8-I99.9

I23.6   **Thrombosis of atrium, auricular appendage, and ventricle as current complications following acute myocardial infarction** 🩺   A
     Excludes1   thrombosis of atrium, auricular appendage, and ventricle not specified as current complication following acute myocardial infarction (I51.3)

I23.7   **Postinfarction angina** 🩺   A
     Coding Clinic: 2015, Q2, P16-17

I23.8   **Other current complications following acute myocardial infarction** 🩺   A

● **I24**   **Other acute ischemic heart diseases**
     Excludes1   angina pectoris (I20.-)
                   transient myocardial ischemia in newborn (P29.4)
     (Ex) **For category I24 CC codes unless otherwise indicated:** I20.0-I22.9, I24.0-I24.9, I25.5-I25.6, I25.89-I25.9, I87.8-I87.9, I99.8-I99.9

I24.0   **Acute coronary thrombosis not resulting in myocardial infarction** 🩺
     Acute coronary (artery) (vein) embolism not resulting in myocardial infarction
     Acute coronary (artery) (vein) occlusion not resulting in myocardial infarction
     Acute coronary (artery) (vein) thromboembolism not resulting in myocardial infarction
     Excludes1   atherosclerotic heart disease (I25.1-)
     Coding Clinic: 2013, Q1, P24

I24.1   **Dressler's syndrome** 🩺
     Postmyocardial infarction syndrome
     Excludes1   postinfarction angina (I23.7)
     (Ex) I24.0-I24.9, I87.8-I87.9, I99.8-I99.9

I24.8   **Other forms of acute ischemic heart disease** 🩺

I24.9   **Acute ischemic heart disease, unspecified** 🩺
     Excludes1   ischemic heart disease (chronic) NOS (I25.9)

● **I25**   **Chronic ischemic heart disease**
     Use additional code to identify:
        chronic total occlusion of coronary artery (I25.82)
        exposure to environmental tobacco smoke (Z77.22)
        history of tobacco dependence (Z87.891) ◀▥
        occupational exposure to environmental tobacco smoke (Z57.31)
        tobacco dependence (F17.-)
        tobacco use (Z72.0)

★ **(See Plates 218 and 219 on pages 74 and 75.)**

   ● **I25.1**   **Atherosclerotic heart disease of native coronary artery**
     Disease in which fatty deposits form on the walls of arteries
     Atherosclerotic cardiovascular disease
     Coronary (artery) atheroma
     Coronary (artery) atherosclerosis
     Coronary (artery) disease
     Coronary (artery) sclerosis
     Use additional code, if applicable, to identify:
        coronary atherosclerosis due to calcified coronary lesion (I25.84)
        coronary atherosclerosis due to lipid rich plaque (I25.83)
     Excludes2   atheroembolism (I75.-)
                  atherosclerosis of coronary artery bypass graft(s) and transplanted heart (I25.7-)

     I25.10   **Atherosclerotic heart disease of native coronary artery without angina pectoris**   A
        Atherosclerotic heart disease NOS
        Coding Clinic: 2015, Q2, P17; 2012, Q4, P92

Item 9-6 Classification is based on the location of the atherosclerosis. **"Of native coronary artery"** indicates the atherosclerosis is within an original heart artery. **"Of autologous vein bypass graft"** indicates that the atherosclerosis is within a vein graft that was taken from within the patient. **"Of nonautologous biological bypass graft"** indicates the atherosclerosis is within a vessel grafted from other than the patient. **"Of artery bypass graft"** indicates the atherosclerosis is within an artery that was grafted from within the patient.

N Newborn Age: 0   **P** Pediatric Age: 0–17   **M** Maternity DX: 12–55   **A** Adult Age: 15–124   ♀ Females Only   ♂ Males Only

🩺 Complication\Comorbidity   🩺 Major C\C   (Ex) CC/MCC Exclusions   🩺 Hospital-Acquired Condition   873

CHAPTER 9 (I00-I99)

CHAPTER 9 (I00-I99)

OGCR See Section I.9.b.

Atherosclerotic Coronary Artery Disease and Angina

ICD-10-CM has combination codes for atherosclerotic heart disease with angina pectoris. The subcategories for these codes are I25.11, Atherosclerotic heart disease of native coronary artery with angina pectoris and I25.7, Atherosclerosis of coronary artery bypass graft(s) and coronary artery of transplanted heart with angina pectoris.

When using one of these combination codes it is not necessary to use an additional code for angina pectoris. A causal relationship can be assumed in a patient with both atherosclerosis and angina pectoris, unless the documentation indicates the angina is due to something other than the atherosclerosis.

If a patient with coronary artery disease is admitted due to an acute myocardial infarction (AMI), the AMI should be sequenced before the coronary artery disease.

See Section I.C.9. Acute myocardial infarction (AMI)

● **I25.11**   **Atherosclerotic heart disease of native coronary artery with angina pectoris**

  I25.110   **Atherosclerotic heart disease of native coronary artery with unstable angina pectoris** 🔊   A

    Excludes1   unstable angina without atherosclerotic heart disease (I20.0)

    CC when PDx is its own CC
    Ⓔⓧ See I20.0

  I25.111   **Atherosclerotic heart disease of native coronary artery with angina pectoris with documented spasm**   A

    Excludes1   angina pectoris with documented spasm without atherosclerotic heart disease (I20.1)

  I25.118   **Atherosclerotic heart disease of native coronary artery with other forms of angina pectoris**   A

    Excludes1   other forms of angina pectoris without atherosclerotic heart disease (I20.8)

    Coding Clinic: 2015, Q2, P16-17

  I25.119   **Atherosclerotic heart disease of native coronary artery with unspecified angina pectoris**   A

    Atherosclerotic heart disease with angina NOS
    Atherosclerotic heart disease with ischemic chest pain

    Excludes1   unspecified angina pectoris without atherosclerotic heart disease (I20.9)

I25.2   **Old myocardial infarction**
  Healed myocardial infarction
  Past myocardial infarction diagnosed by ECG or other investigation, but currently presenting no symptoms

Figure 9-2 Atherosclerotic plaque.

Atherosclerotic plaque (atheromas)

I25.3   **Aneurysm of heart** 🔊
  Mural aneurysm
  Ventricular aneurysm
  Ⓔⓧ I25.3-I25.41

● **I25.4**   **Coronary artery aneurysm and dissection**

  I25.41   **Coronary artery aneurysm**
    Coronary arteriovenous fistula, acquired

    Excludes1   congenital coronary (artery) aneurysm (Q24.5)

  I25.42   **Coronary artery dissection** 🔊
    Ⓔⓧ I25.42, I67.0, I77.2-I77.3, I77.5-I77.6, I77.70, I77.75-I77.79, I77.89-I77.9, M31.8-M31.9

I25.5   **Ischemic cardiomyopathy**
  Excludes2   coronary atherosclerosis (I25.1-, I25.7-)

I25.6   **Silent myocardial ischemia**

● **I25.7**   **Atherosclerosis of coronary artery bypass graft(s) and coronary artery of transplanted heart with angina pectoris**

  Use additional code, if applicable, to identify:
    coronary atherosclerosis due to calcified coronary lesion (I25.84)
    coronary atherosclerosis due to lipid rich plaque (I25.83)

  Excludes1   atherosclerosis of bypass graft(s) of transplanted heart without angina pectoris (I25.812)
    atherosclerosis of coronary artery bypass graft(s) without angina pectoris (I25.810)
    atherosclerosis of native coronary artery of transplanted heart without angina pectoris (I25.811)
    embolism or thrombus of coronary artery bypass graft(s) (T82.8-)

● **I25.70**   **Atherosclerosis of coronary artery bypass graft(s), unspecified, with angina pectoris**

  I25.700   **Atherosclerosis of coronary artery bypass graft(s), unspecified, with unstable angina pectoris** 🔊   A

    Excludes1   unstable angina pectoris without atherosclerosis of coronary artery bypass graft (I20.0)

    CC when PDx is its own CC
    Ⓔⓧ See I20.0

  I25.701   **Atherosclerosis of coronary artery bypass graft(s), unspecified, with angina pectoris with documented spasm**

    Excludes1   angina pectoris with documented spasm without atherosclerosis of coronary artery bypass graft (I20.1)

  I25.708   **Atherosclerosis of coronary artery bypass graft(s), unspecified, with other forms of angina pectoris**   A

    Excludes1   other forms of angina pectoris without atherosclerosis of coronary artery bypass graft (I20.8)

  I25.709   **Atherosclerosis of coronary artery bypass graft(s), unspecified, with unspecified angina pectoris**   A

    Excludes1   unspecified angina pectoris without atherosclerosis of coronary artery bypass graft (I20.9)

◄ New   ◄▥ Revised   ~~deleted~~ Deleted   Excludes 1   Excludes 2   Includes   Use additional   Code first   Code also   Unspecified

OGCR Official Guidelines   ● Unacceptable Principal Diagnosis   X Assign placeholder X   ● Use Additional Character(s)   ▸ Manifestation Code   **Coding Clinic**

● **I25.71**   **Atherosclerosis of autologous vein coronary artery bypass graft(s) with angina pectoris**

> (Ex:) **For category I25.71 CC codes unless otherwise indicated:** I25.10-I25.119, I25.700-I25.739, I25.760-I25.799, I25.812-I25.84

     I25.710   **Atherosclerosis of autologous vein coronary artery bypass graft(s) with unstable angina pectoris** 🦠   **A**

> **Excludes1**   unstable angina without atherosclerosis of autologous vein coronary artery bypass graft(s) (I20.0)

         CC when PDx is its own CC
>
> (Ex:) I09.81, I11.0, I13.0, I13.2, I20.0-I22.9, I24.0, I24.8-I25.119, I25.5-I25.739, I25.760-I25.799, I25.812-I25.9, I50.1, I50.9, I87.8-I87.9, I99.8-I99.9, R57.0, R57.9

     I25.711   **Atherosclerosis of autologous vein coronary artery bypass graft(s) with angina pectoris with documented spasm** 🦠   **A**

> **Excludes1**   angina pectoris with documented spasm without atherosclerosis of autologous vein coronary artery bypass graft(s) (I20.1)

     I25.718   **Atherosclerosis of autologous vein coronary artery bypass graft(s) with other forms of angina pectoris** 🦠   **A**

> **Excludes1**   other forms of angina pectoris without atherosclerosis of autologous vein coronary artery bypass graft(s) (I20.8)

     I25.719   **Atherosclerosis of autologous vein coronary artery bypass graft(s) with unspecified angina pectoris** 🦠   **A**

> **Excludes1**   unspecified angina pectoris without atherosclerosis of autologous vein coronary artery bypass graft(s) (I20.9)

● **I25.72**   **Atherosclerosis of autologous artery coronary artery bypass graft(s) with angina pectoris**

Atherosclerosis of internal mammary artery graft with angina pectoris

> (Ex:) **For category I25.72 CC codes unless otherwise indicated:** See I25.71

     I25.720   **Atherosclerosis of autologous artery coronary artery bypass graft(s) with unstable angina pectoris** 🦠   **A**

> **Excludes1**   unstable angina without atherosclerosis of autologous artery coronary artery bypass graft(s) (I20.0)

         CC when PDx is its own CC
>
> (Ex:) See I25.710

● **I25.721**   **Atherosclerosis of autologous artery coronary artery bypass graft(s) with angina pectoris with documented spasm** 🦠   **A**

> **Excludes1**   angina pectoris with documented spasm without atherosclerosis of autologous artery coronary artery bypass graft(s) (I20.1)

     I25.728   **Atherosclerosis of autologous artery coronary artery bypass graft(s) with other forms of angina pectoris** 🦠   **A**

> **Excludes1**   other forms of angina pectoris without atherosclerosis of autologous artery coronary artery bypass graft(s) (I20.8)

     I25.729   **Atherosclerosis of autologous artery coronary artery bypass graft(s) with unspecified angina pectoris** 🦠   **A**

> **Excludes1**   unspecified angina pectoris without atherosclerosis of autologous artery coronary artery bypass graft(s) (I20.9)

● **I25.73**   **Atherosclerosis of nonautologous biological coronary artery bypass graft(s) with angina pectoris**

> (Ex:) **For category I25.73 CC codes unless otherwise indicated:** See I25.71

     I25.730   **Atherosclerosis of nonautologous biological coronary artery bypass graft(s) with unstable angina pectoris** 🦠   **A**

> **Excludes1**   unstable angina without atherosclerosis of nonautologous biological coronary artery bypass graft(s) (I20.0)

         CC when PDx is its own CC
>
> (Ex:) See I25.710

     I25.731   **Atherosclerosis of nonautologous biological coronary artery bypass graft(s) with angina pectoris with documented spasm** 🦠   **A**

> **Excludes1**   angina pectoris with documented spasm without atherosclerosis of nonautologous biological coronary artery bypass graft(s) (I20.1)

     I25.738   **Atherosclerosis of nonautologous biological coronary artery bypass graft(s) with other forms of angina pectoris** 🦠   **A**

> **Excludes1**   other forms of angina pectoris without atherosclerosis of nonautologous biological coronary artery bypass graft(s) (I20.8)

N Newborn Age: 0   **P** Pediatric Age: 0–17   **M** Maternity DX: 12–55   **A** Adult Age: 15–124   ♀ Females Only   ♂ Males Only

🦠 Complication\Comorbidity   🦠 Major C\C   (Ex:) CC/MCC Exclusions   🦠 Hospital-Acquired Condition

875

I25.739 Atherosclerosis of nonautologous biological coronary artery bypass graft(s) with unspecified angina pectoris 🗐   A

> **Excludes1**   unspecified angina pectoris without atherosclerosis of nonautologous biological coronary artery bypass graft(s) (I20.9)

● **I25.75** Atherosclerosis of native coronary artery of transplanted heart with angina pectoris

> **Excludes1**   atherosclerosis of native coronary artery of transplanted heart without angina pectoris (I25.811)

> Ⓔ **For category I25.75 CC codes unless otherwise indicated:** I25.10-I25.119, I25.700-I25.799, I25.811-I25.84

I25.750 Atherosclerosis of native coronary artery of transplanted heart with unstable angina 🗐

> CC when PDx is its own CC
> Ⓔ I09.81, I11.0, I13.0, I13.2, I20.0-I22.9, I24.0, I24.8-I25.119, I25.5-I25.799, I25.811-I25.9, I50.1, I50.9, I87.8-I87.9, I99.8-I99.9, R57.0, R57.9

I25.751 Atherosclerosis of native coronary artery of transplanted heart with angina pectoris with documented spasm 🗐

I25.758 Atherosclerosis of native coronary artery of transplanted heart with other forms of angina pectoris 🗐

I25.759 Atherosclerosis of native coronary artery of transplanted heart with unspecified angina pectoris 🗐

● **I25.76** Atherosclerosis of bypass graft of coronary artery of transplanted heart with angina pectoris

> **Excludes1**   atherosclerosis of bypass graft of coronary artery of transplanted heart without angina pectoris (I25.812)

> Ⓔ **For category I25.76 CC codes unless otherwise indicated:** I25.10-I25.119, I25.700-I25.759, I25.790-I25.799, I25.811, I25.82-I25.84

I25.760 Atherosclerosis of bypass graft of coronary artery of transplanted heart with unstable angina 🗐   A

> CC when PDx is its own CC
> Ⓔ I09.81, I11.0, I13.0, I13.2, I20.0-I22.9, I24.0, I24.8-I25.119, I25.5-I25.759, I25.790-I25.799, I25.811, I25.82-I25.9, I50.1, I50.9, I87.8-I87.9, I99.8-I99.9, R57.0, R57.9

I25.761 Atherosclerosis of bypass graft of coronary artery of transplanted heart with angina pectoris with documented spasm 🗐   A

I25.768 Atherosclerosis of bypass graft of coronary artery of transplanted heart with other forms of angina pectoris 🗐   A

I25.769 Atherosclerosis of bypass graft of coronary artery of transplanted heart with unspecified angina pectoris 🗐   A

● **I25.79** Atherosclerosis of other coronary artery bypass graft(s) with angina pectoris   A

> Ⓔ **For category I25.79 CC codes unless otherwise indicated:** No exclusions

I25.790 Atherosclerosis of other coronary artery bypass graft(s) with unstable angina pectoris 🗐

> **Excludes1**   unstable angina without atherosclerosis of other coronary artery bypass graft(s) (I20.0)

> CC when PDx is its own CC
> Ⓔ See I20.0

I25.791 Atherosclerosis of other coronary artery bypass graft(s) with angina pectoris with documented spasm 🗐 A

> **Excludes1**   angina pectoris with documented spasm without atherosclerosis of other coronary artery bypass graft(s) (I20.1)

I25.798 Atherosclerosis of other coronary artery bypass graft(s) with other forms of angina pectoris 🗐   A

> **Excludes1**   other forms of angina pectoris without atherosclerosis of other coronary artery bypass graft(s) (I20.8)

I25.799 Atherosclerosis of other coronary artery bypass graft(s) with unspecified angina pectoris 🗐   A

> **Excludes1**   unspecified angina pectoris without atherosclerosis of other coronary artery bypass graft(s) (I20.9)

● **I25.8** Other forms of chronic ischemic heart disease

● **I25.81** Atherosclerosis of other coronary vessels without angina pectoris

> Use additional code, if applicable, to identify:
> coronary atherosclerosis due to calcified coronary lesion (I25.84)
> coronary atherosclerosis due to lipid rich plaque (I25.83)

> **Excludes1**   atherosclerotic heart disease of native coronary artery without angina pectoris (I25.10)

I25.810 Atherosclerosis of coronary artery bypass graft(s) without angina pectoris 🗐   A

> Atherosclerosis of coronary artery bypass graft NOS

> **Excludes1**   atherosclerosis of coronary bypass graft(s) with angina pectoris (I25.70- -I25.73-, I25.79-)

> Ⓔ No exclusions

I25.811 Atherosclerosis of native coronary artery of transplanted heart without angina pectoris 🗐

> Atherosclerosis of native coronary artery of transplanted heart NOS

> **Excludes1**   atherosclerosis of native coronary artery of transplanted heart with angina pectoris (I25.75-)

> Ⓔ See I25.75

I25.812   **Atherosclerosis of bypass graft of coronary artery of transplanted heart without angina pectoris** 🔖   **A**

Atherosclerosis of bypass graft of transplanted heart NOS

> **Excludes1**   atherosclerosis of bypass graft of transplanted heart with angina pectoris (I25.76)

● **I25.82**   **Chronic total occlusion of coronary artery**

Complete occlusion of coronary artery

Total occlusion of coronary artery

Code first coronary atherosclerosis (I25.1-, I25.7-, I25.81-)

> **Excludes1**   acute coronary occlusion with myocardial infarction (I21.-, I22.-)
> acute coronary occlusion without myocardial infarction (I24.0)

(Ex) See I25.76

● **I25.83**   **Coronary atherosclerosis due to lipid rich plaque**   **A**

Code first coronary atherosclerosis (I25.1-, I25.7-, I25.81-)

● **I25.84**   **Coronary atherosclerosis due to calcified coronary lesion**

Coronary atherosclerosis due to severely calcified coronary lesion

Code first coronary atherosclerosis (I25.1-, I25.7-, I25.81-)

I25.89   **Other forms of chronic ischemic heart disease**

I25.9   **Chronic ischemic heart disease, unspecified**

Ischemic heart disease (chronic) NOS

PULMONARY HEART DISEASE AND DISEASES OF PULMONARY CIRCULATION (I26-I28)

● **I26**   **Pulmonary embolism**

> **Includes**   pulmonary (acute)(artery)(vein) infarction
> pulmonary (acute)(artery)(vein) thromboembolism
> pulmonary (acute)(artery)(vein) thrombosis

> **Excludes2**   chronic pulmonary embolism (I27.82)
> personal history of pulmonary embolism (Z86.711)
> pulmonary embolism due to trauma (T79.0, T79.1)
> pulmonary embolism due to complications of surgical and medical care (T80.0, T81.7-, T82.8-)
> pulmonary embolism complicating abortion, ectopic or molar pregnancy (O00-O07, O08.2)
> pulmonary embolism complicating pregnancy, childbirth and the puerperium (O88.-)
> septic (non-pulmonary) arterial embolism (I76)

● **I26.0**   **Pulmonary embolism with acute cor pulmonale**

(Ex) **For category I26.0 CC codes:** I26.01-I26.99, I27.2-I27.9, I74.01-I74.10, I74.19, I87.8-I87.9, I99.8-I99.9

● **I26.01**   **Septic pulmonary embolism with acute cor pulmonale** 🔖

Code first underlying infection

MCC when PDx is its own MCC

I26.02   **Saddle embolus of pulmonary artery with acute cor pulmonale** 🔖 🔖

MCC when PDx is its own MCC

I26.09   **Other pulmonary embolism with acute cor pulmonale** 🔖 🔖

Acute cor pulmonale NOS

MCC when PDx is its own MCC

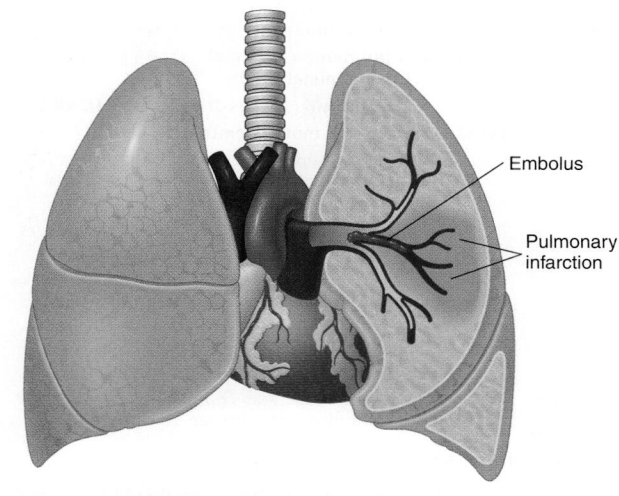

Figure 9-3   Pulmonary Embolism. (From Chabner: The Language of Medicine, ed 8, St. Louis, Saunders, 2007)

Item 9–7   Pulmonary heart disease or **cor pulmonale** is right ventricle hypertrophy or RVH as a result of a respiratory disorder increasing back flow pressure to the right ventricle. Left untreated, cor pulmonale leads to right-heart failure and death.

● **I26.9**   **Pulmonary embolism without acute cor pulmonale**

● **I26.90**   **Septic pulmonary embolism without acute cor pulmonale** 🔖

Code first underlying infection

(Ex) I26.01-I26.99, I27.82, I74.01-I74.10, I74.19, I87.8-I87.9, I99.8-I99.9, T80.0XX[A], T81.718[A], T81.72X[A,] T82.817-T82.818[A]

I26.92   **Saddle embolus of pulmonary artery without acute cor pulmonale** 🔖 🔖

(Ex) I26.01-I26.99, I27.82, I74.01-I74.10, I74.19, I87.8-I87.9, I99.8-I99.9

I26.99   **Other pulmonary embolism without acute cor pulmonale** 🔖 🔖

Acute pulmonary embolism NOS

Pulmonary embolism NOS

(Ex) I26.01-I26.99, I27.82, I74.01-I74.10, I74.19, I87.8-I87.9, I99.8-I99.9, T80.0XX[A], T81.718[A], T81.72X[A], T82.817-T82.818[A]

● **I27**   **Other pulmonary heart diseases**

I27.0   **Primary pulmonary hypertension** 🔖

> **Excludes1**   pulmonary hypertension NOS (I27.2)
> secondary pulmonary hypertension (I27.2)

(Ex) E66.2, I27.0, I27.2-I27.81, I27.89-I27.9, I28.8-I28.9, I87.8-I87.9, I99.8-I99.9

I27.1   **Kyphoscoliotic heart disease** 🔖

(Ex) E66.2, I27.0-I27.81, I27.89-I27.9

I27.2   **Other secondary pulmonary hypertension**

Pulmonary hypertension NOS

Code also associated underlying condition

Coding Clinic: 2016, Q2, P8

N   Newborn Age: 0   **P**   Pediatric Age: 0–17   **M**   Maternity DX: 12–55   **A**   Adult Age: 15–124   ♀   Females Only   ♂   Males Only

🔖   Complication\Comorbidity   🔖   Major C\C   (Ex)   CC/MCC Exclusions   🔖   Hospital-Acquired Condition

877

● **I27.8**   **Other specified pulmonary heart diseases**

    I27.81   **Cor pulmonale (chronic)**
       Cor pulmonale NOS
       Excludes1   acute cor pulmonale (I26.0-)

    I27.82   **Chronic pulmonary embolism** 🔖
       Use additional code, if applicable, for associated long-term (current) use of anticoagulants (Z79.01)
       Excludes1   personal history of pulmonary embolism (Z86.711)
       (Ex:) See I26.92

    I27.89   **Other specified pulmonary heart diseases**
       Eisenmenger's complex
       Eisenmenger's syndrome
       Excludes1   Eisenmenger's defect (Q21.8)

    I27.9   **Pulmonary heart disease, unspecified**
       Chronic cardiopulmonary disease

● **I28**   **Other diseases of pulmonary vessels**
    (Ex:) For category I28 CC codes: I28.0-I28.9

    I28.0   **Arteriovenous fistula of pulmonary vessels** 🔖
       Excludes1   congenital arteriovenous fistula (Q25.72)

    I28.1   **Aneurysm of pulmonary artery** 🔖
       Excludes1   congenital aneurysm (Q25.79)
                   congenital arteriovenous aneurysm (Q25.72)

    I28.8   **Other diseases of pulmonary vessels**
       Pulmonary arteritis
       Pulmonary endarteritis
       Rupture of pulmonary vessels
       Stenosis of pulmonary vessels
       Stricture of pulmonary vessels

    I28.9   **Disease of pulmonary vessels, unspecified**

OTHER FORMS OF HEART DISEASE (I30-I52)

● **I30**   **Acute pericarditis**
Inflammation of pericardium (sac surrounding the heart) caused by an infection

    Includes   acute mediastinopericarditis
               acute myopericarditis
               acute pericardial effusion
               acute pleuropericarditis
               acute pneumopericarditis

    Excludes1   Dressler's syndrome (I24.1)
                 rheumatic pericarditis (acute) (I01.0)
    (Ex:) For category I30 CC codes: I01.0, I09.2, I30.0-I30.9, I31.3-I32, I87.8-I87.9, I99.8-I99.9

    I30.0   **Acute nonspecific idiopathic pericarditis** 🔖

    I30.1   **Infective pericarditis** 🔖
       Pneumococcal pericarditis
       Pneumopyopericardium
       Purulent pericarditis
       Pyopericarditis
       Pyopericardium
       Pyopneumopericardium
       Staphylococcal pericarditis
       Streptococcal pericarditis
       Suppurative pericarditis
       Viral pericarditis
       Use additional code (B95-B97) to identify infectious agent

    I30.8   **Other forms of acute pericarditis** 🔖

    I30.9   **Acute pericarditis, unspecified** 🔖

● **I31**   **Other diseases of pericardium**

    Excludes1   diseases of pericardium specified as rheumatic (I09.2)
                 postcardiotomy syndrome (I97.0)
                 traumatic injury to pericardium (S26.-)
    (Ex:) For category I31 CC codes unless otherwise indicated: B33.23, I01.0, I09.2, I30.0-I30.9, I31.3-I32, I87.8-I87.9, I99.8-I99.9

    I31.0   **Chronic adhesive pericarditis** 🔖
       Accretio cordis
       Adherent pericardium
       Adhesive mediastinopericarditis
       (Ex:) I31.0-I31.9, I87.8, I99.8-I99.9

    I31.1   **Chronic constrictive pericarditis** 🔖
       Concretio cordis
       Pericardial calcification
       (Ex:) I31.0-I31.9, I87.8, I99.8-I99.9

    I31.2   **Hemopericardium, not elsewhere classified** 🔖
       Excludes1   hemopericardium as current complication following acute myocardial infarction (I23.0)
       (Ex:) I31.0-I31.9, I87.8, I99.8-I99.9

    I31.3   **Pericardial effusion (noninflammatory)** 🔖
       Chylopericardium
       Excludes1   acute pericardial effusion (I30.9)

    ● **I31.4**   **Cardiac tamponade** 🔖
       Code first underlying cause

    I31.8   **Other specified diseases of pericardium** 🔖
       Epicardial plaques
       Focal pericardial adhesions

    I31.9   **Disease of pericardium, unspecified** 🔖
       Pericarditis (chronic) NOS

▸ **I32**   *Pericarditis in diseases classified elsewhere* 🔖
    Code first underlying disease

    Excludes1   pericarditis (in):
                 coxsackie (virus) (B33.23)
                 gonococcal (A54.83)
                 meningococcal (A39.53)
                 rheumatoid (arthritis) (M05.31)
                 syphilitic (A52.06)
                 systemic lupus erythematosus (M32.12)
                 tuberculosis (A18.84)
    (Ex:) See I30

● **I33**   **Acute and subacute endocarditis**
Inflammation/infection of lining of heart, affecting heart valves including replacement valves and is usually caused by a bacterial infection

    Excludes1   acute rheumatic endocarditis (I01.1)
                 endocarditis NOS (I38)
    (Ex:) For category I33 CC codes: I01.1, I08.1-I08.3, I09.1, I33.0-I33.9, I38-I39, I87.8-I87.9, I99.8-I99.9

    I33.0   **Acute and subacute infective endocarditis** 🔖
       Bacterial endocarditis (acute) (subacute)
       Infective endocarditis (acute) (subacute) NOS
       Endocarditis lenta (acute) (subacute)
       Malignant endocarditis (acute) (subacute)
       Purulent endocarditis (acute) (subacute)
       Septic endocarditis (acute) (subacute)
       Ulcerative endocarditis (acute) (subacute)
       Vegetative endocarditis (acute) (subacute)
       Use additional code (B95-B97) to identify infectious agent

    I33.9   **Acute and subacute endocarditis, unspecified** 🔖
       Acute endocarditis NOS
       Acute myoendocarditis NOS
       Acute periendocarditis NOS
       Subacute endocarditis NOS
       Subacute myoendocarditis NOS
       Subacute periendocarditis NOS

◀ New   ◀ Revised   ~~deleted~~ Deleted   Excludes 1   Excludes 2   Includes   Use additional   Code first   Code also   Unspecified

OGCR Official Guidelines   ● Unacceptable Principal Diagnosis   X Assign placeholder X   ● Use Additional Character(s)   ▸ Manifestation Code   **Coding Clinic**

878

● **I34**   **Nonrheumatic mitral valve disorders**
     Excludes1   mitral valve disease (I05.9)
                   mitral valve failure (I05.8)
                   mitral valve stenosis (I05.0)
                   mitral valve disorder of unspecified cause with
                         diseases of aortic and/or tricuspid valve(s)
                         (I08.-)
                   mitral valve disorder of unspecified cause with
                         mitral stenosis or obstruction (I05.0)
                   mitral valve disorder specified as congenital
                         (Q23.2, Q23.3)
                   mitral valve disorder specified as rheumatic
                         (I05.-)

   I34.0   **Nonrheumatic mitral (valve) insufficiency**
          Nonrheumatic mitral (valve) incompetence NOS
          Nonrheumatic mitral (valve) regurgitation NOS

   I34.1   **Nonrheumatic mitral (valve) prolapse**
          Floppy nonrheumatic mitral valve syndrome
         Excludes1   Marfan's syndrome (Q87.4-)

   I34.2   **Nonrheumatic mitral (valve) stenosis**
   I34.8   **Other nonrheumatic mitral valve disorders**
   I34.9   **Nonrheumatic mitral valve disorder, unspecified**

● **I35**   **Nonrheumatic aortic valve disorders**
     Excludes1   aortic valve disorder of unspecified cause but
                   with diseases of mitral and/or tricuspid
                   valve(s) (I08.-)
                   aortic valve disorder specified as congenital
                         (Q23.0, Q23.1)
                   aortic valve disorder specified as rheumatic (I06.-)
                   hypertrophic subaortic stenosis (I42.1)

   I35.0   **Nonrheumatic aortic (valve) stenosis**
   I35.1   **Nonrheumatic aortic (valve) insufficiency**
          Nonrheumatic aortic (valve) incompetence NOS
          Nonrheumatic aortic (valve) regurgitation NOS

   I35.2   **Nonrheumatic aortic (valve) stenosis with insufficiency**
   I35.8   **Other nonrheumatic aortic valve disorders**
   I35.9   **Nonrheumatic aortic valve disorder, unspecified**

● **I36**   **Nonrheumatic tricuspid valve disorders**
     Excludes1   tricuspid valve disorders of unspecified cause
                         (I07.-)
                   tricuspid valve disorders specified as congenital
                         (Q22.4, Q22.8, Q22.9)
                   tricuspid valve disorders specified as rheumatic
                         (I07.-)
                   tricuspid valve disorders with aortic and/or
                         mitral valve involvement (I08.-)

   I36.0   **Nonrheumatic tricuspid (valve) stenosis**
   I36.1   **Nonrheumatic tricuspid (valve) insufficiency**
          Nonrheumatic tricuspid (valve) incompetence
          Nonrheumatic tricuspid (valve) regurgitation

   I36.2   **Nonrheumatic tricuspid (valve) stenosis with insufficiency**
   I36.8   **Other nonrheumatic tricuspid valve disorders**
   I36.9   **Nonrheumatic tricuspid valve disorder, unspecified**

● **I37**   **Nonrheumatic pulmonary valve disorders**
     Excludes1   pulmonary valve disorder specified as congenital
                         (Q22.1, Q22.2, Q22.3)
                   pulmonary valve disorder specified as rheumatic
                         (I09.89)

   I37.0   **Nonrheumatic pulmonary valve stenosis**
   I37.1   **Nonrheumatic pulmonary valve insufficiency**
          Nonrheumatic pulmonary valve incompetence
          Nonrheumatic pulmonary valve regurgitation

   I37.2   **Nonrheumatic pulmonary valve stenosis with insufficiency**
   I37.8   **Other nonrheumatic pulmonary valve disorders**
   I37.9   **Nonrheumatic pulmonary valve disorder, unspecified**

● **I38**   **Endocarditis, valve unspecified** 🔧
     Includes   endocarditis (chronic) NOS
                   valvular incompetence NOS
                   valvular insufficiency NOS
                   valvular regurgitation NOS
                   valvular stenosis NOS
                   valvulitis (chronic) NOS
     Excludes1   congenital insufficiency of cardiac valve NOS
                         (Q24.8)
                   congenital stenosis of cardiac valve NOS (Q24.8)
                   endocardial fibroelastosis (I42.4)
                   endocarditis specified as rheumatic (I09.1)
     (Ex) I38-I39, I87.8-I87.9, I99.8-I99.9

▷ **I39**   *Endocarditis and heart valve disorders in diseases classified elsewhere* 🔧
     Code first underlying disease, such as:
       Q fever (A78)
     Excludes1   endocardial involvement in:
                   candidiasis (B37.6)
                   gonococcal infection (A54.83)
                   Libman-Sacks disease (M32.11)
                   listerosis (A32.82)
                   meningococcal infection (A39.51)
                   rheumatoid arthritis (M05.31)
                   syphilis (A52.03)
                   tuberculosis (A18.84)
                   typhoid fever (A01.02)
     (Ex) I38-I39, I87.8-I87.9, I99.8-I99.9

● **I40**   **Acute myocarditis**
     Inflammation of heart muscle due to infection (viral/bacterial)
     Includes   subacute myocarditis
     Excludes1   acute rheumatic myocarditis (I01.2)
     (Ex) **For category I40 CC codes:** I01.2, I09.0, I23.0-I23.3, I23.6-I23.8, I40.0-I41, I51.0,
         I51.4, I87.8-I87.9, I99.8-I99.9

   I40.0   **Infective myocarditis** 🔧
          Septic myocarditis
          Use additional code (B95-B97) to identify infectious
               agent

   I40.1   **Isolated myocarditis** 🔧
          Fiedler's myocarditis
          Giant cell myocarditis
          Idiopathic myocarditis

   I40.8   **Other acute myocarditis** 🔧
   I40.9   **Acute myocarditis, unspecified** 🔧

▷ **I41**   *Myocarditis in diseases classified elsewhere* 🔧
     Code first underlying disease, such as:
       typhus (A75.0-A75.9)
     Excludes1   myocarditis (in):
                   Chagas' disease (chronic) (B57.2)
                   acute (B57.0)
                   coxsackie (virus) infection (B33.22)
                   diphtheritic (A36.81)
                   gonococcal (A54.83)
                   influenzal (J09.X9, J10.82, J11.82)
                   meningococcal (A39.52)
                   mumps (B26.82)
                   rheumatoid arthritis (M05.31)
                   sarcoid (D86.85)
                   syphilis (A52.06)
                   toxoplasmosis (B58.81)
                   tuberculous (A18.84)
     (Ex) See I40

N   Newborn Age: 0   P   Pediatric Age: 0–17   M   Maternity DX: 12–55   A   Adult Age: 15–124   ♀   Females Only   ♂   Males Only

🔧   Complication\Comorbidity   🔧   Major C\C   (Ex)   CC/MCC Exclusions   🔧   Hospital-Acquired Condition

● **I42 Cardiomyopathy**
Disease of the heart muscle resulting in an abnormally enlarged, weakened, thickened, and/or stiffened muscles

Includes myocardiopathy

Code first pre-existing cardiomyopathy complicating pregnancy and puerperium (O99.4)

Excludes2 ischemic cardiomyopathy (I25.5) ◄
peripartum cardiomyopathy (O90.3) ◄
ventricular hypertrophy (I51.7)

(Ex) **For category I42 CC codes:** I09.81, I11.0, I13.0, I13.2, I25.10-I25.119, I25.5-I25.799, I25.811-I25.9, I42.0-I44.1, I44.30-I44.39, I45.2-I45.4, I45.81-I45.89, I48.0-I49.1, I49.3-I49.8, I50.1, I50.9, I87.8-I87.9, I99.8-I99.9, Q24.6, R00.0-R00.2, R57.0, R57.9

I42.0 Dilated cardiomyopathy 🔖
Congestive cardiomyopathy

I42.1 Obstructive hypertrophic cardiomyopathy 🔖
Hypertrophic subaortic stenosis (idiopathic)

I42.2 Other hypertrophic cardiomyopathy 🔖
Nonobstructive hypertrophic cardiomyopathy

I42.3 Endomyocardial (eosinophilic) disease 🔖
Endomyocardial (tropical) fibrosis
Löffler's endocarditis

I42.4 Endocardial fibroelastosis 🔖
Congenital cardiomyopathy
Elastomyofibrosis

I42.5 Other restrictive cardiomyopathy 🔖
Constrictive cardiomyopathy NOS

I42.6 Alcoholic cardiomyopathy 🔖
Code also presence of alcoholism (F10.-)

I42.7 Cardiomyopathy due to drug and external agent 🔖
Code first poisoning due to drug or toxin, if applicable (T36-T65 with fifth or sixth character 1-4 or 6)
Use additional code for adverse effect, if applicable, to identify drug (T36-T50 with fifth or sixth character 5)

I42.8 Other cardiomyopathies 🔖

I42.9 Cardiomyopathy, unspecified 🔖
Cardiomyopathy (primary) (secondary) NOS

▶ **I43 Cardiomyopathy in diseases classified elsewhere** 🔖
Code first underlying disease, such as:
amyloidosis (E85.-)
glycogen storage disease (E74.0)
gout (M10.0-)
thyrotoxicosis (E05.0-E05.9-)

Excludes1 cardiomyopathy (in):
coxsackie (virus) (B33.24)
diphtheria (A36.81)
sarcoidosis (D86.85)
tuberculosis (A18.84)

(Ex) See I42

● **I44 Atrioventricular and left bundle-branch block**
Conduction problem resulting in arrhythmias/dysrhythmias due to a lack of electrical impulses being transmitted normally through the heart

I44.0 Atrioventricular block, first degree

I44.1 Atrioventricular block, second degree
Atrioventricular block, type I and II
Möbitz block, type I and II
Second degree block, type I and II
Wenckebach's block

I44.2 Atrioventricular block, complete 🔖
Complete heart block NOS
Third degree block
(Ex) I44.0-I49.02, I49.2, I49.8, I87.8-I87.9, I99.8-I99.9, R00.1

● **I44.3 Other and unspecified atrioventricular block**
Atrioventricular block NOS

I44.30 Unspecified atrioventricular block

I44.39 Other atrioventricular block

I44.4 Left anterior fascicular block
MCE: Questionable admission when principal dx

I44.5 Left posterior fascicular block
MCE: Questionable admission when principal dx

● **I44.6 Other and unspecified fascicular block**

I44.60 Unspecified fascicular block
Left bundle-branch hemiblock NOS
MCE: Questionable admission when principal dx

I44.69 Other fascicular block
MCE: Questionable admission when principal dx

I44.7 Left bundle-branch block, unspecified
MCE: Questionable admission when principal dx

● **I45 Other conduction disorders**

I45.0 Right fascicular block
MCE: Questionable admission when principal dx

● **I45.1 Other and unspecified right bundle-branch block**

I45.10 Unspecified right bundle-branch block
Right bundle-branch block NOS
MCE: Questionable admission when principal dx

I45.19 Other right bundle-branch block
MCE: Questionable admission when principal dx

I45.2 Bifascicular block 🔖
(Ex) See I44.2

I45.3 Trifascicular block 🔖
(Ex) See I44.2

I45.4 Nonspecific intraventricular block
Bundle-branch block NOS

I45.5 Other specified heart block
Sinoatrial block
Sinoauricular block

Excludes1 heart block NOS (I45.9)

I45.6 Pre-excitation syndrome
Accelerated atrioventricular conduction
Accessory atrioventricular conduction
Anomalous atrioventricular excitation
Lown-Ganong-Levine syndrome
Pre-excitation atrioventricular conduction
Wolff-Parkinson-White syndrome

● **I45.8 Other specified conduction disorders**

I45.81 Long QT syndrome

I45.89 Other specified conduction disorders 🔖
Atrioventricular [AV] dissociation
Interference dissociation
Isorhythmic dissociation
Nonparoxysmal AV nodal tachycardia
(Ex) See I44.2
Coding Clinic: 2013, Q2, P32

I45.9 Conduction disorder, unspecified
Heart block NOS
Stokes-Adams syndrome

● **I46 Cardiac arrest**
Excludes1 cardiogenic shock (R57.0)
(Ex) **For category I46 CC codes:** I46.2-I49.02, I49.2, I87.8-I87.9, I99.8-I99.9

I46.2 Cardiac arrest due to underlying cardiac condition 🔖
Code first underlying cardiac condition
MCC: If patient discharged alive

I46.8 Cardiac arrest due to other underlying condition 🔖
Code first underlying condition
MCC: If patient discharged alive

I46.9 Cardiac arrest, cause unspecified 🔖
MCC: If patient discharged alive

● **I47 Paroxysmal tachycardia**
Code first tachycardia complicating:
abortion or ectopic or molar pregnancy (O00-O07, O08.8)
obstetric surgery and procedures (O75.4)

Excludes1 tachycardia NOS (R00.0)
sinoauricular tachycardia NOS (R00.0)
sinus [sinusal] tachycardia NOS (R00.0)
(Ex) **For category I47 CC codes:** See I44.2

I47.0 Re-entry ventricular arrhythmia 🔖

◄ New   ◄ Revised   ~~deleted~~ Deleted   Excludes 1   Excludes 2   Includes   Use additional   Code first   Code also   Unspecified

OGCR Official Guidelines   ● Unacceptable Principal Diagnosis   X Assign placeholder X   ● Use Additional Character(s)   ▶ Manifestation Code   **Coding Clinic**

880

I47.1   Supraventricular tachycardia 🔧
    Atrial (paroxysmal) tachycardia
    Atrioventricular [AV] (paroxysmal) tachycardia
    Atrioventricular re-entrant (nodal) tachycardia
      [AVNRT] [AVRT]
    Junctional (paroxysmal) tachycardia
    Nodal (paroxysmal) tachycardia

I47.2   Ventricular tachycardia 🔧
    Coding Clinic: 2013, Q3, P23

I47.9   Paroxysmal tachycardia, unspecified
    Bouveret (-Hoffman) syndrome

● **I48   Atrial fibrillation and flutter**
    Most common abnormal heart rhythm (arrhythmia) presenting
      as irregular, rapid beating (tachycardia) of the heart's upper
      chamber.
    (Ex:) For category I48 CC codes: See I44.2

I48.0   Paroxysmal atrial fibrillation

I48.1   Persistent atrial fibrillation 🔧
    Rapid contractions of the upper heart chamber

I48.2   Chronic atrial fibrillation
    Permanent atrial fibrillation

I48.3   Typical atrial flutter 🔧
    Type I atrial flutter

I48.4   Atypical atrial flutter 🔧
    Type II atrial flutter

● **I48.9   Unspecified atrial fibrillation and atrial flutter**

    I48.91   Unspecified atrial fibrillation

    I48.92   Unspecified atrial flutter 🔧

● **I49   Other cardiac arrhythmias**
    Code first cardiac arrhythmia complicating:
      abortion or ectopic or molar pregnancy (O00-O07, O08.8)
      obstetric surgery and procedures (O75.4)

    Excludes1   bradycardia NOS (R00.1)
               neonatal dysrhythmia (P29.1-)
               sinoatrial bradycardia (R00.1)
               sinus bradycardia (R00.1)
               vagal bradycardia (R00.1)

● **I49.0   Ventricular fibrillation and flutter**

    I49.01   Ventricular fibrillation 🔧
       MCC: If patient discharged alive
       (Ex:) See I44.2

    I49.02   Ventricular flutter 🔧
       (Ex:) See I44.2

I49.1   Atrial premature depolarization
    Atrial premature beats

I49.2   Junctional premature depolarization 🔧
    (Ex:) See I44.2

I49.3   Ventricular premature depolarization

● **I49.4   Other and unspecified premature depolarization**

    I49.40   Unspecified premature depolarization
       Premature beats NOS

    I49.49   Other premature depolarization
       Ectopic beats
       Extrasystoles
       Extrasystolic arrhythmias
       Premature contractions

I49.5   Sick sinus syndrome
    Tachycardia-bradycardia syndrome

I49.8   Other specified cardiac arrhythmias
    Coronary sinus rhythm disorder
    Ectopic rhythm disorder
    Nodal rhythm disorder

I49.9   Cardiac arrhythmia, unspecified
    Arrhythmia (cardiac) NOS

● **I50   Heart failure**
    Code first heart failure complicating abortion or ectopic or molar
      pregnancy (O00-O07, O08.8)
      heart failure due to hypertension (I11.0)
      heart failure due to hypertension with chronic kidney disease
        (I13.-)
      heart failure following surgery (I97.13-)
      obstetric surgery and procedures (O75.4)
      rheumatic heart failure (I09.81)

    Excludes1   neonatal cardiac failure (P29.0)

    Excludes2   cardiac arrest (I46.-) ◄

    Coding Clinic: 2016, Q1, P38; 2015, Q2, P15

I50.1   Left ventricular failure 🔧
    Cardiac asthma
    Edema of lung with heart disease NOS
    Edema of lung with heart failure
    Left heart failure
    Pulmonary edema with heart disease NOS
    Pulmonary edema with heart failure

    Excludes1   edema of lung without heart disease or
               heart failure (J81.-)
               pulmonary edema without heart disease
               or failure (J81.-)
    (Ex:) I09.81, I11.0, I50.1-I50.9, I87.8-I87.9, I99.8-I99.9

● **I50.2   Systolic (congestive) heart failure**

    Excludes1   combined systolic (congestive) and
               diastolic (congestive) heart failure
               (I50.4-)
    (Ex:) For category I50.2 CC codes: I09.81, I11.0, I50.1-I50.9, I87.8-I87.9,
       I99.8-I99.9, J81.0

    I50.20   Unspecified systolic (congestive) heart
           failure 🔧

    I50.21   Acute systolic (congestive) heart failure 🔧
       Presenting a short and relatively severe episode

    I50.22   Chronic systolic (congestive) heart failure 🔧
       Long-lasting, presenting over time

    I50.23   Acute on chronic systolic (congestive) heart
           failure 🔧
       Combination code. What was a chronic condition
       now has an acute exacerbation (to make more
       severe).
       Coding Clinic: 2013, Q2, P33

● **I50.3   Diastolic (congestive) heart failure**

    Excludes1   combined systolic (congestive) and
               diastolic (congestive) heart failure
               (I50.4-)
    (Ex:) For category I50.3 CC codes: See I50.2

    I50.30   Unspecified diastolic (congestive) heart
           failure 🔧

    I50.31   Acute diastolic (congestive) heart failure 🔧

    I50.32   Chronic diastolic (congestive) heart failure 🔧

    I50.33   Acute on chronic diastolic (congestive) heart
           failure 🔧

● **I50.4   Combined systolic (congestive) and diastolic**
    (congestive) heart failure
    (Ex:) For category I50.4 CC codes: See I50.2

    I50.40   Unspecified combined systolic (congestive) and
           diastolic (congestive) heart failure 🔧

    I50.41   Acute combined systolic (congestive) and
           diastolic (congestive) heart failure 🔧

    I50.42   Chronic combined systolic (congestive) and
           diastolic (congestive) heart failure 🔧

    I50.43   Acute on chronic combined systolic
           (congestive) and diastolic (congestive) heart
           failure 🔧

Item 9–8 Congestive heart failure (CHF) is a condition in which the left ventricle of the heart cannot pump enough blood to the body. The blood flow from the heart slows or returns to the heart from the venous system back flow resulting in congestion (fluid accumulation) particularly in the abdomen. Most commonly, fluid collects in the lungs and results in shortness of breath, especially when in a reclining position.

N   Newborn Age: 0   **P**   Pediatric Age: 0–17   **M**   Maternity DX: 12–55   **A**   Adult Age: 15–124   ♀   Females Only   ♂   Males Only

🔧   Complication\Comorbidity   🔧   Major C\C   (Ex:)   CC/MCC Exclusions   🔧   Hospital-Acquired Condition

CHAPTER 9 (I00-I99)

I50.9   **Heart failure, unspecified**
Biventricular (heart) failure NOS
Cardiac, heart or myocardial failure NOS
Congestive heart disease
Congestive heart failure NOS
Right ventricular failure (secondary to left heart failure)
> **Excludes2**   fluid overload (E87.70) ◄
> **Coding Clinic: 2015, Q2, P15; 2012, Q4, P92**

● **I51**   **Complications and ill-defined descriptions of heart disease**
> **Excludes1**   any condition in I51.4-I51.9 due to hypertension (I11.-)
> any condition in I51.4-I51.9 due to hypertension and chronic kidney disease (I13.-)
> heart disease specified as rheumatic (I00-I09)

I51.0   **Cardiac septal defect, acquired** 🔍   A
Acquired septal atrial defect (old)
Acquired septal auricular defect (old)
Acquired septal ventricular defect (old)
> **Excludes1**   cardiac septal defect as current complication following acute myocardial infarction (I23.1, I23.2)
> (Ex:) See I23

I51.1   **Rupture of chordae tendineae, not elsewhere classified** 🔍
> **Excludes1**   rupture of chordae tendineae as current complication following acute myocardial infarction (I23.4)
> (Ex:) I23.0-I23.4, I23.6-I23.8, I51.8-I51.1, I87.8-I87.9, I99.8-I99.9

I51.2   **Rupture of papillary muscle, not elsewhere classified** 🔍
> **Excludes1**   rupture of papillary muscle as current complication following acute myocardial infarction (I23.5)
> (Ex:) I23.0-I23.3, I23.5-I23.8, I51.0, I51.2, I87.8-I87.9, I99.8-I99.9

I51.3   **Intracardiac thrombosis, not elsewhere classified**
Apical thrombosis (old)
Atrial thrombosis (old)
Auricular thrombosis (old)
Mural thrombosis (old)
Ventricular thrombosis (old)
> **Excludes1**   intracardiac thrombosis as current complication following acute myocardial infarction (I23.6)
> **Coding Clinic: 2013, Q1, P24**

I51.4   **Myocarditis, unspecified**
Chronic (interstitial) myocarditis
Myocardial fibrosis
Myocarditis NOS
> **Excludes1**   acute or subacute myocarditis (I40.-)

I51.5   **Myocardial degeneration**
Fatty degeneration of heart or myocardium
Myocardial disease
Senile degeneration of heart or myocardium

I51.7   **Cardiomegaly**
Cardiac dilatation
Cardiac hypertrophy
Ventricular dilatation

● **I51.8**   **Other ill-defined heart diseases**
I51.81   **Takotsubo syndrome** 🔍
Reversible left ventricular dysfunction following sudden emotional stress
Stress induced cardiomyopathy
Takotsubo cardiomyopathy
Transient left ventricular apical ballooning syndrome
> (Ex:) I09.81, I11.0, I50.1-I50.9, I51.81, I51.9-I52, I87.8-I87.9, I99.8-I99.9

I51.89   **Other ill-defined heart diseases**
Carditis (acute)(chronic)
Pancarditis (acute)(chronic)

I51.9   **Heart disease, unspecified**

▷ **I52**   *Other heart disorders in diseases classified elsewhere*
Code first underlying disease, such as:
congenital syphilis (A50.5)
mucopolysaccharidosis (E76.3)
schistosomiasis (B65.0-B65.9)
> **Excludes1**   heart disease (in):
> gonococcal infection (A54.83)
> meningococcal infection (A39.50)
> rheumatoid arthritis (M05.31)
> syphilis (A52.06)

CEREBROVASCULAR DISEASES (I60-I69)

Use additional code to identify presence of:
alcohol abuse and dependence (F10.-)
exposure to environmental tobacco smoke (Z77.22)
history of tobacco dependence (Z87.891) ◄▥
hypertension (I10-I15)
occupational exposure to environmental tobacco smoke (Z57.31)
tobacco dependence (F17.-)
tobacco use (Z72.0)
> **Excludes1**   transient cerebral ischemic attacks and related syndromes (G45.-)
> traumatic intracranial hemorrhage (S06.-)
> **Coding Clinic: 2015, Q4, P40**

● **I60**   **Nontraumatic subarachnoid hemorrhage**
> **Includes**   ruptured cerebral aneurysm
> **Excludes1**   syphilitic ruptured cerebral aneurysm (A52.05)
> **Excludes2**   sequelae of subarachnoid hemorrhage (I69.0-) ◄
> (Ex:) For category I60 CC codes: E03.5, G93.82, I60.00-I62.9, I87.8-I87.9, I99.8-I99.9, R40.0-R40.2224, R40.2310-R40.2324, R40.2340-R40.2344, R40.3-R40.4, S02.0XX[A,B], S02.101-S02.102[A,B], S02.109[A,B], S02.110-S02.19X[A,B], S02.91X[A,B], S06.0X0-S06.0X1[A], S06.0X9-S06.9X9[A]

● **I60.0**   **Nontraumatic subarachnoid hemorrhage from carotid siphon and bifurcation**
I60.00   **Nontraumatic subarachnoid hemorrhage from unspecified carotid siphon and bifurcation** 🔍
I60.01   **Nontraumatic subarachnoid hemorrhage from right carotid siphon and bifurcation**
I60.02   **Nontraumatic subarachnoid hemorrhage from left carotid siphon and bifurcation** 🔍

● **I60.1**   **Nontraumatic subarachnoid hemorrhage from middle cerebral artery**
I60.10   **Nontraumatic subarachnoid hemorrhage from unspecified middle cerebral artery** 🔍
I60.11   **Nontraumatic subarachnoid hemorrhage from right middle cerebral artery**
I60.12   **Nontraumatic subarachnoid hemorrhage from left middle cerebral artery** 🔍

● **I60.2**   **Nontraumatic subarachnoid hemorrhage from anterior communicating artery** 🔍
~~I60.20~~   ~~Nontraumatic subarachnoid hemorrhage from unspecified anterior communicating artery~~
~~I60.21~~   ~~Nontraumatic subarachnoid hemorrhage from right anterior communicating artery~~
~~I60.22~~   ~~Nontraumatic subarachnoid hemorrhage from left anterior communicating artery~~

● **I60.3**   **Nontraumatic subarachnoid hemorrhage from posterior communicating artery**
I60.30   **Nontraumatic subarachnoid hemorrhage from unspecified posterior communicating artery** 🔍
I60.31   **Nontraumatic subarachnoid hemorrhage from right posterior communicating artery** 🔍
I60.32   **Nontraumatic subarachnoid hemorrhage from left posterior communicating artery** 🔍

I60.4   **Nontraumatic subarachnoid hemorrhage from basilar artery** 🔍

◄ New   ▥ Revised   ~~deleted~~ Deleted   Excludes 1   Excludes 2   Includes   Use additional   Code first   Code also   Unspecified
OGCR Official Guidelines   ● Unacceptable Principal Diagnosis   X Assign placeholder X   ● Use Additional Character(s)   ▷ Manifestation Code   **Coding Clinic**

- **I60.5** Nontraumatic subarachnoid hemorrhage from vertebral artery
  - **I60.50** Nontraumatic subarachnoid hemorrhage from unspecified vertebral artery 🔖
  - **I60.51** Nontraumatic subarachnoid hemorrhage from right vertebral artery 🔖
  - **I60.52** Nontraumatic subarachnoid hemorrhage from left vertebral artery 🔖
- **I60.6** Nontraumatic subarachnoid hemorrhage from other intracranial arteries 🔖
- **I60.7** Nontraumatic subarachnoid hemorrhage from unspecified intracranial artery 🔖
  - Ruptured (congenital) berry aneurysm
  - Ruptured (congenital) cerebral aneurysm
  - Subarachnoid hemorrhage (nontraumatic) from cerebral artery NOS
  - Subarachnoid hemorrhage (nontraumatic) from communicating artery NOS
  - **Excludes1**   berry aneurysm, nonruptured (I67.1)
- **I60.8** Other nontraumatic subarachnoid hemorrhage 🔖
  - Meningeal hemorrhage
  - Rupture of cerebral arteriovenous malformation
- **I60.9** Nontraumatic subarachnoid hemorrhage, unspecified 🔖

- **I61** Nontraumatic intracerebral hemorrhage
  - **Excludes2**   sequelae of intracerebral hemorrhage (I69.1-) ◀
  - (Ex) **For category I61 CC codes:** See I60
  - **I61.0** Nontraumatic intracerebral hemorrhage in hemisphere, subcortical 🔖
    - Deep intracerebral hemorrhage (nontraumatic)
  - **I61.1** Nontraumatic intracerebral hemorrhage in hemisphere, cortical 🔖
    - Cerebral lobe hemorrhage (nontraumatic)
    - Superficial intracerebral hemorrhage (nontraumatic)
  - **I61.2** Nontraumatic intracerebral hemorrhage in hemisphere, unspecified 🔖
  - **I61.3** Nontraumatic intracerebral hemorrhage in brain stem 🔖
  - **I61.4** Nontraumatic intracerebral hemorrhage in cerebellum 🔖
  - **I61.5** Nontraumatic intracerebral hemorrhage, intraventricular 🔖
  - **I61.6** Nontraumatic intracerebral hemorrhage, multiple localized 🔖
  - **I61.8** Other nontraumatic intracerebral hemorrhage 🔖
  - **I61.9** Nontraumatic intracerebral hemorrhage, unspecified 🔖

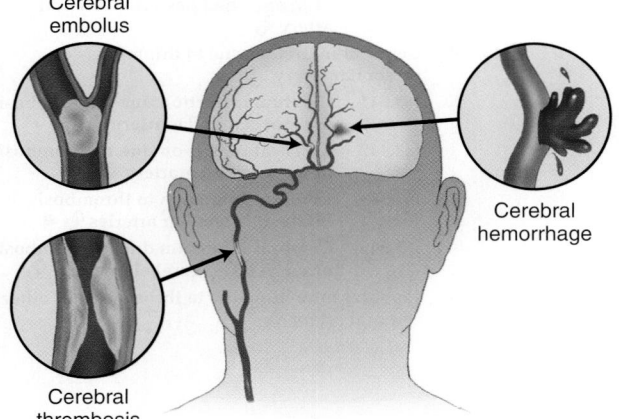

Figure 9-4   Events causing a stroke. (From Shiland: Mastering Healthcare Terminology, ed 1, St. Louis, Mosby, 2003)

- **I62** Other and unspecified nontraumatic intracranial hemorrhage
  - **Excludes2**   sequelae of intracranial hemorrhage (I69.2) ◀
  - (Ex) **For category I62 CC codes:** See I60
  - **I62.0** Nontraumatic subdural hemorrhage
    - **I62.00** Nontraumatic subdural hemorrhage, unspecified 🔖
    - **I62.01** Nontraumatic acute subdural hemorrhage 🔖
    - **I62.02** Nontraumatic subacute subdural hemorrhage 🔖
    - **I62.03** Nontraumatic chronic subdural hemorrhage 🔖
  - **I62.1** Nontraumatic extradural hemorrhage 🔖
    - Nontraumatic epidural hemorrhage
  - **I62.9** Nontraumatic intracranial hemorrhage, unspecified 🔖

⭐**(See Plate 141 on page 76.)**

- **I63** Cerebral infarction
  - **Includes**   occlusion and stenosis of cerebral and precerebral arteries, resulting in cerebral infarction
  - Use additional code, if applicable, to identify status post administration of tPA (rtPA) in a different facility within the last 24 hours prior to admission to current facility (Z92.82)
  - Use additional code, if known, to indicate National Institutes of Health Stroke Scale (NIHSS) score (R29.7-) ◀
  - **Excludes2**   sequelae of cerebral infarction (I69.3-) ◀
  - **I63.0** Cerebral infarction due to thrombosis of precerebral arteries
    - **I63.00** Cerebral infarction due to thrombosis of unspecified precerebral artery 🔖
      - (Ex) E08.51-E08.59, E08.618-E08.638, E08.649-E08.8, E09.51-E09.59, E09.618-E09.638, E09.649-E09.8, E10.51-E10.59, E10.618-E10.638, E10.649, E10.69-E10.8, E11.51-E11.59, E11.618-E11.638, E11.649, E11.69-E11.8, E13.51-E13.59, E13.618-E13.638, E13.649-E13.8, G43.601-G43.619, I63.00-I63.29, I65.01-I65.9, I87.8-I87.9, I99.8, I99.9
    - **I63.01** Cerebral infarction due to thrombosis of vertebral artery
      - (Ex) **For category I63.01 CC codes unless otherwise indicated:** E08.51-E08.59, E08.618-E08.638, E08.649-E08.8, E09.51-E09.59, E09.618-E09.638, E09.649-E09.8, E10.51-E10.59, E10.618-E10.638, E10.649, E10.69-E10.8, E11.51-E11.59, E11.618-E11.638, E11.649, E11.69-E11.8, E13.51-E13.59, E13.618-E13.638, E13.649-E13.8, G43.601-G43.619, I63.00-I63.29, I65.01-I65.9, I87.8-I87.9, I99.8-I99.9
      - **I63.011** Cerebral infarction due to thrombosis of right vertebral artery 🔖
      - **I63.012** Cerebral infarction due to thrombosis of left vertebral artery 🔖
      - **I63.013** Cerebral infarction due to thrombosis of bilateral vertebral arteries 🔖 ◀
      - **I63.019** Cerebral infarction due to thrombosis of unspecified vertebral artery 🔖
    - **I63.02** Cerebral infarction due to thrombosis of basilar artery 🔖
      - (Ex) See I63.00
    - **I63.03** Cerebral infarction due to thrombosis of carotid artery
      - (Ex) **For category I63.03 CC codes:** E08.51-E08.59, E08.618-E08.638, E08.649-E08.8, E09.51-E09.59, E09.618-E09.638, E09.649-E09.8, E10.51-E10.59, E10.618-E10.638, E10.649, E10.69-E10.8, E11.51-E11.59, E11.618-E11.638, E11.649, E11.69-E11.8, E13.51-E13.59, E13.618-E13.638, E13.649-E13.8, G43.601-G43.619, I63.00-I63.29, I65.01-I65.9, I87.8-I87.9, I99.8-I99.9
      - **I63.031** Cerebral infarction due to thrombosis of right carotid artery 🔖
      - **I63.032** Cerebral infarction due to thrombosis of left carotid artery 🔖

CHAPTER 9 (I00-I99)

I63.033   Cerebral infarction due to thrombosis of bilateral carotid arteries 🔲 ◀

I63.039   Cerebral infarction due to thrombosis of unspecified carotid artery 🔲

I63.09   Cerebral infarction due to thrombosis of other precerebral artery 🔲
          Ⓔⓧ See I63.00

● I63.1   Cerebral infarction due to embolism of precerebral arteries

I63.10   Cerebral infarction due to embolism of unspecified precerebral artery 🔲
          Ⓔⓧ See I63.00

● I63.11   Cerebral infarction due to embolism of vertebral artery
          Ⓔⓧ For category I63.11 CC codes: See I63.01

I63.111   Cerebral infarction due to embolism of right vertebral artery 🔲

I63.112   Cerebral infarction due to embolism of left vertebral artery 🔲

I63.113   Cerebral infarction due to embolism of bilateral vertebral arteries 🔲 ◀

I63.119   Cerebral infarction due to embolism of unspecified vertebral artery 🔲

I63.12   Cerebral infarction due to embolism of basilar artery 🔲
          Ⓔⓧ See I63.00

● I63.13   Cerebral infarction due to embolism of carotid artery
          Ⓔⓧ For category I63.13 CC codes: See I63.03

I63.131   Cerebral infarction due to embolism of right carotid artery 🔲

I63.132   Cerebral infarction due to embolism of left carotid artery 🔲

I63.133   Cerebral infarction due to embolism of bilateral carotid arteries 🔲 ◀

I63.139   Cerebral infarction due to embolism of unspecified carotid artery 🔲

I63.19   Cerebral infarction due to embolism of other precerebral artery 🔲
          Ⓔⓧ See I63.00

● I63.2   Cerebral infarction due to unspecified occlusion or stenosis of precerebral arteries

I63.20   Cerebral infarction due to unspecified occlusion or stenosis of unspecified precerebral arteries 🔲
          Ⓔⓧ See I63.00

● I63.21   Cerebral infarction due to unspecified occlusion or stenosis of vertebral arteries
          Ⓔⓧ For category I63.21 CC codes: See I63.01

I63.211   Cerebral infarction due to unspecified occlusion or stenosis of right vertebral arteries 🔲

I63.212   Cerebral infarction due to unspecified occlusion or stenosis of left vertebral arteries 🔲

I63.213   Cerebral infarction due to unspecified occlusion or stenosis of bilateral vertebral arteries 🔲 ◀

I63.219   Cerebral infarction due to unspecified occlusion or stenosis of unspecified vertebral arteries 🔲

I63.22   Cerebral infarction due to unspecified occlusion or stenosis of basilar arteries 🔲
          Ⓔⓧ See I63.00

● I63.23   Cerebral infarction due to unspecified occlusion or stenosis of carotid arteries
          Ⓔⓧ For category I63.23 CC codes: See I63.03

I63.231   Cerebral infarction due to unspecified occlusion or stenosis of right carotid arteries 🔲

I63.232   Cerebral infarction due to unspecified occlusion or stenosis of left carotid arteries 🔲

I63.233   Cerebral infarction due to unspecified occlusion or stenosis of bilateral carotid arteries 🔲 ◀

I63.239   Cerebral infarction due to unspecified occlusion or stenosis of unspecified carotid arteries 🔲

I63.29   Cerebral infarction due to unspecified occlusion or stenosis of other precerebral arteries 🔲
          Ⓔⓧ See I63.00

● I63.3   Cerebral infarction due to thrombosis of cerebral arteries
          Ⓔⓧ For category I63.3 CC codes: E08.51-E08.59, E08.618-E08.638, E08.649-E08.8, E09.51-E09.59, E09.618-E09.638, E09.649-E09.8, E10.51-E10.59, E10.618-E10.638, E10.649, E10.69-E10.8, E11.51-E11.59, E11.618-E11.638, E11.649, E11.69-E11.8, E13.51-E13.59, E13.618-E13.638, E13.649-E13.8, G43.601-G43.619, I63.30-I63.9, I66.01-I66.9, I87.8-I87.9, I99.8-I99.9

I63.30   Cerebral infarction due to thrombosis of unspecified cerebral artery 🔲

● I63.31   Cerebral infarction due to thrombosis of middle cerebral artery

I63.311   Cerebral infarction due to thrombosis of right middle cerebral artery 🔲

I63.312   Cerebral infarction due to thrombosis of left middle cerebral artery 🔲

I63.313   Cerebral infarction due to thrombosis of bilateral middle cerebral arteries 🔲 ◀

I63.319   Cerebral infarction due to thrombosis of unspecified middle cerebral artery 🔲

● I63.32   Cerebral infarction due to thrombosis of anterior cerebral artery

I63.321   Cerebral infarction due to thrombosis of right anterior cerebral artery 🔲

I63.322   Cerebral infarction due to thrombosis of left anterior cerebral artery 🔲

I63.323   Cerebral infarction due to thrombosis of bilateral anterior arteries 🔲 ◀

I63.329   Cerebral infarction due to thrombosis of unspecified anterior cerebral artery 🔲

● I63.33   Cerebral infarction due to thrombosis of posterior cerebral artery

I63.331   Cerebral infarction due to thrombosis of right posterior cerebral artery 🔲

I63.332   Cerebral infarction due to thrombosis of left posterior cerebral artery 🔲

I63.333   Cerebral infarction to thrombosis of bilateral posterior arteries 🔲 ◀

I63.339   Cerebral infarction due to thrombosis of unspecified posterior cerebral artery 🔲

● I63.34   Cerebral infarction due to thrombosis of cerebellar artery

I63.341   Cerebral infarction due to thrombosis of right cerebellar artery 🔲

I63.342   Cerebral infarction due to thrombosis of left cerebellar artery 🔲

I63.343   Cerebral infarction to thrombosis of bilateral cerebellar arteries 🔲 ◀

I63.349   Cerebral infarction due to thrombosis of unspecified cerebellar artery 🔲

I63.39   Cerebral infarction due to thrombosis of other cerebral artery 🔲

◀ New   ◀━ Revised   ~~deleted~~ Deleted   Excludes 1   Excludes 2   Includes   Use additional   Code first   Code also   Unspecified

OGCR Official Guidelines   ● Unacceptable Principal Diagnosis   X Assign placeholder X   ● Use Additional Character(s)   ▶ Manifestation Code   Coding Clinic

● **I63.4**   **Cerebral infarction due to embolism of cerebral arteries**
     (Ex) For category I63.4 CC codes: See I63.3

     I63.40   Cerebral infarction due to embolism of unspecified cerebral artery 🐾

● **I63.41**   Cerebral infarction due to embolism of middle cerebral artery

       I63.411   Cerebral infarction due to embolism of right middle cerebral artery 🐾

       I63.412   Cerebral infarction due to embolism of left middle cerebral artery 🐾

       I63.413   Cerebral infarction due to embolism of bilateral middle cerebral arteries 🐾 ◀

       I63.419   Cerebral infarction due to embolism of unspecified middle cerebral artery 🐾

● **I63.42**   Cerebral infarction due to embolism of anterior cerebral artery

       I63.421   Cerebral infarction due to embolism of right anterior cerebral artery 🐾

       I63.422   Cerebral infarction due to embolism of left anterior cerebral artery 🐾

       I63.423   Cerebral infarction due to embolism of bilateral anterior cerebral arteries 🐾 ◀

       I63.429   Cerebral infarction due to embolism of unspecified anterior cerebral artery 🐾

● **I63.43**   Cerebral infarction due to embolism of posterior cerebral artery

       I63.431   Cerebral infarction due to embolism of right posterior cerebral artery 🐾

       I63.432   Cerebral infarction due to embolism of left posterior cerebral artery 🐾

       I63.433   Cerebral infarction due to embolism of bilateral posterior cerebral arteries 🐾 ◀

       I63.439   Cerebral infarction due to embolism of unspecified posterior cerebral artery 🐾

● **I63.44**   Cerebral infarction due to embolism of cerebellar artery

       I63.441   Cerebral infarction due to embolism of right cerebellar artery 🐾

       I63.442   Cerebral infarction due to embolism of left cerebellar artery 🐾

       I63.443   Cerebral infarction due to embolism of bilateral cerebellar arteries 🐾 ◀

       I63.449   Cerebral infarction due to embolism of unspecified cerebellar artery 🐾

     I63.49   Cerebral infarction due to embolism of other cerebral artery 🐾

● **I63.5**   **Cerebral infarction due to unspecified occlusion or stenosis of cerebral arteries**
     (Ex) For category I63.5 CC codes: See I63.3

     I63.50   Cerebral infarction due to unspecified occlusion or stenosis of unspecified cerebral artery 🐾

● **I63.51**   Cerebral infarction due to unspecified occlusion or stenosis of middle cerebral artery

       I63.511   Cerebral infarction due to unspecified occlusion or stenosis of right middle cerebral artery 🐾

       I63.512   Cerebral infarction due to unspecified occlusion or stenosis of left middle cerebral artery 🐾

       I63.513   Cerebral infarction due to unspecified occlusion or stenosis of bilateral middle arteries 🐾 ◀

       I63.519   Cerebral infarction due to unspecified occlusion or stenosis of unspecified middle cerebral artery 🐾

● **I63.52**   Cerebral infarction due to unspecified occlusion or stenosis of anterior cerebral artery

       I63.521   Cerebral infarction due to unspecified occlusion or stenosis of right anterior cerebral artery 🐾

       I63.522   Cerebral infarction due to unspecified occlusion or stenosis of left anterior cerebral artery 🐾

       I63.523   Cerebral infarction due to unspecified occlusion or stenosis of bilateral anterior arteries 🐾 ◀

       I63.529   Cerebral infarction due to unspecified occlusion or stenosis of unspecified anterior cerebral artery 🐾

● **I63.53**   Cerebral infarction due to unspecified occlusion or stenosis of posterior cerebral artery

       I63.531   Cerebral infarction due to unspecified occlusion or stenosis of right posterior cerebral artery 🐾

       I63.532   Cerebral infarction due to unspecified occlusion or stenosis of left posterior cerebral artery 🐾

       I63.533   Cerebral infarction due to unspecified occlusion or stenosis of bilateral posterior arteries 🐾 ◀

       I63.539   Cerebral infarction due to unspecified occlusion or stenosis of unspecified posterior cerebral artery 🐾

● **I63.54**   Cerebral infarction due to unspecified occlusion or stenosis of cerebellar artery

       I63.541   Cerebral infarction due to unspecified occlusion or stenosis of right cerebellar artery 🐾

       I63.542   Cerebral infarction due to unspecified occlusion or stenosis of left cerebellar artery 🐾

       I63.543   Cerebral infarction due to unspecified occlusion or stenosis of bilateral cerebellar arteries 🐾 ◀

       I63.549   Cerebral infarction due to unspecified occlusion or stenosis of unspecified cerebellar artery 🐾

     I63.59   Cerebral infarction due to unspecified occlusion or stenosis of other cerebral artery 🐾

I63.6   Cerebral infarction due to cerebral venous thrombosis, nonpyogenic 🐾
     (Ex) See I63.3

I63.8   Other cerebral infarction 🐾
     (Ex) See I63.3

I63.9   Cerebral infarction, unspecified 🐾
     Stroke NOS
     (Ex) See I63.3
     Coding Clinic: 2015, Q1, P26

● **I65**   **Occlusion and stenosis of precerebral arteries, not resulting in cerebral infarction**

     Includes   embolism of precerebral artery
                     narrowing of precerebral artery
                     obstruction (complete) (partial) of precerebral artery
                     thrombosis of precerebral artery

     Excludes1   insufficiency, NOS, of precerebral artery (G45.-)
                     insufficiency of precerebral arteries causing cerebral infarction (I63.0-I63.2)

● **I65.0**   Occlusion and stenosis of vertebral artery

     I65.01   Occlusion and stenosis of right vertebral artery

     I65.02   Occlusion and stenosis of left vertebral artery

     I65.03   Occlusion and stenosis of bilateral vertebral arteries

     I65.09   Occlusion and stenosis of unspecified vertebral artery

I65.1   Occlusion and stenosis of basilar artery

N   Newborn Age: 0   **P**   Pediatric Age: 0–17   **M**   Maternity DX: 12–55   **A**   Adult Age: 15–124   ♀   Females Only   ♂   Males Only

 Complication\Comorbidity   🐾   Major C\C   (Ex)   CC/MCC Exclusions   🐾   Hospital-Acquired Condition

885

CHAPTER 9 (I00-I99)

● **I65.2 Occlusion and stenosis of carotid artery**

    I65.21 Occlusion and stenosis of right carotid artery

    I65.22 Occlusion and stenosis of left carotid artery

    I65.23 Occlusion and stenosis of bilateral carotid arteries

    I65.29 Occlusion and stenosis of unspecified carotid artery

I65.8 Occlusion and stenosis of other precerebral arteries

I65.9 Occlusion and stenosis of unspecified precerebral artery
    Occlusion and stenosis of precerebral artery NOS

● **I66 Occlusion and stenosis of cerebral arteries, not resulting in cerebral infarction**

    Includes   embolism of cerebral artery
                  narrowing of cerebral artery
                  obstruction (complete) (partial) of cerebral artery
                  thrombosis of cerebral artery

    Excludes1   occlusion and stenosis of cerebral artery causing cerebral infarction (I63.3-I63.5)

● **I66.0 Occlusion and stenosis of middle cerebral artery**

    I66.01 Occlusion and stenosis of right middle cerebral artery

    I66.02 Occlusion and stenosis of left middle cerebral artery

    I66.03 Occlusion and stenosis of bilateral middle cerebral arteries

    I66.09 Occlusion and stenosis of unspecified middle cerebral artery

● **I66.1 Occlusion and stenosis of anterior cerebral artery**

    I66.11 Occlusion and stenosis of right anterior cerebral artery

    I66.12 Occlusion and stenosis of left anterior cerebral artery

    I66.13 Occlusion and stenosis of bilateral anterior cerebral arteries

    I66.19 Occlusion and stenosis of unspecified anterior cerebral artery

● **I66.2 Occlusion and stenosis of posterior cerebral artery**

    I66.21 Occlusion and stenosis of right posterior cerebral artery

    I66.22 Occlusion and stenosis of left posterior cerebral artery

    I66.23 Occlusion and stenosis of bilateral posterior cerebral arteries

    I66.29 Occlusion and stenosis of unspecified posterior cerebral artery

I66.3 Occlusion and stenosis of cerebellar arteries

I66.8 Occlusion and stenosis of other cerebral arteries
    Occlusion and stenosis of perforating arteries

I66.9 Occlusion and stenosis of unspecified cerebral artery

● **I67 Other cerebrovascular diseases**

    Excludes2   sequelae of the listed conditions (I69.8) ◀

    I67.0 Dissection of cerebral arteries, nonruptured 🖰

        Excludes1   ruptured cerebral arteries (I60.7)
        (Ex) I77.2-I77.3, I77.5-I77.6, I77.89-I77.9, M31.8-M31.9

    I67.1 Cerebral aneurysm, nonruptured
        Cerebral aneurysm NOS
        Cerebral arteriovenous fistula, acquired
        Internal carotid artery aneurysm, intracranial portion
        Internal carotid artery aneurysm, NOS

        Excludes1   congenital cerebral aneurysm, nonruptured (Q28.-)
                  ruptured cerebral aneurysm (I60.7)

    I67.2 Cerebral atherosclerosis   **A**
        Atheroma of cerebral and precerebral arteries

I67.3 Progressive vascular leukoencephalopathy 🖰
    Binswanger's disease
    (Ex) A17.82, A50.42, A52.14, A75.9, A79.9, A81.00-A81.9, A83.0-A85.8, A87.2,
       A88.0, A88.8, A92.1-A92.2, A92.4-A92.8, A93.0, B00.4, B00.82,
       B01.11-B01.12, B04, B06.01, B08.09, B08.20-B08.22, B08.60-B08.79, B09,
       B10.01-B10.09, B26.2, B27.00-B27.99, B33.1, B45.0, B45.2-B45.9, B58.2,
       B75, G04.00-G04.01, G04.31, G04.81-G05.4, G37.0, G37.4-G37.5, I67.3,
       J09.X3-J09.X9, J10.2-J10.89, J11.2-J11.89, L44.4, M1A.10X0-M1A.19X1,
       P35.2-P35.9, P37.0-P37.4, P37.8-P37.9, T56.0X1-T56.0X4[A]

I67.4 Hypertensive encephalopathy 🖰
    (Ex) E08.51-E08.59, E08.618-E08.638, E08.649-E08.8, E09.51-E09.59,
       E09.618-E09.638, E09.649-E09.8, E10.51-E10.59, E10.618-E10.638, E10.649,
       E10.69-E10.8, E11.51-E11.59, E11.618-E11.638, E11.649, E11.69-E11.8,
       E13.51-E13.59, E13.618-E13.638, E13.649-E13.8, I67.4, I87.8-I87.9, I99.8-I99.9

I67.5 Moyamoya disease 🖰
    (Ex) E08.51-E08.59, E08.618-E08.638, E08.649-E08.8, E09.51-E09.59,
       E09.618-E09.638, E09.649-E09.8, E10.51-E10.59, E10.618-E10.638, E10.649,
       E10.69-E10.8, E11.51-E11.59, E11.618-E11.638, E11.649, E11.69-E11.8,
       E13.51-E13.59, E13.618-E13.638, E13.649-E13.8, I67.5, I87.8-I87.9, I99.8-I99.9

I67.6 Nonpyogenic thrombosis of intracranial venous system 🖰
    Nonpyogenic thrombosis of cerebral vein
    Nonpyogenic thrombosis of intracranial venous sinus

    Excludes1   nonpyogenic thrombosis of intracranial venous system causing infarction (I63.6)

    (Ex) E08.51-E08.59, E08.618-E08.638, E08.649-E08.8, E09.51-E09.59,
       E09.618-E09.638, E09.649-E09.8, E10.51-E10.59, E10.618-E10.638, E10.649,
       E10.69-E10.8, E11.51-E11.59, E11.618-E11.638, E11.649, E11.69-E11.8,
       E13.51-E13.59, E13.618-E13.638, E13.649-E13.8, I67.6, I87.8-I87.9, I99.8-I99.9

I67.7 Cerebral arteritis, not elsewhere classified 🖰
    Granulomatous angiitis of the nervous system

    Excludes1   allergic granulomatous angiitis (M30.1)

    (Ex) E08.51-E08.59, E08.618-E08.638, E08.649-E08.8, E09.51-E09.59,
       E09.618-E09.638, E09.649-E09.8, E10.51-E10.59, E10.618-E10.638,
       E10.649, E10.69-E10.8, E11.51-E11.59, E11.618-E11.638, E11.649,
       E11.69-E11.8, E13.51-E13.59, E13.618-E13.638, E13.649-E13.8, I67.7,
       I68.2, I87.8-I87.9, I99.8-I99.9

● **I67.8 Other specified cerebrovascular diseases**

    I67.81 Acute cerebrovascular insufficiency 🖰
        Acute cerebrovascular insufficiency unspecified as to location or reversibility
        (Ex) E08.51-E08.59, E08.618-E08.638, E08.649-E08.8, E09.51-E09.59,
           E09.618-E09.638, E09.649-E09.8, E10.51-E10.59,
           E10.618-E10.638, E10.649, E10.69-E10.8, E11.51-E11.59,
           E11.618-E11.638, E11.649, E11.69-E11.8, E13.51-E13.59,
           E13.618-E13.638, E13.649-E13.8, G45.0-G45.2, G45.8-G46.2,
           I60.00-I62.9, I63.30-I63.9, I66.01-I66.9, I67.81-I67.82,
           I67.841-I67.89, I87.8-I87.9, I99.8-I99.9

    I67.82 Cerebral ischemia 🖰
        Chronic cerebral ischemia
        (Ex) See I67.81

    I67.83 Posterior reversible encephalopathy syndrome 🖰
        PRES
        (Ex) G21.0, G83.5, G93.40-G93.41

    ● **I67.84 Cerebral vasospasm and vasoconstriction**
        (Ex) For category I67.84 CC codes: E08.51-E08.59,
           E08.618-E08.638, E08.649-E08.8, E09.51-E09.59,
           E09.618-E09.638, E09.649-E09.8, E10.51-E10.59,
           E10.618-E10.638, E10.649, E10.69-E10.8, E11.51-E11.59,
           E11.618-E11.638, E11.649, E11.69, E11.8, E13.51-E13.59,
           E13.618-E13.638, E13.649-E13.8, G45.0-G45.2, G45.8-G46.2,
           I63.00-I63.02, I63.033, I63.113, I63.133, I63.213, I63.233,
           I63.039, I63.09, I63.139, I63.19-I63.239, I63.29, I65.01-I65.9,
           I67.841-I67.848, I87.8-I87.9, I99.8-I99.9

        I67.841 Reversible cerebrovascular vasoconstriction syndrome 🖰
            Call-Fleming syndrome

            Code first underlying condition, if applicable, such as eclampsia (O15.00-O15.9)

        I67.848 Other cerebrovascular vasospasm and vasoconstriction 🖰

    I67.89 Other cerebrovascular disease 🖰
        (Ex) See I67.81

I67.9 Cerebrovascular disease, unspecified

◀ New   ◀◀ Revised   ~~deleted~~ Deleted   Excludes 1   Excludes 2   Includes   Use additional   Code first   Code also   Unspecified

OGCR Official Guidelines   ● Unacceptable Principal Diagnosis   X Assign placeholder X   ● Use Additional Character(s)   ▶ Manifestation Code   **Coding Clinic**

● **I68**   **Cerebrovascular disorders in diseases classified elsewhere**

▷ **I68.Ø**   *Cerebral amyloid angiopathy*

   Code first *underlying amyloidosis (E85.-)*

▷ **I68.2**   *Cerebral arteritis in other diseases classified elsewhere* 🔖

   Code first *underlying disease*

Excludes1	cerebral arteritis (in):
	listerosis (A32.89)
	systemic lupus erythematosus (M32.19)
	syphilis (A52.Ø4)
	tuberculosis (A18.89)

   (Ex:) See I67.7

▷ **I68.8**   *Other cerebrovascular disorders in diseases classified elsewhere*

   Code first *underlying disease*

Excludes1	syphilitic cerebral aneurysm (A52.Ø5)

OGCR Section I.c.9.d.

Sequelae of Cerebrovascular Disease

1) Category I69, Sequelae of Cerebrovascular disease

Category I69 is used to indicate conditions classifiable to categories I6Ø-I67 as the causes of sequela (neurologic deficits), themselves classified elsewhere. These "late effects" include neurologic deficits that persist after initial onset of conditions classifiable to categories I6Ø-I67. The neurologic deficits caused by cerebrovascular disease may be present from the onset of may arise at any time after the onset of the condition classifiable to categories I6Ø-I67.

Codes from category I69, Sequelae of cerebrovascular disease, that specify hemiplegia, hemiparesis and monoplegia identify whether the dominant or nondominant side is affected. Should the affected side be documented, but not specified as dominant or nondominant, and the classification system does not indicate a default, code selection is as follows:

For ambidextrous patients, the default should be dominant.

If the left side is affected, the default is non-dominant.

If the right side is affected, the default is dominant.

2) Codes from category I69 with codes from I6Ø-I67

Codes from category I69 may be assigned on a health care record with codes from I6Ø-I67, if the patient has a current cerebrovascular disease and deficits from an old cerebrovascular disease.

● **I69**   **Sequelae of cerebrovascular disease**

   Note: Category I69 is to be used to indicate conditions in I6Ø-I67 as the cause of sequelae. The 'sequelae' include conditions specified as such or as residuals which may occur at any time after the onset of the causal condition.

Excludes1	personal history of cerebral infarction without residual deficit (Z86.73)
	personal history of prolonged reversible ischemic neurologic deficit (PRIND) (Z86.73)
	personal history of reversible ischemic neurologcial deficit (RIND) (Z86.73)
	sequelae of traumatic intracranial injury (SØ6.-)
	transient ischemic attack (TIA) (G45.9)

   Coding Clinic: 2Ø15, Q4, P4Ø; 2Ø12, Q4, P1Ø7

● **I69.Ø**   **Sequelae of nontraumatic subarachnoid hemorrhage**

   I69.ØØ   Unspecified sequelae of nontraumatic subarachnoid hemorrhage

   ● **I69.Ø1**   **Cognitive deficits following nontraumatic subarachnoid hemorrhage**

      I69.Ø1Ø   **Attention and concentration deficit following nontraumatic subarachnoid hemorrhage** ◀

      I69.Ø11   **Memory deficit following nontraumatic subarachnoid hemorrhage** ◀

      I69.Ø12   **Visuospatial deficit and spatial neglect following nontraumatic subarachnoid hemorrhage** ◀

      I69.Ø13   **Psychomotor deficit following nontraumatic subarachnoid hemorrhage** ◀

      I69.Ø14   **Frontal lobe and executive function deficit following nontraumatic subarachnoid hemorrhage** ◀

      I69.Ø15   **Cognitive social or emotional deficit following nontraumatic subarachnoid hemorrhage** ◀

      I69.Ø18   **Other symptoms and signs involving cognitive functions following nontraumatic subarachnoid hemorrhage** ◀

      I69.Ø19   Unspecified **symptoms and signs involving cognitive functions following nontraumatic subarachnoid hemorrhage** ◀

   ● **I69.Ø2**   **Speech and language deficits following nontraumatic subarachnoid hemorrhage**

      I69.Ø2Ø   **Aphasia following nontraumatic subarachnoid hemorrhage**

      I69.Ø21   **Dysphasia following nontraumatic subarachnoid hemorrhage**

      I69.Ø22   **Dysarthria following nontraumatic subarachnoid hemorrhage**

      I69.Ø23   **Fluency disorder following nontraumatic subarachnoid hemorrhage**

         Stuttering following nontraumatic subarachnoid hemorrhage

      I69.Ø28   **Other speech and language deficits following nontraumatic subarachnoid hemorrhage**

   ● **I69.Ø3**   **Monoplegia of upper limb following nontraumatic subarachnoid hemorrhage**

      I69.Ø31   **Monoplegia of upper limb following nontraumatic subarachnoid hemorrhage affecting right dominant side**

      I69.Ø32   **Monoplegia of upper limb following nontraumatic subarachnoid hemorrhage affecting left dominant side**

      I69.Ø33   **Monoplegia of upper limb following nontraumatic subarachnoid hemorrhage affecting right non-dominant side**

      I69.Ø34   **Monoplegia of upper limb following nontraumatic subarachnoid hemorrhage affecting left non-dominant side**

      I69.Ø39   **Monoplegia of upper limb following nontraumatic subarachnoid hemorrhage affecting** unspecified **side**

   ● **I69.Ø4**   **Monoplegia of lower limb following nontraumatic subarachnoid hemorrhage**

      I69.Ø41   **Monoplegia of lower limb following nontraumatic subarachnoid hemorrhage affecting right dominant side**

      I69.Ø42   **Monoplegia of lower limb following nontraumatic subarachnoid hemorrhage affecting left dominant side**

      I69.Ø43   **Monoplegia of lower limb following nontraumatic subarachnoid hemorrhage affecting right non-dominant side**

      I69.Ø44   **Monoplegia of lower limb following nontraumatic subarachnoid hemorrhage affecting left non-dominant side**

      I69.Ø49   **Monoplegia of lower limb following nontraumatic subarachnoid hemorrhage affecting** unspecified **side**

N Newborn Age: Ø   **P** Pediatric Age: Ø–17   **M** Maternity DX: 12–55   **A** Adult Age: 15–124   ♀ Females Only   ♂ Males Only

🔖 Complication\Comorbidity   🔖 Major C\C   (Ex:) CC/MCC Exclusions   🔖 Hospital-Acquired Condition

887

● I69.05 **Hemiplegia and hemiparesis following nontraumatic subarachnoid hemorrhage**

I69.051 **Hemiplegia and hemiparesis following nontraumatic subarachnoid hemorrhage affecting right dominant side** 🔗

Ex: I69.051-I69.052, I69.151-I69.152, I69.251-I69.252, I69.351-I69.352, I69.851-I69.852, I69.951-I69.952

I69.052 **Hemiplegia and hemiparesis following nontraumatic subarachnoid hemorrhage affecting left dominant side** 🔗

Ex: See I69.051

I69.053 **Hemiplegia and hemiparesis following nontraumatic subarachnoid hemorrhage affecting right non-dominant side** 🔗

Ex: I69.053-I69.054, I69.153-I69.154, I69.253-I69.254, I69.353-I69.354, I69.853-I69.854, I69.953-I69.954

I69.054 **Hemiplegia and hemiparesis following nontraumatic subarachnoid hemorrhage affecting left non-dominant side** 🔗

Ex: See I69.053

I69.059 **Hemiplegia and hemiparesis following nontraumatic subarachnoid hemorrhage affecting unspecified side** 🔗

Ex: I69.059, I69.159, I69.259, I69.359, I69.859, I69.959

● I69.06 **Other paralytic syndrome following nontraumatic subarachnoid hemorrhage**

Use additional code to identify type of paralytic syndrome, such as:
locked-in state (G83.5)
quadriplegia (G82.5-)

Excludes 1 hemiplegia/hemiparesis following nontraumatic subarachnoid hemorrhage (I69.05-)
monoplegia of lower limb following nontraumatic subarachnoid hemorrhage (I69.04-)
monoplegia of upper limb following nontraumatic subarachnoid hemorrhage (I69.03-)

I69.061 **Other paralytic syndrome following nontraumatic subarachnoid hemorrhage affecting right dominant side**

I69.062 **Other paralytic syndrome following nontraumatic subarachnoid hemorrhage affecting left dominant side**

I69.063 **Other paralytic syndrome following nontraumatic subarachnoid hemorrhage affecting right non-dominant side**

I69.064 **Other paralytic syndrome following nontraumatic subarachnoid hemorrhage affecting left non-dominant side**

I69.065 **Other paralytic syndrome following nontraumatic subarachnoid hemorrhage, bilateral**

I69.069 **Other paralytic syndrome following nontraumatic subarachnoid hemorrhage affecting unspecified side**

● I69.09 **Other sequelae of nontraumatic subarachnoid hemorrhage**

I69.090 **Apraxia following nontraumatic subarachnoid hemorrhage**

I69.091 **Dysphagia following nontraumatic subarachnoid hemorrhage**

Use additional code to identify the type of dysphagia, if known (R13.1-)

I69.092 **Facial weakness following nontraumatic subarachnoid hemorrhage**

Facial droop following nontraumatic subarachnoid hemorrhage

I69.093 **Ataxia following nontraumatic subarachnoid hemorrhage**

I69.098 **Other sequelae following nontraumatic subarachnoid hemorrhage**

Alterations of sensation following nontraumatic subarachnoid hemorrhage

Disturbance of vision following nontraumatic subarachnoid hemorrhage

Use additional code to identify the sequelae

● I69.1 **Sequelae of nontraumatic intracerebral hemorrhage**

I69.10 **Unspecified sequelae of nontraumatic intracerebral hemorrhage**

● I69.11 **Cognitive deficits following nontraumatic intracerebral hemorrhage**

I69.110 **Attention and concentration deficit following nontraumatic intracerebral hemorrhage** ◀

I69.111 **Memory deficit following nontraumatic intracerebral hemorrhage** ◀

I69.112 **Visuospatial deficit and spatial neglect following nontraumatic intracerebral hemorrhage** ◀

I69.113 **Psychomotor deficit following nontraumatic intracerebral hemorrhage** ◀

I69.114 **Frontal lobe and executive function deficit following nontraumatic intracerebral hemorrhage** ◀

I69.115 **Cognitive social or emotional deficit following nontraumatic intracerebral hemorrhage** ◀

I69.118 **Other symptoms and signs involving cognitive functions following nontraumatic intracerebral hemorrhage** ◀

I69.119 **Unspecified symptoms and signs involving cognitive functions following nontraumatic intracerebral hemorrhage** ◀

● I69.12 **Speech and language deficits following nontraumatic intracerebral hemorrhage**

I69.120 **Aphasia following nontraumatic intracerebral hemorrhage**

I69.121 **Dysphasia following nontraumatic intracerebral hemorrhage**

I69.122 **Dysarthria following nontraumatic intracerebral hemorrhage**

CHAPTER 9 (I00-I99)

I69.123   **Fluency disorder following nontraumatic intracerebral hemorrhage**
Stuttering following nontraumatic intracerebral hemorrhage ◀▥

I69.128   **Other speech and language deficits following nontraumatic intracerebral hemorrhage**

● I69.13   **Monoplegia of upper limb following nontraumatic intracerebral hemorrhage**

I69.131   **Monoplegia of upper limb following nontraumatic intracerebral hemorrhage affecting right dominant side**

I69.132   **Monoplegia of upper limb following nontraumatic intracerebral hemorrhage affecting left dominant side**

I69.133   **Monoplegia of upper limb following nontraumatic intracerebral hemorrhage affecting right non-dominant side**

I69.134   **Monoplegia of upper limb following nontraumatic intracerebral hemorrhage affecting left non-dominant side**

I69.139   **Monoplegia of upper limb following nontraumatic intracerebral hemorrhage affecting unspecified side**

● I69.14   **Monoplegia of lower limb following nontraumatic intracerebral hemorrhage**

I69.141   **Monoplegia of lower limb following nontraumatic intracerebral hemorrhage affecting right dominant side**

I69.142   **Monoplegia of lower limb following nontraumatic intracerebral hemorrhage affecting left dominant side**

I69.143   **Monoplegia of lower limb following nontraumatic intracerebral hemorrhage affecting right non-dominant side**

I69.144   **Monoplegia of lower limb following nontraumatic intracerebral hemorrhage affecting left non-dominant side**

I69.149   **Monoplegia of lower limb following nontraumatic intracerebral hemorrhage affecting unspecified side**

● I69.15   **Hemiplegia and hemiparesis following nontraumatic intracerebral hemorrhage**

I69.151   **Hemiplegia and hemiparesis following nontraumatic intracerebral hemorrhage affecting right dominant side** 🇶
(Ex) See I69.051

I69.152   **Hemiplegia and hemiparesis following nontraumatic intracerebral hemorrhage affecting left dominant side** 🇶
(Ex) See I69.051

I69.153   **Hemiplegia and hemiparesis following nontraumatic intracerebral hemorrhage affecting right non-dominant side** 🇶
(Ex) See I69.053

I69.154   **Hemiplegia and hemiparesis following nontraumatic intracerebral hemorrhage affecting left non-dominant side** 🇶
(Ex) See I69.053

I69.159   **Hemiplegia and hemiparesis following nontraumatic intracerebral hemorrhage affecting unspecified side** 🇶
(Ex) See I69.059

● I69.16   **Other paralytic syndrome following nontraumatic intracerebral hemorrhage**
Use additional code to identify type of paralytic syndrome, such as:
locked-in state (G83.5)
quadriplegia (G82.5-)

Excludes1   hemiplegia/hemiparesis following nontraumatic intracerebral hemorrhage (I69.15-)
monoplegia of lower limb following nontraumatic intracerebral hemorrhage (I69.14-)
monoplegia of upper limb following nontraumatic intracerebral hemorrhage (I69.13-)

I69.161   **Other paralytic syndrome following nontraumatic intracerebral hemorrhage affecting right dominant side**

I69.162   **Other paralytic syndrome following nontraumatic intracerebral hemorrhage affecting left dominant side**

I69.163   **Other paralytic syndrome following nontraumatic intracerebral hemorrhage affecting right non-dominant side**

I69.164   **Other paralytic syndrome following nontraumatic intracerebral hemorrhage affecting left non-dominant side**

I69.165   **Other paralytic syndrome following nontraumatic intracerebral hemorrhage, bilateral**

I69.169   **Other paralytic syndrome following nontraumatic intracerebral hemorrhage affecting unspecified side**

● I69.19   **Other sequelae of nontraumatic intracerebral hemorrhage**

I69.190   **Apraxia following nontraumatic intracerebral hemorrhage**

I69.191   **Dysphagia following nontraumatic intracerebral hemorrhage**
Use additional code to identify the type of dysphagia, if known (R13.1-)

I69.192   **Facial weakness following nontraumatic intracerebral hemorrhage**
Facial droop following nontraumatic intracerebral hemorrhage

I69.193   **Ataxia following nontraumatic intracerebral hemorrhage**

I69.198   **Other sequelae of nontraumatic intracerebral hemorrhage**
Alteration of sensations following nontraumatic intracerebral hemorrhage
Disturbance of vision following nontraumatic intracerebral hemorrhage
Use additional code to identify the sequelae

N Newborn Age: 0   **P** Pediatric Age: 0–17   **M** Maternity DX: 12–55   **A** Adult Age: 15–124   ♀ Females Only   ♂ Males Only

🇶 Complication\Comorbidity   🇶 Major C\C   (Ex) CC/MCC Exclusions   🇶 Hospital-Acquired Condition

889

CHAPTER 9 (I00-I99)

● I69.2   **Sequelae of other nontraumatic intracranial hemorrhage**

I69.20   Unspecified sequelae of other nontraumatic intracranial hemorrhage

● I69.21   Cognitive deficits following other nontraumatic intracranial hemorrhage

I69.210   Attention and concentration deficit following other nontraumatic intracranial hemorrhage ◄

I69.211   Memory deficit following other nontraumatic intracranial hemorrhage ◄

I69.212   Visuospatial deficit and spatial neglect following other nontraumatic intracranial hemorrhage ◄

I69.213   Psychomotor deficit following other nontraumatic intracranial hemorrhage ◄

I69.214   Frontal lobe and executive function deficit following other nontraumatic intracranial hemorrhage ◄

I69.215   Cognitive social or emotional deficit following other nontraumatic intracranial hemorrhage ◄

I69.218   Other symptoms and signs involving cognitive functions following other nontraumatic intracranial hemorrhage ◄

I69.219   Unspecified symptoms and signs involving cognitive functions following other nontraumatic intracranial hemorrhage ◄

● I69.22   Speech and language deficits following other nontraumatic intracranial hemorrhage

I69.220   Aphasia following other nontraumatic intracranial hemorrhage

I69.221   Dysphasia following other nontraumatic intracranial hemorrhage

I69.222   Dysarthria following other nontraumatic intracranial hemorrhage

I69.223   Fluency disorder following other nontraumatic intracranial hemorrhage
Stuttering following other nontraumatic intracranial hemorrhage ◄▪▪

I69.228   Other speech and language deficits following other nontraumatic intracranial hemorrhage

● I69.23   Monoplegia of upper limb following other nontraumatic intracranial hemorrhage

I69.231   Monoplegia of upper limb following other nontraumatic intracranial hemorrhage affecting right dominant side

I69.232   Monoplegia of upper limb following other nontraumatic intracranial hemorrhage affecting left dominant side

I69.233   Monoplegia of upper limb following other nontraumatic intracranial hemorrhage affecting right non-dominant side

I69.234   Monoplegia of upper limb following other nontraumatic intracranial hemorrhage affecting left non-dominant side

I69.239   Monoplegia of upper limb following other nontraumatic intracranial hemorrhage affecting unspecified side

● I69.24   Monoplegia of lower limb following other nontraumatic intracranial hemorrhage

I69.241   Monoplegia of lower limb following other nontraumatic intracranial hemorrhage affecting right dominant side

I69.242   Monoplegia of lower limb following other nontraumatic intracranial hemorrhage affecting left dominant side

I69.243   Monoplegia of lower limb following other nontraumatic intracranial hemorrhage affecting right non-dominant side

I69.244   Monoplegia of lower limb following other nontraumatic intracranial hemorrhage affecting left non-dominant side

I69.249   Monoplegia of lower limb following other nontraumatic intracranial hemorrhage affecting unspecified side

● I69.25   Hemiplegia and hemiparesis following other nontraumatic intracranial hemorrhage

I69.251   Hemiplegia and hemiparesis following other nontraumatic intracranial hemorrhage affecting right dominant side
(Ex) See I69.051

I69.252   Hemiplegia and hemiparesis following other nontraumatic intracranial hemorrhage affecting left dominant side
(Ex) See I69.051

I69.253   Hemiplegia and hemiparesis following other nontraumatic intracranial hemorrhage affecting right non-dominant side
(Ex) See I69.053

I69.254   Hemiplegia and hemiparesis following other nontraumatic intracranial hemorrhage affecting left non-dominant side
(Ex) See I69.053

I69.259   Hemiplegia and hemiparesis following other nontraumatic intracranial hemorrhage affecting unspecified side
(Ex) See I69.059

● I69.26   Other paralytic syndrome following other nontraumatic intracranial hemorrhage

Use additional code to identify type of paralytic syndrome, such as:
locked-in state (G83.5)
quadriplegia (G82.5-)

Excludes 1   hemiplegia/hemiparesis following other nontraumatic intracranial hemorrhage (I69.25-)
monoplegia of lower limb following other nontraumatic intracranial hemorrhage (I69.24-)
monoplegia of upper limb following other nontraumatic intracranial hemorrhage (I69.23-)

I69.261   Other paralytic syndrome following other nontraumatic intracranial hemorrhage affecting right dominant side

I69.262   Other paralytic syndrome following other nontraumatic intracranial hemorrhage affecting left dominant side

I69.263   Other paralytic syndrome following other nontraumatic intracranial hemorrhage affecting right non-dominant side

I69.264   Other paralytic syndrome following other nontraumatic intracranial hemorrhage affecting left non-dominant side

I69.265   Other paralytic syndrome following other nontraumatic intracranial hemorrhage, bilateral

I69.269   Other paralytic syndrome following other nontraumatic intracranial hemorrhage affecting unspecified side

● **I69.29**   Other sequelae of other nontraumatic intracranial hemorrhage

I69.290   Apraxia following other nontraumatic intracranial hemorrhage

I69.291   Dysphagia following other nontraumatic intracranial hemorrhage
> Use additional code to identify the type of dysphagia, if known (R13.1-)

I69.292   Facial weakness following other nontraumatic intracranial hemorrhage
> Facial droop following other nontraumatic intracranial hemorrhage

I69.293   Ataxia following other nontraumatic intracranial hemorrhage

I69.298   Other sequelae of other nontraumatic intracranial hemorrhage
> Alteration of sensation following other nontraumatic intracranial hemorrhage
> Disturbance of vision following other nontraumatic intracranial hemorrhage
> Use additional code to identify the sequelae

● **I69.3**   **Sequelae of cerebral infarction**
Sequelae of stroke NOS
Coding Clinic: 2012, Q4, P92, 95

I69.30   Unspecified sequelae of cerebral infarction

● **I69.31**   Cognitive deficits following cerebral infarction

I69.310   Attention and concentration deficit following cerebral infarction ◀

I69.311   Memory deficit following cerebral infarction ◀

I69.312   Visuospatial deficit and spatial neglect following cerebral infarction ◀

I69.313   Psychomotor deficit following cerebral infarction ◀

I69.314   Frontal lobe and executive function deficit following cerebral infarction ◀

I69.315   Cognitive social or emotional deficit following cerebral infarction ◀

I69.318   Other symptoms and signs involving cognitive functions following cerebral infarction ◀

I69.319   Unspecified symptoms and signs involving cognitive functions following cerebral infarction ◀

● **I69.32**   Speech and language deficits following cerebral infarction

I69.320   Aphasia following cerebral infarction

I69.321   Dysphasia following cerebral infarction
Coding Clinic: 2012, Q4, P91

I69.322   Dysarthria following cerebral infarction

I69.323   Fluency disorder following cerebral infarction
> Stuttering following cerebral infarction ◀

I69.328   Other speech and language deficits following cerebral infarction

● **I69.33**   Monoplegia of upper limb following cerebral infarction

I69.331   Monoplegia of upper limb following cerebral infarction affecting right dominant side

I69.332   Monoplegia of upper limb following cerebral infarction affecting left dominant side

I69.333   Monoplegia of upper limb following cerebral infarction affecting right non-dominant side

I69.334   Monoplegia of upper limb following cerebral infarction affecting left non-dominant side

I69.339   Monoplegia of upper limb following cerebral infarction affecting unspecified side

● **I69.34**   Monoplegia of lower limb following cerebral infarction

I69.341   Monoplegia of lower limb following cerebral infarction affecting right dominant side

I69.342   Monoplegia of lower limb following cerebral infarction affecting left dominant side

I69.343   Monoplegia of lower limb following cerebral infarction affecting right non-dominant side

I69.344   Monoplegia of lower limb following cerebral infarction affecting left non-dominant side

I69.349   Monoplegia of lower limb following cerebral infarction affecting unspecified side

● **I69.35**   Hemiplegia and hemiparesis following cerebral infarction

I69.351   Hemiplegia and hemiparesis following cerebral infarction affecting right dominant side 🏷
> (Ex:) See I69.051
Coding Clinic: 2015, Q1, P25

I69.352   Hemiplegia and hemiparesis following cerebral infarction affecting left dominant side 🏷
> (Ex:) See I69.051

I69.353   Hemiplegia and hemiparesis following cerebral infarction affecting right non-dominant side 🏷
> (Ex:) See I69.053

I69.354   Hemiplegia and hemiparesis following cerebral infarction affecting left non-dominant side 🏷
> (Ex:) See I69.053
Coding Clinic: 2012, Q4, P91

I69.359   Hemiplegia and hemiparesis following cerebral infarction affecting unspecified side 🏷
> (Ex:) See I69.059

N Newborn Age: 0   **P** Pediatric Age: 0–17   **M** Maternity DX: 12–55   **A** Adult Age: 15–124   ♀ Females Only   ♂ Males Only
🏷 Complication\Comorbidity   Major C\C   (Ex:) CC/MCC Exclusions   Hospital-Acquired Condition
891

● **I69.36 Other paralytic syndrome following cerebral infarction**

Use additional code to identify type of paralytic syndrome, such as:
locked-in state (G83.5)
quadriplegia (G82.5-)

Excludes1   hemiplegia/hemiparesis following cerebral infarction (I69.35-)
monoplegia of lower limb following cerebral infarction (I69.34-)
monoplegia of upper limb following cerebral infarction (I69.33-)

I69.361   **Other paralytic syndrome following cerebral infarction affecting right dominant side**

I69.362   **Other paralytic syndrome following cerebral infarction affecting left dominant side**

I69.363   **Other paralytic syndrome following cerebral infarction affecting right non-dominant side**

I69.364   **Other paralytic syndrome following cerebral infarction affecting left non-dominant side**

I69.365   **Other paralytic syndrome following cerebral infarction, bilateral**

I69.369   **Other paralytic syndrome following cerebral infarction affecting unspecified side**

● **I69.39 Other sequelae of cerebral infarction**

I69.390   **Apraxia following cerebral infarction**

I69.391   **Dysphagia following cerebral infarction**

Use additional code to identify the type of dysphagia, if known (R13.1-)

I69.392   **Facial weakness following cerebral infarction**
Facial droop following cerebral infarction

I69.393   **Ataxia following cerebral infarction**

I69.398   **Other sequelae of cerebral infarction**
Alteration of sensation following cerebral infarction
Disturbance of vision following cerebral infarction
Use additional code to identify the sequelae

● **I69.8 Sequelae of other cerebrovascular diseases**

Excludes1   sequelae of traumatic intracranial injury (S06.-)

I69.80   **Unspecified sequelae of other cerebrovascular disease**

● I69.81   **Cognitive deficits following other cerebrovascular disease**

I69.810   **Attention and concentration deficit following other cerebrovascular disease** ◀

I69.811   **Memory deficit following other cerebrovascular disease** ◀

I69.812   **Visuospatial deficit and spatial neglect following other cerebrovascular disease** ◀

I69.813   **Psychomotor deficit following other cerebrovascular disease** ◀

I69.814   **Frontal lobe and executive function deficit following other cerebrovascular disease** ◀

I69.815   **Cognitive social or emotional deficit following other cerebrovascular disease** ◀

I69.818   **Other symptoms and signs involving cognitive functions following other cerebrovascular disease** ◀

I69.819   **Unspecified symptoms and signs involving cognitive functions following other cerebrovascular disease** ◀

● **I69.82 Speech and language deficits following other cerebrovascular disease**

I69.820   **Aphasia following other cerebrovascular disease**

I69.821   **Dysphasia following other cerebrovascular disease**

I69.822   **Dysarthria following other cerebrovascular disease**

I69.823   **Fluency disorder following other cerebrovascular disease**
Stuttering following other cerebrovascular disease ◀||||

I69.828   **Other speech and language deficits following other cerebrovascular disease**

● **I69.83 Monoplegia of upper limb following other cerebrovascular disease**

I69.831   **Monoplegia of upper limb following other cerebrovascular disease affecting right dominant side**

I69.832   **Monoplegia of upper limb following other cerebrovascular disease affecting left dominant side**

I69.833   **Monoplegia of upper limb following other cerebrovascular disease affecting right non-dominant side**

I69.834   **Monoplegia of upper limb following other cerebrovascular disease affecting left non-dominant side**

I69.839   **Monoplegia of upper limb following other cerebrovascular disease affecting unspecified side**

● **I69.84 Monoplegia of lower limb following other cerebrovascular disease**

I69.841   **Monoplegia of lower limb following other cerebrovascular disease affecting right dominant side**

I69.842   **Monoplegia of lower limb following other cerebrovascular disease affecting left dominant side**

I69.843   **Monoplegia of lower limb following other cerebrovascular disease affecting right non-dominant side**

I69.844   **Monoplegia of lower limb following other cerebrovascular disease affecting left non-dominant side**

I69.849   **Monoplegia of lower limb following other cerebrovascular disease affecting unspecified side**

● **I69.85 Hemiplegia and hemiparesis following other cerebrovascular disease**

I69.851   **Hemiplegia and hemiparesis following other cerebrovascular disease affecting right dominant side** 🔗
(Ex:) See I69.051

I69.852   **Hemiplegia and hemiparesis following other cerebrovascular disease affecting left dominant side** 🔗
(Ex:) See I69.051

I69.853　Hemiplegia and hemiparesis following other cerebrovascular disease affecting right non-dominant side 🝛
　　(Ex:) See I69.053

I69.854　Hemiplegia and hemiparesis following other cerebrovascular disease affecting left non-dominant side 🝛
　　(Ex:) See I69.053

I69.859　Hemiplegia and hemiparesis following other cerebrovascular disease affecting unspecified side 🝛
　　(Ex:) See I69.059

● I69.86　Other paralytic syndrome following other cerebrovascular disease

Use additional code to identify type of paralytic syndrome, such as:
locked-in state (G83.5)
quadriplegia (G82.5-)

Excludes1　hemiplegia/hemiparesis following other cerebrovascular disease (I69.85-)
monoplegia of lower limb following other cerebrovascular disease (I69.84-)
monoplegia of upper limb following other cerebrovascular disease (I69.83-)

I69.861　Other paralytic syndrome following other cerebrovascular disease affecting right dominant side

I69.862　Other paralytic syndrome following other cerebrovascular disease affecting left dominant side

I69.863　Other paralytic syndrome following other cerebrovascular disease affecting right non-dominant side

I69.864　Other paralytic syndrome following other cerebrovascular disease affecting left non-dominant side

I69.865　Other paralytic syndrome following other cerebrovascular disease, bilateral

I69.869　Other paralytic syndrome following other cerebrovascular disease affecting unspecified side

● I69.89　Other sequelae of other cerebrovascular disease

I69.890　Apraxia following other cerebrovascular disease

I69.891　Dysphagia following other cerebrovascular disease
Use additional code to identify the type of dysphagia, if known (R13.1-)

I69.892　Facial weakness following other cerebrovascular disease
Facial droop following other cerebrovascular disease

I69.893　Ataxia following other cerebrovascular disease

I69.898　Other sequelae of other cerebrovascular disease
Alteration of sensation following other cerebrovascular disease
Disturbance of vision following other cerebrovascular disease
Use additional code to identify the sequelae

● I69.9　Sequelae of unspecified cerebrovascular diseases

Excludes1　sequelae of stroke (I69.3)
sequelae of traumatic intracranial injury (S06.-)

I69.90　Unspecified sequelae of unspecified cerebrovascular disease

● I69.91　Cognitive deficits following unspecified cerebrovascular disease

I69.910　Attention and concentration deficit following unspecified cerebrovascular disease ◀

I69.911　Memory deficit following unspecified cerebrovascular disease ◀

I69.912　Visuospatial deficit and spatial neglect following unspecified cerebrovascular disease ◀

I69.913　Psychomotor deficit following unspecified cerebrovascular disease ◀

I69.914　Frontal lobe and executive function deficit following unspecified cerebrovascular disease ◀

I69.915　Cognitive social or emotional deficit following unspecified cerebrovascular disease ◀

I69.918　Other symptoms and signs involving cognitive functions following unspecified cerebrovascular disease ◀

I69.919　Unspecified symptoms and signs involving cognitive functions following unspecified cerebrovascular disease ◀

● I69.92　Speech and language deficits following unspecified cerebrovascular disease

I69.920　Aphasia following unspecified cerebrovascular disease

I69.921　Dysphasia following unspecified cerebrovascular disease

I69.922　Dysarthria following unspecified cerebrovascular disease

I69.923　Fluency disorder following unspecified cerebrovascular disease
Stuttering following unspecified cerebrovascular disease ◀

I69.928　Other speech and language deficits following unspecified cerebrovascular disease

● I69.93　Monoplegia of upper limb following unspecified cerebrovascular disease

I69.931　Monoplegia of upper limb following unspecified cerebrovascular disease affecting right dominant side

I69.932　Monoplegia of upper limb following unspecified cerebrovascular disease affecting left dominant side

I69.933　Monoplegia of upper limb following unspecified cerebrovascular disease affecting right non-dominant side

I69.934　Monoplegia of upper limb following unspecified cerebrovascular disease affecting left non-dominant side

I69.939　Monoplegia of upper limb following unspecified cerebrovascular disease affecting unspecified side

CHAPTER 9 (I00-I99)

● **I69.94** **Monoplegia of lower limb following unspecified cerebrovascular disease**

     I69.941 **Monoplegia of lower limb following unspecified cerebrovascular disease affecting right dominant side**

     I69.942 **Monoplegia of lower limb following unspecified cerebrovascular disease affecting left dominant side**

     I69.943 **Monoplegia of lower limb following unspecified cerebrovascular disease affecting right non-dominant side**

     I69.944 **Monoplegia of lower limb following unspecified cerebrovascular disease affecting left non-dominant side**

     I69.949 **Monoplegia of lower limb following unspecified cerebrovascular disease affecting unspecified side**

● **I69.95** **Hemiplegia and hemiparesis following unspecified cerebrovascular disease**

     I69.951 **Hemiplegia and hemiparesis following unspecified cerebrovascular disease affecting right dominant side**
         (Ex:) See I69.051

     I69.952 **Hemiplegia and hemiparesis following unspecified cerebrovascular disease affecting left dominant side**
         (Ex:) See I69.051

     I69.953 **Hemiplegia and hemiparesis following unspecified cerebrovascular disease affecting right non-dominant side**
         (Ex:) See I69.053

     I69.954 **Hemiplegia and hemiparesis following unspecified cerebrovascular disease affecting left non-dominant side**
         (Ex:) See I69.053

     I69.959 **Hemiplegia and hemiparesis following unspecified cerebrovascular disease affecting unspecified side**
         (Ex:) See I69.059

● **I69.96** **Other paralytic syndrome following unspecified cerebrovascular disease**

     Use additional code to identify type of paralytic syndrome, such as:
     locked-in state (G83.5)
     quadriplegia (G82.5-)

     Excludes1   hemiplegia/hemiparesis following unspecified cerebrovascular disease (I69.95-)
         monoplegia of lower limb following unspecified cerebrovascular disease (I69.94-)
         monoplegia of upper limb following unspecified cerebrovascular disease (I69.93-)

     I69.961 **Other paralytic syndrome following unspecified cerebrovascular disease affecting right dominant side**

     I69.962 **Other paralytic syndrome following unspecified cerebrovascular disease affecting left dominant side**

     I69.963 **Other paralytic syndrome following unspecified cerebrovascular disease affecting right non-dominant side**

     I69.964 **Other paralytic syndrome following unspecified cerebrovascular disease affecting left non-dominant side**

     I69.965 **Other paralytic syndrome following unspecified cerebrovascular disease, bilateral**

     I69.969 **Other paralytic syndrome following unspecified cerebrovascular disease affecting unspecified side**

● **I69.99** **Other sequelae of unspecified cerebrovascular disease**

     I69.990 **Apraxia following unspecified cerebrovascular disease**

     I69.991 **Dysphagia following unspecified cerebrovascular disease**
         Use additional code to identify the type of dysphagia, if known (R13.1-)

     I69.992 **Facial weakness following unspecified cerebrovascular disease**
         Facial droop following unspecified cerebrovascular disease

     I69.993 **Ataxia following unspecified cerebrovascular disease**

     I69.998 **Other sequelae following unspecified cerebrovascular disease**
         Alteration in sensation following unspecified cerebrovascular disease
         Disturbance of vision following unspecified cerebrovascular disease
         Use additional code to identify the sequelae

DISEASES OF ARTERIES, ARTERIOLES AND CAPILLARIES (I70-I79)

● **I70** **Atherosclerosis**

     Includes   arteriolosclerosis
         arterial degeneration
         arteriosclerosis
         arteriosclerotic vascular disease
         arteriovascular degeneration
         atheroma
         endarteritis deformans or obliterans
         senile arteritis
         senile endarteritis
         vascular degeneration

     Use additional code to identify:
     exposure to environmental tobacco smoke (Z77.22)
     history of tobacco dependence (Z87.891) ◀▥
     occupational exposure to environmental tobacco smoke (Z57.31)
     tobacco dependence (F17.-)
     tobacco use (Z72.0)

     Excludes2   arteriosclerotic cardiovascular disease (I25.1-)
         arteriosclerotic heart disease (I25.1-)
         atheroembolism (I75.-)
         cerebral atherosclerosis (I67.2)
         coronary atherosclerosis (I25.1-)
         mesenteric atherosclerosis (K55.1)
         precerebral atherosclerosis (I67.2)
         primary pulmonary atherosclerosis (I27.0)

   I70.0 **Atherosclerosis of aorta**   A

   I70.1 **Atherosclerosis of renal artery**   A
     Goldblatt's kidney

     Excludes2   atherosclerosis of renal arterioles (I12.-)

◀ New   ◀▥ Revised   ~~deleted~~ Deleted   Excludes 1   Excludes 2   Includes   Use additional   Code first   Code also   Unspecified

OGCR Official Guidelines   ● Unacceptable Principal Diagnosis   X Assign placeholder X   ● Use Additional Character(s)   ▶ Manifestation Code   **Coding Clinic**

★ **(See Plates 500, 501, and 502 on pages 60 – 62.)**

● **I70.2 Atherosclerosis of native arteries of the extremities**
Mönckeberg's (medial) sclerosis

Use additional code, if applicable, to identify chronic total occlusion of artery of extremity (I70.92)

Excludes2 atherosclerosis of bypass graft of extremities (I70.30-I70.79)

● **I70.20 Unspecified atherosclerosis of native arteries of extremities**
     I70.201 Unspecified atherosclerosis of native arteries of extremities, right leg   A
     I70.202 Unspecified atherosclerosis of native arteries of extremities, left leg   A
     I70.203 Unspecified atherosclerosis of native arteries of extremities, bilateral legs   A
     I70.208 Unspecified atherosclerosis of native arteries of extremities, other extremity   A
     I70.209 Unspecified atherosclerosis of native arteries of extremities, unspecified extremity   A

● **I70.21 Atherosclerosis of native arteries of extremities with intermittent claudication**
     I70.211 Atherosclerosis of native arteries of extremities with intermittent claudication, right leg   A
     I70.212 Atherosclerosis of native arteries of extremities with intermittent claudication, left leg   A
     I70.213 Atherosclerosis of native arteries of extremities with intermittent claudication, bilateral legs   A
     I70.218 Atherosclerosis of native arteries of extremities with intermittent claudication, other extremity   A
     I70.219 Atherosclerosis of native arteries of extremities with intermittent claudication, unspecified extremity   A

● **I70.22 Atherosclerosis of native arteries of extremities with rest pain**
Includes any condition classifiable to I70.21-
     I70.221 Atherosclerosis of native arteries of extremities with rest pain, right leg   A
     I70.222 Atherosclerosis of native arteries of extremities with rest pain, left leg   A
     I70.223 Atherosclerosis of native arteries of extremities with rest pain, bilateral legs   A
     I70.228 Atherosclerosis of native arteries of extremities with rest pain, other extremity   A
     I70.229 Atherosclerosis of native arteries of extremities with rest pain, unspecified extremity   A

● **I70.23 Atherosclerosis of native arteries of right leg with ulceration**
Includes any condition classifiable to I70.211 and I70.221
Use additional code to identify severity of ulcer (L97.-)
     I70.231 Atherosclerosis of native arteries of right leg with ulceration of thigh   A
     I70.232 Atherosclerosis of native arteries of right leg with ulceration of calf   A
     I70.233 Atherosclerosis of native arteries of right leg with ulceration of ankle   A

     I70.234 Atherosclerosis of native arteries of right leg with ulceration of heel and midfoot   A
         Atherosclerosis of native arteries of right leg with ulceration of plantar surface of midfoot
     I70.235 Atherosclerosis of native arteries of right leg with ulceration of other part of foot   A
         Atherosclerosis of native arteries of right leg extremities with ulceration of toe
     I70.238 Atherosclerosis of native arteries of right leg with ulceration of other part of lower right leg   A
     I70.239 Atherosclerosis of native arteries of right leg with ulceration of unspecified site   A

● **I70.24 Atherosclerosis of native arteries of left leg with ulceration**
Includes any condition classifiable to I70.212 and I70.222
Use additional code to identify severity of ulcer (L97.-)
     I70.241 Atherosclerosis of native arteries of left leg with ulceration of thigh   A
     I70.242 Atherosclerosis of native arteries of left leg with ulceration of calf   A
     I70.243 Atherosclerosis of native arteries of left leg with ulceration of ankle   A
     I70.244 Atherosclerosis of native arteries of left leg with ulceration of heel and midfoot   A
         Atherosclerosis of native arteries of left leg with ulceration of plantar surface of midfoot
     I70.245 Atherosclerosis of native arteries of left leg with ulceration of other part of foot   A
         Atherosclerosis of native arteries of left leg extremities with ulceration of toe
     I70.248 Atherosclerosis of native arteries of left leg with ulceration of other part of lower left leg   A
     I70.249 Atherosclerosis of native arteries of left leg with ulceration of unspecified site   A

     I70.25 Atherosclerosis of native arteries of other extremities with ulceration   A
Includes any condition classifiable to I70.218 and I70.228
Use additional code to identify the severity of the ulcer (L98.49-)

● **I70.26 Atherosclerosis of native arteries of extremities with gangrene**
Includes any condition classifiable to I70.21-, I70.22-, I70.23-, I70.24-, and I70.25-
Use additional code to identify the severity of any ulcer (L97.-, L98.49-), if applicable
Ⓔ *For category I70.26 CC codes:* G89.0-G89.4, I70.261-I70.269, I96, R29.700-R29.742, R41.0-R41.3, R41.82, R41.9, R44.8-R44.9, R45.83-R45.84, R46.0-R46.89, R52, R68.0-R68.19, R68.81-R68.83, R68.89-R69
     I70.261 Atherosclerosis of native arteries of extremities with gangrene, right leg 🅒   A
     I70.262 Atherosclerosis of native arteries of extremities with gangrene, left leg 🅒 A
     I70.263 Atherosclerosis of native arteries of extremities with gangrene, bilateral legs 🅒   A

N Newborn Age: 0   **P** Pediatric Age: 0–17   **M** Maternity DX: 12–55   **A** Adult Age: 15–124   ♀ Females Only   ♂ Males Only

🅒 Complication\Comorbidity   🅜 Major C\C   Ⓔ CC/MCC Exclusions   🅗 Hospital-Acquired Condition

895

CHAPTER 9 (I00-I99)

I70.268 **Atherosclerosis of native arteries of extremities with gangrene, other extremity** 🔗   A

I70.269 **Atherosclerosis of native arteries of extremities with gangrene, unspecified extremity** 🔗   A

● **I70.29** **Other atherosclerosis of native arteries of extremities**

I70.291 **Other atherosclerosis of native arteries of extremities, right leg**   A

I70.292 **Other atherosclerosis of native arteries of extremities, left leg**   A

I70.293 **Other atherosclerosis of native arteries of extremities, bilateral legs**   A

I70.298 **Other atherosclerosis of native arteries of extremities, other extremity**   A

I70.299 **Other atherosclerosis of native arteries of extremities, unspecified extremity**   A

● **I70.3** **Atherosclerosis of unspecified type of bypass graft(s) of the extremities**

Use additional code, if applicable, to identify chronic total occlusion of artery of extremity (I70.92)

Excludes1   embolism or thrombus of bypass graft(s) of extremities (T82.8-)

● **I70.30** **Unspecified atherosclerosis of unspecified type of bypass graft(s) of the extremities**

70.301 **Unspecified atherosclerosis of unspecified type of bypass graft(s) of the extremities, right leg**   A

I70.302 **Unspecified atherosclerosis of unspecified type of bypass graft(s) of the extremities, left leg**   A

I70.303 **Unspecified atherosclerosis of unspecified type of bypass graft(s) of the extremities, bilateral legs**   A

I70.308 **Unspecified atherosclerosis of unspecified type of bypass graft(s) of the extremities, other extremity**   A

I70.309 **Unspecified atherosclerosis of unspecified type of bypass graft(s) of the extremities, unspecified extremity**   A

● **I70.31** **Atherosclerosis of unspecified type of bypass graft(s) of the extremities with intermittent claudication**

I70.311 **Atherosclerosis of unspecified type of bypass graft(s) of the extremities with intermittent claudication, right leg**   A

I70.312 **Atherosclerosis of unspecified type of bypass graft(s) of the extremities with intermittent claudication, left leg**   A

I70.313 **Atherosclerosis of unspecified type of bypass graft(s) of the extremities with intermittent claudication, bilateral legs**   A

I70.318 **Atherosclerosis of unspecified type of bypass graft(s) of the extremities with intermittent claudication, other extremity**   A

I70.319 **Atherosclerosis of unspecified type of bypass graft(s) of the extremities with intermittent claudication, unspecified extremity**   A

● **I70.32** **Atherosclerosis of unspecified type of bypass graft(s) of the extremities with rest pain**

Includes   any condition classifiable to I70.31-

I70.321 **Atherosclerosis of unspecified type of bypass graft(s) of the extremities with rest pain, right leg**   A

I70.322 **Atherosclerosis of unspecified type of bypass graft(s) of the extremities with rest pain, left leg**   A

I70.323 **Atherosclerosis of unspecified type of bypass graft(s) of the extremities with rest pain, bilateral legs**   A

I70.328 **Atherosclerosis of unspecified type of bypass graft(s) of the extremities with rest pain, other extremity**   A

I70.329 **Atherosclerosis of unspecified type of bypass graft(s) of the extremities with rest pain, unspecified extremity**   A

● **I70.33** **Atherosclerosis of unspecified type of bypass graft(s) of the right leg with ulceration**

Includes   any condition classifiable to I70.311 and I70.321

Use additional code to identify severity of ulcer (L97.-)

(Ex) **For category I70.33 CC codes:** I70.231-I70.25, L44.8-L45, L94.2, L94.4, L97.101-L97.929, L98.411-L98.499, L98.7, L98.7-L99

I70.331 **Atherosclerosis of unspecified type of bypass graft(s) of the right leg with ulceration of thigh** 🔗
CC when PDx is its own CC

I70.332 **Atherosclerosis of unspecified type of bypass graft(s) of the right leg with ulceration of calf** 🔗   A
CC when PDx is its own CC

I70.333 **Atherosclerosis of unspecified type of bypass graft(s) of the right leg with ulceration of ankle** 🔗   A
CC when PDx is its own CC

I70.334 **Atherosclerosis of unspecified type of bypass graft(s) of the right leg with ulceration of heel and midfoot** 🔗   A
Atherosclerosis of unspecified type of bypass graft(s) of right leg with ulceration of plantar surface of midfoot
CC when PDx is its own CC

I70.335 **Atherosclerosis of unspecified type of bypass graft(s) of the right leg with ulceration of other part of foot**   A
Atherosclerosis of unspecified type of bypass graft(s) of the right leg with ulceration of toe

I70.338 **Atherosclerosis of unspecified type of bypass graft(s) of the right leg with ulceration of other part of lower leg** 🔗
CC when PDx is its own CC

I70.339 **Atherosclerosis of unspecified type of bypass graft(s) of the right leg with ulceration of unspecified site** 🔗   A
CC when PDx is its own CC

◀ New   ◀▥ Revised   ~~deleted~~ Deleted   Excludes 1   Excludes 2   Includes   Use additional   Code first   Code also   Unspecified
OGCR Official Guidelines   ● Unacceptable Principal Diagnosis   X Assign placeholder X   ● Use Additional Character(s)   ▶ Manifestation Code   **Coding Clinic**

● **I70.34** **Atherosclerosis of unspecified type of bypass graft(s) of the left leg with ulceration**

> **Includes** any condition classifiable to I70.312 and I70.322

> Use additional code to identify severity of ulcer (L97.-)

> Ⓔⓧ **For category I70.34 CC codes:** See I70.33

I70.341 Atherosclerosis of unspecified type of bypass graft(s) of the left leg with ulceration of thigh 🔵 A
CC when PDx is its own CC

I70.342 Atherosclerosis of unspecified type of bypass graft(s) of the left leg with ulceration of calf 🔵 A
CC when PDx is its own CC

I70.343 Atherosclerosis of unspecified type of bypass graft(s) of the left leg with ulceration of ankle 🔵 A
CC when PDx is its own CC

I70.344 Atherosclerosis of unspecified type of bypass graft(s) of the left leg with ulceration of heel and midfoot 🔵 A
Atherosclerosis of unspecified type of bypass graft(s) of left leg with ulceration of plantar surface of midfoot
CC when PDx is its own CC

I70.345 Atherosclerosis of unspecified type of bypass graft(s) of the left leg with ulceration of other part of foot A
Atherosclerosis of unspecified type of bypass graft(s) of the left leg with ulceration of toe

I70.348 Atherosclerosis of unspecified type of bypass graft(s) of the left leg with ulceration of other part of lower leg 🔵 A
CC when PDx is its own CC

I70.349 Atherosclerosis of unspecified type of bypass graft(s) of the left leg with ulceration of unspecified site 🔵 A
CC when PDx is its own CC

I70.35 **Atherosclerosis of unspecified type of bypass graft(s) of other extremity with ulceration** A

> **Includes** any condition classifiable to I70.318 and I70.328

> Use additional code to identify severity of ulcer (L98.49-)

● **I70.36** **Atherosclerosis of unspecified type of bypass graft(s) of the extremities with gangrene**

> **Includes** any condition classifiable to I70.31-, I70.32-, I70.33-, I70.34-, I70.35

> Use additional code to identify the severity of any ulcer (L97.-, L98.49-), if applicable

> Ⓔⓧ **For category I70.36 CC codes:** See I70.26

I70.361 Atherosclerosis of unspecified type of bypass graft(s) of the extremities with gangrene, right leg 🔵 A
CC when PDx is its own CC

I70.362 Atherosclerosis of unspecified type of bypass graft(s) of the extremities with gangrene, left leg 🔵 A
CC when PDx is its own CC

I70.363 Atherosclerosis of unspecified type of bypass graft(s) of the extremities with gangrene, bilateral legs 🔵 A
CC when PDx is its own CC

I70.368 Atherosclerosis of unspecified type of bypass graft(s) of the extremities with gangrene, other extremity 🔵 A
CC when PDx is its own CC

I70.369 Atherosclerosis of unspecified type of bypass graft(s) of the extremities with gangrene, unspecified extremity 🔵 A
CC when PDx is its own CC

● **I70.39** **Other atherosclerosis of unspecified type of bypass graft(s) of the extremities**

I70.391 Other atherosclerosis of unspecified type of bypass graft(s) of the extremities, right leg A

I70.392 Other atherosclerosis of unspecified type of bypass graft(s) of the extremities, left leg A

I70.393 Other atherosclerosis of unspecified type of bypass graft(s) of the extremities, bilateral legs A

I70.398 Other atherosclerosis of unspecified type of bypass graft(s) of the extremities, other extremity A

I70.399 Other atherosclerosis of unspecified type of bypass graft(s) of the extremities, unspecified extremity A

● **I70.4** **Atherosclerosis of autologous vein bypass graft(s) of the extremities**

> Use additional code, if applicable, to identify chronic total occlusion of artery of extremity (I70.92)

● **I70.40** **Unspecified atherosclerosis of autologous vein bypass graft(s) of the extremities**

I70.401 Unspecified atherosclerosis of autologous vein bypass graft(s) of the extremities, right leg A

I70.402 Unspecified atherosclerosis of autologous vein bypass graft(s) of the extremities, left leg A

I70.403 Unspecified atherosclerosis of autologous vein bypass graft(s) of the extremities, bilateral legs A

I70.408 Unspecified atherosclerosis of autologous vein bypass graft(s) of the extremities, other extremity A

I70.409 Unspecified atherosclerosis of autologous vein bypass graft(s) of the extremities, unspecified extremity A

● **I70.41** **Atherosclerosis of autologous vein bypass graft(s) of the extremities with intermittent claudication**

I70.411 Atherosclerosis of autologous vein bypass graft(s) of the extremities with intermittent claudication, right leg A

I70.412 Atherosclerosis of autologous vein bypass graft(s) of the extremities with intermittent claudication, left leg A

I70.413 Atherosclerosis of autologous vein bypass graft(s) of the extremities with intermittent claudication, bilateral legs A

I70.418 Atherosclerosis of autologous vein bypass graft(s) of the extremities with intermittent claudication, other extremity A

I70.419 Atherosclerosis of autologous vein bypass graft(s) of the extremities with intermittent claudication, unspecified extremity A

● **I70.42** **Atherosclerosis of autologous vein bypass graft(s) of the extremities with rest pain**

> **Includes** any condition classifiable to I70.41-

I70.421 Atherosclerosis of autologous vein bypass graft(s) of the extremities with rest pain, right leg A

I70.422 Atherosclerosis of autologous vein bypass graft(s) of the extremities with rest pain, left leg A

N Newborn Age: 0 **P** Pediatric Age: 0–17 **M** Maternity DX: 12–55 **A** Adult Age: 15–124 ♀ Females Only ♂ Males Only

🔵 Complication\Comorbidity 🔵 Major C\C Ⓔⓧ CC/MCC Exclusions 🔵 Hospital-Acquired Condition

897

CHAPTER 9 (I00–I99)

CHAPTER 9 (I00-I99)

I70.423   **Atherosclerosis of autologous vein bypass graft(s) of the extremities with rest pain, bilateral legs**   A

I70.428   **Atherosclerosis of autologous vein bypass graft(s) of the extremities with rest pain, other extremity**   A

I70.429   **Atherosclerosis of autologous vein bypass graft(s) of the extremities with rest pain, unspecified extremity**   A

● **I70.43**   **Atherosclerosis of autologous vein bypass graft(s) of the right leg with ulceration**

> **Includes**   any condition classifiable to I70.411 and I70.421

> Use additional code to identify severity of ulcer (L97.-)

> (Ex) For category I70.43 CC codes: See I70.33

I70.431   **Atherosclerosis of autologous vein bypass graft(s) of the right leg with ulceration of thigh**   A
> CC when PDx is its own CC

I70.432   **Atherosclerosis of autologous vein bypass graft(s) of the right leg with ulceration of calf**   A
> CC when PDx is its own CC

I70.433   **Atherosclerosis of autologous vein bypass graft(s) of the right leg with ulceration of ankle**   A
> CC when PDx is its own CC

I70.434   **Atherosclerosis of autologous vein bypass graft(s) of the right leg with ulceration of heel and midfoot**   A
> Atherosclerosis of autologous vein bypass graft(s) of right leg with ulceration of plantar surface of midfoot
> CC when PDx is its own CC

I70.435   **Atherosclerosis of autologous vein bypass graft(s) of the right leg with ulceration of other part of foot**   A
> Atherosclerosis of autologous vein bypass graft(s) of right leg with ulceration of toe

I70.438   **Atherosclerosis of autologous vein bypass graft(s) of the right leg with ulceration of other part of lower leg**   A
> CC when PDx is its own CC

I70.439   **Atherosclerosis of autologous vein bypass graft(s) of the right leg with ulceration of unspecified site**   A
> CC when PDx is its own CC

● **I70.44**   **Atherosclerosis of autologous vein bypass graft(s) of the left leg with ulceration**

> **Includes**   any condition classifiable to I70.412 and I70.422

> Use additional code to identify severity of ulcer (L97.-)

> (Ex) For category I70.44 CC codes: See I70.33

I70.441   **Atherosclerosis of autologous vein bypass graft(s) of the left leg with ulceration of thigh**   A
> CC when PDx is its own CC

I70.442   **Atherosclerosis of autologous vein bypass graft(s) of the left leg with ulceration of calf**   A
> CC when PDx is its own CC

I70.443   **Atherosclerosis of autologous vein bypass graft(s) of the left leg with ulceration of ankle**   A
> CC when PDx is its own CC

I70.444   **Atherosclerosis of autologous vein bypass graft(s) of the left leg with ulceration of heel and midfoot**   A
> Atherosclerosis of autologous vein bypass graft(s) of left leg with ulceration of plantar surface of midfoot
> CC when PDx is its own CC

I70.445   **Atherosclerosis of autologous vein bypass graft(s) of the left leg with ulceration of other part of foot**   A
> Atherosclerosis of autologous vein bypass graft(s) of left leg with ulceration of toe

I70.448   **Atherosclerosis of autologous vein bypass graft(s) of the left leg with ulceration of other part of lower leg**   A
> CC when PDx is its own CC

I70.449   **Atherosclerosis of autologous vein bypass graft(s) of the left leg with ulceration of unspecified site**   A
> CC when PDx is its own CC

I70.45   **Atherosclerosis of autologous vein bypass graft(s) of other extremity with ulceration**   A

> **Includes**   any condition classifiable to I70.418, I70.428, and I70.438

> Use additional code to identify severity of ulcer (L98.49-)

● **I70.46**   **Atherosclerosis of autologous vein bypass graft(s) of the extremities with gangrene**

> **Includes**   any condition classifiable to I70.41-, I70.42-, and I70.43-, I70.44-, I70.45

> Use additional code to identify the severity of any ulcer (L97.-, L98.49-), if applicable

> (Ex) For category I70.46 CC codes: See I70.26

I70.461   **Atherosclerosis of autologous vein bypass graft(s) of the extremities with gangrene, right leg**   A
> CC when PDx is its own CC

I70.462   **Atherosclerosis of autologous vein bypass graft(s) of the extremities with gangrene, left leg**   A
> CC when PDx is its own CC

I70.463   **Atherosclerosis of autologous vein bypass graft(s) of the extremities with gangrene, bilateral legs**   A
> CC when PDx is its own CC

I70.468   **Atherosclerosis of autologous vein bypass graft(s) of the extremities with gangrene, other extremity**   A
> CC when PDx is its own CC

I70.469   **Atherosclerosis of autologous vein bypass graft(s) of the extremities with gangrene, unspecified extremity**   A
> CC when PDx is its own CC

● **I70.49**   **Other atherosclerosis of autologous vein bypass graft(s) of the extremities**

I70.491   **Other atherosclerosis of autologous vein bypass graft(s) of the extremities, right leg**   A

I70.492   **Other atherosclerosis of autologous vein bypass graft(s) of the extremities, left leg**   A

I70.493   **Other atherosclerosis of autologous vein bypass graft(s) of the extremities, bilateral legs**   A

I70.498   **Other atherosclerosis of autologous vein bypass graft(s) of the extremities, other extremity**   A

I70.499   **Other atherosclerosis of autologous vein bypass graft(s) of the extremities, unspecified extremity**   A

◀ New   ◀ Revised   deleted Deleted   Excludes 1   Excludes 2   Includes   Use additional   Code first   Code also   Unspecified

898

OGCR Official Guidelines   ● Unacceptable Principal Diagnosis   X Assign placeholder X   ● Use Additional Character(s)   ▶ Manifestation Code   **Coding Clinic**

● **I70.5**   **Atherosclerosis of nonautologous biological bypass graft(s) of the extremities**

Use additional code, if applicable, to identify chronic total occlusion of artery of extremity (I70.92)

● **I70.50**   **Unspecified atherosclerosis of nonautologous biological bypass graft(s) of the extremities**

I70.501   Unspecified atherosclerosis of nonautologous biological bypass graft(s) of the extremities, right leg   A

I70.502   Unspecified atherosclerosis of nonautologous biological bypass graft(s) of the extremities, left leg   A

I70.503   Unspecified atherosclerosis of nonautologous biological bypass graft(s) of the extremities, bilateral legs   A

I70.508   Unspecified atherosclerosis of nonautologous biological bypass graft(s) of the extremities, other extremity   A

I70.509   Unspecified atherosclerosis of nonautologous biological bypass graft(s) of the extremities, unspecified extremity   A

● **I70.51**   **Atherosclerosis of nonautologous biological bypass graft(s) of the extremities intermittent claudication**

I70.511   Atherosclerosis of nonautologous biological bypass graft(s) of the extremities with intermittent claudication, right leg   A

I70.512   Atherosclerosis of nonautologous biological bypass graft(s) of the extremities with intermittent claudication, left leg   A

I70.513   Atherosclerosis of nonautologous biological bypass graft(s) of the extremities with intermittent claudication, bilateral legs   A

I70.518   Atherosclerosis of nonautologous biological bypass graft(s) of the extremities with intermittent claudication, other extremity   A

I70.519   Atherosclerosis of nonautologous biological bypass graft(s) of the extremities with intermittent claudication, unspecified extremity   A

● **I70.52**   **Atherosclerosis of nonautologous biological bypass graft(s) of the extremities with rest pain**

Includes   any condition classifiable to I70.51-

I70.521   Atherosclerosis of nonautologous biological bypass graft(s) of the extremities with rest pain, right leg   A

I70.522   Atherosclerosis of nonautologous biological bypass graft(s) of the extremities with rest pain, left leg   A

I70.523   Atherosclerosis of nonautologous biological bypass graft(s) of the extremities with rest pain, bilateral legs   A

I70.528   Atherosclerosis of nonautologous biological bypass graft(s) of the extremities with rest pain, other extremity   A

I70.529   Atherosclerosis of nonautologous biological bypass graft(s) of the extremities with rest pain, unspecified extremity   A

● **I70.53**   **Atherosclerosis of nonautologous biological bypass graft(s) of the right leg with ulceration**

Includes   any condition classifiable to I70.511 and I70.521

Use additional code to identify severity of ulcer (L97.-)

Ⓔⓧ **For category I70.53 CC codes:** See I70.33

I70.531   Atherosclerosis of nonautologous biological bypass graft(s) of the right leg with ulceration of thigh 🖥   A
CC when PDx is its own CC

I70.532   Atherosclerosis of nonautologous biological bypass graft(s) of the right leg with ulceration of calf 🖥   A
CC when PDx is its own CC

I70.533   Atherosclerosis of nonautologous biological bypass graft(s) of the right leg with ulceration of ankle 🖥   A
CC when PDx is its own CC

I70.534   Atherosclerosis of nonautologous biological bypass graft(s) of the right leg with ulceration of heel and midfoot 🖥   A
Atherosclerosis of nonautologous biological bypass graft(s) of right leg with ulceration of plantar surface of midfoot
CC when PDx is its own CC

I70.535   Atherosclerosis of nonautologous biological bypass graft(s) of the right leg with ulceration of other part of foot   A
Atherosclerosis of nonautologous biological bypass graft(s) of the right leg with ulceration of toe

I70.538   Atherosclerosis of nonautologous biological bypass graft(s) of the right leg with ulceration of other part of lower leg 🖥   A
CC when PDx is its own CC

I70.539   Atherosclerosis of nonautologous biological bypass graft(s) of the right leg with ulceration of unspecified site 🖥   A
CC when PDx is its own CC

● **I70.54**   **Atherosclerosis of nonautologous biological bypass graft(s) of the left leg with ulceration**

Includes   any condition classifiable to I70.512 and I70.522

Use additional code to identify severity of ulcer (L97.-)

Ⓔⓧ **For category I70.54 CC codes:** See I70.33

I70.541   Atherosclerosis of nonautologous biological bypass graft(s) of the left leg with ulceration of thigh 🖥   A
CC when PDx is its own CC

I70.542   Atherosclerosis of nonautologous biological bypass graft(s) of the left leg with ulceration of calf 🖥   A
CC when PDx is its own CC

I70.543   Atherosclerosis of nonautologous biological bypass graft(s) of the left leg with ulceration of ankle 🖥   A
CC when PDx is its own CC

I70.544   Atherosclerosis of nonautologous biological bypass graft(s) of the left leg with ulceration of heel and midfoot 🖥   A
Atherosclerosis of nonautologous biological bypass graft(s) of left leg with ulceration of plantar surface of midfoot
CC when PDx is its own CC

N Newborn Age: 0   **P** Pediatric Age: 0–17   **M** Maternity DX: 12–55   **A** Adult Age: 15–124   ♀ Females Only   ♂ Males Only

🖥 Complication\Comorbidity   🖥 Major C\C   Ⓔⓧ CC/MCC Exclusions   🖥 Hospital-Acquired Condition

899

CHAPTER 9 (I00-I99)

CHAPTER 9 (I00-I99)

I70.545   **Atherosclerosis of nonautologous biological bypass graft(s) of the left leg with ulceration of other part of foot**   A
     Atherosclerosis of nonautologous biological bypass graft(s) of the left leg with ulceration of toe

I70.548   **Atherosclerosis of nonautologous biological bypass graft(s) of the left leg with ulceration of other part of lower leg**   A
     CC when PDx is its own CC

I70.549   **Atherosclerosis of nonautologous biological bypass graft(s) of the left leg with ulceration of unspecified site**   A
     CC when PDx is its own CC

I70.55   **Atherosclerosis of nonautologous biological bypass graft(s) of other extremity with ulceration**   A
     Includes   any condition classifiable to I70.518, I70.528, and I70.538
     Use additional code to identify severity of ulcer (L98.49)

● **I70.56**   **Atherosclerosis of nonautologous biological bypass graft(s) of the extremities with gangrene**
     Includes   any condition classifiable to I70.51-, I70.52-, and I70.53-, I70.54-, I70.55
     Use additional code to identify the severity of any ulcer (L97.-, L98.49-), if applicable
     (Ex) For category I70.56 CC codes: See I70.26

I70.561   **Atherosclerosis of nonautologous biological bypass graft(s) of the extremities with gangrene, right leg**   A
     CC when PDx is its own CC

I70.562   **Atherosclerosis of nonautologous biological bypass graft(s) of the extremities with gangrene, left leg**   A
     CC when PDx is its own CC

I70.563   **Atherosclerosis of nonautologous biological bypass graft(s) of the extremities with gangrene, bilateral legs**   A
     CC when PDx is its own CC

I70.568   **Atherosclerosis of nonautologous biological bypass graft(s) of the extremities with gangrene, other extremity**   A
     CC when PDx is its own CC

I70.569   **Atherosclerosis of nonautologous biological bypass graft(s) of the extremities with gangrene, unspecified extremity**   A
     CC when PDx is its own CC

● **I70.59**   **Other atherosclerosis of nonautologous biological bypass graft(s) of the extremities**

I70.591   **Other atherosclerosis of nonautologous biological bypass graft(s) of the extremities, right leg**   A

I70.592   **Other atherosclerosis of nonautologous biological bypass graft(s) of the extremities, left leg**   A

I70.593   **Other atherosclerosis of nonautologous biological bypass graft(s) of the extremities, bilateral legs**   A

I70.598   **Other atherosclerosis of nonautologous biological bypass graft(s) of the extremities, other extremity**   A

I70.599   **Other atherosclerosis of nonautologous biological bypass graft(s) of the extremities, unspecified extremity**   A

● **I70.6**   **Atherosclerosis of nonbiological bypass graft(s) of the extremities**
     Use additional code, if applicable, to identify chronic total occlusion of artery of extremity (I70.92)

● **I70.60**   **Unspecified atherosclerosis of nonbiological bypass graft(s) of the extremities**

I70.601   **Unspecified atherosclerosis of nonbiological bypass graft(s) of the extremities, right leg**   A

I70.602   **Unspecified atherosclerosis of nonbiological bypass graft(s) of the extremities, left leg**   A

I70.603   **Unspecified atherosclerosis of nonbiological bypass graft(s) of the extremities, bilateral legs**   A

I70.608   **Unspecified atherosclerosis of nonbiological bypass graft(s) of the extremities, other extremity**   A

I70.609   **Unspecified atherosclerosis of nonbiological bypass graft(s) of the extremities, unspecified extremity**   A

● **I70.61**   **Atherosclerosis of nonbiological bypass graft(s) of the extremities with intermittent claudication**

I70.611   **Atherosclerosis of nonbiological bypass graft(s) of the extremities with intermittent claudication, right leg**   A

I70.612   **Atherosclerosis of nonbiological bypass graft(s) of the extremities with intermittent claudication, left leg**   A

I70.613   **Atherosclerosis of nonbiological bypass graft(s) of the extremities with intermittent claudication, bilateral legs**   A

I70.618   **Atherosclerosis of nonbiological bypass graft(s) of the extremities with intermittent claudication, other extremity**   A

I70.619   **Atherosclerosis of nonbiological bypass graft(s) of the extremities with intermittent claudication, unspecified extremity**   A

● **I70.62**   **Atherosclerosis of nonbiological bypass graft(s) of the extremities with rest pain**
     Includes   any condition classifiable to I70.61-

I70.621   **Atherosclerosis of nonbiological bypass graft(s) of the extremities with rest pain, right leg**   A

I70.622   **Atherosclerosis of nonbiological bypass graft(s) of the extremities with rest pain, left leg**   A

I70.623   **Atherosclerosis of nonbiological bypass graft(s) of the extremities with rest pain, bilateral legs**   A

I70.628   **Atherosclerosis of nonbiological bypass graft(s) of the extremities with rest pain, other extremity**   A

I70.629   **Atherosclerosis of nonbiological bypass graft(s) of the extremities with rest pain, unspecified extremity**   A

◀ New   ◀ Revised   ~~deleted~~ Deleted   Excludes 1   Excludes 2   Includes   Use additional   Code first   Code also   Unspecified
OGCR Official Guidelines   ● Unacceptable Principal Diagnosis   X Assign placeholder X   ● Use Additional Character(s)   ▌ Manifestation Code   **Coding Clinic**

● **I70.63**   **Atherosclerosis of nonbiological bypass graft(s) of the right leg with ulceration**

> **Includes**   any condition classifiable to I70.611 and I70.621
>
> Use additional code to identify severity of ulcer (L97.-)
>
> (Ex:) **For category I70.63 CC codes:** See I70.33

    I70.631   Atherosclerosis of nonbiological bypass graft(s) of the right leg with ulceration of thigh 🖉   A
>
> CC when PDx is its own CC

    I70.632   Atherosclerosis of nonbiological bypass graft(s) of the right leg with ulceration of calf 🖉   A
>
> CC when PDx is its own CC

    I70.633   Atherosclerosis of nonbiological bypass graft(s) of the right leg with ulceration of ankle 🖉   A
>
> CC when PDx is its own CC

    I70.634   Atherosclerosis of nonbiological bypass graft(s) of the right leg with ulceration of heel and midfoot 🖉   A
>
> Atherosclerosis of nonbiological bypass graft(s) of right leg with ulceration of plantar surface of midfoot
>
> CC when PDx is its own CC

    I70.635   Atherosclerosis of nonbiological bypass graft(s) of the right leg with ulceration of other part of foot   A
>
> Atherosclerosis of nonbiological bypass graft(s) of the right leg with ulceration of toe

    I70.638   Atherosclerosis of nonbiological bypass graft(s) of the right leg with ulceration of other part of lower leg 🖉   A
>
> CC when PDx is its own CC

    I70.639   Atherosclerosis of nonbiological bypass graft(s) of the right leg with ulceration of unspecified site 🖉   A
>
> CC when PDx is its own CC

● **I70.64**   **Atherosclerosis of nonbiological bypass graft(s) of the left leg with ulceration**

> **Includes**   any condition classifiable to I70.612 and I70.622
>
> Use additional code to identify severity of ulcer (L97.-)
>
> (Ex:) **For category I70.64 CC codes:** See I70.33

    I70.641   Atherosclerosis of nonbiological bypass graft(s) of the left leg with ulceration of thigh 🖉   A
>
> CC when PDx is its own CC

    I70.642   Atherosclerosis of nonbiological bypass graft(s) of the left leg with ulceration of calf 🖉   A
>
> CC when PDx is its own CC

    I70.643   Atherosclerosis of nonbiological bypass graft(s) of the left leg with ulceration of ankle 🖉   A
>
> CC when PDx is its own CC

    I70.644   Atherosclerosis of nonbiological bypass graft(s) of the left leg with ulceration of heel and midfoot 🖉   A
>
> Atherosclerosis of nonbiological bypass graft(s) of left leg with ulceration of plantar surface of midfoot
>
> CC when PDx is its own CC

    I70.645   Atherosclerosis of nonbiological bypass graft(s) of the left leg with ulceration of other part of foot   A
>
> Atherosclerosis of nonbiological bypass graft(s) of the left leg with ulceration of toe

    I70.648   Atherosclerosis of nonbiological bypass graft(s) of the left leg with ulceration of other part of lower leg 🖉   A
>
> CC when PDx is its own CC

    I70.649   Atherosclerosis of nonbiological bypass graft(s) of the left leg with ulceration of unspecified site 🖉   A
>
> CC when PDx is its own CC

  I70.65   Atherosclerosis of nonbiological bypass graft(s) of other extremity with ulceration   A

> **Includes**   any condition classifiable to I70.618 and I70.628
>
> Use additional code to identify severity of ulcer (L98.49-)

● **I70.66**   **Atherosclerosis of nonbiological bypass graft(s) of the extremities with gangrene**

> **Includes**   any condition classifiable to I70.61-, I70.62-, I70.63-, I70.64-, I70.65
>
> Use additional code to identify the severity of any ulcer (L97.-, L98.49-), if applicable
>
> (Ex:) **For category I70.66 CC codes:** See I70.26

    I70.661   Atherosclerosis of nonbiological bypass graft(s) of the extremities with gangrene, right leg 🖉   A
>
> CC when PDx is its own CC

    I70.662   Atherosclerosis of nonbiological bypass graft(s) of the extremities with gangrene, left leg 🖉   A
>
> CC when PDx is its own CC

    I70.663   Atherosclerosis of nonbiological bypass graft(s) of the extremities with gangrene, bilateral legs 🖉   A
>
> CC when PDx is its own CC

    I70.668   Atherosclerosis of nonbiological bypass graft(s) of the extremities with gangrene, other extremity 🖉   A
>
> CC when PDx is its own CC

    I70.669   Atherosclerosis of nonbiological bypass graft(s) of the extremities with gangrene, unspecified extremity 🖉   A
>
> CC when PDx is its own CC

● **I70.69**   **Other atherosclerosis of nonbiological bypass graft(s) of the extremities**

    I70.691   Other atherosclerosis of nonbiological bypass graft(s) of the extremities, right leg   A

    I70.692   Other atherosclerosis of nonbiological bypass graft(s) of the extremities, left leg   A

    I70.693   Other atherosclerosis of nonbiological bypass graft(s) of the extremities, bilateral legs   A

    I70.698   Other atherosclerosis of nonbiological bypass graft(s) of the extremities, other extremity   A

    I70.699   Other atherosclerosis of nonbiological bypass graft(s) of the extremities, unspecified extremity   A

● **I70.7**   **Atherosclerosis of other type of bypass graft(s) of the extremities**

> Use additional code, if applicable, to identify chronic total occlusion of artery of extremity (I70.92)

● **I70.70**   **Unspecified atherosclerosis of other type of bypass graft(s) of the extremities**

    I70.701   Unspecified atherosclerosis of other type of bypass graft(s) of the extremities, right leg   A

    I70.702   Unspecified atherosclerosis of other type of bypass graft(s) of the extremities, left leg   A

N   Newborn Age: Ø   P   Pediatric Age: Ø–17   M   Maternity DX: 12–55   A   Adult Age: 15–124   ♀   Females Only   ♂   Males Only

🖉 Complication\Comorbidity   🖉 Major C\C   (Ex:) CC/MCC Exclusions   🖉 Hospital-Acquired Condition

I70.703   **Unspecified** atherosclerosis of other type of bypass graft(s) of the extremities, bilateral legs   A

I70.708   **Unspecified** atherosclerosis of other type of bypass graft(s) of the extremities, other extremity   A

I70.709   **Unspecified** atherosclerosis of other type of bypass graft(s) of the extremities, unspecified extremity   A

● I70.71   **Atherosclerosis of other type of bypass graft(s) of the extremities with intermittent claudication**

I70.711   **Atherosclerosis of other type of bypass graft(s) of the extremities with intermittent claudication, right leg**   A

I70.712   **Atherosclerosis of other type of bypass graft(s) of the extremities with intermittent claudication, left leg**   A

I70.713   **Atherosclerosis of other type of bypass graft(s) of the extremities with intermittent claudication, bilateral legs**   A

I70.718   **Atherosclerosis of other type of bypass graft(s) of the extremities with intermittent claudication, other extremity**   A

I70.719   **Atherosclerosis of other type of bypass graft(s) of the extremities with intermittent claudication, unspecified extremity**   A

● I70.72   **Atherosclerosis of other type of bypass graft(s) of the extremities with rest pain**

Includes   any condition classifiable to I70.71-

I70.721   **Atherosclerosis of other type of bypass graft(s) of the extremities with rest pain, right leg**   A

I70.722   **Atherosclerosis of other type of bypass graft(s) of the extremities with rest pain, left leg**   A

I70.723   **Atherosclerosis of other type of bypass graft(s) of the extremities with rest pain, bilateral legs**   A

I70.728   **Atherosclerosis of other type of bypass graft(s) of the extremities with rest pain, other extremity**   A

I70.729   **Atherosclerosis of other type of bypass graft(s) of the extremities with rest pain, unspecified extremity**   A

● I70.73   **Atherosclerosis of other type of bypass graft(s) of the right leg with ulceration**

Includes   any condition classifiable to I70.711 and I70.721

Use additional code to identify severity of ulcer (L97.-)

(Ex) For category I70.73 CC codes: See I70.33

I70.731   **Atherosclerosis of other type of bypass graft(s) of the right leg with ulceration of thigh**   A
CC when PDx is its own CC

I70.732   **Atherosclerosis of other type of bypass graft(s) of the right leg with ulceration of calf**   A
CC when PDx is its own CC

I70.733   **Atherosclerosis of other type of bypass graft(s) of the right leg with ulceration of ankle**   A
CC when PDx is its own CC

I70.734   **Atherosclerosis of other type of bypass graft(s) of the right leg with ulceration of heel and midfoot**   A
Atherosclerosis of other type of bypass graft(s) of right leg with ulceration of plantar surface of midfoot
CC when PDx is its own CC

I70.735   **Atherosclerosis of other type of bypass graft(s) of the right leg with ulceration of other part of foot**   A
Atherosclerosis of other type of bypass graft(s) of right leg with ulceration of toe

I70.738   **Atherosclerosis of other type of bypass graft(s) of the right leg with ulceration of other part of lower leg**   A
CC when PDx is its own CC

I70.739   **Atherosclerosis of other type of bypass graft(s) of the right leg with ulceration of unspecified site**   A
CC when PDx is its own CC

● I70.74   **Atherosclerosis of other type of bypass graft(s) of the left leg with ulceration**

Includes   any condition classifiable to I70.712 and I70.722

Use additional code to identify severity of ulcer (L97.-)

(Ex) For category I70.74 CC codes: See I70.33

I70.741   **Atherosclerosis of other type of bypass graft(s) of the left leg with ulceration of thigh**   A
CC when PDx is its own CC

I70.742   **Atherosclerosis of other type of bypass graft(s) of the left leg with ulceration of calf**   A
CC when PDx is its own CC

I70.743   **Atherosclerosis of other type of bypass graft(s) of the left leg with ulceration of ankle**   A
CC when PDx is its own CC

I70.744   **Atherosclerosis of other type of bypass graft(s) of the left leg with ulceration of heel and midfoot**   A
Atherosclerosis of other type of bypass graft(s) of left leg with ulceration of plantar surface of midfoot
CC when PDx is its own CC

I70.745   **Atherosclerosis of other type of bypass graft(s) of the left leg with ulceration of other part of foot**   A
Atherosclerosis of other type of bypass graft(s) of left leg with ulceration of toe

I70.748   **Atherosclerosis of other type of bypass graft(s) of the left leg with ulceration of other part of lower leg**   A
CC when PDx is its own CC

I70.749   **Atherosclerosis of other type of bypass graft(s) of the left leg with ulceration of unspecified site**   A
CC when PDx is its own CC

I70.75   **Atherosclerosis of other type of bypass graft(s) of other extremity with ulceration**   A
     Includes   any condition classifiable to I70.718 and I70.728
    Use additional code to identify severity of ulcer (L98.49)

● I70.76   **Atherosclerosis of other type of bypass graft(s) of the extremities with gangrene**
     Includes   any condition classifiable to I70.71-, I70.72-, I70.73-, I70.74-, I70.75
    Use additional code to identify the severity of any ulcer (L97.-, L98.49-), if applicable
    (Ex:) **For category I70.76 CC codes:** See I70.26

    I70.761   **Atherosclerosis of other type of bypass graft(s) of the extremities with gangrene, right leg** 🌢   A
        CC when PDx is its own CC

    I70.762   **Atherosclerosis of other type of bypass graft(s) of the extremities with gangrene, left leg** 🌢   A
        CC when PDx is its own CC

    I70.763   **Atherosclerosis of other type of bypass graft(s) of the extremities with gangrene, bilateral legs** 🌢   A
        CC when PDx is its own CC

    I70.768   **Atherosclerosis of other type of bypass graft(s) of the extremities with gangrene, other extremity** 🌢   A
        CC when PDx is its own CC

    I70.769   **Atherosclerosis of other type of bypass graft(s) of the extremities with gangrene, unspecified extremity** 🌢   A
        CC when PDx is its own CC

● I70.79   **Other atherosclerosis of other type of bypass graft(s) of the extremities**
    I70.791   **Other atherosclerosis of other type of bypass graft(s) of the extremities, right leg**   A
    I70.792   **Other atherosclerosis of other type of bypass graft(s) of the extremities, left leg**   A
    I70.793   **Other atherosclerosis of other type of bypass graft(s) of the extremities, bilateral legs**   A
    I70.798   **Other atherosclerosis of other type of bypass graft(s) of the extremities, other extremity**   A
    I70.799   **Other atherosclerosis of other type of bypass graft(s) of the extremities, unspecified extremity**   A

I70.8   **Atherosclerosis of other arteries**   A
● I70.9   **Other and unspecified atherosclerosis**
    I70.90   **Unspecified atherosclerosis**   A
    I70.91   **Generalized atherosclerosis**   A
   ● I70.92   **Chronic total occlusion of artery of the extremities** 🌢   A
        Complete occlusion of artery of the extremities
        Total occlusion of artery of the extremities
        Code first atherosclerosis of arteries of the extremities (I70.2-, I70.3-, I70.4-, I70.5-, I70.6-, I70.7-)
        (Ex:) I70.92, I73.81-I74.19, .I74.2-I77.2, I77.5-I77.6, I77.810-I77.819, I79.1-I79.8, M31.8-M31.9

● I71   **Aortic aneurysm and dissection**
    Excludes1   aortic ectasia (I77.81-)
              syphilitic aortic aneurysm (A52.01)
              traumatic aortic aneurysm (S25.09, S35.09)
    (Ex:) **For category I71 CC codes:** E08.51-E08.59, E08.618-E08.638, E08.649-E08.8, E09.51-E09.59, E09.618-E09.638, E09.649, E09.65-E09.8, E10.51-E10.59, E10.618-E10.638, E10.649, E10.69-E10.8, E11.51-E11.59, E11.618-E11.638, E11.649, E11.69-E11.8, E13.51-E13.59, E13.618-E13.638, E13.649-E13.8, I71.00-I71.9, I77.810-I77.819, I79.0, I87.8-I87.9, I99.8-I99.9

 ● I71.0   **Dissection of aorta**
    I71.00   **Dissection of unspecified site of aorta** 🌢
    I71.01   **Dissection of thoracic aorta** 🌢
    I71.02   **Dissection of abdominal aorta** 🌢
    I71.03   **Dissection of thoracoabdominal aorta** 🌢

I71.1   **Thoracic aortic aneurysm, ruptured** 🌢
I71.2   **Thoracic aortic aneurysm, without rupture**
I71.3   **Abdominal aortic aneurysm, ruptured** 🌢
I71.4   **Abdominal aortic aneurysm, without rupture**
I71.5   **Thoracoabdominal aortic aneurysm, ruptured** 🌢
I71.6   **Thoracoabdominal aortic aneurysm, without rupture**
I71.8   **Aortic aneurysm of unspecified site, ruptured** 🌢
    Rupture of aorta NOS
I71.9   **Aortic aneurysm of unspecified site, without rupture**
    Aneurysm of aorta
    Dilatation of aorta
    Hyaline necrosis of aorta

● I72   **Other aneurysm**
    Includes   aneurysm (cirsoid) (false) (ruptured)
    Excludes2   acquired aneurysm (I77.0)
              aneurysm (of) aorta (I71.-)
              aneurysm (of) arteriovenous NOS (Q27.3-)
              carotid artery dissection (I77.71)
              cerebral (nonruptured) aneurysm (I67.1)
              coronary aneurysm (I25.4)
              coronary artery dissection (I25.42)
              dissection of artery NEC (I77.79)
              dissection of precerebral artery, congenital (nonruptured) (Q28.1) ◄
              heart aneurysm (I25.3)
              iliac artery dissection (I77.72)
              pulmonary artery aneurysm (I28.1)
              renal artery dissection (I77.73)
              retinal aneurysm (H35.0)
              ruptured cerebral aneurysm (I60.7)
              varicose aneurysm (I77.0)
              vertebral artery dissection (I77.74)

I72.0   **Aneurysm of carotid artery**
    Aneurysm of common carotid artery
    Aneurysm of external carotid artery
    Aneurysm of internal carotid artery, extracranial portion
    Excludes1   aneurysm of internal carotid artery, intracranial portion (I67.1)
              aneurysm of internal carotid artery NOS (I67.1)

I72.1   **Aneurysm of artery of upper extremity**
I72.2   **Aneurysm of renal artery**
I72.3   **Aneurysm of iliac artery**
I72.4   **Aneurysm of artery of lower extremity**
I72.5   **Aneurysm of other precerebral arteries** ◄
    Aneurysm of basilar artery (trunk) ◄
    Excludes2   aneurysm of carotid artery (I72.0) ◄
              aneurysm of vertebral artery (I72.6) ◄
              dissection of carotid artery (I77.71) ◄
              dissection of other precerebral arteries (I77.75) ◄
              dissection of vertebral artery (I77.74) ◄

CHAPTER 9 (I00-I99)

I72.6   **Aneurysm of vertebral artery** ◄
       Excludes2   dissection of vertebral artery (I77.74) ◄

I72.8   **Aneurysm of other specified arteries**

I72.9   **Aneurysm of unspecified site**

● **I73**   **Other peripheral vascular diseases**
      Excludes2   chilblains (T69.1)
                  frostbite (T33-T34)
                  immersion hand or foot (T69.0-)
                  spasm of cerebral artery (G45.9)

● **I73.0**   **Raynaud's syndrome**
      Diminishing oxygen supply to fingers, toes, nose, and ears
           when exposed to temperature changes or stress
      Raynaud's disease
      Raynaud's phenomenon (secondary)

      I73.00   **Raynaud's syndrome without gangrene**

      I73.01   **Raynaud's syndrome with gangrene** 🦠
              CC when PDx is its own CC
              (Ex) See I70.26

I73.1   **Thromboangiitis obliterans [Buerger's disease]**
      Inflammatory occlusive disease resulting in poor circulation
      to the legs, feet, and sometimes the hands due to
      progressive inflammatory narrowing and eventually
      obliteration of the small arteries

● **I73.8**   **Other specified peripheral vascular diseases**
      Excludes1   diabetic (peripheral) angiopathy
                    (E08-E13 with .51-.52)

      I73.81   **Erythromelalgia**

      I73.89   **Other specified peripheral vascular diseases**
              Acrocyanosis
              Erythrocyanosis
              Simple acroparesthesia [Schultze's type]
              Vasomotor acroparesthesia [Nothnagel's type]

I73.9   **Peripheral vascular disease, unspecified**
      Intermittent claudication
      Peripheral angiopathy NOS
      Spasm of artery
      Excludes1   atherosclerosis of the extremities
                    (I70.2--I70.7-)

● **I74**   **Arterial embolism and thrombosis**
      Includes   embolic infarction
                embolic occlusion
                thrombotic infarction
                thrombotic occlusion
      Code first embolism and thrombosis complicating abortion or
           ectopic or molar pregnancy (O00-O07, O08.2)
           embolism and thrombosis complicating pregnancy, childbirth
           and the puerperium (O88.-)
      Excludes2   atheroembolism (I75.-)
                  basilar embolism and thrombosis (I63.0-I63.2,
                    I65.1)
                  carotid embolism and thrombosis (I63.0-I63.2,
                    I65.2)
                  cerebral embolism and thrombosis (I63.3-I63.5,
                    I66.-)
                  coronary embolism and thrombosis (I21-I25)
                  mesenteric embolism and thrombosis (K55.0-) ◄
                  ophthalmic embolism and thrombosis (H34.-)
                  precerebral embolism and thrombosis NOS
                    (I63.0-I63.2, I65.9)
                  pulmonary embolism and thrombosis (I26.-)
                  renal embolism and thrombosis (N28.0)
                  retinal embolism and thrombosis (H34.-)
                  septic embolism and thrombosis (I76)
                  vertebral embolism and thrombosis (I63.0-I63.2,
                    I65.0)

● **I74.0**   **Embolism and thrombosis of abdominal aorta**
      (Ex) For category 174.0 CC codes: I26.01-I26.99, I27.82, I74.01-I74.10, I74.19,
      I87.8-I87.9, I99.8-I99.9

      I74.01   **Saddle embolus of abdominal aorta** 🦠

      I74.09   **Other arterial embolism and thrombosis of**
              abdominal aorta 🦠
              Aortic bifurcation syndrome
              Aortoiliac obstruction
              Leriche's syndrome

● **I74.1**   **Embolism and thrombosis of other and unspecified parts**
      of aorta
      (Ex) For category I74.1 CC codes unless otherwise indicated: See I74.0

      I74.10   **Embolism and thrombosis of unspecified parts**
              of aorta 🦠

      I74.11   **Embolism and thrombosis of thoracic aorta** 🦠
              (Ex) E08.51-E08.59, E08.618-E08.638, E08.649-E08.8,
                 E09.51-E09.59, E09.618-E09.638, E09.649, E09.65-E09.8,
                 E10.51-E10.59, E10.618-E10.638, E10.649, E10.69-E10.8,
                 E11.51-E11.59, E11.618-E11.638, E11.649, E11.69-E11.8,
                 E13.51-E13.59, E13.618-E13.638, E13.649-E13.8, I74.11,
                 I74.8-I74.9, I76, I87.8-I87.9, I99.8-I99.9

      I74.19   **Embolism and thrombosis of other parts of**
              aorta 🦠

I74.2   **Embolism and thrombosis of arteries of the upper**
      extremities 🦠
      (Ex) E08.51-E08.59, E08.618-E08.638, E08.649-E08.8, E09.51-E09.59,
      E09.618-E09.638, E09.649, E09.65-E09.8, E10.51-E10.59, E10.618-E10.638,
      E10.649, E10.69-E10.8, E11.51-E11.59, E11.618-E11.638, E11.649,
      E11.69-E11.8, E13.51-E13.59, E13.618-E13.638, E13.649-E13.8, I74.2,
      I74.8-I74.9, I76, I87.8-I87.9, I99.8-I99.9

Item 9–9   An **embolus** is a mass of undissolved matter present in the blood that is transported by the blood current. A **thrombus** is a blood clot that occludes or shuts off a vessel. When a thrombus is dislodged, it becomes an embolus.

Embolus

Figure 9-6   An arterial embolus.

Figure 9-5   Raynaud's syndrome. (From Hallett: Comprehensive Vascular and Endovascular Surgery, ed 2, Philadelphia, Mosby Ltd., 2010)

◄ New   ◄ Revised   ~~deleted~~ Deleted   Excludes 1   Excludes 2   Includes   Use additional   Code first   Code also   Unspecified
OGCR Official Guidelines   ● Unacceptable Principal Diagnosis   X Assign placeholder X   ● Use Additional Character(s)   ▶ Manifestation Code   **Coding Clinic**

I74.3   **Embolism and thrombosis of arteries of the lower extremities** 🦠
(Ex) E08.51-E08.59, E08.618-E08.638, E08.649-E08.8, E09.51-E09.59,
E09.618-E09.638, E09.649, E09.65-E09.8, E10.51-E10.59, E10.618-E10.638,
E10.649, E10.69-E10.8, E11.51-E11.59, E11.618-E11.638, E11.649,
E11.69-E11.8, E13.51-E13.59, E13.618-E13.638, E13.649-E13.8, I74.3-I74.4,
I74.8-I74.9, I76, I87.8-I87.9, I99.8-I99.9

I74.4   **Embolism and thrombosis of arteries of extremities, unspecified** 🦠
Peripheral arterial embolism NOS
(Ex) See I74.3

I74.5   **Embolism and thrombosis of iliac artery** 🦠
(Ex) E08.51-E08.59, E08.618-E08.638, E08.649-E08.8, E09.51-E09.59,
E09.618-E09.638, E09.649, E09.65-E09.8, E10.51-E10.59, E10.618-E10.638,
E10.649, E10.69-E10.8, E11.51-E11.59, E11.618-E11.638, E11.649,
E11.69-E11.8, E13.51-E13.59, E13.618-E13.638, E13.649-E13.8, I74.5-I74.9,
I76, I87.8-I87.9, I99.8-I99.9

I74.8   **Embolism and thrombosis of other arteries** 🦠
(Ex) E08.51-E08.59, E08.618-E08.638, E08.649-E08.8, E09.51-E09.59,
E09.618-E09.638, E09.649, E09.65-E09.8, E10.51-E10.59, E10.618-E10.638,
E10.649, E10.69-E10.8, E11.51-E11.59, E11.618-E11.638, E11.649,
E11.69-E11.8, E13.51-E13.59, E13.618-E13.638, E13.649-E13.8, I74.8-I74.9,
I76, I87.8-I87.9, I99.8-I99.9

I74.9   **Embolism and thrombosis of unspecified artery** 🦠
(Ex) See I74.8

● **I75**   **Atheroembolism**
Includes   atherothrombotic microembolism
cholesterol embolism

● **I75.0**   **Atheroembolism of extremities**
● **I75.01**   **Atheroembolism of upper extremity**
(Ex) For category I75.01 CC codes: E08.51-E08.59,
E08.618-E08.638, E08.649-E08.8, E09.51-E09.59,
E09.618-E09.638, E09.649, E09.65-E09.8, E10.51-E10.59,
E10.618-E10.638, E10.649, E10.69-E10.8, E11.51-E11.59,
E11.618-E11.638, E11.649, E11.69-E11.8, E13.51-E13.59,
E13.618-E13.638, E13.649-E13.8, I74.8-I75.019, I76,
I87.8-I87.9, I99.8-I99.9

I75.011   **Atheroembolism of right upper extremity** 🦠

I75.012   **Atheroembolism of left upper extremity** 🦠

I75.013   **Atheroembolism of bilateral upper extremities** 🦠

I75.019   **Atheroembolism of unspecified upper extremity** 🦠

● **I75.02**   **Atheroembolism of lower extremity**
(Ex) For category I75.02 CC codes: E08.51-E08.59,
E08.618-E08.638, E08.649-E08.8, E09.51-E09.59,
E09.618-E09.638, E09.649, E09.65-E09.8, E10.51-E10.59,
E10.618-E10.638, E10.649, E10.69-E10.8, E11.51-E11.59,
E11.618-E11.638, E11.649, E11.69-E11.8, E13.51-E13.59,
E13.618-E13.638, E13.649-E13.8, I74.8-I74.9,
I75.021-I75.029, I76, I87.8-I87.9, I99.8-I99.9

I75.021   **Atheroembolism of right lower extremity** 🦠

I75.022   **Atheroembolism of left lower extremity** 🦠

I75.023   **Atheroembolism of bilateral lower extremities** 🦠

I75.029   **Atheroembolism of unspecified lower extremity** 🦠

● **I75.8**   **Atheroembolism of other sites**
I75.81   **Atheroembolism of kidney** 🦠
Use additional code for any associated acute
kidney failure and chronic kidney disease
(N17.-, N18.-)
(Ex) E08.51-E08.59, E08.618-E08.638, E08.649-E08.8,
E09.51-E09.59, E09.618-E09.638, E09.649, E09.65-E09.8,
E10.51-E10.59, E10.618-E10.638, E10.649, E10.69-E10.8,
E11.51-E11.59, E11.618-E11.638, E11.649, E11.69-E11.8,
E13.51-E13.59, E13.618-E13.638, E13.649-E13.8, I74.8-I74.9,
I75.81, I76, I87.8-I87.9, I99.8-I99.9

I75.89   **Atheroembolism of other site** 🦠
(Ex) E08.51-E08.59, E08.618-E08.638, E08.649-E08.8,
E09.51-E09.59, E09.618-E09.638, E09.649, E09.65-E09.8,
E10.51-E10.59, E10.618-E10.638, E10.649, E10.69-E10.8,
E11.51-E11.59, E11.618-E11.638, E11.649, E11.69-E11.8,
E13.51-E13.59, E13.618-E13.638, E13.649-E13.8, I74.8-I74.9,
I75.89, I76, I87.8-I87.9, I99.8-I99.9

● **I76**   **Septic arterial embolism** 🦠
Code first underlying infection, such as:
infective endocarditis (I33.0)
lung abscess (J85.-)
Use additional code to identify the site of the embolism (I74.-)
Excludes2   septic pulmonary embolism (I26.01, I26.90)
(Ex) See I74.8

● **I77**   **Other disorders of arteries and arterioles**
Excludes2   collagen (vascular) diseases (M30-M36)
hypersensitivity angiitis (M31.0)
pulmonary artery (I28.-)

I77.0   **Arteriovenous fistula, acquired**
Aneurysmal varix
Arteriovenous aneurysm, acquired
Excludes1   arteriovenous aneurysm NOS (Q27.3-)
presence of arteriovenous shunt (fistula)
for dialysis (Z99.2)
traumatic - see injury of blood vessel by
body region
Excludes2   cerebral (I67.1)
coronary (I25.4)

I77.1   **Stricture of artery**
Narrowing of artery

I77.2   **Rupture of artery** 🦠
Erosion of artery
Fistula of artery
Ulcer of artery
Excludes1   traumatic rupture of artery - see injury of
blood vessel by body region
(Ex) I25.42, I67.0, I77.2, I77.70, I77.72-I77.79

I77.3   **Arterial fibromuscular dysplasia**
Fibromuscular hyperplasia (of) carotid artery
Fibromuscular hyperplasia (of) renal artery

I77.4   **Celiac artery compression syndrome** 🦠
(Ex) I77.4

I77.5   **Necrosis of artery** 🦠
(Ex) I77.5, M31.8-M31.9

I77.6   **Arteritis, unspecified**
Aortitis NOS
Endarteritis NOS
Excludes1   arteritis or endarteritis:
aortic arch (M31.4)
cerebral NEC (I67.7)
coronary (I25.89)
deformans (I70.-)
giant cell (M31.5., M31.6)
obliterans (I70.-)
senile (I70.-)

CHAPTER 9 (I00-I99)

N Newborn Age: 0   **P** Pediatric Age: 0–17   **M** Maternity DX: 12–55   **A** Adult Age: 15–124   ♀ Females Only   ♂ Males Only
🦠 Complication\Comorbidity   🦠 Major C\C   (Ex) CC/MCC Exclusions   🦠 Hospital-Acquired Condition

905

● **I77.7**   **Other arterial dissection**

      Excludes2   dissection of aorta (I71.0-)
                  dissection of coronary artery (I25.42)
      (Ex:) **For category I77.7 CC codes:** I77.2-I77.3, I77.5-I77.6, I77.89-I77.9, M31.8-M31.9

    I77.70   **Dissection of unspecified artery** ◐ ◀

    I77.71   **Dissection of carotid artery** ◐

    I77.72   **Dissection of iliac artery** ◐

    I77.73   **Dissection of renal artery** ◐

    I77.74   **Dissection of vertebral artery** ◐

        Excludes2   aneurysm of vertebral artery (I72.6) ◀

    I77.75   **Dissection of other precerebral arteries** ◐ ◀
        Dissection of basilar artery (trunk) ◀

        Excludes2   aneurysm of carotid artery (I72.0) ◀
                  aneurysm of other precerebral arteries (I72.5) ◀
                  aneurysm of vertebral artery (I72.6) ◀
                  dissection of carotid artery (I77.71) ◀
                  dissection of vertebral artery (I77.74) ◀

    I77.76   **Dissection of artery of upper extremity** ◐ ◀

    I77.77   **Dissection of artery of lower extremity** ◐ ◀

    I77.79   **Dissection of other specified artery** ◐ ◀▬

● **I77.8**   **Other specified disorders of arteries and arterioles**

    I77.81   **Aortic ectasia**
        Ectasis aorta

        Excludes1   aortic aneurysm and dissection (I71.0-)

    I77.810   **Thoracic aortic ectasia**

    I77.811   **Abdominal aortic ectasia**

    I77.812   **Thoracoabdominal aortic ectasia**

    I77.819   **Aortic ectasia, unspecified site**

    I77.89   **Other specified disorders of arteries and arterioles**

  I77.9   **Disorder of arteries and arterioles, unspecified**

● **I78**   **Diseases of capillaries**

  I78.0   **Hereditary hemorrhagic telangiectasia**
    Rendu-Osler-Weber disease

  I78.1   **Nevus, non-neoplastic**
    Araneus nevus   Spider nevus
    Senile nevus   Stellar nevus

    Excludes1   nevus NOS (D22.-)
              vascular NOS (Q82.5)

    Excludes2   blue nevus (D22.-)
              flammeus nevus (Q82.5)
              hairy nevus (D22.-)
              melanocytic nevus (D22.-)
              pigmented nevus (D22.-)
              portwine nevus (Q82.5)
              sanguineous nevus (Q82.5)
              strawberry nevus (Q82.5)
              verrucous nevus (Q82.5)

  I78.8   **Other diseases of capillaries**

  I78.9   **Disease of capillaries, unspecified**

● **I79**   **Disorders of arteries, arterioles and capillaries in diseases classified elsewhere**

  ❱ *I79.0*   *Aneurysm of aorta in diseases classified elsewhere*
    Code first underlying disease

    Excludes1   syphilitic aneurysm (A52.01)

  ❱ *I79.1*   *Aortitis in diseases classified elsewhere*
    Code first underlying disease

    Excludes1   syphilitic aortitis (A52.02)

  ❱ *I79.8*   *Other disorders of arteries, arterioles and capillaries in diseases classified elsewhere*
    Code first underlying disease, such as:
    amyloidosis (E85.-)

    Excludes1   diabetic (peripheral) angiopathy (E08-E13 with .51-.52)
              syphilitic endarteritis (A52.09)
              tuberculous endarteritis (A18.89)

DISEASES OF VEINS, LYMPHATIC VESSELS AND LYMPH NODES, NOT ELSEWHERE CLASSIFIED (I80-I89)

● **I80**   **Phlebitis and thrombophlebitis**
  Inflammation of a vein with infiltration of walls (phlebitis).

    Includes   endophlebitis
              inflammation, vein
              periphlebitis
              suppurative phlebitis

  Code first phlebitis and thrombophlebitis complicating abortion, ectopic or molar pregnancy (O00-O07, O08.7)
    phlebitis and thrombophlebitis complicating pregnancy, childbirth and the puerperium (O22.-, O87.-)

    Excludes1   venous embolism and thrombosis of lower extremities (I82.4-, I82.5-, I82.81-)

● **I80.0**   **Phlebitis and thrombophlebitis of superficial vessels of lower extremities**
    Phlebitis and thrombophlebitis of femoropopliteal vein

    I80.00   **Phlebitis and thrombophlebitis of superficial vessels of unspecified lower extremity**

    I80.01   **Phlebitis and thrombophlebitis of superficial vessels of right lower extremity**

    I80.02   **Phlebitis and thrombophlebitis of superficial vessels of left lower extremity**

    I80.03   **Phlebitis and thrombophlebitis of superficial vessels of lower extremities, bilateral**

● **I80.1**   **Phlebitis and thrombophlebitis of femoral vein**
    (Ex:) **For category I80.1 CC codes:** E08.51-E08.59, E08.618-E08.638, E08.649-E08.8, E09.51-E09.59, E09.618-E09.638, E09.649, E09.65-E09.8, E10.51-E10.59, E10.618-E10.638, E10.649, E10.69-E10.8, E11.51-E11.59, E11.618-E11.638, E11.649, E11.69-E11.8, E13.51-E13.59, E13.618-E13.638, E13.649-E13.8, I80.00-I80.9, I87.8-I87.9, I99.8-I99.9

    I80.10   **Phlebitis and thrombophlebitis of unspecified femoral vein** ◐

    I80.11   **Phlebitis and thrombophlebitis of right femoral vein** ◐

    I80.12   **Phlebitis and thrombophlebitis of left femoral vein** ◐

    I80.13   **Phlebitis and thrombophlebitis of femoral vein, bilateral** ◐

● **I80.2**   **Phlebitis and thrombophlebitis of other and unspecified deep vessels of lower extremities**
    (Ex:) **For category I80.2 CC codes:** See I80.1

  ● **I80.20**   **Phlebitis and thrombophlebitis of unspecified deep vessels of lower extremities**

    I80.201   **Phlebitis and thrombophlebitis of unspecified deep vessels of right lower extremity** ◐

    I80.202   **Phlebitis and thrombophlebitis of unspecified deep vessels of left lower extremity** ◐

    I80.203   **Phlebitis and thrombophlebitis of unspecified deep vessels of lower extremities, bilateral** ◐

    I80.209   **Phlebitis and thrombophlebitis of unspecified deep vessels of unspecified lower extremity** ◐

  ● **I80.21**   **Phlebitis and thrombophlebitis of iliac vein**

    I80.211   **Phlebitis and thrombophlebitis of right iliac vein** ◐

    I80.212   **Phlebitis and thrombophlebitis of left iliac vein** ◐

◀ New   ◀▬ Revised   ~~deleted~~ Deleted   Excludes 1   Excludes 2   Includes   Use additional   Code first   Code also   Unspecified
OGCR Official Guidelines   ● Unacceptable Principal Diagnosis   X Assign placeholder X   ◐ Use Additional Character(s)   ❱ Manifestation Code   **Coding Clinic**

I80.213   Phlebitis and thrombophlebitis of iliac vein, bilateral 🬀

I80.219   Phlebitis and thrombophlebitis of unspecified iliac vein 🬀

● I80.22   Phlebitis and thrombophlebitis of popliteal vein

I80.221   Phlebitis and thrombophlebitis of right popliteal vein 🬀

I80.222   Phlebitis and thrombophlebitis of left popliteal vein 🬀

I80.223   Phlebitis and thrombophlebitis of popliteal vein, bilateral 🬀

I80.229   Phlebitis and thrombophlebitis of unspecified popliteal vein 🬀

● I80.23   Phlebitis and thrombophlebitis of tibial vein

I80.231   Phlebitis and thrombophlebitis of right tibial vein 🬀

I80.232   Phlebitis and thrombophlebitis of left tibial vein 🬀

I80.233   Phlebitis and thrombophlebitis of tibial vein, bilateral 🬀

I80.239   Phlebitis and thrombophlebitis of unspecified tibial vein 🬀

● I80.29   Phlebitis and thrombophlebitis of other deep vessels of lower extremities

I80.291   Phlebitis and thrombophlebitis of other deep vessels of right lower extremity 🬀

I80.292   Phlebitis and thrombophlebitis of other deep vessels of left lower extremity 🬀

I80.293   Phlebitis and thrombophlebitis of other deep vessels of lower extremity, bilateral 🬀

I80.299   Phlebitis and thrombophlebitis of other deep vessels of unspecified lower extremity 🬀

I80.3   Phlebitis and thrombophlebitis of lower extremities, unspecified

I80.8   Phlebitis and thrombophlebitis of other sites

I80.9   Phlebitis and thrombophlebitis of unspecified site

I81   Portal vein thrombosis 🬀
Portal (vein) obstruction

Excludes2   hepatic vein thrombosis (I82.0)
phlebitis of portal vein (K75.1)

(Ex:) E08.51-E08.59, E08.618-E08.638, E08.649-E08.8, E09.51-E09.59, E09.618-E09.638, E09.649, E09.65-E09.8, E10.51-E10.59, E10.618-E10.638, E10.649, E10.69-E10.8, E11.51-E11.59, E11.618-E11.638, E11.649, E11.69-E11.8, E13.51-E13.59, E13.618-E13.638, E13.649-E13.8, I81, I82.210-I82.291, I82.401-I82.729, I82.811-I82.91, I82.A11-I82.C29, I87.8-I87.9, I99.8-I99.9

● I82   Other venous embolism and thrombosis

Code first venous embolism and thrombosis complicating:
abortion, ectopic or molar pregnancy (O00-O07, O08.7)
pregnancy, childbirth and the puerperium (O22.-, O87.-)

Excludes2   venous embolism and thrombosis (of):
cerebral (I63.6, I67.6)
coronary (I21-I25)
intracranial and intraspinal, septic or NOS (G08)
intracranial, nonpyogenic (I67.6)
intraspinal, nonpyogenic (G95.1)
mesenteric (K55.0-) ◀▥
portal (I81)
pulmonary (I26.-)

I82.0   Budd-Chiari syndrome 🬀
Hepatic vein thrombosis
(Ex:) E08.51-E08.59, E08.618-E08.638, E08.649-E08.8, E09.51-E09.59, E09.618-E09.638, E09.649, E09.65-E09.8, E10.51-E10.59, E10.618-E10.638, E10.649, E10.69-E10.8, E11.51-E11.59, E11.618-E11.638, E11.649, E11.69-E11.8, E13.51-E13.59, E13.618-E13.638, E13.649-E13.8, I82.0, I82.210-I82.291, I82.401-I82.729, I82.811-I82.91, I82.A11-I82.C29, I87.8-I87.9, I99.8-I99.9

I82.1   Thrombophlebitis migrans 🬀
"White leg" is the other term to describe a migrating thrombus.
(Ex:) E08.51-E08.59, E08.618-E08.638, E08.649-E08.8, E09.51-E09.59, E09.618-E09.638, E09.649, E09.65-E09.8, E10.51-E10.59, E10.618-E10.638, E10.649, E10.69-E10.8, E11.51-E11.59, E11.618-E11.638, E11.649, E11.69-E11.8, E13.51-E13.59, E13.618-E13.638, E13.649-E13.8, I82.1, I82.210-I82.291, I82.401-I82.729, I82.811-I82.91, I82.A11-I82.C29, I87.8-I87.9, I99.8-I99.9

● I82.2   Embolism and thrombosis of vena cava and other thoracic veins
(Ex:) For category I82.2 CC codes unless otherwise indicated:
E08.51-E08.59, E08.618-E08.638, E08.649-E08.8, E09.51-E09.59, E09.618-E09.638, E09.649, E09.65-E09.8, E10.51-E10.59, E10.618-E10.638, E10.649, E10.69-E10.8, E11.51-E11.59, E11.618-E11.638, E11.649, E11.69-E11.8, E13.51-E13.59, E13.618-E13.638, E13.649-E13.8, I82.210-I82.291, I82.401-I82.729, I82.811-I82.91, I82.A11-I82.C29, I87.8-I87.9, I99.8-I99.9

● I82.21   Embolism and thrombosis of superior vena cava

I82.210   Acute embolism and thrombosis of superior vena cava 🬀
Embolism and thrombosis of superior vena cava NOS

I82.211   Chronic embolism and thrombosis of superior vena cava 🬀

● I82.22   Embolism and thrombosis of inferior vena cava
(Ex:) For category I82.22 CC codes: E08.51-E08.59, E08.618-E08.638, E08.649-E08.8, E09.51-E09.59, E09.618-E09.638, E09.649, E09.65-E09.8, E10.51-E10.59, E10.618-E10.638, E10.649, E10.69-E10.8, E11.51-E11.59, E11.618-E11.638, E11.649, E11.69-E11.8, E13.51-E13.59, E13.618-E13.638, E13.649-E13.8, I82.210-I82.291, I82.401-I82.729, I82.811-I82.91, I82.A11-I82.C29, I87.8-I87.9, I99.8-I99.9

I82.220   Acute embolism and thrombosis of inferior vena cava 🬀
Embolism and thrombosis of inferior vena cava NOS

I82.221   Chronic embolism and thrombosis of inferior vena cava 🬀

● I82.29   Embolism and thrombosis of other thoracic veins
Embolism and thrombosis of brachiocephalic (innominate) vein

I82.290   Acute embolism and thrombosis of other thoracic veins 🬀

I82.291   Chronic embolism and thrombosis of other thoracic veins 🬀

I82.3   Embolism and thrombosis of renal vein 🬀
(Ex:) E08.51-E08.59, E08.618-E08.638, E08.649-E08.8, E09.51-E09.59, E09.618-E09.638, E09.649, E09.65-E09.8, E10.51-E10.59, E10.618-E10.638, E10.649, E10.69-E10.8, E11.51-E11.59, E11.618-E11.638, E11.649, E11.69-E11.8, E13.51-E13.59, E13.618-E13.638, E13.649-E13.8, I82.210-I82.291, I82.3, I82.401-I82.729, I82.811-I82.91, I82.A11-I82.C29, I87.8-I87.9, I99.8-I99.9

CHAPTER 9 (I00-I99)

● **I82.4** **Acute embolism and thrombosis of deep veins of lower extremity**
　　(Ex) **For category I82.4 CC codes:** See I82.2

　I82.40 **Acute embolism and thrombosis of unspecified deep veins of lower extremity**
　　　Deep vein thrombosis NOS
　　　DVT NOS
　　　Excludes1 acute embolism and thrombosis of unspecified deep veins of distal lower extremity (I82.4Z-)
　　　　　　acute embolism and thrombosis of unspecified deep veins of proximal lower extremity (I82.4Y-)

　　I82.401 **Acute embolism and thrombosis of** unspecified **deep veins of right lower extremity** 🕭 🕭

　　I82.402 **Acute embolism and thrombosis of** unspecified **deep veins of left lower extremity** 🕭 🕭

　　I82.403 **Acute embolism and thrombosis of** unspecified **deep veins of lower extremity, bilateral** 🕭 🕭

　　I82.409 **Acute embolism and thrombosis of** unspecified **deep veins of unspecified lower extremity** 🕭 🕭

● **I82.41** **Acute embolism and thrombosis of femoral vein**

　　I82.411 **Acute embolism and thrombosis of right femoral vein** 🕭 🕭

　　I82.412 **Acute embolism and thrombosis of left femoral vein** 🕭 🕭

　　I82.413 **Acute embolism and thrombosis of femoral vein, bilateral** 🕭 🕭

　　I82.419 **Acute embolism and thrombosis of** unspecified **femoral vein** 🕭 🕭

● **I82.42** **Acute embolism and thrombosis of iliac vein**

　　I82.421 **Acute embolism and thrombosis of right iliac vein** 🕭 🕭

　　I82.422 **Acute embolism and thrombosis of left iliac vein** 🕭 🕭

　　I82.423 **Acute embolism and thrombosis of iliac vein, bilateral** 🕭 🕭

　　I82.429 **Acute embolism and thrombosis of** unspecified **iliac vein** 🕭 🕭

● **I82.43** **Acute embolism and thrombosis of popliteal vein**

　　I82.431 **Acute embolism and thrombosis of right popliteal vein** 🕭 🕭

　　I82.432 **Acute embolism and thrombosis of left popliteal vein** 🕭 🕭

　　I82.433 **Acute embolism and thrombosis of popliteal vein, bilateral** 🕭 🕭

　　I82.439 **Acute embolism and thrombosis of** unspecified **popliteal vein** 🕭 🕭

● **I82.44** **Acute embolism and thrombosis of tibial vein**

　　I82.441 **Acute embolism and thrombosis of right tibial vein** 🕭 🕭

　　I82.442 **Acute embolism and thrombosis of left tibial vein** 🕭 🕭

　　I82.443 **Acute embolism and thrombosis of tibial vein, bilateral** 🕭 🕭

　　I82.449 **Acute embolism and thrombosis of** unspecified **tibial vein** 🕭 🕭

● **I82.49** **Acute embolism and thrombosis of other specified deep vein of lower extremity**

　　I82.491 **Acute embolism and thrombosis of other specified deep vein of right lower extremity** 🕭 🕭

　　I82.492 **Acute embolism and thrombosis of other specified deep vein of left lower extremity** 🕭 🕭

　　I82.493 **Acute embolism and thrombosis of other specified deep vein of lower extremity, bilateral** 🕭 🕭

　　I82.499 **Acute embolism and thrombosis of other specified deep vein of** unspecified **lower extremity** 🕭 🕭

● **I82.4Y** **Acute embolism and thrombosis of unspecified deep veins of proximal lower extremity**
　　　Acute embolism and thrombosis of deep vein of thigh NOS
　　　Acute embolism and thrombosis of deep vein of upper leg NOS

　　I82.4Y1 **Acute embolism and thrombosis of** unspecified **deep veins of right proximal lower extremity** 🕭 🕭

　　I82.4Y2 **Acute embolism and thrombosis of** unspecified **deep veins of left proximal lower extremity** 🕭 🕭

　　I82.4Y3 **Acute embolism and thrombosis of** unspecified **deep veins of proximal lower extremity, bilateral** 🕭 🕭

　　I82.4Y9 **Acute embolism and thrombosis of** unspecified **deep veins of unspecified proximal lower extremity** 🕭 🕭

● **I82.4Z** **Acute embolism and thrombosis of unspecified deep veins of distal lower extremity**
　　　Acute embolism and thrombosis of deep vein of calf NOS
　　　Acute embolism and thrombosis of deep vein of lower leg NOS

　　I82.4Z1 **Acute embolism and thrombosis of** unspecified **deep veins of right distal lower extremity** 🕭 🕭

　　I82.4Z2 **Acute embolism and thrombosis of** unspecified **deep veins of left distal lower extremity** 🕭 🕭

　　I82.4Z3 **Acute embolism and thrombosis of** unspecified **deep veins of distal lower extremity, bilateral** 🕭 🕭

　　I82.4Z9 **Acute embolism and thrombosis of** unspecified **deep veins of unspecified distal lower extremity** 🕭 🕭

● **I82.5** **Chronic embolism and thrombosis of deep veins of lower extremity**
　　　Use additional code, if applicable, for associated long-term (current) use of anticoagulants (Z79.01)
　　　Excludes1 personal history of venous embolism and thrombosis (Z86.718)
　　　(Ex) **For category I82.5 CC codes:** See I82.2

　● **I82.50** **Chronic embolism and thrombosis of unspecified deep veins of lower extremity**
　　　Excludes1 chronic embolism and thrombosis of unspecified deep veins of distal lower extremity (I82.5Z-)
　　　　　　chronic embolism and thrombosis of unspecified deep veins of proximal lower extremity (I82.5Y-)

　　I82.501 **Chronic embolism and thrombosis of** unspecified **deep veins of right lower extremity** 🕭

　　I82.502 **Chronic embolism and thrombosis of** unspecified **deep veins of left lower extremity** 🕭

Item 9-10 Varicose/Varicosities (varix = singular, varices = plural): Enlarged, engorged, tortuous, twisted vascular vessels (veins, arteries, lymphatics). As such, the condition can present in various parts of the body, although the most familiar locations are the lower extremities. A common complication of varices is thrombophlebitis. Varicosities of the anus and rectum are called hemorrhoids.

Figure 9-7 Varicose veins of the legs. (From Goldman: Cecil Medicine, ed 23, Saunders, 2008)

I82.503   Chronic embolism and thrombosis of unspecified deep veins of lower extremity, bilateral 🔖

I82.509   Chronic embolism and thrombosis of unspecified deep veins of unspecified lower extremity 🔖

● I82.51   Chronic embolism and thrombosis of femoral vein

I82.511   Chronic embolism and thrombosis of right femoral vein 🔖

I82.512   Chronic embolism and thrombosis of left femoral vein 🔖

I82.513   Chronic embolism and thrombosis of femoral vein, bilateral 🔖

I82.519   Chronic embolism and thrombosis of unspecified femoral vein 🔖

● I82.52   Chronic embolism and thrombosis of iliac vein

I82.521   Chronic embolism and thrombosis of right iliac vein 🔖

I82.522   Chronic embolism and thrombosis of left iliac vein 🔖

I82.523   Chronic embolism and thrombosis of iliac vein, bilateral 🔖

I82.529   Chronic embolism and thrombosis of unspecified iliac vein 🔖

● I82.53   Chronic embolism and thrombosis of popliteal vein

I82.531   Chronic embolism and thrombosis of right popliteal vein 🔖

I82.532   Chronic embolism and thrombosis of left popliteal vein 🔖

I82.533   Chronic embolism and thrombosis of popliteal vein, bilateral 🔖

I82.539   Chronic embolism and thrombosis of unspecified popliteal vein 🔖

● I82.54   Chronic embolism and thrombosis of tibial vein

I82.541   Chronic embolism and thrombosis of right tibial vein 🔖

I82.542   Chronic embolism and thrombosis of left tibial vein 🔖

I82.543   Chronic embolism and thrombosis of tibial vein, bilateral 🔖

I82.549   Chronic embolism and thrombosis of unspecified tibial vein 🔖

● I82.59   Chronic embolism and thrombosis of other specified deep vein of lower extremity

I82.591   Chronic embolism and thrombosis of other specified deep vein of right lower extremity 🔖

I82.592   Chronic embolism and thrombosis of other specified deep vein of left lower extremity 🔖

I82.593   Chronic embolism and thrombosis of other specified deep vein of lower extremity, bilateral 🔖

I82.599   Chronic embolism and thrombosis of other specified deep vein of unspecified lower extremity 🔖

● I82.5Y   Chronic embolism and thrombosis of unspecified deep veins of proximal lower extremity

Chronic embolism and thrombosis of deep veins of thigh NOS

Chronic embolism and thrombosis of deep veins of upper leg NOS

I82.5Y1   Chronic embolism and thrombosis of unspecified deep veins of right proximal lower extremity 🔖

I82.5Y2   Chronic embolism and thrombosis of unspecified deep veins of left proximal lower extremity 🔖

I82.5Y3   Chronic embolism and thrombosis of unspecified deep veins of proximal lower extremity, bilateral 🔖

I82.5Y9   Chronic embolism and thrombosis of unspecified deep veins of unspecified proximal lower extremity 🔖

● I82.5Z   Chronic embolism and thrombosis of unspecified deep veins of distal lower extremity

Chronic embolism and thrombosis of deep veins of calf NOS

Chronic embolism and thrombosis of deep veins of lower leg NOS

I82.5Z1   Chronic embolism and thrombosis of unspecified deep veins of right distal lower extremity 🔖

I82.5Z2   Chronic embolism and thrombosis of unspecified deep veins of left distal lower extremity 🔖

I82.5Z3   Chronic embolism and thrombosis of unspecified deep veins of distal lower extremity, bilateral 🔖

I82.5Z9   Chronic embolism and thrombosis of unspecified deep veins of unspecified distal lower extremity 🔖

● I82.6   Acute embolism and thrombosis of veins of upper extremity

Ex) For category I82.6 CC codes: See I82.2

● I82.60   Acute embolism and thrombosis of unspecified veins of upper extremity

I82.601   Acute embolism and thrombosis of unspecified veins of right upper extremity 🔖

I82.602   Acute embolism and thrombosis of unspecified veins of left upper extremity 🔖

I82.603   Acute embolism and thrombosis of unspecified veins of upper extremity, bilateral 🔖

I82.609   Acute embolism and thrombosis of unspecified veins of unspecified upper extremity 🔖

CHAPTER 9 (I00-I99)

● **I82.61** **Acute embolism and thrombosis of superficial veins of upper extremity**
Acute embolism and thrombosis of antecubital vein
Acute embolism and thrombosis of basilic vein
Acute embolism and thrombosis of cephalic vein

    I82.611 Acute embolism and thrombosis of superficial veins of right upper extremity 🦟

    I82.612 Acute embolism and thrombosis of superficial veins of left upper extremity 🦟

    I82.613 Acute embolism and thrombosis of superficial veins of upper extremity, bilateral 🦟

    I82.619 Acute embolism and thrombosis of superficial veins of unspecified upper extremity 🦟

● **I82.62** **Acute embolism and thrombosis of deep veins of upper extremity**
Acute embolism and thrombosis of brachial vein
Acute embolism and thrombosis of radial vein
Acute embolism and thrombosis of ulnar vein

    I82.621 Acute embolism and thrombosis of deep veins of right upper extremity 🦟

    I82.622 Acute embolism and thrombosis of deep veins of left upper extremity 🦟

    I82.623 Acute embolism and thrombosis of deep veins of upper extremity, bilateral 🦟

    I82.629 Acute embolism and thrombosis of deep veins of unspecified upper extremity 🦟

● **I82.7** **Chronic embolism and thrombosis of veins of upper extremity**
Use additional code, if applicable, for associated long-term (current) use of anticoagulants (Z79.01)
Excludes1   personal history of venous embolism and thrombosis (Z86.718)
(Ex) **For category I82.7 CC codes:** See I82.2

● **I82.70** **Chronic embolism and thrombosis of unspecified veins of upper extremity**

    I82.701 Chronic embolism and thrombosis of unspecified veins of right upper extremity 🦟

    I82.702 Chronic embolism and thrombosis of unspecified veins of left upper extremity 🦟

    I82.703 Chronic embolism and thrombosis of unspecified veins of upper extremity, bilateral 🦟

    I82.709 Chronic embolism and thrombosis of unspecified veins of unspecified upper extremity 🦟

● **I82.71** **Chronic embolism and thrombosis of superficial veins of upper extremity**
Chronic embolism and thrombosis of antecubital vein
Chronic embolism and thrombosis of basilic vein
Chronic embolism and thrombosis of cephalic vein

    I82.711 Chronic embolism and thrombosis of superficial veins of right upper extremity 🦟

    I82.712 Chronic embolism and thrombosis of superficial veins of left upper extremity 🦟

    I82.713 Chronic embolism and thrombosis of superficial veins of upper extremity, bilateral 🦟

    I82.719 Chronic embolism and thrombosis of superficial veins of unspecified upper extremity 🦟

● **I82.72** **Chronic embolism and thrombosis of deep veins of upper extremity**
Chronic embolism and thrombosis of brachial vein
Chronic embolism and thrombosis of radial vein
Chronic embolism and thrombosis of ulnar vein

    I82.721 Chronic embolism and thrombosis of deep veins of right upper extremity 🦟

    I82.722 Chronic embolism and thrombosis of deep veins of left upper extremity 🦟

    I82.723 Chronic embolism and thrombosis of deep veins of upper extremity, bilateral 🦟

    I82.729 Chronic embolism and thrombosis of deep veins of unspecified upper extremity 🦟

● **I82.A** **Embolism and thrombosis of axillary vein**
(Ex) **For category I82.A CC codes:** See I82.2

● **I82.A1** **Acute embolism and thrombosis of axillary vein**

    I82.A11 Acute embolism and thrombosis of right axillary vein 🦟

    I82.A12 Acute embolism and thrombosis of left axillary vein 🦟

    I82.A13 Acute embolism and thrombosis of axillary vein, bilateral 🦟

    I82.A19 Acute embolism and thrombosis of unspecified axillary vein 🦟

● **I82.A2** **Chronic embolism and thrombosis of axillary vein**

    I82.A21 Chronic embolism and thrombosis of right axillary vein 🦟

    I82.A22 Chronic embolism and thrombosis of left axillary vein 🦟

    I82.A23 Chronic embolism and thrombosis of axillary vein, bilateral 🦟

    I82.A29 Chronic embolism and thrombosis of unspecified axillary vein 🦟

● **I82.B** **Embolism and thrombosis of subclavian vein**
(Ex) **For category I82.B CC codes:** See I82.2

● **I82.B1** **Acute embolism and thrombosis of subclavian vein**

    I82.B11 Acute embolism and thrombosis of right subclavian vein 🦟

    I82.B12 Acute embolism and thrombosis of left subclavian vein 🦟

    I82.B13 Acute embolism and thrombosis of subclavian vein, bilateral 🦟

    I82.B19 Acute embolism and thrombosis of unspecified subclavian vein 🦟

● **I82.B2** **Chronic embolism and thrombosis of subclavian vein**

    I82.B21 Chronic embolism and thrombosis of right subclavian vein 🦟

    I82.B22 Chronic embolism and thrombosis of left subclavian vein 🦟

    I82.B23 Chronic embolism and thrombosis of subclavian vein, bilateral 🦟

    I82.B29 Chronic embolism and thrombosis of unspecified subclavian vein 🦟

◀ New   ◀▥ Revised   ~~deleted~~ Deleted   Excludes 1   Excludes 2   Includes   Use additional   Code first   Code also   Unspecified
OGCR Official Guidelines   ● Unacceptable Principal Diagnosis   X Assign placeholder X   ● Use Additional Character(s)   ▶ Manifestation Code   **Coding Clinic**
910

● **I82.C   Embolism and thrombosis of internal jugular vein**
   (Ex) For category I82.C CC codes: See I82.2

 ● **I82.C1   Acute embolism and thrombosis of internal jugular vein**

    I82.C11   Acute embolism and thrombosis of right internal jugular vein 🗪

    I82.C12   Acute embolism and thrombosis of left internal jugular vein 🗪

    I82.C13   Acute embolism and thrombosis of internal jugular vein, bilateral 🗪

    I82.C19   Acute embolism and thrombosis of unspecified internal jugular vein 🗪

 ● **I82.C2   Chronic embolism and thrombosis of internal jugular vein**

    I82.C21   Chronic embolism and thrombosis of right internal jugular vein 🗪

    I82.C22   Chronic embolism and thrombosis of left internal jugular vein 🗪

    I82.C23   Chronic embolism and thrombosis of internal jugular vein, bilateral 🗪

    I82.C29   Chronic embolism and thrombosis of unspecified internal jugular vein 🗪

● **I82.8   Embolism and thrombosis of other specified veins**
   Use additional code, if applicable, for associated long-term (current) use of anticoagulants (Z79.01)
   (Ex) For category I82.8 CC codes: See I82.2

 ● **I82.81   Embolism and thrombosis of superficial veins of lower extremities**
    Embolism and thrombosis of saphenous vein (greater) (lesser)

    I82.811   Embolism and thrombosis of superficial veins of right lower extremities 🗪

    I82.812   Embolism and thrombosis of superficial veins of left lower extremities 🗪

    I82.813   Embolism and thrombosis of superficial veins of lower extremities, bilateral 🗪

    I82.819   Embolism and thrombosis of superficial veins of unspecified lower extremities 🗪

 ● **I82.89   Embolism and thrombosis of other specified veins**

    I82.890   Acute embolism and thrombosis of other specified veins 🗪

    I82.891   Chronic embolism and thrombosis of other specified veins 🗪

● **I82.9   Embolism and thrombosis of unspecified vein**
   (Ex) For category I82.9 CC codes: See I82.2

   I82.90   Acute embolism and thrombosis of unspecified vein 🗪
    Embolism of vein NOS
    Thrombosis (vein) NOS

   I82.91   Chronic embolism and thrombosis of unspecified vein 🗪

● **I83   Varicose veins of lower extremities**
   Excludes1   varicose veins complicating pregnancy (O22.0-)
        varicose veins complicating the puerperium (O87.4)

● **I83.0   Varicose veins of lower extremities with ulcer**
   Use additional code to identify severity of ulcer (L97.-)

 ● **I83.00   Varicose veins of unspecified lower extremity with ulcer**

    I83.001   Varicose veins of unspecified lower extremity with ulcer of thigh   A

    I83.002   Varicose veins of unspecified lower extremity with ulcer of calf   A

    I83.003   Varicose veins of unspecified lower extremity with ulcer of ankle   A

    I83.004   Varicose veins of unspecified lower extremity with ulcer of heel and midfoot   A
     Varicose veins of unspecified lower extremity with ulcer of plantar surface of midfoot

    I83.005   Varicose veins of unspecified lower extremity with ulcer other part of foot   A
     Varicose veins of unspecified lower extremity with ulcer of toe

    I83.008   Varicose veins of unspecified lower extremity with ulcer other part of lower leg   A

    I83.009   Varicose veins of unspecified lower extremity with ulcer of unspecified site   A

 ● **I83.01   Varicose veins of right lower extremity with ulcer**

    I83.011   Varicose veins of right lower extremity with ulcer of thigh   A

    I83.012   Varicose veins of right lower extremity with ulcer of calf   A

    I83.013   Varicose veins of right lower extremity with ulcer of ankle   A

    I83.014   Varicose veins of right lower extremity with ulcer of heel and midfoot   A
     Varicose veins of right lower extremity with ulcer of plantar surface of midfoot

    I83.015   Varicose veins of right lower extremity with ulcer other part of foot   A
     Varicose veins of right lower extremity with ulcer of toe

    I83.018   Varicose veins of right lower extremity with ulcer other part of lower leg   A

    I83.019   Varicose veins of right lower extremity with ulcer of unspecified site   A

 ● **I83.02   Varicose veins of left lower extremity with ulcer**

    I83.021   Varicose veins of left lower extremity with ulcer of thigh   A

    I83.022   Varicose veins of left lower extremity with ulcer of calf   A

    I83.023   Varicose veins of left lower extremity with ulcer of ankle   A

    I83.024   Varicose veins of left lower extremity with ulcer of heel and midfoot   A
     Varicose veins of left lower extremity with ulcer of plantar surface of midfoot

    I83.025   Varicose veins of left lower extremity with ulcer other part of foot   A
     Varicose veins of left lower extremity with ulcer of toe

    I83.028   Varicose veins of left lower extremity with ulcer other part of lower leg   A

    I83.029   Varicose veins of left lower extremity with ulcer of unspecified site   A

● **I83.1   Varicose veins of lower extremities with inflammation**
   ~~Stasis dermatitis~~

   I83.10   Varicose veins of unspecified lower extremity with inflammation   A

   I83.11   Varicose veins of right lower extremity with inflammation   A

   I83.12   Varicose veins of left lower extremity with inflammation   A

N Newborn Age: 0   **P** Pediatric Age: 0–17   **M** Maternity DX: 12–55   **A** Adult Age: 15–124   ♀ Females Only   ♂ Males Only

🗪 Complication\Comorbidity   🗪 Major C\C   (Ex) CC/MCC Exclusions   🗪 Hospital-Acquired Condition

CHAPTER 9 (I00–I99)

911

CHAPTER 9 (I00-I99)

● **I83.2**   **Varicose veins of lower extremities with both ulcer and inflammation**

    Use additional code to identify severity of ulcer (L97.-)

    (Ex) **For category I83.2 CC codes:** I83.001-I83.229, I83.90-I83.93

  ● **I83.20**   **Varicose veins of unspecified lower extremity with both ulcer and inflammation**

      I83.201   **Varicose veins of unspecified lower extremity with both ulcer of thigh and inflammation** 🔖   A

      I83.202   **Varicose veins of unspecified lower extremity with both ulcer of calf and inflammation** 🔖   A

      I83.203   **Varicose veins of unspecified lower extremity with both ulcer of ankle and inflammation** 🔖   A

      I83.204   **Varicose veins of unspecified lower extremity with both ulcer of heel and midfoot and inflammation** 🔖   A

            Varicose veins of unspecified lower extremity with both ulcer of plantar surface of midfoot and inflammation

      I83.205   **Varicose veins of unspecified lower extremity with both ulcer other part of foot and inflammation** 🔖   A

            Varicose veins of unspecified lower extremity with both ulcer of toe and inflammation

      I83.208   **Varicose veins of unspecified lower extremity with both ulcer of other part of lower extremity and inflammation** 🔖   A

      I83.209   **Varicose veins of unspecified lower extremity with both ulcer of unspecified site and inflammation** 🔖 A

  ● **I83.21**   **Varicose veins of right lower extremity with both ulcer and inflammation**

      I83.211   **Varicose veins of right lower extremity with both ulcer of thigh and inflammation** 🔖   A

      I83.212   **Varicose veins of right lower extremity with both ulcer of calf and inflammation** 🔖   A

      I83.213   **Varicose veins of right lower extremity with both ulcer of ankle and inflammation** 🔖   A

      I83.214   **Varicose veins of right lower extremity with both ulcer of heel and midfoot and inflammation** 🔖   A

            Varicose veins of right lower extremity with both ulcer of plantar surface of midfoot and inflammation

      I83.215   **Varicose veins of right lower extremity with both ulcer other part of foot and inflammation** 🔖   A

            Varicose veins of right lower extremity with both ulcer of toe and inflammation

      I83.218   **Varicose veins of right lower extremity with both ulcer of other part of lower extremity and inflammation** 🔖   A

      I83.219   **Varicose veins of right lower extremity with both ulcer of unspecified site and inflammation** 🔖 A

  ● **I83.22**   **Varicose veins of left lower extremity with both ulcer and inflammation**

      I83.221   **Varicose veins of left lower extremity with both ulcer of thigh and inflammation** 🔖   A

      I83.222   **Varicose veins of left lower extremity with both ulcer of calf and inflammation** 🔖   A

      I83.223   **Varicose veins of left lower extremity with both ulcer of ankle and inflammation** 🔖   A

      I83.224   **Varicose veins of left lower extremity with both ulcer of heel and midfoot and inflammation** 🔖   A

            Varicose veins of left lower extremity with both ulcer of plantar surface of midfoot and inflammation

      I83.225   **Varicose veins of left lower extremity with both ulcer other part of foot and inflammation** 🔖   A

            Varicose veins of left lower extremity with both ulcer of toe and inflammation

      I83.228   **Varicose veins of left lower extremity with both ulcer of other part of lower extremity and inflammation** 🔖   A

      I83.229   **Varicose veins of left lower extremity with both ulcer of unspecified site and inflammation** 🔖

● **I83.8**   **Varicose veins of lower extremities with other complications**

  ● **I83.81**   **Varicose veins of lower extremities with pain**

      I83.811   **Varicose veins of right lower extremities with pain**   A

      I83.812   **Varicose veins of left lower extremities with pain**   A

      I83.813   **Varicose veins of bilateral lower extremities with pain**   A

      I83.819   **Varicose veins of unspecified lower extremities with pain**   A

  ● **I83.89**   **Varicose veins of lower extremities with other complications**

            Varicose veins of lower extremities with edema

            Varicose veins of lower extremities with swelling

      I83.891   **Varicose veins of right lower extremities with other complications** A

      I83.892   **Varicose veins of left lower extremities with other complications** A

      I83.893   **Varicose veins of bilateral lower extremities with other complications** A

      I83.899   **Varicose veins of unspecified lower extremities with other complications** A

● **I83.9**   **Asymptomatic varicose veins of lower extremities**

      Phlebectasia of lower extremities
      Varicose veins of lower extremities
      Varix of lower extremities

    I83.90   **Asymptomatic varicose veins of unspecified lower extremity**   A

            Varicose veins NOS

    I83.91   **Asymptomatic varicose veins of right lower extremity**   A

    I83.92   **Asymptomatic varicose veins of left lower extremity**   A

    I83.93   **Asymptomatic varicose veins of bilateral lower extremities**   A

◀ New   ◀ Revised   ~~deleted~~ Deleted   Excludes 1   Excludes 2   Includes   Use additional   Code first   Code also   Unspecified

OGCR Official Guidelines   ● Unacceptable Principal Diagnosis   X Assign placeholder X   ● Use Additional Character(s)   ▶ Manifestation Code   **Coding Clinic**

● **I85** **Esophageal varices**
　　Use additional code to identify:
　　　alcohol abuse and dependence (F10.-)

● **I85.0** **Esophageal varices**
　　Idiopathic esophageal varices
　　Primary esophageal varices

　I85.00 **Esophageal varices without bleeding** 🔹
　　　Esophageal varices NOS
　　　(Ex) E16.4, I85.00-I85.01, I85.11, I87.8-I87.9, I99.8-I99.9, K22.6,
　　　　K25.0-K28.9, K29.01, K29.21, K29.31, K29.41, K29.51,
　　　　K29.61, K29.71, K29.81, K29.91, K31.811, K92.0-K92.2

　I85.01 **Esophageal varices with bleeding** 🔹
　　　(Ex) E16.4, I85.01, I85.11, I87.8-I87.9, I99.8-I99.9, K22.10-K22.11,
　　　　K22.6-K22.70, K22.710-K22.719, K25.0-K28.9, K29.01,
　　　　K29.21, K29.31, K29.41, K29.51, K29.61, K29.71, K29.81,
　　　　K29.91, K31.811, K55.21, K57.01, K57.11, K57.13, K57.21,
　　　　K57.31, K57.33, K57.41, K57.51, K57.53, K57.81, K57.91,
　　　　K57.93, K62.5, K92.0-K92.2

● **I85.1** **Secondary esophageal varices**
　　Esophageal varices secondary to alcoholic liver disease
　　Esophageal varices secondary to cirrhosis of liver
　　Esophageal varices secondary to schistosomiasis
　　Esophageal varices secondary to toxic liver disease
　　Code first underlying disease

　I85.10 **Secondary esophageal varices without
　　　bleeding** 🔹
　　　(Ex) E16.4, I85.01, I85.10-I85.11, I87.8-I87.9, I99.8-I99.9, K22.6,
　　　　K25.0-K28.9, K29.01, K29.21, K29.31, K29.41, K29.51,
　　　　K29.61, K29.71, K29.81, K29.91, K31.811, K92.0-K92.2

　I85.11 **Secondary esophageal varices with bleeding** 🔹
　　　(Ex) I85.01, I85.11, I87.8-I87.9, I99.8-I99.9

● **I86** **Varicose veins of other sites**
　　Excludes1 varicose veins of unspecified site (I83.9-)
　　Excludes2 retinal varices (H35.0-)
　I86.0 **Sublingual varices**
　I86.1 **Scrotal varices** ♂
　　　Varicocele
　I86.2 **Pelvic varices**
　I86.3 **Vulval varices** ♀
　　Excludes1 vulval varices complicating childbirth
　　　　and the puerperium (O87.8)
　　　　vulval varices complicating pregnancy
　　　　　(O22.1-)
　I86.4 **Gastric varices**
　I86.8 **Varicose veins of other specified sites**   A
　　　Varicose ulcer of nasal septum

● **I87** **Other disorders of veins**
● **I87.0** **Postthrombotic syndrome**
　　Chronic venous hypertension due to deep vein
　　　thrombosis
　　Postphlebitic syndrome
　　Excludes1 chronic venous hypertension without
　　　　deep vein thrombosis (I87.3-)

　● **I87.00** **Postthrombotic syndrome without
　　　complications**
　　　Asymptomatic Postthrombotic syndrome
　　I87.001 **Postthrombotic syndrome without
　　　　complications of right lower
　　　　extremity**
　　I87.002 **Postthrombotic syndrome without
　　　　complications of left lower extremity**
　　I87.003 **Postthrombotic syndrome without
　　　　complications of bilateral lower
　　　　extremity**
　　I87.009 **Postthrombotic syndrome without
　　　　complications of unspecified
　　　　extremity**
　　　　Postthrombotic syndrome NOS

● **I87.01** **Postthrombotic syndrome with ulcer**
　　Use additional code to specify site and severity
　　　of ulcer (L97.-)
　　(Ex) For category I87.01 CC codes: I80.00-I80.9
　　I87.011 **Postthrombotic syndrome with ulcer
　　　　of right lower extremity** 🔹
　　I87.012 **Postthrombotic syndrome with ulcer
　　　　of left lower extremity** 🔹
　　I87.013 **Postthrombotic syndrome with ulcer
　　　　of bilateral lower extremity** 🔹
　　I87.019 **Postthrombotic syndrome with ulcer
　　　　of unspecified lower extremity** 🔹

● **I87.02** **Postthrombotic syndrome with inflammation**
　　I87.021 **Postthrombotic syndrome with
　　　　inflammation of right lower extremity**
　　I87.022 **Postthrombotic syndrome with
　　　　inflammation of left lower extremity**
　　I87.023 **Postthrombotic syndrome with
　　　　inflammation of bilateral lower
　　　　extremity**
　　I87.029 **Postthrombotic syndrome with
　　　　inflammation of unspecified lower
　　　　extremity**

● **I87.03** **Postthrombotic syndrome with ulcer and
　　inflammation**
　　Use additional code to specify site and severity
　　　of ulcer (L97.-)
　　(Ex) For category I87.03 CC codes: I80.00-I80.9
　　I87.031 **Postthrombotic syndrome with ulcer
　　　　and inflammation of right lower
　　　　extremity** 🔹
　　I87.032 **Postthrombotic syndrome with ulcer
　　　　and inflammation of left lower
　　　　extremity** 🔹
　　I87.033 **Postthrombotic syndrome with ulcer
　　　　and inflammation of bilateral lower
　　　　extremity** 🔹
　　I87.039 **Postthrombotic syndrome with ulcer
　　　　and inflammation of unspecified
　　　　lower extremity** 🔹

● **I87.09** **Postthrombotic syndrome with other
　　complications**
　　I87.091 **Postthrombotic syndrome with
　　　　other complications of right lower
　　　　extremity**
　　I87.092 **Postthrombotic syndrome with other
　　　　complications of left lower extremity**
　　I87.093 **Postthrombotic syndrome with other
　　　　complications of bilateral lower
　　　　extremity**
　　I87.099 **Postthrombotic syndrome with other
　　　　complications of unspecified lower
　　　　extremity**

　I87.1 **Compression of vein** 🔹
　　　Stricture of vein
　　　Vena cava syndrome (inferior) (superior)
　　Excludes2 compression of pulmonary vein (I28.8)
　　(Ex) I87.1

　I87.2 **Venous insufficiency (chronic) (peripheral)**
　　　Stasis dermatitis ◄
　　Excludes1 stasis dermatitis with varicose veins of
　　　　lower extremities (I83.1-, I83.2-) ◄

N Newborn Age: 0   **P** Pediatric Age: 0–17   **M** Maternity DX: 12–55   **A** Adult Age: 15–124   ♀ Females Only   ♂ Males Only
🔹 Complication\Comorbidity   🔹 Major C\C   (Ex) CC/MCC Exclusions   🔹 Hospital-Acquired Condition

913

● **I87.3**   **Chronic venous hypertension (idiopathic)**
Stasis edema

> **Excludes1**   chronic venous hypertension due to deep vein thrombosis (I87.0-)
> varicose veins of lower extremities (I83.-)

● **I87.30**   **Chronic venous hypertension (idiopathic) without complications**
Asymptomatic chronic venous hypertension (idiopathic)

I87.301   **Chronic venous hypertension (idiopathic) without complications of right lower extremity**

I87.302   **Chronic venous hypertension (idiopathic) without complications of left lower extremity**

I87.303   **Chronic venous hypertension (idiopathic) without complications of bilateral lower extremity**

I87.309   **Chronic venous hypertension (idiopathic) without complications of unspecified lower extremity**
Chronic venous hypertension NOS

● **I87.31**   **Chronic venous hypertension (idiopathic) with ulcer**

> Use additional code to specify site and severity of ulcer (L97.-)
> ⒺⓍ **For category I87.31 CC codes:** I83.001-I83.229, I83.90-I83.93, I87.2, I87.8-I87.9, I99.8-I99.9

I87.311   **Chronic venous hypertension (idiopathic) with ulcer of right lower extremity** 🔗

I87.312   **Chronic venous hypertension (idiopathic) with ulcer of left lower extremity** 🔗

I87.313   **Chronic venous hypertension (idiopathic) with ulcer of bilateral lower extremity** 🔗

I87.319   **Chronic venous hypertension (idiopathic) with ulcer of unspecified lower extremity** 🔗

● **I87.32**   **Chronic venous hypertension (idiopathic) with inflammation**

I87.321   **Chronic venous hypertension (idiopathic) with inflammation of right lower extremity**

I87.322   **Chronic venous hypertension (idiopathic) with inflammation of left lower extremity**

I87.323   **Chronic venous hypertension (idiopathic) with inflammation of bilateral lower extremity**

I87.329   **Chronic venous hypertension (idiopathic) with inflammation of unspecified lower extremity**

● **I87.33**   **Chronic venous hypertension (idiopathic) with ulcer and inflammation**

> Use additional code to specify site and severity of ulcer (L97.-)
> ⒺⓍ **For category I87.33 CC codes:** See I87.31

I87.331   **Chronic venous hypertension (idiopathic) with ulcer and inflammation of right lower extremity** 🔗

I87.332   **Chronic venous hypertension (idiopathic) with ulcer and inflammation of left lower extremity** 🔗

I87.333   **Chronic venous hypertension (idiopathic) with ulcer and inflammation of bilateral lower extremity** 🔗

I87.339   **Chronic venous hypertension (idiopathic) with ulcer and inflammation of unspecified lower extremity** 🔗

● **I87.39**   **Chronic venous hypertension (idiopathic) with other complications**

I87.391   **Chronic venous hypertension (idiopathic) with other complications of right lower extremity**

I87.392   **Chronic venous hypertension (idiopathic) with other complications of left lower extremity**

I87.393   **Chronic venous hypertension (idiopathic) with other complications of bilateral lower extremity**

I87.399   **Chronic venous hypertension (idiopathic) with other complications of unspecified lower extremity**

I87.8   **Other specified disorders of veins**
Phlebosclerosis
Venofibrosis

I87.9   **Disorder of vein, unspecified**

● **I88**   **Nonspecific lymphadenitis**

> **Excludes1**   acute lymphadenitis, except mesenteric (L04.-)
> enlarged lymph nodes NOS (R59.-)
> human immunodeficiency virus [HIV] disease resulting in generalized lymphadenopathy (B20)

I88.0   **Nonspecific mesenteric lymphadenitis**
Mesenteric lymphadenitis (acute)(chronic)

I88.1   **Chronic lymphadenitis, except mesenteric**
Adenitis
Lymphadenitis

I88.8   **Other nonspecific lymphadenitis**

I88.9   **Nonspecific lymphadenitis, unspecified**
Lymphadenitis NOS

● **I89**   **Other noninfective disorders of lymphatic vessels and lymph nodes**

> **Excludes1**   chylocele, tunica vaginalis (nonfilarial) NOS (N50.89) ◀▥
> enlarged lymph nodes NOS (R59.-)
> filarial chylocele (B74.-)
> hereditary lymphedema (Q82.0)

I89.0   **Lymphedema, not elsewhere classified**
Elephantiasis (nonfilarial) NOS
Lymphangiectasis
Obliteration, lymphatic vessel
Praecox lymphedema
Secondary lymphedema

> **Excludes1**   postmastectomy lymphedema (I97.2)

I89.1   **Lymphangitis**
Chronic lymphangitis
Lymphangitis NOS
Subacute lymphangitis

> **Excludes1**   acute lymphangitis (L03.-)

I89.8   **Other specified noninfective disorders of lymphatic vessels and lymph nodes**
Chylocele (nonfilarial)
Chylous ascites
Chylous cyst
Lipomelanotic reticulosis
Lymph node or vessel fistula
Lymph node or vessel infarction
Lymph node or vessel rupture

I89.9   **Noninfective disorder of lymphatic vessels and lymph nodes, unspecified**
Disease of lymphatic vessels NOS

◀ New   ◀▥ Revised   ~~deleted~~ Deleted   Excludes 1   Excludes 2   Includes   Use additional   Code first   Code also   Unspecified

914   OGCR Official Guidelines   ● Unacceptable Principal Diagnosis   X Assign placeholder X   ● Use Additional Character(s)   ▸ Manifestation Code   **Coding Clinic**

OTHER AND UNSPECIFIED DISORDERS OF THE CIRCULATORY SYSTEM (I95-I99)

● **I95** **Hypotension**
Subnormal arterial blood pressure
> **Excludes1** cardiovascular collapse (R57.9)
> maternal hypotension syndrome (O26.5-)
> nonspecific low blood pressure reading NOS
> (R03.1)

I95.0 **Idiopathic hypotension**

I95.1 **Orthostatic hypotension**
Hypotension, postural
> *Moving from a sitting or reclining position to a standing*
> *position precipitates a sudden drop in blood pressure*
> *(hypotension).*
>> **Excludes1** neurogenic orthostatic hypotension [Shy-
>> Drager] (G90.3)
>> orthostatic hypotension due to drugs
>> (I95.2)

I95.2 **Hypotension due to drugs**
Orthostatic hypotension due to drugs
Use additional code for adverse effect, if applicable,
to identify drug (T36-T50 with fifth or sixth
character 5)

I95.3 **Hypotension of hemodialysis**
Intra-dialytic hypotension

● **I95.8** **Other hypotension**
> **I95.81** **Postprocedural hypotension**
> **I95.89** **Other hypotension**
> Chronic hypotension

I95.9 **Hypotension, unspecified**

I96 **Gangrene, not elsewhere classified** 🦠
Gangrenous cellulitis
> **Excludes1** gangrene in atherosclerosis of native arteries of
> the extremities (I70.26)
> gangrene of certain specified sites - *see*
> Alphabetical Index
> gangrene in diabetes mellitus
> (E08-E13 with .52) ◀▥
> gangrene in hernia (K40.1, K40.4, K41.1, K41.4,
> K42.1, K43.1-, K44.1, K45.1, K46.1)
> gangrene in other peripheral vascular diseases
> (I73.-)
> gas gangrene (A48.0)
> pyoderma gangrenosum (L88)
> (Ex.) See I70.26

Coding Clinic: 2013, Q2, P35

● **I97** **Intraoperative and postprocedural complications and disorders
of circulatory system, not elsewhere classified**
> **Excludes2** postprocedural shock (T81.1-)

I97.0 **Postcardiotomy syndrome**

● **I97.1** **Other postprocedural cardiac functional disturbances**
> **Excludes2** acute pulmonary insufficiency following
> thoracic surgery (J95.1)
> intraoperative cardiac functional
> disturbances (I97.7-)
> (Ex.) For category I97.1 CC codes: D78.81-D78.89, E36.8, E89.810-E89.89,
> H59.011-H59.019, H59.031-H59.099, H59.811-H59.89, H95.811-H95.89,
> I97.110-I97.191, I97.3, I97.710-I97.791, I97.88-I97.89, L76.81-L76.82,
> M96.89, N98.1-N98.9, T81.82X[A], T81.89X-T81.9XX[A]

> ● **I97.11** **Postprocedural cardiac insufficiency**
>> **I97.110** **Postprocedural cardiac insufficiency**
>> **following cardiac surgery** 🦠
>> **I97.111** **Postprocedural cardiac insufficiency**
>> **following other surgery** 🦠

> ● **I97.12** **Postprocedural cardiac arrest**
>> **I97.120** **Postprocedural cardiac arrest**
>> **following cardiac surgery** 🦠
>> **I97.121** **Postprocedural cardiac arrest**
>> **following other surgery** 🦠

● **I97.13** **Postprocedural heart failure**
Use additional code to identify the heart
failure (I50.-)
> **I97.130** **Postprocedural heart failure**
> **following cardiac surgery** 🦠
> **I97.131** **Postprocedural heart failure**
> **following other surgery** 🦠

● **I97.19** **Other postprocedural cardiac functional
disturbances**
Use additional code, if applicable, to further
specify disorder
> **I97.190** **Other postprocedural cardiac
> functional disturbances following
> cardiac surgery** 🦠
> **I97.191** **Other postprocedural cardiac
> functional disturbances following
> other surgery** 🦠

I97.2 **Postmastectomy lymphedema syndrome**   A
Elephantiasis due to mastectomy
Obliteration of lymphatic vessels

I97.3 **Postprocedural hypertension**

● **I97.4** **Intraoperative hemorrhage and hematoma of a
circulatory system organ or structure complicating a
procedure**
> **Excludes1** intraoperative hemorrhage and
> hematoma of a circulatory system
> organ or structure due to accidental
> puncture and laceration during a
> procedure (I97.5-)
> **Excludes2** intraoperative cerebrovascular
> hemorrhage complicating a
> procedure (G97.3-)
> (Ex.) For category I97.4 CC codes: H95.811-H95.89, I85.01, I85.11,
> I97.3-I97.42, I97.610-I97.648, K21.9, K22.8, K23-K25.0, K25.2, K25.4,
> K25.6, K26.0, K26.2, K26.4, K26.6, K27.0, K27.2, K27.4, K27.6, K28.0,
> K28.2, K28.4, K28.6, K29.01, K29.21, K29.31, K29.41, K29.51, K29.61,
> K29.71, K29.81, K29.91, K31.811, K55.21, K57.01, K57.11, K57.13,
> K57.21, K57.31, K57.33, K57.41, K57.51, K57.53, K57.81, K57.91, K57.93,
> K62.5, K92.0-K92.2, M96.89, N98.1-N98.9, P54.1-P54.3,
> T81.10X-T81.19X[A], T81.82X[A], T81.89X-T81.9XX[A]

> ● **I97.41** **Intraoperative hemorrhage and hematoma
> of a circulatory system organ or structure
> complicating a circulatory system procedure**
>> **I97.410** **Intraoperative hemorrhage and
>> hematoma of a circulatory system
>> organ or structure complicating a
>> cardiac catheterization** 🦠
>> **I97.411** **Intraoperative hemorrhage and
>> hematoma of a circulatory system
>> organ or structure complicating a
>> cardiac bypass** 🦠
>> **I97.418** **Intraoperative hemorrhage and
>> hematoma of a circulatory system
>> organ or structure complicating other
>> circulatory system procedure** 🦠

> **I97.42** **Intraoperative hemorrhage and hematoma of a
> circulatory system organ or structure
> complicating other procedure**

● **I97.5** **Accidental puncture and laceration of a circulatory
system organ or structure during a procedure**
> **Excludes2** accidental puncture and laceration of
> brain during a procedure (G97.4-)
> (Ex.) For category I97.5 CC codes: D78.11-D78.12, D78.81-D78.89,
> E36.11-E36.8, E89.810-E89.89, G96.11, G97.41-G97.49, H59.011-H59.019,
> H59.031-H59.099, H59.211-H59.229, H59.811-H59.89, H95.31-H95.32,
> H95.811-H95.89, I97.3, I97.51-I97.52, J95.71-J95.72, K91.71-K91.72,
> L76.11-L76.12, L76.81-L76.82, M96.820-M96.821, M96.89, N98.1-N98.9,
> N99.71-N99.72, T81.82X[A], T81.89X-T81.9XX[A]

> **I97.51** **Accidental puncture and laceration of a
> circulatory system organ or structure during a
> circulatory system procedure** 🦠

> **I97.52** **Accidental puncture and laceration of a
> circulatory system organ or structure during
> other procedure** 🦠

N Newborn Age: 0   **P** Pediatric Age: 0–17   **M** Maternity DX: 12–55   **A** Adult Age: 15–124   ♀ Females Only   ♂ Males Only
🦠 Complication\Comorbidity   🦠 Major C\C   (Ex.) CC/MCC Exclusions   🦠 Hospital-Acquired Condition

915

● **I97.6** **Postprocedural hemorrhage, hematoma and seroma of a circulatory system organ or structure following a procedure** ◄⊪

    Excludes2   postprocedural cerebrovascular hemorrhage complicating a procedure (G97.5-)

    (Ex) For category I97.6 CC codes: See I97.4

● **I97.61** Postprocedural hemorrhage of a circulatory system organ or structure following a circulatory system procedure ◄⊪

    I97.610   Postprocedural hemorrhage of a circulatory system organ or structure following a cardiac catheterization 🞉 ◄⊪

    I97.611   Postprocedural hemorrhage of a circulatory system organ or structure following cardiac bypass 🞉 ◄⊪

    I97.618   Postprocedural hemorrhage of a circulatory system organ or structure following other circulatory system procedure 🞉 ◄⊪

● **I97.62** Postprocedural hemorrhage, hematoma and seroma of a circulatory system organ or structure following other procedure ◄⊪

    I97.620   Postprocedural hemorrhage of a circulatory system organ or structure following other procedure 🞉 ◄

    I97.621   Postprocedural hematoma of a circulatory system organ or structure following other procedure 🞉 ◄

    I97.622   Postprocedural seroma of a circulatory system organ or structure following other procedure 🞉 ◄

● **I97.63** Postprocedural hematoma of a circulatory system organ or structure following a circulatory system procedure ◄

    I97.630   Postprocedural hematoma of a circulatory system organ or structure following a cardiac catheterization 🞉 ◄

    I97.631   Postprocedural hematoma of a circulatory system organ or structure following cardiac bypass 🞉 ◄

    I97.638   Postprocedural hematoma of a circulatory system organ or structure following other circulatory system procedure 🞉 ◄

● **I97.64** Postprocedural seroma of a circulatory system organ or structure following a circulatory system procedure ◄

    I97.640   Postprocedural seroma of a circulatory system organ or structure following a cardiac catheterization 🞉 ◄

    I97.641   Postprocedural seroma of a circulatory system organ or structure following cardiac bypass 🞉 ◄

    I97.648   Postprocedural seroma of a circulatory system organ or structure following other procedure 🞉 ◄

● **I97.7** **Intraoperative cardiac functional disturbances**

    Excludes2   acute pulmonary insufficiency following thoracic surgery (J95.1)
postprocedural cardiac functional disturbances (I97.1-)

    (Ex) For category I97.7 CC codes: See I97.1

● **I97.71** Intraoperative cardiac arrest

    I97.710   Intraoperative cardiac arrest during cardiac surgery 🞉

    I97.711   Intraoperative cardiac arrest during other surgery 🞉

● **I97.79** Other intraoperative cardiac functional disturbances

    Use additional code, if applicable, to further specify disorder

    I97.790   Other intraoperative cardiac functional disturbances during cardiac surgery 🞉

    I97.791   Other intraoperative cardiac functional disturbances during other surgery 🞉

● **I97.8** **Other intraoperative and postprocedural complications and disorders of the circulatory system, not elsewhere classified**

    Use additional code, if applicable, to further specify disorder

    (Ex) For category I97.8 CC codes unless otherwise indicated: D78.81-D78.89, E36.8, E89.810-E89.89, G97.0, G97.2-G97.32, G97.81-G97.82, H59.011-H59.019, H59.031-H59.099, H59.811-H59.89, H95.811-H95.89, I97.3, I97.810-I97.821, L76.81-L76.82, M96.89, N98.1-N98.9, T81.82X[A], T81.89X-T81.9XX[A]

● **I97.81** Intraoperative cerebrovascular infarction

    I97.810   Intraoperative cerebrovascular infarction during cardiac surgery 🞉

    I97.811   Intraoperative cerebrovascular infarction during other surgery 🞉

● **I97.82** Postprocedural cerebrovascular infarction

    I97.820   Postprocedural cerebrovascular infarction following cardiac surgery 🞉 ◄⊪

    I97.821   Postprocedural cerebrovascular infarction following other surgery 🞉 ◄⊪

    I97.88   Other intraoperative complications of the circulatory system, not elsewhere classified 🞉
        (Ex) See I97.1

    I97.89   Other postprocedural complications and disorders of the circulatory system, not elsewhere classified 🞉
        (Ex) See I97.1

● **I99** **Other and unspecified disorders of circulatory system**

    I99.8   Other disorder of circulatory system

    I99.9   Unspecified disorder of circulatory system

◄ New   ◄⊪ Revised   ~~deleted~~ Deleted   Excludes 1   Excludes 2   Includes   Use additional   Code first   Code also   Unspecified
OGCR Official Guidelines   ● Unacceptable Principal Diagnosis   X Assign placeholder X   🞉 Use Additional Character(s)   ▶ Manifestation Code   **Coding Clinic**

CHAPTER 10

DISEASES OF THE RESPIRATORY SYSTEM (J00-J99)

OGCR Chapter-Specific Coding Guidelines

10. **Chapter 10: Diseases of the Respiratory System (J00-J99)**

   a. **Chronic Obstructive Pulmonary Disease [COPD] and Asthma**

      1) **Acute exacerbation of chronic obstructive bronchitis and asthma**

The codes in categories J44 and J45 distinguish between uncomplicated cases and those in acute exacerbation. An acute exacerbation is a worsening or a decompensation of a chronic condition. An acute exacerbation is not equivalent to an infection superimposed on a chronic condition, though an exacerbation may be triggered by an infection.

   b. **Acute Respiratory Failure**

      1) **Acute respiratory failure as principal diagnosis**

A code from subcategory J96.0, Acute respiratory failure, or subcategory J96.2, Acute and chronic respiratory failure, may be assigned as a principal diagnosis when it is the condition established after study to be chiefly responsible for occasioning the admission to the hospital, and the selection is supported by the Alphabetic Index and Tabular List. However, chapter-specific coding guidelines (such as obstetrics, poisoning, HIV, newborn) that provide sequencing direction take precedence.

      2) **Acute respiratory failure as secondary diagnosis**

Respiratory failure may be listed as a secondary diagnosis if it occurs after admission, or if it is present on admission, but does not meet the definition of principal diagnosis.

      3) **Sequencing of acute respiratory failure and another acute condition**

When a patient is admitted with respiratory failure and another acute condition, (e.g., myocardial infarction, cerebrovascular accident, aspiration pneumonia), the principal diagnosis will not be the same in every situation. This applies whether the other acute condition is a respiratory or nonrespiratory condition. Selection of the principal diagnosis will be dependent on the circumstances of admission. If both the respiratory failure and the other acute condition are equally responsible for occasioning the admission to the hospital, and there are no chapter-specific sequencing rules, the guideline regarding two or more diagnoses that equally meet the definition for principal diagnosis (*Section II, C.*) may be applied in these situations.

If the documentation is not clear as to whether acute respiratory failure and another condition are equally responsible for occasioning the admission, query the provider for clarification.

   c. **Influenza due to certain identified influenza viruses**

Code only confirmed cases of influenza due to certain identified influenza viruses (category J09), and due to other identified influenza virus (category J10). This is an exception to the hospital inpatient guideline Section II, H. (Uncertain Diagnosis).

In this context, "confirmation" does not require documentation of positive laboratory testing specific for avian or other novel influenza A or other identified influenza virus. However, coding should be based on the provider's diagnostic statement that the patient has avian influenza, or other novel influenza A, for category J09, or has another particular identified strain of influenza, such as H1N1 or H3N2, but not identified as novel or variant, for category J10.

If the provider records "suspected" or "possible" or "probable" avian influenza, or novel influenza, or other identified influenza, then the appropriate influenza code from category J11, Influenza due to unidentified influenza virus, should be assigned. A code from category J09, Influenza due to certain identified influenza viruses, should not be assigned nor should a code from category J10, Influenza due to other identified influenza virus.

   d. **Ventilator associated Pneumonia**

      1) **Documentation of Ventilator associated Pneumonia**

As with all procedural or postprocedural complications, code assignment is based on the provider's documentation of the relationship between the condition and the procedure.

Code J95.851, Ventilator associated pneumonia, should be assigned only when the provider has documented ventilator associated pneumonia (VAP). An additional code to identify the organism (e.g., Pseudomonas aeruginosa, code B96.5) should also be assigned. Do not assign an additional code from categories J12-J18 to identify the type of pneumonia.

Code J95.851 should not be assigned for cases where the patient has pneumonia and is on a mechanical ventilator and the provider has not specifically stated that the pneumonia is ventilator-associated pneumonia. If the documentation is unclear as to whether the patient has a pneumonia that is a complication attributable to the mechanical ventilator, query the provider.

      2) **Ventilator associated Pneumonia Develops after Admission**

A patient may be admitted with one type of pneumonia (e.g., code J13, Pneumonia due to Streptococcus pneumonia) and subsequently develop VAP. In this instance, the principal diagnosis would be the appropriate code from categories J12-J18 for the pneumonia diagnosed at the time of admission. Code J95.851, Ventilator associated pneumonia, would be assigned as an additional diagnosis when the provider has also documented the presence of ventilator associated pneumonia.

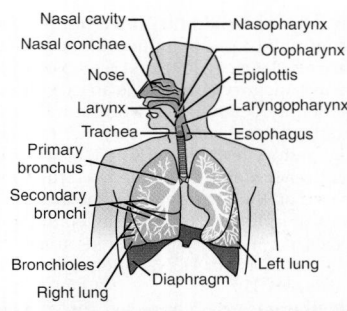

Figure 10-1 Respiratory system. (From Buck CJ: Step-by-Step Medical Coding, ed 2016, St. Louis, Elsevier, 2016)

Figure 10-2 Paranasal sinuses. (From Buck CJ: Step-by-Step Medical Coding, ed 2016, St. Louis, Elsevier, 2016)

Item 10–1 Pharyngitis is painful inflammation of the pharynx (sore throat). Ninety percent of the infections are caused by a virus with the remaining being bacterial and rarely a fungus (candidiasis). Other irritants such as pollutants, chemicals, or smoke may cause similar symptoms.

CHAPTER 10

DISEASES OF THE RESPIRATORY SYSTEM (J00–J99)

Note: When a respiratory condition is described as occurring in more than one site and is not specifically indexed, it should be classified to the lower anatomic site (e.g., tracheobronchitis to bronchitis in J40).

Use additional code, where applicable, to identify:
exposure to environmental tobacco smoke (Z77.22)
exposure to tobacco smoke in the perinatal period (P96.81)
history of tobacco dependence (Z87.891) ◀▥▥
occupational exposure to environmental tobacco smoke (Z57.31)
tobacco dependence (F17.-)
tobacco use (Z72.0)

Excludes2 certain conditions originating in the perinatal period (P04-P96)
certain infectious and parasitic diseases (A00-B99)
complications of pregnancy, childbirth and the puerperium (O00-O99A)
congenital malformations, deformations and chromosomal abnormalities (Q00-Q99)
endocrine, nutritional and metabolic diseases (E00-E88)
injury, poisoning and certain other consequences of external causes (S00-T88)
neoplasms (C00-D49)
smoke inhalation (T59.81-)
symptoms, signs and abnormal clinical and laboratory findings, not elsewhere classified (R00-R94)

This chapter contains the following blocks:

J00-J06	Acute upper respiratory infections
J09-J18	Influenza and pneumonia
J20-J22	Other acute lower respiratory infections
J30-J39	Other diseases of upper respiratory tract
J40-J47	Chronic lower respiratory diseases
J60-J70	Lung diseases due to external agents
J80-J84	Other respiratory diseases principally affecting the interstitium
J85-J86	Suppurative and necrotic conditions of the lower respiratory tract
J90-J94	Other diseases of the pleura
J95	Intraoperative and postprocedural complications and disorders of respiratory system, not elsewhere classified
J96-J99	Other diseases of the respiratory system

ACUTE UPPER RESPIRATORY INFECTIONS (J00-J06)

Excludes1 chronic obstructive pulmonary disease with acute lower respiratory infection (J44.0)
influenza virus with other respiratory manifestations (J09.X2, J10.1, J11.1)

J00   Acute nasopharyngitis [common cold]
Acute rhinitis
Coryza (acute)
Infective nasopharyngitis NOS
Infective rhinitis
Nasal catarrh, acute
Nasopharyngitis NOS

Excludes1 acute pharyngitis (J02.-)
acute sore throat NOS (J02.9)
pharyngitis NOS (J02.9)
rhinitis NOS (J31.0)
sore throat NOS (J02.9)

Excludes2 allergic rhinitis (J30.1-J30.9)
chronic pharyngitis (J31.2)
chronic rhinitis (J31.0)
chronic sore throat (J31.2)
nasopharyngitis, chronic (J31.1)
vasomotor rhinitis (J30.0)

★ **(See Plate 49 on page 72.)**

● **J01   Acute sinusitis**
Includes acute abscess of sinus
acute empyema of sinus
acute infection of sinus
acute inflammation of sinus
acute suppuration of sinus

Use additional code (B95-B97) to identify infectious agent.
Excludes1 sinusitis NOS (J32.9)
Excludes2 chronic sinusitis (J32.0-J32.8)

● **J01.0   Acute maxillary sinusitis**
Acute antritis
J01.00   Acute maxillary sinusitis, unspecified
J01.01   Acute recurrent maxillary sinusitis

● **J01.1   Acute frontal sinusitis**
J01.10   Acute frontal sinusitis, unspecified
J01.11   Acute recurrent frontal sinusitis

● **J01.2   Acute ethmoidal sinusitis**
J01.20   Acute ethmoidal sinusitis, unspecified
J01.21   Acute recurrent ethmoidal sinusitis

● **J01.3   Acute sphenoidal sinusitis**
J01.30   Acute sphenoidal sinusitis, unspecified
J01.31   Acute recurrent sphenoidal sinusitis

● **J01.4   Acute pansinusitis**
J01.40   Acute pansinusitis, unspecified
J01.41   Acute recurrent pansinusitis

◀ New   ◀▥▥ Revised   ~~deleted~~ Deleted   Excludes 1   Excludes 2   Includes   Use additional   Code first   Code also   Unspecified

OGCR Official Guidelines   ● Unacceptable Principal Diagnosis   X Assign placeholder X   ● Use Additional Character(s)   ▶ Manifestation Code   **Coding Clinic**

J01.8   **Other acute sinusitis**

    J01.80   **Other acute sinusitis**

         Acute sinusitis involving more than one sinus but not pansinusitis

    J01.81   **Other acute recurrent sinusitis**

         Acute recurrent sinusitis involving more than one sinus but not pansinusitis

J01.9   **Acute sinusitis, unspecified**

    J01.90   **Acute sinusitis, unspecified**

    J01.91   **Acute recurrent sinusitis, unspecified**

J02   **Acute pharyngitis**

    Includes   acute sore throat

    Excludes1   acute laryngopharyngitis (J06.0)

         peritonsillar abscess (J36)

         pharyngeal abscess (J39.1)

         retropharyngeal abscess (J39.0)

    Excludes2   chronic pharyngitis (J31.2)

    J02.0   **Streptococcal pharyngitis**

       Septic pharyngitis

       Streptococcal sore throat

       Excludes2   scarlet fever (A38.-)

    J02.8   **Acute pharyngitis due to other specified organisms**

       Use additional code (B95-B97) to identify infectious agent

       Excludes1   pharyngitis due to coxsackie virus (B08.5)

           pharyngitis due to gonococcus (A54.5)

           acute pharyngitis due to herpes [simplex] virus (B00.2)

           acute pharyngitis due to infectious mononucleosis (B27.-)

           enteroviral vesicular pharyngitis (B08.5)

    J02.9   **Acute pharyngitis, unspecified**

       Gangrenous pharyngitis (acute)

       Infective pharyngitis (acute) NOS

       Pharyngitis (acute) NOS

       Sore throat (acute) NOS

       Suppurative pharyngitis (acute)

       Ulcerative pharyngitis (acute)

J03   **Acute tonsillitis**

    Inflammation of pharyngeal tonsils caused by virus or bacteria

    Excludes1   acute sore throat (J02.-)

         hypertrophy of tonsils (J35.1)

         peritonsillar abscess (J36)

         sore throat NOS (J02.9)

         streptococcal sore throat (J02.0)

    Excludes2   chronic tonsillitis (J35.0)

    J03.0   **Streptococcal tonsillitis**

      J03.00   **Acute streptococcal tonsillitis, unspecified**

      J03.01   **Acute recurrent streptococcal tonsillitis**

    J03.8   **Acute tonsillitis due to other specified organisms**

       Use additional code (B95-B97) to identify infectious agent.

       Excludes1   diphtheritic tonsillitis (A36.0)

           herpesviral pharyngotonsillitis (B00.2)

           streptococcal tonsillitis (J03.0)

           tuberculous tonsillitis (A15.8)

           Vincent's tonsillitis (A69.1)

      J03.80   **Acute tonsillitis due to other specified organisms**

      J03.81   **Acute recurrent tonsillitis due to other specified organisms**

    J03.9   **Acute tonsillitis, unspecified**

       Follicular tonsillitis (acute)

       Gangrenous tonsillitis (acute)

       Infective tonsillitis (acute)

       Tonsillitis (acute) NOS

       Ulcerative tonsillitis (acute)

      J03.90   **Acute tonsillitis, unspecified**

      J03.91   **Acute recurrent tonsillitis, unspecified**

Item 10–2   **Laryngitis** is an inflammation of the larynx (voice box) resulting in hoarse voice or the complete loss of the voice. **Tracheitis** is an inflammation of the trachea (often following a URI) commonly caused by *staphylococcus aureus* resulting in inspiratory stridor (crowing sound on inspiration) and a croup like cough.

J04   **Acute laryngitis and tracheitis**

    Use additional code (B95-B97) to identify infectious agent.

    Excludes1   acute obstructive laryngitis [croup] and epiglottitis (J05.-)

    Excludes2   laryngismus (stridulus) (J38.5)

    J04.0   **Acute laryngitis**

       Edematous laryngitis (acute)

       Laryngitis (acute) NOS

       Subglottic laryngitis (acute)

       Suppurative laryngitis (acute)

       Ulcerative laryngitis (acute)

       Excludes1   acute obstructive laryngitis (J05.0)

       Excludes2   chronic laryngitis (J37.0)

    J04.1   **Acute tracheitis**

       Acute viral tracheitis

       Catarrhal tracheitis (acute)

       Tracheitis (acute) NOS

       Excludes2   chronic tracheitis (J42)

      J04.10   **Acute tracheitis without obstruction**

      J04.11   **Acute tracheitis with obstruction** 🏥

         (Ex:) A15.8-A15.9, A17.9, A18.82, A18.84, A18.89, J04.10-J04.2, J05.10-J05.11, J22, J98.8-J98.9

    J04.2   **Acute laryngotracheitis**

       Laryngotracheitis NOS

       Tracheitis (acute) with laryngitis (acute)

       Excludes1   acute obstructive laryngotracheitis (J05.0)

       Excludes2   chronic laryngotracheitis (J37.1)

    J04.3   **Supraglottitis, unspecified**

      J04.30   **Supraglottitis, unspecified, without obstruction**

      J04.31   **Supraglottitis, unspecified, with obstruction** 🏥

         (Ex:) A15.8-A15.9, A17.9, A18.82, A18.84, A18.89, J04.0-J04.2, J05.10-J05.11, J22, J98.8-J98.9

J05   **Acute obstructive laryngitis [croup] and epiglottitis**

    Use additional code (B95-B97) to identify infectious agent.

    J05.0   **Acute obstructive laryngitis [croup]**

       Obstructive laryngitis (acute) NOS

       Obstructive laryngotracheitis NOS

    J05.1   **Acute epiglottitis**

       Excludes2   epiglottitis, chronic (J37.0)

      J05.10   **Acute epiglottitis without obstruction** 🏥

         Epiglottitis NOS

         (Ex:) J04.31, J05.10-J05.11

      J05.11   **Acute epiglottitis with obstruction** 🏥

         (Ex:) See J04.10

J06   **Acute upper respiratory infections of multiple and unspecified sites**

    Excludes1   acute respiratory infection NOS (J22)

         streptococcal pharyngitis (J02.0)

    J06.0   **Acute laryngopharyngitis**

    J06.9   **Acute upper respiratory infection, unspecified**

       Upper respiratory disease, acute

       Upper respiratory infection NOS

CHAPTER 10 (J00-J99)

N   Newborn Age: 0   **P**   Pediatric Age: 0–17   **M**   Maternity DX: 12–55   **A**   Adult Age: 15–124   ♀ Females Only   ♂ Males Only

🏥 Complication\Comorbidity   🏥 Major C\C   (Ex:) CC/MCC Exclusions   🏥 Hospital-Acquired Condition

919

CHAPTER 10 (J00-J99)

INFLUENZA AND PNEUMONIA (J09-J18)

Excludes2   allergic or eosinophilic pneumonia (J82)
aspiration pneumonia NOS (J69.0)
meconium pneumonia (P24.01)
neonatal aspiration pneumonia (P24.-)
pneumonia due to solids and liquids (J69.-)
congenital pneumonia (P23.9)
lipid pneumonia (J69.1)
rheumatic pneumonia (I00)
ventilator associated pneumonia (J95.851)

● **J09**   **Influenza due to certain identified influenza viruses**

Excludes1   influenza due to other influenza viruses (J10.-)
influenza due to unidentified influenza virus (J11.-)
seasonal influenza due to other identified influenza virus (J10.-)
seasonal influenza due to unidentified influenza virus (J11.-)

● **J09.X**   **Influenza due to identified novel influenza A virus**
Avian influenza
Bird influenza
Influenza A/H5N1
Influenza of other animal origin, not bird or swine
Swine influenza virus (viruses that normally cause infections in pigs)

J09.X1   **Influenza due to identified novel influenza A virus with pneumonia** 🐾
Code also , if applicable, associated:
lung abscess (J85.1)
other specified type of pneumonia
Ⓔⓧ A15.0-A15.9, A17.9, A18.82, A18.84, A18.89, A21.2, A22.1, A31.0, A37.01, A37.11, A37.81, A37.91, A42.0, A43.0, A48.1, B25.0, B39.0-B39.2, B44.0, B58.3, B59, B67.1, J09.X1-J09.X2, J10.00-J10.1, J11.00-J11.1, J12.0-J12.3, J12.89-J18.1, J18.8-J18.9, J22, J44.9, J47.0-J70.4, J70.8-J70.9, J98.4, J98.8-J98.9, Q33.4, R91.1

J09.X2   **Influenza due to identified novel influenza A virus with other respiratory manifestations**
Influenza due to identified novel influenza A virus NOS
Influenza due to identified novel influenza A virus with laryngitis
Influenza due to identified novel influenza A virus with pharyngitis
Influenza due to identified novel influenza A virus with upper respiratory symptoms
Use additional code, if applicable, for associated:
pleural effusion (J91.8)
sinusitis (J01.-)

J09.X3   **Influenza due to identified novel influenza A virus with gastrointestinal manifestations**
Influenza due to identified novel influenza A virus gastroenteritis
Excludes1   'intestinal flu' [viral gastroenteritis] (A08.-)

J09.X9   **Influenza due to identified novel influenza A virus with other manifestations**
Influenza due to identified novel influenza A virus with encephalopathy
Influenza due to identified novel influenza A virus with myocarditis
Influenza due to identified novel influenza A virus with otitis media
Use additional code to identify manifestation

● **J10**   **Influenza due to other identified influenza virus**

Excludes1   influenza due to avian influenza virus (J09.X-)
influenza due to swine flu (J09.X-)
influenza due to unidentified influenza virus (J11.-)

● **J10.0**   **Influenza due to other identified influenza virus with pneumonia**
Code also associated lung abscess, if applicable (J85.1)

J10.00   **Influenza due to other identified influenza virus with unspecified type of pneumonia** 🐾
Ⓔⓧ See J09.X1

J10.01   **Influenza due to other identified influenza virus with the same other identified influenza virus pneumonia** 🐾
Ⓔⓧ See J09.X1

J10.08   **Influenza due to other identified influenza virus with other specified pneumonia** 🐾
Code also other specified type of pneumonia
Ⓔⓧ A15.0-A15.6, A15.8-A15.9, A17.9, A18.82, A18.84, A18.89, A21.2, A22.1, A31.0, A37.01, A37.11, A37.81, A37.91, A42.0, A43.0, A48.1, B25.0, B39.0-B39.2, B44.0, B58.3, B59, B67.1, J09.X1-J09.X2, J10.00-J10.1, J11.00-J11.1, J12.0-J12.3, J12.89-J18.1, J18.8-J18.9, J22, J44.0-J44.9, J45.21-J45.22, J45.31-J45.32, J45.41-J45.42, J45.51-J45.902, J47.0-J70.4, J70.8-J70.9, J98.4, J98.8-J99, Q33.4, R91.1

J10.1   **Influenza due to other identified influenza virus with other respiratory manifestations**
Influenza due to other identified influenza virus NOS
Influenza due to other identified influenza virus with laryngitis
Influenza due to other identified influenza virus with pharyngitis
Influenza due to other identified influenza virus with upper respiratory symptoms
Use additional code for associated pleural effusion, if applicable (J91.8)
Use additional code for associated sinusitis, if applicable (J01.-)

J10.2   **Influenza due to other identified influenza virus with gastrointestinal manifestations**
Influenza due to other identified influenza virus gastroenteritis
Excludes1   'intestinal flu' [viral gastroenteritis] (A08.-)

● **J10.8**   **Influenza due to other identified influenza virus with other manifestations**

J10.81   **Influenza due to other identified influenza virus with encephalopathy**

J10.82   **Influenza due to other identified influenza virus with myocarditis**

J10.83   **Influenza due to other identified influenza virus with otitis media**
Use additional code for any associated perforated tympanic membrane (H72.-)

J10.89   **Influenza due to other identified influenza virus with other manifestations**
Use additional codes to identify the manifestations

● **J11**   **Influenza due to unidentified influenza virus**

● **J11.0**   **Influenza due to unidentified influenza virus with pneumonia**
Code also associated lung abscess, if applicable (J85.1)
Ⓔⓧ For category J11.0 CC codes: See J09.X1

J11.00   **Influenza due to unidentified influenza virus with unspecified type of pneumonia** 🐾
Influenza with pneumonia NOS

J11.08   **Influenza due to unidentified influenza virus with specified pneumonia** 🐾
Code also other specified type of pneumonia

◄ New   ⟵ Revised   ~~deleted~~ Deleted   Excludes 1   Excludes 2   Includes   Use additional   Code first   Code also   Unspecified
OGCR Official Guidelines   ● Unacceptable Principal Diagnosis   X Assign placeholder X   ● Use Additional Character(s)   ▌ Manifestation Code   **Coding Clinic**

J11.1   **Influenza due to unidentified influenza virus with other respiratory manifestations**
Influenza NOS
Influenzal laryngitis NOS
Influenzal pharyngitis NOS
Influenza with upper respiratory symptoms NOS
Use additional code for associated pleural effusion, if applicable (J91.8)
Use additional code for associated sinusitis, if applicable (J01.-)

J11.2   **Influenza due to unidentified influenza virus with gastrointestinal manifestations**
Influenza gastroenteritis NOS
Excludes1   'intestinal flu' [viral gastroenteritis] (A08.-)

● **J11.8**   **Influenza due to unidentified influenza virus with other manifestations**

     J11.81   **Influenza due to unidentified influenza virus with encephalopathy**
Influenzal encephalopathy NOS

     J11.82   **Influenza due to unidentified influenza virus with myocarditis**
Influenzal myocarditis NOS

     J11.83   **Influenza due to unidentified influenza virus with otitis media**
Influenzal otitis media NOS
Use additional code for any associated perforated tympanic membrane (H72.-)

     J11.89   **Influenza due to unidentified influenza virus with other manifestations**
Use additional codes to identify the manifestations

● **J12**   **Viral pneumonia, not elsewhere classified**
Includes   bronchopneumonia due to viruses other than influenza viruses
Code first associated influenza, if applicable (J09.X1, J10.0-, J11.0-)
Code also associated abscess, if applicable (J85.1)
Excludes1   aspiration pneumonia due to anesthesia during labor and delivery (O74.0)
aspiration pneumonia due to anesthesia during pregnancy (O29)
aspiration pneumonia due to anesthesia during puerperium (O89.0)
aspiration pneumonia due to solids and liquids (J69.-)
aspiration pneumonia NOS (J69.0)
congenital pneumonia (P23.0)
congenital rubella pneumonitis (P35.0)
interstitial pneumonia NOS (J84.9)
lipid pneumonia (J69.1)
neonatal aspiration pneumonia (P24.-)
(Ex) **For category J12 CC codes unless otherwise indicated:** A15.0-A15.6, A15.8-A15.9, A17.9, A18.82, A18.84, A18.89, A20.2, A21.1, A22.1, A31.0, A37.01, A37.11, A37.81, A37.91, A42.0, A43.0, A48.1, B25.0, B39.0-B39.2, B44.0, B58.3, B59, B67.1, J09. X1-J09.X2, J10.00-J10.1, J11.00-J11.1, J12.0-J12.3, J12.81-J18.1, J18.8-J18.9, J22, J60-J70.4, J70.8-J70.9, J98.4, J98.8-J99, R91.1

J12.0   **Adenoviral pneumonia** 🦠
J12.1   **Respiratory syncytial virus pneumonia** 🦠
J12.2   **Parainfluenza virus pneumonia** 🦠
J12.3   **Human metapneumovirus pneumonia** 🦠
● **J12.8**   **Other viral pneumonia**

     J12.81   **Pneumonia due to SARS-associated coronavirus** 🦠
Severe acute respiratory syndrome NOS
(Ex) A15.0-A15.6, A15.8-A15.9, A17.9, A18.82, A18.84, A18.89, A21.2, A22.1, A31.0, A37.01, A37.11, A37.81, A37.91, A42.0, A43.0, A48.1, B25.0, B39.0-B39.2, B44.0, B58.3, B59, B67.1, J09.X1-J09.X2, J10.00-J10.1, J11.00-J11.1, J12.0-J12.3, J12.81-J18.1, J18.8-J18.9, J22, J44.9, J47.0-J70.4, J70.8-J70.9, J98.4, J98.8-J99, Q33.4, R91.1

     J12.89   **Other viral pneumonia** 🦠
J12.9   **Viral pneumonia, unspecified** 🦠

Item 10-3   Pneumonia is an infection of the lungs, caused by a variety of microorganisms, including viruses, most commonly the Streptococcus pneumoniae (pneumococcus) bacteria, fungi, and parasites. Pneumonia occurs when the immune system is weakened, often by a URI or influenza.

J13   **Pneumonia due to Streptococcus pneumoniae** 🦠
Bronchopneumonia due to S. pneumoniae
Code first associated influenza, if applicable (J09.X1, J10.0-, J11.0-)
Code also associated abscess, if applicable (J85.1)
Excludes1   congenital pneumonia due to S. pneumoniae (P23.6)
lobar pneumonia, unspecified organism (J18.1)
pneumonia due to other streptococci (J15.3-J15.4)
(Ex) See J09.X1

J14   **Pneumonia due to Hemophilus influenzae** 🦠
Bronchopneumonia due to H. influenzae
Code first associated influenza, if applicable (J09.X1, J10.0-, J11.0-)
Code also associated abscess, if applicable (J85.1)
Excludes1   congenital pneumonia due to H. influenzae (P23.6)
(Ex) See J09.X1

● **J15**   **Bacterial pneumonia, not elsewhere classified**
Includes   bronchopneumonia due to bacteria other than S. pneumoniae and H. influenzae
Code first associated influenza, if applicable (J09.X1, J10.0-, J11.0-)
Code also associated abscess, if applicable (J85.1)
Excludes1   chlamydial pneumonia (J16.0)
congenital pneumonia (P23.-)
Legionnaires' disease (A48.1)
spirochetal pneumonia (A69.8)
(Ex) **For category J15 CC codes:** See J09.X1

J15.0   **Pneumonia due to Klebsiella pneumoniae** 🦠
J15.1   **Pneumonia due to Pseudomonas** 🦠
● **J15.2**   **Pneumonia due to staphylococcus**

     J15.20   **Pneumonia due to staphylococcus, unspecified** 🦠
     ● **J15.21**   **Pneumonia due to staphylococcus aureus**

         J15.211   **Pneumonia due to Methicillin susceptible Staphylococcus aureus** 🦠
MSSA pneumonia
Pneumonia due to Staphylococcus aureus NOS

         J15.212   **Pneumonia due to Methicillin resistant Staphylococcus aureus** 🦠

     J15.29   **Pneumonia due to other staphylococcus** 🦠
J15.3   **Pneumonia due to streptococcus, group B** 🦠
J15.4   **Pneumonia due to other streptococci** 🦠
     Excludes1   pneumonia due to streptococcus, group B (J15.3)
pneumonia due to Streptococcus pneumoniae (J13)

J15.5   **Pneumonia due to Escherichia coli** 🦠
J15.6   **Pneumonia due to other aerobic Gram-negative bacteria** 🦠
Pneumonia due to Serratia marcescens
J15.7   **Pneumonia due to Mycoplasma pneumoniae** 🦠
J15.8   **Pneumonia due to other specified bacteria** 🦠
J15.9   **Unspecified bacterial pneumonia** 🦠
Pneumonia due to gram-positive bacteria

N   Newborn Age: 0   P   Pediatric Age: 0-17   M   Maternity DX: 12-55   A   Adult Age: 15-124   ♀   Females Only   ♂   Males Only
🦠   Complication\Comorbidity   🦠   Major C\C   (Ex)   CC/MCC Exclusions   🦠   Hospital-Acquired Condition

CHAPTER 10 (J00-J99)

● **J16**   **Pneumonia due to other infectious organisms, not elsewhere classified**

     Code first associated influenza, if applicable (J09.X1, J10.0-, J11.0-)

     Code also associated abscess, if applicable (J85.1)

     Excludes1   congenital pneumonia (P23.-)
                  ornithosis (A70)
                  pneumocystosis (B59)
                  pneumonia NOS (J18.9)

     (Ex) For category J16 CC codes: See J09.X1

   J16.0   **Chlamydial pneumonia** 🐾

   J16.8   **Pneumonia due to other specified infectious organisms** 🐾

▷ **J17**   *Pneumonia in diseases classified elsewhere* 🐾

     Code first underlying disease, such as:
       Q fever (A78)
       rheumatic fever (I00)
       schistosomiasis (B65.0-B65.9)

     Excludes1   candidial pneumonia (B37.1)
                  chlamydial pneumonia (J16.0)
                  gonorrheal pneumonia (A54.84)
                  histoplasmosis pneumonia (B39.0-B39.2)
                  measles pneumonia (B05.2)
                  nocardiosis pneumonia (A43.0)
                  pneumocystosis (B59)
                  pneumonia due to Pneumocystis carinii (B59)
                  pneumonia due to Pneumocystis jiroveci (B59)
                  pneumonia in actinomycosis (A42.0)
                  pneumonia in anthrax (A22.1)
                  pneumonia in ascariasis (B77.81)
                  pneumonia in aspergillosis (B44.0-B44.1)
                  pneumonia in coccidioidomycosis (B38.0-B38.2)
                  pneumonia in cytomegalovirus disease (B25.0)
                  pneumonia in toxoplasmosis (B58.3)
                  rubella pneumonia (B06.81)
                  salmonella pneumonia (A02.22)
                  spirochetal infection NEC with pneumonia (A69.8)
                  tularemia pneumonia (A21.2)
                  typhoid fever with pneumonia (A01.03)
                  varicella pneumonia (B01.2)
                  whooping cough with pneumonia (A37 with fifth-character 1)

     (Ex) See J09.X1

● **J18**   **Pneumonia, unspecified organism**

     Code first associated influenza, if applicable (J09.X1, J10.0-, J11.0-)

     Excludes1   abscess of lung with pneumonia (J85.1)
                  aspiration pneumonia due to anesthesia during labor and delivery (O74.0)
                  aspiration pneumonia due to anesthesia during pregnancy (O29)
                  aspiration pneumonia due to anesthesia during puerperium (O89.0)
                  aspiration pneumonia due to solids and liquids (J69.-)
                  aspiration pneumonia NOS (J69.0)
                  congenital pneumonia (P23.0)
                  drug-induced interstitial lung disorder (J70.2-J70.4)
                  interstitial pneumonia NOS (J84.9)
                  lipid pneumonia (J69.1)
                  neonatal aspiration pneumonia (P24.-)
                  pneumonitis due to external agents (J67-J70)
                  pneumonitis due to fumes and vapors (J68.0)
                  usual interstitial pneumonia (J84.17)

     (Ex) For category J18 CC code unless otherwise indicated: See J09.X1

   J18.0   **Bronchopneumonia, unspecified organism** 🐾

       Excludes1   hypostatic bronchopneumonia (J18.2)
                    lipid pneumonia (J69.1)

       Excludes2   acute bronchiolitis (J21.-)
                    chronic bronchiolitis (J44.9)

   J18.1   **Lobar pneumonia, unspecified organism** 🐾

   J18.2   **Hypostatic pneumonia, unspecified organism** 🐾
       Hypostatic bronchopneumonia
       Passive pneumonia
       (Ex) J18.2, J22, J81.1, J98.4, J98.8-J99, R91.1

   J18.8   **Other pneumonia, unspecified organism** 🐾

   J18.9   **Pneumonia, unspecified organism** 🐾
       Coding Clinic: 2012, Q4, P94

OTHER ACUTE LOWER RESPIRATORY INFECTIONS (J20-J22)

     Excludes2   chronic obstructive pulmonary disease with acute lower respiratory infection (J44.0)

● **J20**   **Acute bronchitis**
     Inflammation/irritation of the bronchial tubes lasting 2-3 weeks, most commonly caused by a virus

     Includes   acute and subacute bronchitis (with) bronchospasm
                acute and subacute bronchitis (with) tracheitis
                acute and subacute bronchitis (with) tracheobronchitis, acute
                acute and subacute fibrinous bronchitis
                acute and subacute membranous bronchitis
                acute and subacute purulent bronchitis
                acute and subacute septic bronchitis

     Excludes1   bronchitis NOS (J40)
                  tracheobronchitis NOS (J40)

     Excludes2   acute bronchitis with bronchiectasis (J47.0)
                  acute bronchitis with chronic obstructive asthma (J44.0)
                  acute bronchitis with chronic obstructive pulmonary disease (J44.0)
                  allergic bronchitis NOS (J45.909-)
                  bronchitis due to chemicals, fumes and vapors (J68.0)
                  chronic bronchitis NOS (J42)
                  chronic mucopurulent bronchitis (J41.1)
                  chronic obstructive bronchitis (J44.-)
                  chronic obstructive tracheobronchitis (J44.-)
                  chronic simple bronchitis (J41.0)
                  chronic tracheobronchitis (J42)

   J20.0   **Acute bronchitis due to Mycoplasma pneumoniae**

   J20.1   **Acute bronchitis due to Hemophilus influenzae**

   J20.2   **Acute bronchitis due to streptococcus**

   J20.3   **Acute bronchitis due to coxsackievirus**

   J20.4   **Acute bronchitis due to parainfluenza virus**

   J20.5   **Acute bronchitis due to respiratory syncytial virus**

   J20.6   **Acute bronchitis due to rhinovirus**

   J20.7   **Acute bronchitis due to echovirus**

   J20.8   **Acute bronchitis due to other specified organisms**

   J20.9   **Acute bronchitis, unspecified**

● **J21**   **Acute bronchiolitis**
     Bronchiolitis obliterans with organizing pneumonia (BOOP) inflammation of bronchioles and surrounding tissue in lung

     Includes   acute bronchiolitis with bronchospasm

     Excludes2   respiratory bronchiolitis interstitial lung disease (J84.115)

     (Ex) For category J21 CC codes unless otherwise indicated: J20.0-J21.9

   J21.0   **Acute bronchiolitis due to respiratory syncytial virus** 🐾
       (Ex) J21.0

   J21.1   **Acute bronchiolitis due to human metapneumovirus** 🐾

   J21.8   **Acute bronchiolitis due to other specified organisms** 🐾

   J21.9   **Acute bronchiolitis, unspecified** 🐾
       Bronchiolitis (acute)

       Excludes1   chronic bronchiolitis (J44.-)

   J22   **Unspecified acute lower respiratory infection**
     Acute (lower) respiratory (tract) infection NOS

     Excludes1   upper respiratory infection (acute) (J06.9)

◀ New   ⬅ Revised   ~~deleted~~ Deleted   Excludes 1   Excludes 2   Includes   Use additional   Code first   Code also   Unspecified

OGCR Official Guidelines   ● Unacceptable Principal Diagnosis   X Assign placeholder X   ● Use Additional Character(s)   ▷ Manifestation Code   **Coding Clinic**

OTHER DISEASES OF UPPER RESPIRATORY TRACT (J30-J39)

● **J30** **Vasomotor and allergic rhinitis**

Includes spasmodic rhinorrhea

Excludes1 allergic rhinitis with asthma (bronchial) (J45.909)
rhinitis NOS (J31.0)

J30.0 **Vasomotor rhinitis**

J30.1 **Allergic rhinitis due to pollen**
Allergy NOS due to pollen
Hay fever
Pollinosis

J30.2 **Other seasonal allergic rhinitis**

J30.5 **Allergic rhinitis due to food**

● **J30.8** **Other allergic rhinitis**

J30.81 **Allergic rhinitis due to animal (cat) (dog) hair and dander**

J30.89 **Other allergic rhinitis**
Perennial allergic rhinitis

J30.9 **Allergic rhinitis, unspecified**

● **J31** **Chronic rhinitis, nasopharyngitis and pharyngitis**

Use additional code to identify:
exposure to environmental tobacco smoke (Z77.22)
exposure to tobacco smoke in the perinatal period (P96.81)
history of tobacco dependence (Z87.891) ◀▥▥
occupational exposure to environmental tobacco smoke (Z57.31)
tobacco dependence (F17.-)
tobacco use (Z72.0)

J31.0 **Chronic rhinitis**
Atrophic rhinitis (chronic)
Granulomatous rhinitis (chronic)
Hypertrophic rhinitis (chronic)
Obstructive rhinitis (chronic)
Ozena
Purulent rhinitis (chronic)
Rhinitis (chronic) NOS
Ulcerative rhinitis (chronic)

Excludes1 allergic rhinitis (J30.1-J30.9)
vasomotor rhinitis (J30.0)

J31.1 **Chronic nasopharyngitis**

Excludes2 acute nasopharyngitis (J00)

J31.2 **Chronic pharyngitis**
Chronic sore throat
Atrophic pharyngitis (chronic)
Granular pharyngitis (chronic)
Hypertrophic pharyngitis (chronic)

Excludes2 acute pharyngitis (J02.9)

● **J32** **Chronic sinusitis**

Includes sinus abscess
sinus empyema
sinus infection
sinus suppuration

Use additional code to identify:
exposure to environmental tobacco smoke (Z77.22)
exposure to tobacco smoke in the perinatal period (P96.81)
history of tobacco dependence (Z87.891) ◀▥▥
infectious agent (B95-B97)
occupational exposure to environmental tobacco smoke (Z57.31)
tobacco dependence (F17.-)
tobacco use (Z72.0)

Excludes2 acute sinusitis (J01.-)

J32.0 **Chronic maxillary sinusitis**
Antritis (chronic)
Maxillary sinusitis NOS

J32.1 **Chronic frontal sinusitis**
Frontal sinusitis NOS

Item 10–4 Nasal polyps are an abnormal growth of tissue (tumor) projecting from a mucous membrane and attached to the surface by a narrow elongated stalk (pedunculated). Nasal polyps usually originate in the ethmoid sinus but also may occur in the maxillary sinus. Symptoms are nasal block, sinusitis, anosmia, and secondary infections.

J32.2 **Chronic ethmoidal sinusitis**
Ethmoidal sinusitis NOS

Excludes1 Woakes' ethmoiditis (J33.1)

J32.3 **Chronic sphenoidal sinusitis**
Sphenoidal sinusitis NOS

J32.4 **Chronic pansinusitis**
Pansinusitis NOS

J32.8 **Other chronic sinusitis**
Sinusitis (chronic) involving more than one sinus but not pansinusitis

J32.9 **Chronic sinusitis, unspecified**
Sinusitis (chronic) NOS

● **J33** **Nasal polyp**

Use additional code to identify:
exposure to environmental tobacco smoke (Z77.22)
exposure to tobacco smoke in the perinatal period (P96.81)
history of tobacco dependence (Z87.891) ◀▥▥
occupational exposure to environmental tobacco smoke (Z57.31)
tobacco dependence (F17.-)
tobacco use (Z72.0)

Excludes1 adenomatous polyps (D14.0)

J33.0 **Polyp of nasal cavity**
Choanal polyp
Nasopharyngeal polyp

J33.1 **Polypoid sinus degeneration**
Woakes' syndrome or ethmoiditis

J33.8 **Other polyp of sinus**
Accessory polyp of sinus
Ethmoidal polyp of sinus
Maxillary polyp of sinus
Sphenoidal polyp of sinus

J33.9 **Nasal polyp, unspecified**

● **J34** **Other and unspecified disorders of nose and nasal sinuses**

Excludes2 varicose ulcer of nasal septum (I86.8)

J34.0 **Abscess, furuncle and carbuncle of nose**
Cellulitis of nose
Necrosis of nose
Ulceration of nose

J34.1 **Cyst and mucocele of nose and nasal sinus**

J34.2 **Deviated nasal septum**
Deflection or deviation of septum (nasal) (acquired)

Excludes1 congenital deviated nasal septum (Q67.4)

J34.3 **Hypertrophy of nasal turbinates**

Deviated septal cartilage

Figure 10-3 Deviated nasal septum.

Item 10–5 A **deviated nasal septum** is the displacement of the septal cartilage that separates the nares. This displacement causes obstructed air flow through the nasal passages. A child can be born with this displacement (congenital), or the condition may be acquired through trauma, such as a sports injury. Symptoms include nasal block, sinusitis, and related secondary infections. Septoplasty is surgical repair of this condition.

CHAPTER 10 (J00-J99)

N Newborn Age: 0 **P** Pediatric Age: 0–17 **M** Maternity DX: 12–55 **A** Adult Age: 15–124 ♀ Females Only ♂ Males Only

🞕 Complication\Comorbidity 🞕 Major C\C Ⓔⓧ CC/MCC Exclusions 🞕 Hospital-Acquired Condition

923

● **J34.8   Other specified disorders of nose and nasal sinuses**

J34.81   Nasal mucositis (ulcerative)

Code also type of associated therapy, such as:
antineoplastic and immunosuppressive
drugs (T45.1X-)
radiological procedure and radiotherapy
(Y84.2)

Excludes2 gastrointestinal mucositis
(ulcerative) (K92.81)
mucositis (ulcerative) of vagina
and vulva (N76.81)
oral mucositis (ulcerative)
(K12.3-)

**J34.89   Other specified disorders of nose and nasal
sinuses**
Perforation of nasal septum NOS
Rhinolith

J34.9   Unspecified disorder of nose and nasal sinuses

● **J35   Chronic diseases of tonsils and adenoids**

Use additional code to identify:
exposure to environmental tobacco smoke (Z77.22)
exposure to tobacco smoke in the perinatal period (P96.81)
history of tobacco dependence (Z87.891) ◀▦
occupational exposure to environmental tobacco smoke
(Z57.31)
tobacco dependence (F17.-)
tobacco use (Z72.0)

● **J35.0   Chronic tonsillitis and adenoiditis**

Excludes2 acute tonsillitis (J03.-)

J35.01   Chronic tonsillitis

J35.02   Chronic adenoiditis

J35.03   Chronic tonsillitis and adenoiditis

J35.1   Hypertrophy of tonsils
Enlargement of tonsils

Excludes1 hypertrophy of tonsils with tonsillitis
(J35.0-)

J35.2   Hypertrophy of adenoids
Enlargement of adenoids

Excludes1 hypertrophy of adenoids with adenoiditis
(J35.0-)

J35.3   Hypertrophy of tonsils with hypertrophy of adenoids

Excludes1 hypertrophy of tonsils and adenoids with
tonsillitis and adenoiditis (J35.03)

J35.8   Other chronic diseases of tonsils and adenoids
Adenoid vegetations
Amygdalolith
Calculus, tonsil
Cicatrix of tonsil (and adenoid)
Tonsillar tag
Ulcer of tonsil

J35.9   Chronic disease of tonsils and adenoids, unspecified
Disease (chronic) of tonsils and adenoids NOS

J36   Peritonsillar abscess ▣

Includes abscess of tonsil
peritonsillar cellulitis
quinsy

Use additional code (B95-B97) to identify infectious agent.

Excludes1 acute tonsillitis (J03.-)
chronic tonsillitis (J35.0)
retropharyngeal abscess (J39.0)
tonsillitis NOS (J03.9-)

(Ex:) J22, J36, J98.8-J98.9

● **J37   Chronic laryngitis and laryngotracheitis**

Use additional code to identify:
exposure to environmental tobacco smoke (Z77.22)
exposure to tobacco smoke in the perinatal period (P96.81)
history of tobacco dependence (Z87.891) ◀▦
infectious agent (B95-B97)
occupational exposure to environmental tobacco smoke
(Z57.31)
tobacco dependence (F17.-)
tobacco use (Z72.0)

J37.0   Chronic laryngitis
Catarrhal laryngitis
Hypertrophic laryngitis
Sicca laryngitis

Excludes2 acute laryngitis (J04.0)
obstructive (acute) laryngitis (J05.0)

J37.1   Chronic laryngotracheitis
Laryngitis, chronic, with tracheitis (chronic)
Tracheitis, chronic, with laryngitis

Excludes1 chronic tracheitis (J42)

Excludes2 acute laryngotracheitis (J04.2)
acute tracheitis (J04.1)

● **J38   Diseases of vocal cords and larynx, not elsewhere classified**

Use additional code to identify:
exposure to environmental tobacco smoke (Z77.22)
exposure to tobacco smoke in the perinatal period (P96.81)
history of tobacco dependence (Z87.891) ◀▦
occupational exposure to environmental tobacco smoke
(Z57.31)
tobacco dependence (F17.-)
tobacco use (Z72.0)

Excludes1 congenital laryngeal stridor (P28.89)
obstructive laryngitis (acute) (J05.0)
postprocedural subglottic stenosis (J95.5)
stridor (R06.1)
ulcerative laryngitis (J04.0)

● **J38.0   Paralysis of vocal cords and larynx**
Laryngoplegia
Paralysis of glottis

J38.00   Paralysis of vocal cords and larynx, unspecified

J38.01   Paralysis of vocal cords and larynx, unilateral

J38.02   Paralysis of vocal cords and larynx, bilateral

J38.1   Polyp of vocal cord and larynx

Excludes1 adenomatous polyps (D14.1)

J38.2   Nodules of vocal cords
Chorditis (fibrinous)(nodosa)(tuberosa)
Singer's nodes
Teacher's nodes

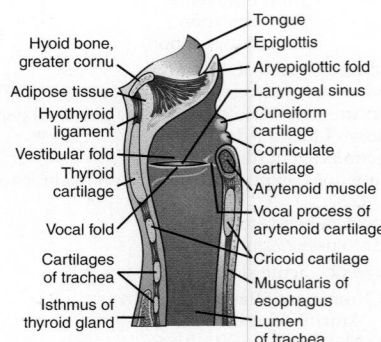

Figure 10-4 Coronal section of the larynx.

Item 10–6 The **larynx** extends from the tongue to the trachea and is divided into an upper and lower portion separated by folds. The framework of the larynx is cartilage composed of the single cricoid, thyroid, and epiglottic cartilages, and the paired arytenoid, cuneiform, and corniculate cartilages.

◀ New   ◀▦ Revised   ~~deleted~~ Deleted   Excludes 1   Excludes 2   Includes   Use additional   Code first   Code also   Unspecified

OGCR Official Guidelines   ● Unacceptable Principal Diagnosis   X Assign placeholder X   ● Use Additional Character(s)   ▸ Manifestation Code   **Coding Clinic**

J38.3   **Other diseases of vocal cords**
Abscess of vocal cords
Cellulitis of vocal cords
Granuloma of vocal cords
Leukokeratosis of vocal cords
Leukoplakia of vocal cords

J38.4   **Edema of larynx**
Edema (of) glottis
Subglottic edema
Supraglottic edema
> **Excludes1**   acute obstructive laryngitis [croup] (J05.0)
> edematous laryngitis (J04.0)

J38.5   **Laryngeal spasm**
Laryngismus (stridulus)

J38.6   **Stenosis of larynx**

J38.7   **Other diseases of larynx**
Abscess of larynx
Cellulitis of larynx
Disease of larynx NOS
Necrosis of larynx
Pachyderma of larynx
Perichondritis of larynx
Ulcer of larynx

● **J39**   **Other diseases of upper respiratory tract**
> **Excludes1**   acute respiratory infection NOS (J22)
> acute upper respiratory infection (J06.9)
> upper respiratory inflammation due to chemicals, gases, fumes or vapors (J68.2)

J39.0   **Retropharyngeal and parapharyngeal abscess** 🜚
Peripharyngeal abscess
> **Excludes1**   peritonsillar abscess (J36)
> (Ex) J22, J39.0-J39.1, J98.8-J98.9

J39.1   **Other abscess of pharynx** 🜚
Cellulitis of pharynx
Nasopharyngeal abscess
(Ex) J22, J39.0-J39.1, J98.8-J98.9

J39.2   **Other diseases of pharynx**
Cyst of pharynx
Edema of pharynx
> **Excludes2**   chronic pharyngitis (J31.2)
> ulcerative pharyngitis (J02.9)

J39.3   **Upper respiratory tract hypersensitivity reaction, site unspecified**
> **Excludes1**   hypersensitivity reaction of upper respiratory tract, such as:
> extrinsic allergic alveolitis (J67.9)
> pneumoconiosis (J60-J67.9)

J39.8   **Other specified diseases of upper respiratory tract**

J39.9   **Disease of upper respiratory tract, unspecified**

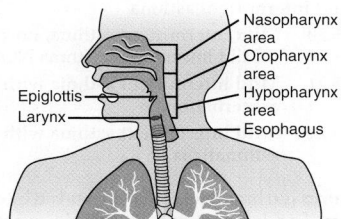

Nasopharynx area
Oropharynx area
Hypopharynx area
Esophagus
Epiglottis
Larynx

Figure 10-5 The pharynx.

Item 10–7 The **pharynx** is the passage for both food and air between the mouth and the esophagus and is divided into three areas: nasopharynx, oropharynx, and hypopharynx. The hypopharynx branches into the esophagus and the voice box.

Item 10–8 **Chronic bronchitis** is usually defined as being present in any patient who has persistent cough with sputum production for at least three months in at least two consecutive years. **Simple chronic bronchitis** is marked by a productive cough but no pathological airflow obstruction. **Chronic obstructive pulmonary disease (COPD)** is a group of conditions—bronchitis, emphysema, asthma, bronchiectasis, allergic alveolitis—marked by dyspnea. **Catarrhal** bronchitis is an acute form of bronchitis marked by profuse mucus and pus production (**mucopurulent** discharge). **Croupous** bronchitis, also known as pseudomembranous, fibrinous, plastic, exudative, or membranous, is marked by a violent cough and dyspnea.

CHRONIC LOWER RESPIRATORY DISEASES (J40-J47)

> **Excludes1**   bronchitis due to chemicals, gases, fumes and vapors (J68.0)
> **Excludes2**   cystic fibrosis (E84.-)

J40   **Bronchitis, not specified as acute or chronic**
Bronchitis NOS
Catarrhal bronchitis
Bronchitis with tracheitis NOS
Tracheobronchitis NOS
Use additional code to identify:
exposure to environmental tobacco smoke (Z77.22)
exposure to tobacco smoke in the perinatal period (P96.81)
history of tobacco dependence (Z87.891) ◄▥
occupational exposure to environmental tobacco smoke (Z57.31)
tobacco dependence (F17.-)
tobacco use (Z72.0)
> **Excludes1**   acute bronchitis (J20.-)
> allergic bronchitis NOS (J45.909-)
> asthmatic bronchitis NOS (J45.9-)
> bronchitis due to chemicals, gases, fumes and vapors (J68.0)

● **J41**   **Simple and mucopurulent chronic bronchitis**
Use additional code to identify:
exposure to environmental tobacco smoke (Z77.22)
exposure to tobacco smoke in the perinatal period (P96.81)
history of tobacco dependence (Z87.891) ◄▥
occupational exposure to environmental tobacco smoke (Z57.31)
tobacco dependence (F17.-)
tobacco use (Z72.0)
> **Excludes1**   chronic bronchitis NOS (J42)
> chronic obstructive bronchitis (J44.-)

J41.0   **Simple chronic bronchitis**

J41.1   **Mucopurulent chronic bronchitis**

J41.8   **Mixed simple and mucopurulent chronic bronchitis**

J42   **Unspecified chronic bronchitis**
Chronic bronchitis NOS
Chronic tracheitis
Chronic tracheobronchitis
Use additional code to identify:
exposure to environmental tobacco smoke (Z77.22)
exposure to tobacco smoke in the perinatal period (P96.81)
history of tobacco dependence (Z87.891) ◄▥
occupational exposure to environmental tobacco smoke (Z57.31)
tobacco dependence (F17.-)
tobacco use (Z72.0)
> **Excludes1**   chronic asthmatic bronchitis (J44.-)
> chronic bronchitis with airways obstruction (J44.-)
> chronic emphysematous bronchitis (J44.-)
> chronic obstructive pulmonary disease NOS (J44.9)
> simple and mucopurulent chronic bronchitis (J41.-)

CHAPTER 10 (J00-J99)

N Newborn Age: 0   P Pediatric Age: 0–17   M Maternity DX: 12–55   A Adult Age: 15–124   ♀ Females Only   ♂ Males Only
🜚 Complication\Comorbidity   🜚 Major C\C   (Ex) CC/MCC Exclusions   🜚 Hospital-Acquired Condition
925

● **J43**   **Emphysema**

Use additional code to identify:
exposure to environmental tobacco smoke (Z77.22)
history of tobacco dependence (Z87.891) ◀▪▪
occupational exposure to environmental tobacco smoke
   (Z57.31)
tobacco dependence (F17.-)
tobacco use (Z72.0)

Excludes1   compensatory emphysema (J98.3)
emphysema due to inhalation of chemicals, gases,
   fumes or vapors (J68.4)
emphysema with chronic (obstructive) bronchitis
   (J44.-)
emphysematous (obstructive) bronchitis (J44.-)
interstitial emphysema (J98.2)
mediastinal emphysema (J98.2)
neonatal interstitial emphysema (P25.0)
surgical (subcutaneous) emphysema (T81.82)
traumatic subcutaneous emphysema (T79.7)

J43.0   **Unilateral pulmonary emphysema [MacLeod's
syndrome]**
Swyer-James syndrome
Unilateral emphysema
Unilateral hyperlucent lung
Unilateral pulmonary artery functional hypoplasia
Unilateral transparency of lung

J43.1   **Panlobular emphysema**
Panacinar emphysema

J43.2   **Centrilobular emphysema**

J43.8   **Other emphysema**

J43.9   **Emphysema, unspecified**
Bullous emphysema (lung)(pulmonary)
Emphysema (lung)(pulmonary) NOS
Emphysematous bleb
Vesicular emphysema (lung)(pulmonary)

● **J44**   **Other chronic obstructive pulmonary disease**

Includes   asthma with chronic obstructive pulmonary
   disease
chronic asthmatic (obstructive) bronchitis
chronic bronchitis with airways obstruction
chronic bronchitis with emphysema
chronic emphysematous bronchitis
chronic obstructive asthma
chronic obstructive bronchitis
chronic obstructive tracheobronchitis

Code also type of asthma, if applicable (J45.-)
Use additional code to identify:
exposure to environmental tobacco smoke (Z77.22)
history of tobacco dependence (Z87.891) ◀▪▪
occupational exposure to environmental tobacco smoke
   (Z57.31)
tobacco dependence (F17.-)
tobacco use (Z72.0)

Excludes1   bronchiectasis (J47.-)
chronic bronchitis NOS (J42)
chronic simple and mucopurulent bronchitis (J41.-)
chronic tracheitis (J42)
chronic tracheobronchitis (J42)
emphysema without chronic bronchitis (J43.-)

Excludes2   lung diseases due to external agents (J60-J70) ◀

J44.0   **Chronic obstructive pulmonary disease with acute lower
respiratory infection** 🅒
Use additional code to identify the infection
   (Ex:) J10.08, J41.1-J42, J44.0-J44.1

Figure 10-6   Emphysema. (From Shiland, BJ: Medical Terminology &
Anatomy for ICD-10 Coding, ed 2, Mosby, 2015)

J44.1   **Chronic obstructive pulmonary disease with (acute)
exacerbation** 🅒
Decompensated COPD
Decompensated COPD with (acute) exacerbation

Excludes2   chronic obstructive pulmonary disease
   [COPD] with acute bronchitis (J44.0)
   (Ex:) J10.08, J41.1-J42, J44.0-J44.1
Coding Clinic: 2016, Q1, P36

J44.9   **Chronic obstructive pulmonary disease, unspecified**
Chronic obstructive airway disease NOS
Chronic obstructive lung disease NOS
Coding Clinic: 2016, Q1, P37

● **J45**   **Asthma**
Allergic (predominantly) asthma
Allergic bronchitis NOS
Allergic rhinitis with asthma
Atopic asthma
Extrinsic allergic asthma
Hay fever with asthma
Idiosyncratic asthma
Intrinsic nonallergic asthma
Nonallergic asthma
Use additional code to identify:
exposure to environmental tobacco smoke (Z77.22)
exposure to tobacco smoke in the perinatal period (P96.81)
history of tobacco dependence (Z87.891) ◀▪▪
occupational exposure to environmental tobacco smoke
   (Z57.31)
tobacco dependence (F17.-)
tobacco use (Z72.0)

Excludes1   detergent asthma (J69.8)
eosinophilic asthma (J82)
lung diseases due to external agents (J60-J70)
miner's asthma (J60)
wheezing NOS (R06.2)
wood asthma (J67.8)

Excludes2   asthma with chronic obstructive pulmonary
   disease (J44.9)
chronic asthmatic (obstructive) bronchitis (J44.9)
chronic obstructive asthma (J44.9)
(Ex:) **For category J45 CC codes:** J10.08, J22, J45.20-J45.998, J98.4, J98.8-J99, R91.1

● **J45.2**   **Mild intermittent asthma**

J45.20   **Mild intermittent asthma, uncomplicated**
Mild intermittent asthma NOS

J45.21   **Mild intermittent asthma with (acute)
exacerbation** 🅒

J45.22   **Mild intermittent asthma with status
asthmaticus** 🅒

Item 10–9   **Asthma** is a bronchial condition marked by airway obstruction,
hyper-responsiveness, and inflammation. **Extrinsic** asthma, also known as
allergic asthma, is characterized by the same symptoms that occur with exposure
to allergens and is divided into the following types: **atopic, occupational,
and allergic bronchopulmonary aspergillosis. Intrinsic** asthma
occurs in patients who have no history of allergy or sensitivities to allergens
and is divided into the following types: **nonreaginic and pharmacologic.
Status asthmaticus** is the most severe form of asthma attack and can last
for days or weeks.

◀ New   ◀▪▪ Revised   ~~deleted~~ Deleted   Excludes 1   Excludes 2   Includes   Use additional   Code first   Code also   Unspecified

926

OGCR Official Guidelines   ● Unacceptable Principal Diagnosis   X Assign placeholder X   🅒 Use Additional Character(s)   ▶ Manifestation Code   **Coding Clinic**

Figure 10-7 Factors causing expiratory obstruction in asthma. **A.** Cross section of a bronchiole occluded by muscle spasm, swollen mucosa, and mucus. **B.** Longitudinal section of an obstructed bronchiole. **C.** Cross-section of a clear bronchiole. (From Shiland: Mastering Healthcare Terminology, ed 1, St. Louis, Mosby, 2003)

● **J45.3** **Mild persistent asthma**

    J45.30 **Mild persistent asthma, uncomplicated**
          Mild persistent asthma NOS

    J45.31 **Mild persistent asthma with (acute) exacerbation** 🔖
          Coding Clinic: 2016, Q1, P35

    J45.32 **Mild persistent asthma with status asthmaticus** 🔖

● **J45.4** **Moderate persistent asthma**

    J45.40 **Moderate persistent asthma, uncomplicated**
          Moderate persistent asthma NOS

    J45.41 **Moderate persistent asthma with (acute) exacerbation** 🔖

    J45.42 **Moderate persistent asthma with status asthmaticus** 🔖

● **J45.5** **Severe persistent asthma**

    J45.50 **Severe persistent asthma, uncomplicated**
          Severe persistent asthma NOS

    J45.51 **Severe persistent asthma with (acute) exacerbation** 🔖

    J45.52 **Severe persistent asthma with status asthmaticus** 🔖

● **J45.9** **Other and unspecified asthma**

  ● **J45.90** **Unspecified asthma**
          Asthmatic bronchitis NOS
          Childhood asthma NOS
          Late onset asthma

    J45.901 Unspecified **asthma with (acute) exacerbation** 🔖

    J45.902 Unspecified **asthma with status asthmaticus** 🔖

    J45.909 Unspecified **asthma, uncomplicated**
          Asthma NOS

  ● **J45.99** **Other asthma**

    J45.990 **Exercise induced bronchospasm**
    J45.991 **Cough variant asthma**
    J45.998 **Other asthma**

● **J47** **Bronchiectasis**

    Includes bronchiolectasis

    Use additional code to identify:
      exposure to environmental tobacco smoke (Z77.22)
      exposure to tobacco smoke in the perinatal period (P96.81)
      history of tobacco dependence (Z87.891) ◄▥
      occupational exposure to environmental tobacco smoke (Z57.31)
      tobacco dependence (F17.-)
      tobacco use (Z72.0)

    Excludes1 congenital bronchiectasis (Q33.4)
          tuberculous bronchiectasis (current disease) (A15.0)

    Ⓔⓧ **For category J47 CC codes:** A17.9, A18.82, A18.84, A18.89, J09.X2, J10.08, J11.1, J44.9, J47.0-J47.1, J68.1, J68.4-J68.9, Q33.4

    J47.0 **Bronchiectasis with acute lower respiratory infection** 🔖
         Bronchiectasis with acute bronchitis
         Use additional code to identify the infection ◄

    J47.1 **Bronchiectasis with (acute) exacerbation** 🔖

    J47.9 **Bronchiectasis, uncomplicated**
         Bronchiectasis NOS

LUNG DISEASES DUE TO EXTERNAL AGENTS (J60-J70)

    Excludes2 asthma (J45.-)
          malignant neoplasm of bronchus and lung (C34.-)

  J60 **Coalworker's pneumoconiosis**   A
      Anthracosilicosis
      Anthracosis
      Black lung disease
      Coalworker's lung

    Excludes1 coalworker pneumoconiosis with tuberculosis, any type in A15 (J65)

  J61 **Pneumoconiosis due to asbestos and other mineral fibers** A
      Asbestosis

    Excludes1 pleural plaque with asbestosis (J92.0)
          pneumoconiosis with tuberculosis, any type in A15 (J65)

● **J62** **Pneumoconiosis due to dust containing silica**

    Includes silicotic fibrosis (massive) of lung
    Excludes1 pneumoconiosis with tuberculosis, any type in A15 (J65)

    J62.0 **Pneumoconiosis due to talc dust**
    J62.8 **Pneumoconiosis due to other dust containing silica**
         Silicosis NOS

● **J63** **Pneumoconiosis due to other inorganic dusts**

    Excludes1 pneumoconiosis with tuberculosis, any type in A15 (J65)

    J63.0 **Aluminosis (of lung)**
    J63.1 **Bauxite fibrosis (of lung)**
    J63.2 **Berylliosis**
    J63.3 **Graphite fibrosis (of lung)**
    J63.4 **Siderosis**
    J63.5 **Stannosis**
    J63.6 **Pneumoconiosis due to other specified inorganic dusts**

Figure 10-8 Progressive massive fibrosis superimposed on coal workers' pneumoconiosis. The large, blackened scars are located principally in the upper lobe. (From Cotran R, Kumar V, Collins T: Robbins Pathologic Basis of Disease, ed 8, Philadelphia, WB Saunders, 2009. Courtesy of Dr. Warner Laquer, Dr. Jerome Kleinerman, and the National Institute of Occupational Safety and Health, Morgantown, WV)

Item 10–10 Pneumoconiosis refers to a lung condition resulting from exposure to inorganic or organic airborne particles, such as coal dust or moldy hay, as well as chemical fumes and vapors, such as insecticides. In this condition, the lungs retain the airborne particles.

CHAPTER 10 (J00-J99)

J64   Unspecified pneumoconiosis

> **Excludes1**   pneumonoconiosis with tuberculosis, any type in A15 (J65)

J65   Pneumoconiosis associated with tuberculosis
> Any condition in J60-J64 with tuberculosis, any type in A15
> Silicotuberculosis

● **J66**   Airway disease due to specific organic dust

> **Excludes2**   allergic alveolitis (J67.-)
> asbestosis (J61)
> bagassosis (J67.1)
> farmer's lung (J67.0)
> hypersensitivity pneumonitis due to organic dust (J67.-)
> reactive airways dysfunction syndrome (J68.3)

J66.0   Byssinosis
> Airway disease due to cotton dust

J66.1   Flax-dressers' disease

J66.2   Cannabinosis

J66.8   Airway disease due to other specific organic dusts

● **J67**   Hypersensitivity pneumonitis due to organic dust

> **Includes**   allergic alveolitis and pneumonitis due to inhaled organic dust and particles of fungal, actinomycetic or other origin

> **Excludes1**   pneumonitis due to inhalation of chemicals, gases, fumes or vapors (J68.0)

J67.0   Farmer's lung
> Harvester's lung
> Haymaker's lung
> Moldy hay disease

J67.1   Bagassosis
> Bagasse disease
> Bagasse pneumonitis

J67.2   Bird fancier's lung
> Budgerigar fancier's disease or lung
> Pigeon fancier's disease or lung

J67.3   Suberosis
> Corkhandler's disease or lung
> Corkworker's disease or lung

J67.4   Maltworker's lung
> Alveolitis due to Aspergillus clavatus

J67.5   Mushroom-worker's lung

J67.6   Maple-bark-stripper's lung
> Alveolitis due to Cryptostroma corticale
> Cryptostromosis

J67.7   Air conditioner and humidifier lung 🔖
> Allergic alveolitis due to fungal, thermophilic actinomycetes and other organisms growing in ventilation [air conditioning] systems
> (Ex) A15.0-A15.9, A17.9, A18.82, A18.84, A18.89, A21.2, A22.1, A31.0, A37.01, A37.11, A37.81, A37.91, A42.0, A43.0, A48.1, B25.0, B39.0-B39.2, B44.0, B58.3, B59, B67.1, J09.X1-J09.X2, J10.00-J10.1, J11.00-J11.1, J12.0-J12.3, J12.89-J18.1, J18.8-J18.9, J22, J44.9, J47.0-J70.4, J70.8-J70.9, J98.4, J98.8-J98.9, Q33.4, R91.1

J67.8   Hypersensitivity pneumonitis due to other organic dusts 🔖
> Cheese-washer's lung
> Coffee-worker's lung
> Fish-meal worker's lung
> Furrier's lung
> Sequoiosis
> (Ex) See J67.7

J67.9   Hypersensitivity pneumonitis due to unspecified organic dust 🔖
> Allergic alveolitis (extrinsic) NOS
> Hypersensitivity pneumonitis NOS
> (Ex) See J67.7

● **J68**   Respiratory conditions due to inhalation of chemicals, gases, fumes and vapors
> *Code first (T51-T65) to identify cause*
> Use additional code to identify associated respiratory conditions, such as:
> acute respiratory failure (J96.0-)

J68.0   Bronchitis and pneumonitis due to chemicals, gases, fumes and vapors 🔖
> Chemical bronchitis (acute)
> (Ex) See J67.7

J68.1   Pulmonary edema due to chemicals, gases, fumes and vapors 🔖
> Chemical pulmonary edema (acute) (chronic)
> > **Excludes1**   pulmonary edema (acute) (chronic) NOS (J81.-)
> (Ex) See J67.7

J68.2   Upper respiratory inflammation due to chemicals, gases, fumes and vapors, not elsewhere classified

J68.3   Other acute and subacute respiratory conditions due to chemicals, gases, fumes and vapors
> Reactive airways dysfunction syndrome

J68.4   Chronic respiratory conditions due to chemicals, gases, fumes and vapors
> Emphysema (diffuse) (chronic) due to inhalation of chemicals, gases, fumes and vapors
> Obliterative bronchiolitis (chronic) (subacute) due to inhalation of chemicals, gases, fumes and vapors
> Pulmonary fibrosis (chronic) due to inhalation of chemicals, gases, fumes and vapors
> > **Excludes1**   chronic pulmonary edema due to chemicals, gases, fumes and vapors (J68.1)

J68.8   Other respiratory conditions due to chemicals, gases, fumes and vapors

J68.9   Unspecified respiratory condition due to chemicals, gases, fumes and vapors

● **J69**   Pneumonitis due to solids and liquids

> **Excludes1**   neonatal aspiration syndromes (P24.-)
> postprocedural pneumonitis (J95.4)
> (Ex) For category J69 CC codes: See J67.7

J69.0   Pneumonitis due to inhalation of food and vomit 🔖
> Aspiration pneumonia NOS
> Aspiration pneumonia (due to) food (regurgitated)
> Aspiration pneumonia (due to) gastric secretions
> Aspiration pneumonia (due to) milk
> Aspiration pneumonia (due to) vomit
> Code also any associated foreign body in respiratory tract (T17.-)
> > **Excludes1**   chemical pneumonitis due to anesthesia (J95.4)
> > obstetric aspiration pneumonia (O74.0)

J69.1   Pneumonitis due to inhalation of oils and essences 🔖
> Exogenous lipoid pneumonia
> Lipid pneumonia NOS
> *Code first (T51-T65) to identify substance*
> > **Excludes1**   endogenous lipoid pneumonia (J84.89)

J69.8   Pneumonitis due to inhalation of other solids and liquids 🔖
> Pneumonitis due to aspiration of blood
> Pneumonitis due to aspiration of detergent
> *Code first (T51-T65) to identify substance*

◀ New   ◀▥ Revised   ~~deleted~~ Deleted   Excludes 1   Excludes 2   Includes   Use additional   Code first   Code also   Unspecified

OGCR Official Guidelines   ● Unacceptable Principal Diagnosis   X Assign placeholder X   ● Use Additional Character(s)   ▶ Manifestation Code   **Coding Clinic**

928

J70 Respiratory conditions due to other external agents

J70.0 Acute pulmonary manifestations due to radiation 🦠
Radiation pneumonitis
Use additional code (W88-W90, X39.0-) to identify the external cause
Ⓔ See J67.7

J70.1 Chronic and other pulmonary manifestations due to radiation 🦠
Fibrosis of lung following radiation
Use additional code (W88-W90, X39.0-) to identify the external cause
Ⓔ See J67.7

J70.2 Acute drug-induced interstitial lung disorders
Use additional code for adverse effect, if applicable, to identify drug (T36-T50 with fifth or sixth character 5)
Excludes1 interstitial pneumonia NOS (J84.9)
lymphoid interstitial pneumonia (J84.2)

J70.3 Chronic drug-induced interstitial lung disorders
Use additional code for adverse effect, if applicable, to identify drug (T36-T50 with fifth or sixth character 5)
Excludes1 interstitial pneumonia NOS (J84.9)
lymphoid interstitial pneumonia (J84.2)

J70.4 Drug-induced interstitial lung disorders, unspecified
Use additional code for adverse effect, if applicable, to identify drug (T36-T50 with fifth or sixth character 5)
Excludes1 interstitial pneumonia NOS (J84.9)
lymphoid interstitial pneumonia (J84.2)

J70.5 Respiratory conditions due to smoke inhalation
Smoke inhalation NOS
Excludes1 smoke inhalation due to chemicals, gases, fumes and vapors (J68.9)

J70.8 Respiratory conditions due to other specified external agents
Code first (T51-T65) to identify the external agent

J70.9 Respiratory conditions due to unspecified external agent
Code first (T51-T65) to identify the external agent

OTHER RESPIRATORY DISEASES PRINCIPALLY AFFECTING THE INTERSTITIUM (J80-J84)

J80 Acute respiratory distress syndrome 🦠
Acute respiratory distress syndrome in adult or child
Adult hyaline membrane disease
Excludes1 respiratory distress syndrome in newborn (perinatal) (P22.0)
Ⓔ J22, J80, J96.00-J96.92, J98.8-J98.9, R09.2

J81 Pulmonary edema
Use additional code to identify:
exposure to environmental tobacco smoke (Z77.22)
history of tobacco dependence (Z87.891) ◀▥
occupational exposure to environmental tobacco smoke (Z57.31)
tobacco dependence (F17.-)
tobacco use (Z72.0)
Excludes1 chemical (acute) pulmonary edema (J68.1)
hypostatic pneumonia (J18.2)
passive pneumonia (J18.2)
pulmonary edema due to external agents (J60-J70)
pulmonary edema with heart disease NOS (I50.1)
pulmonary edema with heart failure (I50.1)

J81.0 Acute pulmonary edema 🦠
Acute edema of lung
Ⓔ I09.81, I50.1-I50.9, J22, J81.0, J98.8-J98.9

J81.1 Chronic pulmonary edema 🦠
Pulmonary congestion (chronic) (passive)
Pulmonary edema NOS
Ⓔ J18.2, J22, J81.1, J98.4, J98.8-J99, R91.1

Figure 10-9 Bullous emphysema with large subpleural bullae *(upper left)*. (From Kumar: Robbins and Cotran: Pathologic Basis of Disease, ed 8, Saunders, An Imprint of Elsevier, 2009)

J82 Pulmonary eosinophilia, not elsewhere classified 🦠
Allergic pneumonia
Eosinophilic asthma
Eosinophilic pneumonia
Löffler's pneumonia
Tropical (pulmonary) eosinophilia NOS
Excludes1 pulmonary eosinophilia due to aspergillosis (B44.-)
pulmonary eosinophilia due to drugs (J70.2-J70.4)
pulmonary eosinophilia due to specified parasitic infection (B50-B83)
pulmonary eosinophilia due to systemic connective tissue disorders (M30-M36)
pulmonary infiltrate NOS (R91.8)
Ⓔ A15.0-A15.6, A15.8-A15.9, A17.9, A18.82, A18.84, A18.89, A20.2, A21.1, A22.1, A31.0, A37.01, A37.11, A37.81, A37.91, A42.0, A43.0, A48.1, B25.0, B39.0-B39.2, B44.0, B58.3, B59, B67.1, J09.X1-J09.X2, J10.00-J10.1, J11.00-J11.1, J12.0-J12.3, J12.89-J18.1, J18.8-J18.9, J22, J47.0-J70.4, J70.8-J70.9, J82, J98.4, J98.8-J99, Q33.4, R91.1

J84 Other interstitial pulmonary diseases
Excludes1 drug-induced interstitial lung disorders (J70.2-J70.4)
interstitial emphysema (J98.2)
lung diseases due to external agents (J60-J70)
Ⓔ For category J84 CC codes unless otherwise indicated: A15.0-A15.6, A15.8-A15.9, A17.9, A18.82, A18.84, A18.89, J22, J44.9, J47.0-J70.4, J70.8-J70.9, J84.01-J84.82, J84.89-J84.9, J98.4, J98.8-J99, Q33.4, R91.1

J84.0 Alveolar and parieto-alveolar conditions

J84.01 Alveolar proteinosis 🦠

J84.02 Pulmonary alveolar microlithiasis 🦠

▶ **J84.03** *Idiopathic pulmonary hemosiderosis* 🦠
Essential brown induration of lung
Code first underlying disease, such as:
disorders of iron metabolism (E83.1-)
Excludes1 acute idiopathic pulmonary hemorrhage in infants [AIPHI] (R04.81)

J84.09 Other alveolar and parieto-alveolar conditions 🦠

J84.1 Other interstitial pulmonary diseases with fibrosis
Excludes1 pulmonary fibrosis (chronic) due to inhalation of chemicals, gases, fumes or vapors (J68.4)
pulmonary fibrosis (chronic) following radiation (J70.1)

J84.10 Pulmonary fibrosis, unspecified
Capillary fibrosis of lung
Cirrhosis of lung (chronic) NOS
Fibrosis of lung (atrophic) (chronic) (confluent) (massive) (perialveolar) (peribronchial) NOS
Induration of lung (chronic) NOS
Postinflammatory pulmonary fibrosis

N Newborn Age: 0 **P** Pediatric Age: 0–17 **M** Maternity DX: 12–55 **A** Adult Age: 15–124 ♀ Females Only ♂ Males Only
🦠 Complication\Comorbidity 🦠 Major C\C Ⓔ CC/MCC Exclusions 🦠 Hospital-Acquired Condition

929

● **J84.11**   **Idiopathic interstitial pneumonia**

> **Excludes1**   lymphoid interstitial pneumonia (J84.2)
> pneumocystis pneumonia (B59)

J84.111   **Idiopathic interstitial pneumonia, not otherwise specified**

J84.112   **Idiopathic pulmonary fibrosis**
Cryptogenic fibrosing alveolitis
Idiopathic fibrosing alveolitis

J84.113   **Idiopathic non-specific interstitial pneumonitis**

> **Excludes1**   non-specific interstitial pneumonia NOS, or due to known underlying cause (J84.89)

J84.114   **Acute interstitial pneumonitis** 🦠
Hamman-Rich syndrome

> **Excludes1**   pneumocystis pneumonia (B59)

J84.115   **Respiratory bronchiolitis interstitial lung disease**

J84.116   **Cryptogenic organizing pneumonia** 🦠

> **Excludes1**   organizing pneumonia NOS, or due to known underlying cause (J84.89)

J84.117   **Desquamative interstitial pneumonia** 🦠

▹ *J84.17*   *Other interstitial pulmonary diseases with fibrosis in diseases classified elsewhere*
Interstitial pneumonia (nonspecific) (usual) due to collagen vascular disease
Interstitial pneumonia (nonspecific) (usual) in diseases classified elsewhere
Organizing pneumonia due to collagen vascular disease
Organizing pneumonia in diseases classified elsewhere

> *Code first* underlying disease, such as:
> progressive systemic sclerosis (M34.0)
> rheumatoid arthritis (M05.00-M06.9)
> systemic lupus erythematosis (M32.0-M32.9)

J84.2   **Lymphoid interstitial pneumonia**
Lymphoid interstitial pneumonitis

● **J84.8**   **Other specified interstitial pulmonary diseases**

> **Excludes1**   exogenous lipoid pneumonia (J69.1)
> unspecified lipoid pneumonia (J69.1)

J84.81   **Lymphangioleiomyomatosis** ♀ 🦠
Lymphangiomyomatosis

J84.82   **Adult pulmonary Langerhans cell histiocytosis** 🦠   A
Adult PLCH

J84.83   **Surfactant mutations of the lung** 🦠
> (Ex:) J84.83-J84.848, P22.0-P28.5, P28.89-P29.2, P29.4,
> P29.89-P29.9, P84, P94.1-P96.0, P96.3-P96.5, P96.82-P96.89

● **J84.84**   **Other interstitial lung diseases of childhood**
> (Ex:) For category J84.84 CC codes: See J84.83

J84.841   **Neuroendocrine cell hyperplasia of infancy** 🦠

J84.842   **Pulmonary interstitial glycogenosis** 🦠

J84.843   **Alveolar capillary dysplasia with vein misalignment** 🦠

J84.848   **Other interstitial lung diseases of childhood** 🦠

J84.89   **Other specified interstitial pulmonary diseases**
Endogenous lipoid pneumonia
Interstitial pneumonitis
Non-specific interstitial pneumonitis NOS
~~Organizing pneumonia due to known underlying cause~~
Organizing pneumonia NOS

> *Code first*, *if applicable:*
> poisoning due to drug or toxin (T51-T65 with fifth or sixth character to indicate intent), for toxic pneumonopathy underlying cause of pneumonopathy, if known

> Use additional code, for adverse effect, to identify drug (T36-T50 with fifth or sixth character 5), if drug-induced

> **Excludes1**   cryptogenic organizing pneumonia (J84.116)
> idiopathic non-specific interstitial pneumonitis (J84.113)
> lipoid pneumonia, exogenous or unspecified (J69.1)
> lymphoid interstitial pneumonia (J84.2)

J84.9   **Interstitial pulmonary disease, unspecified** 🦠
Interstitial pneumonia NOS

SUPPURATIVE AND NECROTIC CONDITIONS OF THE LOWER RESPIRATORY TRACT (J85-J86)

● **J85**   **Abscess of lung and mediastinum**
Use additional code (B95-B97) to identify infectious agent.
> (Ex:) For category J85 CC codes unless otherwise indicated: A06.5, A15.0-A15.6,
> A15.8-A15.9, A17.9, A18.82, A18.84, A18.89, J22, J85.0-J85.2, J98.8-J98.9

J85.0   **Gangrene and necrosis of lung** 🦠

J85.1   **Abscess of lung with pneumonia** 🦠
Code also the type of pneumonia

J85.2   **Abscess of lung without pneumonia** 🦠
Abscess of lung NOS

J85.3   **Abscess of mediastinum** 🦠
> (Ex:) J22, J85.3, J98.8-J98.9

Item 10–11   **Empyema** is a condition in which pus accumulates in a body cavity. Empyema **with fistula** occurs when the pus passes from one cavity to another organ or structure.

● **J86**   **Pyothorax**
Use additional code (B95-B97) to identify infectious agent.
> **Excludes1**   abscess of lung (J85.-)
> pyothorax due to tuberculosis (A15.6)
> (Ex:) For category J86 CC codes: J22, J86.0-J86.9, J98.4, J98.8-J99, R91.1

J86.0   **Pyothorax with fistula** 🦠
Bronchocutaneous fistula
Bronchopleural fistula
Hepatopleural fistula
Mediastinal fistula
Pleural fistula
Thoracic fistula
Any condition classifiable to J86.9 with fistula

J86.9   **Pyothorax without fistula** 🦠
Abscess of pleura
Abscess of thorax
Empyema (chest) (lung) (pleura)
Fibrinopurulent pleurisy
Purulent pleurisy
Pyopneumothorax
Septic pleurisy
Seropurulent pleurisy
Suppurative pleurisy

◀ New   ◀ Revised   ~~deleted~~ Deleted   Excludes 1   Excludes 2   Includes   Use additional   Code first   Code also   Unspecified
OGCR Official Guidelines   ● Unacceptable Principal Diagnosis   X Assign placeholder X   🦠 Use Additional Character(s)   ▹ Manifestation Code   **Coding Clinic**

OTHER DISEASES OF THE PLEURA (J90-J94)

J90   **Pleural effusion, not elsewhere classified** 🔹
Encysted pleurisy
Pleural effusion NOS
Pleurisy with effusion (exudative) (serous)

> **Excludes1**   chylous (pleural) effusion (J94.0)
> malignant pleural effusion (J91.0))
> pleurisy NOS (R09.1)
> tuberculous pleural effusion (A15.6)
> (Ex:) A15.0-A15.6, A15.8-A15.9, A17.9, A18.82, A18.84, A18.89, J22, J90-J92.9, J94.0-J94.9,
> J98.4, J98.8-J99, R09.1, R91.1
> **Coding Clinic: 2015, Q2, P16**

J91   **Pleural effusion in conditions classified elsewhere**

> **Excludes2**   pleural effusion in heart failure (I50.-)
> pleural effusion in systemic lupus erythematosus (M32.13)

   J91.0   *Malignant pleural effusion* 🔹

> *Code first underlying neoplasm*
> (Ex:) C45.7-C45.9, C76.8, C78.2-C78.39, C79.89-C79.9, C7A.00, C7A.098,
> C7A.1-C7B.00, C7B.09-C7B.8, C80.0-C80.2, D49.81-D49.9, J90-J91.0, J94.0,
> J94.2

   J91.8   *Pleural effusion in other conditions classified elsewhere* 🔹

> *Code first underlying disease, such as:*
> filariasis (B74.0-B74.9)
> influenza (J09.X2, J10.1, J11.1)
> (Ex:) See J90
> **Coding Clinic: 2015, Q2, P16**

J92   **Pleural plaque**

> **Includes**   pleural thickening

   J92.0   **Pleural plaque with presence of asbestos**

   J92.9   **Pleural plaque without asbestos**
Pleural plaque NOS

J93   **Pneumothorax and air leak**
Collapsed lung

> **Excludes1**   congenital or perinatal pneumothorax (P25.1)
> postprocedural air leak (J95.812)
> postprocedural pneumothorax (J95.811)
> traumatic pneumothorax (S27.0)
> tuberculous (current disease) pneumothorax (A15.-)
> pyopneumothorax (J86.-)
> (Ex:) **For category J93 CC codes:** J22, J93.0-J93.9, J95.811-J95.812, J98.4, J98.8-J99, R91.1

   J93.0   **Spontaneous tension pneumothorax** 🔹
Tension pneumothorax (most serious type) occurs when air (positive pressure) collects in the pleural space

   J93.1   **Other spontaneous pneumothorax**

     J93.11   **Primary spontaneous pneumothorax** 🔹

     J93.12   **Secondary spontaneous pneumothorax** 🔹

> *Code first underlying condition, such as:*
> catamenial pneumothorax due to endometriosis (N80.8)
> cystic fibrosis (E84.-)
> eosinophilic pneumonia (J82)
> lymphangioleiomyomatosis (J84.81)
> malignant neoplasm of bronchus and lung (C34.-)
> Marfan's syndrome (Q87.4)
> pneumonia due to Pneumocystis carinii (B59)
> secondary malignant neoplasm of lung (C78.0-)
> spontaneous rupture of the esophagus (K22.3)

   J93.8   **Other pneumothorax and air leak**

     J93.81   **Chronic pneumothorax** 🔹

     J93.82   **Other air leak** 🔹
Persistent air leak

     J93.83   **Other pneumothorax** 🔹
Acute pneumothorax
Spontaneous pneumothorax NOS

   J93.9   **Pneumothorax, unspecified** 🔹
Pneumothorax NOS

J94   **Other pleural conditions**

> **Excludes1**   pleurisy NOS (R09.1)
> traumatic hemopneumothorax (S27.2)
> traumatic hemothorax (S27.1)
> tuberculous pleural conditions (current disease) (A15.-)
> (Ex:) **For category J94 CC codes unless otherwise indicated:** See J90

   J94.0   **Chylous effusion** 🔹
Chyliform effusion

   J94.1   **Fibrothorax**

   J94.2   **Hemothorax** 🔹
Hemopneumothorax

   J94.8   **Other specified pleural conditions** 🔹
Hydropneumothorax
Hydrothorax
(Ex:) No exclusions

   J94.9   **Pleural condition, unspecified**

INTRAOPERATIVE AND POSTPROCEDURAL COMPLICATIONS AND DISORDERS OF RESPIRATORY SYSTEM, NOT ELSEWHERE CLASSIFIED (J95)

J95   **Intraoperative and postprocedural complications and disorders of respiratory system, not elsewhere classified**

> **Excludes2**   aspiration pneumonia (J69.-)
> emphysema (subcutaneous) resulting from a procedure (T81.82)
> hypostatic pneumonia (J18.2)
> pulmonary manifestations due to radiation (J70.0- J70.1)

   J95.0   **Tracheostomy complications**
(Ex:) **For category J95.0 CC codes:** J22, J39.8, J95.00-J95.09, J98.01-J98.09, J98.8-J98.9

     J95.00   **Unspecified tracheostomy complication** 🔹

     J95.01   **Hemorrhage from tracheostomy stoma** 🔹

     J95.02   **Infection of tracheostomy stoma** 🔹

> Use additional code to identify type of infection, such as:
> cellulitis of neck (L03.8)
> sepsis (A40, A41.-)

     J95.03   **Malfunction of tracheostomy stoma** 🔹
Mechanical complication of tracheostomy stoma
Obstruction of tracheostomy airway
Tracheal stenosis due to tracheostomy

     J95.04   **Tracheo-esophageal fistula following tracheostomy** 🔹

     J95.09   **Other tracheostomy complication** 🔹

   J95.1   **Acute pulmonary insufficiency following thoracic surgery** 🔹

> **Excludes2**   functional disturbances following cardiac surgery (I97.0, I97.1-)
> (Ex:) J22, J95.1-J95.3, J95.821-J95.822, J98.8-J98.9

   J95.2   **Acute pulmonary insufficiency following nonthoracic surgery** 🔹

> **Excludes2**   functional disturbances following cardiac surgery (I97.0, I97.1-)
> (Ex:) See J95.1

CHAPTER 10 (J00-J99)

N Newborn Age: 0   **P** Pediatric Age: 0–17   **M** Maternity DX: 12–55   **A** Adult Age: 15–124   ♀ Females Only   ♂ Males Only
🔹 Complication\Comorbidity   Major C\C   (Ex:) CC/MCC Exclusions   Hospital-Acquired Condition

931

CHAPTER 10 (J00-J99)

J95.3   **Chronic pulmonary insufficiency following surgery** 🔖
     Excludes2   functional disturbances following cardiac surgery (I97.0, I97.1-)
     (Ex:) See J95.1

J95.4   **Chemical pneumonitis due to anesthesia** 🔖
     Mendelson's syndrome
     Postprocedural aspiration pneumonia
     Use additional code for adverse effect, if applicable, to identify drug (T41.- with fifth or sixth character 5)
     Excludes1   aspiration pneumonitis due to anesthesia complicating labor and delivery (O74.0)
                aspiration pneumonitis due to anesthesia complicating pregnancy (O29)
                aspiration pneumonitis due to anesthesia complicating the puerperium (O89.01)
     (Ex:) D78.81-D78.89, E36.8, E89.810-E89.89, H59.011-H59.019, H59.031-H59.099, H59.811-H59.89, H95.811-H95.89, I97.3, J95.4-J95.5, J95.84, J95.851-J95.89, L76.81-L76.82, M96.89, N98.1-N98.9, T81.82X[A], T81.89X-T81.9XX[A]

J95.5   **Postprocedural subglottic stenosis** 🔖
     (Ex:) See J95.4

● **J95.6**   **Intraoperative hemorrhage and hematoma of a respiratory system organ or structure complicating a procedure**
     Excludes1   intraoperative hemorrhage and hematoma of a respiratory system organ or structure due to accidental puncture and laceration during procedure (J95.7-)
     (Ex:) **For category J95.6 CC codes:** H95.811-H95.89, I85.01, I85.11, I97.3, J95.61-J95.62, J95.830-J95.831, J95.860-J95.863, K21.9, K22.8, K23-K25.0, K25.2, K25.4, K25.6, K26.0, K26.2, K26.4, K26.6, K27.0, K27.2, K27.4, K27.6, K28.0, K28.2, K28.4, K28.6, K29.01, K29.21, K29.31, K29.41, K29.51, K29.61, K29.71, K29.81, K29.91, K31.811, K55.21, K57.01, K57.11, K57.13, K57.21, K57.31, K57.33, K57.41, K57.51, K57.53, K57.81, K57.91, K57.93, K62.5, K92.0-K92.2, M96.89, N98.1-N98.9, P54.1-P54.3, T81.10X-T81.19X[A], T81.82X[A], T81.89X-T81.9XX[A]

     J95.61   **Intraoperative hemorrhage and hematoma of a respiratory system organ or structure complicating a respiratory system procedure** 🔖

     J95.62   **Intraoperative hemorrhage and hematoma of a respiratory system organ or structure complicating other procedure** 🔖

● **J95.7**   **Accidental puncture and laceration of a respiratory system organ or structure during a procedure**
     Excludes2   postprocedural pneumothorax (J95.811)
     (Ex:) **For category J95.7 CC codes:** D78.11-D78.12, D78.81-D78.89, E36.11-E36.8, E89.810-E89.89, G96.11, G97.41-G97.49, H59.011-H59.019, H59.031-H59.099, H59.211-H59.229, H59.811-H59.89, H95.31-H95.32, H95.811-H95.89, I97.3, I97.51-I97.52, J95.71-J95.72, K91.71-K91.72, L76.11-L76.12, L76.81-L76.82, M96.820-M96.821, M96.89, N98.1-N98.9, N99.71-N99.72, T81.82X[A], T81.89X-T81.9XX[A]

     J95.71   **Accidental puncture and laceration of a respiratory system organ or structure during a respiratory system procedure** 🔖

     J95.72   **Accidental puncture and laceration of a respiratory system organ or structure during other procedure** 🔖

● **J95.8**   **Other intraoperative and postprocedural complications and disorders of respiratory system, not elsewhere classified**

● **J95.81**   **Postprocedural pneumothorax and air leak**
     (Ex:) **For category J95.81 CC codes:** J22, J93.0-J93.9, J95.811-J95.812, J98.4, J98.8-J99, R91.1

     J95.811   **Postprocedural pneumothorax** 🔖 🔖

     J95.812   **Postprocedural air leak** 🔖

● **J95.82**   **Postprocedural respiratory failure**
     Excludes1   Respiratory failure in other conditions (J96.-)
     (Ex:) **For category J95.82 CC codes:** See J95.1

     J95.821   **Acute postprocedural respiratory failure** 🔖
         Postprocedural respiratory failure NOS

     J95.822   **Acute and chronic postprocedural respiratory failure** 🔖

● **J95.83**   **Postprocedural hemorrhage of a respiratory system organ or structure following a procedure** ◀
     (Ex:) **For category J95.83 CC codes:** See J95.6

     J95.830   **Postprocedural hemorrhage of a respiratory system organ or structure following a respiratory system procedure** 🔖 ◀

     J95.831   **Postprocedural hemorrhage of a respiratory system organ or structure following other procedure** 🔖 ◀

   J95.84   **Transfusion-related acute lung injury (TRALI)** 🔖
     (Ex:) See J95.4

● **J95.85**   **Complication of respirator [ventilator]**

     J95.850   **Mechanical complication of respirator** 🔖
         Excludes1   encounter for respirator [ventilator] dependence during power failure (Z99.12)
         (Ex:) J95.850, Z99.0-Z99.12, Z99.81-Z99.89

     J95.851   **Ventilator associated pneumonia** 🔖
         Ventilator associated pneumonitis
         Use additional code to identify the organism, if known (B95.-, B96.-, B97.-)
         Excludes1   ventilator lung in newborn (P27.8)
         (Ex:) See J95.4

     J95.859   **Other complication of respirator [ventilator]** 🔖
         (Ex:) See J95.4

● **J95.86** **Postprocedural hematoma and seroma of a respiratory system organ or structure following a procedure** ◀
   (Ex) **For Category J95.86 CC codes:** See J95.6

    J95.860 Postprocedural hematoma of a respiratory system organ or structure following a respiratory system procedure 🔖 ◀

    J95.861 Postprocedural hematoma of a respiratory system organ or structure following other procedure 🔖 ◀

    J95.862 Postprocedural seroma of a respiratory system organ or structure following a respiratory system procedure 🔖 ◀

    J95.863 Postprocedural seroma of a respiratory system organ or structure following other procedure 🔖 ◀

   J95.88 **Other intraoperative complications of respiratory system, not elsewhere classified** 🔖
    (Ex) See J95.4

   J95.89 **Other postprocedural complications and disorders of respiratory system, not elsewhere classified** 🔖
    Use additional code to identify disorder, such as:
    aspiration pneumonia (J69.-)
    bacterial or viral pneumonia (J12-J18)
    Excludes2 acute pulmonary insufficiency following thoracic surgery (J95.1)
        postprocedural subglottic stenosis (J95.5)
    (Ex) See J95.4

OTHER DISEASES OF THE RESPIRATORY SYSTEM (J96-J99)

● **J96** **Respiratory failure, not elsewhere classified**
   Excludes1 acute respiratory distress syndrome (J80)
    cardiorespiratory failure (R09.2)
    newborn respiratory distress syndrome (P22.0)
    postprocedural respiratory failure (J95.82-)
    respiratory arrest (R09.2)
    respiratory arrest of newborn (P28.81)
    respiratory failure of newborn (P28.5)
   (Ex) **For category J96 CC codes:** J22, J80, J96.00-J96.92, J98.8-J98.9, R09.2

● **J96.0** **Acute respiratory failure**
   J96.00 **Acute respiratory failure, unspecified whether with hypoxia or hypercapnia** 🔖
   J96.01 **Acute respiratory failure with hypoxia** 🔖
   J96.02 **Acute respiratory failure with hypercapnia** 🔖

● **J96.1** **Chronic respiratory failure**
   J96.10 **Chronic respiratory failure, unspecified whether with hypoxia or hypercapnia** 🔖
    Coding Clinic: 2016, Q1, P38; 2015, Q1, P21
   J96.11 **Chronic respiratory failure with hypoxia** 🔖
   J96.12 **Chronic respiratory failure with hypercapnia** 🔖

● **J96.2** **Acute and chronic respiratory failure**
   Acute on chronic respiratory failure
   J96.20 **Acute and chronic respiratory failure, unspecified whether with hypoxia or hypercapnia** 🔖
   J96.21 **Acute and chronic respiratory failure with hypoxia** 🔖
   J96.22 **Acute and chronic respiratory failure with hypercapnia** 🔖

● **J96.9** **Respiratory failure, unspecified**
   J96.90 **Respiratory failure, unspecified, unspecified whether with hypoxia or hypercapnia** 🔖
   J96.91 **Respiratory failure, unspecified with hypoxia** 🔖
   J96.92 **Respiratory failure, unspecified with hypercapnia** 🔖

● **J98** **Other respiratory disorders**
   Use additional code to identify:
   exposure to environmental tobacco smoke (Z77.22)
   exposure to tobacco smoke in the perinatal period (P96.81)
   history of tobacco dependence (Z87.891) ◀
   occupational exposure to environmental tobacco smoke (Z57.31)
   tobacco dependence (F17.-)
   tobacco use (Z72.0)
   Excludes1 newborn apnea (P28.4)
    newborn sleep apnea (P28.3)
   Excludes2 apnea NOS (R06.81)
    sleep apnea (G47.3-)

● **J98.0** **Diseases of bronchus, not elsewhere classified**
   J98.01 **Acute bronchospasm**
    Excludes1 acute bronchiolitis with bronchospasm (J21.-)
     acute bronchitis with bronchospasm (J20.-)
     asthma (J45.-)
     exercise induced bronchospasm (J45.990)

   J98.09 **Other diseases of bronchus, not elsewhere classified**
    Broncholithiasis
    Calcification of bronchus
    Stenosis of bronchus
    Tracheobronchial collapse
    Tracheobronchial dyskinesia
    Ulcer of bronchus

● **J98.1** **Pulmonary collapse**
   Excludes1 therapeutic collapse of lung status (Z98.3)
   (Ex) **For category J98.1 CC codes:** J22, J98.11-J98.19, J98.8-J98.9
   J98.11 **Atelectasis** 🔖
    Excludes1 newborn atelectasis
     tuberculous atelectasis (current disease) (A15)
   J98.19 **Other pulmonary collapse** 🔖

   J98.2 **Interstitial emphysema**
   Mediastinal emphysema
   Excludes1 emphysema NOS (J43.9)
    emphysema in newborn (P25.0)
    surgical emphysema (subcutaneous) (T81.82)
    traumatic subcutaneous emphysema (T79.7)

CHAPTER 10 (J00-J99)

J98.3   **Compensatory emphysema**

J98.4   **Other disorders of lung**
              Calcification of lung
              Cystic lung disease (acquired)
              Lung disease NOS
              Pulmolithiasis

              Excludes1   acute interstitial pneumonitis (J84.114)
                                pulmonary insufficiency following
                                surgery (J95.1-J95.2)

● **J98.5**   **Diseases of mediastinum, not elsewhere classified**

              Excludes2   abscess of mediastinum (J85.3)

   J98.51   **Mediastinitis** 🔖🔖 ◄

                  Code first underlying condition, if applicable, such
                  as postoperative mediastinitis (T81.-) ◄
                  (Ex) No Exclusions ◄

   J98.59   **Other diseases of mediastinum, not elsewhere**
                  classified 🔖🔖 ◄
                  Fibrosis of mediastinum ◄
                  Hernia of mediastinum ◄
                  Retraction of mediastinum ◄
                  (Ex) No Exclusions ◄

J98.6   **Disorders of diaphragm**
              Diaphragmatitis
              Paralysis of diaphragm
              Relaxation of diaphragm

              Excludes1   congenital malformation of diaphragm
                                NEC (Q79.1)
                                congenital diaphragmatic hernia (Q79.0)

              Excludes2   diaphragmatic hernia (K44.-)

J98.8   **Other specified respiratory disorders**

J98.9   **Respiratory disorder, unspecified**
              Respiratory disease (chronic) NOS

▶ **J99**   *Respiratory disorders in diseases classified elsewhere*
              Code first underlying disease, such as:
                  amyloidosis (E85.-)
                  ankylosing spondylitis (M45)
                  congenital syphilis (A50.5)
                  cryoglobulinemia (D89.1)
                  early congenital syphilis (A50.0)
                  schistosomiasis (B65.0-B65.9)

              Excludes1   respiratory disorders in:
                                amebiasis (A06.5)
                                blastomycosis (B40.0-B40.2)
                                candidiasis (B37.1)
                                coccidioidomycosis (B38.0-B38.2)
                                cystic fibrosis with pulmonary manifestations
                                    (E84.0)
                                dermatomyositis (M33.01, M33.11)
                                histoplasmosis (B39.0-B39.2)
                                late syphilis (A52.72, A52.73)
                                polymyositis (M33.21)
                                sicca syndrome (M35.02)
                                systemic lupus erythematosus (M32.13)
                                systemic sclerosis (M34.81)
                                Wegener's granulomatosis (M31.30-M31.31)

◄ New   ◄║║║ Revised   ~~deleted~~ Deleted   Excludes 1   Excludes 2   Includes   Use additional   Code first   Code also   Unspecified

OGCR Official Guidelines   ● Unacceptable Principal Diagnosis   X Assign placeholder X   ● Use Additional Character(s)   ▶ Manifestation Code   **Coding Clinic**

CHAPTER 11

DISEASES OF THE DIGESTIVE SYSTEM (K00-K95)

OGCR Chapter-Specific Coding Guidelines

11. Chapter 11: Diseases of the Digestive System (K00-K95)
Reserved for future guideline expansion

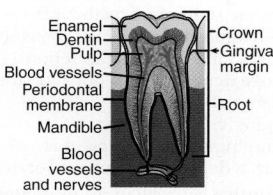

Figure 11-1 Anatomy of a tooth.

Item 11-1 Anodontia is the congenital absence of teeth. **Hypodontia** is partial anodontia. **Oligodontia** is the congenital absence of some teeth, whereas **supernumerary** is having more teeth than the normal number. **Mesiodens** are small extra teeth that often appear in pairs, although single small teeth are not uncommon.

CHAPTER 11

DISEASES OF THE DIGESTIVE SYSTEM (K00-K95)

Excludes2 certain conditions originating in the perinatal period (P04-P96)
certain infectious and parasitic diseases (A00-B99)
complications of pregnancy, childbirth and the puerperium (O00-O9A)
congenital malformations, deformations and chromosomal abnormalities (Q00-Q99)
endocrine, nutritional and metabolic diseases (E00-E88)
injury, poisoning and certain other consequences of external causes (S00-T88)
neoplasms (C00-D49)
symptoms, signs and abnormal clinical and laboratory findings, not elsewhere classified (R00-R94)

This chapter contains the following blocks:

K00-K14	Diseases of oral cavity and salivary glands
K20-K31	Diseases of esophagus, stomach and duodenum
K35-K38	Diseases of appendix
K40-K46	Hernia
K50-K52	Noninfective enteritis and colitis
K55-K64	Other diseases of intestines
K65-K68	Diseases of peritoneum and retroperitoneum
K70-K77	Diseases of liver
K80-K87	Disorders of gallbladder, biliary tract and pancreas
K90-K95	Other diseases of the digestive system

DISEASES OF ORAL CAVITY AND SALIVARY GLANDS (K00-K14)

● **K00 Disorders of tooth development and eruption**
    Excludes2 embedded and impacted teeth (K01.-)
    K00.0 Anodontia
       Hypodontia
       Oligodontia
       Excludes1 acquired absence of teeth (K08.1-)
    K00.1 Supernumerary teeth
       Distomolar
       Fourth molar
       Mesiodens
       Paramolar
       Supplementary teeth
       Excludes2 supernumerary roots (K00.2)

K00.2 Abnormalities of size and form of teeth
    Concrescence of teeth
    Fusion of teeth
    Gemination of teeth
    Dens evaginatus
    Dens in dente
    Dens invaginatus
    Enamel pearls
    Macrodontia
    Microdontia
    Peg-shaped [conical] teeth
    Supernumerary roots
    Taurodontism
    Tuberculum paramolare
    Excludes1 abnormalities of teeth due to congenital syphilis (A50.5)
       tuberculum Carabelli, which is regarded as a normal variation and should not be coded

K00.3 Mottled teeth
    Dental fluorosis
    Mottling of enamel
    Nonfluoride enamel opacities
    Excludes2 deposits [accretions] on teeth (K03.6)

K00.4 Disturbances in tooth formation
    Aplasia and hypoplasia of cementum
    Dilaceration of tooth
    Enamel hypoplasia (neonatal) (postnatal) (prenatal)
    Regional odontodysplasia
    Turner's tooth
    Excludes1 Hutchinson's teeth and mulberry molars in congenital syphilis (A50.5)
    Excludes2 mottled teeth (K00.3)

K00.5 Hereditary disturbances in tooth structure, not elsewhere classified
    Amelogenesis imperfecta
    Dentinogenesis imperfecta
    Odontogenesis imperfecta
    Dentinal dysplasia
    Shell teeth

K00.6 Disturbances in tooth eruption
    Dentia praecox
    Natal tooth
    Neonatal tooth
    Premature eruption of tooth
    Premature shedding of primary [deciduous] tooth
    Prenatal teeth
    Retained [persistent] primary tooth
    Excludes2 embedded and impacted teeth (K01.-)

K00.7 Teething syndrome

K00.8 Other disorders of tooth development
    Color changes during tooth formation
    Intrinsic staining of teeth NOS
    Excludes2 posteruptive color changes (K03.7)

K00.9 Disorder of tooth development, unspecified
    Disorder of odontogenesis NOS

● **K01 Embedded and impacted teeth**
    Excludes1 abnormal position of fully erupted teeth (M26.3-)
    K01.0 Embedded teeth
    K01.1 Impacted teeth

N Newborn Age: 0   P Pediatric Age: 0–17   M Maternity DX: 12–55   A Adult Age: 15–124   ♀ Females Only   ♂ Males Only

🔾 Complication\Comorbidity   🔾 Major C\C   (Ex) CC/MCC Exclusions   🔾 Hospital-Acquired Condition

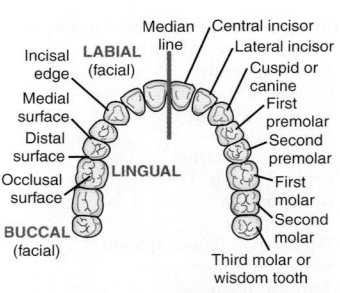

Figure 11-2 The permanent teeth within the dental arch.

Item 11-2 Each dental arch (jaw) normally contains 16 teeth. Tooth decay or **dental caries** is a disease of the enamel, dentin, and cementum of the tooth and can result in a cavity.

CHAPTER 11 (K00-K95)

● **K02 Dental caries**

    Includes   caries of dentine ◄
                  dental cavities
                  early childhood caries ◄
                  pre-eruptive caries ◄
                  recurrent caries (dentino enamel junction)
                      (enamel) (to the pulp) ◄
                  tooth decay

    K02.3 Arrested dental caries
           Arrested coronal and root caries

●   **K02.5 Dental caries on pit and fissure surface**
           Dental caries on chewing surface of tooth

        K02.51 Dental caries on pit and fissure surface limited to enamel
              White spot lesions [initial caries] on pit and fissure surface of tooth

        K02.52 Dental caries on pit and fissure surface penetrating into dentin
              Primary dental caries, cervical origin ◄

        K02.53 Dental caries on pit and fissure surface penetrating into pulp

●   **K02.6 Dental caries on smooth surface**

        K02.61 Dental caries on smooth surface limited to enamel
              White spot lesions [initial caries] on smooth surface of tooth

        K02.62 Dental caries on smooth surface penetrating into dentin

        K02.63 Dental caries on smooth surface penetrating into pulp

    K02.7 Dental root caries

    K02.9 Dental caries, unspecified

● **K03 Other diseases of hard tissues of teeth**

    Excludes2   bruxism (F45.8)
                  dental caries (K02.-)
                  teeth-grinding NOS (F45.8)

    K03.0 Excessive attrition of teeth
           Approximal wear of teeth
           Occlusal wear of teeth

    K03.1 Abrasion of teeth
           Dentifrice abrasion of teeth
           Habitual abrasion of teeth
           Occupational abrasion of teeth
           Ritual abrasion of teeth
           Traditional abrasion of teeth
           Wedge defect NOS

    K03.2 Erosion of teeth
           Erosion of teeth due to diet
           Erosion of teeth due to drugs and medicaments
           Erosion of teeth due to persistent vomiting
           Erosion of teeth NOS
           Idiopathic erosion of teeth
           Occupational erosion of teeth

    K03.3 Pathological resorption of teeth
           Internal granuloma of pulp
           Resorption of teeth (external)

    K03.4 Hypercementosis
           Cementation hyperplasia

    K03.5 Ankylosis of teeth

    K03.6 Deposits [accretions] on teeth
           Betel deposits [accretions] on teeth
           Black deposits [accretions] on teeth
           Extrinsic staining of teeth NOS
           Green deposits [accretions] on teeth
           Materia alba deposits [accretions] on teeth
           Orange deposits [accretions] on teeth
           Staining of teeth NOS
           Subgingival dental calculus
           Supragingival dental calculus
           Tobacco deposits [accretions] on teeth

    K03.7 Posteruptive color changes of dental hard tissues
        Excludes2   deposits [accretions] on teeth (K03.6)

●   **K03.8 Other specified diseases of hard tissues of teeth**

        K03.81 Cracked tooth
             Excludes1   asymptomatic craze lines in enamel - omit code
                        broken or fractured tooth due to trauma (S02.5)

        K03.89 Other specified diseases of hard tissues of teeth

    K03.9 Disease of hard tissues of teeth, unspecified

  K04 Diseases of pulp and periapical tissues

●   **K04.0 Pulpitis**
           Acute pulpitis
           Chronic (hyperplastic) (ulcerative) pulpitis
           (Ex) for category K04.0 CC codes: K00.0-K08.9, M26.00-M26.9, M27.61-M27.69

        K04.01 Reversible pulpitis 🔒 ◄

        K04.02 Irreversible pulpitis 🔒 ◄

    K04.1 Necrosis of pulp
           Pulpal gangrene

    K04.2 Pulp degeneration
           Denticles
           Pulpal calcifications
           Pulpal stones

    K04.3 Abnormal hard tissue formation in pulp
           Secondary or irregular dentine

    K04.4 Acute apical periodontitis of pulpal origin 🔒
           Acute apical periodontitis NOS
         Excludes1   acute periodontitis (K05.2-)
        (Ex) See K04.0

    K04.5 Chronic apical periodontitis
           Apical or periapical granuloma
           Apical periodontitis NOS
         Excludes1   chronic periodontitis (K05.3-)

    K04.6 Periapical abscess with sinus
           Dental abscess with sinus
           Dentoalveolar abscess with sinus

    K04.7 Periapical abscess without sinus
           Dental abscess without sinus
           Dentoalveolar abscess without sinus
           Periapical abscess without sinus

    K04.8 Radicular cyst
           Apical (periodontal) cyst
           Periapical cyst
           Residual radicular cyst
         Excludes2   lateral periodontal cyst (K09.0)

●   **K04.9 Other and unspecified diseases of pulp and periapical tissues**

        K04.90 Unspecified diseases of pulp and periapical tissues

        K04.99 Other diseases of pulp and periapical tissues

◄ New   ◄||| Revised   ~~deleted~~ Deleted   Excludes 1   Excludes 2   Includes   Use additional   Code first   Code also   Unspecified

OGCR Official Guidelines   ● Unacceptable Principal Diagnosis   X Assign placeholder X   ● Use Additional Character(s)   ▶ Manifestation Code   **Coding Clinic**

Item 11–3   **Acute gingivitis,** also known as orilitis or ulitis, is the short-term, severe inflammation of the gums (gingiva) caused by bacteria. **Chronic gingivitis** is persistent inflammation of the gums. When the gingivitis moves into the periodontium it is called periodontitis, also known as paradentitis.

● **K05**   **Gingivitis and periodontal diseases**
    Use additional code to identify:
      alcohol abuse and dependence (F10.-)
      exposure to environmental tobacco smoke (Z77.22)
      exposure to tobacco smoke in the perinatal period (P96.81)
      history of tobacco dependence (Z87.891) ◄▥
      occupational exposure to environmental tobacco smoke
        (Z57.31)
      tobacco dependence (F17.-)
      tobacco use (Z72.0)

● **K05.0**   **Acute gingivitis**
    Excludes1   acute necrotizing ulcerative gingivitis
           (A69.1)
           herpesviral [herpes simplex]
             gingivostomatitis (B00.2)

    K05.00   **Acute gingivitis, plaque induced**
        Acute gingivitis NOS
        Plaque induced gingival disease ◄

    K05.01   **Acute gingivitis, non-plaque induced**

● **K05.1**   **Chronic gingivitis**
    Desquamative gingivitis (chronic)
    Gingivitis (chronic) NOS
    Hyperplastic gingivitis (chronic)
    Pregnancy associated gingivitis ◄
    Simple marginal gingivitis (chronic)
    Ulcerative gingivitis (chronic)
    *Code first, if applicable, diseases of the digestive system
        complicating pregnancy (O99.61-)* ◄

    K05.10   **Chronic gingivitis, plaque induced**
        Chronic gingivitis NOS
        Gingivitis NOS

    K05.11   **Chronic gingivitis, non-plaque induced**

● **K05.2**   **Aggressive periodontitis**
    Acute pericoronitis
    Excludes1   acute apical periodontitis (K04.4)
           periapical abscess (K04.7)
           periapical abscess with sinus (K04.6)

    K05.20   **Aggressive periodontitis, unspecified**
●   **K05.21**   **Aggressive periodontitis, localized**
        Periodontal abscess
        K05.211   **Aggressive periodontitis, localized,
            slight** ◄
        K05.212   **Aggressive periodontitis, localized,
            moderate** ◄
        K05.213   **Aggressive periodontitis, localized,
            severe** ◄
        K05.219   **Aggressive periodontitis, localized,
            unspecified severity** ◄

●   **K05.22**   **Aggressive periodontitis, generalized**
        K05.221   **Aggressive periodontitis, generalized,
            slight** ◄
        K05.222   **Aggressive periodontitis, generalized,
            moderate** ◄
        K05.223   **Aggressive periodontitis, generalized,
            severe** ◄
        K05.229   **Aggressive periodontitis, generalized,
            unspecified severity** ◄

● **K05.3**   **Chronic periodontitis**
    Chronic pericoronitis
    Complex periodontitis
    Periodontitis NOS
    Simplex periodontitis
    Excludes1   chronic apical periodontitis (K04.5)

    K05.30   **Chronic periodontitis, unspecified**
●   **K05.31**   **Chronic periodontitis, localized**
        K05.311   **Chronic periodontitis, localized,
            slight** ◄
        K05.312   **Chronic periodontitis, localized,
            moderate** ◄
        K05.313   **Chronic periodontitis, localized,
            severe** ◄
        K05.319   **Chronic periodontitis, localized,
            unspecified severity** ◄

●   **K05.32**   **Chronic periodontitis, generalized**
        K05.321   **Chronic periodontitis, generalized,
            slight** ◄
        K05.322   **Chronic periodontitis, generalized,
            moderate** ◄
        K05.323   **Chronic periodontitis, generalized,
            severe** ◄
        K05.329   **Chronic periodontitis, generalized,
            unspecified severity** ◄

  K05.4   **Periodontosis**
    Juvenile periodontosis

  K05.5   **Other periodontal diseases**
    Combined periodontic-endodontic lesion ◄
    Narrow gingival width (of periodontal soft tissue) ◄
    Excludes2   leukoplakia of gingiva (K13.21)

  K05.6   **Periodontal disease, unspecified**

● **K06**   **Other disorders of gingiva and edentulous alveolar ridge**
    Excludes2   acute gingivitis (K05.0)
           atrophy of edentulous alveolar ridge (K08.2)
           chronic gingivitis (K05.1)
           gingivitis NOS (K05.1)

  K06.0   **Gingival recession**
    Gingival recession (generalized) (localized)
      (postinfective) (postprocedural)

  K06.1   **Gingival enlargement**
    Gingival fibromatosis

  K06.2   **Gingival and edentulous alveolar ridge lesions
    associated with trauma**
    Irritative hyperplasia of edentulous ridge [denture
      hyperplasia]
    Use additional code (Chapter 20) to identify external
      cause or denture status (Z97.2)

  K06.3   **Horizontal alveolar bone loss** ◄

  K06.8   **Other specified disorders of gingiva and edentulous
    alveolar ridge**
    Fibrous epulis
    Flabby alveolar ridge
    Giant cell epulis
    Peripheral giant cell granuloma of gingiva
    Pyogenic granuloma of gingiva
    Vertical ridge deficiency ◄
    Excludes2   gingival cyst (K09.0)

  K06.9   **Disorder of gingiva and edentulous alveolar ridge,
    unspecified**

● **K08**   **Other disorders of teeth and supporting structures**
    Excludes2   dentofacial anomalies [including malocclusion]
           (M26.-)
           disorders of jaw (M27.-)

  K08.0   **Exfoliation of teeth due to systemic causes**
    Code also underlying systemic condition

N Newborn Age: 0   **P** Pediatric Age: 0–17   **M** Maternity DX: 12–55   **A** Adult Age: 15–124   ♀ Females Only   ♂ Males Only

⬡ Complication\Comorbidity   ⬡ Major C\C   Ⓔⓧ CC/MCC Exclusions   ⬡ Hospital-Acquired Condition   937

● **K08.1 Complete loss of teeth**
    Acquired loss of teeth, complete
    Excludes1   congenital absence of teeth (K00.0)
                    exfoliation of teeth due to systemic causes
                        (K08.0)
                    partial loss of teeth (K08.4-)
  ● **K08.10   Complete loss of teeth, unspecified cause**
        **K08.101   Complete loss of teeth, unspecified
                    cause, class I**
        **K08.102   Complete loss of teeth, unspecified
                    cause, class II**
        **K08.103   Complete loss of teeth, unspecified
                    cause, class III**
        **K08.104   Complete loss of teeth, unspecified
                    cause, class IV**
        **K08.109   Complete loss of teeth, unspecified
                    cause, unspecified class**
                    Edentulism NOS
  ● **K08.11   Complete loss of teeth due to trauma**
        **K08.111   Complete loss of teeth due to trauma,
                    class I**
        **K08.112   Complete loss of teeth due to trauma,
                    class II**
        **K08.113   Complete loss of teeth due to trauma,
                    class III**
        **K08.114   Complete loss of teeth due to trauma,
                    class IV**
        **K08.119   Complete loss of teeth due to trauma,
                    unspecified class**
  ● **K08.12   Complete loss of teeth due to periodontal
              diseases**
        **K08.121   Complete loss of teeth due to
                    periodontal diseases, class I**
        **K08.122   Complete loss of teeth due to
                    periodontal diseases, class II**
        **K08.123   Complete loss of teeth due to
                    periodontal diseases, class III**
        **K08.124   Complete loss of teeth due to
                    periodontal diseases, class IV**
        **K08.129   Complete loss of teeth due to
                    periodontal diseases, unspecified
                    class**
  ● **K08.13   Complete loss of teeth due to caries**
        **K08.131   Complete loss of teeth due to caries,
                    class I**
        **K08.132   Complete loss of teeth due to caries,
                    class II**
        **K08.133   Complete loss of teeth due to caries,
                    class III**
        **K08.134   Complete loss of teeth due to caries,
                    class IV**
        **K08.139   Complete loss of teeth due to caries,
                    unspecified class**
  ● **K08.19   Complete loss of teeth due to other specified
              cause**
        **K08.191   Complete loss of teeth due to other
                    specified cause, class I**
        **K08.192   Complete loss of teeth due to other
                    specified cause, class II**
        **K08.193   Complete loss of teeth due to other
                    specified cause, class III**
        **K08.194   Complete loss of teeth due to other
                    specified cause, class IV**
        **K08.199   Complete loss of teeth due to other
                    specified cause, unspecified class**

● **K08.2 Atrophy of edentulous alveolar ridge**
    **K08.20   Unspecified atrophy of edentulous alveolar
              ridge**
              Atrophy of the mandible NOS
              Atrophy of the maxilla NOS
    K08.21   Minimal atrophy of the mandible
              Minimal atrophy of the edentulous mandible
    K08.22   Moderate atrophy of the mandible
              Moderate atrophy of the edentulous mandible
    K08.23   Severe atrophy of the mandible
              Severe atrophy of the edentulous mandible
    K08.24   Minimal atrophy of maxilla
              Minimal atrophy of the edentulous maxilla
    K08.25   Moderate atrophy of the maxilla
              Moderate atrophy of the edentulous maxilla
    K08.26   Severe atrophy of the maxilla
              Severe atrophy of the edentulous maxilla
  K08.3 Retained dental root
● **K08.4 Partial loss of teeth**
    Acquired loss of teeth, partial
    Excludes1   complete loss of teeth (K08.1-)
                    congenital absence of teeth (K00.0)
    Excludes2   exfoliation of teeth due to systemic causes
                        (K08.0)
  ● **K08.40   Partial loss of teeth, unspecified cause**
        **K08.401   Partial loss of teeth, unspecified
                    cause, class I**
        **K08.402   Partial loss of teeth, unspecified
                    cause, class II**
        **K08.403   Partial loss of teeth, unspecified
                    cause, class III**
        **K08.404   Partial loss of teeth, unspecified
                    cause, class IV**
        **K08.409   Partial loss of teeth, unspecified
                    cause, unspecified class**
                    Tooth extraction status NOS
  ● **K08.41   Partial loss of teeth due to trauma**
        **K08.411   Partial loss of teeth due to trauma,
                    class I**
        **K08.412   Partial loss of teeth due to trauma,
                    class II**
        **K08.413   Partial loss of teeth due to trauma,
                    class III**
        **K08.414   Partial loss of teeth due to trauma,
                    class IV**
        **K08.419   Partial loss of teeth due to trauma,
                    unspecified class**
  ● **K08.42   Partial loss of teeth due to periodontal diseases**
        **K08.421   Partial loss of teeth due to periodontal
                    diseases, class I**
        **K08.422   Partial loss of teeth due to periodontal
                    diseases, class II**
        **K08.423   Partial loss of teeth due to periodontal
                    diseases, class III**
        **K08.424   Partial loss of teeth due to periodontal
                    diseases, class IV**
        **K08.429   Partial loss of teeth due to periodontal
                    diseases, unspecified class**
  ● **K08.43   Partial loss of teeth due to caries**
        **K08.431   Partial loss of teeth due to caries,
                    class I**
        **K08.432   Partial loss of teeth due to caries,
                    class II**
        **K08.433   Partial loss of teeth due to caries,
                    class III**
        **K08.434   Partial loss of teeth due to caries,
                    class IV**
        **K08.439   Partial loss of teeth due to caries,
                    unspecified class**

◀ New   ◀▥ Revised   ~~deleted~~ Deleted   Excludes 1   Excludes 2   Includes   Use additional   Code first   Code also   Unspecified
OGCR Official Guidelines   ● Unacceptable Principal Diagnosis   X Assign placeholder X   ● Use Additional Character(s)   ▸ Manifestation Code   **Coding Clinic**

● **K08.49 Partial loss of teeth due to other specified cause**

    K08.491 Partial loss of teeth due to other specified cause, class I

    K08.492 Partial loss of teeth due to other specified cause, class II

    K08.493 Partial loss of teeth due to other specified cause, class III

    K08.494 Partial loss of teeth due to other specified cause, class IV

    K08.499 Partial loss of teeth due to other specified cause, `unspecified` class

● **K08.5 Unsatisfactory restoration of tooth**
    Defective bridge, crown, filling
    Defective dental restoration

    `Excludes1` dental restoration status (Z98.811)
    `Excludes2` endosseous dental implant failure (M27.6-)
              unsatisfactory endodontic treatment (M27.5-)

    K08.50 Unsatisfactory restoration of tooth, `unspecified`
        Defective dental restoration NOS

    K08.51 Open restoration margins of tooth
        Dental restoration failure of marginal integrity
        Open margin on tooth restoration
        Poor gingival margin to tooth restoration

    K08.52 Unrepairable overhanging of dental restorative materials
        Overhanging of tooth restoration

●   **K08.53 Fractured dental restorative material**
        `Excludes1` cracked tooth (K03.81)
                  traumatic fracture of tooth (S02.5)

    K08.530 Fractured dental restorative material without loss of material

    K08.531 Fractured dental restorative material with loss of material

    K08.539 Fractured dental restorative material, `unspecified`

    K08.54 Contour of existing restoration of tooth biologically incompatible with oral health
        Dental restoration failure of periodontal anatomical integrity
        Unacceptable contours of existing restoration of tooth
        Unacceptable morphology of existing restoration of tooth

    K08.55 Allergy to existing dental restorative material
        Use additional code to identify the specific type of allergy

    K08.56 Poor aesthetic of existing restoration of tooth
        Dental restoration aesthetically inadequate or displeasing

    K08.59 Other unsatisfactory restoration of tooth
        Other defective dental restoration

● **K08.8 Other specified disorders of teeth and supporting structures**

    K08.81 Primary occlusal trauma ◄

    K08.82 Secondary occlusal trauma ◄

    K08.89 Other specified disorders of teeth and supporting structures ◄
        Enlargement of alveolar ridge NOS ◄
        Insufficient anatomic crown height ◄
        Insufficient clinical crown length ◄
        Irregular alveolar process ◄
        Toothache NOS ◄

K08.9 Disorder of teeth and supporting structures, `unspecified`

● **K09 Cysts of oral region, not elsewhere classified**

    `Includes` lesions showing histological features both of aneurysmal cyst and of another fibro-osseous lesion

    `Excludes2` cysts of jaw (M27.0-, M27.4-)
              radicular cyst (K04.8)

    K09.0 Developmental odontogenic cysts
        Dentigerous cyst
        Eruption cyst
        Follicular cyst
        Gingival cyst
        Lateral periodontal cyst
        Primordial cyst

        `Excludes2` keratocysts (D16.4, D16.5)
                 odontogenic keratocystic tumors (D16.4, D16.5)

    K09.1 Developmental (nonodontogenic) cysts of oral region
        Cyst (of) incisive canal
        Cyst (of) palatine of papilla
        Globulomaxillary cyst
        Median palatal cyst
        Nasoalveolar cyst
        Nasolabial cyst
        Nasopalatine duct cyst

    K09.8 Other cysts of oral region, not elsewhere classified
        Dermoid cyst
        Epidermoid cyst
        Lymphoepithelial cyst
        Epstein's pearl

    K09.9 Cyst of oral region, `unspecified`

★ **(See Plate 61 on page 73.)**

● **K11 Diseases of salivary glands**
    Use additional code to identify:
        alcohol abuse and dependence (F10.-)
        exposure to environmental tobacco smoke (Z77.22)
        exposure to tobacco smoke in the perinatal period (P96.81)
        history of tobacco dependence (Z87.891) ◄▥
        occupational exposure to environmental tobacco smoke (Z57.31)
        tobacco dependence (F17.-)
        tobacco use (Z72.0)

    K11.0 Atrophy of salivary gland

    K11.1 Hypertrophy of salivary gland

●   **K11.2 Sialoadenitis**
        Parotitis

        `Excludes1` epidemic parotitis (B26.-)
                 mumps (B26.-)
                 uveoparotid fever [Heerfordt] (D86.89)

    K11.20 Sialoadenitis, `unspecified`

    K11.21 Acute sialoadenitis
        `Excludes1` acute recurrent sialoadenitis (K11.22)

    K11.22 Acute recurrent sialoadenitis

    K11.23 Chronic sialoadenitis

Item 11–4 Atrophy is wasting away of a tissue or organ, whereas **hypertrophy** is overdevelopment or enlargement of a tissue or organ. **Sialoadenitis** is salivary gland inflammation. **Parotitis** is the inflammation of the parotid gland. In the epidemic form, parotitis is also known as mumps. **Sialolithiasis** is the formation of calculus within a salivary gland. **Mucocele** is a polyp composed of mucus.

Figure 11-3 Major salivary glands.

Parotid gland
Sublingual gland
Submandibular gland

CHAPTER 11 (K00-K95)

K11.3   Abscess of salivary gland 🔖
(Ex:) K11.0-K11.9, K31.89-K31.9, K92.81, R68.2

K11.4   Fistula of salivary gland 🔖
> **Excludes1**   congenital fistula of salivary gland
> (Q38.4)

(Ex:) See K11.3

K11.5   Sialolithiasis
Calculus of salivary gland or duct
Stone of salivary gland or duct

K11.6   Mucocele of salivary gland
Mucous extravasation cyst of salivary gland
Mucous retention cyst of salivary gland
Ranula

K11.7   Disturbances of salivary secretion
Hypoptyalism
Ptyalism
Xerostomia
> **Excludes2**   dry mouth NOS (R68.2)

K11.8   Other diseases of salivary glands
Benign lymphoepithelial lesion of salivary gland
Mikulicz' disease
Necrotizing sialometaplasia
Sialectasia
Stenosis of salivary duct
Stricture of salivary duct
> **Excludes1**   sicca syndrome [Sjögren] (M35.0-)

K11.9   Disease of salivary gland, unspecified
Sialoadenopathy NOS

● **K12   Stomatitis and related lesions**
Use additional code to identify:
alcohol abuse and dependence (F10.-)
exposure to environmental tobacco smoke (Z77.22)
exposure to tobacco smoke in the perinatal period (P96.81)
history of tobacco dependence (Z87.891) ◀▦
occupational exposure to environmental tobacco smoke (Z57.31)
tobacco dependence (F17.-)
tobacco use (Z72.0)
> **Excludes1**   cancrum oris (A69.0)
> cheilitis (K13.0)
> gangrenous stomatitis (A69.0)
> herpesviral [herpes simplex] gingivostomatitis (B00.2)
> noma (A69.0)

K12.0   Recurrent oral aphthae
Aphthous stomatitis (major) (minor)
Bednar's aphthae
Periadenitis mucosa necrotica recurrens
Recurrent aphthous ulcer
Stomatitis herpetiformis

K12.1   Other forms of stomatitis
Stomatitis NOS
Denture stomatitis
Ulcerative stomatitis
Vesicular stomatitis
> **Excludes1**   acute necrotizing ulcerative stomatitis (A69.1)
> Vincent's stomatitis (A69.1)

K12.2   Cellulitis and abscess of mouth 🔖
Cellulitis of mouth (floor)
Submandibular abscess
> **Excludes2**   abscess of salivary gland (K11.3)
> abscess of tongue (K14.0)
> periapical abscess (K04.6-K04.7)
> periodontal abscess (K05.21)
> peritonsillar abscess (J36)
(Ex:) K12.1-K12.39, K14.0, K14.2

● **K12.3   Oral mucositis (ulcerative)**
Mucositis (oral) (oropharyneal)
> **Excludes2**   gastrointestinal mucositis (ulcerative) (K92.81)
> mucositis (ulcerative) of vagina and vulva (N76.81)
> nasal mucositis (ulcerative) (J34.81)

K12.30   Oral mucositis (ulcerative), unspecified

K12.31   Oral mucositis (ulcerative) due to antineoplastic therapy
Use additional code for adverse effect, if applicable, to identify antineoplastic and immunosuppressive drugs (T45.1X5)
Use additional code for other antineoplastic therapy, such as:
radiological procedure and radiotherapy (Y84.2)

K12.32   Oral mucositis (ulcerative) due to other drugs
Use additional code for adverse effect, if applicable, to identify drug (T36-T50 with fifth or sixth character 5)

K12.33   Oral mucositis (ulcerative) due to radiation
Use additional external cause code (W88-W90, X39.0-) to identify cause

K12.39   Other oral mucositis (ulcerative)
Viral oral mucositis (ulcerative)

● **K13   Other diseases of lip and oral mucosa**
> **Includes**   epithelial disturbances of tongue
Use additional code to identify:
alcohol abuse and dependence (F10.-)
exposure to environmental tobacco smoke (Z77.22)
exposure to tobacco smoke in the perinatal period (P96.81)
history of tobacco dependence (Z87.891) ◀▦
occupational exposure to environmental tobacco smoke (Z57.31)
tobacco dependence (F17.-)
tobacco use (Z72.0)
> **Excludes2**   certain disorders of gingiva and edentulous alveolar ridge (K05-K06)
> cysts of oral region (K09.-)
> diseases of tongue (K14.-)
> stomatitis and related lesions (K12.-)

K13.0   Diseases of lips

Abscess of lips	Exfoliative cheilitis
Angular cheilitis	Fistula of lips
Cellulitis of lips	Glandular cheilitis
Cheilitis NOS	Hypertrophy of lips
Cheilodynia	Perlèche NEC
Cheilosis	

> **Excludes1**   ariboflavinosis (E53.0)
> cheilitis due to radiation-related disorders (L55-L59)
> congenital fistula of lips (Q38.0)
> congenital hypertrophy of lips (Q18.6)
> Perlèche due to candidiasis (B37.83)
> Perlèche due to riboflavin deficiency (E53.0)

K13.1   Cheek and lip biting

Item 11–5   Stomatitis is the inflammation of the oral mucosa. **Mucositis** is the inflammation of the mucous membranes lining the digestive tract from the mouth to the anus. It is a common side effect of chemotherapy and of radiotherapy that involves any part of the digestive tract.

◀ New   ◀▦ Revised   ~~deleted~~ Deleted   Excludes 1   Excludes 2   Includes   Use additional   Code first   Code also   Unspecified

OGCR Official Guidelines   ● Unacceptable Principal Diagnosis   X Assign placeholder X   ● Use Additional Character(s)   ▌ Manifestation Code   **Coding Clinic**

Figure 11-4 Oral leukoplakia and associated squamous carcinoma. (From Feldman: Sleisenger & Fordtran's Gastrointestinal and Liver Disease, ed 8, Saunders, An Imprint of Elsevier, 2006)

● **K13.2 Leukoplakia and other disturbances of oral epithelium, including tongue**

> **Excludes1** carcinoma in situ of oral epithelium (D00.0-)
> hairy leukoplakia (K13.3)

K13.21 Leukoplakia of oral mucosa, including tongue
> *Considered precancerous and evidenced by thickened white patches of epithelium on mucous membranes*
> Leukokeratosis of oral mucosa
> Leukoplakia of gingiva, lips, tongue
>> **Excludes1** hairy leukoplakia (K13.3)
>> leukokeratosis nicotina palati (K13.24)

K13.22 Minimal keratinized residual ridge mucosa
> Minimal keratinization of alveolar ridge mucosa

K13.23 Excessive keratinized residual ridge mucosa
> Excessive keratinization of alveolar ridge mucosa

K13.24 Leukokeratosis nicotina palati
> Smoker's palate

K13.29 Other disturbances of oral epithelium, including tongue
> Erythroplakia of mouth or tongue
> Focal epithelial hyperplasia of mouth or tongue
> Leukoedema of mouth or tongue
> Other oral epithelium disturbances

K13.3 Hairy leukoplakia

K13.4 Granuloma and granuloma-like lesions of oral mucosa
> Eosinophilic granuloma
> Granuloma pyogenicum
> Verrucous xanthoma

K13.5 Oral submucous fibrosis
> Submucous fibrosis of tongue

K13.6 Irritative hyperplasia of oral mucosa
> **Excludes2** irritative hyperplasia of edentulous ridge [denture hyperplasia] (K06.2)

● **K13.7 Other and unspecified lesions of oral mucosa**
K13.70 Unspecified lesions of oral mucosa
K13.79 Other lesions of oral mucosa
> Focal oral mucinosis

★ **(See Plate 58 on page 71.)**

● **K14 Diseases of tongue**
> Use additional code to identify:
> alcohol abuse and dependence (F10.-)
> exposure to environmental tobacco smoke (Z77.22)
> history of tobacco dependence (Z87.891) ◀◀◀
> occupational exposure to environmental tobacco smoke (Z57.31)
> tobacco dependence (F17.-)
> tobacco use (Z72.0)
> **Excludes2** erythroplakia (K13.29)
> focal epithelial hyperplasia (K13.29)
> leukedema of tongue (K13.29)
> leukoplakia of tongue (K13.21)
> hairy leukoplakia (K13.3)
> macroglossia (congenital) (Q38.2)
> submucous fibrosis of tongue (K13.5)

K14.0 Glossitis
> Abscess of tongue
> Ulceration (traumatic) of tongue
> **Excludes1** atrophic glossitis (K14.4)

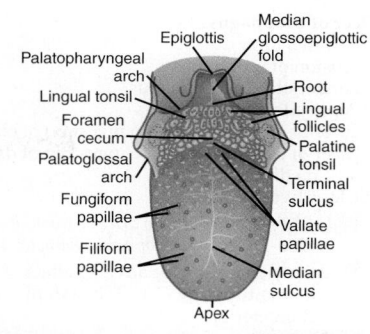

Figure 11-5 Structure of the tongue.

K14.1 Geographic tongue
> Benign migratory glossitis
> Glossitis areata exfoliativa

K14.2 Median rhomboid glossitis

K14.3 Hypertrophy of tongue papillae
> Black hairy tongue
> Coated tongue
> Hypertrophy of foliate papillae
> Lingua villosa nigra

K14.4 Atrophy of tongue papillae
> Atrophic glossitis

K14.5 Plicated tongue
> Fissured tongue   Scrotal tongue
> Furrowed tongue
>> **Excludes1** fissured tongue, congenital (Q38.3)

K14.6 Glossodynia
> Glossopyrosis   Painful tongue

K14.8 Other diseases of tongue
> Atrophy of tongue   Glossocele
> Crenated tongue   Glossoptosis
> Enlargement of tongue   Hypertrophy of tongue

K14.9 Disease of tongue, unspecified
> Glossopathy NOS

DISEASES OF ESOPHAGUS, STOMACH AND DUODENUM (K20-K31)

> **Excludes2** hiatus hernia (K44.-)

● **K20 Esophagitis**
> Use additional code to identify:
> alcohol abuse and dependence (F10.-)
> **Excludes1** erosion of esophagus (K22.1-)
> esophagitis with gastro-esophageal reflux disease (K21.0)
> reflux esophagitis (K21.0)
> ulcerative esophagitis (K22.1-)
> **Excludes2** eosinophilic gastritis or gastroenteritis (K52.81)

K20.0 Eosinophilic esophagitis

K20.8 Other esophagitis
> Abscess of esophagus

K20.9 Esophagitis, unspecified
> Esophagitis NOS

● **K21 Gastro-esophageal reflux disease**
> **Excludes1** newborn esophageal reflux (P78.83)

K21.0 Gastro-esophageal reflux disease with esophagitis
> Reflux esophagitis

K21.9 Gastro-esophageal reflux disease without esophagitis
> Esophageal reflux NOS
> **Coding Clinic: 2016, Q1, P18**

● **K22 Other diseases of esophagus**
> **Excludes2** esophageal varices (I85.-)

K22.0 Achalasia of cardia
> Achalasia NOS
> Cardiospasm
>> **Excludes1** congenital cardiospasm (Q39.5)

N Newborn Age: 0   **P** Pediatric Age: 0–17   **M** Maternity DX: 12–55   **A** Adult Age: 15–124   ♀ Females Only   ♂ Males Only

🔴 Complication\Comorbidity   🔵 Major C\C   (Ex) CC/MCC Exclusions   🔴 Hospital-Acquired Condition

941

CHAPTER 11 (K00-K95)

● **K22.1 Ulcer of esophagus**
Barrett's ulcer
Erosion of esophagus
Fungal ulcer of esophagus
Peptic ulcer of esophagus
Ulcer of esophagus due to ingestion of chemicals
Ulcer of esophagus due to ingestion of drugs and medicaments
Ulcerative esophagitis
Code first poisoning due to drug or toxin, if applicable (T36-T65 with fifth or sixth character 1-4 or 6)
Use additional code for adverse effect, if applicable, to identify drug (T36-T50 with fifth or sixth character 5)
Excludes1 Barrett's esophagus (K22.87-)

K22.10 Ulcer of esophagus without bleeding 🔖
Ulcer of esophagus NOS
Ⓔ K22.11, K22.8-K23, K31.82

K22.11 Ulcer of esophagus with bleeding 🔖
Excludes2 bleeding esophageal varices (I85.01, I85.11)
Ⓔ E16.4, I85.01, K22.10-K22.11, K22.6-K22.719, K25.0-K28.9, K29.01, K29.21, K29.31, K29.41, K29.51, K29.61, K29.71, K29.81, K29.91, K31.811, K31.89-K31.9, K55.21, K57.01, K57.11, K57.13, K57.21, K57.31, K57.33, K57.41, K57.51, K57.53, K57.81, K57.91, K57.93, K62.5, K92.0-K92.81

K22.2 Esophageal obstruction
Compression of esophagus
Constriction of esophagus
Stenosis of esophagus
Stricture of esophagus
Excludes1 congenital stenosis or stricture of esophagus (Q39.3)

K22.3 Perforation of esophagus 🔖
Rupture of esophagus
Excludes1 traumatic perforation of (thoracic) esophagus (S27.8-)
Ⓔ K21.9, K22.3, K22.6, K22.8-K23

K22.4 Dyskinesia of esophagus
Difficulty in moving
Corkscrew esophagus
Diffuse esophageal spasm
Spasm of esophagus
Excludes1 cardiospasm (K22.0)

K22.5 Diverticulum of esophagus, acquired
Esophageal pouch, acquired
Excludes1 diverticulum of esophagus (congenital) (Q39.6)

Item 11–6 Esophageal reflux is the return flow of the contents of the stomach to the esophagus and is referred to as GERD and/or "heartburn." **Gastroesophageal reflux** is the return flow of the contents of the stomach and duodenum to the esophagus. **Esophageal leukoplakia** are white areas on the mucous membrane of the esophagus for which no specific cause can be identified.

CERVICAL ESOPHAGUS
Left subclavian artery
First rib
Arch of aorta
Diaphragm
THORACIC ESOPHAGUS
Stomach
ABDOMINAL ESOPHAGUS

Figure 11-6 The esophagus is the muscular tube that connects the pharynx and the stomach. The 10 inch (25 cm) long esophagus is divided into three parts: **cervical, thoracic,** and **abdominal.**

Item 11–7 Achalasia is a condition in which the smooth muscle fibers of the esophagus do not relax. Most frequently, this condition occurs at the esophagogastric sphincter. **Cardiospasm,** also known as **megaesophagus,** is achalasia of the thoracic esophagus.

K22.6 Gastro-esophageal laceration-hemorrhage syndrome 🔖
Mallory-Weiss syndrome
Ⓔ E16.4, I85.01, K21.9, K22.10-K22.11, K22.3, K22.6-K28.9, K29.01, K29.21, K29.31, K29.41, K29.51, K29.61, K29.71, K29.81, K29.91, K31.811, K55.21, K57.01, K57.11, K57.13, K57.21, K57.31, K57.33, K57.41, K57.51, K57.53, K57.81, K57.91, K57.93, K62.5, K92.0-K92.2

● **K22.7 Barrett's esophagus**
Barrett's disease
Barrett's syndrome
Excludes1 Barrett's ulcer (K22.1)
malignant neoplasm of esophagus (C15.-)

K22.70 Barrett's esophagus without dysplasia
Barrett's esophagus NOS

● **K22.71 Barrett's esophagus with dysplasia**
K22.710 Barrett's esophagus with low grade dysplasia
K22.711 Barrett's esophagus with high grade dysplasia
K22.719 Barrett's esophagus with dysplasia, unspecified

K22.8 Other specified diseases of esophagus
Hemorrhage of esophagus NOS
Excludes2 esophageal varices (I85.-)
Paterson-Kelly syndrome (D50.1)

K22.9 Disease of esophagus, unspecified

▶ *K23 Disorders of esophagus in diseases classified elsewhere*
Code first underlying disease, such as:
congenital syphilis (A50.5)
Excludes1 late syphilis (A52.79)
megaesophagus due to Chagas' disease (B57.31)
tuberculosis (A18.83)

● **K25 Gastric ulcer**
Includes erosion (acute) of stomach
pylorus ulcer (peptic)
stomach ulcer (peptic)
Use additional code to identify:
alcohol abuse and dependence (F10.-)
Excludes1 acute gastritis (K29.0-)
peptic ulcer NOS (K27.-)
Ⓔ For category K25 CC codes: E16.4, I85.01, K22.10-K22.11, K22.6-K22.719, K25.0-K28.9, K29.01, K29.21, K29.31, K29.41, K29.51, K29.61, K29.71, K29.81, K29.91, K31.811, K31.89-K31.9, K55.21, K57.01, K57.11, K57.13, K57.33, K57.41, K57.51, K57.53, K57.81, K57.91, K57.93, K62.5, K92.0-K92.81

K25.0 Acute gastric ulcer with hemorrhage 🔖
K25.1 Acute gastric ulcer with perforation 🔖
K25.2 Acute gastric ulcer with both hemorrhage and perforation 🔖
K25.3 Acute gastric ulcer without hemorrhage or perforation 🔖
K25.4 Chronic or unspecified gastric ulcer with hemorrhage 🔖
K25.5 Chronic or unspecified gastric ulcer with perforation 🔖
K25.6 Chronic or unspecified gastric ulcer with both hemorrhage and perforation 🔖
K25.7 Chronic gastric ulcer without hemorrhage or perforation
K25.9 Gastric ulcer, unspecified as acute or chronic, without hemorrhage or perforation

Figure 11-7 A. Ulcer. **B.** Perforated ulcer. **C.** Laparoscopic view of a perforated duodenal ulcer *(arrow)* with fibrinous exudate on the adjacent peritoneum. (**C** from Feldman: Sleisenger & Fordtran's Gastrointestinal and Liver Disease, ed 8, Saunders, An Imprint of Elsevier, 2006)

Item 11–8 Gastric ulcers are lesions of the stomach that result in the death of the tissue and a defect of the surface. **Perforated ulcers** are those in which the lesion penetrates the gastric wall, leaving a hole. **Peptic ulcers** are lesions of the stomach or the duodenum. **Peptic** refers to the gastric juice, pepsin.

● **K26**   **Duodenal ulcer**

     Includes   erosion (acute) of duodenum
                      duodenum ulcer (peptic)
                      postpyloric ulcer (peptic)

     Use additional code to identify:
         alcohol abuse and dependence (F10.-)

     Excludes1   peptic ulcer NOS (K27.-)

     Ⓔ**x**) **For category K26 CC codes unless otherwise indicated:** E16.4, I85.01, K22.10-K22.11, K22.6-K22.719, K25.0-K28.9, K29.01, K29.21, K29.31, K29.41, K29.51, K29.61, K29.71, K29.81, K29.91, K31.5, K31.811, K31.89-K31.9, K55.21, K57.01, K57.11, K57.13, K57.21, K57.31, K57.33, K57.41, K57.51, K57.53, K57.81, K57.91, K57.93, K62.5, K92.0-K92.81

   K26.0   Acute duodenal ulcer with hemorrhage 🏥
   K26.1   Acute duodenal ulcer with perforation 🏥
   K26.2   Acute duodenal ulcer with both hemorrhage and perforation 🏥
   K26.3   Acute duodenal ulcer without hemorrhage or perforation 🏥
         Ⓔ**x**) E16.4, I85.01, K22.6, K25.0-K28.9, K29.01, K29.21, K29.31, K29.41, K29.51, K29.61, K29.71, K29.81, K29.91, K31.5, K31.811, K31.82, K31.89-K31.9, K55.21, K57.01, K57.11, K57.13, K57.21, K57.31, K57.33, K57.41, K57.51, K57.53, K57.81, K57.91, K57.93, K62.5, K92.0-K92.81
   K26.4   Chronic or unspecified duodenal ulcer with hemorrhage 🏥
         Coding Clinic: 2016, Q1, P14
   K26.5   Chronic or unspecified duodenal ulcer with perforation 🏥
   K26.6   Chronic or unspecified duodenal ulcer with both hemorrhage and perforation 🏥
   K26.7   Chronic duodenal ulcer without hemorrhage or perforation
   K26.9   Duodenal ulcer, unspecified as acute or chronic, without hemorrhage or perforation

● **K27**   **Peptic ulcer, site unspecified**

     Includes   gastroduodenal ulcer NOS
                      peptic ulcer NOS

     Use additional code to identify:
         alcohol abuse and dependence (F10.-)

     Excludes1   peptic ulcer of newborn (P78.82)

     Ⓔ**x**) **For category K27 CC codes:** See K26

   K27.0   Acute peptic ulcer, site unspecified, with hemorrhage 🏥
   K27.1   Acute peptic ulcer, site unspecified, with perforation 🏥
   K27.2   Acute peptic ulcer, site unspecified, with both hemorrhage and perforation 🏥
   K27.3   Acute peptic ulcer, site unspecified, without hemorrhage or perforation 🏥
   K27.4   Chronic or unspecified peptic ulcer, site unspecified, with hemorrhage 🏥
   K27.5   Chronic or unspecified peptic ulcer, site unspecified, with perforation 🏥

   K27.6   Chronic or unspecified peptic ulcer, site unspecified, with both hemorrhage and perforation 🏥
   K27.7   Chronic peptic ulcer, site unspecified, without hemorrhage or perforation
   K27.9   Peptic ulcer, site unspecified, unspecified as acute or chronic, without hemorrhage or perforation

● **K28**   **Gastrojejunal ulcer**

     Includes   anastomotic ulcer (peptic) or erosion
                      gastrocolic ulcer (peptic) or erosion
                      gastrointestinal ulcer (peptic) or erosion
                      gastrojejunal ulcer (peptic) or erosion
                      jejunal ulcer (peptic) or erosion
                      marginal ulcer (peptic) or erosion
                      stomal ulcer (peptic) or erosion

     Use additional code to identify:
         alcohol abuse and dependence (F10.-)

     Excludes1   primary ulcer of small intestine (K63.3)

     Ⓔ**x**) **For category K28 CC codes:** See K25

   K28.0   Acute gastrojejunal ulcer with hemorrhage 🏥
   K28.1   Acute gastrojejunal ulcer with perforation 🏥
   K28.2   Acute gastrojejunal ulcer with both hemorrhage and perforation 🏥
   K28.3   Acute gastrojejunal ulcer without hemorrhage or perforation 🏥
   K28.4   Chronic or unspecified gastrojejunal ulcer with hemorrhage 🏥
   K28.5   Chronic or unspecified gastrojejunal ulcer with perforation 🏥
   K28.6   Chronic or unspecified gastrojejunal ulcer with both hemorrhage and perforation 🏥
   K28.7   Chronic gastrojejunal ulcer without hemorrhage or perforation
   K28.9   Gastrojejunal ulcer, unspecified as acute or chronic, without hemorrhage or perforation

● **K29**   **Gastritis and duodenitis**

     Excludes1   eosinophilic gastritis or gastroenteritis (K52.81)
                          Zollinger-Ellison syndrome (E16.4)

     Ⓔ**x**) **For category K29 CC codes:** E16.4, I85.01, K22.10-K22.11, K22.6-K22.719, K25.0-K28.9, K29.01, K29.21, K29.31, K29.41, K29.51, K29.61, K29.71, K29.81, K29.91, K31.811, K55.21, K57.01, K57.11, K57.13, K57.21, K57.31, K57.33, K57.41, K57.51, K57.53, K57.81, K57.91, K57.93, K62.5, K92.0-K92.2

● **K29.0**   **Acute gastritis**

     Use additional code to identify:
         alcohol abuse and dependence (F10.-)

     Excludes1   erosion (acute) of stomach (K25.-)

   K29.00   Acute gastritis without bleeding
   K29.01   Acute gastritis with bleeding 🏥

● **K29.2**   **Alcoholic gastritis**

     Use additional code to identify:
         alcohol abuse and dependence (F10.-)

   K29.20   Alcoholic gastritis without bleeding
   K29.21   Alcoholic gastritis with bleeding 🏥

● **K29.3**   **Chronic superficial gastritis**

   K29.30   Chronic superficial gastritis without bleeding
   K29.31   Chronic superficial gastritis with bleeding 🏥

● **K29.4**   **Chronic atrophic gastritis**
     Gastric atrophy

   K29.40   Chronic atrophic gastritis without bleeding
   K29.41   Chronic atrophic gastritis with bleeding 🏥

● **K29.5**   **Unspecified chronic gastritis**
     Chronic antral gastritis
     Chronic fundal gastritis

   K29.50   Unspecified chronic gastritis without bleeding
   K29.51   Unspecified chronic gastritis with bleeding 🏥

Item 11–9 Gastritis is a severe inflammation of the stomach. **Atrophic gastritis** is a chronic inflammation of the stomach that results in destruction of the cells of the mucosa of the stomach. Duodenitis is an inflammation of the duodenum, the first section of the small intestine.

N   Newborn Age: 0   **P**   Pediatric Age: 0–17   **M**   Maternity DX: 12–55   **A**   Adult Age: 15–124   ♀ Females Only   ♂ Males Only

🏥   Complication\Comorbidity   🏥 Major C\C   Ⓔx) CC/MCC Exclusions   🏥 Hospital-Acquired Condition

● **K29.6 Other gastritis**
Giant hypertrophic gastritis
Granulomatous gastritis
Ménétrier's disease
     K29.60 Other gastritis without bleeding
     K29.61 Other gastritis with bleeding 🔹

● **K29.7 Gastritis, unspecified**
     K29.70 Gastritis, unspecified, without bleeding
     K29.71 Gastritis, unspecified, with bleeding 🔹

● **K29.8 Duodenitis**
     K29.80 Duodenitis without bleeding
     K29.81 Duodenitis with bleeding 🔹

● **K29.9 Gastroduodenitis, unspecified**
     K29.90 Gastroduodenitis, unspecified, without bleeding
     K29.91 Gastroduodenitis, unspecified, with bleeding 🔹

K30 Functional dyspepsia
Indigestion
> **Excludes1**   dyspepsia NOS (R10.13)
> heartburn (R12)
> nervous dyspepsia (F45.8)
> neurotic dyspepsia (F45.8)
> psychogenic dyspepsia (F45.8)

● **K31 Other diseases of stomach and duodenum**
Includes   functional disorders of stomach
> **Excludes2**   diabetic gastroparesis (E08.43, E09.43, E10.43, E11.43, E13.43)
> diverticulum of duodenum (K57.00-K57.13)

K31.0 Acute dilatation of stomach 🔹
Acute distention of stomach
ⒺⓍ K31.0

K31.1 Adult hypertrophic pyloric stenosis 🔹   A
Pyloric stenosis NOS
> **Excludes1**   congenital or infantile pyloric stenosis (Q40.0)
ⒺⓍ K30-K31.1, K31.5, K31.84, Q38.5, Q40.0, Q40.8-Q41.9, Q43.4-Q43.9

K31.2 Hourglass stricture and stenosis of stomach
> **Excludes1**   congenital hourglass stomach (Q40.2)
> hourglass contraction of stomach (K31.89)

K31.3 Pylorospasm, not elsewhere classified
> **Excludes1**   congenital or infantile pylorospasm (Q40.0)
> neurotic pylorospasm (F45.8)
> psychogenic pylorospasm (F45.8)

K31.4 Gastric diverticulum
> **Excludes1**   congenital diverticulum of stomach (Q40.2)

K31.5 Obstruction of duodenum 🔹
Constriction of duodenum
Duodenal ileus (chronic)
Stenosis of duodenum
     Narrowing
Stricture of duodenum
     Narrowing
Volvulus of duodenum
     Twisting/knotting
> **Excludes1**   congenital stenosis of duodenum (Q41.0)
ⒺⓍ K31.5, Q38.5, Q40.8-Q41.9, Q43.4-Q43.9

K31.6 Fistula of stomach and duodenum 🔹
Gastrocolic fistula
Gastrojejunocolic fistula
ⒺⓍ K31.6, Q38.5, Q40.8-Q40.9, Q43.4-Q43.9

K31.7 Polyp of stomach and duodenum
> **Excludes1**   adenomatous polyp of stomach (D13.1)

Item 11-10 Achlorhydria, also known as gastric anacidity, is the absence of gastric acid.

● **K31.8 Other specified diseases of stomach and duodenum**
● **K31.81 Angiodysplasia of stomach and duodenum**
     K31.811 Angiodysplasia of stomach and duodenum with bleeding 🔹
        ⒺⓍ See K29
     K31.819 Angiodysplasia of stomach and duodenum without bleeding
        Angiodysplasia of stomach and duodenum NOS

     K31.82 Dieulafoy lesion (hemorrhagic) of stomach and duodenum 🔹
> **Excludes2**   Dieulafoy lesion of intestine (K63.81)
ⒺⓍ E16.4, I85.01, K22.10-K22.11, K22.6-K22.719, K25.0-K28.9, K29.01, K29.21, K29.31, K29.41, K29.51, K29.61, K29.71, K29.81, K29.91, K31.811, K31.82, K55.21, K57.01, K57.11, K57.13, K57.21, K57.31, K57.33, K57.41, K57.51, K57.53, K57.81, K57.91, K57.93, K62.5, K92.0-K92.2

     K31.83 Achlorhydria
     K31.84 Gastroparesis
        Gastroparalysis
        Code first underlying disease, if known, such as:
        anorexia nervosa (F50.0-)
        diabetes mellitus (E08.43, E09.43, E10.43, E11.43, E13.43)
        scleroderma (M34.-)
     K31.89 Other diseases of stomach and duodenum
     K31.9 Disease of stomach and duodenum, unspecified

DISEASES OF APPENDIX (K35-K38)

● **K35 Acute appendicitis**
     ⒺⓍ For category K35 CC codes: K31.89-K38.9, K92.81

K35.2 Acute appendicitis with generalized peritonitis 🔹
Appendicitis (acute) with generalized (diffuse) peritonitis following rupture or perforation of appendix
Perforated appendix NOS
Ruptured appendix NOS

K35.3 Acute appendicitis with localized peritonitis 🔹
Acute appendicitis with or without perforation or rupture with peritonitis NOS ◀▥
Acute appendicitis with or without perforation or rupture with localized peritonitis
Acute appendicitis with peritoneal abscess

● **K35.8 Other and unspecified acute appendicitis**
     K35.80 Unspecified acute appendicitis 🔹
        Acute appendicitis NOS
        Acute appendicitis without (localized) (generalized) peritonitis
     K35.89 Other acute appendicitis 🔹

K36 Other appendicitis
Chronic appendicitis
Recurrent appendicitis

K37 Unspecified appendicitis
> **Excludes1**   -unspecified appendicitis with peritonitis (K35.2-K35.3)

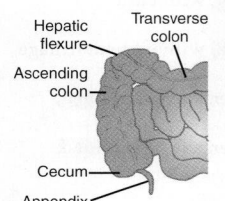

Figure 11-8   Acute appendicitis is the inflammation of the appendix, usually associated with obstruction. Most often this is a disease of adolescents and young adults.

Hepatic flexure   Transverse colon
Ascending colon
Cecum
Appendix

◀ New   ◀▥ Revised   ~~deleted~~ Deleted   Excludes 1   Excludes 2   Includes   Use additional   Code first   Code also   Unspecified
OGCR Official Guidelines   ● Unacceptable Principal Diagnosis   X Assign placeholder X   ● Use Additional Character(s)   🔹 Manifestation Code   **Coding Clinic**

● **K38**   **Other diseases of appendix**

     K38.0   **Hyperplasia of appendix**

     K38.1   **Appendicular concretions**
         Fecalith of appendix
         Stercolith of appendix

     K38.2   **Diverticulum of appendix**

     K38.3   **Fistula of appendix**

     K38.8   **Other specified diseases of appendix**
         Intussusception of appendix

     K38.9   **Disease of appendix, unspecified**

HERNIA (K40-K46)

     Note: Hernia with both gangrene and obstruction is classified to hernia with gangrene.

     Includes   acquired hernia
                   congenital [except diaphragmatic or hiatus] hernia
                   recurrent hernia

● **K40**   **Inguinal hernia**

     Includes   bubonocele
                   direct inguinal hernia
                   double inguinal hernia
                   indirect inguinal hernia
                   inguinal hernia NOS
                   oblique inguinal hernia
                   scrotal hernia

     (Ex) **For category K40 CC codes:** K31.89-K31.9, K40.00-K40.91, K45.0, K45.8-K46.0, K92.81

● **K40.0**   **Bilateral inguinal hernia, with obstruction, without gangrene**
         Inguinal hernia (bilateral) causing obstruction without gangrene
         Incarcerated inguinal hernia (bilateral) without gangrene
         Irreducible inguinal hernia (bilateral) without gangrene
         Strangulated inguinal hernia (bilateral) without gangrene

     K40.00   **Bilateral inguinal hernia, with obstruction, without gangrene, not specified as recurrent** 🔾
         Bilateral inguinal hernia, with obstruction, without gangrene NOS

     K40.01   **Bilateral inguinal hernia, with obstruction, without gangrene, recurrent** 🔾

● **K40.1**   **Bilateral inguinal hernia, with gangrene**

     K40.10   **Bilateral inguinal hernia, with gangrene, not specified as recurrent** 🔾
         Bilateral inguinal hernia, with gangrene NOS

     K40.11   **Bilateral inguinal hernia, with gangrene, recurrent** 🔾

Figure 11-9   Inguinal hernias are those that are located in the inguinal or iliac areas of the abdomen.

● **K40.2**   **Bilateral inguinal hernia, without obstruction or gangrene**

     K40.20   **Bilateral inguinal hernia, without obstruction or gangrene, not specified as recurrent**
         Bilateral inguinal hernia NOS

     K40.21   **Bilateral inguinal hernia, without obstruction or gangrene, recurrent**

● **K40.3**   **Unilateral inguinal hernia, with obstruction, without gangrene**
         Inguinal hernia (unilateral) causing obstruction without gangrene
         Incarcerated inguinal hernia (unilateral) without gangrene
         Irreducible inguinal hernia (unilateral) without gangrene
         Strangulated inguinal hernia (unilateral) without gangrene

     K40.30   **Unilateral inguinal hernia, with obstruction, without gangrene, not specified as recurrent** 🔾
         Inguinal hernia, with obstruction NOS
         Unilateral inguinal hernia, with obstruction, without gangrene NOS

     K40.31   **Unilateral inguinal hernia, with obstruction, without gangrene, recurrent** 🔾

● **K40.4**   **Unilateral inguinal hernia, with gangrene**

     K40.40   **Unilateral inguinal hernia, with gangrene, not specified as recurrent** 🔾
         Inguinal hernia with gangrene NOS
         Unilateral inguinal hernia with gangrene NOS

     K40.41   **Unilateral inguinal hernia, with gangrene, recurrent** 🔾

● **K40.9**   **Unilateral inguinal hernia, without obstruction or gangrene**

     K40.90   **Unilateral inguinal hernia, without obstruction or gangrene, not specified as recurrent**
         Inguinal hernia NOS
         Unilateral inguinal hernia NOS

     K40.91   **Unilateral inguinal hernia, without obstruction or gangrene, recurrent**

● **K41**   **Femoral hernia**

● **K41.0**   **Bilateral femoral hernia, with obstruction, without gangrene**
         Femoral hernia (bilateral) causing obstruction, without gangrene
         Incarcerated femoral hernia (bilateral), without gangrene
         Irreducible femoral hernia (bilateral), without gangrene
         Strangulated femoral hernia (bilateral), without gangrene

     (Ex) **For category K41.0 CC codes:** K31.89-K31.9, K41.00-K41.91, K45.0, K45.8-K46.0, K92.81

     K41.00   **Bilateral femoral hernia, with obstruction, without gangrene, not specified as recurrent** 🔾
         Bilateral femoral hernia, with obstruction, without gangrene NOS

     K41.01   **Bilateral femoral hernia, with obstruction, without gangrene, recurrent** 🔾

Item 11-11   **Hernias** of the groin are the most common type, accounting for 80 percent of all hernias. There are two major types of inguinal hernias: indirect (oblique) affecting men only and direct. **Indirect inguinal hernias** result when the intestines emerge through the abdominal wall in an indirect fashion through the inguinal canal. **Direct inguinal hernias** penetrate through the abdominal wall in a direct fashion. **Femoral hernias** occur at the femoral ring where the femoral vessels enter the thigh and is most common in women. An abdominal wall hernia is also called a ventral or epigastric hernia and occurs in both sexes. Classification is based on location of the hernia and whether there is obstruction or gangrene.

Ventral, epigastric, or incisional hernia occurs on the abdominal surface caused by musculature weakness or a tear at a previous surgical site and is evidenced by a bulge that changes in size, becoming larger with exertion. An **incarcerated** hernia is one in which the intestines become trapped in the hernia. A **strangulated** hernia is one in which the blood supply to the intestines is lost. Hiatal hernia occurs when a loop of the stomach protrudes upward through the small opening in the diaphragm through which the esophagus passes, leaving the abdominal cavity and entering the chest. It occurs in both sexes.

N Newborn Age: 0   **P** Pediatric Age: 0–17   **M** Maternity DX: 12–55   **A** Adult Age: 15–124   ♀ Females Only   ♂ Males Only

🔾 Complication\Comorbidity   🔾 Major C\C   (Ex) CC/MCC Exclusions   🔾 Hospital-Acquired Condition

945

● **K41.1   Bilateral femoral hernia, with gangrene**
(Ex:) For category K41.1 CC codes: K31.89-K31.9, K41.10-K41.21, K41.40-K41.91, K45.0, K45.8-K46.0, K92.81

    K41.10   Bilateral femoral hernia, with gangrene, not specified as recurrent 🔗
        Bilateral femoral hernia, with gangrene NOS

    K41.11   Bilateral femoral hernia, with gangrene, recurrent 🔗

● **K41.2   Bilateral femoral hernia, without obstruction or gangrene**

    K41.20   Bilateral femoral hernia, without obstruction or gangrene, not specified as recurrent
        Bilateral femoral hernia NOS

    K41.21   Bilateral femoral hernia, without obstruction or gangrene, recurrent

● **K41.3   Unilateral femoral hernia, with obstruction, without gangrene**
    Femoral hernia (unilateral) causing obstruction, without gangrene
    Incarcerated femoral hernia (unilateral), without gangrene
    Irreducible femoral hernia (unilateral), without gangrene
    Strangulated femoral hernia (unilateral), without gangrene
    (Ex:) For category K41.3 CC codes: See K41.0

    K41.30   Unilateral femoral hernia, with obstruction, without gangrene, not specified as recurrent 🔗
        Femoral hernia, with obstruction NOS
        Unilateral femoral hernia, with obstruction NOS

    K41.31   Unilateral femoral hernia, with obstruction, without gangrene, recurrent 🔗

● **K41.4   Unilateral femoral hernia, with gangrene**
    (Ex:) For category K41.4 CC codes: K41.1

    K41.40   Unilateral femoral hernia, with gangrene, not specified as recurrent 🔗
        Femoral hernia, with gangrene NOS
        Unilateral femoral hernia, with gangrene NOS

    K41.41   Unilateral femoral hernia, with gangrene, recurrent 🔗

● **K41.9   Unilateral femoral hernia, without obstruction or gangrene**

    K41.90   Unilateral femoral hernia, without obstruction or gangrene, not specified as recurrent
        Femoral hernia NOS
        Unilateral femoral hernia NOS

    K41.91   Unilateral femoral hernia, without obstruction or gangrene, recurrent

● **K42   Umbilical hernia**
    Includes   paraumbilical hernia
    Excludes1 omphalocele (Q79.2)

    K42.0   Umbilical hernia with obstruction, without gangrene 🔗
        Umbilical hernia causing obstruction, without gangrene
        Incarcerated umbilical hernia, without gangrene
        Irreducible umbilical hernia, without gangrene
        Strangulated umbilical hernia, without gangrene
        (Ex:) K42.0-K42.1, K43.0-K43.1, K43.3-K43.4, K43.6-K43.7, K45.0, K45.8-K46.0

    K42.1   Umbilical hernia with gangrene 🔗
        Gangrenous umbilical hernia
        (Ex:) K31.89-K31.9, K42.0-K43.9, K45.0, K45.8-K46.0, K46.9, K92.81

    K42.9   Umbilical hernia without obstruction or gangrene
        Umbilical hernia NOS

● **K43   Ventral hernia**

    K43.0   Incisional hernia with obstruction, without gangrene 🔗
        Incisional hernia causing obstruction, without gangrene
        Incarcerated incisional hernia, without gangrene
        Irreducible incisional hernia, without gangrene
        Strangulated incisional hernia, without gangrene
        (Ex:) See K42.0

    K43.1   Incisional hernia with gangrene 🔗
        Gangrenous incisional hernia
        (Ex:) See K42.1

    K43.2   Incisional hernia without obstruction or gangrene
        Incisional hernia NOS

    K43.3   Parastomal hernia with obstruction, without gangrene 🔗
        Incarcerated parastomal hernia, without gangrene
        Irreducible parastomal hernia, without gangrene
        Parastomal hernia causing obstruction, without gangrene
        Strangulated parastomal hernia, without gangrene
        (Ex:) See K42.0

    K43.4   Parastomal hernia with gangrene 🔗
        Gangrenous parastomal hernia
        (Ex:) See K42.1

    K43.5   Parastomal hernia without obstruction or gangrene
        Parastomal hernia NOS

    K43.6   Other and `unspecified` ventral hernia with obstruction, without gangrene 🔗
        Epigastric hernia causing obstruction, without gangrene
        Hypogastric hernia causing obstruction, without gangrene
        Incarcerated epigastric hernia without gangrene
        Incarcerated hypogastric hernia without gangrene
        Incarcerated midline hernia without gangrene
        Incarcerated spigelian hernia without gangrene
        Incarcerated subxiphoid hernia without gangrene
        Irreducible epigastric hernia without gangrene
        Irreducible hypogastric hernia without gangrene
        Irreducible midline hernia without gangrene
        Irreducible spigelian hernia without gangrene
        Irreducible subxiphoid hernia without gangrene
        Midline hernia causing obstruction, without gangrene
        Spigelian hernia causing obstruction, without gangrene
        Strangulated epigastric hernia without gangrene
        Strangulated hypogastric hernia without gangrene
        Strangulated midline hernia without gangrene
        Strangulated spigelian hernia without gangrene
        Strangulated subxiphoid hernia without gangrene
        Subxiphoid hernia causing obstruction, without gangrene
        (Ex:) See K42.0

    K43.7   Other and `unspecified` ventral hernia with gangrene 🔗
        Any condition listed under K43.6 specified as gangrenous
        (Ex:) See K42.1

    K43.9   Ventral hernia without obstruction or gangrene
        Epigastric hernia
        Ventral hernia NOS

● **K44   Diaphragmatic hernia**
    Includes   hiatus hernia (esophageal) (sliding)
               paraesophageal hernia
    Excludes1 congenital diaphragmatic hernia (Q79.0)
              congenital hiatus hernia (Q40.1)
    (Ex:) For category K44 CC codes: K44.0-K46.0

    K44.0   Diaphragmatic hernia with obstruction, without gangrene 🔗
        Diaphragmatic hernia causing obstruction
        Incarcerated diaphragmatic hernia
        Irreducible diaphragmatic hernia
        Strangulated diaphragmatic hernia

    K44.1   Diaphragmatic hernia with gangrene 🔗
        Gangrenous diaphragmatic hernia

    K44.9   Diaphragmatic hernia without obstruction or gangrene
        Diaphragmatic hernia NOS

◄ New   ◄▥▥ Revised   ~~deleted~~ Deleted | Excludes 1 | | Excludes 2 | | Includes | Use additional | Code first | Code also | Unspecified |

OGCR Official Guidelines   ● Unacceptable Principal Diagnosis   X Assign placeholder X   ● Use Additional Character(s)   ▶ Manifestation Code   **Coding Clinic**

● K45   **Other abdominal hernia**
     Includes   abdominal hernia, specified site NEC
                  lumbar hernia
                  obturator hernia
                  pudendal hernia
                  retroperitoneal hernia
                  sciatic hernia

   K45.0   **Other specified abdominal hernia with obstruction, without gangrene** 🔖
          Other specified abdominal hernia causing obstruction
          Other specified incarcerated abdominal hernia
          Other specified irreducible abdominal hernia
          Other specified strangulated abdominal hernia
          (Ex) K40.00-K46.9

   K45.1   **Other specified abdominal hernia with gangrene** 🔖
          Any condition listed under K45 specified as gangrenous
          (Ex) K31.89-K31.9, K40.00-K46.9, K92.81

   K45.8   **Other specified abdominal hernia without obstruction or gangrene**

● K46   **Unspecified abdominal hernia**
     Includes   enterocele
                  epiplocele
                  hernia NOS
                  interstitial hernia
                  intestinal hernia
                  intra-abdominal hernia
     Excludes1   vaginal enterocele (N81.5)

   K46.0   **Unspecified abdominal hernia with obstruction, without gangrene** 🔖
          Unspecified abdominal hernia causing obstruction
          Unspecified incarcerated abdominal hernia
          Unspecified irreducible abdominal hernia
          Unspecified strangulated abdominal hernia
          (Ex) K40.00-K46.9

   K46.1   **Unspecified abdominal hernia with gangrene** 🔖
          Any condition listed under K46 specified as gangrenous
          (Ex) K31.89-K31.9, K40.00-K46.9, K92.81

   K46.9   **Unspecified abdominal hernia without obstruction or gangrene**
          Abdominal hernia NOS

★ **(See Plate 284 on page 77.)**

NONINFECTIVE ENTERITIS AND COLITIS (K50-K52)

     Includes   noninfective inflammatory bowel disease
     Excludes1   irritable bowel syndrome (K58.-)
                  megacolon (K59.3-) ◀

● K50   **Crohn's disease [regional enteritis]**
     Includes   granulomatous enteritis
     Use additional code to identify manifestations, such as:
     pyoderma gangrenosum (L88)
     Excludes1   ulcerative colitis (K51.-)
     (Ex) For category K50 CC codes unless otherwise indicated: K50.00-K51.919

   ● **K50.0**   **Crohn's disease of small intestine**
          Crohn's disease [regional enteritis] of duodenum
          Crohn's disease [regional enteritis] of ileum
          Crohn's disease [regional enteritis] of jejunum
          Regional ileitis
          Terminal ileitis
       Excludes1   Crohn's disease of both small and large intestine (K50.8-)

     K50.00   **Crohn's disease of small intestine without complications** 🔖

● K50.01   **Crohn's disease of small intestine with complications**

     K50.011   **Crohn's disease of small intestine with rectal bleeding** 🔖

     K50.012   **Crohn's disease of small intestine with intestinal obstruction** 🔖
             CC when PDx is its own CC

     K50.013   **Crohn's disease of small intestine with fistula** 🔖
             CC when PDx is its own CC

     K50.014   **Crohn's disease of small intestine with abscess** 🔖
             CC when PDx is its own CC
             Coding Clinic: 2012, Q4, P104

     K50.018   **Crohn's disease of small intestine with other complication** 🔖

     K50.019   **Crohn's disease of small intestine with unspecified complications** 🔖

● K50.1   **Crohn's disease of large intestine**
     Crohn's disease [regional enteritis] of colon
     Crohn's disease [regional enteritis] of large bowel
     Crohn's disease [regional enteritis] of rectum
     Granulomatous colitis
     Regional colitis
     Excludes1   Crohn's disease of both small and large intestine (K50.8)

     K50.10   **Crohn's disease of large intestine without complications** 🔖

   ● **K50.11**   **Crohn's disease of large intestine with complications**

     K50.111   **Crohn's disease of large intestine with rectal bleeding** 🔖

     K50.112   **Crohn's disease of large intestine with intestinal obstruction** 🔖
             CC when PDx is its own CC

     K50.113   **Crohn's disease of large intestine with fistula** 🔖
             CC when PDx is its own CC

     K50.114   **Crohn's disease of large intestine with abscess** 🔖
             CC when PDx is its own CC
             Coding Clinic: 2012, Q4, P104

     K50.118   **Crohn's disease of large intestine with other complication** 🔖

     K50.119   **Crohn's disease of large intestine with unspecified complications** 🔖

● K50.8   **Crohn's disease of both small and large intestine**

     K50.80   **Crohn's disease of both small and large intestine without complications** 🔖

   ● **K50.81**   **Crohn's disease of both small and large intestine with complications**

     K50.811   **Crohn's disease of both small and large intestine with rectal bleeding** 🔖

     K50.812   **Crohn's disease of both small and large intestine with intestinal obstruction** 🔖
             CC when PDx is its own CC

     K50.813   **Crohn's disease of both small and large intestine with fistula** 🔖
             CC when PDx is its own CC

     K50.814   **Crohn's disease of both small and large intestine with abscess** 🔖
             CC when PDx is its own CC
             Coding Clinic: 2012, Q4, P104

     K50.818   **Crohn's disease of both small and large intestine with other complication** 🔖

     K50.819   **Crohn's disease of both small and large intestine with unspecified complications** 🔖

Item 11-12 Crohn's disease, also known as **regional enteritis,** is a chronic inflammatory disease of the intestines. Classification is based on location in the small (duodenum, ileum, jejunum) or large (cecum, colon, rectum, anal canal) intestine.

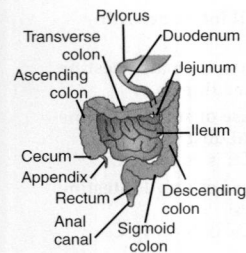

Figure 11-10 Small and large intestines.

CHAPTER 11 (K00-K95)

● **K50.9   Crohn's disease, unspecified**
     Ⓔ **For category K50.9 CC codes:** K50.00-K50.919
     K50.90   Crohn's disease, unspecified, without complications 🔖
         Crohn's disease NOS
         Regional enteritis NOS
●   **K50.91   Crohn's disease, unspecified, with complications**
     K50.911   Crohn's disease, unspecified, with rectal bleeding 🔖
     K50.912   Crohn's disease, unspecified, with intestinal obstruction 🔖
         CC when PDx is its own CC
     K50.913   Crohn's disease, unspecified, with fistula 🔖
         CC when PDx is its own CC
     K50.914   Crohn's disease, unspecified, with abscess 🔖
         CC when PDx is its own CC
         Coding Clinic: 2012, Q4, P104
     K50.918   Crohn's disease, unspecified, with other complication 🔖
     K50.919   Crohn's disease, unspecified, with unspecified complications 🔖

● **K51   Ulcerative colitis**
     Use additional code to identify manifestations, such as:
     pyoderma gangrenosum (L88)
     Excludes1   Crohn's disease [regional enteritis] (K50.-)
     Ⓔ **For category K51 CC codes unless otherwise indicated:** K50.00-K51.919
●   **K51.0   Ulcerative (chronic) pancolitis**
     Backwash ileitis
     K51.00   Ulcerative (chronic) pancolitis without complications 🔖
         Ulcerative (chronic) pancolitis NOS
●   **K51.01   Ulcerative (chronic) pancolitis with complications**
     K51.011   Ulcerative (chronic) pancolitis with rectal bleeding 🔖
     K51.012   Ulcerative (chronic) pancolitis with intestinal obstruction 🔖
         CC when PDx is its own CC
     K51.013   Ulcerative (chronic) pancolitis with fistula 🔖
         CC when PDx is its own CC
     K51.014   Ulcerative (chronic) pancolitis with abscess 🔖
         CC when PDx is its own CC
     K51.018   Ulcerative (chronic) pancolitis with other complication 🔖
     K51.019   Ulcerative (chronic) pancolitis with unspecified complications 🔖

● **K51.2   Ulcerative (chronic) proctitis**
     K51.20   Ulcerative (chronic) proctitis without complications 🔖
         Ulcerative (chronic) proctitis NOS
●   **K51.21   Ulcerative (chronic) proctitis with complications**
     K51.211   Ulcerative (chronic) proctitis with rectal bleeding 🔖
     K51.212   Ulcerative (chronic) proctitis with intestinal obstruction 🔖
         CC when PDx is its own CC
     K51.213   Ulcerative (chronic) proctitis with fistula 🔖
         CC when PDx is its own CC
     K51.214   Ulcerative (chronic) proctitis with abscess 🔖
         CC when PDx is its own CC
     K51.218   Ulcerative (chronic) proctitis with other complication 🔖
     K51.219   Ulcerative (chronic) proctitis with unspecified complications 🔖

● **K51.3   Ulcerative (chronic) rectosigmoiditis**
     K51.30   Ulcerative (chronic) rectosigmoiditis without complications 🔖
         Ulcerative (chronic) rectosigmoiditis NOS
●   **K51.31   Ulcerative (chronic) rectosigmoiditis with complications**
     K51.311   Ulcerative (chronic) rectosigmoiditis with rectal bleeding 🔖
     K51.312   Ulcerative (chronic) rectosigmoiditis with intestinal obstruction 🔖
         CC when PDx is its own CC
     K51.313   Ulcerative (chronic) rectosigmoiditis with fistula 🔖
         CC when PDx is its own CC
     K51.314   Ulcerative (chronic) rectosigmoiditis with abscess 🔖
         CC when PDx is its own CC
     K51.318   Ulcerative (chronic) rectosigmoiditis with other complication 🔖
     K51.319   Ulcerative (chronic) rectosigmoiditis with unspecified complications 🔖

● **K51.4   Inflammatory polyps of colon**
     Excludes1   adenomatous polyp of colon (D12.6)
         polyposis of colon (D12.6)
         polyps of colon NOS (K63.5)
     K51.40   Inflammatory polyps of colon without complications 🔖
         Inflammatory polyps of colon NOS
●   **K51.41   Inflammatory polyps of colon with complications**
     K51.411   Inflammatory polyps of colon with rectal bleeding 🔖
     K51.412   Inflammatory polyps of colon with intestinal obstruction 🔖
         CC when PDx is its own CC
     K51.413   Inflammatory polyps of colon with fistula 🔖
         CC when PDx is its own CC
     K51.414   Inflammatory polyps of colon with abscess 🔖
         CC when PDx is its own CC
     K51.418   Inflammatory polyps of colon with other complication 🔖
     K51.419   Inflammatory polyps of colon with unspecified complications 🔖

Item 11-13   Ulcerative colitis attacks the colonic mucosa and forms abscesses. The disease involves the intestines. Classification is based on the location:
- Enterocolitis: large and small intestine
- Ileocolitis: ileum and colon
- Proctitis: rectum
- Proctosigmoiditis: sigmoid colon and rectum

◀ New   ◀▦ Revised   ~~deleted~~ Deleted   Excludes 1   Excludes 2   Includes   Use additional   Code first   Code also   Unspecified

948
   OGCR Official Guidelines   ● Unacceptable Principal Diagnosis   X Assign placeholder X   ● Use Additional Character(s)   🔖 Manifestation Code   **Coding Clinic**

● **K51.5** **Left sided colitis**
Left hemicolitis
   K51.5Ø   **Left sided colitis without complications** 🝡
      Left sided colitis NOS
  ● **K51.51**   **Left sided colitis with complications**
      K51.511 **Left sided colitis with rectal bleeding** 🝡
      K51.512 **Left sided colitis with intestinal obstruction** 🝡
          CC when PDx is its own CC
      K51.513 **Left sided colitis with fistula** 🝡
          CC when PDx is its own CC
      K51.514 **Left sided colitis with abscess** 🝡
          CC when PDx is its own CC
      K51.518 **Left sided colitis with other complication** 🝡
      K51.519 **Left sided colitis with unspecified complications** 🝡

● **K51.8** **Other ulcerative colitis**
   K51.8Ø   **Other ulcerative colitis without complications** 🝡
  ● **K51.81**   **Other ulcerative colitis with complications**
      K51.811 **Other ulcerative colitis with rectal bleeding** 🝡
      K51.812 **Other ulcerative colitis with intestinal obstruction** 🝡
          CC when PDx is its own CC
      K51.813 **Other ulcerative colitis with fistula** 🝡
          CC when PDx is its own CC
      K51.814 **Other ulcerative colitis with abscess** 🝡
          CC when PDx is its own CC
      K51.818 **Other ulcerative colitis with other complication** 🝡
      K51.819 **Other ulcerative colitis with unspecified complications** 🝡

● **K51.9** **Ulcerative colitis, unspecified**
   (Ex:) For category K51.9 CC codes: K51.ØØ-K51.919
   K51.9Ø   **Ulcerative colitis, unspecified, without complications** 🝡
  ● **K51.91**   **Ulcerative colitis, unspecified, with complications**
      K51.911 **Ulcerative colitis, unspecified with rectal bleeding** 🝡
      K51.912 **Ulcerative colitis, unspecified with intestinal obstruction** 🝡
          CC when PDx is its own CC
      K51.913 **Ulcerative colitis, unspecified with fistula** 🝡
          CC when PDx is its own CC
      K51.914 **Ulcerative colitis, unspecified with abscess** 🝡
          CC when PDx is its own CC
      K51.918 **Ulcerative colitis, unspecified with other complication** 🝡
      K51.919 **Ulcerative colitis, unspecified with unspecified complications** 🝡

● **K52** **Other and unspecified noninfective gastroenteritis and colitis**
   K52.Ø   **Gastroenteritis and colitis due to radiation** 🝡
      (Ex:) K52.Ø
   K52.1   **Toxic gastroenteritis and colitis** 🝡
      Drug-induced gastroenteritis and colitis
      Code first (T51-T65) to identify toxic agent
      Use additional code for adverse effect, if applicable, to identify drug (T36-T5Ø with fifth or sixth character 5)
      (Ex:) K52.1

● **K52.2** **Allergic and dietetic gastroenteritis and colitis**
      Food hypersensitivity gastroenteritis or colitis
      Use additional code to identify type of food allergy (Z91.Ø1-, Z91.Ø2-)
      Excludes2 allergic eosinophilic colitis (K52.82) ◄
          allergic eosinophilic esophagitis (K2Ø.Ø) ◄
          allergic eosinophilic gastritis (K52.81) ◄
          allergic eosinophilic gastroenteritis (K52.81) ◄
          food protein-induced proctocolitis (K52.82) ◄
      K52.21 **Food protein-induced enterocolitis syndrome** ◄
          Use additional code for hypovolemic shock, if present (R57.1) ◄
      K52.22 **Food protein-induced enteropathy** ◄
      K52.29 **Other allergic and dietetic gastroenteritis and colitis**
          Food hypersensitivity gastroenteritis or colitis ◄
          Immediate gastrointestinal hypersensitivity ◄
   K52.3   **Indeterminate colitis** ◄
      Colonic inflammatory bowel disease unclassified (IBDU) ◄
      Excludes1 unspecified colitis (K52.9) ◄
● **K52.8** **Other specified noninfective gastroenteritis and colitis**
      K52.81 **Eosinophilic gastritis or gastroenteritis**
          Eosinophilic enteritis
          Excludes2 eosinophilic esophagitis (K2Ø.Ø) ◄
      K52.82 **Eosinophilic colitis**
          Allergic proctocolitis ◄
          Food-induced eosinophilic proctocolitis ◄
          Food protein-induced proctocolitis ◄
          Milk protein-induced proctocolitis ◄
  ● **K52.83** **Microscopic colitis** ◄
      K52.831 **Collagenous colitis** ◄
      K52.832 **Lymphocytic colitis** ◄
      K52.838 **Other microscopic colitis** ◄
      K52.839 **Microscopic colitis, unspecified** ◄
      K52.89 **Other specified noninfective gastroenteritis and colitis**
   K52.9   **Noninfective gastroenteritis and colitis, unspecified**
      Colitis NOS   Ileitis NOS
      Enteritis NOS   Jejunitis NOS
      Gastroenteritis NOS   Sigmoiditis NOS
      Excludes1 diarrhea NOS (R19.7)
          functional diarrhea (K59.1)
          infectious gastroenteritis and colitis NOS (AØ9)
          neonatal diarrhea (noninfective) (P78.3)
          psychogenic diarrhea (F45.8)

OTHER DISEASES OF INTESTINES (K55-K64)

● **K55** **Vascular disorders of intestine**
   Excludes1 necrotizing enterocolitis of newborn (P77.-)
   (Ex:) For category K55 CC codes unless otherwise indicated: K55.Ø21-K55.1, K55.3Ø-K55.33
● **K55.Ø** **Acute vascular disorders of intestine**
      Infarction of appendices epiploicae
      Mesenteric (artery) (vein) embolism
      Mesenteric (artery) (vein) infarction
      Mesenteric (artery) (vein) thrombosis
  ● **K55.Ø1** **Acute (reversible) ischemia of small intestine** ◄
      K55.Ø11 **Focal (segmental) acute (reversible) ischemia of small intestine** 🝡 ◄
      K55.Ø12 **Diffuse acute (reversible) ischemia of small intestine** 🝡 ◄
      K55.Ø19 **Acute (reversible) ischemia of small intestine, extent unspecified** 🝡 ◄

N Newborn Age: Ø   **P** Pediatric Age: Ø–17   **M** Maternity DX: 12–55   **A** Adult Age: 15–124   ♀ Females Only   ♂ Males Only

🝡 Complication\Comorbidity   🝡 Major C\C   (Ex:) CC/MCC Exclusions   🝡 Hospital-Acquired Condition

949

CHAPTER 11 (K00-K95)

● **K55.02**   **Acute infarction of small intestine** ◀
    Gangrene of small intestine ◀
    Necrosis of small intestine ◀

    K55.021   **Focal (segmental) acute infarction of small intestine** 🐾 ◀

    K55.022   **Diffuse acute infarction of small intestine** 🐾 ◀

    K55.029   **Acute infarction of small intestine, extent** unspecified 🐾 ◀

● **K55.03**   **Acute (reversible) ischemia of large intestine** ◀
    Acute fulminant ischemic colitis ◀
    Subacute ischemic colitis ◀

    K55.031   **Focal (segmental) acute (reversible) ischemia of large intestine** 🐾 ◀

    K55.032   **Diffuse acute (reversible) ischemia of large intestine** 🐾 ◀

    K55.039   **Acute (reversible) ischemia of large intestine, extent** unspecified 🐾 ◀

● **K55.04**   **Acute infarction of large intestine** ◀
    Gangrene of large intestine ◀
    Necrosis of large intestine ◀

    K55.041   **Focal (segmental) acute infarction of large intestine** 🐾 ◀

    K55.042   **Diffuse acute infarction of large intestine** 🐾 ◀

    K55.049   **Acute infarction of large intestine, extent** unspecified 🐾 ◀

● **K55.05**   **Acute (reversible) ischemia of intestine, part** unspecified ◀

    K55.051   **Focal (segmental) acute (reversible) ischemia of intestine, part** unspecified 🐾 ◀

    K55.052   **Diffuse acute (reversible) ischemia of intestine, part** unspecified 🐾 ◀

    K55.059   **Acute (reversible) ischemia of intestine, part and extent** unspecified 🐾 ◀

● **K55.06**   **Acute infarction of intestine, part unspecified** ◀
    Acute intestinal infarction ◀
    Gangrene of intestine ◀
    Necrosis of intestine ◀

    K55.061   **Focal (segmental) acute infarction of intestine, part** unspecified 🐾 ◀

    K55.062   **Diffuse acute infarction of intestine, part** unspecified 🐾 ◀

    K55.069   **Acute infarction of intestine, part and extent** unspecified 🐾 ◀

K55.1   **Chronic vascular disorders of intestine** 🐾
    Chronic ischemic colitis
    Chronic ischemic enteritis
    Chronic ischemic enterocolitis
    Ischemic stricture of intestine
    Mesenteric atherosclerosis
    Mesenteric vascular insufficiency
    (Ex:) K55.012-K55.069, K55.1, K55.30-K55.33, K55.8-K55.9

● **K55.2**   **Angiodysplasia of colon**

    K55.20   **Angiodysplasia of colon without hemorrhage**

    K55.21   **Angiodysplasia of colon with hemorrhage** 🐾
      (Ex:) E16.4, I85.01, K22.10-K22.11, K22.6-K22.719, K25.0-K28.9, K29.01, K29.21, K29.31, K29.41, K29.51, K29.61, K29.71, K29.81, K29.91, K31.811, K55.21, K57.01, K57.11, K57.13, K57.21, K57.31, K57.33, K57.41, K57.51, K57.53, K57.81, K57.91, K57.93, K62.5, K92.0-K92.2

● **K55.3**   **Necrotizing enterocolitis** ◀

    Excludes1   necrotizing enterocolitis of newborn (P77.-) ◀

    Excludes2   necrotizing enterocolitis due to Clostridium difficile (A04.7) ◀

    K55.30   **Necrotizing enterocolitis,** unspecified 🐾 ◀
      Necrotizing enterocolitis, NOS ◀

    K55.31   **Stage 1 necrotizing enterocolitis** 🐾 ◀
      Necrotizing enterocolitis without pneumatosis, without perforation ◀

    K55.32   **Stage 2 necrotizing enterocolitis** 🐾 ◀
      Necrotizing enterocolitis with pneumatosis, without perforation ◀

    K55.33   **Stage 3 necrotizing enterocolitis** 🐾 ◀
      Necrotizing enterocolitis with perforation ◀
      Necrotizing enterocolitis with pneumatosis and perforation ◀

K55.8   **Other vascular disorders of intestine** 🐾
    (Ex:) See K55.1

K55.9   **Vascular disorder of intestine,** unspecified 🐾
    Ischemic colitis
    Ischemic enteritis
    Ischemic enterocolitis
    (Ex:) See K55.1

● **K56**   **Paralytic ileus and intestinal obstruction without hernia**

    Excludes1   congenital stricture or stenosis of intestine (Q41-Q42)
      cystic fibrosis with meconium ileus (E84.11)
      ischemic stricture of intestine (K55.1)
      meconium ileus NOS (P76.0)
      neonatal intestinal obstructions classifiable to P76.-
      obstruction of duodenum (K31.5)
      postprocedural intestinal obstruction (K91.3)
      stenosis of anus or rectum (K62.4)
      intestinal obstruction with hernia (K40-K46)

    (Ex:) **For category K56 CC codes:** K56.0-K56.3, K56.49-K56.7, K63.4, K63.89-K63.9, K92.89-K92.9, R11.13

    K56.0   **Paralytic ileus** 🐾
      Paralysis of bowel
      Paralysis of colon
      Paralysis of intestine

      Excludes1   gallstone ileus (K56.3)
        ileus NOS (K56.7)
        obstructive ileus NOS (K56.69)

    K56.1   **Intussusception** 🐾
      Intussusception or invagination of bowel
      Intussusception or invagination of colon
      Intussusception or invagination of intestine
      Intussusception or invagination of rectum

      Excludes2   intussusception of appendix (K38.8)

SIMPLE TYPES   DOUBLE TYPES

Cecum and appendix

Ileum
Ileocecal valve

Ileum   Ileocecal valve

ILEOCOLIC

ILEOCECAL

Figure 11-11   Types of intussusception.

Item 11-14   **Intussusception** is the prolapse (telescoping) of a part of the intestine into another adjacent part of the intestine. Intussusception may be enteric (ileoileal, jejunoileal, jejunojejunal), colic (colocolic), or intracolic (ileocecal, ileocolic).

◀ New   ◀ Revised   ~~deleted~~ Deleted   Excludes 1   Excludes 2   Includes   Use additional   Code first   Code also   Unspecified

OGCR Official Guidelines   ● Unacceptable Principal Diagnosis   X Assign placeholder X   ● Use Additional Character(s)   ◀ Manifestation Code   **Coding Clinic**

Item 11–15   **Volvulus** is the twisting of a segment of the intestine, resulting in obstruction. Paralytic ileus is paralysis of the intestine. It need not be a complete paralysis, but it must prohibit the passage of food through the intestine and lead to intestinal blockage. It is a common aftermath of some types of surgery.

K56.2   **Volvulus**
     Strangulation of colon or intestine
     Torsion of colon or intestine
     Twist of colon or intestine
     Excludes2   volvulus of duodenum (K31.5)

K56.3   **Gallstone ileus**
     Obstruction of intestine by gallstone

●**K56.4**   **Other impaction of intestine**
     K56.41   **Fecal impaction**
        Excludes1   constipation (K59.0-)
                  incomplete defecation (R15.0)
     K56.49   **Other impaction of intestine**

K56.5   **Intestinal adhesions [bands] with obstruction (postprocedural) (postinfection)**
     Abdominal hernia due to adhesions with obstruction
     Peritoneal adhesions [bands] with intestinal obstruction (postprocedural) (postinfection)

●**K56.6**   **Other and unspecified intestinal obstruction**
     K56.60   **Unspecified intestinal obstruction Intestinal obstruction NOS**
        Excludes1   intestinal obstruction due to specified condition-code to condition
     K56.69   **Other intestinal obstruction**
        Enterostenosis NOS
        Obstructive ileus NOS
        Occlusion of colon or intestine NOS
        Stenosis of colon or intestine NOS
        Stricture of colon or intestine NOS
        Excludes1   intestinal obstruction due to specified condition-code to condition

K56.7   **Ileus, unspecified**
     Excludes1   obstructive ileus (K56.69)

●**K57**   **Diverticular disease of intestine**
     Excludes1   congenital diverticulum of intestine (Q43.8)
                 Meckel's diverticulum (Q43.0)
     Excludes2   diverticulum of appendix (K38.2)
     (Ex:) **For category K57 CC codes unless otherwise indicated:** E16.4, I85.01, K22.10-K22.11, K22.6-K22.719, K25.0-K28.9, K29.01, K29.21, K29.31, K29.41, K29.51, K29.61, K29.71, K29.81, K29.91, K31.811, K55.21, K57.01, K57.11, K57.13, K57.21, K57.31, K57.33, K57.41, K57.51, K57.53, K57.81, K57.91, K57.93, K62.5, K92.0-K92.2

●**K57.0**   **Diverticulitis of small intestine with perforation and abscess**
     Diverticulitis of small intestine with peritonitis
     Excludes1   diverticulitis of both small and large intestine with perforation and abscess (K57.4-)
     K57.00   **Diverticulitis of small intestine with perforation and abscess without bleeding**
        CC when PDx is its own CC
        (Ex:) K57.00-K57.13
     K57.01   **Diverticulitis of small intestine with perforation and abscess with bleeding**
        CC when PDx is its own CC

●**K57.1**   **Diverticular disease of small intestine without perforation or abscess**
     Excludes1   diverticular disease of both small and large intestine without perforation or abscess (K57.5-)
     K57.10   **Diverticulosis of small intestine without perforation or abscess without bleeding**
        Diverticular disease of small intestine NOS
     K57.11   **Diverticulosis of small intestine without perforation or abscess with bleeding**

K57.12   **Diverticulitis of small intestine without perforation or abscess without bleeding**
     (Ex:) K57.00-K57.13

K57.13   **Diverticulitis of small intestine without perforation or abscess with bleeding**

●**K57.2**   **Diverticulitis of large intestine with perforation and abscess**
     Diverticulitis of colon with peritonitis
     Excludes1   diverticulitis of both small and large intestine with perforation and abscess (K57.4-)
     K57.20   **Diverticulitis of large intestine with perforation and abscess without bleeding**
        CC when PDx is its own CC
        (Ex:) K57.20-K57.93
     K57.21   **Diverticulitis of large intestine with perforation and abscess with bleeding**
        CC when PDx is its own CC

●**K57.3**   **Diverticular disease of large intestine without perforation or abscess**
     Excludes1   diverticular disease of both small and large intestine without perforation or abscess (K57.5-)
     K57.30   **Diverticulosis of large intestine without perforation or abscess without bleeding**
        Diverticular disease of colon NOS
     K57.31   **Diverticulosis of large intestine without perforation or abscess with bleeding**
     K57.32   **Diverticulitis of large intestine without perforation or abscess without bleeding**
        (Ex:) K57.20-K57.93
     K57.33   **Diverticulitis of large intestine without perforation or abscess with bleeding**

●**K57.4**   **Diverticulitis of both small and large intestine with perforation and abscess**
     Diverticulitis of both small and large intestine with peritonitis
     K57.40   **Diverticulitis of both small and large intestine with perforation and abscess without bleeding**
        CC when PDx is its own CC
        (Ex:) K57.20-K57.93
     K57.41   **Diverticulitis of both small and large intestine with perforation and abscess with bleeding**
        CC when PDx is its own CC

Figure 11-12   Diverticulosis. (From Shiland: Mastering Healthcare Terminology, ed 4, St. Louis, Mosby, 2012)

Item 11–16   **Diverticula** of the intestines are acquired herniations of the mucosa. Diverticulum (singular): Pocket or pouch that bulges outward through a weak spot (herniation) in the colon. Diverticula (plural). **Diverticulosis** is the condition of having diverticula. **Diverticulitis** is inflammation of these pouches or herniations. Classification is based on location (small intestine or colon) and whether it occurs with or without hemorrhage.

N Newborn Age: 0   **P** Pediatric Age: 0–17   **M** Maternity DX: 12–55   **A** Adult Age: 15–124   ♀ Females Only   ♂ Males Only

Complication\Comorbidity   Major C\C   (Ex:) CC/MCC Exclusions   Hospital-Acquired Condition

951

CHAPTER 11 (K00-K95)

● **K57.5**   **Diverticular disease of both small and large intestine without perforation or abscess**

    K57.50   **Diverticulosis of both small and large intestine without perforation or abscess without bleeding**
       Diverticular disease of both small and large intestine NOS

    K57.51   **Diverticulosis of both small and large intestine without perforation or abscess with bleeding** 🖉

    K57.52   **Diverticulitis of both small and large intestine without perforation or abscess without bleeding** 🖉
       CC when PDx is its own CC
       (Ex) K57.20-K57.93

    K57.53   **Diverticulitis of both small and large intestine without perforation or abscess with bleeding** 🖉

● **K57.8**   **Diverticulitis of intestine, part unspecified, with perforation and abscess**
    Diverticulitis of intestine NOS with peritonitis

    K57.80   **Diverticulitis of intestine, part unspecified, with perforation and abscess without bleeding** 🖉
       CC when PDx is its own CC
       (Ex) K57.20-K57.93

    K57.81   **Diverticulitis of intestine, part unspecified, with perforation and abscess with bleeding** 🖉 🖉
       CC when PDx is its own CC

● **K57.9**   **Diverticular disease of intestine, part unspecified, without perforation or abscess**

    K57.90   **Diverticulosis of intestine, part unspecified, without perforation or abscess without bleeding**
       Diverticular disease of intestine NOS

    K57.91   **Diverticulosis of intestine, part unspecified, without perforation or abscess with bleeding** 🖉

    K57.92   **Diverticulitis of intestine, part unspecified, without perforation or abscess without bleeding** 🖉
       (Ex) K57.20-K57.93

    K57.93   **Diverticulitis of intestine, part unspecified, without perforation or abscess with bleeding** 🖉

● **K58**   **Irritable bowel syndrome**

    Includes   irritable colon
       spastic colon

    K58.0   **Irritable bowel syndrome with diarrhea**

    K58.1   **Irritable bowel syndrome with constipation** ◀

    K58.2   **Mixed irritable bowel syndrome** ◀

    K58.8   **Other irritable bowel syndrome** ◀

    K58.9   **Irritable bowel syndrome without diarrhea**
       Irritable bowel syndrome NOS

● **K59**   **Other functional intestinal disorders**

    Excludes 1   change in bowel habit NOS (R19.4)
       intestinal malabsorption (K90.-)
       psychogenic intestinal disorders (F45.8)

    Excludes 2   functional disorders of stomach (K31.-)

● **K59.0**   **Constipation**
    Use additional code for adverse effect, if applicable, to identify drug (T36-T50 with fifth or sixth character 5) ◀

    Excludes 1   fecal impaction (K56.41)
       incomplete defecation (R15.0)

    K59.00   **Constipation, unspecified**

    K59.01   **Slow transit constipation**

    K59.02   **Outlet dysfunction constipation**

    K59.03   **Drug induced constipation** ◀
       Use additional code for adverse effect, if applicable, to identify drug (T36-T50 with fifth or sixth character 5) ◀

    K59.04   **Chronic idiopathic constipation** ◀
       Functional constipation ◀

    K59.09   **Other constipation**
       Chronic constipation ◀

    K59.1   **Functional diarrhea**

    Excludes 1   diarrhea NOS (R19.7)
       irritable bowel syndrome with diarrhea (K58.0)

    K59.2   **Neurogenic bowel, not elsewhere classified** 🖉
       (Ex) K58.0-K58.9, K59.1-K59.9, K91.0-K91.1

● **K59.3**   **Megacolon, not elsewhere classified**
    Dilatation of colon
    Code first, if applicable (T51-T65) to identify toxic agent ◀⫿

    Excludes 1   congenital megacolon (aganglionic) (Q43.1)
       megacolon (due to) (in) Chagas' disease (B57.32)
       megacolon (due to) (in) Clostridium difficile (A04.7)
       megacolon (due to) (in) Hirschsprung's disease (Q43.1)
    (Ex) For category K59.3 CC codes: See K59.2

    K59.31   **Toxic megacolon** 🖉 ◀

    K59.39   **Other megacolon** 🖉 ◀
       Megacolon NOS ◀

    K59.4   **Anal spasm**
       Proctalgia fugax

    K59.8   **Other specified functional intestinal disorders**
       Atony of colon Pseudo-obstruction (acute) (chronic) of intestine

    K59.9   **Functional intestinal disorder, unspecified**

● **K60**   **Fissure and fistula of anal and rectal regions**

    Excludes 1   fissure and fistula of anal and rectal regions with abscess or cellulitis (K61.-)

    Excludes 2   anal sphincter tear (healed) (nontraumatic) (old) (K62.81)

    K60.0   **Acute anal fissure**

    K60.1   **Chronic anal fissure**

    K60.2   **Anal fissure, unspecified**

    K60.3   **Anal fistula**

    K60.4   **Rectal fistula**
       Fistula of rectum to skin

    Excludes 1   rectovaginal fistula (N82.3)
       vesicorectal fistula (N32.1)

    K60.5   **Anorectal fistula**

● **K61**   **Abscess of anal and rectal regions**

    Includes   abscess of anal and rectal regions
       cellulitis of anal and rectal regions
    (Ex) For category K61 CC codes: K61.0-K61.4

    K61.0   **Anal abscess** 🖉
       Perianal abscess

    Excludes 1   intrasphincteric abscess (K61.4)

    K61.1   **Rectal abscess** 🖉
       Perirectal abscess

    Excludes 1   ischiorectal abscess (K61.3)
    Coding Clinic: 2012, Q4, P104

    K61.2   **Anorectal abscess** 🖉

    K61.3   **Ischiorectal abscess** 🖉
       Abscess of ischiorectal fossa

    K61.4   **Intrasphincteric abscess** 🖉

Item 11-17   A **fissure** is a groove in the surface, whereas a **fistula** is an abnormal passage. An **abscess** is an accumulation of pus in a tissue cavity resulting from a bacterial or parasitic infection.

◀ New   ⫿ Revised   ~~deleted~~ Deleted   Excludes 1   Excludes 2   Includes   Use additional   Code first   Code also   Unspecified

OGCR Official Guidelines   ● Unacceptable Principal Diagnosis   X Assign placeholder X   🖉 Use Additional Character(s)   ▶ Manifestation Code   **Coding Clinic**

● **K62**   **Other diseases of anus and rectum**

     Includes   anal canal

     Excludes2   colostomy and enterostomy malfunction (K94.0-, K91.4-)

                fecal incontinence (R15.-)

                hemorrhoids (K64.-)

    K62.0   **Anal polyp**

    K62.1   **Rectal polyp**

        Excludes1   adenomatous polyp (D12.8)

    K62.2   **Anal prolapse**

        Prolapse of anal canal

    K62.3   **Rectal prolapse**

        Prolapse of rectal mucosa

    K62.4   **Stenosis of anus and rectum**

        Stricture of anus (sphincter)

    K62.5   **Hemorrhage of anus and rectum** 🗪

        Excludes1   gastrointestinal bleeding NOS (K92.2)

                melena (K92.1)

                neonatal rectal hemorrhage (P54.2)

        Ⓔⓧ See K57

    K62.6   **Ulcer of anus and rectum** 🗪

        Solitary ulcer of anus and rectum

        Stercoral ulcer of anus and rectum

        Excludes1   fissure and fistula of anus and rectum (K60.-)

                ulcerative colitis (K51.-)

        Ⓔⓧ K62.6

    K62.7   **Radiation proctitis**

        Use additional code to identify the type of radiation (W90.-)

● **K62.8**   **Other specified diseases of anus and rectum**

        Excludes2   ulcerative proctitis (K51.2)

      K62.81   **Anal sphincter tear (healed) (nontraumatic) (old)**

           Tear of anus, nontraumatic

           Use additional code for any associated fecal incontinence (R15.-)

           Excludes2   anal fissure (K60.-)

                     anal sphincter tear (healed) (old) complicating delivery (O34.7-)

                     traumatic tear of anal sphincter (S31.831)

      K62.82   **Dysplasia of anus**

           Anal intraepithelial neoplasia I and II (AIN I and II) (histologically confirmed)

           Dysplasia of anus NOS

           Mild and moderate dysplasia of anus (histologically confirmed)

           Excludes1   abnormal results from anal cytologic examination without histologic confirmation (R85.61-)

                     anal intraepithelial neoplasia III (D01.3)

                     carcinoma in situ of anus (D01.3)

                     HGSIL of anus (R85.613)

                     severe dysplasia of anus (D01.3)

      K62.89   **Other specified diseases of anus and rectum**

           Proctitis NOS

           Use additional code for any associated fecal incontinence (R15.-)

    K62.9   **Disease of anus and rectum, unspecified**

● **K63**   **Other diseases of intestine**

    K63.0   **Abscess of intestine** 🗪

        Excludes1   abscess of intestine with Crohn's disease (K50.014, K50.114, K50.814, K50.914)

                abscess of intestine with diverticular disease (K57.0, K57.2, K57.4, K57.8)

                abscess of intestine with ulcerative colitis (K51.014, K51.214, K51.314, K51.414, K51.514, K51.814, K51.914)

        Excludes2   abscess of anal and rectal regions (K61.-)

                abscess of appendix (K35.3)

        Ⓔⓧ K63.0

    K63.1   **Perforation of intestine (nontraumatic)** 🗪

        Perforation (nontraumatic) of rectum

        Excludes1   perforation (nontraumatic) of duodenum (K26.-)

                perforation (nontraumatic) of intestine with diverticular disease (K57.0, K57.2, K57.4, K57.8)

        Excludes2   perforation (nontraumatic) of appendix (K35.2, K35.3)

        Ⓔⓧ K63.1

    K63.2   **Fistula of intestine** 🗪

        Excludes1   fistula of duodenum (K31.6)

                fistula of intestine with Crohn's disease (K50.013, K50.113, K50.813, K50.913)

                fistula of intestine with ulcerative colitis (K51.013, K51.213, K51.313, K51.413, K51.513, K51.813, K51.913)

        Excludes2   fistula of anal and rectal regions (K60.-)

                fistula of appendix (K38.3)

                intestinal-genital fistula, female (N82.2-N82.4)

                vesicointestinal fistula (N32.1)

        Ⓔⓧ K63.2

    K63.3   **Ulcer of intestine** 🗪

        Primary ulcer of small intestine

        Excludes1   duodenal ulcer (K26.-)

                gastrointestinal ulcer (K28.-)

                gastrojejunal ulcer (K28.-)

                jejunal ulcer (K28.-)

                peptic ulcer, site unspecified (K27.-)

                ulcer of intestine with perforation (K63.1)

                ulcer of anus or rectum (K62.6)

                ulcerative colitis (K51.-)

        Ⓔⓧ K63.3

    K63.4   **Enteroptosis**

    K63.5   **Polyp of colon**

        Excludes1   adenomatous polyp of colon (D12.6)

                inflammatory polyp of colon (K51.4-)

                polyposis of colon (D12.6)

        Coding Clinic: 2015, Q2, P14

● **K63.8**   **Other specified diseases of intestine**

      K63.81   **Dieulafoy lesion of intestine** 🗪

           Excludes2   Dieulafoy lesion of stomach and duodenum (K31.82)

           Ⓔⓧ E16.4, I85.01, K22.10-K22.11, K22.6-K22.719, K25.0-K28.9, K29.01, K29.21, K29.31, K29.41, K29.51, K29.61, K29.71, K29.81, K29.91, K31.811, K55.21, K57.01, K57.11, K57.13, K57.21, K57.31, K57.33, K57.41, K57.51, K57.53, K57.81, K57.91, K57.93, K62.5, K63.81, K92.0-K92.2

      K63.89   **Other specified diseases of intestine**

           Coding Clinic: 2013, Q2, P31

    K63.9   **Disease of intestine, unspecified**

N Newborn Age: 0   **P** Pediatric Age: 0–17   **M** Maternity DX: 12–55   **A** Adult Age: 15–124   ♀ Females Only   ♂ Males Only

🗪 Complication\Comorbidity   🗪 Major C\C   Ⓔⓧ CC/MCC Exclusions   🗪 Hospital-Acquired Condition

953

CHAPTER 11 (K00-K95)

CHAPTER 11 (K00-K95)

● **K64**   **Hemorrhoids and perianal venous thrombosis**

> **Includes**   piles
>
> **Excludes1**   hemorrhoids complicating childbirth and the puerperium (O87.2)
> hemorrhoids complicating pregnancy (O22.4)

K64.0   **First degree hemorrhoids**
> Grade/stage I hemorrhoids
> Hemorrhoids (bleeding) without prolapse outside of anal canal

K64.1   **Second degree hemorrhoids**
> Grade/stage II hemorrhoids
> Hemorrhoids (bleeding) that prolapse with straining, but retract spontaneously

K64.2   **Third degree hemorrhoids**
> Grade/stage III hemorrhoids
> Hemorrhoids (bleeding) that prolapse with straining and require manual replacement back inside anal canal

K64.3   **Fourth degree hemorrhoids**
> Grade/stage IV hemorrhoids
> Hemorrhoids (bleeding) with prolapsed tissue that cannot be manually replaced

K64.4   **Residual hemorrhoidal skin tags**
> External hemorrhoids, NOS
> Skin tags of anus

K64.5   **Perianal venous thrombosis**
> External hemorrhoids with thrombosis
> Perianal hematoma
> Thrombosed hemorrhoids NOS

K64.8   **Other hemorrhoids**
> Internal hemorrhoids, without mention of degree
> Prolapsed hemorrhoids, degree not specified

K64.9   **Unspecified hemorrhoids**
> Hemorrhoids (bleeding) NOS
> Hemorrhoids (bleeding) without mention of degree

DISEASES OF PERITONEUM AND RETROPERITONEUM (K65-K68)

● **K65**   **Peritonitis**

> Use additional code (B95-B97), to identify infectious agent
>
> **Excludes1**   acute appendicitis with generalized peritonitis (K35.2)
> aseptic peritonitis (T81.6)
> benign paroxysmal peritonitis (E85.0)
> chemical peritonitis (T81.6)
> diverticulitis of both small and large intestine with peritonitis (K57.4-)
> diverticulitis of colon with peritonitis (K57.2-)
> diverticulitis of intestine, NOS, with peritonitis (K57.8-)
> diverticulitis of small intestine with peritonitis (K57.0-)
> gonococcal peritonitis (A54.85)
> neonatal peritonitis (P78.0-P78.1)
> pelvic peritonitis, female (N73.3-N73.5)
> periodic familial peritonitis (E85.0)
> peritonitis due to talc or other foreign substance (T81.6)
> peritonitis in chlamydia (A74.81)
> peritonitis in diphtheria (A36.89)
> peritonitis in syphilis (late) (A52.74)
> peritonitis in tuberculosis (A18.31)
> peritonitis with or following abortion or ectopic or molar pregnancy (O00-O07, O08.0)
> peritonitis with or following appendicitis (K35.-)
> peritonitis with or following diverticular disease of intestine (K57.-)
> puerperal peritonitis (O85)
> retroperitoneal infections (K68.-)

> (Ex:) **For category K65 CC codes:** K63.4, K63.89-K63.9, K65.0-K65.9, K67, K68.19-K68.9, K92.89-K92.9, R11.13

Item 11-19 **Retroperitoneal infections** occur between the posterior parietal peritoneum and posterior abdominal wall where the kidneys, adrenal glands, ureters, duodenum, ascending colon, descending colon, pancreas, and the large vessels and nerves are located.

K65.0   **Generalized (acute) peritonitis** 🔗
> Pelvic peritonitis (acute), male
> Subphrenic peritonitis (acute)
> Suppurative peritonitis (acute)

K65.1   **Peritoneal abscess** 🔗
> Abdominopelvic abscess
> Abscess (of) omentum
> Abscess (of) peritoneum
> Mesenteric abscess
> Retrocecal abscess
> Subdiaphragmatic abscess
> Subhepatic abscess
> Subphrenic abscess

K65.2   **Spontaneous bacterial peritonitis** 🔗
> **Excludes1**   bacterial peritonitis NOS (K65.9)

K65.3   **Choleperitonitis** 🔗
> Peritonitis due to bile

K65.4   **Sclerosing mesenteritis** 🔗
> Fat necrosis of peritoneum
> (Idiopathic) sclerosing mesenteric fibrosis
> Mesenteric lipodystrophy
> Mesenteric panniculitis
> Retractile mesenteritis

K65.8   **Other peritonitis** 🔗
> Chronic proliferative peritonitis
> Peritonitis due to urine

K65.9   **Peritonitis, unspecified** 🔗
> Bacterial peritonitis NOS
> **Coding Clinic: 2013, Q2, P31**

● **K66**   **Other disorders of peritoneum**
> **Excludes2**   ascites (R18.-)
> peritoneal effusion (chronic) (R18.8)

K66.0   **Peritoneal adhesions (postprocedural) (postinfection)**
> Adhesions (of) abdominal (wall)
> Adhesions (of) diaphragm
> Adhesions (of) intestine
> Adhesions (of) male pelvis
> Adhesions (of) omentum
> Adhesions (of) stomach
> Adhesive bands
> Mesenteric adhesions
>
> **Excludes1**   female pelvic adhesions [bands] (N73.6)
> peritoneal adhesions with intestinal obstruction (K56.5)

K66.1   **Hemoperitoneum** 🔗
> **Excludes1**   traumatic hemoperitoneum (S36.8-)
> (Ex:) K66.1

K66.8   **Other specified disorders of peritoneum**

K66.9   **Disorder of peritoneum, unspecified**

▶ **K67**   *Disorders of peritoneum in infectious diseases classified elsewhere* 🔗
> *Code first* underlying disease, such as:
> congenital syphilis (A50.0)
> helminthiasis (B65.0-B83.9)
>
> **Excludes1**   peritonitis in chlamydia (A74.81)
> peritonitis in diphtheria (A36.89)
> peritonitis in gonococcal (A54.85)
> peritonitis in syphilis (late) (A52.74)
> peritonitis in tuberculosis (A18.31)
>
> (Ex:) See K65

Item 11-18 **Peritonitis** is an inflammation of the lining (peritoneum) of the abdominal cavity and surface of the intestines.

◀ New   ◀▥ Revised   ~~deleted~~ Deleted   Excludes 1   Excludes 2   Includes   Use additional   Code first   Code also   Unspecified
OGCR Official Guidelines   ● Unacceptable Principal Diagnosis   X Assign placeholder X   ● Use Additional Character(s)   ▶ Manifestation Code   **Coding Clinic**

● **K68**   **Disorders of retroperitoneum**
  ● **K68.1**   **Retroperitoneal abscess**
     K68.11   **Postprocedural retroperitoneal abscess** 🔖 🔖
       (Ex:) D78.81-D78.89, E36.8, E89.810-E89.89, H59.011-H59.019,
         H59.031-H59.099, H59.811-H59.89, H95.811-H95.89, I97.3,
         K68.11, L76.81-L76.82, M96.89, N98.1-N98.9, T81.4XX[A],
         T81.82X[A], T81.89X-T81.9XX[A]

     K68.12   **Psoas muscle abscess** 🔖
       (Ex:) K68.12, M60.00-M60.19, M61.00-M61.19, M61.30-M61.59,
         M62.3, M62.50-M62.59, M62.84, M62.89, M72.6

     K68.19   **Other retroperitoneal abscess** 🔖
       (Ex:) See K65

   K68.9   **Other disorders of retroperitoneum** 🔖
     (Ex:) See K65

DISEASES OF LIVER (K70-K77)

Excludes1   jaundice NOS (R17)
Excludes2   hemochromatosis (E83.11-)
        Reye's syndrome (G93.7)
        viral hepatitis (B15-B19)
        Wilson's disease (E83.0)

● **K70**   **Alcoholic liver disease**
   Use additional code to identify:
     alcohol abuse and dependence (F10.-)
   K70.0   **Alcoholic fatty liver**   A
  ● **K70.1**   **Alcoholic hepatitis**
     K70.10   **Alcoholic hepatitis without ascites**   A
     K70.11   **Alcoholic hepatitis with ascites**   A
   K70.2   **Alcoholic fibrosis and sclerosis of liver**   A
  ● **K70.3**   **Alcoholic cirrhosis of liver**
     Alcoholic cirrhosis NOS
     K70.30   **Alcoholic cirrhosis of liver without ascites**   A
     K70.31   **Alcoholic cirrhosis of liver with ascites**   A
  ● **K70.4**   **Alcoholic hepatic failure**
     Acute alcoholic hepatic failure
     Alcoholic hepatic failure NOS
     Chronic alcoholic hepatic failure
     Subacute alcoholic hepatic failure
     K70.40   **Alcoholic hepatic failure without coma**   A
     K70.41   **Alcoholic hepatic failure with coma** 🔖   A
       MCC when PDx is its own MCC
       (Ex:) K72.91, K76.5, K76.89-K76.9
   K70.9   **Alcoholic liver disease, unspecified**   A

● **K71**   **Toxic liver disease**
   Includes   drug-induced idiosyncratic (unpredictable) liver
             disease
          drug-induced toxic (predictable) liver disease
   Code first poisoning due to drug or toxin, if applicable (T36-T65 with
   fifth or sixth character 1-4 or 6)
   Use additional code for adverse effect, if applicable, to identify
     drug (T36-T50 with fifth or sixth character 5)
   Excludes2   alcoholic liver disease (K70.-)
           Budd-Chiari syndrome (I82.0)
   K71.0   **Toxic liver disease with cholestasis**
     Cholestasis with hepatocyte injury
     'Pure' cholestasis
  ● **K71.1**   **Toxic liver disease with hepatic necrosis**
     Hepatic failure (acute) (chronic) due to drugs
     K71.10   **Toxic liver disease with hepatic necrosis, without coma**
     K71.11   **Toxic liver disease with hepatic necrosis, with coma** 🔖
       MCC when PDx is its own MCC
       (Ex:) K72.91, K76.5, K76.89-K76.9

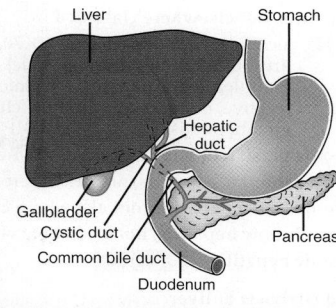

Figure 11-13   Liver and bile ducts.

   K71.2   **Toxic liver disease with acute hepatitis**
   K71.3   **Toxic liver disease with chronic persistent hepatitis**
   K71.4   **Toxic liver disease with chronic lobular hepatitis**
  ● **K71.5**   **Toxic liver disease with chronic active hepatitis**
     Toxic liver disease with lupoid hepatitis
     K71.50   **Toxic liver disease with chronic active hepatitis without ascites**
     K71.51   **Toxic liver disease with chronic active hepatitis with ascites**
   K71.6   **Toxic liver disease with hepatitis, not elsewhere classified**
   K71.7   **Toxic liver disease with fibrosis and cirrhosis of liver**
   K71.8   **Toxic liver disease with other disorders of liver**
     Toxic liver disease with focal nodular hyperplasia
     Toxic liver disease with hepatic granulomas
     Toxic liver disease with peliosis hepatis
     Toxic liver disease with veno-occlusive disease of liver
   K71.9   **Toxic liver disease, unspecified**

● **K72**   **Hepatic failure, not elsewhere classified**
   Includes   ~~acute hepatitis NEC, with hepatic failure~~
          fulminant hepatitis NEC, with hepatic failure
          hepatic encephalopathy NOS
          liver (cell) necrosis with hepatic failure
          malignant hepatitis NEC, with hepatic failure
          yellow liver atrophy or dystrophy
   Excludes1   alcoholic hepatic failure (K70.4)
          hepatic failure with toxic liver disease (K71.1-)
          icterus of newborn (P55-P59)
          postprocedural hepatic failure (K91.82)
   Excludes2   hepatic failure complicating abortion or ectopic
            or molar pregnancy (O00-O07, O08.8)
          hepatic failure complicating pregnancy, childbirth
            and the puerperium (O26.6-)
          viral hepatitis with hepatic coma (B15-B19) ◄
  ● **K72.0**   **Acute and subacute hepatic failure**
     Acute non-viral hepatitis NOS ◄
     (Ex:) **For category K72.0 CC codes:** K72.00-K72.01, K76.2-K76.3, K76.5,
       K76.89-K76.9
     Coding Clinic: 2015, Q2, P17
     K72.00   **Acute and subacute hepatic failure without coma** 🔖
       Coding Clinic: 2015, Q2, P17
     K72.01   **Acute and subacute hepatic failure with coma** 🔖
       MCC when PDx is its own MCC
  ● **K72.1**   **Chronic hepatic failure**
     K72.10   **Chronic hepatic failure without coma**
     K72.11   **Chronic hepatic failure with coma** 🔖
       MCC when PDx is its own MCC
       (Ex:) K72.91, K76.5, K76.89-K76.9
  ● **K72.9**   **Hepatic failure, unspecified**
     K72.90   **Hepatic failure, unspecified without coma**
     K72.91   **Hepatic failure, unspecified with coma** 🔖
       Hepatic coma NOS
       (Ex:) K72.91, K76.5, K76.89-K76.9
       Coding Clinic: 2016, Q2, P35

Item 11-20   Cirrhosis is the progressive fibrosis of the liver resulting in loss of liver function. The main causes of cirrhosis of the liver are alcohol abuse, chronic hepatitis (inflammation of the liver), biliary disease, and excessive amounts of iron. **Alcoholic cirrhosis of the liver** is also called portal, Laënnec's, or fatty nutritional cirrhosis.

N   Newborn Age: 0   **P**   Pediatric Age: 0-17   **M**   Maternity DX: 12-55   **A**   Adult Age: 15-124   ♀   Females Only   ♂   Males Only

🔖   Complication\Comorbidity   🔖   Major C\C   (Ex:)   CC/MCC Exclusions   🔖   Hospital-Acquired Condition   955

CHAPTER 11 (K00-K95)

CHAPTER 11 (K00-K95)

● **K73   Chronic hepatitis, not elsewhere classified**

Excludes1   alcoholic hepatitis (chronic) (K70.1-)
drug-induced hepatitis (chronic) (K71.-)
granulomatous hepatitis (chronic) NEC (K75.3)
reactive, nonspecific hepatitis (chronic) (K75.2)
viral hepatitis (chronic) (B15-B19)

K73.0   Chronic persistent hepatitis, not elsewhere classified

K73.1   Chronic lobular hepatitis, not elsewhere classified

K73.2   Chronic active hepatitis, not elsewhere classified

K73.8   Other chronic hepatitis, not elsewhere classified

K73.9   Chronic hepatitis, unspecified

● **K74   Fibrosis and cirrhosis of liver**

Code also, if applicable, viral hepatitis (acute) (chronic) (B15-B19)

Excludes1   alcoholic cirrhosis (of liver) (K70.3)
alcoholic fibrosis of liver (K70.2)
cardiac sclerosis of liver (K76.1)
cirrhosis (of liver) with toxic liver disease (K71.7)
congenital cirrhosis (of liver) (P78.81)
pigmentary cirrhosis (of liver) (E83.110)

K74.0   Hepatic fibrosis

K74.1   Hepatic sclerosis

K74.2   Hepatic fibrosis with hepatic sclerosis

K74.3   Primary biliary cirrhosis
Chronic nonsuppurative destructive cholangitis

K74.4   Secondary biliary cirrhosis

K74.5   Biliary cirrhosis, unspecified

● **K74.6   Other and unspecified cirrhosis of liver**

K74.60   Unspecified cirrhosis of liver
Cirrhosis (of liver) NOS

K74.69   Other cirrhosis of liver
Cryptogenic cirrhosis (of liver)
Macronodular cirrhosis (of liver)
Micronodular cirrhosis (of liver)
Mixed type cirrhosis (of liver)
Portal cirrhosis (of liver)
Postnecrotic cirrhosis (of liver)

● **K75   Other inflammatory liver diseases**

Excludes2   toxic liver disease (K71.-)

K75.0   Abscess of liver 🦠
Cholangitic hepatic abscess
Hematogenic hepatic abscess
Hepatic abscess NOS
Lymphogenic hepatic abscess
Pylephlebitic hepatic abscess

Excludes1   amebic liver abscess (A06.4)
cholangitis without liver abscess (K83.0)
pylephlebitis without liver abscess
(K75.1)

Excludes2   acute or subacute hepatitis NOS
(B17.9) ◄
acute or subacute non-viral hepatitis
(K72.0) ◄
chronic hepatitis NEC (K73.8) ◄
(Ex:) A06.4, K75.0-K75.1, K76.5, K76.89-K76.9

K75.1   Phlebitis of portal vein 🦠
Pylephlebitis

Excludes1   pylephlebitic liver abscess (K75.0)
(Ex:) A06.4, K75.0-K75.1, K76.5, K76.89-K76.9

K75.2   Nonspecific reactive hepatitis

Excludes1   acute or subacute hepatitis (K72.0-)
chronic hepatitis NEC (K73.-)
viral hepatitis (B15-B19)

K75.3   Granulomatous hepatitis, not elsewhere classified

Excludes1   acute or subacute hepatitis (K72.0-)
chronic hepatitis NEC (K73.-)
viral hepatitis (B15-B19)

K75.4   Autoimmune hepatitis
Lupoid hepatitis NEC

● **K75.8   Other specified inflammatory liver diseases**

K75.81   Nonalcoholic steatohepatitis (NASH)

K75.89   Other specified inflammatory liver diseases

K75.9   Inflammatory liver disease, unspecified
Hepatitis NOS

Excludes1   acute or subacute hepatitis (K72.0-)
chronic hepatitis NEC (K73.-)
viral hepatitis (B15-B19)

Coding Clinic: 2015, Q2, P17

● **K76   Other diseases of liver**

Excludes2   alcoholic liver disease (K70.-)
amyloid degeneration of liver (E85.-)
cystic disease of liver (congenital) (Q44.6)
hepatic vein thrombosis (I82.0)
hepatomegaly NOS (R16.0)
pigmentary cirrhosis (of liver) (E83.110)
portal vein thrombosis (I81)
toxic liver disease (K71.-)

K76.0   Fatty (change of) liver, not elsewhere classified
Nonalcoholic fatty liver disease (NAFLD)

Excludes1   nonalcoholic steatohepatitis (NASH)
(K75.81)

K76.1   Chronic passive congestion of liver
Cardiac cirrhosis
Cardiac sclerosis

K76.2   Central hemorrhagic necrosis of liver 🦠

Excludes1   liver necrosis with hepatic failure (K72.-)
(Ex:) K72.00-K72.01, K76.2-K76.3, K76.5, K76.89-K76.9

K76.3   Infarction of liver 🦠
(Ex:) See K76.2

K76.4   Peliosis hepatis
Hepatic angiomatosis

K76.5   Hepatic veno-occlusive disease

Excludes1   Budd-Chiari syndrome (I82.0)

K76.6   Portal hypertension 🦠

Use additional code for any associated complications,
such as:
portal hypertensive gastropathy (K31.89)
(Ex:) K72.91, K76.5-K76.6, K76.89-K76.9

K76.7   Hepatorenal syndrome 🦠

Excludes1   hepatorenal syndrome following labor
and delivery (O90.4)
postprocedural hepatorenal syndrome
(K91.83) ◄⫿⫿
(Ex:) K76.5, K76.7, K76.89-K76.9

● **K76.8   Other specified diseases of liver**

● **K76.81   Hepatopulmonary syndrome**

Code first underlying liver disease, such as:
alcoholic cirrhosis of liver (K70.3-)
cirrhosis of liver without mention of alcohol
(K74.6-)

K76.89   Other specified diseases of liver
Cyst (simple) of liver
Focal nodular hyperplasia of liver
Hepatoptosis

K76.9   Liver disease, unspecified

▌ K77   *Liver disorders in diseases classified elsewhere* 🦠

Code first underlying disease, such as:
amyloidosis (E85.-)
congenital syphilis (A50.0, A50.5)
congenital toxoplasmosis (P37.1)
schistosomiasis (B65.0-B65.9)

Excludes1   alcoholic hepatitis (K70.1-)
alcoholic liver disease (K70.-)
cytomegaloviral hepatitis (B25.1)
herpesviral [herpes simplex] hepatitis (B00.81)
infectious mononucleosis with liver disease
(B27.0-B27.9 with .9)
mumps hepatitis (B26.81)
sarcoidosis with liver disease (D86.89)
secondary syphilis with liver disease (A51.45)
syphilis (late) with liver disease (A52.74)
toxoplasmosis (acquired) hepatitis (B58.1)
tuberculosis with liver disease (A18.83)

(Ex:) No exclusions

New   ◄⫿⫿ Revised   ~~deleted~~ Deleted   Excludes 1   Excludes 2   Includes   Use additional   Code first   Code also   Unspecified

OGCR Official Guidelines   ● Unacceptable Principal Diagnosis   X Assign placeholder X   🦠 Use Additional Character(s)   ▌ Manifestation Code   Coding Clinic

DISORDERS OF GALLBLADDER, BILIARY TRACT AND PANCREAS (K80–K87)

● **K80**   **Cholelithiasis**
Presence or formation of gallstones

    Excludes1   retained cholelithiasis following cholecystectomy (K91.86)

● **K80.0**   **Calculus of gallbladder with acute cholecystitis**
Any condition listed in K80.2 with acute cholecystitis
Check documentation for acute/chronic gallbladder/common bile duct either with or without obstruction.

    K80.00   **Calculus of gallbladder with acute cholecystitis without obstruction**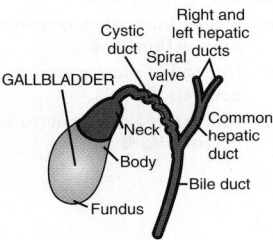
       Ex: K80.00-K80.21, K80.40, K80.44, K80.62-K80.63, K80.66-K80.67, K80.80, K81.0-K81.9, K82.9, K83.5-K83.9, K87

    K80.01   **Calculus of gallbladder with acute cholecystitis with obstruction**
       Ex: K80.00-K80.21, K80.62-K80.63, K80.66-K80.67, K80.80, K81.0-K81.9, K82.9, K83.5-K83.9, K87

● **K80.1**   **Calculus of gallbladder with other cholecystitis**
       Ex: For category K80.1 CC codes unless otherwise indicated: See K80.01

    K80.10   **Calculus of gallbladder with chronic cholecystitis without obstruction**
       Cholelithiasis with cholecystitis NOS

    K80.11   **Calculus of gallbladder with chronic cholecystitis with obstruction**

    K80.12   **Calculus of gallbladder with acute and chronic cholecystitis without obstruction**
       Ex: See K80.00

    K80.13   **Calculus of gallbladder with acute and chronic cholecystitis with obstruction**

    K80.18   **Calculus of gallbladder with other cholecystitis without obstruction**

    K80.19   **Calculus of gallbladder with other cholecystitis with obstruction**

● **K80.2**   **Calculus of gallbladder without cholecystitis**
       Cholecystolithiasis without cholecystitis
       Cholelithiasis (without cholecystitis)
       Colic (recurrent) of gallbladder (without cholecystitis)
       Gallstone (impacted) of cystic duct (without cholecystitis)
       Gallstone (impacted) of gallbladder (without cholecystitis)

    K80.20   **Calculus of gallbladder without cholecystitis without obstruction**

    K80.21   **Calculus of gallbladder without cholecystitis with obstruction**
       Ex: See K80.01

● **K80.3**   **Calculus of bile duct with cholangitis**
       Any condition listed in K80.5 with cholangitis

    K80.30   **Calculus of bile duct with cholangitis, unspecified, without obstruction**
       CC when PDx is its own CC
       Ex: K83.0, K83.5-K83.9, K87

    K80.31   **Calculus of bile duct with cholangitis, unspecified, with obstruction**
       CC when PDx is its own CC
       Ex: K80.30-K80.71, K80.81-K81.9, K83.5-K83.9, K87

    K80.32   **Calculus of bile duct with acute cholangitis without obstruction**
       CC when PDx is its own CC
       Ex: See K80.30

    K80.33   **Calculus of bile duct with acute cholangitis with obstruction**
       CC when PDx is its own CC
       Ex: See K80.31

    K80.34   **Calculus of bile duct with chronic cholangitis without obstruction**
       CC when PDx is its own CC
       Ex: See K80.30

    K80.35   **Calculus of bile duct with chronic cholangitis with obstruction**
       CC when PDx is its own CC
       Ex: See K80.31

    K80.36   **Calculus of bile duct with acute and chronic cholangitis without obstruction**
       CC when PDx is its own CC
       Ex: See K80.30

    K80.37   **Calculus of bile duct with acute and chronic cholangitis with obstruction**
       CC when PDx is its own CC
       Ex: See K80.31

● **K80.4**   **Calculus of bile duct with cholecystitis**
       Any condition listed in K80.5 with cholecystitis (with cholangitis)
       Ex: For category K80.4 CC codes: K80.30-K80.71, K80.81-K81.9, K83.5-K83.9, K87

    K80.40   **Calculus of bile duct with cholecystitis, unspecified, without obstruction**

    K80.41   **Calculus of bile duct with cholecystitis, unspecified, with obstruction**

    K80.42   **Calculus of bile duct with acute cholecystitis without obstruction**

    K80.43   **Calculus of bile duct with acute cholecystitis with obstruction**

    K80.44   **Calculus of bile duct with chronic cholecystitis without obstruction**

    K80.45   **Calculus of bile duct with chronic cholecystitis with obstruction**

    K80.46   **Calculus of bile duct with acute and chronic cholecystitis without obstruction**

    K80.47   **Calculus of bile duct with acute and chronic cholecystitis with obstruction**

● **K80.5**   **Calculus of bile duct without cholangitis or cholecystitis**
       Choledocholithiasis (without cholangitis or cholecystitis)
       Gallstone (impacted) of bile duct NOS (without cholangitis or cholecystitis)
       Gallstone (impacted) of common duct (without cholangitis or cholecystitis)
       Gallstone (impacted) of hepatic duct (without cholangitis or cholecystitis)
       Hepatic cholelithiasis (without cholangitis or cholecystitis)
       Hepatic colic (recurrent) (without cholangitis or cholecystitis)

    K80.50   **Calculus of bile duct without cholangitis or cholecystitis without obstruction**

    K80.51   **Calculus of bile duct without cholangitis or cholecystitis with obstruction**
       Ex: See K80.4

● **K80.6**   **Calculus of gallbladder and bile duct with cholecystitis**

    K80.60   **Calculus of gallbladder and bile duct with cholecystitis, unspecified, without obstruction**
       Ex: See K80.4

    K80.61   **Calculus of gallbladder and bile duct with cholecystitis, unspecified, with obstruction**
       Ex: See K80.4

    K80.62   **Calculus of gallbladder and bile duct with acute cholecystitis without obstruction**
       Ex: K80.62-K80.63, K81.0-K81.9, K82.9, K83.5-K83.9, K87

Figure 11-14   *Gallbladder and bile ducts.*

N   Newborn Age: 0   P   Pediatric Age: 0–17   M   Maternity DX: 12–55   A   Adult Age: 15–124   ♀   Females Only   ♂   Males Only
    🖉 Complication\Comorbidity   🖉 Major C\C   Ex: CC/MCC Exclusions   🖉 Hospital-Acquired Condition

K80.63 Calculus of gallbladder and bile duct with acute cholecystitis with obstruction 🔊
Ex: See K80.62

K80.64 Calculus of gallbladder and bile duct with chronic cholecystitis without obstruction 🔊
Ex: See K80.4

K80.65 Calculus of gallbladder and bile duct with chronic cholecystitis with obstruction 🔊
Ex: See K80.4

K80.66 Calculus of gallbladder and bile duct with acute and chronic cholecystitis without obstruction 🔊
Ex: K80.66-K80.67, K81.0-K81.9, K82.9, K83.5-K83.9, K87

K80.67 Calculus of gallbladder and bile duct with acute and chronic cholecystitis with obstruction 🔊
Ex: See K80.66

● **K80.7** Calculus of gallbladder and bile duct without cholecystitis

K80.70 Calculus of gallbladder and bile duct without cholecystitis without obstruction

K80.71 Calculus of gallbladder and bile duct without cholecystitis with obstruction 🔊
Ex: See K80.4

● **K80.8** Other cholelithiasis

K80.80 Other cholelithiasis without obstruction

K80.81 Other cholelithiasis with obstruction 🔊
Ex: See K80.4

● **K81** Cholecystitis
Chronic or acute inflammation of the gallbladder
Excludes1 cholecystitis with cholelithiasis (K80.-)

K81.0 Acute cholecystitis 🔊
Abscess of gallbladder
Angiocholecystitis
Emphysematous (acute) cholecystitis
Empyema of gallbladder
Gangrene of gallbladder
Gangrenous cholecystitis
Suppurative cholecystitis
Ex: K80.00, K80.12, K80.62-K80.63, K80.66-K80.67, K81.0-K81.9, K82.9, K83.5-K83.9, K87

K81.1 Chronic cholecystitis

K81.2 Acute cholecystitis with chronic cholecystitis 🔊
Ex: K81.0-K81.9, K82.9, K83.5-K83.9, K87

K81.9 Cholecystitis, unspecified

● **K82** Other diseases of gallbladder
Excludes1 nonvisualization of gallbladder (R93.2)
postcholecystectomy syndrome (K91.5)
Ex: For category K82 CC codes: K82.0-K82.9, K83.5-K83.9, K87

K82.0 Obstruction of gallbladder 🔊
Occlusion of cystic duct or gallbladder without cholelithiasis
Stenosis of cystic duct or gallbladder without cholelithiasis
Stricture of cystic duct or gallbladder without cholelithiasis
Excludes1 obstruction of gallbladder with cholelithiasis (K80.-)

K82.1 Hydrops of gallbladder 🔊
Mucocele of gallbladder

K82.2 Perforation of gallbladder 🔊
Rupture of cystic duct or gallbladder

K82.3 Fistula of gallbladder 🔊
Cholecystocolic fistula
Cholecystoduodenal fistula

K82.4 Cholesterolosis of gallbladder
Strawberry gallbladder
Excludes1 cholesterolosis of gallbladder with cholecystitis (K81.-)
cholesterolosis of gallbladder with cholelithiasis (K80.-)

K82.8 Other specified diseases of gallbladder
Adhesions of cystic duct or gallbladder
Atrophy of cystic duct or gallbladder
Cyst of cystic duct or gallbladder
Dyskinesia of cystic duct or gallbladder
Hypertrophy of cystic duct or gallbladder
Nonfunctioning of cystic duct or gallbladder
Ulcer of cystic duct or gallbladder

K82.9 Disease of gallbladder, unspecified

● **K83** Other diseases of biliary tract
Excludes1 postcholecystectomy syndrome (K91.5)
Excludes2 conditions involving the gallbladder (K81-K82)
conditions involving the cystic duct (K81-K82)

K83.0 Cholangitis 🔊
Ascending cholangitis   Sclerosing cholangitis
Cholangitis NOS   Secondary cholangitis
Primary cholangitis   Stenosing cholangitis
Recurrent cholangitis   Suppurative cholangitis
Excludes1 cholangitic liver abscess (K75.0)
cholangitis with choledocholithiasis (K80.3-, K80.4-)
chronic nonsuppurative destructive cholangitis (K74.3)
Ex: K83.0, K83.5-K83.9, K87

K83.1 Obstruction of bile duct 🔊
Occlusion of bile duct without cholelithiasis
Stenosis of bile duct without cholelithiasis
Stricture of bile duct without cholelithiasis
Excludes1 congenital obstruction of bile duct (Q44.3)
obstruction of bile duct with cholelithiasis (K80.-)
Ex: K80.31, K80.33, K80.35, K80.37, K80.41, K80.43, K80.45, K80.47, K80.51, K80.81, K83.1, K83.5-K83.9, K87, Q44.2-Q44.3
Coding Clinic: 2016, Q1, P18

K83.2 Perforation of bile duct 🔊
Rupture of bile duct
Ex: K83.2-K83.3, K83.5-K83.9, K87

K83.3 Fistula of bile duct 🔊
Choledochoduodenal fistula
Ex: K83.2-K83.3, K83.5-K83.9, K87

K83.4 Spasm of sphincter of Oddi

K83.5 Biliary cyst

K83.8 Other specified diseases of biliary tract
Adhesions of biliary tract
Atrophy of biliary tract
Hypertrophy of biliary tract
Ulcer of biliary tract

K83.9 Disease of biliary tract, unspecified

● **K85** Acute pancreatitis
Inflammatory process in which pancreatic enzymes autodigest the gland
Includes ~~abscess of pancreas~~
~~acute necrosis of pancreas~~
acute (recurrent) pancreatitis
~~gangrene of (gangrenous) pancreas~~
~~hemorrhagic pancreatitis~~
~~infective necrosis of pancreas~~
subacute pancreatitis
~~suppurative pancreatitis~~
Ex: For category K85 CC codes: B25.2, K86.0-K86.1, K86.81-K86.9

● **K85.0** Idiopathic acute pancreatitis

K85.00 Idiopathic acute pancreatitis without necrosis or infection 🔊 ◀

K85.01 Idiopathic acute pancreatitis with uninfected necrosis 🔊 ◀

K85.02 Idiopathic acute pancreatitis with infected necrosis 🔊 ◀

◀ New ◀║║ Revised ~~deleted~~ Deleted Excludes 1 Excludes 2 Includes Use additional Code first Code also Unspecified
OGCR Official Guidelines ● Unacceptable Principal Diagnosis X Assign placeholder X 🔊 Use Additional Character(s) ▌ Manifestation Code **Coding Clinic**

- **K85.1   Biliary acute pancreatitis**
  Gallstone pancreatitis
  - **K85.10   Biliary acute pancreatitis without necrosis or infection** 🔹◀
  - **K85.11   Biliary acute pancreatitis with uninfected necrosis** 🔹◀
  - **K85.12   Biliary acute pancreatitis with infected necrosis** 🔹◀
- **K85.2   Alcohol induced acute pancreatitis**
  > **Excludes2**   alcohol induced chronic pancreatitis (K86.0)
  - **K85.20   Alcohol induced acute pancreatitis without necrosis or infection** 🔹◀
  - **K85.21   Alcohol induced acute pancreatitis with uninfected necrosis** 🔹◀
  - **K85.22   Alcohol induced acute pancreatitis with infected necrosis** 🔹◀
- **K85.3   Drug induced acute pancreatitis**
  Use additional code for adverse effect, if applicable, to identify drug (T36-T50 with fifth or sixth character 5)
  Use additional code to identify drug abuse and dependence (F11.-F17.-)
  - **K85.30   Drug induced acute pancreatitis without necrosis or infection** 🔹◀
  - **K85.31   Drug induced acute pancreatitis with uninfected necrosis** 🔹◀
  - **K85.32   Drug induced acute pancreatitis with infected necrosis** 🔹◀
- **K85.8   Other acute pancreatitis**
  - **K85.80   Other acute pancreatitis without necrosis or infection** 🔹◀
  - **K85.81   Other acute pancreatitis with uninfected necrosis** 🔹◀
  - **K85.82   Other acute pancreatitis with infected necrosis** 🔹◀
- **K85.9   Acute pancreatitis, unspecified**
  Pancreatitis NOS
  - **K85.90   Acute pancreatitis without necrosis or infection, unspecified** 🔹◀
  - **K85.91   Acute pancreatitis with uninfected necrosis, unspecified** 🔹◀
  - **K85.92   Acute pancreatitis with infected necrosis, unspecified** 🔹◀
- **K86   Other diseases of pancreas**
  > **Excludes2**   fibrocystic disease of pancreas (E84.-)
  > islet cell tumor (of pancreas) (D13.7)
  > pancreatic steatorrhea (K90.3)
  - **K86.0   Alcohol-induced chronic pancreatitis** 🔹
    Use additional code to identify:
    alcohol abuse and dependence (F10.-)
    Code also exocrine pancreatic insufficiency (K86.81) ◀
    > **Excludes2**   alcohol induced acute pancreatitis (K85.2-) ◀
    (Ex:) B25.2, E16.8, K85.00-K86.9

- **K86.1   Other chronic pancreatitis** 🔹
  Chronic pancreatitis NOS
  Infectious chronic pancreatitis
  Recurrent chronic pancreatitis
  Relapsing chronic pancreatitis
  Code also exocrine pancreatic insufficiency (K86.81) ◀
  (Ex:) B25.2, E16.8, K85.00-K86.9
- **K86.2   Cyst of pancreas** 🔹
  (Ex:) K86.2-K86.9
- **K86.3   Pseudocyst of pancreas** 🔹
  (Ex:) K86.2-K86.9
- **K86.8   Other specified diseases of pancreas**
  - **K86.81   Exocrine pancreatic insufficiency** ◀
  - **K86.89   Other specified diseases of pancreas** ◀
    Aseptic pancreatic necrosis, unrelated to acute pancreatitis ◀
    Atrophy of pancreas ◀
    Calculus of pancreas ◀
    Cirrhosis of pancreas ◀
    Fibrosis of pancreas ◀
    Pancreatic fat necrosis, unrelated to acute pancreatitis ◀
    Pancreatic infantilism ◀
    Pancreatic necrosis NOS, unrelated to acute pancreatitis ◀
- **K86.9   Disease of pancreas, unspecified**

▶ **K87   Disorders of gallbladder, biliary tract and pancreas in diseases classified elsewhere**
  Code first underlying disease
  > **Excludes1**   cytomegaloviral pancreatitis (B25.2)
  > mumps pancreatitis (B26.3)
  > syphilitic gallbladder (A52.74)
  > syphilitic pancreas (A52.74)
  > tuberculosis of gallbladder (A18.83)
  > tuberculosis of pancreas (A18.83)

OTHER DISEASES OF THE DIGESTIVE SYSTEM (K90-K95)

- **K90   Intestinal malabsorption**
  > **Excludes1**   intestinal malabsorption following gastrointestinal surgery (K91.2)
  (Ex:) **For category K90 cc does unless otherwise indicated:** E84.19, K90.0-K90.49, K90.89-K90.9, K91.2
  - **K90.0   Celiac disease**
    Celiac disease with steatorrhea ◀
    Gluten-sensitive enteropathy
    ~~Idiopathic steatorrhea~~
    Nontropical sprue
    Use additional code for associated disorders including:
    dermatitis herpetiformis (L13.0)
    gluten ataxia (G32.81)
    Code also exocrine pancreatic insufficiency (K86.81) ◀
  - **K90.1   Tropical sprue** 🔹
    Sprue NOS
    Tropical steatorrhea
  - **K90.2   Blind loop syndrome, not elsewhere classified** 🔹
    Blind loop syndrome NOS
    > **Excludes1**   congenital blind loop syndrome (Q43.8)
    > postsurgical blind loop syndrome (K91.2)
  - **K90.3   Pancreatic steatorrhea** 🔹
- **K90.4   Other malabsorption due to intolerance** ◀▥
    > **Excludes2**   gluten-sensitive enteropathy (K90.0)
    > lactose intolerance (E73.-)
    (Ex:) **For category K90.4 CC codes:** E84.19, K90.0-K90.3, K90.41, K90.49, K90.89-K90.9, K91.2
  - **K90.41   Non-celiac gluten sensitivity** 🔹◀
    Gluten sensitivity NOS ◀
    Non-celiac gluten sensitive enteropathy ◀
  - **K90.49   Malabsorption due to intolerance, not elsewhere classified** 🔹◀
    Malabsorption due to intolerance to carbohydrate ◀
    Malabsorption due to intolerance to fat ◀
    Malabsorption due to intolerance to protein ◀
    Malabsorption due to intolerance to starch ◀

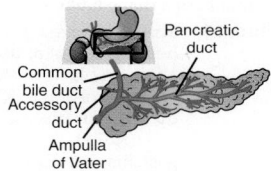

Figure 11-15   Pancreatic ductal system.

CHAPTER 11 (K00-K95)

CHAPTER 11 (K00–K95)

● K90.8   **Other intestinal malabsorption**

 K90.81   **Whipple's disease** 🔖
  (Ex:) K90.81

 K90.89   **Other intestinal malabsorption** 🔖

K90.9   **Intestinal malabsorption, unspecified** 🔖

● K91   **Intraoperative and postprocedural complications and disorders of digestive system, not elsewhere classified**

 Excludes2   complications of artificial opening of digestive system (K94.-)
  complications of bariatric procedures (K95.-)
  gastrojejunal ulcer (K28.-)
  postprocedural (radiation) retroperitoneal abscess (K68.11)
  radiation colitis (K52.0)
  radiation gastroenteritis (K52.0)
  radiation proctitis (K62.7)

K91.0   **Vomiting following gastrointestinal surgery**

K91.1   **Postgastric surgery syndromes**
 Dumping syndrome
 Postgastrectomy syndrome
 Postvagotomy syndrome

K91.2   **Postsurgical malabsorption, not elsewhere classified** 🔖
 Postsurgical blind loop syndrome

 Excludes1   malabsorption osteomalacia in adults (M83.2)
  malabsorption osteoporosis, postsurgical (M80.8-, M81.8)
 (Ex:) K90.3–K90.49, K90.89–K90.9, K91.2

K91.3   **Postprocedural intestinal obstruction** 🔖
 (Ex:) D78.81–D78.89, E36.8, E89.810–E89.89, H59.011–H59.019, H59.031–H59.099, H59.811–H59.89, H95.811–H95.89, I97.3, K91.3, K91.81–K91.83, K91.850–K91.89, K94.20–K95.89, L76.81–L76.82, M96.89, N98.1–N98.9, T81.710[A], T81.82X[A], T81.89X–T81.9XX[A]

K91.5   **Postcholecystectomy syndrome**

● K91.6   **Intraoperative hemorrhage and hematoma of a digestive system organ or structure complicating a procedure**

 Excludes1   intraoperative hemorrhage and hematoma of a digestive system organ or structure due to accidental puncture and laceration during a procedure (K91.7-)
 (Ex:) **For category K91.6 CC codes:** H95.811–H95.89, I85.01, I85.11, I97.3, K21.9, K22.8, K23–K25.0, K25.2, K25.4, K25.6, K26.0, K26.2, K26.4, K26.6, K27.0, K27.2, K27.4, K27.6, K28.0, K28.2, K28.4, K28.6, K29.01, K29.21, K29.31, K29.41, K29.51, K29.61, K29.71, K29.81, K29.91, K31.811, K55.21, K57.01, K57.11, K57.13, K57.21, K57.31, K57.33, K57.41, K57.51, K57.53, K57.81, K57.91, K57.93, K62.5, K91.61–K91.62, K91.840–K91.841, K91.870–K91.873, K92.0–K92.2, M96.89, N98.1–N98.9, P54.1–P54.3, T81.10X–T81.19X[A], T81.82X[A], T81.89X–T81.9XX[A]

 K91.61   **Intraoperative hemorrhage and hematoma of a digestive system organ or structure complicating a digestive system procedure** 🔖 ⬅
 K91.62   **Intraoperative hemorrhage and hematoma of a digestive system organ or structure complicating other procedure** 🔖

● K91.7   **Accidental puncture and laceration of a digestive system organ or structure during a procedure**
 (Ex:) **For category K91.7 CC codes:** D78.11–D78.12, D78.81–D78.89, E36.11–E36.8, E89.810–E89.89, G96.11, G97.41–G97.49, H59.011–H59.019, H59.031–H59.099, H59.211–H59.229, H59.811–H59.89, H95.31–H95.32, H95.811–H95.89, I97.3, I97.51–I97.52, J95.71–J95.72, K91.71–K91.72, L76.11–L76.12, L76.81–L76.82, M96.820–M96.821, M96.89, N98.1–N98.9, N99.71–N99.72, T81.82X[A], T81.89X–T81.9XX[A]

 K91.71   **Accidental puncture and laceration of a digestive system organ or structure during a digestive system procedure** 🔖
 K91.72   **Accidental puncture and laceration of a digestive system organ or structure during other procedure** 🔖

● K91.8   **Other intraoperative and postprocedural complications and disorders of digestive system**
 (Ex:) **For category K91.8 CC codes unless otherwise indicated:** See K91.3

 K91.81   **Other intraoperative complications of digestive system** 🔖
 K91.82   **Postprocedural hepatic failure** 🔖
 K91.83   **Postprocedural hepatorenal syndrome** 🔖

● K91.84   **Postprocedural hemorrhage of a digestive system organ or structure following a procedure** ⬅
 (Ex:) **For category K91.84 CC codes:** K91.6

 K91.840   **Postprocedural hemorrhage of a digestive system organ or structure following a digestive system procedure** 🔖 ⬅
  Coding Clinic: 2016, Q1, P15
 K91.841   **Postprocedural hemorrhage of a digestive system organ or structure following other procedure** 🔖 ⬅

● K91.85   **Complications of intestinal pouch**

 K91.850   **Pouchitis** 🔖
  Inflammation of internal ileoanal pouch
 K91.858   **Other complications of intestinal pouch** 🔖

K91.86   **Retained cholelithiasis following cholecystectomy** 🔖

● K91.87   **Postprocedural hematoma and seroma of a digestive system organ or structure following a procedure** ◀
 (Ex:) **For category K97.87 CC codes:** See K91.6

 K91.870   **Postprocedural hematoma of a digestive system organ or structure following a digestive system procedure** 🔖 ◀
 K91.871   **Postprocedural hematoma of a digestive system organ or structure following other procedure** 🔖 ◀
 K91.872   **Postprocedural seroma of a digestive system organ or structure following a digestive system procedure** 🔖 ◀
 K91.873   **Postprocedural seroma of a digestive system organ or structure following other procedure** 🔖 ◀

K91.89   **Other postprocedural complications and disorders of digestive system** 🔖

 Use additional code, if applicable, to further specify disorder
 Excludes2   postprocedural retroperitoneal abscess (K68.11)

● K92   **Other diseases of digestive system**
 Excludes1   neonatal gastrointestinal hemorrhage (P54.0–P54.3)
 (Ex:) **For category K92 CC codes unless otherwise indicated:** E16.4, I85.01, K22.10–K22.11, K22.6–K22.719, K25.0–K28.9, K29.01, K29.21, K29.31, K29.41, K29.51, K29.61, K29.71, K29.81, K29.91, K31.811, K55.21, K57.01, K57.11, K57.13, K57.21, K57.31, K57.33, K57.41, K57.51, K57.53, K57.81, K57.91, K57.93, K62.5, K92.0–K92.2

K92.0   **Hematemesis** 🔖

K92.1   **Melena** 🔖
 Excludes1   occult blood in feces (R19.5)

K92.2   **Gastrointestinal hemorrhage, unspecified** 🔖
 Gastric hemorrhage NOS
 Intestinal hemorrhage NOS
 Excludes1   acute hemorrhagic gastritis (K29.01)
  hemorrhage of anus and rectum (K62.5)
  angiodysplasia of stomach with hemorrhage (K31.811)
  diverticular disease with hemorrhage (K57.-)
  gastritis and duodenitis with hemorrhage (K29.-)
  peptic ulcer with hemorrhage (K25–K28)

◀ New   ◀▥ Revised   ~~deleted~~ Deleted   Excludes 1   Excludes 2   Includes   Use additional   Code first   Code also   Unspecified
OGCR Official Guidelines   ● Unacceptable Principal Diagnosis   X Assign placeholder X   ● Use Additional Character(s)   ▎ Manifestation Code   **Coding Clinic**

● **K92.8**   **Other specified diseases of the digestive system**

     K92.81   **Gastrointestinal mucositis (ulcerative)** 🗲

         Code also type of associated therapy, such as:
             antineoplastic and immunosuppressive
                drugs (T45.1X-)
             radiological procedure and radiotherapy
                (Y84.2)

         Excludes2   mucositis (ulcerative) of vagina
                   and vulva (N76.81)
                nasal mucositis (ulcerative)
                   (J34.81)
                oral mucositis (ulcerative)
                   (K12.3-)

         (Ex:) E16.4, I85.01, K22.10-K22.11, K22.6-K22.719, K25.0-K28.9,
             K29.01, K29.21, K29.31, K29.41, K29.51, K29.61, K29.71,
             K29.81, K29.91, K31.811, K31.89-K31.9, K55.21, K57.01,
             K57.11, K57.13, K57.21, K57.31, K57.33, K57.41, K57.51,
             K57.53, K57.81, K57.91, K57.93, K62.5, K92.0-K92.81

     K92.89   **Other specified diseases of the digestive system**

     K92.9   **Disease of digestive system, unspecified**

● **K94**   **Complications of artificial openings of the digestive system**

     ● **K94.0**   **Colostomy complications**

         (Ex:) For category K94.0 CC does unless otherwise indicated:
         K94.00-K94.19

         K94.00   **Colostomy complication, unspecified**

         K94.01   **Colostomy hemorrhage** 🗲

         K94.02   **Colostomy infection** 🗲

             Use additional code to specify type of
                infection, such as:
                cellulitis of abdominal wall (L03.311)
                sepsis (A40.-, A41.-)

         K94.03   **Colostomy malfunction** 🗲
             Mechanical complication of colostomy
             (Ex:) D78.81-D78.89, E36.8, E89.810-E89.89, H59.011-H59.019,
                H59.031-H59.099, H59.811-H59.89, H95.811-H95.89, I97.3,
                K91.3, K91.81-K91.83, K91.850-K91.89, K94.00-K95.89,
                L76.81-L76.82, M96.89, N98.1-N98.9, T81.710[A], T81.82X[A],
                T81.89X-T81.9XX[A]

         K94.09   **Other complications of colostomy** 🗲

     ● **K94.1**   **Enterostomy complications**

         (Ex:) For category K94.1 CC does unless otherwise indicated:
         K94.00-K94.19

         K94.10   **Enterostomy complication, unspecified**

         K94.11   **Enterostomy hemorrhage** 🗲

         K94.12   **Enterostomy infection** 🗲

             Use additional code to specify type of
                infection, such as:
                cellulitis of abdominal wall (L03.311)
                sepsis (A40.-, A41.-)

         K94.13   **Enterostomy malfunction** 🗲
             Mechanical complication of enterostomy
             (Ex:) See K94.03

         K94.19   **Other complications of enterostomy** 🗲

     ● **K94.2**   **Gastrostomy complications**

         K94.20   **Gastrostomy complication, unspecified**

         K94.21   **Gastrostomy hemorrhage**

         K94.22   **Gastrostomy infection** 🗲

             Use additional code to specify type of
                infection, such as:
                cellulitis of abdominal wall (L03.311)
                sepsis (A40.-, A41.-)
             (Ex:) See K91.3

         K94.23   **Gastrostomy malfunction** 🗲
             Mechanical complication of gastrostomy
             (Ex:) See K91.3

         K94.29   **Other complications of gastrostomy**

     ● **K94.3**   **Esophagostomy complications**

         (Ex:) For category K94.3 CC codes: See K91.3

         K94.30   **Esophagostomy complications, unspecified** 🗲

         K94.31   **Esophagostomy hemorrhage** 🗲

         K94.32   **Esophagostomy infection** 🗲

             Use additional code to identify the infection

         K94.33   **Esophagostomy malfunction** 🗲
             Mechanical complication of esophagostomy

         K94.39   **Other complications of esophagostomy** 🗲

● **K95**   **Complications of bariatric procedures**

     (Ex:) For category K95 CC codes: See K91.3

     ● **K95.0**   **Complications of gastric band procedure**

         K95.01   **Infection due to gastric band procedure** 🗲🗲

             Use additional code to specify type of infection
                or organism, such as:
                bacterial and viral infectious agents
                   (B95.-, B96.-)
                cellulitis of abdominal wall (L03.311)
                sepsis (A40.-, A41.-)

         K95.09   **Other complications of gastric band
             procedure** 🗲

             Use additional code, if applicable, to further
                specify complication

     ● **K95.8**   **Complications of other bariatric procedure**

         Excludes1   complications of gastric band surgery
                   (K95.0-)

         K95.81   **Infection due to other bariatric procedure** 🗲🗲

             Use additional code to specify type of infection
                or organism, such as:
                bacterial and viral infectious agents
                   (B95.-, B96.-)
                cellulitis of abdominal wall (L03.311)
                sepsis (A40.-, A41.-)

         K95.89   **Other complications of other bariatric
             procedure** 🗲

             Use additional code, if applicable, to further
                specify complication

CHAPTER 11 (K00-K95)

CHAPTER 12

DISEASES OF THE SKIN AND SUBCUTANEOUS TISSUE (L00-L99)

OGCR Chapter-Specific Coding Guidelines

12. **Chapter 12: Diseases of the Skin and Subcutaneous Tissue (L00-L99)**

a. **Pressure ulcer stage codes**

1) **Pressure ulcer stages**

Codes from category L89, Pressure ulcer, identify the site of the pressure ulcer as well as the stage of the ulcer.

The ICD-10-CM classifies pressure ulcer stages based on severity, which is designated by stages 1-4, unspecified stage and unstageable.

Assign as many codes from category L89 as needed to identify all the pressure ulcers the patient has, if applicable.

2) **Unstageable pressure ulcers**

Assignment of the code for unstageable pressure ulcer (L89.--0) should be based on the clinical documentation. These codes are used for pressure ulcers whose stage cannot be clinically determined (e.g., the ulcer is covered by eschar or has been treated with a skin or muscle graft) and pressure ulcers that are documented as deep tissue injury but not documented as due to trauma. This code should not be confused with the codes for unspecified stage (L89.--9). When there is no documentation regarding the stage of the pressure ulcer, assign the appropriate code for unspecified stage (L89.--9).

3) **Documented pressure ulcer stage**

Assignment of the pressure ulcer stage code should be guided by clinical documentation of the stage or documentation of the terms found in the Alphabetic Index. For clinical terms describing the stage that are not found in the Alphabetic Index, and there is no documentation of the stage, the provider should be queried.

4) **Patients admitted with pressure ulcers documented as healed**

No code is assigned if the documentation states that the pressure ulcer is completely healed.

5) **Patients admitted with pressure ulcers documented as healing**

Pressure ulcers described as healing should be assigned the appropriate pressure ulcer stage code based on the documentation in the medical record. If the documentation does not provide information about the stage of the healing pressure ulcer, assign the appropriate code for unspecified stage.

If the documentation is unclear as to whether the patient has a current (new) pressure ulcer or if the patient is being treated for a healing pressure ulcer, query the provider.

For ulcers that were present on admission but healed at the time of discharge, assign the code for the site and stage of the pressure ulcer at the time of admission.

6) **Patient admitted with pressure ulcer evolving into another stage during the admission**

If a patient is admitted with a pressure ulcer at one stage and it progresses to a higher stage, **two separate codes should be assigned: one code for the site and stage of the ulcer on admission and a second code for the same ulcer site and the highest stage reported during the stay.**

Figure 12-1 Furuncle, also known as a boil, is a staphylococcal infection. The organism enters the body through a hair follicle and so furuncles usually appear in hairy areas of the body. A cluster of furuncles is known as a carbuncle and involves infection into the deep subcutaneous fascia. These usually appear on the back and neck. (**B** from Habif: Clinical Dermatology, ed 5, Mosby, 2009)

CHAPTER 12

DISEASES OF THE SKIN AND SUBCUTANEOUS TISSUE (L00-L99)

Excludes2   certain conditions originating in the perinatal period (P04-P96)
certain infectious and parasitic diseases (A00-B99)
complications of pregnancy, childbirth and the puerperium (O00-O9A)
congenital malformations, deformations, and chromosomal abnormalities (Q00-Q99)
endocrine, nutritional and metabolic diseases (E00-E88)
lipomelanotic reticulosis (I89.8)
neoplasms (C00-D49)
symptoms, signs and abnormal clinical and laboratory findings, not elsewhere classified (R00-R94)
systemic connective tissue disorders (M30-M36)
viral warts (B07.-)

This chapter contains the following blocks:

L00-L08	Infections of the skin and subcutaneous tissue
L10-L14	Bullous disorders
L20-L30	Dermatitis and eczema
L40-L45	Papulosquamous disorders
L49-L54	Urticaria and erythema
L55-L59	Radiation-related disorders of the skin and subcutaneous tissue
L60-L75	Disorders of skin appendages
L76	Intraoperative and postprocedural complications of skin and subcutaneous tissue
L80-L99	Other disorders of the skin and subcutaneous tissue

◀ New   ◀▥ Revised   ~~deleted~~ Deleted   Excludes 1   Excludes 2   Includes   Use additional   Code first   Code also   Unspecified
OGCR Official Guidelines   ● Unacceptable Principal Diagnosis   X Assign placeholder X   ● Use Additional Character(s)   ▌ Manifestation Code   **Coding Clinic**

INFECTIONS OF THE SKIN AND SUBCUTANEOUS TISSUE (L00-L08)

Use additional code (B95-B97) to identify infectious agent.

Excludes2 hordeolum (H00.0)
infective dermatitis (L30.3)
local infections of skin classified in Chapter 1
lupus panniculitis (L93.2)
panniculitis NOS (M79.3)
panniculitis of neck and back (M54.0-)
Perlèche NOS (K13.0)
Perlèche due to candidiasis (B37.0)
Perlèche due to riboflavin deficiency (E53.0)
pyogenic granuloma (L98.0)
relapsing panniculitis [Weber-Christian] (M35.6)
viral warts (B07.-)
zoster (B02.-)

L00   Staphylococcal scalded skin syndrome
Ritter's disease
Use additional code to identify percentage of skin exfoliation (L49.-)

Excludes1 bullous impetigo (L01.03)
pemphigus neonatorum (L01.03)
toxic epidermal necrolysis [Lyell] (L51.2)

● **L01   Impetigo**
Contagious skin infection caused by a streptococcus or staphylococcus aureus, common skin infections among children

Excludes1 impetigo herpetiformis (L40.1)

● **L01.0   Impetigo**
Impetigo contagiosa
Impetigo vulgaris

L01.00   Impetigo, unspecified
Impetigo NOS

L01.01   Non-bullous impetigo

L01.02   Bockhart's impetigo
Impetigo follicularis
Perifolliculitis NOS
Superficial pustular perifolliculitis

L01.03   Bullous impetigo
Impetigo neonatorum
Pemphigus neonatorum
Neonate = newborn

L01.09   Other impetigo
Ulcerative impetigo

L01.1   Impetiginization of other dermatoses

● **L02   Cutaneous abscess, furuncle and carbuncle**
Use additional code to identify organism (B95-B96)

Excludes2 abscess of anus and rectal regions (K61.-)
abscess of female genital organs (external) (N76.4)
abscess of male genital organs (external) (N48.2, N49.-)

● **L02.0   Cutaneous abscess, furuncle and carbuncle of face**

Excludes2 abscess of ear, external (H60.0)
abscess of eyelid (H00.0)
abscess of head [any part, except face] (L02.8)
abscess of lacrimal gland (H04.0)
abscess of lacrimal passages (H04.3)
abscess of mouth (K12.2)
abscess of nose (J34.0)
abscess of orbit (H05.0)
submandibular abscess (K12.2)

L02.01   Cutaneous abscess of face 🔹
(Ex): No exclusions

L02.02   Furuncle of face
Boil of face
Folliculitis of face

L02.03   Carbuncle of face

● **L02.1   Cutaneous abscess, furuncle and carbuncle of neck**

L02.11   Cutaneous abscess of neck 🔹
(Ex): A17.9, A18.4, A18.82, A18.84, A18.89, A48.2-A48.4, A48.8-A49.9, B78.1, B95.0-B96.89, E83.2, L02.11, L02.811-L02.818, L02.91, L03.221-L03.222, L03.811-L03.91, L08.0-L08.9, L44.8-L45, L73.2, L88, L92.8, L94.2, L94.4, L98.0, L98.3, L98.7, L98.8, L99, Z16.10-Z16.39

L02.12   Furuncle of neck
Boil of neck
Folliculitis of neck

L02.13   Carbuncle of neck

● **L02.2   Cutaneous abscess, furuncle and carbuncle of trunk**

Excludes1 non-newborn omphalitis (L08.82)
omphalitis of newborn (P38.-)

Excludes2 abscess of breast (N61.1) ◀▥
abscess of buttocks (L02.3)
abscess of female external genital organs (N76.4)
abscess of male external genital organs (N48.2, N49.-)
abscess of hip (L02.4)

● **L02.21   Cutaneous abscess of trunk**
(Ex): For category L02.21 CC codes: A17.9, A18.4, A18.82, A18.84, A18.89, A48.2-A48.4, A48.8-A49.9, B78.1, B95.0-B96.89, E83.2, L02.211-L02.219, L02.811-L02.818, L02.91, L03.311-L03.316, L03.319-L03.326, L03.329-L03.91, L08.0, L08.81-L08.9, L44.8-L45, L73.2, L88, L92.8, L94.2, L94.4, L98.0, L98.3, L98.7, L98.8, L99, Z16.10-Z16.39

L02.211   Cutaneous abscess of abdominal wall 🔹

L02.212   Cutaneous abscess of back [any part, except buttock] 🔹

L02.213   Cutaneous abscess of chest wall 🔹

L02.214   Cutaneous abscess of groin 🔹

L02.215   Cutaneous abscess of perineum 🔹

L02.216   Cutaneous abscess of umbilicus 🔹

L02.219   Cutaneous abscess of trunk, unspecified 🔹

● **L02.22   Furuncle of trunk**
Boil of trunk
Folliculitis of trunk

L02.221   Furuncle of abdominal wall

L02.222   Furuncle of back [any part, except buttock]

L02.223   Furuncle of chest wall

L02.224   Furuncle of groin

L02.225   Furuncle of perineum

L02.226   Furuncle of umbilicus

L02.229   Furuncle of trunk, unspecified

● **L02.23   Carbuncle of trunk**

L02.231   Carbuncle of abdominal wall

L02.232   Carbuncle of back [any part, except buttock]

L02.233   Carbuncle of chest wall

L02.234   Carbuncle of groin

L02.235   Carbuncle of perineum

L02.236   Carbuncle of umbilicus

L02.239   Carbuncle of trunk, unspecified

● **L02.3   Cutaneous abscess, furuncle and carbuncle of buttock**

Excludes1 pilonidal cyst with abscess (L05.01)

L02.31   Cutaneous abscess of buttock 🔹
Cutaneous abscess of gluteal region
(Ex): A17.9, A18.4, A18.82, A18.84, A18.89, A48.2-A48.4, A48.8-A49.9, B78.1, B95.0-B96.89, E83.2, L02.31, L02.811-L02.818, L02.91, L03.317, L03.327, L03.811-L03.91, L08.0, L08.81-L08.9, L44.8-L45, L73.2, L88, L92.8, L94.2, L94.4, L98.0, L98.3, L98.7, L98.8, L99, Z16.10-Z16.39

L02.32   **Furuncle of buttock**
Boil of buttock
Folliculitis of buttock
Furuncle of gluteal region

L02.33   **Carbuncle of buttock**
Carbuncle of gluteal region

● **L02.4**   **Cutaneous abscess, furuncle and carbuncle of limb**

Excludes2   Cutaneous abscess, furuncle and carbuncle of groin (L02.214, L02.224, L02.234)
Cutaneous abscess, furuncle and carbuncle of hand (L02.5-)
Cutaneous abscess, furuncle and carbuncle of foot (L02.6-)

● **L02.41**   **Cutaneous abscess of limb**

L02.411   **Cutaneous abscess of right axilla** 🔗
(Ex:) A17.9, A18.4, A18.82, A18.84, A18.89, A48.2-A48.4, A48.8-A49.9, B78.1, B95.0-B96.89, E83.2, L02.411-L02.414, L02.811-L02.818, L02.91, L03.111-L03.111, L03.121-L03.124, L03.811-L03.91, L08.0, L08.81-L08.9, L44.8-L45, L73.2, L88, L92.8, L94.2, L94.4, L98.0, L98.3, L98.7, L98.8, L99, Z16.10-Z16.39

L02.412   **Cutaneous abscess of left axilla** 🔗
(Ex:) See L02.411

L02.413   **Cutaneous abscess of right upper limb** 🔗
(Ex:) See L02.411

L02.414   **Cutaneous abscess of left upper limb** 🔗
(Ex:) See L02.411

L02.415   **Cutaneous abscess of right lower limb** 🔗
(Ex:) A17.9, A18.4, A18.82, A18.84, A18.89, A48.2-A48.4, A48.8-A49.9, B78.1, B95.0-B96.89, E83.2, L02.415-L02.419, L02.811-L02.818, L02.91, L03.115-L03.119, L03.125-L03.129, L03.811-L03.91, L08.0, L08.81-L08.9, L44.8-L45, L73.2, L88, L92.8, L94.2, L94.4, L98.0, L98.3, L98.7, L98.8, L99, Z16.10-Z16.39

L02.416   **Cutaneous abscess of left lower limb** 🔗
(Ex:) See L02.415

L02.419   **Cutaneous abscess of limb, unspecified** 🔗
(Ex:) See L02.415

● **L02.42**   **Furuncle of limb**
Boil of limb
Folliculitis of limb

L02.421   **Furuncle of right axilla**

L02.422   **Furuncle of left axilla**

L02.423   **Furuncle of right upper limb**

L02.424   **Furuncle of left upper limb**

L02.425   **Furuncle of right lower limb**

L02.426   **Furuncle of left lower limb**

L02.429   **Furuncle of limb, unspecified**

● **L02.43**   **Carbuncle of limb**

L02.431   **Carbuncle of right axilla**

L02.432   **Carbuncle of left axilla**

L02.433   **Carbuncle of right upper limb**

L02.434   **Carbuncle of left upper limb**

L02.435   **Carbuncle of right lower limb**

L02.436   **Carbuncle of left lower limb**

L02.439   **Carbuncle of limb, unspecified**

● **L02.5**   **Cutaneous abscess, furuncle and carbuncle of hand**

● **L02.51**   **Cutaneous abscess of hand**
(Ex:) For category L02.51 CC codes: A17.9, A18.4, A18.82, A18.84, A18.89, A48.2-A48.4, A48.8-A49.9, B78.1, B95.0-B96.89, E83.2, L02.511-L02.519, L02.811-L02.818, L02.91, L03.811-L03.91, L08.0, L08.81-L08.9, L44.8-L45, L73.2, L88, L92.8, L94.2, L94.4, L98.0, L98.3, L98.7, L98.8, L99, Z16.10-Z16.39

L02.511   **Cutaneous abscess of right hand** 🔗

L02.512   **Cutaneous abscess of left hand** 🔗

L02.519   **Cutaneous abscess of unspecified hand** 🔗

● **L02.52**   **Furuncle hand**
Boil of hand
Folliculitis of hand

L02.521   **Furuncle right hand**

L02.522   **Furuncle left hand**

L02.529   **Furuncle unspecified hand**

● **L02.53**   **Carbuncle of hand**

L02.531   **Carbuncle of right hand**

L02.532   **Carbuncle of left hand**

L02.539   **Carbuncle of unspecified hand**

● **L02.6**   **Cutaneous abscess, furuncle and carbuncle of foot**

● **L02.61**   **Cutaneous abscess of foot**
(Ex:) For category L02.61 CC codes: A17.9, A18.4, A18.82, A18.84, A18.89, A48.2-A48.4, A48.8-A49.9, B78.1, B95.0-B96.89, E83.2, L02.611-L02.619, L02.811-L02.818, L02.91, L03.811-L03.91, L08.0, L08.81-L08.9, L44.8-L45, L73.2, L88, L92.8, L94.2, L94.4, L98.0, L98.3, L98.7, L98.8, L99, Z16.10-Z16.39

L02.611   **Cutaneous abscess of right foot** 🔗

L02.612   **Cutaneous abscess of left foot** 🔗

L02.619   **Cutaneous abscess of unspecified foot** 🔗

● **L02.62**   **Furuncle of foot**
Boil of foot
Folliculitis of foot

L02.621   **Furuncle of right foot**

L02.622   **Furuncle of left foot**

L02.629   **Furuncle of unspecified foot**

● **L02.63**   **Carbuncle of foot**

L02.631   **Carbuncle of right foot**

L02.632   **Carbuncle of left foot**

L02.639   **Carbuncle of unspecified foot**

● **L02.8**   **Cutaneous abscess, furuncle and carbuncle of other sites**

● **L02.81**   **Cutaneous abscess of other sites**
(Ex:) For category L02.81 CC codes: A17.9, A18.4, A18.82, A18.84, A18.89, A48.2-A48.4, A48.8-A49.9, B78.1, B95.0-B96.89, E83.2, L02.811-L02.818, L02.91, L03.811-L03.91, L08.0, L08.81-L08.9, L44.8-L45, L73.2, L88, L92.8, L94.2, L94.4, L98.0, L98.3, L98.7, L98.8, L99, Z16.10-Z16.39

L02.811   **Cutaneous abscess of head [any part, except face]** 🔗

L02.818   **Cutaneous abscess of other sites** 🔗

● **L02.82**   **Furuncle of other sites**
Boil of other sites
Folliculitis of other sites

L02.821   **Furuncle of head [any part, except face]**

L02.828   **Furuncle of other sites**

● **L02.83**   **Carbuncle of other sites**

L02.831   **Carbuncle of head [any part, except face]**

L02.838   **Carbuncle of other sites**

● **L02.9**   **Cutaneous abscess, furuncle and carbuncle, unspecified**

L02.91   **Cutaneous abscess, unspecified** 🔗
(Ex:) See L02.81

L02.92   **Furuncle, unspecified**
Boil NOS
Furunculosis NOS

L02.93   **Carbuncle, unspecified**

◀ New   ◀▦ Revised   ~~deleted~~ Deleted   Excludes 1   Excludes 2   Includes   Use additional   Code first   Code also   Unspecified
OGCR Official Guidelines   ● Unacceptable Principal Diagnosis   X Assign placeholder X   ● Use Additional Character(s)   ▸ Manifestation Code   **Coding Clinic**

Item 12-1   **Onychia** is an inflammation of the tissue surrounding the nail with pus accumulation and loss of the nail, resulting from microscopic pathogens entering through small wounds. **Paronychia** is a nail disease also known as felon or whitlow and is a bacterial or fungal infection.

● **L03**   **Cellulitis and acute lymphangitis**
     Excludes2   cellulitis of anal and rectal region (K61.-)
                     cellulitis of external auditory canal (H60.1)
                     cellulitis of eyelid (H00.0)
                     cellulitis of female external genital organs (N76.4)
                     cellulitis of lacrimal apparatus (H04.3)
                     cellulitis of male external genital organs (N48.2, N49.-)
                     cellulitis of mouth (K12.2)
                     cellulitis of nose (J34.0)
                     eosinophilic cellulitis [Wells] (L98.3)
                     febrile neutrophilic dermatosis [Sweet] (L98.2)
                     lymphangitis (chronic) (subacute) (I89.1)

● **L03.0**   **Cellulitis and acute lymphangitis of finger and toe**
     Infection of nail
     Onychia
     Paronychia
     Perionychia

  ● **L03.01**   **Cellulitis of finger**
       Felon
       Whitlow
       Excludes1   herpetic whitlow (B00.89)
       L03.011   **Cellulitis of right finger**
       L03.012   **Cellulitis of left finger**
       L03.019   **Cellulitis of unspecified finger**

  ● **L03.02**   **Acute lymphangitis of finger**
       Hangnail with lymphangitis of finger
       L03.021   **Acute lymphangitis of right finger**
       L03.022   **Acute lymphangitis of left finger**
       L03.029   **Acute lymphangitis of unspecified finger**

  ● **L03.03**   **Cellulitis of toe**
       L03.031   **Cellulitis of right toe**
       L03.032   **Cellulitis of left toe**
       L03.039   **Cellulitis of unspecified toe**

  ● **L03.04**   **Acute lymphangitis of toe**
       Hangnail with lymphangitis of toe
       L03.041   **Acute lymphangitis of right toe**
       L03.042   **Acute lymphangitis of left toe**
       L03.049   **Acute lymphangitis of unspecified toe**

● **L03.1**   **Cellulitis and acute lymphangitis of other parts of limb**
  ● **L03.11**   **Cellulitis of other parts of limb**
       Excludes2   cellulitis of fingers (L03.01-)
                       cellulitis of toes (L03.03-)
                       groin (L03.314)
       L03.111   **Cellulitis of right axilla** 🏥
              Ⓔ See L02.411
       L03.112   **Cellulitis of left axilla** 🏥
              Ⓔ See L02.411
       L03.113   **Cellulitis of right upper limb** 🏥
              Ⓔ See L02.411
       L03.114   **Cellulitis of left upper limb** 🏥
              Ⓔ See L02.411
       L03.115   **Cellulitis of right lower limb** 🏥
              Ⓔ See L02.415
       L03.116   **Cellulitis of left lower limb** 🏥
              Ⓔ See L02.415
       L03.119   **Cellulitis of unspecified part of limb** 🏥
              Ⓔ See L02.415

● **L03.12**   **Acute lymphangitis of other parts of limb**
       Excludes2   acute lymphangitis of fingers (L03.2-)
                       acute lymphangitis of toes (L03.04-)
                       acute lymphangitis of groin (L03.324)
       L03.121   **Acute lymphangitis of right axilla** 🏥
              Ⓔ See L02.411
       L03.122   **Acute lymphangitis of left axilla** 🏥
              Ⓔ See L02.411
       L03.123   **Acute lymphangitis of right upper limb** 🏥
              Ⓔ See L02.411
       L03.124   **Acute lymphangitis of left upper limb** 🏥
              Ⓔ See L02.411
       L03.125   **Acute lymphangitis of right lower limb** 🏥
              Ⓔ See L02.415
       L03.126   **Acute lymphangitis of left lower limb** 🏥
              Ⓔ See L02.415
       L03.129   **Acute lymphangitis of unspecified part of limb** 🏥
              Ⓔ See L02.415

● **L03.2**   **Cellulitis and acute lymphangitis of face and neck**
  ● **L03.21**   **Cellulitis and acute lymphangitis of face**
       L03.211   **Cellulitis of face** 🏥
           Excludes2   abscess of orbit (H05.01-) ◀
                       cellulitis of ear (H60.1-)
                       cellulitis of eyelid (H00.0-)
                       cellulitis of head (L03.81)
                       cellulitis of lacrimal apparatus (H04.3)
                       cellulitis of lip (K13.0)
                       cellulitis of mouth (K12.2)
                       cellulitis of nose (internal) (J34.0)
                       cellulitis of orbit (H05.01-) ◀═
                       cellulitis of scalp (L03.81)
           Ⓔ A17.9, A18.4, A18.82, A18.84, A18.89, A48.2-A48.4, A48.8-A49.9, B78.1, B95.0-B96.89, E83.2, L02.811-L02.818, L02.91, L03.211, L03.213, L03.811-L03.91, L08.0, L08.81-L08.9, L44.8-L45, L73.2, L88, L92.8, L94.2, L94.4, L98.0, L98.3, L98.7, L98.8, L99, Z16.10-Z16.39
       L03.212   **Acute lymphangitis of face** 🏥
              Ⓔ No exclusions
       L03.213   **Periorbital cellulitis** 🏥 ◀
           Preseptal cellulitis ◀
           Ⓔ See L03.211

  ● **L03.22**   **Cellulitis and acute lymphangitis of neck**
       Ⓔ **For category L03.22 CC codes:** See L02.11
       L03.221   **Cellulitis of neck** 🏥
       L03.222   **Acute lymphangitis of neck** 🏥

CHAPTER 12 (L00-L99)

Item 12–2 Cellulitis is an acute spreading bacterial infection below the surface of the skin characterized by redness (erythema), warmth, swelling, pain, fever, chills, and enlarged lymph nodes ("swollen glands").

● **L03.3   Cellulitis and acute lymphangitis of trunk**

● **L03.31   Cellulitis of trunk**

Excludes2   cellulitis of anal and rectal regions (K61.-)
cellulitis of breast NOS (N61.0) ◄▪▪
cellulitis of female external genital organs (N76.4)
cellulitis of male external genital organs (N48.2, N49.-)
omphalitis of newborn (P38.-)
puerperal cellulitis of breast (O91.2)

Ⓔ **For category L03.31 CC codes unless otherwise indicated:** See L02.21

L03.311   **Cellulitis of abdominal wall** 🅒

Excludes2   cellulitis of umbilicus (L03.316)
cellulitis of groin (L03.314)

L03.312   **Cellulitis of back [any part except buttock]** 🅒

L03.313   **Cellulitis of chest wall** 🅒

L03.314   **Cellulitis of groin** 🅒

L03.315   **Cellulitis of perineum** 🅒

L03.316   **Cellulitis of umbilicus** 🅒

L03.317   **Cellulitis of buttock** 🅒
Ⓔ See L02.31

L03.319   **Cellulitis of trunk, unspecified** 🅒

● **L03.32   Acute lymphangitis of trunk**
Ⓔ **For category L03.32 CC codes unless otherwise indicated:** See L02.21

L03.321   **Acute lymphangitis of abdominal wall** 🅒

L03.322   **Acute lymphangitis of back [any part except buttock]** 🅒

L03.323   **Acute lymphangitis of chest wall** 🅒

L03.324   **Acute lymphangitis of groin** 🅒

L03.325   **Acute lymphangitis of perineum** 🅒

L03.326   **Acute lymphangitis of umbilicus** 🅒

L03.327   **Acute lymphangitis of buttock** 🅒
Ⓔ See L02.31

L03.329   **Acute lymphangitis of trunk, unspecified** 🅒

● **L03.8   Cellulitis and acute lymphangitis of other sites**
Ⓔ **For category L03.8 CC codes:** See L02.81

● **L03.81   Cellulitis of other sites**

L03.811   **Cellulitis of head [any part, except face]** 🅒
Cellulitis of scalp

Excludes2   cellulitis of face (L03.211)

L03.818   **Cellulitis of other sites** 🅒

● **L03.89   Acute lymphangitis of other sites**

L03.891   **Acute lymphangitis of head [any part, except face]** 🅒

L03.898   **Acute lymphangitis of other sites** 🅒

● **L03.9   Cellulitis and acute lymphangitis, unspecified**
Ⓔ **For category L03.9 CC codes:** See L02.81

L03.90   **Cellulitis, unspecified** 🅒

L03.91   **Acute lymphangitis, unspecified** 🅒

Excludes1   lymphangitis NOS (I89.1)

● **L04   Acute lymphadenitis**
Short-term inflammation of lymph nodes which can be regionalized to involve a given area of the lymph system or systemic involving much of the body

Includes   abscess (acute) of lymph nodes, except mesenteric
acute lymphadenitis, except mesenteric

Excludes1   chronic or subacute lymphadenitis, except mesenteric (I88.1)
enlarged lymph nodes (R59.-)
human immunodeficiency virus [HIV] disease resulting in generalized lymphadenopathy (B20)
lymphadenitis NOS (I88.9)
nonspecific mesenteric lymphadenitis (I88.0)

L04.0   **Acute lymphadenitis of face, head and neck**

L04.1   **Acute lymphadenitis of trunk**

L04.2   **Acute lymphadenitis of upper limb**
Acute lymphadenitis of axilla
Acute lymphadenitis of shoulder

L04.3   **Acute lymphadenitis of lower limb**
Acute lymphadenitis of hip

Excludes2   acute lymphadenitis of groin (L04.1)

L04.8   **Acute lymphadenitis of other sites**

L04.9   **Acute lymphadenitis, unspecified**

● **L05   Pilonidal cyst and sinus**

● **L05.0   Pilonidal cyst and sinus with abscess**
Ⓔ **For category L05.0 CC codes:** L05.01-L05.92, L44.8-L45, L94.2, L94.4, L98.7, L98.8, L99

L05.01   **Pilonidal cyst with abscess** 🅒
Pilonidal abscess
Pilonidal dimple with abscess
Postanal dimple with abscess

Excludes2   congenital sacral dimple (Q82.6) ◄
parasacral dimple (Q82.6) ◄

L05.02   **Pilonidal sinus with abscess** 🅒
Coccygeal fistula with abscess
Coccygeal sinus with abscess
Pilonidal fistula with abscess

● **L05.9   Pilonidal cyst and sinus without abscess**

L05.91   **Pilonidal cyst without abscess**
Pilonidal dimple
Postanal dimple
Pilonidal cyst NOS

Excludes2   congenital sacral dimple (Q82.6) ◄
parasacral dimple (Q82.6) ◄

L05.92   **Pilonidal sinus without abscess**
Coccygeal fistula
Coccygeal sinus without abscess
Pilonidal fistula

● **L08   Other local infections of skin and subcutaneous tissue**

L08.0   **Pyoderma**
Dermatitis gangrenosa
Purulent dermatitis
Septic dermatitis
Suppurative dermatitis

Excludes1   pyoderma gangrenosum (L88)
pyoderma vegetans (L08.81)

Figure 12-2   Impetigo. A thick, honey-yellow adherent crust covers the entire eroded surface. (From Habif: Clinical Dermatology, ed 4, Mosby, Inc., 2004)

Item 12–3 Abscess is a localized collection of pus in tissues or organs and is a sign of infection resulting in swelling and inflammation.

Item 12–4 Pilonidal cyst, also called a coccygeal cyst, is the result of a disorder called pilonidal disease. The cyst usually contains hair and pus.

◄ New   ◄▪▪ Revised   ~~deleted~~ Deleted | Excludes 1 | | Excludes 2 | | Includes | | Use additional | | Code first | | Code also | | Unspecified |

OGCR Official Guidelines   ● Unacceptable Principal Diagnosis   X Assign placeholder X   ● Use Additional Character(s)   ▶ Manifestation Code   **Coding Clinic**

L08.1   Erythrasma 🏵
> (Ex) A42.81-A42.9, A43.1-A43.9, B47.1, L08.

● **L08.8   Other specified local infections of the skin and subcutaneous tissue**

> **L08.81   Pyoderma vegetans**
>> **Excludes1**   pyoderma gangrenosum (L88)
>> pyoderma NOS (L08.0)
>
> **L08.82   Omphalitis not of newborn**
>> **Excludes1**   omphalitis of newborn (P38.-)
>
> **L08.89   Other specified local infections of the skin and subcutaneous tissue**

L08.9   Local infection of the skin and subcutaneous tissue, unspecified

BULLOUS DISORDERS (L10-L14)

> **Excludes1**   benign familial pemphigus [Hailey-Hailey] (Q82.8)
> staphylococcal scalded skin syndrome (L00)
> toxic epidermal necrolysis [Lyell] (L51.2)

● **L10   Pemphigus**
> **Excludes1**   pemphigus neonatorum (L01.03)
> (Ex) **For category L10 CC codes:** L10.0-L10.9, L12.0-L12.1, L12.8-L12.9, L13.8-L14, L44.8-L45, L94.2, L94.4, L98.7, L98.8, L99

L10.0   Pemphigus vulgaris 🏵
L10.1   Pemphigus vegetans 🏵
L10.2   Pemphigus foliaceous 🏵
L10.3   Brazilian pemphigus [fogo selvagem] 🏵
L10.4   Pemphigus erythematosus 🏵
> Senear-Usher syndrome

L10.5   Drug-induced pemphigus 🏵
> Use additional code for adverse effect, if applicable, to identify drug (T36-T50 with fifth or sixth character 5)

● **L10.8   Other pemphigus**
> **L10.81   Paraneoplastic pemphigus** 🏵
> **L10.89   Other pemphigus** 🏵

L10.9   Pemphigus, unspecified 🏵

● **L11   Other acantholytic disorders**
> **L11.0   Acquired keratosis follicularis**
>> **Excludes1**   keratosis follicularis (congenital) [Darier-White] (Q82.8)
>
> **L11.1   Transient acantholytic dermatosis [Grover]**
> **L11.8   Other specified acantholytic disorders**
> **L11.9   Acantholytic disorder, unspecified**

● **L12   Pemphigoid**
> **Excludes1**   herpes gestationis (O26.4-)
> impetigo herpetiformis (L40.1)

L12.0   Bullous pemphigoid 🏵
> (Ex) See L10

L12.1   Cicatricial pemphigoid
> Benign mucous membrane pemphigoid

L12.2   Chronic bullous disease of childhood   P
> Juvenile dermatitis herpetiformis

● **L12.3   Acquired epidermolysis bullosa**
> **Excludes1**   epidermolysis bullosa (congenital) (Q81.-)
> (Ex) **For category L12.3 CC codes:** L00, L12.30-L12.35, L26, L30.4, L44.8-L45, L51.0-L54, L71.0-L71.9, L92.0, L93.0-L93.2, L94.2, L94.4, L95.1, L98.2, L98.7, L98.8, L99

> **L12.30   Acquired epidermolysis bullosa, unspecified** 🏵
> **L12.31   Epidermolysis bullosa due to drug** 🏵
>> Use additional code for adverse effect, if applicable, to identify drug (T36-T50 with fifth or sixth character 5)
>
> **L12.35   Other acquired epidermolysis bullosa** 🏵

L12.8   Other pemphigoid 🏵
> (Ex) See L10

L12.9   Pemphigoid, unspecified 🏵
> (Ex) See L10

● **L13   Other bullous disorders**
> **L13.0   Dermatitis herpetiformis**
>> Duhring's disease
>> Hydroa herpetiformis
>> **Excludes1**   juvenile dermatitis herpetiformis (L12.2)
>> senile dermatitis herpetiformis (L12.0)
>
> **L13.1   Subcorneal pustular dermatitis**
>> Sneddon-Wilkinson disease
>
> **L13.8   Other specified bullous disorders**
> **L13.9   Bullous disorder, unspecified**

▷ **L14   *Bullous disorders in diseases classified elsewhere***
> *Code first* underlying disease

DERMATITIS AND ECZEMA (L20-L30)

Note: In this block the terms dermatitis and eczema are used synonymously and interchangeably.

> **Excludes2**   chronic (childhood) granulomatous disease (D71)
> dermatitis gangrenosa (L08.0)
> dermatitis herpetiformis (L13.0)
> dry skin dermatitis (L85.3)
> factitial dermatitis (L98.1)
> perioral dermatitis (L71.0)
> radiation-related disorders of the skin and subcutaneous tissue (L55-L59)
> stasis dermatitis (I87.2) ◀▦

● **L20   Atopic dermatitis**
> **L20.0   Besnier's prurigo**

● **L20.8   Other atopic dermatitis**
> **Excludes2**   circumscribed neurodermatitis (L28.0)
>
> **L20.81   Atopic neurodermatitis**
>> Diffuse neurodermatitis
>
> **L20.82   Flexural eczema**
> **L20.83   Infantile (acute) (chronic) eczema**   P
> **L20.84   Intrinsic (allergic) eczema**
> **L20.89   Other atopic dermatitis**

L20.9   Atopic dermatitis, unspecified

● **L21   Seborrheic dermatitis**
> **Excludes2**   infective dermatitis (L30.3)
> seborrheic keratosis (L82.-)

L21.0   Seborrhea capitis   P
> Cradle cap

L21.1   Seborrheic infantile dermatitis   P
L21.8   Other seborrheic dermatitis
L21.9   Seborrheic dermatitis, unspecified
> Seborrhea NOS

Item 12–5   Dermatitis herpetiformis, also known as Duhring's disease, is a systemic disease characterized by small blisters (3 to 5 mm) and occasionally large bullae (> 5 mm).

Figure 12-3   Dermatitis herpetiformis. (From Arnold HL, Odom RB, James WD: Andrews' Diseases of the Skin, Clinical Dermatology, ed 8, Philadelphia, WB Saunders, 1990)

N   Newborn Age: 0   **P**   Pediatric Age: 0–17   **M**   Maternity DX: 12–55   **A**   Adult Age: 15–124   ♀ Females Only   ♂ Males Only

🏵 Complication\Comorbidity   🏵 Major C\C   (Ex) CC/MCC Exclusions   🏵 Hospital-Acquired Condition

Item 12–6 Seborrheic dermatitis is characterized by greasy, scaly, red patches and is associated with oily skin and scalp.

Figure 12-4 Seborrheic dermatitis. (From Cohen BA: Atlas of Pediatric Dermatology, St. Louis, Mosby, 1993)

Item 12–7 Atopic dermatitis, also known as atopic eczema, infantile eczema, disseminated neuro dermatitis, flexural eczema, and *prurigo diathesique* (Besnier), is characterized by intense itching and is often hereditary.

Figure 12-5 Atopic dermatitis. (From Moschella SL, Hurley HJ: Dermatology, ed 3, Philadelphia, WB Saunders, 1993)

L22   Diaper dermatitis
    Diaper erythema
    Diaper rash
    Psoriasiform diaper rash

● **L23   Allergic contact dermatitis**

    Excludes1   allergy NOS (T78.40)
                   contact dermatitis NOS (L25.9)
                   dermatitis NOS (L30.9)

    Excludes2   dermatitis due to substances taken internally (L27.-)
                   dermatitis of eyelid (H01.1-)
                   diaper dermatitis (L22)
                   eczema of external ear (H60.5-)
                   irritant contact dermatitis (L24.-)
                   perioral dermatitis (L71.0)
                   radiation-related disorders of the skin and subcutaneous tissue (L55-L59)

L23.0   Allergic contact dermatitis due to metals
    Allergic contact dermatitis due to chromium
    Allergic contact dermatitis due to nickel

L23.1   Allergic contact dermatitis due to adhesives

L23.2   Allergic contact dermatitis due to cosmetics

L23.3   Allergic contact dermatitis due to drugs in contact with skin
    Use additional code for adverse effect, if applicable, to identify drug (T36-T50 with fifth or sixth character 5)

    Excludes2   dermatitis due to ingested drugs and medicaments (L27.0-L27.1)

L23.4   Allergic contact dermatitis due to dyes

L23.5   Allergic contact dermatitis due to other chemical products
    Allergic contact dermatitis due to cement
    Allergic contact dermatitis due to insecticide
    Allergic contact dermatitis due to plastic
    Allergic contact dermatitis due to rubber

L23.6   Allergic contact dermatitis due to food in contact with the skin
    Excludes2   dermatitis due to ingested food (L27.2)

L23.7   Allergic contact dermatitis due to plants, except food
    Excludes2   allergy NOS due to pollen (J30.1)

● **L23.8   Allergic contact dermatitis due to other agents**

    L23.81   Allergic contact dermatitis due to animal (cat) (dog) dander
           Allergic contact dermatitis due to animal (cat) (dog) hair

    L23.89   Allergic contact dermatitis due to other agents

L23.9   Allergic contact dermatitis, unspecified cause
    Allergic contact eczema NOS

● **L24   Irritant contact dermatitis**

    Excludes1   allergy NOS (T78.40)
                   contact dermatitis NOS (L25.9)
                   dermatitis NOS (L30.9)

    Excludes2   allergic contact dermatitis (L23.-)
                   dermatitis due to substances taken internally (L27.-)
                   dermatitis of eyelid (H01.1-)
                   diaper dermatitis (L22)
                   eczema of external ear (H60.5-)
                   perioral dermatitis (L71.0)
                   radiation-related disorders of the skin and subcutaneous tissue (L55-L59)

L24.0   Irritant contact dermatitis due to detergents

L24.1   Irritant contact dermatitis due to oils and greases

L24.2   Irritant contact dermatitis due to solvents
    Irritant contact dermatitis due to chlorocompound
    Irritant contact dermatitis due to cyclohexane
    Irritant contact dermatitis due to ester
    Irritant contact dermatitis due to glycol
    Irritant contact dermatitis due to hydrocarbon
    Irritant contact dermatitis due to ketone

L24.3   Irritant contact dermatitis due to cosmetics

L24.4   Irritant contact dermatitis due to drugs in contact with skin
    Use additional code for adverse effect, if applicable, to identify drug (T36-T50 with fifth or sixth character 5)

L24.5   Irritant contact dermatitis due to other chemical products
    Irritant contact dermatitis due to cement
    Irritant contact dermatitis due to insecticide
    Irritant contact dermatitis due to plastic
    Irritant contact dermatitis due to rubber

L24.6   Irritant contact dermatitis due to food in contact with skin
    Excludes2   dermatitis due to ingested food (L27.2)

L24.7   Irritant contact dermatitis due to plants, except food
    Excludes2   allergy NOS to pollen (J30.1)

● **L24.8   Irritant contact dermatitis due to other agents**

    L24.81   Irritant contact dermatitis due to metals
           Irritant contact dermatitis due to chromium
           Irritant contact dermatitis due to nickel

    L24.89   Irritant contact dermatitis due to other agents
           Irritant contact dermatitis due to dyes

L24.9   Irritant contact dermatitis, unspecified cause
    Irritant contact eczema NOS

◀ New   ⬛ Revised   ~~deleted~~ Deleted   Excludes 1   Excludes 2   Includes   Use additional   Code first   Code also   Unspecified

OGCR Official Guidelines   ● Unacceptable Principal Diagnosis   X Assign placeholder X   ● Use Additional Character(s)   ▶ Manifestation Code   **Coding Clinic**

● **L25**   **Unspecified contact dermatitis**
> **Excludes1**   allergic contact dermatitis (L23.-)
> allergy NOS (T78.40)
> dermatitis NOS (L30.9)
> irritant contact dermatitis (L24.-)
>
> **Excludes2**   dermatitis due to ingested substances (L27.-)
> dermatitis of eyelid (H01.1-)
> eczema of external ear (H60.5-)
> perioral dermatitis (L71.0)
> radiation-related disorders of the skin and subcutaneous tissue (L55-L59)

  L25.0   Unspecified contact dermatitis due to cosmetics
  L25.1   Unspecified contact dermatitis due to drugs in contact with skin
> Use additional code for adverse effect, if applicable, to identify drug (T36-T50 with fifth or sixth character 5)
>
> **Excludes2**   dermatitis due to ingested drugs and medicaments (L27.0-L27.1)

  L25.2   Unspecified contact dermatitis due to dyes
  L25.3   Unspecified contact dermatitis due to other chemical products
> Unspecified contact dermatitis due to cement
> Unspecified contact dermatitis due to insecticide

  L25.4   Unspecified contact dermatitis due to food in contact with skin
> **Excludes2**   dermatitis due to ingested food (L27.2)

  L25.5   Unspecified contact dermatitis due to plants, except food
> **Excludes1**   nettle rash (L50.9)
> **Excludes2**   allergy NOS due to pollen (J30.1)

  L25.8   Unspecified contact dermatitis due to other agents
  L25.9   Unspecified contact dermatitis, unspecified cause
> Contact dermatitis (occupational) NOS
> Contact eczema (occupational) NOS

 L26   **Exfoliative dermatitis**
> Hebra's pityriasis
> **Excludes1**   Ritter's disease (L00)

● **L27**   **Dermatitis due to substances taken internally**
> **Excludes1**   allergy NOS (T78.40)
> **Excludes2**   adverse food reaction, except dermatitis (T78.0-T78.1)
> contact dermatitis (L23-L25)
> drug photoallergic response (L56.1)
> drug phototoxic response (L56.0)
> urticaria (L50.-)

  L27.0   Generalized skin eruption due to drugs and medicaments taken internally
> Use additional code for adverse effect, if applicable, to identify drug (T36-T50 with fifth or sixth character 5)

  L27.1   Localized skin eruption due to drugs and medicaments taken internally
> Use additional code for adverse effect, if applicable, to identify drug (T36-T50 with fifth or sixth character 5)

  L27.2   Dermatitis due to ingested food
> **Excludes2**   dermatitis due to food in contact with skin (L23.6, L24.6, L25.4)

  L27.8   Dermatitis due to other substances taken internally
  L27.9   Dermatitis due to unspecified substance taken internally

● **L28**   **Lichen simplex chronicus and prurigo**
  L28.0   **Lichen simplex chronicus**
> Circumscribed neurodermatitis
> Lichen NOS

  L28.1   **Prurigo nodularis**
  L28.2   **Other prurigo**

> Prurigo NOS   Prurigo mitis
> Prurigo Hebra   Urticaria papulosa

● **L29**   **Pruritus**
> **Excludes1**   neurotic excoriation (L98.1)
> psychogenic pruritus (F45.8)

  L29.0   **Pruritus ani**
  L29.1   **Pruritus scroti** ♂
  L29.2   **Pruritus vulvae** ♀
  L29.3   **Anogenital pruritus, unspecified**
  L29.8   **Other pruritus**
  L29.9   **Pruritus, unspecified**
> Itch NOS

● **L30**   **Other and unspecified dermatitis**
> **Excludes2**   contact dermatitis (L23-L25)
> dry skin dermatitis (L85.3)
> small plaque parapsoriasis (L41.3)
> stasis dermatitis (I87.2) ◀▥

  L30.0   **Nummular dermatitis**
  L30.1   **Dyshidrosis [pompholyx]**
  L30.2   **Cutaneous autosensitization**
> Candidid [levurid]   Eczematid
> Dermatophytid

  L30.3   **Infective dermatitis**
> Infectious eczematoid dermatitis

  L30.4   **Erythema intertrigo**
  L30.5   **Pityriasis alba**
  L30.8   **Other specified dermatitis**
  L30.9   **Dermatitis, unspecified**
> Eczema NOS

PAPULOSQUAMOUS DISORDERS (L40-L45)

● **L40**   **Psoriasis**
  L40.0   **Psoriasis vulgaris**
> Nummular psoriasis   Plaque psoriasis

  L40.1   **Generalized pustular psoriasis**
> Impetigo herpetiformis
> Von Zumbusch's disease

  L40.2   **Acrodermatitis continua**
  L40.3   **Pustulosis palmaris et plantaris**
  L40.4   **Guttate psoriasis**
● **L40.5**   **Arthropathic psoriasis**
    L40.50   **Arthropathic psoriasis, unspecified**
    L40.51   **Distal interphalangeal psoriatic arthropathy**
    L40.52   **Psoriatic arthritis mutilans**
    L40.53   **Psoriatic spondylitis**
    L40.54   **Psoriatic juvenile arthropathy**
    L40.59   **Other psoriatic arthropathy**
  L40.8   **Other psoriasis**
> Flexural psoriasis

  L40.9   **Psoriasis, unspecified**

CHAPTER 12 (L00-L99)

Item 12-8 Psoriasis is a chronic, recurrent inflammatory skin disease characterized by small patches covered with thick silvery scales. **Parapsoriasis** is a treatment-resistant erythroderma. **Pityriasis rosea** is characterized by a herald patch that is a single large lesion and that usually appears on the trunk and is followed by scattered, smaller lesions.

N   Newborn Age: 0   **P**   Pediatric Age: 0–17   **M**   Maternity DX: 12–55   **A**   Adult Age: 15–124   ♀   Females Only   ♂   Males Only

Complication\Comorbidity   Major C\C   CC/MCC Exclusions   Hospital-Acquired Condition   **969**

● L41　Parapsoriasis
　　　　Excludes1　poikiloderma vasculare atrophicans (L94.5)
　　　L41.0　Pityriasis lichenoides et varioliformis acuta
　　　　　　　Mucha-Habermann disease
　　　L41.1　Pityriasis lichenoides chronica
　　　L41.3　Small plaque parapsoriasis
　　　L41.4　Large plaque parapsoriasis
　　　L41.5　Retiform parapsoriasis
　　　L41.8　Other parapsoriasis
　　　L41.9　Parapsoriasis, unspecified

L42　Pityriasis rosea

● L43　Lichen planus
　　　　Excludes1　lichen planopilaris (L66.1)
　　　L43.0　Hypertrophic lichen planus
　　　L43.1　Bullous lichen planus
　　　L43.2　Lichenoid drug reaction
　　　　　　　Use additional code for adverse effect, if applicable,
　　　　　　　　to identify drug (T36-T50 with fifth or sixth
　　　　　　　　character 5)
　　　L43.3　Subacute (active) lichen planus
　　　　　　　Lichen planus tropicus
　　　L43.8　Other lichen planus
　　　L43.9　Lichen planus, unspecified

● L44　Other papulosquamous disorders
　　　L44.0　Pityriasis rubra pilaris
　　　L44.1　Lichen nitidus
　　　L44.2　Lichen striatus
　　　L44.3　Lichen ruber moniliformis
　　　L44.4　Infantile papular acrodermatitis [Gianotti-Crosti]　　P
　　　L44.8　Other specified papulosquamous disorders
　　　L44.9　Papulosquamous disorder, unspecified

▶ L45　*Papulosquamous disorders in diseases classified elsewhere*
　　　　Code first underlying disease

URTICARIA AND ERYTHEMA (L49-L54)

　　　　Excludes1　Lyme disease (A69.2-)
　　　　　　　　　　rosacea (L71.-)

● L49　Exfoliation due to erythematous conditions according to extent
　　　　of body surface involved
　　　　Code first erythematous condition causing exfoliation, such as:
　　　　　Ritter's disease (L00)
　　　　　(Staphylococcal) scalded skin syndrome (L00)
　　　　　Stevens-Johnson syndrome (L51.1)
　　　　　Stevens-Johnson syndrome-toxic epidermal necrolysis
　　　　　overlap syndrome (L51.3)
　　　　　Toxic epidermal necrolysis (L51.2)
　　● L49.0　Exfoliation due to erythematous condition involving
　　　　　　　less than 10 percent of body surface
　　　　　　　Exfoliation due to erythematous condition NOS
　　● L49.1　Exfoliation due to erythematous condition involving
　　　　　　　10-19 percent of body surface
　　● L49.2　Exfoliation due to erythematous condition involving
　　　　　　　20-29 percent of body surface
　　● L49.3　Exfoliation due to erythematous condition involving
　　　　　　　30-39 percent of body surface �という
　　　　　　　ⒺⓍ L49.3
　　● L49.4　Exfoliation due to erythematous condition involving
　　　　　　　40-49 percent of body surface 🌍
　　　　　　　ⒺⓍ L49.4
　　● L49.5　Exfoliation due to erythematous condition involving
　　　　　　　50-59 percent of body surface 🌍
　　　　　　　ⒺⓍ L49.5

Figure 12-6　Erythematous plaques with silvery scales in a patient with psoriasis. (From Goldman: Cecil Textbook of Medicine, ed 22, Saunders, 2004)

　　● L49.6　Exfoliation due to erythematous condition involving
　　　　　　　60-69 percent of body surface 🌍
　　　　　　　ⒺⓍ L49.6
　　● L49.7　Exfoliation due to erythematous condition involving
　　　　　　　70-79 percent of body surface 🌍
　　　　　　　ⒺⓍ L49.7
　　● L49.8　Exfoliation due to erythematous condition involving
　　　　　　　80-89 percent of body surface 🌍
　　　　　　　ⒺⓍ L49.8
　　● L49.9　Exfoliation due to erythematous condition involving 90
　　　　　　　or more percent of body surface 🌍
　　　　　　　ⒺⓍ L49.9

● L50　Urticaria
　　　　Excludes1　allergic contact dermatitis (L23.-)
　　　　　　　　　　angioneurotic edema (T78.3)
　　　　　　　　　　giant urticaria (T78.3)
　　　　　　　　　　hereditary angio-edema (D84.1)
　　　　　　　　　　Quincke's edema (T78.3)
　　　　　　　　　　serum urticaria (T80.6-)
　　　　　　　　　　solar urticaria (L56.3)
　　　　　　　　　　urticaria neonatorum (P83.8)
　　　　　　　　　　urticaria papulosa (L28.2)
　　　　　　　　　　urticaria pigmentosa (Q82.2)
　　　L50.0　Allergic urticaria
　　　L50.1　Idiopathic urticaria
　　　L50.2　Urticaria due to cold and heat
　　　　　　　Excludes2　familial cold urticaria (M04.2) ◀
　　　L50.3　Dermatographic urticaria
　　　L50.4　Vibratory urticaria
　　　L50.5　Cholinergic urticaria
　　　L50.6　Contact urticaria
　　　L50.8　Other urticaria
　　　　　　　Chronic urticaria
　　　　　　　Recurrent periodic urticaria
　　　L50.9　Urticaria, unspecified

Figure 12-7　Urticaria (hives). *(Courtesy of David Effron, MD.)* (From Marx: Rosen's Emergency Medicine: Concepts and Clinical Practice, ed 6, Mosby, Inc., 2006)

Item 12-9　Urticaria is a vascular reaction in which wheals surrounded by a red halo appear and cause severe itching. The causes of urticaria or hives are extensive and varied (e.g., food, heat, cold, drugs, stress, infections).

◀ New　◀◀◀ Revised　~~deleted~~ Deleted　Excludes 1　Excludes 2　Includes　Use additional　Code first　Code also　Unspecified
OGCR Official Guidelines　● Unacceptable Principal Diagnosis　X Assign placeholder X　● Use Additional Character(s)　▶ Manifestation Code　**Coding Clinic**

● **L51　Erythema multiforme**

> Use additional code for adverse effect, if applicable, to identify drug (T36-T50 with fifth or sixth character 5)
>
> Use additional code to identify associated manifestations, such as:
> > arthropathy associated with dermatological disorders (M14.8-)
> > conjunctival edema (H11.42)
> > conjunctivitis (H10.22-)
> > corneal scars and opacities (H17.-)
> > corneal ulcer (H16.0-)
> > edema of eyelid (H02.84)
> > inflammation of eyelid (H01.8)
> > keratoconjunctivitis sicca (H16.22-)
> > mechanical lagophthalmos (H02.22-)
> > stomatitis (K12.-)
> > symblepharon (H11.23-)
>
> Use additional code to identify percentage of skin exfoliation (L49.-)
>
> **Excludes1**　staphylococcal scalded skin syndrome (L00)
> > Ritter's disease (L00)
>
> (Ex:) For category L51 CC codes: See L12.3

L51.0　Nonbullous erythema multiforme

L51.1　Stevens-Johnson syndrome 🔓

L51.2　Toxic epidermal necrolysis [Lyell] 🔓

L51.3　Stevens-Johnson syndrome-toxic epidermal necrolysis overlap syndrome 🔓
> SJS-TEN overlap syndrome

L51.8　Other erythema multiforme

L51.9　Erythema multiforme, unspecified
> Erythema iris
> Erythema multiforme major NOS
> Erythema multiforme minor NOS
> Herpes iris

L52　Erythema nodosum

> **Excludes1**　tuberculous erythema nodosum (A18.4)

● **L53　Other erythematous conditions**

> **Excludes1**　erythema ab igne (L59.0)
> > erythema due to external agents in contact with skin (L23-L25)
> > erythema intertrigo (L30.4)
>
> (Ex:) For category L53 CC codes: L12.30-L12.35, L44.8-L45, L51.0-L53.3, L71.0-L71.9, L93.0-L93.2, L94.2, L94.4, L98.7, L98.8, L99

L53.0　Toxic erythema 🔓
> *Code first* poisoning due to drug or toxin, if applicable *(T36-T65 with fifth or sixth character 1-4 or 6)*
>
> Use additional code for adverse effect, if applicable, to identify drug (T36-T50 with fifth or sixth character 5)
>
> **Excludes1**　neonatal erythema toxicum (P83.1)

L53.1　Erythema annulare centrifugum 🔓

L53.2　Erythema marginatum 🔓

L53.3　Other chronic figurate erythema 🔓

L53.8　Other specified erythematous conditions

L53.9　Erythematous condition, unspecified
> Erythema NOS
> Erythroderma NOS

▷ *L54　Erythema in diseases classified elsewhere*
> *Code first* underlying disease

RADIATION-RELATED DISORDERS OF THE SKIN AND SUBCUTANEOUS TISSUE (L55-L59)

● **L55　Sunburn**

L55.0　Sunburn of first degree

L55.1　Sunburn of second degree

L55.2　Sunburn of third degree

L55.9　Sunburn, unspecified

● **L56　Other acute skin changes due to ultraviolet radiation**

> Use additional code to identify the source of the ultraviolet radiation (W89, X32)

L56.0　Drug phototoxic response
> Use additional code for adverse effect, if applicable, to identify drug (T36-T50 with fifth or sixth character 5)

L56.1　Drug photoallergic response
> Use additional code for adverse effect, if applicable, to identify drug (T36-T50 with fifth or sixth character 5)

L56.2　Photocontact dermatitis [berloque dermatitis]

L56.3　Solar urticaria

L56.4　Polymorphous light eruption

L56.5　Disseminated superficial actinic porokeratosis (DSAP)

L56.8　Other specified acute skin changes due to ultraviolet radiation

L56.9　Acute skin change due to ultraviolet radiation, unspecified

● **L57　Skin changes due to chronic exposure to nonionizing radiation**

> Use additional code to identify the source of the ultraviolet radiation (W89, X32)

L57.0　Actinic keratosis
> Keratosis NOS　　　Solar keratosis
> Senile keratosis

L57.1　Actinic reticuloid

L57.2　Cutis rhomboidalis nuchae

L57.3　Poikiloderma of Civatte

L57.4　Cutis laxa senilis
> Elastosis senilis

L57.5　Actinic granuloma

L57.8　Other skin changes due to chronic exposure to nonionizing radiation
> Farmer's skin　　　Solar dermatitis
> Sailor's skin

L57.9　Skin changes due to chronic exposure to nonionizing radiation, unspecified

● **L58　Radiodermatitis**

> Use additional code to identify the source of the radiation (W88, W90)

L58.0　Acute radiodermatitis

L58.1　Chronic radiodermatitis

L58.9　Radiodermatitis, unspecified

● **L59　Other disorders of skin and subcutaneous tissue related to radiation**

L59.0　Erythema ab igne [dermatitis ab igne]

L59.8　Other specified disorders of the skin and subcutaneous tissue related to radiation

L59.9　Disorder of the skin and subcutaneous tissue related to radiation, unspecified

DISORDERS OF SKIN APPENDAGES (L60-L75)

> **Excludes1**　congenital malformations of integument (Q84.-)

● **L60　Nail disorders**

> **Excludes2**　clubbing of nails (R68.3)
> > onychia and paronychia (L03.0-)

L60.0　Ingrowing nail

L60.1　Onycholysis

L60.2　Onychogryphosis

L60.3　Nail dystrophy

L60.4　Beau's lines

L60.5　Yellow nail syndrome

L60.8　Other nail disorders

L60.9　Nail disorder, unspecified

CHAPTER 12 (L00-L99)

N　Newborn Age: 0　　**P**　Pediatric Age: 0–17　　**M**　Maternity DX: 12–55　　**A**　Adult Age: 15–124　　♀　Females Only　　♂　Males Only

🔓　Complication\Comorbidity　　🔓　Major C\C　　(Ex:)　CC/MCC Exclusions　　🔓　Hospital-Acquired Condition

Item 12–10 **Alopecia** is lack of hair and takes many forms. The most common is male pattern alopecia, also known as **androgenetic alopecia.** **Telogen effluvium** is early and excessive loss of hair resulting from a trauma to the hair follicle (fever, drugs, surgery, etc.).

Figure 12-8 Male pattern alopecia.

▶ *L62* *Nail disorders in diseases classified elsewhere*
> *Code first* underlying disease, such as:
> pachydermoperiostosis (M89.4-)

● **L63** **Alopecia areata**
    L63.0 Alopecia (capitis) totalis
    L63.1 Alopecia universalis
    L63.2 Ophiasis
    L63.8 Other alopecia areata
    L63.9 Alopecia areata, unspecified

● **L64** **Androgenic alopecia**
    Includes male-pattern baldness
    L64.0 **Drug-induced androgenic alopecia**
        Use additional code for adverse effect, if applicable, to identify drug (T36-T50 with fifth or sixth character 5)
    L64.8 Other androgenic alopecia
    L64.9 Androgenic alopecia, unspecified

● **L65** **Other nonscarring hair loss**
    Use additional code for adverse effect, if applicable, to identify drug (T36-T50 with fifth or sixth character 5)
    Excludes1 trichotillomania (F63.3)
    L65.0 Telogen effluvium
    L65.1 Anagen effluvium
    L65.2 Alopecia mucinosa
    L65.8 Other specified nonscarring hair loss
    L65.9 Nonscarring hair loss, unspecified
        Alopecia NOS

● **L66** **Cicatricial alopecia [scarring hair loss]**
    L66.0 Pseudopelade
    L66.1 Lichen planopilaris
        Follicular lichen planus
    L66.2 Folliculitis decalvans
    L66.3 Perifolliculitis capitis abscedens
    L66.4 Folliculitis ulerythematosa reticulata
    L66.8 Other cicatricial alopecia
        Coding Clinic: 2015, Q1, P19
    L66.9 Cicatricial alopecia, unspecified

● **L67** **Hair color and hair shaft abnormalities**
    Excludes1 monilethrix (Q84.1)
                pili annulati (Q84.1)
                telogen effluvium (L65.0)
    L67.0 Trichorrhexis nodosa
    L67.1 **Variations in hair color**
        Canities
        Greyness, hair (premature)
        Heterochromia of hair
        Poliosis circumscripta, acquired
        Poliosis NOS
    L67.8 **Other hair color and hair shaft abnormalities**
        Fragilitas crinium
    L67.9 **Hair color and hair shaft abnormality,** unspecified

● **L68** **Hypertrichosis**
    Includes excess hair
    Excludes1 congenital hypertrichosis (Q84.2)
                persistent lanugo (Q84.2)
    L68.0 **Hirsutism**
        Excessive growth of hair
    L68.1 Acquired hypertrichosis lanuginosa
    L68.2 Localized hypertrichosis
    L68.3 Polytrichia
    L68.8 Other hypertrichosis
    L68.9 Hypertrichosis, unspecified

● **L70** **Acne**
    Excludes2 acne keloid (L73.0)
    L70.0 Acne vulgaris
    L70.1 Acne conglobata
    L70.2 Acne varioliformis
        Acne necrotica miliaris
    L70.3 Acne tropica
    L70.4 Infantile acne
    L70.5 Acné excoriée ◀▥
        Acné excoriée des jeunes filles ◀
        Picker's acne
    L70.8 Other acne
    L70.9 Acne, unspecified

● **L71** **Rosacea**
    Use additional code for adverse effect, if applicable, to identify drug (T36-T50 with fifth or sixth character 5)
    L71.0 Perioral dermatitis
    L71.1 Rhinophyma
    L71.8 Other rosacea
    L71.9 Rosacea, unspecified

● **L72** **Follicular cysts of skin and subcutaneous tissue**
    L72.0 Epidermal cyst
    ● **L72.1** **Pilar and trichodermal cyst**
        L72.11 **Pilar cyst**
        L72.12 **Trichodermal cyst**
            Trichilemmal (proliferating) cyst
    L72.3 **Sebaceous cyst**
        Excludes2 pilar cyst (L72.11)
                trichilemmal (proliferating) cyst (L72.12)
    L72.2 Steatocystoma multiplex
    L72.8 **Other follicular cysts of the skin and subcutaneous tissue**
    L72.9 **Follicular cyst of the skin and subcutaneous tissue,** unspecified

● **L73** **Other follicular disorders**
    L73.0 Acne keloid
    L73.1 Pseudofolliculitis barbae
    L73.2 Hidradenitis suppurativa
    L73.8 **Other specified follicular disorders**
        Sycosis barbae
    L73.9 **Follicular disorder,** unspecified

P

● **L74** **Eccrine sweat disorders**
> **Excludes2** generalized hyperhidrosis (R61)

L74.0 **Miliaria rubra**

L74.1 **Miliaria crystallina**

L74.2 **Miliaria profunda**
Miliaria tropicalis

L74.3 **Miliaria, unspecified**

L74.4 **Anhidrosis**
Hypohidrosis

● **L74.5** **Focal hyperhidrosis**
> ● **L74.51** **Primary focal hyperhidrosis**
> > **L74.510** **Primary focal hyperhidrosis, axilla**
> > **L74.511** **Primary focal hyperhidrosis, face**
> > **L74.512** **Primary focal hyperhidrosis, palms**
> > **L74.513** **Primary focal hyperhidrosis, soles**
> > **L74.519** **Primary focal hyperhidrosis, unspecified**
> **L74.52** **Secondary focal hyperhidrosis**
> Frey's syndrome

L74.8 **Other eccrine sweat disorders**

L74.9 **Eccrine sweat disorder, unspecified**
Sweat gland disorder NOS

● **L75** **Apocrine sweat disorders**
> **Excludes1** dyshidrosis (L30.1)
> hidradenitis suppurativa (L73.2)

L75.0 **Bromhidrosis**

L75.1 **Chromhidrosis**

L75.2 **Apocrine miliaria**
Fox-Fordyce disease

L75.8 **Other apocrine sweat disorders**

L75.9 **Apocrine sweat disorder, unspecified**
Intraoperative and postprocedural complications of skin and subcutaneous tissue (L76)

INTRAOPERATIVE AND POSTPROCEDURAL COMPLICATIONS OF SKIN AND SUBCUTANEOUS TISSUE (L76)

● **L76** **Intraoperative and postprocedural complications of skin and subcutaneous tissue**
> (Ex) **For category L76 CC codes unless otherwise indicated:** H95.811-H95.89, I85.01, I85.11, I97.3, K21.9, K22.8, K23, K25.0, K25.2, K25.4, K25.6, K26.0, K26.2, K26.4, K26.6, K27.0, K27.2, K27.4, K27.6, K28.0, K28.2, K28.4, K28.6, K29.01, K29.21, K29.31, K29.41, K29.51, K29.61, K29.71, K29.81, K29.91, K31.811, K55.21, K57.01, K57.11, K57.13, K57.21, K57.31, K57.33, K57.41, K57.51, K57.53, K57.81, K57.91, K57.93, K62.5, K92.0-K92.2, L76.01-L76.02, L76.21-L76.82, M96.89, N98.1-N98.9, P54.1-P54.3, T81.10X-T81.19X[A], T81.82X[A], T81.89X-T81.9XX[A]

● **L76.0** **Intraoperative hemorrhage and hematoma of skin and subcutaneous tissue complicating a procedure**
> **Excludes1** intraoperative hemorrhage and hematoma of skin and subcutaneous tissue due to accidental puncture and laceration during a procedure (L76.1-)

> **L76.01** **Intraoperative hemorrhage and hematoma of skin and subcutaneous tissue complicating a dermatologic procedure** 🔖

> **L76.02** **Intraoperative hemorrhage and hematoma of skin and subcutaneous tissue complicating other procedure** 🔖

● **L76.1** **Accidental puncture and laceration of skin and subcutaneous tissue during a procedure**
> (Ex) **For category L76.1 CC codes:** D78.11-D78.12, D78.81-D78.89, E36.11-E36.8, E89.810-E89.89, G96.11, G97.41-G97.49, H59.011-H59.019, H59.031-H59.099, H59.211-H59.229, H59.811-H59.89, H95.31-H95.32, H95.811-H95.89, I97.3, I97.51-I97.52, J95.71-J95.72, K91.71-K91.72, L76.11-L76.12, L76.81-L76.82, M96.820-M96.821, M96.89, N98.1-N98.9, N99.71-N99.72, T81.82X[A], T81.89X-T81.9XX[A]

> **L76.11** **Accidental puncture and laceration of skin and subcutaneous tissue during a dermatologic procedure** 🔖

> **L76.12** **Accidental puncture and laceration of skin and subcutaneous tissue during other procedure** 🔖

● **L76.2** **Postprocedural hemorrhage of skin and subcutaneous tissue following a procedure** ◀▥
> **L76.21** **Postprocedural hemorrhage of skin and subcutaneous tissue following a dermatologic procedure** 🔖 ◀▥
> **L76.22** **Postprocedural hemorrhage of skin and subcutaneous tissue following other procedure** 🔖 ◀▥

● **L76.3** **Postprocedural hematoma and seroma of skin and subcutaneous tissue following a procedure** ◀
> **L76.31** **Postprocedural hematoma of skin and subcutaneous tissue following a dermatologic procedure** 🔖 ◀
> **L76.32** **Postprocedural hematoma of skin and subcutaneous tissue following other procedure** 🔖 ◀
> **L76.33** **Postprocedural seroma of skin and subcutaneous tissue following a dermatologic procedure** 🔖 ◀
> **L76.34** **Postprocedural seroma of skin and subcutaneous tissue following other procedure** 🔖 ◀

● **L76.8** **Other intraoperative and postprocedural complications of skin and subcutaneous tissue**
> **Use additional** code, if applicable, to further specify disorder
> **L76.81** **Other intraoperative complications of skin and subcutaneous tissue**
> **L76.82** **Other postprocedural complications of skin and subcutaneous tissue**

OTHER DISORDERS OF THE SKIN AND SUBCUTANEOUS TISSUE (L80-L99)

L80 **Vitiligo**
> **Excludes2** vitiligo of eyelids (H02.73-)
> vitiligo of vulva (N90.89)

● **L81** **Other disorders of pigmentation**
> **Excludes1** birthmark NOS (Q82.5)
> Peutz-Jeghers syndrome (Q85.8)
> **Excludes2** nevus - see Alphabetical Index

L81.0 **Postinflammatory hyperpigmentation**

L81.1 **Chloasma**

L81.2 **Freckles**

L81.3 **Café au lait spots**

L81.4 **Other melanin hyperpigmentation**
Lentigo

L81.5 **Leukoderma, not elsewhere classified**

L81.6 **Other disorders of diminished melanin formation**

L81.7 **Pigmented purpuric dermatosis**
Angioma serpiginosum

L81.8 **Other specified disorders of pigmentation**
Iron pigmentation
Tattoo pigmentation

L81.9 **Disorder of pigmentation, unspecified**

● **L82** **Seborrheic keratosis**
> **Includes** basal cell papilloma ◀
> dermatosis papulosa nigra
> Leser-Trélat disease
> **Excludes2** seborrheic dermatitis (L21.-)

L82.0 **Inflamed seborrheic keratosis**

L82.1 **Other seborrheic keratosis**
Seborrheic keratosis NOS

L83 **Acanthosis nigricans**
Confluent and reticulated papillomatosis

L84 **Corns and callosities**
Callus
Clavus

● **L85 Other epidermal thickening**

  Excludes2 hypertrophic disorders of the skin (L91.-)

 L85.0 Acquired ichthyosis

   Excludes1 congenital ichthyosis (Q80.-)

 L85.1 Acquired keratosis [keratoderma] palmaris et plantaris

   Excludes1 inherited keratosis palmaris et plantaris (Q82.8)

 L85.2 Keratosis punctata (palmaris et plantaris)

 L85.3 Xerosis cutis

   Dry skin dermatitis

 L85.8 Other specified epidermal thickening

   Cutaneous horn

 L85.9 Epidermal thickening, unspecified

▶ *L86 Keratoderma in diseases classified elsewhere*

  Firm horny papules that have a cobblestone appearance.

  Code first underlying disease, such as:

   Reiter's disease (M02.3-)

  Excludes1 gonococcal keratoderma (A54.89)

      gonococcal keratosis (A54.89)

      keratoderma due to vitamin A deficiency (E50.8)

      keratosis due to vitamin A deficiency (E50.8)

      xeroderma due to vitamin A deficiency (E50.8)

● **L87 Transepidermal elimination disorders**

  Excludes1 granuloma annulare (perforating) (L92.0)

 L87.0 Keratosis follicularis et parafollicularis in cutem penetrans

   Kyrle disease

   Hyperkeratosis follicularis penetrans

 L87.1 Reactive perforating collagenosis

 L87.2 Elastosis perforans serpiginosa

 L87.8 Other transepidermal elimination disorders

 L87.9 Transepidermal elimination disorder, unspecified

L88 Pyoderma gangrenosum 🅒

  Phagedenic pyoderma

  Excludes1 dermatitis gangrenosa (L08.0)

  Ⓔˣ L08.0, L08.81, L88

  OGCR Section I.B.14.

> General Coding Guidelines
>
> Documentation for BMI, *Depth of* Non-pressure ulcers, Pressure Ulcer Stages, **Coma Scale, and** *NIH Stroke Scale*
>
> For the Body Mass Index (BMI), depth of non-pressure chronic ulcers, pressure ulcer stage, **coma scale, and NIH stroke scale (NIHSS) codes,** code assignment may be based on medical record documentation from clinicians who are not the patient's provider (i.e., physician or other qualified healthcare practitioner legally accountable for establishing the patient's diagnosis), since this information is typically documented by other clinicians involved in the care of the patient (e.g., a dietitian often documents the BMI, a nurse often documents the pressure ulcer stages, **and an emergency medical technician often documents the coma scale**). However, the associated diagnosis (such as overweight, obesity, **acute stroke,** or pressure ulcer) must be documented by the patient's provider. If there is conflicting medical record documentation, either from the same clinician or different clinicians, the patient's attending provider should be queried for clarification.
>
> The BMI, **coma scale, and NHSS** codes should only be reported as secondary diagnoses.

● **L89 Pressure ulcer**

  Includes bed sore   pressure area

       decubitus ulcer pressure sore

       plaster ulcer

  Code first any associated gangrene (I96)

  Excludes2 decubitus (trophic) ulcer of cervix (uteri) (N86)

      diabetic ulcers (E08.621, E08.622, E09.621, E09.622, E10.621, E10.622, E11.621, E11.622, E13.621, E13.622)

      non-pressure chronic ulcer of skin (L97.-)

      skin infections (L00-L08)

      varicose ulcer (I83.0, I83.2)

  Ⓔˣ **For category L89 CC codes:** L89.000-L89.95, L97.101-L97.929, L98.411-L98.499

● **L89.0 Pressure ulcer of elbow**

 ● **L89.00 Pressure ulcer of unspecified elbow**

  L89.000 Pressure ulcer of unspecified elbow, unstageable

  L89.001 Pressure ulcer of unspecified elbow, stage 1

   Healing pressure ulcer of unspecified elbow, stage 1

   Pressure pre-ulcer skin changes limited to persistent focal edema, unspecified elbow

  L89.002 Pressure ulcer of unspecified elbow, stage 2

   Healing pressure ulcer of unspecified elbow, stage 2

   Pressure ulcer with abrasion, blister, partial thickness skin loss involving epidermis and/or dermis, unspecified elbow

  L89.003 Pressure ulcer of unspecified elbow, stage 3 🅒 🅒

   Healing pressure ulcer of unspecified elbow, stage 3

   Pressure ulcer with full thickness skin loss involving damage or necrosis of subcutaneous tissue, unspecified elbow

   MCC when PDx is its own MCC

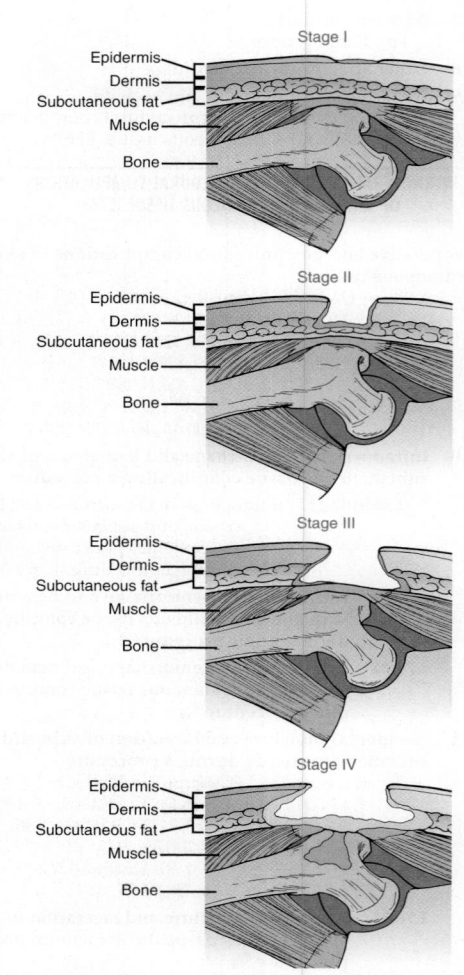

Figure 12-9 Stage I, II, III, and IV of pressure ulcers.

◀ New ◀▦ Revised ~~deleted~~ Deleted Excludes 1 Excludes 2 Includes Use additional Code first Code also Unspecified

OGCR Official Guidelines ● Unacceptable Principal Diagnosis X Assign placeholder X ● Use Additional Character(s) ▶ Manifestation Code **Coding Clinic**

L89.004   **Pressure ulcer of unspecified elbow, stage 4** 🔹🔹
> Healing pressure ulcer of unspecified elbow, stage 4
> Pressure ulcer with necrosis of soft tissues through to underlying muscle, tendon, or bone, unspecified elbow
> MCC when PDx is its own MCC

L89.009   **Pressure ulcer of unspecified elbow, unspecified stage**
> Healing pressure ulcer of elbow NOS
> Healing pressure ulcer of unspecified elbow, unspecified stage

● **L89.01**   **Pressure ulcer of right elbow**

L89.010   **Pressure ulcer of right elbow, unstageable**

L89.011   **Pressure ulcer of right elbow, stage 1**
> Healing pressure ulcer of right elbow, stage 1
> Pressure pre-ulcer skin changes limited to persistent focal edema, right elbow

L89.012   **Pressure ulcer of right elbow, stage 2**
> Healing pressure ulcer of right elbow, stage 2
> Pressure ulcer with abrasion, blister, partial thickness skin loss involving epidermis and/or dermis, right elbow

L89.013   **Pressure ulcer of right elbow, stage 3** 🔹🔹
> Healing pressure ulcer of right elbow, stage 3
> Pressure ulcer with full thickness skin loss involving damage or necrosis of subcutaneous tissue, right elbow
> MCC when PDx is its own MCC

L89.014   **Pressure ulcer of right elbow, stage 4** 🔹🔹
> Healing pressure ulcer of right elbow, stage 4
> Pressure ulcer with necrosis of soft tissues through to underlying muscle, tendon, or bone, right elbow
> MCC when PDx is its own MCC

L89.019   **Pressure ulcer of right elbow, unspecified stage**
> Healing pressure right of elbow NOS
> Healing pressure ulcer of unspecified elbow, unspecified stage

● **L89.02**   **Pressure ulcer of left elbow**

L89.020   **Pressure ulcer of left elbow, unstageable**

L89.021   **Pressure ulcer of left elbow, stage 1**
> Healing pressure ulcer of left elbow, stage 1
> Pressure pre-ulcer skin changes limited to persistent focal edema, left elbow

L89.022   **Pressure ulcer of left elbow, stage 2**
> Healing pressure ulcer of left elbow, stage 2
> Pressure ulcer with abrasion, blister, partial thickness skin loss involving epidermis and/or dermis, left elbow

L89.023   **Pressure ulcer of left elbow, stage 3** 🔹🔹
> Healing pressure ulcer of left elbow, stage 3
> Pressure ulcer with full thickness skin loss involving damage or necrosis of subcutaneous tissue, left elbow
> MCC when PDx is its own MCC

L89.024   **Pressure ulcer of left elbow, stage 4** 🔹🔹
> Healing pressure ulcer of left elbow, stage 4
> Pressure ulcer with necrosis of soft tissues through to underlying muscle, tendon, or bone, left elbow
> MCC when PDx is its own MCC

L89.029   **Pressure ulcer of left elbow, unspecified stage**
> Healing pressure ulcer of left of elbow NOS
> Healing pressure ulcer of unspecified elbow, unspecified stage

● **L89.1**   **Pressure ulcer of back**

● **L89.10**   **Pressure ulcer of unspecified part of back**

L89.100   **Pressure ulcer of unspecified part of back, unstageable**

L89.101   **Pressure ulcer of unspecified part of back, stage 1**
> Healing pressure ulcer of unspecified part of back, stage 1
> Pressure pre-ulcer skin changes limited to persistent focal edema, unspecified part of back

L89.102   **Pressure ulcer of unspecified part of back, stage 2**
> Healing pressure ulcer of unspecified part of back, stage 2
> Pressure ulcer with abrasion, blister, partial thickness skin loss involving epidermis and/or dermis, unspecified part of back

L89.103   **Pressure ulcer of unspecified part of back, stage 3** 🔹🔹
> Healing pressure ulcer of unspecified part of back, stage 3
> Pressure ulcer with full thickness skin loss involving damage or necrosis of subcutaneous tissue, unspecified part of back
> MCC when PDx is its own MCC

L89.104   **Pressure ulcer of unspecified part of back, stage 4** 🔹🔹
> Healing pressure ulcer of unspecified part of back, stage 4
> Pressure ulcer with necrosis of soft tissues through to underlying muscle, tendon, or bone, unspecified part of back
> MCC when PDx is its own MCC

L89.109   **Pressure ulcer of unspecified part of back, unspecified stage**
> Healing pressure ulcer of unspecified part of back NOS
> Healing pressure ulcer of unspecified part of back, unspecified stage

CHAPTER 12 (L00–L99)

N Newborn Age: 0   **P** Pediatric Age: 0–17   **M** Maternity DX: 12–55   **A** Adult Age: 15–124   ♀ Females Only   ♂ Males Only

🔹 Complication\Comorbidity   🔹 Major C\C   (Ex) CC/MCC Exclusions   🔹 Hospital-Acquired Condition

975

● **L89.11** **Pressure ulcer of right upper back**
    Pressure ulcer of right shoulder blade

  L89.110 **Pressure ulcer of right upper back, unstageable**

  L89.111 **Pressure ulcer of right upper back, stage 1**
    Healing pressure ulcer of right upper back, stage 1
    Pressure pre-ulcer skin changes limited to persistent focal edema, right upper back

  L89.112 **Pressure ulcer of right upper back, stage 2**
    Healing pressure ulcer of right upper back, stage 2
    Pressure ulcer with abrasion, blister, partial thickness skin loss involving epidermis and/or dermis, right upper back

  L89.113 **Pressure ulcer of right upper back, stage 3** 🎗🎗
    Healing pressure ulcer of right upper back, stage 3
    Pressure ulcer with full thickness skin loss involving damage or necrosis of subcutaneous tissue, right upper back
    MCC when PDx is its own MCC

  L89.114 **Pressure ulcer of right upper back, stage 4** 🎗🎗
    Healing pressure ulcer of right upper back, stage 4
    Pressure ulcer with necrosis of soft tissues through to underlying muscle, tendon, or bone, right upper back
    MCC when PDx is its own MCC

  L89.119 **Pressure ulcer of right upper back, unspecified stage**
    Healing pressure ulcer of right upper back NOS
    Healing pressure ulcer of right upper back, unspecified stage

● **L89.12** **Pressure ulcer of left upper back**
    Pressure ulcer of left shoulder blade

  L89.120 **Pressure ulcer of left upper back, unstageable**

  L89.121 **Pressure ulcer of left upper back, stage 1**
    Healing pressure ulcer of left upper back, stage 1
    Pressure pre-ulcer skin changes limited to persistent focal edema, left upper back

  L89.122 **Pressure ulcer of left upper back, stage 2**
    Healing pressure ulcer of left upper back, stage 2
    Pressure ulcer with abrasion, blister, partial thickness skin loss involving epidermis and/or dermis, left upper back

  L89.123 **Pressure ulcer of left upper back, stage 3** 🎗🎗
    Healing pressure ulcer of left upper back, stage 3
    Pressure ulcer with full thickness skin loss involving damage or necrosis of subcutaneous tissue, left upper back
    MCC when PDx is its own MCC

  L89.124 **Pressure ulcer of left upper back, stage 4** 🎗🎗
    Healing pressure ulcer of left upper back, stage 4
    Pressure ulcer with necrosis of soft tissues through to underlying muscle, tendon, or bone, left upper back
    MCC when PDx is its own MCC

  L89.129 **Pressure ulcer of left upper back, unspecified stage**
    Healing pressure ulcer of left upper back NOS
    Healing pressure ulcer of left upper back, unspecified stage

● **L89.13** **Pressure ulcer of right lower back**

  L89.130 **Pressure ulcer of right lower back, unstageable**

  L89.131 **Pressure ulcer of right lower back, stage 1**
    Healing pressure ulcer of right lower back, stage 1
    Pressure pre-ulcer skin changes limited to persistent focal edema, right lower back

  L89.132 **Pressure ulcer of right lower back, stage 2**
    Healing pressure ulcer of right lower back, stage 2
    Pressure ulcer with abrasion, blister, partial thickness skin loss involving epidermis and/or dermis, right lower back

  L89.133 **Pressure ulcer of right lower back, stage 3** 🎗🎗
    Healing pressure ulcer of right lower back, stage 3
    Pressure ulcer with full thickness skin loss involving damage or necrosis of subcutaneous tissue, right lower back
    MCC when PDx is its own MCC

  L89.134 **Pressure ulcer of right lower back, stage 4** 🎗🎗
    Healing pressure ulcer of right lower back, stage 4
    Pressure ulcer with necrosis of soft tissues through to underlying muscle, tendon, or bone, right lower back
    MCC when PDx is its own MCC

  L89.139 **Pressure ulcer of right lower back, unspecified stage**
    Healing pressure ulcer of right lower back NOS
    Healing pressure ulcer of right lower back, unspecified stage

● **L89.14** **Pressure ulcer of left lower back**

  L89.140 **Pressure ulcer of left lower back, unstageable**

  L89.141 **Pressure ulcer of left lower back, stage 1**
    Healing pressure ulcer of left lower back, stage 1
    Pressure pre-ulcer skin changes limited to persistent focal edema, left lower back

  L89.142 **Pressure ulcer of left lower back, stage 2**
    Healing pressure ulcer of left lower back, stage 2
    Pressure ulcer with abrasion, blister, partial thickness skin loss involving epidermis and/or dermis, left lower back

L89.143   **Pressure ulcer of left lower back, stage 3** 🔖🔖
  Healing pressure ulcer of left lower back, stage 3
  Pressure ulcer with full thickness skin loss involving damage or necrosis of subcutaneous tissue, left lower back
  MCC when PDx is its own MCC

L89.144   **Pressure ulcer of left lower back, stage 4** 🔖🔖
  Healing pressure ulcer of left lower back, stage 4
  Pressure ulcer with necrosis of soft tissues through to underlying muscle, tendon, or bone, left lower back
  MCC when PDx is its own MCC

L89.149   **Pressure ulcer of left lower back, unspecified stage**
  Healing pressure ulcer of left lower back NOS
  Healing pressure ulcer of left lower back, unspecified stage

⬤ **L89.15**   **Pressure ulcer of sacral region**
  Pressure ulcer of coccyx
  Pressure ulcer of tailbone

L89.150   **Pressure ulcer of sacral region, unstageable**

L89.151   **Pressure ulcer of sacral region, stage 1**
  Healing pressure ulcer of sacral region, stage 1
  Pressure pre-ulcer skin changes limited to persistent focal edema, sacral region

L89.152   **Pressure ulcer of sacral region, stage 2**
  Healing pressure ulcer of sacral region, stage 2
  Pressure ulcer with abrasion, blister, partial thickness skin loss involving epidermis and/or dermis, sacral region

L89.153   **Pressure ulcer of sacral region, stage 3** 🔖🔖
  Healing pressure ulcer of sacral region, stage 3
  Pressure ulcer with full thickness skin loss involving damage or necrosis of subcutaneous tissue, sacral region
  MCC when PDx is its own MCC

L89.154   **Pressure ulcer of sacral region, stage 4** 🔖🔖
  Healing pressure ulcer of sacral region, stage 4
  Pressure ulcer with necrosis of soft tissues through to underlying muscle, tendon, or bone, sacral region
  MCC when PDx is its own MCC

L89.159   **Pressure ulcer of sacral region, unspecified stage**
  Healing pressure ulcer of sacral region NOS
  Healing pressure ulcer of sacral region, unspecified stage

⬤ **L89.2**   **Pressure ulcer of hip**

⬤ **L89.20**   **Pressure ulcer of unspecified hip**

L89.200   **Pressure ulcer of unspecified hip, unstageable**

L89.201   **Pressure ulcer of unspecified hip, stage 1**
  Healing pressure ulcer of unspecified hip back, stage 1
  Pressure pre-ulcer skin changes limited to persistent focal edema, unspecified hip

L89.202   **Pressure ulcer of unspecified hip, stage 2**
  Healing pressure ulcer of unspecified hip, stage 2
  Pressure ulcer with abrasion, blister, partial thickness skin loss involving epidermis and/or dermis, unspecified hip

L89.203   **Pressure ulcer of unspecified hip, stage 3** 🔖🔖
  Healing pressure ulcer of unspecified hip, stage 3
  Pressure ulcer with full thickness skin loss involving damage or necrosis of subcutaneous tissue, unspecified hip
  MCC when PDx is its own MCC

L89.204   **Pressure ulcer of unspecified hip, stage 4** 🔖🔖
  Healing pressure ulcer of unspecified hip, stage 4
  Pressure ulcer with necrosis of soft tissues through to underlying muscle, tendon, or bone, unspecified hip
  MCC when PDx is its own MCC

L89.209   **Pressure ulcer of unspecified hip, unspecified stage**
  Healing pressure ulcer of unspecified hip NOS
  Healing pressure ulcer of unspecified hip, unspecified stage

⬤ **L89.21**   **Pressure ulcer of right hip**

L89.210   **Pressure ulcer of right hip, unstageable**

L89.211   **Pressure ulcer of right hip, stage 1**
  Healing pressure ulcer of right hip back, stage 1
  Pressure pre-ulcer skin changes limited to persistent focal edema, right hip

L89.212   **Pressure ulcer of right hip, stage 2**
  Healing pressure ulcer of right hip, stage 2
  Pressure ulcer with abrasion, blister, partial thickness skin loss involving epidermis and/or dermis, right hip

L89.213   **Pressure ulcer of right hip, stage 3** 🔖🔖
  Healing pressure ulcer of right hip, stage 3
  Pressure ulcer with full thickness skin loss involving damage or necrosis of subcutaneous tissue, right hip
  MCC when PDx is its own MCC

L89.214   **Pressure ulcer of right hip, stage 4** 🔖🔖
  Healing pressure ulcer of right hip, stage 4
  Pressure ulcer with necrosis of soft tissues through to underlying muscle, tendon, or bone, right hip
  MCC when PDx is its own MCC

L89.219   **Pressure ulcer of right hip, unspecified stage**
  Healing pressure ulcer of right hip NOS
  Healing pressure ulcer of right hip, unspecified stage

CHAPTER 12 (L00–L99)

● **L89.22   Pressure ulcer of left hip**
     L89.220   Pressure ulcer of left hip, unstageable
     L89.221   Pressure ulcer of left hip, stage 1
        Healing pressure ulcer of left hip back, stage 1
        Pressure pre-ulcer skin changes limited to persistent focal edema, left hip
     L89.222   Pressure ulcer of left hip, stage 2
        Healing pressure ulcer of left hip, stage 2
        Pressure ulcer with abrasion, blister, partial thickness skin loss involving epidermis and/or dermis, left hip
     L89.223   Pressure ulcer of left hip, stage 3 🔗 🔗
        Healing pressure ulcer of left hip, stage 3
        Pressure ulcer with full thickness skin loss involving damage or necrosis of subcutaneous tissue, left hip
        MCC when PDx is its own MCC
     L89.224   Pressure ulcer of left hip, stage 4 🔗 🔗
        Healing pressure ulcer of left hip, stage 4
        Pressure ulcer with necrosis of soft tissues through to underlying muscle, tendon, or bone, left hip
        MCC when PDx is its own MCC
     L89.229   Pressure ulcer of left hip, unspecified stage
        Healing pressure ulcer of left hip NOS
        Healing pressure ulcer of left hip, unspecified stage

● **L89.3   Pressure ulcer of buttock**
   ● **L89.30   Pressure ulcer of unspecified buttock**
     L89.300   Pressure ulcer of unspecified buttock, unstageable
     L89.301   Pressure ulcer of unspecified buttock, stage 1
        Healing pressure ulcer of unspecified buttock, stage 1
        Pressure pre-ulcer skin changes limited to persistent focal edema, unspecified buttock
     L89.302   Pressure ulcer of unspecified buttock, stage 2
        Healing pressure ulcer of unspecified buttock, stage 2
        Pressure ulcer with abrasion, blister, partial thickness skin loss involving epidermis and/or dermis, unspecified buttock
     L89.303   Pressure ulcer of unspecified buttock, stage 3 🔗 🔗
        Healing pressure ulcer of unspecified buttock, stage 3
        Pressure ulcer with full thickness skin loss involving damage or necrosis of subcutaneous tissue, unspecified buttock
        MCC when PDx is its own MCC

     L89.304   Pressure ulcer of unspecified buttock, stage 4 🔗 🔗
        Healing pressure ulcer of unspecified buttock, stage 4
        Pressure ulcer with necrosis of soft tissues through to underlying muscle, tendon, or bone, unspecified buttock
        MCC when PDx is its own MCC
     L89.309   Pressure ulcer of unspecified buttock, unspecified stage
        Healing pressure ulcer of unspecified buttock NOS
        Healing pressure ulcer of unspecified buttock, unspecified stage

   ● **L89.31   Pressure ulcer of right buttock**
     L89.310   Pressure ulcer of right buttock, unstageable
     L89.311   Pressure ulcer of right buttock, stage 1
        Healing pressure ulcer of right buttock, stage 1
        Pressure pre-ulcer skin changes limited to persistent focal edema, right buttock
     L89.312   Pressure ulcer of right buttock, stage 2
        Healing pressure ulcer of right buttock, stage 2
        Pressure ulcer with abrasion, blister, partial thickness skin loss involving epidermis and/or dermis, right buttock
     L89.313   Pressure ulcer of right buttock, stage 3 🔗 🔗
        Healing pressure ulcer of right buttock, stage 3
        Pressure ulcer with full thickness skin loss involving damage or necrosis of subcutaneous tissue, right buttock
        MCC when PDx is its own MCC
     L89.314   Pressure ulcer of right buttock, stage 4 🔗 🔗
        Healing pressure ulcer of right buttock, stage 4
        Pressure ulcer with necrosis of soft tissues through to underlying muscle, tendon, or bone, right buttock
        MCC when PDx is its own MCC
     L89.319   Pressure ulcer of right buttock, unspecified stage
        Healing pressure ulcer of right buttock NOS
        Healing pressure ulcer of right buttock, unspecified stage

   ● **L89.32   Pressure ulcer of left buttock**
     L89.320   Pressure ulcer of left buttock, unstageable
     L89.321   Pressure ulcer of left buttock, stage 1
        Healing pressure ulcer of left buttock, stage 1
        Pressure pre-ulcer skin changes limited to persistent focal edema, left buttock
     L89.322   Pressure ulcer of left buttock, stage 2
        Healing pressure ulcer of left buttock, stage 2
        Pressure ulcer with abrasion, blister, partial thickness skin loss involving epidermis and/or dermis, left buttock

L89.323   **Pressure ulcer of left buttock, stage 3** 🦠 🦠
> Healing pressure ulcer of left buttock, stage 3
> Pressure ulcer with full thickness skin loss involving damage or necrosis of subcutaneous tissue, left buttock
> MCC when PDx is its own MCC

L89.324   **Pressure ulcer of left buttock, stage 4** 🦠 🦠
> Healing pressure ulcer of left buttock, stage 4
> Pressure ulcer with necrosis of soft tissues through to underlying muscle, tendon, or bone, left buttock
> MCC when PDx is its own MCC

L89.329   **Pressure ulcer of left buttock, unspecified stage**
> Healing pressure ulcer of left buttock NOS
> Healing pressure ulcer of left buttock, unspecified stage

● **L89.4   Pressure ulcer of contiguous site of back, buttock and hip**

L89.40   **Pressure ulcer of contiguous site of back, buttock and hip, unspecified stage**
> Healing pressure ulcer of contiguous site of back, buttock and hip NOS
> Healing pressure ulcer of contiguous site of back, buttock and hip, unspecified stage

L89.41   **Pressure ulcer of contiguous site of back, buttock and hip, stage 1**
> Healing pressure ulcer of contiguous site of back, buttock and hip, stage 1
> Pressure pre-ulcer skin changes limited to persistent focal edema, contiguous site of back, buttock and hip

L89.42   **Pressure ulcer of contiguous site of back, buttock and hip, stage 2**
> Healing pressure ulcer of contiguous site of back, buttock and hip, stage 2
> Pressure ulcer with abrasion, blister, partial thickness skin loss involving epidermis and/or dermis, contiguous site of back, buttock and hip

L89.43   **Pressure ulcer of contiguous site of back, buttock and hip, stage 3** 🦠 🦠
> Healing pressure ulcer of contiguous site of back, buttock and hip, stage 3
> Pressure ulcer with full thickness skin loss involving damage or necrosis of subcutaneous tissue, contiguous site of back, buttock and hip
> MCC when PDx is its own MCC

L89.44   **Pressure ulcer of contiguous site of back, buttock and hip, stage 4** 🦠 🦠
> Healing pressure ulcer of contiguous site of back, buttock and hip, stage 4
> Pressure ulcer with necrosis of soft tissues through to underlying muscle, tendon, or bone, contiguous site of back, buttock and hip
> MCC when PDx is its own MCC

L89.45   **Pressure ulcer of contiguous site of back, buttock and hip, unstageable**

● **L89.5   Pressure ulcer of ankle**

● L89.50   **Pressure ulcer of unspecified ankle**

L89.500   **Pressure ulcer of unspecified ankle, unstageable**

L89.501   **Pressure ulcer of unspecified ankle, stage 1**
> Healing pressure ulcer of unspecified ankle, stage 1
> Pressure pre-ulcer skin changes limited to persistent focal edema, unspecified ankle

L89.502   **Pressure ulcer of unspecified ankle, stage 2**
> Healing pressure ulcer of unspecified ankle, stage 2
> Pressure ulcer with abrasion, blister, partial thickness skin loss involving epidermis and/or dermis, unspecified ankle

L89.503   **Pressure ulcer of unspecified ankle, stage 3** 🦠 🦠
> Healing pressure ulcer of unspecified ankle, stage 3
> Pressure ulcer with full thickness skin loss involving damage or necrosis of subcutaneous tissue, unspecified ankle
> MCC when PDx is its own MCC

L89.504   **Pressure ulcer of unspecified ankle, stage 4** 🦠 🦠
> Healing pressure ulcer of unspecified ankle, stage 4
> Pressure ulcer with necrosis of soft tissues through to underlying muscle, tendon, or bone, unspecified ankle
> MCC when PDx is its own MCC

L89.509   **Pressure ulcer of unspecified ankle, unspecified stage**
> Healing pressure ulcer of unspecified ankle NOS
> Healing pressure ulcer of unspecified ankle, unspecified stage

● **L89.51   Pressure ulcer of right ankle**

L89.510   **Pressure ulcer of right ankle, unstageable**

L89.511   **Pressure ulcer of right ankle, stage 1**
> Healing pressure ulcer of right ankle, stage 1
> Pressure pre-ulcer skin changes limited to persistent focal edema, right ankle

L89.512   **Pressure ulcer of right ankle, stage 2**
> Healing pressure ulcer of right ankle, stage 2
> Pressure ulcer with abrasion, blister, partial thickness skin loss involving epidermis and/or dermis, right ankle

L89.513   **Pressure ulcer of right ankle, stage 3** 🦠 🦠
> Healing pressure ulcer of right ankle, stage 3
> Pressure ulcer with full thickness skin loss involving damage or necrosis of subcutaneous tissue, right ankle
> MCC when PDx is its own MCC

CHAPTER 12 (L00-L99)

N Newborn Age: 0   **P** Pediatric Age: 0–17   **M** Maternity DX: 12–55   **A** Adult Age: 15–124   ♀ Females Only   ♂ Males Only
🦠 Complication\Comorbidity   🦠 Major C\C   (Ex) CC/MCC Exclusions   🦠 Hospital-Acquired Condition

979

L89.514 **Pressure ulcer of right ankle, stage 4** 🔲🔲
> Healing pressure ulcer of right ankle, stage 4
> Pressure ulcer with necrosis of soft tissues through to underlying muscle, tendon, or bone, right ankle
> MCC when PDx is its own MCC

L89.519 **Pressure ulcer of right ankle, unspecified stage**
> Healing pressure ulcer of right ankle NOS
> Healing pressure ulcer of right ankle, unspecified stage

● L89.52 **Pressure ulcer of left ankle**

L89.520 **Pressure ulcer of left ankle, unstageable**

L89.521 **Pressure ulcer of left ankle, stage 1**
> Healing pressure ulcer of left ankle, stage 1
> Pressure pre-ulcer skin changes limited to persistent focal edema, left ankle ◀▥

L89.522 **Pressure ulcer of left ankle, stage 2**
> Healing pressure ulcer of left ankle, stage 2
> Pressure ulcer with abrasion, blister, partial thickness skin loss involving epidermis and/or dermis, left ankle

L89.523 **Pressure ulcer of left ankle, stage 3** 🔲🔲
> Healing pressure ulcer of left ankle, stage 3
> Pressure ulcer with full thickness skin loss involving damage or necrosis of subcutaneous tissue, left ankle
> MCC when PDx is its own MCC

L89.524 **Pressure ulcer of left ankle, stage 4** 🔲🔲
> Healing pressure ulcer of left ankle, stage 4
> Pressure ulcer with necrosis of soft tissues through to underlying muscle, tendon, or bone, left ankle
> MCC when PDx is its own MCC

L89.529 **Pressure ulcer of left ankle, unspecified stage**
> Healing pressure ulcer of left ankle NOS
> Healing pressure ulcer of left ankle, unspecified stage

● L89.6 **Pressure ulcer of heel**

● L89.60 **Pressure ulcer of unspecified heel**

L89.600 **Pressure ulcer of unspecified heel, unstageable**

L89.601 **Pressure ulcer of unspecified heel, stage 1**
> Healing pressure ulcer of unspecified heel, stage 1
> Pressure pre-ulcer skin changes limited to persistent focal edema, unspecified heel

L89.602 **Pressure ulcer of unspecified heel, stage 2**
> Healing pressure ulcer of unspecified heel, stage 2
> Pressure ulcer with abrasion, blister, partial thickness skin loss involving epidermis and/or dermis, unspecified heel

L89.603 **Pressure ulcer of unspecified heel, stage 3** 🔲🔲
> Healing pressure ulcer of unspecified heel, stage 3
> Pressure ulcer with full thickness skin loss involving damage or necrosis of subcutaneous tissue, unspecified heel
> MCC when PDx is its own MCC

L89.604 **Pressure ulcer of unspecified heel, stage 4** 🔲🔲
> Healing pressure ulcer of unspecified heel, stage 4
> Pressure ulcer with necrosis of soft tissues through to underlying muscle, tendon, or bone, unspecified heel
> MCC when PDx is its own MCC

L89.609 **Pressure ulcer of unspecified heel, unspecified stage**
> Healing pressure ulcer of unspecified heel NOS
> Healing pressure ulcer of unspecified heel, unspecified stage

● L89.61 **Pressure ulcer of right heel**

L89.610 **Pressure ulcer of right heel, unstageable**

L89.611 **Pressure ulcer of right heel, stage 1**
> Healing pressure ulcer of right heel, stage 1
> Pressure pre-ulcer skin changes limited to persistent focal edema, right heel

L89.612 **Pressure ulcer of right heel, stage 2**
> Healing pressure ulcer of right heel, stage 2
> Pressure ulcer with abrasion, blister, partial thickness skin loss involving epidermis and/or dermis, right heel

L89.613 **Pressure ulcer of right heel, stage 3** 🔲🔲
> Healing pressure ulcer of right heel, stage 3
> Pressure ulcer with full thickness skin loss involving damage or necrosis of subcutaneous tissue, right heel
> MCC when PDx is its own MCC

L89.614 **Pressure ulcer of right heel, stage 4** 🔲🔲
> Healing pressure ulcer of right heel, stage 4
> Pressure ulcer with necrosis of soft tissues through to underlying muscle, tendon, or bone, right heel
> MCC when PDx is its own MCC

L89.619 **Pressure ulcer of right heel, unspecified stage**
> Healing pressure ulcer of right heel NOS
> Healing pressure ulcer of unspecified heel, right stage

● L89.62 **Pressure ulcer of left heel**

L89.620 **Pressure ulcer of left heel, unstageable**

L89.621 **Pressure ulcer of left heel, stage 1**
> Healing pressure ulcer of left heel, stage 1
> Pressure pre-ulcer skin changes limited to persistent focal edema, left heel

◀ New   ◀▥ Revised   ~~deleted~~ Deleted   Excludes 1   Excludes 2   Includes   Use additional   Code first   Code also   Unspecified

OGCR Official Guidelines   ● Unacceptable Principal Diagnosis   X Assign placeholder X   ● Use Additional Character(s)   ▶ Manifestation Code   **Coding Clinic**

L89.622   **Pressure ulcer of left heel, stage 2**
　　　Healing pressure ulcer of left heel,
　　　　stage 2
　　　Pressure ulcer with abrasion, blister,
　　　　partial thickness skin loss
　　　　involving epidermis and/or
　　　　dermis, left heel

L89.623   **Pressure ulcer of left heel,**
　　　　stage 3 🪙 🪙
　　　Healing pressure ulcer of left heel,
　　　　stage 3
　　　Pressure ulcer with full thickness
　　　　skin loss involving damage or
　　　　necrosis of subcutaneous tissue,
　　　　left heel
　　　MCC when PDx is its own MCC

L89.624   **Pressure ulcer of left heel,**
　　　　stage 4 🪙 🪙
　　　Healing pressure ulcer of left heel,
　　　　stage 4
　　　Pressure ulcer with necrosis of soft
　　　　tissues through to underlying
　　　　muscle, tendon, or bone, left
　　　　heel
　　　MCC when PDx is its own MCC

L89.629   **Pressure ulcer of left heel, unspecified**
　　　　stage
　　　Healing pressure ulcer of left heel
　　　　NOS
　　　Healing pressure ulcer of left heel,
　　　　unspecified stage

● **L89.8** **Pressure ulcer of other site**

　● **L89.81** **Pressure ulcer of head**
　　　Pressure ulcer of face

L89.810   **Pressure ulcer of head, unstageable**

L89.811   **Pressure ulcer of head, stage 1**
　　　Healing pressure ulcer of head,
　　　　stage 1
　　　Pressure pre-ulcer skin changes
　　　　limited to persistent focal
　　　　edema, head

L89.812   **Pressure ulcer of head, stage 2**
　　　Healing pressure ulcer of head,
　　　　stage 2
　　　Pressure ulcer with abrasion, blister,
　　　　partial thickness skin loss
　　　　involving epidermis and/or
　　　　dermis, head

L89.813   **Pressure ulcer of head, stage 3** 🪙 🪙
　　　Healing pressure ulcer of head,
　　　　stage 3
　　　Pressure ulcer with full thickness
　　　　skin loss involving damage or
　　　　necrosis of subcutaneous tissue,
　　　　head
　　　MCC when PDx is its own MCC

L89.814   **Pressure ulcer of head, stage 4** 🪙 🪙
　　　Healing pressure ulcer of head,
　　　　stage 4
　　　Pressure ulcer with necrosis of soft
　　　　tissues through to underlying
　　　　muscle, tendon, or bone, head
　　　MCC when PDx is its own MCC

L89.819   **Pressure ulcer of head, unspecified**
　　　　stage
　　　Healing pressure ulcer of head NOS
　　　Healing pressure ulcer of head,
　　　　unspecified stage

● **L89.89** **Pressure ulcer of other site**

L89.890   **Pressure ulcer of other site,**
　　　　unstageable

L89.891   **Pressure ulcer of other site, stage 1**
　　　Healing pressure ulcer of other site,
　　　　stage 1
　　　Pressure pre-ulcer skin changes
　　　　limited to persistent focal
　　　　edema, other site

L89.892   **Pressure ulcer of other site, stage 2**
　　　Healing pressure ulcer of other site,
　　　　stage 2
　　　Pressure ulcer with abrasion, blister,
　　　　partial thickness skin loss
　　　　involving epidermis and/or
　　　　dermis, other site

L89.893   **Pressure ulcer of other site,**
　　　　stage 3 🪙 🪙
　　　Healing pressure ulcer of other site,
　　　　stage 3
　　　Pressure ulcer with full thickness
　　　　skin loss involving damage or
　　　　necrosis of subcutaneous tissue,
　　　　other site
　　　MCC when PDx is its own MCC

L89.894   **Pressure ulcer of other site,**
　　　　stage 4 🪙 🪙
　　　Healing pressure ulcer of other site,
　　　　stage 4
　　　Pressure ulcer with necrosis of soft
　　　　tissues through to underlying
　　　　muscle, tendon, or bone, other
　　　　site
　　　MCC when PDx is its own MCC

L89.899   **Pressure ulcer of other site,**
　　　　unspecified stage
　　　Healing pressure ulcer of other site
　　　　NOS
　　　Healing pressure ulcer of other site,
　　　　unspecified stage

● **L89.9** **Pressure ulcer of unspecified site**

L89.90   **Pressure ulcer of unspecified site, unspecified**
　　　　stage
　　　Healing pressure ulcer of unspecified site NOS
　　　Healing pressure ulcer of unspecified site,
　　　　unspecified stage

L89.91   **Pressure ulcer of unspecified site, stage 1**
　　　Healing pressure ulcer of unspecified site,
　　　　stage 1
　　　Pressure pre-ulcer skin changes limited to
　　　　persistent focal edema, unspecified site

L89.92   **Pressure ulcer of unspecified site, stage 2**
　　　Healing pressure ulcer of unspecified site,
　　　　stage 2
　　　Pressure ulcer with abrasion, blister, partial
　　　　thickness skin loss involving epidermis
　　　　and/or dermis, unspecified site

L89.93   **Pressure ulcer of unspecified site, stage 3** 🪙 🪙
　　　Healing pressure ulcer of unspecified site,
　　　　stage 3
　　　Pressure ulcer with full thickness skin
　　　　loss involving damage or necrosis of
　　　　subcutaneous tissue, unspecified site
　　　MCC when PDx is its own MCC

L89.94   **Pressure ulcer of unspecified site, stage 4** 🪙 🪙
　　　Healing pressure ulcer of unspecified site,
　　　　stage 4
　　　Pressure ulcer with necrosis of soft tissues
　　　　through to underlying muscle, tendon, or
　　　　bone, unspecified site
　　　MCC when PDx is its own MCC

L89.95   **Pressure ulcer of unspecified site, unstageable**

N Newborn Age: 0   **P** Pediatric Age: 0–17   **M** Maternity DX: 12–55   **A** Adult Age: 15–124   ♀ Females Only   ♂ Males Only

🪙 Complication\Comorbidity   🪙 Major C\C   ⓔ⨯ CC/MCC Exclusions   🪙 Hospital-Acquired Condition

981

CHAPTER 12 (L00-L99)

● **L90**   **Atrophic disorders of skin**

     L90.0   **Lichen sclerosus et atrophicus**

         Excludes2   lichen sclerosus of external female genital organs (N90.4)

                   lichen sclerosus of external male genital organs (N48.0)

     L90.1   **Anetoderma of Schweninger-Buzzi**

     L90.2   **Anetoderma of Jadassohn-Pellizzari**

     L90.3   **Atrophoderma of Pasini and Pierini**

     L90.4   **Acrodermatitis chronica atrophicans**

     L90.5   **Scar conditions and fibrosis of skin**

         Adherent scar (skin)

         Cicatrix

         Disfigurement of skin due to scar

         Fibrosis of skin NOS

         Scar NOS

         Excludes2   hypertrophic scar (L91.0)

                   keloid scar (L91.0)

         Coding Clinic: 2016, Q2, P5; 2015, Q1, P19

     L90.6   **Striae atrophicae**

     L90.8   **Other atrophic disorders of skin**

     L90.9   **Atrophic disorder of skin, unspecified**

● **L91**   **Hypertrophic disorders of skin**

     L91.0   **Keloid scar**

         Hypertrophic scar

         Keloid

         Excludes2   acne keloid (L73.0)

                   scar NOS (L90.5)

     L91.8   **Other hypertrophic disorders of the skin**

     L91.9   **Hypertrophic disorder of the skin, unspecified**

● **L92**   **Granulomatous disorders of skin and subcutaneous tissue**

     Excludes2   actinic granuloma (L57.5)

     L92.0   **Granuloma annulare**

         Perforating granuloma annulare

     L92.1   **Necrobiosis lipoidica, not elsewhere classified**

         Excludes1   necrobiosis lipoidica associated with diabetes mellitus (E08-E13 with .620)

     L92.2   **Granuloma faciale [eosinophilic granuloma of skin]**

     L92.3   **Foreign body granuloma of the skin and subcutaneous tissue**

         Use additional code to identify the type of retained foreign body (Z18.-)

     L92.8   **Other granulomatous disorders of the skin and subcutaneous tissue**

     L92.9   **Granulomatous disorder of the skin and subcutaneous tissue, unspecified**

● **L93**   **Lupus erythematosus**

     Use additional code for adverse effect, if applicable, to identify drug (T36-T50 with fifth or sixth character 5)

     Excludes1   lupus exedens (A18.4)

                   lupus vulgaris (A18.4)

                   scleroderma (M34.-)

                   systemic lupus erythematosus (M32.-)

     L93.0   **Discoid lupus erythematosus**

         Lupus erythematosus NOS

     L93.1   **Subacute cutaneous lupus erythematosus**

     L93.2   **Other local lupus erythematosus**

         Lupus erythematosus profundus

         Lupus panniculitis

● **L94**   **Other localized connective tissue disorders**

     Excludes1   systemic connective tissue disorders (M30-M36)

     L94.0   **Localized scleroderma [morphea]**

         Circumscribed scleroderma

     L94.1   **Linear scleroderma**

         En coup de sabre lesion

     L94.2   **Calcinosis cutis**

     L94.3   **Sclerodactyly**

     L94.4   **Gottron's papules**

     L94.5   **Poikiloderma vasculare atrophicans**

     L94.6   **Ainhum**

     L94.8   **Other specified localized connective tissue disorders**

     L94.9   **Localized connective tissue disorder, unspecified**

● **L95**   **Vasculitis limited to skin, not elsewhere classified**

     Excludes1   angioma serpiginosum (L81.7)

                   Henoch(-Schönlein) purpura (D69.0)

                   hypersensitivity angiitis (M31.0)

                   lupus panniculitis (L93.2)

                   panniculitis NOS (M79.3)

                   panniculitis of neck and back (M54.0-)

                   polyarteritis nodosa (M30.0)

                   relapsing panniculitis (M35.6)

                   rheumatoid vasculitis (M05.2)

                   serum sickness (T80.6-)

                   urticaria (L50.-)

                   Wegener's granulomatosis (M31.3-)

     L95.0   **Livedoid vasculitis**

         Atrophie blanche (en plaque)

     L95.1   **Erythema elevatum diutinum**

     L95.8   **Other vasculitis limited to the skin**

     L95.9   **Vasculitis limited to the skin, unspecified**

● **L97**   **Non-pressure chronic ulcer of lower limb, not elsewhere classified**

     Includes   chronic ulcer of skin of lower limb NOS

                non-healing ulcer of skin

                non-infected sinus of skin

                trophic ulcer NOS

                tropical ulcer NOS

                ulcer of skin of lower limb NOS

     Code first any associated underlying condition, such as:

         any associated gangrene (I96)

         atherosclerosis of the lower extremities (I70.23-, I70.24-, I70.33-, I70.34-, I70.43-, I70.44-, I70.53-, I70.54-, I70.63-, I70.64-, I70.73-, I70.74-)

         chronic venous hypertension (I87.31-, I87.33-)

         diabetic ulcers (E08.621, E08.622, E09.621, E09.622, E10.621, E10.622, E11.621, E11.622, E13.621, E13.622)

         postphlebitic syndrome (I87.01-, I87.03-)

         postthrombotic syndrome (I87.01-, I87.03-)

         varicose ulcer (I83.0-, I83.2-)

     Excludes2   pressure ulcer (pressure area) (L89.-)

                   skin infections (L00-L08)

                   specific infections classified to A00-B99

     (Ex) **For category L97 CC codes:** I70.231-I70.25, L44.8-L45, L94.2, L94.4, L97.101-L97.929, L98.411-L98.499, L98.7-L99

● **L97.1**   **Non-pressure chronic ulcer of thigh**

     ● **L97.10**   **Non-pressure chronic ulcer of unspecified thigh**

         L97.101   **Non-pressure chronic ulcer of unspecified thigh limited to breakdown of skin** 🔎

         L97.102   **Non-pressure chronic ulcer of unspecified thigh with fat layer exposed** 🔎

         L97.103   **Non-pressure chronic ulcer of unspecified thigh with necrosis of muscle** 🔎

Item 12–11   **Scleroderma** means hard skin. It is a group of diseases that causes abnormal growth of connective tissues that support the skin and organs. There are two types: localized scleroderma affecting the skin and systemic scleroderma affecting blood vessels and internal organs and the skin.

◀ New   ◀▥ Revised   ~~deleted~~ Deleted   Excludes 1   Excludes 2   Includes   Use additional   Code first   Code also   Unspecified

OGCR Official Guidelines   ● Unacceptable Principal Diagnosis   **X** Assign placeholder X   ● Use Additional Character(s)   ▶ Manifestation Code   **Coding Clinic**

L97.104   Non-pressure chronic ulcer of unspecified thigh with necrosis of bone 🗞

L97.109   Non-pressure chronic ulcer of unspecified thigh with unspecified severity 🗞

● L97.11   Non-pressure chronic ulcer of right thigh

L97.111   Non-pressure chronic ulcer of right thigh limited to breakdown of skin 🗞

L97.112   Non-pressure chronic ulcer of right thigh with fat layer exposed 🗞

L97.113   Non-pressure chronic ulcer of right thigh with necrosis of muscle 🗞

L97.114   Non-pressure chronic ulcer of right thigh with necrosis of bone 🗞

L97.119   Non-pressure chronic ulcer of right thigh with unspecified severity 🗞

● L97.12   Non-pressure chronic ulcer of left thigh

L97.121   Non-pressure chronic ulcer of left thigh limited to breakdown of skin 🗞

L97.122   Non-pressure chronic ulcer of left thigh with fat layer exposed 🗞

L97.123   Non-pressure chronic ulcer of left thigh with necrosis of muscle 🗞

L97.124   Non-pressure chronic ulcer of left thigh with necrosis of bone 🗞

L97.129   Non-pressure chronic ulcer of left thigh with unspecified severity 🗞

● L97.2   Non-pressure chronic ulcer of calf

● L97.20   Non-pressure chronic ulcer of unspecified calf

L97.201   Non-pressure chronic ulcer of unspecified calf limited to breakdown of skin 🗞

L97.202   Non-pressure chronic ulcer of unspecified calf with fat layer exposed 🗞

L97.203   Non-pressure chronic ulcer of unspecified calf with necrosis of muscle 🗞

L97.204   Non-pressure chronic ulcer of unspecified calf with necrosis of bone 🗞

L97.209   Non-pressure chronic ulcer of unspecified calf with unspecified severity 🗞

● L97.21   Non-pressure chronic ulcer of right calf

L97.211   Non-pressure chronic ulcer of right calf limited to breakdown of skin 🗞

L97.212   Non-pressure chronic ulcer of right calf with fat layer exposed 🗞

L97.213   Non-pressure chronic ulcer of right calf with necrosis of muscle 🗞

L97.214   Non-pressure chronic ulcer of right calf with necrosis of bone 🗞

L97.219   Non-pressure chronic ulcer of right calf with unspecified severity 🗞

● L97.22   Non-pressure chronic ulcer of left calf

L97.221   Non-pressure chronic ulcer of left calf limited to breakdown of skin 🗞

L97.222   Non-pressure chronic ulcer of left calf with fat layer exposed 🗞

L97.223   Non-pressure chronic ulcer of left calf with necrosis of muscle 🗞

L97.224   Non-pressure chronic ulcer of left calf with necrosis of bone 🗞

L97.229   Non-pressure chronic ulcer of left calf with unspecified severity 🗞

● L97.3   Non-pressure chronic ulcer of ankle

● L97.30   Non-pressure chronic ulcer of unspecified ankle

L97.301   Non-pressure chronic ulcer of unspecified ankle limited to breakdown of skin 🗞

L97.302   Non-pressure chronic ulcer of unspecified ankle with fat layer exposed 🗞

L97.303   Non-pressure chronic ulcer of unspecified ankle with necrosis of muscle 🗞

L97.304   Non-pressure chronic ulcer of unspecified ankle with necrosis of bone 🗞

L97.309   Non-pressure chronic ulcer of unspecified ankle with unspecified severity 🗞

● L97.31   Non-pressure chronic ulcer of right ankle

L97.311   Non-pressure chronic ulcer of right ankle limited to breakdown of skin 🗞

L97.312   Non-pressure chronic ulcer of right ankle with fat layer exposed 🗞

L97.313   Non-pressure chronic ulcer of right ankle with necrosis of muscle 🗞

L97.314   Non-pressure chronic ulcer of right ankle with necrosis of bone 🗞

L97.319   Non-pressure chronic ulcer of right ankle with unspecified severity 🗞

● L97.32   Non-pressure chronic ulcer of left ankle

L97.321   Non-pressure chronic ulcer of left ankle limited to breakdown of skin 🗞

L97.322   Non-pressure chronic ulcer of left ankle with fat layer exposed 🗞

L97.323   Non-pressure chronic ulcer of left ankle with necrosis of muscle 🗞

L97.324   Non-pressure chronic ulcer of left ankle with necrosis of bone 🗞

L97.329   Non-pressure chronic ulcer of left ankle with unspecified severity 🗞

● L97.4   Non-pressure chronic ulcer of heel and midfoot
Non-pressure chronic ulcer of plantar surface of midfoot

● L97.40   Non-pressure chronic ulcer of unspecified heel and midfoot

L97.401   Non-pressure chronic ulcer of unspecified heel and midfoot limited to breakdown of skin 🗞

L97.402   Non-pressure chronic ulcer of unspecified heel and midfoot with fat layer exposed 🗞

L97.403   Non-pressure chronic ulcer of unspecified heel and midfoot with necrosis of muscle 🗞

L97.404   Non-pressure chronic ulcer of unspecified heel and midfoot with necrosis of bone 🗞

L97.409   Non-pressure chronic ulcer of unspecified heel and midfoot with unspecified severity 🗞

● L97.41   Non-pressure chronic ulcer of right heel and midfoot

L97.411   Non-pressure chronic ulcer of right heel and midfoot limited to breakdown of skin 🗞

L97.412   Non-pressure chronic ulcer of right heel and midfoot with fat layer exposed 🗞

L97.413   Non-pressure chronic ulcer of right heel and midfoot with necrosis of muscle 🗞

N   Newborn Age: Ø   **P**   Pediatric Age: Ø–17   **M**   Maternity DX: 12–55   **A**   Adult Age: 15–124   ♀   Females Only   ♂   Males Only

🗞   Complication\Comorbidity   🗞   Major C\C   (Ex)   CC/MCC Exclusions   🗞   Hospital-Acquired Condition

CHAPTER 12 (LØØ-L99)

983

L97.414   Non-pressure chronic ulcer of right heel and midfoot with necrosis of bone 🦴

L97.419   Non-pressure chronic ulcer of right heel and midfoot with unspecified severity 🦴

● L97.42   Non-pressure chronic ulcer of left heel and midfoot

L97.421   Non-pressure chronic ulcer of left heel and midfoot limited to breakdown of skin 🦴
Coding Clinic: 2016, Q1, P13

L97.422   Non-pressure chronic ulcer of left heel and midfoot with fat layer exposed 🦴

L97.423   Non-pressure chronic ulcer of left heel and midfoot with necrosis of muscle 🦴

L97.424   Non-pressure chronic ulcer of left heel and midfoot with necrosis of bone 🦴

L97.429   Non-pressure chronic ulcer of left heel and midfoot with unspecified severity 🦴

● L97.5   Non-pressure chronic ulcer of other part of foot
Non-pressure chronic ulcer of toe

● L97.50   Non-pressure chronic ulcer of other part of unspecified foot

L97.501   Non-pressure chronic ulcer of other part of unspecified foot limited to breakdown of skin

L97.502   Non-pressure chronic ulcer of other part of unspecified foot with fat layer exposed

L97.503   Non-pressure chronic ulcer of other part of unspecified foot with necrosis of muscle

L97.504   Non-pressure chronic ulcer of other part of unspecified foot with necrosis of bone

L97.509   Non-pressure chronic ulcer of other part of unspecified foot with unspecified severity

● L97.51   Non-pressure chronic ulcer of other part of right foot

L97.511   Non-pressure chronic ulcer of other part of right foot limited to breakdown of skin

L97.512   Non-pressure chronic ulcer of other part of right foot with fat layer exposed

L97.513   Non-pressure chronic ulcer of other part of right foot with necrosis of muscle

L97.514   Non-pressure chronic ulcer of other part of right foot with necrosis of bone

L97.519   Non-pressure chronic ulcer of other part of right foot with unspecified severity

● L97.52   Non-pressure chronic ulcer of other part of left foot

L97.521   Non-pressure chronic ulcer of other part of left foot limited to breakdown of skin

L97.522   Non-pressure chronic ulcer of other part of left foot with fat layer exposed

L97.523   Non-pressure chronic ulcer of other part of left foot with necrosis of muscle

L97.524   Non-pressure chronic ulcer of other part of left foot with necrosis of bone

L97.529   Non-pressure chronic ulcer of other part of left foot with unspecified severity

● L97.8   Non-pressure chronic ulcer of other part of lower leg

● L97.80   Non-pressure chronic ulcer of other part of unspecified lower leg

L97.801   Non-pressure chronic ulcer of other part of unspecified lower leg limited to breakdown of skin 🦴

L97.802   Non-pressure chronic ulcer of other part of unspecified lower leg with fat layer exposed 🦴

L97.803   Non-pressure chronic ulcer of other part of unspecified lower leg with necrosis of muscle 🦴

L97.804   Non-pressure chronic ulcer of other part of unspecified lower leg with necrosis of bone 🦴

L97.809   Non-pressure chronic ulcer of other part of unspecified lower leg with unspecified severity

● L97.81   Non-pressure chronic ulcer of other part of right lower leg

L97.811   Non-pressure chronic ulcer of other part of right lower leg limited to breakdown of skin 🦴

L97.812   Non-pressure chronic ulcer of other part of right lower leg with fat layer exposed 🦴

L97.813   Non-pressure chronic ulcer of other part of right lower leg with necrosis of muscle 🦴

L97.814   Non-pressure chronic ulcer of other part of right lower leg with necrosis of bone 🦴

L97.819   Non-pressure chronic ulcer of other part of right lower leg with unspecified severity 🦴

● L97.82   Non-pressure chronic ulcer of other part of left lower leg

L97.821   Non-pressure chronic ulcer of other part of left lower leg limited to breakdown of skin 🦴

L97.822   Non-pressure chronic ulcer of other part of left lower leg with fat layer exposed 🦴

L97.823   Non-pressure chronic ulcer of other part of left lower leg with necrosis of muscle 🦴

L97.824   Non-pressure chronic ulcer of other part of left lower leg with necrosis of bone 🦴

L97.829   Non-pressure chronic ulcer of other part of left lower leg with unspecified severity 🦴

● L97.9   Non-pressure chronic ulcer of unspecified part of lower leg

● L97.90   Non-pressure chronic ulcer of unspecified part of unspecified lower leg

L97.901   Non-pressure chronic ulcer of unspecified part of unspecified lower leg limited to breakdown of skin 🦴

L97.902   Non-pressure chronic ulcer of unspecified part of unspecified lower leg with fat layer exposed 🦴

◀ New   ⬅ Revised   ~~deleted~~ Deleted   Excludes 1   Excludes 2   Includes   Use additional   Code first   Code also   Unspecified

OGCR Official Guidelines   ● Unacceptable Principal Diagnosis   X Assign placeholder X   ● Use Additional Character(s)   ▶ Manifestation Code   **Coding Clinic**

L97.903   Non-pressure chronic ulcer of unspecified part of unspecified lower leg with necrosis of muscle 🔖

L97.904   Non-pressure chronic ulcer of unspecified part of unspecified lower leg with necrosis of bone 🔖

L97.909   Non-pressure chronic ulcer of unspecified part of unspecified lower leg with unspecified severity 🔖

● **L97.91**   **Non-pressure chronic ulcer of unspecified part of right lower leg**

L97.911   Non-pressure chronic ulcer of unspecified part of right lower leg limited to breakdown of skin 🔖

L97.912   Non-pressure chronic ulcer of unspecified part of right lower leg with fat layer exposed 🔖

L97.913   Non-pressure chronic ulcer of unspecified part of right lower leg with necrosis of muscle 🔖

L97.914   Non-pressure chronic ulcer of unspecified part of right lower leg with necrosis of bone 🔖

L97.919   Non-pressure chronic ulcer of unspecified part of right lower leg with unspecified severity 🔖

● **L97.92**   **Non-pressure chronic ulcer of unspecified part of left lower leg**

L97.921   Non-pressure chronic ulcer of unspecified part of left lower leg limited to breakdown of skin 🔖

L97.922   Non-pressure chronic ulcer of unspecified part of left lower leg with fat layer exposed 🔖

L97.923   Non-pressure chronic ulcer of unspecified part of left lower leg with necrosis of muscle 🔖

L97.924   Non-pressure chronic ulcer of unspecified part of left lower leg with necrosis of bone 🔖

L97.929   Non-pressure chronic ulcer of unspecified part of left lower leg with unspecified severity 🔖

● **L98**   **Other disorders of skin and subcutaneous tissue, not elsewhere classified**

L98.0   **Pyogenic granuloma**

> **Excludes2**   pyogenic granuloma of gingiva (K06.8)
> pyogenic granuloma of maxillary alveolar ridge (K04.5)
> pyogenic granuloma of oral mucosa (K13.4)

L98.1   **Factitial dermatitis**
Neurotic excoriation

> **Excludes1**   Excoriation (skin-picking) disorder (F42.4) ◄

L98.2   **Febrile neutrophilic dermatosis [Sweet]**

L98.3   **Eosinophilic cellulitis [Wells]** 🔖
    (Ex) See L02.81

● **L98.4**   **Non-pressure chronic ulcer of skin, not elsewhere classified**
Chronic ulcer of skin NOS
Tropical ulcer NOS
Ulcer of skin NOS

> **Excludes2**   pressure ulcer (pressure area) (L89.-)
> gangrene (I96)
> skin infections (L00-L08)
> specific infections classified to A00-B99
> ulcer of lower limb NEC (L97.-)
> varicose ulcer (I83.0-I82.2)

● L98.41   **Non-pressure chronic ulcer of buttock**

L98.411   Non-pressure chronic ulcer of buttock limited to breakdown of skin

L98.412   Non-pressure chronic ulcer of buttock with fat layer exposed

L98.413   Non-pressure chronic ulcer of buttock with necrosis of muscle

L98.414   Non-pressure chronic ulcer of buttock with necrosis of bone

L98.419   Non-pressure chronic ulcer of buttock with unspecified severity

● L98.42   **Non-pressure chronic ulcer of back**

L98.421   Non-pressure chronic ulcer of back limited to breakdown of skin

L98.422   Non-pressure chronic ulcer of back with fat layer exposed

L98.423   Non-pressure chronic ulcer of back with necrosis of muscle

L98.424   Non-pressure chronic ulcer of back with necrosis of bone

L98.429   Non-pressure chronic ulcer of back with unspecified severity

● L98.49   **Non-pressure chronic ulcer of skin of other sites**
Non-pressure chronic ulcer of skin NOS

L98.491   Non-pressure chronic ulcer of skin of other sites limited to breakdown of skin

L98.492   Non-pressure chronic ulcer of skin of other sites with fat layer exposed

L98.493   Non-pressure chronic ulcer of skin of other sites with necrosis of muscle

L98.494   Non-pressure chronic ulcer of skin of other sites with necrosis of bone

L98.499   Non-pressure chronic ulcer of skin of other sites with unspecified severity

L98.5   **Mucinosis of the skin**
Focal mucinosis
Lichen myxedematosus
Reticular erythematous mucinosis

> **Excludes1**   focal oral mucinosis (K13.79)
> myxedema (E03.9)

L98.6   **Other infiltrative disorders of the skin and subcutaneous tissue**

> **Excludes1**   hyalinosis cutis et mucosae (E78.89)

L98.7   **Excessive and redundant skin and subcutaneous tissue** ◄
Loose or sagging skin following bariatric surgery weight loss ◄
Loose or sagging skin following dietary weight loss ◄
Loose or sagging skin, NOS ◄

> **Excludes2**   acquired excess or redundant skin of eyelid (H02.3-) ◄
> congenital excess or redundant skin of eyelid (Q10.3) ◄
> skin changes due to chronic exposure to nonionizing radiation (L57.-) ◄

L98.8   **Other specified disorders of the skin and subcutaneous tissue**
Coding Clinic: 2013, Q2, P32

L98.9   **Disorder of the skin and subcutaneous tissue, unspecified**

▶ **L99**   **Other disorders of skin and subcutaneous tissue in diseases classified elsewhere**

> *Code first* underlying disease, such as:
> amyloidosis (E85.-)

> **Excludes1**   skin disorders in diabetes (E08-E13 with .62)
> skin disorders in gonorrhea (A54.89)
> skin disorders in syphilis (A51.31, A52.79)

CHAPTER 12 (L00-L99)

N   Newborn Age: 0   **P**   Pediatric Age: 0–17   **M**   Maternity DX: 12–55   **A**   Adult Age: 15–124   ♀ Females Only   ♂ Males Only

🔖 Complication\Comorbidity   🔖 Major C\C   (Ex) CC/MCC Exclusions   🔖 Hospital-Acquired Condition

CHAPTER 13

DISEASES OF THE MUSCULOSKELETAL SYSTEM AND CONNECTIVE TISSUE (M00-M99)

OGCR Chapter-Specific Coding Guidelines

13. **Chapter 13: Diseases of the Musculoskeletal System and Connective Tissue (M00-M99)**

a. Site and laterality

Most of the codes within Chapter 13 have site and laterality designations. The site represents the bone, joint or the muscle involved. For some conditions where more than one bone, joint or muscle is usually involved, such as osteoarthritis, there is a "multiple sites" code available. For categories where no multiple site code is provided and more than one bone, joint or muscle is involved, multiple codes should be used to indicate the different sites involved.

1) Bone versus joint

For certain conditions, the bone may be affected at the upper or lower end, (e.g., avascular necrosis of bone, M87, Osteoporosis, M80, M81). Though the portion of the bone affected may be at the joint, the site designation will be the bone, not the joint.

b. Acute traumatic versus chronic or recurrent musculoskeletal conditions

Many musculoskeletal conditions are a result of previous injury or trauma to a site, or are recurrent conditions. Bone, joint or muscle conditions that are the result of a healed injury are usually found in chapter 13. Recurrent bone, joint or muscle conditions are also usually found in chapter 13. Any current, acute injury should be coded to the appropriate injury code from chapter 19. Chronic or recurrent conditions should generally be coded with a code from chapter 13. If it is difficult to determine from the documentation in the record which code is best to describe a condition, query the provider.

c. Coding of Pathologic Fractures

7th character A is for use as long as the patient is receiving active treatment for the fracture. While the patient may be seen by a new or different provider over the course of treatment for a pathological fracture, assignment of the 7th character is based on whether the patient is undergoing active treatment and not whether the provider is seeing the patient for the first time.

7th character, D is to be used for encounters after the patient has completed active treatment. The other 7th characters, listed under each subcategory in the Tabular List, are to be used for subsequent encounters for **routine care of fractures during the healing and recovery phase as well as** treatment of problems associated with the healing, such as malunions, nonunions, and sequelae.

Care for complications of surgical treatment for fracture repairs during the healing or recovery phase should be coded with the appropriate complication codes.

See Section I.C.19. Coding of traumatic fractures.

d. Osteoporosis

Osteoporosis is a systemic condition, meaning that all bones of the musculoskeletal system are affected. Therefore, site is not a component of the codes under category M81, Osteoporosis without current pathological fracture. The site codes under category M80, Osteoporosis with current pathological fracture, identify the site of the fracture, not the osteoporosis.

1) Osteoporosis without pathological fracture

Category M81, Osteoporosis without current pathological fracture, is for use for patients with osteoporosis who do not currently have a pathologic fracture due to the osteoporosis, even if they have had a fracture in the past. For patients with a history of osteoporosis fractures, status code Z87.310, Personal history of (healed) osteoporosis fracture, should follow the code from M81.

2) Osteoporosis with current pathological fracture

Category M80, Osteoporosis with current pathological fracture, is for patients who have a current pathologic fracture at the time of an encounter. The codes under M80 identify the site of the fracture. A code from category M80, not a traumatic fracture code, should be used for any patient with known osteoporosis who suffers a fracture, even if the patient had a minor fall or trauma, if that fall or trauma would not usually break a normal, healthy bone.

CHAPTER 13

DISEASES OF THE MUSCULOSKELETAL SYSTEM AND CONNECTIVE TISSUE (M00-M99)

Note: Use an external cause code following the code for the musculoskeletal condition, if applicable, to identify the cause of the musculoskeletal condition

Excludes2 arthropathic psoriasis (L40.5-)
certain conditions originating in the perinatal period (P04-P96)
certain infectious and parasitic diseases (A00-B99)
compartment syndrome (traumatic) (T79.A-)
complications of pregnancy, childbirth and the puerperium (O00-O9A)
congenital malformations, deformations, and chromosomal abnormalities (Q00-Q99)
endocrine, nutritional and metabolic diseases (E00-E88)
injury, poisoning and certain other consequences of external causes (S00-T88)
neoplasms (C00-D49)
symptoms, signs and abnormal clinical and laboratory findings, not elsewhere classified (R00-R94)

This chapter contains the following blocks:

M00-M02	Infectious arthropathies
M04	Autoinflammatory syndromes ◀
M05-M14	Inflammatory polyarthropathies
M15-M19	Osteoarthritis
M20-M25	Other joint disorders
M26-M27	Dentofacial anomalies [including malocclusion] and other disorders of jaw
M30-M36	Systemic connective tissue disorders
M40-M43	Deforming dorsopathies
M45-M49	Spondylopathies
M50-M54	Other dorsopathies
M60-M63	Disorders of muscles
M65-M67	Disorders of synovium and tendon
M70-M79	Other soft tissue disorders
M80-M85	Disorders of bone density and structure
M86-M90	Other osteopathies
M91-M94	Chondropathies
M95	Other disorders of the musculoskeletal system and connective tissue
M96	Intraoperative and postprocedural complications and disorders of musculoskeletal system, not elsewhere classified
M97	Periprosthetic fracture around internal prosthetic joint ◀
M99	Biomechanical lesions, not elsewhere classified

ARTHROPATHIES (M00-M25)

Includes Disorders affecting predominantly peripheral (limb) joints

INFECTIOUS ARTHROPATHIES (M00-M02)

Note: This block comprises arthropathies due to microbiological agents.

Distinction is made between the following types of etiological relationship:

a) direct infection of joint, where organisms invade synovial tissue and microbial antigen is present in the joint;

b) indirect infection, which may be of two types: a reactive arthropathy, where microbial infection of the body is established but neither organisms nor antigens can be identified in the joint, and a postinfective arthropathy, where microbial antigen is present but recovery of an organism is inconstant and evidence of local multiplication is lacking.

◀ New ◀= Revised ~~deleted~~ Deleted Excludes 1 Excludes 2 Includes Use additional Code first Code also Unspecified

986 OGCR Official Guidelines ● Unacceptable Principal Diagnosis X Assign placeholder X ● Use Additional Character(s) ▶ Manifestation Code **Coding Clinic**

● **M00   Pyogenic arthritis**

  ● **M00.0   Staphylococcal arthritis and polyarthritis**

      Use additional code (B95.61-B95.8) to identify bacterial agent

      Excludes2   infection and inflammatory reaction due to internal joint prosthesis (T84.5-)

     M00.00   Staphylococcal arthritis, unspecified joint 🔹

        (Ex:) A17.9, A18.02, A18.09, A18.82, A18.84, A18.89, A39.83-A39.84, A54.40, A54.42-A54.43, A54.82, A54.84, A54.89-A54.9, B06.82, M00.00-M02.30, M02.319, M02.329, M02.339, M02.349, M02.359, M02.369, M02.379-M02.9, M05.40-M05.59, M05.70-M06.09, M06.20-M07.69, M11.00-M11.9, M12.10-M15.0, M15.3-M15.9, M16.2-M16.9, M17.2-M17.9, M18.2-M19.93, M24.10-M24.176, M25.00, M25.08-M25.18, M25.40-M25.676, M25.80-M25.9, M35.2, M36.1-M36.4, R26.2, R29.4

     ● **M00.01   Staphylococcal arthritis, shoulder**

        (Ex:) **For category M00.01 CC codes:** A17.9, A18.02, A18.09, A18.82, A18.84, A18.89, A39.83-A39.84, A54.40, A54.42-A54.43, A54.82, A54.84, A54.89-A54.9, B06.82, M00.00-M02.30, M02.319, M02.38-M02.819, M02.88-M02.9, M05.40-M05.59, M05.70-M06.09, M06.20-M07.69, M11.00-M11.9, M11.20-M11.219, M11.28-M11.819, M11.88-M11.9, M12.10-M15.0, M15.3-M15.9, M19.011-M19.019, M19.111-M19.119, M19.211-M19.219, M19.90-M19.93, M24.10-M24.119, M25.00, M25.011-M25.019, M25.08-M25.119, M25.18, M25.40-M25.419, M25.48-M25.519, M25.541-M25.549, M25.60-M25.619, M25.80-M25.819, M25.9, M35.2, M36.1-M36.4, R26.2

       M00.011   Staphylococcal arthritis, right shoulder 🔹

       M00.012   Staphylococcal arthritis, left shoulder 🔹

       M00.019   Staphylococcal arthritis, unspecified shoulder 🔹

     ● **M00.02   Staphylococcal arthritis, elbow**

        (Ex:) **For category M00.02 CC codes:** A17.9, A18.02, A18.09, A18.82, A18.84, A18.89, A39.83-A39.84, A54.40, A54.42-A54.43, A54.82, A54.84, A54.89-A54.9, B06.82, M00.00-M02.30, M02.329, M02.38-M02.80, M02.821-M02.829, M02.88-M02.9, M05.40-M05.59, M05.70-M07.60, M07.621-M07.629, M07.68-M07.69, M11.00, M11.021-M11.029, M11.08-M11.10, M11.121-M11.129, M11.18-M11.20, M11.221-M11.229, M11.28-M11.80, M11.821-M11.829, M11.88-M11.9, M12.10, M12.121-M12.129, M12.18-M12.20, M12.221-M12.229, M12.28-M12.30, M12.321-M12.329, M12.38-M12.40, M12.421-M12.429, M12.48-M12.50, M12.521-M12.529, M12.58-M12.80, M12.821-M12.829, M12.88-M12.9, M13.0-M13.10, M13.121-M13.129, M13.80, M13.821-M13.829, M13.88-M13.89, M14.60-M15.9, M19.021-M19.029, M19.121-M19.129, M19.221-M19.229, M19.90-M19.93, M24.10, M24.121-M24.129, M25.00, M25.021-M25.029, M25.08-M25.10, M25.121-M25.129, M25.18, M25.40, M25.421-M25.429, M25.48-M25.50, M25.521-M25.529, M25.541-M25.549, M25.60, M25.621-M25.629, M25.80, M25.821-M25.829, M25.9, M35.2, M36.1-M36.4, R26.2

       M00.021   Staphylococcal arthritis, right elbow 🔹

       M00.022   Staphylococcal arthritis, left elbow 🔹

       M00.029   Staphylococcal arthritis, unspecified elbow 🔹

  ● **M00.03   Staphylococcal arthritis, wrist**

      Staphylococcal arthritis of carpal bones

      (Ex:) **For category M00.03 CC codes:** A17.9, A18.02, A18.09, A18.82, A18.84, A18.89, A39.83-A39.84, A54.40, A54.42-A54.43, A54.82, A54.84, A54.89-A54.9, B06.82, M00.00-M02.30, M02.339, M02.38-M02.80, M02.831-M02.839, M02.88-M02.9, M05.40-M05.59, M05.70-M07.60, M07.631-M07.639, M07.68-M07.69, M11.00, M11.031-M11.039, M11.08-M11.10, M11.131-M11.139, M11.18-M11.20, M11.231-M11.239, M11.28-M11.80, M11.831-M11.839, M11.88-M11.9, M12.10, M12.131-M12.139, M12.18-M12.20, M12.231-M12.239, M12.28-M12.30, M12.331-M12.339, M12.38-M12.40, M12.431-M12.439, M12.48-M12.50, M12.531-M12.539, M12.58-M12.80, M12.831-M12.839, M12.88-M12.9, M13.0-M13.10, M13.131-M13.139, M13.80, M13.831-M13.839, M13.88-M15.9, M19.031-M19.039, M19.131-M19.139, M19.231-M19.239, M19.90-M19.93, M24.10, M24.131-M24.139, M25.00, M25.031-M25.039, M25.08-M25.10, M25.131-M25.139, M25.18, M25.40, M25.431-M25.439, M25.48-M25.50, M25.531-M25.539, M25.541-M25.549, M25.60, M25.631-M25.639, M25.80, M25.831-M25.839, M25.9, M35.2, M36.1-M36.4, R26.2

     M00.031   Staphylococcal arthritis, right wrist 🔹

     M00.032   Staphylococcal arthritis, left wrist 🔹

     M00.039   Staphylococcal arthritis, unspecified wrist 🔹

  ● **M00.04   Staphylococcal arthritis, hand**

      Staphylococcal arthritis of metacarpus and phalanges

      (Ex:) **For category M00.04 CC codes:** A17.9, A18.02, A18.09, A18.82, A18.84, A18.89, A39.83-A39.84, A54.40, A54.42-A54.43, A54.82, A54.84, A54.89-A54.9, B06.82, M00.00, M00.041-M00.049, M00.08-M00.10, M00.141-M00.149, M00.18-M00.20, M00.241-M00.249, M00.28-M00.80, M00.841-M00.849, M00.88-M01.X0, M01.X41-M01.X49, M01.X8-M02.10, M02.141-M02.149, M02.18-M02.30, M02.349, M02.38-M02.80, M02.841-M02.849, M02.88-M02.9, M05.40-M05.59, M05.70-M06.09, M06.20-M07.60, M07.641-M07.649, M07.68-M07.69, M11.00, M11.041-M11.049, M11.08-M11.10, M11.141-M11.149, M11.18-M11.20, M11.241-M11.249, M11.28-M11.80, M11.841-M11.849, M11.88-M11.9, M12.10, M12.141-M12.149, M12.18-M12.20, M12.241-M12.249, M12.28-M12.30, M12.341-M12.349, M12.38-M12.40, M12.441-M12.449, M12.48-M12.50, M12.541-M12.549, M12.58-M12.80, M12.841-M12.849, M12.88-M13.10, M13.141-M13.149, M13.80, M13.841-M13.849, M13.88-M15.9, M18.0-M18.9, M19.041-M19.049, M19.141-M19.149, M19.241-M19.249, M19.90-M19.93, M24.10, M24.141-M24.149, M25.00, M25.041-M25.049, M25.08-M25.10, M25.141-M25.149, M25.18, M25.40, M25.441-M25.449, M25.48-M25.50, M25.541-M25.549, M25.60, M25.641-M25.649, M25.80, M25.841-M25.849, M25.9, M35.2, M36.1-M36.4, R26.2

     M00.041   Staphylococcal arthritis, right hand 🔹

     M00.042   Staphylococcal arthritis, left hand 🔹

     M00.049   Staphylococcal arthritis, unspecified hand 🔹

N   Newborn Age: 0   **P**   Pediatric Age: 0–17   **M**   Maternity DX: 12–55   **A**   Adult Age: 15–124   ♀   Females Only   ♂   Males Only

🔹   Complication\Comorbidity   🔹   Major C\C   (Ex:)   CC/MCC Exclusions   🔹   Hospital-Acquired Condition

● **M00.05** **Staphylococcal arthritis, hip**
ⒺⓍ For category **M00.05** CC codes: A17.9, A18.02, A18.09, A18.82, A18.84, A18.89, A39.83-A39.84, A54.40, A54.42-A54.43, A54.82, A54.84, A54.89-A54.9, B06.82, M00.00, M00.051-M00.059, M00.08-M00.10, M00.151-M00.159, M00.18-M00.20, M00.251-M00.259, M00.28-M00.29, M00.80, M00.851-M00.859, M00.88-M00.9, M01.X0, M01.X51-M01.X59 , M01.X8-M02.10, M02.151-M02.159, M02.18-M02.30, M02.359, M02.38-M02.80, M02.851-M02.9, M05.40-M05.59, M05.70-M06.09, M06.20-M06.39, M06.80-M07.60, M07.651-M07.659, M07.68-M07.69, M11.00, M11.051-M11.059, M11.08-M11.10, M11.151-M11.159, M11.18-M11.20, M11.251-M11.259, M11.28-M11.80, M11.851-M11.859, M11.88-M12.10, M12.151-M12.159, M12.18-M12.20, M12.251-M12.259, M12.28-M12.30, M12.351-M12.359, M12.38-M12.40, M12.451-M12.459, M12.48-M12.50, M12.551-M12.559, M12.58-M12.80, M12.851-M12.859, M12.88-M13.10, M13.151-M13.159, M13.80, M13.851-M13.859, M13.88-M15.0, M15.3-M16.9, M19.90-M19.93, M24.10, M24.151-M24.159, M25.00, M25.051-M25.059, M25.08-M25.10, M25.151-M25.159, M25.18, M25.40, M25.451-M25.459, M25.48-M25.559, M25.60, M25.651-M25.659, M25.80, M25.851-M25.859, M25.9, M35.2, M36.1-M36.4, R26.2, R29.4

　　M00.051 **Staphylococcal arthritis, right hip** Ⓒ

　　M00.052 **Staphylococcal arthritis, left hip** Ⓒ

　　M00.059 **Staphylococcal arthritis, unspecified hip** Ⓒ

● **M00.06** **Staphylococcal arthritis, knee**
ⒺⓍ For category **M00.06** CC codes: A17.9, A18.02, A18.09, A18.82, A18.84, A18.89, A39.83-A39.84, A54.40, A54.42-A54.43, A54.82, A54.84, A54.89-A54.9, B06.82, M00.00, M00.061-M00.069, M00.08-M00.10, M00.161-M00.169, M00.18-M00.20, M00.261-M00.269, M00.28-M00.29, M00.80, M00.861-M00.869, M00.88-M00.9, M01.X0, M01.X61-M01.X69 , M01.X8-M02.10, M02.161-M02.169, M02.18-M02.30, M02.369, M02.38-M02.80, M02.861-M02.869, M02.88-M02.9, M05.40-M05.59, M05.70-M06.09, M06.20-M06.39, M06.80-M07.60, M07.661-M07.669, M07.68-M07.69, M11.00, M11.061-M11.069, M11.08-M11.10, M11.161-M11.169, M11.18-M11.20, M11.261-M11.269, M11.28-M11.80, M11.861-M11.869, M11.88-M12.10, M12.161-M12.169, M12.18-M12.20, M12.261-M12.269, M12.28-M12.30, M12.361-M12.369, M12.38-M12.40, M12.461-M12.469, M12.48-M12.50, M12.561-M12.569, M12.58-M12.80, M12.861-M12.869, M12.88-M13.10, M13.161-M13.169, M13.80, M13.861-M13.869, M13.88-M15.0, M15.3-M15.9, M17.0-M17.9, M19.90-M19.93, M24.10, M25.00, M25.061-M25.069, M25.08-M25.10, M25.161-M25.169, M25.18, M25.40, M25.461-M25.469, M25.48-M25.50, M25.541-M25.549, M25.561-M25.569, M25.60, M25.661-M25.669, M25.80, M25.861-M25.869, M25.9, M35.2, M36.1-M36.4, R26.2

　　M00.061 **Staphylococcal arthritis, right knee** Ⓒ

　　M00.062 **Staphylococcal arthritis, left knee** Ⓒ

　　M00.069 **Staphylococcal arthritis, unspecified knee** Ⓒ

● **M00.07** **Staphylococcal arthritis, ankle and foot**
Staphylococcal arthritis, tarsus, metatarsus and phalanges
ⒺⓍ For category **M00.07** CC codes: A17.9, A18.02, A18.09, A18.82, A18.84, A18.89, A39.83-A39.84, A54.40, A54.42-A54.43, A54.82, A54.84, A54.89-A54.9, B06.82, M00.00, M00.071-M00.079, M00.08-M00.10, M00.171-M00.179, M00.18-M00.20, M00.271-M00.279, M00.28-M00.29, M00.80, M00.871-M00.879, M00.88-M00.9, M01.X0, M01.X71-M01.X79 , M01.X8-M02.10, M02.171-M02.179, M02.18-M02.9, M05.40-M05.59, M05.70-M06.09, M06.20-M06.39, M06.80-M07.60, M07.671-M07.679, M07.68-M07.69, M11.00, M11.071-M11.079, M11.08-M11.10, M11.171-M11.179, M11.18-M11.20, M11.271-M11.279, M11.28-M11.80, M11.871-M11.879, M11.88-M11.9, M12.10, M12.171-M12.179, M12.18-M12.20, M12.271-M12.279, M12.28-M12.30, M12.371-M12.379, M12.38-M12.40, M12.471-M12.479, M12.48-M12.50, M12.571-M12.579, M12.58-M12.80, M12.871-M12.879, M12.88-M13.10, M13.171-M13.179, M13.80, M13.871-M13.879, M13.88-M15.0, M15.3-M15.9, M19.071-M19.079, M19.171-M19.179, M19.271-M19.279, M19.90-M19.93, M24.10, M24.171-M24.176, M25.00, M25.071-M25.10, M25.171-M25.18, M25.40, M25.471-M25.50, M25.541-M25.549, M25.571-M25.60, M25.671-M25.676, M25.80, M25.871-M25.9, M35.2, M36.1-M36.4, R26.2

　　M00.071 **Staphylococcal arthritis, right ankle and foot** Ⓒ

　　M00.072 **Staphylococcal arthritis, left ankle and foot** Ⓒ

　　M00.079 **Staphylococcal arthritis, unspecified ankle and foot** Ⓒ

M00.08 **Staphylococcal arthritis, vertebrae** Ⓒ
ⒺⓍ See M00.00

M00.09 **Staphylococcal polyarthritis** Ⓒ
ⒺⓍ See M00.00

● **M00.1** **Pneumococcal arthritis and polyarthritis**

M00.10 **Pneumococcal arthritis, unspecified joint** Ⓒ
ⒺⓍ See M00.00

● **M00.11** **Pneumococcal arthritis, shoulder**
ⒺⓍ For category **M00.11** CC codes: See M00.01

　　M00.111 **Pneumococcal arthritis, right shoulder** Ⓒ

　　M00.112 **Pneumococcal arthritis, left shoulder** Ⓒ

　　M00.119 **Pneumococcal arthritis, unspecified shoulder** Ⓒ

● **M00.12** **Pneumococcal arthritis, elbow**
ⒺⓍ For category **M00.12** CC codes: See M00.02

　　M00.121 **Pneumococcal arthritis, right elbow** Ⓒ

　　M00.122 **Pneumococcal arthritis, left elbow** Ⓒ

　　M00.129 **Pneumococcal arthritis, unspecified elbow** Ⓒ

● **M00.13** **Pneumococcal arthritis, wrist**
Pneumococcal arthritis of carpal bones
ⒺⓍ For category **M00.13** CC codes: See M00.03

　　M00.131 **Pneumococcal arthritis, right wrist** Ⓒ

　　M00.132 **Pneumococcal arthritis, left wrist** Ⓒ

　　M00.139 **Pneumococcal arthritis, unspecified wrist** Ⓒ

● **M00.14** **Pneumococcal arthritis, hand**
Pneumococcal arthritis of metacarpus and phalanges
ⒺⓍ For category **M00.14** CC codes: See M00.04

　　M00.141 **Pneumococcal arthritis, right hand** Ⓒ

　　M00.142 **Pneumococcal arthritis, left hand** Ⓒ

　　M00.149 **Pneumococcal arthritis, unspecified hand** Ⓒ

◀ New　◀⦙ Revised　deleted Deleted　Excludes 1　Excludes 2　Includes　Use additional　Code first　Code also　Unspecified
OGCR Official Guidelines　● Unacceptable Principal Diagnosis　X Assign placeholder X　● Use Additional Character(s)　▌ Manifestation Code　**Coding Clinic**

● **M00.15** **Pneumococcal arthritis, hip**
     (Ex) **For category M00.15 CC codes:** See M00.05
     M00.151 Pneumococcal arthritis, right hip 🦠
     M00.152 Pneumococcal arthritis, left hip 🦠
     M00.159 Pneumococcal arthritis, unspecified hip 🦠

● **M00.16** **Pneumococcal arthritis, knee**
     (Ex) **For category M00.16 CC codes:** See M00.06
     M00.161 Pneumococcal arthritis, right knee 🦠
     M00.162 Pneumococcal arthritis, left knee 🦠
     M00.169 Pneumococcal arthritis, unspecified knee 🦠

● **M00.17** **Pneumococcal arthritis, ankle and foot**
     Pneumococcal arthritis, tarsus, metatarsus and phalanges
     (Ex) **For category M00.17 CC codes:** See M00.07
     M00.171 Pneumococcal arthritis, right ankle and foot 🦠
     M00.172 Pneumococcal arthritis, left ankle and foot 🦠
     M00.179 Pneumococcal arthritis, unspecified ankle and foot 🦠

M00.18 **Pneumococcal arthritis, vertebrae** 🦠
     (Ex) See M00.00

M00.19 **Pneumococcal polyarthritis** 🦠
     (Ex) See M00.00

● **M00.2** **Other streptococcal arthritis and polyarthritis**
     Use additional code (B95.0-B95.2, B95.4-B95.5) to identify bacterial agent

M00.20 **Other streptococcal arthritis, unspecified joint** 🦠
     (Ex) See M00.00

● **M00.21** **Other streptococcal arthritis, shoulder**
     (Ex) **For category M00.21 CC codes:** See M00.01
     M00.211 Other streptococcal arthritis, right shoulder 🦠
     M00.212 Other streptococcal arthritis, left shoulder 🦠
     M00.219 Other streptococcal arthritis, unspecified shoulder 🦠

● **M00.22** **Other streptococcal arthritis, elbow**
     (Ex) **For category M00.22 CC codes:** See M00.02
     M00.221 Other streptococcal arthritis, right elbow 🦠
     M00.222 Other streptococcal arthritis, left elbow 🦠
     M00.229 Other streptococcal arthritis, unspecified elbow 🦠

● **M00.23** **Other streptococcal arthritis, wrist**
     Other streptococcal arthritis of carpal bones
     (Ex) **For category M00.23 CC codes:** See M00.03
     M00.231 Other streptococcal arthritis, right wrist 🦠
     M00.232 Other streptococcal arthritis, left wrist 🦠
     M00.239 Other streptococcal arthritis, unspecified wrist 🦠

● **M00.24** **Other streptococcal arthritis, hand**
     Other streptococcal arthritis metacarpus and phalanges
     (Ex) **For category M00.24 CC codes:** See M00.04
     M00.241 Other streptococcal arthritis, right hand 🦠
     M00.242 Other streptococcal arthritis, left hand 🦠
     M00.249 Other streptococcal arthritis, unspecified hand 🦠

● **M00.25** **Other streptococcal arthritis, hip**
     (Ex) **For category M00.25 CC codes:** See M00.05
     M00.251 Other streptococcal arthritis, right hip 🦠
     M00.252 Other streptococcal arthritis, left hip 🦠
     M00.259 Other streptococcal arthritis, unspecified hip 🦠

● **M00.26** **Other streptococcal arthritis, knee**
     (Ex) **For category M00.26 CC codes:** See M00.06
     M00.261 Other streptococcal arthritis, right knee 🦠
     M00.262 Other streptococcal arthritis, left knee 🦠
     M00.269 Other streptococcal arthritis, unspecified knee 🦠

● **M00.27** **Other streptococcal arthritis, ankle and foot**
     Other streptococcal arthritis, tarsus, metatarsus and phalanges
     (Ex) **For category M00.27 CC codes:** See M00.07
     M00.271 Other streptococcal arthritis, right ankle and foot 🦠
     M00.272 Other streptococcal arthritis, left ankle and foot 🦠
     M00.279 Other streptococcal arthritis, unspecified ankle and foot 🦠

M00.28 **Other streptococcal arthritis, vertebrae** 🦠
     (Ex) See M00.00

M00.29 **Other streptococcal polyarthritis** 🦠
     (Ex) See M00.00

● **M00.8** **Arthritis and polyarthritis due to other bacteria**
     Use additional code (B96) to identify bacteria

M00.80 **Arthritis due to other bacteria, unspecified joint** 🦠
     (Ex) See M00.00

● **M00.81** **Arthritis due to other bacteria, shoulder**
     (Ex) **For category M00.81 CC codes:** See M00.01
     M00.811 Arthritis due to other bacteria, right shoulder 🦠
     M00.812 Arthritis due to other bacteria, left shoulder 🦠
     M00.819 Arthritis due to other bacteria, unspecified shoulder 🦠

● **M00.82** **Arthritis due to other bacteria, elbow**
     (Ex) **For category M00.82 CC codes:** See M00.02
     M00.821 Arthritis due to other bacteria, right elbow 🦠
     M00.822 Arthritis due to other bacteria, left elbow 🦠
     M00.829 Arthritis due to other bacteria, unspecified elbow 🦠

● **M00.83** **Arthritis due to other bacteria, wrist**
     Arthritis due to other bacteria, carpal bones
     (Ex) **For category M00.83 CC codes:** See M00.03
     M00.831 Arthritis due to other bacteria, right wrist 🦠
     M00.832 Arthritis due to other bacteria, left wrist 🦠
     M00.839 Arthritis due to other bacteria, unspecified wrist 🦠

● **M00.84** **Arthritis due to other bacteria, hand**
     Arthritis due to other bacteria, metacarpus and phalanges
     (Ex) **For category M00.84 CC codes:** See M00.04
     M00.841 Arthritis due to other bacteria, right hand 🦠
     M00.842 Arthritis due to other bacteria, left hand 🦠
     M00.849 Arthritis due to other bacteria, unspecified hand 🦠

CHAPTER 13 (M00-M99)

N   Newborn Age: 0   P   Pediatric Age: 0–17   M   Maternity DX: 12–55   A   Adult Age: 15–124   ♀   Females Only   ♂   Males Only

🦠 Complication\Comorbidity   🦠 Major C\C   (Ex) CC/MCC Exclusions   🦠 Hospital-Acquired Condition

● **M00.85** **Arthritis due to other bacteria, hip**
   (Ex:) For category M00.85 CC codes: See M00.05

   M00.851 **Arthritis due to other bacteria, right hip** 🖑

   M00.852 **Arthritis due to other bacteria, left hip** 🖑

   M00.859 **Arthritis due to other bacteria, unspecified hip** 🖑

● **M00.86** **Arthritis due to other bacteria, knee**
   (Ex:) For category M00.86 CC codes: See M00.06

   M00.861 **Arthritis due to other bacteria, right knee** 🖑

   M00.862 **Arthritis due to other bacteria, left knee** 🖑

   M00.869 **Arthritis due to other bacteria, unspecified knee** 🖑

● **M00.87** **Arthritis due to other bacteria, ankle and foot**
   Arthritis due to other bacteria, tarsus, metatarsus, and phalanges
   (Ex:) For category M00.87 CC codes: See M00.07

   M00.871 **Arthritis due to other bacteria, right ankle and foot** 🖑

   M00.872 **Arthritis due to other bacteria, left ankle and foot** 🖑

   M00.879 **Arthritis due to other bacteria, unspecified ankle and foot** 🖑

   M00.88 **Arthritis due to other bacteria, vertebrae** 🖑
      (Ex:) See M00.00

   M00.89 **Polyarthritis due to other bacteria** 🖑
      (Ex:) See M00.00

M00.9 **Pyogenic arthritis, unspecified** 🖑
   Infective arthritis NOS
   (Ex:) See M00.00

● **M01** **Direct infections of joint in infectious and parasitic diseases classified elsewhere**

   Code first underlying disease, such as:
   leprosy [Hansen's disease] (A30.-)
   mycoses (B35-B49)
   O'nyong-nyong fever (A92.1)
   paratyphoid fever (A01.1-A01.4)

   Excludes1   arthropathy in Lyme disease (A69.23)
              gonococcal arthritis (A54.42)
              meningococcal arthritis (A39.83)
              mumps arthritis (B26.85)
              postinfective arthropathy (M02.-)
              postmeningococcal arthritis (A39.84)
              reactive arthritis (M02.3)
              rubella arthritis (B06.82)
              sarcoidosis arthritis (D86.86)
              typhoid fever arthritis (A01.04)
              tuberculosis arthritis (A18.01-A18.02)

● **M01.X** **Direct infection of joint in infectious and parasitic diseases classified elsewhere**
   (Ex:) For category M01.X CC codes unless otherwise indicated: A02.23, A17.9, A18.02, A18.09, A18.82, A18.84, A18.89, A39.83-A39.84, A54.40, A54.42-A54.43, A54.82, A54.84, A54.89-A54.9, B06.82, M00.00, M00.011-M02.30, M02.319, M02.329, M02.339, M02.349, M02.359, M02.369, M02.379, M02.38-M02.9, M05.40-M05.59, M05.70-M07.69, M11.00-M15.0, M15.3-M15.9, M16.2-M16.9, M17.2-M17.9, M18.2-M18.9, M19.111-M19.93, M24.10-M24.176, M25.00, M25.08-M25.18, M25.40-M25.676, M25.80-M25.9, M35.2, M36.1-M36.4, R29.4

  ❱ *M01.X0* *Direct infection of unspecified joint in infectious and parasitic diseases classified elsewhere* 🖑

● **M01.X1** **Direct infection of shoulder joint in infectious and parasitic diseases classified elsewhere**
   (Ex:) For category M01.X1 CC codes: A02.23, A17.9, A18.02, A18.09, A18.82, A18.84, A18.89, A39.83-A39.84, A54.40, A54.42-A54.43, A54.82, A54.84, A54.89-A54.9, B06.82, M00.00, M00.011-M02.30, M02.319, M02.329, M02.339, M02.349, M02.359, M02.369, M02.379, M02.38-M02.9, M05.40-M05.59, M05.70-M07.69, M11.00-M15.0, M15.3-M15.9, M16.2-M16.9, M17.2-M17.9, M18.2-M18.9, M19.111-M19.93, M24.10-M24.176, M25.00, M25.08-M25.18, M25.40-M25.676, M25.80-M25.9, M35.2, M36.1-M36.4, R29.4

  ❱ *M01.X11* *Direct infection of right shoulder in infectious and parasitic diseases classified elsewhere* 🖑

  ❱ *M01.X12* *Direct infection of left shoulder in infectious and parasitic diseases classified elsewhere* 🖑

  ❱ *M01.X19* *Direct infection of unspecified shoulder in infectious and parasitic diseases classified elsewhere* 🖑

● **M01.X2** **Direct infection of elbow in infectious and parasitic diseases classified elsewhere**

  ❱ *M01.X21* *Direct infection of right elbow in infectious and parasitic diseases classified elsewhere* 🖑

  ❱ *M01.X22* *Direct infection of left elbow in infectious and parasitic diseases classified elsewhere* 🖑

  ❱ *M01.X29* *Direct infection of unspecified elbow in infectious and parasitic diseases classified elsewhere* 🖑

● **M01.X3** **Direct infection of wrist in infectious and parasitic diseases classified elsewhere**
   Direct infection of carpal bones in infectious and parasitic diseases classified elsewhere

  ❱ *M01.X31* *Direct infection of right wrist in infectious and parasitic diseases classified elsewhere* 🖑

  ❱ *M01.X32* *Direct infection of left wrist in infectious and parasitic diseases classified elsewhere* 🖑

  ❱ *M01.X39* *Direct infection of unspecified wrist in infectious and parasitic diseases classified elsewhere* 🖑

● **M01.X4** **Direct infection of hand in infectious and parasitic diseases classified elsewhere**
   Direct infection of metacarpus and phalanges in infectious and parasitic diseases classified elsewhere

  ❱ *M01.X41* *Direct infection of right hand in infectious and parasitic diseases classified elsewhere* 🖑

  ❱ *M01.X42* *Direct infection of left hand in infectious and parasitic diseases classified elsewhere* 🖑

  ❱ *M01.X49* *Direct infection of unspecified hand in infectious and parasitic diseases classified elsewhere* 🖑

● **M01.X5** **Direct infection of hip in infectious and parasitic diseases classified elsewhere**

  ❱ *M01.X51* *Direct infection of right hip in infectious and parasitic diseases classified elsewhere* 🖑

  ❱ *M01.X52* *Direct infection of left hip in infectious and parasitic diseases classified elsewhere* 🖑

  ❱ *M01.X59* *Direct infection of unspecified hip in infectious and parasitic diseases classified elsewhere* 🖑

◄ New   ⬅ Revised   ~~deleted~~ Deleted   Excludes 1   Excludes 2   Includes   Use additional   Code first   Code also   Unspecified
OGCR Official Guidelines   ● Unacceptable Principal Diagnosis   X Assign placeholder X   ● Use Additional Character(s)   ❱ Manifestation Code   **Coding Clinic**

● **M01.X6** **Direct infection of knee in infectious and parasitic diseases classified elsewhere**
  ▸ *M01.X61* *Direct infection of right knee in infectious and parasitic diseases classified elsewhere* 🟡
  ▸ *M01.X62* *Direct infection of left knee in infectious and parasitic diseases classified elsewhere* 🟡
  ▸ *M01.X69* *Direct infection of* unspecified *knee in infectious and parasitic diseases classified elsewhere* 🟡

● **M01.X7** **Direct infection of ankle and foot in infectious and parasitic diseases classified elsewhere**
  Direct infection of tarsus, metatarsus and phalanges in infectious and parasitic diseases classified elsewhere
  ▸ *M01.X71* *Direct infection of right ankle and foot in infectious and parasitic diseases classified elsewhere* 🟡
  ▸ *M01.X72* *Direct infection of left ankle and foot in infectious and parasitic diseases classified elsewhere* 🟡
  ▸ *M01.X79* *Direct infection of* unspecified *ankle and foot in infectious and parasitic diseases classified elsewhere* 🟡

  ▸ *M01.X8* *Direct infection of vertebrae in infectious and parasitic diseases classified elsewhere* 🟡
  ▸ *M01.X9* *Direct infection of multiple joints in infectious and parasitic diseases classified elsewhere* 🟡

● **M02** **Postinfective and reactive arthropathies**
  Code first underlying disease, such as:
    congenital syphilis [Clutton's joints] (A50.5)
    enteritis due to Yersinia enterocolitica (A04.6)
    infective endocarditis (I33.0)
    viral hepatitis (B15-B19)
  Excludes1   Behçet's disease (M35.2)
    direct infections of joint in infectious and parasitic diseases classified elsewhere (M01.-)
    postmeningococcal arthritis (A39.84)
    mumps arthritis (B26.85)
    rubella arthritis (B06.82)
    syphilis arthritis (late) (A52.77)
    rheumatic fever (I00)
    tabetic arthropathy [Charcôt's] (A52.16)
  🅴🆇 For category M02 CC codes unless otherwise indicated: See M01.X

● **M02.0** **Arthropathy following intestinal bypass**
  M02.00 **Arthropathy following intestinal bypass,** unspecified **site**
  ● **M02.01** **Arthropathy following intestinal bypass, shoulder**
    M02.011 **Arthropathy following intestinal bypass, right shoulder**
    M02.012 **Arthropathy following intestinal bypass, left shoulder**
    M02.019 **Arthropathy following intestinal bypass,** unspecified **shoulder**
  ● **M02.02** **Arthropathy following intestinal bypass, elbow**
    M02.021 **Arthropathy following intestinal bypass, right elbow**
    M02.022 **Arthropathy following intestinal bypass, left elbow**
    M02.029 **Arthropathy following intestinal bypass,** unspecified **elbow**
  ● **M02.03** **Arthropathy following intestinal bypass, wrist**
    Arthropathy following intestinal bypass, carpal bones
    M02.031 **Arthropathy following intestinal bypass, right wrist**
    M02.032 **Arthropathy following intestinal bypass, left wrist**
    M02.039 **Arthropathy following intestinal bypass,** unspecified **wrist**

● **M02.04** **Arthropathy following intestinal bypass, hand**
  Arthropathy following intestinal bypass, metacarpals and phalanges
    M02.041 **Arthropathy following intestinal bypass, right hand**
    M02.042 **Arthropathy following intestinal bypass, left hand**
    M02.049 **Arthropathy following intestinal bypass,** unspecified **hand**
● **M02.05** **Arthropathy following intestinal bypass, hip**
    M02.051 **Arthropathy following intestinal bypass, right hip**
    M02.052 **Arthropathy following intestinal bypass, left hip**
    M02.059 **Arthropathy following intestinal bypass,** unspecified **hip**
● **M02.06** **Arthropathy following intestinal bypass, knee**
    M02.061 **Arthropathy following intestinal bypass, right knee**
    M02.062 **Arthropathy following intestinal bypass, left knee**
    M02.069 **Arthropathy following intestinal bypass,** unspecified **knee**
● **M02.07** **Arthropathy following intestinal bypass, ankle and foot**
  Arthropathy following intestinal bypass, tarsus, metatarsus and phalanges
    M02.071 **Arthropathy following intestinal bypass, right ankle and foot**
    M02.072 **Arthropathy following intestinal bypass, left ankle and foot**
    M02.079 **Arthropathy following intestinal bypass,** unspecified **ankle and foot**
  M02.08 **Arthropathy following intestinal bypass, vertebrae**
  M02.09 **Arthropathy following intestinal bypass, multiple sites**
● **M02.1** **Postdysenteric arthropathy**
  M02.10 **Postdysenteric arthropathy,** unspecified **site** 🟡
● **M02.11** **Postdysenteric arthropathy, shoulder**
    M02.111 **Postdysenteric arthropathy, right shoulder** 🟡
    M02.112 **Postdysenteric arthropathy, left shoulder** 🟡
    M02.119 **Postdysenteric arthropathy,** unspecified **shoulder** 🟡
● **M02.12** **Postdysenteric arthropathy, elbow**
    M02.121 **Postdysenteric arthropathy, right elbow** 🟡
    M02.122 **Postdysenteric arthropathy, left elbow** 🟡
    M02.129 **Postdysenteric arthropathy,** unspecified **elbow** 🟡
● **M02.13** **Postdysenteric arthropathy, wrist**
  Postdysenteric arthropathy, carpal bones
    M02.131 **Postdysenteric arthropathy, right wrist** 🟡
    M02.132 **Postdysenteric arthropathy, left wrist** 🟡
    M02.139 **Postdysenteric arthropathy,** unspecified **wrist** 🟡
● **M02.14** **Postdysenteric arthropathy, hand**
  Postdysenteric arthropathy, metacarpus and phalanges
    M02.141 **Postdysenteric arthropathy, right hand** 🟡
    M02.142 **Postdysenteric arthropathy, left hand** 🟡
    M02.149 **Postdysenteric arthropathy,** unspecified **hand** 🟡

N Newborn Age: 0   **P** Pediatric Age: 0–17   **M** Maternity DX: 12–55   **A** Adult Age: 15–124   ♀ Females Only   ♂ Males Only

🟡 Complication\Comorbidity   🟡 Major C\C   🅴🆇 CC/MCC Exclusions   🟡 Hospital-Acquired Condition

991

● **M02.15 Postdysenteric arthropathy, hip**
    M02.151 Postdysenteric arthropathy, right hip 🐾
    M02.152 Postdysenteric arthropathy, left hip 🐾
    M02.159 Postdysenteric arthropathy, unspecified hip 🐾

● **M02.16 Postdysenteric arthropathy, knee**
    Ⓔⓧ **For category M02.16 CC codes:** A02.23, A17.9, A18.02, A18.09, A18.82, A18.84, A18.89, A39.83-A39.84, A54.40, A54.42-A54.43, A54.82, A54.84, A54.89-A54.9, B06.82, M00.00, M00.011-M02.30, M02.319, M02.329, M02.339, M02.349, M02.359, M02.369, M02.379, M02.38-M02.9, M05.40-M05.59, M05.70-M07.69, M11.00-M15.0, M15.3-M15.9, M16.2-M16.9, M17.2-M17.9, M18.2-M18.9, M19.111-M19.93, M24.10-M24.176, M25.00, M25.08-M25.18, M25.40-M25.676, M25.80-M25.9, M35.2, M36.1-M36.4, R29.4
    M02.161 Postdysenteric arthropathy, right knee 🐾
    M02.162 Postdysenteric arthropathy, left knee 🐾
    M02.169 Postdysenteric arthropathy, unspecified knee 🐾

● **M02.17 Postdysenteric arthropathy, ankle and foot**
    Postdysenteric arthropathy, tarsus, metatarsus and phalanges
    M02.171 Postdysenteric arthropathy, right ankle and foot 🐾
    M02.172 Postdysenteric arthropathy, left ankle and foot 🐾
    M02.179 Postdysenteric arthropathy, unspecified ankle and foot 🐾

M02.18 Postdysenteric arthropathy, vertebrae 🐾
    Ⓔⓧ A02.23, A17.9, A18.02, A18.09, A18.82, A18.84, A18.89, A39.83-A39.84, A54.40, A54.42-A54.43, A54.82, A54.84, A54.89-A54.9, B06.82, M00.00, M00.011-M02.30, M02.319, M02.329, M02.339, M02.349, M02.359, M02.369, M02.379, M02.38-M02.9, M05.40-M05.59, M05.70-M07.69, M11.00-M15.0, M15.3-M15.9, M16.2-M16.9, M17.2-M17.9, M18.2-M18.9, M19.111-M19.93, M24.10-M24.176, M25.00, M25.08-M25.18, M25.40-M25.676, M25.80-M25.9, M35.2, M36.1-M36.4, R29.4

M02.19 Postdysenteric arthropathy, multiple sites 🐾

● **M02.2 Postimmunization arthropathy**
    M02.20 Postimmunization arthropathy, unspecified site

● **M02.21 Postimmunization arthropathy, shoulder**
    M02.211 Postimmunization arthropathy, right shoulder
    M02.212 Postimmunization arthropathy, left shoulder
    M02.219 Postimmunization arthropathy, unspecified shoulder

● **M02.22 Postimmunization arthropathy, elbow**
    M02.221 Postimmunization arthropathy, right elbow
    M02.222 Postimmunization arthropathy, left elbow
    M02.229 Postimmunization arthropathy, unspecified elbow

● **M02.23 Postimmunization arthropathy, wrist**
    Postimmunization arthropathy, carpal bones
    M02.231 Postimmunization arthropathy, right wrist
    M02.232 Postimmunization arthropathy, left wrist
    M02.239 Postimmunization arthropathy, unspecified wrist

● **M02.24 Postimmunization arthropathy, hand**
    Postimmunization arthropathy, metacarpus and phalanges
    M02.241 Postimmunization arthropathy, right hand
    M02.242 Postimmunization arthropathy, left hand
    M02.249 Postimmunization arthropathy, unspecified hand

● **M02.25 Postimmunization arthropathy, hip**
    M02.251 Postimmunization arthropathy, right hip
    M02.252 Postimmunization arthropathy, left hip
    M02.259 Postimmunization arthropathy, unspecified hip

● **M02.26 Postimmunization arthropathy, knee**
    M02.261 Postimmunization arthropathy, right knee
    M02.262 Postimmunization arthropathy, left knee
    M02.269 Postimmunization arthropathy, unspecified knee

● **M02.27 Postimmunization arthropathy, ankle and foot**
    Postimmunization arthropathy, tarsus, metatarsus and phalanges
    M02.271 Postimmunization arthropathy, right ankle and foot
    M02.272 Postimmunization arthropathy, left ankle and foot
    M02.279 Postimmunization arthropathy, unspecified ankle and foot

    M02.28 Postimmunization arthropathy, vertebrae
    M02.29 Postimmunization arthropathy, multiple sites

● **M02.3 Reiter's disease**
    Reactive arthritis
    M02.30 Reiter's disease, unspecified site 🐾
       CC when PDx is its own CC

● **M02.31 Reiter's disease, shoulder**
    M02.311 Reiter's disease, right shoulder 🐾
       CC when PDx is its own CC
    M02.312 Reiter's disease, left shoulder 🐾
       CC when PDx is its own CC
    M02.319 Reiter's disease, unspecified shoulder 🐾
       CC when PDx is its own CC

● **M02.32 Reiter's disease, elbow**
    M02.321 Reiter's disease, right elbow 🐾
       CC when PDx is its own CC
    M02.322 Reiter's disease, left elbow 🐾
       CC when PDx is its own CC
    M02.329 Reiter's disease, unspecified elbow 🐾
       CC when PDx is its own CC

● **M02.33 Reiter's disease, wrist**
    Reiter's disease, carpal bones
    M02.331 Reiter's disease, right wrist 🐾
       CC when PDx is its own CC
    M02.332 Reiter's disease, left wrist 🐾
       CC when PDx is its own CC
    M02.339 Reiter's disease, unspecified wrist 🐾
       CC when PDx is its own CC

● **M02.34 Reiter's disease, hand**
    Reiter's disease, metacarpus and phalanges
    M02.341 Reiter's disease, right hand 🐾
       CC when PDx is its own CC
    M02.342 Reiter's disease, left hand 🐾
       CC when PDx is its own CC
    M02.349 Reiter's disease, unspecified hand 🐾
       CC when PDx is its own CC

● **M02.35 Reiter's disease, hip**
    M02.351 Reiter's disease, right hip 🐾
       CC when PDx is its own CC
    M02.352 Reiter's disease, left hip 🐾
       CC when PDx is its own CC
    M02.359 Reiter's disease, unspecified hip 🐾
       CC when PDx is its own CC

CHAPTER 13 (M00-M99)

◄ New   ⬅ Revised   ~~deleted~~ Deleted   Excludes 1   Excludes 2   Includes   Use additional   Code first   Code also   Unspecified
OGCR Official Guidelines   ● Unacceptable Principal Diagnosis   X Assign placeholder X   ● Use Additional Character(s)   🐾 Manifestation Code   **Coding Clinic**

● **M02.36**   Reiter's disease, knee

     M02.361   Reiter's disease, right knee 🔹
         CC when PDx is its own CC

     M02.362   Reiter's disease, left knee 🔹
         CC when PDx is its own CC

     M02.369   Reiter's disease, unspecified knee 🔹
         CC when PDx is its own CC

● **M02.37**   Reiter's disease, ankle and foot
     Reiter's disease, tarsus, metatarsus and phalanges

     M02.371   Reiter's disease, right ankle and foot 🔹
         CC when PDx is its own CC

     M02.372   Reiter's disease, left ankle and foot 🔹
         CC when PDx is its own CC

     M02.379   Reiter's disease, unspecified ankle and foot 🔹
         CC when PDx is its own CC

     M02.38   Reiter's disease, vertebrae 🔹
         CC when PDx is its own CC

     M02.39   Reiter's disease, multiple sites 🔹
         CC when PDx is its own CC

● **M02.8**   Other reactive arthropathies

   ▶ *M02.80*   *Other reactive arthropathies, unspecified site* 🔹

● **M02.81**   Other reactive arthropathies, shoulder
     Ⓔ For category M02.81 CC codes: See M01.X1

   ▶ *M02.811*   *Other reactive arthropathies, right shoulder* 🔹

   ▶ *M02.812*   *Other reactive arthropathies, left shoulder* 🔹

   ▶ *M02.819*   *Other reactive arthropathies, unspecified shoulder* 🔹

● **M02.82**   Other reactive arthropathies, elbow

   ▶ *M02.821*   *Other reactive arthropathies, right elbow* 🔹

   ▶ *M02.822*   *Other reactive arthropathies, left elbow* 🔹

   ▶ *M02.829*   *Other reactive arthropathies, unspecified elbow* 🔹

● **M02.83**   Other reactive arthropathies, wrist
     Other reactive arthropathies, carpal bones

   ▶ *M02.831*   *Other reactive arthropathies, right wrist* 🔹

   ▶ *M02.832*   *Other reactive arthropathies, left wrist* 🔹

   ▶ *M02.839*   *Other reactive arthropathies, unspecified wrist* 🔹

● **M02.84**   Other reactive arthropathies, hand
     Other reactive arthropathies, metacarpus and phalanges

   ▶ *M02.841*   *Other reactive arthropathies, right hand* 🔹

   ▶ *M02.842*   *Other reactive arthropathies, left hand* 🔹

   ▶ *M02.849*   *Other reactive arthropathies, unspecified hand* 🔹

● **M02.85**   Other reactive arthropathies, hip

   ▶ *M02.851*   *Other reactive arthropathies, right hip* 🔹

   ▶ *M02.852*   *Other reactive arthropathies, left hip* 🔹

   ▶ *M02.859*   *Other reactive arthropathies, unspecified hip* 🔹

● **M02.86**   Other reactive arthropathies, knee

   ▶ *M02.861*   *Other reactive arthropathies, right knee* 🔹

   ▶ *M02.862*   *Other reactive arthropathies, left knee* 🔹

   ▶ *M02.869*   *Other reactive arthropathies, unspecified knee* 🔹

● **M02.87**   Other reactive arthropathies, ankle and foot
     Other reactive arthropathies, tarsus, metatarsus and phalanges

   ▶ *M02.871*   *Other reactive arthropathies, right ankle and foot* 🔹

   ▶ *M02.872*   *Other reactive arthropathies, left ankle and foot* 🔹

   ▶ *M02.879*   *Other reactive arthropathies, unspecified ankle and foot* 🔹

   ▶ *M02.88*   *Other reactive arthropathies, vertebrae* 🔹

   ▶ *M02.89*   *Other reactive arthropathies, multiple sites* 🔹

▶ *M02.9*   *Reactive arthropathy, unspecified*

AUTOINFLAMMATORY SYNDROMES (M04) ◀

● **M04**   Autoinflammatory syndromes ◀
     Excludes2   Crohn's disease (K50.-) ◀

   M04.1   Periodic fever syndromes ◀
     Familial Mediterranean fever ◀
     Hyperimmunoglobin D syndrome ◀
     Mevalonate kinase deficiency ◀
     Tumor necrosis factor receptor associated periodic syndrome [TRAPS] ◀

   M04.2   Cryopyrin-associated periodic syndromes ◀
     Chronic infantile neurological, cutaneous and articular syndrome [CINCA] ◀
     Familial cold autoinflammatory syndrome ◀
     Familial cold urticaria ◀
     Muckle-Wells syndrome ◀
     Neonatal onset multisystemic inflammatory disorder [NOMID] ◀

   M04.8   Other autoinflammatory syndromes ◀
     Blau syndrome ◀
     Deficiency of interleukin 1 receptor antagonist [DIRA] ◀
     Majeed syndrome ◀
     Periodic fever, aphthous stomatitis, pharyngitis, and adenopathy syndrome [PFAPA] ◀
     Pyogenic arthritis, pyoderma gangrenosum, and acne syndrome [PAPA] ◀

   M04.9   Autoinflammatory syndrome, unspecified ◀

INFLAMMATORY POLYARTHROPATHIES (M05-M14)

● **M05**   Rheumatoid arthritis with rheumatoid factor
     Excludes1   rheumatic fever (I00)
           juvenile rheumatoid arthritis (M08.-)
           rheumatoid arthritis of spine (M45.-)

● **M05.0**   Felty's syndrome
     Rheumatoid arthritis with splenoadenomegaly and leukopenia

   M05.00   Felty's syndrome, unspecified site

● **M05.01**   Felty's syndrome, shoulder

     M05.011   Felty's syndrome, right shoulder

     M05.012   Felty's syndrome, left shoulder

     M05.019   Felty's syndrome, unspecified shoulder

● **M05.02**   Felty's syndrome, elbow

     M05.021   Felty's syndrome, right elbow

     M05.022   Felty's syndrome, left elbow

     M05.029   Felty's syndrome, unspecified elbow

● **M05.03**   Felty's syndrome, wrist
     Felty's syndrome, carpal bones

     M05.031   Felty's syndrome, right wrist

     M05.032   Felty's syndrome, left wrist

     M05.039   Felty's syndrome, unspecified wrist

Item 13–1   **Rheumatoid arthritis** (RA) is a chronic systemic inflammatory autoimmune disease of undetermined etiology involving primarily the synovial membranes and articular structures of multiple joints. It can also affect other organs, including the eyes, blood vessels, heart, and lungs. The disease is often progressive. In late stages, deformity, ankylosis, and other **inflammatory polyarthropathies** develop.

N   Newborn Age: 0   **P**   Pediatric Age: 0–17   **M**   Maternity DX: 12–55   **A**   Adult Age: 15–124   ♀ Females Only   ♂ Males Only

🔹 Complication\Comorbidity   🔹 Major C\C   Ⓔ CC/MCC Exclusions   🔹 Hospital-Acquired Condition

993

● **M05.04** Felty's syndrome, hand
    Felty's syndrome, metacarpus and phalanges
    M05.041 Felty's syndrome, right hand
    M05.042 Felty's syndrome, left hand
    M05.049 Felty's syndrome, unspecified hand
● **M05.05** Felty's syndrome, hip
    M05.051 Felty's syndrome, right hip
    M05.052 Felty's syndrome, left hip
    M05.059 Felty's syndrome, unspecified hip
● **M05.06** Felty's syndrome, knee
    M05.061 Felty's syndrome, right knee
    M05.062 Felty's syndrome, left knee
    M05.069 Felty's syndrome, unspecified knee
● **M05.07** Felty's syndrome, ankle and foot
    Felty's syndrome, tarsus, metatarsus and phalanges
    M05.071 Felty's syndrome, right ankle and foot
    M05.072 Felty's syndrome, left ankle and foot
    M05.079 Felty's syndrome, unspecified ankle and foot
    M05.09 Felty's syndrome, multiple sites
● **M05.1** Rheumatoid lung disease with rheumatoid arthritis
    M05.10 Rheumatoid lung disease with rheumatoid arthritis of unspecified site
● **M05.11** Rheumatoid lung disease with rheumatoid arthritis of shoulder
    M05.111 Rheumatoid lung disease with rheumatoid arthritis of right shoulder
    M05.112 Rheumatoid lung disease with rheumatoid arthritis of left shoulder
    M05.119 Rheumatoid lung disease with rheumatoid arthritis of unspecified shoulder
● **M05.12** Rheumatoid lung disease with rheumatoid arthritis of elbow
    M05.121 Rheumatoid lung disease with rheumatoid arthritis of right elbow
    M05.122 Rheumatoid lung disease with rheumatoid arthritis of left elbow
    M05.129 Rheumatoid lung disease with rheumatoid arthritis of unspecified elbow
● **M05.13** Rheumatoid lung disease with rheumatoid arthritis of wrist
    Rheumatoid lung disease with rheumatoid arthritis, carpal bones
    M05.131 Rheumatoid lung disease with rheumatoid arthritis of right wrist
    M05.132 Rheumatoid lung disease with rheumatoid arthritis of left wrist
    M05.139 Rheumatoid lung disease with rheumatoid arthritis of unspecified wrist
● **M05.14** Rheumatoid lung disease with rheumatoid arthritis of hand
    Rheumatoid lung disease with rheumatoid arthritis, metacarpus and phalanges
    M05.141 Rheumatoid lung disease with rheumatoid arthritis of right hand
    M05.142 Rheumatoid lung disease with rheumatoid arthritis of left hand
    M05.149 Rheumatoid lung disease with rheumatoid arthritis of unspecified hand

● **M05.15** Rheumatoid lung disease with rheumatoid arthritis of hip
    M05.151 Rheumatoid lung disease with rheumatoid arthritis of right hip
    M05.152 Rheumatoid lung disease with rheumatoid arthritis of left hip
    M05.159 Rheumatoid lung disease with rheumatoid arthritis of unspecified hip
● **M05.16** Rheumatoid lung disease with rheumatoid arthritis of knee
    M05.161 Rheumatoid lung disease with rheumatoid arthritis of right knee
    M05.162 Rheumatoid lung disease with rheumatoid arthritis of left knee
    M05.169 Rheumatoid lung disease with rheumatoid arthritis of unspecified knee
● **M05.17** Rheumatoid lung disease with rheumatoid arthritis of ankle and foot
    Rheumatoid lung disease with rheumatoid arthritis, tarsus, metatarsus and phalanges
    M05.171 Rheumatoid lung disease with rheumatoid arthritis of right ankle and foot
    M05.172 Rheumatoid lung disease with rheumatoid arthritis of left ankle and foot
    M05.179 Rheumatoid lung disease with rheumatoid arthritis of unspecified ankle and foot
    M05.19 Rheumatoid lung disease with rheumatoid arthritis of multiple sites
● **M05.2** Rheumatoid vasculitis with rheumatoid arthritis
    M05.20 Rheumatoid vasculitis with rheumatoid arthritis of unspecified site
● **M05.21** Rheumatoid vasculitis with rheumatoid arthritis of shoulder
    M05.211 Rheumatoid vasculitis with rheumatoid arthritis of right shoulder
    M05.212 Rheumatoid vasculitis with rheumatoid arthritis of left shoulder
    M05.219 Rheumatoid vasculitis with rheumatoid arthritis of unspecified shoulder
● **M05.22** Rheumatoid vasculitis with rheumatoid arthritis of elbow
    M05.221 Rheumatoid vasculitis with rheumatoid arthritis of right elbow
    M05.222 Rheumatoid vasculitis with rheumatoid arthritis of left elbow
    M05.229 Rheumatoid vasculitis with rheumatoid arthritis of unspecified elbow
● **M05.23** Rheumatoid vasculitis with rheumatoid arthritis of wrist
    Rheumatoid vasculitis with rheumatoid arthritis, carpal bones
    M05.231 Rheumatoid vasculitis with rheumatoid arthritis of right wrist
    M05.232 Rheumatoid vasculitis with rheumatoid arthritis of left wrist
    M05.239 Rheumatoid vasculitis with rheumatoid arthritis of unspecified wrist

◀ New ⬅ Revised ~~deleted~~ Deleted Excludes 1 Excludes 2 Includes Use additional Code first Code also Unspecified
OGCR Official Guidelines ● Unacceptable Principal Diagnosis X Assign placeholder X ● Use Additional Character(s) ▶ Manifestation Code Coding Clinic

● **M05.24   Rheumatoid vasculitis with rheumatoid arthritis of hand**
    Rheumatoid vasculitis with rheumatoid arthritis, metacarpus and phalanges
    M05.241   Rheumatoid vasculitis with rheumatoid arthritis of right hand
    M05.242   Rheumatoid vasculitis with rheumatoid arthritis of left hand
    M05.249   Rheumatoid vasculitis with rheumatoid arthritis of unspecified hand

● **M05.25   Rheumatoid vasculitis with rheumatoid arthritis of hip**
    M05.251   Rheumatoid vasculitis with rheumatoid arthritis of right hip
    M05.252   Rheumatoid vasculitis with rheumatoid arthritis of left hip
    M05.259   Rheumatoid vasculitis with rheumatoid arthritis of unspecified hip

● **M05.26   Rheumatoid vasculitis with rheumatoid arthritis of knee**
    M05.261   Rheumatoid vasculitis with rheumatoid arthritis of right knee
    M05.262   Rheumatoid vasculitis with rheumatoid arthritis of left knee
    M05.269   Rheumatoid vasculitis with rheumatoid arthritis of unspecified knee

● **M05.27   Rheumatoid vasculitis with rheumatoid arthritis of ankle and foot**
    Rheumatoid vasculitis with rheumatoid arthritis, tarsus, metatarsus and phalanges
    M05.271   Rheumatoid vasculitis with rheumatoid arthritis of right ankle and foot
    M05.272   Rheumatoid vasculitis with rheumatoid arthritis of left ankle and foot
    M05.279   Rheumatoid vasculitis with rheumatoid arthritis of unspecified ankle and foot

    M05.29   Rheumatoid vasculitis with rheumatoid arthritis of multiple sites

● **M05.3   Rheumatoid heart disease with rheumatoid arthritis**
    Rheumatoid carditis
    Rheumatoid endocarditis
    Rheumatoid myocarditis
    Rheumatoid pericarditis
    M05.30   Rheumatoid heart disease with rheumatoid arthritis of unspecified site

● **M05.31   Rheumatoid heart disease with rheumatoid arthritis of shoulder**
    M05.311   Rheumatoid heart disease with rheumatoid arthritis of right shoulder
    M05.312   Rheumatoid heart disease with rheumatoid arthritis of left shoulder
    M05.319   Rheumatoid heart disease with rheumatoid arthritis of unspecified shoulder

● **M05.32   Rheumatoid heart disease with rheumatoid arthritis of elbow**
    M05.321   Rheumatoid heart disease with rheumatoid arthritis of right elbow
    M05.322   Rheumatoid heart disease with rheumatoid arthritis of left elbow
    M05.329   Rheumatoid heart disease with rheumatoid arthritis of unspecified elbow

● **M05.33   Rheumatoid heart disease with rheumatoid arthritis of wrist**
    Rheumatoid heart disease with rheumatoid arthritis, carpal bones
    M05.331   Rheumatoid heart disease with rheumatoid arthritis of right wrist
    M05.332   Rheumatoid heart disease with rheumatoid arthritis of left wrist
    M05.339   Rheumatoid heart disease with rheumatoid arthritis of unspecified wrist

● **M05.34   Rheumatoid heart disease with rheumatoid arthritis of hand**
    Rheumatoid heart disease with rheumatoid arthritis, metacarpus and phalanges
    M05.341   Rheumatoid heart disease with rheumatoid arthritis of right hand
    M05.342   Rheumatoid heart disease with rheumatoid arthritis of left hand
    M05.349   Rheumatoid heart disease with rheumatoid arthritis of unspecified hand

● **M05.35   Rheumatoid heart disease with rheumatoid arthritis of hip**
    M05.351   Rheumatoid heart disease with rheumatoid arthritis of right hip
    M05.352   Rheumatoid heart disease with rheumatoid arthritis of left hip
    M05.359   Rheumatoid heart disease with rheumatoid arthritis of unspecified hip

● **M05.36   Rheumatoid heart disease with rheumatoid arthritis of knee**
    M05.361   Rheumatoid heart disease with rheumatoid arthritis of right knee
    M05.362   Rheumatoid heart disease with rheumatoid arthritis of left knee
    M05.369   Rheumatoid heart disease with rheumatoid arthritis of unspecified knee

● **M05.37   Rheumatoid heart disease with rheumatoid arthritis of ankle and foot**
    Rheumatoid heart disease with rheumatoid arthritis, tarsus, metatarsus and phalanges
    M05.371   Rheumatoid heart disease with rheumatoid arthritis of right ankle and foot
    M05.372   Rheumatoid heart disease with rheumatoid arthritis of left ankle and foot
    M05.379   Rheumatoid heart disease with rheumatoid arthritis of unspecified ankle and foot

    M05.39   Rheumatoid heart disease with rheumatoid arthritis of multiple sites

CHAPTER 13 (M00-M99)

N   Newborn Age: 0   **P**   Pediatric Age: 0–17   **M**   Maternity DX: 12–55   **A**   Adult Age: 15–124   ♀   Females Only   ♂   Males Only

🔖 Complication\Comorbidity   🔖 Major C\C   (Ex) CC/MCC Exclusions   🔖 Hospital-Acquired Condition   **995**

● **M05.4　Rheumatoid myopathy with rheumatoid arthritis**
　　ⓔ **For category M05.4 CC codes:** E08.40-E08.49, E08.618-E08.638,
　　　E08.649-E08.8, E09.40-E09.49, E09.618-E09.638, E09.649-E09.8,
　　　E10.40-E10.49, E10.618-E10.638, E10.649, E10.69-E10.8, E11.40-E11.49,
　　　E11.618-E11.638, E11.649, E11.69-E11.8, E13.40-E13.49, E13.618-E13.638,
　　　E13.649-E13.8, G32.89, G70.00-G72.3, G72.81-G73.7, G96.8-G96.9,
　　　G98.0-G98.8, G99.8

　　M05.40　Rheumatoid myopathy with rheumatoid arthritis of unspecified site ⓒ
　　　　CC when PDx is its own CC

● **M05.41　Rheumatoid myopathy with rheumatoid arthritis of shoulder**

　　M05.411　Rheumatoid myopathy with rheumatoid arthritis of right shoulder ⓒ
　　　　CC when PDx is its own CC

　　M05.412　Rheumatoid myopathy with rheumatoid arthritis of left shoulder ⓒ
　　　　CC when PDx is its own CC

　　M05.419　Rheumatoid myopathy with rheumatoid arthritis of unspecified shoulder ⓒ
　　　　CC when PDx is its own CC

● **M05.42　Rheumatoid myopathy with rheumatoid arthritis of elbow**

　　M05.421　Rheumatoid myopathy with rheumatoid arthritis of right elbow ⓒ
　　　　CC when PDx is its own CC

　　M05.422　Rheumatoid myopathy with rheumatoid arthritis of left elbow ⓒ
　　　　CC when PDx is its own CC

　　M05.429　Rheumatoid myopathy with rheumatoid arthritis of unspecified elbow ⓒ
　　　　CC when PDx is its own CC

● **M05.43　Rheumatoid myopathy with rheumatoid arthritis of wrist**
　　Rheumatoid myopathy with rheumatoid arthritis, carpal bones

　　M05.431　Rheumatoid myopathy with rheumatoid arthritis of right wrist ⓒ
　　　　CC when PDx is its own CC

　　M05.432　Rheumatoid myopathy with rheumatoid arthritis of left wrist ⓒ
　　　　CC when PDx is its own CC

　　M05.439　Rheumatoid myopathy with rheumatoid arthritis of unspecified wrist ⓒ
　　　　CC when PDx is its own CC

● **M05.44　Rheumatoid myopathy with rheumatoid arthritis of hand**
　　Rheumatoid myopathy with rheumatoid arthritis, metacarpus and phalanges

　　M05.441　Rheumatoid myopathy with rheumatoid arthritis of right hand ⓒ
　　　　CC when PDx is its own CC

　　M05.442　Rheumatoid myopathy with rheumatoid arthritis of left hand ⓒ
　　　　CC when PDx is its own CC

　　M05.449　Rheumatoid myopathy with rheumatoid arthritis of unspecified hand ⓒ
　　　　CC when PDx is its own CC

● **M05.45　Rheumatoid myopathy with rheumatoid arthritis of hip**

　　M05.451　Rheumatoid myopathy with rheumatoid arthritis of right hip ⓒ
　　　　CC when PDx is its own CC

　　M05.452　Rheumatoid myopathy with rheumatoid arthritis of left hip ⓒ
　　　　CC when PDx is its own CC

　　M05.459　Rheumatoid myopathy with rheumatoid arthritis of unspecified hip ⓒ
　　　　CC when PDx is its own CC

● **M05.46　Rheumatoid myopathy with rheumatoid arthritis of knee**

　　M05.461　Rheumatoid myopathy with rheumatoid arthritis of right knee ⓒ
　　　　CC when PDx is its own CC

　　M05.462　Rheumatoid myopathy with rheumatoid arthritis of left knee ⓒ
　　　　CC when PDx is its own CC

　　M05.469　Rheumatoid myopathy with rheumatoid arthritis of unspecified knee ⓒ
　　　　CC when PDx is its own CC

● **M05.47　Rheumatoid myopathy with rheumatoid arthritis of ankle and foot**
　　Rheumatoid myopathy with rheumatoid arthritis, tarsus, metatarsus and phalanges

　　M05.471　Rheumatoid myopathy with rheumatoid arthritis of right ankle and foot ⓒ
　　　　CC when PDx is its own CC

　　M05.472　Rheumatoid myopathy with rheumatoid arthritis of left ankle and foot ⓒ
　　　　CC when PDx is its own CC

　　M05.479　Rheumatoid myopathy with rheumatoid arthritis of unspecified ankle and foot ⓒ
　　　　CC when PDx is its own CC

　　M05.49　Rheumatoid myopathy with rheumatoid arthritis of multiple sites ⓒ
　　　　CC when PDx is its own CC

● **M05.5　Rheumatoid polyneuropathy with rheumatoid arthritis**

　　M05.50　Rheumatoid polyneuropathy with rheumatoid arthritis of unspecified site

● **M05.51　Rheumatoid polyneuropathy with rheumatoid arthritis of shoulder**

　　M05.511　Rheumatoid polyneuropathy with rheumatoid arthritis of right shoulder

　　M05.512　Rheumatoid polyneuropathy with rheumatoid arthritis of left shoulder

　　M05.519　Rheumatoid polyneuropathy with rheumatoid arthritis of unspecified shoulder

● **M05.52　Rheumatoid polyneuropathy with rheumatoid arthritis of elbow**

　　M05.521　Rheumatoid polyneuropathy with rheumatoid arthritis of right elbow

　　M05.522　Rheumatoid polyneuropathy with rheumatoid arthritis of left elbow

　　M05.529　Rheumatoid polyneuropathy with rheumatoid arthritis of unspecified elbow

◀ New　◀▥ Revised　~~deleted~~ Deleted　Excludes 1　Excludes 2　Includes　Use additional　Code first　Code also　Unspecified
OGCR Official Guidelines　● Unacceptable Principal Diagnosis　X Assign placeholder X　● Use Additional Character(s)　▶ Manifestation Code　**Coding Clinic**

● **M05.53　Rheumatoid polyneuropathy with rheumatoid arthritis of wrist**
　　　　Rheumatoid polyneuropathy with rheumatoid arthritis, carpal bones
　　M05.531　Rheumatoid polyneuropathy with rheumatoid arthritis of right wrist
　　M05.532　Rheumatoid polyneuropathy with rheumatoid arthritis of left wrist
　　M05.539　Rheumatoid polyneuropathy with rheumatoid arthritis of unspecified wrist

● **M05.54　Rheumatoid polyneuropathy with rheumatoid arthritis of hand**
　　　　Rheumatoid polyneuropathy with rheumatoid arthritis, metacarpus and phalanges
　　M05.541　Rheumatoid polyneuropathy with rheumatoid arthritis of right hand
　　M05.542　Rheumatoid polyneuropathy with rheumatoid arthritis of left hand
　　M05.549　Rheumatoid polyneuropathy with rheumatoid arthritis of unspecified hand

● **M05.55　Rheumatoid polyneuropathy with rheumatoid arthritis of hip**
　　M05.551　Rheumatoid polyneuropathy with rheumatoid arthritis of right hip
　　M05.552　Rheumatoid polyneuropathy with rheumatoid arthritis of left hip
　　M05.559　Rheumatoid polyneuropathy with rheumatoid arthritis of unspecified hip

● **M05.56　Rheumatoid polyneuropathy with rheumatoid arthritis of knee**
　　M05.561　Rheumatoid polyneuropathy with rheumatoid arthritis of right knee
　　M05.562　Rheumatoid polyneuropathy with rheumatoid arthritis of left knee
　　M05.569　Rheumatoid polyneuropathy with rheumatoid arthritis of unspecified knee

● **M05.57　Rheumatoid polyneuropathy with rheumatoid arthritis of ankle and foot**
　　　　Rheumatoid polyneuropathy with rheumatoid arthritis, tarsus, metatarsus and phalanges
　　M05.571　Rheumatoid polyneuropathy with rheumatoid arthritis of right ankle and foot
　　M05.572　Rheumatoid polyneuropathy with rheumatoid arthritis of left ankle and foot
　　M05.579　Rheumatoid polyneuropathy with rheumatoid arthritis of unspecified ankle and foot

　　M05.59　Rheumatoid polyneuropathy with rheumatoid arthritis of multiple sites

● **M05.6　Rheumatoid arthritis with involvement of other organs and systems**
　　M05.60　Rheumatoid arthritis of unspecified site with involvement of other organs and systems

● **M05.61　Rheumatoid arthritis of shoulder with involvement of other organs and systems**
　　M05.611　Rheumatoid arthritis of right shoulder with involvement of other organs and systems
　　M05.612　Rheumatoid arthritis of left shoulder with involvement of other organs and systems
　　M05.619　Rheumatoid arthritis of unspecified shoulder with involvement of other organs and systems

● **M05.62　Rheumatoid arthritis of elbow with involvement of other organs and systems**
　　M05.621　Rheumatoid arthritis of right elbow with involvement of other organs and systems
　　M05.622　Rheumatoid arthritis of left elbow with involvement of other organs and systems
　　M05.629　Rheumatoid arthritis of unspecified elbow with involvement of other organs and systems

● **M05.63　Rheumatoid arthritis of wrist with involvement of other organs and systems**
　　　　Rheumatoid arthritis of carpal bones with involvement of other organs and systems
　　M05.631　Rheumatoid arthritis of right wrist with involvement of other organs and systems
　　M05.632　Rheumatoid arthritis of left wrist with involvement of other organs and systems
　　M05.639　Rheumatoid arthritis of unspecified wrist with involvement of other organs and systems

● **M05.64　Rheumatoid arthritis of hand with involvement of other organs and systems**
　　　　Rheumatoid arthritis of metacarpus and phalanges with involvement of other organs and systems
　　M05.641　Rheumatoid arthritis of right hand with involvement of other organs and systems
　　M05.642　Rheumatoid arthritis of left hand with involvement of other organs and systems
　　M05.649　Rheumatoid arthritis of unspecified hand with involvement of other organs and systems

● **M05.65　Rheumatoid arthritis of hip with involvement of other organs and systems**
　　M05.651　Rheumatoid arthritis of right hip with involvement of other organs and systems
　　M05.652　Rheumatoid arthritis of left hip with involvement of other organs and systems
　　M05.659　Rheumatoid arthritis of unspecified hip with involvement of other organs and systems

● **M05.66　Rheumatoid arthritis of knee with involvement of other organs and systems**
　　M05.661　Rheumatoid arthritis of right knee with involvement of other organs and systems
　　M05.662　Rheumatoid arthritis of left knee with involvement of other organs and systems
　　M05.669　Rheumatoid arthritis of unspecified knee with involvement of other organs and systems

CHAPTER 13 (M00-M99)

N Newborn Age: 0　　**P** Pediatric Age: 0–17　　**M** Maternity DX: 12–55　　**A** Adult Age: 15–124　　♀ Females Only　　♂ Males Only

🔴 Complication\Comorbidity　　🔵 Major C\C　　Ⓔ CC/MCC Exclusions　　🔴 Hospital-Acquired Condition

997

CHAPTER 13 (M00-M99)

● M05.67 **Rheumatoid arthritis of ankle and foot with involvement of other organs and systems**
Rheumatoid arthritis of tarsus, metatarsus and phalanges with involvement of other organs and systems

M05.671 **Rheumatoid arthritis of right ankle and foot with involvement of other organs and systems**

M05.672 **Rheumatoid arthritis of left ankle and foot with involvement of other organs and systems**

M05.679 **Rheumatoid arthritis of unspecified ankle and foot with involvement of other organs and systems**

M05.69 **Rheumatoid arthritis of multiple sites with involvement of other organs and systems**

● M05.7 **Rheumatoid arthritis with rheumatoid factor without organ or systems involvement**

M05.70 **Rheumatoid arthritis with rheumatoid factor of unspecified site without organ or systems involvement**

● M05.71 **Rheumatoid arthritis with rheumatoid factor of shoulder without organ or systems involvement**

M05.711 **Rheumatoid arthritis with rheumatoid factor of right shoulder without organ or systems involvement**

M05.712 **Rheumatoid arthritis with rheumatoid factor of left shoulder without organ or systems involvement**

M05.719 **Rheumatoid arthritis with rheumatoid factor of unspecified shoulder without organ or systems involvement**

● M05.72 **Rheumatoid arthritis with rheumatoid factor of elbow without organ or systems involvement**

M05.721 **Rheumatoid arthritis with rheumatoid factor of right elbow without organ or systems involvement**

M05.722 **Rheumatoid arthritis with rheumatoid factor of left elbow without organ or systems involvement**

M05.729 **Rheumatoid arthritis with rheumatoid factor of unspecified elbow without organ or systems involvement**

● M05.73 **Rheumatoid arthritis with rheumatoid factor of wrist without organ or systems involvement**

M05.731 **Rheumatoid arthritis with rheumatoid factor of right wrist without organ or systems involvement**

M05.732 **Rheumatoid arthritis with rheumatoid factor of left wrist without organ or systems involvement**

M05.739 **Rheumatoid arthritis with rheumatoid factor of unspecified wrist without organ or systems involvement**

● M05.74 **Rheumatoid arthritis with rheumatoid factor of hand without organ or systems involvement**

M05.741 **Rheumatoid arthritis with rheumatoid factor of right hand without organ or systems involvement**

M05.742 **Rheumatoid arthritis with rheumatoid factor of left hand without organ or systems involvement**

M05.749 **Rheumatoid arthritis with rheumatoid factor of unspecified hand without organ or systems involvement**

● M05.75 **Rheumatoid arthritis with rheumatoid factor of hip without organ or systems involvement**

M05.751 **Rheumatoid arthritis with rheumatoid factor of right hip without organ or systems involvement**

M05.752 **Rheumatoid arthritis with rheumatoid factor of left hip without organ or systems involvement**

M05.759 **Rheumatoid arthritis with rheumatoid factor of unspecified hip without organ or systems involvement**

● M05.76 **Rheumatoid arthritis with rheumatoid factor of knee without organ or systems involvement**

M05.761 **Rheumatoid arthritis with rheumatoid factor of right knee without organ or systems involvement**

M05.762 **Rheumatoid arthritis with rheumatoid factor of left knee without organ or systems involvement**

M05.769 **Rheumatoid arthritis with rheumatoid factor of unspecified knee without organ or systems involvement**

● M05.77 **Rheumatoid arthritis with rheumatoid factor of ankle and foot without organ or systems involvement**

M05.771 **Rheumatoid arthritis with rheumatoid factor of right ankle and foot without organ or systems involvement**

M05.772 **Rheumatoid arthritis with rheumatoid factor of left ankle and foot without organ or systems involvement**

M05.779 **Rheumatoid arthritis with rheumatoid factor of unspecified ankle and foot without organ or systems involvement**

M05.79 **Rheumatoid arthritis with rheumatoid factor of multiple sites without organ or systems involvement**

● M05.8 **Other rheumatoid arthritis with rheumatoid factor**

M05.80 **Other rheumatoid arthritis with rheumatoid factor of unspecified site**

● M05.81 **Other rheumatoid arthritis with rheumatoid factor of shoulder**

M05.811 **Other rheumatoid arthritis with rheumatoid factor of right shoulder**

M05.812 **Other rheumatoid arthritis with rheumatoid factor of left shoulder**

M05.819 **Other rheumatoid arthritis with rheumatoid factor of unspecified shoulder**

◀ New   ◀|||| Revised   ~~deleted~~ Deleted   Excludes 1   Excludes 2   Includes   Use additional   Code first   Code also   Unspecified
OGCR Official Guidelines   ● Unacceptable Principal Diagnosis   X Assign placeholder X   ● Use Additional Character(s)   ▶ Manifestation Code   **Coding Clinic**

● M05.82   Other rheumatoid arthritis with rheumatoid factor of elbow
   M05.821   Other rheumatoid arthritis with rheumatoid factor of right elbow
   M05.822   Other rheumatoid arthritis with rheumatoid factor of left elbow
   M05.829   Other rheumatoid arthritis with rheumatoid factor of unspecified elbow

● M05.83   Other rheumatoid arthritis with rheumatoid factor of wrist
   M05.831   Other rheumatoid arthritis with rheumatoid factor of right wrist
   M05.832   Other rheumatoid arthritis with rheumatoid factor of left wrist
   M05.839   Other rheumatoid arthritis with rheumatoid factor of unspecified wrist

● M05.84   Other rheumatoid arthritis with rheumatoid factor of hand
   M05.841   Other rheumatoid arthritis with rheumatoid factor of right hand
   M05.842   Other rheumatoid arthritis with rheumatoid factor of left hand
   M05.849   Other rheumatoid arthritis with rheumatoid factor of unspecified hand

● M05.85   Other rheumatoid arthritis with rheumatoid factor of hip
   M05.851   Other rheumatoid arthritis with rheumatoid factor of right hip
   M05.852   Other rheumatoid arthritis with rheumatoid factor of left hip
   M05.859   Other rheumatoid arthritis with rheumatoid factor of unspecified hip

● M05.86   Other rheumatoid arthritis with rheumatoid factor of knee
   M05.861   Other rheumatoid arthritis with rheumatoid factor of right knee
   M05.862   Other rheumatoid arthritis with rheumatoid factor of left knee
   M05.869   Other rheumatoid arthritis with rheumatoid factor of unspecified knee

● M05.87   Other rheumatoid arthritis with rheumatoid factor of ankle and foot
   M05.871   Other rheumatoid arthritis with rheumatoid factor of right ankle and foot
   M05.872   Other rheumatoid arthritis with rheumatoid factor of left ankle and foot
   M05.879   Other rheumatoid arthritis with rheumatoid factor of unspecified ankle and foot

  M05.89   Other rheumatoid arthritis with rheumatoid factor of multiple sites

  M05.9   Rheumatoid arthritis with rheumatoid factor, unspecified

● M06   Other rheumatoid arthritis
 ● M06.0   Rheumatoid arthritis without rheumatoid factor
   M06.00   Rheumatoid arthritis without rheumatoid factor, unspecified site
  ● M06.01   Rheumatoid arthritis without rheumatoid factor, shoulder
   M06.011   Rheumatoid arthritis without rheumatoid factor, right shoulder
   M06.012   Rheumatoid arthritis without rheumatoid factor, left shoulder
   M06.019   Rheumatoid arthritis without rheumatoid factor, unspecified shoulder

● M06.02   Rheumatoid arthritis without rheumatoid factor, elbow
   M06.021   Rheumatoid arthritis without rheumatoid factor, right elbow
   M06.022   Rheumatoid arthritis without rheumatoid factor, left elbow
   M06.029   Rheumatoid arthritis without rheumatoid factor, unspecified elbow

● M06.03   Rheumatoid arthritis without rheumatoid factor, wrist
   M06.031   Rheumatoid arthritis without rheumatoid factor, right wrist
   M06.032   Rheumatoid arthritis without rheumatoid factor, left wrist
   M06.039   Rheumatoid arthritis without rheumatoid factor, unspecified wrist

● M06.04   Rheumatoid arthritis without rheumatoid factor, hand
   M06.041   Rheumatoid arthritis without rheumatoid factor, right hand
   M06.042   Rheumatoid arthritis without rheumatoid factor, left hand
   M06.049   Rheumatoid arthritis without rheumatoid factor, unspecified hand

● M06.05   Rheumatoid arthritis without rheumatoid factor, hip
   M06.051   Rheumatoid arthritis without rheumatoid factor, right hip
   M06.052   Rheumatoid arthritis without rheumatoid factor, left hip
   M06.059   Rheumatoid arthritis without rheumatoid factor, unspecified hip

● M06.06   Rheumatoid arthritis without rheumatoid factor, knee
   M06.061   Rheumatoid arthritis without rheumatoid factor, right knee
   M06.062   Rheumatoid arthritis without rheumatoid factor, left knee
   M06.069   Rheumatoid arthritis without rheumatoid factor, unspecified knee

● M06.07   Rheumatoid arthritis without rheumatoid factor, ankle and foot
   M06.071   Rheumatoid arthritis without rheumatoid factor, right ankle and foot
   M06.072   Rheumatoid arthritis without rheumatoid factor, left ankle and foot
   M06.079   Rheumatoid arthritis without rheumatoid factor, unspecified ankle and foot

  M06.08   Rheumatoid arthritis without rheumatoid factor, vertebrae

  M06.09   Rheumatoid arthritis without rheumatoid factor, multiple sites

  M06.1   Adult-onset Still's disease   A
    Excludes1   Still's disease NOS (M08.2-)

● M06.2   Rheumatoid bursitis
  M06.20   Rheumatoid bursitis, unspecified site
 ● M06.21   Rheumatoid bursitis, shoulder
   M06.211   Rheumatoid bursitis, right shoulder
   M06.212   Rheumatoid bursitis, left shoulder
   M06.219   Rheumatoid bursitis, unspecified shoulder
 ● M06.22   Rheumatoid bursitis, elbow
   M06.221   Rheumatoid bursitis, right elbow
   M06.222   Rheumatoid bursitis, left elbow
   M06.229   Rheumatoid bursitis, unspecified elbow

N Newborn Age: 0   **P** Pediatric Age: 0–17   **M** Maternity DX: 12–55   **A** Adult Age: 15–124   ♀ Females Only   ♂ Males Only

🔧 Complication\Comorbidity   🔧 Major C\C   (Ex) CC/MCC Exclusions   🔧 Hospital-Acquired Condition

999

● **M06.23** Rheumatoid bursitis, wrist
    M06.231 Rheumatoid bursitis, right wrist
    M06.232 Rheumatoid bursitis, left wrist
    M06.239 Rheumatoid bursitis, unspecified wrist
● **M06.24** Rheumatoid bursitis, hand
    M06.241 Rheumatoid bursitis, right hand
    M06.242 Rheumatoid bursitis, left hand
    M06.249 Rheumatoid bursitis, unspecified hand
● **M06.25** Rheumatoid bursitis, hip
    M06.251 Rheumatoid bursitis, right hip
    M06.252 Rheumatoid bursitis, left hip
    M06.259 Rheumatoid bursitis, unspecified hip
● **M06.26** Rheumatoid bursitis, knee
    M06.261 Rheumatoid bursitis, right knee
    M06.262 Rheumatoid bursitis, left knee
    M06.269 Rheumatoid bursitis, unspecified knee
● **M06.27** Rheumatoid bursitis, ankle and foot
    M06.271 Rheumatoid bursitis, right ankle and foot
    M06.272 Rheumatoid bursitis, left ankle and foot
    M06.279 Rheumatoid bursitis, unspecified ankle and foot
    M06.28 Rheumatoid bursitis, vertebrae
    M06.29 Rheumatoid bursitis, multiple sites
● **M06.3** Rheumatoid nodule
    M06.30 Rheumatoid nodule, unspecified site
● **M06.31** Rheumatoid nodule, shoulder
    M06.311 Rheumatoid nodule, right shoulder
    M06.312 Rheumatoid nodule, left shoulder
    M06.319 Rheumatoid nodule, unspecified shoulder
● **M06.32** Rheumatoid nodule, elbow
    M06.321 Rheumatoid nodule, right elbow
    M06.322 Rheumatoid nodule, left elbow
    M06.329 Rheumatoid nodule, unspecified elbow
● **M06.33** Rheumatoid nodule, wrist
    M06.331 Rheumatoid nodule, right wrist
    M06.332 Rheumatoid nodule, left wrist
    M06.339 Rheumatoid nodule, unspecified wrist
● **M06.34** Rheumatoid nodule, hand
    M06.341 Rheumatoid nodule, right hand
    M06.342 Rheumatoid nodule, left hand
    M06.349 Rheumatoid nodule, unspecified hand
● **M06.35** Rheumatoid nodule, hip
    M06.351 Rheumatoid nodule, right hip
    M06.352 Rheumatoid nodule, left hip
    M06.359 Rheumatoid nodule, unspecified hip
● **M06.36** Rheumatoid nodule, knee
    M06.361 Rheumatoid nodule, right knee
    M06.362 Rheumatoid nodule, left knee
    M06.369 Rheumatoid nodule, unspecified knee

● **M06.37** Rheumatoid nodule, ankle and foot
    M06.371 Rheumatoid nodule, right ankle and foot
    M06.372 Rheumatoid nodule, left ankle and foot
    M06.379 Rheumatoid nodule, unspecified ankle and foot
    M06.38 Rheumatoid nodule, vertebrae
    M06.39 Rheumatoid nodule, multiple sites
M06.4 Inflammatory polyarthropathy
    Excludes1 polyarthritis NOS (M13.0)
● **M06.8** Other specified rheumatoid arthritis
    M06.80 Other specified rheumatoid arthritis, unspecified site
● **M06.81** Other specified rheumatoid arthritis, shoulder
    M06.811 Other specified rheumatoid arthritis, right shoulder
    M06.812 Other specified rheumatoid arthritis, left shoulder
    M06.819 Other specified rheumatoid arthritis, unspecified shoulder
● **M06.82** Other specified rheumatoid arthritis, elbow
    M06.821 Other specified rheumatoid arthritis, right elbow
    M06.822 Other specified rheumatoid arthritis, left elbow
    M06.829 Other specified rheumatoid arthritis, unspecified elbow
● **M06.83** Other specified rheumatoid arthritis, wrist
    M06.831 Other specified rheumatoid arthritis, right wrist
    M06.832 Other specified rheumatoid arthritis, left wrist
    M06.839 Other specified rheumatoid arthritis, unspecified wrist
● **M06.84** Other specified rheumatoid arthritis, hand
    M06.841 Other specified rheumatoid arthritis, right hand
    M06.842 Other specified rheumatoid arthritis, left hand
    M06.849 Other specified rheumatoid arthritis, unspecified hand
● **M06.85** Other specified rheumatoid arthritis, hip
    M06.851 Other specified rheumatoid arthritis, right hip
    M06.852 Other specified rheumatoid arthritis, left hip
    M06.859 Other specified rheumatoid arthritis, unspecified hip
● **M06.86** Other specified rheumatoid arthritis, knee
    M06.861 Other specified rheumatoid arthritis, right knee
    M06.862 Other specified rheumatoid arthritis, left knee
    M06.869 Other specified rheumatoid arthritis, unspecified knee
● **M06.87** Other specified rheumatoid arthritis, ankle and foot
    M06.871 Other specified rheumatoid arthritis, right ankle and foot
    M06.872 Other specified rheumatoid arthritis, left ankle and foot
    M06.879 Other specified rheumatoid arthritis, unspecified ankle and foot
    M06.88 Other specified rheumatoid arthritis, vertebrae
    M06.89 Other specified rheumatoid arthritis, multiple sites
M06.9 Rheumatoid arthritis, unspecified

◄ New   ◄▬ Revised   ~~deleted~~ Deleted   Excludes 1   Excludes 2   Includes   Use additional   Code first   Code also   Unspecified
OGCR Official Guidelines   ● Unacceptable Principal Diagnosis   X Assign placeholder X   ● Use Additional Character(s)   ▶ Manifestation Code   **Coding Clinic**

● **M07 Enteropathic arthropathies**

    Code also associated enteropathy, such as:
      regional enteritis [Crohn's disease] (K50.-)
      ulcerative colitis (K51.-)

    Excludes 1   psoriatic arthropathies (L40.5-)

● **M07.6 Enteropathic arthropathies**

    M07.60   Enteropathic arthropathies, unspecified site

  ● **M07.61**   Enteropathic arthropathies, shoulder

      M07.611   Enteropathic arthropathies, right shoulder

      M07.612   Enteropathic arthropathies, left shoulder

      M07.619   Enteropathic arthropathies, unspecified shoulder

  ● **M07.62**   Enteropathic arthropathies, elbow

      M07.621   Enteropathic arthropathies, right elbow

      M07.622   Enteropathic arthropathies, left elbow

      M07.629   Enteropathic arthropathies, unspecified elbow

  ● **M07.63**   Enteropathic arthropathies, wrist

      M07.631   Enteropathic arthropathies, right wrist

      M07.632   Enteropathic arthropathies, left wrist

      M07.639   Enteropathic arthropathies, unspecified wrist

  ● **M07.64**   Enteropathic arthropathies, hand

      M07.641   Enteropathic arthropathies, right hand

      M07.642   Enteropathic arthropathies, left hand

      M07.649   Enteropathic arthropathies, unspecified hand

  ● **M07.65**   Enteropathic arthropathies, hip

      M07.651   Enteropathic arthropathies, right hip

      M07.652   Enteropathic arthropathies, left hip

      M07.659   Enteropathic arthropathies, unspecified hip

  ● **M07.66**   Enteropathic arthropathies, knee

      M07.661   Enteropathic arthropathies, right knee

      M07.662   Enteropathic arthropathies, left knee

      M07.669   Enteropathic arthropathies, unspecified knee

  ● **M07.67**   Enteropathic arthropathies, ankle and foot

      M07.671   Enteropathic arthropathies, right ankle and foot

      M07.672   Enteropathic arthropathies, left ankle and foot

      M07.679   Enteropathic arthropathies, unspecified ankle and foot

    M07.68   Enteropathic arthropathies, vertebrae

    M07.69   Enteropathic arthropathies, multiple sites

● **M08 Juvenile arthritis**

    Code also any associated underlying condition, such as:
      regional enteritis [Crohn's disease] (K50.-)
      ulcerative colitis (K51.-)

    Excludes 1   arthropathy in Whipple's disease (M14.8)
      Felty's syndrome (M05.0)
      juvenile dermatomyositis (M33.0-)
      psoriatic juvenile arthropathy (L40.54)

● **M08.0 Unspecified juvenile rheumatoid arthritis**

    Juvenile rheumatoid arthritis with or without rheumatoid factor

    M08.00   Unspecified juvenile rheumatoid arthritis of unspecified site

  ● **M08.01**   Unspecified juvenile rheumatoid arthritis, shoulder

      M08.011   Unspecified juvenile rheumatoid arthritis, right shoulder

      M08.012   Unspecified juvenile rheumatoid arthritis, left shoulder

      M08.019   Unspecified juvenile rheumatoid arthritis, unspecified shoulder

  ● **M08.02**   Unspecified juvenile rheumatoid arthritis of elbow

      M08.021   Unspecified juvenile rheumatoid arthritis, right elbow

      M08.022   Unspecified juvenile rheumatoid arthritis, left elbow

      M08.029   Unspecified juvenile rheumatoid arthritis, unspecified elbow

  ● **M08.03**   Unspecified juvenile rheumatoid arthritis, wrist

      M08.031   Unspecified juvenile rheumatoid arthritis, right wrist

      M08.032   Unspecified juvenile rheumatoid arthritis, left wrist

      M08.039   Unspecified juvenile rheumatoid arthritis, unspecified wrist

  ● **M08.04**   Unspecified juvenile rheumatoid arthritis, hand

      M08.041   Unspecified juvenile rheumatoid arthritis, right hand

      M08.042   Unspecified juvenile rheumatoid arthritis, left hand

      M08.049   Unspecified juvenile rheumatoid arthritis, unspecified hand

  ● **M08.05**   Unspecified juvenile rheumatoid arthritis, hip

      M08.051   Unspecified juvenile rheumatoid arthritis, right hip

      M08.052   Unspecified juvenile rheumatoid arthritis, left hip

      M08.059   Unspecified juvenile rheumatoid arthritis, unspecified hip

  ● **M08.06**   Unspecified juvenile rheumatoid arthritis, knee

      M08.061   Unspecified juvenile rheumatoid arthritis, right knee

      M08.062   Unspecified juvenile rheumatoid arthritis, left knee

      M08.069   Unspecified juvenile rheumatoid arthritis, unspecified knee

  ● **M08.07**   Unspecified juvenile rheumatoid arthritis, ankle and foot

      M08.071   Unspecified juvenile rheumatoid arthritis, right ankle and foot

      M08.072   Unspecified juvenile rheumatoid arthritis, left ankle and foot

      M08.079   Unspecified juvenile rheumatoid arthritis, unspecified ankle and foot

    M08.08   Unspecified juvenile rheumatoid arthritis, vertebrae

    M08.09   Unspecified juvenile rheumatoid arthritis, multiple sites

M08.1 Juvenile ankylosing spondylitis

    Excludes 1   ankylosing spondylitis in adults (M45.0-)

● **M08.2 Juvenile rheumatoid arthritis with systemic onset**

    Still's disease NOS

    Excludes 1   adult-onset Still's disease (M06.1-)

    M08.20   Juvenile rheumatoid arthritis with systemic onset, unspecified site

  ● **M08.21**   Juvenile rheumatoid arthritis with systemic onset, shoulder

      M08.211   Juvenile rheumatoid arthritis with systemic onset, right shoulder

      M08.212   Juvenile rheumatoid arthritis with systemic onset, left shoulder

      M08.219   Juvenile rheumatoid arthritis with systemic onset, unspecified shoulder

CHAPTER 13 (M00-M99)

- **M08.22** Juvenile rheumatoid arthritis with systemic onset, elbow
  - M08.221 Juvenile rheumatoid arthritis with systemic onset, right elbow
  - M08.222 Juvenile rheumatoid arthritis with systemic onset, left elbow
  - M08.229 Juvenile rheumatoid arthritis with systemic onset, unspecified elbow
- **M08.23** Juvenile rheumatoid arthritis with systemic onset, wrist
  - M08.231 Juvenile rheumatoid arthritis with systemic onset, right wrist
  - M08.232 Juvenile rheumatoid arthritis with systemic onset, left wrist
  - M08.239 Juvenile rheumatoid arthritis with systemic onset, unspecified wrist
- **M08.24** Juvenile rheumatoid arthritis with systemic onset, hand
  - M08.241 Juvenile rheumatoid arthritis with systemic onset, right hand
  - M08.242 Juvenile rheumatoid arthritis with systemic onset, left hand
  - M08.249 Juvenile rheumatoid arthritis with systemic onset, unspecified hand
- **M08.25** Juvenile rheumatoid arthritis with systemic onset, hip
  - M08.251 Juvenile rheumatoid arthritis with systemic onset, right hip
  - M08.252 Juvenile rheumatoid arthritis with systemic onset, left hip
  - M08.259 Juvenile rheumatoid arthritis with systemic onset, unspecified hip
- **M08.26** Juvenile rheumatoid arthritis with systemic onset, knee
  - M08.261 Juvenile rheumatoid arthritis with systemic onset, right knee
  - M08.262 Juvenile rheumatoid arthritis with systemic onset, left knee
  - M08.269 Juvenile rheumatoid arthritis with systemic onset, unspecified knee
- **M08.27** Juvenile rheumatoid arthritis with systemic onset, ankle and foot
  - M08.271 Juvenile rheumatoid arthritis with systemic onset, right ankle and foot
  - M08.272 Juvenile rheumatoid arthritis with systemic onset, left ankle and foot
  - M08.279 Juvenile rheumatoid arthritis with systemic onset, unspecified ankle and foot
- **M08.28** Juvenile rheumatoid arthritis with systemic onset, vertebrae
- **M08.29** Juvenile rheumatoid arthritis with systemic onset, multiple sites
- **M08.3** Juvenile rheumatoid polyarthritis (seronegative)
- **M08.4** Pauciarticular juvenile rheumatoid arthritis
  - M08.40 Pauciarticular juvenile rheumatoid arthritis, unspecified site
- **M08.41** Pauciarticular juvenile rheumatoid arthritis, shoulder
  - M08.411 Pauciarticular juvenile rheumatoid arthritis, right shoulder
  - M08.412 Pauciarticular juvenile rheumatoid arthritis, left shoulder
  - M08.419 Pauciarticular juvenile rheumatoid arthritis, unspecified shoulder

- **M08.42** Pauciarticular juvenile rheumatoid arthritis, elbow
  - M08.421 Pauciarticular juvenile rheumatoid arthritis, right elbow
  - M08.422 Pauciarticular juvenile rheumatoid arthritis, left elbow
  - M08.429 Pauciarticular juvenile rheumatoid arthritis, unspecified elbow
- **M08.43** Pauciarticular juvenile rheumatoid arthritis, wrist
  - M08.431 Pauciarticular juvenile rheumatoid arthritis, right wrist
  - M08.432 Pauciarticular juvenile rheumatoid arthritis, left wrist
  - M08.439 Pauciarticular juvenile rheumatoid arthritis, unspecified wrist
- **M08.44** Pauciarticular juvenile rheumatoid arthritis, hand
  - M08.441 Pauciarticular juvenile rheumatoid arthritis, right hand
  - M08.442 Pauciarticular juvenile rheumatoid arthritis, left hand
  - M08.449 Pauciarticular juvenile rheumatoid arthritis, unspecified hand
- **M08.45** Pauciarticular juvenile rheumatoid arthritis, hip
  - M08.451 Pauciarticular juvenile rheumatoid arthritis, right hip
  - M08.452 Pauciarticular juvenile rheumatoid arthritis, left hip
  - M08.459 Pauciarticular juvenile rheumatoid arthritis, unspecified hip
- **M08.46** Pauciarticular juvenile rheumatoid arthritis, knee
  - M08.461 Pauciarticular juvenile rheumatoid arthritis, right knee
  - M08.462 Pauciarticular juvenile rheumatoid arthritis, left knee
  - M08.469 Pauciarticular juvenile rheumatoid arthritis, unspecified knee
- **M08.47** Pauciarticular juvenile rheumatoid arthritis, ankle and foot
  - M08.471 Pauciarticular juvenile rheumatoid arthritis, right ankle and foot
  - M08.472 Pauciarticular juvenile rheumatoid arthritis, left ankle and foot
  - M08.479 Pauciarticular juvenile rheumatoid arthritis, unspecified ankle and foot
- **M08.48** Pauciarticular juvenile rheumatoid arthritis, vertebrae
- **M08.8** Other juvenile arthritis
  - M08.80 Other juvenile arthritis, unspecified site
- **M08.81** Other juvenile arthritis, shoulder
  - M08.811 Other juvenile arthritis, right shoulder
  - M08.812 Other juvenile arthritis, left shoulder
  - M08.819 Other juvenile arthritis, unspecified shoulder
- **M08.82** Other juvenile arthritis, elbow
  - M08.821 Other juvenile arthritis, right elbow
  - M08.822 Other juvenile arthritis, left elbow
  - M08.829 Other juvenile arthritis, unspecified elbow
- **M08.83** Other juvenile arthritis, wrist
  - M08.831 Other juvenile arthritis, right wrist
  - M08.832 Other juvenile arthritis, left wrist
  - M08.839 Other juvenile arthritis, unspecified wrist

◄ New   ◄█ Revised   ~~deleted~~ Deleted   Excludes 1   Excludes 2   Includes   Use additional   Code first   Code also   Unspecified

OGCR Official Guidelines   ● Unacceptable Principal Diagnosis   X Assign placeholder X   ● Use Additional Character(s)   ▶ Manifestation Code   **Coding Clinic**

● **M08.84   Other juvenile arthritis, hand**
    M08.841   Other juvenile arthritis, right hand
    M08.842   Other juvenile arthritis, left hand
    M08.849   Other juvenile arthritis, unspecified hand

● **M08.85   Other juvenile arthritis, hip**
    M08.851   Other juvenile arthritis, right hip
    M08.852   Other juvenile arthritis, left hip
    M08.859   Other juvenile arthritis, unspecified hip

● **M08.86   Other juvenile arthritis, knee**
    M08.861   Other juvenile arthritis, right knee
    M08.862   Other juvenile arthritis, left knee
    M08.869   Other juvenile arthritis, unspecified knee

● **M08.87   Other juvenile arthritis, ankle and foot**
    M08.871   Other juvenile arthritis, right ankle and foot
    M08.872   Other juvenile arthritis, left ankle and foot
    M08.879   Other juvenile arthritis, unspecified ankle and foot

    M08.88   Other juvenile arthritis, other specified site
       Other juvenile arthritis, vertebrae

    M08.89   Other juvenile arthritis, multiple sites

● **M08.9   Juvenile arthritis, unspecified**
    Excludes1   juvenile rheumatoid arthritis, unspecified (M08.0-)

    M08.90   Juvenile arthritis, unspecified, unspecified site

● **M08.91   Juvenile arthritis, unspecified, shoulder**
    M08.911   Juvenile arthritis, unspecified, right shoulder
    M08.912   Juvenile arthritis, unspecified, left shoulder
    M08.919   Juvenile arthritis, unspecified, unspecified shoulder

● **M08.92   Juvenile arthritis, unspecified, elbow**
    M08.921   Juvenile arthritis, unspecified, right elbow
    M08.922   Juvenile arthritis, unspecified, left elbow
    M08.929   Juvenile arthritis, unspecified, unspecified elbow

● **M08.93   Juvenile arthritis, unspecified, wrist**
    M08.931   Juvenile arthritis, unspecified, right wrist
    M08.932   Juvenile arthritis, unspecified, left wrist
    M08.939   Juvenile arthritis, unspecified, unspecified wrist

● **M08.94   Juvenile arthritis, unspecified, hand**
    M08.941   Juvenile arthritis, unspecified, right hand
    M08.942   Juvenile arthritis, unspecified, left hand
    M08.949   Juvenile arthritis, unspecified, unspecified hand

● **M08.95   Juvenile arthritis, unspecified, hip**
    M08.951   Juvenile arthritis, unspecified, right hip
    M08.952   Juvenile arthritis, unspecified, left hip
    M08.959   Juvenile arthritis, unspecified, unspecified hip

● **M08.96   Juvenile arthritis, unspecified, knee**
    M08.961   Juvenile arthritis, unspecified, right knee
    M08.962   Juvenile arthritis, unspecified, left knee
    M08.969   Juvenile arthritis, unspecified, unspecified knee

● **M08.97   Juvenile arthritis, unspecified, ankle and foot**
    M08.971   Juvenile arthritis, unspecified, right ankle and foot
    M08.972   Juvenile arthritis, unspecified, left ankle and foot
    M08.979   Juvenile arthritis, unspecified, unspecified ankle and foot

    M08.98   Juvenile arthritis, unspecified, vertebrae

    M08.99   Juvenile arthritis, unspecified, multiple sites

● **M1A   Chronic gout**
    Use additional code to identify:
       Autonomic neuropathy in diseases classified elsewhere (G99.0)
       Calculus of urinary tract in diseases classified elsewhere (N22)
       Cardiomyopathy in diseases classified elsewhere (I43)
       Disorders of external ear in diseases classified elsewhere (H61.1-, H62.8-)
       Disorders of iris and ciliary body in diseases classified elsewhere (H22)
       Glomerular disorders in diseases classified elsewhere (N08)

    Excludes1   gout NOS (M10.-)

    Excludes2   acute gout (M10.-) ◀

    The appropriate 7th character is to be added to each code from category M1A

0	without tophus (tophi)
1	with tophus (tophi)

● **M1A.0   Idiopathic chronic gout**
       Chronic gouty bursitis
       Primary chronic gout

   X ● **M1A.00   Idiopathic chronic gout, unspecified site**
    ● **M1A.01   Idiopathic chronic gout, shoulder**
       ● M1A.011   Idiopathic chronic gout, right shoulder
       ● M1A.012   Idiopathic chronic gout, left shoulder
       ● M1A.019   Idiopathic chronic gout, unspecified shoulder

    ● **M1A.02   Idiopathic chronic gout, elbow**
       ● M1A.021   Idiopathic chronic gout, right elbow
       ● M1A.022   Idiopathic chronic gout, left elbow
       ● M1A.029   Idiopathic chronic gout, unspecified elbow

    ● **M1A.03   Idiopathic chronic gout, wrist**
       ● M1A.031   Idiopathic chronic gout, right wrist
       ● M1A.032   Idiopathic chronic gout, left wrist
       ● M1A.039   Idiopathic chronic gout, unspecified wrist

    ● **M1A.04   Idiopathic chronic gout, hand**
       ● M1A.041   Idiopathic chronic gout, right hand
       ● M1A.042   Idiopathic chronic gout, left hand
       ● M1A.049   Idiopathic chronic gout, unspecified hand

    ● **M1A.05   Idiopathic chronic gout, hip**
       ● M1A.051   Idiopathic chronic gout, right hip
       ● M1A.052   Idiopathic chronic gout, left hip
       ● M1A.059   Idiopathic chronic gout, unspecified hip

    ● **M1A.06   Idiopathic chronic gout, knee**
       ● M1A.061   Idiopathic chronic gout, right knee
       ● M1A.062   Idiopathic chronic gout, left knee
       ● M1A.069   Idiopathic chronic gout, unspecified knee

CHAPTER 13 (M00-M99)

- ● M1A.07 Idiopathic chronic gout, ankle and foot
  - ● M1A.071 Idiopathic chronic gout, right ankle and foot
  - ● M1A.072 Idiopathic chronic gout, left ankle and foot
  - ● M1A.079 Idiopathic chronic gout, unspecified ankle and foot
- X ● M1A.08 Idiopathic chronic gout, vertebrae
- X ● M1A.09 Idiopathic chronic gout, multiple sites
- ● M1A.1 Lead-induced chronic gout
  - *Code first toxic effects of lead and its compounds (T56.0-)*
  - X ● M1A.10 Lead-induced chronic gout, unspecified site
  - ● M1A.11 Lead-induced chronic gout, shoulder
    - ● M1A.111 Lead-induced chronic gout, right shoulder
    - ● M1A.112 Lead-induced chronic gout, left shoulder
    - ● M1A.119 Lead-induced chronic gout, unspecified shoulder
  - ● M1A.12 Lead-induced chronic gout, elbow
    - ● M1A.121 Lead-induced chronic gout, right elbow
    - ● M1A.122 Lead-induced chronic gout, left elbow
    - ● M1A.129 Lead-induced chronic gout, unspecified elbow
  - ● M1A.13 Lead-induced chronic gout, wrist
    - ● M1A.131 Lead-induced chronic gout, right wrist
    - ● M1A.132 Lead-induced chronic gout, left wrist
    - ● M1A.139 Lead-induced chronic gout, unspecified wrist
  - ● M1A.14 Lead-induced chronic gout, hand
    - ● M1A.141 Lead-induced chronic gout, right hand
    - ● M1A.142 Lead-induced chronic gout, left hand
    - ● M1A.149 Lead-induced chronic gout, unspecified hand
  - ● M1A.15 Lead-induced chronic gout, hip
    - ● M1A.151 Lead-induced chronic gout, right hip
    - ● M1A.152 Lead-induced chronic gout, left hip
    - ● M1A.159 Lead-induced chronic gout, unspecified hip
  - ● M1A.16 Lead-induced chronic gout, knee
    - ● M1A.161 Lead-induced chronic gout, right knee
    - ● M1A.162 Lead-induced chronic gout, left knee
    - ● M1A.169 Lead-induced chronic gout, unspecified knee
  - ● M1A.17 Lead-induced chronic gout, ankle and foot
    - ● M1A.171 Lead-induced chronic gout, right ankle and foot
    - ● M1A.172 Lead-induced chronic gout, left ankle and foot
    - ● M1A.179 Lead-induced chronic gout, unspecified ankle and foot
  - X ● M1A.18 Lead-induced chronic gout, vertebrae
  - X ● M1A.19 Lead-induced chronic gout, multiple sites
- ● M1A.2 Drug-induced chronic gout
  - Use additional code for adverse effect, if applicable, to identify drug (T36-T50 with fifth or sixth character 5)
  - X ● M1A.20 Drug-induced chronic gout, unspecified site
  - ● M1A.21 Drug-induced chronic gout, shoulder
    - ● M1A.211 Drug-induced chronic gout, right shoulder
    - ● M1A.212 Drug-induced chronic gout, left shoulder
    - ● M1A.219 Drug-induced chronic gout, unspecified shoulder

- ● M1A.22 Drug-induced chronic gout, elbow
  - ● M1A.221 Drug-induced chronic gout, right elbow
  - ● M1A.222 Drug-induced chronic gout, left elbow
  - ● M1A.229 Drug-induced chronic gout, unspecified elbow
- ● M1A.23 Drug-induced chronic gout, wrist
  - ● M1A.231 Drug-induced chronic gout, right wrist
  - ● M1A.232 Drug-induced chronic gout, left wrist
  - ● M1A.239 Drug-induced chronic gout, unspecified wrist
- ● M1A.24 Drug-induced chronic gout, hand
  - ● M1A.241 Drug-induced chronic gout, right hand
  - ● M1A.242 Drug-induced chronic gout, left hand
  - ● M1A.249 Drug-induced chronic gout, unspecified hand
- ● M1A.25 Drug-induced chronic gout, hip
  - ● M1A.251 Drug-induced chronic gout, right hip
  - ● M1A.252 Drug-induced chronic gout, left hip
  - ● M1A.259 Drug-induced chronic gout, unspecified hip
- ● M1A.26 Drug-induced chronic gout, knee
  - ● M1A.261 Drug-induced chronic gout, right knee
  - ● M1A.262 Drug-induced chronic gout, left knee
  - ● M1A.269 Drug-induced chronic gout, unspecified knee
- ● M1A.27 Drug-induced chronic gout, ankle and foot
  - ● M1A.271 Drug-induced chronic gout, right ankle and foot
  - ● M1A.272 Drug-induced chronic gout, left ankle and foot
  - ● M1A.279 Drug-induced chronic gout, unspecified ankle and foot
- X ● M1A.28 Drug-induced chronic gout, vertebrae
- X ● M1A.29 Drug-induced chronic gout, multiple sites
- ● M1A.3 Chronic gout due to renal impairment
  - *Code first associated renal disease*
  - X ● M1A.30 Chronic gout due to renal impairment, unspecified site
  - ● M1A.31 Chronic gout due to renal impairment, shoulder
    - ● M1A.311 Chronic gout due to renal impairment, right shoulder
    - ● M1A.312 Chronic gout due to renal impairment, left shoulder
    - ● M1A.319 Chronic gout due to renal impairment, unspecified shoulder
  - ● M1A.32 Chronic gout due to renal impairment, elbow
    - ● M1A.321 Chronic gout due to renal impairment, right elbow
    - ● M1A.322 Chronic gout due to renal impairment, left elbow
    - ● M1A.329 Chronic gout due to renal impairment, unspecified elbow
  - ● M1A.33 Chronic gout due to renal impairment, wrist
    - ● M1A.331 Chronic gout due to renal impairment, right wrist
    - ● M1A.332 Chronic gout due to renal impairment, left wrist
    - ● M1A.339 Chronic gout due to renal impairment, unspecified wrist

◄ New   ◄ Revised   ~~deleted~~ Deleted   Excludes 1   Excludes 2   Includes   Use additional   Code first   Code also   Unspecified

OGCR Official Guidelines   ● Unacceptable Principal Diagnosis   X Assign placeholder X   ● Use Additional Character(s)   ▶ Manifestation Code   **Coding Clinic**

● M1A.34 Chronic gout due to renal impairment, hand
  ● M1A.341 Chronic gout due to renal impairment, right hand
  ● M1A.342 Chronic gout due to renal impairment, left hand
  ● M1A.349 Chronic gout due to renal impairment, unspecified hand
● M1A.35 Chronic gout due to renal impairment, hip
  ● M1A.351 Chronic gout due to renal impairment, right hip
  ● M1A.352 Chronic gout due to renal impairment, left hip
  ● M1A.359 Chronic gout due to renal impairment, unspecified hip
● M1A.36 Chronic gout due to renal impairment, knee
  ● M1A.361 Chronic gout due to renal impairment, right knee
  ● M1A.362 Chronic gout due to renal impairment, left knee
  ● M1A.369 Chronic gout due to renal impairment, unspecified knee
● M1A.37 Chronic gout due to renal impairment, ankle and foot
  ● M1A.371 Chronic gout due to renal impairment, right ankle and foot
  ● M1A.372 Chronic gout due to renal impairment, left ankle and foot
  ● M1A.379 Chronic gout due to renal impairment, unspecified ankle and foot
X ● M1A.38 Chronic gout due to renal impairment, vertebrae
X ● M1A.39 Chronic gout due to renal impairment, multiple sites
● M1A.4 Other secondary chronic gout
  Code first associated condition
X ● M1A.40 Other secondary chronic gout, unspecified site
● M1A.41 Other secondary chronic gout, shoulder
  ● M1A.411 Other secondary chronic gout, right shoulder
  ● M1A.412 Other secondary chronic gout, left shoulder
  ● M1A.419 Other secondary chronic gout, unspecified shoulder
● M1A.42 Other secondary chronic gout, elbow
  ● M1A.421 Other secondary chronic gout, right elbow
  ● M1A.422 Other secondary chronic gout, left elbow
  ● M1A.429 Other secondary chronic gout, unspecified elbow
● M1A.43 Other secondary chronic gout, wrist
  ● M1A.431 Other secondary chronic gout, right wrist
  ● M1A.432 Other secondary chronic gout, left wrist
  ● M1A.439 Other secondary chronic gout, unspecified wrist
● M1A.44 Other secondary chronic gout, hand
  ● M1A.441 Other secondary chronic gout, right hand
  ● M1A.442 Other secondary chronic gout, left hand
  ● M1A.449 Other secondary chronic gout, unspecified hand

● M1A.45 Other secondary chronic gout, hip
  ● M1A.451 Other secondary chronic gout, right hip
  ● M1A.452 Other secondary chronic gout, left hip
  ● M1A.459 Other secondary chronic gout, unspecified hip
● M1A.46 Other secondary chronic gout, knee
  ● M1A.461 Other secondary chronic gout, right knee
  ● M1A.462 Other secondary chronic gout, left knee
  ● M1A.469 Other secondary chronic gout, unspecified knee
● M1A.47 Other secondary chronic gout, ankle and foot
  ● M1A.471 Other secondary chronic gout, right ankle and foot
  ● M1A.472 Other secondary chronic gout, left ankle and foot
  ● M1A.479 Other secondary chronic gout, unspecified ankle and foot
X ● M1A.48 Other secondary chronic gout, vertebrae
X ● M1A.49 Other secondary chronic gout, multiple sites
X ● M1A.9 Chronic gout, unspecified

● **M10** **Gout**
  Accumulation of uric acid that results in swollen, red, hot, painful, stiff joints
  Acute gout
  Gout attack
  Gout flare
  Podagra
  Use additional code to identify:
    Autonomic neuropathy in diseases classified elsewhere (G99.0)
    Calculus of urinary tract in diseases classified elsewhere (N22)
    Cardiomyopathy in diseases classified elsewhere (I43)
    Disorders of external ear in diseases classified elsewhere (H61.1-, H62.8-)
    Disorders of iris and ciliary body in diseases classified elsewhere (H22)
    Glomerular disorders in diseases classified elsewhere (N08)
  Excludes2 chronic gout (M1A.-) ◄
  ● M10.0 Idiopathic gout
    Gouty bursitis
    Primary gout
    M10.00 Idiopathic gout, unspecified site
    ● M10.01 Idiopathic gout, shoulder
      M10.011 Idiopathic gout, right shoulder
      M10.012 Idiopathic gout, left shoulder
      M10.019 Idiopathic gout, unspecified shoulder
    ● M10.02 Idiopathic gout, elbow
      M10.021 Idiopathic gout, right elbow
      M10.022 Idiopathic gout, left elbow
      M10.029 Idiopathic gout, unspecified elbow
    ● M10.03 Idiopathic gout, wrist
      M10.031 Idiopathic gout, right wrist
      M10.032 Idiopathic gout, left wrist
      M10.039 Idiopathic gout, unspecified wrist
    ● M10.04 Idiopathic gout, hand
      M10.041 Idiopathic gout, right hand
      M10.042 Idiopathic gout, left hand
      M10.049 Idiopathic gout, unspecified hand
    ● M10.05 Idiopathic gout, hip
      M10.051 Idiopathic gout, right hip
      M10.052 Idiopathic gout, left hip
      M10.059 Idiopathic gout, unspecified hip

CHAPTER 13 (M00-M99)

N Newborn Age: 0   P Pediatric Age: 0–17   M Maternity DX: 12–55   A Adult Age: 15–124   ♀ Females Only   ♂ Males Only
🔹 Complication\Comorbidity   🔹 Major C\C   (Ex) CC/MCC Exclusions   🔹 Hospital-Acquired Condition
1005

● M10.06   Idiopathic gout, knee
    M10.061   Idiopathic gout, right knee
    M10.062   Idiopathic gout, left knee
    M10.069   Idiopathic gout, unspecified knee
● M10.07   Idiopathic gout, ankle and foot
    M10.071   Idiopathic gout, right ankle and foot
    M10.072   Idiopathic gout, left ankle and foot
    M10.079   Idiopathic gout, unspecified ankle and foot
  M10.08   Idiopathic gout, vertebrae
  M10.09   Idiopathic gout, multiple sites
● M10.1   Lead-induced gout
Code first toxic effects of lead and its compounds (T56.0-)
  M10.10   Lead-induced gout, unspecified site
● M10.11   Lead-induced gout, shoulder
    M10.111   Lead-induced gout, right shoulder
    M10.112   Lead-induced gout, left shoulder
    M10.119   Lead-induced gout, unspecified shoulder
● M10.12   Lead-induced gout, elbow
    M10.121   Lead-induced gout, right elbow
    M10.122   Lead-induced gout, left elbow
    M10.129   Lead-induced gout, unspecified elbow
● M10.13   Lead-induced gout, wrist
    M10.131   Lead-induced gout, right wrist
    M10.132   Lead-induced gout, left wrist
    M10.139   Lead-induced gout, unspecified wrist
● M10.14   Lead-induced gout, hand
    M10.141   Lead-induced gout, right hand
    M10.142   Lead-induced gout, left hand
    M10.149   Lead-induced gout, unspecified hand
● M10.15   Lead-induced gout, hip
    M10.151   Lead-induced gout, right hip
    M10.152   Lead-induced gout, left hip
    M10.159   Lead-induced gout, unspecified hip
● M10.16   Lead-induced gout, knee
    M10.161   Lead-induced gout, right knee
    M10.162   Lead-induced gout, left knee
    M10.169   Lead-induced gout, unspecified knee
● M10.17   Lead-induced gout, ankle and foot
    M10.171   Lead-induced gout, right ankle and foot
    M10.172   Lead-induced gout, left ankle and foot
    M10.179   Lead-induced gout, unspecified ankle and foot
  M10.18   Lead-induced gout, vertebrae
  M10.19   Lead-induced gout, multiple sites
● M10.2   Drug-induced gout
Use additional code for adverse effect, if applicable, to identify drug (T36-T50 with fifth or sixth character 5)
  M10.20   Drug-induced gout, unspecified site
● M10.21   Drug-induced gout, shoulder
    M10.211   Drug-induced gout, right shoulder
    M10.212   Drug-induced gout, left shoulder
    M10.219   Drug-induced gout, unspecified shoulder
● M10.22   Drug-induced gout, elbow
    M10.221   Drug-induced gout, right elbow
    M10.222   Drug-induced gout, left elbow
    M10.229   Drug-induced gout, unspecified elbow

● M10.23   Drug-induced gout, wrist
    M10.231   Drug-induced gout, right wrist
    M10.232   Drug-induced gout, left wrist
    M10.239   Drug-induced gout, unspecified wrist
● M10.24   Drug-induced gout, hand
    M10.241   Drug-induced gout, right hand
    M10.242   Drug-induced gout, left hand
    M10.249   Drug-induced gout, unspecified hand
● M10.25   Drug-induced gout, hip
    M10.251   Drug-induced gout, right hip
    M10.252   Drug-induced gout, left hip
    M10.259   Drug-induced gout, unspecified hip
● M10.26   Drug-induced gout, knee
    M10.261   Drug-induced gout, right knee
    M10.262   Drug-induced gout, left knee
    M10.269   Drug-induced gout, unspecified knee
● M10.27   Drug-induced gout, ankle and foot
    M10.271   Drug-induced gout, right ankle and foot
    M10.272   Drug-induced gout, left ankle and foot
    M10.279   Drug-induced gout, unspecified ankle and foot
  M10.28   Drug-induced gout, vertebrae
  M10.29   Drug-induced gout, multiple sites
● M10.3   Gout due to renal impairment
Code also associated renal disease
  M10.30   Gout due to renal impairment, unspecified site
● M10.31   Gout due to renal impairment, shoulder
    M10.311   Gout due to renal impairment, right shoulder
    M10.312   Gout due to renal impairment, left shoulder
    M10.319   Gout due to renal impairment, unspecified shoulder
● M10.32   Gout due to renal impairment, elbow
    M10.321   Gout due to renal impairment, right elbow
    M10.322   Gout due to renal impairment, left elbow
    M10.329   Gout due to renal impairment, unspecified elbow
● M10.33   Gout due to renal impairment, wrist
    M10.331   Gout due to renal impairment, right wrist
    M10.332   Gout due to renal impairment, left wrist
    M10.339   Gout due to renal impairment, unspecified wrist
● M10.34   Gout due to renal impairment, hand
    M10.341   Gout due to renal impairment, right hand
    M10.342   Gout due to renal impairment, left hand
    M10.349   Gout due to renal impairment, unspecified hand
● M10.35   Gout due to renal impairment, hip
    M10.351   Gout due to renal impairment, right hip
    M10.352   Gout due to renal impairment, left hip
    M10.359   Gout due to renal impairment, unspecified hip
● M10.36   Gout due to renal impairment, knee
    M10.361   Gout due to renal impairment, right knee
    M10.362   Gout due to renal impairment, left knee
    M10.369   Gout due to renal impairment, unspecified knee

● M10.37 Gout due to renal impairment, ankle and foot
    M10.371 Gout due to renal impairment, right ankle and foot
    M10.372 Gout due to renal impairment, left ankle and foot
    M10.379 Gout due to renal impairment, unspecified ankle and foot
  M10.38 Gout due to renal impairment, vertebrae
  M10.39 Gout due to renal impairment, multiple sites
● M10.4 Other secondary gout
    Code first associated condition
  M10.40 Other secondary gout, unspecified site
● M10.41 Other secondary gout, shoulder
    M10.411 Other secondary gout, right shoulder
    M10.412 Other secondary gout, left shoulder
    M10.419 Other secondary gout, unspecified shoulder
● M10.42 Other secondary gout, elbow
    M10.421 Other secondary gout, right elbow
    M10.422 Other secondary gout, left elbow
    M10.429 Other secondary gout, unspecified elbow
● M10.43 Other secondary gout, wrist
    M10.431 Other secondary gout, right wrist
    M10.432 Other secondary gout, left wrist
    M10.439 Other secondary gout, unspecified wrist
● M10.44 Other secondary gout, hand
    M10.441 Other secondary gout, right hand
    M10.442 Other secondary gout, left hand
    M10.449 Other secondary gout, unspecified hand
● M10.45 Other secondary gout, hip
    M10.451 Other secondary gout, right hip
    M10.452 Other secondary gout, left hip
    M10.459 Other secondary gout, unspecified hip
● M10.46 Other secondary gout, knee
    M10.461 Other secondary gout, right knee
    M10.462 Other secondary gout, left knee
    M10.469 Other secondary gout, unspecified knee
● M10.47 Other secondary gout, ankle and foot
    M10.471 Other secondary gout, right ankle and foot
    M10.472 Other secondary gout, left ankle and foot
    M10.479 Other secondary gout, unspecified ankle and foot
  M10.48 Other secondary gout, vertebrae
  M10.49 Other secondary gout, multiple sites
M10.9 Gout, unspecified
    Gout NOS

● M11 Other crystal arthropathies
● M11.0 Hydroxyapatite deposition disease
  M11.00 Hydroxyapatite deposition disease, unspecified site
● M11.01 Hydroxyapatite deposition disease, shoulder
    M11.011 Hydroxyapatite deposition disease, right shoulder
    M11.012 Hydroxyapatite deposition disease, left shoulder
    M11.019 Hydroxyapatite deposition disease, unspecified shoulder
● M11.02 Hydroxyapatite deposition disease, elbow
    M11.021 Hydroxyapatite deposition disease, right elbow
    M11.022 Hydroxyapatite deposition disease, left elbow
    M11.029 Hydroxyapatite deposition disease, unspecified elbow
● M11.03 Hydroxyapatite deposition disease, wrist
    M11.031 Hydroxyapatite deposition disease, right wrist
    M11.032 Hydroxyapatite deposition disease, left wrist
    M11.039 Hydroxyapatite deposition disease, unspecified wrist
● M11.04 Hydroxyapatite deposition disease, hand
    M11.041 Hydroxyapatite deposition disease, right hand
    M11.042 Hydroxyapatite deposition disease, left hand
    M11.049 Hydroxyapatite deposition disease, unspecified hand
● M11.05 Hydroxyapatite deposition disease, hip
    M11.051 Hydroxyapatite deposition disease, right hip
    M11.052 Hydroxyapatite deposition disease, left hip
    M11.059 Hydroxyapatite deposition disease, unspecified hip
● M11.06 Hydroxyapatite deposition disease, knee
    M11.061 Hydroxyapatite deposition disease, right knee
    M11.062 Hydroxyapatite deposition disease, left knee
    M11.069 Hydroxyapatite deposition disease, unspecified knee
● M11.07 Hydroxyapatite deposition disease, ankle and foot
    M11.071 Hydroxyapatite deposition disease, right ankle and foot
    M11.072 Hydroxyapatite deposition disease, left ankle and foot
    M11.079 Hydroxyapatite deposition disease, unspecified ankle and foot
  M11.08 Hydroxyapatite deposition disease, vertebrae
  M11.09 Hydroxyapatite deposition disease, multiple sites
● M11.1 Familial chondrocalcinosis
  M11.10 Familial chondrocalcinosis, unspecified site
● M11.11 Familial chondrocalcinosis, shoulder
    M11.111 Familial chondrocalcinosis, right shoulder
    M11.112 Familial chondrocalcinosis, left shoulder
    M11.119 Familial chondrocalcinosis, unspecified shoulder
● M11.12 Familial chondrocalcinosis, elbow
    M11.121 Familial chondrocalcinosis, right elbow
    M11.122 Familial chondrocalcinosis, left elbow
    M11.129 Familial chondrocalcinosis, unspecified elbow
● M11.13 Familial chondrocalcinosis, wrist
    M11.131 Familial chondrocalcinosis, right wrist
    M11.132 Familial chondrocalcinosis, left wrist
    M11.139 Familial chondrocalcinosis, unspecified wrist

CHAPTER 13 (M00–M99)

N Newborn Age: 0 P Pediatric Age: 0–17 M Maternity DX: 12–55 A Adult Age: 15–124 ♀ Females Only ♂ Males Only
Complication\Comorbidity Major C\C CC/MCC Exclusions Hospital-Acquired Condition
1007

● **M11.14**   Familial chondrocalcinosis, hand
    M11.141   Familial chondrocalcinosis, right hand
    M11.142   Familial chondrocalcinosis, left hand
    M11.149   Familial chondrocalcinosis, unspecified hand
● **M11.15**   Familial chondrocalcinosis, hip
    M11.151   Familial chondrocalcinosis, right hip
    M11.152   Familial chondrocalcinosis, left hip
    M11.159   Familial chondrocalcinosis, unspecified hip
● **M11.16**   Familial chondrocalcinosis, knee
    M11.161   Familial chondrocalcinosis, right knee
    M11.162   Familial chondrocalcinosis, left knee
    M11.169   Familial chondrocalcinosis, unspecified knee
● **M11.17**   Familial chondrocalcinosis, ankle and foot
    M11.171   Familial chondrocalcinosis, right ankle and foot
    M11.172   Familial chondrocalcinosis, left ankle and foot
    M11.179   Familial chondrocalcinosis, unspecified ankle and foot
   M11.18   Familial chondrocalcinosis, vertebrae
   M11.19   Familial chondrocalcinosis, multiple sites
● **M11.2**   Other chondrocalcinosis
    Chondrocalcinosis NOS
   M11.20   Other chondrocalcinosis, unspecified site
● **M11.21**   Other chondrocalcinosis, shoulder
    M11.211   Other chondrocalcinosis, right shoulder
    M11.212   Other chondrocalcinosis, left shoulder
    M11.219   Other chondrocalcinosis, unspecified shoulder
● **M11.22**   Other chondrocalcinosis, elbow
    M11.221   Other chondrocalcinosis, right elbow
    M11.222   Other chondrocalcinosis, left elbow
    M11.229   Other chondrocalcinosis, unspecified elbow
● **M11.23**   Other chondrocalcinosis, wrist
    M11.231   Other chondrocalcinosis, right wrist
    M11.232   Other chondrocalcinosis, left wrist
    M11.239   Other chondrocalcinosis, unspecified wrist
● **M11.24**   Other chondrocalcinosis, hand
    M11.241   Other chondrocalcinosis, right hand
    M11.242   Other chondrocalcinosis, left hand
    M11.249   Other chondrocalcinosis, unspecified hand
● **M11.25**   Other chondrocalcinosis, hip
    M11.251   Other chondrocalcinosis, right hip
    M11.252   Other chondrocalcinosis, left hip
    M11.259   Other chondrocalcinosis, unspecified hip
● **M11.26**   Other chondrocalcinosis, knee
    M11.261   Other chondrocalcinosis, right knee
    M11.262   Other chondrocalcinosis, left knee
    M11.269   Other chondrocalcinosis, unspecified knee
● **M11.27**   Other chondrocalcinosis, ankle and foot
    M11.271   Other chondrocalcinosis, right ankle and foot
    M11.272   Other chondrocalcinosis, left ankle and foot
    M11.279   Other chondrocalcinosis, unspecified ankle and foot

   M11.28   Other chondrocalcinosis, vertebrae
   M11.29   Other chondrocalcinosis, multiple sites
● **M11.8**   Other specified crystal arthropathies
   M11.80   Other specified crystal arthropathies, unspecified site
● **M11.81**   Other specified crystal arthropathies, shoulder
    M11.811   Other specified crystal arthropathies, right shoulder
    M11.812   Other specified crystal arthropathies, left shoulder
    M11.819   Other specified crystal arthropathies, unspecified shoulder
● **M11.82**   Other specified crystal arthropathies, elbow
    M11.821   Other specified crystal arthropathies, right elbow
    M11.822   Other specified crystal arthropathies, left elbow
    M11.829   Other specified crystal arthropathies, unspecified elbow
● **M11.83**   Other specified crystal arthropathies, wrist
    M11.831   Other specified crystal arthropathies, right wrist
    M11.832   Other specified crystal arthropathies, left wrist
    M11.839   Other specified crystal arthropathies, unspecified wrist
● **M11.84**   Other specified crystal arthropathies, hand
    M11.841   Other specified crystal arthropathies, right hand
    M11.842   Other specified crystal arthropathies, left hand
    M11.849   Other specified crystal arthropathies, unspecified hand
● **M11.85**   Other specified crystal arthropathies, hip
    M11.851   Other specified crystal arthropathies, right hip
    M11.852   Other specified crystal arthropathies, left hip
    M11.859   Other specified crystal arthropathies, unspecified hip
● **M11.86**   Other specified crystal arthropathies, knee
    M11.861   Other specified crystal arthropathies, right knee
    M11.862   Other specified crystal arthropathies, left knee
    M11.869   Other specified crystal arthropathies, unspecified knee
● **M11.87**   Other specified crystal arthropathies, ankle and foot
    M11.871   Other specified crystal arthropathies, right ankle and foot
    M11.872   Other specified crystal arthropathies, left ankle and foot
    M11.879   Other specified crystal arthropathies, unspecified ankle and foot
   M11.88   Other specified crystal arthropathies, vertebrae
   M11.89   Other specified crystal arthropathies, multiple sites
   M11.9   Crystal arthropathy, unspecified

● **M12**   Other and unspecified arthropathy
   Excludes1   arthrosis (M15-M19)
            cricoarytenoid arthropathy (J38.7)
● **M12.0**   Chronic postrheumatic arthropathy [Jaccoud]
    M12.00   Chronic postrheumatic arthropathy [Jaccoud], unspecified site

◀ New   ◀▥ Revised   ~~deleted~~ Deleted   Excludes 1   Excludes 2   Includes   Use additional   Code first   Code also   Unspecified
OGCR Official Guidelines   ● Unacceptable Principal Diagnosis   X Assign placeholder X   ● Use Additional Character(s)   ▶ Manifestation Code   Coding Clinic

● M12.01 Chronic postrheumatic arthropathy [Jaccoud], shoulder

    M12.011 Chronic postrheumatic arthropathy [Jaccoud], right shoulder

    M12.012 Chronic postrheumatic arthropathy [Jaccoud], left shoulder

    M12.019 Chronic postrheumatic arthropathy [Jaccoud], unspecified shoulder

● M12.02 Chronic postrheumatic arthropathy [Jaccoud], elbow

    M12.021 Chronic postrheumatic arthropathy [Jaccoud], right elbow

    M12.022 Chronic postrheumatic arthropathy [Jaccoud], left elbow

    M12.029 Chronic postrheumatic arthropathy [Jaccoud], unspecified elbow

● M12.03 Chronic postrheumatic arthropathy [Jaccoud], wrist

    M12.031 Chronic postrheumatic arthropathy [Jaccoud], right wrist

    M12.032 Chronic postrheumatic arthropathy [Jaccoud], left wrist

    M12.039 Chronic postrheumatic arthropathy [Jaccoud], unspecified wrist

● M12.04 Chronic postrheumatic arthropathy [Jaccoud], hand

    M12.041 Chronic postrheumatic arthropathy [Jaccoud], right hand

    M12.042 Chronic postrheumatic arthropathy [Jaccoud], left hand

    M12.049 Chronic postrheumatic arthropathy [Jaccoud], unspecified hand

● M12.05 Chronic postrheumatic arthropathy [Jaccoud], hip

    M12.051 Chronic postrheumatic arthropathy [Jaccoud], right hip

    M12.052 Chronic postrheumatic arthropathy [Jaccoud], left hip

    M12.059 Chronic postrheumatic arthropathy [Jaccoud], unspecified hip

● M12.06 Chronic postrheumatic arthropathy [Jaccoud], knee

    M12.061 Chronic postrheumatic arthropathy [Jaccoud], right knee

    M12.062 Chronic postrheumatic arthropathy [Jaccoud], left knee

    M12.069 Chronic postrheumatic arthropathy [Jaccoud], unspecified knee

● M12.07 Chronic postrheumatic arthropathy [Jaccoud], ankle and foot

    M12.071 Chronic postrheumatic arthropathy [Jaccoud], right ankle and foot

    M12.072 Chronic postrheumatic arthropathy [Jaccoud], left ankle and foot

    M12.079 Chronic postrheumatic arthropathy [Jaccoud], unspecified ankle and foot

    M12.08 Chronic postrheumatic arthropathy [Jaccoud], other specified site

        Chronic postrheumatic arthropathy [Jaccoud], vertebrae

    M12.09 Chronic postrheumatic arthropathy [Jaccoud], multiple sites

● M12.1 Kaschin-Beck disease

    Osteochondroarthrosis deformans endemica

    M12.10 Kaschin-Beck disease, unspecified site

● M12.11 Kaschin-Beck disease, shoulder

    M12.111 Kaschin-Beck disease, right shoulder

    M12.112 Kaschin-Beck disease, left shoulder

    M12.119 Kaschin-Beck disease, unspecified shoulder

● M12.12 Kaschin-Beck disease, elbow

    M12.121 Kaschin-Beck disease, right elbow

    M12.122 Kaschin-Beck disease, left elbow

    M12.129 Kaschin-Beck disease, unspecified elbow

● M12.13 Kaschin-Beck disease, wrist

    M12.131 Kaschin-Beck disease, right wrist

    M12.132 Kaschin-Beck disease, left wrist

    M12.139 Kaschin-Beck disease, unspecified wrist

● M12.14 Kaschin-Beck disease, hand

    M12.141 Kaschin-Beck disease, right hand

    M12.142 Kaschin-Beck disease, left hand

    M12.149 Kaschin-Beck disease, unspecified hand

● M12.15 Kaschin-Beck disease, hip

    M12.151 Kaschin-Beck disease, right hip

    M12.152 Kaschin-Beck disease, left hip

    M12.159 Kaschin-Beck disease, unspecified hip

● M12.16 Kaschin-Beck disease, knee

    M12.161 Kaschin-Beck disease, right knee

    M12.162 Kaschin-Beck disease, left knee

    M12.169 Kaschin-Beck disease, unspecified knee

● M12.17 Kaschin-Beck disease, ankle and foot

    M12.171 Kaschin-Beck disease, right ankle and foot

    M12.172 Kaschin-Beck disease, left ankle and foot

    M12.179 Kaschin-Beck disease, unspecified ankle and foot

    M12.18 Kaschin-Beck disease, vertebrae

    M12.19 Kaschin-Beck disease, multiple sites

● M12.2 Villonodular synovitis (pigmented)

    M12.20 Villonodular synovitis (pigmented), unspecified site

● M12.21 Villonodular synovitis (pigmented), shoulder

    M12.211 Villonodular synovitis (pigmented), right shoulder

    M12.212 Villonodular synovitis (pigmented), left shoulder

    M12.219 Villonodular synovitis (pigmented), unspecified shoulder

● M12.22 Villonodular synovitis (pigmented), elbow

    M12.221 Villonodular synovitis (pigmented), right elbow

    M12.222 Villonodular synovitis (pigmented), left elbow

    M12.229 Villonodular synovitis (pigmented), unspecified elbow

● M12.23 Villonodular synovitis (pigmented), wrist

    M12.231 Villonodular synovitis (pigmented), right wrist

    M12.232 Villonodular synovitis (pigmented), left wrist

    M12.239 Villonodular synovitis (pigmented), unspecified wrist

● M12.24 Villonodular synovitis (pigmented), hand

    M12.241 Villonodular synovitis (pigmented), right hand

    M12.242 Villonodular synovitis (pigmented), left hand

    M12.249 Villonodular synovitis (pigmented), unspecified hand

CHAPTER 13 (M00-M99)

● M12.25   Villonodular synovitis (pigmented), hip
     M12.251   Villonodular synovitis (pigmented), right hip
     M12.252   Villonodular synovitis (pigmented), left hip
     M12.259   Villonodular synovitis (pigmented), unspecified hip
● M12.26   Villonodular synovitis (pigmented), knee
     M12.261   Villonodular synovitis (pigmented), right knee
     M12.262   Villonodular synovitis (pigmented), left knee
     M12.269   Villonodular synovitis (pigmented), unspecified knee
● M12.27   Villonodular synovitis (pigmented), ankle and foot
     M12.271   Villonodular synovitis (pigmented), right ankle and foot
     M12.272   Villonodular synovitis (pigmented), left ankle and foot
     M12.279   Villonodular synovitis (pigmented), unspecified ankle and foot
   M12.28   Villonodular synovitis (pigmented), other specified site
        Villonodular synovitis (pigmented), vertebrae
   M12.29   Villonodular synovitis (pigmented), multiple sites
● M12.3   Palindromic rheumatism
   M12.30   Palindromic rheumatism, unspecified site
● M12.31   Palindromic rheumatism, shoulder
     M12.311   Palindromic rheumatism, right shoulder
     M12.312   Palindromic rheumatism, left shoulder
     M12.319   Palindromic rheumatism, unspecified shoulder
● M12.32   Palindromic rheumatism, elbow
     M12.321   Palindromic rheumatism, right elbow
     M12.322   Palindromic rheumatism, left elbow
     M12.329   Palindromic rheumatism, unspecified elbow
● M12.33   Palindromic rheumatism, wrist
     M12.331   Palindromic rheumatism, right wrist
     M12.332   Palindromic rheumatism, left wrist
     M12.339   Palindromic rheumatism, unspecified wrist
● M12.34   Palindromic rheumatism, hand
     M12.341   Palindromic rheumatism, right hand
     M12.342   Palindromic rheumatism, left hand
     M12.349   Palindromic rheumatism, unspecified hand
● M12.35   Palindromic rheumatism, hip
     M12.351   Palindromic rheumatism, right hip
     M12.352   Palindromic rheumatism, left hip
     M12.359   Palindromic rheumatism, unspecified hip
● M12.36   Palindromic rheumatism, knee
     M12.361   Palindromic rheumatism, right knee
     M12.362   Palindromic rheumatism, left knee
     M12.369   Palindromic rheumatism, unspecified knee
● M12.37   Palindromic rheumatism, ankle and foot
     M12.371   Palindromic rheumatism, right ankle and foot
     M12.372   Palindromic rheumatism, left ankle and foot
     M12.379   Palindromic rheumatism, unspecified ankle and foot

   M12.38   Palindromic rheumatism, other specified site
        Palindromic rheumatism, vertebrae
   M12.39   Palindromic rheumatism, multiple sites
● M12.4   Intermittent hydrarthrosis
   M12.40   Intermittent hydrarthrosis, unspecified site
● M12.41   Intermittent hydrarthrosis, shoulder
     M12.411   Intermittent hydrarthrosis, right shoulder
     M12.412   Intermittent hydrarthrosis, left shoulder
     M12.419   Intermittent hydrarthrosis, unspecified shoulder
● M12.42   Intermittent hydrarthrosis, elbow
     M12.421   Intermittent hydrarthrosis, right elbow
     M12.422   Intermittent hydrarthrosis, left elbow
     M12.429   Intermittent hydrarthrosis, unspecified elbow
● M12.43   Intermittent hydrarthrosis, wrist
     M12.431   Intermittent hydrarthrosis, right wrist
     M12.432   Intermittent hydrarthrosis, left wrist
     M12.439   Intermittent hydrarthrosis, unspecified wrist
● M12.44   Intermittent hydrarthrosis, hand
     M12.441   Intermittent hydrarthrosis, right hand
     M12.442   Intermittent hydrarthrosis, left hand
     M12.449   Intermittent hydrarthrosis, unspecified hand
● M12.45   Intermittent hydrarthrosis, hip
     M12.451   Intermittent hydrarthrosis, right hip
     M12.452   Intermittent hydrarthrosis, left hip
     M12.459   Intermittent hydrarthrosis, unspecified hip
● M12.46   Intermittent hydrarthrosis, knee
     M12.461   Intermittent hydrarthrosis, right knee
     M12.462   Intermittent hydrarthrosis, left knee
     M12.469   Intermittent hydrarthrosis, unspecified knee
● M12.47   Intermittent hydrarthrosis, ankle and foot
     M12.471   Intermittent hydrarthrosis, right ankle and foot
     M12.472   Intermittent hydrarthrosis, left ankle and foot
     M12.479   Intermittent hydrarthrosis, unspecified ankle and foot
   M12.48   Intermittent hydrarthrosis, other site
   M12.49   Intermittent hydrarthrosis, multiple sites
● M12.5   Traumatic arthropathy
   Excludes1   current injury-see Alphabetic Index
       post-traumatic osteoarthritis of first carpometacarpal joint (M18.2-M18.3)
       post-traumatic osteoarthritis of hip (M16.4-M16.5)
       post-traumatic osteoarthritis of knee (M17.2-M17.3)
       post-traumatic osteoarthritis NOS (M19.1-)
       post-traumatic osteoarthritis of other single joints (M19.1-)
   M12.50   Traumatic arthropathy, unspecified site
● M12.51   Traumatic arthropathy, shoulder
     M12.511   Traumatic arthropathy, right shoulder
     M12.512   Traumatic arthropathy, left shoulder
     M12.519   Traumatic arthropathy, unspecified shoulder

◄ New   ◄ Revised   ~~deleted~~ Deleted   Excludes 1   Excludes 2   Includes   Use additional   Code first   Code also   Unspecified
OGCR Official Guidelines   ● Unacceptable Principal Diagnosis   X Assign placeholder X   ● Use Additional Character(s)   ▌Manifestation Code   **Coding Clinic**

● **M12.52**   Traumatic arthropathy, elbow
     M12.521   Traumatic arthropathy, right elbow
     M12.522   Traumatic arthropathy, left elbow
     M12.529   Traumatic arthropathy, unspecified elbow

● **M12.53**   Traumatic arthropathy, wrist
     M12.531   Traumatic arthropathy, right wrist
     M12.532   Traumatic arthropathy, left wrist
     M12.539   Traumatic arthropathy, unspecified wrist

● **M12.54**   Traumatic arthropathy, hand
     M12.541   Traumatic arthropathy, right hand
     M12.542   Traumatic arthropathy, left hand
     M12.549   Traumatic arthropathy, unspecified hand

● **M12.55**   Traumatic arthropathy, hip
     M12.551   Traumatic arthropathy, right hip
     M12.552   Traumatic arthropathy, left hip
         Coding Clinic: 2015, Q1, P17
     M12.559   Traumatic arthropathy, unspecified hip

● **M12.56**   Traumatic arthropathy, knee
     M12.561   Traumatic arthropathy, right knee
     M12.562   Traumatic arthropathy, left knee
     M12.569   Traumatic arthropathy, unspecified knee

● **M12.57**   Traumatic arthropathy, ankle and foot
     M12.571   Traumatic arthropathy, right ankle and foot
     M12.572   Traumatic arthropathy, left ankle and foot
     M12.579   Traumatic arthropathy, unspecified ankle and foot

     M12.58   Traumatic arthropathy, other specified site
         Traumatic arthropathy, vertebrae

     M12.59   Traumatic arthropathy, multiple sites

● **M12.8**   Other specific arthropathies, not elsewhere classified
     Transient arthropathy
     M12.80   Other specific arthropathies, not elsewhere classified, unspecified site

● **M12.81**   Other specific arthropathies, not elsewhere classified, shoulder
     M12.811   Other specific arthropathies, not elsewhere classified, right shoulder
     M12.812   Other specific arthropathies, not elsewhere classified, left shoulder
     M12.819   Other specific arthropathies, not elsewhere classified, unspecified shoulder

● **M12.82**   Other specific arthropathies, not elsewhere classified, elbow
     M12.821   Other specific arthropathies, not elsewhere classified, right elbow
     M12.822   Other specific arthropathies, not elsewhere classified, left elbow
     M12.829   Other specific arthropathies, not elsewhere classified, unspecified elbow

● **M12.83**   Other specific arthropathies, not elsewhere classified, wrist
     M12.831   Other specific arthropathies, not elsewhere classified, right wrist
     M12.832   Other specific arthropathies, not elsewhere classified, left wrist
     M12.839   Other specific arthropathies, not elsewhere classified, unspecified wrist

● **M12.84**   Other specific arthropathies, not elsewhere classified, hand
     M12.841   Other specific arthropathies, not elsewhere classified, right hand
     M12.842   Other specific arthropathies, not elsewhere classified, left hand
     M12.849   Other specific arthropathies, not elsewhere classified, unspecified hand

● **M12.85**   Other specific arthropathies, not elsewhere classified, hip
     M12.851   Other specific arthropathies, not elsewhere classified, right hip
     M12.852   Other specific arthropathies, not elsewhere classified, left hip
     M12.859   Other specific arthropathies, not elsewhere classified, unspecified hip

● **M12.86**   Other specific arthropathies, not elsewhere classified, knee
     M12.861   Other specific arthropathies, not elsewhere classified, right knee
     M12.862   Other specific arthropathies, not elsewhere classified, left knee
     M12.869   Other specific arthropathies, not elsewhere classified, unspecified knee

● **M12.87**   Other specific arthropathies, not elsewhere classified, ankle and foot
     M12.871   Other specific arthropathies, not elsewhere classified, right ankle and foot
     M12.872   Other specific arthropathies, not elsewhere classified, left ankle and foot
     M12.879   Other specific arthropathies, not elsewhere classified, unspecified ankle and foot

     M12.88   Other specific arthropathies, not elsewhere classified, other specified site
         Other specific arthropathies, not elsewhere classified, vertebrae

     M12.89   Other specific arthropathies, not elsewhere classified, multiple sites

     M12.9   Arthropathy, unspecified

● **M13**   Other arthritis
     Excludes1   arthrosis (M15-M19)
               osteoarthritis (M15-M19)

     M13.0   Polyarthritis, unspecified

● **M13.1**   Monoarthritis, not elsewhere classified
     M13.10   Monoarthritis, not elsewhere classified, unspecified site

● **M13.11**   Monoarthritis, not elsewhere classified, shoulder
     M13.111   Monoarthritis, not elsewhere classified, right shoulder
     M13.112   Monoarthritis, not elsewhere classified, left shoulder
     M13.119   Monoarthritis, not elsewhere classified, unspecified shoulder

● **M13.12**   Monoarthritis, not elsewhere classified, elbow
     M13.121   Monoarthritis, not elsewhere classified, right elbow
     M13.122   Monoarthritis, not elsewhere classified, left elbow
     M13.129   Monoarthritis, not elsewhere classified, unspecified elbow

● **M13.13**   Monoarthritis, not elsewhere classified, wrist
     M13.131   Monoarthritis, not elsewhere classified, right wrist
     M13.132   Monoarthritis, not elsewhere classified, left wrist
     M13.139   Monoarthritis, not elsewhere classified, unspecified wrist

CHAPTER 13 (M00-M99)

N   Newborn Age: 0   **P**   Pediatric Age: 0–17   **M**   Maternity DX: 12–55   **A**   Adult Age: 15–124   ♀   Females Only   ♂   Males Only

🍭   Complication\Comorbidity   🍭   Major C\C   (Ex)   CC/MCC Exclusions   🍭   Hospital-Acquired Condition   **1011**

● M13.14 Monoarthritis, not elsewhere classified, hand
    M13.141 Monoarthritis, not elsewhere classified, right hand
    M13.142 Monoarthritis, not elsewhere classified, left hand
    M13.149 Monoarthritis, not elsewhere classified, unspecified hand
● M13.15 Monoarthritis, not elsewhere classified, hip
    M13.151 Monoarthritis, not elsewhere classified, right hip
    M13.152 Monoarthritis, not elsewhere classified, left hip
    M13.159 Monoarthritis, not elsewhere classified, unspecified hip
● M13.16 Monoarthritis, not elsewhere classified, knee
    M13.161 Monoarthritis, not elsewhere classified, right knee
    M13.162 Monoarthritis, not elsewhere classified, left knee
    M13.169 Monoarthritis, not elsewhere classified, unspecified knee
● M13.17 Monoarthritis, not elsewhere classified, ankle and foot
    M13.171 Monoarthritis, not elsewhere classified, right ankle and foot
    M13.172 Monoarthritis, not elsewhere classified, left ankle and foot
    M13.179 Monoarthritis, not elsewhere classified, unspecified ankle and foot
● M13.8 Other specified arthritis
    Allergic arthritis
    Excludes1 osteoarthritis (M15-M19)
    M13.80 Other specified arthritis, unspecified site
● M13.81 Other specified arthritis, shoulder
    M13.811 Other specified arthritis, right shoulder
    M13.812 Other specified arthritis, left shoulder
    M13.819 Other specified arthritis, unspecified shoulder
● M13.82 Other specified arthritis, elbow
    M13.821 Other specified arthritis, right elbow
    M13.822 Other specified arthritis, left elbow
    M13.829 Other specified arthritis, unspecified elbow
● M13.83 Other specified arthritis, wrist
    M13.831 Other specified arthritis, right wrist
    M13.832 Other specified arthritis, left wrist
    M13.839 Other specified arthritis, unspecified wrist
● M13.84 Other specified arthritis, hand
    M13.841 Other specified arthritis, right hand
    M13.842 Other specified arthritis, left hand
    M13.849 Other specified arthritis, unspecified hand
● M13.85 Other specified arthritis, hip
    M13.851 Other specified arthritis, right hip
    M13.852 Other specified arthritis, left hip
    M13.859 Other specified arthritis, unspecified hip
● M13.86 Other specified arthritis, knee
    M13.861 Other specified arthritis, right knee
    M13.862 Other specified arthritis, left knee
    M13.869 Other specified arthritis, unspecified knee

● M13.87 Other specified arthritis, ankle and foot
    M13.871 Other specified arthritis, right ankle and foot
    M13.872 Other specified arthritis, left ankle and foot
    M13.879 Other specified arthritis, unspecified ankle and foot
    M13.88 Other specified arthritis, other site
    M13.89 Other specified arthritis, multiple sites
● M14 Arthropathies in other diseases classified elsewhere
    Excludes1 arthropathy in:
        diabetes mellitus (E08-E13 with .61-)
        hematological disorders (M36.2-M36.3)
        hypersensitivity reactions (M36.4)
        neoplastic disease (M36.1)
        neurosyphillis (A52.16)
        sarcoidosis (D86.86)
       enteropathic arthropathies (M07.0-)
       juvenile psoriatic arthropathy (L40.54)
       lipoid dermatoarthritis (E78.81)
● M14.6 Charcôt's joint
    Neuropathic arthropathy
    Excludes1 Charcôt's joint in diabetes mellitus (E08-E13 with .610)
        Charcôt's joint in tabes dorsalis (A52.16)
    M14.60 Charcôt's joint, unspecified site
● M14.61 Charcôt's joint, shoulder
    M14.611 Charcôt's joint, right shoulder
    M14.612 Charcôt's joint, left shoulder
    M14.619 Charcôt's joint, unspecified shoulder
● M14.62 Charcôt's joint, elbow
    M14.621 Charcôt's joint, right elbow
    M14.622 Charcôt's joint, left elbow
    M14.629 Charcôt's joint, unspecified elbow
● M14.63 Charcôt's joint, wrist
    M14.631 Charcôt's joint, right wrist
    M14.632 Charcôt's joint, left wrist
    M14.639 Charcôt's joint, unspecified wrist
● M14.64 Charcôt's joint, hand
    M14.641 Charcôt's joint, right hand
    M14.642 Charcôt's joint, left hand
    M14.649 Charcôt's joint, unspecified hand
● M14.65 Charcôt's joint, hip
    M14.651 Charcôt's joint, right hip
    M14.652 Charcôt's joint, left hip
    M14.659 Charcôt's joint, unspecified hip
● M14.66 Charcôt's joint, knee
    M14.661 Charcôt's joint, right knee
    M14.662 Charcôt's joint, left knee
    M14.669 Charcôt's joint, unspecified knee
● M14.67 Charcôt's joint, ankle and foot
    M14.671 Charcôt's joint, right ankle and foot
    M14.672 Charcôt's joint, left ankle and foot
    M14.679 Charcôt's joint, unspecified ankle and foot
    M14.68 Charcôt's joint, vertebrae
    M14.69 Charcôt's joint, multiple sites

CHAPTER 13 (M00-M99)

◀ New   ◀ Revised   ~~deleted~~ Deleted   Excludes 1   Excludes 2   Includes   Use additional   Code first   Code also   Unspecified
OGCR Official Guidelines   ● Unacceptable Principal Diagnosis   X Assign placeholder X   ● Use Additional Character(s)   ▷ Manifestation Code   **Coding Clinic**

● **M14.8   Arthropathies in other specified diseases classified elsewhere**

> *Code first* underlying disease, such as:
> amyloidosis (E85.-)
> erythema multiforme (L51.-)
> erythema nodosum (L52)
> hemochromatosis (E83.11-)
> hyperparathyroidism (E21.-)
> hypothyroidism (E00-E03)
> sickle-cell disorders (D57.-)
> thyrotoxicosis [hyperthyroidism] (E05.-)
> Whipple's disease (K90.81)

▌*M14.80   Arthropathies in other specified diseases classified elsewhere, unspecified site*

● **M14.81   Arthropathies in other specified diseases classified elsewhere, shoulder**

    ▌*M14.811   Arthropathies in other specified diseases classified elsewhere, right shoulder*

    ▌*M14.812   Arthropathies in other specified diseases classified elsewhere, left shoulder*

    ▌*M14.819   Arthropathies in other specified diseases classified elsewhere, unspecified shoulder*

● **M14.82   Arthropathies in other specified diseases classified elsewhere, elbow**

    ▌*M14.821   Arthropathies in other specified diseases classified elsewhere, right elbow*

    ▌*M14.822   Arthropathies in other specified diseases classified elsewhere, left elbow*

    ▌*M14.829   Arthropathies in other specified diseases classified elsewhere, unspecified elbow*

● **M14.83   Arthropathies in other specified diseases classified elsewhere, wrist**

    ▌*M14.831   Arthropathies in other specified diseases classified elsewhere, right wrist*

    ▌*M14.832   Arthropathies in other specified diseases classified elsewhere, left wrist*

    ▌*M14.839   Arthropathies in other specified diseases classified elsewhere, unspecified wrist*

● **M14.84   Arthropathies in other specified diseases classified elsewhere, hand**

    ▌*M14.841   Arthropathies in other specified diseases classified elsewhere, right hand*

    ▌*M14.842   Arthropathies in other specified diseases classified elsewhere, left hand*

    ▌*M14.849   Arthropathies in other specified diseases classified elsewhere, unspecified hand*

● **M14.85   Arthropathies in other specified diseases classified elsewhere, hip**

    ▌*M14.851   Arthropathies in other specified diseases classified elsewhere, right hip*

    ▌*M14.852   Arthropathies in other specified diseases classified elsewhere, left hip*

    ▌*M14.859   Arthropathies in other specified diseases classified elsewhere, unspecified hip*

● **M14.86   Arthropathies in other specified diseases classified elsewhere, knee**

    ▌*M14.861   Arthropathies in other specified diseases classified elsewhere, right knee*

    ▌*M14.862   Arthropathies in other specified diseases classified elsewhere, left knee*

    ▌*M14.869   Arthropathies in other specified diseases classified elsewhere, unspecified knee*

● **M14.87   Arthropathies in other specified diseases classified elsewhere, ankle and foot**

    ▌*M14.871   Arthropathies in other specified diseases classified elsewhere, right ankle and foot*

    ▌*M14.872   Arthropathies in other specified diseases classified elsewhere, left ankle and foot*

    ▌*M14.879   Arthropathies in other specified diseases classified elsewhere, unspecified ankle and foot*

▌*M14.88   Arthropathies in other specified diseases classified elsewhere, vertebrae*

▌*M14.89   Arthropathies in other specified diseases classified elsewhere, multiple sites*

OSTEOARTHRITIS (M15-M19)

Osteoarthritis is the most common degenerative joint disease and form of arthritis that breaks down the cartilage causing pain, swelling, and reduced motion in the joints.

    Excludes2   osteoarthritis of spine (M47.-)

● **M15   Polyosteoarthritis**

    Includes   arthritis of multiple sites
    Excludes1   bilateral involvement of single joint (M16-M19)

    M15.0   Primary generalized (osteo)arthritis

    M15.1   Heberden's nodes (with arthropathy)
       Interphalangeal distal osteoarthritis

    M15.2   Bouchard's nodes (with arthropathy)
       Juxtaphalangeal distal osteoarthritis

    M15.3   Secondary multiple arthritis
       Post-traumatic polyosteoarthritis

    M15.4   Erosive (osteo)arthritis

    M15.8   Other polyosteoarthritis

    M15.9   Polyosteoarthritis, unspecified
       Generalized osteoarthritis NOS

● **M16   Osteoarthritis of hip**

    M16.0   Bilateral primary osteoarthritis of hip

    ● **M16.1   Unilateral primary osteoarthritis of hip**
       Primary osteoarthritis of hip NOS

       M16.10   Unilateral primary osteoarthritis, unspecified hip

       M16.11   Unilateral primary osteoarthritis, right hip

       M16.12   Unilateral primary osteoarthritis, left hip

    M16.2   Bilateral osteoarthritis resulting from hip dysplasia

    ● **M16.3   Unilateral osteoarthritis resulting from hip dysplasia**
       Dysplastic osteoarthritis of hip NOS

       M16.30   Unilateral osteoarthritis resulting from hip dysplasia, unspecified hip

       M16.31   Unilateral osteoarthritis resulting from hip dysplasia, right hip

       M16.32   Unilateral osteoarthritis resulting from hip dysplasia, left hip

    M16.4   Bilateral post-traumatic osteoarthritis of hip

CHAPTER 13 (M00-M99)

N   Newborn Age: 0   **P**   Pediatric Age: 0–17   **M**   Maternity DX: 12–55   **A**   Adult Age: 15–124   ♀   Females Only   ♂   Males Only

🔖 Complication\Comorbidity   🔖 Major C\C   (Ex) CC/MCC Exclusions   🔖 Hospital-Acquired Condition   **1013**

● **M16.5 Unilateral post-traumatic osteoarthritis of hip**
Post-traumatic osteoarthritis of hip NOS

    M16.50 Unilateral post-traumatic osteoarthritis, unspecified hip

    M16.51 Unilateral post-traumatic osteoarthritis, right hip

    M16.52 Unilateral post-traumatic osteoarthritis, left hip

M16.6 Other bilateral secondary osteoarthritis of hip

M16.7 Other unilateral secondary osteoarthritis of hip
Secondary osteoarthritis of hip NOS

M16.9 Osteoarthritis of hip, unspecified

● **M17 Osteoarthritis of knee**

M17.0 Bilateral primary osteoarthritis of knee

● **M17.1 Unilateral primary osteoarthritis of knee**
Primary osteoarthritis of knee NOS

    M17.10 Unilateral primary osteoarthritis, unspecified knee

    M17.11 Unilateral primary osteoarthritis, right knee

    M17.12 Unilateral primary osteoarthritis, left knee

M17.2 Bilateral post-traumatic osteoarthritis of knee

● **M17.3 Unilateral post-traumatic osteoarthritis of knee**
Post-traumatic osteoarthritis of knee NOS

    M17.30 Unilateral post-traumatic osteoarthritis, unspecified knee

    M17.31 Unilateral post-traumatic osteoarthritis, right knee

    M17.32 Unilateral post-traumatic osteoarthritis, left knee

M17.4 Other bilateral secondary osteoarthritis of knee

M17.5 Other unilateral secondary osteoarthritis of knee
Secondary osteoarthritis of knee NOS

M17.9 Osteoarthritis of knee, unspecified

● **M18 Osteoarthritis of first carpometacarpal joint**

M18.0 Bilateral primary osteoarthritis of first carpometacarpal joints

● **M18.1 Unilateral primary osteoarthritis of first carpometacarpal joint**
Primary osteoarthritis of first carpometacarpal joint NOS

    M18.10 Unilateral primary osteoarthritis of first carpometacarpal joint, unspecified hand

    M18.11 Unilateral primary osteoarthritis of first carpometacarpal joint, right hand

    M18.12 Unilateral primary osteoarthritis of first carpometacarpal joint, left hand

M18.2 Bilateral post-traumatic osteoarthritis of first carpometacarpal joints

● **M18.3 Unilateral post-traumatic osteoarthritis of first carpometacarpal joint**
Post-traumatic osteoarthritis of first carpometacarpal joint NOS

    M18.30 Unilateral post-traumatic osteoarthritis of first carpometacarpal joint, unspecified hand

    M18.31 Unilateral post-traumatic osteoarthritis of first carpometacarpal joint, right hand

    M18.32 Unilateral post-traumatic osteoarthritis of first carpometacarpal joint, left hand

M18.4 Other bilateral secondary osteoarthritis of first carpometacarpal joints

● **M18.5 Other unilateral secondary osteoarthritis of first carpometacarpal joint**
Secondary osteoarthritis of first carpometacarpal joint NOS

    M18.50 Other unilateral secondary osteoarthritis of first carpometacarpal joint, unspecified hand

    M18.51 Other unilateral secondary osteoarthritis of first carpometacarpal joint, right hand

    M18.52 Other unilateral secondary osteoarthritis of first carpometacarpal joint, left hand

M18.9 Osteoarthritis of first carpometacarpal joint, unspecified

● **M19 Other and unspecified osteoarthritis**

    Excludes1 polyarthritis (M15.-)

    Excludes2 arthrosis of spine (M47.-)
           hallux rigidus (M20.2)
           osteoarthritis of spine (M47.-)

● **M19.0 Primary osteoarthritis of other joints**

● **M19.01 Primary osteoarthritis, shoulder**

    M19.011 Primary osteoarthritis, right shoulder

    M19.012 Primary osteoarthritis, left shoulder

    M19.019 Primary osteoarthritis, unspecified shoulder

● **M19.02 Primary osteoarthritis, elbow**

    M19.021 Primary osteoarthritis, right elbow

    M19.022 Primary osteoarthritis, left elbow

    M19.029 Primary osteoarthritis, unspecified elbow

● **M19.03 Primary osteoarthritis, wrist**

    M19.031 Primary osteoarthritis, right wrist

    M19.032 Primary osteoarthritis, left wrist

    M19.039 Primary osteoarthritis, unspecified wrist

● **M19.04 Primary osteoarthritis, hand**

    Excludes2 primary osteoarthritis of first carpometacarpal joint (M18.0-, M18.1-)

    M19.041 Primary osteoarthritis, right hand

    M19.042 Primary osteoarthritis, left hand

    M19.049 Primary osteoarthritis, unspecified hand

● **M19.07 Primary osteoarthritis ankle and foot**

    M19.071 Primary osteoarthritis, right ankle and foot

    M19.072 Primary osteoarthritis, left ankle and foot

    M19.079 Primary osteoarthritis, unspecified ankle and foot

● **M19.1 Post-traumatic osteoarthritis of other joints**

● **M19.11 Post-traumatic osteoarthritis, shoulder**

    M19.111 Post-traumatic osteoarthritis, right shoulder

    M19.112 Post-traumatic osteoarthritis, left shoulder

    M19.119 Post-traumatic osteoarthritis, unspecified shoulder

● **M19.12 Post-traumatic osteoarthritis, elbow**

    M19.121 Post-traumatic osteoarthritis, right elbow

    M19.122 Post-traumatic osteoarthritis, left elbow

    M19.129 Post-traumatic osteoarthritis, unspecified elbow

● **M19.13 Post-traumatic osteoarthritis, wrist**

    M19.131 Post-traumatic osteoarthritis, right wrist

    M19.132 Post-traumatic osteoarthritis, left wrist

    M19.139 Post-traumatic osteoarthritis, unspecified wrist

● **M19.14 Post-traumatic osteoarthritis, hand**

    Excludes2 post-traumatic osteoarthritis of first carpometacarpal joint (M18.2-, M18.3-)

    M19.141 Post-traumatic osteoarthritis, right hand

    M19.142 Post-traumatic osteoarthritis, left hand

    M19.149 Post-traumatic osteoarthritis, unspecified hand

◀ New   ◀■■ Revised   ~~deleted~~ Deleted   Excludes 1   Excludes 2   Includes   Use additional   Code first   Code also   Unspecified

 OGCR Official Guidelines   ● Unacceptable Principal Diagnosis   X Assign placeholder X   ● Use Additional Character(s)   ▌ Manifestation Code   **Coding Clinic**

● **M19.17 Post-traumatic osteoarthritis, ankle and foot**
     M19.171   Post-traumatic osteoarthritis, right ankle and foot
     M19.172   Post-traumatic osteoarthritis, left ankle and foot
     M19.179   Post-traumatic osteoarthritis, unspecified ankle and foot

● **M19.2 Secondary osteoarthritis of other joints**
   ● **M19.21 Secondary osteoarthritis, shoulder**
     M19.211   Secondary osteoarthritis, right shoulder
     M19.212   Secondary osteoarthritis, left shoulder
     M19.219   Secondary osteoarthritis, unspecified shoulder
   ● **M19.22 Secondary osteoarthritis, elbow**
     M19.221   Secondary osteoarthritis, right elbow
     M19.222   Secondary osteoarthritis, left elbow
     M19.229   Secondary osteoarthritis, unspecified elbow
   ● **M19.23 Secondary osteoarthritis, wrist**
     M19.231   Secondary osteoarthritis, right wrist
     M19.232   Secondary osteoarthritis, left wrist
     M19.239   Secondary osteoarthritis, unspecified wrist
   ● **M19.24 Secondary osteoarthritis, hand**
     M19.241   Secondary osteoarthritis, right hand
     M19.242   Secondary osteoarthritis, left hand
     M19.249   Secondary osteoarthritis, unspecified hand
   ● **M19.27 Secondary osteoarthritis, ankle and foot**
     M19.271   Secondary osteoarthritis, right ankle and foot
     M19.272   Secondary osteoarthritis, left ankle and foot
     M19.279   Secondary osteoarthritis, unspecified ankle and foot

● **M19.9 Osteoarthritis, unspecified site**
   M19.90 Unspecified osteoarthritis, unspecified site
     Arthrosis NOS
     Arthritis NOS
     Osteoarthritis NOS
   M19.91 Primary osteoarthritis, unspecified site
     Primary osteoarthritis NOS
   M19.92 Post-traumatic osteoarthritis, unspecified site
     Post-traumatic osteoarthritis NOS
   M19.93 Secondary osteoarthritis, unspecified site
     Secondary osteoarthritis NOS

OTHER JOINT DISORDERS (M20-M25)

Excludes2   joints of the spine (M40-M54)

● **M20 Acquired deformities of fingers and toes**
   Excludes1   acquired absence of fingers and toes (Z89.-)
     congenital absence of fingers and toes (Q71.3-, Q72.3-)
     congenital deformities and malformations of fingers and toes (Q66.-, Q68-Q70, Q74.-)

● **M20.0 Deformity of finger(s)**
   Excludes1   clubbing of fingers (R68.3)
     palmar fascial fibromatosis [Dupuytren] (M72.0)
     trigger finger (M65.3)
   ● **M20.00 Unspecified deformity of finger(s)**
     M20.001   Unspecified deformity of right finger(s)
     M20.002   Unspecified deformity of left finger(s)
     M20.009   Unspecified deformity of unspecified finger(s)

   ● **M20.01 Mallet finger**
     M20.011   Mallet finger of right finger(s)
     M20.012   Mallet finger of left finger(s)
     M20.019   Mallet finger of unspecified finger(s)
   ● **M20.02 Boutonnière deformity**
     M20.021   Boutonnière deformity of right finger(s)
     M20.022   Boutonnière deformity of left finger(s)
     M20.029   Boutonnière deformity of unspecified finger(s)
   ● **M20.03 Swan-neck deformity**
     M20.031   Swan-neck deformity of right finger(s)
     M20.032   Swan-neck deformity of left finger(s)
     M20.039   Swan-neck deformity of unspecified finger(s)
   ● **M20.09 Other deformity of finger(s)**
     M20.091   Other deformity of right finger(s)
     M20.092   Other deformity of left finger(s)
     M20.099   Other deformity of finger(s), unspecified finger(s)

● **M20.1 Hallux valgus (acquired)**
   Excludes2   bunion (M21.6-) ◀
   M20.10 Hallux valgus (acquired), unspecified foot
   M20.11 Hallux valgus (acquired), right foot
   M20.12 Hallux valgus (acquired), left foot

● **M20.2 Hallux rigidus**
   M20.20 Hallux rigidus, unspecified foot
   M20.21 Hallux rigidus, right foot
   M20.22 Hallux rigidus, left foot

● **M20.3 Hallux varus (acquired)**
   M20.30 Hallux varus (acquired), unspecified foot
   M20.31 Hallux varus (acquired), right foot
   M20.32 Hallux varus (acquired), left foot

● **M20.4 Other hammer toe(s) (acquired)**
   M20.40 Other hammer toe(s) (acquired), unspecified foot
   M20.41 Other hammer toe(s) (acquired), right foot
   M20.42 Other hammer toe(s) (acquired), left foot

Figure 13-1   Hallux valgus or bunion.

Item 13-2   Hallux valgus or bunion is a sometimes painful structural deformity caused by an inflammation of the bursal sac at the base of the metatarsophalangeal joint (big toe). **Hallus varus** is a deviation of the great toe to the inner side of the foot or away from the next toe.

CHAPTER 13 (M00-M99)

N Newborn Age: Ø   **P** Pediatric Age: Ø-17   **M** Maternity DX: 12-55   **A** Adult Age: 15-124   ♀ Females Only   ♂ Males Only

🗪 Complication\Comorbidity   🗪 Major C\C   (Ex) CC/MCC Exclusions   🗪 Hospital-Acquired Condition   **1015**

● **M20.5   Other deformities of toe(s) (acquired)**

    ● **M20.5X   Other deformities of toe(s) (acquired)**

         M20.5X1   Other deformities of toe(s) (acquired), right foot

         M20.5X2   Other deformities of toe(s) (acquired), left foot

         M20.5X9   Other deformities of toe(s) (acquired), unspecified foot

● **M20.6   Acquired deformities of toe(s), unspecified**

     M20.60   Acquired deformities of toe(s), unspecified, unspecified foot

     M20.61   Acquired deformities of toe(s), unspecified, right foot

     M20.62   Acquired deformities of toe(s), unspecified, left foot

● **M21   Other acquired deformities of limbs**

     Excludes1   acquired absence of limb (Z89.-)
                     congenital absence of limbs (Q71-Q73)
                     congenital deformities and malformations of limbs (Q65-Q66, Q68-Q74)

     Excludes2   acquired deformities of fingers or toes (M20.-)
                     coxa plana (M91.2)

● **M21.0   Valgus deformity, not elsewhere classified**

     Excludes1   metatarsus valgus (Q66.6)
                     talipes calcaneovalgus (Q66.4)

     M21.00   Valgus deformity, not elsewhere classified, unspecified site

    ● **M21.02   Valgus deformity, not elsewhere classified, elbow**
                   Cubitus valgus

         M21.021   Valgus deformity, not elsewhere classified, right elbow

         M21.022   Valgus deformity, not elsewhere classified, left elbow

         M21.029   Valgus deformity, not elsewhere classified, unspecified elbow

    ● **M21.05   Valgus deformity, not elsewhere classified, hip**

         M21.051   Valgus deformity, not elsewhere classified, right hip

         M21.052   Valgus deformity, not elsewhere classified, left hip

         M21.059   Valgus deformity, not elsewhere classified, unspecified hip

    ● **M21.06   Valgus deformity, not elsewhere classified, knee**
                   Genu valgum
                   Knock knee

         M21.061   Valgus deformity, not elsewhere classified, right knee

         M21.062   Valgus deformity, not elsewhere classified, left knee

         M21.069   Valgus deformity, not elsewhere classified, unspecified knee

    ● **M21.07   Valgus deformity, not elsewhere classified, ankle**

         M21.071   Valgus deformity, not elsewhere classified, right ankle

         M21.072   Valgus deformity, not elsewhere classified, left ankle

         M21.079   Valgus deformity, not elsewhere classified, unspecified ankle

Item 13–3   Cubitus valgus is a deformity of the elbow resulting in an increased carrying angle in which the arm extends at the side and the palm faces forward, which results in the forearm and hand extended at a greater than 15 degrees.

Item 13–4   Cubitus varus is a deformity of the elbow resulting in the arm extended at the side and the palm facing forward so that the forearm and hand are held at less than 5 degrees, decreasing the carrying angle.

● **M21.1   Varus deformity, not elsewhere classified**

     Excludes1   metatarsus varus (Q66.22) ◄▥
                     tibia vara (M92.5)

     M21.10   Varus deformity, not elsewhere classified, unspecified site

    ● **M21.12   Varus deformity, not elsewhere classified, elbow**
                   Cubitus varus, elbow

         M21.121   Varus deformity, not elsewhere classified, right elbow

         M21.122   Varus deformity, not elsewhere classified, left elbow

         M21.129   Varus deformity, not elsewhere classified, unspecified elbow

    ● **M21.15   Varus deformity, not elsewhere classified, hip**

         M21.151   Varus deformity, not elsewhere classified, right hip

         M21.152   Varus deformity, not elsewhere classified, left hip

         M21.159   Varus deformity, not elsewhere classified, unspecified

    ● **M21.16   Varus deformity, not elsewhere classified, knee**
                   Bow leg
                   Genu varum

         M21.161   Varus deformity, not elsewhere classified, right knee

         M21.162   Varus deformity, not elsewhere classified, left knee

         M21.169   Varus deformity, not elsewhere classified, unspecified knee

    ● **M21.17   Varus deformity, not elsewhere classified, ankle**

         M21.171   Varus deformity, not elsewhere classified, right ankle

         M21.172   Varus deformity, not elsewhere classified, left ankle

         M21.179   Varus deformity, not elsewhere classified, unspecified ankle

● **M21.2   Flexion deformity**

     M21.20   Flexion deformity, unspecified site

    ● **M21.21   Flexion deformity, shoulder**

         M21.211   Flexion deformity, right shoulder

         M21.212   Flexion deformity, left shoulder

         M21.219   Flexion deformity, unspecified shoulder

    ● **M21.22   Flexion deformity, elbow**

         M21.221   Flexion deformity, right elbow

         M21.222   Flexion deformity, left elbow

         M21.229   Flexion deformity, unspecified elbow

    ● **M21.23   Flexion deformity, wrist**

         M21.231   Flexion deformity, right wrist

         M21.232   Flexion deformity, left wrist

         M21.239   Flexion deformity, unspecified wrist

    ● **M21.24   Flexion deformity, finger joints**

         M21.241   Flexion deformity, right finger joints

         M21.242   Flexion deformity, left finger joints

         M21.249   Flexion deformity, unspecified finger joints

    ● **M21.25   Flexion deformity, hip**

         M21.251   Flexion deformity, right hip

         M21.252   Flexion deformity, left hip

         M21.259   Flexion deformity, unspecified hip

    ● **M21.26   Flexion deformity, knee**

         M21.261   Flexion deformity, right knee

         M21.262   Flexion deformity, left knee

         M21.269   Flexion deformity, unspecified knee

◄ New   ◄▥ Revised   ~~deleted~~ Deleted   Excludes 1   Excludes 2   Includes   Use additional   Code first   Code also   Unspecified

OGCR Official Guidelines   ● Unacceptable Principal Diagnosis   X Assign placeholder X   ● Use Additional Character(s)   ▶ Manifestation Code   **Coding Clinic**

- M21.27　Flexion deformity, ankle and toes

  M21.271　Flexion deformity, right ankle and toes

  M21.272　Flexion deformity, left ankle and toes

  M21.279　Flexion deformity, unspecified ankle and toes

- M21.3　Wrist or foot drop (acquired)

  - M21.33　Wrist drop (acquired)

    M21.331　Wrist drop, right wrist

    M21.332　Wrist drop, left wrist

    M21.339　Wrist drop, unspecified wrist

  - M21.37　Foot drop (acquired)

    M21.371　Foot drop, right foot

    M21.372　Foot drop, left foot

    M21.379　Foot drop, unspecified foot

- M21.4　Flat foot [pes planus] (acquired)

  Excludes1　congenital pes planus (Q66.5-)

  M21.40　Flat foot [pes planus] (acquired), unspecified foot

  M21.41　Flat foot [pes planus] (acquired), right foot

  M21.42　Flat foot [pes planus] (acquired), left foot

- M21.5　Acquired clawhand, clubhand, clawfoot and clubfoot

  Excludes1　clubfoot, not specified as acquired (Q66.89)

  - M21.51　Acquired clawhand

    M21.511　Acquired clawhand, right hand

    M21.512　Acquired clawhand, left hand

    M21.519　Acquired clawhand, unspecified hand

  - M21.52　Acquired clubhand

    M21.521　Acquired clubhand, right hand

    M21.522　Acquired clubhand, left hand

    M21.529　Acquired clubhand, unspecified hand

  - M21.53　Acquired clawfoot

    M21.531　Acquired clawfoot, right foot

    M21.532　Acquired clawfoot, left foot

    M21.539　Acquired clawfoot, unspecified foot

  - M21.54　Acquired clubfoot

    M21.541　Acquired clubfoot, right foot

    M21.542　Acquired clubfoot, left foot

    M21.549　Acquired clubfoot, unspecified foot

- M21.6　Other acquired deformities of foot

  Excludes2　deformities of toe (acquired) (M20.1-M20.6-) ◀

  - M21.61　Bunion ◀

    M21.611　Bunion of right foot ◀

    M21.612　Bunion of left foot ◀

    M21.619　Bunion of unspecified foot ◀

  - M21.62　Bunionette ◀

    M21.621　Bunionette of right foot ◀

    M21.622　Bunionette of left foot ◀

    M21.629　Bunionette of unspecified foot ◀

  - M21.6X　Other acquired deformities of foot

    M21.6X1　Other acquired deformities of right foot

    M21.6X2　Other acquired deformities of left foot

    M21.6X9　Other acquired deformities of unspecified foot

- M21.7　Unequal limb length (acquired)

  Note: The site used should correspond to the shorter limb.

  M21.70　Unequal limb length (acquired), unspecified site

  - M21.72　Unequal limb length (acquired), humerus

    M21.721　Unequal limb length (acquired), right humerus

    M21.722　Unequal limb length (acquired), left humerus

    M21.729　Unequal limb length (acquired), unspecified humerus

  - M21.73　Unequal limb length (acquired), ulna and radius

    M21.731　Unequal limb length (acquired), right ulna

    M21.732　Unequal limb length (acquired), left ulna

    M21.733　Unequal limb length (acquired), right radius

    M21.734　Unequal limb length (acquired), left radius

    M21.739　Unequal limb length (acquired), unspecified ulna and radius

  - M21.75　Unequal limb length (acquired), femur

    M21.751　Unequal limb length (acquired), right femur

    M21.752　Unequal limb length (acquired), left femur

    M21.759　Unequal limb length (acquired), unspecified femur

  - M21.76　Unequal limb length (acquired), tibia and fibula

    M21.761　Unequal limb length (acquired), right tibia

    M21.762　Unequal limb length (acquired), left tibia

    M21.763　Unequal limb length (acquired), right fibula

    M21.764　Unequal limb length (acquired), left fibula

    M21.769　Unequal limb length (acquired), unspecified tibia and fibula

- M21.8　Other specified acquired deformities of limbs

  Excludes2　coxa plana (M91.2)

  M21.80　Other specified acquired deformities of unspecified limb

  - M21.82　Other specified acquired deformities of upper arm

    M21.821　Other specified acquired deformities of right upper arm

    M21.822　Other specified acquired deformities of left upper arm

    M21.829　Other specified acquired deformities of unspecified upper arm

  - M21.83　Other specified acquired deformities of forearm

    M21.831　Other specified acquired deformities of right forearm

    M21.832　Other specified acquired deformities of left forearm

    M21.839　Other specified acquired deformities of unspecified forearm

  - M21.85　Other specified acquired deformities of thigh

    M21.851　Other specified acquired deformities of right thigh

    M21.852　Other specified acquired deformities of left thigh

    M21.859　Other specified acquired deformities of unspecified thigh

CHAPTER 13 (M00-M99)

N Newborn Age: 0　　**P** Pediatric Age: 0–17　　**M** Maternity DX: 12–55　　**A** Adult Age: 15–124　　♀ Females Only　　♂ Males Only

Complication\Comorbidity　　　Major C\C　　(Ex) CC/MCC Exclusions　　Hospital-Acquired Condition

1017

CHAPTER 13 (M00-M99)

● M21.86 Other specified acquired deformities of lower leg
    M21.861 Other specified acquired deformities of right lower leg
    M21.862 Other specified acquired deformities of left lower leg
    M21.869 Other specified acquired deformities of `unspecified` lower leg
● M21.9 Unspecified acquired deformity of limb and hand
    M21.90 `Unspecified` acquired deformity of unspecified limb
 ● M21.92 Unspecified acquired deformity of upper arm
    M21.921 `Unspecified` acquired deformity of right upper arm
    M21.922 `Unspecified` acquired deformity of left upper arm
    M21.929 `Unspecified` acquired deformity of unspecified upper arm
 ● M21.93 Unspecified acquired deformity of forearm
    M21.931 `Unspecified` acquired deformity of right forearm
    M21.932 `Unspecified` acquired deformity of left forearm
    M21.939 `Unspecified` acquired deformity of unspecified forearm
 ● M21.94 Unspecified acquired deformity of hand
    M21.941 `Unspecified` acquired deformity of hand, right hand
    M21.942 `Unspecified` acquired deformity of hand, left hand
    M21.949 `Unspecified` acquired deformity of hand, unspecified hand
 ● M21.95 Unspecified acquired deformity of thigh
    M21.951 `Unspecified` acquired deformity of right thigh
    M21.952 `Unspecified` acquired deformity of left thigh
    M21.959 `Unspecified` acquired deformity of unspecified thigh
 ● M21.96 Unspecified acquired deformity of lower leg
    M21.961 `Unspecified` acquired deformity of right lower leg
    M21.962 `Unspecified` acquired deformity of left lower leg
    M21.969 `Unspecified` acquired deformity of unspecified lower leg

● **M22** **Disorder of patella**
   Excludes1   traumatic dislocation of patella (S83.0-)
 ● M22.0 Recurrent dislocation of patella
    M22.00 Recurrent dislocation of patella, `unspecified` knee
    M22.01 Recurrent dislocation of patella, right knee
    M22.02 Recurrent dislocation of patella, left knee
 ● M22.1 Recurrent subluxation of patella
    Incomplete dislocation of patella
    M22.10 Recurrent subluxation of patella, `unspecified` knee
    M22.11 Recurrent subluxation of patella, right knee
    M22.12 Recurrent subluxation of patella, left knee
 ● M22.2 Patellofemoral disorders
  ● M22.2X Patellofemoral disorders
    M22.2X1 Patellofemoral disorders, right knee
    M22.2X2 Patellofemoral disorders, left knee
    M22.2X9 Patellofemoral disorders, `unspecified` knee

 ● M22.3 Other derangements of patella
  ● M22.3X Other derangements of patella
    M22.3X1 Other derangements of patella, right knee
    M22.3X2 Other derangements of patella, left knee
    M22.3X9 Other derangements of patella, `unspecified` knee
 ● M22.4 Chondromalacia patellae
    M22.40 Chondromalacia patellae, `unspecified` knee
    M22.41 Chondromalacia patellae, right knee
    M22.42 Chondromalacia patellae, left knee
 ● M22.8 Other disorders of patella
  ● M22.8X Other disorders of patella
    M22.8X1 Other disorders of patella, right knee
    M22.8X2 Other disorders of patella, left knee
    M22.8X9 Other disorders of patella, `unspecified` knee
 ● M22.9 Unspecified disorder of patella
    M22.90 `Unspecified` disorder of patella, unspecified knee
    M22.91 `Unspecified` disorder of patella, right knee
    M22.92 `Unspecified` disorder of patella, left knee

● **M23** **Internal derangement of knee**
   Excludes1   ankylosis (M24.66)
         current injury - see injury of knee and lower leg (S80-S89)
         deformity of knee (M21.-)
         osteochondritis dissecans (M93.2)
         recurrent dislocation or subluxation of joints (M24.4)
         recurrent dislocation or subluxation of patella (M22.0-M22.1)
 ● M23.0 Cystic meniscus
  ● M23.00 Cystic meniscus, unspecified meniscus
    Cystic meniscus, unspecified lateral meniscus
    Cystic meniscus, unspecified medial meniscus
    M23.000 Cystic meniscus, `unspecified` lateral meniscus, right knee
    M23.001 Cystic meniscus, `unspecified` lateral meniscus, left knee
    M23.002 Cystic meniscus, `unspecified` lateral meniscus, unspecified knee
    M23.003 Cystic meniscus, `unspecified` medial meniscus, right knee
    M23.004 Cystic meniscus, `unspecified` medial meniscus, left knee
    M23.005 Cystic meniscus, `unspecified` medial meniscus, unspecified knee
    M23.006 Cystic meniscus, `unspecified` meniscus, right knee
    M23.007 Cystic meniscus, `unspecified` meniscus, left knee
    M23.009 Cystic meniscus, `unspecified` meniscus, unspecified knee
  ● M23.01 Cystic meniscus, anterior horn of medial meniscus
    M23.011 Cystic meniscus, anterior horn of medial meniscus, right knee
    M23.012 Cystic meniscus, anterior horn of medial meniscus, left knee
    M23.019 Cystic meniscus, anterior horn of medial meniscus, `unspecified` knee

● M23.02 **Cystic meniscus, posterior horn of medial meniscus**
  M23.021 **Cystic meniscus, posterior horn of medial meniscus, right knee**
  M23.022 **Cystic meniscus, posterior horn of medial meniscus, left knee**
  M23.029 **Cystic meniscus, posterior horn of medial meniscus, unspecified knee**
● M23.03 **Cystic meniscus, other medial meniscus**
  M23.031 **Cystic meniscus, other medial meniscus, right knee**
  M23.032 **Cystic meniscus, other medial meniscus, left knee**
  M23.039 **Cystic meniscus, other medial meniscus, unspecified knee**
● M23.04 **Cystic meniscus, anterior horn of lateral meniscus**
  M23.041 **Cystic meniscus, anterior horn of lateral meniscus, right knee**
  M23.042 **Cystic meniscus, anterior horn of lateral meniscus, left knee**
  M23.049 **Cystic meniscus, anterior horn of lateral meniscus, unspecified knee**
● M23.05 **Cystic meniscus, posterior horn of lateral meniscus**
  M23.051 **Cystic meniscus, posterior horn of lateral meniscus, right knee**
  M23.052 **Cystic meniscus, posterior horn of lateral meniscus, left knee**
  M23.059 **Cystic meniscus, posterior horn of lateral meniscus, unspecified knee**
● M23.06 **Cystic meniscus, other lateral meniscus**
  M23.061 **Cystic meniscus, other lateral meniscus, right knee**
  M23.062 **Cystic meniscus, other lateral meniscus, left knee**
  M23.069 **Cystic meniscus, other lateral meniscus, unspecified knee**

★ **(See Plate 509 on page 79.)**
● M23.2 **Derangement of meniscus due to old tear or injury**
  Old bucket-handle tear
● M23.20 **Derangement of unspecified meniscus due to old tear or injury**
  Derangement of unspecified lateral meniscus due to old tear or injury
  Derangement of unspecified medial meniscus due to old tear or injury
  M23.200 **Derangement of unspecified lateral meniscus due to old tear or injury, right knee**
  M23.201 **Derangement of unspecified lateral meniscus due to old tear or injury, left knee**
  M23.202 **Derangement of unspecified lateral meniscus due to old tear or injury, unspecified knee**
  M23.203 **Derangement of unspecified medial meniscus due to old tear or injury, right knee**
  M23.204 **Derangement of unspecified medial meniscus due to old tear or injury, left knee**
  M23.205 **Derangement of unspecified medial meniscus due to old tear or injury, unspecified knee**
  M23.206 **Derangement of unspecified meniscus due to old tear or injury, right knee**

  M23.207 **Derangement of unspecified meniscus due to old tear or injury, left knee**
  M23.209 **Derangement of unspecified meniscus due to old tear or injury, unspecified knee**
● M23.21 **Derangement of anterior horn of medial meniscus due to old tear or injury**
  M23.211 **Derangement of anterior horn of medial meniscus due to old tear or injury, right knee**
  M23.212 **Derangement of anterior horn of medial meniscus due to old tear or injury, left knee**
  M23.219 **Derangement of anterior horn of medial meniscus due to old tear or injury, unspecified knee**
● M23.22 **Derangement of posterior horn of medial meniscus due to old tear or injury**
  M23.221 **Derangement of posterior horn of medial meniscus due to old tear or injury, right knee**
  M23.222 **Derangement of posterior horn of medial meniscus due to old tear or injury, left knee**
  M23.229 **Derangement of posterior horn of medial meniscus due to old tear or injury, unspecified knee**
● M23.23 **Derangement of other medial meniscus due to old tear or injury**
  M23.231 **Derangement of other medial meniscus due to old tear or injury, right knee**
  M23.232 **Derangement of other medial meniscus due to old tear or injury, left knee**
  M23.239 **Derangement of other medial meniscus due to old tear or injury, unspecified knee**
● M23.24 **Derangement of anterior horn of lateral meniscus due to old tear or injury**
  M23.241 **Derangement of anterior horn of lateral meniscus due to old tear or injury, right knee**
  M23.242 **Derangement of anterior horn of lateral meniscus due to old tear or injury, left knee**
  M23.249 **Derangement of anterior horn of lateral meniscus due to old tear or injury, unspecified knee**
● M23.25 **Derangement of posterior horn of lateral meniscus due to old tear or injury**
  M23.251 **Derangement of posterior horn of lateral meniscus due to old tear or injury, right knee**
  M23.252 **Derangement of posterior horn of lateral meniscus due to old tear or injury, left knee**
  M23.259 **Derangement of posterior horn of lateral meniscus due to old tear or injury, unspecified knee**
● M23.26 **Derangement of other lateral meniscus due to old tear or injury**
  M23.261 **Derangement of other lateral meniscus due to old tear or injury, right knee**
  M23.262 **Derangement of other lateral meniscus due to old tear or injury, left knee**
  M23.269 **Derangement of other lateral meniscus due to old tear or injury, unspecified knee**

CHAPTER 13 (M00–M99)

● **M23.3 Other meniscus derangements**
  Degenerate meniscus
  Detached meniscus
  Retained meniscus

● **M23.30 Other meniscus derangements, unspecified meniscus**
  Other meniscus derangements, unspecified lateral meniscus
  Other meniscus derangements, unspecified medial meniscus

    M23.300 Other meniscus derangements, unspecified lateral meniscus, right knee

    M23.301 Other meniscus derangements, unspecified lateral meniscus, left knee

    M23.302 Other meniscus derangements, unspecified lateral meniscus, unspecified knee

    M23.303 Other meniscus derangements, unspecified medial meniscus, right knee

    M23.304 Other meniscus derangements, unspecified medial meniscus, left knee

    M23.305 Other meniscus derangements, unspecified medial meniscus, unspecified knee

    M23.306 Other meniscus derangements, unspecified meniscus, right knee

    M23.307 Other meniscus derangements, unspecified meniscus, left knee

    M23.309 Other meniscus derangements, unspecified meniscus, unspecified knee

● **M23.31 Other meniscus derangements, anterior horn of medial meniscus**

    M23.311 Other meniscus derangements, anterior horn of medial meniscus, right knee

    M23.312 Other meniscus derangements, anterior horn of medial meniscus, left knee

    M23.319 Other meniscus derangements, anterior horn of medial meniscus, unspecified knee

● **M23.32 Other meniscus derangements, posterior horn of medial meniscus**

    M23.321 Other meniscus derangements, posterior horn of medial meniscus, right knee

    M23.322 Other meniscus derangements, posterior horn of medial meniscus, left knee

    M23.329 Other meniscus derangements, posterior horn of medial meniscus, unspecified knee

● **M23.33 Other meniscus derangements, other medial meniscus**

    M23.331 Other meniscus derangements, other medial meniscus, right knee

    M23.332 Other meniscus derangements, other medial meniscus, left knee

    M23.339 Other meniscus derangements, other medial meniscus, unspecified knee

● **M23.34 Other meniscus derangements, anterior horn of lateral meniscus**

    M23.341 Other meniscus derangements, anterior horn of lateral meniscus, right knee

    M23.342 Other meniscus derangements, anterior horn of lateral meniscus, left knee

    M23.349 Other meniscus derangements, anterior horn of lateral meniscus, unspecified knee

● **M23.35 Other meniscus derangements, posterior horn of lateral meniscus**

    M23.351 Other meniscus derangements, posterior horn of lateral meniscus, right knee

    M23.352 Other meniscus derangements, posterior horn of lateral meniscus, left knee

    M23.359 Other meniscus derangements, posterior horn of lateral meniscus, unspecified knee

● **M23.36 Other meniscus derangements, other lateral meniscus**

    M23.361 Other meniscus derangements, other lateral meniscus, right knee

    M23.362 Other meniscus derangements, other lateral meniscus, left knee

    M23.369 Other meniscus derangements, other lateral meniscus, unspecified knee

● **M23.4 Loose body in knee**
    M23.40 Loose body in knee, unspecified knee
    M23.41 Loose body in knee, right knee
    M23.42 Loose body in knee, left knee

● **M23.5 Chronic instability of knee**
    M23.50 Chronic instability of knee, unspecified knee
    M23.51 Chronic instability of knee, right knee
    M23.52 Chronic instability of knee, left knee

● **M23.6 Other spontaneous disruption of ligament(s) of knee**

  ● **M23.60 Other spontaneous disruption of unspecified ligament of knee**

    M23.601 Other spontaneous disruption of unspecified ligament of right knee

    M23.602 Other spontaneous disruption of unspecified ligament of left knee

    M23.609 Other spontaneous disruption of unspecified ligament of unspecified knee

  ● **M23.61 Other spontaneous disruption of anterior cruciate ligament of knee**

    M23.611 Other spontaneous disruption of anterior cruciate ligament of right knee

    M23.612 Other spontaneous disruption of anterior cruciate ligament of left knee

    M23.619 Other spontaneous disruption of anterior cruciate ligament of unspecified knee

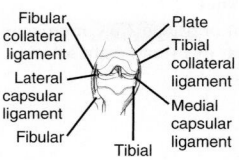

Figure 13-2 Collateral and cruciate ligament of knee. (From DeLee: DeLee and Drez's Orthopaedic Sports Medicine, ed 3, Saunders, 2009)

◄ New   ◄ Revised   ~~deleted~~ Deleted   Excludes 1   Excludes 2   Includes   Use additional   Code first   Code also   Unspecified

OGCR Official Guidelines   ● Unacceptable Principal Diagnosis   X Assign placeholder X   ● Use Additional Character(s)   ▶ Manifestation Code   **Coding Clinic**

● **M23.62** Other spontaneous disruption of posterior cruciate ligament of knee
  M23.621 Other spontaneous disruption of posterior cruciate ligament of right knee
  M23.622 Other spontaneous disruption of posterior cruciate ligament of left knee
  M23.629 Other spontaneous disruption of posterior cruciate ligament of unspecified knee

● **M23.63** Other spontaneous disruption of medial collateral ligament of knee
  M23.631 Other spontaneous disruption of medial collateral ligament of right knee
  M23.632 Other spontaneous disruption of medial collateral ligament of left knee
  M23.639 Other spontaneous disruption of medial collateral ligament of unspecified knee

● **M23.64** Other spontaneous disruption of lateral collateral ligament of knee
  M23.641 Other spontaneous disruption of lateral collateral ligament of right knee
  M23.642 Other spontaneous disruption of lateral collateral ligament of left knee
  M23.649 Other spontaneous disruption of lateral collateral ligament of unspecified knee

● **M23.67** Other spontaneous disruption of capsular ligament of knee
  M23.671 Other spontaneous disruption of capsular ligament of right knee
  M23.672 Other spontaneous disruption of capsular ligament of left knee
  M23.679 Other spontaneous disruption of capsular ligament of unspecified knee

● **M23.8** Other internal derangements of knee
  Laxity of ligament of knee
  Snapping knee
  ● **M23.8X** Other internal derangements of knee
    M23.8X1 Other internal derangements of right knee
    M23.8X2 Other internal derangements of left knee
    M23.8X9 Other internal derangements of unspecified knee

● **M23.9** Unspecified internal derangement of knee
  M23.90 Unspecified internal derangement of unspecified knee
  M23.91 Unspecified internal derangement of right knee
  M23.92 Unspecified internal derangement of left knee

● **M24** Other specific joint derangements
  Excludes1 current injury - see injury of joint by body region
  Excludes2 ganglion (M67.4)
    snapping knee (M23.8-)
    temporomandibular joint disorders (M26.6-)

● **M24.0** Loose body in joint
  Excludes2 loose body in knee (M23.4)
  M24.00 Loose body in unspecified joint
  ● **M24.01** Loose body in shoulder
    M24.011 Loose body in right shoulder
    M24.012 Loose body in left shoulder
    M24.019 Loose body in unspecified shoulder

● **M24.02** Loose body in elbow
  M24.021 Loose body in right elbow
  M24.022 Loose body in left elbow
  M24.029 Loose body in unspecified elbow

● **M24.03** Loose body in wrist
  M24.031 Loose body in right wrist
  M24.032 Loose body in left wrist
  M24.039 Loose body in unspecified wrist

● **M24.04** Loose body in finger joints
  M24.041 Loose body in right finger joint(s)
  M24.042 Loose body in left finger joint(s)
  M24.049 Loose body in unspecified finger joint(s)

● **M24.05** Loose body in hip
  M24.051 Loose body in right hip
  M24.052 Loose body in left hip
  M24.059 Loose body in unspecified hip

● **M24.07** Loose body in ankle and toe joints
  M24.071 Loose body in right ankle
  M24.072 Loose body in left ankle
  M24.073 Loose body in unspecified ankle
  M24.074 Loose body in right toe joint(s)
  M24.075 Loose body in left toe joint(s)
  M24.076 Loose body in unspecified toe joints

  M24.08 Loose body, other site

● **M24.1** Other articular cartilage disorders
  Excludes2 chondrocalcinosis (M11.1, M11.2-)
    internal derangement of knee (M23.-)
    metastatic calcification (E83.5)
    ochronosis (E70.2)
  M24.10 Other articular cartilage disorders, unspecified site
● **M24.11** Other articular cartilage disorders, shoulder
  M24.111 Other articular cartilage disorders, right shoulder
  M24.112 Other articular cartilage disorders, left shoulder
  M24.119 Other articular cartilage disorders, unspecified shoulder
● **M24.12** Other articular cartilage disorders, elbow
  M24.121 Other articular cartilage disorders, right elbow
  M24.122 Other articular cartilage disorders, left elbow
  M24.129 Other articular cartilage disorders, unspecified elbow
● **M24.13** Other articular cartilage disorders, wrist
  M24.131 Other articular cartilage disorders, right wrist
  M24.132 Other articular cartilage disorders, left wrist
  M24.139 Other articular cartilage disorders, unspecified wrist
● **M24.14** Other articular cartilage disorders, hand
  M24.141 Other articular cartilage disorders, right hand
  M24.142 Other articular cartilage disorders, left hand
  M24.149 Other articular cartilage disorders, unspecified hand

CHAPTER 13 (M00-M99)

N Newborn Age: 0   **P** Pediatric Age: 0–17   **M** Maternity DX: 12–55   **A** Adult Age: 15–124   ♀ Females Only   ♂ Males Only

● Complication\Comorbidity   ● Major C\C   Ⓔ CC/MCC Exclusions   ● Hospital-Acquired Condition

1021

● M24.15 Other articular cartilage disorders, hip
    M24.151 Other articular cartilage disorders, right hip
    M24.152 Other articular cartilage disorders, left hip
    M24.159 Other articular cartilage disorders, unspecified hip

● M24.17 Other articular cartilage disorders, ankle and foot
    M24.171 Other articular cartilage disorders, right ankle
    M24.172 Other articular cartilage disorders, left ankle
    M24.173 Other articular cartilage disorders, unspecified ankle
    M24.174 Other articular cartilage disorders, right foot
    M24.175 Other articular cartilage disorders, left foot
    M24.176 Other articular cartilage disorders, unspecified foot

● M24.2 Disorder of ligament
    Instability secondary to old ligament injury
    Ligamentous laxity NOS
    Excludes1 familial ligamentous laxity (M35.7)
    Excludes2 internal derangement of knee (M23.5-M23.89)

    M24.20 Disorder of ligament, unspecified site
● M24.21 Disorder of ligament, shoulder
    M24.211 Disorder of ligament, right shoulder
    M24.212 Disorder of ligament, left shoulder
    M24.219 Disorder of ligament, unspecified shoulder
● M24.22 Disorder of ligament, elbow
    M24.221 Disorder of ligament, right elbow
    M24.222 Disorder of ligament, left elbow
    M24.229 Disorder of ligament, unspecified elbow
● M24.23 Disorder of ligament, wrist
    M24.231 Disorder of ligament, right wrist
    M24.232 Disorder of ligament, left wrist
    M24.239 Disorder of ligament, unspecified wrist
● M24.24 Disorder of ligament, hand
    M24.241 Disorder of ligament, right hand
    M24.242 Disorder of ligament, left hand
    M24.249 Disorder of ligament, unspecified hand
● M24.25 Disorder of ligament, hip
    M24.251 Disorder of ligament, right hip
    M24.252 Disorder of ligament, left hip
    M24.259 Disorder of ligament, unspecified hip
● M24.27 Disorder of ligament, ankle and foot
    M24.271 Disorder of ligament, right ankle
    M24.272 Disorder of ligament, left ankle
    M24.273 Disorder of ligament, unspecified ankle
    M24.274 Disorder of ligament, right foot
    M24.275 Disorder of ligament, left foot
    M24.276 Disorder of ligament, unspecified foot
    M24.28 Disorder of ligament, vertebrae

● M24.3 Pathological dislocation of joint, not elsewhere classified
    Excludes1 congenital dislocation or displacement of joint - see congenital malformations and deformations of the musculoskeletal system (Q65-Q79)
    current injury - see injury of joints and ligaments by body region
    recurrent dislocation of joint (M24.4-)

    M24.30 Pathological dislocation of unspecified joint, not elsewhere classified
● M24.31 Pathological dislocation of shoulder, not elsewhere classified
    M24.311 Pathological dislocation of right shoulder, not elsewhere classified
    M24.312 Pathological dislocation of left shoulder, not elsewhere classified
    M24.319 Pathological dislocation of unspecified shoulder, not elsewhere classified
● M24.32 Pathological dislocation of elbow, not elsewhere classified
    M24.321 Pathological dislocation of right elbow, not elsewhere classified
    M24.322 Pathological dislocation of left elbow, not elsewhere classified
    M24.329 Pathological dislocation of unspecified elbow, not elsewhere classified
● M24.33 Pathological dislocation of wrist, not elsewhere classified
    M24.331 Pathological dislocation of right wrist, not elsewhere classified
    M24.332 Pathological dislocation of left wrist, not elsewhere classified
    M24.339 Pathological dislocation of unspecified wrist, not elsewhere classified
● M24.34 Pathological dislocation of hand, not elsewhere classified
    M24.341 Pathological dislocation of right hand, not elsewhere classified
    M24.342 Pathological dislocation of left hand, not elsewhere classified
    M24.349 Pathological dislocation of unspecified hand, not elsewhere classified
● M24.35 Pathological dislocation of hip, not elsewhere classified
    M24.351 Pathological dislocation of right hip, not elsewhere classified
    M24.352 Pathological dislocation of left hip, not elsewhere classified
    M24.359 Pathological dislocation of unspecified hip, not elsewhere classified
● M24.36 Pathological dislocation of knee, not elsewhere classified
    M24.361 Pathological dislocation of right knee, not elsewhere classified
    M24.362 Pathological dislocation of left knee, not elsewhere classified
    M24.369 Pathological dislocation of unspecified knee, not elsewhere classified
● M24.37 Pathological dislocation of ankle and foot, not elsewhere classified
    M24.371 Pathological dislocation of right ankle, not elsewhere classified
    M24.372 Pathological dislocation of left ankle, not elsewhere classified

M24.373 Pathological dislocation of unspecified ankle, not elsewhere classified

M24.374 Pathological dislocation of right foot, not elsewhere classified

M24.375 Pathological dislocation of left foot, not elsewhere classified

M24.376 Pathological dislocation of unspecified foot, not elsewhere classified

● M24.4 **Recurrent dislocation of joint**
Recurrent subluxation of joint

Excludes2   recurrent dislocation of patella (M22.0-M22.1)
recurrent vertebral dislocation (M43.3-, M43.4, M43.5-)

M24.40 Recurrent dislocation, unspecified joint

● M24.41 Recurrent dislocation, shoulder

M24.411 Recurrent dislocation, right shoulder

M24.412 Recurrent dislocation, left shoulder

M24.419 Recurrent dislocation, unspecified shoulder

● M24.42 Recurrent dislocation, elbow

M24.421 Recurrent dislocation, right elbow

M24.422 Recurrent dislocation, left elbow

M24.429 Recurrent dislocation, unspecified elbow

● M24.43 Recurrent dislocation, wrist

M24.431 Recurrent dislocation, right wrist

M24.432 Recurrent dislocation, left wrist

M24.439 Recurrent dislocation, unspecified wrist

● M24.44 Recurrent dislocation, hand and finger(s)

M24.441 Recurrent dislocation, right hand

M24.442 Recurrent dislocation, left hand

M24.443 Recurrent dislocation, unspecified hand

M24.444 Recurrent dislocation, right finger

M24.445 Recurrent dislocation, left finger

M24.446 Recurrent dislocation, unspecified finger

● M24.45 Recurrent dislocation, hip

M24.451 Recurrent dislocation, right hip

M24.452 Recurrent dislocation, left hip

M24.459 Recurrent dislocation, unspecified hip

● M24.46 Recurrent dislocation, knee

M24.461 Recurrent dislocation, right knee

M24.462 Recurrent dislocation, left knee

M24.469 Recurrent dislocation, unspecified knee

● M24.47 Recurrent dislocation, ankle, foot and toes

M24.471 Recurrent dislocation, right ankle

M24.472 Recurrent dislocation, left ankle

M24.473 Recurrent dislocation, unspecified ankle

M24.474 Recurrent dislocation, right foot

M24.475 Recurrent dislocation, left foot

M24.476 Recurrent dislocation, unspecified foot

M24.477 Recurrent dislocation, right toe(s)

M24.478 Recurrent dislocation, left toe(s)

M24.479 Recurrent dislocation, unspecified toe(s)

● M24.5 **Contracture of joint**

Excludes1   contracture of muscle without contracture of joint (M62.4-)
contracture of tendon (sheath) without contracture of joint (M62.4-)
Dupuytren's contracture (M72.0)

Excludes2   acquired deformities of limbs (M20-M21)

M24.50 Contracture, unspecified joint

● M24.51 Contracture, shoulder

M24.511 Contracture, right shoulder

M24.512 Contracture, left shoulder

M24.519 Contracture, unspecified shoulder

● M24.52 Contracture, elbow

M24.521 Contracture, right elbow

M24.522 Contracture, left elbow

M24.529 Contracture, unspecified elbow

● M24.53 Contracture, wrist

M24.531 Contracture, right wrist

M24.532 Contracture, left wrist

M24.539 Contracture, unspecified wrist

● M24.54 Contracture, hand

M24.541 Contracture, right hand

M24.542 Contracture, left hand

M24.549 Contracture, unspecified hand

● M24.55 Contracture, hip

M24.551 Contracture, right hip
Coding Clinic: 2016, Q2, P6

M24.552 Contracture, left hip
Coding Clinic: 2016, Q2, P6

M24.559 Contracture, unspecified hip

● M24.56 Contracture, knee

M24.561 Contracture, right knee
Coding Clinic: 2016, Q2, P6

M24.562 Contracture, left knee
Coding Clinic: 2016, Q2, P6

M24.569 Contracture, unspecified knee

● M24.57 Contracture, ankle and foot

M24.571 Contracture, right ankle

M24.572 Contracture, left ankle

M24.573 Contracture, unspecified ankle

M24.574 Contracture, right foot

M24.575 Contracture, left foot

M24.576 Contracture, unspecified foot

● M24.6 **Ankylosis of joint**

Excludes1   stiffness of joint without ankylosis (M25.6-)

Excludes2   spine (M43.2-)

M24.60 Ankylosis, unspecified joint

● M24.61 Ankylosis, shoulder

M24.611 Ankylosis, right shoulder

M24.612 Ankylosis, left shoulder

M24.619 Ankylosis, unspecified shoulder

● M24.62 Ankylosis, elbow

M24.621 Ankylosis, right elbow

M24.622 Ankylosis, left elbow

M24.629 Ankylosis, unspecified elbow

● M24.63 Ankylosis, wrist

M24.631 Ankylosis, right wrist

M24.632 Ankylosis, left wrist

M24.639 Ankylosis, unspecified wrist

Item 13–5 Ankylosis or arthrokleisis is a consolidation of a joint due to disease, injury, or surgical procedure. Spondylosis is the degeneration of the vertebral processes and formation of osteophytes and commonly occurs with age. **Spondylitis** or ankylosing spondylitis is a type of arthritis that affects the spine or backbone causing back pain and stiffness.

CHAPTER 13 (M00-M99)

N Newborn Age: 0   **P** Pediatric Age: 0–17   **M** Maternity DX: 12–55   **A** Adult Age: 15–124   ♀ Females Only   ♂ Males Only

● Complication\Comorbidity   ● Major C\C   (Ex) CC/MCC Exclusions   ● Hospital-Acquired Condition

1023

● M24.64   Ankylosis, hand
      M24.641   Ankylosis, right hand
      M24.642   Ankylosis, left hand
      M24.649   Ankylosis, unspecified hand
● M24.65   Ankylosis, hip
      M24.651   Ankylosis, right hip
      M24.652   Ankylosis, left hip
      M24.659   Ankylosis, unspecified hip
● M24.66   Ankylosis, knee
      M24.661   Ankylosis, right knee
      M24.662   Ankylosis, left knee
      M24.669   Ankylosis, unspecified knee
● M24.67   Ankylosis, ankle and foot
      M24.671   Ankylosis, right ankle
      M24.672   Ankylosis, left ankle
      M24.673   Ankylosis, unspecified ankle
      M24.674   Ankylosis, right foot
      M24.675   Ankylosis, left foot
      M24.676   Ankylosis, unspecified foot

M24.7   Protrusio acetabuli

● M24.8   Other specific joint derangements, not elsewhere classified

      Excludes2   iliotibial band syndrome (M76.3)

      M24.80   Other specific joint derangements of unspecified joint, not elsewhere classified
● M24.81   Other specific joint derangements of shoulder, not elsewhere classified
      M24.811   Other specific joint derangements of right shoulder, not elsewhere classified
      M24.812   Other specific joint derangements of left shoulder, not elsewhere classified
      M24.819   Other specific joint derangements of unspecified shoulder, not elsewhere classified
● M24.82   Other specific joint derangements of elbow, not elsewhere classified
      M24.821   Other specific joint derangements of right elbow, not elsewhere classified
      M24.822   Other specific joint derangements of left elbow, not elsewhere classified
      M24.829   Other specific joint derangements of unspecified elbow, not elsewhere classified
● M24.83   Other specific joint derangements of wrist, not elsewhere classified
      M24.831   Other specific joint derangements of right wrist, not elsewhere classified
      M24.832   Other specific joint derangements of left wrist, not elsewhere classified
      M24.839   Other specific joint derangements of unspecified wrist, not elsewhere classified
● M24.84   Other specific joint derangements of hand, not elsewhere classified
      M24.841   Other specific joint derangements of right hand, not elsewhere classified
      M24.842   Other specific joint derangements of left hand, not elsewhere classified
      M24.849   Other specific joint derangements of unspecified hand, not elsewhere classified

● M24.85   Other specific joint derangements of hip, not elsewhere classified
      Irritable hip
      M24.851   Other specific joint derangements of right hip, not elsewhere classified
      M24.852   Other specific joint derangements of left hip, not elsewhere classified
      M24.859   Other specific joint derangements of unspecified hip, not elsewhere classified
● M24.87   Other specific joint derangements of ankle and foot, not elsewhere classified
      M24.871   Other specific joint derangements of right ankle, not elsewhere classified
      M24.872   Other specific joint derangements of left ankle, not elsewhere classified
      M24.873   Other specific joint derangements of unspecified ankle, not elsewhere classified
      M24.874   Other specific joint derangements of right foot, not elsewhere classified
      M24.875   Other specific joint derangements left foot, not elsewhere classified
      M24.876   Other specific joint derangements of unspecified foot, not elsewhere classified

M24.9   Joint derangement, unspecified

● M25   Other joint disorder, not elsewhere classified

      Excludes2   abnormality of gait and mobility (R26.-)
                    acquired deformities of limb (M20-M21)
                    calcification of bursa (M71.4-)
                    calcification of shoulder (joint) (M75.3)
                    calcification of tendon (M65.2-)
                    difficulty in walking (R26.2)
                    temporomandibular joint disorder (M26.6-)

● M25.0   Hemarthrosis

      Excludes1   current injury - see injury of joint by body region
                    hemophilic arthropathy (M36.2)

      ● M25.00   Hemarthrosis, unspecified joint 🔧
         (Ex) M25.00-M25.08, T79.A11A-T79.A29A
      ● M25.01   Hemarthrosis, shoulder
         (Ex) For category M25.01 CC codes: M25.00-M25.039, M25.08, T79.A11-T79.A19[A]
         M25.011   Hemarthrosis, right shoulder 🔧
         M25.012   Hemarthrosis, left shoulder 🔧
         M25.019   Hemarthrosis, unspecified shoulder 🔧
      ● M25.02   Hemarthrosis, elbow
         (Ex) For category M25.02 CC codes: M25.00-M25.029, M25.08, T79.A11-T79.A19[A]
         M25.021   Hemarthrosis, right elbow 🔧
         M25.022   Hemarthrosis, left elbow 🔧
         M25.029   Hemarthrosis, unspecified elbow 🔧
      ● M25.03   Hemarthrosis, wrist
         (Ex) For category M25.03 CC codes: M25.00-M25.049, M25.08, T79.A11-T79.A19[A]
         M25.031   Hemarthrosis, right wrist 🔧
         M25.032   Hemarthrosis, left wrist 🔧
         M25.039   Hemarthrosis, unspecified wrist 🔧
      ● M25.04   Hemarthrosis, hand
         (Ex) For category M25.04 CC codes: M25.00, M25.031-M25.049, M25.08, T79.A11-T79.A19[A]
         M25.041   Hemarthrosis, right hand 🔧
         M25.042   Hemarthrosis, left hand 🔧
         M25.049   Hemarthrosis, unspecified hand 🔧

● M25.05 Hemarthrosis, hip
    (Ex) **For category M25.05 CC codes:** See M25.00
    M25.051 Hemarthrosis, right hip 🔗
    M25.052 Hemarthrosis, left hip 🔗
    M25.059 Hemarthrosis, unspecified hip 🔗
● M25.06 Hemarthrosis, knee
    (Ex) **For category M25.06 CC codes:** M25.00, M25.061-M25.08,
        T79.A21-T79.A29[A]
    M25.061 Hemarthrosis, right knee 🔗
    M25.062 Hemarthrosis, left knee 🔗
    M25.069 Hemarthrosis, unspecified knee 🔗
● M25.07 Hemarthrosis, ankle and foot
    (Ex) **For category M25.07 CC codes:** See M25.06
    M25.071 Hemarthrosis, right ankle 🔗
    M25.072 Hemarthrosis, left ankle 🔗
    M25.073 Hemarthrosis, unspecified ankle 🔗
    M25.074 Hemarthrosis, right foot 🔗
    M25.075 Hemarthrosis, left foot 🔗
    M25.076 Hemarthrosis, unspecified foot 🔗
  M25.08 Hemarthrosis, other specified site 🔗
    Hemarthrosis, vertebrae
    (Ex) See M25.00
● M25.1 Fistula of joint
  M25.10 Fistula, unspecified joint
● M25.11 Fistula, shoulder
    M25.111 Fistula, right shoulder
    M25.112 Fistula, left shoulder
    M25.119 Fistula, unspecified shoulder
● M25.12 Fistula, elbow
    M25.121 Fistula, right elbow
    M25.122 Fistula, left elbow
    M25.129 Fistula, unspecified elbow
● M25.13 Fistula, wrist
    M25.131 Fistula, right wrist
    M25.132 Fistula, left wrist
    M25.139 Fistula, unspecified wrist
● M25.14 Fistula, hand
    M25.141 Fistula, right hand
    M25.142 Fistula, left hand
    M25.149 Fistula, unspecified hand
● M25.15 Fistula, hip
    M25.151 Fistula, right hip
    M25.152 Fistula, left hip
    M25.159 Fistula, unspecified hip
● M25.16 Fistula, knee
    M25.161 Fistula, right knee
    M25.162 Fistula, left knee
    M25.169 Fistula, unspecified knee
● M25.17 Fistula, ankle and foot
    M25.171 Fistula, right ankle
    M25.172 Fistula, left ankle
    M25.173 Fistula, unspecified ankle
    M25.174 Fistula, right foot
    M25.175 Fistula, left foot
    M25.176 Fistula, unspecified foot
  M25.18 Fistula, other specified site
    Fistula, vertebrae
● M25.2 Flail joint
  M25.20 Flail joint, unspecified joint
● M25.21 Flail joint, shoulder
    M25.211 Flail joint, right shoulder
    M25.212 Flail joint, left shoulder
    M25.219 Flail joint, unspecified shoulder

● M25.22 Flail joint, elbow
    M25.221 Flail joint, right elbow
    M25.222 Flail joint, left elbow
    M25.229 Flail joint, unspecified elbow
● M25.23 Flail joint, wrist
    M25.231 Flail joint, right wrist
    M25.232 Flail joint, left wrist
    M25.239 Flail joint, unspecified wrist
● M25.24 Flail joint, hand
    M25.241 Flail joint, right hand
    M25.242 Flail joint, left hand
    M25.249 Flail joint, unspecified hand
● M25.25 Flail joint, hip
    M25.251 Flail joint, right hip
    M25.252 Flail joint, left hip
    M25.259 Flail joint, unspecified hip
● M25.26 Flail joint, knee
    M25.261 Flail joint, right knee
    M25.262 Flail joint, left knee
    M25.269 Flail joint, unspecified knee
● M25.27 Flail joint, ankle and foot
    M25.271 Flail joint, right ankle and foot
    M25.272 Flail joint, left ankle and foot
    M25.279 Flail joint, unspecified ankle and foot
  M25.28 Flail joint, other site
● M25.3 Other instability of joint
    Excludes1 instability of joint secondary to old
            ligament injury (M24.2-)
            instability of joint secondary to removal
            of joint prosthesis (M96.8-)
    Excludes2 spinal instabilities (M53.2-)
  M25.30 Other instability, unspecified joint
● M25.31 Other instability, shoulder
    M25.311 Other instability, right shoulder
    M25.312 Other instability, left shoulder
    M25.319 Other instability, unspecified
          shoulder
● M25.32 Other instability, elbow
    M25.321 Other instability, right elbow
    M25.322 Other instability, left elbow
    M25.329 Other instability, unspecified elbow
● M25.33 Other instability, wrist
    M25.331 Other instability, right wrist
    M25.332 Other instability, left wrist
    M25.339 Other instability, unspecified wrist
● M25.34 Other instability, hand
    M25.341 Other instability, right hand
    M25.342 Other instability, left hand
    M25.349 Other instability, unspecified hand
● M25.35 Other instability, hip
    M25.351 Other instability, right hip
    M25.352 Other instability, left hip
    M25.359 Other instability, unspecified hip
● M25.36 Other instability, knee
    M25.361 Other instability, right knee
    M25.362 Other instability, left knee
    M25.369 Other instability, unspecified knee
● M25.37 Other instability, ankle and foot
    M25.371 Other instability, right ankle
    M25.372 Other instability, left ankle
    M25.373 Other instability, unspecified ankle
    M25.374 Other instability, right foot
    M25.375 Other instability, left foot
    M25.376 Other instability, unspecified foot

CHAPTER 13 (M00–M99)

CHAPTER 13 (M00–M99)

● **M25.4　Effusion of joint**

　　Excludes1　hydrarthrosis in yaws (A66.6)
　　　　　　　　　intermittent hydrarthrosis (M12.4-)
　　　　　　　　　other infective (teno)synovitis (M65.1-)

　　M25.40　Effusion, unspecified joint

● M25.41　Effusion, shoulder
　　　　M25.411　Effusion, right shoulder
　　　　M25.412　Effusion, left shoulder
　　　　M25.419　Effusion, unspecified shoulder

● M25.42　Effusion, elbow
　　　　M25.421　Effusion, right elbow
　　　　M25.422　Effusion, left elbow
　　　　M25.429　Effusion, unspecified elbow

● M25.43　Effusion, wrist
　　　　M25.431　Effusion, right wrist
　　　　M25.432　Effusion, left wrist
　　　　M25.439　Effusion, unspecified wrist

● M25.44　Effusion, hand
　　　　M25.441　Effusion, right hand
　　　　M25.442　Effusion, left hand
　　　　M25.449　Effusion, unspecified hand

● M25.45　Effusion, hip
　　　　M25.451　Effusion, right hip
　　　　M25.452　Effusion, left hip
　　　　M25.459　Effusion, unspecified hip

● M25.46　Effusion, knee
　　　　M25.461　Effusion, right knee
　　　　M25.462　Effusion, left knee
　　　　M25.469　Effusion, unspecified knee

● M25.47　Effusion, ankle and foot
　　　　M25.471　Effusion, right ankle
　　　　M25.472　Effusion, left ankle
　　　　M25.473　Effusion, unspecified ankle
　　　　M25.474　Effusion, right foot
　　　　M25.475　Effusion, left foot
　　　　M25.476　Effusion, unspecified foot

　　M25.48　Effusion, other site

● **M25.5　Pain in joint**

　　Excludes2　pain in hand (M79.64-)
　　　　　　　　　pain in fingers (M79.64-)
　　　　　　　　　pain in foot (M79.67-)
　　　　　　　　　pain in limb (M79.6-)
　　　　　　　　　pain in toes (M79.67-)

　　M25.50　Pain in unspecified joint

● M25.51　Pain in shoulder
　　　　M25.511　Pain in right shoulder
　　　　M25.512　Pain in left shoulder
　　　　M25.519　Pain in unspecified shoulder

● M25.52　Pain in elbow
　　　　M25.521　Pain in right elbow
　　　　M25.522　Pain in left elbow
　　　　M25.529　Pain in unspecified elbow

● M25.53　Pain in wrist
　　　　M25.531　Pain in right wrist
　　　　M25.532　Pain in left wrist
　　　　M25.539　Pain in unspecified wrist

● M25.54　Pain in joints of hand ◀
　　　　M25.541　Pain in joints of right hand ◀
　　　　M25.542　Pain in joints of left hand ◀
　　　　M25.549　Pain in joints of unspecified hand ◀
　　　　　　　　Pain in joints of hand NOS ◀

● M25.55　Pain in hip
　　　　M25.551　Pain in right hip
　　　　M25.552　Pain in left hip
　　　　M25.559　Pain in unspecified hip

● M25.56　Pain in knee
　　　　M25.561　Pain in right knee
　　　　M25.562　Pain in left knee
　　　　M25.569　Pain in unspecified knee

● M25.57　Pain in ankle and joints of foot
　　　　M25.571　Pain in right ankle and joints of right foot
　　　　M25.572　Pain in left ankle and joints of left foot
　　　　M25.579　Pain in unspecified ankle and joints of unspecified foot

● **M25.6　Stiffness of joint, not elsewhere classified**

　　Excludes1　ankylosis of joint (M24.6-)
　　　　　　　　　contracture of joint (M24.5-)

　　M25.60　Stiffness of unspecified joint, not elsewhere classified

● M25.61　Stiffness of shoulder, not elsewhere classified
　　　　M25.611　Stiffness of right shoulder, not elsewhere classified
　　　　M25.612　Stiffness of left shoulder, not elsewhere classified
　　　　M25.619　Stiffness of unspecified shoulder, not elsewhere classified

● M25.62　Stiffness of elbow, not elsewhere classified
　　　　M25.621　Stiffness of right elbow, not elsewhere classified
　　　　M25.622　Stiffness of left elbow, not elsewhere classified
　　　　M25.629　Stiffness of unspecified elbow, not elsewhere classified

● M25.63　Stiffness of wrist, not elsewhere classified
　　　　M25.631　Stiffness of right wrist, not elsewhere classified
　　　　M25.632　Stiffness of left wrist, not elsewhere classified
　　　　M25.639　Stiffness of unspecified wrist, not elsewhere classified

● M25.64　Stiffness of hand, not elsewhere classified
　　　　M25.641　Stiffness of right hand, not elsewhere classified
　　　　M25.642　Stiffness of left hand, not elsewhere classified
　　　　M25.649　Stiffness of unspecified hand, not elsewhere classified

● M25.65　Stiffness of hip, not elsewhere classified
　　　　M25.651　Stiffness of right hip, not elsewhere classified
　　　　M25.652　Stiffness of left hip, not elsewhere classified
　　　　M25.659　Stiffness of unspecified hip, not elsewhere classified

● M25.66　Stiffness of knee, not elsewhere classified
　　　　M25.661　Stiffness of right knee, not elsewhere classified
　　　　M25.662　Stiffness of left knee, not elsewhere classified
　　　　M25.669　Stiffness of unspecified knee, not elsewhere classified

● M25.67　Stiffness of ankle and foot, not elsewhere classified
　　　　M25.671　Stiffness of right ankle, not elsewhere classified
　　　　M25.672　Stiffness of left ankle, not elsewhere classified
　　　　M25.673　Stiffness of unspecified ankle, not elsewhere classified
　　　　M25.674　Stiffness of right foot, not elsewhere classified

M25.675   Stiffness of left foot, not elsewhere classified

M25.676   Stiffness of unspecified foot, not elsewhere classified

● M25.7   **Osteophyte**

    M25.70   Osteophyte, unspecified joint

● M25.71   Osteophyte, shoulder

    M25.711   Osteophyte, right shoulder

    M25.712   Osteophyte, left shoulder

    M25.719   Osteophyte, unspecified shoulder

● M25.72   Osteophyte, elbow

    M25.721   Osteophyte, right elbow

    M25.722   Osteophyte, left elbow

    M25.729   Osteophyte, unspecified elbow

● M25.73   Osteophyte, wrist

    M25.731   Osteophyte, right wrist

    M25.732   Osteophyte, left wrist

    M25.739   Osteophyte, unspecified wrist

● M25.74   Osteophyte, hand

    M25.741   Osteophyte, right hand

    M25.742   Osteophyte, left hand

    M25.749   Osteophyte, unspecified hand

● M25.75   Osteophyte, hip

    M25.751   Osteophyte, right hip

    M25.752   Osteophyte, left hip

    M25.759   Osteophyte, unspecified hip

● M25.76   Osteophyte, knee

    M25.761   Osteophyte, right knee

    M25.762   Osteophyte, left knee

    M25.769   Osteophyte, unspecified knee

● M25.77   Osteophyte, ankle and foot

    M25.771   Osteophyte, right ankle

    M25.772   Osteophyte, left ankle

    M25.773   Osteophyte, unspecified ankle

    M25.774   Osteophyte, right foot

    M25.775   Osteophyte, left foot

    M25.776   Osteophyte, unspecified foot

    M25.78   Osteophyte, vertebrae

● M25.8   **Other specified joint disorders**

    M25.80   Other specified joint disorders, unspecified joint

● M25.81   Other specified joint disorders, shoulder

    M25.811   Other specified joint disorders, right shoulder

    M25.812   Other specified joint disorders, left shoulder

    M25.819   Other specified joint disorders, unspecified shoulder

● M25.82   Other specified joint disorders, elbow

    M25.821   Other specified joint disorders, right elbow

    M25.822   Other specified joint disorders, left elbow

    M25.829   Other specified joint disorders, unspecified elbow

● M25.83   Other specified joint disorders, wrist

    M25.831   Other specified joint disorders, right wrist

    M25.832   Other specified joint disorders, left wrist

    M25.839   Other specified joint disorders, unspecified wrist

● M25.84   Other specified joint disorders, hand

    M25.841   Other specified joint disorders, right hand

    M25.842   Other specified joint disorders, left hand

    M25.849   Other specified joint disorders, unspecified hand

● M25.85   Other specified joint disorders, hip

    M25.851   Other specified joint disorders, right hip

    M25.852   Other specified joint disorders, left hip

    M25.859   Other specified joint disorders, unspecified hip

● M25.86   Other specified joint disorders, knee

    M25.861   Other specified joint disorders, right knee

    M25.862   Other specified joint disorders, left knee

    M25.869   Other specified joint disorders, unspecified knee

● M25.87   Other specified joint disorders, ankle and foot

    M25.871   Other specified joint disorders, right ankle and foot

    M25.872   Other specified joint disorders, left ankle and foot

    M25.879   Other specified joint disorders, unspecified ankle and foot

   M25.9   Joint disorder, unspecified

DENTOFACIAL ANOMALIES [INCLUDING MALOCCLUSION] AND OTHER DISORDERS OF JAW (M26-M27)

    Excludes1   hemifacial atrophy or hypertrophy (Q67.4)

       unilateral condylar hyperplasia or hypoplasia (M27.8)

● M26   **Dentofacial anomalies [including malocclusion]**

● M26.0   **Major anomalies of jaw size**

    Excludes1   acromegaly (E22.0)

       Robin's syndrome (Q87.0)

    M26.00   Unspecified anomaly of jaw size

    M26.01   Maxillary hyperplasia

    M26.02   Maxillary hypoplasia

    M26.03   Mandibular hyperplasia

    M26.04   Mandibular hypoplasia

    M26.05   Macrogenia

    M26.06   Microgenia

    M26.07   Excessive tuberosity of jaw

       Entire maxillary tuberosity

    M26.09   Other specified anomalies of jaw size

● M26.1   **Anomalies of jaw-cranial base relationship**

    M26.10   Unspecified anomaly of jaw-cranial base relationship

    M26.11   Maxillary asymmetry

    M26.12   Other jaw asymmetry

    M26.19   Other specified anomalies of jaw-cranial base relationship

Figure 13-3   Dentofacial malocclusion.

Item 13–6 Hyperplasia is a condition of overdevelopment, whereas **hypoplasia** is a condition of underdevelopment. **Macrogenia** is overdevelopment of the chin, whereas **microgenia** is underdevelopment of the chin.

N Newborn Age: Ø   **P** Pediatric Age: Ø–17   **M** Maternity DX: 12–55   **A** Adult Age: 15–124   ♀ Females Only   ♂ Males Only

Complication\Comorbidity   Major C\C   (Ex) CC/MCC Exclusions   Hospital-Acquired Condition

1027

● **M26.2 Anomalies of dental arch relationship**

　M26.20 Unspecified anomaly of dental arch relationship

　● **M26.21 Malocclusion, Angle's class**

　　M26.211 Malocclusion, Angle's class I
　　　Neutro-occlusion

　　M26.212 Malocclusion, Angle's class II
　　　Disto-occlusion Division I
　　　Disto-occlusion Division II

　　M26.213 Malocclusion, Angle's class III
　　　Mesio-occlusion

　　M26.219 Malocclusion, Angle's class, unspecified

　● **M26.22 Open occlusal relationship**

　　M26.220 Open anterior occlusal relationship
　　　Anterior openbite

　　M26.221 Open posterior occlusal relationship
　　　Posterior openbite

　M26.23 Excessive horizontal overlap
　　Excessive horizontal overjet

　M26.24 Reverse articulation
　　Crossbite (anterior) (posterior)

　M26.25 Anomalies of interarch distance

　M26.29 Other anomalies of dental arch relationship
　　Midline deviation of dental arch
　　Overbite (excessive) deep
　　Overbite (excessive) horizontal
　　Overbite (excessive) vertical
　　Posterior lingual occlusion of mandibular teeth

● **M26.3 Anomalies of tooth position of fully erupted tooth or teeth**

　Excludes2 embedded and impacted teeth (K01.-)

　M26.30 Unspecified anomaly of tooth position of fully erupted tooth or teeth
　　Abnormal spacing of fully erupted tooth or teeth NOS
　　Displacement of fully erupted tooth or teeth NOS
　　Transposition of fully erupted tooth or teeth NOS

　M26.31 Crowding of fully erupted teeth

　M26.32 Excessive spacing of fully erupted teeth
　　Diastema of fully erupted tooth or teeth NOS

　M26.33 Horizontal displacement of fully erupted tooth or teeth
　　Tipped tooth or teeth
　　Tipping of fully erupted tooth

　M26.34 Vertical displacement of fully erupted tooth or teeth
　　Extruded tooth
　　Infraeruption of tooth or teeth
　　Supraeruption of tooth or teeth

　M26.35 Rotation of fully erupted tooth or teeth

　M26.36 Insufficient interocclusal distance of fully erupted teeth (ridge)
　　Lack of adequate intermaxillary vertical dimension of fully erupted teeth

　M26.37 Excessive interocclusal distance of fully erupted teeth
　　Excessive intermaxillary vertical dimension of fully erupted teeth
　　Loss of occlusal vertical dimension of fully erupted teeth

　M26.39 Other anomalies of tooth position of fully erupted tooth or teeth

M26.4 Malocclusion, unspecified

● **M26.5 Dentofacial functional abnormalities**

　Excludes1 bruxism (F45.8)
　　　teeth-grinding NOS (F45.8)

　M26.50 Dentofacial functional abnormalities, unspecified

　M26.51 Abnormal jaw closure

M26.52 Limited mandibular range of motion

M26.53 Deviation in opening and closing of the mandible

M26.54 Insufficient anterior guidance
　Insufficient anterior occlusal guidance

M26.55 Centric occlusion maximum intercuspation discrepancy
　Excludes1 centric occlusion NOS (M26.59)

M26.56 Non-working side interference
　Balancing side interference

M26.57 Lack of posterior occlusal support

M26.59 Other dentofacial functional abnormalities
　Centric occlusion (of teeth) NOS
　Malocclusion due to abnormal swallowing
　Malocclusion due to mouth breathing
　Malocclusion due to tongue, lip or finger habits

● **M26.6 Temporomandibular joint disorders**

　Excludes2 current temporomandibular joint dislocation (S03.0)
　　　current temporomandibular joint sprain (S03.4)

　● **M26.60 Temporomandibular joint disorder, unspecified**

　　M26.601 Right temporomandibular joint disorder, unspecified ◄

　　M26.602 Left temporomandibular joint disorder, unspecified ◄

　　M26.603 Bilateral temporomandibular joint disorder, unspecified ◄

　　M26.609 Unspecified temporomandibular joint disorder, unspecified side ◄
　　　Temporomandibular joint disorder NOS ◄

　● **M26.61 Adhesions and ankylosis of temporomandibular joint**

　　M26.611 Adhesions and ankylosis of right temporomandibular joint ◄

　　M26.612 Adhesions and ankylosis of left temporomandibular joint ◄

　　M26.613 Adhesions and ankylosis of bilateral temporomandibular joint ◄

　　M26.619 Adhesions and ankylosis of temporomandibular joint, unspecified side ◄

　● **M26.62 Arthralgia of temporomandibular joint**

　　M26.621 Arthralgia of right temporomandibular joint ◄

　　M26.622 Arthralgia of left temporomandibular joint ◄

　　M26.623 Arthralgia of bilateral temporomandibular joint ◄

　　M26.629 Arthralgia of temporomandibular joint, unspecified side ◄

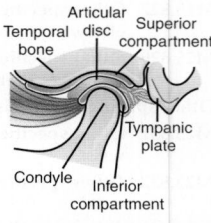

Figure 13-4 Temporomandibular joint.

Item 13–7 Dysfunction of the temporomandibular joint is termed **temporomandibular joint (TMJ) syndrome** and is characterized by pain and tenderness/spasm of the muscles of mastication, joint noise, and in the later stages, limited mandibular movement.

◄ New ◀▦ Revised ~~deleted~~ Deleted | Excludes 1 | Excludes 2 | Includes | Use additional | Code first | Code also | Unspecified

OGCR Official Guidelines ● Unacceptable Principal Diagnosis X Assign placeholder X ▶ Use Additional Character(s) ▶ Manifestation Code **Coding Clinic**

● M26.63   **Articular disc disorder of temporomandibular joint**

    M26.631   **Articular disc disorder of right temporomandibular joint** ◄

    M26.632   **Articular disc disorder of left temporomandibular joint** ◄

    M26.633   **Articular disc disorder of bilateral temporomandibular joint** ◄

    M26.639   **Articular disc disorder of temporomandibular joint, unspecified side** ◄

   M26.69   **Other specified disorders of temporomandibular joint**

● M26.7   **Dental alveolar anomalies**

   M26.70   **Unspecified alveolar anomaly**

   M26.71   **Alveolar maxillary hyperplasia**

   M26.72   **Alveolar mandibular hyperplasia**

   M26.73   **Alveolar maxillary hypoplasia**

   M26.74   **Alveolar mandibular hypoplasia**

   M26.79   **Other specified alveolar anomalies**

● M26.8   **Other dentofacial anomalies**

   M26.81   **Anterior soft tissue impingement**
      Anterior soft tissue impingement on teeth

   M26.82   **Posterior soft tissue impingement**
      Posterior soft tissue impingement on teeth

   M26.89   **Other dentofacial anomalies**

● M26.9   **Dentofacial anomaly, unspecified**

● M27   **Other diseases of jaws**

   M27.0   **Developmental disorders of jaws**
      Latent bone cyst of jaw
      Stafne's cyst
      Torus mandibularis
      Torus palatinus

   M27.1   **Giant cell granuloma, central**
      Giant cell granuloma NOS

     Excludes1   peripheral giant cell granuloma (K06.8)

   M27.2   **Inflammatory conditions of jaws**
      Osteitis of jaw(s)
      Osteomyelitis (neonatal) jaw(s)
      Osteoradionecrosis jaw(s)
      Periostitis jaw(s)
      Sequestrum of jaw bone

     Use additional code (W88-W90, X39.0) to identify radiation, if radiation-induced

     Excludes2   osteonecrosis of jaw due to drug (M87.180)

   M27.3   **Alveolitis of jaws**
      Alveolar osteitis
      Dry socket

● M27.4   **Other and unspecified cysts of jaw**

     Excludes1   cysts of oral region (K09.-)
        latent bone cyst of jaw (M27.0)
        Stafne's cyst (M27.0)

   M27.40   **Unspecified cyst of jaw**
      Cyst of jaw NOS

   M27.49   **Other cysts of jaw**
      Aneurysmal cyst of jaw
      Hemorrhagic cyst of jaw
      Traumatic cyst of jaw

● M27.5   **Periradicular pathology associated with previous endodontic treatment**

   M27.51   **Perforation of root canal space due to endodontic treatment**

   M27.52   **Endodontic overfill**

   M27.53   **Endodontic underfill**

   M27.59   **Other periradicular pathology associated with previous endodontic treatment**

● M27.6   **Endosseous dental implant failure**

   M27.61   **Osseointegration failure of dental implant**
      Hemorrhagic complications of dental implant placement
      Iatrogenic osseointegration failure of dental implant
      Osseointegration failure of dental implant due to complications of systemic disease
      Osseointegration failure of dental implant due to poor bone quality
      Pre-integration failure of dental implant NOS
      Pre-osseointegration failure of dental implant

   M27.62   **Post-osseointegration biological failure of dental implant**
      Failure of dental implant due to lack of attached gingiva
      Failure of dental implant due to occlusal trauma (caused by poor prosthetic design)
      Failure of dental implant due to parafunctional habits
      Failure of dental implant due to periodontal infection (peri–implantitis)
      Failure of dental implant due to poor oral hygiene
      Iatrogenic post-osseointegration failure of dental implant
      Post-osseointegration failure of dental implant due to complications of systemic disease

   M27.63   **Post-osseointegration mechanical failure of dental implant**
      Failure of dental prosthesis causing loss of dental implant
      Fracture of dental implant

     Excludes2   cracked tooth (K03.81)
        fractured dental restorative material with loss of material (K08.531)
        fractured dental restorative material without loss of material (K08.530)
        fractured tooth (S02.5)

   M27.69   **Other endosseous dental implant failure**
      Dental implant failure NOS

● M27.8   **Other specified diseases of jaws**
      Cherubism
      Exostosis
      Fibrous dysplasia
      Unilateral condylar hyperplasia
      Unilateral condylar hypoplasia

     Excludes1   jaw pain (R68.84)

● M27.9   **Disease of jaws, unspecified**

SYSTEMIC CONNECTIVE TISSUE DISORDERS (M30-M36)

   Includes   autoimmune disease NOS
       collagen (vascular) disease NOS
       systemic autoimmune disease
       systemic collagen (vascular) disease

   Excludes1   autoimmune disease, single organ or single cell-type - code to relevant condition category

● M30   **Polyarteritis nodosa and related conditions**

   Excludes1   microscopic polyarteritis (M31.7)

   (Ex) **For category M30 CC codes unless otherwise indicated:** E08.51-E08.59, E08.618-E08.638, E08.649-E08.8, E09.51-E09.59, E09.618-E09.638, E09.649-E09.8, E10.51-E10.59, E10.618-E10.638, E10.649, E10.69-E10.8, E11.51-E11.59, E11.618-E11.638, E11.649, E11.69-E11.8, E13.51-E13.59, E13.618-E13.638, E13.649-E13.8, I87.8-I87.9, I99.8-I99.9, M30.0-M31.7

   M30.0   **Polyarteritis nodosa** 🅲

   M30.1   **Polyarteritis with lung involvement [Churg-Strauss]** 🅲
      Allergic granulomatous angiitis

   M30.2   **Juvenile polyarteritis** 🅲

   M30.3   **Mucocutaneous lymph node syndrome [Kawasaki]** 🅲
      (Ex) I87.8-I87.9, I99.8-I99.9, M30.0-M31.7

   M30.8   **Other conditions related to polyarteritis nodosa** 🅲
      Polyangiitis overlap syndrome

CHAPTER 13 (M00-M99)

● **M31   Other necrotizing vasculopathies**
> ⒺⓍ **For category M31 CC codes unless otherwise indicated:** See M30

     M31.0   Hypersensitivity angiitis 🔍
         Goodpasture's syndrome

     M31.1   Thrombotic microangiopathy 🔍
         Thrombotic thrombocytopenic purpura

     M31.2   Lethal midline granuloma 🔍

●   **M31.3   Wegener's granulomatosis**
         Necrotizing respiratory granulomatosis

         M31.30   Wegener's granulomatosis without renal involvement 🔍
                 Wegener's granulomatosis NOS

         M31.31   Wegener's granulomatosis with renal involvement 🔍

     M31.4   Aortic arch syndrome [Takayasu] 🔍

     M31.5   Giant cell arteritis with polymyalgia rheumatica

     M31.6   Other giant cell arteritis

     M31.7   Microscopic polyangiitis 🔍
         Microscopic polyarteritis
         Excludes1   polyarteritis nodosa (M30.0)

     M31.8   Other specified necrotizing vasculopathies 🔍
         Hypocomplementemic vasculitis
         Septic vasculitis
         ⒺⓍ I77.5, M31.8-M31.9

     M31.9   Necrotizing vasculopathy, unspecified 🔍
         ⒺⓍ I77.5, M31.8-M31.9

● **M32   Systemic lupus erythematosus (SLE)**
     Autoimmune inflammatory connective tissue disease of unknown cause that occurs most often in women
     Excludes1   lupus erythematosus (discoid) (NOS) (L93.0)

     M32.0   Drug-induced systemic lupus erythematosus
         Use additional code for adverse effect, if applicable, to identify drug (T36-T50 with fifth or sixth character 5)

●   **M32.1   Systemic lupus erythematosus with organ or system involvement**
         M32.10   Systemic lupus erythematosus, organ or system involvement unspecified

         M32.11   Endocarditis in systemic lupus erythematosus 🔍
                 Libman-Sacks disease
                 CC when PDx is its own CC
                 ⒺⓍ I38-I39, I87.8-I87.9, I99.8-I99.9

         M32.12   Pericarditis in systemic lupus erythematosus 🔍
                 Lupus pericarditis
                 CC when PDx is its own CC
                 ⒺⓍ I01.0, I09.2, I30.0-I30.9, I31.3-I32, I87.8-I87.9, I99.8-I99.9

         M32.13   Lung involvement in systemic lupus erythematosus
                 Pleural effusion due to systemic lupus erythematosus

         M32.14   Glomerular disease in systemic lupus erythematosus
                 Lupus renal disease NOS

         M32.15   Tubulo-interstitial nephropathy in systemic lupus erythematosus

         M32.19   Other organ or system involvement in systemic lupus erythematosus

     M32.8   Other forms of systemic lupus erythematosus

     M32.9   Systemic lupus erythematosus, unspecified
         SLE NOS
         Systemic lupus erythematosus NOS
         Systemic lupus erythematosus without organ involvement

● **M33   Dermatopolymyositis**
     ⒺⓍ **For category M33 CC codes unless otherwise indicated:** M33.00-M33.19, M33.90-M33.99, M36.0

●   **M33.0   Juvenile dermatopolymyositis**
         M33.00   Juvenile dermatopolymyositis, organ involvement unspecified 🔍

         M33.01   Juvenile dermatopolymyositis with respiratory involvement 🔍

         M33.02   Juvenile dermatopolymyositis with myopathy 🔍
                 CC when PDx is its own CC
                 ⒺⓍ E08.40-E08.49, E08.618-E08.638, E08.649-E08.8,
                     E09.40-E09.49, E09.618-E09.638, E09.649-E09.8,
                     E10.40-E10.49, E10.618-E10.638, E10.649, E10.69-E10.8,
                     E11.40-E11.49, E11.618-E11.638, E11.649, E11.69-E11.8,
                     E13.40-E13.49, E13.618-E13.638, E13.649-E13.8, G32.89,
                     G70.00-G72.3, G72.81-G73.7, G96.8-G96.9, G98.0-G98.8,
                     G99.8, M33.00-M33.19, M33.90-M33.99, M36.0

         M33.09   Juvenile dermatopolymyositis with other organ involvement 🔍

●   **M33.1   Other dermatopolymyositis**
         M33.10   Other dermatopolymyositis, organ involvement unspecified 🔍

         M33.11   Other dermatopolymyositis with respiratory involvement 🔍

         M33.12   Other dermatopolymyositis with myopathy 🔍
                 CC when PDx is its own CC
                 ⒺⓍ See M33.02

         M33.19   Other dermatopolymyositis with other organ involvement 🔍

●   **M33.2   Polymyositis**
         M33.20   Polymyositis, organ involvement unspecified 🔍
                 ⒺⓍ M33.20-M33.29

         M33.21   Polymyositis with respiratory involvement 🔍
                 ⒺⓍ M33.20-M33.29

         M33.22   Polymyositis with myopathy 🔍
                 CC when PDx is its own CC
                 ⒺⓍ E08.40-E08.49, E08.618-E08.638, E08.649-E08.8,
                     E09.40-E09.49, E09.618-E09.638, E09.649-E09.8,
                     E10.40-E10.49, E10.618-E10.638, E10.649, E10.69-E10.8,
                     E11.40-E11.49, E11.618-E11.638, E11.649, E11.69-E11.8,
                     E13.40-E13.49, E13.618-E13.638, E13.649-E13.8, G32.89,
                     G70.00-G72.3, G72.81-G73.7, G96.8-G96.9, G98.0-G98.8,
                     G99.8, M33.20-M33.29

         M33.29   Polymyositis with other organ involvement 🔍
                 ⒺⓍ M33.20-M33.29

●   **M33.9   Dermatopolymyositis, unspecified**
         M33.90   Dermatopolymyositis, unspecified, organ involvement unspecified 🔍

         M33.91   Dermatopolymyositis, unspecified with respiratory involvement 🔍

         M33.92   Dermatopolymyositis, unspecified with myopathy 🔍
                 CC when PDx is its own CC
                 ⒺⓍ See M33.02

         M33.99   Dermatopolymyositis, unspecified with other organ involvement 🔍

● **M34   Systemic sclerosis [scleroderma]**
     Excludes1   circumscribed scleroderma (L94.0)
                   neonatal scleroderma (P83.8)

     M34.0   Progressive systemic sclerosis

     M34.1   CR(E)ST syndrome
         Combination of calcinosis, Raynaud's phenomenon, esophageal dysfunction, sclerodactyly, telangiectasia

     M34.2   Systemic sclerosis induced by drug and chemical
         Code first poisoning due to drug or toxin, if applicable (T36-T65 with fifth or sixth character 1-4 or 6)
         Use additional code for adverse effect, if applicable, to identify drug (T36-T50 with fifth or sixth character 5)

◀ New   ◀◀ Revised   ~~deleted~~ Deleted   Excludes 1   Excludes 2   Includes   Use additional   Code first   Code also   Unspecified
OGCR Official Guidelines   ● Unacceptable Principal Diagnosis   X Assign placeholder X   ● Use Additional Character(s)   🔍 Manifestation Code   **Coding Clinic**

Item 13–8 Polymyalgia rheumatica is a syndrome characterized by aching and morning stiffness and is related to aging and hereditary predisposition.

● **M34.8 Other forms of systemic sclerosis**

 M34.81 Systemic sclerosis with lung involvement 🔹
  CC when PDx is its own CC
  (Ex:) No exclusions

 M34.82 Systemic sclerosis with myopathy 🔹
  CC when PDx is its own CC
  (Ex:) E08.40-E08.49, E08.618-E08.638, E08.649-E08.8,
   E09.40-E09.49, E09.618-E09.638, E09.649-E09.8,
   E10.40-E10.49, E10.618-E10.638, E10.649, E10.69-E10.8,
   E11.40-E11.49, E11.618-E11.638, E11.649, E11.69-E11.8,
   E13.40-E13.49, E13.618-E13.638, E13.649-E13.8, G32.89,
   G70.00-G72.3, G72.81-G73.7, G96.8-G96.9, G98.0-G98.8,
   G99.8

 M34.83 Systemic sclerosis with polyneuropathy

 M34.89 Other systemic sclerosis

 M34.9 Systemic sclerosis, unspecified

● **M35 Other systemic involvement of connective tissue**
  Excludes1 reactive perforating collagenosis (L87.1)

● **M35.0 Sicca syndrome [Sjögren]**

 M35.00 Sicca syndrome, unspecified

 M35.01 Sicca syndrome with keratoconjunctivitis

 M35.02 Sicca syndrome with lung involvement

 M35.03 Sicca syndrome with myopathy 🔹
  CC when PDx is its own CC
  (Ex:) See M34.82

 M35.04 Sicca syndrome with tubulo-interstitial nephropathy
  Renal tubular acidosis in sicca syndrome

 M35.09 Sicca syndrome with other organ involvement

 M35.1 Other overlap syndromes 🔹
  Mixed connective tissue disease
  Excludes1 polyangiitis overlap syndrome (M30.8)
  (Ex:) G72.41-G72.49, M35.1, M35.5, M35.8

 M35.2 Behçet's disease 🔹
  (Ex:) See M01.X

 M35.3 Polymyalgia rheumatica
  Excludes1 polymyalgia rheumatica with giant cell arteritis (M31.5)

 M35.4 Diffuse (eosinophilic) fasciitis

 M35.5 Multifocal fibrosclerosis 🔹
  (Ex:) G72.41-G72.49, M35.1, M35.5, M35.8

 M35.6 Relapsing panniculitis [Weber-Christian]
  Excludes1 lupus panniculitis (L93.2)
   panniculitis NOS (M79.3-)

 M35.7 Hypermobility syndrome
  Familial ligamentous laxity
  Excludes1 Ehlers-Danlos syndrome (Q79.6)
   ligamentous laxity, NOS (M24.2-)

 M35.8 Other specified systemic involvement of connective tissue 🔹
  (Ex:) G72.41-G72.49, M35.1, M35.5, M35.8

 M35.9 Systemic involvement of connective tissue, unspecified
  Autoimmune disease (systemic) NOS
  Collagen (vascular) disease NOS

● **M36 Systemic disorders of connective tissue in diseases classified elsewhere**
  Excludes2 arthropathies in diseases classified elsewhere (M14.-)

▶ *M36.0 Dermato(poly)myositis in neoplastic disease* 🔹
  Code first underlying neoplasm (C00-D49)
  (Ex:) M33.00-M33.19, M33.90-M33.99, M36.0

▶ *M36.1 Arthropathy in neoplastic disease*
  Code first underlying neoplasm, such as:
   leukemia (C91-C95)
   malignant histiocytosis (C96.A)
   multiple myeloma (C90.0)

▶ *M36.2 Hemophilic arthropathy*
  Hemarthrosis in hemophilic arthropathy
  Code first underlying disease, such as:
   factor VIII deficiency (D66)
   with vascular defect (D68.0)
   factor IX deficiency (D67)
   hemophilia (classical) (D66)
   hemophilia B (D67)
   hemophilia C (D68.1)

▶ *M36.3 Arthropathy in other blood disorders*

▶ *M36.4 Arthropathy in hypersensitivity reactions classified elsewhere*
  Code first underlying disease, such as:
   Henoch (-Schönlein) purpura (D69.0)
   serum sickness (T80.6-)

▶ *M36.8 Systemic disorders of connective tissue in other diseases classified elsewhere*
  Code first underlying disease, such as:
   alkaptonuria (E70.2)
   hypogammaglobulinemia (D80.-)
   ochronosis (E70.2)

DORSOPATHIES (M40-M54)

DEFORMING DORSOPATHIES (M40-M43)

● **M40 Kyphosis and lordosis**
  Excludes1 congenital kyphosis and lordosis (Q76.4)
   kyphoscoliosis (M41.-)
   postprocedural kyphosis and lordosis (M96.-)

● **M40.0 Postural kyphosis**
  Excludes1 osteochondrosis of spine (M42.-)

 M40.00 Postural kyphosis, site unspecified

 M40.03 Postural kyphosis, cervicothoracic region

 M40.04 Postural kyphosis, thoracic region

 M40.05 Postural kyphosis, thoracolumbar region

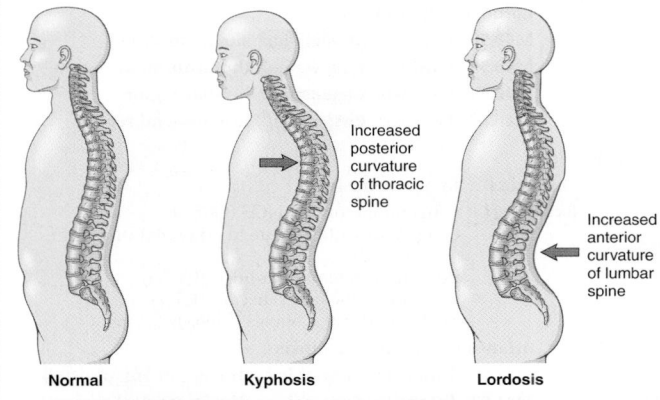

Increased posterior curvature of thoracic spine

Increased anterior curvature of lumbar spine

Normal   Kyphosis   Lordosis

Figure 13-5 Kyphosis, Lordosis, Scoliosis. (From Chabner: The Language of Medicine, ed 8, St. Louis, Saunders, 2007)

Item 13–9 Kyphosis is an abnormal curvature of the spine. **Senile kyphosis** is a result of disc degeneration causing ossification (turning to bone). **Adolescent** or **juvenile** kyphosis is also known as **Scheuermann's disease,** a condition in which the discs of the lower thoracic spine herniate, causing the disc space to narrow and the spine to tilt forward. This condition is attributed to poor posture. Lordosis or swayback is an abnormal curvature of the spine resulting in an inward curve of the lumbar spine just above the buttocks. Scoliosis causes a sideways curve to the spine. The curves are S- or C-shaped, and it is most commonly acquired in late childhood and early teen years, when growth is fast.

● **M40.1   Other secondary kyphosis**
   M40.10   Other secondary kyphosis, site unspecified
   M40.12   Other secondary kyphosis, cervical region
   M40.13   Other secondary kyphosis, cervicothoracic region
   M40.14   Other secondary kyphosis, thoracic region
   M40.15   Other secondary kyphosis, thoracolumbar region
● **M40.2   Other and unspecified kyphosis**
   ● **M40.20   Unspecified kyphosis**
      M40.202   Unspecified kyphosis, cervical region
      M40.203   Unspecified kyphosis, cervicothoracic region
      M40.204   Unspecified kyphosis, thoracic region
      M40.205   Unspecified kyphosis, thoracolumbar region
      M40.209   Unspecified kyphosis, site unspecified
   ● **M40.29   Other kyphosis**
      M40.292   Other kyphosis, cervical region
      M40.293   Other kyphosis, cervicothoracic region
      M40.294   Other kyphosis, thoracic region
      M40.295   Other kyphosis, thoracolumbar region
      M40.299   Other kyphosis, site unspecified
● **M40.3   Flatback syndrome**
   M40.30   Flatback syndrome, site unspecified
   M40.35   Flatback syndrome, thoracolumbar region
   M40.36   Flatback syndrome, lumbar region
   M40.37   Flatback syndrome, lumbosacral region
● **M40.4   Postural lordosis**
      Abnormal increase in the normal curvature of the lumbar spine (sway back)
      Acquired lordosis
   M40.40   Postural lordosis, site unspecified
   M40.45   Postural lordosis, thoracolumbar region
   M40.46   Postural lordosis, lumbar region
   M40.47   Postural lordosis, lumbosacral region
● **M40.5   Lordosis, unspecified**
   M40.50   Lordosis, unspecified, site unspecified
   M40.55   Lordosis, unspecified, thoracolumbar region
   M40.56   Lordosis, unspecified, lumbar region
   M40.57   Lordosis, unspecified, lumbosacral region

● **M41   Scoliosis**
Includes	kyphoscoliosis
Excludes1	congenital scoliosis NOS (Q67.5)
	congenital scoliosis due to bony malformation (Q76.3)
	postural congenital scoliosis (Q67.5)
	kyphoscoliotic heart disease (I27.1)
	postprocedural scoliosis (M96.-)
   ● **M41.0   Infantile idiopathic scoliosis**
      M41.00   Infantile idiopathic scoliosis, site unspecified
      M41.02   Infantile idiopathic scoliosis, cervical region
      M41.03   Infantile idiopathic scoliosis, cervicothoracic region

   M41.04   Infantile idiopathic scoliosis, thoracic region
   M41.05   Infantile idiopathic scoliosis, thoracolumbar region
   M41.06   Infantile idiopathic scoliosis, lumbar region
   M41.07   Infantile idiopathic scoliosis, lumbosacral region
   M41.08   Infantile idiopathic scoliosis, sacral and sacrococcygeal region
● **M41.1   Juvenile and adolescent idiopathic scoliosis**
   ● **M41.11   Juvenile idiopathic scoliosis**
      M41.112   Juvenile idiopathic scoliosis, cervical region
      M41.113   Juvenile idiopathic scoliosis, cervicothoracic region
      M41.114   Juvenile idiopathic scoliosis, thoracic region
      M41.115   Juvenile idiopathic scoliosis, thoracolumbar region
      M41.116   Juvenile idiopathic scoliosis, lumbar region
      M41.117   Juvenile idiopathic scoliosis, lumbosacral region
      M41.119   Juvenile idiopathic scoliosis, site unspecified
   ● **M41.12   Adolescent scoliosis**
      M41.122   Adolescent idiopathic scoliosis, cervical region
      M41.123   Adolescent idiopathic scoliosis, cervicothoracic region
      M41.124   Adolescent idiopathic scoliosis, thoracic region
      M41.125   Adolescent idiopathic scoliosis, thoracolumbar region
      M41.126   Adolescent idiopathic scoliosis, lumbar region
      M41.127   Adolescent idiopathic scoliosis, lumbosacral region
      M41.129   Adolescent idiopathic scoliosis, site unspecified
● **M41.2   Other idiopathic scoliosis**
   M41.20   Other idiopathic scoliosis, site unspecified
   M41.22   Other idiopathic scoliosis, cervical region
   M41.23   Other idiopathic scoliosis, cervicothoracic region
   M41.24   Other idiopathic scoliosis, thoracic region
   M41.25   Other idiopathic scoliosis, thoracolumbar region
   M41.26   Other idiopathic scoliosis, lumbar region
   M41.27   Other idiopathic scoliosis, lumbosacral region
● **M41.3   Thoracogenic scoliosis**
   M41.30   Thoracogenic scoliosis, site unspecified
   M41.34   Thoracogenic scoliosis, thoracic region
   M41.35   Thoracogenic scoliosis, thoracolumbar region
● **M41.4   Neuromuscular scoliosis**
      Scoliosis secondary to cerebral palsy, Friedreich's ataxia, poliomyelitis and other neuromuscular disorders
      Code also underlying condition
   M41.40   Neuromuscular scoliosis, site unspecified
   M41.41   Neuromuscular scoliosis, occipito-atlanto-axial region
   M41.42   Neuromuscular scoliosis, cervical region
   M41.43   Neuromuscular scoliosis, cervicothoracic region
   M41.44   Neuromuscular scoliosis, thoracic region
   M41.45   Neuromuscular scoliosis, thoracolumbar region
   M41.46   Neuromuscular scoliosis, lumbar region
   M41.47   Neuromuscular scoliosis, lumbosacral region

◀ New   ◀■ Revised   ~~deleted~~ Deleted   Excludes 1   Excludes 2   Includes   Use additional   Code first   Code also   Unspecified
OGCR Official Guidelines   ● Unacceptable Principal Diagnosis   X Assign placeholder X   ● Use Additional Character(s)   ▶ Manifestation Code   Coding Clinic
1032

● M41.5 Other secondary scoliosis
    M41.50 Other secondary scoliosis, site unspecified
    M41.52 Other secondary scoliosis, cervical region
    M41.53 Other secondary scoliosis, cervicothoracic region
    M41.54 Other secondary scoliosis, thoracic region
    M41.55 Other secondary scoliosis, thoracolumbar region
    M41.56 Other secondary scoliosis, lumbar region
    M41.57 Other secondary scoliosis, lumbosacral region
● M41.8 Other forms of scoliosis
    M41.80 Other forms of scoliosis, site unspecified
    M41.82 Other forms of scoliosis, cervical region
    M41.83 Other forms of scoliosis, cervicothoracic region
    M41.84 Other forms of scoliosis, thoracic region
    M41.85 Other forms of scoliosis, thoracolumbar region
    M41.86 Other forms of scoliosis, lumbar region
    M41.87 Other forms of scoliosis, lumbosacral region
  M41.9 Scoliosis, unspecified

● M42 Spinal osteochondrosis
● M42.0 Juvenile osteochondrosis of spine
    Calvé's disease
    Scheuermann's disease
    Excludes1 postural kyphosis (M40.0)
    M42.00 Juvenile osteochondrosis of spine, site unspecified
    M42.01 Juvenile osteochondrosis of spine, occipito-atlanto-axial region
    M42.02 Juvenile osteochondrosis of spine, cervical region
    M42.03 Juvenile osteochondrosis of spine, cervicothoracic region
    M42.04 Juvenile osteochondrosis of spine, thoracic region
    M42.05 Juvenile osteochondrosis of spine, thoracolumbar region
    M42.06 Juvenile osteochondrosis of spine, lumbar region
    M42.07 Juvenile osteochondrosis of spine, lumbosacral region
    M42.08 Juvenile osteochondrosis of spine, sacral and sacrococcygeal region
    M42.09 Juvenile osteochondrosis of spine, multiple sites in spine
● M42.1 Adult osteochondrosis of spine
    M42.10 Adult osteochondrosis of spine, site unspecified   A
    M42.11 Adult osteochondrosis of spine, occipitoatlanto-axial region   A
    M42.12 Adult osteochondrosis of spine, cervical region   A
    M42.13 Adult osteochondrosis of spine, cervicothoracic region   A
    M42.14 Adult osteochondrosis of spine, thoracic region   A
    M42.15 Adult osteochondrosis of spine, thoracolumbar region   A
    M42.16 Adult osteochondrosis of spine, lumbar region   A
    M42.17 Adult osteochondrosis of spine, lumbosacral region   A
    M42.18 Adult osteochondrosis of spine, sacral and sacrococcygeal region   A
    M42.19 Adult osteochondrosis of spine, multiple sites in spine   A
  M42.9 Spinal osteochondrosis, unspecified

Item 13–10 Spondylolisthesis is a condition caused by the slipping forward of one disc over another.

● M43 Other deforming dorsopathies
    Excludes1 congenital spondylolysis and spondylolisthesis (Q76.2)
      hemivertebra (Q76.3-Q76.4)
      Klippel-Feil syndrome (Q76.1)
      lumbarization and sacralization (Q76.4)
      platyspondylisis (Q76.4)
      spina bifida occulta (Q76.0)
      spinal curvature in osteoporosis (M80.-)
      spinal curvature in Paget's disease of bone [osteitis deformans] (M88.-)
● M43.0 Spondylolysis
    Excludes1 congenital spondylolysis (Q76.2)
      spondylolisthesis (M43.1)
    M43.00 Spondylolysis, site unspecified
    M43.01 Spondylolysis, occipito-atlanto-axial region
    M43.02 Spondylolysis, cervical region
    M43.03 Spondylolysis, cervicothoracic region
    M43.04 Spondylolysis, thoracic region
    M43.05 Spondylolysis, thoracolumbar region
    M43.06 Spondylolysis, lumbar region
    M43.07 Spondylolysis, lumbosacral region
    M43.08 Spondylolysis, sacral and sacrococcygeal region
    M43.09 Spondylolysis, multiple sites in spine
● M43.1 Spondylolisthesis
    Excludes1 acute traumatic of lumbosacral region (S33.1)
      acute traumatic of sites other than lumbosacral - code to Fracture, vertebra, by region
      congenital spondylolisthesis (Q76.2)
    M43.10 Spondylolisthesis, site unspecified
    M43.11 Spondylolisthesis, occipito-atlanto-axial region
    M43.12 Spondylolisthesis, cervical region
    M43.13 Spondylolisthesis, cervicothoracic region
    M43.14 Spondylolisthesis, thoracic region
    M43.15 Spondylolisthesis, thoracolumbar region
    M43.16 Spondylolisthesis, lumbar region
    M43.17 Spondylolisthesis, lumbosacral region
    M43.18 Spondylolisthesis, sacral and sacrococcygeal region
    M43.19 Spondylolisthesis, multiple sites in spine
● M43.2 Fusion of spine
    Ankylosis of spinal joint
    Excludes1 ankylosing spondylitis (M45.0-)
      congenital fusion of spine (Q76.4)
    Excludes2 arthrodesis status (Z98.1)
      pseudoarthrosis after fusion or arthrodesis (M96.0)
    M43.20 Fusion of spine, site unspecified
    M43.21 Fusion of spine, occipito-atlanto-axial region
    M43.22 Fusion of spine, cervical region
    M43.23 Fusion of spine, cervicothoracic region
    M43.24 Fusion of spine, thoracic region
    M43.25 Fusion of spine, thoracolumbar region
    M43.26 Fusion of spine, lumbar region
    M43.27 Fusion of spine, lumbosacral region
    M43.28 Fusion of spine, sacral and sacrococcygeal region
  M43.3 Recurrent atlantoaxial dislocation with myelopathy
  M43.4 Other recurrent atlantoaxial dislocation

CHAPTER 13 (M00-M99)

● **M43.5 Other recurrent vertebral dislocation**
> **Excludes1**   biomechanical lesions NEC (M99.-)

  ● **M43.5X Other recurrent vertebral dislocation**

    M43.5X2 Other recurrent vertebral dislocation, cervical region

    M43.5X3 Other recurrent vertebral dislocation, cervicothoracic region

    M43.5X4 Other recurrent vertebral dislocation, thoracic region

    M43.5X5 Other recurrent vertebral dislocation, thoracolumbar region

    M43.5X6 Other recurrent vertebral dislocation, lumbar region

    M43.5X7 Other recurrent vertebral dislocation, lumbosacral region

    M43.5X8 Other recurrent vertebral dislocation, sacral and sacrococcygeal region

    M43.5X9 Other recurrent vertebral dislocation, site unspecified

● **M43.6 Torticollis**
> **Excludes1**   congenital (sternomastoid) torticollis (Q68.0)
> current injury - see Injury, of spine, by body region ocular torticollis (R29.891)
> psychogenic torticollis (F45.8)
> spasmodic torticollis (G24.3)
> torticollis due to birth injury (P15.2)

● **M43.8 Other specified deforming dorsopathies**
> **Excludes2**   kyphosis and lordosis (M40.-)
> scoliosis (M41.-)

  ● **M43.8X Other specified deforming dorsopathies**

    M43.8X1 Other specified deforming dorsopathies, occipito-atlanto-axial region

    M43.8X2 Other specified deforming dorsopathies, cervical region

    M43.8X3 Other specified deforming dorsopathies, cervicothoracic region

    M43.8X4 Other specified deforming dorsopathies, thoracic region

    M43.8X5 Other specified deforming dorsopathies, thoracolumbar region

    M43.8X6 Other specified deforming dorsopathies, lumbar region

    M43.8X7 Other specified deforming dorsopathies, lumbosacral region

    M43.8X8 Other specified deforming dorsopathies, sacral and sacrococcygeal region

    M43.8X9 Other specified deforming dorsopathies, site unspecified

M43.9 Deforming dorsopathy, unspecified
> Curvature of spine NOS

SPONDYLOPATHIES (M45-M49)

● **M45 Ankylosing spondylitis**
> Rheumatoid arthritis of spine
> **Excludes1**   arthropathy in Reiter's disease (M02.3-)
> juvenile (ankylosing) spondylitis (M08.1)
> **Excludes2**   Behçet's disease (M35.2)

M45.0 Ankylosing spondylitis of multiple sites in spine

M45.1 Ankylosing spondylitis of occipito-atlanto-axial region

M45.2 Ankylosing spondylitis of cervical region

M45.3 Ankylosing spondylitis of cervicothoracic region

M45.4 Ankylosing spondylitis of thoracic region

M45.5 Ankylosing spondylitis of thoracolumbar region

M45.6 Ankylosing spondylitis lumbar region

M45.7 Ankylosing spondylitis of lumbosacral region

M45.8 Ankylosing spondylitis sacral and sacrococcygeal region

M45.9 Ankylosing spondylitis of unspecified sites in spine

● **M46 Other inflammatory spondylopathies**

  ● **M46.0 Spinal enthesopathy**
> Disorder of ligamentous or muscular attachments of spine

    M46.00 Spinal enthesopathy, site unspecified

    M46.01 Spinal enthesopathy, occipito-atlanto-axial region

    M46.02 Spinal enthesopathy, cervical region

    M46.03 Spinal enthesopathy, cervicothoracic region

    M46.04 Spinal enthesopathy, thoracic region

    M46.05 Spinal enthesopathy, thoracolumbar region

    M46.06 Spinal enthesopathy, lumbar region

    M46.07 Spinal enthesopathy, lumbosacral region

    M46.08 Spinal enthesopathy, sacral and sacrococcygeal region

    M46.09 Spinal enthesopathy, multiple sites in spine

M46.1 Sacroiliitis, not elsewhere classified

● **M46.2 Osteomyelitis of vertebra**
> (Ex) For category **M46.2** CC codes: A02.24, A17.9, A18.03, A18.09, A18.82, A18.84, A18.89, M46.20-M46.39, M86.00-M86.9

    M46.20 Osteomyelitis of vertebra, site unspecified

    M46.21 Osteomyelitis of vertebra, occipito-atlanto-axial region

    M46.22 Osteomyelitis of vertebra, cervical region

    M46.23 Osteomyelitis of vertebra, cervicothoracic region

    M46.24 Osteomyelitis of vertebra, thoracic region

    M46.25 Osteomyelitis of vertebra, thoracolumbar region

    M46.26 Osteomyelitis of vertebra, lumbar region

    M46.27 Osteomyelitis of vertebra, lumbosacral region

    M46.28 Osteomyelitis of vertebra, sacral and sacrococcygeal region

● **M46.3 Infection of intervertebral disc (pyogenic)**
> Use additional code (B95-B97) to identify infectious agent
> (Ex) For category **M46.3** CC codes: A17.9, A18.01, A18.03, A18.09, A18.82, A18.84, A18.89, M46.20-M46.39, M86.00-M86.9

    M46.30 Infection of intervertebral disc (pyogenic), site unspecified

    M46.31 Infection of intervertebral disc (pyogenic), occipito-atlanto-axial region

    M46.32 Infection of intervertebral disc (pyogenic), cervical region

    M46.33 Infection of intervertebral disc (pyogenic), cervicothoracic region

    M46.34 Infection of intervertebral disc (pyogenic), thoracic region

    M46.35 Infection of intervertebral disc (pyogenic), thoracolumbar region

    M46.36 Infection of intervertebral disc (pyogenic), lumbar region

    M46.37 Infection of intervertebral disc (pyogenic), lumbosacral region

    M46.38 Infection of intervertebral disc (pyogenic), sacral and sacrococcygeal region

    M46.39 Infection of intervertebral disc (pyogenic), multiple sites in spine

● **M46.4 Discitis, unspecified**

    M46.40 Discitis, unspecified, site unspecified

    M46.41 Discitis, unspecified, occipito-atlanto-axial region

    M46.42 Discitis, unspecified, cervical region

    M46.43 Discitis, unspecified, cervicothoracic region

    M46.44 Discitis, unspecified, thoracic region

M46.45   Discitis, unspecified, thoracolumbar region

M46.46   Discitis, unspecified, lumbar region

M46.47   Discitis, unspecified, lumbosacral region

M46.48   Discitis, unspecified, sacral and sacrococcygeal region

M46.49   Discitis, unspecified, multiple sites in spine

● M46.5   Other infective spondylopathies

M46.50   **Other infective spondylopathies, site unspecified**

M46.51   **Other infective spondylopathies, occipitoatlanto-axial region**

M46.52   **Other infective spondylopathies, cervical region**

M46.53   **Other infective spondylopathies, cervicothoracic region**

M46.54   **Other infective spondylopathies, thoracic region**

M46.55   **Other infective spondylopathies, thoracolumbar region**

M46.56   **Other infective spondylopathies, lumbar region**

M46.57   **Other infective spondylopathies, lumbosacral region**

M46.58   **Other infective spondylopathies, sacral and sacrococcygeal region**

M46.59   **Other infective spondylopathies, multiple sites in spine**

● M46.8   Other specified inflammatory spondylopathies

M46.80   **Other specified inflammatory spondylopathies, site unspecified**

M46.81   **Other specified inflammatory spondylopathies, occipito-atlanto-axial region**

M46.82   **Other specified inflammatory spondylopathies, cervical region**

M46.83   **Other specified inflammatory spondylopathies, cervicothoracic region**

M46.84   **Other specified inflammatory spondylopathies, thoracic region**

M46.85   **Other specified inflammatory spondylopathies, thoracolumbar region**

M46.86   **Other specified inflammatory spondylopathies, lumbar region**

M46.87   **Other specified inflammatory spondylopathies, lumbosacral region**

M46.88   **Other specified inflammatory spondylopathies, sacral and sacrococcygeal region**

M46.89   **Other specified inflammatory spondylopathies, multiple sites in spine**

● M46.9   Unspecified inflammatory spondylopathy

M46.90   **Unspecified inflammatory spondylopathy, site unspecified**

M46.91   **Unspecified inflammatory spondylopathy, occipito-atlanto-axial region**

M46.92   **Unspecified inflammatory spondylopathy, cervical region**

M46.93   **Unspecified inflammatory spondylopathy, cervicothoracic region**

M46.94   **Unspecified inflammatory spondylopathy, thoracic region**

M46.95   **Unspecified inflammatory spondylopathy, thoracolumbar region**

M46.96   **Unspecified inflammatory spondylopathy, lumbar region**

M46.97   **Unspecified inflammatory spondylopathy, lumbosacral region**

M46.98   **Unspecified inflammatory spondylopathy, sacral and sacrococcygeal region**

M46.99   **Unspecified inflammatory spondylopathy, multiple sites in spine**

● M47   Spondylosis

Includes   arthrosis or osteoarthritis of spine
degeneration of facet joints

● M47.0   Anterior spinal and vertebral artery compression syndromes

Ex: For category M47.0 CC codes: M47.011-M47.029, M47.11-M47.13, M47.21-M47.23, M47.811-M47.813, M47.891-M47.893

● M47.01   Anterior spinal artery compression syndromes

M47.011   **Anterior spinal artery compression syndromes, occipito-atlanto-axial region** 🔗

M47.012   **Anterior spinal artery compression syndromes, cervical region** 🔗

M47.013   **Anterior spinal artery compression syndromes, cervicothoracic region** 🔗

M47.014   **Anterior spinal artery compression syndromes, thoracic region** 🔗

M47.015   **Anterior spinal artery compression syndromes, thoracolumbar region** 🔗

M47.016   **Anterior spinal artery compression syndromes, lumbar region** 🔗

M47.019   **Anterior spinal artery compression syndromes, site unspecified** 🔗

● M47.02   Vertebral artery compression syndromes

M47.021   **Vertebral artery compression syndromes, occipito-atlanto-axial region** 🔗

M47.022   **Vertebral artery compression syndromes, cervical region** 🔗

M47.029   **Vertebral artery compression syndromes, site unspecified** 🔗

● M47.1   Other spondylosis with myelopathy

Spondylogenic compression of spinal cord

Excludes1   vertebral subluxation (M43.3-M43.59)

M47.10   **Other spondylosis with myelopathy, site unspecified** 🔗

Ex: M25.78, M47.011-M47.16, M47.20-M47.9, M48.10-M48.38, M48.9

M47.11   **Other spondylosis with myelopathy, occipito-atlanto-axial region** 🔗

Ex: See M47.0

M47.12   **Other spondylosis with myelopathy, cervical region** 🔗

Ex: See M47.0

M47.13   **Other spondylosis with myelopathy, cervicothoracic region** 🔗

Ex: See M47.0

M47.14   **Other spondylosis with myelopathy, thoracic region** 🔗

Ex: M47.14-M47.15

M47.15   **Other spondylosis with myelopathy, thoracolumbar region** 🔗

Ex: M47.14-M47.15

M47.16   **Other spondylosis with myelopathy, lumbar region** 🔗

Ex: M46.40, M46.46-M46.49, M47.16, M47.26-M47.28, M47.816-M47.818, M47.896-M47.898, M51.06, M51.26-M51.27, M51.36-M51.37, M51.46-M51.47, M51.86-M51.9

● M47.2   Other spondylosis with radiculopathy

M47.20   **Other spondylosis with radiculopathy, site unspecified**

M47.21   **Other spondylosis with radiculopathy, occipito-atlanto-axial region**

M47.22   **Other spondylosis with radiculopathy, cervical region**

M47.23   **Other spondylosis with radiculopathy, cervicothoracic region**

M47.24   **Other spondylosis with radiculopathy, thoracic region**

N Newborn Age: 0   **P** Pediatric Age: 0–17   **M** Maternity DX: 12–55   **A** Adult Age: 15–124   ♀ Females Only   ♂ Males Only

🔗 Complication\Comorbidity   🔗 Major C\C   Ex: CC/MCC Exclusions   🔗 Hospital-Acquired Condition

1035

M47.25   Other spondylosis with radiculopathy, thoracolumbar region

M47.26   Other spondylosis with radiculopathy, lumbar region

M47.27   Other spondylosis with radiculopathy, lumbosacral region

M47.28   Other spondylosis with radiculopathy, sacral and sacrococcygeal region

● M47.8   Other spondylosis

  ● M47.81   Spondylosis without myelopathy or radiculopathy

    M47.811   Spondylosis without myelopathy or radiculopathy, occipito-atlanto-axial region

    M47.812   Spondylosis without myelopathy or radiculopathy, cervical region

    M47.813   Spondylosis without myelopathy or radiculopathy, cervicothoracic region

    M47.814   Spondylosis without myelopathy or radiculopathy, thoracic region

    M47.815   Spondylosis without myelopathy or radiculopathy, thoracolumbar region

    M47.816   Spondylosis without myelopathy or radiculopathy, lumbar region

    M47.817   Spondylosis without myelopathy or radiculopathy, lumbosacral region

    M47.818   Spondylosis without myelopathy or radiculopathy, sacral and sacrococcygeal region

    M47.819   Spondylosis without myelopathy or radiculopathy, site unspecified

  ● M47.89   Other spondylosis

    M47.891   Other spondylosis, occipito-atlanto-axial region

    M47.892   Other spondylosis, cervical region

    M47.893   Other spondylosis, cervicothoracic region

    M47.894   Other spondylosis, thoracic region

    M47.895   Other spondylosis, thoracolumbar region

    M47.896   Other spondylosis, lumbar region

    M47.897   Other spondylosis, lumbosacral region

    M47.898   Other spondylosis, sacral and sacrococcygeal region

    M47.899   Other spondylosis, site unspecified

M47.9   Spondylosis, unspecified

● M48   Other spondylopathies

  ● M48.0   Spinal stenosis
    Caudal stenosis

    M48.00   Spinal stenosis, site unspecified

    M48.01   Spinal stenosis, occipito-atlanto-axial region

    M48.02   Spinal stenosis, cervical region

    M48.03   Spinal stenosis, cervicothoracic region

    M48.04   Spinal stenosis, thoracic region

    M48.05   Spinal stenosis, thoracolumbar region

    M48.06   Spinal stenosis, lumbar region

    M48.07   Spinal stenosis, lumbosacral region

    M48.08   Spinal stenosis, sacral and sacrococcygeal region

  ● M48.1   Ankylosing hyperostosis [Forestier]
    Diffuse idiopathic skeletal hyperostosis [DISH]

    M48.10   Ankylosing hyperostosis [Forestier], site unspecified

    M48.11   Ankylosing hyperostosis [Forestier], occipito-atlanto-axial region

    M48.12   Ankylosing hyperostosis [Forestier], cervical region

M48.13   Ankylosing hyperostosis [Forestier], cervicothoracic region

M48.14   Ankylosing hyperostosis [Forestier], thoracic region

M48.15   Ankylosing hyperostosis [Forestier], thoracolumbar region

M48.16   Ankylosing hyperostosis [Forestier], lumbar region

M48.17   Ankylosing hyperostosis [Forestier], lumbosacral region

M48.18   Ankylosing hyperostosis [Forestier], sacral and sacrococcygeal region

M48.19   Ankylosing hyperostosis [Forestier], multiple sites in spine

● M48.2   Kissing spine

  M48.20   Kissing spine, site unspecified

  M48.21   Kissing spine, occipito-atlanto-axial region

  M48.22   Kissing spine, cervical region

  M48.23   Kissing spine, cervicothoracic region

  M48.24   Kissing spine, thoracic region

  M48.25   Kissing spine, thoracolumbar region

  M48.26   Kissing spine, lumbar region

  M48.27   Kissing spine, lumbosacral region

● M48.3   Traumatic spondylopathy
  Ex For category M48.3 CC codes: M48.30–M48.38

  M48.30   Traumatic spondylopathy, site unspecified

  M48.31   Traumatic spondylopathy, occipito-atlanto-axial region

  M48.32   Traumatic spondylopathy, cervical region

  M48.33   Traumatic spondylopathy, cervicothoracic region

  M48.34   Traumatic spondylopathy, thoracic region

  M48.35   Traumatic spondylopathy, thoracolumbar region

  M48.36   Traumatic spondylopathy, lumbar region

  M48.37   Traumatic spondylopathy, lumbosacral region

  M48.38   Traumatic spondylopathy, sacral and sacrococcygeal region

● M48.4   Fatigue fracture of vertebra
  Stress fracture of vertebra

  Excludes1   pathological fracture NOS (M84.4-)
    pathological fracture of vertebra due to neoplasm (M84.58)
    pathological fracture of vertebra due to other diagnosis (M84.68)
    pathological fracture of vertebra due to osteoporosis (M80.-)
    traumatic fracture of vertebrae (S12.0-S12.3-, S22.0-, S32.0-)

The appropriate 7th character is to be added to each code from subcategory M48.4:

A	initial encounter for fracture
D	subsequent encounter for fracture with routine healing
G	subsequent encounter for fracture with delayed healing
S	sequela of fracture

X ● M48.40   Fatigue fracture of vertebra, site unspecified

X ● M48.41   Fatigue fracture of vertebra, occipitoatlanto-axial region

X ● M48.42   Fatigue fracture of vertebra, cervical region

X ● M48.43   Fatigue fracture of vertebra, cervicothoracic region

X ● M48.44   Fatigue fracture of vertebra, thoracic region

X ● M48.45   Fatigue fracture of vertebra, thoracolumbar region

◀ New   ◀▥ Revised   ~~deleted~~ Deleted   Excludes 1   Excludes 2   Includes   Use additional   Code first   Code also   Unspecified

OGCR Official Guidelines   ● Unacceptable Principal Diagnosis   X Assign placeholder X   ● Use Additional Character(s)   ▶ Manifestation Code   **Coding Clinic**

X● **M48.46**   **Fatigue fracture of vertebra, lumbar region**

X● **M48.47**   **Fatigue fracture of vertebra, lumbosacral region**

X● **M48.48**   **Fatigue fracture of vertebra, sacral and sacrococcygeal region**

● **M48.5**   **Collapsed vertebra, not elsewhere classified**
Collapsed vertebra NOS
Compression fracture of vertebra NOS ◄
Wedging of vertebra NOS

> **Excludes1**   current injury - see Injury of spine, by body region
> fatigue fracture of vertebra (M48.4)
> pathological fracture of vertebra due to neoplasm (M84.58)
> pathological fracture of vertebra due to other diagnosis (M84.68)
> pathological fracture of vertebra due to osteoporosis (M80.-)
> pathological fracture NOS (M84.4-)
> stress fracture of vertebra (M48.4-)
> traumatic fracture of vertebra (S12.-, S22.-, S32.-)

The appropriate 7th character is to be added to each code from subcategory M48.5:

> A   initial encounter for fracture
> D   subsequent encounter for fracture with routine healing
> G   subsequent encounter for fracture with delayed healing
> S   sequela of fracture

(Ex) **For category M48.5 CC codes:** M48.40X-M48.58X[A], M80.00X-M80.88X[A], M84.30X-M84.68X[A], M84.750-M84.759[A]

X● **M48.50**   **Collapsed vertebra, not elsewhere classified, site unspecified** A 🐾

X● **M48.51**   **Collapsed vertebra, not elsewhere classified, occipito-atlanto-axial region** A 🐾

X● **M48.52**   **Collapsed vertebra, not elsewhere classified, cervical region** A 🐾

X● **M48.53**   **Collapsed vertebra, not elsewhere classified, cervicothoracic region** A 🐾

X● **M48.54**   **Collapsed vertebra, not elsewhere classified, thoracic region** A 🐾

X● **M48.55**   **Collapsed vertebra, not elsewhere classified, thoracolumbar region** A 🐾

X● **M48.56**   **Collapsed vertebra, not elsewhere classified, lumbar region** A 🐾

X● **M48.57**   **Collapsed vertebra, not elsewhere classified, lumbosacral region** A 🐾

X● **M48.58**   **Collapsed vertebra, not elsewhere classified, sacral and sacrococcygeal region** A 🐾

● **M48.8**   **Other specified spondylopathies**
Ossification of posterior longitudinal ligament

  ● **M48.8X**   **Other specified spondylopathies**

     M48.8X1   **Other specified spondylopathies, occipito-atlanto-axial region**

     M48.8X2   **Other specified spondylopathies, cervical region**

     M48.8X3   **Other specified spondylopathies, cervicothoracic region**

     M48.8X4   **Other specified spondylopathies, thoracic region**

     M48.8X5   **Other specified spondylopathies, thoracolumbar region**

     M48.8X6   **Other specified spondylopathies, lumbar region**

     M48.8X7   **Other specified spondylopathies, lumbosacral region**

     M48.8X8   **Other specified spondylopathies, sacral and sacrococcygeal region**

     M48.8X9   **Other specified spondylopathies, site unspecified**

M48.9   **Spondylopathy, unspecified**

● **M49**   **Spondylopathies in diseases classified elsewhere**

> **Includes**   curvature of spine in diseases classified elsewhere
> deformity of spine in diseases classified elsewhere
> kyphosis in diseases classified elsewhere
> scoliosis in diseases classified elsewhere
> spondylopathy in diseases classified elsewhere

Code first underlying disease, such as:
   brucellosis (A23.-)
   Charcot-Marie-Tooth disease (G60.0)
   enterobacterial infections (A01-A04)
   osteitis fibrosa cystica (E21.0)

> **Excludes1**   curvature of spine in tuberculosis [Pott's] (A18.01)
> enteropathic arthropathies (M07.-)
> gonococcal spondylitis (A54.41)
> neuropathic [tabes dorsalis] spondylitis (A52.11)
> neuropathic spondylopathy in syringomyelia (G95.0)
> neuropathic spondylopathy in tabes dorsalis (A52.11)
> nonsyphilitic neuropathic spondylopathy NEC (G98.0)
> spondylitis in syphilis (acquired) (A52.77)
> tuberculous spondylitis (A18.01)
> typhoid fever spondylitis (A01.05)

● **M49.8**   **Spondylopathy in diseases classified elsewhere**

  ▷ *M49.80*   *Spondylopathy in diseases classified elsewhere, site unspecified*

  ▷ *M49.81*   *Spondylopathy in diseases classified elsewhere, occipito-atlanto-axial region*

  ▷ *M49.82*   *Spondylopathy in diseases classified elsewhere, cervical region*

  ▷ *M49.83*   *Spondylopathy in diseases classified elsewhere, cervicothoracic region*

  ▷ *M49.84*   *Spondylopathy in diseases classified elsewhere, thoracic region*

  ▷ *M49.85*   *Spondylopathy in diseases classified elsewhere, thoracolumbar region*

  ▷ *M49.86*   *Spondylopathy in diseases classified elsewhere, lumbar region*

  ▷ *M49.87*   *Spondylopathy in diseases classified elsewhere, lumbosacral region*

  ▷ *M49.88*   *Spondylopathy in diseases classified elsewhere, sacral and sacrococcygeal region*

  ▷ *M49.89*   *Spondylopathy in diseases classified elsewhere, multiple sites in spine*

OTHER DORSOPATHIES (M50-M54)

> **Excludes1**   current injury - see injury of spine by body region
> discitis NOS (M46.4-)

● **M50**   **Cervical disc disorders**
Note: Code to the most superior level of disorder.

> **Includes**   cervicothoracic disc disorders with cervicalgia
> cervicothoracic disc disorders

Coding Clinic: 2016, Q1, P17

● **M50.0**   **Cervical disc disorder with myelopathy**
(Ex) **For category M50.0 CC codes:** M50.00-M50.03, M50.20-M50.23

     M50.00   **Cervical disc disorder with myelopathy, unspecified cervical region** 🐾

     M50.01   **Cervical disc disorder with myelopathy, high cervical region** 🐾
C2-C3 disc disorder with myelopathy
C3-C4 disc disorder with myelopathy
Coding Clinic: 2016, Q1, P17

● M50.02 Cervical disc disorder with myelopathy, mid-cervical region
    M50.020 Cervical disc disorder with myelopathy, mid-cervical region, unspecified level ◐ ◀
    M50.021 Cervical disc disorder at C4-C5 level with myelopathy ◐ ◀
        C4-C5 disc disorder with myelopathy ◀
    M50.022 Cervical disc disorder at C5-C6 level with myelopathy ◐ ◀
        C5-C6 disc disorder with myelopathy ◀
    M50.023 Cervical disc disorder at C6-C7 level with myelopathy ◐ ◀
        C6-C7 disc disorder with myelopathy ◀
  M50.03 Cervical disc disorder with myelopathy, cervicothoracic region ◐
    C7-T1 disc disorder with myelopathy

● M50.1 Cervical disc disorder with radiculopathy
    Excludes2 brachial radiculitis NOS (M54.13)
  M50.10 Cervical disc disorder with radiculopathy, unspecified cervical region
  M50.11 Cervical disc disorder with radiculopathy, high cervical region
    C2-C3 disc disorder with radiculopathy
    C3 radiculopathy due to disc disorder
    C3-C4 disc disorder with radiculopathy
    C4 radiculopathy due to disc disorder
● M50.12 Cervical disc disorder with radiculopathy, mid-cervical region
    M50.120 Mid-cervical disc disorder, unspecified ◀
    M50.121 Cervical disc disorder at C4-C5 level with radiculopathy ◀
        C4-C5 disc disorder with radiculopathy ◀
        C5 radiculopathy due to disc disorder ◀
    M50.122 Cervical disc disorder at C5-C6 level with radiculopathy ◀
        C5-C6 disc disorder with radiculopathy ◀
        C6 radiculopathy due to disc disorder ◀
    M50.123 Cervical disc disorder at C6-C7 level with radiculopathy ◀
        C6-C7 disc disorder with radiculopathy ◀
        C7 radiculopathy due to disc disorder ◀
  M50.13 Cervical disc disorder with radiculopathy, cervicothoracic region
    C7-T1 disc disorder with radiculopathy
    C8 radiculopathy due to disc disorder

● M50.2 Other cervical disc displacement
  M50.20 Other cervical disc displacement, unspecified cervical region
  M50.21 Other cervical disc displacement, high cervical region
    Other C2-C3 cervical disc displacement
    Other C3-C4 cervical disc displacement
● M50.22 Other cervical disc displacement, mid-cervical region
    M50.220 Other cervical disc displacement, mid-cervical region, unspecified level ◀
    M50.221 Other cervical disc displacement at C4-C5 level ◀
        Other C4-C5 cervical disc displacement ◀
    M50.222 Other cervical disc displacement at C5-C6 level ◀
        Other C5-C6 cervical disc displacement ◀
    M50.223 Other cervical disc displacement at C6-C7 level ◀
        Other C6-C7 cervical disc displacement ◀
  M50.23 Other cervical disc displacement, cervicothoracic region
    Other C7-T1 cervical disc displacement

● M50.3 Other cervical disc degeneration
  M50.30 Other cervical disc degeneration, unspecified cervical region
  M50.31 Other cervical disc degeneration, high cervical region
    Other C2-C3 cervical disc degeneration
    Other C3-C4 cervical disc degeneration
● M50.32 Other cervical disc degeneration, mid-cervical region
    M50.320 Other cervical disc degeneration, mid-cervical region, unspecified level ◀
    M50.321 Other cervical disc degeneration at C4-C5 level ◀
        Other C4-C5 cervical disc degeneration ◀
    M50.322 Other cervical disc degeneration at C5-C6 level ◀
        Other C5-C6 cervical disc degeneration ◀
    M50.323 Other cervical disc degeneration at C6-C7 level ◀
        Other C6-C7 cervical disc degeneration ◀
  M50.33 Other cervical disc degeneration, cervicothoracic region
    Other C7-T1 cervical disc degeneration

● M50.8 Other cervical disc disorders
  M50.80 Other cervical disc disorders, unspecified cervical region
  M50.81 Other cervical disc disorders, high cervical region
    Other C2-C3 cervical disc disorders
    Other C3-C4 cervical disc disorders
● M50.82 Other cervical disc disorders, mid-cervical region
    M50.820 Other cervical disc disorders, mid-cervical region, unspecified level ◀
    M50.821 Other cervical disc disorders at C4-C5 level ◀
        Other C4-C5 cervical disc disorders ◀
    M50.822 Other cervical disc disorders at C5-C6 level ◀
        Other C5-C6 cervical disc disorders ◀
    M50.823 Other cervical disc disorders at C6-C7 level ◀
        Other C6-C7 cervical disc disorders ◀
  M50.83 Other cervical disc disorders, cervicothoracic region
    Other C7-T1 cervical disc disorders

◀ New   ◀▬ Revised   d̶e̶l̶e̶t̶e̶d̶ Deleted   Excludes 1   Excludes 2   Includes   Use additional   Code first   Code also   Unspecified
OGCR Official Guidelines   ● Unacceptable Principal Diagnosis   X Assign placeholder X   ◐ Use Additional Character(s)   ▶ Manifestation Code   **Coding Clinic**

● **M50.9   Cervical disc disorder, unspecified**

     M50.90   Cervical disc disorder, unspecified, unspecified cervical region

     M50.91   Cervical disc disorder, unspecified, high cervical region

         C2-C3 cervical disc disorder, unspecified

         C3-C4 cervical disc disorder, unspecified

     ● **M50.92   Cervical disc disorder, unspecified, mid-cervical region**

         M50.920   Unspecified cervical disc disorder, mid-cervical region, unspecified level ◄

         M50.921   Unspecified cervical disc disorder at C4-C5 level ◄

             Unspecified C4-C5 cervical disc disorder ◄

         M50.922   Unspecified cervical disc disorder at C5-C6 level ◄

             Unspecified C5-C6 cervical disc disorder ◄

         M50.923   Unspecified cervical disc disorder at C6-C7 level ◄

             Unspecified C6-C7 cervical disc disorder ◄

     M50.93   Cervical disc disorder, unspecified, cervicothoracic region

         C7-T1 cervical disc disorder, unspecified

● **M51   Thoracic, thoracolumbar, and lumbosacral intervertebral disc disorders**

     Excludes2   cervical and cervicothoracic disc disorders (M50.-)

                 sacral and sacrococcygeal disorders (M53.3)

   ● **M51.0   Thoracic, thoracolumbar and lumbosacral intervertebral disc disorders with myelopathy**

     (Ex) **For category M51.0 CC codes unless otherwise indicated:** M51.04-M51.05, M51.24-M51.25

     M51.04   Intervertebral disc disorders with myelopathy, thoracic region 🔖

     M51.05   Intervertebral disc disorders with myelopathy, thoracolumbar region 🔖

     M51.06   Intervertebral disc disorders with myelopathy, lumbar region 🔖

         (Ex) M51.06, M51.24-M51.25

   ● **M51.1   Thoracic, thoracolumbar and lumbosacral intervertebral disc disorders with radiculopathy**

     Sciatica due to intervertebral disc disorder

     Excludes1   lumbar radiculitis NOS (M54.16)

                 sciatica NOS (M54.3)

     M51.14   Intervertebral disc disorders with radiculopathy, thoracic region

     M51.15   Intervertebral disc disorders with radiculopathy, thoracolumbar region

     M51.16   Intervertebral disc disorders with radiculopathy, lumbar region

     M51.17   Intervertebral disc disorders with radiculopathy, lumbosacral region

   ● **M51.2   Other thoracic, thoracolumbar and lumbosacral intervertebral disc displacement**

     Lumbago due to displacement of intervertebral disc

     M51.24   Other intervertebral disc displacement, thoracic region

     M51.25   Other intervertebral disc displacement, thoracolumbar region

     M51.26   Other intervertebral disc displacement, lumbar region

     M51.27   Other intervertebral disc displacement, lumbosacral region

   ● **M51.3   Other thoracic, thoracolumbar and lumbosacral intervertebral disc degeneration**

     Coding Clinic: 2013, Q3, P22

     M51.34   Other intervertebral disc degeneration, thoracic region

     M51.35   Other intervertebral disc degeneration, thoracolumbar region

     M51.36   Other intervertebral disc degeneration, lumbar region

     M51.37   Other intervertebral disc degeneration, lumbosacral region

   ● **M51.4   Schmorl's nodes**

     M51.44   Schmorl's nodes, thoracic region

     M51.45   Schmorl's nodes, thoracolumbar region

     M51.46   Schmorl's nodes, lumbar region

     M51.47   Schmorl's nodes, lumbosacral region

   ● **M51.8   Other thoracic, thoracolumbar and lumbosacral intervertebral disc disorders**

     M51.84   Other intervertebral disc disorders, thoracic region

     M51.85   Other intervertebral disc disorders, thoracolumbar region

     M51.86   Other intervertebral disc disorders, lumbar region

     M51.87   Other intervertebral disc disorders, lumbosacral region

     M51.9   Unspecified thoracic, thoracolumbar and lumbosacral intervertebral disc disorder

● **M53   Other and unspecified dorsopathies, not elsewhere classified**

     M53.0   Cervicocranial syndrome

         Posterior cervical sympathetic syndrome

     M53.1   Cervicobrachial syndrome

         Excludes2   cervical disc disorder (M50.-)

                     thoracic outlet syndrome (G54.0)

   ● **M53.2   Spinal instabilities**

     ● **M53.2X   Spinal instabilities**

         M53.2X1   Spinal instabilities, occipito-atlanto-axial region

         M53.2X2   Spinal instabilities, cervical region

         M53.2X3   Spinal instabilities, cervicothoracic region

         M53.2X4   Spinal instabilities, thoracic region

         M53.2X5   Spinal instabilities, thoracolumbar region

         M53.2X6   Spinal instabilities, lumbar region

         M53.2X7   Spinal instabilities, lumbosacral region

         M53.2X8   Spinal instabilities, sacral and sacrococcygeal region

         M53.2X9   Spinal instabilities, site unspecified

     M53.3   Sacrococcygeal disorders, not elsewhere classified

         Coccygodynia

   ● **M53.8   Other specified dorsopathies**

     M53.80   Other specified dorsopathies, site unspecified

     M53.81   Other specified dorsopathies, occipito-atlanto-axial region

     M53.82   Other specified dorsopathies, cervical region

     M53.83   Other specified dorsopathies, cervicothoracic region

     M53.84   Other specified dorsopathies, thoracic region

     M53.85   Other specified dorsopathies, thoracolumbar region

     M53.86   Other specified dorsopathies, lumbar region

     M53.87   Other specified dorsopathies, lumbosacral region

     M53.88   Other specified dorsopathies, sacral and sacrococcygeal region

     M53.9   Dorsopathy, unspecified

CHAPTER 13 (M00-M99)

N   Newborn Age: 0   P   Pediatric Age: 0–17   M   Maternity DX: 12–55   A   Adult Age: 15–124   ♀   Females Only   ♂   Males Only

🔖   Complication\Comorbidity   🔖   Major C\C   (Ex)   CC/MCC Exclusions   🔖   Hospital-Acquired Condition

● **M54   Dorsalgia**
    Excludes1   psychogenic dorsalgia (F45.41)
● **M54.0   Panniculitis affecting regions of neck and back**
      Excludes1   lupus panniculitis (L93.2)
                panniculitis NOS (M79.3)
                relapsing [Weber-Christian] panniculitis
                   (M35.6)

    M54.00   Panniculitis affecting regions of neck and back, site unspecified

    M54.01   Panniculitis affecting regions of neck and back, occipito-atlanto-axial region

    M54.02   Panniculitis affecting regions of neck and back, cervical region

    M54.03   Panniculitis affecting regions of neck and back, cervicothoracic region

    M54.04   Panniculitis affecting regions of neck and back, thoracic region

    M54.05   Panniculitis affecting regions of neck and back, thoracolumbar region

    M54.06   Panniculitis affecting regions of neck and back, lumbar region

    M54.07   Panniculitis affecting regions of neck and back, lumbosacral region

    M54.08   Panniculitis affecting regions of neck and back, sacral and sacrococcygeal region

    M54.09   Panniculitis affecting regions, neck and back, multiple sites in spine

● **M54.1   Radiculopathy**
    Brachial neuritis or radiculitis NOS
    Lumbar neuritis or radiculitis NOS
    Lumbosacral neuritis or radiculitis NOS
    Thoracic neuritis or radiculitis NOS
    Radiculitis NOS
    Excludes1   neuralgia and neuritis NOS (M79.2)
                radiculopathy with cervical disc disorder
                  (M50.1)
                radiculopathy with lumbar and other
                  intervertebral disc disorder (M51.1-)
                radiculopathy with spondylosis (M47.2-)

    M54.10   Radiculopathy, site unspecified
    M54.11   Radiculopathy, occipito-atlanto-axial region
    M54.12   Radiculopathy, cervical region
    M54.13   Radiculopathy, cervicothoracic region
    M54.14   Radiculopathy, thoracic region
    M54.15   Radiculopathy, thoracolumbar region
    M54.16   Radiculopathy, lumbar region
    M54.17   Radiculopathy, lumbosacral region
    M54.18   Radiculopathy, sacral and sacrococcygeal region

● **M54.2   Cervicalgia**
    Excludes1   cervicalgia due to intervertebral cervical
                disc disorder (M50.-)

● **M54.3   Sciatica**
    Excludes1   lesion of sciatic nerve (G57.0)
                sciatica due to intervertebral disc disorder
                  (M51.1-)
                sciatica with lumbago (M54.4-)

    M54.30   Sciatica, unspecified side
    M54.31   Sciatica, right side
    M54.32   Sciatica, left side

● **M54.4   Lumbago with sciatica**
    Excludes1   lumbago with sciatica due to
                intervertebral disc disorder (M51.1-)

    M54.40   Lumbago with sciatica, unspecified side
    M54.41   Lumbago with sciatica, right side
    M54.42   Lumbago with sciatica, left side
            Coding Clinic: 2016, Q2, P7

M54.5   Low back pain
    Loin pain
    Lumbago NOS
    Excludes1   low back strain (S39.012)
                lumbago due to intervertebral disc
                  displacement (M51.2-)
                lumbago with sciatica (M54.4-)

M54.6   Pain in thoracic spine
    Excludes1   pain in thoracic spine due to
                intervertebral disc disorder (M51.)

● **M54.8   Other dorsalgia**
    Excludes1   dorsalgia in thoracic region (M54.6)
                low back pain (M54.5)

    M54.81   Occipital neuralgia
    M54.89   Other dorsalgia

M54.9   Dorsalgia, unspecified
    Backache NOS
    Back pain NOS

SOFT TISSUE DISORDERS (M60-M79)

DISORDERS OF MUSCLES (M60-M63)

Excludes1   dermatopolymyositis (M33.-)
            muscular dystrophies and myopathies (G71-G72)
            myopathy in amyloidosis (E85.-)
            myopathy in polyarteritis nodosa (M30.0)
            myopathy in rheumatoid arthritis (M05.32)
            myopathy in scleroderma (M34.-)
            myopathy in Sjögren's syndrome (M35.03)
            myopathy in systemic lupus erythematosus
              (M32.-)

● **M60   Myositis**
    Excludes2   inclusion body myositis [IBM] (G72.41)
● **M60.0   Infective myositis**
    Tropical pyomyositis
    Use additional code (B95-B97) to identify infectious
    agent
    Ex: **For category M60.0 CC codes:** K68.12, M60.000-M60.19, M61.00-M61.19,
    M61.30-M61.59, M62.3, M62.50-M62.59, M62.84, M62.89, M72.6

    ● **M60.00   Infective myositis, unspecified site**

      M60.000   Infective myositis, unspecified right arm 🔵
          Infective myositis, right upper limb NOS

      M60.001   Infective myositis, unspecified left arm 🔵
          Infective myositis, left upper limb NOS

      M60.002   Infective myositis, unspecified arm 🔵
          Infective myositis, upper limb NOS

      M60.003   Infective myositis, unspecified right leg 🔵
          Infective myositis, right lower limb NOS

      M60.004   Infective myositis, unspecified left leg 🔵
          Infective myositis, left lower limb NOS

      M60.005   Infective myositis, unspecified leg 🔵
          Infective myositis, lower limb NOS

      M60.009   Infective myositis, unspecified site 🔵

    ● **M60.01   Infective myositis, shoulder**
      M60.011   Infective myositis, right shoulder 🔵
      M60.012   Infective myositis, left shoulder 🔵
      M60.019   Infective myositis, unspecified shoulder 🔵

    ● **M60.02   Infective myositis, upper arm**
      M60.021   Infective myositis, right upper arm 🔵
      M60.022   Infective myositis, left upper arm 🔵
      M60.029   Infective myositis, unspecified upper arm 🔵

● **M60.03** Infective myositis, forearm
　　M60.031 Infective myositis, right forearm 🗐
　　M60.032 Infective myositis, left forearm 🗐
　　M60.039 Infective myositis, unspecified
　　　　　　forearm 🗐
● **M60.04** Infective myositis, hand and fingers
　　M60.041 Infective myositis, right hand 🗐
　　M60.042 Infective myositis, left hand 🗐
　　M60.043 Infective myositis, unspecified
　　　　　　hand 🗐
　　M60.044 Infective myositis, right finger(s) 🗐
　　M60.045 Infective myositis, left finger(s) 🗐
　　M60.046 Infective myositis, unspecified
　　　　　　finger(s) 🗐
● **M60.05** Infective myositis, thigh
　　M60.051 Infective myositis, right thigh 🗐
　　M60.052 Infective myositis, left thigh 🗐
　　M60.059 Infective myositis, unspecified
　　　　　　thigh 🗐
● **M60.06** Infective myositis, lower leg
　　M60.061 Infective myositis, right lower leg 🗐
　　M60.062 Infective myositis, left lower leg 🗐
　　M60.069 Infective myositis, unspecified lower
　　　　　　leg 🗐
● **M60.07** Infective myositis, ankle, foot and toes
　　M60.070 Infective myositis, right ankle 🗐
　　M60.071 Infective myositis, left ankle 🗐
　　M60.072 Infective myositis, unspecified
　　　　　　ankle 🗐
　　M60.073 Infective myositis, right foot 🗐
　　M60.074 Infective myositis, left foot 🗐
　　M60.075 Infective myositis, unspecified foot 🗐
　　M60.076 Infective myositis, right toe(s) 🗐
　　M60.077 Infective myositis, left toe(s) 🗐
　　M60.078 Infective myositis, unspecified
　　　　　　toe(s) 🗐
　　M60.08 Infective myositis, other site 🗐
　　M60.09 Infective myositis, multiple sites 🗐
● **M60.1** Interstitial myositis
　　M60.10 Interstitial myositis of unspecified site
● **M60.11** Interstitial myositis, shoulder
　　M60.111 Interstitial myositis, right shoulder
　　M60.112 Interstitial myositis, left shoulder
　　M60.119 Interstitial myositis, unspecified
　　　　　　shoulder
● **M60.12** Interstitial myositis, upper arm
　　M60.121 Interstitial myositis, right upper arm
　　M60.122 Interstitial myositis, left upper arm
　　M60.129 Interstitial myositis, unspecified
　　　　　　upper arm
● **M60.13** Interstitial myositis, forearm
　　M60.131 Interstitial myositis, right forearm
　　M60.132 Interstitial myositis, left forearm
　　M60.139 Interstitial myositis, unspecified
　　　　　　forearm
● **M60.14** Interstitial myositis, hand
　　M60.141 Interstitial myositis, right hand
　　M60.142 Interstitial myositis, left hand
　　M60.149 Interstitial myositis, unspecified hand
● **M60.15** Interstitial myositis, thigh
　　M60.151 Interstitial myositis, right thigh
　　M60.152 Interstitial myositis, left thigh
　　M60.159 Interstitial myositis, unspecified thigh

● **M60.16** Interstitial myositis, lower leg
　　M60.161 Interstitial myositis, right lower leg
　　M60.162 Interstitial myositis, left lower leg
　　M60.169 Interstitial myositis, unspecified
　　　　　　lower leg
● **M60.17** Interstitial myositis, ankle and foot
　　M60.171 Interstitial myositis, right ankle and
　　　　　　foot
　　M60.172 Interstitial myositis, left ankle and
　　　　　　foot
　　M60.179 Interstitial myositis, unspecified
　　　　　　ankle and foot
　　M60.18 Interstitial myositis, other site
　　M60.19 Interstitial myositis, multiple sites
● **M60.2** Foreign body granuloma of soft tissue, not elsewhere
classified
　　　Use additional code to identify the type of retained
　　　foreign body (Z18.-)
　　　Excludes1　　foreign body granuloma of skin and
　　　　　　　　　　　subcutaneous tissue (L92.3)
　　M60.20 Foreign body granuloma of soft tissue, not
　　　　　　elsewhere classified, unspecified site
● **M60.21** Foreign body granuloma of soft tissue, not
elsewhere classified, shoulder
　　M60.211 Foreign body granuloma of soft
　　　　　　tissue, not elsewhere classified, right
　　　　　　shoulder
　　M60.212 Foreign body granuloma of soft
　　　　　　tissue, not elsewhere classified, left
　　　　　　shoulder
　　M60.219 Foreign body granuloma of soft
　　　　　　tissue, not elsewhere classified,
　　　　　　unspecified shoulder
● **M60.22** Foreign body granuloma of soft tissue, not
elsewhere classified, upper arm
　　M60.221 Foreign body granuloma of soft
　　　　　　tissue, not elsewhere classified, right
　　　　　　upper arm
　　M60.222 Foreign body granuloma of soft
　　　　　　tissue, not elsewhere classified, left
　　　　　　upper arm
　　M60.229 Foreign body granuloma of soft
　　　　　　tissue, not elsewhere classified,
　　　　　　unspecified upper arm
● **M60.23** Foreign body granuloma of soft tissue, not
elsewhere classified, forearm
　　M60.231 Foreign body granuloma of soft
　　　　　　tissue, not elsewhere classified, right
　　　　　　forearm
　　M60.232 Foreign body granuloma of soft
　　　　　　tissue, not elsewhere classified, left
　　　　　　forearm
　　M60.239 Foreign body granuloma of soft
　　　　　　tissue, not elsewhere classified,
　　　　　　unspecified forearm
● **M60.24** Foreign body granuloma of soft tissue, not
elsewhere classified, hand
　　M60.241 Foreign body granuloma of soft tissue,
　　　　　　not elsewhere classified, right hand
　　M60.242 Foreign body granuloma of soft
　　　　　　tissue, not elsewhere classified, left
　　　　　　hand
　　M60.249 Foreign body granuloma of soft
　　　　　　tissue, not elsewhere classified,
　　　　　　unspecified hand

CHAPTER 13 (M00-M99)

N Newborn Age: 0　　**P** Pediatric Age: 0–17　　**M** Maternity DX: 12–55　　**A** Adult Age: 15–124　　♀ Females Only　　♂ Males Only
🗐 Complication\Comorbidity　　🗐 Major C\C　　(Ex) CC/MCC Exclusions　　🗐 Hospital-Acquired Condition

1041

● M60.25   Foreign body granuloma of soft tissue, not elsewhere classified, thigh

     M60.251   Foreign body granuloma of soft tissue, not elsewhere classified, right thigh

     M60.252   Foreign body granuloma of soft tissue, not elsewhere classified, left thigh

     M60.259   Foreign body granuloma of soft tissue, not elsewhere classified, unspecified thigh

● M60.26   Foreign body granuloma of soft tissue, not elsewhere classified, lower leg

     M60.261   Foreign body granuloma of soft tissue, not elsewhere classified, right lower leg

     M60.262   Foreign body granuloma of soft tissue, not elsewhere classified, left lower leg

     M60.269   Foreign body granuloma of soft tissue, not elsewhere classified, unspecified lower leg

● M60.27   Foreign body granuloma of soft tissue, not elsewhere classified, ankle and foot

     M60.271   Foreign body granuloma of soft tissue, not elsewhere classified, right ankle and foot

     M60.272   Foreign body granuloma of soft tissue, not elsewhere classified, left ankle and foot

     M60.279   Foreign body granuloma of soft tissue, not elsewhere classified, unspecified ankle and foot

   M60.28   Foreign body granuloma of soft tissue, not elsewhere classified, other site

● M60.8   Other myositis

   M60.80   Other myositis, unspecified site

● M60.81   Other myositis shoulder

     M60.811   Other myositis, right shoulder

     M60.812   Other myositis, left shoulder

     M60.819   Other myositis, unspecified shoulder

● M60.82   Other myositis, upper arm

     M60.821   Other myositis, right upper arm

     M60.822   Other myositis, left upper arm

     M60.829   Other myositis, unspecified upper arm

● M60.83   Other myositis, forearm

     M60.831   Other myositis, right forearm

     M60.832   Other myositis, left forearm

     M60.839   Other myositis, unspecified forearm

● M60.84   Other myositis, hand

     M60.841   Other myositis, right hand

     M60.842   Other myositis, left hand

     M60.849   Other myositis, unspecified hand

● M60.85   Other myositis, thigh

     M60.851   Other myositis, right thigh

     M60.852   Other myositis, left thigh

     M60.859   Other myositis, unspecified thigh

● M60.86   Other myositis, lower leg

     M60.861   Other myositis, right lower leg

     M60.862   Other myositis, left lower leg

     M60.869   Other myositis, unspecified lower leg

● M60.87   Other myositis, ankle and foot

     M60.871   Other myositis, right ankle and foot

     M60.872   Other myositis, left ankle and foot

     M60.879   Other myositis, unspecified ankle and foot

   M60.88   Other myositis, other site

   M60.89   Other myositis, multiple sites

● M60.9   Myositis, unspecified

● M61   Calcification and ossification of muscle

● M61.0   Myositis ossificans traumatica

   M61.00   Myositis ossificans traumatica, unspecified site

● M61.01   Myositis ossificans traumatica, shoulder

     M61.011   Myositis ossificans traumatica, right shoulder

     M61.012   Myositis ossificans traumatica, left shoulder

     M61.019   Myositis ossificans traumatica, unspecified shoulder

● M61.02   Myositis ossificans traumatica, upper arm

     M61.021   Myositis ossificans traumatica, right upper arm

     M61.022   Myositis ossificans traumatica, left upper arm

     M61.029   Myositis ossificans traumatica, unspecified upper arm

● M61.03   Myositis ossificans traumatica, forearm

     M61.031   Myositis ossificans traumatica, right forearm

     M61.032   Myositis ossificans traumatica, left forearm

     M61.039   Myositis ossificans traumatica, unspecified forearm

● M61.04   Myositis ossificans traumatica, hand

     M61.041   Myositis ossificans traumatica, right hand

     M61.042   Myositis ossificans traumatica, left hand

     M61.049   Myositis ossificans traumatica, unspecified hand

● M61.05   Myositis ossificans traumatica, thigh

     M61.051   Myositis ossificans traumatica, right thigh

     M61.052   Myositis ossificans traumatica, left thigh

     M61.059   Myositis ossificans traumatica, unspecified thigh

● M61.06   Myositis ossificans traumatica, lower leg

     M61.061   Myositis ossificans traumatica, right lower leg

     M61.062   Myositis ossificans traumatica, left lower leg

     M61.069   Myositis ossificans traumatica, unspecified lower leg

● M61.07   Myositis ossificans traumatica, ankle and foot

     M61.071   Myositis ossificans traumatica, right ankle and foot

     M61.072   Myositis ossificans traumatica, left ankle and foot

     M61.079   Myositis ossificans traumatica, unspecified ankle and foot

   M61.08   Myositis ossificans traumatica, other site

   M61.09   Myositis ossificans traumatica, multiple sites

● M61.1   Myositis ossificans progressiva

     Fibrodysplasia ossificans progressiva

   M61.10   Myositis ossificans progressiva, unspecified site

● M61.11   Myositis ossificans progressiva, shoulder

     M61.111   Myositis ossificans progressiva, right shoulder

     M61.112   Myositis ossificans progressiva, left shoulder

     M61.119   Myositis ossificans progressiva, unspecified shoulder

◀ New   ◀▥ Revised   ~~deleted~~ Deleted   Excludes 1   Excludes 2   Includes   Use additional   Code first   Code also   Unspecified

OGCR Official Guidelines   ● Unacceptable Principal Diagnosis   X Assign placeholder X   ● Use Additional Character(s)   ▶ Manifestation Code   **Coding Clinic**

● **M61.12** Myositis ossificans progressiva, upper arm
     M61.121 Myositis ossificans progressiva, right upper arm
     M61.122 Myositis ossificans progressiva, left upper arm
     M61.129 Myositis ossificans progressiva, unspecified arm

● **M61.13** Myositis ossificans progressiva, forearm
     M61.131 Myositis ossificans progressiva, right forearm
     M61.132 Myositis ossificans progressiva, left forearm
     M61.139 Myositis ossificans progressiva, unspecified forearm

● **M61.14** Myositis ossificans progressiva, hand and finger(s)
     M61.141 Myositis ossificans progressiva, right hand
     M61.142 Myositis ossificans progressiva, left hand
     M61.143 Myositis ossificans progressiva, unspecified hand
     M61.144 Myositis ossificans progressiva, right finger(s)
     M61.145 Myositis ossificans progressiva, left finger(s)
     M61.146 Myositis ossificans progressiva, unspecified finger(s)

● **M61.15** Myositis ossificans progressiva, thigh
     M61.151 Myositis ossificans progressiva, right thigh
     M61.152 Myositis ossificans progressiva, left thigh
     M61.159 Myositis ossificans progressiva, unspecified thigh

● **M61.16** Myositis ossificans progressiva, lower leg
     M61.161 Myositis ossificans progressiva, right lower leg
     M61.162 Myositis ossificans progressiva, left lower leg
     M61.169 Myositis ossificans progressiva, unspecified lower leg

● **M61.17** Myositis ossificans progressiva, ankle, foot and toe(s)
     M61.171 Myositis ossificans progressiva, right ankle
     M61.172 Myositis ossificans progressiva, left ankle
     M61.173 Myositis ossificans progressiva, unspecified ankle
     M61.174 Myositis ossificans progressiva, right foot
     M61.175 Myositis ossificans progressiva, left foot
     M61.176 Myositis ossificans progressiva, unspecified foot
     M61.177 Myositis ossificans progressiva, right toe(s)
     M61.178 Myositis ossificans progressiva, left toe(s)
     M61.179 Myositis ossificans progressiva, unspecified toe(s)

M61.18 Myositis ossificans progressiva, other site
M61.19 Myositis ossificans progressiva, multiple sites

● **M61.2** Paralytic calcification and ossification of muscle
     Myositis ossificans associated with quadriplegia or paraplegia
     M61.20 Paralytic calcification and ossification of muscle, unspecified site
●   **M61.21** Paralytic calcification and ossification of muscle, shoulder
         M61.211 Paralytic calcification and ossification of muscle, right shoulder
         M61.212 Paralytic calcification and ossification of muscle, left shoulder
         M61.219 Paralytic calcification and ossification of muscle, unspecified shoulder
●   **M61.22** Paralytic calcification and ossification of muscle, upper arm
         M61.221 Paralytic calcification and ossification of muscle, right upper arm
         M61.222 Paralytic calcification and ossification of muscle, left upper arm
         M61.229 Paralytic calcification and ossification of muscle, unspecified upper arm
●   **M61.23** Paralytic calcification and ossification of muscle, forearm
         M61.231 Paralytic calcification and ossification of muscle, right forearm
         M61.232 Paralytic calcification and ossification of muscle, left forearm
         M61.239 Paralytic calcification and ossification of muscle, unspecified forearm
●   **M61.24** Paralytic calcification and ossification of muscle, hand
         M61.241 Paralytic calcification and ossification of muscle, right hand
         M61.242 Paralytic calcification and ossification of muscle, left hand
         M61.249 Paralytic calcification and ossification of muscle, unspecified hand
●   **M61.25** Paralytic calcification and ossification of muscle, thigh
         M61.251 Paralytic calcification and ossification of muscle, right thigh
         M61.252 Paralytic calcification and ossification of muscle, left thigh
         M61.259 Paralytic calcification and ossification of muscle, unspecified thigh
●   **M61.26** Paralytic calcification and ossification of muscle, lower leg
         M61.261 Paralytic calcification and ossification of muscle, right lower leg
         M61.262 Paralytic calcification and ossification of muscle, left lower leg
         M61.269 Paralytic calcification and ossification of muscle, unspecified lower leg
●   **M61.27** Paralytic calcification and ossification of muscle, ankle and foot
         M61.271 Paralytic calcification and ossification of muscle, right ankle and foot
         M61.272 Paralytic calcification and ossification of muscle, left ankle and foot
         M61.279 Paralytic calcification and ossification of muscle, unspecified ankle and foot
     M61.28 Paralytic calcification and ossification of muscle, other site
     M61.29 Paralytic calcification and ossification of muscle, multiple sites

N Newborn Age: 0   **P** Pediatric Age: 0–17   **M** Maternity DX: 12–55   **A** Adult Age: 15–124   ♀ Females Only   ♂ Males Only

 Complication\Comorbidity   Major C\C   Ⓔₓ CC/MCC Exclusions   Hospital-Acquired Condition

1043

● M61.3 Calcification and ossification of muscles associated with burns
> Myositis ossificans associated with burns

M61.30 Calcification and ossification of muscles associated with burns, unspecified site

● M61.31 Calcification and ossification of muscles associated with burns, shoulder

M61.311 Calcification and ossification of muscles associated with burns, right shoulder

M61.312 Calcification and ossification of muscles associated with burns, left shoulder

M61.319 Calcification and ossification of muscles associated with burns, unspecified shoulder

● M61.32 Calcification and ossification of muscles associated with burns, upper arm

M61.321 Calcification and ossification of muscles associated with burns, right upper arm

M61.322 Calcification and ossification of muscles associated with burns, left upper arm

M61.329 Calcification and ossification of muscles associated with burns, unspecified upper arm

● M61.33 Calcification and ossification of muscles associated with burns, forearm

M61.331 Calcification and ossification of muscles associated with burns, right forearm

M61.332 Calcification and ossification of muscles associated with burns, left forearm

M61.339 Calcification and ossification of muscles associated with burns, unspecified forearm

● M61.34 Calcification and ossification of muscles associated with burns, hand

M61.341 Calcification and ossification of muscles associated with burns, right hand

M61.342 Calcification and ossification of muscles associated with burns, left hand

M61.349 Calcification and ossification of muscles associated with burns, unspecified hand

● M61.35 Calcification and ossification of muscles associated with burns, thigh

M61.351 Calcification and ossification of muscles associated with burns, right thigh

M61.352 Calcification and ossification of muscles associated with burns, left thigh

M61.359 Calcification and ossification of muscles associated with burns, unspecified thigh

● M61.36 Calcification and ossification of muscles associated with burns, lower leg

M61.361 Calcification and ossification of muscles associated with burns, right lower leg

M61.362 Calcification and ossification of muscles associated with burns, left lower leg

M61.369 Calcification and ossification of muscles associated with burns, unspecified lower leg

● M61.37 Calcification and ossification of muscles associated with burns, ankle and foot

M61.371 Calcification and ossification of muscles associated with burns, right ankle and foot

M61.372 Calcification and ossification of muscles associated with burns, left ankle and foot

M61.379 Calcification and ossification of muscles associated with burns, unspecified ankle and foot

M61.38 Calcification and ossification of muscles associated with burns, other site

M61.39 Calcification and ossification of muscles associated with burns, multiple sites

● M61.4 Other calcification of muscle

> **Excludes1** calcific tendinitis NOS (M65.2-)
> calcific tendinitis of shoulder (M75.3)

M61.40 Other calcification of muscle, unspecified site

● M61.41 Other calcification of muscle, shoulder

M61.411 Other calcification of muscle, right shoulder

M61.412 Other calcification of muscle, left shoulder

M61.419 Other calcification of muscle, unspecified shoulder

● M61.42 Other calcification of muscle, upper arm

M61.421 Other calcification of muscle, right upper arm

M61.422 Other calcification of muscle, left upper arm

M61.429 Other calcification of muscle, unspecified upper arm

● M61.43 Other calcification of muscle, forearm

M61.431 Other calcification of muscle, right forearm

M61.432 Other calcification of muscle, left forearm

M61.439 Other calcification of muscle, unspecified forearm

● M61.44 Other calcification of muscle, hand

M61.441 Other calcification of muscle, right hand

M61.442 Other calcification of muscle, left hand

M61.449 Other calcification of muscle, unspecified hand

● M61.45 Other calcification of muscle, thigh

M61.451 Other calcification of muscle, right thigh

M61.452 Other calcification of muscle, left thigh

M61.459 Other calcification of muscle, unspecified thigh

● M61.46 Other calcification of muscle, lower leg

M61.461 Other calcification of muscle, right lower leg

M61.462 Other calcification of muscle, left lower leg

M61.469 Other calcification of muscle, unspecified lower leg

● M61.47 Other calcification of muscle, ankle and foot

M61.471 Other calcification of muscle, right ankle and foot

M61.472 Other calcification of muscle, left ankle and foot

M61.479 Other calcification of muscle, unspecified ankle and foot

M61.48 Other calcification of muscle, other site

M61.49 Other calcification of muscle, multiple sites

◀ New   ◀▥ Revised   ~~deleted~~ Deleted   Excludes 1   Excludes 2   Includes   Use additional   Code first   Code also   Unspecified
OGCR Official Guidelines   ● Unacceptable Principal Diagnosis   X Assign placeholder X   ● Use Additional Character(s)   ▶ Manifestation Code   **Coding Clinic**

● M61.5 Other ossification of muscle

   M61.50 Other ossification of muscle, unspecified site

● M61.51 Other ossification of muscle, shoulder

   M61.511 Other ossification of muscle, right shoulder

   M61.512 Other ossification of muscle, left shoulder

   M61.519 Other ossification of muscle, unspecified shoulder

● M61.52 Other ossification of muscle, upper arm

   M61.521 Other ossification of muscle, right upper arm

   M61.522 Other ossification of muscle, left upper arm

   M61.529 Other ossification of muscle, unspecified upper arm

● M61.53 Other ossification of muscle, forearm

   M61.531 Other ossification of muscle, right forearm

   M61.532 Other ossification of muscle, left forearm

   M61.539 Other ossification of muscle, unspecified forearm

● M61.54 Other ossification of muscle, hand

   M61.541 Other ossification of muscle, right hand

   M61.542 Other ossification of muscle, left hand

   M61.549 Other ossification of muscle, unspecified hand

● M61.55 Other ossification of muscle, thigh

   M61.551 Other ossification of muscle, right thigh

   M61.552 Other ossification of muscle, left thigh

   M61.559 Other ossification of muscle, unspecified thigh

● M61.56 Other ossification of muscle, lower leg

   M61.561 Other ossification of muscle, right lower leg

   M61.562 Other ossification of muscle, left lower leg

   M61.569 Other ossification of muscle, unspecified lower leg

● M61.57 Other ossification of muscle, ankle and foot

   M61.571 Other ossification of muscle, right ankle and foot

   M61.572 Other ossification of muscle, left ankle and foot

   M61.579 Other ossification of muscle, unspecified ankle and foot

   M61.58 Other ossification of muscle, other site

   M61.59 Other ossification of muscle, multiple sites

   M61.9 Calcification and ossification of muscle, unspecified

● M62 Other disorders of muscle

   Excludes1 alcoholic myopathy (G72.1)
   cramp and spasm (R25.2)
   drug-induced myopathy (G72.0)
   myalgia (M79.1)
   stiff-man syndrome (G25.82)

   Excludes2 nontraumatic hematoma of muscle (M79.81)

● M62.0 Separation of muscle (nontraumatic)

   Diastasis of muscle

   Excludes1 diastasis recti complicating pregnancy, labor and delivery (O71.8)
   traumatic separation of muscle - see strain of muscle by body region

   M62.00 Separation of muscle (nontraumatic), unspecified site

● M62.01 Separation of muscle (nontraumatic), shoulder

   M62.011 Separation of muscle (nontraumatic), right shoulder

   M62.012 Separation of muscle (nontraumatic), left shoulder

   M62.019 Separation of muscle (nontraumatic), unspecified shoulder

● M62.02 Separation of muscle (nontraumatic), upper arm

   M62.021 Separation of muscle (nontraumatic), right upper arm

   M62.022 Separation of muscle (nontraumatic), left upper arm

   M62.029 Separation of muscle (nontraumatic), unspecified upper arm

● M62.03 Separation of muscle (nontraumatic), forearm

   M62.031 Separation of muscle (nontraumatic), right forearm

   M62.032 Separation of muscle (nontraumatic), left forearm

   M62.039 Separation of muscle (nontraumatic), unspecified forearm

● M62.04 Separation of muscle (nontraumatic), hand

   M62.041 Separation of muscle (nontraumatic), right hand

   M62.042 Separation of muscle (nontraumatic), left hand

   M62.049 Separation of muscle (nontraumatic), unspecified hand

● M62.05 Separation of muscle (nontraumatic), thigh

   M62.051 Separation of muscle (nontraumatic), right thigh

   M62.052 Separation of muscle (nontraumatic), left thigh

   M62.059 Separation of muscle (nontraumatic), unspecified thigh

● M62.06 Separation of muscle (nontraumatic), lower leg

   M62.061 Separation of muscle (nontraumatic), right lower leg

   M62.062 Separation of muscle (nontraumatic), left lower leg

   M62.069 Separation of muscle (nontraumatic), unspecified lower leg

● M62.07 Separation of muscle (nontraumatic), ankle and foot

   M62.071 Separation of muscle (nontraumatic), right ankle and foot

   M62.072 Separation of muscle (nontraumatic), left ankle and foot

   M62.079 Separation of muscle (nontraumatic), unspecified ankle and foot

   M62.08 Separation of muscle (nontraumatic), other site

● M62.1 Other rupture of muscle (nontraumatic)

   Excludes1 traumatic rupture of muscle - see strain of muscle by body region

   Excludes2 rupture of tendon (M66.-)

   M62.10 Other rupture of muscle (nontraumatic), unspecified site

● M62.11 Other rupture of muscle (nontraumatic), shoulder

   M62.111 Other rupture of muscle (nontraumatic), right shoulder

   M62.112 Other rupture of muscle (nontraumatic), left shoulder

   M62.119 Other rupture of muscle (nontraumatic), unspecified shoulder

CHAPTER 13 (M00-M99)

● M62.12 Other rupture of muscle (nontraumatic), upper arm
  M62.121 Other rupture of muscle (nontraumatic), right upper arm
  M62.122 Other rupture of muscle (nontraumatic), left upper arm
  M62.129 Other rupture of muscle (nontraumatic), unspecified upper arm
● M62.13 Other rupture of muscle (nontraumatic), forearm
  M62.131 Other rupture of muscle (nontraumatic), right forearm
  M62.132 Other rupture of muscle (nontraumatic), left forearm
  M62.139 Other rupture of muscle (nontraumatic), unspecified forearm
● M62.14 Other rupture of muscle (nontraumatic), hand
  M62.141 Other rupture of muscle (nontraumatic), right hand
  M62.142 Other rupture of muscle (nontraumatic), left hand
  M62.149 Other rupture of muscle (nontraumatic), unspecified hand
● M62.15 Other rupture of muscle (nontraumatic), thigh
  M62.151 Other rupture of muscle (nontraumatic), right thigh
  M62.152 Other rupture of muscle (nontraumatic), left thigh
  M62.159 Other rupture of muscle (nontraumatic), unspecified thigh
● M62.16 Other rupture of muscle (nontraumatic), lower leg
  M62.161 Other rupture of muscle (nontraumatic), right lower leg
  M62.162 Other rupture of muscle (nontraumatic), left lower leg
  M62.169 Other rupture of muscle (nontraumatic), unspecified lower leg
● M62.17 Other rupture of muscle (nontraumatic), ankle and foot
  M62.171 Other rupture of muscle (nontraumatic), right ankle and foot
  M62.172 Other rupture of muscle (nontraumatic), left ankle and foot
  M62.179 Other rupture of muscle (nontraumatic), unspecified ankle and foot
  M62.18 Other rupture of muscle (nontraumatic), other site
● M62.2 Nontraumatic ischemic infarction of muscle
  Excludes1   compartment syndrome (traumatic) (T79.A-)
               nontraumatic compartment syndrome (M79.A-)
               traumatic ischemia of muscle (T79.6)
               rhabdomyolysis (M62.82)
               Volkmann's ischemic contracture (T79.6)
  M62.20 Nontraumatic ischemic infarction of muscle, unspecified site
● M62.21 Nontraumatic ischemic infarction of muscle, shoulder
  M62.211 Nontraumatic ischemic infarction of muscle, right shoulder
  M62.212 Nontraumatic ischemic infarction of muscle, left shoulder
  M62.219 Nontraumatic ischemic infarction of muscle, unspecified shoulder

● M62.22 Nontraumatic ischemic infarction of muscle, upper arm
  M62.221 Nontraumatic ischemic infarction of muscle, right upper arm
  M62.222 Nontraumatic ischemic infarction of muscle, left upper arm
  M62.229 Nontraumatic ischemic infarction of muscle, unspecified upper arm
● M62.23 Nontraumatic ischemic infarction of muscle, forearm
  M62.231 Nontraumatic ischemic infarction of muscle, right forearm
  M62.232 Nontraumatic ischemic infarction of muscle, left forearm
  M62.239 Nontraumatic ischemic infarction of muscle, unspecified forearm
● M62.24 Nontraumatic ischemic infarction of muscle, hand
  M62.241 Nontraumatic ischemic infarction of muscle, right hand
  M62.242 Nontraumatic ischemic infarction of muscle, left hand
  M62.249 Nontraumatic ischemic infarction of muscle, unspecified hand
● M62.25 Nontraumatic ischemic infarction of muscle, thigh
  M62.251 Nontraumatic ischemic infarction of muscle, right thigh
  M62.252 Nontraumatic ischemic infarction of muscle, left thigh
  M62.259 Nontraumatic ischemic infarction of muscle, unspecified thigh
● M62.26 Nontraumatic ischemic infarction of muscle, lower leg
  M62.261 Nontraumatic ischemic infarction of muscle, right lower leg
  M62.262 Nontraumatic ischemic infarction of muscle, left lower leg
  M62.269 Nontraumatic ischemic infarction of muscle, unspecified lower leg
● M62.27 Nontraumatic ischemic infarction of muscle, ankle and foot
  M62.271 Nontraumatic ischemic infarction of muscle, right ankle and foot
  M62.272 Nontraumatic ischemic infarction of muscle, left ankle and foot
  M62.279 Nontraumatic ischemic infarction of muscle, unspecified ankle and foot
  M62.28 Nontraumatic ischemic infarction of muscle, other site
M62.3 Immobility syndrome (paraplegic)
M62.4 Contracture of muscle

CONTRACTURE OF TENDON (SHEATH)

Excludes1   contracture of joint (M24.5-)
  M62.40 Contracture of muscle, unspecified site
● M62.41 Contracture of muscle, shoulder
  M62.411 Contracture of muscle, right shoulder
  M62.412 Contracture of muscle, left shoulder
  M62.419 Contracture of muscle, unspecified shoulder
● M62.42 Contracture of muscle, upper arm
  M62.421 Contracture of muscle, right upper arm
  M62.422 Contracture of muscle, left upper arm
  M62.429 Contracture of muscle, unspecified upper arm

◀ New   ◀▦ Revised   deleted Deleted   Excludes 1   Excludes 2   Includes   Use additional   Code first   Code also   Unspecified
OGCR Official Guidelines   ● Unacceptable Principal Diagnosis   X Assign placeholder X   ● Use Additional Character(s)   ▶ Manifestation Code   Coding Clinic

● M62.43 Contracture of muscle, forearm
  M62.431 Contracture of muscle, right forearm
  M62.432 Contracture of muscle, left forearm
  M62.439 Contracture of muscle, unspecified forearm
● M62.44 Contracture of muscle, hand
  M62.441 Contracture of muscle, right hand
  M62.442 Contracture of muscle, left hand
  M62.449 Contracture of muscle, unspecified hand
● M62.45 Contracture of muscle, thigh
  M62.451 Contracture of muscle, right thigh
  M62.452 Contracture of muscle, left thigh
  M62.459 Contracture of muscle, unspecified thigh
● M62.46 Contracture of muscle, lower leg
  M62.461 Contracture of muscle, right lower leg
  M62.462 Contracture of muscle, left lower leg
  M62.469 Contracture of muscle, unspecified lower leg
● M62.47 Contracture of muscle, ankle and foot
  M62.471 Contracture of muscle, right ankle and foot
  M62.472 Contracture of muscle, left ankle and foot
  M62.479 Contracture of muscle, unspecified ankle and foot
  M62.48 Contracture of muscle, other site
  M62.49 Contracture of muscle, multiple sites
● M62.5 Muscle wasting and atrophy, not elsewhere classified
  Disuse atrophy NEC
  Excludes1 neuralgic amyotrophy (G54.5)
        progressive muscular atrophy (G12.29)
        sarcopenia (M62.84) ◄
  Excludes2 pelvic muscle wasting (N81.84)
  M62.50 Muscle wasting and atrophy, not elsewhere classified, unspecified site
● M62.51 Muscle wasting and atrophy, not elsewhere classified, shoulder
  M62.511 Muscle wasting and atrophy, not elsewhere classified, right shoulder
  M62.512 Muscle wasting and atrophy, not elsewhere classified, left shoulder
  M62.519 Muscle wasting and atrophy, not elsewhere classified, unspecified shoulder
● M62.52 Muscle wasting and atrophy, not elsewhere classified, upper arm
  M62.521 Muscle wasting and atrophy, not elsewhere classified, right upper arm
  M62.522 Muscle wasting and atrophy, not elsewhere classified, left upper arm
  M62.529 Muscle wasting and atrophy, not elsewhere classified, unspecified upper arm
● M62.53 Muscle wasting and atrophy, not elsewhere classified, forearm
  M62.531 Muscle wasting and atrophy, not elsewhere classified, right forearm
  M62.532 Muscle wasting and atrophy, not elsewhere classified, left forearm
  M62.539 Muscle wasting and atrophy, not elsewhere classified, unspecified forearm

● M62.54 Muscle wasting and atrophy, not elsewhere classified, hand
  M62.541 Muscle wasting and atrophy, not elsewhere classified, right hand
  M62.542 Muscle wasting and atrophy, not elsewhere classified, left hand
  M62.549 Muscle wasting and atrophy, not elsewhere classified, unspecified hand
● M62.55 Muscle wasting and atrophy, not elsewhere classified, thigh
  M62.551 Muscle wasting and atrophy, not elsewhere classified, right thigh
  M62.552 Muscle wasting and atrophy, not elsewhere classified, left thigh
  M62.559 Muscle wasting and atrophy, not elsewhere classified, unspecified thigh
● M62.56 Muscle wasting and atrophy, not elsewhere classified, lower leg
  M62.561 Muscle wasting and atrophy, not elsewhere classified, right lower leg
  M62.562 Muscle wasting and atrophy, not elsewhere classified, left lower leg
  M62.569 Muscle wasting and atrophy, not elsewhere classified, unspecified lower leg
● M62.57 Muscle wasting and atrophy, not elsewhere classified, ankle and foot
  M62.571 Muscle wasting and atrophy, not elsewhere classified, right ankle and foot
  M62.572 Muscle wasting and atrophy, not elsewhere classified, left ankle and foot
  M62.579 Muscle wasting and atrophy, not elsewhere classified, unspecified ankle and foot
  M62.58 Muscle wasting and atrophy, not elsewhere classified, other site
  M62.59 Muscle wasting and atrophy, not elsewhere classified, multiple sites
● M62.8 Other specified disorders of muscle
  Excludes2 nontraumatic hematoma of muscle (M79.81)
  M62.81 Muscle weakness (generalized)
    Excludes1 muscle weakness in sarcopenia (M62.84) ◄
  M62.82 Rhabdomyolysis 🅒
    Excludes1 traumatic rhabdomyolysis (T79.6)
    Ⓔ K68.12, M60.000-M60.19, M61.00-M61.19, M61.30-M61.59, M62.3, M62.50-M62.59, M62.82, M62.84, M62.89, M72.6
● M62.83 Muscle spasm
  M62.830 Muscle spasm of back
  M62.831 Muscle spasm of calf
        Charley-horse
  M62.838 Other muscle spasm
  M62.84 Sarcopenia ◄
      Age-related sarcopenia ◄
      Code first underlying disease, if applicable, such as:
        disorders of myoneural junction and muscle disease in diseases classified elsewhere (G73.-) ◄
        other and unspecified myopathies (G72.-) ◄
        primary disorders of muscles (G71.-) ◄
  M62.89 Other specified disorders of muscle
        Muscle (sheath) hernia
  M62.9 Disorder of muscle, unspecified

CHAPTER 13 (M00-M99)

N Newborn Age: 0   **P** Pediatric Age: 0–17   **M** Maternity DX: 12–55   **A** Adult Age: 15–124   ♀ Females Only   ♂ Males Only
🅒 Complication\Comorbidity   🅜 Major C\C   Ⓔ CC/MCC Exclusions   🅗 Hospital-Acquired Condition

● **M63   Disorders of muscle in diseases classified elsewhere**

Code first underlying disease, such as:

leprosy (A3Ø.-)

neoplasm (C49.-, C79.89, D21.-, D48.1)

schistosomiasis (B65.-)

trichinellosis (B75)

Excludes1   myopathy in cysticercosis (B69.81)

myopathy in endocrine diseases (G73.7)

myopathy in metabolic diseases (G73.7)

myopathy in sarcoidosis (D86.87)

myopathy in secondary syphilis (A51.49)

myopathy in syphilis (late) (A52.78)

myopathy in toxoplasmosis (B58.82)

myopathy in tuberculosis (A18.Ø9)

● **M63.8   Disorders of muscle in diseases classified elsewhere**

◗ *M63.80   Disorders of muscle in diseases classified elsewhere, unspecified site*

● **M63.81   Disorders of muscle in diseases classified elsewhere, shoulder**

◗ *M63.811   Disorders of muscle in diseases classified elsewhere, right shoulder*

◗ *M63.812   Disorders of muscle in diseases classified elsewhere, left shoulder*

◗ *M63.819   Disorders of muscle in diseases classified elsewhere, unspecified shoulder*

● **M63.82   Disorders of muscle in diseases classified elsewhere, upper arm**

◗ *M63.821   Disorders of muscle in diseases classified elsewhere, right upper arm*

◗ *M63.822   Disorders of muscle in diseases classified elsewhere, left upper arm*

◗ *M63.829   Disorders of muscle in diseases classified elsewhere, unspecified upper arm*

● **M63.83   Disorders of muscle in diseases classified elsewhere, forearm**

◗ *M63.831   Disorders of muscle in diseases classified elsewhere, right forearm*

◗ *M63.832   Disorders of muscle in diseases classified elsewhere, left forearm*

◗ *M63.839   Disorders of muscle in diseases classified elsewhere, unspecified forearm*

● **M63.84   Disorders of muscle in diseases classified elsewhere, hand**

◗ *M63.841   Disorders of muscle in diseases classified elsewhere, right hand*

◗ *M63.842   Disorders of muscle in diseases classified elsewhere, left hand*

◗ *M63.849   Disorders of muscle in diseases classified elsewhere, unspecified hand*

● **M63.85   Disorders of muscle in diseases classified elsewhere, thigh**

◗ *M63.851   Disorders of muscle in diseases classified elsewhere, right thigh*

◗ *M63.852   Disorders of muscle in diseases classified elsewhere, left thigh*

◗ *M63.859   Disorders of muscle in diseases classified elsewhere, unspecified thigh*

● **M63.86   Disorders of muscle in diseases classified elsewhere, lower leg**

◗ *M63.861   Disorders of muscle in diseases classified elsewhere, right lower leg*

◗ *M63.862   Disorders of muscle in diseases classified elsewhere, left lower leg*

◗ *M63.869   Disorders of muscle in diseases classified elsewhere, unspecified lower leg*

● **M63.87   Disorders of muscle in diseases classified elsewhere, ankle and foot**

◗ *M63.871   Disorders of muscle in diseases classified elsewhere, right ankle and foot*

◗ *M63.872   Disorders of muscle in diseases classified elsewhere, left ankle and foot*

◗ *M63.879   Disorders of muscle in diseases classified elsewhere, unspecified ankle and foot*

◗ *M63.88   Disorders of muscle in diseases classified elsewhere, other site*

◗ *M63.89   Disorders of muscle in diseases classified elsewhere, multiple sites*

DISORDERS OF SYNOVIUM AND TENDON (M65-M67)

● **M65   Synovitis and tenosynovitis**

Excludes1   chronic crepitant synovitis of hand and wrist (M70.Ø-)

current injury - see injury of ligament or tendon by body region

soft tissue disorders related to use, overuse and pressure (M70.-)

● **M65.Ø   Abscess of tendon sheath**

Use additional code (B95-B96) to identify bacterial agent

M65.ØØ   Abscess of tendon sheath, unspecified site

● **M65.Ø1   Abscess of tendon sheath, shoulder**

M65.Ø11   Abscess of tendon sheath, right shoulder

M65.Ø12   Abscess of tendon sheath, left shoulder

M65.Ø19   Abscess of tendon sheath, unspecified shoulder

● **M65.Ø2   Abscess of tendon sheath, upper arm**

M65.Ø21   Abscess of tendon sheath, right upper arm

M65.Ø22   Abscess of tendon sheath, left upper arm

M65.Ø29   Abscess of tendon sheath, unspecified upper arm

● **M65.Ø3   Abscess of tendon sheath, forearm**

M65.Ø31   Abscess of tendon sheath, right forearm

M65.Ø32   Abscess of tendon sheath, left forearm

M65.Ø39   Abscess of tendon sheath, unspecified forearm

● **M65.Ø4   Abscess of tendon sheath, hand**

M65.Ø41   Abscess of tendon sheath, right hand

M65.Ø42   Abscess of tendon sheath, left hand

M65.Ø49   Abscess of tendon sheath, unspecified hand

● **M65.Ø5   Abscess of tendon sheath, thigh**

M65.Ø51   Abscess of tendon sheath, right thigh

M65.Ø52   Abscess of tendon sheath, left thigh

M65.Ø59   Abscess of tendon sheath, unspecified thigh

Item 13–11   Synovitis is an inflammation of a synovial membrane resulting in pain on motion and is characterized by fluctuating swelling due to effusion in a synovial sac. **Tenosynovitis** is an inflammation of a tendon sheath and occurs most commonly in the wrists, hands, and feet. Bursitis is inflammation of a bursa (fluid filled sac) caused by repetitive use, trauma, infection, or systemic inflammatory disease. Bursae act as protectors and facilitate movement between bones and overlapping muscles (deep bursae) or between bones and tendons/skin (superficial bursae).

◀ New   ◀ Revised   ~~deleted~~ Deleted   Excludes 1   Excludes 2   Includes   Use additional   Code first   Code also   Unspecified

1Ø48   OGCR Official Guidelines   ● Unacceptable Principal Diagnosis   X Assign placeholder X   ● Use Additional Character(s)   ◗ Manifestation Code   **Coding Clinic**

● M65.06   Abscess of tendon sheath, lower leg
    M65.061   Abscess of tendon sheath, right lower leg
    M65.062   Abscess of tendon sheath, left lower leg
    M65.069   Abscess of tendon sheath, unspecified lower leg
● M65.07   Abscess of tendon sheath, ankle and foot
    M65.071   Abscess of tendon sheath, right ankle and foot
    M65.072   Abscess of tendon sheath, left ankle and foot
    M65.079   Abscess of tendon sheath, unspecified ankle and foot
   M65.08   Abscess of tendon sheath, other site
● M65.1   Other infective (teno)synovitis
   M65.10   Other infective (teno)synovitis, unspecified site
● M65.11   Other infective (teno)synovitis, shoulder
    M65.111   Other infective (teno)synovitis, right shoulder
    M65.112   Other infective (teno)synovitis, left shoulder
    M65.119   Other infective (teno)synovitis, unspecified shoulder
● M65.12   Other infective (teno)synovitis, elbow
    M65.121   Other infective (teno)synovitis, right elbow
    M65.122   Other infective (teno)synovitis, left elbow
    M65.129   Other infective (teno)synovitis, unspecified elbow
● M65.13   Other infective (teno)synovitis, wrist
    M65.131   Other infective (teno)synovitis, right wrist
    M65.132   Other infective (teno)synovitis, left wrist
    M65.139   Other infective (teno)synovitis, unspecified wrist
● M65.14   Other infective (teno)synovitis, hand
    M65.141   Other infective (teno)synovitis, right hand
    M65.142   Other infective (teno)synovitis, left hand
    M65.149   Other infective (teno)synovitis, unspecified hand
● M65.15   Other infective (teno)synovitis, hip
    M65.151   Other infective (teno)synovitis, right hip
    M65.152   Other infective (teno)synovitis, left hip
    M65.159   Other infective (teno)synovitis, unspecified hip
● M65.16   Other infective (teno)synovitis, knee
    M65.161   Other infective (teno)synovitis, right knee
    M65.162   Other infective (teno)synovitis, left knee
    M65.169   Other infective (teno)synovitis, unspecified knee
● M65.17   Other infective (teno)synovitis, ankle and foot
    M65.171   Other infective (teno)synovitis, right ankle and foot
    M65.172   Other infective (teno)synovitis, left ankle and foot
    M65.179   Other infective (teno)synovitis, unspecified ankle and foot
   M65.18   Other infective (teno)synovitis, other site
   M65.19   Other infective (teno)synovitis, multiple sites

● M65.2   Calcific tendinitis
    Excludes1   tendinitis as classified in M75-M77
              calcified tendinitis of shoulder (M75.3)
   M65.20   Calcific tendinitis, unspecified site
● M65.22   Calcific tendinitis, upper arm
    M65.221   Calcific tendinitis, right upper arm
    M65.222   Calcific tendinitis, left upper arm
    M65.229   Calcific tendinitis, unspecified upper arm
● M65.23   Calcific tendinitis, forearm
    M65.231   Calcific tendinitis, right forearm
    M65.232   Calcific tendinitis, left forearm
    M65.239   Calcific tendinitis, unspecified forearm
● M65.24   Calcific tendinitis, hand
    M65.241   Calcific tendinitis, right hand
    M65.242   Calcific tendinitis, left hand
    M65.249   Calcific tendinitis, unspecified hand
● M65.25   Calcific tendinitis, thigh
    M65.251   Calcific tendinitis, right thigh
    M65.252   Calcific tendinitis, left thigh
    M65.259   Calcific tendinitis, unspecified thigh
● M65.26   Calcific tendinitis, lower leg
    M65.261   Calcific tendinitis, right lower leg
    M65.262   Calcific tendinitis, left lower leg
    M65.269   Calcific tendinitis, unspecified lower leg
● M65.27   Calcific tendinitis, ankle and foot
    M65.271   Calcific tendinitis, right ankle and foot
    M65.272   Calcific tendinitis, left ankle and foot
    M65.279   Calcific tendinitis, unspecified ankle and foot
   M65.28   Calcific tendinitis, other site
   M65.29   Calcific tendinitis, multiple sites
● M65.3   Trigger finger
    Nodular tendinous disease
   M65.30   Trigger finger, unspecified finger
● M65.31   Trigger thumb
    M65.311   Trigger thumb, right thumb
    M65.312   Trigger thumb, left thumb
    M65.319   Trigger thumb, unspecified thumb
● M65.32   Trigger finger, index finger
    M65.321   Trigger finger, right index finger
    M65.322   Trigger finger, left index finger
    M65.329   Trigger finger, unspecified index finger
● M65.33   Trigger finger, middle finger
    M65.331   Trigger finger, right middle finger
    M65.332   Trigger finger, left middle finger
    M65.339   Trigger finger, unspecified middle finger
● M65.34   Trigger finger, ring finger
    M65.341   Trigger finger, right ring finger
    M65.342   Trigger finger, left ring finger
    M65.349   Trigger finger, unspecified ring finger
● M65.35   Trigger finger, little finger
    M65.351   Trigger finger, right little finger
    M65.352   Trigger finger, left little finger
    M65.359   Trigger finger, unspecified little finger
M65.4   Radial styloid tenosynovitis [de Quervain]

CHAPTER 13 (M00-M99)

CHAPTER 13 (M00-M99)

● M65.8   Other synovitis and tenosynovitis

   M65.80   Other synovitis and tenosynovitis, unspecified site

● M65.81   Other synovitis and tenosynovitis, shoulder

   M65.811   Other synovitis and tenosynovitis, right shoulder

   M65.812   Other synovitis and tenosynovitis, left shoulder

   M65.819   Other synovitis and tenosynovitis, unspecified shoulder

● M65.82   Other synovitis and tenosynovitis, upper arm

   M65.821   Other synovitis and tenosynovitis, right upper arm

   M65.822   Other synovitis and tenosynovitis, left upper arm

   M65.829   Other synovitis and tenosynovitis, unspecified upper arm

● M65.83   Other synovitis and tenosynovitis, forearm

   M65.831   Other synovitis and tenosynovitis, right forearm

   M65.832   Other synovitis and tenosynovitis, left forearm

   M65.839   Other synovitis and tenosynovitis, unspecified forearm

● M65.84   Other synovitis and tenosynovitis, hand

   M65.841   Other synovitis and tenosynovitis, right hand

   M65.842   Other synovitis and tenosynovitis, left hand

   M65.849   Other synovitis and tenosynovitis, unspecified hand

● M65.85   Other synovitis and tenosynovitis, thigh

   M65.851   Other synovitis and tenosynovitis, right thigh

   M65.852   Other synovitis and tenosynovitis, left thigh

   M65.859   Other synovitis and tenosynovitis, unspecified thigh

● M65.86   Other synovitis and tenosynovitis, lower leg

   M65.861   Other synovitis and tenosynovitis, right lower leg

   M65.862   Other synovitis and tenosynovitis, left lower leg

   M65.869   Other synovitis and tenosynovitis, unspecified lower leg

● M65.87   Other synovitis and tenosynovitis, ankle and foot

   M65.871   Other synovitis and tenosynovitis, right ankle and foot

   M65.872   Other synovitis and tenosynovitis, left ankle and foot

   M65.879   Other synovitis and tenosynovitis, unspecified ankle and foot

   M65.88   Other synovitis and tenosynovitis, other site

   M65.89   Other synovitis and tenosynovitis, multiple sites

M65.9   Synovitis and tenosynovitis, unspecified

● M66   Spontaneous rupture of synovium and tendon

   Includes   rupture that occurs when a normal force is applied to tissues that are inferred to have less than normal strength

   Excludes2   rotator cuff syndrome (M75.1-)

      rupture where an abnormal force is applied to normal tissue - see injury of tendon by body region

   M66.0   Rupture of popliteal cyst

● M66.1   Rupture of synovium

   Rupture of synovial cyst

   Excludes2   rupture of popliteal cyst (M66.0)

   M66.10   Rupture of synovium, unspecified joint

● M66.11   Rupture of synovium, shoulder

   M66.111   Rupture of synovium, right shoulder

   M66.112   Rupture of synovium, left shoulder

   M66.119   Rupture of synovium, unspecified shoulder

● M66.12   Rupture of synovium, elbow

   M66.121   Rupture of synovium, right elbow

   M66.122   Rupture of synovium, left elbow

   M66.129   Rupture of synovium, unspecified elbow

● M66.13   Rupture of synovium, wrist

   M66.131   Rupture of synovium, right wrist

   M66.132   Rupture of synovium, left wrist

   M66.139   Rupture of synovium, unspecified wrist

● M66.14   Rupture of synovium, hand and fingers

   M66.141   Rupture of synovium, right hand

   M66.142   Rupture of synovium, left hand

   M66.143   Rupture of synovium, unspecified hand

   M66.144   Rupture of synovium, right finger(s)

   M66.145   Rupture of synovium, left finger(s)

   M66.146   Rupture of synovium, unspecified finger(s)

● M66.15   Rupture of synovium, hip

   M66.151   Rupture of synovium, right hip

   M66.152   Rupture of synovium, left hip

   M66.159   Rupture of synovium, unspecified hip

● M66.17   Rupture of synovium, ankle, foot and toes

   M66.171   Rupture of synovium, right ankle

   M66.172   Rupture of synovium, left ankle

   M66.173   Rupture of synovium, unspecified ankle

   M66.174   Rupture of synovium, right foot

   M66.175   Rupture of synovium, left foot

   M66.176   Rupture of synovium, unspecified foot

   M66.177   Rupture of synovium, right toe(s)

   M66.178   Rupture of synovium, left toe(s)

   M66.179   Rupture of synovium, unspecified toe(s)

   M66.18   Rupture of synovium, other site

● M66.2   Spontaneous rupture of extensor tendons

   M66.20   Spontaneous rupture of extensor tendons, unspecified site

● M66.21   Spontaneous rupture of extensor tendons, shoulder

   M66.211   Spontaneous rupture of extensor tendons, right shoulder

   M66.212   Spontaneous rupture of extensor tendons, left shoulder

   M66.219   Spontaneous rupture of extensor tendons, unspecified shoulder

◄ New   ◄◄◄ Revised   ~~deleted~~ Deleted   Excludes 1   Excludes 2   Includes   Use additional   Code first   Code also   Unspecified

OGCR Official Guidelines   ● Unacceptable Principal Diagnosis   X Assign placeholder X   ● Use Additional Character(s)   ▷ Manifestation Code   **Coding Clinic**

● M66.22 Spontaneous rupture of extensor tendons, upper arm
   M66.221 Spontaneous rupture of extensor tendons, right upper arm
   M66.222 Spontaneous rupture of extensor tendons, left upper arm
   M66.229 Spontaneous rupture of extensor tendons, unspecified upper arm
● M66.23 Spontaneous rupture of extensor tendons, forearm
   M66.231 Spontaneous rupture of extensor tendons, right forearm
   M66.232 Spontaneous rupture of extensor tendons, left forearm
   M66.239 Spontaneous rupture of extensor tendons, unspecified forearm
● M66.24 Spontaneous rupture of extensor tendons, hand
   M66.241 Spontaneous rupture of extensor tendons, right hand
   M66.242 Spontaneous rupture of extensor tendons, left hand
   M66.249 Spontaneous rupture of extensor tendons, unspecified hand
● M66.25 Spontaneous rupture of extensor tendons, thigh
   M66.251 Spontaneous rupture of extensor tendons, right thigh
   M66.252 Spontaneous rupture of extensor tendons, left thigh
   M66.259 Spontaneous rupture of extensor tendons, unspecified thigh
● M66.26 Spontaneous rupture of extensor tendons, lower leg
   M66.261 Spontaneous rupture of extensor tendons, right lower leg
   M66.262 Spontaneous rupture of extensor tendons, left lower leg
   M66.269 Spontaneous rupture of extensor tendons, unspecified lower leg
● M66.27 Spontaneous rupture of extensor tendons, ankle and foot
   M66.271 Spontaneous rupture of extensor tendons, right ankle and foot
   M66.272 Spontaneous rupture of extensor tendons, left ankle and foot
   M66.279 Spontaneous rupture of extensor tendons, unspecified ankle and foot
   M66.28 Spontaneous rupture of extensor tendons, other site
   M66.29 Spontaneous rupture of extensor tendons, multiple sites
● M66.3 Spontaneous rupture of flexor tendons
   M66.30 Spontaneous rupture of flexor tendons, unspecified site
● M66.31 Spontaneous rupture of flexor tendons, shoulder
   M66.311 Spontaneous rupture of flexor tendons, right shoulder
   M66.312 Spontaneous rupture of flexor tendons, left shoulder
   M66.319 Spontaneous rupture of flexor tendons, unspecified shoulder
● M66.32 Spontaneous rupture of flexor tendons, upper arm
   M66.321 Spontaneous rupture of flexor tendons, right upper arm
   M66.322 Spontaneous rupture of flexor tendons, left upper arm
   M66.329 Spontaneous rupture of flexor tendons, unspecified upper arm

● M66.33 Spontaneous rupture of flexor tendons, forearm
   M66.331 Spontaneous rupture of flexor tendons, right forearm
   M66.332 Spontaneous rupture of flexor tendons, left forearm
   M66.339 Spontaneous rupture of flexor tendons, unspecified forearm
● M66.34 Spontaneous rupture of flexor tendons, hand
   M66.341 Spontaneous rupture of flexor tendons, right hand
   M66.342 Spontaneous rupture of flexor tendons, left hand
   M66.349 Spontaneous rupture of flexor tendons, unspecified hand
● M66.35 Spontaneous rupture of flexor tendons, thigh
   M66.351 Spontaneous rupture of flexor tendons, right thigh
   M66.352 Spontaneous rupture of flexor tendons, left thigh
   M66.359 Spontaneous rupture of flexor tendons, unspecified thigh
● M66.36 Spontaneous rupture of flexor tendons, lower leg
   M66.361 Spontaneous rupture of flexor tendons, right lower leg
   M66.362 Spontaneous rupture of flexor tendons, left lower leg
   M66.369 Spontaneous rupture of flexor tendons, unspecified lower leg
● M66.37 Spontaneous rupture of flexor tendons, ankle and foot
   M66.371 Spontaneous rupture of flexor tendons, right ankle and foot
   M66.372 Spontaneous rupture of flexor tendons, left ankle and foot
   M66.379 Spontaneous rupture of flexor tendons, unspecified ankle and foot
   M66.38 Spontaneous rupture of flexor tendons, other site
   M66.39 Spontaneous rupture of flexor tendons, multiple sites
● M66.8 Spontaneous rupture of other tendons
   M66.80 Spontaneous rupture of other tendons, unspecified site
● M66.81 Spontaneous rupture of other tendons, shoulder
   M66.811 Spontaneous rupture of other tendons, right shoulder
   M66.812 Spontaneous rupture of other tendons, left shoulder
   M66.819 Spontaneous rupture of other tendons, unspecified shoulder
● M66.82 Spontaneous rupture of other tendons, upper arm
   M66.821 Spontaneous rupture of other tendons, right upper arm
   M66.822 Spontaneous rupture of other tendons, left upper arm
   M66.829 Spontaneous rupture of other tendons, unspecified upper arm
● M66.83 Spontaneous rupture of other tendons, forearm
   M66.831 Spontaneous rupture of other tendons, right forearm
   M66.832 Spontaneous rupture of other tendons, left forearm
   M66.839 Spontaneous rupture of other tendons, unspecified forearm

CHAPTER 13 (M00-M99)

● **M66.84**   **Spontaneous rupture of other tendons, hand**
- M66.841   Spontaneous rupture of other tendons, right hand
- M66.842   Spontaneous rupture of other tendons, left hand
- M66.849   Spontaneous rupture of other tendons, unspecified hand

● **M66.85**   **Spontaneous rupture of other tendons, thigh**
- M66.851   Spontaneous rupture of other tendons, right thigh
- M66.852   Spontaneous rupture of other tendons, left thigh
- M66.859   Spontaneous rupture of other tendons, unspecified thigh

● **M66.86**   **Spontaneous rupture of other tendons, lower leg**
- M66.861   Spontaneous rupture of other tendons, right lower leg
- M66.862   Spontaneous rupture of other tendons, left lower leg
- M66.869   Spontaneous rupture of other tendons, unspecified lower leg

● **M66.87**   **Spontaneous rupture of other tendons, ankle and foot**
- M66.871   Spontaneous rupture of other tendons, right ankle and foot
- M66.872   Spontaneous rupture of other tendons, left ankle and foot
- M66.879   Spontaneous rupture of other tendons, unspecified ankle and foot

M66.88   Spontaneous rupture of other tendons, other

M66.89   Spontaneous rupture of other tendons, multiple sites

M66.9   **Spontaneous rupture of unspecified tendon**
Rupture at musculotendinous junction, nontraumatic

● **M67**   **Other disorders of synovium and tendon**
> **Excludes1**   palmar fascial fibromatosis [Dupuytren] (M72.0)
> tendinitis NOS (M77.9-)
> xanthomatosis localized to tendons (E78.2)

● **M67.0**   **Short Achilles tendon (acquired)**
- **M67.00**   Short Achilles tendon (acquired), unspecified ankle
- **M67.01**   Short Achilles tendon (acquired), right ankle
- **M67.02**   Short Achilles tendon (acquired), left ankle

● **M67.2**   **Synovial hypertrophy, not elsewhere classified**
> **Excludes1**   villonodular synovitis (pigmented) (M12.2-)

- **M67.20**   Synovial hypertrophy, not elsewhere classified, unspecified site

● **M67.21**   Synovial hypertrophy, not elsewhere classified, shoulder
- M67.211   Synovial hypertrophy, not elsewhere classified, right shoulder
- M67.212   Synovial hypertrophy, not elsewhere classified, left shoulder
- M67.219   Synovial hypertrophy, not elsewhere classified, unspecified shoulder

● **M67.22**   Synovial hypertrophy, not elsewhere classified, upper arm
- M67.221   Synovial hypertrophy, not elsewhere classified, right upper arm
- M67.222   Synovial hypertrophy, not elsewhere classified, left upper arm
- M67.229   Synovial hypertrophy, not elsewhere classified, unspecified upper arm

● **M67.23**   Synovial hypertrophy, not elsewhere classified, forearm
- M67.231   Synovial hypertrophy, not elsewhere classified, right forearm
- M67.232   Synovial hypertrophy, not elsewhere classified, left forearm
- M67.239   Synovial hypertrophy, not elsewhere classified, unspecified forearm

● **M67.24**   Synovial hypertrophy, not elsewhere classified, hand
- M67.241   Synovial hypertrophy, not elsewhere classified, right hand
- M67.242   Synovial hypertrophy, not elsewhere classified, left hand
- M67.249   Synovial hypertrophy, not elsewhere classified, unspecified hand

● **M67.25**   Synovial hypertrophy, not elsewhere classified, thigh
- M67.251   Synovial hypertrophy, not elsewhere classified, right thigh
- M67.252   Synovial hypertrophy, not elsewhere classified, left thigh
- M67.259   Synovial hypertrophy, not elsewhere classified, unspecified thigh

● **M67.26**   Synovial hypertrophy, not elsewhere classified, lower leg
- M67.261   Synovial hypertrophy, not elsewhere classified, right lower leg
- M67.262   Synovial hypertrophy, not elsewhere classified, left lower leg
- M67.269   Synovial hypertrophy, not elsewhere classified, unspecified lower leg

● **M67.27**   Synovial hypertrophy, not elsewhere classified, ankle and foot
- M67.271   Synovial hypertrophy, not elsewhere classified, right ankle and foot
- M67.272   Synovial hypertrophy, not elsewhere classified, left ankle and foot
- M67.279   Synovial hypertrophy, not elsewhere classified, unspecified ankle and foot

M67.28   Synovial hypertrophy, not elsewhere classified, other site

M67.29   Synovial hypertrophy, not elsewhere classified, multiple sites

● **M67.3**   **Transient synovitis**
Toxic synovitis
> **Excludes1**   palindromic rheumatism (M12.3-)

M67.30   Transient synovitis, unspecified site

● **M67.31**   Transient synovitis, shoulder
- M67.311   Transient synovitis, right shoulder
- M67.312   Transient synovitis, left shoulder
- M67.319   Transient synovitis, unspecified shoulder

● **M67.32**   Transient synovitis, elbow
- M67.321   Transient synovitis, right elbow
- M67.322   Transient synovitis, left elbow
- M67.329   Transient synovitis, unspecified elbow

● **M67.33**   Transient synovitis, wrist
- M67.331   Transient synovitis, right wrist
- M67.332   Transient synovitis, left wrist
- M67.339   Transient synovitis, unspecified wrist

● **M67.34**   Transient synovitis, hand
- M67.341   Transient synovitis, right hand
- M67.342   Transient synovitis, left hand
- M67.349   Transient synovitis, unspecified hand

◀ New   ⬅ Revised   ~~deleted~~ Deleted   Excludes 1   Excludes 2   Includes   Use additional   Code first   Code also   Unspecified

OGCR Official Guidelines   ● Unacceptable Principal Diagnosis   X Assign placeholder X   ● Use Additional Character(s)   ▶ Manifestation Code   **Coding Clinic**

- M67.35 **Transient synovitis, hip**
  - M67.351 **Transient synovitis, right hip**
  - M67.352 **Transient synovitis, left hip**
  - M67.359 **Transient synovitis, unspecified hip**
- M67.36 **Transient synovitis, knee**
  - M67.361 **Transient synovitis, right knee**
  - M67.362 **Transient synovitis, left knee**
  - M67.369 **Transient synovitis, unspecified knee**
- M67.37 **Transient synovitis, ankle and foot**
  - M67.371 **Transient synovitis, right ankle and foot**
  - M67.372 **Transient synovitis, left ankle and foot**
  - M67.379 **Transient synovitis, unspecified ankle and foot**
  - M67.38 **Transient synovitis, other site**
  - M67.39 **Transient synovitis, multiple sites**
- M67.4 **Ganglion**
  Ganglion of joint or tendon (sheath)
  Excludes1 ganglion in yaws (A66.6)
  Excludes2 cyst of bursa (M71.2-M71.3)
              cyst of synovium (M71.2-M71.3)
  - M67.40 **Ganglion, unspecified site**
- M67.41 **Ganglion, shoulder**
  - M67.411 **Ganglion, right shoulder**
  - M67.412 **Ganglion, left shoulder**
  - M67.419 **Ganglion, unspecified shoulder**
- M67.42 **Ganglion, elbow**
  - M67.421 **Ganglion, right elbow**
  - M67.422 **Ganglion, left elbow**
  - M67.429 **Ganglion, unspecified elbow**
- M67.43 **Ganglion, wrist**
  - M67.431 **Ganglion, right wrist**
  - M67.432 **Ganglion, left wrist**
  - M67.439 **Ganglion, unspecified wrist**
- M67.44 **Ganglion, hand**
  - M67.441 **Ganglion, right hand**
  - M67.442 **Ganglion, left hand**
  - M67.449 **Ganglion, unspecified hand**
- M67.45 **Ganglion, hip**
  - M67.451 **Ganglion, right hip**
  - M67.452 **Ganglion, left hip**
  - M67.459 **Ganglion, unspecified hip**
- M67.46 **Ganglion, knee**
  - M67.461 **Ganglion, right knee**
  - M67.462 **Ganglion, left knee**
  - M67.469 **Ganglion, unspecified knee**
- M67.47 **Ganglion, ankle and foot**
  - M67.471 **Ganglion, right ankle and foot**
  - M67.472 **Ganglion, left ankle and foot**
  - M67.479 **Ganglion, unspecified ankle and foot**
  - M67.48 **Ganglion, other site**
  - M67.49 **Ganglion, multiple sites**
- M67.5 **Plica syndrome**
  Plica knee
  - M67.50 **Plica syndrome, unspecified knee**
  - M67.51 **Plica syndrome, right knee**
  - M67.52 **Plica syndrome, left knee**
- M67.8 **Other specified disorders of synovium and tendon**
  - M67.80 **Other specified disorders of synovium and tendon, unspecified site**
- M67.81 **Other specified disorders of synovium and tendon, shoulder**
  - M67.811 **Other specified disorders of synovium, right shoulder**
  - M67.812 **Other specified disorders of synovium, left shoulder**

  - M67.813 **Other specified disorders of tendon, right shoulder**
  - M67.814 **Other specified disorders of tendon, left shoulder**
  - M67.819 **Other specified disorders of synovium and tendon, unspecified shoulder**
- M67.82 **Other specified disorders of synovium and tendon, elbow**
  - M67.821 **Other specified disorders of synovium, right elbow**
  - M67.822 **Other specified disorders of synovium, left elbow**
  - M67.823 **Other specified disorders of tendon, right elbow**
  - M67.824 **Other specified disorders of tendon, left elbow**
  - M67.829 **Other specified disorders of synovium and tendon, unspecified elbow**
- M67.83 **Other specified disorders of synovium and tendon, wrist**
  - M67.831 **Other specified disorders of synovium, right wrist**
  - M67.832 **Other specified disorders of synovium, left wrist**
  - M67.833 **Other specified disorders of tendon, right wrist**
  - M67.834 **Other specified disorders of tendon, left wrist**
  - M67.839 **Other specified disorders of synovium and tendon, unspecified forearm**
- M67.84 **Other specified disorders of synovium and tendon, hand**
  - M67.841 **Other specified disorders of synovium, right hand**
  - M67.842 **Other specified disorders of synovium, left hand**
  - M67.843 **Other specified disorders of tendon, right hand**
  - M67.844 **Other specified disorders of tendon, left hand**
  - M67.849 **Other specified disorders of synovium and tendon, unspecified hand**
- M67.85 **Other specified disorders of synovium and tendon, hip**
  - M67.851 **Other specified disorders of synovium, right hip**
  - M67.852 **Other specified disorders of synovium, left hip**
  - M67.853 **Other specified disorders of tendon, right hip**
  - M67.854 **Other specified disorders of tendon, left hip**
  - M67.859 **Other specified disorders of synovium and tendon, unspecified hip**
- M67.86 **Other specified disorders of synovium and tendon, knee**
  - M67.861 **Other specified disorders of synovium, right knee**
  - M67.862 **Other specified disorders of synovium, left knee**
  - M67.863 **Other specified disorders of tendon, right knee**
  - M67.864 **Other specified disorders of tendon, left knee**
  - M67.869 **Other specified disorders of synovium and tendon, unspecified knee**

CHAPTER 13 (M00-M99)

- M67.87 Other specified disorders of synovium and tendon, ankle and foot
  - M67.871 Other specified disorders of synovium, right ankle and foot
  - M67.872 Other specified disorders of synovium, left ankle and foot
  - M67.873 Other specified disorders of tendon, right ankle and foot
  - M67.874 Other specified disorders of tendon, left ankle and foot
  - M67.879 Other specified disorders of synovium and tendon, unspecified ankle and foot
- M67.88 Other specified disorders of synovium and tendon, other site
- M67.89 Other specified disorders of synovium and tendon, multiple sites
- M67.9 Unspecified disorder of synovium and tendon
  - M67.90 Unspecified disorder of synovium and tendon, unspecified site
  - M67.91 Unspecified disorder of synovium and tendon, shoulder
    - M67.911 Unspecified disorder of synovium and tendon, right shoulder
    - M67.912 Unspecified disorder of synovium and tendon, left shoulder
    - M67.919 Unspecified disorder of synovium and tendon, unspecified shoulder
  - M67.92 Unspecified disorder of synovium and tendon, upper arm
    - M67.921 Unspecified disorder of synovium and tendon, right upper arm
    - M67.922 Unspecified disorder of synovium and tendon, left upper arm
    - M67.929 Unspecified disorder of synovium and tendon, unspecified upper arm
  - M67.93 Unspecified disorder of synovium and tendon, forearm
    - M67.931 Unspecified disorder of synovium and tendon, right forearm
    - M67.932 Unspecified disorder of synovium and tendon, left forearm
    - M67.939 Unspecified disorder of synovium and tendon, unspecified forearm
  - M67.94 Unspecified disorder of synovium and tendon, hand
    - M67.941 Unspecified disorder of synovium and tendon, right hand
    - M67.942 Unspecified disorder of synovium and tendon, left hand
    - M67.949 Unspecified disorder of synovium and tendon, unspecified hand
  - M67.95 Unspecified disorder of synovium and tendon, thigh
    - M67.951 Unspecified disorder of synovium and tendon, right thigh
    - M67.952 Unspecified disorder of synovium and tendon, left thigh
    - M67.959 Unspecified disorder of synovium and tendon, unspecified thigh
  - M67.96 Unspecified disorder of synovium and tendon, lower leg
    - M67.961 Unspecified disorder of synovium and tendon, right lower leg
    - M67.962 Unspecified disorder of synovium and tendon, left lower leg
    - M67.969 Unspecified disorder of synovium and tendon, unspecified lower leg

- M67.97 Unspecified disorder of synovium and tendon, ankle and foot
  - M67.971 Unspecified disorder of synovium and tendon, right ankle and foot
  - M67.972 Unspecified disorder of synovium and tendon, left ankle and foot
  - M67.979 Unspecified disorder of synovium and tendon, unspecified ankle and foot
- M67.98 Unspecified disorder of synovium and tendon, other site
- M67.99 Unspecified disorder of synovium and tendon, multiple sites

OTHER SOFT TISSUE DISORDERS (M70-M79)

- M70 Soft tissue disorders related to use, overuse and pressure
  - **Includes** soft tissue disorders of occupational origin
  - Use additional external cause code to identify activity causing disorder (Y93.-)
  - **Excludes1** bursitis NOS (M71.9-)
  - **Excludes2** bursitis of shoulder (M75.5)
    enthesopathies (M76-M77)
    pressure ulcer (pressure area) (L89.-)
- M70.0 Crepitant synovitis (acute) (chronic) of hand and wrist
  - M70.03 Crepitant synovitis (acute) (chronic), wrist
    - M70.031 Crepitant synovitis (acute) (chronic), right wrist
    - M70.032 Crepitant synovitis (acute) (chronic), left wrist
    - M70.039 Crepitant synovitis (acute) (chronic), unspecified wrist
  - M70.04 Crepitant synovitis (acute) (chronic), hand
    - M70.041 Crepitant synovitis (acute) (chronic), right hand
    - M70.042 Crepitant synovitis (acute) (chronic), left hand
    - M70.049 Crepitant synovitis (acute) (chronic), unspecified hand
- M70.1 Bursitis of hand
  - M70.10 Bursitis, unspecified hand
  - M70.11 Bursitis, right hand
  - M70.12 Bursitis, left hand
- M70.2 Olecranon bursitis
  - M70.20 Olecranon bursitis, unspecified elbow
  - M70.21 Olecranon bursitis, right elbow
  - M70.22 Olecranon bursitis, left elbow
- M70.3 Other bursitis of elbow
  - M70.30 Other bursitis of elbow, unspecified elbow
  - M70.31 Other bursitis of elbow, right elbow
  - M70.32 Other bursitis of elbow, left elbow
- M70.4 Prepatellar bursitis
  - M70.40 Prepatellar bursitis, unspecified knee
  - M70.41 Prepatellar bursitis, right knee
  - M70.42 Prepatellar bursitis, left knee
- M70.5 Other bursitis of knee
  - M70.50 Other bursitis of knee, unspecified knee
  - M70.51 Other bursitis of knee, right knee
  - M70.52 Other bursitis of knee, left knee
- M70.6 Trochanteric bursitis
  - Trochanteric tendinitis
  - M70.60 Trochanteric bursitis, unspecified hip
  - M70.61 Trochanteric bursitis, right hip
  - M70.62 Trochanteric bursitis, left hip

● **M70.7**   Other bursitis of hip
     Ischial bursitis
     M70.70   Other bursitis of hip, unspecified hip
     M70.71   Other bursitis of hip, right hip
     M70.72   Other bursitis of hip, left hip

● **M70.8**   Other soft tissue disorders related to use, overuse and pressure
     M70.80   Other soft tissue disorders related to use, overuse and pressure of unspecified site

 ● **M70.81**   Other soft tissue disorders related to use, overuse and pressure of shoulder
       M70.811   Other soft tissue disorders related to use, overuse and pressure, right shoulder
       M70.812   Other soft tissue disorders related to use, overuse and pressure, left shoulder
       M70.819   Other soft tissue disorders related to use, overuse and pressure, unspecified shoulder

 ● **M70.82**   Other soft tissue disorders related to use, overuse and pressure of upper arm
       M70.821   Other soft tissue disorders related to use, overuse and pressure, right upper arm
       M70.822   Other soft tissue disorders related to use, overuse and pressure, left upper arm
       M70.829   Other soft tissue disorders related to use, overuse and pressure, unspecified upper arms

 ● **M70.83**   Other soft tissue disorders related to use, overuse and pressure of forearm
       M70.831   Other soft tissue disorders related to use, overuse and pressure, right forearm
       M70.832   Other soft tissue disorders related to use, overuse and pressure, left forearm
       M70.839   Other soft tissue disorders related to use, overuse and pressure, unspecified forearm

 ● **M70.84**   Other soft tissue disorders related to use, overuse and pressure of hand
       M70.841   Other soft tissue disorders related to use, overuse and pressure, right hand
       M70.842   Other soft tissue disorders related to use, overuse and pressure, left hand
       M70.849   Other soft tissue disorders related to use, overuse and pressure, unspecified hand

 ● **M70.85**   Other soft tissue disorders related to use, overuse and pressure of thigh
       M70.851   Other soft tissue disorders related to use, overuse and pressure, right thigh
       M70.852   Other soft tissue disorders related to use, overuse and pressure, left thigh
       M70.859   Other soft tissue disorders related to use, overuse and pressure, unspecified thigh

 ● **M70.86**   Other soft tissue disorders related to use, overuse and pressure lower leg
       M70.861   Other soft tissue disorders related to use, overuse and pressure, right lower leg
       M70.862   Other soft tissue disorders related to use, overuse and pressure, left lower leg
       M70.869   Other soft tissue disorders related to use, overuse and pressure, unspecified leg

 ● **M70.87**   Other soft tissue disorders related to use, overuse and pressure of ankle and foot
       M70.871   Other soft tissue disorders related to use, overuse and pressure, right ankle and foot
       M70.872   Other soft tissue disorders related to use, overuse and pressure, left ankle and foot
       M70.879   Other soft tissue disorders related to use, overuse and pressure, unspecified ankle and foot

     M70.88   Other soft tissue disorders related to use, overuse and pressure other site
     M70.89   Other soft tissue disorders related to use, overuse and pressure multiple sites

● **M70.9**   Unspecified soft tissue disorder related to use, overuse and pressure
     M70.90   Unspecified soft tissue disorder related to use, overuse and pressure of unspecified site

 ● **M70.91**   Unspecified soft tissue disorder related to use, overuse and pressure of shoulder
       M70.911   Unspecified soft tissue disorder related to use, overuse and pressure, right shoulder
       M70.912   Unspecified soft tissue disorder related to use, overuse and pressure, left shoulder
       M70.919   Unspecified soft tissue disorder related to use, overuse and pressure, unspecified shoulder

 ● **M70.92**   Unspecified soft tissue disorder related to use, overuse and pressure of upper arm
       M70.921   Unspecified soft tissue disorder related to use, overuse and pressure, right upper arm
       M70.922   Unspecified soft tissue disorder related to use, overuse and pressure, left upper arm
       M70.929   Unspecified soft tissue disorder related to use, overuse and pressure, unspecified upper arm

 ● **M70.93**   Unspecified soft tissue disorder related to use, overuse and pressure of forearm
       M70.931   Unspecified soft tissue disorder related to use, overuse and pressure, right forearm
       M70.932   Unspecified soft tissue disorder related to use, overuse and pressure, left forearm
       M70.939   Unspecified soft tissue disorder related to use, overuse and pressure, unspecified forearm

 ● **M70.94**   Unspecified soft tissue disorder related to use, overuse and pressure of hand
       M70.941   Unspecified soft tissue disorder related to use, overuse and pressure, right hand
       M70.942   Unspecified soft tissue disorder related to use, overuse and pressure, left hand
       M70.949   Unspecified soft tissue disorder related to use, overuse and pressure, unspecified hand

CHAPTER 13 (M00–M99)

N   Newborn Age: 0   **P**   Pediatric Age: 0–17   **M**   Maternity DX: 12–55   **A**   Adult Age: 15–124   ♀   Females Only   ♂   Males Only

   Complication\Comorbidity   Major C\C   (Ex) CC/MCC Exclusions   Hospital-Acquired Condition

1055

● M70.95   Unspecified soft tissue disorder related to use, overuse and pressure of thigh

    M70.951   Unspecified soft tissue disorder related to use, overuse and pressure, right thigh

    M70.952   Unspecified soft tissue disorder related to use, overuse and pressure, left thigh

    M70.959   Unspecified soft tissue disorder related to use, overuse and pressure, unspecified thigh

● M70.96   Unspecified soft tissue disorder related to use, overuse and pressure lower leg

    M70.961   Unspecified soft tissue disorder related to use, overuse and pressure, right lower leg

    M70.962   Unspecified soft tissue disorder related to use, overuse and pressure, left lower leg

    M70.969   Unspecified soft tissue disorder related to use, overuse and pressure, unspecified lower leg

● M70.97   Unspecified soft tissue disorder related to use, overuse and pressure of ankle and foot

    M70.971   Unspecified soft tissue disorder related to use, overuse and pressure, right ankle and foot

    M70.972   Unspecified soft tissue disorder related to use, overuse and pressure, left ankle and foot

    M70.979   Unspecified soft tissue disorder related to use, overuse and pressure, unspecified ankle and foot

  M70.98   Unspecified soft tissue disorder related to use, overuse and pressure other

  M70.99   Unspecified soft tissue disorder related to use, overuse and pressure multiple sites

● **M71**   **Other bursopathies**

    Excludes1   bunion (M20.1)

            bursitis related to use, overuse or pressure (M70.-)

            enthesopathies (M76-M77)

● M71.0   Abscess of bursa

    Use additional code (B95.-, B96.-) to identify causative organism

  M71.00   Abscess of bursa, unspecified site

● M71.01   Abscess of bursa, shoulder

    M71.011   Abscess of bursa, right shoulder

    M71.012   Abscess of bursa, left shoulder

    M71.019   Abscess of bursa, unspecified shoulder

● M71.02   Abscess of bursa, elbow

    M71.021   Abscess of bursa, right elbow

    M71.022   Abscess of bursa, left elbow

    M71.029   Abscess of bursa, unspecified elbow

● M71.03   Abscess of bursa, wrist

    M71.031   Abscess of bursa, right wrist

    M71.032   Abscess of bursa, left wrist

    M71.039   Abscess of bursa, unspecified wrist

● M71.04   Abscess of bursa, hand

    M71.041   Abscess of bursa, right hand

    M71.042   Abscess of bursa, left hand

    M71.049   Abscess of bursa, unspecified hand

● M71.05   Abscess of bursa, hip

    M71.051   Abscess of bursa, right hip

    M71.052   Abscess of bursa, left hip

    M71.059   Abscess of bursa, unspecified hip

● M71.06   Abscess of bursa, knee

    M71.061   Abscess of bursa, right knee

    M71.062   Abscess of bursa, left knee

    M71.069   Abscess of bursa, unspecified knee

● M71.07   Abscess of bursa, ankle and foot

    M71.071   Abscess of bursa, right ankle and foot

    M71.072   Abscess of bursa, left ankle and foot

    M71.079   Abscess of bursa, unspecified ankle and foot

  M71.08   Abscess of bursa, other site

  M71.09   Abscess of bursa, multiple sites

● M71.1   Other infective bursitis

    Use additional code (B95.-, B96.-) to identify causative organism

  M71.10   Other infective bursitis, unspecified site

● M71.11   Other infective bursitis, shoulder

    M71.111   Other infective bursitis, right shoulder

    M71.112   Other infective bursitis, left shoulder

    M71.119   Other infective bursitis, unspecified shoulder

● M71.12   Other infective bursitis, elbow

    M71.121   Other infective bursitis, right elbow

    M71.122   Other infective bursitis, left elbow

    M71.129   Other infective bursitis, unspecified elbow

● M71.13   Other infective bursitis, wrist

    M71.131   Other infective bursitis, right wrist

    M71.132   Other infective bursitis, left wrist

    M71.139   Other infective bursitis, unspecified wrist

● M71.14   Other infective bursitis, hand

    M71.141   Other infective bursitis, right hand

    M71.142   Other infective bursitis, left hand

    M71.149   Other infective bursitis, unspecified hand

● M71.15   Other infective bursitis, hip

    M71.151   Other infective bursitis, right hip

    M71.152   Other infective bursitis, left hip

    M71.159   Other infective bursitis, unspecified hip

● M71.16   Other infective bursitis, knee

    M71.161   Other infective bursitis, right knee

    M71.162   Other infective bursitis, left knee

    M71.169   Other infective bursitis, unspecified knee

● M71.17   Other infective bursitis, ankle and foot

    M71.171   Other infective bursitis, right ankle and foot

    M71.172   Other infective bursitis, left ankle and foot

    M71.179   Other infective bursitis, unspecified ankle and foot

  M71.18   Other infective bursitis, other site

  M71.19   Other infective bursitis, multiple sites

● M71.2   Synovial cyst of popliteal space [Baker]

    Popliteal space = popliteal cavity, popliteal fossa. Depression in the posterior aspect of the knee (behind the knee).

    Excludes1   synovial cyst of popliteal space with rupture (M66.0)

  M71.20   Synovial cyst of popliteal space [Baker], unspecified knee

  M71.21   Synovial cyst of popliteal space [Baker], right knee

  M71.22   Synovial cyst of popliteal space [Baker], left knee

---

◀ New   ◀▥ Revised   ~~deleted~~ Deleted   Excludes 1   Excludes 2   Includes   Use additional   Code first   Code also   Unspecified

OGCR Official Guidelines   ● Unacceptable Principal Diagnosis   X Assign placeholder X   ● Use Additional Character(s)   ▶ Manifestation Code   **Coding Clinic**

- **M71.3　Other bursal cyst**
  Synovial cyst NOS
  > **Excludes1**　synovial cyst with rupture (M66.1-)
  - M71.30　Other bursal cyst, unspecified site
  - M71.31　Other bursal cyst, shoulder
    - M71.311　Other bursal cyst, right shoulder
    - M71.312　Other bursal cyst, left shoulder
    - M71.319　Other bursal cyst, unspecified shoulder
  - M71.32　Other bursal cyst, elbow
    - M71.321　Other bursal cyst, right elbow
    - M71.322　Other bursal cyst, left elbow
    - M71.329　Other bursal cyst, unspecified elbow
  - M71.33　Other bursal cyst, wrist
    - M71.331　Other bursal cyst, right wrist
    - M71.332　Other bursal cyst, left wrist
    - M71.339　Other bursal cyst, unspecified wrist
  - M71.34　Other bursal cyst, hand
    - M71.341　Other bursal cyst, right hand
    - M71.342　Other bursal cyst, left hand
    - M71.349　Other bursal cyst, unspecified hand
  - M71.35　Other bursal cyst, hip
    - M71.351　Other bursal cyst, right hip
    - M71.352　Other bursal cyst, left hip
    - M71.359　Other bursal cyst, unspecified hip
  - M71.37　Other bursal cyst, ankle and foot
    - M71.371　Other bursal cyst, right ankle and foot
    - M71.372　Other bursal cyst, left ankle and foot
    - M71.379　Other bursal cyst, unspecified ankle and foot
  - M71.38　Other bursal cyst, other site
  - M71.39　Other bursal cyst, multiple sites
- **M71.4　Calcium deposit in bursa**
  > **Excludes2**　calcium deposit in bursa of shoulder (M75.3)
  - M71.40　Calcium deposit in bursa, unspecified site
  - M71.42　Calcium deposit in bursa, elbow
    - M71.421　Calcium deposit in bursa, right elbow
    - M71.422　Calcium deposit in bursa, left elbow
    - M71.429　Calcium deposit in bursa, unspecified elbow
  - M71.43　Calcium deposit in bursa, wrist
    - M71.431　Calcium deposit in bursa, right wrist
    - M71.432　Calcium deposit in bursa, left wrist
    - M71.439　Calcium deposit in bursa, unspecified wrist
  - M71.44　Calcium deposit in bursa, hand
    - M71.441　Calcium deposit in bursa, right hand
    - M71.442　Calcium deposit in bursa, left hand
    - M71.449　Calcium deposit in bursa, unspecified hand
  - M71.45　Calcium deposit in bursa, hip
    - M71.451　Calcium deposit in bursa, right hip
    - M71.452　Calcium deposit in bursa, left hip
    - M71.459　Calcium deposit in bursa, unspecified hip
  - M71.46　Calcium deposit in bursa, knee
    - M71.461　Calcium deposit in bursa, right knee
    - M71.462　Calcium deposit in bursa, left knee
    - M71.469　Calcium deposit in bursa, unspecified knee
  - M71.47　Calcium deposit in bursa, ankle and foot
    - M71.471　Calcium deposit in bursa, right ankle and foot
    - M71.472　Calcium deposit in bursa, left ankle and foot
    - M71.479　Calcium deposit in bursa, unspecified ankle and foot
  - M71.48　Calcium deposit in bursa, other site
  - M71.49　Calcium deposit in bursa, multiple sites
- **M71.5　Other bursitis, not elsewhere classified**
  > **Excludes1**　bursitis NOS (M71.9-)
  > **Excludes2**　bursitis of shoulder (M75.5)
  > 　　　　　　　bursitis of tibial collateral [Pellegrini-Stieda] (M76.4-) ◀
  - M71.50　Other bursitis, not elsewhere classified, unspecified site
  - M71.52　Other bursitis, not elsewhere classified, elbow
    - M71.521　Other bursitis, not elsewhere classified, right elbow
    - M71.522　Other bursitis, not elsewhere classified, left elbow
    - M71.529　Other bursitis, not elsewhere classified, unspecified elbow
  - M71.53　Other bursitis, not elsewhere classified, wrist
    - M71.531　Other bursitis, not elsewhere classified, right wrist
    - M71.532　Other bursitis, not elsewhere classified, left wrist
    - M71.539　Other bursitis, not elsewhere classified, unspecified wrist
  - M71.54　Other bursitis, not elsewhere classified, hand
    - M71.541　Other bursitis, not elsewhere classified, right hand
    - M71.542　Other bursitis, not elsewhere classified, left hand
    - M71.549　Other bursitis, not elsewhere classified, unspecified hand
  - M71.55　Other bursitis, not elsewhere classified, hip
    - M71.551　Other bursitis, not elsewhere classified, right hip
    - M71.552　Other bursitis, not elsewhere classified, left hip
    - M71.559　Other bursitis, not elsewhere classified, unspecified hip
  - M71.56　Other bursitis, not elsewhere classified, knee
    - M71.561　Other bursitis, not elsewhere classified, right knee
    - M71.562　Other bursitis, not elsewhere classified, left knee
    - M71.569　Other bursitis, not elsewhere classified, unspecified knee
  - M71.57　Other bursitis, not elsewhere classified, ankle and foot
    - M71.571　Other bursitis, not elsewhere classified, right ankle and foot
    - M71.572　Other bursitis, not elsewhere classified, left ankle and foot
    - M71.579　Other bursitis, not elsewhere classified, unspecified ankle and foot
  - M71.58　Other bursitis, not elsewhere classified, other site

CHAPTER 13 (M00-M99)

● **M71.8   Other specified bursopathies**

     M71.80   Other specified bursopathies, unspecified site

     ● M71.81   Other specified bursopathies, shoulder

         M71.811   Other specified bursopathies, right shoulder

         M71.812   Other specified bursopathies, left shoulder

         M71.819   Other specified bursopathies, unspecified shoulder

     ● M71.82   Other specified bursopathies, elbow

         M71.821   Other specified bursopathies, right elbow

         M71.822   Other specified bursopathies, left elbow

         M71.829   Other specified bursopathies, unspecified elbow

     ● M71.83   Other specified bursopathies, wrist

         M71.831   Other specified bursopathies, right wrist

         M71.832   Other specified bursopathies, left wrist

         M71.839   Other specified bursopathies, unspecified wrist

     ● M71.84   Other specified bursopathies, hand

         M71.841   Other specified bursopathies, right hand

         M71.842   Other specified bursopathies, left hand

         M71.849   Other specified bursopathies, unspecified hand

     ● M71.85   Other specified bursopathies, hip

         M71.851   Other specified bursopathies, right hip

         M71.852   Other specified bursopathies, left hip

         M71.859   Other specified bursopathies, unspecified hip

     ● M71.86   Other specified bursopathies, knee

         M71.861   Other specified bursopathies, right knee

         M71.862   Other specified bursopathies, left knee

         M71.869   Other specified bursopathies, unspecified knee

     ● M71.87   Other specified bursopathies, ankle and foot

         M71.871   Other specified bursopathies, right ankle and foot

         M71.872   Other specified bursopathies, left ankle and foot

         M71.879   Other specified bursopathies, unspecified ankle and foot

     M71.88   Other specified bursopathies, other site

     M71.89   Other specified bursopathies, multiple sites

     M71.9   **Bursopathy, unspecified**

         Bursitis NOS

● **M72   Fibroblastic disorders**

     Excludes2   retroperitoneal fibromatosis (D48.3)

     M72.0   Palmar fascial fibromatosis [Dupuytren]   A

     M72.1   Knuckle pads

     M72.2   Plantar fascial fibromatosis

         Plantar fasciitis

     M72.4   Pseudosarcomatous fibromatosis

         Nodular fasciitis

     M72.6   Necrotizing fasciitis 🦠

         Use additional code (B95.-, B96.-) to identify causative organism

         (Ex) See M60.0

     M72.8   Other fibroblastic disorders

         Abscess of fascia

         Fasciitis NEC

         Other infective fasciitis

         Use additional code to (B95.-, B96.-) identify causative organism

         Excludes1   diffuse (eosinophilic) fasciitis (M35.4)

                 necrotizing fasciitis (M72.6)

                 nodular fasciitis (M72.4)

                 perirenal fasciitis NOS (N13.5)

                 perirenal fasciitis with infection (N13.6)

                 plantar fasciitis (M72.2)

     M72.9   Fibroblastic disorder, unspecified

         Fasciitis NOS

         Fibromatosis NOS

● **M75   Shoulder lesions**

     Excludes2   shoulder-hand syndrome (M89.0-)

     ● **M75.0   Adhesive capsulitis of shoulder**

         Frozen shoulder

         Periarthritis of shoulder

         M75.00   **Adhesive capsulitis of unspecified shoulder**

         M75.01   **Adhesive capsulitis of right shoulder**

         M75.02   **Adhesive capsulitis of left shoulder**

            Coding Clinic: 2015, Q2, P23

     ● **M75.1   Rotator cuff tear or rupture, not specified as traumatic**

         Rotator cuff syndrome

         Supraspinatus syndrome

         Supraspinatus tear or rupture, not specified as traumatic

         Excludes1   tear of rotator cuff, traumatic (S46.01-)

         Gradual onset due to repetitive stress to rotator cuff

       ● M75.10   **Unspecified rotator cuff tear or rupture, not specified as traumatic**

         M75.100   Unspecified rotator cuff tear or rupture of unspecified shoulder, not specified as traumatic

         M75.101   Unspecified rotator cuff tear or rupture of right shoulder, not specified as traumatic

         M75.102   Unspecified rotator cuff tear or rupture of left shoulder, not specified as traumatic

       ● M75.11   **Incomplete rotator cuff tear or rupture not specified as traumatic**

         M75.110   Incomplete rotator cuff tear or rupture of unspecified shoulder, not specified as traumatic

         M75.111   Incomplete rotator cuff tear or rupture of right shoulder, not specified as traumatic

         M75.112   Incomplete rotator cuff tear or rupture of left shoulder, not specified as traumatic

       ● M75.12   **Complete rotator cuff tear or rupture not specified as traumatic**

         M75.120   Complete rotator cuff tear or rupture of unspecified shoulder, not specified as traumatic

         M75.121   Complete rotator cuff tear or rupture of right shoulder, not specified as traumatic

         M75.122   Complete rotator cuff tear or rupture of left shoulder, not specified as traumatic

● **M75.2 Bicipital tendinitis**
    M75.20   Bicipital tendinitis, unspecified shoulder
    M75.21   Bicipital tendinitis, right shoulder
    M75.22   Bicipital tendinitis, left shoulder

● **M75.3 Calcific tendinitis of shoulder**
    Calcified bursa of shoulder
    M75.30   Calcific tendinitis of unspecified shoulder
    M75.31   Calcific tendinitis of right shoulder
    M75.32   Calcific tendinitis of left shoulder

● **M75.4 Impingement syndrome of shoulder**
    M75.40   Impingement syndrome of unspecified shoulder
    M75.41   Impingement syndrome of right shoulder
    M75.42   Impingement syndrome of left shoulder

● **M75.5 Bursitis of shoulder**
    M75.50   Bursitis of unspecified shoulder
    M75.51   Bursitis of right shoulder
    M75.52   Bursitis of left shoulder

● **M75.8 Other shoulder lesions**
    M75.80   Other shoulder lesions, unspecified shoulder
    M75.81   Other shoulder lesions, right shoulder
    M75.82   Other shoulder lesions, left shoulder

● **M75.9 Shoulder lesion, unspecified**
    M75.90   Shoulder lesion, unspecified, unspecified shoulder
    M75.91   Shoulder lesion, unspecified, right shoulder
    M75.92   Shoulder lesion, unspecified, left shoulder

● **M76 Enthesopathies, lower limb, excluding foot**
    Excludes2   bursitis due to use, overuse and pressure (M70.-)
              enthesopathies of ankle and foot (M77.5-)

● **M76.0 Gluteal tendinitis**
    M76.00   Gluteal tendinitis, unspecified hip
    M76.01   Gluteal tendinitis, right hip
    M76.02   Gluteal tendinitis, left hip

● **M76.1 Psoas tendinitis**
    M76.10   Psoas tendinitis, unspecified hip
    M76.11   Psoas tendinitis, right hip
    M76.12   Psoas tendinitis, left hip

● **M76.2 Iliac crest spur**
    M76.20   Iliac crest spur, unspecified hip
    M76.21   Iliac crest spur, right hip
    M76.22   Iliac crest spur, left hip

● **M76.3 Iliotibial band syndrome**
    M76.30   Iliotibial band syndrome, unspecified leg
    M76.31   Iliotibial band syndrome, right leg
    M76.32   Iliotibial band syndrome, left leg

● **M76.4 Tibial collateral bursitis [Pellegrini-Stieda]**
    M76.40   Tibial collateral bursitis [Pellegrini-Stieda], unspecified leg
    M76.41   Tibial collateral bursitis [Pellegrini-Stieda], right leg
    M76.42   Tibial collateral bursitis [Pellegrini-Stieda], left leg

● **M76.5 Patellar tendinitis**
    M76.50   Patellar tendinitis, unspecified knee
    M76.51   Patellar tendinitis, right knee
    M76.52   Patellar tendinitis, left knee

● **M76.6 Achilles tendinitis**
    Achilles bursitis
    M76.60   Achilles tendinitis, unspecified leg
    M76.61   Achilles tendinitis, right leg
    M76.62   Achilles tendinitis, left leg

● **M76.7 Peroneal tendinitis**
    M76.70   Peroneal tendinitis, unspecified leg
    M76.71   Peroneal tendinitis, right leg
    M76.72   Peroneal tendinitis, left leg

● **M76.8 Other specified enthesopathies of lower limb, excluding foot**
  ● **M76.81 Anterior tibial syndrome**
    M76.811   Anterior tibial syndrome, right leg
    M76.812   Anterior tibial syndrome, left leg
    M76.819   Anterior tibial syndrome, unspecified leg
  ● **M76.82 Posterior tibial tendinitis**
    M76.821   Posterior tibial tendinitis, right leg
    M76.822   Posterior tibial tendinitis, left leg
    M76.829   Posterior tibial tendinitis, unspecified leg
  ● **M76.89 Other specified enthesopathies of lower limb, excluding foot**
    M76.891   Other specified enthesopathies of right lower limb, excluding foot
    M76.892   Other specified enthesopathies of left lower limb, excluding foot
    M76.899   Other specified enthesopathies of unspecified lower limb, excluding foot

  M76.9 Unspecified enthesopathy, lower limb, excluding foot

● **M77 Other enthesopathies**
    Excludes1   bursitis NOS (M71.9-)
    Excludes2   bursitis due to use, overuse and pressure (M70.-)
              osteophyte (M25.7)
              spinal enthesopathy (M46.0-)

● **M77.0 Medial epicondylitis**
    M77.00   Medial epicondylitis, unspecified elbow
    M77.01   Medial epicondylitis, right elbow
    M77.02   Medial epicondylitis, left elbow

● **M77.1 Lateral epicondylitis**
    Tennis elbow
    M77.10   Lateral epicondylitis, unspecified elbow
    M77.11   Lateral epicondylitis, right elbow
    M77.12   Lateral epicondylitis, left elbow

● **M77.2 Periarthritis of wrist**
    M77.20   Periarthritis, unspecified wrist
    M77.21   Periarthritis, right wrist
    M77.22   Periarthritis, left wrist

● **M77.3 Calcaneal spur**
    M77.30   Calcaneal spur, unspecified foot
    M77.31   Calcaneal spur, right foot
    M77.32   Calcaneal spur, left foot

● **M77.4 Metatarsalgia**
    Excludes1   Morton's metatarsalgia (G57.6)
    M77.40   Metatarsalgia, unspecified foot
    M77.41   Metatarsalgia, right foot
    M77.42   Metatarsalgia, left foot

● **M77.5 Other enthesopathy of foot**
    M77.50   Other enthesopathy of unspecified foot
    M77.51   Other enthesopathy of right foot
    M77.52   Other enthesopathy of left foot

  M77.8 Other enthesopathies, not elsewhere classified

  M77.9 Enthesopathy, unspecified
    Bone spur NOS
    Capsulitis NOS
    Periarthritis NOS
    Tendinitis NOS

CHAPTER 13 (M00-M99)

N Newborn Age: 0   **P** Pediatric Age: 0–17   **M** Maternity DX: 12–55   **A** Adult Age: 15–124   ♀ Females Only   ♂ Males Only

 Complication\Comorbidity   Major C\C   (Ex) CC/MCC Exclusions   Hospital-Acquired Condition

1059

● **M79   Other and unspecified soft tissue disorders, not elsewhere classified**

> **Excludes1**   psychogenic rheumatism (F45.8)
> soft tissue pain, psychogenic (F45.41)

M79.0   Rheumatism, unspecified

> **Excludes1**   fibromyalgia (M79.7)
> palindromic rheumatism (M12.3-)

M79.1   Myalgia
Myofascial pain syndrome

> **Excludes1**   fibromyalgia (M79.7)
> myositis (M60.-)

M79.2   Neuralgia and neuritis, unspecified

> **Excludes1**   brachial radiculitis NOS (M54.1)
> lumbosacral radiculitis NOS (M54.1)
> mononeuropathies (G56-G58)
> radiculitis NOS (M54.1)
> sciatica (M54.3-M54.4)

M79.3   Panniculitis, unspecified

> **Excludes1**   lupus panniculitis (L93.2)
> neck and back panniculitis (M54.0-)
> relapsing [Weber-Christian] panniculitis (M35.6)

M79.4   Hypertrophy of (infrapatellar) fat pad

M79.5   Residual foreign body in soft tissue

> **Excludes1**   foreign body granuloma of skin and subcutaneous tissue (L92.3)
> foreign body granuloma of soft tissue (M60.2-)

● **M79.6   Pain in limb, hand, foot, fingers and toes**

> **Excludes2**   pain in joint (M25.5-)

   ● **M79.60   Pain in limb, unspecified**

     M79.601   Pain in right arm
       Pain in right upper limb NOS

     M79.602   Pain in left arm
       Pain in left upper limb NOS

     M79.603   Pain in arm, unspecified
       Pain in upper limb NOS

     M79.604   Pain in right leg
       Pain in right lower limb NOS

     M79.605   Pain in left leg
       Pain in left lower limb NOS

     M79.606   Pain in leg, unspecified
       Pain in lower limb NOS

     M79.609   Pain in unspecified limb
       Pain in limb NOS

   ● **M79.62   Pain in upper arm**
     Pain in axillary region

     M79.621   Pain in right upper arm
     M79.622   Pain in left upper arm
     M79.629   Pain in unspecified upper arm

   ● **M79.63   Pain in forearm**

     M79.631   Pain in right forearm
     M79.632   Pain in left forearm
     M79.639   Pain in unspecified forearm

   ● **M79.64   Pain in hand and fingers**

     M79.641   Pain in right hand
     M79.642   Pain in left hand
     M79.643   Pain in unspecified hand
     M79.644   Pain in right finger(s)
     M79.645   Pain in left finger(s)
     M79.646   Pain in unspecified finger(s)

   ● **M79.65   Pain in thigh**

     M79.651   Pain in right thigh
     M79.652   Pain in left thigh
     M79.659   Pain in unspecified thigh

● **M79.66   Pain in lower leg**

     M79.661   Pain in right lower leg
     M79.662   Pain in left lower leg
     M79.669   Pain in unspecified lower leg

● **M79.67   Pain in foot and toes**

     M79.671   Pain in right foot
     M79.672   Pain in left foot
     M79.673   Pain in unspecified foot
     M79.674   Pain in right toe(s)
     M79.675   Pain in left toe(s)
     M79.676   Pain in unspecified toe(s)

M79.7   Fibromyalgia
Fibromyositis
Fibrositis
Myofibrositis

● **M79.A   Nontraumatic compartment syndrome**

> *Code first, if applicable, associated postprocedural complication*

> **Excludes1**   compartment syndrome NOS (T79.A-)
> fibromyalgia (M79.7) nontraumatic ischemic infarction of muscle (M62.2-)
> traumatic compartment syndrome (T79.A-)

● **M79.A1   Nontraumatic compartment syndrome of upper extremity**
Nontraumatic compartment syndrome of shoulder, arm, forearm, wrist, hand, and fingers
> (Ex) For category **M79.A1** CC codes: M70.80-M70.99, M79.81-M79.9, R29.898, S45.301-S45.899[A], S55.201-S55.899[A], S65.801-S65.899[A]

     M79.A11   Nontraumatic compartment syndrome of right upper extremity 🔸

     M79.A12   Nontraumatic compartment syndrome of left upper extremity 🔸

     M79.A19   Nontraumatic compartment syndrome of unspecified upper extremity 🔸

● **M79.A2   Nontraumatic compartment syndrome of lower extremity**
Nontraumatic compartment syndrome of hip, buttock, thigh, leg, foot, and toes
> (Ex) For category **M79.A2** CC codes: M70.80-M70.99, M79.81-M79.9, R29.898, S75.801-S75.899[A], S85.201-S85.899[A], S95.001-S95.099[A], S95.201-S95.899[A]

     M79.A21   Nontraumatic compartment syndrome of right lower extremity 🔸

     M79.A22   Nontraumatic compartment syndrome of left lower extremity 🔸

     M79.A29   Nontraumatic compartment syndrome of unspecified lower extremity 🔸

   M79.A3   Nontraumatic compartment syndrome of abdomen 🔸
> (Ex) S31.001[A], S31.011[A], S31.021[A], S31.031[A], S31.041[A], S31.051-S31.159[A], S31.600-S31.659[A], S31.831-S31.839[A], S36.00X-S37.599[A], S37.812-S37.99X[A], S38.3XX[A], S39.021-S39.023[A], T14.90-T14.91, T79.8XX-T79.9XX[A]

   M79.A9   Nontraumatic compartment syndrome of other sites 🔸
> (Ex) S31.001[A], S31.011[A], S31.021[A], S31.031[A], S31.041[A], S31.051[A], S31.600-S31.659[A], S36.81X-S36.899[A]

● **M79.8   Other specified soft tissue disorders**

   M79.81   Nontraumatic hematoma of soft tissue
Nontraumatic hematoma of muscle
Nontraumatic seroma of muscle and soft tissue

   M79.89   Other specified soft tissue disorders
Polyalgia

M79.9   Soft tissue disorder, unspecified

OGCR See Section I.C., Chapter 13.d.

> **Osteoporosis**
>
> Osteoporosis is a systemic condition, meaning that all bones of the musculoskeletal system are affected. Therefore, site is not a component of the codes under category M81, Osteoporosis without current pathological fracture. The site codes under category M80, Osteoporosis with current pathological fracture, identify the site of the fracture, not the osteoporosis.
>
> **1) Osteoporosis without pathological fracture**
>
> Category M81, Osteoporosis without current pathological fracture, is for use for patients with osteoporosis who do not currently have a pathologic fracture due to the osteoporosis, even if they have had a fracture in the past. For patients with a history of osteoporosis fractures, status code Z87.310, Personal history of (healed) osteoporosis fracture, should follow the code from M81.
>
> **2) Osteoporosis with current pathological fracture**
>
> Category M80, Osteoporosis with current pathological fracture, is for patients who have a current pathologic fracture at the time of an encounter. The codes under M80 identify the site of the fracture. A code from category M80, not a traumatic fracture code, should be used for any patient with known osteoporosis who suffers a fracture, even if the patient had a minor fall or trauma, if that fall or trauma would not usually break a normal, healthy bone.

OSTEOPATHIES AND CHONDROPATHIES (M80-M94)

DISORDERS OF BONE DENSITY AND STRUCTURE (M80-M85)

M80 Osteoporosis with current pathological fracture
Excessive skeletal fragility (porous bone) resulting in bone fractures

> **Includes**   osteoporosis with current fragility fracture

Use additional code to identify major osseous defect, if applicable (M89.7-)

> **Excludes1**   collapsed vertebra NOS (M48.5)
> pathological fracture NOS (M84.4)
> wedging of vertebra NOS (M48.5)

> **Excludes2**   personal history of (healed) osteoporosis fracture (Z87.310)

The appropriate 7th character is to be added to each code from category M80:

> A   initial encounter for fracture
>   *All encounters involving diagnosis and treatment*
> D   subsequent encounter for fracture with routine healing
> G   subsequent encounter for fracture with delayed healing
>   *Encounters for attention to casting or fixation devices, medication, and follow-up visits during the healing phase*
> K   subsequent encounter for fracture with nonunion
>   *Total failure of fracture healing*
> P   subsequent encounter for fracture with malunion
>   *Fracture ends do not heal together correctly.*
> S   sequela

(Ex:) **For category M80[A] CC codes:** M48.40X-M48.58X[A], M80.00X-M80.88X[A], M84.30X-M84.68X[A], M84.750-M84.759[A] **For category M80[K,P] CC codes:** M80.00X-M80.88X[K,P], M84.30X-M84.68X[K,P], M84.750-M84.759[K,P], S02.0XX-S02.92X[K], S12.000-S12.691[K], S22.000-S22.9XX[K], S32.000-S32.9XX[K], S42.001-S42.92X[K,P], S49.001-S49.199[K,P], S52.001-S52.92X[K,M,N,P,Q,R], S59.001-S59.299[K,P], S62.001-S62.92X[K,P], S72.001-S72.92X[K,M,N,P,Q,R], S79.001-S79.199[K,P], S82.001-S82.92X[K,M,N,P,Q,R], S89.001-S89.399[K,P], S92.001-S92.919[K,P]

● **M80.0 Age-related osteoporosis with current pathological fracture**
     Involutional osteoporosis with current pathological fracture
     Osteoporosis NOS with current pathological fracture
     Postmenopausal osteoporosis with current pathological fracture
     Senile osteoporosis with current pathological fracture

X ● **M80.00 Age-related osteoporosis with current pathological fracture, unspecified site**
     A, K, P 🖐   A

● **M80.01 Age-related osteoporosis with current pathological fracture, shoulder**

● **M80.011 Age-related osteoporosis with current pathological fracture, right shoulder**
     A, K, P 🖐   A

● **M80.012 Age-related osteoporosis with current pathological fracture, left shoulder**
     A, K, P 🖐   A

● **M80.019 Age-related osteoporosis with current pathological fracture, unspecified shoulder** A, K, P 🖐   A

● **M80.02 Age-related osteoporosis with current pathological fracture, humerus**

● **M80.021 Age-related osteoporosis with current pathological fracture, right humerus**
     A, K, P 🖐   A

● **M80.022 Age-related osteoporosis with current pathological fracture, left humerus**
     A, K, P 🖐   A

● **M80.029 Age-related osteoporosis with current pathological fracture, unspecified humerus** A, K, P 🖐   A

● **M80.03 Age-related osteoporosis with current pathological fracture, forearm**
     Age-related osteoporosis with current pathological fracture of wrist

● **M80.031 Age-related osteoporosis with current pathological fracture, right forearm**
     A, K, P 🖐   A

● **M80.032 Age-related osteoporosis with current pathological fracture, left forearm**
     A, K, P 🖐   A

● **M80.039 Age-related osteoporosis with current pathological fracture, unspecified forearm** A, K, P 🖐   A

● **M80.04 Age-related osteoporosis with current pathological fracture, hand**

● **M80.041 Age-related osteoporosis with current pathological fracture, right hand**
     A, K, P 🖐   A

● **M80.042 Age-related osteoporosis with current pathological fracture, left hand**
     A, K, P 🖐   A

● **M80.049 Age-related osteoporosis with current pathological fracture, unspecified hand** A, K, P 🖐   A

● **M80.05 Age-related osteoporosis with current pathological fracture, femur**
     Age-related osteoporosis with current pathological fracture of hip

● **M80.051 Age-related osteoporosis with current pathological fracture, right femur**
     A, K, P 🖐   A

● **M80.052 Age-related osteoporosis with current pathological fracture, left femur**
     A, K, P 🖐   A

● **M80.059 Age-related osteoporosis with current pathological fracture, unspecified femur** A, K, P 🖐   A

● **M80.06 Age-related osteoporosis with current pathological fracture, lower leg**

● **M80.061 Age-related osteoporosis with current pathological fracture, right lower leg**
     A, K, P 🖐   A

● **M80.062 Age-related osteoporosis with current pathological fracture, left lower leg**
     A, K, P 🖐   A

● **M80.069 Age-related osteoporosis with current pathological fracture, unspecified lower leg** A, K, P 🖐   A

CHAPTER 13 (M00-M99)

CHAPTER 13 (M00–M99)

● **M80.07** **Age-related osteoporosis with current pathological fracture, ankle and foot**

   ● **M80.071** Age-related osteoporosis with current pathological fracture, right ankle and foot A, K, P 🔖   A

   ● **M80.072** Age-related osteoporosis with current pathological fracture, left ankle and foot A, K, P 🔖   A

   ● **M80.079** Age-related osteoporosis with current pathological fracture, unspecified ankle and foot A, K, P 🔖   A

X ● **M80.08** **Age-related osteoporosis with current pathological fracture, vertebra(e)** A, K, P 🔖   A

● **M80.8** **Other osteoporosis with current pathological fracture**

   Drug-induced osteoporosis with current pathological fracture

   Idiopathic osteoporosis with current pathological fracture

   Osteoporosis of disuse with current pathological fracture

   Postoophorectomy osteoporosis with current pathological fracture

   Postsurgical malabsorption osteoporosis with current pathological fracture

   Post-traumatic osteoporosis with current pathological fracture

   Use additional code for adverse effect, if applicable, to identify drug (T36-T50 with fifth or sixth character 5)

X ● **M80.80** **Other osteoporosis with current pathological fracture, unspecified site** A, K, P 🔖   A

● **M80.81** **Other osteoporosis with pathological fracture, shoulder**

   ● **M80.811** Other osteoporosis with current pathological fracture, right shoulder A, K, P 🔖

   ● **M80.812** Other osteoporosis with current pathological fracture, left shoulder A, K, P 🔖

   ● **M80.819** Other osteoporosis with current pathological fracture, unspecified shoulder A, K, P 🔖

● **M80.82** **Other osteoporosis with current pathological fracture, humerus**

   ● **M80.821** Other osteoporosis with current pathological fracture, right humerus A, K, P 🔖

   ● **M80.822** Other osteoporosis with current pathological fracture, left humerus A, K, P 🔖

   ● **M80.829** Other osteoporosis with current pathological fracture, unspecified humerus A, K, P 🔖

● **M80.83** **Other osteoporosis with current pathological fracture, forearm**

   Other osteoporosis with current pathological fracture of wrist

   ● **M80.831** Other osteoporosis with current pathological fracture, right forearm A, K, P 🔖

   ● **M80.832** Other osteoporosis with current pathological fracture, left forearm A, K, P 🔖

   ● **M80.839** Other osteoporosis with current pathological fracture, unspecified forearm A, K, P 🔖

● **M80.84** **Other osteoporosis with current pathological fracture, hand**

   ● **M80.841** Other osteoporosis with current pathological fracture, right hand A, K, P 🔖

   ● **M80.842** Other osteoporosis with current pathological fracture, left hand A, K, P 🔖

   ● **M80.849** Other osteoporosis with current pathological fracture, unspecified hand A, K, P 🔖

● **M80.85** **Other osteoporosis with current pathological fracture, femur**

   Other osteoporosis with current pathological fracture of hip

   ● **M80.851** Other osteoporosis with current pathological fracture, right femur A, K, P 🔖

   ● **M80.852** Other osteoporosis with current pathological fracture, left femur A, K, P 🔖

   ● **M80.859** Other osteoporosis with current pathological fracture, unspecified femur A, K, P 🔖

● **M80.86** **Other osteoporosis with current pathological fracture, lower leg**

   ● **M80.861** Other osteoporosis with current pathological fracture, right lower leg A, K, P 🔖

   ● **M80.862** Other osteoporosis with current pathological fracture, left lower leg A, K, P 🔖

   ● **M80.869** Other osteoporosis with current pathological fracture, unspecified lower leg A, K, P 🔖

● **M80.87** **Other osteoporosis with current pathological fracture, ankle and foot**

   ● **M80.871** Other osteoporosis with current pathological fracture, right ankle and foot A, K, P 🔖

   ● **M80.872** Other osteoporosis with current pathological fracture, left ankle and foot A, K, P 🔖

   ● **M80.879** Other osteoporosis with current pathological fracture, unspecified ankle and foot A, K, P 🔖

X ● **M80.88** **Other osteoporosis with current pathological fracture, vertebra(e)** A, K, P 🔖

● **M81** **Osteoporosis without current pathological fracture**

   Use additional code to identify:
     major osseous defect, if applicable (M89.7-)
     personal history of (healed) osteoporosis fracture, if applicable (Z87.310)

   Excludes1   osteoporosis with current pathological fracture (M80.-)
               Sudeck's atrophy (M89.0)

M81.0 **Age-related osteoporosis without current pathological fracture**   A

   Involutional osteoporosis without current pathological fracture

   Osteoporosis NOS

   Postmenopausal osteoporosis without current pathological fracture

   Senile osteoporosis without current pathological fracture

M81.6 **Localized osteoporosis [Lequesne]**

   Excludes1   Sudeck's atrophy (M89.0)

◀ New   ⬅ Revised   ~~deleted~~ Deleted   Excludes 1   Excludes 2   Includes   Use additional   Code first   Code also   Unspecified

OGCR Official Guidelines   ● Unacceptable Principal Diagnosis   X Assign placeholder X   ● Use Additional Character(s)   ▌ Manifestation Code   **Coding Clinic**

M81.8 Other osteoporosis without current pathological fracture
Drug-induced osteoporosis without current pathological fracture
Idiopathic osteoporosis without current pathological fracture
Osteoporosis of disuse without current pathological fracture
Postoophorectomy osteoporosis without current pathological fracture
Postsurgical malabsorption osteoporosis without current pathological fracture
Post-traumatic osteoporosis without current pathological fracture
Use additional code for adverse effect, if applicable, to identify drug (T36-T50 with fifth or sixth character 5)

● **M83 Adult osteomalacia**
Excludes1 infantile and juvenile osteomalacia (E55.0)
renal osteodystrophy (N25.0)
rickets (active) (E55.0)
rickets (active) sequelae (E64.3)
vitamin D-resistant osteomalacia (E83.3)
vitamin D-resistant rickets (active) (E83.3)

M83.0 Puerperal osteomalacia ♀   M
M83.1 Senile osteomalacia   A
M83.2 Adult osteomalacia due to malabsorption   A
Postsurgical malabsorption osteomalacia in adults
M83.3 Adult osteomalacia due to malnutrition   A
M83.4 Aluminum bone disease
M83.5 Other drug-induced osteomalacia in adults   A
Use additional code for adverse effect, if applicable, to identify drug (T36-T50 with fifth or sixth character 5)
M83.8 Other adult osteomalacia   A
M83.9 Adult osteomalacia, unspecified   A

● **M84 Disorder of continuity of bone**
Excludes2 traumatic fracture of bone-see fracture, by site
(Ex) **For category M84[A] CC codes:** M48.40X-M48.58X[A], M80.00X-M80.88X[A], M84.30X-M84.68X[A], M84.750-M84.759[A] **For category M84[K,P] CC codes:** See M80[K,P]

● **M84.3 Stress fracture**
Fatigue fracture
March fracture
Stress fracture NOS
Stress reaction
Use additional external cause code(s) to identify the cause of the stress fracture
Excludes1 pathological fracture NOS (M84.4.-)
pathological fracture due to osteoporosis (M80.-)
traumatic fracture (S12.-, S22.-, S32.-, S42.-, S52.-, S62.-, S72.-, S82.-, S92.-)
Excludes2 personal history of (healed) stress (fatigue) fracture (Z87.312)
stress fracture of vertebra (M48.4-)
The appropriate 7th character is to be added to each code from subcategory M84.3:

A	initial encounter for fracture
D	subsequent encounter for fracture with routine healing
G	subsequent encounter for fracture with delayed healing
K	subsequent encounter for fracture with nonunion
P	subsequent encounter for fracture with malunion
S	sequela

(Ex) See M84

X ● **M84.30 Stress fracture, unspecified site** K, P 🏥

● **M84.31 Stress fracture, shoulder**
● M84.311 Stress fracture, right shoulder K, P 🏥
● M84.312 Stress fracture, left shoulder K, P 🏥
● M84.319 Stress fracture, unspecified shoulder K, P 🏥
● **M84.32 Stress fracture, humerus**
● M84.321 Stress fracture, right humerus K, P 🏥
● M84.322 Stress fracture, left humerus K, P 🏥
● M84.329 Stress fracture, unspecified humerus K, P 🏥
● **M84.33 Stress fracture, ulna and radius**
● M84.331 Stress fracture, right ulna K, P 🏥
● M84.332 Stress fracture, left ulna K, P 🏥
● M84.333 Stress fracture, right radius K, P 🏥
● M84.334 Stress fracture, left radius K, P 🏥
● M84.339 Stress fracture, unspecified ulna and radius K, P 🏥
● **M84.34 Stress fracture, hand and fingers**
● M84.341 Stress fracture, right hand K, P 🏥
● M84.342 Stress fracture, left hand K, P 🏥
● M84.343 Stress fracture, unspecified hand K, P 🏥
● M84.344 Stress fracture, right finger(s) K, P 🏥
● M84.345 Stress fracture, left finger(s) K, P 🏥
● M84.346 Stress fracture, unspecified finger(s) K, P 🏥
● **M84.35 Stress fracture, pelvis and femur**
Stress fracture, hip
● M84.350 Stress fracture, pelvis K, P 🏥
● M84.351 Stress fracture, right femur K, P 🏥
● M84.352 Stress fracture, left femur K, P 🏥
● M84.353 Stress fracture, unspecified femur K, P 🏥
● M84.359 Stress fracture, hip, unspecified K, P 🏥
● **M84.36 Stress fracture, tibia and fibula**
● M84.361 Stress fracture, right tibia K, P 🏥
● M84.362 Stress fracture, left tibia K, P 🏥
● M84.363 Stress fracture, right fibula K, P 🏥
● M84.364 Stress fracture, left fibula K, P 🏥
● M84.369 Stress fracture, unspecified tibia and fibula K, P 🏥
● **M84.37 Stress fracture, ankle, foot and toes**
● M84.371 Stress fracture, right ankle K, P 🏥
● M84.372 Stress fracture, left ankle K, P 🏥
● M84.373 Stress fracture, unspecified ankle K, P 🏥
● M84.374 Stress fracture, right foot K, P 🏥
● M84.375 Stress fracture, left foot K, P 🏥
● M84.376 Stress fracture, unspecified foot K, P 🏥
● M84.377 Stress fracture, right toe(s) K, P 🏥
● M84.378 Stress fracture, left toe(s) K, P 🏥
● M84.379 Stress fracture, unspecified toe(s) K, P 🏥
X ● **M84.38 Stress fracture, other site** K, P 🏥
Excludes2 stress fracture of vertebra (M48.4-)

N Newborn Age: 0   P Pediatric Age: 0–17   M Maternity DX: 12–55   A Adult Age: 15–124   ♀ Females Only   ♂ Males Only
🏥 Complication\Comorbidity   Major C\C   (Ex) CC/MCC Exclusions   Hospital-Acquired Condition

1063

CHAPTER 13 (M00-M99)

● **M84.4** **Pathological fracture, not elsewhere classified**
Chronic fracture
Pathological fracture NOS

Excludes1 collapsed vertebra NEC (M48.5)
pathological fracture in neoplastic disease
(M84.5-)
pathological fracture in osteoporosis
(M80.-)
pathological fracture in other disease
(M84.6-)
stress fracture (M84.3-)
traumatic fracture (S12.-, S22.-, S32.-, S42.-
, S52.-, S62.-, S72.-, S82.-, S92.-)

Excludes2 personal history of (healed) pathological
fracture (Z87.311)

The appropriate 7th character is to be added to each
code from subcategory M84.4:

> A   initial encounter for fracture
> D   subsequent encounter for fracture with routine
>   healing
> G   subsequent encounter for fracture with
>   delayed healing
> K   subsequent encounter for fracture with
>   nonunion
> P   subsequent encounter for fracture with
>   malunion
> S   sequela

Ex: See M80

X ● **M84.40** Pathological fracture, unspecified site A, K, P
● **M84.41** **Pathological fracture, shoulder**
  ● **M84.411** Pathological fracture, right shoulder
    A, K, P
  ● **M84.412** Pathological fracture, left shoulder
    A, K, P
  ● **M84.419** Pathological fracture, unspecified
    shoulder A, K, P
● **M84.42** **Pathological fracture, humerus**
  ● **M84.421** Pathological fracture, right humerus
    A, K, P
  ● **M84.422** Pathological fracture, left humerus
    A, K, P
  ● **M84.429** Pathological fracture, unspecified
    humerus A, K, P
● **M84.43** **Pathological fracture, ulna and radius**
  ● **M84.431** Pathological fracture, right ulna
    A, K, P
  ● **M84.432** Pathological fracture, left ulna
    A, K, P
  ● **M84.433** Pathological fracture, right radius
    A, K, P
  ● **M84.434** Pathological fracture, left radius
    A, K, P
  ● **M84.439** Pathological fracture, unspecified
    ulna and radius A, K, P

● **M84.44** **Pathological fracture, hand and fingers**
  ● **M84.441** Pathological fracture, right hand
    A, K, P
  ● **M84.442** Pathological fracture, left hand
    A, K, P
  ● **M84.443** Pathological fracture, unspecified
    hand A, K, P
  ● **M84.444** Pathological fracture, right finger(s)
    A, K, P
  ● **M84.445** Pathological fracture, left finger(s)
    A, K, P
  ● **M84.446** Pathological fracture, unspecified
    finger(s) A, K, P
● **M84.45** **Pathological fracture, femur and pelvis**
  ● **M84.451** Pathological fracture, right femur
    A, K, P
  ● **M84.452** Pathological fracture, left femur
    A, K, P
  ● **M84.453** Pathological fracture, unspecified
    femur A, K, P
  ● **M84.454** Pathological fracture, pelvis A, K, P
  ● **M84.459** Pathological fracture, hip, unspecified
    A, K, P
● **M84.46** **Pathological fracture, tibia and fibula**
  ● **M84.461** Pathological fracture, right tibia
    A, K, P
  ● **M84.462** Pathological fracture, left tibia
    A, K, P
  ● **M84.463** Pathological fracture, right fibula
    A, K, P
  ● **M84.464** Pathological fracture, left fibula
    A, K, P
  ● **M84.469** Pathological fracture, unspecified
    tibia and fibula A, K, P
● **M84.47** **Pathological fracture, ankle, foot and toes**
  ● **M84.471** Pathological fracture, right ankle
    A, K, P
  ● **M84.472** Pathological fracture, left ankle
    A, K, P
  ● **M84.473** Pathological fracture, unspecified
    ankle A, K, P
  ● **M84.474** Pathological fracture, right foot
    A, K, P
  ● **M84.475** Pathological fracture, left foot
    A, K, P
  ● **M84.476** Pathological fracture, unspecified foot
    A, K, P
  ● **M84.477** Pathological fracture, right toe(s)
    A, K, P
  ● **M84.478** Pathological fracture, left toe(s)
    A, K, P
  ● **M84.479** Pathological fracture, unspecified
    toe(s) A, K, P
X ● **M84.48** Pathological fracture, other site A, K, P

OGCR Section I.a, Chapter 13.C.

Coding of Pathologic Fractures

7th character A is for use as long as the patient is receiving active treatment for the fracture. While the patient may be seen by a new or different provider over the course of treatment for a pathological fracture, assignment of the 7th character is based on whether the patient is undergoing active treatment and not whether the provider is seeing the patient for the first time.3. 7th character, D is to be used for encounters after the patient has completed active treatment. The other 7th characters, listed under each subcategory in the Tabular List, are to be used for subsequent encounters for **routine care of fractures during the healing and recovery phase as well as** treatment of problems associated with the healing, such as malunions, nonunions, and sequelae.

Care for complications of surgical treatment for fracture repairs during the healing or recovery phase should be coded with the appropriate complication codes.

See Section I.C.19. Coding of traumatic fractures.

● **M84.5 Pathological fracture in neoplastic disease**

    Code also underlying neoplasm

    The appropriate 7th character is to be added to each code from subcategory M84.5:

A	initial encounter for fracture
D	subsequent encounter for fracture with routine healing
G	subsequent encounter for fracture with delayed healing
K	subsequent encounter for fracture with nonunion
P	subsequent encounter for fracture with malunion
S	sequela

Ⓔⓧ See M80

X ● **M84.50 Pathological fracture in neoplastic disease, unspecified site** A, K, P Ⓖ

● **M84.51 Pathological fracture in neoplastic disease, shoulder**
    ● **M84.511 Pathological fracture in neoplastic disease, right shoulder** A, K, P Ⓖ
    ● **M84.512 Pathological fracture in neoplastic disease, left shoulder** A, K, P Ⓖ
    ● **M84.519 Pathological fracture in neoplastic disease, unspecified shoulder** A, K, P Ⓖ

● **M84.52 Pathological fracture in neoplastic disease, humerus**
    ● **M84.521 Pathological fracture in neoplastic disease, right humerus** A, K, P Ⓖ
    ● **M84.522 Pathological fracture in neoplastic disease, left humerus** A, K, P Ⓖ
    ● **M84.529 Pathological fracture in neoplastic disease, unspecified humerus** A, K, P Ⓖ

● **M84.53 Pathological fracture in neoplastic disease, ulna and radius**
    ● **M84.531 Pathological fracture in neoplastic disease, right ulna** A, K, P Ⓖ
    ● **M84.532 Pathological fracture in neoplastic disease, left ulna** A, K, P Ⓖ
    ● **M84.533 Pathological fracture in neoplastic disease, right radius** A, K, P Ⓖ
    ● **M84.534 Pathological fracture in neoplastic disease, left radius** A, K, P Ⓖ
    ● **M84.539 Pathological fracture in neoplastic disease, unspecified ulna and radius** A, K, P Ⓖ

● **M84.54 Pathological fracture in neoplastic disease, hand**
    ● **M84.541 Pathological fracture in neoplastic disease, right hand** A, K, P Ⓖ
    ● **M84.542 Pathological fracture in neoplastic disease, left hand** A, K, P Ⓖ
    ● **M84.549 Pathological fracture in neoplastic disease, unspecified hand** A, K, P Ⓖ

● **M84.55 Pathological fracture in neoplastic disease, pelvis and femur**
    ● **M84.550 Pathological fracture in neoplastic disease, pelvis** A, K, P Ⓖ
    ● **M84.551 Pathological fracture in neoplastic disease, right femur** A, K, P Ⓖ
    ● **M84.552 Pathological fracture in neoplastic disease, left femur** A, K, P Ⓖ
    ● **M84.553 Pathological fracture in neoplastic disease, unspecified femur** A, K, P Ⓖ
    ● **M84.559 Pathological fracture in neoplastic disease, hip, unspecified** A, K, P Ⓖ

● **M84.56 Pathological fracture in neoplastic disease, tibia and fibula**
    ● **M84.561 Pathological fracture in neoplastic disease, right tibia** A, K, P Ⓖ
    ● **M84.562 Pathological fracture in neoplastic disease, left tibia** A, K, P Ⓖ
    ● **M84.563 Pathological fracture in neoplastic disease, right fibula** A, K, P Ⓖ
    ● **M84.564 Pathological fracture in neoplastic disease, left fibula** A, K, P Ⓖ
    ● **M84.569 Pathological fracture in neoplastic disease, unspecified tibia and fibula** A, K, P Ⓖ

● **M84.57 Pathological fracture in neoplastic disease, ankle and foot**
    ● **M84.571 Pathological fracture in neoplastic disease, right ankle** A, K, P Ⓖ
    ● **M84.572 Pathological fracture in neoplastic disease, left ankle** A, K, P Ⓖ
    ● **M84.573 Pathological fracture in neoplastic disease, unspecified ankle** A, K, P Ⓖ
    ● **M84.574 Pathological fracture in neoplastic disease, right foot** A, K, P Ⓖ
    ● **M84.575 Pathological fracture in neoplastic disease, left foot** A, K, P Ⓖ
    ● **M84.576 Pathological fracture in neoplastic disease, unspecified foot** A, K, P Ⓖ

X ● **M84.58 Pathological fracture in neoplastic disease, other specified site** A, K, P Ⓖ
    Pathological fracture in neoplastic disease, vertebrae

● **M84.6 Pathological fracture in other disease**
    Code also underlying condition
    Excludes1   pathological fracture in osteoporosis (M80.-)
    The appropriate 7th character is to be added to each code from subcategory M84.6:

A	initial encounter for fracture
D	subsequent encounter for fracture with routine healing
G	subsequent encounter for fracture with delayed healing
K	subsequent encounter for fracture with nonunion
P	subsequent encounter for fracture with malunion
S	sequela

Ⓔⓧ See M80

X ● **M84.60 Pathological fracture in other disease, unspecified site** A, K, P Ⓖ

N Newborn Age: 0   **P** Pediatric Age: 0–17   **M** Maternity DX: 12–55   **A** Adult Age: 15–124   ♀ Females Only   ♂ Males Only

 Complication\Comorbidity   Major C\C   Ⓔⓧ CC/MCC Exclusions   Hospital-Acquired Condition

1065

CHAPTER 13 (M00-M99)

● **M84.61** Pathological fracture in other disease, shoulder
  ● **M84.611** Pathological fracture in other disease, right shoulder A, K, P 🔒
  ● **M84.612** Pathological fracture in other disease, left shoulder A, K, P 🔒
  ● **M84.619** Pathological fracture in other disease, unspecified shoulder A, K, P 🔒
● **M84.62** Pathological fracture in other disease, humerus
  ● **M84.621** Pathological fracture in other disease, right humerus A, K, P 🔒
  ● **M84.622** Pathological fracture in other disease, left humerus A, K, P 🔒
  ● **M84.629** Pathological fracture in other disease, unspecified humerus A, K, P 🔒
● **M84.63** Pathological fracture in other disease, ulna and radius
  ● **M84.631** Pathological fracture in other disease, right ulna A, K, P 🔒
  ● **M84.632** Pathological fracture in other disease, left ulna A, K, P 🔒
  ● **M84.633** Pathological fracture in other disease, right radius A, K, P 🔒
  ● **M84.634** Pathological fracture in other disease, left radius A, K, P 🔒
  ● **M84.639** Pathological fracture in other disease, unspecified ulna and radius A, K, P 🔒
● **M84.64** Pathological fracture in other disease, hand
  ● **M84.641** Pathological fracture in other disease, right hand A, K, P 🔒
  ● **M84.642** Pathological fracture in other disease, left hand A, K, P 🔒
  ● **M84.649** Pathological fracture in other disease, unspecified hand A, K, P 🔒
● **M84.65** Pathological fracture in other disease, pelvis and femur
  ● **M84.650** Pathological fracture in other disease, pelvis A, K, P 🔒
  ● **M84.651** Pathological fracture in other disease, right femur A, K, P 🔒
  ● **M84.652** Pathological fracture in other disease, left femur A, K, P 🔒
  ● **M84.653** Pathological fracture in other disease, unspecified femur A, K, P 🔒
  ● **M84.659** Pathological fracture in other disease, hip, unspecified A, K, P 🔒
● **M84.66** Pathological fracture in other disease, tibia and fibula
  ● **M84.661** Pathological fracture in other disease, right tibia A, K, P 🔒
  ● **M84.662** Pathological fracture in other disease, left tibia A, K, P 🔒
  ● **M84.663** Pathological fracture in other disease, right fibula A, K, P 🔒
  ● **M84.664** Pathological fracture in other disease, left fibula A, K, P 🔒
  ● **M84.669** Pathological fracture in other disease, unspecified tibia and fibula A, K, P 🔒
● **M84.67** Pathological fracture in other disease, ankle and foot
  ● **M84.671** Pathological fracture in other disease, right ankle A, K, P 🔒
  ● **M84.672** Pathological fracture in other disease, left ankle A, K, P 🔒
  ● **M84.673** Pathological fracture in other disease, unspecified ankle A, K, P 🔒

  ● **M84.674** Pathological fracture in other disease, right foot A, K, P 🔒
  ● **M84.675** Pathological fracture in other disease, left foot A, K, P 🔒
  ● **M84.676** Pathological fracture in other disease, unspecified foot A, K, P 🔒
X ● **M84.68** Pathological fracture in other disease, other site A, K, P 🔒
● **M84.7** Nontraumatic fracture, not elsewhere classified ◀
  ● **M84.75** Atypical femoral fracture ◀

The appropriate 7th character is to be added to each code from M84.75: ◀

A	initial encounter for fracture ◀
D	subsequent encounter for fracture with routine healing ◀
G	subsequent encounter for fracture with delayed healing ◀
K	subsequent encounter for fracture with nonunion ◀
P	subsequent encounter for fracture with malunion ◀
S	sequela ◀

(Ex:) See M80 ◀

  ● **M84.750** Atypical femoral fracture, unspecified A, K, P 🔒 ◀
  ● **M84.751** Incomplete atypical femoral fracture, right leg A, K, P 🔒 ◀
  ● **M84.752** Incomplete atypical femoral fracture, left leg A, K, P 🔒 ◀
  ● **M84.753** Incomplete atypical femoral fracture, unspecified leg A, K, P 🔒 ◀
  ● **M84.754** Complete transverse atypical femoral fracture, right leg A, K, P 🔒 ◀
  ● **M84.755** Complete transverse atypical femoral fracture, left leg A, K, P 🔒 ◀
  ● **M84.756** Complete transverse atypical femoral fracture, unspecified leg A, K, P 🔒 ◀
  ● **M84.757** Complete oblique atypical femoral fracture, right leg A, K, P 🔒 ◀
  ● **M84.758** Complete oblique atypical femoral fracture, left leg A, K, P 🔒 ◀
  ● **M84.759** Complete oblique atypical femoral fracture, unspecified leg A, K, P 🔒 ◀
● **M84.8** Other disorders of continuity of bone
  M84.80 Other disorders of continuity of bone, unspecified site
  ● **M84.81** Other disorders of continuity of bone, shoulder
    M84.811 Other disorders of continuity of bone, right shoulder
    M84.812 Other disorders of continuity of bone, left shoulder
    M84.819 Other disorders of continuity of bone, unspecified shoulder
  ● **M84.82** Other disorders of continuity of bone, humerus
    M84.821 Other disorders of continuity of bone, right humerus
    M84.822 Other disorders of continuity of bone, left humerus
    M84.829 Other disorders of continuity of bone, unspecified humerus

● **M84.83** Other disorders of continuity of bone, ulna and radius

     M84.831   Other disorders of continuity of bone, right ulna

     M84.832   Other disorders of continuity of bone, left ulna

     M84.833   Other disorders of continuity of bone, right radius

     M84.834   Other disorders of continuity of bone, left radius

     M84.839   Other disorders of continuity of bone, unspecified ulna and radius

● **M84.84** Other disorders of continuity of bone, hand

     M84.841   Other disorders of continuity of bone, right hand

     M84.842   Other disorders of continuity of bone, left hand

     M84.849   Other disorders of continuity of bone, unspecified hand

● **M84.85** Other disorders of continuity of bone, pelvic region and thigh

     M84.851   Other disorders of continuity of bone, right pelvic region and thigh

     M84.852   Other disorders of continuity of bone, left pelvic region and thigh

     M84.859   Other disorders of continuity of bone, unspecified pelvic region and thigh

● **M84.86** Other disorders of continuity of bone, tibia and fibula

     M84.861   Other disorders of continuity of bone, right tibia

     M84.862   Other disorders of continuity of bone, left tibia

     M84.863   Other disorders of continuity of bone, right fibula

     M84.864   Other disorders of continuity of bone, left fibula

     M84.869   Other disorders of continuity of bone, unspecified tibia and fibula

● **M84.87** Other disorders of continuity of bone, ankle and foot

     M84.871   Other disorders of continuity of bone, right ankle and foot

     M84.872   Other disorders of continuity of bone, left ankle and foot

     M84.879   Other disorders of continuity of bone, unspecified ankle and foot

     M84.88   Other disorders of continuity of bone, other site

   M84.9   Disorder of continuity of bone, unspecified

● **M85**   Other disorders of bone density and structure

     Excludes1   osteogenesis imperfecta (Q78.0)
                 osteopetrosis (Q78.2)
                 osteopoikilosis (Q78.8)
                 polyostotic fibrous dysplasia (Q78.1)

● **M85.0**   Fibrous dysplasia (monostotic)

     Excludes2   fibrous dysplasia of jaw (M27.8)

     M85.00   Fibrous dysplasia (monostotic), unspecified site

● **M85.01** Fibrous dysplasia (monostotic), shoulder

     M85.011   Fibrous dysplasia (monostotic), right shoulder

     M85.012   Fibrous dysplasia (monostotic), left shoulder

     M85.019   Fibrous dysplasia (monostotic), unspecified shoulder

● **M85.02** Fibrous dysplasia (monostotic), upper arm

     M85.021   Fibrous dysplasia (monostotic), right upper arm

     M85.022   Fibrous dysplasia (monostotic), left upper arm

     M85.029   Fibrous dysplasia (monostotic), unspecified upper arm

● **M85.03** Fibrous dysplasia (monostotic), forearm

     M85.031   Fibrous dysplasia (monostotic), right forearm

     M85.032   Fibrous dysplasia (monostotic), left forearm

     M85.039   Fibrous dysplasia (monostotic), unspecified forearm

● **M85.04** Fibrous dysplasia (monostotic), hand

     M85.041   Fibrous dysplasia (monostotic), right hand

     M85.042   Fibrous dysplasia (monostotic), left hand

     M85.049   Fibrous dysplasia (monostotic), unspecified hand

● **M85.05** Fibrous dysplasia (monostotic), thigh

     M85.051   Fibrous dysplasia (monostotic), right thigh

     M85.052   Fibrous dysplasia (monostotic), left thigh

     M85.059   Fibrous dysplasia (monostotic), unspecified thigh

● **M85.06** Fibrous dysplasia (monostotic), lower leg

     M85.061   Fibrous dysplasia (monostotic), right lower leg

     M85.062   Fibrous dysplasia (monostotic), left lower leg

     M85.069   Fibrous dysplasia (monostotic), unspecified lower leg

● **M85.07** Fibrous dysplasia (monostotic), ankle and foot

     M85.071   Fibrous dysplasia (monostotic), right ankle and foot

     M85.072   Fibrous dysplasia (monostotic), left ankle and foot

     M85.079   Fibrous dysplasia (monostotic), unspecified ankle and foot

     M85.08   Fibrous dysplasia (monostotic), other site

     M85.09   Fibrous dysplasia (monostotic), multiple sites

● **M85.1**   Skeletal fluorosis

     M85.10   Skeletal fluorosis, unspecified site

● **M85.11** Skeletal fluorosis, shoulder

     M85.111   Skeletal fluorosis, right shoulder

     M85.112   Skeletal fluorosis, left shoulder

     M85.119   Skeletal fluorosis, unspecified shoulder

● **M85.12** Skeletal fluorosis, upper arm

     M85.121   Skeletal fluorosis, right upper arm

     M85.122   Skeletal fluorosis, left upper arm

     M85.129   Skeletal fluorosis, unspecified upper arm

● **M85.13** Skeletal fluorosis, forearm

     M85.131   Skeletal fluorosis, right forearm

     M85.132   Skeletal fluorosis, left forearm

     M85.139   Skeletal fluorosis, unspecified forearm

● **M85.14** Skeletal fluorosis, hand

     M85.141   Skeletal fluorosis, right hand

     M85.142   Skeletal fluorosis, left hand

     M85.149   Skeletal fluorosis, unspecified hand

CHAPTER 13 (M00-M99)

● M85.15 Skeletal fluorosis, thigh
  M85.151 Skeletal fluorosis, right thigh
  M85.152 Skeletal fluorosis, left thigh
  M85.159 Skeletal fluorosis, unspecified thigh
● M85.16 Skeletal fluorosis, lower leg
  M85.161 Skeletal fluorosis, right lower leg
  M85.162 Skeletal fluorosis, left lower leg
  M85.169 Skeletal fluorosis, unspecified lower leg
● M85.17 Skeletal fluorosis, ankle and foot
  M85.171 Skeletal fluorosis, right ankle and foot
  M85.172 Skeletal fluorosis, left ankle and foot
  M85.179 Skeletal fluorosis, unspecified ankle and foot
  M85.18 Skeletal fluorosis, other site
  M85.19 Skeletal fluorosis, multiple sites
M85.2 Hyperostosis of skull
● M85.3 Osteitis condensans
  M85.30 Osteitis condensans, unspecified site
● M85.31 Osteitis condensans, shoulder
  M85.311 Osteitis condensans, right shoulder
  M85.312 Osteitis condensans, left shoulder
  M85.319 Osteitis condensans, unspecified shoulder
● M85.32 Osteitis condensans, upper arm
  M85.321 Osteitis condensans, right upper arm
  M85.322 Osteitis condensans, left upper arm
  M85.329 Osteitis condensans, unspecified upper arm
● M85.33 Osteitis condensans, forearm
  M85.331 Osteitis condensans, right forearm
  M85.332 Osteitis condensans, left forearm
  M85.339 Osteitis condensans, unspecified forearm
● M85.34 Osteitis condensans, hand
  M85.341 Osteitis condensans, right hand
  M85.342 Osteitis condensans, left hand
  M85.349 Osteitis condensans, unspecified hand
● M85.35 Osteitis condensans, thigh
  M85.351 Osteitis condensans, right thigh
  M85.352 Osteitis condensans, left thigh
  M85.359 Osteitis condensans, unspecified thigh
● M85.36 Osteitis condensans, lower leg
  M85.361 Osteitis condensans, right lower leg
  M85.362 Osteitis condensans, left lower leg
  M85.369 Osteitis condensans, unspecified lower leg
● M85.37 Osteitis condensans, ankle and foot
  M85.371 Osteitis condensans, right ankle and foot
  M85.372 Osteitis condensans, left ankle and foot
  M85.379 Osteitis condensans, unspecified ankle and foot
  M85.38 Osteitis condensans, other site
  M85.39 Osteitis condensans, multiple sites
● M85.4 Solitary bone cyst
  Excludes2 solitary cyst of jaw (M27.4)
  M85.40 Solitary bone cyst, unspecified site
● M85.41 Solitary bone cyst, shoulder
  M85.411 Solitary bone cyst, right shoulder
  M85.412 Solitary bone cyst, left shoulder
  M85.419 Solitary bone cyst, unspecified shoulder

● M85.42 Solitary bone cyst, humerus
  M85.421 Solitary bone cyst, right humerus
  M85.422 Solitary bone cyst, left humerus
  M85.429 Solitary bone cyst, unspecified humerus
● M85.43 Solitary bone cyst, ulna and radius
  M85.431 Solitary bone cyst, right ulna and radius
  M85.432 Solitary bone cyst, left ulna and radius
  M85.439 Solitary bone cyst, unspecified ulna and radius
● M85.44 Solitary bone cyst, hand
  M85.441 Solitary bone cyst, right hand
  M85.442 Solitary bone cyst, left hand
  M85.449 Solitary bone cyst, unspecified hand
● M85.45 Solitary bone cyst, pelvis
  M85.451 Solitary bone cyst, right pelvis
  M85.452 Solitary bone cyst, left pelvis
  M85.459 Solitary bone cyst, unspecified pelvis
● M85.46 Solitary bone cyst, tibia and fibula
  M85.461 Solitary bone cyst, right tibia and fibula
  M85.462 Solitary bone cyst, left tibia and fibula
  M85.469 Solitary bone cyst, unspecified tibia and fibula
● M85.47 Solitary bone cyst, ankle and foot
  M85.471 Solitary bone cyst, right ankle and foot
  M85.472 Solitary bone cyst, left ankle and foot
  M85.479 Solitary bone cyst, unspecified ankle and foot
  M85.48 Solitary bone cyst, other site
● M85.5 Aneurysmal bone cyst
  Excludes2 aneurysmal cyst of jaw (M27.4)
  M85.50 Aneurysmal bone cyst, unspecified site
● M85.51 Aneurysmal bone cyst, shoulder
  M85.511 Aneurysmal bone cyst, right shoulder
  M85.512 Aneurysmal bone cyst, left shoulder
  M85.519 Aneurysmal bone cyst, unspecified shoulder
● M85.52 Aneurysmal bone cyst, upper arm
  M85.521 Aneurysmal bone cyst, right upper arm
  M85.522 Aneurysmal bone cyst, left upper arm
  M85.529 Aneurysmal bone cyst, unspecified upper arm
● M85.53 Aneurysmal bone cyst, forearm
  M85.531 Aneurysmal bone cyst, right forearm
  M85.532 Aneurysmal bone cyst, left forearm
  M85.539 Aneurysmal bone cyst, unspecified forearm
● M85.54 Aneurysmal bone cyst, hand
  M85.541 Aneurysmal bone cyst, right hand
  M85.542 Aneurysmal bone cyst, left hand
  M85.549 Aneurysmal bone cyst, unspecified hand
● M85.55 Aneurysmal bone cyst, thigh
  M85.551 Aneurysmal bone cyst, right thigh
  M85.552 Aneurysmal bone cyst, left thigh
  M85.559 Aneurysmal bone cyst, unspecified thigh

● M85.56   Aneurysmal bone cyst, lower leg

     M85.561   Aneurysmal bone cyst, right lower leg

     M85.562   Aneurysmal bone cyst, left lower leg

     M85.569   Aneurysmal bone cyst, unspecified lower leg

● M85.57   Aneurysmal bone cyst, ankle and foot

     M85.571   Aneurysmal bone cyst, right ankle and foot

     M85.572   Aneurysmal bone cyst, left ankle and foot

     M85.579   Aneurysmal bone cyst, unspecified ankle and foot

     M85.58   Aneurysmal bone cyst, other site

     M85.59   Aneurysmal bone cyst, multiple sites

● M85.6   Other cyst of bone

     Excludes1   cyst of jaw NEC (M27.4)
         osteitis fibrosa cystica generalisata [von Recklinghausen's disease of bone] (E21.0)

     M85.60   Other cyst of bone, unspecified site

●   M85.61   Other cyst of bone, shoulder

     M85.611   Other cyst of bone, right shoulder

     M85.612   Other cyst of bone, left shoulder

     M85.619   Other cyst of bone, unspecified shoulder

● M85.62   Other cyst of bone, upper arm

     M85.621   Other cyst of bone, right upper arm

     M85.622   Other cyst of bone, left upper arm

     M85.629   Other cyst of bone, unspecified upper arm

● M85.63   Other cyst of bone, forearm

     M85.631   Other cyst of bone, right forearm

     M85.632   Other cyst of bone, left forearm

     M85.639   Other cyst of bone, unspecified forearm

● M85.64   Other cyst of bone, hand

     M85.641   Other cyst of bone, right hand

     M85.642   Other cyst of bone, left hand

     M85.649   Other cyst of bone, unspecified hand

● M85.65   Other cyst of bone, thigh

     M85.651   Other cyst of bone, right thigh

     M85.652   Other cyst of bone, left thigh

     M85.659   Other cyst of bone, unspecified thigh

● M85.66   Other cyst of bone, lower leg

     M85.661   Other cyst of bone, right lower leg

     M85.662   Other cyst of bone, left lower leg

     M85.669   Other cyst of bone, unspecified lower leg

● M85.67   Other cyst of bone, ankle and foot

     M85.671   Other cyst of bone, right ankle and foot

     M85.672   Other cyst of bone, left ankle and foot

     M85.679   Other cyst of bone, unspecified ankle and foot

     M85.68   Other cyst of bone, other site

     M85.69   Other cyst of bone, multiple sites

● M85.8   Other specified disorders of bone density and structure

     Hyperostosis of bones, except skull
     Osteosclerosis, acquired

     Excludes1   diffuse idiopathic skeletal hyperostosis [DISH] (M48.1)
         osteosclerosis congenita (Q77.4)
         osteosclerosis fragilitas (generalista) (Q78.2)
         osteosclerosis myelofibrosis (D75.81)

     M85.80   Other specified disorders of bone density and structure, unspecified site

● M85.81   Other specified disorders of bone density and structure, shoulder

     M85.811   Other specified disorders of bone density and structure, right shoulder

     M85.812   Other specified disorders of bone density and structure, left shoulder

     M85.819   Other specified disorders of bone density and structure, unspecified shoulder

● M85.82   Other specified disorders of bone density and structure, upper arm

     M85.821   Other specified disorders of bone density and structure, right upper arm

     M85.822   Other specified disorders of bone density and structure, left upper arm

     M85.829   Other specified disorders of bone density and structure, unspecified upper arm

● M85.83   Other specified disorders of bone density and structure, forearm

     M85.831   Other specified disorders of bone density and structure, right forearm

     M85.832   Other specified disorders of bone density and structure, left forearm

     M85.839   Other specified disorders of bone density and structure, unspecified forearm

● M85.84   Other specified disorders of bone density and structure, hand

     M85.841   Other specified disorders of bone density and structure, right hand

     M85.842   Other specified disorders of bone density and structure, left hand

     M85.849   Other specified disorders of bone density and structure, unspecified hand

● M85.85   Other specified disorders of bone density and structure, thigh

     M85.851   Other specified disorders of bone density and structure, right thigh

     M85.852   Other specified disorders of bone density and structure, left thigh

     M85.859   Other specified disorders of bone density and structure, unspecified thigh

● M85.86   Other specified disorders of bone density and structure, lower leg

     M85.861   Other specified disorders of bone density and structure, right lower leg

     M85.862   Other specified disorders of bone density and structure, left lower leg

     M85.869   Other specified disorders of bone density and structure, unspecified lower leg

● M85.87   Other specified disorders of bone density and structure, ankle and foot

     M85.871   Other specified disorders of bone density and structure, right ankle and foot

     M85.872   Other specified disorders of bone density and structure, left ankle and foot

     M85.879   Other specified disorders of bone density and structure, unspecified ankle and foot

     M85.88   Other specified disorders of bone density and structure, other site

     M85.89   Other specified disorders of bone density and structure, multiple sites

M85.9   Disorder of bone density and structure, unspecified

CHAPTER 13 (M00-M99)

CHAPTER 13 (M00-M99)

OTHER OSTEOPATHIES (M86-M90)

> **Excludes1**   postprocedural osteopathies (M96.-)

● **M86 Osteomyelitis**

Use additional code (B95-B97) to identify infectious agent

Use additional code to identify major osseous defect, if applicable (M89.7-)

> **Excludes1**   osteomyelitis due to:
> echinococcus (B67.2)
> gonococcus (A54.43)
> salmonella (A02.24)

> **Excludes2**   ostemyelitis of:
> orbit (H05.0-)
> petrous bone (H70.2-)
> vertebra (M46.2-)

● **M86.0   Acute hematogenous osteomyelitis**

     M86.00   Acute hematogenous osteomyelitis, unspecified site 🔍

         ⓔⓧ A17.9, A18.03-A18.09, A18.82, A18.84, A18.89, M46.20-M46.39, M86.00-M86.9

     ● **M86.01   Acute hematogenous osteomyelitis, shoulder**

         ⓔⓧ **For category M86.01 CC codes:** A17.9, A18.03-A18.09, A18.82, A18.84, A18.89, M46.20-M46.39, M86.00, M86.08-M86.10, M86.18-M86.20, M86.28-M86.319, M86.38-M86.419, M86.48-M86.519, M86.58-M86.619, M86.68-M86.8X1, M86.8X8-M86.9

         M86.011   Acute hematogenous osteomyelitis, right shoulder 🔍

         M86.012   Acute hematogenous osteomyelitis, left shoulder 🔍

         M86.019   Acute hematogenous osteomyelitis, unspecified shoulder 🔍

     ● **M86.02   Acute hematogenous osteomyelitis, humerus**

         ⓔⓧ **For category M86.02 CC codes:** A17.9, A18.03-A18.09, A18.82, A18.84, A18.89, M46.20-M46.39, M86.00, M86.08-M86.10, M86.18-M86.20, M86.28-M86.30, M86.321-M86.329, M86.38-M86.40, M86.421-M86.429, M86.48-M86.50, M86.521-M86.529, M86.58-M86.60, M86.621-M86.629, M86.68-M86.69, M86.8X0, M86.8X2, M86.8X8-M86.9

         M86.021   Acute hematogenous osteomyelitis, right humerus 🔍

         M86.022   Acute hematogenous osteomyelitis, left humerus 🔍

         M86.029   Acute hematogenous osteomyelitis, unspecified humerus 🔍

Figure 13-6   Osteomyelitis of the spine. A lateral view of the lower thoracic spine demonstrates destruction of the disk space *(arrow)* as well as destruction of the adjoining vertebral bodies. (From Mettler: Essentials of Radiology, ed 2, Saunders, An Imprint of Elsevier, 2005)

Item 13–12 Osteomyelitis is an inflammation of the bone. **Acute osteomyelitis** is a rapidly destructive, pus-producing infection capable of causing severe bone destruction. **Chronic osteomyelitis** can remain long after the initial acute episode has passed and may lead to a recurrence of the acute phase. **Brodie's abscess** is an encapsulated focal abscess that must be surgically drained. Periostitis is an inflammation of the periosteum, a dense membrane composed of fibrous connective tissue that closely wraps all bone, except those with articulating surfaces in joints, which are covered by synovial membranes.

● **M86.03   Acute hematogenous osteomyelitis, radius and ulna**

     ⓔⓧ **For category M86.03 CC codes:** A17.9, A18.03-A18.09, A18.82, A18.84, A18.89, M46.20-M46.39, M86.00, M86.08-M86.10, M86.18-M86.20, M86.28-M86.30, M86.331-M86.339, M86.38-M86.40, M86.431-M86.439, M86.48-M86.50, M86.531-M86.539, M86.58-M86.60, M86.631-M86.639, M86.68-M86.8X0, M86.8X3, M86.8X8-M86.9

     M86.031   Acute hematogenous osteomyelitis, right radius and ulna 🔍

     M86.032   Acute hematogenous osteomyelitis, left radius and ulna 🔍

     M86.039   Acute hematogenous osteomyelitis, unspecified radius and ulna 🔍

● **M86.04   Acute hematogenous osteomyelitis, hand**

     ⓔⓧ **For category M86.04 CC codes:** A17.9, A18.03-A18.09, A18.82, A18.84, A18.89, M46.20-M46.39, M86.00, M86.08-M86.10, M86.18-M86.20, M86.28-M86.30, M86.341-M86.349, M86.38-M86.40, M86.441-M86.449, M86.48-M86.50, M86.541-M86.549, M86.58-M86.60, M86.41-M86.649, M86.68-M86.69, M86.8X0, M86.8X4, M86.8X8-M86.9

     M86.041   Acute hematogenous osteomyelitis, right hand 🔍

     M86.042   Acute hematogenous osteomyelitis, left hand 🔍

     M86.049   Acute hematogenous osteomyelitis, unspecified hand 🔍

● **M86.05   Acute hematogenous osteomyelitis, femur**

     ⓔⓧ **For category M86.05 CC codes:** A17.9, A18.03-A18.09, A18.82, A18.84, A18.89, M46.20-M46.39, M86.00, M86.08-M86.10, M86.18-M86.20, M86.28-M86.30, M86.351-M86.359, M86.38-M86.40, M86.451-M86.459, M86.48-M86.50, M86.551-M86.559, M86.58-M86.60, M86.651-M86.659, M86.68-M86.8X0, M86.8X5, M86.8X8-M86.9

     M86.051   Acute hematogenous osteomyelitis, right femur 🔍

     M86.052   Acute hematogenous osteomyelitis, left femur 🔍

     M86.059   Acute hematogenous osteomyelitis, unspecified femur 🔍

● **M86.06   Acute hematogenous osteomyelitis, tibia and fibula**

     ⓔⓧ **For category M86.06 CC codes:** A17.9, A18.03-A18.09, A18.82, A18.84, A18.89, M46.20-M46.39, M86.00, M86.08-M86.10, M86.18-M86.20, M86.28-M86.30, M86.361-M86.369, M86.38-M86.40, M86.461-M86.469, M86.48-M86.50, M86.561-M86.569, M86.58-M86.60, M86.661-M86.669, M86.68-M86.8X0, M86.8X6, M86.8X8-M86.9

     M86.061   Acute hematogenous osteomyelitis, right tibia and fibula 🔍

     M86.062   Acute hematogenous osteomyelitis, left tibia and fibula 🔍

     M86.069   Acute hematogenous osteomyelitis, unspecified tibia and fibula 🔍

● **M86.07   Acute hematogenous osteomyelitis, ankle and foot**

     ⓔⓧ **For category M86.07 CC codes:** A17.9, A18.03-A18.09, A18.82, A18.84, A18.89, M46.20-M46.39, M86.00, M86.08-M86.10, M86.18-M86.20, M86.28-M86.30, M86.371-M86.379, M86.38-M86.40, M86.471-M86.479, M86.48-M86.50, M86.571-M86.579, M86.58-M86.60, M86.671-M86.679, M86.68-M86.8X0, M86.8X7-M86.9

     M86.071   Acute hematogenous osteomyelitis, right ankle and foot 🔍

     M86.072   Acute hematogenous osteomyelitis, left ankle and foot 🔍

     M86.079   Acute hematogenous osteomyelitis, unspecified ankle and foot 🔍

◀ New   ◀ Revised   ~~deleted~~ Deleted   Excludes 1   Excludes 2   Includes   Use additional   Code first   Code also   Unspecified
OGCR Official Guidelines   ● Unacceptable Principal Diagnosis   X Assign placeholder X   ● Use Additional Character(s)   ▶ Manifestation Code   **Coding Clinic**

M86.08   Acute hematogenous osteomyelitis, other sites 🖢
     Ⓔⓧ A17.9, A18.01, A18.03, A18.09, A18.82, A18.84, A18.89, M46.20-M46.39, M86.00-M86.9

M86.09   Acute hematogenous osteomyelitis, multiple sites 🖢
     Ⓔⓧ See M86.00

● M86.1   Other acute osteomyelitis

     M86.10   Other acute osteomyelitis, unspecified site 🖢
         Ⓔⓧ See M86.00

   ● M86.11   Other acute osteomyelitis, shoulder
         Ⓔⓧ For category M86.11 CC codes: See M86.01

         M86.111   Other acute osteomyelitis, right shoulder 🖢
         M86.112   Other acute osteomyelitis, left shoulder 🖢
         M86.119   Other acute osteomyelitis, unspecified shoulder 🖢

   ● M86.12   Other acute osteomyelitis, humerus
         Ⓔⓧ For category M86.12 CC codes: See M86.02

         M86.121   Other acute osteomyelitis, right humerus 🖢
         M86.122   Other acute osteomyelitis, left humerus 🖢
         M86.129   Other acute osteomyelitis, unspecified humerus 🖢

   ● M86.13   Other acute osteomyelitis, radius and ulna
         Ⓔⓧ For category M86.13 CC codes: See M86.03

         M86.131   Other acute osteomyelitis, right radius and ulna 🖢
         M86.132   Other acute osteomyelitis, left radius and ulna 🖢
         M86.139   Other acute osteomyelitis, unspecified radius and ulna 🖢

   ● M86.14   Other acute osteomyelitis, hand
         Ⓔⓧ For category M86.14 CC codes: See M86.04

         M86.141   Other acute osteomyelitis, right hand 🖢
         M86.142   Other acute osteomyelitis, left hand 🖢
         M86.149   Other acute osteomyelitis, unspecified hand 🖢

   ● M86.15   Other acute osteomyelitis, femur
         Ⓔⓧ For category M86.15 CC codes: See M86.05

         M86.151   Other acute osteomyelitis, right femur 🖢
         M86.152   Other acute osteomyelitis, left femur 🖢
         M86.159   Other acute osteomyelitis, unspecified femur 🖢

   ● M86.16   Other acute osteomyelitis, tibia and fibula
         Ⓔⓧ For category M86.16 CC codes: See M86.06

         M86.161   Other acute osteomyelitis, right tibia and fibula 🖢
         M86.162   Other acute osteomyelitis, left tibia and fibula 🖢
         M86.169   Other acute osteomyelitis, unspecified tibia and fibula 🖢

   ● M86.17   Other acute osteomyelitis, ankle and foot
         Ⓔⓧ For category M86.17 CC codes: See M86.07

         M86.171   Other acute osteomyelitis, right ankle and foot 🖢
         M86.172   Other acute osteomyelitis, left ankle and foot 🖢
         M86.179   Other acute osteomyelitis, unspecified ankle and foot 🖢

     M86.18   Other acute osteomyelitis, other site 🖢
         Ⓔⓧ See M86.08

     M86.19   Other acute osteomyelitis, multiple sites 🖢
         Ⓔⓧ See M86.00

● M86.2   Subacute osteomyelitis

     M86.20   Subacute osteomyelitis, unspecified site 🖢
         Ⓔⓧ See M86.00

   ● M86.21   Subacute osteomyelitis, shoulder
         Ⓔⓧ For category M86.21 CC codes: See M86.01

         M86.211   Subacute osteomyelitis, right shoulder 🖢
         M86.212   Subacute osteomyelitis, left shoulder 🖢
         M86.219   Subacute osteomyelitis, unspecified shoulder 🖢

   ● M86.22   Subacute osteomyelitis, humerus
         Ⓔⓧ For category M86.22 CC codes: See M86.02

         M86.221   Subacute osteomyelitis, right humerus 🖢
         M86.222   Subacute osteomyelitis, left humerus 🖢
         M86.229   Subacute osteomyelitis, unspecified humerus 🖢

   ● M86.23   Subacute osteomyelitis, radius and ulna
         Ⓔⓧ For category M86.23 CC codes: See M86.03

         M86.231   Subacute osteomyelitis, right radius and ulna 🖢
         M86.232   Subacute osteomyelitis, left radius and ulna 🖢
         M86.239   Subacute osteomyelitis, unspecified radius and ulna 🖢

   ● M86.24   Subacute osteomyelitis, hand
         Ⓔⓧ For category M86.24 CC codes: See M86.04

         M86.241   Subacute osteomyelitis, right hand 🖢
         M86.242   Subacute osteomyelitis, left hand 🖢
         M86.249   Subacute osteomyelitis, unspecified hand 🖢

   ● M86.25   Subacute osteomyelitis, femur
         Ⓔⓧ For category M86.25 CC codes: See M86.05

         M86.251   Subacute osteomyelitis, right femur 🖢
         M86.252   Subacute osteomyelitis, left femur 🖢
         M86.259   Subacute osteomyelitis, unspecified femur 🖢

   ● M86.26   Subacute osteomyelitis, tibia and fibula
         Ⓔⓧ For category M86.26 CC codes: See M86.06

         M86.261   Subacute osteomyelitis, right tibia and fibula 🖢
         M86.262   Subacute osteomyelitis, left tibia and fibula 🖢
         M86.269   Subacute osteomyelitis, unspecified tibia and fibula 🖢

   ● M86.27   Subacute osteomyelitis, ankle and foot
         Ⓔⓧ For category M86.27 CC codes: See M86.07

         M86.271   Subacute osteomyelitis, right ankle and foot 🖢
         M86.272   Subacute osteomyelitis, left ankle and foot 🖢
         M86.279   Subacute osteomyelitis, unspecified ankle and foot 🖢

     M86.28   Subacute osteomyelitis, other site 🖢
         Ⓔⓧ See M86.08

     M86.29   Subacute osteomyelitis, multiple sites 🖢
         Ⓔⓧ See M86.00

● M86.3   Chronic multifocal osteomyelitis
     Ⓔⓧ For category M86.3 CC codes unless otherwise indicated: A02.24, A17.9, A18.03, A18.09, A18.82, A18.84, A18.89, M46.20-M46.39, M86.00-M86.9

     M86.30   Chronic multifocal osteomyelitis, unspecified site 🖢
         Ⓔⓧ M46.20-M46.39, M86.30-M86.9, M88.0-M88.9, M90.60-M90.69

N   Newborn Age: 0   **P**   Pediatric Age: 0–17   **M**   Maternity DX: 12–55   **A**   Adult Age: 15–124   ♀ Females Only   ♂ Males Only

🖢 Complication\Comorbidity   🖢 Major C\C   Ⓔⓧ CC/MCC Exclusions   🖢 Hospital-Acquired Condition

1071

CHAPTER 13 (M00-M99)

● M86.31   Chronic multifocal osteomyelitis, shoulder
    M86.311   Chronic multifocal osteomyelitis, right shoulder 🔵
    M86.312   Chronic multifocal osteomyelitis, left shoulder 🔵
    M86.319   Chronic multifocal osteomyelitis, unspecified shoulder 🔵

● M86.32   Chronic multifocal osteomyelitis, humerus
    M86.321   Chronic multifocal osteomyelitis, right humerus 🔵
    M86.322   Chronic multifocal osteomyelitis, left humerus 🔵
    M86.329   Chronic multifocal osteomyelitis, unspecified humerus 🔵

● M86.33   Chronic multifocal osteomyelitis, radius and ulna
    M86.331   Chronic multifocal osteomyelitis, right radius and ulna 🔵
    M86.332   Chronic multifocal osteomyelitis, left radius and ulna 🔵
    M86.339   Chronic multifocal osteomyelitis, unspecified radius and ulna 🔵

● M86.34   Chronic multifocal osteomyelitis, hand
    M86.341   Chronic multifocal osteomyelitis, right hand 🔵
    M86.342   Chronic multifocal osteomyelitis, left hand 🔵
    M86.349   Chronic multifocal osteomyelitis, unspecified hand 🔵

● M86.35   Chronic multifocal osteomyelitis, femur
    M86.351   Chronic multifocal osteomyelitis, right femur 🔵
    M86.352   Chronic multifocal osteomyelitis, left femur 🔵
    M86.359   Chronic multifocal osteomyelitis, unspecified femur 🔵

● M86.36   Chronic multifocal osteomyelitis, tibia and fibula
    M86.361   Chronic multifocal osteomyelitis, right tibia and fibula 🔵
    M86.362   Chronic multifocal osteomyelitis, left tibia and fibula 🔵
    M86.369   Chronic multifocal osteomyelitis, unspecified tibia and fibula 🔵

● M86.37   Chronic multifocal osteomyelitis, ankle and foot
    M86.371   Chronic multifocal osteomyelitis, right ankle and foot 🔵
    M86.372   Chronic multifocal osteomyelitis, left ankle and foot 🔵
    M86.379   Chronic multifocal osteomyelitis, unspecified ankle and foot 🔵

    M86.38   Chronic multifocal osteomyelitis, other site 🔵
    M86.39   Chronic multifocal osteomyelitis, multiple sites 🔵

● M86.4   Chronic osteomyelitis with draining sinus
    Ⓔⓧ For category M86.4 CC codes unless otherwise indicated: See M86.3
    M86.40   Chronic osteomyelitis with draining sinus, unspecified site 🔵
       Ⓔⓧ See M86.30

● M86.41   Chronic osteomyelitis with draining sinus, shoulder
    M86.411   Chronic osteomyelitis with draining sinus, right shoulder 🔵
    M86.412   Chronic osteomyelitis with draining sinus, left shoulder 🔵
    M86.419   Chronic osteomyelitis with draining sinus, unspecified shoulder 🔵

● M86.42   Chronic osteomyelitis with draining sinus, humerus
    M86.421   Chronic osteomyelitis with draining sinus, right humerus 🔵
    M86.422   Chronic osteomyelitis with draining sinus, left humerus 🔵
    M86.429   Chronic osteomyelitis with draining sinus, unspecified humerus 🔵

● M86.43   Chronic osteomyelitis with draining sinus, radius and ulna
    M86.431   Chronic osteomyelitis with draining sinus, right radius and ulna 🔵
    M86.432   Chronic osteomyelitis with draining sinus, left radius and ulna 🔵
    M86.439   Chronic osteomyelitis with draining sinus, unspecified radius and ulna 🔵

● M86.44   Chronic osteomyelitis with draining sinus, hand
    M86.441   Chronic osteomyelitis with draining sinus, right hand 🔵
    M86.442   Chronic osteomyelitis with draining sinus, left hand 🔵
    M86.449   Chronic osteomyelitis with draining sinus, unspecified hand 🔵

● M86.45   Chronic osteomyelitis with draining sinus, femur
    M86.451   Chronic osteomyelitis with draining sinus, right femur 🔵
    M86.452   Chronic osteomyelitis with draining sinus, left femur 🔵
    M86.459   Chronic osteomyelitis with draining sinus, unspecified femur 🔵

● M86.46   Chronic osteomyelitis with draining sinus, tibia and fibula
    M86.461   Chronic osteomyelitis with draining sinus, right tibia and fibula 🔵
    M86.462   Chronic osteomyelitis with draining sinus, left tibia and fibula 🔵
    M86.469   Chronic osteomyelitis with draining sinus, unspecified tibia and fibula 🔵

● M86.47   Chronic osteomyelitis with draining sinus, ankle and foot
    M86.471   Chronic osteomyelitis with draining sinus, right ankle and foot 🔵
    M86.472   Chronic osteomyelitis with draining sinus, left ankle and foot 🔵
    M86.479   Chronic osteomyelitis with draining sinus, unspecified ankle and foot 🔵

    M86.48   Chronic osteomyelitis with draining sinus, other site 🔵
    M86.49   Chronic osteomyelitis with draining sinus, multiple sites 🔵

● M86.5   Other chronic hematogenous osteomyelitis
    Ⓔⓧ For category M86.5 CC codes unless otherwise indicated: See M86.3
    M86.50   Other chronic hematogenous osteomyelitis, unspecified site 🔵
       Ⓔⓧ See M86.30

● M86.51   Other chronic hematogenous osteomyelitis, shoulder
    M86.511   Other chronic hematogenous osteomyelitis, right shoulder 🔵
    M86.512   Other chronic hematogenous osteomyelitis, left shoulder 🔵
    M86.519   Other chronic hematogenous osteomyelitis, unspecified shoulder 🔵

◀ New   ◀▥ Revised   ~~deleted~~ Deleted   Excludes 1   Excludes 2   Includes   Use additional   Code first   Code also   Unspecified
OGCR Official Guidelines   ● Unacceptable Principal Diagnosis   X Assign placeholder X   ● Use Additional Character(s)   ▶ Manifestation Code   Coding Clinic

● **M86.52**   Other chronic hematogenous osteomyelitis, humerus
    M86.521   Other chronic hematogenous osteomyelitis, right humerus 🏥
    M86.522   Other chronic hematogenous osteomyelitis, left humerus 🏥
    M86.529   Other chronic hematogenous osteomyelitis, <mark>unspecified</mark> humerus 🏥

● **M86.53**   Other chronic hematogenous osteomyelitis, radius and ulna
    M86.531   Other chronic hematogenous osteomyelitis, right radius and ulna 🏥
    M86.532   Other chronic hematogenous osteomyelitis, left radius and ulna 🏥
    M86.539   Other chronic hematogenous osteomyelitis, <mark>unspecified</mark> radius and ulna 🏥

● **M86.54**   Other chronic hematogenous osteomyelitis, hand
    M86.541   Other chronic hematogenous osteomyelitis, right hand 🏥
    M86.542   Other chronic hematogenous osteomyelitis, left hand 🏥
    M86.549   Other chronic hematogenous osteomyelitis, <mark>unspecified</mark> hand 🏥

● **M86.55**   Other chronic hematogenous osteomyelitis, femur
    M86.551   Other chronic hematogenous osteomyelitis, right femur 🏥
    M86.552   Other chronic hematogenous osteomyelitis, left femur 🏥
    M86.559   Other chronic hematogenous osteomyelitis, <mark>unspecified</mark> femur 🏥

● **M86.56**   Other chronic hematogenous osteomyelitis, tibia and fibula
    M86.561   Other chronic hematogenous osteomyelitis, right tibia and fibula 🏥
    M86.562   Other chronic hematogenous osteomyelitis, left tibia and fibula 🏥
    M86.569   Other chronic hematogenous osteomyelitis, <mark>unspecified</mark> tibia and fibula 🏥

● **M86.57**   Other chronic hematogenous osteomyelitis, ankle and foot
    M86.571   Other chronic hematogenous osteomyelitis, right ankle and foot 🏥
    M86.572   Other chronic hematogenous osteomyelitis, left ankle and foot 🏥
    M86.579   Other chronic hematogenous osteomyelitis, <mark>unspecified</mark> ankle and foot 🏥

    M86.58   Other chronic hematogenous osteomyelitis, other site 🏥
    M86.59   Other chronic hematogenous osteomyelitis, multiple sites 🏥

● **M86.6**   Other chronic osteomyelitis
    (Ex) **For category M86.6 CC codes unless otherwise indicated:** See M86.3
    M86.60   Other chronic osteomyelitis, <mark>unspecified</mark> site 🏥
       (Ex) See M86.30

● **M86.61**   Other chronic osteomyelitis, shoulder
    M86.611   Other chronic osteomyelitis, right shoulder 🏥
    M86.612   Other chronic osteomyelitis, left shoulder 🏥
    M86.619   Other chronic osteomyelitis, <mark>unspecified</mark> shoulder 🏥

● **M86.62**   Other chronic osteomyelitis, humerus
    M86.621   Other chronic osteomyelitis, right humerus 🏥
    M86.622   Other chronic osteomyelitis, left humerus 🏥
    M86.629   Other chronic osteomyelitis, <mark>unspecified</mark> humerus 🏥

● **M86.63**   Other chronic osteomyelitis, radius and ulna
    M86.631   Other chronic osteomyelitis, right radius and ulna 🏥
    M86.632   Other chronic osteomyelitis, left radius and ulna 🏥
    M86.639   Other chronic osteomyelitis, <mark>unspecified</mark> radius and ulna 🏥

● **M86.64**   Other chronic osteomyelitis, hand
    M86.641   Other chronic osteomyelitis, right hand 🏥
    M86.642   Other chronic osteomyelitis, left hand 🏥
    M86.649   Other chronic osteomyelitis, <mark>unspecified</mark> hand 🏥

● **M86.65**   Other chronic osteomyelitis, thigh
    M86.651   Other chronic osteomyelitis, right thigh 🏥
    M86.652   Other chronic osteomyelitis, left thigh 🏥
    M86.659   Other chronic osteomyelitis, <mark>unspecified</mark> thigh 🏥

● **M86.66**   Other chronic osteomyelitis, tibia and fibula
    M86.661   Other chronic osteomyelitis, right tibia and fibula 🏥
    M86.662   Other chronic osteomyelitis, left tibia and fibula 🏥
    M86.669   Other chronic osteomyelitis, <mark>unspecified</mark> tibia and fibula 🏥

● **M86.67**   Other chronic osteomyelitis, ankle and foot
    M86.671   Other chronic osteomyelitis, right ankle and foot 🏥
       Coding Clinic: 2016, Q1, P13
    M86.672   Other chronic osteomyelitis, left ankle and foot 🏥
    M86.679   Other chronic osteomyelitis, <mark>unspecified</mark> ankle and foot 🏥

    M86.68   Other chronic osteomyelitis, other site 🏥
    M86.69   Other chronic osteomyelitis, multiple sites 🏥

● **M86.8**   Other osteomyelitis
    Brodie's abscess
    (Ex) **For category M86.8 CC codes unless otherwise indicated:** See M86.3
    ● **M86.8X**   Other osteomyelitis
       M86.8X0   Other osteomyelitis, multiple sites 🏥
       M86.8X1   Other osteomyelitis, shoulder 🏥
       M86.8X2   Other osteomyelitis, upper arm 🏥
       M86.8X3   Other osteomyelitis, forearm 🏥
       M86.8X4   Other osteomyelitis, hand 🏥
       M86.8X5   Other osteomyelitis, thigh 🏥
       M86.8X6   Other osteomyelitis, lower leg 🏥
       M86.8X7   Other osteomyelitis, ankle and foot 🏥
       M86.8X8   Other osteomyelitis, other site 🏥
       M86.8X9   Other osteomyelitis, <mark>unspecified</mark> sites 🏥
          (Ex) See M86.30

   M86.9   Osteomyelitis, <mark>unspecified</mark> 🏥
     Infection of bone NOS
     Periostitis without osteomyelitis
     (Ex) See M86.30

N   Newborn Age: 0   **P**   Pediatric Age: 0–17   **M**   Maternity DX: 12–55   **A**   Adult Age: 15–124   ♀   Females Only   ♂   Males Only

🏥   Complication\Comorbidity   🏥   Major C\C   (Ex)   CC/MCC Exclusions   🏥   Hospital-Acquired Condition

CHAPTER 13 (M00-M99)

● **M87   Osteonecrosis**
> **Includes**   avascular necrosis of bone
> Use additional code to identify major osseous defect, if applicable (M89.7-)
> **Excludes1**   juvenile osteonecrosis (M91-M92)
>   osteochondropathies (M90-M93)
> (Ex:) For category M87 CC codes unless otherwise indicated: M87.00-M87.9, M90.50-M90.59

  ● **M87.0   Idiopathic aseptic necrosis of bone**
      M87.00   Idiopathic aseptic necrosis of unspecified bone 🔁
    ● **M87.01   Idiopathic aseptic necrosis of shoulder**
          Idiopathic aseptic necrosis of clavicle and scapula
          (Ex:) For category M87.01 CC codes: M87.00-M87.9, M90.50-M90.59
        M87.011   Idiopathic aseptic necrosis of right shoulder 🔁
        M87.012   Idiopathic aseptic necrosis of left shoulder 🔁
        M87.019   Idiopathic aseptic necrosis of unspecified shoulder 🔁
    ● **M87.02   Idiopathic aseptic necrosis of humerus**
          (Ex:) For category M87.02 CC codes: See M87.01
        M87.021   Idiopathic aseptic necrosis of right humerus 🔁
        M87.022   Idiopathic aseptic necrosis of left humerus 🔁
        M87.029   Idiopathic aseptic necrosis of unspecified humerus 🔁
    ● **M87.03   Idiopathic aseptic necrosis of radius, ulna and carpus**
        M87.031   Idiopathic aseptic necrosis of right radius 🔁
        M87.032   Idiopathic aseptic necrosis of left radius 🔁
        M87.033   Idiopathic aseptic necrosis of unspecified radius 🔁
        M87.034   Idiopathic aseptic necrosis of right ulna 🔁
        M87.035   Idiopathic aseptic necrosis of left ulna 🔁
        M87.036   Idiopathic aseptic necrosis of unspecified ulna 🔁
        M87.037   Idiopathic aseptic necrosis of right carpus 🔁
        M87.038   Idiopathic aseptic necrosis of left carpus 🔁
        M87.039   Idiopathic aseptic necrosis of unspecified carpus 🔁
    ● **M87.04   Idiopathic aseptic necrosis of hand and fingers**
          Idiopathic aseptic necrosis of metacarpals and phalanges of hands
        M87.041   Idiopathic aseptic necrosis of right hand 🔁
        M87.042   Idiopathic aseptic necrosis of left hand 🔁
        M87.043   Idiopathic aseptic necrosis of unspecified hand 🔁
        M87.044   Idiopathic aseptic necrosis of right finger(s) 🔁
        M87.045   Idiopathic aseptic necrosis of left finger(s) 🔁
        M87.046   Idiopathic aseptic necrosis of unspecified finger(s) 🔁

  ● **M87.05   Idiopathic aseptic necrosis of pelvis and femur**
        M87.050   Idiopathic aseptic necrosis of pelvis 🔁
        M87.051   Idiopathic aseptic necrosis of right femur 🔁
           (Ex:) M87.00-M87.9, M90.50-M90.59
        M87.052   Idiopathic aseptic necrosis of left femur 🔁
           (Ex:) See M87.501
        M87.059   Idiopathic aseptic necrosis of unspecified femur 🔁
          Idiopathic aseptic necrosis of hip NOS
           (Ex:) See M87.501
  ● **M87.06   Idiopathic aseptic necrosis of tibia and fibula**
        M87.061   Idiopathic aseptic necrosis of right tibia 🔁
        M87.062   Idiopathic aseptic necrosis of left tibia 🔁
        M87.063   Idiopathic aseptic necrosis of unspecified tibia 🔁
        M87.064   Idiopathic aseptic necrosis of right fibula 🔁
        M87.065   Idiopathic aseptic necrosis of left fibula 🔁
        M87.066   Idiopathic aseptic necrosis of unspecified fibula 🔁
  ● **M87.07   Idiopathic aseptic necrosis of ankle, foot and toes**
          Idiopathic aseptic necrosis of metatarsus, tarsus, and phalanges of toes
        M87.071   Idiopathic aseptic necrosis of right ankle 🔁
        M87.072   Idiopathic aseptic necrosis of left ankle 🔁
        M87.073   Idiopathic aseptic necrosis of unspecified ankle 🔁
        M87.074   Idiopathic aseptic necrosis of right foot 🔁
           (Ex:) M87.00, M87.031-M87.819, M87.831-M87.849, M87.861-M87.9, M90.50, M90.521-M90.549, M90.561-M90.59
        M87.075   Idiopathic aseptic necrosis of left foot 🔁
           (Ex:) See M87.074
        M87.076   Idiopathic aseptic necrosis of unspecified foot 🔁
           (Ex:) See M87.074
        M87.077   Idiopathic aseptic necrosis of right toe(s) 🔁
        M87.078   Idiopathic aseptic necrosis of left toe(s) 🔁
        M87.079   Idiopathic aseptic necrosis of unspecified toe(s) 🔁
      M87.08   Idiopathic aseptic necrosis of bone, other site 🔁
      M87.09   Idiopathic aseptic necrosis of bone, multiple sites 🔁
  ● **M87.1   Osteonecrosis due to drugs**
          Use additional code for adverse effect, if applicable, to identify drug (T36-T50 with fifth or sixth character 5)
           (Ex:) See M87
      M87.10   Osteonecrosis due to drugs, unspecified bone 🔁
    ● **M87.11   Osteonecrosis due to drugs, shoulder**
        M87.111   Osteonecrosis due to drugs, right shoulder 🔁
        M87.112   Osteonecrosis due to drugs, left shoulder 🔁
        M87.119   Osteonecrosis due to drugs, unspecified shoulder 🔁

◀ New   ◀◀ Revised   ~~deleted~~ Deleted   Excludes 1   Excludes 2   Includes   Use additional   Code first   Code also   Unspecified
OGCR Official Guidelines   ● Unacceptable Principal Diagnosis   X Assign placeholder X   🔁 Use Additional Character(s)   ▶ Manifestation Code   **Coding Clinic**

● **M87.12** **Osteonecrosis due to drugs, humerus**
(Ex) For category M87.12 CC codes: See M87.01

     M87.121 Osteonecrosis due to drugs, right humerus 🦴

     M87.122 Osteonecrosis due to drugs, left humerus 🦴

     M87.129 Osteonecrosis due to drugs, unspecified humerus 🦴

● **M87.13** **Osteonecrosis due to drugs of radius, ulna and carpus**

     M87.131 Osteonecrosis due to drugs of right radius 🦴

     M87.132 Osteonecrosis due to drugs of left radius 🦴

     M87.133 Osteonecrosis due to drugs of unspecified radius 🦴

     M87.134 Osteonecrosis due to drugs of right ulna 🦴

     M87.135 Osteonecrosis due to drugs of left ulna 🦴

     M87.136 Osteonecrosis due to drugs of unspecified ulna 🦴

     M87.137 Osteonecrosis due to drugs of right carpus 🦴

     M87.138 Osteonecrosis due to drugs of left carpus 🦴

     M87.139 Osteonecrosis due to drugs of unspecified carpus 🦴

● **M87.14** **Osteonecrosis due to drugs, hand and fingers**

     M87.141 Osteonecrosis due to drugs, right hand 🦴

     M87.142 Osteonecrosis due to drugs, left hand 🦴

     M87.143 Osteonecrosis due to drugs, unspecified hand 🦴

     M87.144 Osteonecrosis due to drugs, right finger(s) 🦴

     M87.145 Osteonecrosis due to drugs, left finger(s) 🦴

     M87.146 Osteonecrosis due to drugs, unspecified finger(s) 🦴

● **M87.15** **Osteonecrosis due to drugs, pelvis and femur**
(Ex) For category M87.15 CC codes: See M87.051

     M87.150 Osteonecrosis due to drugs, pelvis 🦴

     M87.151 Osteonecrosis due to drugs, right femur 🦴

     M87.152 Osteonecrosis due to drugs, left femur 🦴

     M87.159 Osteonecrosis due to drugs, unspecified femur 🦴

● **M87.16** **Osteonecrosis due to drugs, tibia and fibula**

     M87.161 Osteonecrosis due to drugs, right tibia 🦴

     M87.162 Osteonecrosis due to drugs, left tibia 🦴

     M87.163 Osteonecrosis due to drugs, unspecified tibia 🦴

     M87.164 Osteonecrosis due to drugs, right fibula 🦴

     M87.165 Osteonecrosis due to drugs, left fibula 🦴

     M87.166 Osteonecrosis due to drugs, unspecified fibula 🦴

● **M87.17** **Osteonecrosis due to drugs, ankle, foot and toes**

     M87.171 Osteonecrosis due to drugs, right ankle 🦴

     M87.172 Osteonecrosis due to drugs, left ankle 🦴

     M87.173 Osteonecrosis due to drugs, unspecified ankle 🦴

     M87.174 Osteonecrosis due to drugs, right foot 🦴
         (Ex) See M87.074

     M87.175 Osteonecrosis due to drugs, left foot 🦴
         (Ex) See M87.074

     M87.176 Osteonecrosis due to drugs, unspecified foot 🦴
         (Ex) See M87.074

     M87.177 Osteonecrosis due to drugs, right toe(s) 🦴

     M87.178 Osteonecrosis due to drugs, left toe(s) 🦴

     M87.179 Osteonecrosis due to drugs, unspecified toe(s) 🦴

● **M87.18** **Osteonecrosis due to drugs, other site**

     M87.180 Osteonecrosis due to drugs, jaw 🦴

     M87.188 Osteonecrosis due to drugs, other site 🦴

     M87.19 Osteonecrosis due to drugs, multiple sites 🦴

● **M87.2** **Osteonecrosis due to previous trauma**
(Ex) See M87

     M87.20 Osteonecrosis due to previous trauma, unspecified bone 🦴

● **M87.21** **Osteonecrosis due to previous trauma, shoulder**

     M87.211 Osteonecrosis due to previous trauma, right shoulder 🦴

     M87.212 Osteonecrosis due to previous trauma, left shoulder 🦴

     M87.219 Osteonecrosis due to previous trauma, unspecified shoulder 🦴

● **M87.22** **Osteonecrosis due to previous trauma, humerus**
(Ex) For category M87.22 CC codes: See M87.01

     M87.221 Osteonecrosis due to previous trauma, right humerus 🦴

     M87.222 Osteonecrosis due to previous trauma, left humerus 🦴

     M87.229 Osteonecrosis due to previous trauma, unspecified humerus 🦴

● **M87.23** **Osteonecrosis due to previous trauma of radius, ulna and carpus**

     M87.231 Osteonecrosis due to previous trauma of right radius 🦴

     M87.232 Osteonecrosis due to previous trauma of left radius 🦴

     M87.233 Osteonecrosis due to previous trauma of unspecified radius 🦴

     M87.234 Osteonecrosis due to previous trauma of right ulna 🦴

     M87.235 Osteonecrosis due to previous trauma of left ulna 🦴

     M87.236 Osteonecrosis due to previous trauma of unspecified ulna 🦴

     M87.237 Osteonecrosis due to previous trauma of right carpus 🦴

     M87.238 Osteonecrosis due to previous trauma of left carpus 🦴

     M87.239 Osteonecrosis due to previous trauma of unspecified carpus 🦴

CHAPTER 13 (M00–M99)

N   Newborn Age: 0   **P**   Pediatric Age: 0–17   **M**   Maternity DX: 12–55   **A**   Adult Age: 15–124   ♀   Females Only   ♂   Males Only

🦴   Complication\Comorbidity   🦴   Major C\C   (Ex)   CC/MCC Exclusions   🦴   Hospital-Acquired Condition   **1075**

● **M87.24 Osteonecrosis due to previous trauma, hand and fingers**

    M87.241 Osteonecrosis due to previous trauma, right hand 🦴

    M87.242 Osteonecrosis due to previous trauma, left hand 🦴

    M87.243 Osteonecrosis due to previous trauma, `unspecified` hand 🦴

    M87.244 Osteonecrosis due to previous trauma, right finger(s) 🦴

    M87.245 Osteonecrosis due to previous trauma, left finger(s) 🦴

    M87.246 Osteonecrosis due to previous trauma, `unspecified` finger(s) 🦴

● **M87.25 Osteonecrosis due to previous trauma, pelvis and femur**

    M87.250 Osteonecrosis due to previous trauma, pelvis 🦴

    M87.251 Osteonecrosis due to previous trauma, right femur 🦴
        Ex: See M87.051

    M87.252 Osteonecrosis due to previous trauma, left femur 🦴
        Ex: See M87.051

    M87.256 Osteonecrosis due to previous trauma, `unspecified` femur 🦴
        Ex: See M87.051

● **M87.26 Osteonecrosis due to previous trauma, tibia and fibula**

    M87.261 Osteonecrosis due to previous trauma, right tibia 🦴

    M87.262 Osteonecrosis due to previous trauma, left tibia 🦴

    M87.263 Osteonecrosis due to previous trauma, `unspecified` tibia 🦴

    M87.264 Osteonecrosis due to previous trauma, right fibula 🦴

    M87.265 Osteonecrosis due to previous trauma, left fibula 🦴

    M87.266 Osteonecrosis due to previous trauma, `unspecified` fibula 🦴

● **M87.27 Osteonecrosis due to previous trauma, ankle, foot and toes**

    M87.271 Osteonecrosis due to previous trauma, right ankle 🦴

    M87.272 Osteonecrosis due to previous trauma, left ankle 🦴

    M87.273 Osteonecrosis due to previous trauma, `unspecified` ankle 🦴

    M87.274 Osteonecrosis due to previous trauma, right foot 🦴
        Ex: See M87.074

    M87.275 Osteonecrosis due to previous trauma, left foot 🦴
        Ex: See M87.074

    M87.276 Osteonecrosis due to previous trauma, `unspecified` foot 🦴
        Ex: See M87.074

    M87.277 Osteonecrosis due to previous trauma, right toe(s) 🦴

    M87.278 Osteonecrosis due to previous trauma, left toe(s) 🦴

    M87.279 Osteonecrosis due to previous trauma, `unspecified` toe(s) 🦴

  M87.28 Osteonecrosis due to previous trauma, other site 🦴

  M87.29 Osteonecrosis due to previous trauma, multiple sites 🦴

● **M87.3 Other secondary osteonecrosis**
    Ex: See M87

  M87.30 Other secondary osteonecrosis, `unspecified` bone 🦴

● **M87.31 Other secondary osteonecrosis, shoulder**

    M87.311 Other secondary osteonecrosis, right shoulder 🦴

    M87.312 Other secondary osteonecrosis, left shoulder 🦴

    M87.319 Other secondary osteonecrosis, `unspecified` shoulder 🦴

● **M87.32 Other secondary osteonecrosis, humerus**
    Ex: For category M87.32 CC codes: See M87.01

    M87.321 Other secondary osteonecrosis, right humerus 🦴

    M87.322 Other secondary osteonecrosis, left humerus 🦴

    M87.329 Other secondary osteonecrosis, `unspecified` humerus 🦴

● **M87.33 Other secondary osteonecrosis of radius, ulna and carpus**

    M87.331 Other secondary osteonecrosis of right radius 🦴

    M87.332 Other secondary osteonecrosis of left radius 🦴

    M87.333 Other secondary osteonecrosis of `unspecified` radius 🦴

    M87.334 Other secondary osteonecrosis of right ulna 🦴

    M87.335 Other secondary osteonecrosis of left ulna 🦴

    M87.336 Other secondary osteonecrosis of `unspecified` ulna 🦴

    M87.337 Other secondary osteonecrosis of right carpus 🦴

    M87.338 Other secondary osteonecrosis of left carpus 🦴

    M87.339 Other secondary osteonecrosis of `unspecified` carpus 🦴

● **M87.34 Other secondary osteonecrosis, hand and fingers**

    M87.341 Other secondary osteonecrosis, right hand 🦴

    M87.342 Other secondary osteonecrosis, left hand 🦴

    M87.343 Other secondary osteonecrosis, `unspecified` hand 🦴

    M87.344 Other secondary osteonecrosis, right finger(s) 🦴

    M87.345 Other secondary osteonecrosis, left finger(s) 🦴

    M87.346 Other secondary osteonecrosis, `unspecified` finger(s) 🦴

● **M87.35 Other secondary osteonecrosis, pelvis and femur**
    Ex: For category M87.35 CC codes: See M87.051

    M87.350 Other secondary osteonecrosis, pelvis 🦴

    M87.351 Other secondary osteonecrosis, right femur 🦴

    M87.352 Other secondary osteonecrosis, left femur 🦴

    M87.353 Other secondary osteonecrosis, `unspecified` femur 🦴

◀ New   ◀▥ Revised   ~~deleted~~ Deleted   `Excludes 1`   `Excludes 2`   `Includes`   `Use additional`   `Code first`   `Code also`   `Unspecified`
OGCR Official Guidelines   ● Unacceptable Principal Diagnosis   X Assign placeholder X   ● Use Additional Character(s)   ▶ Manifestation Code   **Coding Clinic**

● M87.36　Other secondary osteonecrosis, tibia and fibula
　　　　M87.361　Other secondary osteonecrosis, right tibia 🦠
　　　　M87.362　Other secondary osteonecrosis, left tibia 🦠
　　　　M87.363　Other secondary osteonecrosis, unspecified tibia 🦠
　　　　M87.364　Other secondary osteonecrosis, right fibula 🦠
　　　　M87.365　Other secondary osteonecrosis, left fibula 🦠
　　　　M87.366　Other secondary osteonecrosis, unspecified fibula 🦠
● M87.37　Other secondary osteonecrosis, ankle and foot
　　　　M87.371　Other secondary osteonecrosis, right ankle 🦠
　　　　M87.372　Other secondary osteonecrosis, left ankle 🦠
　　　　M87.373　Other secondary osteonecrosis, unspecified ankle 🦠
　　　　M87.374　Other secondary osteonecrosis, right foot 🦠
　　　　　　　　(Ex:) See M87.074
　　　　M87.375　Other secondary osteonecrosis, left foot 🦠
　　　　　　　　(Ex:) See M87.074
　　　　M87.376　Other secondary osteonecrosis, unspecified foot 🦠
　　　　　　　　(Ex:) See M87.074
　　　　M87.377　Other secondary osteonecrosis, right toe(s) 🦠
　　　　M87.378　Other secondary osteonecrosis, left toe(s) 🦠
　　　　M87.379　Other secondary osteonecrosis, unspecified toe(s) 🦠
　　M87.38　Other secondary osteonecrosis, other site 🦠
　　M87.39　Other secondary osteonecrosis, multiple sites 🦠
● M87.8　Other osteonecrosis
　　　　(Ex:) See M87
　　M87.80　Other osteonecrosis, unspecified bone 🦠
● M87.81　Other osteonecrosis, shoulder
　　　　M87.811　Other osteonecrosis, right shoulder 🦠
　　　　M87.812　Other osteonecrosis, left shoulder 🦠
　　　　M87.819　Other osteonecrosis, unspecified shoulder 🦠
● M87.82　Other osteonecrosis, humerus
　　　　(Ex:) For category M87.82 CC codes: See M87.01
　　　　M87.821　Other osteonecrosis, right humerus 🦠
　　　　M87.822　Other osteonecrosis, left humerus 🦠
　　　　M87.829　Other osteonecrosis, unspecified humerus 🦠
● M87.83　Other osteonecrosis of radius, ulna and carpus
　　　　M87.831　Other osteonecrosis of right radius 🦠
　　　　M87.832　Other osteonecrosis of left radius 🦠
　　　　M87.833　Other osteonecrosis of unspecified radius 🦠
　　　　M87.834　Other osteonecrosis of right ulna 🦠
　　　　M87.835　Other osteonecrosis of left ulna 🦠
　　　　M87.836　Other osteonecrosis of unspecified ulna 🦠
　　　　M87.837　Other osteonecrosis of right carpus 🦠
　　　　M87.838　Other osteonecrosis of left carpus 🦠
　　　　M87.839　Other osteonecrosis of unspecified carpus 🦠

● M87.84　Other osteonecrosis, hand and fingers
　　　　M87.841　Other osteonecrosis, right hand 🦠
　　　　M87.842　Other osteonecrosis, left hand 🦠
　　　　M87.843　Other osteonecrosis, unspecified hand 🦠
　　　　M87.844　Other osteonecrosis, right finger(s) 🦠
　　　　M87.845　Other osteonecrosis, left finger(s) 🦠
　　　　M87.849　Other osteonecrosis, unspecified finger(s) 🦠
● M87.85　Other osteonecrosis, pelvis and femur
　　　　(Ex:) For category M87.85 CC codes: See M87.051
　　　　M87.850　Other osteonecrosis, pelvis 🦠
　　　　M87.851　Other osteonecrosis, right femur 🦠
　　　　M87.852　Other osteonecrosis, left femur 🦠
　　　　M87.859　Other osteonecrosis, unspecified femur 🦠
● M87.86　Other osteonecrosis, tibia and fibula
　　　　M87.861　Other osteonecrosis, right tibia 🦠
　　　　M87.862　Other osteonecrosis, left tibia 🦠
　　　　M87.863　Other osteonecrosis, unspecified tibia 🦠
　　　　M87.864　Other osteonecrosis, right fibula 🦠
　　　　M87.865　Other osteonecrosis, left fibula 🦠
　　　　M87.869　Other osteonecrosis, unspecified fibula 🦠
● M87.87　Other osteonecrosis, ankle, foot and toes
　　　　M87.871　Other osteonecrosis, right ankle 🦠
　　　　M87.872　Other osteonecrosis, left ankle 🦠
　　　　M87.873　Other osteonecrosis, unspecified ankle 🦠
　　　　M87.874　Other osteonecrosis, right foot 🦠
　　　　　　　　(Ex:) See M87.074
　　　　M87.875　Other osteonecrosis, left foot 🦠
　　　　　　　　(Ex:) See M87.074
　　　　M87.876　Other osteonecrosis, unspecified foot 🦠
　　　　　　　　(Ex:) See M87.074
　　　　M87.877　Other osteonecrosis, right toe(s) 🦠
　　　　M87.878　Other osteonecrosis, left toe(s) 🦠
　　　　M87.879　Other osteonecrosis, unspecified toe(s) 🦠
　　M87.88　Other osteonecrosis, other site 🦠
　　M87.89　Other osteonecrosis, multiple sites 🦠
　M87.9　Osteonecrosis, unspecified 🦠
　　　　Necrosis of bone NOS
　　　　(Ex:) See M87

● M88　Osteitis deformans [Paget's disease of bone]
　　　Chronic disorder that results in enlarged and deformed bones. The excessive breakdown and formation of bone tissue causes bones to weaken and results in bone pain, arthritis, deformities, and fractures.
　　　Excludes1　osteitis deformans in neoplastic disease (M90.6)
　M88.0　Osteitis deformans of skull
　M88.1　Osteitis deformans of vertebrae
● M88.8　Osteitis deformans of other bones
　● M88.81　Osteitis deformans of shoulder
　　　　M88.811　Osteitis deformans of right shoulder
　　　　M88.812　Osteitis deformans of left shoulder
　　　　M88.819　Osteitis deformans of unspecified shoulder
　● M88.82　Osteitis deformans of upper arm
　　　　M88.821　Osteitis deformans of right upper arm
　　　　M88.822　Osteitis deformans of left upper arm
　　　　M88.829　Osteitis deformans of unspecified upper arm

CHAPTER 13 (M00-M99)

CHAPTER 13 (M00–M99)

● M88.83   Osteitis deformans of forearm
    M88.831   Osteitis deformans of right forearm
    M88.832   Osteitis deformans of left forearm
    M88.839   Osteitis deformans of unspecified
              forearm
● M88.84   Osteitis deformans of hand
    M88.841   Osteitis deformans of right hand
    M88.842   Osteitis deformans of left hand
    M88.849   Osteitis deformans of unspecified
              hand
● M88.85   Osteitis deformans of thigh
    M88.851   Osteitis deformans of right thigh
    M88.852   Osteitis deformans of left thigh
    M88.859   Osteitis deformans of unspecified
              thigh
● M88.86   Osteitis deformans of lower leg
    M88.861   Osteitis deformans of right lower leg
    M88.862   Osteitis deformans of left lower leg
    M88.869   Osteitis deformans of unspecified
              lower leg
● M88.87   Osteitis deformans of ankle and foot
    M88.871   Osteitis deformans of right ankle and
              foot
    M88.872   Osteitis deformans of left ankle and
              foot
    M88.879   Osteitis deformans of unspecified
              ankle and foot
  M88.88   Osteitis deformans of other bones
           Excludes2   osteitis deformans of skull
                       (M88.0)
                       osteitis deformans of vertebrae
                       (M88.1)
  M88.89   Osteitis deformans of multiple sites
  M88.9   Osteitis deformans of unspecified bone

● M89   Other disorders of bone
  ● M89.0   Algoneurodystrophy
            Shoulder-hand syndrome
            Sudeck's atrophy
            Excludes1   causalgia, lower limb (G57.7-)
                        causalgia, upper limb (G56.4-)
                        complex regional pain syndrome II, lower
                          limb (G57.7-)
                        complex regional pain syndrome II,
                          upper limb (G56.4-)
                        reflex sympathetic dystrophy (G90.5-)
    M89.00   Algoneurodystrophy, unspecified site
  ● M89.01   Algoneurodystrophy, shoulder
    M89.011   Algoneurodystrophy, right shoulder
    M89.012   Algoneurodystrophy, left shoulder
    M89.019   Algoneurodystrophy, unspecified
              shoulder
  ● M89.02   Algoneurodystrophy, upper arm
    M89.021   Algoneurodystrophy, right upper arm
    M89.022   Algoneurodystrophy, left upper arm
    M89.029   Algoneurodystrophy, unspecified
              upper arm
  ● M89.03   Algoneurodystrophy, forearm
    M89.031   Algoneurodystrophy, right forearm
    M89.032   Algoneurodystrophy, left forearm
    M89.039   Algoneurodystrophy, unspecified
              forearm
  ● M89.04   Algoneurodystrophy, hand
    M89.041   Algoneurodystrophy, right hand
    M89.042   Algoneurodystrophy, left hand
    M89.049   Algoneurodystrophy, unspecified
              hand

● M89.05   Algoneurodystrophy, thigh
    M89.051   Algoneurodystrophy, right thigh
    M89.052   Algoneurodystrophy, left thigh
    M89.059   Algoneurodystrophy, unspecified
              thigh
● M89.06   Algoneurodystrophy, lower leg
    M89.061   Algoneurodystrophy, right lower leg
    M89.062   Algoneurodystrophy, left lower leg
    M89.069   Algoneurodystrophy, unspecified
              lower leg
● M89.07   Algoneurodystrophy, ankle and foot
    M89.071   Algoneurodystrophy, right ankle and
              foot
    M89.072   Algoneurodystrophy, left ankle and
              foot
    M89.079   Algoneurodystrophy, unspecified
              ankle and foot
  M89.08   Algoneurodystrophy, other site
  M89.09   Algoneurodystrophy, multiple sites
● M89.1   Physeal arrest
          Arrest of growth plate
          Epiphyseal arrest
          Growth plate arrest
  ● M89.12   Physeal arrest, humerus
    M89.121   Complete physeal arrest, right
              proximal humerus
    M89.122   Complete physeal arrest, left proximal
              humerus
    M89.123   Partial physeal arrest, right proximal
              humerus
    M89.124   Partial physeal arrest, left proximal
              humerus
    M89.125   Complete physeal arrest, right distal
              humerus
    M89.126   Complete physeal arrest, left distal
              humerus
    M89.127   Partial physeal arrest, right distal
              humerus
    M89.128   Partial physeal arrest, left distal
              humerus
    M89.129   Physeal arrest, humerus, unspecified
  ● M89.13   Physeal arrest, forearm
    M89.131   Complete physeal arrest, right distal
              radius
    M89.132   Complete physeal arrest, left distal
              radius
    M89.133   Partial physeal arrest, right distal
              radius
    M89.134   Partial physeal arrest, left distal
              radius
    M89.138   Other physeal arrest of forearm
    M89.139   Physeal arrest, forearm, unspecified
  ● M89.15   Physeal arrest, femur
    M89.151   Complete physeal arrest, right
              proximal femur
    M89.152   Complete physeal arrest, left proximal
              femur
    M89.153   Partial physeal arrest, right proximal
              femur
    M89.154   Partial physeal arrest, left proximal
              femur
    M89.155   Complete physeal arrest, right distal
              femur
    M89.156   Complete physeal arrest, left distal
              femur
    M89.157   Partial physeal arrest, right distal
              femur
    M89.158   Partial physeal arrest, left distal femur
    M89.159   Physeal arrest, femur, unspecified

◄ New   ◄▥ Revised   ~~deleted~~ Deleted   Excludes 1   Excludes 2   Includes   Use additional   Code first   Code also   Unspecified
OGCR Official Guidelines   ● Unacceptable Principal Diagnosis   X Assign placeholder X   ● Use Additional Character(s)   ▶ Manifestation Code   **Coding Clinic**

● M89.16   Physeal arrest, lower leg

     M89.160   Complete physeal arrest, right proximal tibia

     M89.161   Complete physeal arrest, left proximal tibia

     M89.162   Partial physeal arrest, right proximal tibia

     M89.163   Partial physeal arrest, left proximal tibia

     M89.164   Complete physeal arrest, right distal tibia

     M89.165   Complete physeal arrest, left distal tibia

     M89.166   Partial physeal arrest, right distal tibia

     M89.167   Partial physeal arrest, left distal tibia

     M89.168   Other physeal arrest of lower leg

     M89.169   Physeal arrest, lower leg, unspecified

   M89.18   Physeal arrest, other site

● M89.2   Other disorders of bone development and growth

   M89.20   Other disorders of bone development and growth, unspecified site

● M89.21   Other disorders of bone development and growth, shoulder

     M89.211   Other disorders of bone development and growth, right shoulder

     M89.212   Other disorders of bone development and growth, left shoulder

     M89.219   Other disorders of bone development and growth, unspecified shoulder

● M89.22   Other disorders of bone development and growth, humerus

     M89.221   Other disorders of bone development and growth, right humerus

     M89.222   Other disorders of bone development and growth, left humerus

     M89.229   Other disorders of bone development and growth, unspecified humerus

● M89.23   Other disorders of bone development and growth, ulna and radius

     M89.231   Other disorders of bone development and growth, right ulna

     M89.232   Other disorders of bone development and growth, left ulna

     M89.233   Other disorders of bone development and growth, right radius

     M89.234   Other disorders of bone development and growth, left radius

     M89.239   Other disorders of bone development and growth, unspecified ulna and radius

● M89.24   Other disorders of bone development and growth, hand

     M89.241   Other disorders of bone development and growth, right hand

     M89.242   Other disorders of bone development and growth, left hand

     M89.249   Other disorders of bone development and growth, unspecified hand

● M89.25   Other disorders of bone development and growth, femur

     M89.251   Other disorders of bone development and growth, right femur

     M89.252   Other disorders of bone development and growth, left femur

     M89.259   Other disorders of bone development and growth, unspecified femur

● M89.26   Other disorders of bone development and growth, tibia and fibula

     M89.261   Other disorders of bone development and growth, right tibia

     M89.262   Other disorders of bone development and growth, left tibia

     M89.263   Other disorders of bone development and growth, right fibula

     M89.264   Other disorders of bone development and growth, left fibula

     M89.269   Other disorders of bone development and growth, unspecified lower leg

● M89.27   Other disorders of bone development and growth, ankle and foot

     M89.271   Other disorders of bone development and growth, right ankle and foot

     M89.272   Other disorders of bone development and growth, left ankle and foot

     M89.279   Other disorders of bone development and growth, unspecified ankle and foot

   M89.28   Other disorders of bone development and growth, other site

   M89.29   Other disorders of bone development and growth, multiple sites

● M89.3   Hypertrophy of bone

   M89.30   Hypertrophy of bone, unspecified site

● M89.31   Hypertrophy of bone, shoulder

     M89.311   Hypertrophy of bone, right shoulder

     M89.312   Hypertrophy of bone, left shoulder

     M89.319   Hypertrophy of bone, unspecified shoulder

● M89.32   Hypertrophy of bone, humerus

     M89.321   Hypertrophy of bone, right humerus

     M89.322   Hypertrophy of bone, left humerus

     M89.329   Hypertrophy of bone, unspecified humerus

● M89.33   Hypertrophy of bone, ulna and radius

     M89.331   Hypertrophy of bone, right ulna

     M89.332   Hypertrophy of bone, left ulna

     M89.333   Hypertrophy of bone, right radius

     M89.334   Hypertrophy of bone, left radius

     M89.339   Hypertrophy of bone, unspecified ulna and radius

● M89.34   Hypertrophy of bone, hand

     M89.341   Hypertrophy of bone, right hand

     M89.342   Hypertrophy of bone, left hand

     M89.349   Hypertrophy of bone, unspecified hand

● M89.35   Hypertrophy of bone, femur

     M89.351   Hypertrophy of bone, right femur

     M89.352   Hypertrophy of bone, left femur

     M89.359   Hypertrophy of bone, unspecified femur

● M89.36   Hypertrophy of bone, tibia and fibula

     M89.361   Hypertrophy of bone, right tibia

     M89.362   Hypertrophy of bone, left tibia

     M89.363   Hypertrophy of bone, right fibula

     M89.364   Hypertrophy of bone, left fibula

     M89.369   Hypertrophy of bone, unspecified tibia and fibula

CHAPTER 13 (M00-M99)

- M89.37 Hypertrophy of bone, ankle and foot
  - M89.371 Hypertrophy of bone, right ankle and foot
  - M89.372 Hypertrophy of bone, left ankle and foot
  - M89.379 Hypertrophy of bone, unspecified ankle and foot
  - M89.38 Hypertrophy of bone, other site
  - M89.39 Hypertrophy of bone, multiple sites
- M89.4 Other hypertrophic osteoarthropathy
  - Marie-Bamberger disease
  - Pachydermoperiostosis
  - M89.40 Other hypertrophic osteoarthropathy, unspecified site
- M89.41 Other hypertrophic osteoarthropathy, shoulder
  - M89.411 Other hypertrophic osteoarthropathy, right shoulder
  - M89.412 Other hypertrophic osteoarthropathy, left shoulder
  - M89.419 Other hypertrophic osteoarthropathy, unspecified shoulder
- M89.42 Other hypertrophic osteoarthropathy, upper arm
  - M89.421 Other hypertrophic osteoarthropathy, right upper arm
  - M89.422 Other hypertrophic osteoarthropathy, left upper arm
  - M89.429 Other hypertrophic osteoarthropathy, unspecified upper arm
- M89.43 Other hypertrophic osteoarthropathy, forearm
  - M89.431 Other hypertrophic osteoarthropathy, right forearm
  - M89.432 Other hypertrophic osteoarthropathy, left forearm
  - M89.439 Other hypertrophic osteoarthropathy, unspecified forearm
- M89.44 Other hypertrophic osteoarthropathy, hand
  - M89.441 Other hypertrophic osteoarthropathy, right hand
  - M89.442 Other hypertrophic osteoarthropathy, left hand
  - M89.449 Other hypertrophic osteoarthropathy, unspecified hand
- M89.45 Other hypertrophic osteoarthropathy, thigh
  - M89.451 Other hypertrophic osteoarthropathy, right thigh
  - M89.452 Other hypertrophic osteoarthropathy, left thigh
  - M89.459 Other hypertrophic osteoarthropathy, unspecified thigh
- M89.46 Other hypertrophic osteoarthropathy, lower leg
  - M89.461 Other hypertrophic osteoarthropathy, right lower leg
  - M89.462 Other hypertrophic osteoarthropathy, left lower leg
  - M89.469 Other hypertrophic osteoarthropathy, unspecified lower leg
- M89.47 Other hypertrophic osteoarthropathy, ankle and foot
  - M89.471 Other hypertrophic osteoarthropathy, right ankle and foot
  - M89.472 Other hypertrophic osteoarthropathy, left ankle and foot
  - M89.479 Other hypertrophic osteoarthropathy, unspecified ankle and foot
  - M89.48 Other hypertrophic osteoarthropathy, other site
  - M89.49 Other hypertrophic osteoarthropathy, multiple sites

- M89.5 Osteolysis
  - Use additional code to identify major osseous defect, if applicable (M89.7-)
  - **Excludes2** periprosthetic osteolysis of internal prosthetic joint (T84.05-)
  - M89.50 Osteolysis, unspecified site
- M89.51 Osteolysis, shoulder
  - M89.511 Osteolysis, right shoulder
  - M89.512 Osteolysis, left shoulder
  - M89.519 Osteolysis, unspecified shoulder
- M89.52 Osteolysis, upper arm
  - M89.521 Osteolysis, right upper arm
  - M89.522 Osteolysis, left upper arm
  - M89.529 Osteolysis, unspecified upper arm
- M89.53 Osteolysis, forearm
  - M89.531 Osteolysis, right forearm
  - M89.532 Osteolysis, left forearm
  - M89.539 Osteolysis, unspecified forearm
- M89.54 Osteolysis, hand
  - M89.541 Osteolysis, right hand
  - M89.542 Osteolysis, left hand
  - M89.549 Osteolysis, unspecified hand
- M89.55 Osteolysis, thigh
  - M89.551 Osteolysis, right thigh
  - M89.552 Osteolysis, left thigh
  - M89.559 Osteolysis, unspecified thigh
- M89.56 Osteolysis, lower leg
  - M89.561 Osteolysis, right lower leg
  - M89.562 Osteolysis, left lower leg
  - M89.569 Osteolysis, unspecified lower leg
- M89.57 Osteolysis, ankle and foot
  - M89.571 Osteolysis, right ankle and foot
  - M89.572 Osteolysis, left ankle and foot
  - M89.579 Osteolysis, unspecified ankle and foot
  - M89.58 Osteolysis, other site
  - M89.59 Osteolysis, multiple sites
- M89.6 Osteopathy after poliomyelitis
  - Use additional code (B91) to identify previous poliomyelitis
  - **Excludes1** postpolio syndrome (G14)
  - M89.60 Osteopathy after poliomyelitis, unspecified site
- M89.61 Osteopathy after poliomyelitis, shoulder
  - M89.611 Osteopathy after poliomyelitis, right shoulder
  - M89.612 Osteopathy after poliomyelitis, left shoulder
  - M89.619 Osteopathy after poliomyelitis, unspecified shoulder
- M89.62 Osteopathy after poliomyelitis, upper arm
  - M89.621 Osteopathy after poliomyelitis, right upper arm
  - M89.622 Osteopathy after poliomyelitis, left upper arm
  - M89.629 Osteopathy after poliomyelitis, unspecified upper arm
- M89.63 Osteopathy after poliomyelitis, forearm
  - M89.631 Osteopathy after poliomyelitis, right forearm
  - M89.632 Osteopathy after poliomyelitis, left forearm
  - M89.639 Osteopathy after poliomyelitis, unspecified forearm

◀ New ◀▥▥ Revised ~~deleted~~ Deleted | Excludes 1 | Excludes 2 | Includes | Use additional | Code first | Code also | Unspecified
OGCR Official Guidelines ● Unacceptable Principal Diagnosis X Assign placeholder X ▶ Use Additional Character(s) ▶ Manifestation Code **Coding Clinic**

● **M89.64 Osteopathy after poliomyelitis, hand**
     M89.641 Osteopathy after poliomyelitis, right hand
     M89.642 Osteopathy after poliomyelitis, left hand
     M89.649 Osteopathy after poliomyelitis, unspecified hand

● **M89.65 Osteopathy after poliomyelitis, thigh**
     M89.651 Osteopathy after poliomyelitis, right thigh
     M89.652 Osteopathy after poliomyelitis, left thigh
     M89.659 Osteopathy after poliomyelitis, unspecified thigh

● **M89.66 Osteopathy after poliomyelitis, lower leg**
     M89.661 Osteopathy after poliomyelitis, right lower leg
     M89.662 Osteopathy after poliomyelitis, left lower leg
     M89.669 Osteopathy after poliomyelitis, unspecified lower leg

● **M89.67 Osteopathy after poliomyelitis, ankle and foot**
     M89.671 Osteopathy after poliomyelitis, right ankle and foot
     M89.672 Osteopathy after poliomyelitis, left ankle and foot
     M89.679 Osteopathy after poliomyelitis, unspecified ankle and foot

     M89.68 Osteopathy after poliomyelitis, other site
     M89.69 Osteopathy after poliomyelitis, multiple sites

● **M89.7 Major osseous defect**
     Code first underlying disease, if known, such as:
       aseptic necrosis of bone (M87.-)
       malignant neoplasm of bone (C40.-)
       osteolysis (M89.5)
       osteomyelitis (M86.-)
       osteonecrosis (M87.-)
       osteoporosis (M80.-, M81.-)
       periprosthetic osteolysis (T84.05-)

     M89.70 Major osseous defect, unspecified site
● **M89.71 Major osseous defect, shoulder region**
     Major osseous defect clavicle or scapula
     M89.711 Major osseous defect, right shoulder region
     M89.712 Major osseous defect, left shoulder region
     M89.719 Major osseous defect, unspecified shoulder region

● **M89.72 Major osseous defect, humerus**
     M89.721 Major osseous defect, right humerus
     M89.722 Major osseous defect, left humerus
     M89.729 Major osseous defect, unspecified humerus

● **M89.73 Major osseous defect, forearm**
     Major osseous defect of radius and ulna
     M89.731 Major osseous defect, right forearm
     M89.732 Major osseous defect, left forearm
     M89.739 Major osseous defect, unspecified forearm

● **M89.74 Major osseous defect, hand**
     Major osseous defect of carpus, fingers, metacarpus
     M89.741 Major osseous defect, right hand
     M89.742 Major osseous defect, left hand
     M89.749 Major osseous defect, unspecified hand

● **M89.75 Major osseous defect, pelvic region and thigh**
     Major osseous defect of femur and pelvis
     M89.751 Major osseous defect, right pelvic region and thigh
     M89.752 Major osseous defect, left pelvic region and thigh
     M89.759 Major osseous defect, unspecified pelvic region and thigh

● **M89.76 Major osseous defect, lower leg**
     Major osseous defect of fibula and tibia
     M89.761 Major osseous defect, right lower leg
     M89.762 Major osseous defect, left lower leg
     M89.769 Major osseous defect, unspecified lower leg

● **M89.77 Major osseous defect, ankle and foot**
     Major osseous defect of metatarsus, tarsus, toes
     M89.771 Major osseous defect, right ankle and foot
     M89.772 Major osseous defect, left ankle and foot
     M89.779 Major osseous defect, unspecified ankle and foot

     M89.78 Major osseous defect, other site
     M89.79 Major osseous defect, multiple sites

● **M89.8 Other specified disorders of bone**
     Infantile cortical hyperostoses
     Post-traumatic subperiosteal ossification
     ● **M89.8X Other specified disorders of bone**
       M89.8X0 Other specified disorders of bone, multiple sites
       M89.8X1 Other specified disorders of bone, shoulder
       M89.8X2 Other specified disorders of bone, upper arm
       M89.8X3 Other specified disorders of bone, forearm
       M89.8X4 Other specified disorders of bone, hand
       M89.8X5 Other specified disorders of bone, thigh
       M89.8X6 Other specified disorders of bone, lower leg
       M89.8X7 Other specified disorders of bone, ankle and foot
       M89.8X8 Other specified disorders of bone, other site
       M89.8X9 Other specified disorders of bone, unspecified site

     M89.9 Disorder of bone, unspecified

● **M90 Osteopathies in diseases classified elsewhere**
     Excludes1   osteochondritis, osteomyelitis, and osteopathy (in):
       cryptococcosis (B45.3)
       diabetes mellitus (E08-E13 with .69-) ◄▥
       gonococcal (A54.43)
       neurogenic syphilis (A52.11)
       renal osteodystrophy (N25.0)
       salmonellosis (A02.24)
       secondary syphilis (A51.46)
       syphilis (late) (A52.77)

● **M90.5 Osteonecrosis in diseases classified elsewhere**
     Code first underlying disease, such as:
       caisson disease (T70.3)
       hemoglobinopathy (D50-D64)
     (Ex:) **For category M90.5 CC codes unless otherwise indicated:**
       M87.00-M87.9, M90.50-M90.59

     ▶ *M90.50 Osteonecrosis in diseases classified elsewhere, unspecified site* 🔖
       CC when PDx is its own CC

CHAPTER 13 (M00-M99)

- **M90.51** **Osteonecrosis in diseases classified elsewhere, shoulder**
  - (Ex) For category **M90.51** CC codes: M87.00-M87.9, M90.50-M90.59
  - *M90.511* *Osteonecrosis in diseases classified elsewhere, right shoulder* 🦴
    CC when PDx is its own CC
  - *M90.512* *Osteonecrosis in diseases classified elsewhere, left shoulder* 🦴
    CC when PDx is its own CC
  - *M90.519* *Osteonecrosis in diseases classified elsewhere, unspecified shoulder* 🦴
    CC when PDx is its own CC
- **M90.52** **Osteonecrosis in diseases classified elsewhere, upper arm**
  - *M90.521* *Osteonecrosis in diseases classified elsewhere, right upper arm* 🦴
    CC when PDx is its own CC
  - *M90.522* *Osteonecrosis in diseases classified elsewhere, left upper arm* 🦴
    CC when PDx is its own CC
  - *M90.529* *Osteonecrosis in diseases classified elsewhere, unspecified upper arm* 🦴
    CC when PDx is its own CC
- **M90.53** **Osteonecrosis in diseases classified elsewhere, forearm**
  - *M90.531* *Osteonecrosis in diseases classified elsewhere, right forearm* 🦴
    CC when PDx is its own CC
  - *M90.532* *Osteonecrosis in diseases classified elsewhere, left forearm* 🦴
    CC when PDx is its own CC
  - *M90.539* *Osteonecrosis in diseases classified elsewhere, unspecified forearm* 🦴
    CC when PDx is its own CC
- **M90.54** **Osteonecrosis in diseases classified elsewhere, hand**
  - *M90.541* *Osteonecrosis in diseases classified elsewhere, right hand* 🦴
    CC when PDx is its own CC
  - *M90.542* *Osteonecrosis in diseases classified elsewhere, left hand* 🦴
    CC when PDx is its own CC
  - *M90.549* *Osteonecrosis in diseases classified elsewhere, unspecified hand* 🦴
    CC when PDx is its own CC
- **M90.55** **Osteonecrosis in diseases classified elsewhere, thigh**
  - (Ex) For category **M90.55** CC codes: M87.00-M87.9, M90.50-M90.59, M87.9
  - *M90.551* *Osteonecrosis in diseases classified elsewhere, right thigh* 🦴
    CC when PDx is its own CC
  - *M90.552* *Osteonecrosis in diseases classified elsewhere, left thigh* 🦴
    CC when PDx is its own CC
  - *M90.559* *Osteonecrosis in diseases classified elsewhere, unspecified thigh* 🦴
    CC when PDx is its own CC
- **M90.56** **Osteonecrosis in diseases classified elsewhere, lower leg**
  - *M90.561* *Osteonecrosis in diseases classified elsewhere, right lower leg* 🦴
    CC when PDx is its own CC
  - *M90.562* *Osteonecrosis in diseases classified elsewhere, left lower leg* 🦴
    CC when PDx is its own CC
  - *M90.569* *Osteonecrosis in diseases classified elsewhere, unspecified lower leg* 🦴
    CC when PDx is its own CC

- **M90.57** **Osteonecrosis in diseases classified elsewhere, ankle and foot**
  - *M90.571* *Osteonecrosis in diseases classified elsewhere, right ankle and foot* 🦴
    CC when PDx is its own CC
  - *M90.572* *Osteonecrosis in diseases classified elsewhere, left ankle and foot* 🦴
    CC when PDx is its own CC
  - *M90.579* *Osteonecrosis in diseases classified elsewhere, unspecified ankle and foot* 🦴
    CC when PDx is its own CC
  - *M90.58* *Osteonecrosis in diseases classified elsewhere, other site* 🦴
    CC when PDx is its own CC
  - *M90.59* *Osteonecrosis in diseases classified elsewhere, multiple sites* 🦴
    CC when PDx is its own CC
- **M90.6** **Osteitis deformans in neoplastic diseases**
  Osteitis deformans in malignant neoplasm of bone
  Code first the neoplasm (C40.-, C41.-)
  Excludes1   osteitis deformans [Paget's disease of bone] (M88.-)
  - *M90.60* *Osteitis deformans in neoplastic diseases, unspecified site*
  - **M90.61** **Osteitis deformans in neoplastic diseases, shoulder**
    - *M90.611* *Osteitis deformans in neoplastic diseases, right shoulder*
    - *M90.612* *Osteitis deformans in neoplastic diseases, left shoulder*
    - *M90.619* *Osteitis deformans in neoplastic diseases, unspecified shoulder*
  - **M90.62** **Osteitis deformans in neoplastic diseases, upper arm**
    - *M90.621* *Osteitis deformans in neoplastic diseases, right upper arm*
    - *M90.622* *Osteitis deformans in neoplastic diseases, left upper arm*
    - *M90.629* *Osteitis deformans in neoplastic diseases, unspecified upper arm*
  - **M90.63** **Osteitis deformans in neoplastic diseases, forearm**
    - *M90.631* *Osteitis deformans in neoplastic diseases, right forearm*
    - *M90.632* *Osteitis deformans in neoplastic diseases, left forearm*
    - *M90.639* *Osteitis deformans in neoplastic diseases, unspecified forearm*
  - **M90.64** **Osteitis deformans in neoplastic diseases, hand**
    - *M90.641* *Osteitis deformans in neoplastic diseases, right hand*
    - *M90.642* *Osteitis deformans in neoplastic diseases, left hand*
    - *M90.649* *Osteitis deformans in neoplastic diseases, unspecified hand*
  - **M90.65** **Osteitis deformans in neoplastic diseases, thigh**
    - *M90.651* *Osteitis deformans in neoplastic diseases, right thigh*
    - *M90.652* *Osteitis deformans in neoplastic diseases, left thigh*
    - *M90.659* *Osteitis deformans in neoplastic diseases, unspecified thigh*
  - **M90.66** **Osteitis deformans in neoplastic diseases, lower leg**
    - *M90.661* *Osteitis deformans in neoplastic diseases, right lower leg*
    - *M90.662* *Osteitis deformans in neoplastic diseases, left lower leg*
    - *M90.669* *Osteitis deformans in neoplastic diseases, unspecified lower leg*

◀ New   ◀▥ Revised   ~~deleted~~ Deleted   Excludes 1   Excludes 2   Includes   Use additional   Code first   Code also   Unspecified
OGCR Official Guidelines   ● Unacceptable Principal Diagnosis   X Assign placeholder X   ● Use Additional Character(s)   ▌ Manifestation Code   **Coding Clinic**

● **M90.67 Osteitis deformans in neoplastic diseases, ankle and foot**

  ▷ *M90.671 Osteitis deformans in neoplastic diseases, right ankle and foot*

  ▷ *M90.672 Osteitis deformans in neoplastic diseases, left ankle and foot*

  ▷ *M90.679 Osteitis deformans in neoplastic diseases, unspecified ankle and foot*

 ▷ *M90.68 Osteitis deformans in neoplastic diseases, other site*

 ▷ *M90.69 Osteitis deformans in neoplastic diseases, multiple sites*

● **M90.8 Osteopathy in diseases classified elsewhere**

  Code first underlying disease, such as:
  rickets (E55.0)
  vitamin-D-resistant rickets (E83.3)

 ▷ *M90.80 Osteopathy in diseases classified elsewhere, unspecified site*

● **M90.81 Osteopathy in diseases classified elsewhere, shoulder**

  ▷ *M90.811 Osteopathy in diseases classified elsewhere, right shoulder*

  ▷ *M90.812 Osteopathy in diseases classified elsewhere, left shoulder*

  ▷ *M90.819 Osteopathy in diseases classified elsewhere, unspecified shoulder*

● **M90.82 Osteopathy in diseases classified elsewhere, upper arm**

  ▷ *M90.821 Osteopathy in diseases classified elsewhere, right upper arm*

  ▷ *M90.822 Osteopathy in diseases classified elsewhere, left upper arm*

  ▷ *M90.829 Osteopathy in diseases classified elsewhere, unspecified upper arm*

● **M90.83 Osteopathy in diseases classified elsewhere, forearm**

  ▷ *M90.831 Osteopathy in diseases classified elsewhere, right forearm*

  ▷ *M90.832 Osteopathy in diseases classified elsewhere, left forearm*

  ▷ *M90.839 Osteopathy in diseases classified elsewhere, unspecified forearm*

● **M90.84 Osteopathy in diseases classified elsewhere, hand**

  ▷ *M90.841 Osteopathy in diseases classified elsewhere, right hand*

  ▷ *M90.842 Osteopathy in diseases classified elsewhere, left hand*

  ▷ *M90.849 Osteopathy in diseases classified elsewhere, unspecified hand*

● **M90.85 Osteopathy in diseases classified elsewhere, thigh**

  ▷ *M90.851 Osteopathy in diseases classified elsewhere, right thigh*

  ▷ *M90.852 Osteopathy in diseases classified elsewhere, left thigh*

  ▷ *M90.859 Osteopathy in diseases classified elsewhere, unspecified thigh*

● **M90.86 Osteopathy in diseases classified elsewhere, lower leg**

  ▷ *M90.861 Osteopathy in diseases classified elsewhere, right lower leg*

  ▷ *M90.862 Osteopathy in diseases classified elsewhere, left lower leg*

  ▷ *M90.869 Osteopathy in diseases classified elsewhere, unspecified lower leg*

● **M90.87 Osteopathy in diseases classified elsewhere, ankle and foot**

  ▷ *M90.871 Osteopathy in diseases classified elsewhere, right ankle and foot*

  ▷ *M90.872 Osteopathy in diseases classified elsewhere, left ankle and foot*

  ▷ *M90.879 Osteopathy in diseases classified elsewhere, unspecified ankle and foot*

 ▷ *M90.88 Osteopathy in diseases classified elsewhere, other site*

 ▷ *M90.89 Osteopathy in diseases classified elsewhere, multiple sites*

CHONDROPATHIES (M91-M94)

Excludes1 postprocedural chondropathies (M96.-)

● **M91 Juvenile osteochondrosis of hip and pelvis**

  Excludes1 slipped upper femoral epiphysis (nontraumatic) (M93.0)

  M91.0 Juvenile osteochondrosis of pelvis
  Osteochondrosis (juvenile) of acetabulum
  Osteochondrosis (juvenile) of iliac crest [Buchanan]
  Osteochondrosis (juvenile) of ischiopubic synchondrosis [van Neck]
  Osteochondrosis (juvenile) of symphysis pubis [Pierson]

 ● **M91.1 Juvenile osteochondrosis of head of femur [Legg-Calvé-Perthes]**

  M91.10 Juvenile osteochondrosis of head of femur [Legg-Calvé-Perthes], unspecified leg

  M91.11 Juvenile osteochondrosis of head of femur [Legg-Calvé-Perthes], right leg

  M91.12 Juvenile osteochondrosis of head of femur [Legg-Calvé-Perthes], left leg

 ● **M91.2 Coxa plana**
  Hip deformity due to previous juvenile osteochondrosis

  M91.20 Coxa plana, unspecified hip

  M91.21 Coxa plana, right hip

  M91.22 Coxa plana, left hip

 ● **M91.3 Pseudocoxalgia**

  M91.30 Pseudocoxalgia, unspecified hip

  M91.31 Pseudocoxalgia, right hip

  M91.32 Pseudocoxalgia, left hip

 ● **M91.4 Coxa magna**

  M91.40 Coxa magna, unspecified hip

  M91.41 Coxa magna, right hip

  M91.42 Coxa magna, left hip

 ● **M91.8 Other juvenile osteochondrosis of hip and pelvis**
  Juvenile osteochondrosis after reduction of congenital dislocation of hip

  M91.80 Other juvenile osteochondrosis of hip and pelvis, unspecified leg

  M91.81 Other juvenile osteochondrosis of hip and pelvis, right leg

  M91.82 Other juvenile osteochondrosis of hip and pelvis, left leg

 ● **M91.9 Juvenile osteochondrosis of hip and pelvis, unspecified**

  M91.90 Juvenile osteochondrosis of hip and pelvis, unspecified, unspecified leg

  M91.91 Juvenile osteochondrosis of hip and pelvis, unspecified, right leg

  M91.92 Juvenile osteochondrosis of hip and pelvis, unspecified, left leg

CHAPTER 13 (M00-M99)

CHAPTER 13 (M00-M99)

● **M92**   **Other juvenile osteochondrosis**

  ● **M92.0**   **Juvenile osteochondrosis of humerus**
Osteochondrosis (juvenile) of capitulum of humerus [Panner]
Osteochondrosis (juvenile) of head of humerus [Haas]

    M92.00   **Juvenile osteochondrosis of humerus, unspecified arm**
    M92.01   **Juvenile osteochondrosis of humerus, right arm**
    M92.02   **Juvenile osteochondrosis of humerus, left arm**

  ● **M92.1**   **Juvenile osteochondrosis of radius and ulna**
Osteochondrosis (juvenile) of lower ulna [Burns]
Osteochondrosis (juvenile) of radial head [Brailsford]

    M92.10   **Juvenile osteochondrosis of radius and ulna, unspecified arm**
    M92.11   **Juvenile osteochondrosis of radius and ulna, right arm**
    M92.12   **Juvenile osteochondrosis of radius and ulna, left arm**

  ● **M92.2**   **Juvenile osteochondrosis, hand**

    ● **M92.20**   **Unspecified juvenile osteochondrosis, hand**
      M92.201   **Unspecified juvenile osteochondrosis, right hand**
      M92.202   **Unspecified juvenile osteochondrosis, left hand**
      M92.209   **Unspecified juvenile osteochondrosis, unspecified hand**

    ● **M92.21**   **Osteochondrosis (juvenile) of carpal lunate [Kienböck]**
      M92.211   **Osteochondrosis (juvenile) of carpal lunate [Kienböck], right hand**
      M92.212   **Osteochondrosis (juvenile) of carpal lunate [Kienböck], left hand**
      M92.219   **Osteochondrosis (juvenile) of carpal lunate [Kienböck], unspecified hand**

    ● **M92.22**   **Osteochondrosis (juvenile) of metacarpal heads [Mauclaire]**
      M92.221   **Osteochondrosis (juvenile) of metacarpal heads [Mauclaire], right hand**
      M92.222   **Osteochondrosis (juvenile) of metacarpal heads [Mauclaire], left hand**
      M92.229   **Osteochondrosis (juvenile) of metacarpal heads [Mauclaire], unspecified hand**

    ● **M92.29**   **Other juvenile osteochondrosis, hand**
      M92.291   **Other juvenile osteochondrosis, right hand**
      M92.292   **Other juvenile osteochondrosis, left hand**
      M92.299   **Other juvenile osteochondrosis, unspecified hand**

  ● **M92.3**   **Other juvenile osteochondrosis, upper limb**
    M92.30   **Other juvenile osteochondrosis, unspecified upper limb**
    M92.31   **Other juvenile osteochondrosis, right upper limb**
    M92.32   **Other juvenile osteochondrosis, left upper limb**

  ● **M92.4**   **Juvenile osteochondrosis of patella**
Osteochondrosis (juvenile) of primary patellar center [Köhler]
Osteochondrosis (juvenile) of secondary patellar center [Sinding Larsen]

    M92.40   **Juvenile osteochondrosis of patella, unspecified knee**
    M92.41   **Juvenile osteochondrosis of patella, right knee**
    M92.42   **Juvenile osteochondrosis of patella, left knee**

  ● **M92.5**   **Juvenile osteochondrosis of tibia and fibula**
Osteochondrosis (juvenile) of proximal tibia [Blount]
Osteochondrosis (juvenile) of tibial tubercle [Osgood-Schlatter]
Tibia vara

    M92.50   **Juvenile osteochondrosis of tibia and fibula, unspecified leg**
    M92.51   **Juvenile osteochondrosis of tibia and fibula, right leg**
    M92.52   **Juvenile osteochondrosis of tibia and fibula, left leg**

  ● **M92.6**   **Juvenile osteochondrosis of tarsus**
Osteochondrosis (juvenile) of calcaneum [Sever]
Osteochondrosis (juvenile) of os tibiale externum [Haglund]
Osteochondrosis (juvenile) of talus [Diaz]
Osteochondrosis (juvenile) of tarsal navicular [Köhler]

    M92.60   **Juvenile osteochondrosis of tarsus, unspecified ankle**
    M92.61   **Juvenile osteochondrosis of tarsus, right ankle**
    M92.62   **Juvenile osteochondrosis of tarsus, left ankle**

  ● **M92.7**   **Juvenile osteochondrosis of metatarsus**
Osteochondrosis (juvenile) of fifth metatarsus [Iselin]
Osteochondrosis (juvenile) of second metatarsus [Freiberg]

    M92.70   **Juvenile osteochondrosis of metatarsus, unspecified foot**
    M92.71   **Juvenile osteochondrosis of metatarsus, right foot**
    M92.72   **Juvenile osteochondrosis of metatarsus, left foot**

  M92.8   **Other specified juvenile osteochondrosis**
Calcaneal apophysitis

  M92.9   **Juvenile osteochondrosis, unspecified**
Juvenile apophysitis NOS
Juvenile epiphysitis NOS
Juvenile osteochondritis NOS
Juvenile osteochondrosis NOS

● **M93**   **Other osteochondropathies**
  Excludes2   osteochondrosis of spine (M42.-)

  ● **M93.0**   **Slipped upper femoral epiphysis (nontraumatic)**
Use additional code for associated chondrolysis (M94.3)

    ● **M93.00**   **Unspecified slipped upper femoral epiphysis (nontraumatic)**
      M93.001   **Unspecified slipped upper femoral epiphysis (nontraumatic), right hip**
      M93.002   **Unspecified slipped upper femoral epiphysis (nontraumatic), left hip**
      M93.003   **Unspecified slipped upper femoral epiphysis (nontraumatic), unspecified hip**

    ● **M93.01**   **Acute slipped upper femoral epiphysis (nontraumatic)**
      M93.011   **Acute slipped upper femoral epiphysis (nontraumatic), right hip**
      M93.012   **Acute slipped upper femoral epiphysis (nontraumatic), left hip**
      M93.013   **Acute slipped upper femoral epiphysis (nontraumatic), unspecified hip**

    ● **M93.02**   **Chronic slipped upper femoral epiphysis (nontraumatic)**
      M93.021   **Chronic slipped upper femoral epiphysis (nontraumatic), right hip**
      M93.022   **Chronic slipped upper femoral epiphysis (nontraumatic), left hip**
      M93.023   **Chronic slipped upper femoral epiphysis (nontraumatic), unspecified hip**

◄ New   ◄▥ Revised   ~~deleted~~ Deleted   Excludes 1   Excludes 2   Includes   Use additional   Code first   Code also   Unspecified
OGCR Official Guidelines   ● Unacceptable Principal Diagnosis   X Assign placeholder X   ● Use Additional Character(s)   ▌ Manifestation Code   **Coding Clinic**

- **M93.03** Acute on chronic slipped upper femoral epiphysis (nontraumatic)
  - M93.031 Acute on chronic slipped upper femoral epiphysis (nontraumatic), right hip
  - M93.032 Acute on chronic slipped upper femoral epiphysis (nontraumatic), left hip
  - M93.033 Acute on chronic slipped upper femoral epiphysis (nontraumatic), unspecified hip
- M93.1 **Kienböck's disease of adults**   A
  - Adult osteochondrosis of carpal lunates
- **M93.2 Osteochondritis dissecans**
  - M93.20 Osteochondritis dissecans of unspecified site
  - **M93.21** Osteochondritis dissecans of shoulder
    - M93.211 Osteochondritis dissecans, right shoulder
    - M93.212 Osteochondritis dissecans, left shoulder
    - M93.219 Osteochondritis dissecans, unspecified shoulder
  - **M93.22** Osteochondritis dissecans of elbow
    - M93.221 Osteochondritis dissecans, right elbow
    - M93.222 Osteochondritis dissecans, left elbow
    - M93.229 Osteochondritis dissecans, unspecified elbow
  - **M93.23** Osteochondritis dissecans of wrist
    - M93.231 Osteochondritis dissecans, right wrist
    - M93.232 Osteochondritis dissecans, left wrist
    - M93.239 Osteochondritis dissecans, unspecified wrist
  - **M93.24** Osteochondritis dissecans of joints of hand
    - M93.241 Osteochondritis dissecans, joints of right hand
    - M93.242 Osteochondritis dissecans, joints of left hand
    - M93.249 Osteochondritis dissecans, joints of unspecified hand
  - **M93.25** Osteochondritis dissecans of hip
    - M93.251 Osteochondritis dissecans, right hip
    - M93.252 Osteochondritis dissecans, left hip
    - M93.259 Osteochondritis dissecans, unspecified hip
  - **M93.26** Osteochondritis dissecans knee
    - M93.261 Osteochondritis dissecans, right knee
    - M93.262 Osteochondritis dissecans, left knee
    - M93.269 Osteochondritis dissecans, unspecified knee
  - **M93.27** Osteochondritis dissecans of ankle and joints of foot
    - M93.271 Osteochondritis dissecans, right ankle and joints of right foot
    - M93.272 Osteochondritis dissecans, left ankle and joints of left foot
    - M93.279 Osteochondritis dissecans, unspecified ankle and joints of foot
  - M93.28 Osteochondritis dissecans other site
  - M93.29 Osteochondritis dissecans multiple sites

- **M93.8 Other specified osteochondropathies**
  - M93.80 Other specified osteochondropathies of unspecified site
  - **M93.81** Other specified osteochondropathies of shoulder
    - M93.811 Other specified osteochondropathies, right shoulder
    - M93.812 Other specified osteochondropathies, left shoulder
    - M93.819 Other specified osteochondropathies, unspecified shoulder
  - **M93.82** Other specified osteochondropathies of upper arm
    - M93.821 Other specified osteochondropathies, right upper arm
    - M93.822 Other specified osteochondropathies, left upper arm
    - M93.829 Other specified osteochondropathies, unspecified upper arm
  - **M93.83** Other specified osteochondropathies of forearm
    - M93.831 Other specified osteochondropathies, right forearm
    - M93.832 Other specified osteochondropathies, left forearm
    - M93.839 Other specified osteochondropathies, unspecified forearm
  - **M93.84** Other specified osteochondropathies of hand
    - M93.841 Other specified osteochondropathies, right hand
    - M93.842 Other specified osteochondropathies, left hand
    - M93.849 Other specified osteochondropathies, unspecified hand
  - **M93.85** Other specified osteochondropathies of thigh
    - M93.851 Other specified osteochondropathies, right thigh
    - M93.852 Other specified osteochondropathies, left thigh
    - M93.859 Other specified osteochondropathies, unspecified thigh
  - **M93.86** Other specified osteochondropathies lower leg
    - M93.861 Other specified osteochondropathies, right lower leg
    - M93.862 Other specified osteochondropathies, left lower leg
    - M93.869 Other specified osteochondropathies, unspecified lower leg
  - **M93.87** Other specified osteochondropathies of ankle and foot
    - M93.871 Other specified osteochondropathies, right ankle and foot
    - M93.872 Other specified osteochondropathies, left ankle and foot
    - M93.879 Other specified osteochondropathies, unspecified ankle and foot
  - M93.88 Other specified osteochondropathies other
  - M93.89 Other specified osteochondropathies multiple sites

CHAPTER 13 (M00-M99)

CHAPTER 13 (M00-M99)

M93.9   Osteochondropathy, unspecified
    Apophysitis NOS
    Epiphysitis NOS
    Osteochondritis NOS
    Osteochondrosis NOS
    M93.90   Osteochondropathy, unspecified of unspecified site
    ● M93.91   Osteochondropathy, unspecified of shoulder
        M93.911   Osteochondropathy, unspecified, right shoulder
        M93.912   Osteochondropathy, unspecified, left shoulder
        M93.919   Osteochondropathy, unspecified, unspecified shoulder
    ● M93.92   Osteochondropathy, unspecified of upper arm
        M93.921   Osteochondropathy, unspecified, right upper arm
        M93.922   Osteochondropathy, unspecified, left upper arm
        M93.929   Osteochondropathy, unspecified, unspecified upper arm
    ● M93.93   Osteochondropathy, unspecified of forearm
        M93.931   Osteochondropathy, unspecified, right forearm
        M93.932   Osteochondropathy, unspecified, left forearm
        M93.939   Osteochondropathy, unspecified, unspecified forearm
    ● M93.94   Osteochondropathy, unspecified of hand
        M93.941   Osteochondropathy, unspecified, right hand
        M93.942   Osteochondropathy, unspecified, left hand
        M93.949   Osteochondropathy, unspecified, unspecified hand
    ● M93.95   Osteochondropathy, unspecified of thigh
        M93.951   Osteochondropathy, unspecified, right thigh
        M93.952   Osteochondropathy, unspecified, left thigh
        M93.959   Osteochondropathy, unspecified, unspecified thigh
    ● M93.96   Osteochondropathy, unspecified lower leg
        M93.961   Osteochondropathy, unspecified, right lower leg
        M93.962   Osteochondropathy, unspecified, left lower leg
        M93.969   Osteochondropathy, unspecified, unspecified lower leg
    ● M93.97   Osteochondropathy, unspecified of ankle and foot
        M93.971   Osteochondropathy, unspecified, right ankle and foot
        M93.972   Osteochondropathy, unspecified, left ankle and foot
        M93.979   Osteochondropathy, unspecified, unspecified ankle and foot
    M93.98   Osteochondropathy, unspecified other
    M93.99   Osteochondropathy, unspecified multiple sites
● M94   Other disorders of cartilage
    M94.0   Chondrocostal junction syndrome [Tietze]
        Costochondritis
    M94.1   Relapsing polychondritis
    ● M94.2   Chondromalacia
        Excludes1   chondromalacia patellae (M22.4)
        M94.20   Chondromalacia, unspecified site

● M94.21   Chondromalacia, shoulder
    M94.211   Chondromalacia, right shoulder
    M94.212   Chondromalacia, left shoulder
    M94.219   Chondromalacia, unspecified shoulder
● M94.22   Chondromalacia, elbow
    M94.221   Chondromalacia, right elbow
    M94.222   Chondromalacia, left elbow
    M94.229   Chondromalacia, unspecified elbow
● M94.23   Chondromalacia, wrist
    M94.231   Chondromalacia, right wrist
    M94.232   Chondromalacia, left wrist
    M94.239   Chondromalacia, unspecified wrist
● M94.24   Chondromalacia, joints of hand
    M94.241   Chondromalacia, joints of right hand
    M94.242   Chondromalacia, joints of left hand
    M94.249   Chondromalacia, joints of unspecified hand
● M94.25   Chondromalacia, hip
    M94.251   Chondromalacia, right hip
    M94.252   Chondromalacia, left hip
    M94.259   Chondromalacia, unspecified hip
● M94.26   Chondromalacia, knee
    M94.261   Chondromalacia, right knee
    M94.262   Chondromalacia, left knee
    M94.269   Chondromalacia, unspecified knee
● M94.27   Chondromalacia, ankle and joints of foot
    M94.271   Chondromalacia, right ankle and joints of right foot
    M94.272   Chondromalacia, left ankle and joints of left foot
    M94.279   Chondromalacia, unspecified ankle and joints of foot
    M94.28   Chondromalacia, other site
    M94.29   Chondromalacia, multiple sites
● M94.3   Chondrolysis
    Code first any associated slipped upper femoral epiphysis (nontraumatic) (M93.0-)
    ● M94.35   Chondrolysis, hip
        M94.351   Chondrolysis, right hip
        M94.352   Chondrolysis, left hip
        M94.359   Chondrolysis, unspecified hip
● M94.8   Other specified disorders of cartilage
    ● M94.8X   Other specified disorders of cartilage
        M94.8X0   Other specified disorders of cartilage, multiple sites
        M94.8X1   Other specified disorders of cartilage, shoulder
        M94.8X2   Other specified disorders of cartilage, upper arm
        M94.8X3   Other specified disorders of cartilage, forearm
        M94.8X4   Other specified disorders of cartilage, hand
        M94.8X5   Other specified disorders of cartilage, thigh
        M94.8X6   Other specified disorders of cartilage, lower leg
        M94.8X7   Other specified disorders of cartilage, ankle and foot
        M94.8X8   Other specified disorders of cartilage, other site
        M94.8X9   Other specified disorders of cartilage, unspecified sites
    M94.9   Disorder of cartilage, unspecified

◀ New   ⬅ Revised   ~~deleted~~ Deleted   Excludes 1   Excludes 2   Includes   Use additional   Code first   Code also   Unspecified

OGCR Official Guidelines   ● Unacceptable Principal Diagnosis   X Assign placeholder X   ● Use Additional Character(s)   ▷ Manifestation Code   **Coding Clinic**

OTHER DISORDERS OF THE MUSCULOSKELETAL SYSTEM AND CONNECTIVE TISSUE (M95)

● **M95**   **Other acquired deformities of musculoskeletal system and connective tissue**
> **Excludes2**   acquired absence of limbs and organs (Z89-Z90)
> acquired deformities of limbs (M20-M21)
> congenital malformations and deformations of the musculoskeletal system (Q65-Q79)
> deforming dorsopathies (M40-M43)
> dentofacial anomalies [including malocclusion] (M26.-)
> postprocedural musculoskeletal disorders (M96.-)

    M95.0   **Acquired deformity of nose**
> **Excludes2**   deviated nasal septum (J34.2)

    ● **M95.1**   **Cauliflower ear**
> **Excludes2**   other acquired deformities of ear (H61.1)

       M95.10   Cauliflower ear, unspecified ear
       M95.11   Cauliflower ear, right ear
       M95.12   Cauliflower ear, left ear

    M95.2   **Other acquired deformity of head**
    M95.3   **Acquired deformity of neck**
    M95.4   **Acquired deformity of chest and rib**
    M95.5   **Acquired deformity of pelvis**
> **Excludes1**   maternal care for known or suspected disproportion (O33.-)

    M95.8   **Other specified acquired deformities of musculoskeletal system**
    M95.9   **Acquired deformity of musculoskeletal system, unspecified**

INTRAOPERATIVE AND POSTPROCEDURAL COMPLICATIONS AND DISORDERS OF MUSCULOSKELETAL SYSTEM, NOT ELSEWHERE CLASSIFIED (M96)

● **M96**   **Intraoperative and postprocedural complications and disorders of musculoskeletal system, not elsewhere classified**
> **Excludes2**   arthropathy following intestinal bypass (M02.0-)
> complications of internal orthopedic prosthetic devices, implants and grafts (T84.-)
> disorders associated with osteoporosis (M80)
> periprosthetic fracture around internal prosthetic joint (M97.-) ◀
> presence of functional implants and other devices (Z96-Z97)

    M96.0   **Pseudarthrosis after fusion or arthrodesis** 🔊
> (Ex) No exclusions

    M96.1   **Postlaminectomy syndrome, not elsewhere classified**
    M96.2   **Postradiation kyphosis**
    M96.3   **Postlaminectomy kyphosis**
    M96.4   **Postsurgical lordosis**
    M96.5   **Postradiation scoliosis**
    ● **M96.6**   **Fracture of bone following insertion of orthopedic implant, joint prosthesis, or bone plate**
> Intraoperative fracture of bone during insertion of orthopedic implant, joint prosthesis, or bone plate
> **Excludes2**   complication of internal orthopedic devices, implants or grafts (T84.-)

> (Ex) **For category M96.6 CC codes:** D78.81, D78.89, E36.8, E89.810-E89.89, H59.011-H59.019, H59.031-H59.819, H59.88-H59.89, H95.811-H95.89, I97.3, L76.81-L76.82, M96.621-M96.69, M96.89, M97.01X-M97.9XX[A], N98.1-N98.9, T81.82X[A], T81.89X-T81.9XX[A], T84.010-T84.039[A], T84.050-T84.9XX[A]

    ● **M96.62**   **Fracture of humerus following insertion of orthopedic implant, joint prosthesis, or bone plate**
       M96.621   **Fracture of humerus following insertion of orthopedic implant, joint prosthesis, or bone plate, right arm** 🔊
       M96.622   **Fracture of humerus following insertion of orthopedic implant, joint prosthesis, or bone plate, left arm** 🔊
       M96.629   **Fracture of humerus following insertion of orthopedic implant, joint prosthesis, or bone plate, unspecified arm** 🔊

    ● **M96.63**   **Fracture of radius or ulna following insertion of orthopedic implant, joint prosthesis, or bone plate**
       M96.631   **Fracture of radius or ulna following insertion of orthopedic implant, joint prosthesis, or bone plate, right arm** 🔊
       M96.632   **Fracture of radius or ulna following insertion of orthopedic implant, joint prosthesis, or bone plate, left arm** 🔊
       M96.639   **Fracture of radius or ulna following insertion of orthopedic implant, joint prosthesis, or bone plate, unspecified arm** 🔊

    M96.65   **Fracture of pelvis following insertion of orthopedic implant, joint prosthesis, or bone plate** 🔊

    ● **M96.66**   **Fracture of femur following insertion of orthopedic implant, joint prosthesis, or bone plate**
       M96.661   **Fracture of femur following insertion of orthopedic implant, joint prosthesis, or bone plate, right leg** 🔊
       M96.662   **Fracture of femur following insertion of orthopedic implant, joint prosthesis, or bone plate, left leg** 🔊
       M96.669   **Fracture of femur following insertion of orthopedic implant, joint prosthesis, or bone plate, unspecified leg** 🔊

    ● **M96.67**   **Fracture of tibia or fibula following insertion of orthopedic implant, joint prosthesis, or bone plate**
       M96.671   **Fracture of tibia or fibula following insertion of orthopedic implant, joint prosthesis, or bone plate, right leg** 🔊
       M96.672   **Fracture of tibia or fibula following insertion of orthopedic implant, joint prosthesis, or bone plate, left leg** 🔊
       M96.679   **Fracture of tibia or fibula following insertion of orthopedic implant, joint prosthesis, or bone plate, unspecified leg** 🔊

    M96.69   **Fracture of other bone following insertion of orthopedic implant, joint prosthesis, or bone plate** 🔊

N Newborn Age: 0   **P** Pediatric Age: 0-17   **M** Maternity DX: 12-55   **A** Adult Age: 15-124   ♀ Females Only   ♂ Males Only
🔊 Complication\Comorbidity   🔊 Major C\C   (Ex) CC/MCC Exclusions   🔊 Hospital-Acquired Condition

1087

● **M96.8**   **Other intraoperative and postprocedural complications and disorders of musculoskeletal system, not elsewhere classified**

● **M96.81**   **Intraoperative hemorrhage and hematoma of a musculoskeletal structure complicating a procedure**

> **Excludes1**   intraoperative hemorrhage and hematoma of a musculoskeletal structure due to accidental puncture and laceration during a procedure (M96.82-)

> (Ex) **For category M96.81 CC codes:** H95.811-H95.89, I85.01, I85.11, I97.3, K21.9, K22.8, K23-K25.2, K25.4, K25.6, K26.0, K26.2, K26.4, K26.6, K27.0, K27.2, K27.4, K27.6, K28.0, K28.2, K28.4, K28.6, K29.01, K29.21, K29.31, K29.41, K29.51, K29.61, K29.71, K29.81, K29.91, K31.811, K55.21, K57.01, K57.11, K57.13, K57.21, K57.31, K57.33, K57.41, K57.51, K57.53, K57.81, K57.91, K57.93, K62.5, K92.0-K92.2, M96.810-M96.811, M96.830-M96.89, N98.1-N98.9, P54.1-P54.3, T81.10X-T81.19X[A], T81.82X[A], T81.89X-T81.9XX[A]

M96.810   **Intraoperative hemorrhage and hematoma of a musculoskeletal structure complicating a musculoskeletal system procedure** ✪

M96.811   **Intraoperative hemorrhage and hematoma of a musculoskeletal structure complicating other procedure** ✪

● **M96.82**   **Accidental puncture and laceration of a musculoskeletal structure during a procedure**

> (Ex) **For category M96.82 CC codes:** D78.11-D78.12, D78.81-D78.89, E36.11-E36.8, E89.810-E89.89, G96.11, G97.41-G97.49, H59.011-H59.019, H59.031-H59.099, H59.211-H59.229, H59.811-H59.89, H95.31-H95.32, H95.811-H95.89, I97.3, I97.51-I97.52, J95.71-J95.72, K91.71-K91.72, L76.11-L76.12, L76.81-L76.82, M96.820-M96.821, M96.89, N98.1-N98.9, N99.71-N99.72, T81.82X[A], T81.89X-T81.9XX[A]

M96.820   **Accidental puncture and laceration of a musculoskeletal structure during a musculoskeletal system procedure** ✪

M96.821   **Accidental puncture and laceration of a musculoskeletal structure during other procedure** ✪

● **M96.83**   **Postprocedural hemorrhage of a musculoskeletal structure following a procedure** ◀▥

> (Ex) **For category M96.83 CC codes:** See M96.81

M96.830   **Postprocedural hemorrhage of a musculoskeletal structure following a musculoskeletal system procedure** ✪ ◀▥

M96.831   **Postprocedural hemorrhage of a musculoskeletal structure following other procedure** ✪ ◀▥

● **M96.84**   **Postprocedural hematoma and seroma of a musculoskeletal structure following a procedure** ◀

> (Ex) **For category M96.84 CC codes:** See M96.81

M96.840   **Postprocedural hematoma of a musculoskeletal structure following a musculoskeletal system procedure** ✪ ◀

M96.841   **Postprocedural hematoma of a musculoskeletal structure following other procedure** ✪ ◀

M96.842   **Postprocedural seroma of a musculoskeletal structure following a musculoskeletal system procedure** ✪ ◀

M96.843   **Postprocedural seroma of a musculoskeletal structure following other procedure** ✪ ◀

● **M96.89**   **Other intraoperative and postprocedural complications and disorders of the musculoskeletal system** ✪

Instability of joint secondary to removal of joint prosthesis

Use additional code, if applicable, to further specify disorder

> (Ex) D78.81-D78.89, E36.8, E89.810-E89.89, H59.011-H59.019, H59.031-H59.099, H59.811-H59.89, H95.811-H95.89, I97.3, L76.81-L76.82, M96.89, N98.1-N98.9, T81.82X[A], T81.89X-T81.9XX[A]

PERIPROSTHETIC FRACTURE AROUND INTERNAL PROSTHETIC JOINT (M97) ◀

● **M97**   **Periprosthetic fracture around internal prosthetic joint** ◀

> **Excludes2**   fracture of bone following insertion of orthopedic implant, joint prosthesis or bone plate (M96.6-) ◀
>
> breakage (fracture) of prosthetic joint (T84.01-) ◀

The appropriate 7th character is to be added to each code from category M97: ◀

A	initial encounter ◀
D	subsequent encounter ◀
S	sequela ◀

> (Ex) **For category M97 CC codes:** See M96.6

● **M97.0**   **Periprosthetic fracture around internal prosthetic hip joint**

X ● **M97.01**   **Periprosthetic fracture around internal prosthetic right hip joint** A ✪ ◀

X ● **M97.02**   **Periprosthetic fracture around internal prosthetic left hip joint** A ✪ ◀

● **M97.1**   **Periprosthetic fracture around internal prosthetic knee joint** ◀

X ● **M97.11**   **Periprosthetic fracture around internal prosthetic right knee joint** A ✪ ◀

X ● **M97.12**   **Periprosthetic fracture around internal prosthetic left knee joint** A ✪ ◀

● **M97.2**   **Periprosthetic fracture around internal prosthetic ankle joint** ◀

X ● **M97.21**   **Periprosthetic fracture around internal prosthetic right ankle joint** A ✪ ◀

X ● **M97.22**   **Periprosthetic fracture around internal prosthetic left ankle joint** A ✪ ◀

● **M97.3**   **Periprosthetic fracture around internal prosthetic shoulder joint** ◀

X ● **M97.31**   **Periprosthetic fracture around internal prosthetic right shoulder joint** A ✪ ◀

X ● **M97.32**   **Periprosthetic fracture around internal prosthetic left shoulder joint** A ✪ ◀

● **M97.4**   **Periprosthetic fracture around internal prosthetic elbow joint** ◀

X ● **M97.41**   **Periprosthetic fracture around internal prosthetic right elbow joint** A ✪ ◀

X ● **M97.42**   **Periprosthetic fracture around internal prosthetic left elbow joint** A ✪ ◀

◀ New   ◀▥ Revised   ~~deleted~~ Deleted   Excludes 1   Excludes 2   Includes   Use additional   Code first   Code also   Unspecified

OGCR Official Guidelines   ● Unacceptable Principal Diagnosis   X Assign placeholder X   ✪ Use Additional Character(s)   ▣ Manifestation Code   **Coding Clinic**

X ● **M97.8　Periprosthetic fracture around other internal prosthetic joint** A 🌣 ◄

　　　Periprosthetic fracture around internal prosthetic finger joint ◄

　　　Periprosthetic fracture around internal prosthetic spinal joint ◄

　　　Periprosthetic fracture around internal prosthetic toe joint ◄

　　　Periprosthetic fracture around internal prosthetic wrist joint ◄

　　　Use additional code to identify the joint (Z96.6-) ◄

X ● **M97.9　Periprosthetic fracture around unspecified internal prosthetic joint** A 🌣 ◄

BIOMECHANICAL LESIONS, NOT ELSEWHERE CLASSIFIED (M99)

● **M99　Biomechanical lesions, not elsewhere classified**

　　Note: This category should not be used if the condition can be classified elsewhere.

● **M99.0　Segmental and somatic dysfunction**

　M99.00　Segmental and somatic dysfunction of head region

　M99.01　Segmental and somatic dysfunction of cervical region

　M99.02　Segmental and somatic dysfunction of thoracic region

　M99.03　Segmental and somatic dysfunction of lumbar region

　M99.04　Segmental and somatic dysfunction of sacral region

　M99.05　Segmental and somatic dysfunction of pelvic region

　M99.06　Segmental and somatic dysfunction of lower extremity

　M99.07　Segmental and somatic dysfunction of upper extremity

　M99.08　Segmental and somatic dysfunction of rib cage

　M99.09　Segmental and somatic dysfunction of abdomen and other regions

● **M99.1　Subluxation complex (vertebral)**

　M99.10　Subluxation complex (vertebral) of head region 🌣 🌣
　　Ex: M99.10-M99.11, S03.8XX-S03.9XX[A], S12.000-S12.691[A,B], S12.9XX-S13.4XX[A], S13.8XX[A], S14.0XX-S14.108[A], S14.111-S14.118[A], S14.121-S14.128[A], S14.131-S14.138[A], S14.141-S14.148[A], S14.151-S14.158[A], S16.1XX[A], S29.011-S29.019[A], S38.3XX[A], S39.011-S39.013[A], T14.90-T14.91, T79.A0X-T79.9XX[A]

　M99.11　Subluxation complex (vertebral) of cervical region 🌣 🌣
　　Ex: See M99.10

　M99.12　Subluxation complex (vertebral) of thoracic region

　M99.13　Subluxation complex (vertebral) of lumbar region

　M99.14　Subluxation complex (vertebral) of sacral region

　M99.15　Subluxation complex (vertebral) of pelvic region

　M99.16　Subluxation complex (vertebral) of lower extremity

　M99.17　Subluxation complex (vertebral) of upper extremity

　M99.18　Subluxation complex (vertebral) of rib cage 🌣 🌣
　　Ex: M99.18, S43.201A-S43.226[A]

　M99.19　Subluxation complex (vertebral) of abdomen and other regions

● **M99.2　Subluxation stenosis of neural canal**

　M99.20　Subluxation stenosis of neural canal of head region

　M99.21　Subluxation stenosis of neural canal of cervical region

　M99.22　Subluxation stenosis of neural canal of thoracic region

　M99.23　Subluxation stenosis of neural canal of lumbar region

　M99.24　Subluxation stenosis of neural canal of sacral region

　M99.25　Subluxation stenosis of neural canal of pelvic region

　M99.26　Subluxation stenosis of neural canal of lower extremity

　M99.27　Subluxation stenosis of neural canal of upper extremity

　M99.28　Subluxation stenosis of neural canal of rib cage

　M99.29　Subluxation stenosis of neural canal of abdomen and other regions

● **M99.3　Osseous stenosis of neural canal**

　M99.30　Osseous stenosis of neural canal of head region

　M99.31　Osseous stenosis of neural canal of cervical region

　M99.32　Osseous stenosis of neural canal of thoracic region

　M99.33　Osseous stenosis of neural canal of lumbar region

　M99.34　Osseous stenosis of neural canal of sacral region

　M99.35　Osseous stenosis of neural canal of pelvic region

　M99.36　Osseous stenosis of neural canal of lower extremity

　M99.37　Osseous stenosis of neural canal of upper extremity

　M99.38　Osseous stenosis of neural canal of rib cage

　M99.39　Osseous stenosis of neural canal of abdomen and other regions

● **M99.4　Connective tissue stenosis of neural canal**

　M99.40　Connective tissue stenosis of neural canal of head region

　M99.41　Connective tissue stenosis of neural canal of cervical region

　M99.42　Connective tissue stenosis of neural canal of thoracic region

　M99.43　Connective tissue stenosis of neural canal of lumbar region

　M99.44　Connective tissue stenosis of neural canal of sacral region

　M99.45　Connective tissue stenosis of neural canal of pelvic region

　M99.46　Connective tissue stenosis of neural canal of lower extremity

　M99.47　Connective tissue stenosis of neural canal of upper extremity

　M99.48　Connective tissue stenosis of neural canal of rib cage

　M99.49　Connective tissue stenosis of neural canal of abdomen and other regions

● M99.5   Intervertebral disc stenosis of neural canal

M99.50   Intervertebral disc stenosis of neural canal of head region

M99.51   Intervertebral disc stenosis of neural canal of cervical region

M99.52   Intervertebral disc stenosis of neural canal of thoracic region

M99.53   Intervertebral disc stenosis of neural canal of lumbar region

M99.54   Intervertebral disc stenosis of neural canal of sacral region

M99.55   Intervertebral disc stenosis of neural canal of pelvic region

M99.56   Intervertebral disc stenosis of neural canal of lower extremity

M99.57   Intervertebral disc stenosis of neural canal of upper extremity

M99.58   Intervertebral disc stenosis of neural canal of rib cage

M99.59   Intervertebral disc stenosis of neural canal of abdomen and other regions

● M99.6   Osseous and subluxation stenosis of intervertebral foramina

M99.60   Osseous and subluxation stenosis of intervertebral foramina of head region

M99.61   Osseous and subluxation stenosis of intervertebral foramina of cervical region

M99.62   Osseous and subluxation stenosis of intervertebral foramina of thoracic region

M99.63   Osseous and subluxation stenosis of intervertebral foramina of lumbar region

M99.64   Osseous and subluxation stenosis of intervertebral foramina of sacral region

M99.65   Osseous and subluxation stenosis of intervertebral foramina of pelvic region

M99.66   Osseous and subluxation stenosis of intervertebral foramina of lower extremity

M99.67   Osseous and subluxation stenosis of intervertebral foramina of upper extremity

M99.68   Osseous and subluxation stenosis of intervertebral foramina of rib cage

M99.69   Osseous and subluxation stenosis of intervertebral foramina of abdomen and other regions

● M99.7   Connective tissue and disc stenosis of intervertebral foramina

M99.70   Connective tissue and disc stenosis of intervertebral foramina of head region

M99.71   Connective tissue and disc stenosis of intervertebral foramina of cervical region

M99.72   Connective tissue and disc stenosis of intervertebral foramina of thoracic region

M99.73   Connective tissue and disc stenosis of intervertebral foramina of lumbar region

M99.74   Connective tissue and disc stenosis of intervertebral foramina of sacral region

M99.75   Connective tissue and disc stenosis of intervertebral foramina of pelvic region

M99.76   Connective tissue and disc stenosis of intervertebral foramina of lower extremity

M99.77   Connective tissue and disc stenosis of intervertebral foramina of upper extremity

M99.78   Connective tissue and disc stenosis of intervertebral foramina of rib cage

M99.79   Connective tissue and disc stenosis of intervertebral foramina of abdomen and other regions

● M99.8   Other biomechanical lesions

M99.80   Other biomechanical lesions of head region

M99.81   Other biomechanical lesions of cervical region

M99.82   Other biomechanical lesions of thoracic region

M99.83   Other biomechanical lesions of lumbar region

M99.84   Other biomechanical lesions of sacral region

M99.85   Other biomechanical lesions of pelvic region

M99.86   Other biomechanical lesions of lower extremity

M99.87   Other biomechanical lesions of upper extremity

M99.88   Other biomechanical lesions of rib cage

M99.89   Other biomechanical lesions of abdomen and other regions

M99.9   Biomechanical lesion, unspecified

◄ New   ◄▥ Revised   ~~deleted~~ Deleted   Excludes 1   Excludes 2   Includes   Use additional   Code first   Code also   Unspecified

OGCR Official Guidelines   ● Unacceptable Principal Diagnosis   X Assign placeholder X   ● Use Additional Character(s)   ▶ Manifestation Code   Coding Clinic

CHAPTER 14

DISEASES OF THE GENITOURINARY SYSTEM (N00-N99)

OGCR Chapter-Specific Coding Guidelines

> 14. Chapter 14: Diseases of Genitourinary System (N00-N99)
>
>   a. Chronic kidney disease
>
>   1) **Stages of chronic kidney disease (CKD)**
> The ICD-10-CM classifies CKD based on severity. The severity of CKD is designated by stages 1-5. Stage 2, code N18.2, equates to mild CKD; stage 3, code N18.3, equates to moderate CKD; and stage 4, code N18.4, equates to severe CKD. Code N18.6, End stage renal disease (ESRD), is assigned when the provider has documented end-stage-renal disease (ESRD).
>
>   If both a stage of CKD and ESRD are documented, assign code N18.6 only.
>
>   2) **Chronic kidney disease and kidney transplant status**
> Patients who have undergone kidney transplant may still have some form of chronic kidney disease CKD because the kidney transplant may not fully restore kidney function. Therefore, the presence of CKD alone does not constitute a transplant complication. Assign the appropriate N18 code for the patient's stage of CKD and code Z94.0, Kidney transplant status. If a transplant complication such as failure or rejection or other transplant complication is documented, see section I.C.19.g for information on coding complications of a kidney transplant. If the documentation is unclear as to whether the patient has a complication of the transplant, query the provider.
>
>   3) **Chronic kidney disease with other conditions**
> Patients with CKD may also suffer from other serious conditions, most commonly diabetes mellitus and hypertension. The sequencing of the CKD code in relationship to codes for other contributing conditions is based on the conventions in the Tabular List.
> *See I.C.9. Hypertensive chronic kidney disease.*
> *See I.C.19. Chronic kidney disease and kidney transplant complications.*

Item 14–1 Nephritis (inflammation) or **nephropathy** (disease) **with lesion of proliferative glomerulonephritis** results from a streptococcal infection.

  Nephritis (inflammation) or **nephropathy** (disease) **with lesion of membranous glomerulonephritis** is characterized by deposits along the epithelial side of the basement membrane.

  Nephritis (inflammation) or **nephropathy** (disease) **with lesion of membranoproliferative glomerulonephritis** is characterized by alterations in the basement membranes of the kidney and the glomerular cells.

  Nephritis (inflammation) or **nephropathy** (disease) **with lesion of rapidly progressive glomerulonephritis** is characterized by rapid and progressive decline in renal function.

  Nephritis (inflammation) or **nephropathy** (disease) **with lesion of renal cortical necrosis** is characterized by death of the cortical tissues.

  Nephritis (inflammation) or **nephropathy** (disease) **with lesion of renal medullary necrosis** is characterized by death of the tissues that collect urine.

Figure 14-1 Kidneys within the urinary system.

Item 14–2 Glomerulonephritis is nephritis accompanied by inflammation of the glomeruli of the kidney, resulting in the degeneration of the glomeruli and the nephrons.

  Acute glomerulonephritis primarily affects children and young adults and is usually a result of a streptococcal infection.

  Proliferative glomerulonephritis is the acute form of the disease resulting from a streptococcal infection.

  Rapidly progressive glomerulonephritis, also known as **crescentic** or **malignant glomerulonephritis**, is the acute form of the disease, which leads quickly to rapid and progressive decline in renal function.

CHAPTER 14

DISEASES OF THE GENITOURINARY SYSTEM (N00-N99)

Excludes2	certain conditions originating in the perinatal period (P04-P96)
	certain infectious and parasitic diseases (A00-B99)
	complications of pregnancy, childbirth and the puerperium (O00-O9A)
	congenital malformations, deformations and chromosomal abnormalities (Q00-Q99)
	endocrine, nutritional and metabolic diseases (E00-E88)
	injury, poisoning and certain other consequences of external causes (S00-T88)
	neoplasms (C00-D49)
	symptoms, signs and abnormal clinical and laboratory findings, not elsewhere classified (R00-R94)

This chapter contains the following blocks:

N00-N08	Glomerular diseases
N10-N16	Renal tubulo-interstitial diseases
N17-N19	Acute kidney failure and chronic kidney disease
N20-N23	Urolithiasis
N25-N29	Other disorders of kidney and ureter
N30-N39	Other diseases of the urinary system
N40-N53	Diseases of male genital organs
N60-N65	Disorders of breast
N70-N77	Inflammatory diseases of female pelvic organs
N80-N98	Noninflammatory disorders of female genital tract
N99	Intraoperative and postprocedural complications and disorders of genitourinary system, not elsewhere classified

GLOMERULAR DISEASES (N00-N08)

Code also any associated kidney failure (N17-N19)

Excludes1	hypertensive chronic kidney disease (I12.-)

● **N00**   **Acute nephritic syndrome**

Includes	acute glomerular disease
	acute glomerulonephritis
	acute nephritis

Excludes1	acute tubulo-interstitial nephritis (N10)
	nephritic syndrome NOS (N05.-)

(Ex:) **For category N00 CC codes unless otherwise indicated:** A17.9, A18.10-A18.11, A18.13, A18.82, A18.84, A18.89, A54.21, A54.29, A54.82, A54.84, A54.89-A54.9, A59.00, A59.8-A59.9, B37.41-B37.49, E08.21-E08.29, E08.618-E08.638, E08.649, E08.65-E08.8, E09.21-E09.29, E09.618-E09.638, E09.649-E09.8, E10.21-E10.29, E10.618-E10.638, E10.649, E10.69-E10.8, E11.21-E11.29, E11.618-E11.638, E11.649, E11.69-E11.8, E13.21-E13.29, E13.618-E13.638, E13.649-E13.69, E13.8, E88.3, M10.30-M10.39, N10, N11.10, N11.8, N11.9, N13.0-N13.39, N13.6, N14.0-N19, N25.0-N27.9, N28.1-N29, N36.41-N36.43, N36.8-N36.9, N39.8-N39.9, R31.0-R31.9

N00.0   **Acute nephritic syndrome with minor glomerular abnormality** 🔹
    Acute nephritic syndrome with minimal change lesion

N00.1   **Acute nephritic syndrome with focal and segmental glomerular lesions** 🔹
    Acute nephritic syndrome with focal and segmental hyalinosis
    Acute nephritic syndrome with focal and segmental sclerosis
    Acute nephritic syndrome with focal glomerulonephritis

N00.2   **Acute nephritic syndrome with diffuse membranous glomerulonephritis** 🔍

N00.3   **Acute nephritic syndrome with diffuse mesangial proliferative glomerulonephritis** 🔍

N00.4   **Acute nephritic syndrome with diffuse endocapillary proliferative glomerulonephritis** 🔍

N00.5   **Acute nephritic syndrome with diffuse mesangiocapillary glomerulonephritis** 🔍

     Acute nephritic syndrome with membranoproliferative glomerulonephritis, types 1 and 3, or NOS

N00.6   **Acute nephritic syndrome with dense deposit disease** 🔍

     Acute nephritic syndrome with membranoproliferative glomerulonephritis, type 2

N00.7   **Acute nephritic syndrome with diffuse crescentic glomerulonephritis** 🔍

     Acute nephritic syndrome with extracapillary glomerulonephritis

N00.8   **Acute nephritic syndrome with other morphologic changes** 🔍

     Acute nephritic syndrome with proliferative glomerulonephritis NOS

     (Ex:) A17.9, A18.10-A18.11, A18.13, A18.82, A18.84, A18.89, A54.21, A54.29, A54.82, A54.84, A54.89-A54.9, A59.00, A59.8-A59.9, B37.41-B37.49, E08.21-E08.29, E09.21-E09.29, E88.3, M10.30-M10.39, N00.0-N13.39, N13.6, N14.0-N19, N25.0-N27.9, N28.1-N29, N36.41-N36.43, N36.8-N36.9, N39.8-N39.9, R31.0-R31.9

N00.9   **Acute nephritic syndrome with** `unspecified` **morphologic changes** 🔍

🔴 **N01**   **Rapidly progressive nephritic syndrome**

     `Includes`   rapidly progressive glomerular disease
                   rapidly progressive glomerulonephritis
                   rapidly progressive nephritis

     `Excludes1`   nephritic syndrome NOS (N05.-)

     (Ex:) For category N01 CC codes: See N00

N01.0   **Rapidly progressive nephritic syndrome with minor glomerular abnormality** 🔍

     Rapidly progressive nephritic syndrome with minimal change lesion

N01.1   **Rapidly progressive nephritic syndrome with focal and segmental glomerular lesions** 🔍

     Rapidly progressive nephritic syndrome with focal and segmental hyalinosis
     Rapidly progressive nephritic syndrome with focal and segmental sclerosis
     Rapidly progressive nephritic syndrome with focal glomerulonephritis

N01.2   **Rapidly progressive nephritic syndrome with diffuse membranous glomerulonephritis** 🔍

N01.3   **Rapidly progressive nephritic syndrome with diffuse mesangial proliferative glomerulonephritis** 🔍

N01.4   **Rapidly progressive nephritic syndrome with diffuse endocapillary proliferative glomerulonephritis** 🔍

N01.5   **Rapidly progressive nephritic syndrome with diffuse mesangiocapillary glomerulonephritis** 🔍

     Rapidly progressive nephritic syndrome with membranoproliferative glomerulonephritis, types 1 and 3, or NOS

N01.6   **Rapidly progressive nephritic syndrome with dense deposit disease** 🔍

     Rapidly progressive nephritic syndrome with membranoproliferative glomerulonephritis, type 2

N01.7   **Rapidly progressive nephritic syndrome with diffuse crescentic glomerulonephritis** 🔍

     Rapidly progressive nephritic syndrome with extracapillary glomerulonephritis

N01.8   **Rapidly progressive nephritic syndrome with other morphologic changes** 🔍

     Rapidly progressive nephritic syndrome with proliferative glomerulonephritis NOS

N01.9   **Rapidly progressive nephritic syndrome with** `unspecified` **morphologic changes** 🔍

🔴 **N02**   **Recurrent and persistent hematuria**

     `Excludes1`   acute cystitis with hematuria (N30.01)
                   hematuria NOS (R31.9)
                   hematuria not associated with specified morphologic lesions (R31.-)

     (Ex:) For category N02 CC codes unless otherwise indicated: A17.9, A18.10-A18.11, A18.13, A18.82, A18.84, A18.89, A54.21, A54.29, A54.82, A54.84, A54.89-A54.9, A59.00, A59.8-A59.9, B37.41-B37.49, E08.21-E08.29, E08.618-E08.638, E08.649, E08.65-E08.8, E09.21-E09.29, E09.618-E09.638, E09.649-E09.8, E10.21-E10.29, E10.618-E10.638, E10.649, E10.69-E10.8, E11.21-E11.29, E11.618-E11.638, E11.649, E11.69-E11.8, E13.21-E13.29, E13.618-E13.638, E13.649-E13.69, E13.8, M10.30-M10.39, N00.0-N13.39, N13.6, N14.0-N19, N25.0-N27.9, N28.1-N29, N36.41-N36.43, N36.8-N36.9, N39.8-N39.9, R31.0-R31.9

N02.0   **Recurrent and persistent hematuria with minor glomerular abnormality** 🔍

     Recurrent and persistent hematuria with minimal change lesion

N02.1   **Recurrent and persistent hematuria with focal and segmental glomerular lesions** 🔍

     Recurrent and persistent hematuria with focal and segmental hyalinosis
     Recurrent and persistent hematuria with focal and segmental sclerosis
     Recurrent and persistent hematuria with focal glomerulonephritis

N02.2   **Recurrent and persistent hematuria with diffuse membranous glomerulonephritis** 🔍

N02.3   **Recurrent and persistent hematuria with diffuse mesangial proliferative glomerulonephritis** 🔍

N02.4   **Recurrent and persistent hematuria with diffuse endocapillary proliferative glomerulonephritis** 🔍

N02.5   **Recurrent and persistent hematuria with diffuse mesangiocapillary glomerulonephritis** 🔍

     Recurrent and persistent hematuria with membranoproliferative glomerulonephritis, types 1 and 3, or NOS

N02.6   **Recurrent and persistent hematuria with dense deposit disease** 🔍

     Recurrent and persistent hematuria with membranoproliferative glomerulonephritis, type 2

N02.7   **Recurrent and persistent hematuria with diffuse crescentic glomerulonephritis** 🔍

     Recurrent and persistent hematuria with extracapillary glomerulonephritis

N02.8   **Recurrent and persistent hematuria with other morphologic changes** 🔍

     Recurrent and persistent hematuria with proliferative glomerulonephritis NOS

     (Ex:) See N00

N02.9   **Recurrent and persistent hematuria with** `unspecified` **morphologic changes** 🔍

     (Ex:) See N00

🔴 **N03**   **Chronic nephritic syndrome**

     `Includes`   chronic glomerular disease
                   chronic glomerulonephritis
                   chronic nephritis

     `Excludes1`   chronic tubulo-interstitial nephritis (N11.-)
                   diffuse sclerosing glomerulonephritis (N05.8-)
                   nephritic syndrome NOS (N05.-)

     (Ex:) For category N03 CC codes: A17.9, A18.10-A18.11, A18.13, A18.82, A18.84, A18.89, A54.21, A54.29, A54.82, A54.84, A54.89-A54.9, A59.00, A59.8-A59.9, A98.5, B37.41-B37.49, E08.21-E08.29, E08.618-E08.638, E08.649, E08.65-E08.8, E09.21-E09.29, E09.618-E09.638, E09.649-E09.8, E10.21-E10.29, E10.618-E10.638, E10.649, E10.69-E10.8, E11.21-E11.29, E11.618-E11.638, E11.649, E11.69-E11.8, E13.21-E13.29, E13.618-E13.638, E13.649-E13.69, E13.8, M10.30-M10.39, N00.0-N13.39, N13.6, N14.0-N19, N25.0-N27.9, N28.1-N29, N36.41-N36.43, N36.8-N36.9, N39.8-N39.9, R31.0-R31.9

N03.0   **Chronic nephritic syndrome with minor glomerular abnormality** 🔍

     Chronic nephritic syndrome with minimal change lesion

◀ New   ◀ Revised   ~~deleted~~ Deleted   `Excludes 1`   `Excludes 2`   `Includes`   `Use additional`   `Code first`   `Code also`   `Unspecified`

OGCR Official Guidelines   ● Unacceptable Principal Diagnosis   X Assign placeholder X   ● Use Additional Character(s)   ▶ Manifestation Code   **Coding Clinic**

Item 14–3 Chronic glomerulonephritis (GN) persists over a period of years, with remissions and exacerbation.

Chronic GN with lesion of proliferative glomerulonephritis results from a streptococcal infection.

Chronic GN with lesion of membranous glomerulonephritis, also known as membranous nephropathy, is characterized by deposits along the epithelial side of the basement membrane.

Chronic GN with lesion of membrano-proliferative glomerulonephritis (MPGN) is a group of disorders characterized by alterations in the basement membranes of the kidney and the glomerular cells.

Chronic GN with lesion of rapidly progressive glomerulonephritis is characterized by necrosis, endothelial proliferation, and mesangial proliferation. The condition is marked by rapid and progressive decline in renal function.

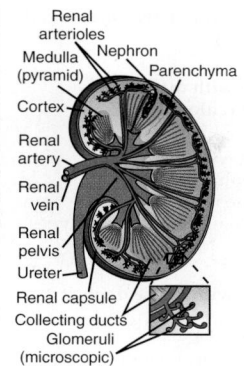

Figure 14-2 Kidney cross section.

N03.1 **Chronic nephritic syndrome with focal and segmental glomerular lesions** 🔖
    Chronic nephritic syndrome with focal and segmental hyalinosis
    Chronic nephritic syndrome with focal and segmental sclerosis
    Chronic nephritic syndrome with focal glomerulonephritis

N03.2 **Chronic nephritic syndrome with diffuse membranous glomerulonephritis** 🔖

N03.3 **Chronic nephritic syndrome with diffuse mesangial proliferative glomerulonephritis** 🔖

N03.4 **Chronic nephritic syndrome with diffuse endocapillary proliferative glomerulonephritis** 🔖

N03.5 **Chronic nephritic syndrome with diffuse mesangiocapillary glomerulonephritis** 🔖
    Chronic nephritic syndrome with membranoproliferative glomerulonephritis, types 1 and 3, or NOS

N03.6 **Chronic nephritic syndrome with dense deposit disease** 🔖
    Chronic nephritic syndrome with membranoproliferative glomerulonephritis, type 2

N03.7 **Chronic nephritic syndrome with diffuse crescentic glomerulonephritis** 🔖
    Chronic nephritic syndrome with extracapillary glomerulonephritis

N03.8 **Chronic nephritic syndrome with other morphologic changes** 🔖
    Chronic nephritic syndrome with proliferative glomerulonephritis NOS

N03.9 **Chronic nephritic syndrome with unspecified morphologic changes** 🔖

● **N04** **Nephrotic syndrome**
    Includes   congenital nephrotic syndrome
                lipoid nephrosis
    Ⓔⓧ For category N04 CC codes unless otherwise indicated: See N02

N04.0 **Nephrotic syndrome with minor glomerular abnormality** 🔖
    Nephrotic syndrome with minimal change lesion

N04.1 **Nephrotic syndrome with focal and segmental glomerular lesions** 🔖
    Nephrotic syndrome with focal and segmental hyalinosis
    Nephrotic syndrome with focal and segmental sclerosis
    Nephrotic syndrome with focal glomerulonephritis

N04.2 **Nephrotic syndrome with diffuse membranous glomerulonephritis** 🔖

N04.3 **Nephrotic syndrome with diffuse mesangial proliferative glomerulonephritis** 🔖

N04.4 **Nephrotic syndrome with diffuse endocapillary proliferative glomerulonephritis** 🔖

Item 14–4 Nephrotic syndrome (NS) is marked by massive proteinuria (protein in the urine) and water retention. Patients with NS are particularly vulnerable to staphylococcal and pneumococcal infections. NS with lesion of proliferative glomerulonephritis results from a streptococcal infection. NS with lesion of membranous glomerulonephritis results in thickening of the capillary walls. NS with lesion of minimal change glomerulonephritis is usually a benign disorder that occurs mostly in children and requires electron microscopy (biopsy) to verify changes in the glomeruli.

N04.5 **Nephrotic syndrome with diffuse mesangiocapillary glomerulonephritis** 🔖
    Nephrotic syndrome with membranoproliferative glomerulonephritis, types 1 and 3, or NOS

N04.6 **Nephrotic syndrome with dense deposit disease** 🔖
    Nephrotic syndrome with membranoproliferative glomerulonephritis, type 2

N04.7 **Nephrotic syndrome with diffuse crescentic glomerulonephritis** 🔖
    Nephrotic syndrome with extracapillary glomerulonephritis
    Ⓔⓧ See N00

N04.8 **Nephrotic syndrome with other morphologic changes** 🔖
    Nephrotic syndrome with proliferative glomerulonephritis NOS
    Ⓔⓧ See N00

N04.9 **Nephrotic syndrome with unspecified morphologic changes** 🔖
    Ⓔⓧ See N00

● **N05** **Unspecified nephritic syndrome**
    Includes   glomerular disease NOS
                glomerulonephritis NOS
                nephritis NOS
                nephropathy NOS and renal disease NOS with morphological lesion specified in .0-.8

    Excludes1   nephropathy NOS with no stated morphological lesion (N28.9)
                renal disease NOS with no stated morphological lesion (N28.9)
                tubulo-interstitial nephritis NOS (N12)

N05.0 **Unspecified nephritic syndrome with minor glomerular abnormality**
    Unspecified nephritic syndrome with minimal change lesion

N05.1 **Unspecified nephritic syndrome with focal and segmental glomerular lesions**
    Unspecified nephritic syndrome with focal and segmental hyalinosis
    Unspecified nephritic syndrome with focal and segmental sclerosis
    Unspecified nephritic syndrome with focal glomerulonephritis

N05.2 **Unspecified nephritic syndrome with diffuse membranous glomerulonephritis** 🔖
    Ⓔⓧ See N03

N Newborn Age: 0   **P** Pediatric Age: 0–17   **M** Maternity DX: 12–55   **A** Adult Age: 15–124   ♀ Females Only   ♂ Males Only

🔖 Complication\Comorbidity   🔖 Major C\C   Ⓔⓧ CC/MCC Exclusions   🔖 Hospital-Acquired Condition   **1093**

N05.3   Unspecified nephritic syndrome with diffuse mesangial proliferative glomerulonephritis
     (Ex) See N03

N05.4   Unspecified nephritic syndrome with diffuse endocapillary proliferative glomerulonephritis
     (Ex) See N03

N05.5   Unspecified nephritic syndrome with diffuse mesangiocapillary glomerulonephritis
     Unspecified nephritic syndrome with membranoproliferative glomerulonephritis, types 1 and 3, or NOS
     (Ex) See N03

N05.6   Unspecified nephritic syndrome with dense deposit disease
     Unspecified nephritic syndrome with membranoproliferative glomerulonephritis, type 2

N05.7   Unspecified nephritic syndrome with diffuse crescentic glomerulonephritis
     Unspecified nephritic syndrome with extracapillary glomerulonephritis

N05.8   Unspecified nephritic syndrome with other morphologic changes
     Unspecified nephritic syndrome with proliferative glomerulonephritis NOS

N05.9   Unspecified nephritic syndrome with unspecified morphologic changes

● **N06**   **Isolated proteinuria with specified morphological lesion**
     Excludes1   proteinuria not associated with specific morphologic lesions (R80.0)

N06.0   Isolated proteinuria with minor glomerular abnormality
     Isolated proteinuria with minimal change lesion

N06.1   Isolated proteinuria with focal and segmental glomerular lesions
     Isolated proteinuria with focal and segmental hyalinosis
     Isolated proteinuria with focal and segmental sclerosis
     Isolated proteinuria with focal glomerulonephritis

N06.2   Isolated proteinuria with diffuse membranous glomerulonephritis
     (Ex) See N03

N06.3   Isolated proteinuria with diffuse mesangial proliferative glomerulonephritis
     (Ex) See N03

N06.4   Isolated proteinuria with diffuse endocapillary proliferative glomerulonephritis
     (Ex) See N03

N06.5   Isolated proteinuria with diffuse mesangiocapillary glomerulonephritis
     Isolated proteinuria with membranoproliferative glomerulonephritis, types 1 and 3, or NOS
     (Ex) See N03

N06.6   Isolated proteinuria with dense deposit disease
     Isolated proteinuria with membranoproliferative glomerulonephritis, type 2

N06.7   Isolated proteinuria with diffuse crescentic glomerulonephritis
     Isolated proteinuria with extracapillary glomerulonephritis

N06.8   Isolated proteinuria with other morphologic lesion
     Isolated proteinuria with proliferative glomerulonephritis NOS

N06.9   Isolated proteinuria with unspecified morphologic lesion

● **N07**   **Hereditary nephropathy, not elsewhere classified**
     Excludes2   Alport's syndrome (Q87.81-)
         hereditary amyloid nephropathy (E85.-)
         nail patella syndrome (Q87.2)
         non-neuropathic heredofamilial amyloidosis (E85.-)

N07.0   Hereditary nephropathy, not elsewhere classified with minor glomerular abnormality
     Hereditary nephropathy, not elsewhere classified with minimal change lesion

N07.1   Hereditary nephropathy, not elsewhere classified with focal and segmental glomerular lesions
     Hereditary nephropathy, not elsewhere classified with focal and segmental hyalinosis
     Hereditary nephropathy, not elsewhere classified with focal and segmental sclerosis
     Hereditary nephropathy, not elsewhere classified with focal glomerulonephritis

N07.2   Hereditary nephropathy, not elsewhere classified with diffuse membranous glomerulonephritis
     (Ex) See N03

N07.3   Hereditary nephropathy, not elsewhere classified with diffuse mesangial proliferative glomerulonephritis
     (Ex) See N03

N07.4   Hereditary nephropathy, not elsewhere classified with diffuse endocapillary proliferative glomerulonephritis
     (Ex) See N03

N07.5   Hereditary nephropathy, not elsewhere classified with diffuse mesangiocapillary glomerulonephritis
     Hereditary nephropathy, not elsewhere classified with membranoproliferative glomerulonephritis, types 1 and 3, or NOS
     (Ex) See N03

N07.6   Hereditary nephropathy, not elsewhere classified with dense deposit disease
     Hereditary nephropathy, not elsewhere classified with membranoproliferative glomerulonephritis, type 2

N07.7   Hereditary nephropathy, not elsewhere classified with diffuse crescentic glomerulonephritis
     Hereditary nephropathy, not elsewhere classified with extracapillary glomerulonephritis

N07.8   Hereditary nephropathy, not elsewhere classified with other morphologic lesions
     Hereditary nephropathy, not elsewhere classified with proliferative glomerulonephritis NOS

N07.9   Hereditary nephropathy, not elsewhere classified with unspecified morphologic lesions

▷ **N08**   *Glomerular disorders in diseases classified elsewhere*
     Glomerulonephritis
     Nephritis
     Nephropathy
     Code first underlying disease, such as:
         amyloidosis (E85.-)
         congenital syphilis (A50.5)
         cryoglobulinemia (D89.1)
         disseminated intravascular coagulation (D65)
         gout (M1A.-, M10.-)
         microscopic polyangiitis (M31.7)
         multiple myeloma (C90.0-)
         sepsis (A40.0-A41.9)
         sickle-cell disease (D57.0-D57.8)
     Excludes1   glomerulonephritis, nephritis and nephropathy (in):
         antiglomerular basement membrane disease (M31.0)
         diabetes (E08-E13 with .21)
         gonococcal (A54.21)
         Goodpasture's syndrome (M31.0)
         hemolytic-uremic syndrome (D59.3)
         lupus (M32.14)
         mumps (B26.83)
         syphilis (A52.75)
         systemic lupus erythematosus (M32.14)
         Wegener's granulomatosis (M31.31)
         pyelonephritis in diseases classified elsewhere (N16)
         renal tubulo-interstitial disorders classified elsewhere (N16)

◀ New   ⬅ Revised   ~~deleted~~ Deleted   Excludes 1   Excludes 2   Includes   Use additional   Code first   Code also   Unspecified

OGCR Official Guidelines   ● Unacceptable Principal Diagnosis   X Assign placeholder X   ● Use Additional Character(s)   ▷ Manifestation Code   **Coding Clinic**

Figure 14-3 Acute pyelonephritis. Cortical surface exhibits grayish white areas of inflammation and abscess formation. (From Kumar: Robbins and Cotran: Pathologic Basis of Disease, ed 8, Saunders, An Imprint of Elsevier, 2009)

Item 14–5 Pyelonephritis is an infection of the kidneys and ureters and may be chronic or acute in one or both kidneys.

RENAL TUBULO-INTERSTITIAL DISEASES (N10-N16)

| **Includes** | pyelonephritis |
| **Excludes1** | pyeloureteritis cystica (N28.85) |

N10 Acute pyelonephritis 🕹️🕹️◀▥
Acute infectious interstitial nephritis
Acute pyelitis
Acute tubulo-interstitial nephritis ◀▥
Hemoglobin nephrosis
Myoglobin nephrosis
Use additional code (B95-B97), to identify infectious agent
(Ex:) A17.9, A18.10-A18.11, A18.13, A18.82, A18.84, A18.89, A54.21, A54.29, A54.82, A54.84, A54.89-A54.9, A59.00, A59.8-A59.9, B37.41-B37.49, E08.21-E08.29, E08.618-E08.638, E08.649, E08.65-E08.8, E09.21-E09.29, E09.618-E09.638, E09.649-E09.8, E10.21-E10.29, E10.618-E10.638, E10.649, E10.69-E10.8, E11.21-E11.29, E11.618-E11.638, E11.649, E11.69-E11.8, E13.21-E13.29, E13.618-E13.638, E13.649-E13.69, E13.8, M10.30-M10.39, N00.0-N13.39, N13.6, N14.0-N19, N25.0-N27.9, N28.1-N29, N36.41-N36.43, N36.8-N36.9, N39.0, N39.8-N39.9, R31.0-R31.9, R82.71

● **N11 Chronic tubulo-interstitial nephritis**
Includes	chronic infectious interstitial nephritis
	chronic pyelitis
	chronic pyelonephritis
Use additional code (B95-B97), to identify infectious agent

N11.0 Nonobstructive reflux-associated chronic pyelonephritis
Pyelonephritis (chronic) associated with (vesicoureteral) reflux
| **Excludes1** | vesicoureteral reflux NOS (N13.70) |

N11.1 Chronic obstructive pyelonephritis 🕹️
Pyelonephritis (chronic) associated with anomaly of pelviureteric junction
Pyelonephritis (chronic) associated with anomaly of pyeloureteric junction
Pyelonephritis (chronic) associated with crossing of vessel
Pyelonephritis (chronic) associated with kinking of ureter
Pyelonephritis (chronic) associated with obstruction of ureter
Pyelonephritis (chronic) associated with stricture of pelviureteric junction
Pyelonephritis (chronic) associated with stricture of ureter
| **Excludes1** | calculous pyelonephritis (N20.9) |
| | obstructive uropathy (N13.-) |
CC when PDx is its own CC
(Ex:) N11.1, N13.4-N13.5, N13.8-N13.9, N28.82, N28.89-N30.91, N32.89-N33, N36.41-N36.43, N36.8-N36.9, N39.0, N39.8-N39.9, Q62.4-Q62.8, Q64.10-Q64.19, Q64.8-Q64.9, R31.0-R31.9, R82.71, Z90.6

N11.8 Other chronic tubulo-interstitial nephritis 🕹️
Nonobstructive chronic pyelonephritis NOS
(Ex:) A17.9, A18.10-A18.11, A18.13, A18.82, A18.84, A18.89, A54.21, A54.29, A54.82, A54.84, A54.89-A54.9, A59.00, A59.8-A59.9, A98.5, B37.41-B37.49, E08.21-E08.29, E08.618-E08.638, E08.649, E08.65-E08.8, E09.21-E09.29, E09.618-E09.638, E09.649-E09.8, E10.21-E10.29, E10.618-E10.638, E10.649, E10.69-E10.8, E11.21-E11.29, E11.618-E11.638, E11.649, E11.69-E11.8, E13.21-E13.29, E13.618-E13.638, E13.649-E13.69, E13.8, M10.30-M10.39, N00.0-N13.39, N13.6, N14.0-N19, N25.0-N27.9, N28.1-N29, N36.41-N36.43, N36.8-N36.9, N39.8-N39.9, O23.01-O23.03, O23.11-O23.13, O23.21-O23.23, O23.31-O23.33, O23.41-O23.43, O23.511-O23.513, O23.521-O23.523, O23.591-O23.593, O23.91-O23.93, O86.11, O86.13-O86.29, R31.0-R31.9

N11.9 Chronic tubulo-interstitial nephritis, unspecified 🕹️🕹️
Chronic interstitial nephritis NOS
Chronic pyelitis NOS
Chronic pyelonephritis NOS
(Ex:) A17.9, A18.10-A18.11, A18.13, A18.82, A18.84, A18.89, A54.21, A54.29, A54.82, A54.84, A54.89-A54.9, A59.00, A59.8-A59.9, B37.41-B37.49, E08.21-E08.29, E09.21-E09.29, M10.30-M10.39, N00.0-N13.39, N13.6, N14.0-N19, N25.0-N27.9, N28.1-N29, N36.41-N36.43, N36.8-N36.9, N39.0, N39.8-N39.9, R31.0-R31.9, R82.71

N12 Tubulo-interstitial nephritis, not specified as acute or chronic 🕹️🕹️
Interstitial nephritis NOS
Pyelitis NOS
Pyelonephritis NOS
| **Excludes1** | calculous pyelonephritis (N20.9) |
(Ex:) See N11.9

● **N13 Obstructive and reflux uropathy**
Excludes2	calculus of kidney and ureter without hydronephrosis (N20.-)
	congenital obstructive defects of renal pelvis and ureter (Q62.0-Q62.3)
	hydronephrosis with ureteropelvic junction obstruction (Q62.1)
	obstructive pyelonephritis (N11.1)
(Ex:) **For category N13 CC codes unless otherwise indicated:** See N11.9

N13.0 Hydronephrosis with ureteropelvic junction obstruction 🕹️◀
Hydronephrosis due to acquired occlusion of ureteropelvic junction ◀
| **Excludes2** | Hydronephrosis with ureteropelvic junction obstruction due to calculus (N13.2) ◀ |
CC when PDx is its own CC

N13.1 Hydronephrosis with ureteral stricture, not elsewhere classified 🕹️
| **Excludes1** | hydronephrosis with ureteral stricture with infection (N13.6) |
CC when PDx is its own CC

N13.2 Hydronephrosis with renal and ureteral calculous obstruction 🕹️
| **Excludes1** | hydronephrosis with renal and ureteral calculous obstruction with infection (N13.6) |
CC when PDx is its own CC

● **N13.3 Other and unspecified hydronephrosis**
| **Excludes1** | hydronephrosis with infection (N13.6) |
N13.30 Unspecified hydronephrosis 🕹️
N13.39 Other hydronephrosis 🕹️

N13.4 Hydroureter 🕹️
Excludes1	congenital hydroureter (Q62.3-)
	hydroureter with infection (N13.6)
	vesicoureteral-reflux with hydroureter (N13.73-)
(Ex:) N11.1, N13.4-N13.5, N13.8-N13.9, N28.82, N28.89-N30.91, N32.89-N33, N36.41-N36.43, N36.8-N36.9, N39.0, N39.8-N39.9, Q62.4-Q62.8, Q64.10-Q64.19, Q64.8-Q64.9, R31.0-R31.9, R82.71

Figure 14-4 Hydronephrosis of the kidney, with marked dilatation of pelvis and calyces and thinning of renal parenchyma. (From Kumar: Robbins and Cotran: Pathologic Basis of Disease, ed 8, Saunders, An Imprint of Elsevier, 2009)

CHAPTER 14 (N00-N99)

N13.5 **Crossing vessel and stricture of ureter without hydronephrosis**

    Kinking and stricture of ureter without hydronephrosis

    Excludes1   crossing vessel and stricture of ureter without hydronephrosis with infection (N13.6)

N13.6 **Pyonephrosis** 🔊 🔊

    Conditions in N13.0-N13.5 with infection ◀▥

    Obstructive uropathy with infection

    Use additional code (B95-B97), to identify infectious agent

● **N13.7** **Vesicoureteral-reflux**

    Excludes1   reflux-associated pyelonephritis (N11.0)

    N13.70 **Vesicoureteral-reflux, unspecified**

        Occurs when urine flows from bladder back into ureters

        Vesicoureteral-reflux NOS

    N13.71 **Vesicoureteral-reflux without reflux nephropathy**

  ● **N13.72** **Vesicoureteral-reflux with reflux nephropathy without hydroureter**

        N13.721 **Vesicoureteral-reflux with reflux nephropathy without hydroureter, unilateral**

        N13.722 **Vesicoureteral-reflux with reflux nephropathy without hydroureter, bilateral**

        N13.729 **Vesicoureteral-reflux with reflux nephropathy without hydroureter, unspecified**

  ● **N13.73** **Vesicoureteral-reflux with reflux nephropathy with hydroureter**

        N13.731 **Vesicoureteral-reflux with reflux nephropathy with hydroureter, unilateral**

        N13.732 **Vesicoureteral-reflux with reflux nephropathy with hydroureter, bilateral**

        N13.739 **Vesicoureteral-reflux with reflux nephropathy with hydroureter, unspecified**

N13.8 **Other obstructive and reflux uropathy** 🔊

    Urinary tract obstruction due to specified cause

    Code first, if applicable, any causal condition first, such as:

        enlarged prostate (N40.1)

        (Ex) See N11.1

N13.9 **Obstructive and reflux uropathy, unspecified**

    Urinary tract obstruction NOS

● **N14** **Drug- and heavy-metal-induced tubulo-interstitial and tubular conditions**

    Code first poisoning due to drug or toxin, if applicable (T36-T65 with fifth or sixth character 1-4 or 6)

    Use additional code for adverse effect, if applicable, to identify drug (T36-T50 with fifth or sixth character 5)

  N14.0 **Analgesic nephropathy**

  N14.1 **Nephropathy induced by other drugs, medicaments and biological substances**

  N14.2 **Nephropathy induced by unspecified drug, medicament or biological substance**

  N14.3 **Nephropathy induced by heavy metals**

  N14.4 **Toxic nephropathy, not elsewhere classified**

● **N15** **Other renal tubulo-interstitial diseases**

  N15.0 **Balkan nephropathy**

    Balkan endemic nephropathy

  N15.1 **Renal and perinephric abscess** 🔊 🔊

    (Ex) See N10

  N15.8 **Other specified renal tubulo-interstitial diseases**

  N15.9 **Renal tubulo-interstitial disease, unspecified**

    Infection of kidney NOS

    Excludes1   urinary tract infection NOS (N39.0)

▌ ● **N16** *Renal tubulo-interstitial disorders in diseases classified elsewhere*

    Pyelonephritis

    Tubulo-interstitial nephritis

    Code first underlying disease, such as:

        brucellosis (A23.0-A23.9)

        cryoglobulinemia (D89.1)

        glycogen storage disease (E74.0)

        leukemia (C91-C95)

        lymphoma (C81.0-C85.9, C96.0-C96.9)

        multiple myeloma (C90.0-)

        sepsis (A40.0-A41.9)

        Wilson's disease (E83.0)

    Excludes1   diphtheritic pyelonephritis and tubulo-interstitial nephritis (A36.84)

        pyelonephritis and tubulo-interstitial nephritis in candidiasis (B37.49)

        pyelonephritis and tubulo-interstitial nephritis in cystinosis (E72.04)

        pyelonephritis and tubulo-interstitial nephritis in salmonella infection (A02.25)

        pyelonephritis and tubulo-interstitial nephritis in sarcoidosis (D86.84)

        pyelonephritis and tubulo-interstitial nephritis in sicca syndrome [Sjogren's] (M35.04)

        pyelonephritis and tubulo-interstitial nephritis in systemic lupus erythematosus (M32.15)

        pyelonephritis and tubulo-interstitial nephritis in toxoplasmosis (B58.83)

        renal tubular degeneration in diabetes (E08-E13 with .29)

        syphilitic pyelonephritis and tubulo-interstitial nephritis (A52.75)

ACUTE KIDNEY FAILURE AND CHRONIC KIDNEY DISEASE (N17-N19)

    Excludes2   congenital renal failure (P96.0)

        drug- and heavy-metal-induced tubulo-interstitial and tubular conditions (N14.-)

        extrarenal uremia (R39.2)

        hemolytic-uremic syndrome (D59.3)

        hepatorenal syndrome (K76.7)

        postpartum hepatorenal syndrome (O90.4)

        posttraumatic renal failure (T79.5)

        prerenal uremia (R39.2)

        renal failure complicating abortion or ectopic or molar pregnancy (O00-O07, O08.4)

        renal failure following labor and delivery (O90.4)

        renal failure postprocedural (N99.0)

● **N17** **Acute kidney failure**

    Code also associated underlying condition

    Excludes1   posttraumatic renal failure (T79.5)

    (Ex) **For category N17 CC codes unless otherwise indicated:** E08.21-E08.29, E08.618-E08.638, E08.649-E08.8, E09.21-E09.29, E09.618-E09.638, E09.649-E09.8, E10.21-E10.29, E10.618-E10.638, E10.649, E10.69-E10.8, E11.21-E11.29, E11.618-E11.638, E11.649, E11.69-E11.8, E13.21-E13.29, E13.618-E13.638, E13.649-E13.8, E88.3, M10.30-M10.39, N00.0-N13.39, N13.6, N14.0-N19, N25.0-N27.9, N28.1-N29, N36.41-N36.43, N36.8-N36.9, N39.8-N39.9, Q60.0-Q62.39, Q63.0-Q63.9, Q64.8-Q64.9, R31.0-R31.9

  N17.0 **Acute kidney failure with tubular necrosis** 🔊

    Acute tubular necrosis

    Renal tubular necrosis

    Tubular necrosis NOS

  N17.1 **Acute kidney failure with acute cortical necrosis** 🔊

    Acute cortical necrosis

    Cortical necrosis NOS

    Renal cortical necrosis

  N17.2 **Acute kidney failure with medullary necrosis** 🔊

    Medullary [papillary] necrosis NOS

    Acute medullary [papillary] necrosis

    Renal medullary [papillary] necrosis

◀ New   ◀▥ Revised   ~~deleted~~ Deleted   Excludes 1   Excludes 2   Includes   Use additional   Code first   Code also   Unspecified

OGCR Official Guidelines   ● Unacceptable Principal Diagnosis   X Assign placeholder X   ● Use Additional Character(s)   ▌ Manifestation Code   **Coding Clinic**

Item 14–6 Decreased blood flow is the usual cause of **acute renal failure** that offers a good prognosis for recovery.

    Chronic renal failure is usually the result of long-standing kidney disease and is a very serious condition that generally results in death.

    N17.8   Other acute kidney failure 🔖
      (Ex:) E08.21-E08.29, E08.618-E08.638, E08.649-E08.8, E09.21-E09.29,
      E09.618-E09.638, E09.649-E09.8, E10.21-E10.29, E10.618-E10.638,
      E10.649, E10.69-E10.8, E11.21-E11.29, E11.618-E11.638, E11.649,
      E11.69-E11.8, E13.21-E13.29, E13.618-E13.638, E13.649-E13.8, E88.3,
      M10.30-M10.39, N00.0-N13.39, N13.6, N14.0-N19, N25.0-N27.9,
      N28.1-N29, N36.41-N36.43, N36.8-N36.9, N39.8-N39.9, R31.0-R31.9

    N17.9   Acute kidney failure, `unspecified` 🔖
      Acute kidney injury (nontraumatic)
      Excludes2   traumatic kidney injury (S37.0-)

🔴**N18   Chronic kidney disease (CKD)**
    Code first any associated:
      diabetic chronic kidney disease (E08.22, E09.22, E10.22,
        E11.22, E13.22)
      hypertensive chronic kidney disease (I12.-, I13.-)
    Use additional code to identify kidney transplant status, if
      applicable, (Z94.0)
    N18.1   Chronic kidney disease, stage 1
    N18.2   Chronic kidney disease, stage 2 (mild)
    N18.3   Chronic kidney disease, stage 3 (moderate)
    N18.4   Chronic kidney disease, stage 4 (severe) 🔖
      (Ex:) E08.21-E08.29, E08.618-E08.638, E08.649-E08.8, E09.21-E09.29,
      E09.618-E09.638, E09.649-E09.8, E10.21-E10.29, E10.618-E10.638,
      E10.649, E10.69-E10.8, E11.21-E11.29, E11.618-E11.638, E11.649,
      E11.69-E11.8, E13.21-E13.29, E13.618-E13.638, E13.649-E13.8,
      M10.30-M10.39, N00.0-N13.39, N13.6, N14.0-N19, N25.0-N27.9,
      N28.1-N29, N36.41-N36.43, N36.8-N36.9, N39.8-N39.9, Q60.0-Q62.39,
      Q63.0-Q63.9, Q64.8-Q64.9, R31.0-R31.9
      Coding Clinic: 2013, Q1, P24
    N18.5   Chronic kidney disease, stage 5 🔖
      Excludes1   chronic kidney disease, stage 5 requiring
                 chronic dialysis (N18.6)
      (Ex:) See N18.4
    N18.6   End stage renal disease 🔖
      Chronic kidney disease requiring chronic dialysis
      Use additional code to identify dialysis status (Z99.2)
      (Ex:) E08.21-E08.29, E08.618-E08.638, E08.649-E08.8, E09.21-E09.29,
      E09.618-E09.638, E09.649-E09.8, E10.21-E10.29, E10.618-E10.638,
      E10.649, E10.69-E10.8, E11.21-E11.29, E11.618-E11.638, E11.649,
      E11.69-E11.8, E13.21-E13.29, E13.618-E13.638, E13.649-E13.69, I12.9,
      M10.30-M10.39, N00.0-N13.39, N13.6, N14.0-N19, N25.0-N27.9,
      N28.1-N29, N36.41-N36.43, N36.8-N36.9, N39.8-N39.9, Q60.0-Q62.39,
      Q63.0-Q63.9, Q64.8-Q64.9, R31.0-R31.9
      Coding Clinic: 2016, Q1, P13
    N18.9   Chronic kidney disease, `unspecified`
      Chronic renal disease
      Chronic renal failure NOS
      Chronic renal insufficiency
      Chronic uremia

N19   `Unspecified` kidney failure
    Uremia NOS
    Excludes1   acute kidney failure (N17.-)
                 chronic kidney disease (N18.-)
                 chronic uremia (N18.9)
                 extrarenal uremia (R39.2)
                 prerenal uremia (R39.2)
                 renal insufficiency (acute) (N28.9)
                 uremia of newborn (P96.0)

Figure 14-5   Multiple urinary calculi.

Multiple calculi

UROLITHIASIS (N20-N23)

🔴**N20   Calculus of kidney and ureter**
    Calculous pyelonephritis
    Excludes1   nephrocalcinosis (E83.5)
                 that with hydronephrosis (N13.2)
    N20.0   Calculus of kidney
      Nephrolithiasis NOS   Staghorn calculus
      Renal calculus   Stone in kidney
      Renal stone
    N20.1   Calculus of ureter 🔖
      Ureteric stone
      (Ex:) N11.1, N13.4-N13.5, N13.8-N13.9, N20.0-N22, N28.82, N28.89-N29,
      N36.41-N36.43, N36.8-N36.9, N39.8-N39.9, R31.0-R31.9
    N20.2   Calculus of kidney with calculus of ureter 🔖
      (Ex:) See N20.1
    N20.9   Urinary calculus, `unspecified`

🔴**N21   Calculus of lower urinary tract**
    Includes   calculus of lower urinary tract with cystitis and
                    urethritis
    N21.0   Calculus in bladder
      Calculus in diverticulum of bladder
      Urinary bladder stone
      Excludes2   staghorn calculus (N20.0)
      Coding Clinic: 2015, Q2, P9
    N21.1   Calculus in urethra
      Excludes2   calculus of prostate (N42.0)
    N21.8   Other lower urinary tract calculus
    N21.9   Calculus of lower urinary tract, `unspecified`
      Excludes1   calculus of urinary tract NOS (N20.9)

▷*N22   Calculus of urinary tract in diseases classified elsewhere*
    Code first underlying disease, such as:
      gout (M1A.-, M10.-)
      schistosomiasis (B65.0-B65.9)

N23   `Unspecified` renal colic

OTHER DISORDERS OF KIDNEY AND URETER (N25-N29)

    Excludes2   disorders of kidney and ureter with urolithiasis
                 (N20-N23)

🔴**N25   Disorders resulting from impaired renal tubular function**
    Excludes1   metabolic disorders classifiable to E70-E88
    N25.0   Renal osteodystrophy
      Azotemic osteodystrophy
      Phosphate-losing tubular disorders
      Renal rickets
      Renal short stature
    N25.1   Nephrogenic diabetes insipidus 🔖
      Excludes1   diabetes insipidus NOS (E23.2)
      (Ex:) A17.9, A18.10-A18.11, A18.13, A18.82, A18.84, A18.89, A54.21, A54.29,
      A54.82, A54.84, A54.89-A54.9, A59.00, A59.8-A59.9, A98.5,
      B37.41-B37.49, E08.21-E08.29, E08.618-E08.638, E08.649, E08.65-E08.8,
      E09.21-E09.29, E09.618-E09.638, E09.649-E09.8, E10.21-E10.29,
      E10.618-E10.638, E10.649, E10.69-E10.8, E11.21-E11.29, E11.618-E11.638,
      E11.649, E11.69-E11.8, E13.21-E13.29, E13.618-E13.638, E13.649-E13.69,
      E13.8, M10.30-M10.39, N00.0-N13.39, N13.6, N14.0-N19, N25.0-N27.9,
      N28.1-N29, N36.41-N36.43, N36.8-N36.9, N39.8-N39.9, R31.0-R31.9

N   Newborn Age: 0   **P**   Pediatric Age: 0–17   **M**   Maternity DX: 12–55   **A**   Adult Age: 15–124   ♀   Females Only   ♂   Males Only

🔖   Complication\Comorbidity   🔖   Major C\C   (Ex:)   CC/MCC Exclusions   🔖   Hospital-Acquired Condition

● **N25.8**   **Other disorders resulting from impaired renal tubular function**

     N25.81   **Secondary hyperparathyroidism of renal origin** 🔗

         Excludes1   secondary hyperparathyroidism, non-renal (E21.1)

         (Ex:) A17.9, A18.10-A18.11, A18.13, A18.82, A18.84, A18.89, A54.21, A54.29, A54.82, A54.84, A54.89-A54.9, A59.00, A59.8-A59.9, A98.5, B37.41-B37.49, E08.21-E08.29, E08.618-E08.638, E08.649, E08.65-E08.8, E09.21-E09.29, E09.618-E09.638, E09.649-E09.8, E10.21-E10.29, E10.618-E10.638, E10.649, E10.69-E10.8, E11.21-E11.29, E11.618-E11.638, E11.649, E11.69-E11.8, E13.21-E13.29, E13.618-E13.638, E13.649-E13.69, E13.8, M10.30-M10.39, N00.0-N13.39, N13.6, N14.0-N19, N25.0-N27.9, N28.1-N29, N36.41-N36.43, N36.8-N36.9, N39.8-N39.9, R31.0-R31.9

     N25.89   **Other disorders resulting from impaired renal tubular function**
         Hypokalemic nephropathy
         Lightwood-Albright syndrome
         Renal tubular acidosis NOS

     N25.9   **Disorder resulting from impaired renal tubular function, unspecified**

● **N26**   **Unspecified contracted kidney**

     Excludes1   contracted kidney due to hypertension (I12.-)
         diffuse sclerosing glomerulonephritis (N05.8.-)
         hypertensive nephrosclerosis (arteriolar) (arteriosclerotic) (I12.-)
         small kidney of unknown cause (N27.-)

     N26.1   **Atrophy of kidney (terminal)**

     N26.2   **Page kidney**

     N26.9   **Renal sclerosis, unspecified**

● **N27**   **Small kidney of unknown cause**

     Includes   oligonephronia

     N27.0   **Small kidney, unilateral**

     N27.1   **Small kidney, bilateral**

     N27.9   **Small kidney, unspecified**

● **N28**   **Other disorders of kidney and ureter, not elsewhere classified**

     N28.0   **Ischemia and infarction of kidney** 🔗
         Renal artery embolism
         Renal artery obstruction
         Renal artery occlusion
         Renal artery thrombosis
         Renal infarct

         Excludes1   atherosclerosis of renal artery (extrarenal part) (I70.1)
           congenital stenosis of renal artery (Q27.1)
           Goldblatt's kidney (I70.1)
         (Ex:) N13.70-N13.739, N28.0, N28.9-N29

     N28.1   **Cyst of kidney, acquired**
         Cyst (multiple)(solitary) of kidney, acquired

         Excludes1   cystic kidney disease (congenital) (Q61.-)

     N28.8   **Other specified disorders of kidney and ureter**

         Excludes1   hydroureter (N13.4)
           ureteric stricture with hydronephrosis (N13.1)
           ureteric stricture without hydronephrosis (N13.5)

     N28.81   **Hypertrophy of kidney**

     N28.82   **Megaloureter**

     N28.83   **Nephroptosis**

     N28.84   **Pyelitis cystica** 🔗 🔗
         (Ex:) See N11.9

     N28.85   **Pyeloureteritis cystica** 🔗 🔗
         (Ex:) See N11.9

     N28.86   **Ureteritis cystica** 🔗 🔗
         (Ex:) See N11.9

     N28.89   **Other specified disorders of kidney and ureter**

● **N28.9**   **Disorder of kidney and ureter, unspecified**
     Nephropathy NOS
     Renal disease (acute) NOS
     Renal insufficiency (acute)

     Excludes1   chronic renal insufficiency (N18.9)
         unspecified nephritic syndrome (N05.-)

     Coding Clinic: 2016, Q1, P13

▶ **N29**   *Other disorders of kidney and ureter in diseases classified elsewhere*
     Code first underlying disease, such as:
         amyloidosis (E85.-)
         nephrocalcinosis (E83.5)
         schistosomiasis (B65.0-B65.9)

     Excludes1   disorders of kidney and ureter in:
         cystinosis (E72.0)
         gonorrhea (A54.21)
         syphilis (A52.75)
         tuberculosis (A18.11)

OTHER DISEASES OF THE URINARY SYSTEM (N30-N39)

     Excludes1   urinary infection (complicating):
         abortion or ectopic or molar pregnancy (O00-O07, O08.8)
         pregnancy, childbirth and the puerperium (O23.-, O75.3, O86.2-)

● **N30**   **Cystitis**
     Infection of bladder and irritation in lower urinary tract
     Use additional code to identify infectious agent (B95-B97)

     Excludes1   prostatocystitis (N41.3)

     ● **N30.0**   **Acute cystitis**

         Excludes1   irradiation cystitis (N30.4-)
           trigonitis (N30.3-)

         (Ex:) For category N30.0 CC codes: A17.9, A18.10, A18.12-A18.13, A18.82, A18.84, A18.89, A54.00-A54.02, A54.09-A54.1, A54.82, A54.84, A54.89-A54.9, A59.00, A59.8-A59.9, B37.41-B37.49, N11.1, N13.4-N13.5, N13.8-N13.9, N28.82, N28.89-N30.91, N32.89-N33, N36.41-N36.43, N36.8-N36.9, N39.0, N39.8-N39.9, R31.0-R31.9

         N30.00   **Acute cystitis without hematuria** 🔗 🔗

         N30.01   **Acute cystitis with hematuria** 🔗 🔗

     ● **N30.1**   **Interstitial cystitis (chronic)**
         Ongoing infection of kidney glomeruli and tubules

         N30.10   **Interstitial cystitis (chronic) without hematuria**

         N30.11   **Interstitial cystitis (chronic) with hematuria**

     ● **N30.2**   **Other chronic cystitis**

         N30.20   **Other chronic cystitis without hematuria**

         N30.21   **Other chronic cystitis with hematuria**

     ● **N30.3**   **Trigonitis**
         Inflammation of triangular area of bladder (where the ureters and urethra come together)
         Urethrotrigonitis

         N30.30   **Trigonitis without hematuria**

         N30.31   **Trigonitis with hematuria**

     ● **N30.4**   **Irradiation cystitis**
         (Ex:) For category N30.4 CC codes: See N30.0

         N30.40   **Irradiation cystitis without hematuria** 🔗

         N30.41   **Irradiation cystitis with hematuria** 🔗

     ● **N30.8**   **Other cystitis**
         Abscess of bladder

         N30.80   **Other cystitis without hematuria**

         N30.81   **Other cystitis with hematuria**

     ● **N30.9**   **Cystitis, unspecified**

         N30.90   **Cystitis, unspecified without hematuria**

         N30.91   **Cystitis, unspecified with hematuria**

◀ New   ◀━ Revised   ~~deleted~~ Deleted   Excludes 1   Excludes 2   Includes   Use additional   Code first   Code also   Unspecified

OGCR Official Guidelines   ● Unacceptable Principal Diagnosis   X Assign placeholder X   🔗 Use Additional Character(s)   ▶ Manifestation Code   **Coding Clinic**

N31 **Neuromuscular dysfunction of bladder, not elsewhere classified**

Use additional code to identify any associated urinary incontinence (N39.3-N39.4-)

> **Excludes1** cord bladder NOS (G95.89)
> neurogenic bladder due to cauda equina syndrome (G83.4)
> neuromuscular dysfunction due to spinal cord lesion (G95.89)

N31.0 **Uninhibited neuropathic bladder, not elsewhere classified**

N31.1 **Reflex neuropathic bladder, not elsewhere classified**

N31.2 **Flaccid neuropathic bladder, not elsewhere classified**
Atonic (motor) (sensory) neuropathic bladder
Diminished tone of bladder muscle
Autonomous neuropathic bladder
Nonreflex neuropathic bladder

N31.8 **Other neuromuscular dysfunction of bladder**

N31.9 **Neuromuscular dysfunction of bladder, unspecified**
Neurogenic bladder dysfunction NOS

N32 **Other disorders of bladder**

> **Excludes2** calculus of bladder (N21.0)
> cystocele (N81.1-)
> hernia or prolapse of bladder, female (N81.1-)

N32.0 **Bladder-neck obstruction**
Bladder-neck stenosis (acquired)

> **Excludes1** congenital bladder-neck obstruction (Q64.3-)

N32.1 **Vesicointestinal fistula** 🅒
Vesicorectal fistula
(Ex) A54.00-A54.02, A54.09-A54.1, A54.82, A54.84, A54.89-A54.9, N32.1-N32.2, N32.89-N33, N36.41-N36.43, N36.8-N36.9, N39.8-N39.9, R30.0, R30.9, R31.0-R31.9

N32.2 **Vesical fistula, not elsewhere classified** 🅒

> **Excludes1** fistula between bladder and female genital tract (N82.0-N82.1)

(Ex) See N32.1

N32.3 **Diverticulum of bladder**
Formation of sac from a herniation of wall of bladder

> **Excludes1** congenital diverticulum of bladder (Q64.6)
> diverticulitis of bladder (N30.8-)

N32.8 **Other specified disorders of bladder**

N32.81 **Overactive bladder**
Detrusor muscle hyperactivity

> **Excludes1** frequent urination due to specified bladder condition-code to condition

N32.89 **Other specified disorders of bladder**
Bladder hemorrhage
Bladder hypertrophy
Calcified bladder
Contracted bladder

N32.9 **Bladder disorder, unspecified**

▷ *N33* *Bladder disorders in diseases classified elsewhere*
Code first underlying disease, such as:
schistosomiasis (B65.0-B65.9)

> **Excludes1** bladder disorder in syphilis (A52.76)
> bladder disorder in tuberculosis (A18.12)
> candidal cystitis (B37.41)
> chlamydial cystitis(A56.01)
> cystitis in gonorrhea (A54.01)
> cystitis in neurogenic bladder (N31.-)
> diphtheritic cystitis (A36.85)
> syphilitic cystitis (A52.76)
> trichomonal cystitis (A59.03)

N34 **Urethritis and urethral syndrome**

Use additional code (B95-B97), to identify infectious agent

> **Excludes2** Reiter's disease (M02.3-)
> urethritis in diseases with a predominantly sexual mode of transmission (A50-A64)
> urethrotrigonitis (N30.3-)

N34.0 **Urethral abscess** 🅒 🅒
Abscess (of) Cowper's gland
Abscess (of) Littré's gland
Abscess (of) urethral (gland)
Periurethral abscess

> **Excludes1** urethral caruncle (N36.2)

(Ex) A54.00-A54.02, A54.09-A54.1, A54.82, A54.84, A54.89-A54.9, A59.00, A59.03, A59.8-A59.9, B37.41-B37.49, N13.9, N34.0-N34.3, N35.111-N35.9, N36.41-N36.43, N36.8-N39.0, N39.8-N39.9, N44.1-N44.8, N47.6, N48.1-N48.9, N49.1-N49.9, N50.3-N50.89, N51, N53.11-N53.9, Q54.0-Q55.9, Q64.0, Q64.2-Q64.9, R30.0, R30.9-R31.9, R82.71

N34.1 **Nonspecific urethritis**
Nongonococcal urethritis
Nonvenereal urethritis

N34.2 **Other urethritis**
Inflammation of urethra
Meatitis, urethral
Postmenopausal urethritis
Ulcer of urethra (meatus)
Urethritis NOS

N34.3 **Urethral syndrome, unspecified**

N35 **Urethral stricture**
Narrowing of lumen of urethra caused by scarring due to infection or injury

> **Excludes1** congenital urethral stricture (Q64.3-)
> postprocedural urethral stricture (N99.1-)

N35.0 **Post-traumatic urethral stricture**
Urethral stricture due to injury

> **Excludes1** postprocedural urethral stricture (N99.1-)

N35.01 **Post-traumatic urethral stricture, male**

N35.010 **Post-traumatic urethral stricture, male, meatal** ♂

N35.011 **Post-traumatic bulbous urethral stricture**

N35.012 **Post-traumatic membranous urethral stricture**

N35.013 **Post-traumatic anterior urethral stricture**

N35.014 **Post-traumatic urethral stricture, male, unspecified** ♂

N35.02 **Post-traumatic urethral stricture, female**

N35.021 **Urethral stricture due to childbirth** ♀

N35.028 **Other post-traumatic urethral stricture, female** ♀

N35.1 **Postinfective urethral stricture, not elsewhere classified**

> **Excludes1** urethral stricture associated with schistosomiasis (B65.-, N29)
> gonococcal urethral stricture (A54.01)
> syphilitic urethral stricture (A52.76)

N35.11 **Postinfective urethral stricture, not elsewhere classified, male**

N35.111 **Postinfective urethral stricture, not elsewhere classified, male, meatal** ♂

N35.112 **Postinfective bulbous urethral stricture, not elsewhere classified**

N35.113 **Postinfective membranous urethral stricture, not elsewhere classified**

N35.114 **Postinfective anterior urethral stricture, not elsewhere classified**

N35.119 **Postinfective urethral stricture, not elsewhere classified, male, unspecified** ♂

N35.12 **Postinfective urethral stricture, not elsewhere classified, female** ♀

CHAPTER 14 (N00-N99)

N Newborn Age: 0   **P** Pediatric Age: 0–17   **M** Maternity DX: 12–55   **A** Adult Age: 15–124   ♀ Females Only   ♂ Males Only

🅒 Complication\Comorbidity   🅒 Major C\C   (Ex) CC/MCC Exclusions   🅒 Hospital-Acquired Condition

1099

N35.8 **Other urethral stricture**
> **Excludes1** postprocedural urethral stricture (N99.1-)

N35.9 **Urethral stricture, unspecified**

●**N36** **Other disorders of urethra**

N36.0 **Urethral fistula** 🔗
> Urethroperineal fistula
> Urethrorectal fistula
> Urinary fistula NOS
> **Excludes1** urethroscrotal fistula (N50.89) ◀▥
> urethrovaginal fistula (N82.1)
> urethrovesicovaginal fistula (N82.1)
> (Ex) N13.9, N34.0, N34.2-N36.43, N36.5-N37, N39.8-N39.9, N44.1-N44.8, N47.6,
> N48.1-N48.9, N49.1-N49.9, N50.3-N50.89, N51, N53.11-N53.9,
> N99.110-N99.115, Q54.0-Q55.21, Q55.23-Q55.9, Q64.0, Q64.8-Q64.9,
> R30.0, R30.9-R31.9

N36.1 **Urethral diverticulum**

N36.2 **Urethral caruncle**

●**N36.4** **Urethral functional and muscular disorders**
> Use additional code to identify associated urinary stress
> incontinence (N39.3)

N36.41 **Hypermobility of urethra**

N36.42 **Intrinsic sphincter deficiency (ISD)**

N36.43 **Combined hypermobility of urethra and
intrinsic sphincter deficiency**

N36.44 **Muscular disorders of urethra**
> Bladder sphincter dyssynergy

N36.5 **Urethral false passage**

N36.8 **Other specified disorders of urethra**
> **Excludes1** congenital urethrocele (Q64.7) ◀
> female urethrocele (N81.0) ◀

N36.9 **Urethral disorder, unspecified**

▷**N37** *Urethral disorders in diseases classified elsewhere*
> *Code first underlying disease*
> **Excludes1** urethritis (in):
> candidal infection (B37.41)
> chlamydial (A56.01)
> gonorrhea (A54.01)
> syphilis (A52.76)
> trichomonal infection (A59.03)
> tuberculosis (A18.13)

●**N39** **Other disorders of urinary system**
> **Excludes2** hematuria NOS (R31.-)
> recurrent or persistent hematuria (N02.-)
> recurrent or persistent hematuria with specified
> morphological lesion (N02.-)
> proteinuria NOS (R80.-)

N39.0 **Urinary tract infection, site not specified** 🔗🔗
> Use additional code (B95-B97), to identify infectious
> agent
> **Excludes1** candidiasis of urinary tract (B37.4-)
> neonatal urinary tract infection (P39.3)
> urinary tract infection of specified site,
> such as:
> cystitis (N30.-)
> urethritis (N34.-)
> (Ex) A54.82, A54.84, A54.89-A54.9, A59.00, A59.8-A59.9, B37.41-B37.49, N10,
> N11.9-N13.39, N13.6, N13.9, N15.1, N28.82, N28.84-N30.91, N34.1,
> N36.41-N36.43, N36.8-N36.9, N39.0, N39.8-N39.9, N99.511, R30.0,
> R30.9-R31.9, T83.511A
> **Coding Clinic: 2012, Q4, P94**

N39.3 **Stress incontinence (female) (male)**
> Code also any associated overactive bladder (N32.81)
> **Excludes1** mixed incontinence (N39.46)

●**N39.4** **Other specified urinary incontinence**
> Code also any associated overactive bladder (N32.81)
> **Excludes1** enuresis NOS (R32)
> functional urinary incontinence (R39.81)
> urinary incontinence associated with
> cognitive impairment (R39.81)
> urinary incontinence NOS (R32)
> urinary incontinence of nonorganic origin
> (F98.0)

N39.41 **Urge incontinence**
> **Excludes1** mixed incontinence (N39.46)

N39.42 **Incontinence without sensory awareness**
> Insensible (urinary) incontinence ◀

N39.43 **Post-void dribbling**

N39.44 **Nocturnal enuresis**

N39.45 **Continuous leakage**

N39.46 **Mixed incontinence**
> Urge and stress incontinence

●**N39.49** **Other specified urinary incontinence**

N39.490 **Overflow incontinence**

N39.491 **Coital incontinence** ◀

N39.492 **Postural (urinary) incontinence** ◀

N39.498 **Other specified urinary incontinence**
> Reflex incontinence
> Total incontinence

N39.8 **Other specified disorders of urinary system**

N39.9 **Disorder of urinary system, unspecified**

DISEASES OF MALE GENITAL ORGANS (N40-N53)

★**(See Plate 387 on page 53.)**

●**N40** **Benign prostatic hyperplasia** ◀▥
> **Includes** adenofibromatous hypertrophy of prostate
> benign hypertrophy of the prostate
> *Enlargement of prostate gland usually occurring
> with age and causing obstructed urine flow*
> benign prostatic hypertrophy
> BPH
> enlarged prostate ◀
> nodular prostate
> polyp of prostate
> **Excludes1** benign neoplasms of prostate (adenoma, benign)
> (fibroadenoma) (fibroma) (myoma) (D29.1)
> malignant neoplasm of prostate (C61)

N40.0 **Benign prostatic hyperplasia without lower urinary tract
symptoms** ♂◀▥   A
> Enlarged prostate without LUTS
> Enlarged prostate NOS

Figure 14-6 Benign prostatic hyperplasia. (From Shiland: Mastering
Healthcare Terminology, ed 3, St. Louis, Mosby, 2010)

◀ New ◀▥ Revised ~~deleted~~ Deleted Excludes 1 Excludes 2 Includes Use additional Code first Code also Unspecified
OGCR Official Guidelines ● Unacceptable Principal Diagnosis X Assign placeholder X ● Use Additional Character(s) ▷ Manifestation Code **Coding Clinic**

N40.1 **Benign prostatic hyperplasia with lower urinary tract symptoms** ♂ ◀▥▥▥   A
　　　　Enlarged prostate with LUTS
　　　　Use additional code for associated symptoms, when specified:
　　　　　　incomplete bladder emptying (R39.14)
　　　　　　nocturia (R35.1)
　　　　　　straining on urination (R39.16)
　　　　　　urinary frequency (R35.0)
　　　　　　urinary hesitancy (R39.11)
　　　　　　urinary incontinence (N39.4-)
　　　　　　urinary obstruction (N13.8)
　　　　　　urinary retention (R33.8)
　　　　　　urinary urgency (R39.15)
　　　　　　weak urinary stream (R39.12)

N40.2 **Nodular prostate without lower urinary tract symptoms** ♂   A
　　　　Nodular prostate without LUTS

N40.3 **Nodular prostate with lower urinary tract symptoms** ♂   A
　　　　Use additional code for associated symptoms, when specified:
　　　　　　incomplete bladder emptying (R39.14)
　　　　　　nocturia (R35.1)
　　　　　　straining on urination (R39.16)
　　　　　　urinary frequency (R35.0)
　　　　　　urinary hesitancy (R39.11)
　　　　　　urinary incontinence (N39.4-)
　　　　　　urinary obstruction (N13.8)
　　　　　　urinary retention (R33.8)
　　　　　　urinary urgency (R39.15)
　　　　　　weak urinary stream (R39.12)

● **N41** **Inflammatory diseases of prostate**
　　　Use additional code (B95-B97), to identify infectious agent

N41.0 **Acute prostatitis** ♂ 🦠   A
　　　　(Ex:) A18.14, A54.22, A54.82, A54.84, A54.89-A54.9, A59.00, A59.02,
　　　　　　A59.8-A59.9, B37.41-B37.49, N40.0-N42.9

N41.1 **Chronic prostatitis** ♂   A

N41.2 **Abscess of prostate** ♂ 🦠   A
　　　　(Ex:) See N41.0

N41.3 **Prostatocystitis** ♂   A

N41.4 **Granulomatous prostatitis** ♂   A

N41.8 **Other inflammatory diseases of prostate** ♂   A

N41.9 **Inflammatory disease of prostate, unspecified** ♂   A
　　　　Prostatitis NOS

● **N42** **Other and unspecified disorders of prostate**

N42.0 **Calculus of prostate** ♂   A
　　　　Prostatic stone

N42.1 **Congestion and hemorrhage of prostate** ♂   A
　　　　Excludes1   enlarged prostate (N40.-)
　　　　　　　　hematuria (R31.-)
　　　　　　　　hyperplasia of prostate (N40.-)
　　　　　　　　inflammatory diseases of prostate (N41.-)

● **N42.3** **Dysplasia of prostate**

N42.30 **Unspecified dysplasia of prostate** ♂ ◀

N42.31 **Prostatic intraepithelial neoplasia** ♂ ◀
　　　　PIN ◀
　　　　Prostatic intraepithelial neoplasia I (PIN I) ◀
　　　　Prostatic intraepithelial neoplasia II (PIN II) ◀
　　　　Excludes1   prostatic intraepithelial neoplasia III (PIN III) (D07.5) ◀

N42.32 **Atypical small acinar proliferation of prostate** ♂ ◀

N42.39 **Other dysplasia of prostate** ♂ ◀

● **N42.8** **Other specified disorders of prostate**

N42.81 **Prostatodynia syndrome** ♂   A
　　　　Painful prostate syndrome

N42.82 **Prostatosis syndrome** ♂   A

N42.83 **Cyst of prostate** ♂   A

N42.89 **Other specified disorders of prostate** ♂   A

N42.9 **Disorder of prostate, unspecified** ♂   A

Item 14–7 **Hydrocele** is a sac of fluid accumulating in the testes membrane.

Blood vessels
Vas deferens
Epididymis
Testis
A   Hydrocele   B

Figure 14-7 **A.** Hydrocele. **B.** Newborn with large right hydrocele. (**B** from Behrman: Nelson Textbook of Pediatrics, ed 18, Saunders, An Imprint of Elsevier, 2007)

● **N43** **Hydrocele and spermatocele**
　　　Includes   hydrocele of spermatic cord, testis or tunica vaginalis
　　　Excludes1   congenital hydrocele (P83.5)

N43.0 **Encysted hydrocele** ♂

N43.1 **Infected hydrocele** ♂ 🦠
　　　　Use additional code (B95-B97), to identify infectious agent
　　　　(Ex:) A59.00, A59.8-A59.9, B37.41-B37.49, N43.0-N43.3

N43.2 **Other hydrocele** ♂

N43.3 **Hydrocele, unspecified** ♂

● **N43.4** **Spermatocele of epididymis**
　　　　Spermatic cyst

N43.40 **Spermatocele of epididymis, unspecified** ♂

N43.41 **Spermatocele of epididymis, single** ♂

N43.42 **Spermatocele of epididymis, multiple** ♂

● **N44** **Noninflammatory disorders of testis**

● **N44.0** **Torsion of testis**
　　　　(Ex:) For category N44.0 CC codes: N44.00-N44.04

N44.00 **Torsion of testis, unspecified** ♂ 🦠

N44.01 **Extravaginal torsion of spermatic cord** ♂ 🦠

N44.02 **Intravaginal torsion of spermatic cord** ♂ 🦠
　　　　Torsion of spermatic cord NOS

N44.03 **Torsion of appendix testis** ♂ 🦠

N44.04 **Torsion of appendix epididymis** ♂ 🦠

N44.1 **Cyst of tunica albuginea testis** ♂

N44.2 **Benign cyst of testis** ♂

N44.8 **Other noninflammatory disorders of the testis** ♂

● **N45** **Orchitis and epididymitis**
　　　*Orchitis is inflammation of one or both of the testes as a result of mumps or other infection, trauma, or metastasis. **Epididymitis** is inflammation of the tubular structure that connects the testicle with the vas deferens.*
　　　Use additional code (B95-B97), to identify infectious agent

N45.1 **Epididymitis** ♂

N45.2 **Orchitis** ♂

N45.3 **Epididymo-orchitis** ♂

N45.4 **Abscess of epididymis or testis** ♂ 🦠
　　　　(Ex:) A54.23, A54.82, A54.84, A54.89-A54.9, A59.00, A59.8-A59.9, B26.0,
　　　　　　B37.41-B37.49, N45.1-N45.4

N Newborn Age: 0   **P** Pediatric Age: 0–17   **M** Maternity DX: 12–55   **A** Adult Age: 15–124   ♀ Females Only   ♂ Males Only

🦠 Complication\Comorbidity   🦠 Major C\C   (Ex:) CC/MCC Exclusions   🦠 Hospital-Acquired Condition

Item 14-8 Male infertility is the inability of the female sex partner to conceive after one year of unprotected intercourse.

Azoospermia is no sperm ejaculated and **oligospermia** is few sperm ejaculated—both resulting in infertility. Extratesticular causes such as injury, infections, radiation, and chemotherapy may also cause male infertility.

N46   Male infertility

Excludes1   vasectomy status (Z98.52)

N46.0 Azoospermia
     Absolute male infertility
     Male infertility due to germinal (cell) aplasia
     Male infertility due to spermatogenic arrest (complete)

    N46.01   Organic azoospermia ♂   A
          Azoospermia NOS

    N46.02   Azoospermia due to extratesticular causes
          Code also associated cause

        N46.021   Azoospermia due to drug therapy ♂ A
        N46.022   Azoospermia due to infection ♂   A
        N46.023   Azoospermia due to obstruction of efferent ducts ♂   A
        N46.024   Azoospermia due to radiation ♂   A
        N46.025   Azoospermia due to systemic disease ♂   A
        N46.029   Azoospermia due to other extratesticular causes ♂   A

N46.1 Oligospermia
     Male infertility due to germinal cell desquamation
     Male infertility due to hypospermatogenesis
     Male infertility due to incomplete spermatogenic arrest

    N46.11   Organic oligospermia ♂   A
          Oligospermia NOS

    N46.12   Oligospermia due to extratesticular causes
          Code also associated cause

        N46.121   Oligospermia due to drug therapy ♂ A
         N46.122   Oligospermia due to infection ♂   A
         N46.123   Oligospermia due to obstruction of efferent ducts ♂   A
         N46.124   Oligospermia due to radiation ♂   A
         N46.125   Oligospermia due to systemic disease ♂   A
         N46.129   Oligospermia due to other extratesticular causes ♂   A

    N46.8   Other male infertility ♂   A
    N46.9   Male infertility, unspecified ♂   A

N47 Disorders of prepuce
    N47.0   Adherent prepuce, newborn ♂   N
    N47.1   Phimosis ♂
    N47.2   Paraphimosis ♂
    N47.3   Deficient foreskin ♂
    N47.4   Benign cyst of prepuce ♂
    N47.5   Adhesions of prepuce and glans penis ♂
    N47.6   Balanoposthitis ♂
         Use additional code (B95-B97), to identify infectious agent
         Excludes1   balanitis (N48.1)
    N47.7   Other inflammatory diseases of prepuce ♂
         Use additional code (B95-B97), to identify infectious agent
    N47.8   Other disorders of prepuce ♂

N48 Other disorders of penis
    N48.0   Leukoplakia of penis ♂
         Balanitis xerotica obliterans
         Kraurosis of penis
         Lichen sclerosus of external male genital organs
         Excludes1   carcinoma in situ of penis (D07.4)
    N48.1   Balanitis ♂
         Use additional code (B95-B97), to identify infectious agent
         Excludes1   amebic balanitis (A06.8)
                   balanitis xerotica obliterans (N48.0)
                   candidal balanitis (B37.42)
                   gonococcal balanitis (A54.23)
                   herpesviral [herpes simplex] balanitis (A60.01)
    N48.2   Other inflammatory disorders of penis
         Use additional code (B95-B97), to identify infectious agent
         Excludes1   balanitis (N48.1)
                   balanitis xerotica obliterans (N48.0)
                   balanoposthitis (N47.6)
        N48.21   Abscess of corpus cavernosum and penis ♂
        N48.22   Cellulitis of corpus cavernosum and penis ♂
        N48.29   Other inflammatory disorders of penis ♂
    N48.3   Priapism
         Painful erection
         Code first underlying cause
         (Ex) **For category N48.3 CC codes:** N47.6, N48.0-N48.9, N52.01-N52.9
        N48.30   Priapism, unspecified ♂
        N48.31   Priapism due to trauma ♂
        N48.32   *Priapism due to disease classified elsewhere* ♂
        N48.33   Priapism, drug-induced ♂
        N48.39   Other priapism ♂
    N48.5   Ulcer of penis ♂
    N48.6   Induration penis plastica ♂
         Peyronie's disease
         Plastic induration of penis
    N48.8   Other specified disorders of penis
        N48.81   Thrombosis of superficial vein of penis ♂
        N48.82   Acquired torsion of penis ♂
            Acquired torsion of penis NOS
            Excludes1   congenital torsion of penis (Q55.63)
        N48.83   Acquired buried penis ♂
            Excludes1   congenital hidden penis (Q55.64)
        N48.89   Other specified disorders of penis ♂
    N48.9   Disorder of penis, unspecified ♂

N49 Inflammatory disorders of male genital organs, not elsewhere classified
         Use additional code (B95-B97), to identify infectious agent
         Excludes1   inflammation of penis (N48.1, N48.2-)
                   orchitis and epididymitis (N45.-)
    N49.0   Inflammatory disorders of seminal vesicle ♂
         Vesiculitis NOS
    N49.1   Inflammatory disorders of spermatic cord, tunica vaginalis and vas deferens ♂
         Vasitis
    N49.2   Inflammatory disorders of scrotum ♂
    N49.3   Fournier gangrene ♂
    N49.8   Inflammatory disorders of other specified male genital organs ♂
         Inflammation of multiple sites in male genital organs
    N49.9   Inflammatory disorder of unspecified male genital organ ♂
         Abscess of unspecified male genital organ
         Boil of unspecified male genital organ
         Carbuncle of unspecified male genital organ
         Cellulitis of unspecified male genital organ

◀ New   ◀ Revised   ~~deleted~~ Deleted   Excludes 1   Excludes 2   Includes   Use additional   Code first   Code also   Unspecified
OGCR Official Guidelines   ● Unacceptable Principal Diagnosis   X Assign placeholder X   ● Use Additional Character(s)   ▶ Manifestation Code   **Coding Clinic**

Item 14–9 Seminal vesiculitis is an inflammation of the seminal vesicle. Spermatocele is a benign cystic accumulation of sperm arising from the head of the epididymis. Torsion of the testis is a medical emergency occurring most commonly in boys 7 to 12 years of age and results from a congenital abnormality of the covering of the testis allowing the testis to twist within its sac and cutting off the blood supply to the testis.

Figure 14-8 A. Torsion of testis. **B.** Torsion of the testis. (**B** from Kumar: Robbins and Cotran: Pathologic Basis of Disease, ed 8, Saunders, An Imprint of Elsevier, 2009)

● N50   Other and unspecified disorders of male genital organs
     Excludes2   torsion of testis (N44.0-)
  N50.0   Atrophy of testis ♂
  N50.1   Vascular disorders of male genital organs ♂
          Hematocele, NOS, of male genital organs
          Hemorrhage of male genital organs
          Thrombosis of male genital organs
  N50.3   Cyst of epididymis ♂
● N50.8   Other specified disorders of male genital organs
     ● N50.81   Testicular pain ◀
          N50.811   Right testicular pain ♂ ◀
          N50.812   Left testicular pain ♂ ◀
          N50.819   Testicular pain, unspecified ♂ ◀
       N50.82   Scrotal pain ♂ ◀
       N50.89   Other specified disorders of the male genital
                organs ♂ ◀
          Atrophy of scrotum, seminal vesicle, spermatic
            cord, tunica vaginalis and vas deferens ◀
          Chylocele, tunica vaginalis (nonfilarial)
            NOS ◀
          Edema of scrotum, seminal vesicle, spermatic
            cord, tunica vaginalis and vas deferens ◀
          Hypertrophy of scrotum, seminal vesicle,
            spermatic cord, tunica vaginalis and vas
            deferens ◀
          Stricture of spermatic cord, tunica vaginalis,
            and vas deferens ◀
          Ulcer of scrotum, seminal vesicle, spermatic
            cord, testis, tunica vaginalis and vas
            deferens ◀
          Urethroscrotal fistula ◀
  N50.9   Disorder of male genital organs, unspecified ♂

▶ N51   Disorders of male genital organs in diseases classified
        elsewhere ♂
     Code first underlying disease, such as:
          filariasis (B74.0-B74.9)
     Excludes1   amebic balanitis (A06.8)
                    candidal balanitis (B37.42)
                    gonococcal balanitis (A54.23)
                    gonococcal prostatitis (A54.22)
                    herpesviral [herpes simplex] balanitis (A60.01)
                    trichomonal prostatitis (A59.02)
                    tuberculous prostatitis (A18.14)

● N52   Male erectile dysfunction
     Excludes1   psychogenic impotence (F52.21)
  ● N52.0   Vasculogenic erectile dysfunction
          N52.01   Erectile dysfunction due to arterial
                   insufficiency ♂   A
          N52.02   Corporo-venous occlusive erectile
                   dysfunction ♂   A
          N52.03   Combined arterial insufficiency and corporo-
                   venous occlusive erectile
                   dysfunction ♂   A
  ▶ N52.1   Erectile dysfunction due to diseases classified
            elsewhere ♂   A
             Code first underlying disease
    N52.2   Drug-induced erectile dysfunction ♂   A
  ● N52.3   Postprocedural erectile dysfunction ◀▥
          N52.31   Erectile dysfunction following radical
                   prostatectomy ♂   A
          N52.32   Erectile dysfunction following radical
                   cystectomy ♂   A
          N52.33   Erectile dysfunction following urethral
                   surgery ♂   A
          N52.34   Erectile dysfunction following simple
                   prostatectomy ♂   A
          N52.35   Erectile dysfunction following radiation
                   therapy ♂ ◀   A
          N52.36   Erectile dysfunction following interstitial seed
                   therapy ♂ ◀   A
          N52.37   Erectile dysfunction following prostate ablative
                   therapy ♂ ◀   A
                   Erectile dysfunction following cryotherapy ◀
                   Erectile dysfunction following other prostate
                     ablative therapies ◀
                   Erectile dysfunction following ultrasound
                     ablative therapies ◀
          N52.39   Other and unspecified postprocedural erectile
                   dysfunction ♂ ◀▥   A
    N52.8   Other male erectile dysfunction ♂   A
    N52.9   Male erectile dysfunction, unspecified ♂   A
             Impotence NOS

● N53   Other male sexual dysfunction
     Excludes1   psychogenic sexual dysfunction (F52.-)
  ● N53.1   Ejaculatory dysfunction
     Excludes1   premature ejaculation (F52.4)
          N53.11   Retarded ejaculation ♂
          N53.12   Painful ejaculation ♂
          N53.13   Anejaculatory orgasm ♂
          N53.14   Retrograde ejaculation ♂
          N53.19   Other ejaculatory dysfunction ♂
                   Ejaculatory dysfunction NOS
    N53.8   Other male sexual dysfunction ♂
    N53.9   Unspecified male sexual dysfunction ♂

DISORDERS OF BREAST (N60-N65)

     Excludes1   disorders of breast associated with childbirth
                    (O91-O92)

● N60   Benign mammary dysplasia
        Benign lumpiness of breast
     Includes   fibrocystic mastopathy
  ● N60.0   Solitary cyst of breast
             Cyst of breast
          N60.01   Solitary cyst of right breast
          N60.02   Solitary cyst of left breast
          N60.09   Solitary cyst of unspecified breast

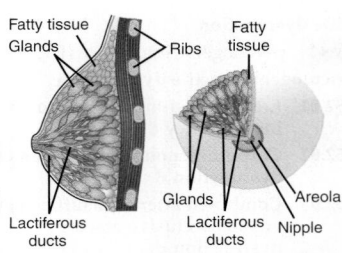

Figure 14-9 Breast.

● **N60.1 Diffuse cystic mastopathy**
Cystic breast
Fibrocystic disease of breast

> **Excludes1** diffuse cystic mastopathy with epithelial proliferation (N60.3-)

N60.11 Diffuse cystic mastopathy of right breast   A
N60.12 Diffuse cystic mastopathy of left breast   A
N60.19 Diffuse cystic mastopathy of unspecified breast   A

● **N60.2 Fibroadenosis of breast**
Adenofibrosis of breast

> **Excludes2** fibroadenoma of breast (D24.-)

N60.21 Fibroadenosis of right breast
N60.22 Fibroadenosis of left breast
N60.29 Fibroadenosis of unspecified breast

● **N60.3 Fibrosclerosis of breast**
Cystic mastopathy with epithelial proliferation

N60.31 Fibrosclerosis of right breast
N60.32 Fibrosclerosis of left breast
N60.39 Fibrosclerosis of unspecified breast

● **N60.4 Mammary duct ectasia**
N60.41 Mammary duct ectasia of right breast
N60.42 Mammary duct ectasia of left breast
N60.49 Mammary duct ectasia of unspecified breast

● **N60.8 Other benign mammary dysplasias**
N60.81 Other benign mammary dysplasias of right breast
N60.82 Other benign mammary dysplasias of left breast
N60.89 Other benign mammary dysplasias of unspecified breast

● **N60.9 Unspecified benign mammary dysplasia**
N60.91 Unspecified benign mammary dysplasia of right breast
N60.92 Unspecified benign mammary dysplasia of left breast
N60.99 Unspecified benign mammary dysplasia of unspecified breast

● **N61 Inflammatory disorders of breast**

> **Excludes1** inflammatory carcinoma of breast (C50.9)
> inflammatory disorder of breast associated with childbirth (O91.-)
> neonatal infective mastitis (P39.0)
> thrombophlebitis of breast [Mondor's disease] (I80.8)

N61.0 **Mastitis without abscess** ◀
Infective mastitis (acute) (nonpuerperal) (subacute) ◀
Mastitis (acute) (nonpuerperal) (subacute) NOS ◀
Cellulitis (acute) (nonpuerperal) (subacute) of breast NOS ◀
Cellulitis (acute) (nonpuerperal) (subacute) of nipple NOS ◀

N61.1 **Abscess of the breast and nipple** ◀
Abscess (acute) (chronic) (nonpuerperal) of areola ◀
Abscess (acute) (chronic) (nonpuerperal) of breast ◀
Carbuncle of breast ◀
Mastitis with abscess ◀

N62 **Hypertrophy of breast**
Gynecomastia
Hypertrophy of breast NOS
Massive pubertal hypertrophy of breast

> **Excludes1** breast engorgement of newborn (P83.4)
> disproportion of reconstructed breast (N65.1)

N63 **Unspecified lump in breast**
Nodule(s) NOS in breast

● **N64 Other disorders of breast**

> **Excludes2** mechanical complication of breast prosthesis and implant (T85.4-)

N64.0 **Fissure and fistula of nipple**

● **N64.1 Fat necrosis of breast**
Fat necrosis (segmental) of breast
Code first breast necrosis due to breast graft (T85.898) ◀▥

N64.2 **Atrophy of breast**

N64.3 **Galactorrhea not associated with childbirth**
Excessive or spontaneous flow of milk

N64.4 **Mastodynia**

● **N64.5 Other signs and symptoms in breast**

> **Excludes2** abnormal findings on diagnostic imaging of breast (R92.-)

N64.51 **Induration of breast**
N64.52 **Nipple discharge**

> **Excludes1** abnormal findings in nipple discharge (R89.-)

N64.53 **Retraction of nipple**
N64.59 **Other signs and symptoms in breast**

● **N64.8 Other specified disorders of breast**
N64.81 **Ptosis of breast**   A

> **Excludes1** ptosis of native breast in relation to reconstructed breast (N65.1)

N64.82 **Hypoplasia of breast**   A
Micromastia

> **Excludes1** congenital absence of breast (Q83.0)
> hypoplasia of native breast in relation to reconstructed breast (N65.1)

N64.89 **Other specified disorders of breast**
Galactocele
Subinvolution of breast (postlactational)

N64.9 **Disorder of breast, unspecified**

● **N65 Deformity and disproportion of reconstructed breast**
N65.0 **Deformity of reconstructed breast**   A
Contour irregularity in reconstructed breast
Excess tissue in reconstructed breast
Misshapen reconstructed breast

N65.1 **Disproportion of reconstructed breast**   A
Breast asymmetry between native breast and reconstructed breast
Disproportion between native breast and reconstructed breast

CHAPTER 14 (N00-N99)

INFLAMMATORY DISEASES OF FEMALE PELVIC ORGANS (N70-N77)

Excludes1   inflammatory diseases of female pelvic organs
                complicating:
                abortion or ectopic or molar pregnancy
                (O00-O07, O08.0)
                pregnancy, childbirth and the puerperium
                (O23.-, O75.3, O85, O86.-)

★ **(See Plate 360 on page 80.)**

● **N70   Salpingitis and oophoritis**
   Oophoritis = inflammation of ovary
   Salpingitis = inflammation of falloplan tube

   Includes   abscess (of) fallopian tube
                  abscess (of) ovary
                  pyosalpinx
                  salpingo-oophoritis
                  tubo-ovarian abscess
                  tubo-ovarian inflammatory disease

   Use additional code (B95-B97), to identify infectious agent

   Excludes1   gonococcal infection (A54.24)
                   tuberculous infection (A18.17)

● **N70.0   Acute salpingitis and oophoritis**
   Ex: **For category N70.0 CC codes:** A17.9, A18.10, A18.16-A18.18, A18.82,
   A18.84, A18.89, A54.03, A54.24, A54.82, A54.84, A54.89-A54.9, A59.00,
   A59.8-A59.9, B37.41-B37.49, N70.01-N71.9, N73.0-N74, N75.9, N76.5,
   N76.81-N76.89, N90.810-N90.818, N94.818-N94.9, N96, Q55.0-Q55.4,
   Q55.7-Q55.9

   N70.01   Acute salpingitis ♀ 🦠
   N70.02   Acute oophoritis ♀ 🦠
   N70.03   Acute salpingitis and oophoritis ♀ 🦠

● **N70.1   Chronic salpingitis and oophoritis**
   Hydrosalpinx

   N70.11   Chronic salpingitis ♀
   N70.12   Chronic oophoritis ♀
   N70.13   Chronic salpingitis and oophoritis ♀

● **N70.9   Salpingitis and oophoritis, unspecified**
   N70.91   Salpingitis, unspecified ♀
   N70.92   Oophoritis, unspecified ♀
   N70.93   Salpingitis and oophoritis, unspecified ♀

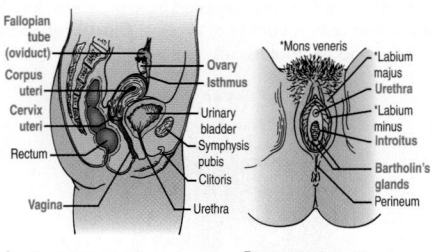

Fallopian
tube
(oviduct)
Corpus
uteri   *Mons veneris   *Labium
Cervix   majus
uteri   Ovary   Urethra
                               Isthmus   *Labium
Rectum   Urinary   minus
                               bladder   Introitus
                               Symphysis
                               pubis   Bartholin's
Vagina   Clitoris   glands
                               Urethra   Perineum

A   Female Genital System   B   *The three parts of the vulva

Figure 14-10   A. Female genital system. **B.** External female genital
system. (From Buck CJ: Step-by-Step Medical Coding, ed 2016, St. Louis,
Elsevier, 2016)

Item 14–10 Salpingitis is an infection of one or both fallopian tubes.
Oophoritis is an infection of one or both ovaries.

● **N71   Inflammatory disease of uterus, except cervix**

   Includes   endo (myo) metritis
                  metritis
                  myometritis
                  pyometra
                  uterine abscess

   Use additional code (B95-B97), to identify infectious agent

   Excludes1   hyperplastic endometritis (N85.0-)
                   infection of uterus following delivery (O85, O86.-)

   N71.0   Acute inflammatory disease of uterus ♀ 🦠
      Ex: A17.9, A18.10, A18.16-A18.18, A18.82, A18.84, A18.89, A54.03, A54.24,
      A54.82, A54.84, A54.89-A54.9, A59.00, A59.8-A59.9, B37.41-B37.49,
      N70.01-N71.9, N72, N73.0-N74, N75.9, N76.5, N76.81-N76.89, N85.8-N85.9,
      N90.810-N90.818, N94.818-N94.9, N96, Q55.0-Q55.4, Q55.7-Q55.9

   N71.1   Chronic inflammatory disease of uterus ♀
   N71.9   Inflammatory disease of uterus, unspecified ♀

   N72   Inflammatory disease of cervix uteri ♀

   Includes   cervicitis (with or without erosion or ectropion)
                  endocervicitis (with or without erosion or
                  ectropion)
                  exocervicitis (with or without erosion or ectropion)

   Use additional code (B95-B97), to identify infectious agent

   Excludes1   erosion and ectropion of cervix without cervicitis
                   (N86)

● **N73   Other female pelvic inflammatory diseases**
   Use additional code (B95-B97), to identify infectious agent

   N73.0   Acute parametritis and pelvic cellulitis ♀ 🦠
      Abscess of broad ligament
      Abscess of parametrium
      Pelvic cellulitis, female
      Ex: See N70.0

   N73.1   Chronic parametritis and pelvic cellulitis ♀
      Any condition in N73.0 specified as chronic
      Excludes1   tuberculous parametritis and pelvic
                      cellultis (A18.17)

   N73.2   Unspecified parametritis and pelvic cellulitis ♀
      Any condition in N73.0 unspecified whether acute or
      chronic

   N73.3   Female acute pelvic peritonitis ♀ 🦠
      Ex: See N70.0

   N73.4   Female chronic pelvic peritonitis ♀ 🦠
      Excludes1   tuberculous pelvic (female) peritonitis
                      (A18.17)
      Ex: See N70.0

   N73.5   Female pelvic peritonitis, unspecified ♀

   N73.6   Female pelvic peritoneal adhesions (postinfective) ♀
      Excludes2   postprocedural pelvic peritoneal
                      adhesions (N99.4)

   N73.8   Other specified female pelvic inflammatory diseases ♀
   N73.9   Female pelvic inflammatory disease, unspecified ♀
      Female pelvic infection or inflammation NOS

▷ **N74   Female pelvic inflammatory disorders in diseases classified
   elsewhere** ♀

   Code first underlying disease

   Excludes1   chlamydial cervicitis (A56.02)
                   chlamydial pelvic inflammatory disease (A56.11)
                   gonococcal cervicitis (A54.03)
                   gonococcal pelvic inflammatory disease (A54.24)
                   herpesviral [herpes simplex] cervicitis (A60.03)
                   herpesviral [herpes simplex] pelvic inflammatory
                   disease (A60.09)
                   syphilitic cervicitis (A52.76)
                   syphilitic pelvic inflammatory disease (A52.76)
                   trichomonal cervicitis (A59.09)
                   tuberculous cervicitis (A18.16)
                   tuberculous pelvic inflammatory disease (A18.17)

CHAPTER 14 (N00-N99)

● **N75**   **Diseases of Bartholin's gland**

    N75.0   **Cyst of Bartholin's gland** ♀
       Cysts filled with liquid or semisolid material

    N75.1   **Abscess of Bartholin's gland** ♀ 🔗
       Localized collection of pus
       (Ex) A17.9, A18.10, A18.16-A18.18, A18.82, A18.84, A18.89, A59.00-A59.01,
           A59.8-A59.9, B37.3-B37.49, N75.0-N77.1, N84.3, N90.3, N90.60-N90.9,
           N94.810-N94.9, N96, Q55.0-Q55.4, Q55.7-Q55.9

    N75.8   **Other diseases of Bartholin's gland** ♀
       Bartholinitis

    N75.9   **Disease of Bartholin's gland,** unspecified ♀

● **N76**   **Other inflammation of vagina and vulva**
       Use additional code (B95-B97), to identify infectious agent
       Excludes2   senile (atrophic) vaginitis (N95.2)
                 vulvar vestibulitis (N94.810)

    N76.0   **Acute vaginitis** ♀
       Acute vulvovaginitis
       Vaginitis NOS
       Vulvovaginitis NOS

    N76.1   **Subacute and chronic vaginitis** ♀
       Chronic vulvovaginitis
       Subacute vulvovaginitis

    N76.2   **Acute vulvitis** ♀
       Vulvitis NOS

    N76.3   **Subacute and chronic vulvitis** ♀

    N76.4   **Abscess of vulva** ♀ 🔗
       Furuncle of vulva
       (Ex) See N75.1

    N76.5   **Ulceration of vagina** ♀

    N76.6   **Ulceration of vulva** ♀

●   **N76.8**   **Other specified inflammation of vagina and vulva**

       N76.81   **Mucositis (ulcerative) of vagina and vulva** ♀ 🔗
              Code also type of associated therapy, such as:
                 antineoplastic and immunosuppressive
                    drugs (T45.1X-)
                 radiological procedure and radiotherapy
                    (Y84.2)
              Excludes2   gastrointestinal mucositis
                        (ulcerative) (K92.81)
                        nasal mucositis (ulcerative)
                        (J34.81)
                        oral mucositis (ulcerative) (K12.3-)
              (Ex) N72, N75.9, N76.5, N76.81-N76.89

       N76.89   **Other specified inflammation of vagina and
              vulva** ♀

● **N77**   **Vulvovaginal ulceration and inflammation in diseases classified
       elsewhere**

▷   **N77.0**   *Ulceration of vulva in diseases classified elsewhere* ♀
       Code first underlying disease, such as:
       Behçet's disease (M35.2)
       Excludes1   ulceration of vulva in gonococcal
                  infection (A54.02)
                 ulceration of vulva in herpesviral [herpes
                  simplex] infection (A60.04)
                 ulceration of vulva in syphilis (A51.0)
                 ulceration of vulva in tuberculosis (A18.18)

▷   **N77.1**   *Vaginitis, vulvitis and vulvovaginitis in diseases
       classified elsewhere* ♀
       Code first underlying disease, such as:
       pinworm (B80)
       Excludes1   candidial vulvovaginitis (B37.3)
                  chlamydial vulvovaginitis (A56.02)
                 gonococcal vulvovaginitis (A54.02)
                 herpesviral [herpes simplex]
                  vulvovaginitis (A60.04)
                 trichomonal vulvovaginitis (A59.01)
                 tuberculous vulvovaginitis (A18.18)
                 vulvovaginitis in early syphilis (A51.0)
                 vulvovaginitis in late syphilis (A52.76)

NONINFLAMMATORY DISORDERS OF FEMALE GENITAL TRACT (N80-N98)

● **N80**   **Endometriosis**

    N80.0   **Endometriosis of uterus** ♀
       Adenomyosis
       Excludes1   stromal endometriosis (D39.0)

    N80.1   **Endometriosis of ovary** ♀

    N80.2   **Endometriosis of fallopian tube** ♀

    N80.3   **Endometriosis of pelvic peritoneum** ♀

    N80.4   **Endometriosis of rectovaginal septum and vagina** ♀

    N80.5   **Endometriosis of intestine** ♀

    N80.6   **Endometriosis in cutaneous scar** ♀

    N80.8   **Other endometriosis** ♀

    N80.9   **Endometriosis,** unspecified ♀

● **N81**   **Female genital prolapse**
       Excludes1   genital prolapse complicating pregnancy, labor or
                  delivery (O34.5-)
                 prolapse and hernia of ovary and fallopian tube
                  (N83.4-) ◀▥
                 prolapse of vaginal vault after hysterectomy (N99.3)

    N81.0   **Urethrocele** ♀
       Excludes1   urethrocele with cystocele (N81.1-)
                  urethrocele with prolapse of uterus
                    (N81.2-N81.4)

●   **N81.1**   **Cystocele**
       Cystocele with urethrocele
       Cystourethrocele
       Excludes1   cystocele with prolapse of uterus
                  (N81.2-N81.4)

       N81.10   **Cystocele,** unspecified ♀
              Prolapse of (anterior) vaginal wall NOS

       N81.11   **Cystocele, midline** ♀

       N81.12   **Cystocele, lateral** ♀
              Paravaginal cystocele

    N81.2   **Incomplete uterovaginal prolapse** ♀
       First degree uterine prolapse
       Prolapse of cervix NOS
       Second degree uterine prolapse
       Excludes1   cervical stump prolaspe (N81.85)

    N81.3   **Complete uterovaginal prolapse** ♀
       Procidentia (uteri) NOS
       Third degree uterine prolapse

    N81.4   **Uterovaginal prolapse,** unspecified ♀
       Prolapse of uterus NOS

Item 14-11 Endometriosis is a condition for which no clear cause has
been identified. Endometrial tissue is expelled from the uterus into the abdominal
cavity and can implant onto a variety of organs. Classification is based on the
site of implant of the endometrial tissue.

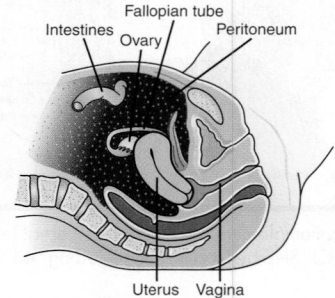

Figure 14-11   Sites of potential endometrial implants.

◀ New   ◀▥ Revised   ~~deleted~~ Deleted   Excludes 1   Excludes 2   Includes   Use additional   Code first   Code also   Unspecified

OGCR Official Guidelines   ● Unacceptable Principal Diagnosis   X Assign placeholder X   ● Use Additional Character(s)   ▷ Manifestation Code   **Coding Clinic**

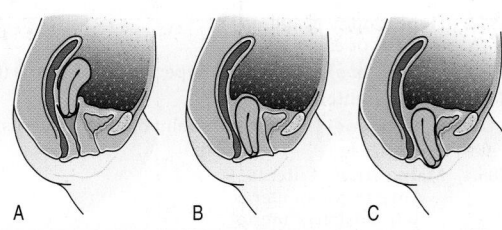

Figure 14-12   Three stages of uterine prolapse. **A.** Uterus is prolapsed. **B.** Vagina and uterus are prolapsed (incomplete uterovaginal prolapse). **C.** Vagina and uterus are completely prolapsed and are exposed through the external genitalia (complete uterovaginal prolapse).

N81.5   **Vaginal enterocele** ♀
      Excludes1   enterocele with prolapse of uterus (N81.2-N81.4)

N81.6   **Rectocele** ♀
      Prolapse of posterior vaginal wall
      Use additional code for any associated fecal incontinence, if applicable (R15.-)
      Excludes2   perineocele (N81.81)
                 rectal prolapse (K62.3)
                 rectocele with prolapse of uterus (N81.2-N81.4)

● **N81.8**   **Other female genital prolapse**
     N81.81   **Perineocele** ♀
     N81.82   **Incompetence or weakening of pubocervical tissue** ♀
     N81.83   **Incompetence or weakening of rectovaginal tissue** ♀
     N81.84   **Pelvic muscle wasting** ♀
             Disuse atrophy of pelvic muscles and anal sphincter
     N81.85   **Cervical stump prolapse** ♀
     N81.89   **Other female genital prolapse** ♀
             Deficient perineum
             Old laceration of muscles of pelvic floor
   N81.9   **Female genital prolapse, unspecified** ♀

● **N82**   **Fistulae involving female genital tract**
      Excludes1   vesicointestinal fistulae (N32.1)
      (Ex) **For category N82 CC codes: N82.0-N82.9**
   N82.0   **Vesicovaginal fistula** ♀
   N82.1   **Other female urinary-genital tract fistulae** ♀
           Cervicovesical fistula
           Ureterovaginal fistula
           Urethrovaginal fistula
           Uteroureteric fistula
           Uterovesical fistula
   N82.2   **Fistula of vagina to small intestine** ♀
   N82.3   **Fistula of vagina to large intestine** ♀
           Rectovaginal fistula
   N82.4   **Other female intestinal-genital tract fistulae** ♀
           Intestinouterine fistula
   N82.5   **Female genital tract-skin fistulae** ♀
           Uterus to abdominal wall fistula
           Vaginoperineal fistula
   N82.8   **Other female genital tract fistulae** ♀
   N82.9   **Female genital tract fistula, unspecified** ♀

● **N83**   **Noninflammatory disorders of ovary, fallopian tube and broad ligament**
      Excludes2   hydrosalpinx (N70.1-)
   ● **N83.0**   **Follicular cyst of ovary**
           Cyst of graafian follicle
           Hemorrhagic follicular cyst (of ovary)
     N83.00   **Follicular cyst of ovary, unspecified side** ♀ ◄
     N83.01   **Follicular cyst of right ovary** ♀ ◄
     N83.02   **Follicular cyst of left ovary** ♀ ◄
   ● **N83.1**   **Corpus luteum cyst**
           Hemorrhagic corpus luteum cyst
     N83.10   **Corpus luteum cyst of ovary, unspecified side** ♀ ◄
     N83.11   **Corpus luteum cyst of right ovary** ♀ ◄
     N83.12   **Corpus luteum cyst of left ovary** ♀ ◄
   ● **N83.2**   **Other and unspecified ovarian cysts**
      Excludes1   developmental ovarian cyst (Q50.1)
                 neoplastic ovarian cyst (D27.-)
                 polycystic ovarian syndrome (E28.2)
                 Stein-Leventhal syndrome (E28.2)
    ● **N83.20**   **Unspecified ovarian cysts**
      N83.201   **Unspecified ovarian cyst, right side** ♀ ◄
      N83.202   **Unspecified ovarian cyst, left side** ♀ ◄
      N83.209   **Unspecified ovarian cyst, unspecified side** ♀ ◄
             Ovarian cyst, NOS ◄
    ● **N83.29**   **Other ovarian cysts**
           Retention cyst of ovary
           Simple cyst of ovary
      N83.291   **Other ovarian cyst, right side** ♀ ◄
      N83.292   **Other ovarian cyst, left side** ♀ ◄
      N83.299   **Other ovarian cyst, unspecified side** ♀ ◄
   ● **N83.3**   **Acquired atrophy of ovary and fallopian tube**
    ● **N83.31**   **Acquired atrophy of ovary**
      N83.311   **Acquired atrophy of right ovary** ♀ ◄
      N83.312   **Acquired atrophy of left ovary** ♀ ◄
      N83.319   **Acquired atrophy of ovary, unspecified side** ♀ ◄
             Acquired atrophy of ovary, NOS ◄
    ● **N83.32**   **Acquired atrophy of fallopian tube**
      N83.321   **Acquired atrophy of right fallopian tube** ♀ ◄
      N83.322   **Acquired atrophy of left fallopian tube** ♀ ◄
      N83.329   **Acquired atrophy of fallopian tube, unspecified side** ♀ ◄
             Acquired atrophy of fallopian tube, NOS ◄
    ● **N83.33**   **Acquired atrophy of ovary and fallopian tube**
      N83.331   **Acquired atrophy of right ovary and fallopian tube** ♀ ◄
      N83.332   **Acquired atrophy of left ovary and fallopian tube** ♀ ◄
      N83.339   **Acquired atrophy of ovary and fallopian tube, unspecified side** ♀ ◄
             Acquired atrophy of ovary and fallopian tube, NOS ◄
   ● **N83.4**   **Prolapse and hernia of ovary and fallopian tube**
     N83.40   **Prolapse and hernia of ovary and fallopian tube, unspecified side** ♀ ◄
             Prolapse and hernia of ovary and fallopian tube, NOS ◄
     N83.41   **Prolapse and hernia of right ovary and fallopian tube** ♀ ◄
     N83.42   **Prolapse and hernia of left ovary and fallopian tube** ♀ ◄

● **N83.5** **Torsion of ovary, ovarian pedicle and fallopian tube**
    Torsion of accessory tube
    (Ex) **For category N83.5 CC codes:** N83.00-N83.53, N83.6-N83.9, N99.83

  ● **N83.51** **Torsion of ovary and ovarian pedicle**

    N83.511 **Torsion of right ovary and ovarian pedicle** ♀ 🐾 ◀

    N83.512 **Torsion of left ovary and ovarian pedicle** ♀ 🐾 ◀

    N83.519 **Torsion of ovary and ovarian pedicle, unspecified side** ♀ 🐾 ◀
        Torsion of ovary and ovarian pedicle, NOS ◀

  ● **N83.52** **Torsion of fallopian tube**
    Torsion of hydatid of Morgagni

    N83.521 **Torsion of right fallopian tube** ♀ 🐾 ◀

    N83.522 **Torsion of left fallopian tube** ♀ 🐾 ◀

    N83.529 **Torsion of fallopian tube, unspecified side** ♀ 🐾 ◀
        Torsion of fallopian tube, NOS ◀

  N83.53 **Torsion of ovary, ovarian pedicle and fallopian tube** ♀ 🐾

N83.6 **Hematosalpinx** ♀

  Excludes1   hematosalpinx (with) (in):
      hematocolpos (N89.7)
      hematometra (N85.7)
      tubal pregnancy (O00.1-) ◀▥

N83.7 **Hematoma of broad ligament** ♀

N83.8 **Other noninflammatory disorders of ovary, fallopian tube and broad ligament** ♀
  Broad ligament laceration syndrome [Allen-Masters]

N83.9 **Noninflammatory disorder of ovary, fallopian tube and broad ligament, unspecified** ♀

● **N84** **Polyp of female genital tract**
  Excludes1   adenomatous polyp (D28.-)
    placental polyp (O90.89)

N84.0 **Polyp of corpus uteri** ♀
  Polyp of endometrium
  Polyp of uterus NOS
  Excludes1   polypoid endometrial hyperplasia (N85.0-)

N84.1 **Polyp of cervix uteri** ♀
  Mucous polyp of cervix

N84.2 **Polyp of vagina** ♀

N84.3 **Polyp of vulva** ♀
  Polyp of labia

N84.8 **Polyp of other parts of female genital tract** ♀

N84.9 **Polyp of female genital tract, unspecified** ♀

● **N85** **Other noninflammatory disorders of uterus, except cervix**
  Excludes1   endometriosis (N80.-)
    inflammatory diseases of uterus (N71.-)
    noninflammatory disorders of cervix, except malposition (N86-N88)
    polyp of corpus uteri (N84.0)
    uterine prolapse (N81.-)

● **N85.0** **Endometrial hyperplasia**

  N85.00 **Endometrial hyperplasia, unspecified** ♀
    Hyperplasia (adenomatous) (cystic) (glandular) of endometrium
    Hyperplastic endometritis

  N85.01 **Benign endometrial hyperplasia** ♀
    Endometrial hyperplasia (complex) (simple) without atypia

  N85.02 **Endometrial intraepithelial neoplasia [EIN]** ♀
    Endometrial hyperplasia with atypia
    Excludes1   malignant neoplasm of endometrium (with endometrial intraepithelial neoplasia [EIN]) (C54.1)

N85.2 **Hypertrophy of uterus** ♀
  Bulky or enlarged uterus
  Excludes1   puerperal hypertrophy of uterus (O90.89)

N85.3 **Subinvolution of uterus** ♀
  Excludes1   puerperal subinvolution of uterus (O90.89)

N85.4 **Malposition of uterus** ♀
  Anteversion of uterus
  Retroflexion of uterus
  Retroversion of uterus
  Excludes1   malposition of uterus complicating pregnancy, labor or delivery (O34.5-, O65.5)

N85.5 **Inversion of uterus** ♀
  Excludes1   current obstetric trauma (O71.2)
    postpartum inversion of uterus (O71.2)

N85.6 **Intrauterine synechiae** ♀

N85.7 **Hematometra** ♀
  Hematosalpinx with hematometra
  Excludes1   hematometra with hematocolpos (N89.7)

N85.8 **Other specified noninflammatory disorders of uterus** ♀
  Atrophy of uterus, acquired
  Fibrosis of uterus NOS

N85.9 **Noninflammatory disorder of uterus, unspecified** ♀
  Disorder of uterus NOS

● **N86** **Erosion and ectropion of cervix uteri** ♀
  Decubitus (trophic) ulcer of cervix
  Eversion of cervix
  Excludes1   erosion and ectropion of cervix with cervicitis (N72)

● **N87** **Dysplasia of cervix uteri**
  Excludes1   abnormal results from cervical cytologic examination without histologic confirmation (R87.61-)
    carcinoma in situ of cervix uteri (D06.-)
    cervical intraepithelial neoplasia III [CIN III] (D06.-)
    HGSIL of cervix (R87.613)
    severe dysplasia of cervix uteri (D06.-)

N87.0 **Mild cervical dysplasia** ♀
  Cervical intraepithelial neoplasia I [CIN I]

N87.1 **Moderate cervical dysplasia** ♀
  Cervical intraepithelial neoplasia II [CIN II]

N87.9 **Dysplasia of cervix uteri, unspecified** ♀
  Anaplasia of cervix
  Cervical atypism
  Cervical dysplasia NOS

● **N88** **Other noninflammatory disorders of cervix uteri**
  Excludes2   inflammatory disease of cervix (N72)
    polyp of cervix (N84.1)

N88.0 **Leukoplakia of cervix uteri** ♀

N88.1 **Old laceration of cervix uteri** ♀
  Adhesions of cervix
  Excludes1   current obstetric trauma (O71.3)

N88.2 **Stricture and stenosis of cervix uteri** ♀
  Excludes1   stricture and stenosis of cervix uteri complicating labor (O65.5)

N88.3 **Incompetence of cervix uteri** ♀
  Investigation and management of (suspected) cervical incompetence in a nonpregnant woman
  Excludes1   cervical incompetence complicating pregnancy (O34.3-)

N88.4 **Hypertrophic elongation of cervix uteri** ♀

N88.8 **Other specified noninflammatory disorders of cervix uteri** ♀
  Excludes1   current obstetric trauma (O71.3)

N88.9 **Noninflammatory disorder of cervix uteri, unspecified** ♀

◀ New   ◀▥ Revised   ~~deleted~~ Deleted   Excludes 1   Excludes 2   Includes   Use additional   Code first   Code also   Unspecified

OGCR Official Guidelines   ● Unacceptable Principal Diagnosis   X Assign placeholder X   🐾 Use Additional Character(s)   ▥ Manifestation Code   **Coding Clinic**

● **N89**   **Other noninflammatory disorders of vagina**

> **Excludes1**   abnormal results from vaginal cytologic examination without histologic confirmation (R87.62-)
> carcinoma in situ of vagina (D07.2)
> HGSIL of vagina (R87.623)
> inflammation of vagina (N76.-)
> senile (atrophic) vaginitis (N95.2)
> severe dysplasia of vagina (D07.2)
> trichomonal leukorrhea (A59.00)
> vaginal intraepithelial neoplasia [VAIN], grade III (D07.2)

N89.0   **Mild vaginal dysplasia** ♀
> Vaginal intraepithelial neoplasia [VAIN], grade I

N89.1   **Moderate vaginal dysplasia** ♀
> Vaginal intraepithelial neoplasia [VAIN], grade II

N89.3   **Dysplasia of vagina, unspecified** ♀

N89.4   **Leukoplakia of vagina** ♀

N89.5   **Stricture and atresia of vagina** ♀
> Vaginal adhesions   Vaginal stenosis

> **Excludes1**   congenital atresia or stricture (Q52.4)
> postprocedural adhesions of vagina (N99.2)

N89.6   **Tight hymenal ring** ♀
> Rigid hymen   Tight introitus

> **Excludes1**   imperforate hymen (Q52.3)

N89.7   **Hematocolpos**
> Hematocolpos with hematometra or hematosalpinx

N89.8   **Other specified noninflammatory disorders of vagina** ♀
> Leukorrhea NOS
> Old vaginal laceration
> Pessary ulcer of vagina

> **Excludes1**   current obstetric trauma (O70.-, O71.4, O71.7-O71.8)
> old laceration involving muscles of pelvic floor (N81.8)

N89.9   **Noninflammatory disorder of vagina, unspecified** ♀

● **N90**   **Other noninflammatory disorders of vulva and perineum**

> **Excludes1**   anogenital (venereal) warts (A63.0)
> carcinoma in situ of vulva (D07.1)
> condyloma acuminatum (A63.0)
> current obstetric trauma (O70.-, O71.7-O71.8)
> inflammation of vulva (N76.-)
> severe dysplasia of vulva (D07.1)
> vulvar intraepithelial neoplasm III [VIN III] (D07.1)

N90.0   **Mild vulvar dysplasia** ♀
> Vulvar intraepithelial neoplasia [VIN], grade I

N90.1   **Moderate vulvar dysplasia** ♀
> Vulvar intraepithelial neoplasia [VIN], grade II

N90.3   **Dysplasia of vulva, unspecified** ♀

N90.4   **Leukoplakia of vulva** ♀
> Dystrophy of vulva
> Kraurosis of vulva
> Lichen sclerosus of external female genital organs

N90.5   **Atrophy of vulva** ♀
> Stenosis of vulva

● **N90.6**   **Hypertrophy of vulva**

> **N90.60**   **Unspecified hypertrophy of vulva** ♀ ◄
> Unspecified hypertrophy of labia ◄

> **N90.61**   **Childhood asymmetric labium majus enlargement** ♀ ◄
> CALME ◄

> **N90.69**   **Other specified hypertrophy of vulva** ♀ ◄
> Other specified hypertrophy of labia ◄

N90.7   **Vulvar cyst** ♀

● **N90.8**   **Other specified noninflammatory disorders of vulva and perineum**

> ● **N90.81**   **Female genital mutilation status**
> Female genital cutting status

> > **N90.810**   **Female genital mutilation status, unspecified** ♀
> > Female genital cutting status, unspecified
> > Female genital mutilation status NOS

> > **N90.811**   **Female genital mutilation Type I status** ♀
> > Clitorectomy status
> > Female genital cutting Type I status

> > **N90.812**   **Female genital mutilation Type II status** ♀
> > Clitorectomy with excision of labia minora status
> > Female genital cutting Type II status

> > **N90.813**   **Female genital mutilation Type III status** ♀
> > Female genital cutting Type III status
> > Infibulation status

> > **N90.818**   **Other female genital mutilation status** ♀
> > Female genital cutting Type IV status
> > Female genital mutilation Type IV status
> > Other female genital cutting status

> **N90.89**   **Other specified noninflammatory disorders of vulva and perineum** ♀
> Adhesions of vulva
> Hypertrophy of clitoris

N90.9   **Noninflammatory disorder of vulva and perineum, unspecified** ♀

● **N91**   **Absent, scanty and rare menstruation**

> **Excludes1**   ovarian dysfunction (E28.-)

N91.0   **Primary amenorrhea** ♀

N91.1   **Secondary amenorrhea** ♀

N91.2   **Amenorrhea, unspecified** ♀

N91.3   **Primary oligomenorrhea** ♀

N91.4   **Secondary oligomenorrhea** ♀

N91.5   **Oligomenorrhea, unspecified** ♀
> Hypomenorrhea NOS

● **N92**   **Excessive, frequent and irregular menstruation**

> **Excludes1**   postmenopausal bleeding (N95.0)
> precocious puberty (menstruation) (E30.1)

N92.0   **Excessive and frequent menstruation with regular cycle** ♀
> Heavy periods NOS   Polymenorrhea
> Menorrhagia NOS

N92.1   **Excessive and frequent menstruation with irregular cycle** ♀
> Irregular intermenstrual bleeding
> Irregular, shortened intervals between menstrual bleeding
> Menometrorrhagia
> Metrorrhagia

N92.2   **Excessive menstruation at puberty** ♀   P
> Excessive bleeding associated with onset of menstrual periods
> Pubertal menorrhagia
> Puberty bleeding

N92.3   **Ovulation bleeding** ♀
> Regular intermenstrual bleeding

N92.4   **Excessive bleeding in the premenopausal period** ♀
> Climacteric menorrhagia or metrorrhagia
> Menopausal menorrhagia or metrorrhagia
> Preclimacteric menorrhagia or metrorrhagia
> Premenopausal menorrhagia or metrorrhagia

CHAPTER 14 (N00-N99)

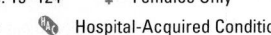

N Newborn Age: 0   **P** Pediatric Age: 0–17   **M** Maternity DX: 12–55   **A** Adult Age: 15–124   ♀ Females Only   ♂ Males Only
   Complication\Comorbidity   Major C\C   (Ex) CC/MCC Exclusions   Hospital-Acquired Condition

1109

N92.5   **Other specified irregular menstruation** ♀

N92.6   **Irregular menstruation, unspecified** ♀
Irregular bleeding NOS
Irregular periods NOS

> **Excludes1**   irregular menstruation with:
> lengthened intervals or scanty bleeding (N91.3-N91.5)
> shortened intervals or excessive bleeding (N92.1)

● **N93**   **Other abnormal uterine and vaginal bleeding**

> **Excludes1**   neonatal vaginal hemorrhage (P54.6)
> precocious puberty (menstruation) (E30.1)
> pseudomenses (P54.6)

N93.0   **Postcoital and contact bleeding** ♀

N93.1   **Pre-pubertal vaginal bleeding** ♀ ◀

N93.8   **Other specified abnormal uterine and vaginal bleeding** ♀
Dysfunctional or functional uterine or vaginal bleeding NOS

N93.9   **Abnormal uterine and vaginal bleeding, unspecified** ♀

● **N94**   **Pain and other conditions associated with female genital organs and menstrual cycle**

N94.0   **Mittelschmerz** ♀
Ovulation pain

● **N94.1**   **Dyspareunia**
Painful intercourse/coitus

> **Excludes1**   psychogenic dyspareunia (F52.6)

N94.10   **Unspecified dyspareunia** ♀ ◀

N94.11   **Superficial (introital) dyspareunia** ♀ ◀

N94.12   **Deep dyspareunia** ♀ ◀

N94.19   **Other specified dyspareunia** ♀ ◀

N94.2   **Vaginismus** ♀
Vagina tightness

> **Excludes1**   psychogenic vaginismus (F52.5)

N94.3   **Premenstrual tension syndrome** ♀
AKA: PMS
Premenstrual dysphoric disorder

> Code also associated menstrual migraine (G43.82-, G43.83-)

> **Excludes1**   Premenstrual dysphoric disorder (F32.81) ◀

N94.4   **Primary dysmenorrhea** ♀
Lifelong painful menstruation

N94.5   **Secondary dysmenorrhea** ♀
Later onset of painful menstruation

N94.6   **Dysmenorrhea, unspecified** ♀

> **Excludes1**   psychogenic dysmenorrhea (F45.8)

● **N94.8**   **Other specified conditions associated with female genital organs and menstrual cycle**

● **N94.81**   **Vulvodynia**

N94.810   **Vulvar vestibulitis** ♀

N94.818   **Other vulvodynia** ♀

N94.819   **Vulvodynia, unspecified** ♀
Vulvodynia NOS

N94.89   **Other specified conditions associated with female genital organs and menstrual cycle** ♀

N94.9   **Unspecified condition associated with female genital organs and menstrual cycle** ♀

● **N95**   **Menopausal and other perimenopausal disorders**
Menopausal and other perimenopausal disorders due to naturally occurring (age-related) menopause and perimenopause

> **Excludes1**   excessive bleeding in the premenopausal period (N92.4)
> menopausal and perimenopausal disorders due to artificial or premature menopause (E89.4-, E28.31-)
> premature menopause (E28.31-)

> **Excludes2**   postmenopausal osteoporosis (M81.0-)
> postmenopausal osteoporosis with current pathological fracture (M80.0-)
> postmenopausal urethritis (N34.2)

N95.0   **Postmenopausal bleeding** ♀

N95.1   **Menopausal and female climacteric states** ♀
Symptoms such as flushing, sleeplessness, headache, lack of concentration, associated with natural (age-related) menopause

> Use additional code for associated symptoms

> **Excludes1**   asymptomatic menopausal state (Z78.0)
> symptoms associated with artificial menopause (E89.41)
> symptoms associated with premature menopause (E28.310)

N95.2   **Postmenopausal atrophic vaginitis** ♀
Senile (atrophic) vaginitis

N95.8   **Other specified menopausal and perimenopausal disorders** ♀

N95.9   **Unspecified menopausal and perimenopausal disorder** ♀

N96   **Recurrent pregnancy loss** ♀
Investigation or care in a nonpregnant woman with history of recurrent pregnancy loss

> **Excludes1**   recurrent pregnancy loss with current pregnancy (O26.2-)

● **N97**   **Female infertility**

> **Includes**   inability to achieve a pregnancy
> sterility, female NOS

> **Excludes1**   female infertility associated with:
> hypopituitarism (E23.0)
> Stein-Leventhal syndrome (E28.2)

> **Excludes2**   incompetence of cervix uteri (N88.3)

N97.0   **Female infertility associated with anovulation** ♀

N97.1   **Female infertility of tubal origin** ♀
Female infertility associated with congenital anomaly of tube
Female infertility due to tubal block
Female infertility due to tubal occlusion
Female infertility due to tubal stenosis

N97.2   **Female infertility of uterine origin** ♀
Female infertility associated with congenital anomaly of uterus
Female infertility due to nonimplantation of ovum

N97.8   **Female infertility of other origin** ♀

N97.9   **Female infertility, unspecified** ♀

● **N98   Complications associated with artificial fertilization**
> (Ex:) For category N98 CC codes unless otherwise indicated: D78.81-D78.89, E36.8,
> E89.810-E89.89, H59.011-H59.019, H59.031-H59.099, H59.811-H59.89,
> H95.811-H95.89, I97.3, L76.81-L76.82, M96.89, N98.1-N98.9, T81.82X[A],
> T81.89X-T81.9XX[A]

  N98.0   Infection associated with artificial insemination ♀ 🦠
  > (Ex:) N98.0, T80.211-T80.29X[A], T82.7XX[A], T88.0XX[A]

  N98.1   Hyperstimulation of ovaries ♀ 🦠
  > Hyperstimulation of ovaries NOS
  > Hyperstimulation of ovaries associated with induced
  >   ovulation

  **N98.2   Complications of attempted introduction of fertilized
             ovum following in vitro fertilization** ♀ 🦠

  **N98.3   Complications of attempted introduction of embryo in
             embryo transfer** ♀ 🦠

  **N98.8   Other complications associated with artificial
             fertilization** ♀ 🦠

  **N98.9   Complication associated with artificial fertilization,
             unspecified** ♀ 🦠

INTRAOPERATIVE AND POSTPROCEDURAL COMPLICATIONS AND DISORDERS OF GENITOURINARY SYSTEM, NOT ELSEWHERE CLASSIFIED (N99)

● **N99   Intraoperative and postprocedural complications and disorders
           of genitourinary system, not elsewhere classified**
  > **Excludes2**   irradiation cystitis (N30.4-)
  >   postoophorectomy osteoporosis with current
  >   pathological fracture (M80.8-)
  >   postoophorectomy osteoporosis without current
  >   pathological fracture (M81.8)

  N99.0   Postprocedural (acute) (chronic) kidney failure
  > Use additional code to type of kidney disease

● **N99.1   Postprocedural urethral stricture**
  > Postcatheterization urethral stricture

  ● **N99.11   Postprocedural urethral stricture, male**

    **N99.110   Postprocedural urethral stricture,
                 male, meatal** ♂

    **N99.111   Postprocedural bulbous urethral
                 stricture** ♂

    **N99.112   Postprocedural membranous urethral
                 stricture** ♂

    **N99.113   Postprocedural anterior bulbous
                 urethral stricture** ♂ ◀▥

    **N99.114   Postprocedural urethral stricture,
                 male, unspecified** ♂

    **N99.115   Postprocedural fossa navicularis
                 urethral stricture** ◀

  N99.12   Postprocedural urethral stricture, female ♀

  N99.2   Postprocedural adhesions of vagina ♀

  N99.3   Prolapse of vaginal vault after hysterectomy ♀

  N99.4   Postprocedural pelvic peritoneal adhesions
  > **Excludes2**   pelvic peritoneal adhesions NOS (N73.6)
  >   postinfective pelvic peritoneal adhesions
  >   (N73.6)

● **N99.5   Complications of stoma of urinary tract**
  > **Excludes2**   mechanical complication of urinary
  >   catheter (T83.0-) ◀▥

  ● **N99.51   Complication of cystostomy**

    N99.510   Cystostomy hemorrhage 🦠
    > (Ex:) D78.81-D78.89, E36.8, E89.810-E89.89,
    > H59.011-H59.019, H59.031-H59.099,
    > H59.811-H59.89, H95.811-H95.89, I97.3,
    > L76.81-L76.82, M96.89, N32.89, N33,
    > N98.1-N98.9, N99.510-N99.518, T81.82X[A],
    > T81.89X-T81.9XX[A], T83.010[A], T83.020[A],
    > T83.030[A], T83.090[A], T83.110-T83.29X[A],
    > T83.410-T83.69X[A], T83.712-T83.714[A],
    > T83.718[A], T83.719A, T83.722-T83.724[A],
    > T83.728-T83.9XX[A], T85.310-T85.311[A],
    > T85.320-T85.321[A], T85.390-T85.391[A],
    > T85.510-T85.9XX[A], T85.810D, T85.820D,
    > T85.830D, T85.840D, T85.850D, T85.860D,
    > T85.890D, T86.820-T86.829, T86.842-T86.849

    N99.511   Cystostomy infection 🦠
    > (Ex:) D78.81-D78.89, E36.8, E89.810-E89.89,
    > H59.011-H59.019, H59.031-H59.099,
    > H59.811-H59.89, H95.811-H95.89, I97.3,
    > L76.81-L76.82, M96.89, N32.89, N33, N39.0,
    > N98.1-N98.9, N99.510-N99.518, R82.71,
    > T81.82X[A], T81.89X-T81.9XX[A], T83.010[A],
    > T83.020[A], T83.030[A], T83.090[A],
    > T83.110-T83.29X[A], T83.410-T83.69X[A],
    > T83.712-T83.714[A], T83.718[A], T83.719A,
    > T83.722A-T83.724A, T83.728-T83.9XX[A],
    > T85.310-T85.311[A], T85.320-T85.321[A],
    > T85.390-T85.391[A], T85.510-T85.9XX[A],
    > T85.810D, T85.820D, T85.830D, T85.840D,
    > T85.850D, T85.860D, T85.890D,
    > T86.842-T86.849

    N99.512   Cystostomy malfunction 🦠
    > (Ex:) D78.81-D78.89, E36.8, E89.810-E89.89,
    > H59.011-H59.019, H59.031-H59.099,
    > H59.811-H59.89, H95.811-H95.89, I97.3,
    > L76.81-L76.82, M96.89, N32.89, N33,
    > N98.1-N98.9, N99.510-N99.518, T81.82XA,
    > T81.89XA-T81.9XXA, T83.010[A], T83.020[A],
    > T83.030[A], T83.090[A], T83.110-T83.29X[A],
    > T83.410-T83.69X[A], T83.712-T83.714[A],
    > T83.718[A], T83.719A, T83.722A-T83.724A,
    > T83.728-T83.9XX[A]

    N99.518   Other cystostomy complication 🦠
    > (Ex:) See N99.510

  ● **N99.52   Complication of incontinent external stoma of
                urinary tract** ◀▥

    **N99.520   Hemorrhage of incontinent external
                 stoma of urinary tract** ◀▥

    **N99.521   Infection of incontinent external
                 stoma of urinary tract** ◀▥

    **N99.522   Malfunction of incontinent external
                 stoma of urinary tract** ◀▥

    **N99.523   Herniation of incontinent stoma of
                 urinary tract** ◀

    **N99.524   Stenosis of incontinent stoma of
                 urinary tract** ◀

    **N99.528   Other complication of incontinent
                 external stoma of urinary tract** ◀▥

N Newborn Age: 0   **P** Pediatric Age: 0–17   **M** Maternity DX: 12–55   **A** Adult Age: 15–124   ♀ Females Only   ♂ Males Only

🦠 Complication\Comorbidity   🦠 Major C\C   (Ex:) CC/MCC Exclusions   🦠 Hospital-Acquired Condition

1111

● **N99.53**   **Complication of continent stoma of urinary tract** ◀▥

    N99.530   Hemorrhage of continent stoma of urinary tract ◀▥

    N99.531   Infection of continent stoma of urinary tract ◀▥

    N99.532   Malfunction of continent stoma of urinary tract ◀▥

    N99.533   Herniation of continent stoma of urinary tract ◀

    N99.534   Stenosis of continent stoma of urinary tract ◀

    N99.538   Other complication of continent stoma of urinary tract ◀▥

● **N99.6**   **Intraoperative hemorrhage and hematoma of a genitourinary system organ or structure complicating a procedure**

> **Excludes1**   intraoperative hemorrhage and hematoma of a genitourinary system organ or structure due to accidental puncture or laceration during a procedure (N99.7-)

Ex) **For category N99.6 CC codes:** H95.811-H95.89, I85.01, I85.11, I97.3, K21.9, K22.8, K23-K25.0, K25.2, K25.4, K25.6, K26.0, K26.2, K26.4, K26.6, K27.0, K27.2, K27.4, K27.6, K28.0, K28.2, K28.4, K28.6, K29.01, K29.21, K29.31, K29.41, K29.51, K29.61, K29.71, K29.81, K29.91, K31.811, K55.21, K57.01, K57.11, K57.13, K57.21, K57.31, K57.33, K57.41, K57.51, K57.53, K57.81, K57.91, K57.93, K62.5, K92.0-K92.2, M96.89, N98.1-N98.9, N99.61-N99.62, N99.820-N99.821, N99.840-N99.843, P54.1-P54.3, T81.10X-T81.19X[A], T81.82X[A], T81.89X-T81.9XX[A]

   N99.61   Intraoperative hemorrhage and hematoma of a genitourinary system organ or structure complicating a genitourinary system procedure 🔖

   N99.62   Intraoperative hemorrhage and hematoma of a genitourinary system organ or structure complicating other procedure 🔖

● **N99.7**   **Accidental puncture and laceration of a genitourinary system organ or structure during a procedure**

Ex) **For category N99.7 CC codes:** D78.11-D78.12, D78.81-D78.89, E36.11-E36.8, E89.810-E89.89, G96.11, G97.41-G97.49, H59.011-H59.019, H59.031-H59.099, H59.211-H59.229, H59.811-H59.89, H95.31-H95.32, H95.811-H95.89, I97.3, I97.51-I97.52, J95.71-J95.72, K91.71-K91.72, L76.11-L76.12, L76.81-L76.82, M96.820-M96.821, M96.89, N98.1-N98.9, N99.71-N99.72, T81.82X[A], T81.89X-T81.9XX[A]

   N99.71   Accidental puncture and laceration of a genitourinary system organ or structure during a genitourinary system procedure 🔖

   N99.72   Accidental puncture and laceration of a genitourinary system organ or structure during other procedure 🔖

● **N99.8**   **Other intraoperative and postprocedural complications and disorders of genitourinary system**

   N99.81   Other intraoperative complications of genitourinary system

● **N99.82**   Postprocedural hemorrhage of a genitourinary system organ or structure following a procedure ◀▥

> Ex) **For category N99.82 CC codes:** See N99.6

    N99.820   Postprocedural hemorrhage of a genitourinary system organ or structure following a genitourinary system procedure 🔖 ◀▥

    N99.821   Postprocedural hemorrhage of a genitourinary system organ or structure following other procedure 🔖 ◀▥

   N99.83   Residual ovary syndrome ♀

● **N99.84**   Postprocedural hematoma and seroma of a genitourinary system organ or structure following a procedure ◀

> Ex) **For category N99.84 CC codes:** See N99.6

    N99.840   Postprocedural hematoma of a genitourinary system organ or structure following a genitourinary system procedure 🔖 ◀

    N99.841   Postprocedural hematoma of a genitourinary system organ or structure following other procedure 🔖 ◀

    N99.842   Postprocedural seroma of a genitourinary system organ or structure following a genitourinary system procedure 🔖 ◀

    N99.843   Postprocedural seroma of a genitourinary system organ or structure following other procedure 🔖 ◀

   N99.89   Other postprocedural complications and disorders of genitourinary system

◀ New   ◀▥ Revised   ~~deleted~~ Deleted   Excludes 1   Excludes 2   Includes   Use additional   Code first   Code also   Unspecified

OGCR Official Guidelines   ● Unacceptable Principal Diagnosis   X Assign placeholder X   ● Use Additional Character(s)   ▶ Manifestation Code   **Coding Clinic**

CHAPTER 15

PREGNANCY, CHILDBIRTH AND THE PUERPERIUM (O00-O9A)

OGCR Chapter-Specific Coding Guidelines

15. Chapter 15: Pregnancy, Childbirth, and the Puerperium (O00-O9A)

a. General Rules for Obstetric Cases

1) Codes from chapter 15 and sequencing priority

Obstetric cases require codes from chapter 15, codes in the range O00-O9A, Pregnancy, Childbirth, and the Puerperium. Chapter 15 codes have sequencing priority over codes from other chapters. Additional codes from other chapters may be used in conjunction with chapter 15 codes to further specify conditions. Should the provider document that the pregnancy is incidental to the encounter, then code Z33.1, Pregnant state, incidental, should be used in place of any chapter 15 codes. It is the provider's responsibility to state that the condition being treated is not affecting the pregnancy.

2) Chapter 15 codes used only on the maternal record

Chapter 15 codes are to be used only on the maternal record, never on the record of the newborn.

3) Final character for trimester

The majority of codes in Chapter 15 have a final character indicating the trimester of pregnancy. The timeframes for the trimesters are indicated at the beginning of the chapter. If trimester is not a component of a code it is because the condition always occurs in a specific trimester, or the concept of trimester of pregnancy is not applicable. Certain codes have characters for only certain trimesters because the condition does not occur in all trimesters, but it may occur in more than just one.

Assignment of the final character for trimester should be based on the provider's documentation of the trimester (or number of weeks) for the current admission/encounter. This applies to the assignment of trimester for pre-existing conditions as well as those that develop during or are due to the pregnancy. The provider's documentation of the number of weeks may be used to assign the appropriate code identifying the trimester.

Whenever delivery occurs during the current admission, and there is an "in childbirth" option for the obstetric complication being coded, the "in childbirth" code should be assigned.

4) Selection of trimester for inpatient admissions that encompass more than one trimester

In instances when a patient is admitted to a hospital for complications of pregnancy during one trimester and remains in the hospital into a subsequent trimester, the trimester character for the antepartum complication code should be assigned on the basis of the trimester when the complication developed, not the trimester of the discharge. If the condition developed prior to the current admission/encounter or represents a pre-existing condition, the trimester character for the trimester at the time of the admission/encounter should be assigned.

5) Unspecified trimester

Each category that includes codes for trimester has a code for "unspecified trimester." The "unspecified trimester" code should rarely be used, such as when the documentation in the record is insufficient to determine the trimester and it is not possible to obtain clarification.

6) 7th character for Fetus Identification

Where applicable, a 7th character is to be assigned for certain categories (O31, O32, O33.3 - O33.6, O35, O36, O40, O41, O60.1, O60.2, O64, and O69) to identify the fetus for which the complication code applies.

Assign 7th character "0":
- For single gestations
- When the documentation in the record is insufficient to determine the fetus affected and it is not possible to obtain clarification.
- When it is not possible to clinically determine which fetus is affected.

b. Selection of OB Principal or First-listed Diagnosis

1) Routine outpatient prenatal visits

For routine outpatient prenatal visits when no complications are present, a code from category Z34, Encounter for supervision of normal pregnancy, should be used as the first-listed diagnosis. These codes should not be used in conjunction with chapter 15 codes.

2) *Supervision of High-Risk Pregnancy*

Codes from category O09, Supervision of high-risk pregnancy, are intended for use only during the prenatal period. For complications during the labor or delivery episode as a result of a high-risk pregnancy, assign the applicable complication codes from Chapter 15. If there are no complications during the labor or delivery episode, assign code O80, Encounter for full-term uncomplicated delivery.

For routine prenatal outpatient visits for patients with high-risk pregnancies, a code from category O09, Supervision of high-risk pregnancy, should be used as the first-listed diagnosis. Secondary chapter 15 codes may be used in conjunction with these codes if appropriate.

3) Episodes when no delivery occurs

In episodes when no delivery occurs, the principal diagnosis should correspond to the principal complication of the pregnancy which necessitated the encounter. Should more than one complication exist, all of which are treated or monitored, any of the complications codes may be sequenced first.

4) When a delivery occurs

When an obstetric patient is admitted and delivers during that admission, the condition that prompted the admission should be sequenced as the principal diagnosis. If multiple conditions prompted the admission, sequence the one most related to the delivery as the principal diagnosis. A code for any complication of the delivery should be assigned as an additional diagnosis. In cases of cesarean delivery, if the patient was admitted with a condition that resulted in the performance of a cesarean procedure, that condition should be selected as the principal diagnosis. If the reason for the admission was unrelated to the condition resulting in the cesarean delivery, the condition related to the reason for the admission should be selected as the principal diagnosis.

5) Outcome of delivery

A code from category Z37, Outcome of delivery, should be included on every maternal record when a delivery has occurred. These codes are not to be used on subsequent records or on the newborn record.

c. Pre-existing conditions versus conditions due to the pregnancy

Certain categories in Chapter 15 distinguish between conditions of the mother that existed prior to pregnancy (pre-existing) and those that are a direct result of pregnancy. When assigning codes from Chapter 15, it is important to assess if a condition was pre-existing prior to pregnancy or developed during or due to the pregnancy in order to assign the correct code.

Categories that do not distinguish between pre-existing and pregnancy-related conditions may be used for either. It is acceptable to use codes specifically for the puerperium with codes complicating pregnancy and childbirth if a condition arises postpartum during the delivery encounter.

d. Pre-existing hypertension in pregnancy

Category O10, Pre-existing hypertension complicating pregnancy, childbirth and the puerperium, includes codes for hypertensive heart and hypertensive chronic kidney disease. When assigning one of the O10 codes that includes hypertensive heart disease or hypertensive chronic kidney disease, it is necessary to add a secondary code from the appropriate hypertension category to specify the type of heart failure or chronic kidney disease.

See Section I.C.9. Hypertension.

e. Fetal Conditions Affecting the Management of the Mother

1) Codes from categories O35 and O36

Codes from categories O35, Maternal care for known or suspected fetal abnormality and damage, and O36, Maternal care for other fetal problems, are assigned only when the fetal condition is actually responsible for modifying the management of the mother, i.e., by requiring diagnostic studies, additional observation, special care, or termination of pregnancy. The fact that the fetal condition exists does not justify assigning a code from this series to the mother's record.

2) In utero surgery

In cases when surgery is performed on the fetus, a diagnosis code from category O35, Maternal care for known or suspected fetal abnormality and damage, should be assigned identifying the fetal condition. Assign the appropriate procedure code for the procedure performed.

No code from Chapter 16, the perinatal codes, should be used on the mother's record to identify fetal conditions. Surgery performed in utero on a fetus is still to be coded as an obstetric encounter.

f. HIV Infection in Pregnancy, Childbirth and the Puerperium

During pregnancy, childbirth or the puerperium, a patient admitted because of an HIV-related illness should receive a principal diagnosis from subcategory O98.7-, Human immunodeficiency [HIV] disease complicating pregnancy, childbirth and the puerperium, followed by the code(s) for the HIV-related illness(es).

Patients with asymptomatic HIV infection status admitted during pregnancy, childbirth, or the puerperium should receive codes of O98.7- and Z21, Asymptomatic human immunodeficiency virus [HIV] infection status.

g. Diabetes mellitus in pregnancy

Diabetes mellitus is a significant complicating factor in pregnancy. Pregnant women who are diabetic should be assigned a code from category O24, Diabetes mellitus in pregnancy, childbirth, and the puerperium, first, followed by the appropriate diabetes code(s) (E08-E13) from Chapter 4.

h. Long term use of insulin and oral hypoglycemics
Code Z79.4, Long-term (current) use of insulin **or code Z79.84, Long-term (current) use of oral hypoglycemic drugs,** should also be assigned if the diabetes mellitus is being treated with insulin **or oral medications. If the patient is treated with both oral medications and insulin, only the code for insulin-controlled should be assigned.**

i. Gestational (pregnancy induced) diabetes
Gestational (pregnancy induced) diabetes can occur during the second and third trimester of pregnancy in women who were not diabetic prior to pregnancy. Gestational diabetes can cause complications in the pregnancy similar to those of pre-existing diabetes mellitus. It also puts the woman at greater risk of developing diabetes after the pregnancy. Codes for gestational diabetes are in subcategory O24.4, Gestational diabetes mellitus. No other code from category O24, Diabetes mellitus in pregnancy, childbirth, and the puerperium, should be used with a code from O24.4.

The codes under subcategory O24.4 include diet controlled, insulin controlled**, and controlled by oral hypoglycemic drugs.** If a patient with gestational diabetes is treated with both diet and insulin, only the code for insulin-controlled is required. **If a patient with gestational diabetes is treated with both diet and oral hypoglycemic medications, only the code for "controlled by oral hypoglycemic drugs" is required.** Code Z79.4, Long-term (current) use of insulin **or code Z79.84, Long-term (current) use of oral hypoglycemic drugs,** should not be assigned with codes from subcategory O24.4.

An abnormal glucose tolerance in pregnancy is assigned a code from subcategory O99.81, Abnormal glucose complicating pregnancy, childbirth, and the puerperium.

j. Sepsis and septic shock complicating abortion, pregnancy, childbirth and the puerperium
When assigning a chapter 15 code for sepsis complicating abortion, pregnancy, childbirth, and the puerperium, a code for the specific type of infection should be assigned as an additional diagnosis. If severe sepsis is present, a code from subcategory R65.2, Severe sepsis, and code(s) for associated organ dysfunction(s) should also be assigned as additional diagnoses.

k. Puerperal sepsis
Code O85, Puerperal sepsis, should be assigned with a secondary code to identify the causal organism (e.g., for a bacterial infection, assign a code from category B95-B96, Bacterial infections in conditions classified elsewhere). A code from category A40, Streptococcal sepsis, or A41, Other sepsis, should not be used for puerperal sepsis. If applicable, use additional codes to identify severe sepsis (R65.2-) and any associated acute organ dysfunction.

l. Alcohol and tobacco use during pregnancy, childbirth and the puerperium

1) Alcohol use during pregnancy, childbirth and the puerperium
Codes under subcategory O99.31, Alcohol use complicating pregnancy, childbirth, and the puerperium, should be assigned for any pregnancy case when a mother uses alcohol during the pregnancy or postpartum. A secondary code from category F10, Alcohol related disorders, should also be assigned to identify manifestations of the alcohol use.

2) Tobacco use during pregnancy, childbirth and the puerperium
Codes under subcategory O99.33, Smoking (tobacco) complicating pregnancy, childbirth, and the puerperium, should be assigned for any pregnancy case when a mother uses any type of tobacco product during the pregnancy or postpartum. A secondary code from category F17, Nicotine dependence, should also be assigned to identify the type of nicotine dependence.

m. Poisoning, toxic effects, adverse effects and underdosing in a pregnant patient
A code from subcategory O9A.2, Injury, poisoning and certain other consequences of external causes complicating pregnancy, childbirth, and the puerperium, should be sequenced first, followed by the appropriate injury, poisoning, toxic effect, adverse effect or underdosing code, and then the additional code(s) that specifies the condition caused by the poisoning, toxic effect, adverse effect or underdosing.
See Section I.C.19. Adverse effects, poisoning, underdosing and toxic effects.

n. Normal Delivery, Code O80

1) Encounter for full term uncomplicated delivery
Code O80 should be assigned when a woman is admitted for a full-term normal delivery and delivers a single, healthy infant without any complications antepartum, during the delivery, or postpartum during the delivery episode. Code O80 is always a principal diagnosis. It is not to be used if any other code from chapter 15 is needed to describe a current complication of the antenatal, delivery, or perinatal period. Additional codes from other chapters may be used with code O80 if they are not related to or are in any way complicating the pregnancy.

2) Uncomplicated delivery with resolved antepartum complication
Code O80 may be used if the patient had a complication at some point during the pregnancy, but the complication is not present at the time of the admission for delivery.

3) Outcome of delivery for O80
Z37.0, Single live birth, is the only outcome of delivery code appropriate for use with O80.

o. The Peripartum and Postpartum Periods

1) Peripartum and Postpartum periods
The postpartum period begins immediately after delivery and continues for six weeks following delivery. The peripartum period is defined as the last month of pregnancy to five months postpartum.

2) Peripartum and postpartum complication
A postpartum complication is any complication occurring within the six-week period.

3) Pregnancy-related complications after 6 week period
Chapter 15 codes may also be used to describe pregnancy-related complications after the peripartum or postpartum period if the provider documents that a condition is pregnancy related.

4) Admission for routine postpartum care following delivery outside hospital
When the mother delivers outside the hospital prior to admission and is admitted for routine postpartum care and no complications are noted, code Z39.0, Encounter for care and examination of mother immediately after delivery, should be assigned as the principal diagnosis.

5) Pregnancy associated cardiomyopathy
Pregnancy associated cardiomyopathy, code O90.3, is unique in that it may be diagnosed in the third trimester of pregnancy but may continue to progress months after delivery. For this reason, it is referred to as peripartum cardiomyopathy. Code O90.3 is only for use when the cardiomyopathy develops as a result of pregnancy in a woman who did not have pre-existing heart disease.

p. Code O94, Sequelae of complication of pregnancy, childbirth, and the puerperium

1) Code O94
Code O94, Sequelae of complication of pregnancy, childbirth, and the puerperium, is for use in those cases when an initial complication of a pregnancy develops a sequelae requiring care or treatment at a future date.

2) After the initial postpartum period
This code may be used at any time after the initial postpartum period.

3) Sequencing of Code O94
This code, like all sequela codes, is to be sequenced following the code describing the sequelae of the complication.

q. *Termination of Pregnancy and Spontaneous abortions*

1) Abortion with Liveborn Fetus
When an attempted termination of pregnancy results in a liveborn fetus assign code Z33.2, Encounter for elective termination of pregnancy and a code from category Z37, Outcome of Delivery.

2) Retained Products of Conception following an abortion
Subsequent encounters for retained products of conception following a spontaneous abortion or elective termination of pregnancy are assigned the appropriate code from category O03, Spontaneous abortion, or codes O07.4, Failed attempted termination of pregnancy without complication and Z33.2, Encounter for elective termination of pregnancy. This advice is appropriate even when the patient was discharged previously with a discharge diagnosis of complete abortion.

3) Complications leading to abortion
Codes from Chapter 15 may be used as additional codes to identify any documented complications of the pregnancy in conjunction with codes in categories in O07 and O08.

r. Abuse in a pregnant patient
For suspected or confirmed cases of abuse of a pregnant patient, a code(s) from subcategories O9A.3, Physical abuse complicating pregnancy, childbirth, and the puerperium, O9A.4, Sexual abuse complicating pregnancy, childbirth, and the puerperium, and O9A.5, Psychological abuse complicating pregnancy, childbirth, and the puerperium, should be sequenced first, followed by the appropriate codes (if applicable) to identify any associated current injury due to physical abuse, sexual abuse, and the perpetrator of abuse.
See Section I.C.19. Adult and child abuse, neglect and other maltreatment.

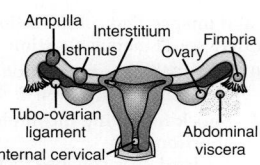

Figure 15-1   Implantation sites of ectopic pregnancy.

Item 15–1 Ectopic pregnancy most often occurs in the fallopian tube. Pregnancy outside the uterus may end in a lifethreatening rupture.

★**(See Plate 375 on page 52.)**

CHAPTER 15

PREGNANCY, CHILDBIRTH AND THE PUERPERIUM (O00-O9A)

Note: CODES FROM THIS CHAPTER ARE FOR USE ONLY ON MATERNAL RECORDS, NEVER ON NEWBORN RECORDS

Codes from this chapter are for use for conditions related to or aggravated by the pregnancy, childbirth, or by the puerperium (maternal causes or obstetric causes)

Trimesters are counted from the first day of the last menstrual period. They are defined as follows:

1st trimester - less than 14 weeks 0 days

2nd trimester - 14 weeks 0 days to less than 28 weeks 0 days

3rd trimester - 28 weeks 0 days until delivery

Use additional code from category Z3A, Weeks of gestation, to identify the specific week of the pregnancy, if known. ◄▥

Excludes1   supervision of normal pregnancy (Z34.-)

Excludes2   mental and behavioral disorders associated with the puerperium (F53)
obstetrical tetanus (A34)
postpartum necrosis of pituitary gland (E23.0)
puerperal osteomalacia (M83.0)

This chapter contains the following blocks:

O00-O08	Pregnancy with abortive outcome
O09	Supervision of high risk pregnancy
O10-O16	Edema, proteinuria and hypertensive disorders in pregnancy, childbirth and the puerperium
O20-O29	Other maternal disorders predominantly related to pregnancy
O30-O48	Maternal care related to the fetus and amniotic cavity and possible delivery problems
O60-O77	Complications of labor and delivery
O80, O82	Encounter for delivery
O85-O92	Complications predominantly related to the puerperium
O94-O9A	Other obstetric conditions, not elsewhere classified

PREGNANCY WITH ABORTIVE OUTCOME (O00-O08)

Excludes1   continuing pregnancy in multiple gestation after abortion of one fetus or more (O31.1-, O31.3-)

● **O00   Ectopic pregnancy**

    Includes   ruptured ectopic pregnancy

    Use additional code from category O08 to identify any associated complication

    (Ex) **For category O00 CC codes:** O00.00-O00.91

 ● **O00.0   Abdominal pregnancy**

      Excludes1   maternal care for viable fetus in abdominal pregnancy (O36.7-)

      O00.00   Abdominal pregnancy without intrauterine pregnancy ♀ 🦠 ◄   M
Abdominal pregnancy NOS ◄

      O00.01   Abdominal pregnancy with intrauterine pregnancy ♀ 🦠 ◄   M

Item 15–2 A **hydatidiform** mole is an overproduction of placental tissue. The tumor secretes a hormone, chorionic gonadotropic hormone (CGH), that indicates a positive pregnancy test. There is no viable fetus. More than 80% of hydatidiform moles are noncancerous.

 ● **O00.1   Tubal pregnancy**
Fallopian pregnancy
Rupture of (fallopian) tube due to pregnancy
Tubal abortion

      O00.10   Tubal pregnancy without intrauterine pregnancy ♀ 🦠 ◄   M
Tubal pregnancy NOS ◄

      O00.11   Tubal pregnancy with intrauterine pregnancy ♀ 🦠 ◄   M

 ● **O00.2   Ovarian pregnancy**

      O00.20   Ovarian pregnancy without intrauterine pregnancy ♀ 🦠 ◄   M
Ovarian pregnancy NOS ◄

      O00.21   Ovarian pregnancy with intrauterine pregnancy ♀ 🦠 ◄   M

 ● **O00.8   Other ectopic pregnancy**
Cervical pregnancy
Cornual pregnancy
Intraligamentous pregnancy
Mural pregnancy

      O00.80   Other ectopic pregnancy without intrauterine pregnancy ♀ 🦠 ◄   M
Other ectopic pregnancy NOS ◄

      O00.81   Other ectopic pregnancy with intrauterine pregnancy ♀ 🦠 ◄   M

 ● **O00.9   Ectopic pregnancy, unspecified**

      O00.90   Unspecified ectopic pregnancy without intrauterine pregnancy ♀ 🦠 ◄   M
Ectopic pregnancy NOS ◄

      O00.91   Unspecified ectopic pregnancy with intrauterine pregnancy ♀ 🦠 ◄   M

● **O01   Hydatidiform mole**

    Use additional code from category O08 to identify any associated complication

    Excludes1   chorioadenoma (destruens) (D39.2)
malignant hydatidiform mole (D39.2)

    O01.0   Classical hydatidiform mole ♀   M
Complete hydatidiform mole

    O01.1   Incomplete and partial hydatidiform mole ♀   M

    O01.9   Hydatidiform mole, unspecified ♀   M
Trophoblastic disease NOS
Vesicular mole NOS

● **O02   Other abnormal products of conception**

    Use additional code from category O08 to identify any associated complication

    Excludes1   papyraceous fetus (O31.0-)

    O02.0   Blighted ovum and nonhydatidiform mole ♀   M
Carneous mole   Molar pregnancy NEC
Fleshy mole   Pathological ovum
Intrauterine mole NOS

    O02.1   Missed abortion ♀   M
Early fetal death, before completion of 20 weeks of gestation, with retention of dead fetus

      Excludes1   failed induced abortion (O07.-)
fetal death (intrauterine) (late) (O36.4)
missed abortion with blighted ovum (O02.0)
missed abortion with hydatidiform mole (O01.-)
missed abortion with nonhydatidiform (O02.0)
missed abortion with other abnormal products of conception (O02.8-)
missed delivery (O36.4)
stillbirth (P95)

N   Newborn Age: 0   **P**   Pediatric Age: 0–17   **M**   Maternity DX: 12–55   **A**   Adult Age: 15–124   ♀   Females Only   ♂   Males Only

🦠 Complication\Comorbidity   🦠 Major C\C   (Ex) CC/MCC Exclusions   🦠 Hospital-Acquired Condition   **1115**

● **O02.8**   **Other specified abnormal products of conception**
     Excludes1   abnormal products of conception with blighted ovum (O02.0)
           abnormal products of conception with hydatidiform mole (O01.-)
           abnormal products of conception with nonhydatidiform mole (O02.0)

     O02.81   **Inappropriate change in quantitative human chorionic gonadotropin (hCG) in early pregnancy** ♀   M
           Biochemical pregnancy
           Chemical pregnancy
           Inappropriate level of quantitative human chorionic gonadotropin (hCG) for gestational age in early pregnancy

     O02.89   **Other abnormal products of conception** ♀   M

   O02.9   **Abnormal product of conception, unspecified** ♀   M

● **O03**   **Spontaneous abortion**
     (Ex) For category **O03** CC codes: G70.1-G72.3, G72.81-G73.7, O11.4, O11.5, O12.04, O12.05, O12.14, O12.15, O12.24, O12.25, O13.4, O13.5, O14.04, O14.05, O14.14, O14.15, O14.24, O14.25, O14.94, O14.95, O16.4, O16.5, O20.0, O20.8, O20.9, O25.10-O25.3, O26.10-O26.93, O29.011-O26.63, O29.8X1-O29.93, O35.7XX0-O35.7XX9, O44.00, O44.53, O45.8X1-O45.93, O75.4, O75.81-O75.9, O80, O90.111-O99.355, O99.511-O99.73, O99.820, O99.824, O99.825, O99.840-O99.845, O99.89, O9A.111-O9A.53, Z33.2

     Note: Incomplete abortion includes retained products of conception following spontaneous abortion.
     Includes   miscarriage

   O03.0   **Genital tract and pelvic infection following incomplete spontaneous abortion** ♀ 🦠   M
           Endometritis following incomplete spontaneous abortion
           Oophoritis following incomplete spontaneous abortion
           Parametritis following incomplete spontaneous abortion
           Pelvic peritonitis following incomplete spontaneous abortion
           Salpingitis following incomplete spontaneous abortion
           Salpingo-oophoritis following incomplete spontaneous abortion
     Excludes1   sepsis following incomplete spontaneous abortion (O03.37)
           urinary tract infection following incomplete spontaneous abortion (O03.38)

   O03.1   **Delayed or excessive hemorrhage following incomplete spontaneous abortion** ♀   M
           Afibrinogenemia following incomplete spontaneous abortion
           Defibrination syndrome following incomplete spontaneous abortion
           Hemolysis following incomplete spontaneous abortion
           Intravascular coagulation following incomplete spontaneous abortion

   O03.2   **Embolism following incomplete spontaneous abortion** ♀ 🦠   M
           Air embolism following incomplete spontaneous abortion
           Amniotic fluid embolism following incomplete spontaneous abortion
           Blood-clot embolism following incomplete spontaneous abortion
           Embolism NOS following incomplete spontaneous abortion
           Fat embolism following incomplete spontaneous abortion
           Pulmonary embolism following incomplete spontaneous abortion
           Pyemic embolism following incomplete spontaneous abortion
           Septic or septicopyemic embolism following incomplete spontaneous abortion
           Soap embolism following incomplete spontaneous abortion

● **O03.3**   **Other and unspecified complications following incomplete spontaneous abortion**
     O03.30   **Unspecified complication following incomplete spontaneous abortion** ♀ 🦠   M
     O03.31   **Shock following incomplete spontaneous abortion** ♀ 🦠   M
           Circulatory collapse following incomplete spontaneous abortion
           Shock (postprocedural) following incomplete spontaneous abortion
         Excludes1   shock due to infection following incomplete spontaneous abortion (O03.37)
     O03.32   **Renal failure following incomplete spontaneous abortion** ♀ 🦠   M
           Kidney failure (acute) following incomplete spontaneous abortion
           Oliguria following incomplete spontaneous abortion
           Renal shutdown following incomplete spontaneous abortion
           Renal tubular necrosis following incomplete spontaneous abortion
           Uremia following incomplete spontaneous abortion
     O03.33   **Metabolic disorder following incomplete spontaneous abortion** ♀ 🦠   M
     O03.34   **Damage to pelvic organs following incomplete spontaneous abortion** ♀ 🦠   M
           Laceration, perforation, tear or chemical damage of bladder following incomplete spontaneous abortion
           Laceration, perforation, tear or chemical damage of bowel following incomplete spontaneous abortion
           Laceration, perforation, tear or chemical damage of broad ligament following incomplete spontaneous abortion
           Laceration, perforation, tear or chemical damage of cervix following incomplete spontaneous abortion
           Laceration, perforation, tear or chemical damage of periurethral tissue following incomplete spontaneous abortion
           Laceration, perforation, tear or chemical damage of uterus following incomplete spontaneous abortion
           Laceration, perforation, tear or chemical damage of vagina following incomplete spontaneous abortion
     O03.35   **Other venous complications following incomplete spontaneous abortion** ♀ 🦠   M
     O03.36   **Cardiac arrest following incomplete spontaneous abortion** ♀ 🦠   M
     O03.37   **Sepsis following incomplete spontaneous abortion** ♀ 🦠   M
         Use additional code to identify infectious agent (B95-B97)
         Use additional code to identify severe sepsis, if applicable (R65.2-)
         Excludes1   septic or septicopyemic embolism following incomplete spontaneous abortion (O03.2)
     O03.38   **Urinary tract infection following incomplete spontaneous abortion** ♀ 🦠   M
           Cystitis following incomplete spontaneous abortion
     O03.39   **Incomplete spontaneous abortion with other complications** ♀ 🦠   M
   O03.4   **Incomplete spontaneous abortion without complication** ♀   M

◀ New   ◀▪▪ Revised   ~~deleted~~ Deleted   Excludes 1   Excludes 2   Includes   Use additional   Code first   Code also   Unspecified
OGCR Official Guidelines   ● Unacceptable Principal Diagnosis   X Assign placeholder X   ● Use Additional Character(s)   ▶ Manifestation Code   **Coding Clinic**

O03.5 **Genital tract and pelvic infection following complete or unspecified spontaneous abortion** ♀ 🦠   **M**

     Endometritis following complete or unspecified spontaneous abortion

     Oophoritis following complete or unspecified spontaneous abortion

     Parametritis following complete or unspecified spontaneous abortion

     Pelvic peritonitis following complete or unspecified spontaneous abortion

     Salpingitis following complete or unspecified spontaneous abortion

     Salpingo-oophoritis following complete or unspecified spontaneous abortion

     Excludes1   sepsis following complete or unspecified spontaneous abortion (O03.87)

           urinary tract infection following complete or unspecified spontaneous abortion (O03.88)

O03.6 **Delayed or excessive hemorrhage following complete or unspecified spontaneous abortion** ♀   **M**

     Afibrinogenemia following complete or unspecified spontaneous abortion

     Defibrination syndrome following complete or unspecified spontaneous abortion

     Hemolysis following complete or unspecified spontaneous abortion

     Intravascular coagulation following complete or unspecified spontaneous abortion

O03.7 **Embolism following complete or unspecified spontaneous abortion** ♀ 🦠   **M**

     Air embolism following complete or unspecified spontaneous abortion

     Amniotic fluid embolism following complete or unspecified spontaneous abortion

     Blood-clot embolism following complete or unspecified spontaneous abortion

     Embolism NOS following complete or unspecified spontaneous abortion

     Fat embolism following complete or unspecified spontaneous abortion

     Pulmonary embolism following complete or unspecified spontaneous abortion

     Pyemic embolism following complete or unspecified spontaneous abortion

     Septic or septicopyemic embolism following complete or unspecified spontaneous abortion

     Soap embolism following complete or unspecified spontaneous abortion

● O03.8 **Other and unspecified complications following complete or unspecified spontaneous abortion**

    O03.80 **Unspecified complication following complete or unspecified spontaneous abortion** ♀ 🦠   **M**

    O03.81 **Shock following complete or unspecified spontaneous abortion** ♀ 🦠   **M**

        Circulatory collapse following complete or unspecified spontaneous abortion

        Shock (postprocedural) following complete or unspecified spontaneous abortion

        Excludes1   shock due to infection following complete or unspecified spontaneous abortion (O03.87)

O03.82 **Renal failure following complete or unspecified spontaneous abortion** ♀ 🦠   **M**

     Kidney failure (acute) following complete or unspecified spontaneous abortion

     Oliguria following complete or unspecified spontaneous abortion

     Renal shutdown following complete or unspecified spontaneous abortion

     Renal tubular necrosis following complete or unspecified spontaneous abortion

     Uremia following complete or unspecified spontaneous abortion

O03.83 **Metabolic disorder following complete or unspecified spontaneous abortion** ♀ 🦠   **M**

O03.84 **Damage to pelvic organs following complete or unspecified spontaneous abortion** ♀ 🦠   **M**

     Laceration, perforation, tear or chemical damage of bladder following complete or unspecified spontaneous abortion

     Laceration, perforation, tear or chemical damage of bowel following complete or unspecified spontaneous abortion

     Laceration, perforation, tear or chemical damage of broad ligament following complete or unspecified spontaneous abortion

     Laceration, perforation, tear or chemical damage of cervix following complete or unspecified spontaneous abortion

     Laceration, perforation, tear or chemical damage of periurethral tissue following complete or unspecified spontaneous abortion

     Laceration, perforation, tear or chemical damage of uterus following complete or unspecified spontaneous abortion

     Laceration, perforation, tear or chemical damage of vagina following complete or unspecified spontaneous abortion

O03.85 **Other venous complications following complete or unspecified spontaneous abortion** ♀ 🦠   **M**

O03.86 **Cardiac arrest following complete or unspecified spontaneous abortion** ♀ 🦠   **M**

O03.87 **Sepsis following complete or unspecified spontaneous abortion** ♀ 🦠   **M**

     Use additional code to identify infectious agent (B95-B97)

     Use additional code to identify severe sepsis, if applicable (R65.2-)

     Excludes1   septic or septicopyemic embolism following complete or unspecified spontaneous abortion (O03.7)

O03.88 **Urinary tract infection following complete or unspecified spontaneous abortion** ♀ 🦠   **M**

     Cystitis following complete or unspecified spontaneous abortion

O03.89 **Complete or unspecified spontaneous abortion with other complications** ♀ 🦠   **M**

O03.9 **Complete or unspecified spontaneous abortion without complication** ♀   **M**

     Miscarriage NOS

     Spontaneous abortion NOS

N Newborn Age: 0   **P** Pediatric Age: 0–17   **M** Maternity DX: 12–55   **A** Adult Age: 15–124   ♀ Females Only   ♂ Males Only

🦠 Complication\Comorbidity   🦠 Major C\C   Ⓔ⁓ CC/MCC Exclusions   🦠 Hospital-Acquired Condition   **1117**

● **O04   Complications following (induced) termination of pregnancy**

    Includes   complications following (induced) termination of pregnancy

    Excludes1   encounter for elective termination of pregnancy, uncomplicated (Z33.2)

                     failed attempted termination of pregnancy (O07.-)

    (Ex:) For category O04 CC codes unless otherwise indicated: See O03

O04.5   Genital tract and pelvic infection following (induced) termination of pregnancy ♀ 🔹   M

     Endometritis following (induced) termination of pregnancy

     Oophoritis following (induced) termination of pregnancy

     Parametritis following (induced) termination of pregnancy

     Pelvic peritonitis following (induced) termination of pregnancy

     Salpingitis following (induced) termination of pregnancy

     Salpingo-oophoritis following (induced) termination of pregnancy

    Excludes1   sepsis following (induced) termination of pregnancy (O04.87)

                     urinary tract infection following (induced) termination of pregnancy (O04.88)

O04.6   Delayed or excessive hemorrhage following (induced) termination of pregnancy ♀   M

     Afibrinogenemia following (induced) termination of pregnancy

     Defibrination syndrome following (induced) termination of pregnancy

     Hemolysis following (induced) termination of pregnancy

     Intravascular coagulation following (induced) termination of pregnancy

O04.7   Embolism following (induced) termination of pregnancy ♀ 🔹   M

     Air embolism following (induced) termination of pregnancy

     Amniotic fluid embolism following (induced) termination of pregnancy

     Blood-clot embolism following (induced) termination of pregnancy

     Embolism NOS following (induced) termination of pregnancy

     Fat embolism following (induced) termination of pregnancy

     Pulmonary embolism following (induced) termination of pregnancy

     Pyemic embolism following (induced) termination of pregnancy

     Septic or septicopyemic embolism following (induced) termination of pregnancy

     Soap embolism following (induced) termination of pregnancy

● **O04.8   (Induced) termination of pregnancy with other and unspecified complications**

    O04.80   (Induced) termination of pregnancy with unspecified complications ♀ 🔹   M

    O04.81   Shock following (induced) termination of pregnancy ♀ 🔹   M

         Circulatory collapse following (induced) termination of pregnancy

         Shock (postprocedural) following (induced) termination of pregnancy

        Excludes1   shock due to infection following (induced) termination of pregnancy (O04.87)

O04.82   Renal failure following (induced) termination of pregnancy ♀ 🔹   M

     Kidney failure (acute) following (induced) termination of pregnancy

     Oliguria following (induced) termination of pregnancy

     Renal shutdown following (induced) termination of pregnancy

     Renal tubular necrosis following (induced) termination of pregnancy

     Uremia following (induced) termination of pregnancy

O04.83   Metabolic disorder following (induced) termination of pregnancy ♀ 🔹   M

O04.84   Damage to pelvic organs following (induced) termination of pregnancy ♀ 🔹   M

     Laceration, perforation, tear or chemical damage of bladder following (induced) termination of pregnancy

     Laceration, perforation, tear or chemical damage of bowel following (induced) termination of pregnancy

     Laceration, perforation, tear or chemical damage of broad ligament following (induced) termination of pregnancy

     Laceration, perforation, tear or chemical damage of cervix following (induced) termination of pregnancy

     Laceration, perforation, tear or chemical damage of periurethral tissue following (induced) termination of pregnancy

     Laceration, perforation, tear or chemical damage of uterus following (induced) termination of pregnancy

     Laceration, perforation, tear or chemical damage of vagina following (induced) termination of pregnancy

O04.85   Other venous complications following (induced) termination of pregnancy ♀ 🔹   M

O04.86   Cardiac arrest following (induced) termination of pregnancy ♀ 🔹   M

O04.87   Sepsis following (induced) termination of pregnancy ♀ 🔹   M

    Use additional code to identify infectious agent (B95-B97)

    Use additional code to identify severe sepsis, if applicable (R65.2-)

    Excludes1   septic or septicopyemic embolism following (induced) termination of pregnancy (O04.7)

    (Ex:) O03.0-O07.4, O11.4, O11.5, O12.04, O12.05, O12.14, O12.15, O12.24, O12.25, O13.4, O13.5, O14.04, O14.05, O14.14, O14.15, O14.24, O14.25, O14.94, O14.95, O16.4, O16.5, O20.0-O20.9, O25.10-O25.3, O26.10-O26.13, O26.30-O26.43, O26.63-O26.819, O26.841-O26.86, O26.891-O26.93, O29.011-O29.93, O35.7XX0-O35.7XX9, O44.00-O44.13, O44.20-O44.53, O45.8X1-O45.93, O75.4, O75.81, O75.89-O75.9, O80, O90.89, O99.111-O99.285, O99.330-O99.335, O99.350-O99.355, O99.511-O99.73, O99.820-O99.825, O99.840-O9A.53, Z33.2

O04.88   Urinary tract infection following (induced) termination of pregnancy ♀ 🔹   M

     Cystitis following (induced) termination of pregnancy

O04.89   (Induced) termination of pregnancy with other complications ♀ 🔹   M

◀ New   ◀▦ Revised   ~~deleted~~ Deleted   Excludes 1   Excludes 2   Includes   Use additional   Code first   Code also   Unspecified

OGCR Official Guidelines   ● Unacceptable Principal Diagnosis   X Assign placeholder X   ● Use Additional Character(s)   ▶ Manifestation Code   **Coding Clinic**

● **O07**   **Failed attempted termination of pregnancy**

> | **Includes** | failure of attempted induction of termination of pregnancy |
> | --- | --- |
> | | incomplete elective abortion |

> | **Excludes1** | incomplete spontaneous abortion (O03.0-) |
> | --- | --- |

O07.0   **Genital tract and pelvic infection following failed attempted termination of pregnancy** ♀ 🦠   **M**

Endometritis following failed attempted termination of pregnancy

Oophoritis following failed attempted termination of pregnancy

Parametritis following failed attempted termination of pregnancy

Pelvic peritonitis following failed attempted termination of pregnancy

Salpingitis following failed attempted termination of pregnancy

Salpingo-oophoritis following failed attempted termination of pregnancy

> | **Excludes1** | sepsis following failed attempted termination of pregnancy (O07.37) |
> | --- | --- |
> | | urinary tract infection following failed attempted termination of pregnancy (O07.38) |

(Ex:) O03.0-O07.4, O11.4, O11.5, O12.04, O12.05, O12.14, O12.15, O12.24, O12.25, O13.4, O13.5, O14.04, O14.05, O14.14, O14.15, O14.24, O14.25, O14.94, O14.95, O16.4, O16.5, O20.0-O20.9, O25.10-O25.3, O26.10-O26.13, O26.30-O26.43, O26.63-O26.819, O26.841-O26.86, O26.891-O26.93, O29.011-O29.93, O35.7XX0-O35.7XX9, O44.00-O44.13, O44.20-O44.53, O45.8X1-O45.93, O75.4, O75.81, O75.89-O75.9, O80, O90.89, O99.111-O99.285, O99.330-O99.335, O99.350-O99.355, O99.511-O99.73, O99.820-O99.825, O99.840-O9A.53, Z33.2

O07.1   **Delayed or excessive hemorrhage following failed attempted termination of pregnancy** ♀ 🦠   **M**

Afibrinogenemia following failed attempted termination of pregnancy

Defibrination syndrome following failed attempted termination of pregnancy

Hemolysis following failed attempted termination of pregnancy

Intravascular coagulation following failed attempted termination of pregnancy

(Ex:) O03.0-O07.4, O11.4, O11.5, O12.04, O12.05, O12.14, O12.15, O12.24, O12.25, O13.4, O13.5, O14.04, O14.05, O14.14, O14.15, O14.24, O14.25, O14.94, O14.95, O16.4, O16.5, O20.0-O20.9, O25.10-O25.3, O26.10-O26.13, O26.30-O26.43, O26.63-O26.819, O26.841-O26.86, O26.891-O26.93, O29.011-O29.93, O35.7XX0-O35.7XX9, O44.00-O44.13, O44.20-O44.53, O45.8X1-O45.93, O75.4, O75.81, O75.89-O75.9, O80, O90.89, O99.111-O99.285, O99.330-O99.335, O99.350-O99.355, O99.511-O99.73, O99.820-O99.825, O99.840-O9A.53, Z33.2

O07.2   **Embolism following failed attempted termination of pregnancy** ♀ 🦠   **M**

Air embolism following failed attempted termination of pregnancy

Amniotic fluid embolism following failed attempted termination of pregnancy

Blood-clot embolism following failed attempted termination of pregnancy

Embolism NOS following failed attempted termination of pregnancy

Fat embolism following failed attempted termination of pregnancy

Pulmonary embolism following failed attempted termination of pregnancy

Pyemic embolism following failed attempted termination of pregnancy

Septic or septicopyemic embolism following failed attempted termination of pregnancy

Soap embolism following failed attempted termination of pregnancy

(Ex:) O03.0-O07.4, O11.4, O11.5, O12.04, O12.05, O12.14, O12.15, O12.24, O12.25, O13.4, O13.5, O14.04, O14.05, O14.14, O14.15, O14.24, O14.25, O14.94, O14.95, O16.4, O16.5, O20.0-O20.9, O25.10-O25.3, O26.10-O26.13, O26.30-O26.43, O26.63-O26.819, O26.841-O26.86, O26.891-O26.93, O29.011-O29.93, O35.7XX0-O35.7XX9, O44.00-O44.13, O44.20-O44.53, O45.8X1-O45.93, O75.4, O75.81, O75.89-O75.9, O80, O90.89, O99.111-O99.285, O99.330-O99.335, O99.350-O99.355, O99.511-O99.73, O99.820-O99.825, O99.840-O9A.53, Z33.2

● **O07.3**   **Failed attempted termination of pregnancy with other and unspecified complications**

O07.30   **Failed attempted termination of pregnancy with unspecified complications** ♀ 🦠   **M**

(Ex:) See O03

O07.31   **Shock following failed attempted termination of pregnancy** ♀ 🦠   **M**

Circulatory collapse following failed attempted termination of pregnancy

Shock (postprocedural) following failed attempted termination of pregnancy

> | **Excludes1** | shock due to infection following failed attempted termination of pregnancy (O07.37) |
> | --- | --- |

(Ex:) O03.0-O07.4, O11.4, O11.5, O12.04, O12.05, O12.14, O12.15, O12.24, O12.25, O13.4, O13.5, O14.04, O14.05, O14.14, O14.15, O14.24, O14.25, O14.94, O14.95, O16.4, O16.5, O20.0-O20.9, O25.10-O25.3, O26.10-O26.13, O26.30-O26.43, O26.63-O26.819, O26.841-O26.86, O26.891-O26.93, O29.011-O29.93, O35.7XX0-O35.7XX9, O44.00-O44.13, O44.20-O44.53, O45.8X1-O45.93, O75.4, O75.81, O75.89-O75.9, O80, O90.89, O99.111-O99.285, O99.330-O99.335, O99.350-O99.355, O99.511-O99.73, O99.820-O99.825, O99.840-O9A.53, Z33.2

O07.32   **Renal failure following failed attempted termination of pregnancy** ♀ 🦠   **M**

Kidney failure (acute) following failed attempted termination of pregnancy

Oliguria following failed attempted termination of pregnancy

Renal shutdown following failed attempted termination of pregnancy

Renal tubular necrosis following failed attempted termination of pregnancy

Uremia following failed attempted termination of pregnancy

(Ex:) O03.0-O07.4, O11.4, O11.5, O12.04, O12.05, O12.14, O12.15, O12.24, O12.25, O13.4, O13.5, O14.04, O14.05, O14.14, O14.15, O14.24, O14.25, O14.94, O14.95, O16.4, O16.5, O20.0-O20.9, O25.10-O25.3, O26.10-O26.13, O26.30-O26.43, O26.63-O26.819, O26.841-O26.86, O26.891-O26.93, O29.011-O29.93, O35.7XX0-O35.7XX9, O44.00-O44.13, O44.20-O44.53, O45.8X1-O45.93, O75.4, O75.81, O75.89-O75.9, O80, O90.89, O99.111-O99.285, O99.330-O99.335, O99.350-O99.355, O99.511-O99.73, O99.820-O99.825, O99.840-O9A.53, Z33.2

O07.33   **Metabolic disorder following failed attempted termination of pregnancy** ♀ 🦠   **M**

(Ex:) See O03

O07.34   **Damage to pelvic organs following failed attempted termination of pregnancy** ♀ 🦠   **M**

Laceration, perforation, tear or chemical damage of bladder following failed attempted termination of pregnancy

Laceration, perforation, tear or chemical damage of bowel following failed attempted termination of pregnancy

Laceration, perforation, tear or chemical damage of broad ligament following failed attempted termination of pregnancy

Laceration, perforation, tear or chemical damage of cervix following failed attempted termination of pregnancy

Laceration, perforation, tear or chemical damage of periurethral tissue following failed attempted termination of pregnancy

Laceration, perforation, tear or chemical damage of uterus following failed attempted termination of pregnancy

Laceration, perforation, tear or chemical damage of vagina following failed attempted termination of pregnancy

(Ex:) O03.0-O07.4, O11.4, O11.5, O12.04, O12.05, O12.14, O12.15, O12.24, O12.25, O13.4, O13.5, O14.04, O14.05, O14.14, O14.15, O14.24, O14.25, O14.94, O14.95, O16.4, O16.5, O20.0-O20.9, O25.10-O25.3, O26.10-O26.13, O26.30-O26.43, O26.63-O26.819, O26.841-O26.86, O26.891-O26.93, O29.011-O29.93, O35.7XX0-O35.7XX9, O44.00-O44.13, O44.20-O44.53, O45.8X1-O45.93, O75.4, O75.81, O75.89-O75.9, O80, O90.89, O99.111-O99.285, O99.330-O99.335, O99.350-O99.355, O99.511-O99.73, O99.820-O99.825, O99.840-O9A.53, Z33.2

N Newborn Age: 0   **P** Pediatric Age: 0–17   **M** Maternity DX: 12–55   **A** Adult Age: 15–124   ♀ Females Only   ♂ Males Only

🦠 Complication\Comorbidity   🦠 Major C\C   (Ex:) CC/MCC Exclusions   🦠 Hospital-Acquired Condition

O07.35   **Other venous complications following failed attempted termination of pregnancy** ♀ 🦠   M
     (Ex) See O03

O07.36   **Cardiac arrest following failed attempted termination of pregnancy** ♀ 🦠   M
     (Ex) See O03

O07.37   **Sepsis following failed attempted termination of pregnancy** ♀ 🦠   M
     Use additional code (B95-B97), to identify infectious agent
     Use additional code (R65.2-) to identify severe sepsis, if applicable

> **Excludes1**   septic or septicopyemic embolism following failed attempted termination of pregnancy (O07.2)

     (Ex) See O07.0

O07.38   **Urinary tract infection following failed attempted termination of pregnancy** ♀ 🦠   M
     Cystitis following failed attempted termination of pregnancy
     (Ex) See O03

O07.39   **Failed attempted termination of pregnancy with other complications** ♀ 🦠   M
     (Ex) See O03

O07.4   **Failed attempted termination of pregnancy without complication** ♀   M

● **O08**   **Complications following ectopic and molar pregnancy**
This category is for use with categories O00-O02 to identify any associated complications.

     (Ex) **For category O08 CC codes unless otherwise indicated:** O08.2-O08.81, O08.83-O08.9, O11.4, O11.5, O12.04, O12.05, O12.14, O12.15, O12.24, O12.25, O13.4, O13.5, O14.04, O14.05, O14.14, O14.15, O14.24, O14.25, O14.94, O14.95, O16.4, O16.5, O20.0-O20.9, O25.10-O25.3, O26.10-O26.13, O26.30-O26.43, O26.63-O26.819, O26.841-O26.86, O26.891-O26.93, O29.011-O29.93, O35.7XX0-O35.7XX9, O44.00-O44.13, O44.20-O44.53, O45.8X1-O45.93, O75.4, O75.81, O75.89-O75.9, O80, O90.89, O99.111-O99.285, O99.330-O99.335, O99.350-O99.355, O99.511-O99.73, O99.820-O99.825, O99.840-O9A.53

O08.0   **Genital tract and pelvic infection following ectopic and molar pregnancy** ♀   M
     Endometritis following ectopic and molar pregnancy
     Oophoritis following ectopic and molar pregnancy
     Parametritis following ectopic and molar pregnancy
     Pelvic peritonitis following ectopic and molar pregnancy
     Salpingitis following ectopic and molar pregnancy
     Salpingo-oophoritis following ectopic and molar pregnancy

> **Excludes1**   sepsis following ectopic and molar pregnancy (O08.82)
>   urinary tract infection (O08.83)

     (Ex) A34, O08.0, O08.2-O08.9, O11.4, O11.5, O12.04, O12.05, O12.14, O12.15, O12.24, O12.25, O13.4, O13.5, O14.04, O14.05, O14.14, O14.15, O14.24, O14.25, O14.94, O14.95, O16.4, O16.5, O20.0-O20.9, O25.10-O25.3, O26.10-O26.13, O26.30-O26.43, O26.63-O26.819, O26.841-O26.86, O26.891-O26.93, O29.011-O29.93, O35.7XX0-O35.7XX9, O44.00-O44.13, O44.20-O44.53, O45.8X1-O45.93, O75.4, O75.81, O75.89-O75.9, O80, O90.89, O99.111-O99.285, O99.330-O99.335, O99.350-O99.355, O99.511-O99.73, O99.820-O99.825, O99.840-O9A.53

O08.1   **Delayed or excessive hemorrhage following ectopic and molar pregnancy** ♀ 🦠   M
     Afibrinogenemia following ectopic and molar pregnancy
     Defibrination syndrome following ectopic and molar pregnancy
     Hemolysis following ectopic and molar pregnancy
     Intravascular coagulation following ectopic and molar pregnancy

> **Excludes1**   delayed or excessive hemorrhage due to incomplete abortion (O03.1)

     (Ex) O08.1-O08.81, O08.83-O08.9, O11.4, O11.5, O12.04, O12.05, O12.14, O12.15, O12.24, O12.25, O13.4, O13.5, O14.04, O14.05, O14.14, O14.15, O14.24, O14.25, O14.94, O14.95, O16.4, O16.5, O20.0-O20.9, O25.10-O25.3, O26.10-O26.13, O26.30-O26.43, O26.63-O26.819, O26.841-O26.86, O26.891-O26.93, O29.011-O29.93, O35.7XX0-O35.7XX9, O44.00-O44.13, O44.20-O44.53, O45.8X1-O45.93, O75.4, O75.81, O75.89-O75.9, O80, O90.89, O99.111-O99.285, O99.330-O99.335, O99.350-O99.355, O99.511-O99.73, O99.820-O99.825, O99.840-O9A.53

O08.2   **Embolism following ectopic and molar pregnancy** ♀ 🦠 M
     Air embolism following ectopic and molar pregnancy
     Amniotic fluid embolism following ectopic and molar pregnancy
     Blood-clot embolism following ectopic and molar pregnancy
     Embolism NOS following ectopic and molar pregnancy
     Fat embolism following ectopic and molar pregnancy
     Pulmonary embolism following ectopic and molar pregnancy
     Pyemic embolism following ectopic and molar pregnancy
     Septic or septicopyemic embolism following ectopic and molar pregnancy
     Soap embolism following ectopic and molar pregnancy

O08.3   **Shock following ectopic and molar pregnancy** ♀ 🦠   M
     Circulatory collapse following ectopic and molar pregnancy
     Shock (postprocedural) following ectopic and molar pregnancy

> **Excludes1**   shock due to infection following ectopic and molar pregnancy (O08.82)

O08.4   **Renal failure following ectopic and molar pregnancy** ♀ 🦠   M
     Kidney failure (acute) following ectopic and molar pregnancy
     Oliguria following ectopic and molar pregnancy
     Renal shutdown following ectopic and molar pregnancy
     Renal tubular necrosis following ectopic and molar pregnancy
     Uremia following ectopic and molar pregnancy

O08.5   **Metabolic disorders following an ectopic and molar pregnancy** ♀ 🦠   M

O08.6   **Damage to pelvic organs and tissues following an ectopic and molar pregnancy** ♀ 🦠   M
     Laceration, perforation, tear or chemical damage of bladder following an ectopic and molar pregnancy
     Laceration, perforation, tear or chemical damage of bowel following an ectopic and molar pregnancy
     Laceration, perforation, tear or chemical damage of broad ligament following an ectopic and molar pregnancy
     Laceration, perforation, tear or chemical damage of cervix following an ectopic and molar pregnancy
     Laceration, perforation, tear or chemical damage of periurethral tissue following an ectopic and molar pregnancy
     Laceration, perforation, tear or chemical damage of uterus following an ectopic and molar pregnancy
     Laceration, perforation, tear or chemical damage of vagina following an ectopic and molar pregnancy

O08.7   Other venous complications following an ectopic and molar pregnancy ♀ 🝊   **M**

● **O08.8**   Other complications following an ectopic and molar pregnancy

     O08.81   Cardiac arrest following an ectopic and molar pregnancy ♀ 🝊   **M**

     O08.82   Sepsis following ectopic and molar pregnancy ♀ 🝊   **M**

         Use additional code (B95-B97), to identify infectious agent

         Use additional code (R65.2-) to identify severe sepsis, if applicable

         Excludes1   septic or septicopyemic embolism following ectopic and molar pregnancy (O08.2)

         (Ex) See O08.0

     O08.83   Urinary tract infection following an ectopic and molar pregnancy ♀ 🝊   **M**

         Cystitis following an ectopic and molar pregnancy

     O08.89   Other complications following an ectopic and molar pregnancy ♀ 🝊   **M**

O08.9   Unspecified complication following an ectopic and molar pregnancy ♀ 🝊   **M**

SUPERVISION OF HIGH RISK PREGNANCY (O09)

● **O09**   Supervision of high risk pregnancy

   ● **O09.0**   Supervision of pregnancy with history of infertility

     ● **O09.00**   Supervision of pregnancy with history of infertility, unspecified trimester ♀   **M**

     ● **O09.01**   Supervision of pregnancy with history of infertility, first trimester ♀   **M**

     ● **O09.02**   Supervision of pregnancy with history of infertility, second trimester ♀   **M**

     ● **O09.03**   Supervision of pregnancy with history of infertility, third trimester ♀   **M**

   ● **O09.1**   Supervision of pregnancy with history of ectopic pregnancy ◀▥

     ● **O09.10**   Supervision of pregnancy with history of ectopic pregnancy, unspecified trimester ♀ ◀▥ **M**

     ● **O09.11**   Supervision of pregnancy with history of ectopic pregnancy, first trimester ♀ ◀▥ **M**

     ● **O09.12**   Supervision of pregnancy with history of ectopic pregnancy, second trimester ♀ ◀▥ **M**

     ● **O09.13**   Supervision of pregnancy with history of ectopic pregnancy, third trimester ♀ ◀▥ **M**

   ● **O09.A**   Supervision of pregnancy with history of molar pregnancy ◀

     ● **O09.A0**   Supervision of pregnancy with history of molar pregnancy, unspecified trimester ♀ ◀ **M**

     ● **O09.A1**   Supervision of pregnancy with history of molar pregnancy, first trimester ♀ ◀ **M**

     ● **O09.A2**   Supervision of pregnancy with history of molar pregnancy, second trimester ♀ ◀ **M**

     ● **O09.A3**   Supervision of pregnancy with history of molar pregnancy, third trimester ♀ ◀ **M**

● **O09.2**   Supervision of pregnancy with other poor reproductive or obstetric history

     Excludes2   pregnancy care for patient with history of recurrent pregnancy loss (O26.2-)

   ● **O09.21**   Supervision of pregnancy with history of pre-term labor

     ● **O09.211**   Supervision of pregnancy with history of pre-term labor, first trimester ♀   **M**

     ● **O09.212**   Supervision of pregnancy with history of pre-term labor, second trimester ♀ **M**

     ● **O09.213**   Supervision of pregnancy with history of pre-term labor, third trimester ♀ **M**

     ● **O09.219**   Supervision of pregnancy with history of pre-term labor, unspecified trimester ♀ **M**

   ● **O09.29**   Supervision of pregnancy with other poor reproductive or obstetric history

         Supervision of pregnancy with history of neonatal death

         Supervision of pregnancy with history of stillbirth

     ● **O09.291**   Supervision of pregnancy with other poor reproductive or obstetric history, first trimester ♀ **M**

     ● **O09.292**   Supervision of pregnancy with other poor reproductive or obstetric history, second trimester ♀ **M**

     ● **O09.293**   Supervision of pregnancy with other poor reproductive or obstetric history, third trimester ♀ **M**

     ● **O09.299**   Supervision of pregnancy with other poor reproductive or obstetric history, unspecified trimester ♀ **M**

● **O09.3**   Supervision of pregnancy with insufficient antenatal care

     Supervision of concealed pregnancy

     Supervision of hidden pregnancy

   ● **O09.30**   Supervision of pregnancy with insufficient antenatal care, unspecified trimester ♀ **M**

   ● **O09.31**   Supervision of pregnancy with insufficient antenatal care, first trimester ♀ **M**

   ● **O09.32**   Supervision of pregnancy with insufficient antenatal care, second trimester ♀ **M**

   ● **O09.33**   Supervision of pregnancy with insufficient antenatal care, third trimester ♀ **M**

● **O09.4**   Supervision of pregnancy with grand multiparity

   ● **O09.40**   Supervision of pregnancy with grand multiparity, unspecified trimester ♀ **M**

   ● **O09.41**   Supervision of pregnancy with grand multiparity, first trimester ♀ **M**

   ● **O09.42**   Supervision of pregnancy with grand multiparity, second trimester ♀ **M**

   ● **O09.43**   Supervision of pregnancy with grand multiparity, third trimester ♀ **M**

● **O09.5**   Supervision of elderly primigravida and multigravida

     Pregnancy for a female 35 years and older at expected date of delivery

   ● **O09.51**   Supervision of elderly primigravida

     ● **O09.511**   Supervision of elderly primigravida, first trimester ♀ **M**

     ● **O09.512**   Supervision of elderly primigravida, second trimester ♀ **M**

     ● **O09.513**   Supervision of elderly primigravida, third trimester ♀ **M**

     ● **O09.519**   Supervision of elderly primigravida, unspecified trimester ♀ **M**

CHAPTER 15 (O00-O9A)

N   Newborn Age: Ø   **P**   Pediatric Age: Ø–17   **M**   Maternity DX: 12–55   **A**   Adult Age: 15–124   ♀   Females Only   ♂   Males Only

🝊   Complication\Comorbidity   🝊   Major C\C   (Ex)   CC/MCC Exclusions   🝊   Hospital-Acquired Condition

1121

- O09.52   Supervision of elderly multigravida
  - O09.521   Supervision of elderly multigravida, first trimester ♀   M
  - O09.522   Supervision of elderly multigravida, second trimester ♀   M
  - O09.523   Supervision of elderly multigravida, third trimester ♀   M
  - O09.529   Supervision of elderly multigravida, unspecified trimester ♀   M
- O09.6   Supervision of young primigravida and multigravida
  - Supervision of pregnancy for a female less than 16 years old at expected date of delivery
  - O09.61   Supervision of young primigravida
    - O09.611   Supervision of young primigravida, first trimester ♀   M
    - O09.612   Supervision of young primigravida, second trimester ♀   M
    - O09.613   Supervision of young primigravida, third trimester ♀   M
    - O09.619   Supervision of young primigravida, unspecified trimester ♀   M
  - O09.62   Supervision of young multigravida
    - O09.621   Supervision of young multigravida, first trimester ♀   M
    - O09.622   Supervision of young multigravida, second trimester ♀   M
    - O09.623   Supervision of young multigravida, third trimester ♀   M
    - O09.629   Supervision of young multigravida, unspecified trimester ♀   M
- O09.7   Supervision of high risk pregnancy due to social problems
  - O09.70   Supervision of high risk pregnancy due to social problems, unspecified trimester ♀   M
  - O09.71   Supervision of high risk pregnancy due to social problems, first trimester ♀   M
  - O09.72   Supervision of high risk pregnancy due to social problems, second trimester ♀   M
  - O09.73   Supervision of high risk pregnancy due to social problems, third trimester ♀   M
- O09.8   Supervision of other high risk pregnancies
  - O09.81   Supervision of pregnancy resulting from assisted reproductive technology
    - Supervision of pregnancy resulting from in-vitro fertilization
    - Excludes2   gestational carrier status (Z33.3) ◄
    - O09.811   Supervision of pregnancy resulting from assisted reproductive technology, first trimester ♀   M
    - O09.812   Supervision of pregnancy resulting from assisted reproductive technology, second trimester ♀   M
    - O09.813   Supervision of pregnancy resulting from assisted reproductive technology, third trimester ♀   M
    - O09.819   Supervision of pregnancy resulting from assisted reproductive technology, unspecified trimester ♀   M
  - O09.82   Supervision of pregnancy with history of in utero procedure during previous pregnancy
    - O09.821   Supervision of pregnancy with history of in utero procedure during previous pregnancy, first trimester ♀   M
    - O09.822   Supervision of pregnancy with history of in utero procedure during previous pregnancy, second trimester ♀   M

- O09.823   Supervision of pregnancy with history of in utero procedure during previous pregnancy, third trimester ♀   M
- O09.829   Supervision of pregnancy with history of in utero procedure during previous pregnancy, unspecified trimester ♀   M
  - Excludes1   supervision of pregnancy affected by in utero procedure during current pregnancy (O35.7)
- O09.89   Supervision of other high risk pregnancies
  - O09.891   Supervision of other high risk pregnancies, first trimester ♀   M
  - O09.892   Supervision of other high risk pregnancies, second trimester ♀   M
  - O09.893   Supervision of other high risk pregnancies, third trimester ♀   M
  - O09.899   Supervision of other high risk pregnancies, unspecified trimester ♀   M
- O09.9   Supervision of high risk pregnancy, unspecified
  - O09.90   Supervision of high risk pregnancy, unspecified, unspecified trimester ♀   M
  - O09.91   Supervision of high risk pregnancy, unspecified, first trimester ♀   M
  - O09.92   Supervision of high risk pregnancy, unspecified, second trimester ♀   M
  - O09.93   Supervision of high risk pregnancy, unspecified, third trimester ♀   M

EDEMA, PROTEINURIA AND HYPERTENSIVE DISORDERS IN PREGNANCY, CHILDBIRTH AND THE PUERPERIUM (O10-O16)

- O10   Pre-existing hypertension complicating pregnancy, childbirth and the puerperium
  - Includes   pre-existing hypertension with pre-existing proteinuria complicating pregnancy, childbirth and the puerperium
  - Excludes2   pre-existing hypertension with superimposed pre-eclampsia complicating pregnancy, childbirth and the puerperium (O11.-)
  - (Ex:) For category O10 CC codes: O10.011-O12.03, O12.04, O12.05, O12.14, O12.15, O12.20-O16.9, O25.10-O26.13, O26.30-O26.43, O26.63-O26.819, O26.841-O26.86, O26.891-O26.93, O29.011-O29.93, O35.7XX0-O35.7XX9, O75.4, O75.81, O75.89-O75.9, O80, O90.89, O99.111-O99.285, O99.330-O99.335, O99.350-O99.355, O99.511-O99.73, O99.820-O99.825, O99.840-O9A.53
  - O10.0   Pre-existing essential hypertension complicating pregnancy, childbirth and the puerperium
    - Any condition in I10 specified as a reason for obstetric care during pregnancy, childbirth or the puerperium
    - O10.01   Pre-existing essential hypertension complicating pregnancy
      - O10.011   Pre-existing essential hypertension complicating pregnancy, first trimester ♀ 🔒   M
      - O10.012   Pre-existing essential hypertension complicating pregnancy, second trimester ♀ 🔒   M
      - O10.013   Pre-existing essential hypertension complicating pregnancy, third trimester ♀ 🔒   M
      - O10.019   Pre-existing essential hypertension complicating pregnancy, unspecified trimester ♀   M
    - O10.02   Pre-existing essential hypertension complicating childbirth ♀ 🔒   M
    - O10.03   Pre-existing essential hypertension complicating the puerperium ♀   M

◄ New   ◄▬ Revised   ~~deleted~~ Deleted   Excludes 1   Excludes 2   Includes   Use additional   Code first   Code also   Unspecified

OGCR Official Guidelines   ● Unacceptable Principal Diagnosis   X Assign placeholder X   ● Use Additional Character(s)   ▶ Manifestation Code   Coding Clinic

● **O10.1** **Pre-existing hypertensive heart disease complicating pregnancy, childbirth and the puerperium**
Any condition in I11 specified as a reason for obstetric care during pregnancy, childbirth or the puerperium
Use additional code from I11 to identify the type of hypertensive heart disease

  ● **O10.11** **Pre-existing hypertensive heart disease complicating pregnancy**

     O10.111 **Pre-existing hypertensive heart disease complicating pregnancy, first trimester** ♀   **M**

     O10.112 **Pre-existing hypertensive heart disease complicating pregnancy, second trimester** ♀   **M**

     O10.113 **Pre-existing hypertensive heart disease complicating pregnancy, third trimester** ♀   **M**

     O10.119 **Pre-existing hypertensive heart disease complicating pregnancy, unspecified trimester** ♀   **M**

     O10.12 **Pre-existing hypertensive heart disease complicating childbirth** ♀   **M**

     O10.13 **Pre-existing hypertensive heart disease complicating the puerperium** ♀   **M**

● **O10.2** **Pre-existing hypertensive chronic kidney disease complicating pregnancy, childbirth and the puerperium**
Any condition in I12 specified as a reason for obstetric care during pregnancy, childbirth or the puerperium
Use additional code from I12 to identify the type of hypertensive chronic kidney disease

  ● **O10.21** **Pre-existing hypertensive chronic kidney disease complicating pregnancy**

     O10.211 **Pre-existing hypertensive chronic kidney disease complicating pregnancy, first trimester** ♀   **M**

     O10.212 **Pre-existing hypertensive chronic kidney disease complicating pregnancy, second trimester** ♀   **M**

     O10.213 **Pre-existing hypertensive chronic kidney disease complicating pregnancy, third trimester** ♀   **M**

     O10.219 **Pre-existing hypertensive chronic kidney disease complicating pregnancy, unspecified trimester** ♀   **M**

     O10.22 **Pre-existing hypertensive chronic kidney disease complicating childbirth** ♀   **M**

     O10.23 **Pre-existing hypertensive chronic kidney disease complicating the puerperium** ♀   **M**

● **O10.3** **Pre-existing hypertensive heart and chronic kidney disease complicating pregnancy, childbirth and the puerperium**
Any condition in I13 specified as a reason for obstetric care during pregnancy, childbirth or the puerperium
Use additional code from I13 to identify the type of hypertensive heart and chronic kidney disease

  ● **O10.31** **Pre-existing hypertensive heart and chronic kidney disease complicating pregnancy**

     O10.311 **Pre-existing hypertensive heart and chronic kidney disease complicating pregnancy, first trimester** ♀   **M**

     O10.312 **Pre-existing hypertensive heart and chronic kidney disease complicating pregnancy, second trimester** ♀   **M**

     O10.313 **Pre-existing hypertensive heart and chronic kidney disease complicating pregnancy, third trimester** ♀   **M**

     O10.319 **Pre-existing hypertensive heart and chronic kidney disease complicating pregnancy, unspecified trimester** ♀   **M**

     O10.32 **Pre-existing hypertensive heart and chronic kidney disease complicating childbirth** ♀   **M**

     O10.33 **Pre-existing hypertensive heart and chronic kidney disease complicating the puerperium** ♀   **M**

● **O10.4** **Pre-existing secondary hypertension complicating pregnancy, childbirth and the puerperium**
Any condition in I15 specified as a reason for obstetric care during pregnancy, childbirth or the puerperium
Use additional code from I15 to identify the type of secondary hypertension

  ● **O10.41** **Pre-existing secondary hypertension complicating pregnancy**

     O10.411 **Pre-existing secondary hypertension complicating pregnancy, first trimester** ♀ 🗘   **M**

     O10.412 **Pre-existing secondary hypertension complicating pregnancy, second trimester** ♀ 🗘   **M**

     O10.413 **Pre-existing secondary hypertension complicating pregnancy, third trimester** ♀ 🗘   **M**

     O10.419 **Pre-existing secondary hypertension complicating pregnancy, unspecified trimester** ♀   **M**

     O10.42 **Pre-existing secondary hypertension complicating childbirth** ♀ 🗘   **M**

     O10.43 **Pre-existing secondary hypertension complicating the puerperium** ♀ 🗘   **M**

● **O10.9** **Unspecified pre-existing hypertension complicating pregnancy, childbirth and the puerperium**

  ● **O10.91** **Unspecified pre-existing hypertension complicating pregnancy**

     O10.911 **Unspecified pre-existing hypertension complicating pregnancy, first trimester** ♀ 🗘   **M**

     O10.912 **Unspecified pre-existing hypertension complicating pregnancy, second trimester** ♀ 🗘   **M**

     O10.913 **Unspecified pre-existing hypertension complicating pregnancy, third trimester** ♀ 🗘   **M**

     O10.919 **Unspecified pre-existing hypertension complicating pregnancy, unspecified trimester** ♀   **M**

     O10.92 **Unspecified pre-existing hypertension complicating childbirth** ♀ 🗘   **M**

     O10.93 **Unspecified pre-existing hypertension complicating the puerperium** ♀   **M**

● **O11** **Pre-existing hypertension with pre-eclampsia**

  Includes   conditions in O10 complicated by pre-eclampsia
pre-eclampsia superimposed pre-existing hypertension

Use additional code from O10 to identify the type of hypertension
(Ex) **For category O11 CC codes:** See O10

  O11.1 **Pre-existing hypertension with pre-eclampsia, first trimester** ♀ 🗘   **M**

  O11.2 **Pre-existing hypertension with pre-eclampsia, second trimester** ♀ 🗘   **M**

  O11.3 **Pre-existing hypertension with pre-eclampsia, third trimester** ♀ 🗘   **M**

  O11.4 **Pre-existing hypertension with pre-eclampsia, complicating childbirth** ♀ ◀   **M**

  O11.5 **Pre-existing hypertension with pre-eclampsia, complicating the puerperium** ♀ ◀   **M**

  O11.9 **Pre-existing hypertension with pre-eclampsia, unspecified trimester** ♀   **M**

N Newborn Age: 0   **P** Pediatric Age: 0–17   **M** Maternity DX: 12–55   **A** Adult Age: 15–124   ♀ Females Only   ♂ Males Only

🗘 Complication\Comorbidity   🗘 Major C\C   (Ex) CC/MCC Exclusions   🗘 Hospital-Acquired Condition

CHAPTER 15 (O00-O9A)

1123

● **O12   Gestational [pregnancy-induced] edema and proteinuria without hypertension**
  (Ex) For category **O12** CC codes: O11.5, O12.05, O12.11-O12.13, O12.15, O12.21-O12.23, O12.25, O13.5, O14.05, O14.15, O14.25, O14.95, O16.5, O26.831-O26.833, O90.89

  ● **O12.0   Gestational edema**
    O12.00   Gestational edema, unspecified trimester ♀   M
    O12.01   Gestational edema, first trimester ♀   M
    O12.02   Gestational edema, second trimester ♀   M
    O12.03   Gestational edema, third trimester ♀   M
    O12.04   Gestational edema, complicating childbirth ♀ ◄   M
    O12.05   Gestational edema, complicating the puerperium ♀ ◄   M

  ● **O12.1   Gestational proteinuria**
    O12.10   Gestational proteinuria, unspecified trimester ♀   M
    O12.11   Gestational proteinuria, first trimester ♀ 🔖   M
    O12.12   Gestational proteinuria, second trimester ♀ 🔖 M
    O12.13   Gestational proteinuria, third trimester ♀ 🔖 M
    O12.14   Gestational proteinuria, complicating childbirth ♀ ◄   M
    O12.15   Gestational proteinuria, complicating the puerperium ♀ ◄   M

  ● **O12.2   Gestational edema with proteinuria**
    O12.20   Gestational edema with proteinuria, unspecified trimester ♀   M
    O12.21   Gestational edema with proteinuria, first trimester ♀ 🔖   M
             CC when PDx is its own CC
    O12.22   Gestational edema with proteinuria, second trimester ♀ 🔖   M
             CC when PDx is its own CC
    O12.23   Gestational edema with proteinuria, third trimester ♀ 🔖   M
             CC when PDx is its own CC
    O12.24   Gestational edema with proteinuria, complicating childbirth ♀ ◄   M
    O12.25   Gestational edema with proteinuria, complicating the puerperium ♀ ◄   M

● **O13   Gestational [pregnancy-induced] hypertension without significant proteinuria**
    Includes   gestational hypertension NOS
                   transient hypertension of pregnancy ◄
    O13.1   Gestational [pregnancy-induced] hypertension without significant proteinuria, first trimester ♀   M
    O13.2   Gestational [pregnancy-induced] hypertension without significant proteinuria, second trimester ♀   M
    O13.3   Gestational [pregnancy-induced] hypertension without significant proteinuria, third trimester ♀   M
    O13.4   Gestational [pregnancy-induced] hypertension without significant proteinuria, complicating childbirth ♀ ◄   M
    O13.5   Gestational [pregnancy-induced] hypertension without significant proteinuria, complicating the puerperium ♀ ◄   M
    O13.9   Gestational [pregnancy-induced] hypertension without significant proteinuria, unspecified trimester ♀   M

● **O14   Pre-eclampsia**
    Excludes1   pre-existing hypertension with pre-eclampsia (O11)
    (Ex) For category **O14** CC codes: See O10
  ● **O14.0   Mild to moderate pre-eclampsia**
    O14.00   Mild to moderate pre-eclampsia, unspecified trimester ♀   M
    O14.02   Mild to moderate pre-eclampsia, second trimester ♀ 🔖   M
    O14.03   Mild to moderate pre-eclampsia, third trimester ♀ 🔖   M

    O14.04   Mild to moderate pre-eclampsia, complicating childbirth ♀ ◄
    O14.05   Mild to moderate pre-eclampsia, complicating the puerperium ♀ ◄   M

  ● **O14.1   Severe pre-eclampsia**
    Excludes1   HELLP syndrome (O14.2-)
    H=hemolysis, EL=elevated liver enzymes, LP=low platelet count
    O14.10   Severe pre-eclampsia, unspecified trimester ♀   M
    O14.12   Severe pre-eclampsia, second trimester ♀ 🔖   M
    O14.13   Severe pre-eclampsia, third trimester ♀ 🔖   M
    O14.14   Severe pre-eclampsia complicating childbirth ♀ ◄   M
    O14.15   Severe pre-eclampsia, complicating the puerperium ♀ ◄   M

  ● **O14.2   HELLP syndrome**
    Severe pre-eclampsia with hemolysis, elevated liver enzymes and low platelet count (HELLP)
    O14.20   HELLP syndrome (HELLP), unspecified trimester ♀   M
    O14.22   HELLP syndrome (HELLP), second trimester ♀ 🔖   M
    O14.23   HELLP syndrome (HELLP), third trimester ♀ 🔖   M
    O14.24   HELLP syndrome, complicating childbirth ♀ ◄   M
    O14.25   HELLP syndrome, complicating the puerperium ♀ ◄   M

  ● **O14.9   Unspecified pre-eclampsia**
    O14.90   Unspecified pre-eclampsia, unspecified trimester ♀   M
    O14.92   Unspecified pre-eclampsia, second trimester ♀ 🔖   M
    O14.93   Unspecified pre-eclampsia, third trimester ♀ 🔖   M
    O14.94   Unspecified pre-eclampsia, complicating childbirth ♀ ◄   M
    O14.95   Unspecified pre-eclampsia, complicating the puerperium ♀ ◄   M

● **O15   Eclampsia**
    Includes   convulsions following conditions in O10-O14 and O16
    (Ex) For category **O15** CC codes: See O10
  ● **O15.0   Eclampsia complicating pregnancy** ◄▥
    O15.00   Eclampsia complicating pregnancy, unspecified trimester ♀ ◄▥   M
    O15.02   Eclampsia complicating pregnancy, second trimester ♀ 🔖 ◄▥   M
    O15.03   Eclampsia complicating pregnancy, third trimester ♀ 🔖 ◄▥   M
    O15.1   Eclampsia complicating labor ♀ 🔖 ◄▥   M
    O15.2   Eclampsia complicating the puerperium ♀ 🔖 ◄▥   M
    O15.9   Eclampsia, unspecified as to time period ♀   M
            Eclampsia NOS

● **O16   Unspecified maternal hypertension**
    (Ex) For category **O16** CC codes: See O10
    O16.1   Unspecified maternal hypertension, first trimester ♀ 🔖 M
    O16.2   Unspecified maternal hypertension, second trimester ♀ 🔖   M
    O16.3   Unspecified maternal hypertension, third trimester ♀ 🔖   M
    O16.4   Unspecified maternal hypertension, complicating childbirth ♀ ◄   M
    O16.5   Unspecified maternal hypertension, complicating the puerperium ♀ ◄   M
    O16.9   Unspecified maternal hypertension, unspecified trimester ♀   M

◄ New   ◄▥ Revised   ~~deleted~~ Deleted   Excludes 1   Excludes 2   Includes   Use additional   Code first   Code also   Unspecified
OGCR Official Guidelines   ● Unacceptable Principal Diagnosis   X Assign placeholder X   ● Use Additional Character(s)   ▶ Manifestation Code   **Coding Clinic**

OTHER MATERNAL DISORDERS PREDOMINANTLY RELATED TO PREGNANCY (O20-O29)

Excludes2   maternal care related to the fetus and amniotic cavity and possible delivery problems (O30-O48)
maternal diseases classifiable elsewhere but complicating pregnancy, labor and delivery, and the puerperium (O98-O99)

● **O20**   **Hemorrhage in early pregnancy**

Includes   hemorrhage before completion of 20 weeks gestation

Excludes1   pregnancy with abortive outcome (O00-O08)

(Ex) **For category O20 CC codes:** O11.4, O11.5, O12.04, O12.05, O12.14, O12.15, O12.24, O12.25, O13.4, O13.5, O14.04, O14.05, O14.14, O14.15, O14.24, O14.25, O14.94, O14.95, O16.4, O16.5, O20.0-O20.9, O25.10-O25.3, O26.10-O26.13, O26.30-O26.43, O26.63-O26.819, O26.841-O26.86, O26.891-O26.93, O29.011-O29.93, O35.7XX0-O35.7XX9, O44.00-O44.13, O44.20-O44.53, O75.4, O75.81, O75.89-O75.9, O80, O90.89, O99.111-O99.119, O99.12-O99.285, O99.330-O99.335, O99.350-O99.355, O99.511-O99.73, O99.820-O99.825, O99.840-O9A.53

O20.0   **Threatened abortion** ♀ 💊   M
Hemorrhage specified as due to threatened abortion

O20.8   **Other hemorrhage in early pregnancy** ♀   M

O20.9   **Hemorrhage in early pregnancy, unspecified** ♀ 💊   M

● **O21**   **Excessive vomiting in pregnancy**

O21.0   **Mild hyperemesis gravidarum** ♀   M
Hyperemesis gravidarum, mild or unspecified, starting before the end of the 20th week of gestation

O21.1   **Hyperemesis gravidarum with metabolic disturbance** ♀   M
Hyperemesis gravidarum, starting before the end of the 20th week of gestation, with metabolic disturbance such as carbohydrate depletion
Hyperemesis gravidarum, starting before the end of the 20th week of gestation, with metabolic disturbance such as dehydration
Hyperemesis gravidarum, starting before the end of the 20th week of gestation, with metabolic disturbance such as electrolyte imbalance

O21.2   **Late vomiting of pregnancy** ♀   M
Excessive vomiting starting after 20 completed weeks of gestation

O21.8   **Other vomiting complicating pregnancy** ♀   M
Vomiting due to diseases classified elsewhere, complicating pregnancy

Use additional code, to identify cause

O21.9   **Vomiting of pregnancy, unspecified** ♀   M

● **O22**   **Venous complications and hemorrhoids in pregnancy**

Excludes1   venous complications of:
     abortion NOS (O03.9)
     ectopic or molar pregnancy (O08.7)
     failed attempted abortion (O07.35)
     induced abortion (O04.85)
     spontaneous abortion (O03.89)

Excludes2   obstetric pulmonary embolism (O88.-)
venous complications and hemorrhoids of childbirth and the puerperium (O87.-)

(Ex) **For category O22 CC codes unless otherwise indicated:** O22.20-O22.93, O25.10-O25.3, O26.10-O26.13, O26.30-O26.43, O26.63-O26.819, O26.841-O26.86, O26.891-O26.93, O29.011-O29.93, O35.7XX0-O35.7XX9, O75.4, O75.81, O75.89-O75.9, O80, O87.0-O87.9, O90.89, O99.111-O99.119, O99.12-O99.285, O99.330-O99.335, O99.350-O99.355, O99.511-O99.73, O99.820-O99.825, O99.840-O9A.53

● **O22.0**   **Varicose veins of lower extremity in pregnancy**
Varicose veins NOS in pregnancy

O22.00   **Varicose veins of lower extremity in pregnancy, unspecified trimester** ♀   M

O22.01   **Varicose veins of lower extremity in pregnancy, first trimester** ♀   M

O22.02   **Varicose veins of lower extremity in pregnancy, second trimester** ♀   M

O22.03   **Varicose veins of lower extremity in pregnancy, third trimester** ♀   M

● **O22.1**   **Genital varices in pregnancy**
Perineal varices in pregnancy
Vaginal varices in pregnancy
Vulval varices in pregnancy

O22.10   **Genital varices in pregnancy, unspecified trimester** ♀   M

O22.11   **Genital varices in pregnancy, first trimester** ♀   M

O22.12   **Genital varices in pregnancy, second trimester** ♀   M

O22.13   **Genital varices in pregnancy, third trimester** ♀ M

● **O22.2**   **Superficial thrombophlebitis in pregnancy**
Phlebitis in pregnancy NOS
Thrombophlebitis of legs in pregnancy
Thrombosis in pregnancy NOS

Use additional code to identify the superficial thrombophlebitis (I80.0-)

(Ex) **For category O22.2 CC codes:** O11.4, O11.5, O12.04, O12.05, O12.14, O12.15, O12.24, O12.25, O13.4, O13.5, O14.04, O14.05, O14.14, O14.15, O14.24, O14.25, O14.94, O14.95, O16.4, O16.5, O22.20-O22.93, O25.10-O25.3, O26.10-O26.13, O26.30-O26.43, O26.63-O26.819, O26.841-O26.86, O26.891-O26.93, O29.011-O29.93, O35.7XX0-O35.7XX9, O75.4, O75.81, O75.89-O75.9, O80, O87.0-O87.9, O90.89, O99.111-O99.119, O99.12-O99.285, O99.330-O99.335, O99.350-O99.355, O99.511-O99.73, O99.820-O99.825, O99.840-O9A.53

O22.20   **Superficial thrombophlebitis in pregnancy, unspecified trimester** ♀ 💊   M

O22.21   **Superficial thrombophlebitis in pregnancy, first trimester** ♀ 💊   M

O22.22   **Superficial thrombophlebitis in pregnancy, second trimester** ♀ 💊   M

O22.23   **Superficial thrombophlebitis in pregnancy, third trimester** ♀ 💊   M

● **O22.3**   **Deep phlebothrombosis in pregnancy**
Deep vein thrombosis, antepartum

Use additional code to identify the deep vein thrombosis (I82.4-, I82.5-, I82.62-. I82.72-)

Use additional code, if applicable, for associated long-term (current) use of anticoagulants (Z79.01)

(Ex) **For category O22.3 CC codes:** See O22.2

O22.30   **Deep phlebothrombosis in pregnancy, unspecified trimester** ♀ 💊   M

O22.31   **Deep phlebothrombosis in pregnancy, first trimester** ♀ 💊   M

O22.32   **Deep phlebothrombosis in pregnancy, second trimester** ♀ 💊   M

O22.33   **Deep phlebothrombosis in pregnancy, third trimester** ♀ 💊   M

● **O22.4**   **Hemorrhoids in pregnancy**

(Ex) **For category O22.4 CC codes:** See O22.2

O22.40   **Hemorrhoids in pregnancy, unspecified trimester** ♀ 💊   M

O22.41   **Hemorrhoids in pregnancy, first trimester** ♀ 💊 M

O22.42   **Hemorrhoids in pregnancy, second trimester** ♀ 💊   M

O22.43   **Hemorrhoids in pregnancy, third trimester** ♀ 💊   M

● **O22.5**   **Cerebral venous thrombosis in pregnancy**
Cerebrovenous sinus thrombosis in pregnancy

(Ex) **For category O22.5 CC codes:** See O22.2

O22.50   **Cerebral venous thrombosis in pregnancy, unspecified trimester** ♀ 💊   M

O22.51   **Cerebral venous thrombosis in pregnancy, first trimester** ♀ 💊   M

O22.52   **Cerebral venous thrombosis in pregnancy, second trimester** ♀ 💊   M

O22.53   **Cerebral venous thrombosis in pregnancy, third trimester** ♀ 💊   M

CHAPTER 15 (O00-O9A)

N   Newborn Age: 0   **P**   Pediatric Age: 0–17   **M**   Maternity DX: 12–55   **A**   Adult Age: 15–124   ♀   Females Only   ♂   Males Only

💊   Complication\Comorbidity   💊   Major C\C   (Ex)   CC/MCC Exclusions   💊   Hospital-Acquired Condition

● **O22.8** **Other venous complications in pregnancy**
　Ⓔⓧ For category O22.8 CC codes: See O22.2

　● **O22.8X** **Other venous complications in pregnancy**
　　O22.8X1 **Other venous complications in pregnancy, first trimester** ♀ 🦠　　M
　　O22.8X2 **Other venous complications in pregnancy, second trimester** ♀ 🦠　　M
　　O22.8X3 **Other venous complications in pregnancy, third trimester** ♀ 🦠　　M
　　O22.8X9 **Other venous complications in pregnancy, unspecified trimester** ♀ 🦠　　M

● **O22.9** **Venous complication in pregnancy, unspecified**
　Gestational phlebitis NOS
　Gestational phlebopathy NOS
　Gestational thrombosis NOS
　Ⓔⓧ For category O22.9 CC codes: See O22.2

　O22.90 **Venous complication in pregnancy, unspecified, unspecified trimester** ♀ 🦠　　M
　O22.91 **Venous complication in pregnancy, unspecified, first trimester** ♀　　M
　O22.92 **Venous complication in pregnancy, unspecified, second trimester** ♀　　M
　O22.93 **Venous complication in pregnancy, unspecified, third trimester** ♀　　M

● **O23** **Infections of genitourinary tract in pregnancy**
　Use additional code to identify organism (B95.-, B96.-)
　Excludes2　gonococcal infections complicating pregnancy, childbirth and the puerperium (O98.2)
　　　infections with a predominantly sexual mode of transmission NOS complicating pregnancy, childbirth and the puerperium (O98.3)
　　　syphilis complicating pregnancy, childbirth and the puerperium (O98.1)
　　　tuberculosis of genitourinary system complicating pregnancy, childbirth and the puerperium (O98.0)
　　　venereal disease NOS complicating pregnancy, childbirth and the puerperium (O98.3)
　Ⓔⓧ For category O23 CC codes: O11.4, O11.5, O12.04, O12.05, O12.14, O12.15, O12.24, O12.25, O13.4, O13.5, O14.04, O14.05, O14.14, O14.15, O14.24, O14.25, O14.94, O14.95, O16.4, O16.5, O23.00-O23.93, O25.10-O25.3, O26.10-O26.13, O26.30-O26.43, O26.63-O26.819, O26.841-O26.86, O26.891-O26.93, O29.011-O29.93, O35.7XX0-O35.7XX9, O75.4, O75.81, O75.89-O75.9, O80, O86.11, O86.13-O86.29, O90.89, O99.111-O99.285, O99.330-O99.335, O99.350-O99.355, O99.511-O99.73, O99.820-O99.825, O99.840-O9A.53

　● **O23.0** **Infections of kidney in pregnancy**
　　Pyelonephritis in pregnancy
　　O23.00 **Infections of kidney in pregnancy, unspecified trimester** ♀　　M
　　O23.01 **Infections of kidney in pregnancy, first trimester** ♀ 🦠　　M
　　O23.02 **Infections of kidney in pregnancy, second trimester** ♀ 🦠　　M
　　O23.03 **Infections of kidney in pregnancy, third trimester** ♀ 🦠　　M

　● **O23.1** **Infections of bladder in pregnancy**
　　O23.10 **Infections of bladder in pregnancy, unspecified trimester** ♀　　M
　　O23.11 **Infections of bladder in pregnancy, first trimester** ♀ 🦠　　M
　　O23.12 **Infections of bladder in pregnancy, second trimester** ♀ 🦠　　M
　　O23.13 **Infections of bladder in pregnancy, third trimester** ♀ 🦠　　M

● **O23.2** **Infections of urethra in pregnancy**
　O23.20 **Infections of urethra in pregnancy, unspecified trimester** ♀　　M
　O23.21 **Infections of urethra in pregnancy, first trimester** ♀ 🦠　　M
　O23.22 **Infections of urethra in pregnancy, second trimester** ♀ 🦠　　M
　O23.23 **Infections of urethra in pregnancy, third trimester** ♀ 🦠　　M

● **O23.3** **Infections of other parts of urinary tract in pregnancy**
　O23.30 **Infections of other parts of urinary tract in pregnancy, unspecified trimester** ♀　　M
　O23.31 **Infections of other parts of urinary tract in pregnancy, first trimester** ♀ 🦠　　M
　O23.32 **Infections of other parts of urinary tract in pregnancy, second trimester** ♀ 🦠　　M
　O23.33 **Infections of other parts of urinary tract in pregnancy, third trimester** ♀ 🦠　　M

● **O23.4** **Unspecified infection of urinary tract in pregnancy**
　O23.40 **Unspecified infection of urinary tract in pregnancy, unspecified trimester** ♀　　M
　O23.41 **Unspecified infection of urinary tract in pregnancy, first trimester** ♀ 🦠　　M
　O23.42 **Unspecified infection of urinary tract in pregnancy, second trimester** ♀ 🦠　　M
　O23.43 **Unspecified infection of urinary tract in pregnancy, third trimester** ♀ 🦠　　M

● **O23.5** **Infections of the genital tract in pregnancy**
　● **O23.51** **Infection of cervix in pregnancy**
　　O23.511 **Infections of cervix in pregnancy, first trimester** ♀ 🦠　　M
　　O23.512 **Infections of cervix in pregnancy, second trimester** ♀ 🦠　　M
　　O23.513 **Infections of cervix in pregnancy, third trimester** ♀ 🦠　　M
　　O23.519 **Infections of cervix in pregnancy, unspecified trimester** ♀　　M

　● **O23.52** **Salpingo-oophoritis in pregnancy**
　　Oophoritis = inflammation of ovary
　　Salpingitis = inflammation of fallopian tube
　　Oophoritis in pregnancy
　　Salpingitis in pregnancy
　　O23.521 **Salpingo-oophoritis in pregnancy, first trimester** ♀ 🦠　　M
　　O23.522 **Salpingo-oophoritis in pregnancy, second trimester** ♀ 🦠　　M
　　O23.523 **Salpingo-oophoritis in pregnancy, third trimester** ♀ 🦠　　M
　　O23.529 **Salpingo-oophoritis in pregnancy, unspecified trimester** ♀　　M

　● **O23.59** **Infection of other part of genital tract in pregnancy**
　　O23.591 **Infection of other part of genital tract in pregnancy, first trimester** ♀ 🦠　　M
　　O23.592 **Infection of other part of genital tract in pregnancy, second trimester** ♀ 🦠　　M
　　O23.593 **Infection of other part of genital tract in pregnancy, third trimester** ♀ 🦠　　M
　　O23.599 **Infection of other part of genital tract in pregnancy, unspecified trimester** ♀　　M

● **O23.9** **Unspecified genitourinary tract infection in pregnancy**
　Genitourinary tract infection in pregnancy NOS
　O23.90 **Unspecified genitourinary tract infection in pregnancy, unspecified trimester** ♀　　M
　O23.91 **Unspecified genitourinary tract infection in pregnancy, first trimester** ♀ 🦠　　M
　O23.92 **Unspecified genitourinary tract infection in pregnancy, second trimester** ♀ 🦠　　M
　O23.93 **Unspecified genitourinary tract infection in pregnancy, third trimester** ♀ 🦠　　M

◀ New　◀ⅲ Revised　deleted Deleted　Excludes 1　Excludes 2　Includes　Use additional　Code first　Code also　Unspecified
OGCR Official Guidelines　● Unacceptable Principal Diagnosis　X Assign placeholder X　● Use Additional Character(s)　▶ Manifestation Code　**Coding Clinic**

OGCR Section I.C.15.g.

Diabetes mellitus in pregnancy
Diabetes mellitus is a significant complicating factor in pregnancy. Pregnant women who are diabetic should be assigned a code from category O24, Diabetes mellitus in pregnancy, childbirth, and the puerperium, first, followed by the appropriate diabetes code(s) (E08-E13) from Chapter 4.

● O24   **Diabetes mellitus in pregnancy, childbirth, and the puerperium**
    (Ex:) **For category O24 CC codes:** 011.4, 011.5, 012.04, 012.05, 012.14, 012.15, 012.24, 012.25, 013.4, 013.5, 014.04, 014.05, 014.14, 014.15, 014.24, 014.25, 014.94, 014.95, 016.4, 016.5, 024.011-024.33, 024.811-025.3, 026.10-026.13, 026.30-026.43, 026.63-026.819, 026.841-026.86, 026.891-026.93, 029.011-029.93, 035.7XX0-035.7XX9, 075.4, 075.81, 075.89-075.9, 080, 090.89, 099.111-099.285, 099.330-099.335, 099.350-099.355, 099.511-099.73, 099.820-099.825, 099.840-09A.53

   ● O24.0   **Pre-existing type 1 diabetes mellitus, in pregnancy, childbirth and the puerperium** ◄▥
       Juvenile onset diabetes mellitus, in pregnancy, childbirth and the puerperium
       Ketosis-prone diabetes mellitus in pregnancy, childbirth and the puerperium
       Use additional code from category E10 to further identify any manifestations

     ● O24.01   **Pre-existing type 1 diabetes mellitus, in pregnancy** ◄▥
       O24.011   **Pre-existing type 1 diabetes mellitus, in pregnancy, first trimester** ♀ 🗇 ◄▥ M
       O24.012   **Pre-existing type 1 diabetes mellitus, in pregnancy, second trimester** ♀ 🗇 M
       O24.013   **Pre-existing type 1 diabetes mellitus, in pregnancy, third trimester** ♀ 🗇 ◄▥ M
       O24.019   **Pre-existing type 1 diabetes mellitus, in pregnancy, unspecified trimester** ♀ 🗇 ◄▥ M

     O24.02   **Pre-existing type 1 diabetes mellitus, in childbirth** ♀ 🗇 ◄▥ M

     O24.03   **Pre-existing type 1 diabetes mellitus, in the puerperium** ♀ 🗇 ◄▥ M

   ● O24.1   **Pre-existing type 2 diabetes mellitus, in pregnancy, childbirth and the puerperium** ◄▥
       Insulin-resistant diabetes mellitus in pregnancy, childbirth and the puerperium
       Use additional code (for):
         from category E11 to further identify any manifestations
         long-term (current) use of insulin (Z79.4)

     ● O24.11   **Pre-existing type 2 diabetes mellitus, in pregnancy** ◄▥
       O24.111   **Pre-existing type 2 diabetes mellitus, in pregnancy, first trimester** ♀ 🗇 ◄▥ M
       O24.112   **Pre-existing type 2 diabetes mellitus, in pregnancy, second trimester** ♀ 🗇 ◄▥ M
       O24.113   **Pre-existing type 2 diabetes mellitus, in pregnancy, third trimester** ♀ 🗇 ◄▥ M
       O24.119   **Pre-existing type 2 diabetes mellitus, in pregnancy, unspecified trimester** ♀ 🗇 ◄▥ M

     O24.12   **Pre-existing type 2 diabetes mellitus, in childbirth** ♀ 🗇 ◄▥ M

     O24.13   **Pre-existing type 2 diabetes mellitus, in the puerperium** ♀ 🗇 ◄▥ M

   ● O24.3   **Unspecified pre-existing diabetes mellitus in pregnancy, childbirth and the puerperium**
       Use additional code (for):
         from category E11 to further identify any manifestation
         long-term (current) use of insulin (Z79.4)

     ● O24.31   **Unspecified pre-existing diabetes mellitus in pregnancy**
       O24.311   **Unspecified pre-existing diabetes mellitus in pregnancy, first trimester** ♀ 🗇 M

       O24.312   **Unspecified pre-existing diabetes mellitus in pregnancy, second trimester** ♀ 🗇 M
       O24.313   **Unspecified pre-existing diabetes mellitus in pregnancy, third trimester** ♀ 🗇 M
       O24.319   **Unspecified pre-existing diabetes mellitus in pregnancy, unspecified trimester** ♀ 🗇 M

     O24.32   **Unspecified pre-existing diabetes mellitus in childbirth** ♀ 🗇 M

     O24.33   **Unspecified pre-existing diabetes mellitus in the puerperium** ♀ 🗇 M

   ● O24.4   **Gestational diabetes mellitus**
       Diabetes mellitus arising in pregnancy
       Gestational diabetes mellitus NOS

     ● O24.41   **Gestational diabetes mellitus in pregnancy**
       O24.410   **Gestational diabetes mellitus in pregnancy, diet controlled** ♀ M
       O24.414   **Gestational diabetes mellitus in pregnancy, insulin controlled** ♀ M
       O24.415   **Gestational diabetes mellitus in pregnancy, controlled by oral hypoglycemic drugs** ♀ ◄ M
         Gestational diabetes mellitus in pregnancy, controlled by oral antidiabetic drugs ◄
       O24.419   **Gestational diabetes mellitus in pregnancy, unspecified control** ♀ M
         Coding Clinic: 2015, Q4, P34

     ● O24.42   **Gestational diabetes mellitus in childbirth**
       O24.420   **Gestational diabetes mellitus in childbirth, diet controlled** ♀ M
       O24.424   **Gestational diabetes mellitus in childbirth, insulin controlled** ♀ M
       O24.425   **Gestational diabetes mellitus in childbirth, controlled by oral hypoglycemic drugs** ♀ ◄ M
         Gestational diabetes mellitus in childbirth, controlled by oral antidiabetic drugs ◄
       O24.429   **Gestational diabetes mellitus in childbirth, unspecified control** ♀ M

OGCR Section I.C.15.i.

Gestational (pregnancy induced) diabetes
Gestational (pregnancy induced) diabetes can occur during the second and third trimester of pregnancy in women who were not diabetic prior to pregnancy. Gestational diabetes can cause complications in the pregnancy similar to those of pre-existing diabetes mellitus. It also puts the woman at greater risk of developing diabetes after the pregnancy. Codes for gestational diabetes are in subcategory O24.4, Gestational diabetes mellitus. No other code from category O24, Diabetes mellitus in pregnancy, childbirth, and the puerperium, should be used with a code from O24.4

The codes under subcategory O24.4 include diet controlled, insulin controlled, **and controlled by oral hypoglycemic drugs.** If a patient with gestational diabetes is treated with both diet and insulin, only the code for insulin-controlled is required. **If a patient with gestational diabetes is treated with both diet and oral hypoglycemic medications, only the code for "controlled by oral hypoglycemic drugs" is required.** Code Z79.4, Long-term (current) use of insulin or code Z79.84, Long-term (current) use of oral hypoglycemic drugs, should not be assigned with codes from subcategory O24.4.

An abnormal glucose tolerance in pregnancy is assigned a code from subcategory O99.81, Abnormal glucose complicating pregnancy, childbirth, and the puerperium.

CHAPTER 15 (O00-O9A)

● **O24.43 Gestational diabetes mellitus in the puerperium**

     O24.430   Gestational diabetes mellitus in the puerperium, diet controlled ♀   M

     O24.434   Gestational diabetes mellitus in the puerperium, insulin controlled ♀   M

     O24.435   Gestational diabetes mellitus in puerperium, controlled by oral hypoglycemic drugs ♀ ◀   M
         Gestational diabetes mellitus in puerperium, controlled by oral antidiabetic drugs ◀

     O24.439   Gestational diabetes mellitus in the puerperium, unspecified control ♀   M

● **O24.8 Other pre-existing diabetes mellitus in pregnancy, childbirth, and the puerperium**

     Use additional code (for):
       from categories E08, E09 and E13 to further identify any manifestation
       long-term (current) use of insulin (Z79.4)

  ● **O24.81 Other pre-existing diabetes mellitus in pregnancy**

     O24.811   Other pre-existing diabetes mellitus in pregnancy, first trimester ♀ 🐾   M

     O24.812   Other pre-existing diabetes mellitus in pregnancy, second trimester ♀ 🐾   M

     O24.813   Other pre-existing diabetes mellitus in pregnancy, third trimester ♀ 🐾   M

     O24.819   Other pre-existing diabetes mellitus in pregnancy, unspecified trimester ♀ 🐾   M

   O24.82   Other pre-existing diabetes mellitus in childbirth ♀ 🐾   M

   O24.83   Other pre-existing diabetes mellitus in the puerperium ♀ 🐾   M

● **O24.9 Unspecified diabetes mellitus in pregnancy, childbirth and the puerperium**

     Use additional code for long-term (current) use of insulin (Z79.4)
     Unknown whether patient was diabetic before pregnancy occurred

  ● **O24.91 Unspecified diabetes mellitus in pregnancy**

     O24.911   Unspecified diabetes mellitus in pregnancy, first trimester ♀ 🐾   M

     O24.912   Unspecified diabetes mellitus in pregnancy, second trimester ♀ 🐾   M

     O24.913   Unspecified diabetes mellitus in pregnancy, third trimester ♀ 🐾   M

     O24.919   Unspecified diabetes mellitus in pregnancy, unspecified trimester ♀ 🐾   M

   O24.92   Unspecified diabetes mellitus in childbirth ♀   M

   O24.93   Unspecified diabetes mellitus in the puerperium ♀ 🐾   M

● **O25 Malnutrition in pregnancy, childbirth and the puerperium**

  ● **O25.1 Malnutrition in pregnancy**

     O25.10   Malnutrition in pregnancy, unspecified trimester ♀   M

     O25.11   Malnutrition in pregnancy, first trimester ♀   M

     O25.12   Malnutrition in pregnancy, second trimester ♀ M

     O25.13   Malnutrition in pregnancy, third trimester ♀   M

   O25.2   Malnutrition in childbirth ♀   M

   O25.3   Malnutrition in the puerperium ♀   M

● **O26 Maternal care for other conditions predominantly related to pregnancy**

  ● **O26.0 Excessive weight gain in pregnancy**

     Excludes2   gestational edema (O12.0, O12.2)

     O26.00   Excessive weight gain in pregnancy, unspecified trimester ♀   M

     O26.01   Excessive weight gain in pregnancy, first trimester ♀   M

     O26.02   Excessive weight gain in pregnancy, second trimester ♀   M

     O26.03   Excessive weight gain in pregnancy, third trimester ♀   M

  ● **O26.1 Low weight gain in pregnancy**

     O26.10   Low weight gain in pregnancy, unspecified trimester ♀   M

     O26.11   Low weight gain in pregnancy, first trimester ♀   M

     O26.12   Low weight gain in pregnancy, second trimester ♀   M

     O26.13   Low weight gain in pregnancy, third trimester ♀   M

  ● **O26.2 Pregnancy care for patient with recurrent pregnancy loss**

     O26.20   Pregnancy care for patient with recurrent pregnancy loss, unspecified trimester ♀   M

     O26.21   Pregnancy care for patient with recurrent pregnancy loss, first trimester ♀   M

     O26.22   Pregnancy care for patient with recurrent pregnancy loss, second trimester ♀   M

     O26.23   Pregnancy care for patient with recurrent pregnancy loss, third trimester ♀   M

  ● **O26.3 Retained intrauterine contraceptive device in pregnancy**

     O26.30   Retained intrauterine contraceptive device in pregnancy, unspecified trimester ♀   M

     O26.31   Retained intrauterine contraceptive device in pregnancy, first trimester ♀   M

     O26.32   Retained intrauterine contraceptive device in pregnancy, second trimester ♀   M

     O26.33   Retained intrauterine contraceptive device in pregnancy, third trimester ♀   M

  ● **O26.4 Herpes gestationis**

     O26.40   Herpes gestationis, unspecified trimester ♀   M

     O26.41   Herpes gestationis, first trimester ♀   M

     O26.42   Herpes gestationis, second trimester ♀   M

     O26.43   Herpes gestationis, third trimester ♀   M

  ● **O26.5 Maternal hypotension syndrome**
     Supine hypotensive syndrome

     O26.50   Maternal hypotension syndrome, unspecified trimester ♀   M

     O26.51   Maternal hypotension syndrome, first trimester ♀   M

     O26.52   Maternal hypotension syndrome, second trimester ♀   M

     O26.53   Maternal hypotension syndrome, third trimester ♀   M

◀ New   ◀|||| Revised   ~~deleted~~ Deleted   Excludes 1   Excludes 2   Includes   Use additional   Code first   Code also   Unspecified
OGCR Official Guidelines   ● Unacceptable Principal Diagnosis   X Assign placeholder X   ● Use Additional Character(s)   ▶ Manifestation Code   **Coding Clinic**

● **O26.6** **Liver and biliary tract disorders in pregnancy, childbirth and the puerperium**

    Use additional code to identify the specific disorder

    Excludes2 hepatorenal syndrome following labor and delivery (O90.4)

  ● **O26.61** **Liver and biliary tract disorders in pregnancy**

    (Ex) **For category O26.61 CC codes:** 011.4, 011.5, 012.04, 012.05, 012.14, 012.15, 012.24, 012.25, 013.4, 013.5, 014.04, 014.05, 014.14, 014.15, 014.24, 014.25, 014.94, 014.95, 016.4, 016.5, 025.10-025.3, 026.10-026.13, 026.30-026.43, 026.611-026.819, 026.841-026.86, 026.891-026.93, 029.011-029.93, 035.7XX0-035.7XX9, 075.4, 075.81, 075.89-075.9, 080, 090.89, 099.111-099.285, 099.330-099.335, 099.350-099.355, 099.511-099.73, 099.820-099.825, 099.840-09A.53

    O26.611 **Liver and biliary tract disorders in pregnancy, first trimester** ♀ 🔗   **M**

    O26.612 **Liver and biliary tract disorders in pregnancy, second trimester** ♀ 🔗   **M**

    O26.613 **Liver and biliary tract disorders in pregnancy, third trimester** ♀ 🔗   **M**

    O26.619 **Liver and biliary tract disorders in pregnancy,** unspecified **trimester** ♀ **M**

  ● **O26.62** **Liver and biliary tract disorders in childbirth** ♀ 🔗   **M**

    (Ex) See 026.61

  ● **O26.63** **Liver and biliary tract disorders in the puerperium** ♀   **M**

● **O26.7** **Subluxation of symphysis (pubis) in pregnancy, childbirth and the puerperium**

    Excludes1 traumatic separation of symphysis (pubis) during childbirth (O71.6)

  ● **O26.71** **Subluxation of symphysis (pubis) in pregnancy**

    O26.711 **Subluxation of symphysis (pubis) in pregnancy, first trimester** ♀ **M**

    O26.712 **Subluxation of symphysis (pubis) in pregnancy, second trimester** ♀ **M**

    O26.713 **Subluxation of symphysis (pubis) in pregnancy, third trimester** ♀ **M**

    O26.719 **Subluxation of symphysis (pubis) in pregnancy,** unspecified **trimester** ♀ **M**

  ● **O26.72** **Subluxation of symphysis (pubis) in childbirth** ♀   **M**

  ● **O26.73** **Subluxation of symphysis (pubis) in the puerperium** ♀   **M**

● **O26.8** **Other specified pregnancy related conditions**

  ● **O26.81** **Pregnancy related exhaustion and fatigue**

    O26.811 **Pregnancy related exhaustion and fatigue, first trimester** ♀ **M**

    O26.812 **Pregnancy related exhaustion and fatigue, second trimester** ♀ **M**

    O26.813 **Pregnancy related exhaustion and fatigue, third trimester** ♀ **M**

    O26.819 **Pregnancy related exhaustion and fatigue,** unspecified **trimester** ♀ **M**

  ● **O26.82** **Pregnancy related peripheral neuritis**

    O26.821 **Pregnancy related peripheral neuritis, first trimester** ♀ **M**

    O26.822 **Pregnancy related peripheral neuritis, second trimester** ♀ **M**

    O26.823 **Pregnancy related peripheral neuritis, third trimester** ♀ **M**

    O26.829 **Pregnancy related peripheral neuritis,** unspecified **trimester** ♀ **M**

  ● **O26.83** **Pregnancy related renal disease**

    Use additional code to identify the specific disorder

    (Ex) **For category O26.83 CC codes:** 011.5, 012.05, 012.11-012.13, 012.15, 012.21-012.23, 012.25, 013.5, 014.05, 014.15, 014.25, 014.95, 016.5, 026.831-026.833, 090.89

    O26.831 **Pregnancy related renal disease, first trimester** ♀ 🔗   **M**

    O26.832 **Pregnancy related renal disease, second trimester** ♀ 🔗   **M**

    O26.833 **Pregnancy related renal disease, third trimester** ♀ 🔗   **M**

    O26.839 **Pregnancy related renal disease,** unspecified **trimester** ♀   **M**

  ● **O26.84** **Uterine size-date discrepancy complicating pregnancy**

    Excludes1 encounter for suspected problem with fetal growth ruled out (Z03.74)

    O26.841 **Uterine size-date discrepancy, first trimester** ♀ **M**

    O26.842 **Uterine size-date discrepancy, second trimester** ♀ **M**

    O26.843 **Uterine size-date discrepancy, third trimester** ♀ **M**

    O26.849 **Uterine size-date discrepancy,** unspecified **trimester** ♀ **M**

  ● **O26.85** **Spotting complicating pregnancy**

    O26.851 **Spotting complicating pregnancy, first trimester** ♀ **M**

    O26.852 **Spotting complicating pregnancy, second trimester** ♀ **M**

    O26.853 **Spotting complicating pregnancy, third trimester** ♀ **M**

    O26.859 **Spotting complicating pregnancy,** unspecified **trimester** ♀ **M**

   O26.86 **Pruritic urticarial papules and plaques of pregnancy (PUPPP)** ♀   **M**

    Polymorphic eruption of pregnancy

  ● **O26.87** **Cervical shortening**

    Excludes1 encounter for suspected cervical shortening ruled out (Z03.75)

    (Ex) **For category O26.87 CC codes:** 026.872-026.879, 034.31-034.33

    O26.872 **Cervical shortening, second trimester** ♀ 🔗   **M**

    O26.873 **Cervical shortening, third trimester** ♀ 🔗   **M**

    O26.879 **Cervical shortening,** unspecified **trimester** ♀ 🔗   **M**

  ● **O26.89** **Other specified pregnancy related conditions**

    O26.891 **Other specified pregnancy related conditions, first trimester** ♀ **M**

    O26.892 **Other specified pregnancy related conditions, second trimester** ♀ **M**

    O26.893 **Other specified pregnancy related conditions, third trimester** ♀ **M**

      Coding Clinic: 2015, Q3, P40

    O26.899 **Other specified pregnancy related conditions,** unspecified **trimester** ♀ **M**

● **O26.9** **Pregnancy related conditions, unspecified**

    O26.90 **Pregnancy related conditions,** unspecified, **unspecified trimester** ♀   **M**

    O26.91 **Pregnancy related conditions,** unspecified, **first trimester** ♀   **M**

    O26.92 **Pregnancy related conditions,** unspecified, **second trimester** ♀   **M**

    O26.93 **Pregnancy related conditions,** unspecified, **third trimester** ♀   **M**

N Newborn Age: 0   **P** Pediatric Age: 0–17   **M** Maternity DX: 12–55   **A** Adult Age: 15–124   ♀ Females Only   ♂ Males Only

🔗 Complication\Comorbidity   🔗 Major C\C   (Ex) CC/MCC Exclusions   🔗 Hospital-Acquired Condition

● O28   **Abnormal findings on antenatal screening of mother**

     Excludes1   diagnostic findings classified elsewhere - see Alphabetical Index

  O28.0   Abnormal hematological finding on antenatal screening of mother ♀   **M**

  O28.1   Abnormal biochemical finding on antenatal screening of mother ♀   **M**

  O28.2   Abnormal cytological finding on antenatal screening of mother ♀   **M**

  O28.3   Abnormal ultrasonic finding on antenatal screening of mother ♀   **M**

  O28.4   Abnormal radiological finding on antenatal screening of mother ♀   **M**

  O28.5   Abnormal chromosomal and genetic finding on antenatal screening of mother ♀   **M**

  O28.8   Other abnormal findings on antenatal screening of mother ♀   **M**

  O28.9   Unspecified abnormal findings on antenatal screening of mother ♀   **M**

● O29   **Complications of anesthesia during pregnancy**

     Includes   maternal complications arising from the administration of a general, regional or local anesthetic, analgesic or other sedation during pregnancy

     Use additional code, if necessary, to identify the complication

     Excludes2   complications of anesthesia during labor and delivery (O74.-)

                        complications of anesthesia during the puerperium (O89.-)

  ● O29.0   **Pulmonary complications of anesthesia during pregnancy**

    ● O29.01   Aspiration pneumonitis due to anesthesia during pregnancy

       Inhalation of stomach contents or secretions NOS due to anesthesia during pregnancy

       Mendelson's syndrome due to anesthesia during pregnancy

      O29.011   Aspiration pneumonitis due to anesthesia during pregnancy, first trimester ♀   **M**

      O29.012   Aspiration pneumonitis due to anesthesia during pregnancy, second trimester ♀   **M**

      O29.013   Aspiration pneumonitis due to anesthesia during pregnancy, third trimester ♀   **M**

      O29.019   Aspiration pneumonitis due to anesthesia during pregnancy, unspecified trimester ♀   **M**

    ● O29.02   Pressure collapse of lung due to anesthesia during pregnancy

      O29.021   Pressure collapse of lung due to anesthesia during pregnancy, first trimester ♀   **M**

      O29.022   Pressure collapse of lung due to anesthesia during pregnancy, second trimester ♀   **M**

      O29.023   Pressure collapse of lung due to anesthesia during pregnancy, third trimester ♀   **M**

      O29.029   Pressure collapse of lung due to anesthesia during pregnancy, unspecified trimester ♀   **M**

    ● O29.09   Other pulmonary complications of anesthesia during pregnancy

      O29.091   Other pulmonary complications of anesthesia during pregnancy, first trimester ♀   **M**

      O29.092   Other pulmonary complications of anesthesia during pregnancy, second trimester ♀   **M**

      O29.093   Other pulmonary complications of anesthesia during pregnancy, third trimester ♀   **M**

      O29.099   Other pulmonary complications of anesthesia during pregnancy, unspecified trimester ♀   **M**

  ● O29.1   **Cardiac complications of anesthesia during pregnancy**

    ● O29.11   Cardiac arrest due to anesthesia during pregnancy

      O29.111   Cardiac arrest due to anesthesia during pregnancy, first trimester ♀   **M**

      O29.112   Cardiac arrest due to anesthesia during pregnancy, second trimester ♀   **M**

      O29.113   Cardiac arrest due to anesthesia during pregnancy, third trimester ♀   **M**

      O29.119   Cardiac arrest due to anesthesia during pregnancy, unspecified trimester ♀   **M**

    ● O29.12   Cardiac failure due to anesthesia during pregnancy

      O29.121   Cardiac failure due to anesthesia during pregnancy, first trimester ♀   **M**

      O29.122   Cardiac failure due to anesthesia during pregnancy, second trimester ♀   **M**

      O29.123   Cardiac failure due to anesthesia during pregnancy, third trimester ♀   **M**

      O29.129   Cardiac failure due to anesthesia during pregnancy, unspecified trimester ♀   **M**

    ● O29.19   Other cardiac complications of anesthesia during pregnancy

      O29.191   Other cardiac complications of anesthesia during pregnancy, first trimester ♀   **M**

      O29.192   Other cardiac complications of anesthesia during pregnancy, second trimester ♀   **M**

      O29.193   Other cardiac complications of anesthesia during pregnancy, third trimester ♀   **M**

      O29.199   Other cardiac complications of anesthesia during pregnancy, unspecified trimester ♀   **M**

  ● O29.2   **Central nervous system complications of anesthesia during pregnancy**

    ● O29.21   Cerebral anoxia due to anesthesia during pregnancy

      O29.211   Cerebral anoxia due to anesthesia during pregnancy, first trimester ♀   **M**

      O29.212   Cerebral anoxia due to anesthesia during pregnancy, second trimester ♀   **M**

      O29.213   Cerebral anoxia due to anesthesia during pregnancy, third trimester ♀   **M**

      O29.219   Cerebral anoxia due to anesthesia during pregnancy, unspecified trimester ♀   **M**

    ● O29.29   Other central nervous system complications of anesthesia during pregnancy

      O29.291   Other central nervous system complications of anesthesia during pregnancy, first trimester ♀   **M**

      O29.292   Other central nervous system complications of anesthesia during pregnancy, second trimester ♀   **M**

      O29.293   Other central nervous system complications of anesthesia during pregnancy, third trimester ♀   **M**

      O29.299   Other central nervous system complications of anesthesia during pregnancy, unspecified trimester ♀   **M**

◀ New   ◀▥ Revised   ~~deleted~~ Deleted   Excludes 1   Excludes 2   Includes   Use additional   Code first   Code also   Unspecified

OGCR Official Guidelines   ● Unacceptable Principal Diagnosis   X Assign placeholder X   ● Use Additional Character(s)   ▶ Manifestation Code   **Coding Clinic**

● O29.3   Toxic reaction to local anesthesia during pregnancy
   ● O29.3X   Toxic reaction to local anesthesia during pregnancy
      O29.3X1   Toxic reaction to local anesthesia during pregnancy, first trimester ♀   M
      O29.3X2   Toxic reaction to local anesthesia during pregnancy, second trimester ♀   M
      O29.3X3   Toxic reaction to local anesthesia during pregnancy, third trimester ♀   M
      O29.3X9   Toxic reaction to local anesthesia during pregnancy, unspecified trimester ♀   M

● O29.4   Spinal and epidural anesthesia induced headache during pregnancy
      O29.40   Spinal and epidural anesthesia induced headache during pregnancy, unspecified trimester ♀   M
      O29.41   Spinal and epidural anesthesia induced headache during pregnancy, first trimester ♀   M
      O29.42   Spinal and epidural anesthesia induced headache during pregnancy, second trimester ♀   M
      O29.43   Spinal and epidural anesthesia induced headache during pregnancy, third trimester ♀   M

● O29.5   Other complications of spinal and epidural anesthesia during pregnancy
   ● O29.5X   Other complications of spinal and epidural anesthesia during pregnancy
      O29.5X1   Other complications of spinal and epidural anesthesia during pregnancy, first trimester ♀   M
      O29.5X2   Other complications of spinal and epidural anesthesia during pregnancy, second trimester ♀   M
      O29.5X3   Other complications of spinal and epidural anesthesia during pregnancy, third trimester ♀   M
      O29.5X9   Other complications of spinal and epidural anesthesia during pregnancy, unspecified trimester ♀   M

● O29.6   Failed or difficult intubation for anesthesia during pregnancy
      O29.60   Failed or difficult intubation for anesthesia during pregnancy, unspecified trimester ♀   M
      O29.61   Failed or difficult intubation for anesthesia during pregnancy, first trimester ♀   M
      O29.62   Failed or difficult intubation for anesthesia during pregnancy, second trimester ♀   M
      O29.63   Failed or difficult intubation for anesthesia during pregnancy, third trimester ♀   M

● O29.8   Other complications of anesthesia during pregnancy
   ● O29.8X   Other complications of anesthesia during pregnancy
      O29.8X1   Other complications of anesthesia during pregnancy, first trimester ♀   M
      O29.8X2   Other complications of anesthesia during pregnancy, second trimester ♀   M
      O29.8X3   Other complications of anesthesia during pregnancy, third trimester ♀   M
      O29.8X9   Other complications of anesthesia during pregnancy, unspecified trimester ♀   M

● O29.9   Unspecified complication of anesthesia during pregnancy
      O29.90   Unspecified complication of anesthesia during pregnancy, unspecified trimester ♀   M
      O29.91   Unspecified complication of anesthesia during pregnancy, first trimester ♀   M
      O29.92   Unspecified complication of anesthesia during pregnancy, second trimester ♀   M
      O29.93   Unspecified complication of anesthesia during pregnancy, third trimester ♀   M

MATERNAL CARE RELATED TO THE FETUS AND AMNIOTIC CAVITY AND POSSIBLE DELIVERY PROBLEMS (O30-O48)

● O30   Multiple gestation
   Code also any complications specific to multiple gestation
   ● O30.0   Twin pregnancy
      ● O30.00   Twin pregnancy, unspecified number of placenta and unspecified number of amniotic sacs
         O30.001   Twin pregnancy, unspecified number of placenta and unspecified number of amniotic sacs, first trimester ♀   M
         O30.002   Twin pregnancy, unspecified number of placenta and unspecified number of amniotic sacs, second trimester ♀   M
         O30.003   Twin pregnancy, unspecified number of placenta and unspecified number of amniotic sacs, third trimester ♀   M
         O30.009   Twin pregnancy, unspecified number of placenta and unspecified number of amniotic sacs, unspecified trimester ♀   M

      ● O30.01   Twin pregnancy, monochorionic/monoamniotic
         Twin pregnancy, one placenta, one amniotic sac
         Excludes1   conjoined twins (O30.02-)
         O30.011   Twin pregnancy, monochorionic/monoamniotic, first trimester ♀   M
         O30.012   Twin pregnancy, monochorionic/monoamniotic, second trimester ♀   M
         O30.013   Twin pregnancy, monochorionic/monoamniotic, third trimester ♀   M
         O30.019   Twin pregnancy, monochorionic/monoamniotic, unspecified trimester ♀   M

      ● O30.02   Conjoined twin pregnancy
         O30.021   Conjoined twin pregnancy, first trimester ♀   M
         O30.022   Conjoined twin pregnancy, second trimester ♀   M
         O30.023   Conjoined twin pregnancy, third trimester ♀   M
         O30.029   Conjoined twin pregnancy, unspecified trimester ♀   M

      ● O30.03   Twin pregnancy, monochorionic/diamniotic
         Twin pregnancy, one placenta, two amniotic sacs
         O30.031   Twin pregnancy, monochorionic/diamniotic, first trimester ♀   M
         O30.032   Twin pregnancy, monochorionic/diamniotic, second trimester ♀   M
         O30.033   Twin pregnancy, monochorionic/diamniotic, third trimester ♀   M
         O30.039   Twin pregnancy, monochorionic/diamniotic, unspecified trimester ♀   M

● O30.04   Twin pregnancy, dichorionic/diamniotic
       Twin pregnancy, two placentae, two amniotic sacs

    O30.041   Twin pregnancy, dichorionic/diamniotic, first trimester ♀   M

    O30.042   Twin pregnancy, dichorionic/diamniotic, second trimester ♀   M

    O30.043   Twin pregnancy, dichorionic/diamniotic, third trimester ♀   M

    O30.049   Twin pregnancy, dichorionic/diamniotic, unspecified trimester ♀   M

● O30.09   Twin pregnancy, unable to determine number of placenta and number of amniotic sacs

    O30.091   Twin pregnancy, unable to determine number of placenta and number of amniotic sacs, first trimester ♀   M

    O30.092   Twin pregnancy, unable to determine number of placenta and number of amniotic sacs, second trimester ♀   M

    O30.093   Twin pregnancy, unable to determine number of placenta and number of amniotic sacs, third trimester ♀   M

    O30.099   Twin pregnancy, unable to determine number of placenta and number of amniotic sacs, unspecified trimester ♀   M

● O30.1   Triplet pregnancy
    Ⓔⓧ **For category O30.1 CC codes:** O30.001-O30.019, O30.031-O31.23X9, O31.31X0-O32.9XX9, O80

● O30.10   Triplet pregnancy, unspecified number of placenta and unspecified number of amniotic sacs

    O30.101   Triplet pregnancy, unspecified number of placenta and unspecified number of amniotic sacs, first trimester ♀ 🦠   M

    O30.102   Triplet pregnancy, unspecified number of placenta and unspecified number of amniotic sacs, second trimester ♀ 🦠   M

    O30.103   Triplet pregnancy, unspecified number of placenta and unspecified number of amniotic sacs, third trimester ♀ 🦠   M
       Coding Clinic: 2016, Q2, P8

    O30.109   Triplet pregnancy, unspecified number of placenta and unspecified number of amniotic sacs, unspecified trimester ♀   M

● O30.11   Triplet pregnancy with two or more monochorionic fetuses

    O30.111   Triplet pregnancy with two or more monochorionic fetuses, first trimester ♀ 🦠   M

    O30.112   Triplet pregnancy with two or more monochorionic fetuses, second trimester ♀ 🦠   M

    O30.113   Triplet pregnancy with two or more monochorionic fetuses, third trimester ♀ 🦠   M

    O30.119   Triplet pregnancy with two or more monochorionic fetuses, unspecified trimester ♀   M

● O30.12   Triplet pregnancy with two or more monoamniotic fetuses

    O30.121   Triplet pregnancy with two or more monoamniotic fetuses, first trimester ♀ 🦠   M

    O30.122   Triplet pregnancy with two or more monoamniotic fetuses, second trimester ♀ 🦠   M

    O30.123   Triplet pregnancy with two or more monoamniotic fetuses, third trimester ♀ 🦠   M

    O30.129   Triplet pregnancy with two or more monoamniotic fetuses, unspecified trimester ♀   M

● O30.19   Triplet pregnancy, unable to determine number of placenta and number of amniotic sacs

    O30.191   Triplet pregnancy, unable to determine number of placenta and number of amniotic sacs, first trimester ♀ 🦠   M

    O30.192   Triplet pregnancy, unable to determine number of placenta and number of amniotic sacs, second trimester ♀ 🦠   M

    O30.193   Triplet pregnancy, unable to determine number of placenta and number of amniotic sacs, third trimester ♀   M

    O30.199   Triplet pregnancy, unable to determine number of placenta and number of amniotic sacs, unspecified trimester ♀   M

● O30.2   Quadruplet pregnancy
    Ⓔⓧ **For category O30.2 CC codes:** See O30.1

● O30.20   Quadruplet pregnancy, unspecified number of placenta and unspecified number of amniotic sacs

    O30.201   Quadruplet pregnancy, unspecified number of placenta and unspecified number of amniotic sacs, first trimester ♀ 🦠   M

    O30.202   Quadruplet pregnancy, unspecified number of placenta and unspecified number of amniotic sacs, second trimester ♀ 🦠   M

    O30.203   Quadruplet pregnancy, unspecified number of placenta and unspecified number of amniotic sacs, third trimester ♀ 🦠   M

    O30.209   Quadruplet pregnancy, unspecified number of placenta and unspecified number of amniotic sacs, unspecified trimester ♀   M

● O30.21   Quadruplet pregnancy with two or more monochorionic fetuses

    O30.211   Quadruplet pregnancy with two or more monochorionic fetuses, first trimester ♀ 🦠   M

    O30.212   Quadruplet pregnancy with two or more monochorionic fetuses, second trimester ♀ 🦠   M

    O30.213   Quadruplet pregnancy with two or more monochorionic fetuses, third trimester ♀ 🦠   M

    O30.219   Quadruplet pregnancy with two or more monochorionic fetuses, unspecified trimester ♀   M

● O30.22   Quadruplet pregnancy with two or more monoamniotic fetuses

    O30.221   Quadruplet pregnancy with two or more monoamniotic fetuses, first trimester ♀ 🦠   M

    O30.222   Quadruplet pregnancy with two or more monoamniotic fetuses, second trimester ♀ 🦠   M

    O30.223   Quadruplet pregnancy with two or more monoamniotic fetuses, third trimester ♀ 🦠   M

    O30.229   Quadruplet pregnancy with two or more monoamniotic fetuses, unspecified trimester ♀   M

◀ New   ◀⁞ Revised   ~~deleted~~ Deleted   Excludes 1   Excludes 2   Includes   Use additional   Code first   Code also   Unspecified
OGCR Official Guidelines   ● Unacceptable Principal Diagnosis   X Assign placeholder X   ● Use Additional Character(s)   ▶ Manifestation Code   **Coding Clinic**

● **O30.29** Quadruplet pregnancy, unable to determine number of placenta and number of amniotic sacs

     O30.291 Quadruplet pregnancy, unable to determine number of placenta and number of amniotic sacs, first trimester ♀ 🏷   M

     O30.292 Quadruplet pregnancy, unable to determine number of placenta and number of amniotic sacs, second trimester ♀   M

     O30.293 Quadruplet pregnancy, unable to determine number of placenta and number of amniotic sacs, third trimester ♀ 🏷   M

     O30.299 Quadruplet pregnancy, unable to determine number of placenta and number of amniotic sacs, unspecified trimester ♀   M

● **O30.8** Other specified multiple gestation
     Multiple gestation pregnancy greater then quadruplets
     Ⓔ For category O30.8 CC codes: See O30.1

● **O30.80** Other specified multiple gestation, unspecified number of placenta and unspecified number of amniotic sacs

     O30.801 Other specified multiple gestation, unspecified number of placenta and unspecified number of amniotic sacs, first trimester ♀ 🏷   M

     O30.802 Other specified multiple gestation, unspecified number of placenta and unspecified number of amniotic sacs, second trimester ♀ 🏷   M

     O30.803 Other specified multiple gestation, unspecified number of placenta and unspecified number of amniotic sacs, third trimester ♀ 🏷   M

     O30.809 Other specified multiple gestation, unspecified number of placenta and unspecified number of amniotic sacs, unspecified trimester ♀   M

● **O30.81** Other specified multiple gestation with two or more monochorionic fetuses

     O30.811 Other specified multiple gestation with two or more monochorionic fetuses, first trimester ♀ 🏷   M

     O30.812 Other specified multiple gestation with two or more monochorionic fetuses, second trimester ♀ 🏷   M

     O30.813 Other specified multiple gestation with two or more monochorionic fetuses, third trimester ♀ 🏷   M

     O30.819 Other specified multiple gestation with two or more monochorionic fetuses, unspecified trimester ♀   M

● **O30.82** Other specified multiple gestation with two or more monoamniotic fetuses

     O30.821 Other specified multiple gestation with two or more monoamniotic fetuses, first trimester ♀ 🏷   M

     O30.822 Other specified multiple gestation with two or more monoamniotic fetuses, second trimester ♀ 🏷   M

     O30.823 Other specified multiple gestation with two or more monoamniotic fetuses, third trimester ♀ 🏷   M

     O30.829 Other specified multiple gestation with two or more monoamniotic fetuses, unspecified trimester ♀   M

● **O30.89** Other specified multiple gestation, unable to determine number of placenta and number of amniotic sacs

     O30.891 Other specified multiple gestation, unable to determine number of placenta and number of amniotic sacs, first trimester ♀ 🏷   M

     O30.892 Other specified multiple gestation, unable to determine number of placenta and number of amniotic sacs, second trimester ♀ 🏷   M

     O30.893 Other specified multiple gestation, unable to determine number of placenta and number of amniotic sacs, third trimester ♀ 🏷   M

     O30.899 Other specified multiple gestation, unable to determine number of placenta and number of amniotic sacs, unspecified trimester ♀   M

● **O30.9** Multiple gestation, unspecified
     Multiple pregnancy NOS

     O30.90 Multiple gestation, unspecified, unspecified trimester ♀   M

     O30.91 Multiple gestation, unspecified, first trimester ♀   M

     O30.92 Multiple gestation, unspecified, second trimester ♀   M

     O30.93 Multiple gestation, unspecified, third trimester ♀   M

● **O31** Complications specific to multiple gestation

     Excludes2   delayed delivery of second twin, triplet, etc. (O63.2)
                 malpresentation of one fetus or more (O32.9)
                 placental transfusion syndromes (O43.0-)

     Coding Clinic: 2012, Q4, P107

     One of the following 7th characters is to be assigned to each code under category O31. 7th character 0 is for single gestations and multiple gestations where the fetus is unspecified. 7th characters 1 through 9 are for cases of multiple gestations to identify the fetus for which the code applies. The appropriate code from category O30, Multiple gestation, must also be assigned when assigning a code from category O31 that has a 7th character of 1 through 9.

     | 0 | not applicable or unspecified |
     | 1 | fetus 1 |
     | 2 | fetus 2 |
     | 3 | fetus 3 |
     | 4 | fetus 4 |
     | 5 | fetus 5 |
     | 9 | other fetus |

● **O31.0** Papyraceous fetus
     Fetus compressus

     X● O31.00 Papyraceous fetus, unspecified trimester ♀   M
     X● O31.01 Papyraceous fetus, first trimester ♀   M
     X● O31.02 Papyraceous fetus, second trimester ♀   M
     X● O31.03 Papyraceous fetus, third trimester ♀   M

● **O31.1** Continuing pregnancy after spontaneous abortion of one fetus or more

     X● O31.10 Continuing pregnancy after spontaneous abortion of one fetus or more, unspecified trimester ♀   M

     X● O31.11 Continuing pregnancy after spontaneous abortion of one fetus or more, first trimester ♀ M

     X● O31.12 Continuing pregnancy after spontaneous abortion of one fetus or more, second trimester ♀   M

     X● O31.13 Continuing pregnancy after spontaneous abortion of one fetus or more, third trimester ♀   M

N Newborn Age: 0   **P** Pediatric Age: 0–17   **M** Maternity DX: 12–55   **A** Adult Age: 15–124   ♀ Females Only   ♂ Males Only

🏷 Complication\Comorbidity   🏷 Major C\C   Ⓔ CC/MCC Exclusions   🏷 Hospital-Acquired Condition   **1133**

CHAPTER 15 (O00-O9A)

CHAPTER 15 (O00-O9A)

● O31.2   **Continuing pregnancy after intrauterine death of one fetus or more**

    X ● O31.20   Continuing pregnancy after intrauterine death of one fetus or more, unspecified trimester ♀   M

    X ● O31.21   Continuing pregnancy after intrauterine death of one fetus or more, first trimester ♀   M

    X ● O31.22   Continuing pregnancy after intrauterine death of one fetus or more, second trimester ♀   M

    X ● O31.23   Continuing pregnancy after intrauterine death of one fetus or more, third trimester ♀   M

● O31.3   **Continuing pregnancy after elective fetal reduction of one fetus or more**

    Continuing pregnancy after selective termination of one fetus or more

    X ● O31.30   Continuing pregnancy after elective fetal reduction of one fetus or more, unspecified trimester ♀   M

    X ● O31.31   Continuing pregnancy after elective fetal reduction of one fetus or more, first trimester ♀   M

    X ● O31.32   Continuing pregnancy after elective fetal reduction of one fetus or more, second trimester ♀   M

    X ● O31.33   Continuing pregnancy after elective fetal reduction of one fetus or more, third trimester ♀   M

● O31.8   **Other complications specific to multiple gestation**

    (Ex) **For category O31.8 CC codes:** See O30.1

    ● O31.8X   Other complications specific to multiple gestation

       ● O31.8X1   Other complications specific to multiple gestation, first trimester ♀ 🔖   M

       ● O31.8X2   Other complications specific to multiple gestation, second trimester ♀ 🔖   M

       ● O31.8X3   Other complications specific to multiple gestation, third trimester ♀ 🔖   M

       ● O31.8X9   Other complications specific to multiple gestation, unspecified trimester ♀   M

● O32   **Maternal care for malpresentation of fetus**

    Includes   the listed conditions as a reason for observation, hospitalization or other obstetric care of the mother, or for cesarean delivery before onset of labor

    Excludes1   malpresentation of fetus with obstructed labor (O64.-)

    Coding Clinic: 2012, Q4, P107

    One of the following 7th characters is to be assigned to each code under category O32. 7th character Ø is for single gestations and multiple gestations where the fetus is unspecified. 7th characters 1 through 9 are for cases of multiple gestations to identify the fetus for which the code applies. The appropriate code from category O30, Multiple gestation, must also be assigned when assigning a code from category O32 that has a 7th character of 1 through 9.

Ø	not applicable or unspecified
1	fetus 1
2	fetus 2
3	fetus 3
4	fetus 4
5	fetus 5
9	other fetus

    X ● O32.0   **Maternal care for unstable lie** ♀   M

    X ● O32.1   **Maternal care for breech presentation** ♀   M

       Maternal care for buttocks presentation
       Maternal care for complete breech
       Maternal care for frank breech

       Excludes1   footling presentation (O32.8)
               incomplete breech (O32.8)

X ● O32.2   **Maternal care for transverse and oblique lie** ♀   M

    Maternal care for oblique presentation
    Maternal care for transverse presentation

X ● O32.3   **Maternal care for face, brow and chin presentation** ♀   M

X ● O32.4   **Maternal care for high head at term** ♀   M

    Maternal care for failure of head to enter pelvic brim

X ● O32.6   **Maternal care for compound presentation** ♀   M

X ● O32.8   **Maternal care for other malpresentation of fetus** ♀   M

    Maternal care for footling presentation
    Maternal care for incomplete breech

X ● O32.9   **Maternal care for malpresentation of fetus, unspecified** ♀   M

● O33   **Maternal care for disproportion**

    Includes   the listed conditions as a reason for observation, hospitalization or other obstetric care of the mother, or for cesarean delivery before onset of labor

    Excludes1   disproportion with obstructed labor (O65-O66)

    O33.0   **Maternal care for disproportion due to deformity of maternal pelvic bones** ♀ 🔖   M

       Maternal care for disproportion due to pelvic deformity causing disproportion NOS
       (Ex) O33.0

    O33.1   **Maternal care for disproportion due to generally contracted pelvis** ♀   M

       Maternal care for disproportion due to contracted pelvis NOS causing disproportion

    O33.2   **Maternal care for disproportion due to inlet contraction of pelvis** ♀   M

       Maternal care for disproportion due to inlet contraction (pelvis) causing disproportion

    X ● O33.3   **Maternal care for disproportion due to outlet contraction of pelvis** ♀   M

       Maternal care for disproportion due to mid-cavity contraction (pelvis)
       Maternal care for disproportion due to outlet contraction (pelvis)

       One of the following 7th characters is to be assigned to code O33.3. 7th character Ø is for single gestations and multiple gestations where the fetus is unspecified. 7th characters 1 through 9 are for cases of multiple gestations to identify the fetus for which the code applies. The appropriate code from category O30, Multiple gestation, must also be assigned when assigning code O33.3 with a 7th character of 1 through 9.

Ø	not applicable or unspecified
1	fetus 1
2	fetus 2
3	fetus 3
4	fetus 4
5	fetus 5
9	other fetus

X ● O33.4   **Maternal care for disproportion of mixed maternal and fetal origin** ♀   M

       One of the following 7th characters is to be assigned to code O33.4. 7th character Ø is for single gestations and multiple gestations where the fetus is unspecified. 7th characters 1 through 9 are for cases of multiple gestations to identify the fetus for which the code applies. The appropriate code from category O30, Multiple gestation, must also be assigned when assigning code O33.4 with a 7th character of 1 through 9.

Ø	not applicable or unspecified
1	fetus 1
2	fetus 2
3	fetus 3
4	fetus 4
5	fetus 5
9	other fetus

◄ New   ◄▦ Revised   ~~deleted~~ Deleted   Excludes 1   Excludes 2   Includes   Use additional   Code first   Code also   Unspecified

OGCR Official Guidelines   ● Unacceptable Principal Diagnosis   X Assign placeholder X   ● Use Additional Character(s)   ▶ Manifestation Code   **Coding Clinic**

X ● **O33.5** **Maternal care for disproportion due to unusually large fetus** ♀ **M**

    Maternal care for disproportion due to disproportion of fetal origin with normally formed fetus

    Maternal care for disproportion due to fetal disproportion NOS

    One of the following 7th characters is to be assigned to code O33.5. 7th character Ø is for single gestations and multiple gestations where the fetus is unspecified. 7th characters 1 through 9 are for cases of multiple gestations to identify the fetus for which the code applies. The appropriate code from category O30, Multiple gestation, must also be assigned when assigning code O33.5 with a 7th character of 1 through 9.

Ø	not applicable or unspecified
1	fetus 1
2	fetus 2
3	fetus 3
4	fetus 4
5	fetus 5
9	other fetus

X ● **O33.6** **Maternal care for disproportion due to hydrocephalic fetus** ♀ **M**

    One of the following 7th characters is to be assigned to code O33.6. 7th character Ø is for single gestations and multiple gestations where the fetus is unspecified. 7th characters 1 through 9 are for cases of multiple gestations to identify the fetus for which the code applies. The appropriate code from category O30, Multiple gestation, must also be assigned when assigning code O33.6 with a 7th character of 1 through 9.

Ø	not applicable or unspecified
1	fetus 1
2	fetus 2
3	fetus 3
4	fetus 4
5	fetus 5
9	other fetus

X ● **O33.7** **Maternal care for disproportion due to other fetal deformities** ♀ **M**

    Maternal care for disproportion due to fetal ascites

    Maternal care for disproportion due to fetal hydrops

    Maternal care for disproportion due to fetal meningomyelocele

    Maternal care for disproportion due to fetal sacral teratoma

    Maternal care for disproportion due to fetal tumor

    Excludes1   obstructed labor due to other fetal deformities (O66.3)

    One of the following 7th characters is to be assigned to code O33.7. 7th character Ø is for single gestations and multiple gestations where the fetus is unspecified. 7th characters 1 through 9 are for cases of multiple gestations to identify the fetus for which the code applies. The appropriate code from category O30, Multiple gestation, must also be assigned when assigning code O33.7 with a 7th character of 1 through 9. ◄

Ø	not applicable or unspecified ◄
1	fetus 1 ◄
2	fetus 2 ◄
3	fetus 3 ◄
4	fetus 4 ◄
5	fetus 5 ◄
9	other fetus ◄

O33.8 **Maternal care for disproportion of other origin** ♀ **M**

O33.9 **Maternal care for disproportion, unspecified** ♀ **M**

    Maternal care for disproportion due to cephalopelvic disproportion NOS

    Maternal care for disproportion due to fetopelvic disproportion NOS

● **O34** **Maternal care for abnormality of pelvic organs**

    Includes   the listed conditions as a reason for hospitalization or other obstetric care of the mother, or for cesarean delivery before onset of labor

    Code first any associated obstructed labor (O65.5)

    Use additional code for specific condition

● **O34.0** **Maternal care for congenital malformation of uterus**

    Maternal care for double uterus ◄

    Maternal care for uterus bicornis ◄

    O34.00 **Maternal care for unspecified congenital malformation of uterus, unspecified trimester** ♀ **M**

    O34.01 **Maternal care for unspecified congenital malformation of uterus, first trimester** ♀ **M**

    O34.02 **Maternal care for unspecified congenital malformation of uterus, second trimester** ♀ **M**

    O34.03 **Maternal care for unspecified congenital malformation of uterus, third trimester** ♀ **M**

● **O34.1** **Maternal care for benign tumor of corpus uteri**

    Excludes2   maternal care for benign tumor of cervix (O34.4-)

        maternal care for malignant neoplasm of uterus (O9A.1-)

    O34.10 **Maternal care for benign tumor of corpus uteri, unspecified trimester** ♀ **M**

    O34.11 **Maternal care for benign tumor of corpus uteri, first trimester** ♀ **M**

    O34.12 **Maternal care for benign tumor of corpus uteri, second trimester** ♀ **M**

    O34.13 **Maternal care for benign tumor of corpus uteri, third trimester** ♀ **M**

● **O34.2** **Maternal care due to uterine scar from previous surgery**

    ● **O34.21** **Maternal care for scar from previous cesarean delivery**

        O34.211 **Maternal care for low transverse scar from previous cesarean delivery** ♀ ◄ **M**

        O34.212 **Maternal care for vertical scar from previous cesarean delivery** ♀ ◄ **M**

            Maternal care for classical scar from previous cesarean delivery ◄

        O34.219 **Maternal care for unspecified type scar from previous cesarean delivery** ♀ ◄ **M**

    O34.29 **Maternal care due to uterine scar from other previous surgery** ♀ **M**

        Maternal care due to uterine scar from other transmural uterine incision ◄

● **O34.3** **Maternal care for cervical incompetence**

    Maternal care for cerclage with or without cervical incompetence

    Maternal care for Shirodkar suture with or without cervical incompetence

    (Ex) **For category O34.3 CC codes:** O26.872-O26.879, O34.31-O34.33

    O34.30 **Maternal care for cervical incompetence, unspecified trimester** ♀ **M**

    O34.31 **Maternal care for cervical incompetence, first trimester** ♀ 🔹 **M**

    O34.32 **Maternal care for cervical incompetence, second trimester** ♀ 🔹 **M**

    O34.33 **Maternal care for cervical incompetence, third trimester** ♀ 🔹 **M**

● **O34.4** **Maternal care for other abnormalities of cervix**

    O34.40 **Maternal care for other abnormalities of cervix, unspecified trimester** ♀ **M**

    O34.41 **Maternal care for other abnormalities of cervix, first trimester** ♀ **M**

    O34.42 **Maternal care for other abnormalities of cervix, second trimester** ♀ **M**

    O34.43 **Maternal care for other abnormalities of cervix, third trimester** ♀ **M**

N Newborn Age: 0   **P** Pediatric Age: 0–17   **M** Maternity DX: 12–55   **A** Adult Age: 15–124   ♀ Females Only   ♂ Males Only

🔹 Complication\Comorbidity   🔹 Major C\C   (Ex) CC/MCC Exclusions   🔹 Hospital-Acquired Condition

1135

CHAPTER 15 (O00-O9A)

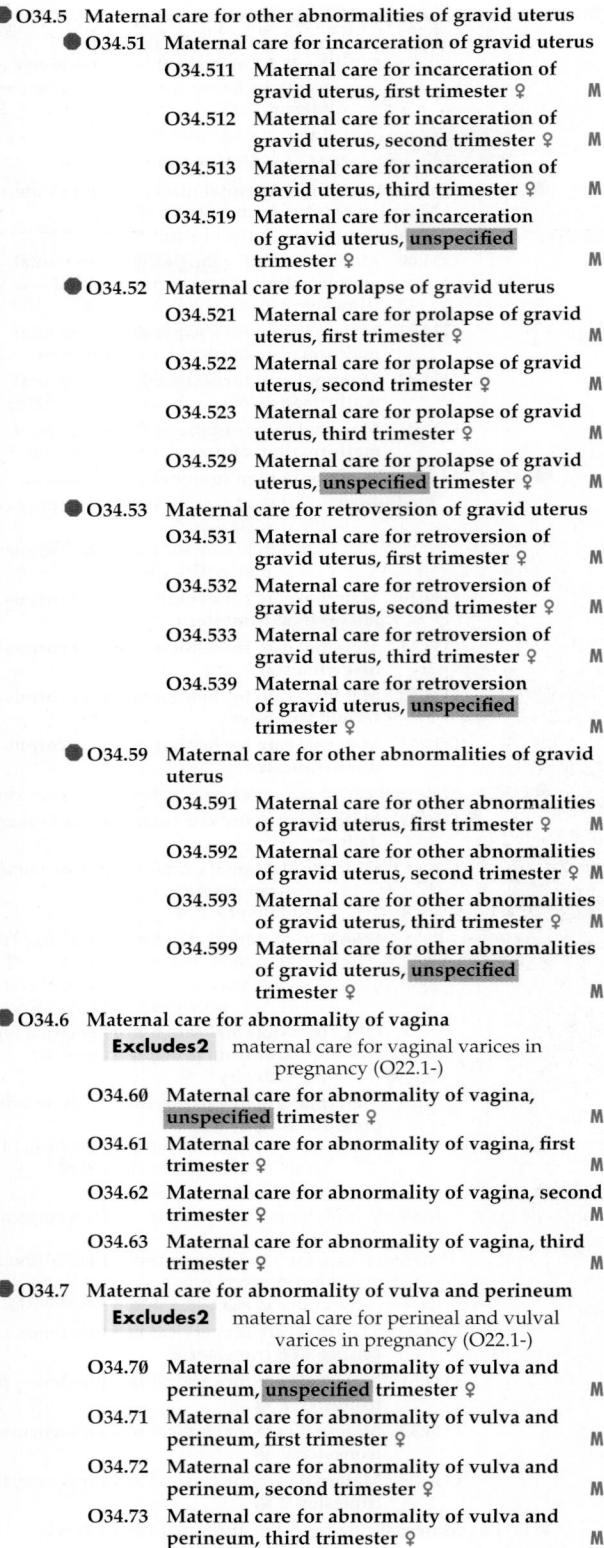

● O34.5   Maternal care for other abnormalities of gravid uterus
 ● O34.51   Maternal care for incarceration of gravid uterus
  O34.511   Maternal care for incarceration of gravid uterus, first trimester ♀   M
  O34.512   Maternal care for incarceration of gravid uterus, second trimester ♀   M
  O34.513   Maternal care for incarceration of gravid uterus, third trimester ♀   M
  O34.519   Maternal care for incarceration of gravid uterus, unspecified trimester ♀   M
 ● O34.52   Maternal care for prolapse of gravid uterus
  O34.521   Maternal care for prolapse of gravid uterus, first trimester ♀   M
  O34.522   Maternal care for prolapse of gravid uterus, second trimester ♀   M
  O34.523   Maternal care for prolapse of gravid uterus, third trimester ♀   M
  O34.529   Maternal care for prolapse of gravid uterus, unspecified trimester ♀   M
 ● O34.53   Maternal care for retroversion of gravid uterus
  O34.531   Maternal care for retroversion of gravid uterus, first trimester ♀   M
  O34.532   Maternal care for retroversion of gravid uterus, second trimester ♀   M
  O34.533   Maternal care for retroversion of gravid uterus, third trimester ♀   M
  O34.539   Maternal care for retroversion of gravid uterus, unspecified trimester ♀   M
 ● O34.59   Maternal care for other abnormalities of gravid uterus
  O34.591   Maternal care for other abnormalities of gravid uterus, first trimester ♀   M
  O34.592   Maternal care for other abnormalities of gravid uterus, second trimester ♀   M
  O34.593   Maternal care for other abnormalities of gravid uterus, third trimester ♀   M
  O34.599   Maternal care for other abnormalities of gravid uterus, unspecified trimester ♀   M
● O34.6   Maternal care for abnormality of vagina
  Excludes2   maternal care for vaginal varices in pregnancy (O22.1-)
  O34.60   Maternal care for abnormality of vagina, unspecified trimester ♀   M
  O34.61   Maternal care for abnormality of vagina, first trimester ♀   M
  O34.62   Maternal care for abnormality of vagina, second trimester ♀   M
  O34.63   Maternal care for abnormality of vagina, third trimester ♀   M
● O34.7   Maternal care for abnormality of vulva and perineum
  Excludes2   maternal care for perineal and vulval varices in pregnancy (O22.1-)
  O34.70   Maternal care for abnormality of vulva and perineum, unspecified trimester ♀   M
  O34.71   Maternal care for abnormality of vulva and perineum, first trimester ♀   M
  O34.72   Maternal care for abnormality of vulva and perineum, second trimester ♀   M
  O34.73   Maternal care for abnormality of vulva and perineum, third trimester ♀

● O34.8   Maternal care for other abnormalities of pelvic organs
  O34.80   Maternal care for other abnormalities of pelvic organs, unspecified trimester ♀   M
  O34.81   Maternal care for other abnormalities of pelvic organs, first trimester ♀   M
  O34.82   Maternal care for other abnormalities of pelvic organs, second trimester ♀   M
  O34.83   Maternal care for other abnormalities of pelvic organs, third trimester ♀   M
● O34.9   Maternal care for abnormality of pelvic organ, unspecified
  O34.90   Maternal care for abnormality of pelvic organ, unspecified, unspecified trimester ♀   M
  O34.91   Maternal care for abnormality of pelvic organ, unspecified, first trimester ♀   M
  O34.92   Maternal care for abnormality of pelvic organ, unspecified, second trimester ♀   M
  O34.93   Maternal care for abnormality of pelvic organ, unspecified, third trimester ♀   M
● O35   Maternal care for known or suspected fetal abnormality and damage
  Includes   the listed conditions in the fetus as a reason for hospitalization or other obstetric care to the mother, or for termination of pregnancy
  Code also any associated maternal condition
  Excludes1   encounter for suspected maternal and fetal conditions ruled out (Z03.7-)
  One of the following 7th characters is to be assigned to each code under category O35. 7th character 0 is for single gestations and multiple gestations where the fetus is unspecified. 7th characters 1 through 9 are for cases of multiple gestations to identify the fetus for which the code applies. The appropriate code from category O30, Multiple gestation, must also be assigned when assigning a code from category O35 that has a 7th character of 1 through 9.

0	not applicable or unspecified
1	fetus 1
2	fetus 2
3	fetus 3
4	fetus 4
5	fetus 5
9	other fetus

  X ● O35.0   Maternal care for (suspected) central nervous system malformation in fetus ♀   M
    Maternal care for fetal anencephaly
    Maternal care for fetal hydrocephalus
    Maternal care for fetal spina bifida
    Excludes2   chromosomal abnormality in fetus (O35.1)
  X ● O35.1   Maternal care for (suspected) chromosomal abnormality in fetus ♀   M
  X ● O35.2   Maternal care for (suspected) hereditary disease in fetus ♀   M
    Excludes2   chromosomal abnormality in fetus (O35.1)

OGCR   Section I.C.15.e.l.

Fetal Conditions Affecting the Management of the Mother
1) Code from categories O35 and O36
Codes from categories O35, Maternal care for known or suspected fetal abnormality and damage, and O36, Maternal care for other fetal problems, are assigned only when the fetal condition is actually responsible for modifying the management of the mother, i.e., by requiring diagnostic studies, additional observation, special care, or termination of pregnancy. The fact that the fetal condition exists does not justify assigning a code from this series to the mother's record.
2) In utero surgery
In cases when surgery is performed on the fetus, a diagnosis code from category O35, Maternal care for known or suspected fetal abnormality and damage, should be assigned identifying the fetal condition. Assign the appropriate procedure code for the procedure performed.
No code from Chapter 16, the perinatal codes, should be used on the mother's record to identify fetal conditions. Surgery performed in utero on a fetus is still to be coded as an obstetric encounter.

◄ New   ◄═ Revised   ~~deleted~~ Deleted   Excludes 1   Excludes 2   Includes   Use additional   Code first   Code also   Unspecified
OGCR Official Guidelines   ● Unacceptable Principal Diagnosis   X Assign placeholder X   ● Use Additional Character(s)   ▷ Manifestation Code   Coding Clinic

CHAPTER 15 (O00-O9A)

X⬤ **O35.3** **Maternal care for (suspected) damage to fetus from viral disease in mother** ♀   M
     Maternal care for damage to fetus from maternal cytomegalovirus infection
     Maternal care for damage to fetus from maternal rubella

X⬤ **O35.4** **Maternal care for (suspected) damage to fetus from alcohol** ♀   M

X⬤ **O35.5** **Maternal care for (suspected) damage to fetus by drugs** ♀   M
     Maternal care for damage to fetus from drug addiction

X⬤ **O35.6** **Maternal care for (suspected) damage to fetus by radiation** ♀   M

X⬤ **O35.7** **Maternal care for (suspected) damage to fetus by other medical procedures** ♀   M
     Maternal care for damage to fetus by amniocentesis
     Maternal care for damage to fetus by biopsy procedures
     Maternal care for damage to fetus by hematological investigation
     Maternal care for damage to fetus by intrauterine contraceptive device
     Maternal care for damage to fetus by intrauterine surgery

X⬤ **O35.8** **Maternal care for other (suspected) fetal abnormality and damage** ♀   M
     Maternal care for damage to fetus from maternal listeriosis
     Maternal care for damage to fetus from maternal toxoplasmosis

X⬤ **O35.9** **Maternal care for (suspected) fetal abnormality and damage, unspecified** ♀   M

⬤ **O36** **Maternal care for other fetal problems**

Includes   the listed conditions in the fetus as a reason for hospitalization or other obstetric care of the mother, or for termination of pregnancy

Excludes1   encounter for suspected maternal and fetal conditions ruled out (Z03.7-)
     placental transfusion syndromes (O43.0-)

Excludes2   labor and delivery complicated by fetal stress (O77.-)

One of the following 7th characters is to be assigned to each code under category O36. 7th character Ø is for single gestations and multiple gestations where the fetus is unspecified. 7th characters 1 through 9 are for cases of multiple gestations to identify the fetus for which the code applies. The appropriate code from category O30, Multiple gestation, must also be assigned when assigning a code from category O36 that has a 7th character of 1 through 9.

Ø	not applicable or unspecified
1	fetus 1
2	fetus 2
3	fetus 3
4	fetus 4
5	fetus 5
9	other fetus

Coding Clinic: 2015, Q3, P40

⬤ **O36.0** **Maternal care for rhesus isoimmunization**
     Maternal care for Rh incompatibility (with hydrops fetalis)
     (Ex) For category O36.0 CC codes: O36.0110-O36.0139, O36.0910-O36.0939

⬤ **O36.01** **Maternal care for anti-D [Rh] antibodies**

     ⬤ **O36.011** **Maternal care for anti-D [Rh] antibodies, first trimester** ♀ 🦠   M

     ⬤ **O36.012** **Maternal care for anti-D [Rh] antibodies, second trimester** ♀ 🦠   M

     ⬤ **O36.013** **Maternal care for anti-D [Rh] antibodies, third trimester** ♀ 🦠   M

     ⬤ **O36.019** **Maternal care for anti-D [Rh] antibodies, unspecified trimester** ♀   M

⬤ **O36.09** **Maternal care for other rhesus isoimmunization**

     ⬤ **O36.091** **Maternal care for other rhesus isoimmunization, first trimester** ♀ 🦠   M

     ⬤ **O36.092** **Maternal care for other rhesus isoimmunization, second trimester** ♀ 🦠   M

     ⬤ **O36.093** **Maternal care for other rhesus isoimmunization, third trimester** ♀ 🦠   M
         Coding Clinic: 2015, Q3, P40

     ⬤ **O36.099** **Maternal care for other rhesus isoimmunization, unspecified trimester** ♀   M

⬤ **O36.1** **Maternal care for other isoimmunization**
     Maternal care for ABO isoimmunization

     ⬤ **O36.11** **Maternal care for Anti-A sensitization**
         Maternal care for isoimmunization NOS (with hydrops fetalis)

         ⬤ **O36.111** **Maternal care for Anti-A sensitization, first trimester** ♀   M

         ⬤ **O36.112** **Maternal care for Anti-A sensitization, second trimester** ♀   M

         ⬤ **O36.113** **Maternal care for Anti-A sensitization, third trimester** ♀   M

         ⬤ **O36.119** **Maternal care for Anti-A sensitization, unspecified trimester** ♀   M

     ⬤ **O36.19** **Maternal care for other isoimmunization**
         Maternal care for Anti-B sensitization

         ⬤ **O36.191** **Maternal care for other isoimmunization, first trimester** ♀   M

         ⬤ **O36.192** **Maternal care for other isoimmunization, second trimester** ♀   M

         ⬤ **O36.193** **Maternal care for other isoimmunization, third trimester** ♀   M

         ⬤ **O36.199** **Maternal care for other isoimmunization, unspecified trimester** ♀   M

⬤ **O36.2** **Maternal care for hydrops fetalis**
     Maternal care for hydrops fetalis NOS
     Maternal care for hydrops fetalis not associated with isoimmunization

     Excludes1   hydrops fetalis associated with ABO isoimmunization (O36.1-)
         hydrops fetalis associated with rhesus isoimmunization (O36.0-)

     ⬤ **O36.20** **Maternal care for hydrops fetalis, unspecified trimester** ♀   M

     ⬤ **O36.21** **Maternal care for hydrops fetalis, first trimester** ♀   M

     ⬤ **O36.22** **Maternal care for hydrops fetalis, second trimester** ♀   M

     ⬤ **O36.23** **Maternal care for hydrops fetalis, third trimester** ♀   M

⬤ **O36.4** **Maternal care for intrauterine death** ♀ 🦠   M
     Maternal care for intrauterine fetal death NOS
     Maternal care for intrauterine fetal death after completion of 20 weeks of gestation
     Maternal care for late fetal death
     Maternal care for missed delivery

     Excludes1   missed abortion (O02.1)
         stillbirth (P95)
     (Ex) O36.4XX0-O36.4XX9

CHAPTER 15 (O00-O9A)

● O36.5   **Maternal care for known or suspected poor fetal growth**

  ● O36.51   **Maternal care for known or suspected placental insufficiency**

    ● O36.511   **Maternal care for known or suspected placental insufficiency, first trimester** ♀   M

    ● O36.512   **Maternal care for known or suspected placental insufficiency, second trimester** ♀   M

    ● O36.513   **Maternal care for known or suspected placental insufficiency, third trimester** ♀   M

    ● O36.519   **Maternal care for known or suspected placental insufficiency, unspecified trimester** ♀   M

  ● O36.59   **Maternal care for other known or suspected poor fetal growth**

    Maternal care for known or suspected light-for-dates NOS

    Maternal care for known or suspected small-for-dates NOS

    ● O36.591   **Maternal care for other known or suspected poor fetal growth, first trimester** ♀   M

    ● O36.592   **Maternal care for other known or suspected poor fetal growth, second trimester** ♀   M

    ● O36.593   **Maternal care for other known or suspected poor fetal growth, third trimester** ♀   M

    ● O36.599   **Maternal care for other known or suspected poor fetal growth, unspecified trimester** ♀   M

● O36.6   **Maternal care for excessive fetal growth**

  Maternal care for known or suspected large-for-dates

  X ● O36.60   **Maternal care for excessive fetal growth, unspecified trimester** ♀   M

  X ● O36.61   **Maternal care for excessive fetal growth, first trimester** ♀   M

  X ● O36.62   **Maternal care for excessive fetal growth, second trimester** ♀   M

  X ● O36.63   **Maternal care for excessive fetal growth, third trimester** ♀   M

● O36.7   **Maternal care for viable fetus in abdominal pregnancy**

  X ● O36.70   **Maternal care for viable fetus in abdominal pregnancy, unspecified trimester** ♀   M

  X ● O36.71   **Maternal care for viable fetus in abdominal pregnancy, first trimester** ♀   M

  X ● O36.72   **Maternal care for viable fetus in abdominal pregnancy, second trimester** ♀   M

  X ● O36.73   **Maternal care for viable fetus in abdominal pregnancy, third trimester** ♀   M

● O36.8   **Maternal care for other specified fetal problems**

  ● X ● O36.80   **Pregnancy with inconclusive fetal viability** ♀   M

    Encounter to determine fetal viability of pregnancy

  ● O36.81   **Decreased fetal movements**

    ● O36.812   **Decreased fetal movements, second trimester** ♀   M

    ● O36.813   **Decreased fetal movements, third trimester** ♀   M

    ● O36.819   **Decreased fetal movements, unspecified trimester** ♀   M

  ● O36.82   **Fetal anemia and thrombocytopenia**

    ● O36.821   **Fetal anemia and thrombocytopenia, first trimester** ♀   M

    ● O36.822   **Fetal anemia and thrombocytopenia, second trimester** ♀   M

    ● O36.823   **Fetal anemia and thrombocytopenia, third trimester** ♀   M

    ● O36.829   **Fetal anemia and thrombocytopenia, unspecified trimester** ♀   M

  ● O36.89   **Maternal care for other specified fetal problems**

    ● O36.891   **Maternal care for other specified fetal problems, first trimester** ♀   M

    ● O36.892   **Maternal care for other specified fetal problems, second trimester** ♀   M

    ● O36.893   **Maternal care for other specified fetal problems, third trimester** ♀   M

    ● O36.899   **Maternal care for other specified fetal problems, unspecified trimester** ♀   M

● O36.9   **Maternal care for fetal problem, unspecified**

  X ● O36.90   **Maternal care for fetal problem, unspecified, unspecified trimester** ♀   M

  X ● O36.91   **Maternal care for fetal problem, unspecified, first trimester** ♀   M

  X ● O36.92   **Maternal care for fetal problem, unspecified, second trimester** ♀   M

  X ● O36.93   **Maternal care for fetal problem, unspecified, third trimester** ♀   M

● O40   **Polyhydramnios**

  Overabundance of amniotic fluid

  Includes   hydramnios

  Excludes1   encounter for suspected maternal and fetal conditions ruled out (Z03.7-)

  One of the following 7th characters is to be assigned to each code under category O40. 7th character Ø is for single gestations and multiple gestations where the fetus is unspecified. 7th characters 1 through 9 are for cases of multiple gestations to identify the fetus for which the code applies. The appropriate code from category O30, Multiple gestation, must also be assigned when assigning a code from category O40 that has a 7th character of 1 through 9.

Ø	not applicable or unspecified
1	fetus 1
2	fetus 2
3	fetus 3
4	fetus 4
5	fetus 5
9	other fetus

  X ● O40.1   **Polyhydramnios, first trimester** ♀   M

  X ● O40.2   **Polyhydramnios, second trimester** ♀   M

  X ● O40.3   **Polyhydramnios, third trimester** ♀   M

  X ● O40.9   **Polyhydramnios, unspecified trimester** ♀   M

● O41   **Other disorders of amniotic fluid and membranes**

  Excludes1   encounter for suspected maternal and fetal conditions ruled out (Z03.7-)

  One of the following 7th characters is to be assigned to each code under category O41. 7th character Ø is for single gestations and multiple gestations where the fetus is unspecified. 7th characters 1 through 9 are for cases of multiple gestations to identify the fetus for which the code applies. The appropriate code from category O30, Multiple gestation, must also be assigned when assigning a code from category O41 that has a 7th character of 1 through 9.

Ø	not applicable or unspecified
1	fetus 1
2	fetus 2
3	fetus 3
4	fetus 4
5	fetus 5
9	other fetus

● O41.0   **Oligohydramnios**

  Scant volume of amniotic fluid

  Oligohydramnios without rupture of membranes

  Ⓔⓧ For category O41.0 CC codes: O41.01X0-O41.03X9

  X ● O41.00   **Oligohydramnios, unspecified trimester** ♀   M

  X ● O41.01   **Oligohydramnios, first trimester** 🔗   M

  X ● O41.02   **Oligohydramnios, second trimester** ♀ 🔗   M

  X ● O41.03   **Oligohydramnios, third trimester** ♀ 🔗   M

◀ New   ◀ Revised   ~~deleted~~ Deleted   Excludes 1   Excludes 2   Includes   Use additional   Code first   Code also   Unspecified

OGCR Official Guidelines   ● Unacceptable Principal Diagnosis   X Assign placeholder X   ● Use Additional Character(s)   ▶ Manifestation Code   **Coding Clinic**

● O41.1   **Infection of amniotic sac and membranes**
    (Ex): **For category O41.1 CC codes:** 041.1010-041.1039, 041.1210-041.1239, 041.1410-041.1439

   ● O41.10   **Infection of amniotic sac and membranes, unspecified**
     ● O41.101   Infection of amniotic sac and membranes, unspecified, first trimester ♀   M
     ● O41.102   Infection of amniotic sac and membranes, unspecified, second trimester ♀ 🐾   M
     ● O41.103   Infection of amniotic sac and membranes, unspecified, third trimester ♀ 🐾   M
     ● O41.109   Infection of amniotic sac and membranes, unspecified, unspecified trimester ♀   M

   ● O41.12   **Chorioamnionitis**
     ● O41.121   Chorioamnionitis, first trimester ♀ 🐾   M
     ● O41.122   Chorioamnionitis, second trimester ♀ 🐾   M
     ● O41.123   Chorioamnionitis, third trimester ♀ 🐾   M
     ● O41.129   Chorioamnionitis, unspecified trimester ♀   M

   ● O41.14   **Placentitis**
     ● O41.141   Placentitis, first trimester ♀ 🐾   M
     ● O41.142   Placentitis, second trimester ♀ 🐾   M
     ● O41.143   Placentitis, third trimester ♀ 🐾   M
     ● O41.149   Placentitis, unspecified trimester ♀   M

● O41.8   **Other specified disorders of amniotic fluid and membranes**
   ● O41.8X   **Other specified disorders of amniotic fluid and membranes**
     ● O41.8X1   Other specified disorders of amniotic fluid and membranes, first trimester ♀   M
     ● O41.8X2   Other specified disorders of amniotic fluid and membranes, second trimester ♀   M
     ● O41.8X3   Other specified disorders of amniotic fluid and membranes, third trimester ♀   M
     ● O41.8X9   Other specified disorders of amniotic fluid and membranes, unspecified trimester ♀   M

● O41.9   **Disorder of amniotic fluid and membranes, unspecified**
  X ● O41.90   Disorder of amniotic fluid and membranes, unspecified, unspecified trimester ♀   M
  X ● O41.91   Disorder of amniotic fluid and membranes, unspecified, first trimester ♀   M
  X ● O41.92   Disorder of amniotic fluid and membranes, unspecified, second trimester ♀   M
  X ● O41.93   Disorder of amniotic fluid and membranes, unspecified, third trimester ♀   M

● O42   **Premature rupture of membranes**
   ● O42.0   **Premature rupture of membranes, onset of labor within 24 hours of rupture**
     ● O42.00   Premature rupture of membranes, onset of labor within 24 hours of rupture, unspecified weeks of gestation ♀   M
     ● O42.01   Preterm premature rupture of membranes, onset of labor within 24 hours of rupture
       Premature rupture of membranes before 37 completed weeks of gestation
       O42.011   Preterm premature rupture of membranes, onset of labor within 24 hours of rupture, first trimester ♀   M
       O42.012   Preterm premature rupture of membranes, onset of labor within 24 hours of rupture, second trimester ♀ M
       O42.013   Preterm premature rupture of membranes, onset of labor within 24 hours of rupture, third trimester ♀   M
       O42.019   Preterm premature rupture of membranes, onset of labor within 24 hours of rupture, unspecified trimester ♀   M
     O42.02   Full-term premature rupture of membranes, onset of labor within 24 hours of rupture ♀   M
       Premature rupture of membranes at or after 37 completed weeks of gestation, onset of labor within 24 hours of rupture ◀▬

   ● O42.1   **Premature rupture of membranes, onset of labor more than 24 hours following rupture**
     O42.10   Premature rupture of membranes, onset of labor more than 24 hours following rupture, unspecified weeks of gestation ♀   M
     ● O42.11   Preterm premature rupture of membranes, onset of labor more than 24 hours following rupture
       Premature rupture of membranes before 37 completed weeks of gestation
       O42.111   Preterm premature rupture of membranes, onset of labor more than 24 hours following rupture, first trimester ♀   M
       O42.112   Preterm premature rupture of membranes, onset of labor more than 24 hours following rupture, second trimester ♀   M
       O42.113   Preterm premature rupture of membranes, onset of labor more than 24 hours following rupture, third trimester ♀   M
       O42.119   Preterm premature rupture of membranes, onset of labor more than 24 hours following rupture, unspecified trimester ♀   M
     O42.12   Full-term premature rupture of membranes, onset of labor more than 24 hours following rupture ♀   M
       Premature rupture of membranes at or after 37 completed weeks of gestation, onset of labor more than 24 hours following rupture ◀▬

● **O42.9**   **Premature rupture of membranes, unspecified as to length of time between rupture and onset of labor**

    O42.90   Premature rupture of membranes, unspecified as to length of time between rupture and onset of labor, unspecified weeks of gestation ♀   M

   ● **O42.91**   Preterm premature rupture of membranes, unspecified as to length of time between rupture and onset of labor
        Premature rupture of membranes before 37 completed weeks of gestation

         O42.911   Preterm premature rupture of membranes, unspecified as to length of time between rupture and onset of labor, first trimester ♀   M

         O42.912   Preterm premature rupture of membranes, unspecified as to length of time between rupture and onset of labor, second trimester ♀   M

         O42.913   Preterm premature rupture of membranes, unspecified as to length of time between rupture and onset of labor, third trimester ♀   M

         O42.919   Preterm premature rupture of membranes, unspecified as to length of time between rupture and onset of labor, unspecified trimester ♀   M

    O42.92   Full-term premature rupture of membranes, unspecified as to length of time between rupture and onset of labor ♀   M
        Premature rupture of membranes at or after 37 completed weeks of gestation, unspecified as to length of time between rupture and onset of labor ◀◀◀

● **O43**   **Placental disorders**
    Excludes2   maternal care for poor fetal growth due to placental insufficiency (O36.5-)
         placenta previa (O44.-)
         placental polyp (O90.89)
         placentitis (O41.14-)
         premature separation of placenta [abruptio placentae] (O45.-)

 ● **O43.0**   **Placental transfusion syndromes**
   ● **O43.01**   Fetomaternal placental transfusion syndrome
        Maternofetal placental transfusion syndrome

         O43.011   Fetomaternal placental transfusion syndrome, first trimester ♀   M

         O43.012   Fetomaternal placental transfusion syndrome, second trimester ♀   M

         O43.013   Fetomaternal placental transfusion syndrome, third trimester ♀   M

         O43.019   Fetomaternal placental transfusion syndrome, unspecified trimester ♀   M

   ● **O43.02**   Fetus-to-fetus placental transfusion syndrome

         O43.021   Fetus-to-fetus placental transfusion syndrome, first trimester ♀   M

         O43.022   Fetus-to-fetus placental transfusion syndrome, second trimester ♀   M

         O43.023   Fetus-to-fetus placental transfusion syndrome, third trimester ♀   M

         O43.029   Fetus-to-fetus placental transfusion syndrome, unspecified trimester ♀   M

 ● **O43.1**   **Malformation of placenta**
   ● **O43.10**   Malformation of placenta, unspecified
        Abnormal placenta NOS

         O43.101   Malformation of placenta, unspecified, first trimester ♀   M

         O43.102   Malformation of placenta, unspecified, second trimester ♀   M

         O43.103   Malformation of placenta, unspecified, third trimester ♀   M

         O43.109   Malformation of placenta, unspecified, unspecified trimester ♀   M

   ● **O43.11**   Circumvallate placenta

         O43.111   Circumvallate placenta, first trimester ♀   M

         O43.112   Circumvallate placenta, second trimester ♀   M

         O43.113   Circumvallate placenta, third trimester ♀   M

         O43.119   Circumvallate placenta, unspecified trimester ♀   M

   ● **O43.12**   Velamentous insertion of umbilical cord

         O43.121   Velamentous insertion of umbilical cord, first trimester ♀   M

         O43.122   Velamentous insertion of umbilical cord, second trimester ♀   M

         O43.123   Velamentous insertion of umbilical cord, third trimester ♀   M

         O43.129   Velamentous insertion of umbilical cord, unspecified trimester ♀   M

   ● **O43.19**   Other malformation of placenta

         O43.191   Other malformation of placenta, first trimester ♀   M

         O43.192   Other malformation of placenta, second trimester ♀   M

         O43.193   Other malformation of placenta, third trimester ♀   M

         O43.199   Other malformation of placenta, unspecified trimester ♀   M

 ● **O43.2**   **Morbidly adherent placenta**
    Code also associated third stage postpartum hemorrhage, if applicable (O72.0)
      Excludes1   retained placenta (O73.-)

   ● **O43.21**   Placenta accreta

         O43.211   Placenta accreta, first trimester ♀   M

         O43.212   Placenta accreta, second trimester ♀   M

         O43.213   Placenta accreta, third trimester ♀   M

         O43.219   Placenta accreta, unspecified trimester ♀   M

   ● **O43.22**   Placenta increta

         O43.221   Placenta increta, first trimester ♀   M

         O43.222   Placenta increta, second trimester ♀   M

         O43.223   Placenta increta, third trimester ♀   M

         O43.229   Placenta increta, unspecified trimester ♀   M

   ● **O43.23**   Placenta percreta

         O43.231   Placenta percreta, first trimester ♀   M

         O43.232   Placenta percreta, second trimester ♀ M

         O43.233   Placenta percreta, third trimester ♀   M

         O43.239   Placenta percreta, unspecified trimester ♀   M

 ● **O43.8**   **Other placental disorders**
   ● **O43.81**   Placental infarction

         O43.811   Placental infarction, first trimester ♀ M

         O43.812   Placental infarction, second trimester ♀   M

         O43.813   Placental infarction, third trimester ♀   M

         O43.819   Placental infarction, unspecified trimester ♀   M

   ● **O43.89**   Other placental disorders
        Placental dysfunction

         O43.891   Other placental disorders, first trimester ♀   M

         O43.892   Other placental disorders, second trimester ♀   M

         O43.893   Other placental disorders, third trimester ♀   M

         O43.899   Other placental disorders, unspecified trimester ♀   M

Figure 15-2 **A.** Marginal placento previa. **B.** Partial placenta previa. **C.** Total placento previa.

Item 15–3 Placenta previa is a condition in which the opening of the cervix is obstructed by the displaced placenta. The three types, marginal, partial, and total, are varying degrees of placenta displacement. Placenta abruption is the premature breaking away of the placenta from the site of the uterine implant before the delivery of the fetus.

● **O43.9 Unspecified placental disorder**

     O43.90 Unspecified placental disorder, unspecified trimester ♀   M

     O43.91 Unspecified placental disorder, first trimester ♀   M

     O43.92 Unspecified placental disorder, second trimester ♀   M

     O43.93 Unspecified placental disorder, third trimester ♀   M

● **O44 Placenta previa**

   (Ex) **For category O44 CC codes:** See O20

● **O44.0 Complete placenta previa NOS or without hemorrhage** ◀▥▥

     Placenta previa NOS ◀

     O44.00 Complete placenta previa NOS or without hemorrhage, unspecified trimester ♀ ◀▥▥   M

     O44.01 Complete placenta previa NOS or without hemorrhage, first trimester ♀ 🦠 ◀▥▥   M

     O44.02 Complete placenta previa NOS or without hemorrhage, second trimester ♀ 🦠 ◀▥▥   M

     O44.03 Complete placenta previa NOS or without hemorrhage, third trimester ♀ 🦠 ◀▥▥   M

● **O44.1 Complete placenta previa with hemorrhage** ◀▥▥

     Excludes1 labor and delivery complicated by hemorrhage from vasa previa (O69.4)

     O44.10 Complete placenta previa with hemorrhage, unspecified trimester ♀ ◀▥▥   M

     O44.11 Complete placenta previa with hemorrhage, first trimester ♀ 🦠 ◀▥▥   M

     O44.12 Complete placenta previa with hemorrhage, second trimester ♀ 🦠 ◀▥▥   M

     O44.13 Complete placenta previa with hemorrhage, third trimester ♀ 🦠 ◀▥▥   M

● **O44.2 Partial placenta previa without hemorrhage** ◀

     Marginal placenta previa, NOS or without hemorrhage ◀

     O44.20 Partial placenta previa NOS or without hemorrhage, unspecified trimester ♀ ◀   M

     O44.21 Partial placenta previa NOS or without hemorrhage, first trimester ♀ 🦠 ◀   M

     O44.22 Partial placenta previa NOS or without hemorrhage, second trimester ♀ 🦠 ◀   M

     O44.23 Partial placenta previa NOS or without hemorrhage, third trimester ♀ 🦠 ◀   M

● **O44.3 Partial placenta previa with hemorrhage** ◀

     Marginal placenta previa with hemorrhage ◀

     O44.30 Partial placenta previa with hemorrhage, unspecified trimester ♀ ◀   M

     O44.31 Partial placenta previa with hemorrhage, first trimester ♀ 🦠 ◀   M

     O44.32 Partial placenta previa with hemorrhage, second trimester ♀ 🦠 ◀   M

     O44.33 Partial placenta previa with hemorrhage, third trimester ♀ 🦠 ◀   M

● **O44.4 Low lying placenta NOS or without hemorrhage** ◀

     Low implantation of placenta NOS or without hemorrhage ◀

     O44.40 Low lying placenta NOS or without hemorrhage, unspecified trimester ♀ ◀   M

     O44.41 Low lying placenta NOS or without hemorrhage, first trimester ♀ 🦠 ◀   M

     O44.42 Low lying placenta NOS or without hemorrhage, second trimester ♀ 🦠 ◀   M

     O44.43 Low lying placenta NOS or without hemorrhage, third trimester ♀ 🦠 ◀   M

● **O44.5 Low lying placenta with hemorrhage** ◀

     Low implantation of placenta with hemorrhage ◀

     O44.50 Low lying placenta with hemorrhage, unspecified trimester ♀ ◀   M

     O44.51 Low lying placenta with hemorrhage, first trimester ♀ 🦠 ◀   M

     O44.52 Low lying placenta with hemorrhage, second trimester ♀ 🦠 ◀   M

     O44.53 Low lying placenta with hemorrhage, third trimester ♀ 🦠 ◀   M

● **O45 Premature separation of placenta [abruptio placentae]**

● **O45.0 Premature separation of placenta with coagulation defect**

   (Ex) **For category O45.0 CC codes:** O11.4, O11.5, O12.04, O12.05, O12.14, O12.15, O12.24, O12.25, O13.4, O13.5, O14.04, O14.05, O14.14, O14.15, O14.24, O14.25, O14.94, O14.95, O16.4, O16.5, O25.10-O25.3, O26.10-O26.13, O26.30-O26.43, O26.63-O26.819, O26.841-O26.86, O26.891-O26.93, O29.011-O29.93, O35.7XX0-O35.7XX9, O45.001-O45.099, O46.001-O46.93, O67.0-O67.9, O75.4, O75.81, O75.89-O75.9, O80, O90.89, O99.111-O99.285, O99.330-O99.335, O99.350-O99.355, O99.511-O99.73, O99.820-O99.825, O99.840-O9A.53

● **O45.00 Premature separation of placenta with coagulation defect, unspecified**

     O45.001 Premature separation of placenta with coagulation defect, unspecified, first trimester ♀ 🦠   M

     O45.002 Premature separation of placenta with coagulation defect, unspecified, second trimester ♀ 🦠   M

Figure 15-3 Abruptio placentae is classified according to the grade of separation of the placenta from the uterine wall. **A.** Mild separation in which hemorrhage is internal. **B.** Moderate separation in which there is external hemorrhage. **C.** Severe separation in which there is external hemorrhage and extreme separation.

CHAPTER 15 (O00-O9A)

CHAPTER 15 (O00-O9A)

O45.003   Premature separation of placenta with coagulation defect, unspecified, third trimester ♀ 🦠   M

O45.009   Premature separation of placenta with coagulation defect, unspecified, unspecified trimester ♀   M

● O45.01   Premature separation of placenta with afibrinogenemia
Premature separation of placenta with hypofibrinogenemia

O45.011   Premature separation of placenta with afibrinogenemia, first trimester ♀ 🦠 M

O45.012   Premature separation of placenta with afibrinogenemia, second trimester ♀ 🦠   M

O45.013   Premature separation of placenta with afibrinogenemia, third trimester ♀ 🦠   M

O45.019   Premature separation of placenta with afibrinogenemia, unspecified trimester ♀   M

● O45.02   Premature separation of placenta with disseminated intravascular coagulation

O45.021   Premature separation of placenta with disseminated intravascular coagulation, first trimester ♀ 🦠   M

O45.022   Premature separation of placenta with disseminated intravascular coagulation, second trimester ♀ 🦠   M

O45.023   Premature separation of placenta with disseminated intravascular coagulation, third trimester ♀ 🦠   M

O45.029   Premature separation of placenta with disseminated intravascular coagulation, unspecified trimester ♀ M

● O45.09   Premature separation of placenta with other coagulation defect

O45.091   Premature separation of placenta with other coagulation defect, first trimester ♀ 🦠   M

O45.092   Premature separation of placenta with other coagulation defect, second trimester ♀ 🦠   M

O45.093   Premature separation of placenta with other coagulation defect, third trimester ♀ 🦠   M

O45.099   Premature separation of placenta with other coagulation defect, unspecified trimester ♀   M

● O45.8   Other premature separation of placenta
Ⓔⓧ For category O45.8 CC codes: O11.4, O11.5, O12.04, O12.05, O12.14, O12.15, O12.24, O12.25, O13.4, O13.5, O14.04, O14.05, O14.14, O14.15, O14.24, O14.25, O14.94, O14.95, O16.4, O16.5, O20.0-O20.9, O25.10-O25.3, O26.10-O26.13, O26.30-O26.43, O26.63-O26.819, O26.841-O26.86, O26.891-O26.93, O29.011-O29.93, O35.7XX0-O35.7XX9, O44.00-O44.13, O44.20-O44.53, O45.8X1-O45.8X3, O45.91-O45.93, O75.4, O75.81, O75.89-O75.9, O80, O90.89, O99.111-O99.285, O99.330-O99.335, O99.350-O99.355, O99.511-O99.73, O99.820-O99.825, O99.840-O9A.53

● O45.8X   Other premature separation of placenta

O45.8X1   Other premature separation of placenta, first trimester ♀ 🦠   M

O45.8X2   Other premature separation of placenta, second trimester ♀ 🦠   M

O45.8X3   Other premature separation of placenta, third trimester ♀ 🦠   M

O45.8X9   Other premature separation of placenta, unspecified trimester ♀   M

● O45.9   Premature separation of placenta, unspecified
Abruptio placentae NOS
Ⓔⓧ For category O45.9 CC codes: See O45.8

O45.90   Premature separation of placenta, unspecified, unspecified trimester ♀   M

O45.91   Premature separation of placenta, unspecified, first trimester ♀ 🦠   M

O45.92   Premature separation of placenta, unspecified, second trimester ♀ 🦠   M

O45.93   Premature separation of placenta, unspecified, third trimester ♀ 🦠   M

● O46   Antepartum hemorrhage, not elsewhere classified
Excludes1   hemorrhage in early pregnancy (O20.-)
intrapartum hemorrhage NEC (O67.-)
placenta previa (O44.-)
premature separation of placenta [abruptio placentae] (O45.-)

● O46.0   Antepartum hemorrhage with coagulation defect
Ⓔⓧ For category O46.0 CC codes: See O45.0

● O46.00   Antepartum hemorrhage with coagulation defect, unspecified

O46.001   Antepartum hemorrhage with coagulation defect, unspecified, first trimester ♀   M

O46.002   Antepartum hemorrhage with coagulation defect, unspecified, second trimester ♀ 🦠   M

O46.003   Antepartum hemorrhage with coagulation defect, unspecified, third trimester ♀ 🦠   M

O46.009   Antepartum hemorrhage with coagulation defect, unspecified, unspecified trimester ♀   M

● O46.01   Antepartum hemorrhage with afibrinogenemia
Antepartum hemorrhage with hypofibrinogenemia

O46.011   Antepartum hemorrhage with afibrinogenemia, first trimester ♀ 🦠 M

O46.012   Antepartum hemorrhage with afibrinogenemia, second trimester ♀ 🦠   M

O46.013   Antepartum hemorrhage with afibrinogenemia, third trimester ♀ 🦠   M

O46.019   Antepartum hemorrhage with afibrinogenemia, unspecified trimester ♀   M

● O46.02   Antepartum hemorrhage with disseminated intravascular coagulation

O46.021   Antepartum hemorrhage with disseminated intravascular coagulation, first trimester ♀ 🦠   M

O46.022   Antepartum hemorrhage with disseminated intravascular coagulation, second trimester ♀ 🦠   M

O46.023   Antepartum hemorrhage with disseminated intravascular coagulation, third trimester ♀ 🦠   M

O46.029   Antepartum hemorrhage with disseminated intravascular coagulation, unspecified trimester ♀ M

◀ New   ◀▥ Revised   ̶d̶e̶l̶e̶t̶e̶d̶ Deleted   Excludes 1   Excludes 2   Includes   Use additional   Code first   Code also   Unspecified
OGCR Official Guidelines   ● Unacceptable Principal Diagnosis   X Assign placeholder X   ● Use Additional Character(s)   ▸ Manifestation Code   Coding Clinic

● O46.09   **Antepartum hemorrhage with other coagulation defect**

     O46.091   **Antepartum hemorrhage with other coagulation defect, first trimester** ♀ 🦠   M

     O46.092   **Antepartum hemorrhage with other coagulation defect, second trimester** ♀ 🦠   M

     O46.093   **Antepartum hemorrhage with other coagulation defect, third trimester** ♀ 🦠   M

     O46.099   **Antepartum hemorrhage with other coagulation defect, unspecified trimester** ♀   M

● O46.8   **Other antepartum hemorrhage**

   ● O46.8x   **Other antepartum hemorrhage**

     O46.8x1   **Other antepartum hemorrhage, first trimester** ♀   M

     O46.8x2   **Other antepartum hemorrhage, second trimester** ♀   M

     O46.8x3   **Other antepartum hemorrhage, third trimester** ♀   M

     O46.8x9   **Other antepartum hemorrhage, unspecified trimester** ♀   M

● O46.9   **Antepartum hemorrhage, unspecified**

     O46.90   **Antepartum hemorrhage, unspecified, unspecified trimester** ♀   M

     O46.91   **Antepartum hemorrhage, unspecified, first trimester** ♀   M

     O46.92   **Antepartum hemorrhage, unspecified, second trimester** ♀   M

     O46.93   **Antepartum hemorrhage, unspecified, third trimester** ♀   M

● O47   **False labor**

   Includes   Braxton Hicks contractions
               threatened labor

   Excludes1   preterm labor (O60.-)

   (Ex:) **For category O47 CC codes:** O11.4, O11.5, O12.04, O12.05, O12.14, O12.15, O12.24, O12.25, O13.4, O13.5, O14.04, O14.05, O14.14, O14.15, O14.24, O14.25, O14.94, O14.95, O16.4, O16.5, O25.10-O25.3, O26.10-O26.13, O26.30-O26.43, O26.63-O26.819, O26.841-O26.86, O26.891-O26.93, O29.011-O29.93, O35.7XX0-O35.7XX9, O47.00-O47.9, O60.00-O60.23X9, O75.4, O75.81, O75.89-O75.9, O80, O90.89, O99.111-O99.285, O99.330-O99.335, O99.350-O99.355, O99.511-O99.73, O99.820-O99.825, O99.840-O9A.53

● O47.0   **False labor before 37 completed weeks of gestation**

     O47.00   **False labor before 37 completed weeks of gestation, unspecified trimester** ♀   M

     O47.02   **False labor before 37 completed weeks of gestation, second trimester** ♀ 🦠   M

     O47.03   **False labor before 37 completed weeks of gestation, third trimester** ♀ 🦠   M

   O47.1   **False labor at or after 37 completed weeks of gestation** ♀ 🦠   M

   O47.9   **False labor, unspecified** ♀   M

● O48   **Late pregnancy**

   O48.0   **Post-term pregnancy** ♀   M
       Pregnancy over 40 completed weeks to 42 completed weeks gestation

   O48.1   **Prolonged pregnancy** ♀   M
       Pregnancy which has advanced beyond 42 completed weeks gestation

---

COMPLICATIONS OF LABOR AND DELIVERY (O60-O77)

● O60   **Preterm labor**

   Includes   onset (spontaneous) of labor before 37 completed weeks of gestation

   Excludes1   false labor (O47.0-)
               threatened labor NOS (O47.0-)

   (Ex:) **For category O60 CC codes:** See O47

● O60.0   **Preterm labor without delivery**

     O60.00   **Preterm labor without delivery, unspecified trimester** ♀   M

     O60.02   **Preterm labor without delivery, second trimester** ♀ 🦠   M

     O60.03   **Preterm labor without delivery, third trimester** ♀ 🦠   M

● O60.1   **Preterm labor with preterm delivery**

     One of the following 7th characters is to be assigned to each code under subcategory O60.1. 7th character 0 is for single gestations and multiple gestations where the fetus is unspecified. 7th characters 1 through 9 are for cases of multiple gestations to identify the fetus for which the code applies. The appropriate code from category O30, Multiple gestation, must also be assigned when assigning a code from subcategory O60.1 that has a 7th character of 1 through 9.

0	not applicable or unspecified
1	fetus 1
2	fetus 2
3	fetus 3
4	fetus 4
5	fetus 5
9	other fetus

   Coding Clinic: 2016, Q2, P11

X ● O60.10   **Preterm labor with preterm delivery, unspecified trimester** ♀ 🦠   M
       Preterm labor with delivery NOS

X ● O60.12   **Preterm labor second trimester with preterm delivery second trimester** ♀ 🦠   M

X ● O60.13   **Preterm labor second trimester with preterm delivery third trimester** ♀ 🦠   M

X ● O60.14   **Preterm labor third trimester with preterm delivery third trimester** ♀ 🦠   M
       Coding Clinic: 2016, Q2, P10

N   Newborn Age: 0   **P**   Pediatric Age: 0–17   **M**   Maternity DX: 12–55   **A**   Adult Age: 15–124   ♀   Females Only   ♂   Males Only

🦠   Complication\Comorbidity   🦠   Major C\C   (Ex:)   CC/MCC Exclusions   🦠   Hospital-Acquired Condition   **1143**

● **O60.2**   **Term delivery with preterm labor**

One of the following 7th characters is to be assigned to each code under subcategory O60.2. 7th character Ø is for single gestations and multiple gestations where the fetus is unspecified. 7th characters 1 through 9 are for cases of multiple gestations to identify the fetus for which the code applies. The appropriate code from category O30, Multiple gestation, must also be assigned when assigning a code from subcategory O60.2 that has a 7th character of 1 through 9.

Ø	not applicable or unspecified
1	fetus 1
2	fetus 2
3	fetus 3
4	fetus 4
5	fetus 5
9	other fetus

X ● **O60.20**   **Term delivery with preterm labor, unspecified trimester** ♀ 🖑   **M**

X ● **O60.22**   **Term delivery with preterm labor, second trimester** ♀ 🖑   **M**

X ● **O60.23**   **Term delivery with preterm labor, third trimester** ♀ 🖑   **M**

● **O61**   **Failed induction of labor**

O61.0   **Failed medical induction of labor** ♀   **M**
Failed induction (of labor) by oxytocin
Failed induction (of labor) by prostaglandins

O61.1   **Failed instrumental induction of labor** ♀   **M**
Failed mechanical induction (of labor)
Failed surgical induction (of labor)

O61.8   **Other failed induction of labor** ♀   **M**

O61.9   **Failed induction of labor, unspecified** ♀   **M**

● **O62**   **Abnormalities of forces of labor**

O62.0   **Primary inadequate contractions** ♀   **M**
Failure of cervical dilatation
Primary hypotonic uterine dysfunction
Uterine inertia during latent phase of labor

O62.1   **Secondary uterine inertia** ♀   **M**
Arrested active phase of labor
Secondary hypotonic uterine dysfunction

O62.2   **Other uterine inertia** ♀   **M**
Atony of uterus without hemorrhage
Atony of uterus NOS
Desultory labor
Hypotonic uterine dysfunction NOS
Irregular labor
Poor contractions
Slow slope active phase of labor
Uterine inertia NOS

     Excludes1   atony of uterus with hemorrhage (postpartum) (O72.1)
postpartum atony of uterus without hemorrhage (O75.89)

O62.3   **Precipitate labor** ♀   **M**

O62.4   **Hypertonic, incoordinate, and prolonged uterine contractions** ♀   **M**
Cervical spasm
Contraction ring dystocia
Dyscoordinate labor
Hour-glass contraction of uterus
Hypertonic uterine dysfunction
Incoordinate uterine action
Tetanic contractions
Uterine dystocia NOS
Uterine spasm

     Excludes1   dystocia (fetal) (maternal) NOS (O66.9)

O62.8   **Other abnormalities of forces of labor** ♀   **M**

O62.9   **Abnormality of forces of labor, unspecified** ♀   **M**

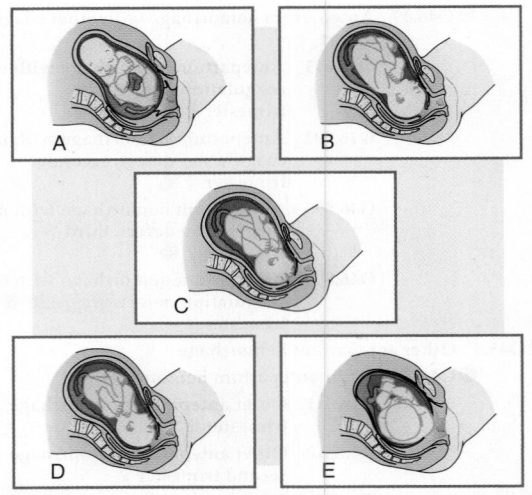

Figure 15-4   Five types of malposition and malpresentation of the fetus: **A.** Breech. **B.** Vertex. **C.** Face. **D.** Brow. **E.** Shoulder.

● **O63**   **Long labor**

O63.0   **Prolonged first stage (of labor)** ♀   **M**

O63.1   **Prolonged second stage (of labor)** ♀   **M**

O63.2   **Delayed delivery of second twin, triplet, etc.** ♀   **M**

O63.9   **Long labor, unspecified** ♀ 🖑   **M**
Prolonged labor NOS
Ⓔⓧ O11.4, O11.5, O12.04, O12.05, O12.14, O12.15, O12.24, O12.25, O13.4, O13.5, O14.04, O14.05, O14.14, O14.15, O14.24, O14.25, O14.94, O14.95, O16.4, O16.5, O25.10-O25.3, O26.10-O26.13, O26.30-O26.43, O26.63-O26.819, O26.841-O26.86, O26.891-O26.93, O29.011-O29.93, O35.7XX0-O35.7XX9, O36.8120-O36.8199, O63.9, O71.00-O71.1, O71.5, O71.81, O71.89-O71.9, O75.4, O75.81, O75.89-O75.9, O80, O90.89, O99.111-O99.285, O99.330-O99.335, O99.350-O99.355, O99.511-O99.73, O99.820-O99.825, O99.840-O9A.53

● **O64**   **Obstructed labor due to malposition and malpresentation of fetus**

One of the following 7th characters is to be assigned to each code under category O64. 7th character Ø is for single gestations and multiple gestations where the fetus is unspecified. 7th characters 1 through 9 are for cases of multiple gestations to identify the fetus for which the code applies. The appropriate code from category O30, Multiple gestation, must also be assigned when assigning a code from category O64 that has a 7th character of 1 through 9.

Ø	not applicable or unspecified
1	fetus 1
2	fetus 2
3	fetus 3
4	fetus 4
5	fetus 5
9	other fetus

X ● **O64.0**   **Obstructed labor due to incomplete rotation of fetal head** ♀   **M**
Deep transverse arrest
Obstructed labor due to persistent occipitoiliac (position)
Obstructed labor due to persistent occipitoposterior (position)
Obstructed labor due to persistent occipitosacral (position)
Obstructed labor due to persistent occipitotransverse (position)

X ● **O64.1**   **Obstructed labor due to breech presentation** ♀   **M**
Obstructed labor due to buttocks presentation
Obstructed labor due to complete breech presentation
Obstructed labor due to frank breech presentation

◀ New   ⬅ Revised   ~~deleted~~ Deleted   Excludes 1   Excludes 2   Includes   Use additional   Code first   Code also   Unspecified

1144   OGCR Official Guidelines   ● Unacceptable Principal Diagnosis   X Assign placeholder X   ● Use Additional Character(s)   🟤 Manifestation Code   **Coding Clinic**

X ● **O64.2** **Obstructed labor due to face presentation** ♀   M
     Obstructed labor due to chin presentation

X ● **O64.3** **Obstructed labor due to brow presentation** ♀   M

X ● **O64.4** **Obstructed labor due to shoulder presentation** ♀   M
     Prolapsed arm
     Excludes1   impacted shoulders (O66.0)
                 shoulder dystocia (O66.0)

X ● **O64.5** **Obstructed labor due to compound presentation** ♀   M

X ● **O64.8** **Obstructed labor due to other malposition and malpresentation** ♀   M
     Obstructed labor due to footling presentation
     Obstructed labor due to incomplete breech presentation

X ● **O64.9** **Obstructed labor due to malposition and malpresentation, unspecified** ♀   M

● **O65** **Obstructed labor due to maternal pelvic abnormality**

     O65.0 **Obstructed labor due to deformed pelvis** ♀   M

     O65.1 **Obstructed labor due to generally contracted pelvis** ♀   M

     O65.2 **Obstructed labor due to pelvic inlet contraction** ♀   M

     O65.3 **Obstructed labor due to pelvic outlet and mid-cavity contraction** ♀   M

     O65.4 **Obstructed labor due to fetopelvic disproportion, unspecified** ♀   M
         Excludes1   dystocia due to abnormality of fetus (O66.2-O66.3)

     O65.5 **Obstructed labor due to abnormality of maternal pelvic organs** ♀   M
         Obstructed labor due to conditions listed in O34.-
         Use additional code to identify abnormality of pelvic organs O34.-

     O65.8 **Obstructed labor due to other maternal pelvic abnormalities** ♀   M

     O65.9 **Obstructed labor due to maternal pelvic abnormality, unspecified** ♀   M

● **O66** **Other obstructed labor**

     O66.0 **Obstructed labor due to shoulder dystocia** ♀   M
         Impacted shoulders

     O66.1 **Obstructed labor due to locked twins** ♀   M

     O66.2 **Obstructed labor due to unusually large fetus** ♀   M

     O66.3 **Obstructed labor due to other abnormalities of fetus** ♀   M
         Dystocia due to fetal ascites
         Dystocia due to fetal hydrops
         Dystocia due to fetal meningomyelocele
         Dystocia due to fetal sacral teratoma
         Dystocia due to fetal tumor
         Dystocia due to hydrocephalic fetus
         Use additional code to identify cause of obstruction

   ● **O66.4** **Failed trial of labor**
         O66.40 **Failed trial of labor, unspecified** ♀   M
         O66.41 **Failed attempted vaginal birth after previous cesarean delivery** ♀   M
             Code first rupture of uterus, if applicable (O71.0-, O71.1)

     O66.5 **Attempted application of vacuum extractor and forceps** ♀   M
         Attempted application of vacuum or forceps, with subsequent delivery by forceps or cesarean delivery

     O66.6 **Obstructed labor due to other multiple fetuses** ♀   M

     O66.8 **Other specified obstructed labor** ♀   M
         Use additional code to identify cause of obstruction

     O66.9 **Obstructed labor, unspecified** ♀   M
         Dystocia NOS
         Fetal dystocia NOS
         Maternal dystocia NOS

Figure 15-5 Hydrocephalic fetus causing disproportion.

● **O67** **Labor and delivery complicated by intrapartum hemorrhage, not elsewhere classified**
     Excludes1   antepartum hemorrhage NEC (O46.-)
                  placenta previa (O44.-)
                  premature separation of placenta [abruptio placentae] (O45.-)
     Excludes2   postpartum hemorrhage (O72.-)

     O67.0 **Intrapartum hemorrhage with coagulation defect** ♀ 🖧 M
         Intrapartum hemorrhage (excessive) associated with afibrinogenemia
         Intrapartum hemorrhage (excessive) associated with disseminated intravascular coagulation
         Intrapartum hemorrhage (excessive) associated with hyperfibrinolysis
         Intrapartum hemorrhage (excessive) associated with hypofibrinogenemia
         (Ex:) See O45.0

     O67.8 **Other intrapartum hemorrhage** ♀   M
         Excessive intrapartum hemorrhage

     O67.9 **Intrapartum hemorrhage, unspecified** ♀   M

● **O68** **Labor and delivery complicated by abnormality of fetal acid-base balance** ♀ 🖧   M
     Fetal acidemia complicating labor and delivery
     Fetal acidosis complicating labor and delivery
     Fetal alkalosis complicating labor and delivery
     Fetal metabolic acidemia complicating labor and delivery
     Excludes1   fetal stress NOS (O77.9)
                  labor and delivery complicated by electrocardiographic evidence of fetal stress (O77.8)
                  labor and delivery complicated by ultrasonic evidence of fetal stress (O77.8)
     Excludes2   abnormality in fetal heart rate or rhythm (O76)
                  labor and delivery complicated by meconium in amniotic fluid (O77.0)
     (Ex:) 068, 076, P03.811

● **O69** **Labor and delivery complicated by umbilical cord complications**
     One of the following 7th characters is to be assigned to each code under category O69. 7th character Ø is for single gestations and multiple gestations where the fetus is unspecified. 7th characters 1 through 9 are for cases of multiple gestations to identify the fetus for which the code applies. The appropriate code from category O30, Multiple gestation, must also be assigned when assigning a code from category O69 that has a 7th character of 1 through 9.

Ø	not applicable or unspecified
1	fetus 1
2	fetus 2
3	fetus 3
4	fetus 4
5	fetus 5
9	other fetus

X ● **O69.0** **Labor and delivery complicated by prolapse of cord** ♀   M

X ● **O69.1** **Labor and delivery complicated by cord around neck, with compression** ♀   M
     Excludes1   labor and delivery complicated by cord around neck, without compression (O69.81)

X ● **O69.2** **Labor and delivery complicated by other cord entanglement, with compression** ♀   M
     Labor and delivery complicated by compression of cord NOS
     Labor and delivery complicated by entanglement of cords of twins in monoamniotic sac
     Labor and delivery complicated by knot in cord
     Excludes1   labor and delivery complicated by other cord entanglement, without compression (O69.82)

X ● **O69.3** **Labor and delivery complicated by short cord** ♀   M

N   Newborn Age: Ø   P   Pediatric Age: Ø–17   M   Maternity DX: 12–55   A   Adult Age: 15–124   ♀   Females Only   ♂   Males Only
🖧   Complication\Comorbidity   🖧   Major C\C   (Ex:)   CC/MCC Exclusions   🖧   Hospital-Acquired Condition

1145

X ● **O69.4** **Labor and delivery complicated by vasa previa** ♀   **M**
　　　　Labor and delivery complicated by hemorrhage from vasa previa

X ● **O69.5** **Labor and delivery complicated by vascular lesion of cord** ♀   **M**
　　　　Labor and delivery complicated by cord bruising
　　　　Labor and delivery complicated by cord hematoma
　　　　Labor and delivery complicated by thrombosis of umbilical vessels

● **O69.8** **Labor and delivery complicated by other cord complications**

　X ● **O69.81** **Labor and delivery complicated by cord around neck, without compression** ♀   **M**

　X ● **O69.82** **Labor and delivery complicated by other cord entanglement, without compression** ♀   **M**

　X ● **O69.89** **Labor and delivery complicated by other cord complications** ♀   **M**

X ● **O69.9** **Labor and delivery complicated by cord complication, unspecified** ♀   **M**

● **O70** **Perineal laceration during delivery**

    Includes   episiotomy extended by laceration
    Excludes1   obstetric high vaginal laceration alone (O71.4)

　O70.0 **First degree perineal laceration during delivery** ♀   **M**
　　　Perineal laceration, rupture or tear involving fourchette during delivery
　　　Perineal laceration, rupture or tear involving labia during delivery
　　　Perineal laceration, rupture or tear involving skin during delivery
　　　Perineal laceration, rupture or tear involving vagina during delivery
　　　Perineal laceration, rupture or tear involving vulva during delivery
　　　Slight perineal laceration, rupture or tear during delivery

　O70.1 **Second degree perineal laceration during delivery** ♀   **M**
　　　Perineal laceration, rupture or tear during delivery as in O70.0, also involving pelvic floor
　　　Perineal laceration, rupture or tear during delivery as in O70.0, also involving perineal muscles
　　　Perineal laceration, rupture or tear during delivery as in O70.0, also involving vaginal muscles

    Excludes1   perineal laceration involving anal sphincter (O70.2)

    Coding Clinic: 2016, Q2, P34

● **O70.2** **Third degree perineal laceration during delivery**
　　　Perineal laceration, rupture or tear during delivery as in O70.1, also involving anal sphincter
　　　Perineal laceration, rupture or tear during delivery as in O70.1, also involving rectovaginal septum
　　　Perineal laceration, rupture or tear during delivery as in O70.1, also involving sphincter NOS

    Excludes1   anal sphincter tear during delivery without third degree perineal laceration (O70.4)
　　　　　perineal laceration involving anal or rectal mucosa (O70.3)

    (Ex) For category O70.2 CC codes: 011.4, 011.5, 012.04, 012.05, 012.14, 012.15, 012.24, 012.25, 013.4, 013.5, 014.04, 014.05, 014.14, 014.15, 014.24, 014.25, 014.94, 014.95, 016.4, 016.5, 025.10-025.3, 026.10-026.13, 026.30-026.43, 026.63-026.819, 026.841-026.86, 026.891-026.93, 029.011-029.93, 035.7XX0-035.7XX9, 036.8120-036.8199, 070.4, 071.00-071.1, 071.5, 071.81, 071.89-071.9, 075.4, 075.81, 075.89-075.9, 080, 090.89, 099.111-099.285, 099.330-099.335, 099.350-099.355, 099.511-099.73, 099.820-099.825, 099.840-09A.53

　O70.20 **Third degree perineal laceration during delivery, unspecified** ♀ 🔧 ◄   **M**

　O70.21 **Third degree perineal laceration during delivery, IIIa** ♀ 🔧 ◄   **M**
　　　Third degree perineal laceration during delivery with less than 50% of external anal sphincter (EAS) thickness torn ◄

                     Vaginal   Urethral
                    opening   opening

Figure 15-6   Perineal lacerations: **A.** First-degree is laceration of superficial tissues. **B.** Second-degree is limited to the pelvic floor and may involve the perineal or vaginal muscles. **C.** Third-degree involves the anal sphincter. **D.** Fourth-degree involves anal or rectal mucosa.

　O70.22 **Third degree perineal laceration during delivery, IIIb** ♀ 🔧 ◄   **M**
　　　Third degree perineal laceration during delivery with more than 50% external anal sphincter (EAS) thickness torn ◄

　O70.23 **Third degree perineal laceration during delivery, IIIc** ♀ 🔧 ◄   **M**
　　　Third degree perineal laceration during delivery with both external anal sphincter (EAS) and internal anal sphincter (IAS) torn ◄

　O70.3 **Fourth degree perineal laceration during delivery** ♀ 🔧 **M**
　　　Perineal laceration, rupture or tear during delivery as in O70.2, also involving anal mucosa
　　　Perineal laceration, rupture or tear during delivery as in O70.2, also involving rectal mucosa
　　　(Ex) 011.4, 011.5, 012.04, 012.05, 012.14, 012.15, 012.24, 012.25, 013.4, 013.5, 014.04, 014.05, 014.14, 014.15, 014.24, 014.25, 014.94, 014.95, 016.4, 016.5, 025.10-025.3, 026.10-026.13, 026.30-026.43, 026.63-026.819, 026.841-026.86, 026.891-026.93, 029.011-029.93, 035.7XX0-035.7XX9, 036.8120-036.8199, 070.3, 071.00-071.1, 071.5, 071.81, 071.89-071.9, 075.4, 075.81, 075.89-075.9, 080, 090.89, 099.111-099.285, 099.330-099.335, 099.350-099.355, 099.511-099.73, 099.820-099.825, 099.840-09A.53

　O70.4 **Anal sphincter tear complicating delivery, not associated with third degree laceration** ♀ 🔧   **M**

    Excludes1   anal sphincter tear with third degree perineal laceration (O70.2)
　　　　(Ex) 011.4, 011.5, 012.04, 012.05, 012.14, 012.15, 012.24, 012.25, 013.4, 013.5, 014.04, 014.05, 014.14, 014.15, 014.24, 014.25, 014.94, 014.95, 016.4, 016.5, 025.10-025.3, 026.10-026.13, 026.30-026.43, 026.63-026.819, 026.841-026.86, 026.891-026.93, 029.011-029.93, 035.7XX0-035.7XX9, 036.8120-036.8199, 070.20-070.23, 070.4, 071.00-071.1, 071.5, 071.81, 071.89-071.9, 075.4, 075.81, 075.89-075.9, 080, 090.89, 099.111-099.285, 099.330-099.335, 099.350-099.355, 099.511-099.73, 099.820-099.825, 099.840-09A.53

　O70.9 **Perineal laceration during delivery, unspecified** ♀   **M**

● **O71** **Other obstetric trauma**

    Includes   obstetric damage from instruments

● **O71.0** **Rupture of uterus (spontaneous) before onset of labor**

    Excludes1   disruption of (current) cesarean delivery wound (O90.0)
　　　　laceration of uterus, NEC (O71.81)
　　　　(Ex) For category O71.0 CC codes: 011.4, 011.5, 012.04, 012.05, 012.14, 012.15, 012.24, 012.25, 013.4, 013.5, 014.04, 014.05, 014.14, 014.15, 014.24, 014.25, 014.94, 014.95, 016.4, 016.5, 025.10-025.3, 026.10-026.13, 026.30-026.43, 026.63-026.819, 026.841-026.86, 026.891-026.93, 029.011-029.93, 035.7XX0-035.7XX9, 036.8120-036.8199, 071.00-071.1, 071.5, 071.81, 071.89-071.9, 075.4, 075.81, 075.89-075.9, 080, 090.89, 099.111-099.285, 099.330-099.335, 099.350-099.355, 099.511-099.73, 099.820-099.825, 099.840-09A.53

　O71.00 **Rupture of uterus before onset of labor, unspecified trimester** ♀   **M**

　O71.02 **Rupture of uterus before onset of labor, second trimester** ♀ 🔧   **M**

　O71.03 **Rupture of uterus before onset of labor, third trimester** ♀ 🔧   **M**

◄ New   ◄ᴵᴵᴵ Revised   ~~deleted~~ Deleted   Excludes 1   Excludes 2   Includes   Use additional   Code first   Code also   Unspecified
OGCR Official Guidelines   ● Unacceptable Principal Diagnosis   X Assign placeholder X   ● Use Additional Character(s)   ▶ Manifestation Code   **Coding Clinic**

O71.1 **Rupture of uterus during labor** ♀   **M**
Rupture of uterus not stated as occurring before onset of labor

     Excludes1   disruption of cesarean delivery wound (O90.0)
                 laceration of uterus, NEC (O71.81)
     (Ex:) See O71.0

O71.2 **Postpartum inversion of uterus** ♀   **M**
     (Ex:) O11.4, O11.5, O12.04, O12.05, O12.14, O12.15, O12.24, O12.25, O13.4, O13.5, O14.04, O14.05, O14.14, O14.15, O14.24, O14.25, O14.94, O14.95, O16.4, O16.5, O25.10-O25.3, O26.10-O26.13, O26.30-O26.43, O26.63-O26.819, O26.841-O26.86, O26.891-O26.93, O29.011-O29.93, O35.7XX0-O35.7XX9, O36.8120-O36.8199, O71.00-O71.1, O71.5, O71.81, O71.89-O71.9, O75.4, O75.81, O75.89-O75.9, O80, O90.89, O99.111-O99.285, O99.330-O99.335, O99.350-O99.355, O99.511-O99.73, O99.820-O99.825, O99.840-O9A.53

O71.3 **Obstetric laceration of cervix** ♀   **M**
Annular detachment of cervix
     (Ex:) O11.4, O11.5, O12.04, O12.05, O12.14, O12.15, O12.24, O12.25, O13.4, O13.5, O14.04, O14.05, O14.14, O14.15, O14.24, O14.25, O14.94, O14.95, O16.4, O16.5, O25.10-O25.3, O26.10-O26.13, O26.30-O26.43, O26.63-O26.819, O26.841-O26.86, O26.891-O26.93, O29.011-O29.93, O35.7XX0-O35.7XX9, O36.8120-O36.8199, O71.00-O71.1, O71.5, O71.81, O71.89-O71.9, O75.4, O75.81, O75.89-O75.9, O80, O90.89, O99.111-O99.285, O99.330-O99.335, O99.350-O99.355, O99.511-O99.73, O99.820-O99.825, O99.840-O9A.53

O71.4 **Obstetric high vaginal laceration alone** ♀   **M**
Laceration of vaginal wall without perineal laceration

     Excludes1   obstetric high vaginal laceration with perineal laceration (O70.-)
     (Ex:) O11.4, O11.5, O12.04, O12.05, O12.14, O12.15, O12.24, O12.25, O13.4, O13.5, O14.04, O14.05, O14.14, O14.15, O14.24, O14.25, O14.94, O14.95, O16.4, O16.5, O25.10-O25.3, O26.10-O26.13, O26.30-O26.43, O26.63-O26.819, O26.841-O26.86, O26.891-O26.93, O29.011-O29.93, O35.7XX0-O35.7XX9, O36.8120-O36.8199, O71.00-O71.1, O71.4, O71.5, O71.81, O71.89-O71.9, O75.4, O75.81, O75.89-O75.9, O80, O90.89, O99.111-O99.285, O99.330-O99.335, O99.350-O99.355, O99.511-O99.73, O99.820-O99.825, O99.840-O9A.53

O71.5 **Other obstetric injury to pelvic organs** ♀   **M**
Obstetric injury to bladder
Obstetric injury to urethra

     Excludes2   obstetric periurethral trauma (O71.82)
     (Ex:) See O71.0

O71.6 **Obstetric damage to pelvic joints and ligaments** ♀   **M**
Obstetric avulsion of inner symphyseal cartilage
Obstetric damage to coccyx
Obstetric traumatic separation of symphysis (pubis)
     (Ex:) O11.4, O11.5, O12.04, O12.05, O12.14, O12.15, O12.24, O12.25, O13.4, O13.5, O14.04, O14.05, O14.14, O14.15, O14.24, O14.25, O14.94, O14.95, O16.4, O16.5, O25.10-O25.3, O26.10-O26.13, O26.30-O26.43, O26.63-O26.819, O26.841-O26.86, O26.891-O26.93, O29.011-O29.93, O35.7XX0-O35.7XX9, O36.8120-O36.8199, O71.00-O71.1, O71.5-O71.6, O71.81, O71.89-O71.9, O75.4, O75.81, O75.89-O75.9, O80, O90.89, O99.111-O99.285, O99.330-O99.335, O99.350-O99.355, O99.511-O99.73, O99.820-O99.825, O99.840-O9A.53

O71.7 **Obstetric hematoma of pelvis** ♀   **M**
Obstetric hematoma of perineum
Obstetric hematoma of vagina
Obstetric hematoma of vulva
     (Ex:) O11.4, O11.5, O12.04, O12.05, O12.14, O12.15, O12.24, O12.25, O13.4, O13.5, O14.04, O14.05, O14.14, O14.15, O14.24, O14.25, O14.94, O14.95, O16.4, O16.5, O25.10-O25.3, O26.10-O26.13, O26.30-O26.43, O26.63-O26.819, O26.841-O26.86, O26.891-O26.93, O29.011-O29.93, O35.7XX0-O35.7XX9, O36.8120-O36.8199, O71.00-O71.1, O71.5, O71.7, O71.81, O71.89-O71.9, O75.4, O75.81, O75.89-O75.9, O80, O90.89, O99.111-O99.285, O99.330-O99.335, O99.350-O99.355, O99.511-O99.73, O99.820-O99.825, O99.840-O9A.53

● **O71.8** **Other specified obstetric trauma**

     O71.81 **Laceration of uterus, not elsewhere classified** ♀   **M**

     O71.82 **Other specified trauma to perineum and vulva** ♀   **M**
              Obstetric periurethral trauma

     O71.89 **Other specified obstetric trauma** ♀   **M**

O71.9 **Obstetric trauma, unspecified** ♀   **M**

● **O72** **Postpartum hemorrhage**

     Includes   hemorrhage after delivery of fetus or infant

O72.0 **Third-stage hemorrhage** ♀   **M**
Hemorrhage associated with retained, trapped or adherent placenta
Retained placenta NOS

     Code also type of adherent placenta (O43.2-)
     (Ex:) O11.4, O11.5, O12.04, O12.05, O12.14, O12.15, O12.24, O12.25, O13.4, O13.5, O14.04, O14.05, O14.14, O14.15, O14.24, O14.25, O14.94, O14.95, O16.4, O16.5, O25.10-O25.3, O26.10-O26.13, O26.30-O26.43, O26.63-O26.819, O26.841-O26.86, O26.891-O26.93, O29.011-O29.93, O35.7XX0-O35.7XX9, O36.8120-O36.8199, O71.00-O71.1, O71.5, O71.81, O71.89-O71.9, O72.0, O75.4, O75.81, O75.89-O75.9, O80, O90.89, O99.111-O99.285, O99.330-O99.335, O99.350-O99.355, O99.511-O99.73, O99.820-O99.825, O99.840-O9A.53

O72.1 **Other immediate postpartum hemorrhage** ♀   **M**
Hemorrhage following delivery of placenta
Postpartum hemorrhage (atonic) NOS
Uterine atony with hemorrhage

     Excludes1   uterine atony NOS (O62.2)
               uterine atony without hemorrhage (O62.2)
               postpartum atony of uterus without hemorrhage (O75.89)
     (Ex:) O11.4, O11.5, O12.04, O12.05, O12.14, O12.15, O12.24, O12.25, O13.4, O13.5, O14.04, O14.05, O14.14, O14.15, O14.24, O14.25, O14.94, O14.95, O16.4, O16.5, O25.10-O25.3, O26.10-O26.13, O26.30-O26.43, O26.63-O26.819, O26.841-O26.86, O26.891-O26.93, O29.011-O29.93, O35.7XX0-O35.7XX9, O36.8120-O36.8199, O71.00-O71.1, O71.5, O71.81, O71.89-O71.9, O72.1, O75.4, O75.81, O75.89-O75.9, O80, O90.89, O99.111-O99.285, O99.330-O99.335, O99.350-O99.355, O99.511-O99.73, O99.820-O99.825, O99.840-O9A.53

O72.2 **Delayed and secondary postpartum hemorrhage** ♀   **M**
Hemorrhage associated with retained portions of placenta or membranes after the first 24 hours following delivery of placenta
Retained products of conception NOS, following delivery
     (Ex:) O11.4, O11.5, O12.04, O12.05, O12.14, O12.15, O12.24, O12.25, O13.4, O13.5, O14.04, O14.05, O14.14, O14.15, O14.24, O14.25, O14.94, O14.95, O16.4, O16.5, O25.10-O25.3, O26.10-O26.13, O26.30-O26.43, O26.63-O26.819, O26.841-O26.86, O26.891-O26.93, O29.011-O29.93, O35.7XX0-O35.7XX9, O36.8120-O36.8199, O71.00-O71.1, O71.5, O71.81, O71.89-O71.9, O72.2, O75.4, O75.81, O75.89-O75.9, O80, O90.89, O99.111-O99.285, O99.330-O99.335, O99.350-O99.355, O99.511-O99.73, O99.820-O99.825, O99.840-O9A.53

O72.3 **Postpartum coagulation defects** ♀   **M**
Postpartum afibrinogenemia
Postpartum fibrinolysis

● **O73** **Retained placenta and membranes, without hemorrhage**

     Excludes1   placenta accreta (O43.21-)
               placenta increta (O43.22-)
               placenta percreta (O43.23-)

O73.0 **Retained placenta without hemorrhage** ♀   **M**
Adherent placenta, without hemorrhage
Trapped placenta without hemorrhage

O73.1 **Retained portions of placenta and membranes, without hemorrhage** ♀   **M**
Retained products of conception following delivery, without hemorrhage

N   Newborn Age: 0   **P**   Pediatric Age: 0–17   **M**   Maternity DX: 12–55   **A**   Adult Age: 15–124   ♀   Females Only   ♂   Males Only
 Complication\Comorbidity   Major C\C   (Ex:) CC/MCC Exclusions   Hospital-Acquired Condition

1147

● **O74 Complications of anesthesia during labor and delivery**
> **Includes**   maternal complications arising from the administration of a general, regional or local anesthetic, analgesic or other sedation during labor and delivery

Use additional code, if applicable, to identify specific complication

O74.0 Aspiration pneumonitis due to anesthesia during labor and delivery ♀   M
> Inhalation of stomach contents or secretions NOS due to anesthesia during labor and delivery
> Mendelson's syndrome due to anesthesia during labor and delivery

O74.1 Other pulmonary complications of anesthesia during labor and delivery ♀   M

O74.2 Cardiac complications of anesthesia during labor and delivery ♀   M

O74.3 Central nervous system complications of anesthesia during labor and delivery ♀   M

O74.4 Toxic reaction to local anesthesia during labor and delivery ♀   M

O74.5 Spinal and epidural anesthesia-induced headache during labor and delivery ♀   M

O74.6 Other complications of spinal and epidural anesthesia during labor and delivery ♀   M

O74.7 Failed or difficult intubation for anesthesia during labor and delivery ♀   M

O74.8 Other complications of anesthesia during labor and delivery ♀   M

O74.9 Complication of anesthesia during labor and delivery, unspecified ♀   M

● **O75 Other complications of labor and delivery, not elsewhere classified**
> **Excludes2**   puerperal (postpartum) infection (O86.-)
> puerperal (postpartum) sepsis (O85)

O75.0 Maternal distress during labor and delivery ♀   M

O75.1 Shock during or following labor and delivery ♀ 🐾   M
> Obstetric shock following labor and delivery
> (Ex) 011.4, 011.5, 012.04, 012.05, 012.14, 012.15, 012.24, 012.25, 013.4, 013.5, 014.04, 014.05, 014.14, 014.15, 014.24, 014.25, 014.94, 014.95, 016.4, 016.5, 025.10-025.3, 026.10-026.13, 026.30-026.43, 026.63-026.819, 026.841-026.86, 026.891-026.93, 029.011-029.93, 035.7XX0-035.7XX9, 075.1, 075.4, 075.81, 075.89-075.9, 080, 090.89, 099.111-099.285, 099.330-099.335, 099.350-099.355, 099.511-099.73, 099.820-099.825, 099.840-09A.53

O75.2 Pyrexia during labor, not elsewhere classified ♀ 🐾   M
> (Ex) 075.2

O75.3 Other infection during labor ♀ 🐾   M
> Sepsis during labor
> Use additional code (B95-B97), to identify infectious agent
> (Ex) 011.4, 011.5, 012.04, 012.05, 012.14, 012.15, 012.24, 012.25, 013.4, 013.5, 014.04, 014.05, 014.14, 014.15, 014.24, 014.25, 014.94, 014.95, 016.4, 016.5, 025.10-025.3, 026.10-026.13, 026.30-026.43, 026.63-026.819, 026.841-026.86, 026.891-026.93, 029.011-029.93, 035.7XX0-035.7XX9, 075.3-075.4, 075.81, 075.89-075.9, 080, 090.89, 099.111-099.285, 099.330-099.335, 099.350-099.355, 099.511-099.73, 099.820-099.825, 099.840-09A.53

O75.4 Other complications of obstetric surgery and procedures ♀   M
> Cardiac arrest following obstetric surgery or procedures
> Cardiac failure following obstetric surgery or procedures
> Cerebral anoxia following obstetric surgery or procedures
> Pulmonary edema following obstetric surgery or procedures

Use additional code to identify specific complication
> **Excludes2**   complications of anesthesia during labor and delivery (O74.-)
> disruption of obstetrical (surgical) wound (O90.0-O90.1)
> hematoma of obstetrical (surgical) wound (O90.2)
> infection of obstetrical (surgical) wound (O86.0)

O75.5 Delayed delivery after artificial rupture of membranes ♀   M

● **O75.8 Other specified complications of labor and delivery**

O75.81 Maternal exhaustion complicating labor and delivery ♀   M

O75.82 Onset (spontaneous) of labor after 37 completed weeks of gestation but before 39 completed weeks gestation, with delivery by (planned) cesarean section ♀   M
> Delivery by (planned) cesarean section occurring after 37 completed weeks of gestation but before 39 completed weeks gestation due to (spontaneous) onset of labor
> *Code first to specify reason for planned cesarean section such as:*
> cephalopelvic disproportion (normally formed fetus) (O33.9)
> previous cesarean delivery (O34.21)

O75.89 Other specified complications of labor and delivery ♀   M

O75.9 Complication of labor and delivery, unspecified ♀   M

O76 Abnormality in fetal heart rate and rhythm complicating labor and delivery ♀   M
> Depressed fetal heart rate tones complicating labor and delivery
> Fetal bradycardia complicating labor and delivery
> Fetal heart rate decelerations complicating labor and delivery
> Fetal heart rate irregularity complicating labor and delivery
> Fetal heart rate abnormal variability complicating labor and delivery
> Fetal tachycardia complicating labor and delivery
> Non-reassuring fetal heart rate or rhythm complicating labor and delivery

> **Excludes1**   fetal stress NOS (O77.9)
> labor and delivery complicated by electrocardiographic evidence of fetal stress (O77.8)
> labor and delivery complicated by ultrasonic evidence of fetal stress (O77.8)

> **Excludes2**   fetal metabolic acidemia (O68)
> other fetal stress (O77.0-O77.1)

● **O77 Other fetal stress complicating labor and delivery**

O77.0 Labor and delivery complicated by meconium in amniotic fluid ♀   M

O77.1 Fetal stress in labor or delivery due to drug administration ♀   M

◀ New   ◀╴ Revised   ~~deleted~~ Deleted   Excludes 1   Excludes 2   Includes   Use additional   Code first   Code also   Unspecified
OGCR Official Guidelines   ● Unacceptable Principal Diagnosis   X Assign placeholder X   ● Use Additional Character(s)   ▷ Manifestation Code   **Coding Clinic**

Figure 15-7 The four stages of normal delivery: **I.** Lightening, which occurs 2 to 4 weeks before birth, at which time the fetus turns with head toward the vagina. **II.** Regular contractions begin, the amniotic sac ruptures, and dilation is complete. **III.** Delivery of the head and rotation. **IV.** Expulsion of placenta.

O77.8 **Labor and delivery complicated by other evidence of fetal stress** ♀ M
  Labor and delivery complicated by electrocardiographic evidence of fetal stress
  Labor and delivery complicated by ultrasonic evidence of fetal stress
  Excludes1 abnormality of fetal acid-base balance (O68)
    abnormality in fetal heart rate or rhythm (O76)
    fetal metabolic acidemia (O68)

O77.9 **Labor and delivery complicated by fetal stress, unspecified** ♀ M
  Excludes1 abnormality of fetal acid-base balance (O68)
    abnormality in fetal heart rate or rhythm (O76)
    fetal metabolic acidemia (O68)

OGCR Section I.C., Chapter 15.n.

Normal Delivery, Code O80

1) Encounter for full term uncomplicated delivery

Code O80 should be assigned when a woman is admitted for a full-term normal delivery and delivers a single, healthy infant without any complications antepartum, during the delivery, or postpartum during the delivery episode. Code O80 is always a principal diagnosis. It is not to be used if any other code from chapter 15 is needed to describe a current complication of the antenatal, delivery, or perinatal period. Additional codes from other chapters may be used with code O80 if they are not related to or are in any way complicating the pregnancy.

2) Uncomplicated delivery with resolved antepartum complication

Code O80 may be used if the patient had a complication at some point during the pregnancy, but the complication is not present at the time of the admission for delivery.

3) Outcome of delivery for O80

Z37.0, Single live birth, is the only outcome of delivery code appropriate for use with O80.

ENCOUNTER FOR DELIVERY (O80-O82)

O80 **Encounter for full-term uncomplicated delivery** ♀ M
  Delivery requiring minimal or no assistance, with or without episiotomy, without fetal manipulation [e.g., rotation version] or instrumentation [forceps] of a spontaneous, cephalic, vaginal, full-term, single, live-born infant. This code is for use as a single diagnosis code and is not to be used with any other code from chapter 15.
  Use additional code to indicate outcome of delivery (Z37.0)

O82 **Encounter for cesarean delivery without indication** ♀ M
  Use additional code to indicate outcome of delivery (Z37.0)

COMPLICATIONS PREDOMINANTLY RELATED TO THE PUERPERIUM (O85-O92)

  Excludes2 mental and behavioral disorders associated with the puerperium (F53)
    obstetrical tetanus (A34)
    puerperal osteomalacia (M83.0)

O85 **Puerperal sepsis** ♀ M
  Postpartum sepsis
  Puerperal peritonitis
  Puerperal pyemia
  Use additional code (B95-B97), to identify infectious agent
  Use additional code (R65.2-) to identify severe sepsis, if applicable
  Excludes1 fever of unknown origin following delivery (O86.4)
    genital tract infection following delivery (O86.1-)
    obstetric pyemic and septic embolism (O88.3-)
    puerperal septic thrombophlebitis (O86.81)
    urinary tract infection following delivery (O86.2-)
  Excludes2 sepsis during labor (O75.3)
  (Ex) 011.4, 011.5, 012.04, 012.05, 012.14, 012.15, 012.24, 012.25, 013.4, 013.5, 014.04, 014.05, 014.14, 014.15, 014.24, 014.25, 014.94, 014.95, 016.4, 016.5, 025.10-025.3, 026.10-026.13, 026.30-026.43, 026.63-026.819, 026.841-026.86, 026.891-026.93, 026.899-026.93, 029.011-029.93, 035.7XX0-035.7XX9, 075.4, 075.81, 075.89, 075.9, 080, 085, 086.12, 086.81-086.89, 090.89, 099.111-099.285, 099.330-099.335, 099.350-099.355, 099.511-099.73, 099.820-099.825, 099.840-09A.53

● O86 **Other puerperal infections**
  Use additional code (B95-B97), to identify infectious agent
  Excludes2 infection during labor (O75.3)
    obstetrical tetanus (A34)
  (Ex) For category O86 CC codes unless otherwise indicated: See O23

  O86.0 **Infection of obstetric surgical wound** ♀ M
    Infected cesarean delivery wound following delivery
    Infected perineal repair following delivery

● O86.1 **Other infection of genital tract following delivery**
  O86.11 **Cervicitis following delivery** ♀ M
  O86.12 **Endometritis following delivery** ♀ M
    (Ex) See O85
  O86.13 **Vaginitis following delivery** ♀ M
  O86.19 **Other infection of genital tract following delivery** ♀ M

● O86.2 **Urinary tract infection following delivery**
  O86.20 **Urinary tract infection following delivery, unspecified** ♀ M
    Puerperal urinary tract infection NOS
  O86.21 **Infection of kidney following delivery** ♀ M
  O86.22 **Infection of bladder following delivery** ♀ M
    Infection of urethra following delivery
  O86.29 **Other urinary tract infection following delivery** ♀ M

  O86.4 **Pyrexia of unknown origin following delivery** ♀ M
    Puerperal infection NOS following delivery
    Puerperal pyrexia NOS following delivery
    Excludes2 pyrexia during labor (O75.2)
    (Ex) 011.4, 011.5, 012.04, 012.05, 012.14, 012.15, 012.24, 012.25, 013.4, 013.5, 014.04, 014.05, 014.14, 014.15, 014.24, 014.25, 014.94, 014.95, 016.4, 016.5, 022.20-022.93, 025.10-025.3, 026.10-026.13, 026.30-026.43, 026.63-026.819, 026.841-026.86, 026.891-026.93, 029.011-029.93, 035.7XX0-035.7XX9, 075.4, 075.81, 075.89-075.9, 080, 086.4-087.9, 090.89, 099.111-099.285, 099.330-099.335, 099.350-099.355, 099.511-099.73, 099.820-099.825, 099.840-09A.53

● O86.8 **Other specified puerperal infections**
  (Ex) For category O86.8 CC codes: See O85
  O86.81 **Puerperal septic thrombophlebitis** ♀ M
  O86.89 **Other specified puerperal infections** ♀ M

CHAPTER 15 (O00-O9A)

CHAPTER 15 (O00-O9A)

● **O87** **Venous complications and hemorrhoids in the puerperium**
    Includes   venous complications in labor, delivery and the puerperium
    Excludes2   obstetric embolism (O88.-)
        puerperal septic thrombophlebitis (O86.81)
        venous complications in pregnancy (O22.-)
    Ⓔⓧ **For category O87 CC codes:** See O22.2

    O87.0 **Superficial thrombophlebitis in the puerperium** ♀ 🦠 M
        Puerperal phlebitis NOS
        Puerperal thrombosis NOS

    O87.1 **Deep phlebothrombosis in the puerperium** ♀ 🦠 M
        Deep vein thrombosis, postpartum
        Pelvic thrombophlebitis, postpartum
        Use additional code to identify the deep vein thrombosis (I82.4-, I82.5-, I82.62-. I82.72-)
        Use additional code, if applicable, for associated long-term (current) use of anticoagulants (Z79.01)

    O87.2 **Hemorrhoids in the puerperium** ♀ 🦠 M

    O87.3 **Cerebral venous thrombosis in the puerperium** ♀ 🦠 M
        Cerebrovenous sinus thrombosis in the puerperium

    O87.4 **Varicose veins of lower extremity in the puerperium** ♀ M

    O87.8 **Other venous complications in the puerperium** ♀ 🦠 M
        Genital varices in the puerperium

    O87.9 **Venous complication in the puerperium, unspecified** ♀ M
        Puerperal phlebopathy NOS

O88 **Obstetric embolism**
    Excludes1   embolism complicating abortion NOS (O03.2)
        embolism complicating ectopic or molar pregnancy (O08.2)
        embolism complicating failed attempted abortion (O07.2)
        embolism complicating induced abortion (O04.7)
        embolism complicating spontaneous abortion (O03.2, O03.7)
    Ⓔⓧ **For category O88 CC codes:** O11.4, O11.5, O12.04, O12.05, O12.14, O12.15, O12.24, O12.25, O13.4, O13.5, O14.04, O14.05, O14.14, O14.15, O14.24, O14.25, O14.94, O14.95, O16.4, O16.5, O25.10-O25.3, O26.10-O26.93, O29.011-O29.93, O35.7XX0-O35.7XX9, O75.4, O75.81-O80, O88.011-O88.83, O90.89, O99.111-O9A.53

  ● **O88.0** **Obstetric air embolism**
    ● **O88.01** **Obstetric air embolism in pregnancy**
        O88.011 **Air embolism in pregnancy, first trimester** ♀ 🦠 M
        O88.012 **Air embolism in pregnancy, second trimester** ♀ 🦠 M
        O88.013 **Air embolism in pregnancy, third trimester** ♀ 🦠 M
        O88.019 **Air embolism in pregnancy, unspecified trimester** ♀ M
    O88.02 **Air embolism in childbirth** ♀ 🦠 M
    O88.03 **Air embolism in the puerperium** ♀ 🦠 M

  ● **O88.1** **Amniotic fluid embolism**
    Anaphylactoid syndrome in pregnancy
    ● **O88.11** **Amniotic fluid embolism in pregnancy**
        O88.111 **Amniotic fluid embolism in pregnancy, first trimester** ♀ 🦠 M
        O88.112 **Amniotic fluid embolism in pregnancy, second trimester** ♀ 🦠 M
        O88.113 **Amniotic fluid embolism in pregnancy, third trimester** ♀ 🦠 M
        O88.119 **Amniotic fluid embolism in pregnancy, unspecified trimester** ♀ M
    O88.12 **Amniotic fluid embolism in childbirth** ♀ 🦠 M
    O88.13 **Amniotic fluid embolism in the puerperium** ♀ 🦠 M

● **O88.2** **Obstetric thromboembolism**
  ● **O88.21** **Thromboembolism in pregnancy**
    Obstetric (pulmonary) embolism NOS
        O88.211 **Thromboembolism in pregnancy, first trimester** ♀ 🦠 M
        O88.212 **Thromboembolism in pregnancy, second trimester** ♀ 🦠 M
        O88.213 **Thromboembolism in pregnancy, third trimester** ♀ 🦠 M
        O88.219 **Thromboembolism in pregnancy, unspecified trimester** ♀ M
    O88.22 **Thromboembolism in childbirth** ♀ 🦠 M
    O88.23 **Thromboembolism in the puerperium** ♀ 🦠 M
        Puerperal (pulmonary) embolism NOS

● **O88.3** **Obstetric pyemic and septic embolism**
  ● **O88.31** **Pyemic and septic embolism in pregnancy**
        O88.311 **Pyemic and septic embolism in pregnancy, first trimester** ♀ 🦠 M
        O88.312 **Pyemic and septic embolism in pregnancy, second trimester** ♀ 🦠 M
        O88.313 **Pyemic and septic embolism in pregnancy, third trimester** ♀ 🦠 M
        O88.319 **Pyemic and septic embolism in pregnancy, unspecified trimester** ♀ M
    O88.32 **Pyemic and septic embolism in childbirth** ♀ 🦠 M
    O88.33 **Pyemic and septic embolism in the puerperium** ♀ 🦠 M

● **O88.8** **Other obstetric embolism**
    Obstetric fat embolism
  ● **O88.81** **Other embolism in pregnancy**
        O88.811 **Other embolism in pregnancy, first trimester** ♀ 🦠 M
        O88.812 **Other embolism in pregnancy, second trimester** ♀ 🦠 M
        O88.813 **Other embolism in pregnancy, third trimester** ♀ 🦠 M
        O88.819 **Other embolism in pregnancy, unspecified trimester** ♀ M
    O88.82 **Other embolism in childbirth** ♀ 🦠 M
    O88.83 **Other embolism in the puerperium** ♀ 🦠 M

● **O89** **Complications of anesthesia during the puerperium**
    Includes   maternal complications arising from the administration of a general, regional or local anesthetic, analgesic or other sedation during the puerperium
    Use additional code, if applicable, to identify specific complication

  ● **O89.0** **Pulmonary complications of anesthesia during the puerperium**
    O89.01 **Aspiration pneumonitis due to anesthesia during the puerperium** ♀ M
        Inhalation of stomach contents or secretions NOS due to anesthesia during the puerperium
        Mendelson's syndrome due to anesthesia during the puerperium
    O89.09 **Other pulmonary complications of anesthesia during the puerperium** ♀ M

    O89.1 **Cardiac complications of anesthesia during the puerperium** ♀ M

    O89.2 **Central nervous system complications of anesthesia during the puerperium** ♀ M

    O89.3 **Toxic reaction to local anesthesia during the puerperium** ♀ M

◀ New   ◀▥ Revised   d̶e̶l̶e̶t̶e̶d̶ Deleted   Excludes 1   Excludes 2   Includes   Use additional   Code first   Code also   Unspecified
OGCR Official Guidelines   ● Unacceptable Principal Diagnosis   X Assign placeholder X   ● Use Additional Character(s)   ▶ Manifestation Code   **Coding Clinic**

O89.4   **Spinal and epidural anesthesia-induced headache during the puerperium** ♀   M

O89.5   **Other complications of spinal and epidural anesthesia during the puerperium** ♀   M

O89.6   **Failed or difficult intubation for anesthesia during the puerperium** ♀   M

O89.8   **Other complications of anesthesia during the puerperium** ♀   M

O89.9   **Complication of anesthesia during the puerperium, unspecified** ♀   M

● **O90**   **Complications of the puerperium, not elsewhere classified**

     O90.0   **Disruption of cesarean delivery wound** ♀   M
       Dehiscence of cesarean delivery wound

       Excludes1   rupture of uterus (spontaneous) before onset of labor (O71.0-)
             rupture of uterus during labor (O71.1)

     O90.1   **Disruption of perineal obstetric wound** ♀   M
       Disruption of wound of episiotomy
       Disruption of wound of perineal laceration
       Secondary perineal tear

     O90.2   **Hematoma of obstetric wound** ♀   M

     O90.3   **Peripartum cardiomyopathy** ♀ 🔾   M
       Conditions in I42.- arising during pregnancy and the puerperium

       Excludes1   pre-existing heart disease complicating pregnancy and the puerperium (O99.4-)
       (Ex) 011.4, 011.5, 012.04, 012.05, 012.14, 012.15, 012.24, 012.25, 013.4, 013.5, 014.04, 014.05, 014.14, 014.15, 014.24, 014.25, 014.94, 014.95, 016.4, 016.5, 025.10-025.3, 026.10-026.13, 026.30-026.43, 026.63-026.819, 026.841-026.86, 026.891-026.93, 029.011-029.93, 035.7XX0-035.7XX9, 075.4, 075.81, 075.89-075.9, 080, 090.3, 090.89, 099.111-099.285, 099.330-099.335, 099.350-099.73, 099.820-099.825, 099.840-09A.53

     O90.4   **Postpartum acute kidney failure** ♀ 🔾   M
       Hepatorenal syndrome following labor and delivery
       (Ex) 011.4, 011.5, 012.04, 012.05, 012.14, 012.15, 012.24, 012.25, 013.4, 013.5, 014.04, 014.05, 014.14, 014.15, 014.24, 014.25, 014.94, 014.95, 016.4, 016.5, 025.10-025.3, 026.10-026.13, 026.30-026.43, 026.63-026.819, 026.841-026.86, 026.891-026.93, 029.011-029.93, 035.7XX0-035.7XX9, 075.4, 075.81, 075.89-075.9, 080, 090.4, 090.89, 099.111-099.285, 099.330-099.335, 099.350-099.355, 099.511-099.73, 099.820-099.825, 099.840-09A.53

     O90.5   **Postpartum thyroiditis** ♀   M

     O90.6   **Postpartum mood disturbance** ♀   M
       Postpartum blues   Postpartum sadness
       Postpartum dysphoria

       Excludes1   postpartum depression (F53)
             puerperal psychosis (F53)

● **O90.8**   **Other complications of the puerperium, not elsewhere classified**

     O90.81   **Anemia of the puerperium** ♀   M
       Postpartum anemia NOS

       Excludes1   pre-existing anemia complicating the puerperium (O99.03)

     O90.89   **Other complications of the puerperium, not elsewhere classified** ♀   M
       Placental polyp

     O90.9   **Complication of the puerperium, unspecified** ♀   M

● **O91**   **Infections of breast associated with pregnancy, the puerperium and lactation**
     Use additional code to identify infection

     ● **O91.0**   **Infection of nipple associated with pregnancy, the puerperium and lactation**

       ● **O91.01**   **Infection of nipple associated with pregnancy**
          Gestational abscess of nipple

          O91.011   **Infection of nipple associated with pregnancy, first trimester** ♀   M

          O91.012   **Infection of nipple associated with pregnancy, second trimester** ♀   M

          O91.013   **Infection of nipple associated with pregnancy, third trimester** ♀   M

          O91.019   **Infection of nipple associated with pregnancy, unspecified trimester** ♀   M

       O91.02   **Infection of nipple associated with the puerperium** ♀   M
          Puerperal abscess of nipple

       O91.03   **Infection of nipple associated with lactation** ♀ M
          Abscess of nipple associated with lactation

     ● **O91.1**   **Abscess of breast associated with pregnancy, the puerperium and lactation**

       ● **O91.11**   **Abscess of breast associated with pregnancy**
          Gestational mammary abscess
          Gestational purulent mastitis
          Gestational subareolar abscess

          O91.111   **Abscess of breast associated with pregnancy, first trimester** ♀   M

          O91.112   **Abscess of breast associated with pregnancy, second trimester** ♀   M

          O91.113   **Abscess of breast associated with pregnancy, third trimester** ♀   M

          O91.119   **Abscess of breast associated with pregnancy, unspecified trimester** ♀   M

       O91.12   **Abscess of breast associated with the puerperium** ♀   M
          Puerperal mammary abscess
          Puerperal purulent mastitis
          Puerperal subareolar abscess

       O91.13   **Abscess of breast associated with lactation** ♀ M
          Mammary abscess associated with lactation
          Purulent mastitis associated with lactation
          Subareolar abscess associated with lactation

     ● **O91.2**   **Nonpurulent mastitis associated with pregnancy, the puerperium and lactation**

       ● **O91.21**   **Nonpurulent mastitis associated with pregnancy**
          Gestational interstitial mastitis
          Gestational lymphangitis of breast
          Gestational mastitis NOS
          Gestational parenchymatous mastitis

          O91.211   **Nonpurulent mastitis associated with pregnancy, first trimester** ♀   M

          O91.212   **Nonpurulent mastitis associated with pregnancy, second trimester** ♀   M

          O91.213   **Nonpurulent mastitis associated with pregnancy, third trimester** ♀   M

          O91.219   **Nonpurulent mastitis associated with pregnancy, unspecified trimester** ♀   M

       O91.22   **Nonpurulent mastitis associated with the puerperium** ♀   M
          Puerperal interstitial mastitis
          Puerperal lymphangitis of breast
          Puerperal mastitis NOS
          Puerperal parenchymatous mastitis

       O91.23   **Nonpurulent mastitis associated with lactation** ♀   M
          Interstitial mastitis associated with lactation
          Lymphangitis of breast associated with lactation
          Mastitis NOS associated with lactation
          Parenchymatous mastitis associated with lactation

CHAPTER 15 (O00-O9A)

N Newborn Age: 0   **P** Pediatric Age: 0–17   **M** Maternity DX: 12–55   **A** Adult Age: 15–124   ♀ Females Only   ♂ Males Only

🔾 Complication\Comorbidity   🔾 Major C\C   (Ex) CC/MCC Exclusions   🔾 Hospital-Acquired Condition

1151

● **O92**   **Other disorders of breast and disorders of lactation associated with pregnancy and the puerperium**

  ● **O92.0**   **Retracted nipple associated with pregnancy, the puerperium, and lactation**

    ● **O92.01**   **Retracted nipple associated with pregnancy**

       O92.011   **Retracted nipple associated with pregnancy, first trimester** ♀   **M**

       O92.012   **Retracted nipple associated with pregnancy, second trimester** ♀   **M**

       O92.013   **Retracted nipple associated with pregnancy, third trimester** ♀   **M**

       O92.019   **Retracted nipple associated with pregnancy, unspecified trimester** ♀   **M**

     O92.02   **Retracted nipple associated with the puerperium** ♀   **M**

     O92.03   **Retracted nipple associated with lactation** ♀   **M**

  ● **O92.1**   **Cracked nipple associated with pregnancy, the puerperium, and lactation**
     Fissure of nipple, gestational or puerperal

    ● **O92.11**   **Cracked nipple associated with pregnancy**

       O92.111   **Cracked nipple associated with pregnancy, first trimester** ♀   **M**

       O92.112   **Cracked nipple associated with pregnancy, second trimester** ♀   **M**

       O92.113   **Cracked nipple associated with pregnancy, third trimester** ♀   **M**

       O92.119   **Cracked nipple associated with pregnancy, unspecified trimester** ♀   **M**

     O92.12   **Cracked nipple associated with the puerperium** ♀   **M**

     O92.13   **Cracked nipple associated with lactation** ♀   **M**

  ● **O92.2**   **Other and unspecified disorders of breast associated with pregnancy and the puerperium**

     O92.20   **Unspecified disorder of breast associated with pregnancy and the puerperium** ♀   **M**

     O92.29   **Other disorders of breast associated with pregnancy and the puerperium** ♀   **M**

   O92.3   **Agalactia** ♀   **M**
     Primary agalactia

     Excludes1   elective agalactia (O92.5)
              secondary agalactia (O92.5)
              therapeutic agalactia (O92.5)

   O92.4   **Hypogalactia** ♀   **M**

   O92.5   **Suppressed lactation** ♀   **M**
     Elective agalactia   Therapeutic agalactia
     Secondary agalactia

     Excludes1   primary agalactia (O92.3)

   O92.6   **Galactorrhea** ♀   **M**

  ● **O92.7**   **Other and unspecified disorders of lactation**

     O92.70   **Unspecified disorders of lactation** ♀   **M**

     O92.79   **Other disorders of lactation** ♀   **M**
       Puerperal galactocele

OTHER OBSTETRIC CONDITIONS, NOT ELSEWHERE CLASSIFIED (O94-O9A)

O94   **Sequelae of complication of pregnancy, childbirth, and the puerperium** ♀   **M**

   Note: This category is to be used to indicate conditions in O00-O77.-, O85-O94 and O98-O9A.- as the cause of late effects. The 'sequelae' include conditions specified as such, or as late effects, which may occur at any time after the puerperium.

   Code first condition resulting from (sequela) of complication of pregnancy, childbirth, and the puerperium

O98   **Maternal infectious and parasitic diseases classifiable elsewhere but complicating pregnancy, childbirth and the puerperium**

   Includes   the listed conditions when complicating the pregnant state, when aggravated by the pregnancy, or as a reason for obstetric care

   Use additional code (Chapter 1), to identify specific infectious or parasitic disease

   Excludes2   herpes gestationis (O26.4-)
              infectious carrier state (O99.82-, O99.83-)
              obstetrical tetanus (A34)
              puerperal infection (O86.-)
              puerperal sepsis (O85)
              when the reason for maternal care is that the disease is known or suspected to have affected the fetus (O35-O36)

  ● **O98.0**   **Tuberculosis complicating pregnancy, childbirth and the puerperium**
     Conditions in A15-A19
     (Ex) **For category O98.0 CC codes:** 011.4, 011.5, 012.04, 012.05, 012.14, 012.15, 012.24, 012.25, 013.4, 013.5, 014.04, 014.05, 014.14, 014.15, 014.24, 014.25, 014.94, 014.95, 016.4, 016.5, 025.10-025.3, 026.10-026.13, 026.30-026.43, 026.63-026.819, 026.841-026.86, 026.891-026.93, 029.011-029.93, 035.7XX0-035.7XX9, 075.4, 075.81, 075.89-075.9, 080, 090.89, 098.011-098.03, 099.111-099.285, 099.330-099.335, 099.350-099.355, 099.511-099.73, 099.820-099.825, 099.840-09A.53

    ● **O98.01**   **Tuberculosis complicating pregnancy**

       O98.011   **Tuberculosis complicating pregnancy, first trimester** ♀ 🔗   **M**

       O98.012   **Tuberculosis complicating pregnancy, second trimester** ♀ 🔗   **M**

       O98.013   **Tuberculosis complicating pregnancy, third trimester** ♀ 🔗   **M**

       O98.019   **Tuberculosis complicating pregnancy, unspecified trimester** ♀   **M**

     O98.02   **Tuberculosis complicating childbirth** ♀ 🔗   **M**

     O98.03   **Tuberculosis complicating the puerperium** ♀ 🔗   **M**

  ● **O98.1**   **Syphilis complicating pregnancy, childbirth and the puerperium**
     Conditions in A50-A53
     (Ex) **For category O98.1 CC codes:** 011.4, 012.04, 012.14, 012.24, 013.4, 014.04, 014.14, 014.24, 014.94, 016.4, 026.11-026.13, 026.31-026.33, 026.41-026.43, 026.63-026.713, 026.72-026.813, 026.86, 026.891-026.893, 026.90-026.93, 029.011-029.013, 029.021-029.023, 029.091-029.093, 029.111-029.113, 029.121-029.123, 029.191-029.193, 029.211-029.213, 029.291-029.293, 029.3X1-029.3X3, 029.41-029.5X3, 029.61-029.8X3, 029.91-029.93, 035.7XX0-035.7XX9, 098.111-098.33, 099.351-099.353, 099.355, 099.89

    ● **O98.11**   **Syphilis complicating pregnancy**

       O98.111   **Syphilis complicating pregnancy, first trimester** ♀ 🔗   **M**

       O98.112   **Syphilis complicating pregnancy, second trimester** ♀ 🔗   **M**

       O98.113   **Syphilis complicating pregnancy, third trimester** ♀ 🔗   **M**

       O98.119   **Syphilis complicating pregnancy, unspecified trimester** ♀   **M**

     O98.12   **Syphilis complicating childbirth** ♀ 🔗   **M**

     O98.13   **Syphilis complicating the puerperium** ♀ 🔗   **M**

◀ New   ◀━ Revised   ~~deleted~~ Deleted   Excludes 1   Excludes 2   Includes   Use additional   Code first   Code also   Unspecified

OGCR Official Guidelines   ● Unacceptable Principal Diagnosis   X Assign placeholder X   ● Use Additional Character(s)   ▌ Manifestation Code   **Coding Clinic**

● **O98.2 Gonorrhea complicating pregnancy, childbirth and the puerperium**
Conditions in A54.-
Ⓔ For category O98.2 CC codes: See O98.1

  ● **O98.21 Gonorrhea complicating pregnancy**

    O98.211 Gonorrhea complicating pregnancy, first trimester ♀ 🔹   **M**

    O98.212 Gonorrhea complicating pregnancy, second trimester ♀ 🔹   **M**

    O98.213 Gonorrhea complicating pregnancy, third trimester ♀ 🔹   **M**

    O98.219 Gonorrhea complicating pregnancy, unspecified trimester ♀   **M**

  O98.22 Gonorrhea complicating childbirth ♀ 🔹   **M**

  O98.23 Gonorrhea complicating the puerperium ♀ 🔹 **M**

● **O98.3 Other infections with a predominantly sexual mode of transmission complicating pregnancy, childbirth and the puerperium**
Conditions in A55-A64
Ⓔ For category O98.3 CC codes: See O98.1

  ● **O98.31 Other infections with a predominantly sexual mode of transmission complicating pregnancy**

    O98.311 Other infections with a predominantly sexual mode of transmission complicating pregnancy, first trimester ♀ 🔹   **M**

    O98.312 Other infections with a predominantly sexual mode of transmission complicating pregnancy, second trimester ♀ 🔹   **M**

    O98.313 Other infections with a predominantly sexual mode of transmission complicating pregnancy, third trimester ♀ 🔹   **M**

    O98.319 Other infections with a predominantly sexual mode of transmission complicating pregnancy, unspecified trimester ♀   **M**

  O98.32 Other infections with a predominantly sexual mode of transmission complicating childbirth ♀ 🔹   **M**

  O98.33 Other infections with a predominantly sexual mode of transmission complicating the puerperium ♀ 🔹   **M**

● **O98.4 Viral hepatitis complicating pregnancy, childbirth and the puerperium**
Conditions in B15-B19
Ⓔ For category O98.4 CC codes: O98.411-O98.613, O98.711-O98.93, O99.830-O99.835

  ● **O98.41 Viral hepatitis complicating pregnancy**

    O98.411 Viral hepatitis complicating pregnancy, first trimester ♀ 🔹   **M**

    O98.412 Viral hepatitis complicating pregnancy, second trimester ♀ 🔹   **M**

    O98.413 Viral hepatitis complicating pregnancy, third trimester ♀ 🔹   **M**

    O98.419 Viral hepatitis complicating pregnancy, unspecified trimester ♀   **M**

  O98.42 Viral hepatitis complicating childbirth ♀ 🔹   **M**

  O98.43 Viral hepatitis complicating the puerperium ♀ 🔹   **M**

● **O98.5 Other viral diseases complicating pregnancy, childbirth and the puerperium**
Conditions in A80-B09, B25-B34, R87.81-, R87.82-

  Excludes:1 human immunodeficiency virus [HIV] disease complicating pregnancy, childbirth and the puerperium (O98.7-)
Ⓔ For category O98.5 CC codes: See O98.4

  ● **O98.51 Other viral diseases complicating pregnancy**

    O98.511 Other viral diseases complicating pregnancy, first trimester ♀ 🔹   **M**

    O98.512 Other viral diseases complicating pregnancy, second trimester ♀ 🔹   **M**

    O98.513 Other viral diseases complicating pregnancy, third trimester ♀ 🔹   **M**

    O98.519 Other viral diseases complicating pregnancy, unspecified trimester ♀   **M**

  O98.52 Other viral diseases complicating childbirth ♀ 🔹   **M**

  O98.53 Other viral diseases complicating the puerperium ♀ 🔹   **M**

● **O98.6 Protozoal diseases complicating pregnancy, childbirth and the puerperium**
Conditions in B50-B64

  ● **O98.61 Protozoal diseases complicating pregnancy**
Ⓔ For category O98.61 CC codes: O11.4, O11.5, O12.04, O12.05, O12.14, O12.15, O12.24, O12.25, O13.4, O13.5, O14.04, O14.05, O14.14, O14.15, O14.24, O14.25, O14.94, O14.95, O16.4, O16.5, O25.10-O25.3, O26.10-O26.13, O26.30-O26.43, O26.63-O26.819, O26.841-O26.86, O26.891-O26.93, O29.011-O29.93, O35.7XX0-O35.7XX9, O75.4, O75.81, O75.89-O75.9, O80, O90.89, O98.411-O98.93, O99.111-O99.285, O99.330-O99.335, O99.350-O99.355, O99.511-O99.73, O99.820-O9A.53

    O98.611 Protozoal diseases complicating pregnancy, first trimester ♀ 🔹   **M**

    O98.612 Protozoal diseases complicating pregnancy, second trimester ♀ 🔹   **M**

    O98.613 Protozoal diseases complicating pregnancy, third trimester ♀ 🔹   **M**

    O98.619 Protozoal diseases complicating pregnancy, unspecified trimester ♀   **M**

  O98.62 Protozoal diseases complicating childbirth ♀ 🔹   **M**
Ⓔ O11.4, O11.5, O12.04, O12.05, O12.14, O12.15, O12.24, O12.25, O13.4, O13.5, O14.04, O14.05, O14.14, O14.15, O14.24, O14.25, O14.94, O14.95, O16.4, O16.5, O25.10-O25.3, O26.10-O26.13, O26.30-O26.43, O26.63-O26.819, O26.841-O26.86, O26.891-O26.93, O29.011-O29.93, O35.7XX0-O35.7XX9, O75.4, O75.81, O75.89-O75.9, O80, O90.89, O98.611-O98.63, O99.111-O99.285, O99.330-O99.335, O99.350-O99.355, O99.511-O99.73, O99.820-O9A.53

  O98.63 Protozoal diseases complicating the puerperium ♀ 🔹   **M**
Ⓔ See O98.62

N Newborn Age: Ø   P Pediatric Age: Ø–17   M Maternity DX: 12–55   A Adult Age: 15–124   ♀ Females Only   ♂ Males Only
🔹 Complication\Comorbidity   🔹 Major C\C   Ⓔ CC/MCC Exclusions   🔹 Hospital-Acquired Condition

CHAPTER 15 (OØØ-O9A)

1153

● O98.7 **Human immunodeficiency virus [HIV] disease complicating pregnancy, childbirth and the puerperium**

Use additional code to identify the type of HIV disease:
Acquired immune deficiency syndrome (AIDS) (B2Ø)
Asymptomatic HIV status (Z21)
HIV positive NOS (Z21)
Symptomatic HIV disease (B2Ø)

OGCR Section I.C.15.f.

HIV Infection in Pregnancy, Childbirth and the Puerperium

During pregnancy, childbirth or the puerperium, a patient admitted because of an HIV-related illness should receive a principal diagnosis from subcategory O98.7-. Human immunodeficiency [HIV] disease complicating pregnancy, childbirth and the puerperium, followed by the code(s) for the HIV-related illness(es).

Patients with asymptomatic HIV infection status admitted during pregnancy, childbirth, or the puerperium should receive codes of O98.7- and Z21, Asymptomatic human immunodeficiency virus [HIV] infection status.

(Ex) For category O98.7 CC codes: See O98.4

● O98.71 **Human immunodeficiency virus [HIV] disease complicating pregnancy**

O98.711 Human immunodeficiency virus [HIV] disease complicating pregnancy, first trimester ♀ 🕮 M

O98.712 Human immunodeficiency virus [HIV] disease complicating pregnancy, second trimester ♀ 🕮 M

O98.713 Human immunodeficiency virus [HIV] disease complicating pregnancy, third trimester ♀ 🕮 M

O98.719 Human immunodeficiency virus [HIV] disease complicating pregnancy, unspecified trimester ♀ M

O98.72 Human immunodeficiency virus [HIV] disease complicating childbirth ♀ 🕮 M

O98.73 Human immunodeficiency virus [HIV] disease complicating the puerperium ♀ 🕮 M

● O98.8 **Other maternal infectious and parasitic diseases complicating pregnancy, childbirth and the puerperium**

(Ex) For category O98.8 CC codes: See O98.4

● O98.81 **Other maternal infectious and parasitic diseases complicating pregnancy**

O98.811 Other maternal infectious and parasitic diseases complicating pregnancy, first trimester ♀ 🕮 M

O98.812 Other maternal infectious and parasitic diseases complicating pregnancy, second trimester ♀ 🕮 M

O98.813 Other maternal infectious and parasitic diseases complicating pregnancy, third trimester ♀ 🕮 M

O98.819 Other maternal infectious and parasitic diseases complicating pregnancy, unspecified trimester ♀ M

O98.82 Other maternal infectious and parasitic diseases complicating childbirth ♀ 🕮 M

O98.83 Other maternal infectious and parasitic diseases complicating the puerperium ♀ 🕮 M

● O98.9 **Unspecified maternal infectious and parasitic disease complicating pregnancy, childbirth and the puerperium**

(Ex) For category O98.9 CC codes: See O98.4

● O98.91 **Unspecified maternal infectious and parasitic disease complicating pregnancy**

O98.911 Unspecified maternal infectious and parasitic disease complicating pregnancy, first trimester ♀ 🕮 M

O98.912 Unspecified maternal infectious and parasitic disease complicating pregnancy, second trimester ♀ 🕮 M

O98.913 Unspecified maternal infectious and parasitic disease complicating pregnancy, third trimester ♀ 🕮 M

O98.919 Unspecified maternal infectious and parasitic disease complicating pregnancy, unspecified trimester ♀ M

O98.92 Unspecified maternal infectious and parasitic disease complicating childbirth ♀ 🕮 M

O98.93 Unspecified maternal infectious and parasitic disease complicating the puerperium ♀ 🕮 M

● O99 **Other maternal diseases classifiable elsewhere but complicating pregnancy, childbirth and the puerperium**

Includes: conditions which complicate the pregnant state, are aggravated by the pregnancy or are a main reason for obstetric care

Use additional code to identify specific condition

Excludes2 when the reason for maternal care is that the condition is known or suspected to have affected the fetus (O35-O36)

● O99.0 **Anemia complicating pregnancy, childbirth and the puerperium**

Conditions in D50-D64

Excludes1 anemia arising in the puerperium (O9Ø.81)
postpartum anemia NOS (O9Ø.81)

● O99.01 **Anemia complicating pregnancy**

O99.011 Anemia complicating pregnancy, first trimester ♀ M

O99.012 Anemia complicating pregnancy, second trimester ♀ M

O99.013 Anemia complicating pregnancy, third trimester ♀ M

O99.019 Anemia complicating pregnancy, unspecified trimester ♀ M

O99.02 Anemia complicating childbirth ♀ M

O99.03 Anemia complicating the puerperium ♀ M

Excludes1 postpartum anemia not pre-existing prior to delivery (O9Ø.81)

● O99.1 **Other diseases of the blood and blood-forming organs and certain disorders involving the immune mechanism complicating pregnancy, childbirth and the puerperium**

Conditions in D65-D89

Excludes2 hemorrhage with coagulation defects (O45.-, O46.Ø-, O67.Ø, O72.3)

(Ex) For category O99.1 CC codes unless otherwise indicated: O25.11-O25.3, O99.281-O99.285, O99.511-O99.513, O99.52-O99.613, O99.62-O99.713, O99.72-O99.73, O99.82Ø-O99.825, O9A.111-O9A.113, O9A.12-O9A.213, O9A.22-O9A.313, O9A.32-O9A.413, O9A.42-O9A.513, O9A.52-O9A.53

● O99.11 **Other diseases of the blood and blood-forming organs and certain disorders involving the immune mechanism complicating pregnancy**

O99.111 Other diseases of the blood and blood-forming organs and certain disorders involving the immune mechanism complicating pregnancy, first trimester ♀ 🕮 M

O99.112 Other diseases of the blood and blood-forming organs and certain disorders involving the immune mechanism complicating pregnancy, second trimester ♀ 🕮 M

O99.113 Other diseases of the blood and blood-forming organs and certain disorders involving the immune mechanism complicating pregnancy, third trimester ♀ 🕮 M

O99.119 Other diseases of the blood and blood-forming organs and certain disorders involving the immune mechanism complicating pregnancy, unspecified trimester ♀ 🕮 M

(Ex) O25.1Ø, O99.28Ø, O99.519, O99.619, O99.719, O9A.119, O9A.219, O9A.319, O9A.419, O9A.519

◄ New ◄▥ Revised ~~deleted~~ Deleted | Excludes 1 | Excludes 2 | Includes | Use additional | Code first | Code also | Unspecified

OGCR Official Guidelines ● Unacceptable Principal Diagnosis X Assign placeholder X ● Use Additional Character(s) ▶ Manifestation Code **Coding Clinic**

O99.12   **Other diseases of the blood and blood-forming organs and certain disorders involving the immune mechanism complicating childbirth** ♀ 🏥   M

O99.13   **Other diseases of the blood and blood-forming organs and certain disorders involving the immune mechanism complicating the puerperium** ♀ 🏥   M

● O99.2   **Endocrine, nutritional and metabolic diseases complicating pregnancy, childbirth and the puerperium**
Conditions in E00-E88

> **Excludes2**   diabetes mellitus (O24.-)
> malnutrition (O25.-)
> postpartum thyroiditis (O90.5)

● O99.21   **Obesity complicating pregnancy, childbirth, and the puerperium**
Use additional code to identify the type of obesity (E66.-)

O99.210   **Obesity complicating pregnancy, unspecified trimester** ♀   M

O99.211   **Obesity complicating pregnancy, first trimester** ♀   M

O99.212   **Obesity complicating pregnancy, second trimester** ♀   M

O99.213   **Obesity complicating pregnancy, third trimester** ♀   M

O99.214   **Obesity complicating childbirth** ♀   M

O99.215   **Obesity complicating the puerperium** ♀   M

● O99.28   **Other endocrine, nutritional and metabolic diseases complicating pregnancy, childbirth and the puerperium**

O99.280   **Endocrine, nutritional and metabolic diseases complicating pregnancy, unspecified trimester** ♀   M

O99.281   **Endocrine, nutritional and metabolic diseases complicating pregnancy, first trimester** ♀   M

O99.282   **Endocrine, nutritional and metabolic diseases complicating pregnancy, second trimester** ♀   M

O99.283   **Endocrine, nutritional and metabolic diseases complicating pregnancy, third trimester** ♀   M

O99.284   **Endocrine, nutritional and metabolic diseases complicating childbirth** ♀   M

O99.285   **Endocrine, nutritional and metabolic diseases complicating the puerperium** ♀   M

● O99.3   **Mental disorders and diseases of the nervous system complicating pregnancy, childbirth and the puerperium**

● O99.31   **Alcohol use complicating pregnancy, childbirth, and the puerperium**
Use additional code(s) from F10 to identify manifestations of the alcohol use

O99.310   **Alcohol use complicating pregnancy, unspecified trimester** ♀   M

O99.311   **Alcohol use complicating pregnancy, first trimester** ♀   M

O99.312   **Alcohol use complicating pregnancy, second trimester** ♀   M

O99.313   **Alcohol use complicating pregnancy, third trimester** ♀   M

O99.314   **Alcohol use complicating childbirth** ♀   M

O99.315   **Alcohol use complicating the puerperium** ♀   M

● O99.32   **Drug use complicating pregnancy, childbirth, and the puerperium**
Use additional code(s) from F11-F16 and F18-F19 to identify manifestations of the drug use

Ⓔⓧ **For category O99.32 CC codes:** 011.4, 011.5, 012.04, 012.05, 012.14, 012.15, 012.24, 012.25, 013.4, 013.5, 014.04, 014.05, 014.14, 014.15, 014.24, 014.25, 014.94, 014.95, 016.4, 016.5, 025.10-025.3, 026.10-026.13, 026.30-026.43, 026.63-026.819, 026.841-026.86, 026.891-026.93, 029.011-029.93, 035.7XX0-035.7XX9, 075.4, 075.81, 075.89-075.9, 080, 090.89, 099.111-099.285, 099.320-099.335, 099.350-099.355, 099.511-099.73, 099.820-099.825, 099.840-09A.53

O99.320   **Drug use complicating pregnancy, unspecified trimester** ♀   M

O99.321   **Drug use complicating pregnancy, first trimester** ♀ 🏥   M

O99.322   **Drug use complicating pregnancy, second trimester** ♀ 🏥   M

O99.323   **Drug use complicating pregnancy, third trimester** ♀ 🏥   M

O99.324   **Drug use complicating childbirth** ♀ 🏥   M

O99.325   **Drug use complicating the puerperium** ♀ 🏥   M

● O99.33   **Tobacco use disorder complicating pregnancy, childbirth, and the puerperium** ◀▥
Smoking complicating pregnancy, childbirth, and the puerperium ◀
Use additional code from category F17 to identify type of tobacco nicotine dependence ◀

O99.330   **Smoking (tobacco) complicating pregnancy, unspecified trimester** ♀   M

O99.331   **Smoking (tobacco) complicating pregnancy, first trimester** ♀   M

O99.332   **Smoking (tobacco) complicating pregnancy, second trimester** ♀   M

O99.333   **Smoking (tobacco) complicating pregnancy, third trimester** ♀   M

O99.334   **Smoking (tobacco) complicating childbirth** ♀   M

O99.335   **Smoking (tobacco) complicating the puerperium** ♀   M

● O99.34   **Other mental disorders complicating pregnancy, childbirth, and the puerperium**
Conditions in F01-F09 and F20-F99

> **Excludes2**   postpartum mood disturbance (O90.6)
> postnatal psychosis (F53)
> puerperal psychosis (F53)

O99.340   **Other mental disorders complicating pregnancy, unspecified trimester** ♀   M

O99.341   **Other mental disorders complicating pregnancy, first trimester** ♀   M

O99.342   **Other mental disorders complicating pregnancy, second trimester** ♀   M

O99.343   **Other mental disorders complicating pregnancy, third trimester** ♀   M

O99.344   **Other mental disorders complicating childbirth** ♀   M

O99.345   **Other mental disorders complicating the puerperium** ♀   M

CHAPTER 15 (O00-O9A)

● **O99.35 Diseases of the nervous system complicating pregnancy, childbirth, and the puerperium**
Conditions in G00-G99

> **Excludes2** pregnancy related peripheral neuritis (O26.8-)

O99.350 Diseases of the nervous system complicating pregnancy, unspecified trimester ♀ M

O99.351 Diseases of the nervous system complicating pregnancy, first trimester ♀ M

O99.352 Diseases of the nervous system complicating pregnancy, second trimester ♀ M

O99.353 Diseases of the nervous system complicating pregnancy, third trimester ♀ M

O99.354 Diseases of the nervous system complicating childbirth ♀ ⊘ M
Ex: See O99.1

O99.355 Diseases of the nervous system complicating the puerperium ♀ ⊘ M
Ex: See O99.1

● **O99.4 Diseases of the circulatory system complicating pregnancy, childbirth and the puerperium**
Conditions in I00-I99

> **Excludes1** peripartum cardiomyopathy (O90.3)
> **Excludes2** hypertensive disorders (O10-O16)
> obstetric embolism (O88.-)
> venous complications and cerebrovenous sinus thrombosis in labor, childbirth and the puerperium (O87.-)
> venous complications and cerebrovenous sinus thrombosis in pregnancy (O22.-)

Ex: **For category O99.4 CC codes unless otherwise indicated:** O11.4, O11.5, O12.04, O12.05, O12.14, O12.15, O12.24, O12.25, O13.4, O13.5, O14.04, O14.05, O14.14, O14.15, O14.24, O14.25, O14.94, O14.95, O16.4, O16.5, O25.10-O25.3, O26.10-O26.13, O26.30-O26.43, O26.63-O26.819, O26.841-O26.86, O26.891-O26.93, O29.011-O29.93, O35.7XX0-O35.7XX9, O75.4, O75.81, O75.89-O75.9, O80, O90.3, O90.89, O99.111-O99.285, O99.330-O99.335, O99.350-O99.73, O99.820-O99.825, O99.840-O9A.53

● **O99.41 Diseases of the circulatory system complicating pregnancy**
Coding Clinic: 2016, Q2, P8

O99.411 Diseases of the circulatory system complicating pregnancy, first trimester ♀ ⊘ M

O99.412 Diseases of the circulatory system complicating pregnancy, second trimester ♀ ⊘ M

O99.413 Diseases of the circulatory system complicating pregnancy, third trimester ♀ ⊘ M

O99.419 Diseases of the circulatory system complicating pregnancy, unspecified trimester ♀ M

O99.42 Diseases of the circulatory system complicating childbirth ♀ ⊘ M
Ex: O25.10-O25.3, O26.10-O26.13, O26.30-O26.43, O26.63-O26.819, O26.841-O26.86, O26.891-O26.93, O29.011-O29.93, O35.7XX0-O35.7XX9, O75.4, O75.81, O75.89-O75.9, O80, O90.3, O90.89, O99.111-O99.285, O99.330-O99.335, O99.350-O99.73, O99.820-O99.825, O99.840-O9A.53

O99.43 Diseases of the circulatory system complicating the puerperium ♀ ⊘ M

● **O99.5 Diseases of the respiratory system complicating pregnancy, childbirth and the puerperium**
Conditions in J00-J99

● **O99.51 Diseases of the respiratory system complicating pregnancy**

O99.511 Diseases of the respiratory system complicating pregnancy, first trimester ♀ M

O99.512 Diseases of the respiratory system complicating pregnancy, second trimester ♀ M

O99.513 Diseases of the respiratory system complicating pregnancy, third trimester ♀ M

O99.519 Diseases of the respiratory system complicating pregnancy, unspecified trimester ♀ M

O99.52 Diseases of the respiratory system complicating childbirth ♀ M

O99.53 Diseases of the respiratory system complicating the puerperium ♀ M

● **O99.6 Diseases of the digestive system complicating pregnancy, childbirth and the puerperium**
Conditions in K00-K93

> **Excludes2** hemorrhoids in pregnancy (O22.4-) ◀
> liver and biliary tract disorders in pregnancy, childbirth and the puerperium (O26.6-)

● **O99.61 Diseases of the digestive system complicating pregnancy**

O99.611 Diseases of the digestive system complicating pregnancy, first trimester ♀ M

O99.612 Diseases of the digestive system complicating pregnancy, second trimester ♀ M

O99.613 Diseases of the digestive system complicating pregnancy, third trimester ♀ M

O99.619 Diseases of the digestive system complicating pregnancy, unspecified trimester ♀ M

O99.62 Diseases of the digestive system complicating childbirth ♀ M

O99.63 Diseases of the digestive system complicating the puerperium ♀ M

● **O99.7 Diseases of the skin and subcutaneous tissue complicating pregnancy, childbirth and the puerperium**
Conditions in L00-L99

> **Excludes2** herpes gestationis (O26.4)
> pruritic urticarial papules and plaques of pregnancy (PUPPP) (O26.86)

● **O99.71 Diseases of the skin and subcutaneous tissue complicating pregnancy**

O99.711 Diseases of the skin and subcutaneous tissue complicating pregnancy, first trimester ♀ M

O99.712 Diseases of the skin and subcutaneous tissue complicating pregnancy, second trimester ♀ M

O99.713 Diseases of the skin and subcutaneous tissue complicating pregnancy, third trimester ♀ M

O99.719 Diseases of the skin and subcutaneous tissue complicating pregnancy, unspecified trimester ♀ M

O99.72 Diseases of the skin and subcutaneous tissue complicating childbirth ♀ M

O99.73 Diseases of the skin and subcutaneous tissue complicating the puerperium ♀ M

◀ New   ◀▥ Revised   ~~deleted~~ Deleted   Excludes 1   Excludes 2   Includes   Use additional   Code first   Code also   Unspecified
OGCR Official Guidelines   ● Unacceptable Principal Diagnosis   X Assign placeholder X   ● Use Additional Character(s)   ▷ Manifestation Code   **Coding Clinic**

● **O99.8** **Other specified diseases and conditions complicating pregnancy, childbirth and the puerperium**
　　Conditions in D00-D48, H00-H95, M00-N99, and Q00-Q99

　　Use additional code to identify condition

　　Excludes2　genitourinary infections in pregnancy (O23.-)
　　　　infection of genitourinary tract following delivery (O86.1-O86.3)
　　　　malignant neoplasm complicating pregnancy, childbirth and the puerperium (O9A.1-)
　　　　maternal care for known or suspected abnormality of maternal pelvic organs (O34.-)
　　　　postpartum acute kidney failure (O90.4)
　　　　traumatic injuries in pregnancy (O9A.2-)

● **O99.81** **Abnormal glucose complicating pregnancy, childbirth and the puerperium**

　　Excludes1　gestational diabetes (O24.4-)

　　O99.810　**Abnormal glucose complicating pregnancy** ♀ 　M

　　O99.814　**Abnormal glucose complicating childbirth** ♀ 　M

　　O99.815　**Abnormal glucose complicating the puerperium** ♀ 　M

● **O99.82** **Streptococcus B carrier state complicating pregnancy, childbirth and the puerperium**

　　Excludes1　Carrier of streptococcus group B (GBS) in a nonpregnant woman (Z22.330) ◄

　　● **O99.820**　**Streptococcus B carrier state complicating pregnancy** ♀ 　M

　　O99.824　**Streptococcus B carrier state complicating childbirth** ♀ 　M

　　● **O99.825**　**Streptococcus B carrier state complicating the puerperium** ♀ 　M

● **O99.83** **Other infection carrier state complicating pregnancy, childbirth and the puerperium**

　　Use additional code to identify the carrier state (Z22.-)

　　(Ex) **For category O99.83 CC codes:** 098.411-098.613, 098.711-098.93, 099.830-099.835

　　O99.830　**Other infection carrier state complicating pregnancy** ♀ 🦠 　M

　　O99.834　**Other infection carrier state complicating childbirth** ♀ 🦠 　M

　　O99.835　**Other infection carrier state complicating the puerperium** ♀ 🦠 　M

● **O99.84** **Bariatric surgery status complicating pregnancy, childbirth and the puerperium**
　　Gastric banding status complicating pregnancy, childbirth and the puerperium
　　Gastric bypass status for obesity complicating pregnancy, childbirth and the puerperium
　　Obesity surgery status complicating pregnancy, childbirth and the puerperium

　　O99.840　**Bariatric surgery status complicating pregnancy, unspecified trimester** ♀ 　M

　　O99.841　**Bariatric surgery status complicating pregnancy, first trimester** ♀ 　M

　　O99.842　**Bariatric surgery status complicating pregnancy, second trimester** ♀ 　M

　　O99.843　**Bariatric surgery status complicating pregnancy, third trimester** ♀ 　M

　　O99.844　**Bariatric surgery status complicating childbirth** ♀ 　M

　　O99.845　**Bariatric surgery status complicating the puerperium** ♀ 　M

　　O99.89　**Other specified diseases and conditions complicating pregnancy, childbirth and the puerperium** ♀ 　M

OGCR Section I.C.2.I.3.

Malignant neoplasm in a pregnant patient
When a pregnant woman has a malignant neoplasm, a code from subcategory O9A.1-, Malignant neoplasm complicating pregnancy, childbirth, and the puerperium, should be sequenced first, followed by the appropriate code from Chapter 2 to indicate the type of neoplasm.

● **O9A** **Maternal malignant neoplasms, traumatic injuries and abuse classifiable elsewhere but complicating pregnancy, childbirth and the puerperium**

　● **O9A.1** **Malignant neoplasm complicating pregnancy, childbirth and the puerperium**
　　Conditions in C00-C96

　　Use additional code to identify neoplasm

　　Excludes2　maternal care for benign tumor of corpus uteri (O34.1-)
　　　　maternal care for benign tumor of cervix (O34.4-)

　　● **O9A.11** **Malignant neoplasm complicating pregnancy**

　　　O9A.111　**Malignant neoplasm complicating pregnancy, first trimester** ♀ 　M

　　　O9A.112　**Malignant neoplasm complicating pregnancy, second trimester** ♀ 　M

　　　O9A.113　**Malignant neoplasm complicating pregnancy, third trimester** ♀ 　M

　　　O9A.119　**Malignant neoplasm complicating pregnancy, unspecified trimester** ♀ 　M

　　O9A.12　**Malignant neoplasm complicating childbirth** ♀ 　M

　　O9A.13　**Malignant neoplasm complicating the puerperium** ♀ 　M
　　　　Coding Clinic: 2015, Q3, P19

　● **O9A.2** **Injury, poisoning and certain other consequences of external causes complicating pregnancy, childbirth and the puerperium**
　　Conditions in S00-T88, except T74 and T76

　　Use additional code(s) to identify the injury or poisoning

　　Excludes2　physical, sexual and psychological abuse complicating pregnancy, childbirth and the puerperium (O9A.3-, O9A.4-, O9A.5-)

　　● **O9A.21** **Injury, poisoning and certain other consequences of external causes complicating pregnancy**

　　　O9A.211　**Injury, poisoning and certain other consequences of external causes complicating pregnancy, first trimester** ♀ 　M

　　　O9A.212　**Injury, poisoning and certain other consequences of external causes complicating pregnancy, second trimester** ♀ 　M

　　　O9A.213　**Injury, poisoning and certain other consequences of external causes complicating pregnancy, third trimester** ♀ 　M

　　　O9A.219　**Injury, poisoning and certain other consequences of external causes complicating pregnancy, unspecified trimester** ♀ 　M

　　O9A.22　**Injury, poisoning and certain other consequences of external causes complicating childbirth** ♀ 　M

　　O9A.23　**Injury, poisoning and certain other consequences of external causes complicating the puerperium** ♀ 　M

CHAPTER 15 (O00-O9A)

N Newborn Age: 0　　**P** Pediatric Age: 0–17　　**M** Maternity DX: 12–55　　**A** Adult Age: 15–124　　♀ Females Only　　♂ Males Only

🦠 Complication\Comorbidity　　🦠 Major C\C　　(Ex) CC/MCC Exclusions　　🦠 Hospital-Acquired Condition

● **O9A.3 Physical abuse complicating pregnancy, childbirth and the puerperium**
    Conditions in T74.11 or T76.11

    Use additional code (if applicable):
      to identify any associated current injury due to physical abuse
      to identify the perpetrator of abuse (Y07.-)

    Excludes2   sexual abuse complicating pregnancy, childbirth and the puerperium (O9A.4)

  ● **O9A.31 Physical abuse complicating pregnancy**
      O9A.311 Physical abuse complicating pregnancy, first trimester ♀   M
      O9A.312 Physical abuse complicating pregnancy, second trimester ♀   M
      O9A.313 Physical abuse complicating pregnancy, third trimester ♀   M
      O9A.319 Physical abuse complicating pregnancy, unspecified trimester ♀   M
    O9A.32 Physical abuse complicating childbirth ♀   M
    O9A.33 Physical abuse complicating the puerperium ♀   M

● **O9A.4 Sexual abuse complicating pregnancy, childbirth and the puerperium**
    Conditions in T74.21 or T76.21

    Use additional code (if applicable):
      to identify any associated current injury due to sexual abuse
      to identify the perpetrator of abuse (Y07.-)

  ● **O9A.41 Sexual abuse complicating pregnancy**
      O9A.411 Sexual abuse complicating pregnancy, first trimester ♀   M
      O9A.412 Sexual abuse complicating pregnancy, second trimester ♀   M
      O9A.413 Sexual abuse complicating pregnancy, third trimester ♀   M
      O9A.419 Sexual abuse complicating pregnancy, unspecified trimester ♀   M
    O9A.42 Sexual abuse complicating childbirth ♀   M
    O9A.43 Sexual abuse complicating the puerperium ♀   M

● **O9A.5 Psychological abuse complicating pregnancy, childbirth and the puerperium**
    Conditions in T74.31 or T76.31

    Use additional code to identify the perpetrator of abuse (Y07.-)

  ● **O9A.51 Psychological abuse complicating pregnancy**
      O9A.511 Psychological abuse complicating pregnancy, first trimester ♀   M
      O9A.512 Psychological abuse complicating pregnancy, second trimester ♀   M
      O9A.513 Psychological abuse complicating pregnancy, third trimester ♀   M
      O9A.519 Psychological abuse complicating pregnancy, unspecified trimester ♀   M
    O9A.52 Psychological abuse complicating childbirth ♀ M
    O9A.53 Psychological abuse complicating the puerperium ♀   M

CHAPTER 16

CERTAIN CONDITIONS ORIGINATING IN THE PERINATAL PERIOD (P00-P96)

OGCR Chapter-Specific Coding Guidelines

16. **Chapter 16: Certain Conditions Originating in the Perinatal Period (P00-P96)**

For coding and reporting purposes the perinatal period is defined as before birth through the 28th day following birth. The following guidelines are provided for reporting purposes

a. **General Perinatal Rules**

1) **Use of Chapter 16 Codes**

Codes in this chapter are never for use on the maternal record. Codes from Chapter 15, the obstetric chapter, are never permitted on the newborn record. Chapter 16 codes may be used throughout the life of the patient if the condition is still present.

2) **Principal Diagnosis for Birth Record**

When coding the birth episode in a newborn record, assign a code from category Z38, Liveborn infants according to place of birth and type of delivery, as the principal diagnosis. A code from category Z38 is assigned only once, to a newborn at the time of birth. If a newborn is transferred to another institution, a code from category Z38 should not be used at the receiving hospital.

A code from category Z38 is used only on the newborn record, not on the mother's record.

3) **Use of Codes from other Chapters with Codes from Chapter 16**

Codes from other chapters may be used with codes from chapter 16 if the codes from the other chapters provide more specific detail. Codes for signs and symptoms may be assigned when a definitive diagnosis has not been established. If the reason for the encounter is a perinatal condition, the code from chapter 16 should be sequenced first.

4) **Use of Chapter 16 Codes after the Perinatal Period**

Should a condition originate in the perinatal period, and continue throughout the life of the patient, the perinatal code should continue to be used regardless of the patient's age.

5) **Birth process or community acquired conditions**

If a newborn has a condition that may be either due to the birth process or community acquired and the documentation does not indicate which it is, the default is due to the birth process and the code from Chapter 16 should be used. If the condition is community-acquired, a code from Chapter 16 should not be assigned.

6) **Code all clinically significant conditions**

All clinically significant conditions noted on routine newborn examination should be coded. A condition is clinically significant if it requires:
- clinical evaluation; or
- therapeutic treatment; or
- diagnostic procedures; or
- extended length of hospital stay; or
- increased nursing care and/or monitoring; or
- has implications for future health care needs

Note: The perinatal guidelines listed above are the same as the general coding guidelines for "additional diagnoses", except for the final point regarding implications for future health care needs. Codes should be assigned for conditions that have been specified by the provider as having implications for future health care needs.

b. **Observation and Evaluation of Newborns for Suspected Conditions not Found**

1) **Assign a code from category Z05, Observation and evaluation of newborns and infants for suspected** conditions ruled out, to identify those instances when a healthy newborn is evaluated for a suspected condition that is determined after study not to be present. Do not use a code from category Z05 when the patient has identified signs or symptoms of a suspected problem; in such cases code the sign or symptom.

2) A code from category Z05 may also be assigned as a principal or first-listed code for readmissions or encounters when the code from category Z38 code no longer applies. Codes from category Z05 are for use only for healthy newborns and infants for which no condition after study is found to be present.

3) **Z05 on a birth record**

A code from category Z05 is to be used as a secondary code after the code from category Z38, Liveborn infants according to place of birth and type of delivery.

c. **Coding Additional Perinatal Diagnoses**

1) **Assigning codes for conditions that require treatment**

Assign codes for conditions that require treatment or further investigation, prolong the length of stay, or require resource utilization.

2) **Codes for conditions specified as having implications for future health care needs**

Assign codes for conditions that have been specified by the provider as having implications for future health care needs.

Note: This guideline should not be used for adult patients.

d. **Prematurity and Fetal Growth Retardation**

Providers utilize different criteria in determining prematurity. A code for prematurity should not be assigned unless it is documented. Assignment of codes in categories P05, Disorders of newborn related to slow fetal growth and fetal malnutrition, and P07, Disorders of newborn related to short gestation and low birth weight, not elsewhere classified, should be based on the recorded birth weight and estimated gestational age. Codes from category P05 should not be assigned with codes from category P07.

When both birth weight and gestational age are available, two codes from category P07 should be assigned, with the code for birth weight sequenced before the code for gestational age.

e. **Low birth weight and immaturity status**

Codes from category P07, Disorders of newborn related to short gestation and low birth weight, not elsewhere classified, are for use for a child or adult who was premature or had a low birth weight as a newborn and this is affecting the patient's current health status.

See Section I.C.21. Factors influencing health status and contact with health services, Status.

f. **Bacterial Sepsis of Newborn**

Category P36, Bacterial sepsis of newborn, includes congenital sepsis. If a perinate is documented as having sepsis without documentation of congenital or community acquired, the default is congenital and a code from category P36 should be assigned. If the P36 code includes the causal organism, an additional code from category B95, Streptococcus, Staphylococcus, and Enterococcus as the cause of diseases classified elsewhere, or B96, Other bacterial agents as the cause of diseases classified elsewhere, should not be assigned. If the P36 code does not include the causal organism, assign an additional code from category B96. If applicable, use additional codes to identify severe sepsis (R65.2-) and any associated acute organ dysfunction.

g. **Stillbirth**

Code P95, Stillbirth, is only for use in institutions that maintain separate records for stillbirths. No other code should be used with P95. Code P95 should not be used on the mother's record.

CHAPTER 16

CERTAIN CONDITIONS ORIGINATING IN THE PERINATAL PERIOD (P00-P96)

Note: Codes from this chapter are for use on newborn records only, never on maternal records.

Includes   conditions that have their origin in the fetal or perinatal period (before birth through the first 28 days after birth) even if morbidity occurs later

Excludes2   congenital malformations, deformations and chromosomal abnormalities (Q00-Q99)
endocrine, nutritional and metabolic diseases (E00-E88)
injury, poisoning and certain other consequences of external causes (S00-T88)
neoplasms (C00-D49)
tetanus neonatorum (A33)

This chapter contains the following blocks:

P00-P04	Newborn affected by maternal factors and by complications of pregnancy, labor, and delivery
P05-P08	Disorders of newborns related to length of gestation and fetal growth
P09	Abnormal findings on neonatal screening
P10-P15	Birth trauma
P19-P29	Respiratory and cardiovascular disorders specific to the perinatal period
P35-P39	Infections specific to the perinatal period
P50-P61	Hemorrhagic and hematological disorders of newborn
P70-P74	Transitory endocrine and metabolic disorders specific to newborn
P76-P78	Digestive system disorders of newborn
P80-P83	Conditions involving the integument and temperature regulation of newborn
P84	Other problems with newborn
P90-P96	Other disorders originating in the perinatal period

NEWBORN AFFECTED BY MATERNAL FACTORS AND BY COMPLICATIONS OF PREGNANCY, LABOR, AND DELIVERY (P00–P04)

Note: These codes are for use when the listed maternal conditions are specified as the cause of confirmed morbidity or potential morbidity which have their origin in the perinatal period (before birth through the first 28 days after birth). ◄▥▥

● **P00**   **Newborn affected by maternal conditions that may be unrelated to present pregnancy** ◄▥▥

Code first any current condition in newborn

Excludes2   encounter for observation of newborn for suspected diseases and conditions ruled out (Z05.-) ◄
newborn affected by maternal complications of pregnancy (P01.-) ◄
newborn affected by maternal endocrine and metabolic disorders (P70–P74)
newborn affected by noxious substances transmitted via placenta or breast milk (P04.-)

P00.0   **Newborn affected by maternal hypertensive disorders** ◄▥▥
Newborn affected by maternal conditions classifiable to O10-O11, O13-O16 ◄▥▥

P00.1   **Newborn affected by maternal renal and urinary tract diseases** ◄▥▥
Newborn affected by maternal conditions classifiable to N00-N39 ◄▥▥

P00.2   **Newborn affected by maternal infectious and parasitic diseases** ◄▥▥
Newborn affected by maternal infectious disease classifiable to A00-B99, J09 and J10 ◄▥▥

     Excludes1   infections specific to the perinatal period (P35-P39)
maternal genital tract or other localized infections (P00.8)

     Coding Clinic: 2015, Q3, P21

P00.3   **Newborn affected by other maternal circulatory and respiratory diseases** ◄▥▥
Newborn affected by maternal conditions classifiable to I00-I99, J00-J99, Q20-Q34 and not included in P00.0, P00.2 ◄▥▥

P00.4   **Newborn affected by maternal nutritional disorders** ◄▥▥
Newborn affected by maternal disorders classifiable to E40-E64 ◄▥▥
Maternal malnutrition NOS

P00.5   **Newborn affected by maternal injury** ◄▥▥
Newborn affected by maternal conditions classifiable to O9A.2- ◄▥▥

P00.6   **Newborn affected by surgical procedure on mother** ◄▥▥
Newborn affected by amniocentesis ◄▥▥

     Excludes1   Cesarean delivery for present delivery (P03.4)
damage to placenta from amniocentesis, cesarean delivery or surgical induction (P02.1)
previous surgery to uterus or pelvic organs (P03.89)

     Excludes2   newborn affected by complication of (fetal) intrauterine procedure (P96.5)

P00.7   **Newborn affected by other medical procedures on mother, not elsewhere classified** ◄▥▥
Newborn affected by radiation to mother ◄▥▥

     Excludes1   damage to placenta from amniocentesis, cesarean delivery or surgical induction (P02.1)
newborn affected by other complications of labor and delivery (P03.-)

● **P00.8**   **Newborn affected by other maternal conditions** ◄▥▥

P00.81   **Newborn affected by periodontal disease in mother** ◄▥▥

P00.89   **Newborn affected by other maternal conditions** ◄▥▥
Newborn affected by conditions classifiable to T80-T88 ◄▥▥
Newborn affected by maternal genital tract or other localized infections ◄▥▥
Newborn affected by maternal systemic lupus erythematosus ◄▥▥

P00.9   **Newborn affected by unspecified maternal condition** ◄▥▥

● **P01**   **Newborn affected by maternal complications of pregnancy** ◄▥▥

Code first any current condition in newborn

     Excludes2   encounter for observation of newborn for suspected diseases and conditions ruled out (Z05.-) ◄

P01.0   **Newborn affected by incompetent cervix** ◄▥▥

P01.1   **Newborn affected by premature rupture of membranes** ◄▥▥

P01.2   **Newborn affected by oligohydramnios** ◄▥▥

     Excludes1   oligohydramnios due to premature rupture of membranes (P01.1)

P01.3   **Newborn affected by polyhydramnios** ◄▥▥
Excess of amniotic fluid, usually > 2000 mL
Newborn affected by hydramnios ◄▥▥

P01.4   **Newborn affected by ectopic pregnancy** ◄▥▥
Newborn affected by abdominal pregnancy ◄▥▥

P01.5   **Newborn affected by multiple pregnancy** ◄▥▥
Newborn affected by triplet (pregnancy) ◄▥▥
Newborn affected by twin (pregnancy) ◄▥▥

P01.6   **Newborn affected by maternal death** ◄▥▥

P01.7   **Newborn affected by malpresentation before labor** ◄▥▥
Newborn affected by breech presentation before labor ◄▥▥
Newborn affected by external version before labor ◄▥▥
Newborn affected by face presentation before labor ◄▥▥
Newborn affected by transverse lie before labor ◄▥▥
Newborn affected by unstable lie before labor ◄▥▥

P01.8   **Newborn affected by other maternal complications of pregnancy** ◄▥▥

P01.9   **Newborn affected by maternal complication of pregnancy, unspecified** ◄▥▥

◄ New   ◄▥▥ Revised   ~~deleted~~ Deleted   Excludes 1   Excludes 2   Includes   Use additional   Code first   Code also   Unspecified

OGCR Official Guidelines   ● Unacceptable Principal Diagnosis   X Assign placeholder X   ● Use Additional Character(s)   ▶ Manifestation Code   **Coding Clinic**

● **P02** **Newborn affected by complications of placenta, cord and membranes** ◀▥

     Code first any current condition in newborn

     Excludes2   encounter for observation of newborn for suspected diseases and conditions ruled out (Z05.-) ◀

   P02.0   **Newborn affected by placenta previa** ◀▥

   P02.1   **Newborn affected by other forms of placental separation and hemorrhage** ◀▥
       Newborn affected by abruptio placenta ◀▥
       Newborn affected by accidental hemorrhage ◀▥
       Newborn affected by antepartum hemorrhage ◀▥
       Newborn affected by damage to placenta from amniocentesis, cesarean delivery or surgical induction ◀▥
       Newborn affected by maternal blood loss ◀▥
       Newborn affected by premature separation of placenta ◀▥

 ● **P02.2**   **Newborn affected by other and unspecified morphological and functional abnormalities of placenta** ◀▥

     P02.20   **Newborn affected by unspecified morphological and functional abnormalities of placenta** ◀▥

     P02.29   **Newborn affected by other morphological and functional abnormalities of placenta** ◀▥
         Newborn affected by placental dysfunction ◀▥
         Newborn affected by placental infarction ◀▥
         Newborn affected by placental insufficiency ◀▥

   P02.3   **Newborn affected by placental transfusion syndromes** ◀▥
       Newborn affected by placental and cord abnormalities resulting in twin-to-twin or other transplacental transfusion ◀▥

   P02.4   **Newborn affected by prolapsed cord** ◀▥

   P02.5   **Newborn affected by other compression of umbilical cord** ◀▥
       Newborn affected by umbilical cord (tightly) around neck ◀▥
       Newborn affected by entanglement of umbilical cord ◀▥
       Newborn affected by knot in umbilical cord ◀▥

 ● **P02.6**   **Newborn affected by other and unspecified conditions of umbilical cord** ◀▥

     P02.60   **Newborn affected by unspecified conditions of umbilical cord** ◀▥

     P02.69   **Newborn affected by other conditions of umbilical cord** ◀▥
         Newborn affected by short umbilical cord ◀▥
         Newborn affected by vasa previa ◀▥

         Excludes1   newborn affected by single umbilical artery (Q27.0)

   P02.7   **Newborn affected by chorioamnionitis** ◀▥
       Inflammation of chorion and amnion
       Newborn affected by amnionitis ◀▥
       Newborn affected by membranitis ◀▥
       Newborn affected by placentitis ◀▥

   P02.8   **Newborn affected by other abnormalities of membranes** ◀▥

   P02.9   **Newborn affected by abnormality of membranes, unspecified** ◀▥

● **P03** **Newborn affected by other complications of labor and delivery** ◀▥

     Code first any current condition in newborn

     Excludes2   encounter for observation of newborn for suspected diseases and conditions ruled out (Z05.-) ◀

   P03.0   **Newborn affected by breech delivery and extraction** ◀▥

   P03.1   **Newborn affected by other malpresentation, malposition and disproportion during labor and delivery** ◀▥
       Newborn affected by contracted pelvis ◀▥
       Newborn affected by conditions classifiable to O64-O66 ◀▥
       Newborn affected by persistent occipitoposterior ◀▥
       Newborn affected by transverse lie ◀▥

   P03.2   **Newborn affected by forceps delivery** ◀▥

   P03.3   **Newborn affected by delivery by vacuum extractor [ventouse]** ◀▥

   P03.4   **Newborn affected by Cesarean delivery** ◀▥

   P03.5   **Newborn affected by precipitate delivery** ◀▥
       Newborn affected by rapid second stage ◀▥

   P03.6   **Newborn affected by abnormal uterine contractions** ◀▥
       Newborn affected by conditions classifiable to O62.-, except O62.3 ◀▥
       Newborn affected by hypertonic labor ◀▥
       Newborn affected by uterine inertia ◀▥

 ● **P03.8**   **Newborn affected by other specified complications of labor and delivery** ◀▥

  ● **P03.81**   **Newborn affected by abnormality in fetal (intrauterine) heart rate or rhythm** ◀▥

       Excludes1   neonatal cardiac dysrhythmia (P29.1-)

     P03.810   **Newborn affected by abnormality in fetal (intrauterine) heart rate or rhythm before the onset of labor** ◀▥

     P03.811   **Newborn affected by abnormality in fetal (intrauterine) heart rate or rhythm during labor** ◀▥

     P03.819   **Newborn affected by abnormality in fetal (intrauterine) heart rate or rhythm, unspecified as to time of onset** ◀▥

     P03.82   **Meconium passage during delivery**

       Excludes1   meconium aspiration (P24.00, P24.01)
           meconium staining (P96.83)

     P03.89   **Newborn affected by other specified complications of labor and delivery** ◀▥
         Newborn affected by abnormality of maternal soft tissues ◀▥
         Newborn affected by conditions classifiable to O60-O75 and by procedures used in labor and delivery not included in P02.- and P03.0-P03.6 ◀▥
         Newborn affected by induction of labor ◀▥

   P03.9   **Newborn affected by complication of labor and delivery, unspecified** ◀▥

● **P04** **Newborn affected by noxious substances transmitted via placenta or breast milk** ◀▥

     Includes   nonteratogenic effects of substances transmitted via placenta

     Excludes2   congenital malformations (Q00-Q99)
         encounter for observation of newborn for suspected diseases and conditions ruled out (Z05.-) ◀
         neonatal jaundice from excessive hemolysis due to drugs or toxins transmitted from mother (P58.4)
         newborn in contact with and (suspected) exposures hazardous to health not transmitted via placenta or breast milk (Z77.-)

   P04.0   **Newborn affected by maternal anesthesia and analgesia in pregnancy, labor and delivery** ◀▥
       Newborn affected by reactions and intoxications from maternal opiates and tranquilizers administered during labor and delivery ◀▥

   P04.1   **Newborn affected by other maternal medication** ◀▥
       Newborn affected by cancer chemotherapy ◀▥
       Newborn affected by cytotoxic drugs ◀▥

       Excludes1   dysmorphism due to warfarin (Q86.2)
           fetal hydantoin syndrome (Q86.1)
           maternal use of drugs of addiction (P04.4-)

CHAPTER 16 (P00-P96)

P04.2　**Newborn affected by maternal use of tobacco** ◀▦
　　　Newborn affected by exposure in utero to tobacco smoke ◀▦

　　　　Excludes2　newborn exposure to environmental tobacco smoke (P96.81)

P04.3　**Newborn affected by maternal use of alcohol** ◀▦

　　　　Excludes1　fetal alcohol syndrome (Q86.0)

● P04.4　**Newborn affected by maternal use of drugs of addiction** ◀▦

　　P04.41　**Newborn affected by maternal use of cocaine** ◀▦
　　　　　'Crack baby'

　　P04.49　**Newborn affected by maternal use of other drugs of addiction** ◀▦

　　　　　Excludes2　newborn affected by maternal anesthesia and analgesia (P04.0) ◀▦
　　　　　　　　　withdrawal symptoms from maternal use of drugs of addiction (P96.1)

P04.5　**Newborn affected by maternal use of nutritional chemical substances** ◀▦

P04.6　**Newborn affected by maternal exposure to environmental chemical substances** ◀▦

P04.8　**Newborn affected by other maternal noxious substances** ◀▦

P04.9　**Newborn affected by maternal noxious substance, unspecified** ◀▦

OGCR Section I.C.16.d.

Prematurity and Fetal Growth Retardation

Providers utilize different criteria in determining prematurity. A code for prematurity should not be assigned unless it is documented. Assignment of codes in categories P05, Disorders of newborn related to slow fetal growth and fetal malnutrition, and P07, Disorders of newborn related to short gestation and low birth weight, not elsewhere classified, should be based on the recorded birth weight and estimated gestational age. Codes from category P05 should not be assigned with codes from category P07.

When both birth weight and gestational age are available, two codes from category P07 should be assigned, with the code for birth weight sequenced before the code for gestational age.

A code from P05 and codes from P07.2 and P07.3 may be used to specify weeks of gestation as documented by the provider in the record.

DISORDERS OF NEWBORN RELATED TO LENGTH OF GESTATION AND FETAL GROWTH (P05-P08)

● P05　**Disorders of newborn related to slow fetal growth and fetal malnutrition**

● P05.0　**Newborn light for gestational age**
　　　Newborn light-for-dates
　　　Weight below but length above 10th percentile for gestational age ◀

　　P05.00　**Newborn light for gestational age, unspecified weight**

　　P05.01　**Newborn light for gestational age, less than 500 grams**

　　P05.02　**Newborn light for gestational age, 500-749 grams**

　　P05.03　**Newborn light for gestational age, 750-999 grams**

　　P05.04　**Newborn light for gestational age, 1000-1249 grams**

　　P05.05　**Newborn light for gestational age, 1250-1499 grams**

　　P05.06　**Newborn light for gestational age, 1500-1749 grams**

　　P05.07　**Newborn light for gestational age, 1750-1999 grams**

　　P05.08　**Newborn light for gestational age, 2000-2499 grams**

　　P05.09　**Newborn light for gestational age, 2500 grams and over** ◀
　　　　　Newborn light for gestational age, other ◀

● P05.1　**Newborn small for gestational age**
　　　Newborn small-and-light-for-dates
　　　Newborn small-for-dates
　　　Weight and length below 10th percentile for gestational age ◀

　　P05.10　**Newborn small for gestational age, unspecified weight**

　　P05.11　**Newborn small for gestational age, less than 500 grams**

　　P05.12　**Newborn small for gestational age, 500-749 grams**

　　P05.13　**Newborn small for gestational age, 750-999 grams**

　　P05.14　**Newborn small for gestational age, 1000-1249 grams**

　　P05.15　**Newborn small for gestational age, 1250-1499 grams**

　　P05.16　**Newborn small for gestational age, 1500-1749 grams**

　　P05.17　**Newborn small for gestational age, 1750-1999 grams**

　　P05.18　**Newborn small for gestational age, 2000-2499 grams**

　　P05.19　**Newborn small for gestational age, other** ◀
　　　　　Newborn small for gestational age, 2500 grams and over ◀

P05.2　**Newborn affected by fetal (intrauterine) malnutrition not light or small for gestational age**
　　　Infant, not light or small for gestational age, showing signs of fetal malnutrition, such as dry, peeling skin and loss of subcutaneous tissue

　　　　Excludes1　newborn affected by fetal malnutrition with light for gestational age (P05.0-)
　　　　　　　　newborn affected by fetal malnutrition with small for gestational age (P05.1-)

P05.9　**Newborn affected by slow intrauterine growth, unspecified**
　　　Newborn affected by fetal growth retardation NOS

● P07　**Disorders of newborn related to short gestation and low birth weight, not elsewhere classified**

　　Note: When both birth weight and gestational age of the newborn are available, both should be coded with birth weight sequenced before gestational age.

　　　Includes　the listed conditions, without further specification, as the cause of morbidity or additional care, in newborn

● P07.0　**Extremely low birth weight newborn**
　　　Newborn birth weight 999 g. or less

　　　　Excludes1　low birth weight due to slow fetal growth and fetal malnutrition (P05.-) ◀

　　P07.00　**Extremely low birth weight newborn, unspecified weight**

　　P07.01　**Extremely low birth weight newborn, less than 500 grams**

　　P07.02　**Extremely low birth weight newborn, 500-749 grams**

　　P07.03　**Extremely low birth weight newborn, 750-999 grams**

◀ New　◀▦ Revised　~~deleted~~ Deleted　Excludes 1　Excludes 2　Includes　Use additional　Code first　Code also　Unspecified
OGCR Official Guidelines　● Unacceptable Principal Diagnosis　X Assign placeholder X　● Use Additional Character(s)　▸ Manifestation Code　**Coding Clinic**

● **P07.1** **Other low birth weight newborn**
Newborn birth weight 1000-2499 g.
Excludes1 low birth weight due to slow fetal growth and fetal malnutrition (P05.-) ◄

P07.10 **Other low birth weight newborn, unspecified weight**

P07.14 **Other low birth weight newborn, 1000-1249 grams**

P07.15 **Other low birth weight newborn, 1250-1499 grams**

P07.16 **Other low birth weight newborn, 1500-1749 grams**

P07.17 **Other low birth weight newborn, 1750-1999 grams**

P07.18 **Other low birth weight newborn, 2000-2499 grams**

● **P07.2** **Extreme immaturity of newborn**
Less than 28 completed weeks (less than 196 completed days) of gestation

P07.20 **Extreme immaturity of newborn, unspecified weeks of gestation**
Gestational age less than 28 completed weeks NOS

P07.21 **Extreme immaturity of newborn, gestational age less than 23 completed weeks**
Extreme immaturity of newborn, gestational age less than 23 weeks, 0 days

P07.22 **Extreme immaturity of newborn, gestational age 23 completed weeks**
Extreme immaturity of newborn, gestational age 23 weeks, 0 days through 23 weeks, 6 days

P07.23 **Extreme immaturity of newborn, gestational age 24 completed weeks**
Extreme immaturity of newborn, gestational age 24 weeks, 0 days through 24 weeks, 6 days

P07.24 **Extreme immaturity of newborn, gestational age 25 completed weeks**
Extreme immaturity of newborn, gestational age 25 weeks, 0 days through 25 weeks, 6 days

P07.25 **Extreme immaturity of newborn, gestational age 26 completed weeks**
Extreme immaturity of newborn, gestational age 26 weeks, 0 days through 26 weeks, 6 days

P07.26 **Extreme immaturity of newborn, gestational age 27 completed weeks**
Extreme immaturity of newborn, gestational age 27 weeks, 0 days through 27 weeks, 6 days

● **P07.3** **Preterm [premature] newborn [other]**
28 completed weeks or more but less than 37 completed weeks (196 completed days but less than 259 completed days) of gestation
Prematurity NOS

P07.30 **Preterm newborn, unspecified weeks of gestation**

P07.31 **Preterm newborn, gestational age 28 completed weeks**
Preterm newborn, gestational age 28 weeks, 0 days through 28 weeks, 6 days

P07.32 **Preterm newborn, gestational age 29 completed weeks**
Preterm newborn, gestational age 29 weeks, 0 days through 29 weeks, 6 days

P07.33 **Preterm newborn, gestational age 30 completed weeks**
Preterm newborn, gestational age 30 weeks, 0 days through 30 weeks, 6 days

P07.34 **Preterm newborn, gestational age 31 completed weeks**
Preterm newborn, gestational age 31 weeks, 0 days through 31 weeks, 6 days

P07.35 **Preterm newborn, gestational age 32 completed weeks**
Preterm newborn, gestational age 32 weeks, 0 days through 32 weeks, 6 days

P07.36 **Preterm newborn, gestational age 33 completed weeks**
Preterm newborn, gestational age 33 weeks, 0 days through 33 weeks, 6 days

P07.37 **Preterm newborn, gestational age 34 completed weeks**
Preterm newborn, gestational age 34 weeks, 0 days through 34 weeks, 6 days

P07.38 **Preterm newborn, gestational age 35 completed weeks**
Preterm newborn, gestational age 35 weeks, 0 days through 35 weeks, 6 days

P07.39 **Preterm newborn, gestational age 36 completed weeks**
Preterm newborn, gestational age 36 weeks, 0 days through 36 weeks, 6 days

● **P08** **Disorders of newborn related to long gestation and high birth weight**
Note: When both birth weight and gestational age of the newborn are available, priority of assignment should be given to birth weight.
Includes the listed conditions, without further specification, as causes of morbidity or additional care, in newborn

P08.0 **Exceptionally large newborn baby**
Usually implies a birth weight of 4500 g. or more
Excludes1 syndrome of infant of diabetic mother (P70.1)
syndrome of infant of mother with gestational diabetes (P70.0)

P08.1 **Other heavy for gestational age newborn**
Other newborn heavy- or large-for-dates regardless of period of gestation
Usually implies a birth weight of 4000 g. to 4499 g.
Excludes1 newborn with a birth weight of 4500 or more (P08.0)
syndrome of infant of diabetic mother (P70.1)
syndrome of infant of mother with gestational diabetes (P70.0)

● **P08.2** **Late newborn, not heavy for gestational age**

P08.21 **Post-term newborn**
Newborn with gestation period over 40 completed weeks to 42 completed weeks

P08.22 **Prolonged gestation of newborn**
Newborn with gestation period over 42 completed weeks (294 days or more), not heavy- or large-for-dates
Postmaturity NOS

ABNORMAL FINDINGS ON NEONATAL SCREENING (P09)

P09 **Abnormal findings on neonatal screening**
Use additional code to identify signs, symptoms and conditions associated with the screening
Excludes2 nonspecific serologic evidence of human immunodeficiency virus [HIV] (R75)

BIRTH TRAUMA (P10-P15)

● **P10**   **Intracranial laceration and hemorrhage due to birth injury**

> **Excludes1**   intracranial hemorrhage of newborn NOS (P52.9)
> intracranial hemorrhage of newborn due to anoxia or hypoxia (P52.-)
> nontraumatic intracranial hemorrhage of newborn (P52.-)

> (Ex) **For category P10 CC codes unless otherwise indicated:** P10.0-P10.1, P10.4-P11.2, P11.9, P15.0-P15.9, P29.0-P29.2, P29.4, P29.89-P29.9, P52.4, P52.6-P52.9, P94.1-P94.9, P96.0, P96.3-P96.5, P96.82-P96.89

    P10.0   **Subdural hemorrhage due to birth injury** 🔍
> Subdural hematoma (localized) due to birth injury

> > **Excludes1**   subdural hemorrhage accompanying tentorial tear (P10.4)

    P10.1   **Cerebral hemorrhage due to birth injury** 🔍

    P10.2   **Intraventricular hemorrhage due to birth injury** 🔍
> (Ex) P10.2-P10.3, P29.0-P29.2, P29.4, P29.89-P29.9, P50.0-P50.9, P52.0-P52.3, P52.5, P53-P54.0, P54.6-P54.9, P60-P61.9, P94.1-P94.9, P96.0, P96.3-P96.5, P96.82-P96.89

    P10.3   **Subarachnoid hemorrhage due to birth injury** 🔍
> (Ex) P10.2-P10.3, P29.0-P29.2, P29.4, P29.89-P29.9, P50.0-P50.9, P52.0-P52.3, P52.5, P53-P54.0, P54.6-P54.9, P60-P61.9, P91.2, P94.1-P94.9, P96.0, P96.3-P96.5, P96.82-P96.89

Item 16–1   The **peripheral nervous system** consists of 31 pairs of spinal nerves, 12 pairs of cranial nerves, and the autonomic nerves, which are divided into the parasympathetic and sympathetic nerves. The cranial nerves are: olfactory (I), optic (II), oculomotor (III), trochlear (IV), trigeminal (V), abducens (VI), facial (VII), vestibulocochlear (VIII), glossopharyngeal (IX), vagus (X), accessory (XI), and hypoglossal (XII).

Central Nervous System
- Brain
- Spinal cord

Peripheral Nervous System
- Cranial nerves (12)
- Spinal nerves
   cervical (8)
   thoracic (12)
   lumbar (5)
   sacral (5)
   coccyx (1)

Figure 16-1   The central nervous system consists of the brain and spinal cord. The peripheral nervous system consists of nerves that lie outside the skull and spinal cord. (From Stoy: Mosby's EMT-Basic Textbook, ed 2, St. Louis, Mosby, 2007)

    P10.4   **Tentorial tear due to birth injury** 🔍
> *Pertaining to tentorium of cerebellum (extension of dura mater that separates cerebellum from inferior portion of occipital lobes)*

    P10.8   **Other intracranial lacerations and hemorrhages due to birth injury** 🔍

    P10.9   **Unspecified intracranial laceration and hemorrhage due to birth injury** 🔍

● **P11**   **Other birth injuries to central nervous system**

    P11.0   **Cerebral edema due to birth injury** 🔍
> (Ex) See P10

    P11.1   **Other specified brain damage due to birth injury**

    P11.2   **Unspecified brain damage due to birth injury** 🔍
> (Ex) See P10

    P11.3   **Birth injury to facial nerve**
> Facial palsy due to birth injury

    P11.4   **Birth injury to other cranial nerves**

    P11.5   **Birth injury to spine and spinal cord**
> Fracture of spine due to birth injury

    P11.9   **Birth injury to central nervous system, unspecified** 🔍
> (Ex) See P10

● **P12**   **Birth injury to scalp**

    P12.0   **Cephalhematoma due to birth injury**

    P12.1   **Chignon (from vacuum extraction) due to birth injury**

    P12.2   **Epicranial subaponeurotic hemorrhage due to birth injury** 🔍
> Subgaleal hemorrhage
> (Ex) P10.0-P10.1, P10.4-P11.2, P11.9-P12.2, P15.0-P15.9, P29.0-P29.2, P29.4, P29.89-P29.9, P52.4, P52.6-P52.9, P94.1-P94.9, P96.0, P96.3-P96.5, P96.82-P96.89

    P12.3   **Bruising of scalp due to birth injury**

    P12.4   **Injury of scalp of newborn due to monitoring equipment**
> Sampling incision of scalp of newborn
> Scalp clip (electrode) injury of newborn

   ● **P12.8**   **Other birth injuries to scalp**

      P12.81   **Caput succedaneum**

      P12.89   **Other birth injuries to scalp**

    P12.9   **Birth injury to scalp, unspecified**

● **P13**   **Birth injury to skeleton**

> **Excludes2**   birth injury to spine (P11.5)

    P13.0   **Fracture of skull due to birth injury**

    P13.1   **Other birth injuries to skull**

> > **Excludes1**   cephalhematoma (P12.0)

    P13.2   **Birth injury to femur**

    P13.3   **Birth injury to other long bones**

    P13.4   **Fracture of clavicle due to birth injury**

    P13.8   **Birth injuries to other parts of skeleton**

    P13.9   **Birth injury to skeleton, unspecified**

● **P14**   **Birth injury to peripheral nervous system**

    P14.0   **Erb's paralysis due to birth injury**

    P14.1   **Klumpke's paralysis due to birth injury**

    P14.2   **Phrenic nerve paralysis due to birth injury**

    P14.3   **Other brachial plexus birth injuries**

    P14.8   **Birth injuries to other parts of peripheral nervous system**

    P14.9   **Birth injury to peripheral nervous system, unspecified**

● **P15**   **Other birth injuries**

    P15.0   **Birth injury to liver**
> Rupture of liver due to birth injury

    P15.1   **Birth injury to spleen**
> Rupture of spleen due to birth injury

    P15.2   **Sternomastoid injury due to birth injury**

    P15.3   **Birth injury to eye**
> Subconjunctival hemorrhage due to birth injury
> Traumatic glaucoma due to birth injury

◀ New   ◀▬ Revised   ~~deleted~~ Deleted   Excludes 1   Excludes 2   Includes   Use additional   Code first   Code also   Unspecified

OGCR Official Guidelines   ● Unacceptable Principal Diagnosis   X Assign placeholder X   🔍 Use Additional Character(s)   ▶ Manifestation Code   **Coding Clinic**

P15.4   **Birth injury to face**
     Facial congestion due to birth injury

P15.5   **Birth injury to external genitalia**

P15.6   **Subcutaneous fat necrosis due to birth injury**

P15.8   **Other specified birth injuries**

P15.9   **Birth injury, unspecified**

RESPIRATORY AND CARDIOVASCULAR DISORDERS SPECIFIC TO THE PERINATAL PERIOD (P19-P29)

● **P19**   **Metabolic acidemia in newborn**
     Includes   metabolic acidemia in newborn

P19.0   **Metabolic acidemia in newborn first noted before onset of labor**

P19.1   **Metabolic acidemia in newborn first noted during labor**

P19.2   **Metabolic acidemia noted at birth**

P19.9   **Metabolic acidemia, unspecified**

● **P22**   **Respiratory distress of newborn**
     Excludes1   respiratory arrest of newborn (P28.81)
                  respiratory failure of newborn NOS (P28.5)

P22.0   **Respiratory distress syndrome of newborn** 🦠
     Cardiorespiratory distress syndrome of newborn
     Hyaline membrane disease
     Idiopathic respiratory distress syndrome [IRDS or RDS] of newborn
     Pulmonary hypoperfusion syndrome
     Respiratory distress syndrome, type I
     (Ex) J84.83-J84.848, P22.0-P28.5, P28.89-P29.2, P29.4, P29.89-P29.9, P84, P94.1-P96.0, P96.3-P96.5, P96.82-P96.89

P22.1   **Transient tachypnea of newborn**
     Idiopathic tachypnea of newborn
     Respiratory distress syndrome, type II
     Wet lung syndrome

P22.8   **Other respiratory distress of newborn**

P22.9   **Respiratory distress of newborn, unspecified**

● **P23**   **Congenital pneumonia**
     Includes   infective pneumonia acquired in utero or during birth
     Excludes1   neonatal pneumonia resulting from aspiration (P24.-)
     (Ex) For category P23 CC codes: See P22.0

P23.0   **Congenital pneumonia due to viral agent** 🦠
     Use additional code (B97) to identify organism
     Excludes1   congenital rubella pneumonitis (P35.0)

P23.1   **Congenital pneumonia due to Chlamydia** 🦠

P23.2   **Congenital pneumonia due to staphylococcus** 🦠

P23.3   **Congenital pneumonia due to streptococcus, group B** 🦠

P23.4   **Congenital pneumonia due to Escherichia coli** 🦠

P23.5   **Congenital pneumonia due to Pseudomonas** 🦠

P23.6   **Congenital pneumonia due to other bacterial agents** 🦠
     Congenital pneumonia due to Hemophilus influenzae
     Congenital pneumonia due to Klebsiella pneumoniae
     Congenital pneumonia due to Mycoplasma
     Congenital pneumonia due to Streptococcus, except group B
     Use additional code (B95-B96) to identify organism

P23.8   **Congenital pneumonia due to other organisms** 🦠

P23.9   **Congenital pneumonia, unspecified** 🦠

● **P24**   **Neonatal aspiration**
     Includes   aspiration in utero and during delivery

● **P24.0**   **Meconium aspiration**
     Excludes1   meconium passage (without aspiration) during delivery (P03.82)
                  meconium staining (P96.83)

P24.00   **Meconium aspiration without respiratory symptoms**
     Meconium aspiration NOS

P24.01   **Meconium aspiration with respiratory symptoms** 🦠
     Meconium aspiration pneumonia
     Meconium aspiration pneumonitis
     Meconium aspiration syndrome NOS
     Use additional code to identify any secondary pulmonary hypertension, if applicable (I27.2)
     (Ex) See P22.0

● **P24.1**   **Neonatal aspiration of (clear) amniotic fluid and mucus**
     Neonatal aspiration of liquor (amnii)

P24.10   **Neonatal aspiration of (clear) amniotic fluid and mucus without respiratory symptoms**
     Neonatal aspiration of amniotic fluid and mucus NOS

P24.11   **Neonatal aspiration of (clear) amniotic fluid and mucus with respiratory symptoms** 🦠
     Neonatal aspiration of amniotic fluid and mucus with pneumonia
     Neonatal aspiration of amniotic fluid and mucus with pneumonitis
     Use additional code to identify any secondary pulmonary hypertension, if applicable (I27.2)
     (Ex) See P22.0

● **P24.2**   **Neonatal aspiration of blood**

P24.20   **Neonatal aspiration of blood without respiratory symptoms**
     Neonatal aspiration of blood NOS

P24.21   **Neonatal aspiration of blood with respiratory symptoms** 🦠
     Neonatal aspiration of blood with pneumonia
     Neonatal aspiration of blood with pneumonitis
     Use additional code to identify any secondary pulmonary hypertension, if applicable (I27.2)
     (Ex) See P22.0

● **P24.3**   **Neonatal aspiration of milk and regurgitated food**
     Neonatal aspiration of stomach contents

P24.30   **Neonatal aspiration of milk and regurgitated food without respiratory symptoms**
     Neonatal aspiration of milk and regurgitated food NOS

P24.31   **Neonatal aspiration of milk and regurgitated food with respiratory symptoms** 🦠
     Neonatal aspiration of milk and regurgitated food with pneumonia
     Neonatal aspiration of milk and regurgitated food with pneumonitis
     Use additional code to identify any secondary pulmonary hypertension, if applicable (I27.2)
     (Ex) See P22.0

N   Newborn Age: 0   **P**   Pediatric Age: 0–17   **M**   Maternity DX: 12–55   **A**   Adult Age: 15–124   ♀   Females Only   ♂   Males Only

🦠   Complication\Comorbidity   🦠   Major C\C   (Ex)   CC/MCC Exclusions   🦠   Hospital-Acquired Condition   **1165**

CHAPTER 16 (P00-P96)

● **P24.8   Other neonatal aspiration**

P24.80   **Other neonatal aspiration without respiratory symptoms**
Neonatal aspiration NEC

P24.81   **Other neonatal aspiration with respiratory symptoms** 🐾
Neonatal aspiration pneumonia NEC
Neonatal aspiration with pneumonitis NEC
Neonatal aspiration with pneumonia NOS
Neonatal aspiration with pneumonitis NOS
Use additional code to identify any secondary pulmonary hypertension, if applicable (I27.2)
Ⓔⓧ See P22.0

P24.9   **Neonatal aspiration, unspecified**

● **P25   Interstitial emphysema and related conditions originating in the perinatal period**
Ⓔⓧ For category P25 CC codes: See P22.0

P25.0   **Interstitial emphysema originating in the perinatal period** 🐾

P25.1   **Pneumothorax originating in the perinatal period** 🐾

P25.2   **Pneumomediastinum originating in the perinatal period** 🐾

P25.3   **Pneumopericardium originating in the perinatal period** 🐾

P25.8   **Other conditions related to interstitial emphysema originating in the perinatal period** 🐾

● **P26   Pulmonary hemorrhage originating in the perinatal period**
Excludes1   acute idiopathic hemorrhage in infants over 28 days old (R04.81)
Ⓔⓧ For category P26 CC codes: See P22.0

P26.0   **Tracheobronchial hemorrhage originating in the perinatal period** 🐾

P26.1   **Massive pulmonary hemorrhage originating in the perinatal period** 🐾

P26.8   **Other pulmonary hemorrhages originating in the perinatal period** 🐾

P26.9   **Unspecified pulmonary hemorrhage originating in the perinatal period** 🐾

● **P27   Chronic respiratory disease originating in the perinatal period**
Excludes1   respiratory distress of newborn (P22.0-P22.9)
Ⓔⓧ For category P27 CC codes: See P22.0

P27.0   **Wilson-Mikity syndrome** 🐾
Pulmonary dysmaturity

P27.1   **Bronchopulmonary dysplasia originating in the perinatal period** 🐾

P27.8   **Other chronic respiratory diseases originating in the perinatal period** 🐾
Congenital pulmonary fibrosis
Ventilator lung in newborn

P27.9   **Unspecified chronic respiratory disease originating in the perinatal period** 🐾

● **P28   Other respiratory conditions originating in the perinatal period**
Excludes1   congenital malformations of the respiratory system (Q30-Q34)

P28.0   **Primary atelectasis of newborn** 🐾
Failure of lungs to expand properly at birth
Primary failure to expand terminal respiratory units
Pulmonary hypoplasia associated with short gestation
Pulmonary immaturity NOS
Ⓔⓧ See P22.0

● **P28.1   Other and unspecified atelectasis of newborn**
Ⓔⓧ For category P28.1 CC codes: See P22.0

P28.10   **Unspecified atelectasis of newborn** 🐾
Atelectasis of newborn NOS

P28.11   **Resorption atelectasis without respiratory distress syndrome** 🐾
Excludes1   resorption atelectasis with respiratory distress syndrome (P22.0)

P28.19   **Other atelectasis of newborn** 🐾
Partial atelectasis of newborn
Secondary atelectasis of newborn

P28.2   **Cyanotic attacks of newborn** 🐾
Excludes1   apnea of newborn (P28.3-P28.4)
Ⓔⓧ P22.8-P22.9, P28.2-P28.4, P28.81-P28.9, R06.81, R23.0

P28.3   **Primary sleep apnea of newborn** 🐾
Central sleep apnea of newborn
Obstructive sleep apnea of newborn
Sleep apnea of newborn NOS
Ⓔⓧ P22.8-P22.9, P28.2, P28.4, P28.81-P28.9, R06.81

P28.4   **Other apnea of newborn** 🐾
Apnea of prematurity
Obstructive apnea of newborn
Excludes1   obstructive sleep apnea of newborn (P28.3)
Ⓔⓧ P22.8-P22.9, P28.2-P28.4, P28.81-P28.9, R06.81

P28.5   **Respiratory failure of newborn** 🐾
Excludes1   respiratory arrest of newborn (P28.81)
respiratory distress of newborn (P22.0-)
Ⓔⓧ See P22.0

● **P28.8   Other specified respiratory conditions of newborn**

P28.81   **Respiratory arrest of newborn** 🐾
Ⓔⓧ P22.1-P22.9, P24.00, P24.10, P24.20, P24.30, P24.80, P28.2-P28.5, P28.89-P28.9, P29.81, R06.81, R09.2

P28.89   **Other specified respiratory conditions of newborn**
Congenital laryngeal stridor
Sniffles in newborn
Snuffles in newborn
Excludes1   early congenital syphilitic rhinitis (A50.05)

P28.9   **Respiratory condition of newborn, unspecified**
Respiratory depression in newborn

● **P29   Cardiovascular disorders originating in the perinatal period**
Excludes1   congenital malformations of the circulatory system (Q20-Q28)

P29.0   **Neonatal cardiac failure**

● **P29.1   Neonatal cardiac dysrhythmia**

P29.11   **Neonatal tachycardia**

P29.12   **Neonatal bradycardia**

P29.2   **Neonatal hypertension**

P29.3   **Persistent fetal circulation** 🐾
Delayed closure of ductus arteriosus
(Persistent) pulmonary hypertension of newborn
Ⓔⓧ I27.0, I27.2-I27.81, I27.89-I27.9

P29.4   **Transient myocardial ischemia in newborn**

● **P29.8   Other cardiovascular disorders originating in the perinatal period**

P29.81   **Cardiac arrest of newborn** 🐾
Ⓔⓧ P29.81

P29.89   **Other cardiovascular disorders originating in the perinatal period**

P29.9   **Cardiovascular disorder originating in the perinatal period, unspecified**

◄ New   ◄═ Revised   ~~deleted~~ Deleted   Excludes 1   Excludes 2   Includes   Use additional   Code first   Code also   Unspecified
OGCR Official Guidelines   ● Unacceptable Principal Diagnosis   X Assign placeholder X   ● Use Additional Character(s)   ▌ Manifestation Code   **Coding Clinic**

INFECTIONS SPECIFIC TO THE PERINATAL PERIOD (P35-P39)

Infections acquired in utero, during birth via the umbilicus, or during the first 28 days after birth

Excludes2   asymptomatic human immunodeficiency virus [HIV] infection status (Z21)
congenital gonococcal infection (A54.-)
congenital pneumonia (P23.-)
congenital syphilis (A50.-)
human immunodeficiency virus [HIV] disease (B20)
infant botulism (A48.51)
infectious diseases not specific to the perinatal period (A00-B99, J09, J10.-)
intestinal infectious disease (A00-A09)
laboratory evidence of human immunodeficiency virus [HIV] (R75)
tetanus neonatorum (A33)

● **P35**   Congenital viral diseases

Includes   infections acquired in utero or during birth

Ⓔ **For category P35 CC codes unless otherwise indicated:** A17.82, A28.1, A50.42, A52.14, A75.9, A79.9, A81.1, A81.82-A81.89, A83.0-A85.8, A87.2, A88.0, A88.8, A92.1-A92.8, A93.0, B00.4, B00.82, B01.11-B01.12, B04, B06.01, B08.09, B08.20-B08.22, B08.60-B08.79, B09, B10.01-B10.09, B26.2, B27.00-B27.99, B33.1, B45.0, B45.2-B45.9, B54, B58.2, B75, B97.10, B97.21, G04.00-G04.01, G04.31, G04.81-G05.4, G37.0, G37.4-G37.5, H66.40-H66.43, J09.X3-J09.X9, J10.2-J10.89, J11.2-J11.89, L44.4, M1A.10X0-M1A.19X1, M32.0-M32.9, P35.2-P35.9, P37.0-P37.9, T56.0X1-T56.0X4[A]

P35.0   Congenital rubella syndrome 🔖
Congenital rubella pneumonitis
Ⓔ P29.0-P29.2, P29.4, P29.89-P35.9, P37.0-P37.4, P37.8-P37.9, P94.1-P94.9, P96.0, P96.3-P96.5, P96.82-P96.89

P35.1   Congenital cytomegalovirus infection 🔖
Viruses transmitted by multiple routes that cause mild/subclinical infection
Ⓔ See P35.0

P35.2   Congenital herpesviral [herpes simplex] infection 🔖

P35.3   Congenital viral hepatitis 🔖

P35.8   Other congenital viral diseases 🔖
Congenital varicella [chickenpox]

P35.9   Congenital viral disease, unspecified 🔖

● **P36**   Bacterial sepsis of newborn

Includes   congenital sepsis

Use additional code(s), if applicable, to identify severe sepsis (R65.2-) and associated acute organ dysfunction(s)
Ⓔ **For category P36 CC codes:** P29.0-P29.2, P29.4, P29.89-P29.9, P36.0-P36.9, P37.5, P38.1-P39.9, P53, P60-P61.9, P94.1-P94.9, P96.0, P96.3-P96.5, P96.82-P96.89

P36.0   Sepsis of newborn due to streptococcus, group B 🔖

● **P36.1**   Sepsis of newborn due to other and unspecified streptococci

P36.10   Sepsis of newborn due to unspecified streptococci 🔖

P36.19   Sepsis of newborn due to other streptococci 🔖

P36.2   Sepsis of newborn due to Staphylococcus aureus 🔖

● **P36.3**   Sepsis of newborn due to other and unspecified staphylococci

P36.30   Sepsis of newborn due to unspecified staphylococci 🔖

P36.39   Sepsis of newborn due to other staphylococci 🔖

P36.4   Sepsis of newborn due to Escherichia coli 🔖

P36.5   Sepsis of newborn due to anaerobes 🔖

P36.8   Other bacterial sepsis of newborn 🔖
Use additional code from category B96 to identify organism

P36.9   Bacterial sepsis of newborn, unspecified 🔖

● **P37**   Other congenital infectious and parasitic diseases

Excludes2   congenital syphilis (A50.-)
infectious neonatal diarrhea (A00-A09)
necrotizing enterocolitis in newborn (P77.-)
noninfectious neonatal diarrhea (P78.3)
ophthalmia neonatorum due to gonococcus (A54.31)
tetanus neonatorum (A33)

Ⓔ **For category P37 CC codes:** See P35

P37.0   Congenital tuberculosis 🔖

P37.1   Congenital toxoplasmosis 🔖
Parasitic infection, often causing mild flu-like illness
Hydrocephalus due to congenital toxoplasmosis

P37.2   Neonatal (disseminated) listeriosis 🔖
Acquired transplacentally or during/after parturition in which symptoms are those of sepsis

P37.3   Congenital falciparum malaria 🔖

P37.4   Other congenital malaria 🔖

P37.5   Neonatal candidiasis 🔖

P37.8   Other specified congenital infectious and parasitic diseases 🔖

P37.9   Congenital infectious or parasitic disease, unspecified 🔖

● **P38**   Omphalitis of newborn
Inflammation of umbilicus

Excludes1   omphalitis not of newborn (L08.82)
tetanus omphalitis (A33)
umbilical hemorrhage of newborn (P51.-)

Ⓔ **For category P38 CC codes:** P39.2, P39.4-P39.9

P38.1   Omphalitis with mild hemorrhage 🔖

P38.9   Omphalitis without hemorrhage 🔖
Omphalitis of newborn NOS

● **P39**   Other infections specific to the perinatal period
Use additional code to identify organism or specific infection
Ⓔ **For category P39 CC codes unless otherwise indicated:** A02.1, A20.7, A22.7, A39.2-A39.4, A40.9-A41.59, A41.81-A41.9, A42.7, A48.2, A48.4, A48.8-A49.9, B00.7, B92, B94.2-B96.89, P39.2-P39.9, P95, P96.9, R78.81

P39.0   Neonatal infective mastitis 🔖

Excludes1   breast engorgement of newborn (P83.4)
noninfective mastitis of newborn (P83.4)

Ⓔ See P38

P39.1   Neonatal conjunctivitis and dacryocystitis
Neonatal chlamydial conjunctivitis
Ophthalmia neonatorum NOS
Neonate = newborn

Excludes1   gonococcal conjunctivitis (A54.31)

P39.2   Intra-amniotic infection affecting newborn, not elsewhere classified 🔖

P39.3   Neonatal urinary tract infection 🔖
Ⓔ A49.9, N10-N11.0, N11.8-N12, N13.6, N15.1, N28.82, N28.84-N30.31, N30.80-N30.91, N36.9-N39.0, N39.9, N99.511, P39.2, P39.4-P39.9, R30.0, R30.9, T83.511A

P39.4   Neonatal skin infection 🔖
Neonatal pyoderma

Excludes1   pemphigus neonatorum (L00)
staphylococcal scalded skin syndrome (L00)

P39.8   Other specified infections specific to the perinatal period 🔖

P39.9   Infection specific to the perinatal period, unspecified 🔖

CHAPTER 16 (P00-P96)

N   Newborn Age: 0   P   Pediatric Age: 0–17   M   Maternity DX: 12–55   A   Adult Age: 15–124   ♀   Females Only   ♂   Males Only
🔖   Complication\Comorbidity   🔖   Major C\C   Ⓔ   CC/MCC Exclusions   🔖   Hospital-Acquired Condition

HEMORRHAGIC AND HEMATOLOGICAL DISORDERS OF NEWBORN (P50-P61)

> **Excludes1**   congenital stenosis and stricture of bile ducts
> (Q44.3)
> Crigler-Najjar syndrome (E80.5)
> Dubin-Johnson syndrome (E80.6)
> Gilbert syndrome (E80.4)
> hereditary hemolytic anemias (D55-D58)

● **P50   Newborn affected by intrauterine (fetal) blood loss**

> **Excludes1**   congenital anemia from intrauterine (fetal) blood
> loss (P61.3)

P50.0   Newborn affected by intrauterine (fetal) blood loss from
vasa previa

P50.1   Newborn affected by intrauterine (fetal) blood loss from
ruptured cord

P50.2   Newborn affected by intrauterine (fetal) blood loss from
placenta

P50.3   Newborn affected by hemorrhage into co-twin

P50.4   Newborn affected by hemorrhage into maternal
circulation

P50.5   Newborn affected by intrauterine (fetal) blood loss from
cut end of co-twin's cord

P50.8   Newborn affected by other intrauterine (fetal) blood
loss

P50.9   Newborn affected by intrauterine (fetal) blood loss,
unspecified
Newborn affected by fetal hemorrhage NOS

● **P51   Umbilical hemorrhage of newborn**

> **Excludes1**   omphalitis with mild hemorrhage (P38.1)
> umbilical hemorrhage from cut end of co-twins
> cord (P50.5)

P51.0   Massive umbilical hemorrhage of newborn

P51.8   Other umbilical hemorrhages of newborn
Slipped umbilical ligature NOS

P51.9   Umbilical hemorrhage of newborn, unspecified

● **P52   Intracranial nontraumatic hemorrhage of newborn**

> **Includes**   intracranial hemorrhage due to anoxia or hypoxia
> **Excludes1**   intracranial hemorrhage due to birth injury
> (P10.-)
> intracranial hemorrhage due to other injury
> (S06.-)

P52.0   Intraventricular (nontraumatic) hemorrhage, grade 1,
of newborn
Subependymal hemorrhage (without intraventricular
extension)
Bleeding into germinal matrix
(Ex) P10.2-P10.3, P29.0-P29.2, P29.4, P29.89-P29.9, P50.0-P50.9, P52.0-P52.3,
P52.5, P53-P54.0, P54.6-P54.9, P60-P61.9, P94.1-P94.9, P96.0,
P96.3-P96.5, P96.82-P96.89

P52.1   Intraventricular (nontraumatic) hemorrhage, grade 2,
of newborn
Subependymal hemorrhage with intraventricular
extension
Bleeding into ventricle
(Ex) See P52.0

● **P52.2**   Intraventricular (nontraumatic) hemorrhage, grade 3
and grade 4, of newborn

P52.21   Intraventricular (nontraumatic) hemorrhage,
grade 3, of newborn
Subependymal hemorrhage with
intraventricular extension with
enlargement of ventricle
(Ex) See P52.0

P52.22   Intraventricular (nontraumatic) hemorrhage,
grade 4, of newborn
Bleeding into cerebral cortex
Subependymal hemorrhage with intracerebral
extension
(Ex) See P52.0

P52.3   Unspecified intraventricular (nontraumatic) hemorrhage
of newborn
(Ex) See P52.0

P52.4   Intracerebral (nontraumatic) hemorrhage of newborn
(Ex) P10.0-P10.1, P10.4-P11.2, P11.9, P15.0-P15.9, P29.0-P29.2, P29.4,
P29.89-P29.9, P52.4, P52.6-P52.9, P94.1-P94.9, P96.0, P96.3-P96.5,
P96.82-P96.89

P52.5   Subarachnoid (nontraumatic) hemorrhage of
newborn
(Ex) P10.2-P10.3, P29.0-P29.2, P29.4, P29.89-P29.9, P50.0-P50.9, P52.0-P52.3,
P52.5, P53-P54.0, P54.6-P54.9, P60-P61.9, P91.2, P94.1-P94.9, P96.0,
P96.3-P96.5, P96.82-P96.89

P52.6   Cerebellar (nontraumatic) and posterior fossa
hemorrhage of newborn
(Ex) See P52.4

P52.8   Other intracranial (nontraumatic) hemorrhages
of newborn
(Ex) See P52.4

P52.9   Intracranial (nontraumatic) hemorrhage of newborn,
unspecified
(Ex) See P52.4

P53   Hemorrhagic disease of newborn
Vitamin K deficiency of newborn
(Ex) P29.0-P29.2, P29.4, P29.89-P29.9, P53, P60-P61.9, P94.1-P96.0, P96.3-P96.5,
P96.82-P96.89

● **P54   Other neonatal hemorrhages**

> **Excludes1**   newborn affected by (intrauterine) blood loss
> (P50.-)
> pulmonary hemorrhage originating in the
> perinatal period (P26.-)

P54.0   Neonatal hematemesis
Vomiting of blood

> **Excludes1**   neonatal hematemesis due to swallowed
> maternal blood (P78.2)

P54.1   Neonatal melena
Dark-colored feces stained with blood pigments

> **Excludes1**   neonatal melena due to swallowed
> maternal blood (P78.2)
> (Ex) P29.0-P29.2, P29.4, P29.89-P29.9, P50.0-P50.9, P53-P54.9, P60-P61.9,
> P94.1-P96.0, P96.3-P96.5, P96.82-P96.89

P54.2   Neonatal rectal hemorrhage
(Ex) See P54.1

P54.3   Other neonatal gastrointestinal hemorrhage
(Ex) See P54.1

P54.4   Neonatal adrenal hemorrhage
(Ex) See P54.1

P54.5   Neonatal cutaneous hemorrhage
Neonatal bruising
Neonatal ecchymoses
Neonatal petechiae
Neonatal superficial hematomata

> **Excludes2**   bruising of scalp due to birth injury
> (P12.3)
> cephalhematoma due to birth injury
> (P12.0)

P54.6   Neonatal vaginal hemorrhage ♀
Neonatal pseudomenses

P54.8   Other specified neonatal hemorrhages

P54.9   Neonatal hemorrhage, unspecified

● **P55   Hemolytic disease of newborn**
*AKA erythroblastosis fetalis and is due to Rh isoimmunization,
result of Rh blood factor incompatibilities between mother (Rh
negative) and fetus (Rh positive)*

P55.0   Rh isoimmunization of newborn

P55.1   ABO isoimmunization of newborn
Coding Clinic: 2015, Q3, P20

P55.8   Other hemolytic diseases of newborn

P55.9   Hemolytic disease of newborn, unspecified

CHAPTER 16 (P00-P96)

● **P56**   **Hydrops fetalis due to hemolytic disease**
Caused by maternal sensitization to fetal blood group antigen

> **Excludes1**   hydrops fetalis NOS (P83.2)

> (Ex) **For category P56 CC codes:** P29.0-P29.2, P29.4, P29.89-P29.9, P55.0-P57.0, P94.1-P96.0, P96.3-P96.5, P96.82-P96.89

     P56.0   Hydrops fetalis due to isoimmunization

●   **P56.9**   Hydrops fetalis due to other and unspecified hemolytic disease

         P56.90   Hydrops fetalis due to **unspecified** hemolytic disease

         P56.99   Hydrops fetalis due to other hemolytic disease

● **P57**   **Kernicterus**
High levels of bilirubin in blood, with severe neural symptoms

> (Ex) **For category P57 CC codes unless otherwise indicated:** P29.0-P29.2, P29.4, P29.89-P29.9, P57.8-P59.9, P94.1-P96.0, P96.3-P96.5, P96.82-P96.89

     P57.0   Kernicterus due to isoimmunization
> (Ex) See P56

     P57.8   Other specified kernicterus

> **Excludes1**   Crigler-Najjar syndrome (E80.5)

     P57.9   Kernicterus, **unspecified**

● **P58**   **Neonatal jaundice due to other excessive hemolysis**

> **Excludes1**   jaundice due to isoimmunization (P55-P57)

     P58.0   Neonatal jaundice due to bruising
     P58.1   Neonatal jaundice due to bleeding
     P58.2   Neonatal jaundice due to infection
     P58.3   Neonatal jaundice due to polycythemia

●   **P58.4**   Neonatal jaundice due to drugs or toxins transmitted from mother or given to newborn
Code first poisoning due to drug or toxin, if applicable (T36-T65 with fifth or sixth character 1-4 or 6)
Use additional code for adverse effect, if applicable, to identify drug (T36-T50 with fifth or sixth character 5)

     ● **P58.41**   Neonatal jaundice due to drugs or toxins transmitted from mother

     ● **P58.42**   Neonatal jaundice due to drugs or toxins given to newborn

     P58.5   Neonatal jaundice due to swallowed maternal blood

     P58.8   Neonatal jaundice due to other specified excessive hemolysis

     P58.9   Neonatal jaundice due to excessive hemolysis, **unspecified**

● **P59**   **Neonatal jaundice from other and unspecified causes**

> **Excludes1**   jaundice due to inborn errors of metabolism (E70-E88)
> kernicterus (P57.-)

     P59.0   Neonatal jaundice associated with preterm delivery
Hyperbilirubinemia of prematurity
Jaundice due to delayed conjugation associated with preterm delivery

     P59.1   Inspissated bile syndrome
> (Ex) See P57

●   **P59.2**   Neonatal jaundice from other and unspecified hepatocellular damage

> **Excludes1**   congenital viral hepatitis (P35.3)

> (Ex) **For category P59.2 CC codes unless otherwise indicated:** See P57

     P59.20   Neonatal jaundice from **unspecified** hepatocellular damage

     P59.29   Neonatal jaundice from other hepatocellular damage
Neonatal giant cell hepatitis
Neonatal (idiopathic) hepatitis

     P59.3   Neonatal jaundice from breast milk inhibitor
     P59.8   Neonatal jaundice from other specified causes
     P59.9   Neonatal jaundice, **unspecified**
Neonatal physiological jaundice (intense)(prolonged) NOS
Coding Clinic: 2015, Q3, P20

● **P60**   **Disseminated intravascular coagulation of newborn**
Defibrination syndrome of newborn
> (Ex) See P53

● **P61**   **Other perinatal hematological disorders**

> **Excludes1**   transient hypogammaglobulinemia of infancy (D80.7)

     P61.0   Transient neonatal thrombocytopenia
Lack of sufficient numbers of circulating thrombocytes (platelets)
Neonatal thrombocytopenia due to exchange transfusion
Neonatal thrombocytopenia due to idiopathic maternal thrombocytopenia
Neonatal thrombocytopenia due to isoimmunization
> (Ex) See P53

     P61.1   Polycythemia neonatorum
Neonate = newborn

     P61.2   Anemia of prematurity
> (Ex) D50.0-D55.9, D56.4, D57.00-D57.3, D57.80-D64.9, D75.9, P61.2-P61.4

     P61.3   Congenital anemia from fetal blood loss
> (Ex) See P61.2

     P61.4   Other congenital anemias, not elsewhere classified
Congenital anemia NOS
> (Ex) See P61.2

     P61.5   Transient neonatal neutropenia
Low levels of granulocytic neutrophilic white blood cells

> **Excludes1**   congenital neutropenia (nontransient) (D70.0)

> (Ex) D50.1-D53.9, D56.4, D57.00-D57.20, D57.3, D57.811-D57.819, D58.2, D59.0-D59.1, D59.3, D60.0-D61.9, D63.0-D64.9, D75.9, P61.5, P61.8-P61.9

     P61.6   Other transient neonatal disorders of coagulation
> (Ex) See P53

     P61.8   Other specified perinatal hematological disorders
     P61.9   Perinatal hematological disorder, **unspecified**

TRANSITORY ENDOCRINE AND METABOLIC DISORDERS SPECIFIC TO NEWBORN (P70-P74)

> **Includes**   transitory endocrine and metabolic disturbances caused by the infant's response to maternal endocrine and metabolic factors, or its adjustment to extrauterine environment

● **P70**   **Transitory disorders of carbohydrate metabolism specific to newborn**

     P70.0   Syndrome of infant of mother with gestational diabetes
Newborn (with hypoglycemia) affected by maternal gestational diabetes

> **Excludes1**   newborn (with hypoglycemia) affected by maternal (pre-existing) diabetes mellitus (P70.1)
> syndrome of infant of a diabetic mother (P70.1)

     P70.1   Syndrome of infant of a diabetic mother
Newborn (with hypoglycemia) affected by maternal (pre-existing) diabetes mellitus

> **Excludes1**   newborn (with hypoglycemia) affected by maternal gestational diabetes (P70.0)
> syndrome of infant of mother with gestational diabetes (P70.0)

     P70.2   Neonatal diabetes mellitus
> (Ex) P29.0-P29.2, P29.4, P29.89-P29.9, P70.0-P71.9, P72.1, P72.9-P74.4, P74.9, P94.0-P94.9, P96.0, P96.3-P96.5, P96.82-P96.89

     P70.3   Iatrogenic neonatal hypoglycemia
     P70.4   Other neonatal hypoglycemia
Transitory neonatal hypoglycemia

     P70.8   Other transitory disorders of carbohydrate metabolism of newborn
> (Ex) P70.0-P70.4, P70.9-P71.9, P72.1, P72.9-P74.4, P74.9, P94.0

     P70.9   Transitory disorder of carbohydrate metabolism of newborn, **unspecified**

CHAPTER 16 (P00-P96)

● **P71**   **Transitory neonatal disorders of calcium and magnesium metabolism**
    (Ex) For category P71 CC codes: See 70.2

   P71.0   **Cow's milk hypocalcemia in newborn** 🔷

   P71.1   **Other neonatal hypocalcemia** 🔷
      Excludes1   neonatal hypoparathyroidism (P71.4)

   P71.2   **Neonatal hypomagnesemia** 🔷

   P71.3   **Neonatal tetany without calcium or magnesium deficiency** 🔷
     Neonatal tetany NOS

   P71.4   **Transitory neonatal hypoparathyroidism** 🔷

   P71.8   **Other transitory neonatal disorders of calcium and magnesium metabolism** 🔷

   P71.9   **Transitory neonatal disorder of calcium and magnesium metabolism, unspecified** 🔷

● **P72**   **Other transitory neonatal endocrine disorders**
    Excludes1   congenital hypothyroidism with or without goiter (E03.0-E03.1)
       dyshormogenetic goiter (E07.1)
       Pendred's syndrome (E07.1)
    (Ex) For category P72 CC codes unless otherwise noted: See P70.8

   P72.0   **Neonatal goiter, not elsewhere classified** 🔷
     Transitory congenital goiter with normal functioning

   P72.1   **Transitory neonatal hyperthyroidism** 🔷
     Neonatal thyrotoxicosis
     (Ex) See 70.2

   P72.2   **Other transitory neonatal disorders of thyroid function, not elsewhere classified** 🔷
     Transitory neonatal hypothyroidism

   P72.8   **Other specified transitory neonatal endocrine disorders** 🔷

   P72.9   **Transitory neonatal endocrine disorder, unspecified**

● **P74**   **Other transitory neonatal electrolyte and metabolic disturbances**

   P74.0   **Late metabolic acidosis of newborn** 🔷
      Excludes1   (fetal) metabolic acidosis of newborn (P19)
     (Ex) See 70.2

   P74.1   **Dehydration of newborn**

   P74.2   **Disturbances of sodium balance of newborn**

   P74.3   **Disturbances of potassium balance of newborn**

   P74.4   **Other transitory electrolyte disturbances of newborn**

   P74.5   **Transitory tyrosinemia of newborn** 🔷
     (Ex) See 70.8

   P74.6   **Transitory hyperammonemia of newborn** 🔷
     (Ex) See 70.8

   P74.8   **Other transitory metabolic disturbances of newborn** 🔷
     Amino-acid metabolic disorders described as transitory
     (Ex) See 70.8

   P74.9   **Transitory metabolic disturbance of newborn, unspecified**

DIGESTIVE SYSTEM DISORDERS OF NEWBORN (P76-P78)

● **P76**   **Other intestinal obstruction of newborn**

   P76.0   **Meconium plug syndrome**
     Fetal stool obstruction in large intestine, present at birth; may be symptom of organic disease.
     Meconium ileus NOS
      Excludes1   meconium ileus in cystic fibrosis (E84.11)

   P76.1   **Transitory ileus of newborn** 🔷
     Temporary obstruction of ileus (small intestine)
      Excludes1   Hirschsprung's disease (Q43.1)
     (Ex) P76.0-P78.9

   P76.2   **Intestinal obstruction due to inspissated milk**
     Being thickened, dried, or made less fluid

   P76.8   **Other specified intestinal obstruction of newborn**
      Excludes1   intestinal obstruction classifiable to K56.-

   P76.9   **Intestinal obstruction of newborn, unspecified**

● **P77**   **Necrotizing enterocolitis of newborn**
    (Ex) For category P77 CC codes: P29.0-P29.2, P29.4-P29.9, P76.0-P78.9, P94.1-P96.0, P96.3-P96.5, P96.82-P96.89

   P77.1   **Stage 1 necrotizing enterocolitis in newborn** 🔷
     Necrotizing enterocolitis without pneumatosis, without perforation

   P77.2   **Stage 2 necrotizing enterocolitis in newborn** 🔷
     Necrotizing enterocolitis with pneumatosis, without perforation

   P77.3   **Stage 3 necrotizing enterocolitis in newborn** 🔷
     Necrotizing enterocolitis with perforation
     Necrotizing enterocolitis with pneumatosis and perforation

   P77.9   **Necrotizing enterocolitis in newborn, unspecified** 🔷
     Necrotizing enterocolitis in newborn, NOS

● **P78**   **Other perinatal digestive system disorders**
    Excludes1   cystic fibrosis (E84.0-E84.9)
       neonatal gastrointestinal hemorrhages (P54.0-P54.3)

   P78.0   **Perinatal intestinal perforation** 🔷
     Meconium peritonitis
     (Ex) See P77

   P78.1   **Other neonatal peritonitis**
     Neonatal peritonitis NOS

   P78.2   **Neonatal hematemesis and melena due to swallowed maternal blood**

   P78.3   **Noninfective neonatal diarrhea**
     Neonatal diarrhea NOS

 ● **P78.8**   **Other specified perinatal digestive system disorders**

    P78.81   **Congenital cirrhosis (of liver)**

    P78.82   **Peptic ulcer of newborn**

    P78.83   **Newborn esophageal reflux**
      Neonatal esophageal reflux

    P78.89   **Other specified perinatal digestive system disorders**

   P78.9   **Perinatal digestive system disorder, unspecified**

CONDITIONS INVOLVING THE INTEGUMENT AND TEMPERATURE REGULATION OF NEWBORN (P80-P83)

● **P80**   **Hypothermia of newborn**

   P80.0   **Cold injury syndrome**
     Severe and usually chronic hypothermia associated with a pink flushed appearance, edema and neurological and biochemical abnormalities.
      Excludes1   mild hypothermia of newborn (P80.8)

   P80.8   **Other hypothermia of newborn**
     Mild hypothermia of newborn

   P80.9   **Hypothermia of newborn, unspecified**

● **P81**   **Other disturbances of temperature regulation of newborn**

   P81.0   **Environmental hyperthermia of newborn**

   P81.8   **Other specified disturbances of temperature regulation of newborn**

   P81.9   **Disturbance of temperature regulation of newborn, unspecified**
     Fever of newborn NOS

◀ New   ◀▬ Revised   ~~deleted~~ Deleted   Excludes 1   Excludes 2   Includes   Use additional   Code first   Code also   Unspecified
OGCR Official Guidelines   ● Unacceptable Principal Diagnosis   X Assign placeholder X   🔷 Use Additional Character(s)   ▷ Manifestation Code   **Coding Clinic**

● P83   **Other conditions of integument specific to newborn**
    Excludes 1   congenital malformations of skin and integument
                  (Q80-Q84)
                  hydrops fetalis due to hemolytic disease (P56.-)
                  neonatal skin infection (P39.4)
                  staphylococcal scalded skin syndrome (L00)
    Excludes 2   cradle cap (L21.0)
                  diaper [napkin] dermatitis (L22)
    P83.0   **Sclerema neonatorum** 🞄
          Neonate = newborn
          (Ex:) P83.0, P83.30-P83.39
    P83.1   **Neonatal erythema toxicum**
          *Benign, generalized, transient pustules that become firm
              vesicles*
    P83.2   **Hydrops fetalis not due to hemolytic disease** 🞄
          *Severe, life-threatening problem of severe edema (swelling)
              as result of too much fluid leaving blood and entering
              tissue*
          Hydrops fetalis NOS
          (Ex:) P29.0-P29.2, P29.4, P29.89-P29.9, P83.2, P94.1-P96.0, P96.3-P96.5,
          P96.82-P96.89
    ● P83.3   **Other and unspecified edema specific to newborn**
          (Ex:) For category P83.3 CC codes: P80.0-P83.0, P83.30-P83.39
          P83.30   **Unspecified** edema specific to newborn 🞄
          P83.39   **Other edema specific to newborn** 🞄
    P83.4   **Breast engorgement of newborn**
          Noninfective mastitis of newborn
    P83.5   **Congenital hydrocele** ♂
    P83.6   **Umbilical polyp of newborn**
    P83.8   **Other specified conditions of integument specific to
          newborn**
          Bronze baby syndrome
          Neonatal scleroderma
          Urticaria neonatorum
    P83.9   **Condition of the integument specific to newborn,
          unspecified**

OTHER PROBLEMS WITH NEWBORN (P84)

P84   **Other problems with newborn**
    Acidemia of newborn
    Acidosis of newborn
    Anoxia of newborn NOS
    Asphyxia of newborn NOS
    Hypercapnia of newborn
    Hypoxemia of newborn
    Hypoxia of newborn NOS
    Mixed metabolic and respiratory acidosis of newborn
    Excludes 1   intracranial hemorrhage due to anoxia or hypoxia
                  (P52.-)
                  hypoxic ischemic encephalopathy [HIE] (P91.6-)
                  late metabolic acidosis of newborn (P74.0)

OTHER DISORDERS ORIGINATING IN THE PERINATAL PERIOD (P90-P96)

P90   **Convulsions of newborn** 🞄
    Excludes 1   benign myoclonic epilepsy in infancy (G40.3-)
                  benign neonatal convulsions (familial) (G40.3-)
    (Ex:) P29.0-P29.2, P29.4, P29.89-P29.9, P90, P91.8-P91.9, P94.1-P96.0, P96.3-P96.5,
    P96.82-P96.89
● P91   **Other disturbances of cerebral status of newborn**
    P91.0   **Neonatal cerebral ischemia** 🞄
          (Ex:) P90-P91.1, P91.3-P91.5, P91.8-P91.9
    P91.1   **Acquired periventricular cysts of newborn** 🞄
          (Ex:) See P91.0
    P91.2   **Neonatal cerebral leukomalacia** 🞄
          *Degeneration of white matter adjacent to cerebral ventricles
              following cerebral hypoxia or brain ischemia in neonates*
          Periventricular leukomalacia
          (Ex:) P10.2-P10.3, P29.0-P29.2, P29.4, P29.89-P29.9, P50.0-P50.9, P52.0-P52.3,
          P52.5, P53-P54.0, P54.6-P54.9, P60-P61.9, P91.2, P94.1-P94.9, P96.0,
          P96.3-P96.5, P96.82-P96.89
    P91.3   **Neonatal cerebral irritability** 🞄
          (Ex:) See P91.0
    P91.4   **Neonatal cerebral depression** 🞄
          (Ex:) See P91.0
    P91.5   **Neonatal coma** 🞄
          (Ex:) See P91.0
    ● P91.6   **Hypoxic ischemic encephalopathy [HIE]**
          (Ex:) For category P91.6 CC codes: P84, P91.60-P91.63
          P91.60   **Hypoxic ischemic encephalopathy [HIE],
                  unspecified** 🞄
          P91.61   **Mild hypoxic ischemic encephalopathy
                  [HIE]** 🞄
          P91.62   **Moderate hypoxic ischemic encephalopathy
                  [HIE]** 🞄
          P91.63   **Severe hypoxic ischemic encephalopathy
                  [HIE]** 🞄
    P91.8   **Other specified disturbances of cerebral status of
          newborn**
    P91.9   **Disturbance of cerebral status of newborn, unspecified**
● P92   **Feeding problems of newborn**
    Excludes 1   feeding problems in child over 28 days old
                  (R63.3)
    ● P92.0   **Vomiting of newborn**
          Excludes 1   vomiting of child over 28 days old (R11.-)
          P92.01   **Bilious vomiting of newborn** 🞄
                  Excludes 1   bilious vomiting in child over
                              28 days old (R11.14)
                  (Ex:) P92.01-P92.09
          P92.09   **Other vomiting of newborn**
                  Excludes 1   regurgitation of food in newborn
                              (P92.1)
    P92.1   **Regurgitation and rumination of newborn**
    P92.2   **Slow feeding of newborn**
    P92.3   **Underfeeding of newborn**
    P92.4   **Overfeeding of newborn**
    P92.5   **Neonatal difficulty in feeding at breast**
    P92.6   **Failure to thrive in newborn**
          Excludes 1   failure to thrive in child over 28 days old
                      (R62.51)
    P92.8   **Other feeding problems of newborn**
    P92.9   **Feeding problem of newborn, unspecified**

CHAPTER 16 (P00-P96)

● **P93** **Reactions and intoxications due to drugs administered to newborn**

> **Includes** reactions and intoxications due to drugs administered to fetus affecting newborn
>
> **Excludes1** jaundice due to drugs or toxins transmitted from mother or given to newborn (P58.4-)
> reactions and intoxications from maternal opiates, tranquilizers and other medication (P04.0-P04.1, P04.4)
> withdrawal symptoms from maternal use of drugs of addiction (P96.1)
> withdrawal symptoms from therapeutic use of drugs in newborn (P96.2)

(Ex:) For category P93 CC codes: P93.0-P93.8, P96.1-P96.2

P93.0 **Grey baby syndrome** 🦠
> Grey syndrome from chloramphenicol administration in newborn

P93.8 **Other reactions and intoxications due to drugs administered to newborn** 🦠
> Use additional code for adverse effect, if applicable, to identify drug (T36-T50 with fifth or sixth character 5)

● **P94** **Disorders of muscle tone of newborn**

P94.0 **Transient neonatal myasthenia gravis** 🦠
> **Excludes1** myasthenia gravis (G70.0)
>
> (Ex:) P29.0-P29.2, P29.4, P29.89-P29.9, P70.0-P71.9, P72.1, P72.9-P74.4, P74.9, P94.0-P94.9, P96.0, P96.3-P96.5, P96.82-P96.89

P94.1 **Congenital hypertonia**

P94.2 **Congenital hypotonia**
> Floppy baby syndrome, unspecified

P94.8 **Other disorders of muscle tone of newborn**

P94.9 **Disorder of muscle tone of newborn, unspecified**

P95 **Stillbirth**
> Deadborn fetus NOS
> Fetal death of unspecified cause
> Stillbirth NOS
>
> **Excludes1** maternal care for intrauterine death (O36.4)
> missed abortion (O02.1)
> outcome of delivery, stillbirth (Z37.1, Z37.3, Z37.4, Z37.7)

OGCR Section I.C.16.g.

> Stillbirth
>
> Code P95, Stillbirth, is only for use for institutions that maintain separate records for stillbirths. No other code should be used with P95. Code P95 should not be used on the mother's record.

● **P96** **Other conditions originating in the perinatal period**

P96.0 **Congenital renal failure**
> Uremia of newborn

P96.1 **Neonatal withdrawal symptoms from maternal use of drugs of addiction** 🦠
> Drug withdrawal syndrome in infant of dependent mother
> Neonatal abstinence syndrome
>
> **Excludes1** reactions and intoxications from maternal opiates and tranquilizers administered during labor and delivery (P04.0)

(Ex:) See P93

P96.2 **Withdrawal symptoms from therapeutic use of drugs in newborn** 🦠
(Ex:) See P93

P96.3 **Wide cranial sutures of newborn**
> Neonatal craniotabes

P96.5 **Complication to newborn due to (fetal) intrauterine procedure**
> **Excludes2** newborn affected by amniocentesis (P00.6) ◀▥▥

● **P96.8** **Other specified conditions originating in the perinatal period**

P96.81 **Exposure to (parental) (environmental) tobacco smoke in the perinatal period**
> **Excludes2** newborn affected by in utero exposure to tobacco (P04.2)
> exposure to environmental tobacco smoke after the perinatal period (Z77.22)

P96.82 **Delayed separation of umbilical cord**

P96.83 **Meconium staining**
> **Excludes1** meconium aspiration (P24.00, P24.01)
> meconium passage during delivery (P03.82)

P96.89 **Other specified conditions originating in the perinatal period**
> Use additional code to specify condition

P96.9 **Condition originating in the perinatal period, unspecified**
> Congenital debility NOS

◀ New   ◀▥▥ Revised   ~~deleted~~ Deleted   Excludes 1   Excludes 2   Includes   Use additional   Code first   Code also   Unspecified
OGCR Official Guidelines   ● Unacceptable Principal Diagnosis   X Assign placeholder X   ● Use Additional Character(s)   ▶ Manifestation Code   **Coding Clinic**

CHAPTER 17

CONGENITAL MALFORMATIONS, DEFORMATIONS AND CHROMOSOMAL ABNORMALITIES (Q00-Q99)

OGCR Chapter-Specific Coding Guidelines

> 17. **Chapter 17: Congenital malformations, deformations, and chromosomal abnormalities (Q00-Q99)**
> Assign an appropriate code(s) from categories Q00-Q99, Congenital malformations, deformations, and chromosomal abnormalities when a malformation/deformation or chromosomal abnormality is documented. A malformation/deformation/ or chromosomal abnormality may be the principal/first-listed diagnosis on a record or a secondary diagnosis.
>
> When a malformation/deformation/or chromosomal abnormality does not have a unique code assignment, assign additional code(s) for any manifestations that may be present.
>
> When the code assignment specifically identifies the malformation/deformation/or chromosomal abnormality, manifestations that are an inherent component of the anomaly should not be coded separately. Additional codes should be assigned for manifestations that are not an inherent component.
>
> Codes from Chapter 17 may be used throughout the life of the patient. If a congenital malformation or deformity has been corrected, a personal history code should be used to identify the history of the malformation or deformity. Although present at birth, malformation/deformation/or chromosomal abnormality may not be identified until later in life. Whenever the condition is diagnosed by the physician, it is appropriate to assign a code from codes Q00-Q99.
>
> For the birth admission, the appropriate code from category Z38, Liveborn infants, according to place of birth and type of delivery, should be sequenced as the principal diagnosis, followed by any congenital anomaly codes, Q00-Q99.

CHAPTER 17

CONGENITAL MALFORMATIONS, DEFORMATIONS AND CHROMOSOMAL ABNORMALITIES (Q00-Q99)

Note: Codes from this chapter are not for use on maternal or fetal records

Excludes2 inborn errors of metabolism (E70-E88)

This chapter contains the following blocks:

Q00-Q07	Congenital malformations of the nervous system
Q10-Q18	Congenital malformations of eye, ear, face and neck
Q20-Q28	Congenital malformations of the circulatory system
Q30-Q34	Congenital malformations of the respiratory system
Q35-Q37	Cleft lip and cleft palate
Q38-Q45	Other congenital malformations of the digestive system
Q50-Q56	Congenital malformations of genital organs
Q60-Q64	Congenital malformations of the urinary system
Q65-Q79	Congenital malformations and deformations of the musculoskeletal system
Q80-Q89	Other congenital malformations
Q90-Q99	Chromosomal abnormalities, not elsewhere classified

Figure 17-1 An infant with a large occipital encephalocele. The large skin-covered encephalocele is visible. (From Townsend: Sabiston Textbook of Surgery, ed 19, Saunders, An Imprint of Elsevier, 2012)

CONGENITAL MALFORMATIONS OF THE NERVOUS SYSTEM (Q00–Q07)

● **Q00   Anencephaly and similar malformations**
     Ex: For category Q00 CC codes: Q00.0-Q00.2

   Q00.0   Anencephaly 🔹
      Absence of skull with cerebral hemispheres missing or reduced to small masses attached to base of cranium
      Acephaly
      Acrania
      Amyelencephaly
      Hemianencephaly
      Hemicephaly

   Q00.1   Craniorachischisis 🔹
      Developmental anomaly consisting of fissure of cranium and vertebral column

   Q00.2   Iniencephaly 🔹
      Developmental anomaly characterized by enlargement of foramen magnum and absence of laminae and spinous processes of cervical, dorsal

● **Q01   Encephalocele**
     Sac-like protrusions of brain and membranes visible through an opening in skull

     Includes   Arnold-Chiari syndrome, type III
                   encephalocystocele
                   encephalomyelocele
                   hydroencephalocele
                   hydromeningocele, cranial
                   meningocele, cerebral
                   meningoencephalocele

     Excludes1   Meckel-Gruber syndrome (Q61.9)
     Ex: For category Q01 CC codes: Q01.0-Q02, Q04.0-Q04.8

   Q01.0   Frontal encephalocele 🔹
   Q01.1   Nasofrontal encephalocele 🔹
   Q01.2   Occipital encephalocele 🔹
   Q01.8   Encephalocele of other sites 🔹
   Q01.9   Encephalocele, unspecified 🔹

  Q02   Microcephaly
     Head size measures significantly below normal based on standardized charts

     Includes   hydromicrocephaly
                   micrencephalon

     Excludes1   Meckel-Gruber syndrome (Q61.9)

● **Q03   Congenital hydrocephalus**
     Accumulation of cerebrospinal fluid in ventricles resulting in swelling and enlargement

     Includes   hydrocephalus in newborn

     Excludes1   Arnold-Chiari syndrome, type II (Q07.0-)
                 acquired hydrocephalus (G91.-)
                 hydrocephalus due to congenital toxoplasmosis (P37.1)
                 hydrocephalus with spina bifida (Q05.0-Q05.4)

   Q03.0   Malformations of aqueduct of Sylvius
      Anomaly of aqueduct of Sylvius
      Obstruction of aqueduct of Sylvius, congenital
      Stenosis of aqueduct of Sylvius

   Q03.1   Atresia of foramina of Magendie and Luschka
      Dandy-Walker syndrome

   Q03.8   Other congenital hydrocephalus
   Q03.9   Congenital hydrocephalus, unspecified

N   Newborn Age: 0   **P**   Pediatric Age: 0–17   **M**   Maternity DX: 12–55   **A**   Adult Age: 15–124   ♀   Females Only   ♂   Males Only

🔹 Complication\Comorbidity   Major C\C   Ex: CC/MCC Exclusions   Hospital-Acquired Condition

1173

CHAPTER 17 (Q00-Q99)

● **Q04　Other congenital malformations of brain**

　　Excludes1　cyclopia (Q87.0)
　　　　　　　　　macrocephaly (Q75.3)
　　(Ex:) For category Q04 CC codes Q04.0-Q04.3: Q01.0-Q02, Q04.0-Q04.8
　　　　For category Q04 CC codes Q04.4-Q04.8: Q04.4-Q04.8

　Q04.0　Congenital malformations of corpus callosum
　　　　　Agenesis of corpus callosum

　Q04.1　Arhinencephaly 🔗
　　　　　Congenital absence of olfactory bulbs, tract, or nerves

　Q04.2　Holoprosencephaly 🔗
　　　　　*Failure of cleavage of forebrain (prosencephalon) resulting in
　　　　　incomplete or absent cortical separation and deficits in
　　　　　midline facial development*

　Q04.3　Other reduction deformities of brain 🔗
　　　　　Absence of part of brain　　　　Agyria
　　　　　Agenesis of part of brain
　　　　　　*Cerebral cortex are not fully formed, brain surface is
　　　　　　smooth*
　　　　　Aplasia of part of brain
　　　　　Hydranencephaly
　　　　　Hypoplasia of part of brain
　　　　　Lissencephaly
　　　　　　*Congenital malformation or absence of convolutions of
　　　　　　cerebral cortex*
　　　　　Microgyria
　　　　　　*Malformation of brain characterized by excessive number
　　　　　　of small convolutions (gyri) on surface*
　　　　　Pachygyria
　　　　　　Reduction in number of sulci of cerebrum
　　　　　Excludes1　congenital malformations of corpus
　　　　　　　　　　　callosum (Q04.0)

　Q04.4　Septo-optic dysplasia of brain 🔗

　Q04.5　Megalencephaly 🔗
　　　　　Abnormally large brain

　Q04.6　Congenital cerebral cysts 🔗
　　　　　Porencephaly　　　　Schizencephaly
　　　　　Excludes1　acquired porencephalic cyst (G93.0)

　Q04.8　Other specified congenital malformations of brain 🔗
　　　　　Arnold-Chiari syndrome, type IV
　　　　　Macrogyria

　Q04.9　Congenital malformation of brain, unspecified
　　　　　Congenital anomaly NOS of brain
　　　　　Congenital deformity NOS of brain
　　　　　Congenital disease or lesion NOS of brain
　　　　　Multiple anomalies NOS of brain, congenital

● **Q05　Spina bifida**
　　*Developmental anomaly characterized by defective closure of vertebral
　　arch, through which spinal cord and meninges may protrude*

　　Includes　hydromeningocele (spinal)
　　　　　　　　meningocele (spinal)
　　　　　　　　meningomyelocele
　　　　　　　　myelocele
　　　　　　　　myelomeningocele
　　　　　　　　rachischisis
　　　　　　　　spina bifida (aperta)(cystica)
　　　　　　　　syringomyelocele

　Use additional code for any associated paraplegia (paraparesis)
　(G82.2-)

　　Excludes1　Arnold-Chiari syndrome, type II (Q07.0-)
　　　　　　　　spina bifida occulta (Q76.0)
　　(Ex:) For category Q05 CC codes: E78.71-E78.72, G90.1, Q05.0-Q06.1, Q06.3, Q06.8-Q07.9,
　　　　Q87.1-Q87.89, Q89.7-Q89.8, Q99.2

　Q05.0　Cervical spina bifida with hydrocephalus 🔗

　Q05.1　Thoracic spina bifida with hydrocephalus 🔗
　　　　　Dorsal spina bifida with hydrocephalus
　　　　　Thoracolumbar spina bifida with hydrocephalus

　Q05.2　Lumbar spina bifida with hydrocephalus 🔗
　　　　　Lumbosacral spina bifida with hydrocephalus

　Q05.3　Sacral spina bifida with hydrocephalus 🔗

　Q05.4　Unspecified spina bifida with hydrocephalus 🔗

　Q05.5　Cervical spina bifida without hydrocephalus

　Q05.6　Thoracic spina bifida without hydrocephalus
　　　　　Dorsal spina bifida NOS
　　　　　Thoracolumbar spina bifida NOS

　Q05.7　Lumbar spina bifida without hydrocephalus
　　　　　Lumbosacral spina bifida NOS

　Q05.8　Sacral spina bifida without hydrocephalus

　Q05.9　Spina bifida, unspecified

● **Q06　Other congenital malformations of spinal cord**

　Q06.0　Amyelia
　　　　　Congenital absence of spinal cord

　Q06.1　Hypoplasia and dysplasia of spinal cord
　　　　　Underdevelopment of spinal cord
　　　　　Atelomyelia
　　　　　　Congenitally incomplete development of spinal cord
　　　　　Myelatelia
　　　　　Myelodysplasia of spinal cord
　　　　　　*Defective development of spinal cord, especially lower
　　　　　　segments*

　Q06.2　Diastematomyelia
　　　　　*Congenital anomaly, associated with spina bifida, in which
　　　　　spinal cord is split into halves and surrounded by dural
　　　　　sac*

　Q06.3　Other congenital cauda equina malformations

　Q06.4　Hydromyelia
　　　　　*Dilation of central canal of spinal cord with increased fluid
　　　　　accumulation*
　　　　　Hydrorachis

　Q06.8　Other specified congenital malformations of spinal cord

　Q06.9　Congenital malformation of spinal cord, unspecified
　　　　　Congenital anomaly NOS of spinal cord
　　　　　Congenital deformity NOS of spinal cord
　　　　　Congenital disease or lesion NOS of spinal cord

● **Q07　Other congenital malformations of nervous system**

　　Excludes2　congenital central alveolar hypoventilation
　　　　　　　　syndrome (G47.35)
　　　　　　　　familial dysautonomia [Riley-Day] (G90.1)
　　　　　　　　neurofibromatosis (nonmalignant) (Q85.0-)

● **Q07.0　Arnold-Chiari syndrome**
　　　　　*Herniation of cerebellar tonsils and vermis through foramen
　　　　　magnum into spinal canal*
　　　　　Arnold-Chiari syndrome, type II

　　Excludes1　Arnold-Chiari syndrome, type III (Q01.-)
　　　　　　　　Arnold-Chiari syndrome, type IV (Q04.8)

　**Q07.00　Arnold-Chiari syndrome without spina bifida
　　　　　　or hydrocephalus**

　**Q07.01　Arnold-Chiari syndrome with spina
　　　　　　bifida**

　Q07.02　Arnold-Chiari syndrome with hydrocephalus 🔗
　　　　　(Ex:) See Q05

　**Q07.03　Arnold-Chiari syndrome with spina
　　　　　　bifida and hydrocephalus** 🔗
　　　　　(Ex:) See Q05

　**Q07.8　Other specified congenital malformations of nervous
　　　　　system**
　　　　　Agenesis of nerve
　　　　　Displacement of brachial plexus
　　　　　Jaw-winking syndrome
　　　　　Marcus Gunn's syndrome

　Q07.9　Congenital malformation of nervous system, unspecified
　　　　　Congenital anomaly NOS of nervous system
　　　　　Congenital deformity NOS of nervous system
　　　　　Congenital disease or lesion NOS of nervous system

◀ New　◀┅ Revised　ᵈᵉˡᵉᵗᵉᵈ Deleted　Excludes 1　Excludes 2　Includes　Use additional　Code first　Code also　Unspecified
OGCR Official Guidelines　● Unacceptable Principal Diagnosis　X Assign placeholder X　● Use Additional Character(s)　▶ Manifestation Code　**Coding Clinic**

1174

CONGENITAL MALFORMATIONS OF EYE, EAR, FACE AND NECK (Q10-Q18)

    Excludes2   cleft lip and cleft palate (Q35-Q37)
            congenital malformation of cervical spine (Q05.0, Q05.5, Q67.5, Q76.0-Q76.4)
            congenital malformation of larynx (Q31.-)
            congenital malformation of lip NEC (Q38.0)
            congenital malformation of nose (Q30.-)
            congenital malformation of parathyroid gland (Q89.2)
            congenital malformation of thyroid gland (Q89.2)

● **Q10   Congenital malformations of eyelid, lacrimal apparatus and orbit**
    Excludes1   cryptophthalmos NOS (Q11.2)
            cryptophthalmos syndrome (Q87.0)

  Q10.0   Congenital ptosis
      Prolapse or drooping of upper eyelid from paralysis of third nerve or from sympathetic innervations

  Q10.1   Congenital ectropion
      Outward turning of eyelid

  Q10.2   Congenital entropion
      Inward turning of eyelid

  Q10.3   Other congenital malformations of eyelid
      Ablepharon
      Blepharophimosis, congenital
      Coloboma of eyelid
      Congenital absence or agenesis of cilia
      Congenital absence or agenesis of eyelid
      Congenital accessory eyelid
      Congenital accessory eye muscle
      Congenital malformation of eyelid NOS

  Q10.4   Absence and agenesis of lacrimal apparatus
      Congenital absence of punctum lacrimale

  Q10.5   Congenital stenosis and stricture of lacrimal duct

  Q10.6   Other congenital malformations of lacrimal apparatus
      Congenital malformation of lacrimal apparatus NOS

  Q10.7   Congenital malformation of orbit

● **Q11   Anophthalmos, microphthalmos and macrophthalmos**
  Absence of eye and optic pit

  Q11.0   Cystic eyeball

  Q11.1   Other anophthalmos
      Anophthalmos NOS
      Agenesis of eye
        Absence of eye
      Aplasia of eye

  Q11.2   Microphthalmos
      Partial absence of eye and optic pit
      Cryptophthalmos NOS
      Dysplasia of eye
      Hypoplasia of eye
      Rudimentary eye
    Excludes1   cryptophthalmos syndrome (Q87.0)

  Q11.3   Macrophthalmos
      Congenital enlargement of eyes
    Excludes1   macrophthalmos in congenital glaucoma (Q15.0)

● **Q12   Congenital lens malformations**
  Q12.0   Congenital cataract
  Q12.1   Congenital displaced lens
  Q12.2   Coloboma of lens
  Q12.3   Congenital aphakia
  Q12.4   Spherophakia
      Smaller, more spherical optic lens than normal
  Q12.8   Other congenital lens malformations
      Microphakia
  Q12.9   Congenital lens malformation, unspecified

Figure 17-2   Bilateral congenital **hydrophthalmia,** in which the eyes are very large in comparison to the other facial features due to glaucoma.

● **Q13   Congenital malformations of anterior segment of eye**
  Q13.0   Coloboma of iris
      Coloboma NOS

  Q13.1   Absence of iris
      Aniridia
      Use additional code for associated glaucoma (H42)

  Q13.2   Other congenital malformations of iris
      Anisocoria, congenital
      Atresia of pupil
      Congenital malformation of iris NOS
      Corectopia

  Q13.3   Congenital corneal opacity

  Q13.4   Other congenital corneal malformations
      Congenital malformation of cornea NOS
      Microcornea
      Peter's anomaly

  Q13.5   Blue sclera
      Condition of unusual blueness of sclera; not harmful

● **Q13.8   Other congenital malformations of anterior segment of eye**
    Q13.81   Rieger's anomaly
        Use additional code for associated glaucoma (H42)
    Q13.89   Other congenital malformations of anterior segment of eye

  Q13.9   Congenital malformation of anterior segment of eye, unspecified

● **Q14   Congenital malformations of posterior segment of eye**
    Excludes2   optic nerve hypoplasia (H47.03-)
  Q14.0   Congenital malformation of vitreous humor
      Congenital vitreous opacity
  Q14.1   Congenital malformation of retina
      Congenital retinal aneurysm
  Q14.2   Congenital malformation of optic disc
      Coloboma of optic disc
  Q14.3   Congenital malformation of choroid
  Q14.8   Other congenital malformations of posterior segment of eye
      Coloboma of the fundus
  Q14.9   Congenital malformation of posterior segment of eye, unspecified

● **Q15   Other congenital malformations of eye**
    Excludes1   congenital nystagmus (H55.01)
            ocular albinism (E70.31-)
            optic nerve hypoplasia (H47.03-)
            retinitis pigmentosa (H35.52)

  Q15.0   Congenital glaucoma
      Axenfeld's anomaly
      Buphthalmos
        Congenital syndrome characterized by port-wine nevus covering portions of face and cranium
      Glaucoma of childhood
      Glaucoma of newborn
      Hydrophthalmos
      Keratoglobus, congenital, with glaucoma
      Macrocornea with glaucoma
      Macrophthalmos in congenital glaucoma
      Megalocornea with glaucoma

N Newborn Age: 0   **P** Pediatric Age: 0–17   **M** Maternity DX: 12–55   **A** Adult Age: 15–124   ♀ Females Only   ♂ Males Only

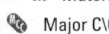 Complication\Comorbidity   Major C\C   (Ex) CC/MCC Exclusions   Hospital-Acquired Condition   **1175**

CHAPTER 17 (Q00-Q99)

Q15.8   **Other specified congenital malformations of eye**

Q15.9   **Congenital malformation of eye, unspecified**
    Congenital anomaly of eye
    Congenital deformity of eye

● **Q16   Congenital malformations of ear causing impairment of hearing**
    Excludes1   congenital deafness (H90.-)

Q16.0   **Congenital absence of (ear) auricle**

Q16.1   **Congenital absence, atresia and stricture of auditory canal (external)**
    Congenital atresia or stricture of osseous meatus

Q16.2   **Absence of eustachian tube**

Q16.3   **Congenital malformation of ear ossicles**
    Congenital fusion of ear ossicles

Q16.4   **Other congenital malformations of middle ear**
    Congenital malformation of middle ear NOS

Q16.5   **Congenital malformation of inner ear**
    Congenital anomaly of membranous labyrinth
    Congenital anomaly of organ of Corti

Q16.9   **Congenital malformation of ear causing impairment of hearing, unspecified**
    Congenital absence of ear NOS

● **Q17   Other congenital malformations of ear**
    Excludes1   congenital malformations of ear with impairment of hearing (Q16.0-Q16.9)
               preauricular sinus (Q18.1)

Q17.0   **Accessory auricle**
    Accessory tragus
    Polyotia
    Preauricular appendage or tag
    Supernumerary ear
    Supernumerary lobule

Q17.1   **Macrotia**
    Enlarged ears

Q17.2   **Microtia**
    An abnormally small or underdeveloped external ear

Q17.3   **Other misshapen ear**
    Pointed ear

Q17.4   **Misplaced ear**
    Low-set ears
    Excludes1   cervical auricle (Q18.2)

Q17.5   **Prominent ear**
    Bat ear

Q17.8   **Other specified congenital malformations of ear**
    Congenital absence of lobe of ear

Q17.9   **Congenital malformation of ear, unspecified**
    Congenital anomaly of ear NOS

● **Q18   Other congenital malformations of face and neck**
    Excludes1   cleft lip and cleft palate (Q35-Q37)
               conditions classified to Q67.0-Q67.4
               congenital malformations of skull and face bones (Q75.-)
               cyclopia (Q87.0)
               dentofacial anomalies [including malocclusion] (M26.-)
               malformation syndromes affecting facial appearance (Q87.0)
               persistent thyroglossal duct (Q89.2)

Q18.0   **Sinus, fistula and cyst of branchial cleft**
    Branchial vestige
    Brachial remnants (cysts, fistula, skin tags) that are developmental anomalies

Q18.1   **Preauricular sinus and cyst**
    Fistula of auricle, congenital
    Cervicoaural fistula
    Abnormal passage in neck originating from first branchial cleft

Q18.2   **Other branchial cleft malformations**
    Branchial cleft malformation NOS
    Cervical auricle
    Otocephaly

Q18.3   **Webbing of neck**
    Pterygium colli
    Thick fold of skin on side of neck

Q18.4   **Macrostomia**
    Results from failure of union of maxillary and mandibular processes, results in abnormally large mouth

Q18.5   **Microstomia**

Q18.6   **Macrocheilia**
    Excessive size of lips
    Hypertrophy of lip, congenital

Q18.7   **Microcheilia**
    Abnormal smallness of lips

Q18.8   **Other specified congenital malformations of face and neck**
    Medial cyst of face and neck
    Medial fistula of face and neck
    Medial sinus of face and neck

Q18.9   **Congenital malformation of face and neck, unspecified**
    Congenital anomaly NOS of face and neck

CONGENITAL MALFORMATIONS OF THE CIRCULATORY SYSTEM (Q20-Q28)

● **Q20   Congenital malformations of cardiac chambers and connections**
    Excludes1   dextrocardia with situs inversus (Q89.3)
               mirror-image atrial arrangement with situs inversus (Q89.3)
    (Ex) For category Q20 CC codes: E78.71-E78.72, I23.0-I23.3, I23.6-I23.8, I51.0, P29.3, Q20.0-Q21.9, Q23.8-Q23.9, Q24.8-Q24.9, Q27.30, Q27.4, Q28.0-Q28.1, Q28.8-Q28.9, Q87.1-Q87.89, Q89.7-Q89.8, Q99.2

Q20.0   **Common arterial trunk** 🔗
    Persistent truncus arteriosus
    Excludes1   aortic septal defect (Q21.4)

Q20.1   **Double outlet right ventricle** 🔗
    Taussig-Bing syndrome

Q20.2   **Double outlet left ventricle** 🔗

Q20.3   **Discordant ventriculoarterial connection** 🔗
    Dextrotransposition of aorta
    Transposition of great vessels (complete)

Q20.4   **Double inlet ventricle** 🔗
    Common ventricle
    Cor triloculare biatriatum
    Single ventricle

Q20.5   **Discordant atrioventricular connection** 🔗
    Corrected transposition
    Levotransposition
    Ventricular inversion

Q20.6   **Isomerism of atrial appendages**
    Isomerism of atrial appendages with asplenia or polysplenia

Q20.8   **Other congenital malformations of cardiac chambers and connections**
    Cor binoculare

Q20.9   **Congenital malformation of cardiac chambers and connections, unspecified**

● **Q21   Congenital malformations of cardiac septa**
    Excludes1   acquired cardiac septal defect (I51.0)

Q21.0   **Ventricular septal defect** 🔗
    Roger's disease
    (Ex) See Q20

Q21.1   **Atrial septal defect** 🔗
    Coronary sinus defect
    Patent or persistent foramen ovale
    Patent or persistent ostium secundum defect (type II)
    Patent or persistent sinus venosus defect
    (Ex) E78.71-E78.72, I23.0-I23.3, I23.6-I23.8, I51.0, Q20.0-Q20.9, Q21.1-Q21.9, Q23.8-Q23.9, Q24.8-Q24.9, Q27.30, Q27.4, Q28.0-Q28.1, Q28.8-Q28.9, Q87.2-Q87.3, Q87.5-Q87.89, Q89.7-Q89.8

Q21.2   **Atrioventricular septal defect** 🔗
    Common atrioventricular canal
    Endocardial cushion defect
    Ostium primum atrial septal defect (type I)
    (Ex) See Q20

CHAPTER 17 (Q00-Q99)

◀ New   ◀▥ Revised   ~~deleted~~ Deleted | Excludes 1 | | Excludes 2 | | Includes | | Use additional | | Code first | | Code also | | Unspecified |

OGCR Official Guidelines   ● Unacceptable Principal Diagnosis   X Assign placeholder X   ● Use Additional Character(s)   ▶ Manifestation Code   **Coding Clinic**

Q21.3 Tetralogy of Fallot 🐾
 Ventricular septal defect with pulmonary stenosis or atresia, dextroposition of aorta and hypertrophy of right ventricle.
 (Ex) See Q20

Q21.4 Aortopulmonary septal defect
 Aortic septal defect
 Aortopulmonary window

Q21.8 Other congenital malformations of cardiac septa
 Eisenmenger's defect
 Pentalogy of Fallot
 Excludes1   Eisenmenger's complex (I27.8)
                Eisenmenger's syndrome (I27.8)

Q21.9 Congenital malformation of cardiac septum, unspecified
 Septal (heart) defect NOS

● **Q22 Congenital malformations of pulmonary and tricuspid valves**
 (Ex) For category Q22 CC codes unless otherwise indicated: E78.71-E78.72, P29.3, Q20.9, Q22.4-Q23.9, Q24.8-Q24.9, Q27.30, Q27.4, Q28.0-Q28.1, Q28.8-Q28.9, Q87.1-Q87.89, Q89.7-Q89.8, Q99.2

Q22.0 Pulmonary valve atresia 🐾
 (Ex) E78.71-E78.72, P29.3, Q20.9, Q22.0-Q22.3, Q23.8-Q23.9, Q24.8-Q24.9, Q27.4, Q28.0-Q28.1, Q28.8-Q28.9, Q87.1-Q87.89, Q89.7-Q89.8, Q99.2

Q22.1 Congenital pulmonary valve stenosis 🐾
 (Ex) See Q22.0

Q22.2 Congenital pulmonary valve insufficiency 🐾
 Congenital pulmonary valve regurgitation
 (Ex) E78.71-E78.72, Q20.9, Q22.0-Q22.3, Q23.8-Q23.9, Q24.8-Q24.9, Q27.30, Q27.4, Q28.0-Q28.1, Q28.8-Q28.9, Q87.2-Q87.3, Q87.5-Q87.89, Q89.7-Q89.8

Q22.3 Other congenital malformations of pulmonary valve 🐾
 Congenital malformation of pulmonary valve NOS
 Supernumerary cusps of pulmonary valve
 (Ex) See Q22.2

Q22.4 Congenital tricuspid stenosis 🐾
 Congenital tricuspid atresia

Q22.5 Ebstein's anomaly 🐾
 Malformation of tricuspid valve

Q22.6 Hypoplastic right heart syndrome 🐾

Q22.8 Other congenital malformations of tricuspid valve 🐾

Q22.9 Congenital malformation of tricuspid valve, unspecified 🐾

● **Q23 Congenital malformations of aortic and mitral valves**
 (Ex) For category Q23 CC codes unless otherwise indicated: See Q22

Q23.0 Congenital stenosis of aortic valve 🐾
 Congenital aortic atresia
 Congenital aortic stenosis NOS
 Excludes1   congenital stenosis of aortic valve in hypoplastic left heart syndrome (Q23.4)
                congenital subaortic stenosis (Q24.4)
                supravalvular aortic stenosis (congenital) (Q25.3)

Q23.1 Congenital insufficiency of aortic valve 🐾
 Bicuspid aortic valve
 Congenital aortic insufficiency

Q23.2 Congenital mitral stenosis 🐾
 Congenital mitral atresia

Q23.3 Congenital mitral insufficiency 🐾

Q23.4 Hypoplastic left heart syndrome 🐾

Q23.8 Other congenital malformations of aortic and mitral valves

Q23.9 Congenital malformation of aortic and mitral valves, unspecified

● **Q24 Other congenital malformations of heart**
 Excludes1   endocardial fibroelastosis (I42.4)

Q24.0 Dextrocardia 🐾
 Heart is located in right hemithorax
 Excludes1   dextrocardia with situs inversus (Q89.3)
                isomerism of atrial appendages (with asplenia or polysplenia) (Q20.6)
                mirror-image atrial arrangement with situs inversus (Q89.3)
 (Ex) E78.71-E78.72, Q20.9, Q23.8-Q24.4, Q24.8-Q24.9, Q27.30, Q27.4, Q28.0-Q28.1, Q28.8-Q28.9, Q87.2-Q87.3, Q87.5-Q87.89, Q89.7-Q89.8

Q24.1 Levocardia 🐾
 Normal position of heart but related structures on wrong side
 (Ex) See Q24.0

Q24.2 Cor triatriatum 🐾
 Congenital heart defect; left atrium is subdivided
 (Ex) E78.71-E78.72, P29.3, Q20.9, Q23.8-Q23.9, Q24.2-Q24.4, Q24.8-Q24.9, Q27.30, Q27.4, Q28.0-Q28.1, Q28.8-Q28.9, Q87.1-Q87.89, Q89.7-Q89.8, Q99.2

Q24.3 Pulmonary infundibular stenosis 🐾
 Subvalvular pulmonic stenosis
 (Ex) See Q24.3

Q24.4 Congenital subaortic stenosis 🐾
 (Ex) See Q24.3

Q24.5 Malformation of coronary vessels 🐾
 Congenital coronary (artery) aneurysm
 (Ex) Q20.9, Q23.8-Q23.9, Q24.5, Q24.8-Q24.9

Q24.6 Congenital heart block 🐾
 (Ex) E78.71-E78.72, P29.3, Q20.9, Q23.8-Q23.9, Q24.6-Q24.9, Q27.30, Q27.4, Q28.0-Q28.1, Q28.8-Q28.9, Q87.1-Q87.89, Q89.7-Q89.8, Q99.2

Q24.8 Other specified congenital malformations of heart
 Congenital diverticulum of left ventricle
 Congenital malformation of myocardium
 Congenital malformation of pericardium
 Malposition of heart
 Uhl's disease

Q24.9 Congenital malformation of heart, unspecified
 Congenital anomaly of heart
 Congenital disease of heart

● **Q25 Congenital malformations of great arteries**

Q25.0 Patent ductus arteriosus 🐾
 Fetal blood vessel connecting left pulmonary artery directly to descending aorta
 Patent ductus Botallo
 Persistent ductus arteriosus
 (Ex) Q25.0, Q27.30, Q27.4, Q28.0-Q28.1, Q28.8

Q25.1 Coarctation of aorta 🐾
 Coarctation of aorta (preductal) (postductal)
 Stenosis of aorta ◄
 (Ex) E78.71-E78.72, Q25.1-Q25.3, Q27.30, Q27.4, Q28.0-Q28.1, Q28.8-Q28.9, Q87.2-Q87.3, Q87.5-Q87.89, Q89.7-Q89.8

● **Q25.2 Atresia of aorta**
 (Ex) For category Q25.2 CC codes: E78.71-E78.72, P29.3, Q25.1-Q25.3, Q27.30, Q27.4, Q28.0-Q28.1, Q28.8-Q28.9, Q87.1-Q87.89, Q89.7-Q89.8, Q99.2

Q25.21 Interruption of aortic arch 🐾 ◄
 Atresia of aortic arch ◄

Q25.29 Other atresia of aorta 🐾 ◄
 Atresia of aorta ◄

Q25.3 Supravalvular aortic stenosis 🐾
 Excludes1   congenital aortic stenosis NOS (Q23.0)
                congenital stenosis of aortic valve (Q23.0)
 (Ex) See Q25.2

● **Q25.4 Other congenital malformations of aorta**
 Excludes1   hypoplasia of aorta in hypoplastic left heart syndrome (Q23.4)
 (Ex) For category Q25.4 CC codes: E78.71-E78.72, Q25.1-Q25.49, Q25.8-Q25.9, Q27.30, Q27.4, Q28.0-Q28.1, Q28.8-Q28.9, Q87.2-Q87.3, Q87.5-Q87.89, Q89.7-Q89.8

Q25.40 Congenital malformation of aorta unspecified 🐾 ◄

Q25.41 Absence and aplasia of aorta 🐾 ◄

Q25.42 Hypoplasia of aorta 🐾 ◄

CHAPTER 17 (Q00-Q99)

CHAPTER 17 (Q00-Q99)

Q25.43 **Congenital aneurysm of aorta** ◕ ◀
    Congenital aneurysm of aortic root ◀
    Congenital aneurysm of aortic sinus ◀

Q25.44 **Congenital dilation of aorta** ◕ ◀

Q25.45 **Double aortic arch** ◕ ◀
    Vascular ring of aorta ◀

Q25.46 **Tortuous aortic arch** ◕ ◀
    Persistent convolutions of aortic arch ◀

Q25.47 **Right aortic arch** ◕ ◀
    Persistent right aortic arch ◀

Q25.48 **Anomalous origin of subclavian artery** ◕ ◀

Q25.49 **Other congenital malformations of aorta** ◕ ◀

Q25.5 **Atresia of pulmonary artery** ◕
    Ⓔⓧ Q25.5-Q25.79, Q27.30, Q27.4, Q28.0-Q28.1, Q28.8-Q28.9

Q25.6 **Stenosis of pulmonary artery** ◕
    Supravalvular pulmonary stenosis
    Ⓔⓧ See Q25.5

● Q25.7 **Other congenital malformations of pulmonary artery**
    Ⓔⓧ For category Q25.7 CC codes: See Q25.5

Q25.71 **Coarctation of pulmonary artery** ◕

Q25.72 **Congenital pulmonary arteriovenous malformation** ◕
    Congenital pulmonary arteriovenous aneurysm

Q25.79 **Other congenital malformations of pulmonary artery** ◕
    Aberrant pulmonary artery
    Agenesis of pulmonary artery
    Congenital aneurysm of pulmonary artery
    Congenital anomaly of pulmonary artery
    Hypoplasia of pulmonary artery

Q25.8 **Other congenital malformations of other great arteries** ◕
    Ⓔⓧ See Q25.4

Q25.9 **Congenital malformation of great arteries, unspecified** ◕
    Ⓔⓧ See Q25.4

● Q26 **Congenital malformations of great veins**

Q26.0 **Congenital stenosis of vena cava** ◕
    Congenital stenosis of vena cava (inferior)(superior)
    Ⓔⓧ Q26.0-Q26.1, Q26.8, Q27.30, Q27.4, Q28.0-Q28.1, Q28.8-Q28.9

Q26.1 **Persistent left superior vena cava** ◕
    Ⓔⓧ See Q26.0

Q26.2 **Total anomalous pulmonary venous connection** ◕
    Total anomalous pulmonary venous return [TAPVR], subdiaphragmatic
    Total anomalous pulmonary venous return [TAPVR], supradiaphragmatic
    Ⓔⓧ Q26.2, Q27.30, Q27.4, Q28.0-Q28.1, Q28.8-Q28.9

Q26.3 **Partial anomalous pulmonary venous connection** ◕
    Partial anomalous pulmonary venous return
    Ⓔⓧ Q26.3-Q26.4, Q27.30, Q27.4, Q28.0-Q28.1, Q28.8-Q28.9

Q26.4 **Anomalous pulmonary venous connection, unspecified** ◕
    Ⓔⓧ See Q26.3

Q26.5 **Anomalous portal venous connection**

Q26.6 **Portal vein-hepatic artery fistula**

Q26.8 **Other congenital malformations of great veins** ◕
    Absence of vena cava (inferior) (superior)
    Azygos continuation of inferior vena cava
    Persistent left posterior cardinal vein
    Scimitar syndrome
    Ⓔⓧ See Q26.0

Q26.9 **Congenital malformation of great vein, unspecified** ◕
    Congenital anomaly of vena cava (inferior) (superior) NOS
    Ⓔⓧ Q26.9, Q27.30, Q27.4, Q28.0-Q28.1, Q28.8-Q28.9

● Q27 **Other congenital malformations of peripheral vascular system**
    Excludes2 anomalies of cerebral and precerebral vessels (Q28.0-Q28.3)
                anomalies of coronary vessels (Q24.5)
                anomalies of pulmonary artery (Q25.5-Q25.7)
                congenital retinal aneurysm (Q14.1)
                hemangioma and lymphangioma (D18.-)

Q27.0 **Congenital absence and hypoplasia of umbilical artery**
    Single umbilical artery

Q27.1 **Congenital renal artery stenosis**

Q27.2 **Other congenital malformations of renal artery**
    Congenital malformation of renal artery NOS
    Multiple renal arteries

● Q27.3 **Arteriovenous malformation (peripheral)**
    Arteriovenous aneurysm
    Excludes1 acquired arteriovenous aneurysm (I77.0)
    Excludes2 arteriovenous malformation of cerebral vessels (Q28.2)
                arteriovenous malformation of precerebral vessels (Q28.0)

Q27.30 **Arteriovenous malformation, site unspecified** ◕
    Ⓔⓧ Q20.0-Q20.8, Q21.0-Q21.9, Q27.30, Q27.4, Q28.0-Q28.1, Q28.8

Q27.31 **Arteriovenous malformation of vessel of upper limb**

Q27.32 **Arteriovenous malformation of vessel of lower limb**

Q27.33 **Arteriovenous malformation of digestive system vessel**

Q27.34 **Arteriovenous malformation of renal vessel**

Q27.39 **Arteriovenous malformation, other site**

Q27.4 **Congenital phlebectasia** ◕
    Ⓔⓧ See Q27.30

Q27.8 **Other specified congenital malformations of peripheral vascular system**
    Absence of peripheral vascular system
    Atresia of peripheral vascular system
    Congenital aneurysm (peripheral)
    Congenital stricture, artery
    Congenital varix
    Excludes1 arteriovenous malformation (Q27.3-)

Q27.9 **Congenital malformation of peripheral vascular system, unspecified**
    Anomaly of artery or vein NOS

● Q28 **Other congenital malformations of circulatory system**
    Excludes1 congenital aneurysm NOS (Q27.8)
                congenital coronary aneurysm (Q24.5)
                ruptured cerebral arteriovenous malformation (I60.8)
                ruptured malformation of precerebral vessels (I72.0)
    Excludes2 congenital peripheral aneurysm (Q27.8)
                congenital pulmonary aneurysm (Q25.79)
                congenital retinal aneurysm (Q14.1)

Q28.0 **Arteriovenous malformation of precerebral vessels** ◕
    Congenital arteriovenous precerebral aneurysm (nonruptured)
    Ⓔⓧ See Q27.30

Q28.1 **Other malformations of precerebral vessels** ◕
    Congenital malformation of precerebral vessels NOS
    Congenital precerebral aneurysm (nonruptured)
    Ⓔⓧ See Q27.30

Q28.2 **Arteriovenous malformation of cerebral vessels** ◕
    Arteriovenous malformation of brain NOS
    Congenital arteriovenous cerebral aneurysm (nonruptured)
    Ⓔⓧ Q27.30, Q27.4, Q28.0-Q28.9

Q28.3 **Other malformations of cerebral vessels** ◕
    Congenital cerebral aneurysm (nonruptured)
    Congenital malformation of cerebral vessels NOS
    Developmental venous anomaly
    Ⓔⓧ See Q28.2

◀ New   ◀▥ Revised   ~~deleted~~ Deleted   Excludes 1   Excludes 2   Includes   Use additional   Code first   Code also   Unspecified

OGCR Official Guidelines   ● Unacceptable Principal Diagnosis   X Assign placeholder X   ◕ Use Additional Character(s)   ▮ Manifestation Code   **Coding Clinic**

Q28.8 **Other specified congenital malformations of circulatory system** 🔖
> Congenital aneurysm, specified site NEC
> Spinal vessel anomaly
> (Ex) See Q27.30

Q28.9 **Congenital malformation of circulatory system, unspecified** 🔖
> (Ex) Q20.0-Q28.9

CONGENITAL MALFORMATIONS OF THE RESPIRATORY SYSTEM (Q30-Q34)

⬤ **Q30** **Congenital malformations of nose**
> **Excludes1** congenital deviation of nasal septum (Q67.4)

Q30.0 **Choanal atresia**
> Atresia of nares (anterior) (posterior)
> Congenital stenosis of nares (anterior) (posterior)

Q30.1 **Agenesis and underdevelopment of nose**
> Congenital absent of nose

Q30.2 **Fissured, notched and cleft nose**

Q30.3 **Congenital perforated nasal septum**

Q30.8 **Other congenital malformations of nose**
> Accessory nose
> Congenital anomaly of nasal sinus wall

Q30.9 **Congenital malformation of nose, unspecified**

⬤ **Q31** **Congenital malformations of larynx**
> **Excludes1** congenital laryngeal stridor NOS (P28.89)
> (Ex) **For category Q31 CC codes:** J39.8, J45.990, J98.09, Q31.1-Q32.4, Q34.0-Q34.9

Q31.0 **Web of larynx**
> Glottic web of larynx
> Subglottic web of larynx
> Web of larynx NOS

Q31.1 **Congenital subglottic stenosis** 🔖

Q31.2 **Laryngeal hypoplasia** 🔖

Q31.3 **Laryngocele** 🔖

Q31.5 **Congenital laryngomalacia** 🔖

Q31.8 **Other congenital malformations of larynx** 🔖
> Absence of larynx
> Agenesis of larynx
> Atresia of larynx
> Congenital cleft thyroid cartilage
> Congenital fissure of epiglottis
> Congenital stenosis of larynx NEC
> Posterior cleft of cricoid cartilage

Q31.9 **Congenital malformation of larynx, unspecified** 🔖

⬤ **Q32** **Congenital malformations of trachea and bronchus**
> **Excludes1** congenital bronchiectasis (Q33.4)
> (Ex) **For category Q32 CC codes:** See Q31

Q32.0 **Congenital tracheomalacia** 🔖

Q32.1 **Other congenital malformations of trachea** 🔖
> Atresia of trachea
> Congenital anomaly of tracheal cartilage
> Congenital dilatation of trachea
> Congenital malformation of trachea
> Congenital stenosis of trachea
> Congenital tracheocele

Q32.2 **Congenital bronchomalacia** 🔖

Q32.3 **Congenital stenosis of bronchus** 🔖

Q32.4 **Other congenital malformations of bronchus** 🔖
> Absence of bronchus
> Agenesis of bronchus
> Atresia of bronchus
> Congenital diverticulum of bronchus
> Congenital malformation of bronchus NOS

⬤ **Q33** **Congenital malformations of lung**

Q33.0 **Congenital cystic lung** 🔖
> Congenital cystic lung disease
> Congenital honeycomb lung
> Congenital polycystic lung disease
> **Excludes1** cystic fibrosis (E84.0)
> cystic lung disease, acquired or unspecified (J98.4)
> (Ex) Q33.0-Q34.9

Q33.1 **Accessory lobe of lung**
> Azygos lobe (fissured), lung

Q33.2 **Sequestration of lung** 🔖
> (Ex) Q33.0-Q34.9

Q33.3 **Agenesis of lung** 🔖
> Congenital absence of lung (lobe)
> (Ex) Q33.0-Q34.9

Q33.4 **Congenital bronchiectasis** 🔖
> (Ex) J44.9, J47.0-J47.9, J68.1, J68.4-J68.9, Q33.4

Q33.5 **Ectopic tissue in lung**

Q33.6 **Congenital hypoplasia and dysplasia of lung** 🔖
> **Excludes1** pulmonary hypoplasia associated with short gestation (P28.0)
> (Ex) Q33.0-Q34.9

Q33.8 **Other congenital malformations of lung**

Q33.9 **Congenital malformation of lung, unspecified**

⬤ **Q34** **Other congenital malformations of respiratory system**
> **Excludes2** congenital central alveolar hypoventilation syndrome (G47.35)

Q34.0 **Anomaly of pleura**

Q34.1 **Congenital cyst of mediastinum**

Q34.8 **Other specified congenital malformations of respiratory system**
> Atresia of nasopharynx

Q34.9 **Congenital malformation of respiratory system, unspecified**
> Congenital absence of respiratory system
> Congenital anomaly of respiratory system NOS

CLEFT LIP AND CLEFT PALATE (Q35-Q37)

Use additional code to identify associated malformation of the nose (Q30.2)
> **Excludes1** Robin's syndrome (Q87.0)

⬤ **Q35** **Cleft palate**
> **Includes** fissure of palate
> palatoschisis
> **Excludes1** cleft palate with cleft lip (Q37.-)

Q35.1 **Cleft hard palate**

Q35.3 **Cleft soft palate**

Q35.5 **Cleft hard palate with cleft soft palate**

Q35.7 **Cleft uvula**

Q35.9 **Cleft palate, unspecified**
> Cleft palate NOS

Figure 17-3 Cleft palate.

CHAPTER 17 (Q00-Q99)

● **Q36**   **Cleft lip**

> **Includes**   cheiloschisis
>   congenital fissure of lip
>   harelip
>   labium leporinum
>
> **Excludes1**   cleft lip with cleft palate (Q37.-)

  Q36.0   Cleft lip, bilateral

  Q36.1   Cleft lip, median

  Q36.9   Cleft lip, unilateral
>   Cleft lip NOS

● **Q37**   **Cleft palate with cleft lip**

> **Includes**   cheilopalatoschisis

  Q37.0   Cleft hard palate with bilateral cleft lip

  Q37.1   Cleft hard palate with unilateral cleft lip
>   Cleft hard palate with cleft lip NOS

  Q37.2   Cleft soft palate with bilateral cleft lip

  Q37.3   Cleft soft palate with unilateral cleft lip
>   Cleft soft palate with cleft lip NOS

  Q37.4   Cleft hard and soft palate with bilateral cleft lip

  Q37.5   Cleft hard and soft palate with unilateral cleft lip
>   Cleft hard and soft palate with cleft lip NOS

  Q37.8   Unspecified cleft palate with bilateral cleft lip

  Q37.9   Unspecified cleft palate with unilateral cleft lip
>   Cleft palate with cleft lip NOS

OTHER CONGENITAL MALFORMATIONS OF THE DIGESTIVE SYSTEM (Q38-Q45)

● **Q38**   **Other congenital malformations of tongue, mouth and pharynx**

> **Excludes1**   dentofacial anomalies (M26.-)
>   macrostomia (Q18.4)
>   microstomia (Q18.5)

  Q38.0   **Congenital malformations of lips, not elsewhere classified**
>   Congenital fistula of lip
>   Congenital malformation of lip NOS
>   Van der Woude's syndrome
>
> **Excludes1**   cleft lip (Q36.-)
>   cleft lip with cleft palate (Q37.-)
>   macrocheilia (Q18.6)
>   microcheilia (Q18.7)

  Q38.1   **Ankyloglossia**
>   *Restricted movement of tongue resulting in speech difficulty*
>   Tongue tie

  Q38.2   **Macroglossia**
>   *Excessive size of tongue*
>   Congenital hypertrophy of tongue

  Q38.3   **Other congenital malformations of tongue**
>   Aglossia
>   Bifid tongue
>   Congenital adhesion of tongue
>   Congenital fissure of tongue
>   Congenital malformation of tongue NOS
>   Double tongue
>   Hypoglossia
>   Hypoplasia of tongue
>   Microglossia

  Q38.4   **Congenital malformations of salivary glands and ducts**
>   Atresia of salivary glands and ducts
>   Congenital absence of salivary glands and ducts
>   Congenital accessory salivary glands and ducts
>   Congenital fistula of salivary gland

  Q38.5   **Congenital malformations of palate, not elsewhere classified**
>   Congenital absence of uvula
>   Congenital malformation of palate NOS
>   Congenital high arched palate
>
> **Excludes1**   cleft palate (Q35.-)
>   cleft palate with cleft lip (Q37.-)

  Q38.6   **Other congenital malformations of mouth**
>   Congenital malformation of mouth NOS

  Q38.7   **Congenital pharyngeal pouch**
>   Congenital diverticulum of pharynx
>
> **Excludes1**   pharyngeal pouch syndrome (D82.1)

  Q38.8   **Other congenital malformations of pharynx**
>   Congenital malformation of pharynx NOS
>   Imperforate pharynx

● **Q39**   **Congenital malformations of esophagus**

> (Ex) **For category Q39 CC codes Q39.0-Q39.4:** Q39.0-Q39.9, Q45.8-Q45.9
>   **For category Q39 CC codes Q39.5-Q39.9:** Q39.5-Q39.9, Q45.8-Q45.9

  Q39.0   **Atresia of esophagus without fistula** 🔖
>   Atresia of esophagus NOS

  Q39.1   **Atresia of esophagus with tracheo-esophageal fistula** 🔖
>   Atresia of esophagus with broncho-esophageal fistula

  Q39.2   **Congenital tracheo-esophageal fistula without atresia** 🔖
>   Congenital tracheo-esophageal fistula NOS

  Q39.3   **Congenital stenosis and stricture of esophagus** 🔖

  Q39.4   **Esophageal web** 🔖

  Q39.5   **Congenital dilatation of esophagus** 🔖
>   Congenital cardiospasm

  Q39.6   **Congenital diverticulum of esophagus** 🔖
>   Congenital esophageal pouch

  Q39.8   **Other congenital malformations of esophagus** 🔖
>   Congenital absence of esophagus
>   Congenital displacement of esophagus
>   Congenital duplication of esophagus

  Q39.9   **Congenital malformation of esophagus, unspecified** 🔖

● **Q40**   **Other congenital malformations of upper alimentary tract**

  Q40.0   **Congenital hypertrophic pyloric stenosis**
>   Congenital or infantile constriction
>   Congenital or infantile hypertrophy
>   Congenital or infantile spasm
>   Congenital or infantile stenosis
>   Congenital or infantile stricture

  Q40.1   **Congenital hiatus hernia**
>   Congenital displacement of cardia through esophageal hiatus
>
> **Excludes1**   congenital diaphragmatic hernia (Q79.0)

  Q40.2   **Other specified congenital malformations of stomach**
>   Congenital displacement of stomach
>   Congenital diverticulum of stomach
>   Congenital hourglass stomach
>   Congenital duplication of stomach
>   Megalogastria
>   Microgastria

  Q40.3   **Congenital malformation of stomach, unspecified**

  Q40.8   **Other specified congenital malformations of upper alimentary tract**

  Q40.9   **Congenital malformation of upper alimentary tract, unspecified**
>   Congenital anomaly of upper alimentary tract
>   Congenital deformity of upper alimentary tract

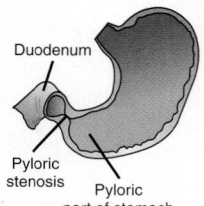

Figure 17-4   Pyloric stenosis.

Duodenum

Pyloric stenosis

Pyloric part of stomach

◀ New   ◀▬ Revised   ~~deleted~~ Deleted   Excludes 1   Excludes 2   Includes   Use additional   Code first   Code also   Unspecified

OGCR Official Guidelines   ● Unacceptable Principal Diagnosis   X Assign placeholder X   🔖 Use Additional Character(s)   ▌ Manifestation Code   **Coding Clinic**

● **Q41 Congenital absence, atresia and stenosis of small intestine**

Includes   congenital obstruction, occlusion or stricture of small intestine or intestine NOS

Excludes1   cystic fibrosis with intestinal manifestation (E84.11)
meconium ileus NOS (without cystic fibrosis) (P76.0)

(Ex) For category Q41 CC codes: Q41.0-Q41.9, Q45.8-Q45.9

Q41.0 Congenital absence, atresia and stenosis of duodenum 🦠

Q41.1 Congenital absence, atresia and stenosis of jejunum 🦠
Apple peel syndrome
Imperforate jejunum

Q41.2 Congenital absence, atresia and stenosis of ileum 🦠

Q41.8 Congenital absence, atresia and stenosis of other specified parts of small intestine 🦠

Q41.9 Congenital absence, atresia and stenosis of small intestine, part unspecified 🦠
Congenital absence, atresia and stenosis of intestine NOS

● **Q42 Congenital absence, atresia and stenosis of large intestine**

Includes   congenital obstruction, occlusion and stricture of large intestine

(Ex) For category Q42 CC codes: Q42.0-Q42.9, Q45.8-Q45.9

Q42.0 Congenital absence, atresia and stenosis of rectum with fistula 🦠

Q42.1 Congenital absence, atresia and stenosis of rectum without fistula 🦠
Imperforate rectum

Q42.2 Congenital absence, atresia and stenosis of anus with fistula 🦠

Q42.3 Congenital absence, atresia and stenosis of anus without fistula 🦠
Imperforate anus

Q42.8 Congenital absence, atresia and stenosis of other parts of large intestine 🦠

Q42.9 Congenital absence, atresia and stenosis of large intestine, part unspecified 🦠

● **Q43 Other congenital malformations of intestine**

(Ex) For category Q43 CC codes unless otherwise indicated: Q41.0-Q43.9

Q43.0 Meckel's diverticulum (displaced) (hypertrophic)
Congenital abnormality in which a pouch remains on the lower end of the small intestine
Persistent omphalomesenteric duct
Persistent vitelline duct

Q43.1 Hirschsprung's disease 🦠
Developmental disorder of enteric nervous system characterized by absence of ganglion cells in distal colon resulting in functional obstruction
Aganglionosis
Congenital (aganglionic) megacolon
(Ex) Q43.1-Q43.2, Q45.8-Q45.9

Q43.2 Other congenital functional disorders of colon 🦠
Congenital dilatation of colon
(Ex) Q43.1-Q43.2, Q45.8-Q45.9

Q43.3 Congenital malformations of intestinal fixation 🦠
Congenital omental, anomalous adhesions [bands]
Congenital peritoneal adhesions [bands]
Incomplete rotation of cecum and colon
Insufficient rotation of cecum and colon
Jackson's membrane
Malrotation of colon
Rotation failure of cecum and colon
Universal mesentery
(Ex) Q43.3-Q43.9

Q43.4 Duplication of intestine 🦠

Q43.5 Ectopic anus 🦠
Anal opening in abnormal location

Q43.6 Congenital fistula of rectum and anus 🦠

Excludes1   congenital fistula of anus with absence, atresia and stenosis (Q42.2)
congenital fistula of rectum with absence, atresia and stenosis (Q42.0)
congenital rectovaginal fistula (Q52.2)
congenital urethrorectal fistula (Q64.73)
pilonidal fistula or sinus (L05.-)

Q43.7 Persistent cloaca 🦠
Malformation in which rectum, vagina, and urinary tract form one channel AKA congenital cloaca
Cloaca NOS

Q43.8 Other specified congenital malformations of intestine 🦠
Congenital blind loop syndrome
Congenital diverticulitis, colon
Congenital diverticulum, intestine
Dolichocolon
Megaloappendix
Megaloduodenum
Microcolon
Transposition of appendix
Transposition of colon
Transposition of intestine

Q43.9 Congenital malformation of intestine, unspecified 🦠

● **Q44 Congenital malformations of gallbladder, bile ducts and liver**

(Ex) For category Q44 CC codes unless otherwise indicated: Q44.0-Q44.7

Q44.0 Agenesis, aplasia and hypoplasia of gallbladder 🦠
Congenital absence of gallbladder

Q44.1 Other congenital malformations of gallbladder 🦠
Congenital malformation of gallbladder NOS
Intrahepatic gallbladder

Q44.2 Atresia of bile ducts 🦠
(Ex) Q44.2-Q44.3, Q45.8-Q45.9

Q44.3 Congenital stenosis and stricture of bile ducts 🦠
(Ex) Q44.2-Q44.3, Q45.8-Q45.9

Q44.4 Choledochal cyst 🦠

Q44.5 Other congenital malformations of bile ducts 🦠
Accessory hepatic duct
Biliary duct duplication
Congenital malformation of bile duct NOS
Cystic duct duplication

Q44.6 Cystic disease of liver 🦠
Fibrocystic disease of liver
(Ex) Q44.0-Q44.1, Q44.4-Q44.7

Q44.7 Other congenital malformations of liver 🦠
Accessory liver
Alagille's syndrome
Congenital absence of liver
Congenital hepatomegaly
Congenital malformation of liver NOS

● **Q45 Other congenital malformations of digestive system**

Excludes2   congenital diaphragmatic hernia (Q79.0)
congenital hiatus hernia (Q40.1)

(Ex) For category Q45 CC codes: Q45.0-Q45.9

Q45.0 Agenesis, aplasia and hypoplasia of pancreas 🦠
Congenital absence of pancreas

Q45.1 Annular pancreas 🦠

Q45.2 Congenital pancreatic cyst 🦠

Q45.3 Other congenital malformations of pancreas and pancreatic duct 🦠
Accessory pancreas
Congenital malformation of pancreas or pancreatic duct NOS

Excludes1   congenital diabetes mellitus (E10.-)
cystic fibrosis (E84.0-E84.9)
fibrocystic disease of pancreas (E84.-)
neonatal diabetes mellitus (P70.2)

CHAPTER 17 (Q00-Q99)

N Newborn Age: 0   **P** Pediatric Age: 0–17   **M** Maternity DX: 12–55   **A** Adult Age: 15–124   ♀ Females Only   ♂ Males Only

🦠 Complication\Comorbidity   🦠 Major C\C   (Ex) CC/MCC Exclusions   🦠 Hospital-Acquired Condition   **1181**

Q45.8   **Other specified congenital malformations of digestive system**
    Absence (complete) (partial) of alimentary tract NOS
    Duplication of digestive system
    Malposition, congenital of digestive system

Q45.9   **Congenital malformation of digestive system, unspecified**
    Congenital anomaly of digestive system
    Congenital deformity of digestive system

CONGENITAL MALFORMATIONS OF GENITAL ORGANS (Q50-Q56)

Excludes1   androgen insensitivity syndrome (E34.5-)
    syndromes associated with anomalies in the number and form of chromosomes (Q90-Q99)

● Q50   **Congenital malformations of ovaries, fallopian tubes and broad ligaments**

  ● Q50.0   **Congenital absence of ovary**
    Excludes1   Turner's syndrome (Q96.-)
    Q50.01   Congenital absence of ovary, unilateral ♀
    Q50.02   Congenital absence of ovary, bilateral ♀

  Q50.1   Developmental ovarian cyst ♀

  Q50.2   Congenital torsion of ovary ♀

  ● Q50.3   **Other congenital malformations of ovary**
    Q50.31   Accessory ovary ♀
    Q50.32   Ovarian streak ♀
      Inadequate ovaries with absent follicular and hormonal function
      46, XX with streak gonads
    Q50.39   Other congenital malformation of ovary ♀
      Congenital malformation of ovary NOS

  Q50.4   **Embryonic cyst of fallopian tube ♀**
    Fimbrial cyst

  Q50.5   **Embryonic cyst of broad ligament ♀**
    Epoophoron cyst
    Parovarian cyst

  Q50.6   **Other congenital malformations of fallopian tube and broad ligament ♀**
    Absence of fallopian tube and broad ligament
    Accessory fallopian tube and broad ligament
    Atresia of fallopian tube and broad ligament
    Congenital malformation of fallopian tube or broad ligament NOS

● Q51   **Congenital malformations of uterus and cervix**

  Q51.0   **Agenesis and aplasia of uterus ♀**
    Congenital absence of uterus

  ● Q51.1   **Doubling of uterus with doubling of cervix and vagina**
    Q51.10   **Doubling of uterus with doubling of cervix and vagina without obstruction ♀**
      Doubling of uterus with doubling of cervix and vagina NOS
    Q51.11   **Doubling of uterus with doubling of cervix and vagina with obstruction ♀**

  Q51.2   **Other doubling of uterus ♀**
    Doubling of uterus NOS
    Septate uterus, complete or partial

  Q51.3   **Bicornate uterus ♀**
    Bicornate uterus, complete or partial
    Birth defect in which uterus has two separate 'horns' that form top of uterus

  Q51.4   **Unicornate uterus ♀**
    Unicornate uterus with or without a separate uterine horn
    Uterus with only one functioning horn
    Uterus with half being undeveloped

  Q51.5   **Agenesis and aplasia of cervix ♀**
    Congenital absence of cervix

  Q51.6   **Embryonic cyst of cervix ♀**

  Q51.7   **Congenital fistulae between uterus and digestive and urinary tracts ♀**

  ● Q51.8   **Other congenital malformations of uterus and cervix**
    ● Q51.81   **Other congenital malformations of uterus**
      Q51.810   **Arcuate uterus ♀**
        Arcuatus uterus
      Q51.811   **Hypoplasia of uterus ♀**
      Q51.818   **Other congenital malformations of uterus ♀**
        Müllerian anomaly of uterus NEC
    ● Q51.82   **Other congenital malformations of cervix**
      Q51.820   **Cervical duplication ♀**
      Q51.821   **Hypoplasia of cervix ♀**
      Q51.828   **Other congenital malformations of cervix ♀**

  Q51.9   **Congenital malformation of uterus and cervix, unspecified ♀**

● Q52   **Other congenital malformations of female genitalia**

  Q52.0   **Congenital absence of vagina ♀**
    Vaginal agenesis, total or partial

  ● Q52.1   **Doubling of vagina**
    Excludes1   doubling of vagina with doubling of uterus and cervix (Q51.1-)
    Q52.10   **Doubling of vagina, unspecified ♀**
      Septate vagina NOS
    Q52.11   **Transverse vaginal septum ♀**
    ● Q52.12   **Longitudinal vaginal septum**
      ~~Longitudinal vaginal septum with or without obstruction~~
      Q52.120   **Longitudinal vaginal septum, nonobstructing ♀ ◄**
      Q52.121   **Longitudinal vaginal septum, obstructing, right side ♀ ◄**
      Q52.122   **Longitudinal vaginal septum, obstructing, left side ♀ ◄**
      Q52.123   **Longitudinal vaginal septum, microperforate, right side ♀ ◄**
      Q52.124   **Longitudinal vaginal septum, microperforate, left side ♀ ◄**
      Q52.129   **Other and unspecified longitudinal vaginal septum ♀ ◄**

  Q52.2   **Congenital rectovaginal fistula ♀**
    Excludes1   cloaca (Q43.7)

  Q52.3   **Imperforate hymen ♀**
    Membrane (hymen) completely closes vaginal orifice

  Q52.4   **Other congenital malformations of vagina ♀**
    Canal of Nuck cyst, congenital
    Congenital malformation of vagina NOS
    Embryonic vaginal cyst
    Gartner's duct cyst

  Q52.5   **Fusion of labia ♀**

  Q52.6   **Congenital malformation of clitoris ♀**

  ● Q52.7   **Other and unspecified congenital malformations of vulva**
    Q52.70   **Unspecified congenital malformations of vulva ♀**
      Congenital malformation of vulva NOS
    Q52.71   **Congenital absence of vulva ♀**
    Q52.79   **Other congenital malformations of vulva ♀**
      Congenital cyst of vulva

  Q52.8   **Other specified congenital malformations of female genitalia ♀**

  Q52.9   **Congenital malformation of female genitalia, unspecified ♀**

● Q53   **Undescended and ectopic testicle**

  ● Q53.0   **Ectopic testis**
    Q53.00   **Ectopic testis, unspecified ♂**
    Q53.01   **Ectopic testis, unilateral ♂**
    Q53.02   **Ectopic testes, bilateral ♂**

◄ New   ◄▦ Revised   ~~deleted~~ Deleted   Excludes 1   Excludes 2   Includes   Use additional   Code first   Code also   Unspecified

OGCR Official Guidelines   ● Unacceptable Principal Diagnosis   X Assign placeholder X   ● Use Additional Character(s)   ▸ Manifestation Code   **Coding Clinic**

1182

Item 17–1 Testes form in the abdomen of the male and only descend into the scrotum during normal embryonic development. "Ectopic" testes are out of their normal place or "retained" (left behind) in the abdomen. Crypto (hidden) orchism (testicle) is a major risk factor for testicular cancer.

ECTOPIC TESTES	CRYPTORCHID TESTES
Penile	Abdominal
Superficial inguinal	Inguinal
(most common)	Prepubic
Femoral	(most common)

Figure 17-5 Undescended testes and the positions of the testes in various types of cryptorchidism or abnormal paths of descent.

- ● **Q53.1 Undescended testicle, unilateral**
  - **Q53.10** Unspecified undescended testicle, unilateral ♂
  - **Q53.11 Abdominal testis, unilateral** ♂
  - **Q53.12 Ectopic perineal testis, unilateral** ♂
- ● **Q53.2 Undescended testicle, bilateral**
  - **Q53.20 Undescended testicle, unspecified, bilateral** ♂
  - **Q53.21 Abdominal testis, bilateral** ♂
  - **Q53.22 Ectopic perineal testis, bilateral** ♂
- **Q53.9 Undescended testicle, unspecified** ♂
  - Cryptorchism NOS
- ● **Q54 Hypospadias**
  - *Birth defect of male; urethra opens in abnormal location on shaft*
  - **Excludes1** epispadias (Q64.0)
  - **Q54.0 Hypospadias, balanic** ♂
    - Hypospadias, coronal
    - Hypospadias, glandular
  - **Q54.1 Hypospadias, penile** ♂
  - **Q54.2 Hypospadias, penoscrotal** ♂
  - **Q54.3 Hypospadias, perineal** ♂
  - **Q54.4 Congenital chordee** ♂
    - Chordee without hypospadias
  - **Q54.8 Other hypospadias** ♂
    - Hypospadias with intersex state
  - **Q54.9 Hypospadias, unspecified** ♂
- ● **Q55 Other congenital malformations of male genital organs**
  - **Excludes1** congenital hydrocele (P83.5)
    - hypospadias (Q54.-)
  - **Q55.0 Absence and aplasia of testis** ♂
    - Monorchism
  - **Q55.1 Hypoplasia of testis and scrotum** ♂
    - Fusion of testes
  - ● **Q55.2 Other and unspecified congenital malformations of testis and scrotum**
    - **Q55.20 Unspecified congenital malformations of testis and scrotum** ♂
      - Congenital malformation of testis or scrotum NOS
    - **Q55.21 Polyorchism** ♂
      - *Developmental anomaly characterized by presence of more than two testes*
    - **Q55.22 Retractile testis** ♂
    - **Q55.23 Scrotal transposition** ♂
    - **Q55.29 Other congenital malformations of testis and scrotum** ♂
  - **Q55.3 Atresia of vas deferens** ♂
    - *Code first any associated cystic fibrosis (E84.-)*

- **Q55.4 Other congenital malformations of vas deferens, epididymis, seminal vesicles and prostate** ♂
  - Absence or aplasia of prostate
  - Absence or aplasia of spermatic cord
  - Congenital malformation of vas deferens, epididymis, seminal vesicles or prostate NOS
- **Q55.5 Congenital absence and aplasia of penis** ♂
- ● **Q55.6 Other congenital malformations of penis**
  - **Q55.61 Curvature of penis (lateral)** ♂
  - **Q55.62 Hypoplasia of penis** ♂
    - *Underdevelopment penis*
    - Micropenis
  - **Q55.63 Congenital torsion of penis** ♂
    - **Excludes1** acquired torsion of penis (N48.82)
  - **Q55.64 Hidden penis** ♂
    - Buried penis
    - Concealed penis
    - **Excludes1** acquired buried penis (N48.83)
  - **Q55.69 Other congenital malformation of penis** ♂
    - Congenital malformation of penis NOS
- **Q55.7 Congenital vasocutaneous fistula** ♂
  - *Abnormal opening between vas deferens and skin*
- **Q55.8 Other specified congenital malformations of male genital organs** ♂
- **Q55.9 Congenital malformation of male genital organ, unspecified** ♂
  - Congenital anomaly of male genital organ
  - Congenital deformity of male genital organ
- ● **Q56 Indeterminate sex and pseudohermaphroditism**
  - *Internal reproductive organs are opposite external physical characteristics.*
  - **Excludes1** 46,XX true hermaphrodite (Q99.1)
    - androgen insensitivity syndrome (E34.5-)
    - chimera 46,XX/46,XY true hermaphrodite (Q99.0)
    - female pseudohermaphroditism with adrenocortical disorder (E25.-)
    - pseudohermaphroditism with specified chromosomal anomaly (Q96-Q99)
    - pure gonadal dysgenesis (Q99.1)
  - **Q56.0 Hermaphroditism, not elsewhere classified**
    - Ovotestis
  - **Q56.1 Male pseudohermaphroditism, not elsewhere classified** ♂
    - 46, XY with streak gonads
    - Male pseudohermaphroditism NOS
  - **Q56.2 Female pseudohermaphroditism, not elsewhere classified** ♀
    - Female pseudohermaphroditism NOS
  - **Q56.3 Pseudohermaphroditism, unspecified**
  - **Q56.4 Indeterminate sex, unspecified**
    - Ambiguous genitalia

CONGENITAL MALFORMATIONS OF THE URINARY SYSTEM (Q60-Q64)

- ● **Q60 Renal agenesis and other reduction defects of kidney**
  - **Includes** congenital absence of kidney
    - congenital atrophy of kidney
    - infantile atrophy of kidney
  - (Ex:) **For category Q60 CC codes: N13.9, Q60.0-Q60.6**
  - **Q60.0 Renal agenesis, unilateral** 🦠
  - **Q60.1 Renal agenesis, bilateral** 🦠
  - **Q60.2 Renal agenesis, unspecified** 🦠
  - **Q60.3 Renal hypoplasia, unilateral** 🦠
  - **Q60.4 Renal hypoplasia, bilateral** 🦠
  - **Q60.5 Renal hypoplasia, unspecified** 🦠
  - **Q60.6 Potter's syndrome** 🦠

CHAPTER 17 (Q00-Q99)

N Newborn Age: 0   **P** Pediatric Age: 0–17   **M** Maternity DX: 12–55   **A** Adult Age: 15–124   ♀ Females Only   ♂ Males Only

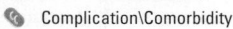 Complication\Comorbidity   🦠 Major C\C   (Ex:) CC/MCC Exclusions   🦠 Hospital-Acquired Condition

1183

● **Q61　Cystic kidney disease**
　Cysts that develop in failing kidney due to end-stage renal disease
　　Excludes1　acquired cyst of kidney (N28.1)
　　　　　　　　　　Potter's syndrome (Q60.6)

● **Q61.0　Congenital renal cyst**
　　Q61.00　Congenital renal cyst, unspecified 🔖
　　　　　Cyst of kidney NOS (congenital)
　　　　　(Ex) N13.9, Q61.00, Q61.9
　　Q61.01　Congenital single renal cyst 🔖
　　　　　(Ex) N13.9, Q61.01
　　Q61.02　Congenital multiple renal cysts 🔖
　　　　　(Ex) N13.9, Q61.02, Q61.5-Q61.8

● **Q61.1　Polycystic kidney, infantile type**
　　　Polycystic kidney, autosomal recessive
　　　(Ex) For category Q61.1 CC codes: N13.9, Q61.11-Q61.3
　　Q61.11　Cystic dilatation of collecting ducts 🔖
　　Q61.19　Other polycystic kidney, infantile type 🔖

Q61.2　Polycystic kidney, adult type 🔖
　　Polycystic kidney, autosomal dominant
　　(Ex) N13.9, Q61.11-Q61.3

Q61.3　Polycystic kidney, unspecified 🔖
　　(Ex) N13.9, Q61.11-Q61.3

Q61.4　Renal dysplasia 🔖
　　Multicystic dysplastic kidney
　　Multicystic kidney (development)
　　Multicystic kidney disease
　　Multicystic renal dysplasia
　　Excludes1　polycystic kidney disease (Q61.11-Q61.3)
　　(Ex) N13.9, Q61.4

Q61.5　Medullary cystic kidney 🔖
　　Nephronopthisis
　　Sponge kidney NOS
　　(Ex) N13.9, Q61.02, Q61.5-Q61.8

Q61.8　Other cystic kidney diseases 🔖
　　Fibrocystic kidney
　　Fibrocystic renal degeneration or disease
　　(Ex) N13.9, Q61.02, Q61.5-Q61.8

Q61.9　Cystic kidney disease, unspecified 🔖
　　Meckel-Gruber syndrome
　　(Ex) N13.9, Q61.00, Q61.9

● **Q62　Congenital obstructive defects of renal pelvis and congenital malformations of ureter**
　　Q62.0　Congenital hydronephrosis 🔖
　　　　(Ex) N13.9, Q62.0-Q62.2, Q62.39

● **Q62.1　Congenital occlusion of ureter**
　　　Atresia and stenosis of ureter
　　　(Ex) For category Q62.1 CC codes: See Q62.0
　　Q62.10　Congenital occlusion of ureter, unspecified 🔖
　　Q62.11　Congenital occlusion of ureteropelvic junction 🔖
　　Q62.12　Congenital occlusion of ureterovesical orifice 🔖

Q62.2　Congenital megaureter 🔖
　　Congenital dilatation of ureter
　　(Ex) See Q62.0

● **Q62.3　Other obstructive defects of renal pelvis and ureter**
　　　(Ex) For category Q62.3 CC codes: See Q62.0
　　Q62.31　Congenital ureterocele, orthotopic 🔖
　　Q62.32　Cecoureterocele 🔖
　　　　Ectopic ureterocele
　　Q62.39　Other obstructive defects of renal pelvis and ureter 🔖
　　　　Ureteropelvic junction obstruction NOS

Q62.4　Agenesis of ureter
　　Congenital absence ureter

Q62.5　Duplication of ureter
　　Accessory ureter
　　Double ureter

Q62.6　Malposition of ureter
　　Q62.60　Malposition of ureter, unspecified
　　Q62.61　Deviation of ureter
　　Q62.62　Displacement of ureter
　　Q62.63　Anomalous implantation of ureter
　　　　Ectopia of ureter
　　　　Ectopic ureter
　　Q62.69　Other malposition of ureter

Q62.7　Congenital vesico-uretero-renal reflux

Q62.8　Other congenital malformations of ureter
　　Anomaly of ureter NOS

● **Q63　Other congenital malformations of kidney**
　　Excludes1　congenital nephrotic syndrome (N04.-)
　　Q63.0　Accessory kidney
　　Q63.1　Lobulated, fused and horseshoe kidney
　　Q63.2　Ectopic kidney
　　　　Congenital displaced kidney
　　　　Malrotation of kidney
　　Q63.3　Hyperplastic and giant kidney
　　　　Compensatory hypertrophy of kidney
　　Q63.8　Other specified congenital malformations of kidney
　　　　Congenital renal calculi
　　Q63.9　Congenital malformation of kidney, unspecified

● **Q64　Other congenital malformations of urinary system**
　　Q64.0　Epispadias ♂
　　　Urethral opening somewhere on dorsum of penis
　　　　Excludes1　hypospadias (Q54.-)

● **Q64.1　Exstrophy of urinary bladder**
　　　Bladder is exposed, inside out, and protrudes through abdominal wall
　　　(Ex) For category Q64.1 CC codes: N13.9, Q64.10-Q64.19, Q64.8-Q64.9
　　Q64.10　Exstrophy of urinary bladder, unspecified 🔖
　　　　Ectopia vesicae
　　Q64.11　Supravesical fissure of urinary bladder 🔖
　　Q64.12　Cloacal extrophy of urinary bladder 🔖
　　Q64.19　Other exstrophy of urinary bladder 🔖
　　　　Extroversion of bladder

Q64.2　Congenital posterior urethral valves 🔖
　　(Ex) N13.9, Q64.2-Q64.39, Q64.8-Q64.9

● **Q64.3　Other atresia and stenosis of urethra and bladder neck**
　　　(Ex) For category Q64.3 CC codes: See Q64.2
　　Q64.31　Congenital bladder neck obstruction 🔖
　　　　Congenital obstruction of vesicourethral orifice
　　Q64.32　Congenital stricture of urethra 🔖
　　Q64.33　Congenital stricture of urinary meatus 🔖
　　Q64.39　Other atresia and stenosis of urethra and bladder neck 🔖
　　　　Atresia and stenosis of urethra and bladder neck NOS

Q64.4　Malformation of urachus
　　Cyst of urachus
　　Patent urachus
　　Prolapse of urachus

Q64.5　Congenital absence of bladder and urethra

Q64.6　Congenital diverticulum of bladder

● **Q64.7　Other and unspecified congenital malformations of bladder and urethra**
　　　Excludes1　congenital prolapse of bladder (mucosa) (Q79.4)
　　Q64.70　Unspecified congenital malformation of bladder and urethra
　　　　Malformation of bladder or urethra NOS
　　Q64.71　Congenital prolapse of urethra
　　Q64.72　Congenital prolapse of urinary meatus
　　Q64.73　Congenital urethrorectal fistula
　　Q64.74　Double urethra
　　Q64.75　Double urinary meatus
　　Q64.79　Other congenital malformations of bladder and urethra

◀ New　◀▥ Revised　~~deleted~~ Deleted　Excludes 1　Excludes 2　Includes　Use additional　Code first　Code also　Unspecified
OGCR Official Guidelines　● Unacceptable Principal Diagnosis　X Assign placeholder X　● Use Additional Character(s)　▶ Manifestation Code　**Coding Clinic**

Q64.8　**Other specified congenital malformations of urinary system**

Q64.9　**Congenital malformation of urinary system, unspecified**
　　　　Congenital anomaly NOS of urinary system
　　　　Congenital deformity NOS of urinary system

CONGENITAL MALFORMATIONS AND DEFORMATIONS OF THE MUSCULOSKELETAL SYSTEM (Q65-Q79)

● Q65　**Congenital deformities of hip**

　　Excludes1　clicking hip (R29.4)

● Q65.0　**Congenital dislocation of hip, unilateral**

　　Q65.00　**Congenital dislocation of unspecified hip, unilateral**

　　Q65.01　**Congenital dislocation of right hip, unilateral**

　　Q65.02　**Congenital dislocation of left hip, unilateral**

　Q65.1　**Congenital dislocation of hip, bilateral**

　Q65.2　**Congenital dislocation of hip, unspecified**

● Q65.3　**Congenital partial dislocation of hip, unilateral**

　　Q65.30　**Congenital partial dislocation of unspecified hip, unilateral**

　　Q65.31　**Congenital partial dislocation of right hip, unilateral**

　　Q65.32　**Congenital partial dislocation of left hip, unilateral**

　Q65.4　**Congenital partial dislocation of hip, bilateral**

　Q65.5　**Congenital partial dislocation of hip, unspecified**

　Q65.6　**Congenital unstable hip**
　　　　Congenital dislocatable hip

● Q65.8　**Other congenital deformities of hip**

　　Q65.81　**Congenital coxa valga**

　　Q65.82　**Congenital coxa vara**

　　Q65.89　**Other specified congenital deformities of hip**
　　　　　　Anteversion of femoral neck
　　　　　　Congenital acetabular dysplasia

　Q65.9　**Congenital deformity of hip, unspecified**

● Q66　**Congenital deformities of feet**

　　Excludes1　reduction defects of feet (Q72.-)
　　　　　　valgus deformities (acquired) (M21.0-)
　　　　　　varus deformities (acquired) (M21.1-)

　Q66.0　**Congenital talipes equinovarus**
　　　　Heel is turned inward from midline and foot is plantar flexed; AKA clubfoot

　Q66.1　**Congenital talipes calcaneovarus**
　　　　Deformity of foot in which heel is turned toward midline of body and anterior of foot is elevated

● Q66.2　**Congenital metatarsus (primus) varus**
　　　　Angulation of first metatarsal bone toward midline of body

　　Q66.21　**Congenital metatarsus primus varus** ◄

　　Q66.22　**Congenital metatarsus adductus** ◄
　　　　　　Congenital metatarsus varus ◄

　Q66.3　**Other congenital varus deformities of feet**
　　　　Hallux varus, congenital

　Q66.4　**Congenital talipes calcaneovalgus**

● Q66.5　**Congenital pes planus**
　　　　Congenital flat foot
　　　　Congenital rigid flat foot
　　　　Congenital spastic (everted) flat foot

　　Excludes1　pes planus, acquired (M21.4)

　　Q66.50　**Congenital pes planus, unspecified foot**

　　Q66.51　**Congenital pes planus, right foot**

　　Q66.52　**Congenital pes planus, left foot**

　Q66.6　**Other congenital valgus deformities of feet**
　　　　Inward angulation
　　　　Congenital metatarsus valgus

　Q66.7　**Congenital pes cavus**

Item 17–2　Equinus foot is a term referring to the hoof of a horse. The deformity is usually congenital or spastic. Talipes equinovarus is referred to as clubfoot. The foot tends to be smaller than normal, with the heel pointing downward and the forefoot turning inward. The heel cord (Achilles tendon) is tight, causing the heel to be drawn up toward the leg.

Figure 17-6　Supination and cavus deformity of forefoot. *(Courtesy Jay Cummings, MD.)* (From Canale: Campbell's Operative Orthopaedics, ed 11, Mosby, Inc., 2007)

Figure 17-7　Talipes. (From Dorland: Dorland's Illustrated Medical Dictionary, ed 31, Saunders, 2007, p 1893)

● Q66.8　**Other congenital deformities of feet**

　　Q66.80　**Congenital vertical talus deformity, unspecified foot**

　　Q66.81　**Congenital vertical talus deformity, right foot**

　　Q66.82　**Congenital vertical talus deformity, left foot**

　　Q66.89　**Other specified congenital deformities of feet**
　　　　　　Congenital asymmetric talipes
　　　　　　Congenital clubfoot NOS
　　　　　　Congenital talipes NOS
　　　　　　Congenital tarsal coalition
　　　　　　Hammer toe, congenital

　Q66.9　**Congenital deformity of feet, unspecified**

● Q67　**Congenital musculoskeletal deformities of head, face, spine and chest**

　　Excludes1　congenital malformation syndromes classified to Q87.-
　　　　　　Potter's syndrome (Q60.6)

　Q67.0　**Congenital facial asymmetry**

　Q67.1　**Congenital compression facies**

　Q67.2　**Dolichocephaly**
　　　　Long head dimension

　Q67.3　**Plagiocephaly**
　　　　Asymmetric shape of head resulting from irregular closure of cranial sutures

　Q67.4　**Other congenital deformities of skull, face and jaw**
　　　　Congenital depressions in skull
　　　　Congenital hemifacial atrophy or hypertrophy
　　　　Deviation of nasal septum, congenital
　　　　Squashed or bent nose, congenital

　　Excludes1　dentofacial anomalies [including malocclusion] (M26.-)
　　　　　　syphilitic saddle nose (A50.5)

Figure 17-8 Mild to moderate inbowing of the lower leg. (From Jones KL: Smith's Recognizable Patterns of Human Malformation, ed 6, Philadelphia, Saunders, 2005)

Figure 17-9 Polydactyly, congenital duplicated thumb. (From DeLee: DeLee and Drez's Orthopaedic Sports Medicine, ed 3, Saunders, An Imprint of Elsevier, 2009)

Q67.5 **Congenital deformity of spine** 🔧
    Congenital postural scoliosis
    Congenital scoliosis NOS
    Excludes1 infantile idiopathic scoliosis (M41.0)
        scoliosis due to congenital bony
        malformation (Q76.3)
    (Ex) Q67.5, Q76.3, Q76.425-Q76.429

Q67.6 **Pectus excavatum**
    Congenital funnel chest
    Funnel-shaped chest depression

Q67.7 **Pectus carinatum**
    Congenital pigeon chest

Q67.8 **Other congenital deformities of chest** 🔧
    Congenital deformity of chest wall NOS
    (Ex) Q67.6-Q67.8, Q68.1, Q74.3

● Q68 **Other congenital musculoskeletal deformities**
    Excludes1 reduction defects of limb(s) (Q71-Q73)
    Excludes2 congenital myotonic chondrodystrophy (G71.13)

Q68.0 **Congenital deformity of sternocleidomastoid muscle**
    Congenital contracture of sternocleidomastoid (muscle)
    Congenital (sternomastoid) torticollis
    Sternomastoid tumor (congenital)

Q68.1 **Congenital deformity of finger(s) and hand** 🔧
    Congenital clubfinger
    Spade-like hand (congenital)
    (Ex) Q67.6-Q67.8, Q68.1, Q74.3

Q68.2 **Congenital deformity of knee**
    Congenital dislocation of knee
    Congenital genu recurvatum
    Hyperextension of knee resulting from hypermobility

Q68.3 **Congenital bowing of femur**
    Excludes1 anteversion of femur (neck) (Q65.89)

Q68.4 **Congenital bowing of tibia and fibula**

Q68.5 **Congenital bowing of long bones of leg, unspecified**

Q68.6 **Discoid meniscus**

Q68.8 **Other specified congenital musculoskeletal deformities**
    Congenital deformity of clavicle
    Congenital deformity of elbow
    Congenital deformity of forearm
    Congenital deformity of scapula
    Congenital deformity of wrist
    Congenital dislocation of elbow
    Congenital dislocation of shoulder
    Congenital dislocation of wrist

● Q69 **Polydactyly**
    AKA hyperdactyly, consists of supernumerary fingers or toes

Q69.0 **Accessory finger(s)**

Q69.1 **Accessory thumb(s)**

Q69.2 **Accessory toe(s)**
    Accessory hallux

Q69.9 **Polydactyly, unspecified**
    Supernumerary digit(s) NOS

● Q70 **Syndactyly**
    Webbing between distal phalanges of adjacent digits

● Q70.0 **Fused fingers**
    Complex syndactyly of fingers with synostosis
    Q70.00 **Fused fingers, unspecified hand**
    Q70.01 **Fused fingers, right hand**
    Q70.02 **Fused fingers, left hand**
    Q70.03 **Fused fingers, bilateral**

● Q70.1 **Webbed fingers**
    Simple syndactyly of fingers without synostosis
    Q70.10 **Webbed fingers, unspecified hand**
    Q70.11 **Webbed fingers, right hand**
    Q70.12 **Webbed fingers, left hand**
    Q70.13 **Webbed fingers, bilateral**

● Q70.2 **Fused toes**
    Complex syndactyly of toes with synostosis
    Q70.20 **Fused toes, unspecified foot**
    Q70.21 **Fused toes, right foot**
    Q70.22 **Fused toes, left foot**
    Q70.23 **Fused toes, bilateral**

● Q70.3 **Webbed toes**
    Simple syndactyly of toes without synostosis
    Q70.30 **Webbed toes, unspecified foot**
    Q70.31 **Webbed toes, right foot**
    Q70.32 **Webbed toes, left foot**
    Q70.33 **Webbed toes, bilateral**

Q70.4 **Polysyndactyly, unspecified**
    Excludes1 specified syndactyly of hand and
        feet - code to specified conditions
        (Q70.0- -Q70.3-)
    Extra and webbed digits

Q70.9 **Syndactyly, unspecified**
    Symphalangy NOS

● Q71 **Reduction defects of upper limb**

● Q71.0 **Congenital complete absence of upper limb**
    Q71.00 **Congenital complete absence of unspecified upper limb**
    Q71.01 **Congenital complete absence of right upper limb**
    Q71.02 **Congenital complete absence of left upper limb**
    Q71.03 **Congenital complete absence of upper limb, bilateral**

● Q71.1 **Congenital absence of upper arm and forearm with hand present**
    Q71.10 **Congenital absence of unspecified upper arm and forearm with hand present**
    Q71.11 **Congenital absence of right upper arm and forearm with hand present**
    Q71.12 **Congenital absence of left upper arm and forearm with hand present**
    Q71.13 **Congenital absence of upper arm and forearm with hand present, bilateral**

● Q71.2 **Congenital absence of both forearm and hand**
    Q71.20 **Congenital absence of both forearm and hand, unspecified upper limb**
    Q71.21 **Congenital absence of both forearm and hand, right upper limb**
    Q71.22 **Congenital absence of both forearm and hand, left upper limb**
    Q71.23 **Congenital absence of both forearm and hand, bilateral**

● Q71.3 **Congenital absence of hand and finger**
    Q71.30 **Congenital absence of unspecified hand and finger**
    Q71.31 **Congenital absence of right hand and finger**
    Q71.32 **Congenital absence of left hand and finger**
    Q71.33 **Congenital absence of hand and finger, bilateral**

CHAPTER 17 (Q00-Q99)

◀ New   ◀═ Revised   ~~deleted~~ Deleted   Excludes 1   Excludes 2   Includes   Use additional   Code first   Code also   Unspecified

OGCR Official Guidelines   ● Unacceptable Principal Diagnosis   X Assign placeholder X   ● Use Additional Character(s)   ▶ Manifestation Code   **Coding Clinic**

● Q71.4　Longitudinal reduction defect of radius
　　　　Clubhand (congenital)
　　　　Radial clubhand
　　　Q71.40　Longitudinal reduction defect of unspecified radius
　　　Q71.41　Longitudinal reduction defect of right radius
　　　Q71.42　Longitudinal reduction defect of left radius
　　　Q71.43　Longitudinal reduction defect of radius, bilateral
● Q71.5　Longitudinal reduction defect of ulna
　　　Q71.50　Longitudinal reduction defect of unspecified ulna
　　　Q71.51　Longitudinal reduction defect of right ulna
　　　Q71.52　Longitudinal reduction defect of left ulna
　　　Q71.53　Longitudinal reduction defect of ulna, bilateral
● Q71.6　Lobster-claw hand
　　　Q71.60　Lobster-claw hand, unspecified hand
　　　Q71.61　Lobster-claw right hand
　　　Q71.62　Lobster-claw left hand
　　　Q71.63　Lobster-claw hand, bilateral
● Q71.8　Other reduction defects of upper limb
　　● Q71.81　Congenital shortening of upper limb
　　　　　Q71.811　Congenital shortening of right upper limb
　　　　　Q71.812　Congenital shortening of left upper limb
　　　　　Q71.813　Congenital shortening of upper limb, bilateral
　　　　　Q71.819　Congenital shortening of unspecified upper limb
　　● Q71.89　Other reduction defects of upper limb
　　　　　Q71.891　Other reduction defects of right upper limb
　　　　　Q71.892　Other reduction defects of left upper limb
　　　　　Q71.893　Other reduction defects of upper limb, bilateral
　　　　　Q71.899　Other reduction defects of unspecified upper limb
● Q71.9　Unspecified reduction defect of upper limb
　　　Q71.90　Unspecified reduction defect of unspecified upper limb
　　　Q71.91　Unspecified reduction defect of right upper limb
　　　Q71.92　Unspecified reduction defect of left upper limb
　　　Q71.93　Unspecified reduction defect of upper limb, bilateral

● Q72　Reduction defects of lower limb
　● Q72.0　Congenital complete absence of lower limb
　　　Q72.00　Congenital complete absence of unspecified lower limb
　　　Q72.01　Congenital complete absence of right lower limb
　　　Q72.02　Congenital complete absence of left lower limb
　　　Q72.03　Congenital complete absence of lower limb, bilateral
　● Q72.1　Congenital absence of thigh and lower leg with foot present
　　　Q72.10　Congenital absence of unspecified thigh and lower leg with foot present
　　　Q72.11　Congenital absence of right thigh and lower leg with foot present
　　　Q72.12　Congenital absence of left thigh and lower leg with foot present
　　　Q72.13　Congenital absence of thigh and lower leg with foot present, bilateral

● Q72.2　Congenital absence of both lower leg and foot
　　　Q72.20　Congenital absence of both lower leg and foot, unspecified lower limb
　　　Q72.21　Congenital absence of both lower leg and foot, right lower limb
　　　Q72.22　Congenital absence of both left lower leg and foot, left lower limb
　　　Q72.23　Congenital absence of both lower leg and foot, bilateral
● Q72.3　Congenital absence of foot and toe(s)
　　　Q72.30　Congenital absence of unspecified foot and toe(s)
　　　Q72.31　Congenital absence of right foot and toe(s)
　　　Q72.32　Congenital absence of left foot and toe(s)
　　　Q72.33　Congenital absence of foot and toe(s), bilateral
● Q72.4　Longitudinal reduction defect of femur
　　　　Proximal femoral focal deficiency
　　　Q72.40　Longitudinal reduction defect of unspecified femur
　　　Q72.41　Longitudinal reduction defect of right femur
　　　Q72.42　Longitudinal reduction defect of left femur
　　　Q72.43　Longitudinal reduction defect of femur, bilateral
● Q72.5　Longitudinal reduction defect of tibia
　　　Q72.50　Longitudinal reduction defect of unspecified tibia
　　　Q72.51　Longitudinal reduction defect of right tibia
　　　Q72.52　Longitudinal reduction defect of left tibia
　　　Q72.53　Longitudinal reduction defect of tibia, bilateral
● Q72.6　Longitudinal reduction defect of fibula
　　　Q72.60　Longitudinal reduction defect of unspecified fibula
　　　Q72.61　Longitudinal reduction defect of right fibula
　　　Q72.62　Longitudinal reduction defect of left fibula
　　　Q72.63　Longitudinal reduction defect of fibula, bilateral
● Q72.7　Split foot
　　　Q72.70　Split foot, unspecified lower limb
　　　Q72.71　Split foot, right lower limb
　　　Q72.72　Split foot, left lower limb
　　　Q72.73　Split foot, bilateral
● Q72.8　Other reduction defects of lower limb
　　● Q72.81　Congenital shortening of lower limb
　　　　　Q72.811　Congenital shortening of right lower limb
　　　　　Q72.812　Congenital shortening of left lower limb
　　　　　Q72.813　Congenital shortening of lower limb, bilateral
　　　　　Q72.819　Congenital shortening of unspecified lower limb
　　● Q72.89　Other reduction defects of lower limb
　　　　　Q72.891　Other reduction defects of right lower limb
　　　　　Q72.892　Other reduction defects of left lower limb
　　　　　Q72.893　Other reduction defects of lower limb, bilateral
　　　　　Q72.899　Other reduction defects of unspecified lower limb
● Q72.9　Unspecified reduction defect of lower limb
　　　Q72.90　Unspecified reduction defect of unspecified lower limb
　　　Q72.91　Unspecified reduction defect of right lower limb
　　　Q72.92　Unspecified reduction defect of left lower limb
　　　Q72.93　Unspecified reduction defect of lower limb, bilateral

CHAPTER 17 (Q00-Q99)

N Newborn Age: 0　**P** Pediatric Age: 0–17　**M** Maternity DX: 12–55　**A** Adult Age: 15–124　♀ Females Only　♂ Males Only

🅒 Complication\Comorbidity　🅜 Major C\C　(Ex) CC/MCC Exclusions　🅗 Hospital-Acquired Condition

1187

● **Q73   Reduction defects of unspecified limb**

Q73.0   Congenital absence of unspecified **limb(s)**
Amelia NOS

Q73.1   Phocomelia, unspecified **limb(s)**
Phocomelia NOS
Absence/shortening of long bones primarily as a result of thalidomide

Q73.8   Other reduction defects of unspecified **limb(s)**
Longitudinal reduction deformity of unspecified limb(s)
Ectromelia of limb NOS
Gross hypoplasia or aplasia of one or more long bones of limb(s)
Hemimelia of limb NOS
Absence of one-half of long bone
Reduction defect of limb NOS

● **Q74   Other congenital malformations of limb(s)**

Excludes1   polydactyly (Q69.-)
reduction defect of limb (Q71-Q73)
syndactyly (Q70.-)

Q74.0   Other congenital malformations of upper limb(s), including shoulder girdle
Accessory carpal bones
Cleidocranial dysostosis
Congenital pseudarthrosis of clavicle
Macrodactylia (fingers)
Madelung's deformity
Radioulnar synostosis
Sprengel's deformity
Triphalangeal thumb

Q74.1   Congenital malformation of knee
Congenital absence of patella
Congenital dislocation of patella
Congenital genu valgum
Congenital genu varum
Rudimentary patella

Excludes1   congenital dislocation of knee (Q68.2)
congenital genu recurvatum (Q68.2)
nail patella syndrome (Q87.2)

Q74.2   Other congenital malformations of lower limb(s), including pelvic girdle
Congenital fusion of sacroiliac joint
Congenital malformation of ankle joint
Congenital malformation of sacroiliac joint

Excludes1   anteversion of femur (neck) (Q65.89)

Q74.3   Arthrogryposis multiplex congenita 🔗
ⒺⓍ Q67.6-Q67.8, Q68.1, Q74.3

Q74.8   Other specified congenital malformations of limb(s)

Q74.9   Unspecified congenital malformation of limb(s)
Congenital anomaly of limb(s) NOS

● **Q75   Other congenital malformations of skull and face bones**

Excludes1   congenital malformation of face NOS (Q18.-)
congenital malformation syndromes classified to Q87.-
dentofacial anomalies [including malocclusion] (M26.-)
musculoskeletal deformities of head and face (Q67.0-Q67.4)
skull defects associated with congenital anomalies of brain such as:
anencephaly (Q00.0)
encephalocele (Q01.-)
hydrocephalus (Q03.-)
microcephaly (Q02)

Q75.0   Craniosynostosis
Premature closure of sutures of skull
Acrocephaly
Imperfect fusion of skull
Oxycephaly
Trigonocephaly

Q75.1   Craniofacial dysostosis
Congenital deformity of head
Crouzon's disease

Item 17-3   Anencephalus is a congenital deformity of the cranial vault. **Craniosynostosis,** also known as craniostenosis and stenocephaly, signifies any form of congenital deformity of the skull that results from the premature closing of the sutures of the skull. **Iniencephaly** is a deformity in which the head and neck are flexed backward to a great extent and the head is very large in comparison to the shortened body.

Figure 17-10 Generalized craniosynostosis in a 4-year-old girl without symptoms or signs of increased intracranial pressure. (From Bell WE, McCormick WF: Increased Intracranial Pressure in Children, ed 2, Philadelphia, WB Saunders, 1978, p 116)

Q75.2   Hypertelorism

Q75.3   Macrocephaly
Unusually large size of head; AKA megalocephaly

Q75.4   Mandibulofacial dysostosis
Franceschetti syndrome
Treacher Collins syndrome

Q75.5   Oculomandibular dysostosis
Ossification of occular and mandibular bones

Q75.8   Other specified congenital malformations of skull and face bones
Absence of skull bone, congenital
Congenital deformity of forehead
Platybasia

Q75.9   Congenital malformation of skull and face bones, unspecified
Congenital anomaly of face bones NOS
Congenital anomaly of skull NOS

● **Q76   Congenital malformations of spine and bony thorax**

Excludes1   congenital musculoskeletal deformities of spine and chest (Q67.5-Q67.8)

Q76.0   Spina bifida occulta

Excludes1   meningocele (spinal) (Q05.-)
spina bifida (aperta) (cystica) (Q05.-)

Q76.1   Klippel-Feil syndrome
Cervical fusion syndrome

Q76.2   Congenital spondylolisthesis
Congenital spondylolysis

Excludes1   spondylolisthesis (acquired) (M43.1-)
spondylolysis (acquired) (M43.0-)

Q76.3   Congenital scoliosis due to congenital bony malformation 🔗
Hemivertebra fusion or failure of segmentation with scoliosis
ⒺⓍ Q67.5, Q76.3, Q76.425-Q76.429

● **Q76.4   Other congenital malformations of spine, not associated with scoliosis**

● **Q76.41   Congenital kyphosis**
Abnormal increase in convexity curvature of thoracic spinal column; AKA humpback

Q76.411   Congenital kyphosis, occipito-atlanto-axial region

Q76.412   Congenital kyphosis, cervical region

Q76.413   Congenital kyphosis, cervicothoracic region

Q76.414   Congenital kyphosis, thoracic region

Q76.415   Congenital kyphosis, thoracolumbar region

Q76.419   Congenital kyphosis, unspecified **region**

◀ New   ◀━ Revised   ~~deleted~~ Deleted   Excludes 1   Excludes 2   Includes   Use additional   Code first   Code also   Unspecified

1188   OGCR Official Guidelines   ● Unacceptable Principal Diagnosis   X Assign placeholder X   ● Use Additional Character(s)   ▶ Manifestation Code   **Coding Clinic**

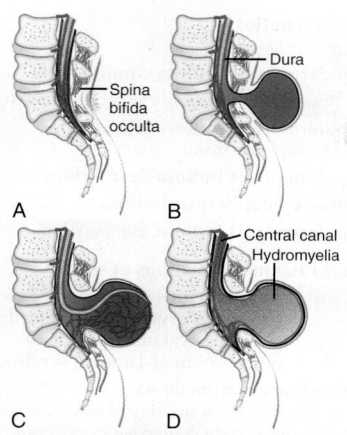

Figure 17-11   A. Spina bifida occulta. **B.** Meningocele.
C. Myelomeningocele. **D.** Myelocystocele (syringomyelocele)
or hydromyelia.

Item 17–4   Spina bifida is a midline spinal defect in which one or more vertebrae fail to fuse, leaving an opening in the vertebral canal. When the defect is not visible, it is called spina bifida occulta, and when it is visible, it is called spina bifida cystica.

● **Q76.42   Congenital lordosis**
   An abnormal increase in curvature of lumbar spine (sway back)
   (Ex) **For category Q76.42 CC codes:** Q67.5, Q76.3, Q76.425-Q76.429

   Q76.425   Congenital lordosis, thoracolumbar region 🔹

   Q76.426   Congenital lordosis, lumbar region 🔹

   Q76.427   Congenital lordosis, lumbosacral region 🔹

   Q76.428   Congenital lordosis, sacral and sacrococcygeal region 🔹

   Q76.429   Congenital lordosis, unspecified region 🔹

   Q76.49   Other congenital malformations of spine, not associated with scoliosis
   Congenital absence of vertebra NOS
   Congenital fusion of spine NOS
   Congenital malformation of lumbosacral (joint) (region) NOS
   Congenital malformation of spine NOS
   Hemivertebra NOS
   Malformation of spine NOS
   Platyspondylisis NOS
   Supernumerary vertebra NOS

Q76.5   Cervical rib
   Supernumerary rib in cervical region

Q76.6   Other congenital malformations of ribs 🔹
   Accessory rib
   Congenital absence of rib
   Congenital fusion of ribs
   Congenital malformation of ribs NOS
   Excludes1   short rib syndrome (Q77.2)
   (Ex) Q76.5-Q76.9, Q77.2

Q76.7   Congenital malformation of sternum 🔹
   Congenital absence of sternum
   Sternum bifidum
   (Ex) Q76.5-Q76.9, Q77.2

Q76.8   Other congenital malformations of bony thorax 🔹
   (Ex) Q76.5-Q76.9, Q77.2

Q76.9   Congenital malformation of bony thorax, unspecified 🔹
   (Ex) Q76.5-Q76.9, Q77.2

● **Q77   Osteochondrodysplasia with defects of growth of tubular bones and spine**
   Excludes1   mucopolysaccharidosis (E76.0-E76.3)
   Excludes2   congenital myotonic chondrodystrophy (G71.13)

Q77.0   Achondrogenesis
   Hypochondrogenesis

Q77.1   Thanatophoric short stature

Q77.2   Short rib syndrome 🔹
   Asphyxiating thoracic dysplasia [Jeune]
   (Ex) Q76.5-Q76.9, Q77.2

Q77.3   Chondrodysplasia punctata
   Benign cartilaginous neoplasms
   Excludes1   rhizomelic chondrodysplasia punctata (E71.43)

Q77.4   Achondroplasia
   Disturbance of epiphyseal chondroblastic growth and maturation, results in dwarfism
   Hypochondroplasia
   Osteosclerosis congenita

Q77.5   Diastrophic dysplasia

Q77.6   Chondroectodermal dysplasia
   Defective development of skin, hair, teeth, with polydactyly and defect of cardiac septum
   Ellis-van Creveld syndrome

Q77.7   Spondyloepiphyseal dysplasia

Q77.8   Other osteochondrodysplasia with defects of growth of tubular bones and spine

Q77.9   Osteochondrodysplasia with defects of growth of tubular bones and spine, unspecified

● **Q78   Other osteochondrodysplasias**
   Disorder of development of bone and cartilage; common cause of dwarfism
   Excludes2   congenital myotonic chondrodystrophy (G71.13)

Q78.0   Osteogenesis imperfecta 🔹
   Fragilitas ossium
   Osteopsathyrosis
   (Ex) Q77.3, Q77.6, Q78.0-Q78.3, Q78.5-Q78.9

Q78.1   Polyostotic fibrous dysplasia
   Albright(-McCune)(-Sternberg) syndrome
   (Ex) See Q78.0

Q78.2   Osteopetrosis 🔹
   Abnormally dense bone; AKA marble bones disease, ivory bones
   Albers-Schönberg syndrome
   Osteosclerosis NOS

Q78.3   Progressive diaphyseal dysplasia
   Camurati-Engelmann syndrome

Q78.4   Enchondromatosis
   Thinning of overlying cortex of bone and distorted length
   Maffucci's syndrome
   Ollier's disease

Q78.5   Metaphyseal dysplasia
   Disturbance in enchondral bone growth, causing ends of shafts to remain larger than normal in circumference
   Pyle's syndrome

Q78.6   Multiple congenital exostoses
   Diaphyseal aclasis

Q78.8   Other specified osteochondrodysplasias
   Osteopoikilosis

Q78.9   Osteochondrodysplasia, unspecified
   Chondrodystrophy NOS
   AKA skeletal dysplasia (dwarfism) caused by genetic mutations affecting hyaline cartilage capping long bones and vertebrae
   Osteodystrophy NOS

CHAPTER 17 (Q00-Q99)

N Newborn Age: Ø   **P** Pediatric Age: Ø–17   **M** Maternity DX: 12–55   **A** Adult Age: 15–124   ♀ Females Only   ♂ Males Only
🔹 Complication\Comorbidity   🔹 Major C\C   (Ex) CC/MCC Exclusions   🔹 Hospital-Acquired Condition

● **Q79 Congenital malformations of musculoskeletal system, not elsewhere classified**

     Excludes2   congenital (sternomastoid) torticollis (Q68.0)

   Q79.0 Congenital diaphragmatic hernia 🔧

       Excludes1   congenital hiatus hernia (Q40.1)

       (Ex) Q40.1, Q79.0-Q79.1

   Q79.1 Other congenital malformations of diaphragm 🔧

       Absence of diaphragm

       Congenital malformation of diaphragm NOS

       Eventration of diaphragm

       (Ex) Q40.1, Q79.0-Q79.1

   Q79.2 Exomphalos 🔧

       Abdominal hernia in which part of intestine protrudes at umbilicus; AKA exomphalos and exumbilication

       Omphalocele

       Excludes1   umbilical hernia (K42.-)

       (Ex) Q79.2-Q79.59

   Q79.3 Gastroschisis 🔧

       Congenital fissure of anterior abdominal wall often with protrusion of small/large intestine

       (Ex) Q79.2-Q79.59

   Q79.4 Prune belly syndrome 🔧

       Congenital prolapse of bladder mucosa

       Eagle-Barrett syndrome

       (Ex) Q79.2-Q79.59

●   **Q79.5 Other congenital malformations of abdominal wall**

       Excludes1   umbilical hernia (K42.-)

       (Ex) For category Q79.5 CC codes: Q79.2-Q79.59

     Q79.51 Congenital hernia of bladder 🔧

     Q79.59 Other congenital malformations of abdominal wall 🔧

   Q79.6 Ehlers-Danlos syndrome 🔧

       (Ex) Q79.6

       Group of inherited disorders of connective tissue; AKA cutis hyperelastica

   Q79.8 Other congenital malformations of musculoskeletal system

       Absence of muscle

       Absence of tendon

       Accessory muscle

       Amyotrophia congenita

       Congenital constricting bands

       Congenital shortening of tendon

       Poland syndrome

   Q79.9 Congenital malformation of musculoskeletal system, unspecified

       Congenital anomaly of musculoskeletal system NOS

       Congenital deformity of musculoskeletal system NOS

OTHER CONGENITAL MALFORMATIONS (Q80-Q89)

● **Q80 Congenital ichthyosis**

     Characterized by increased keratinization, resulting in noninflammatory scaling of skin

     Excludes1   Refsum's disease (G60.1)

   Q80.0 Ichthyosis vulgaris

   Q80.1 X-linked ichthyosis

   Q80.2 Lamellar ichthyosis

       Collodion baby

   Q80.3 Congenital bullous ichthyosiform erythroderma

   Q80.4 Harlequin fetus

   Q80.8 Other congenital ichthyosis

   Q80.9 Congenital ichthyosis, unspecified

● **Q81 Epidermolysis bullosa**

     Loosening of epidermis

   Q81.0 Epidermolysis bullosa simplex

       Excludes1   Cockayne's syndrome (Q87.1)

   Q81.1 Epidermolysis bullosa letalis

       Herlitz' syndrome

   Q81.2 Epidermolysis bullosa dystrophica

   Q81.8 Other epidermolysis bullosa

   Q81.9 Epidermolysis bullosa, unspecified

● **Q82 Other congenital malformations of skin**

     Excludes1   acrodermatitis enteropathica (E83.2)

               congenital erythropoietic porphyria (E80.0)

               pilonidal cyst or sinus (L05.-)

               Sturge-Weber (-Dimitri) syndrome (Q85.8)

   Q82.0 Hereditary lymphedema

       Characterized by swelling of subcutaneous tissue caused by obstruction of lymphatic vessels and resulting edema of lymph fluid

   Q82.1 Xeroderma pigmentosum

       Dry, rough, discolored state of skin, and formation of scaly desquamation

   Q82.2 Mastocytosis

       Characterized by infiltrates of mast cells in tissues/organs

       Urticaria pigmentosa

       Excludes1   malignant mastocytosis (C96.2)

   Q82.3 Incontinentia pigmenti

       Characterized by hyperpigmented cutaneous

   Q82.4 Ectodermal dysplasia (anhidrotic)

       Absence/deficiency of tissues/structures, including teeth, hair, nails, and certain glands

       Excludes1   Ellis-van Creveld syndrome (Q77.6)

   Q82.5 Congenital non-neoplastic nevus

       Birthmark NOS

       Flammeus Nevus

       Portwine Nevus

       Sanguineous Nevus

       Strawberry Nevus

       Vascular Nevus NOS

       Verrucous Nevus

       Excludes2   Café au lait spots (L81.3)

               lentigo (L81.4)

               nevus NOS (D22.-)

               araneus nevus (I78.1)

               melanocytic nevus (D22.-)

               pigmented nevus (D22.-)

               spider nevus (I78.1)

               stellar nevus (I78.1)

   Q82.6 Congenital sacral dimple ◀

       Parasacral dimple ◀

       Excludes2   pilonidal cyst with abscess (L05.01) ◀

               pilonidal cyst without abscess (L05.91) ◀

   Q82.8 Other specified congenital malformations of skin

       Abnormal palmar creases

       Accessory skin tags

       Benign familial pemphigus [Hailey-Hailey]

       Congenital poikiloderma

       Cutis laxa (hyperelastica)

       Dermatoglyphic anomalies

       Inherited keratosis palmaris et plantaris

       Keratosis follicularis [Darier-White]

       Excludes1   Ehlers-Danlos syndrome (Q79.6)

       Coding Clinic: 2016, Q1, P17

   Q82.9 Congenital malformation of skin, unspecified

◀ New   ◀▦▦ Revised   ~~deleted~~ Deleted   Excludes 1   Excludes 2   Includes   Use additional   Code first   Code also   Unspecified

OGCR Official Guidelines   ● Unacceptable Principal Diagnosis   X Assign placeholder X   ● Use Additional Character(s)   ▶ Manifestation Code   **Coding Clinic**

Q83   Congenital malformations of breast
> Excludes2   absence of pectoral muscle (Q79.8)
> hypoplasia of breast (N64.82)
> micromastia (N64.82)

Q83.0   **Congenital absence of breast with absent nipple**

Q83.1   **Accessory breast**
Supernumerary breast

Q83.2   **Absent nipple**

Q83.3   **Accessory nipple**
Supernumerary nipple

Q83.8   **Other congenital malformations of breast**

Q83.9   **Congenital malformation of breast, unspecified**

Q84   Other congenital malformations of integument

Q84.0   **Congenital alopecia**
Congenital atrichosis

Q84.1   **Congenital morphological disturbances of hair, not elsewhere classified**
Beaded hair
Monilethrix
Pili annulati
> Excludes1   Menkes' kinky hair syndrome (E83.0)

Q84.2   **Other congenital malformations of hair**
Congenital hypertrichosis
Congenital malformation of hair NOS
Persistent lanugo

Q84.3   **Anonychia**
Absence of nail
> Excludes1   nail patella syndrome (Q87.2)

Q84.4   **Congenital leukonychia**
Opaque, whitish discoloration of nails; AKA leukopathia unguium

Q84.5   **Enlarged and hypertrophic nails**
Congenital onychauxis
Pachyonychia

Q84.6   **Other congenital malformations of nails**
Congenital clubnail
Congenital koilonychia
Congenital malformation of nail NOS

Q84.8   **Other specified congenital malformations of integument**
Aplasia cutis congenita

Q84.9   **Congenital malformation of integument, unspecified**
Congenital anomaly of integument NOS
Congenital deformity of integument NOS

Q85   Phakomatoses, not elsewhere classified
> Excludes1   ataxia telangiectasia [Louis-Bar] (G11.3)
> familial dysautonomia [Riley-Day] (G90.1)

Q85.0   **Neurofibromatosis (nonmalignant)**
Developmental changes in nervous system and other structures, with formation of neurofibromas

Q85.00   **Neurofibromatosis, unspecified**

Q85.01   **Neurofibromatosis, type 1**
Von Recklinghausen disease

Q85.02   **Neurofibromatosis, type 2**
Acoustic neurofibromatosis

Q85.03   **Schwannomatosis**

Q85.09   **Other neurofibromatosis**

Q85.1   **Tuberous sclerosis** 🔹
Bourneville's disease
Epiloia
> Ⓔ Q85.1-Q85.9, Q89.7, Q89.9

Q85.8   **Other phakomatoses, not elsewhere classified** 🔹
Peutz-Jeghers Syndrome
Sturge-Weber(-Dimitri) syndrome
von Hippel-Lindau syndrome
> Excludes1   Meckel-Gruber syndrome (Q61.9)
> Ⓔ Q85.8-Q85.9, Q89.9

Q85.9   **Phakomatosis, unspecified** 🔹
Hamartosis NOS
> Ⓔ Q85.8-Q85.9, Q89.9

Q86   Congenital malformation syndromes due to known exogenous causes, not elsewhere classified
> Excludes2   iodine-deficiency-related hypothyroidism (E00-E02)
> nonteratogenic effects of substances transmitted via placenta or breast milk (P04.-)

Q86.0   **Fetal alcohol syndrome (dysmorphic)**

Q86.1   **Fetal hydantoin syndrome**
Meadow's syndrome

Q86.2   **Dysmorphism due to warfarin**

Q86.8   **Other congenital malformation syndromes due to known exogenous causes**

Q87   Other specified congenital malformation syndromes affecting multiple systems
Use additional code(s) to identify all associated manifestations

Q87.0   **Congenital malformation syndromes predominantly affecting facial appearance**
Acrocephalopolysyndactyly
Acrocephalosyndactyly [Apert]
Cryptophthalmos syndrome
Cyclopia
Goldenhar syndrome
Moebius syndrome
Oro-facial-digital syndrome
Robin syndrome
Whistling face

Q87.1   **Congenital malformation syndromes predominantly associated with short stature** 🔹
Aarskog syndrome
Cockayne syndrome
De Lange syndrome
Dubowitz syndrome
Noonan syndrome
Prader-Willi syndrome
Robinow-Silverman-Smith syndrome
Russell-Silver syndrome
Seckel syndrome
> Excludes1   Ellis-van Creveld syndrome (Q77.6)
> Smith-Lemli-Opitz syndrome (E78.72)
> Ⓔ E78.71-E78.72, Q85.8-Q85.9, Q87.1-Q87.89, Q89.7-Q89.9, Q99.2

Q87.2   **Congenital malformation syndromes predominantly involving limbs** 🔹
Holt-Oram syndrome
Klippel-Trenaunay-Weber syndrome
Nail patella syndrome
Rubinstein-Taybi syndrome
Sirenomelia syndrome
Thrombocytopenia with absent radius [TAR] syndrome
VATER syndrome
> Ⓔ E78.71-E78.72, Q87.1-Q87.89, Q89.8, Q99.2

Q87.3   **Congenital malformation syndromes involving early overgrowth** 🔹
Beckwith-Wiedemann syndrome
Sotos' syndrome
Weaver syndrome
> Ⓔ See Q87.2

Q87.4   **Marfan's syndrome**
> Ⓔ For category Q87.4 CC codes: See Q87.1

Q87.40   **Marfan's syndrome, unspecified** 🔹

Q87.41   **Marfan's syndrome with cardiovascular manifestations**

Q87.410   **Marfan's syndrome with aortic dilation** 🔹

Q87.418   **Marfan's syndrome with other cardiovascular manifestations** 🔹

Q87.42   **Marfan's syndrome with ocular manifestations** 🔹

Q87.43   **Marfan's syndrome with skeletal manifestation** 🔹

Q87.5 Other congenital malformation syndromes with other skeletal changes 🔗
> (Ex) See Q87.2

● **Q87.8 Other specified congenital malformation syndromes, not elsewhere classified**
> **Excludes1** Zellweger syndrome (E71.510)
> (Ex) For category Q87.8 CC codes: See Q87.2

Q87.81 Alport syndrome 🔗
> *Progressive sensorineural hearing loss, progressive pyelonephritis or glomerulonephritis, and ocular defects*
> Use additional code to identify stage of chronic kidney disease (N18.1-N18.6)

Q87.82 Arterial tortuosity syndrome 🔗 ◀

Q87.89 Other specified congenital malformation syndromes, not elsewhere classified 🔗
> Laurence-Moon (-Bardet)-Biedl syndrome

● **Q89 Other congenital malformations, not elsewhere classified**

● **Q89.0 Congenital absence and malformations of spleen**
> **Excludes1** isomerism of atrial appendages (with asplenia or polysplenia) (Q20.6)
> (Ex) For category Q87.8 CC codes: Q89.01-Q89.09, Q89.9

Q89.01 Asplenia (congenital) 🔗

Q89.09 Congenital malformations of spleen 🔗
> Congenital splenomegaly

Q89.1 Congenital malformations of adrenal gland
> **Excludes1** adrenogenital disorders (E25.-)
> congenital adrenal hyperplasia (E25.0)

Q89.2 Congenital malformations of other endocrine glands
> Congenital malformation of parathyroid or thyroid gland
> Persistent thyroglossal duct
> Thyroglossal cyst
> **Excludes1** congenital goiter (E03.0)
> congenital hypothyroidism (E03.1)

Q89.3 Situs inversus 🔗
> *Lateral transposition of viscera of thorax and abdomen*
> Dextrocardia with situs inversus
> Mirror-image atrial arrangement with situs inversus
> Situs inversus or transversus abdominalis
> Situs inversus or transversus thoracis
> Transposition of abdominal viscera
> Transposition of thoracic viscera
> **Excludes1** dextrocardia NOS (Q24.0)
> (Ex) Q89.3, Q89.7, Q89.9

Q89.4 Conjoined twins 🔗
> Craniopagus
> Dicephaly
> Pygopagus
> Thoracopagus
> (Ex) Q89.4-Q89.7, Q89.9

Q89.7 Multiple congenital malformations, not elsewhere classified 🔗
> Multiple congenital anomalies NOS
> Multiple congenital deformities NOS
> **Excludes1** congenital malformation syndromes affecting multiple systems (Q87.-)
> (Ex) Q89.3, Q89.7, Q89.9

Q89.8 Other specified congenital malformations 🔗
> Use additional code(s) to identify all associated manifestations
> (Ex) See Q87.2

Q89.9 Congenital malformation, unspecified
> Congenital anomaly NOS
> Congenital deformity NOS

CHROMOSOMAL ABNORMALITIES, NOT ELSEWHERE CLASSIFIED (Q90-Q99)
> **Excludes2** mitochondrial metabolic disorders (E88.4-)

● **Q90 Down syndrome**
> Use additional code(s) to identify any associated physical conditions and degree of intellectual disabilities (F70-F79)

Q90.0 Trisomy 21, nonmosaicism (meiotic nondisjunction)
> *Trisomy 21, nondisjunction, accounts for 95% of Downs syndrome cases*

Q90.1 Trisomy 21, mosaicism (mitotic nondisjunction)

Q90.2 Trisomy 21, translocation

Q90.9 Down syndrome, unspecified
> Trisomy 21 NOS

● **Q91 Trisomy 18 and Trisomy 13**
> (Ex) For category Q91 CC codes: Q90.0-Q99.1, Q99.8-Q99.9

Q91.0 Trisomy 18, nonmosaicism (meiotic nondisjunction) 🔗

Q91.1 Trisomy 18, mosaicism (mitotic nondisjunction) 🔗

Q91.2 Trisomy 18, translocation 🔗

Q91.3 Trisomy 18, unspecified 🔗

Q91.4 Trisomy 13, nonmosaicism (meiotic nondisjunction) 🔗

Q91.5 Trisomy 13, mosaicism (mitotic nondisjunction) 🔗

Q91.6 Trisomy 13, translocation 🔗

Q91.7 Trisomy 13, unspecified 🔗

● **Q92 Other trisomies and partial trisomies of the autosomes, not elsewhere classified**
> **Includes** unbalanced translocations and insertions
> **Excludes1** trisomies of chromosomes 13, 18, 21 (Q90-Q91)

Q92.0 Whole chromosome trisomy, nonmosaicism (meiotic nondisjunction)

Q92.1 Whole chromosome trisomy, mosaicism (mitotic nondisjunction)

Q92.2 Partial trisomy
> Less than whole arm duplicated
> Whole arm or more duplicated
> **Excludes1** partial trisomy due to unbalanced translocation (Q92.5)

Q92.5 Duplications with other complex rearrangements
> Partial trisomy due to unbalanced translocations
> Code also any associated deletions due to unbalanced translocations, inversions and insertions (Q93.7)

● **Q92.6 Marker chromosomes**
> Trisomies due to dicentrics
> Trisomies due to extra rings
> Trisomies due to isochromosomes
> Individual with marker heterochromatin

Q92.61 Marker chromosomes in normal individual

Q92.62 Marker chromosomes in abnormal individual

Q92.7 Triploidy and polyploidy

Q92.8 Other specified trisomies and partial trisomies of autosomes
> Duplications identified by fluorescence in situ hybridization (FISH)
> Duplications identified by in situ hybridization (ISH)
> Duplications seen only at prometaphase

Q92.9 Trisomy and partial trisomy of autosomes, unspecified

● **Q93 Monosomies and deletions from the autosomes, not elsewhere classified**
> (Ex) For category Q93 CC codes unless otherwise indicated: Q90.0-Q99.1, Q99.8-Q99.9

Q93.0 Whole chromosome monosomy, nonmosaicism (meiotic nondisjunction)

Q93.1 Whole chromosome monosomy, mosaicism (mitotic nondisjunction)

Q93.2 Chromosome replaced with ring, dicentric or isochromosome

Q93.3 Deletion of short arm of chromosome 4 🔗
> Wolff-Hirschorn syndrome

◀ New   ◀▪▪ Revised   ~~deleted~~ Deleted   Excludes 1   Excludes 2   Includes   Use additional   Code first   Code also   Unspecified
OGCR Official Guidelines   ● Unacceptable Principal Diagnosis   X Assign placeholder X   ● Use Additional Character(s)   ▷ Manifestation Code   **Coding Clinic**

Q93.4　**Deletion of short arm of chromosome 5** 🗘
　　　　Cri-du-chat syndrome
　　　　(Ex) Q90.0–Q99.1, Q99.8–Q99.9

Q93.5　**Other deletions of part of a chromosome** 🗘
　　　　Angelman syndrome

Q93.7　**Deletions with other complex rearrangements** 🗘
　　　　Deletions due to unbalanced translocations, inversions and insertions
　　　　Code also any associated duplications due to unbalanced translocations, inversions and insertions (Q92.5)

● **Q93.8**　**Other deletions from the autosomes**

　　Q93.81　**Velo-cardio-facial syndrome** 🗘
　　　　　Deletion 22q11.2
　　　　　(Ex) Q90.0–Q99.1, Q99.8–Q99.9

　　Q93.88　**Other microdeletions Miller-Dieker syndrome** 🗘
　　　　　Smith-Magenis syndrome
　　　　　(Ex) Q90.0–Q99.1, Q99.8–Q99.9

　　Q93.89　**Other deletions from the autosomes** 🗘
　　　　　Deletions identified by fluorescence in situ hybridization (FISH)
　　　　　Deletions identified by in situ hybridization (ISH)
　　　　　Deletions seen only at prometaphase

Q93.9　**Deletion from autosomes, unspecified** 🗘

● **Q95**　**Balanced rearrangements and structural markers, not elsewhere classified**

　　Includes　Robertsonian and balanced reciprocal translocations and insertions

Q95.0　**Balanced translocation and insertion in normal individual**

Q95.1　**Chromosome inversion in normal individual**

Q95.2　**Balanced autosomal rearrangement in abnormal individual**

Q95.3　**Balanced sex/autosomal rearrangement in abnormal individual**

Q95.5　**Individual with autosomal fragile site**

Q95.8　**Other balanced rearrangements and structural markers**

Q95.9　**Balanced rearrangement and structural marker, unspecified**

● **Q96**　**Turner's syndrome**
　　Caused by missing or incomplete X chromosome affecting growth and sexual development

　　Excludes1　Noonan syndrome (Q87.1)

Q96.0　**Karyotype 45, X** ♀

Q96.1　**Karyotype 46, X iso (Xq)** ♀
　　　　Karyotype 46, isochromosome Xq

Q96.2　**Karyotype 46, X with abnormal sex chromosome, except iso (Xq)** ♀
　　　　Karyotype 46, X with abnormal sex chromosome, except isochromosome Xq

Q96.3　**Mosaicism, 45, X/46, XX or XY** ♀

Q96.4　**Mosaicism, 45, X/other cell line(s) with abnormal sex chromosome** ♀

Q96.8　**Other variants of Turner's syndrome** ♀

Q96.9　**Turner's syndrome, unspecified** ♀

● **Q97**　**Other sex chromosome abnormalities, female phenotype, not elsewhere classified**

　　Excludes1　Turner's syndrome (Q96.-)

Q97.0　**Karyotype 47, XXX** ♀

Q97.1　**Female with more than three X chromosomes** ♀

Q97.2　**Mosaicism, lines with various numbers of X chromosomes** ♀

Q97.3　**Female with 46, XY karyotype** ♀

Q97.8　**Other specified sex chromosome abnormalities, female phenotype** ♀

Q97.9　**Sex chromosome abnormality, female phenotype, unspecified** ♀

● **Q98**　**Other sex chromosome abnormalities, male phenotype, not elsewhere classified**

Q98.0　**Klinefelter syndrome karyotype 47, XXY** ♂

Q98.1　**Klinefelter syndrome, male with more than two X chromosomes** ♂

Q98.3　**Other male with 46, XX karyotype** ♂

Q98.4　**Klinefelter syndrome, unspecified** ♂

Q98.5　**Karyotype 47, XYY** ♂

Q98.6　**Male with structurally abnormal sex chromosome** ♂

Q98.7　**Male with sex chromosome mosaicism** ♂

Q98.8　**Other specified sex chromosome abnormalities, male phenotype** ♂

Q98.9　**Sex chromosome abnormality, male phenotype, unspecified** ♂

● **Q99**　**Other chromosome abnormalities, not elsewhere classified**

Q99.0　**Chimera 46, XX/46, XY**
　　　　Chimera 46, XX/46, XY true hermaphrodite

Q99.1　**46, XX true hermaphrodite**
　　　　46, XX with streak gonads
　　　　46, XY with streak gonads
　　　　Pure gonadal dysgenesis

Q99.2　**Fragile X chromosome**
　　　　Fragile X syndrome

Q99.8　**Other specified chromosome abnormalities**

Q99.9　**Chromosomal abnormality, unspecified**

CHAPTER 18

SYMPTOMS, SIGNS AND ABNORMAL CLINICAL AND LABORATORY FINDINGS, NOT ELSEWHERE CLASSIFIED (R00-R99)

OGCR Chapter-Specific Coding Guidelines

18. **Chapter 18: Symptoms, signs, and abnormal clinical and laboratory findings, not elsewhere classified (R00-R99)**

Chapter 18 includes symptoms, signs, abnormal results of clinical or other investigative procedures, and ill-defined conditions regarding which no diagnosis classifiable elsewhere is recorded. Signs and symptoms that point to a specific diagnosis have been assigned to a category in other chapters of the classification.

a. Use of symptom codes

Codes that describe symptoms and signs are acceptable for reporting purposes when a related definitive diagnosis has not been established (confirmed) by the provider.

b. Use of a symptom code with a definitive diagnosis code

Codes for signs and symptoms may be reported in addition to a related definitive diagnosis when the sign or symptom is not routinely associated with that diagnosis, such as the various signs and symptoms associated with complex syndromes. The definitive diagnosis code should be sequenced before the symptom code.

Signs or symptoms that are associated routinely with a disease process should not be assigned as additional codes, unless otherwise instructed by the classification.

c. Combination codes that include symptoms

ICD-10-CM contains a number of combination codes that identify both the definitive diagnosis and common symptoms of that diagnosis. When using one of these combination codes, an additional code should not be assigned for the symptom.

d. Repeated falls

Code R29.6, Repeated falls, is for use for encounters when a patient has recently fallen and the reason for the fall is being investigated.

Code Z91.81, History of falling, is for use when a patient has fallen in the past and is at risk for future falls. When appropriate, both codes R29.6 and Z91.81 may be assigned together.

e. Coma scale

The coma scale codes (R40.2-) can be used in conjunction with traumatic brain injury codes, acute cerebrovascular disease or sequelae of cerebrovascular disease codes. These codes are primarily for use by trauma registries, but they may be used in any setting where this information is collected. **The coma scale may also be used to assess the status of the central nervous system for other non-trauma conditions, such as monitoring patients in the intensive care unit regardless of medical condition.** The coma scale codes should be sequenced after the diagnosis code(s).

These codes, one from each subcategory, are needed to complete the scale. The 7th character indicates when the scale was recorded. The 7th character should match for all three codes.

At a minimum, report the initial score documented on presentation at your facility. This may be a score from the emergency medicine technician (EMT) or in the emergency department. If desired, a facility may choose to capture multiple coma scale scores.

Assign code R40.24, Glasgow coma scale, total score, when only the total score is documented in the medical record and not the individual score(s).

f. Functional quadriplegia

Functional quadriplegia (code R53.2) is the lack of ability to use one's limbs or to ambulate due to extreme debility. It is not associated with neurologic deficit or injury, and code R53.2 should not be used for cases of neurologic quadriplegia. It should only be assigned if functional quadriplegia is specifically documented in the medical record.

g. SIRS due to Non-Infectious Process

The systemic inflammatory response syndrome (SIRS) can develop as a result of certain non-infectious disease processes, such as trauma, malignant neoplasm, or pancreatitis. When SIRS is documented with a noninfectious condition, and no subsequent infection is documented, the code for the underlying condition, such as an injury, should be assigned, followed by code R65.10, Systemic inflammatory response syndrome (SIRS) of non-infectious origin without acute organ dysfunction, or code R65.11, Systemic inflammatory response syndrome (SIRS) of non-infectious origin with acute organ dysfunction. If an associated acute organ dysfunction is documented, the appropriate code(s) for the specific type of organ dysfunction(s) should be assigned in addition to code R65.11. If acute organ dysfunction is documented, but it cannot be determined if the acute organ dysfunction is associated with SIRS or due to another condition (e.g., directly due to the trauma), the provider should be queried.

h. Death NOS

Code R99, Ill-defined and unknown cause of mortality, is only for use in the very limited circumstance when a patient who has already died is brought into an emergency department or other healthcare facility and is pronounced dead upon arrival. It does not represent the discharge disposition of death.

i. NIHSS Stroke Scale

The NIH stroke scale (NIHSS) codes (R29.7- -) can be used in conjunction with acute stroke codes (I63) to identify the patient's neurological status and the severity of the stroke. The stroke scale codes should be sequenced after the acute stroke diagnosis code(s).

At a minimum, report the initial score documented. If desired, a facility may choose to capture multiple stroke scale scores.

See Section I.B.14. for information concerning the medical record documentation that may be used for assignment of the NIHSS codes.

OGCR Section I.B.4.

Signs and symptoms

Codes that describe symptoms and signs, as opposed to diagnoses, are acceptable for reporting purposes when a related definitive diagnosis has not been established (confirmed) by the provider. Chapter 18 of ICD-10-CM, Symptoms, Signs, and Abnormal Clinical and Laboratory Findings, Not Elsewhere Classified (codes R00.0-R99) contains many, but not all codes for symptoms.

CHAPTER 18

SYMPTOMS, SIGNS AND ABNORMAL CLINICAL AND LABORATORY FINDINGS, NOT ELSEWHERE CLASSIFIED (R00-R99)

Note: This chapter includes symptoms, signs, abnormal results of clinical or other investigative procedures, and ill-defined conditions regarding which no diagnosis classifiable elsewhere is recorded.

Signs and symptoms that point rather definitely to a given diagnosis have been assigned to a category in other chapters of the classification. In general, categories in this chapter include the less well-defined conditions and symptoms that, without the necessary study of the case to establish a final diagnosis, point perhaps equally to two or more diseases or to two or more systems of the body. Practically all categories in the chapter could be designated 'not otherwise specified', 'unknown etiology' or 'transient'. The Alphabetical Index should be consulted to determine which symptoms and signs are to be allocated here and which to other chapters. The residual subcategories, numbered .8, are generally provided for other relevant symptoms that cannot be allocated elsewhere in the classification.

The conditions and signs or symptoms included in categories R00-R94 consist of:

(a) cases for which no more specific diagnosis can be made even after all the facts bearing on the case have been investigated;

(b) signs or symptoms existing at the time of initial encounter that proved to be transient and whose causes could not be determined;

(c) provisional diagnosis in a patient who failed to return for further investigation or care;

(d) cases referred elsewhere for investigation or treatment before the diagnosis was made;

(e) cases in which a more precise diagnosis was not available for any other reason;

(f) certain symptoms, for which supplementary information is provided, that represent important problems in medical care in their own right.

Excludes2   abnormal findings on antenatal screening of mother (O28.-)

certain conditions originating in the perinatal period (P04-P96)

signs and symptoms classified in the body system chapters

signs and symptoms of breast (N63, N64.5)

This chapter contains the following blocks:

R00-R09	Symptoms and signs involving the circulatory and respiratory systems
R10-R19	Symptoms and signs involving the digestive system and abdomen
R20-R23	Symptoms and signs involving the skin and subcutaneous tissue
R25-R29	Symptoms and signs involving the nervous and musculoskeletal systems
R30-R39	Symptoms and signs involving the genitourinary system
R40-R46	Symptoms and signs involving cognition, perception, emotional state and behavior
R47-R49	Symptoms and signs involving speech and voice
R50-R69	General symptoms and signs
R70-R79	Abnormal findings on examination of blood, without diagnosis
R80-R82	Abnormal findings on examination of urine, without diagnosis
R83-R89	Abnormal findings on examination of other body fluids, substances and tissues, without diagnosis
R90-R94	Abnormal findings on diagnostic imaging and in function studies, without diagnosis
R97	Abnormal tumor markers
R99	Ill-defined and unknown cause of mortality

SYMPTOMS AND SIGNS INVOLVING THE CIRCULATORY AND RESPIRATORY SYSTEMS (R00-R09)

● **R00**   **Abnormalities of heart beat**

     Excludes1   abnormalities originating in the perinatal period (P29.1-)

     Excludes2   specified arrhythmias (I47-I49) ◀

   R00.0   **Tachycardia,** **unspecified**

     Rapid heart rate >100 beats

     Rapid heart beat

     Sinoauricular tachycardia NOS

     Sinus [sinusal] tachycardia NOS

     Excludes1   neonatal tachycardia (P29.11)

         paroxysmal tachycardia (I47.-)

   R00.1   **Bradycardia,** **unspecified**

     Slow heart rate, <60

     Sinoatrial bradycardia

     Sinus bradycardia

     Slow heart beat

     Vagal bradycardia

     Use additional code for adverse effect, if applicable, to identify drug (T36-T50 with fifth or sixth character 5)

     Excludes1   neonatal bradycardia (P29.12)

   R00.2   **Palpitations**

     Awareness of heart beat

   R00.8   **Other abnormalities of heart beat**

   R00.9   **Unspecified abnormalities of heart beat**

N Newborn Age: 0   **P** Pediatric Age: 0–17   **M** Maternity DX: 12–55   **A** Adult Age: 15–124   ♀ Females Only   ♂ Males Only

Complication\Comorbidity   Major C\C   Ⓔ CC/MCC Exclusions   Hospital-Acquired Condition   **1195**

● **R01**   **Cardiac murmurs and other cardiac sounds**

> **Excludes1**   cardiac murmurs and sounds originating in the perinatal period (P29.8)

R01.0   **Benign and innocent cardiac murmurs**
Functional cardiac murmur

R01.1   **Cardiac murmur, unspecified**
Cardiac bruit NOS
Heart murmur NOS
Systolic murmur NOS ◀

R01.2   **Other cardiac sounds**
Cardiac dullness, increased or decreased
Precordial friction

OGCR   Section I.C.9.a.7.

> Hypertension, Transient
> Assign code R03.0, Elevated blood pressure reading without diagnosis of hypertension, unless patient has an established diagnosis of hypertension. Assign code O13.-, Gestational [pregnancy-induced] hypertension with significant proteinuria, or O14.-, Pre-eclampsia, for transient hypertension of pregnancy.

● **R03**   **Abnormal blood-pressure reading, without diagnosis**

R03.0   **Elevated blood-pressure reading, without diagnosis of hypertension**
Note: This category is to be used to record an episode of elevated blood pressure in a patient in whom no formal diagnosis of hypertension has been made, or as an isolated incidental finding.
MCE: Questionable admission when principal dx

R03.1   **Nonspecific low blood-pressure reading**

> **Excludes1**   hypotension (I95.-)
> maternal hypotension syndrome (O26.5-)
> neurogenic orthostatic hypotension (G90.3)

● **R04**   **Hemorrhage from respiratory passages**
Ⓔ **For category R04 CC codes:** R04.2-R04.9, R09.3, R68.13

R04.0   **Epistaxis**
Hemorrhage from nose
Nosebleed

R04.1   **Hemorrhage from throat**

> **Excludes2**   hemoptysis (R04.2)

R04.2   **Hemoptysis** 🔖
Blood-stained sputum
Cough with hemorrhage

● **R04.8**   **Hemorrhage from other sites in respiratory passages**

R04.81   **Acute idiopathic pulmonary hemorrhage in infants** 🔖   P
AIPHI
Acute idiopathic hemorrhage in infants over 28 days old

> **Excludes1**   perinatal pulmonary hemorrhage (P26.-)
> von Willebrand's disease (D68.0)

R04.89   **Hemorrhage from other sites in respiratory passages** 🔖
Pulmonary hemorrhage NOS

R04.9   **Hemorrhage from respiratory passages, unspecified** 🔖

R05   **Cough**

> **Excludes1**   cough with hemorrhage (R04.2)
> smoker's cough (J41.0)

● **R06**   **Abnormalities of breathing**

> **Excludes1**   acute respiratory distress syndrome (J80)
> respiratory arrest (R09.2)
> respiratory arrest of newborn (P28.81)
> respiratory distress syndrome of newborn (P22.-)
> respiratory failure (J96.-)
> respiratory failure of newborn (P28.5)

● **R06.0**   **Dyspnea**

> **Excludes1**   tachypnea NOS (R06.82)
> transient tachypnea of newborn (P22.1)

R06.00   **Dyspnea, unspecified**

R06.01   **Orthopnea**

R06.02   **Shortness of breath**

R06.09   **Other forms of dyspnea**

R06.1   **Stridor**
Harsh, high-pitched breath sound

> **Excludes1**   congenital laryngeal stridor (P28.89)
> laryngismus (stridulus) (J38.5)

R06.2   **Wheezing**

> **Excludes1**   Asthma (J45.-)

Coding Clinic: 2016, Q2, P34

R06.3   **Periodic breathing** 🔖
Cheyne-Stokes breathing
An abnormal pattern of breathing with gradually increasing and decreasing tidal volume with some periods of apnea
Ⓔ J22, J80, I96.00-I96.92, J98.8-J98.9, R06.3, R06.81, R09.2

R06.4   **Hyperventilation**

> **Excludes1**   psychogenic hyperventilation (F45.8)

R06.5   **Mouth breathing**

> **Excludes2**   dry mouth NOS (R68.2)

R06.6   **Hiccough**

> **Excludes1**   psychogenic hiccough (F45.8)

R06.7   **Sneezing**

● **R06.8**   **Other abnormalities of breathing**

R06.81   **Apnea, not elsewhere classified**
Apnea NOS

> **Excludes1**   apnea (of) newborn (P28.4)
> sleep apnea (G47.3-)
> sleep apnea of newborn (primary) (P28.3)

R06.82   **Tachypnea, not elsewhere classified**
Tachypnea NOS

> **Excludes1**   transitory tachypnea of newborn (P22.1)

R06.83   **Snoring**

R06.89   **Other abnormalities of breathing**
Breath-holding (spells)
Sighing

R06.9   **Unspecified abnormalities of breathing**

● **R07**   **Pain in throat and chest**

> **Excludes1**   epidemic myalgia (B33.0)
> **Excludes2**   jaw pain R68.84
> pain in breast (N64.4)

R07.0   **Pain in throat**

> **Excludes1**   chronic sore throat (J31.2)
> sore throat (acute) NOS (J02.9)
> **Excludes2**   dysphagia (R13.1-)
> pain in neck (M54.2)

R07.1   **Chest pain on breathing**
Painful respiration

R07.2   **Precordial pain**

● **R07.8**   **Other chest pain**

R07.81   **Pleurodynia**
Pleurodynia NOS

> **Excludes1**   epidemic pleurodynia (B33.0)

R07.82   **Intercostal pain**

R07.89   **Other chest pain**
Anterior chest-wall pain NOS

R07.9   **Chest pain, unspecified**

◀ New   ◀◀ Revised   ~~deleted~~ Deleted   Excludes 1   Excludes 2   Includes   Use additional   Code first   Code also   Unspecified

1196   OGCR Official Guidelines   ● Unacceptable Principal Diagnosis   X Assign placeholder X   ● Use Additional Character(s)   ▶ Manifestation Code   **Coding Clinic**

● **R09   Other symptoms and signs involving the circulatory and respiratory system**

   Excludes1   acute respiratory distress syndrome (J80)
                   respiratory arrest of newborn (P28.81)
                   respiratory distress syndrome of newborn (P22.0)
                   respiratory failure (J96.-)
                   respiratory failure of newborn (P28.5)

● **R09.0   Asphyxia and hypoxemia**

   Excludes1   asphyxia due to carbon monoxide (T58.-)
                   asphyxia due to foreign body in
                       respiratory tract (T17.-)
                   birth (intrauterine) asphyxia (P84)
                   hypercapnia (R06.4)
                   hyperventilation (R06.4)
                   traumatic asphyxia (T71.-)

   R09.01   Asphyxia 🔧
      (Ex) G89.0-G89.4, J80, J96.00-J96.92, R09.01-R09.02, R09.2,
           R29.700-R29.742, R41.0-R41.3, R41.82, R41.9, R44.8-R44.9,
           R45.83-R45.84, R46.0-R46.89, R52, R68.0-R68.19,
           R68.81-R68.83, R68.89-R69

   R09.02   Hypoxemia

R09.1   Pleurisy
   *Occurs when double membrane (pleura) lining chest cavity
       and lung surface becomes inflamed causing sharp pain
       on inspiration/expiration*

   Excludes1   pleurisy with effusion (J90)

R09.2   Respiratory arrest 🔧
   Cardiorespiratory failure

   Excludes1   cardiac arrest (I46.-)
                   respiratory arrest of newborn (P28.81)
                   respiratory distress of newborn (P22.0)
                   respiratory failure (J96.-)
                   respiratory failure of newborn (P28.5)
                   respiratory insufficiency (R06.89)
                   respiratory insufficiency of newborn
                       (P28.5)

   MCC: Only if patient discharged alive
   (Ex) See R09.01

R09.3   Abnormal sputum
   Abnormal amount of sputum
   Abnormal color of sputum
   Abnormal odor of sputum
   Excessive sputum

   Excludes1   blood-stained sputum (R04.2)

● **R09.8   Other specified symptoms and signs involving the circulatory and respiratory systems**

   R09.81   Nasal congestion

   R09.82   Postnasal drip

   **R09.89   Other specified symptoms and signs involving
               the circulatory and respiratory systems**
      Bruit (arterial)
      Abnormal chest percussion
      Feeling of foreign body in throat
      Friction sounds in chest
      Chest tympany
      Choking sensation
      Rales
         *Wet rattling, clicking, crackling sounds on
             auscultation*
      Weak pulse

      Excludes2   foreign body in throat (T17.2-)
                      wheezing (R06.2)

**SYMPTOMS AND SIGNS INVOLVING THE DIGESTIVE
SYSTEM AND ABDOMEN (R10-R19)**

   Excludes2   congenital or infantile pylorospasm (Q40.0) ◀
                   gastrointestinal hemorrhage (K92.0-K92.2) ◀
                   intestinal obstruction (K56.-) ◀
                   newborn gastrointestinal hemorrhage
                       (P54.0-P54.3) ◀
                   newborn intestinal obstruction (P76.-) ◀
                   pylorospasm (K31.3) ◀
                   signs and symptoms involving the urinary
                       system (R30-R39) ◀
                   symptoms referable to female genital organs
                       (N94.-) ◀
                   symptoms referable to male genital organs
                       (N48-N50) ◀

● **R10   Abdominal and pelvic pain**

   Excludes1   renal colic (N23)
   Excludes2   dorsalgia (M54.-)
                   flatulence and related conditions (R14.-)

R10.0   Acute abdomen
   Severe abdominal pain (generalized) (with abdominal
       rigidity)

   Excludes1   abdominal rigidity NOS (R19.3)
                   generalized abdominal pain NOS (R10.84)
                   localized abdominal pain (R10.1-R10.3-)

● **R10.1   Pain localized to upper abdomen**

   R10.10   Upper abdominal pain, unspecified

   R10.11   Right upper quadrant pain

   R10.12   Left upper quadrant pain

   R10.13   Epigastric pain
      Dyspepsia

      Excludes1   functional dyspepsia (K30)

R10.2   Pelvic and perineal pain
   Excludes1   vulvodynia (N94.81)

● **R10.3   Pain localized to other parts of lower abdomen**

   R10.30   Lower abdominal pain, unspecified

   R10.31   Right lower quadrant pain

   R10.32   Left lower quadrant pain

   R10.33   Periumbilical pain

● **R10.8   Other abdominal pain**

   ● **R10.81   Abdominal tenderness**
      Abdominal tenderness NOS

      **R10.811   Right upper quadrant abdominal
                   tenderness**

      **R10.812   Left upper quadrant abdominal
                   tenderness**

      **R10.813   Right lower quadrant abdominal
                   tenderness**

      **R10.814   Left lower quadrant abdominal
                   tenderness**

      R10.815   Periumbilic abdominal tenderness

      R10.816   Epigastric abdominal tenderness

      R10.817   Generalized abdominal tenderness

      **R10.819   Abdominal tenderness, unspecified
                   site**

   ● **R10.82   Rebound abdominal tenderness**

      **R10.821   Right upper quadrant rebound
                   abdominal tenderness**

      **R10.822   Left upper quadrant rebound
                   abdominal tenderness**

      **R10.823   Right lower quadrant rebound
                   abdominal tenderness**

N Newborn Age: 0   **P** Pediatric Age: 0–17   **M** Maternity DX: 12–55   **A** Adult Age: 15–124   ♀ Females Only   ♂ Males Only

   🔧 Complication\Comorbidity   🔧 Major C\C   (Ex) CC/MCC Exclusions   🔧 Hospital-Acquired Condition

1197

R10.824　Left lower quadrant rebound abdominal tenderness

R10.825　Periumbilic rebound abdominal tenderness

R10.826　Epigastric rebound abdominal tenderness

R10.827　Generalized rebound abdominal tenderness

R10.829　Rebound abdominal tenderness, **unspecified** site

R10.83　Colic　　　　　　　　　　　　　　　　　　P
　　　　Colic NOS
　　　　Infantile colic
　　　　Excludes1　colic in adult and child over 12 months old (R10.84)

R10.84　Generalized abdominal pain
　　　　Excludes1　generalized abdominal pain associated with acute abdomen (R10.0)

R10.9　**Unspecified** abdominal pain

● R11　Nausea and vomiting
　　　Excludes1　cyclical vomiting associated with migraine (G43.A-)
　　　　　　　　　　excessive vomiting in pregnancy (O21.-)
　　　　　　　　　　hematemesis (K92.0)
　　　　　　　　　　neonatal hematemesis (P54.0)
　　　　　　　　　　newborn vomiting (P92.0-)
　　　　　　　　　　psychogenic vomiting (F50.89) ◄▥
　　　　　　　　　　vomiting associated with bulimia nervosa (F50.2)
　　　　　　　　　　vomiting following gastrointestinal surgery (K91.0)

● R11.0　Nausea
　　　　Nausea NOS
　　　　Nausea without vomiting

● R11.1　Vomiting
　　　R11.10　Vomiting, **unspecified**
　　　　　　　Vomiting NOS
　　　R11.11　Vomiting without nausea
　　　R11.12　Projectile vomiting
　　　R11.13　Vomiting of fecal matter
　　　R11.14　Bilious vomiting
　　　　　　　Bilious emesis

R11.2　Nausea with vomiting, **unspecified**
　　　　Persistent nausea with vomiting NOS

R12　Heartburn
　　　Excludes1　dyspepsia NOS (R10.13)
　　　　　　　　　　functional dyspepsia (K30)

● R13　Aphagia and dysphagia
　　R13.0　Aphagia
　　　　　Inability to swallow
　　　　　Excludes1　psychogenic aphagia (F50.9)

● R13.1　Dysphagia
　　　Difficulty swallowing
　　　Code first, if applicable, dysphagia following cerebrovascular disease (I69. with final characters -91)
　　　Excludes1　psychogenic dysphagia (F45.8)
　　R13.10　Dysphagia, **unspecified**
　　　　　　Difficulty in swallowing NOS
　　R13.11　Dysphagia, oral phase
　　R13.12　Dysphagia, oropharyngeal phase
　　R13.13　Dysphagia, pharyngeal phase
　　R13.14　Dysphagia, pharyngoesophageal phase
　　R13.19　Other dysphagia
　　　　　　Cervical dysphagia
　　　　　　Neurogenic dysphagia

● R14　Flatulence and related conditions
　　　Excludes1　psychogenic aerophagy (F45.8)
　　R14.0　Abdominal distension (gaseous)
　　　　　Bloating
　　　　　Tympanites (abdominal) (intestinal)
　　R14.1　Gas pain
　　R14.2　Eructation
　　　　　Belching air from stomach through mouth
　　R14.3　Flatulence

● R15　Fecal incontinence
　　　Includes　encopresis NOS
　　　Excludes1　fecal incontinence of nonorganic origin (F98.1)
　　R15.0　Incomplete defecation
　　　　　Excludes1　constipation (K59.0-)
　　　　　　　　　　　fecal impaction (K56.41)
　　R15.1　Fecal smearing
　　　　　Fecal soiling
　　R15.2　Fecal urgency
　　R15.9　Full incontinence of feces
　　　　　Fecal incontinence NOS

● R16　Hepatomegaly and splenomegaly, not elsewhere classified
　　　Enlargement of liver or spleen
　　R16.0　Hepatomegaly, not elsewhere classified
　　　　　Hepatomegaly NOS
　　R16.1　Splenomegaly, not elsewhere classified
　　　　　Splenomegaly NOS
　　R16.2　Hepatomegaly with splenomegaly, not elsewhere classified
　　　　　Hepatosplenomegaly NOS

R17　**Unspecified** jaundice 🏷
　　　Excludes1　neonatal jaundice (P55, P57-P59)
　　　(Ex) P57.8-P59.9, R17, R23.8-R23.9

● R18　Ascites
　　　Includes　fluid in peritoneal cavity
　　　Excludes1　ascites in alcoholic cirrhosis (K70.31)
　　　　　　　　　　ascites in alcoholic hepatitis (K70.11)
　　　　　　　　　　ascites in toxic liver disease with chronic active hepatitis (K71.51)
　　　(Ex) **For category R18 CC codes:** G89.0-G89.4, R18.0-R19.09, R19.30-R19.37, R29.700-R29.742, R41.0-R41.3, R41.82, R41.9, R44.8-R44.9, R45.83-R45.84, R46.0-R46.89, R52, R68.0-R68.19, R68.81-R68.83, R68.89-R69

● R18.0　Malignant ascites 🏷
　　　　Code first malignancy, such as:
　　　　　malignant neoplasm of ovary (C56.-)
　　　　　secondary malignant neoplasm of retroperitoneum and peritoneum (C78.6)

● R18.8　Other ascites 🏷
　　　　Ascites NOS
　　　　Peritoneal effusion (chronic)

● R19　Other symptoms and signs involving the digestive system and abdomen
　　　Excludes1　acute abdomen (R10.0)
● R19.0　Intra-abdominal and pelvic swelling, mass and lump
　　　Excludes1　abdominal distension (gaseous) (R14.-)
　　　　　　　　　　ascites (R18.-)
　　R19.00　Intra-abdominal and pelvic swelling, mass and lump, **unspecified** site
　　R19.01　Right upper quadrant abdominal swelling, mass and lump
　　R19.02　Left upper quadrant abdominal swelling, mass and lump
　　R19.03　Right lower quadrant abdominal swelling, mass and lump
　　R19.04　Left lower quadrant abdominal swelling, mass and lump

◄ New　◄▥ Revised　~~deleted~~ Deleted　**Excludes 1**　Excludes 2　Includes　Use additional　Code first　Code also　**Unspecified**
OGCR Official Guidelines　● Unacceptable Principal Diagnosis　**X** Assign placeholder X　🏷 Use Additional Character(s)　▶ Manifestation Code　**Coding Clinic**

R19.05   **Periumbilic swelling, mass or lump**
Diffuse or generalized umbilical swelling or mass

R19.06   **Epigastric swelling, mass or lump**

R19.07   **Generalized intra-abdominal and pelvic swelling, mass and lump**
Diffuse or generalized intra-abdominal swelling or mass NOS
Diffuse or generalized pelvic swelling or mass NOS

R19.09   **Other intra-abdominal and pelvic swelling, mass and lump**

● **R19.1**   **Abnormal bowel sounds**

R19.11   **Absent bowel sounds**

R19.12   **Hyperactive bowel sounds**

R19.15   **Other abnormal bowel sounds**
Abnormal bowel sounds NOS

R19.2   **Visible peristalsis**
Hyperperistalsis

● **R19.3**   **Abdominal rigidity**
> **Excludes1**   abdominal rigidity with severe abdominal pain (R10.0)

R19.30   **Abdominal rigidity, unspecified site**

R19.31   **Right upper quadrant abdominal rigidity**

R19.32   **Left upper quadrant abdominal rigidity**

R19.33   **Right lower quadrant abdominal rigidity**

R19.34   **Left lower quadrant abdominal rigidity**

R19.35   **Periumbilic abdominal rigidity**

R19.36   **Epigastric abdominal rigidity**

R19.37   **Generalized abdominal rigidity**

R19.4   **Change in bowel habit**
> **Excludes1**   constipation (K59.0-)
> functional diarrhea (K59.1)

R19.5   **Other fecal abnormalities**
Abnormal stool color
Bulky stools
Mucus in stools
Occult blood in feces
Occult blood in stools
> **Excludes1**   melena (K92.1)
> neonatal melena (P54.1)

R19.6   **Halitosis**

R19.7   **Diarrhea, unspecified**
Diarrhea NOS
> **Excludes1**   functional diarrhea (K59.1)
> neonatal diarrhea (P78.3)
> psychogenic diarrhea (F45.8)

R19.8   **Other specified symptoms and signs involving the digestive system and abdomen**

SYMPTOMS AND SIGNS INVOLVING THE SKIN AND SUBCUTANEOUS TISSUE (R20-R23)

> **Excludes2**   symptoms relating to breast (N64.4-N64.5)

● **R20**   **Disturbances of skin sensation**
> **Excludes1**   dissociative anesthesia and sensory loss (F44.6)
> psychogenic disturbances (F45.8)

R20.0   **Anesthesia of skin**
Loss of sensation

R20.1   **Hypoesthesia of skin**
Unpleasant abnormal sensation

R20.2   **Paresthesia of skin**
Abnormal touch sensation, including burning, prickling, often in absence of external stimulus
Formication   Tingling skin
Pins and needles
> **Excludes1**   acroparesthesia (I73.8)

R20.3   **Hyperesthesia**

R20.8   **Other disturbances of skin sensation**

R20.9   **Unspecified disturbances of skin sensation**

R21   **Rash and other nonspecific skin eruption**
> **Includes**   rash NOS
> **Excludes1**   specified type of rash- code to condition
> vesicular eruption (R23.8)

● **R22**   **Localized swelling, mass and lump of skin and subcutaneous tissue**
> **Includes**   subcutaneous nodules (localized) (superficial)
> **Excludes1**   abnormal findings on diagnostic imaging (R90-R93)
> edema (R60.-)
> enlarged lymph nodes (R59.-)
> localized adiposity (E65)
> swelling of joint (M25.4-)

R22.0   **Localized swelling, mass and lump, head**

R22.1   **Localized swelling, mass and lump, neck**

R22.2   **Localized swelling, mass and lump, trunk**
> **Excludes1**   intra-abdominal or pelvic mass and lump (R19.0-)
> intra-abdominal or pelvic swelling (R19.0-)
> **Excludes2**   breast mass and lump (N63)

● **R22.3**   **Localized swelling, mass and lump, upper limb**

R22.30   **Localized swelling, mass and lump, unspecified upper limb**

R22.31   **Localized swelling, mass and lump, right upper limb**

R22.32   **Localized swelling, mass and lump, left upper limb**

R22.33   **Localized swelling, mass and lump, upper limb, bilateral**

● **R22.4**   **Localized swelling, mass and lump, lower limb**

R22.40   **Localized swelling, mass and lump, unspecified lower limb**

R22.41   **Localized swelling, mass and lump, right lower limb**

R22.42   **Localized swelling, mass and lump, left lower limb**

R22.43   **Localized swelling, mass and lump, lower limb, bilateral**

R22.9   **Localized swelling, mass and lump, unspecified**

● **R23**   **Other skin changes**

R23.0   **Cyanosis**
> **Excludes1**   acrocyanosis (I73.8)
> cyanotic attacks of newborn (P28.2)

R23.1   **Pallor**
Clammy skin

R23.2   **Flushing**
Excessive blushing
Code first, if applicable, menopausal and female climacteric states (N95.1)

R23.3   **Spontaneous ecchymoses**
Small hemorrhagic spot of skin; AKA black and blue spot
Petechiae
> **Excludes1**   ecchymoses of newborn (P54.5)
> purpura (D69.-)

R23.4   **Changes in skin texture**
Desquamation of skin   Scaling of skin
Induration of skin
> **Excludes1**   epidermal thickening NOS (L85.9)

R23.8   **Other skin changes**

R23.9   **Unspecified skin changes**

CHAPTER 18 (R00-R99)

SYMPTOMS AND SIGNS INVOLVING THE NERVOUS AND MUSCULOSKELETAL SYSTEMS (R25-R29)

● **R25** **Abnormal involuntary movements**
> **Excludes1** specific movement disorders (G20-G26)
> stereotyped movement disorders (F98.4)
> tic disorders (F95.-)

R25.0 **Abnormal head movements**

R25.1 **Tremor, unspecified**
> **Excludes1** chorea NOS (G25.5)
> essential tremor (G25.0)
> hysterical tremor (F44.4)
> intention tremor (G25.2)

R25.2 **Cramp and spasm**
> **Excludes2** carpopedal spasm (R29.0)
> charley-horse (M62.831)
> infantile spasms (G40.4-)
> muscle spasm of back (M62.830)
> muscle spasm of calf (M62.831)

R25.3 **Fasciculation**
Twitching NOS

R25.8 **Other abnormal involuntary movements**

R25.9 **Unspecified abnormal involuntary movements**

● **R26** **Abnormalities of gait and mobility**
> **Excludes1** ataxia NOS (R27.0)
> hereditary ataxia (G11.-)
> locomotor (syphilitic) ataxia (A52.11)
> immobility syndrome (paraplegic) (M62.3)

R26.0 **Ataxic gait**
Staggering gait

R26.1 **Paralytic gait**
Spastic gait

R26.2 **Difficulty in walking, not elsewhere classified**
> **Excludes1** falling (R29.6)
> unsteadiness on feet (R26.81)
> Coding Clinic: 2016, Q2, P7

● **R26.8** **Other abnormalities of gait and mobility**

R26.81 **Unsteadiness on feet**

R26.89 **Other abnormalities of gait and mobility**

R26.9 **Unspecified abnormalities of gait and mobility**

● **R27** **Other lack of coordination**
> **Excludes1** ataxic gait (R26.0)
> hereditary ataxia (G11.-)
> vertigo NOS (R42)

R27.0 **Ataxia, unspecified**
> **Excludes1** ataxia following cerebrovascular disease
> (I69. with final characters -93)

R27.8 **Other lack of coordination**

R27.9 **Unspecified lack of coordination**

● **R29** **Other symptoms and signs involving the nervous and musculoskeletal systems**

R29.0 **Tetany** 🔗
> *Hyperexcitability of nerves and muscles characterized by spasm, twitching, and cramps*
> Carpopedal spasm
> **Excludes1** hysterical tetany (F44.5)
> neonatal tetany (P71.3)
> parathyroid tetany (E20.9)
> post-thyroidectomy tetany (E89.2)
> (Ex:) A33, A35, G10-G11.2, G11.4, G20-G25.79, G25.82-G26, G32.81, G80.3, G81.10-G81.14, G89.0-G89.4, G90.3, R29.0, R29.700-R29.742, R41.0-R41.3, R41.82, R41.9, R44.8-R44.9, R45.83-R45.84, R46.0-R46.89, R52, R68.0-R68.19, R68.81-R68.83, R68.89-R69

R29.1 **Meningismus** 🔗
> (Ex:) R29.1, R29.810

R29.2 **Abnormal reflex**
> **Excludes2** abnormal pupillary reflex (H57.0)
> hyperactive gag reflex (J39.2)
> vasovagal reaction or syncope (R55)

R29.3 **Abnormal posture**

R29.4 **Clicking hip**
> **Excludes1** congenital deformities of hip (Q65.-)

R29.5 **Transient paralysis** 🔗
> *Code first any associated spinal cord injury (S14.0, S14.1-, S24.0, S24.1-, S34.0-, S34.1-)*
> **Excludes1** transient ischemic attack (G45.9)
> (Ex:) R29.5, R29.810

R29.6 **Repeated falls**
Falling
Tendency to fall
> **Excludes2** at risk for falling (Z91.81)
> history of falling (Z91.81)

> **OGCR** Section I.C.18.d.
> Repeated falls
> Code R29.6, Repeated falls, is for use for encounters when a patient has recently fallen and the reason for the fall is being investigated.
> Code Z91.81, History of falling, is for use when a patient has fallen in the past and is at risk for future falls. When appropriate, both codes R29.6 and Z91.81 may be assigned together.

> **Coding Clinic: 2016, Q2, P7**

● **R29.7** **National Institutes of Health Stroke Scale (NIHSS) score** ◀
> *Code first the type of cerebral infarction (I63-)* ◀

● **R29.70** **NIHSS score 0-9** ◀
> ● **R29.700** NIHSS score 0 ◀
> ● **R29.701** NIHSS score 1 ◀
> ● **R29.702** NIHSS score 2 ◀
> ● **R29.703** NIHSS score 3 ◀
> ● **R29.704** NIHSS score 4 ◀
> ● **R29.705** NIHSS score 5 ◀
> ● **R29.706** NIHSS score 6 ◀
> ● **R29.707** NIHSS score 7 ◀
> ● **R29.708** NIHSS score 8 ◀
> ● **R29.709** NIHSS score 9 ◀

● **R29.71** **NIHSS score 10-19** ◀
> ● **R29.710** NIHSS score 10 ◀
> ● **R29.711** NIHSS score 11 ◀
> ● **R29.712** NIHSS score 12 ◀
> ● **R29.713** NIHSS score 13 ◀
> ● **R29.714** NIHSS score 14 ◀
> ● **R29.715** NIHSS score 15 ◀
> ● **R29.716** NIHSS score 16 ◀
> ● **R29.717** NIHSS score 17 ◀
> ● **R29.718** NIHSS score 18 ◀
> ● **R29.719** NIHSS score 19 ◀

● **R29.72** **NIHSS score 20-29** ◀
> ● **R29.720** NIHSS score 20 ◀
> ● **R29.721** NIHSS score 21 ◀
> ● **R29.722** NIHSS score 22 ◀
> ● **R29.723** NIHSS score 23 ◀
> ● **R29.724** NIHSS score 24 ◀
> ● **R29.725** NIHSS score 25 ◀
> ● **R29.726** NIHSS score 26 ◀
> ● **R29.727** NIHSS score 27 ◀
> ● **R29.728** NIHSS score 28 ◀
> ● **R29.729** NIHSS score 29 ◀

> **OGCR** Section I.C.18.i.
> NIHSS Stroke Scale
> The NIH stroke scale (NIHSS) codes (R29.7- -) can be used in conjunction with acute stroke codes (I63) to identify the patient's neurological status and the severity of the stroke. The stroke scale codes should be sequenced after the acute stroke diagnosis code(s).
> At a minimum, report the initial score documented. If desired, a facility may choose to capture multiple stroke scale scores.

◀ New   ◀‖‖ Revised   ~~deleted~~ Deleted   Excludes 1   Excludes 2   Includes   Use additional   Code first   Code also   Unspecified
OGCR Official Guidelines   ● Unacceptable Principal Diagnosis   X Assign placeholder X   ● Use Additional Character(s)   ▶ Manifestation Code   Coding Clinic

● R29.73   NIHSS score 30-39 ◄
- ● R29.730   NIHSS score 30 ◄
- ● R29.731   NIHSS score 31 ◄
- ● R29.732   NIHSS score 32 ◄
- ● R29.733   NIHSS score 33 ◄
- ● R29.734   NIHSS score 34 ◄
- ● R29.735   NIHSS score 35 ◄
- ● R29.736   NIHSS score 36 ◄
- ● R29.737   NIHSS score 37 ◄
- ● R29.738   NIHSS score 38 ◄
- ● R29.739   NIHSS score 39 ◄

● R29.74   NIHSS score 40-42 ◄
- ● R29.740   NIHSS score 40 ◄
- ● R29.741   NIHSS score 41 ◄
- ● R29.742   NIHSS score 42 ◄

● **R29.8**   **Other symptoms and signs involving the nervous and musculoskeletal systems**

● **R29.81**   **Other symptoms and signs involving the nervous system**

    R29.810   **Facial weakness**
    Facial droop
    Excludes1   Bell's palsy (G51.0) facial weakness following cerebrovascular disease (I69. with final characters -92)

    R29.818   **Other symptoms and signs involving the nervous system**

● **R29.89**   **Other symptoms and signs involving the musculoskeletal system**
    Excludes2   pain in limb (M79.6-)

    R29.890   **Loss of height**
    Excludes1   osteoporosis (M80-M81)

    R29.891   **Ocular torticollis**
    Excludes1   congenital (sterno-mastoid) torticollis Q68.0 psychogenic torticollis (F45.8) spasmodic torticollis (G24.3) torticollis due to birth injury (P15.8) torticollis NOS M43.6

    R29.898   **Other symptoms and signs involving the musculoskeletal system**

● **R29.9**   **Unspecified symptoms and signs involving the nervous and musculoskeletal systems**

    R29.90   **Unspecified symptoms and signs involving the nervous system**

    R29.91   **Unspecified symptoms and signs involving the musculoskeletal system**

SYMPTOMS AND SIGNS INVOLVING THE GENITOURINARY SYSTEM (R30-R39)

● **R30**   **Pain associated with micturition**
    Excludes1   psychogenic pain associated with micturition (F45.8)

    R30.0   **Dysuria**
    Painful urination
    Strangury

    R30.1   **Vesical tenesmus**
    Straining to urinate

    R30.9   **Painful micturition, unspecified**
    Painful urination NOS

● **R31**   **Hematuria**
    Excludes1   hematuria included with underlying conditions, such as:
    acute cystitis with hematuria (N30.01) recurrent and persistent hematuria in glomerular diseases (N02.-)

    R31.0   **Gross hematuria**
    R31.1   **Benign essential microscopic hematuria**
●   **R31.2**   **Other microscopic hematuria**
    R31.21   **Asymptomatic microscopic hematuria** ◄
    AMH ◄
    R31.29   **Other microscopic hematuria** ◄
    R31.9   **Hematuria, unspecified**

● **R32**   **Unspecified urinary incontinence**
    Enuresis NOS
    Excludes1   functional urinary incontinence (R39.81) nonorganic enuresis (F98.0) stress incontinence and other specified urinary incontinence (N39.3-N39.4-) urinary incontinence associated with cognitive impairment (R39.81)

● **R33**   **Retention of urine**
    Excludes1   psychogenic retention of urine (F45.8)

    R33.0   **Drug induced retention of urine**
    Use additional code for adverse effect, if applicable, to identify drug (T36-T50 with fifth or sixth character 5)

    R33.8   **Other retention of urine**
    Code first, if applicable, any causal condition, such as: enlarged prostate (N40.1)

    R33.9   **Retention of urine, unspecified**

● **R34**   **Anuria and oliguria**
    Excludes1   anuria and oliguria complicating abortion or ectopic or molar pregnancy (O00-O07, O08.4) anuria and oliguria complicating pregnancy (O26.83-) anuria and oliguria complicating the puerperium (O90.4)

● **R35**   **Polyuria**
    Passage of excessive volume of urine
    Code first, if applicable, any causal condition, such as: enlarged prostate (N40.1)
    Excludes1   psychogenic polyuria (F45.8)

    R35.0   **Frequency of micturition**
    Discharge or passage of urine; AKA uresis

    R35.1   **Nocturia**
    Urinary frequency at night

    R35.8   **Other polyuria**
    Polyuria NOS

● **R36**   **Urethral discharge**
    R36.0   **Urethral discharge without blood**
    R36.1   **Hematospermia** ♂
    Presence of blood in semen
    R36.9   **Urethral discharge, unspecified**
    Penile discharge NOS
    Urethrorrhea

● **R37**   **Sexual dysfunction, unspecified**

N   Newborn Age: 0   **P**   Pediatric Age: 0–17   **M**   Maternity DX: 12–55   **A**   Adult Age: 15–124   ♀   Females Only   ♂   Males Only

🅒   Complication\Comorbidity   🅜   Major C\C   Ⓔⓧ   CC/MCC Exclusions   🅗   Hospital-Acquired Condition   1201

● R39   Other and unspecified symptoms and signs involving the genitourinary system

R39.0   **Extravasation of urine** 🔗
Leakage, discharge
(Ex:) R30.1, R39.0, R39.2-R39.9

● R39.1   Other difficulties with micturition
Code first, if applicable, any causal condition, such as:
enlarged prostate (N40.1)

R39.11   **Hesitancy of micturition**

R39.12   **Poor urinary stream**
Weak urinary steam

R39.13   **Splitting of urinary stream**

R39.14   **Feeling of incomplete bladder emptying**

R39.15   **Urgency of urination**
Excludes1   urge incontinence (N39.41, N39.46)

R39.16   **Straining to void**

● R39.19   Other difficulties with micturition
R39.191   **Need to immediately re-void** ◄
R39.192   **Position dependent micturition** ◄
R39.198   **Other difficulties with micturition** ◄

R39.2   **Extrarenal uremia**
Prerenal uremia
Excludes1   uremia NOS (N19)

● R39.8   Other symptoms and signs involving the genitourinary system

R39.81   **Functional urinary incontinence**
Urinary incontinence due to cognitive impairment, or severe physical disability or immobility
Excludes1   stress incontinence and other specified urinary incontinence (N39.3-N39.4-)
urinary incontinence NOS (R32)

R39.82   **Chronic bladder pain** ◄

R39.89   **Other symptoms and signs involving the genitourinary system**

R39.9   **Unspecified symptoms and signs involving the genitourinary system**

SYMPTOMS AND SIGNS INVOLVING COGNITION, PERCEPTION, EMOTIONAL STATE AND BEHAVIOR (R40-R46)

Excludes2   symptoms and signs constituting part of a pattern of mental disorder (F01-F99) ◄
Coding Clinic: 2015, Q4, P40

● R40   Somnolence, stupor and coma
Excludes1   neonatal coma (P91.5)
somnolence, stupor and coma in diabetes (E08-E13)
somnolence, stupor and coma in hepatic failure (K72.-)
somnolence, stupor and coma in hypoglycemia (nondiabetic) (E15)

R40.0   **Somnolence**
Drowsiness
Excludes1   coma (R40.2-)

R40.1   **Stupor**
Lowered level of consciousness
Catatonic stupor
Semicoma
Excludes1   catatonic schizophrenia (F20.2)
coma (R40.2-)
depressive stupor (F31-F33)
dissociative stupor (F44.2)
manic stupor (F30.2)

Coma scale

The coma scale codes (R40.2-) can be used in conjunction with traumatic brain injury codes, acute cerebrovascular disease or sequelae of cerebrovascular disease codes. These codes are primarily for use by trauma registries, but they may be used in any setting where this information is collected. **The coma scale may also be used to assess the status of the central nervous system for other non-trauma conditions, such as monitoring patients in the intensive care unit regardless of medical condition.** The coma scale codes should be sequenced after the diagnosis code(s).

These codes, one from each subcategory, are needed to complete the scale. The 7th character indicates when the scale was recorded. The 7th character should match for all three codes.

At a minimum, report the initial score documented on presentation at your facility. This may be a score from the emergency medicine technician (EMT) or in the emergency department. If desired, a facility may choose to capture multiple coma scale scores.

Assign code R40.24, Glasgow coma scale, total score, when only the total score is documented in the medical record and not the individual score(s).

● R40.2   Coma
Code first any associated:
fracture of skull (S02.-)
intracranial injury (S06.-)
Note: One code from each subcategory R40.21-R40-23 is required to complete the coma scale ◄▥▥
(Ex:) **For category R40.2 CC codes:** B15.0-B19.9, E03.5, E08.00-E08.59, E08.618-E09.59, E09.618-E10.59, E10.618-E10.649, E10.69-E11.59, E11.618-E11.649, E11.69-E13.59, E13.618-E16.2, E89.1, G32.89, G89.0-G89.4, G93.81-G93.9, G96.8-G96.9, G98.0-G98.8, G99.8, I60.00-I62.9, K72.91, R29.700-R29.742, R40.0-R40.2124, R40.2210-R40.2224, R40.2310-R40.2324, R40.2340-R40.2344, R40.3-R41.3, R41.82, R41.9-R42, R44.8-R44.9, R45.83-R45.84, R46.0-R46.89, R52, R55, R68.0-R68.83, R68.89-R69, S02.0XX-S02.19X[A,B], S02.91X[A,B], S06.0X0-S06.0X1[A], S06.0X9-S06.9X9[A]

R40.20   **Unspecified coma** 🔗
Coma NOS
Unconsciousness NOS

● R40.21   Coma scale, eyes open
The following appropriate 7th character is to be added to subcategory R40.21-:

0	unspecified time
1	in the field [EMT or ambulance]
2	at arrival to emergency department
3	at hospital admission
4	24 hours or more after hospital admission

Coding Clinic: 2015, Q2, P18

● R40.211   Coma scale, eyes open, never 🔗
● R40.212   Coma scale, eyes open, to pain 🔗
● R40.213   Coma scale, eyes open, to sound
● R40.214   Coma scale, eyes open, spontaneous

● R40.22   Coma scale, best verbal response
The following appropriate 7th character is to be added to subcategory R40.22-:

0	unspecified time
1	in the field [EMT or ambulance]
2	at arrival to emergency department
3	at hospital admission
4	24 hours or more after hospital admission

Coding Clinic: 2015, Q2, P18

● R40.221   Coma scale, best verbal response, none 🔗
● R40.222   Coma scale, best verbal response, incomprehensible words 🔗

Glasgow Coma Scale

Eye Opening Response	
• Spontaneous--open with blinking at baseline	4 points
• To verbal stimuli, command, speech	3 points
• To pain only (not applied to face)	2 points
• No response	1 point
Verbal Response	
• Oriented	5 points
• Confused conversation, but able to answer questions	4 points
• Inappropriate words	3 points
• Incomprehensible speech	2 points
• No response	1 point
Motor Response	
• Obeys commands for movement	6 points
• Purposeful movement to painful stimulus	5 points
• Withdraws in response to pain	4 points
• Flexion in response to pain (decorticate posturing)	3 points
• Extension response in response to pain (decerebrate posturing)	2 points
• No response	1 point
Categorization: Coma: No eye opening, no ability to follow commands, no word verbalizations (3-8)	
Head Injury Classification: Severe Head Injury--GCS score of 8 or less Moderate Head Injury--GCS score of 9 to 12 Mild head injury--GCS score of 13 to 15	
(Adapted from: Advanced Trauma Life Support: Course for Physicians, American College of Surgeons, 1993). http://www.bt.cdc.gov/masscasulatires/gscale.asp	

Figure 18-1

● **R40.223   Coma scale, best verbal response, inappropriate words**

● **R40.224   Coma scale, best verbal response, confused conversation**

● **R40.225   Coma scale, best verbal response, oriented**

● **R40.23   Coma scale, best motor response**

The following appropriate 7th character is to be added to subcategory R40.23-:

0	unspecified time
1	in the field [EMT or ambulance]
2	at arrival to emergency department
3	at hospital admission
4	24 hours or more after hospital admission

Coding Clinic: 2015, Q2, P18

● **R40.231   Coma scale, best motor response, none** 🔖

● **R40.232   Coma scale, best motor response, extension** 🔖

● **R40.233   Coma scale, best motor response, abnormal**

● **R40.234   Coma scale, best motor response, flexion withdrawal** 🔖

● **R40.235   Coma scale, best motor response, localizes pain**

● **R40.236   Coma scale, best motor response, obeys commands**

● **R40.24   Glasgow coma scale, total score**

Note: Assign a code from subcategory R40.24, when only the total coma score is documented ◄

The following appropriate 7th character is to be added to subcategory R40.24-: ◄

0	unspecified time ◄
1	in the field [EMT or ambulance] ◄
2	at arrival to emergency department ◄
3	at hospital admission ◄
4	24 hours or more after hospital admission ◄

Coding Clinic: 2015, Q2, P18

● **R40.241   Glasgow coma scale score 13-15**

● **R40.242   Glasgow coma scale score 9-12**

● **R40.243   Glasgow coma scale score 3-8**

● **R40.244   Other coma, without documented Glasgow coma scale score, or with partial score reported**

R40.3   Persistent vegetative state 🔖
  (Ex.) See R40.2

R40.4   Transient alteration of awareness

● **R41   Other symptoms and signs involving cognitive functions and awareness**

Excludes1   dissociative [conversion] disorders (F44.-)
                mild cognitive impairment, so stated (G31.84)

R41.0   Disorientation, unspecified
  Confusion NOS   Delirium NOS

R41.1   Anterograde amnesia

R41.2   Retrograde amnesia

R41.3   Other amnesia
  Amnesia NOS
  Memory loss NOS

Excludes1   amnestic disorder due to known physiologic condition (F04)
                amnestic syndrome due to psychoactive substance use (F10-F19 with 5th character .6)
                mild memory disturbance due to known physiological condition (F06.8)
                transient global amnesia (G45.4)

R41.4   Neurologic neglect syndrome 🔖
  Asomatognosia   Left-sided neglect
  Hemi-akinesia   Sensory neglect
  Hemi-inattention   Visuospatial neglect
  Hemispatial neglect

Excludes1   visuospatial deficit (R41.842)
  (Ex.) R29.3, R29.6-R29.890, R29.90-R29.91, R41.4

● **R41.8   Other symptoms and signs involving cognitive functions and awareness**

R41.81   Age-related cognitive decline   A
  Senility NOS

R41.82   Altered mental status, unspecified
  Change in mental status NOS

Excludes1   altered level of consciousness (R40.-)
                altered mental status due to known condition - code to condition
                delirium NOS (R41.0)
  Coding Clinic: 2012, Q4, P98

● **R41.83   Borderline intellectual functioning**
  IQ level 71 to 84

Excludes1   intellectual disabilities (F70-F79)

N Newborn Age: 0	P Pediatric Age: 0–17	M Maternity DX: 12–55	A Adult Age: 15–124	♀ Females Only	♂ Males Only	
🔖 Complication\Comorbidity	🔖 Major C\C	(Ex.) CC/MCC Exclusions	🔖 Hospital-Acquired Condition			

CHAPTER 18 (R00-R99)

● R41.84   **Other specified cognitive deficit**

     Excludes1   cognitive deficits as sequelae of cerebrovascular disease (I69.01-, I69.11-, I69.21-, I69.31-, I69.81-, I69.91-) ◀

     R41.840   **Attention and concentration deficit**

         Excludes1   attention-deficit hyperactivity disorders (F90.-)

     R41.841   **Cognitive communication deficit**

     R41.842   **Visuospatial deficit**

     R41.843   **Psychomotor deficit**

     R41.844   **Frontal lobe and executive function deficit**

     R41.89   **Other symptoms and signs involving cognitive functions and awareness**

         Anosognosia

   R41.9   **Unspecified symptoms and signs involving cognitive functions and awareness**

● R42   **Dizziness and giddiness**

     Light-headedness

     Vertigo NOS

     Excludes1   vertiginous syndromes (H81.-)

         vertigo from infrasound (T75.23)

     Coding Clinic: 2015, Q4, P40

● R43   **Disturbances of smell and taste**

     R43.0   **Anosmia**

         Absence of sense of smell; AKA anosphresia and olfactory anesthesia

     R43.1   **Parosmia**

     R43.2   **Parageusia**

         Perversion of sense of taste or bad taste in mouth; AKA dysgeusia

     R43.8   **Other disturbances of smell and taste**

         Mixed disturbance of smell and taste

     R43.9   **Unspecified disturbances of smell and taste**

● R44   **Other symptoms and signs involving general sensations and perceptions**

     Excludes1   alcoholic hallucinations (F1.5)

         hallucinations in drug psychosis (F11-F19 with .5)

         hallucinations in mood disorders with psychotic symptoms (F30.2, F31.5, F32.3, F33.3)

         hallucinations in schizophrenia, schizotypal and delusional disorders (F20-F29)

     Excludes2   disturbances of skin sensation (R20.-)

     R44.0   **Auditory hallucinations**

         (Ex) G89.0-G89.4, R29.700-R29.742, R41.0-R41.3, R41.82, R41.9-R42, R44.0, R44.2-R44.9, R45.83-R45.84, R46.0-R46.89, R52, R68.0-R68.19, R68.81-R68.83, R68.89-R69

     R44.1   **Visual hallucinations**

     R44.2   **Other hallucinations**

         (Ex) See R44.0

     R44.3   **Hallucinations, unspecified**

         (Ex) See R44.0

     R44.8   **Other symptoms and signs involving general sensations and perceptions**

     R44.9   **Unspecified symptoms and signs involving general sensations and perceptions**

● R45   **Symptoms and signs involving emotional state**

     R45.0   **Nervousness**

         Nervous tension

     R45.1   **Restlessness and agitation**

     R45.2   **Unhappiness**

     R45.3   **Demoralization and apathy**

         Excludes1   anhedonia (R45.84)

     R45.4   **Irritability and anger**

     R45.5   **Hostility**

     R45.6   **Violent behavior**

     R45.7   **State of emotional shock and stress, unspecified**

● R45.8   **Other symptoms and signs involving emotional state**

     R45.81   **Low self-esteem**

     R45.82   **Worries**

     R45.83   **Excessive crying of child, adolescent or adult**

         Excludes1   excessive crying of infant (baby) R68.11

     R45.84   **Anhedonia**

         Total loss of feeling of pleasure in pleasurable acts

● R45.85   **Homicidal and suicidal ideations**

     Excludes1   suicide attempt (T14.91)

     ● R45.850   **Homicidal ideations**

     R45.851   **Suicidal ideations**

         (Ex) F05

     R45.86   **Emotional lability**

     R45.87   **Impulsiveness**

     R45.89   **Other symptoms and signs involving emotional state**

● R46   **Symptoms and signs involving appearance and behavior**

     Excludes1   appearance and behavior in schizophrenia, schizotypal and delusional disorders (F20-F29)

         mental and behavioral disorders (F01-F99)

     R46.0   **Very low level of personal hygiene**

     R46.1   **Bizarre personal appearance**

     R46.2   **Strange and inexplicable behavior**

     R46.3   **Overactivity**

     R46.4   **Slowness and poor responsiveness**

         Excludes1   stupor (R40.1)

     R46.5   **Suspiciousness and marked evasiveness**

     R46.6   **Undue concern and preoccupation with stressful events**

     R46.7   **Verbosity and circumstantial detail obscuring reason for contact**

● R46.8   **Other symptoms and signs involving appearance and behavior**

     ● R46.81   **Obsessive-compulsive behavior**

         Excludes1   obsessive-compulsive disorder (F42-) ◀

     ● R46.89   **Other symptoms and signs involving appearance and behavior**

SYMPTOMS AND SIGNS INVOLVING SPEECH AND VOICE (R47-R49)

● R47   **Speech disturbances, not elsewhere classified**

     Excludes1   autism (F84.0)

         cluttering (F80.81)

         specific developmental disorders of speech and language (F80.-)

         stuttering (F80.81)

● R47.0   **Dysphasia and aphasia**

     R47.01   **Aphasia**

         Excludes1   aphasia following cerebrovascular disease (I69. with final characters -20)

         progressive isolated aphasia (G31.01)

         (Ex) F80.1, F80.81, I62.00-I66.9, R47.01-R47.9, R49.0-R49.9

     R47.02   **Dysphasia**

         Impairment in comprehension of speech, caused by left-sided brain damage

         Excludes1   dysphasia following cerebrovascular disease (I69. with final characters -21)

   R47.1   **Dysarthria and anarthria**

     Motor speech disorder

     Excludes1   dysarthria following cerebrovascular disease (I69. with final characters -22)

◀ New   ◀■ Revised   ~~deleted~~ Deleted   Excludes 1   Excludes 2   Includes   Use additional   Code first   Code also   Unspecified

OGCR Official Guidelines   ● Unacceptable Principal Diagnosis   X Assign placeholder X   ● Use Additional Character(s)   ▸ Manifestation Code   **Coding Clinic**

- **R47.8   Other speech disturbances**
    - **Excludes1**   dysarthria following cerebrovascular disease (I69. with final characters -28)
    - **R47.81   Slurred speech**
    - ▶ *R47.82   Fluency disorder in conditions classified elsewhere*
        - Stuttering in conditions classified elsewhere
        - *Code first* underlying disease or condition, such as: Parkinson's disease (G20)
        - **Excludes1**   adult onset fluency disorder (F98.5)
            - childhood onset fluency disorder (F80.81)
            - fluency disorder (stuttering) following cerebrovascular disease (I69. with final characters -23)
    - **R47.89   Other speech disturbances**
    - **R47.9   Unspecified speech disturbances**

- **R48   Dyslexia and other symbolic dysfunctions, not elsewhere classified**
    - **Excludes1**   specific developmental disorders of scholastic skills (F81.-)
    - **R48.0   Dyslexia and alexia**
    - **R48.1   Agnosia**
        - *Loss of ability to recognize objects, persons, sounds, shapes, or smells*
        - Astereognosia (astereognosis)
        - Autotopagnosia
        - **Excludes1**   visual object agnosia (R48.3)
    - **R48.2   Apraxia**
        - *Loss of ability to execute or carry out learned purposeful movements*
        - **Excludes1**   apraxia following cerebrovascular disease (I69. with final characters -90)
    - **R48.3   Visual agnosia**
        - Prosopagnosia
        - Simultanagnosia (asimultagnosia)
    - **R48.8   Other symbolic dysfunctions**
        - Acalculia
            - *Difficulty performing simple mathematical tasks resulting from neurological injury*
        - Agraphia
    - **R48.9   Unspecified symbolic dysfunctions**

- **R49   Voice and resonance disorders**
    - **Excludes1**   psychogenic voice and resonance disorders (F44.4)
    - **R49.0   Dysphonia**
        - Hoarseness
    - **R49.1   Aphonia**
        - Loss of voice
    - **R49.2   Hypernasality and hyponasality**
        - **R49.21   Hypernasality**
        - **R49.22   Hyponasality**
    - **R49.8   Other voice and resonance disorders**
    - **R49.9   Unspecified voice and resonance disorder**
        - Change in voice NOS
        - Resonance disorder NOS

GENERAL SYMPTOMS AND SIGNS (R50-R69)

- **R50   Fever of other and unknown origin**
    - **Excludes1**   chills without fever (R68.83)
        - febrile convulsions (R56.0-)
        - fever of unknown origin during labor (O75.2)
        - fever of unknown origin in newborn (P81.9)
        - hypothermia due to illness (R68.0)
        - malignant hyperthermia due to anesthesia (T88.3)
        - puerperal pyrexia NOS (O86.4)

- **R50.2   Drug induced fever**
    - Use additional code for adverse effect, if applicable, to identify drug (T36-T50 with fifth or sixth character 5)
    - **Excludes1**   postvaccination (postimmunization) fever (R50.83)
- **R50.8   Other specified fever**
    - ▶ *R50.81   Fever presenting with conditions classified elsewhere*
        - *Code first* underlying condition when associated fever is present, such as with:
        - leukemia (C91-C95)
        - neutropenia (D70.-)
        - sickle-cell disease (D57.-)
    - **R50.82   Postprocedural fever**
        - **Excludes1**   postprocedural infection (T81.4-) ◀▥
            - posttransfusion fever (R50.84)
            - postvaccination (postimmunization) fever (R50.83)
    - **R50.83   Postvaccination fever**
        - Postimmunization fever
    - **R50.84   Febrile nonhemolytic transfusion reaction**
        - FNHTR
        - Posttransfusion fever
- **R50.9   Fever, unspecified**
    - Fever NOS
    - Fever of unknown origin [FUO]
    - Fever with chills
    - Fever with rigors
    - Hyperpyrexia NOS
    - Persistent fever
    - Pyrexia NOS

R51   Headache
- Facial pain NOS
- **Excludes1**   atypical face pain (G50.1)
    - migraine and other headache syndromes (G43-G44)
    - trigeminal neuralgia (G50.0)

R52   Pain, unspecified
- Acute pain NOS   Pain NOS
- Generalized pain NOS
- **Excludes1**   acute and chronic pain, not elsewhere classified (G89.-)
    - localized pain, unspecified type - code to pain by site, such as:
        - abdomen pain (R10.-)
        - back pain (M54.9)
        - breast pain (N64.4)
        - chest pain (R07.1-R07.9)
        - ear pain (H92.0-)
        - eye pain (H57.1)
        - headache (R51)
        - joint pain (M25.5-)
        - limb pain (M79.6-)
        - lumbar region pain (M54.5)
        - pelvic and perineal pain (R10.2)
        - shoulder pain (M25.51-)
        - spine pain (M54.-)
        - throat pain (R07.0)
        - tongue pain (K14.6)
        - tooth pain (K08.8)
        - renal colic (N23)
    - pain disorders exclusively related to psychological factors (F45.41)

CHAPTER 18 (R00-R99)

● **R53**   **Malaise and fatigue**

     R53.0   **Neoplastic (malignant) related fatigue**
         Code first associated neoplasm

     R53.1   **Weakness**
         Asthenia NOS
         Excludes1   age-related weakness (R54)
                     muscle weakness (M62.8-)
                     sarcopenia (M62.84) ◀
                     senile asthenia (R54)

     R53.2   **Functional quadriplegia** 🔖
         Complete immobility due to severe physical disability
           or frailty
         Excludes1   frailty NOS (R54)
                     hysterical paralysis (F44.4)
                     immobility syndrome (M62.3)
                     neurologic quadriplegia (G82.5-)
                     quadriplegia (G82.50)

         (Ex:) E08.40-E08.49, E08.618-E08.638, E08.649-E08.8, E09.40-E09.49,
              E09.618-E09.638, E09.649-E09.8, E10.40-E10.49, E10.618-E10.638,
              E10.649, E10.69-E10.8, E11.40-E11.49, E11.618-E11.638, E11.649,
              E11.69-E11.8, E13.40-E13.49, E13.618-E13.638, E13.649-E13.8, G04.1,
              G32.89, G80.0-G80.2, G80.4-G83.9, G90.1, G93.81, G93.89-G93.9,
              G96.8-G96.9, G98.0-G98.8, G99.8, Q06.0-Q06.1, Q06.3, Q06.8-Q06.9,
              Q07.8-Q07.9, R53.2

         Coding Clinic: 2016, Q2, P6

     ● **R53.8**   **Other malaise and fatigue**
         Excludes1   combat exhaustion and fatigue (F43.0)
                     congenital debility (P96.9)
                     exhaustion and fatigue due to depressive
                         episode (F32.-)
                     exhaustion and fatigue due to excessive
                         exertion (T73.3)
                     exhaustion and fatigue due to exposure
                       (T73.2)
                     exhaustion and fatigue due to heat (T67.-)
                     exhaustion and fatigue due to pregnancy
                       (O26.8-)
                     exhaustion and fatigue due to recurrent
                       depressive episode (F33)
                     exhaustion and fatigue due to senile
                       debility (R54)

         R53.81   **Other malaise**
             Chronic debility
             Debility NOS
             General physical deterioration
             Malaise NOS
             Nervous debility
             Excludes1   age-related physical debility
                           (R54)

         R53.82   **Chronic fatigue, unspecified**
             Chronic fatigue syndrome NOS
             Excludes1   postviral fatigue syndrome
                           (G93.3)

         R53.83   **Other fatigue**
             Fatigue NOS   Lethargy
             Lack of energy   Tiredness

  R54   **Age-related physical debility**   A
        Frailty   Senile asthenia
        Old age   Senile debility
        Senescence
        Excludes1   age-related cognitive decline (R41.81)
                    sarcopenia (M62.84) ◀
                    senile psychosis (F03)
                    senility NOS (R41.81)

  R55   **Syncope and collapse**
        Blackout
        Fainting
        Vasovagal attack
        Excludes1   cardiogenic shock (R57.0)
                    carotid sinus syncope (G90.01)
                    heat syncope (T67.1)
                    neurocirculatory asthenia (F45.8)
                    neurogenic orthostatic hypotension (G90.3)
                    orthostatic hypotension (I95.1)
                    postprocedural shock (T81.1-)
                    psychogenic syncope (F48.8)
                    shock NOS (R57.9)
                    shock complicating or following abortion or
                       ectopic or molar pregnancy (O00-O07, O08.3)
                    shock complicating or following labor and
                       delivery (O75.1)
                    Stokes-Adams attack (I45.9)
                    unconsciousness NOS (R40.2-)

● **R56**   **Convulsions, not elsewhere classified**
        Excludes1   dissociative convulsions and seizures (F44.5)
                    epileptic convulsions and seizures (G40.-)
                    newborn convulsions and seizures (P90)

     ● **R56.0**   **Febrile convulsions**
         (Ex:) **For category R56.0 CC codes:** G32.89, G40.001-G40.319,
            G40.401-G40.919, G40.A01-G40.B19, G89.0-G89.4, G93.81, G93.89-G93.9,
            G96.8-G96.9, G98.0-G98.8, P90, P91.8-P91.9, R29.700-R29.742,
            R41.0-R41.3, R41.82, R41.9, R44.8-R44.9, R45.83-R45.84, R46.0-R46.89,
            R52, R56.00-R56.9, R68.0-R68.19, R68.81-R68.83, R68.89-R69

         R56.00   **Simple febrile convulsions** 🔖
             Febrile convulsion NOS
             Febrile seizure NOS

         R56.01   **Complex febrile convulsions** 🔖
             Atypical febrile seizure
             Complex febrile seizure
             Complicated febrile seizure
             Excludes1   status epilepticus (G40.901)

     R56.1   **Post traumatic seizures** 🔖
         Excludes1   post traumatic epilepsy (G40.-)
         (Ex:) E08.40-E08.49, E09.40-E09.49, E10.40-E10.49, E11.40-E11.49,
            E13.40-E13.49, G32.89, G40.001-G40.319, G40.401-G40.919, G40.
            A01-G40.A19, G40.B01-G40.B19, G93.81, G93.89-G93.9, G96.8-G96.9,
            G98.0-G98.8, G99.8, R56.1

     R56.9   **Unspecified convulsions**
         Convulsion disorder   Recurrent convulsions
         Fit NOS   Seizure(s) (convulsive) NOS

● **R57**   **Shock, not elsewhere classified**
        Excludes1   anaphylactic shock NOS (T78.2)
                    anaphylactic reaction or shock due to adverse
                       food reaction (T78.0-)
                    anaphylactic shock due to adverse effect of
                       correct drug or medicament properly
                       administered (T88.6)
                    anaphylactic shock due to serum (T80.5-)
                    anesthetic shock (T88.3)
                    electric shock (T75.4)
                    obstetric shock (O75.1)
                    postprocedural shock (T81.1-)
                    psychic shock (F43.0)
                    septic shock (R65.21)
                    shock complicating or following ectopic or molar
                       pregnancy (O00-O07, O08.3)
                    shock due to lightning (T75.01)
                    traumatic shock (T79.4)
                    toxic shock syndrome (A48.3)
        (Ex:) **For category R57 CC codes:** G89.0-G89.4, R09.89, R29.700-R29.742, R41.0-R41.3,
           R41.82, R41.9, R44.8-R44.9, R45.83-R45.84, R46.0-R46.89, R52, R57.0-R57.9, R65.21,
           R68.0-R68.19, R68.81-R68.83, R68.89-R69

     R57.0   **Cardiogenic shock** 🔖
         MCC: Only if patient discharged alive

     R57.1   **Hypovolemic shock** 🔖
         Decreased blood volume (loss)
         MCC: Only if patient discharged alive

R57.8   **Other shock** 🩸
     MCC: Only if patient discharged alive

R57.9   **Shock, unspecified** 🩸
     Failure of peripheral circulation NOS
     Resulting in significant blood pressure drop

R58   **Hemorrhage, not elsewhere classified**
     Hemorrhage NOS
     Excludes1   hemorrhage included with underlying
           conditions, such as:
           acute duodenal ulcer with hemorrhage (K26.0)
           acute gastritis with bleeding (K29.01)
           ulcerative enterocolitis with rectal bleeding
              (K51.01)

● **R59**   **Enlarged lymph nodes**
     Includes   swollen glands
     Excludes1   lymphadenitis NOS (I88.9)
           acute lymphadenitis (L04.-)
           chronic lymphadenitis (I88.1)
           mesenteric (acute) (chronic) lymphadenitis (I88.0)

R59.0   **Localized enlarged lymph nodes**

R59.1   **Generalized enlarged lymph nodes**
     Lymphadenopathy NOS

R59.9   **Enlarged lymph nodes, unspecified**

● **R60**   **Edema, not elsewhere classified**
     Excludes1   angioneurotic edema (T78.3)
           ascites (R18.-)
           cerebral edema (G93.6)
           cerebral edema due to birth injury (P11.0)
           edema of larynx (J38.4)
           edema of nasopharynx (J39.2)
           edema of pharynx (J39.2)
           gestational edema (O12.0-)
           hereditary edema (Q82.0)
           hydrops fetalis NOS (P83.2)
           hydrothorax (J94.8)
           nutritional edema (E40-E46)
           hydrops fetalis NOS (P83.2)
           newborn edema (P83.3)
           pulmonary edema (J81.-)

R60.0   **Localized edema**

R60.1   **Generalized edema**

R60.9   **Edema, unspecified**
     Fluid retention NOS

R61   **Generalized hyperhidrosis**
     Excessive sweating
     Night sweats
     Secondary hyperhidrosis
     Code first, if applicable, menopausal and female climacteric states (N95.1)
     Excludes1   focal (primary) (secondary) hyperhidrosis (L74.5-)
           Frey's syndrome (L74.52)
           localized (primary) (secondary) hyperhidrosis (L74.5-)

● **R62**   **Lack of expected normal physiological development in childhood and adults**
     Excludes1   delayed puberty (E30.0)
           gonadal dysgenesis (Q99.1)
           hypopituitarism (E23.0)

R62.0   **Delayed milestone in childhood**   P
     Delayed attainment of expected physiological
         developmental stage
     Late talker
     Late walker

● **R62.5**   **Other and unspecified lack of expected normal physiological development in childhood**
     Excludes1   HIV disease resulting in failure to thrive (B20)
           physical retardation due to malnutrition (E45)

     R62.50   **Unspecified lack of expected normal physiological development in childhood**
         Infantilism NOS

R62.51   **Failure to thrive (child)**   P
     Failure to gain weight
     Excludes1   failure to thrive in child under 28 days old (P92.6)

R62.52   **Short stature (child)**
     Lack of growth   Short stature NOS
     Physical retardation
     Excludes1   short stature due to endocrine disorder (E34.3)

R62.59   **Other lack of expected normal physiological development in childhood**

R62.7   **Adult failure to thrive**   A

● **R63**   **Symptoms and signs concerning food and fluid intake**
     Excludes1   bulimia NOS (F50.2)
           eating disorders of nonorganic origin (F50.-)
           malnutrition (E40-E46)

R63.0   **Anorexia**
     Loss of appetite
     Excludes1   anorexia nervosa (F50.0-)
           loss of appetite of nonorganic origin (F50.89) ◀▬

R63.1   **Polydipsia**
     Excessive thirst

R63.2   **Polyphagia**
     Excessive eating   Hyperalimentation NOS

R63.3   **Feeding difficulties**
     Feeding problem (elderly) (infant) NOS
     Excludes1   feeding problems of newborn (P92.-)
           infant feeding disorder of nonorganic origin (F98.2-)

R63.4   **Abnormal weight loss**

R63.5   **Abnormal weight gain**
     Excludes1   excessive weight gain in pregnancy (O26.0-)
           obesity (E66.-)

R63.6   **Underweight**
     Use additional code to identify body mass index (BMI), if known (Z68.-)
     Excludes1   abnormal weight loss (R63.4)
           anorexia nervosa (F50.0-)
           malnutrition (E40-E46)

R63.8   **Other symptoms and signs concerning food and fluid intake**

R64   **Cachexia** 🩸
     Wasting syndrome
     Code first underlying condition, if known
     Excludes1   abnormal weight loss (R63.4)
           nutritional marasmus (E41)
     (Ex) G89.0-G89.4, R29.700-R29.742, R41.0-R41.3, R41.82, R41.9, R44.8-R44.9, R45.83-R45.84, R46.0-R46.89, R52, R64, R68.0-R68.19, R68.81-R68.83, R68.89-R69

OGCR   Section I.C.18.g.

SIRS due to Non-Infectious Process

The systemic inflammatory response syndrome (SIRS) can develop as a result of certain non-infectious disease processes, such as trauma, malignant neoplasm, or pancreatitis. When SIRS is documented with a noninfectious condition, and no subsequent infection is documented, the code for the underlying condition, such as an injury, should be assigned, followed by code R65.10. Systemic inflammatory response syndrome (SIRS) of non-infectious origin without acute organ dysfunction, or code R65.11, Systemic inflammatory response syndrome (SIRS) of non-infectious origin with acute organ dysfunction. If an associated acute organ dysfunction is documented, the appropriate code(s) for the specific type of organ dysfunction(s) should be assigned in addition to code R65.11. If acute organ dysfunction is documented, but it cannot be determined if the acute organ dysfunction is associated with SIRS or due to another condition (e.g., directly due to the trauma), the provider should be queried.

N Newborn Age: 0   **P** Pediatric Age: 0–17   **M** Maternity DX: 12–55   **A** Adult Age: 15–124   ♀ Females Only   ♂ Males Only

🩸 Complication\Comorbidity   🩸 Major C\C   (Ex) CC/MCC Exclusions   🩸 Hospital-Acquired Condition

1207

CHAPTER 18 (R00-R99)

● **R65 Symptoms and signs specifically associated with systemic inflammation and infection**

(Ex) For category R65 CC codes unless otherwise indicated: A02.1, A20.7, A22.7, A26.7, A32.7, A39.2-A39.4, A40.0-A40.1, A40.8-A41.9, A42.7, A48.2-A48.4, A48.8-A49.9, A54.86, B00.7, B3.77, B92, B94.2-B96.89, R65.10-R65.20, Z16.10-Z16.39

● **R65.1 Systemic inflammatory response syndrome (SIRS) of non-infectious origin**

Code first underlying condition, such as:
heatstroke (T67.0)
injury and trauma (S00-T88)

Excludes1   sepsis - code to infection
severe sepsis (R65.2)

R65.10 Systemic inflammatory response syndrome (SIRS) of non-infectious origin without acute organ dysfunction 🔎
Systemic inflammatory response syndrome (SIRS) NOS

R65.11 Systemic inflammatory response syndrome (SIRS) of non-infectious origin with acute organ dysfunction 🔎
Use additional code to identify specific acute organ dysfunction, such as:
acute kidney failure (N17.-)
acute respiratory failure (J96.0-)
critical illness myopathy (G72.81)
critical illness polyneuropathy (G62.81)
disseminated intravascular coagulopathy [DIC] (D65)
encephalopathy (metabolic) (septic) (G93.41)
hepatic failure (K72.0-)

● **R65.2 Severe sepsis**
Infection with associated acute organ dysfunction
Sepsis with acute organ dysfunction
Sepsis with multiple organ dysfunction
Systemic inflammatory response syndrome due to infectious process with acute organ dysfunction

Code first underlying infection, such as:
infection following a procedure (T81.4-) ◀▥
infections following infusion, transfusion and therapeutic injection (T80.2-)
puerperal sepsis (O85)
sepsis following complete or unspecified spontaneous abortion (O03.87)
sepsis following ectopic and molar pregnancy (O08.82)
sepsis following incomplete spontaneous abortion (O03.37)
sepsis following (induced) termination of pregnancy (O04.87)
sepsis NOS (A41.9)

Use additional code to identify specific acute organ dysfunction, such as:
acute kidney failure (N17.-)
acute respiratory failure (J96.0-)
critical illness myopathy (G72.81)
critical illness polyneuropathy (G62.81)
disseminated intravascular coagulopathy [DIC] (D65)
encephalopathy (metabolic) (septic) (G93.41)
hepatic failure (K72.0-)

R65.20 Severe sepsis without septic shock 🔎
Severe sepsis NOS

R65.21 Severe sepsis with septic shock 🔎
MCC when PDx is its own MCC
(Ex) See R57

● **R68 Other general symptoms and signs**

R68.0 Hypothermia, not associated with low environmental temperature
Excludes1   hypothermia NOS (accidental) (T68)
hypothermia due to anesthesia (T88.51)
hypothermia due to low environmental temperature (T68)
newborn hypothermia (P80.-)

● **R68.1 Nonspecific symptoms peculiar to infancy**
Excludes1   colic, infantile (R10.83)
neonatal cerebral irritability (P91.3)
teething syndrome (K00.7)

R68.11 Excessive crying of infant (baby)   P
Excludes1   excessive crying of child, adolescent, or adult (R45.83)

R68.12 Fussy infant (baby)   P
Irritable infant

R68.13 Apparent life threatening event in infant (ALTE)   P
Apparent life threatening event in newborn
Code first confirmed diagnosis, if known
Use additional code(s) for associated signs and symptoms if no confirmed diagnosis established, or if signs and symptoms are not associated routinely with confirmed diagnosis, or provide additional information for cause of ALTE

R68.19 Other nonspecific symptoms peculiar to infancy   P

R68.2 Dry mouth, unspecified
Excludes1   dry mouth due to dehydration (E86.0)
dry mouth due to sicca syndrome [Sjögren] (M35.0-)
salivary gland hyposecretion (K11.7)

R68.3 Clubbing of fingers
Clubbing of nails
Excludes1   congenital clubfinger (Q68.1)

● **R68.8 Other general symptoms and signs**

R68.81 Early satiety

R68.82 Decreased libido   A
Decreased sexual desire

R68.83 Chills (without fever)
Chills NOS
Excludes1   chills with fever (R50.9)

R68.84 Jaw pain
Mandibular pain
Maxilla pain
Excludes1   temporomandibular joint arthralgia (M26.62-) ◀▥

R68.89 Other general symptoms and signs

R69 Illness, unspecified
Unknown and unspecified cases of morbidity

ABNORMAL FINDINGS ON EXAMINATION OF BLOOD, WITHOUT DIAGNOSIS (R70-R79)

Excludes2   abnormal findings on antenatal screening of mother (O28.-) ◀
abnormalities of lipids (E78.-) ◀
abnormalities of platelets and thrombocytes (D69.-) ◀
abnormalities of white blood cells classified elsewhere (D70-D72) ◀
coagulation hemorrhagic disorders (D65-D68) ◀
diagnostic abnormal findings classified elsewhere —*see* Alphabetical Index ◀
hemorrhagic and hematological disorders of newborn (P50-P61) ◀

● **R70 Elevated erythrocyte sedimentation rate and abnormality of plasma viscosity**
R70.0 Elevated erythrocyte sedimentation rate
R70.1 Abnormal plasma viscosity

◀ New   ◀▥ Revised   ~~deleted~~ Deleted   Excludes 1   Excludes 2   Includes   Use additional   Code first   Code also   Unspecified
OGCR Official Guidelines   ● Unacceptable Principal Diagnosis   X Assign placeholder X   ● Use Additional Character(s)   ▸ Manifestation Code   **Coding Clinic**

● **R71**   **Abnormality of red blood cells**

     Excludes1   anemias (D50-D64)
         anemia of premature infant (P61.2)
         benign (familial) polycythemia (D75.0)
         congenital anemias (P61.2-P61.4)
         newborn anemia due to isoimmunization (P55.-)
         polycythemia neonatorum (P61.1)
         polycythemia NOS (D75.1)
         polycythemia vera (D45)
         secondary polycythemia (D75.1)

   R71.0   **Precipitous drop in hematocrit** 🏥
       Drop (precipitous) in hemoglobin
       Drop in hematocrit
       Blood volume that is red blood cells
       ⓔ D62, D64.4-D64.9

   R71.8   **Other abnormality of red blood cells**
       Abnormal red-cell morphology NOS
       Abnormal red-cell volume NOS
       Anisocytosis
       Red blood cells of unequal size
       Poikilocytosis
       Red blood cells of abnormal shape

● **R73**   **Elevated blood glucose level**

     Excludes1   diabetes mellitus (E08-E13)
         diabetes mellitus in pregnancy, childbirth and the puerperium (O24.-)
         neonatal disorders (P70.0-P70.2)
         postsurgical hypoinsulinemia (E89.1)

   ● **R73.0**   **Abnormal glucose**
       Excludes1   abnormal glucose in pregnancy (O99.81-)
           diabetes mellitus (E08-E13)
           dysmetabolic syndrome X (E88.81)
           gestational diabetes (O24.4-)
           glycosuria (R81)
           hypoglycemia (E16.2)

     R73.01   **Impaired fasting glucose**
         Elevated fasting glucose

     R73.02   **Impaired glucose tolerance (oral)**
         Elevated glucose tolerance

     R73.03   **Prediabetes** ◀
         Latent diabetes ◀

     R73.09   **Other abnormal glucose**
         Abnormal glucose NOS
         Abnormal non-fasting glucose tolerance
         ~~Prediabetes~~

   R73.9   **Hyperglycemia, unspecified**

● **R74**   **Abnormal serum enzyme levels**

   R74.0   **Nonspecific elevation of levels of transaminase and lactic acid dehydrogenase [LDH]**

   R74.8   **Abnormal levels of other serum enzymes**
       Abnormal level of acid phosphatase
       Abnormal level of alkaline phosphatase
       Abnormal level of amylase
       Abnormal level of lipase [triacylglycerol lipase]

   R74.9   **Abnormal serum enzyme level, unspecified**

OGCR   Section I.C.1.2.e and f.

Patients with inconclusive HIV serology

e. Patients with inconclusive HIV serology, but no definitive diagnosis or manifestations of the illness, may be assigned code R75, Inconclusive laboratory evidence of human immunodeficiency virus [HIV].

f. Previously diagnosed HIV-related illness

Patients with any known prior diagnosis of an HIV-related illness should be coded to B20. Once a patient has developed an HIV-related illness, the patient should always be assigned code B20 on every subsequent admission/encounter. Patients previously diagnosed with any HIV illness (B20) should never be assigned to R75 or Z21, Asymptomatic human immunodeficiency virus [HIV] infection status.

● **R75**   **Inconclusive laboratory evidence of human immunodeficiency virus [HIV]**
     Nonconclusive HIV-test finding in infants

     Excludes1   asymptomatic human immunodeficiency virus [HIV] infection status (Z21)
         human immunodeficiency virus [HIV] disease (B20)

● **R76**   **Other abnormal immunological findings in serum**

   R76.0   **Raised antibody titer**
       Excludes1   isoimmunization in pregnancy (O36.0-O36.1)
           isoimmunization affecting newborn (P55.-)

   ● **R76.1**   **Nonspecific reaction to test for tuberculosis**

     R76.11   **Nonspecific reaction to tuberculin skin test without active tuberculosis**
         Abnormal result of Mantoux test
         PPD positive
         Tuberculin (skin test) positive
         Tuberculin (skin test) reactor
         Excludes1   nonspecific reaction to cell mediated immunity measurement of gamma interferon antigen response without active tuberculosis (R76.12)

     R76.12   **Nonspecific reaction to cell mediated immunity measurement of gamma interferon antigen response without active tuberculosis**
         Nonspecific reaction to QuantiFERON-TB test (QFT) without active tuberculosis
         Excludes1   nonspecific reaction to tuberculin skin test without active tuberculosis (R76.11)
           positive tuberculin skin test (R76.11)

   R76.8   **Other specified abnormal immunological findings in serum**
       Raised level of immunoglobulins NOS

   R76.9   **Abnormal immunological finding in serum, unspecified**

● **R77**   **Other abnormalities of plasma proteins**

     Excludes1   disorders of plasma-protein metabolism (E88.0)

   R77.0   **Abnormality of albumin**

   R77.1   **Abnormality of globulin**
       Hyperglobulinemia NOS

   R77.2   **Abnormality of alphafetoprotein**

   R77.8   **Other specified abnormalities of plasma proteins**

   R77.9   **Abnormality of plasma protein, unspecified**

● **R78**   **Findings of drugs and other substances, not normally found in blood**

     Use additional code to identify any retained foreign body, if applicable (Z18.-)

     Excludes1   mental or behavioral disorders due to psychoactive substance use (F10-F19)

   R78.0   **Finding of alcohol in blood**
       Use additional external cause code (Y90.-), for detail regarding alcohol level.

   R78.1   **Finding of opiate drug in blood**

   R78.2   **Finding of cocaine in blood**

   R78.3   **Finding of hallucinogen in blood**

   R78.4   **Finding of other drugs of addictive potential in blood**

   R78.5   **Finding of other psychotropic drug in blood**

   R78.6   **Finding of steroid agent in blood**

   ● **R78.7**   **Finding of abnormal level of heavy metals in blood**

     R78.71   **Abnormal lead level in blood**
         Excludes1   lead poisoning (T56.0-)

     R78.79   **Finding of abnormal level of heavy metals in blood**

CHAPTER 18 (R00-R99)

N Newborn Age: 0   **P** Pediatric Age: 0–17   **M** Maternity DX: 12–55   **A** Adult Age: 15–124   ♀ Females Only   ♂ Males Only

🏥 Complication\Comorbidity   🏥 Major C\C   ⓔ CC/MCC Exclusions   🏥 Hospital-Acquired Condition

1209

● **R78.8 Finding of other specified substances, not normally found in blood**

    R78.81 Bacteremia 🔖

      Blood poisoning/bacteremia

      Excludes1   sepsis-code to specified infection ◄▥▥

        ⒺⓍ B34.9, E07.81, G89.0-G89.4, R29.700-R29.742, R41.0-R41.3, R41.82, R41.9, R44.8-R44.9, R45.83-R45.84, R46.0-R46.89, R52, R68.0-R68.19, R68.81-R68.83, R68.89-R69, R70.1, R77.0-R77.9, R78.1-R78.6, R78.81, R78.9, R79.1-R79.89, R97.20, R97.21

    R78.89 Finding of other specified substances, not normally found in blood

      Finding of abnormal level of lithium in blood

  R78.9 Finding of unspecified substance, not normally found in blood

● **R79 Other abnormal findings of blood chemistry**

  Use additional code to identify any retained foreign body, if applicable (Z18.-)

  Excludes1   abnormality of fluid, electrolyte or acid-base balance (E86-E87)

      asymptomatic hyperuricemia (E79.0)

      hyperglycemia NOS (R73.9)

      hypoglycemia NOS (E16.2)

      neonatal hypoglycemia (P70.3-P70.4)

      specific findings indicating disorder of amino-acid metabolism (E70-E72)

      specific findings indicating disorder of carbohydrate metabolism (E73-E74)

      specific findings indicating disorder of lipid metabolism (E75.-)

  R79.0 Abnormal level of blood mineral

    Abnormal blood level of cobalt

    Abnormal blood level of copper

    Abnormal blood level of iron

    Abnormal blood level of magnesium

    Abnormal blood level of mineral NEC

    Abnormal blood level of zinc

    Excludes1   abnormal level of lithium (R78.89)

      disorders of mineral metabolism (E83.-)

      neonatal hypomagnesemia (P71.2)

      nutritional mineral deficiency (E58-E61)

  R79.1 Abnormal coagulation profile

    Abnormal or prolonged bleeding time

    Abnormal or prolonged coagulation time

    Abnormal or prolonged partial thromboplastin time [PTT]

    Abnormal or prolonged prothrombin time [PT]

    Excludes1   coagulation defects (D68.-)

● **R79.8 Other specified abnormal findings of blood chemistry**

  R79.81 Abnormal blood-gas level

  R79.82 Elevated C-reactive protein (CRP)

  R79.89 Other specified abnormal findings of blood chemistry

  R79.9 Abnormal finding of blood chemistry, unspecified

ABNORMAL FINDINGS ON EXAMINATION OF URINE, WITHOUT DIAGNOSIS (R80-R82)

Excludes1   abnormal findings on antenatal screening of mother (O28.-)

    diagnostic abnormal findings classified elsewhere - see Alphabetical Index

    specific findings indicating disorder of amino-acid metabolism (E70-E72)

    specific findings indicating disorder of carbohydrate metabolism (E73-E74)

● **R80 Proteinuria**

  Excludes1   gestational proteinuria (O12.1-)

  R80.0 Isolated proteinuria

    Idiopathic proteinuria

    Excludes1   isolated proteinuria with specific morphological lesion (N06.-)

  R80.1 Persistent proteinuria, unspecified

  R80.2 Orthostatic proteinuria, unspecified

    Postural proteinuria

  R80.3 Bence Jones proteinuria

  R80.8 Other proteinuria

  R80.9 Proteinuria, unspecified

    Albuminuria NOS

R81 Glycosuria

  Excludes1   renal glycosuria (E74.8)

● **R82 Other and unspecified abnormal findings in urine**

  Includes   chromoabnormalities in urine

  Use additional code to identify any retained foreign body, if applicable (Z18.-)

  Excludes2   hematuria (R31.-)

  R82.0 Chyluria 🔖

    White milky urine

    Excludes1   filarial chyluria (B74.-)

      ⒺⓍ G89.0-G89.4, R29.700-R29.742, R41.0-R41.3, R41.82, R41.9, R44.8-R44.9, R45.83-R45.84, R46.0-R46.89, R52, R68.0-R68.19, R68.81-R68.83, R68.89-R69, R82.0, R82.5-R82.99

  R82.1 Myoglobinuria 🔖

    Presence of myoglobin (iron containing protein) in urine

    ⒺⓍ G89.0-G89.4, R29.700-R29.742, R41.0-R41.3, R41.82, R41.9, R44.8-R44.9, R45.83-R45.84, R46.0-R46.89, R52, R68.0-R68.19, R68.81-R68.83, R68.89-R69, R82.1, R82.3, R82.5-R82.99

  R82.2 Biliuria

    Presence of bile pigments/salts in urine

  R82.3 Hemoglobinuria

    Presence of hemoglobin in urine

    Excludes1   hemoglobinuria due to hemolysis from external causes NEC (D59.6)

      hemoglobinuria due to paroxysmal nocturnal [Marchiafava-Micheli] (D59.5)

  R82.4 Acetonuria

    Ketonuria

  R82.5 Elevated urine levels of drugs, medicaments and biological substances

    Elevated urine levels of catecholamines

    Elevated urine levels of indoleacetic acid

    Elevated urine levels of 17-ketosteroids

    Elevated urine levels of steroids

  R82.6 Abnormal urine levels of substances chiefly nonmedicinal as to source

    Abnormal urine level of heavy metals

● **R82.7 Abnormal findings on microbiological examination of urine**

  Excludes1   colonization status (Z22.-)

  R82.71 Bacteriuria ◄

  R82.79 Other abnormal findings on microbiological examination of urine ◄

    Positive culture findings of urine ◄

  R82.8 Abnormal findings on cytological and histological examination of urine

● R82.9   **Other and unspecified abnormal findings in urine**

     R82.90   Unspecified **abnormal findings in urine**

     R82.91   **Other chromoabnormalities of urine**
Chromoconversion (dipstick)
Idiopathic dipstick converts positive for blood
with no cellular forms in sediment

         Excludes1   hemoglobinuria (R82.3)
myoglobinuria (R82.1)

     R82.99   **Other abnormal findings in urine**
Cells and casts in urine
Crystalluria
Melanuria

ABNORMAL FINDINGS ON EXAMINATION OF OTHER BODY FLUIDS, SUBSTANCES AND TISSUES, WITHOUT DIAGNOSIS (R83-R89)

     Excludes1   abnormal findings on antenatal screening of
mother (O28.-)
diagnostic abnormal findings classified elsewhere
- see Alphabetical Index

     Excludes2   abnormal findings on examination of blood,
without diagnosis (R70-R79)
abnormal findings on examination of urine,
without diagnosis (R80-R82)
abnormal tumor markers (R97.-)

● R83   **Abnormal findings in cerebrospinal fluid**

     R83.0   **Abnormal level of enzymes in cerebrospinal fluid**

     R83.1   **Abnormal level of hormones in cerebrospinal fluid**

     R83.2   **Abnormal level of other drugs, medicaments and biological substances in cerebrospinal fluid**

     R83.3   **Abnormal level of substances chiefly nonmedicinal as to source in cerebrospinal fluid**

     R83.4   **Abnormal immunological findings in cerebrospinal fluid**

     R83.5   **Abnormal microbiological findings in cerebrospinal fluid**
Positive culture findings in cerebrospinal fluid

         Excludes1   colonization status (Z22.-)

     R83.6   **Abnormal cytological findings in cerebrospinal fluid**

     R83.8   **Other abnormal findings in cerebrospinal fluid**
Abnormal chromosomal findings in cerebrospinal fluid

     R83.9   Unspecified **abnormal finding in cerebrospinal fluid**

● R84   **Abnormal findings in specimens from respiratory organs and thorax**

     Includes   abnormal findings in bronchial washings
abnormal findings in nasal secretions
abnormal findings in pleural fluid
abnormal findings in sputum
abnormal findings in throat scrapings

     Excludes1   blood-stained sputum (R04.2)

     R84.0   **Abnormal level of enzymes in specimens from respiratory organs and thorax**

     R84.1   **Abnormal level of hormones in specimens from respiratory organs and thorax**

     R84.2   **Abnormal level of other drugs, medicaments and biological substances in specimens from respiratory organs and thorax**

     R84.3   **Abnormal level of substances chiefly nonmedicinal as to source in specimens from respiratory organs and thorax**

     R84.4   **Abnormal immunological findings in specimens from respiratory organs and thorax**

     R84.5   **Abnormal microbiological findings in specimens from respiratory organs and thorax**
Positive culture findings in specimens from respiratory organs and thorax

         Excludes1   colonization status (Z22.-)

     R84.6   **Abnormal cytological findings in specimens from respiratory organs and thorax**

     R84.7   **Abnormal histological findings in specimens from respiratory organs and thorax**

     R84.8   **Other abnormal findings in specimens from respiratory organs and thorax**
Abnormal chromosomal findings in specimens from respiratory organs and thorax

     R84.9   Unspecified **abnormal finding in specimens from respiratory organs and thorax**

● R85   **Abnormal findings in specimens from digestive organs and abdominal cavity**

     Includes   abnormal findings in peritoneal fluid
abnormal findings in saliva

     Excludes1   cloudy peritoneal dialysis effluent (R88.0)
fecal abnormalities (R19.5)

     R85.0   **Abnormal level of enzymes in specimens from digestive organs and abdominal cavity**

     R85.1   **Abnormal level of hormones in specimens from digestive organs and abdominal cavity**

     R85.2   **Abnormal level of other drugs, medicaments and biological substances in specimens from digestive organs and abdominal cavity**

     R85.3   **Abnormal level of substances chiefly nonmedicinal as to source in specimens from digestive organs and abdominal cavity**

     R85.4   **Abnormal immunological findings in specimens from digestive organs and abdominal cavity**

     R85.5   **Abnormal microbiological findings in specimens from digestive organs and abdominal cavity**
Positive culture findings in specimens from digestive organs and abdominal cavity

         Excludes1   colonization status (Z22.-)

● R85.6   **Abnormal cytological findings in specimens from digestive organs and abdominal cavity**

     ● R85.61   **Abnormal cytologic smear of anus**

         Excludes1   abnormal cytological findings
in specimens from other
digestive organs and
abdominal cavity (R85.69)
carcinoma in situ of anus
(histologically confirmed)
(D01.3)
anal intraepithelial neoplasia I
[AIN I] (K62.82)
anal intraepithelial neoplasia II
[AIN II] (K62.82)
anal intraepithelial neoplasia III
[AIN III] (D01.3)
dysplasia (mild) (moderate)
of anus (histologically
confirmed) (K62.82)
severe dysplasia of anus
(histologically confirmed)
(D01.3)

         Excludes2   anal high risk human
papillomavirus (HPV) DNA
test positive (R85.81)
anal low risk human
papillomavirus (HPV) DNA
test positive (R85.82)

         R85.610   **Atypical squamous cells of undetermined significance on cytologic smear of anus (ASC-US)**

         R85.611   **Atypical squamous cells cannot exclude high grade squamous intraepithelial lesion on cytologic smear of anus (ASC-H)**

         R85.612   **Low grade squamous intraepithelial lesion on cytologic smear of anus (LGSIL)**

         R85.613   **High grade squamous intraepithelial lesion on cytologic smear of anus (HGSIL)**

         R85.614   **Cytologic evidence of malignancy on smear of anus**

CHAPTER 18 (R00-R99)

N Newborn Age: 0   **P** Pediatric Age: 0–17   **M** Maternity DX: 12–55   **A** Adult Age: 15–124   ♀ Females Only   ♂ Males Only

🔧 Complication\Comorbidity   🔧 Major C\C   (Ex) CC/MCC Exclusions   🔧 Hospital-Acquired Condition   **1211**

R85.615 **Unsatisfactory cytologic smear of anus**
  Inadequate sample of cytologic smear of anus

R85.616 **Satisfactory anal smear but lacking transformation zone**

R85.618 **Other abnormal cytological findings on specimens from anus**

R85.619 **Unspecified abnormal cytological findings in specimens from anus**
  Abnormal anal cytology NOS
  Atypical glandular cells of anus NOS

R85.69 **Abnormal cytological findings in specimens from other digestive organs and abdominal cavity**

R85.7 **Abnormal histological findings in specimens from digestive organs and abdominal cavity**

● **R85.8** **Other abnormal findings in specimens from digestive organs and abdominal cavity**

R85.81 **Anal high risk human papillomavirus (HPV) DNA test positive**
  Excludes1 anogenital warts due to human papillomavirus (HPV) (A63.0)
    condyloma acuminatum (A63.0)

R85.82 **Anal low risk human papillomavirus (HPV) DNA test positive**
  Use additional code for associated human papillomavirus (B97.7)

R85.89 **Other abnormal findings in specimens from digestive organs and abdominal cavity**
  Abnormal chromosomal findings in specimens from digestive organs and abdominal cavity

R85.9 **Unspecified abnormal finding in specimens from digestive organs and abdominal cavity**

● **R86** **Abnormal findings in specimens from male genital organs**
  Includes abnormal findings in prostatic secretions
    abnormal findings in semen, seminal fluid
    abnormal spermatozoa
  Excludes1 azoospermia (N46.0-)
    oligospermia (N46.1-)

R86.0 **Abnormal level of enzymes in specimens from male genital organs** ♂

R86.1 **Abnormal level of hormones in specimens from male genital organs** ♂

R86.2 **Abnormal level of other drugs, medicaments and biological substances in specimens from male genital organs** ♂

R86.3 **Abnormal level of substances chiefly nonmedicinal as to source in specimens from male genital organs** ♂

R86.4 **Abnormal immunological findings in specimens from male genital organs** ♂

R86.5 **Abnormal microbiological findings in specimens from male genital organs** ♂
  Positive culture findings in specimens from male genital organs
  Excludes1 colonization status (Z22.-)

R86.6 **Abnormal cytological findings in specimens from male genital organs** ♂

R86.7 **Abnormal histological findings in specimens from male genital organs** ♂

R86.8 **Other abnormal findings in specimens from male genital organs** ♂
  Abnormal chromosomal findings in specimens from male genital organs

R86.9 **Unspecified abnormal finding in specimens from male genital organs** ♂

● **R87** **Abnormal findings in specimens from female genital organs**
  Includes abnormal findings in secretion and smears from cervix uteri
    abnormal findings in secretion and smears from vagina
    abnormal findings in secretion and smears from vulva

R87.0 **Abnormal level of enzymes in specimens from female genital organs** ♀

R87.1 **Abnormal level of hormones in specimens from female genital organs** ♀

R87.2 **Abnormal level of other drugs, medicaments and biological substances in specimens from female genital organs** ♀

R87.3 **Abnormal level of substances chiefly nonmedicinal as to source in specimens from female genital organs** ♀

R87.4 **Abnormal immunological findings in specimens from female genital organs** ♀

R87.5 **Abnormal microbiological findings in specimens from female genital organs** ♀
  Positive culture findings in specimens from female genital organs
  Excludes1 colonization status (Z22.-)

● **R87.6** **Abnormal cytological findings in specimens from female genital organs**

● **R87.61** **Abnormal cytological findings in specimens from cervix uteri**
  Excludes1 abnormal cytological findings in specimens from other female genital organs (R87.69)
    abnormal cytological findings in specimens from vagina (R87.62-)
    carcinoma in situ of cervix uteri (histologically confirmed) (D06.-)
    cervical intraepithelial neoplasia I [CIN I] (N87.0)
    cervical intraepithelial neoplasia II [CIN II] (N87.1)
    cervical intraepithelial neoplasia III [CIN III] (D06.-)
    dysplasia (mild) (moderate) of cervix uteri (histologically confirmed) (N87.-)
    severe dysplasia of cervix uteri (histologically confirmed) (D06.-)

  Excludes2 cervical high risk human papillomavirus (HPV) DNA test positive (R87.810)
    cervical low risk human papillomavirus (HPV) DNA test positive (R87.820)

R87.610 **Atypical squamous cells of undetermined significance on cytologic smear of cervix (ASC-US)** ♀

R87.611 **Atypical squamous cells cannot exclude high grade squamous intraepithelial lesion on cytologic smear of cervix (ASC-H)** ♀

R87.612 **Low grade squamous intraepithelial lesion on cytologic smear of cervix (LGSIL)** ♀

R87.613 **High grade squamous intraepithelial lesion on cytologic smear of cervix (HGSIL)** ♀

R87.614 **Cytologic evidence of malignancy on smear of cervix** ♀

R87.615 **Unsatisfactory cytologic smear of cervix** ♀
  Inadequate sample of cytologic smear of cervix

    R87.616   **Satisfactory cervical smear but lacking transformation zone** ♀

    R87.618   **Other abnormal cytological findings on specimens from cervix uteri** ♀

    R87.619   Unspecified **abnormal cytological findings in specimens from cervix uteri** ♀

         Abnormal cervical cytology NOS

         Abnormal Papanicolaou smear of cervix NOS

         Abnormal thin preparation smear of cervix NOS

         Atypical endocervial cells of cervix NOS

         Atypical endometrial cells of cervix NOS

         Atypical glandular cells of cervix NOS

● R87.62   **Abnormal cytological findings in specimens from vagina**

     Use additional code to identify acquired absence of uterus and cervix, if applicable (Z90.71-)

     Excludes1   abnormal cytological findings in specimens from cervix uteri (R87.61-)

         abnormal cytological findings in specimens from other female genital organs (R87.69)

         carcinoma in situ of vagina (histologically confirmed) (D07.2)

         vaginal intraepithelial neoplasia I [VAIN I] (N89.0)

         vaginal intraepithelial neoplasia II [VAIN II] (N89.1)

         vaginal intraepithelial neoplasia III [VAIN III] (D07.2)

         dysplasia (mild) (moderate) of vagina (histologically confirmed) (N89.-)

         severe dysplasia of vagina (histologically confirmed) (D07.2)

     Excludes2   vaginal high risk human papillomavirus (HPV) DNA test positive (R87.811)

         vaginal low risk human papillomavirus (HPV) DNA test positive (R87.821)

    R87.620   **Atypical squamous cells of undetermined significance on cytologic smear of vagina (ASC-US)** ♀

    R87.621   **Atypical squamous cells cannot exclude high grade squamous intraepithelial lesion on cytologic smear of vagina (ASC-H)** ♀

    R87.622   **Low grade squamous intraepithelial lesion on cytologic smear of vagina (LGSIL)** ♀

    R87.623   **High grade squamous intraepithelial lesion on cytologic smear of vagina (HGSIL)** ♀

    R87.624   **Cytologic evidence of malignancy on smear of vagina** ♀

    R87.625   **Unsatisfactory cytologic smear of vagina** ♀

         Inadequate sample of cytologic smear of vagina

    R87.628   **Other abnormal cytological findings on specimens from vagina** ♀

    R87.629   Unspecified **abnormal cytological findings in specimens from vagina** ♀

         Abnormal Papanicolaou smear of vagina NOS

         Abnormal thin preparation smear of vagina NOS

         Abnormal vaginal cytology NOS

         Atypical endocervical cells of vagina NOS

         Atypical endometrial cells of vagina NOS

         Atypical glandular cells of vagina NOS

    R87.69   **Abnormal cytological findings in specimens from other female genital organs** ♀

         Abnormal cytological findings in specimens from female genital organs NOS

     Excludes1   dysplasia of vulva (histologically confirmed) (N90.0-N90.3)

R87.7   **Abnormal histological findings in specimens from female genital organs** ♀

     Excludes1   carcinoma in situ (histologically confirmed) of female genital organs (D06-D07.3)

         cervical intraepithelial neoplasia I [CIN I] (N87.0)

         cervical intraepithelial neoplasia II [CIN II] (N87.1)

         cervical intraepithelial neoplasia III [CIN III] (D06.-)

         dysplasia (mild) (moderate) of cervix uteri (histologically confirmed) (N87.-)

         dysplasia (mild) (moderate) of vagina (histologically confirmed) (N89.-)

         vaginal intraepithelial neoplasia I [VAIN I] (N89.0)

         vaginal intraepithelial neoplasia II [VAIN II] (N89.1)

         vaginal intraepithelial neoplasia III [VAIN III] (D07.2)

         severe dysplasia of cervix uteri (histologically confirmed) (D06.-)

         severe dysplasia of vagina (histologically confirmed) (D07.2)

● R87.8   **Other abnormal findings in specimens from female genital organs**

  ● R87.81   **High risk human papillomavirus (HPV) DNA test positive from female genital organs**

     Excludes1   anogenital warts due to human papillomavirus (HPV) (A63.0)

         condyloma acuminatum (A63.0)

    R87.810   **Cervical high risk human papillomavirus (HPV) DNA test positive** ♀

    R87.811   **Vaginal high risk human papillomavirus (HPV) DNA test positive** ♀

  ● R87.82   **Low risk human papillomavirus (HPV) DNA test positive from female genital organs**

     Use additional code for associated human papillomavirus (B97.7)

    R87.820   **Cervical low risk human papillomavirus (HPV) DNA test positive** ♀

    R87.821   **Vaginal low risk human papillomavirus (HPV) DNA test positive** ♀

    R87.89   **Other abnormal findings in specimens from female genital organs** ♀

         Abnormal chromosomal findings in specimens from female genital organs

R87.9   Unspecified **abnormal finding in specimens from female genital organs** ♀

CHAPTER 18 (R00-R99)

N Newborn Age: 0   **P** Pediatric Age: 0–17   **M** Maternity DX: 12–55   **A** Adult Age: 15–124   ♀ Females Only   ♂ Males Only

🔹 Complication\Comorbidity   🔹 Major C\C   (Ex) CC/MCC Exclusions   🔹 Hospital-Acquired Condition   **1213**

● **R88**   **Abnormal findings in other body fluids and substances**
    R88.0   Cloudy (hemodialysis) (peritoneal) dialysis effluent
    R88.8   Abnormal findings in other body fluids and substances

● **R89**   **Abnormal findings in specimens from other organs, systems and tissues**
    | **Includes** | abnormal findings in nipple discharge |
                      abnormal findings in synovial fluid
                      abnormal findings in wound secretions
    R89.0   Abnormal level of enzymes in specimens from other organs, systems and tissues
    R89.1   Abnormal level of hormones in specimens from other organs, systems and tissues
    R89.2   Abnormal level of other drugs, medicaments and biological substances in specimens from other organs, systems and tissues
    R89.3   Abnormal level of substances chiefly nonmedicinal as to source in specimens from other organs, systems and tissues
    R89.4   Abnormal immunological findings in specimens from other organs, systems and tissues
    R89.5   Abnormal microbiological findings in specimens from other organs, systems and tissues
        Positive culture findings in specimens from other organs, systems and tissues
        Excludes1   colonization status (Z22.-)
    R89.6   Abnormal cytological findings in specimens from other organs, systems and tissues
    R89.7   Abnormal histological findings in specimens from other organs, systems and tissues
    R89.8   Other abnormal findings in specimens from other organs, systems and tissues
        Abnormal chromosomal findings in specimens from other organs, systems and tissues
    R89.9   **Unspecified** abnormal finding in specimens from other organs, systems and tissues

---

ABNORMAL FINDINGS ON DIAGNOSTIC IMAGING AND IN FUNCTION STUDIES, WITHOUT DIAGNOSIS (R90-R94)

    | **Includes** | nonspecific abnormal findings on diagnostic imaging by computerized axial tomography [CAT scan] |
              nonspecific abnormal findings on diagnostic imaging by magnetic resonance imaging [MRI][NMR]
              nonspecific abnormal findings on diagnostic imaging by positron emission tomography [PET scan]
              nonspecific abnormal findings on diagnostic imaging by thermography
              nonspecific abnormal findings on diagnostic imaging by ultrasound [echogram]
              nonspecific abnormal findings on diagnostic imaging by X-ray examination
        Excludes1   abnormal findings on antenatal screening of mother (O28.-)
              diagnostic abnormal findings classified elsewhere - see Alphabetical Index

● **R90**   **Abnormal findings on diagnostic imaging of central nervous system**
    R90.0   Intracranial space-occupying lesion found on diagnostic imaging of central nervous system
  ● **R90.8**   Other abnormal findings on diagnostic imaging of central nervous system
        R90.81   Abnormal echoencephalogram
        R90.82   White matter disease, **unspecified**
        R90.89   Other abnormal findings on diagnostic imaging of central nervous system
              Other cerebrovascular abnormality found on diagnostic imaging of central nervous system

● **R91**   **Abnormal findings on diagnostic imaging of lung**
    R91.1   Solitary pulmonary nodule
        Coin lesion lung
        Solitary pulmonary nodule, subsegmental branch of the bronchial tree
    R91.8   Other nonspecific abnormal finding of lung field
        Lung mass NOS found on diagnostic imaging of lung
        Pulmonary infiltrate NOS
        Shadow, lung

● **R92**   **Abnormal and inconclusive findings on diagnostic imaging of breast**
    R92.0   Mammographic microcalcification found on diagnostic imaging of breast
        Excludes2   mammographic calcification (calculus) found on diagnostic imaging of breast (R92.1)
    R92.1   Mammographic calcification found on diagnostic imaging of breast
        Mammographic calculus found on diagnostic imaging of breast
    R92.2   Inconclusive mammogram
        Dense breasts NOS
        Inconclusive mammogram NEC
        Inconclusive mammography due to dense breasts
        Inconclusive mammography NEC
        Coding Clinic: 2015, Q1, P24
    R92.8   Other abnormal and inconclusive findings on diagnostic imaging of breast

● **R93**   **Abnormal findings on diagnostic imaging of other body structures**
    R93.0   Abnormal findings on diagnostic imaging of skull and head, not elsewhere classified
        Excludes1   intracranial space-occupying lesion found on diagnostic imaging (R90.0)
    R93.1   Abnormal findings on diagnostic imaging of heart and coronary circulation
        Abnormal echocardiogram NOS
        Abnormal heart shadow
    R93.2   Abnormal findings on diagnostic imaging of liver and biliary tract
        Nonvisualization of gallbladder
    R93.3   Abnormal findings on diagnostic imaging of other parts of digestive tract
  ● **R93.4**   Abnormal findings on diagnostic imaging of urinary organs
        Excludes2   hypertrophy of kidney (N28.81) ◀
        R93.41   Abnormal radiologic findings on diagnostic imaging of renal pelvis, ureter, or bladder ◀
            Filling defect of bladder found on diagnostic imaging ◀
            Filling defect of renal pelvis found on diagnostic imaging ◀
            Filling defect of ureter found on diagnostic imaging ◀
      ● **R93.42**   Abnormal radiologic findings on diagnostic imaging of kidney ◀
            R93.421   Abnormal radiologic findings on diagnostic imaging of right kidney ◀
            R93.422   Abnormal radiologic findings on diagnostic imaging of left kidney ◀
            R93.429   Abnormal radiologic findings on diagnostic imaging of **unspecified** kidney ◀
        R93.49   Abnormal radiologic findings on diagnostic imaging of other urinary organs ◀

Trochlear nerve (IV)

Optic nerve (II)

Olfactory nerve (I)

Abducens nerve (VI)

Oculomotor nerve (III)

Trigeminal nerve (V)

Facial nerve (VII)

Vestibulocochlear nerve (VIII)

Glossopharyngeal nerve (IX)

Vagus nerve (X)

Accessory nerve (XI)

Hypoglossal nerve (XII)

Figure 18-2 Cranial nerves. (From Patton and Thibodeau: Anatomy and physiology, ed 7, St. Louis, Mosby, 2009)

R93.5   **Abnormal findings on diagnostic imaging of other abdominal regions, including retroperitoneum**

R93.6   **Abnormal findings on diagnostic imaging of limbs**

    Excludes2   abnormal finding in skin and subcutaneous tissue (R93.8)

R93.7   **Abnormal findings on diagnostic imaging of other parts of musculoskeletal system**

    Excludes2   abnormal findings on diagnostic imaging of skull (R93.0)

R93.8   **Abnormal findings on diagnostic imaging of other specified body structures**

    Abnormal finding by radioisotope localization of placenta

    Abnormal radiological finding in skin and subcutaneous tissue

    Mediastinal shift

R93.9   **Diagnostic imaging inconclusive due to excess body fat of patient**

● **R94**   **Abnormal results of function studies**

    Includes   abnormal results of radionuclide [radioisotope] uptake studies

       abnormal results of scintigraphy

● **R94.0**   **Abnormal results of function studies of central nervous system**

    R94.01   **Abnormal electroencephalogram [EEG]**

    R94.02   **Abnormal brain scan**

    R94.09   **Abnormal results of other function studies of central nervous system**

● **R94.1**   **Abnormal results of function studies of peripheral nervous system and special senses**

● **R94.11**   **Abnormal results of function studies of eye**

    R94.110   **Abnormal electro-oculogram [EOG]**

    R94.111   **Abnormal electroretinogram [ERG]**

       Abnormal retinal function study

    R94.112   **Abnormal visually evoked potential [VEP]**

    R94.113   **Abnormal oculomotor study**

    R94.118   **Abnormal results of other function studies of eye**

● **R94.12**   **Abnormal results of function studies of ear and other special senses**

    R94.120   **Abnormal auditory function study**

    R94.121   **Abnormal vestibular function study**

    R94.128   **Abnormal results of other function studies of ear and other special senses**

● **R94.13**   **Abnormal results of function studies of peripheral nervous system**

    R94.130   **Abnormal response to nerve stimulation, unspecified**

    R94.131   **Abnormal electromyogram [EMG]**

       Excludes1   electromyogram of eye (R94.113)

    R94.138   **Abnormal results of other function studies of peripheral nervous system**

R94.2   **Abnormal results of pulmonary function studies**

    Reduced ventilatory capacity

    Reduced vital capacity

Item 18–1 The **peripheral nervous system** consists of 31 pairs of spinal nerves, 12 pairs of cranial nerves, and the autonomic nerves, which are divided into the parasympathetic and sympathetic nerves. The cranial nerves are: olfactory (I), optic (II), oculomotor (III), trochlear (IV), trigeminal (V), abducens (VI), facial (VII), vestibulocochlear (VIII), glossopharyngeal (IX), vagus (X), accessory (XI), and hypoglossal (XII).

N   Newborn Age: 0   **P**   Pediatric Age: 0–17   **M**   Maternity DX: 12–55   **A**   Adult Age: 15–124   ♀   Females Only   ♂   Males Only

🍇 Complication\Comorbidity   🍇 Major C\C   ⓔ CC/MCC Exclusions   🍇 Hospital-Acquired Condition   **1215**

● **R94.3**   **Abnormal results of cardiovascular function studies**

    R94.30   **Abnormal result of cardiovascular function study, unspecified**

    R94.31   **Abnormal electrocardiogram [ECG] [EKG]**

        Excludes1   long QT syndrome (I45.81)

    R94.39   **Abnormal result of other cardiovascular function study**

        Abnormal electrophysiological intracardiac studies

        Abnormal phonocardiogram

        Abnormal vectorcardiogram

R94.4   **Abnormal results of kidney function studies**

    Abnormal renal function test

R94.5   **Abnormal results of liver function studies**

R94.6   **Abnormal results of thyroid function studies**

R94.7   **Abnormal results of other endocrine function studies**

    Excludes2   abnormal glucose (R73.0-)

R94.8   **Abnormal results of function studies of other organs and systems**

    Abnormal basal metabolic rate [BMR]

    Abnormal bladder function test

    Abnormal splenic function test

ABNORMAL TUMOR MARKERS (R97)

● **R97**   **Abnormal tumor markers**

    Elevated tumor associated antigens [TAA]

    Elevated tumor specific antigens [TSA]

    R97.0   **Elevated carcinoembryonic antigen [CEA]**

    R97.1   **Elevated cancer antigen 125 [CA 125]** ♀

●   **R97.2**   **Elevated prostate specific antigen [PSA]**

        R97.20   **Elevated prostate specific antigen [PSA]** ♂ ◀   **A**

            MCE: Questionable admission when principal dx

        R97.21   **Rising PSA following treatment for malignant neoplasm of prostate** ♂ ◀   **A**

            MCE: Questionable admission when principal dx

    R97.8   **Other abnormal tumor markers**

ILL-DEFINED AND UNKNOWN CAUSE OF MORTALITY (R99)

R99   **Ill-defined and unknown cause of mortality**

    Death (unexplained) NOS

    Unspecified cause of mortality

OGCR Section I.C.18.h.

    Death NOS

    Code R99, Ill-defined and unknown cause of mortality, is only for use in the very limited circumstance when a patient who has already died is brought into the emergency department or other healthcare facility and is pronounced dead upon arrival. It does not represent the discharge disposition of death.

◀ New   ◀▥ Revised   ~~deleted~~ Deleted   Excludes 1   Excludes 2   Includes   Use additional   Code first   Code also   Unspecified

OGCR Official Guidelines   ● Unacceptable Principal Diagnosis   X Assign placeholder X   ● Use Additional Character(s)   ▶ Manifestation Code   **Coding Clinic**

CHAPTER 19

INJURY, POISONING AND CERTAIN OTHER CONSEQUENCES OF EXTERNAL CAUSES (S00-T88)

OGCR Chapter-Specific Coding Guidelines

19. **Chapter 19: Injury, poisoning, and certain other consequences of external causes (S00-T88)**

a. Application of 7th Characters in Chapter 19

Most categories in chapter 19 have a 7th character requirement for each applicable code. Most categories in this chapter have three 7th character values (with the exception of fractures): A, initial encounter, D, subsequent encounter and S, sequela. Categories for traumatic fractures have additional 7th character values. **While the patient may be seen by a new or different provider over the course of treatment for an injury, assignment of the 7th character is based on whether the patient is undergoing active treatment and not whether the provider is seeing the patient for the first time.**

For complication codes, active treatment refers to treatment for the condition described by the code, even though it may be related to an earlier precipitating problem. For example, code T84.50XA, Infection and inflammatory reaction due to unspecified internal joint prosthesis, initial encounter, is used when active treatment is provided for the infection, even though the condition relates to the prosthetic device, implant or graft that was placed at a previous encounter.

7th character "A", initial encounter is used **for each encounter where** the patient is receiving active treatment for the condition.

7th character "D" subsequent encounter is used for encounters after the patient has **completed** active treatment of the condition and is receiving routine care for the condition during the healing or recovery phase.

The aftercare Z codes should not be used for aftercare for conditions such as injuries or poisonings, where 7th characters are provided to identify subsequent care. For example, for aftercare of an injury, assign the acute injury code with the 7th character "D" (subsequent encounter).

7th character "S", sequela, is for use for complications or conditions that arise as a direct result of a condition, such as scar formation after a burn. The scars are sequelae of the burn. When using 7th character "S", it is necessary to use both the injury code that precipitated the sequela and the code for the sequela itself. The "S" is added only to the injury code, not the sequela code. The 7th character "S" identifies the injury responsible for the sequela. The specific type of sequela (e.g. scar) is sequenced first, followed by the injury code.

See Section I.B.10. Sequelae, (Late Effects)

b. Coding of Injuries

When coding injuries, assign separate codes for each injury unless a combination code is provided, in which case the combination code is assigned. Code T07, Unspecified multiple injuries should not be assigned in the inpatient setting unless information for a more specific code is not available. Traumatic injury codes (S00-T14.9) are not to be used for normal, healing surgical wounds or to identify complications of surgical wounds.

The code for the most serious injury, as determined by the provider and the focus of treatment, is sequenced first.

1) Superficial injuries

Superficial injuries such as abrasions or contusions are not coded when associated with more severe injuries of the same site.

2) Primary injury with damage to nerves/blood vessels

When a primary injury results in minor damage to peripheral nerves or blood vessels, the primary injury is sequenced first with additional code(s) for injuries to nerves and spinal cord (such as category S04), and/or injury to blood vessels (such as category S15). When the primary injury is to the blood vessels or nerves, that injury should be sequenced first.

c. Coding of Traumatic Fractures

The principles of multiple coding of injuries should be followed in coding fractures. Fractures of specified sites are coded individually by site in accordance with both the provisions within categories S02, S12, S22, S32, S42, S49, S52, S59, S62, S72, S79, S82, S89, S92 and the level of detail furnished by medical record content.

A fracture not indicated as open or closed should be coded to closed. A fracture not indicated whether displaced or not displaced should be coded to displaced.

More specific guidelines are as follows:

1) Initial vs. Subsequent Encounter for Fractures

Traumatic fractures are coded using the appropriate 7th character for initial encounter (A, B, C) **for each encounter where** the patient is receiving active treatment for the fracture. The appropriate 7th character for initial encounter should also be assigned for a patient who delayed seeking treatment for the fracture or nonunion.

Fractures are coded using the appropriate 7th character for subsequent care for encounters after the patient has completed active treatment of the fracture and is receiving routine care for the fracture during the healing or recovery phase.

Care for complications of surgical treatment for fracture repairs during the healing or recovery phase should be coded with the appropriate complication codes.

Care of complications of fractures, such as malunion and nonunion, should be reported with the appropriate 7th character for subsequent care with nonunion (K, M, N,) or subsequent care with malunion (P, Q, R).

Malunion/nonunion: The appropriate 7th character for initial encounter should also be assigned for a patient who delayed seeking treatment for the fracture or nonunion.

The open fracture designations in the assignment of the 7th character for fractures of the forearm, femur and lower leg, including ankle are based on the Gustilo open fracture classification. When the Gustilo classification type is not specified for an open fracture, the 7th character for open fracture type I or II should be assigned (B, E, H, M, Q).

A code from category M80, not a traumatic fracture code, should be used for any patient with known osteoporosis who suffers a fracture, even if the patient had a minor fall or trauma, if that fall or trauma would not usually break a normal, healthy bone.

See Section I.C.13. Osteoporosis.

The aftercare Z codes should not be used for aftercare for traumatic fractures. For aftercare of a traumatic fracture, assign the acute fracture code with the appropriate 7th character.

2) Multiple fractures sequencing

Multiple fractures are sequenced in accordance with the severity of the fracture.

d. Coding of Burns and Corrosions

The ICD-10-CM makes a distinction between burns and corrosions. The burn codes are for thermal burns, except sunburns, that come from a heat source, such as a fire or hot appliance. The burn codes are also for burns resulting from electricity and radiation. Corrosions are burns due to chemicals. The guidelines are the same for burns and corrosions.

Current burns (T20-T25) are classified by depth, extent and by agent (X code). Burns are classified by depth as first degree (erythema), second degree (blistering), and third degree (full-thickness involvement). Burns of the eye and internal organs (T26-T28) are classified by site, but not by degree.

1) Sequencing of burn and related condition codes

Sequence first the code that reflects the highest degree of burn when more than one burn is present.

   a. When the reason for the admission or encounter is for treatment of external multiple burns, sequence first the code that reflects the burn of the highest degree.

   b. When a patient has both internal and external burns, the circumstances of admission govern the selection of the principal diagnosis or first-listed diagnosis.

   c. When a patient is admitted for burn injuries and other related conditions such as smoke inhalation and/or respiratory failure, the circumstances of admission govern the selection of the principal or first-listed diagnosis.

N Newborn Age: 0   **P** Pediatric Age: 0–17   **M** Maternity DX: 12–55   **A** Adult Age: 15–124   ♀ Females Only   ♂ Males Only

Complication\Comorbidity   Major C\C   (Ex) CC/MCC Exclusions   Hospital-Acquired Condition

1217

2) Burns of the same local site

Classify burns of the same local site (three-character category level, T20-T28) but of different degrees to the subcategory identifying the highest degree recorded in the diagnosis.

3) Non-healing burns

Non-healing burns are coded as acute burns.

Necrosis of burned skin should be coded as a non-healed burn.

4) Infected Burn

For any documented infected burn site, use an additional code for the infection.

5) Assign separate codes for each burn site

When coding burns, assign separate codes for each burn site. Category T30, Burn and corrosion, body region unspecified is extremely vague and should rarely be used.

6) Burns and Corrosions Classified According to Extent of Body Surface Involved

Assign codes from category T31, Burns classified according to extent of body surface involved, or T32, Corrosions classified according to extent of body surface involved, when the site of the burn is not specified or when there is a need for additional data. It is advisable to use category T31 as additional coding when needed to provide data for evaluating burn mortality, such as that needed by burn units. It is also advisable to use category T31 as an additional code for reporting purposes when there is mention of a third-degree burn involving 20 percent or more of the body surface.

Categories T31 and T32 are based on the classic "rule of nines" in estimating body surface involved: head and neck are assigned nine percent, each arm nine percent, each leg 18 percent, the anterior trunk 18 percent, posterior trunk 18 percent, and genitalia one percent. Providers may change these percentage assignments where necessary to accommodate infants and children who have proportionately larger heads than adults, and patients who have large buttocks, thighs, or abdomen that involve burns.

7) Encounters for treatment of sequela of burns

Encounters for the treatment of the late effects of burns or corrosions (i.e., scars or joint contractures) should be coded with a burn or corrosion code with the 7th character "S" for sequela.

8) Sequelae with a late effect code and current burn

When appropriate, both a code for a current burn or corrosion with 7th character "A" or "D" and a burn or corrosion code with 7th character "S" may be assigned on the same record (when both a current burn and sequelae of an old burn exist). Burns and corrosions do not heal at the same rate and a current healing wound may still exist with sequela of a healed burn or corrosion.

See Section I.B.10. Sequela, (Late Effects)

9) Use of an external cause code with burns and corrosions

An external cause code should be used with burns and corrosions to identify the source and intent of the burn, as well as the place where it occurred.

e. Adverse Effects, Poisoning , Underdosing and Toxic Effects

Codes in categories T36-T65 are combination codes that include the substance that was taken as well as the intent. No additional external cause code is required for poisonings, toxic effects, adverse effects and underdosing codes.

1) Do not code directly from the Table of Drugs

Do not code directly from the Table of Drugs and Chemicals. Always refer back to the Tabular List.

2) Use as many codes as necessary to describe

Use as many codes as necessary to describe completely all drugs, medicinal or biological substances.

3) If the same code would describe the causative agent

If the same code would describe the causative agent for more than one adverse reaction, poisoning, toxic effect or underdosing, assign the code only once.

4) If two or more drugs, medicinal or biological substances

If two or more drugs, medicinal or biological substances are reported, code each individually unless a combination code is listed in the Table of Drugs and Chemicals.

5) The occurrence of drug toxicity is classified in ICD-10-CM as follows:

(a) Adverse Effect

When coding an adverse effect of a drug that has been correctly prescribed and properly administered, assign the appropriate code for the nature of the adverse effect followed by the appropriate code for the adverse effect of the drug (T36-T50). The code for the drug should have a 5th or 6th character "5" (for example T36.0X5-) Examples of the nature of an adverse effect are tachycardia, delirium, gastrointestinal hemorrhaging, vomiting, hypokalemia, hepatitis, renal failure, or respiratory failure.

(b) Poisoning

When coding a poisoning or reaction to the improper use of a medication (e.g., overdose, wrong substance given or taken in error, wrong route of administration), first assign the appropriate code from categories T36-T50. The poisoning codes have an associated intent as their 5th or 6th character (accidental, intentional self-harm, assault and undetermined). **If the intent of the poisoning is unknown or unspecified, code the intent as accidental intent. The undetermined intent is only for use if the documentation in the record specifies that the intent cannot be determined.** Use additional code(s) for all manifestations of poisonings.

If there is also a diagnosis of abuse or dependence of the substance, the abuse or dependence is assigned as an additional code.

Examples of poisoning include:

(i) Error was made in drug prescription

Errors made in drug prescription or in the administration of the drug by provider, nurse, patient, or other person.

(ii) Overdose of a drug intentionally taken If an overdose of a drug was intentionally taken or administered and resulted in drug toxicity, it would be coded as a poisoning.

(iii) Nonprescribed drug taken with correctly prescribed and properly administered drug. If a nonprescribed drug or medicinal agent was taken in combination with a correctly prescribed and properly administered drug, any drug toxicity or other reaction resulting from the interaction of the two drugs would be classified as a poisoning.

(iv) Interaction of drug(s) and alcohol. When a reaction results from the interaction of a drug(s) and alcohol, this would be classified as a poisoning.

See Section I.C.4. if poisoning is the result of insulin pump malfunctions.

(c) Underdosing

Underdosing refers to taking less of a medication than is prescribed by a provider or a manufacturer's instruction. For

◀ New ◀▥ Revised ~~deleted~~ Deleted Excludes 1 Excludes 2 Includes Use additional Code first Code also Unspecified

OGCR Official Guidelines ● Unacceptable Principal Diagnosis X Assign placeholder X ● Use Additional Character(s) ▷ Manifestation Code **Coding Clinic**

underdosing, assign the code from categories T36-T50 (fifth or sixth character "6").

Codes for underdosing should never be assigned as principal or first-listed codes. If a patient has a relapse or exacerbation of the medical condition for which the drug is prescribed because of the reduction in dose, then the medical condition itself should be coded.

Noncompliance (Z91.12-, Z91.13-) or complication of care (Y63.6-Y63.9) codes are to be used with an underdosing code to indicate intent, if known.

(d) Toxic Effects

When a harmful substance is ingested or comes in contact with a person, this is classified as a toxic effect. The toxic effect codes are in categories T51-T65.

Toxic effect codes have an associated intent: accidental, intentional self-harm, assault and undetermined.

f. Adult and child abuse, neglect and other maltreatment

Sequence first the appropriate code from categories T74.- (Adult and child abuse, neglect and other maltreatment, confirmed) or T76.- (Adult and child abuse, neglect and other maltreatment, suspected) for abuse, neglect and other maltreatment, followed by any accompanying mental health or injury code(s).

If the documentation in the medical record states abuse or neglect it is coded as confirmed (T74.-). It is coded as suspected if it is documented as suspected (T76.-).

For cases of confirmed abuse or neglect an external cause code from the assault section (X92-**Y09**) should be added to identify the cause of any physical injuries. A perpetrator code (Y07) should be added when the perpetrator of the abuse is known. For suspected cases of abuse or neglect, do not report external cause or perpetrator code.

If a suspected case of abuse, neglect or mistreatment is ruled out during an encounter code Z04.71, Encounter for examination and observation following alleged physical adult abuse, ruled out, or code Z04.72, Encounter for examination and observation following alleged child physical abuse, ruled out, should be used, not a code from T76.

If a suspected case of alleged rape or sexual abuse is ruled out during an encounter code Z04.41, Encounter for examination and observation following alleged **adult rape** or code Z04.42, Encounter for examination and observation following alleged **child rape**, should be used, not a code from T76.

See Section I.C.15. Abuse in a pregnant patient.

g. Complications of care

1) General guidelines for complications of care

(a) Documentation of complications of care

See Section I.B.16. for information on documentation of complications of care.

2) Pain due to medical devices

Pain associated with devices, implants or grafts left in a surgical site (for example painful hip prosthesis) is assigned to the appropriate code(s) found in Chapter 19, Injury, poisoning, and certain other consequences of external causes. Specific codes for pain due to medical devices are found in the T code section of the ICD-10-CM. Use additional code(s) from category G89 to identify acute or chronic pain due to presence of the device, implant or graft (G89.18 or G89.28).

3) Transplant complications

(a) Transplant complications other than kidney

Codes under category T86, Complications of transplanted organs and tissues, are for use for both complications and rejection of transplanted organs. A transplant complication code is only assigned if the complication affects the function of the transplanted organ. Two codes are required to fully describe a transplant complication: the appropriate code from category T86 and a secondary code that identifies the complication.

Pre-existing conditions or conditions that develop after the transplant are not coded as complications unless they affect the function of the transplanted organs.

See I.C.21. for transplant organ removal status

See I.C.2. for malignant neoplasm associated with transplanted organ.

(b) Kidney transplant complications

Patients who have undergone kidney transplant may still have some form of chronic kidney disease (CKD) because the kidney transplant may not fully restore kidney function. Code T86.1- should be assigned for documented complications of a kidney transplant, such as transplant failure or rejection or other transplant complication. Code T86.1- should not be assigned for post kidney transplant patients who have chronic kidney (CKD) unless a transplant complication such as transplant failure or rejection is documented. If the documentation is unclear as to whether the patient has a complication of the transplant, query the provider.

Conditions that affect the function of the transplanted kidney, other than CKD, should be assigned a code from subcategory T86.1, Complications of transplanted organ, Kidney, and a secondary code that identifies the complication.

For patients with CKD following a kidney transplant, but who do not have a complication such as failure or rejection, *see section I.C.14. Chronic kidney disease and kidney transplant status.*

4) Complication codes that include the external cause

As with certain other T codes, some of the complications of care codes have the external cause included in the code. The code includes the nature of the complication as well as the type of procedure that caused the complication. No external cause code indicating the type of procedure is necessary for these codes.

5) Complications of care codes within the body system chapters

Intraoperative and postprocedural complication codes are found within the body system chapters with codes specific to the organs and structures of that body system. These codes should be sequenced first, followed by a code(s) for the specific complication, if applicable.

N Newborn Age: 0   **P** Pediatric Age: 0–17   **M** Maternity DX: 12–55   **A** Adult Age: 15–124   ♀ Females Only   ♂ Males Only

Complication\Comorbidity   Major C\C   (Ex) CC/MCC Exclusions   Hospital-Acquired Condition

1219

CHAPTER 19 (S00-T88)

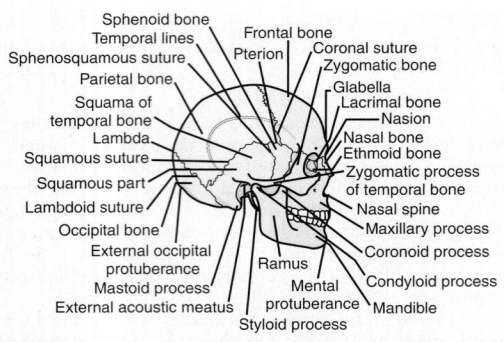

Figure 19-1 Lateral view of skull.

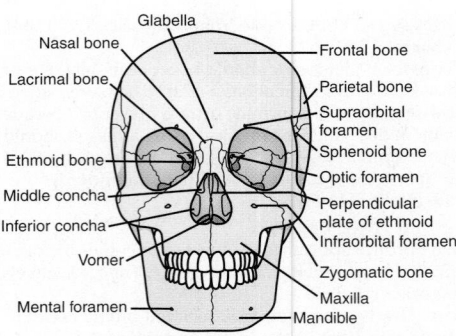

Figure 19-2 Frontal view of skull.

Figure 19-3 Anterior view of vertebral column.

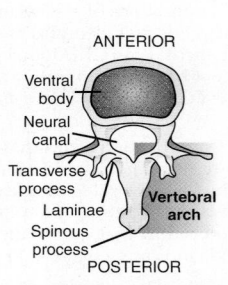

Figure 19-4 Vertebra viewed from above.

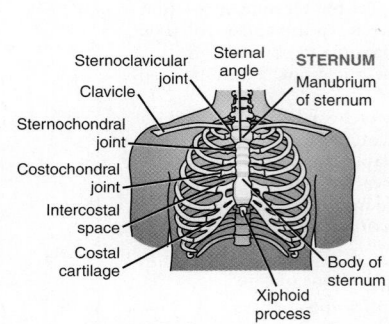

Figure 19-5 Anterior view of rib cage.

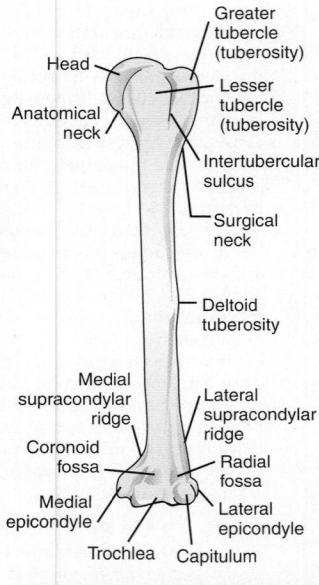

Figure 19-6 Anterior aspect of left humerus.

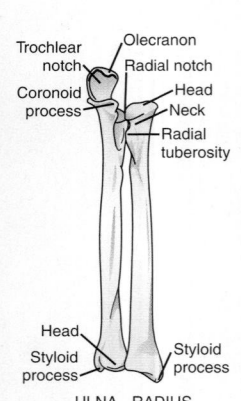

Figure 19-7 Anterior aspect of left radius and ulna.

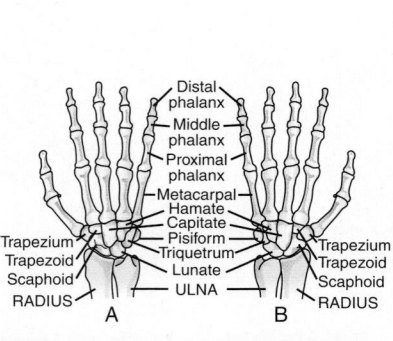

Figure 19-8 Right hand and wrist: **A.** Dorsal surface. **B.** Palmar surface.

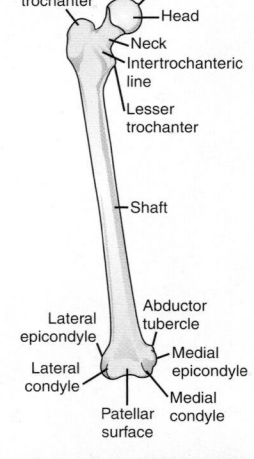

Figure 19-9 Anterior aspect of right femur.

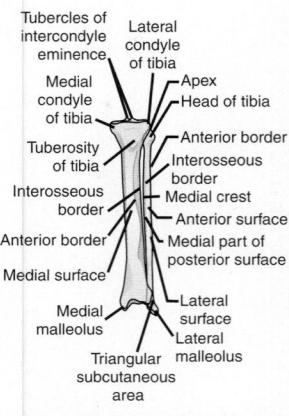

Figure 19-10 Anterior aspect of left tibia and fibula.

◀ New ◀ Revised ~~deleted~~ Deleted | Excludes 1 | Excludes 2 | Includes | Use additional | Code first | Code also | Unspecified

1220 OGCR Official Guidelines ● Unacceptable Principal Diagnosis X Assign placeholder X ● Use Additional Character(s) ▶ Manifestation Code **Coding Clinic**

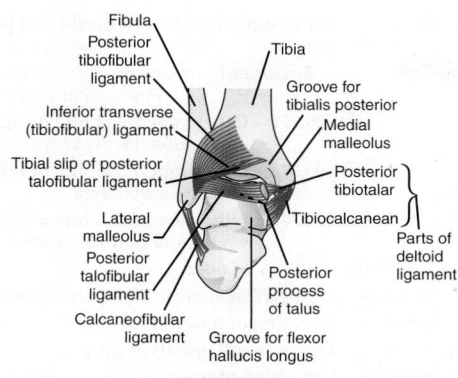

Figure 19-11   Posterior aspect of the left ankle joint.

Figure 19-12   Right foot viewed from above.

CHAPTER 19

INJURY, POISONING AND CERTAIN OTHER CONSEQUENCES OF EXTERNAL CAUSES (S00-T88)

Note: Use secondary code(s) from Chapter 20, External causes of morbidity, to indicate cause of injury. Codes within the T section that include the external cause do not require an additional external cause code.

Use additional code to identify any retained foreign body, if applicable (Z18.-)

Excludes1   birth trauma (P10-P15)
           obstetric trauma (O70-O71)

Note: The chapter uses the S-section for coding different types of injuries related to single body regions and the T-section to cover injuries to unspecified body regions as well as poisoning and certain other consequences of external causes.

This chapter contains the following blocks:

S00-S09	Injuries to the head
S10-S19	Injuries to the neck
S20-S29	Injuries to the thorax
S30-S39	Injuries to the abdomen, lower back, lumbar spine, pelvis and external genitals
S40-S49	Injuries to the shoulder and upper arm
S50-S59	Injuries to the elbow and forearm
S60-S69	Injuries to the wrist, hand, and fingers
S70-S79	Injuries to the hip and thigh
S80-S89	Injuries to the knee and lower leg
S90-S99	Injuries to the ankle and foot

T07	Injuries involving multiple body regions
T14	Injury of unspecified body region
T15-T19	Effects of foreign body entering through natural orifice
T20-T32	Burns and corrosions
T20-T25	Burns and corrosions of external body surface, specified by site
T26-T28	Burns and corrosions confined to eye and internal organs
T30-T32	Burns and corrosions of multiple and unspecified body regions
T33-T34	Frostbite
T36-T50	Poisoning by, adverse effect of and underdosing of drugs, medicaments and biological substances
T51-T65	Toxic effects of substances chiefly nonmedicinal as to source
T66-T78	Other and unspecified effects of external causes
T79	Certain early complications of trauma
T80-T88	Complications of surgical and medical care, not elsewhere classified

INJURIES TO THE HEAD (S00-S09)

Includes   injuries of ear
                injuries of eye
                injuries of face [any part]
                injuries of gum
                injuries of jaw
                injuries of oral cavity
                injuries of palate
                injuries of periocular area
                injuries of scalp
                injuries of temporomandibular joint area
                injuries of tongue
                injuries of tooth

Code also for any associated infection

Excludes2   burns and corrosions (T20-T32)
             effects of foreign body in ear (T16)
             effects of foreign body in larynx (T17.3)
             effects of foreign body in mouth NOS (T18.0)
             effects of foreign body in nose (T17.0-T17.1)
             effects of foreign body in pharynx (T17.2)
             effects of foreign body on external eye (T15.-)
             frostbite (T33-T34)
             insect bite or sting, venomous (T63.4)

● **S00**   **Superficial injury of head**

     Excludes1   diffuse cerebral contusion (S06.2-)
                    focal cerebral contusion (S06.3-)
                    injury of eye and orbit (S05.-)
                    open wound of head (S01.-)

The appropriate 7th character is to be added to each code from category S00

A	initial encounter
	All encounters involving diagnosis and treatment
D	subsequent encounter
	Encounters during the healing phase
S	sequela

● **S00.0**   **Superficial injury of scalp**

   X ● **S00.00**   **Unspecified superficial injury of scalp**

   X ● **S00.01**   **Abrasion of scalp**

   X ● **S00.02**   **Blister (nonthermal) of scalp**

   X ● **S00.03**   **Contusion of scalp**
                     Bruise of scalp
                     Hematoma of scalp

   X ● **S00.04**   **External constriction of part of scalp**

   X ● **S00.05**   **Superficial foreign body of scalp**
                     Splinter in the scalp

   X ● **S00.06**   **Insect bite (nonvenomous) of scalp**

   X ● **S00.07**   **Other superficial bite of scalp**
         Excludes1   open bite of scalp (S01.05)

N Newborn Age: 0   **P** Pediatric Age: 0–17   **M** Maternity DX: 12–55   **A** Adult Age: 15–124   ♀ Females Only   ♂ Males Only

Complication\Comorbidity   Major C\C   (Ex:) CC/MCC Exclusions   Hospital-Acquired Condition   **1221**

- S00.1 **Contusion of eyelid and periocular area**
  Black eye

  Excludes2   contusion of eyeball and orbital tissues (S05.1)

  X- S00.10 Contusion of unspecified eyelid and periocular area

  X- S00.11 Contusion of right eyelid and periocular area

  X- S00.12 Contusion of left eyelid and periocular area

- S00.2 **Other and unspecified superficial injuries of eyelid and periocular area**

  Excludes2   superficial injury of conjunctiva and cornea (S05.0-)

  - S00.20 Unspecified superficial injury of eyelid and periocular area
    - S00.201 Unspecified superficial injury of right eyelid and periocular area
    - S00.202 Unspecified superficial injury of left eyelid and periocular area
    - S00.209 Unspecified superficial injury of unspecified eyelid and periocular area

  - S00.21 Abrasion of eyelid and periocular area
    - S00.211 Abrasion of right eyelid and periocular area
    - S00.212 Abrasion of left eyelid and periocular area
    - S00.219 Abrasion of unspecified eyelid and periocular area

  - S00.22 Blister (nonthermal) of eyelid and periocular area
    - S00.221 Blister (nonthermal) of right eyelid and periocular area
    - S00.222 Blister (nonthermal) of left eyelid and periocular area
    - S00.229 Blister (nonthermal) of unspecified eyelid and periocular area

  - S00.24 External constriction of eyelid and periocular area
    - S00.241 External constriction of right eyelid and periocular area
    - S00.242 External constriction of left eyelid and periocular area
    - S00.249 External constriction of unspecified eyelid and periocular area

  - S00.25 Superficial foreign body of eyelid and periocular area
    Splinter of eyelid and periocular area

    Excludes2   retained foreign body in eyelid (H02.81-)

    - S00.251 Superficial foreign body of right eyelid and periocular area
    - S00.252 Superficial foreign body of left eyelid and periocular area
    - S00.259 Superficial foreign body of unspecified eyelid and periocular area

  - S00.26 Insect bite (nonvenomous) of eyelid and periocular area
    - S00.261 Insect bite (nonvenomous) of right eyelid and periocular area
    - S00.262 Insect bite (nonvenomous) of left eyelid and periocular area
    - S00.269 Insect bite (nonvenomous) of unspecified eyelid and periocular area

- S00.27 Other superficial bite of eyelid and periocular area

  Excludes1   open bite of eyelid and periocular area (S01.15)

  - S00.271 Other superficial bite of right eyelid and periocular area
  - S00.272 Other superficial bite of left eyelid and periocular area
  - S00.279 Other superficial bite of unspecified eyelid and periocular area

- S00.3 **Superficial injury of nose**

  X- S00.30 Unspecified superficial injury of nose

  X- S00.31 Abrasion of nose

  X- S00.32 Blister (nonthermal) of nose

  X- S00.33 Contusion of nose
    Bruise of nose
    Hematoma of nose

  X- S00.34 External constriction of nose

  X- S00.35 Superficial foreign body of nose
    Splinter in the nose

  X- S00.36 Insect bite (nonvenomous) of nose

  X- S00.37 Other superficial bite of nose

    Excludes1   open bite of nose (S01.25)

- S00.4 **Superficial injury of ear**

  - S00.40 Unspecified superficial injury of ear
    - S00.401 Unspecified superficial injury of right ear
    - S00.402 Unspecified superficial injury of left ear
    - S00.409 Unspecified superficial injury of unspecified ear

  - S00.41 Abrasion of ear
    - S00.411 Abrasion of right ear
    - S00.412 Abrasion of left ear
    - S00.419 Abrasion of unspecified ear

  - S00.42 Blister (nonthermal) of ear
    - S00.421 Blister (nonthermal) of right ear
    - S00.422 Blister (nonthermal) of left ear
    - S00.429 Blister (nonthermal) of unspecified ear

  - S00.43 Contusion of ear
    Bruise of ear
    Hematoma of ear
    - S00.431 Contusion of right ear
    - S00.432 Contusion of left ear
    - S00.439 Contusion of unspecified ear

  - S00.44 External constriction of ear
    - S00.441 External constriction of right ear
    - S00.442 External constriction of left ear
    - S00.449 External constriction of unspecified ear

  - S00.45 Superficial foreign body of ear
    Splinter in the ear
    - S00.451 Superficial foreign body of right ear
    - S00.452 Superficial foreign body of left ear
    - S00.459 Superficial foreign body of unspecified ear

  - S00.46 Insect bite (nonvenomous) of ear
    - S00.461 Insect bite (nonvenomous) of right ear
    - S00.462 Insect bite (nonvenomous) of left ear
    - S00.469 Insect bite (nonvenomous) of unspecified ear

◀ New   ◀⋯ Revised   ~~deleted~~ Deleted   Excludes 1   Excludes 2   Includes   Use additional   Code first   Code also   Unspecified

1222   OGCR Official Guidelines   ● Unacceptable Principal Diagnosis   X Assign placeholder X   ● Use Additional Character(s)   ▶ Manifestation Code   **Coding Clinic**

● **S00.47　Other superficial bite of ear**
　　Excludes1　open bite of ear (S01.35)
　　● S00.471　Other superficial bite of right ear
　　● S00.472　Other superficial bite of left ear
　　● S00.479　Other superficial bite of unspecified ear
● **S00.5　Superficial injury of lip and oral cavity**
　● **S00.50　Unspecified superficial injury of lip and oral cavity**
　　● S00.501　Unspecified superficial injury of lip
　　● S00.502　Unspecified superficial injury of oral cavity
　● **S00.51　Abrasion of lip and oral cavity**
　　● S00.511　Abrasion of lip
　　● S00.512　Abrasion of oral cavity
　● **S00.52　Blister (nonthermal) of lip and oral cavity**
　　● S00.521　Blister (nonthermal) of lip
　　● S00.522　Blister (nonthermal) of oral cavity
　● **S00.53　Contusion of lip and oral cavity**
　　● S00.531　Contusion of lip
　　　　Bruise of lip
　　　　Hematoma of oral cavity
　　● S00.532　Contusion of oral cavity
　　　　Bruise of lip
　　　　Hematoma of oral cavity
　● **S00.54　External constriction of lip and oral cavity**
　　● S00.541　External constriction of lip
　　● S00.542　External constriction of oral cavity
　● **S00.55　Superficial foreign body of lip and oral cavity**
　　● S00.551　Superficial foreign body of lip
　　　　Splinter of lip and oral cavity
　　● S00.552　Superficial foreign body of oral cavity
　　　　Splinter of lip and oral cavity
　● **S00.56　Insect bite (nonvenomous) of lip and oral cavity**
　　● S00.561　Insect bite (nonvenomous) of lip
　　● S00.562　Insect bite (nonvenomous) of oral cavity
　● **S00.57　Other superficial bite of lip and oral cavity**
　　● S00.571　Other superficial bite of lip
　　　　Excludes1　open bite of lip (S01.551)
　　● S00.572　Other superficial bite of oral cavity
　　　　Excludes1　open bite of oral cavity (S01.552)
● **S00.8　Superficial injury of other parts of head**
　　Superficial injuries of face [any part] ◀
　X● **S00.80　Unspecified superficial injury of other part of head**
　X● **S00.81　Abrasion of other part of head**
　X● **S00.82　Blister (nonthermal) of other part of head**
　X● **S00.83　Contusion of other part of head**
　　　Bruise of other part of head
　　　Hematoma of other part of head
　X● **S00.84　External constriction of other part of head**
　X● **S00.85　Superficial foreign body of other part of head**
　　　Splinter in other part of head
　X● **S00.86　Insect bite (nonvenomous) of other part of head**
　X● **S00.87　Other superficial bite of other part of head**
　　　Excludes1　open bite of other part of head (S01.85)
● **S00.9　Superficial injury of unspecified part of head**
　X● **S00.90　Unspecified superficial injury of unspecified part of head**
　X● **S00.91　Abrasion of unspecified part of head**
　X● **S00.92　Blister (nonthermal) of unspecified part of head**
　X● **S00.93　Contusion of unspecified part of head**
　　　Bruise of head
　　　Hematoma of head

X● **S00.94　External constriction of unspecified part of head**
X● **S00.95　Superficial foreign body of unspecified part of head**
　　Splinter of head
X● **S00.96　Insect bite (nonvenomous) of unspecified part of head**
X● **S00.97　Other superficial bite of unspecified part of head**
　　Excludes1　open bite of head (S01.95)

● **S01　Open wound of head**
　Code also any associated:
　　injury of cranial nerve (S04.-)
　　injury of muscle and tendon of head (S09.1-)
　　intracranial injury (S06.-)
　　wound infection
　　Excludes1　open skull fracture (S02.- with 7th character B)
　　Excludes2　injury of eye and orbit (S05.-)
　　　　　　traumatic amputation of part of head (S08.-)
　The appropriate 7th character is to be added to each code from category S01

A	initial encounter
D	subsequent encounter
S	sequela

　● **S01.0　Open wound of scalp**
　　　Excludes1　avulsion of scalp (S08.0)
　X● **S01.00　Unspecified open wound of scalp**
　X● **S01.01　Laceration without foreign body of scalp**
　X● **S01.02　Laceration with foreign body of scalp**
　　　Coding Clinic: 2015, Q1, P5-7
　X● **S01.03　Puncture wound without foreign body of scalp**
　X● **S01.04　Puncture wound with foreign body of scalp**
　X● **S01.05　Open bite of scalp**
　　　Bite of scalp NOS
　　　Excludes1　superficial bite of scalp (S00.06, S00.07-)
　● **S01.1　Open wound of eyelid and periocular area**
　　Open wound of eyelid and periocular area with or without involvement of lacrimal passages
　　● **S01.10　Unspecified open wound of eyelid and periocular area**
　　　Ⓔ **For category S01.10 CC codes:** S01.101-S01.159[A], S05.20X-S05.8X9[A], S05.91X-S05.92X[A], S38.3XX[A], T14.90-T14.91, T79.A0X-T79.9XX[A]
　　　● S01.101　Unspecified open wound of right eyelid and periocular area A ☃
　　　● S01.102　Unspecified open wound of left eyelid and periocular area A ☃
　　　● S01.109　Unspecified open wound of unspecified eyelid and periocular area A ☃
　　● **S01.11　Laceration without foreign body of eyelid and periocular area**
　　　● S01.111　Laceration without foreign body of right eyelid and periocular area
　　　● S01.112　Laceration without foreign body of left eyelid and periocular area
　　　● S01.119　Laceration without foreign body of unspecified eyelid and periocular area
　　● **S01.12　Laceration with foreign body of eyelid and periocular area**
　　　● S01.121　Laceration with foreign body of right eyelid and periocular area
　　　● S01.122　Laceration with foreign body of left eyelid and periocular area
　　　● S01.129　Laceration with foreign body of unspecified eyelid and periocular area

N Newborn Age: 0　　**P** Pediatric Age: 0–17　　**M** Maternity DX: 12–55　　**A** Adult Age: 15–124　　♀ Females Only　　♂ Males Only

☃ Complication\Comorbidity　　☒ Major C\C　　Ⓔ CC/MCC Exclusions　　☃ Hospital-Acquired Condition

1223

CHAPTER 19 (S00-T88)

- S01.13   Puncture wound without foreign body of eyelid and periocular area
  - S01.131   Puncture wound without foreign body of right eyelid and periocular area
  - S01.132   Puncture wound without foreign body of left eyelid and periocular area
  - S01.139   Puncture wound without foreign body of unspecified eyelid and periocular area
- S01.14   Puncture wound with foreign body of eyelid and periocular area
  - S01.141   Puncture wound with foreign body of right eyelid and periocular area
  - S01.142   Puncture wound with foreign body of left eyelid and periocular area
  - S01.149   Puncture wound with foreign body of unspecified eyelid and periocular area
- S01.15   Open bite of eyelid and periocular area
  Bite of eyelid and periocular area NOS
  > **Excludes1**   superficial bite of eyelid and periocular area (S00.26, S00.27)
  - S01.151   Open bite of right eyelid and periocular area
  - S01.152   Open bite of left eyelid and periocular area
  - S01.159   Open bite of unspecified eyelid and periocular area
- S01.2   Open wound of nose
  - X● S01.20   Unspecified open wound of nose
  - X● S01.21   Laceration without foreign body of nose
    Coding Clinic: 2015, Q1, P5-6
  - X● S01.22   Laceration with foreign body of nose
  - X● S01.23   Puncture wound without foreign body of nose
  - X● S01.24   Puncture wound with foreign body of nose
  - X● S01.25   Open bite of nose
    Bite of nose NOS
    > **Excludes1**   superficial bite of nose (S00.36, S00.37)
- S01.3   Open wound of ear
  - S01.30   Unspecified open wound of ear
    - S01.301   Unspecified open wound of right ear
    - S01.302   Unspecified open wound of left ear
    - S01.309   Unspecified open wound of unspecified ear
  - S01.31   Laceration without foreign body of ear
    - S01.311   Laceration without foreign body of right ear
    - S01.312   Laceration without foreign body of left ear
    - S01.319   Laceration without foreign body of unspecified ear
  - S01.32   Laceration with foreign body of ear
    - S01.321   Laceration with foreign body of right ear
    - S01.322   Laceration with foreign body of left ear
    - S01.329   Laceration with foreign body of unspecified ear
  - S01.33   Puncture wound without foreign body of ear
    - S01.331   Puncture wound without foreign body of right ear
    - S01.332   Puncture wound without foreign body of left ear
    - S01.339   Puncture wound without foreign body of unspecified ear

- S01.34   Puncture wound with foreign body of ear
  - S01.341   Puncture wound with foreign body of right ear
  - S01.342   Puncture wound with foreign body of left ear
  - S01.349   Puncture wound with foreign body of unspecified ear
- S01.35   Open bite of ear
  Bite of ear NOS
  > **Excludes1**   superficial bite of ear (S00.46, S00.47)
  - S01.351   Open bite of right ear
  - S01.352   Open bite of left ear
  - S01.359   Open bite of unspecified ear
- S01.4   Open wound of cheek and temporomandibular area
  - S01.40   Unspecified open wound of cheek and temporomandibular area
    - S01.401   Unspecified open wound of right cheek and temporomandibular area
    - S01.402   Unspecified open wound of left cheek and temporomandibular area
    - S01.409   Unspecified open wound of unspecified cheek and temporomandibular area
  - S01.41   Laceration without foreign body of cheek and temporomandibular area
    - S01.411   Laceration without foreign body of right cheek and temporomandibular area
      Coding Clinic: 2015, Q1, P5-7
    - S01.412   Laceration without foreign body of left cheek and temporomandibular area
    - S01.419   Laceration without foreign body of unspecified cheek and temporomandibular area
  - S01.42   Laceration with foreign body of cheek and temporomandibular area
    - S01.421   Laceration with foreign body of right cheek and temporomandibular area
    - S01.422   Laceration with foreign body of left cheek and temporomandibular area
    - S01.429   Laceration with foreign body of unspecified cheek and temporomandibular area
  - S01.43   Puncture wound without foreign body of cheek and temporomandibular area
    - S01.431   Puncture wound without foreign body of right cheek and temporomandibular area
    - S01.432   Puncture wound without foreign body of left cheek and temporomandibular area
    - S01.439   Puncture wound without foreign body of unspecified cheek and temporomandibular area
  - S01.44   Puncture wound with foreign body of cheek and temporomandibular area
    - S01.441   Puncture wound with foreign body of right cheek and temporomandibular area
    - S01.442   Puncture wound with foreign body of left cheek and temporomandibular area
    - S01.449   Puncture wound with foreign body of unspecified cheek and temporomandibular area

◀ New   ⬅ Revised   ~~deleted~~ Deleted   Excludes 1   Excludes 2   Includes   Use additional   Code first   Code also   Unspecified

OGCR Official Guidelines   ● Unacceptable Principal Diagnosis   X Assign placeholder X   ● Use Additional Character(s)   ▷ Manifestation Code   **Coding Clinic**

● **S01.45** **Open bite of cheek and temporomandibular area**
     Bite of cheek and temporomandibular area NOS

     Excludes2   superficial bite of cheek and temporomandibular area (S00.86, S00.87)

  ● **S01.451** **Open bite of right cheek and temporomandibular area**

  ● **S01.452** **Open bite of left cheek and temporomandibular area**

  ● **S01.459** **Open bite of unspecified cheek and temporomandibular area**

● **S01.5** **Open wound of lip and oral cavity**

     Excludes2   tooth dislocation (S03.2)
                 tooth fracture (S02.5)

 ● **S01.50** **Unspecified open wound of lip and oral cavity**

  ● **S01.501** **Unspecified open wound of lip**

  ● **S01.502** **Unspecified open wound of oral cavity**

 ● **S01.51** **Laceration of lip and oral cavity without foreign body**

  ● **S01.511** **Laceration without foreign body of lip**

  ● **S01.512** **Laceration without foreign body of oral cavity**

 ● **S01.52** **Laceration of lip and oral cavity with foreign body**

  ● **S01.521** **Laceration with foreign body of lip**

  ● **S01.522** **Laceration with foreign body of oral cavity**

 ● **S01.53** **Puncture wound of lip and oral cavity without foreign body**

  ● **S01.531** **Puncture wound without foreign body of lip**

  ● **S01.532** **Puncture wound without foreign body of oral cavity**

 ● **S01.54** **Puncture wound of lip and oral cavity with foreign body**

  ● **S01.541** **Puncture wound with foreign body of lip**

  ● **S01.542** **Puncture wound with foreign body of oral cavity**

 ● **S01.55** **Open bite of lip and oral cavity**

  ● **S01.551** **Open bite of lip**
          Bite of lip NOS

        Excludes1   superficial bite of lip (S00.571)

  ● **S01.552** **Open bite of oral cavity**
          Bite of oral cavity NOS

        Excludes1   superficial bite of oral cavity (S00.572)

● **S01.8** **Open wound of other parts of head**

 X● **S01.80** **Unspecified open wound of other part of head**

 X● **S01.81** **Laceration without foreign body of other part of head**

 X● **S01.82** **Laceration with foreign body of other part of head**

 X● **S01.83** **Puncture wound without foreign body of other part of head**

 X● **S01.84** **Puncture wound with foreign body of other part of head**

 X● **S01.85** **Open bite of other part of head**
       Bite of other part of head NOS

     Excludes1   superficial bite of other part of head (S00.85)

● **S01.9** **Open wound of unspecified part of head**

 X● **S01.90** **Unspecified open wound of unspecified part of head**

 X● **S01.91** **Laceration without foreign body of unspecified part of head**

 X● **S01.92** **Laceration with foreign body of unspecified part of head**

 X● **S01.93** **Puncture wound without foreign body of unspecified part of head**

 X● **S01.94** **Puncture wound with foreign body of unspecified part of head**

 X● **S01.95** **Open bite of unspecified part of head**
      Bite of head NOS

     Excludes1   superficial bite of head NOS (S00.97)

● **S02** **Fracture of skull and facial bones**

    Note: A fracture not indicated as open or closed should be coded to closed

      The appropriate 7th character is to be added to each code from category S02

A	initial encounter for closed fracture
B	initial encounter for open fracture
D	subsequent encounter for fracture with routine healing
G	subsequent encounter for fracture with delayed healing
K	subsequent encounter for fracture with nonunion
S	sequela

    Code also any associated intracranial injury (S06.-)

 X● **S02.0** **Fracture of vault of skull** A, K 🐾, B 🐾, A, B 🐾
      Fracture of frontal bone
      Fracture of parietal bone

     (Ex.) **For category S02.0 CC codes S02.0[A,B]:** S01.90X-S01.95X[A], S02.0XX-S02.19X[A,B,S], S02.2XX-S02.82X[S], S02.91X[A,B,S], S02.92XS, S06.0X0-S07.9XX[A], S08.89X[A], S09.10X-S09.19X[A], S09.8XX-S09.90X[A], S09.92X-S09.93X[A], S16.8XX-S19.9XX[A], S38.3XX[A], T14.90-T14.91, T79.A0XA-T79.9XX[A] **For S02.0[K]:** M80.00X-M80.88X[K,P], M84.30X-M84.68X[K,P], M84.750-M84.759[K,P], S02.0XXK, S02.110-S02.2X[K], S02.400-S02.609[K], S02.63XK, S02.66XK, S02.69XK, S02.19X-S02.92X[K], S12.000-S12.691[K], S22.000-S22.9XX[K], S32.000-S32.9XX[K], S42.001-S42.92X[K,P], S49.001-S49.199[K,P], S52.001-S52.92X[K,M,N,P,Q,R], S59.001-S59.299[K,P], S62.001-S62.92X[K,P], S72.001-S72.92X[K,M,N,P,Q,R], S79.001-S79.199[K,P], S82.001-S82.92X[K,M,N,P,Q,R], S89.001-S89.399[K,P], S92.001-S92.919[K,P]

 ● **S02.1** **Fracture of base of skull**

     Excludes1   orbit NOS (S02.8)
     Excludes2   orbital floor (S02.3-)

     (Ex.) **For category S02.1 CC codes S02.1[A,B]: For S02.1[A,B] CC codes:** See S02.0[A,B] **For S02.1[K] CC codes:** See S02.0[K]

 ● **S02.10** **Unspecified fracture of base of skull**

  ● **S02.101** **Fracture of base of skull, right side** A, K 🐾, B 🐾, A, B 🐾 ◀

  ● **S02.102** **Fracture of base of skull, left side** A, K 🐾, B 🐾, A, B 🐾 ◀

  ● **S02.109** **Fracture of base of skull, unspecified side** A, K 🐾, B 🐾, A, B 🐾 ◀

CHAPTER 19 (S00-T88)

● **S02.11 Fracture of occiput**

● **S02.110** Type I occipital condyle fracture, unspecified side A, K 🐾, B 🐾, A, B 🐾 ◀▥

● **S02.111** Type II occipital condyle fracture, unspecified side A, K 🐾, B 🐾, A, B 🐾 ◀▥

● **S02.112** Type III occipital condyle fracture, unspecified side A, K 🐾, B 🐾, A, B 🐾 ◀▥

● **S02.113** Unspecified occipital condyle fracture A, K 🐾, B 🐾, A, B 🐾

● **S02.118** Other fracture of occiput, unspecified side A, K 🐾, B 🐾, A, B 🐾 ◀▥

● **S02.119** Unspecified fracture of occiput A, K 🐾, B 🐾, A, B 🐾

● **S02.11A** Type I occipital condyle fracture, right side A, K 🐾, B 🐾, A, B 🐾 ◀

● **S02.11B** Type I occipital condyle fracture, left side A, K 🐾, B 🐾, A, B 🐾 ◀

● **S02.11C** Type II occipital condyle fracture, right side A, K 🐾, B 🐾, A, B 🐾 ◀

● **S02.11D** Type II occipital condyle fracture, left side A, K 🐾, B 🐾, A, B 🐾 ◀

● **S02.11E** Type III occipital condyle fracture, right side A, K 🐾, B 🐾, A, B 🐾 ◀

● **S02.11F** Type III occipital condyle fracture, left side A, K 🐾, B 🐾, A, B 🐾 ◀

● **S02.11G** Other fracture of occiput, right side A, K 🐾, B 🐾, A, B 🐾 ◀

● **S02.11H** Other fracture of occiput, left side A, K 🐾, B 🐾, A, B 🐾 ◀

X ● **S02.19** Other fracture of base of skull A, K 🐾, B 🐾, A, B 🐾

Fracture of anterior fossa of base of skull
Fracture of ethmoid sinus
Fracture of frontal sinus
Fracture of middle fossa of base of skull
Fracture of orbital roof
Fracture of posterior fossa of base of skull
Fracture of sphenoid
Fracture of temporal bone

X ● **S02.2 Fracture of nasal bones** B, K 🐾, B 🐾

Ⓔ **For category S02.2 CC codes S02.2[B]:** S01.90X-S01.95X[A], S02.0XX-S02.2XX[A,B,S], S02.30X-S02.413[S], S02.42XS-S02.82X[S], S02.91X[A,B,S], S02.92X[S], S06.0X0-S07.9XX[A], S08.89X[A], S09.10X-S09.19X[A], S09.8XX-S09.90X[A], S09.92XA-S09.93X[A], S16.8XX-S19.9XX[A], S38.3XX[A], S92.811-S92.819X[A,B], T14.90-T14.91, T79.A0X-T79.8XX[A] **For S02.2[K]:** See S02.0[K]

● **S02.3 Fracture of orbital floor**

Excludes1 orbit NOS (S02.8)
Excludes2 orbital roof (S02.1-)

Ⓔ **For category S02.3 CC codes S02.3[A,B]:** S01.90X-S01.95X[A], S02.0XX[A,B,S], S02.101-S02.2XX[A,B,S], S02.30X-S02.32X[A,B,S], S02.400-S02.413[S], S02.42X[A,B,S], S02.5XX-S02.69X[S], S02.80X-S02.92X[A,B,S], S06.0X0-S07.9XX[A], S08.89X[A], S09.10X-S09.19X[A], S09.8XX-S09.919X[A], S09.8XX-S09.90X[A]-S09.3X[A], S16.8XX-S19.9XX[A], S38.3XX[A], T14.90-T14.91, T79.8XX-T79.9XX[A], T79.A0X-T79.A9X[A] **For S02.3[K]:** See S02.0[K]

X ● **S02.30** Fracture of orbital floor, unspecified side A, B, K 🐾, A, B 🐾 ◀

X ● **S02.31** Fracture of orbital floor, right side A, B, K 🐾, A, B 🐾 ◀

X ● **S02.32** Fracture of orbital floor, left side A, B, K 🐾, A, B 🐾 ◀

● **S02.4 Fracture of malar, maxillary and zygoma bones**

Fracture of superior maxilla
Fracture of upper jaw (bone)
Fracture of zygomatic process of temporal bone

Ⓔ **For category S02.4 CC codes S02.4[A,B]:** N13.0, S01.90X- S01.95X[A], S02.0XX[A,B,S], S02.101-S02.413[A,B,S], S02.42XS, S02.5XXS, S02.600[A,B,S]-S02.69X[A,B,S], S02.91[A,B,S], S02.92X[A,B,S], S06.0X0-S07.9XX[A], S08.89X[A], S09.10X-S09.19X[A], S09.8XX-S09.90X[A], S09.92X-S09.93X[A], S16.8XX-S19.9XX[A], S38.3XX[A], T14.90-T14.91, T79.8XX-T79.9XX[A], T79.A0X-T79.A9X[A] **For S02.4[K]:** See S02.0[K] **unless otherwise indicated**

● **S02.40** Fracture of malar, maxillary and zygoma bones, unspecified

● **S02.400** Malar fracture unspecified side A, B, K 🐾, A, B 🐾 ◀▥

● **S02.401** Maxillary fracture, unspecified side A, B, K 🐾, A, B 🐾 ◀▥

● **S02.402** Zygomatic fracture, unspecified side A, B, K 🐾, A, B 🐾 ◀▥

● **S02.40A** Malar fracture, right side A, B, K 🐾, A, B 🐾 ◀

● **S02.40B** Malar fracture, left side A, B, K 🐾, A, B 🐾 ◀

● **S02.40C** Maxillary fracture, right side A, B, K 🐾, A, B 🐾 ◀

● **S02.40D** Maxillary fracture, left side A, B, K 🐾, A, B 🐾 ◀

● **S02.40E** Zygomatic fracture, right side A, B, K 🐾, A, B 🐾 ◀

● **S02.40F** Zygomatic fracture, left side A, B, K 🐾, A, B 🐾 ◀

● **S02.41** LeFort fracture

● **S02.411** LeFort I fracture A, B, K 🐾, A, B 🐾

● **S02.412** LeFort II fracture A, B, K 🐾, A, B 🐾

● **S02.413** LeFort III fracture A, B, K 🐾, A, B 🐾

X ● **S02.42** Fracture of alveolus of maxilla A, B, K 🐾, A, B 🐾

Ⓔ **For S02.42[A,B]:** See S02.3[A,B] **For S02.42[K]:** See S02.0[K]

X ● **S02.5 Fracture of tooth (traumatic) Broken tooth** K 🐾

Excludes1 cracked tooth (nontraumatic) (K03.81)

Ⓔ See S02.0[K]

● **S02.6 Fracture of mandible**

Fracture of lower jaw (bone)

Ⓔ **For category S02.6 CC codes S02.6[A,B]:** See S02.4[A,B] **For S02.6[K]:** See S02.0[K]

● **S02.60** Fracture of mandible of unspecified site

● **S02.600** Fracture of unspecified part of body of mandible, unspecified side A, B, K 🐾, A, B 🐾 ◀▥

● **S02.601** Fracture of unspecified part of body of right mandible A, B, K 🐾, A, B 🐾 ◀

● **S02.602** Fracture of unspecified part of body of left mandible A, B, K 🐾, A, B 🐾 ◀

● **S02.609** Fracture of mandible, unspecified A, B, K 🐾, A, B 🐾

● **S02.61** Fracture of condylar process of mandible

● **S02.610** Fracture of condylar process of mandible, unspecified side A, B, K 🐾, A, B 🐾 ◀

● **S02.611** Fracture of condylar process of right mandible A, B, K 🐾, A, B 🐾 ◀

● **S02.612** Fracture of condylar process of left mandible A, B, K 🐾, A, B 🐾 ◀

● **S02.62** Fracture of subcondylar process of mandible

● **S02.620** Fracture of subcondylar process of mandible, unspecified side A, B, K 🐾, A, B 🐾 ◀

● **S02.621** Fracture of subcondylar process of right mandible A, B, K 🐾, A, B 🐾 ◀

● **S02.622** Fracture of subcondylar process of left mandible A, B, K 🐾, A, B 🐾

◀ New ◀▥ Revised ~~deleted~~ Deleted Excludes 1 Excludes 2 Includes Use additional Code first Code also Unspecified
OGCR Official Guidelines ● Unacceptable Principal Diagnosis X Assign placeholder X ● Use Additional Character(s) ▷ Manifestation Code **Coding Clinic**

● **S02.63**   Fracture of coronoid process of mandible

   ● **S02.630**   Fracture of coronoid process of mandible, unspecified side A, B, K 🐾, A, B 🐾 ◀

   ● **S02.631**   Fracture of coronoid process of right mandible A, B, K 🐾, A, B 🐾 ◀

   ● **S02.632**   Fracture of coronoid process of left mandible A, B, K 🐾, A, B 🐾 ◀

● **S02.64**   Fracture of ramus of mandible

   ● **S02.640**   Fracture of ramus of mandible, unspecified side A, B, K 🐾, A, B 🐾 ◀

   ● **S02.641**   Fracture of ramus of right mandible A, B, K 🐾, A, B 🐾 ◀

   ● **S02.642**   Fracture of ramus of left mandible A, B, K 🐾, A, B 🐾 ◀

● **S02.65**   Fracture of angle of mandible

   ● **S02.650**   Fracture of angle of mandible, unspecified side A, B, K 🐾, A, B 🐾 ◀

   ● **S02.651**   Fracture of angle of right mandible A, B, K 🐾, A, B 🐾 ◀

   ● **S02.652**   Fracture of angle of left mandible A, B, K 🐾, A, B 🐾 ◀

X ● **S02.66**   Fracture of symphysis of mandible A, B, K 🐾, A, B 🐾

● **S02.67**   Fracture of alveolus of mandible

   ● **S02.670**   Fracture of alveolus of mandible, unspecified side A, B, K 🐾, A, B 🐾 ◀

   ● **S02.671**   Fracture of alveolus of right mandible A, B, K 🐾, A, B 🐾 ◀

   ● **S02.672**   Fracture of alveolus of left mandible A, B, K 🐾, A, B 🐾 ◀

X ● **S02.69**   Fracture of mandible of other specified site A, B, K 🐾, A, B 🐾

● **S02.8**   Fractures of other specified skull and facial bones
Fracture of orbit NOS
Fracture of palate

   Excludes1   fracture of orbital floor (S02.3-)
              fracture of orbital roof (S02.1-)

   (Ex) For category S02.8 CC codes S02.8[A,B]: See S02.3[A,B] For S02.8[K]: See S02.0[K]

X ● **S02.80**   Fracture of other specified skull and facial bones, unspecified side A, B, K 🐾, A, B 🐾 ◀

X ● **S02.81**   Fracture of other specified skull and facial bones, right side A, B, K 🐾, A, B 🐾 ◀

X ● **S02.82**   Fracture of other specified skull and facial bones, left side A, B, K 🐾, A, B 🐾 ◀

● **S02.9**   Fracture of unspecified skull and facial bones

X ● **S02.91**   Unspecified fracture of skull A, K 🐾, B 🐾, A, B 🐾

     (Ex) For category S02.91 CC codes S02.91[A,B]: See S02.0[A,B] For S02.91[K]: See S02.0[K]

X ● **S02.92**   Unspecified fracture of facial bones A, B, K 🐾, A, B 🐾

     (Ex) For category S02.92 CC codes S02.92[A,B]: See S02.3[A,B] For S02.92[K]: See S02.0[K]

● **S03**   Dislocation and sprain of joints and ligaments of head

   Includes   avulsion of joint (capsule) or ligament of head
          laceration of cartilage, joint (capsule) or ligament of head
          sprain of cartilage, joint (capsule) or ligament of head
          traumatic hemarthrosis of joint or ligament of head
          traumatic rupture of joint or ligament of head
          traumatic subluxation of joint or ligament of head
          traumatic tear of joint or ligament of head

Code also any associated open wound

   Excludes2   Strain of muscle or tendon of head (S09.1)

The appropriate 7th character is to be added to each code from category S03

A	initial encounter
D	subsequent encounter
S	sequela

● **S03.0**   Dislocation of jaw
Dislocation of jaw (cartilage) (meniscus)
Dislocation of mandible
Dislocation of temporomandibular (joint)

  X ● **S03.00**   Dislocation of jaw, unspecified side ◀

  X ● **S03.01**   Dislocation of jaw, right side ◀

  X ● **S03.02**   Dislocation of jaw, left side ◀

  X ● **S03.03**   Dislocation of jaw, bilateral side ◀

X ● **S03.1**   Dislocation of septal cartilage of nose

X ● **S03.2**   Dislocation of tooth

● **S03.4**   Sprain of jaw
Sprain of temporomandibular (joint) (ligament)

  X ● **S03.40**   Sprain of jaw, unspecified side ◀

  X ● **S03.41**   Sprain of jaw, right side ◀

  X ● **S03.42**   Sprain of jaw, left side ◀

  X ● **S03.43**   Sprain of jaw, bilateral side ◀

X ● **S03.8**   Sprain of joints and ligaments of other parts of head

X ● **S03.9**   Sprain of joints and ligaments of unspecified parts of head

● **S04**   Injury of cranial nerve
The selection of side should be based on the side of the body being affected

Code first any associated intracranial injury (S06.-)

Code also any associated:
   open wound of head (S01.-)
   skull fracture (S02.-)

The appropriate 7th character is to be added to each code from category S04

A	initial encounter
D	subsequent encounter
S	sequela

● **S04.0**   Injury of optic nerve and pathways
Use additional code to identify any visual field defect or blindness (H53.4-, H54)

   (Ex) For category S04.0 CC codes: S04.011-S04.049[A], S04.811A-S04.9XX[A]

  ● **S04.01**   Injury of optic nerve
Injury of 2nd cranial nerve

   ● **S04.011**   Injury of optic nerve, right eye A 🐾

   ● **S04.012**   Injury of optic nerve, left eye A 🐾

   ● **S04.019**   Injury of optic nerve, unspecified eye A 🐾
       Injury of optic nerve NOS

CHAPTER 19 (S00-T88)

Trochlear nerve (IV)
Optic nerve (II)
Olfactory nerve (I)
Abducens nerve (VI)
Oculomotor nerve (III)
Facial nerve (VII)
Trigeminal nerve (V)
Vestibulocochlear nerve (VIII)
Glossopharyngeal nerve (IX)
Vagus nerve (X)
Accessory nerve (XI)
Hypoglossal nerve (XII)

Figure 19-13 Cranial nerves. (From Patton and Thibodeau: Anatomy and physiology, ed 7, St. Louis, Mosby, 2009)

X● **S04.02** **Injury of optic chiasm** A ⦿

● **S04.03** **Injury of optic tract and pathways**
Injury of optic radiation

● **S04.031** **Injury of optic tract and pathways, right eye** A ⦿

● **S04.032** **Injury of optic tract and pathways, left eye** A ⦿

● **S04.039** **Injury of optic tract and pathways, unspecified eye** A ⦿
Injury of optic tract and pathways NOS

● **S04.04** **Injury of visual cortex**

● **S04.041** **Injury of visual cortex, right eye** A ⦿

● **S04.042** **Injury of visual cortex, left eye** A ⦿

● **S04.049** **Injury of visual cortex, unspecified eye** A ⦿
Injury of visual cortex NOS

● **S04.1** **Injury of oculomotor nerve**
Injury of 3rd cranial nerve
Ⓔ⦁ For category S04.1 CC codes: S04.10X-S04.12X[A], S04.811-S04.9XX[A]

X● **S04.10** **Injury of oculomotor nerve, unspecified side** A ⦿

X● **S04.11** **Injury of oculomotor nerve, right side** A ⦿

X● **S04.12** **Injury of oculomotor nerve, left side** A ⦿

● **S04.2** **Injury of trochlear nerve**
Injury of 4th cranial nerve
Ⓔ⦁ For category S04.2 CC codes: S04.20X-S04.22X[A], S04.811-S04.9XX[A]

X● **S04.20** **Injury of trochlear nerve, unspecified side** A ⦿

X● **S04.21** **Injury of trochlear nerve, right side** A ⦿

X● **S04.22** **Injury of trochlear nerve, left side** A ⦿

● **S04.3** **Injury of trigeminal nerve**
Injury of 5th cranial nerve
Ⓔ⦁ For category S04.3 CC codes: S04.30XA-S04.32X[A], S04.811-S04.9XX[A]

X● **S04.30** **Injury of trigeminal nerve, unspecified side** A ⦿

X● **S04.31** **Injury of trigeminal nerve, right side** A ⦿

X● **S04.32** **Injury of trigeminal nerve, left side** A ⦿

● **S04.4** **Injury of abducent nerve**
Injury of 6th cranial nerve
Ⓔ⦁ For category S04.4 CC codes: S04.40X-S04.42X[A], S04.811-S04.9XX[A]

X● **S04.40** **Injury of abducent nerve, unspecified side** A ⦿

X● **S04.41** **Injury of abducent nerve, right side** A ⦿

X● **S04.42** **Injury of abducent nerve, left side** A ⦿

● **S04.5** **Injury of facial nerve**
Injury of 7th cranial nerve
Ⓔ⦁ For category S04.5 CC codes: S04.50X-S04.52X[A], S04.811-S04.9XX[A]

X● **S04.50** **Injury of facial nerve, unspecified side** A ⦿

X● **S04.51** **Injury of facial nerve, right side** A ⦿

X● **S04.52** **Injury of facial nerve, left side** A ⦿

● **S04.6** **Injury of acoustic nerve**
Injury of auditory nerve
Injury of 8th cranial nerve
Ⓔ⦁ For category S04.6 CC codes: S04.60X-S04.62X[A], S04.811-S04.9XX[A]

X● **S04.60** **Injury of acoustic nerve, unspecified side** A ⦿

X● **S04.61** **Injury of acoustic nerve, right side** A ⦿

X● **S04.62** **Injury of acoustic nerve, left side** A ⦿

● **S04.7** **Injury of accessory nerve**
Injury of 11th cranial nerve
Ⓔ⦁ For category S04.7 CC codes: S04.70X-S04.9XX[A]

X● **S04.70** **Injury of accessory nerve, unspecified side** A ⦿

X● **S04.71** **Injury of accessory nerve, right side** A ⦿

X● **S04.72** **Injury of accessory nerve, left side** A ⦿

◀ New   ◀━ Revised   ~~deleted~~ Deleted   Excludes 1   Excludes 2   Includes   Use additional   Code first   Code also   Unspecified
OGCR Official Guidelines   ● Unacceptable Principal Diagnosis   X Assign placeholder X   ● Use Additional Character(s)   ▸ Manifestation Code   **Coding Clinic**

● **S04.8   Injury of other cranial nerves**
⮡ (Ex) **For category S04.8 CC codes:** S04.811-S04.9XX[A]

　● **S04.81   Injury of olfactory [1st] nerve**

　　● **S04.811   Injury of olfactory [1st] nerve, right side** A 🔧

　　● **S04.812   Injury of olfactory [1st] nerve, left side** A 🔧

　　● **S04.819   Injury of olfactory [1st] nerve, unspecified side** A 🔧

　● **S04.89   Injury of other cranial nerves**
　　Injury of vagus [10th] nerve

　　● **S04.891   Injury of other cranial nerves, right side** A 🔧

　　● **S04.892   Injury of other cranial nerves, left side** A 🔧

　　● **S04.899   Injury of other cranial nerves, unspecified side** A 🔧

X ● **S04.9   Injury of unspecified cranial nerve** A 🔧
⮡ (Ex) S04.811-S04.9XX[A]

● **S05   Injury of eye and orbit**
　Includes   open wound of eye and orbit
　Excludes2   2nd cranial [optic] nerve injury (S04.0-)
　　　　　　　3rd cranial [oculomotor] nerve injury (S04.1-)
　　　　　　　open wound of eyelid and periocular area (S01.1-)
　　　　　　　orbital bone fracture (S02.1-, S02.3-, S02.8-)
　　　　　　　superficial injury of eyelid (S00.1-S00.2)

　The appropriate 7th character is to be added to each code from category S05

```
A    initial encounter
D    subsequent encounter
S    sequela
```

● **S05.0   Injury of conjunctiva and corneal abrasion without foreign body**
　Excludes1   foreign body in conjunctival sac (T15.1)
　　　　　　　foreign body in cornea (T15.0)
⮡ (Ex) **For category S05 CC codes unless otherwise indicated:**
　　S01.101-S01.159[A], S05.20X-S05.8X9[A], S05.91X-S05.92X[A],
　　S38.3XX[A], T14.90-T14.91, T79.A0X-T79.9XX[A]

X ● **S05.00   Injury of conjunctiva and corneal abrasion without foreign body, unspecified eye**

X ● **S05.01   Injury of conjunctiva and corneal abrasion without foreign body, right eye**

X ● **S05.02   Injury of conjunctiva and corneal abrasion without foreign body, left eye**

● **S05.1   Contusion of eyeball and orbital tissues**
　Traumatic hyphema
　Excludes2   black eye NOS (S00.1)
　　　　　　　contusion of eyelid and periocular area (S00.1)

X ● **S05.10   Contusion of eyeball and orbital tissues, unspecified eye**

X ● **S05.11   Contusion of eyeball and orbital tissues, right eye**

X ● **S05.12   Contusion of eyeball and orbital tissues, left eye**

● **S05.2   Ocular laceration and rupture with prolapse or loss of intraocular tissue**

X ● **S05.20   Ocular laceration and rupture with prolapse or loss of intraocular tissue, unspecified eye** A 🔧

X ● **S05.21   Ocular laceration and rupture with prolapse or loss of intraocular tissue, right eye** A 🔧

X ● **S05.22   Ocular laceration and rupture with prolapse or loss of intraocular tissue, left eye** A 🔧

● **S05.3   Ocular laceration without prolapse or loss of intraocular tissue**
　Laceration of eye NOS

X ● **S05.30   Ocular laceration without prolapse or loss of intraocular tissue, unspecified eye** A 🔧

X ● **S05.31   Ocular laceration without prolapse or loss of intraocular tissue, right eye** A 🔧

X ● **S05.32   Ocular laceration without prolapse or loss of intraocular tissue, left eye** A 🔧

● **S05.4   Penetrating wound of orbit with or without foreign body**
　Excludes2   retained (old) foreign body following penetrating wound in orbit (H05.5-)

X ● **S05.40   Penetrating wound of orbit with or without foreign body, unspecified eye** A 🔧

X ● **S05.41   Penetrating wound of orbit with or without foreign body, right eye** A 🔧

X ● **S05.42   Penetrating wound of orbit with or without foreign body, left eye** A 🔧

● **S05.5   Penetrating wound with foreign body of eyeball**
　Excludes2   retained (old) intraocular foreign body (H44.6-, H44.7)
⮡ (Ex) **For category S05.5 CC codes:** S01.101-S01.159[A], S05.20X-S05.8X9[A],
　　S05.91X-S05.92X[A], S38.3XX[A], T14.90-T14.91, T79.8XX-T79.9XX[A]

X ● **S05.50   Penetrating wound with foreign body of unspecified eyeball** A 🔧

X ● **S05.51   Penetrating wound with foreign body of right eyeball** A 🔧

X ● **S05.52   Penetrating wound with foreign body of left eyeball** A 🔧

● **S05.6   Penetrating wound without foreign body of eyeball**
　Ocular penetration NOS

X ● **S05.60   Penetrating wound without foreign body of unspecified eyeball**

X ● **S05.61   Penetrating wound without foreign body of right eyeball**

X ● **S05.62   Penetrating wound without foreign body of left eyeball**

● **S05.7   Avulsion of eye**
　Traumatic enucleation

X ● **S05.70   Avulsion of unspecified eye** A 🔧

X ● **S05.71   Avulsion of right eye** A 🔧

X ● **S05.72   Avulsion of left eye** A 🔧

● **S05.8   Other injuries of eye and orbit**
　Lacrimal duct injury

　● **S05.8X   Other injuries of eye and orbit**

　　● **S05.8X1   Other injuries of right eye and orbit** A 🔧

　　● **S05.8X2   Other injuries of left eye and orbit** A 🔧

　　● **S05.8X9   Other injuries of unspecified eye and orbit** A 🔧

● **S05.9   Unspecified injury of eye and orbit**
　Injury of eye NOS

X ● **S05.90   Unspecified injury of unspecified eye and orbit**

X ● **S05.91   Unspecified injury of right eye and orbit** A 🔧

X ● **S05.92   Unspecified injury of left eye and orbit** A 🔧

● **S06   Intracranial injury**

> **Includes**   traumatic brain injury

> Code also any associated:
> > open wound of head (S01.-)
> > skull fracture (S02.-)

> **Excludes1**   head injury NOS (S09.90)

> The appropriate 7th character is to be added to each code from category S06

> | | |
> |---|---|
> | A | initial encounter |
> | D | subsequent encounter |
> | S | sequela |

> (Ex:) For category S06 CC codes unless otherwise indicated: For S06[A,B]: See S02.4[A,B] For S06[S]: See S02.0[K]

> **Coding Clinic: 2015, Q4, P40**

● **S06.0   Concussion**

> Commotio cerebri

> > **Excludes1**   concussion with other intracranial injuries classified in subcategories S06.1- to S06.6- , S06.81- and S06.82- code to specified intracranial injury ◄▥

> ● **S06.0X   Concussion**

> > ● **S06.0X0   Concussion without loss of consciousness**

> > ● **S06.0X1   Concussion with loss of consciousness of 30 minutes or less** A 🔊, A 🔊

> > S06.0X2   Concussion with loss of consciousness of 31 minutes to 59 minutes

> > S06.0X3   Concussion with loss of consciousness of 1 hour to 5 hours 59 minutes

> > S06.0X4   Concussion with loss of consciousness of 6 hours to 24 hours

> > S06.0X5   Concussion with loss of consciousness greater than 24 hours with return to pre-existing conscious level

> > S06.0X6   Concussion with loss of consciousness greater than 24 hours without return to pre-existing conscious level with patient surviving

> > S06.0X7   Concussion with loss of consciousness of any duration with death due to brain injury prior to regaining consciousness

> > S06.0X8   Concussion with loss of consciousness of any duration with death due to other cause prior to regaining consciousness

> > ● **S06.0X9   Concussion with loss of consciousness of unspecified duration** A 🔊, A 🔊

> > > Concussion NOS

● **S06.1   Traumatic cerebral edema**

> Diffuse traumatic cerebral edema
> Focal traumatic cerebral edema

> ● **S06.1X   Traumatic cerebral edema**

> > ● **S06.1X0   Traumatic cerebral edema without loss of consciousness** A 🔊

> > > MCC when PDx is its own MCC
> > > (Ex:) G93.6, G93.82
> > > **Coding Clinic: 2015, Q1, P12**

● **S06.1X1   Traumatic cerebral edema with loss of consciousness of 30 minutes or less** A 🔊, A 🔊

> MCC when PDx is its own MCC
> (Ex:) G93.6, G93.82, S01.90X-S01.95X[A], S02.0XX-S02.19X[A,B,S], S02.2XXS-S02.82X[S], S02.91X[A,B,S], S02.92X[S], S06.0X0-S07.9XX[A], S08.89X-S09.19X[A], S09.8XX-S09.90X[A], S09.92X-S09.93X[A], S16.8XX-S19.9XX[A], S38.3XX[A], T14.90-T14.91, T79.8XX-T79.9XX[A], T79.A0X-T79.A9X[A]

● **S06.1X2   Traumatic cerebral edema with loss of consciousness of 31 minutes to 59 minutes** A 🔊, A 🔊

> MCC when PDx is its own MCC
> (Ex:) See S06.1X1

● **S06.1X3   Traumatic cerebral edema with loss of consciousness of 1 hour to 5 hours 59 minutes** A 🔊, A 🔊

> MCC when PDx is its own MCC
> (Ex:) See S06.1X1

● **S06.1X4   Traumatic cerebral edema with loss of consciousness of 6 hours to 24 hours** A 🔊, A 🔊

> MCC when PDx is its own MCC
> (Ex:) See S06.1X1

● **S06.1X5   Traumatic cerebral edema with loss of consciousness greater than 24 hours with return to pre-existing conscious level** A 🔊, A 🔊

> MCC when PDx is its own MCC
> (Ex:) See S06.1X1

● **S06.1X6   Traumatic cerebral edema with loss of consciousness greater than 24 hours without return to pre-existing conscious level with patient surviving** A 🔊, A 🔊

> MCC when PDx is its own MCC

● **S06.1X7   Traumatic cerebral edema with loss of consciousness of any duration with death due to brain injury prior to regaining consciousness** A 🔊, A 🔊

> MCC when PDx is its own MCC

● **S06.1X8   Traumatic cerebral edema with loss of consciousness of any duration with death due to other cause prior to regaining consciousness** A 🔊, A 🔊

> MCC when PDx is its own MCC

● **S06.1X9   Traumatic cerebral edema with loss of consciousness of unspecified duration** A 🔊, A 🔊

> Traumatic cerebral edema NOS
> MCC when PDx is its own MCC
> (Ex:) See S06.1X1

● **S06.2   Diffuse traumatic brain injury**

> Diffuse axonal brain injury

> > **Excludes1**   traumatic diffuse cerebral edema (S06.1X-)

> ● **S06.2X   Diffuse traumatic brain injury**

> > ● **S06.2X0   Diffuse traumatic brain injury without loss of consciousness**

> > ● **S06.2X1   Diffuse traumatic brain injury with loss of consciousness of 30 minutes or less** A 🔊, A 🔊

> > ● **S06.2X2   Diffuse traumatic brain injury with loss of consciousness of 31 minutes to 59 minutes** A 🔊, A 🔊

> > ● **S06.2X3   Diffuse traumatic brain injury with loss of consciousness of 1 hour to 5 hours 59 minutes** A 🔊, A 🔊

> > ● **S06.2X4   Diffuse traumatic brain injury with loss of consciousness of 6 hours to 24 hours** A 🔊, A 🔊

◄ New   ◄▥ Revised   ~~deleted~~ Deleted   Excludes 1   Excludes 2   Includes   Use additional   Code first   Code also   Unspecified

OGCR Official Guidelines   ● Unacceptable Principal Diagnosis   X Assign placeholder X   ● Use Additional Character(s)   ▌ Manifestation Code   Coding Clinic

1230

● **S06.2X5** Diffuse traumatic brain injury with loss of consciousness greater than 24 hours with return to pre-existing conscious levels A 🐷, A 🐷

● **S06.2X6** Diffuse traumatic brain injury with loss of consciousness greater than 24 hours without return to pre-existing conscious level with patient surviving A 🐷, A 🐷

● **S06.2X7** Diffuse traumatic brain injury with loss of consciousness of any duration with death due to brain injury prior to regaining consciousness A 🐷, A 🐷

● **S06.2X8** Diffuse traumatic brain injury with loss of consciousness of any duration with death due to other cause prior to regaining consciousness A 🐷, A 🐷

● **S06.2X9** Diffuse traumatic brain injury with loss of consciousness of unspecified duration A 🐷, A 🐷
     Diffuse traumatic brain injury NOS

● **S06.3**   **Focal traumatic brain injury**
     Excludes1   any condition classifiable to S06.4–S06.6
                focal cerebral edema (S06.1)

● **S06.30**   Unspecified focal traumatic brain injury

● **S06.300** Unspecified focal traumatic brain injury without loss of consciousness

● **S06.301** Unspecified focal traumatic brain injury with loss of consciousness of 30 minutes or less A 🐷, A 🐷

● **S06.302** Unspecified focal traumatic brain injury with loss of consciousness of 31 minutes to 59 minutes A 🐷, A 🐷

● **S06.303** Unspecified focal traumatic brain injury with loss of consciousness of 1 hour to 5 hours 59 minutes A 🐷, A 🐷

● **S06.304** Unspecified focal traumatic brain injury with loss of consciousness of 6 hours to 24 hours A 🐷, A 🐷

● **S06.305** Unspecified focal traumatic brain injury with loss of consciousness greater than 24 hours with return to pre-existing conscious level A 🐷, A 🐷

● **S06.306** Unspecified focal traumatic brain injury with loss of consciousness greater than 24 hours without return to pre-existing conscious level with patient surviving A 🐷, A 🐷

● **S06.307** Unspecified focal traumatic brain injury with loss of consciousness of any duration with death due to brain injury prior to regaining consciousness A 🐷, A 🐷

● **S06.308** Unspecified focal traumatic brain injury with loss of consciousness of any duration with death due to other cause prior to regaining consciousness A 🐷, A 🐷

● **S06.309** Unspecified focal traumatic brain injury with loss of consciousness of unspecified duration A 🐷, A 🐷
     Unspecified focal traumatic brain injury NOS

● **S06.31**   Contusion and laceration of right cerebrum

● **S06.310** Contusion and laceration of right cerebrum without loss of consciousness A 🐷, A 🐷

● **S06.311** Contusion and laceration of right cerebrum with loss of consciousness of 30 minutes or less A 🐷, A 🐷

● **S06.312** Contusion and laceration of right cerebrum with loss of consciousness of 31 minutes to 59 minutes A 🐷, A 🐷

● **S06.313** Contusion and laceration of right cerebrum with loss of consciousness of 1 hour to 5 hours 59 minutes A 🐷, A 🐷

● **S06.314** Contusion and laceration of right cerebrum with loss of consciousness of 6 hours to 24 hours A 🐷, A 🐷

● **S06.315** Contusion and laceration of right cerebrum with loss of consciousness greater than 24 hours with return to pre-existing conscious level A 🐷, A 🐷

● **S06.316** Contusion and laceration of right cerebrum with loss of consciousness greater than 24 hours without return to pre-existing conscious level with patient surviving A 🐷, A 🐷

● **S06.317** Contusion and laceration of right cerebrum with loss of consciousness of any duration with death due to brain injury prior to regaining consciousness A 🐷, A 🐷

● **S06.318** Contusion and laceration of right cerebrum with loss of consciousness of any duration with death due to other cause prior to regaining consciousness A 🐷, A 🐷

● **S06.319** Contusion and laceration of right cerebrum with loss of consciousness of unspecified duration A 🐷, A 🐷
     Contusion and laceration of right cerebrum NOS

● **S06.32**   Contusion and laceration of left cerebrum

● **S06.320** Contusion and laceration of left cerebrum without loss of consciousness A 🐷, A 🐷

● **S06.321** Contusion and laceration of left cerebrum with loss of consciousness of 30 minutes or less A 🐷, A 🐷

● **S06.322** Contusion and laceration of left cerebrum with loss of consciousness of 31 minutes to 59 minutes A 🐷, A 🐷

● **S06.323** Contusion and laceration of left cerebrum with loss of consciousness of 1 hour to 5 hours 59 minutes A 🐷, A 🐷

● **S06.324** Contusion and laceration of left cerebrum with loss of consciousness of 6 hours to 24 hours A 🐷, A 🐷

● **S06.325** Contusion and laceration of left cerebrum with loss of consciousness greater than 24 hours with return to pre-existing conscious level A 🐷, A 🐷

● **S06.326** Contusion and laceration of left cerebrum with loss of consciousness greater than 24 hours without return to pre-existing conscious level with patient surviving A 🐷, A 🐷

● **S06.327** Contusion and laceration of left cerebrum with loss of consciousness of any duration with death due to brain injury prior to regaining consciousness A 🐷, A 🐷

N Newborn Age: 0   **P** Pediatric Age: 0–17   **M** Maternity DX: 12–55   **A** Adult Age: 15–124   ♀ Females Only   ♂ Males Only

🐷 Complication\Comorbidity   🐷 Major C\C   Ⓔⓧ CC/MCC Exclusions   🐷 Hospital-Acquired Condition

1231

● S06.328   Contusion and laceration of left cerebrum with loss of consciousness of any duration with death due to other cause prior to regaining consciousness A 🔖, A 🔖

● S06.329   Contusion and laceration of left cerebrum with loss of consciousness of unspecified duration A 🔖, A 🔖
Contusion and laceration of left cerebrum NOS

● S06.33   Contusion and laceration of cerebrum, unspecified

● S06.330   Contusion and laceration of cerebrum, unspecified, without loss of consciousness A 🔖, A 🔖

● S06.331   Contusion and laceration of cerebrum, unspecified, with loss of consciousness of 30 minutes or less A 🔖, A 🔖

● S06.332   Contusion and laceration of cerebrum, unspecified, with loss of consciousness of 31 minutes to 59 minutes A 🔖, A 🔖

● S06.333   Contusion and laceration of cerebrum, unspecified, with loss of consciousness of 1 hour to 5 hours 59 minutes A 🔖, A 🔖

● S06.334   Contusion and laceration of cerebrum, unspecified, with loss of consciousness of 6 hours to 24 hours A 🔖, A 🔖

● S06.335   Contusion and laceration of cerebrum, unspecified, with loss of consciousness greater than 24 hours with return to pre-existing conscious level A 🔖, A 🔖

● S06.336   Contusion and laceration of cerebrum, unspecified, with loss of consciousness greater than 24 hours without return to pre-existing conscious level with patient surviving A 🔖, A 🔖

● S06.337   Contusion and laceration of cerebrum, unspecified, with loss of consciousness of any duration with death due to brain injury prior to regaining consciousness A 🔖, A 🔖

● S06.338   Contusion and laceration of cerebrum, unspecified, with loss of consciousness of any duration with death due to other cause prior to regaining consciousness A 🔖, A 🔖

● S06.339   Contusion and laceration of cerebrum, unspecified, with loss of consciousness of unspecified duration A 🔖, A 🔖
Contusion and laceration of cerebrum NOS

● S06.34   Traumatic hemorrhage of right cerebrum
Traumatic intracerebral hemorrhage and hematoma of right cerebrum

● S06.340   Traumatic hemorrhage of right cerebrum without loss of consciousness A 🔖, A 🔖
Coding Clinic: 2015, Q1, P12

● S06.341   Traumatic hemorrhage of right cerebrum with loss of consciousness of 30 minutes or less A 🔖, A 🔖

● S06.342   Traumatic hemorrhage of right cerebrum with loss of consciousness of 31 minutes to 59 minutes A 🔖, A 🔖

● S06.343   Traumatic hemorrhage of right cerebrum with loss of consciousness of 1 hours to 5 hours 59 minutes A 🔖, A 🔖

● S06.344   Traumatic hemorrhage of right cerebrum with loss of consciousness of 6 hours to 24 hours A 🔖, A 🔖

● S06.345   Traumatic hemorrhage of right cerebrum with loss of consciousness greater than 24 hours with return to pre-existing conscious level A 🔖, A 🔖

● S06.346   Traumatic hemorrhage of right cerebrum with loss of consciousness greater than 24 hours without return to pre-existing conscious level with patient surviving A 🔖, A 🔖

● S06.347   Traumatic hemorrhage of right cerebrum with loss of consciousness of any duration with death due to brain injury prior to regaining consciousness A 🔖, A 🔖

● S06.348   Traumatic hemorrhage of right cerebrum with loss of consciousness of any duration with death due to other cause prior to regaining consciousness A 🔖, A 🔖

● S06.349   Traumatic hemorrhage of right cerebrum with loss of consciousness of unspecified duration A 🔖, A 🔖
Traumatic hemorrhage of right cerebrum NOS

● S06.35   Traumatic hemorrhage of left cerebrum
Traumatic intracerebral hemorrhage and hematoma of left cerebrum

● S06.350   Traumatic hemorrhage of left cerebrum without loss of consciousness A 🔖, A 🔖

● S06.351   Traumatic hemorrhage of left cerebrum with loss of consciousness of 30 minutes or less A 🔖, A 🔖

● S06.352   Traumatic hemorrhage of left cerebrum with loss of consciousness of 31 minutes to 59 minutes A 🔖, A 🔖

● S06.353   Traumatic hemorrhage of left cerebrum with loss of consciousness of 1 hours to 5 hours 59 minutes A 🔖, A 🔖

● S06.354   Traumatic hemorrhage of left cerebrum with loss of consciousness of 6 hours to 24 hours A 🔖, A 🔖

● S06.355   Traumatic hemorrhage of left cerebrum with loss of consciousness greater than 24 hours with return to pre-existing conscious level A 🔖, A 🔖

● S06.356   Traumatic hemorrhage of left cerebrum with loss of consciousness greater than 24 hours without return to pre-existing conscious level with patient surviving A 🔖, A 🔖

● S06.357   Traumatic hemorrhage of left cerebrum with loss of consciousness of any duration with death due to brain injury prior to regaining consciousness A 🔖, A 🔖

● S06.358   Traumatic hemorrhage of left cerebrum with loss of consciousness of any duration with death due to other cause prior to regaining consciousness A 🔖, A 🔖

◀ New   ◀▥ Revised   ~~deleted~~ Deleted   Excludes 1   Excludes 2   Includes   Use additional   Code first   Code also   Unspecified
OGCR Official Guidelines   ● Unacceptable Principal Diagnosis   X Assign placeholder X   ● Use Additional Character(s)   ▶ Manifestation Code   **Coding Clinic**

● S06.359 Traumatic hemorrhage of left cerebrum with loss of consciousness of unspecified duration A 🔹, A 🔹
Traumatic hemorrhage of left cerebrum NOS

● S06.36 Traumatic hemorrhage of cerebrum, unspecified
Traumatic intracerebral hemorrhage and hematoma, unspecified

● S06.360 Traumatic hemorrhage of cerebrum, unspecified, without loss of consciousness A 🔹, A 🔹

● S06.361 Traumatic hemorrhage of cerebrum, unspecified, with loss of consciousness of 30 minutes or less A 🔹, A 🔹

● S06.362 Traumatic hemorrhage of cerebrum, unspecified, with loss of consciousness of 31 minutes to 59 minutes A 🔹, A 🔹

● S06.363 Traumatic hemorrhage of cerebrum, unspecified, with loss of consciousness of 1 hours to 5 hours 59 minutes A 🔹, A 🔹

● S06.364 Traumatic hemorrhage of cerebrum, unspecified, with loss of consciousness of 6 hours to 24 hours A 🔹, A 🔹

● S06.365 Traumatic hemorrhage of cerebrum, unspecified, with loss of consciousness greater than 24 hours with return to pre-existing conscious level A 🔹, A 🔹

● S06.366 Traumatic hemorrhage of cerebrum, unspecified, with loss of consciousness greater than 24 hours without return to pre-existing conscious level with patient surviving A 🔹, A 🔹

● S06.367 Traumatic hemorrhage of cerebrum, unspecified, with loss of consciousness of any duration with death due to brain injury prior to regaining consciousness A 🔹, A 🔹

● S06.368 Traumatic hemorrhage of cerebrum, unspecified, with loss of consciousness of any duration with death due to other cause prior to regaining consciousness A 🔹, A 🔹

● S06.369 Traumatic hemorrhage of cerebrum, unspecified, with loss of consciousness of unspecified duration A 🔹, A 🔹
Traumatic hemorrhage of cerebrum NOS

● S06.37 Contusion, laceration, and hemorrhage of cerebellum

● S06.370 Contusion, laceration, and hemorrhage of cerebellum without loss of consciousness A 🔹, A 🔹
(Ex) No exclusions

● S06.371 Contusion, laceration, and hemorrhage of cerebellum with loss of consciousness of 30 minutes or less A 🔹, A 🔹

● S06.372 Contusion, laceration, and hemorrhage of cerebellum with loss of consciousness of 31 minutes to 59 minutes A 🔹, A 🔹

● S06.373 Contusion, laceration, and hemorrhage of cerebellum with loss of consciousness of 1 hour to 5 hours 59 minutes A 🔹, A 🔹

● S06.374 Contusion, laceration, and hemorrhage of cerebellum with loss of consciousness of 6 hours to 24 hours A 🔹, A 🔹

● S06.375 Contusion, laceration, and hemorrhage of cerebellum with loss of consciousness greater than 24 hours with return to pre-existing conscious level A 🔹, A 🔹

● S06.376 Contusion, laceration, and hemorrhage of cerebellum with loss of consciousness greater than 24 hours without return to pre-existing conscious level with patient surviving A 🔹, A 🔹

● S06.377 Contusion, laceration, and hemorrhage of cerebellum with loss of consciousness of any duration with death due to brain injury prior to regaining consciousness A 🔹, A 🔹

● S06.378 Contusion, laceration, and hemorrhage of cerebellum with loss of consciousness of any duration with death due to other cause prior to regaining consciousness A 🔹, A 🔹

● S06.379 Contusion, laceration, and hemorrhage of cerebellum with loss of consciousness of unspecified duration A 🔹, A 🔹
Contusion, laceration, and hemorrhage of cerebellum NOS

● S06.38 Contusion, laceration, and hemorrhage of brainstem

● S06.380 Contusion, laceration, and hemorrhage of brainstem without loss of consciousness A 🔹, A 🔹
(Ex) No exclusions

● S06.381 Contusion, laceration, and hemorrhage of brainstem with loss of consciousness of 30 minutes or less A 🔹, A 🔹

● S06.382 Contusion, laceration, and hemorrhage of brainstem with loss of consciousness of 31 minutes to 59 minutes A 🔹, A 🔹

● S06.383 Contusion, laceration, and hemorrhage of brainstem with loss of consciousness of 1 hour to 5 hours 59 minutes A 🔹, A 🔹

● S06.384 Contusion, laceration, and hemorrhage of brainstem with loss of consciousness of 6 hours to 24 hours A 🔹, A 🔹

● S06.385 Contusion, laceration, and hemorrhage of brainstem with loss of consciousness greater than 24 hours with return to pre-existing conscious level A 🔹, A 🔹

● S06.386 Contusion, laceration, and hemorrhage of brainstem with loss of consciousness greater than 24 hours without return to pre-existing conscious level with patient surviving A 🔹, A 🔹

● S06.387 Contusion, laceration, and hemorrhage of brainstem with loss of consciousness of any duration with death due to brain injury prior to regaining consciousness A 🔹, A 🔹

CHAPTER 19 (S00-T88)

N Newborn Age: 0　　**P** Pediatric Age: 0–17　　**M** Maternity DX: 12–55　　**A** Adult Age: 15–124　　♀ Females Only　　♂ Males Only

🔹 Complication\Comorbidity　　🔹 Major C\C　　(Ex) CC/MCC Exclusions　　🔹 Hospital-Acquired Condition

1233

● S06.388   Contusion, laceration, and
             hemorrhage of brainstem with loss of
             consciousness of any duration with
             death due to other cause prior to
             regaining consciousness A 🐾, A 🐾

● S06.389   Contusion, laceration, and
             hemorrhage of brainstem with loss of
             consciousness of unspecified duration
             A 🐾, A 🐾
                 Contusion, laceration, and
                     hemorrhage of brainstem NOS

● S06.4 Epidural hemorrhage
         Situated outside dura mater
         Extradural hemorrhage NOS
         Intracranial hemorrhage due to trauma
         Extradural hemorrhage (traumatic)

   ● S06.4X Epidural hemorrhage

      ● S06.4X0   Epidural hemorrhage without loss of
                  consciousness A 🐾, A 🐾

      ● S06.4X1   Epidural hemorrhage with loss of
                  consciousness of 30 minutes or less
                  A 🐾, A 🐾

      ● S06.4X2   Epidural hemorrhage with loss of
                  consciousness of 31 minutes to
                  59 minutes A 🐾, A 🐾

      ● S06.4X3   Epidural hemorrhage with loss of
                  consciousness of 1 hour to 5 hours
                  59 minutes A 🐾, A 🐾

      ● S06.4X4   Epidural hemorrhage with loss of
                  consciousness of 6 hours to 24 hours
                  A 🐾, A 🐾

      ● S06.4X5   Epidural hemorrhage with loss of
                  consciousness greater than 24 hours
                  with return to pre-existing conscious
                  level A 🐾, A 🐾

      ● S06.4X6   Epidural hemorrhage with loss of
                  consciousness greater than 24 hours
                  without return to pre-existing
                  conscious level with patient surviving
                  A 🐾, A 🐾

      ● S06.4X7   Epidural hemorrhage with loss of
                  consciousness of any duration with
                  death due to brain injury prior to
                  regaining consciousness A 🐾, A 🐾

      ● S06.4X8   Epidural hemorrhage with loss of
                  consciousness of any duration with
                  death due to other causes prior to
                  regaining consciousness A 🐾, A 🐾

      ● S06.4X9   Epidural hemorrhage with loss of
                  consciousness of unspecified duration
                  A 🐾, A 🐾
                      Epidural hemorrhage NOS

● S06.5 Traumatic subdural hemorrhage

   ● S06.5X Traumatic subdural hemorrhage

      ● S06.5X0   Traumatic subdural hemorrhage
                  without loss of consciousness A 🐾,
                  A 🐾
                      Coding Clinic: 2015, Q3, P37

      ● S06.5X1   Traumatic subdural hemorrhage with
                  loss of consciousness of 30 minutes or
                  less A 🐾, A 🐾

      ● S06.5X2   Traumatic subdural hemorrhage with
                  loss of consciousness of 31 minutes to
                  59 minutes A 🐾, A 🐾

      ● S06.5X3   Traumatic subdural hemorrhage with
                  loss of consciousness of 1 hour to
                  5 hours 59 minutes A 🐾, A 🐾

      ● S06.5X4   Traumatic subdural hemorrhage with
                  loss of consciousness of 6 hours to
                  24 hours A 🐾, A 🐾

      ● S06.5X5   Traumatic subdural hemorrhage with
                  loss of consciousness greater than
                  24 hours with return to pre-existing
                  conscious level A 🐾, A 🐾

● S06.5X6   Traumatic subdural hemorrhage
             with loss of consciousness greater
             than 24 hours without return to
             pre-existing conscious level with
             patient surviving A 🐾, A 🐾

● S06.5X7   Traumatic subdural hemorrhage with
             loss of consciousness of any duration
             with death due to brain injury before
             regaining consciousness A 🐾, A 🐾

● S06.5X8   Traumatic subdural hemorrhage with
             loss of consciousness of any duration
             with death due to other cause before
             regaining consciousness A 🐾, A 🐾

● S06.5X9   Traumatic subdural hemorrhage with
             loss of consciousness of unspecified
             duration A 🐾, A 🐾
                 Traumatic subdural hemorrhage
                     NOS

● S06.6 Traumatic subarachnoid hemorrhage
         Between arachnoid and pia mater

   ● S06.6X Traumatic subarachnoid hemorrhage

      ● S06.6X0   Traumatic subarachnoid hemorrhage
                  without loss of consciousness A 🐾,
                  A 🐾
                      Coding Clinic: 2015, Q3, P37

      ● S06.6X1   Traumatic subarachnoid hemorrhage
                  with loss of consciousness of
                  30 minutes or less A 🐾, A 🐾

      ● S06.6X2   Traumatic subarachnoid hemorrhage
                  with loss of consciousness of
                  31 minutes to 59 minutes A 🐾, A 🐾

      ● S06.6X3   Traumatic subarachnoid hemorrhage
                  with loss of consciousness of
                  1 hour to 5 hours 59 minutes A 🐾,
                  A 🐾

      ● S06.6X4   Traumatic subarachnoid hemorrhage
                  with loss of consciousness of 6 hours
                  to 24 hours A 🐾, A 🐾

      ● S06.6X5   Traumatic subarachnoid hemorrhage
                  with loss of consciousness greater
                  than 24 hours with return to
                  pre-existing conscious level A 🐾,
                  A 🐾

      ● S06.6X6   Traumatic subarachnoid hemorrhage
                  with loss of consciousness greater
                  than 24 hours without return to
                  pre-existing conscious level with
                  patient surviving A 🐾, A 🐾

      ● S06.6X7   Traumatic subarachnoid hemorrhage
                  with loss of consciousness of any
                  duration with death due to brain
                  injury prior to regaining
                  consciousness A 🐾, A 🐾

      ● S06.6X8   Traumatic subarachnoid hemorrhage
                  with loss of consciousness of any
                  duration with death due to other
                  cause prior to regaining consciousness
                  A 🐾, A 🐾

      ● S06.6X9   Traumatic subarachnoid hemorrhage
                  with loss of consciousness of
                  unspecified duration A 🐾, A 🐾
                      Traumatic subarachnoid hemorrhage
                          NOS

● S06.8 Other specified intracranial injuries

   ● S06.81 Injury of right internal carotid artery,
             intracranial portion, not elsewhere classified

      ● S06.810   Injury of right internal carotid
                  artery, intracranial portion, not
                  elsewhere classified without loss of
                  consciousness

      ● S06.811   Injury of right internal carotid artery,
                  intracranial portion, not elsewhere
                  classified with loss of consciousness
                  of 30 minutes or less A 🐾, A 🐾

◀ New   ◀▥ Revised   ~~deleted~~ Deleted   Excludes 1   Excludes 2   Includes   Use additional   Code first   Code also   Unspecified
OGCR Official Guidelines   ● Unacceptable Principal Diagnosis   X Assign placeholder X   ● Use Additional Character(s)   ▌ Manifestation Code   **Coding Clinic**

CHAPTER 19 (S00-T88)

● **S06.812**   Injury of right internal carotid artery, intracranial portion, not elsewhere classified with loss of consciousness of 31 minutes to 59 minutes A 🅰, A 🅰

● **S06.813**   Injury of right internal carotid artery, intracranial portion, not elsewhere classified with loss of consciousness of 1 hour to 5 hours 59 minutes A 🅰, A 🅰

● **S06.814**   Injury of right internal carotid artery, intracranial portion, not elsewhere classified with loss of consciousness of 6 hours to 24 hours A 🅰, A 🅰

● **S06.815**   Injury of right internal carotid artery, intracranial portion, not elsewhere classified with loss of consciousness greater than 24 hours with return to pre-existing conscious level A 🅰, A 🅰

● **S06.816**   Injury of right internal carotid artery, intracranial portion, not elsewhere classified with loss of consciousness greater than 24 hours without return to pre-existing conscious level with patient surviving A 🅰, A 🅰

● **S06.817**   Injury of right internal carotid artery, intracranial portion, not elsewhere classified with loss of consciousness of any duration with death due to brain injury prior to regaining consciousness A 🅰, A 🅰

● **S06.818**   Injury of right internal carotid artery, intracranial portion, not elsewhere classified with loss of consciousness of any duration with death due to other cause prior to regaining consciousness A 🅰, A 🅰

● **S06.819**   Injury of right internal carotid artery, intracranial portion, not elsewhere classified with loss of consciousness of unspecified duration A 🅰, A 🅰
     Injury of right internal carotid artery, intracranial portion, not elsewhere classified NOS

● **S06.82**   Injury of left internal carotid artery, intracranial portion, not elsewhere classified

● **S06.820**   Injury of left internal carotid artery, intracranial portion, not elsewhere classified without loss of consciousness

● **S06.821**   Injury of left internal carotid artery, intracranial portion, not elsewhere classified with loss of consciousness of 30 minutes or less A 🅰, A 🅰

● **S06.822**   Injury of left internal carotid artery, intracranial portion, not elsewhere classified with loss of consciousness of 31 minutes to 59 minutes A 🅰, A 🅰

● **S06.823**   Injury of left internal carotid artery, intracranial portion, not elsewhere classified with loss of consciousness of 1 hour to 5 hours 59 minutes A 🅰, A 🅰

● **S06.824**   Injury of left internal carotid artery, intracranial portion, not elsewhere classified with loss of consciousness of 6 hours to 24 hours A 🅰, A 🅰

● **S06.825**   Injury of left internal carotid artery, intracranial portion, not elsewhere classified with loss of consciousness greater than 24 hours with return to pre-existing conscious level A 🅰, A 🅰

● **S06.826**   Injury of left internal carotid artery, intracranial portion, not elsewhere classified with loss of consciousness greater than 24 hours without return to pre-existing conscious level with patient surviving A 🅰, A 🅰

● **S06.827**   Injury of left internal carotid artery, intracranial portion, not elsewhere classified with loss of consciousness of any duration with death due to brain injury prior to regaining consciousness A 🅰, A 🅰

● **S06.828**   Injury of left internal carotid artery, intracranial portion, not elsewhere classified with loss of consciousness of any duration with death due to other cause prior to regaining consciousness A 🅰, A 🅰

● **S06.829**   Injury of left internal carotid artery, intracranial portion, not elsewhere classified with loss of consciousness of unspecified duration A 🅰, A 🅰
     Injury of left internal carotid artery, intracranial portion, not elsewhere classified NOS

● **S06.89**   Other specified intracranial injury
    Excludes1   concussion (S06.0X-) ◄

● **S06.890**   Other specified intracranial injury without loss of consciousness

● **S06.891**   Other specified intracranial injury with loss of consciousness of 30 minutes or less A 🅰, A 🅰

● **S06.892**   Other specified intracranial injury with loss of consciousness of 31 minutes to 59 minutes A 🅰, A 🅰

● **S06.893**   Other specified intracranial injury with loss of consciousness of 1 hour to 5 hours 59 minutes A 🅰, A 🅰

● **S06.894**   Other specified intracranial injury with loss of consciousness of 6 hours to 24 hours A 🅰, A 🅰

● **S06.895**   Other specified intracranial injury with loss of consciousness greater than 24 hours with return to pre-existing conscious level A 🅰, A 🅰

● **S06.896**   Other specified intracranial injury with loss of consciousness greater than 24 hours without return to pre-existing conscious level with patient surviving A 🅰, A 🅰

● **S06.897**   Other specified intracranial injury with loss of consciousness of any duration with death due to brain injury prior to regaining consciousness A 🅰, A 🅰

● **S06.898**   Other specified intracranial injury with loss of consciousness of any duration with death due to other cause prior to regaining consciousness A 🅰, A 🅰

● **S06.899**   Other specified intracranial injury with loss of consciousness of unspecified duration A 🅰, A 🅰

CHAPTER 19 (S00–T88)

N Newborn Age: 0   **P** Pediatric Age: 0–17   **M** Maternity DX: 12–55   **A** Adult Age: 15–124   ♀ Females Only   ♂ Males Only

🅰 Complication\Comorbidity   🅰 Major C\C   Ⓔ CC/MCC Exclusions   🅰 Hospital-Acquired Condition

1235

● **S06.9** **Unspecified intracranial injury**
　　Brain injury NOS
　　Head injury NOS with loss of consciousness
　　Traumatic brain injury NOS ◄
　　　Excludes1　conditions classifiable to S06.0- to
　　　　　　　　　S06.8-code to specified intracranial
　　　　　　　　　injury ◄
　　　　　　head injury NOS (S09.90)
　● **S06.9X** **Unspecified intracranial injury**
　　● **S06.9X0** Unspecified intracranial injury
　　　　　　　　without loss of consciousness
　　● **S06.9X1** Unspecified intracranial injury with
　　　　　　　　loss of consciousness of 30 minutes or
　　　　　　　　less A 🪙, A 🪙
　　● **S06.9X2** Unspecified intracranial injury with
　　　　　　　　loss of consciousness of 31 minutes to
　　　　　　　　59 minutes A 🪙, A 🪙
　　● **S06.9X3** Unspecified intracranial injury with
　　　　　　　　loss of consciousness of 1 hour to
　　　　　　　　5 hours 59 minutes A 🪙, A 🪙
　　● **S06.9X4** Unspecified intracranial injury with
　　　　　　　　loss of consciousness of 6 hours to
　　　　　　　　24 hours A 🪙, A 🪙
　　● **S06.9X5** Unspecified intracranial injury with
　　　　　　　　loss of consciousness greater than
　　　　　　　　24 hours with return to pre-existing
　　　　　　　　conscious level A 🪙, A 🪙
　　● **S06.9X6** Unspecified intracranial injury with
　　　　　　　　loss of consciousness greater than
　　　　　　　　24 hours without return to pre-
　　　　　　　　existing conscious level with patient
　　　　　　　　surviving A 🪙, A 🪙
　　● **S06.9X7** Unspecified intracranial injury with
　　　　　　　　loss of consciousness of any duration
　　　　　　　　with death due to brain injury prior
　　　　　　　　to regaining consciousness A 🪙, A 🪙
　　● **S06.9X8** Unspecified intracranial injury with
　　　　　　　　loss of consciousness of any duration
　　　　　　　　with death due to other cause prior to
　　　　　　　　regaining consciousness A 🪙, A 🪙
　　● **S06.9X9** Unspecified intracranial injury with
　　　　　　　　loss of consciousness of unspecified
　　　　　　　　duration A 🪙, A 🪙

● **S07** **Crushing injury of head**
　　Use additional code for all associated injuries, such as:
　　　intracranial injuries (S06.-)
　　　skull fractures (S02.-)
　　The appropriate 7th character is to be added to each code from
　　　category S07

A	initial encounter
D	subsequent encounter
S	sequela

　　(Ex:) **For category S07 CC codes:** S01.90X-S01.95X[A], S02.0XX-S02.92X[S],
　　　S07.0XX-S07.9XX[A], S08.89X-S09.19X[A], S09.8XXA-S09.90X[A], S09.92XA-S09.93X[A],
　　　S16.8XX-S19.9XX[A], T14.90-T14.91, T79.8XX-T79.9XX[A], T79.A0X-T79.A9X[A]

X● **S07.0** Crushing injury of face A 🪙, A 🪙
X● **S07.1** Crushing injury of skull A 🪙, A 🪙
X● **S07.8** Crushing injury of other parts of head A 🪙, A 🪙
X● **S07.9** Crushing injury of head, part unspecified A 🪙, A 🪙

● **S08** **Avulsion and traumatic amputation of part of head**
　　An amputation not identified as partial or complete should be
　　　coded to complete
　　The appropriate 7th character is to be added to each code from
　　　category S08

A	initial encounter
D	subsequent encounter
S	sequela

X● **S08.0** **Avulsion of scalp**
　● **S08.1** **Traumatic amputation of ear**
　　● **S08.11** Complete traumatic amputation of ear
　　　● **S08.111** Complete traumatic amputation of
　　　　　　　　　right ear
　　　● **S08.112** Complete traumatic amputation of
　　　　　　　　　left ear
　　　● **S08.119** Complete traumatic amputation of
　　　　　　　　　unspecified ear
　　● **S08.12** Partial traumatic amputation of ear
　　　● **S08.121** Partial traumatic amputation of right
　　　　　　　　　ear
　　　● **S08.122** Partial traumatic amputation of left
　　　　　　　　　ear
　　　● **S08.129** Partial traumatic amputation of
　　　　　　　　　unspecified ear
　● **S08.8** **Traumatic amputation of other parts of head**
　　● **S08.81** Traumatic amputation of nose
　　　● **S08.811** Complete traumatic amputation of
　　　　　　　　　nose
　　　● **S08.812** Partial traumatic amputation of nose
　　X● **S08.89** Traumatic amputation of other parts of head

● **S09** **Other and unspecified injuries of head**
　　The appropriate 7th character is to be added to each code from
　　　category S09

A	initial encounter
D	subsequent encounter
S	sequela

X● **S09.0** **Injury of blood vessels of head, not elsewhere classified**
　　A 🪙
　　　Excludes1　injury of cerebral blood vessels (S06.-)
　　　　　　　　　injury of precerebral blood vessels (S15.-)
　　　(Ex:) S09.0XX[A], S15.101-S15.199[A], S15.8XX-S15.9XX[A], T14.90-T14.91,
　　　　T79.8XX-T79.9XX[A], T79.A0X-T79.A9X[A]

● **S09.1** **Injury of muscle and tendon of head**
　　Code also any associated open wound (S01.-)
　　　Excludes2　sprain to joints and ligament of head
　　　　　　　　　(S03.9)
　X● **S09.10** Unspecified injury of muscle and tendon of
　　　　　　　head
　　　　　　　Injury of muscle and tendon of head NOS
　X● **S09.11** Strain of muscle and tendon of head
　X● **S09.12** Laceration of muscle and tendon of head
　X● **S09.19** Other specified injury of muscle and tendon of
　　　　　　　head

● **S09.2** **Traumatic rupture of ear drum**
　　　Excludes1　traumatic rupture of ear drum due to
　　　　　　　　　blast injury (S09.31-)
　　(Ex:) **For category S09.2 CC codes:** S01.301-S01.359[A], S08.111-S08.129[A],
　　　S09.20X-S09.399[A], S09.91X[A], S38.3XX[A], T14.90-T14.91,
　　　T79.8XX-T79.9XX[A]

　X● **S09.20** Traumatic rupture of unspecified ear drum A 🪙
　X● **S09.21** Traumatic rupture of right ear drum A 🪙
　X● **S09.22** Traumatic rupture of left ear drum A 🪙

● **S09.3**   **Other specified and unspecified injury of middle and inner ear**

> **Excludes1**   injury to ear NOS (S09.91-)
> **Excludes2**   injury to external ear (S00.4-, S01.3-, S08.1-)
> (Ex) For category S09.3 CC codes: See S09.2

   ● **S09.30**   Unspecified injury of middle and inner ear

     ● **S09.301**   Unspecified **injury of right middle and inner ear** A 🅒

     ● **S09.302**   Unspecified **injury of left middle and inner ear** A 🅒

     ● **S09.309**   Unspecified **injury of unspecified middle and inner ear** A 🅒

   ● **S09.31**   **Primary blast injury of ear**
       Blast injury of ear NOS

     ● **S09.311**   **Primary blast injury of right ear** A 🅒

     ● **S09.312**   **Primary blast injury of left ear** A 🅒

     ● **S09.313**   **Primary blast injury of ear, bilateral** A 🅒

     ● **S09.319**   **Primary blast injury of unspecified ear** A 🅒

   ● **S09.39**   **Other specified injury of middle and inner ear**
       Secondary blast injury to ear

     ● **S09.391**   **Other specified injury of right middle and inner ear** A 🅒

     ● **S09.392**   **Other specified injury of left middle and inner ear** A 🅒

     ● **S09.399**   **Other specified injury of unspecified middle and inner ear** A 🅒

X ● **S09.8**   **Other specified injuries of head**

● **S09.9**   **Unspecified injury of face and head**

   X ● **S09.90**   Unspecified **injury of head**
       Head injury NOS

> **Excludes1**   brain injury NOS (S06.9-)
>   head injury NOS with loss of consciousness (S06.9-)
>   intracranial injury NOS (S06.9-)

   X ● **S09.91**   Unspecified **injury of ear**
       Injury of ear NOS

   X ● **S09.92**   Unspecified **injury of nose**
       Injury of nose NOS

   X ● **S09.93**   Unspecified **injury of face**
       Injury of face NOS

INJURIES TO THE NECK (S10-S19)

> **Includes**   injuries of nape
>   injuries of supraclavicular region
>   injuries of throat
>
> **Excludes2**   burns and corrosions (T20-T32)
>   effects of foreign body in esophagus (T18.1)
>   effects of foreign body in larynx (T17.3)
>   effects of foreign body in pharynx (T17.2)
>   effects of foreign body in trachea (T17.4)
>   frostbite (T33-T34)
>   insect bite or sting, venomous (T63.4)

● **S10**   **Superficial injury of neck**

The appropriate 7th character is to be added to each code from category S10

> | A | initial encounter |
> | D | subsequent encounter |
> | S | sequela |

X ● **S10.0**   **Contusion of throat**
       Contusion of cervical esophagus
       Contusion of larynx
       Contusion of pharynx
       Contusion of trachea

● **S10.1**   **Other and unspecified superficial injuries of throat**

   X ● **S10.10**   Unspecified **superficial injuries of throat**

   X ● **S10.11**   **Abrasion of throat**

   X ● **S10.12**   **Blister (nonthermal) of throat**

   X ● **S10.14**   **External constriction of part of throat**

   X ● **S10.15**   **Superficial foreign body of throat**
       Splinter in the throat

   X ● **S10.16**   **Insect bite (nonvenomous) of throat**

   X ● **S10.17**   **Other superficial bite of throat**

> **Excludes1**   open bite of throat (S11.85)

● **S10.8**   **Superficial injury of other specified parts of neck**

   X ● **S10.80**   Unspecified **superficial injury of other specified part of neck**

   X ● **S10.81**   **Abrasion of other specified part of neck**

   X ● **S10.82**   **Blister (nonthermal) of other specified part of neck**

   X ● **S10.83**   **Contusion of other specified part of neck**

   X ● **S10.84**   **External constriction of other specified part of neck**

   X ● **S10.85**   **Superficial foreign body of other specified part of neck**
       Splinter in other part of neck

   X ● **S10.86**   **Insect bite of other specified part of neck**

   X ● **S10.87**   **Other superficial bite of other specified part of neck**

> **Excludes1**   open bite of other specified parts of neck (S11.85)

● **S10.9**   **Superficial injury of unspecified part of neck**

   X ● **S10.90**   **Unspecified superficial injury of unspecified part of neck**

   X ● **S10.91**   **Abrasion of unspecified part of neck**

   X ● **S10.92**   **Blister (nonthermal) of unspecified part of neck**

   X ● **S10.93**   **Contusion of unspecified part of neck**

   X ● **S10.94**   **External constriction of unspecified part of neck**

   X ● **S10.95**   **Superficial foreign body of unspecified part of neck**

   X ● **S10.96**   **Insect bite of unspecified part of neck**

   X ● **S10.97**   **Other superficial bite of unspecified part of neck**

● **S11**   **Open wound of neck**

Code also any associated:
       spinal cord injury (S14.0, S14.1-)
       wound infection

> **Excludes2**   open fracture of vertebra (S12.- with 7th character B)

The appropriate 7th character is to be added to each code from category S11

> | A | initial encounter |
> | D | subsequent encounter |
> | S | sequela |

● **S11.0**   **Open wound of larynx and trachea**
       (Ex) For category S11.0 CC codes: S11.011-S11.039[A], S11.80X-S11.95X[A], S13.4XX[A], S13.8XX[A], S16.1XX-S16.2XX[A], S38.3XX[A], T14.90-T14.91, T79.8XX-T79.9XX[A], T79.A0X-T79.A9X[A]

   ● **S11.01**   **Open wound of larynx**

> **Excludes2**   open wound of vocal cord (S11.03)

     ● **S11.011**   **Laceration without foreign body of larynx** A 🅒

     ● **S11.012**   **Laceration with foreign body of larynx** A 🅒

     ● **S11.013**   **Puncture wound without foreign body of larynx** A 🅒

     ● **S11.014**   **Puncture wound with foreign body of larynx** A 🅒

     ● **S11.015**   **Open bite of larynx** A 🅒
       Bite of larynx NOS

     ● **S11.019**   Unspecified **open wound of larynx** A 🅒

CHAPTER 19 (S00-T88)

● **S11.02   Open wound of trachea**
Open wound of cervical trachea
Open wound of trachea NOS

Excludes2   open wound of thoracic trachea (S27.5-)

● S11.021   **Laceration without foreign body of trachea** A 🔗

● S11.022   **Laceration with foreign body of trachea** A 🔗

● S11.023   **Puncture wound without foreign body of trachea** A 🔗

● S11.024   **Puncture wound with foreign body of trachea** A 🔗

● S11.025   **Open bite of trachea** A 🔗
Bite of trachea NOS

● S11.029   **Unspecified open wound of trachea** A 🔗

● **S11.03   Open wound of vocal cord**

● S11.031   **Laceration without foreign body of vocal cord** A 🔗

● S11.032   **Laceration with foreign body of vocal cord** A 🔗

● S11.033   **Puncture wound without foreign body of vocal cord** A 🔗

● S11.034   **Puncture wound with foreign body of vocal cord** A 🔗

● S11.035   **Open bite of vocal cord** A 🔗
Bite of vocal cord NOS

● S11.039   **Unspecified open wound of vocal cord** A 🔗

● **S11.1   Open wound of thyroid gland**

(Ex:) **For category S11.1 CC codes unless otherwise indicated:** S11.10X-S11.15X[A], S11.80X-S11.95X[A], S13.4XX[A], S13.8XX[A], S16.1XX-S16.2XX[A], S38.3XX[A], T14.90-T14.91, T79.8XX-T79.9XX[A]

X● S11.10   **Unspecified open wound of thyroid gland** A 🔗

X● S11.11   **Laceration without foreign body of thyroid gland** A 🔗

X● S11.12   **Laceration with foreign body of thyroid gland** A 🔗
(Ex:) S11.10X-S11.15X[A], S11.80X-S11.95X[A], S13.4XX[A], S13.8XX[A], S16.1XX-S16.2XX[A], S38.3XX[A], T14.90-T14.91, T79.8XX-T79.9XX[A], T79.A0XA-T79.A9X[A]

X● S11.13   **Puncture wound without foreign body of thyroid gland** A 🔗

X● S11.14   **Puncture wound with foreign body of thyroid gland** A 🔗
(Ex:) See S11.12

X● S11.15   **Open bite of thyroid gland** A 🔗
Bite of thyroid gland NOS

● **S11.2   Open wound of pharynx and cervical esophagus**

Excludes1   open wound of esophagus NOS (S27.8-)

(Ex:) **For category S11.2 CC codes unless otherwise indicated:** S11.20X-S11.95X[A], S13.4XX[A], S13.8XX[A], S16.1XX-S16.2XX[A], S38.3XX[A], T14.90-T14.91, T79.8XX-T79.9XX[A]

X● S11.20   **Unspecified open wound of pharynx and cervical esophagus** A 🔗

X● S11.21   **Laceration without foreign body of pharynx and cervical esophagus** A 🔗

X● S11.22   **Laceration with foreign body of pharynx and cervical esophagus** A 🔗
(Ex:) S11.20X-S11.95X[A], S13.4XX[A], S13.8XX[A], S16.1XX-S16.2XX[A], S38.3XX[A], T14.90-T14.91, T79.8XX-T79.9XX[A], T79.A0X-T79.A9X[A]

X● S11.23   **Puncture wound without foreign body of pharynx and cervical esophagus** A 🔗

X● S11.24   **Puncture wound with foreign body of pharynx and cervical esophagus** A 🔗
(Ex:) See S11.22

X● S11.25   **Open bite of pharynx and cervical esophagus** A 🔗
Bite of pharynx and cervical esophagus NOS

● **S11.8   Open wound of other specified parts of neck**

X● S11.80   **Unspecified open specified wound of other part of neck**

X● S11.81   **Laceration without foreign body of other specified part of neck**

X● S11.82   **Laceration with foreign body of other specified part of neck**

X● S11.83   **Puncture wound without foreign body of other specified part of neck**

X● S11.84   **Puncture wound with foreign body of other specified part of neck**

X● S11.85   **Open bite of other specified part of neck**
Bite of other part of neck NOS

Excludes1   superficial bite of other specified part of neck (S10.87)

X● S11.89   **Other open wound of other part of neck**

● **S11.9   Open wound of unspecified part of neck**

X● S11.90   **Unspecified open wound of unspecified part of neck**

X● S11.91   **Laceration without foreign body of unspecified part of neck**

X● S11.92   **Laceration with foreign body of unspecified part of neck**

X● S11.93   **Puncture wound without foreign body of unspecified part of neck**

X● S11.94   **Puncture wound with foreign body of unspecified part of neck**

X● S11.95   **Open bite of unspecified part of neck**
Bite of neck NOS

Excludes1   superficial bite of neck (S10.97)

● **S12   Fracture of cervical vertebra and other parts of neck**

Note: A fracture not indicated as displaced or nondisplaced should be coded to displaced

A fracture not indicated as open or closed should be coded to closed

Includes   fracture of cervical neural arch
fracture of cervical spine
fracture of cervical spinous process
fracture of cervical transverse process
fracture of cervical vertebral arch
fracture of neck

Code first any associated cervical spinal cord injury (S14.0, S14.1-)

The appropriate 7th character is to be added to all codes from subcategories S12.0-S12.6

A	initial encounter for closed fracture
B	initial encounter for open fracture
D	subsequent encounter for fracture with routine healing
G	subsequent encounter for fracture with delayed healing
K	subsequent encounter for fracture with nonunion
S	sequela

(Ex:) **For category S12 CC codes S12[A,B]:** M48.40X-M48.58X[S], M80.08X[S], M80.88X[S], M84.350[S], M84.454[S], M84.550[S], M84.58X[S], M84.650[S], M99.10-M99.11, M99.15-M99.17, M99.19, S03.1XX[A], S03.8XX-S03.9XX[A], S12.000-S12.691{A,B,S], S12.8XX[S], S12.9XX{A,S], S13.0XX-S13.4XX[A], S13.8XXA-S14.159[A], S16.1XX[A], S22.000-S22.9XX[S], S23.20X-S23.29X[A], S23.9XX[A], S24.109[A], S24.119[A], S24.139[A], S24.149[A], S24.159[A], S29.001-S29.019[A], S29.091-S29.9XX[A], S32.000-S32.9XX[S], S33.30X-S33.39X[A], S33.9XX[A], S38.1XX[A], S38.3XX-S39.013[A], S39.091-S39.94X[A], T14.90-T14.91, T79.8XX-T79.9XX[A], T79.A0X-T79.A9X[A] **For S12[K]:** See S02.0[K] **unless otherwise indicated**

● **S12.0   Fracture of first cervical vertebra**
Atlas

● S12.00   **Unspecified fracture of first cervical vertebra**

● S12.000   **Unspecified displaced fracture of first cervical vertebra** A, K 🔗, B 🔗, A, B 🔗

● S12.001   **Unspecified nondisplaced fracture of first cervical vertebra** A, K 🔗, B 🔗, A, B 🔗

X● **S12.01**   Stable burst fracture of first cervical vertebra
A, K 🪙, B 🪙, A, B 🪙

X● **S12.02**   Unstable burst fracture of first cervical vertebra
A, K 🪙, B 🪙, A, B 🪙

● **S12.03**   Posterior arch fracture of first cervical vertebra

  ● **S12.030**   Displaced posterior arch fracture of first cervical vertebra A, K 🪙, B 🪙, A, B 🪙

  ● **S12.031**   Nondisplaced posterior arch fracture of first cervical vertebra A, K 🪙, B 🪙, A, B 🪙

● **S12.04**   Lateral mass fracture of first cervical vertebra

  ● **S12.040**   Displaced lateral mass fracture of first cervical vertebra A, K 🪙, B 🪙, A, B 🪙

  ● **S12.041**   Nondisplaced lateral mass fracture of first cervical vertebra A, K 🪙, B 🪙, A, B 🪙

● **S12.09**   Other fracture of first cervical vertebra

  ● **S12.090**   Other displaced fracture of first cervical vertebra A, K 🪙, B 🪙, A, B 🪙

  ● **S12.091**   Other nondisplaced fracture of first cervical vertebra A, K 🪙, B 🪙, A, B 🪙

● **S12.1**   Fracture of second cervical vertebra
Axis

● **S12.10**   Unspecified fracture of second cervical vertebra

  ● **S12.100**   Unspecified displaced fracture of second cervical vertebra A, K 🪙, B 🪙, A, B 🪙

  ● **S12.101**   Unspecified nondisplaced fracture of second cervical vertebra A, K 🪙, B 🪙, A, B 🪙

● **S12.11**   Type II dens fracture

  ● **S12.110**   Anterior displaced Type II dens fracture A, K 🪙, B 🪙, A, B 🪙

  ● **S12.111**   Posterior displaced Type II dens fracture A, K 🪙, B 🪙, A, B 🪙

  ● **S12.112**   Nondisplaced Type II dens fracture A, K 🪙, B 🪙, A, B 🪙

● **S12.12**   Other dens fracture

  ● **S12.120**   Other displaced dens fracture A, K 🪙, B 🪙, A, B 🪙

  ● **S12.121**   Other nondisplaced dens fracture A, K 🪙, B 🪙, A, B 🪙

● **S12.13**   Unspecified traumatic spondylolisthesis of second cervical vertebra

  ● **S12.130**   Unspecified traumatic displaced spondylolisthesis of second cervical vertebra A, K 🪙, B 🪙, A, B 🪙

  ● **S12.131**   Unspecified traumatic nondisplaced spondylolisthesis of second cervical vertebra A, K 🪙, B 🪙, A, B 🪙

X● **S12.14**   Type III traumatic spondylolisthesis of second cervical vertebra A, K 🪙, B 🪙, A, B 🪙

● **S12.15**   Other traumatic spondylolisthesis of second cervical vertebra

  ● **S12.150**   Other traumatic displaced spondylolisthesis of second cervical vertebra A, K 🪙, B 🪙, A, B 🪙

  ● **S12.151**   Other traumatic nondisplaced spondylolisthesis of second cervical vertebra A, K 🪙, B 🪙, A, B 🪙

● **S12.19**   Other fracture of second cervical vertebra

  ● **S12.190**   Other displaced fracture of second cervical vertebra A, K 🪙, B 🪙, A, B 🪙

  ● **S12.191**   Other nondisplaced fracture of second cervical vertebra A, K 🪙, B 🪙, A, B 🪙

● **S12.2**   Fracture of third cervical vertebra

● **S12.20**   Unspecified fracture of third cervical vertebra

  ● **S12.200**   Unspecified displaced fracture of third cervical vertebra A, K 🪙, B 🪙, A, B 🪙

  ● **S12.201**   Unspecified nondisplaced fracture of third cervical vertebra A, K 🪙, B 🪙, A, B 🪙

● **S12.23**   Unspecified traumatic spondylolisthesis of third cervical vertebra

  ● **S12.230**   Unspecified traumatic displaced spondylolisthesis of third cervical vertebra A, K 🪙, B 🪙, A, B 🪙

  ● **S12.231**   Unspecified traumatic nondisplaced spondylolisthesis of third cervical vertebra A, K 🪙, B 🪙, A, B 🪙

X● **S12.24**   Type III traumatic spondylolisthesis of third cervical vertebra A, K 🪙, B 🪙, A, B 🪙

● **S12.25**   Other traumatic spondylolisthesis of third cervical vertebra

  ● **S12.250**   Other traumatic displaced spondylolisthesis of third cervical vertebra A, K 🪙, B 🪙, A, B 🪙

  ● **S12.251**   Other traumatic nondisplaced spondylolisthesis of third cervical vertebra A, K 🪙, B 🪙, A, B 🪙

● **S12.29**   Other fracture of third cervical vertebra

  ● **S12.290**   Other displaced fracture of third cervical vertebra A, K 🪙, B 🪙, A, B 🪙

  ● **S12.291**   Other nondisplaced fracture of third cervical vertebra A, K 🪙, B 🪙, A, B 🪙

● **S12.3**   Fracture of fourth cervical vertebra

● **S12.30**   Unspecified fracture of fourth cervical vertebra

  ● **S12.300**   Unspecified displaced fracture of fourth cervical vertebra A, K 🪙, B 🪙, A, B 🪙

  ● **S12.301**   Unspecified nondisplaced fracture of fourth cervical vertebra A, K 🪙, B 🪙, A, B 🪙

● **S12.33**   Unspecified traumatic spondylolisthesis of fourth cervical vertebra

  ● **S12.330**   Unspecified traumatic displaced spondylolisthesis of fourth cervical vertebra A, K 🪙, B 🪙, A, B 🪙

  ● **S12.331**   Unspecified traumatic nondisplaced spondylolisthesis of fourth cervical vertebra A, K 🪙, B 🪙, A, B 🪙

X● **S12.34**   Type III traumatic spondylolisthesis of fourth cervical vertebra A, K 🪙, B 🪙, A, B 🪙

● **S12.35**   Other traumatic spondylolisthesis of fourth cervical vertebra

  ● **S12.350**   Other traumatic displaced spondylolisthesis of fourth cervical vertebra A, K 🪙, B 🪙, A, B 🪙

  ● **S12.351**   Other traumatic nondisplaced spondylolisthesis of fourth cervical vertebra A, K 🪙, B 🪙, A, B 🪙

● **S12.39**   Other fracture of fourth cervical vertebra

  ● **S12.390**   Other displaced fracture of fourth cervical vertebra A, K 🪙, B 🪙, A, B 🪙

  ● **S12.391**   Other nondisplaced fracture of fourth cervical vertebra A, K 🪙, B 🪙, A, B 🪙

CHAPTER 19 (SØØ-T88)

N Newborn Age: Ø   **P** Pediatric Age: Ø–17   **M** Maternity DX: 12–55   **A** Adult Age: 15–124   ♀ Females Only   ♂ Males Only

🪙 Complication\Comorbidity   🪙 Major C\C   Ⓔ CC/MCC Exclusions   🪙 Hospital-Acquired Condition

1239

CHAPTER 19 (S00-T88)

- S12.4   Fracture of fifth cervical vertebra
  - S12.40   Unspecified fracture of fifth cervical vertebra
    - S12.400   Unspecified displaced fracture of fifth cervical vertebra A, K, B, A, B
    - S12.401   Unspecified nondisplaced fracture of fifth cervical vertebra A, K, B, A, B
  - S12.43   Unspecified traumatic spondylolisthesis of fifth cervical vertebra
    - S12.430   Unspecified traumatic displaced spondylolisthesis of fifth cervical vertebra A, K, B, A, B
    - S12.431   Unspecified traumatic nondisplaced spondylolisthesis of fifth cervical vertebra A, K, B, A, B
  - X S12.44   Type III traumatic spondylolisthesis of fifth cervical vertebra A, K, B, A, B
  - S12.45   Other traumatic spondylolisthesis of fifth cervical vertebra
    - S12.450   Other traumatic displaced spondylolisthesis of fifth cervical vertebra A, K, B, A, B
    - S12.451   Other traumatic nondisplaced spondylolisthesis of fifth cervical vertebra A, K, B, A, B
  - S12.49   Other fracture of fifth cervical vertebra
    - S12.490   Other displaced fracture of fifth cervical vertebra A, K, B, A, B
    - S12.491   Other nondisplaced fracture of fifth cervical vertebra A, K, B, A, B
- S12.5   Fracture of sixth cervical vertebra
  - S12.50   Unspecified fracture of sixth cervical vertebra
    - S12.500   Unspecified displaced fracture of sixth cervical vertebra A, K, B, A, B
    - S12.501   Unspecified nondisplaced fracture of sixth cervical vertebra A, K, B, A, B
  - S12.53   Unspecified traumatic spondylolisthesis of sixth cervical vertebra
    - S12.530   Unspecified traumatic displaced spondylolisthesis of sixth cervical vertebra A, K, B, A, B
    - S12.531   Unspecified traumatic nondisplaced spondylolisthesis of sixth cervical vertebra A, K, B, A, B
  - X S12.54   Type III traumatic spondylolisthesis of sixth cervical vertebra A, K, B, A, B
  - S12.55   Other traumatic spondylolisthesis of sixth cervical vertebra
    - S12.550   Other traumatic displaced spondylolisthesis of sixth cervical vertebra A, K, B, A, B
    - S12.551   Other traumatic nondisplaced spondylolisthesis of sixth cervical vertebra A, K, B, A, B
  - S12.59   Other fracture of sixth cervical vertebra
    - S12.590   Other displaced fracture of sixth cervical vertebra A, K, B, A, B
    - S12.591   Other nondisplaced fracture of sixth cervical vertebra A, K, B, A, B

- S12.6   Fracture of seventh cervical vertebra
  - S12.60   Unspecified fracture of seventh cervical vertebra
    - S12.600   Unspecified displaced fracture of seventh cervical vertebra A, K, B, A, B
    - S12.601   Unspecified nondisplaced fracture of seventh cervical vertebra A, K, B, A, B
  - S12.63   Unspecified traumatic spondylolisthesis of seventh cervical vertebra
    - S12.630   Unspecified traumatic displaced spondylolisthesis of seventh cervical vertebra A, K, B, A, B
    - S12.631   Unspecified traumatic nondisplaced spondylolisthesis of seventh cervical vertebra A, K, B, A, B
  - X S12.64   Type III traumatic spondylolisthesis of seventh cervical vertebra A, K, B, A, B
  - S12.65   Other traumatic spondylolisthesis of seventh cervical vertebra
    - S12.650   Other traumatic displaced spondylolisthesis of seventh cervical vertebra A, K, B, A, B
    - S12.651   Other traumatic nondisplaced spondylolisthesis of seventh cervical vertebra A, K, B, A, B
  - S12.69   Other fracture of seventh cervical vertebra
    - S12.690   Other displaced fracture of seventh cervical vertebra A, K, B, A, B
    - S12.691   Other nondisplaced fracture of seventh cervical vertebra A, K, B, A, B
- X S12.8   **Fracture of other parts of neck** A, A

Hyoid bone	Thyroid cartilage
Larynx	Trachea

The appropriate 7th character is to be added to code S12.8

A	initial encounter
D	subsequent encounter
S	sequela

Ex: S03.8XX-S03.9XX[A], S12.8XX[A], S29.011-S29.019[A], S38.3XX[A] S39.011-S39.013[A], T14.90-T14.91, T79.8XX-T79.9XX[A] T79.A0XA-T79.A9X[A]

- X S12.9   **Fracture of neck, unspecified** A, A

Fracture of neck NOS
Fracture of cervical spine NOS
Fracture of cervical vertebra NOS

The appropriate 7th character is to be added to code S12.9

A	initial encounter
D	subsequent encounter
S	sequela

◀ New   ◀ Revised   ~~deleted~~ Deleted   Excludes 1   Excludes 2   Includes   Use additional   Code first   Code also   Unspecified

OGCR Official Guidelines   ● Unacceptable Principal Diagnosis   X Assign placeholder X   ● Use Additional Character(s)   ▶ Manifestation Code   **Coding Clinic**

● **S13**   **Dislocation and sprain of joints and ligaments at neck level**

     Includes   avulsion of joint or ligament at neck level
           laceration of cartilage, joint or ligament at neck level
           sprain of cartilage, joint or ligament at neck level
           traumatic hemarthrosis of joint or ligament at neck level
           traumatic rupture of joint or ligament at neck level
           traumatic subluxation of joint or ligament at neck level
           traumatic tear of joint or ligament at neck level

     Code also any associated open wound

     Excludes2   strain of muscle or tendon at neck level (S16.1)

     The appropriate 7th character is to be added to each code from category S13

       A   initial encounter
       D   subsequent encounter
       S   sequela

     (Ex) **For category S13 CC codes:** M99.10-M99.11, S03.8XX-S03.9XX[A], S12.000-S12.691[A,B], S12.9XX-S13.4XX[A], S13.8XX[A], S14.0XX-S14.108[A], S14.111-S14.118[A], S14.121-S14.128[A], S14.131-S14.138[A], S14.141-S14.148[A], S14.151-S14.158[A], S16.1XX[A], S29.011-S29.019[A], S38.3XX[A], S39.011-S39.013[A], T14.90-T14.91, T79.A0X-T79.9XX[A]

X ● **S13.0**   **Traumatic rupture of cervical intervertebral disc** A 🔴, A 🔴

       Excludes1   rupture or displacement (nontraumatic) of cervical intervertebral disc NOS (M50.-)

● **S13.1**   **Subluxation and dislocation of cervical vertebrae**

     Code also any associated:
       open wound of neck (S11.-)
       spinal cord injury (S14.1-)

       Excludes2   fracture of cervical vertebrae (S12.0-S12.3-)

   ● **S13.10**   **Subluxation and dislocation of unspecified cervical vertebrae**

     ● **S13.100**   **Subluxation of unspecified cervical vertebrae** A 🔴, A 🔴

     ● **S13.101**   **Dislocation of unspecified cervical vertebrae** A 🔴, A 🔴

   ● **S13.11**   **Subluxation and dislocation of C_0/C_1 cervical vertebrae**

       Subluxation and dislocation of atlantooccipital joint
       Subluxation and dislocation of atloidooccipital joint
       Subluxation and dislocation of occipitoatloid joint

     ● **S13.110**   **Subluxation of C_0/C_1 cervical vertebrae** A 🔴, A 🔴

     ● **S13.111**   **Dislocation of C_0/C_1 cervical vertebrae** A 🔴, A 🔴

   ● **S13.12**   **Subluxation and dislocation of C_1/C_2 cervical vertebrae**

       Subluxation and dislocation of atlantoaxial joint

     ● **S13.120**   **Subluxation of C_1/C_2 cervical vertebrae** A 🔴, A 🔴

     ● **S13.121**   **Dislocation of C_1/C_2 cervical vertebrae** A 🔴, A 🔴

● **S13.13**   **Subluxation and dislocation of C_2/C_3 cervical vertebrae**

     ● **S13.130**   **Subluxation of C_2/C_3 cervical vertebrae** A 🔴, A 🔴

     ● **S13.131**   **Dislocation of C_2/C_3 cervical vertebrae** A 🔴, A 🔴

● **S13.14**   **Subluxation and dislocation of C_3/C_4 cervical vertebrae**

     ● **S13.140**   **Subluxation of C_3/C_4 cervical vertebrae** A 🔴, A 🔴

     ● **S13.141**   **Dislocation of C_3/C_4 cervical vertebrae** A 🔴, A 🔴

● **S13.15**   **Subluxation and dislocation of C_4/C_5 cervical vertebrae**

     ● **S13.150**   **Subluxation of C_4/C_5 cervical vertebrae** A 🔴, A 🔴

     ● **S13.151**   **Dislocation of C_4/C_5 cervical vertebrae** A 🔴, A 🔴

● **S13.16**   **Subluxation and dislocation of C_5/C_6 cervical vertebrae**

     ● **S13.160**   **Subluxation of C_5/C_6 cervical vertebrae** A 🔴, A 🔴

     ● **S13.161**   **Dislocation of C_5/C_6 cervical vertebrae** A 🔴, A 🔴

● **S13.17**   **Subluxation and dislocation of C_6/C_7 cervical vertebrae**

     ● **S13.170**   **Subluxation of C_6/C_7 cervical vertebrae** A 🔴, A 🔴

     ● **S13.171**   **Dislocation of C_6/C_7 cervical vertebrae** A 🔴, A 🔴

● **S13.18**   **Subluxation and dislocation of C_7/T_1 cervical vertebrae**

     ● **S13.180**   **Subluxation of C_7/T_1 cervical vertebrae** A 🔴, A 🔴

     ● **S13.181**   **Dislocation of C_7/T_1 cervical vertebrae** A 🔴, A 🔴

● **S13.2**   **Dislocation of other and unspecified parts of neck**

   X ● **S13.20**   **Dislocation of unspecified parts of neck** A 🔴, A 🔴

   X ● **S13.29**   **Dislocation of other parts of neck** A 🔴, A 🔴

X ● **S13.4**   **Sprain of ligaments of cervical spine**
       Sprain of anterior longitudinal (ligament), cervical
       Sprain of atlanto-axial (joints)
       Sprain of atlanto-occipital (joints)
       Whiplash injury of cervical spine

X ● **S13.5**   **Sprain of thyroid region**
       Sprain of cricoarytenoid (joint) (ligament)
       Sprain of cricothyroid (joint) (ligament)
       Sprain of thyroid cartilage

X ● **S13.8**   **Sprain of joints and ligaments of other parts of neck**

X ● **S13.9**   **Sprain of joints and ligaments of unspecified parts of neck**

N Newborn Age: 0   **P** Pediatric Age: 0–17   **M** Maternity DX: 12–55   **A** Adult Age: 15–124   ♀ Females Only   ♂ Males Only

🔴 Complication\Comorbidity   🔴 Major C\C   (Ex) CC/MCC Exclusions   🔴 Hospital-Acquired Condition   **1241**

● **S14**   **Injury of nerves and spinal cord at neck level**

    Note: Code to highest level of cervical cord injury

     Code also any associated:
       fracture of cervical vertebra (S12.0--S12.6.-)
       open wound of neck (S11.-)
       transient paralysis (R29.5)

     The appropriate 7th character is to be added to each code from
       category S14

       A   initial encounter
       D   subsequent encounter
       S   sequela

     Ex: **For category S14 CC codes:** M48.40X-M48.58X[S], M80.08X[S], M80.88X[S],
       M84.350[S], M84.454[S], M84.550[S], M84.58X[S], M84.650[S], M99.10-M99.11,
       M99.15-M99.17, M99.19, S03.1XX[A], S12.000-S12.691[A,B,S], S12.8XX[S], S12.9XX[A,
       S], S13.0XX-S13.29X[A], S13.9XX-S14.159[A], S22.000-S22.9XX[S],
       S23.20X-S23.29X[A], S23.9XX[A], S24.109[A], S24.119[A], S24.139[A], S24.149[A],
       S24.159[A], S29.001-S29.009[A], S29.091-S29.9XX[A], S32.000-S32.9XX[S],
       S33.30X-S33.39X[A], S33.9XX[A], S38.1XX[A], S39.001-S39.003[A],
       S39.091-S39.94X[A], T14.90-T14.91, T79.8XX-T79.9XX[A], T79.A0X-T79.A9X[A]

X ● **S14.0**   Concussion and edema of cervical spinal cord A 🖐

● **S14.1**   Other and unspecified injuries of cervical spinal cord

   ● **S14.10**   Unspecified injury of cervical spinal cord

     ● **S14.101**   Unspecified injury at C₁ level of
cervical spinal cord A 🖐, A 🖐

     ● **S14.102**   Unspecified injury at C₂ level of
cervical spinal cord A 🖐, A 🖐

     ● **S14.103**   Unspecified injury at C₃ level of
cervical spinal cord A 🖐, A 🖐

     ● **S14.104**   Unspecified injury at C₄ level of
cervical spinal cord A 🖐, A 🖐

     ● **S14.105**   Unspecified injury at C₅ level of
cervical spinal cord A 🖐, A 🖐

     ● **S14.106**   Unspecified injury at C₆ level of
cervical spinal cord A 🖐, A 🖐

     ● **S14.107**   Unspecified injury at C₇ level of
cervical spinal cord A 🖐, A 🖐

     ● **S14.108**   Unspecified injury at C₈ level of
cervical spinal cord A 🖐

     ● **S14.109**   Unspecified injury at unspecified
level of cervical spinal cord A 🖐
Injury of cervical spinal cord NOS

   ● **S14.11**   Complete lesion of cervical spinal cord

     ● **S14.111**   Complete lesion at C₁ level of cervical
spinal cord A 🖐, A 🖐

     ● **S14.112**   Complete lesion at C₂ level of cervical
spinal cord A 🖐, A 🖐

     ● **S14.113**   Complete lesion at C₃ level of cervical
spinal cord A 🖐, A 🖐

     ● **S14.114**   Complete lesion at C₄ level of cervical
spinal cord A 🖐, A 🖐

     ● **S14.115**   Complete lesion at C₅ level of cervical
spinal cord A 🖐, A 🖐

     ● **S14.116**   Complete lesion at C₆ level of cervical
spinal cord A 🖐, A 🖐

     ● **S14.117**   Complete lesion at C₇ level of cervical
spinal cord A 🖐, A 🖐

     ● **S14.118**   Complete lesion at C₈ level of cervical
spinal cord A 🖐

     ● **S14.119**   Complete lesion at unspecified level
of cervical spinal cord

   ● **S14.12**   Central cord syndrome of cervical spinal cord

     ● **S14.121**   Central cord syndrome at C₁ level of
cervical spinal cord A 🖐, A 🖐

     ● **S14.122**   Central cord syndrome at C₂ level of
cervical spinal cord A 🖐, A 🖐

     ● **S14.123**   Central cord syndrome at C₃ level of
cervical spinal cord A 🖐, A 🖐

     ● **S14.124**   Central cord syndrome at C₄ level of
cervical spinal cord A 🖐, A 🖐

     ● **S14.125**   Central cord syndrome at C₅ level of
cervical spinal cord A 🖐, A 🖐

     ● **S14.126**   Central cord syndrome at C₆ level of
cervical spinal cord A 🖐, A 🖐

     ● **S14.127**   Central cord syndrome at C₇ level of
cervical spinal cord A 🖐, A 🖐

     ● **S14.128**   Central cord syndrome at C₈ level of
cervical spinal cord A 🖐

     ● **S14.129**   Central cord syndrome at unspecified
level of cervical spinal cord

   ● **S14.13**   Anterior cord syndrome of cervical spinal cord

     ● **S14.131**   Anterior cord syndrome at C₁ level of
cervical spinal cord A 🖐, A 🖐

     ● **S14.132**   Anterior cord syndrome at C₂ level of
cervical spinal cord A 🖐, A 🖐

     ● **S14.133**   Anterior cord syndrome at C₃ level of
cervical spinal cord A 🖐, A 🖐

     ● **S14.134**   Anterior cord syndrome at C₄ level of
cervical spinal cord A 🖐, A 🖐

     ● **S14.135**   Anterior cord syndrome at C₅ level of
cervical spinal cord A 🖐, A 🖐

     ● **S14.136**   Anterior cord syndrome at C₆ level of
cervical spinal cord A 🖐, A 🖐

     ● **S14.137**   Anterior cord syndrome at C₇ level of
cervical spinal cord A 🖐, A 🖐

     ● **S14.138**   Anterior cord syndrome at C₈ level of
cervical spinal cord A 🖐

     ● **S14.139**   Anterior cord syndrome at unspecified
level of cervical spinal cord

   ● **S14.14**   Brown-Séquard syndrome of cervical spinal
cord

     ● **S14.141**   Brown-Séquard syndrome at C₁ level
of cervical spinal cord A 🖐

     ● **S14.142**   Brown-Séquard syndrome at C₂ level
of cervical spinal cord A 🖐

     ● **S14.143**   Brown-Séquard syndrome at C₃ level
of cervical spinal cord A 🖐

     ● **S14.144**   Brown-Séquard syndrome at C₄ level
of cervical spinal cord A 🖐

     ● **S14.145**   Brown-Séquard syndrome at C₅ level
of cervical spinal cord A 🖐

     ● **S14.146**   Brown-Séquard syndrome at C₆ level
of cervical spinal cord A 🖐

     ● **S14.147**   Brown-Séquard syndrome at C₇ level
of cervical spinal cord A 🖐

     ● **S14.148**   Brown-Séquard syndrome at C₈ level
of cervical spinal cord A 🖐

     ● **S14.149**   Brown-Séquard syndrome at
unspecified level of cervical spinal
cord

   ● **S14.15**   Other incomplete lesions of cervical spinal cord
Incomplete lesion of cervical spinal cord NOS
Posterior cord syndrome of cervical spinal cord

     ● **S14.151**   Other incomplete lesion at C₁ level of
cervical spinal cord A 🖐, A 🖐

     ● **S14.152**   Other incomplete lesion at C₂ level of
cervical spinal cord A 🖐, A 🖐

     ● **S14.153**   Other incomplete lesion at C₃ level of
cervical spinal cord A 🖐, A 🖐

     ● **S14.154**   Other incomplete lesion at C₄ level of
cervical spinal cord A 🖐, A 🖐

     ● **S14.155**   Other incomplete lesion at C₅ level of
cervical spinal cord A 🖐, A 🖐

     ● **S14.156**   Other incomplete lesion at C₆ level of
cervical spinal cord A 🖐, A 🖐

     ● **S14.157**   Other incomplete lesion at C₇ level of
cervical spinal cord A 🖐, A 🖐

     ● **S14.158**   Other incomplete lesion at C₈ level of
cervical spinal cord A 🖐

     ● **S14.159**   Other incomplete lesion at unspecified
level of cervical spinal cord

◀ New   ◀⁐ Revised   ~~deleted~~ Deleted   Excludes 1   Excludes 2   Includes   Use additional   Code first   Code also   Unspecified

OGCR Official Guidelines   ● Unacceptable Principal Diagnosis   X Assign placeholder X   ● Use Additional Character(s)   ▶ Manifestation Code   **Coding Clinic**

X● **S14.2**   **Injury of nerve root of cervical spine**

X● **S14.3**   **Injury of brachial plexus**

X● **S14.4**   **Injury of peripheral nerves of neck**

X● **S14.5**   **Injury of cervical sympathetic nerves**

X● **S14.8**   **Injury of other specified nerves of neck**

X● **S14.9**   **Injury of unspecified nerves of neck**

● **S15**   **Injury of blood vessels at neck level**

> Code also any associated open wound (S11.-)
>
> The appropriate 7th character is to be added to each code from category S15

> | | |
> |---|---|
> | A | initial encounter |
> | D | subsequent encounter |
> | S | sequela |

● **S15.0**   **Injury of carotid artery of neck**

> Injury of carotid artery (common) (external) (internal, extracranial portion)
> Injury of carotid artery NOS

> **Excludes1**   injury of internal carotid artery, intracranial portion (S06.8)

> (Ex) **For category S15.0 CC codes:** S09.0XX[A], S15.009[A], S15.029[A], S15.099-S15.199[A], S15.8XX-S15.9XX[A], T14.90-T14.91, T79.8XX-T79.9XX[A], T79.A0X-T79.A9X[A]

   ● **S15.00**   **Unspecified injury of carotid artery**

      ● **S15.001**   **Unspecified injury of right carotid artery** A ⌖

      ● **S15.002**   **Unspecified injury of left carotid artery** A ⌖

      ● **S15.009**   **Unspecified injury of unspecified carotid artery** A ⌖

   ● **S15.01**   **Minor laceration of carotid artery**

> Incomplete transection of carotid artery
> Laceration of carotid artery NOS
> Superficial laceration of carotid artery

      ● **S15.011**   **Minor laceration of right carotid artery** A ⌖

      ● **S15.012**   **Minor laceration of left carotid artery** A ⌖

      ● **S15.019**   **Minor laceration of unspecified carotid artery** A ⌖

   ● **S15.02**   **Major laceration of carotid artery**

> Complete transection of carotid artery
> Traumatic rupture of carotid artery

      ● **S15.021**   **Major laceration of right carotid artery** A ⌖

      ● **S15.022**   **Major laceration of left carotid artery** A ⌖

      ● **S15.029**   **Major laceration of unspecified carotid artery** A ⌖

   ● **S15.09**   **Other specified injury of carotid artery**

      ● **S15.091**   **Other specified injury of right carotid artery** A ⌖

      ● **S15.092**   **Other specified injury of left carotid artery** A ⌖

      ● **S15.099**   **Other specified injury of unspecified carotid artery** A ⌖

● **S15.1**   **Injury of vertebral artery**

> (Ex) **For category S15.1 CC codes:** S09.0XX[A], S15.101-S15.199[A] S15.8XX-S15.9XX[A], T14.90-T14.91, T79.8XX-T79.9XX[A] T79.A0X-T79.A9X[A]

   ● **S15.10**   **Unspecified injury of vertebral artery**

      ● **S15.101**   **Unspecified injury of right vertebral artery** A ⌖

      ● **S15.102**   **Unspecified injury of left vertebral artery** A ⌖

      ● **S15.109**   **Unspecified injury of unspecified vertebral artery** A ⌖

   ● **S15.11**   **Minor laceration of vertebral artery**

> Incomplete transection of vertebral artery
> Laceration of vertebral artery NOS
> Superficial laceration of vertebral artery

      ● **S15.111**   **Minor laceration of right vertebral artery** A ⌖

      ● **S15.112**   **Minor laceration of left vertebral artery** A ⌖

      ● **S15.119**   **Minor laceration of unspecified vertebral artery** A ⌖

   ● **S15.12**   **Major laceration of vertebral artery**

> Complete transection of vertebral artery
> Traumatic rupture of vertebral artery

      ● **S15.121**   **Major laceration of right vertebral artery** A ⌖

      ● **S15.122**   **Major laceration of left vertebral artery** A ⌖

      ● **S15.129**   **Major laceration of unspecified vertebral artery** A ⌖

   ● **S15.19**   **Other specified injury of vertebral artery**

      ● **S15.191**   **Other specified injury of right vertebral artery** A ⌖

      ● **S15.192**   **Other specified injury of left vertebral artery** A ⌖

      ● **S15.199**   **Other specified injury of unspecified vertebral artery** A ⌖

● **S15.2**   **Injury of external jugular vein**

> (Ex) **For category S15.2 CC codes:** See S15.1

   ● **S15.20**   **Unspecified injury of external jugular vein**

      ● **S15.201**   **Unspecified injury of right external jugular vein** A ⌖

      ● **S15.202**   **Unspecified injury of left external jugular vein** A ⌖

      ● **S15.209**   **Unspecified injury of unspecified external jugular vein** A ⌖

   ● **S15.21**   **Minor laceration of external jugular vein**

> Incomplete transection of external jugular vein
> Laceration of external jugular vein NOS
> Superficial laceration of external jugular vein

      ● **S15.211**   **Minor laceration of right external jugular vein** A ⌖

      ● **S15.212**   **Minor laceration of left external jugular vein** A ⌖

      ● **S15.219**   **Minor laceration of unspecified external jugular vein** A ⌖

   ● **S15.22**   **Major laceration of external jugular vein**

> Complete transection of external jugular vein
> Traumatic rupture of external jugular vein

      ● **S15.221**   **Major laceration of right external jugular vein** A ⌖

      ● **S15.222**   **Major laceration of left external jugular vein** A ⌖

      ● **S15.229**   **Major laceration of unspecified external jugular vein** A ⌖

   ● **S15.29**   **Other specified injury of external jugular vein**

      ● **S15.291**   **Other specified injury of right external jugular vein** A ⌖

      ● **S15.292**   **Other specified injury of left external jugular vein** A ⌖

      ● **S15.299**   **Other specified injury of unspecified external jugular vein** A ⌖

● **S15.3**   **Injury of internal jugular vein**

> (Ex) **For category S15.3 CC codes:** See S15.1

   ● **S15.30**   **Unspecified injury of internal jugular vein**

      ● **S15.301**   **Unspecified injury of right internal jugular vein** A ⌖

      ● **S15.302**   **Unspecified injury of left internal jugular vein** A ⌖

      ● **S15.309**   **Unspecified injury of unspecified internal jugular vein** A ⌖

CHAPTER 19 (S00-T88)

N Newborn Age: 0   **P** Pediatric Age: 0–17   **M** Maternity DX: 12–55   **A** Adult Age: 15–124   ♀ Females Only   ♂ Males Only

⌖ Complication\Comorbidity   ⌖ Major C\C   (Ex) CC/MCC Exclusions   ⌖ Hospital-Acquired Condition

1243

● **S15.31**   **Minor laceration of internal jugular vein**
Incomplete transection of internal jugular vein
Laceration of internal jugular vein NOS
Superficial laceration of internal jugular vein

     ● **S15.311**   **Minor laceration of right internal jugular vein** A 🦠

     ● **S15.312**   **Minor laceration of left internal jugular vein** A 🦠

     ● **S15.319**   **Minor laceration of unspecified internal jugular vein** A 🦠

● **S15.32**   **Major laceration of internal jugular vein**
Complete transection of internal jugular vein
Traumatic rupture of internal jugular vein

     ● **S15.321**   **Major laceration of right internal jugular vein** A 🦠

     ● **S15.322**   **Major laceration of left internal jugular vein** A 🦠

     ● **S15.329**   **Major laceration of unspecified internal jugular vein** A 🦠

● **S15.39**   **Other specified injury of internal jugular vein**

     ● **S15.391**   **Other specified injury of right internal jugular vein** A 🦠

     ● **S15.392**   **Other specified injury of left internal jugular vein** A 🦠

     ● **S15.399**   **Other specified injury of unspecified internal jugular vein** A 🦠

X ● **S15.8**   **Injury of other specified blood vessels at neck level** A 🦠
     (Ex:) See S15.1

X ● **S15.9**   **Injury of unspecified blood vessel at neck level** A 🦠
     (Ex:) See S15.1

● **S16**   **Injury of muscle, fascia and tendon at neck level**
Code also any associated open wound (S11.-)

     Excludes2   sprain of joint or ligament at neck level (S13.9)

The appropriate 7th character is to be added to each code from category S16

A	initial encounter
D	subsequent encounter
S	sequela

X ● **S16.1**   **Strain of muscle, fascia and tendon at neck level**

X ● **S16.2**   **Laceration of muscle, fascia and tendon at neck level**

X ● **S16.8**   **Other specified injury of muscle, fascia and tendon at neck level**

X ● **S16.9**   **Unspecified injury of muscle, fascia and tendon at neck level**

● **S17**   **Crushing injury of neck**
Use additional code for all associated injuries, such as:
injury of blood vessels (S15.-)
open wound of neck (S11.-)
spinal cord injury (S14.0, S14.1-)
vertebral fracture (S12.0--S12.3-)

The appropriate 7th character is to be added to each code from category S17

A	initial encounter
D	subsequent encounter
S	sequela

     (Ex:) For category S17 CC codes: See S07

X ● **S17.0**   **Crushing injury of larynx and trachea** A 🦠, A 🦠

X ● **S17.8**   **Crushing injury of other specified parts of neck** A 🦠, A 🦠

X ● **S17.9**   **Crushing injury of neck, part unspecified** A 🦠, A 🦠

● **S19**   **Other and unspecified injuries of neck**
The appropriate 7th character is to be added to each code from category S19

A	initial encounter
D	subsequent encounter
S	sequela

● **S19.8**   **Other specified injuries of neck**

   X ● **S19.80**   **Other specified injuries of unspecified part of neck**

   X ● **S19.81**   **Other specified injuries of larynx**

   X ● **S19.82**   **Other specified injuries of cervical trachea**

     Excludes2   other specified injury of thoracic trachea (S27.5-)

   X ● **S19.83**   **Other specified injuries of vocal cord**

   X ● **S19.84**   **Other specified injuries of thyroid gland**

   X ● **S19.85**   **Other specified injuries of pharynx and cervical esophagus**

   X ● **S19.89**   **Other specified injuries of other specified part of neck**

X ● **S19.9**   **Unspecified injury of neck**

INJURIES TO THE THORAX (S20-S29)

Includes	injuries of breast
	injuries of chest (wall)
	injuries of interscapular area

Excludes2	burns and corrosions (T20-T32)
	effects of foreign body in bronchus (T17.5)
	effects of foreign body in esophagus (T18.1)
	effects of foreign body in lung (T17.8)
	effects of foreign body in trachea (T17.4)
	frostbite (T33-T34)
	injuries of axilla
	injuries of clavicle
	injuries of scapular region
	injuries of shoulder
	insect bite or sting, venomous (T63.4)

● **S20**   **Superficial injury of thorax**
The appropriate 7th character is to be added to each code from category S20

A	initial encounter
D	subsequent encounter
S	sequela

● **S20.0**   **Contusion of breast**

   X ● **S20.00**   **Contusion of breast, unspecified breast**

   X ● **S20.01**   **Contusion of right breast**

   X ● **S20.02**   **Contusion of left breast**

● **S20.1**   **Other and unspecified superficial injuries of breast**

   ● **S20.10**   **Unspecified superficial injuries of breast**

     ● **S20.101**   **Unspecified superficial injuries of breast, right breast**

     ● **S20.102**   **Unspecified superficial injuries of breast, left breast**

     ● **S20.109**   **Unspecified superficial injuries of breast, unspecified breast**

   ● **S20.11**   **Abrasion of breast**

     ● **S20.111**   **Abrasion of breast, right breast**

     ● **S20.112**   **Abrasion of breast, left breast**

     ● **S20.119**   **Abrasion of breast, unspecified breast**

   ● **S20.12**   **Blister (nonthermal) of breast**

     ● **S20.121**   **Blister (nonthermal) of breast, right breast**

     ● **S20.122**   **Blister (nonthermal) of breast, left breast**

     ● **S20.129**   **Blister (nonthermal) of breast, unspecified breast**

◀ New   ◀▥ Revised   ~~deleted~~ Deleted   Excludes 1   Excludes 2   Includes   Use additional   Code first   Code also   Unspecified

OGCR Official Guidelines   ● Unacceptable Principal Diagnosis   X Assign placeholder X   ● Use Additional Character(s)   🦠 Manifestation Code   **Coding Clinic**

- S20.14   External constriction of part of breast
  - S20.141   External constriction of part of breast, right breast
  - S20.142   External constriction of part of breast, left breast
  - S20.149   External constriction of part of breast, unspecified breast
- S20.15   Superficial foreign body of breast
    Splinter in the breast
  - S20.151   Superficial foreign body of breast, right breast
  - S20.152   Superficial foreign body of breast, left breast
  - S20.159   Superficial foreign body of breast, unspecified breast
- S20.16   Insect bite (nonvenomous) of breast
  - S20.161   Insect bite (nonvenomous) of breast, right breast
  - S20.162   Insect bite (nonvenomous) of breast, left breast
  - S20.169   Insect bite (nonvenomous) of breast, unspecified breast
- S20.17   Other superficial bite of breast
    Excludes1   open bite of breast (S21.05-)
  - S20.171   Other superficial bite of breast, right breast
  - S20.172   Other superficial bite of breast, left breast
  - S20.179   Other superficial bite of breast, unspecified breast
- S20.2   Contusion of thorax
  - X S20.20   Contusion of thorax, unspecified
  - S20.21   Contusion of front wall of thorax
    - S20.211   Contusion of right front wall of thorax
    - S20.212   Contusion of left front wall of thorax
    - S20.219   Contusion of unspecified front wall of thorax
  - S20.22   Contusion of back wall of thorax
    - S20.221   Contusion of right back wall of thorax
    - S20.222   Contusion of left back wall of thorax
    - S20.229   Contusion of unspecified back wall of thorax
- S20.3   Other and unspecified superficial injuries of front wall of thorax
  - S20.30   Unspecified superficial injuries of front wall of thorax
    - S20.301   Unspecified superficial injuries of right front wall of thorax
    - S20.302   Unspecified superficial injuries of left front wall of thorax
    - S20.309   Unspecified superficial injuries of unspecified front wall of thorax
  - S20.31   Abrasion of front wall of thorax
    - S20.311   Abrasion of right front wall of thorax
    - S20.312   Abrasion of left front wall of thorax
    - S20.319   Abrasion of unspecified front wall of thorax
  - S20.32   Blister (nonthermal) of front wall of thorax
    - S20.321   Blister (nonthermal) of right front wall of thorax
    - S20.322   Blister (nonthermal) of left front wall of thorax
    - S20.329   Blister (nonthermal) of unspecified front wall of thorax

- S20.34   External constriction of front wall of thorax
  - S20.341   External constriction of right front wall of thorax
  - S20.342   External constriction of left front wall of thorax
  - S20.349   External constriction of unspecified front wall of thorax
- S20.35   Superficial foreign body of front wall of thorax
    Splinter in front wall of thorax
  - S20.351   Superficial foreign body of right front wall of thorax
  - S20.352   Superficial foreign body of left front wall of thorax
  - S20.359   Superficial foreign body of unspecified front wall of thorax
- S20.36   Insect bite (nonvenomous) of front wall of thorax
  - S20.361   Insect bite (nonvenomous) of right front wall of thorax
  - S20.362   Insect bite (nonvenomous) of left front wall of thorax
  - S20.369   Insect bite (nonvenomous) of unspecified front wall of thorax
- S20.37   Other superficial bite of front wall of thorax
    Excludes1   open bite of front wall of thorax (S21.14)
  - S20.371   Other superficial bite of right front wall of thorax
  - S20.372   Other superficial bite of left front wall of thorax
  - S20.379   Other superficial bite of unspecified front wall of thorax
- S20.4   Other and unspecified superficial injuries of back wall of thorax
  - S20.40   Unspecified superficial injuries of back wall of thorax
    - S20.401   Unspecified superficial injuries of right back wall of thorax
    - S20.402   Unspecified superficial injuries of left back wall of thorax
    - S20.409   Unspecified superficial injuries of unspecified back wall of thorax
  - S20.41   Abrasion of back wall of thorax
    - S20.411   Abrasion of right back wall of thorax
    - S20.412   Abrasion of left back wall of thorax
    - S20.419   Abrasion of unspecified back wall of thorax
  - S20.42   Blister (nonthermal) of back wall of thorax
    - S20.421   Blister (nonthermal) of right back wall of thorax
    - S20.422   Blister (nonthermal) of left back wall of thorax
    - S20.429   Blister (nonthermal) of unspecified back wall of thorax
  - S20.44   External constriction of back wall of thorax
    - S20.441   External constriction of right back wall of thorax
    - S20.442   External constriction of left back wall of thorax
    - S20.449   External constriction of unspecified back wall of thorax
  - S20.45   Superficial foreign body of back wall of thorax
      Splinter of back wall of thorax
    - S20.451   Superficial foreign body of right back wall of thorax
    - S20.452   Superficial foreign body of left back wall of thorax
    - S20.459   Superficial foreign body of unspecified back wall of thorax

CHAPTER 19 (S00-T88)

● **S20.46**   **Insect bite (nonvenomous) of back wall of thorax**
   ● **S20.461**   Insect bite (nonvenomous) of right back wall of thorax
   ● **S20.462**   Insect bite (nonvenomous) of left back wall of thorax
   ● **S20.469**   Insect bite (nonvenomous) of unspecified back wall of thorax
● **S20.47**   **Other superficial bite of back wall of thorax**
   Excludes1   open bite of back wall of thorax (S21.24)
   ● **S20.471**   Other superficial bite of right back wall of thorax
   ● **S20.472**   Other superficial bite of left back wall of thorax
   ● **S20.479**   Other superficial bite of unspecified back wall of thorax
● **S20.9**   **Superficial injury of unspecified parts of thorax**
   Excludes1   contusion of thorax NOS (S20.20)
X ● **S20.90**   Unspecified superficial injury of unspecified parts of thorax
     Superficial injury of thoracic wall NOS
X ● **S20.91**   Abrasion of unspecified parts of thorax
X ● **S20.92**   Blister (nonthermal) of unspecified parts of thorax
X ● **S20.94**   External constriction of unspecified parts of thorax
X ● **S20.95**   Superficial foreign body of unspecified parts of thorax
     Splinter in thorax NOS
X ● **S20.96**   Insect bite (nonvenomous) of unspecified parts of thorax
X ● **S20.97**   Other superficial bite of unspecified parts of thorax
     Excludes1   open bite of thorax NOS (S21.95)

● **S21**   **Open wound of thorax**
   Code also any associated injury such as:
     injury of heart (S26.-)
     injury of intrathoracic organs (S27.-)
     rib fracture (S22.3-, S22.4-)
     spinal cord injury (S24.0-, S24.1-)
     traumatic hemothorax (S27.1)
     traumatic hemopneumothorax (S27.3)
     traumatic pneumothorax (S27.0)
     wound infection
   Excludes1   traumatic amputation (partial) of thorax (S28.1)
   The appropriate 7th character is to be added to each code from category S21

A	initial encounter
D	subsequent encounter
S	sequela

● **S21.0**   **Open wound of breast**
   ● **S21.00**   Unspecified open wound of breast
     ● **S21.001**   Unspecified open wound of right breast
     ● **S21.002**   Unspecified open wound of left breast
     ● **S21.009**   Unspecified open wound of unspecified breast

● **S21.01**   **Laceration without foreign body of breast**
   ● **S21.011**   Laceration without foreign body of right breast
   ● **S21.012**   Laceration without foreign body of left breast
   ● **S21.019**   Laceration without foreign body of unspecified breast
● **S21.02**   **Laceration with foreign body of breast**
   ● **S21.021**   Laceration with foreign body of right breast
   ● **S21.022**   Laceration with foreign body of left breast
   ● **S21.029**   Laceration with foreign body of unspecified breast
● **S21.03**   **Puncture wound without foreign body of breast**
   ● **S21.031**   Puncture wound without foreign body of right breast
   ● **S21.032**   Puncture wound without foreign body of left breast
   ● **S21.039**   Puncture wound without foreign body of unspecified breast
● **S21.04**   **Puncture wound with foreign body of breast**
   ● **S21.041**   Puncture wound with foreign body of right breast
   ● **S21.042**   Puncture wound with foreign body of left breast
   ● **S21.049**   Puncture wound with foreign body of unspecified breast
● **S21.05**   **Open bite of breast**
     Bite of breast NOS
   Excludes1   superficial bite of breast (S20.17)
   ● **S21.051**   Open bite of right breast
   ● **S21.052**   Open bite of left breast
   ● **S21.059**   Open bite of unspecified breast

● **S21.1**   **Open wound of front wall of thorax without penetration into thoracic cavity**
   Open wound of chest without penetration into thoracic cavity
   Ⓔⓧ **For category S21.1 CC codes:** S21.101-S21.159[A], S21.301-S21.95X[A], S23.3XX[A], S23.8XX[A], S27.50X-S27.69X[A], S27.892A-S28.1XX[A], S29.021[A], S29.029[A], S38.3XX[A], T14.90-T14.91, T79.7XX[A] T79.8XX-T79.9XX[A], T79.A0X-T79.A9X[A]

   ● **S21.10**   Unspecified open wound of front wall of thorax without penetration into thoracic cavity
     ● **S21.101**   Unspecified open wound of right front wall of thorax without penetration into thoracic cavity A 🐾
     ● **S21.102**   Unspecified open wound of left front wall of thorax without penetration into thoracic cavity A 🐾
     ● **S21.109**   Unspecified open wound of unspecified front wall of thorax without penetration into thoracic cavity A 🐾
   ● **S21.11**   Laceration without foreign body of front wall of thorax without penetration into thoracic cavity
     ● **S21.111**   Laceration without foreign body of right front wall of thorax without penetration into thoracic cavity A 🐾
     ● **S21.112**   Laceration without foreign body of left front wall of thorax without penetration into thoracic cavity A 🐾
     ● **S21.119**   Laceration without foreign body of unspecified front wall of thorax without penetration into thoracic cavity A 🐾

Item 19–1   **Pneumothorax** is a collection of gas (positive air pressure) in the pleural space resulting in the lung collapsing. A tension pneumothorax is life-threatening and is a result of air in the pleural space causing a displacement in the mediastinal structures and cardiopulmonary function compromise. A traumatic pneumothorax results from blunt or penetrating injury that disrupts the parietal/visceral pleura. **Hemothorax** is blood or bloody fluid in the pleural cavity as a result of traumatic blood vessel rupture or inflammation of the lungs from pneumonia.

◀ New   ◀▥ Revised   ~~deleted~~ Deleted   Excludes 1   Excludes 2   Includes   Use additional   Code first   Code also   Unspecified
OGCR Official Guidelines   ● Unacceptable Principal Diagnosis   X Assign placeholder X   ● Use Additional Character(s)   ▷ Manifestation Code   **Coding Clinic**

● **S21.12** **Laceration with foreign body of front wall of thorax without penetration into thoracic cavity**

  ● **S21.121** Laceration with foreign body of right front wall of thorax without penetration into thoracic cavity A 🦠

  ● **S21.122** Laceration with foreign body of left front wall of thorax without penetration into thoracic cavity A 🦠

  ● **S21.129** Laceration with foreign body of unspecified front wall of thorax without penetration into thoracic cavity A 🦠

● **S21.13** **Puncture wound without foreign body of front wall of thorax without penetration into thoracic cavity**

  ● **S21.131** Puncture wound without foreign body of right front wall of thorax without penetration into thoracic cavity A 🦠

  ● **S21.132** Puncture wound without foreign body of left front wall of thorax without penetration into thoracic cavity A 🦠

  ● **S21.139** Puncture wound without foreign body of unspecified front wall of thorax without penetration into thoracic cavity A 🦠

● **S21.14** **Puncture wound with foreign body of front wall of thorax without penetration into thoracic cavity**

  ● **S21.141** Puncture wound with foreign body of right front wall of thorax without penetration into thoracic cavity A 🦠

  ● **S21.142** Puncture wound with foreign body of left front wall of thorax without penetration into thoracic cavity A 🦠

  ● **S21.149** Puncture wound with foreign body of unspecified front wall of thorax without penetration into thoracic cavity A 🦠

● **S21.15** **Open bite of front wall of thorax without penetration into thoracic cavity**
  Bite of front wall of thorax NOS

  Excludes1 superficial bite of front wall of thorax (S20.37)

  ● **S21.151** Open bite of right front wall of thorax without penetration into thoracic cavity A 🦠

  ● **S21.152** Open bite of left front wall of thorax without penetration into thoracic cavity A 🦠

  ● **S21.159** Open bite of unspecified front wall of thorax without penetration into thoracic cavity A 🦠

● **S21.2** **Open wound of back wall of thorax without penetration into thoracic cavity**

  ● **S21.20** Unspecified open wound of back wall of thorax without penetration into thoracic cavity

    ● **S21.201** Unspecified open wound of right back wall of thorax without penetration into thoracic cavity

    ● **S21.202** Unspecified open wound of left back wall of thorax without penetration into thoracic cavity

    ● **S21.209** Unspecified open wound of unspecified back wall of thorax without penetration into thoracic cavity

● **S21.21** **Laceration without foreign body of back wall of thorax without penetration into thoracic cavity**

  ● **S21.211** Laceration without foreign body of right back wall of thorax without penetration into thoracic cavity

  ● **S21.212** Laceration without foreign body of left back wall of thorax without penetration into thoracic cavity

  ● **S21.219** Laceration without foreign body of unspecified back wall of thorax without penetration into thoracic cavity

● **S21.22** **Laceration with foreign body of back wall of thorax without penetration into thoracic cavity**

  ● **S21.221** Laceration with foreign body of right back wall of thorax without penetration into thoracic cavity

  ● **S21.222** Laceration with foreign body of left back wall of thorax without penetration into thoracic cavity

  ● **S21.229** Laceration with foreign body of unspecified back wall of thorax without penetration into thoracic cavity

● **S21.23** **Puncture wound without foreign body of back wall of thorax without penetration into thoracic cavity**

  ● **S21.231** Puncture wound without foreign body of right back wall of thorax without penetration into thoracic cavity

  ● **S21.232** Puncture wound without foreign body of left back wall of thorax without penetration into thoracic cavity

  ● **S21.239** Puncture wound without foreign body of unspecified back wall of thorax without penetration into thoracic cavity

● **S21.24** **Puncture wound with foreign body of back wall of thorax without penetration into thoracic cavity**

  ● **S21.241** Puncture wound with foreign body of right back wall of thorax without penetration into thoracic cavity

  ● **S21.242** Puncture wound with foreign body of left back wall of thorax without penetration into thoracic cavity

  ● **S21.249** Puncture wound with foreign body of unspecified back wall of thorax without penetration into thoracic cavity

● **S21.25** **Open bite of back wall of thorax without penetration into thoracic cavity**
  Bite of back wall of thorax NOS

  Excludes1 superficial bite of back wall of thorax (S20.47)

  ● **S21.251** Open bite of right back wall of thorax without penetration into thoracic cavity

  ● **S21.252** Open bite of left back wall of thorax without penetration into thoracic cavity

  ● **S21.259** Open bite of unspecified back wall of thorax without penetration into thoracic cavity

N Newborn Age: 0 **P** Pediatric Age: 0–17 **M** Maternity DX: 12–55 **A** Adult Age: 15–124 ♀ Females Only ♂ Males Only

🦠 Complication\Comorbidity 🦠 Major C\C (Ex) CC/MCC Exclusions 🦠 Hospital-Acquired Condition

1247

● **S21.3**   **Open wound of front wall of thorax with penetration into thoracic cavity**
Open wound of chest with penetration into thoracic cavity

(Ex:) **For category S21.3 CC codes unless otherwise indicated:** S21.101-S21.159[A], S21.301A-S21.95X[A], S27.50X-S27.69X[A] S27.892-S27.9XX[A], S28.1XX[A], S29.021[A], S29.029[A], S38.3XX[A], T14.90-T14.91, T79.7XX[A], T79.8XX-T79.9XX[A], T79.A0X-T79.A9X[A]

● **S21.30**   Unspecified open wound of front wall of thorax with penetration into thoracic cavity

   ● **S21.301**   Unspecified open wound of right front wall of thorax with penetration into thoracic cavity A 🐾

   ● **S21.302**   Unspecified open wound of left front wall of thorax with penetration into thoracic cavity A 🐾

   ● **S21.309**   Unspecified open wound of unspecified front wall of thorax with penetration into thoracic cavity A 🐾

       (Ex:) S21.101A-S21.159[A], S21.301-S21.95X[A], S27.0XX-S27.2XX[A], S27.309[A], S27.329[A], S27.339[A], S27.409[A], S27.50X-S27.69X[A], S27.803[A], S27.892-S28.1XX[A], S29.021[A], S29.029[A], S38.3XX[A], T14.90-T14.91, T79.7XX[A], T79.8XX-T79.9XX[A] T79.A0X-T79.A9X[A]

● **S21.31**   Laceration without foreign body of front wall of thorax with penetration into thoracic cavity

   ● **S21.311**   Laceration without foreign body of right front wall of thorax with penetration into thoracic cavity A 🐾

   ● **S21.312**   Laceration without foreign body of left front wall of thorax with penetration into thoracic cavity A 🐾

   ● **S21.319**   Laceration without foreign body of unspecified front wall of thorax with penetration into thoracic cavity A 🐾

● **S21.32**   Laceration with foreign body of front wall of thorax with penetration into thoracic cavity

   ● **S21.321**   Laceration with foreign body of right front wall of thorax with penetration into thoracic cavity A 🐾

   ● **S21.322**   Laceration with foreign body of left front wall of thorax with penetration into thoracic cavity A 🐾

   ● **S21.329**   Laceration with foreign body of unspecified front wall of thorax with penetration into thoracic cavity A 🐾

● **S21.33**   Puncture wound without foreign body of front wall of thorax with penetration into thoracic cavity

   ● **S21.331**   Puncture wound without foreign body of right front wall of thorax with penetration into thoracic cavity A 🐾

   ● **S21.332**   Puncture wound without foreign body of left front wall of thorax with penetration into thoracic cavity A 🐾

   ● **S21.339**   Puncture wound without foreign body of unspecified front wall of thorax with penetration into thoracic cavity A 🐾

● **S21.34**   Puncture wound with foreign body of front wall of thorax with penetration into thoracic cavity

   ● **S21.341**   Puncture wound with foreign body of right front wall of thorax with penetration into thoracic cavity A 🐾

   ● **S21.342**   Puncture wound with foreign body of left front wall of thorax with penetration into thoracic cavity A 🐾

   ● **S21.349**   Puncture wound with foreign body of unspecified front wall of thorax with penetration into thoracic cavity A 🐾

● **S21.35**   Open bite of front wall of thorax with penetration into thoracic cavity

   Excludes1   superficial bite of front wall of thorax (S20.37)

   ● **S21.351**   Open bite of right front wall of thorax with penetration into thoracic cavity A 🐾

   ● **S21.352**   Open bite of left front wall of thorax with penetration into thoracic cavity A 🐾

   ● **S21.359**   Open bite of unspecified front wall of thorax with penetration into thoracic cavity A 🐾

● **S21.4**   **Open wound of back wall of thorax with penetration into thoracic cavity**

(Ex:) **For category S21.4 CC codes:** See S21.3

● **S21.40**   Unspecified open wound of back wall of thorax with penetration into thoracic cavity

   ● **S21.401**   Unspecified open wound of right back wall of thorax with penetration into thoracic cavity A 🐾

   ● **S21.402**   Unspecified open wound of left back wall of thorax with penetration into thoracic cavity A 🐾

   ● **S21.409**   Unspecified open wound of unspecified back wall of thorax with penetration into thoracic cavity A 🐾

● **S21.41**   Laceration without foreign body of back wall of thorax with penetration into thoracic cavity

   ● **S21.411**   Laceration without foreign body of right back wall of thorax with penetration into thoracic cavity A 🐾

   ● **S21.412**   Laceration without foreign body of left back wall of thorax with penetration into thoracic cavity A 🐾

   ● **S21.419**   Laceration without foreign body of unspecified back wall of thorax with penetration into thoracic cavity A 🐾

● **S21.42**   Laceration with foreign body of back wall of thorax with penetration into thoracic cavity

   ● **S21.421**   Laceration with foreign body of right back wall of thorax with penetration into thoracic cavity A 🐾

   ● **S21.422**   Laceration with foreign body of left back wall of thorax with penetration into thoracic cavity A 🐾

   ● **S21.429**   Laceration with foreign body of unspecified back wall of thorax with penetration into thoracic cavity A 🐾

CHAPTER 19 (S00-T88)

● **S21.43** **Puncture wound without foreign body of back wall of thorax with penetration into thoracic cavity**

    ● **S21.431** Puncture wound without foreign body of right back wall of thorax with penetration into thoracic cavity A 🐾

    ● **S21.432** Puncture wound without foreign body of left back wall of thorax with penetration into thoracic cavity A 🐾

    ● **S21.439** Puncture wound without foreign body of unspecified back wall of thorax with penetration into thoracic cavity A 🐾

● **S21.44** **Puncture wound with foreign body of back wall of thorax with penetration into thoracic cavity**

    ● **S21.441** Puncture wound with foreign body of right back wall of thorax with penetration into thoracic cavity A 🐾

    ● **S21.442** Puncture wound with foreign body of left back wall of thorax with penetration into thoracic cavity A 🐾

    ● **S21.449** Puncture wound with foreign body of unspecified back wall of thorax with penetration into thoracic cavity A 🐾

● **S21.45** **Open bite of back wall of thorax with penetration into thoracic cavity**
    Bite of back wall of thorax NOS

    Excludes1   superficial bite of back wall of thorax (S20.47)

    ● **S21.451** Open bite of right back wall of thorax with penetration into thoracic cavity A 🐾

    ● **S21.452** Open bite of left back wall of thorax with penetration into thoracic cavity A 🐾

    ● **S21.459** Open bite of unspecified back wall of thorax with penetration into thoracic cavity A 🐾

● **S21.9** **Open wound of unspecified part of thorax**
    Open wound of thoracic wall NOS
    (Ex) **For category S21.9 CC codes:** See S21.1

X ● **S21.90** Unspecified open wound of unspecified part of thorax A 🐾

X ● **S21.91** Laceration without foreign body of unspecified part of thorax A 🐾

X ● **S21.92** Laceration with foreign body of unspecified part of thorax A 🐾

X ● **S21.93** Puncture wound without foreign body of unspecified part of thorax A 🐾

X ● **S21.94** Puncture wound with foreign body of unspecified part of thorax A 🐾

X ● **S21.95** Open bite of unspecified part of thorax A 🐾

    Excludes1   superficial bite of thorax (S20.97)

● **S22** **Fracture of rib(s), sternum and thoracic spine**

Note: A fracture not indicated as displaced or nondisplaced should be coded to displaced

    A fracture not indicated as open or closed should be coded to closed

Includes   fracture of thoracic neural arch
          fracture of thoracic spinous process
          fracture of thoracic transverse process
          fracture of thoracic vertebra
          fracture of thoracic vertebral arch

Code first any associated:
    injury of intrathoracic organ (S27.-)
    spinal cord injury (S24.0-, S24.1-)

Excludes1   transection of thorax (S28.1)

Excludes2   fracture of clavicle (S42.0-)
               fracture of scapula (S42.1-)

The appropriate 7th character is to be added to each code from category S22

A	initial encounter for closed fracture
B	initial encounter for open fracture
D	subsequent encounter for fracture with routine healing
G	subsequent encounter for fracture with delayed healing
K	subsequent encounter for fracture with nonunion
S	sequela

● **S22.0** **Fracture of thoracic vertebra**

    (Ex) **For category S22.0 CC codes S22.0[A,B]:** M48.40X-M48.58X[S], M80.08X[S], M80.88X[S], M83.50[S], M84.454[S], M84.550[S], M84.58X[S], M84.650[S], M99.12, M99.15-M99.17, M99.19, S03.1XX[A], S03.8XX-S03.9XX[A], S12.000-S12.9XX[S], S13.9XX[A], S14.109[A], S14.119[A], S14.129[A], S14.139[A], S14.149[A], S14.159[A], S22.000-S22.089[A,B,S], S22.20XS-S23.3XX[A], S23.8XX-S24.159[A], S29.001-S29.019[A], S29.091-S29.9XX[A], S32.000-S32.9XX[S], S32.9XX[S], S33.30X-S33.39X[A], S33.9XX[A], S38.1XX[A], S38.3XX[A], S39.001-S39.013[A], S39.091A-S39.94X[A], T14.90-T14.91, T79.8XX-T79.9XX[A], T79.A0X-T79.A9X[A] **For S22.0[K]:** See S02.0[K]

    ● **S22.00** **Fracture of unspecified thoracic vertebra**

       ● **S22.000** Wedge compression fracture of unspecified thoracic vertebra A, K 🐾, B 🐾, A, B 🐾

       ● **S22.001** Stable burst fracture of unspecified thoracic vertebra A, K 🐾, B 🐾, A, B 🐾

       ● **S22.002** Unstable burst fracture of unspecified thoracic vertebra A, K 🐾, B 🐾, A, B 🐾

       ● **S22.008** Other fracture of unspecified thoracic vertebra A, K 🐾, B 🐾, A, B 🐾

       ● **S22.009** Unspecified fracture of unspecified thoracic vertebra A, K 🐾, B 🐾, A, B 🐾

    ● **S22.01** **Fracture of first thoracic vertebra**

       ● **S22.010** Wedge compression fracture of first thoracic vertebra A, K 🐾, B 🐾, A, B 🐾

       ● **S22.011** Stable burst fracture of first thoracic vertebra A, K 🐾, B 🐾, A, B 🐾

       ● **S22.012** Unstable burst fracture of first thoracic vertebra A, K 🐾, B 🐾, A, B 🐾

       ● **S22.018** Other fracture of first thoracic vertebra A, K 🐾, B 🐾, A, B 🐾

       ● **S22.019** Unspecified fracture of first thoracic vertebra A, K 🐾, B 🐾, A, B 🐾

CHAPTER 19 (S00–T88)

N Newborn Age: 0   **P** Pediatric Age: 0–17   **M** Maternity DX: 12–55   **A** Adult Age: 15–124   ♀ Females Only   ♂ Males Only

🐾 Complication\Comorbidity   🐾 Major C\C   (Ex) CC/MCC Exclusions   🐾 Hospital-Acquired Condition

1249

- S22.02   Fracture of second thoracic vertebra
  - S22.020   Wedge compression fracture of second thoracic vertebra A, K, B, A, B
  - S22.021   Stable burst fracture of second thoracic vertebra A, K, B, A, B
  - S22.022   Unstable burst fracture of second thoracic vertebra A, K, B, A, B
  - S22.028   Other fracture of second thoracic vertebra A, K, B, A, B
  - S22.029   **Unspecified** fracture of second thoracic vertebra A, K, B, A, B
- S22.03   Fracture of third thoracic vertebra
  - S22.030   Wedge compression fracture of third thoracic vertebra A, K, B, A, B
  - S22.031   Stable burst fracture of third thoracic vertebra A, K, B, A, B
  - S22.032   Unstable burst fracture of third thoracic vertebra A, K, B, A, B
  - S22.038   Other fracture of third thoracic vertebra A, K, B, A, B
  - S22.039   **Unspecified** fracture of third thoracic vertebra A, K, B, A, B
- S22.04   Fracture of fourth thoracic vertebra
  - S22.040   Wedge compression fracture of fourth thoracic vertebra A, K, B, A, B
  - S22.041   Stable burst fracture of fourth thoracic vertebra A, K, B, A, B
  - S22.042   Unstable burst fracture of fourth thoracic vertebra A, K, B, A, B
  - S22.048   Other fracture of fourth thoracic vertebra A, K, B, A, B
  - S22.049   **Unspecified** fracture of fourth thoracic vertebra A, K, B, A, B
- S22.05   Fracture of T_5-T_6 vertebra
  - S22.050   Wedge compression fracture of T_5-T_6 vertebra A, K, B, A, B
  - S22.051   Stable burst fracture of T_5-T_6 vertebra A, K, B, A, B
  - S22.052   Unstable burst fracture of T_5-T_6 vertebra A, K, B, A, B
  - S22.058   Other fracture of T_5-T_6 vertebra A, K, B, A, B
  - S22.059   **Unspecified** fracture of T_5-T_6 vertebra A, K, B, A, B
- S22.06   Fracture of T_7-T_8 vertebra
  - S22.060   Wedge compression fracture of T_7-T_8 vertebra A, K, B, A, B
  - S22.061   Stable burst fracture of T_7-T_8 vertebra A, K, B, A, B
  - S22.062   Unstable burst fracture of T_7-T_8 vertebra A, K, B, A, B
  - S22.068   Other fracture of T_7-T_8 thoracic vertebra A, K, B, A, B
  - S22.069   **Unspecified** fracture of T_7-T_8 vertebra A, K, B, A, B

- S22.07   Fracture of T_9-T_{10} vertebra
  - S22.070   Wedge compression fracture of T_9-T_{10} vertebra A, K, B, A, B
  - S22.071   Stable burst fracture of T_9-T_{10} vertebra A, K, B, A, B
  - S22.072   Unstable burst fracture of T_9-T_{10} vertebra A, K, B, A, B
  - S22.078   Other fracture of T_9-T_{10} vertebra A, K, B, A, B
  - S22.079   **Unspecified** fracture of T_9-T_{10} vertebra A, K, B, A, B
- S22.08   Fracture of T_{11}-T_{12} vertebra
  - S22.080   Wedge compression fracture of T_{11}-T_{12} vertebra A, K, B, A, B
  - S22.081   Stable burst fracture of T_{11}-T_{12} vertebra A, K, B, A, B
  - S22.082   Unstable burst fracture of T_{11}-T_{12} vertebra A, K, B, A, B
  - S22.088   Other fracture of T_{11}-T_{12} vertebra A, K, B, A, B
  - S22.089   **Unspecified** fracture of T_{11}-T_{12} vertebra A, K, B, A, B
- S22.2   Fracture of sternum
  - (Ex) For category S22.2 CC codes S22.2[A,B]: S03.8XX-S03.9XX[A], S22.20X-S22.24X[A,B], S29.011-S29.019[A], S38.3XX[A], S39.011-S39.013[A], T14.90-T14.91, T79.8XX-T79.9XX[A], T79.A0X-T79.A9X[A] For S22.2[K]: See S02.0[K]

  - X S22.20   **Unspecified** fracture of sternum A, K, B, A, B
  - X S22.21   Fracture of manubrium A, K, B, A, B
  - X S22.22   Fracture of body of sternum A, K, B, A, B
  - X S22.23   Sternal manubrial dissociation A, K, B, A, B
  - X S22.24   Fracture of xiphoid process A, K, B, A, B
- S22.3   Fracture of one rib
  - (Ex) For category S22.3 CC codes S22.3[A]: S03.8XX-S03.9XX[A], S22.20X-S22.24X[A], S29.011-S29.019[A], S38.3XX[A], S39.011-S39.013[A], T14.90-T14.91, T79.8XX-T79.9XX[A], T79.A0X-T79.A9X[A] For S22.3[B]: S03.8XX-S03.9XX[A], S22.31X-S22.5XX[A,B], S29.011-S29.019[A], S38.3XX[A], S39.011-S39.013[A], T14.90-T14.91, T79.8XX-T79.9XX[A], T79.A0X-T79.A9X[A] For S22.3[K]: See S02.0[K]

  - X S22.31   Fracture of one rib, right side A, K, B, A, B
  - X S22.32   Fracture of one rib, left side A, K, B, A, B
  - X S22.39   Fracture of one rib, **unspecified** side A, K, B, A, B
- S22.4   Multiple fractures of ribs
  - Fractures of two or more ribs
  - **Excludes1**   flail chest (S22.5-)
  - (Ex) For category S22.4 CC codes S22.4[A,B]: See S22.3[B] For S22.49[B]: No exclusions For S22.4[K]: See S02.0[K]

  - X S22.41   Multiple fractures of ribs, right side A, K, B, A, B
  - X S22.42   Multiple fractures of ribs, left side A, K, B, A, B
  - X S22.43   Multiple fractures of ribs, bilateral A, K, B, A, B
  - X S22.49   Multiple fractures of ribs, **unspecified** side A, K, B, A, B

◀ New   ◀▥ Revised   ~~deleted~~ Deleted   Excludes 1   Excludes 2   Includes   Use additional   Code first   Code also   Unspecified

OGCR Official Guidelines   ● Unacceptable Principal Diagnosis   X Assign placeholder X   ● Use Additional Character(s)   ▶ Manifestation Code   **Coding Clinic**

X ● **S22.5**   **Flail chest** K 🔾, A, B 🔾, A, B 🔾
     Unstable chest due to sternum and/or rib fracture
     ⓔ **For category S22.5 CC codes S22.5[A,B]:** S03.8XX-S03.9XX[A],
     S22.20X-S22.5XX[A,B], S29.011-S29.019[A], S38.3XX[A],
     S39.011-S39.013[A], T14.90-T14.91, T79.8XX-T79.9XX[A], T79.A0X-T79.
     A9X[A] **For S22.5[K]:** See S02.0[K]

X ● **S22.9**   **Fracture of bony thorax, part** unspecified A, K 🔾, B 🔾,
     A, B 🔾
     ⓔ **For category S22.9 CC codes S22.9[A,B]:** M80.00X-M80.019[A],
     M80.041A-M80.049[A], M80.80X-M80.819[A], M80.841-M80.849[A],
     M84.40X-M84.419[A], M84.441-M84.446[A], M84.454[A],
     M84.474-M84.519[A], M84.541-M84.550[A], M84.574-M84.576[A],
     M84.60X-M84.619[A], M84.641-M84.650[A], M84.674-M84.68[A],
     S03.8XX-S03.9XX[A], S22.9XX-S22.9XX[A,B], S29.011A-S29.019[A],
     S32.301-S32.9XX[A,B], S33.4XX[A], S33.6XX-S33.8XX[A], S38.3XX[A],
     S39.011-S39.013[A], S73.001-S73.199[A], S76.001-S76.019[A],
     S76.091-S76.119[A], S76.191-S76.219[A], S76.291-S76.319[A],
     S76.391-S76.819[A], S76.891-S76.919[A], S76.991-S76.999[A],
     S79.811-S79.929[A], T14.90-T14.91, T79.8XX-T79.9XX[A], T79.A9X[A] **For**
     S22.9[K]: See S02.0[K]

● **S23**   **Dislocation and sprain of joints and ligaments of thorax**
    Includes   avulsion of joint or ligament of thorax
               laceration of cartilage, joint or ligament of thorax
               sprain of cartilage, joint or ligament of thorax
               traumatic hemarthrosis of joint or ligament of
                   thorax
               traumatic rupture of joint or ligament of thorax
               traumatic subluxation of joint or ligament of
                   thorax
               traumatic tear of joint or ligament of thorax

    Code also any associated open wound
    Excludes2   dislocation, sprain of sternoclavicular joint (S43.2,
               S43.6)
               strain of muscle or tendon of thorax (S29.01-)
    The appropriate 7th character is to be added to each code from
        category S23

> A   initial encounter
> D   subsequent encounter
> S   sequela

X ● **S23.0**   **Traumatic rupture of thoracic intervertebral disc**
      Excludes1   rupture or displacement (nontraumatic)
                     of thoracic intervertebral disc NOS
                     (M51.- with fifth character 4)

● **S23.1**   **Subluxation and dislocation of thoracic vertebra**
      Code also any associated
        open wound of thorax (S21.-)
        spinal cord injury (S24.0-, S24.1-)
      Excludes2   fracture of thoracic vertebrae (S22.0-)
   ● **S23.10**   **Subluxation and dislocation of unspecified**
          thoracic vertebra
     ● **S23.100**   Subluxation of unspecified thoracic
              vertebra
     ● **S23.101**   Dislocation of unspecified thoracic
              vertebra
   ● **S23.11**   **Subluxation and dislocation of T_1/T_2 thoracic**
          vertebra
     ● **S23.110**   Subluxation of T_1/T_2 thoracic vertebra
     ● **S23.111**   Dislocation of T_1/T_2 thoracic vertebra

● **S23.12**   **Subluxation and dislocation of T_2/T_3-T_3/T_4**
         thoracic vertebra
   ● **S23.120**   Subluxation of T_2/T_3 thoracic vertebra
   ● **S23.121**   Dislocation of T_2/T_3 thoracic vertebra
   ● **S23.122**   Subluxation of T_3/T_4 thoracic vertebra
   ● **S23.123**   Dislocation of T_3/T_4 thoracic vertebra
● **S23.13**   **Subluxation and dislocation of T_4/T_5-T_5/T_6**
         thoracic vertebra
   ● **S23.130**   Subluxation of T_4/T_5 thoracic vertebra
   ● **S23.131**   Dislocation of T_4/T_5 thoracic vertebra
   ● **S23.132**   Subluxation of T_5/T_6 thoracic vertebra
   ● **S23.133**   Dislocation of T_5/T_6 thoracic vertebra
● **S23.14**   **Subluxation and dislocation of T_6/T_7-T_7/T_8**
         thoracic vertebra
   ● **S23.140**   Subluxation of T_6/T_7 thoracic vertebra
   ● **S23.141**   Dislocation of T_6/T_7 thoracic vertebra
   ● **S23.142**   Subluxation of T_7/T_8 thoracic vertebra
   ● **S23.143**   Dislocation of T_7/T_8 thoracic vertebra
● **S23.15**   **Subluxation and dislocation of T_8/T_9-T_9/T_{10}**
         thoracic vertebra
   ● **S23.150**   Subluxation of T_8/T_9 thoracic vertebra
   ● **S23.151**   Dislocation of T_8/T_9 thoracic vertebra
   ● **S23.152**   Subluxation of T_9/T_{10} thoracic
              vertebra
   ● **S23.153**   Dislocation of T_9/T_{10} thoracic vertebra
● **S23.16**   **Subluxation and dislocation of T_{10}/T_{11}-T_{11}/T_{12}**
         thoracic vertebra
   ● **S23.160**   Subluxation of T_{10}/T_{11} thoracic
              vertebra
   ● **S23.161**   Dislocation of T_{10}/T_{11} thoracic vertebra
   ● **S23.162**   Subluxation of T_{11}/T_{12} thoracic
              vertebra
   ● **S23.163**   Dislocation of T_{11}/T_{12} thoracic vertebra
● **S23.17**   **Subluxation and dislocation of T_{12}/L_1 thoracic**
         vertebra
   ● **S23.170**   Subluxation of T_{12}/L_1 thoracic vertebra
   ● **S23.171**   Dislocation of T_{12}/L_1 thoracic vertebra
● **S23.2**   **Dislocation of other and unspecified parts of thorax**
   X ● **S23.20**   **Dislocation of** unspecified **part of thorax**
   X ● **S23.29**   **Dislocation of other parts of thorax**
X ● **S23.3**   **Sprain of ligaments of thoracic spine**
● **S23.4**   **Sprain of ribs and sternum**
   X ● **S23.41**   **Sprain of ribs**
   ● **S23.42**   **Sprain of sternum**
     ● **S23.420**   Sprain of sternoclavicular (joint)
              (ligament)
     ● **S23.421**   Sprain of chondrosternal joint
     ● **S23.428**   Other sprain of sternum
     ● **S23.429**   Unspecified sprain of sternum
X ● **S23.8**   **Sprain of other specified parts of thorax**
X ● **S23.9**   **Sprain of** unspecified **parts of thorax**

● **S24 Injury of nerves and spinal cord at thorax level**

Note: Code to highest level of thoracic spinal cord injury.

Injuries to the spinal cord (S24.0 and S24.1) refer to the cord level and not bone level injury, and can affect nerve roots at and below the level given.

Code also any associated:
    fracture of thoracic vertebra (S22.0-)
    open wound of thorax (S21.-)
    transient paralysis (R29.5)

Excludes2 injury of brachial plexus (S14.3)

The appropriate 7th character is to be added to each code from category S24

A	initial encounter
D	subsequent encounter
S	sequela

(Ex) **For category S24 CC codes:** M48.40X-M48.58X[S], M80.08X[S], M80.88X[S], M84.350[S], M84.454[S], M84.550[S], M84.58[S], M84.650[S], M99.15-M99.17, M99.19, S03.1XX[A], S12.000-S12.9XX[S], S13.9XX[A], S14.109[A], S14.119[A], S14.129[A], S14.139[A], S14.149[A], S14.159[A], S22.000-S22.9XX[S], S23.20X-S23.29X[A], S23.9XX-S24.159[A], S29.001-S29.009[A], S29.091-S29.9XX[A], S32.000-S32.9XX[S], S33.30X-S33.39X[A], S33.9XX[A], S38.1XX[A], S39.001-S39.003[A], S39.091-S39.94X[A], T14.90-T14.91, T79.8XX-T79.9XX[A], T79.A0X-T79.A9X[A]

X ● **S24.0 Concussion and edema of thoracic spinal cord** A 🐾

● **S24.1 Other and unspecified injuries of thoracic spinal cord**

  ● **S24.10 Unspecified injury of thoracic spinal cord**

    ● **S24.101 Unspecified injury at T$_1$ level of thoracic spinal cord** A 🐾, A 🐾

    ● **S24.102 Unspecified injury at T$_2$-T$_6$ level of thoracic spinal cord** A 🐾, A 🐾

    ● **S24.103 Unspecified injury at T$_7$-T$_{10}$ level of thoracic spinal cord** A 🐾, A 🐾

    ● **S24.104 Unspecified injury at T$_{11}$-T$_{12}$ level of thoracic spinal cord** A 🐾, A 🐾

    ● **S24.109 Unspecified injury at unspecified level of thoracic spinal cord** A 🐾
           Injury of thoracic spinal cord NOS

  ● **S24.11 Complete lesion of thoracic spinal cord**

    ● **S24.111 Complete lesion at T$_1$ level of thoracic spinal cord** A 🐾, A 🐾

    ● **S24.112 Complete lesion at T$_2$-T$_6$ level of thoracic spinal cord** A 🐾, A 🐾

    ● **S24.113 Complete lesion at T$_7$-T$_{10}$ level of thoracic spinal cord** A 🐾, A 🐾

    ● **S24.114 Complete lesion at T$_{11}$-T$_{12}$ level of thoracic spinal cord** A 🐾, A 🐾

    ● **S24.119 Complete lesion at unspecified level of thoracic spinal cord**

  ● **S24.13 Anterior cord syndrome of thoracic spinal cord**

    ● **S24.131 Anterior cord syndrome at T$_1$ level of thoracic spinal cord** A 🐾, A 🐾

    ● **S24.132 Anterior cord syndrome at T$_2$-T$_6$ level of thoracic spinal cord** A 🐾, A 🐾

    ● **S24.133 Anterior cord syndrome at T$_7$-T$_{10}$ level of thoracic spinal cord** A 🐾, A 🐾

    ● **S24.134 Anterior cord syndrome at T$_{11}$-T$_{12}$ level of thoracic spinal cord** A 🐾, A 🐾

    ● **S24.139 Anterior cord syndrome at unspecified level of thoracic spinal cord**

  ● **S24.14 Brown-Séquard syndrome of thoracic spinal cord**

    ● **S24.141 Brown-Séquard syndrome at T$_1$ level of thoracic spinal cord** A 🐾

    ● **S24.142 Brown-Séquard syndrome at T$_2$-T$_6$ level of thoracic spinal cord** A 🐾

    ● **S24.143 Brown-Séquard syndrome at T$_7$-T$_{10}$ level of thoracic spinal cord** A 🐾

    ● **S24.144 Brown-Séquard syndrome at T$_{11}$-T$_{12}$ level of thoracic spinal cord** A 🐾

    ● **S24.149 Brown-Séquard syndrome at unspecified level of thoracic spinal cord**

  ● **S24.15 Other incomplete lesions of thoracic spinal cord**
         Incomplete lesion of thoracic spinal cord NOS
         Posterior cord syndrome of thoracic spinal cord

    ● **S24.151 Other incomplete lesion at T$_1$ level of thoracic spinal cord** A 🐾, A 🐾

    ● **S24.152 Other incomplete lesion at T$_2$-T$_6$ level of thoracic spinal cord** A 🐾, A 🐾

    ● **S24.153 Other incomplete lesion at T$_7$-T$_{10}$ level of thoracic spinal cord** A 🐾, A 🐾

    ● **S24.154 Other incomplete lesion at T$_{11}$-T$_{12}$ level of thoracic spinal cord** A 🐾, A 🐾

    ● **S24.159 Other incomplete lesion at unspecified level of thoracic spinal cord**

X ● **S24.2 Injury of nerve root of thoracic spine**

X ● **S24.3 Injury of peripheral nerves of thorax**

X ● **S24.4 Injury of thoracic sympathetic nervous system**
     Injury of cardiac plexus
     Injury of esophageal plexus
     Injury of pulmonary plexus
     Injury of stellate ganglion
     Injury of thoracic sympathetic ganglion

X ● **S24.8 Injury of other specified nerves of thorax**

X ● **S24.9 Injury of unspecified nerve of thorax**

● **S25 Injury of blood vessels of thorax**

The appropriate 7th character is to be added to each code from category S25

A	initial encounter
D	subsequent encounter
S	sequela

Code also any associated open wound (S21.-)

● **S25.0 Injury of thoracic aorta**
     Injury of aorta NOS
    (Ex) **For category S25.0 CC codes:** S25.00XA-S25.09X[A], T14.90-T14.91, T79.8XX-T79.9XX[A], T79.A0X-T79.A9X[A]

X ● **S25.00 Unspecified injury of thoracic aorta** A 🐾

X ● **S25.01 Minor laceration of thoracic aorta** A 🐾
     Incomplete transection of thoracic aorta
     Laceration of thoracic aorta NOS
     Superficial laceration of thoracic aorta

X ● **S25.02 Major laceration of thoracic aorta** A 🐾
     Complete transection of thoracic aorta
     Traumatic rupture of thoracic aorta

X ● **S25.09 Other specified injury of thoracic aorta** A 🐾

◀ New   ◀▥ Revised   ~~deleted~~ Deleted   Excludes 1   Excludes 2   Includes   Use additional   Code first   Code also   Unspecified

OGCR Official Guidelines   ● Unacceptable Principal Diagnosis   X Assign placeholder X   ● Use Additional Character(s)   ▸ Manifestation Code   **Coding Clinic**

● **S25.1**   **Injury of innominate or subclavian artery**
   (Ex) **For category S25.1 CC codes:** S25.101-S25.199[A], T14.90-T14.91,
      T79.8XX-T79.9XX[A], T79.A0X-T79.A9X[A]

  ● **S25.10**   **Unspecified injury of innominate or subclavian artery**
    ● **S25.101**   Unspecified injury of right innominate or subclavian artery A 🐾
    ● **S25.102**   Unspecified injury of left innominate or subclavian artery A 🐾
    ● **S25.109**   Unspecified injury of unspecified innominate or subclavian artery A 🐾

  ● **S25.11**   **Minor laceration of innominate or subclavian artery**
      Incomplete transection of innominate or subclavian artery
      Laceration of innominate or subclavian artery NOS
      Superficial laceration of innominate or subclavian artery
    ● **S25.111**   Minor laceration of right innominate or subclavian artery A 🐾
    ● **S25.112**   Minor laceration of left innominate or subclavian artery A 🐾
    ● **S25.119**   Minor laceration of unspecified innominate or subclavian artery A 🐾

  ● **S25.12**   **Major laceration of innominate or subclavian artery**
      Complete transection of innominate or subclavian artery
      Traumatic rupture of innominate or subclavian artery
    ● **S25.121**   Major laceration of right innominate or subclavian artery A 🐾
    ● **S25.122**   Major laceration of left innominate or subclavian artery A 🐾
    ● **S25.129**   Major laceration of unspecified innominate or subclavian artery A 🐾

  ● **S25.19**   **Other specified injury of innominate or subclavian artery**
    ● **S25.191**   Other specified injury of right innominate or subclavian artery A 🐾
    ● **S25.192**   Other specified injury of left innominate or subclavian artery A 🐾
    ● **S25.199**   Other specified injury of unspecified innominate or subclavian artery A 🐾

● **S25.2**   **Injury of superior vena cava**
     Injury of vena cava NOS
   (Ex) **For category S25.2 CC codes:** S25.20X-S25.29X[A], T14.90-T14.91,
      T79.8XX-T79.9XX[A], T79.A0XA-T79.A9X[A]

  X ● **S25.20**   Unspecified injury of superior vena cava A 🐾
  X ● **S25.21**   Minor laceration of superior vena cava A 🐾
      Incomplete transection of superior vena cava
      Laceration of superior vena cava NOS
      Superficial laceration of superior vena cava
  X ● **S25.22**   Major laceration of superior vena cava A 🐾
      Complete transection of superior vena cava
      Traumatic rupture of superior vena cava
  X ● **S25.29**   Other specified injury of superior vena cava A 🐾

● **S25.3**   **Injury of innominate or subclavian vein**
   (Ex) **For category S25.3 CC codes:** S25.301-S25.399[A], T14.90-T14.91,
      T79.8XX-T79.9XX[A], T79.A0X-T79.A9X[A]

  ● **S25.30**   **Unspecified injury of innominate or subclavian vein**
    ● **S25.301**   Unspecified injury of right innominate or subclavian vein A 🐾
    ● **S25.302**   Unspecified injury of left innominate or subclavian vein A 🐾
    ● **S25.309**   Unspecified injury of unspecified innominate or subclavian vein A 🐾

● **S25.31**   **Minor laceration of innominate or subclavian vein**
     Incomplete transection of innominate or subclavian vein
     Laceration of innominate or subclavian vein NOS
     Superficial laceration of innominate or subclavian vein
    ● **S25.311**   Minor laceration of right innominate or subclavian vein A 🐾
    ● **S25.312**   Minor laceration of left innominate or subclavian vein A 🐾
    ● **S25.319**   Minor laceration of unspecified innominate or subclavian vein A 🐾

● **S25.32**   **Major laceration of innominate or subclavian vein**
     Complete transection of innominate or subclavian vein
     Traumatic rupture of innominate or subclavian vein
    ● **S25.321**   Major laceration of right innominate or subclavian vein A 🐾
    ● **S25.322**   Major laceration of left innominate or subclavian vein A 🐾
    ● **S25.329**   Major laceration of unspecified innominate or subclavian vein A 🐾

● **S25.39**   **Other specified injury of innominate or subclavian vein**
    ● **S25.391**   Other specified injury of right innominate or subclavian vein A 🐾
    ● **S25.392**   Other specified injury of left innominate or subclavian vein A 🐾
    ● **S25.399**   Other specified injury of unspecified innominate or subclavian vein A 🐾

● **S25.4**   **Injury of pulmonary blood vessels**
   (Ex) **For category S25.4 CC codes unless otherwise indicated:**
      S25.401-S25.499[A], T14.90-T14.91, T79.8XX-T79.9XX[A], T79.A0X-T79.A9X[A]

  ● **S25.40**   **Unspecified injury of pulmonary blood vessels**
    ● **S25.401**   Unspecified injury of right pulmonary blood vessels A 🐾
    ● **S25.402**   Unspecified injury of left pulmonary blood vessels A 🐾
    ● **S25.409**   Unspecified injury of unspecified pulmonary blood vessels A 🐾

● **S25.41**   **Minor laceration of pulmonary blood vessels**
     Incomplete transection of pulmonary blood vessels
     Laceration of pulmonary blood vessels NOS
     Superficial laceration of pulmonary blood vessels
    ● **S25.411**   Minor laceration of right pulmonary blood vessels A 🐾
    ● **S25.412**   Minor laceration of left pulmonary blood vessels A 🐾
    ● **S25.419**   Minor laceration of unspecified pulmonary blood vessels A 🐾

● **S25.42**   **Major laceration of pulmonary blood vessels**
     Complete transection of pulmonary blood vessels
     Traumatic rupture of pulmonary blood vessels
    ● **S25.421**   Major laceration of right pulmonary blood vessels A 🐾
      (Ex) S25.401[A]-S25.499[A], T14.90-T14.91, T79.A0X[A]-T79.9XX[A]
    ● **S25.422**   Major laceration of left pulmonary blood vessels A 🐾
    ● **S25.429**   Major laceration of unspecified pulmonary blood vessels A 🐾

N Newborn Age: 0   **P** Pediatric Age: 0–17   **M** Maternity DX: 12–55   **A** Adult Age: 15–124   ♀ Females Only   ♂ Males Only

🐾 Complication\Comorbidity   🐾 Major C\C   (Ex) CC/MCC Exclusions   🐾 Hospital-Acquired Condition   **1253**

CHAPTER 19 (S00-T88)

● **S25.49** **Other specified injury of pulmonary blood vessels**
  ● S25.491 Other specified injury of right pulmonary blood vessels A 🔖
  ● S25.492 Other specified injury of left pulmonary blood vessels A 🔖
  ● S25.499 Other specified injury of unspecified pulmonary blood vessels A 🔖

● **S25.5** **Injury of intercostal blood vessels**
  Ex: For category S25.5 CC codes: S25.501-S25.899[A]
  ● **S25.50** Unspecified injury of intercostal blood vessels
    ● S25.501 Unspecified injury of intercostal blood vessels, right side A 🔖
    ● S25.502 Unspecified injury of intercostal blood vessels, left side A 🔖
    ● S25.509 Unspecified injury of intercostal blood vessels, unspecified side A 🔖
  ● **S25.51** Laceration of intercostal blood vessels
    ● S25.511 Laceration of intercostal blood vessels, right side A 🔖
    ● S25.512 Laceration of intercostal blood vessels, left side A 🔖
    ● S25.519 Laceration of intercostal blood vessels, unspecified side A 🔖
  ● **S25.59** Other specified injury of intercostal blood vessels
    ● S25.591 Other specified injury of intercostal blood vessels, right side A 🔖
    ● S25.592 Other specified injury of intercostal blood vessels, left side A 🔖
    ● S25.599 Other specified injury of intercostal blood vessels, unspecified side A 🔖

● **S25.8** **Injury of other blood vessels of thorax**
  Injury of azygos vein
  Injury of mammary artery or vein
  Ex: For category S25.8 CC codes: S25.00X-S25.99X[A]
  ● **S25.80** Unspecified injury of other blood vessels of thorax
    ● S25.801 Unspecified injury of other blood vessels of thorax, right side A 🔖
    ● S25.802 Unspecified injury of other blood vessels of thorax, left side A 🔖
    ● S25.809 Unspecified injury of other blood vessels of thorax, unspecified side A 🔖
  ● **S25.81** Laceration of other blood vessels of thorax
    ● S25.811 Laceration of other blood vessels of thorax, right side A 🔖
    ● S25.812 Laceration of other blood vessels of thorax, left side A 🔖
    ● S25.819 Laceration of other blood vessels of thorax, unspecified side A 🔖
  ● **S25.89** Other specified injury of other blood vessels of thorax
    ● S25.891 Other specified injury of other blood vessels of thorax, right side A 🔖
    ● S25.892 Other specified injury of other blood vessels of thorax, left side A 🔖
    ● S25.899 Other specified injury of other blood vessels of thorax, unspecified side A 🔖

● **S25.9** **Injury of unspecified blood vessel of thorax**
  Ex: For category S25.9 CC codes: S25.00X-S25.99X[A]
  X ● S25.90 Unspecified injury of unspecified blood vessel of thorax A 🔖
  X ● S25.91 Laceration of unspecified blood vessel of thorax A 🔖
  X ● S25.99 Other specified injury of unspecified blood vessel of thorax A 🔖

● **S26** **Injury of heart**
  The appropriate 7th character is to be added to each code from category S26

A	initial encounter
D	subsequent encounter
S	sequela

  Code also any associated:
    open wound of thorax (S21.-)
    traumatic hemopneumothorax (S27.2)
    traumatic hemothorax (S27.1)
    traumatic pneumothorax (S27.0)

● **S26.0** **Injury of heart with hemopericardium**
  Hemopericardium: effusion of blood within pericardium
  Ex: For category S26.0 CC codes unless otherwise indicated:
    S21.101-S21.159[A], S21.301-S21.95X[A], S26.00X-S26.99X[A],
    S27.50X-S27.69X[A], S27.892-S27.9XX[A], S28.1XX[A], S29.021[A],
    S29.029[A], S38.3XX[A], T14.90-T14.91, T79.7XX-T79.9XX[A],
    T79.A0X-T79.A9X[A]
  X ● S26.00 Unspecified injury of heart with hemopericardium A 🔖
    Ex: S21.301-S21.459[A], S26.00X-S26.99X[A], S27.50X-S27.69X[A],
    S27.892-S27.9XX[A], T14.90-T14.91
  X ● S26.01 Contusion of heart with hemopericardium A 🔖
  ● S26.02 Laceration of heart with hemopericardium
    ● S26.020 Mild laceration of heart with hemopericardium A 🔖
      Laceration of heart without penetration of heart chamber
    ● S26.021 Moderate laceration of heart with hemopericardium A 🔖
      Laceration of heart with penetration of heart chamber
    ● S26.022 Major laceration of heart with hemopericardium A 🔖
      Laceration of heart with penetration of multiple heart chambers
  X ● S26.09 Other injury of heart with hemopericardium A 🔖
    Ex: See 26.00

● **S26.1** **Injury of heart without hemopericardium**
  Hemopericardium: effusion of blood within pericardium
  X ● S26.10 Unspecified injury of heart without hemopericardium A 🔖
    Ex: See S26.00
  X ● S26.11 Contusion of heart without hemopericardium A 🔖
  X ● S26.12 Laceration of heart without hemopericardium A 🔖
  X ● S26.19 Other injury of heart without hemopericardium A 🔖
    Ex: See S26.00

Item 19–2 **Pneumothorax** is a collection of gas (positive air pressure) in the pleural space resulting in the lung collapsing. A tension pneumothorax is life-threatening and is a result of air in the pleural space causing a displacement in the mediastinal structures and cardiopulmonary function compromise. A traumatic pneumothorax results from blunt or penetrating injury that disrupts the parietal/visceral pleura. **Hemothorax** is blood or bloody fluid in the pleural cavity as a result of traumatic blood vessel rupture or inflammation of the lungs from pneumonia.

◀ New   ◀▬ Revised   ~~deleted~~ Deleted   Excludes 1   Excludes 2   Includes   Use additional   Code first   Code also   Unspecified
OGCR Official Guidelines   ● Unacceptable Principal Diagnosis   X Assign placeholder X   ● Use Additional Character(s)   ▶ Manifestation Code   **Coding Clinic**

X ● **S26.9** **Injury of heart, unspecified with or without hemopericardium**
Hemopericardium: effusion of blood within pericardium

X ● **S26.90** **Unspecified injury of heart, unspecified with or without hemopericardium** A 🔒
Ⓔ See S26.00

X ● **S26.91** **Contusion of heart, unspecified with or without hemopericardium** A 🔒

X ● **S26.92** **Laceration of heart, unspecified with or without hemopericardium** A 🔒
Laceration of heart NOS

X ● **S26.99** **Other injury of heart, unspecified with or without hemopericardium** A 🔒
Ⓔ See S26.00

● **S27** **Injury of other and unspecified intrathoracic organs**
Code also any associated open wound of thorax (S21.-)
Excludes2 injury of cervical esophagus (S10–S19)
injury of trachea (cervical) (S10–S19)

The appropriate 7th character is to be added to each code from category S27.

A	initial encounter
D	subsequent encounter
S	sequela

X ● **S27.0** **Traumatic pneumothorax** A 🔒
Excludes1 spontaneous pneumothorax (J93.-)
Ⓔ S21.101–S21.159[A], S21.301–S21.95X[A], S27.0XX–S27.399[A],
S27.50X–S27.69X[A], S27.892–S27.9XX[A], S28.1XX[A], S29.021[A],
S29.029[A], S38.3XX[A], T14.90–T14.91, T79.7XX–T79.9XX[A],
T79.A0X–T79.A9X[A]

X ● **S27.1** **Traumatic hemothorax** A 🔒
Ⓔ See S27.0

X ● **S27.2** **Traumatic hemopneumothorax** A 🔒
Ⓔ See S27.0

● **S27.3** **Other and unspecified injuries of lung**
Ⓔ **For category S27.3 CC codes unless otherwise indicated:**
S21.101–S21.159[A], S21.301–S21.95X[A], S27.301–S27.399[A]
S27.50X–S27.69X[A], S27.892–S27.9XX[A], S28.1XX[A], S29.021[A],
S29.029[A], S38.3XX[A], T14.90–T14.91, T79.7XX–T79.9XX[A], T79.A9X[A]

● **S27.30** **Unspecified injury of lung**

● **S27.301** **Unspecified injury of lung, unilateral** A 🔒

● **S27.302** **Unspecified injury of lung, bilateral** A 🔒

● **S27.309** **Unspecified injury of lung, unspecified** A 🔒

● **S27.31** **Primary blast injury of lung**
Blast injury of lung NOS

● **S27.311** **Primary blast injury of lung, unilateral** A 🔒

● **S27.312** **Primary blast injury of lung, bilateral** A 🔒

● **S27.319** **Primary blast injury of lung, unspecified** A 🔒

● **S27.32** **Contusion of lung**

● **S27.321** **Contusion of lung, unilateral** A 🔒

● **S27.322** **Contusion of lung, bilateral** A 🔒

● **S27.329** **Contusion of lung, unspecified** A 🔒

● **S27.33** **Laceration of lung**
Ⓔ **For category S27.33 CC codes:** S21.101–S21.159[A],
S21.301–S21.95X[A], S27.301–S27.399[A],
S27.50X–S27.69X[A], S27.892–S27.9XX[A], S28.1XX[A],
S29.021[A], S29.029[A], S38.3XX[A], T14.90–T14.91,
T79.7XX–T79.9XX[A], T79.A0X–T79.A9X[A]

● **S27.331** **Laceration of lung, unilateral** A 🔒

● **S27.332** **Laceration of lung, bilateral** A 🔒

● **S27.339** **Laceration of lung, unspecified** A 🔒

● **S27.39** **Other injuries of lung**
Secondary blast injury of lung

● **S27.391** **Other injuries of lung, unilateral** A 🔒

● **S27.392** **Other injuries of lung, bilateral** A 🔒

● **S27.399** **Other injuries of lung, unspecified** A 🔒

● **S27.4** **Injury of bronchus**
Ⓔ **For category S27.4 CC codes:** S21.101–S21.159[A], S21.301–S21.95X[A],
S27.401–S27.69X[A], S27.892–S27.9XX[A], S28.1XX[A], S29.021[A],
S29.029[A], S38.3XX[A], T14.90–T14.91, T79.7XX–T79.9XX[A],
T79.A0X–T79.A9X[A]

● **S27.40** **Unspecified injury of bronchus**

● **S27.401** **Unspecified injury of bronchus, unilateral** A 🔒

● **S27.402** **Unspecified injury of bronchus, bilateral** A 🔒

● **S27.409** **Unspecified injury of bronchus, unspecified** A 🔒

● **S27.41** **Primary blast injury of bronchus**
Blast injury of bronchus NOS

● **S27.411** **Primary blast injury of bronchus, unilateral** A 🔒

● **S27.412** **Primary blast injury of bronchus, bilateral** A 🔒

● **S27.419** **Primary blast injury of bronchus, unspecified** A 🔒

● **S27.42** **Contusion of bronchus**

● **S27.421** **Contusion of bronchus, unilateral** A 🔒

● **S27.422** **Contusion of bronchus, bilateral** A 🔒

● **S27.429** **Contusion of bronchus, unspecified** A 🔒

● **S27.43** **Laceration of bronchus**

● **S27.431** **Laceration of bronchus, unilateral** A 🔒

● **S27.432** **Laceration of bronchus, bilateral** A 🔒

● **S27.439** **Laceration of bronchus, unspecified** A 🔒

● **S27.49** **Other injury of bronchus**
Secondary blast injury of bronchus

● **S27.491** **Other injury of bronchus, unilateral** A 🔒

● **S27.492** **Other injury of bronchus, bilateral** A 🔒

● **S27.499** **Other injury of bronchus, unspecified** A 🔒

N Newborn Age: 0   P Pediatric Age: 0–17   M Maternity DX: 12–55   A Adult Age: 15–124   ♀ Females Only   ♂ Males Only
🔒 Complication\Comorbidity   🔒 Major C\C   Ⓔ CC/MCC Exclusions   🔒 Hospital-Acquired Condition

1255

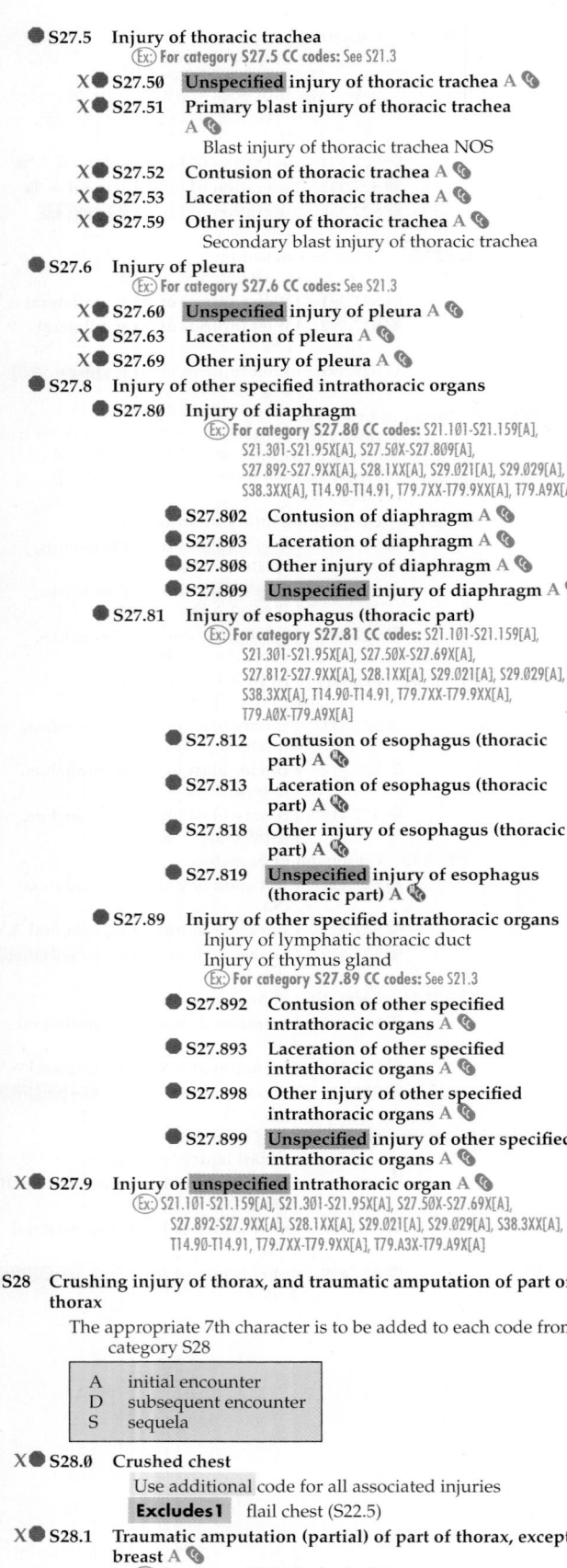

● **S27.5   Injury of thoracic trachea**
  Ⓔⓧ For category S27.5 CC codes: See S21.3

X● **S27.50   Unspecified injury of thoracic trachea** A 🐾

X● **S27.51   Primary blast injury of thoracic trachea** A 🐾
          Blast injury of thoracic trachea NOS

X● **S27.52   Contusion of thoracic trachea** A 🐾

X● **S27.53   Laceration of thoracic trachea** A 🐾

X● **S27.59   Other injury of thoracic trachea** A 🐾
          Secondary blast injury of thoracic trachea

● **S27.6   Injury of pleura**
  Ⓔⓧ For category S27.6 CC codes: See S21.3

X● **S27.60   Unspecified injury of pleura** A 🐾

X● **S27.63   Laceration of pleura** A 🐾

X● **S27.69   Other injury of pleura** A 🐾

● **S27.8   Injury of other specified intrathoracic organs**

  ● **S27.80   Injury of diaphragm**
      Ⓔⓧ For category S27.80 CC codes: S21.101-S21.159[A],
            S21.301-S21.95X[A], S27.50X-S27.809[A],
            S27.892-S27.9XX[A], S28.1XX[A], S29.021[A], S29.029[A],
            S38.3XX[A], T14.90-T14.91, T79.7XX-T79.9XX[A], T79.A9X[A]

      ● **S27.802   Contusion of diaphragm** A 🐾

      ● **S27.803   Laceration of diaphragm** A 🐾

      ● **S27.808   Other injury of diaphragm** A 🐾

      ● **S27.809   Unspecified injury of diaphragm** A 🐾

  ● **S27.81   Injury of esophagus (thoracic part)**
      Ⓔⓧ For category S27.81 CC codes: S21.101-S21.159[A],
            S21.301-S21.95X[A], S27.50X-S27.69X[A],
            S27.812-S27.9XX[A], S28.1XX[A], S29.021[A], S29.029[A],
            S38.3XX[A], T14.90-T14.91, T79.7XX-T79.9XX[A],
            T79.A0X-T79.A9X[A]

      ● **S27.812   Contusion of esophagus (thoracic part)** A 🐾

      ● **S27.813   Laceration of esophagus (thoracic part)** A 🐾

      ● **S27.818   Other injury of esophagus (thoracic part)** A 🐾

      ● **S27.819   Unspecified injury of esophagus (thoracic part)** A 🐾

  ● **S27.89   Injury of other specified intrathoracic organs**
          Injury of lymphatic thoracic duct
          Injury of thymus gland
      Ⓔⓧ For category S27.89 CC codes: See S21.3

      ● **S27.892   Contusion of other specified intrathoracic organs** A 🐾

      ● **S27.893   Laceration of other specified intrathoracic organs** A 🐾

      ● **S27.898   Other injury of other specified intrathoracic organs** A 🐾

      ● **S27.899   Unspecified injury of other specified intrathoracic organs** A 🐾

X● **S27.9   Injury of unspecified intrathoracic organ** A 🐾
      Ⓔⓧ S21.101-S21.159[A], S21.301-S21.95X[A], S27.50X-S27.69X[A],
            S27.892-S27.9XX[A], S28.1XX[A], S29.021[A], S29.029[A], S38.3XX[A],
            T14.90-T14.91, T79.7XX-T79.9XX[A], T79.A3X-T79.A9X[A]

● **S28   Crushing injury of thorax, and traumatic amputation of part of thorax**

      The appropriate 7th character is to be added to each code from category S28

      | A | initial encounter |
      | D | subsequent encounter |
      | S | sequela |

X● **S28.0   Crushed chest**
          Use additional code for all associated injuries
          Excludes1   flail chest (S22.5)

X● **S28.1   Traumatic amputation (partial) of part of thorax, except breast** A 🐾
      Ⓔⓧ For category S28.1 CC codes: See S21.1

● **S28.2   Traumatic amputation of breast**

  ● **S28.21   Complete traumatic amputation of breast**
          Traumatic amputation of breast NOS

      ● **S28.211   Complete traumatic amputation of right breast**

      ● **S28.212   Complete traumatic amputation of left breast**

      ● **S28.219   Complete traumatic amputation of unspecified breast**

  ● **S28.22   Partial traumatic amputation of breast**

      ● **S28.221   Partial traumatic amputation of right breast**

      ● **S28.222   Partial traumatic amputation of left breast**

      ● **S28.229   Partial traumatic amputation of unspecified breast**

● **S29   Other and unspecified injuries of thorax**
      Code also any associated open wound (S21.-)
      The appropriate 7th character is to be added to each code from category S29

      | A | initial encounter |
      | D | subsequent encounter |
      | S | sequela |

● **S29.0   Injury of muscle and tendon at thorax level**

  ● **S29.00   Unspecified injury of muscle and tendon of thorax**

      ● **S29.001   Unspecified injury of muscle and tendon of front wall of thorax**

      ● **S29.002   Unspecified injury of muscle and tendon of back wall of thorax**

      ● **S29.009   Unspecified injury of muscle and tendon of unspecified wall of thorax**

  ● **S29.01   Strain of muscle and tendon of thorax**

      ● **S29.011   Strain of muscle and tendon of front wall of thorax**

      ● **S29.012   Strain of muscle and tendon of back wall of thorax**

      ● **S29.019   Strain of muscle and tendon of unspecified wall of thorax**

  ● **S29.02   Laceration of muscle and tendon of thorax**
      Ⓔⓧ For category S29.02 CC codes: See S21.1

      ● **S29.021   Laceration of muscle and tendon of front wall of thorax** A 🐾

      ● **S29.022   Laceration of muscle and tendon of back wall of thorax**

      ● **S29.029   Laceration of muscle and tendon of unspecified wall of thorax** A 🐾

  ● **S29.09   Other injury of muscle and tendon of thorax**

      ● **S29.091   Other injury of muscle and tendon of front wall of thorax**

      ● **S29.092   Other injury of muscle and tendon of back wall of thorax**

      ● **S29.099   Other injury of muscle and tendon of unspecified wall of thorax**

X● **S29.8   Other specified injuries of thorax**

X● **S29.9   Unspecified injury of thorax**

INJURIES TO THE ABDOMEN, LOWER BACK, LUMBAR SPINE PELVIS AND EXTERNAL GENITALS (S30-S39)

Includes	injuries to the abdominal wall
	injuries to the anus
	injuries to the buttock
	injuries to the external genitalia
	injuries to the flank
	injuries to the groin
Excludes2	burns and corrosions (T20-T32)
	effects of foreign body in anus and rectum (T18.5)
	effects of foreign body in genitourinary tract (T19.-)
	effects of foreign body in stomach, small intestine and colon (T18.2-T18.4)
	frostbite (T33-T34)
	insect bite or sting, venomous (T63.4)

● **S30   Superficial injury of abdomen, lower back, pelvis and external genitals**

Excludes2   superficial injury of hip (S70.-)

The appropriate 7th character is to be added to each code from category S30

A	initial encounter
D	subsequent encounter
S	sequela

X● **S30.0   Contusion of lower back and pelvis**
Contusion of buttock

X● **S30.1   Contusion of abdominal wall**
Contusion of flank
Contusion of groin

● **S30.2   Contusion of external genital organs**
  ● **S30.20   Contusion of unspecified external genital organ**
    ● **S30.201   Contusion of unspecified external genital organ, male ♂**
    ● **S30.202   Contusion of unspecified external genital organ, female ♀**
  X● **S30.21   Contusion of penis ♂**
  X● **S30.22   Contusion of scrotum and testes ♂**
  X● **S30.23   Contusion of vagina and vulva ♀**

X● **S30.3   Contusion of anus**

● **S30.8   Other superficial injuries of abdomen, lower back, pelvis and external genitals**
  ● **S30.81   Abrasion of abdomen, lower back, pelvis and external genitals**
    ● **S30.810   Abrasion of lower back and pelvis**
    ● **S30.811   Abrasion of abdominal wall**
    ● **S30.812   Abrasion of penis ♂**
    ● **S30.813   Abrasion of scrotum and testes ♂**
    ● **S30.814   Abrasion of vagina and vulva ♀**
    ● **S30.815   Abrasion of unspecified external genital organs, male ♂**
    ● **S30.816   Abrasion of unspecified external genital organs, female ♀**
    ● **S30.817   Abrasion of anus**
  ● **S30.82   Blister (nonthermal) of abdomen, lower back, pelvis and external genitals**
    ● **S30.820   Blister (nonthermal) of lower back and pelvis**
    ● **S30.821   Blister (nonthermal) of abdominal wall**
    ● **S30.822   Blister (nonthermal) of penis ♂**
    ● **S30.823   Blister (nonthermal) of scrotum and testes ♂**
    ● **S30.824   Blister (nonthermal) of vagina and vulva ♀**
    ● **S30.825   Blister (nonthermal) of unspecified external genital organs, male ♂**
    ● **S30.826   Blister (nonthermal) of unspecified external genital organs, female ♀**
    ● **S30.827   Blister (nonthermal) of anus**

● **S30.84   External constriction of abdomen, lower back, pelvis and external genitals**
  ● **S30.840   External constriction of lower back and pelvis**
  ● **S30.841   External constriction of abdominal wall**
  ● **S30.842   External constriction of penis ♂**
    Hair tourniquet syndrome of penis
    Use additional cause code to identify the constricting item (W49.0-)
  ● **S30.843   External constriction of scrotum and testes ♂**
  ● **S30.844   External constriction of vagina and vulva ♀**
  ● **S30.845   External constriction of unspecified external genital organs, male ♂**
  ● **S30.846   External constriction of unspecified external genital organs, female ♀**

● **S30.85   Superficial foreign body of abdomen, lower back, pelvis and external genitals**
    Splinter in the abdomen, lower back, pelvis and external genitals
  ● **S30.850   Superficial foreign body of lower back and pelvis**
  ● **S30.851   Superficial foreign body of abdominal wall**
  ● **S30.852   Superficial foreign body of penis ♂**
  ● **S30.853   Superficial foreign body of scrotum and testes ♂**
  ● **S30.854   Superficial foreign body of vagina and vulva ♀**
  ● **S30.855   Superficial foreign body of unspecified external genital organs, male ♂**
  ● **S30.856   Superficial foreign body of unspecified external genital organs, female ♀**
  ● **S30.857   Superficial foreign body of anus**

● **S30.86   Insect bite (nonvenomous) of abdomen, lower back, pelvis and external genitals**
  ● **S30.860   Insect bite (nonvenomous) of lower back and pelvis**
  ● **S30.861   Insect bite (nonvenomous) of abdominal wall**
  ● **S30.862   Insect bite (nonvenomous) of penis ♂**
  ● **S30.863   Insect bite (nonvenomous) of scrotum and testes ♂**
  ● **S30.864   Insect bite (nonvenomous) of vagina and vulva ♀**
  ● **S30.865   Insect bite (nonvenomous) of unspecified external genital organs, male ♂**
  ● **S30.866   Insect bite (nonvenomous) of unspecified external genital organs, female ♀**
  ● **S30.867   Insect bite (nonvenomous) of anus**

CHAPTER 19 (S00-T88)

N Newborn Age: 0   **P** Pediatric Age: 0–17   **M** Maternity DX: 12–55   **A** Adult Age: 15–124   ♀ Females Only   ♂ Males Only

🔹 Complication\Comorbidity   🔹 Major C\C   (Ex) CC/MCC Exclusions   🔹 Hospital-Acquired Condition

1257

● **S30.87** **Other superficial bite of abdomen, lower back, pelvis and external genitals**

> **Excludes1** open bite of abdomen, lower back, pelvis and external genitals (S31.05, S31.15, S31.25, S31.35, S31.45, S31.55)

　● **S30.870** **Other superficial bite of lower back and pelvis**

　● **S30.871** **Other superficial bite of abdominal wall**

　● **S30.872** **Other superficial bite of penis** ♂

　● **S30.873** **Other superficial bite of scrotum and testes** ♂

　● **S30.874** **Other superficial bite of vagina and vulva** ♀

　● **S30.875** **Other superficial bite of unspecified external genital organs, male** ♂

　● **S30.876** **Other superficial bite of unspecified external genital organs, female** ♀

　● **S30.877** **Other superficial bite of anus**

● **S30.9** **Unspecified superficial injury of abdomen, lower back, pelvis and external genitals**

X ● **S30.91** **Unspecified superficial injury of lower back and pelvis**

X ● **S30.92** **Unspecified superficial injury of abdominal wall**

X ● **S30.93** **Unspecified superficial injury of penis** ♂

X ● **S30.94** **Unspecified superficial injury of scrotum and testes** ♂

X ● **S30.95** **Unspecified superficial injury of vagina and vulva** ♀

X ● **S30.96** **Unspecified superficial injury of unspecified external genital organs, male** ♂

X ● **S30.97** **Unspecified superficial injury of unspecified external genital organs, female** ♀

X ● **S30.98** **Unspecified superficial injury of anus**

● **S31** **Open wound of abdomen, lower back, pelvis and external genitals**

> Code also any associated:
> spinal cord injury (S24.0, S24.1-, S34.0-, S34.1-)
> wound infection
>
> **Excludes1** traumatic amputation of part of abdomen, lower back and pelvis (S38.2-, S38.3)
>
> **Excludes2** open wound of hip (S71.00-S71.02)
> open fracture of pelvis (S32.1--S32.9 with 7th character B)

The appropriate 7th character is to be added to each code from category S31

A	initial encounter
D	subsequent encounter
S	sequela

● **S31.0** **Open wound of lower back and pelvis**

> (Ex) **For category S31.0 CC codes:** S31.001[A], S31.011[A], S31.021[A], S31.031[A], S31.041[A], S31.051[A], S31.100-S31.159[A] S31.600-S31.659[A], S31.831-S31.839[A], S36.81X-S36.99X[A], S38.3XX[A], S39.021-S39.023[A], T14.90-T14.91, T79.8XX-T79.9XX[A] T79.A0X-T79.A9X[A]

● **S31.00** **Unspecified open wound of lower back and pelvis**

　● **S31.000** **Unspecified open wound of lower back and pelvis without penetration into retroperitoneum**
　　　Unspecified open wound of lower back and pelvis NOS

　● **S31.001** **Unspecified open wound of lower back and pelvis with penetration into retroperitoneum** A ✇

● **S31.01** **Laceration without foreign body of lower back and pelvis**

　● **S31.010** **Laceration without foreign body of lower back and pelvis without penetration into retroperitoneum**
　　　Laceration without foreign body of lower back and pelvis NOS

　● **S31.011** **Laceration without foreign body of lower back and pelvis with penetration into retroperitoneum** A ✇

● **S31.02** **Laceration with foreign body of lower back and pelvis**

　● **S31.020** **Laceration with foreign body of lower back and pelvis without penetration into retroperitoneum**
　　　Laceration with foreign body of lower back and pelvis NOS

　● **S31.021** **Laceration with foreign body of lower back and pelvis with penetration into retroperitoneum** A ✇

● **S31.03** **Puncture wound without foreign body of lower back and pelvis**

　● **S31.030** **Puncture wound without foreign body of lower back and pelvis without penetration into retroperitoneum**
　　　Puncture wound without foreign body of lower back and pelvis NOS

　● **S31.031** **Puncture wound without foreign body of lower back and pelvis with penetration into retroperitoneum** A ✇

● **S31.04** **Puncture wound with foreign body of lower back and pelvis**

　● **S31.040** **Puncture wound with foreign body of lower back and pelvis without penetration into retroperitoneum**
　　　Puncture wound with foreign body of lower back and pelvis NOS

　● **S31.041** **Puncture wound with foreign body of lower back and pelvis with penetration into retroperitoneum** A ✇

● **S31.05** **Open bite of lower back and pelvis**
　　Bite of lower back and pelvis NOS

> **Excludes1** superficial bite of lower back and pelvis (S30.860, S30.870)

　● **S31.050** **Open bite of lower back and pelvis without penetration into retroperitoneum**
　　　Open bite of lower back and pelvis NOS

　● **S31.051** **Open bite of lower back and pelvis with penetration into retroperitoneum** A ✇

● **S31.1** **Open wound of abdominal wall without penetration into peritoneal cavity**
　　Open wound of abdominal wall NOS

> **Excludes2** open wound of abdominal wall with penetration into peritoneal cavity (S31.6-)

● **S31.10** **Unspecified open wound of abdominal wall without penetration into peritoneal cavity**

　● **S31.100** **Unspecified open wound of abdominal wall, right upper quadrant without penetration into peritoneal cavity**

　● **S31.101** **Unspecified open wound of abdominal wall, left upper quadrant without penetration into peritoneal cavity**

- S31.102 Unspecified open wound of abdominal wall, epigastric region without penetration into peritoneal cavity
- S31.103 Unspecified open wound of abdominal wall, right lower quadrant without penetration into peritoneal cavity
- S31.104 Unspecified open wound of abdominal wall, left lower quadrant without penetration into peritoneal cavity
- S31.105 Unspecified open wound of abdominal wall, periumbilic region without penetration into peritoneal cavity
- S31.109 Unspecified open wound of abdominal wall, unspecified quadrant without penetration into peritoneal cavity

    Unspecified open wound of abdominal wall NOS

- S31.11 Laceration without foreign body of abdominal wall without penetration into peritoneal cavity
  - S31.110 Laceration without foreign body of abdominal wall, right upper quadrant without penetration into peritoneal cavity
  - S31.111 Laceration without foreign body of abdominal wall, left upper quadrant without penetration into peritoneal cavity
  - S31.112 Laceration without foreign body of abdominal wall, epigastric region without penetration into peritoneal cavity
  - S31.113 Laceration without foreign body of abdominal wall, right lower quadrant without penetration into peritoneal cavity
  - S31.114 Laceration without foreign body of abdominal wall, left lower quadrant without penetration into peritoneal cavity
  - S31.115 Laceration without foreign body of abdominal wall, periumbilic region without penetration into peritoneal cavity
  - S31.119 Laceration without foreign body of abdominal wall, unspecified quadrant without penetration into peritoneal cavity
- S31.12 Laceration with foreign body of abdominal wall without penetration into peritoneal cavity
  - S31.120 Laceration of abdominal wall with foreign body, right upper quadrant without penetration into peritoneal cavity
  - S31.121 Laceration of abdominal wall with foreign body, left upper quadrant without penetration into peritoneal cavity
  - S31.122 Laceration of abdominal wall with foreign body, epigastric region without penetration into peritoneal cavity
  - S31.123 Laceration of abdominal wall with foreign body, right lower quadrant without penetration into peritoneal cavity
  - S31.124 Laceration of abdominal wall with foreign body, left lower quadrant without penetration into peritoneal cavity

- S31.125 Laceration of abdominal wall with foreign body, periumbilic region without penetration into peritoneal cavity
- S31.129 Laceration of abdominal wall with foreign body, unspecified quadrant without penetration into peritoneal cavity
- S31.13 Puncture wound of abdominal wall without foreign body without penetration into peritoneal cavity
  - S31.130 Puncture wound of abdominal wall without foreign body, right upper quadrant without penetration into peritoneal cavity
  - S31.131 Puncture wound of abdominal wall without foreign body, left upper quadrant without penetration into peritoneal cavity
  - S31.132 Puncture wound of abdominal wall without foreign body, epigastric region without penetration into peritoneal cavity
  - S31.133 Puncture wound of abdominal wall without foreign body, right lower quadrant without penetration into peritoneal cavity
  - S31.134 Puncture wound of abdominal wall without foreign body, left lower quadrant without penetration into peritoneal cavity
  - S31.135 Puncture wound of abdominal wall without foreign body, periumbilic region without penetration into peritoneal cavity
  - S31.139 Puncture wound of abdominal wall without foreign body, unspecified quadrant without penetration into peritoneal cavity
- S31.14 Puncture wound of abdominal wall with foreign body without penetration into peritoneal cavity
  - S31.140 Puncture wound of abdominal wall with foreign body, right upper quadrant without penetration into peritoneal cavity
  - S31.141 Puncture wound of abdominal wall with foreign body, left upper quadrant without penetration into peritoneal cavity
  - S31.142 Puncture wound of abdominal wall with foreign body, epigastric region without penetration into peritoneal cavity
  - S31.143 Puncture wound of abdominal wall with foreign body, right lower quadrant without penetration into peritoneal cavity
  - S31.144 Puncture wound of abdominal wall with foreign body, left lower quadrant without penetration into peritoneal cavity
  - S31.145 Puncture wound of abdominal wall with foreign body, periumbilic region without penetration into peritoneal cavity
  - S31.149 Puncture wound of abdominal wall with foreign body, unspecified quadrant without penetration into peritoneal cavity

- S31.15 **Open bite of abdominal wall without penetration into peritoneal cavity**
  Bite of abdominal wall NOS
  > **Excludes1** superficial bite of abdominal wall (S30.871)

  - S31.150 **Open bite of abdominal wall, right upper quadrant without penetration into peritoneal cavity**
  - S31.151 **Open bite of abdominal wall, left upper quadrant without penetration into peritoneal cavity**
  - S31.152 **Open bite of abdominal wall, epigastric region without penetration into peritoneal cavity**
  - S31.153 **Open bite of abdominal wall, right lower quadrant without penetration into peritoneal cavity**
  - S31.154 **Open bite of abdominal wall, left lower quadrant without penetration into peritoneal cavity**
  - S31.155 **Open bite of abdominal wall, periumbilic region without penetration into peritoneal cavity**
  - S31.159 **Open bite of abdominal wall, unspecified quadrant without penetration into peritoneal cavity**

- S31.2 **Open wound of penis**
  - X● S31.20 **Unspecified open wound of penis** ♂
  - X● S31.21 **Laceration without foreign body of penis** ♂
  - X● S31.22 **Laceration with foreign body of penis** ♂
  - X● S31.23 **Puncture wound without foreign body of penis** ♂
  - X● S31.24 **Puncture wound with foreign body of penis** ♂
  - X● S31.25 **Open bite of penis** ♂
    Bite of penis NOS
    > **Excludes1** superficial bite of penis (S30.862, S30.872)

- S31.3 **Open wound of scrotum and testes**
  - X● S31.30 **Unspecified open wound of scrotum and testes** ♂
  - X● S31.31 **Laceration without foreign body of scrotum and testes** ♂
  - X● S31.32 **Laceration with foreign body of scrotum and testes** ♂
  - X● S31.33 **Puncture wound without foreign body of scrotum and testes** ♂
  - X● S31.34 **Puncture wound with foreign body of scrotum and testes** ♂
  - X● S31.35 **Open bite of scrotum and testes** ♂
    Bite of scrotum and testes NOS
    > **Excludes1** superficial bite of scrotum and testes (S30.863, S30.873)

- S31.4 **Open wound of vagina and vulva**
  > **Excludes1** injury to vagina and vulva during delivery (O70.-, O71.4)

  - X● S31.40 **Unspecified open wound of vagina and vulva** ♀
  - X● S31.41 **Laceration without foreign body of vagina and vulva** ♀
  - X● S31.42 **Laceration with foreign body of vagina and vulva** ♀
  - X● S31.43 **Puncture wound without foreign body of vagina and vulva** ♀
  - X● S31.44 **Puncture wound with foreign body of vagina and vulva** ♀
  - X● S31.45 **Open bite of vagina and vulva** ♀
    Bite of vagina and vulva NOS
    > **Excludes1** superficial bite of vagina and vulva (S30.864, S30.874)

- S31.5 **Open wound of unspecified external genital organs**
  > **Excludes1** traumatic amputation of external genital organs (S38.21, S38.22)

  - S31.50 **Unspecified open wound of unspecified external genital organs**
    - S31.501 **Unspecified open wound of unspecified external genital organs, male** ♂
    - S31.502 **Unspecified open wound of unspecified external genital organs, female** ♀
  - S31.51 **Laceration without foreign body of unspecified external genital organs**
    - S31.511 **Laceration without foreign body of unspecified external genital organs, male** ♂
    - S31.512 **Laceration without foreign body of unspecified external genital organs, female** ♀
  - S31.52 **Laceration with foreign body of unspecified external genital organs**
    - S31.521 **Laceration with foreign body of unspecified external genital organs, male** ♂
    - S31.522 **Laceration with foreign body of unspecified external genital organs, female** ♀
  - S31.53 **Puncture wound without foreign body of unspecified external genital organs**
    - S31.531 **Puncture wound without foreign body of unspecified external genital organs, male** ♂
    - S31.532 **Puncture wound without foreign body of unspecified external genital organs, female** ♀
  - S31.54 **Puncture wound with foreign body of unspecified external genital organs**
    - S31.541 **Puncture wound with foreign body of unspecified external genital organs, male** ♂
    - S31.542 **Puncture wound with foreign body of unspecified external genital organs, female** ♀
  - S31.55 **Open bite of unspecified external genital organs**
    Bite of unspecified external genital organs NOS
    > **Excludes1** superficial bite of unspecified external genital organs (S30.865, S30.866, S30.875, S30.876)

    - S31.551 **Open bite of unspecified external genital organs, male** ♂
    - S31.552 **Open bite of unspecified external genital organs, female** ♀

- S31.6 **Open wound of abdominal wall with penetration into peritoneal cavity**
  > (Ex) For category S31.6 CC codes: See S31.0

  - S31.60 **Unspecified open wound of abdominal wall with penetration into peritoneal cavity**
    - S31.600 **Unspecified open wound of abdominal wall, right upper quadrant with penetration into peritoneal cavity** A
    - S31.601 **Unspecified open wound of abdominal wall, left upper quadrant with penetration into peritoneal cavity** A
    - S31.602 **Unspecified open wound of abdominal wall, epigastric region with penetration into peritoneal cavity** A

◀ New   ◀▥ Revised   ~~deleted~~ Deleted   Excludes 1   Excludes 2   Includes   Use additional   Code first   Code also   Unspecified
OGCR Official Guidelines   ● Unacceptable Principal Diagnosis   X Assign placeholder X   ● Use Additional Character(s)   ▶ Manifestation Code   **Coding Clinic**

● S31.603   Unspecified open wound of
             abdominal wall, right lower quadrant
             with penetration into peritoneal
             cavity A 🔓

● S31.604   Unspecified open wound of
             abdominal wall, left lower quadrant
             with penetration into peritoneal
             cavity A 🔓

● S31.605   Unspecified open wound of
             abdominal wall, periumbilic region
             with penetration into peritoneal
             cavity A 🔓

● S31.609   Unspecified open wound of
             abdominal wall, unspecified quadrant
             with penetration into peritoneal
             cavity A 🔓

● S31.61   Laceration without foreign body of abdominal
           wall with penetration into peritoneal cavity

● S31.610   Laceration without foreign body of
             abdominal wall, right upper quadrant
             with penetration into peritoneal
             cavity A 🔓

● S31.611   Laceration without foreign body of
             abdominal wall, left upper quadrant
             with penetration into peritoneal
             cavity A 🔓

● S31.612   Laceration without foreign body of
             abdominal wall, epigastric region
             with penetration into peritoneal
             cavity A 🔓

● S31.613   Laceration without foreign body of
             abdominal wall, right lower quadrant
             with penetration into peritoneal
             cavity A 🔓,
                Coding Clinic: 2015, Q4, P37

● S31.614   Laceration without foreign body of
             abdominal wall, left lower quadrant
             with penetration into peritoneal
             cavity A 🔓

● S31.615   Laceration without foreign body of
             abdominal wall, periumbilic region
             with penetration into peritoneal
             cavity A 🔓

● S31.619   Laceration without foreign body of
             abdominal wall, unspecified quadrant
             with penetration into peritoneal
             cavity A 🔓

● S31.62   Laceration with foreign body of abdominal
           wall with penetration into peritoneal cavity

● S31.620   Laceration with foreign body of
             abdominal wall, right upper quadrant
             with penetration into peritoneal
             cavity A 🔓

● S31.621   Laceration with foreign body of
             abdominal wall, left upper quadrant
             with penetration into peritoneal
             cavity A 🔓

● S31.622   Laceration with foreign body of
             abdominal wall, epigastric region
             with penetration into peritoneal
             cavity A 🔓

● S31.623   Laceration with foreign body of
             abdominal wall, right lower quadrant
             with penetration into peritoneal
             cavity A 🔓

● S31.624   Laceration with foreign body of
             abdominal wall, left lower quadrant
             with penetration into peritoneal
             cavity A 🔓

● S31.625   Laceration with foreign body of
             abdominal wall, periumbilic region
             with penetration into peritoneal
             cavity A 🔓

● S31.629   Laceration with foreign body of
             abdominal wall, unspecified quadrant
             with penetration into peritoneal
             cavity A 🔓

● S31.63   Puncture wound without foreign body
           of abdominal wall with penetration into
           peritoneal cavity

● S31.630   Puncture wound without foreign
             body of abdominal wall, right upper
             quadrant with penetration into
             peritoneal cavity A 🔓

● S31.631   Puncture wound without foreign
             body of abdominal wall, left upper
             quadrant with penetration into
             peritoneal cavity A 🔓

● S31.632   Puncture wound without foreign
             body of abdominal wall, epigastric
             region with penetration into
             peritoneal cavity A 🔓

● S31.633   Puncture wound without foreign
             body of abdominal wall, right lower
             quadrant with penetration into
             peritoneal cavity A 🔓

● S31.634   Puncture wound without foreign
             body of abdominal wall, left lower
             quadrant with penetration into
             peritoneal cavity A 🔓

● S31.635   Puncture wound without foreign
             body of abdominal wall, periumbilic
             region with penetration into
             peritoneal cavity A 🔓

● S31.639   Puncture wound without foreign
             body of abdominal wall, unspecified
             quadrant with penetration into
             peritoneal cavity A 🔓

● S31.64   Puncture wound with foreign body of
           abdominal wall with penetration into
           peritoneal cavity

● S31.640   Puncture wound with foreign body of
             abdominal wall, right upper quadrant
             with penetration into peritoneal
             cavity A 🔓

● S31.641   Puncture wound with foreign body of
             abdominal wall, left upper quadrant
             with penetration into peritoneal
             cavity A 🔓

● S31.642   Puncture wound with foreign body of
             abdominal wall, epigastric region
             with penetration into peritoneal
             cavity A 🔓

● S31.643   Puncture wound with foreign body of
             abdominal wall, right lower quadrant
             with penetration into peritoneal
             cavity A 🔓

● S31.644   Puncture wound with foreign body of
             abdominal wall, left lower quadrant
             with penetration into peritoneal
             cavity A 🔓

● S31.645   Puncture wound with foreign body of
             abdominal wall, periumbilic region
             with penetration into peritoneal
             cavity A 🔓

● S31.649   Puncture wound with foreign body of
             abdominal wall, unspecified quadrant
             with penetration into peritoneal
             cavity A 🔓

CHAPTER 19 (S00-T88)

N Newborn Age: 0   **P** Pediatric Age: 0–17   **M** Maternity DX: 12–55   **A** Adult Age: 15–124   ♀ Females Only   ♂ Males Only

🔓 Complication\Comorbidity   🔓 Major C\C   Ⓔ🆇 CC/MCC Exclusions   🔓 Hospital-Acquired Condition

1261

- **S31.65** **Open bite of abdominal wall with penetration into peritoneal cavity**
  - **Excludes1** superficial bite of abdominal wall (S30.861, S30.871)
  - **S31.650** Open bite of abdominal wall, right upper quadrant with penetration into peritoneal cavity A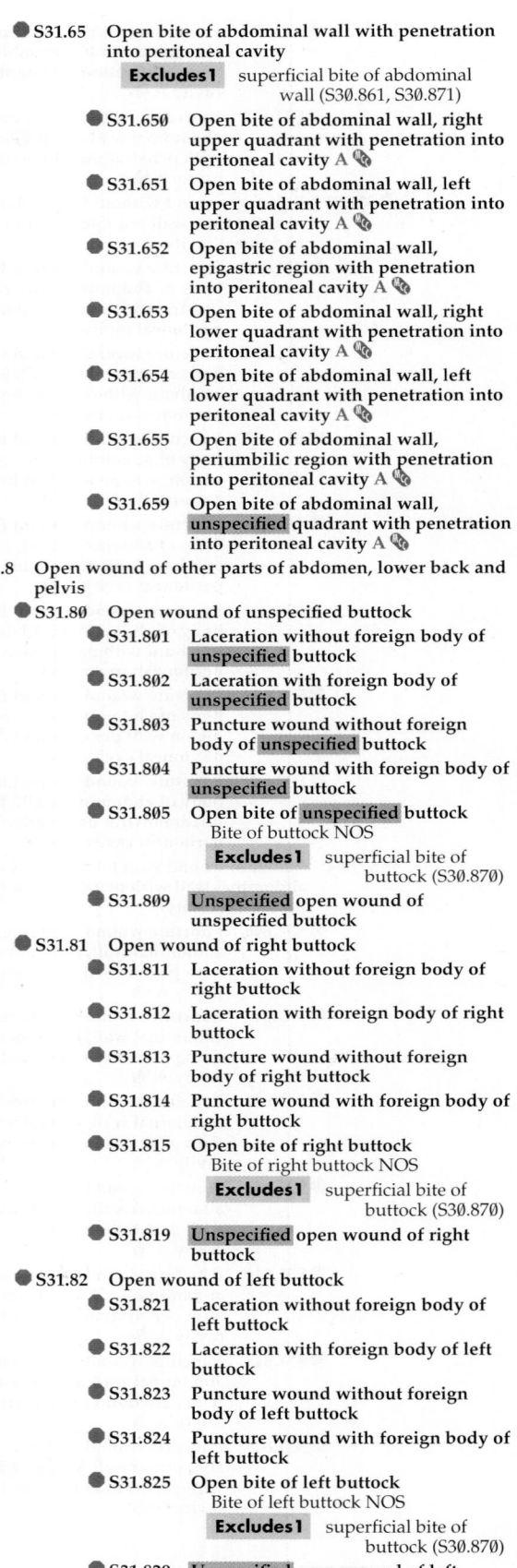
  - **S31.651** Open bite of abdominal wall, left upper quadrant with penetration into peritoneal cavity A
  - **S31.652** Open bite of abdominal wall, epigastric region with penetration into peritoneal cavity A
  - **S31.653** Open bite of abdominal wall, right lower quadrant with penetration into peritoneal cavity A
  - **S31.654** Open bite of abdominal wall, left lower quadrant with penetration into peritoneal cavity A
  - **S31.655** Open bite of abdominal wall, periumbilic region with penetration into peritoneal cavity A
  - **S31.659** Open bite of abdominal wall, unspecified quadrant with penetration into peritoneal cavity A
- **S31.8** **Open wound of other parts of abdomen, lower back and pelvis**
  - **S31.80** **Open wound of unspecified buttock**
    - **S31.801** Laceration without foreign body of unspecified buttock
    - **S31.802** Laceration with foreign body of unspecified buttock
    - **S31.803** Puncture wound without foreign body of unspecified buttock
    - **S31.804** Puncture wound with foreign body of unspecified buttock
    - **S31.805** Open bite of unspecified buttock
      Bite of buttock NOS
      - **Excludes1** superficial bite of buttock (S30.870)
    - **S31.809** Unspecified open wound of unspecified buttock
  - **S31.81** **Open wound of right buttock**
    - **S31.811** Laceration without foreign body of right buttock
    - **S31.812** Laceration with foreign body of right buttock
    - **S31.813** Puncture wound without foreign body of right buttock
    - **S31.814** Puncture wound with foreign body of right buttock
    - **S31.815** Open bite of right buttock
      Bite of right buttock NOS
      - **Excludes1** superficial bite of buttock (S30.870)
    - **S31.819** Unspecified open wound of right buttock
  - **S31.82** **Open wound of left buttock**
    - **S31.821** Laceration without foreign body of left buttock
    - **S31.822** Laceration with foreign body of left buttock
    - **S31.823** Puncture wound without foreign body of left buttock
    - **S31.824** Puncture wound with foreign body of left buttock
    - **S31.825** Open bite of left buttock
      Bite of left buttock NOS
      - **Excludes1** superficial bite of buttock (S30.870)
    - **S31.829** Unspecified open wound of left buttock

- **S31.83** **Open wound of anus**
  - **S31.831** Laceration without foreign body of anus
  - **S31.832** Laceration with foreign body of anus
  - **S31.833** Puncture wound without foreign body of anus
  - **S31.834** Puncture wound with foreign body of anus
  - **S31.835** Open bite of anus
    Bite of anus NOS
    - **Excludes1** superficial bite of anus (S30.877)
  - **S31.839** Unspecified open wound of anus
- **S32** **Fracture of lumbar spine and pelvis**
  - **Note:** A fracture not indicated as displaced or nondisplaced should be coded to displaced

    A fracture not indicated as opened or closed should be coded to closed
  - **Includes** fracture of lumbosacral neural arch
    fracture of lumbosacral spinous process
    fracture of lumbosacral transverse process
    fracture of lumbosacral vertebra
    fracture of lumbosacral vertebral arch

  Code first any associated spinal cord and spinal nerve injury (S34.-)
  - **Excludes1** transection of abdomen (S38.3)
  - **Excludes2** fracture of hip NOS (S72.0-)

  The appropriate 7th character is to be added to each code from category S32

A	initial encounter for closed fracture
B	initial encounter for open fracture
D	subsequent encounter for fracture with routine healing
G	subsequent encounter for fracture with delayed healing
K	subsequent encounter for fracture with nonunion
S	sequela

  - **S32.0** **Fracture of lumbar vertebra**
    Fracture of lumbar spine NOS
    - (Ex) **For category S32.0 CC codes S32.0[A,B]:** M48.40X-M48.58X[S], M80.08X[S], M80.88X[S], M84.350[S], M84.454[S], M84.550[S], M84.58X[S], M84.650[S], M99.13, M99.15-M99.17, M99.19, S03.1XX[A], S03.8XX-S03.9XX[A], S12.000-S12.9XX[S], S13.9XX[A], S14.109[A], S14.119[A], S14.129[A], S14.139[A], S14.149[A], S14.159[A], S22.000-S22.9XX[S], S23.20X-S23.29X[A], S23.9XX[A], S24.109[A], S24.119[A], S24.139[A], S24.149[A], S24.159[A], S29.001-S29.019[A], S29.091-S29.9XX[A], S32.000-S32.059[A,B,S], S32.10X-S32.9XX[S], S33.0XX-S33.141[A], S33.30X-S33.39X[A], S33.5XX[A], S33.9XX[A], S34.01X[A], S34.101-S34.129[A], S38.1XX[A], S38.3XX-S39.013[A], S39.091-S39.94X[A], T14.90-T14.91, T79.8XX-T79.9XX[A], T79.A0X-T79.A9X[A] **For S32.0[K]:** See S02.0[K]
    - **S32.00** **Fracture of unspecified lumbar vertebra**
      - **S32.000** Wedge compression fracture of unspecified lumbar vertebra A, K, B, A, B
      - **S32.001** Stable burst fracture of unspecified lumbar vertebra A, K, B, A, B
      - **S32.002** Unstable burst fracture of unspecified lumbar vertebra A, K, B, A, B
      - **S32.008** Other fracture of unspecified lumbar vertebra A, K, B, A, B
      - **S32.009** Unspecified fracture of unspecified lumbar vertebra A, K, B, A, B

- S32.01   Fracture of first lumbar vertebra
  - S32.010   Wedge compression fracture of first lumbar vertebra A, K 🜨, B 🜨, A, B 🜨
  - S32.011   Stable burst fracture of first lumbar vertebra A, K 🜨, B 🜨, A, B 🜨
  - S32.012   Unstable burst fracture of first lumbar vertebra A, K 🜨, B 🜨, A, B 🜨
  - S32.018   Other fracture of first lumbar vertebra A, K 🜨, B 🜨, A, B 🜨
  - S32.019   Unspecified fracture of first lumbar vertebra A, K 🜨, B 🜨, A, B 🜨
- S32.02   Fracture of second lumbar vertebra
  - S32.020   Wedge compression fracture of second lumbar vertebra A, K 🜨, B 🜨, A, B 🜨
  - S32.021   Stable burst fracture of second lumbar vertebra A, K 🜨, B 🜨, A, B 🜨
  - S32.022   Unstable burst fracture of second lumbar vertebra A, K 🜨, B 🜨, A, B 🜨
  - S32.028   Other fracture of second lumbar vertebra A, K 🜨, B 🜨, A, B 🜨
  - S32.029   Unspecified fracture of second lumbar vertebra A, K 🜨, B 🜨, A, B 🜨
- S32.03   Fracture of third lumbar vertebra
  - S32.030   Wedge compression fracture of third lumbar vertebra A, K 🜨, B 🜨, A, B 🜨
  - S32.031   Stable burst fracture of third lumbar vertebra A, K 🜨, B 🜨, A, B 🜨
  - S32.032   Unstable burst fracture of third lumbar vertebra A, K 🜨, B 🜨, A, B 🜨
  - S32.038   Other fracture of third lumbar vertebra A, K 🜨, B 🜨, A, B 🜨
  - S32.039   Unspecified fracture of third lumbar vertebra A, K 🜨, B 🜨, A, B 🜨
- S32.04   Fracture of fourth lumbar vertebra
  - S32.040   Wedge compression fracture of fourth lumbar vertebra A, K 🜨, B 🜨, A, B 🜨
  - S32.041   Stable burst fracture of fourth lumbar vertebra A, K 🜨, B 🜨, A, B 🜨
  - S32.042   Unstable burst fracture of fourth lumbar vertebra A, K 🜨, B 🜨, A, B 🜨
  - S32.048   Other fracture of fourth lumbar vertebra A, K 🜨, B 🜨, A, B 🜨
  - S32.049   Unspecified fracture of fourth lumbar vertebra A, K 🜨, B 🜨, A, B 🜨
- S32.05   Fracture of fifth lumbar vertebra
  - S32.050   Wedge compression fracture of fifth lumbar vertebra A, K 🜨, B 🜨, A, B 🜨
  - S32.051   Stable burst fracture of fifth lumbar vertebra A, K 🜨, B 🜨, A, B 🜨
  - S32.052   Unstable burst fracture of fifth lumbar vertebra A, K 🜨, B 🜨, A, B 🜨
  - S32.058   Other fracture of fifth lumbar vertebra A, K 🜨, B 🜨, A, B 🜨
  - S32.059   Unspecified fracture of fifth lumbar vertebra A, K 🜨, B 🜨, A, B 🜨

- S32.1   Fracture of sacrum
  For vertical fractures, code to most medial fracture extension
  Use two codes if both a vertical and transverse fracture are present
  Code also any associated fracture of pelvic ring (S32.8-)
  Ⓔₓ **For category S32.1 CC codes S32.1[A,B]:** M48.40X-M48.58X[S], M80.08X[S], M80.88X[S], M84.350[S], M84.454[S], M84.550[S], M84.58X[S], M84.650[S], M99.14-M99.17, M99.19, S03.1XX[A], S03.8XX-S03.9XX[A], S12.000-S12.9XX[S], S13.9XX[A], S14.109[A], S14.119[A], S14.129[A], S14.139[A], S14.149[A], S14.159[A], S22.000-S22.9XX[S], S23.20X[A], S23.29X[A], S23.9XX[A], S24.109[A], S24.119[A], S24.139[A], S24.149[A], S24.159[A], S29.001-S29.019[A], S29.091-S29.9XX[A], S32.000-S32.059[S], S32.10X-S32.2XX[A,B,S], S32.301-S32.9XX[S], S33.2XX-S33.4XX[A], S33.6XX-S33.9XX[A], S34.02X[A], S34.131-S34.3XX[A], S38.1XX[A], S38.3XX[A], S39.001-S39.013[A], S39.091-39.94X[A], T14.90-T14.91, T79.8XX-T79.9XX[A], T79.A0X-T79.A9X[A] **For S32.1[K]:** See S02.0[K]
  - X S32.10   Unspecified fracture of sacrum A, K 🜨, B 🜨, A, B 🜨
  - S32.11   Zone I fracture of sacrum
    Vertical sacral ala fracture of sacrum
    - S32.110   Nondisplaced Zone I fracture of sacrum A, K 🜨, B 🜨, A, B 🜨
    - S32.111   Minimally displaced Zone I fracture of sacrum A, K 🜨, B 🜨, A, B 🜨
    - S32.112   Severely displaced Zone I fracture of sacrum A, K 🜨, B 🜨, A, B 🜨
    - S32.119   Unspecified Zone I fracture of sacrum A, K 🜨, B 🜨, A, B 🜨
  - S32.12   Zone II fracture of sacrum
    Vertical foraminal region fracture of sacrum
    - S32.120   Nondisplaced Zone II fracture of sacrum A, K 🜨, B 🜨, A, B 🜨
    - S32.121   Minimally displaced Zone II fracture of sacrum A, K 🜨, B 🜨, A, B 🜨
    - S32.122   Severely displaced Zone II fracture of sacrum A, K 🜨, B 🜨, A, B 🜨
    - S32.129   Unspecified Zone II fracture of sacrum A, K 🜨, B 🜨, A, B 🜨
  - S32.13   Zone III fracture of sacrum
    Vertical fracture into spinal canal region of sacrum
    - S32.130   Nondisplaced Zone III fracture of sacrum A, K 🜨, B 🜨, A, B 🜨
    - S32.131   Minimally displaced Zone III fracture of sacrum A, K 🜨, B 🜨, A, B 🜨
    - S32.132   Severely displaced Zone III fracture of sacrum A, K 🜨, B 🜨, A, B 🜨
    - S32.139   Unspecified Zone III fracture of sacrum A, K 🜨, B 🜨, A, B 🜨
  - X S32.14   Type 1 fracture of sacrum A, K 🜨, B 🜨, A, B 🜨
    Transverse flexion fracture of sacrum without displacement
  - X S32.15   Type 2 fracture of sacrum A, K 🜨, B 🜨, A, B 🜨
    Transverse flexion fracture of sacrum with posterior displacement
  - X S32.16   Type 3 fracture of sacrum A, K 🜨, B 🜨, A, B 🜨
    Transverse extension fracture of sacrum with anterior displacement
  - X S32.17   Type 4 fracture of sacrum A, K 🜨, B 🜨, A, B 🜨
    Transverse segmental comminution of upper sacrum
  - X S32.19   Other fracture of sacrum A, K 🜨, B 🜨, A, B 🜨
- X S32.2   Fracture of coccyx A, K 🜨, B 🜨, A, B 🜨
  Ⓔₓ **For category S32.2 CC codes S32.2[A,B]:** See S32.1 [A,B]
  For S32.2[K]: See S02.0[K]

● **S32.3**   Fracture of ilium

> **Excludes1**   fracture of ilium with associated disruption of pelvic ring (S32.8-)

> (Ex) For category S32.3 CC codes **S32.3[A]:** See S22.9 For **S32.3[B]:**
> M48.40X-M48.58X[A], M80.00X-M80.88X[A], M84.30X-M84.68X[A],
> M84.750-M84.759[A], S03.8XX-S03.9XX[A], S22.9XX[A,B],
> S29.011-S29.019[A], S32.301-S32.399[A,B], S32.810-S32.9XX[A,B],
> S33.4XX[A], S33.6XX-S33.8XX[A], S38.3XX[A], S39.011-S39.013[A],
> S73.001-S73.199[A], S76.001-S76.019[A], S76.091-S76.119[A],
> S76.191-S76.219[A], S76.291-S76.319[A], S76.391-S76.819[A],
> S76.891-S76.919[A], S76.991-S76.999[A], S79.811-S79.929[A],
> T14.90-T14.91, T79.8XX-T79.9XX[A], T79.A0X-T79.A9X[A]
> For **S32.3[K]:** See S02.0[K]

  ● **S32.30**   Unspecified fracture of ilium

    ● **S32.301**   Unspecified fracture of right ilium A, K 🗪, B 🗪, A, B 🗪

    ● **S32.302**   Unspecified fracture of left ilium A, K 🗪, B 🗪, A, B 🗪

    ● **S32.309**   Unspecified fracture of unspecified ilium A, K 🗪, B 🗪, A, B 🗪

  ● **S32.31**   Avulsion fracture of ilium

    ● **S32.311**   Displaced avulsion fracture of right ilium A, K 🗪, B 🗪, A, B 🗪

    ● **S32.312**   Displaced avulsion fracture of left ilium A, K 🗪, B 🗪, A, B 🗪

    ● **S32.313**   Displaced avulsion fracture of unspecified ilium A, K 🗪, B 🗪, A, B 🗪

    ● **S32.314**   Nondisplaced avulsion fracture of right ilium A, K 🗪, B 🗪, A, B 🗪

    ● **S32.315**   Nondisplaced avulsion fracture of left ilium A, K 🗪, B 🗪, A, B 🗪

    ● **S32.316**   Nondisplaced avulsion fracture of unspecified ilium A, K 🗪, B 🗪, A, B 🗪

  ● **S32.39**   Other fracture of ilium

    ● **S32.391**   Other fracture of right ilium A, K 🗪, B 🗪, A, B 🗪

    ● **S32.392**   Other fracture of left ilium A, K 🗪, B 🗪, A, B 🗪

    ● **S32.399**   Other fracture of unspecified ilium A, K 🗪, B 🗪, A, B 🗪

● **S32.4**   Fracture of acetabulum

> Code also any associated fracture of pelvic ring (S32.8-)

> (Ex) For category S32.4 CC codes **S32.4[A]:** M48.40X-M48.58X[A],
> M80.00X-M80.88X[A], M84.30X-M84.68X[A], M84.750-M84.759[A],
> S03.8XX-S03.9XX[A], S22.9XX [A,B], S29.011-S29.019[A], S32.401-S32.499[A,B],
> S32.810-S32.811[A,B], S32.89X-S32.9XX[A,B], S33.4XX[A], S33.6XX-S33.8XX[A],
> S38.3XX[A], S39.011-S39.013[A], S73.001-S73.199[A], S76.001-S76.019[A],
> S76.091-S76.119[A], S76.191-S76.219[A], S76.291-S76.319[A],
> S76.391-S76.819[A], S76.891-S76.919[A], S76.991-S76.999[A],
> S79.811-S79.829[A], S79.911-S79.929[A], T14.90-T14.91, T79.8XX-T79.9XX[A],
> T79.A0X-T79.A9X[A] For **S32.4[B]:** S03.8XX-S03.9XX[A], S22.9XX [A,B],
> S29.011-S29.019[A], S32.401-S32.499[A,B], S32.810-S32.811[A,B],
> S32.89X-S32.9XX[A,B], S33.4XX[A], S33.6XX-S33.8XX[A], S38.3XX[A],
> S39.011-S39.013[A], S73.001-S73.199[A], S76.001-S76.019[A],
> S76.091-S76.119[A], S76.191-S76.219[A], S76.291-S76.319[A],
> S76.391-S76.819[A], S76.891-S76.919[A], S76.991-S76.999[A],
> S79.811-S79.929[A], T14.90-T14.91, T79.A0X-T79.A9X[A], T79.8XX-T79.9XX[A]
> For **S32.4[K]:** See S02.0[K]

  ● **S32.40**   Unspecified fracture of acetabulum

    ● **S32.401**   Unspecified fracture of right acetabulum K 🗪, A, B 🗪, A, B 🗪

    ● **S32.402**   Unspecified fracture of left acetabulum K 🗪, A, B 🗪, A, B 🗪

    ● **S32.409**   Unspecified fracture of unspecified acetabulum K 🗪, A, B 🗪, A, B 🗪

  ● **S32.41**   Fracture of anterior wall of acetabulum

    ● **S32.411**   Displaced fracture of anterior wall of right acetabulum K 🗪, A, B 🗪, A, B 🗪

    ● **S32.412**   Displaced fracture of anterior wall of left acetabulum K 🗪, A, B 🗪, A, B 🗪

    ● **S32.413**   Displaced fracture of anterior wall of unspecified acetabulum K 🗪, A, B 🗪, A, B 🗪

    ● **S32.414**   Nondisplaced fracture of anterior wall of right acetabulum K 🗪, A, B 🗪, A, B 🗪

    ● **S32.415**   Nondisplaced fracture of anterior wall of left acetabulum K 🗪, A, B 🗪, A, B 🗪

    ● **S32.416**   Nondisplaced fracture of anterior wall of unspecified acetabulum K 🗪, A, B 🗪, A, B 🗪

  ● **S32.42**   Fracture of posterior wall of acetabulum

    ● **S32.421**   Displaced fracture of posterior wall of right acetabulum K 🗪, A, B 🗪, A, B 🗪

    ● **S32.422**   Displaced fracture of posterior wall of left acetabulum K 🗪, A, B 🗪, A, B 🗪

    ● **S32.423**   Displaced fracture of posterior wall of unspecified acetabulum K 🗪, A, B 🗪, A, B 🗪

    ● **S32.424**   Nondisplaced fracture of posterior wall of right acetabulum K 🗪, A, B 🗪, A, B 🗪

    ● **S32.425**   Nondisplaced fracture of posterior wall of left acetabulum K 🗪, A, B 🗪, A, B 🗪

    ● **S32.426**   Nondisplaced fracture of posterior wall of unspecified acetabulum K 🗪, A, B 🗪, A, B 🗪

  ● **S32.43**   Fracture of anterior column [iliopubic] of acetabulum

    ● **S32.431**   Displaced fracture of anterior column [iliopubic] of right acetabulum K 🗪, A, B 🗪, A, B 🗪

    ● **S32.432**   Displaced fracture of anterior column [iliopubic] of left acetabulum K 🗪, A, B 🗪, A, B 🗪

    ● **S32.433**   Displaced fracture of anterior column [iliopubic] of unspecified acetabulum K 🗪, A, B 🗪, A, B 🗪

    ● **S32.434**   Nondisplaced fracture of anterior column [iliopubic] of right acetabulum K 🗪, A, B 🗪, A, B 🗪

    ● **S32.435**   Nondisplaced fracture of anterior column [iliopubic] of left acetabulum K 🗪, A, B 🗪, A, B 🗪

    ● **S32.436**   Nondisplaced fracture of anterior column [iliopubic] of unspecified acetabulum K 🗪, A, B 🗪, A, B 🗪

  ● **S32.44**   Fracture of posterior column [ilioischial] of acetabulum

    ● **S32.441**   Displaced fracture of posterior column [ilioischial] of right acetabulum K 🗪, A, B 🗪, A, B 🗪

    ● **S32.442**   Displaced fracture of posterior column [ilioischial] of left acetabulum K 🗪, A, B 🗪, A, B 🗪

    ● **S32.443**   Displaced fracture of posterior column [ilioischial] of unspecified acetabulum K 🗪, A, B 🗪, A, B 🗪

    ● **S32.444**   Nondisplaced fracture of posterior column [ilioischial] of right acetabulum K 🗪, A, B 🗪, A, B 🗪

    ● **S32.445**   Nondisplaced fracture of posterior column [ilioischial] of left acetabulum K 🗪, A, B 🗪, A, B 🗪

    ● **S32.446**   Nondisplaced fracture of posterior column [ilioischial] of unspecified acetabulum K 🗪, A, B 🗪, A, B 🗪

◀ New   ◀▦ Revised   ~~deleted~~ Deleted   Excludes 1   Excludes 2   Includes   Use additional   Code first   Code also   Unspecified

OGCR Official Guidelines   ● Unacceptable Principal Diagnosis   X Assign placeholder X   ● Use Additional Character(s)   🗪 Manifestation Code   **Coding Clinic**

● **S32.45**   **Transverse fracture of acetabulum**
- ● **S32.451**   Displaced transverse fracture of right acetabulum K 🔹, A, B 🔹, A, B 🔹
- ● **S32.452**   Displaced transverse fracture of left acetabulum K 🔹, A, B 🔹, A, B 🔹
- ● **S32.453**   Displaced transverse fracture of unspecified acetabulum K 🔹, A, B 🔹, A, B 🔹
- ● **S32.454**   Nondisplaced transverse fracture of right acetabulum K 🔹, A, B 🔹, A, B 🔹
- ● **S32.455**   Nondisplaced transverse fracture of left acetabulum K 🔹, A, B 🔹, A, B 🔹
- ● **S32.456**   Nondisplaced transverse fracture of unspecified acetabulum K 🔹, A, B 🔹, A, B 🔹

● **S32.46**   **Associated transverse-posterior fracture of acetabulum**
- ● **S32.461**   Displaced associated transverse-posterior fracture of right acetabulum K 🔹, A, B 🔹, A, B 🔹
- ● **S32.462**   Displaced associated transverse-posterior fracture of left acetabulum K 🔹, A, B 🔹, A, B 🔹
- ● **S32.463**   Displaced associated transverse-posterior fracture of unspecified acetabulum K 🔹, A, B 🔹, A, B 🔹
- ● **S32.464**   Nondisplaced associated transverse-posterior fracture of right acetabulum K 🔹, A, B 🔹, A, B 🔹
- ● **S32.465**   Nondisplaced associated transverse-posterior fracture of left acetabulum K 🔹, A, B 🔹, A, B 🔹
- ● **S32.466**   Nondisplaced associated transverse-posterior fracture of unspecified acetabulum K 🔹, A, B 🔹, A, B 🔹

● **S32.47**   **Fracture of medial wall of acetabulum**
- ● **S32.471**   Displaced fracture of medial wall of right acetabulum K 🔹, A, B 🔹, A, B 🔹
- ● **S32.472**   Displaced fracture of medial wall of left acetabulum K 🔹, A, B 🔹, A, B 🔹
- ● **S32.473**   Displaced fracture of medial wall of unspecified acetabulum K 🔹, A, B 🔹, A, B 🔹
- ● **S32.474**   Nondisplaced fracture of medial wall of right acetabulum K 🔹, A, B 🔹, A, B 🔹
- ● **S32.475**   Nondisplaced fracture of medial wall of left acetabulum K 🔹, A, B 🔹, A, B 🔹
- ● **S32.476**   Nondisplaced fracture of medial wall of unspecified acetabulum K 🔹, A, B 🔹, A, B 🔹

● **S32.48**   **Dome fracture of acetabulum**
- ● **S32.481**   Displaced dome fracture of right acetabulum K 🔹, A, B 🔹, A, B 🔹
- ● **S32.482**   Displaced dome fracture of left acetabulum K 🔹, A, B 🔹, A, B 🔹
- ● **S32.483**   Displaced dome fracture of unspecified acetabulum K 🔹, A, B 🔹, A, B 🔹
- ● **S32.484**   Nondisplaced dome fracture of right acetabulum K 🔹, A, B 🔹, A, B 🔹
- ● **S32.485**   Nondisplaced dome fracture of left acetabulum K 🔹, A, B 🔹, A, B 🔹
- ● **S32.486**   Nondisplaced dome fracture of unspecified acetabulum K 🔹, A, B 🔹, A, B 🔹

● **S32.49**   **Other fracture of acetabulum**
- ● **S32.491**   Other fracture of right acetabulum K 🔹, A, B 🔹, A, B 🔹
- ● **S32.492**   Other fracture of left acetabulum K 🔹, A, B 🔹, A, B 🔹
- ● **S32.499**   Other fracture of unspecified acetabulum K 🔹, A, B 🔹, A, B 🔹

● **S32.5**   **Fracture of pubis**

> **Excludes1**   fracture of pubis with associated disruption of pelvic ring (S32.8-)
>
> ⒺⓍ **For category S32.5 CC codes S32.5[A,B]:** M48.40X-M48.58X[A], M80.00X-M80.88X[A], M84.30X-M84.68X[A], M84.750-M84.759[A], S03.8XX-S03.9XX[A], S22.9XX [A,B], S29.011-S29.019[A], S32.501A-S32.599[A,B], S32.810-S32.811[A,B], S32.89X-S32.9XX[A,B], S33.4XX[A], S33.6XX-S33.8XX[A], S38.3XX-S39.013[A], S73.001-S73.199[A], S76.001-S76.019[A], S76.091-S76.119[A], S76.191-S76.219[A], S76.291-S76.319[A], S76.391-S76.819[A], S76.891-S76.919[A], S76.991-S76.999[A], T14.90-T14.91, T79.A0X-T79.A9X[A], T79.8XX-T79.9XX[A] **For S32.5[K]:** See S02.0[K]

● **S32.50**   **Unspecified fracture of pubis**
- ● **S32.501**   Unspecified fracture of right pubis A, K 🔹, B 🔹, A, B 🔹
- ● **S32.502**   Unspecified fracture of left pubis A, K 🔹, B 🔹, A, B 🔹
- ● **S32.509**   Unspecified fracture of unspecified pubis A, K 🔹, B 🔹, A, B 🔹

● **S32.51**   **Fracture of superior rim of pubis**
- ● **S32.511**   Fracture of superior rim of right pubis A, K 🔹, B 🔹, A, B 🔹
- ● **S32.512**   Fracture of superior rim of left pubis A, K 🔹, B 🔹, A, B 🔹
- ● **S32.519**   Fracture of superior rim of unspecified pubis A, K 🔹, B 🔹, A, B 🔹

● **S32.59**   **Other specified fracture of pubis**
- ● **S32.591**   Other specified fracture of right pubis A, K 🔹, B 🔹, A, B 🔹
- ● **S32.592**   Other specified fracture of left pubis A, K 🔹, B 🔹, A, B 🔹
- ● **S32.599**   Other specified fracture of unspecified pubis A, K 🔹, B 🔹, A, B 🔹

● **S32.6**   **Fracture of ischium**

> **Excludes1**   fracture of ischium with associated disruption of pelvic ring (S32.8-)
>
> ⒺⓍ **For category S32.6 CC codes S32.6[A]:** S32.601-S32.699[A] **For S32.6[B]:** M48.40X-M48.58X[A], M80.00X-M80.88X[A], M84.30X-M84.68X[A], M84.750-M84.759[A], S03.8XX-S03.9XX[A], S22.9XX[A,B], S29.011-S29.019[A], S32.601-S32.811[A,B], S32.89X-S32.9XX[A,B], S33.4XX[A], S33.6XX-S33.8XX[A], S38.3XX[A], S39.011-S39.013[A], S73.001-S73.199[A], S76.001-S76.019[A], S76.091-S76.119[A], S76.191-S76.219[A], S76.291-S76.319[A], S76.391-S76.819[A], S76.891-S76.919[A], S76.991-S76.999[A], S79.811-S79.929[A], T14.90-T14.91, T79.A0X-T79.A9X[A], T79.8XX-T79.9XX[A] **For S32.5[K]:** See S02.0[K]

● **S32.60**   **Unspecified fracture of ischium**
- ● **S32.601**   Unspecified fracture of right ischium A, K 🔹, B 🔹, A, B 🔹
- ● **S32.602**   Unspecified fracture of left ischium A, K 🔹, B 🔹, A, B 🔹
- ● **S32.609**   Unspecified fracture of unspecified ischium A, K 🔹, B 🔹, A, B 🔹

● S32.61   **Avulsion fracture of ischium**
    ● S32.611   **Displaced avulsion fracture of right ischium** A, K 🖑, B 🖑, A, B 🖑
    ● S32.612   **Displaced avulsion fracture of left ischium** A, K 🖑, B 🖑, A, B 🖑
    ● S32.613   **Displaced avulsion fracture of unspecified ischium** A, K 🖑, B 🖑, A, B 🖑
    ● S32.614   **Nondisplaced avulsion fracture of right ischium** A, K 🖑, B 🖑, A, B 🖑
    ● S32.615   **Nondisplaced avulsion fracture of left ischium** A, K 🖑, B 🖑, A, B 🖑
    ● S32.616   **Nondisplaced avulsion fracture of unspecified ischium** A, K 🖑, B 🖑, A, B 🖑

● S32.69   **Other specified fracture of ischium**
    ● S32.691   **Other specified fracture of right ischium** A, K 🖑, B 🖑, A, B 🖑
    ● S32.692   **Other specified fracture of left ischium** A, K 🖑, B 🖑, A, B 🖑
    ● S32.699   **Other specified fracture of unspecified ischium** A, K 🖑, B 🖑, A, B 🖑

● S32.8   **Fracture of other parts of pelvis**
   Code also any associated:
     fracture of acetabulum (S32.4-)
     sacral fracture (S32.1-)

   ● S32.81   **Multiple fractures of pelvis with disruption of pelvic ring**
       Multiple pelvic fractures with disruption of pelvic circle
      (Ex) **For category S32.81 CC codes S32.81[A,B]:** M48.40X-M48.58X[A], M80.00X-M80.88X[A], M84.30X-M84.68X[A], M84.750-M84.759[A], S03.8XX-S03.9XX[A,B], S22.9XX[A,B], S29.011-S29.019[A], S32.301-S32.811[A,B], S32.89X-S32.9XX[A,B], S33.4XX[A], S33.6XX-S33.8XX[A], S38.3XX[A], S39.011-S39.013[A], S73.001-S73.199[A], S76.001-S76.019[A], S76.091-S76.119[A], S76.191-S76.219[A], S76.291-S76.319[A], S76.391-S76.819[A], S76.891-S76.919[A], S76.991-S76.999[A], S79.811-S79.929[A], T14.90-T14.91, T79.A0X-T79.A9X[A], T79.8XX-T79.9XX[A] **For S32.81[K]:** See S02.0[K]

    ● S32.810   **Multiple fractures of pelvis with stable disruption of pelvic ring** A, K 🖑, B 🖑, A, B 🖑
    ● S32.811   **Multiple fractures of pelvis with unstable disruption of pelvic ring** A, K 🖑, B 🖑, A, B 🖑

   X ● S32.82   **Multiple fractures of pelvis without disruption of pelvic ring** A, K 🖑, B 🖑, A, B 🖑
       Multiple pelvic fractures without disruption of pelvic circle
      (Ex) **For category S32.82 CC codes S32.82[A,B]:** S32.89X[A] **For S32.81[K]:** See S32.0[K]

   X ● S32.89   **Fracture of other parts of pelvis** A, K 🖑, B 🖑, A, B 🖑
      (Ex) **For category S32.89 CC codes S32.89[A,B]:** M48.40X-M48.58X[A], M80.00X-M80.88X[A], M84.30X-M84.68X[A], M84.750-M84.759[A], S03.8XX-S03.9XX[A], S22.9XX[A,B], S29.011-S29.019[A], S32.301-S32.9XX[A,B], S33.4XX[A], S33.6XX-S33.8XX[A], S38.3XX[A], S39.011-S39.013[A], S73.001-S73.199[A], S76.001-S76.019[A], S76.091-S76.119[A], S76.191-S76.219[A], 76.291-S76.319[A], S76.391-S76.819[A], S76.891-S76.919[A], S76.991-S76.999[A], S79.811-S79.929[A], T14.90-T14.91, T79.A0X-T79.A9X[A], T79.8XX-T79.9XX[A] **For S32.89[K]:** See S02.0[K]

  X ● S32.9   **Fracture of unspecified parts of lumbosacral spine and pelvis** A, K 🖑, B 🖑, A, B 🖑
     Fracture of lumbosacral spine NOS
     Fracture of pelvis NOS
    (Ex) **For category S32.9 CC codes S32.9[A,B]:** See S32.81 **For S32.9[K]:** See S32.0[K]
    Coding Clinic: 2012, Q4, P93

● S33   **Dislocation and sprain of joints and ligaments of lumbar spine and pelvis**
   Includes   avulsion of joint or ligament of lumbar spine and pelvis
          laceration of cartilage, joint or ligament of lumbar spine and pelvis
          sprain of cartilage, joint or ligament of lumbar spine and pelvis
          traumatic hemarthrosis of joint or ligament of lumbar spine and pelvis
          traumatic rupture of joint or ligament of lumbar spine and pelvis
          traumatic subluxation of joint or ligament of lumbar spine and pelvis
          traumatic tear of joint or ligament of lumbar spine and pelvis
   Code also any associated open wound
   Excludes1   nontraumatic rupture or displacement of lumbar intervertebral disc NOS (M51.-)
          obstetric damage to pelvic joints and ligaments (O71.6)
   Excludes2   dislocation and sprain of joints and ligaments of hip (S73.-)
          strain of muscle of lower back and pelvis (S39.01-)
   The appropriate 7th character is to be added to each code from category S33

A	initial encounter
D	subsequent encounter
S	sequela

  X ● S33.0   **Traumatic rupture of lumbar intervertebral disc**
    Excludes1   rupture or displacement (nontraumatic) of lumbar intervertebral disc NOS (M51.- with fifth character 6)

  ● S33.1   **Subluxation and dislocation of lumbar vertebra**
    Code also any associated:
      open wound of abdomen, lower back and pelvis (S31)
      spinal cord injury (S24.0, S24.1-, S34.0-, S34.1-)
    Excludes2   fracture of lumbar vertebrae (S32.0-)
   ● S33.10   **Subluxation and dislocation of unspecified lumbar vertebra**
    ● S33.100   **Subluxation of unspecified lumbar vertebra**
    ● S33.101   **Dislocation of unspecified lumbar vertebra**
   ● S33.11   **Subluxation and dislocation of L_1/L_2 lumbar vertebra**
    ● S33.110   **Subluxation of L_1/L_2 lumbar vertebra**
    ● S33.111   **Dislocation of L_1/L_2 lumbar vertebra**
   ● S33.12   **Subluxation and dislocation of L_2/L_3 lumbar vertebra**
    ● S33.120   **Subluxation of L_2/L_3 lumbar vertebra**
    ● S33.121   **Dislocation of L_2/L_3 lumbar vertebra**
   ● S33.13   **Subluxation and dislocation of L_3/L_4 lumbar vertebra**
    ● S33.130   **Subluxation of L_3/L_4 lumbar vertebra**
    ● S33.131   **Dislocation of L_3/L_4 lumbar vertebra**
   ● S33.14   **Subluxation and dislocation of L_4/L_5 lumbar vertebra**
    ● S33.140   **Subluxation of L_4/L_5 lumbar vertebra**
    ● S33.141   **Dislocation of L_4/L_5 lumbar vertebra**

  X ● S33.2   **Dislocation of sacroiliac and sacrococcygeal joint**
  ● S33.3   **Dislocation of other and unspecified parts of lumbar spine and pelvis**
   X ● S33.30   **Dislocation of unspecified parts of lumbar spine and pelvis**
   X ● S33.39   **Dislocation of other parts of lumbar spine and pelvis**

◀ New   ◀▥ Revised   ~~deleted~~ Deleted   Excludes 1   Excludes 2   Includes   Use additional   Code first   Code also   Unspecified
OGCR Official Guidelines   ● Unacceptable Principal Diagnosis   X Assign placeholder X   ● Use Additional Character(s)   ▶ Manifestation Code   **Coding Clinic**

X ● S33.4   **Traumatic rupture of symphysis pubis**
X ● S33.5   **Sprain of ligaments of lumbar spine**
X ● S33.6   **Sprain of sacroiliac joint**
X ● S33.8   **Sprain of other parts of lumbar spine and pelvis**
X ● S33.9   **Sprain of** unspecified **parts of lumbar spine and pelvis**

● S34   **Injury of lumbar and sacral spinal cord and nerves at abdomen, lower back and pelvis level**

Note: Code to highest level of lumbar cord injury

Injuries to the spinal cord (S34.0 and S34.1) refer to the cord level and not bone level injury, and can affect nerve roots at and below the level given.

The appropriate 7th character is to be added to each code from category S34

> A   initial encounter
> D   subsequent encounter
> S   sequela

Code also any associated:
    fracture of vertebra (S22.0-, S32.0-)
    open wound of abdomen, lower back and pelvis (S31.-)
    transient paralysis (R29.5)
Ⓔⓧ **For category S34 CC codes unless otherwise indicated:** M48.40X-M48.58X[S], M80.08X[S], M80.88X[S], M84.350[S], M84.454[S], M84.550[S], M84.58X[S], M84.650[S], M99.15-M99.17, M99.19, S03.1XX[A], S12.000-S12.9XX[S], S13.9XX[A], S14.109[A], S14.119[A], S14.129[A], S14.139[A], S14.149[A], S14.159[A], S22.000-S22.9XX[S], S23.20X[A], S23.29X[A], S23.9XX[A], S24.109[A], S24.119[A], S24.139[A], S24.149[A]c, S24.159[A], S29.001-S29.009[A], S29.091-S29.9XX[A], S32.000-S32.9XX[S], S33.30X-S33.39X[A], S33.9XX-S34.01X[A], S34.101-S34.129[A], S38.1XX[A], S39.001-S39.003[A], S39.091-S39.94X[A], T14.90-T14.91, T79.A0X-T79.A9X[A], T79.8XX-T79.9XX[A]

● S34.0   **Concussion and edema of lumbar and sacral spinal cord**

   X ● S34.01   **Concussion and edema of lumbar spinal cord** A 🔖

   X ● S34.02   **Concussion and edema of sacral spinal cord** A 🔖

      Concussion and edema of conus medullaris
      Ⓔⓧ M48.40X-M48.58X[S], M80.08X[S], M80.88X[S], M84.350[S], M84.454[S], M84.550[S], M84.58X[S], M84.650[S], M99.15-M99.17, M99.19, S03.1XX[A], S12.000-S12.9XX[S], S13.9XX[A], S14.109[A], S14.119[A], S14.129[A], S14.139[A], S14.149[A], S14.159[A], S22.000-S22.9XX[S], S23.20X-S23.29X[A], S23.9XX[A], S24.109[A], S24.119[A], S24.139[A], S24.149[A], S24.159[A], S29.001-S29.009[A], S29.091-S29.9XX[A], S32.000-S32.9XX[S], S33.30X-S33.39X[A], S33.9XX[A], S34.02X[A], S34.131-S34.139[A], S34.3XX[A], S38.1XX[A], S39.001-S39.003[A], S39.091-S39.94X[A], T14.90-T14.91, T79.A0X-T79.A9X[A], T79.8XX-T79.9XX[A]

● S34.1   **Other and unspecified injury of lumbar and sacral spinal cord**

   ● S34.10   **Unspecified injury to lumbar spinal cord**

     ● S34.101   Unspecified **injury to L₁ level of lumbar spinal cord** A 🔖, A 🔖
       Unspecified injury to lumbar spinal cord level 1 ◀

     ● S34.102   Unspecified **injury to L₂ level of lumbar spinal cord** A 🔖, A 🔖
       Unspecified injury to lumbar spinal cord level 2 ◀

     ● S34.103   Unspecified **injury to L₃ level of lumbar spinal cord** A 🔖, A 🔖
       Unspecified injury to lumbar spinal cord level 3 ◀

     ● S34.104   Unspecified **injury to L₄ level of lumbar spinal cord** A 🔖, A 🔖
       Unspecified injury to lumbar spinal cord level 4 ◀

     ● S34.105   Unspecified **injury to L₅ level of lumbar spinal cord** A 🔖, A 🔖
       Unspecified injury to lumbar spinal cord level 5 ◀

     ● S34.109   Unspecified **injury to unspecified level of lumbar spinal cord** A 🔖, A 🔖

   ● S34.11   **Complete lesion of lumbar spinal cord**

     ● S34.111   **Complete lesion of L₁ level of lumbar spinal cord** A 🔖, A 🔖
       Complete lesion of lumbar spinal cord level 1 ◀

     ● S34.112   **Complete lesion of L₂ level of lumbar spinal cord** A 🔖, A 🔖
       Complete lesion of lumbar spinal cord level 2 ◀

     ● S34.113   **Complete lesion of L₃ level of lumbar spinal cord** A 🔖, A 🔖
       Complete lesion of lumbar spinal cord level 3 ◀

     ● S34.114   **Complete lesion of L₄ level of lumbar spinal cord** A 🔖, A 🔖
       Complete lesion of lumbar spinal cord level 4 ◀

     ● S34.115   **Complete lesion of L₅ level of lumbar spinal cord** A 🔖, A 🔖
       Complete lesion of lumbar spinal cord level 5 ◀

     ● S34.119   **Complete lesion of** unspecified **level of lumbar spinal cord** A 🔖, A 🔖

   ● S34.12   **Incomplete lesion of lumbar spinal cord**

     ● S34.121   **Incomplete lesion of L₁ level of lumbar spinal cord** A 🔖, A 🔖
       Incomplete lesion of lumbar spinal cord level 1 ◀

     ● S34.122   **Incomplete lesion of L₂ level of lumbar spinal cord** A 🔖, A 🔖
       Incomplete lesion of lumbar spinal cord level 2 ◀

     ● S34.123   **Incomplete lesion of L₃ level of lumbar spinal cord** A 🔖, A 🔖
       Incomplete lesion of lumbar spinal cord level 3 ◀

     ● S34.124   **Incomplete lesion of L₄ level of lumbar spinal cord** A 🔖, A 🔖
       Incomplete lesion of lumbar spinal cord level 4 ◀

     ● S34.125   **Incomplete lesion of L₅ level of lumbar spinal cord** A 🔖, A 🔖
       Incomplete lesion of lumbar spinal cord level 5 ◀

     ● S34.129   **Incomplete lesion of** unspecified **level of lumbar spinal cord** A 🔖, A 🔖

   ● S34.13   **Other and unspecified injury to sacral spinal cord**
      Other injury to conus medullaris
      Ⓔⓧ **For category S34.13 CC codes:** See S32.04

     ● S34.131   **Complete lesion of sacral spinal cord** A 🔖, A 🔖
       Complete lesion of conus medullaris

     ● S34.132   **Incomplete lesion of sacral spinal cord** A 🔖, A 🔖
       Incomplete lesion of conus medullaris

     ● S34.139   Unspecified **injury to sacral spinal cord** A 🔖, A 🔖
       Unspecified injury of conus medullaris

CHAPTER 19 (S00-T88)

● S34.2   **Injury of nerve root of lumbar and sacral spine**
X ● S34.21   **Injury of nerve root of lumbar spine**
X ● S34.22   **Injury of nerve root of sacral spine**
X ● **S34.3   Injury of cauda equina** A 🔣, A 🔣
Ex: See S32.04
X ● **S34.4   Injury of lumbosacral plexus**
X ● **S34.5   Injury of lumbar, sacral and pelvic sympathetic nerves**
Injury of celiac ganglion or plexus
Injury of hypogastric plexus
Injury of mesenteric plexus (inferior) (superior)
Injury of splanchnic nerve
X ● **S34.6   Injury of peripheral nerve(s) at abdomen, lower back and pelvis level**
X ● **S34.8   Injury of other nerves at abdomen, lower back and pelvis level**
X ● **S34.9   Injury of** unspecified **nerves at abdomen, lower back and pelvis level**

● **S35   Injury of blood vessels at abdomen, lower back and pelvis level**
The appropriate 7th character is to be added to each code from category S35

A	initial encounter
D	subsequent encounter
S	sequela

Code also any associated open wound (S31.-)
● **S35.0   Injury of abdominal aorta**
Excludes1   injury of aorta NOS (S25.0)
Ex: **For category S35.0 CC codes:** S35.00X-S35.09X[A], S35.8X1-S35.99X[A], T14.90-T14.91, T79.A0X-T79.A9X[A], T79.8XX-T79.9XX[A]
X ● S35.00   Unspecified **injury of abdominal aorta** A 🔣
X ● S35.01   **Minor laceration of abdominal aorta** A 🔣
Incomplete transection of abdominal aorta
Laceration of abdominal aorta NOS
Superficial laceration of abdominal aorta
X ● S35.02   **Major laceration of abdominal aorta** A 🔣
Complete transection of abdominal aorta
Traumatic rupture of abdominal aorta
X ● S35.09   **Other injury of abdominal aorta** A 🔣
● **S35.1   Injury of inferior vena cava**
Injury of hepatic vein
Excludes1   injury of vena cava NOS (S25.2)
Ex: **For category S35.1 CC codes:** S35.10X-S35.19X[A], S35.8X1-S35.99X[A], T14.90-T14.91, T79.A0X-T79.A9X[A], T79.8XX-T79.9XX[A]
X ● S35.10   Unspecified **injury of inferior vena cava** A 🔣
X ● S35.11   **Minor laceration of inferior vena cava** A 🔣
Incomplete transection of inferior vena cava
Laceration of inferior vena cava NOS
Superficial laceration of inferior vena cava
X ● S35.12   **Major laceration of inferior vena cava** A 🔣
Complete transection of inferior vena cava
Traumatic rupture of inferior vena cava
X ● S35.19   **Other injury of inferior vena cava** A 🔣
● **S35.2   Injury of celiac or mesenteric artery and branches**
● S35.21   **Injury of celiac artery**
Ex: **For category S35.21 CC codes:** S35.211-S35.219[A], S35.8X1-S35.99X[A], T14.90-T14.91, T79.A0X-T79.A9X[A], T79.8XX-T79.9XX[A]
● S35.211   **Minor laceration of celiac artery** A 🔣
Incomplete transection of celiac artery
Laceration of celiac artery NOS
Superficial laceration of celiac artery
● S35.212   **Major laceration of celiac artery** A 🔣
Complete transection of celiac artery
Traumatic rupture of celiac artery
● S35.218   **Other injury of celiac artery** A 🔣
● S35.219   Unspecified **injury of celiac artery** A 🔣

● S35.22   **Injury of superior mesenteric artery**
Ex: **For category S35.22 CC codes:** S35.221-S35.229[A], S35.8X1-S35.99X[A], T14.90-T14.91, T79.A0X-T79.A9X[A], T79.8XX-T79.9XX[A]
● S35.221   **Minor laceration of superior mesenteric artery** A 🔣
Incomplete transection of superior mesenteric artery
Laceration of superior mesenteric artery NOS
Superficial laceration of superior mesenteric artery
● S35.222   **Major laceration of superior mesenteric artery** A 🔣
Complete transection of superior mesenteric artery
Traumatic rupture of superior mesenteric artery
● S35.228   **Other injury of superior mesenteric artery** A 🔣
● S35.229   Unspecified **injury of superior mesenteric artery** A 🔣
● S35.23   **Injury of inferior mesenteric artery**
Ex: **For category S35.23 CC codes:** S35.231-S35.239[A], S35.8X1-S35.99X[A], T14.90-T14.91, T79.A0X-T79.A9X[A], T79.8XX-T79.9XX[A]
● S35.231   **Minor laceration of inferior mesenteric artery** A 🔣
Incomplete transection of inferior mesenteric artery
Laceration of inferior mesenteric artery NOS
Superficial laceration of inferior mesenteric artery
● S35.232   **Major laceration of inferior mesenteric artery** A 🔣
Complete transection of inferior mesenteric artery
Traumatic rupture of inferior mesenteric artery
● S35.238   **Other injury of inferior mesenteric artery** A 🔣
● S35.239   Unspecified **injury of inferior mesenteric artery** A 🔣
● S35.29   **Injury of branches of celiac and mesenteric artery**
Injury of gastric artery
Injury of gastroduodenal artery
Injury of hepatic artery
Injury of splenic artery
Ex: **For category S35.29 CC codes unless otherwise indicated:** S35.292-S35.298[A], S35.8X1-S35.99X[A], T14.90-T14.91, T79.A0X-T79.A9X[A], T79.8XX-T79.9XX[A]
● S35.291   **Minor laceration of branches of celiac and mesenteric artery** A 🔣
Incomplete transection of branches of celiac and mesenteric artery
Laceration of branches of celiac and mesenteric artery NOS
Superficial laceration of branches of celiac and mesenteric artery
Ex: S35.291[A], S35.8X1-S35.99X[A], T14.90-T14.91, T79.8XX-T79.9XX[A], T79.A0X[A], T79.A3X-T79.A9X[A]
● S35.292   **Major laceration of branches of celiac and mesenteric artery** A 🔣
Complete transection of branches of celiac and mesenteric artery
Traumatic rupture of branches of celiac and mesenteric artery

◄ New   ◄|||| Revised   ~~deleted~~ Deleted   Excludes 1   Excludes 2   Includes   Use additional   Code first   Code also   Unspecified
OGCR Official Guidelines   ● Unacceptable Principal Diagnosis   X Assign placeholder X   ● Use Additional Character(s)   🔣 Manifestation Code   **Coding Clinic**

● S35.298   Other injury of branches of celiac and mesenteric artery A 🔖

● S35.299   Unspecified injury of branches of celiac and mesenteric artery A 🔖
Ⓔⓧ S35.299[A], S35.8X1-S35.99X[A], T14.90-T14.91, T79.A0X-T79.A9X[A], T79.8XX-T79.9XX[A]

● S35.3   Injury of portal or splenic vein and branches

   ● S35.31   Injury of portal vein
Ⓔⓧ **For category S35.31 CC codes:** S35.311-S35.319[A], S35.8X1-S35.99X[A], T14.90-T14.91, T79.A0X-T79.A9X[A], T79.8XX-T79.9XX[A]

     ● S35.311   Laceration of portal vein A 🔖

     ● S35.318   Other specified injury of portal vein A 🔖

     ● S35.319   Unspecified injury of portal vein A 🔖

   ● S35.32   Injury of splenic vein
Ⓔⓧ **For category S35.32 CC codes:** S35.321-S35.329[A], S35.8X1-S35.99X[A], T14.90-T14.91, T79.A0X-T79.A9X[A], T79.8XX-T79.9XX[A]

     ● S35.321   Laceration of splenic vein A 🔖

     ● S35.328   Other specified injury of splenic vein A 🔖

     ● S35.329   Unspecified injury of splenic vein A 🔖

   ● S35.33   Injury of superior mesenteric vein
Ⓔⓧ **For category S35.33 CC codes:** S35.331-S35.339[A], S35.8X1-S35.99X[A], T14.90-T14.91, T79.A0X-T79.A9X[A], T79.8XX-T79.9XX[A]

     ● S35.331   Laceration of superior mesenteric vein A 🔖

     ● S35.338   Other specified injury of superior mesenteric vein A 🔖

     ● S35.339   Unspecified injury of superior mesenteric vein A 🔖

   ● S35.34   Injury of inferior mesenteric vein
Ⓔⓧ **For category S35.34 CC codes:** S35.341-S35.349[A], S35.8X1-S35.99X[A], T14.90-T14.91, T79.A0X-T79.A9X[A], T79.8XX-T79.9XX[A]

     ● S35.341   Laceration of inferior mesenteric vein A 🔖

     ● S35.348   Other specified injury of inferior mesenteric vein A 🔖

     ● S35.349   Unspecified injury of inferior mesenteric vein A 🔖

● S35.4   Injury of renal blood vessels

   ● S35.40   Unspecified injury of renal blood vessel
Ⓔⓧ **For category S35.40 CC codes S35.401-S35.403:** S35.401-S35.403[A], S35.411-S35.413[A], S35.491-S35.493[A], S35.8X1-S35.99X[A], T14.90-T14.91, T79.A0X-T79.A9X[A], T79.8XX-T79.9XX[A] **For category S35.40 CC codes S35.404-S35.406:** S35.404-S35.406[A], S35.414-S35.416[A], S35.494-S35.496[A], S35.8X1-S35.99X[A], T14.90-T14.91, T79.A0X-T79.A9X[A], T79.8XX-T79.9XX[A]

     ● S35.401   Unspecified injury of right renal artery A 🔖

     ● S35.402   Unspecified injury of left renal artery A 🔖

     ● S35.403   Unspecified injury of unspecified renal artery A 🔖

     ● S35.404   Unspecified injury of right renal vein A 🔖

     ● S35.405   Unspecified injury of left renal vein A 🔖

     ● S35.406   Unspecified injury of unspecified renal vein A 🔖

● S35.41   Laceration of renal blood vessel
Ⓔⓧ **For category S35.41 CC codes S35.411-S35.413:** See S35.401-S35.403 **For category S35.41 CC codes S35.414-S35.416:** See 35.404-S35.406

     ● S35.411   Laceration of right renal artery A 🔖

     ● S35.412   Laceration of left renal artery A 🔖

     ● S35.413   Laceration of unspecified renal artery A 🔖

     ● S35.414   Laceration of right renal vein A 🔖

     ● S35.415   Laceration of left renal vein A 🔖

     ● S35.416   Laceration of unspecified renal vein A 🔖

● S35.49   Other specified injury of renal blood vessel
Ⓔⓧ **For category S35.49 CC codes S35.491-S35.493:** See S35.401-S35.403 **For category S35.49 CC codes S35.494-S35.496:** See 35.404-S35.406

     ● S35.491   Other specified injury of right renal artery A 🔖

     ● S35.492   Other specified injury of left renal artery A 🔖

     ● S35.493   Other specified injury of unspecified renal artery A 🔖

     ● S35.494   Other specified injury of right renal vein A 🔖

     ● S35.495   Other specified injury of left renal vein A 🔖

     ● S35.496   Other specified injury of unspecified renal vein A 🔖

● S35.5   Injury of iliac blood vessels

   X ● S35.50   Injury of unspecified iliac blood vessel(s) A 🔖
Ⓔⓧ S35.50X-S35.516[A], S35.59X-S35.99X[A], T14.90-T14.91, T79.A0X-T79.A9X[A], T79.8XX-T79.9XX[A]

   ● S35.51   Injury of iliac artery or vein
     Injury of hypogastric artery or vein
Ⓔⓧ **For category S35.51 CC codes S35.511-S35.513:** S35.50X-S35.513[A], S35.59X-S35.99X[A], T14.90-T14.91, T79.A0X-T79.A9X[A], T79.8XX-T79.9XX[A] **For category S35.51 CC codes S35.514-S35.516:** S35.50X[A], S35.514-S35.516[A], S35.59X-S35.99X[A], T14.90-T14.91, T79.A0X-T79.A9X[A], T79.8XX-T79.9XX[A]

     ● S35.511   Injury of right iliac artery A 🔖

     ● S35.512   Injury of left iliac artery A 🔖

     ● S35.513   Injury of unspecified iliac artery A 🔖

     ● S35.514   Injury of right iliac vein A 🔖

     ● S35.515   Injury of left iliac vein A 🔖

     ● S35.516   Injury of unspecified iliac vein A 🔖

   ● S35.53   Injury of uterine artery or vein
Ⓔⓧ **For category S35.53 CC codes S35.531-S35.533:** S35.50X[A], S35.531-S35.533[A], S35.59X-S35.99X[A], T14.90-T14.91, T79.8XX-T79.9XX[A], T79.A0X[A], T79.A3X-T79.A9X[A] **For category S35.53 CC codes S35.534-S35.536:** S35.50X[A], S35.534-S35.536[A], S35.59X-S35.99X[A], T14.90-T14.91, T79.8XX-T79.9XX[A], T79.A0X[A], T79.A3X-T79.A9X[A]

     ● S35.531   Injury of right uterine artery ♀ A 🔖

     ● S35.532   Injury of left uterine artery ♀ A 🔖

     ● S35.533   Injury of unspecified uterine artery ♀ A 🔖

     ● S35.534   Injury of right uterine vein ♀ A 🔖

     ● S35.535   Injury of left uterine vein ♀ A 🔖

     ● S35.536   Injury of unspecified uterine vein ♀ A 🔖

   X ● S35.59   Injury of other iliac blood vessels A 🔖
Ⓔⓧ See S35.50

CHAPTER 19 (S00-T88)

CHAPTER 19 (S00–T88)

● **S35.8**   **Injury of other blood vessels at abdomen, lower back and pelvis level**
     Injury of ovarian artery or vein
     (Ex) **For category S35.8 CC codes:** S35.8X1-S35.99X[A], T14.90-T14.91, T79.8XX-T79.9XX[A], T79.A0X[A], T79.A9X[A]

   ● **S35.8X**   **Injury of other blood vessels at abdomen, lower back and pelvis level**

     ● **S35.8X1**   **Laceration of other blood vessels at abdomen, lower back and pelvis level** A 🔓

     ● **S35.8X8**   **Other specified injury of other blood vessels at abdomen, lower back and pelvis level** A 🔓

     ● **S35.8X9**   **Unspecified injury of other blood vessels at abdomen, lower back and pelvis level** A 🔓

● **S35.9**   **Injury of unspecified blood vessel at abdomen, lower back and pelvis level**
     (Ex) **For category S35.9 CC codes:** S35.00X-S35.99X[A], T14.90-T14.91, T79.8XX-T79.9XX[A], T79.A0X[A], T79.A3X-T79.A9X[A]

   X ● **S35.90**   **Unspecified injury of unspecified blood vessel at abdomen, lower back and pelvis level** A 🔓

   X ● **S35.91**   **Laceration of unspecified blood vessel at abdomen, lower back and pelvis level** A 🔓

   X ● **S35.99**   **Other specified injury of unspecified blood vessel at abdomen, lower back and pelvis level** A 🔓

● **S36**   **Injury of intra-abdominal organs**
     The appropriate 7th character is to be added to each code from category S36

A	initial encounter
D	subsequent encounter
S	sequela

     Code also any associated open wound (S31.-)

● **S36.0**   **Injury of spleen**
     (Ex) **For category S36.0 CC codes:** S31.001[A], S31.011[A], S31.021[A], S31.031[A], S31.041[A], S31.051[A], S31.100-S31.159[A], S31.600-S31.659[A], S31.831-S31.839[A], S36.00X-S36.09X[A], S36.81X-S36.99X[A], S38.3XX[A], S39.021-S39.023[A], T14.90-T14.91, T79.8XX-T79.9XX[A], T79.A0X-T79.A9X[A]

   X ● **S36.00**   **Unspecified injury of spleen** A 🔓

   ● **S36.02**   **Contusion of spleen**

     ● **S36.020**   **Minor contusion of spleen** A 🔓
       Contusion of spleen less than 2 cm

     ● **S36.021**   **Major contusion of spleen** A 🔓
       Contusion of spleen greater than 2 cm

     ● **S36.029**   **Unspecified contusion of spleen** A 🔓
       Coding Clinic: 2015, Q2, P36, Q1, P11

   ● **S36.03**   **Laceration of spleen**

     ● **S36.030**   **Superficial (capsular) laceration of spleen** A 🔓
       Laceration of spleen less than 1 cm
       Minor laceration of spleen

     ● **S36.031**   **Moderate laceration of spleen** A 🔓
       Laceration of spleen 1 to 3 cm
       Coding Clinic: 2015, Q2, P36, Q1, P11

     ● **S36.032**   **Major laceration of spleen** A 🔓
       Avulsion of spleen
       Laceration of spleen greater than 3 cm
       Massive laceration of spleen
       Multiple moderate lacerations of spleen
       Stellate laceration of spleen

     ● **S36.039**   **Unspecified laceration of spleen** A 🔓

   X ● **S36.09**   **Other injury of spleen** A 🔓

● **S36.1**   **Injury of liver and gallbladder and bile duct**

   ● **S36.11**   **Injury of liver**
     (Ex) **For category S36.11 CC codes:** S31.001[A], S31.011[A], S31.021[A], S31.031[A], S31.041[A], S31.051[A], S31.100-S31.159[A], S31.600-S31.659[A], S31.831-S31.839[A], S36.112-S36.119[A], S36.81X-S36.99X[A], S38.3XX[A], S39.021-S39.023[A], T14.90-T14.91, T79.8XX-T79.9XX[A], T79.A0XA-T79.A9X[A]

     ● **S36.112**   **Contusion of liver** A 🔓

     ● **S36.113**   **Laceration of liver, unspecified degree** A 🔓

     ● **S36.114**   **Minor laceration of liver** A 🔓
       Laceration involving capsule only, or, without significant involvement of hepatic parenchyma [i.e., less than 1 cm deep]

     ● **S36.115**   **Moderate laceration of liver** A 🔓
       Laceration involving parenchyma but without major disruption of parenchyma [i.e., less than 10 cm long and less than 3 cm deep]

     ● **S36.116**   **Major laceration of liver** A 🔓
       Laceration with significant disruption of hepatic parenchyma [i.e., greater than 10 cm long and 3 cm deep]
       Multiple moderate lacerations, with or without hematoma
       Stellate laceration of liver

     ● **S36.118**   **Other injury of liver** A 🔓

     ● **S36.119**   **Unspecified injury of liver** A 🔓
       Coding Clinic: 2015, Q2, P17

   ● **S36.12**   **Injury of gallbladder**
     (Ex) **For category S36.12 CC codes:** S31.001[A], S31.011[A], S31.021[A], S31.031[A], S31.041[A], S31.051[A], S31.100-S31.159[A], S31.600-S31.659[A], S31.831-S31.839[A], S36.122-S36.13X[A], S36.81X-S36.99X[A], S38.3XX[A], S39.021-S39.023[A], T14.90-T14.91, T79.8XX-T79.9XX[A], T79.A0X-T79.A9X[A]

     ● **S36.122**   **Contusion of gallbladder** A 🔓

     ● **S36.123**   **Laceration of gallbladder** A 🔓

     ● **S36.128**   **Other injury of gallbladder** A 🔓

     ● **S36.129**   **Unspecified injury of gallbladder** A 🔓

   X ● **S36.13**   **Injury of bile duct** A 🔓
     (Ex) See S36.12

● **S36.2**   **Injury of pancreas**
     (Ex) **For category S36.2 CC codes:** M79.A3, S31.001[A], S31.011[A], S31.021[A], S31.031[A], S31.041[A], S31.051[A], S31.100-S31.159[A], S31.600-S31.659[A], S31.831-S31.839[A], S36.200-S36.299[A], S36.81X-S36.99X[A], S38.3XX[A], S39.021-S39.023[A], T14.90-T14.91, T79.8XX-T79.9XX[A], T79.A3X-T79.A9X[A]

   ● **S36.20**   **Unspecified injury of pancreas**

     ● **S36.200**   **Unspecified injury of head of pancreas** A 🔓

     ● **S36.201**   **Unspecified injury of body of pancreas** A 🔓

     ● **S36.202**   **Unspecified injury of tail of pancreas** A 🔓

     ● **S36.209**   **Unspecified injury of unspecified part of pancreas** A 🔓

   ● **S36.22**   **Contusion of pancreas**

     ● **S36.220**   **Contusion of head of pancreas** A 🔓

     ● **S36.221**   **Contusion of body of pancreas** A 🔓

     ● **S36.222**   **Contusion of tail of pancreas** A 🔓

     ● **S36.229**   **Contusion of unspecified part of pancreas** A 🔓

◀ New   ◀ Revised   ~~deleted~~ Deleted   Excludes 1   Excludes 2   Includes   Use additional   Code first   Code also   Unspecified
OGCR Official Guidelines   ● Unacceptable Principal Diagnosis   X Assign placeholder X   ● Use Additional Character(s)   ▶ Manifestation Code   **Coding Clinic**

● S36.23　Laceration of pancreas, unspecified degree
　● S36.230　Laceration of head of pancreas, unspecified degree A 🦠
　● S36.231　Laceration of body of pancreas, unspecified degree A 🦠
　● S36.232　Laceration of tail of pancreas, unspecified degree A 🦠
　● S36.239　Laceration of unspecified part of pancreas, unspecified degree A 🦠
● S36.24　Minor laceration of pancreas
　● S36.240　Minor laceration of head of pancreas A 🦠
　● S36.241　Minor laceration of body of pancreas A 🦠
　● S36.242　Minor laceration of tail of pancreas A 🦠
　● S36.249　Minor laceration of unspecified part of pancreas A 🦠
● S36.25　Moderate laceration of pancreas
　● S36.250　Moderate laceration of head of pancreas A 🦠
　● S36.251　Moderate laceration of body of pancreas A 🦠
　● S36.252　Moderate laceration of tail of pancreas A 🦠
　● S36.259　Moderate laceration of unspecified part of pancreas A 🦠
● S36.26　Major laceration of pancreas
　● S36.260　Major laceration of head of pancreas A 🦠
　● S36.261　Major laceration of body of pancreas A 🦠
　● S36.262　Major laceration of tail of pancreas A 🦠
　● S36.269　Major laceration of unspecified part of pancreas A 🦠
● S36.29　Other injury of pancreas
　● S36.290　Other injury of head of pancreas A 🦠
　● S36.291　Other injury of body of pancreas A 🦠
　● S36.292　Other injury of tail of pancreas A 🦠
　● S36.299　Other injury of unspecified part of pancreas A 🦠
● S36.3　Injury of stomach
　Ⓔⓧ For category S36.3 CC codes: M79.A3, S31.001[A], S31.011[A], S31.021[A], S31.031[A], S31.041[A], S31.051[A], S31.100-S31.159[A], S31.600-S31.659[A], S31.831-S31.839[A], S36.30X-S36.39X[A], S36.81X-S36.99X[A], S38.3XX[A], S39.021-S39.023[A], T14.90-T14.91, T79.8XX-T799.XX[A], T79.A3X-T79.A9X[A]
X ● S36.30　Unspecified injury of stomach A 🦠
X ● S36.32　Contusion of stomach A 🦠
X ● S36.33　Laceration of stomach A 🦠
X ● S36.39　Other injury of stomach A 🦠
● S36.4　Injury of small intestine
　Ⓔⓧ For category S36.4 CC codes: M79.A3, S31.001[A], S31.011[A], S31.021[A], S31.031[A], S31.041[A], S31.051[A], S31.100-S31.159[A], S31.600-S31.659[A], S31.831-S31.839[A], S36.400-S36.499[A], S36.81X-S36.99X[A], S38.3XX[A], S39.021-S39.023[A], T14.90-T14.91, T79.8XX-T79.9XX[A], T79.A3X-T79.A9X[A]
　● S36.40　Unspecified injury of small intestine
　　● S36.400　Unspecified injury of duodenum A 🦠
　　● S36.408　Unspecified injury of other part of small intestine A 🦠
　　● S36.409　Unspecified injury of unspecified part of small intestine A 🦠

● S36.41　Primary blast injury of small intestine
　Blast injury of small intestine NOS
　● S36.410　Primary blast injury of duodenum A 🦠
　● S36.418　Primary blast injury of other part of small intestine A 🦠
　● S36.419　Primary blast injury of unspecified part of small intestine A 🦠
● S36.42　Contusion of small intestine
　● S36.420　Contusion of duodenum A 🦠
　● S36.428　Contusion of other part of small intestine A 🦠
　● S36.429　Contusion of unspecified part of small intestine A 🦠
● S36.43　Laceration of small intestine
　● S36.430　Laceration of duodenum A 🦠
　● S36.438　Laceration of other part of small intestine A 🦠
　● S36.439　Laceration of unspecified part of small intestine A 🦠
● S36.49　Other injury of small intestine
　● S36.490　Other injury of duodenum A 🦠
　● S36.498　Other injury of other part of small intestine A 🦠
　● S36.499　Other injury of unspecified part of small intestine A 🦠
● S36.5　Injury of colon
　Excludes2　injury of rectum (S36.6-)
　Ⓔⓧ For category S36.5 CC codes: M79.A3, S31.001[A], S31.011[A], S31.021[A], S31.031[A], S31.041[A], S31.051[A], S31.100-S31.159[A], S31.600-S31.659[A], S31.831-S31.839[A], S36.500-S36.99X[A], S38.3XX[A], S39.021-S39.023[A], T14.90-T14.91, T79.8XX-T79.9XX[A], T79.A3X-T79.A9X[A]
　● S36.50　Unspecified injury of colon
　　● S36.500　Unspecified injury of ascending [right] colon A 🦠
　　● S36.501　Unspecified injury of transverse colon A 🦠
　　● S36.502　Unspecified injury of descending [left] colon A 🦠
　　● S36.503　Unspecified injury of sigmoid colon A 🦠
　　● S36.508　Unspecified injury of other part of colon A 🦠
　　● S36.509　Unspecified injury of unspecified part of colon A 🦠
　● S36.51　Primary blast injury of colon
　　Blast injury of colon NOS
　　● S36.510　Primary blast injury of ascending [right] colon A 🦠
　　● S36.511　Primary blast injury of transverse colon A 🦠
　　● S36.512　Primary blast injury of descending [left] colon A 🦠
　　● S36.513　Primary blast injury of sigmoid colon A 🦠
　　● S36.518　Primary blast injury of other part of colon A 🦠
　　● S36.519　Primary blast injury of unspecified part of colon A 🦠
　● S36.52　Contusion of colon
　　● S36.520　Contusion of ascending [right] colon A 🦠
　　● S36.521　Contusion of transverse colon A 🦠
　　● S36.522　Contusion of descending [left] colon A 🦠
　　● S36.523　Contusion of sigmoid colon A 🦠
　　● S36.528　Contusion of other part of colon A 🦠
　　● S36.529　Contusion of unspecified part of colon A 🦠

N　Newborn Age: 0　　P　Pediatric Age: 0–17　　M　Maternity DX: 12–55　　A　Adult Age: 15–124　　♀　Females Only　　♂　Males Only
🦠　Complication\Comorbidity　　🦠　Major C\C　　Ⓔⓧ　CC/MCC Exclusions　　🦠　Hospital-Acquired Condition

CHAPTER 19 (S00-T88)

- S36.53   Laceration of colon
  - S36.530   Laceration of ascending [right] colon A
  - S36.531   Laceration of transverse colon A
  - S36.532   Laceration of descending [left] colon A
  - S36.533   Laceration of sigmoid colon A
  - S36.538   Laceration of other part of colon A
  - S36.539   Laceration of unspecified part of colon A
- S36.59   Other injury of colon
  - Secondary blast injury of colon
  - S36.590   Other injury of ascending [right] colon A
  - S36.591   Other injury of transverse colon A
  - S36.592   Other injury of descending [left] colon A
  - S36.593   Other injury of sigmoid colon A
  - S36.598   Other injury of other part of colon A
  - S36.599   Other injury of unspecified part of colon A
- S36.6   Injury of rectum
  - Ⓔⓧ **For category S36.6 CC codes:** See S36.5
  - X● S36.60   Unspecified injury of rectum A
  - X● S36.61   Primary blast injury of rectum A
    - Blast injury of rectum NOS
  - X● S36.62   Contusion of rectum A
  - X● S36.63   Laceration of rectum A
  - X● S36.69   Other injury of rectum A
    - Secondary blast injury of rectum
- S36.8   Injury of other intra-abdominal organs
  - Ⓔⓧ **For category S36.8 CC codes:** See S31.0
  - X● S36.81   Injury of peritoneum A
  - S36.89   Injury of other intra-abdominal organs
    - Injury of retroperitoneum
    - S36.892   Contusion of other intra-abdominal organs A
    - S36.893   Laceration of other intra-abdominal organs A
    - S36.898   Other injury of other intra-abdominal organs A
    - S36.899   Unspecified injury of other intra-abdominal organs A
- S36.9   Injury of unspecified intra-abdominal organ
  - Ⓔⓧ **For category S36.9 CC codes:** See S31.0
  - X● S36.90   Unspecified injury of unspecified intra-abdominal organ A
  - X● S36.92   Contusion of unspecified intra-abdominal organ A
  - X● S36.93   Laceration of unspecified intra-abdominal organ A
  - X● S36.99   Other injury of unspecified intra-abdominal organ A

- ● S37   Injury of urinary and pelvic organs
  - Code also any associated open wound (S31.-)
  - **Excludes1**   obstetric trauma to pelvic organs (O71.-)
  - **Excludes2**   injury of peritoneum (S36.81)
    - injury of retroperitoneum (S36.89-)
  - The appropriate 7th character is to be added to each code from category S37

A	initial encounter
D	subsequent encounter
S	sequela

- ● S37.0   Injury of kidney
  - **Excludes2**   acute kidney injury (nontraumatic) (N17.9)
  - Ⓔⓧ **For category S37.0 CC codes:** S31.001[A], S31.011[A], S31.021[A], S31.031[A], S31.041[A], S31.051[A], S31.100-S31.159[A], S31.600-S31.659[A], S31.831-S31.839[A], S36.81X-S37.099[A], S38.3XX[A], S39.021-S39.023[A], T14.90-T14.91, T79.8XX-T79.9XX[A], T79.A0X-T79.A9X[A]
  - S37.00   Unspecified injury of kidney
    - S37.001   Unspecified injury of right kidney A
    - S37.002   Unspecified injury of left kidney A
    - S37.009   Unspecified injury of unspecified kidney A
  - S37.01   Minor contusion of kidney
    - Contusion of kidney less than 2 cm
    - Contusion of kidney NOS
    - S37.011   Minor contusion of right kidney A
    - S37.012   Minor contusion of left kidney A
    - S37.019   Minor contusion of unspecified kidney A
  - S37.02   Major contusion of kidney
    - Contusion of kidney greater than 2 cm
    - S37.021   Major contusion of right kidney A
    - S37.022   Major contusion of left kidney A
    - S37.029   Major contusion of unspecified kidney A
  - S37.03   Laceration of kidney, unspecified degree
    - S37.031   Laceration of right kidney, unspecified degree A
    - S37.032   Laceration of left kidney, unspecified degree A
    - S37.039   Laceration of unspecified kidney, unspecified degree A
  - S37.04   Minor laceration of kidney
    - Laceration of kidney less than 1 cm
    - S37.041   Minor laceration of right kidney A
    - S37.042   Minor laceration of left kidney A
    - S37.049   Minor laceration of unspecified kidney A
  - S37.05   Moderate laceration of kidney
    - Laceration of kidney 1 to 3 cm
    - S37.051   Moderate laceration of right kidney A
    - S37.052   Moderate laceration of left kidney A
    - S37.059   Moderate laceration of unspecified kidney A
  - S37.06   Major laceration of kidney
    - Avulsion of kidney
    - Laceration of kidney greater than 3 cm
    - Massive laceration of kidney
    - Multiple moderate lacerations of kidney
    - Stellate laceration of kidney
    - S37.061   Major laceration of right kidney A
    - S37.062   Major laceration of left kidney A
    - S37.069   Major laceration of unspecified kidney A
  - S37.09   Other injury of kidney
    - S37.091   Other injury of right kidney A
    - S37.092   Other injury of left kidney A
    - S37.099   Other injury of unspecified kidney A

◀ New   ◀▟ Revised   ~~deleted~~ Deleted   Excludes 1   Excludes 2   Includes   Use additional   Code first   Code also   Unspecified

OGCR Official Guidelines   ● Unacceptable Principal Diagnosis   X Assign placeholder X   ● Use Additional Character(s)   ◀ Manifestation Code   **Coding Clinic**

● **S37.1** **Injury of ureter**
　　(Ex) **For category S37.1 CC codes:** S31.001[A], S31.011[A], S31.021[A],
　　　　S31.031[A], S31.041[A], S31.051[A], S31.100-S31.159[A],
　　　　S31.600-S31.659[A], S31.831-S31.839[A], S36.81X-S36.99X[A],
　　　　S37.10X-S37.19X[A], S37.401-S37.599[A], S37.822-S37.99X[A],
　　　　S38.3XX[A], S39.021-S39.023[A], T14.90-T14.91, T79.8XX-T79.9XX[A],
　　　　T79.A0X-T79.A9X[A]

X ● **S37.10** ▨Unspecified▨ **injury of ureter** A 🈸

X ● **S37.12** **Contusion of ureter** A 🈸

X ● **S37.13** **Laceration of ureter** A 🈸

X ● **S37.19** **Other injury of ureter** A 🈸

● **S37.2** **Injury of bladder**
　　(Ex) **For category S37.2 CC codes:** S31.001[A], S31.011[A], S31.021[A],
　　　　S31.031[A], S31.041[A], S31.051[A], S31.100-S31.159[A],
　　　　S31.600-S31.659[A], S31.831-S31.839[A], S36.81X-S36.99X[A],
　　　　S37.20X-S37.599[A], S37.822-S37.99X[A], S38.3XX[A],
　　　　S39.021-S39.023[A], T14.90-T14.91, T79.8XX-T79.9XX[A],
　　　　T79.A0X-T79.A9X[A]

X ● **S37.20** ▨Unspecified▨ **injury of bladder** A 🈸

X ● **S37.22** **Contusion of bladder** A 🈸

X ● **S37.23** **Laceration of bladder** A 🈸

X ● **S37.29** **Other injury of bladder** A 🈸

● **S37.3** **Injury of urethra**
　　(Ex) **For category S37.3 CC codes:** See S37.2

X ● **S37.30** ▨Unspecified▨ **injury of urethra** A 🈸

X ● **S37.32** **Contusion of urethra** A 🈸

X ● **S37.33** **Laceration of urethra** A 🈸

X ● **S37.39** **Other injury of urethra** A 🈸

● **S37.4** **Injury of ovary**
　● **S37.40** **Unspecified injury of ovary**
　　● **S37.401** ▨Unspecified▨ **injury of ovary,
　　　　unilateral** ♀
　　● **S37.402** ▨Unspecified▨ **injury of ovary,
　　　　bilateral** ♀
　　● **S37.409** ▨Unspecified▨ **injury of ovary,
　　　　unspecified** ♀
　● **S37.42** **Contusion of ovary**
　　● **S37.421** **Contusion of ovary, unilateral** ♀
　　● **S37.422** **Contusion of ovary, bilateral** ♀
　　● **S37.429** **Contusion of ovary, ▨unspecified▨** ♀
　● **S37.43** **Laceration of ovary**
　　● **S37.431** **Laceration of ovary, unilateral** ♀
　　● **S37.432** **Laceration of ovary, bilateral** ♀
　　● **S37.439** **Laceration of ovary, ▨unspecified▨** ♀
　● **S37.49** **Other injury of ovary**
　　● **S37.491** **Other injury of ovary, unilateral** ♀
　　● **S37.492** **Other injury of ovary, bilateral** ♀
　　● **S37.499** **Other injury of ovary, ▨unspecified▨** ♀

● **S37.5** **Injury of fallopian tube**
　● **S37.50** **Unspecified injury of fallopian tube**
　　● **S37.501** ▨Unspecified▨ **injury of fallopian tube,
　　　　unilateral** ♀
　　● **S37.502** ▨Unspecified▨ **injury of fallopian tube,
　　　　bilateral** ♀
　　● **S37.509** ▨Unspecified▨ **injury of fallopian tube,
　　　　unspecified** ♀
　● **S37.51** **Primary blast injury of fallopian tube**
　　　　Blast injury of fallopian tube NOS
　　● **S37.511** **Primary blast injury of fallopian tube,
　　　　unilateral** ♀
　　● **S37.512** **Primary blast injury of fallopian tube,
　　　　bilateral** ♀
　　● **S37.519** **Primary blast injury of fallopian tube,
　　　　▨unspecified▨** ♀

● **S37.52** **Contusion of fallopian tube**
　● **S37.521** **Contusion of fallopian tube,
　　　　unilateral** ♀
　● **S37.522** **Contusion of fallopian tube,
　　　　bilateral** ♀
　● **S37.529** **Contusion of fallopian tube,
　　　　▨unspecified▨** ♀

● **S37.53** **Laceration of fallopian tube**
　● **S37.531** **Laceration of fallopian tube,
　　　　unilateral** ♀
　● **S37.532** **Laceration of fallopian tube,
　　　　bilateral** ♀
　● **S37.539** **Laceration of fallopian tube,
　　　　▨unspecified▨** ♀

● **S37.59** **Other injury of fallopian tube**
　　　　Secondary blast injury of fallopian tube
　● **S37.591** **Other injury of fallopian tube,
　　　　unilateral** ♀
　● **S37.592** **Other injury of fallopian tube,
　　　　bilateral** ♀
　● **S37.599** **Other injury of fallopian tube,
　　　　▨unspecified▨** ♀

● **S37.6** **Injury of uterus**
　Excludes1　injury to gravid uterus (O9A.2-)
　　　　　　　injury to uterus during delivery (O71.-)
　　(Ex) **For category S37.6 CC codes:** S31.001[A], S31.011[A], S31.021[A],
　　　　S31.031[A], S31.041[A], S31.051[A], S31.100-S31.159[A],
　　　　S31.600-S31.659[A], S31.831-S31.839[A], S36.81X-S36.99X[A],
　　　　S37.401-S37.69X[A], S37.822-S37.99X[A], S38.3XX[A], S39.021-S39.023[A],
　　　　T14.90-T14.91, T79.8XX-T79.9XX[A], T79.A0X-T79.A9X[A]

X ● **S37.60** ▨Unspecified▨ **injury of uterus** ♀ A 🈸

X ● **S37.62** **Contusion of uterus** ♀ A 🈸

X ● **S37.63** **Laceration of uterus** ♀ A 🈸

X ● **S37.69** **Other injury of uterus** ♀ A 🈸

● **S37.8** **Injury of other urinary and pelvic organs**
　● **S37.81** **Injury of adrenal gland**
　　(Ex) **For category S37.81 CC codes:** S31.001[A], S31.011[A],
　　　　S31.021[A], S31.031[A], S31.041[A], S31.051[A],
　　　　S31.100-S31.159[A], S31.600-S31.659[A],
　　　　S31.831-S31.839[A], S36.81X-S36.99X[A],
　　　　S37.812-S37.819[A], S38.3XX[A], S39.021-S39.023[A],
　　　　T14.90-T14.91, T79.8XX-T79.9XX[A], T79.A0X-T79.A9X[A]
　　● **S37.812** **Contusion of adrenal gland** A 🈸
　　● **S37.813** **Laceration of adrenal gland** A 🈸
　　● **S37.818** **Other injury of adrenal gland** A 🈸
　　● **S37.819** ▨Unspecified▨ **injury of adrenal gland**
　　　　A 🈸

　● **S37.82** **Injury of prostate**
　　● **S37.822** **Contusion of prostate** ♂
　　● **S37.823** **Laceration of prostate** ♂
　　● **S37.828** **Other injury of prostate** ♂
　　● **S37.829** ▨Unspecified▨ **injury of prostate** ♂

　● **S37.89** **Injury of other urinary and pelvic organ**
　　(Ex) **For category S37.89 CC codes:** S31.001[A], S31.011[A],
　　　　S31.021[A], S31.031[A], S31.041[A], S31.051[A],
　　　　S31.100-S31.159[A], S31.600-S31.659[A],
　　　　S31.831-S31.839[A], S36.81X-S36.99X[A],
　　　　S37.401-S37.599[A], S37.822-S37.99X[A], S38.3XX[A],
　　　　S39.021-S39.023[A], T14.90-T14.91, T79.8XX-T79.9XX[A],
　　　　T79.A0X-T79.A9X[A]
　　● **S37.892** **Contusion of other urinary and pelvic
　　　　organ** A 🈸
　　● **S37.893** **Laceration of other urinary and pelvic
　　　　organ** A 🈸
　　● **S37.898** **Other injury of other urinary and
　　　　pelvic organ** A 🈸
　　● **S37.899** ▨Unspecified▨ **injury of other urinary
　　　　and pelvic organ** A 🈸

CHAPTER 19 (S00-T88)

N　Newborn Age: 0　　**P**　Pediatric Age: 0–17　　**M**　Maternity DX: 12–55　　**A**　Adult Age: 15–124　　♀　Females Only　　♂　Males Only

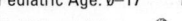　Complication\Comorbidity　　🈳　Major C\C　　(Ex)　CC/MCC Exclusions　　🈸　Hospital-Acquired Condition

1273

S37.9 **Injury of unspecified urinary and pelvic organ**
(Ex) For category S37.9 CC codes: See S37.89

X● S37.90 **Unspecified injury of unspecified urinary and pelvic organ** A 🖉

X● S37.92 **Contusion of unspecified urinary and pelvic organ** A 🖉

X● S37.93 **Laceration of unspecified urinary and pelvic organ** A 🖉

X● S37.99 **Other injury of unspecified urinary and pelvic organ** A 🖉

● S38 **Crushing injury and traumatic amputation of abdomen, lower back, pelvis and external genitals**
An amputation not identified as partial or complete should be coded to complete

The appropriate 7th character is to be added to each code from category S38

A	initial encounter
D	subsequent encounter
S	sequela

● S38.0 **Crushing injury of external genital organs**
Use additional code for any associated injuries

● S38.00 **Crushing injury of unspecified external genital organs**

● S38.001 **Crushing injury of unspecified external genital organs, male** ♂

● S38.002 **Crushing injury of unspecified external genital organs, female** ♀

X● S38.01 **Crushing injury of penis** ♂

X● S38.02 **Crushing injury of scrotum and testis** ♂

X● S38.03 **Crushing injury of vulva** ♀

X● S38.1 **Crushing injury of abdomen, lower back, and pelvis**
Use additional code for all associated injuries, such as:
fracture of thoracic or lumbar spine and pelvis (S22.0-, S32.-)
injury to intra-abdominal organs (S36.-)
injury to urinary and pelvic organs (S37.-)
open wound of abdominal wall (S31.-)
spinal cord injury (S34.0, S34.1-)

Excludes2 crushing injury of external genital organs (S38.0-)

● S38.2 **Traumatic amputation of external genital organs**

● S38.21 **Traumatic amputation of female external genital organs**
Traumatic amputation of clitoris
Traumatic amputation of labium (majus) (minus)
Traumatic amputation of vulva

● S38.211 **Complete traumatic amputation of female external genital organs** ♀

● S38.212 **Partial traumatic amputation of female external genital organs** ♀

● S38.22 **Traumatic amputation of penis**

● S38.221 **Complete traumatic amputation of penis** ♂

● S38.222 **Partial traumatic amputation of penis** ♂

● S38.23 **Traumatic amputation of scrotum and testis**

● S38.231 **Complete traumatic amputation of scrotum and testis** ♂

● S38.232 **Partial traumatic amputation of scrotum and testis** ♂

X● S38.3 **Transection (partial) of abdomen**

● S39 **Other and unspecified injuries of abdomen, lower back, pelvis and external genitals**
Code also any associated open wound (S31.-)

Excludes2 sprain of joints and ligaments of lumbar spine and pelvis (S33.-)

The appropriate 7th character is to be added to each code from category S39

A	initial encounter
D	subsequent encounter
S	sequela

● S39.0 **Injury of muscle, fascia and tendon of abdomen, lower back and pelvis**

● S39.00 **Unspecified injury of muscle, fascia and tendon of abdomen, lower back and pelvis**

● S39.001 **Unspecified injury of muscle, fascia and tendon of abdomen**

● S39.002 **Unspecified injury of muscle, fascia and tendon of lower back**

● S39.003 **Unspecified injury of muscle, fascia and tendon of pelvis**

● S39.01 **Strain of muscle, fascia and tendon of abdomen, lower back and pelvis**

● S39.011 **Strain of muscle, fascia and tendon of abdomen**

● S39.012 **Strain of muscle, fascia and tendon of lower back**

● S39.013 **Strain of muscle, fascia and tendon of pelvis**

● S39.02 **Laceration of muscle, fascia and tendon of abdomen, lower back and pelvis**

● S39.021 **Laceration of muscle, fascia and tendon of abdomen**

● S39.022 **Laceration of muscle, fascia and tendon of lower back**

● S39.023 **Laceration of muscle, fascia and tendon of pelvis**

● S39.09 **Other injury of muscle, fascia and tendon of abdomen, lower back and pelvis**

● S39.091 **Other injury of muscle, fascia and tendon of abdomen**

● S39.092 **Other injury of muscle, fascia and tendon of lower back**

● S39.093 **Other injury of muscle, fascia and tendon of pelvis**

● S39.8 **Other specified injuries of abdomen, lower back, pelvis and external genitals**

X● S39.81 **Other specified injuries of abdomen**

X● S39.82 **Other specified injuries of lower back**

X● S39.83 **Other specified injuries of pelvis**

● S39.84 **Other specified injuries of external genitals**

● S39.840 **Fracture of corpus cavernosum penis** ♂

● S39.848 **Other specified injuries of external genitals**

● S39.9 **Unspecified injury of abdomen, lower back, pelvis and external genitals**

X● S39.91 **Unspecified injury of abdomen**

X● S39.92 **Unspecified injury of lower back**

X● S39.93 **Unspecified injury of pelvis**

X● S39.94 **Unspecified injury of external genitals**

INJURIES TO THE SHOULDER AND UPPER ARM (S40-S49)

Includes	injuries of axilla injuries of scapular region
Excludes2	burns and corrosions (T20-T32)
	frostbite (T33-T34)
	injuries of elbow (S50-S59)
	insect bite or sting, venomous (T63.4)

● S40   Superficial injury of shoulder and upper arm

The appropriate 7th character is to be added to each code from category S40

A	initial encounter
D	subsequent encounter
S	sequela

● S40.0   Contusion of shoulder and upper arm
  ● S40.01   Contusion of shoulder
    ● S40.011   Contusion of right shoulder
    ● S40.012   Contusion of left shoulder
    ● S40.019   Contusion of unspecified shoulder
  ● S40.02   Contusion of upper arm
    ● S40.021   Contusion of right upper arm
    ● S40.022   Contusion of left upper arm
    ● S40.029   Contusion of unspecified upper arm

● S40.2   Other superficial injuries of shoulder
  ● S40.21   Abrasion of shoulder
    ● S40.211   Abrasion of right shoulder
    ● S40.212   Abrasion of left shoulder
    ● S40.219   Abrasion of unspecified shoulder
  ● S40.22   Blister (nonthermal) of shoulder
    ● S40.221   Blister (nonthermal) of right shoulder
    ● S40.222   Blister (nonthermal) of left shoulder
    ● S40.229   Blister (nonthermal) of unspecified shoulder
  ● S40.24   External constriction of shoulder
    ● S40.241   External constriction of right shoulder
    ● S40.242   External constriction of left shoulder
    ● S40.249   External constriction of unspecified shoulder
  ● S40.25   Superficial foreign body of shoulder
    Splinter in the shoulder
    ● S40.251   Superficial foreign body of right shoulder
    ● S40.252   Superficial foreign body of left shoulder
    ● S40.259   Superficial foreign body of unspecified shoulder
  ● S40.26   Insect bite (nonvenomous) of shoulder
    ● S40.261   Insect bite (nonvenomous) of right shoulder
    ● S40.262   Insect bite (nonvenomous) of left shoulder
    ● S40.269   Insect bite (nonvenomous) of unspecified shoulder
  ● S40.27   Other superficial bite of shoulder

Excludes1	open bite of shoulder (S41.05)

    ● S40.271   Other superficial bite of right shoulder
    ● S40.272   Other superficial bite of left shoulder
    ● S40.279   Other superficial bite of unspecified shoulder

● S40.8   Other superficial injuries of upper arm
  ● S40.81   Abrasion of upper arm
    ● S40.811   Abrasion of right upper arm
    ● S40.812   Abrasion of left upper arm
    ● S40.819   Abrasion of unspecified upper arm
  ● S40.82   Blister (nonthermal) of upper arm
    ● S40.821   Blister (nonthermal) of right upper arm
    ● S40.822   Blister (nonthermal) of left upper arm
    ● S40.829   Blister (nonthermal) of unspecified upper arm
  ● S40.84   External constriction of upper arm
    ● S40.841   External constriction of right upper arm
    ● S40.842   External constriction of left upper arm
    ● S40.849   External constriction of unspecified upper arm
  ● S40.85   Superficial foreign body of upper arm
    Splinter in the upper arm
    ● S40.851   Superficial foreign body of right upper arm
    ● S40.852   Superficial foreign body of left upper arm
    ● S40.859   Superficial foreign body of unspecified upper arm
  ● S40.86   Insect bite (nonvenomous) of upper arm
    ● S40.861   Insect bite (nonvenomous) of right upper arm
    ● S40.862   Insect bite (nonvenomous) of left upper arm
    ● S40.869   Insect bite (nonvenomous) of unspecified upper arm
  ● S40.87   Other superficial bite of upper arm

Excludes1	open bite of upper arm (S41.14)
Excludes2	other superficial bite of shoulder (S40.27-)

    ● S40.871   Other superficial bite of right upper arm
    ● S40.872   Other superficial bite of left upper arm
    ● S40.879   Other superficial bite of unspecified upper arm

● S40.9   Unspecified superficial injury of shoulder and upper arm
  ● S40.91   Unspecified superficial injury of shoulder
    ● S40.911   Unspecified superficial injury of right shoulder
    ● S40.912   Unspecified superficial injury of left shoulder
    ● S40.919   Unspecified superficial injury of unspecified shoulder
  ● S40.92   Unspecified superficial injury of upper arm
    ● S40.921   Unspecified superficial injury of right upper arm
    ● S40.922   Unspecified superficial injury of left upper arm
    ● S40.929   Unspecified superficial injury of unspecified upper arm

CHAPTER 19 (S00-T88)

● **S41**   **Open wound of shoulder and upper arm**

Code also any associated wound infection

Excludes1   traumatic amputation of shoulder and upper arm (S48.-)

Excludes2   open fracture of shoulder and upper arm (S42.- with 7th character B or C)

The appropriate 7th character is to be added to each code from category S41

> A   initial encounter
> D   subsequent encounter
> S   sequela

● **S41.0**   **Open wound of shoulder**

  ● **S41.00**   Unspecified open wound of shoulder

    ● **S41.001**   Unspecified open wound of right shoulder

    ● **S41.002**   Unspecified open wound of left shoulder

    ● **S41.009**   Unspecified open wound of unspecified shoulder

  ● **S41.01**   Laceration without foreign body of shoulder

    ● **S41.011**   Laceration without foreign body of right shoulder

    ● **S41.012**   Laceration without foreign body of left shoulder

    ● **S41.019**   Laceration without foreign body of unspecified shoulder

  ● **S41.02**   Laceration with foreign body of shoulder

    ● **S41.021**   Laceration with foreign body of right shoulder

    ● **S41.022**   Laceration with foreign body of left shoulder

    ● **S41.029**   Laceration with foreign body of unspecified shoulder

  ● **S41.03**   Puncture wound without foreign body of shoulder

    ● **S41.031**   Puncture wound without foreign body of right shoulder

    ● **S41.032**   Puncture wound without foreign body of left shoulder

    ● **S41.039**   Puncture wound without foreign body of unspecified shoulder

  ● **S41.04**   Puncture wound with foreign body of shoulder

    ● **S41.041**   Puncture wound with foreign body of right shoulder

    ● **S41.042**   Puncture wound with foreign body of left shoulder

    ● **S41.049**   Puncture wound with foreign body of unspecified shoulder

  ● **S41.05**   Open bite of shoulder

Bite of shoulder NOS

Excludes1   superficial bite of shoulder (S40.27)

    ● **S41.051**   Open bite of right shoulder

    ● **S41.052**   Open bite of left shoulder

    ● **S41.059**   Open bite of unspecified shoulder

● **S41.1**   **Open wound of upper arm**

  ● **S41.10**   Unspecified open wound of upper arm

    ● **S41.101**   Unspecified open wound of right upper arm

    ● **S41.102**   Unspecified open wound of left upper arm

    ● **S41.109**   Unspecified open wound of unspecified upper arm

  ● **S41.11**   Laceration without foreign body of upper arm

    ● **S41.111**   Laceration without foreign body of right upper arm

    ● **S41.112**   Laceration without foreign body of left upper arm

    ● **S41.119**   Laceration without foreign body of unspecified upper arm

  ● **S41.12**   Laceration with foreign body of upper arm

    ● **S41.121**   Laceration with foreign body of right upper arm

    ● **S41.122**   Laceration with foreign body of left upper arm

    ● **S41.129**   Laceration with foreign body of unspecified upper arm

  ● **S41.13**   Puncture wound without foreign body of upper arm

    ● **S41.131**   Puncture wound without foreign body of right upper arm

    ● **S41.132**   Puncture wound without foreign body of left upper arm

    ● **S41.139**   Puncture wound without foreign body of unspecified upper arm

  ● **S41.14**   Puncture wound with foreign body of upper arm

    ● **S41.141**   Puncture wound with foreign body of right upper arm

    ● **S41.142**   Puncture wound with foreign body of left upper arm

    ● **S41.149**   Puncture wound with foreign body of unspecified upper arm

  ● **S41.15**   Open bite of upper arm

Bite of upper arm NOS

Excludes1   superficial bite of upper arm (S40.87)

    ● **S41.151**   Open bite of right upper arm

    ● **S41.152**   Open bite of left upper arm

    ● **S41.159**   Open bite of unspecified upper arm

● **S42**   **Fracture of shoulder and upper arm**

Note: A fracture not indicated as displaced or nondisplaced should be coded to displaced

A fracture not indicated as open or closed should be coded to closed

Excludes1   traumatic amputation of shoulder and upper arm (S48.-)

The appropriate 7th character is to be added to all codes from category S42

> A   initial encounter for closed fracture
> B   initial encounter for open fracture
> D   subsequent encounter for fracture with routine healing
> G   subsequent encounter for fracture with delayed healing
> K   subsequent encounter for fracture with nonunion
> P   subsequent encounter for fracture with malunion
> S   sequela

● **S42.0**   **Fracture of clavicle**

(Ex) For S42.0[B]: S42.001-S42.036[A,B], S62.90X[B] For S42.0[K,P]: See S02.0[K]

  ● **S42.00**   Fracture of unspecified part of clavicle

    ● **S42.001**   Fracture of unspecified part of right clavicle B, K, P ⬙, B ⬙

    ● **S42.002**   Fracture of unspecified part of left clavicle B, K, P ⬙, B ⬙

    ● **S42.009**   Fracture of unspecified part of unspecified clavicle B, K, P ⬙, B ⬙
      Coding Clinic: 2012, Q4, P3

  ● **S42.01**   Fracture of sternal end of clavicle

    ● **S42.011**   Anterior displaced fracture of sternal end of right clavicle B, K, P ⬙, B ⬙

    ● **S42.012**   Anterior displaced fracture of sternal end of left clavicle B, K, P ⬙, B ⬙

    ● **S42.013**   Anterior displaced fracture of sternal end of unspecified clavicle B, K, P ⬙, B ⬙

Displaced fracture of sternal end of clavicle NOS

◀ New   ◀⊪ Revised   ~~deleted~~ Deleted   Excludes 1   Excludes 2   Includes   Use additional   Code first   Code also   Unspecified

OGCR Official Guidelines   ● Unacceptable Principal Diagnosis   X Assign placeholder X   ● Use Additional Character(s)   ▷ Manifestation Code   **Coding Clinic**

● S42.014 Posterior displaced fracture of sternal end of right clavicle B, K, P 🍪, B 🍪

● S42.015 Posterior displaced fracture of sternal end of left clavicle B, K, P 🍪, B 🍪

● S42.016 Posterior displaced fracture of sternal end of unspecified clavicle B, K, P 🍪, B 🍪

● S42.017 Nondisplaced fracture of sternal end of right clavicle B, K, P 🍪, B 🍪

● S42.018 Nondisplaced fracture of sternal end of left clavicle B, K, P 🍪, B 🍪

● S42.019 Nondisplaced fracture of sternal end of unspecified clavicle B, K, P 🍪, B 🍪

● S42.02 Fracture of shaft of clavicle

● S42.021 Displaced fracture of shaft of right clavicle B, K, P 🍪, B 🍪

● S42.022 Displaced fracture of shaft of left clavicle B, K, P 🍪, B 🍪

● S42.023 Displaced fracture of shaft of unspecified clavicle B, K, P 🍪, B 🍪

● S42.024 Nondisplaced fracture of shaft of right clavicle B, K, P 🍪, B 🍪

● S42.025 Nondisplaced fracture of shaft of left clavicle B, K, P 🍪, B 🍪

● S42.026 Nondisplaced fracture of shaft of unspecified clavicle B, K, P 🍪, B 🍪

● S42.03 Fracture of lateral end of clavicle
Fracture of acromial end of clavicle

● S42.031 Displaced fracture of lateral end of right clavicle B, K, P 🍪, B 🍪

● S42.032 Displaced fracture of lateral end of left clavicle B, K, P 🍪, B 🍪

● S42.033 Displaced fracture of lateral end of unspecified clavicle B, K, P 🍪, B 🍪

● S42.034 Nondisplaced fracture of lateral end of right clavicle B, K, P 🍪, B 🍪

● S42.035 Nondisplaced fracture of lateral end of left clavicle B, K, P 🍪, B 🍪

● S42.036 Nondisplaced fracture of lateral end of unspecified clavicle B, K, P 🍪, B 🍪

● S42.1 Fracture of scapula
(Ex) For S42.1[B]: S42.101-S42.199[A,B], S62.90X[B] For S42.1[K,P]: See S02.0[K]

● S42.10 Fracture of unspecified part of scapula

● S42.101 Fracture of unspecified part of scapula, right shoulder B, K, P 🍪, B 🍪

● S42.102 Fracture of unspecified part of scapula, left shoulder B, K, P 🍪, B 🍪

● S42.109 Fracture of unspecified part of scapula, unspecified shoulder B, K, P 🍪, B 🍪

● S42.11 Fracture of body of scapula

● S42.111 Displaced fracture of body of scapula, right shoulder B, K, P 🍪, B 🍪

● S42.112 Displaced fracture of body of scapula, left shoulder B, K, P 🍪, B 🍪

● S42.113 Displaced fracture of body of scapula, unspecified shoulder B, K, P 🍪, B 🍪

● S42.114 Nondisplaced fracture of body of scapula, right shoulder B, K, P 🍪, B 🍪

● S42.115 Nondisplaced fracture of body of scapula, left shoulder B, K, P 🍪, B 🍪

● S42.116 Nondisplaced fracture of body of scapula, unspecified shoulder B, K, P 🍪, B 🍪

● S42.12 Fracture of acromial process

● S42.121 Displaced fracture of acromial process, right shoulder B, K, P 🍪, B 🍪

● S42.122 Displaced fracture of acromial process, left shoulder B, K, P 🍪, B 🍪

● S42.123 Displaced fracture of acromial process, unspecified shoulder B, K, P 🍪, B 🍪

● S42.124 Nondisplaced fracture of acromial process, right shoulder B, K, P 🍪, B 🍪

● S42.125 Nondisplaced fracture of acromial process, left shoulder B, K, P 🍪, B 🍪

● S42.126 Nondisplaced fracture, of acromial process, unspecified shoulder B, K, P 🍪, B 🍪

● S42.13 Fracture of coracoid process

● S42.131 Displaced fracture of coracoid process, right shoulder B, K, P 🍪, B 🍪

● S42.132 Displaced fracture of coracoid process, left shoulder B, K, P 🍪, B 🍪

● S42.133 Displaced fracture of coracoid process, unspecified shoulder B, K, P 🍪, B 🍪

● S42.134 Nondisplaced fracture of coracoid process, right shoulder B, K, P 🍪, B 🍪

● S42.135 Nondisplaced fracture of coracoid process, left shoulder B, K, P 🍪, B 🍪

● S42.136 Nondisplaced fracture of coracoid process, unspecified shoulder B, K, P 🍪, B 🍪

● S42.14 Fracture of glenoid cavity of scapula

● S42.141 Displaced fracture of glenoid cavity of scapula, right shoulder B, K, P 🍪, B 🍪

● S42.142 Displaced fracture of glenoid cavity of scapula, left shoulder B, K, P 🍪, B 🍪

● S42.143 Displaced fracture of glenoid cavity of scapula, unspecified shoulder B, K, P 🍪, B 🍪

● S42.144 Nondisplaced fracture of glenoid cavity of scapula, right shoulder B, K, P 🍪, B 🍪

● S42.145 Nondisplaced fracture of glenoid cavity of scapula, left shoulder B, K, P 🍪, B 🍪

● S42.146 Nondisplaced fracture of glenoid cavity of scapula, unspecified shoulder B, K, P 🍪, B 🍪

● S42.15 Fracture of neck of scapula

● S42.151 Displaced fracture of neck of scapula, right shoulder B, K, P 🍪, B 🍪

● S42.152 Displaced fracture of neck of scapula, left shoulder B, K, P 🍪, B 🍪

● S42.153 Displaced fracture of neck of scapula, unspecified shoulder B, K, P 🍪, B 🍪

● S42.154 Nondisplaced fracture of neck of scapula, right shoulder B, K, P 🍪, B 🍪

● S42.155 Nondisplaced fracture of neck of scapula, left shoulder B, K, P 🍪, B 🍪

● S42.156 Nondisplaced fracture of neck of scapula, unspecified shoulder B, K, P 🍪, B 🍪

● S42.19 Fracture of other part of scapula

● S42.191 Fracture of other part of scapula, right shoulder B, K, P 🍪, B 🍪

● S42.192 Fracture of other part of scapula, left shoulder B, K, P 🍪, B 🍪

● S42.199 Fracture of other part of scapula, unspecified shoulder B, K, P 🍪, B 🍪

● **S42.2**   **Fracture of upper end of humerus**
       Fracture of proximal end of humerus
         Excludes2   fracture of shaft of humerus (S42.3-)
                 physeal fracture of upper end of humerus
                 (S49.0-)

  ● **S42.20**   **Unspecified fracture of upper end of humerus**

    ● **S42.201**   **Unspecified fracture of upper end of right humerus** A, K, P ◐, B ◑, A, B ◑

       Ⓔⓧ **For S42.201[A]:** S42.201[A,B], S42.202[B], S42.209-S42.211[A,B], S42.212[B], S42.213-S42.214[A,B], S42.215[B], S42.216-S42.221[A,B], S42.222[B], S42.223-S42.224[A,B], S42.225[B], S42.226-S42.231[A,B], S42.232[B], S42.239-S42.241[A,B], S42.242[B], S42.249-S42.251[A,B], S42.252[B], S42.253-S42.254[A,B], S42.255[B], S42.256-S42.261[A,B], S42.262[B], S42.263-S42.264[A,B], S42.265[B], S42.266[A,B], S42.271[A], S42.279[A], S42.291[A,B], S42.292[B], S42.293-S42.294[A,B], S42.295[B], S42.296-S42.301[A,B], S42.302[B], S42.309[A,B], S42.311[A], S42.319[A], S42.321[A,B], S42.322[B], S42.323-S42.324[A,B], S42.325[B], S42.326-S42.331[A,B], S42.332[B], S42.333-S42.334[A,B], S42.335[B], S42.336-S42.341[A,B], S42.342[B], S42.343-S42.344[A,B], S42.345[B], S42.346-S42.351[A,B], S42.352[B], S42.353-S42.354[A,B], S42.355[B], S42.356-S42.361[A,B], S42.362[B], S42.363-S42.364[A,B], S42.365[B], S42.366-S42.391[A,B], S42.392[B], S42.399-S42.401[A,B], S42.402[B], S42.409-S42.411[A,B], S42.412[B], S42.413-S42.414[A,B], S42.415[B], S42.416-S42.421[A,B], S42.422[B], S42.423-S42.424[A,B], S42.425[B], S42.426-S42.431[A,B], S42.432[B], S42.433-S42.434[A,B], S42.435[B], S42.436-S42.441[A,B], S42.442[B], S42.443-S42.444[A,B], S42.445[B], S42.446-S42.447[A,B], S42.448[B], S42.449-S42.451[A,B], S42.452[B], S42.453-S42.454[A,B], S42.455[B], S42.456-S42.461[A,B], S42.462[B], S42.463-S42.464[A,B], S42.465[B], S42.466-S42.471[A,B], S42.472[B], S42.473-S42.474[A,B], S42.475[B], S42.476 [A,B], S42.481[A], S42.489[A], S42.491[A,B], S42.492[B], S42.493-S42.494[A,B], S42.495[B], S42.496-S42.92X[A,B], S49.001[A], S49.009-S49.011[A], S49.019-S49.021[A], S49.029-S49.031[A], S49.039-S49.041[A], S49.049-S49.091[A], S49.099-S49.101[A], S49.109-S49.111[A], S49.119-S49.121[A], S49.129-S49.131[A], S49.139-S49.141[A], S49.149-S49.191[A], S49.199[A]
       For S42.201[B]: S42.201-S42.266[B], S42.291-S42.296[B], S42.301-S42.309[A,B], S42.311-S42.319[A], S42.321-S42.476[A,B], S42.481-S42.489[A], S42.491-S42.92X[A,B], S49.101-S49.199[A], S62.90X[B]
       For S42.201[K,P]: See S02.0[K]

    ● **S42.202**   **Unspecified fracture of upper end of left humerus** A, K, P ◐, B ◑, A, B ◑

       Ⓔⓧ **For category S42.202 CC codes**
       S42.202[A]: S42.201[B], S42.202-S42.209[A,B], S42.211[B], S42.212-S42.213[A,B], S42.214[B], S42.215-S42.216[A,B], S42.221[B], S42.222-S42.223[A,B], S42.224[B], S42.225-S42.226[A,B], S42.231[B], S42.232-S42.239[A,B], S42.241[B], S42.242-S42.249[A,B], S42.251[B], S42.252-S42.253[A,B], S42.254[B], S42.255-S42.256[A,B], S42.261[B], S42.262-S42.263[A,B], S42.264[B], S42.265-S42.266[A,B], S42.272-S42.279[A], S42.291[B], S42.292-S42.293[A,B], S42.294[B], S42.295-S42.296[A,B], S42.301[B], S42.302-S42.309[A,B], S42.312-S42.319[A], S42.321[B], S42.322-S42.323[A,B], S42.324[B], S42.325-S42.326[A,B], S42.331[B], S42.332-S42.333[A,B], S42.334[B], S42.335-S42.336[A,B], S42.341[B], S42.342-S42.343[A,B], S42.344[B], S42.345-S42.346[A,B], S42.351[B], S42.352-S42.353[A,B], S42.354[B], S42.355-S42.356[A,B], S42.361[B], S42.362-S42.363[A,B], S42.364[B], S42.365-S42.366[A,B], S42.391[B], S42.392-S42.399[A,B], S42.401[B], S42.402-S42.409[A,B], S42.411[B], S42.412-S42.413[A,B], S42.414[B], S42.415-S42.416[A,B], S42.421[B], S42.422-S42.423[A,B], S42.424[B], S42.425-S42.426[A,B], S42.431[B], S42.432-S42.433[A,B], S42.434[B], S42.435-S42.436[A,B], S42.441[B], S42.442-S42.443[A,B], S42.444[B], S42.445-S42.446[A,B], S42.447[B], S42.448-S42.449[A,B], S42.451[B], S42.452-S42.453[A,B], S42.454[B], S42.455-S42.456[A,B], S42.461[B], S42.462-S42.463[A,B], S42.464[B], S42.465-S42.466[A,B], S42.471[B], S42.472-S42.473[A,B], S42.474[B], S42.475-S42.476[A,B], S42.482-S42.489[A], S42.491[B], S42.492-S42.493[A,B], S42.494[B], S42.495-S42.92X[A,B], S49.002-S49.009[A], S49.012-S49.019[A], S49.022-S49.029[A], S49.032-S49.039[A], S49.042-S49.049[A], S49.092-S49.099[A], S49.102-S49.109[A], S49.112-S49.119[A], S49.122-S49.129[A], S49.132-S49.139[A], S49.142-S49.149[A], S49.192-S49.199[A]
       For S42.202[B]: See S42.201[B]
       For S42.202[K,P]: See S02.0[K]

    ● **S42.209**   **Unspecified fracture of upper end of unspecified humerus** A, K, P ◐, B ◑, A, B ◑

       Ⓔⓧ **For S42.209[A]:** S42.201-S42.266[A,B], S42.271-S42.279[A], S42.291-S42.309[A,B], S42.311-S42.319[A], S42.321-S42.476[A,B], S42.481-S42.489[A], S42.491-S42.92X[A,B], S49.001-S49.199[A] **For S42.202[B]:** See S42.201[B] **For S42.202[K,P]:** See S02.0[K]

◀ New   ◀▬ Revised   ~~deleted~~ Deleted   Excludes 1   Excludes 2   Includes   Use additional   Code first   Code also   Unspecified
OGCR Official Guidelines   ● Unacceptable Principal Diagnosis   X Assign placeholder X   ● Use Additional Character(s)   ▶ Manifestation Code   **Coding Clinic**

● **S42.21** Unspecified fracture of surgical neck of humerus
Fracture of neck of humerus NOS

● **S42.211** Unspecified displaced fracture of surgical neck of right humerus A, K, P 🔹, B 🔹, A, B 🔹
Ⓔⓧ For S42.211[A]: See S42.201[A]
For S42.211[B]: See S42.201[B]
For S42.211[K,P]: See S02.0[K]

● **S42.212** Unspecified displaced fracture of surgical neck of left humerus A, K, P 🔹, B 🔹, A, B 🔹
Ⓔⓧ For S42.212[A]: See S42.202[A]
For S42.212[B]: See S42.201[B]
For S42.212[K,P]: See S02.0[K]

● **S42.213** Unspecified displaced fracture of surgical neck of unspecified humerus A, K, P 🔹, B 🔹, A, B 🔹
Ⓔⓧ For S42.213[A]: See S42.209[A]
For S42.213[B]: See S42.201[B]
For S42.213[K,P]: See S02.0[K]

● **S42.214** Unspecified nondisplaced fracture of surgical neck of right humerus A, K, P 🔹, B 🔹, A, B 🔹
Ⓔⓧ For S42.214[A]: See S42.201[A]
For S42.214[B]: See S42.201[B]
For S42.214[K,P]: See S02.0[K]

● **S42.215** Unspecified nondisplaced fracture of surgical neck of left humerus A, K, P 🔹, B 🔹, A, B 🔹
Ⓔⓧ For S42.215[A]: See S42.202[A]
For S42.215[B]: See S42.201[B]
For S42.215[K,P]: See S02.0[K]

● **S42.216** Unspecified nondisplaced fracture of surgical neck of unspecified humerus A, K, P 🔹, B 🔹, A, B 🔹
Ⓔⓧ For S42.216[A]: See S42.209[A]
For S42.216[B]: See S42.201[B]
For S42.216[K,P]: See S02.0[K]

● **S42.22** 2-part fracture of surgical neck of humerus

● **S42.221** 2-part displaced fracture of surgical neck of right humerus A, K, P 🔹, B 🔹, A, B 🔹
Ⓔⓧ For S42.221[A]: See S42.201[A]
For S42.221[B]: See S42.201[B]
For S42.221[K,P]: See S02.0[K]

● **S42.222** 2-part displaced fracture of surgical neck of left humerus A, K, P 🔹, B 🔹, A, B 🔹
Ⓔⓧ For S42.222[A]: See S42.202[A]
For S42.222[B]: See S42.201[B]
For S42.222[K,P]: See S02.0[K]

● **S42.223** 2-part displaced fracture of surgical neck of unspecified humerus A, K, P 🔹, B 🔹, A, B 🔹
Ⓔⓧ For S42.223[A]: See S42.209[A]
For S42.223[B]: See S42.201[B]
For S42.223[K,P]: See S02.0[K]

● **S42.224** 2-part nondisplaced fracture of surgical neck of right humerus A, K, P 🔹, B 🔹, A, B 🔹
Ⓔⓧ For S42.224[A]: See S42.201[A]
For S42.224[B]: See S42.201[B]
For S42.224[K,P]: See S02.0[K]

● **S42.225** 2-part nondisplaced fracture of surgical neck of left humerus A, K, P 🔹, B 🔹, A, B 🔹
Ⓔⓧ For S42.225[A]: See S42.202[A]
For S42.225[B]: See S42.201[B]
For S42.225[K,P]: See S02.0[K]

● **S42.226** 2-part nondisplaced fracture of surgical neck of unspecified humerus A, K, P 🔹, B 🔹, A, B 🔹
Ⓔⓧ For S42.226[A]: See S42.209[A]
For S42.226[B]: See S42.201[B]
For S42.226[K,P]: See S02.0[K]

● **S42.23** 3-part fracture of surgical neck of humerus

● **S42.231** 3-part fracture of surgical neck of right humerus A, K, P 🔹, B 🔹, A, B 🔹
Ⓔⓧ For S42.231[A]: See S42.201[A]
For S42.231[B]: See S42.201[B]
For S42.231[K,P]: See S02.0[K]

● **S42.232** 3-part fracture of surgical neck of left humerus A, K, P 🔹, B 🔹, A, B 🔹
Ⓔⓧ For S42.232[A]: See S42.202[A]
For S42.232[B]: See S42.201[B]
For S42.232[K,P]: See S02.0[K]

● **S42.239** 3-part fracture of surgical neck of unspecified humerus A, K, P 🔹, B 🔹, A, B 🔹
Ⓔⓧ For S42.239[A]: See S42.209[A]
For S42.239[B]: See S42.201[B]
For S42.239[K,P]: See S02.0[K]

● **S42.24** 4-part fracture of surgical neck of humerus

● **S42.241** 4-part fracture of surgical neck of right humerus A, K, P 🔹, B 🔹, A, B 🔹
Ⓔⓧ For S42.241[A]: See S42.201[A]
For S42.241[B]: See S42.201[B]
For S42.241[K,P]: See S02.0[K]

● **S42.242** 4-part fracture of surgical neck of left humerus A, K, P 🔹, B 🔹, A, B 🔹
Ⓔⓧ For S42.242[A]: See S42.202[A]
For S42.242[B]: See S42.201[B]
For S42.242[K,P]: See S02.0[K]

● **S42.249** 4-part fracture of surgical neck of unspecified humerus A, K, P 🔹, B 🔹, A, B 🔹
Ⓔⓧ For S42.249[A]: See S42.209[A]
For S42.249[B]: See S42.201[B]
For S42.249[K,P]: See S02.0[K]

● **S42.25** Fracture of greater tuberosity of humerus

● **S42.251** Displaced fracture of greater tuberosity of right humerus A, K, P 🔹, B 🔹, A, B 🔹
Ⓔⓧ For S42.251[A]: See S42.201[A]
For S42.251[B]: See S42.201[B]
For S42.251[K,P]: See S02.0[K]

● **S42.252** Displaced fracture of greater tuberosity of left humerus A, K, P 🔹, B 🔹, A, B 🔹
Ⓔⓧ For S42.252[A]: See S42.202[A]
For S42.252[B]: See S42.201[B]
For S42.252[K,P]: See S02.0[K]

● **S42.253** Displaced fracture of greater tuberosity of unspecified humerus A, K, P 🔹, B 🔹, A, B 🔹
Ⓔⓧ For category S42.253 CC codes
S42.253[A]: See S42.209[A]
For S42.253[B]: See S42.201[B]
For S42.253[K,P]: See S02.0[K]

● **S42.254** Nondisplaced fracture of greater tuberosity of right humerus A, K, P 🔹, B 🔹, A, B 🔹
Ⓔⓧ For S42.254[A]: See S42.201[A]
For S42.254[B]: See S42.201[B]
For S42.254[K,P]: See S02.0[K]

● **S42.255** Nondisplaced fracture of greater tuberosity of left humerus A, K, P 🔹, B 🔹, A, B 🔹
Ⓔⓧ For S42.255[A]: See S42.202[A]
For S42.255[B]: See S42.201[B]
For S42.255[K,P]: See S02.0[K]

● **S42.256** Nondisplaced fracture of greater tuberosity of unspecified humerus A, K, P 🔹, B 🔹, A, B 🔹
Ⓔⓧ For S42.256[A]: See S42.209[A]
For S42.256[B]: See S42.201[B]
For S42.256[K,P]: See S02.0[K]

CHAPTER 19 (S00-T88)

N Newborn Age: 0 **P** Pediatric Age: 0–17 **M** Maternity DX: 12–55 **A** Adult Age: 15–124 ♀ Females Only ♂ Males Only

🔹 Complication\Comorbidity 🔹 Major C\C Ⓔⓧ CC/MCC Exclusions 🔹 Hospital-Acquired Condition

1279

● **S42.26**   **Fracture of lesser tuberosity of humerus**
  ● **S42.261**   **Displaced fracture of lesser tuberosity of right humerus** A, K, P 🔾, B 🔾, A, B 🔾
    (Ex) **For S42.261[A]:** See S42.201[A]
    For S42.261[B]: See S42.201[B]
    For S42.261[K,P]: See S02.0[K]

  ● **S42.262**   **Displaced fracture of lesser tuberosity of left humerus** A, K, P 🔾, B 🔾, A, B 🔾
    (Ex) **For S42.262[A]:** See S42.202[A]
    For S42.262[B]: See S42.201[B]
    For S42.262[K,P]: See S02.0[K]

  ● **S42.263**   **Displaced fracture of lesser tuberosity of unspecified humerus** A, K, P 🔾, B 🔾, A, B 🔾
    (Ex) **For S42.263[A]:** See S42.209[A]
    For S42.263[B]: See S42.201[B]
    For S42.263[K,P]: See S02.0[K]

  ● **S42.264**   **Nondisplaced fracture of lesser tuberosity of right humerus** A, K, P 🔾, B 🔾, A, B 🔾
    (Ex) **For S42.264[A]:** See S42.201[A]
    For S42.264[B]: See S42.201[B]
    For S42.264[K,P]: See S02.0[K]

  ● **S42.265**   **Nondisplaced fracture of lesser tuberosity of left humerus** A, K, P 🔾, B 🔾, A, B 🔾
    (Ex) **For S42.265[A]:** See S42.202[A]
    For S42.265[B]: See S42.201[B]
    For S42.265[K,P]: See S02.0[K]

  ● **S42.266**   **Nondisplaced fracture of lesser tuberosity of unspecified humerus** A, K, P 🔾, B 🔾, A, B 🔾
    (Ex) **For S42.266[A]:** See S42.209[A]
    For S42.266[B]: See S42.201[B]
    For S42.266[K,P]: See S02.0[K]

● **S42.27**   **Torus fracture of upper end of humerus**
The appropriate 7th character is to be added to all codes in subcategory S42.27

A	initial encounter for closed fracture
D	subsequent encounter for fracture with routine healing
G	subsequent encounter for fracture with delayed healing
K	subsequent encounter for fracture with nonunion
P	subsequent encounter for fracture with malunion
S	sequela

  ● **S42.271**   **Torus fracture of upper end of right humerus** A, K, P 🔾, A 🔾
    (Ex) **For S42.271[A]:** See S42.201[A]
    For S42.271[K,P]: See S02.0[K]

  ● **S42.272**   **Torus fracture of upper end of left humerus** A, K, P 🔾, A 🔾
    (Ex) **For S42.272[A]:** See S42.202[A]
    For S42.272[K,P]: See S02.0[K]

  ● **S42.279**   **Torus fracture of upper end of unspecified humerus** A, K, P 🔾, A 🔾
    (Ex) **For S42.279[A]:** See S42.209[A]
    For S42.279[K,P]: See S02.0[K]

● **S42.29**   **Other fracture of upper end of humerus**
Fracture of anatomical neck of humerus
Fracture of articular head of humerus
  ● **S42.291**   **Other displaced fracture of upper end of right humerus** A, K, P 🔾, B 🔾, A, B 🔾
    (Ex) **For S42.291[A]:** See S42.201[A]
    For S42.291[B]: See S42.201[B]
    For S42.291[K,P]: See S02.0[K]

  ● **S42.292**   **Other displaced fracture of upper end of left humerus** A, K, P 🔾, B 🔾, A, B 🔾
    (Ex) **For S42.292[A]:** See S42.202[A]
    For S42.292[B]: See S42.201[B]
    For S42.292[K,P]: See S02.0[K]

  ● **S42.293**   **Other displaced fracture of upper end of unspecified humerus** A, K, P 🔾, B 🔾, A, B 🔾
    (Ex) **For S42.293[A]:** See S42.209[A]
    For S42.293[B]: See S42.201[B]
    For S42.293[K,P]: See S02.0[K]

  ● **S42.294**   **Other nondisplaced fracture of upper end of right humerus** A, K, P 🔾, B 🔾, A, B 🔾
    (Ex) **For S42.294[A]:** See S42.201[A]
    For S42.294[B]: See S42.201[B]
    For S42.294[K,P]: See S02.0[K]

  ● **S42.295**   **Other nondisplaced fracture of upper end of left humerus** A, K, P 🔾, B 🔾, A, B 🔾
    (Ex) **For S42.295[A]:** See S42.202[A]
    For S42.295[B]: See S42.201[B]
    For S42.295[K,P]: See S02.0[K]

  ● **S42.296**   **Other nondisplaced fracture of upper end of unspecified humerus** A, K, P 🔾, B 🔾, A, B 🔾
    (Ex) **For S42.296[A]:** See S42.209[A]
    For S42.296[B]: See S42.201[B]
    For S42.296[K,P]: See S02.0[K]

● **S42.3**   **Fracture of shaft of humerus**
Fracture of humerus NOS
Fracture of upper arm NOS
Excludes2   physeal fractures of upper end of humerus (S49.0-)
physeal fractures of lower end of humerus (S49.1-)

  ● **S42.30**   **Unspecified fracture of shaft of humerus**
    ● **S42.301**   **Unspecified fracture of shaft of humerus, right arm** A, K, P 🔾, B 🔾, A, B 🔾
      (Ex) **For S42.301[A]:** See S42.201[A]
      For S42.301[B]: See S42.201[B]
      For S42.301[K,P]: See S02.0[K]

    ● **S42.302**   **Unspecified fracture of shaft of humerus, left arm** A, K, P 🔾, B 🔾, A, B 🔾
      (Ex) **For S42.302[A]:** See S42.202[A]
      For S42.302[B]: See S42.201[B]
      For S42.302[K,P]: See S02.0[K]

    ● **S42.309**   **Unspecified fracture of shaft of humerus, unspecified arm** A, K, P 🔾, B 🔾, A, B 🔾
      (Ex) **For S42.309[A]:** See S42.209[A]
      For S42.309[B]: See S42.201[B]
      For S42.309[K,P]: See S02.0[K]

◀ New   ◀▥ Revised   ~~deleted~~ Deleted   Excludes 1   Excludes 2   Includes   Use additional   Code first   Code also   Unspecified
OGCR Official Guidelines   ● Unacceptable Principal Diagnosis   X Assign placeholder X   ● Use Additional Character(s)   ▶ Manifestation Code   **Coding Clinic**

● **S42.31**   **Greenstick fracture of shaft of humerus**

> The appropriate 7th character is to be added to all codes in subcategory S42.31

A	initial encounter for closed fracture
D	subsequent encounter for fracture with routine healing
G	subsequent encounter for fracture with delayed healing
K	subsequent encounter for fracture with nonunion
P	subsequent encounter for fracture with malunion
S	sequela

● **S42.311**   **Greenstick fracture of shaft of humerus, right arm** A, K, P 🐾, A 🐾

> (Ex:) **For category S42.311 CC codes**
> S42.311[A]: S42.311[A],
> S42.319-S42.321[A], S42.323-S42.324[A],
> S42.326-S42.331[A], S42.333-S42.334[A],
> S42.336-S42.341[A], S42.343-S42.344[A],
> S42.346-S42.351[A], S42.353-S42.354[A],
> S42.356-S42.361[A], S42.363-S42.364[A],
> S42.366-S42.391[A], S42.399[A]
> **For S42.311[K,P]:** See S02.0[K]

● **S42.312**   **Greenstick fracture of shaft of humerus, left arm** A, K, P 🐾, A 🐾

> (Ex:) **For category S42.312 CC codes**
> S42.312[A]: S42.312-S42.319[A],
> S42.322-S42.323[A], S42.325-S42.326[A],
> S42.332-S42.333[A], S42.335-S42.336[A],
> S42.342-S42.343[A], S42.345-S42.346[A],
> S42.352-S42.353[A], S42.355-S42.356[A],
> S42.362-S42.363[A], S42.365-S42.366[A],
> S42.392-S42.399[A] **For S42.312[K,P]:** See
> S02.0[K]

● **S42.319**   **Greenstick fracture of shaft of humerus, unspecified arm** A, K, P 🐾, A 🐾

> (Ex:) **For category S42.319 CC codes**
> S42.319[A]: S42.311-S42.399[A]
> **For S42.319[K,P]:** See S02.0[K]

● **S42.32**   **Transverse fracture of shaft of humerus**

● **S42.321**   **Displaced transverse fracture of shaft of humerus, right arm** A, K, P 🐾, B 🐾, A, B 🐾

> (Ex:) **For category S42.321 CC codes**
> S42.321[A]: See S42.311[A]
> **For S42.321[B]:** See S42.201[B]
> **For S42.321[K,P]:** See S02.0[K]

● **S42.322**   **Displaced transverse fracture of shaft of humerus, left arm** A, K, P 🐾, B 🐾, A, B 🐾

> (Ex:) **For category S42.322 CC codes**
> S42.322[A]: See S42.312[A]
> **For S42.322[B]:** See S42.201[B]
> **For S42.322[K,P]:** See S02.0[K]

● **S42.323**   **Displaced transverse fracture of shaft of humerus, unspecified arm** A, K, P 🐾, B 🐾, A, B 🐾

> (Ex:) **For category S42.323 CC codes**
> S42.323[A]: S42.311-S42.399[A]
> **For S42.323[B]:** See S42.201[B]
> **For S42.313[K,P]:** See S02.0[K]

● **S42.324**   **Nondisplaced transverse fracture of shaft of humerus, right arm** A, K, P 🐾, B 🐾, A, B 🐾

> (Ex:) **For category S42.324 CC codes**
> S42.324[A]: See S42.311[A]
> **For S42.324[B]:** See S42.201[B]
> **For S42.324[K,P]:** See S02.0[K]

● **S42.325**   **Nondisplaced transverse fracture of shaft of humerus, left arm** A, K, P 🐾, B 🐾, A, B 🐾

> (Ex:) **For category S42.325 CC codes**
> S42.325[A]: See S42.312[A]
> **For S42.325[B]:** See S42.201[B]
> **For S42.325[K,P]:** See S02.0[K]

● **S42.326**   **Nondisplaced transverse fracture of shaft of humerus, unspecified arm** A, K, P 🐾, B 🐾, A, B 🐾

> (Ex:) **For category S42.326 CC codes**
> S42.326[A]: S42.311-S42.399[A]
> **For S42.326[B]:** See S42.201[B]
> **For S42.316[K,P]:** See S02.0[K]

● **S42.33**   **Oblique fracture of shaft of humerus**

● **S42.331**   **Displaced oblique fracture of shaft of humerus, right arm** A, K, P 🐾, B 🐾, A, B 🐾

> (Ex:) **For category S42.331 CC codes**
> S42.331[A]: See S42.311[A]
> **For S42.331[B]:** See S42.201[B]
> **For S42.331[K,P]:** See S02.0[K]

● **S42.332**   **Displaced oblique fracture of shaft of humerus, left arm** A, K, P 🐾, B 🐾, A, B 🐾

> (Ex:) **For category S42.332 CC codes**
> S42.332[A]: See S42.312[A]
> **For S42.332[B]:** See S42.201[B]
> **For S42.332[K,P]:** See S02.0[K]

● **S42.333**   **Displaced oblique fracture of shaft of humerus, unspecified arm** A, K, P 🐾, B 🐾, A, B 🐾

> (Ex:) **For category S42.333 CC codes**
> S42.333[A]: S42.311-S42.399[A]
> **For S42.333[B]:** See S42.201[B]
> **For S42.333[K,P]:** See S02.0[K]

● **S42.334**   **Nondisplaced oblique fracture of shaft of humerus, right arm** A, K, P 🐾, B 🐾, A, B 🐾

> (Ex:) **For category S42.334 CC codes**
> S42.334[A]: See S42.311[A]
> **For S42.334[B]:** See S42.201[B]
> **For S42.334[K,P]:** See S02.0[K]

● **S42.335**   **Nondisplaced oblique fracture of shaft of humerus, left arm** A, K, P 🐾, B 🐾, A, B 🐾

> (Ex:) **For category S42.335 CC codes**
> S42.335[A]: See S42.312[A]
> **For S42.335[B]:** See S42.201[B]
> **For S42.335[K,P]:** See S02.0[K]

● **S42.336**   **Nondisplaced oblique fracture of shaft of humerus, unspecified arm** A, K, P 🐾, B 🐾, A, B 🐾

> (Ex:) **For category S42.336 CC codes**
> S42.336[A]: S42.311-S42.399[A]
> **For S42.336[B]:** See S42.201[B]
> **For S42.336[K,P]:** See S02.0[K]

● **S42.34**   **Spiral fracture of shaft of humerus**

● **S42.341**   **Displaced spiral fracture of shaft of humerus, right arm** A, K, P 🐾, B 🐾, A, B 🐾

> (Ex:) **For category S42.341 CC codes**
> S42.341[A]: See S42.311[A]
> **For S42.341[B]:** See S42.201[B]
> **For S42.341[K,P]:** See S02.0[K]

● **S42.342**   **Displaced spiral fracture of shaft of humerus, left arm** A, K, P 🐾, B 🐾, A, B 🐾

> (Ex:) **For category S42.342 CC codes**
> S42.342[A]: See S42.312[A]
> **For S42.342[B]:** See S42.201[B]
> **For S42.342[K,P]:** See S02.0[K]

CHAPTER 19 (S00-T88)

N Newborn Age: 0   **P** Pediatric Age: 0–17   **M** Maternity DX: 12–55   **A** Adult Age: 15–124   ♀ Females Only   ♂ Males Only

🐾 Complication\Comorbidity   🐾 Major C\C   (Ex:) CC/MCC Exclusions   🐾 Hospital-Acquired Condition

1281

● **S42.343** Displaced spiral fracture of shaft of humerus, unspecified arm A, K, P ⬤, B ⬤, A, B ⬤
 (Ex:) For category S42.343 CC codes
  S42.343[A]: S42.311-S42.399[A]
  For S42.343[B]: See S42.201[B]
  For S42.343[K,P]: See S02.0[K]

● **S42.344** Nondisplaced spiral fracture of shaft of humerus, right arm A, K, P ⬤, B ⬤, A, B ⬤
 (Ex:) For category S42.344 CC codes
  S42.344[A]: See S42.311[A]
  For S42.344[B]: See S42.201[B]
  For S42.344[K,P]: See S02.0[K]

● **S42.345** Nondisplaced spiral fracture of shaft of humerus, left arm A, K, P ⬤, B ⬤, A, B ⬤
 (Ex:) For category S42.345 CC codes
  S42.345[A]: See S42.312[A]
  For S42.345[B]: See S42.201[B]
  For S42.345[K,P]: See S02.0[K]

● **S42.346** Nondisplaced spiral fracture of shaft of humerus, unspecified arm A, K, P ⬤, B ⬤, A, B ⬤
 (Ex:) For category S42.346 CC codes
  S42.346[A]: S42.311-S42.399[A]
  For S42.346[B]: See S42.201[B]
  For S42.346[K,P]: See S02.0[K]

● **S42.35** Comminuted fracture of shaft of humerus

● **S42.351** Displaced comminuted fracture of shaft of humerus, right arm A, K, P ⬤, B ⬤, A, B ⬤
 (Ex:) For category S42.351 CC codes
  S42.351[A]: See S42.311[A]
  For S42.351[B]: See S42.201[B]
  For S42.351[K,P]: See S02.0[K]

● **S42.352** Displaced comminuted fracture of shaft of humerus, left arm A, K, P ⬤, B ⬤, A, B ⬤
 (Ex:) For category S42.352 CC codes
  S42.352[A]: See S42.312[A]
  For S42.352[B]: See S42.201[B]
  For S42.352[K,P]: See S02.0[K]

● **S42.353** Displaced comminuted fracture of shaft of humerus, unspecified arm A, K, P ⬤, B ⬤, A, B ⬤
 (Ex:) For category S42.353 CC codes
  S42.353[A]: S42.311-S42.399[A]
  For S42.353[B]: See S42.201[B]
  For S42.353[K,P]: See S02.0[K]

● **S42.354** Nondisplaced comminuted fracture of shaft of humerus, right arm A, K, P ⬤, B ⬤, A, B ⬤
 (Ex:) For category S42.354 CC codes
  S42.354[A]: See S42.311[A]
  For S42.354[B]: See S42.201[B]
  For S42.354[K,P]: See S02.0[K]

● **S42.355** Nondisplaced comminuted fracture of shaft of humerus, left arm A, K, P ⬤, B ⬤, A, B ⬤
 (Ex:) For category S42.355 CC codes
  S42.355[A]: See S42.312[A]
  For S42.355[B]: See S42.201[B]
  For S42.355[K,P]: See S02.0[K]

● **S42.356** Nondisplaced comminuted fracture of shaft of humerus, unspecified arm A, K, P ⬤, B ⬤, A, B ⬤
 (Ex:) For category S42.356 CC codes
  S42.356[A]: S42.311-S42.399[A]
  For S42.356[B]: See S42.201[B]
  For S42.356[K,P]: See S02.0[K]

● **S42.36** Segmental fracture of shaft of humerus

● **S42.361** Displaced segmental fracture of shaft of humerus, right arm A, K, P ⬤, B ⬤, A, B ⬤
 (Ex:) For category S42.361 CC codes
  S42.361[A]: See S42.311[A]
  For S42.361[B]: See S42.201[B]
  For S42.361[K,P]: See S02.0[K]

● **S42.362** Displaced segmental fracture of shaft of humerus, left arm A, K, P ⬤, B ⬤, A, B ⬤
 (Ex:) For category S42.362 CC codes
  S42.362[A]: See S42.312[A]
  For S42.362[B]: See S42.201[B]
  For S42.362[K,P]: See S02.0[K]

● **S42.363** Displaced segmental fracture of shaft of humerus, unspecified arm A, K, P ⬤, B ⬤, A, B ⬤
 (Ex:) For category S42.363 CC codes
  S42.363[A]: S42.311-S42.399[A]
  For S42.363[B]: See S42.201[B]
  For S42.363[K,P]: See S02.0[K]

● **S42.364** Nondisplaced segmental fracture of shaft of humerus, right arm A, K, P ⬤, B ⬤, A, B ⬤
 (Ex:) For category S42.364 CC codes
  S42.364[A]: See S42.311[A]
  For S42.364[B]: See S42.201[B]
  For S42.364[K,P]: See S02.0[K]

● **S42.365** Nondisplaced segmental fracture of shaft of humerus, left arm A, K, P ⬤, B ⬤, A, B ⬤
 (Ex:) For category S42.365 CC codes
  S42.365[A]: See S42.312[A]
  For S42.365[B]: See S42.201[B]
  For S42.365[K,P]: See S02.0[K]

● **S42.366** Nondisplaced segmental fracture of shaft of humerus, unspecified arm A, K, P ⬤, B ⬤, A, B ⬤
 (Ex:) For category S42.366 CC codes
  S42.366[A]: S42.311-S42.399[A]
  For S42.366[B]: See S42.201[B]
  For S42.366[K,P]: See S02.0[K]

● **S42.39** Other fracture of shaft of humerus

● **S42.391** Other fracture of shaft of right humerus A, K, P ⬤, B ⬤, A, B ⬤
 (Ex:) For category S42.391 CC codes
  S42.391[A]: See S42.311[A]
  For S42.391[B]: See S42.201[B]
  For S42.391[K,P]: See S02.0[K]

● **S42.392** Other fracture of shaft of left humerus A, K, P ⬤, B ⬤, A, B ⬤
 (Ex:) For category S42.392 CC codes
  S42.392[A]: See S42.312[A]
  For S42.392[B]: See S42.201[B]
  For S42.392[K,P]: See S02.0[K]

● **S42.399** Other fracture of shaft of unspecified humerus A, K, P ⬤, B ⬤, A, B ⬤
 (Ex:) For category S42.399 CC codes
  S42.399[A]: S42.311-S42.399[A]
  For S42.399[B]: See S42.201[B]
  For S42.399[K,P]: See S02.0[K]

◀ New   ◀▥ Revised   ~~deleted~~ Deleted   Excludes 1   Excludes 2   Includes   Use additional   Code first   Code also   Unspecified
OGCR Official Guidelines   ● Unacceptable Principal Diagnosis   X Assign placeholder X   ● Use Additional Character(s)   ▸ Manifestation Code   **Coding Clinic**

● **S42.4**   **Fracture of lower end of humerus**
Fracture of distal end of humerus

> **Excludes2**   fracture of shaft of humerus (S42.3-)
> physeal fracture of lower end of humerus
> (S49.1-)

  ● **S42.40**   **Unspecified fracture of lower end of humerus**
Fracture of elbow NOS

    ● **S42.401**   Unspecified **fracture of lower end of right humerus** A, K, P 🐾, B 🐾, A, B 🐾
> Ⓔ **For S42.401[A]:** See S42.201[A]
> **For S42.401[B]:** See S42.201[B]
> **For S42.401[K,P]:** See S02.0[K]

    ● **S42.402**   Unspecified **fracture of lower end of left humerus** A, K, P 🐾, B 🐾, A, B 🐾
> Ⓔ **For S42.402[A]:** See S42.202[A]
> **For S42.402[B]:** See S42.201[B]
> **For S42.402[K,P]:** See S02.0[K]

    ● **S42.409**   Unspecified **fracture of lower end of unspecified humerus** A, K, P 🐾, B 🐾, A, B 🐾
> Ⓔ **For S42.409[A]:** See S42.209[A]
> **For S42.409[B]:** See S42.201[B]
> **For S42.409[K,P]:** See S02.0[K]

  ● **S42.41**   **Simple supracondylar fracture without intercondylar fracture of humerus**

    ● **S42.411**   Displaced simple supracondylar fracture without intercondylar fracture of right humerus A, K, P 🐾, B 🐾, A, B 🐾
> Ⓔ **For S42.411[A]:** See S42.201[A]
> **For S42.411[B]:** See S42.201[B]
> **For S42.411[K,P]:** See S02.0[K]

    ● **S42.412**   Displaced simple supracondylar fracture without intercondylar fracture of left humerus A, K, P 🐾, B 🐾, A, B 🐾
> Ⓔ **For S42.412[A]:** See S42.202[A]
> **For S42.412[B]:** See S42.201[B]
> **For S42.412[K,P]:** See S02.0[K]

    ● **S42.413**   Displaced simple supracondylar fracture without intercondylar fracture of unspecified humerus A, K, P 🐾, B 🐾, A, B 🐾
> Ⓔ **For S42.413[A]:** See S42.209[A]
> **For S42.413[B]:** See S42.201[B]
> **For S42.413[K,P]:** See S02.0[K]

    ● **S42.414**   Nondisplaced simple supracondylar fracture without intercondylar fracture of right humerus A, K, P 🐾, B 🐾, A, B 🐾
> Ⓔ **For S42.414[A]:** See S42.201[A]
> **For S42.414[B]:** See S42.201[B]
> **For S42.414[K,P]:** See S02.0[K]

    ● **S42.415**   Nondisplaced simple supracondylar fracture without intercondylar fracture of left humerus A, K, P 🐾, B 🐾, A, B 🐾
> Ⓔ **For S42.415[A]:** See S42.202[A]
> **For S42.415[B]:** See S42.201[B]
> **For S42.415[K,P]:** See S02.0[K]

    ● **S42.416**   Nondisplaced simple supracondylar fracture without intercondylar fracture of unspecified humerus A, K, P 🐾, B 🐾, A, B 🐾
> Ⓔ **For S42.416[A]:** See S42.209[A]
> **For S42.416[B]:** See S42.201[B]
> **For S42.416[K,P]:** See S02.0[K]

  ● **S42.42**   **Comminuted supracondylar fracture without intercondylar fracture of humerus**

    ● **S42.421**   Displaced comminuted supracondylar fracture without intercondylar fracture of right humerus A, K, P 🐾, B 🐾, A, B 🐾
> Ⓔ **For S42.421[A]:** See S42.201[A]
> **For S42.421[B]:** See S42.201[B]
> **For S42.421[K,P]:** See S02.0[K]

    ● **S42.422**   Displaced comminuted supracondylar fracture without intercondylar fracture of left humerus A, K, P 🐾, B 🐾, A, B 🐾
> Ⓔ **For S42.422[A]:** See S42.202[A]
> **For S42.422[B]:** See S42.201[B]
> **For S42.422[K,P]:** See S02.0[K]

    ● **S42.423**   Displaced comminuted supracondylar fracture without intercondylar fracture of unspecified humerus A, K, P 🐾, B 🐾, A, B 🐾
> Ⓔ **For S42.423[A]:** See S42.209[A]
> **For S42.423[B]:** See S42.201[B]
> **For S42.423[K,P]:** See S02.0[K]

    ● **S42.424**   Nondisplaced comminuted supracondylar fracture without intercondylar fracture of right humerus A, K, P 🐾, B 🐾, A, B 🐾
> Ⓔ **For S42.424[A]:** See S42.201[A]
> **For S42.424[B]:** See S42.201[B]
> **For S42.424[K,P]:** See S02.0[K]

    ● **S42.425**   Nondisplaced comminuted supracondylar fracture without intercondylar fracture of left humerus A, K, P 🐾, B 🐾, A, B 🐾
> Ⓔ **For S42.425[A]:** See S42.202[A]
> **For S42.425[B]:** See S42.201[B]
> **For S42.425[K,P]:** See S02.0[K]

    ● **S42.426**   Nondisplaced comminuted supracondylar fracture without intercondylar fracture of unspecified humerus A, K, P 🐾, B 🐾, A, B 🐾
> Ⓔ **For S42.426[A]:** See S42.209[A]
> **For S42.426[B]:** See S42.201[B]
> **For S42.426[K,P]:** See S02.0[K]

  ● **S42.43**   **Fracture (avulsion) of lateral epicondyle of humerus**

    ● **S42.431**   Displaced fracture (avulsion) of lateral epicondyle of right humerus A, K, P 🐾, B 🐾, A, B 🐾
> Ⓔ **For S42.431[A]:** See S42.201[A]
> **For S42.431[B]:** See S42.201[B]
> **For S42.431[K,P]:** See S02.0[K]

    ● **S42.432**   Displaced fracture (avulsion) of lateral epicondyle of left humerus A, K, P 🐾, B 🐾, A, B 🐾
> Ⓔ **For S42.432[A]:** See S42.202[A]
> **For S42.432[B]:** See S42.201[B]
> **For S42.432[K,P]:** See S02.0[K]

    ● **S42.433**   Displaced fracture (avulsion) of lateral epicondyle of unspecified humerus A, K, P 🐾, B 🐾, A, B 🐾
> Ⓔ **For S42.433[A]:** See S42.209[A]
> **For S42.433[B]:** See S42.201[B]
> **For S42.433[K,P]:** See S02.0[K]

    ● **S42.434**   Nondisplaced fracture (avulsion) of lateral epicondyle of right humerus A, K, P 🐾, B 🐾, A, B 🐾
> Ⓔ **For S42.434[A]:** See S42.201[A]
> **For S42.434[B]:** See S42.201[B]
> **For S42.434[K,P]:** See S02.0[K]

CHAPTER 19 (S00–T88)

N   Newborn Age: 0   **P**   Pediatric Age: 0–17   **M**   Maternity DX: 12–55   **A**   Adult Age: 15–124   ♀   Females Only   ♂   Males Only
🐾 Complication\Comorbidity   🐾 Major C\C   Ⓔ CC/MCC Exclusions   🐾 Hospital-Acquired Condition

1283

● S42.435   Nondisplaced fracture (avulsion) of
             lateral epicondyle of left humerus
             A, K, P 🔾, B 🔾, A, B 🔾
             (Ex:) For S42.435[A]: See S42.202[A]
                   For S42.435[B]: See S42.201[B]
                   For S42.435[K,P]: See S02.0[K]

● S42.436   Nondisplaced fracture (avulsion) of
             lateral epicondyle of unspecified
             humerus A, K, P 🔾, B 🔾, A, B 🔾
             (Ex:) For S42.436[A]: See S42.209[A]
                   For S42.436[B]: See S42.201[B]
                   For S42.436[K,P]: See S02.0[K]

● S42.44   Fracture (avulsion) of medial epicondyle of
           humerus

● S42.441   Displaced fracture (avulsion) of
             medial epicondyle of right humerus
             A, K, P 🔾, B 🔾, A, B 🔾
             (Ex:) For S42.441[A]: See S42.201[A]
                   For S42.441[B]: See S42.201[B]
                   For S42.441[K,P]: See S02.0[K]

● S42.442   Displaced fracture (avulsion) of
             medial epicondyle of left humerus
             A, K, P 🔾, B 🔾, A, B 🔾
             (Ex:) For S42.442[A]: See S42.202[A]
                   For S42.442[B]: See S42.201[B]
                   For S42.442[K,P]: See S02.0[K]

● S42.443   Displaced fracture (avulsion) of
             medial epicondyle of unspecified
             humerus A, K, P 🔾, B 🔾, A, B 🔾
             (Ex:) For S42.443[A]: See S42.209[A]
                   For S42.443[B]: See S42.201[B]
                   For S42.443[K,P]: See S02.0[K]

● S42.444   Nondisplaced fracture (avulsion) of
             medial epicondyle of right humerus
             A, K, P 🔾, B 🔾, A, B 🔾
             (Ex:) For S42.444[A]: See S42.201[A]
                   For S42.444[B]: See S42.201[B]
                   For S42.444[K,P]: See S02.0[K]

● S42.445   Nondisplaced fracture (avulsion) of
             medial epicondyle of left humerus
             A, K, P 🔾, B 🔾, A, B 🔾
             (Ex:) For S42.445[A]: See S42.202[A]
                   For S42.445[B]: See S42.201[B]
                   For S42.445[K,P]: See S02.0[K]

● S42.446   Nondisplaced fracture (avulsion) of
             medial epicondyle of unspecified
             humerus A, K, P 🔾, B 🔾, A, B 🔾
             (Ex:) For S42.446[A]: See S42.209[A]
                   For S42.446[B]: See S42.201[B]
                   For S42.446[K,P]: See S02.0[K]

● S42.447   Incarcerated fracture (avulsion) of
             medial epicondyle of right humerus
             A, K, P 🔾, B 🔾, A, B 🔾
             (Ex:) For S42.447[A]: See S42.201[A]
                   For S42.447[B]: See S42.201[B]
                   For S42.447[K,P]: See S02.0[K]

● S42.448   Incarcerated fracture (avulsion) of
             medial epicondyle of left humerus
             A, K, P 🔾, B 🔾, A, B 🔾
             (Ex:) For S42.448[A]: See S42.202[A]
                   For S42.448[B]: See S42.201[B]
                   For S42.448[K,P]: See S02.0[K]

● S42.449   Incarcerated fracture (avulsion) of
             medial epicondyle of unspecified
             humerus A, K, P 🔾, B 🔾, A, B 🔾
             (Ex:) For S42.449[A]: See S42.209[A]
                   For S42.449[B]: See S42.201[B]
                   For S42.449[K,P]: See S02.0[K]

● S42.45   Fracture of lateral condyle of humerus
           Fracture of capitellum of humerus

● S42.451   Displaced fracture of lateral condyle
             of right humerus A, K, P 🔾, B 🔾,
             A, B 🔾
             (Ex:) For S42.451[A]: See S42.201[A]
                   For S42.451[B]: See S42.201[B]
                   For S42.451[K,P]: See S02.0[K]

● S42.452   Displaced fracture of lateral condyle
             of left humerus A, K, P 🔾, B 🔾,
             A, B 🔾
             (Ex:) For S42.452[A]: See S42.202[A]
                   For S42.452[B]: See S42.201[B]
                   For S42.452[K,P]: See S02.0[K]

● S42.453   Displaced fracture of lateral condyle
             of unspecified humerus A, K, P 🔾,
             B 🔾, A, B 🔾
             (Ex:) For S42.453[A]: See S42.209[A]
                   For S42.453[B]: See S42.201[B]
                   For S42.453[K,P]: See S02.0[K]

● S42.454   Nondisplaced fracture of lateral
             condyle of right humerus A, K, P 🔾,
             B 🔾, A, B 🔾
             (Ex:) For S42.454[A]: See S42.201[A]
                   For S42.454[B]: See S42.201[B]
                   For S42.454[K,P]: See S02.0[K]

● S42.455   Nondisplaced fracture of lateral
             condyle of left humerus A, K, P 🔾,
             B 🔾, A, B 🔾
             (Ex:) For S42.455[A]: See S42.202[A]
                   For S42.455[B]: See S42.201[B]
                   For S42.455[K,P]: See S02.0[K]

● S42.456   Nondisplaced fracture of lateral
             condyle of unspecified humerus
             A, K, P 🔾, B 🔾, A, B 🔾
             (Ex:) For S42.456[A]: See S42.209[A]
                   For S42.456[B]: See S42.201[B]
                   For S42.456[K,P]: See S02.0[K]

● S42.46   Fracture of medial condyle of humerus
           Trochlea fracture of humerus

● S42.461   Displaced fracture of medial condyle
             of right humerus A, K, P 🔾, B 🔾,
             A, B 🔾
             (Ex:) For S42.461[A]: See S42.201[A]
                   For S42.461[B]: See S42.201[B]
                   For S42.461[K,P]: See S02.0[K]

● S42.462   Displaced fracture of medial condyle
             of left humerus A, K, P 🔾, B 🔾,
             A, B 🔾
             (Ex:) For S42.462[A]: See S42.202[A]
                   For S42.462[B]: See S42.201[B]
                   For S42.462[K,P]: See S02.0[K]

● S42.463   Displaced fracture of medial condyle
             of unspecified humerus A, K, P 🔾,
             B 🔾, A, B 🔾
             (Ex:) For S42.463[A]: See S42.209[A]
                   For S42.463[B]: See S42.201[B]
                   For S42.463[K,P]: See S02.0[K]

● S42.464   Nondisplaced fracture of medial
             condyle of right humerus A, K, P 🔾,
             B 🔾, A, B 🔾
             (Ex:) For S42.464[A]: See S42.201[A]
                   For S42.464[B]: See S42.201[B]
                   For S42.464[K,P]: See S02.0[K]

● S42.465   Nondisplaced fracture of medial
             condyle of left humerus A, K, P 🔾,
             B 🔾, A, B 🔾
             (Ex:) For S42.465[A]: See S42.202[A]
                   For S42.465[B]: See S42.201[B]
                   For S42.465[K,P]: See S02.0[K]

● S42.466   Nondisplaced fracture of medial
             condyle of unspecified humerus
             A, K, P 🔾, B 🔾, A, B 🔾
             (Ex:) For S42.466[A]: See S42.209[A]
                   For S42.466[B]: See S42.201[B]
                   For S42.466[K,P]: See S02.0[K]

◀ New   ◀▦ Revised   ~~deleted~~ Deleted   Excludes 1   Excludes 2   Includes   Use additional   Code first   Code also   Unspecified

OGCR Official Guidelines   ● Unacceptable Principal Diagnosis   X Assign placeholder X   🔾 Use Additional Character(s)   ▸ Manifestation Code   Coding Clinic

● **S42.47**   **Transcondylar fracture of humerus**

   ● **S42.471**   Displaced transcondylar fracture of right humerus A, K, P 🪙, B 🪙, A, B 🪙
     (Ex) **For S42.471[A]:** See S42.209[A]
       For S42.471[B]: See S42.201[B]
       For S42.471[K,P]: See S02.0[K]

   ● **S42.472**   Displaced transcondylar fracture of left humerus A, K, P 🪙, B 🪙, A, B 🪙
     (Ex) **For S42.472[A]:** See S42.202[A]
       For S42.472[B]: See S42.201[B]
       For S42.472[K,P]: See S02.0[K]

   ● **S42.473**   Displaced transcondylar fracture of unspecified humerus A, K, P 🪙, B 🪙, A, B 🪙
     (Ex) **For S42.473[A]:** See S42.209[A]
       For S42.473[B]: See S42.201[B]
       For S42.473[K,P]: See S02.0[K]

   ● **S42.474**   Nondisplaced transcondylar fracture of right humerus A, K, P 🪙, B 🪙, A, B 🪙
     (Ex) **For S42.474[A]:** See S42.201[A]
       For S42.474[B]: See S42.201[B]
       For S42.474[K,P]: See S02.0[K]

   ● **S42.475**   Nondisplaced transcondylar fracture of left humerus A, K, P 🪙, B 🪙, A, B 🪙
     (Ex) **For S42.475[A]:** See S42.202[A]
       For S42.475[B]: See S42.201[B]
       For S42.475[K,P]: See S02.0[K]

   ● **S42.476**   Nondisplaced transcondylar fracture of unspecified humerus A, K, P 🪙, B 🪙, A, B 🪙
     (Ex) **For S42.476[A]:** See S42.209[A]
       For S42.476[B]: See S42.201[B]
       For S42.476[K,P]: See S02.0[K]

● **S42.48**   **Torus fracture of lower end of humerus**

   The appropriate 7th character is to be added to all codes in subcategory S42.48

A	initial encounter for closed fracture
D	subsequent encounter for fracture with routine healing
G	subsequent encounter for fracture with delayed healing
K	subsequent encounter for fracture with nonunion
P	subsequent encounter for fracture with malunion
S	sequela

   ● **S42.481**   Torus fracture of lower end of right humerus A, K, P 🪙, A 🪙
     (Ex) **For S42.481[A]:** See S42.201[A]
       For S42.481[K,P]: See S02.0[K]

   ● **S42.482**   Torus fracture of lower end of left humerus A, K, P 🪙, A 🪙
     (Ex) **For S42.482[A]:** See S42.202[A]
       For S42.482[K,P]: See S02.0[K]

   ● **S42.489**   Torus fracture of lower end of unspecified humerus A, K, P 🪙, A 🪙
     (Ex) **For S42.489[A]:** See S42.209[A]
       For S42.489[K,P]: See S02.0[K]

● **S42.49**   **Other fracture of lower end of humerus**

   ● **S42.491**   Other displaced fracture of lower end of right humerus A, K, P 🪙, B 🪙, A, B 🪙
     (Ex) **For S42.491[A]:** See S42.201[A]
       For S42.491[B]: See S42.201[B]
       For S42.491[K,P]: See S02.0[K]

   ● **S42.492**   Other displaced fracture of lower end of left humerus A, K, P 🪙, B 🪙, A, B 🪙
     (Ex) **For S42.492[A]:** See S42.202[A]
       For S42.492[B]: See S42.201[B]
       For S42.492[K,P]: See S02.0[K]

   ● **S42.493**   Other displaced fracture of lower end of unspecified humerus A, K, P 🪙, B 🪙, A, B 🪙
     (Ex) **For S42.493[A]:** See S42.209[A]
       For S42.493[B]: See S42.201[B]
       For S42.493[K,P]: See S02.0[K]

   ● **S42.494**   Other nondisplaced fracture of lower end of right humerus A, K, P 🪙, B 🪙, A, B 🪙
     (Ex) **For S42.494[A]:** See S42.201[A]
       For S42.494[B]: See S42.201[B]
       For S42.494[K,P]: See S02.0[K]

   ● **S42.495**   Other nondisplaced fracture of lower end of left humerus A, K, P 🪙, B 🪙, A, B 🪙
     (Ex) **For S42.495[A]:** See S42.202[A]
       For S42.495[B]: See S42.201[B]
       For S42.495[K,P]: See S02.0[K]

   ● **S42.496**   Other nondisplaced fracture of lower end of unspecified humerus A, K, P 🪙, B 🪙, A, B 🪙
     (Ex) **For S42.496[A]:** See S42.209[A]
       For S42.496[B]: See S42.201[B]
       For S42.496[K,P]: See S02.0[K]

● **S42.9**   **Fracture of shoulder girdle, part unspecified**
   Fracture of shoulder NOS
   (Ex) **For category S42.9 CC codes S42.9[A]:** See S42.209[A] **For S42.9[B]:** See S42.201[B] **For S42.9[K,P]:** See S02.0[K]

   X ● **S42.90**   Fracture of unspecified shoulder girdle, part unspecified A, K, P 🪙, B 🪙, A, B 🪙

   X ● **S42.91**   Fracture of right shoulder girdle, part unspecified A, K, P 🪙, B 🪙, A, B 🪙

   X ● **S42.92**   Fracture of left shoulder girdle, part unspecified A, K, P 🪙, B 🪙, A, B 🪙

● **S43**   **Dislocation and sprain of joints and ligaments of shoulder girdle**

   Includes   avulsion of joint or ligament of shoulder girdle
       laceration of cartilage, joint or ligament of shoulder girdle
       sprain of cartilage, joint or ligament of shoulder girdle
       traumatic hemarthrosis of joint or ligament of shoulder girdle
       traumatic rupture of joint or ligament of shoulder girdle
       traumatic subluxation of joint or ligament of shoulder girdle
       traumatic tear of joint or ligament of shoulder girdle

   Code also any associated open wound

   Excludes2   strain of muscle, fascia and tendon of shoulder and upper arm (S46.-)

   The appropriate 7th character is to be added to each code from category S43

A	initial encounter
D	subsequent encounter
S	sequela

● **S43.0**   **Subluxation and dislocation of shoulder joint**
   Dislocation of glenohumeral joint
   Subluxation of glenohumeral joint

   ● **S43.00**   Unspecified subluxation and dislocation of shoulder joint
     Dislocation of humerus NOS
     Subluxation of humerus NOS

     ● **S43.001**   Unspecified subluxation of right shoulder joint

     ● **S43.002**   Unspecified subluxation of left shoulder joint

     ● **S43.003**   Unspecified subluxation of unspecified shoulder joint

     ● **S43.004**   Unspecified dislocation of right shoulder joint

---

● S43.005   Unspecified dislocation of left shoulder joint

● S43.006   Unspecified dislocation of unspecified shoulder joint

● S43.01   Anterior subluxation and dislocation of humerus

    ● S43.011   Anterior subluxation of right humerus

    ● S43.012   Anterior subluxation of left humerus

    ● S43.013   Anterior subluxation of unspecified humerus

    ● S43.014   Anterior dislocation of right humerus

    ● S43.015   Anterior dislocation of left humerus

    ● S43.016   Anterior dislocation of unspecified humerus

● S43.02   Posterior subluxation and dislocation of humerus

    ● S43.021   Posterior subluxation of right humerus

    ● S43.022   Posterior subluxation of left humerus

    ● S43.023   Posterior subluxation of unspecified humerus

    ● S43.024   Posterior dislocation of right humerus

    ● S43.025   Posterior dislocation of left humerus

    ● S43.026   Posterior dislocation of unspecified humerus

● S43.03   Inferior subluxation and dislocation of humerus

    ● S43.031   Inferior subluxation of right humerus

    ● S43.032   Inferior subluxation of left humerus

    ● S43.033   Inferior subluxation of unspecified humerus

    ● S43.034   Inferior dislocation of right humerus

    ● S43.035   Inferior dislocation of left humerus

    ● S43.036   Inferior dislocation of unspecified humerus

● S43.08   Other subluxation and dislocation of shoulder joint

    ● S43.081   Other subluxation of right shoulder joint

    ● S43.082   Other subluxation of left shoulder joint

    ● S43.083   Other subluxation of unspecified shoulder joint

    ● S43.084   Other dislocation of right shoulder joint

    ● S43.085   Other dislocation of left shoulder joint

    ● S43.086   Other dislocation of unspecified shoulder joint

● S43.1   Subluxation and dislocation of acromioclavicular joint

    ● S43.10   Unspecified dislocation of acromioclavicular joint

       ● S43.101   Unspecified dislocation of right acromioclavicular joint

       ● S43.102   Unspecified dislocation of left acromioclavicular joint

       ● S43.109   Unspecified dislocation of unspecified acromioclavicular joint

    ● S43.11   Subluxation of acromioclavicular joint

       ● S43.111   Subluxation of right acromioclavicular joint

       ● S43.112   Subluxation of left acromioclavicular joint

       ● S43.119   Subluxation of unspecified acromioclavicular joint

    ● S43.12   Dislocation of acromioclavicular joint, 100%-200% displacement

       ● S43.121   Dislocation of right acromioclavicular joint, 100%-200% displacement

       ● S43.122   Dislocation of left acromioclavicular joint, 100%-200% displacement

       ● S43.129   Dislocation of unspecified acromioclavicular joint, 100%-200% displacement

    ● S43.13   Dislocation of acromioclavicular joint, greater than 200% displacement

       ● S43.131   Dislocation of right acromioclavicular joint, greater than 200% displacement

       ● S43.132   Dislocation of left acromioclavicular joint, greater than 200% displacement

       ● S43.139   Dislocation of unspecified acromioclavicular joint, greater than 200% displacement

    ● S43.14   Inferior dislocation of acromioclavicular joint

       ● S43.141   Inferior dislocation of right acromioclavicular joint

       ● S43.142   Inferior dislocation of left acromioclavicular joint

       ● S43.149   Inferior dislocation of unspecified acromioclavicular joint

    ● S43.15   Posterior dislocation of acromioclavicular joint

       ● S43.151   Posterior dislocation of right acromioclavicular joint

       ● S43.152   Posterior dislocation of left acromioclavicular joint

       ● S43.159   Posterior dislocation of unspecified acromioclavicular joint

● S43.2   Subluxation and dislocation of sternoclavicular joint

    ● S43.20   Unspecified subluxation and dislocation of sternoclavicular joint

       ● S43.201   Unspecified subluxation of right sternoclavicular joint A, A
          Ex: M99.18, S43.201[A], S43.203-S43.204[A], S43.206[A], S43.211[A], S43.213-S43.214[A], S43.216[A], S43.221[A], S43.223-S43.224[A], S43.226[A]

       ● S43.202   Unspecified subluxation of left sternoclavicular joint A, A
          Ex: M99.18, S43.202-S43.203[A], S43.205-S43.206[A], S43.212-S43.213[A], S43.215-S43.216[A], S43.222-S43.223[A], S43.225-S43.226[A]

       ● S43.203   Unspecified subluxation of unspecified sternoclavicular joint A, A
          Ex: M99.18, S43.201-S43.226[A]

       ● S43.204   Unspecified dislocation of right sternoclavicular joint A, A
          Ex: See S43.201

       ● S43.205   Unspecified dislocation of left sternoclavicular joint A, A
          Ex: See S43.202

       ● S43.206   Unspecified dislocation of unspecified sternoclavicular joint A, A
          Ex: See S43.203

    ● S43.21   Anterior subluxation and dislocation of sternoclavicular joint

       ● S43.211   Anterior subluxation of right sternoclavicular joint A, A
          Ex: See S43.201

       ● S43.212   Anterior subluxation of left sternoclavicular joint A, A
          Ex: See S43.202

       ● S43.213   Anterior subluxation of unspecified sternoclavicular joint A, A
          Ex: See S43.203

● S43.214 Anterior dislocation of right sternoclavicular joint A 🦠, A 🦠
(Ex) See S43.201

● S43.215 Anterior dislocation of left sternoclavicular joint A 🦠, A 🦠
(Ex) See S43.202

● S43.216 Anterior dislocation of unspecified sternoclavicular joint A 🦠, A 🦠
(Ex) See S43.203

● S43.22 Posterior subluxation and dislocation of sternoclavicular joint

● S43.221 Posterior subluxation of right sternoclavicular joint A 🦠, A 🦠
(Ex) See S43.201

● S43.222 Posterior subluxation of left sternoclavicular joint A 🦠, A 🦠
(Ex) See S43.202

● S43.223 Posterior subluxation of unspecified sternoclavicular joint A 🦠, A 🦠
(Ex) See S43.203

● S43.224 Posterior dislocation of right sternoclavicular joint A 🦠, A 🦠
(Ex) See S43.201

● S43.225 Posterior dislocation of left sternoclavicular joint A 🦠, A 🦠
(Ex) See S43.202

● S43.226 Posterior dislocation of unspecified sternoclavicular joint A 🦠, A 🦠
(Ex) See S43.203

● S43.3 Subluxation and dislocation of other and unspecified parts of shoulder girdle

● S43.30 Subluxation and dislocation of unspecified parts of shoulder girdle
Dislocation of shoulder girdle NOS
Subluxation of shoulder girdle NOS

● S43.301 Subluxation of unspecified parts of right shoulder girdle

● S43.302 Subluxation of unspecified parts of left shoulder girdle

● S43.303 Subluxation of unspecified parts of unspecified shoulder girdle

● S43.304 Dislocation of unspecified parts of right shoulder girdle

● S43.305 Dislocation of unspecified parts of left shoulder girdle

● S43.306 Dislocation of unspecified parts of unspecified shoulder girdle

● S43.31 Subluxation and dislocation of scapula

● S43.311 Subluxation of right scapula

● S43.312 Subluxation of left scapula

● S43.313 Subluxation of unspecified scapula

● S43.314 Dislocation of right scapula

● S43.315 Dislocation of left scapula

● S43.316 Dislocation of unspecified scapula

● S43.39 Subluxation and dislocation of other parts of shoulder girdle

● S43.391 Subluxation of other parts of right shoulder girdle

● S43.392 Subluxation of other parts of left shoulder girdle

● S43.393 Subluxation of other parts of unspecified shoulder girdle

● S43.394 Dislocation of other parts of right shoulder girdle

● S43.395 Dislocation of other parts of left shoulder girdle

● S43.396 Dislocation of other parts of unspecified shoulder girdle

● S43.4 Sprain of shoulder joint

● S43.40 Unspecified sprain of shoulder joint

● S43.401 Unspecified sprain of right shoulder joint

● S43.402 Unspecified sprain of left shoulder joint

● S43.409 Unspecified sprain of unspecified shoulder joint

● S43.41 Sprain of coracohumeral (ligament)

● S43.411 Sprain of right coracohumeral (ligament)

● S43.412 Sprain of left coracohumeral (ligament)

● S43.419 Sprain of unspecified coracohumeral (ligament)

● S43.42 Sprain of rotator cuff capsule
Encounters during the healing phase

Excludes1 rotator cuff syndrome (complete) (incomplete), not specified as traumatic (M75.1-)

Excludes2 injury of tendon of rotator cuff (S46.0-)

● S43.421 Sprain of right rotator cuff capsule

● S43.422 Sprain of left rotator cuff capsule

● S43.429 Sprain of unspecified rotator cuff capsule

● S43.43 Superior glenoid labrum lesion
SLAP lesion

● S43.431 Superior glenoid labrum lesion of right shoulder

● S43.432 Superior glenoid labrum lesion of left shoulder

● S43.439 Superior glenoid labrum lesion of unspecified shoulder

● S43.49 Other sprain of shoulder joint

● S43.491 Other sprain of right shoulder joint

● S43.492 Other sprain of left shoulder joint

● S43.499 Other sprain of unspecified shoulder joint

● S43.5 Sprain of acromioclavicular joint
Sprain of acromioclavicular ligament

X ● S43.50 Sprain of unspecified acromioclavicular joint

X ● S43.51 Sprain of right acromioclavicular joint

X ● S43.52 Sprain of left acromioclavicular joint

● S43.6 Sprain of sternoclavicular joint

X ● S43.60 Sprain of unspecified sternoclavicular joint

X ● S43.61 Sprain of right sternoclavicular joint

X ● S43.62 Sprain of left sternoclavicular joint

● S43.8 Sprain of other specified parts of shoulder girdle

X ● S43.80 Sprain of other specified parts of unspecified shoulder girdle

X ● S43.81 Sprain of other specified parts of right shoulder girdle

X ● S43.82 Sprain of other specified parts of left shoulder girdle

● S43.9 Sprain of unspecified parts of shoulder girdle

X ● S43.90 Sprain of unspecified parts of unspecified shoulder girdle
Sprain of shoulder girdle NOS

X ● S43.91 Sprain of unspecified parts of right shoulder girdle

X ● S43.92 Sprain of unspecified parts of left shoulder girdle

CHAPTER 19 (S00-T88)

● **S44**   **Injury of nerves at shoulder and upper arm level**

     Code also any associated open wound (S41.-)

     Excludes2   injury of brachial plexus (S14.3-)

     The appropriate 7th character is to be added to each code from category S44

     A   initial encounter
     D   subsequent encounter
     S   sequela

   ● **S44.0**   **Injury of ulnar nerve at upper arm level**

     Excludes1   ulnar nerve NOS (S54.0)

     X ● **S44.00**   Injury of ulnar nerve at upper arm level, unspecified arm

     X ● **S44.01**   Injury of ulnar nerve at upper arm level, right arm

     X ● **S44.02**   Injury of ulnar nerve at upper arm level, left arm

   ● **S44.1**   **Injury of median nerve at upper arm level**

     Excludes1   median nerve NOS (S54.1)

     X ● **S44.10**   Injury of median nerve at upper arm level, unspecified arm

     X ● **S44.11**   Injury of median nerve at upper arm level, right arm

     X ● **S44.12**   Injury of median nerve at upper arm level, left arm

   ● **S44.2**   **Injury of radial nerve at upper arm level**

     Excludes1   radial nerve NOS (S54.2)

     X ● **S44.20**   Injury of radial nerve at upper arm level, unspecified arm

     X ● **S44.21**   Injury of radial nerve at upper arm level, right arm

     X ● **S44.22**   Injury of radial nerve at upper arm level, left arm

   ● **S44.3**   **Injury of axillary nerve**

     X ● **S44.30**   Injury of axillary nerve, unspecified arm

     X ● **S44.31**   Injury of axillary nerve, right arm

     X ● **S44.32**   Injury of axillary nerve, left arm

   ● **S44.4**   **Injury of musculocutaneous nerve**

     X ● **S44.40**   Injury of musculocutaneous nerve, unspecified arm

     X ● **S44.41**   Injury of musculocutaneous nerve, right arm

     X ● **S44.42**   Injury of musculocutaneous nerve, left arm

   ● **S44.5**   **Injury of cutaneous sensory nerve at shoulder and upper arm level**

     X ● **S44.50**   Injury of cutaneous sensory nerve at shoulder and upper arm level, unspecified arm

     X ● **S44.51**   Injury of cutaneous sensory nerve at shoulder and upper arm level, right arm

     X ● **S44.52**   Injury of cutaneous sensory nerve at shoulder and upper arm level, left arm

   ● **S44.8**   **Injury of other nerves at shoulder and upper arm level**

     ● **S44.8X**   Injury of other nerves at shoulder and upper arm level

       ● **S44.8X1**   Injury of other nerves at shoulder and upper arm level, right arm

       ● **S44.8X2**   Injury of other nerves at shoulder and upper arm level, left arm

       ● **S44.8X9**   Injury of other nerves at shoulder and upper arm level, unspecified arm

   ● **S44.9**   **Injury of unspecified nerve at shoulder and upper arm level**

     X ● **S44.90**   Injury of unspecified nerve at shoulder and upper arm level, unspecified arm

     X ● **S44.91**   Injury of unspecified nerve at shoulder and upper arm level, right arm

     X ● **S44.92**   Injury of unspecified nerve at shoulder and upper arm level, left arm

● **S45**   **Injury of blood vessels at shoulder and upper arm level**

     Code also any associated open wound (S41.-)

     Excludes2   injury of subclavian artery (S25.1)
                    injury of subclavian vein (S25.3)

     The appropriate 7th character is to be added to each code from category S45

     A   initial encounter
     D   subsequent encounter
     S   sequela

   ● **S45.0**   **Injury of axillary artery**

     ● **S45.00**   **Unspecified injury of axillary artery**

       ● **S45.001**   Unspecified injury of axillary artery, right side A

         (Ex) S45.001[A], S45.009-S45.011[A], S45.019-S45.091[A], S45.099[A], S45.301[A], S45.309-S45.311[A], S45.319-S45.391[A], S45.399-S45.801[A], S45.809-S45.811[A], S45.819-S45.891[A], S45.899-S45.901[A], S45.909-S45.911[A], S45.919-S45.991[A], S45.999[A], S55.201[A], S55.209-S55.211[A], S55.219-S55.291[A], S55.299-S55.801[A], S55.809-S55.811[A], S55.819-S55.891[A], S55.899-S55.901[A], S55.909-S55.911[A], S55.919-S55.991[A], S55.999[A], S65.801[A], S65.809-S65.811[A], S65.819-S65.891[A], S65.899-S65.901[A], S65.909-S65.911[A], S65.919-S65.991[A], S65.999[A]

       ● **S45.002**   Unspecified injury of axillary artery, left side A

         (Ex) S45.002-S45.009[A], S45.012-S45.019[A], S45.092-S45.099[A], S45.302-S45.309[A], S45.312-S45.319[A], S45.392-S45.399[A], S45.802-S45.809[A], S45.812-S45.819[A], S45.892-S45.899[A], S45.902-S45.909[A], S45.912-S45.919[A], S45.992-S45.999[A], S55.202-S55.209[A], S55.212-S55.219[A], S55.292-S55.299[A], S55.802-S55.809[A], S55.812-S55.819[A], S55.892-S55.899[A], S55.902-S55.909[A], S55.912-S55.919[A], S55.992-S55.999[A], S65.802-S65.809[A], S65.812-S65.819[A], S65.892-S65.899[A], S65.902-S65.909[A], S65.912-S65.919[A], S65.992-S65.999[A]

       ● **S45.009**   Unspecified injury of axillary artery, unspecified side A

         (Ex) S45.001-S45.099[A], S45.301-S45.399[A], S45.801-S45.999[A], S55.201-S55.999[A], S65.801-S65.999[A]

     ● **S45.01**   **Laceration of axillary artery**

       ● **S45.011**   Laceration of axillary artery, right side A

         (Ex) See S45.001

       ● **S45.012**   Laceration of axillary artery, left side A

         (Ex) See S45.002

       ● **S45.019**   Laceration of axillary artery, unspecified side A

         (Ex) See S45.009

     ● **S45.09**   **Other specified injury of axillary artery**

       ● **S45.091**   Other specified injury of axillary artery, right side A

         (Ex) See S45.001

       ● **S45.092**   Other specified injury of axillary artery, left side A

         (Ex) See S45.002

       ● **S45.099**   Other specified injury of axillary artery, unspecified side A

         (Ex) See S45.009

◀ New   ◀▥ Revised   ~~deleted~~ Deleted   Excludes 1   Excludes 2   Includes   Use additional   Code first   Code also   Unspecified

OGCR Official Guidelines   ● Unacceptable Principal Diagnosis   X Assign placeholder X   ● Use Additional Character(s)   ▶ Manifestation Code   **Coding Clinic**

● **S45.1   Injury of brachial artery**
  ● **S45.10   Unspecified injury of brachial artery**
    ● **S45.101   Unspecified** injury of brachial artery, right side A 🔾
      (Ex) S45.101[A], S45.109-S45.111[A], S45.119-S45.191[A], S45.199-S45.201[A], S45.209A-S45.211[A], S45.219-S45.291[A], S45.299-S45.301[A], S45.309-S45.311[A], S45.319-S45.391[A], S45.399-S45.801[A], S45.809-S45.811[A], S45.819-S45.891[A], S45.899-S45.901[A], S45.909-S45.911[A], S45.919-S45.991[A], S45.999[A], S55.201[A], S55.209-S55.211[A], S55.219-S55.291[A], S55.299-S55.801[A], S55.809-S55.811[A], S55.819-S55.891[A], S55.899-S55.901[A], S55.909-S55.911[A], S55.919-S55.991[A], S55.999[A], S65.801[A], S65.809-S65.811[A], S65.819-S65.891[A], S65.899-S65.901[A], S65.909-S65.911[A], S65.919-S65.991[A], S65.999[A]

    ● **S45.102   Unspecified** injury of brachial artery, left side A 🔾
      (Ex) S45.102-S45.109[A], S45.112-S45.119[A], S45.192-S45.199[A], S45.202-S45.209[A], S45.212-S45.219[A], S45.292-S45.299[A], S45.302-S45.309[A], S45.312-S45.319[A], S45.392-S45.399[A], S45.802-S45.809[A], S45.812-S45.819[A], S45.892-S45.899[A], S45.902-S45.909[A], S45.912-S45.919[A], S45.992-S45.999[A], S55.202-S55.209[A], S55.212-S55.219[A], S55.292-S55.299[A], S55.802-S55.809[A], S55.812-S55.819[A], S55.892-S55.899[A], S55.902-S55.909[A], S55.912-S55.919[A], S55.992-S55.999[A], S65.802-S65.809[A], S65.812-S65.819[A], S65.892-S65.899[A], S65.902-S65.909[A], S65.912-S65.919[A], S65.992-S65.999[A]

    ● **S45.109   Unspecified** injury of brachial artery, unspecified side A 🔾
      (Ex) S45.101-S45.999[A], S55.201-S55.999[A], S65.801-S65.999[A]

  ● **S45.11   Laceration of brachial artery**
    ● **S45.111   Laceration of brachial artery, right side** A 🔾
      (Ex) See S45.101
    ● **S45.112   Laceration of brachial artery, left side** A 🔾
      (Ex) See S45.102
    ● **S45.119   Laceration of brachial artery, unspecified side** A 🔾
      (Ex) See S45.109

  ● **S45.19   Other specified injury of brachial artery**
    ● **S45.191   Other specified injury of brachial artery, right side** A 🔾
      (Ex) See S45.101
    ● **S45.192   Other specified injury of brachial artery, left side** A 🔾
      (Ex) See S45.102
    ● **S45.199   Other specified injury of brachial artery, unspecified side** A 🔾
      (Ex) See S45.109

● **S45.2   Injury of axillary or brachial vein**
  ● **S45.20   Unspecified injury of axillary or brachial vein**
    ● **S45.201   Unspecified** injury of axillary or brachial vein, right side A 🔾
      (Ex) See S45.101
    ● **S45.202   Unspecified** injury of axillary or brachial vein, left side A 🔾
      (Ex) See S45.102
    ● **S45.209   Unspecified** injury of axillary or brachial vein, unspecified side A 🔾
      (Ex) See S45.109

● **S45.21   Laceration of axillary or brachial vein**
  ● **S45.211   Laceration of axillary or brachial vein, right side** A 🔾
    (Ex) See S45.101
  ● **S45.212   Laceration of axillary or brachial vein, left side** A 🔾
    (Ex) See S45.102
  ● **S45.219   Laceration of axillary or brachial vein, unspecified side** A 🔾
    (Ex) See S45.109

● **S45.29   Other specified injury of axillary or brachial vein**
  ● **S45.291   Other specified injury of axillary or brachial vein, right side** A 🔾
    (Ex) See S45.101
  ● **S45.292   Other specified injury of axillary or brachial vein, left side** A 🔾
    (Ex) See S45.102
  ● **S45.299   Other specified injury of axillary or brachial vein, unspecified** side A 🔾
    (Ex) See S45.109

● **S45.3   Injury of superficial vein at shoulder and upper arm level**
  ● **S45.30   Unspecified injury of superficial vein at shoulder and upper arm level**
    ● **S45.301   Unspecified** injury of superficial vein at shoulder and upper arm level, right arm A 🔾
      (Ex) S45.301[A], S45.309-S45.311[A], S45.319-S45.391[A], S45.399-S45.801[A], S45.809-S45.811[A], S45.819-S45.891[A], S45.899-S45.901[A], S45.909-S45.911[A], S45.919-S45.991[A], S45.999[A], S55.001[A], S55.009-S55.011[A], S55.019-S55.091[A], S55.099[A], S55.201[A], S55.209-S55.211[A], S55.219-S55.291[A], S55.299-S55.801[A], S55.809-S55.811[A], S55.819-S55.891[A], S55.899-S55.901[A], S55.909-S55.911[A], S55.919-S55.991[A], S55.999[A], S65.001[A], S65.009-S65.011[A], S65.019-S65.091[A], S65.099[A], S65.201[A], S65.209-S65.211[A], S65.219-S65.291[A], S65.299-S65.301[A], S65.309-S65.311[A], S65.319-S65.391[A], S65.399-S65.401[A], S65.409-S65.411[A], S65.419-S65.491[A], S65.499-S65.500[A], S65.502[A], S65.504[A], S65.506[A], S65.508-S65.510[A], S65.512[A], S65.514[A], S65.516[A], S65.518-S65.590[A], S65.592[A], S65.594[A], S65.596[A], S65.598-S65.801[A], S65.809-S65.811[A], S65.819-S65.891[A], S65.899-S65.901[A], S65.909-S65.911[A], S65.919-S65.991[A], S65.999[A]

    ● **S45.302   Unspecified** injury of superficial vein at shoulder and upper arm level, left arm A 🔾
      (Ex) S45.302-S45.309[A], S45.312-S45.319[A], S45.392-S45.399[A], S45.802-S45.809[A], S45.812-S45.819[A], S45.892-S45.899[A], S45.902-S45.909[A], S45.912-S45.919[A], S45.992-S45.999[A], S55.002-S55.009[A], S55.012-S55.019[A], S55.092-S55.099[A], S55.202-S55.209[A], S55.212-S55.219[A], S55.292-S55.299[A], S55.802-S55.809[A], S55.812-S55.819[A], S55.892-S55.899[A], S55.902-S55.909[A], S55.912-S55.919[A], S55.992-S55.999[A], S65.002-S65.009[A], S65.012-S65.019[A], S65.092-S65.099[A], S65.202-S65.209[A], S65.212-S65.219[A], S65.292-S65.299[A], S65.302-S65.309[A], S65.312-S65.319[A], S65.392-S65.399[A], S65.402-S65.409[A], S65.412-S65.419[A], S65.492-S65.499[A], S65.501[A], S65.503[A], S65.505[A], S65.507-S65.509[A], S65.511[A], S65.513[A], S65.515[A], S65.517-S65.519[A], S65.591[A], S65.593[A], S65.595[A], S65.597-S65.599[A], S65.802-S65.809[A], S65.812-S65.819[A], S65.892-S65.899[A], S65.902-S65.909[A], S65.912-S65.919[A], S65.992-S65.999[A]

N Newborn Age: Ø   **P** Pediatric Age: Ø–17   **M** Maternity DX: 12–55   **A** Adult Age: 15–124   ♀ Females Only   ♂ Males Only

🔾 Complication\Comorbidity   🔾 Major C\C   (Ex) CC/MCC Exclusions   🔾 Hospital-Acquired Condition

CHAPTER 19 (SØØ-T88)

1289

● S45.309 **Unspecified** injury of superficial vein at shoulder and upper arm level, unspecified arm A 🗲
　　　　(Ex:) S45.301-S45.999[A], S55.001-S55.099[A], S55.201-S55.999[A], S65.001-S65.099[A], S65.201-S65.999[A]

● S45.31 Laceration of superficial vein at shoulder and upper arm level
　● S45.311 Laceration of superficial vein at shoulder and upper arm level, right arm A 🗲
　　　　(Ex:) See S45.301
　● S45.312 Laceration of superficial vein at shoulder and upper arm level, left arm A 🗲
　　　　(Ex:) See S45.302
　● S45.319 Laceration of superficial vein at shoulder and upper arm level, **unspecified** arm A 🗲
　　　　(Ex:) See S45.309

● S45.39 Other specified injury of superficial vein at shoulder and upper arm level
　● S45.391 Other specified injury of superficial vein at shoulder and upper arm level, right arm A 🗲
　　　　(Ex:) See S45.301
　● S45.392 Other specified injury of superficial vein at shoulder and upper arm level, left arm A 🗲
　　　　(Ex:) See S45.302
　● S45.399 Other specified injury of superficial vein at shoulder and upper arm level, **unspecified** arm A 🗲
　　　　(Ex:) See S45.309

● S45.8 Injury of other specified blood vessels at shoulder and upper arm level
　● S45.80 Unspecified injury of other specified blood vessels at shoulder and upper arm level
　　● S45.801 **Unspecified** injury of other specified blood vessels at shoulder and upper arm level, right arm A 🗲
　　　　(Ex:) See S45.301
　　● S45.802 **Unspecified** injury of other specified blood vessels at shoulder and upper arm level, left arm A 🗲
　　　　(Ex:) See S45.302
　　● S45.809 **Unspecified** injury of other specified blood vessels at shoulder and upper arm level, unspecified arm A 🗲
　　　　(Ex:) See S45.309

　● S45.81 Laceration of other specified blood vessels at shoulder and upper arm level
　　● S45.811 Laceration of other specified blood vessels at shoulder and upper arm level, right arm A 🗲
　　　　(Ex:) See S45.301
　　● S45.812 Laceration of other specified blood vessels at shoulder and upper arm level, left arm A 🗲
　　　　(Ex:) See S45.302
　　● S45.819 Laceration of other specified blood vessels at shoulder and upper arm level, **unspecified** arm A 🗲
　　　　(Ex:) See S45.309

● S45.89 Other specified injury of other specified blood vessels at shoulder and upper arm level
　● S45.891 Other specified injury of other specified blood vessels at shoulder and upper arm level, right arm A 🗲
　　　　(Ex:) See S45.301
　● S45.892 Other specified injury of other specified blood vessels at shoulder and upper arm level, left arm A 🗲
　　　　(Ex:) See S45.302
　● S45.899 Other specified injury of other specified blood vessels at shoulder and upper arm level, **unspecified** arm A 🗲
　　　　(Ex:) See S45.309

● S45.9 Injury of unspecified blood vessel at shoulder and upper arm level
　● S45.90 Unspecified injury of unspecified blood vessel at shoulder and upper arm level
　　● S45.901 **Unspecified** injury of unspecified blood vessel at shoulder and upper arm level, right arm A 🗲
　　　　(Ex:) See S45.301
　　● S45.902 **Unspecified** injury of unspecified blood vessel at shoulder and upper arm level, left arm A 🗲
　　　　(Ex:) See S45.302
　　● S45.909 **Unspecified** injury of unspecified blood vessel at shoulder and upper arm level, unspecified arm A 🗲
　　　　(Ex:) See S45.309

　● S45.91 Laceration of unspecified blood vessel at shoulder and upper arm level
　　● S45.911 Laceration of **unspecified** blood vessel at shoulder and upper arm level, right arm A 🗲
　　　　(Ex:) See S45.301
　　● S45.912 Laceration of **unspecified** blood vessel at shoulder and upper arm level, left arm A 🗲
　　　　(Ex:) See S45.302
　　● S45.919 Laceration of **unspecified** blood vessel at shoulder and upper arm level, unspecified arm A 🗲
　　　　(Ex:) See S45.309

　● S45.99 Other specified injury of unspecified blood vessel at shoulder and upper arm level
　　● S45.991 Other specified injury of **unspecified** blood vessel at shoulder and upper arm level, right arm A 🗲
　　　　(Ex:) See S45.301
　　● S45.992 Other specified injury of **unspecified** blood vessel at shoulder and upper arm level, left arm A 🗲
　　　　(Ex:) See S45.302
　　● S45.999 Other specified injury of **unspecified** blood vessel at shoulder and upper arm level, unspecified arm A 🗲
　　　　(Ex:) See S45.309

● **S46** **Injury of muscle, fascia and tendon at shoulder and upper arm level**

     Code also any associated open wound (S41.-)

     Excludes2   injury of muscle, fascia and tendon at elbow (S56.-)

                 sprain of joints and ligaments of shoulder girdle (S43.9)

     The appropriate 7th character is to be added to each code from category S46

A	initial encounter
D	subsequent encounter
S	sequela

● **S46.0** **Injury of muscle(s) and tendon(s) of the rotator cuff of shoulder**

   ● **S46.00** **Unspecified injury of muscle(s) and tendon(s) of the rotator cuff of shoulder**

     ● **S46.001** Unspecified injury of muscle(s) and tendon(s) of the rotator cuff of right shoulder

     ● **S46.002** Unspecified injury of muscle(s) and tendon(s) of the rotator cuff of left shoulder

     ● **S46.009** Unspecified injury of muscle(s) and tendon(s) of the rotator cuff of unspecified shoulder

   ● **S46.01** **Strain of muscle(s) and tendon(s) of the rotator cuff of shoulder**

     Acute onset due to trauma to rotator cuff muscle/tendon

     ● **S46.011** Strain of muscle(s) and tendon(s) of the rotator cuff of right shoulder

     ● **S46.012** Strain of muscle(s) and tendon(s) of the rotator cuff of left shoulder

     ● **S46.019** Strain of muscle(s) and tendon(s) of the rotator cuff of unspecified shoulder

   ● **S46.02** **Laceration of muscle(s) and tendon(s) of the rotator cuff of shoulder**

     ● **S46.021** Laceration of muscle(s) and tendon(s) of the rotator cuff of right shoulder A 🐾
         (Ex:) S41.001[A], S41.009-S41.011[A], S41.019-S41.021[A], S41.029-S41.031[A], S41.039-S41.041[A], S41.049-S41.051[A], S41.059-S41.101[A], S41.109-S41.111[A], S41.119-S41.121[A], S41.129-S41.131[A], S41.139-S41.141[A], S41.149-S41.151[A], S41.159[A], S46.021[A], S46.029[A], S46.121[A], S46.129[A], S46.221[A], S46.229[A], S46.321[A], S46.329[A], S46.821[A], S46.829[A], S46.921[A], S46.929[A]

     ● **S46.022** Laceration of muscle(s) and tendon(s) of the rotator cuff of left shoulder A 🐾
         (Ex:) S41.002-S41.009[A], S41.012-S41.019[A], S41.022-S41.029[A], S41.032-S41.039[A], S41.042-S41.049[A], S41.052-S41.059[A], S41.102-S41.109[A], S41.112-S41.119[A], S41.122-S41.129[A], S41.132-S41.139[A], S41.142-S41.149[A], S41.152-S41.159[A], S46.022-S46.029[A], S46.122-S46.129[A], S46.222-S46.229[A], S46.322-S46.329[A], S46.822-S46.829[A], S46.922-S46.929[A]

     ● **S46.029** Laceration of muscle(s) and tendon(s) of the rotator cuff of unspecified shoulder A 🐾
         (Ex:) S41.001-S41.159[A], S46.021-S46.029[A], S46.121-S46.129[A], S46.221-S46.229[A], S46.321-S46.329[A], S46.821-S46.829[A], S46.921-S46.929[A]

● **S46.09** **Other injury of muscle(s) and tendon(s) of the rotator cuff of shoulder**

     ● **S46.091** Other injury of muscle(s) and tendon(s) of the rotator cuff of right shoulder

     ● **S46.092** Other injury of muscle(s) and tendon(s) of the rotator cuff of left shoulder

     ● **S46.099** Other injury of muscle(s) and tendon(s) of the rotator cuff of unspecified shoulder

● **S46.1** **Injury of muscle, fascia and tendon of long head of biceps**

   ● **S46.10** **Unspecified injury of muscle, fascia and tendon of long head of biceps**

     ● **S46.101** Unspecified injury of muscle, fascia and tendon of long head of biceps, right arm

     ● **S46.102** Unspecified injury of muscle, fascia and tendon of long head of biceps, left arm

     ● **S46.109** Unspecified injury of muscle, fascia and tendon of long head of biceps, unspecified arm

   ● **S46.11** **Strain of muscle, fascia and tendon of long head of biceps**

     ● **S46.111** Strain of muscle, fascia and tendon of long head of biceps, right arm

     ● **S46.112** Strain of muscle, fascia and tendon of long head of biceps, left arm

     ● **S46.119** Strain of muscle, fascia and tendon of long head of biceps, unspecified arm

   ● **S46.12** **Laceration of muscle, fascia and tendon of long head of biceps**

     ● **S46.121** Laceration of muscle, fascia and tendon of long head of biceps, right arm A 🐾
         (Ex:) See S46.021

     ● **S46.122** Laceration of muscle, fascia and tendon of long head of biceps, left arm A 🐾
         (Ex:) See S46.022

     ● **S46.129** Laceration of muscle, fascia and tendon of long head of biceps, unspecified arm A 🐾
         (Ex:) See S46.029

   ● **S46.19** **Other injury of muscle, fascia and tendon of long head of biceps**

     ● **S46.191** Other injury of muscle, fascia and tendon of long head of biceps, right arm

     ● **S46.192** Other injury of muscle, fascia and tendon of long head of biceps, left arm

     ● **S46.199** Other injury of muscle, fascia and tendon of long head of biceps, unspecified arm

● **S46.2** **Injury of muscle, fascia and tendon of other parts of biceps**

   ● **S46.20** **Unspecified injury of muscle, fascia and tendon of other parts of biceps**

     ● **S46.201** Unspecified injury of muscle, fascia and tendon of other parts of biceps, right arm

     ● **S46.202** Unspecified injury of muscle, fascia and tendon of other parts of biceps, left arm

     ● **S46.209** Unspecified injury of muscle, fascia and tendon of other parts of biceps, unspecified arm

N   Newborn Age: 0   **P**   Pediatric Age: 0–17   **M**   Maternity DX: 12–55   **A**   Adult Age: 15–124   ♀   Females Only   ♂   Males Only

🐾   Complication\Comorbidity   🐾   Major C\C   (Ex:)   CC/MCC Exclusions   🐾   Hospital-Acquired Condition

1291

● S46.21   Strain of muscle, fascia and tendon of other parts of biceps
  ● S46.211   Strain of muscle, fascia and tendon of other parts of biceps, right arm
  ● S46.212   Strain of muscle, fascia and tendon of other parts of biceps, left arm
  ● S46.219   Strain of muscle, fascia and tendon of other parts of biceps, unspecified arm
● S46.22   Laceration of muscle, fascia and tendon of other parts of biceps
  ● S46.221   Laceration of muscle, fascia and tendon of other parts of biceps, right arm A 🔗
    Ex: See S46.021
  ● S46.222   Laceration of muscle, fascia and tendon of other parts of biceps, left arm A 🔗
    Ex: See S46.022
  ● S46.229   Laceration of muscle, fascia and tendon of other parts of biceps, unspecified arm A 🔗
    Ex: See S46.029
● S46.29   Other injury of muscle, fascia and tendon of other parts of biceps
  ● S46.291   Other injury of muscle, fascia and tendon of other parts of biceps, right arm
  ● S46.292   Other injury of muscle, fascia and tendon of other parts of biceps, left arm
  ● S46.299   Other injury of muscle, fascia and tendon of other parts of biceps, unspecified arm

● S46.3   Injury of muscle, fascia and tendon of triceps
  ● S46.30   Unspecified injury of muscle, fascia and tendon of triceps
    ● S46.301   Unspecified injury of muscle, fascia and tendon of triceps, right arm
    ● S46.302   Unspecified injury of muscle, fascia and tendon of triceps, left arm
    ● S46.309   Unspecified injury of muscle, fascia and tendon of triceps, unspecified arm
  ● S46.31   Strain of muscle, fascia and tendon of triceps
    ● S46.311   Strain of muscle, fascia and tendon of triceps, right arm
    ● S46.312   Strain of muscle, fascia and tendon of triceps, left arm
    ● S46.319   Strain of muscle, fascia and tendon of triceps, unspecified arm
  ● S46.32   Laceration of muscle, fascia and tendon of triceps
    ● S46.321   Laceration of muscle, fascia and tendon of triceps, right arm A 🔗
      Ex: See S46.021
    ● S46.322   Laceration of muscle, fascia and tendon of triceps, left arm A 🔗
      Ex: See S46.022
    ● S46.329   Laceration of muscle, fascia and tendon of triceps, unspecified arm A 🔗
      Ex: See S46.029
  ● S46.39   Other injury of muscle, fascia and tendon of triceps
    ● S46.391   Other injury of muscle, fascia and tendon of triceps, right arm
    ● S46.392   Other injury of muscle, fascia and tendon of triceps, left arm
    ● S46.399   Other injury of muscle, fascia and tendon of triceps, unspecified arm

● S46.8   Injury of other muscles, fascia and tendons at shoulder and upper arm level
  ● S46.80   Unspecified injury of other muscles, fascia and tendons at shoulder and upper arm level
    ● S46.801   Unspecified injury of other muscles, fascia and tendons at shoulder and upper arm level, right arm
    ● S46.802   Unspecified injury of other muscles, fascia and tendons at shoulder and upper arm level, left arm
    ● S46.809   Unspecified injury of other muscles, fascia and tendons at shoulder and upper arm level, unspecified arm
  ● S46.81   Strain of other muscles, fascia and tendons at shoulder and upper arm level
    ● S46.811   Strain of other muscles, fascia and tendons at shoulder and upper arm level, right arm
    ● S46.812   Strain of other muscles, fascia and tendons at shoulder and upper arm level, left arm
    ● S46.819   Strain of other muscles, fascia and tendons at shoulder and upper arm level, unspecified arm
  ● S46.82   Laceration of other muscles, fascia and tendons at shoulder and upper arm level
    ● S46.821   Laceration of other muscles, fascia and tendons at shoulder and upper arm level, right arm A 🔗
      Ex: See S46.021
    ● S46.822   Laceration of other muscles, fascia and tendons at shoulder and upper arm level, left arm A 🔗
      Ex: See S46.022
    ● S46.829   Laceration of other muscles, fascia and tendons at shoulder and upper arm level, unspecified arm A 🔗
      Ex: See S46.029
  ● S46.89   Other injury of other muscles, fascia and tendons at shoulder and upper arm level
    ● S46.891   Other injury of other muscles, fascia and tendons at shoulder and upper arm level, right arm
    ● S46.892   Other injury of other muscles, fascia and tendons at shoulder and upper arm level, left arm
    ● S46.899   Other injury of other muscles, fascia and tendons at shoulder and upper arm level, unspecified arm

● S46.9   Injury of unspecified muscle, fascia and tendon at shoulder and upper arm level
  ● S46.90   Unspecified injury of unspecified muscle, fascia and tendon at shoulder and upper arm level
    ● S46.901   Unspecified injury of unspecified muscle, fascia and tendon at shoulder and upper arm level, right arm
    ● S46.902   Unspecified injury of unspecified muscle, fascia and tendon at shoulder and upper arm level, left arm
    ● S46.909   Unspecified injury of unspecified muscle, fascia and tendon at shoulder and upper arm level, unspecified arm
  ● S46.91   Strain of unspecified muscle, fascia and tendon at shoulder and upper arm level
    ● S46.911   Strain of unspecified muscle, fascia and tendon at shoulder and upper arm level, right arm
    ● S46.912   Strain of unspecified muscle, fascia and tendon at shoulder and upper arm level, left arm
    ● S46.919   Strain of unspecified muscle, fascia and tendon at shoulder and upper arm level, unspecified arm

◀ New   ◀▥ Revised   ~~deleted~~ Deleted   Excludes 1   Excludes 2   Includes   Use additional   Code first   Code also   Unspecified
OGCR Official Guidelines   ● Unacceptable Principal Diagnosis   X Assign placeholder X   ● Use Additional Character(s)   ▶ Manifestation Code   Coding Clinic

● **S46.92** **Laceration of unspecified muscle, fascia and tendon at shoulder and upper arm level**

  ● **S46.921** **Laceration of unspecified muscle, fascia and tendon at shoulder and upper arm level, right arm** A ◔

    (Ex:) See S46.021

  ● **S46.922** **Laceration of unspecified muscle, fascia and tendon at shoulder and upper arm level, left arm** A ◔

    (Ex:) See S46.022

  ● **S46.929** **Laceration of unspecified muscle, fascia and tendon at shoulder and upper arm level, unspecified arm** A ◔

    (Ex:) See S46.029

● **S46.99** **Other injury of unspecified muscle, fascia and tendon at shoulder and upper arm level**

  ● **S46.991** **Other injury of unspecified muscle, fascia and tendon at shoulder and upper arm level, right arm**

  ● **S46.992** **Other injury of unspecified muscle, fascia and tendon at shoulder and upper arm level, left arm**

  ● **S46.999** **Other injury of unspecified muscle, fascia and tendon at shoulder and upper arm level, unspecified arm**

● **S47** **Crushing injury of shoulder and upper arm**

Use additional code for all associated injuries

Excludes2 crushing injury of elbow (S57.0-)

The appropriate 7th character is to be added to each code from category S47

A	initial encounter
D	subsequent encounter
S	sequela

X ● **S47.1** **Crushing injury of right shoulder and upper arm**

X ● **S47.2** **Crushing injury of left shoulder and upper arm**

X ● **S47.9** **Crushing injury of shoulder and upper arm, unspecified arm**

● **S48** **Traumatic amputation of shoulder and upper arm**

An amputation not identified as partial or complete should be coded to complete

Excludes1 traumatic amputation at elbow level (S58.0)

The appropriate 7th character is to be added to each code from category S48

A	initial encounter
D	subsequent encounter
S	sequela

● **S48.0** **Traumatic amputation at shoulder joint**

  ● **S48.01** **Complete traumatic amputation at shoulder joint**

    ● **S48.011** **Complete traumatic amputation at right shoulder joint** A ◔

      (Ex:) S41.001[A], S41.009-S41.011[A], S41.019-S41.021[A], S41.029-S41.031[A], S41.039-S41.041[A], S41.049-S41.051[A], S41.059-S41.101[A], S41.109-S41.111[A], S41.119-S41.121[A], S41.129-S41.131[A], S41.139-S41.141[A], S41.149-S41.151[A], S41.159[A], S46.021[A], S46.029[A], S46.121[A], S46.129[A], S46.221[A], S46.229[A], S46.321[A], S46.329[A], S46.821[A], S46.829[A], S46.921[A],

S46.929[A], S48.011[A], S48.019-S48.021[A], S48.029-S48.111[A], S48.119-S48.121[A], S48.129-S48.911[A], S48.919-S48.921[A], S48.929[A], S51.001[A], S51.009-S51.011[A], S51.019-S51.021[A], S51.029-S51.031[A], S51.039-S51.041[A], S51.049-S51.051[A], S51.059-S51.801[A], S51.809-S51.811[A], S51.819-S51.821[A], S51.829-S51.831[A], S51.839-S51.841[A], S51.849-S51.851[A], S51.859[A], S56.021[A], S56.029[A], S56.121[A], S56.123[A], S56.125[A], S56.127[A], S56.129[A], S56.221[A], S56.229[A], S56.321[A], S56.329[A], S56.421[A], S56.423[A], S56.425[A], S56.427[A], S56.429[A], S56.521[A], S56.529[A], S56.821[A], S56.829[A], S56.921[A], S56.929[A], S58.011[A], S58.019-S58.021[A], S58.029-S58.111[A], S58.119-S58.121[A], S58.129-S58.911[A], S58.919-S58.921[A], S58.929[A], S61.001[A], S61.009-S61.011[A], S61.019-S61.021[A], S61.029-S61.031[A], S61.039-S61.041[A], S61.049-S61.051[A], S61.059-S61.101[A], S61.109-S61.111[A], S61.119-S61.121[A], S61.129-S61.131[A], S61.139-S61.141[A], S61.149-S61.151[A], S61.159-S61.200[A], S61.202[A], S61.204[A], S61.206[A], S61.208-S61.210[A], S61.212[A], S61.214[A], S61.216[A], S61.218-S61.220[A], S61.222[A], S61.224[A], S61.226[A], S61.228-S61.230[A], S61.232[A], S61.234[A], S61.236[A], S61.238-S61.240[A], S61.242[A], S61.244[A], S61.246[A], S61.248-S61.250[A], S61.252[A], S61.254[A], S61.256[A], S61.258-S61.300[A], S61.302[A], S61.304[A], S61.306[A], S61.308-S61.310[A], S61.312[A], S61.314[A], S61.316[A], S61.318-S61.320[A], S61.322[A], S61.324[A], S61.326[A], S61.328-S61.330[A], S61.332[A], S61.334[A], S61.336[A], S61.338-S61.340[A], S61.342[A], S61.344[A], S61.346[A], S61.348-S61.350[A], S61.352[A], S61.354[A], S61.356[A], S61.358-S61.401[A], S61.409-S61.411[A], S61.419-S61.421[A], S61.429-S61.431[A], S61.439-S61.441[A], S61.449-S61.451[A], S61.459-S61.501[A], S61.509-S61.511[A], S61.519-S61.521[A], S61.529-S61.531[A], S61.539-S61.541[A], S61.549-S61.551[A], S61.559[A], S66.021[A], S66.029[A], S66.120[A], S66.122[A], S66.124[A], S66.126[A], S66.128-S66.129[A], S66.221[A], S66.229[A], S66.320[A], S66.322[A], S66.324[A], S66.326[A], S66.328-S66.329[A], S66.421[A], S66.429[A], S66.520[A], S66.522[A], S66.524[A], S66.526[A], S66.528-S66.529[A], S66.821[A], S66.829[A], S66.921[A], S66.929[A], S68.011[A], S68.019-S68.021[A], S68.029-S68.110[A], S68.112[A], S68.114[A], S68.116[A], S68.118-S68.120[A], S68.122[A], S68.124[A], S68.126[A], S68.128-S68.411[A], S68.419-S68.421[A], S68.429-S68.511[A], S68.519-S68.521[A], S68.529-S68.610[A], S68.612[A], S68.614[A], S68.616[A], S68.618-S68.620[A], S68.622[A], S68.624[A], S68.626[A], S68.628-S68.711[A], S68.719-S68.721[A], S68.729[A], T14.90-T14.91, T79.A0X-T79.9XX[A]

● **S48.012** **Complete traumatic amputation at left shoulder joint** A 🔋
Ex: S41.002-S41.009[A], S41.012-S41.019[A],
S41.022-S41.029[A], S41.032-S41.039[A],
S41.042-S41.049[A], S41.052-S41.059[A],
S41.102-S41.109[A], S41.112-S41.119[A],
S41.122-S41.129[A], S41.132-S41.139[A],
S41.142-S41.149[A], S41.152-S41.159[A],
S46.022-S46.029[A], S46.122-S46.129[A],
S46.222-S46.229[A], S46.322-S46.329[A],
S46.822-S46.829[A], S46.922-S46.929[A],
S48.012-S48.019[A], S48.022-S48.029[A],
S48.112-S48.119[A], S48.122-S48.129[A],
S48.912-S48.919[A], S48.922-S48.929[A],
S51.002-S51.009[A], S51.012-S51.019[A],
S51.022-S51.029[A], S51.032-S51.039[A],
S51.042-S51.049[A], S51.052-S51.059[A],
S51.802-S51.809[A], S51.812-S51.819[A],
S51.822-S51.829[A], S51.832-S51.839[A],
S51.842-S51.849[A], S51.852-S51.859[A],
S56.022-S56.029[A], S56.122[A], S56.124[A],
S56.126[A], S56.128-S56.129[A],
S56.222-S56.229[A], S56.322-S56.329[A],
S56.422[A], S56.424[A], S56.426[A],
S56.428-S56.429[A], S56.522-S56.529[A],
S56.822-S56.829[A], S56.922-S56.929[A],
S58.012-S58.019[A], S58.022-S58.029[A],
S58.112-S58.119[A], S58.122-S58.129[A],
S58.912-S58.919[A], S58.922-S58.929[A],
S61.002-S61.009[A], S61.012-S61.019[A],
S61.022-S61.029[A], S61.032-S61.039[A],
S61.042-S61.049[A], S61.052-S61.059[A],
S61.102-S61.109[A], S61.112-S61.119[A],
S61.122-S61.129[A], S61.132-S61.139[A],
S61.142-S61.149[A], S61.152-S61.159[A],
S61.201[A], S61.203[A], S61.205[A],
S61.207-S61.209[A], S61.211[A], S61.213[A],
S61.215[A], S61.217-S61.219[A], S61.221[A],
S61.223[A], S61.225[A], S61.227-S61.229[A],
S61.231[A], S61.233[A], S61.235[A],
S61.237-S61.239[A], S61.241[A], S61.243[A],
S61.245[A], S61.247-S61.249[A], S61.251[A],
S61.253[A], S61.255[A], S61.257-S61.259[A],
S61.301[A], S61.303[A], S61.305[A],
S61.307-S61.309[A], S61.311[A], S61.313[A],
S61.315[A], S61.317-S61.319[A], S61.321[A],
S61.323[A], S61.325[A], S61.327-S61.329[A],
S61.331[A], S61.333[A], S61.335[A],
S61.337-S61.339[A], S61.341[A], S61.343[A],
S61.345[A], S61.347-S61.349[A], S61.351[A],
S61.353[A], S61.355[A], S61.357-S61.359[A],
S61.402-S61.409[A], S61.412-S61.419[A],
S61.422-S61.429[A], S61.432-S61.439[A],
S61.442-S61.449[A], S61.452-S61.459[A],
S61.502-S61.509[A], S61.512-S61.519[A],
S61.522-S61.529[A], S61.532-S61.539[A],
S61.542-S61.549[A], S61.552-S61.559[A],
S66.022-S66.029[A], S66.121[A], S66.123[A],
S66.125[A], S66.127-S66.129[A],
S66.222-S66.229[A], S66.321[A], S66.323[A],
S66.325[A], S66.327-S66.329[A],
S66.422-S66.429[A], S66.521[A], S66.523[A],
S66.525[A], S66.527-S66.529[A],
S66.822-S66.829[A], S66.922-S66.929[A],
S68.012-S68.019[A], S68.022-S68.029[A],
S68.111[A], S68.113[A], S68.115[A],
S68.117-S68.119[A], S68.121[A], S68.123[A],
S68.125[A], S68.127-S68.129[A],
S68.412-S68.419[A], S68.422-S68.429[A],
S68.512-S68.519[A], S68.522-S68.529[A],
S68.611[A], S68.613[A], S68.615[A],
S68.617-S68.619[A], S68.621[A], S68.623[A],
S68.625[A], S68.627-S68.629[A],
S68.712-S68.719[A], S68.722-S68.729[A],
T14.90-T14.91, T79.A0X-T79.9XX[A]

● **S48.019** **Complete traumatic amputation at unspecified shoulder joint** A 🔋
Ex: S41.001-S41.159[A], S46.021-S46.029[A],
S46.121-S46.129[A], S46.221-S46.229[A],
S46.321-S46.329[A], S46.821-S46.829[A],
S46.921-S46.929[A], S48.011-S48.929[A],
S51.001-S51.859[A], S56.021-S56.029[A],
S56.121-S56.129[A], S56.221-S56.229[A],
S56.321-S56.329[A], S56.421-S56.429[A],
S56.521-S56.529[A], S56.821-S56.829[A],
S56.921-S56.929[A], S58.011-S58.929[A],
S61.001-S61.559[A], S66.021-S66.029[A],
S66.120-S66.129[A], S66.221-S66.229[A],
S66.320-S66.329[A], S66.421-S66.429[A],
S66.520-S66.529[A], S66.821-S66.829[A],
S66.921-S66.929[A], S68.011-S68.729[A],
T14.90-T14.91, T79.A0X-T79.9XX[A]

● **S48.02** **Partial traumatic amputation at shoulder joint**

● **S48.021** **Partial traumatic amputation at right shoulder joint** A 🔋
Ex: See S48.011

● **S48.022** **Partial traumatic amputation at left shoulder joint** A 🔋
Ex: See S48.012

● **S48.029** **Partial traumatic amputation at unspecified shoulder joint** A 🔋
Ex: See S48.019

● **S48.1** **Traumatic amputation at level between shoulder and elbow**

● **S48.11** **Complete traumatic amputation at level between shoulder and elbow**

● **S48.111** **Complete traumatic amputation at level between right shoulder and elbow** A 🔋
Ex: See S48.011

● **S48.112** **Complete traumatic amputation at level between left shoulder and elbow** A 🔋
Ex: See S48.012

● **S48.119** **Complete traumatic amputation at level between unspecified shoulder and elbow** A 🔋
Ex: See S48.019

● **S48.12** **Partial traumatic amputation at level between shoulder and elbow**

● **S48.121** **Partial traumatic amputation at level between right shoulder and elbow** A 🔋
Ex: See S48.011

● **S48.122** **Partial traumatic amputation at level between left shoulder and elbow** A 🔋
Ex: See S48.012

● **S48.129** **Partial traumatic amputation at level between unspecified shoulder and elbow** A 🔋
Ex: See S48.019

● **S48.9** **Traumatic amputation of shoulder and upper arm, level unspecified**

● **S48.91** **Complete traumatic amputation of shoulder and upper arm, level unspecified**

● **S48.911** **Complete traumatic amputation of right shoulder and upper arm, level unspecified** A 🔋
Ex: See S48.011

● **S48.912** **Complete traumatic amputation of left shoulder and upper arm, level unspecified** A 🔋
Ex: See S48.012

● **S48.919** **Complete traumatic amputation of unspecified shoulder and upper arm, level unspecified** A 🔋
Ex: See S48.019

● S48.92   Partial traumatic amputation of shoulder and upper arm, level unspecified

   ● S48.921   Partial traumatic amputation of right shoulder and upper arm, level unspecified A 🦠
          Ⓔⓧ See S48.011

   ● S48.922   Partial traumatic amputation of left shoulder and upper arm, level unspecified A 🦠
          Ⓔⓧ See S48.012

   ● S48.929   Partial traumatic amputation of unspecified shoulder and upper arm, level unspecified A 🦠
          Ⓔⓧ See S48.019

● S49   Other and unspecified injuries of shoulder and upper arm

   The appropriate 7th character is to be added to each code from subcategories S49.0 and S49.1

A	initial encounter for closed fracture
D	subsequent encounter for fracture with routine healing
G	subsequent encounter for fracture with delayed healing
K	subsequent encounter for fracture with nonunion
P	subsequent encounter for fracture with malunion
S	sequela

● S49.0   Physeal fracture of upper end of humerus

   ● S49.00   Unspecified physeal fracture of upper end of humerus

      ● S49.001   Unspecified physeal fracture of upper end of humerus, right arm A, K, P 🦠, A 🦠
             Ⓔⓧ For S49.001[A]: See S42.201[A]
                 For S49.001[K,P]: See S02.0[K]

      ● S49.002   Unspecified physeal fracture of upper end of humerus, left arm A, K, P 🦠, A 🦠
             Ⓔⓧ For S49.002[A]: See S42.202[A]
                 For S49.002[K,P]: See S02.0[K]

      ● S49.009   Unspecified physeal fracture of upper end of humerus, unspecified arm A, K, P 🦠, A 🦠
             Ⓔⓧ For S49.009[A]: See S42.209[A]
                 For S49.009[K,P]: See S02.0[K]

   ● S49.01   Salter-Harris Type I physeal fracture of upper end of humerus

      ● S49.011   Salter-Harris Type I physeal fracture of upper end of humerus, right arm A, K, P 🦠, A 🦠
             Ⓔⓧ For S49.011[A]: See S42.201[A]
                 For S49.011[K,P]: See S02.0[K]

      ● S49.012   Salter-Harris Type I physeal fracture of upper end of humerus, left arm A, K, P 🦠, A 🦠
             Ⓔⓧ For S49.012[A]: See S42.202[A]
                 For S49.012[K,P]: See S02.0[K]

      ● S49.019   Salter-Harris Type I physeal fracture of upper end of humerus, unspecified arm A, K, P 🦠, A 🦠
             Ⓔⓧ For S49.019[A]: See S42.209[A]
                 For S49.019[K,P]: See S02.0[K]

● S49.02   Salter-Harris Type II physeal fracture of upper end of humerus

   ● S49.021   Salter-Harris Type II physeal fracture of upper end of humerus, right arm A, K, P 🦠, A 🦠
          Ⓔⓧ For S49.021[A]: See S42.201[A]
              For S49.021[K,P]: See S02.0[K]

   ● S49.022   Salter-Harris Type II physeal fracture of upper end of humerus, left arm A, K, P 🦠, A 🦠
          Ⓔⓧ For S49.022[A]: See S42.202[A]
              For S49.022[K,P]: See S02.0[K]

   ● S49.029   Salter-Harris Type II physeal fracture of upper end of humerus, unspecified arm A, K, P 🦠, A 🦠
          Ⓔⓧ For S49.029[A]: See S42.209[A]
              For S49.029[K,P]: See S02.0[K]

● S49.03   Salter-Harris Type III physeal fracture of upper end of humerus

   ● S49.031   Salter-Harris Type III physeal fracture of upper end of humerus, right arm A, K, P 🦠, A 🦠 ◀▥
          Ⓔⓧ For S49.031[A]: See S42.201[A]
              For S49.031[K,P]: See S02.0[K]

   ● S49.032   Salter-Harris Type III physeal fracture of upper end of humerus, left arm A, K, P 🦠, A 🦠 ◀▥
          Ⓔⓧ For S49.032[A]: See S42.202[A]
              For S49.032[K,P]: See S02.0[K]

   ● S49.039   Salter-Harris Type III physeal fracture of upper end of humerus, unspecified arm A, K, P 🦠, A 🦠 ◀▥
          Ⓔⓧ For S49.039[A]: See S42.209[A]
              For S49.039[K,P]: See S02.0[K]

● S49.04   Salter-Harris Type IV physeal fracture of upper end of humerus

   ● S49.041   Salter-Harris Type IV physeal fracture of upper end of humerus, right arm A, K, P 🦠, A 🦠
          Ⓔⓧ For S49.041[A]: See S42.201[A]
              For S49.041[K,P]: See S02.0[K]

   ● S49.042   Salter-Harris Type IV physeal fracture of upper end of humerus, left arm A, K, P 🦠, A 🦠
          Ⓔⓧ For S49.042[A]: See S42.202[A]
              For S49.042[K,P]: See S02.0[K]

   ● S49.049   Salter-Harris Type IV physeal fracture of upper end of humerus, unspecified arm A, K, P 🦠, A 🦠
          Ⓔⓧ For S49.049[A]: See S42.209[A]
              For S49.049[K,P]: See S02.0[K]

● S49.09   Other physeal fracture of upper end of humerus

   ● S49.091   Other physeal fracture of upper end of humerus, right arm A, K, P 🦠, A 🦠
          Ⓔⓧ For S49.091[A]: See S42.201[A]
              For S49.091[K,P]: See S02.0[K]

   ● S49.092   Other physeal fracture of upper end of humerus, left arm A, K, P 🦠, A 🦠
          Ⓔⓧ For S49.092[A]: See S42.202[A]
              For S49.092[K,P]: See S02.0[K]

   ● S49.099   Other physeal fracture of upper end of humerus, unspecified arm A, K, P 🦠, A 🦠
          Ⓔⓧ For S49.099[A]: See S42.209[A]
              For S49.099[K,P]: See S02.0[K]

Item 19-3 SALTER-HARRIS TYPE 1: epiphysis is completely separated from end of bone, or metaphysic growth plate remains attached to epiphysis

   SALTER-HARRIS TYPE 2: epiphysis and growth plate are partially separated from metaphysis, which is cracked—most common type

   SALTER-HARRIS TYPE 3: fracture occurring through epiphysis and separates part of epiphysis and growth plate from metaphysis fracture, usually at distal end of tibia

   SALTER-HARRIS TYPE 4: fracture runs through epiphysis, across growth plate, into metaphysic, surgery is required to restore joint surface to normal and align growth plate

N Newborn Age: 0   P Pediatric Age: 0–17   M Maternity DX: 12–55   A Adult Age: 15–124   ♀ Females Only   ♂ Males Only

🦠 Complication\Comorbidity   🦠 Major C\C   Ⓔⓧ CC/MCC Exclusions   🦠 Hospital-Acquired Condition

● **S49.1**   **Physeal fracture of lower end of humerus**
  ● **S49.10**   Unspecified physeal fracture of lower end of humerus
    ● **S49.101**   Unspecified physeal fracture of lower end of humerus, right arm A, K, P 🖼, A 🖼
      (Ex:) **For S49.101[A]:** See S42.201[A]
      For S49.101[K,P]: See S02.0[K]
    ● **S49.102**   Unspecified physeal fracture of lower end of humerus, left arm A, K, P 🖼, A 🖼
      (Ex:) **For S49.102[A]:** See S42.202[A]
      For S49.102[K,P]: See S02.0[K]
    ● **S49.109**   Unspecified physeal fracture of lower end of humerus, unspecified arm A, K, P 🖼, A 🖼
      (Ex:) **For S49.109[A]:** See S42.209[A]
      For S49.109[K,P]: See S02.0[K]
  ● **S49.11**   Salter-Harris Type I physeal fracture of lower end of humerus
    ● **S49.111**   Salter-Harris Type I physeal fracture of lower end of humerus, right arm A, K, P 🖼, A 🖼
      (Ex:) **For S49.111[A]:** See S42.201[A]
      For S49.111[K,P]: See S02.0[K]
    ● **S49.112**   Salter-Harris Type I physeal fracture of lower end of humerus, left arm A, K, P 🖼, A 🖼
      (Ex:) **For S49.112[A]:** See S42.202[A]
      For S49.112[K,P]: See S02.0[K]
    ● **S49.119**   Salter-Harris Type I physeal fracture of lower end of humerus, unspecified arm A, K, P 🖼, A 🖼
      (Ex:) **For S49.119[A]:** See S42.209[A]
      For S49.119[K,P]: See S02.0[K]
  ● **S49.12**   Salter-Harris Type II physeal fracture of lower end of humerus
    ● **S49.121**   Salter-Harris Type II physeal fracture of lower end of humerus, right arm A, K, P 🖼, A 🖼
      (Ex:) **For S49.121[A]:** See S42.201[A]
      For S49.121[K,P]: See S02.0[K]
    ● **S49.122**   Salter-Harris Type II physeal fracture of lower end of humerus, left arm A, K, P 🖼, A 🖼
      (Ex:) **For S49.122[A]:** See S42.202[A]
      For S49.122[K,P]: See S02.0[K]
    ● **S49.129**   Salter-Harris Type II physeal fracture of lower end of humerus, unspecified arm A, K, P 🖼, A 🖼
      (Ex:) **For S49.129[A]:** See S42.209[A]
      For S49.129[K,P]: See S02.0[K]
  ● **S49.13**   Salter-Harris Type III physeal fracture of lower end of humerus ◀▥
    ● **S49.131**   Salter-Harris Type III physeal fracture of lower end of humerus, right arm A, K, P 🖼, A 🖼 ◀▥
      (Ex:) **For S49.131[A]:** See S42.201[A]
      For S49.131[K,P]: See S02.0[K]
    ● **S49.132**   Salter-Harris Type III physeal fracture of lower end of humerus, left arm A, K, P 🖼, A 🖼 ◀▥
      (Ex:) **For S49.132[A]:** See S42.202[A]
      For S49.132[K,P]: See S02.0[K]
    ● **S49.139**   Salter-Harris Type III physeal fracture of lower end of humerus, unspecified arm A, K, P 🖼, A 🖼 ◀▥
      (Ex:) **For S49.139[A]:** See S42.209[A]
      For S49.139[K,P]: See S02.0[K]

● **S49.14**   Salter-Harris Type IV physeal fracture of lower end of humerus
    ● **S49.141**   Salter-Harris Type IV physeal fracture of lower end of humerus, right arm A, K, P 🖼, A 🖼
      (Ex:) **For S49.141[A]:** See S42.201[A]
      For S49.141[K,P]: See S02.0[K]
    ● **S49.142**   Salter-Harris Type IV physeal fracture of lower end of humerus, left arm A, K, P 🖼, A 🖼
      (Ex:) **For S49.142[A]:** See S42.202[A]
      For S49.142[K,P]: See S02.0[K]
    ● **S49.149**   Salter-Harris Type IV physeal fracture of lower end of humerus, unspecified arm A, K, P 🖼, A 🖼
      (Ex:) **For S49.149[A]:** See S42.209[A]
      For S49.149[K,P]: See S02.0[K]
  ● **S49.19**   Other physeal fracture of lower end of humerus
    ● **S49.191**   Other physeal fracture of lower end of humerus, right arm A, K, P 🖼, A 🖼
      (Ex:) **For S49.191[A]:** See S42.201[A]
      For S49.191[K,P]: See S02.0[K]
    ● **S49.192**   Other physeal fracture of lower end of humerus, left arm A, K, P 🖼, A 🖼
      (Ex:) **For S49.192[A]:** See S42.202[A]
      For S49.192[K,P]: See S02.0[K]
    ● **S49.199**   Other physeal fracture of lower end of humerus, unspecified arm A, K, P 🖼, A 🖼
      (Ex:) **For S49.199[A]:** See S42.209[A]
      For S49.199[K,P]: See S02.0[K]

● **S49.8**   **Other specified injuries of shoulder and upper arm**
  The appropriate 7th character is to be added to each code in subcategory S49.8

> A   initial encounter
> D   subsequent encounter
> S   sequela

  X ● **S49.80**   Other specified injuries of shoulder and upper arm, unspecified arm
  X ● **S49.81**   Other specified injuries of right shoulder and upper arm
  X ● **S49.82**   Other specified injuries of left shoulder and upper arm

● **S49.9**   **Unspecified injury of shoulder and upper arm**
  The appropriate 7th character is to be added to each code in subcategory S49.9

> A   initial encounter
> D   subsequent encounter
> S   sequela

  X ● **S49.90**   Unspecified injury of shoulder and upper arm, unspecified arm
  X ● **S49.91**   Unspecified injury of right shoulder and upper arm
  X ● **S49.92**   Unspecified injury of left shoulder and upper arm

◀ New   ◀▥ Revised   ~~deleted~~ Deleted   Excludes 1   Excludes 2   Includes   Use additional   Code first   Code also   Unspecified
OGCR Official Guidelines   ● Unacceptable Principal Diagnosis   X Assign placeholder X   ● Use Additional Character(s)   ▶ Manifestation Code   **Coding Clinic**

INJURIES TO THE ELBOW AND FOREARM (S50-S59)

Excludes2   burns and corrosions (T20-T32)
frostbite (T33-T34)
injuries of wrist and hand (S60-S69)
insect bite or sting, venomous (T63.4)

● **S50**   **Superficial injury of elbow and forearm**
      Excludes2   superficial injury of wrist and hand (S60.-)
      The appropriate 7th character is to be added to each code from
      category S50

> A   initial encounter
> D   subsequent encounter
> S   sequela

 ● **S50.0**   **Contusion of elbow**
   X● **S50.00**   Contusion of unspecified elbow
   X● **S50.01**   Contusion of right elbow
   X● **S50.02**   Contusion of left elbow
 ● **S50.1**   **Contusion of forearm**
   X● **S50.10**   Contusion of unspecified forearm
   X● **S50.11**   Contusion of right forearm
   X● **S50.12**   Contusion of left forearm
 ● **S50.3**   **Other superficial injuries of elbow**
  ● **S50.31**   **Abrasion of elbow**
   ● S50.311   Abrasion of right elbow
   ● S50.312   Abrasion of left elbow
   ● S50.319   Abrasion of unspecified elbow
  ● **S50.32**   **Blister (nonthermal) of elbow**
   ● S50.321   Blister (nonthermal) of right elbow
   ● S50.322   Blister (nonthermal) of left elbow
   ● S50.329   Blister (nonthermal) of unspecified elbow
  ● **S50.34**   **External constriction of elbow**
   ● S50.341   External constriction of right elbow
   ● S50.342   External constriction of left elbow
   ● S50.349   External constriction of unspecified elbow
  ● **S50.35**   **Superficial foreign body of elbow**
     Splinter in the elbow
   ● S50.351   Superficial foreign body of right elbow
   ● S50.352   Superficial foreign body of left elbow
   ● S50.359   Superficial foreign body of unspecified elbow
  ● **S50.36**   **Insect bite (nonvenomous) of elbow**
   ● S50.361   Insect bite (nonvenomous) of right elbow
   ● S50.362   Insect bite (nonvenomous) of left elbow
   ● S50.369   Insect bite (nonvenomous) of unspecified elbow
  ● **S50.37**   **Other superficial bite of elbow**
     Excludes1   open bite of elbow (S51.04)
   ● S50.371   Other superficial bite of right elbow
   ● S50.372   Other superficial bite of left elbow
   ● S50.379   Other superficial bite of unspecified elbow
 ● **S50.8**   **Other superficial injuries of forearm**
  ● **S50.81**   **Abrasion of forearm**
   ● S50.811   Abrasion of right forearm
   ● S50.812   Abrasion of left forearm
   ● S50.819   Abrasion of unspecified forearm
  ● **S50.82**   **Blister (nonthermal) of forearm**
   ● S50.821   Blister (nonthermal) of right forearm
   ● S50.822   Blister (nonthermal) of left forearm
   ● S50.829   Blister (nonthermal) of unspecified forearm

  ● **S50.84**   **External constriction of forearm**
   ● S50.841   External constriction of right forearm
   ● S50.842   External constriction of left forearm
   ● S50.849   External constriction of unspecified forearm
  ● **S50.85**   **Superficial foreign body of forearm**
     Splinter in the forearm
   ● S50.851   Superficial foreign body of right forearm
   ● S50.852   Superficial foreign body of left forearm
   ● S50.859   Superficial foreign body of unspecified forearm
  ● **S50.86**   **Insect bite (nonvenomous) of forearm**
   ● S50.861   Insect bite (nonvenomous) of right forearm
   ● S50.862   Insect bite (nonvenomous) of left forearm
   ● S50.869   Insect bite (nonvenomous) of unspecified forearm
  ● **S50.87**   **Other superficial bite of forearm**
     Excludes1   open bite of forearm (S51.84)
   ● S50.871   Other superficial bite of right forearm
   ● S50.872   Other superficial bite of left forearm
   ● S50.879   Other superficial bite of unspecified forearm
 ● **S50.9**   **Unspecified superficial injury of elbow and forearm**
  ● **S50.90**   **Unspecified superficial injury of elbow**
   ● S50.901   Unspecified superficial injury of right elbow
   ● S50.902   Unspecified superficial injury of left elbow
   ● S50.909   Unspecified superficial injury of unspecified elbow
  ● **S50.91**   **Unspecified superficial injury of forearm**
   ● S50.911   Unspecified superficial injury of right forearm
   ● S50.912   Unspecified superficial injury of left forearm
   ● S50.919   Unspecified superficial injury of unspecified forearm

● **S51**   **Open wound of elbow and forearm**
    Code also any associated wound infection
    Excludes1   open fracture of elbow and forearm (S52.- with
                open fracture 7th character)
                traumatic amputation of elbow and forearm
                (S58.-)
    Excludes2   open wound of wrist and hand (S61.-)
    The appropriate 7th character is to be added to each code from
    category S51

> A   initial encounter
> D   subsequent encounter
> S   sequela

 ● **S51.0**   **Open wound of elbow**
  ● **S51.00**   **Unspecified open wound of elbow**
   ● S51.001   Unspecified open wound of right elbow
         Coding Clinic: 2012, Q4, P108
   ● S51.002   Unspecified open wound of left elbow
   ● S51.009   Unspecified open wound of unspecified elbow
        Open wound of elbow NOS

● **S51.01** Laceration without foreign body of elbow
  ● **S51.011** Laceration without foreign body of right elbow
  ● **S51.012** Laceration without foreign body of left elbow
  ● **S51.019** Laceration without foreign body of **unspecified** elbow

● **S51.02** Laceration with foreign body of elbow
  ● **S51.021** Laceration with foreign body of right elbow
  ● **S51.022** Laceration with foreign body of left elbow
  ● **S51.029** Laceration with foreign body of **unspecified** elbow

● **S51.03** Puncture wound without foreign body of elbow
  ● **S51.031** Puncture wound without foreign body of right elbow
  ● **S51.032** Puncture wound without foreign body of left elbow
  ● **S51.039** Puncture wound without foreign body of **unspecified** elbow

● **S51.04** Puncture wound with foreign body of elbow
  ● **S51.041** Puncture wound with foreign body of right elbow
  ● **S51.042** Puncture wound with foreign body of left elbow
  ● **S51.049** Puncture wound with foreign body of **unspecified** elbow

● **S51.05** Open bite of elbow
  Bite of elbow NOS
    Excludes1 superficial bite of elbow (S50.36, S50.37)
  ● **S51.051** Open bite, right elbow
  ● **S51.052** Open bite, left elbow
  ● **S51.059** Open bite, **unspecified** elbow

● **S51.8** Open wound of forearm
  Excludes2 open wound of elbow (S51.0-)
  ● **S51.80** Unspecified open wound of forearm
    ● **S51.801** **Unspecified** open wound of right forearm
    ● **S51.802** **Unspecified** open wound of left forearm
    ● **S51.809** **Unspecified** open wound of unspecified forearm
      Open wound of forearm NOS
  ● **S51.81** Laceration without foreign body of forearm
    ● **S51.811** Laceration without foreign body of right forearm
    ● **S51.812** Laceration without foreign body of left forearm
    ● **S51.819** Laceration without foreign body of **unspecified** forearm
  ● **S51.82** Laceration with foreign body of forearm
    ● **S51.821** Laceration with foreign body of right forearm
    ● **S51.822** Laceration with foreign body of left forearm
    ● **S51.829** Laceration with foreign body of **unspecified** forearm

● **S51.83** Puncture wound without foreign body of forearm
  ● **S51.831** Puncture wound without foreign body of right forearm
  ● **S51.832** Puncture wound without foreign body of left forearm
  ● **S51.839** Puncture wound without foreign body of **unspecified** forearm

● **S51.84** Puncture wound with foreign body of forearm
  ● **S51.841** Puncture wound with foreign body of right forearm
  ● **S51.842** Puncture wound with foreign body of left forearm
  ● **S51.849** Puncture wound with foreign body of **unspecified** forearm

● **S51.85** Open bite of forearm
  Bite of forearm NOS
    Excludes1 superficial bite of forearm (S50.86, S50.87)
  ● **S51.851** Open bite of right forearm
  ● **S51.852** Open bite of left forearm
  ● **S51.859** Open bite of **unspecified** forearm

● **S52** Fracture of forearm
  Note: A fracture not identified as displaced or nondisplaced should be coded to displaced
  A fracture not designated as open or closed should be coded to closed
  The open fracture designations are based on the Gustilo open fracture classification
  Excludes1 traumatic amputation of forearm (S58.-)
  Excludes2 fracture at wrist and hand level (S62.-)
  The appropriate 7th character is to be added to all codes from category S52

A	initial encounter for closed fracture
B	initial encounter for open fracture type I or II
	initial encounter for open fracture NOS
C	initial encounter for open fracture type IIIA, IIIB, or IIIC
D	subsequent encounter for closed fracture with routine healing
E	subsequent encounter for open fracture type I or II with routine healing
F	subsequent encounter for open fracture type IIIA, IIIB, or IIIC with routine healing
G	subsequent encounter for closed fracture with delayed healing
H	subsequent encounter for open fracture type I or II with delayed healing
J	subsequent encounter for open fracture type IIIA, IIIB, or IIIC with delayed healing
K	subsequent encounter for closed fracture with nonunion
M	subsequent encounter for open fracture type I or II with nonunion
N	subsequent encounter for open fracture type IIIA, IIIB, or IIIC with nonunion
P	subsequent encounter for closed fracture with malunion
Q	subsequent encounter for open fracture type I or II with malunion
R	subsequent encounter for open fracture type IIIA, IIIB, or IIIC with malunion
S	sequela

Coding Clinic: 2016, Q1, P33

◀ New ◀ Revised ~~deleted~~ Deleted Excludes 1 Excludes 2 Includes Use additional Code first Code also Unspecified
OGCR Official Guidelines ● Unacceptable Principal Diagnosis X Assign placeholder X ● Use Additional Character(s) ▶ Manifestation Code **Coding Clinic**

● **S52.0** **Fracture of upper end of ulna**
  Fracture of proximal end of ulna
  Excludes2 fracture of elbow NOS (S42.40-)
  fractures of shaft of ulna (S52.2-)

● **S52.00** **Unspecified fracture of upper end of ulna**
  Ⓔ❌ **For category S52.00 CC codes S52.00[B,C]:**
  S52.001-S52.009[B,C], S52.021-S52.109[B,C],
  S52.121-S52.189[B,C], S52.201-S52.209[A,B,C],
  S52.211-S52.219[A], S52.221-S52.266[A,B,C],
  S52.271-S52.279[B,C], S52.281-S52.309[A,B,C],
  S52.311-S52.319[A], S52.321-S52.516[A,B,C],
  S52.531-S52.616[A,B,C], S52.691-S52.92X[A,B,C],
  S59.001-S59.099[A], S59.201-S59.299[A], S62.90X[B]
  For S52.00[K,M,N,P,Q,R]: See S02.0[K]

  ● **S52.001** **Unspecified** fracture of upper end of
    right ulna K, M, N, P, Q, R 🔗, B, C 🔗,
    B, C 🔗

  ● **S52.002** **Unspecified** fracture of upper end of
    left ulna K, M, N, P, Q, R 🔗, B, C 🔗,
    B, C 🔗

  ● **S52.009** **Unspecified** fracture of upper end of
    unspecified ulna K, M, N, P, Q, R 🔗,
    B, C 🔗, B, C 🔗

● **S52.01** **Torus fracture of upper end of ulna**
  The appropriate 7th character is to be added to
  all codes in subcategory S52.01

A	initial encounter for closed fracture
D	subsequent encounter for fracture with routine healing
G	subsequent encounter for fracture with delayed healing
K	subsequent encounter for fracture with nonunion
P	subsequent encounter for fracture with malunion
S	sequela

  ● **S52.011** **Torus fracture of upper end of right
    ulna** A, K, P 🔗, A 🔗
    Ⓔ❌ **For code S52.011[A]:** S52.001 [A,B,C], S52.002
    [B,C], S52.009 [A,B,C], S52.011[A], S52.019[A],
    S52.021[A,B,C], S52.022[B,C],
    S52.023-S52.024[A,B,C], S52.025[B,C],
    S52.026-S52.031[A,B,C], S52.032[B,C],
    S52.033-S52.034[A,B,C], S52.035[B,C],
    S52.036-S59.041[A,B,C], S52.042[B,C],
    S52.043-S52.044[A,B,C], S52.045[B,C],
    S52.046-S52.091[A,B,C], S52.092[B,C],
    S52.099-S52.101[A,B,C], S52.102[B,C],
    S52.109[A,B,C], S52.111[A], S52.119[A],
    S52.121[A,B,C], S52.122[B,C],
    S52.123-S52.124[A,B,C], S52.125[B,C],
    S52.126-S52.131[A,B,C], S52.132[B,C],
    S52.133-S52.134[A,B,C], S52.135[B, C],

S52.136-S52.181[A,B,C], S52.182[B,C],
S52.189-S52.201[A,B,C], S52.202[B,C],
S52.209[A,B,C], S52.211[A], S52.219[A],
S52.221[A,B,C], S52.222[B,C],
S52.223-S52.224[A,B,C], S52.225[B,C],
S52.226-S52.231[C], S52.232[B,C],
S52.233-S52.234[A,B,C], S52.235[B,C],
S52.236-S52.241[C], S52.242[B,C],
S52.243-S52.244[A,B,C], S52.245[B,C],
S52.246-S52.251[A,B,C], S52.252[B,C],
S52.253-S52.254[A,B,C], S52.255[B,C],
S52.256-S52.261[A,B,C], S52.262[BC],
S52.263-S52.264[A,B,C], S52.265[B,C],
S52.266-S52.271[A,B,C], S52.272[B,C],
S52.279-S52.281[A,B,C], S52.282[B,C],
S52.283-S52.291[A,B,C], S52.292[B,C],
S52.299-S52.301[A,B,C], S52.302[B,C],
S52.309[A,B,C], S52.311[A], S52.319[A],
S52.321[A,B,C], S52.322[B,C],
S52.323-S52.324[A,B,C], S52.325[B,C],
S52.326-S52.331[A,B,C], S52.332[B,C],
S52.333-S52.334[A,B,C], S52.335[B,C],
S52.336-S52.341[A,B,C], S52.342[B,C],
S52.343-S52.344[A,B,C], S52.345[B,C],
S52.346-S52.351[A,B,C], S52.352[B,C],
S52.353-S52.354[A,B,C], S52.355[B,C],
S52.356-S52.361[A,B,C], S52.362[B,C],
S52.363-S52.364[A,B,C], S52.365[B,C],
S52.366-S52.371[A,B,C], S52.372[B,C],
S52.379-S52.381[A,B,C], S52.382[B,C],
S52.389-S52.391[A,B,C], S52.392[B,C],
S52.399-S52.501[A,B,C], S52.502[B,C],
S52.509-S52.511[A,B,C], S52.512[B,C],
S52.513-S52.514[A,B,C], S52.515[B,C],
S52.16[A,B,C], S52.521[A], S52.529[A],
S52.531[A,B,C], S52.532[B,C],
S52.539-S52.541[A,B,C], S52.542[B,C],
S52.549-S52.551[A,B,C], S52.552[B,C],
S52.559-S52.561[A,B,C], S52.562[B,C],
S52.569-S52.571[A,B,C], S52.572[B,C],
S52.579-S52.591[A,B,C], S52.592[B,C],
S52.599-S52.601[A,B,C], S52.602[B,C],
S52.609-S52.611[A,B,C], S52.612[B,C],
S52.613-S52.614[A,B,C], S52.615[B,C],
S52.616[A,B,C], S52.621[A], S52.629[A],
S52.691[A,B,C], S52.692[B,C],
S52.699-S52.92X[A,B,C], S59.001[A],
S59.009-S59.011[A], S59.019-S59.021[A],
S59.029-S59.031[A], S59.039-S59.041[A],
S59.049-S59.091[A], S59.099-S59.101[A],
S59.109-S59.111[A], S59.119-S59.121[A],
S59.129-S59.131[A], S59.139-S59.141[A],
S59.149-S59.191[A], S59.199-S59.201[A],
S59.209-S59.211[A], S59.219-S59.221[A],
S59.229-S59.231[A], S59.239-S59.241[A],
S59.249-S59.291[A], S59.299[A]
For S52.011[K,P]: See S02.0[K]

● **S52.012** Torus fracture of upper end of left ulna A, K, P 🩺, A 🩺

(Ex) **For code S52.012[A]:** S52.001[B,C], S52.002-S52.009[A,B,C], S52.012-S52.019[A], S52.021[B,C], S52.022-S52.023[A,B,C], S52.024[B,C], S52.025-S52.026[A,B,C], S52.031[B,C], S52.032-S52.033[A,B,C], S52.034[B,C], S52.035-S52.036[A,B,C], S52.041[B,C], S52.042-S52.043[A,B,C], S52.044[B,C], S52.045-S52.046[A,B,C], S52.091[B,C], S52.092-S52.099[A,B,C], S52.101[B,C], S52.102-S52.109[A,B,C], S52.112-S52.119[A], S52.121[B,C], S52.122-S52.123[A,B,C], S52.124[B,C], S52.125-S52.126[A,B,C], S52.131[B,C], S52.132-S52.133[A,B,C], S52.134[B,C], S52.135-S52.136[A,B,C], S52.181[B,C], S52.182-S52.189[A,B,C], S52.201[B,C], S52.202-S52.209[A,B,C], S52.212-S52.219[A], S52.221[B,C], S52.222-S52.223[A,B,C], S52.224[B,C], S52.225-S52.226[A,B,C], S52.231[B,C], S52.232-S52.233[A,B,C], S52.234[B,C], S52.235-S52.236[A,B,C], S52.241[B,C], S52.242-S52.243[A,B,C], S52.244[B,C], S52.245-S52.246[A,B,C], S52.251[B,C], S52.252-S52.253[A,B,C], S52.254[B,C], S52.255-S52.256[A,B,C], S52.261[B,C], S52.262-S52.263[A,B,C], S52.264[B,C], S52.265-S52.266[A,B,C], S52.271[B,C], S52.272-S52.279[A,B,C], S52.281[B,C], S52.282-S52.283[A,B,C], S52.291[B,C], S52.292-S52.299[A,B,C], S52.301[B,C], S52.302-S52.309[A,B,C], S52.312-S52.319[A], S52.321[B,C], S52.322-S52.323[A,B,C], S52.324[B,C], S52.325-S52.326[A,B,C], S52.331[B,C], S52.332-S52.333[A,B,C], S52.334[B,C], S52.335-S52.336[A,B,C], S52.341[B,C], S52.342-S52.343[A,B,C], S52.344[B,C], S52.345-S52.346[A,B,C], S52.351[B,C], S52.352-S52.353[A,B,C], S52.354[B,C], S52.355-S52.356[A,B,C], S52.361[B,C], S52.362-S52.363[A,B,C], S52.364[B,C], S52.365-S52.366[A,B,C], S52.371[B,C], S52.372-S52.379[A,B,C], S52.381[B,C], S52.382-S52.389[A,B,C], S52.391[B,C], S52.392-S52.399[A,B,C], S52.501[B,C], S52.502-S52.509[A,B,C], S52.511[B,C], S52.512-S52.513[A,B,C], S52.514[B,C], S52.515-S52.516[A,B,C], S52.522-S52.529[A], S52.531[B,C], S52.532-S52.539[A,B,C], S52.541[B,C], S52.542-S52.549[A,B,C], S52.551[B,C], S52.552-S52.559[A,B,C], S52.561[B,C], S52.562-S52.569[A,B,C], S52.571[B,C], S52.572-S52.579[A,B,C], S52.591[B,C], S52.592-S52.599[A,B,C], S52.601[B,C], S52.602-S52.609[A,B,C], S52.611[B,C], S52.612-S52.613[A,B,C], S52.614[B,C], S52.615-S52.616[A,B,C], S52.622-S52.629[A], S52.691[B,C], S52.692-S52.92X[A,B,C], S59.002-S59.009[A], S59.012-S59.019[A], S59.022-S59.029[A], S59.032-S59.039[A], S59.042-S59.049[A], S59.092-S59.099[A], S59.102-S59.109[A], S59.112-S59.119[A], S59.122-S59.129[A], S59.132-S59.139[A], S59.142-S59.149[A], S59.192-S59.199[A], S59.202-S59.209[A], S59.212-S59.219[A], S59.222-S59.229[A], S59.232-S59.239[A], S59.242-S59.249[A], S59.292-S59.299[A] **For S52.012[K,P]:** See S02.0[K]

● **S52.019** Torus fracture of upper end of unspecified ulna A, K, P 🩺, A 🩺

(Ex) **For code S52.019[A]:** S52.001-S52.009[A,B,C], S52.011-S52.019[A], S52.021-S52.109[A,B,C], S52.111-S52.119[A], S52.121-S52.209[A,B,C], S52.211-S52.219[A], S52.221-S52.309[A,B,C], S52.311-S52.319[A], S52.321-S52.516[A,B,C], S52.521-S52.529[A], S52.531-S52.616[A,B,C], S52.621-S52.629[A], S52.691-S52.92X[A,B,C], S59.001-S59.299[A] **For S52.019[K,P]:** See S02.0[K]

● **S52.02** Fracture of olecranon process without intraarticular extension of ulna

(Ex) **For category S52.02 CC codes S52.02[B,C]:** S52.001-S52.009[B,C], S52.021-S52.109[B,C], S52.121-S52.189[B,C], S52.201-S52.209[A,B,C], S52.211-S52.219[A], S52.221-S52.266[A,B,C], S52.271-S52.279[B,C], S52.281-S52.309[A,B,C], S52.311-S52.319[A], S52.321-S52.516[A,B,C], S52.531-S52.549[B,C], S52.551-S52.616[A,B,C], S52.691-S52.92X[A,B,C], S59.001-S59.099[A], S59.201-S59.299[A], S62.90X[B] **For S52.02[K,M,N,P,Q,R]:** See S02.0[K]

● **S52.021** Displaced fracture of olecranon process without intraarticular extension of right ulna K, M, N, P, Q, R 🩺, B, C 🩺, B, C 🩺

● **S52.022** Displaced fracture of olecranon process without intraarticular extension of left ulna K, M, N, P, Q, R 🩺, B, C 🩺, B, C 🩺

● **S52.023** Displaced fracture of olecranon process without intraarticular extension of unspecified ulna K, M, N, P, Q, R 🩺, B, C 🩺, B, C 🩺

● **S52.024** Nondisplaced fracture of olecranon process without intraarticular extension of right ulna K, M, N, P, Q, R 🩺, B, C 🩺, B, C 🩺

● **S52.025** Nondisplaced fracture of olecranon process without intraarticular extension of left ulna K, M, N, P, Q, R 🩺, B, C 🩺, B, C 🩺

● **S52.026** Nondisplaced fracture of olecranon process without intraarticular extension of unspecified ulna K, M, N, P, Q, R 🩺, B, C 🩺, B, C 🩺

● **S52.03** Fracture of olecranon process with intraarticular extension of ulna

(Ex) **For category S52.03 CC codes S52.03[B,C]:** See S52.02[B,C] **For S52.03[K,M,N,P,Q,R]:** See S02.0[K]

● **S52.031** Displaced fracture of olecranon process with intraarticular extension of right ulna K, M, N, P, Q, R 🩺, B, C 🩺, B, C 🩺

● **S52.032** Displaced fracture of olecranon process with intraarticular extension of left ulna K, M, N, P, Q, R 🩺, B, C 🩺, B, C 🩺

● **S52.033** Displaced fracture of olecranon process with intraarticular extension of unspecified ulna K, M, N, P, Q, R 🩺, B, C 🩺, B, C 🩺

● **S52.034** Nondisplaced fracture of olecranon process with intraarticular extension of right ulna K, M, N, P, Q, R 🩺, B, C 🩺, B, C 🩺

● **S52.035** Nondisplaced fracture of olecranon process with intraarticular extension of left ulna K, M, N, P, Q, R 🩺, B, C 🩺, B, C 🩺

● **S52.036** Nondisplaced fracture of olecranon process with intraarticular extension of unspecified ulna K, M, N, P, Q, R 🩺, B, C 🩺, B, C 🩺

◀ New ◀ Revised ~~deleted~~ Deleted Excludes 1 Excludes 2 Includes Use additional Code first Code also Unspecified
OGCR Official Guidelines ● Unacceptable Principal Diagnosis X Assign placeholder X ● Use Additional Character(s) ▶ Manifestation Code Coding Clinic

● **S52.04**   **Fracture of coronoid process of ulna**
   (Ex) *For category S52.04 CC codes S52.04[B,C]:* See
     S52.00[B,C] *For S52.04[K,M,N,P,Q,R]:* See S02.0[K]

   ● **S52.041**   Displaced fracture of coronoid process of right ulna
     K, M, N, P, Q, R 🅒, B, C 🅒, B, C 🅒

   ● **S52.042**   Displaced fracture of coronoid process of left ulna
     K, M, N, P, Q, R 🅒, B, C 🅒, B, C 🅒

   ● **S52.043**   Displaced fracture of coronoid process of unspecified ulna
     K, M, N, P, Q, R 🅒, B, C 🅒, B, C 🅒

   ● **S52.044**   Nondisplaced fracture of coronoid process of right ulna
     K, M, N, P, Q, R 🅒, B, C 🅒, B, C 🅒

   ● **S52.045**   Nondisplaced fracture of coronoid process of left ulna
     K, M, N, P, Q, R 🅒, B, C 🅒, B, C 🅒

   ● **S52.046**   Nondisplaced fracture of coronoid process of unspecified ulna
     K, M, N, P, Q, R 🅒, B, C 🅒, B, C 🅒

● **S52.09**   **Other fracture of upper end of ulna**
   (Ex) *For category S52.09 CC codes S52.09[B,C]:* See
     S52.00[B,C] *For S52.09[K,M,N,P,Q,R]:* See S02.0[K]

   ● **S52.091**   Other fracture of upper end of right ulna K, M, N, P, Q, R 🅒, B, C 🅒, B, C 🅒

   ● **S52.092**   Other fracture of upper end of left ulna K, M, N, P, Q, R 🅒, B, C 🅒, B, C 🅒

   ● **S52.099**   Other fracture of upper end of unspecified ulna K, M, N, P, Q, R 🅒, B, C 🅒, B, C 🅒

● **S52.1**   **Fracture of upper end of radius**
   Fracture of proximal end of radius
   Excludes2   physeal fractures of upper end of radius (S59.2-)
             fracture of shaft of radius (S52.3-)

   ● **S52.10**   **Unspecified fracture of upper end of radius**
     (Ex) *For category S52.10 CC codes S52.10[B,C]:* See
       S52.00[B,C] *For S52.10[K,M,N,P,Q,R]:* See S02.0[K]

     ● **S52.101**   Unspecified fracture of upper end of right radius K, M, N, P, Q, R 🅒, B, C 🅒, B, C 🅒

     ● **S52.102**   Unspecified fracture of upper end of left radius K, M, N, P, Q, R 🅒, B, C 🅒, B, C 🅒

     ● **S52.109**   Unspecified fracture of upper end of unspecified radius K, M, N, P, Q, R 🅒, B, C 🅒, B, C 🅒

   ● **S52.11**   **Torus fracture of upper end of radius**
     The appropriate 7th character is to be added to all codes in subcategory S52.11

> | | |
> |---|---|
> | A | initial encounter for closed fracture |
> | D | subsequent encounter for fracture with routine healing |
> | G | subsequent encounter for fracture with delayed healing |
> | K | subsequent encounter for fracture with nonunion |
> | P | subsequent encounter for fracture with malunion |
> | S | sequela |

     ● **S52.111**   Torus fracture of upper end of right radius A, K, P 🅒, A 🅒
       (Ex) *For code S52.111[A]:* See S52.011[A]
       For S52.111[K,P]: See S02.0[K]

     ● **S52.112**   Torus fracture of upper end of left radius A, K, P 🅒, A 🅒
       (Ex) *For code S52.112[A]:* See S52.012[A]
       For S52.112[K,P]: See S02.0[K]

     ● **S52.119**   Torus fracture of upper end of unspecified radius A, K, P 🅒, A 🅒
       (Ex) *For code S52.119[A]:* See S52.019[A]
       For S52.119[K,P]: See S02.0[K]

   ● **S52.12**   **Fracture of head of radius**
     (Ex) *For category S52.12 CC codes S52.12[B,C]:* See
       S52.00[B,C] *For S52.12[K,M,N,P,Q,R]:* See S02.0[K]

     ● **S52.121**   Displaced fracture of head of right radius K, M, N, P, Q, R 🅒, B, C 🅒, B, C 🅒

     ● **S52.122**   Displaced fracture of head of left radius K, M, N, P, Q, R 🅒, B, C 🅒, B, C 🅒

     ● **S52.123**   Displaced fracture of head of unspecified radius K, M, N, P, Q, R 🅒, B, C 🅒, B, C 🅒

     ● **S52.124**   Nondisplaced fracture of head of right radius K, M, N, P, Q, R 🅒, B, C 🅒, B, C 🅒

     ● **S52.125**   Nondisplaced fracture of head of left radius K, M, N, P, Q, R 🅒, B, C 🅒, B, C 🅒

     ● **S52.126**   Nondisplaced fracture of head of unspecified radius K, M, N, P, Q, R 🅒, B, C 🅒, B, C 🅒

   ● **S52.13**   **Fracture of neck of radius**
     (Ex) *For category S52.13 CC codes S52.13[B,C]:* See
       S52.00[B,C] *For S52.13[K,M,N,P,Q,R]:* See S02.0[K]

     ● **S52.131**   Displaced fracture of neck of right radius K, M, N, P, Q, R 🅒, B, C 🅒, B, C 🅒

     ● **S52.132**   Displaced fracture of neck of left radius K, M, N, P, Q, R 🅒, B, C 🅒, B, C 🅒

     ● **S52.133**   Displaced fracture of neck of unspecified radius K, M, N, P, Q, R 🅒, B, C 🅒, B, C 🅒

     ● **S52.134**   Nondisplaced fracture of neck of right radius K, M, N, P, Q, R 🅒, B, C 🅒, B, C 🅒

     ● **S52.135**   Nondisplaced fracture of neck of left radius K, M, N, P, Q, R 🅒, B, C 🅒, B, C 🅒

     ● **S52.136**   Nondisplaced fracture of neck of unspecified radius K, M, N, P, Q, R 🅒, B, C 🅒, B, C 🅒

   ● **S52.18**   **Other fracture of upper end of radius**
     (Ex) *For category S52.18 CC codes S52.18[B,C]:* See
       S52.00[B,C] *For S52.18[K,M,N,P,Q,R]:* See S02.0[K]

     ● **S52.181**   Other fracture of upper end of right radius K, M, N, P, Q, R 🅒, B, C 🅒, B, C 🅒

     ● **S52.182**   Other fracture of upper end of left radius K, M, N, P, Q, R 🅒, B, C 🅒, B, C 🅒

     ● **S52.189**   Other fracture of upper end of unspecified radius K, M, N, P, Q, R 🅒, B, C 🅒, B, C 🅒

CHAPTER 19 (S00–T88)

● **S52.2**   **Fracture of shaft of ulna**

  ● **S52.20**   **Unspecified fracture of shaft of ulna**
         Fracture of ulna NOS

    ● **S52.201**   **Unspecified fracture of shaft of right ulna** A, K, M, N, P, Q, R 🔵, B, C 🔵, A, B, C 🔵
            (Ex:) For code S52.201[A]: See S52.011[A]
               For S52.201[B,C]: See S52.00[B,C]
               For S52.201[K,M,N,P,Q,R]: See S02.0[K]

    ● **S52.202**   **Unspecified fracture of shaft of left ulna** A, K, M, N, P, Q, R 🔵, B, C 🔵, A, B, C 🔵
            (Ex:) For code S52.202[A]: See S52.012[A] For code S52.202[B,C]: See S52.00[B,C]
               For S52.202[K,M,N,P,Q,R]: See S02.0[K]

    ● **S52.209**   **Unspecified fracture of shaft of unspecified ulna** A, K, M, N, P, Q, R 🔵, B, C 🔵, A, B, C 🔵
            (Ex:) For code S52.209[A]: See S52.019[A] For code S52.209[B,C]: See S52.00[B,C]
               For S52.209[K,M,N,P,Q,R]: See S02.0[K]

  ● **S52.21**   **Greenstick fracture of shaft of ulna**
         The appropriate 7th character is to be added to all codes in subcategory S52.21

A	initial encounter for closed fracture
D	subsequent encounter for fracture with routine healing
G	subsequent encounter for fracture with delayed healing
K	subsequent encounter for fracture with nonunion
P	subsequent encounter for fracture with malunion
S	sequela

    ● **S52.211**   **Greenstick fracture of shaft of right ulna** A, K, P 🔵, A 🔵
            (Ex:) For code S52.211[A]: See S52.011[A]
               For S52.211[K,P]: See S02.0[K]

    ● **S52.212**   **Greenstick fracture of shaft of left ulna** A, K, P 🔵, A 🔵
            (Ex:) For code S52.212[A]: See S52.012[A]
               For S52.202[K,P]: See S02.0[K]

    ● **S52.219**   **Greenstick fracture of shaft of unspecified ulna** A, K, P 🔵, A 🔵
            (Ex:) For code S52.219[A]: See S52.019[A]
               For S52.219[K,P]: See S02.0[K]

  ● **S52.22**   **Transverse fracture of shaft of ulna**

    ● **S52.221**   **Displaced transverse fracture of shaft of right ulna** A, K, M, N, P, Q, R 🔵, B, C 🔵, A, B, C 🔵
            (Ex:) For code S52.221[A]: See S52.011[A]
               For S52.221[B,C]: See S52.00[B,C]
               For S52.221[K,M,N,P,Q,R]: See S02.0[K]

    ● **S52.222**   **Displaced transverse fracture of shaft of left ulna** A, K, M, N, P, Q, R 🔵, B, C 🔵, A, B, C 🔵
            (Ex:) For code S52.222[A]: See S52.012[A] For code S52.222[B,C]: See S52.00[B,C]
               For S52.222[K,M,N,P,Q,R]: See S02.0[K]

    ● **S52.223**   **Displaced transverse fracture of shaft of unspecified ulna** A, K, M, N, P, Q, R 🔵, B, C 🔵, A, B, C 🔵
            (Ex:) For code S52.223[A]: See S52.019[A] For code S52.223[B,C]: See S52.00[B,C]
               For S52.223[K,M,N,P,Q,R]: See S02.0[K]

    ● **S52.224**   **Nondisplaced transverse fracture of shaft of right ulna** A, K, M, N, P, Q, R 🔵, B, C 🔵, A, B, C 🔵
            (Ex:) For code S52.224[A]: See S52.011[A]
               For S52.224[B,C]: See S52.00[B,C]
               For S52.224[K,M,N,P,Q,R]: See S02.0[K]

    ● **S52.225**   **Nondisplaced transverse fracture of shaft of left ulna** A, K, M, N, P, Q, R 🔵, B, C 🔵, A, B, C 🔵
            (Ex:) For code S52.225[A]: See S52.012[A] For code S52.225[B,C]: See S52.00[B,C]
               For S52.225[K,M,N,P,Q,R]: See S02.0[K]

    ● **S52.226**   **Nondisplaced transverse fracture of shaft of unspecified ulna** A, K, M, N, P, Q, R 🔵, B, C 🔵, A, B, C 🔵
            (Ex:) For code S52.226[A]: See S52.019[A] For code S52.226[B,C]: See S52.00[B,C]
               For S52.226[K,M,N,P,Q,R]: See S02.0[K]

  ● **S52.23**   **Oblique fracture of shaft of ulna**

    ● **S52.231**   **Displaced oblique fracture of shaft of right ulna** A, K, M, N, P, Q, R 🔵, B, C 🔵, A, B, C 🔵
            (Ex:) For code S52.231[A]: See S52.011[A]
               For S52.231[B,C]: See S52.00[B,C]
               For S52.231[K,M,N,P,Q,R]: See S02.0[K]

    ● **S52.232**   **Displaced oblique fracture of shaft of left ulna** A, K, M, N, P, Q, R 🔵, B, C 🔵, A, B, C 🔵
            (Ex:) For code S52.232[A]: See S52.012[A] For code S52.232[B,C]: See S52.00[B,C]
               For S52.232[K,M,N,P,Q,R]: See S02.0[K]

    ● **S52.233**   **Displaced oblique fracture of shaft of unspecified ulna** A, K, M, N, P, Q, R 🔵, B, C 🔵, A, B, C 🔵
            (Ex:) For code S52.233[A]: See S52.019[A] For code S52.233[B,C]: See S52.00[B,C]
               For S52.233[K,M,N,P,Q,R]: See S02.0[K]

    ● **S52.234**   **Nondisplaced oblique fracture of shaft of right ulna** A, K, M, N, P, Q, R 🔵, B, C 🔵, A, B, C 🔵
            (Ex:) For code S52.234[A]: See S52.011[A]
               For S52.234[B,C]: See S52.00[B,C]
               For S52.234[K,M,N,P,Q,R]: See S02.0[K]

    ● **S52.235**   **Nondisplaced oblique fracture of shaft of left ulna** A, K, M, N, P, Q, R 🔵, B, C 🔵, A, B, C 🔵
            (Ex:) For code S52.235[A]: See S52.012[A] For code S52.235[B,C]: See S52.00[B,C]
               For S52.235[K,M,N,P,Q,R]: See S02.0[K]

    ● **S52.236**   **Nondisplaced oblique fracture of shaft of unspecified ulna** A, K, M, N, P, Q, R 🔵, B, C 🔵, A, B, C 🔵
            (Ex:) For code S52.236[A]: See S52.019[A] For code S52.236[B,C]: See S52.00[B,C]
               For S52.236[K,M,N,P,Q,R]: See S02.0[K]

● **S52.24**   **Spiral fracture of shaft of ulna**
     ● **S52.241**   **Displaced spiral fracture of shaft of ulna, right arm** A, K, M, N, P, Q, R 🪙, B, C 🪙, A, B, C 🪙
         Ⓔⓧ For code S52.241[A]: See S52.011[A] For code S52.241[B,C]: See S52.00[B,C] For S52.241[K,M,N,P,Q,R]: See S02.0[K]

     ● **S52.242**   **Displaced spiral fracture of shaft of ulna, left arm** A, K, M, N, P, Q, R 🪙, B, C 🪙, A, B, C 🪙
         Ⓔⓧ For code S52.242[A]: See S52.012[A] For code S52.242[B,C]: See S52.00[B,C] For S52.242[K,M,N,P,Q,R]: See S02.0[K]

     ● **S52.243**   **Displaced spiral fracture of shaft of ulna, unspecified arm** A, K, M, N, P, Q, R 🪙, B, C 🪙, A, B, C 🪙
         Ⓔⓧ For code S52.243[A]: See S52.019[A] For code S52.243[B,C]: See S52.00[B,C] For S52.243[K,M,N,P,Q,R]: See S02.0[K]

     ● **S52.244**   **Nondisplaced spiral fracture of shaft of ulna, right arm** A, K, M, N, P, Q, R 🪙, B, C 🪙, A, B, C 🪙
         Ⓔⓧ For code S52.244[A]: See S52.011[A] For code S52.244[B,C]: See S52.00[B,C] For S52.244[K,M,N,P,Q,R]: See S02.0[K]

     ● **S52.245**   **Nondisplaced spiral fracture of shaft of ulna, left arm** A, K, M, N, P, Q, R 🪙, B, C 🪙, A, B, C 🪙
         Ⓔⓧ For code S52.245[A]: See S52.012[A] For code S52.245[B,C]: See S52.00[B,C] For S52.245[K,M,N,P,Q,R]: See S02.0[K]

     ● **S52.246**   **Nondisplaced spiral fracture of shaft of ulna, unspecified arm** A, K, M, N, P, Q, R 🪙, B, C 🪙, A, B, C 🪙
         Ⓔⓧ For code S52.246[A]: See S52.019[A] For code S52.246[B,C]: See S52.00[B,C] For S52.246[K,M,N,P,Q,R]: See S02.0[K]

● **S52.25**   **Comminuted fracture of shaft of ulna**
     ● **S52.251**   **Displaced comminuted fracture of shaft of ulna, right arm** A, K, M, N, P, Q, R 🪙, B, C 🪙, A, B, C 🪙
         Ⓔⓧ For code S52.251[A]: See S52.011[A] For code S52.251[B,C]: See S52.00[B,C] For S52.251[K,M,N,P,Q,R]: See S02.0[K]

     ● **S52.252**   **Displaced comminuted fracture of shaft of ulna, left arm** A, K, M, N, P, Q, R 🪙, B, C 🪙, A, B, C 🪙
         Ⓔⓧ For code S52.252[A]: See S52.012[A] For code S52.252[B,C]: See S52.00[B,C] For S52.252[K,M,N,P,Q,R]: See S02.0[K]

     ● **S52.253**   **Displaced comminuted fracture of shaft of ulna, unspecified arm** A, K, M, N, P, Q, R 🪙, B, C 🪙, A, B, C 🪙
         Ⓔⓧ For code S52.253[A]: See S52.019[A] For code S52.253[B,C]: See S52.00[B,C] For S52.253[K,M,N,P,Q,R]: See S02.0[K]

     ● **S52.254**   **Nondisplaced comminuted fracture of shaft of ulna, right arm** A, K, M, N, P, Q, R 🪙, B, C 🪙, A, B, C 🪙
         Ⓔⓧ For code S52.254[A]: See S52.011[A] For code S52.254[B,C]: See S52.00[B,C] For S52.254[K,M,N,P,Q,R]: See S02.0[K]

     ● **S52.255**   **Nondisplaced comminuted fracture of shaft of ulna, left arm** A, K, M, N, P, Q, R 🪙, B, C 🪙, A, B, C 🪙
         Ⓔⓧ For code S52.255[A]: See S52.012[A] For code S52.255[B,C]: See S52.00[B,C] For S52.255[K,M,N,P,Q,R]: See S02.0[K]

     ● **S52.256**   **Nondisplaced comminuted fracture of shaft of ulna, unspecified arm** A, K, M, N, P, Q, R 🪙, B, C 🪙, A, B, C 🪙
         Ⓔⓧ For code S52.256[A]: See S52.019[A] For code S52.256[B,C]: See S52.00[B,C] For S52.256[K,M,N,P,Q,R]: See S02.0[K]

● **S52.26**   **Segmental fracture of shaft of ulna**
     ● **S52.261**   **Displaced segmental fracture of shaft of ulna, right arm** A, K, M, N, P, Q, R 🪙, B, C 🪙, A, B, C 🪙
         Ⓔⓧ For code S52.261[A]: See S52.011[A] For S52.261[B,C]: See S52.00[B,C] For S52.261[K,M,N,P,Q,R]: S02.0[K]

     ● **S52.262**   **Displaced segmental fracture of shaft of ulna, left arm** A, K, M, N, P, Q, R 🪙, B, C 🪙, A, B, C 🪙
         Ⓔⓧ For code S52.262[A]: See S52.012[A] For code S52.262[B,C]: See S52.00[B,C] For S52.262[K,M,N,P,Q,R]: See S02.0[K]

     ● **S52.263**   **Displaced segmental fracture of shaft of ulna, unspecified arm** A, K, M, N, P, Q, R 🪙, B, C 🪙, A, B, C 🪙
         Ⓔⓧ For code S52.263[A]: See S52.019[A] For code S52.263[B,C]: See S52.00[B,C] For S52.263[K,M,N,P,Q,R]: See S02.0[K]

     ● **S52.264**   **Nondisplaced segmental fracture of shaft of ulna, right arm** A, K, M, N, P, Q, R 🪙, B, C 🪙, A, B, C 🪙
         Ⓔⓧ For code S52.264[A]: See S52.011[A] For S52.264[B,C]: See S52.00[B,C] For S52.264[K,M,N,P,Q,R]: See S02.0[K]

     ● **S52.265**   **Nondisplaced segmental fracture of shaft of ulna, left arm** A, K, M, N, P, Q, R 🪙, B, C 🪙, A, B, C 🪙
         Ⓔⓧ For code S52.265[A]: See S52.012[A] For code S52.265[B,C]: See S52.00[B,C] For S52.265[K,M,N,P,Q,R]: See S02.0[K]

     ● **S52.266**   **Nondisplaced segmental fracture of shaft of ulna, unspecified arm** A, K, M, N, P, Q, R 🪙, B, C 🪙, A, B, C 🪙
         Ⓔⓧ For code S52.266[A]: See S52.019[A] For code S52.266[B,C]: See S52.00[B,C] For S52.266[K,M,N,P,Q,R]: See S02.0[K]

● **S52.27**   **Monteggia's fracture of ulna**
     Fracture of upper shaft of ulna with dislocation of radial head
         Ⓔⓧ For category S52.27 CC codes S52.27[B,C]: See S52.00[B,C] For S52.27[K,M,N,P,Q,R]: See S02.0[K]

     ● **S52.271**   **Monteggia's fracture of right ulna** K, M, N, P, Q, R 🪙, B, C 🪙, B, C 🪙

     ● **S52.272**   **Monteggia's fracture of left ulna** K, M, N, P, Q, R 🪙, B, C 🪙, B, C 🪙

     ● **S52.279**   **Monteggia's fracture of unspecified ulna** K, M, N, P, Q, R 🪙, B, C 🪙, B, C 🪙

N   Newborn Age: 0   **P**   Pediatric Age: 0–17   **M**   Maternity DX: 12–55   **A**   Adult Age: 15–124   ♀   Females Only   ♂   Males Only
🪙   Complication\Comorbidity   🪙   Major C\C   Ⓔⓧ   CC/MCC Exclusions   🪙   Hospital-Acquired Condition

● **S52.28**   Bent bone of ulna
  ● **S52.281**   **Bent bone of right ulna**
      A, K, M, N, P, Q, R 🏷, B, C 🏷,
      A, B, C 🏷
       (Ex:) For code S52.281[A]: See S52.011[A]
        For S52.281[B,C]: See S52.00[B,C]
        For S52.281[K,M,N,P,Q,R]: See S02.0[K]

  ● **S52.282**   **Bent bone of left ulna**
      A, K, M, N, P, Q, R 🏷, B, C 🏷,
      A, B, C 🏷
       (Ex:) For code S52.282[A]: See S52.012[A] For
        code S52.282[B,C]: See S52.00[B,C]
        For S52.282[K,M,N,P,Q,R]: See S02.0[K]

  ● **S52.283**   **Bent bone of** <mark>unspecified</mark> **ulna**
      A, K, M, N, P, Q, R 🏷, B, C 🏷,
      A, B, C 🏷
       (Ex:) For code S52.283[A]: See S52.019[A] For
        For S52.283[B,C]: See S52.00[B,C]
        For S52.283[K,M,N,P,Q,R]: See S02.0[K]

● **S52.29**   Other fracture of shaft of ulna
  ● **S52.291**   **Other fracture of shaft of right ulna**
      A, K, M, N, P, Q, R 🏷, B, C 🏷,
      A, B, C 🏷
       (Ex:) For code S52.291[A]: See S52.011[A]
        For S52.291[B,C]: See S52.00[B,C]
        For S52.291[K,M,N,P,Q,R]: See S02.0[K]

  ● **S52.292**   **Other fracture of shaft of left ulna**
      A, K, M, N, P, Q, R 🏷, B, C 🏷,
      A, B, C 🏷
       (Ex:) For code S52.292[A]: See S52.012[A] For
        code S52.292[B,C]: See S52.00[B,C]
        For S52.292[K,M,N,P,Q,R]: See S02.0[K]

  ● **S52.299**   **Other fracture of shaft of** <mark>unspecified</mark>
      ulna A, K, M, N, P, Q, R 🏷, B, C 🏷,
      A, B, C 🏷
       (Ex:) For code S52.299[A]: See S52.019[A] For
        code S52.299[B,C]: See S52.00[B,C]
        For S52.299[K,M,N,P,Q,R]: See S02.0[K]

● **S52.3**   Fracture of shaft of radius
  ● **S52.30**   Unspecified fracture of shaft of radius
    ● **S52.301**   <mark>Unspecified</mark> **fracture of shaft of right**
       radius A, K, M, N, P, Q, R 🏷, B, C 🏷,
       A, B, C 🏷
        (Ex:) For code S52.301[A]: See S52.011[A]
         For S52.301[B,C]: See S52.00[B,C]
         For S52.301[K,M,N,P,Q,R]: See S02.0[K]

    ● **S52.302**   <mark>Unspecified</mark> **fracture of shaft of left**
       radius A, K, M, N, P, Q, R 🏷, B, C 🏷,
       A, B, C 🏷
        (Ex:) For code S52.302[A]: See S52.012[A] For
         code S52.302[B,C]: See S52.00[B,C]
         For S52.302[K,M,N,P,Q,R]: See S02.0[K]

    ● **S52.309**   <mark>Unspecified</mark> **fracture of shaft of**
       unspecified radius
       A, K, M, N, P, Q, R 🏷, B, C 🏷,
       A, B, C 🏷
        (Ex:) For code S52.309[A]: See S52.019[A] For
         code S52.309[B,C]: See S52.00[B,C]
         For S52.309[K,M,N,P,Q,R]: See S02.0[K]

● **S52.31**   Greenstick fracture of shaft of radius
   The appropriate 7th character is to be added to
   all codes in subcategory S52.31

A	initial encounter for closed fracture
D	subsequent encounter for fracture with routine healing
G	subsequent encounter for fracture with delayed healing
K	subsequent encounter for fracture with nonunion
P	subsequent encounter for fracture with malunion
S	sequela

  ● **S52.311**   **Greenstick fracture of shaft of radius,**
      right arm A, K, P 🏷, A 🏷
       (Ex:) For code S52.311[A]: See S52.011[A]
        For S52.311[K,P]: See S02.0[K]

  ● **S52.312**   **Greenstick fracture of shaft of radius,**
      left arm A, K, P 🏷, A 🏷
       (Ex:) For code S52.312[A]: See S52.012[A]
        For S52.312[K,P]: See S02.0[K]

  ● **S52.319**   **Greenstick fracture of shaft of radius,**
      <mark>unspecified</mark> **arm** A, K, P 🏷, A 🏷
       (Ex:) For code S52.319[A]: See S52.019[A]
        For S52.319[K,P]: See S02.0[K]

● **S52.32**   Transverse fracture of shaft of radius
  ● **S52.321**   **Displaced transverse fracture of shaft**
      of right radius A, K, M, N, P, Q, R 🏷,
      B, C 🏷, A, B, C 🏷
       (Ex:) For code S52.321[A]: See S52.011[A]
        For S52.321[B,C]: See S52.00[B,C]
        For S52.321[K,M,N,P,Q,R]: See S02.0[K]

  ● **S52.322**   **Displaced transverse fracture of shaft**
      of left radius A, K, M, N, P, Q, R 🏷,
      B, C 🏷, A, B, C 🏷
       (Ex:) For code S52.322[A]: See S52.012[A] For
        code S52.322[B,C]: See S52.00[B,C]
        For S52.322[K,M,N,P,Q,R]: See S02.0[K]

  ● **S52.323**   **Displaced transverse fracture of shaft**
      of <mark>unspecified</mark> **radius**
      A, K, M, N, P, Q, R 🏷, B, C 🏷,
      A, B, C 🏷
       (Ex:) For code S52.323[A]: See S52.019[A] For
        code S52.323[B,C]: See S52.00[B,C]
        For S52.323[K,M,N,P,Q,R]: See S02.0[K]

  ● **S52.324**   **Nondisplaced transverse fracture of**
      shaft of right radius
      A, K, M, N, P, Q, R 🏷, B, C 🏷,
      A, B, C 🏷
       (Ex:) For code S52.324[A]: See S52.011[A]
        For S52.324[B,C]: See S52.00[B,C]
        For S52.324[K,M,N,P,Q,R]: See S02.0[K]

  ● **S52.325**   **Nondisplaced transverse fracture of**
      shaft of left radius
      A, K, M, N, P, Q, R 🏷, B, C 🏷,
      A, B, C 🏷
       (Ex:) For code S52.325[A]: See S52.012[A] For
        code S52.325[B,C]: See S52.00[B,C]
        For S52.325[K,M,N,P,Q,R]: See S02.0[K]

  ● **S52.326**   **Nondisplaced transverse fracture of**
      shaft of <mark>unspecified</mark> **radius**
      A, K, M, N, P, Q, R 🏷, B, C 🏷,
      A, B, C 🏷
       (Ex:) For code S52.326[A]: See S52.019[A] For
        code S52.326[B,C]: See S52.00[B,C]
        For S52.326[K,M,N,P,Q,R]: See S02.0[K]

◀ New   ◀≡ Revised   ~~deleted~~ Deleted   Excludes 1   Excludes 2   Includes   Use additional   Code first   Code also   Unspecified
OGCR Official Guidelines   ● Unacceptable Principal Diagnosis   X Assign placeholder X   ● Use Additional Character(s)   ▶ Manifestation Code   **Coding Clinic**

● S52.33　Oblique fracture of shaft of radius
　● S52.331　Displaced oblique fracture of shaft of right radius A, K, M, N, P, Q, R 🔴 B, C 🔴, A, B, C 🔴
　　　Ⓔ **For code S52.331[A]:** See S52.011[A]
　　　For S52.331[B,C]: See S52.00[B,C]
　　　For S52.331[K,M,N,P,Q,R]: See S02.0[K]

　● S52.332　Displaced oblique fracture of shaft of left radius A, K, M, N, P, Q, R 🔴, B, C 🔴, A, B, C 🔴
　　　Ⓔ **For code S52.332[A]:** See S52.012[A] **For code S52.332[B,C]:** See S52.00[B,C]
　　　For S52.332[K,M,N,P,Q,R]: See S02.0[K]

　● S52.333　Displaced oblique fracture of shaft of unspecified radius
　　　A, K, M, N, P, Q, R 🔴, B, C 🔴, A, B, C 🔴
　　　Ⓔ **For code S52.333[A]:** See S52.019[A] **For code S52.333[B,C]:** See S52.00[B,C]
　　　For S52.333[K,M,N,P,Q,R]: See S02.0[K]

　● S52.334　Nondisplaced oblique fracture of shaft of right radius
　　　A, K, M, N, P, Q, R 🔴, B, C 🔴, A, B, C 🔴
　　　Ⓔ **For code S52.334[A]:** See S52.011[A]
　　　For S52.334[B,C]: See S52.00[B,C]
　　　For S52.334[K,M,N,P,Q,R]: See S02.0[K]

　● S52.335　Nondisplaced oblique fracture of shaft of left radius
　　　A, K, M, N, P, Q, R 🔴, B, C 🔴, A, B, C 🔴
　　　Ⓔ **For code S52.335[A]:** See S52.012[A] **For code S52.335[B,C]:** See S52.00[B,C]
　　　For S52.335[K,M,N,P,Q,R]: See S02.0[K]

　● S52.336　Nondisplaced oblique fracture of shaft of unspecified radius
　　　A, K, M, N, P, Q, R 🔴, B, C 🔴, A, B, C 🔴
　　　Ⓔ **For code S52.336[A]:** See S52.019[A] **For code S52.336[B,C]:** See S52.00[B,C]
　　　For S52.336[K,M,N,P,Q,R]: See S02.0[K]

● S52.34　Spiral fracture of shaft of radius
　● S52.341　Displaced spiral fracture of shaft of radius, right arm
　　　A, K, M, N, P, Q, R 🔴, B, C 🔴, A, B, C 🔴
　　　Ⓔ **For code S52.341[A]:** See S52.011[A]
　　　For S52.341[B,C]: See S52.00[B,C]
　　　For S52.341[K,M,N,P,Q,R]: See S02.0[K]

　● S52.342　Displaced spiral fracture of shaft of radius, left arm A, K, M, N, P, Q, R 🔴, B, C 🔴, A, B, C 🔴
　　　Ⓔ **For code S52.342[A]:** See S52.012[A] **For code S52.342[B,C]:** See S52.00[B,C]
　　　For S52.342[K,M,N,P,Q,R]: See S02.0[K]

　● S52.343　Displaced spiral fracture of shaft of radius, unspecified arm
　　　A, K, M, N, P, Q, R 🔴, B, C 🔴, A, B, C 🔴
　　　Ⓔ **For code S52.343[A]:** See S52.019[A] **For code S52.343[B,C]:** See S52.00[B,C]
　　　For S52.343[K,M,N,P,Q,R]: See S02.0[K]

　● S52.344　Nondisplaced spiral fracture of shaft of radius, right arm
　　　A, K, M, N, P, Q, R 🔴, B, C 🔴, A, B, C 🔴
　　　Ⓔ **For code S52.344[A]:** See S52.011[A]
　　　For S52.344[B,C]: See S52.00[B,C]
　　　For S52.344[K,M,N,P,Q,R]: See S02.0[K]

　● S52.345　Nondisplaced spiral fracture of shaft of radius, left arm
　　　A, K, M, N, P, Q, R 🔴, B, C 🔴, A, B, C 🔴
　　　Ⓔ **For code S52.345[A]:** See S52.012[A] **For code S52.345[B,C]:** See S52.00[B,C]
　　　For S52.345[K,M,N,P,Q,R]: See S02.0[K]

　● S52.346　Nondisplaced spiral fracture of shaft of radius, unspecified arm
　　　A, K, M, N, P, Q, R 🔴, B, C 🔴, A, B, C 🔴
　　　Ⓔ **For code S52.346[A]:** See S52.019[A] **For code S52.346[B,C]:** See S52.00[B,C]
　　　For S52.346[K,M,N,P,Q,R]: See S02.0[K]

● S52.35　Comminuted fracture of shaft of radius
　● S52.351　Displaced comminuted fracture of shaft of radius, right arm
　　　A, K, M, N, P, Q, R 🔴, B, C 🔴, A, B, C 🔴
　　　Ⓔ **For code S52.351[A]:** See S52.011[A]
　　　For S52.351[B,C]: See S52.00[B,C]
　　　For S52.351[K,M,N,P,Q,R]: See S02.0[K]

　● S52.352　Displaced comminuted fracture of shaft of radius, left arm
　　　A, K, M, N, P, Q, R 🔴, B, C 🔴, A, B, C 🔴
　　　Ⓔ **For code S52.352[A]:** See S52.012[A] **For code S52.352[B,C]:** See S52.00[B,C]
　　　For S52.352[K,M,N,P,Q,R]: See S02.0[K]

　● S52.353　Displaced comminuted fracture of shaft of radius, unspecified arm
　　　A, K, M, N, P, Q, R 🔴, B, C 🔴, A, B, C 🔴
　　　Ⓔ **For code S52.353[A]:** See S52.019[A] **For code S52.353[B,C]:** See S52.00[B,C]
　　　For S52.353[K,M,N,P,Q,R]: See S02.0[K]

　● S52.354　Nondisplaced comminuted fracture of shaft of radius, right arm
　　　A, K, M, N, P, Q, R 🔴, B, C 🔴, A, B, C 🔴
　　　Ⓔ **For code S52.354[A]:** See S52.011[A]
　　　For S52.354[B,C]: See S52.00[B,C]
　　　For S52.354[K,M,N,P,Q,R]: See S02.0[K]

　● S52.355　Nondisplaced comminuted fracture of shaft of radius, left arm
　　　A, K, M, N, P, Q, R 🔴, B, C 🔴, A, B, C 🔴
　　　Ⓔ **For code S52.355[A]:** See S52.012[A] **For code S52.355[B,C]:** See S52.00[B,C]
　　　For S52.355[K,M,N,P,Q,R]: See S02.0[K]

　● S52.356　Nondisplaced comminuted fracture of shaft of radius, unspecified arm
　　　A, K, M, N, P, Q, R 🔴, B, C 🔴, A, B, C 🔴
　　　Ⓔ **For code S52.356[A]:** See S52.019[A] **For code S52.356[B,C]:** See S52.00[B,C]
　　　For S52.356[K,M,N,P,Q,R]: See S02.0[K]

● **S52.36   Segmental fracture of shaft of radius**

  ● **S52.361   Displaced segmental fracture of shaft of radius, right arm**
A, K, M, N, P, Q, R 🔧, B, C 🔧,
A, B, C 🔧
   (Ex:) For code S52.361[A]: See S52.011[A]
   For S52.361[B,C]: See S52.00[B,C]
   For S52.361[K,M,N,P,Q,R]: See S02.0[K]

  ● **S52.362   Displaced segmental fracture of shaft of radius, left arm**
A, K, M, N, P, Q, R 🔧, B, C 🔧,
A, B, C 🔧
   (Ex:) For code S52.362[A]: See S52.012[A] For
   code S52.362[B,C]: See S52.00[B,C]
   For S52.362[K,M,N,P,Q,R]: See S02.0[K]

  ● **S52.363   Displaced segmental fracture of shaft of radius, unspecified arm**
A, K, M, N, P, Q, R 🔧, B, C 🔧,
A, B, C 🔧
   (Ex:) For code S52.363[A]: See S52.019[A] For
   code S52.363[B,C]: See S52.00[B,C]
   For S52.363[K,M,N,P,Q,R]: See S02.0[K]

  ● **S52.364   Nondisplaced segmental fracture of shaft of radius, right arm**
A, K, M, N, P, Q, R 🔧, B, C 🔧,
A, B, C 🔧
   (Ex:) For code S52.364[A]: See S52.011[A]
   For S52.364[B,C]: See S52.00[B,C]
   For S52.364[K,M,N,P,Q,R]: See S02.0[K]

  ● **S52.365   Nondisplaced segmental fracture of shaft of radius, left arm**
A, K, M, N, P, Q, R 🔧, B, C 🔧,
A, B, C 🔧
   (Ex:) For code S52.365[A]: See S52.012[A] For
   code S52.365[B,C]: See S52.00[B,C]
   For S52.365[K,M,N,P,Q,R]: See S02.0[K]

  ● **S52.366   Nondisplaced segmental fracture of shaft of radius, unspecified arm**
A, K, M, N, P, Q, R 🔧, B, C 🔧,
A, B, C 🔧
   (Ex:) For code S52.366[A]: See S52.019[A] For
   code S52.366[B,C]: See S52.00[B,C]
   For S52.366[K,M,N,P,Q,R]: See S02.0[K]

● **S52.37   Galeazzi's fracture**
Fracture of lower shaft of radius with
radioulnar joint dislocation

  ● **S52.371   Galeazzi's fracture of right radius**
A, K, M, N, P, Q, R 🔧, B, C 🔧,
A, B, C 🔧
   (Ex:) For code S52.371[A]: See S52.011[A]
   For S52.371[B,C]: See S52.00[B,C]
   For S52.371[K,M,N,P,Q,R]: See S02.0[K]

  ● **S52.372   Galeazzi's fracture of left radius**
A, K, M, N, P, Q, R 🔧, B, C 🔧,
A, B, C 🔧
   (Ex:) For code S52.372[A]: See S52.012[A] For
   code S52.372[B,C]: See S52.00[B,C]
   For S52.372[K,M,N,P,Q,R]: See S02.0[K]

  ● **S52.379   Galeazzi's fracture of unspecified radius** A, K, M, N, P, Q, R 🔧, B, C 🔧,
A, B, C 🔧
   (Ex:) For code S52.379[A]: See S52.019[A] For
   code S52.379[B,C]: See S52.00[B,C]
   For S52.379[K,M,N,P,Q,R]: See S02.0[K]

● **S52.38   Bent bone of radius**

  ● **S52.381   Bent bone of right radius**
A, K, M, N, P, Q, R 🔧, B, C 🔧,
A, B, C 🔧
   (Ex:) For code S52.381[A]: See S52.011[A]
   For S52.381[B,C]: See S52.00[B,C]
   For S52.381[K,M,N,P,Q,R]: See S02.0[K]

  ● **S52.382   Bent bone of left radius**
A, K, M, N, P, Q, R 🔧, B, C 🔧,
A, B, C 🔧
   (Ex:) For code S52.382[A]: See S52.012[A] For
   code S52.382[B,C]: See S52.00[B,C]
   For S52.382[K,M,N,P,Q,R]: See S02.0[K]

  ● **S52.389   Bent bone of unspecified radius**
A, K, M, N, P, Q, R 🔧, B, C 🔧,
A, B, C 🔧
   (Ex:) For code S52.389[A]: See S52.019[A] For
   code S52.389[B,C]: See S52.00[B,C]
   For S52.389[K,M,N,P,Q,R]: See S02.0[K]

● **S52.39   Other fracture of shaft of radius**

  ● **S52.391   Other fracture of shaft of radius, right arm** A, K, M, N, P, Q, R 🔧, B, C 🔧,
A, B, C 🔧
   (Ex:) For code S52.391[A]: See S52.011[A]
   For S52.391[B,C]: See S52.00[B,C]
   For S52.391[K,M,N,P,Q,R]: See S02.0[K]

  ● **S52.392   Other fracture of shaft of radius, left arm** A, K, M, N, P, Q, R 🔧, B, C 🔧,
A, B, C 🔧
   (Ex:) For code S52.392[A]: See S52.012[A] For
   code S52.392[B,C]: See S52.00[B,C]
   For S52.392[K,M,N,P,Q,R]: See S02.0[K]

  ● **S52.399   Other fracture of shaft of radius, unspecified arm** A, K, M, N, P, Q, R 🔧,
B, C 🔧, A, B, C 🔧
   (Ex:) For code S52.399[A]: See S52.019[A] For
   code S52.399[B,C]: See S52.00[B,C]
   For S52.399[K,M,N,P,Q,R]: See S02.0[K]

● **S52.5   Fracture of lower end of radius**
Fracture of distal end of radius
Excludes2   physeal fractures of lower end of radius
(S59.2-)

● **S52.50   Unspecified fracture of the lower end of radius**

  ● **S52.501   Unspecified fracture of the lower end of right radius** A, K, M, N, P, Q, R 🔧,
B, C 🔧, A, B, C 🔧
   (Ex:) For code S52.501[A]: See S52.011[A]
   For S52.501[B,C]: See S52.00[B,C]
   For S52.501[K,M,N,P,Q,R]: See S02.0[K]

  ● **S52.502   Unspecified fracture of the lower end of left radius** A, K, M, N, P, Q, R 🔧,
B, C 🔧, A, B, C 🔧
   (Ex:) For code S52.502[A]: See S52.012[A] For
   code S52.502[B,C]: See S52.00[B,C]
   For S52.502[K,M,N,P,Q,R]: See S02.0[K]

  ● **S52.509   Unspecified fracture of the lower end of unspecified radius**
A, K, M, N, P, Q, R 🔧, B, C 🔧,
A, B, C 🔧
   (Ex:) For code S52.509[A]: See S52.019[A] For
   code S52.509[B,C]: See S52.00[B,C]
   For S52.509[K,M,N,P,Q,R]: See S02.0[K]

◀ New   ◀▥ Revised   d̶e̶l̶e̶t̶e̶d̶ Deleted   Excludes 1   Excludes 2   Includes   Use additional   Code first   Code also   Unspecified
OGCR Official Guidelines   ● Unacceptable Principal Diagnosis   X Assign placeholder X   ● Use Additional Character(s)   ▶ Manifestation Code   Coding Clinic

● **S52.51**   **Fracture of radial styloid process**

  ● **S52.511**   Displaced fracture of right radial styloid process A, K, M, N, P, Q, R 🝪, B, C 🝪, A, B, C 🝪
       (Ex) **For code S52.511[A]:** See S52.011[A]
       For S52.511[B,C]: See S52.00[B,C]
       For S52.511[K,M,N,P,Q,R]: See S02.0[K]

  ● **S52.512**   Displaced fracture of left radial styloid process A, K, M, N, P, Q, R 🝪, B, C 🝪, A, B, C 🝪
       (Ex) **For code S52.512[A]:** See S52.012[A] **For code S52.512[B,C]:** See S52.00[B,C]
       For S52.512[K,M,N,P,Q,R]: See S02.0[K]

  ● **S52.513**   Displaced fracture of unspecified radial styloid process A, K, M, N, P, Q, R 🝪, B, C 🝪, A, B, C 🝪
       (Ex) **For code S52.513[A]:** See S52.019[A] **For code S52.513[B,C]:** See S52.00[B,C]
       For S52.513[K,M,N,P,Q,R]: See S02.0[K]

  ● **S52.514**   Nondisplaced fracture of right radial styloid process A, K, M, N, P, Q, R 🝪, B, C 🝪, A, B, C 🝪
       (Ex) **For code S52.514[A]:** See S52.011[A]
       For S52.514[B,C]: See S52.00[B,C]
       For S52.514[K,M,N,P,Q,R]: See S02.0[K]

  ● **S52.515**   Nondisplaced fracture of left radial styloid process A, K, M, N, P, Q, R 🝪, B, C 🝪, A, B, C 🝪
       (Ex) **For code S52.515[A]:** See S52.012[A] **For code S52.515[B,C]:** See S52.00[B,C]
       For S52.515[K,M,N,P,Q,R]: See S02.0[K]

  ● **S52.516**   Nondisplaced fracture of unspecified radial styloid process A, K, M, N, P, Q, R 🝪, B, C 🝪, A, B, C 🝪
       (Ex) **For code S52.516[A]:** See S52.019[A] **For code S52.516[B,C]:** See S52.00[B,C]
       For S52.516[K,M,N,P,Q,R]: See S02.0[K]

● **S52.52**   **Torus fracture of lower end of radius**

     The appropriate 7th character is to be added to all codes in subcategory S52.52

A	initial encounter for closed fracture
D	subsequent encounter for fracture with routine healing
G	subsequent encounter for fracture with delayed healing
K	subsequent encounter for fracture with nonunion
P	subsequent encounter for fracture with malunion
S	sequela

  ● **S52.521**   Torus fracture of lower end of right radius A, K, P 🝪, A 🝪
       (Ex) **For code S52.521[A]:** See S52.011[A]
       For S52.521[K,P]: See S02.0[K]

  ● **S52.522**   Torus fracture of lower end of left radius A, K, P 🝪, A 🝪
       (Ex) **For code S52.522[A]:** See S52.012[A]
       For S52.522[K,P]: See S02.0[K]

  ● **S52.529**   Torus fracture of lower end of unspecified radius A, K, P 🝪, A 🝪
       (Ex) **For code S52.529[A]:** See S52.019[A]
       For S52.529[K,P]: See S02.0[K]

● **S52.53**   **Colles' fracture**

  ● **S52.531**   Colles' fracture of right radius A, K, M, N, P, Q, R 🝪, B, C 🝪, A, B, C 🝪
       (Ex) **For code S52.531[A]:** See S52.011[A]
       For S52.531[B,C]: See S52.00[B,C]
       For S52.531[K,M,N,P,Q,R]: See S02.0[K]

  ● **S52.532**   Colles' fracture of left radius A, K, M, N, P, Q, R 🝪, B, C 🝪, A, B, C 🝪
       (Ex) **For code S52.532[A]:** See S52.012[A] **For code S52.532[B,C]:** See S52.00[B,C]
       For S52.532[K,M,N,P,Q,R]: See S02.0[K]
       Coding Clinic: 2016, Q2, P5

  ● **S52.539**   Colles' fracture of unspecified radius A, K, M, N, P, Q, R 🝪, B, C 🝪, A, B, C 🝪
       (Ex) **For code S52.539[A]:** See S52.019[A] **For code S52.539[B,C]:** See S52.00[B,C]
       For S52.539[K,M,N,P,Q,R]: See S02.0[K]

● **S52.54**   **Smith's fracture**

  ● **S52.541**   Smith's fracture of right radius A, K, M, N, P, Q, R 🝪, B, C 🝪, A, B, C 🝪
       (Ex) **For code S52.541[A]:** See S52.011[A]
       For S52.541[B,C]: See S52.00[B,C]
       For S52.541[K,M,N,P,Q,R]: See S02.0[K]

  ● **S52.542**   Smith's fracture of left radius A, K, M, N, P, Q, R 🝪, B, C 🝪, A, B, C 🝪
       (Ex) **For code S52.542[A]:** See S52.012[A] **For code S52.542[B,C]:** See S52.00[B,C]
       For S52.542[K,M,N,P,Q,R]: See S02.0[K]

  ● **S52.549**   Smith's fracture of unspecified radius A, K, M, N, P, Q, R 🝪, B, C 🝪, A, B, C 🝪
       (Ex) **For code S52.549[A]:** See S52.019[A] **For code S52.549[B,C]:** See S52.00[B,C]
       For S52.549[K,M,N,P,Q,R]: See S02.0[K]

● **S52.55**   **Other extraarticular fracture of lower end of radius**

  ● **S52.551**   Other extraarticular fracture of lower end of right radius A, K, M, N, P, Q, R 🝪, B, C 🝪, A, B, C 🝪
       (Ex) **For code S52.551[A]:** See S52.011[A]
       For S52.551[B,C]: See S52.00[B,C]
       For S52.551[K,M,N,P,Q,R]: See S02.0[K]

  ● **S52.552**   Other extraarticular fracture of lower end of left radius A, K, M, N, P, Q, R 🝪, B, C 🝪, A, B, C 🝪
       (Ex) **For code S52.552[A]:** See S52.012[A] **For code S52.552[B,C]:** See S52.00[B,C]
       For S52.552[K,M,N,P,Q,R]: See S02.0[K]

  ● **S52.559**   Other extraarticular fracture of lower end of unspecified radius A, K, M, N, P, Q, R 🝪, B, C 🝪, A, B, C 🝪
       (Ex) **For code S52.559[A]:** See S52.019[A] **For code S52.559[B,C]:** See S52.00[B,C]
       For S52.559[K,M,N,P,Q,R]: See S02.0[K]

CHAPTER 19 (S00-T88)

CHAPTER 19 (S00-T88)

● **S52.56**   Barton's fracture
  ● **S52.561**   Barton's fracture of right radius
     A, K, M, N, P, Q, R 🔧, B, C 🔧,
     A, B, C 🔧
      Ⓔⓧ **For code S52.561[A]:** See S52.011[A]
       For S52.561[B,C]: See S52.00[B,C]
       For S52.561[K,M,N,P,Q,R]: See S02.0[K]
  ● **S52.562**   Barton's fracture of left radius
     A, K, M, N, P, Q, R 🔧, B, C 🔧,
     A, B, C 🔧
      Ⓔⓧ **For code S52.562[A]:** See S52.012[A] **For**
       code S52.562[B,C]: See S52.00[B,C]
       For S52.562[K,M,N,P,Q,R]: See S02.0[K]
  ● **S52.569**   Barton's fracture of unspecified radius
     A, K, M, N, P, Q, R 🔧, B, C 🔧,
     A, B, C 🔧
      Ⓔⓧ **For code S52.569[A]:** See S52.019[A] **For**
       code S52.569[B,C]: See S52.00[B,C]
       For S52.569[K,M,N,P,Q,R]: See S02.0[K]

● **S52.57**   Other intraarticular fracture of lower end of radius
  ● **S52.571**   Other intraarticular fracture of lower end of right radius
     A, K, M, N, P, Q, R 🔧, B, C 🔧,
     A, B, C 🔧
      Ⓔⓧ **For code S52.571[A]:** See S52.011[A]
       For S52.571[B,C]: See S52.00[B,C]
       For S52.571[K,M,N,P,Q,R]: See S02.0[K]
  ● **S52.572**   Other intraarticular fracture of lower end of left radius
     A, K, M, N, P, Q, R 🔧, B, C 🔧,
     A, B, C 🔧
      Ⓔⓧ **For code S52.572[A]:** See S52.012[A] **For**
       code S52.572[B,C]: See S52.00[B,C]
       For S52.572[K,M,N,P,Q,R]: See S02.0[K]
  ● **S52.579**   Other intraarticular fracture of lower end of unspecified radius
     A, K, M, N, P, Q, R 🔧, B, C 🔧,
     A, B, C 🔧
      Ⓔⓧ **For code S52.579[A]:** See S52.019[A] **For**
       code S52.579[B,C]: See S52.00[B,C]
       For S52.579[K,M,N,P,Q,R]: See S02.0[K]

● **S52.59**   Other fractures of lower end of radius
  ● **S52.591**   Other fractures of lower end of right radius A, K, M, N, P, Q, R 🔧, B, C 🔧,
     A, B, C 🔧
      Ⓔⓧ **For code S52.591[A]:** See S52.011[A]
       For S52.591[B,C]: See S52.00[B,C]
       For S52.591[K,M,N,P,Q,R]: See S02.0[K]
  ● **S52.592**   Other fractures of lower end of left radius A, K, M, N, P, Q, R 🔧, B, C 🔧,
     A, B, C 🔧
      Ⓔⓧ **For code S52.592[A]:** See S52.012[A] **For**
       code S52.592[B,C]: See S52.00[B,C]
       For S52.592[K,M,N,P,Q,R]: See S02.0[K]
  ● **S52.599**   Other fractures of lower end of unspecified radius
     A, K, M, N, P, Q, R 🔧, B, C 🔧,
     A, B, C 🔧
      Ⓔⓧ **For code S52.599[A]:** See S52.019[A] **For**
       code S52.599[B,C]: See S52.00[B,C]
       For S52.599[K,M,N,P,Q,R]: See S02.0[K]

● **S52.6**   Fracture of lower end of ulna
  ● **S52.60**   Unspecified fracture of lower end of ulna
    ● **S52.601**   Unspecified fracture of lower end of right ulna A, K, M, N, P, Q, R 🔧,
       B, C 🔧, A, B, C 🔧
        Ⓔⓧ **For code S52.601[A]:** See S52.011[A]
         For S52.601[B,C]: See S52.00[B,C]
         For S52.601[K,M,N,P,Q,R]: See S02.0[K]
    ● **S52.602**   Unspecified fracture of lower end of left ulna A, K, M, N, P, Q, R 🔧,
       B, C 🔧, A, B, C 🔧
        Ⓔⓧ **For code S52.602[A]:** See S52.012[A] **For**
         code S52.602[B,C]: See S52.00[B,C]
         For S52.602[K,M,N,P,Q,R]: See S02.0[K]
    ● **S52.609**   Unspecified fracture of lower end of unspecified ulna
       A, K, M, N, P, Q, R 🔧, B, C 🔧,
       A, B, C 🔧
        Ⓔⓧ **For code S52.609[A]:** See S52.019[A] **For**
         code S52.609[B,C]: See S52.00[B,C]
         For S52.609[K,M,N,P,Q,R]: See S02.0[K]

  ● **S52.61**   Fracture of ulna styloid process
    ● **S52.611**   Displaced fracture of right ulna styloid process A, K, M, N, P, Q, R 🔧,
       B, C 🔧, A, B, C 🔧
        Ⓔⓧ **For code S52.611[A]:** See S52.011[A]
         For S52.611[B,C]: See S52.00[B,C]
         For S52.611[K,M,N,P,Q,R]: See S02.0[K]
    ● **S52.612**   Displaced fracture of left ulna styloid process A, K, M, N, P, Q, R 🔧, B, C 🔧,
       A, B, C 🔧
        Ⓔⓧ **For code S52.612[A]:** See S52.012[A] **For**
         code S52.612[B,C]: See S52.00[B,C]
         For S52.612[K,M,N,P,Q,R]: See S02.0[K]
    ● **S52.613**   Displaced fracture of unspecified ulna styloid process A, K, M, N, P, Q, R 🔧,
       B, C 🔧, A, B, C 🔧
        Ⓔⓧ **For code S52.613[A]:** See S52.019[A] **For**
         code S52.613[B,C]: See S52.00[B,C]
         For S52.613[K,M,N,P,Q,R]: See S02.0[K]
    ● **S52.614**   Nondisplaced fracture of right ulna styloid process A, K, M, N, P, Q, R 🔧,
       B, C 🔧, A, B, C 🔧
        Ⓔⓧ **For code S52.614[A]:** See S52.011[A]
         For S52.614[B,C]: See S52.00[B,C]
         For S52.614[K,M,N,P,Q,R]: See S02.0[K]
    ● **S52.615**   Nondisplaced fracture of left ulna styloid process A, K, M, N, P, Q, R 🔧,
       B, C 🔧, A, B, C 🔧
        Ⓔⓧ **For code S52.615[A]:** See S52.012[A] **For**
         code S52.615[B,C]: See S52.00[B,C]
         For S52.615[K,M,N,P,Q,R]: See S02.0[K]
    ● **S52.616**   Nondisplaced fracture of unspecified ulna styloid process
       A, K, M, N, P, Q, R 🔧, B, C 🔧,
       A, B, C 🔧
        Ⓔⓧ **For code S52.616[A]:** See S52.019[A] **For**
         code S52.616[B,C]: See S52.00[B,C]
         For S52.616[K,M,N,P,Q,R]: See S02.0[K]

◄ New   ◄═ Revised   ~~deleted~~ Deleted   Excludes 1   Excludes 2   Includes   Use additional   Code first   Code also   Unspecified
OGCR Official Guidelines   ● Unacceptable Principal Diagnosis   X Assign placeholder X   ● Use Additional Character(s)   ▶ Manifestation Code   **Coding Clinic**

● S52.62   **Torus fracture of lower end of ulna**

The appropriate 7th character is to be added to all codes in subcategory S52.62

A	initial encounter for closed fracture
D	subsequent encounter for fracture with routine healing
G	subsequent encounter for fracture with delayed healing
K	subsequent encounter for fracture with nonunion
P	subsequent encounter for fracture with malunion
S	sequela

● S52.621   **Torus fracture of lower end of right ulna** A, K, P 🏷, A 🏷
(Ex) **For code S52.621[A]:** See S52.011[A]
For S52.621[K,P]: See S02.0[K]

● S52.622   **Torus fracture of lower end of left ulna** A, K, P 🏷, A 🏷
(Ex) **For code S52.622[A]:** See S52.012[A]
For S52.622[K,P]: See S02.0[K]

● S52.629   **Torus fracture of lower end of unspecified ulna** A, K, P 🏷, A 🏷
(Ex) **For code S52.629[A]:** See S52.019[A]
For S52.629[K,P]: See S02.0[K]

● S52.69   **Other fracture of lower end of ulna**

● S52.691   **Other fracture of lower end of right ulna** A, K, M, N, P, Q, R 🏷, B, C 🏷, A, B, C 🏷
(Ex) **For code S52.691[A]:** See S52.011[A]
For S52.691[B,C]: See S52.00[B,C]
For S52.691[K,M,N,P,Q,R]: See S02.0[K]

● S52.692   **Other fracture of lower end of left ulna** A, K, M, N, P, Q, R 🏷, B, C 🏷, A, B, C 🏷
(Ex) **For code S52.692[A]:** See S52.012[A] **For code S52.692[B,C]:** See S52.00[B,C]
For S52.692[K,M,N,P,Q,R]: See S02.0[K]

● S52.699   **Other fracture of lower end of unspecified ulna**
A, K, M, N, P, Q, R 🏷, B, C 🏷, A, B, C 🏷
(Ex) **For code S52.699[A]:** See S52.019[A] **For code S52.699[B,C]:** See S52.00[B,C]
For S52.699[K,M,N,P,Q,R]: See S02.0[K]

● S52.9   **Unspecified fracture of forearm**
(Ex) **For category S52.9 CC codes S52.9[A]:** See S52.019[A] **For code S52.9[B,C]:** See S52.00[B,C] **For S52.9[K,M,N,P,Q,R]:** See S02.0[K]

X ● S52.90   **Unspecified fracture of unspecified forearm** A, K, M, N, P, Q, R 🏷, B, C 🏷, A, B, C 🏷

X ● S52.91   **Unspecified fracture of right forearm** A, K, M, N, P, Q, R 🏷, B, C 🏷, A, B, C 🏷

X ● S52.92   **Unspecified fracture of left forearm** A, K, M, N, P, Q, R 🏷, B, C 🏷, A, B, C 🏷

● S53   **Dislocation and sprain of joints and ligaments of elbow**

Includes   avulsion of joint or ligament of elbow
laceration of cartilage, joint or ligament of elbow
sprain of cartilage, joint or ligament of elbow
traumatic hemarthrosis of joint or ligament of elbow
traumatic rupture of joint or ligament of elbow
traumatic subluxation of joint or ligament of elbow
traumatic tear of joint or ligament of elbow

Code also any associated open wound

Excludes2   strain of muscle, fascia and tendon at forearm level (S56.-)

The appropriate 7th character is to be added to each code from category S53

A	initial encounter
D	subsequent encounter
S	sequela

● S53.0   **Subluxation and dislocation of radial head**
Dislocation of radiohumeral joint
Subluxation of radiohumeral joint

Excludes1   Monteggia's fracture-dislocation (S52.27-)

● S53.00   **Unspecified subluxation and dislocation of radial head**

● S53.001   **Unspecified subluxation of right radial head**

● S53.002   **Unspecified subluxation of left radial head**

● S53.003   **Unspecified subluxation of unspecified radial head**

● S53.004   **Unspecified dislocation of right radial head**

● S53.005   **Unspecified dislocation of left radial head**

● S53.006   **Unspecified dislocation of unspecified radial head**

● S53.01   **Anterior subluxation and dislocation of radial head**
Anteriomedial subluxation and dislocation of radial head

● S53.011   **Anterior subluxation of right radial head**

● S53.012   **Anterior subluxation of left radial head**

● S53.013   **Anterior subluxation of unspecified radial head**

● S53.014   **Anterior dislocation of right radial head**

● S53.015   **Anterior dislocation of left radial head**

● S53.016   **Anterior dislocation of unspecified radial head**

CHAPTER 19 (S00-T88)

CHAPTER 19 (S00-T88)

● S53.02   **Posterior subluxation and dislocation of radial head**
    Posteriolateral subluxation and dislocation of radial head

   ● S53.021   **Posterior subluxation of right radial head**

   ● S53.022   **Posterior subluxation of left radial head**

   ● S53.023   **Posterior subluxation of** <mark>unspecified</mark> **radial head**

   ● S53.024   **Posterior dislocation of right radial head**

   ● S53.025   **Posterior dislocation of left radial head**

   ● S53.026   **Posterior dislocation of** <mark>unspecified</mark> **radial head**

● S53.03   **Nursemaid's elbow**

   ● S53.031   **Nursemaid's elbow, right elbow**
      Coding Clinic: 2015, Q1, P7-8

   ● S53.032   **Nursemaid's elbow, left elbow**

   ● S53.033   **Nursemaid's elbow,** <mark>unspecified</mark> **elbow**

● S53.09   **Other subluxation and dislocation of radial head**

   ● S53.091   **Other subluxation of right radial head**

   ● S53.092   **Other subluxation of left radial head**

   ● S53.093   **Other subluxation of** <mark>unspecified</mark> **radial head**

   ● S53.094   **Other dislocation of right radial head**

   ● S53.095   **Other dislocation of left radial head**

   ● S53.096   **Other dislocation of** <mark>unspecified</mark> **radial head**

● S53.1   **Subluxation and dislocation of ulnohumeral joint**
   Subluxation and dislocation of elbow NOS

   Excludes1   dislocation of radial head alone (S53.0-)

● S53.10   **Unspecified subluxation and dislocation of ulnohumeral joint**

   ● S53.101   <mark>Unspecified</mark> **subluxation of right ulnohumeral joint**

   ● S53.102   <mark>Unspecified</mark> **subluxation of left ulnohumeral joint**

   ● S53.103   <mark>Unspecified</mark> **subluxation of unspecified ulnohumeral joint**

   ● S53.104   <mark>Unspecified</mark> **dislocation of right ulnohumeral joint**

   ● S53.105   <mark>Unspecified</mark> **dislocation of left ulnohumeral joint**

   ● S53.106   <mark>Unspecified</mark> **dislocation of unspecified ulnohumeral joint**

● S53.11   **Anterior subluxation and dislocation of ulnohumeral joint**

   ● S53.111   **Anterior subluxation of right ulnohumeral joint**

   ● S53.112   **Anterior subluxation of left ulnohumeral joint**

   ● S53.113   **Anterior subluxation of** <mark>unspecified</mark> **ulnohumeral joint**

   ● S53.114   **Anterior dislocation of right ulnohumeral joint**
      Coding Clinic: 2012, Q4, P108

   ● S53.115   **Anterior dislocation of left ulnohumeral joint**

   ● S53.116   **Anterior dislocation of** <mark>unspecified</mark> **ulnohumeral joint**

● S53.12   **Posterior subluxation and dislocation of ulnohumeral joint**

   ● S53.121   **Posterior subluxation of right ulnohumeral joint**

   ● S53.122   **Posterior subluxation of left ulnohumeral joint**

   ● S53.123   **Posterior subluxation of** <mark>unspecified</mark> **ulnohumeral joint**

   ● S53.124   **Posterior dislocation of right ulnohumeral joint**

   ● S53.125   **Posterior dislocation of left ulnohumeral joint**

   ● S53.126   **Posterior dislocation of** <mark>unspecified</mark> **ulnohumeral joint**

● S53.13   **Medial subluxation and dislocation of ulnohumeral joint**

   ● S53.131   **Medial subluxation of right ulnohumeral joint**

   ● S53.132   **Medial subluxation of left ulnohumeral joint**

   ● S53.133   **Medial subluxation of** <mark>unspecified</mark> **ulnohumeral joint**

   ● S53.134   **Medial dislocation of right ulnohumeral joint**

   ● S53.135   **Medial dislocation of left ulnohumeral joint**

   ● S53.136   **Medial dislocation of** <mark>unspecified</mark> **ulnohumeral joint**

● S53.14   **Lateral subluxation and dislocation of ulnohumeral joint**

   ● S53.141   **Lateral subluxation of right ulnohumeral joint**

   ● S53.142   **Lateral subluxation of left ulnohumeral joint**

   ● S53.143   **Lateral subluxation of** <mark>unspecified</mark> **ulnohumeral joint**

   ● S53.144   **Lateral dislocation of right ulnohumeral joint**

   ● S53.145   **Lateral dislocation of left ulnohumeral joint**

   ● S53.146   **Lateral dislocation of** <mark>unspecified</mark> **ulnohumeral joint**

● S53.19   **Other subluxation and dislocation of ulnohumeral joint**

   ● S53.191   **Other subluxation of right ulnohumeral joint**

   ● S53.192   **Other subluxation of left ulnohumeral joint**

   ● S53.193   **Other subluxation of** <mark>unspecified</mark> **ulnohumeral joint**

   ● S53.194   **Other dislocation of right ulnohumeral joint**

   ● S53.195   **Other dislocation of left ulnohumeral joint**

   ● S53.196   **Other dislocation of** <mark>unspecified</mark> **ulnohumeral joint**

● S53.2   **Traumatic rupture of radial collateral ligament**

   Excludes1   sprain of radial collateral ligament NOS (S53.43-)

X ● S53.20   **Traumatic rupture of** <mark>unspecified</mark> **radial collateral ligament**

X ● S53.21   **Traumatic rupture of right radial collateral ligament**

X ● S53.22   **Traumatic rupture of left radial collateral ligament**

● **S53.3** **Traumatic rupture of ulnar collateral ligament**
    Excludes1 sprain of ulnar collateral ligament (S53.44-)
X ● **S53.30** **Traumatic rupture of unspecified ulnar collateral ligament**
X ● **S53.31** **Traumatic rupture of right ulnar collateral ligament**
X ● **S53.32** **Traumatic rupture of left ulnar collateral ligament**

● **S53.4** **Sprain of elbow**
    Excludes2 traumatic rupture of radial collateral ligament (S53.2-)
            traumatic rupture of ulnar collateral ligament (S53.3-)
  ● **S53.40** **Unspecified sprain of elbow**
    ● **S53.401** **Unspecified sprain of right elbow**
    ● **S53.402** **Unspecified sprain of left elbow**
    ● **S53.409** **Unspecified sprain of unspecified elbow**
           Sprain of elbow NOS
  ● **S53.41** **Radiohumeral (joint) sprain**
    ● **S53.411** **Radiohumeral (joint) sprain of right elbow**
    ● **S53.412** **Radiohumeral (joint) sprain of left elbow**
    ● **S53.419** **Radiohumeral (joint) sprain of unspecified elbow**
  ● **S53.42** **Ulnohumeral (joint) sprain**
    ● **S53.421** **Ulnohumeral (joint) sprain of right elbow**
    ● **S53.422** **Ulnohumeral (joint) sprain of left elbow**
    ● **S53.429** **Ulnohumeral (joint) sprain of unspecified elbow**
  ● **S53.43** **Radial collateral ligament sprain**
    ● **S53.431** **Radial collateral ligament sprain of right elbow**
    ● **S53.432** **Radial collateral ligament sprain of left elbow**
    ● **S53.439** **Radial collateral ligament sprain of unspecified elbow**
  ● **S53.44** **Ulnar collateral ligament sprain**
    ● **S53.441** **Ulnar collateral ligament sprain of right elbow**
    ● **S53.442** **Ulnar collateral ligament sprain of left elbow**
    ● **S53.449** **Ulnar collateral ligament sprain of unspecified elbow**
  ● **S53.49** **Other sprain of elbow**
    ● **S53.491** **Other sprain of right elbow**
    ● **S53.492** **Other sprain of left elbow**
    ● **S53.499** **Other sprain of unspecified elbow**

● **S54** **Injury of nerves at forearm level**
    Code also any associated open wound (S51.-)
    Excludes2 injury of nerves at wrist and hand level (S64.-)
    The appropriate 7th character is to be added to each code from category S54

A	initial encounter
D	subsequent encounter
S	sequela

● **S54.0** **Injury of ulnar nerve at forearm level**
    Injury of ulnar nerve NOS
  X ● **S54.00** **Injury of ulnar nerve at forearm level, unspecified arm**
  X ● **S54.01** **Injury of ulnar nerve at forearm level, right arm**
  X ● **S54.02** **Injury of ulnar nerve at forearm level, left arm**
● **S54.1** **Injury of median nerve at forearm level**
    Injury of median nerve NOS
  X ● **S54.10** **Injury of median nerve at forearm level, unspecified arm**
  X ● **S54.11** **Injury of median nerve at forearm level, right arm**
  X ● **S54.12** **Injury of median nerve at forearm level, left arm**
● **S54.2** **Injury of radial nerve at forearm level**
    Injury of radial nerve NOS
  X ● **S54.20** **Injury of radial nerve at forearm level, unspecified arm**
  X ● **S54.21** **Injury of radial nerve at forearm level, right arm**
  X ● **S54.22** **Injury of radial nerve at forearm level, left arm**
● **S54.3** **Injury of cutaneous sensory nerve at forearm level**
  X ● **S54.30** **Injury of cutaneous sensory nerve at forearm level, unspecified arm**
  X ● **S54.31** **Injury of cutaneous sensory nerve at forearm level, right arm**
  X ● **S54.32** **Injury of cutaneous sensory nerve at forearm level, left arm**
● **S54.8** **Injury of other nerves at forearm level**
  ● **S54.8X** **Injury of other nerves at forearm level** ◄▥
    ● **S54.8X1** **Injury of other nerves at forearm level, right arm** ◄▥
    ● **S54.8X2** **Injury of other nerves at forearm level, left arm** ◄▥
    ● **S54.8X9** **Injury of other nerves at forearm level, unspecified arm** ◄▥
● **S54.9** **Injury of unspecified nerve at forearm level**
  X ● **S54.90** **Injury of unspecified nerve at forearm level, unspecified arm**
  X ● **S54.91** **Injury of unspecified nerve at forearm level, right arm**
  X ● **S54.92** **Injury of unspecified nerve at forearm level, left arm**

● **S55** **Injury of blood vessels at forearm level**
Code also any associated open wound (S51.-)
Excludes2 injury of blood vessels at wrist and hand level (S65.-)
injury of brachial vessels (S45.1-S45.2)

The appropriate 7th character is to be added to each code from category S55

> A initial encounter
> D subsequent encounter
> S sequela

● **S55.0** **Injury of ulnar artery at forearm level**

● **S55.00** Unspecified injury of ulnar artery at forearm level

● **S55.001** Unspecified injury of ulnar artery at forearm level, right arm A 🔧
(Ex:) S45.301[A], S45.309-S45.311[A], S45.319-S45.391[A], S45.399-S45.801[A], S45.809-S45.811[A], S45.819-S45.891[A], S45.899-S45.901[A], S45.909-S45.911[A], S45.919-S45.991[A], S45.999[A], S55.001[A], S55.009-S55.011[A], S55.019-S55.091[A], S55.099[A], S55.201[A], S55.209-S55.211[A], S55.219-S55.291[A], S55.299-S55.801[A], S55.809-S55.811[A], S55.819-S55.891[A], S55.899-S55.901[A], S55.909-S55.911[A], S55.919-S55.991[A], S55.999[A], S65.001[A], S65.009-S65.011[A], S65.019-S65.091[A], S65.099[A], S65.801[A], S65.809-S65.811[A], S65.819-S65.891[A], S65.899-S65.901[A], S65.909-S65.911[A], S65.919-S65.991[A], S65.999[A]

● **S55.002** Unspecified injury of ulnar artery at forearm level, left arm A 🔧
(Ex:) S45.302-S45.309[A], S45.312-S45.319[A], S45.392-S45.399[A], S45.802-S45.809[A], S45.812-S45.819[A], S45.892-S45.899[A], S45.902-S45.909[A], S45.912-S45.919[A], S45.992-S45.999[A], S55.002-S55.009[A], S55.012-S55.019[A], S55.092-S55.099[A], S55.202-S55.209[A], S55.212-S55.219[A], S55.292-S55.299[A], S55.802-S55.809[A], S55.812-S55.819[A], S55.892-S55.899[A], S55.902-S55.909[A], S55.912-S55.919[A], S55.992-S55.999[A], S65.002-S65.009[A], S65.012-S65.019[A], S65.092-S65.099[A], S65.802-S65.809[A] S65.812-S65.819[A], S65.892-S65.899[A], S65.902-S65.909[A], S65.912-S65.919[A], S65.992-S65.999[A]

● **S55.009** Unspecified injury of ulnar artery at forearm level, unspecified arm A 🔧
(Ex:) S45.301-S45.999[A], S55.001-S55.099[A], S55.201-S55.999[A], S65.001-S65.099[A], S65.801-S65.999[A]

● **S55.01** Laceration of ulnar artery at forearm level

● **S55.011** Laceration of ulnar artery at forearm level, right arm A 🔧
(Ex:) See S55.001

● **S55.012** Laceration of ulnar artery at forearm level, left arm A 🔧
(Ex:) See S55.002

● **S55.019** Laceration of ulnar artery at forearm level, unspecified arm A 🔧
(Ex:) See S55.009

● **S55.09** Other specified injury of ulnar artery at forearm level

● **S55.091** Other specified injury of ulnar artery at forearm level, right arm A 🔧
(Ex:) See S55.001

● **S55.092** Other specified injury of ulnar artery at forearm level, left arm A 🔧
(Ex:) See S55.002

● **S55.099** Other specified injury of ulnar artery at forearm level, unspecified arm A 🔧
(Ex:) See S55.009

● **S55.1** **Injury of radial artery at forearm level**

● **S55.10** Unspecified injury of radial artery at forearm level

● **S55.101** Unspecified injury of radial artery at forearm level, right arm A 🔧
(Ex:) S45.301[A], S45.309-S45.311[A], S45.319-S45.391[A], S45.399-S45.801[A], S45.809-S45.811[A], S45.819-S45.891[A], S45.899-S45.901[A], S45.909-S45.911[A], S45.919-S45.991[A], S45.999[A], S55.101[A], S55.109-S55.111[A], S55.119-S55.191[A], S55.199-S55.201[A], S55.209-S55.211[A], S55.219-S55.291[A], S55.299-S55.801[A], S55.809-S55.811[A], S55.819-S55.891[A], S55.899-S55.901[A], S55.909-S55.911[A], S55.919-S55.991[A], S55.999[A], S65.101[A], S65.109-S65.111[A], S65.119-S65.191[A], S65.199[A], S65.801[A], S65.809-S65.811[A], S65.819-S65.891[A], S65.899-S65.901[A], S65.909-S65.911[A], S65.919-S65.991[A], S65.999[A]

● **S55.102** Unspecified injury of radial artery at forearm level, left arm A 🔧
(Ex:) S45.302-S45.309[A], S45.312-S45.319[A], S45.392-S45.399[A], S45.802-S45.809[A], S45.812-S45.819[A], S45.892-S45.899[A], S45.902-S45.909[A], S45.912-S45.919[A], S45.992-S45.999[A], S55.102-S55.109[A], S55.112-S55.119[A], S55.192-S55.199[A], S55.202-S55.209[A], S55.212-S55.219[A], S55.292-S55.299[A], S55.802A-S55.809[A], S55.812-S55.819[A], S55.892-S55.899[A], S55.902-S55.909[A], S55.912-S55.919[A], S55.992-S55.999[A], S65.102-S65.109[A], S65.112-S65.119[A], S65.192-S65.199[A], S65.802-S65.809[A], S65.812-S65.819[A], S65.892-S65.899[A], S65.902-S65.909[A], S65.912-S65.919[A], S65.992-S65.999[A]

● **S55.109** Unspecified injury of radial artery at forearm level, unspecified arm A 🔧
(Ex:) S45.301-S45.999[A], S55.101-S55.999[A], S65.101-S65.199[A], S65.801-S65.999[A]

● **S55.11** Laceration of radial artery at forearm level

● **S55.111** Laceration of radial artery at forearm level, right arm A 🔧
(Ex:) See S55.101

● **S55.112** Laceration of radial artery at forearm level, left arm A 🔧
(Ex:) See S55.102

● **S55.119** Laceration of radial artery at forearm level, unspecified arm A 🔧
(Ex:) See S55.109

◀ New ◀▦ Revised ~~deleted~~ Deleted Excludes 1 Excludes 2 Includes Use additional Code first Code also Unspecified
OGCR Official Guidelines ● Unacceptable Principal Diagnosis X Assign placeholder X ● Use Additional Character(s) ▌ Manifestation Code **Coding Clinic**

● **S55.19** Other specified injury of radial artery at forearm level

  ● **S55.191** Other specified injury of radial artery at forearm level, right arm A 🗞
      Ex: See S55.101

  ● **S55.192** Other specified injury of radial artery at forearm level, left arm A 🗞
      Ex: See S55.102

  ● **S55.199** Other specified injury of radial artery at forearm level, unspecified arm A 🗞
      Ex: See S55.109

● **S55.2** Injury of vein at forearm level

  ● **S55.20** Unspecified injury of vein at forearm level

    ● **S55.201** Unspecified injury of vein at forearm level, right arm A 🗞
       Ex: See S45.301

    ● **S55.202** Unspecified injury of vein at forearm level, left arm A 🗞
       Ex: See S45.302

    ● **S55.209** Unspecified injury of vein at forearm level, unspecified arm A 🗞
       Ex: See S45.309

  ● **S55.21** Laceration of vein at forearm level

    ● **S55.211** Laceration of vein at forearm level, right arm A 🗞
       Ex: See S45.301

    ● **S55.212** Laceration of vein at forearm level, left arm A 🗞
       Ex: See S45.302

    ● **S55.219** Laceration of vein at forearm level, unspecified arm A 🗞
       Ex: See S45.309

  ● **S55.29** Other specified injury of vein at forearm level

    ● **S55.291** Other specified injury of vein at forearm level, right arm A 🗞
       Ex: See S45.301

    ● **S55.292** Other specified injury of vein at forearm level, left arm A 🗞
       Ex: See S45.302

    ● **S55.299** Other specified injury of vein at forearm level, unspecified arm A 🗞
       Ex: See S45.309

● **S55.8** Injury of other blood vessels at forearm level

  ● **S55.80** Unspecified injury of other blood vessels at forearm level

    ● **S55.801** Unspecified injury of other blood vessels at forearm level, right arm A 🗞
       Ex: See S45.301

    ● **S55.802** Unspecified injury of other blood vessels at forearm level, left arm A 🗞
       Ex: See S45.302

    ● **S55.809** Unspecified injury of other blood vessels at forearm level, unspecified arm A 🗞
       Ex: See S45.309

● **S55.81** Laceration of other blood vessels at forearm level

  ● **S55.811** Laceration of other blood vessels at forearm level, right arm A 🗞
      Ex: See S45.301

  ● **S55.812** Laceration of other blood vessels at forearm level, left arm A 🗞
      Ex: See S45.302

  ● **S55.819** Laceration of other blood vessels at forearm level, unspecified arm A 🗞
      Ex: See S45.309

● **S55.89** Other specified injury of other blood vessels at forearm level

  ● **S55.891** Other specified injury of other blood vessels at forearm level, right arm A 🗞
      Ex: See S45.301

  ● **S55.892** Other specified injury of other blood vessels at forearm level, left arm A 🗞
      Ex: See S45.302

  ● **S55.899** Other specified injury of other blood vessels at forearm level, unspecified arm A 🗞
      Ex: See S45.309

● **S55.9** Injury of unspecified blood vessel at forearm level

  ● **S55.90** Unspecified injury of unspecified blood vessel at forearm level

    ● **S55.901** Unspecified injury of unspecified blood vessel at forearm level, right arm A 🗞
       Ex: See S45.301

    ● **S55.902** Unspecified injury of unspecified blood vessel at forearm level, left arm A 🗞
       Ex: See S45.302

    ● **S55.909** Unspecified injury of unspecified blood vessel at forearm level, unspecified arm A 🗞
       Ex: See S45.309

  ● **S55.91** Laceration of unspecified blood vessel at forearm level

    ● **S55.911** Laceration of unspecified blood vessel at forearm level, right arm A 🗞
       Ex: See S45.301

    ● **S55.912** Laceration of unspecified blood vessel at forearm level, left arm A 🗞
       Ex: See S45.302

    ● **S55.919** Laceration of unspecified blood vessel at forearm level, unspecified arm A 🗞
       Ex: See S45.309

  ● **S55.99** Other specified injury of unspecified blood vessel at forearm level

    ● **S55.991** Other specified injury of unspecified blood vessel at forearm level, right arm A 🗞
       Ex: See S45.301

    ● **S55.992** Other specified injury of unspecified blood vessel at forearm level, left arm A 🗞
       Ex: See S45.302

    ● **S55.999** Other specified injury of unspecified blood vessel at forearm level, unspecified arm A 🗞
       Ex: See S45.309

CHAPTER 19 (S00-T88)

● **S56   Injury of muscle, fascia and tendon at forearm level**
　　Code also any associated open wound (S51.-)
　　Excludes2　injury of muscle, fascia and tendon at or below
　　　　　　　　wrist (S66.-)
　　　　　　　　sprain of joints and ligaments of elbow (S53.4-)
　　The appropriate 7th character is to be added to each code from
　　　category S56

> A　initial encounter
> D　subsequent encounter
> S　sequela

● **S56.0　Injury of flexor muscle, fascia and tendon of thumb at
　　forearm level**
　　● **S56.00　Unspecified injury of flexor muscle, fascia and
　　　　tendon of thumb at forearm level**
　　　　● **S56.001　Unspecified injury of flexor muscle,
　　　　　　fascia and tendon of right thumb at
　　　　　　forearm level**
　　　　● **S56.002　Unspecified injury of flexor muscle,
　　　　　　fascia and tendon of left thumb at
　　　　　　forearm level**
　　　　● **S56.009　Unspecified injury of flexor muscle,
　　　　　　fascia and tendon of unspecified
　　　　　　thumb at forearm level**
　　● **S56.01　Strain of flexor muscle, fascia and tendon of
　　　　thumb at forearm level**
　　　　● **S56.011　Strain of flexor muscle, fascia and
　　　　　　tendon of right thumb at forearm
　　　　　　level**
　　　　● **S56.012　Strain of flexor muscle, fascia and
　　　　　　tendon of left thumb at forearm level**
　　　　● **S56.019　Strain of flexor muscle, fascia and
　　　　　　tendon of unspecified thumb at
　　　　　　forearm level**
　　● **S56.02　Laceration of flexor muscle, fascia and tendon
　　　　of thumb at forearm level**
　　　　● **S56.021　Laceration of flexor muscle, fascia and
　　　　　　tendon of right thumb at forearm
　　　　　　level** A 🏷
　　　　　　Ex: S51.001[A], S51.009-S51.011[A],
　　　　　　S51.019-S51.021[A], S51.029-S51.031[A],
　　　　　　S51.039-S51.041[A], S51.049-S51.051[A],
　　　　　　S51.059-S51.801[A], S51.809-S51.811[A],
　　　　　　S51.819-S51.821[A]. S51.829-S51.831[A],
　　　　　　S51.839-S51.841[A], S51.849-S51.851[A],
　　　　　　S51.859[A], S56.021[A], S56.029[A],
　　　　　　S56.121[A], S56.123[A], S56.125[A],
　　　　　　S56.127[A], S56.129[A], S56.221[A],
　　　　　　S56.229[A], S56.321[A], S56.329[A],
　　　　　　S56.421[A], S56.423[A], S56.425[A],
　　　　　　S56.427[A], S56.429[A], S56.521[A],
　　　　　　S56.529[A], S56.821[A], S56.829[A],
　　　　　　S56.921[A], S56.929[A], S61.501[A],
　　　　　　S61.509-S61.511[A], S61.519-S61.521[A],
　　　　　　S61.529-S61.531[A], S61.539-S61.541[A],
　　　　　　S61.549-S61.551[A], S61.559[A]

● **S56.022　Laceration of flexor muscle, fascia and
　　tendon of left thumb at forearm level**
　　A 🏷
　　Ex: S51.002-S51.009[A], S51.012-S51.019[A],
　　S51.022-S51.029[A], S51.032-S51.039[A],
　　S51.042-S51.049[A], S51.052-S51.059[A],
　　S51.802-S51.809[A], S51.812-S51.819[A],
　　S51.822-S51.829[A], S51.832-S51.839[A],
　　S51.842-S51.849[A], S51.852-S51.859[A],
　　S56.022-S56.029[A], S56.122[A], S56.124[A],
　　S56.126[A], S56.128-S56.129[A],
　　S56.222-S56.229[A], S56.322-S56.329[A],
　　S56.422[A], S56.424[A], S56.426[A],
　　S56.428-S56.429[A], S56.522-S56.529[A],
　　S56.822-S56.829[A], S56.922-S56.929[A],
　　S61.502-S61.509[A], S61.512-S61.519[A],
　　S61.522-S61.529[A], S61.532-S61.539[A],
　　S61.542-S61.549[A], S61.552-S61.559[A]

● **S56.029　Laceration of flexor muscle, fascia and
　　tendon of unspecified thumb at
　　forearm level** A 🏷
　　Ex: S51.001-S51.859[A], S56.021-S56.029[A],
　　S56.121-S56.129[A], S56.221-S56.229[A],
　　S56.321-S56.329[A], S56.421-S56.429[A],
　　S56.521-S56.529[A], S56.821-S56.829[A],
　　S56.921-S56.929[A], S61.501-S61.559[A]

● **S56.09　Other injury of flexor muscle, fascia and tendon
　　of thumb at forearm level**
　　● **S56.091　Other injury of flexor muscle, fascia
　　　　and tendon of right thumb at forearm
　　　　level**
　　● **S56.092　Other injury of flexor muscle, fascia
　　　　and tendon of left thumb at forearm
　　　　level**
　　● **S56.099　Other injury of flexor muscle, fascia
　　　　and tendon of unspecified thumb at
　　　　forearm level**

● **S56.1　Injury of flexor muscle, fascia and tendon of other and
　　unspecified finger at forearm level**
　　● **S56.10　Unspecified injury of flexor muscle, fascia
　　　　and tendon of other and unspecified finger at
　　　　forearm level**
　　　　● **S56.101　Unspecified injury of flexor muscle,
　　　　　　fascia and tendon of right index finger
　　　　　　at forearm level**
　　　　● **S56.102　Unspecified injury of flexor muscle,
　　　　　　fascia and tendon of left index finger
　　　　　　at forearm level**
　　　　● **S56.103　Unspecified injury of flexor muscle,
　　　　　　fascia and tendon of right middle
　　　　　　finger at forearm level**
　　　　● **S56.104　Unspecified injury of flexor muscle,
　　　　　　fascia and tendon of left middle
　　　　　　finger at forearm level**
　　　　● **S56.105　Unspecified injury of flexor muscle,
　　　　　　fascia and tendon of right ring finger
　　　　　　at forearm level**
　　　　● **S56.106　Unspecified injury of flexor muscle,
　　　　　　fascia and tendon of left ring finger at
　　　　　　forearm level**
　　　　● **S56.107　Unspecified injury of flexor muscle,
　　　　　　fascia and tendon of right little finger
　　　　　　at forearm level**
　　　　● **S56.108　Unspecified injury of flexor muscle,
　　　　　　fascia and tendon of left little finger
　　　　　　at forearm level**
　　　　● **S56.109　Unspecified injury of flexor muscle,
　　　　　　fascia and tendon of unspecified
　　　　　　finger at forearm level**

● S56.11   Strain of flexor muscle, fascia and tendon of other and unspecified finger at forearm level

     ● S56.111   Strain of flexor muscle, fascia and tendon of right index finger at forearm level

     ● S56.112   Strain of flexor muscle, fascia and tendon of left index finger at forearm level

     ● S56.113   Strain of flexor muscle, fascia and tendon of right middle finger at forearm level

     ● S56.114   Strain of flexor muscle, fascia and tendon of left middle finger at forearm level

     ● S56.115   Strain of flexor muscle, fascia and tendon of right ring finger at forearm level

     ● S56.116   Strain of flexor muscle, fascia and tendon of left ring finger at forearm level

     ● S56.117   Strain of flexor muscle, fascia and tendon of right little finger at forearm level

     ● S56.118   Strain of flexor muscle, fascia and tendon of left little finger at forearm level

     ● S56.119   Strain of flexor muscle, fascia and tendon of finger of unspecified finger at forearm level

● S56.12   Laceration of flexor muscle, fascia and tendon of other and unspecified finger at forearm level

     ● S56.121   Laceration of flexor muscle, fascia and tendon of right index finger at forearm level A 🗫
         Ex: See S56.021

     ● S56.122   Laceration of flexor muscle, fascia and tendon of left index finger at forearm level A 🗫
         Ex: See S56.022

     ● S56.123   Laceration of flexor muscle, fascia and tendon of right middle finger at forearm level A 🗫
         Ex: See S56.021

     ● S56.124   Laceration of flexor muscle, fascia and tendon of left middle finger at forearm level A 🗫
         Ex: See S56.022

     ● S56.125   Laceration of flexor muscle, fascia and tendon of right ring finger at forearm level A 🗫
         Ex: See S56.021

     ● S56.126   Laceration of flexor muscle, fascia and tendon of left ring finger at forearm level A 🗫
         Ex: See S56.022

     ● S56.127   Laceration of flexor muscle, fascia and tendon of right little finger at forearm level A 🗫
         Ex: See S56.021

     ● S56.128   Laceration of flexor muscle, fascia and tendon of left little finger at forearm level A 🗫
         Ex: See S56.022

     ● S56.129   Laceration of flexor muscle, fascia and tendon of unspecified finger at forearm level A 🗫
         Ex: See S56.029

● S56.19   Other injury of flexor muscle, fascia and tendon of other and unspecified finger at forearm level

     ● S56.191   Other injury of flexor muscle, fascia and tendon of right index finger at forearm level

     ● S56.192   Other injury of flexor muscle, fascia and tendon of left index finger at forearm level

     ● S56.193   Other injury of flexor muscle, fascia and tendon of right middle finger at forearm level

     ● S56.194   Other injury of flexor muscle, fascia and tendon of left middle finger at forearm level

     ● S56.195   Other injury of flexor muscle, fascia and tendon of right ring finger at forearm level

     ● S56.196   Other injury of flexor muscle, fascia and tendon of left ring finger at forearm level

     ● S56.197   Other injury of flexor muscle, fascia and tendon of right little finger at forearm level

     ● S56.198   Other injury of flexor muscle, fascia and tendon of left little finger at forearm level

     ● S56.199   Other injury of flexor muscle, fascia and tendon of unspecified finger at forearm level

● S56.2   Injury of other flexor muscle, fascia and tendon at forearm level

     ● S56.20   Unspecified injury of other flexor muscle, fascia and tendon at forearm level

         ● S56.201   Unspecified injury of other flexor muscle, fascia and tendon at forearm level, right arm

         ● S56.202   Unspecified injury of other flexor muscle, fascia and tendon at forearm level, left arm

         ● S56.209   Unspecified injury of other flexor muscle, fascia and tendon at forearm level, unspecified arm

     ● S56.21   Strain of other flexor muscle, fascia and tendon at forearm level

         ● S56.211   Strain of other flexor muscle, fascia and tendon at forearm level, right arm

         ● S56.212   Strain of other flexor muscle, fascia and tendon at forearm level, left arm

         ● S56.219   Strain of other flexor muscle, fascia and tendon at forearm level, unspecified arm

     ● S56.22   Laceration of other flexor muscle, fascia and tendon at forearm level

         ● S56.221   Laceration of other flexor muscle, fascia and tendon at forearm level, right arm A 🗫
             Ex: See S56.021

         ● S56.222   Laceration of other flexor muscle, fascia and tendon at forearm level, left arm A 🗫
             Ex: See S56.022

         ● S56.229   Laceration of other flexor muscle, fascia and tendon at forearm level, unspecified arm A 🗫
             Ex: See S56.029

CHAPTER 19 (S00-T88)

● **S56.29** Other injury of other flexor muscle, fascia and tendon at forearm level

   ● **S56.291** Other injury of other flexor muscle, fascia and tendon at forearm level, right arm

   ● **S56.292** Other injury of other flexor muscle, fascia and tendon at forearm level, left arm

   ● **S56.299** Other injury of other flexor muscle, fascia and tendon at forearm level, unspecified arm

● **S56.3** Injury of extensor or abductor muscles, fascia and tendons of thumb at forearm level

  ● **S56.30** Unspecified injury of extensor or abductor muscles, fascia and tendons of thumb at forearm level

   ● **S56.301** Unspecified injury of extensor or abductor muscles, fascia and tendons of right thumb at forearm level

   ● **S56.302** Unspecified injury of extensor or abductor muscles, fascia and tendons of left thumb at forearm level

   ● **S56.309** Unspecified injury of extensor or abductor muscles, fascia and tendons of unspecified thumb at forearm level

  ● **S56.31** Strain of extensor or abductor muscles, fascia and tendons of thumb at forearm level

   ● **S56.311** Strain of extensor or abductor muscles, fascia and tendons of right thumb at forearm level

   ● **S56.312** Strain of extensor or abductor muscles, fascia and tendons of left thumb at forearm level

   ● **S56.319** Strain of extensor or abductor muscles, fascia and tendons of unspecified thumb at forearm level

  ● **S56.32** Laceration of extensor or abductor muscles, fascia and tendons of thumb at forearm level

   ● **S56.321** Laceration of extensor or abductor muscles, fascia and tendons of right thumb at forearm level A ⊗
     (Ex) See S56.021

   ● **S56.322** Laceration of extensor or abductor muscles, fascia and tendons of left thumb at forearm level A ⊗
     (Ex) See S56.022

   ● **S56.329** Laceration of extensor or abductor muscles, fascia and tendons of unspecified thumb at forearm level A ⊗
     (Ex) See S56.029

  ● **S56.39** Other injury of extensor or abductor muscles, fascia and tendons of thumb at forearm level

   ● **S56.391** Other injury of extensor or abductor muscles, fascia and tendons of right thumb at forearm level

   ● **S56.392** Other injury of extensor or abductor muscles, fascia and tendons of left thumb at forearm level

   ● **S56.399** Other injury of extensor or abductor muscles, fascia and tendons of unspecified thumb at forearm level

● **S56.4** Injury of extensor muscle, fascia and tendon of other and unspecified finger at forearm level

  ● **S56.40** Unspecified injury of extensor muscle, fascia and tendon of other and unspecified finger at forearm level

   ● **S56.401** Unspecified injury of extensor muscle, fascia and tendon of right index finger at forearm level

   ● **S56.402** Unspecified injury of extensor muscle, fascia and tendon of left index finger at forearm level

   ● **S56.403** Unspecified injury of extensor muscle, fascia and tendon of right middle finger at forearm level

   ● **S56.404** Unspecified injury of extensor muscle, fascia and tendon of left middle finger at forearm level

   ● **S56.405** Unspecified injury of extensor muscle, fascia and tendon of right ring finger at forearm level

   ● **S56.406** Unspecified injury of extensor muscle, fascia and tendon of left ring finger at forearm level

   ● **S56.407** Unspecified injury of extensor muscle, fascia and tendon of right little finger at forearm level

   ● **S56.408** Unspecified injury of extensor muscle, fascia and tendon of left little finger at forearm level

   ● **S56.409** Unspecified injury of extensor muscle, fascia and tendon of unspecified finger at forearm level

  ● **S56.41** Strain of extensor muscle, fascia and tendon of other and unspecified finger at forearm level

   ● **S56.411** Strain of extensor muscle, fascia and tendon of right index finger at forearm level

   ● **S56.412** Strain of extensor muscle, fascia and tendon of left index finger at forearm level

   ● **S56.413** Strain of extensor muscle, fascia and tendon of right middle finger at forearm level

   ● **S56.414** Strain of extensor muscle, fascia and tendon of left middle finger at forearm level

   ● **S56.415** Strain of extensor muscle, fascia and tendon of right ring finger at forearm level

   ● **S56.416** Strain of extensor muscle, fascia and tendon of left ring finger at forearm level

   ● **S56.417** Strain of extensor muscle, fascia and tendon of right little finger at forearm level

   ● **S56.418** Strain of extensor muscle, fascia and tendon of left little finger at forearm level

   ● **S56.419** Strain of extensor muscle, fascia and tendon of finger, unspecified finger at forearm level

◀ New   ◀═ Revised   ~~deleted~~ Deleted   Excludes 1   Excludes 2   Includes   Use additional   Code first   Code also   Unspecified

OGCR Official Guidelines   ● Unacceptable Principal Diagnosis   X Assign placeholder X   ● Use Additional Character(s)   ▶ Manifestation Code   **Coding Clinic**

- S56.42   Laceration of extensor muscle, fascia and tendon of other and unspecified finger at forearm level
  - S56.421   Laceration of extensor muscle, fascia and tendon of right index finger at forearm level A 🍂
    Ex: See S56.021
  - S56.422   Laceration of extensor muscle, fascia and tendon of left index finger at forearm level A 🍂
    Ex: See S56.022
  - S56.423   Laceration of extensor muscle, fascia and tendon of right middle finger at forearm level A 🍂
    Ex: See S56.021
  - S56.424   Laceration of extensor muscle, fascia and tendon of left middle finger at forearm level A 🍂
    Ex: See S56.022
  - S56.425   Laceration of extensor muscle, fascia and tendon of right ring finger at forearm level A 🍂
    Ex: See S56.021
  - S56.426   Laceration of extensor muscle, fascia and tendon of left ring finger at forearm level A 🍂
    Ex: See S56.022
  - S56.427   Laceration of extensor muscle, fascia and tendon of right little finger at forearm level A 🍂
    Ex: See S56.021
  - S56.428   Laceration of extensor muscle, fascia and tendon of left little finger at forearm level A 🍂
    Ex: See S56.022
  - S56.429   Laceration of extensor muscle, fascia and tendon of unspecified finger at forearm level A 🍂
    Ex: See S56.029
- S56.49   Other injury of extensor muscle, fascia and tendon of other and unspecified finger at forearm level
  - S56.491   Other injury of extensor muscle, fascia and tendon of right index finger at forearm level
  - S56.492   Other injury of extensor muscle, fascia and tendon of left index finger at forearm level
  - S56.493   Other injury of extensor muscle, fascia and tendon of right middle finger at forearm level
  - S56.494   Other injury of extensor muscle, fascia and tendon of left middle finger at forearm level
  - S56.495   Other injury of extensor muscle, fascia and tendon of right ring finger at forearm level
  - S56.496   Other injury of extensor muscle, fascia and tendon of left ring finger at forearm level
  - S56.497   Other injury of extensor muscle, fascia and tendon of right little finger at forearm level
  - S56.498   Other injury of extensor muscle, fascia and tendon of left little finger at forearm level
  - S56.499   Other injury of extensor muscle, fascia and tendon of unspecified finger at forearm level

- S56.5   Injury of other extensor muscle, fascia and tendon at forearm level
  - S56.50   Unspecified injury of other extensor muscle, fascia and tendon at forearm level
    - S56.501   Unspecified injury of other extensor muscle, fascia and tendon at forearm level, right arm
    - S56.502   Unspecified injury of other extensor muscle, fascia and tendon at forearm level, left arm
    - S56.509   Unspecified injury of other extensor muscle, fascia and tendon at forearm level, unspecified arm
  - S56.51   Strain of other extensor muscle, fascia and tendon at forearm level
    - S56.511   Strain of other extensor muscle, fascia and tendon at forearm level, right arm
    - S56.512   Strain of other extensor muscle, fascia and tendon at forearm level, left arm
    - S56.519   Strain of other extensor muscle, fascia and tendon at forearm level, unspecified arm
  - S56.52   Laceration of other extensor muscle, fascia and tendon at forearm level
    - S56.521   Laceration of other extensor muscle, fascia and tendon at forearm level, right arm A 🍂
      Ex: See S56.021
    - S56.522   Laceration of other extensor muscle, fascia and tendon at forearm level, left arm A 🍂
      Ex: See S56.022
    - S56.529   Laceration of other extensor muscle, fascia and tendon at forearm level, unspecified arm A 🍂
      Ex: See S56.029
  - S56.59   Other injury of other extensor muscle, fascia and tendon at forearm level
    - S56.591   Other injury of other extensor muscle, fascia and tendon at forearm level, right arm
    - S56.592   Other injury of other extensor muscle, fascia and tendon at forearm level, left arm
    - S56.599   Other injury of other extensor muscle, fascia and tendon at forearm level, unspecified arm
- S56.8   Injury of other muscles, fascia and tendons at forearm level
  - S56.80   Unspecified injury of other muscles, fascia and tendons at forearm level
    - S56.801   Unspecified injury of other muscles, fascia and tendons at forearm level, right arm
    - S56.802   Unspecified injury of other muscles, fascia and tendons at forearm level, left arm
    - S56.809   Unspecified injury of other muscles, fascia and tendons at forearm level, unspecified arm
  - S56.81   Strain of other muscles, fascia and tendons at forearm level
    - S56.811   Strain of other muscles, fascia and tendons at forearm level, right arm
    - S56.812   Strain of other muscles, fascia and tendons at forearm level, left arm
    - S56.819   Strain of other muscles, fascia and tendons at forearm level, unspecified arm

● **S56.82**   **Laceration of other muscles, fascia and tendons at forearm level**

    ● **S56.821**   Laceration of other muscles, fascia and tendons at forearm level, right arm A 🔗
       (Ex:) See S56.021

    ● **S56.822**   Laceration of other muscles, fascia and tendons at forearm level, left arm A 🔗
       (Ex:) See S56.022

    ● **S56.829**   Laceration of other muscles, fascia and tendons at forearm level, unspecified arm A 🔗
       (Ex:) See S56.029

● **S56.89**   **Other injury of other muscles, fascia and tendons at forearm level**

    ● **S56.891**   Other injury of other muscles, fascia and tendons at forearm level, right arm

    ● **S56.892**   Other injury of other muscles, fascia and tendons at forearm level, left arm

    ● **S56.899**   Other injury of other muscles, fascia and tendons at forearm level, unspecified arm

● **S56.9**   **Injury of unspecified muscles, fascia and tendons at forearm level**

   ● **S56.90**   **Unspecified injury of unspecified muscles, fascia and tendons at forearm level**

    ● **S56.901**   Unspecified injury of unspecified muscles, fascia and tendons at forearm level, right arm

    ● **S56.902**   Unspecified injury of unspecified muscles, fascia and tendons at forearm level, left arm

    ● **S56.909**   Unspecified injury of unspecified muscles, fascia and tendons at forearm level, unspecified arm

   ● **S56.91**   **Strain of unspecified muscles, fascia and tendons at forearm level**

    ● **S56.911**   Strain of unspecified muscles, fascia and tendons at forearm level, right arm

    ● **S56.912**   Strain of unspecified muscles, fascia and tendons at forearm level, left arm

    ● **S56.919**   Strain of unspecified muscles, fascia and tendons at forearm level, unspecified arm

   ● **S56.92**   **Laceration of unspecified muscles, fascia and tendons at forearm level**

    ● **S56.921**   Laceration of unspecified muscles, fascia and tendons at forearm level, right arm A 🔗
       (Ex:) See S56.021

    ● **S56.922**   Laceration of unspecified muscles, fascia and tendons at forearm level, left arm A 🔗
       (Ex:) See S56.022

    ● **S56.929**   Laceration of unspecified muscles, fascia and tendons at forearm level, unspecified arm A 🔗
       (Ex:) See S56.029

● **S56.99**   **Other injury of unspecified muscles, fascia and tendons at forearm level**

    ● **S56.991**   Other injury of unspecified muscles, fascia and tendons at forearm level, right arm

    ● **S56.992**   Other injury of unspecified muscles, fascia and tendons at forearm level, left arm

    ● **S56.999**   Other injury of unspecified muscles, fascia and tendons at forearm level, unspecified arm

● **S57**   **Crushing injury of elbow and forearm**

   Use additional code(s) for all associated injuries

   Excludes2   crushing injury of wrist and hand (S67.-)

   The appropriate 7th character is to be added to each code from category S57

    | | |
    A   initial encounter
    D   subsequent encounter
    S   sequela

   ● **S57.0**   **Crushing injury of elbow**
    X ● **S57.00**   Crushing injury of unspecified elbow
    X ● **S57.01**   Crushing injury of right elbow
    X ● **S57.02**   Crushing injury of left elbow

   ● **S57.8**   **Crushing injury of forearm**
    X ● **S57.80**   Crushing injury of unspecified forearm
    X ● **S57.81**   Crushing injury of right forearm
    X ● **S57.82**   Crushing injury of left forearm

● **S58**   **Traumatic amputation of elbow and forearm**

   An amputation not identified as partial or complete should be coded to complete

   Excludes1   traumatic amputation of wrist and hand (S68.-)

   The appropriate 7th character is to be added to each code from category S58

    A   initial encounter
    D   subsequent encounter
    S   sequela

   ● **S58.0**   **Traumatic amputation at elbow level**

    ● **S58.01**   **Complete traumatic amputation at elbow level**

     ● **S58.011**   Complete traumatic amputation at elbow level, right arm A 🔗
        (Ex:) See S48.011

     ● **S58.012**   Complete traumatic amputation at elbow level, left arm A 🔗
        (Ex:) See S48.012

     ● **S58.019**   Complete traumatic amputation at elbow level, unspecified arm A 🔗
        (Ex:) See S48.019

    ● **S58.02**   **Partial traumatic amputation at elbow level**

     ● **S58.021**   Partial traumatic amputation at elbow level, right arm A 🔗
        (Ex:) See S48.011

     ● **S58.022**   Partial traumatic amputation at elbow level, left arm A 🔗
        (Ex:) See S48.012

     ● **S58.029**   Partial traumatic amputation at elbow level, unspecified arm A 🔗
        (Ex:) See S48.019

◀ New   ⬅ Revised   ~~deleted~~ Deleted   Excludes 1   Excludes 2   Includes   Use additional   Code first   Code also   Unspecified

OGCR Official Guidelines   ● Unacceptable Principal Diagnosis   X Assign placeholder X   ● Use Additional Character(s)   ▌ Manifestation Code   **Coding Clinic**

● **S58.1   Traumatic amputation at level between elbow and wrist**
  ● **S58.11   Complete traumatic amputation at level between elbow and wrist**
    ● **S58.111   Complete traumatic amputation at level between elbow and wrist, right arm** A
      (Ex:) See S48.011
    ● **S58.112   Complete traumatic amputation at level between elbow and wrist, left arm** A
      (Ex:) See S48.012
    ● **S58.119   Complete traumatic amputation at level between elbow and wrist, unspecified arm** A
      (Ex:) See S48.019
  ● **S58.12   Partial traumatic amputation at level between elbow and wrist**
    ● **S58.121   Partial traumatic amputation at level between elbow and wrist, right arm** A
      (Ex:) See S48.011
    ● **S58.122   Partial traumatic amputation at level between elbow and wrist, left arm** A
      (Ex:) See S48.012
    ● **S58.129   Partial traumatic amputation at level between elbow and wrist, unspecified arm** A
      (Ex:) See S48.019

● **S58.9   Traumatic amputation of forearm, level unspecified**
  Excludes1   traumatic amputation of wrist (S68.-)
  ● **S58.91   Complete traumatic amputation of forearm, level unspecified**
    ● **S58.911   Complete traumatic amputation of right forearm, level unspecified** A
      (Ex:) See S48.011
    ● **S58.912   Complete traumatic amputation of left forearm, level unspecified** A
      (Ex:) See S48.012
    ● **S58.919   Complete traumatic amputation of unspecified forearm, level unspecified** A
      (Ex:) See S48.019
  ● **S58.92   Partial traumatic amputation of forearm, level unspecified**
    ● **S58.921   Partial traumatic amputation of right forearm, level unspecified** A
      (Ex:) See S48.011
    ● **S58.922   Partial traumatic amputation of left forearm, level unspecified** A
      (Ex:) See S48.012
    ● **S58.929   Partial traumatic amputation of unspecified forearm, level unspecified** A
      (Ex:) See S48.019

● **S59   Other and unspecified injuries of elbow and forearm**
  Excludes2   other and unspecified injuries of wrist and hand (S69.-)
  The appropriate 7th character is to be added to each code from subcategories S59.0, S59.1, and S59.2

A	initial encounter for closed fracture
D	subsequent encounter for fracture with routine healing
G	subsequent encounter for fracture with delayed healing
K	subsequent encounter for fracture with nonunion
P	subsequent encounter for fracture with malunion
S	sequela

● **S59.0   Physeal fracture of lower end of ulna**
  ● **S59.00   Unspecified physeal fracture of lower end of ulna**
    ● **S59.001   Unspecified physeal fracture of lower end of ulna, right arm** A, K, P , A
      (Ex:) For code S59.001[A]: See S52.011[A]
      For S59.001[K,P]: See S02.0[K]
    ● **S59.002   Unspecified physeal fracture of lower end of ulna, left arm** A, K, P , A
      (Ex:) For code S59.002[A]: See S52.012[A]
      For S59.002[K,P]: See S02.0[K]
    ● **S59.009   Unspecified physeal fracture of lower end of ulna, unspecified arm** A, K, P , A
      (Ex:) For code S59.009[A]: See S52.019[A]
      For S59.009[K,P]: See S02.0[K]
  ● **S59.01   Salter-Harris Type I physeal fracture of lower end of ulna**
    ● **S59.011   Salter-Harris Type I physeal fracture of lower end of ulna, right arm** A, K, P , A
      (Ex:) For code S59.011[A]: See S52.011[A]
      For S59.011[K,P]: See S02.0[K]
    ● **S59.012   Salter-Harris Type I physeal fracture of lower end of ulna, left arm** A, K, P , A
      (Ex:) For code S59.012[A]: See S52.012[A]
      For S59.012[K,P]: See S02.0[K]
    ● **S59.019   Salter-Harris Type I physeal fracture of lower end of ulna, unspecified arm** A, K, P , A
      (Ex:) For code S59.019[A]: See S52.019[A]
      For S59.019[K,P]: See S02.0[K]

Item 19-4 SALTER-HARRIS TYPE 1: epiphysis is completely separated from end of bone, or metaphysic growth plate remains attached to epiphysis
  SALTER-HARRIS TYPE 2: epiphysis and growth plate are partially separated from metaphysis, which is cracked—most common type
  SALTER-HARRIS TYPE 3: fracture occurring through epiphysis and separates part of epiphysis and growth plate from metaphysis fracture, usually at distal end of tibia
  SALTER-HARRIS TYPE 4: fracture runs through epiphysis, across growth plate, into metaphysic, surgery is required to restore joint surface to normal and align growth plate

CHAPTER 19 (S00-T88)

● **S59.02**   Salter-Harris Type II physeal fracture of lower end of ulna

    ● **S59.021**   Salter-Harris Type II physeal fracture of lower end of ulna, right arm
      A, K, P 🔄, A 🔄
      (Ex) For code S59.021[A]: See S52.011[A]
       For S59.021[K,P]: See S02.0[K]

    ● **S59.022**   Salter-Harris Type II physeal fracture of lower end of ulna, left arm
      A, K, P 🔄, A 🔄
      (Ex) For code S59.022[A]: See S52.012[A]
       For S59.022[K,P]: See S02.0[K]

    ● **S59.029**   Salter-Harris Type II physeal fracture of lower end of ulna, unspecified arm
      A, K, P 🔄, A 🔄
      (Ex) For code S59.029[A]: See S52.019[A]
       For S59.029[K,P]: See S02.0[K]

● **S59.03**   Salter-Harris Type III physeal fracture of lower end of ulna

    ● **S59.031**   Salter-Harris Type III physeal fracture of lower end of ulna, right arm
      A, K, P 🔄, A 🔄
      (Ex) For code S59.031[A]: See S52.011[A]
       For S59.031[K,P]: See S02.0[K]

    ● **S59.032**   Salter-Harris Type III physeal fracture of lower end of ulna, left arm
      A, K, P 🔄, A 🔄
      (Ex) For code S59.032[A]: See S52.012[A]
       For S59.032[K,P]: See S02.0[K]

    ● **S59.039**   Salter-Harris Type III physeal fracture of lower end of ulna, unspecified arm
      A, K, P 🔄, A 🔄
      (Ex) For code S59.039[A]: See S52.019[A]
       For S59.039[K,P]: See S02.0[K]

● **S59.04**   Salter-Harris Type IV physeal fracture of lower end of ulna

    ● **S59.041**   Salter-Harris Type IV physeal fracture of lower end of ulna, right arm
      A, K, P 🔄, A 🔄
      (Ex) For code S59.041[A]: See S52.011[A]
       For S59.041[K,P]: See S02.0[K]

    ● **S59.042**   Salter-Harris Type IV physeal fracture of lower end of ulna, left arm
      A, K, P 🔄, A 🔄
      (Ex) For code S59.042[A]: See S52.012[A]
       For S59.042[K,P]: See S02.0[K]

    ● **S59.049**   Salter-Harris Type IV physeal fracture of lower end of ulna, unspecified arm
      A, K, P 🔄, A 🔄
      (Ex) For code S59.049[A]: See S52.019[A]
       For S59.049[K,P]: See S02.0[K]

● **S59.09**   Other physeal fracture of lower end of ulna

    ● **S59.091**   Other physeal fracture of lower end of ulna, right arm A, K, P 🔄, A 🔄
      (Ex) For code S59.091[A]: See S52.011[A]
       For S59.091[K,P]: See S02.0[K]

    ● **S59.092**   Other physeal fracture of lower end of ulna, left arm A, K, P 🔄, A 🔄
      (Ex) For code S59.092[A]: See S52.012[A]
       For S59.092[K,P]: See S02.0[K]

    ● **S59.099**   Other physeal fracture of lower end of ulna, unspecified arm A, K, P 🔄, A 🔄
      (Ex) For code S59.099[A]: See S52.019[A]
       For S59.099[K,P]: See S02.0[K]

● **S59.1**   Physeal fracture of upper end of radius
    (Ex) For category S59.1 CC codes: See S02.0[K]

    ● **S59.10**   Unspecified physeal fracture of upper end of radius

      ● **S59.101**   Unspecified physeal fracture of upper end of radius, right arm K, P 🔄

      ● **S59.102**   Unspecified physeal fracture of upper end of radius, left arm K, P 🔄

      ● **S59.109**   Unspecified physeal fracture of upper end of radius, unspecified arm K, P 🔄

    ● **S59.11**   Salter-Harris Type I physeal fracture of upper end of radius

      ● **S59.111**   Salter-Harris Type I physeal fracture of upper end of radius, right arm K, P 🔄

      ● **S59.112**   Salter-Harris Type I physeal fracture of upper end of radius, left arm K, P 🔄

      ● **S59.119**   Salter-Harris Type I physeal fracture of upper end of radius, unspecified arm K, P 🔄

    ● **S59.12**   Salter-Harris Type II physeal fracture of upper end of radius

      ● **S59.121**   Salter-Harris Type II physeal fracture of upper end of radius, right arm K, P 🔄

      ● **S59.122**   Salter-Harris Type II physeal fracture of upper end of radius, left arm K, P 🔄

      ● **S59.129**   Salter-Harris Type II physeal fracture of upper end of radius, unspecified arm K, P 🔄

    ● **S59.13**   Salter-Harris Type III physeal fracture of upper end of radius

      ● **S59.131**   Salter-Harris Type III physeal fracture of upper end of radius, right arm K, P 🔄

      ● **S59.132**   Salter-Harris Type III physeal fracture of upper end of radius, left arm K, P 🔄

      ● **S59.139**   Salter-Harris Type III physeal fracture of upper end of radius, unspecified arm K, P 🔄

    ● **S59.14**   Salter-Harris Type IV physeal fracture of upper end of radius

      ● **S59.141**   Salter-Harris Type IV physeal fracture of upper end of radius, right arm K, P 🔄

      ● **S59.142**   Salter-Harris Type IV physeal fracture of upper end of radius, left arm K, P 🔄

      ● **S59.149**   Salter-Harris Type IV physeal fracture of upper end of radius, unspecified arm K, P 🔄

    ● **S59.19**   Other physeal fracture of upper end of radius

      ● **S59.191**   Other physeal fracture of upper end of radius, right arm K, P 🔄

      ● **S59.192**   Other physeal fracture of upper end of radius, left arm K, P 🔄

      ● **S59.199**   Other physeal fracture of upper end of radius, unspecified arm K, P 🔄

◀ New   ◀◀ Revised   ~~deleted~~ Deleted   Excludes 1   Excludes 2   Includes   Use additional   Code first   Code also   Unspecified
OGCR Official Guidelines   ● Unacceptable Principal Diagnosis   X Assign placeholder X   ● Use Additional Character(s)   ▶ Manifestation Code   **Coding Clinic**

● **S59.2 Physeal fracture of lower end of radius**
  ● **S59.20 Unspecified physeal fracture of lower end of radius**
    ● **S59.201** Unspecified physeal fracture of lower end of radius, right arm A, K, P 🅒, A 🅜
      ⓔ For code S59.201[A]: See S52.011[A]
      For S59.201[K,P]: See S02.0[K]
    ● **S59.202** Unspecified physeal fracture of lower end of radius, left arm A, K, P 🅒, A 🅜
      ⓔ For code S59.202[A]: See S52.012[A]
      For S59.202[K,P]: See S02.0[K]
    ● **S59.209** Unspecified physeal fracture of lower end of radius, unspecified arm A, K, P 🅒, A 🅜
      ⓔ For code S59.209[A]: See S52.019[A]
      For S59.209[K,P]: See S02.0[K]
  ● **S59.21 Salter-Harris Type I physeal fracture of lower end of radius**
    ● **S59.211** Salter-Harris Type I physeal fracture of lower end of radius, right arm A, K, P 🅒, A 🅜
      ⓔ For code S59.211[A]: See S52.011[A]
      For S59.211[K,P]: See S02.0[K]
    ● **S59.212** Salter-Harris Type I physeal fracture of lower end of radius, left arm A, K, P 🅒, A 🅜
      ⓔ For code S59.212[A]: See S52.012[A]
      For S59.212[K,P]: See S02.0[K]
    ● **S59.219** Salter-Harris Type I physeal fracture of lower end of radius, unspecified arm A, K, P 🅒, A 🅜
      ⓔ For code S59.219[A]: See S52.019[A]
      For S59.219[K,P]: See S02.0[K]
  ● **S59.22 Salter-Harris Type II physeal fracture of lower end of radius**
    ● **S59.221** Salter-Harris Type II physeal fracture of lower end of radius, right arm A, K, P 🅒, A 🅜
      ⓔ For code S59.221[A]: See S52.011[A]
      For S59.221[K,P]: See S02.0[K]
    ● **S59.222** Salter-Harris Type II physeal fracture of lower end of radius, left arm A, K, P 🅒, A 🅜
      ⓔ For code S59.222[A]: See S52.012[A]
      For S59.222[K,P]: See S02.0[K]
    ● **S59.229** Salter-Harris Type II physeal fracture of lower end of radius, unspecified arm A, K, P 🅒, A 🅜
      ⓔ For code S59.229[A]: See S52.019[A]
      For S59.229[K,P]: See S02.0[K]
  ● **S59.23 Salter-Harris Type III physeal fracture of lower end of radius**
    ● **S59.231** Salter-Harris Type III physeal fracture of lower end of radius, right arm A, K, P 🅒, A 🅜
      ⓔ For code S59.231[A]: See S52.011[A]
      For S59.231[K,P]: See S02.0[K]
    ● **S59.232** Salter-Harris Type III physeal fracture of lower end of radius, left arm A, K, P 🅒, A 🅜
      ⓔ For code S59.232[A]: See S52.012[A]
      For S59.232[K,P]: See S02.0[K]
    ● **S59.239** Salter-Harris Type III physeal fracture of lower end of radius, unspecified arm A, K, P 🅒, A 🅜
      ⓔ For code S59.239[A]: See S52.019[A]
      For S59.239[K,P]: See S02.0[K]

● **S59.24 Salter-Harris Type IV physeal fracture of lower end of radius**
  ● **S59.241** Salter-Harris Type IV physeal fracture of lower end of radius, right arm A, K, P 🅒, A 🅜
    ⓔ For code S59.241[A]: See S52.011[A]
    For S59.241[K,P]: See S02.0[K]
  ● **S59.242** Salter-Harris Type IV physeal fracture of lower end of radius, left arm A, K, P 🅒, A 🅜
    ⓔ For code S59.242[A]: See S52.012[A]
    For S59.242[K,P]: See S02.0[K]
  ● **S59.249** Salter-Harris Type IV physeal fracture of lower end of radius, unspecified arm A, K, P 🅒, A 🅜
    ⓔ For code S59.249[A]: See S52.019[A]
    For S59.249[K,P]: See S02.0[K]
● **S59.29 Other physeal fracture of lower end of radius**
  ● **S59.291** Other physeal fracture of lower end of radius, right arm A, K, P 🅒, A 🅜
    ⓔ For code S59.291[A]: See S52.011[A]
    For S59.291[K,P]: See S02.0[K]
  ● **S59.292** Other physeal fracture of lower end of radius, left arm A, K, P 🅒, A 🅜
    ⓔ For code S59.292[A]: See S52.012[A]
    For S59.292[K,P]: See S02.0[K]
  ● **S59.299** Other physeal fracture of lower end of radius, unspecified arm A, K, P 🅒, A 🅜
    ⓔ For code S59.299[A]: See S52.019[A]
    For S59.299[K,P]: See S02.0[K]

● **S59.8 Other specified injuries of elbow and forearm**
  The appropriate 7th character is to be added to each code in subcategory S59.8

A	initial encounter
D	subsequent encounter
S	sequela

  ● **S59.80 Other specified injuries of elbow**
    ● **S59.801** Other specified injuries of right elbow
    ● **S59.802** Other specified injuries of left elbow
    ● **S59.809** Other specified injuries of unspecified elbow
  ● **S59.81 Other specified injuries of forearm**
    ● **S59.811** Other specified injuries right forearm
    ● **S59.812** Other specified injuries left forearm
    ● **S59.819** Other specified injuries unspecified forearm
● **S59.9 Unspecified injury of elbow and forearm**
  The appropriate 7th character is to be added to each code in subcategory S59.9

A	initial encounter
D	subsequent encounter
S	sequela

  ● **S59.90 Unspecified injury of elbow**
    ● **S59.901** Unspecified injury of right elbow
    ● **S59.902** Unspecified injury of left elbow
    ● **S59.909** Unspecified injury of unspecified elbow
  ● **S59.91 Unspecified injury of forearm**
    ● **S59.911** Unspecified injury of right forearm
    ● **S59.912** Unspecified injury of left forearm
    ● **S59.919** Unspecified injury of unspecified forearm

CHAPTER 19 (S00-T88)

INJURIES TO THE WRIST, HAND AND FINGERS (S60-S69)

Excludes2　burns and corrosions (T20-T32)
frostbite (T33-T34)
insect bite or sting, venomous (T63.4)

● S60　**Superficial injury of wrist, hand and fingers**

The appropriate 7th character is to be added to each code from category S60

> A　initial encounter
> D　subsequent encounter
> S　sequela

● S60.0　**Contusion of finger without damage to nail**
Excludes1　contusion involving nail (matrix) (S60.1)

X ● S60.00　**Contusion of unspecified finger without damage to nail**
Contusion of finger(s) NOS

● S60.01　**Contusion of thumb without damage to nail**

● S60.011　**Contusion of right thumb without damage to nail**

● S60.012　**Contusion of left thumb without damage to nail**

● S60.019　**Contusion of unspecified thumb without damage to nail**

● S60.02　**Contusion of index finger without damage to nail**

● S60.021　**Contusion of right index finger without damage to nail**

● S60.022　**Contusion of left index finger without damage to nail**

● S60.029　**Contusion of unspecified index finger without damage to nail**

● S60.03　**Contusion of middle finger without damage to nail**

● S60.031　**Contusion of right middle finger without damage to nail**

● S60.032　**Contusion of left middle finger without damage to nail**

● S60.039　**Contusion of unspecified middle finger without damage to nail**

● S60.04　**Contusion of ring finger without damage to nail**

● S60.041　**Contusion of right ring finger without damage to nail**

● S60.042　**Contusion of left ring finger without damage to nail**

● S60.049　**Contusion of unspecified ring finger without damage to nail**

● S60.05　**Contusion of little finger without damage to nail**

● S60.051　**Contusion of right little finger without damage to nail**

● S60.052　**Contusion of left little finger without damage to nail**

● S60.059　**Contusion of unspecified little finger without damage to nail**

● S60.1　**Contusion of finger with damage to nail**

X ● S60.10　**Contusion of unspecified finger with damage to nail**

● S60.11　**Contusion of thumb with damage to nail**

● S60.111　**Contusion of right thumb with damage to nail**

● S60.112　**Contusion of left thumb with damage to nail**

● S60.119　**Contusion of unspecified thumb with damage to nail**

● S60.12　**Contusion of index finger with damage to nail**

● S60.121　**Contusion of right index finger with damage to nail**

● S60.122　**Contusion of left index finger with damage to nail**

● S60.129　**Contusion of unspecified index finger with damage to nail**

● S60.13　**Contusion of middle finger with damage to nail**

● S60.131　**Contusion of right middle finger with damage to nail**

● S60.132　**Contusion of left middle finger with damage to nail**

● S60.139　**Contusion of unspecified middle finger with damage to nail**

● S60.14　**Contusion of ring finger with damage to nail**

● S60.141　**Contusion of right ring finger with damage to nail**

● S60.142　**Contusion of left ring finger with damage to nail**

● S60.149　**Contusion of unspecified ring finger with damage to nail**

● S60.15　**Contusion of little finger with damage to nail**

● S60.151　**Contusion of right little finger with damage to nail**

● S60.152　**Contusion of left little finger with damage to nail**

● S60.159　**Contusion of unspecified little finger with damage to nail**

● S60.2　**Contusion of wrist and hand**
Excludes2　contusion of fingers (S60.0-, S60.1-)

● S60.21　**Contusion of wrist**

● S60.211　**Contusion of right wrist**

● S60.212　**Contusion of left wrist**

● S60.219　**Contusion of unspecified wrist**

● S60.22　**Contusion of hand**

● S60.221　**Contusion of right hand**

● S60.222　**Contusion of left hand**

● S60.229　**Contusion of unspecified hand**

● S60.3　**Other superficial injuries of thumb**

● S60.31　**Abrasion of thumb**

● S60.311　**Abrasion of right thumb**

● S60.312　**Abrasion of left thumb**

● S60.319　**Abrasion of unspecified thumb**

● S60.32　**Blister (nonthermal) of thumb**

● S60.321　**Blister (nonthermal) of right thumb**

● S60.322　**Blister (nonthermal) of left thumb**

● S60.329　**Blister (nonthermal) of unspecified thumb**

● S60.34　**External constriction of thumb**
Hair tourniquet syndrome of thumb
Use additional cause code to identify the constricting item (W49.0-)

● S60.341　**External constriction of right thumb**

● S60.342　**External constriction of left thumb**

● S60.349　**External constriction of unspecified thumb**

● S60.35　**Superficial foreign body of thumb**
Splinter in the thumb

● S60.351　**Superficial foreign body of right thumb**

● S60.352　**Superficial foreign body of left thumb**

● S60.359　**Superficial foreign body of unspecified thumb**

◀ New　◀▬ Revised　~~deleted~~ Deleted　Excludes 1　Excludes 2　Includes　Use additional　Code first　Code also　Unspecified
OGCR Official Guidelines　● Unacceptable Principal Diagnosis　X Assign placeholder X　● Use Additional Character(s)　▌ Manifestation Code　**Coding Clinic**

● **S60.36   Insect bite (nonvenomous) of thumb**

    ● **S60.361   Insect bite (nonvenomous) of right thumb**

    ● **S60.362   Insect bite (nonvenomous) of left thumb**

    ● **S60.369   Insect bite (nonvenomous) of unspecified thumb**

● **S60.37   Other superficial bite of thumb**

    Excludes1 open bite of thumb (S61.05-, S61.15-)

    ● **S60.371   Other superficial bite of right thumb**

    ● **S60.372   Other superficial bite of left thumb**

    ● **S60.379   Other superficial bite of unspecified thumb**

● **S60.39   Other superficial injuries of thumb**

    ● **S60.391   Other superficial injuries of right thumb**

    ● **S60.392   Other superficial injuries of left thumb**

    ● **S60.399   Other superficial injuries of unspecified thumb**

● **S60.4   Other superficial injuries of other fingers**

  ● **S60.41   Abrasion of fingers**

    ● **S60.410   Abrasion of right index finger**

    ● **S60.411   Abrasion of left index finger**

    ● **S60.412   Abrasion of right middle finger**

    ● **S60.413   Abrasion of left middle finger**

    ● **S60.414   Abrasion of right ring finger**

    ● **S60.415   Abrasion of left ring finger**

    ● **S60.416   Abrasion of right little finger**

    ● **S60.417   Abrasion of left little finger**

    ● **S60.418   Abrasion of other finger**

        Abrasion of specified finger with unspecified laterality

    ● **S60.419   Abrasion of unspecified finger**

  ● **S60.42   Blister (nonthermal) of fingers**

    ● **S60.420   Blister (nonthermal) of right index finger**

    ● **S60.421   Blister (nonthermal) of left index finger**

    ● **S60.422   Blister (nonthermal) of right middle finger**

    ● **S60.423   Blister (nonthermal) of left middle finger**

    ● **S60.424   Blister (nonthermal) of right ring finger**

    ● **S60.425   Blister (nonthermal) of left ring finger**

    ● **S60.426   Blister (nonthermal) of right little finger**

    ● **S60.427   Blister (nonthermal) of left little finger**

    ● **S60.428   Blister (nonthermal) of other finger**

        Blister (nonthermal) of specified finger with unspecified laterality

    ● **S60.429   Blister (nonthermal) of unspecified finger**

  ● **S60.44   External constriction of fingers**

    Hair tourniquet syndrome of finger

    Use additional cause code to identify the constricting item (W49.0-)

    ● **S60.440   External constriction of right index finger**

    ● **S60.441   External constriction of left index finger**

    ● **S60.442   External constriction of right middle finger**

    ● **S60.443   External constriction of left middle finger**

    ● **S60.444   External constriction of right ring finger**

    ● **S60.445   External constriction of left ring finger**

    ● **S60.446   External constriction of right little finger**

    ● **S60.447   External constriction of left little finger**

    ● **S60.448   External constriction of other finger**

        External constriction of specified finger with unspecified laterality

    ● **S60.449   External constriction of unspecified finger**

  ● **S60.45   Superficial foreign body of fingers**

    Splinter in the finger(s)

    ● **S60.450   Superficial foreign body of right index finger**

    ● **S60.451   Superficial foreign body of left index finger**

    ● **S60.452   Superficial foreign body of right middle finger**

    ● **S60.453   Superficial foreign body of left middle finger**

    ● **S60.454   Superficial foreign body of right ring finger**

    ● **S60.455   Superficial foreign body of left ring finger**

    ● **S60.456   Superficial foreign body of right little finger**

    ● **S60.457   Superficial foreign body of left little finger**

    ● **S60.458   Superficial foreign body of other finger**

        Superficial foreign body of specified finger with unspecified laterality

    ● **S60.459   Superficial foreign body of unspecified finger**

  ● **S60.46   Insect bite (nonvenomous) of fingers**

    ● **S60.460   Insect bite (nonvenomous) of right index finger**

    ● **S60.461   Insect bite (nonvenomous) of left index finger**

    ● **S60.462   Insect bite (nonvenomous) of right middle finger**

    ● **S60.463   Insect bite (nonvenomous) of left middle finger**

    ● **S60.464   Insect bite (nonvenomous) of right ring finger**

    ● **S60.465   Insect bite (nonvenomous) of left ring finger**

    ● **S60.466   Insect bite (nonvenomous) of right little finger**

    ● **S60.467   Insect bite (nonvenomous) of left little finger**

    ● **S60.468   Insect bite (nonvenomous) of other finger**

        Insect bite (nonvenomous) of specified finger with unspecified laterality

    ● **S60.469   Insect bite (nonvenomous) of unspecified finger**

CHAPTER 19 (S00-T88)

● **S60.47**   **Other superficial bite of fingers**
>   **Excludes1**   open bite of fingers (S61.25-, S61.35-)

● S60.470   Other superficial bite of right index finger

● S60.471   Other superficial bite of left index finger

● S60.472   Other superficial bite of right middle finger

● S60.473   Other superficial bite of left middle finger

● S60.474   Other superficial bite of right ring finger

● S60.475   Other superficial bite of left ring finger

● S60.476   Other superficial bite of right little finger

● S60.477   Other superficial bite of left little finger

● S60.478   Other superficial bite of other finger
>   Other superficial bite of specified finger with unspecified laterality

● S60.479   Other superficial bite of unspecified finger

● **S60.5**   **Other superficial injuries of hand**
>   **Excludes2**   superficial injuries of fingers (S60.3-, S60.4-)

● **S60.51**   **Abrasion of hand**

● S60.511   Abrasion of right hand

● S60.512   Abrasion of left hand

● S60.519   Abrasion of unspecified hand

● **S60.52**   **Blister (nonthermal) of hand**

● S60.521   Blister (nonthermal) of right hand

● S60.522   Blister (nonthermal) of left hand

● S60.529   Blister (nonthermal) of unspecified hand

● **S60.54**   **External constriction of hand**

● S60.541   External constriction of right hand

● S60.542   External constriction of left hand

● S60.549   External constriction of unspecified hand

● **S60.55**   **Superficial foreign body of hand**
>   Splinter in the hand

● S60.551   Superficial foreign body of right hand

● S60.552   Superficial foreign body of left hand

● S60.559   Superficial foreign body of unspecified hand

● **S60.56**   **Insect bite (nonvenomous) of hand**

● S60.561   Insect bite (nonvenomous) of right hand

● S60.562   Insect bite (nonvenomous) of left hand

● S60.569   Insect bite (nonvenomous) of unspecified hand

● **S60.57**   **Other superficial bite of hand**
>   **Excludes1**   open bite of hand (S61.45-)

● S60.571   Other superficial bite of hand of right hand

● S60.572   Other superficial bite of hand of left hand

● S60.579   Other superficial bite of hand of unspecified hand

● **S60.8**   **Other superficial injuries of wrist**

● **S60.81**   **Abrasion of wrist**

● S60.811   Abrasion of right wrist

● S60.812   Abrasion of left wrist

● S60.819   Abrasion of unspecified wrist

● **S60.82**   **Blister (nonthermal) of wrist**

● S60.821   Blister (nonthermal) of right wrist

● S60.822   Blister (nonthermal) of left wrist

● S60.829   Blister (nonthermal) of unspecified wrist

● **S60.84**   **External constriction of wrist**

● S60.841   External constriction of right wrist

● S60.842   External constriction of left wrist

● S60.849   External constriction of unspecified wrist

● **S60.85**   **Superficial foreign body of wrist**
>   Splinter in the wrist

● S60.851   Superficial foreign body of right wrist

● S60.852   Superficial foreign body of left wrist

● S60.859   Superficial foreign body of unspecified wrist

● **S60.86**   **Insect bite (nonvenomous) of wrist**

● S60.861   Insect bite (nonvenomous) of right wrist

● S60.862   Insect bite (nonvenomous) of left wrist

● S60.869   Insect bite (nonvenomous) of unspecified wrist

● **S60.87**   **Other superficial bite of wrist**
>   **Excludes1**   open bite of wrist (S61.55)

● S60.871   Other superficial bite of right wrist

● S60.872   Other superficial bite of left wrist

● S60.879   Other superficial bite of unspecified wrist

● **S60.9**   **Unspecified superficial injury of wrist, hand and fingers**

● **S60.91**   **Unspecified superficial injury of wrist**

● S60.911   Unspecified superficial injury of right wrist

● S60.912   Unspecified superficial injury of left wrist

● S60.919   Unspecified superficial injury of unspecified wrist

● **S60.92**   **Unspecified superficial injury of hand**

● S60.921   Unspecified superficial injury of right hand

● S60.922   Unspecified superficial injury of left hand

● S60.929   Unspecified superficial injury of unspecified hand

● **S60.93**   **Unspecified superficial injury of thumb**

● S60.931   Unspecified superficial injury of right thumb

● S60.932   Unspecified superficial injury of left thumb

● S60.939   Unspecified superficial injury of unspecified thumb

● **S60.94**   **Unspecified superficial injury of other fingers**

● S60.940   Unspecified superficial injury of right index finger

● S60.941   Unspecified superficial injury of left index finger

● S60.942   Unspecified superficial injury of right middle finger

● S60.943   Unspecified superficial injury of left middle finger

● S60.944 Unspecified superficial injury of right ring finger

● S60.945 Unspecified superficial injury of left ring finger

● S60.946 Unspecified superficial injury of right little finger

● S60.947 Unspecified superficial injury of left little finger

● S60.948 Unspecified superficial injury of other finger

         Unspecified superficial injury of specified finger with unspecified laterality

● S60.949 Unspecified superficial injury of unspecified finger

● **S61 Open wound of wrist, hand and fingers**

     Code also any associated wound infection

     Excludes1   open fracture of wrist, hand and finger (S62.- with 7th character B)

               traumatic amputation of wrist and hand (S68.-)

     The appropriate 7th character is to be added to each code from category S61

A	initial encounter
D	subsequent encounter
S	sequela

● **S61.0 Open wound of thumb without damage to nail**

     Excludes1   open wound of thumb with damage to nail (S61.1-)

   ● S61.00 Unspecified open wound of thumb without damage to nail

     ● S61.001 Unspecified open wound of right thumb without damage to nail

     ● S61.002 Unspecified open wound of left thumb without damage to nail

     ● S61.009 Unspecified open wound of unspecified thumb without damage to nail

   ● S61.01 Laceration without foreign body of thumb without damage to nail

     ● S61.011 Laceration without foreign body of right thumb without damage to nail

     ● S61.012 Laceration without foreign body of left thumb without damage to nail

     ● S61.019 Laceration without foreign body of unspecified thumb without damage to nail

   ● S61.02 Laceration with foreign body of thumb without damage to nail

     ● S61.021 Laceration with foreign body of right thumb without damage to nail

     ● S61.022 Laceration with foreign body of left thumb without damage to nail

     ● S61.029 Laceration with foreign body of unspecified thumb without damage to nail

   ● S61.03 Puncture wound without foreign body of thumb without damage to nail

     ● S61.031 Puncture wound without foreign body of right thumb without damage to nail

     ● S61.032 Puncture wound without foreign body of left thumb without damage to nail

     ● S61.039 Puncture wound without foreign body of unspecified thumb without damage to nail

● S61.04 Puncture wound with foreign body of thumb without damage to nail

   ● S61.041 Puncture wound with foreign body of right thumb without damage to nail

   ● S61.042 Puncture wound with foreign body of left thumb without damage to nail

   ● S61.049 Puncture wound with foreign body of unspecified thumb without damage to nail

● S61.05 Open bite of thumb without damage to nail

     Bite of thumb NOS

     Excludes1   superficial bite of thumb (S60.36-, S60.37-)

   ● S61.051 Open bite of right thumb without damage to nail

   ● S61.052 Open bite of left thumb without damage to nail

   ● S61.059 Open bite of unspecified thumb without damage to nail

● **S61.1 Open wound of thumb with damage to nail**

   ● S61.10 Unspecified open wound of thumb with damage to nail

     ● S61.101 Unspecified open wound of right thumb with damage to nail

     ● S61.102 Unspecified open wound of left thumb with damage to nail

     ● S61.109 Unspecified open wound of unspecified thumb with damage to nail

   ● S61.11 Laceration without foreign body of thumb with damage to nail

     ● S61.111 Laceration without foreign body of right thumb with damage to nail

     ● S61.112 Laceration without foreign body of left thumb with damage to nail

     ● S61.119 Laceration without foreign body of unspecified thumb with damage to nail

   ● S61.12 Laceration with foreign body of thumb with damage to nail

     ● S61.121 Laceration with foreign body of right thumb with damage to nail

     ● S61.122 Laceration with foreign body of left thumb with damage to nail

     ● S61.129 Laceration with foreign body of unspecified thumb with damage to nail

   ● S61.13 Puncture wound without foreign body of thumb with damage to nail

     ● S61.131 Puncture wound without foreign body of right thumb with damage to nail

     ● S61.132 Puncture wound without foreign body of left thumb with damage to nail

     ● S61.139 Puncture wound without foreign body of unspecified thumb with damage to nail

   ● S61.14 Puncture wound with foreign body of thumb with damage to nail

     ● S61.141 Puncture wound with foreign body of right thumb with damage to nail

     ● S61.142 Puncture wound with foreign body of left thumb with damage to nail

     ● S61.149 Puncture wound with foreign body of unspecified thumb with damage to nail

CHAPTER 19 (S00-T88)

● S61.15   **Open bite of thumb with damage to nail**
     Bite of thumb with damage to nail NOS
     Excludes1   superficial bite of thumb
                (S60.36-, S60.37-)

   ● S61.151   **Open bite of right thumb with damage to nail**

   ● S61.152   **Open bite of left thumb with damage to nail**

   ● S61.159   **Open bite of unspecified thumb with damage to nail**

● S61.2   **Open wound of other finger without damage to nail**
     Excludes1   open wound of finger involving nail
                (matrix) (S61.3-)
     Excludes2   open wound of thumb without damage
                to nail (S61.0-)

   ● S61.20   **Unspecified open wound of other finger without damage to nail**

     ● S61.200   **Unspecified open wound of right index finger without damage to nail**

     ● S61.201   **Unspecified open wound of left index finger without damage to nail**

     ● S61.202   **Unspecified open wound of right middle finger without damage to nail**

     ● S61.203   **Unspecified open wound of left middle finger without damage to nail**

     ● S61.204   **Unspecified open wound of right ring finger without damage to nail**

     ● S61.205   **Unspecified open wound of left ring finger without damage to nail**

     ● S61.206   **Unspecified open wound of right little finger without damage to nail**

     ● S61.207   **Unspecified open wound of left little finger without damage to nail**

     ● S61.208   **Unspecified open wound of other finger without damage to nail**
         Unspecified open wound of
            specified finger with
            unspecified laterality without
            damage to nail

     ● S61.209   **Unspecified open wound of unspecified finger without damage to nail**

   ● S61.21   **Laceration without foreign body of finger without damage to nail**

     ● S61.210   **Laceration without foreign body of right index finger without damage to nail**

     ● S61.211   **Laceration without foreign body of left index finger without damage to nail**

     ● S61.212   **Laceration without foreign body of right middle finger without damage to nail**

     ● S61.213   **Laceration without foreign body of left middle finger without damage to nail**

     ● S61.214   **Laceration without foreign body of right ring finger without damage to nail**

     ● S61.215   **Laceration without foreign body of left ring finger without damage to nail**

     ● S61.216   **Laceration without foreign body of right little finger without damage to nail**

     ● S61.217   **Laceration without foreign body of left little finger without damage to nail**

     ● S61.218   **Laceration without foreign body of other finger without damage to nail**
         Laceration without foreign body
            of specified finger with
            unspecified laterality without
            damage to nail

     ● S61.219   **Laceration without foreign body of unspecified finger without damage to nail**

   ● S61.22   **Laceration with foreign body of finger without damage to nail**

     ● S61.220   **Laceration with foreign body of right index finger without damage to nail**

     ● S61.221   **Laceration with foreign body of left index finger without damage to nail**

     ● S61.222   **Laceration with foreign body of right middle finger without damage to nail**

     ● S61.223   **Laceration with foreign body of left middle finger without damage to nail**

     ● S61.224   **Laceration with foreign body of right ring finger without damage to nail**

     ● S61.225   **Laceration with foreign body of left ring finger without damage to nail**

     ● S61.226   **Laceration with foreign body of right little finger without damage to nail**

     ● S61.227   **Laceration with foreign body of left little finger without damage to nail**

     ● S61.228   **Laceration with foreign body of other finger without damage to nail**
         Laceration with foreign body
            of specified finger with
            unspecified laterality without
            damage to nail

     ● S61.229   **Laceration with foreign body of unspecified finger without damage to nail**

   ● S61.23   **Puncture wound without foreign body of finger without damage to nail**

     ● S61.230   **Puncture wound without foreign body of right index finger without damage to nail**

     ● S61.231   **Puncture wound without foreign body of left index finger without damage to nail**

     ● S61.232   **Puncture wound without foreign body of right middle finger without damage to nail**

     ● S61.233   **Puncture wound without foreign body of left middle finger without damage to nail**

     ● S61.234   **Puncture wound without foreign body of right ring finger without damage to nail**

     ● S61.235   **Puncture wound without foreign body of left ring finger without damage to nail**

     ● S61.236   **Puncture wound without foreign body of right little finger without damage to nail**

     ● S61.237   **Puncture wound without foreign body of left little finger without damage to nail**

     ● S61.238   **Puncture wound without foreign body of other finger without damage to nail**
         Puncture wound without foreign
            body of specified finger with
            unspecified laterality without
            damage to nail

     ● S61.239   **Puncture wound without foreign body of unspecified finger without damage to nail**

◄ New   ◄═ Revised   ~~deleted~~ Deleted   Excludes 1   Excludes 2   Includes   Use additional   Code first   Code also   Unspecified

OGCR Official Guidelines   ● Unacceptable Principal Diagnosis   X Assign placeholder X   ● Use Additional Character(s)   ▶ Manifestation Code   **Coding Clinic**

● S61.24   Puncture wound with foreign body of finger without damage to nail

    ● S61.240   Puncture wound with foreign body of right index finger without damage to nail

    ● S61.241   Puncture wound with foreign body of left index finger without damage to nail

    ● S61.242   Puncture wound with foreign body of right middle finger without damage to nail

    ● S61.243   Puncture wound with foreign body of left middle finger without damage to nail

    ● S61.244   Puncture wound with foreign body of right ring finger without damage to nail

    ● S61.245   Puncture wound with foreign body of left ring finger without damage to nail

    ● S61.246   Puncture wound with foreign body of right little finger without damage to nail

    ● S61.247   Puncture wound with foreign body of left little finger without damage to nail

    ● S61.248   Puncture wound with foreign body of other finger without damage to nail
         Puncture wound with foreign body of specified finger with unspecified laterality without damage to nail

    ● S61.249   Puncture wound with foreign body of unspecified finger without damage to nail

● S61.25   Open bite of finger without damage to nail
      Bite of finger without damage to nail NOS
      Excludes1   superficial bite of finger (S60.46-, S60.47-)

    ● S61.250   Open bite of right index finger without damage to nail

    ● S61.251   Open bite of left index finger without damage to nail

    ● S61.252   Open bite of right middle finger without damage to nail

    ● S61.253   Open bite of left middle finger without damage to nail

    ● S61.254   Open bite of right ring finger without damage to nail

    ● S61.255   Open bite of left ring finger without damage to nail

    ● S61.256   Open bite of right little finger without damage to nail

    ● S61.257   Open bite of left little finger without damage to nail

    ● S61.258   Open bite of other finger without damage to nail
         Open bite of specified finger with unspecified laterality without damage to nail

    ● S61.259   Open bite of unspecified finger without damage to nail

● S61.3   Open wound of other finger with damage to nail

    ● S61.30   Unspecified open wound of finger with damage to nail

    ● S61.300   Unspecified open wound of right index finger with damage to nail

    ● S61.301   Unspecified open wound of left index finger with damage to nail

    ● S61.302   Unspecified open wound of right middle finger with damage to nail

    ● S61.303   Unspecified open wound of left middle finger with damage to nail

    ● S61.304   Unspecified open wound of right ring finger with damage to nail

    ● S61.305   Unspecified open wound of left ring finger with damage to nail

    ● S61.306   Unspecified open wound of right little finger with damage to nail

    ● S61.307   Unspecified open wound of left little finger with damage to nail

    ● S61.308   Unspecified open wound of other finger with damage to nail
         Unspecified open wound of specified finger with unspecified laterality with damage to nail

    ● S61.309   Unspecified open wound of unspecified finger with damage to nail

● S61.31   Laceration without foreign body of finger with damage to nail

    ● S61.310   Laceration without foreign body of right index finger with damage to nail

    ● S61.311   Laceration without foreign body of left index finger with damage to nail

    ● S61.312   Laceration without foreign body of right middle finger with damage to nail

    ● S61.313   Laceration without foreign body of left middle finger with damage to nail

    ● S61.314   Laceration without foreign body of right ring finger with damage to nail

    ● S61.315   Laceration without foreign body of left ring finger with damage to nail

    ● S61.316   Laceration without foreign body of right little finger with damage to nail

    ● S61.317   Laceration without foreign body of left little finger with damage to nail

    ● S61.318   Laceration without foreign body of other finger with damage to nail
         Laceration without foreign body of specified finger with unspecified laterality with damage to nail

    ● S61.319   Laceration without foreign body of unspecified finger with damage to nail

● S61.32   Laceration with foreign body of finger with damage to nail

    ● S61.320   Laceration with foreign body of right index finger with damage to nail

    ● S61.321   Laceration with foreign body of left index finger with damage to nail

    ● S61.322   Laceration with foreign body of right middle finger with damage to nail

    ● S61.323   Laceration with foreign body of left middle finger with damage to nail

    ● S61.324   Laceration with foreign body of right ring finger with damage to nail

    ● S61.325   Laceration with foreign body of left ring finger with damage to nail

    ● S61.326   Laceration with foreign body of right little finger with damage to nail

    ● S61.327   Laceration with foreign body of left little finger with damage to nail

    ● S61.328   Laceration with foreign body of other finger with damage to nail
         Laceration with foreign body of specified finger with unspecified laterality with damage to nail

    ● S61.329   Laceration with foreign body of unspecified finger with damage to nail

CHAPTER 19 (S00–T88)

N Newborn Age: 0   **P** Pediatric Age: 0–17   **M** Maternity DX: 12–55   **A** Adult Age: 15–124   ♀ Females Only   ♂ Males Only

 Complication\Comorbidity   Major C\C   (Ex) CC/MCC Exclusions   Hospital-Acquired Condition

1327

● **S61.33**   **Puncture wound without foreign body of finger with damage to nail**

  ● **S61.330**   Puncture wound without foreign body of right index finger with damage to nail

  ● **S61.331**   Puncture wound without foreign body of left index finger with damage to nail

  ● **S61.332**   Puncture wound without foreign body of right middle finger with damage to nail

  ● **S61.333**   Puncture wound without foreign body of left middle finger with damage to nail

  ● **S61.334**   Puncture wound without foreign body of right ring finger with damage to nail

  ● **S61.335**   Puncture wound without foreign body of left ring finger with damage to nail

  ● **S61.336**   Puncture wound without foreign body of right little finger with damage to nail

  ● **S61.337**   Puncture wound without foreign body of left little finger with damage to nail

  ● **S61.338**   Puncture wound without foreign body of other finger with damage to nail
     Puncture wound without foreign body of specified finger with unspecified laterality with damage to nail

  ● **S61.339**   Puncture wound without foreign body of unspecified finger with damage to nail

● **S61.34**   **Puncture wound with foreign body of finger with damage to nail**

  ● **S61.340**   Puncture wound with foreign body of right index finger with damage to nail

  ● **S61.341**   Puncture wound with foreign body of left index finger with damage to nail

  ● **S61.342**   Puncture wound with foreign body of right middle finger with damage to nail

  ● **S61.343**   Puncture wound with foreign body of left middle finger with damage to nail

  ● **S61.344**   Puncture wound with foreign body of right ring finger with damage to nail

  ● **S61.345**   Puncture wound with foreign body of left ring finger with damage to nail

  ● **S61.346**   Puncture wound with foreign body of right little finger with damage to nail

  ● **S61.347**   Puncture wound with foreign body of left little finger with damage to nail

  ● **S61.348**   Puncture wound with foreign body of other finger with damage to nail
     Puncture wound with foreign body of specified finger with unspecified laterality with damage to nail

  ● **S61.349**   Puncture wound with foreign body of unspecified finger with damage to nail

● **S61.35**   **Open bite of finger with damage to nail**
     Bite of finger with damage to nail NOS

     Excludes1   superficial bite of finger (S60.46-, S60.47-)

  ● **S61.350**   Open bite of right index finger with damage to nail

  ● **S61.351**   Open bite of left index finger with damage to nail

  ● **S61.352**   Open bite of right middle finger with damage to nail

  ● **S61.353**   Open bite of left middle finger with damage to nail

  ● **S61.354**   Open bite of right ring finger with damage to nail

  ● **S61.355**   Open bite of left ring finger with damage to nail

  ● **S61.356**   Open bite of right little finger with damage to nail

  ● **S61.357**   Open bite of left little finger with damage to nail

  ● **S61.358**   Open bite of other finger with damage to nail
     Open bite of specified finger with unspecified laterality with damage to nail

  ● **S61.359**   Open bite of unspecified finger with damage to nail

● **S61.4**   **Open wound of hand**

  ● **S61.40**   **Unspecified open wound of hand**

    ● **S61.401**   Unspecified open wound of right hand

    ● **S61.402**   Unspecified open wound of left hand

    ● **S61.409**   Unspecified open wound of unspecified hand

  ● **S61.41**   **Laceration without foreign body of hand**

    ● **S61.411**   Laceration without foreign body of right hand

    ● **S61.412**   Laceration without foreign body of left hand

    ● **S61.419**   Laceration without foreign body of unspecified hand

  ● **S61.42**   **Laceration with foreign body of hand**

    ● **S61.421**   Laceration with foreign body of right hand

    ● **S61.422**   Laceration with foreign body of left hand

    ● **S61.429**   Laceration with foreign body of unspecified hand

  ● **S61.43**   **Puncture wound without foreign body of hand**

    ● **S61.431**   Puncture wound without foreign body of right hand

    ● **S61.432**   Puncture wound without foreign body of left hand

    ● **S61.439**   Puncture wound without foreign body of unspecified hand

  ● **S61.44**   **Puncture wound with foreign body of hand**

    ● **S61.441**   Puncture wound with foreign body of right hand

    ● **S61.442**   Puncture wound with foreign body of left hand

    ● **S61.449**   Puncture wound with foreign body of unspecified hand

  ● **S61.45**   **Open bite of hand**
     Bite of hand NOS

     Excludes1   superficial bite of hand (S60.56-, S60.57-)

    ● **S61.451**   Open bite of right hand

    ● **S61.452**   Open bite of left hand

    ● **S61.459**   Open bite of unspecified hand

● **S61.5**   **Open wound of wrist**

  ● **S61.50**   **Unspecified open wound of wrist**

    ● **S61.501**   Unspecified open wound of right wrist

    ● **S61.502**   Unspecified open wound of left wrist

    ● **S61.509**   Unspecified open wound of unspecified wrist

◀ New   ◀▥ Revised   ~~deleted~~ Deleted   Excludes 1   Excludes 2   Includes   Use additional   Code first   Code also   Unspecified

OGCR Official Guidelines   ● Unacceptable Principal Diagnosis   X Assign placeholder X   ● Use Additional Character(s)   ▶ Manifestation Code   **Coding Clinic**

- ● **S61.51**   Laceration without foreign body of wrist
  - ● **S61.511**   Laceration without foreign body of right wrist
  - ● **S61.512**   Laceration without foreign body of left wrist
  - ● **S61.519**   Laceration without foreign body of <mark>unspecified</mark> wrist
- ● **S61.52**   Laceration with foreign body of wrist
  - ● **S61.521**   Laceration with foreign body of right wrist
  - ● **S61.522**   Laceration with foreign body of left wrist
  - ● **S61.529**   Laceration with foreign body of <mark>unspecified</mark> wrist
- ● **S61.53**   Puncture wound without foreign body of wrist
  - ● **S61.531**   Puncture wound without foreign body of right wrist
  - ● **S61.532**   Puncture wound without foreign body of left wrist
  - ● **S61.539**   Puncture wound without foreign body of <mark>unspecified</mark> wrist
- ● **S61.54**   Puncture wound with foreign body of wrist
  - ● **S61.541**   Puncture wound with foreign body of right wrist
  - ● **S61.542**   Puncture wound with foreign body of left wrist
  - ● **S61.549**   Puncture wound with foreign body of <mark>unspecified</mark> wrist
- ● **S61.55**   Open bite of wrist

  Bite of wrist NOS

  Excludes1   superficial bite of wrist (S60.86-, S60.87-)
  - ● **S61.551**   Open bite of right wrist
  - ● **S61.552**   Open bite of left wrist
  - ● **S61.559**   Open bite of <mark>unspecified</mark> wrist

● **S62**   **Fracture at wrist and hand level**

     Note: A fracture not indicated as displaced or nondisplaced should be coded to displaced

     A fracture not indicated as open or closed should be coded to closed

     Excludes1   traumatic amputation of wrist and hand (S68.-)

     Excludes2   fracture of distal parts of ulna and radius (S52.-)

     The appropriate 7th character is to be added to each code from category S62

A	initial encounter for closed fracture
B	initial encounter for open fracture
D	subsequent encounter for fracture with routine healing
G	subsequent encounter for fracture with delayed healing
K	subsequent encounter for fracture with nonunion
P	subsequent encounter for fracture with malunion
S	sequela

- ● **S62.0**   **Fracture of navicular [scaphoid] bone of wrist**

  (Ex) For category S62.0 CC codes S62.0[B]: S62.001-S62.186[A,B]

       For S62.0[K,P]: See S02.0[K]
  - ● **S62.00**   Unspecified fracture of navicular [scaphoid] bone of wrist
    - ● **S62.001**   <mark>Unspecified</mark> fracture of navicular [scaphoid] bone of right wrist B, K, P 🅒, B 🅜
    - ● **S62.002**   <mark>Unspecified</mark> fracture of navicular [scaphoid] bone of left wrist B, K, P 🅒, B 🅜

      Coding Clinic: 2012, Q4, P106
    - ● **S62.009**   <mark>Unspecified</mark> fracture of navicular [scaphoid] bone of unspecified wrist B, K, P 🅒, B 🅜

- ● **S62.01**   Fracture of distal pole of navicular [scaphoid] bone of wrist

  Fracture of volar tuberosity of navicular [scaphoid] bone of wrist
  - ● **S62.011**   Displaced fracture of distal pole of navicular [scaphoid] bone of right wrist B, K, P 🅒, B 🅜
  - ● **S62.012**   Displaced fracture of distal pole of navicular [scaphoid] bone of left wrist B, K, P 🅒, B 🅜
  - ● **S62.013**   Displaced fracture of distal pole of navicular [scaphoid] bone of <mark>unspecified</mark> wrist B, K, P 🅒, B 🅜
  - ● **S62.014**   Nondisplaced fracture of distal pole of navicular [scaphoid] bone of right wrist B, K, P 🅒, B 🅜
  - ● **S62.015**   Nondisplaced fracture of distal pole of navicular [scaphoid] bone of left wrist B, K, P 🅒, B 🅜
  - ● **S62.016**   Nondisplaced fracture of distal pole of navicular [scaphoid] bone of <mark>unspecified</mark> wrist B, K, P 🅒, B 🅜
- ● **S62.02**   Fracture of middle third of navicular [scaphoid] bone of wrist
  - ● **S62.021**   Displaced fracture of middle third of navicular [scaphoid] bone of right wrist B, K, P 🅒, B 🅜
  - ● **S62.022**   Displaced fracture of middle third of navicular [scaphoid] bone of left wrist B, K, P 🅒, B 🅜
  - ● **S62.023**   Displaced fracture of middle third of navicular [scaphoid] bone of <mark>unspecified</mark> wrist B, K, P 🅒, B 🅜
  - ● **S62.024**   Nondisplaced fracture of middle third of navicular [scaphoid] bone of right wrist B, K, P 🅒, B 🅜
  - ● **S62.025**   Nondisplaced fracture of middle third of navicular [scaphoid] bone of left wrist B, K, P 🅒, B 🅜
  - ● **S62.026**   Nondisplaced fracture of middle third of navicular [scaphoid] bone of <mark>unspecified</mark> wrist B, K, P 🅒, B 🅜
- ● **S62.03**   Fracture of proximal third of navicular [scaphoid] bone of wrist
  - ● **S62.031**   Displaced fracture of proximal third of navicular [scaphoid] bone of right wrist B, K, P 🅒, B 🅜
  - ● **S62.032**   Displaced fracture of proximal third of navicular [scaphoid] bone of left wrist B, K, P 🅒, B 🅜
  - ● **S62.033**   Displaced fracture of proximal third of navicular [scaphoid] bone of <mark>unspecified</mark> wrist B, K, P 🅒, B 🅜
  - ● **S62.034**   Nondisplaced fracture of proximal third of navicular [scaphoid] bone of right wrist B, K, P 🅒, B 🅜
  - ● **S62.035**   Nondisplaced fracture of proximal third of navicular [scaphoid] bone of left wrist B, K, P 🅒, B 🅜
  - ● **S62.036**   Nondisplaced fracture of proximal third of navicular [scaphoid] bone of <mark>unspecified</mark> wrist B, K, P 🅒, B 🅜

N   Newborn Age: 0   **P**   Pediatric Age: 0–17   **M**   Maternity DX: 12–55   **A**   Adult Age: 15–124   ♀   Females Only   ♂   Males Only

🅒   Complication\Comorbidity   🅜   Major C\C   (Ex)   CC/MCC Exclusions   🅗   Hospital-Acquired Condition

1329

CHAPTER 19 (S00-T88)

● S62.1   Fracture of other and unspecified carpal bone(s)
           Excludes2   fracture of scaphoid of wrist (S62.0-)
           (Ex) For category S62.1 CC codes S62.1[B]: S62.001-S62.186[A,B]
                For S62.0[K,P]: See S02.0[K]
    ● S62.10   Fracture of unspecified carpal bone
               Fracture of wrist NOS
        ● S62.101   Fracture of unspecified carpal bone,
                     right wrist B, K, P 🐾, B 🐾
        ● S62.102   Fracture of unspecified carpal bone,
                     left wrist B, K, P 🐾, B 🐾
                     Coding Clinic: 2012, Q4, P95
        ● S62.109   Fracture of unspecified carpal bone,
                     unspecified wrist B, K, P 🐾, B 🐾
    ● S62.11   Fracture of triquetrum [cuneiform] bone of wrist
        ● S62.111   Displaced fracture of triquetrum
                     [cuneiform] bone, right wrist
                     B, K, P 🐾, B 🐾
        ● S62.112   Displaced fracture of triquetrum
                     [cuneiform] bone, left wrist B, K, P 🐾,
                     B 🐾
        ● S62.113   Displaced fracture of triquetrum
                     [cuneiform] bone, unspecified wrist
                     B, K, P 🐾, B 🐾
        ● S62.114   Nondisplaced fracture of triquetrum
                     [cuneiform] bone, right wrist
                     B, K, P 🐾, B 🐾
        ● S62.115   Nondisplaced fracture of triquetrum
                     [cuneiform] bone, left wrist B, K, P 🐾,
                     B 🐾
        ● S62.116   Nondisplaced fracture of triquetrum
                     [cuneiform] bone, unspecified wrist
                     B, K, P 🐾, B 🐾
    ● S62.12   Fracture of lunate [semilunar]
        ● S62.121   Displaced fracture of lunate
                     [semilunar], right wrist B, K, P 🐾,
                     B 🐾
        ● S62.122   Displaced fracture of lunate
                     [semilunar], left wrist B, K, P 🐾, B 🐾
        ● S62.123   Displaced fracture of lunate
                     [semilunar], unspecified wrist
                     B, K, P 🐾, B 🐾
        ● S62.124   Nondisplaced fracture of lunate
                     [semilunar], right wrist B, K, P 🐾,
                     B 🐾
        ● S62.125   Nondisplaced fracture of lunate
                     [semilunar], left wrist B, K, P 🐾, B 🐾
        ● S62.126   Nondisplaced fracture of lunate
                     [semilunar], unspecified wrist
                     B, K, P 🐾, B 🐾
    ● S62.13   Fracture of capitate [os magnum] bone
        ● S62.131   Displaced fracture of capitate
                     [os magnum] bone, right wrist
                     B, K, P 🐾, B 🐾
        ● S62.132   Displaced fracture of capitate
                     [os magnum] bone, left wrist
                     B, K, P 🐾, B 🐾
        ● S62.133   Displaced fracture of capitate
                     [os magnum] bone, unspecified wrist
                     B, K, P 🐾, B 🐾
        ● S62.134   Nondisplaced fracture of capitate
                     [os magnum] bone, right wrist
                     B, K, P 🐾, B 🐾
        ● S62.135   Nondisplaced fracture of capitate
                     [os magnum] bone, left wrist
                     B, K, P 🐾, B 🐾
        ● S62.136   Nondisplaced fracture of capitate
                     [os magnum] bone, unspecified wrist
                     B, K, P 🐾, B 🐾

● S62.14   Fracture of body of hamate [unciform] bone
           Fracture of hamate [unciform] bone NOS
        ● S62.141   Displaced fracture of body of hamate
                     [unciform] bone, right wrist
                     B, K, P 🐾, B 🐾
        ● S62.142   Displaced fracture of body of hamate
                     [unciform] bone, left wrist B, K, P 🐾,
                     B 🐾
        ● S62.143   Displaced fracture of body of hamate
                     [unciform] bone, unspecified wrist
                     B, K, P 🐾, B 🐾
        ● S62.144   Nondisplaced fracture of body of
                     hamate [unciform] bone, right wrist
                     B, K, P 🐾, B 🐾
        ● S62.145   Nondisplaced fracture of body of
                     hamate [unciform] bone, left wrist
                     B, K, P 🐾, B 🐾
        ● S62.146   Nondisplaced fracture of body of
                     hamate [unciform] bone, unspecified
                     wrist B, K, P 🐾, B 🐾
    ● S62.15   Fracture of hook process of hamate [unciform]
               bone
               Fracture of unciform process of hamate
               [unciform] bone
        ● S62.151   Displaced fracture of hook process of
                     hamate [unciform] bone, right wrist
                     B, K, P 🐾, B 🐾
        ● S62.152   Displaced fracture of hook process of
                     hamate [unciform] bone, left wrist
                     B, K, P 🐾, B 🐾
        ● S62.153   Displaced fracture of hook process of
                     hamate [unciform] bone, unspecified
                     wrist B, K, P 🐾, B 🐾
        ● S62.154   Nondisplaced fracture of hook process
                     of hamate [unciform] bone, right wrist
                     B, K, P 🐾, B 🐾
        ● S62.155   Nondisplaced fracture of hook process
                     of hamate [unciform] bone, left wrist
                     B, K, P 🐾, B 🐾
        ● S62.156   Nondisplaced fracture of hook
                     process of hamate [unciform] bone,
                     unspecified wrist B, K, P 🐾, B 🐾
    ● S62.16   Fracture of pisiform
        ● S62.161   Displaced fracture of pisiform, right
                     wrist B, K, P 🐾, B 🐾
        ● S62.162   Displaced fracture of pisiform, left
                     wrist B, K, P 🐾, B 🐾
        ● S62.163   Displaced fracture of pisiform,
                     unspecified wrist B, K, P 🐾, B 🐾
        ● S62.164   Nondisplaced fracture of pisiform,
                     right wrist B, K, P 🐾, B 🐾
        ● S62.165   Nondisplaced fracture of pisiform,
                     left wrist B, K, P 🐾, B 🐾
        ● S62.166   Nondisplaced fracture of pisiform,
                     unspecified wrist B, K, P 🐾, B 🐾
    ● S62.17   Fracture of trapezium [larger multangular]
        ● S62.171   Displaced fracture of trapezium
                     [larger multangular], right wrist
                     B, K, P 🐾, B 🐾
        ● S62.172   Displaced fracture of trapezium
                     [larger multangular], left wrist
                     B, K, P 🐾, B 🐾
        ● S62.173   Displaced fracture of trapezium
                     [larger multangular], unspecified
                     wrist B, K, P 🐾, B 🐾

◀ New   ⬅ Revised   ~~deleted~~ Deleted   Excludes 1   Excludes 2   Includes   Use additional   Code first   Code also   Unspecified
OGCR Official Guidelines   ● Unacceptable Principal Diagnosis   X Assign placeholder X   ● Use Additional Character(s)   ▶ Manifestation Code   **Coding Clinic**

CHAPTER 19 (S00-T88)

● **S62.174** Nondisplaced fracture of trapezium [larger multangular], right wrist B, K, P 🔵, B 🔵

● **S62.175** Nondisplaced fracture of trapezium [larger multangular], left wrist B, K, P 🔵, B 🔵

● **S62.176** Nondisplaced fracture of trapezium [larger multangular], unspecified wrist B, K, P 🔵, B 🔵

● **S62.18** Fracture of trapezoid [smaller multangular]

● **S62.181** Displaced fracture of trapezoid [smaller multangular], right wrist B, K, P 🔵, B 🔵

● **S62.182** Displaced fracture of trapezoid [smaller multangular], left wrist B, K, P 🔵, B 🔵

● **S62.183** Displaced fracture of trapezoid [smaller multangular], unspecified wrist B, K, P 🔵, B 🔵

● **S62.184** Nondisplaced fracture of trapezoid [smaller multangular], right wrist B, K, P 🔵, B 🔵

● **S62.185** Nondisplaced fracture of trapezoid [smaller multangular], left wrist B, K, P 🔵, B 🔵

● **S62.186** Nondisplaced fracture of trapezoid [smaller multangular], unspecified wrist B, K, P 🔵, B 🔵

● **S62.2** Fracture of first metacarpal bone

ⒺⓍ **For category S62.2 CC codes S62.2[B]:** S62.201-S62.399[B], S62.90X[A]
For S62.2[K,P]: See S02.0[K]

● **S62.20** Unspecified fracture of first metacarpal bone

● **S62.201** Unspecified fracture of first metacarpal bone, right hand B, K, P 🔵, B 🔵

● **S62.202** Unspecified fracture of first metacarpal bone, left hand B, K, P 🔵, B 🔵

● **S62.209** Unspecified fracture of first metacarpal bone, unspecified hand B, K, P 🔵, B 🔵

● **S62.21** Bennett's fracture

● **S62.211** Bennett's fracture, right hand B, K, P 🔵, B 🔵

● **S62.212** Bennett's fracture, left hand B, K, P 🔵, B 🔵

● **S62.213** Bennett's fracture, unspecified hand B, K, P 🔵, B 🔵

● **S62.22** Rolando's fracture

● **S62.221** Displaced Rolando's fracture, right hand B, K, P 🔵, B 🔵

● **S62.222** Displaced Rolando's fracture, left hand B, K, P 🔵, B 🔵

● **S62.223** Displaced Rolando's fracture, unspecified hand B, K, P 🔵, B 🔵

● **S62.224** Nondisplaced Rolando's fracture, right hand B, K, P 🔵, B 🔵

● **S62.225** Nondisplaced Rolando's fracture, left hand B, K, P 🔵, B 🔵

● **S62.226** Nondisplaced Rolando's fracture, unspecified hand B, K, P 🔵, B 🔵

● **S62.23** Other fracture of base of first metacarpal bone

● **S62.231** Other displaced fracture of base of first metacarpal bone, right hand B, K, P 🔵, B 🔵

● **S62.232** Other displaced fracture of base of first metacarpal bone, left hand B, K, P 🔵, B 🔵

● **S62.233** Other displaced fracture of base of first metacarpal bone, unspecified hand B, K, P 🔵, B 🔵

● **S62.234** Other nondisplaced fracture of base of first metacarpal bone, right hand B, K, P 🔵, B 🔵

● **S62.235** Other nondisplaced fracture of base of first metacarpal bone, left hand B, K, P 🔵, B 🔵

● **S62.236** Other nondisplaced fracture of base of first metacarpal bone, unspecified hand B, K, P 🔵, B 🔵

● **S62.24** Fracture of shaft of first metacarpal bone

● **S62.241** Displaced fracture of shaft of first metacarpal bone, right hand B, K, P 🔵, B 🔵

● **S62.242** Displaced fracture of shaft of first metacarpal bone, left hand B, K, P 🔵, B 🔵

● **S62.243** Displaced fracture of shaft of first metacarpal bone, unspecified hand B, K, P 🔵, B 🔵

● **S62.244** Nondisplaced fracture of shaft of first metacarpal bone, right hand B, K, P 🔵, B 🔵

● **S62.245** Nondisplaced fracture of shaft of first metacarpal bone, left hand B, K, P 🔵, B 🔵

● **S62.246** Nondisplaced fracture of shaft of first metacarpal bone, unspecified hand B, K, P 🔵, B 🔵

● **S62.25** Fracture of neck of first metacarpal bone

● **S62.251** Displaced fracture of neck of first metacarpal bone, right hand B, K, P 🔵, B 🔵

● **S62.252** Displaced fracture of neck of first metacarpal bone, left hand B, K, P 🔵, B 🔵

● **S62.253** Displaced fracture of neck of first metacarpal bone, unspecified hand B, K, P 🔵, B 🔵

● **S62.254** Nondisplaced fracture of neck of first metacarpal bone, right hand B, K, P 🔵, B 🔵

● **S62.255** Nondisplaced fracture of neck of first metacarpal bone, left hand B, K, P 🔵, B 🔵

● **S62.256** Nondisplaced fracture of neck of first metacarpal bone, unspecified hand B, K, P 🔵, B 🔵

● **S62.29** Other fracture of first metacarpal bone

● **S62.291** Other fracture of first metacarpal bone, right hand B, K, P 🔵, B 🔵

● **S62.292** Other fracture of first metacarpal bone, left hand B, K, P 🔵, B 🔵

● **S62.299** Other fracture of first metacarpal bone, unspecified hand B, K, P 🔵, B 🔵

CHAPTER 19 (S00-T88)

N Newborn Age: 0   **P** Pediatric Age: 0–17   **M** Maternity DX: 12–55   **A** Adult Age: 15–124   ♀ Females Only   ♂ Males Only

🔵 Complication\Comorbidity   🔵 Major C\C   ⒺⓍ CC/MCC Exclusions   🔵 Hospital-Acquired Condition

1331

● **S62.3**   **Fracture of other and unspecified metacarpal bone**

     Excludes2   fracture of first metacarpal bone (S62.2-)

     (Ex) For category S62.3 CC codes S62.3[B]: See S62.2[B] For S62.3[K,P]: See S02.0[K]

  ● **S62.30**   **Unspecified fracture of other metacarpal bone**

    ● **S62.300**   Unspecified fracture of second metacarpal bone, right hand B, K, P 🏷, B 🏷

    ● **S62.301**   Unspecified fracture of second metacarpal bone, left hand B, K, P 🏷, B 🏷

    ● **S62.302**   Unspecified fracture of third metacarpal bone, right hand B, K, P 🏷, B 🏷

    ● **S62.303**   Unspecified fracture of third metacarpal bone, left hand B, K, P 🏷, B 🏷

    ● **S62.304**   Unspecified fracture of fourth metacarpal bone, right hand B, K, P 🏷, B 🏷

    ● **S62.305**   Unspecified fracture of fourth metacarpal bone, left hand B, K, P 🏷, B 🏷

    ● **S62.306**   Unspecified fracture of fifth metacarpal bone, right hand B, K, P 🏷, B 🏷

    ● **S62.307**   Unspecified fracture of fifth metacarpal bone, left hand B, K, P 🏷, B 🏷

    ● **S62.308**   Unspecified fracture of other metacarpal bone B, K, P 🏷, B 🏷
          Unspecified fracture of specified metacarpal bone with unspecified laterality

    ● **S62.309**   Unspecified fracture of unspecified metacarpal bone B, K, P 🏷, B 🏷

  ● **S62.31**   Displaced fracture of base of other metacarpal bone

    ● **S62.310**   Displaced fracture of base of second metacarpal bone, right hand B, K, P 🏷, B 🏷

    ● **S62.311**   Displaced fracture of base of second metacarpal bone, left hand B, K, P 🏷, B 🏷

    ● **S62.312**   Displaced fracture of base of third metacarpal bone, right hand B, K, P 🏷, B 🏷

    ● **S62.313**   Displaced fracture of base of third metacarpal bone, left hand B, K, P 🏷, B 🏷

    ● **S62.314**   Displaced fracture of base of fourth metacarpal bone, right hand B, K, P 🏷, B 🏷

    ● **S62.315**   Displaced fracture of base of fourth metacarpal bone, left hand B, K, P 🏷, B 🏷

    ● **S62.316**   Displaced fracture of base of fifth metacarpal bone, right hand B, K, P 🏷, B 🏷

    ● **S62.317**   Displaced fracture of base of fifth metacarpal bone, left hand B, K, P 🏷, B 🏷

    ● **S62.318**   Displaced fracture of base of other metacarpal bone B, K, P 🏷, B 🏷
          Displaced fracture of base of specified metacarpal bone with unspecified laterality

    ● **S62.319**   Displaced fracture of base of unspecified metacarpal bone B, K, P 🏷, B 🏷

  ● **S62.32**   Displaced fracture of shaft of other metacarpal bone

    ● **S62.320**   Displaced fracture of shaft of second metacarpal bone, right hand B, K, P 🏷, B 🏷

    ● **S62.321**   Displaced fracture of shaft of second metacarpal bone, left hand B, K, P 🏷, B 🏷

    ● **S62.322**   Displaced fracture of shaft of third metacarpal bone, right hand B, K, P 🏷, B 🏷

    ● **S62.323**   Displaced fracture of shaft of third metacarpal bone, left hand B, K, P 🏷, B 🏷

    ● **S62.324**   Displaced fracture of shaft of fourth metacarpal bone, right hand B, K, P 🏷, B 🏷

    ● **S62.325**   Displaced fracture of shaft of fourth metacarpal bone, left hand B, K, P 🏷, B 🏷

    ● **S62.326**   Displaced fracture of shaft of fifth metacarpal bone, right hand B, K, P 🏷, B 🏷

    ● **S62.327**   Displaced fracture of shaft of fifth metacarpal bone, left hand B, K, P 🏷, B 🏷

    ● **S62.328**   Displaced fracture of shaft of other metacarpal bone B, K, P 🏷, B 🏷
          Displaced fracture of shaft of specified metacarpal bone with unspecified laterality

    ● **S62.329**   Displaced fracture of shaft of unspecified metacarpal bone B, K, P 🏷, B 🏷

  ● **S62.33**   Displaced fracture of neck of other metacarpal bone

    ● **S62.330**   Displaced fracture of neck of second metacarpal bone, right hand B, K, P 🏷, B 🏷

    ● **S62.331**   Displaced fracture of neck of second metacarpal bone, left hand B, K, P 🏷, B 🏷

    ● **S62.332**   Displaced fracture of neck of third metacarpal bone, right hand B, K, P 🏷, B 🏷

    ● **S62.333**   Displaced fracture of neck of third metacarpal bone, left hand B, K, P 🏷, B 🏷

    ● **S62.334**   Displaced fracture of neck of fourth metacarpal bone, right hand B, K, P 🏷, B 🏷

    ● **S62.335**   Displaced fracture of neck of fourth metacarpal bone, left hand B, K, P 🏷, B 🏷

    ● **S62.336**   Displaced fracture of neck of fifth metacarpal bone, right hand B, K, P 🏷, B 🏷

    ● **S62.337**   Displaced fracture of neck of fifth metacarpal bone, left hand B, K, P 🏷, B 🏷

    ● **S62.338**   Displaced fracture of neck of other metacarpal bone B, K, P 🏷, B 🏷
          Displaced fracture of neck of specified metacarpal bone with unspecified laterality

    ● **S62.339**   Displaced fracture of neck of unspecified metacarpal bone B, K, P 🏷, B 🏷

- ● **S62.34**   Nondisplaced fracture of base of other metacarpal bone
  - ● **S62.340**   Nondisplaced fracture of base of second metacarpal bone, right hand
    B, K, P 🔵, B 🔵
  - ● **S62.341**   Nondisplaced fracture of base of second metacarpal bone, left hand
    B, K, P 🔵, B 🔵
  - ● **S62.342**   Nondisplaced fracture of base of third metacarpal bone, right hand
    B, K, P 🔵, B 🔵
  - ● **S62.343**   Nondisplaced fracture of base of third metacarpal bone, left hand B, K, P 🔵, B 🔵
  - ● **S62.344**   Nondisplaced fracture of base of fourth metacarpal bone, right hand
    B, K, P 🔵, B 🔵
  - ● **S62.345**   Nondisplaced fracture of base of fourth metacarpal bone, left hand
    B, K, P 🔵, B 🔵
  - ● **S62.346**   Nondisplaced fracture of base of fifth metacarpal bone, right hand
    B, K, P 🔵, B 🔵
  - ● **S62.347**   Nondisplaced fracture of base of fifth metacarpal bone, left hand B, K, P 🔵, B 🔵
  - ● **S62.348**   Nondisplaced fracture of base of other metacarpal bone B, K, P 🔵, B 🔵
    Nondisplaced fracture of base of specified metacarpal bone with unspecified laterality
  - ● **S62.349**   Nondisplaced fracture of base of unspecified metacarpal bone
    B, K, P 🔵, B 🔵
- ● **S62.35**   Nondisplaced fracture of shaft of other metacarpal bone
  - ● **S62.350**   Nondisplaced fracture of shaft of second metacarpal bone, right hand
    B, K, P 🔵, B 🔵
  - ● **S62.351**   Nondisplaced fracture of shaft of second metacarpal bone, left hand
    B, K, P 🔵, B 🔵
  - ● **S62.352**   Nondisplaced fracture of shaft of third metacarpal bone, right hand
    B, K, P 🔵, B 🔵
  - ● **S62.353**   Nondisplaced fracture of shaft of third metacarpal bone, left hand
    B, K, P 🔵, B 🔵
  - ● **S62.354**   Nondisplaced fracture of shaft of fourth metacarpal bone, right hand
    B, K, P 🔵, B 🔵
  - ● **S62.355**   Nondisplaced fracture of shaft of fourth metacarpal bone, left hand
    B, K, P 🔵, B 🔵
  - ● **S62.356**   Nondisplaced fracture of shaft of fifth metacarpal bone, right hand
    B, K, P 🔵, B 🔵
  - ● **S62.357**   Nondisplaced fracture of shaft of fifth metacarpal bone, left hand B, K, P 🔵, B 🔵
  - ● **S62.358**   Nondisplaced fracture of shaft of other metacarpal bone B, K, P 🔵, B 🔵
    Nondisplaced fracture of shaft of specified metacarpal bone with unspecified laterality
  - ● **S62.359**   Nondisplaced fracture of shaft of unspecified metacarpal bone
    B, K, P 🔵, B 🔵

- ● **S62.36**   Nondisplaced fracture of neck of other metacarpal bone
  - ● **S62.360**   Nondisplaced fracture of neck of second metacarpal bone, right hand
    B, K, P 🔵, B 🔵
  - ● **S62.361**   Nondisplaced fracture of neck of second metacarpal bone, left hand
    B, K, P 🔵, B 🔵
  - ● **S62.362**   Nondisplaced fracture of neck of third metacarpal bone, right hand
    B, K, P 🔵, B 🔵
  - ● **S62.363**   Nondisplaced fracture of neck of third metacarpal bone, left hand
    B, K, P 🔵, B 🔵
  - ● **S62.364**   Nondisplaced fracture of neck of fourth metacarpal bone, right hand
    B, K, P 🔵, B 🔵
  - ● **S62.365**   Nondisplaced fracture of neck of fourth metacarpal bone, left hand
    B, K, P 🔵, B 🔵
  - ● **S62.366**   Nondisplaced fracture of neck of fifth metacarpal bone, right hand
    B, K, P 🔵, B 🔵
  - ● **S62.367**   Nondisplaced fracture of neck of fifth metacarpal bone, left hand B, K, P 🔵, B 🔵
  - ● **S62.368**   Nondisplaced fracture of neck of other metacarpal bone B, K, P 🔵, B 🔵
    Nondisplaced fracture of neck of specified metacarpal bone with unspecified laterality
  - ● **S62.369**   Nondisplaced fracture of neck of unspecified metacarpal bone
    B, K, P 🔵, B 🔵
- ● **S62.39**   Other fracture of other metacarpal bone
  - ● **S62.390**   Other fracture of second metacarpal bone, right hand B, K, P 🔵, B 🔵
  - ● **S62.391**   Other fracture of second metacarpal bone, left hand B, K, P 🔵, B 🔵
  - ● **S62.392**   Other fracture of third metacarpal bone, right hand B, K, P 🔵, B 🔵
  - ● **S62.393**   Other fracture of third metacarpal bone, left hand B, K, P 🔵, B 🔵
  - ● **S62.394**   Other fracture of fourth metacarpal bone, right hand B, K, P 🔵, B 🔵
  - ● **S62.395**   Other fracture of fourth metacarpal bone, left hand B, K, P 🔵, B 🔵
  - ● **S62.396**   Other fracture of fifth metacarpal bone, right hand B, K, P 🔵, B 🔵
  - ● **S62.397**   Other fracture of fifth metacarpal bone, left hand B, K, P 🔵, B 🔵
  - ● **S62.398**   Other fracture of other metacarpal bone B, K, P 🔵, B 🔵
    Other fracture of specified metacarpal bone with unspecified laterality
  - ● **S62.399**   Other fracture of unspecified metacarpal bone B, K, P 🔵, B 🔵
- ● **S62.5**   **Fracture of thumb**
  - (Ex) **For category S62.5 CC codes S62.5[B]:** S62.501-S62.669[A,B], S62.90X[A], S62.91X-S62.92X[A,B] **For S62.5[K,P]:** See S02.0[K]
  - ● **S62.50**   Fracture of unspecified phalanx of thumb
    - ● **S62.501**   Fracture of unspecified phalanx of right thumb B, K, P 🔵, B 🔵
    - ● **S62.502**   Fracture of unspecified phalanx of left thumb B, K, P 🔵, B 🔵
    - ● **S62.509**   Fracture of unspecified phalanx of unspecified thumb B, K, P 🔵, B 🔵

N Newborn Age: 0   **P** Pediatric Age: 0–17   **M** Maternity DX: 12–55   **A** Adult Age: 15–124   ♀ Females Only   ♂ Males Only

🔵 Complication\Comorbidity   🔵 Major C\C   (Ex) CC/MCC Exclusions   🔵 Hospital-Acquired Condition

1333

CHAPTER 19 (S00-T88)

● **S62.51**   Fracture of proximal phalanx of thumb

   ● **S62.511**   Displaced fracture of proximal phalanx of right thumb B, K, P 🔶, B 🔷

   ● **S62.512**   Displaced fracture of proximal phalanx of left thumb B, K, P 🔶, B 🔷

   ● **S62.513**   Displaced fracture of proximal phalanx of unspecified thumb B, K, P 🔶, B 🔷

   ● **S62.514**   Nondisplaced fracture of proximal phalanx of right thumb B, K, P 🔶, B 🔷

   ● **S62.515**   Nondisplaced fracture of proximal phalanx of left thumb B, K, P 🔶, B 🔷

   ● **S62.516**   Nondisplaced fracture of proximal phalanx of unspecified thumb B, K, P 🔶, B 🔷

● **S62.52**   Fracture of distal phalanx of thumb

   ● **S62.521**   Displaced fracture of distal phalanx of right thumb B, K, P 🔶, B 🔷

   ● **S62.522**   Displaced fracture of distal phalanx of left thumb B, K, P 🔶, B 🔷

   ● **S62.523**   Displaced fracture of distal phalanx of unspecified thumb B, K, P 🔶, B 🔷

   ● **S62.524**   Nondisplaced fracture of distal phalanx of right thumb B, K, P 🔶, B 🔷

   ● **S62.525**   Nondisplaced fracture of distal phalanx of left thumb B, K, P 🔶, B 🔷

   ● **S62.526**   Nondisplaced fracture of distal phalanx of unspecified thumb B, K, P 🔶, B 🔷

● **S62.6**   Fracture of other and unspecified finger(s)

   Excludes2   fracture of thumb (S62.5-)

   Ⓔⓧ **For category S62.6 CC codes S62.6[B]: See S62.5[B] For S62.5[K,P]: See S02.0[K]**

  ● **S62.60**   Fracture of unspecified phalanx of finger

    ● **S62.600**   Fracture of unspecified phalanx of right index finger B, K, P 🔶, B 🔷

    ● **S62.601**   Fracture of unspecified phalanx of left index finger B, K, P 🔶, B 🔷

    ● **S62.602**   Fracture of unspecified phalanx of right middle finger B, K, P 🔶, B 🔷

    ● **S62.603**   Fracture of unspecified phalanx of left middle finger B, K, P 🔶, B 🔷

    ● **S62.604**   Fracture of unspecified phalanx of right ring finger B, K, P 🔶, B 🔷

    ● **S62.605**   Fracture of unspecified phalanx of left ring finger B, K, P 🔶, B 🔷

    ● **S62.606**   Fracture of unspecified phalanx of right little finger B, K, P 🔶, B 🔷

    ● **S62.607**   Fracture of unspecified phalanx of left little finger B, K, P 🔶, B 🔷

    ● **S62.608**   Fracture of unspecified phalanx of other finger B, K, P 🔶, B 🔷

       Fracture of unspecified phalanx of specified finger with unspecified laterality

    ● **S62.609**   Fracture of unspecified phalanx of unspecified finger B, K, P 🔶, B 🔷

● **S62.61**   Displaced fracture of proximal phalanx of finger

   ● **S62.610**   Displaced fracture of proximal phalanx of right index finger B, K, P 🔶, B 🔷

   ● **S62.611**   Displaced fracture of proximal phalanx of left index finger B, K, P 🔶, B 🔷

   ● **S62.612**   Displaced fracture of proximal phalanx of right middle finger B, K, P 🔶, B 🔷

   ● **S62.613**   Displaced fracture of proximal phalanx of left middle finger B, K, P 🔶, B 🔷

   ● **S62.614**   Displaced fracture of proximal phalanx of right ring finger B, K, P 🔶, B 🔷

   ● **S62.615**   Displaced fracture of proximal phalanx of left ring finger B, K, P 🔶, B 🔷

   ● **S62.616**   Displaced fracture of proximal phalanx of right little finger B, K, P 🔶, B 🔷

   ● **S62.617**   Displaced fracture of proximal phalanx of left little finger B, K, P 🔶, B 🔷

   ● **S62.618**   Displaced fracture of proximal phalanx of other finger B, K, P 🔶, B 🔷

      Displaced fracture of proximal phalanx of specified finger with unspecified laterality

   ● **S62.619**   Displaced fracture of proximal phalanx of unspecified finger B, K, P 🔶, B 🔷

● **S62.62**   Displaced fracture of medial phalanx of finger

   ● **S62.620**   Displaced fracture of medial phalanx of right index finger B, K, P 🔶, B 🔷

   ● **S62.621**   Displaced fracture of medial phalanx of left index finger B, K, P 🔶, B 🔷

   ● **S62.622**   Displaced fracture of medial phalanx of right middle finger B, K, P 🔶, B 🔷

   ● **S62.623**   Displaced fracture of medial phalanx of left middle finger B, K, P 🔶, B 🔷

   ● **S62.624**   Displaced fracture of medial phalanx of right ring finger B, K, P 🔶, B 🔷

   ● **S62.625**   Displaced fracture of medial phalanx of left ring finger B, K, P 🔶, B 🔷

   ● **S62.626**   Displaced fracture of medial phalanx of right little finger B, K, P 🔶, B 🔷

   ● **S62.627**   Displaced fracture of medial phalanx of left little finger B, K, P 🔶, B 🔷

   ● **S62.628**   Displaced fracture of medial phalanx of other finger B, K, P 🔶, B 🔷

      Displaced fracture of medial phalanx of specified finger with unspecified laterality

   ● **S62.629**   Displaced fracture of medial phalanx of unspecified finger B, K, P 🔶, B 🔷

● **S62.63**   Displaced fracture of distal phalanx of finger

   ● **S62.630**   Displaced fracture of distal phalanx of right index finger B, K, P 🔶, B 🔷

   ● **S62.631**   Displaced fracture of distal phalanx of left index finger B, K, P 🔶, B 🔷

   ● **S62.632**   Displaced fracture of distal phalanx of right middle finger B, K, P 🔶, B 🔷

   ● **S62.633**   Displaced fracture of distal phalanx of left middle finger B, K, P 🔶, B 🔷

◀ New   ◀ Revised   ~~deleted~~ Deleted   Excludes 1   Excludes 2   Includes   Use additional   Code first   Code also   Unspecified

OGCR Official Guidelines   ● Unacceptable Principal Diagnosis   X Assign placeholder X   ● Use Additional Character(s)   🔷 Manifestation Code   **Coding Clinic**

● S62.634   Displaced fracture of distal phalanx of right ring finger B, K, P 🪙, B 🪙

● S62.635   Displaced fracture of distal phalanx of left ring finger B, K, P 🪙, B 🪙

● S62.636   Displaced fracture of distal phalanx of right little finger B, K, P 🪙, B 🪙

● S62.637   Displaced fracture of distal phalanx of left little finger B, K, P 🪙, B 🪙

● S62.638   Displaced fracture of distal phalanx of other finger B, K, P 🪙, B 🪙

    Displaced fracture of distal phalanx of specified finger with unspecified laterality

● S62.639   Displaced fracture of distal phalanx of unspecified finger B, K, P 🪙, B 🪙

● S62.64   Nondisplaced fracture of proximal phalanx of finger

● S62.640   Nondisplaced fracture of proximal phalanx of right index finger B, K, P 🪙, B 🪙

● S62.641   Nondisplaced fracture of proximal phalanx of left index finger B, K, P 🪙, B 🪙

● S62.642   Nondisplaced fracture of proximal phalanx of right middle finger B, K, P 🪙, B 🪙

● S62.643   Nondisplaced fracture of proximal phalanx of left middle finger B, K, P 🪙, B 🪙

● S62.644   Nondisplaced fracture of proximal phalanx of right ring finger B, K, P 🪙, B 🪙

● S62.645   Nondisplaced fracture of proximal phalanx of left ring finger B, K, P 🪙, B 🪙

● S62.646   Nondisplaced fracture of proximal phalanx of right little finger B, K, P 🪙, B 🪙

● S62.647   Nondisplaced fracture of proximal phalanx of left little finger B, K, P 🪙, B 🪙

● S62.648   Nondisplaced fracture of proximal phalanx of other finger B, K, P 🪙, B 🪙

    Nondisplaced fracture of proximal phalanx of specified finger with unspecified laterality

● S62.649   Nondisplaced fracture of proximal phalanx of unspecified finger B, K, P 🪙, B 🪙

● S62.65   Nondisplaced fracture of medial phalanx of finger

● S62.650   Nondisplaced fracture of medial phalanx of right index finger B, K, P 🪙, B 🪙

● S62.651   Nondisplaced fracture of medial phalanx of left index finger B, K, P 🪙, B 🪙

● S62.652   Nondisplaced fracture of medial phalanx of right middle finger B, K, P 🪙, B 🪙

● S62.653   Nondisplaced fracture of medial phalanx of left middle finger B, K, P 🪙, B 🪙

● S62.654   Nondisplaced fracture of medial phalanx of right ring finger B, K, P 🪙, B 🪙

● S62.655   Nondisplaced fracture of medial phalanx of left ring finger B, K, P 🪙, B 🪙

● S62.656   Nondisplaced fracture of medial phalanx of right little finger B, K, P 🪙, B 🪙

● S62.657   Nondisplaced fracture of medial phalanx of left little finger B, K, P 🪙, B 🪙

● S62.658   Nondisplaced fracture of medial phalanx of other finger B, K, P 🪙, B 🪙

    Nondisplaced fracture of medial phalanx of specified finger with unspecified laterality

● S62.659   Nondisplaced fracture of medial phalanx of unspecified finger B, K, P 🪙, B 🪙

● S62.66   Nondisplaced fracture of distal phalanx of finger

● S62.660   Nondisplaced fracture of distal phalanx of right index finger B, K, P 🪙, B 🪙

● S62.661   Nondisplaced fracture of distal phalanx of left index finger B, K, P 🪙, B 🪙

● S62.662   Nondisplaced fracture of distal phalanx of right middle finger B, K, P 🪙, B 🪙

● S62.663   Nondisplaced fracture of distal phalanx of left middle finger B, K, P 🪙, B 🪙

● S62.664   Nondisplaced fracture of distal phalanx of right ring finger B, K, P 🪙, B 🪙

● S62.665   Nondisplaced fracture of distal phalanx of left ring finger B, K, P 🪙, B 🪙

● S62.666   Nondisplaced fracture of distal phalanx of right little finger B, K, P 🪙, B 🪙

● S62.667   Nondisplaced fracture of distal phalanx of left little finger B, K, P 🪙, B 🪙

● S62.668   Nondisplaced fracture of distal phalanx of other finger B, K, P 🪙, B 🪙

    Nondisplaced fracture of distal phalanx of specified finger with unspecified laterality

● S62.669   Nondisplaced fracture of distal phalanx of unspecified finger B, K, P 🪙, B 🪙

● S62.9   Unspecified fracture of wrist and hand

X ● S62.90   Unspecified fracture of unspecified wrist and hand B, K, P 🪙, B 🪙

    ⒺⓍ For S62.90[B]: S42.201-S42.266[A,B], S42.271-S42.279[A], S42.291-S42.309[A,B], S42.311-S42.319[A], S42.321-S42.476[A,B], S42.481-S42.489[A], S42.491-S42.92X[A,B], S49.001-S49.199[A], S52.001-S52.009[A,B,C], S52.021-S52.109[A,B,C], S52.121-S52.209[A,B,C], S52.211-S52.219[A], S52.221-S52.309[A,B,C], S52.311-S52.319[A], S52.321-S52.616[A,B,C], S52.691-S52.92X[A,B,C], S59.001-S59.299[A], S62.001-S62.92X[A,B]

    For S62.90[K,P]: See S02.0[K]

X ● S62.91   Unspecified fracture of right wrist and hand B, K, P 🪙, B 🪙

    ⒺⓍ For S62.91[B]: S62.501-S62.669[A,B], S62.90X[B], S62.91X-S62.92X[A,B] For S62.91[K,P]: See S02.0[K]

X ● S62.92   Unspecified fracture of left wrist and hand B, K, P 🪙, B 🪙

    ⒺⓍ For S62.92[B]: S62.91[B] For S62.92[K,P]: See S02.0[K]

N Newborn Age: 0   **P** Pediatric Age: 0–17   **M** Maternity DX: 12–55   **A** Adult Age: 15–124   ♀ Females Only   ♂ Males Only

🪙 Complication\Comorbidity   🪙 Major C\C   ⒺⓍ CC/MCC Exclusions   🪙 Hospital-Acquired Condition

1335

CHAPTER 19 (S00-T88)

A   B

Figure 19-14 Dislocation including displacement and subluxation. (From Grainger & Allison's Diagnostic Radiology: A Textbook of Medical Imaging, ed 4, Churchill Livingstone, 2001)

● S63   **Dislocation and sprain of joints and ligaments at wrist and hand level**

        Includes   avulsion of joint or ligament at wrist and hand level

                       laceration of cartilage, joint or ligament at wrist and hand level

                       sprain of cartilage, joint or ligament at wrist and hand level

                       traumatic hemarthrosis of joint or ligament at wrist and hand level

                       traumatic rupture of joint or ligament at wrist and hand level

                       traumatic subluxation of joint or ligament at wrist and hand level

                       traumatic tear of joint or ligament at wrist and hand level

    Code also any associated open wound

        Excludes2   strain of muscle, fascia and tendon of wrist and hand (S66.-)

    The appropriate 7th character is to be added to each code from category S63

> A   initial encounter
> D   subsequent encounter
> S   sequela

● S63.0   **Subluxation and dislocation of wrist and hand joints**

    ● S63.00   **Unspecified subluxation and dislocation of wrist and hand**
                 Dislocation of carpal bone NOS
                 Dislocation of distal end of radius NOS
                 Subluxation of carpal bone NOS
                 Subluxation of distal end of radius NOS

       ● S63.001   **Unspecified subluxation of right wrist and hand**

       ● S63.002   **Unspecified subluxation of left wrist and hand**

       ● S63.003   **Unspecified subluxation of unspecified wrist and hand**

       ● S63.004   **Unspecified dislocation of right wrist and hand**

       ● S63.005   **Unspecified dislocation of left wrist and hand**

       ● S63.006   **Unspecified dislocation of unspecified wrist and hand**

    ● S63.01   **Subluxation and dislocation of distal radioulnar joint**

       ● S63.011   **Subluxation of distal radioulnar joint of right wrist**

       ● S63.012   **Subluxation of distal radioulnar joint of left wrist**

       ● S63.013   **Subluxation of distal radioulnar joint of unspecified wrist**

       ● S63.014   **Dislocation of distal radioulnar joint of right wrist**

       ● S63.015   **Dislocation of distal radioulnar joint of left wrist**

       ● S63.016   **Dislocation of distal radioulnar joint of unspecified wrist**

    ● S63.02   **Subluxation and dislocation of radiocarpal joint**

       ● S63.021   **Subluxation of radiocarpal joint of right wrist**

       ● S63.022   **Subluxation of radiocarpal joint of left wrist**

       ● S63.023   **Subluxation of radiocarpal joint of unspecified wrist**

       ● S63.024   **Dislocation of radiocarpal joint of right wrist**

       ● S63.025   **Dislocation of radiocarpal joint of left wrist**

       ● S63.026   **Dislocation of radiocarpal joint of unspecified wrist**

    ● S63.03   **Subluxation and dislocation of midcarpal joint**

       ● S63.031   **Subluxation of midcarpal joint of right wrist**

       ● S63.032   **Subluxation of midcarpal joint of left wrist**

       ● S63.033   **Subluxation of midcarpal joint of unspecified wrist**

       ● S63.034   **Dislocation of midcarpal joint of right wrist**

       ● S63.035   **Dislocation of midcarpal joint of left wrist**

       ● S63.036   **Dislocation of midcarpal joint of unspecified wrist**

    ● S63.04   **Subluxation and dislocation of carpometacarpal joint of thumb**

        Excludes2   interphalangeal subluxation and dislocation of thumb (S63.1-)

       ● S63.041   **Subluxation of carpometacarpal joint of right thumb**

       ● S63.042   **Subluxation of carpometacarpal joint of left thumb**

       ● S63.043   **Subluxation of carpometacarpal joint of unspecified thumb**

       ● S63.044   **Dislocation of carpometacarpal joint of right thumb**

       ● S63.045   **Dislocation of carpometacarpal joint of left thumb**

       ● S63.046   **Dislocation of carpometacarpal joint of unspecified thumb**

    ● S63.05   **Subluxation and dislocation of other carpometacarpal joint**

        Excludes2   subluxation and dislocation of carpometacarpal joint of thumb (S63.04-)

       ● S63.051   **Subluxation of other carpometacarpal joint of right hand**

       ● S63.052   **Subluxation of other carpometacarpal joint of left hand**

       ● S63.053   **Subluxation of other carpometacarpal joint of unspecified hand**

       ● S63.054   **Dislocation of other carpometacarpal joint of right hand**

       ● S63.055   **Dislocation of other carpometacarpal joint of left hand**

       ● S63.056   **Dislocation of other carpometacarpal joint of unspecified hand**

◀ New   ◀▦ Revised   ~~deleted~~ Deleted   Excludes 1   Excludes 2   Includes   Use additional   Code first   Code also   Unspecified

1336   OGCR Official Guidelines   ● Unacceptable Principal Diagnosis   X Assign placeholder X   ● Use Additional Character(s)   ▸ Manifestation Code   **Coding Clinic**

- ● **S63.06**   Subluxation and dislocation of metacarpal (bone), proximal end
  - ● **S63.061**   Subluxation of metacarpal (bone), proximal end of right hand
  - ● **S63.062**   Subluxation of metacarpal (bone), proximal end of left hand
  - ● **S63.063**   Subluxation of metacarpal (bone), proximal end of unspecified hand
  - ● **S63.064**   Dislocation of metacarpal (bone), proximal end of right hand
  - ● **S63.065**   Dislocation of metacarpal (bone), proximal end of left hand
  - ● **S63.066**   Dislocation of metacarpal (bone), proximal end of unspecified hand
- ● **S63.07**   Subluxation and dislocation of distal end of ulna
  - ● **S63.071**   Subluxation of distal end of right ulna
  - ● **S63.072**   Subluxation of distal end of left ulna
  - ● **S63.073**   Subluxation of distal end of unspecified ulna
  - ● **S63.074**   Dislocation of distal end of right ulna
  - ● **S63.075**   Dislocation of distal end of left ulna
  - ● **S63.076**   Dislocation of distal end of unspecified ulna
- ● **S63.09**   Other subluxation and dislocation of wrist and hand
  - ● **S63.091**   Other subluxation of right wrist and hand
  - ● **S63.092**   Other subluxation of left wrist and hand
  - ● **S63.093**   Other subluxation of unspecified wrist and hand
  - ● **S63.094**   Other dislocation of right wrist and hand
  - ● **S63.095**   Other dislocation of left wrist and hand
  - ● **S63.096**   Other dislocation of unspecified wrist and hand
- ● **S63.1**   Subluxation and dislocation of thumb
  - ● **S63.10**   Unspecified subluxation and dislocation of thumb
    - ● **S63.101**   Unspecified subluxation of right thumb
    - ● **S63.102**   Unspecified subluxation of left thumb
    - ● **S63.103**   Unspecified subluxation of unspecified thumb
    - ● **S63.104**   Unspecified dislocation of right thumb
    - ● **S63.105**   Unspecified dislocation of left thumb
    - ● **S63.106**   Unspecified dislocation of unspecified thumb
  - ● **S63.11**   Subluxation and dislocation of metacarpophalangeal joint of thumb
    - ● **S63.111**   Subluxation of metacarpophalangeal joint of right thumb
    - ● **S63.112**   Subluxation of metacarpophalangeal joint of left thumb
    - ● **S63.113**   Subluxation of metacarpophalangeal joint of unspecified thumb
    - ● **S63.114**   Dislocation of metacarpophalangeal joint of right thumb
    - ● **S63.115**   Dislocation of metacarpophalangeal joint of left thumb
    - ● **S63.116**   Dislocation of metacarpophalangeal joint of unspecified thumb
  - ● **S63.12**   Subluxation and dislocation of unspecified interphalangeal joint of thumb
    - ● **S63.121**   Subluxation of unspecified interphalangeal joint of right thumb
    - ● **S63.122**   Subluxation of unspecified interphalangeal joint of left thumb
    - ● **S63.123**   Subluxation of unspecified interphalangeal joint of unspecified thumb
    - ● **S63.124**   Dislocation of unspecified interphalangeal joint of right thumb
    - ● **S63.125**   Dislocation of unspecified interphalangeal joint of left thumb
    - ● **S63.126**   Dislocation of unspecified interphalangeal joint of unspecified thumb
  - ● **S63.13**   Subluxation and dislocation of proximal interphalangeal joint of thumb
    - ● **S63.131**   Subluxation of proximal interphalangeal joint of right thumb
    - ● **S63.132**   Subluxation of proximal interphalangeal joint of left thumb
    - ● **S63.133**   Subluxation of proximal interphalangeal joint of unspecified thumb
    - ● **S63.134**   Dislocation of proximal interphalangeal joint of right thumb
    - ● **S63.135**   Dislocation of proximal interphalangeal joint of left thumb
    - ● **S63.136**   Dislocation of proximal interphalangeal joint of unspecified thumb
  - ● **S63.14**   Subluxation and dislocation of distal interphalangeal joint of thumb
    - ● **S63.141**   Subluxation of distal interphalangeal joint of right thumb
    - ● **S63.142**   Subluxation of distal interphalangeal joint of left thumb
    - ● **S63.143**   Subluxation of distal interphalangeal joint of unspecified thumb
    - ● **S63.144**   Dislocation of distal interphalangeal joint of right thumb
    - ● **S63.145**   Dislocation of distal interphalangeal joint of left thumb
    - ● **S63.146**   Dislocation of distal interphalangeal joint of unspecified thumb
- ● **S63.2**   Subluxation and dislocation of other finger(s)
  - **Excludes2**   subluxation and dislocation of thumb (S63.1-)
  - ● **S63.20**   Unspecified subluxation of other finger
    - ● **S63.200**   Unspecified subluxation of right index finger
    - ● **S63.201**   Unspecified subluxation of left index finger
    - ● **S63.202**   Unspecified subluxation of right middle finger
    - ● **S63.203**   Unspecified subluxation of left middle finger
    - ● **S63.204**   Unspecified subluxation of right ring finger
    - ● **S63.205**   Unspecified subluxation of left ring finger
    - ● **S63.206**   Unspecified subluxation of right little finger
    - ● **S63.207**   Unspecified subluxation of left little finger
    - ● **S63.208**   Unspecified subluxation of other finger
      Unspecified subluxation of specified finger with unspecified laterality
    - ● **S63.209**   Unspecified subluxation of unspecified finger

N Newborn Age: 0   P Pediatric Age: 0–17   M Maternity DX: 12–55   A Adult Age: 15–124   ♀ Females Only   ♂ Males Only

🅒 Complication\Comorbidity   🅜 Major C\C   (Ex) CC/MCC Exclusions   🅗 Hospital-Acquired Condition

● **S63.21** Subluxation of metacarpophalangeal joint of finger

　● **S63.210** Subluxation of metacarpophalangeal joint of right index finger

　● **S63.211** Subluxation of metacarpophalangeal joint of left index finger

　● **S63.212** Subluxation of metacarpophalangeal joint of right middle finger

　● **S63.213** Subluxation of metacarpophalangeal joint of left middle finger

　● **S63.214** Subluxation of metacarpophalangeal joint of right ring finger

　● **S63.215** Subluxation of metacarpophalangeal joint of left ring finger

　● **S63.216** Subluxation of metacarpophalangeal joint of right little finger

　● **S63.217** Subluxation of metacarpophalangeal joint of left little finger

　● **S63.218** Subluxation of metacarpophalangeal joint of other finger

　　　Subluxation of metacarpophalangeal joint of specified finger with unspecified laterality

　● **S63.219** Subluxation of metacarpophalangeal joint of unspecified finger

● **S63.22** Subluxation of unspecified interphalangeal joint of finger

　● **S63.220** Subluxation of unspecified interphalangeal joint of right index finger

　● **S63.221** Subluxation of unspecified interphalangeal joint of left index finger

　● **S63.222** Subluxation of unspecified interphalangeal joint of right middle finger

　● **S63.223** Subluxation of unspecified interphalangeal joint of left middle finger

　● **S63.224** Subluxation of unspecified interphalangeal joint of right ring finger

　● **S63.225** Subluxation of unspecified interphalangeal joint of left ring finger

　● **S63.226** Subluxation of unspecified interphalangeal joint of right little finger

　● **S63.227** Subluxation of unspecified interphalangeal joint of left little finger

　● **S63.228** Subluxation of unspecified interphalangeal joint of other finger

　　　Subluxation of unspecified interphalangeal joint of specified finger with unspecified laterality

　● **S63.229** Subluxation of unspecified interphalangeal joint of unspecified finger

● **S63.23** Subluxation of proximal interphalangeal joint of finger

　● **S63.230** Subluxation of proximal interphalangeal joint of right index finger

　● **S63.231** Subluxation of proximal interphalangeal joint of left index finger

● **S63.232** Subluxation of proximal interphalangeal joint of right middle finger

● **S63.233** Subluxation of proximal interphalangeal joint of left middle finger

● **S63.234** Subluxation of proximal interphalangeal joint of right ring finger

● **S63.235** Subluxation of proximal interphalangeal joint of left ring finger

● **S63.236** Subluxation of proximal interphalangeal joint of right little finger

● **S63.237** Subluxation of proximal interphalangeal joint of left little finger

● **S63.238** Subluxation of proximal interphalangeal joint of other finger

　　Subluxation of proximal interphalangeal joint of specified finger with unspecified laterality

● **S63.239** Subluxation of proximal interphalangeal joint of unspecified finger

● **S63.24** Subluxation of distal interphalangeal joint of finger

● **S63.240** Subluxation of distal interphalangeal joint of right index finger

● **S63.241** Subluxation of distal interphalangeal joint of left index finger

● **S63.242** Subluxation of distal interphalangeal joint of right middle finger

● **S63.243** Subluxation of distal interphalangeal joint of left middle finger

● **S63.244** Subluxation of distal interphalangeal joint of right ring finger

● **S63.245** Subluxation of distal interphalangeal joint of left ring finger

● **S63.246** Subluxation of distal interphalangeal joint of right little finger

● **S63.247** Subluxation of distal interphalangeal joint of left little finger

● **S63.248** Subluxation of distal interphalangeal joint of other finger

　　Subluxation of distal interphalangeal joint of specified finger with unspecified laterality

● **S63.249** Subluxation of distal interphalangeal joint of unspecified finger

● **S63.25** Unspecified dislocation of other finger

● **S63.250** Unspecified dislocation of right index finger

● **S63.251** Unspecified dislocation of left index finger

● **S63.252** Unspecified dislocation of right middle finger

● **S63.253** Unspecified dislocation of left middle finger

● **S63.254** Unspecified dislocation of right ring finger

● **S63.255** Unspecified dislocation of left ring finger

● **S63.256** Unspecified dislocation of right little finger

● **S63.257** Unspecified dislocation of left little finger

CHAPTER 19 (S00-T88)

● S63.258   Unspecified dislocation of other
finger
     Unspecified dislocation of specified
finger with unspecified
laterality

● S63.259   Unspecified dislocation of unspecified
finger
     Unspecified dislocation of specified
finger with unspecified
laterality

● S63.26   Dislocation of metacarpophalangeal joint of
finger

   ● S63.260   Dislocation of metacarpophalangeal
joint of right index finger

   ● S63.261   Dislocation of metacarpophalangeal
joint of left index finger

   ● S63.262   Dislocation of metacarpophalangeal
joint of right middle finger

   ● S63.263   Dislocation of metacarpophalangeal
joint of left middle finger

   ● S63.264   Dislocation of metacarpophalangeal
joint of right ring finger

   ● S63.265   Dislocation of metacarpophalangeal
joint of left ring finger

   ● S63.266   Dislocation of metacarpophalangeal
joint of right little finger

   ● S63.267   Dislocation of metacarpophalangeal
joint of left little finger

   ● S63.268   Dislocation of metacarpophalangeal
joint of other finger
     Dislocation of metacarpophalangeal
joint of specified finger with
unspecified laterality

   ● S63.269   Dislocation of metacarpophalangeal
joint of unspecified finger

● S63.27   Dislocation of unspecified interphalangeal joint
of finger

   ● S63.270   Dislocation of unspecified
interphalangeal joint of right index
finger

   ● S63.271   Dislocation of unspecified
interphalangeal joint of left index
finger

   ● S63.272   Dislocation of unspecified
interphalangeal joint of right middle
finger

   ● S63.273   Dislocation of unspecified
interphalangeal joint of left middle
finger

   ● S63.274   Dislocation of unspecified
interphalangeal joint of right ring
finger

   ● S63.275   Dislocation of unspecified
interphalangeal joint of left ring
finger

   ● S63.276   Dislocation of unspecified
interphalangeal joint of right little
finger

   ● S63.277   Dislocation of unspecified
interphalangeal joint of left little
finger

   ● S63.278   Dislocation of unspecified
interphalangeal joint of other finger
     Dislocation of unspecified
interphalangeal joint
of specified finger with
unspecified laterality

   ● S63.279   Dislocation of unspecified
interphalangeal joint of unspecified
finger
     Dislocation of unspecified
interphalangeal joint of specified
finger without specified laterality

● S63.28   Dislocation of proximal interphalangeal joint
of finger

   ● S63.280   Dislocation of proximal
interphalangeal joint of right index
finger

   ● S63.281   Dislocation of proximal
interphalangeal joint of left index
finger

   ● S63.282   Dislocation of proximal
interphalangeal joint of right middle
finger

   ● S63.283   Dislocation of proximal
interphalangeal joint of left middle
finger

   ● S63.284   Dislocation of proximal
interphalangeal joint of right ring
finger

   ● S63.285   Dislocation of proximal
interphalangeal joint of left ring
finger

   ● S63.286   Dislocation of proximal
interphalangeal joint of right little
finger

   ● S63.287   Dislocation of proximal
interphalangeal joint of left little
finger

   ● S63.288   Dislocation of proximal
interphalangeal joint of other finger
     Dislocation of proximal
interphalangeal joint
of specified finger with
unspecified laterality

   ● S63.289   Dislocation of proximal
interphalangeal joint of unspecified
finger

● S63.29   Dislocation of distal interphalangeal joint of
finger

   ● S63.290   Dislocation of distal interphalangeal
joint of right index finger

   ● S63.291   Dislocation of distal interphalangeal
joint of left index finger

   ● S63.292   Dislocation of distal interphalangeal
joint of right middle finger

   ● S63.293   Dislocation of distal interphalangeal
joint of left middle finger

   ● S63.294   Dislocation of distal interphalangeal
joint of right ring finger

   ● S63.295   Dislocation of distal interphalangeal
joint of left ring finger

   ● S63.296   Dislocation of distal interphalangeal
joint of right little finger

   ● S63.297   Dislocation of distal interphalangeal
joint of left little finger

   ● S63.298   Dislocation of distal interphalangeal
joint of other finger
     Dislocation of distal interphalangeal
joint of specified finger with
unspecified laterality

   ● S63.299   Dislocation of distal interphalangeal
joint of unspecified finger

● S63.3   Traumatic rupture of ligament of wrist

   ● S63.30   Traumatic rupture of unspecified ligament of
wrist

     ● S63.301   Traumatic rupture of unspecified
ligament of right wrist

     ● S63.302   Traumatic rupture of unspecified
ligament of left wrist

     ● S63.309   Traumatic rupture of unspecified
ligament of unspecified wrist

N   Newborn Age: 0   **P**   Pediatric Age: 0–17   **M**   Maternity DX: 12–55   **A**   Adult Age: 15–124   ♀   Females Only   ♂   Males Only

🦚   Complication\Comorbidity   🦚   Major C\C   (Ex)   CC/MCC Exclusions   🦚   Hospital-Acquired Condition   **1339**

● S63.31 Traumatic rupture of collateral ligament of wrist
  ● S63.311 Traumatic rupture of collateral ligament of right wrist
  ● S63.312 Traumatic rupture of collateral ligament of left wrist
  ● S63.319 Traumatic rupture of collateral ligament of unspecified wrist
● S63.32 Traumatic rupture of radiocarpal ligament
  ● S63.321 Traumatic rupture of right radiocarpal ligament
  ● S63.322 Traumatic rupture of left radiocarpal ligament
  ● S63.329 Traumatic rupture of unspecified radiocarpal ligament
● S63.33 Traumatic rupture of ulnocarpal (palmar) ligament
  ● S63.331 Traumatic rupture of right ulnocarpal (palmar) ligament
  ● S63.332 Traumatic rupture of left ulnocarpal (palmar) ligament
  ● S63.339 Traumatic rupture of unspecified ulnocarpal (palmar) ligament
● S63.39 Traumatic rupture of other ligament of wrist
  ● S63.391 Traumatic rupture of other ligament of right wrist
  ● S63.392 Traumatic rupture of other ligament of left wrist
  ● S63.399 Traumatic rupture of other ligament of unspecified wrist
● S63.4 Traumatic rupture of ligament of finger at metacarpophalangeal and interphalangeal joint(s)
● S63.40 Traumatic rupture of unspecified ligament of finger at metacarpophalangeal and interphalangeal joint
  ● S63.400 Traumatic rupture of unspecified ligament of right index finger at metacarpophalangeal and interphalangeal joint
  ● S63.401 Traumatic rupture of unspecified ligament of left index finger at metacarpophalangeal and interphalangeal joint
  ● S63.402 Traumatic rupture of unspecified ligament of right middle finger at metacarpophalangeal and interphalangeal joint
  ● S63.403 Traumatic rupture of unspecified ligament of left middle finger at metacarpophalangeal and interphalangeal joint
  ● S63.404 Traumatic rupture of unspecified ligament of right ring finger at metacarpophalangeal and interphalangeal joint
  ● S63.405 Traumatic rupture of unspecified ligament of left ring finger at metacarpophalangeal and interphalangeal joint
  ● S63.406 Traumatic rupture of unspecified ligament of right little finger at metacarpophalangeal and interphalangeal joint

● S63.407 Traumatic rupture of unspecified ligament of left little finger at metacarpophalangeal and interphalangeal joint
● S63.408 Traumatic rupture of unspecified ligament of other finger at metacarpophalangeal and interphalangeal joint
    Traumatic rupture of unspecified ligament of specified finger with unspecified laterality at metacarpophalangeal and interphalangeal joint
● S63.409 Traumatic rupture of unspecified ligament of unspecified finger at metacarpophalangeal and interphalangeal joint
● S63.41 Traumatic rupture of collateral ligament of finger at metacarpophalangeal and interphalangeal joint
  ● S63.410 Traumatic rupture of collateral ligament of right index finger at metacarpophalangeal and interphalangeal joint
  ● S63.411 Traumatic rupture of collateral ligament of left index finger at metacarpophalangeal and interphalangeal joint
  ● S63.412 Traumatic rupture of collateral ligament of right middle finger at metacarpophalangeal and interphalangeal joint
  ● S63.413 Traumatic rupture of collateral ligament of left middle finger at metacarpophalangeal and interphalangeal joint
  ● S63.414 Traumatic rupture of collateral ligament of right ring finger at metacarpophalangeal and interphalangeal joint
  ● S63.415 Traumatic rupture of collateral ligament of left ring finger at metacarpophalangeal and interphalangeal joint
  ● S63.416 Traumatic rupture of collateral ligament of right little finger at metacarpophalangeal and interphalangeal joint
  ● S63.417 Traumatic rupture of collateral ligament of left little finger at metacarpophalangeal and interphalangeal joint
  ● S63.418 Traumatic rupture of collateral ligament of other finger at metacarpophalangeal and interphalangeal joint
    Traumatic rupture of collateral ligament of specified finger with unspecified laterality at metacarpophalangeal and interphalangeal joint
  ● S63.419 Traumatic rupture of collateral ligament of unspecified finger at metacarpophalangeal and interphalangeal joint

● **S63.42**   **Traumatic rupture of palmar ligament of finger at metacarpophalangeal and interphalangeal joint**

    ● **S63.420**   Traumatic rupture of palmar ligament of right index finger at metacarpophalangeal and interphalangeal joint

    ● **S63.421**   Traumatic rupture of palmar ligament of left index finger at metacarpophalangeal and interphalangeal joint

    ● **S63.422**   Traumatic rupture of palmar ligament of right middle finger at metacarpophalangeal and interphalangeal joint

    ● **S63.423**   Traumatic rupture of palmar ligament of left middle finger at metacarpophalangeal and interphalangeal joint

    ● **S63.424**   Traumatic rupture of palmar ligament of right ring finger at metacarpophalangeal and interphalangeal joint

    ● **S63.425**   Traumatic rupture of palmar ligament of left ring finger at metacarpophalangeal and interphalangeal joint

    ● **S63.426**   Traumatic rupture of palmar ligament of right little finger at metacarpophalangeal and interphalangeal joint

    ● **S63.427**   Traumatic rupture of palmar ligament of left little finger at metacarpophalangeal and interphalangeal joint

    ● **S63.428**   Traumatic rupture of palmar ligament of other finger at metacarpophalangeal and interphalangeal joint

        Traumatic rupture of palmar ligament of specified finger with unspecified laterality at metacarpophalangeal and interphalangeal joint

    ● **S63.429**   Traumatic rupture of palmar ligament of unspecified finger at metacarpophalangeal and interphalangeal joint

● **S63.43**   **Traumatic rupture of volar plate of finger at metacarpophalangeal and interphalangeal joint**

    ● **S63.430**   Traumatic rupture of volar plate of right index finger at metacarpophalangeal and interphalangeal joint

    ● **S63.431**   Traumatic rupture of volar plate of left index finger at metacarpophalangeal and interphalangeal joint

    ● **S63.432**   Traumatic rupture of volar plate of right middle finger at metacarpophalangeal and interphalangeal joint

    ● **S63.433**   Traumatic rupture of volar plate of left middle finger at metacarpophalangeal and interphalangeal joint

    ● **S63.434**   Traumatic rupture of volar plate of right ring finger at metacarpophalangeal and interphalangeal joint

    ● **S63.435**   Traumatic rupture of volar plate of left ring finger at metacarpophalangeal and interphalangeal joint

    ● **S63.436**   Traumatic rupture of volar plate of right little finger at metacarpophalangeal and interphalangeal joint

    ● **S63.437**   Traumatic rupture of volar plate of left little finger at metacarpophalangeal and interphalangeal joint

    ● **S63.438**   Traumatic rupture of volar plate of other finger at metacarpophalangeal and interphalangeal joint

        Traumatic rupture of volar plate of specified finger with unspecified laterality at metacarpophalangeal and interphalangeal joint

    ● **S63.439**   Traumatic rupture of volar plate of unspecified finger at metacarpophalangeal and interphalangeal joint

● **S63.49**   **Traumatic rupture of other ligament of finger at metacarpophalangeal and interphalangeal joint**

    ● **S63.490**   Traumatic rupture of other ligament of right index finger at metacarpophalangeal and interphalangeal joint

    ● **S63.491**   Traumatic rupture of other ligament of left index finger at metacarpophalangeal and interphalangeal joint

    ● **S63.492**   Traumatic rupture of other ligament of right middle finger at metacarpophalangeal and interphalangeal joint

    ● **S63.493**   Traumatic rupture of other ligament of left middle finger at metacarpophalangeal and interphalangeal joint

    ● **S63.494**   Traumatic rupture of other ligament of right ring finger at metacarpophalangeal and interphalangeal joint

    ● **S63.495**   Traumatic rupture of other ligament of left ring finger at metacarpophalangeal and interphalangeal joint

    ● **S63.496**   Traumatic rupture of other ligament of right little finger at metacarpophalangeal and interphalangeal joint

    ● **S63.497**   Traumatic rupture of other ligament of left little finger at metacarpophalangeal and interphalangeal joint

    ● **S63.498**   Traumatic rupture of other ligament of other finger at metacarpophalangeal and interphalangeal joint

        Traumatic rupture of ligament of specified finger with unspecified laterality at metacarpophalangeal and interphalangeal joint

    ● **S63.499**   Traumatic rupture of other ligament of unspecified finger at metacarpophalangeal and interphalangeal joint

CHAPTER 19 (S00-T88)

- S63.5 Other and unspecified sprain of wrist
  - S63.50 Unspecified sprain of wrist
    - S63.501 Unspecified sprain of right wrist
    - S63.502 Unspecified sprain of left wrist
    - S63.509 Unspecified sprain of unspecified wrist
  - S63.51 Sprain of carpal (joint)
    - S63.511 Sprain of carpal joint of right wrist
    - S63.512 Sprain of carpal joint of left wrist
    - S63.519 Sprain of carpal joint of unspecified wrist
  - S63.52 Sprain of radiocarpal joint
    - Excludes1 traumatic rupture of radiocarpal ligament (S63.32-)
    - S63.521 Sprain of radiocarpal joint of right wrist
    - S63.522 Sprain of radiocarpal joint of left wrist
    - S63.529 Sprain of radiocarpal joint of unspecified wrist
  - S63.59 Other specified sprain of wrist
    - S63.591 Other specified sprain of right wrist
    - S63.592 Other specified sprain of left wrist
    - S63.599 Other specified sprain of unspecified wrist
- S63.6 Other and unspecified sprain of finger(s)
  - Excludes1 traumatic rupture of ligament of finger at metacarpophalangeal and interphalangeal joint(s) (S63.4-)
  - S63.60 Unspecified sprain of thumb
    - S63.601 Unspecified sprain of right thumb
    - S63.602 Unspecified sprain of left thumb
    - S63.609 Unspecified sprain of unspecified thumb
  - S63.61 Unspecified sprain of other and unspecified finger(s)
    - S63.610 Unspecified sprain of right index finger
    - S63.611 Unspecified sprain of left index finger
    - S63.612 Unspecified sprain of right middle finger
    - S63.613 Unspecified sprain of left middle finger
    - S63.614 Unspecified sprain of right ring finger
    - S63.615 Unspecified sprain of left ring finger
    - S63.616 Unspecified sprain of right little finger
    - S63.617 Unspecified sprain of left little finger
    - S63.618 Unspecified sprain of other finger
      Unspecified sprain of specified finger with unspecified laterality
    - S63.619 Unspecified sprain of unspecified finger
  - S63.62 Sprain of interphalangeal joint of thumb
    - S63.621 Sprain of interphalangeal joint of right thumb
    - S63.622 Sprain of interphalangeal joint of left thumb
    - S63.629 Sprain of interphalangeal joint of unspecified thumb
  - S63.63 Sprain of interphalangeal joint of other and unspecified finger(s)
    - S63.630 Sprain of interphalangeal joint of right index finger
    - S63.631 Sprain of interphalangeal joint of left index finger
    - S63.632 Sprain of interphalangeal joint of right middle finger
    - S63.633 Sprain of interphalangeal joint of left middle finger
    - S63.634 Sprain of interphalangeal joint of right ring finger
    - S63.635 Sprain of interphalangeal joint of left ring finger
    - S63.636 Sprain of interphalangeal joint of right little finger
    - S63.637 Sprain of interphalangeal joint of left little finger
    - S63.638 Sprain of interphalangeal joint of other finger
    - S63.639 Sprain of interphalangeal joint of unspecified finger
  - S63.64 Sprain of metacarpophalangeal joint of thumb
    - S63.641 Sprain of metacarpophalangeal joint of right thumb
    - S63.642 Sprain of metacarpophalangeal joint of left thumb
    - S63.649 Sprain of metacarpophalangeal joint of unspecified thumb
  - S63.65 Sprain of metacarpophalangeal joint of other and unspecified finger(s)
    - S63.650 Sprain of metacarpophalangeal joint of right index finger
    - S63.651 Sprain of metacarpophalangeal joint of left index finger
    - S63.652 Sprain of metacarpophalangeal joint of right middle finger
    - S63.653 Sprain of metacarpophalangeal joint of left middle finger
    - S63.654 Sprain of metacarpophalangeal joint of right ring finger
    - S63.655 Sprain of metacarpophalangeal joint of left ring finger
    - S63.656 Sprain of metacarpophalangeal joint of right little finger
    - S63.657 Sprain of metacarpophalangeal joint of left little finger
    - S63.658 Sprain of metacarpophalangeal joint of other finger
      Sprain of metacarpophalangeal joint of specified finger with unspecified laterality
    - S63.659 Sprain of metacarpophalangeal joint of unspecified finger
  - S63.68 Other sprain of thumb
    - S63.681 Other sprain of right thumb
    - S63.682 Other sprain of left thumb
    - S63.689 Other sprain of unspecified thumb

CHAPTER 19 (S00-T88)

◀ New   ◀‖‖ Revised   deleted Deleted   Excludes 1   Excludes 2   Includes   Use additional   Code first   Code also   Unspecified
OGCR Official Guidelines   ● Unacceptable Principal Diagnosis   X Assign placeholder X   ● Use Additional Character(s)   ▸ Manifestation Code   Coding Clinic

● S63.69   Other sprain of other and unspecified finger(s)
  ● S63.690   Other sprain of right index finger
  ● S63.691   Other sprain of left index finger
  ● S63.692   Other sprain of right middle finger
  ● S63.693   Other sprain of left middle finger
  ● S63.694   Other sprain of right ring finger
  ● S63.695   Other sprain of left ring finger
  ● S63.696   Other sprain of right little finger
  ● S63.697   Other sprain of left little finger
  ● S63.698   Other sprain of other finger
                Other sprain of specified finger with
                unspecified laterality
  ● S63.699   Other sprain of unspecified finger
● S63.8   Sprain of other part of wrist and hand
  ● S63.8X   Sprain of other part of wrist and hand
    ● S63.8X1   Sprain of other part of right wrist and
                hand
    ● S63.8X2   Sprain of other part of left wrist and
                hand
    ● S63.8X9   Sprain of other part of unspecified
                wrist and hand
● S63.9   Sprain of unspecified part of wrist and hand
  X ● S63.90   Sprain of unspecified part of unspecified wrist
              and hand
  X ● S63.91   Sprain of unspecified part of right wrist and
              hand
  X ● S63.92   Sprain of unspecified part of left wrist and
              hand

● S64   Injury of nerves at wrist and hand level
        The appropriate 7th character is to be added to each code from
        category S64

        | A | initial encounter |
        | D | subsequent encounter |
        | S | sequela |

        Code also any associated open wound (S61.-)
● S64.0   Injury of ulnar nerve at wrist and hand level
  X ● S64.00   Injury of ulnar nerve at wrist and hand level of
              unspecified arm
  X ● S64.01   Injury of ulnar nerve at wrist and hand level of
              right arm
  X ● S64.02   Injury of ulnar nerve at wrist and hand level of
              left arm
● S64.1   Injury of median nerve at wrist and hand level
  X ● S64.10   Injury of median nerve at wrist and hand level
              of unspecified arm
  X ● S64.11   Injury of median nerve at wrist and hand level
              of right arm
  X ● S64.12   Injury of median nerve at wrist and hand level
              of left arm
● S64.2   Injury of radial nerve at wrist and hand level
  X ● S64.20   Injury of radial nerve at wrist and hand level of
              unspecified arm
  X ● S64.21   Injury of radial nerve at wrist and hand level of
              right arm
  X ● S64.22   Injury of radial nerve at wrist and hand level of
              left arm
● S64.3   Injury of digital nerve of thumb
  X ● S64.30   Injury of digital nerve of unspecified thumb
  X ● S64.31   Injury of digital nerve of right thumb
  X ● S64.32   Injury of digital nerve of left thumb

● S64.4   Injury of digital nerve of other and unspecified finger
  X ● S64.40   Injury of digital nerve of unspecified finger
  ● S64.49   Injury of digital nerve of other finger
    ● S64.490   Injury of digital nerve of right index
                finger
    ● S64.491   Injury of digital nerve of left index
                finger
    ● S64.492   Injury of digital nerve of right middle
                finger
    ● S64.493   Injury of digital nerve of left middle
                finger
    ● S64.494   Injury of digital nerve of right ring
                finger
    ● S64.495   Injury of digital nerve of left ring
                finger
    ● S64.496   Injury of digital nerve of right little
                finger
    ● S64.497   Injury of digital nerve of left little
                finger
    ● S64.498   Injury of digital nerve of other finger
                Injury of digital nerve of specified
                finger with unspecified
                laterality
● S64.8   Injury of other nerves at wrist and hand level
  ● S64.8X   Injury of other nerves at wrist and hand level
    ● S64.8X1   Injury of other nerves at wrist and
                hand level of right arm
    ● S64.8X2   Injury of other nerves at wrist and
                hand level of left arm
    ● S64.8X9   Injury of other nerves at wrist and
                hand level of unspecified arm
● S64.9   Injury of unspecified nerve at wrist and hand level
  X ● S64.90   Injury of unspecified nerve at wrist and hand
              level of unspecified arm
  X ● S64.91   Injury of unspecified nerve at wrist and hand
              level of right arm
  X ● S64.92   Injury of unspecified nerve at wrist and hand
              level of left arm

● S65   Injury of blood vessels at wrist and hand level
        The appropriate 7th character is to be added to each code from
        category S65

        | A | initial encounter |
        | D | subsequent encounter |
        | S | sequela |

        Code also any associated open wound (S61.-)
● S65.0   Injury of ulnar artery at wrist and hand level
  ● S65.00   Unspecified injury of ulnar artery at wrist and
            hand level
    ● S65.001   Unspecified injury of ulnar artery at
                wrist and hand level of right arm A ⊘
                (Ex:) See S55.001
    ● S65.002   Unspecified injury of ulnar artery at
                wrist and hand level of left arm A ⊘
                (Ex:) See S55.002
    ● S65.009   Unspecified injury of ulnar artery at
                wrist and hand level of unspecified
                arm A ⊘
                (Ex:) See S55.009

● **S65.01** Laceration of ulnar artery at wrist and hand level
  ● **S65.011** Laceration of ulnar artery at wrist and hand level of right arm A 🌐
      (Ex) See S55.001
  ● **S65.012** Laceration of ulnar artery at wrist and hand level of left arm A 🌐
      (Ex) See S55.002
  ● **S65.019** Laceration of ulnar artery at wrist and hand level of <mark>unspecified</mark> arm A 🌐
      (Ex) See S55.009
● **S65.09** Other specified injury of ulnar artery at wrist and hand level
  ● **S65.091** Other specified injury of ulnar artery at wrist and hand level of right arm A 🌐
      (Ex) See S55.001
  ● **S65.092** Other specified injury of ulnar artery at wrist and hand level of left arm A 🌐
      (Ex) See S55.002
  ● **S65.099** Other specified injury of ulnar artery at wrist and hand level of <mark>unspecified</mark> arm A 🌐
      (Ex) See S55.009
● **S65.1** Injury of radial artery at wrist and hand level
  ● **S65.10** Unspecified injury of radial artery at wrist and hand level
    ● **S65.101** <mark>Unspecified</mark> injury of radial artery at wrist and hand level of right arm A 🌐
        (Ex) See S55.101
    ● **S65.102** <mark>Unspecified</mark> injury of radial artery at wrist and hand level of left arm A 🌐
        (Ex) See S55.102
    ● **S65.109** <mark>Unspecified</mark> injury of radial artery at wrist and hand level of unspecified arm A 🌐
        (Ex) See S55.109
  ● **S65.11** Laceration of radial artery at wrist and hand level
    ● **S65.111** Laceration of radial artery at wrist and hand level of right arm A 🌐
        (Ex) See S55.101
    ● **S65.112** Laceration of radial artery at wrist and hand level of left arm A 🌐
        (Ex) See S55.102
    ● **S65.119** Laceration of radial artery at wrist and hand level of <mark>unspecified</mark> arm A 🌐
        (Ex) See S55.109
  ● **S65.19** Other specified injury of radial artery at wrist and hand level
    ● **S65.191** Other specified injury of radial artery at wrist and hand level of right arm A 🌐
        (Ex) See S55.101
    ● **S65.192** Other specified injury of radial artery at wrist and hand level of left arm A 🌐
        (Ex) See S55.102
    ● **S65.199** Other specified injury of radial artery at wrist and hand level of <mark>unspecified</mark> arm A 🌐
        (Ex) See S55.109

● **S65.2** Injury of superficial palmar arch
  ● **S65.20** Unspecified injury of superficial palmar arch
    ● **S65.201** <mark>Unspecified</mark> injury of superficial palmar arch of right hand A 🌐
        (Ex) S45.301[A], S45.309-S45.311[A], S45.319-S45.391[A], S45.399-S45.801[A], S45.809-S45.811[A], S45.819-S45.891[A], S45.899-S45.901[A], S45.909-S45.911[A], S45.919-S45.991[A], S45.999[A], S55.201[A], S55.209-S55.211[A], S55.219-S55.291[A], S55.299-S55.801[A], S55.809-S55.811[A], S55.819-S55.891[A], S55.899-S55.901[A], S55.909-S55.911[A], S55.919-S55.991[A], S55.999[A], S65.201[A], S65.209-S65.211[A], S65.219-S65.291[A], S65.299-S65.301[A], S65.309-S65.311[A], S65.319- S65.391[A], S65.399[A], S65.801[A], S65.809-S65.811[A], S65.819-S65.891[A], S65.899-S65.901[A], S65.909-S65.911[A], S65.919-S65.991[A], S65.999[A]
    ● **S65.202** <mark>Unspecified</mark> injury of superficial palmar arch of left hand A 🌐
        (Ex) S45.302-S45.309[A], S45.312-S45.319[A], S45.392-S45.399[A], S45.802-S45.809[A], S45.812-S45.819[A], S45.892-S45.899[A], S45.902-S45.909[A], S45.912-S45.919[A], S45.992-S45.999[A], S55.202-S55.209[A], S55.212-S55.219[A], S55.292-S55.299[A], S55.802-S55.809[A], S55.812-S55.819[A], S55.892-S55.899[A], S55.902-S55.909[A], S55.912-S55.919[A], S55.992-S55.999[A], S65.202-S65.209[A], S65.212-S65.219[A], S65.292-S65.299[A], S65.302-S65.309[A], S65.312-S65.319[A], S65.392-S65.399[A], S65.802-S65.809[A], S65.812-S65.819[A], S65.892-S65.899[A], S65.902-S65.909[A], S65.912-S65.919[A], S65.992-S65.999[A]
    ● **S65.209** <mark>Unspecified</mark> injury of superficial palmar arch of unspecified hand A 🌐
        (Ex) S45.301-S45.999[A], S55.201-S55.999[A], S65.201-S65.399[A], S65.801-S65.999[A]
  ● **S65.21** Laceration of superficial palmar arch
    ● **S65.211** Laceration of superficial palmar arch of right hand A 🌐
        (Ex) See S65.201
    ● **S65.212** Laceration of superficial palmar arch of left hand A 🌐
        (Ex) See S65.202
    ● **S65.219** Laceration of superficial palmar arch of <mark>unspecified</mark> hand A 🌐
        (Ex) See S65.209
  ● **S65.29** Other specified injury of superficial palmar arch
    ● **S65.291** Other specified injury of superficial palmar arch of right hand A 🌐
        (Ex) See S65.201
    ● **S65.292** Other specified injury of superficial palmar arch of left hand A 🌐
        (Ex) See S65.202
    ● **S65.299** Other specified injury of superficial palmar arch of <mark>unspecified</mark> hand A 🌐
        (Ex) See S65.209
● **S65.3** Injury of deep palmar arch
  ● **S65.30** Unspecified injury of deep palmar arch
    ● **S65.301** <mark>Unspecified</mark> injury of deep palmar arch of right hand A 🌐
        (Ex) See S65.201
    ● **S65.302** <mark>Unspecified</mark> injury of deep palmar arch of left hand A 🌐
        (Ex) See S65.202
    ● **S65.309** <mark>Unspecified</mark> injury of deep palmar arch of unspecified hand A 🌐
        (Ex) See S65.209

● **S65.31**   Laceration of deep palmar arch
  ● **S65.311**   Laceration of deep palmar arch of right hand A 🐾
    (Ex:) See S65.201
  ● **S65.312**   Laceration of deep palmar arch of left hand A 🐾
    (Ex:) See S65.202
  ● **S65.319**   Laceration of deep palmar arch of unspecified hand A 🐾
    (Ex:) See S65.209

● **S65.39**   Other specified injury of deep palmar arch
  ● **S65.391**   Other specified injury of deep palmar arch of right hand A 🐾
    (Ex:) See S65.201
  ● **S65.392**   Other specified injury of deep palmar arch of left hand A 🐾
    (Ex:) See S65.202
  ● **S65.399**   Other specified injury of deep palmar arch of unspecified hand A 🐾
    (Ex:) See S65.209

● **S65.4**   Injury of blood vessel of thumb
 ● **S65.40**   Unspecified injury of blood vessel of thumb
  ● **S65.401**   Unspecified injury of blood vessel of right thumb A 🐾
    (Ex:) S45.301[A], S45.309-S45.311[A],
    S45.319-S45.391[A], S45.399-S45.801[A],
    S45.809-S45.811[A], S45.819-S45.891[A],
    S45.899-S45.901[A], S45.909-S45.911[A],
    S45.919-S45.991[A], S45.999[A], S55.201[A],
    S55.209-S55.211[A], S55.219-S55.291[A],
    S55.299-S55.801[A], S55.809-S55.811[A],
    S55.819-S55.891[A], S55.899-S55.901[A],
    S55.909-S55.911[A], S55.919-S55.991[A],
    S55.999[A], S65.401[A], S65.409-S65.411[A],
    S65.419-S65.491[A], S65.499-S65.500[A],
    S65.502[A], S65.504[A], S65.506[A],
    S65.508-S65.510[A], S65.512[A], S65.514[A],
    S65.516[A], S65.518-S65.590[A], S65.592[A],
    S65.594[A], S65.596[A], S65.598-S65.801[A],
    S65.809-S65.811[A], S65.819-S65.891[A],
    S65.899-S65.901[A], S65.909-S65.911[A],
    S65.919-S65.991[A], S65.999[A]
  ● **S65.402**   Unspecified injury of blood vessel of left thumb A 🐾
    (Ex:) S45.302-S45.309[A], S45.312-S45.319[A],
    S45.392-S45.399[A], S45.802-S45.809[A],
    S45.812-S45.819[A], S45.892-S45.899[A],
    S45.902-S45.909[A], S45.912-S45.919[A],
    S45.992-S45.999[A], S55.202-S55.209[A],
    S55.212-S55.219[A], S55.292-S55.299[A],
    S55.802-S55.809[A], S55.812-S55.819[A],
    S55.892-S55.899[A], S55.902-S55.909[A],
    S55.912-S55.919[A], S55.992-S55.999[A],
    S65.402-S65.409[A], S65.412-S65.419[A],
    S65.492-S65.499[A], S65.501[A], S65.503[A],
    S65.505[A], S65.507-S65.509[A], S65.511[A],
    S65.513[A], S65.515[A], S65.517-S65.519[A],
    S65.591[A], S65.593[A], S65.595[A],
    S65.597-S65.599[A], S65.802-S65.809[A],
    S65.812-S65.819[A], S65.892-S65.899[A],
    S65.902-S65.909[A], S65.912-S65.919[A],
    S65.992-S65.999[A]
  ● **S65.409**   Unspecified injury of blood vessel of unspecified thumb A 🐾
    (Ex:) S45.301-S45.999[A], S55.201-S55.999[A],
    S65.401-S65.999[A]

● **S65.41**   Laceration of blood vessel of thumb
  ● **S65.411**   Laceration of blood vessel of right thumb A 🐾
    (Ex:) See S65.401
  ● **S65.412**   Laceration of blood vessel of left thumb A 🐾
    (Ex:) See S65.402
  ● **S65.419**   Laceration of blood vessel of unspecified thumb A 🐾
    (Ex:) See S65.409

● **S65.49**   Other specified injury of blood vessel of thumb
  ● **S65.491**   Other specified injury of blood vessel of right thumb A 🐾
    (Ex:) See S65.401
  ● **S65.492**   Other specified injury of blood vessel of left thumb A 🐾
    (Ex:) See S65.402
  ● **S65.499**   Other specified injury of blood vessel of unspecified thumb A 🐾
    (Ex:) See S65.409

● **S65.5**   Injury of blood vessel of other and unspecified finger
 ● **S65.50**   Unspecified injury of blood vessel of other and unspecified finger
  ● **S65.500**   Unspecified injury of blood vessel of right index finger A 🐾
    (Ex:) See S65.401
  ● **S65.501**   Unspecified injury of blood vessel of left index finger A 🐾
    (Ex:) See S65.402
  ● **S65.502**   Unspecified injury of blood vessel of right middle finger A 🐾
    (Ex:) See S65.401
  ● **S65.503**   Unspecified injury of blood vessel of left middle finger A 🐾
    (Ex:) See S65.402
  ● **S65.504**   Unspecified injury of blood vessel of right ring finger A 🐾
    (Ex:) See S65.401
  ● **S65.505**   Unspecified injury of blood vessel of left ring finger A 🐾
    (Ex:) See S65.409
  ● **S65.506**   Unspecified injury of blood vessel of right little finger A 🐾
    (Ex:) See S65.401
  ● **S65.507**   Unspecified injury of blood vessel of left little finger A 🐾
    (Ex:) See S65.402
  ● **S65.508**   Unspecified injury of blood vessel of other finger A 🐾
    Unspecified injury of blood vessel of specified finger with unspecified laterality
    (Ex:) See S65.409
  ● **S65.509**   Unspecified injury of blood vessel of unspecified finger A 🐾
    (Ex:) See S65.409

● **S65.51**   Laceration of blood vessel of other and unspecified finger

    ● **S65.510**   Laceration of blood vessel of right index finger A 🦠
        (Ex:) See S65.401

    ● **S65.511**   Laceration of blood vessel of left index finger A 🦠
        (Ex:) See S65.402

    ● **S65.512**   Laceration of blood vessel of right middle finger A 🦠
        (Ex:) See S65.401

    ● **S65.513**   Laceration of blood vessel of left middle finger A 🦠
        (Ex:) See S65.402

    ● **S65.514**   Laceration of blood vessel of right ring finger A 🦠
        (Ex:) See S65.401

    ● **S65.515**   Laceration of blood vessel of left ring finger A 🦠
        (Ex:) See S65.402

    ● **S65.516**   Laceration of blood vessel of right little finger A 🦠
        (Ex:) See S65.401

    ● **S65.517**   Laceration of blood vessel of left little finger A 🦠
        (Ex:) See S65.402

    ● **S65.518**   Laceration of blood vessel of other finger A 🦠
        Laceration of blood vessel of specified finger with unspecified laterality
        (Ex:) See S65.409

    ● **S65.519**   Laceration of blood vessel of unspecified finger A 🦠
        (Ex:) See S65.409

● **S65.59**   Other specified injury of blood vessel of other and unspecified finger

    ● **S65.590**   Other specified injury of blood vessel of right index finger A 🦠
        (Ex:) See S65.401

    ● **S65.591**   Other specified injury of blood vessel of left index finger A 🦠
        (Ex:) See S65.402

    ● **S65.592**   Other specified injury of blood vessel of right middle finger A 🦠
        (Ex:) See S65.401

    ● **S65.593**   Other specified injury of blood vessel of left middle finger A 🦠
        (Ex:) See S65.402

    ● **S65.594**   Other specified injury of blood vessel of right ring finger A 🦠
        (Ex:) See S65.401

    ● **S65.595**   Other specified injury of blood vessel of left ring finger A 🦠
        (Ex:) See S65.402

    ● **S65.596**   Other specified injury of blood vessel of right little finger A 🦠
        (Ex:) See S65.401

    ● **S65.597**   Other specified injury of blood vessel of left little finger A 🦠
        (Ex:) See S65.402

    ● **S65.598**   Other specified injury of blood vessel of other finger A 🦠
        Other specified injury of blood vessel of specified finger with unspecified laterality
        (Ex:) See S65.409

    ● **S65.599**   Other specified injury of blood vessel of unspecified finger A 🦠
        (Ex:) See S65.409

● **S65.8**   Injury of other blood vessels at wrist and hand level

   ● **S65.80**   Unspecified injury of other blood vessels at wrist and hand level

    ● **S65.801**   Unspecified injury of other blood vessels at wrist and hand level of right arm A 🦠
        (Ex:) See S45.301

    ● **S65.802**   Unspecified injury of other blood vessels at wrist and hand level of left arm A 🦠
        (Ex:) See S45.302

    ● **S65.809**   Unspecified injury of other blood vessels at wrist and hand level of unspecified arm A 🦠
        (Ex:) See S45.309

   ● **S65.81**   Laceration of other blood vessels at wrist and hand level

    ● **S65.811**   Laceration of other blood vessels at wrist and hand level of right arm A 🦠
        (Ex:) See S45.301

    ● **S65.812**   Laceration of other blood vessels at wrist and hand level of left arm A 🦠
        (Ex:) See S45.302

    ● **S65.819**   Laceration of other blood vessels at wrist and hand level of unspecified arm A 🦠
        (Ex:) See S45.309

   ● **S65.89**   Other specified injury of other blood vessels at wrist and hand level

    ● **S65.891**   Other specified injury of other blood vessels at wrist and hand level of right arm A 🦠
        (Ex:) See S45.301

    ● **S65.892**   Other specified injury of other blood vessels at wrist and hand level of left arm A 🦠
        (Ex:) See S45.302

    ● **S65.899**   Other specified injury of other blood vessels at wrist and hand level of unspecified arm A 🦠
        (Ex:) See S45.309

● **S65.9**   Injury of unspecified blood vessel at wrist and hand level

   ● **S65.90**   Unspecified injury of unspecified blood vessel at wrist and hand level

    ● **S65.901**   Unspecified injury of unspecified blood vessel at wrist and hand level of right arm A 🦠
        (Ex:) See S45.301

    ● **S65.902**   Unspecified injury of unspecified blood vessel at wrist and hand level of left arm A 🦠
        (Ex:) See S45.302

    ● **S65.909**   Unspecified injury of unspecified blood vessel at wrist and hand level of unspecified arm A 🦠
        (Ex:) See S45.309

- **S65.91** Laceration of unspecified blood vessel at wrist and hand level
  - **S65.911** Laceration of unspecified blood vessel at wrist and hand level of right arm A 🔖
    - (Ex:) See S45.301
  - **S65.912** Laceration of unspecified blood vessel at wrist and hand level of left arm A 🔖
    - (Ex:) See S45.302
  - **S65.919** Laceration of unspecified blood vessel at wrist and hand level of unspecified arm A 🔖
    - (Ex:) See S45.309
- **S65.99** Other specified injury of unspecified blood vessel at wrist and hand level
  - **S65.991** Other specified injury of unspecified blood vessel at wrist and hand of right arm A 🔖
    - (Ex:) See S45.301
  - **S65.992** Other specified injury of unspecified blood vessel at wrist and hand of left arm A 🔖
    - (Ex:) See S45.302
  - **S65.999** Other specified injury of unspecified blood vessel at wrist and hand of unspecified arm A 🔖
    - (Ex:) See S45.309

- **S66** Injury of muscle, fascia and tendon at wrist and hand level

  Code also any associated open wound (S61.-)

  Excludes2   sprain of joints and ligaments of wrist and hand (S63.-)

  The appropriate 7th character is to be added to each code from category S66

A	initial encounter
D	subsequent encounter
S	sequela

- **S66.0** Injury of long flexor muscle, fascia and tendon of thumb at wrist and hand level
  - **S66.00** Unspecified injury of long flexor muscle, fascia and tendon of thumb at wrist and hand level
    - **S66.001** Unspecified injury of long flexor muscle, fascia and tendon of right thumb at wrist and hand level
    - **S66.002** Unspecified injury of long flexor muscle, fascia and tendon of left thumb at wrist and hand level
    - **S66.009** Unspecified injury of long flexor muscle, fascia and tendon of unspecified thumb at wrist and hand level
  - **S66.01** Strain of long flexor muscle, fascia and tendon of thumb at wrist and hand level
    - **S66.011** Strain of long flexor muscle, fascia and tendon of right thumb at wrist and hand level
    - **S66.012** Strain of long flexor muscle, fascia and tendon of left thumb at wrist and hand level
    - **S66.019** Strain of long flexor muscle, fascia and tendon of unspecified thumb at wrist and hand level

- **S66.02** Laceration of long flexor muscle, fascia and tendon of thumb at wrist and hand level
  - **S66.021** Laceration of long flexor muscle, fascia and tendon of right thumb at wrist and hand level A 🔖
    - (Ex:) S61.401[A], S61.409-S61.411[A], S61.419-S61.421[A], S61.429-S61.431[A], S61.439-S61.441[A], S61.449-S61.451[A], S61.459[A], S66.021[A], S66.029[A], S66.120[A], S66.122[A], S66.124[A], S66.126[A], S66.128-S66.129[A], S66.221[A], S66.229[A], S66.320[A], S66.322[A], S66.324[A], S66.326[A], S66.328-S66.329[A], S66.421[A], S66.429[A], S66.520[A], S66.522[A], S66.524[A], S66.526[A], S66.528-S66.529[A], S66.821[A], S66.829[A], S66.921[A], S66.929[A]
  - **S66.022** Laceration of long flexor muscle, fascia and tendon of left thumb at wrist and hand level A 🔖
    - (Ex:) S61.402-S61.409[A], S61.412-S61.419[A], S61.422-S61.429[A], S61.432-S61.439[A], S61.442-S61.449[A], S61.452-S61.459[A], S66.022-S66.029[A], S66.121[A], S66.123[A], S66.125[A], S66.127-S66.129[A], S66.222-S66.229[A], S66.321[A], S66.323[A], S66.325[A], S66.327-S66.329[A], S66.422-S66.429[A], S66.521[A], S66.523[A], S66.525[A], S66.527-S66.529[A], S66.822-S66.829[A], S66.922-S66.929[A]
  - **S66.029** Laceration of long flexor muscle, fascia and tendon of unspecified thumb at wrist and hand level A 🔖
    - (Ex:) S61.401-S61.459[A], S66.021-S66.029[A], S66.120-S66.129[A], S66.221-S66.229[A], S66.320-S66.329[A], S66.421-S66.429[A], S66.520-S66.529[A], S66.821-S66.829[A], S66.921-S66.929[A]
- **S66.09** Other specified injury of long flexor muscle, fascia and tendon of thumb at wrist and hand level
  - **S66.091** Other specified injury of long flexor muscle, fascia and tendon of right thumb at wrist and hand level
  - **S66.092** Other specified injury of long flexor muscle, fascia and tendon of left thumb at wrist and hand level
  - **S66.099** Other specified injury of long flexor muscle, fascia and tendon of unspecified thumb at wrist and hand level
- **S66.1** Injury of flexor muscle, fascia and tendon of other and unspecified finger at wrist and hand level

  Excludes2   injury of long flexor muscle, fascia and tendon of thumb at wrist and hand level (S66.0-)

  - **S66.10** Unspecified injury of flexor muscle, fascia and tendon of other and unspecified finger at wrist and hand level
    - **S66.100** Unspecified injury of flexor muscle, fascia and tendon of right index finger at wrist and hand level
    - **S66.101** Unspecified injury of flexor muscle, fascia and tendon of left index finger at wrist and hand level
    - **S66.102** Unspecified injury of flexor muscle, fascia and tendon of right middle finger at wrist and hand level

● S66.103   **Unspecified** injury of flexor muscle, fascia and tendon of left middle finger at wrist and hand level

● S66.104   **Unspecified** injury of flexor muscle, fascia and tendon of right ring finger at wrist and hand level

● S66.105   **Unspecified** injury of flexor muscle, fascia and tendon of left ring finger at wrist and hand level

● S66.106   **Unspecified** injury of flexor muscle, fascia and tendon of right little finger at wrist and hand level

● S66.107   **Unspecified** injury of flexor muscle, fascia and tendon of left little finger at wrist and hand level

● S66.108   **Unspecified** injury of flexor muscle, fascia and tendon of other finger at wrist and hand level

      Unspecified injury of flexor muscle, fascia and tendon of specified finger with unspecified laterality at wrist and hand level

● S66.109   **Unspecified** injury of flexor muscle, fascia and tendon of unspecified finger at wrist and hand level

● S66.11   Strain of flexor muscle, fascia and tendon of other and unspecified finger at wrist and hand level

● S66.110   Strain of flexor muscle, fascia and tendon of right index finger at wrist and hand level

● S66.111   Strain of flexor muscle, fascia and tendon of left index finger at wrist and hand level

● S66.112   Strain of flexor muscle, fascia and tendon of right middle finger at wrist and hand level

● S66.113   Strain of flexor muscle, fascia and tendon of left middle finger at wrist and hand level

● S66.114   Strain of flexor muscle, fascia and tendon of right ring finger at wrist and hand level

● S66.115   Strain of flexor muscle, fascia and tendon of left ring finger at wrist and hand level

● S66.116   Strain of flexor muscle, fascia and tendon of right little finger at wrist and hand level

● S66.117   Strain of flexor muscle, fascia and tendon of left little finger at wrist and hand level

● S66.118   Strain of flexor muscle, fascia and tendon of other finger at wrist and hand level

      Strain of flexor muscle, fascia and tendon of specified finger with unspecified laterality at wrist and hand level

● S66.119   Strain of flexor muscle, fascia and tendon of **unspecified** finger at wrist and hand level

● S66.12   Laceration of flexor muscle, fascia and tendon of other and unspecified finger at wrist and hand level

● S66.120   Laceration of flexor muscle, fascia and tendon of right index finger at wrist and hand level A 📞
    (Ex:) See S65.021

● S66.121   Laceration of flexor muscle, fascia and tendon of left index finger at wrist and hand level A 📞
    (Ex:) See S65.022

● S66.122   Laceration of flexor muscle, fascia and tendon of right middle finger at wrist and hand level A 📞
    (Ex:) See S65.021

● S66.123   Laceration of flexor muscle, fascia and tendon of left middle finger at wrist and hand level A 📞
    (Ex:) See S65.022

● S66.124   Laceration of flexor muscle, fascia and tendon of right ring finger at wrist and hand level A 📞
    (Ex:) See S65.021

● S66.125   Laceration of flexor muscle, fascia and tendon of left ring finger at wrist and hand level A 📞
    (Ex:) See S65.022

● S66.126   Laceration of flexor muscle, fascia and tendon of right little finger at wrist and hand level A 📞
    (Ex:) See S65.021

● S66.127   Laceration of flexor muscle, fascia and tendon of left little finger at wrist and hand level A 📞
    (Ex:) See S65.022

● S66.128   Laceration of flexor muscle, fascia and tendon of other finger at wrist and hand level A 📞

      Laceration of flexor muscle, fascia and tendon of specified finger with unspecified laterality at wrist and hand level
    (Ex:) See S65.029

● S66.129   Laceration of flexor muscle, fascia and tendon of **unspecified** finger at wrist and hand level A 📞
    (Ex:) See S65.029

● S66.19   Other injury of flexor muscle, fascia and tendon of other and unspecified finger at wrist and hand level

● S66.190   Other injury of flexor muscle, fascia and tendon of right index finger at wrist and hand level

● S66.191   Other injury of flexor muscle, fascia and tendon of left index finger at wrist and hand level

● S66.192   Other injury of flexor muscle, fascia and tendon of right middle finger at wrist and hand level

● S66.193   Other injury of flexor muscle, fascia and tendon of left middle finger at wrist and hand level

● S66.194   Other injury of flexor muscle, fascia and tendon of right ring finger at wrist and hand level

● S66.195   Other injury of flexor muscle, fascia and tendon of left ring finger at wrist and hand level

◀ New   ◀▥ Revised   ~~deleted~~ Deleted   Excludes 1   Excludes 2   Includes   Use additional   Code first   Code also   Unspecified

OGCR Official Guidelines   ● Unacceptable Principal Diagnosis   X Assign placeholder X   ● Use Additional Character(s)   ▶ Manifestation Code   **Coding Clinic**

● **S66.196**   Other injury of flexor muscle, fascia and tendon of right little finger at wrist and hand level

● **S66.197**   Other injury of flexor muscle, fascia and tendon of left little finger at wrist and hand level

● **S66.198**   Other injury of flexor muscle, fascia and tendon of other finger at wrist and hand level
  Other injury of flexor muscle, fascia and tendon of specified finger with unspecified laterality at wrist and hand level

● **S66.199**   Other injury of flexor muscle, fascia and tendon of unspecified finger at wrist and hand level

● **S66.2**   Injury of extensor muscle, fascia and tendon of thumb at wrist and hand level

● **S66.20**   Unspecified injury of extensor muscle, fascia and tendon of thumb at wrist and hand level

● **S66.201**   Unspecified injury of extensor muscle, fascia and tendon of right thumb at wrist and hand level

● **S66.202**   Unspecified injury of extensor muscle, fascia and tendon of left thumb at wrist and hand level

● **S66.209**   Unspecified injury of extensor muscle, fascia and tendon of unspecified thumb at wrist and hand level

● **S66.21**   Strain of extensor muscle, fascia and tendon of thumb at wrist and hand level

● **S66.211**   Strain of extensor muscle, fascia and tendon of right thumb at wrist and hand level

● **S66.212**   Strain of extensor muscle, fascia and tendon of left thumb at wrist and hand level

● **S66.219**   Strain of extensor muscle, fascia and tendon of unspecified thumb at wrist and hand level

● **S66.22**   Laceration of extensor muscle, fascia and tendon of thumb at wrist and hand level

● **S66.221**   Laceration of extensor muscle, fascia and tendon of right thumb at wrist and hand level A 🗞
  (Ex) See S65.021

● **S66.222**   Laceration of extensor muscle, fascia and tendon of left thumb at wrist and hand level A 🗞
  (Ex) See S65.022

● **S66.229**   Laceration of extensor muscle, fascia and tendon of unspecified thumb at wrist and hand level A 🗞
  (Ex) See S65.029

● **S66.29**   Other specified injury of extensor muscle, fascia and tendon of thumb at wrist and hand level

● **S66.291**   Other specified injury of extensor muscle, fascia and tendon of right thumb at wrist and hand level

● **S66.292**   Other specified injury of extensor muscle, fascia and tendon of left thumb at wrist and hand level

● **S66.299**   Other specified injury of extensor muscle, fascia and tendon of unspecified thumb at wrist and hand level

● **S66.3**   Injury of extensor muscle, fascia and tendon of other and unspecified finger at wrist and hand level

  Excludes2   injury of extensor muscle, fascia and tendon of thumb at wrist and hand level (S66.2-)

● **S66.30**   Unspecified injury of extensor muscle, fascia and tendon of other and unspecified finger at wrist and hand level

● **S66.300**   Unspecified injury of extensor muscle, fascia and tendon of right index finger at wrist and hand level

● **S66.301**   Unspecified injury of extensor muscle, fascia and tendon of left index finger at wrist and hand level

● **S66.302**   Unspecified injury of extensor muscle, fascia and tendon of right middle finger at wrist and hand level

● **S66.303**   Unspecified injury of extensor muscle, fascia and tendon of left middle finger at wrist and hand level

● **S66.304**   Unspecified injury of extensor muscle, fascia and tendon of right ring finger at wrist and hand level

● **S66.305**   Unspecified injury of extensor muscle, fascia and tendon of left ring finger at wrist and hand level

● **S66.306**   Unspecified injury of extensor muscle, fascia and tendon of right little finger at wrist and hand level

● **S66.307**   Unspecified injury of extensor muscle, fascia and tendon of left little finger at wrist and hand level

● **S66.308**   Unspecified injury of extensor muscle, fascia and tendon of other finger at wrist and hand level
  Unspecified injury of extensor muscle, fascia and tendon of specified finger with unspecified laterality at wrist and hand level

● **S66.309**   Unspecified injury of extensor muscle, fascia and tendon of unspecified finger at wrist and hand level

● **S66.31**   Strain of extensor muscle, fascia and tendon of other and unspecified finger at wrist and hand level

● **S66.310**   Strain of extensor muscle, fascia and tendon of right index finger at wrist and hand level

● **S66.311**   Strain of extensor muscle, fascia and tendon of left index finger at wrist and hand level

● **S66.312**   Strain of extensor muscle, fascia and tendon of right middle finger at wrist and hand level

● **S66.313**   Strain of extensor muscle, fascia and tendon of left middle finger at wrist and hand level

● **S66.314**   Strain of extensor muscle, fascia and tendon of right ring finger at wrist and hand level

● **S66.315**   Strain of extensor muscle, fascia and tendon of left ring finger at wrist and hand level

CHAPTER 19 (S00-T88)

● **S66.316**   Strain of extensor muscle, fascia and tendon of right little finger at wrist and hand level

● **S66.317**   Strain of extensor muscle, fascia and tendon of left little finger at wrist and hand level

● **S66.318**   Strain of extensor muscle, fascia and tendon of other finger at wrist and hand level

     Strain of extensor muscle, fascia and tendon of specified finger with unspecified laterality at wrist and hand level

● **S66.319**   Strain of extensor muscle, fascia and tendon of unspecified finger at wrist and hand level

● **S66.32**   Laceration of extensor muscle, fascia and tendon of other and unspecified finger at wrist and hand level

● **S66.320**   Laceration of extensor muscle, fascia and tendon of right index finger at wrist and hand level A
     (Ex:) See S65.021

● **S66.321**   Laceration of extensor muscle, fascia and tendon of left index finger at wrist and hand level A
     (Ex:) See S65.022

● **S66.322**   Laceration of extensor muscle, fascia and tendon of right middle finger at wrist and hand level A
     (Ex:) See S65.021

● **S66.323**   Laceration of extensor muscle, fascia and tendon of left middle finger at wrist and hand level A
     (Ex:) See S65.022

● **S66.324**   Laceration of extensor muscle, fascia and tendon of right ring finger at wrist and hand level A
     (Ex:) See S65.021

● **S66.325**   Laceration of extensor muscle, fascia and tendon of left ring finger at wrist and hand level A
     (Ex:) See S65.022

● **S66.326**   Laceration of extensor muscle, fascia and tendon of right little finger at wrist and hand level A
     (Ex:) See S65.021

● **S66.327**   Laceration of extensor muscle, fascia and tendon of left little finger at wrist and hand level A
     (Ex:) See S65.022

● **S66.328**   Laceration of extensor muscle, fascia and tendon of other finger at wrist and hand level A
     Laceration of extensor muscle, fascia and tendon of specified finger with unspecified laterality at wrist and hand level
     (Ex:) See S65.029

● **S66.329**   Laceration of extensor muscle, fascia and tendon of unspecified finger at wrist and hand level A
     (Ex:) See S65.029

● **S66.39**   Other injury of extensor muscle, fascia and tendon of other and unspecified finger at wrist and hand level

● **S66.390**   Other injury of extensor muscle, fascia and tendon of right index finger at wrist and hand level

● **S66.391**   Other injury of extensor muscle, fascia and tendon of left index finger at wrist and hand level

● **S66.392**   Other injury of extensor muscle, fascia and tendon of right middle finger at wrist and hand level

● **S66.393**   Other injury of extensor muscle, fascia and tendon of left middle finger at wrist and hand level

● **S66.394**   Other injury of extensor muscle, fascia and tendon of right ring finger at wrist and hand level

● **S66.395**   Other injury of extensor muscle, fascia and tendon of left ring finger at wrist and hand level

● **S66.396**   Other injury of extensor muscle, fascia and tendon of right little finger at wrist and hand level

● **S66.397**   Other injury of extensor muscle, fascia and tendon of left little finger at wrist and hand level

● **S66.398**   Other injury of extensor muscle, fascia and tendon of other finger at wrist and hand level
     Other injury of extensor muscle, fascia and tendon of specified finger with unspecified laterality at wrist and hand level

● **S66.399**   Other injury of extensor muscle, fascia and tendon of unspecified finger at wrist and hand level

● **S66.4**   Injury of intrinsic muscle, fascia and tendon of thumb at wrist and hand level

● **S66.40**   Unspecified injury of intrinsic muscle, fascia and tendon of thumb at wrist and hand level

● **S66.401**   Unspecified injury of intrinsic muscle, fascia and tendon of right thumb at wrist and hand level

● **S66.402**   Unspecified injury of intrinsic muscle, fascia and tendon of left thumb at wrist and hand level

● **S66.409**   Unspecified injury of intrinsic muscle, fascia and tendon of unspecified thumb at wrist and hand level

● **S66.41**   Strain of intrinsic muscle, fascia and tendon of thumb at wrist and hand level

● **S66.411**   Strain of intrinsic muscle, fascia and tendon of right thumb at wrist and hand level

● **S66.412**   Strain of intrinsic muscle, fascia and tendon of left thumb at wrist and hand level

● **S66.419**   Strain of intrinsic muscle, fascia and tendon of unspecified thumb at wrist and hand level

- ● S66.42   Laceration of intrinsic muscle, fascia and tendon of thumb at wrist and hand level
  - ● S66.421   Laceration of intrinsic muscle, fascia and tendon of right thumb at wrist and hand level A 🦠
    (Ex:) See S65.021
  - ● S66.422   Laceration of intrinsic muscle, fascia and tendon of left thumb at wrist and hand level A 🦠
    (Ex:) See S65.022
  - ● S66.429   Laceration of intrinsic muscle, fascia and tendon of unspecified thumb at wrist and hand level A 🦠
    (Ex:) See S65.029
- ● S66.49   Other specified injury of intrinsic muscle, fascia and tendon of thumb at wrist and hand level
  - ● S66.491   Other specified injury of intrinsic muscle, fascia and tendon of right thumb at wrist and hand level
  - ● S66.492   Other specified injury of intrinsic muscle, fascia and tendon of left thumb at wrist and hand level
  - ● S66.499   Other specified injury of intrinsic muscle, fascia and tendon of unspecified thumb at wrist and hand level
- ● S66.5   Injury of intrinsic muscle, fascia and tendon of other and unspecified finger at wrist and hand level
  - **Excludes2**   injury of intrinsic muscle, fascia and tendon of thumb at wrist and hand level (S66.4-)
  - ● S66.50   Unspecified injury of intrinsic muscle, fascia and tendon of other and unspecified finger at wrist and hand level
    - ● S66.500   Unspecified injury of intrinsic muscle, fascia and tendon of right index finger at wrist and hand level
    - ● S66.501   Unspecified injury of intrinsic muscle, fascia and tendon of left index finger at wrist and hand level
    - ● S66.502   Unspecified injury of intrinsic muscle, fascia and tendon of right middle finger at wrist and hand level
    - ● S66.503   Unspecified injury of intrinsic muscle, fascia and tendon of left middle finger at wrist and hand level
    - ● S66.504   Unspecified injury of intrinsic muscle, fascia and tendon of right ring finger at wrist and hand level
    - ● S66.505   Unspecified injury of intrinsic muscle, fascia and tendon of left ring finger at wrist and hand level
    - ● S66.506   Unspecified injury of intrinsic muscle, fascia and tendon of right little finger at wrist and hand level
    - ● S66.507   Unspecified injury of intrinsic muscle, fascia and tendon of left little finger at wrist and hand level
    - ● S66.508   Unspecified injury of intrinsic muscle, fascia and tendon of other finger at wrist and hand level
      Unspecified injury of intrinsic muscle, fascia and tendon of specified finger with unspecified laterality at wrist and hand level
    - ● S66.509   Unspecified injury of intrinsic muscle, fascia and tendon of unspecified finger at wrist and hand level

- ● S66.51   Strain of intrinsic muscle, fascia and tendon of other and unspecified finger at wrist and hand level
  - ● S66.510   Strain of intrinsic muscle, fascia and tendon of right index finger at wrist and hand level
  - ● S66.511   Strain of intrinsic muscle, fascia and tendon of left index finger at wrist and hand level
  - ● S66.512   Strain of intrinsic muscle, fascia and tendon of right middle finger at wrist and hand level
  - ● S66.513   Strain of intrinsic muscle, fascia and tendon of left middle finger at wrist and hand level
  - ● S66.514   Strain of intrinsic muscle, fascia and tendon of right ring finger at wrist and hand level
  - ● S66.515   Strain of intrinsic muscle, fascia and tendon of left ring finger at wrist and hand level
  - ● S66.516   Strain of intrinsic muscle, fascia and tendon of right little finger at wrist and hand level
  - ● S66.517   Strain of intrinsic muscle, fascia and tendon of left little finger at wrist and hand level
  - ● S66.518   Strain of intrinsic muscle, fascia and tendon of other finger at wrist and hand level
    Strain of intrinsic muscle, fascia and tendon of specified finger with unspecified laterality at wrist and hand level
  - ● S66.519   Strain of intrinsic muscle, fascia and tendon of unspecified finger at wrist and hand level
- ● S66.52   Laceration of intrinsic muscle, fascia and tendon of other and unspecified finger at wrist and hand level
  - ● S66.520   Laceration of intrinsic muscle, fascia and tendon of right index finger at wrist and hand level A 🦠
    (Ex:) See S65.021
  - ● S66.521   Laceration of intrinsic muscle, fascia and tendon of left index finger at wrist and hand level A 🦠
    (Ex:) See S65.022
  - ● S66.522   Laceration of intrinsic muscle, fascia and tendon of right middle finger at wrist and hand level A 🦠
    (Ex:) See S65.021
  - ● S66.523   Laceration of intrinsic muscle, fascia and tendon of left middle finger at wrist and hand level A 🦠
    (Ex:) See S65.022
  - ● S66.524   Laceration of intrinsic muscle, fascia and tendon of right ring finger at wrist and hand level A 🦠
    (Ex:) See S65.021
  - ● S66.525   Laceration of intrinsic muscle, fascia and tendon of left ring finger at wrist and hand level A 🦠
    (Ex:) See S65.022
  - ● S66.526   Laceration of intrinsic muscle, fascia and tendon of right little finger at wrist and hand level A 🦠
    (Ex:) See S65.021
  - ● S66.527   Laceration of intrinsic muscle, fascia and tendon of left little finger at wrist and hand level A 🦠
    (Ex:) See S65.022

CHAPTER 19 (S00-T88)

● **S66.528**   Laceration of intrinsic muscle, fascia and tendon of other finger at wrist and hand level A 🔗

     Laceration of intrinsic muscle, fascia and tendon of specified finger with unspecified laterality at wrist and hand level

     (Ex:) See S65.029

● **S66.529**   Laceration of intrinsic muscle, fascia and tendon of **unspecified** finger at wrist and hand level A 🔗

     (Ex:) See S65.029

● **S66.59**   Other injury of intrinsic muscle, fascia and tendon of other and unspecified finger at wrist and hand level

● **S66.590**   Other injury of intrinsic muscle, fascia and tendon of right index finger at wrist and hand level

● **S66.591**   Other injury of intrinsic muscle, fascia and tendon of left index finger at wrist and hand level

● **S66.592**   Other injury of intrinsic muscle, fascia and tendon of right middle finger at wrist and hand level

● **S66.593**   Other injury of intrinsic muscle, fascia and tendon of left middle finger at wrist and hand level

● **S66.594**   Other injury of intrinsic muscle, fascia and tendon of right ring finger at wrist and hand level

● **S66.595**   Other injury of intrinsic muscle, fascia and tendon of left ring finger at wrist and hand level

● **S66.596**   Other injury of intrinsic muscle, fascia and tendon of right little finger at wrist and hand level

● **S66.597**   Other injury of intrinsic muscle, fascia and tendon of left little finger at wrist and hand level

● **S66.598**   Other injury of intrinsic muscle, fascia and tendon of other finger at wrist and hand level

     Other injury of intrinsic muscle, fascia and tendon of specified finger with unspecified laterality at wrist and hand level

● **S66.599**   Other injury of intrinsic muscle, fascia and tendon of **unspecified** finger at wrist and hand level

● **S66.8**   Injury of other specified muscles, fascia and tendons at wrist and hand level

● **S66.80**   Unspecified injury of other specified muscles, fascia and tendons at wrist and hand level

● **S66.801**   **Unspecified** injury of other specified muscles, fascia and tendons at wrist and hand level, right hand

● **S66.802**   **Unspecified** injury of other specified muscles, fascia and tendons at wrist and hand level, left hand

● **S66.809**   **Unspecified** injury of other specified muscles, fascia and tendons at wrist and hand level, unspecified hand

● **S66.81**   Strain of other specified muscles, fascia and tendons at wrist and hand level

● **S66.811**   Strain of other specified muscles, fascia and tendons at wrist and hand level, right hand

● **S66.812**   Strain of other specified muscles, fascia and tendons at wrist and hand level, left hand

● **S66.819**   Strain of other specified muscles, fascia and tendons at wrist and hand level, **unspecified** hand

● **S66.82**   Laceration of other specified muscles, fascia and tendons at wrist and hand level

● **S66.821**   Laceration of other specified muscles, fascia and tendons at wrist and hand level, right hand A 🔗

     (Ex:) See S65.021

● **S66.822**   Laceration of other specified muscles, fascia and tendons at wrist and hand level, left hand A 🔗

     (Ex:) See S65.022

● **S66.829**   Laceration of other specified muscles, fascia and tendons at wrist and hand level, **unspecified** hand A 🔗

     (Ex:) See S65.029

● **S66.89**   Other injury of other specified muscles, fascia and tendons at wrist and hand level

● **S66.891**   Other injury of other specified muscles, fascia and tendons at wrist and hand level, right hand

● **S66.892**   Other injury of other specified muscles, fascia and tendons at wrist and hand level, left hand

● **S66.899**   Other injury of other specified muscles, fascia and tendons at wrist and hand level, **unspecified** hand

● **S66.9**   Injury of unspecified muscle, fascia and tendon at wrist and hand level

● **S66.90**   Unspecified injury of unspecified muscle, fascia and tendon at wrist and hand level

● **S66.901**   **Unspecified** injury of unspecified muscle, fascia and tendon at wrist and hand level, right hand

● **S66.902**   **Unspecified** injury of unspecified muscle, fascia and tendon at wrist and hand level, left hand

● **S66.909**   **Unspecified** injury of unspecified muscle, fascia and tendon at wrist and hand level, unspecified hand

● **S66.91**   Strain of unspecified muscle, fascia and tendon at wrist and hand level

● **S66.911**   Strain of **unspecified** muscle, fascia and tendon at wrist and hand level, right hand

● **S66.912**   Strain of **unspecified** muscle, fascia and tendon at wrist and hand level, left hand

● **S66.919**   Strain of **unspecified** muscle, fascia and tendon at wrist and hand level, unspecified hand

◀ New   ◀▥ Revised   ~~deleted~~ Deleted   Excludes 1   Excludes 2   Includes   Use additional   Code first   Code also   Unspecified

OGCR Official Guidelines   ● Unacceptable Principal Diagnosis   X Assign placeholder X   ● Use Additional Character(s)   ▶ Manifestation Code   **Coding Clinic**

● **S66.92**   **Laceration of unspecified muscle, fascia and tendon at wrist and hand level**
> ● **S66.921**   Laceration of unspecified muscle, fascia and tendon at wrist and hand level, right hand A 🔗
> > (Ex) See S65.021
> ● **S66.922**   Laceration of unspecified muscle, fascia and tendon at wrist and hand level, left hand A 🔗
> > (Ex) See S65.022
> ● **S66.929**   Laceration of unspecified muscle, fascia and tendon at wrist and hand level, unspecified hand A 🔗
> > (Ex) See S65.029

● **S66.99**   **Other injury of unspecified muscle, fascia and tendon at wrist and hand level**
> ● **S66.991**   Other injury of unspecified muscle, fascia and tendon at wrist and hand level, right hand
> ● **S66.992**   Other injury of unspecified muscle, fascia and tendon at wrist and hand level, left hand
> ● **S66.999**   Other injury of unspecified muscle, fascia and tendon at wrist and hand level, unspecified hand

● **S67**   **Crushing injury of wrist, hand and fingers**
> Use additional code for all associated injuries, such as:
> fracture of wrist and hand (S62.-)
> open wound of wrist and hand (S61.-)
>
> The appropriate 7th character is to be added to each code from category S67

> | | |
> |---|---|
> | A | initial encounter |
> | D | subsequent encounter |
> | S | sequela |

● **S67.0**   **Crushing injury of thumb**
> X ● **S67.00**   Crushing injury of unspecified thumb
> X ● **S67.01**   Crushing injury of right thumb
> X ● **S67.02**   Crushing injury of left thumb

● **S67.1**   **Crushing injury of other and unspecified finger(s)**
> **Excludes2**   crushing injury of thumb (S67.0-)
> X ● **S67.10**   Crushing injury of unspecified finger(s)
> ● **S67.19**   Crushing injury of other finger(s)
> > ● **S67.190**   Crushing injury of right index finger
> > ● **S67.191**   Crushing injury of left index finger
> > ● **S67.192**   Crushing injury of right middle finger
> > ● **S67.193**   Crushing injury of left middle finger
> > ● **S67.194**   Crushing injury of right ring finger
> > ● **S67.195**   Crushing injury of left ring finger
> > ● **S67.196**   Crushing injury of right little finger
> > ● **S67.197**   Crushing injury of left little finger
> > ● **S67.198**   Crushing injury of other finger
> > > Crushing injury of specified finger with unspecified laterality

● **S67.2**   **Crushing injury of hand**
> **Excludes2**   crushing injury of fingers (S67.1-)
> crushing injury of thumb (S67.0-)
> X ● **S67.20**   Crushing injury of unspecified hand
> X ● **S67.21**   Crushing injury of right hand
> X ● **S67.22**   Crushing injury of left hand

● **S67.3**   **Crushing injury of wrist**
> X ● **S67.30**   Crushing injury of unspecified wrist
> X ● **S67.31**   Crushing injury of right wrist
> X ● **S67.32**   Crushing injury of left wrist

● **S67.4**   **Crushing injury of wrist and hand**
> **Excludes1**   crushing injury of hand alone (S67.2-)
> crushing injury of wrist alone (S67.3-)
>
> **Excludes2**   crushing injury of fingers (S67.1-)
> crushing injury of thumb (S67.0-)
> X ● **S67.40**   Crushing injury of unspecified wrist and hand
> X ● **S67.41**   Crushing injury of right wrist and hand
> X ● **S67.42**   Crushing injury of left wrist and hand

● **S67.9**   **Crushing injury of unspecified part(s) of wrist, hand and fingers**
> X ● **S67.90**   Crushing injury of unspecified part(s) of unspecified wrist, hand and fingers
> X ● **S67.91**   Crushing injury of unspecified part(s) of right wrist, hand and fingers
> X ● **S67.92**   Crushing injury of unspecified part(s) of left wrist, hand and fingers

● **S68**   **Traumatic amputation of wrist, hand and fingers**
> An amputation not identified as partial or complete should be coded to complete
>
> The appropriate 7th character is to be added to each code from category S68

> | | |
> |---|---|
> | A | initial encounter |
> | D | subsequent encounter |
> | S | sequela |

● **S68.0**   **Traumatic metacarpophalangeal amputation of thumb**
> Traumatic amputation of thumb NOS
> ● **S68.01**   Complete traumatic metacarpophalangeal amputation of thumb
> > ● **S68.011**   Complete traumatic metacarpophalangeal amputation of right thumb
> > ● **S68.012**   Complete traumatic metacarpophalangeal amputation of left thumb
> > ● **S68.019**   Complete traumatic metacarpophalangeal amputation of unspecified thumb
> ● **S68.02**   Partial traumatic metacarpophalangeal amputation of thumb
> > ● **S68.021**   Partial traumatic metacarpophalangeal amputation of right thumb
> > ● **S68.022**   Partial traumatic metacarpophalangeal amputation of left thumb
> > ● **S68.029**   Partial traumatic metacarpophalangeal amputation of unspecified thumb

● **S68.1**   **Traumatic metacarpophalangeal amputation of other and unspecified finger**
> Traumatic amputation of finger NOS
> **Excludes2**   traumatic metacarpophalangeal amputation of thumb (S68.0-)
> ● **S68.11**   Complete traumatic metacarpophalangeal amputation of other and unspecified finger
> > ● **S68.110**   Complete traumatic metacarpophalangeal amputation of right index finger
> > ● **S68.111**   Complete traumatic metacarpophalangeal amputation of left index finger
> > ● **S68.112**   Complete traumatic metacarpophalangeal amputation of right middle finger
> > ● **S68.113**   Complete traumatic metacarpophalangeal amputation of left middle finger
> > ● **S68.114**   Complete traumatic metacarpophalangeal amputation of right ring finger

CHAPTER 19 (S00-T88)

N   Newborn Age: 0   **P**   Pediatric Age: 0–17   **M**   Maternity DX: 12–55   **A**   Adult Age: 15–124   ♀   Females Only   ♂   Males Only

🔗   Complication\Comorbidity   🔗   Major C\C   (Ex)   CC/MCC Exclusions   🔗   Hospital-Acquired Condition

1353

● S68.115　Complete traumatic metacarpophalangeal amputation of left ring finger

● S68.116　Complete traumatic metacarpophalangeal amputation of right little finger

● S68.117　Complete traumatic metacarpophalangeal amputation of left little finger

● S68.118　Complete traumatic metacarpophalangeal amputation of other finger
　　　　　　Complete traumatic metacarpophalangeal amputation of specified finger with unspecified laterality

● S68.119　Complete traumatic metacarpophalangeal amputation of unspecified finger

● S68.12　Partial traumatic metacarpophalangeal amputation of other and unspecified finger

● S68.120　Partial traumatic metacarpophalangeal amputation of right index finger

● S68.121　Partial traumatic metacarpophalangeal amputation of left index finger

● S68.122　Partial traumatic metacarpophalangeal amputation of right middle finger

● S68.123　Partial traumatic metacarpophalangeal amputation of left middle finger

● S68.124　Partial traumatic metacarpophalangeal amputation of right ring finger

● S68.125　Partial traumatic metacarpophalangeal amputation of left ring finger

● S68.126　Partial traumatic metacarpophalangeal amputation of right little finger

● S68.127　Partial traumatic metacarpophalangeal amputation of left little finger

● S68.128　Partial traumatic metacarpophalangeal amputation of other finger
　　　　　　Partial traumatic metacarpophalangeal amputation of specified finger with unspecified laterality

● S68.129　Partial traumatic metacarpophalangeal amputation of unspecified finger

● S68.4　Traumatic amputation of hand at wrist level
　　　　Traumatic amputation of hand NOS
　　　　Traumatic amputation of wrist

● S68.41　Complete traumatic amputation of hand at wrist level

● S68.411　Complete traumatic amputation of right hand at wrist level A 🅒
　　　　　　Ex: See S48.011

● S68.412　Complete traumatic amputation of left hand at wrist level A 🅒
　　　　　　Ex: See S48.012

● S68.419　Complete traumatic amputation of unspecified hand at wrist level A 🅒
　　　　　　Ex: See S48.019

● S68.42　Partial traumatic amputation of hand at wrist level

● S68.421　Partial traumatic amputation of right hand at wrist level A 🅒
　　　　　　Ex: See S48.011

● S68.422　Partial traumatic amputation of left hand at wrist level A 🅒
　　　　　　Ex: See S48.012

● S68.429　Partial traumatic amputation of unspecified hand at wrist level A 🅒
　　　　　　Ex: See S48.019

● S68.5　Traumatic transphalangeal amputation of thumb
　　　　Traumatic interphalangeal joint amputation of thumb

● S68.51　Complete traumatic transphalangeal amputation of thumb

● S68.511　Complete traumatic transphalangeal amputation of right thumb

● S68.512　Complete traumatic transphalangeal amputation of left thumb

● S68.519　Complete traumatic transphalangeal amputation of unspecified thumb

● S68.52　Partial traumatic transphalangeal amputation of thumb

● S68.521　Partial traumatic transphalangeal amputation of right thumb

● S68.522　Partial traumatic transphalangeal amputation of left thumb

● S68.529　Partial traumatic transphalangeal amputation of unspecified thumb

● S68.6　Traumatic transphalangeal amputation of other and unspecified finger

● S68.61　Complete traumatic transphalangeal amputation of other and unspecified finger(s)

● S68.610　Complete traumatic transphalangeal amputation of right index finger

● S68.611　Complete traumatic transphalangeal amputation of left index finger

● S68.612　Complete traumatic transphalangeal amputation of right middle finger

● S68.613　Complete traumatic transphalangeal amputation of left middle finger

● S68.614　Complete traumatic transphalangeal amputation of right ring finger

● S68.615　Complete traumatic transphalangeal amputation of left ring finger

● S68.616　Complete traumatic transphalangeal amputation of right little finger

● S68.617　Complete traumatic transphalangeal amputation of left little finger

● S68.618　Complete traumatic transphalangeal amputation of other finger
　　　　　　Complete traumatic transphalangeal amputation of specified finger with unspecified laterality

● S68.619　Complete traumatic transphalangeal amputation of unspecified finger

● S68.62　Partial traumatic transphalangeal amputation of other and unspecified finger

● S68.620　Partial traumatic transphalangeal amputation of right index finger

● S68.621　Partial traumatic transphalangeal amputation of left index finger

● S68.622　Partial traumatic transphalangeal amputation of right middle finger

● S68.623　Partial traumatic transphalangeal amputation of left middle finger

◀ New　◀▥ Revised　deleted Deleted　Excludes 1　Excludes 2　Includes　Use additional　Code first　Code also　Unspecified
OGCR Official Guidelines　● Unacceptable Principal Diagnosis　X Assign placeholder X　● Use Additional Character(s)　▶ Manifestation Code　Coding Clinic

● S68.624 Partial traumatic transphalangeal amputation of right ring finger
● S68.625 Partial traumatic transphalangeal amputation of left ring finger
● S68.626 Partial traumatic transphalangeal amputation of right little finger
● S68.627 Partial traumatic transphalangeal amputation of left little finger
● S68.628 Partial traumatic transphalangeal amputation of other finger
> Partial traumatic transphalangeal amputation of specified finger with unspecified laterality
● S68.629 Partial traumatic transphalangeal amputation of unspecified finger

● S68.7 Traumatic transmetacarpal amputation of hand
  ● S68.71 Complete traumatic transmetacarpal amputation of hand
    ● S68.711 Complete traumatic transmetacarpal amputation of right hand A 🔗
       (Ex) See S48.011
    ● S68.712 Complete traumatic transmetacarpal amputation of left hand A 🔗
       (Ex) See S48.012
    ● S68.719 Complete traumatic transmetacarpal amputation of unspecified hand A 🔗
       (Ex) See S48.019
  ● S68.72 Partial traumatic transmetacarpal amputation of hand
    ● S68.721 Partial traumatic transmetacarpal amputation of right hand A 🔗
       (Ex) See S48.011
    ● S68.722 Partial traumatic transmetacarpal amputation of left hand A 🔗
       (Ex) See S48.012
    ● S68.729 Partial traumatic transmetacarpal amputation of unspecified hand A 🔗
       (Ex) See S48.019

● S69 Other and unspecified injuries of wrist, hand and finger(s)
> The appropriate 7th character is to be added to each code from category S69

A	initial encounter
D	subsequent encounter
S	sequela

  ● S69.8 Other specified injuries of wrist, hand and finger(s)
  X ● S69.80 Other specified injuries of unspecified wrist, hand and finger(s)
  X ● S69.81 Other specified injuries of right wrist, hand and finger(s)
  X ● S69.82 Other specified injuries of left wrist, hand and finger(s)
  ● S69.9 Unspecified injury of wrist, hand and finger(s)
  X ● S69.90 Unspecified injury of unspecified wrist, hand and finger(s)
  X ● S69.91 Unspecified injury of right wrist, hand and finger(s)
  X ● S69.92 Unspecified injury of left wrist, hand and finger(s)

INJURIES TO THE HIP AND THIGH (S70-S79)

Excludes2 burns and corrosions (T20-T32)
          frostbite (T33-T34)
          snake bite (T63.0-)
          venomous insect bite or sting (T63.4-)

● S70 Superficial injury of hip and thigh
> The appropriate 7th character is to be added to each code from category S70

A	initial encounter
D	subsequent encounter
S	sequela

  ● S70.0 Contusion of hip
  X ● S70.00 Contusion of unspecified hip
  X ● S70.01 Contusion of right hip
  X ● S70.02 Contusion of left hip
  ● S70.1 Contusion of thigh
  X ● S70.10 Contusion of unspecified thigh
  X ● S70.11 Contusion of right thigh
  X ● S70.12 Contusion of left thigh
  ● S70.2 Other superficial injuries of hip
    ● S70.21 Abrasion of hip
      ● S70.211 Abrasion, right hip
      ● S70.212 Abrasion, left hip
      ● S70.219 Abrasion, unspecified hip
    ● S70.22 Blister (nonthermal) of hip
      ● S70.221 Blister (nonthermal), right hip
      ● S70.222 Blister (nonthermal), left hip
      ● S70.229 Blister (nonthermal), unspecified hip
    ● S70.24 External constriction of hip
      ● S70.241 External constriction, right hip
      ● S70.242 External constriction, left hip
      ● S70.249 External constriction, unspecified hip
    ● S70.25 Superficial foreign body of hip
> Splinter in the hip
      ● S70.251 Superficial foreign body, right hip
      ● S70.252 Superficial foreign body, left hip
      ● S70.259 Superficial foreign body, unspecified hip
    ● S70.26 Insect bite (nonvenomous) of hip
      ● S70.261 Insect bite (nonvenomous), right hip
      ● S70.262 Insect bite (nonvenomous), left hip
      ● S70.269 Insect bite (nonvenomous), unspecified hip
    ● S70.27 Other superficial bite of hip
> **Excludes1** open bite of hip (S71.05-)
      ● S70.271 Other superficial bite of hip, right hip
      ● S70.272 Other superficial bite of hip, left hip
      ● S70.279 Other superficial bite of hip, unspecified hip
  ● S70.3 Other superficial injuries of thigh
    ● S70.31 Abrasion of thigh
      ● S70.311 Abrasion, right thigh
      ● S70.312 Abrasion, left thigh
      ● S70.319 Abrasion, unspecified thigh
    ● S70.32 Blister (nonthermal) of thigh
      ● S70.321 Blister (nonthermal), right thigh
      ● S70.322 Blister (nonthermal), left thigh
      ● S70.329 Blister (nonthermal), unspecified thigh

CHAPTER 19 (S00-T88)

N Newborn Age: 0   P Pediatric Age: 0–17   M Maternity DX: 12–55   A Adult Age: 15–124   ♀ Females Only   ♂ Males Only
🔗 Complication\Comorbidity   🔗 Major C\C   (Ex) CC/MCC Exclusions   🔗 Hospital-Acquired Condition
1355

● **S70.34   External constriction of thigh**
  ● S70.341   External constriction, right thigh
  ● S70.342   External constriction, left thigh
  ● S70.349   External constriction, unspecified thigh
● **S70.35   Superficial foreign body of thigh**
    Splinter in the thigh
  ● S70.351   Superficial foreign body, right thigh
  ● S70.352   Superficial foreign body, left thigh
  ● S70.359   Superficial foreign body, unspecified thigh
● **S70.36   Insect bite (nonvenomous) of thigh**
  ● S70.361   Insect bite (nonvenomous), right thigh
  ● S70.362   Insect bite (nonvenomous), left thigh
  ● S70.369   Insect bite (nonvenomous), unspecified thigh
● **S70.37   Other superficial bite of thigh**
    Excludes1   open bite of thigh (S71.15)
  ● S70.371   Other superficial bite of right thigh
  ● S70.372   Other superficial bite of left thigh
  ● S70.379   Other superficial bite of unspecified thigh
● **S70.9   Unspecified superficial injury of hip and thigh**
  ● **S70.91   Unspecified superficial injury of hip**
    ● S70.911   Unspecified superficial injury of right hip
    ● S70.912   Unspecified superficial injury of left hip
    ● S70.919   Unspecified superficial injury of unspecified hip
  ● **S70.92   Unspecified superficial injury of thigh**
    ● S70.921   Unspecified superficial injury of right thigh
    ● S70.922   Unspecified superficial injury of left thigh
    ● S70.929   Unspecified superficial injury of unspecified thigh

● **S71   Open wound of hip and thigh**
    Code also any associated wound infection
    Excludes1   open fracture of hip and thigh (S72.-)
                    traumatic amputation of hip and thigh (S78.-)
    Excludes2   bite of venomous animal (T63.-)
                    open wound of ankle, foot and toes (S91.-)
                    open wound of knee and lower leg (S81.-)
    The appropriate 7th character is to be added to each code from category S71

A	initial encounter
D	subsequent encounter
S	sequela

  ● **S71.0   Open wound of hip**
    ● **S71.00   Unspecified open wound of hip**
      ● S71.001   Unspecified open wound, right hip
      ● S71.002   Unspecified open wound, left hip
      ● S71.009   Unspecified open wound, unspecified hip
    ● **S71.01   Laceration without foreign body of hip**
      ● S71.011   Laceration without foreign body, right hip
      ● S71.012   Laceration without foreign body, left hip
      ● S71.019   Laceration without foreign body, unspecified hip

● **S71.02   Laceration with foreign body of hip**
  ● S71.021   Laceration with foreign body, right hip
  ● S71.022   Laceration with foreign body, left hip
  ● S71.029   Laceration with foreign body, unspecified hip
● **S71.03   Puncture wound without foreign body of hip**
  ● S71.031   Puncture wound without foreign body, right hip
  ● S71.032   Puncture wound without foreign body, left hip
  ● S71.039   Puncture wound without foreign body, unspecified hip
● **S71.04   Puncture wound with foreign body of hip**
  ● S71.041   Puncture wound with foreign body, right hip
  ● S71.042   Puncture wound with foreign body, left hip
  ● S71.049   Puncture wound with foreign body, unspecified hip
● **S71.05   Open bite of hip**
    Bite of hip NOS
    Excludes1   superficial bite of hip (S70.26, S70.27)
  ● S71.051   Open bite, right hip
  ● S71.052   Open bite, left hip
  ● S71.059   Open bite, unspecified hip
● **S71.1   Open wound of thigh**
  ● **S71.10   Unspecified open wound of thigh**
    ● S71.101   Unspecified open wound, right thigh
    ● S71.102   Unspecified open wound, left thigh
    ● S71.109   Unspecified open wound, unspecified thigh
  ● **S71.11   Laceration without foreign body of thigh**
    ● S71.111   Laceration without foreign body, right thigh
    ● S71.112   Laceration without foreign body, left thigh
    ● S71.119   Laceration without foreign body, unspecified thigh
  ● **S71.12   Laceration with foreign body of thigh**
    ● S71.121   Laceration with foreign body, right thigh
    ● S71.122   Laceration with foreign body, left thigh
    ● S71.129   Laceration with foreign body, unspecified thigh
  ● **S71.13   Puncture wound without foreign body of thigh**
    ● S71.131   Puncture wound without foreign body, right thigh
    ● S71.132   Puncture wound without foreign body, left thigh
    ● S71.139   Puncture wound without foreign body, unspecified thigh
  ● **S71.14   Puncture wound with foreign body of thigh**
    ● S71.141   Puncture wound with foreign body, right thigh
    ● S71.142   Puncture wound with foreign body, left thigh
    ● S71.149   Puncture wound with foreign body, unspecified thigh
  ● **S71.15   Open bite of thigh**
    Bite of thigh NOS
    Excludes1   superficial bite of thigh (S70.37-)
    ● S71.151   Open bite, right thigh
    ● S71.152   Open bite, left thigh
    ● S71.159   Open bite, unspecified thigh

◀ New   ◀▦ Revised   ~~deleted~~ Deleted   Excludes 1   Excludes 2   Includes   Use additional   Code first   Code also   Unspecified
OGCR Official Guidelines   ● Unacceptable Principal Diagnosis   X Assign placeholder X   ● Use Additional Character(s)   ▌ Manifestation Code   **Coding Clinic**

● **S72   Fracture of femur**

Note: A fracture not indicated as displaced or nondisplaced should be coded to displaced

A fracture not indicated as open or closed should be coded to closed

The open fracture designations are based on the Gustilo open fracture classification

Excludes1	traumatic amputation of hip and thigh (S78.-)
Excludes2	fracture of lower leg and ankle (S82.-)
	fracture of foot (S92.-)
	periprosthetic fracture of prosthetic implant of hip (T84.040, T84.041)

The appropriate 7th character is to be added to all codes from category S72

A	initial encounter for closed fracture
B	initial encounter for open fracture type I or II
	initial encounter for open fracture NOS
C	initial encounter for open fracture type IIIA, IIIB, or IIIC
D	subsequent encounter for closed fracture with routine healing
E	subsequent encounter for open fracture type I or II with routine healing
F	subsequent encounter for open fracture type IIIA, IIIB, or IIIC with routine healing
G	subsequent encounter for closed fracture with delayed healing
H	subsequent encounter for open fracture type I or II with delayed healing
J	subsequent encounter for open fracture type IIIA, IIIB, or IIIC with delayed healing
K	subsequent encounter for closed fracture with nonunion
M	subsequent encounter for open fracture type I or II with nonunion
N	subsequent encounter for open fracture type IIIA, IIIB, or IIIC with nonunion
P	subsequent encounter for closed fracture with malunion
Q	subsequent encounter for open fracture type I or II with malunion
R	subsequent encounter for open fracture type IIIA, IIIB, or IIIC with malunion
S	sequela

● **S72.0   Fracture of head and neck of femur**

Excludes2   physeal fracture of upper end of femur (S79.0-)

● **S72.00   Fracture of unspecified part of neck of femur**
Fracture of hip NOS
Fracture of neck of femur NOS

● **S72.001   Fracture of unspecified part of neck of right femur** K, M, N, P, Q, R 🦠, A, B, C 🦠, A, B, C 🦠

Ex: **For S72.001[A]:** M48.40X-M48.58X[A], M80.00X-M80.88X[A], M84.30X-M84.68X[A], M84.750-M84.759[A], S03.8XX-S03.9XX[A], S29.011-S29.019[A], S38.3XX[A], S39.011-S39.013[A], S72.001[A,B,C], S72.002[B,C], S72.009-S72.011[A,B,C], S72.012[B,C], S72.019-S72.021[A,B,C], S72.022[B,C], S72.023-S72.024[A,B,C], S72.025[B,C], S72.026-S72.031[A,B,C], S72.032[B,C], S72.033-S72.034[A,B,C], S72.035[B,C], S72.036-S72.041[A,B,C], S72.042[B,C], S72.043-S72.044[A,B,C], S72.045[B,C], S72.046-S72.051[A,B,C], S72.052[B,C], S72.059-S72.061[A,B,C], S72.062[B,C], S72.063-S72.064[A,B,C],

S72.065[B,C], S72.066-S72.091[A,B,C], S72.092[B,C], S72.099-S72.101[A,B,C], S72.102[B,C], S72.109-S72.111[A,B,C], S72.112[B,C], S72.113-S72.114[A,B,C], S72.115[B,C], S72.116-S72.121[A,B,C], S72.122[B,C], S72.123-S72.124[A,B,C], S72.125[B,C], S72.126-S72.131[A,B,C], S72.132[B,C], S72.133-S72.134[A,B,C], S72.135[B,C], S72.136-S72.141[A,B,C], S72.142[B,C], S72.143-S72.144[A,B,C], S72.145[B,C], S72.146-S72.301[A,B,C], S72.302[B,C], S72.309-S72.321[A,B,C], S72.322[B,C], S72.323-S72.324[A,B,C], S72.325[B,C], S72.326-S72.331[A,B,C], S72.332[B,C], S72.333-S72.334[A,B,C], S72.335[B,C], S72.336-S72.341[A,B,C], S72.342[B,C], S72.343-S72.344[A,B,C], S72.345[B,C], S72.346-S72.351[A,B,C], S72.352[B,C], S72.353-S72.354[A,B,C], S72.355[B,C], S72.356-S72.361[A,B,C], S72.362[B,C], S72.363-S72.364[A,B,C], S72.365[B,C], S72.366-S72.391[A,B,C], S72.392[B,C], S72.399-S72.401[A,B,C], S72.402[B,C], S72.409-S72.411[A,B,C], S72.412[B,C], S72.413-S72.414[A,B,C], S72.415[B,C], S72.416-S72.421[A,B,C], S72.422[B,C], S72.423-S72.424[A,B,C], S72.425[B,C], S72.426-S72.431[A,B,C], S72.432[B,C], S72.433-S72.434[A,B,C], S72.435[B,C], S72.436-S72.441[A,B,C], S72.442[B,C], S72.443-S72.444[A,B,C], S72.445[B,C], S72.446-S72.451[A,B,C], S72.452[B,C], S72.453-S72.454[A,B,C], S72.455[B,C], S72.456-S72.461[A,B,C], S72.462[B,C], S72.463-S72.464[A,B,C], S72.465[B,C], S72.466[A,B,C], S72.471[A], S72.479[A], S72.491[A,B,C], S72.492[B,C], S72.499-S72.92X[A,B,C], S73.101[A], S73.109-S73.111[A], S73.119-S73.121[A], S73.129-S73.191[A], S73.199[A], S76.001[A], S76.009-S76.011[A], S76.019[A], S76.091[A], S76.099-S76.101[A], S76.109-S76.111[A], S76.119[A], S76.191[A], S76.199-S76.201[A], S76.209-S76.211[A], S76.219[A], S76.291[A], S76.299-S76.301[A], S76.309-S76.311[A], S76.319[A], S76.391[A], S76.399-S76.801[A], S76.809-S76.811[A], S76.819[A], S76.891[A], S76.899-S76.901[A], S76.909-S76.911[A], S76.919[A], S76.991[A], S76.999[A], S79.001[A], S79.009-S79.011[A], S79.019-S79.091[A], S79.099-S79.101[A], S79.109-S79.111[A], S79.119-S79.121[A], S79.129-S79.131[A], S79.139-S79.141[A], S79.149-S79.191[A], S79.199-S79.811[A], S79.819-S79.821[A], S79.829-S79.911[A], S79.919-S79.921[A], S79.929[A], S82.90X-S82.92X[A,B,C], T14.90-T14.91, T79.A0X-T79.9XX[A] **For S72.001[B,C]:** M48.40X-M48.58X[A], M80.00X-M80.88X[A], M84.30X-M84.68X[A], M84.750-M84.759[A], S03.8XX-S03.9XX[A], S29.011-S29.019[A], S38.3XX[A], S39.011-S39.013[A], S72.001-S72.466[A,B,C], S72.471-S72.479[A], S72.491-S72.92X[A,B,C], S73.101-S73.199[A], S76.001-S76.019[A], S76.091-S76.119[A], S76.191-S76.219[A], S76.291-S76.319[A], S76.391-S76.819[A], S76.891-S76.919[A], S76.991-S76.999[A], S79.001-S79.929[A], S82.90X-S82.92X[A,B,C], T14.90-T14.91, T79.A0X-T79.9XX[A] **For S72.001[K,M,N,P,Q,R]:** See S02.0[K]

CHAPTER 19 (S00–T88)

● **S72.002**   **Fracture of** unspecified **part of neck of left femur** K, M, N, P, Q, R 🔵, A, B, C 🔵, A, B, C 🔵
  (Ex) **For S72.002[A]:** M48.40X-M48.58X[A], M80.00X-M80.88X[A], M84.30X-M84.68X[A], M84.750-M84.759[A], S03.8XX-S03.9XX[A], S29.011-S29.019[A], S38.3XX[A], S39.011-S39.013[A], S72.001[B,C], S72.002-S72.009[A,B,C], S72.011[B,C], S72.012-S72.019[A,B,C], S72.021[B,C], S72.022-S72.023[A,B,C], S72.024[B,C], S72.025-S72.026[A,B,C], S72.031[B,C], S72.032-S72.033[A,B,C], S72.034[B,C], S72.035-S72.036[A,B,C], S72.041[B,C], S72.042-S72.043[A,B,C], S72.044[B,C], S72.045-S72.046[A,B,C], S72.051[B,C], S72.052-S72.059[A,B,C], S72.061[B,C], S72.062-S72.063[A,B,C], S72.064[B,C], S72.065-S72.066[A,B,C], S72.091[B,C], S72.092-S72.099[A,B,C], S72.101[B,C], S72.102-S72.109[A,B,C], S72.111[B,C], S72.112-S72.113[A,B,C], S72.114[B,C], S72.115-S72.116[A,B,C], S72.121[B,C], S72.122-S72.123[A,B,C], S72.124[B,C], S72.125-S72.126[A,B,C], S72.131[B,C], S72.132-S72.133[A,B,C], S72.134[B,C], S72.135-S72.136[A,B,C], S72.141[B,C], S72.142-S72.143[C], S72.144[B,C], S72.145-S72.146[A,B,C], S72.21X-S72.26X[A], S72.301[B,C], S72.302-S72.309[A,B,C], S72.321[B,C], S72.322-S72.323[A,B,C], S72.324[B,C], S72.325-S72.326[A,B,C], S72.331[B,C], S72.332-S72.333[A,B,C], S72.334[B,C], S72.335-S72.336[A,B,C], S72.341[B,C], S72.342-S72.343[A,B,C], S72.344[B,C], S72.345-S72.346[A,B,C], S72.351[B,C], S72.352-S72.353[A,B,C], S72.354[B,C], S72.355-S72.356[A,B,C], S72.361[B,C], S72.362-S72.363[A,B,C], S72.364[B,C], S72.365-S72.366[A,B,C], S72.391[B,C], S72.392-S72.399[A,B,C], S72.401[B,C], S72.402-S72.409[A,B,C], S72.411[B,C], S72.412-S72.413[A,B,C], S72.414[B,C], S72.415-S72.416[A,B,C], S72.421[B,C], S72.422-S72.423[A,B,C], S72.424[B,C], S72.425-S72.426[A,B,C], S72.431[B,C], S72.432-S72.433[A,B,C], S72.434[B,C], S72.435-S72.436[A,B,C], S72.441[B,C], S72.442-S72.443[A,B,C], S72.444[B,C], S72.445-S72.446[A,B,C], S72.451[B,C], S72.452-S72.453[A,B,C], S72.454[B,C], S72.455-S72.456[A,B,C], S72.461[B,C], S72.462-S72.463[A,B,C], S72.464[B,C], S72.465-S72.466[A,B,C], S72.472-S72.479[A], S72.491[B,C], S72.492-S72.92X[A,B,C], S73.102-S73.109[A], S73.112-S73.119[A], S73.122-S73.129[A], S73.192-S73.199[A], S76.002-S76.009[A], S76.012-S76.019[A], S76.092-S76.099[A], S76.102-S76.109[A], S76.112-S76.119[A], S76.192-S76.199[A], S76.202-S76.209[A], S76.212-S76.219[A], S76.292-S76.299[A], S76.302-S76.309[A], S76.312-S76.319[A], S76.392-S76.399[A], S76.802-S76.809[A], S76.812-S76.819[A], S76.892-S76.899[A], S76.902-S76.909[A], S76.912-S76.919[A], S76.992-S76.999[A], S79.002-S79.009[A], S79.012-S79.019[A], S79.092-S79.099[A], S79.102-S79.109[A], S79.112-S79.119[A], S79.122-S79.129[A], S79.132-S79.139[A], S79.142-S79.149[A], S79.192-S79.199[A], S79.812-S79.819[A], S79.822-S79.829[A], S79.912-S79.919[A], S79.922-S79.929[A], S82.90X-S82.92X[A,B,C], T14.90-T14.91, T79.8XXA T79.A0X-T79.9XX[A]
      For S72.002[B,C]: See S72.001[B,C]
      For S72.002[K,M,N,P,Q,R]: See S02.0[K]
    Coding Clinic: 2015, Q4, P37, Q1, P17

● **S72.009**   **Fracture of** unspecified **part of neck of unspecified femur** K, M, N, P, Q, R 🔵, A, B, C 🔵, A, B, C 🔵
  (Ex) **For S72.009[A,B,C]:** See S72.001[B,C]
      For S72.009[K,M,N,P,Q,R]: See S02.0[K]

● **S72.01**   **Unspecified intracapsular fracture of femur**
    Subcapital fracture of femur

  ● **S72.011**   Unspecified **intracapsular fracture of right femur** K, M, N, P, Q, R 🔵, A, B, C 🔵, A, B, C 🔵
    (Ex) **For S72.011[A]:** See S72.001 [A]
        For S72.011[B,C]: See S72.001[B,C]
        For S72.011[K,M,N,P,Q,R]: See S02.0[K]

  ● **S72.012**   Unspecified **intracapsular fracture of left femur** K, M, N, P, Q, R 🔵, A, B, C 🔵, A, B, C 🔵
    (Ex) **For S72.012[A]:** See S72.002[A]
        For S72.012[B,C]: See S72.001[B,C]
        For S72.012[K,M,N,P,Q,R]: See S02.0[K]

  ● **S72.019**   Unspecified **intracapsular fracture of unspecified femur** K, M, N, P, Q, R 🔵, A, B, C 🔵, A, B, C 🔵
    (Ex) **For S72.019[A,B,C]:** See S72.001[B,C]
        For S72.019[K,M,N,P,Q,R]: See S02.0[K]

● **S72.02**   **Fracture of epiphysis (separation) (upper) of femur**
    Transepiphyseal fracture of femur
    Fracture and separation across growth plate
    Excludes1   capital femoral epiphyseal fracture (pediatric) of femur (S79.01-)
    Salter-Harris Type I physeal fracture of upper end of femur (S79.01-)

  ● **S72.021**   **Displaced fracture of epiphysis (separation) (upper) of right femur** K, M, N, P, Q, R 🔵, A, B, C 🔵, A, B, C 🔵
    (Ex) **For S72.021[A]:** See S72.001[A]
        For S72.021[B,C]: See S72.001[B,C]
        For S72.021[K,M,N,P,Q,R]: See S02.0[K]

  ● **S72.022**   **Displaced fracture of epiphysis (separation) (upper) of left femur** K, M, N, P, Q, R 🔵, A, B, C 🔵, A, B, C 🔵
    (Ex) **For S72.022[A]:** See S72.002[A]
        For S72.022[B,C]: See S72.001[B,C]
        For S72.022[K,M,N,P,Q,R]: See S02.0[K]

  ● **S72.023**   **Displaced fracture of epiphysis (separation) (upper) of** unspecified **femur** K, M, N, P, Q, R 🔵, A, B, C 🔵, A, B, C 🔵
    (Ex) **For S72.023[A,B,C]:** See S72.001[B,C]
        For S72.023[K,M,N,P,Q,R]: See S02.0[K]

  ● **S72.024**   **Nondisplaced fracture of epiphysis (separation) (upper) of right femur** K, M, N, P, Q, R 🔵, A, B, C 🔵, A, B, C 🔵
    (Ex) **For S72.024[A]:** See S72.001[A]
        For S72.024[B,C]: See S72.001[B,C]
        For S72.024[K,M,N,P,Q,R]: See S02.0[K]

  ● **S72.025**   **Nondisplaced fracture of epiphysis (separation) (upper) of left femur** K, M, N, P, Q, R 🔵, A, B, C 🔵, A, B, C 🔵
    (Ex) **For S72.025[A]:** See S72.002[A]
        For S72.025[B,C]: See S72.001[B,C]
        For S72.025[K,M,N,P,Q,R]: See S02.0[K]

  ● **S72.026**   **Nondisplaced fracture of epiphysis (separation) (upper) of** unspecified **femur** K, M, N, P, Q, R 🔵, A, B, C 🔵, A, B, C 🔵
    (Ex) **For S72.026[A,B,C]:** See S72.001[B,C]
        For S72.026[K,M,N,P,Q,R]: See S02.0[K]

◀ New   ◀ Revised   ~~deleted~~ Deleted   Excludes 1   Excludes 2   Includes   Use additional   Code first   Code also   Unspecified
OGCR Official Guidelines   ● Unacceptable Principal Diagnosis   X Assign placeholder X   ● Use Additional Character(s)   ▸ Manifestation Code   **Coding Clinic**

● **S72.03**   **Midcervical fracture of femur**
     Transcervical fracture of femur NOS

   ● **S72.031**   **Displaced midcervical fracture of right femur** K, M, N, P, Q, R 🦠, A, B, C 🦠, A, B, C 🦠
      Ⓔⓧ For S72.031[A]: See S72.001[A]
        For S72.031[B,C]: See S72.001[B,C]
        For S72.031[K,M,N,P,Q,R]: See S02.0[K]

   ● **S72.032**   **Displaced midcervical fracture of left femur** K, M, N, P, Q, R 🦠, A, B, C 🦠, A, B, C 🦠
      Ⓔⓧ For S72.032[A]: See S72.002[A]
        For S72.032[B,C]: See S72.001[B,C]
        For S72.032[K,M,N,P,Q,R]: See S02.0[K]

   ● **S72.033**   **Displaced midcervical fracture of unspecified femur** K, M, N, P, Q, R 🦠, A, B, C 🦠, A, B, C 🦠
      Ⓔⓧ For S72.033[A,B,C]: See S72.001[B,C]
        For S72.033[K,M,N,P,Q,R]: See S02.0[K]

   ● **S72.034**   **Nondisplaced midcervical fracture of right femur** K, M, N, P, Q, R 🦠, A, B, C 🦠, A, B, C 🦠
      Ⓔⓧ For S72.034[A]: See S72.001[A]
        For S72.034[B,C]: See S72.001[B,C]
        For S72.034[K,M,N,P,Q,R]: See S02.0[K]

   ● **S72.035**   **Nondisplaced midcervical fracture of left femur** K, M, N, P, Q, R 🦠, A, B, C 🦠, A, B, C 🦠
      Ⓔⓧ For S72.035[A]: See S72.002[A]
        For S72.035[B,C]: See S72.001[B,C]
        For S72.035[K,M,N,P,Q,R]: See S02.0[K]

   ● **S72.036**   **Nondisplaced midcervical fracture of unspecified femur** K, M, N, P, Q, R 🦠, A, B, C 🦠, A, B, C 🦠
      Ⓔⓧ For S72.036[A,B,C]: See S72.001[B,C]
        For S72.036[K,M,N,P,Q,R]: See S02.0[K]

● **S72.04**   **Fracture of base of neck of femur**
     Cervicotrochanteric fracture of femur

   ● **S72.041**   **Displaced fracture of base of neck of right femur** K, M, N, P, Q, R 🦠, A, B, C 🦠, A, B, C 🦠
      Ⓔⓧ For S72.041[A]: See S72.001[A]
        For S72.041[B,C]: See S72.001[B,C]
        For S72.041[K,M,N,P,Q,R]: See S02.0[K]

   ● **S72.042**   **Displaced fracture of base of neck of left femur** K, M, N, P, Q, R 🦠, A, B, C 🦠, A, B, C 🦠
      Ⓔⓧ For S72.042[A]: See S72.002[A]
        For S72.042[B,C]: See S72.001[B,C]
        For S72.042[K,M,N,P,Q,R]: See S02.0[K]

   ● **S72.043**   **Displaced fracture of base of neck of unspecified femur** K, M, N, P, Q, R 🦠, A, B, C 🦠, A, B, C 🦠
      Ⓔⓧ For S72.043[A,B,C]: See S72.001[B,C]
        For S72.043[K,M,N,P,Q,R]: See S02.0[K]

   ● **S72.044**   **Nondisplaced fracture of base of neck of right femur** K, M, N, P, Q, R 🦠, A, B, C 🦠, A, B, C 🦠
      Ⓔⓧ For S72.044[A]: See S72.001[A]
        For S72.044[B,C]: See S72.001[B,C]
        For S72.044[K,M,N,P,Q,R]: See S02.0[K]

   ● **S72.045**   **Nondisplaced fracture of base of neck of left femur** K, M, N, P, Q, R 🦠, A, B, C 🦠, A, B, C 🦠
      Ⓔⓧ For S72.045[A]: See S72.002[A]
        For S72.045[B,C]: See S72.001[B,C]
        For S72.045[K,M,N,P,Q,R]: See S02.0[K]

   ● **S72.046**   **Nondisplaced fracture of base of neck of unspecified femur** K, M, N, P, Q, R 🦠, A, B, C 🦠, A, B, C 🦠
      Ⓔⓧ For S72.046[A,B,C]: See S72.001[B,C]
        For S72.046[K,M,N,P,Q,R]: See S02.0[K]

● **S72.05**   **Unspecified fracture of head of femur**
     Fracture of head of femur NOS

   ● **S72.051**   **Unspecified fracture of head of right femur** K, M, N, P, Q, R 🦠, A, B, C 🦠, A, B, C 🦠
      Ⓔⓧ For S72.051[A]: See S72.001[A]
        For S72.051[B,C]: See S72.001[B,C]
        For S72.051[K,M,N,P,Q,R]: See S02.0[K]

   ● **S72.052**   **Unspecified fracture of head of left femur** K, M, N, P, Q, R 🦠, A, B, C 🦠, A, B, C 🦠
      Ⓔⓧ For S72.052[A]: See S72.002[A]
        For S72.052[B,C]: See S72.001[B,C]
        For S72.052[K,M,N,P,Q,R]: See S02.0[K]

   ● **S72.059**   **Unspecified fracture of head of unspecified femur** K, M, N, P, Q, R 🦠, A, B, C 🦠, A, B, C 🦠
      Ⓔⓧ For S72.059[A,B,C]: See S72.001[B,C]
        For S72.059[K,M,N,P,Q,R]: See S02.0[K]

● **S72.06**   **Articular fracture of head of femur**

   ● **S72.061**   **Displaced articular fracture of head of right femur** K, M, N, P, Q, R 🦠, A, B, C 🦠, A, B, C 🦠
      Ⓔⓧ For S72.061[A]: See S72.001[A]
        For S72.061[B,C]: See S72.001[B,C]
        For S72.061[K,M,N,P,Q,R]: See S02.0[K]

   ● **S72.062**   **Displaced articular fracture of head of left femur** K, M, N, P, Q, R 🦠, A, B, C 🦠, A, B, C 🦠
      Ⓔⓧ For S72.062[A]: See S72.002[A]
        For S72.062[B,C]: See S72.001[B,C]
        For S72.062[K,M,N,P,Q,R]: See S02.0[K]

   ● **S72.063**   **Displaced articular fracture of head of unspecified femur** K, M, N, P, Q, R 🦠, A, B, C 🦠, A, B, C 🦠
      Ⓔⓧ For S72.063[A,B,C]: See S72.001[B,C]
        For S72.063[K,M,N,P,Q,R]: See S02.0[K]

   ● **S72.064**   **Nondisplaced articular fracture of head of right femur** K, M, N, P, Q, R 🦠, A, B, C 🦠, A, B, C 🦠
      Ⓔⓧ For S72.064[A]: See S72.001[A]
        For S72.064[B,C]: See S72.001[B,C]
        For S72.064[K,M,N,P,Q,R]: See S02.0[K]

   ● **S72.065**   **Nondisplaced articular fracture of head of left femur** K, M, N, P, Q, R 🦠, A, B, C 🦠, A, B, C 🦠
      Ⓔⓧ For S72.065[A]: See S72.002[A]
        For S72.065[B,C]: See S72.001[B,C]
        For S72.065[K,M,N,P,Q,R]: See S02.0[K]

   ● **S72.066**   **Nondisplaced articular fracture of head of unspecified femur** K, M, N, P, Q, R 🦠, A, B, C 🦠, A, B, C 🦠
      Ⓔⓧ For S72.066[A,B,C]: See S72.001[B,C]
        For S72.066[K,M,N,P,Q,R]: See S02.0[K]

● **S72.09**   **Other fracture of head and neck of femur**

   ● **S72.091**   **Other fracture of head and neck of right femur** K, M, N, P, Q, R 🦠, A, B, C 🦠, A, B, C 🦠
      Ⓔⓧ For S72.091[A]: See S72.001[A]
        For S72.091[B,C]: See S72.001[B,C]
        For S72.091[K,M,N,P,Q,R]: See S02.0[K]

   ● **S72.092**   **Other fracture of head and neck of left femur** K, M, N, P, Q, R 🦠, A, B, C 🦠, A, B, C 🦠
      Ⓔⓧ For S72.092[A]: See S72.002[A]
        For S72.092[B,C]: See S72.001[B,C]
        For S72.092[K,M,N,P,Q,R]: See S02.0[K]

   ● **S72.099**   **Other fracture of head and neck of unspecified femur** K, M, N, P, Q, R 🦠, A, B, C 🦠, A, B, C 🦠
      Ⓔⓧ For S72.099[A,B,C]: See S72.001[B,C]
        For S72.099[K,M,N,P,Q,R]: See S02.0[K]

CHAPTER 19 (S00-T88)

N Newborn Age: 0   **P** Pediatric Age: 0–17   **M** Maternity DX: 12–55   **A** Adult Age: 15–124   ♀ Females Only   ♂ Males Only

🦠 Complication\Comorbidity   🦠 Major C\C   Ⓔⓧ CC/MCC Exclusions   🦠 Hospital-Acquired Condition

1359

● **S72.1   Pertrochanteric fracture**
Fracture extending close to, but not into, joint

● **S72.10   Unspecified trochanteric fracture of femur**
Fracture of trochanter NOS

● **S72.101   Unspecified trochanteric fracture of right femur** K, M, N, P, Q, R 🔧, A, B, C 🔧, A, B, C 🔧
Ⓔⓧ **For S72.101[A]:** See S72.001[A]
For S72.101[B,C]: See S72.001[B,C]
For S72.101[K,M,N,P,Q,R]: See S02.0[K]

● **S72.102   Unspecified trochanteric fracture of left femur** K, M, N, P, Q, R 🔧, A, B, C 🔧, A, B, C 🔧
Ⓔⓧ **For S72.102[A]:** See S72.002[A]
For S72.102[B,C]: See S72.001[B,C]
For S72.102[K,M,N,P,Q,R]: See S02.0[K]

● **S72.109   Unspecified trochanteric fracture of unspecified femur** K, M, N, P, Q, R 🔧, A, B, C 🔧, A, B, C 🔧
Ⓔⓧ **For S72.109[A,B,C]:** See S72.001[B,C]
For S72.109[K,M,N,P,Q,R]: See S02.0[K]

● **S72.11   Fracture of greater trochanter of femur**

● **S72.111   Displaced fracture of greater trochanter of right femur** K, M, N, P, Q, R 🔧, A, B, C 🔧, A, B, C 🔧
Ⓔⓧ **For S72.111[A]:** See S72.001[A]
For S72.111[B,C]: See S72.001[B,C]
For S72.111[K,M,N,P,Q,R]: See S02.0[K]

● **S72.112   Displaced fracture of greater trochanter of left femur** K, M, N, P, Q, R 🔧, A, B, C 🔧, A, B, C 🔧
Ⓔⓧ **For S72.112[A]:** See S72.002[A]
For S72.112[B,C]: See S72.001[B,C]
For S72.112[K,M,N,P,Q,R]: See S02.0[K]

● **S72.113   Displaced fracture of greater trochanter of unspecified femur** K, M, N, P, Q, R 🔧, A, B, C 🔧, A, B, C 🔧
Ⓔⓧ **For S72.113[A,B,C]:** See S72.001[B,C]
For S72.113[K,M,N,P,Q,R]: See S02.0[K]

● **S72.114   Nondisplaced fracture of greater trochanter of right femur** K, M, N, P, Q, R 🔧, A, B, C 🔧, A, B, C 🔧
Ⓔⓧ **For S72.114[A]:** See S72.001[A]
For S72.114[B,C]: See S72.001[B,C]
For S72.114[K,M,N,P,Q,R]: See S02.0[K]

● **S72.115   Nondisplaced fracture of greater trochanter of left femur** K, M, N, P, Q, R 🔧, A, B, C 🔧, A, B, C 🔧
Ⓔⓧ **For S72.115[A]:** See S72.002[A]
For S72.115[B,C]: See S72.001[B,C]
For S72.115[K,M,N,P,Q,R]: See S02.0[K]

● **S72.116   Nondisplaced fracture of greater trochanter of unspecified femur** K, M, N, P, Q, R 🔧, A, B, C 🔧, A, B, C 🔧
Ⓔⓧ **For S72.116[A,B,C]:** See S72.001[B,C]
For S72.116[K,M,N,P,Q,R]: See S02.0[K]

● **S72.12   Fracture of lesser trochanter of femur**

● **S72.121   Displaced fracture of lesser trochanter of right femur** K, M, N, P, Q, R 🔧, A, B, C 🔧, A, B, C 🔧
Ⓔⓧ **For S72.121[A]:** See S72.001[A]
For S72.121[B,C]: See S72.001[B,C]
For S72.121[K,M,N,P,Q,R]: See S02.0[K]

● **S72.122   Displaced fracture of lesser trochanter of left femur** K, M, N, P, Q, R 🔧, A, B, C 🔧, A, B, C 🔧
Ⓔⓧ **For S72.122[A]:** See S72.002[A]
For S72.122[B,C]: See S72.001[B,C]
For S72.122[K,M,N,P,Q,R]: See S02.0[K]

● **S72.123   Displaced fracture of lesser trochanter of unspecified femur** K, M, N, P, Q, R 🔧, A, B, C 🔧, A, B, C 🔧
Ⓔⓧ **For S72.123[A,B,C]:** See S72.001[B,C]
For S72.123[K,M,N,P,Q,R]: See S02.0[K]

● **S72.124   Nondisplaced fracture of lesser trochanter of right femur** K, M, N, P, Q, R 🔧, A, B, C 🔧, A, B, C 🔧
Ⓔⓧ **For S72.124[A]:** See S72.001[A]
For S72.124[B,C]: See S72.001[B,C]
For S72.124[K,M,N,P,Q,R]: See S02.0[K]

● **S72.125   Nondisplaced fracture of lesser trochanter of left femur** K, M, N, P, Q, R 🔧, A, B, C 🔧, A, B, C 🔧
Ⓔⓧ **For S72.125[A]:** See S72.002[A]
For S72.125[B,C]: See S72.001[B,C]
For S72.125[K,M,N,P,Q,R]: See S02.0[K]

● **S72.126   Nondisplaced fracture of lesser trochanter of unspecified femur** K, M, N, P, Q, R 🔧, A, B, C 🔧, A, B, C 🔧
Ⓔⓧ **For S72.126[A,B,C]:** See S72.001[B,C]
For S72.126[K,M,N,P,Q,R]: See S02.0[K]

● **S72.13   Apophyseal fracture of femur**
Pertaining to articulations between articular facets of adjacent vertebrae
Excludes1   chronic (nontraumatic) slipped upper femoral epiphysis (M93.0-)

● **S72.131   Displaced apophyseal fracture of right femur** K, M, N, P, Q, R 🔧, A, B, C 🔧, A, B, C 🔧
Ⓔⓧ **For S72.131[A]:** See S72.001[A]
For S72.131[B,C]: See S72.001[B,C]
For S72.131[K,M,N,P,Q,R]: See S02.0[K]

● **S72.132   Displaced apophyseal fracture of left femur** K, M, N, P, Q, R 🔧, A, B, C 🔧, A, B, C 🔧
Ⓔⓧ **For S72.132[A]:** See S72.002[A]
For S72.132[B,C]: See S72.001[B,C]
For S72.132[K,M,N,P,Q,R]: See S02.0[K]

● **S72.133   Displaced apophyseal fracture of unspecified femur** K, M, N, P, Q, R 🔧, A, B, C 🔧, A, B, C 🔧
Ⓔⓧ **For S72.133[A,B,C]:** See S72.001[B,C]
For S72.133[K,M,N,P,Q,R]: See S02.0[K]

● **S72.134   Nondisplaced apophyseal fracture of right femur** K, M, N, P, Q, R 🔧, A, B, C 🔧, A, B, C 🔧
Ⓔⓧ **For S72.134[A]:** See S72.001[A]
For S72.134[B,C]: See S72.001[B,C]
For S72.134[K,M,N,P,Q,R]: See S02.0[K]

● **S72.135   Nondisplaced apophyseal fracture of left femur** K, M, N, P, Q, R 🔧, A, B, C 🔧, A, B, C 🔧
Ⓔⓧ **For S72.135[A]:** See S72.002[A]
For S72.135[B,C]: See S72.001[B,C]
For S72.135[K,M,N,P,Q,R]: See S02.0[K]

● **S72.136   Nondisplaced apophyseal fracture of unspecified femur** K, M, N, P, Q, R 🔧, A, B, C 🔧, A, B, C 🔧
Ⓔⓧ **For S72.136[A,B,C]:** See S72.001[B,C]
For S72.136[K,M,N,P,Q,R]: See S02.0[K]

◀ New   ◀ⅢⅢ Revised   d̶e̶l̶e̶t̶e̶d̶ Deleted   Excludes 1   Excludes 2   Includes   Use additional   Code first   Code also   Unspecified
OGCR Official Guidelines   ● Unacceptable Principal Diagnosis   X Assign placeholder X   ● Use Additional Character(s)   ▶ Manifestation Code   **Coding Clinic**

● **S72.14** Intertrochanteric fracture of femur

  ● **S72.141** Displaced intertrochanteric fracture of right femur K, M, N, P, Q, R 🔖, A, B, C 🔖, A, B, C 🔖
    Ⓔⓧ For S72.141[A]: See S72.001[A]
    For S72.141[B,C]: See S72.001[B,C]
    For S72.141[K,M,N,P,Q,R]: See S02.0[K]

  ● **S72.142** Displaced intertrochanteric fracture of left femur K, M, N, P, Q, R 🔖, A, B, C 🔖, A, B, C 🔖
    Ⓔⓧ For S72.142[A]: See S72.002[A]
    For S72.142[B,C]: See S72.001[B,C]
    For S72.142[K,M,N,P,Q,R]: See S02.0[K]

  ● **S72.143** Displaced intertrochanteric fracture of unspecified femur K, M, N, P, Q, R 🔖, A, B, C 🔖, A, B, C 🔖
    Ⓔⓧ For S72.143[A,B,C]: See S72.001[B,C]
    For S72.143[K,M,N,P,Q,R]: See S02.0[K]

  ● **S72.144** Nondisplaced intertrochanteric fracture of right femur K, M, N, P, Q, R 🔖, A, B, C 🔖, A, B, C 🔖
    Ⓔⓧ For S72.144[A]: See S72.001[A]
    For S72.324[B,C]: See S72.001[B,C]
    For S72.324[K,M,N,P,Q,R]: See S02.0[K]

  ● **S72.145** Nondisplaced intertrochanteric fracture of left femur K, M, N, P, Q, R 🔖, A, B, C 🔖, A, B, C 🔖
    Ⓔⓧ For S72.145[A]: See S72.002[A]
    For S72.145[B,C]: See S72.001[B,C]
    For S72.145[K,M,N,P,Q,R]: See S02.0[K]

  ● **S72.146** Nondisplaced intertrochanteric fracture of unspecified femur K, M, N, P, Q, R 🔖, A, B, C 🔖, A, B, C 🔖
    Ⓔⓧ For S72.146[A,B,C]: See S72.001[B,C]
    For S72.146[K,M,N,P,Q,R]: See S02.0[K]

● **S72.2** Subtrochanteric fracture of femur
  Subtrochanteric: inferior to trochanter
    Ⓔⓧ For category S72.2 CC codes S72.2[A,B,C]: See S72.001[B,C]
    For S72.2[K,M,N,P,Q,R]: See S02.0[K]

  X● **S72.21** Displaced subtrochanteric fracture of right femur K, M, N, P, Q, R 🔖, A, B, C 🔖, A, B, C 🔖

  X● **S72.22** Displaced subtrochanteric fracture of left femur K, M, N, P, Q, R 🔖, A, B, C 🔖, A, B, C 🔖

  X● **S72.23** Displaced subtrochanteric fracture of unspecified femur K, M, N, P, Q, R 🔖, A, B, C 🔖, A, B, C 🔖

  X● **S72.24** Nondisplaced subtrochanteric fracture of right femur K, M, N, P, Q, R 🔖, A, B, C 🔖, A, B, C 🔖

  X● **S72.25** Nondisplaced subtrochanteric fracture of left femur K, M, N, P, Q, R 🔖, A, B, C 🔖, A, B, C 🔖

  X● **S72.26** Nondisplaced subtrochanteric fracture of unspecified femur K, M, N, P, Q, R 🔖, A, B, C 🔖, A, B, C 🔖

● **S72.3** Fracture of shaft of femur
  ● **S72.30** Unspecified fracture of shaft of femur

    ● **S72.301** Unspecified fracture of shaft of right femur K, M, N, P, Q, R 🔖, A, B, C 🔖, A, B, C 🔖
      Ⓔⓧ For S72.301[A]: See S72.001[A]
      For S72.301[B,C]: See S72.001[B,C]
      For S72.301[K,M,N,P,Q,R]: See S02.0[K]

    ● **S72.302** Unspecified fracture of shaft of left femur K, M, N, P, Q, R 🔖, A, B, C 🔖, A, B, C 🔖
      Ⓔⓧ For S72.302[A]: See S72.002[A]
      For S72.302[B,C]: See S72.001[B,C]
      For S72.302[K,M,N,P,Q,R]: See S02.0[K]

    ● **S72.309** Unspecified fracture of shaft of unspecified femur K, M, N, P, Q, R 🔖, A, B, C 🔖, A, B, C 🔖
      Ⓔⓧ For S72.309[A,B,C]: See S72.001[B,C]
      For S72.309[K,M,N,P,Q,R]: See S02.0[K]

● **S72.32** Transverse fracture of shaft of femur

  ● **S72.321** Displaced transverse fracture of shaft of right femur K, M, N, P, Q, R 🔖, A, B, C 🔖, A, B, C 🔖
    Ⓔⓧ For S72.321[A]: See S72.001[A]
    For S72.321[B,C]: See S72.001[B,C]
    For S72.321[K,M,N,P,Q,R]: See S02.0[K]

  ● **S72.322** Displaced transverse fracture of shaft of left femur K, M, N, P, Q, R 🔖, A, B, C 🔖, A, B, C 🔖
    Ⓔⓧ For S72.322[A]: See S72.002[A]
    For S72.322[B,C]: See S72.001[B,C]
    For S72.322[K,M,N,P,Q,R]: See S02.0[K]

  ● **S72.323** Displaced transverse fracture of shaft of unspecified femur K, M, N, P, Q, R 🔖, A, B, C 🔖, A, B, C 🔖
    Ⓔⓧ For S72.323[A,B,C]: See S72.001[B,C]
    For S72.323[K,M,N,P,Q,R]: See S02.0[K]

  ● **S72.324** Nondisplaced transverse fracture of shaft of right femur K, M, N, P, Q, R 🔖, A, B, C 🔖, A, B, C 🔖
    Ⓔⓧ For S72.324[A]: See S72.001[A]
    For S72.324[B,C]: See S72.001[B,C]
    For S72.324[K,M,N,P,Q,R]: See S02.0[K]

  ● **S72.325** Nondisplaced transverse fracture of shaft of left femur K, M, N, P, Q, R 🔖, A, B, C 🔖, A, B, C 🔖
    Ⓔⓧ For S72.325[A]: See S72.002[A]
    For S72.325[B,C]: See S72.001[B,C]
    For S72.325[K,M,N,P,Q,R]: See S02.0[K]

  ● **S72.326** Nondisplaced transverse fracture of shaft of unspecified femur K, M, N, P, Q, R 🔖, A, B, C 🔖, A, B, C 🔖
    Ⓔⓧ For S72.326[A,B,C]: See S72.001[B,C]
    For S72.326[K,M,N,P,Q,R]: See S02.0[K]

● **S72.33** Oblique fracture of shaft of femur

  ● **S72.331** Displaced oblique fracture of shaft of right femur K, M, N, P, Q, R 🔖, A, B, C 🔖, A, B, C 🔖
    Ⓔⓧ For S72.331[A]: See S72.001[A]
    For S72.331[B,C]: See S72.001[B,C]
    For S72.331[K,M,N,P,Q,R]: See S02.0[K]

  ● **S72.332** Displaced oblique fracture of shaft of left femur K, M, N, P, Q, R 🔖, A, B, C 🔖, A, B, C 🔖
    Ⓔⓧ For S72.332[A]: See S72.002[A]
    For S72.332[B,C]: See S72.001[B,C]
    For S72.332[K,M,N,P,Q,R]: See S02.0[K]

  ● **S72.333** Displaced oblique fracture of shaft of unspecified femur K, M, N, P, Q, R 🔖, A, B, C 🔖, A, B, C 🔖
    Ⓔⓧ For S72.333[A,B,C]: See S72.001[B,C]
    For S72.333[K,M,N,P,Q,R]: See S02.0[K]

  ● **S72.334** Nondisplaced oblique fracture of shaft of right femur K, M, N, P, Q, R 🔖, A, B, C 🔖, A, B, C 🔖
    Ⓔⓧ For S72.334[A]: See S72.001[A]
    For S72.334[B,C]: See S72.001[B,C]
    For S72.334[K,M,N,P,Q,R]: See S02.0[K]

  ● **S72.335** Nondisplaced oblique fracture of shaft of left femur K, M, N, P, Q, R 🔖, A, B, C 🔖, A, B, C 🔖
    Ⓔⓧ For S72.335[A]: See S72.002[A]
    For S72.335[B,C]: See S72.001[B,C]
    For S72.335[K,M,N,P,Q,R]: See S02.0[K]

  ● **S72.336** Nondisplaced oblique fracture of shaft of unspecified femur K, M, N, P, Q, R 🔖, A, B, C 🔖, A, B, C 🔖
    Ⓔⓧ For S72.336[A,B,C]: See S72.001 [B,C]
    For S72.336[K,M,N,P,Q,R]: See S02.0[K]

N Newborn Age: 0   **P** Pediatric Age: 0–17   **M** Maternity DX: 12–55   **A** Adult Age: 15–124   ♀ Females Only   ♂ Males Only

🔖 Complication\Comorbidity   🔖 Major C\C   Ⓔⓧ CC/MCC Exclusions   🔖 Hospital-Acquired Condition

● **S72.34**   **Spiral fracture of shaft of femur**
    ● **S72.341**   **Displaced spiral fracture of shaft of right femur** K, M, N, P, Q, R 🔵, A, B, C 🔵, A, B, C 🔵
       (Ex:) For S72.341[A]: See S72.001[A]
             For S72.341[B,C]: See S72.001[B,C]
             For S72.341[K,M,N,P,Q,R]: See S02.0[K]

    ● **S72.342**   **Displaced spiral fracture of shaft of left femur** K, M, N, P, Q, R 🔵, A, B, C 🔵, A, B, C 🔵
       (Ex:) For S72.342[A]: See S72.002[A]
             For S72.342[B,C]: See S72.001[B,C]
             For S72.342[K,M,N,P,Q,R]: See S02.0[K]

    ● **S72.343**   **Displaced spiral fracture of shaft of unspecified femur** K, M, N, P, Q, R 🔵, A, B, C 🔵, A, B, C 🔵
       (Ex:) For S72.343[A,B,C]: See S72.001[B,C]
             For S72.343[K,M,N,P,Q,R]: See S02.0[K]

    ● **S72.344**   **Nondisplaced spiral fracture of shaft of right femur** K, M, N, P, Q, R, A, B, C 🔵, A, B, C 🔵
       (Ex:) For S72.344[A]: See S72.001[A]
             For S72.344[B,C]: See S72.001[B,C]
             For S72.344[K,M,N,P,Q,R]: See S02.0[K]

    ● **S72.345**   **Nondisplaced spiral fracture of shaft of left femur** K, M, N, P, Q, R 🔵, A, B, C 🔵, A, B, C 🔵
       (Ex:) For S72.345[A]: See S72.002[A]
             For S72.345[B,C]: See S72.001[B,C]
             For S72.345[K,M,N,P,Q,R]: See S02.0[K]

    ● **S72.346**   **Nondisplaced spiral fracture of shaft of unspecified femur** K, M, N, P, Q, R 🔵, A, B, C 🔵, A, B, C 🔵
       (Ex:) For S72.346[A,B,C]: See S72.001[B,C]
             For S72.346[K,M,N,P,Q,R]: See S02.0[K]

● **S72.35**   **Comminuted fracture of shaft of femur**
    ● **S72.351**   **Displaced comminuted fracture of shaft of right femur** K, M, N, P, Q, R 🔵, A, B, C 🔵, A, B, C 🔵
       (Ex:) For S72.351[A]: See S72.001[A]
             For S72.351[B,C]: See S72.001[B,C]
             For S72.351[K,M,N,P,Q,R]: See S02.0[K]

    ● **S72.352**   **Displaced comminuted fracture of shaft of left femur** K, M, N, P, Q, R 🔵, A, B, C 🔵, A, B, C 🔵
       (Ex:) For S72.352[A]: See S72.002[A]
             For S72.352[B,C]: See S72.001[B,C]
             For S72.352[K,M,N,P,Q,R]: See S02.0[K]

    ● **S72.353**   **Displaced comminuted fracture of shaft of unspecified femur** K, M, N, P, Q, R 🔵, A, B, C 🔵, A, B, C 🔵
       (Ex:) For S72.353[A,B,C]: See S72.001[B,C]
             For S72.353[K,M,N,P,Q,R]: See S02.0[K]

    ● **S72.354**   **Nondisplaced comminuted fracture of shaft of right femur** K, M, N, P, Q, R 🔵, A, B, C 🔵, A, B, C 🔵
       (Ex:) For S72.354[A]: See S72.001[A]
             For S72.354[B,C]: See S72.001[B,C]
             For S72.354[K,M,N,P,Q,R]: See S02.0[K]

    ● **S72.355**   **Nondisplaced comminuted fracture of shaft of left femur** K, M, N, P, Q, R 🔵, A, B, C 🔵, A, B, C 🔵
       (Ex:) For S72.355[A]: See S72.002[A]
             For S72.355[B,C]: See S72.001[B,C]
             For S72.355[K,M,N,P,Q,R]: See S02.0[K]

    ● **S72.356**   **Nondisplaced comminuted fracture of shaft of unspecified femur** K, M, N, P, Q, R 🔵, A, B, C 🔵, A, B, C 🔵
       (Ex:) For S72.356[A,B,C]: See S72.001[B,C]
             For S72.356[K,M,N,P,Q,R]: See S02.0[K]

● **S72.36**   **Segmental fracture of shaft of femur**
    ● **S72.361**   **Displaced segmental fracture of shaft of right femur** K, M, N, P, Q, R 🔵, A, B, C 🔵, A, B, C 🔵
       (Ex:) For S72.361[A]: See S72.001[A]
             For S72.361[B,C]: See S72.001[B,C]
             For S72.361[K,M,N,P,Q,R]: See S02.0[K]

    ● **S72.362**   **Displaced segmental fracture of shaft of left femur** K, M, N, P, Q, R 🔵, A, B, C 🔵, A, B, C 🔵
       (Ex:) For S72.362[A]: See S72.002[A]
             For S72.362[B,C]: See S72.001[B,C]
             For S72.362[K,M,N,P,Q,R]: See S02.0[K]

    ● **S72.363**   **Displaced segmental fracture of shaft of unspecified femur** K, M, N, P, Q, R 🔵, A, B, C 🔵, A, B, C 🔵
       (Ex:) For S72.363[A,B,C]: See S72.001[B,C]
             For S72.363[K,M,N,P,Q,R]: See S02.0[K]

    ● **S72.364**   **Nondisplaced segmental fracture of shaft of right femur** K, M, N, P, Q, R 🔵, A, B, C 🔵, A, B, C 🔵
       (Ex:) For S72.364[A]: See S72.001[A]
             For S72.364[B,C]: See S72.001[B,C]
             For S72.364[K,M,N,P,Q,R]: See S02.0[K]

    ● **S72.365**   **Nondisplaced segmental fracture of shaft of left femur** K, M, N, P, Q, R 🔵, A, B, C 🔵, A, B, C 🔵
       (Ex:) For S72.365[A]: See S72.002[A]
             For S72.365[B,C]: See S72.001[B,C]
             For S72.365[K,M,N,P,Q,R]: See S02.0[K]

    ● **S72.366**   **Nondisplaced segmental fracture of shaft of unspecified femur** K, M, N, P, Q, R 🔵, A, B, C 🔵, A, B, C 🔵
       (Ex:) For S72.366[A,B,C]: See S72.001[B,C]
             For S72.366[K,M,N,P,Q,R]: See S02.0[K]

● **S72.39**   **Other fracture of shaft of femur**
    ● **S72.391**   **Other fracture of shaft of right femur** K, M, N, P, Q, R 🔵, A, B, C 🔵, A, B, C 🔵
       (Ex:) For S72.391[A]: See S72.001[A]
             For S72.391[B,C]: See S72.001[B,C]
             For S72.391[K,M,N,P,Q,R]: See S02.0[K]

    ● **S72.392**   **Other fracture of shaft of left femur** K, M, N, P, Q, R 🔵, A, B, C 🔵, A, B, C 🔵
       (Ex:) For S72.392[A]: See S72.002[A]
             For S72.392[B,C]: See S72.001[B,C]
             For S72.392[K,M,N,P,Q,R]: See S02.0[K]

    ● **S72.399**   **Other fracture of shaft of unspecified femur** K, M, N, P, Q, R 🔵, A, B, C 🔵, A, B, C 🔵
       (Ex:) For S72.399[A,B,C]: See S72.001[B,C]
             For S72.399[K,M,N,P,Q,R]: See S02.0[K]

● **S72.4**   **Fracture of lower end of femur**
    Fracture of distal end of femur
    Excludes2   fracture of shaft of femur (S72.3-)
             physeal fracture of lower end of femur (S79.1-)

● **S72.40**   **Unspecified fracture of lower end of femur**
    ● **S72.401**   **Unspecified fracture of lower end of right femur** A, K, M, N, P, Q, R 🔵, B, C 🔵, A, B, C 🔵
       (Ex:) For S72.401[A]: M80.00X-M80.019[A],
           M80.041-M80.059[A], M80.80X-M80.819[A],
           M80.841-M80.859[A], M84.40X-M84.419[A],
           M84.441-M84.459[A], M84.474-M84.519[A],
           M84.541-M84.559[A], M84.574-M84.576[A],
           M84.60X-M84.619[A], M84.641-M84.659[A],
           M84.674-M84.68X[A], M84.750-M84.759[A],
           S03.8XX-S03.9XX[A], S29.011-S29.019[A],
           S38.3XX[A], S39.011-S39.013[A],
           S72.001[A,B,C], S72.002[B,C],
           S72.009-S72.011[A,B,C], S72.012[B,C],
           S72.019-S72.021[A,B,C], S72.022[B,C],
           S72.023-S72.024[A,B,C], S72.025[B,C],
           S72.026-S72.031[A,B,C], S72.032[B,C],

◀ New   ◀▥ Revised   ~~deleted~~ Deleted   Excludes 1   Excludes 2   Includes   Use additional   Code first   Code also   Unspecified
OGCR Official Guidelines   ● Unacceptable Principal Diagnosis   X Assign placeholder X   ● Use Additional Character(s)   ▶ Manifestation Code   **Coding Clinic**

S72.033-S72.034[A,B,C], S72.035[B,C],
S72.036-S72.041[A,B,C], S72.042[B,C],
S72.043-S72.044[A,B,C], S72.045[B,C],
S72.046-S72.051[A,B,C], S72.052[B,C],
S72.059-S72.061[A,B,C], S72.062[B,C],
S72.063-S72.064[A,B,C], S72.065[B,C],
S72.066-S72.091[A,B,C], S72.092[B,C],
S72.099-S72.101[C], S72.102[B,C],
S72.109-S72.111[A,B,C], S72.112[B,C],
S72.113-S72.114[A,B,C], S72.115[B,C],
S72.116-S72.121[A,B,C], S72.122[B,C],
S72.123-S72.124[A,B,C], S72.125[B,C],
S72.126-S72.131[A,B,C], S72.132[B,C],
S72.133-S72.134[A,B,C], S72.135[B,C],
S72.136-S72.141[A,B,C], S72.142[B,C],
S72.143-S72.144[A,B,C], S72.145[B,C],
S72.146-S72.301[A,B,C], S72.302[B,C],
S72.309-S72.321[A,B,C], S72.322[B,C],
S72.323-S72.324[A,B,C], S72.325[B,C],
S72.326-S72.331[A,B,C], S72.332[B,C],
S72.333-S72.334[A,B,C], S72.335[B,C],
S72.336-S72.341[A,B,C], S72.342[B,C],
S72.343-S72.344[A,B,C], S72.345[B,C],
S72.346-S72.351[A,B,C], S72.352[B,C],
S72.353-S72.354[A,B,C], S72.355[B,C],
S72.356-S72.361[A,B,C], S72.362[B,C],
S72.363-S72.364[A,B,C], S72.365[B,C],
S72.366-S72.391[A,B,C], S72.392[B,C],
S72.399-S72.401[A,B,C], S72.402[B,C],
S72.409-S72.411[A,B,C], S72.412[B,C],
S72.413-S72.414[A,B,C], S72.415[B,C],
S72.416-S72.421[A,B,C], S72.422[B,C],
S72.423-S72.424[A,B,C], S72.425[B,C],
S72.426-S72.431[A,B,C], S72.432[B,C],
S72.433-S72.434[A,B,C], S72.435[B,C],
S72.436-S72.441[A,B,C], S72.442[B,C],
S72.443-S72.444[A,B,C], S72.445[B,C],
S72.446-S72.451[A,B,C], S72.452[B,C],
S72.453-S72.454[A,B,C], S72.455[B,C],
S72.456-S72.461[A,B,C], S72.462[B,C],
S72.463-S72.464[A,B,C], S72.465[B,C],
S72.466[A,B,C], S72.471[A], S72.479[A],
S72.491[A,B,C], S72.492[B,C],
S72.499-S72.92X[A,B,C], S73.101[A],
S73.109-S73.111[A], S73.119-S73.121[A],
S73.129-S73.191[A], S73.199[A], S76.001[A],
S76.009-S76.011[A], S76.019[A], S76.091[A],
S76.099-S76.101[A], S76.109-S76.111[A],
S76.119[A], S76.191[A], S76.199-S76.201[A],
S76.209-S76.211[A], S76.219[A], S76.291[A],
S76.299-S76.301[A], S76.309-S76.311[A],
S76.319[A], S76.391[A], S76.399-S76.801[A],
S76.809-S76.811[A], S76.819[A], S76.891[A],
S76.899-S76.901[A], S76.909-S76.911[A],
S76.919[A], S76.991[A], S76.999[A], S79.001[A],
S79.009-S79.011[A], S79.019-S79.091[A],
S79.099-S79.101[A], S79.109-S79.111[A],
S79.119-S79.121[A], S79.129-S79.131[A],
S79.139-S79.141[A], S79.149-S79.191[A],
S79.199-S79.811[A], S79.819-S79.821[A],
S79.829-S79.911[A], S79.919-S79.921[A],
S79.929[A], S82.90X-S82.92X[A,B,C],
T14.90-T14.91, T79.A9X-T79.9XX[A]
For S72.401[B,C]: M80.00X-M80.019[A],
M80.041-M80.059[A], M80.80X-M80.819[A],
M80.841-M80.859[A], M84.40X-M84.419[A],
M84.441-M84.459[A], M84.474-M84.519[A],
M84.541-M84.559[A], M84.574-M84.576[A],
M84.60X-M84.619[A], M84.641-M84.659[A],
M84.674-M84.68X[A], M84.750-M84.759[A],
S03.8XX-S03.9XX[A], S29.011-S29.019[A],
S38.3XX[A], S39.011-S39.013[A],
S72.001-S72.466[A,B,C], S72.471-S72.479[A],
S72.491-S72.92X[A,B,C], S73.101-S73.199[A],
S76.001-S76.019[A], S76.091-S76.119[A],
S76.191-S76.219[A], S76.291-S76.319[A],
S76.391-S76.819[A], S76.891-S76.919[A],
S76.991-S76.999[A], S79.001-S79.929[A],
S82.90X-S82.92X[A,B,C], T14.90-T14.91,
T79.A9X-T79.9XX[A]
For S72.401[K,M,N,P,Q,R]: See S02.0[K]

● **S72.402　Unspecified fracture of lower end of
　　　　　　left femur** A, K, M, N, P, Q, R 🔵,
　　　　　　B, C 🔴, A, B, C 🔴
　　　Ⓔ **For S72.402[A]:** M80.00X-M80.019[A],
　　　M80.041-M80.059[A], M80.80X-M80.819[A],
　　　M80.841-M80.859[A], M84.40X-M84.419[A],
　　　M84.441-M84.459[A], M84.474-M84.519[A],
　　　M84.541-M84.559[A], M84.574-M84.576[A],
　　　M84.60X-M84.619[A], M84.641-M84.659[A],
　　　M84.674-M84.68X[A], M84.750-M84.759[A],
　　　S03.8XX-S03.9XX[A], S29.011-S29.019[A],
　　　S38.3XX[A], S39.011-S39.013[A],
　　　S72.001[B,C], S72.002-S72.009[A,B,C],
　　　S72.011[B,C], S72.012-S72.019[A,B,C],
　　　S72.021[B,C], S72.022-S72.023[A,B,C],
　　　S72.024[B,C], S72.025-S72.026[A,B,C],
　　　S72.031[B,C], S72.032-S72.033[A,B,C],
　　　S72.034[B,C], S72.035-S72.036[A,B,C],
　　　S72.041[B,C], S72.042-S72.043[A,B,C],
　　　S72.044[B,C], S72.045-S72.046[A,B,C],
　　　S72.051[B,C], S72.052-S72.059[A,B,C],
　　　S72.061[B,C], S72.062-S72.063[A,B,C],
　　　S72.064[B,C], S72.065-S72.066[A,B,C],
　　　S72.091[B,C], S72.092-S72.099[A,B,C],
　　　S72.101[B,C], S72.102-S72.109[A,B,C],
　　　S72.111[B,C], S72.112-S72.113[A,B,C],
　　　S72.114[B,C], S72.115-S72.116[A,B,C],
　　　S72.121[B,C], S72.122-S72.123[A,B,C],
　　　S72.124[B,C], S72.125-S72.126[A,B,C],
　　　S72.131[B,C], S72.132-S72.133[A,B,C],
　　　S72.134[B,C], S72.135-S72.136[A,B,C],
　　　S72.141[B,C], S72.142-S72.143[A,B,C],
　　　S72.144[B,C], S72.145-S72.146[A,B,C],
　　　S72.21X-S72.26X[A,B,C], S72.301[B,C],
　　　S72.302-S72.309[A,B,C], S72.321[B,C],
　　　S72.322-S72.323[A,B,C], S72.324[B,C],
　　　S72.325-S72.326[A,B,C], S72.331[B,C],
　　　S72.332-S72.333[A,B,C], S72.334[B,C],
　　　S72.335-S72.336[A,B,C], S72.341[B,C],
　　　S72.342-S72.343[A,B,C], S72.344[B,C],
　　　S72.345-S72.346[A,B,C], S72.351[B,C],
　　　S72.352-S72.353[A,B,C], S72.354[B,C],
　　　S72.355-S72.356[A,B,C], S72.361[B,C],
　　　S72.362-S72.363[A,B,C], S72.364[B,C],
　　　S72.365-S72.366[A,B,C], S72.391[B,C],
　　　S72.392-S72.399[A,B,C], S72.401[B,C],
　　　S72.402-S72.409[A,B,C], S72.411[B,C],
　　　S72.412-S72.413[A,B,C], S72.414[B,C],
　　　S72.415-S72.416[A,B,C], S72.421[B,C],
　　　S72.422-S72.423[A,B,C], S72.424[B,C],
　　　S72.425-S72.426[A,B,C], S72.431[B,C],
　　　S72.432-S72.433[A,B,C], S72.434[B,C],
　　　S72.435-S72.436[A,B,C], S72.441[B,C],
　　　S72.442-S72.443[A,B,C], S72.444[B,C],
　　　S72.445-S72.446[A,B,C], S72.451[B,C],
　　　S72.452-S72.453[A,B,C], S72.454[B,C],
　　　S72.455-S72.456[A,B,C], S72.461[B,C],
　　　S72.462-S72.463[A,B,C], S72.464[B,C],
　　　S72.465-S72.466[A,B,C], S72.472-S72.479[A],
　　　S72.491[B,C], S72.492-S72.92X[A,B,C],
　　　S73.102-S73.109[A], S73.112-S73.119[A],
　　　S73.122-S73.129[A], S73.192-S73.199[A],
　　　S76.002-S76.009[A], S76.012-S76.019[A],
　　　S76.092-S76.099[A], S76.102-S76.109[A],
　　　S76.112-S76.119[A], S76.192-S76.199[A],
　　　S76.202-S76.209[A], S76.212-S76.219[A],
　　　S76.292-S76.299[A], S76.302-S76.309[A],
　　　S76.312-S76.319[A], S76.392-S76.399[A],
　　　S76.802-S76.809[A], S76.812-S76.819[A],
　　　S76.892-S76.899[A], S76.902-S76.909[A],
　　　S76.912-S76.919[A], S76.992-S76.999[A],
　　　S79.002-S79.009[A], S79.012-S79.019[A],
　　　S79.092-S79.099[A], S79.102-S79.109[A],
　　　S79.112-S79.119[A], S79.122-S79.129[A],
　　　S79.132-S79.139[A], S79.142-S79.149[A],
　　　S79.192-S79.199[A], S79.812-S79.819[A],
　　　S79.822-S79.829[A], S79.912-S79.919[A],
　　　S79.922-S79.929[A], S82.90X-S82.92X[A,B,C],
　　　T14.90-T14.91, T79.A9X-T79.9XX[A]
　　For S72.402[B,C]: See S72.401[B,C]
　　For S72.401[K,M,N,P,Q,R]: See S02.0[K]

● S72.409   Unspecified fracture of lower end of unspecified femur
A, K, M, N, P, Q, R 🐾, B, C 🐾, A, B, C 🐾
   (Ex:) **For S72.409[A,B,C]:** See S72.401[B,C]
     For S72.401[K,M,N,P,Q,R]: See S02.0[K]

● S72.41   Unspecified condyle fracture of lower end of femur
   Condyle fracture of femur NOS

   ● S72.411   Displaced unspecified condyle fracture of lower end of right femur
A, K, M, N, P, Q, R 🐾, B, C 🐾, A, B, C 🐾
    (Ex:) **For S72.411[A]:** See S72.401[A]
     For S72.411[B,C]: See S72.401[B,C]
     For S72.411[K,M,N,P,Q,R]: See S02.0[K]

   ● S72.412   Displaced unspecified condyle fracture of lower end of left femur
A, K, M, N, P, Q, R 🐾, B, C 🐾, A, B, C 🐾
    (Ex:) **For S72.412[A]:** See S72.402[A]
     For S72.412[B,C]: See S72.401[B,C]
     For S72.411[K,M,N,P,Q,R]: See S02.0[K]

   ● S72.413   Displaced unspecified condyle fracture of lower end of unspecified femur A, K, M, N, P, Q, R 🐾, B, C 🐾, A, B, C 🐾
    (Ex:) **For S72.413[A,B,C]:** See S72.401[B,C]
     For S72.413[K,M,N,P,Q,R]: See S02.0[K]

   ● S72.414   Nondisplaced unspecified condyle fracture of lower end of right femur
A, K, M, N, P, Q, R 🐾, B, C 🐾, A, B, C 🐾
    (Ex:) **For S72.414[A]:** See S72.401[A]
     For S72.414[B,C]: See S72.401[B,C]
     For S72.414[K,M,N,P,Q,R]: See S02.0[K]

   ● S72.415   Nondisplaced unspecified condyle fracture of lower end of left femur
A, K, M, N, P, Q, R 🐾, B, C 🐾, A, B, C 🐾
    (Ex:) **For S72.415[A]:** See S72.402[A]
     For S72.415[B,C]: See S72.401[B,C]
     For S72.415[K,M,N,P,Q,R]: See S02.0[K]

   ● S72.416   Nondisplaced unspecified condyle fracture of lower end of unspecified femur A, K, M, N, P, Q, R 🐾, B, C 🐾, A, B, C 🐾
    (Ex:) **For S72.416[A,B,C]:** See S72.401[B,C]
     For S72.416[K,M,N,P,Q,R]: See S02.0[K]

● S72.42   Fracture of lateral condyle of femur

   ● S72.421   Displaced fracture of lateral condyle of right femur A, K, M, N, P, Q, R 🐾, B, C 🐾, A, B, C 🐾
    (Ex:) **For S72.421[A]:** See S72.401[A]
     For S72.421[B,C]: See S72.401[B,C]
     For S72.421[K,M,N,P,Q,R]: See S02.0[K]

   ● S72.422   Displaced fracture of lateral condyle of left femur A, K, M, N, P, Q, R 🐾, B, C 🐾, A, B, C 🐾
    (Ex:) **For S72.422[A]:** See S72.402[A]
     For S72.422[B,C]: See S72.401[B,C]
     For S72.422[K,M,N,P,Q,R]: See S02.0[K]

● S72.423   Displaced fracture of lateral condyle of unspecified femur
A, K, M, N, P, Q, R 🐾, B, C 🐾, A, B, C 🐾
    (Ex:) **For S72.423[A,B,C]:** See S72.401[B,C]
     For S72.423[K,M,N,P,Q,R]: See S02.0[K]

● S72.424   Nondisplaced fracture of lateral condyle of right femur
A, K, M, N, P, Q, R 🐾, B, C 🐾, A, B, C 🐾
    (Ex:) **For S72.424[A]:** See S72.401[A]
     For S72.424[B,C]: See S72.401[B,C]
     For S72.424[K,M,N,P,Q,R]: See S02.0[K]

● S72.425   Nondisplaced fracture of lateral condyle of left femur
A, K, M, N, P, Q, R 🐾, B, C 🐾, A, B, C 🐾
    (Ex:) **For S72.425[A]:** See S72.402[A]
     For S72.425[B,C]: See S72.401[B,C]
     For S72.425[K,M,N,P,Q,R]: See S02.0[K]

● S72.426   Nondisplaced fracture of lateral condyle of unspecified femur
A, K, M, N, P, Q, R 🐾, B, C 🐾, A, B, C 🐾
    (Ex:) **For S72.426[A,B,C]:** See S72.401[B,C]
     For S72.426[K,M,N,P,Q,R]: See S02.0[K]

● S72.43   Fracture of medial condyle of femur

   ● S72.431   Displaced fracture of medial condyle of right femur A, K, M, N, P, Q, R 🐾, B, C 🐾, A, B, C 🐾
    (Ex:) **For S72.431[A]:** See S72.401[A]
     For S72.431[B,C]: See S72.401[B,C]
     For S72.431[K,M,N,P,Q,R]: See S02.0[K]

   ● S72.432   Displaced fracture of medial condyle of left femur A, K, M, N, P, Q, R 🐾, B, C 🐾, A, B, C 🐾
    (Ex:) **For S72.432[A]:** See S72.402[A]
     For S72.432[B,C]: See S72.401[B,C]
     For S72.432[K,M,N,P,Q,R]: See S02.0[K]

   ● S72.433   Displaced fracture of medial condyle of unspecified femur
A, K, M, N, P, Q, R 🐾, B, C 🐾, A, B, C 🐾
    (Ex:) **For S72.433[A,B,C]:** See S72.401[B,C]
     For S72.433[K,M,N,P,Q,R]: See S02.0[K]

   ● S72.434   Nondisplaced fracture of medial condyle of right femur
A, K, M, N, P, Q, R 🐾, B, C 🐾, A, B, C 🐾
    (Ex:) **For S72.434[A]:** See S72.401[A]
     For S72.434[B,C]: See S72.401[B,C]
     For S72.434[K,M,N,P,Q,R]: See S02.0[K]

   ● S72.435   Nondisplaced fracture of medial condyle of left femur
A, K, M, N, P, Q, R 🐾, B, C 🐾, A, B, C 🐾
    (Ex:) **For S72.435[A]:** See S72.402[A]
     For S72.435[B,C]: See S72.401[B,C]
     For S72.435[K,M,N,P,Q,R]: See S02.0[K]

   ● S72.436   Nondisplaced fracture of medial condyle of unspecified femur
A, K, M, N, P, Q, R 🐾, B, C 🐾, A, B, C 🐾
    (Ex:) **For S72.436[A,B,C]:** See S72.401[B,C]
     For S72.436[K,M,N,P,Q,R]: See S02.0[K]

◀ New   ◀▥▥ Revised   ~~deleted~~ Deleted   Excludes 1   Excludes 2   Includes   Use additional   Code first   Code also   Unspecified
OGCR Official Guidelines   ● Unacceptable Principal Diagnosis   X Assign placeholder X   🐾 Use Additional Character(s)   ▶ Manifestation Code   **Coding Clinic**

● **S72.44**　Fracture of lower epiphysis (separation) of femur

　　Excludes1　Salter-Harris Type I physeal fracture of lower end of femur (S79.11-)

　● **S72.441**　Displaced fracture of lower epiphysis (separation) of right femur
　　　A, K, M, N, P, Q, R 🅒, B, C 🅒, A, B, C 🅒
　　　　Ⓔ For S72.441[A]: See S72.401[A]
　　　　For S72.441[B,C]: See S72.401[B,C]
　　　　For S72.441[K,M,N,P,Q,R]: See S02.0[K]

　● **S72.442**　Displaced fracture of lower epiphysis (separation) of left femur
　　　A, K, M, N, P, Q, R 🅒, B, C 🅒, A, B, C 🅒
　　　　Ⓔ For S72.442[A]: See S72.402[A]
　　　　For S72.442[B,C]: See S72.401[B,C]
　　　　For S72.442[K,M,N,P,Q,R]: See S02.0[K]

　● **S72.443**　Displaced fracture of lower epiphysis (separation) of unspecified femur
　　　A, K, M, N, P, Q, R 🅒, B, C 🅒, A, B, C 🅒
　　　　Ⓔ For S72.443[A,B,C]: See S72.401[B,C]
　　　　For S72.443[K,M,N,P,Q,R]: See S02.0[K]

　● **S72.444**　Nondisplaced fracture of lower epiphysis (separation) of right femur
　　　A, K, M, N, P, Q, R 🅒, B, C 🅒, A, B, C 🅒
　　　　Ⓔ For S72.444[A]: See S72.401[A]
　　　　For S72.444[B,C]: See S72.401[B,C]
　　　　For S72.444[K,M,N,P,Q,R]: See S02.0[K]

　● **S72.445**　Nondisplaced fracture of lower epiphysis (separation) of left femur
　　　A, K, M, N, P, Q, R 🅒, B, C 🅒, A, B, C 🅒
　　　　Ⓔ For S72.445[A]: See S72.402[A]
　　　　For S72.445[B,C]: See S72.401[B,C]
　　　　For S72.445[K,M,N,P,Q,R]: See S02.0[K]

　● **S72.446**　Nondisplaced fracture of lower epiphysis (separation) of unspecified femur A, K, M, N, P, Q, R 🅒, B, C 🅒, A, B, C 🅒
　　　　Ⓔ For S72.446[A,B,C]: See S72.401[B,C]
　　　　For S72.446[K,M,N,P,Q,R]: See S02.0[K]

● **S72.45**　Supracondylar fracture without intracondylar extension of lower end of femur
　　Supracondylar fracture of lower end of femur NOS

　　Excludes1　supracondylar fracture with intracondylar extension of lower end of femur (S72.46-)

　● **S72.451**　Displaced supracondylar fracture without intracondylar extension of lower end of right femur
　　　A, K, M, N, P, Q, R 🅒, B, C 🅒, A, B, C 🅒
　　　　Ⓔ For S72.451[A]: See S72.401[A]
　　　　For S72.451[B,C]: See S72.401[B,C]
　　　　For S72.451[K,M,N,P,Q,R]: See S02.0[K]

　● **S72.452**　Displaced supracondylar fracture without intracondylar extension of lower end of left femur
　　　A, K, M, N, P, Q, R 🅒, B, C 🅒, A, B, C 🅒
　　　　Ⓔ For S72.452[A]: See S72.402[A]
　　　　For S72.452[B,C]: See S72.401[B,C]
　　　　For S72.452[K,M,N,P,Q,R]: See S02.0[K]

　● **S72.453**　Displaced supracondylar fracture without intracondylar extension of lower end of unspecified femur
　　　A, K, M, N, P, Q, R 🅒, B, C 🅒, A, B, C 🅒
　　　　Ⓔ For S72.453[A,B,C]: See S72.401[B,C]
　　　　For S72.453[K,M,N,P,Q,R]: See S02.0[K]

　● **S72.454**　Nondisplaced supracondylar fracture without intracondylar extension of lower end of right femur
　　　A, K, M, N, P, Q, R 🅒, B, C 🅒, A, B, C 🅒
　　　　Ⓔ For S72.454[A]: See S72.401[A]
　　　　For S72.454[B,C]: See S72.401[B,C]
　　　　For S72.454[K,M,N,P,Q,R]: See S02.0[K]

　● **S72.455**　Nondisplaced supracondylar fracture without intracondylar extension of lower end of left femur
　　　A, K, M, N, P, Q, R 🅒, B, C 🅒, A, B, C 🅒
　　　　Ⓔ For S72.455[A]: See S72.402[A]
　　　　For S72.455[B,C]: See S72.401[B,C]
　　　　For S72.455[K,M,N,P,Q,R]: See S02.0[K]

　● **S72.456**　Nondisplaced supracondylar fracture without intracondylar extension of lower end of unspecified femur
　　　A, K, M, N, P, Q, R 🅒, B, C 🅒, A, B, C 🅒
　　　　Ⓔ For S72.456[A,B,C]: See S72.401[B,C]
　　　　For S72.456[K,M,N,P,Q,R]: See S02.0[K]

● **S72.46**　Supracondylar fracture with intracondylar extension of lower end of femur

　　Excludes1　supracondylar fracture without intracondylar extension of lower end of femur (S72.45-)

　● **S72.461**　Displaced supracondylar fracture with intracondylar extension of lower end of right femur
　　　A, K, M, N, P, Q, R 🅒, B, C 🅒, A, B, C 🅒
　　　　Ⓔ For S72.461[A]: See S72.401[A]
　　　　For S72.461[B,C]: See S72.401[B,C]
　　　　For S72.461[K,M,N,P,Q,R]: See S02.0[K]

　● **S72.462**　Displaced supracondylar fracture with intracondylar extension of lower end of left femur
　　　A, K, M, N, P, Q, R 🅒, B, C 🅒, A, B, C 🅒
　　　　Ⓔ For S72.462[A]: See S72.402[A]
　　　　For S72.462[B,C]: See S72.401[B,C]
　　　　For S72.462[K,M,N,P,Q,R]: See S02.0[K]

　● **S72.463**　Displaced supracondylar fracture with intracondylar extension of lower end of unspecified femur
　　　A, K, M, N, P, Q, R 🅒, B, C 🅒, A, B, C 🅒
　　　　Ⓔ For S72.463[A,B,C]: See S72.401[B,C]
　　　　For S72.463[K,M,N,P,Q,R]: See S02.0[K]

　● **S72.464**　Nondisplaced supracondylar fracture with intracondylar extension of lower end of right femur
　　　A, K, M, N, P, Q, R 🅒, B, C 🅒, A, B, C 🅒
　　　　Ⓔ For S72.464[A]: See S72.401[A]
　　　　For S72.464[B,C]: See S72.401[B,C]
　　　　For S72.464[K,M,N,P,Q,R]: See S02.0[K]

　● **S72.465**　Nondisplaced supracondylar fracture with intracondylar extension of lower end of left femur
　　　A, K, M, N, P, Q, R 🅒, B, C 🅒, A, B, C 🅒
　　　　Ⓔ For S72.465[A]: See S72.402[A]
　　　　For S72.465[B,C]: See S72.401[B,C]
　　　　For S72.465[K,M,N,P,Q,R]: See S02.0[K]

　● **S72.466**　Nondisplaced supracondylar fracture with intracondylar extension of lower end of unspecified femur
　　　A, K, M, N, P, Q, R 🅒, B, C 🅒, A, B, C 🅒
　　　　Ⓔ For S72.466[A,B,C]: See S72.401[B,C]
　　　　For S72.466[K,M,N,P,Q,R]: See S02.0[K]

CHAPTER 19 (S00-T88)

● **S72.47 Torus fracture of lower end of femur**

The appropriate 7th character is to be added to all codes in subcategory S72.47

A	initial encounter for closed fracture
D	subsequent encounter for fracture with routine healing
G	subsequent encounter for fracture with delayed healing
K	subsequent encounter for fracture with nonunion
P	subsequent encounter for fracture with malunion
S	sequela

● **S72.471 Torus fracture of lower end of right femur** A, K, P 🔁, A 🔁
    Ⓔⓧ **For S72.471[A]:** See S72.401[A]
    For S72.471[K,P]: See S02.0[K]

● **S72.472 Torus fracture of lower end of left femur** A, K, P 🔁, A 🔁
    Ⓔⓧ **For S72.472[A]:** See S72.402[A]
    For S72.472[K,P]: See S02.0[K]

● **S72.479 Torus fracture of lower end of unspecified femur** A, K, P 🔁, A 🔁
    Ⓔⓧ **For S72.479[A]:** See S72.401[B,C]
    For S72.479[K,P]: See S02.0[K]

● **S72.49 Other fracture of lower end of femur**

● **S72.491 Other fracture of lower end of right femur** A, K, M, N, P, Q, R 🔁, B, C 🔁, A, B, C 🔁
    Ⓔⓧ **For S72.491[A]:** See S72.401[A]
    For S72.491[B,C]: M80.00X-M80.019[A], M80.041-M80.059[A], M80.80X-M80.819[A], M80.841-M80.859[A], M84.40X-M84.419[A], M84.441-M84.459[A], M84.474-M84.519[A], M84.541-M84.559[A], M84.574-M84.619[A], M84.641-M84.659[A], M84.674-M84.68X[A], M84.750-M84.759[A], S03.8XX-S03.9XX[A], S29.011-S29.019[A], S38.3XX[A], S39.011-S39.013[A], S72.491-S72.499[B,C], S73.101-S73.199[A], S76.001-S76.019[A], S76.091-S76.119[A], S76.191-S76.219[A], S76.291-S76.319[A], S76.391-S76.819[A], S76.891-S76.919[A], S76.991-S76.999[A], S79.811-S79.929[A], S82.001-S82.099[A,B,C], S82.90X-S82.92X[A,B,C], T14.90-T14.91, T79.A9X-T79.9XX[A]
    For S72.491[K,M,N,P,Q,R]: See S02.0[K]

● **S72.492 Other fracture of lower end of left femur** A, K, M, N, P, Q, R 🔁, B, C 🔁, A, B, C 🔁
    Ⓔⓧ **For S72.492[A]:** See S72.402[A]
    For S72.492[B,C]: See S72.491[B,C]
    For S72.492[K,M,N,P,Q,R]: See S02.0[K]

● **S72.499 Other fracture of lower end of unspecified femur** A, K, M, N, P, Q, R 🔁, B, C 🔁, A, B, C 🔁
    Ⓔⓧ **For S72.499[A]:** See S72.401[B,C]
    For S72.499[B,C]: See S72.491[B,C]
    For S72.499[K,M,N,P,Q,R]: See S02.0[K]

● **S72.8 Other fracture of femur**
    Ⓔⓧ **For category S72.8 CC codes S72.8[A,B,C]:** See S72.001[B,C]
    For S72.8[K,M,N,P,Q,R]: See S02.0[K]

● **S72.8X Other fracture of femur**

● **S72.8X1 Other fracture of right femur** K, M, N, P, Q, R 🔁, A, B, C 🔁, A, B, C 🔁

● **S72.8X2 Other fracture of left femur** K, M, N, P, Q, R 🔁, A, B, C 🔁, A, B, C 🔁

● **S72.8X9 Other fracture of unspecified femur** K, M, N, P, Q, R 🔁, A, B, C 🔁, A, B, C 🔁

● **S72.9 Unspecified fracture of femur**
Fracture of thigh NOS
Fracture of upper leg NOS
  Excludes1 fracture of hip NOS (S72.00-, S72.01-)
    Ⓔⓧ **For category S72.9 CC codes S72.9[A,B,C]:** See S72.001[B,C]
    For S72.9[K,M,N,P,Q,R]: See S02.0[K]

X ● **S72.90 Unspecified fracture of unspecified femur** K, M, N, P, Q, R 🔁, A, B, C 🔁, A, B, C 🔁
    Coding Clinic: 2012, Q4, P94

X ● **S72.91 Unspecified fracture of right femur** K, M, N, P, Q, R 🔁, A, B, C 🔁, A, B, C 🔁

X ● **S72.92 Unspecified fracture of left femur** K, M, N, P, Q, R 🔁, A, B, C 🔁, A, B, C 🔁

● **S73 Dislocation and sprain of joint and ligaments of hip**
  Includes avulsion of joint or ligament of hip
laceration of cartilage, joint or ligament of hip
sprain of cartilage, joint or ligament of hip
traumatic hemarthrosis of joint or ligament of hip
traumatic rupture of joint or ligament of hip
traumatic subluxation of joint or ligament of hip
traumatic tear of joint or ligament of hip

Code also any associated open wound
  Excludes2 strain of muscle, fascia and tendon of hip and thigh (S76.-)

The appropriate 7th character is to be added to each code from category S73

A	initial encounter
D	subsequent encounter
S	sequela

● **S73.0 Subluxation and dislocation of hip**
Out of position
  Excludes2 dislocation and subluxation of hip prosthesis (T84.020, T84.021)

● **S73.00 Unspecified subluxation and dislocation of hip**
Dislocation of hip NOS
Subluxation of hip NOS

● **S73.001 Unspecified subluxation of right hip** A 🔁, A 🔁
    Ⓔⓧ M99.16-M99.17, M99.19, S03.1XX[A], S33.30X-S33.39X[A], S73.001[A], S73.003-S73.004[A], S73.006[A], S73.041[A], S73.043-S73.044[A], S73.046[A]

● **S73.002 Unspecified subluxation of left hip** A 🔁, A 🔁
    Ⓔⓧ M99.16-M99.17, M99.19, S03.1XX[A], S33.30X-S33.39X[A], S73.002-S73.003[A], S73.005-S73.006[A], S73.042-S73.043[A], S73.045-S73.046[A]

● **S73.003 Unspecified subluxation of unspecified hip** A 🔁, A 🔁
    Ⓔⓧ M99.16-M99.17, M99.19, S03.1XX[A], S33.30X-S33.39X[A], S73.001-S73.006[A], S73.041-S73.046[A]

● **S73.004 Unspecified dislocation of right hip** A 🔁, A 🔁
    Ⓔⓧ See S73.001

● **S73.005 Unspecified dislocation of left hip** A 🔁, A 🔁
    Ⓔⓧ See S73.002

● **S73.006 Unspecified dislocation of unspecified hip** A 🔁, A 🔁
    Ⓔⓧ See S73.003

- S73.01   **Posterior subluxation and dislocation of hip**
  - S73.011   **Posterior subluxation of right hip** A 🦠, A 🦠
    - Ex: M99.16-M99.17, M99.19, S03.1XX[A], S33.30X-S33.39X[A], S73.011[A], S73.013-S73.014[A], S73.016[A]
  - S73.012   **Posterior subluxation of left hip** A 🦠, A 🦠
    - Ex: M99.16-M99.17, M99.19, S03.1XX[A], S33.30X-S33.39X[A], S73.012-S73.013[A], S73.015-S73.016[A]
  - S73.013   **Posterior subluxation of** unspecified **hip** A 🦠, A 🦠
    - Ex: M99.16-M99.17, M99.19, S03.1XX[A], S33.30X-S33.39X[A], S73.011-S73.016[A]
  - S73.014   **Posterior dislocation of right hip** A 🦠, A 🦠
    - Ex: See S73.011
  - S73.015   **Posterior dislocation of left hip** A 🦠, A 🦠
    - Ex: See S73.012
  - S73.016   **Posterior dislocation of** unspecified **hip** A 🦠, A 🦠
    - Ex: See S73.013
- S73.02   **Obturator subluxation and dislocation of hip**
  - S73.021   **Obturator subluxation of right hip** A 🦠, A 🦠
    - Ex: M99.16-M99.17, M99.19, S03.1XX[A], S33.30X-S33.39X[A], S73.021[A], S73.023-S73.024[A], S73.026[A]
  - S73.022   **Obturator subluxation of left hip** A 🦠, A 🦠
    - Ex: M99.16-M99.17, M99.19, S03.1XX[A], S33.30X-S33.39X[A], S73.022-S73.023[A], S73.025-S73.026[A]
  - S73.023   **Obturator subluxation of** unspecified **hip** A 🦠, A 🦠
    - Ex: M99.16-M99.17, M99.19, S03.1XX[A], S33.30X-S33.39X[A], S73.021-S73.026[A]
  - S73.024   **Obturator dislocation of right hip** A 🦠, A 🦠
    - Ex: See S73.021
  - S73.025   **Obturator dislocation of left hip** A 🦠, A 🦠
    - Ex: See S73.022
  - S73.026   **Obturator dislocation of** unspecified **hip** A 🦠, A 🦠
    - Ex: See S73.023
- S73.03   **Other anterior dislocation of hip**
  - S73.031   **Other anterior subluxation of right hip** A 🦠, A 🦠
    - Ex: M99.16-M99.17, M99.19, S03.1XX[A], S33.30X-S33.39X[A], S73.031[A], S73.033-S73.034[A], S73.036[A]
  - S73.032   **Other anterior subluxation of left hip** A 🦠, A 🦠
    - Ex: M99.16-M99.17, M99.19, S03.1XX[A], S33.30X-S33.39X[A], S73.032-S73.033[A], S73.035-S73.036[A]
  - S73.033   **Other anterior subluxation of** unspecified **hip** A 🦠, A 🦠
    - Ex: M99.16-M99.17, M99.19, S03.1XX[A], S33.30X-S33.39X[A], S73.031-S73.036[A]
  - S73.034   **Other anterior dislocation of right hip** A 🦠, A 🦠
    - Ex: See S73.031
  - S73.035   **Other anterior dislocation of left hip** A 🦠, A 🦠
    - Ex: See S73.032
  - S73.036   **Other anterior dislocation of** unspecified **hip** A 🦠, A 🦠
    - Ex: See S73.033

- S73.04   **Central dislocation of hip**
  - S73.041   **Central subluxation of right hip** A 🦠, A 🦠
    - Ex: See S73.001
  - S73.042   **Central subluxation of left hip** A 🦠, A 🦠
    - Ex: See S73.002
  - S73.043   **Central subluxation of** unspecified **hip** A 🦠, A 🦠
    - Ex: See S73.003
  - S73.044   **Central dislocation of right hip** A 🦠, A 🦠
    - Ex: See S73.001
  - S73.045   **Central dislocation of left hip** A 🦠, A 🦠
    - Ex: See S73.002
  - S73.046   **Central dislocation of** unspecified **hip** A 🦠, A 🦠
    - Ex: See S73.003
- S73.1   **Sprain of hip**
  - S73.10   **Unspecified sprain of hip**
    - S73.101   Unspecified **sprain of right hip**
    - S73.102   Unspecified **sprain of left hip**
    - S73.109   Unspecified **sprain of unspecified hip**
  - S73.11   **Iliofemoral ligament sprain of hip**
    - S73.111   **Iliofemoral ligament sprain of right hip**
    - S73.112   **Iliofemoral ligament sprain of left hip**
    - S73.119   **Iliofemoral ligament sprain of** unspecified **hip**
  - S73.12   **Ischiocapsular (ligament) sprain of hip**
    - S73.121   **Ischiocapsular ligament sprain of right hip**
    - S73.122   **Ischiocapsular ligament sprain of left hip**
    - S73.129   **Ischiocapsular ligament sprain of** unspecified **hip**
  - S73.19   **Other sprain of hip**
    - S73.191   **Other sprain of right hip**
    - S73.192   **Other sprain of left hip**
    - S73.199   **Other sprain of** unspecified **hip**
- S74   **Injury of nerves at hip and thigh level**

  Code also any associated open wound (S71.-)

  Excludes2   injury of nerves at ankle and foot level (S94.-)
  injury of nerves at lower leg level (S84.-)

  The appropriate 7th character is to be added to each code from category S74

A	initial encounter
D	subsequent encounter
S	sequela

  - S74.0   **Injury of sciatic nerve at hip and thigh level**
    - X ● S74.00   **Injury of sciatic nerve at hip and thigh level,** unspecified **leg**
    - X ● S74.01   **Injury of sciatic nerve at hip and thigh level, right leg**
    - X ● S74.02   **Injury of sciatic nerve at hip and thigh level, left leg**
  - S74.1   **Injury of femoral nerve at hip and thigh level**
    - X ● S74.10   **Injury of femoral nerve at hip and thigh level,** unspecified **leg**
    - X ● S74.11   **Injury of femoral nerve at hip and thigh level, right leg**
    - X ● S74.12   **Injury of femoral nerve at hip and thigh level, left leg**

N Newborn Age: 0   **P** Pediatric Age: 0–17   **M** Maternity DX: 12–55   **A** Adult Age: 15–124   ♀ Females Only   ♂ Males Only

🦠 Complication\Comorbidity   🦠 Major C\C   Ex: CC/MCC Exclusions   🦠 Hospital-Acquired Condition

1367

CHAPTER 19 (S00-T88)

- ● S74.2   Injury of cutaneous sensory nerve at hip and thigh level
  - X ● S74.20   Injury of cutaneous sensory nerve at hip and thigh level, `unspecified` leg
  - X ● S74.21   Injury of cutaneous sensory nerve at hip and high level, right leg
  - X ● S74.22   Injury of cutaneous sensory nerve at hip and thigh level, left leg
- ● S74.8   Injury of other nerves at hip and thigh level
  - ● S74.8X   Injury of other nerves at hip and thigh level
    - ● S74.8X1   Injury of other nerves at hip and thigh level, right leg
    - ● S74.8X2   Injury of other nerves at hip and thigh level, left leg
    - ● S74.8X9   Injury of other nerves at hip and thigh level, `unspecified` leg
- ● S74.9   Injury of unspecified nerve at hip and thigh level
  - X ● S74.90   Injury of `unspecified` nerve at hip and thigh level, unspecified leg
  - X ● S74.91   Injury of `unspecified` nerve at hip and thigh level, right leg
  - X ● S74.92   Injury of `unspecified` nerve at hip and thigh level, left leg

- ● S75   **Injury of blood vessels at hip and thigh level**

  Code also any associated open wound (S71.-)

  Excludes2   injury of blood vessels at lower leg level (S85.-)
             injury of popliteal artery (S85.0)

  The appropriate 7th character is to be added to each code from category S75

A	initial encounter
D	subsequent encounter
S	sequela

  - ● S75.0   Injury of femoral artery
    - ● S75.00   Unspecified injury of femoral artery
      - ● S75.001   `Unspecified` injury of femoral artery, right leg A
        (Ex:) S75.001[A], S75.009-S75.021[A], S75.029-S75.091[A], S75.099[A], S75.801[A], S75.809-S75.811[A], S75.819-S75.891[A], S75.899-S75.901[A], S75.909-S75.911[A], S75.919-S75.991[A], S75.999[A], S85.201[A], S85.209-S85.211[A], S85.219-S85.291[A], S85.299[A], S85.801[A], S85.809-S85.811[A], S85.819-S85.891[A], S85.899-S85.901[A], S85.909-S85.911[A], S85.919-S85.991[A], S85.999[A], S95.001[A], S95.009-S95.011[A], S95.019-S95.091[A], S95.099[A], S95.201[A], S95.209-S95.211[A], S95.219-S95.291[A], S95.299[A], S95.801[A], S95.809-S95.811[A], S95.819-S95.891[A], S95.899-S95.901[A], S95.909-S95.911[A], S95.919-S95.991[A], S95.999[A]
      - ● S75.002   `Unspecified` injury of femoral artery, left leg A
        (Ex:) S75.002-S75.009[A], S75.012-S75.019[A], S75.022-S75.029[A], S75.092[A], S75.099[A], S75.802-S75.809[A], S75.812-S75.819[A], S75.892-S75.899[A], S75.902-S75.909[A], S75.912-S75.919[A], S75.992-S75.999[A], S85.202-S85.209[A], S85.212-S85.219[A], S85.292-S85.299[A], S85.802-S85.809[A], S85.812-S85.819[A], S85.892-S85.899[A], S85.902-S85.909[A], S85.912-S85.919[A], S85.992-S85.999[A], S95.002-S95.009[A], S95.012-S95.019[A], S95.092-S95.099[A], S95.202-S95.209[A], S95.212-S95.219[A], S95.292-S95.299[A], S95.802-S95.809[A], S95.812-S95.819[A], S95.892-S95.899[A], S95.902-S95.909[A], S95.912-S95.919[A], S95.992-S95.999[A]

    - ● S75.009   `Unspecified` injury of femoral artery, unspecified leg A
      (Ex:) S75.001-S75.099[A], S75.801-S75.999[A], S85.201-S85.299[A], S85.801-S85.999[A], S95.001-S95.099[A], S95.201-S95.999[A]
  - ● S75.01   Minor laceration of femoral artery
    Incomplete transection of femoral artery
    Laceration of femoral artery NOS
    Superficial laceration of femoral artery
    - ● S75.011   Minor laceration of femoral artery, right leg A
      (Ex:) See S75.001
    - ● S75.012   Minor laceration of femoral artery, left leg A
      (Ex:) See S75.002
    - ● S75.019   Minor laceration of femoral artery, `unspecified` leg A
      (Ex:) See S75.009
  - ● S75.02   Major laceration of femoral artery
    Complete transection of femoral artery
    Traumatic rupture of femoral artery
    - ● S75.021   Major laceration of femoral artery, right leg A
      (Ex:) See S75.001
    - ● S75.022   Major laceration of femoral artery, left leg A
      (Ex:) See S75.002
    - ● S75.029   Major laceration of femoral artery, `unspecified` leg A
      (Ex:) See S75.009
  - ● S75.09   Other specified injury of femoral artery
    - ● S75.091   Other specified injury of femoral artery, right leg A
      (Ex:) See S75.001
    - ● S75.092   Other specified injury of femoral artery, left leg A
      (Ex:) See S75.002
    - ● S75.099   Other specified injury of femoral artery, `unspecified` leg A
      (Ex:) See S75.009
  - ● S75.1   Injury of femoral vein at hip and thigh level
    - ● S75.10   Unspecified injury of femoral vein at hip and thigh level
      - ● S75.101   `Unspecified` injury of femoral vein at hip and thigh level, right leg A
        (Ex:) S75.101[A], S75.109-S75.111[A], S75.119-S75.121[A], S75.129-S75.191[A], S75.199[A], S75.801[A], S75.809-S75.811[A], S75.819-S75.891[A], S75.899-S75.901[A], S75.909-S75.911[A], S75.919-S75.991[A], S75.999[A], S85.201[A], S85.209-S85.211[A], S85.219-S85.291[A], S85.299[A], S85.801[A], S85.809-S85.811[A], S85.819-S85.891[A], S85.899-S85.901[A], S85.909-S85.911[A], S85.919-S85.991[A], S85.999[A], S95.001[A], S95.009-S95.011[A], S95.019-S95.091[A], S95.099[A], S95.201[A], S95.209-S95.211[A], S95.219-S95.291[A], S95.299-S95.801[A], S95.809-S95.811[A], S95.819-S95.891[A], S95.899-S95.901[A], S95.909-S95.911[A], S95.919-S95.991[A], S95.999[A]

◀ New   ◀▥ Revised   ~~deleted~~ Deleted   `Excludes 1`   `Excludes 2`   `Includes`   `Use additional`   `Code first`   `Code also`   `Unspecified`

OGCR Official Guidelines   ● Unacceptable Principal Diagnosis   X Assign placeholder X   ● Use Additional Character(s)   ▶ Manifestation Code   **Coding Clinic**

● **S75.102**   Unspecified injury of femoral vein at hip and thigh level, left leg A 🔖
     Ⓔ�� S75.102-S75.109[A], S75.112-S75.119[A], S75.122-S75.129[A], S75.192-S75.199[A], S75.802-S75.809[A], S75.812-S75.819[A], S75.892-S75.899[A], S75.902-S75.909[A], S75.912-S75.919[A], S75.992-S75.999[A], S85.202-S85.209[A], S85.212-S85.219[A], S85.292-S85.299[A], S85.802-S85.809[A], S85.812-S85.819[A], S85.892-S85.899[A], S85.902-S85.909[A], S85.912-S85.919[A], S85.992-S85.999[A], S95.002-S95.009[A], S95.012-S95.019[A], S95.092-S95.099[A], S95.202-S95.209[A], S95.212-S95.219[A], S95.292-S95.299[A], S95.802-S95.809[A], S95.812-S95.819[A], S95.892-S95.899[A], S95.902-S95.909[A], S95.912-S95.919[A], S95.992-S95.999[A]

● **S75.109**   Unspecified injury of femoral vein at hip and thigh level, unspecified leg A 🔖
     ⒺⓍ S75.101-S75.199[A], S75.801-S75.999[A], S85.201-S85.299[A], S85.801-S85.999[A], S95.001-S95.099[A], S95.201-S95.999[A]

● **S75.11**   Minor laceration of femoral vein at hip and thigh level
     Incomplete transection of femoral vein at hip and thigh level
     Laceration of femoral vein at hip and thigh level NOS
     Superficial laceration of femoral vein at hip and thigh level

● **S75.111**   Minor laceration of femoral vein at hip and thigh level, right leg A 🔖
     ⒺⓍ See S75.101

● **S75.112**   Minor laceration of femoral vein at hip and thigh level, left leg A 🔖
     ⒺⓍ See S75.102

● **S75.119**   Minor laceration of femoral vein at hip and thigh level, unspecified leg A 🔖
     ⒺⓍ See S75.109

● **S75.12**   Major laceration of femoral vein at hip and thigh level
     Complete transection of femoral vein at hip and thigh level
     Traumatic rupture of femoral vein at hip and thigh level

● **S75.121**   Major laceration of femoral vein at hip and thigh level, right leg A 🔖
     ⒺⓍ See S75.101

● **S75.122**   Major laceration of femoral vein at hip and thigh level, left leg A 🔖
     ⒺⓍ See S75.102

● **S75.129**   Major laceration of femoral vein at hip and thigh level, unspecified leg A 🔖
     ⒺⓍ See S75.109

● **S75.19**   Other specified injury of femoral vein at hip and thigh level

● **S75.191**   Other specified injury of femoral vein at hip and thigh level, right leg A 🔖
     ⒺⓍ See S75.101

● **S75.192**   Other specified injury of femoral vein at hip and thigh level, left leg A 🔖
     ⒺⓍ See S75.102

● **S75.199**   Other specified injury of femoral vein at hip and thigh level, unspecified leg A 🔖
     ⒺⓍ See S75.109

● **S75.2**   Injury of greater saphenous vein at hip and thigh level
     Excludes1   greater saphenous vein NOS (S85.3)

● **S75.20**   Unspecified injury of greater saphenous vein at hip and thigh level

● **S75.201**   Unspecified injury of greater saphenous vein at hip and thigh level, right leg A 🔖
     ⒺⓍ S75.201[A], S75.209-S75.211[A], S75.219-S75.221[A], S75.229-S75.291[A], S75.299-S75.801[A], S75.809-S75.811[A], S75.819-S75.891[A], S75.899-S75.901[A], S75.909-S75.911[A], S75.919-S75.991[A], S75.999[A], S85.201[A], S85.209[A], S85.211[A], S85.219-S85.291[A], S85.299-S85.301[A], S85.309-S85.311[A], S85.319-S85.391[A], S85.399-S85.401[A], S85.409-S85.411[A], S85.419-S85.491[A], S85.499[A], S85.801[A], S85.809[A], S85.811[A], S85.819-S85.891[A], S85.899-S85.901[A], S85.909-S85.911[A], S85.919-S85.991[A], S85.999[A], S95.001[A], S95.009-S95.011[A], S95.019-S95.091[A], S95.099[A], S95.201[A], S95.209-S95.211[A], S95.219-S95.291[A], S95.299-S95.801[A], S95.809-S95.811[A], S95.819-S95.891[A], S95.899-S95.901[A], S95.909-S95.911[A], S95.919-S95.991[A], S95.999[A]

● **S75.202**   Unspecified injury of greater saphenous vein at hip and thigh level, left leg A 🔖
     ⒺⓍ S75.202-S75.209[A], S75.212-S75.219[A], S75.222-S75.229[A], S75.292-S75.299[A], S75.802-S75.809[A], S75.812-S75.819[A], S75.892-S75.899[A], S75.902-S75.909[A], S75.912-S75.919[A], S75.992-S75.999[A], S85.202-S85.209[A], S85.212-S85.219[A], S85.292-S85.299[A], S85.302-S85.309[A], S85.312-S85.319[A], S85.392-S85.399[A], S85.402-S85.409[A], S85.412-S85.419[A], S85.492-S85.499[A], S85.802-S85.809[A], S85.812-S85.819[A], S85.892-S85.899[A], S85.902-S85.909[A], S85.912-S85.919[A], S85.992-S85.999[A], S95.002-S95.009[A], S95.012-S95.019[A], S95.092-S95.099[A], S95.202-S95.209[A], S95.212-S95.219[A], S95.292-S95.299[A], S95.802-S95.809[A], S95.812-S95.819[A], S95.892-S95.899[A], S95.902-S95.909[A], S95.912-S95.919[A], S95.992-S95.999[A]

● **S75.209**   Unspecified injury of greater saphenous vein at hip and thigh level, unspecified leg A 🔖
     ⒺⓍ S75.201-S75.999[A], S85.201-S85.499[A], S85.801-S85.999[A], S95.001-S95.099[A], S95.201-S95.999[A]

● **S75.21**   Minor laceration of greater saphenous vein at hip and thigh level
     Incomplete transection of greater saphenous vein at hip and thigh level
     Laceration of greater saphenous vein at hip and thigh level NOS
     Superficial laceration of greater saphenous vein at hip and thigh level

● **S75.211**   Minor laceration of greater saphenous vein at hip and thigh level, right leg A 🔖
     ⒺⓍ See S75.201

● **S75.212**   Minor laceration of greater saphenous vein at hip and thigh level, left leg A 🔖
     ⒺⓍ See S75.202

● **S75.219**   Minor laceration of greater saphenous vein at hip and thigh level, unspecified leg A 🔖
     ⒺⓍ See S75.209

CHAPTER 19 (S00–T88)

● **S75.22 Major laceration of greater saphenous vein at hip and thigh level**
> Complete transection of greater saphenous vein at hip and thigh level
> Traumatic rupture of greater saphenous vein at hip and thigh level

　● **S75.221 Major laceration of greater saphenous vein at hip and thigh level, right leg**
　　A 🔍
　　Ex: See S75.201

　● **S75.222 Major laceration of greater saphenous vein at hip and thigh level, left leg**
　　A 🔍
　　Ex: See S75.202

　● **S75.229 Major laceration of greater saphenous vein at hip and thigh level, unspecified leg** A 🔍
　　Ex: See S75.209

● **S75.29 Other specified injury of greater saphenous vein at hip and thigh level**

　● **S75.291 Other specified injury of greater saphenous vein at hip and thigh level, right leg** A 🔍
　　Ex: See S75.201

　● **S75.292 Other specified injury of greater saphenous vein at hip and thigh level, left leg** A 🔍
　　Ex: See S75.202

　● **S75.299 Other specified injury of greater saphenous vein at hip and thigh level, unspecified leg** A 🔍
　　Ex: See S75.209

● **S75.8 Injury of other blood vessels at hip and thigh level**

　● **S75.80 Unspecified injury of other blood vessels at hip and thigh level**

　　● **S75.801 Unspecified injury of other blood vessels at hip and thigh level, right leg** A 🔍
　　　Ex: M79.A21-M79.A29, S75.001[A],
　　　S75.009-S75.011[A], S75.019-S7.021[A],
　　　S75.029-S75.091[A], S75.099-S75.101[A],
　　　S75.109-S75.111[A], S75.119-S75.121[A],
　　　S75.129-S75.191[A], S75.199-S75.201[A],
　　　S75.209-S75.211[A], S75.219-S75.221[A],
　　　S75.229-S75.291[A], S75.299-S75.801[A],
　　　S75.809-S75.891[A], S75.899-S75.901[A],
　　　S75.909-S75.911[A], S75.919-S75.991[A],
　　　S75.999[A], S85.001[A], S85.009-S85.011[A],
　　　S85.019-S85.091[A], S85.099-S85.101[A],
　　　S85.109-S85.111[A], S85.119-S85.121[A],
　　　S85.129-S85.131[A], S85.139-S85.141[A],
　　　S85.149-S85.151[A], S85.159-S85.161[A],
　　　S85.169-S85.171[A], S85.179-S85.181[A],
　　　S85.189-S85.201[A], S85.209-S85.211[A],
　　　S85.219-S85.291[A], S85.299-S85.301[A],
　　　S85.309-S85.311[A], S85.319-S85.391[A],
　　　S85.399-S85.401[A], S85.409-S85.411[A],
　　　S85.419-S85.491[A], S85.499-S85.501[A],
　　　S85.509-S85.511[A], S85.519-S85.591[A],
　　　S85.599-S85.801[A], S85.809-S85.811[A],
　　　S85.819-S85.891[A], S85.899-S85.901[A]
　　　S85.909-S85.911[A], S85.919-S85.991[A],
　　　S85.999[A], S95.001[A], S95.009-S95.011[A],
　　　S95.019[A], S95.091[A], S95.099-S95.101[A],
　　　S95.109-S95.111[A], S95.119-S95.191[A],
　　　S95.199-S95.201[A], S95.209-S95.211[A],
　　　S95.219-S95.291[A], S95.299-S95.801[A],
　　　S95.809-S95.811[A], S95.819-S95.891[A],
　　　S95.899-S95.901[A], S95.909-S95.911[A],
　　　S95.919-S95.991[A], S95.999[A]

　　● **S75.802 Unspecified injury of other blood vessels at hip and thigh level, left leg**
　　　A 🔍
　　　Ex: M79.A21-M79.A29, S75.002-S75.009[A],
　　　S75.012-S75.019[A], S75.022-S75.029[A],
　　　S75.092-S75.099[A], S75.102-S75.109[A],
　　　S75.112-S75.119[A], S75.122-S75.129[A],
　　　S75.192-S75.199[A], S75.202-S75.209[A],
　　　S75.212-S75.219[A], S75.222-S75.229[A],
　　　S75.292-S75.299[A], S75.802-S75.809[A]
　　　S75.812-S75.819[A], S75.892-S75.899[A],
　　　S75.902-S75.909[A], S75.912-S75.919[A],
　　　S75.992-S75.999[A], S85.002-S85.009[A],
　　　S85.012-S85.019[A], S85.092-S85.099[A],
　　　S85.102-S85.109[A], S85.112-S85.119[A],
　　　S85.122-S85.129[A], S85.132-S85.139[A],
　　　S85.142-S85.149[A], S85.152-S85.159[A],
　　　S85.162-S85.169[A], S85.172-S85.179[A],
　　　S85.182-S85.189[A], S85.202-S85.209[A],
　　　S85.212-S85.219[A], S85.292-S85.299[A],
　　　S85.302-S85.309[A], S85.312-S85.319[A],
　　　S85.392-S85.399[A], S85.402-S85.409[A],
　　　S85.412-S85.419[A], S85.492-S85.499[A],
　　　S85.502-S85.509[A], S85.512-S85.519[A],
　　　S85.592-S85.599[A], S85.802-S85.809[A],
　　　S85.812-S85.819[A], S85.892-S85.899[A],
　　　S85.902-S85.909[A], S85.912-S85.919[A],
　　　S85.992-S85.999[A], S95.002-S95.009[A],
　　　S95.012-S95.019[A], S95.092-S95.099[A],
　　　S95.102-S95.109[A], S95.112-S95.119[A],
　　　S95.192-S95.199[A], S95.202-S95.209[A],
　　　S95.212-S95.219[A], S95.292-S95.299[A],
　　　S95.802-S95.809[A], S95.812-S95.819[A],
　　　S95.892-S95.899[A], S95.902-S95.909[A],
　　　S95.912-S95.919[A], S95.992-S95.999[A]

　　● **S75.809 Unspecified injury of other blood vessels at hip and thigh level, unspecified leg** A 🔍
　　　Ex: M79.A21-M79.A29, S75.001-S75.999[A],
　　　S85.001-S85.999[A], S95.001-S95.999[A]

　● **S75.81 Laceration of other blood vessels at hip and thigh level**

　　● **S75.811 Laceration of other blood vessels at hip and thigh level, right leg** A 🔍
　　　Ex: See S75.801

　　● **S75.812 Laceration of other blood vessels at hip and thigh level, left leg** A 🔍
　　　Ex: See S75.802

　　● **S75.819 Laceration of other blood vessels at hip and thigh level, unspecified leg**
　　　A 🔍
　　　Ex: See S75.809

　● **S75.89 Other specified injury of other blood vessels at hip and thigh level**

　　● **S75.891 Other specified injury of other blood vessels at hip and thigh level, right leg** A 🔍
　　　Ex: See S75.801

　　● **S75.892 Other specified injury of other blood vessels at hip and thigh level, left leg**
　　　A 🔍
　　　Ex: See S75.802

　　● **S75.899 Other specified injury of other blood vessels at hip and thigh level, unspecified leg** A 🔍
　　　Ex: See S75.809

● **S75.9**   **Injury of unspecified blood vessel at hip and thigh level**
  ● **S75.90**   Unspecified injury of unspecified blood vessel at hip and thigh level
    ● **S75.901**   Unspecified injury of unspecified blood vessel at hip and thigh level, right leg A 🦠
       Ex: See S75.801
    ● **S75.902**   Unspecified injury of unspecified blood vessel at hip and thigh level, left leg A 🦠
       Ex: See S75.802
    ● **S75.909**   Unspecified injury of unspecified blood vessel at hip and thigh level, unspecified leg A 🦠
       Ex: See S75.809
  ● **S75.91**   Laceration of unspecified blood vessel at hip and thigh level
    ● **S75.911**   Laceration of unspecified blood vessel at hip and thigh level, right leg A 🦠
       Ex: See S75.801
    ● **S75.912**   Laceration of unspecified blood vessel at hip and thigh level, left leg A 🦠
       Ex: See S75.802
    ● **S75.919**   Laceration of unspecified blood vessel at hip and thigh level, unspecified leg A 🦠
       Ex: See S75.809
  ● **S75.99**   Other specified injury of unspecified blood vessel at hip and thigh level
    ● **S75.991**   Other specified injury of unspecified blood vessel at hip and thigh level, right leg A 🦠
       Ex: See S75.801
    ● **S75.992**   Other specified injury of unspecified blood vessel at hip and thigh level, left leg A 🦠
       Ex: See S75.802
    ● **S75.999**   Other specified injury of unspecified blood vessel at hip and thigh level, unspecified leg A 🦠
       Ex: See S75.809

● **S76**   **Injury of muscle, fascia and tendon at hip and thigh level**
   Code also any associated open wound (S71.-)
   Excludes2   injury of muscle, fascia and tendon at lower leg level (S86)
       sprain of joint and ligament of hip (S73.1)
   The appropriate 7th character is to be added to each code from category S76

     A   initial encounter
     D   subsequent encounter
     S   sequela

  ● **S76.0**   **Injury of muscle, fascia and tendon of hip**
    ● **S76.00**   Unspecified injury of muscle, fascia and tendon of hip
      ● **S76.001**   Unspecified injury of muscle, fascia and tendon of right hip
      ● **S76.002**   Unspecified injury of muscle, fascia and tendon of left hip
      ● **S76.009**   Unspecified injury of muscle, fascia and tendon of unspecified hip
    ● **S76.01**   Strain of muscle, fascia and tendon of hip
      ● **S76.011**   Strain of muscle, fascia and tendon of right hip
      ● **S76.012**   Strain of muscle, fascia and tendon of left hip
      ● **S76.019**   Strain of muscle, fascia and tendon of unspecified hip

● **S76.02**   Laceration of muscle, fascia and tendon of hip
  ● **S76.021**   Laceration of muscle, fascia and tendon of right hip A 🦠
     Ex: S71.001[A], S71.009-S71.011[A], S71.019-S71.021[A], S71.029-S71.031[A], S71.039-S71.041[A], S71.049-S71.051[A], S71.059-S71.101[A], S71.109-S71.111[A], S71.119-S71.121[A], S71.129-S71.131[A], S71.139-S71.141[A], S71.149-S71.151[A], S71.159[A], S76.021[A], S76.029[A], S76.121[A], S76.129[A], S76.221[A], S76.229[A], S76.321[A], S76.329[A], S76.821[A], S76.829[A], S76.921[A], S76.929[A]
  ● **S76.022**   Laceration of muscle, fascia and tendon of left hip A 🦠
     Ex: S71.002-S71.009[A], S71.012-S71.019[A], S71.022-S71.029[A], S71.032-S71.039[A], S71.042-S71.049[A], S71.052-S71.059[A], S71.102-S71.109[A], S71.112-S71.119[A], S71.122-S71.129[A], S71.132-S71.139[A],S71.142-S71.149[A], S71.152-S71.159[A], S76.022-S76.029[A], S76.122-S76.129[A], S76.222-S76.229[A],S76.322-S76.329[A], S76.822-S76.829[A], S76.922-S76.929[A]
  ● **S76.029**   Laceration of muscle, fascia and tendon of unspecified hip A 🦠
     Ex: S71.001-S71.159[A], S76.021-S76.029[A], S76.121-S76.129[A], S76.221-S76.229[A], S76.321-S76.329[A], S76.821-S76.829[A], S76.921-S76.929[A]
● **S76.09**   Other specified injury of muscle, fascia and tendon of hip
  ● **S76.091**   Other specified injury of muscle, fascia and tendon of right hip
  ● **S76.092**   Other specified injury of muscle, fascia and tendon of left hip
  ● **S76.099**   Other specified injury of muscle, fascia and tendon of unspecified hip
● **S76.1**   **Injury of quadriceps muscle, fascia and tendon**
   Injury of patellar ligament (tendon)
  ● **S76.10**   Unspecified injury of quadriceps muscle, fascia and tendon
    ● **S76.101**   Unspecified injury of right quadriceps muscle, fascia and tendon
    ● **S76.102**   Unspecified injury of left quadriceps muscle, fascia and tendon
    ● **S76.109**   Unspecified injury of unspecified quadriceps muscle, fascia and tendon
  ● **S76.11**   Strain of quadriceps muscle, fascia and tendon
    ● **S76.111**   Strain of right quadriceps muscle, fascia and tendon
    ● **S76.112**   Strain of left quadriceps muscle, fascia and tendon
    ● **S76.119**   Strain of unspecified quadriceps muscle, fascia and tendon
  ● **S76.12**   Laceration of quadriceps muscle, fascia and tendon
    ● **S76.121**   Laceration of right quadriceps muscle, fascia and tendon A 🦠
       Ex: See S76.021
    ● **S76.122**   Laceration of left quadriceps muscle, fascia and tendon A 🦠
       Ex: See S76.022
    ● **S76.129**   Laceration of unspecified quadriceps muscle, fascia and tendon A 🦠
       Ex: See S76.029
  ● **S76.19**   Other specified injury of quadriceps muscle, fascia and tendon
    ● **S76.191**   Other specified injury of right quadriceps muscle, fascia and tendon
    ● **S76.192**   Other specified injury of left quadriceps muscle, fascia and tendon
    ● **S76.199**   Other specified injury of unspecified quadriceps muscle, fascia and tendon

CHAPTER 19 (S00-T88)

N   Newborn Age: 0   P   Pediatric Age: 0–17   M   Maternity DX: 12–55   A   Adult Age: 15–124   ♀   Females Only   ♂   Males Only
🦠 Complication\Comorbidity   ☤ Major C\C   Ex: CC/MCC Exclusions   🦠 Hospital-Acquired Condition

1371

CHAPTER 19 (S00-T88)

- S76.2   Injury of adductor muscle, fascia and tendon of thigh
  - S76.20   Unspecified injury of adductor muscle, fascia and tendon of thigh
    - S76.201   Unspecified injury of adductor muscle, fascia and tendon of right thigh
    - S76.202   Unspecified injury of adductor muscle, fascia and tendon of left thigh
    - S76.209   Unspecified injury of adductor muscle, fascia and tendon of unspecified thigh
  - S76.21   Strain of adductor muscle, fascia and tendon of thigh
    - S76.211   Strain of adductor muscle, fascia and tendon of right thigh
    - S76.212   Strain of adductor muscle, fascia and tendon of left thigh
    - S76.219   Strain of adductor muscle, fascia and tendon of unspecified thigh
  - S76.22   Laceration of adductor muscle, fascia and tendon of thigh
    - S76.221   Laceration of adductor muscle, fascia and tendon of right thigh A
      - (Ex:) See S76.021
    - S76.222   Laceration of adductor muscle, fascia and tendon of left thigh A
      - (Ex:) See S76.022
    - S76.229   Laceration of adductor muscle, fascia and tendon of unspecified thigh A
      - (Ex:) See S76.029
  - S76.29   Other injury of adductor muscle, fascia and tendon of thigh
    - S76.291   Other injury of adductor muscle, fascia and tendon of right thigh
    - S76.292   Other injury of adductor muscle, fascia and tendon of left thigh
    - S76.299   Other injury of adductor muscle, fascia and tendon of unspecified thigh
- S76.3   Injury of muscle, fascia and tendon of the posterior muscle group at thigh level
  - S76.30   Unspecified injury of muscle, fascia and tendon of the posterior muscle group at thigh level
    - S76.301   Unspecified injury of muscle, fascia and tendon of the posterior muscle group at thigh level, right thigh
    - S76.302   Unspecified injury of muscle, fascia and tendon of the posterior muscle group at thigh level, left thigh
    - S76.309   Unspecified injury of muscle, fascia and tendon of the posterior muscle group at thigh level, unspecified thigh
  - S76.31   Strain of muscle, fascia and tendon of the posterior muscle group at thigh level
    - S76.311   Strain of muscle, fascia and tendon of the posterior muscle group at thigh level, right thigh
    - S76.312   Strain of muscle, fascia and tendon of the posterior muscle group at thigh level, left thigh
    - S76.319   Strain of muscle, fascia and tendon of the posterior muscle group at thigh level, unspecified thigh
  - S76.32   Laceration of muscle, fascia and tendon of the posterior muscle group at thigh level
    - S76.321   Laceration of muscle, fascia and tendon of the posterior muscle group at thigh level, right thigh A
      - (Ex:) See S76.021

- S76.322   Laceration of muscle, fascia and tendon of the posterior muscle group at thigh level, left thigh A
  - (Ex:) See S76.022
- S76.329   Laceration of muscle, fascia and tendon of the posterior muscle group at thigh level, unspecified thigh A
  - (Ex:) See S76.029
- S76.39   Other specified injury of muscle, fascia and tendon of the posterior muscle group at thigh level
  - S76.391   Other specified injury of muscle, fascia and tendon of the posterior muscle group at thigh level, right thigh
  - S76.392   Other specified injury of muscle, fascia and tendon of the posterior muscle group at thigh level, left thigh
  - S76.399   Other specified injury of muscle, fascia and tendon of the posterior muscle group at thigh level, unspecified thigh
- S76.8   Injury of other specified muscles, fascia and tendons at thigh level
  - S76.80   Unspecified injury of other specified muscles, fascia and tendons at thigh level
    - S76.801   Unspecified injury of other specified muscles, fascia and tendons at thigh level, right thigh
    - S76.802   Unspecified injury of other specified muscles, fascia and tendons at thigh level, left thigh
    - S76.809   Unspecified injury of other specified muscles, fascia and tendons at thigh level, unspecified thigh
  - S76.81   Strain of other specified specified muscles, fascia and tendons at thigh level
    - S76.811   Strain of other specified muscles, fascia and tendons at thigh level, right thigh
    - S76.812   Strain of other specified muscles, fascia and tendons at thigh level, left thigh
    - S76.819   Strain of other specified muscles, fascia and tendons at thigh level, unspecified thigh
  - S76.82   Laceration of other specified muscles, fascia and tendons at thigh level
    - S76.821   Laceration of other specified muscles, fascia and tendons at thigh level, right thigh A
      - (Ex:) See S76.021
    - S76.822   Laceration of other specified muscles, fascia and tendons at thigh level, left thigh A
      - (Ex:) See S76.022
    - S76.829   Laceration of other specified muscles, fascia and tendons at thigh level, unspecified thigh A
      - (Ex:) See S76.029
  - S76.89   Other injury of other specified muscles, fascia and tendons at thigh level
    - S76.891   Other injury of other specified muscles, fascia and tendons at thigh level, right thigh
    - S76.892   Other injury of other specified muscles, fascia and tendons at thigh level, left thigh
    - S76.899   Other injury of other specified muscles, fascia and tendons at thigh level, unspecified thigh

◀ New   ◀ Revised   ~~deleted~~ Deleted   Excludes 1   Excludes 2   Includes   Use additional   Code first   Code also   Unspecified

OGCR Official Guidelines   ● Unacceptable Principal Diagnosis   X Assign placeholder X   ● Use Additional Character(s)   ▶ Manifestation Code   **Coding Clinic**

- ● **S76.9**   **Injury of unspecified muscles, fascia and tendons at thigh level**
  - ● **S76.90**   Unspecified injury of unspecified muscles, fascia and tendons at thigh level
    - ● **S76.901**   Unspecified injury of unspecified muscles, fascia and tendons at thigh level, right thigh
    - ● **S76.902**   Unspecified injury of unspecified muscles, fascia and tendons at thigh level, left thigh
    - ● **S76.909**   Unspecified injury of unspecified muscles, fascia and tendons at thigh level, unspecified thigh
  - ● **S76.91**   Strain of unspecified muscles, fascia and tendons at thigh level
    - ● **S76.911**   Strain of unspecified muscles, fascia and tendons at thigh level, right thigh
    - ● **S76.912**   Strain of unspecified muscles, fascia and tendons at thigh level, left thigh
    - ● **S76.919**   Strain of unspecified muscles fascia and tendons at thigh level, unspecified thigh
  - ● **S76.92**   Laceration of unspecified muscles, fascia and tendons at thigh level
    - ● **S76.921**   Laceration of unspecified muscles, fascia and tendons at thigh level, right thigh A 🗞
      - (Ex) See S76.021
    - ● **S76.922**   Laceration of unspecified muscles, fascia and tendons at thigh level, left thigh A 🗞
      - (Ex) See S76.022
    - ● **S76.929**   Laceration of unspecified muscles, fascia and tendons at thigh level, unspecified thigh A 🗞
      - (Ex) See S76.029
  - ● **S76.99**   Other specified injury of unspecified muscles, fascia and tendons at thigh level
    - ● **S76.991**   Other specified injury of unspecified muscles, fascia and tendons at thigh level, right thigh
    - ● **S76.992**   Other specified injury of unspecified muscles, fascia and tendons at thigh level, left thigh
    - ● **S76.999**   Other specified injury of unspecified muscles, fascia and tendons at thigh level, unspecified thigh

- ● **S77**   **Crushing injury of hip and thigh**

  Use additional code(s) for all associated injuries

  Excludes2   crushing injury of ankle and foot (S97.-)
              crushing injury of lower leg (S87.-)

  The appropriate 7th character is to be added to each code from category S77

A	initial encounter
D	subsequent encounter
S	sequela

  - ● **S77.0**   Crushing injury of hip
    - (Ex) For category S77.0 CC codes: S77.00X-S77.02X[A], S77.20X-S77.22X[A]
    - X ● **S77.00**   Crushing injury of unspecified hip A 🗞, A 🗞
    - X ● **S77.01**   Crushing injury of right hip A 🗞, A 🗞
    - X ● **S77.02**   Crushing injury of left hip A 🗞, A 🗞
  - ● **S77.1**   Crushing injury of thigh
    - (Ex) For category S77.1 CC codes: S77.10X-S77.22X[A]
    - X ● **S77.10**   Crushing injury of unspecified thigh A 🗞, A 🗞
    - X ● **S77.11**   Crushing injury of right thigh A 🗞, A 🗞
    - X ● **S77.12**   Crushing injury of left thigh A 🗞, A 🗞

- ● **S77.2**   Crushing injury of hip with thigh
  - X ● **S77.20**   Crushing injury of unspecified hip with thigh
  - X ● **S77.21**   Crushing injury of right hip with thigh
  - X ● **S77.22**   Crushing injury of left hip with thigh

- ● **S78**   **Traumatic amputation of hip and thigh**

  An amputation not identified as partial or complete should be coded to complete

  Excludes1   traumatic amputation of knee (S88.0-)

  The appropriate 7th character is to be added to each code from category S78

A	initial encounter
D	subsequent encounter
S	sequela

  - ● **S78.0**   Traumatic amputation at hip joint
    - ● **S78.01**   Complete traumatic amputation at hip joint
      - ● **S78.011**   Complete traumatic amputation at right hip joint A 🗞
        - (Ex) S71.001[A], S71.009-S71.011[A], S71.019-S71.021[A], S71.029-S71.031[A], S71.039-S71.041[A], S71.049-S71.051[A], S71.059-S71.101[A], S71.109-S71.111[A], S71.119-S71.121[A], S71.129-S71.131[A], S71.139-S71.141[A], S71.149-S71.151[A], S71.159[A], S76.021[A], S76.029[A], S76.121[A], S76.129[A], S76.221[A], S76.229[A], S76.321[A], S76.329[A], S76.821[A], S76.829[A], S76.921[A], S76.929[A], S78.011[A], S78.019-S78.021[A], S78.029-S78.111[A], S78.119-S78.121[A], S78.129-S78.911[A], S78.919-S78.921[A], S78.929[A], S81.001[A], S81.009-S81.011[A], S81.019-S81.021[A], S81.029-S81.031[A], S81.039-S81.041[A], S81.049-S81.051[A], S81.059-S81.801[A], S81.809-S81.811[A], S81.819-S81.821[A], S81.829-S81.831[A], S81.839-S81.841[A], S81.849-S81.851[A], S81.859[A], S86.021[A], S86.029[A], S86.121[A], S86.129[A], S86.221[A], S86.229[A], S86.321[A], S86.329[A], S86.821[A], S86.829[A], S86.921[A], S86.929[A], S88.011[A], S88.019-S88.021[A], S88.029-S88.111[A], S88.119-S88.121[A], S88.129-S88.911[A], S88.919-S88.921[A], S88.929[A], S91.001[A], S91.009-S91.011[A], S91.019-S91.021[A], S91.029-S91.031[A], S91.039-S91.041[A], S91.049-S91.051[A], S91.059-S91.101[A], S91.103-S91.104[A], S91.106-S91.111[A], S91.113-S91.114[A], S91.116-S91.121[A], S91.123-S91.124[A], S91.126-S91.131[A], S91.133-S91.134[A], S91.136-S91.141[A], S91.143-S91.144[A], S91.146-S91.151[A], S91.153-S91.154[A], S91.156-S91.201[A], S91.203-S91.204[A], S91.206-S91.211[A], S91.213-S91.214[A], S91.216-S91.221[A], S91.223-S91.224[A], S91.226-S91.231[A], S91.233-S91.234[A], S91.236-S91.241[A], S91.243-S91.244[A], S91.246-S91.251[A], S91.253-S91.254[A], S91.256-S91.301[A], S91.309-S91.311[A], S91.319-S91.321[A], S91.329-S91.331[A], S91.339-S91.341[A], S91.349-S91.351[A], S91.359[A], S96.021[A], S96.029[A], S96.121[A], S96.129[A], S96.221[A], S96.229[A], S96.821[A], S96.829[A], S96.921[A], S96.929[A], S98.011[A], S98.019-S98.021[A], S98.029-S98.111[A], S98.119-S98.121[A], S98.129-S98.131[A], S98.139-S98.141[A], S98.149-S98.211[A], S98.219-S98.221[A], S98.229-S98.311[A], S98.319-S98.321[A], S98.329-S98.911[A], S98.919-S98.921[A], S98.929[A], T14.90-T14.91, T79.8XX-T79.9XX[A], T79.A0X-T79.A9X[A]

● **S78.012** **Complete traumatic amputation at left hip joint** A 🦠

(Ex:) S71.002-S71.009[A], S71.012-S71.019[A], S71.022-S71.029[A], S71.032-S71.039[A], S71.042-S71.049[A], S71.052-S71.059[A],S71.102-S71.109[A], S71.112-S71.119[A], S71.122-S71.129[A], S71.132-S71.139[A], S71.142-S71.149[A], S71.152-S71.159[A], S76.022-S76.029[A], S76.122-S76.129[A], S76.222-S76.229[A], S76.322-S76.329[A], S76.822-S76.829[A], S76.922-S76.929[A], S78.012-S78.019[A], S78.022-S78.029[A], S78.112-S78.119[A], S78.122-S78.129[A], S78.912-S78.919[A], S78.922-S78.929[A], S81.002-S81.009[A], S81.012-S81.019[A], S81.022-S81.029[A], S81.032-S81.039[A], S81.042-S81.049[A], S81.052-S81.059[A], S81.802-S81.809[A], S81.812-S81.819[A], S81.822-S81.829[A], S81.832-S81.839[A], S81.842-S81.849[A], S81.852-S81.859[A], S86.022-S86.029[A], S86.122-S86.129[A], S86.222-S86.229[A], S86.322-S86.329[A], S86.822-S86.829[A], S86.922-S86.929[A], S88.012-S88.019[A], S88.022-S88.029[A], S88.112-S88.119[A], S88.122-S88.129[A], S88.912-S88.919[A], S88.922-S88.929[A], S91.002-S91.009[A], S91.012-S91.019[A], S91.022-S91.029[A], S91.032-S91.039[A], S91.042-S91.049[A], S91.052-S91.059[A], S91.102-S91.103[A], S91.105-S91.109[A], S91.112-S91.113[A], S91.115-S91.119[A], S91.122-S91.123[A], S91.125-S91.129[A], S91.132-S91.133[A], S91.135-S91.139[A], S91.142-S91.143[A], S91.145-S91.149[A], S91.152-S91.153[A], S91.155-S91.159[A], S91.202-S91.203[A], S91.205-S91.209[A], S91.212-S91.213[A], S91.215-S91.219[A], S91.222-S91.223[A], S91.225-S91.229[A], S91.232-S91.233[A], S91.235-S91.239[A], S91.242-S91.243[A], S91.245-S91.249[A], S91.252-S91.253[A], S91.255-S91.259[A], S91.302-S91.309[A], S91.312-S91.319[A], S91.322-S91.329[A], S91.332-S91.339[A], S91.342-S91.349[A], S91.352-S91.359[A], S96.022-S96.029[A], S96.122-S96.129[A], S96.222-S96.229[A], S96.822-S96.829[A], S96.922-S96.929[A], S98.012-S98.019[A], S98.022-S98.029[A], S98.112-S98.119[A], S98.122-S98.129[A], S98.132-S98.139[A], S98.142-S98.149[A], S98.212-S98.219[A], S98.222-S98.229[A], S98.312-S98.319[A], S98.322-S98.329[A], S98.912-S98.919[A], S98.922-S98.929[A], T14.90-T14.91, T79.8XX-T79.9XX[A], T79.A0X-T79.A9X[A]

● **S78.019** **Complete traumatic amputation at unspecified hip joint** A 🦠

(Ex:) S71.001-S71.159[A], S76.021-S76.029[A], S76.121-S76.129[A], S76.221-S76.229[A], S76.321-S76.329[A], S76.821-S76.829[A], S76.921-S76.929[A], S78.011-S78.929[A], S81.001-S81.859[A], S86.021-S86.029[A], S86.121-S86.129[A], S86.221-S86.229[A], S86.321-S86.329[A], S86.821-S86.829[A], S86.921-S86.929[A], S88.011-S88.929[A], S91.001-S91.359[A], S96.021-S96.029[A], S96.121-S96.129[A], S96.221-S96.229[A], S96.821-S96.829[A], S96.921-S96.929[A], S98.011-S98.929[A], T14.90-T14.91, T79.8XX-T79.9XX[A], T79.A0X-T79.A9X[A]

● **S78.02** **Partial traumatic amputation at hip joint**

    ● **S78.021** **Partial traumatic amputation at right hip joint** A 🦠
        (Ex:) See S78.011

    ● **S78.022** **Partial traumatic amputation at left hip joint** A 🦠
        (Ex:) See S78.012

    ● **S78.029** **Partial traumatic amputation at unspecified hip joint** A 🦠
        (Ex:) See S78.019

● **S78.1** **Traumatic amputation at level between hip and knee**

  Excludes1   traumatic amputation of knee (S88.0-)

  ● **S78.11** **Complete traumatic amputation at level between hip and knee**

    ● **S78.111** **Complete traumatic amputation at level between right hip and knee** A 🦠
        (Ex:) See S78.011

    ● **S78.112** **Complete traumatic amputation at level between left hip and knee** A 🦠
        (Ex:) See S78.012

    ● **S78.119** **Complete traumatic amputation at level between unspecified hip and knee** A 🦠
        (Ex:) See S78.019

  ● **S78.12** **Partial traumatic amputation at level between hip and knee**

    ● **S78.121** **Partial traumatic amputation at level between right hip and knee** A 🦠
        (Ex:) See S78.011

    ● **S78.122** **Partial traumatic amputation at level between left hip and knee** A 🦠
        (Ex:) See S78.012

    ● **S78.129** **Partial traumatic amputation at level between unspecified hip and knee** A 🦠
        (Ex:) See S78.019

● **S78.9** **Traumatic amputation of hip and thigh, level unspecified**

  ● **S78.91** **Complete traumatic amputation of hip and thigh, level unspecified**

    ● **S78.911** **Complete traumatic amputation of right hip and thigh, level unspecified** A 🦠
        (Ex:) See S78.011

    ● **S78.912** **Complete traumatic amputation of left hip and thigh, level unspecified** A 🦠
        (Ex:) See S78.012

    ● **S78.919** **Complete traumatic amputation of unspecified hip and thigh, level unspecified** A 🦠
        (Ex:) See S78.019

  ● **S78.92** **Partial traumatic amputation of hip and thigh, level unspecified**

    ● **S78.921** **Partial traumatic amputation of right hip and thigh, level unspecified** A 🦠
        (Ex:) See S78.011

    ● **S78.922** **Partial traumatic amputation of left hip and thigh, level unspecified** A 🦠
        (Ex:) See S78.012

    ● **S78.929** **Partial traumatic amputation of unspecified hip and thigh, level unspecified** A 🦠
        (Ex:) See S78.019

◀ New   ◀ᴵ Revised   ~~deleted~~ Deleted   Excludes 1   Excludes 2   Includes   Use additional   Code first   Code also   Unspecified

OGCR Official Guidelines   ● Unacceptable Principal Diagnosis   X Assign placeholder X   ● Use Additional Character(s)   ▶ Manifestation Code   **Coding Clinic**

● **S79** **Other and unspecified injuries of hip and thigh**

Note: A fracture not indicated as open or closed should be coded to closed

The appropriate 7th character is to be added to each code from subcategories S79.0 and S79.1

A	initial encounter for closed fracture
D	subsequent encounter for fracture with routine healing
G	subsequent encounter for fracture with delayed healing
K	subsequent encounter for fracture with nonunion
P	subsequent encounter for fracture with malunion
S	sequela

● **S79.0** **Physeal fracture of upper end of femur**

   Excludes1 apophyseal fracture of upper end of femur (S72.13-)

      nontraumatic slipped upper femoral epiphysis (M93.0-)

● **S79.00** **Unspecified physeal fracture of upper end of femur**

● **S79.001** Unspecified physeal fracture of upper end of right femur K, P 🦠, A 🦠, A 🦠
(Ex) For S79.001[A]: See S72.001[A]
For S79.001[K,P]: See S02.0[K]

● **S79.002** Unspecified physeal fracture of upper end of left femur K, P 🦠, A 🦠, A 🦠
(Ex) For S79.002[A]: See S72.002[A]
For S79.002[K,P]: See S02.0[K]

● **S79.009** Unspecified physeal fracture of upper end of unspecified femur K, P 🦠, A 🦠, A 🦠
(Ex) For S79.009[A]: See S72.001[B,C]
For S79.009[K,P]: See S02.0[K]

● **S79.01** **Salter-Harris Type I physeal fracture of upper end of femur**

Acute on chronic slipped capital femoral epiphysis (traumatic)

Acute slipped capital femoral epiphysis (traumatic)

Capital femoral epiphyseal fracture

   Excludes1 chronic slipped upper femoral epiphysis (nontraumatic) (M93.02-)

● **S79.011** Salter-Harris Type I physeal fracture of upper end of right femur K, P 🦠, A 🦠, A 🦠
(Ex) For S79.011[A]: See S72.001[A]
For S79.011[K,P]: See S02.0[K]

● **S79.012** Salter-Harris Type I physeal fracture of upper end of left femur K, P 🦠, A 🦠, A 🦠
(Ex) For S79.012[A]: See S72.002[A]
For S79.012[K,P]: See S02.0[K]

● **S79.019** Salter-Harris Type I physeal fracture of upper end of unspecified femur K, P 🦠, A 🦠, A 🦠
(Ex) For S79.019[A]: See S72.001[B,C]
For S79.019[K,P]: See S02.0[K]

● **S79.09** **Other physeal fracture of upper end of femur**

● **S79.091** Other physeal fracture of upper end of right femur K, P 🦠, A 🦠, A 🦠
(Ex) For S79.091[A]: See S72.001[A]
For S79.091[K,P]: See S02.0[K]

● **S79.092** Other physeal fracture of upper end of left femur K, P 🦠, A 🦠, A 🦠
(Ex) For S79.092[A]: See S72.002[A]
For S79.092[K,P]: See S02.0[K]

● **S79.099** Other physeal fracture of upper end of unspecified femur K, P 🦠, A 🦠, A 🦠
(Ex) For S79.099[A]: See S72.001[B,C]
For S79.099[K,P]: See S02.0[K]

● **S79.1** **Physeal fracture of lower end of femur**

● **S79.10** **Unspecified physeal fracture of lower end of femur**

● **S79.101** Unspecified physeal fracture of lower end of right femur A, K, P 🦠, A 🦠
(Ex) For S79.101[A]: See S72.401[A]
For S79.101[K,P]: See S02.0[K]

● **S79.102** Unspecified physeal fracture of lower end of left femur A, K, P 🦠, A 🦠
(Ex) For S79.102[A]: See S72.402[A]
For S72.102[K,P]: See S02.0[K]

● **S79.109** Unspecified physeal fracture of lower end of unspecified femur A, K, P 🦠, A 🦠
(Ex) For S79.109[A]: See S72.401[B,C]
For S79.109[K,P]: See S02.0[K]

● **S79.11** **Salter-Harris Type I physeal fracture of lower end of femur**

● **S79.111** Salter-Harris Type I physeal fracture of lower end of right femur A, K, P 🦠, A 🦠
(Ex) For S79.111[A]: See S72.401[A]
For S79.111[K,P]: See S02.0[K]

● **S79.112** Salter-Harris Type I physeal fracture of lower end of left femur A, K, P 🦠, A 🦠
(Ex) For S79.112[A]: See S72.402[A]
For S72.112[K,P]: See S02.0[K]

● **S79.119** Salter-Harris Type I physeal fracture of lower end of unspecified femur A, K, P 🦠, A 🦠
(Ex) For S79.119[A]: See S72.401[B,C]
For S79.119[K,P]: See S02.0[K]

● **S79.12** **Salter-Harris Type II physeal fracture of lower end of femur**

● **S79.121** Salter-Harris Type II physeal fracture of lower end of right femur A, K, P 🦠, A 🦠
(Ex) For S79.121[A]: See S72.401[A]
For S79.121[K,P]: See S72.001[K,M,N,P,Q,R]

● **S79.122** Salter-Harris Type II physeal fracture of lower end of left femur A, K, P 🦠, A 🦠
(Ex) For S79.122[A]: See S72.402[A]
For S72.122[K,P]: See S72.001[K,M,N,P,Q,R]

● **S79.129** Salter-Harris Type II physeal fracture of lower end of unspecified femur A, K, P 🦠, A 🦠
(Ex) For S79.129[A]: See S72.401[B,C]
For S79.129[K,P]: See S72.001[K,M,N,P,Q,R]

Item 19–5 **SALTER-HARRIS TYPE 1:** epiphysis is completely separated from end of bone, or metaphysic growth plate remains attached to epiphysis
  SALTER-HARRIS TYPE 2: epiphysis and growth plate are partially separated from metaphysis, which is cracked—most common type
  SALTER-HARRIS TYPE 3: fracture occurring through epiphysis and separates part of epiphysis and growth plate from metaphysis fracture, usually at distal end of tibia
  SALTER-HARRIS TYPE 4: fracture runs through epiphysis, across growth plate, into metaphysic, surgery is required to restore joint surface to normal and align growth plate

CHAPTER 19 (S00-T88)

N Newborn Age: 0   P Pediatric Age: 0–17   M Maternity DX: 12–55   A Adult Age: 15–124   ♀ Females Only   ♂ Males Only
🦠 Complication\Comorbidity   🦠 Major C\C   (Ex) CC/MCC Exclusions   🦠 Hospital-Acquired Condition

1375

● **S79.13** Salter-Harris Type III physeal fracture of lower end of femur

   ● **S79.131** Salter-Harris Type III physeal fracture of lower end of right femur A, K, P 🔵, A 🔵

      Ⓔⓧ **For S79.131[A]:** See S72.401[A]
      For S79.131[K,P]: See S02.0[K]

   ● **S79.132** Salter-Harris Type III physeal fracture of lower end of left femur A, K, P 🔵, A 🔵

      Ⓔⓧ **For S79.132[A]:** See S72.402[A]
      For S72.132[K,P]: See S02.0[K]

   ● **S79.139** Salter-Harris Type III physeal fracture of lower end of unspecified femur A, K, P 🔵, A 🔵

      Ⓔⓧ **For S79.139[A]:** See S72.401[B,C]
      For S79.139[K,P]: See S02.0[K]

● **S79.14** Salter-Harris Type IV physeal fracture of lower end of femur

   ● **S79.141** Salter-Harris Type IV physeal fracture of lower end of right femur A, K, P 🔵, A 🔵

      Ⓔⓧ **For S79.141[A]:** See S72.401[A]
      For S79.141[K,P]: See S02.0[K]

   ● **S79.142** Salter-Harris Type IV physeal fracture of lower end of left femur A, K, P 🔵, A 🔵

      Ⓔⓧ **For S79.142[A]:** See S72.402[A]
      For S72.142[K,P]: See S02.0[K]

   ● **S79.149** Salter-Harris Type IV physeal fracture of lower end of unspecified femur A, K, P 🔵, A 🔵

      Ⓔⓧ **For S79.149[A]:** See S72.401[B,C]
      For S79.149[K,P]: See S02.0[K]

● **S79.19** Other physeal fracture of lower end of femur

   ● **S79.191** Other physeal fracture of lower end of right femur A, K, P 🔵, A 🔵

      Ⓔⓧ **For S79.191[A]:** See S72.401[A]
      For S79.191[K,P]: See S02.0[K]

   ● **S79.192** Other physeal fracture of lower end of left femur A, K, P 🔵, A 🔵

      Ⓔⓧ **For S79.192[A]:** See S72.402[A]
      For S72.192[K,P]: See S02.0[K]

   ● **S79.199** Other physeal fracture of lower end of unspecified femur A, K, P 🔵, A 🔵

      Ⓔⓧ **For S79.199[A]:** See S72.401[B,C]
      For S79.199[K,P]: See S02.0[K]

● **S79.8** Other specified injuries of hip and thigh

The appropriate 7th character is to be added to each code in subcategory S79.8

A	initial encounter
D	subsequent encounter
S	sequela

● **S79.81** Other specified injuries of hip

   ● **S79.811** Other specified injuries of right hip
   ● **S79.812** Other specified injuries of left hip
   ● **S79.819** Other specified injuries of unspecified hip

● **S79.82** Other specified injuries of thigh

   ● **S79.821** Other specified injuries of right thigh
   ● **S79.822** Other specified injuries of left thigh
   ● **S79.829** Other specified injuries of unspecified thigh

● **S79.9** Unspecified injury of hip and thigh

The appropriate 7th character is to be added to each code in subcategory S79.9

A	initial encounter
D	subsequent encounter
S	sequela

● **S79.91** Unspecified injury of hip

   ● **S79.911** Unspecified injury of right hip
   ● **S79.912** Unspecified injury of left hip
   ● **S79.919** Unspecified injury of unspecified hip

● **S79.92** Unspecified injury of thigh

   ● **S79.921** Unspecified injury of right thigh
   ● **S79.922** Unspecified injury of left thigh
   ● **S79.929** Unspecified injury of unspecified thigh

INJURIES TO THE KNEE AND LOWER LEG (S80-S89)

Excludes2   burns and corrosions (T20-T32)
       frostbite (T33-T34)
       injuries of ankle and foot, except fracture of ankle and malleolus (S90-S99)
       insect bite or sting, venomous (T63.4)

● **S80** Superficial injury of knee and lower leg

Excludes2   superficial injury of ankle and foot (S90.-)

The appropriate 7th character is to be added to each code from category S80

A	initial encounter
D	subsequent encounter
S	sequela

● **S80.0** Contusion of knee

  X ● **S80.00** Contusion of unspecified knee
  X ● **S80.01** Contusion of right knee
  X ● **S80.02** Contusion of left knee

● **S80.1** Contusion of lower leg

  X ● **S80.10** Contusion of unspecified lower leg
  X ● **S80.11** Contusion of right lower leg
  X ● **S80.12** Contusion of left lower leg

● **S80.2** Other superficial injuries of knee

   ● **S80.21** Abrasion of knee

      ● **S80.211** Abrasion, right knee
      ● **S80.212** Abrasion, left knee
      ● **S80.219** Abrasion, unspecified knee

   ● **S80.22** Blister (nonthermal) of knee

      ● **S80.221** Blister (nonthermal), right knee
      ● **S80.222** Blister (nonthermal), left knee
      ● **S80.229** Blister (nonthermal), unspecified knee

   ● **S80.24** External constriction of knee

      ● **S80.241** External constriction, right knee
      ● **S80.242** External constriction, left knee
      ● **S80.249** External constriction, unspecified knee

◀ New   ◀⁞ Revised   ~~deleted~~ Deleted   Excludes 1   Excludes 2   Includes   Use additional   Code first   Code also   Unspecified

1376   OGCR Official Guidelines   ● Unacceptable Principal Diagnosis   X Assign placeholder X   ● Use Additional Character(s)   ▶ Manifestation Code   **Coding Clinic**

● **S80.25**   **Superficial foreign body of knee**
Splinter in the knee
  - ● **S80.251**   **Superficial foreign body, right knee**
  - ● **S80.252**   **Superficial foreign body, left knee**
  - ● **S80.259**   **Superficial foreign body, unspecified knee**

● **S80.26**   **Insect bite (nonvenomous) of knee**
  - ● **S80.261**   **Insect bite (nonvenomous), right knee**
  - ● **S80.262**   **Insect bite (nonvenomous), left knee**
  - ● **S80.269**   **Insect bite (nonvenomous), unspecified knee**

● **S80.27**   **Other superficial bite of knee**
> **Excludes1**   open bite of knee (S81.05-)
  - ● **S80.271**   **Other superficial bite of right knee**
  - ● **S80.272**   **Other superficial bite of left knee**
  - ● **S80.279**   **Other superficial bite of unspecified knee**

● **S80.8**   **Other superficial injuries of lower leg**
  - ● **S80.81**   **Abrasion of lower leg**
    - ● **S80.811**   **Abrasion, right lower leg**
    - ● **S80.812**   **Abrasion, left lower leg**
    - ● **S80.819**   **Abrasion, unspecified lower leg**
  - ● **S80.82**   **Blister (nonthermal) of lower leg**
    - ● **S80.821**   **Blister (nonthermal), right lower leg**
    - ● **S80.822**   **Blister (nonthermal), left lower leg**
    - ● **S80.829**   **Blister (nonthermal), unspecified lower leg**
  - ● **S80.84**   **External constriction of lower leg**
    - ● **S80.841**   **External constriction, right lower leg**
    - ● **S80.842**   **External constriction, left lower leg**
    - ● **S80.849**   **External constriction, unspecified lower leg**
  - ● **S80.85**   **Superficial foreign body of lower leg**
    Splinter in the lower leg
    - ● **S80.851**   **Superficial foreign body, right lower leg**
    - ● **S80.852**   **Superficial foreign body, left lower leg**
    - ● **S80.859**   **Superficial foreign body, unspecified lower leg**
  - ● **S80.86**   **Insect bite (nonvenomous) of lower leg**
    - ● **S80.861**   **Insect bite (nonvenomous), right lower leg**
    - ● **S80.862**   **Insect bite (nonvenomous), left lower leg**
    - ● **S80.869**   **Insect bite (nonvenomous), unspecified lower leg**
  - ● **S80.87**   **Other superficial bite of lower leg**
    > **Excludes1**   open bite of lower leg (S81.85-)
    - ● **S80.871**   **Other superficial bite, right lower leg**
    - ● **S80.872**   **Other superficial bite, left lower leg**
    - ● **S80.879**   **Other superficial bite, unspecified lower leg**

● **S80.9**   **Unspecified superficial injury of knee and lower leg**
  - ● **S80.91**   **Unspecified superficial injury of knee**
    - ● **S80.911**   **Unspecified superficial injury of right knee**
    - ● **S80.912**   **Unspecified superficial injury of left knee**
    - ● **S80.919**   **Unspecified superficial injury of unspecified knee**
  - ● **S80.92**   **Unspecified superficial injury of lower leg**
    - ● **S80.921**   **Unspecified superficial injury of right lower leg**
    - ● **S80.922**   **Unspecified superficial injury of left lower leg**
    - ● **S80.929**   **Unspecified superficial injury of unspecified lower leg**

● **S81**   **Open wound of knee and lower leg**
Code also any associated wound infection
> **Excludes1**   open fracture of knee and lower leg (S82.-)
> traumatic amputation of lower leg (S88.-)

> **Excludes2**   open wound of ankle and foot (S91.-)

The appropriate 7th character is to be added to each code from category S81

A	initial encounter
D	subsequent encounter
S	sequela

● **S81.0**   **Open wound of knee**
  - ● **S81.00**   **Unspecified open wound of knee**
    - ● **S81.001**   **Unspecified open wound, right knee**
    - ● **S81.002**   **Unspecified open wound, left knee**
    - ● **S81.009**   **Unspecified open wound, unspecified knee**
  - ● **S81.01**   **Laceration without foreign body of knee**
    - ● **S81.011**   **Laceration without foreign body, right knee**
    - ● **S81.012**   **Laceration without foreign body, left knee**
    - ● **S81.019**   **Laceration without foreign body, unspecified knee**
  - ● **S81.02**   **Laceration with foreign body of knee**
    - ● **S81.021**   **Laceration with foreign body, right knee**
    - ● **S81.022**   **Laceration with foreign body, left knee**
    - ● **S81.029**   **Laceration with foreign body, unspecified knee**
  - ● **S81.03**   **Puncture wound without foreign body of knee**
    - ● **S81.031**   **Puncture wound without foreign body, right knee**
    - ● **S81.032**   **Puncture wound without foreign body, left knee**
    - ● **S81.039**   **Puncture wound without foreign body, unspecified knee**
  - ● **S81.04**   **Puncture wound with foreign body of knee**
    - ● **S81.041**   **Puncture wound with foreign body, right knee**
    - ● **S81.042**   **Puncture wound with foreign body, left knee**
    - ● **S81.049**   **Puncture wound with foreign body, unspecified knee**
  - ● **S81.05**   **Open bite of knee**
    Bite of knee NOS
    > **Excludes1**   superficial bite of knee (S80.27-)
    - ● **S81.051**   **Open bite, right knee**
    - ● **S81.052**   **Open bite, left knee**
    - ● **S81.059**   **Open bite, unspecified knee**

N   Newborn Age: 0   **P**   Pediatric Age: 0–17   **M**   Maternity DX: 12–55   **A**   Adult Age: 15–124   ♀ Females Only   ♂ Males Only

� Complication\Comorbidity   🌀 Major C\C   (Ex) CC/MCC Exclusions   🌀 Hospital-Acquired Condition

CHAPTER 19 (S00-T88)

1377

● **S81.8**   **Open wound of lower leg**
  ● **S81.80**   **Unspecified open wound of lower leg**
    ● **S81.801**   `Unspecified` **open wound, right lower leg**
    ● **S81.802**   `Unspecified` **open wound, left lower leg**
    ● **S81.809**   `Unspecified` **open wound, unspecified lower leg**
  ● **S81.81**   **Laceration without foreign body of lower leg**
    ● **S81.811**   **Laceration without foreign body, right lower leg**
    ● **S81.812**   **Laceration without foreign body, left lower leg**
    ● **S81.819**   **Laceration without foreign body, `unspecified` lower leg**
  ● **S81.82**   **Laceration with foreign body of lower leg**
    ● **S81.821**   **Laceration with foreign body, right lower leg**
    ● **S81.822**   **Laceration with foreign body, left lower leg**
    ● **S81.829**   **Laceration with foreign body, `unspecified` lower leg**
  ● **S81.83**   **Puncture wound without foreign body of lower leg**
    ● **S81.831**   **Puncture wound without foreign body, right lower leg**
    ● **S81.832**   **Puncture wound without foreign body, left lower leg**
    ● **S81.839**   **Puncture wound without foreign body, `unspecified` lower leg**
  ● **S81.84**   **Puncture wound with foreign body of lower leg**
    ● **S81.841**   **Puncture wound with foreign body, right lower leg**
    ● **S81.842**   **Puncture wound with foreign body, left lower leg**
    ● **S81.849**   **Puncture wound with foreign body, `unspecified` lower leg**
  ● **S81.85**   **Open bite of lower leg**
    Bite of lower leg NOS
    `Excludes1`   superficial bite of lower leg (S80.86-, S80.87-)
    ● **S81.851**   **Open bite, right lower leg**
    ● **S81.852**   **Open bite, left lower leg**
    ● **S81.859**   **Open bite, `unspecified` lower leg**

● **S82**   **Fracture of lower leg, including ankle**
  Note: A fracture not indicated as displaced or nondisplaced should be coded to displaced
    A fracture not indicated as open or closed should be coded to closed
    The open fracture designations are based on the Gustilo open fracture classification
  `Includes`   fracture of malleolus
  `Excludes1`   traumatic amputation of lower leg (S88.-)
  `Excludes2`   fracture of foot, except ankle (S92.-)
    periprosthetic fracture of prosthetic implant of knee (T84.042, T84.043)

The appropriate 7th character is to be added to all codes from category S82

A	initial encounter for closed fracture
B	initial encounter for open fracture type I or II initial encounter for open fracture NOS
C	initial encounter for open fracture type IIIA, IIIB, or IIIC
D	subsequent encounter for closed fracture with routine healing
E	subsequent encounter for open fracture type I or II with routine healing
F	subsequent encounter for open fracture type IIIA, IIIB, or IIIC with routine healing
G	subsequent encounter for closed fracture with delayed healing
H	subsequent encounter for open fracture type I or II with delayed healing
J	subsequent encounter for open fracture type IIIA, IIIB, or IIIC with delayed healing
K	subsequent encounter for closed fracture with nonunion
M	subsequent encounter for open fracture type I or II with nonunion
N	subsequent encounter for open fracture type IIIA, IIIB, or IIIC with nonunion
P	subsequent encounter for closed fracture with malunion
Q	subsequent encounter for open fracture type I or II with malunion
R	subsequent encounter for open fracture type IIIA, IIIB, or IIIC with malunion
S	sequela

● **S82.0**   **Fracture of patella**
  Knee cap
  ● **S82.00**   **Unspecified fracture of patella**
    ● **S82.001**   `Unspecified` **fracture of right patella**
      A, B, C,K,M, N, P, Q, R ⊘, A, B, C ⊘
      Ⓔₓ For **S82.001[A]:** S82.001-S82.099[A,B,C]
      For **S82.001[B,C]:** M80.00X-M80.019[A],
      M80.041-M80.049[A], M80.80X-M80.819[A],
      M80.841-M80.849[A], M84.40X-M84.419[A],
      M84.441-M84.446[A], M84.454[A],
      M84.474-M84.519[A], M84.541-M84.550[A],
      M84.574-M84.576[A], M84.60X-M84.619[A],
      M84.641-M84.650[A], M84.674-M84.68X[A],
      S03.8XX-S03.9XX[A], S29.011-S29.019[A],
      S38.3XX[A], S39.011-S39.013[A],
      S73.101-S73.199[A], S76.001-S76.019[A],
      S76.091-S76.119[A], S76.191-S76.219[A],
      S76.291-S76.319[A], S76.391-S76.819[A],
      S76.891-S76.919[A], S76.991-S76.999[A],
      S79.811-S79.929[A], S82.001-S82.099[B,C],
      S82.101-S82.156[A,B,C], S82.191-S82.299[A,B,C],
      S82.401-S82.499[A,B,C], S82.831-S82.839[A,B,C],
      S82.861-S82.866[A,B,C], S82.90X-S82.92X[A,B,C],
      S89.001-S89.099[A], S89.201-S89.299[A],
      T14.90-T14.91, T79.8XX-T79.9XX[A], T79.A9X[A]
      For **S82.001[K,M,N,P,Q,R]:** See S02.0[K]

◀ New   ◀⁓ Revised   ~~deleted~~ Deleted   `Excludes 1`   `Excludes 2`   `Includes`   `Use additional`   `Code first`   `Code also`   `Unspecified`

1378   `OGCR` Official Guidelines   ● Unacceptable Principal Diagnosis   X Assign placeholder X   ● Use Additional Character(s)   ▌ Manifestation Code   **Coding Clinic**

● **S82.002** <mark>Unspecified</mark> **fracture of left patella**
A, B, C,K,M, N, P, Q, R 🦠, A, B, C 🦠
    (Ex:) For S82.002[A]: S82.001[B,C],
      S82.002-S82.009[A,B,C], S82.011[B,C],
      S82.012-S82.013[A,B,C], S82.014-S82.021[B,C],
      S82.022-S82.023[A,B,C], S82.024[B,C],
      S82.025-S82.026[A,B,C], S82.031-S82.033[A,B,C],
      S82.034[B,C], S82.035-S82.036[A,B,C],
      S82.041[B,C], S82.042-S82.043[A,B,C],
      S82.044[B,C], S82.045-S82.046[A,B,C],
      S82.091[B,C], S82.092-S82.099[A,B,C]
    For S82.002[B,C]: See S82.001[B,C]
    For S82.002[K,M,N,P,Q,R]: See S02.0[K]

● **S82.009** <mark>Unspecified</mark> **fracture of unspecified patella** A, B, C,K,M, N, P, Q, R 🦠, A, B, C 🦠
    (Ex:) For S82.009[A]: S82.001-S82.099[A,B,C]
    For S82.009[B,C]: See S82.001[B,C]
    For S82.009[K,M,N,P,Q,R]: See S02.0[K]

● **S82.01**   **Osteochondral fracture of patella**

● **S82.011** **Displaced osteochondral fracture of right patella**
A, B, C,K,M, N, P, Q, R 🦠, A, B, C 🦠
    (Ex:) For S82.011[A]: See S82.001[A]
    For S82.011[B,C]: See S82.001[B,C]
    For S82.011[K,M,N,P,Q,R]: See S02.0[K]

● **S82.012** **Displaced osteochondral fracture of left patella** A, B, C,K,M, N, P, Q, R 🦠, A, B, C 🦠
    (Ex:) For S82.012[A]: See S82.002[A]
    For S82.012[B,C]: See S82.001[B,C]
    For S82.012[K,M,N,P,Q,R]: See S02.0[K]

● **S82.013** **Displaced osteochondral fracture of** <mark>unspecified</mark> **patella**
A, B, C,K,M, N, P, Q, R 🦠, A, B, C 🦠
    (Ex:) For S82.013[A]: See S82.003
    For S82.013[B,C]: See S82.001[B,C]
    For S82.013[K,M,N,P,Q,R]: See S02.0[K]

● **S82.014** **Nondisplaced osteochondral fracture of right patella** A, B, C,K,M, N, P, Q, R 🦠, A, B, C 🦠
    (Ex:) For S82.014[A]: See S82.001[A]
    For S82.014[B,C]: See S82.001[B,C]
    For S82.014[K,M,N,P,Q,R]: See S02.0[K]

● **S82.015** **Nondisplaced osteochondral fracture of left patella** A, B, C,K,M, N, P, Q, R 🦠, A, B, C 🦠
    (Ex:) For S82.015[A]: See S82.002[A]
    For S82.015[B,C]: See S82.001[B,C]
    For S82.015[K,M,N,P,Q,R]: See S02.0[K]

● **S82.016** **Nondisplaced osteochondral fracture of** <mark>unspecified</mark> **patella** A, B, C,K,M, N, P, Q, R 🦠, A, B, C 🦠
    (Ex:) For S82.016[A]: S82.001-S82.099[A,B,C]
    For S82.016[B,C]: See S82.001[B,C]
    For S82.016[K,M,N,P,Q,R]: See S02.0[K]

● **S82.02**   **Longitudinal fracture of patella**

● **S82.021** **Displaced longitudinal fracture of right patella** A, B, C,K,M, N, P, Q, R 🦠, A, B, C 🦠
    (Ex:) For S82.021[A]: See S82.001[A]
    For S82.021[B,C]: See S82.001[B,C]
    For S82.021[K,M,N,P,Q,R]: See S02.0[K]

● **S82.022** **Displaced longitudinal fracture of left patella** A, B, C,K,M, N, P, Q, R 🦠, A, B, C 🦠
    (Ex:) For S82.022[A]: See S82.002[A]
    For S82.022[B,C]: See S82.001[B,C]
    For S82.022[K,M,N,P,Q,R]: See S02.0[K]

● **S82.023** **Displaced longitudinal fracture of** <mark>unspecified</mark> **patella** A, B, C,K,M, N, P, Q, R 🦠, A, B, C 🦠
    (Ex:) For S82.023[A]: S82.001-S82.099[A,B,C]
    For S82.023[B,C]: See S82.001[B,C]
    For S82.023[K,M,N,P,Q,R]: See S02.0[K]

● **S82.024** **Nondisplaced longitudinal fracture of right patella** A, B, C,K,M, N, P, Q, R 🦠, A, B, C 🦠
    (Ex:) For S82.024[A]: See S82.001[A]
    For S82.024[B,C]: See S82.001[B,C]
    For S82.024[K,M,N,P,Q,R]: See S02.0[K]

● **S82.025** **Nondisplaced longitudinal fracture of left patella** A, B, C,K,M, N, P, Q, R 🦠, A, B, C 🦠
    (Ex:) For S82.025[A]: See S82.002[A]
    For S82.025[B,C]: See S82.001[B,C]
    For S82.025[K,M,N,P,Q,R]: See S02.0[K]

● **S82.026** **Nondisplaced longitudinal fracture of** <mark>unspecified</mark> **patella** A, B, C,K,M, N, P, Q, R 🦠, A, B, C 🦠
    (Ex:) For S82.026[A]: S82.001-S82.099[A,B,C]
    For S82.026[B,C]: See S82.001[B,C]
    For S82.026[K,M,N,P,Q,R]: See S02.0[K]

● **S82.03**   **Transverse fracture of patella**

● **S82.031** **Displaced transverse fracture of right patella** A, B, C,K,M, N, P, Q, R 🦠, A, B, C 🦠
    (Ex:) For S82.031[A]: See S82.001[A]
    For S82.031[B,C]: See S82.001[B,C]
    For S82.031[K,M,N,P,Q,R]: See S02.0[K]

● **S82.032** **Displaced transverse fracture of left patella** A, B, C,K,M, N, P, Q, R 🦠, A, B, C 🦠
    (Ex:) For S82.032[A]: See S82.002[A]
    For S82.032[B,C]: See S82.001[B,C]
    For S82.032[K,M,N,P,Q,R]: See S02.0[K]

● **S82.033** **Displaced transverse fracture of** <mark>unspecified</mark> **patella** A, B, C,K,M, N, P, Q, R 🦠, A, B, C 🦠
    (Ex:) For S82.033[A]: S82.001-S82.099[A,B,C]
    For S82.033[B,C]: See S82.001[B,C]
    For S82.033[K,M,N,P,Q,R]: See S02.0[K]

● **S82.034** **Nondisplaced transverse fracture of right patella** A, B, C,K,M, N, P, Q, R 🦠, A, B, C 🦠
    (Ex:) For S82.034[A]: See S82.001[A]
    For S82.034[B,C]: See S82.001[B,C]
    For S82.034[K,M,N,P,Q,R]: See S02.0[K]

● **S82.035** **Nondisplaced transverse fracture of left patella** A, B, C,K,M, N, P, Q, R 🦠, A, B, C 🦠
    (Ex:) For S82.035[A]: See S82.002[A]
    For S82.035[B,C]: See S82.001[B,C]
    For S82.035[K,M,N,P,Q,R]: See S02.0[K]

● **S82.036** **Nondisplaced transverse fracture of** <mark>unspecified</mark> **patella** A, B, C,K,M, N, P, Q, R 🦠, A, B, C 🦠
    (Ex:) For S82.036[A]: S82.001-S82.099[A,B,C]
    For S82.036[B,C]: See S82.001[B,C]
    For S82.036[K,M,N,P,Q,R]: See S02.0[K]

CHAPTER 19 (S00-T88)

N   Newborn Age: 0   P   Pediatric Age: 0–17   M   Maternity DX: 12–55   A   Adult Age: 15–124   ♀   Females Only   ♂   Males Only
🦠   Complication\Comorbidity   🦠   Major C\C   (Ex:)   CC/MCC Exclusions   🦠   Hospital-Acquired Condition

CHAPTER 19 (S00-T88)

● **S82.04   Comminuted fracture of patella**
     ● **S82.041   Displaced comminuted fracture of right patella** A, B, C,K,M, N, P, Q, R 🏷, A, B, C 🏷
         (Ex:) **For S82.041[A]:** See S82.001[A]
             For S82.041[B,C]: See S82.001[B,C]
             For S82.041[K,M,N,P,Q,R]: See S02.0[K]

     ● **S82.042   Displaced comminuted fracture of left patella** A, B, C,K,M, N, P, Q, R 🏷, A, B, C 🏷
         (Ex:) **For S82.042[A]:** See S82.002[A]
             For S82.042[B,C]: See S82.001[B,C]
             For S82.042[K,M,N,P,Q,R]: See S02.0[K]

     ● **S82.043   Displaced comminuted fracture of** unspecified **patella** A, B, C,K,M, N, P, Q, R 🏷, A, B, C 🏷
         (Ex:) **For S82.043[A]:** S82.001-S82.099[A,B,C]
             For S82.043[B,C]: See S82.001[B,C]
             For S82.043[K,M,N,P,Q,R]: See S02.0[K]

     ● **S82.044   Nondisplaced comminuted fracture of right patella** A, B, C,K,M, N, P, Q, R 🏷, A, B, C 🏷
         (Ex:) **For S82.044[A]:** See S82.001[A]
             For S82.044[B,C]: See S82.001[B,C]
             For S82.044[K,M,N,P,Q,R]: See S02.0[K]

     ● **S82.045   Nondisplaced comminuted fracture of left patella** A, B, C,K,M, N, P, Q, R 🏷, A, B, C 🏷
         (Ex:) **For S82.045[A]:** See S82.002[A]
             For S82.045[B,C]: See S82.001[B,C]
             For S82.045[K,M,N,P,Q,R]: See S02.0[K]

     ● **S82.046   Nondisplaced comminuted fracture of** unspecified **patella** A, B, C,K,M, N, P, Q, R 🏷, A, B, C 🏷
         (Ex:) **For S82.046[A]:** S82.001-S82.099[A,B,C]
             For S82.046[B,C]: See S82.001[B,C]
             For S82.046[K,M,N,P,Q,R]: See S02.0[K]

● **S82.09   Other fracture of patella**
     ● **S82.091   Other fracture of right patella** A, B, C,K,M, N, P, Q, R 🏷, A, B, C 🏷
         (Ex:) **For S82.091[A]:** See S82.001[A]
             For S82.091[B,C]: See S82.001[B,C]
             For S82.091[K,M,N,P,Q,R]: See S02.0[K]

     ● **S82.092   Other fracture of left patella** A, B, C,K,M, N, P, Q, R 🏷, A, B, C 🏷
         (Ex:) **For S82.092[A]:** See S82.002[A]
             For S82.092[B,C]: See S82.001[B,C]
             For S82.092[K,M,N,P,Q,R]: See S02.0[K]

     ● **S82.099   Other fracture of** unspecified **patella** A, B, C,K,M, N, P, Q, R 🏷, A, B, C 🏷
         (Ex:) **For S82.099[A]:** S82.001-S82.099[A,B,C]
             For S82.099[B,C]: See S82.001[B,C]
             For S82.099[K,M,N,P,Q,R]: See S02.0[K]

● **S82.1   Fracture of upper end of tibia**
     Fracture of proximal end of tibia
     Excludes2   fracture of shaft of tibia (S82.2-)
               physeal fracture of upper end of tibia (S89.0-)

● **S82.10   Unspecified fracture of upper end of tibia**
     ● **S82.101 ** Unspecified **fracture of upper end of right tibia** A, K, M, N, P, Q, R 🏷, B, C 🏷, A, B, C 🏷
         (Ex:) **For S82.101[A]:** M80.00X-M80.019[A], M80.041-M80.049[A], M80.061-M80.819[A], M80.841-M80.849[A], M80.861-M80.879[A], M84.40X-M84.419[A], M84.441-M84.446[A], M84.454[A], M84.461-M84.519[A], M84.541-M84.550[A], M84.561-M84.619[A], M84.641-M84.650[A], M84.661-M84.68X[A], S03.8XX-S03.9XX[A], S29.011-S29.019[A], S38.3XX[A], S39.011-S39.013[A], S73.101[A], S73.109-S73.111[A], S73.119-S73.121[A], S73.129-S73.191[A], S73.199[A], S76.001[A], S76.009-S76.011[A], S76.019[A], S76.091[A],

S76.099-S76.101[A], S76.109-S76.111[A], S76.119[A], S76.191[A], S76.199-S76.201[A], S76.209-S76.211[A], S76.219[A], S76.291[A], S76.299-S76.301[A], S76.309-S76.311[A], S76.319[A], S76.391[A], S76.399-S76.801[A], S76.809-S76.811[A], S76.819[A], S76.891[A], S76.899-S76.901[A], S76.909-S76.911[A], S76.919[A], S76.991[A], S76.999[A], S79.811[A], S79.819-S79.821[A], S79.829[A], S79.911[A], S79.919-S79.921[A], S79.929[A], S82.101[A,B,C], S82.102[B,C], S82.109-S82.111[A,B,C], S82.112[B,C], S82.113-S82.114[A,B,C], S82.115[B,C], S82.116-S82.121[A,B,C], S82.122[B,C], S82.123-S82.124[A,B,C], S82.125[B,C], S82.126-S82.131[A,B,C], S82.132[B,C], S82.133-S82.134[A,B,C], S82.135[B,C], S82.136-S82.141[A,B,C], S82.142[B,C], S82.143-S82.144[A,B,C], S82.145[B,C], S82.146-S82.151[A,B,C], S82.152[B,C], S82.153-S82.154[A,B,C], S82.155[B,C], S82.156[A,B,C], S82.191[A,B,C], S82.192[B,C], S82.199-S82.201[A,B,C], S82.202[B,C], S82.209-S82.221[A,B,C], S82.222[B,C], S82.223-S82.224[A,B,C], S82.225[B,C], S82.226-S82.231[A,B,C], S82.232[B,C], S82.233-S82.234[A,B,C], S82.235[B,C], S82.236-S82.241[A,B,C], S82.242[B,C], S82.243-S82.244[A,B,C], S82.245[B,C], S82.246-S82.251[A,B,C], S82.252[B,C], S82.253-S82.254[A,B,C], S82.255[B,C], S82.256-S82.261[A,B,C], S82.262[B,C], S82.263-S82.264[A,B,C], S82.265[B,C], S82.266-S82.291[A,B,C], S82.292[B,C], S82.299[A,B,C], S82.401[A,B,C], S82.402[B,C], S82.409-S82.421[A,B,C], S82.422[B,C], S82.423-S82.424[A,B,C], S82.425[B,C], S82.426-S82.431[A,B,C], S82.432[B,C], S82.433-S82.434[A,B,C], S82.435[B,C], S82.436-S82.441[A,B,C], S82.442[B,C], S82.443-S82.444[A,B,C], S82.445[B,C], S82.446-S82.451[A,B,C], S82.452[B,C], S82.453-S82.454[A,B,C], S82.455[B,C], S82.456-S82.461[A,B,C], S82.462[B,C], S82.463-S82.464[A,B,C], S82.465[B,C], S82.466-S82.491[A,B,C], S82.492[B,C], S82.499[A,B,C], S82.831[A,B,C], S82.831-S82.832[B,C], S82.839[A,B,C], S82.861[A,B,C], S82.862[B,C], S82.863-S82.864[A,B,C], S82.865[B,C], S82.866[A,B,C], S82.90X-S82.92X[A,B,C], S89.001[A], S89.009-S89.011[A], S89.019-S89.021[A], S89.029-S89.031[A], S89.039-S89.041[A], S89.049-S89.091[A], S89.099[A], S89.201[A], S89.209-S89.211[A], S89.219-S89.221[A], S89.229-S89.291[A], S89.299[A], T14.90-T14.91, T79.8XX-T79.9XX[A], T79.A9X[A] **For S82.101[B,C]:** M80.00X-M80.019[A], M80.041-M80.049[A], M80.061-M80.819[A], M80.841-M80.849[A], M80.861-M80.879[A], M84.40X-M84.419[A], M84.441-M84.446[A], M84.454[A], M84.461-M84.519[A], M84.541-M84.550[A], M84.561-M84.619[A], M84.641-M84.650[A], M84.661-M84.68X[A], S03.8XX-S03.9XX[A], S29.011-S29.019[A], S38.3XX[A], S39.011-S39.013[A], S73.101-S73.199[A], S76.001-S76.019[A], S76.091-S76.119[A], S76.191-S76.219[A], S76.291-S76.319[A], S76.391-S76.819[A], S76.891-S76.919[A], S76.991-S76.999[A], S79.811-S79.929[A], S82.101-S82.156[A,B,C], S82.191-S82.299[A,B,C], S82.401-S82.499[A,B,C], S82.831-S82.839[A,B,C], S82.861-S82.866[A,B,C], S82.90X-S82.92X[A,B,C], S89.001-S89.099[A], S89.201-S89.299[A], T14.90-T14.91, T79.8XX-T79.9XX[A], T79.A9X[A]
         For S82.101[K,M,N,P,Q,R]: See S02.0[K]

◀ New   ◀▥ Revised   ~~deleted~~ Deleted   Excludes 1   Excludes 2   Includes   Use additional   Code first   Code also   Unspecified

1380   OGCR Official Guidelines   ● Unacceptable Principal Diagnosis   X Assign placeholder X   ● Use Additional Character(s)   ▶ Manifestation Code   **Coding Clinic**

● S82.102　Unspecified fracture of upper end of left tibia A, K, M, N, P, Q, R ⬤, B, C ⬤, A, B, C ⬤

　　Ⓔⓧ For S82.102[A]: M80.00X-M80.019[A], M80.041-M80.049[A], M80.061-M80.819[A], M80.841-M80.849[A], M80.861-M80.879[A], M84.40X-M84.419[A], M84.441-M84.446[A], M84.454[A], M84.461-M84.519[A], M84.541-M84.550[A], M84.561-M84.619[A], M84.641-M84.650[A], M84.661-M84.68X[A], S03.8XX-S03.9XX[A], S29.011-S29.019[A], S38.3XX[A], S39.011-S39.013[A], S73.102-S73.109[A], S73.112-S73.119[A], S73.122-S73.129[A], S73.192-S73.199[A], S76.002-S76.009[A], S76.012-S76.019[A], S76.092-S76.099[A], S76.102-S76.109[A], S76.112-S76.119[A], S76.192-S76.199[A], S76.202-S76.209[A], S76.212-S76.219[A], S76.292-S76.299[A], S76.302-S76.309[A], S76.312-S76.319[A], S76.392-S76.399[A], S76.802-S76.809[A], S76.812-S76.819[A], S76.892-S76.899[A], S76.902-S76.909[A], S76.912-S76.919[A], S76.992-S76.999[A], S79.812-S79.819[A], S79.822-S79.829[A], S79.912-S79.919[A], S79.922-S79.929[A], S82.101[B,C], S82.102-S82.109[A,B,C], S82.111[B,C], S82.112-S82.113[A,B,C], S82.114[B,C], S82.115-S82.116[A,B,C], S82.121[B,C], S82.122-S82.123[A,B,C], S82.124[B,C], S82.125-S82.126[A,B,C], S82.131[B,C], S82.132-S82.133[A,B,C], S82.134[B,C], S82.135-S82.136[A,B,C], S82.141[B,C], S82.142-S82.143[A,B,C], S82.144[B,C], S82.145-S82.146[A,B,C], S82.151[B,C], S82.152-S82.153[A,B,C], S82.154[B,C], S82.155-S82.156[A,B,C], S82.191[B,C], S82.192-S82.199[A,B,C], S82.201[B,C], S82.202-S82.209[A,B,C], S82.221[B,C], S82.222-S82.223[A,B,C], S82.224[B,C], S82.225-S82.226[A,B,C], S82.231[B,C], S82.232-S82.233[A,B,C], S82.234[B,C], S82.235-S82.236[A,B,C], S82.241[B,C], S82.242-S82.243[A,B,C], S82.244[B,C], S82.245-S82.246[A,B,C], S82.251[B,C], S82.252-S82.253[A,B,C], S82.254[B,C], S82.255-S82.256[A,B,C], S82.261[B,C], S82.262-S82.263[A,B,C], S82.264[B,C], S82.265-S82.266[A,B,C], S82.291[B,C], S82.292-S82.299[A,B,C], S82.401[B,C], S82.402-S82.409[A,B,C], S82.421[B,C], S82.422-S82.423[A,B,C], S82.424[B,C], S82.425-S82.426[A,B,C], S82.431[B,C], S82.432-S82.433[A,B,C], S82.434[B,C], S82.435-S82.436[A,B,C], S82.441[B,C], S82.442-S82.443[A,B,C], S82.444[B,C], S82.445-S82.446[A,B,C], S82.451[B,C], S82.452-S82.453[A,B,C], S82.454[B,C], S82.455-S82.456[A,B,C], S82.461[B,C], S82.462-S82.463[A,B,C], S82.464[B,C], S82.465-S82.466[A,B,C], S82.491[B,C], S82.492-S82.499[A,B,C], S82.831[B,C], S82.832-S82.839[A,B,C], S82.861[B,C], S82.862-S82.863[A,B,C], S82.864[B,C], S82.865-S82.866[A,B,C], S82.90X-S82.92X[A,B,C], S89.002-S89.009[A], S89.012-S89.019[A], S89.022-S89.029[A], S89.032-S89.039[A], S89.042-S89.049[A], S89.092-S89.099[A], S89.202-S89.209[A], S89.212-S89.219[A], S89.222-S89.229[A], S89.292-S89.299[A], T14.90-T14.91, T79.8XX-T79.9XX[A], T79.A9X[A]

　　For S82.102[B,C]: See S82.101[B,C]
　　For S82.102[K,M,N,P,Q,R]: See S02.0[K]

● S82.109　Unspecified fracture of upper end of unspecified tibia A, K, M, N, P, Q, R ⬤, B, C ⬤, A, B, C ⬤

　　Ⓔⓧ For S82.109[A,B,C]: See S82.101[B,C]
　　For S82.109[K,M,N,P,Q,R]: See S02.0[K]

● S82.11　Fracture of tibial spine

● S82.111　Displaced fracture of right tibial spine A, K, M, N, P, Q, R ⬤, B, C ⬤, A, B, C ⬤

　　Ⓔⓧ For S82.111[A]: See S82.101[A]
　　For S82.111[B,C]: See S82.101[B,C]
　　For S82.111[K,M,N,P,Q,R]: See S02.0[K]

● S82.112　Displaced fracture of left tibial spine A, K, M, N, P, Q, R ⬤, B, C ⬤, A, B, C ⬤

　　Ⓔⓧ For S82.112[A]: See S82.102[A]
　　For S82.112[B,C]: See S82.101[B,C]
　　For S82.112[K,M,N,P,Q,R]: See S02.0[K]

● S82.113　Displaced fracture of unspecified tibial spine A, K, M, N, P, Q, R ⬤, B, C ⬤, A, B, C ⬤

　　Ⓔⓧ For S82.113 [A,B,C]: See S82.101[B,C]
　　For S82.113[K,M,N,P,Q,R]: See S02.0[K]

● S82.114　Nondisplaced fracture of right tibial spine A, K, M, N, P, Q, R ⬤, B, C ⬤, A, B, C ⬤

　　Ⓔⓧ For S82.114[A]: See S82.101[A]
　　For S82.114[B,C]: See S82.101[B,C]
　　For S82.114[K,M,N,P,Q,R]: See S02.0[K]

● S82.115　Nondisplaced fracture of left tibial spine A, K, M, N, P, Q, R ⬤, B, C ⬤, A, B, C ⬤

　　Ⓔⓧ For S82.115[A]: See S82.102[A]
　　For S82.115[B,C]: See S82.101[B,C]
　　For S82.115[K,M,N,P,Q,R]: See S02.0[K]

● S82.116　Nondisplaced fracture of unspecified tibial spine A, K, M, N, P, Q, R ⬤, B, C ⬤, A, B, C ⬤

　　Ⓔⓧ For S82.116[A,B,C]: See S82.101[B,C]
　　For S82.116[K,M,N,P,Q,R]: See S02.0[K]

● S82.12　Fracture of lateral condyle of tibia

● S82.121　Displaced fracture of lateral condyle of right tibia A, K, M, N, P, Q, R ⬤, B, C ⬤, A, B, C ⬤

　　Ⓔⓧ For S82.121[A]: See S82.101[A]
　　For S82.121[B,C]: See S82.101[B,C]
　　For S82.121[K,M,N,P,Q,R]: See S02.0[K]

● S82.122　Displaced fracture of lateral condyle of left tibia A, K, M, N, P, Q, R ⬤, B, C ⬤, A, B, C ⬤

　　Ⓔⓧ For S82.122[A]: See S82.102[A]
　　For S82.122[B,C]: See S82.101[B,C]
　　For S82.122[K,M,N,P,Q,R]: See S02.0[K]

● S82.123　Displaced fracture of lateral condyle of unspecified tibia A, K, M, N, P, Q, R ⬤, B, C ⬤, A, B, C ⬤

　　Ⓔⓧ For S82.123[A,B,C]: See S82.101[B,C]
　　For S82.123[K,M,N,P,Q,R]: See S02.0[K]

● S82.124　Nondisplaced fracture of lateral condyle of right tibia A, K, M, N, P, Q, R ⬤, B, C ⬤, A, B, C ⬤

　　Ⓔⓧ For S82.124[A]: See S82.101[A]
　　For S82.124[B,C]: See S82.101[B,C]
　　For S82.124[K,M,N,P,Q,R]: See S02.0[K]

● S82.125　Nondisplaced fracture of lateral condyle of left tibia A, K, M, N, P, Q, R ⬤, B, C ⬤, A, B, C ⬤

　　Ⓔⓧ For S82.125[A]: See S82.102[A]
　　For S82.125[B,C]: See S82.101[B,C]
　　For S82.125[K,M,N,P,Q,R]: See S02.0[K]

● S82.126　Nondisplaced fracture of lateral condyle of unspecified tibia A, K, M, N, P, Q, R ⬤, B, C ⬤, A, B, C ⬤

　　Ⓔⓧ For S82.126[A,B,C]: See S82.101[B,C]
　　For S82.126[K,M,N,P,Q,R]: See S02.0[K]

CHAPTER 19 (S00-T88)

● S82.13   Fracture of medial condyle of tibia
   ● S82.131   Displaced fracture of medial condyle
              of right tibia A, K, M, N, P, Q, R 🔊,
              B, C 🔊, A, B, C 🔊
              Ⓔⓧ For S82.131[A]: See S82.101[A]
                     For S82.131[B,C]: See S82.101[B,C]
                     For S82.131[K,M,N,P,Q,R]: See S02.0[K]
   ● S82.132   Displaced fracture of medial condyle
              of left tibia A, K, M, N, P, Q, R 🔊,
              B, C 🔊, A, B, C 🔊
              Ⓔⓧ For S82.132[A]: See S82.102[A]
                     For S82.132[B,C]: See S82.101[B,C]
                     For S82.132[K,M,N,P,Q,R]: See S02.0[K]
   ● S82.133   Displaced fracture of medial condyle
              of unspecified tibia A, K, M,
              N, P, Q, R 🔊, B, C 🔊, A, B, C 🔊
              Ⓔⓧ For S82.133[A,B,C]: See S82.101[B,C]
                     For S82.133[K,M,N,P,Q,R]: See S02.0[K]
   ● S82.134   Nondisplaced fracture of medial
              condyle of right tibia A, K, M,
              N, P, Q, R 🔊, B, C 🔊, A, B, C 🔊
              Ⓔⓧ For S82.134[A]: See S82.101[A]
                     For S82.134[B,C]: See S82.101[B,C]
                     For S82.134[K,M,N,P,Q,R]: See S02.0[K]
   ● S82.135   Nondisplaced fracture of medial
              condyle of left tibia A, K, M,
              N, P, Q, R 🔊, B, C 🔊, A, B, C 🔊
              Ⓔⓧ For S82.135[A]: See S82.102[A]
                     For S82.135[B,C]: See S82.101[B,C]
                     For S82.135[K,M,N,P,Q,R]: See S02.0[K]
   ● S82.136   Nondisplaced fracture of medial
              condyle of unspecified tibia A, K, M,
              N, P, Q, R 🔊, B, C 🔊, A, B, C 🔊
              Ⓔⓧ For S82.136[A,B,C]: See S82.101[B,C]
                     For S82.136[K,M,N,P,Q,R]: See S02.0[K]
● S82.14   Bicondylar fracture of tibia
           Fracture of tibial plateau NOS
   ● S82.141   Displaced bicondylar fracture of right
              tibia A, K, M, N, P, Q, R 🔊, B, C 🔊,
              A, B, C 🔊
              Ⓔⓧ For S82.141[A]: See S82.101[A]
                     For S82.141[B,C]: See S82.101[B,C]
                     For S82.141[K,M,N,P,Q,R]: See S02.0[K]
   ● S82.142   Displaced bicondylar fracture of left
              tibia A, K, M, N, P, Q, R 🔊, B, C 🔊,
              A, B, C 🔊
              Ⓔⓧ For S82.142[A]: See S82.102[A]
                     For S82.142[B,C]: See S82.101[B,C]
                     For S82.142[K,M,N,P,Q,R]: See S02.0[K]
   ● S82.143   Displaced bicondylar fracture of
              unspecified tibia A, K, M,
              N, P, Q, R 🔊, B, C 🔊, A, B, C 🔊
              Ⓔⓧ For S82.143[A,B,C]: See S82.101[B,C]
                     For S82.143[K,M,N,P,Q,R]: See S02.0[K]

   ● S82.144   Nondisplaced bicondylar fracture of
              right tibia A, K, M, N, P, Q, R 🔊,
              B, C 🔊, A, B, C 🔊
              Ⓔⓧ For S82.144[A]: See S82.101[A]
                     For S82.144[B,C]: See S82.101[B,C]
                     For S82.144[K,M,N,P,Q,R]: See S02.0[K]
   ● S82.145   Nondisplaced bicondylar fracture of
              left tibia A, K, M, N, P, Q, R 🔊,
              B, C 🔊, A, B, C 🔊
              Ⓔⓧ For S82.145[A]: See S82.102[A]
                     For S82.145[B,C]: See S82.101[B,C]
                     For S82.145[K,M,N,P,Q,R]: See S02.0[K]
   ● S82.146   Nondisplaced bicondylar fracture of
              unspecified tibia A, K, M,
              N, P, Q, R 🔊, B, C 🔊, A, B, C 🔊
              Ⓔⓧ For S82.146[A,B,C]: See S82.101[B,C]
                     For S82.146[K,M,N,P,Q,R]: See S02.0[K]
● S82.15   Fracture of tibial tuberosity
   ● S82.151   Displaced fracture of right tibial
              tuberosity A, K, M, N, P, Q, R 🔊,
              B, C 🔊, A, B, C 🔊
              Ⓔⓧ For S82.151[A]: See S82.101[A]
                     For S82.151[B,C]: See S82.101[B,C]
                     For S82.151[K,M,N,P,Q,R]: See S02.0[K]
   ● S82.152   Displaced fracture of left tibial
              tuberosity A, K, M, N, P, Q, R 🔊,
              B, C 🔊, A, B, C 🔊
              Ⓔⓧ For S82.152[A]: See S82.102[A]
                     For S82.152[B,C]: See S82.101[B,C]
                     For S82.152[K,M,N,P,Q,R]: See S02.0[K]
   ● S82.153   Displaced fracture of unspecified
              tibial tuberosity A, K, M,
              N, P, Q, R 🔊, B, C 🔊, A, B, C 🔊
              Ⓔⓧ For S82.153[A,B,C]: See S82.101[B,C]
                     For S82.153[K,M,N,P,Q,R]: See S02.0[K]
   ● S82.154   Nondisplaced fracture of right tibial
              tuberosity A, K, M, N, P, Q, R 🔊,
              B, C 🔊, A, B, C 🔊
              Ⓔⓧ For S82.154[A]: See S82.101[A]
                     For S82.154[B,C]: See S82.101[B,C]
                     For S82.154[K,M,N,P,Q,R]: See S02.0[K]
   ● S82.155   Nondisplaced fracture of left tibial
              tuberosity A, K, M, N, P, Q, R 🔊,
              B, C 🔊, A, B, C 🔊
              Ⓔⓧ For S82.155[A]: See S82.102[A]
                     For S82.155[B,C]: See S82.101[B,C]
                     For S82.155[K,M,N,P,Q,R]: See S02.0[K]
   ● S82.156   Nondisplaced fracture of unspecified
              tibial tuberosity A, K, M,
              N, P, Q, R 🔊, B, C 🔊, A, B, C 🔊
              Ⓔⓧ For S82.156[A,B,C]: See S82.101[B,C]
                     For S82.156[K,M,N,P,Q,R]: See S02.0[K]

CHAPTER 19 (S00-T88)

◀ New   ◀▥ Revised   deleted Deleted   Excludes 1   Excludes 2   Includes   Use additional   Code first   Code also   Unspecified
OGCR Official Guidelines   ● Unacceptable Principal Diagnosis   X Assign placeholder X   ● Use Additional Character(s)   ▶ Manifestation Code   Coding Clinic

● **S82.16**   **Torus fracture of upper end of tibia**

The appropriate 7th character is to be added to all codes in subcategory S82.16

A	initial encounter for closed fracture
D	subsequent encounter for fracture with routine healing
G	subsequent encounter for fracture with delayed healing
K	subsequent encounter for fracture with nonunion
P	subsequent encounter for fracture with malunion
S	sequela

● **S82.161**   **Torus fracture of upper end of right tibia** A, K, P 🞉, A 🞉

🄴🅇 **For S82.161[A]:** S82.101[A,B,C], S82.102[B,C], S82.109-S82.111[A,B,C], S82.112[A,B], S82.113-S82.114[A,B,C], S82.115[B,C], S82.116-S82.121[A,B,C], S82.122[B,C], S82.123-S82.124[A,B,C], S82.125[B,C], S82.126-S82.131[A,B,C], S82.132[B,C], S82.133-S82.134[A,B,C], S82.135[B,C], S82.136-S82.141[A,B,C], S82.142[B,C], S82.143-S82.144[A,B,C], S82.145[B,C], S82.146-S82.151[A,B,C], S82.152[B,C], S82.153-S82.154[A,B,C], S82.155[B,C], S82.156[A,B,C], S82.161[A], S82.169[A], S82.191[A,B,C], S82.192[B,C], S82.199-S82.201[A,B,C], S82.202[B,C], S82.209-S82.221[A,B,C], S82.222[B,C], S82.223-S82.224[A,B,C], S82.225[B,C], S82.226-S82.231[A,B,C], S82.232[B,C], S82.233-S82.234[A,B,C], S82.235[B,C], S82.236-S82.241[A,B,C], S82.242[B,C], S82.243-S82.244[A,B,C], S82.245[B,C], S82.246-S82.251[A,B,C], S82.252[B,C], S82.253-S82.254[A,B,C], S82.255[B,C], S82.256-S82.261[A,B,C], S82.262[B,C], S82.263-S82.264[A,B,C], S82.265[B,C], S82.266-S82.291[A,B,C], S82.292[B,C], S82.299[A,B,C], S82.311[A], S82.319[A], S82.401[A,B,C], S82.402[B,C], S82.409-S82.421[A,B,C], S82.422[B,C], S82.423-S82.424[A,B,C], S82.425[B,C], S82.426-S82.431[A,B,C], S82.432[B,C], S82.433-S82.434[A,B,C], S82.435[B,C], S82.436-S82.441[A,B,C], S82.442[B,C], S82.443-S82.444[A,B,C], S82.445[B,C], S82.446-S82.451[A,B,C], S82.452[B,C], S82.453-S82.454[A,B,C], S82.455[B,C], S82.456-S82.461[A,B,C], S82.462[B,C], S82.463-S82.464[A,B,C], S82.465[B,C], S82.466-S82.491[A,B,C], S82.492[B,C], S82.499[A,B,C], S82.811[A], S82.819-S82.821[A], S82.829[A], S82.831[A,B,C], S82.832[B,C], S82.839[A,B,C], S82.861[A,B,C], S82.862[B,C], S82.863-S82.864[A,B,C], S82.865[B,C], S82.866[A,B,C], S89.001[A], S89.009-S89.011[A], S89.019-S89.021[A], S89.029-S89.031[A], S89.039-S89.041[A], S89.049-S89.091[A], S89.099[A], S89.201[A], S89.209-S89.211[A], S89.219-S89.221[A], S89.229-S89.291[A], S89.299[A] **For S82.161[K,P]:** See S02.0[K]

● **S82.162**   **Torus fracture of upper end of left tibia** A, K, P 🞉, A 🞉

🄴🅇 **For S82.162[A]:** S82.101[B,C], S82.102-S82.109[A,B,C], S82.111[B,C], S82.112-S82.113[A,B,C], S82.114[B,C], S82.115-S82.116[A,B,C], S82.121[B,C], S82.122-S82.123[A,B,C], S82.124[B,C], S82.125-S82.126[A,B,C], S82.131[B,C], S82.132-S82.133[A,B,C], S82.134[B,C], S82.135-S82.136[A,B,C], S82.141[B,C], S82.142-S82.143[A,B,C], S82.144[B,C], S82.145-S82.146[A,B,C], S82.151[B,C], S82.152-S82.153[A,B,C], S82.154[B,C], S82.155-S82.156[A,B,C], S82.162-S82.169[A], S82.191[B,C], S82.192-S82.199[A,B,C], S82.201[B,C], S82.202-S82.209[A,B,C], S82.221[B,C], S82.222-S82.223[A,B,C], S82.224[B,C], S82.225-S82.226[A,B,C], S82.231[B,C], S82.232-S82.233[A,B,C], S82.234[B,C], S82.235-S82.236[A,B,C], S82.241[B,C], S82.242-S82.243[A,B,C], S82.244[B,C], S82.245-S82.246[A,B,C], S82.251[B,C], S82.252-S82.253[A,B,C], S82.254[B,C], S82.255-S82.256[A,B,C], S82.261[B,C], S82.262-S82.263[A,B,C], S82.264[B,C], S82.265-S82.266[A,B,C], S82.291[B,C], S82.292-S82.299[A,B,C], S82.312-S82.319[A], S82.401[B,C], S82.402-S82.409[A,B,C], S82.421[B,C], S82.422-S82.423[A,B,C], S82.424[B,C], S82.425-S82.426[A,B,C], S82.431[B,C], S82.432-S82.433[A,B,C], S82.434[B,C], S82.435-S82.436[A,B,C], S82.441[B,C], S82.442-S82.443[A,B,C], S82.444[B,C], S82.445-S82.446[A,B,C], S82.451[B,C], S82.452-S82.453[A,B,C], S82.454[B,C], S82.455-S82.456[A,B,C], S82.461[B,C], S82.462-S82.463[A,B,C], S82.464[B,C], S82.465-S82.466[A,B,C], S82.491[B,C], S82.492-S82.499[A,B,C], S82.812-S82.819[A], S82.822-S82.829[A], S82.831[B,C], S82.832-S82.839[A,B,C], S82.861[B,C], S82.862-S82.863[A,B,C], S82.864[B,C], S82.865-S82.866[A,B,C], S89.002-S89.009[A], S89.012-S89.019[A], S89.022-S89.029[A], S89.032-S89.039[A], S89.042-S89.049[A], S89.092-S89.099[A], S89.202-S89.209[A], S89.212-S89.219[A], S89.222-S89.229[A], S89.292-S89.299[A] **For S82.162[K,P]:** See S02.0[K]

● **S82.169**   **Torus fracture of upper end of unspecified tibia** A, K, P 🞉, A 🞉

🄴🅇 **For S82.169[A]:** S82.101-S82.156[A,B,C], S82.161-S82.169[A], S82.191-S82.299[A,B,C], S82.311-S82.319[A], S82.401-S82.499[A,B,C], S82.811-S82.829[A], S82.831-S82.839[A,B,C], S82.861-S82.866[A,B,C], S89.001-S89.099[A], S89.201-S89.299[A] **S82.169[K,P]:** See S02.0[K]

N Newborn Age: 0   **P** Pediatric Age: 0–17   **M** Maternity DX: 12–55   **A** Adult Age: 15–124   ♀ Females Only   ♂ Males Only

🞉 Complication\Comorbidity   🞉 Major C\C   🄴🅇 CC/MCC Exclusions   🞉 Hospital-Acquired Condition

● S82.19 Other fracture of upper end of tibia
   ● S82.191 Other fracture of upper end of right tibia A, K, M, N, P, Q, R 🪙, B, C 🪙, A, B, C 🪙
      Ⓔⓧ For S82.191[A]: See S82.101[A]
         For S82.191[B,C]: See S82.101[B,C]
         For S82.191[K,M,N,P,Q,R]: See S02.0[K]
   ● S82.192 Other fracture of upper end of left tibia A, K, M, N, P, Q, R 🪙, B, C 🪙, A, B, C 🪙
      Ⓔⓧ For S82.192[A]: See S82.102[A]
         For S82.192[B,C]: See S82.101[B,C]
         For S82.192[K,M,N,P,Q,R]: See S02.0[K]
   ● S82.199 Other fracture of upper end of unspecified tibia A, K, M, N, P, Q, R 🪙, B, C 🪙, A, B, C 🪙
      Ⓔⓧ For S82.199[A,B,C]: See S82.101[B,C]
         For S82.199[K,M,N,P,Q,R]: See S02.0[K]

● S82.2 Fracture of shaft of tibia
   ● S82.20 Unspecified fracture of shaft of tibia
      Fracture of tibia NOS
      ● S82.201 Unspecified fracture of shaft of right tibia A, K, M, N, P, Q, R 🪙, B, C 🪙, A, B, C 🪙
         Ⓔⓧ For S82.201[A]: M80.00X-M80.019[A], M80.041-M80.049[A], M80.061-M80.819[A], M80.841-M80.849[A], M80.861-M80.879[A], M84.40X-M84.419[A], M84.441-M84.446[A], M84.454[A], M84.461-M84.519[A], M84.541-M84.550[A], M84.561-M84.576[A], M84.60X-M84.619[A], M84.641-M84.650[A], M84.661-M84.68X[A], S03.8XX-S03.9XX[A], S29.011-S29.019[A], S38.3XX[A], S39.011-S39.013[A], S73.101[A], S73.109-S73.111[A], S73.119-S73.121[A], S73.129-S73.191[A], S73.199[A], S76.001[A], S76.009-S76.011[A], S76.019[A], S76.091[A], S76.099-S76.101[A], S76.109-S76.111[A], S76.119[A], S76.191[A], S76.199-S76.201[A], S76.209-S76.211[A], S76.219[A], S76.291[A], S76.299-S76.301[A], S76.309-S76.311[A], S76.319[A], S76.391[A], S76.399-S76.801[A], S76.809-S76.811[A], S76.819[A], S76.891[A], S76.899-S76.901[A], S76.909-S76.911[A], S76.919[A], S76.991[A], S76.999[A], S79.811[A], S79.819-S79.821[A], S79.829-S79.911[A], S79.919-S79.921[A], S79.929[A], S82.101[A,B,C], S82.102[B,C], S82.109-S82.111[A,B,C], S82.112[B,C], S82.113-S82.114[A,B,C], S82.115[B,C], S82.116-S82.121[A,B,C], S82.122[B,C], S82.123-S82.124[A,B,C], S82.125[B,C], S82.126-S82.131[A,B,C], S82.132[B,C], S82.133-S82.134[A,B,C], S82.135[B,C], S82.136-S82.141[A,B,C], S82.142[B,C], S82.143-S82.144[A,B,C], S82.145[B,C], S82.146-S82.151[A,B,C], S82.152[B,C], S82.153-S82.154[A,B,C], S82.155[B,C], S82.156[A,B,C], S82.161[A], S82.169[A], S82.191[A,B,C], S82.192[B,C], S82.199-S82.201[A,B,C], S82.202[B,C], S82.209-S82.221[A,B,C], S82.222[B,C], S82.223-S82.224[A,B,C], S82.225[B,C], S82.226-S82.231[A,B,C], S82.232[B,C], S82.233-S82.234[A,B,C], S82.235[B,C], S82.236-S82.241[A,B,C], S82.242[B,C], S82.243-S82.244[A,B,C], S82.245[B,C], S82.246-S82.251[A,B,C], S82.252[B,C], S82.253-S82.254[A,B,C], S82.255[B,C], S82.256-S82.261[A,B,C], S82.262[B,C], S82.263-S82.264[A,B,C], S82.265[B,C], S82.266-S82.291[A,B,C], S82.292[B,C], S82.299[A,B,C], S82.311[A], S82.319[A],

S82.401[A,B,C], S82.402[B,C], S82.409-S82.421[A,B,C], S82.422[B,C], S82.423-S82.424[A,B,C], S82.425[B,C], S82.426-S82.431[A,B,C], S82.432[B,C], S82.433-S82.434[A,B,C], S82.435[B,C], S82.436-S82.441[A,B,C], S82.442[B,C], S82.443-S82.444[A,B,C], S82.445[B,C], S82.446-S82.451[A,B,C], S82.452[B,C], S82.453-S82.454[A,B,C], S82.455[B,C], S82.456-S82.461[A,B,C], S82.462[B,C], S82.463-S82.464[A,B,C], S82.465[B,C], S82.466-S82.491[A,B,C], S82.492[B,C], S82.499[A,B,C], S82.811[A], S82.819-S82.821[A], S82.829[A], S82.831[A,B,C], S82.832[B,C], S82.839[A,B,C], S82.861[A,B,C], S82.862[B,C], S82.863-S82.864[A,B,C], S82.865[B,C], S82.866[A,B,C], S82.90X-S82.92X[A,B,C], S89.001[A], S89.009-S89.011[A], S89.019-S89.021[A], S89.029-S89.031[A], S89.039-S89.041[A], S89.049-S89.091[A], S89.099[A], S89.201[A], S89.209[A], S89.211-S89.219[A], S89.221-S89.229[A], S89.291-S89.299[A], T14.90-T14.91, T79.A9X-T79.9XX[A] For S82.201[B,C]: See S82.101[B,C] For S82.201[K,M,N,P,Q,R]: See S02.0[K]
      ● S82.202 Unspecified fracture of shaft of left tibia A, K, M, N, P, Q, R 🪙, B, C 🪙, A, B, C 🪙
         Ⓔⓧ For S82.202[A]: See S82.102[A]
            For S82.202[B,C]: See S82.101[B,C]
            For S82.202[K,M,N,P,Q,R]: See S02.0[K]
      ● S82.209 Unspecified fracture of shaft of unspecified tibia A, K, M, N, P, Q, R 🪙, B, C 🪙, A, B, C 🪙
         Ⓔⓧ For S82.209[A,B,C]: See S82.101[B,C]
            For S82.209[K,M,N,P,Q,R]: See S02.0[K]

   ● S82.22 Transverse fracture of shaft of tibia
      ● S82.221 Displaced transverse fracture of shaft of right tibia A, K, M, N, P, Q, R 🪙, B, C 🪙, A, B, C 🪙
         Ⓔⓧ For S82.221[A]: See S82.101[A]
            For S82.221[B,C]: See S82.101[B,C]
            For S82.221[K,M,N,P,Q,R]: See S02.0[K]
      ● S82.222 Displaced transverse fracture of shaft of left tibia A, K, M, N, P, Q, R 🪙, B, C 🪙, A, B, C 🪙
         Ⓔⓧ For S82.222[A]: See S82.102[A]
            For S82.222[B,C]: See S82.101[B,C]
            For S82.222[K,M,N,P,Q,R]: See S02.0[K]
      ● S82.223 Displaced transverse fracture of shaft of unspecified tibia A, K, M, N, P, Q, R 🪙, B, C 🪙, A, B, C 🪙
         Ⓔⓧ For S82.223[A,B,C]: See S82.101[B,C]
            For S82.223[K,M,N,P,Q,R]: See S02.0[K]
      ● S82.224 Nondisplaced transverse fracture of shaft of right tibia A, K, M, N, P, Q, R 🪙, B, C 🪙, A, B, C 🪙
         Ⓔⓧ For S82.224[A]: See S82.101[A]
            For S82.224[B,C]: See S82.101[B,C]
            For S82.224[K,M,N,P,Q,R]: See S02.0[K]
      ● S82.225 Nondisplaced transverse fracture of shaft of left tibia A, K, M, N, P, Q, R 🪙, B, C 🪙, A, B, C 🪙
         Ⓔⓧ For S82.225[A]: See S82.102[A]
            For S82.225[B,C]: See S82.101[B,C]
            For S82.225[K,M,N,P,Q,R]: See S02.0[K]
      ● S82.226 Nondisplaced transverse fracture of shaft of unspecified tibia A, K, M, N, P, Q, R 🪙, B, C 🪙, A, B, C 🪙
         Ⓔⓧ For S82.226[A,B,C]: See S82.101[B,C]
            For S82.226[K,M,N,P,Q,R]: See S02.0[K]

◀ New   ◀≡ Revised   d̶e̶l̶e̶t̶e̶d̶ Deleted   Excludes 1   Excludes 2   Includes   Use additional   Code first   Code also   Unspecified
OGCR Official Guidelines   ● Unacceptable Principal Diagnosis   X Assign placeholder X   ● Use Additional Character(s)   ▶ Manifestation Code   Coding Clinic

● S82.23   **Oblique fracture of shaft of tibia**

   ● S82.231   **Displaced oblique fracture of shaft of right tibia** A, K, M, N, P, Q, R , B, C , A, B, C
      (Ex:) **For S82.231[A]:** See S82.101[A]
        For S82.231[B,C]: See S82.101[B,C]
        For S82.231[K,M,N,P,Q,R]: See S02.0[K]

   ● S82.232   **Displaced oblique fracture of shaft of left tibia** A, K, M, N, P, Q, R , B, C , A, B, C
      (Ex:) **For S82.232[A]:** See S82.102[A]
        For S82.232[B,C]: See S82.101[B,C]
        For S82.232[K,M,N,P,Q,R]: See S02.0[K]

   ● S82.233   **Displaced oblique fracture of shaft of unspecified tibia** A, K, M, N, P, Q, R , B, C , A, B, C
      (Ex:) **For S82.233[A,B,C]:** See S82.101[B,C]
        For S82.233[K,M,N,P,Q,R]: See S02.0[K]

   ● S82.234   **Nondisplaced oblique fracture of shaft of right tibia** A, K, M, N, P, Q, R , B, C , A, B, C
      (Ex:) **For S82.234[A]:** See S82.101[A]
        For S82.234[B,C]: See S82.101[B,C]
        For S82.234[K,M,N,P,Q,R]: See S02.0[K]

      Coding Clinic: 2015, Q1, P9-10

   ● S82.235   **Nondisplaced oblique fracture of shaft of left tibia** A, K, M, N, P, Q, R , B, C , A, B, C
      (Ex:) **For S82.235[A]:** See S82.102[A]
        For S82.235[B,C]: See S82.101[B,C]
        For S82.235[K,M,N,P,Q,R]: See S02.0[K]

   ● S82.236   **Nondisplaced oblique fracture of shaft of unspecified tibia** A, K, M, N, P, Q, R , B, C , A, B, C
      (Ex:) **For S82.236[A,B,C]:** See S82.101[B,C]
        For S82.236[K,M,N,P,Q,R]: See S02.0[K]

● S82.24   **Spiral fracture of shaft of tibia**
      Toddler fracture

   ● S82.241   **Displaced spiral fracture of shaft of right tibia** A, K, M, N, P, Q, R , B, C , A, B, C
      (Ex:) **For S82.241[A]:** See S82.101[A]
        For S82.241[B,C]: See S82.101[B,C]
        For S82.241[K,M,N,P,Q,R]: See S02.0[K]

   ● S82.242   **Displaced spiral fracture of shaft of left tibia** A, K, M, N, P, Q, R , B, C , A, B, C
      (Ex:) **For S82.242[A]:** See S82.102[A]
        For S82.242[B,C]: See S82.101[B,C]
        For S82.242[K,M,N,P,Q,R]: See S02.0[K]

   ● S82.243   **Displaced spiral fracture of shaft of unspecified tibia** A, K, M, N, P, Q, R , B, C , A, B, C
      (Ex:) **For S82.243[A,B,C]:** See S82.101[B,C]
        For S82.243[K,M,N,P,Q,R]: See S02.0[K]

   ● S82.244   **Nondisplaced spiral fracture of shaft of right tibia** A, K, M, N, P, Q, R , B, C , A, B, C
      (Ex:) **For S82.244[A]:** See S82.101[A]
        For S82.244[B,C]: See S82.101[B,C]
        For S82.244[K,M,N,P,Q,R]: See S02.0[K]

   ● S82.245   **Nondisplaced spiral fracture of shaft of left tibia** A, K, M, N, P, Q, R , B, C , A, B, C
      (Ex:) **For S82.245[A]:** See S82.102[A]
        For S82.245[B,C]: See S82.101[B,C]
        For S82.245[K,M,N,P,Q,R]: See S02.0[K]

   ● S82.246   **Nondisplaced spiral fracture of shaft of unspecified tibia** A, K, M, N, P, Q, R , B, C , A, B, C
      (Ex:) **For S82.246[A,B,C]:** See S82.101[B,C]
        For S82.246[K,M,N,P,Q,R]: See S02.0[K]

● S82.25   **Comminuted fracture of shaft of tibia**

   ● S82.251   **Displaced comminuted fracture of shaft of right tibia** A, K, M, N, P, Q, R , B, C , A, B, C
      (Ex:) **For S82.251[A]:** See S82.101[A]
        For S82.251[B,C]: See S82.101[B,C]
        For S82.251[K,M,N,P,Q,R]: See S02.0[K]

      Coding Clinic: 2015, Q2, P6

   ● S82.252   **Displaced comminuted fracture of shaft of left tibia** A, K, M, N, P, Q, R , B, C , A, B, C
      (Ex:) **For S82.252[A]:** See S82.102[A]
        For S82.252[B,C]: See S82.101[B,C]
        For S82.252[K,M,N,P,Q,R]: See S02.0[K]

   ● S82.253   **Displaced comminuted fracture of shaft of unspecified tibia** A, K, M, N, P, Q, R , B, C , A, B, C
      (Ex:) **For S82.253[A,B,C]:** See S82.101[B,C]
        For S82.253[K,M,N,P,Q,R]: See S02.0[K]

   ● S82.254   **Nondisplaced comminuted fracture of shaft of right tibia** A, K, M, N, P, Q, R , B, C , A, B, C
      (Ex:) **For S82.254[A]:** See S82.101[A]
        For S82.254[B,C]: See S82.101[B,C]
        For S82.254[K,M,N,P,Q,R]: See S02.0[K]

   ● S82.255   **Nondisplaced comminuted fracture of shaft of left tibia** A, K, M, N, P, Q, R , B, C , A, B, C
      (Ex:) **For S82.255[A]:** See S82.102[A]
        For S82.255[B,C]: See S82.101[B,C]
        For S82.255[K,M,N,P,Q,R]: See S02.0[K]

   ● S82.256   **Nondisplaced comminuted fracture of shaft of unspecified tibia** A, K, M, N, P, Q, R , B, C , A, B, C
      (Ex:) **For S82.256[A,B,C]:** See S82.101[B,C]
        For S82.256[K,M,N,P,Q,R]: See S02.0[K]

● S82.26   **Segmental fracture of shaft of tibia**

   ● S82.261   **Displaced segmental fracture of shaft of right tibia** A, K, M, N, P, Q, R , B, C , A, B, C
      (Ex:) **For S82.261[A]:** See S82.101[A]
        For S82.261[B,C]: See S82.101[B,C]
        For S82.261[K,M,N,P,Q,R]: See S02.0[K]

   ● S82.262   **Displaced segmental fracture of shaft of left tibia** A, K, M, N, P, Q, R , B, C , A, B, C
      (Ex:) **For S82.262[A]:** See S82.102[A]
        For S82.262[B,C]: See S82.101[B,C]
        For S82.262[K,M,N,P,Q,R]: See S02.0[K]

   ● S82.263   **Displaced segmental fracture of shaft of unspecified tibia** A, K, M, N, P, Q, R , B, C , A, B, C
      (Ex:) **For S82.263[A,B,C]:** See S82.101[B,C]
        For S82.263[K,M,N,P,Q,R]: See S02.0[K]

   ● S82.264   **Nondisplaced segmental fracture of shaft of right tibia** A, K, M, N, P, Q, R , B, C , A, B, C
      (Ex:) **For S82.264[A]:** See S82.101[A]
        For S82.264[B,C]: See S82.101[B,C]
        For S82.264[K,M,N,P,Q,R]: See S02.0[K]

   ● S82.265   **Nondisplaced segmental fracture of shaft of left tibia** A, K, M, N, P, Q, R , B, C , A, B, C
      (Ex:) **For S82.265[A]:** See S82.102[A]
        For S82.265[B,C]: See S82.101[B,C]
        For S82.265[K,M,N,P,Q,R]: See S02.0[K]

   ● S82.266   **Nondisplaced segmental fracture of shaft of unspecified tibia** A, K, M, N, P, Q, R , B, C , A, B, C
      (Ex:) **For S82.266[A,B,C]:** See S82.101[B,C]
        For S82.266[K,M,N,P,Q,R]: See S02.0[K]

CHAPTER 19 (S00-T88)

N Newborn Age: 0   **P** Pediatric Age: 0–17   **M** Maternity DX: 12–55   **A** Adult Age: 15–124   ♀ Females Only   ♂ Males Only

 Complication\Comorbidity   Major C\C   (Ex:) CC/MCC Exclusions   Hospital-Acquired Condition

1385

● S82.29   Other fracture of shaft of tibia

  ● S82.291   Other fracture of shaft of right tibia A, K, M, N, P, Q, R 🝙, B, C 🝙, A, B, C 🝙
     Ⓔⓧ For S82.291[A]: See S82.101[A]
     For S82.291[B,C]: See S82.101[B,C]
     For S82.291[K,M,N,P,Q,R]: See S02.0[K]

  ● S82.292   Other fracture of shaft of left tibia A, K, M, N, P, Q, R 🝙, B, C 🝙, A, B, C 🝙
     Ⓔⓧ For S82.292[A]: See S82.102[A]
     For S82.292[B,C]: See S82.101[B,C]
     For S82.292[K,M,N,P,Q,R]: See S02.0[K]

  ● S82.299   Other fracture of shaft of unspecified tibia A, K, M, N, P, Q, R 🝙, B, C 🝙, A, B, C 🝙
     Ⓔⓧ For S82.299[A,B,C]: See S82.101[B,C]
     For S82.299[K,M,N,P,Q,R]: See S02.0[K]

● S82.3   Fracture of lower end of tibia

   Excludes1   bimalleolar fracture of lower leg (S82.84-)
       fracture of medial malleolus alone (S82.5-)
       Maisonneuve's fracture (S82.86-)
       pilon fracture of distal tibia (S82.87-)
       trimalleolar fractures of lower leg (S82.85-)

  ● S82.30   Unspecified fracture of lower end of tibia
     Ⓔⓧ For category S82.30 CC codes S82.30[B,C]:
     M80.00X-M80.019[A], M80.041-M80.049[A],
     M80.061-M80.819[A], M80.841-M80.849[A],
     M80.861-M80.879[A], M84.40X-M84.419[A],
     M84.441-M84.446[A], M84.454[A], M84.461-M84.519[A],
     M84.541-M84.550[A], M84.561-M84.576[A],
     M84.60X-M84.619[A], M84.641-M84.650[A],
     M84.661-M84.68X[A], S03.8XX-S03.9XX[A],
     S29.011-S29.019[A], S38.3XX[A], S39.011-S39.013[A],
     S73.101-S73.199[A], S76.001-S76.019[A],
     S76.091-S76.119[A], S76.191-S76.219[A],
     S76.291-S76.319[A], S76.391-S76.819[A],
     S76.891-S76.919[A], S76.991-S76.999[A],
     S79.811-S79.929[A], S82.301-S82.309[A,B,C],
     S82.391-S82.399[A,B,C], S82.51X-S82.56X[B,C],
     S82.61X-S82.66X[A,B,C], S82.841-S82.856[A,B,C],
     S82.871-S82.876[B,C], S82.891-S82.92X[A,B,C],
     S89.101-S89.199[A], S89.301-S89.399[A], T14.90-T14.91, T79.
     A9X-T79.9XX[A] For S82.30[K,M,N,P,Q,R]: See S02.0[K]

    ● S82.301   Unspecified fracture of lower end of right tibia B, C, K, M, N, P, Q, R 🝙, B, C 🝙

    ● S82.302   Unspecified fracture of lower end of left tibia B, C, K, M, N, P, Q, R 🝙, B, C 🝙

    ● S82.309   Unspecified fracture of lower end of unspecified tibia B, C, K, M, N, P, Q, R 🝙, B, C 🝙

  ● S82.31   Torus fracture of lower end of tibia
     The appropriate 7th character is to be added to all codes in subcategory S82.31

     | | |
     A   initial encounter for closed fracture
     D   subsequent encounter for fracture with routine healing
     G   subsequent encounter for fracture with delayed healing
     K   subsequent encounter for fracture with nonunion
     P   subsequent encounter for fracture with malunion
     S   sequela

    ● S82.311   Torus fracture of lower end of right tibia A, K, P 🝙, A 🝙
       Ⓔⓧ For S82.311[A]: See S82.161[A]
       For S82.311[K,P]: See S02.0[K]

    ● S82.312   Torus fracture of lower end of left tibia A, K, P 🝙, A 🝙
       Ⓔⓧ For S82.312[A]: See S82.162[A]
       For S82.312[K,P]: See S02.0[K]

    ● S82.319   Torus fracture of lower end of unspecified tibia A, K, P 🝙, A 🝙
       Ⓔⓧ For S82.319[A]: See S82.169[A]
       S82.319[K,P]: See S02.0[K]

  ● S82.39   Other fracture of lower end of tibia
     Ⓔⓧ For category S82.39 CC codes S82.39[B,C]:
     See S82.30[B,C] For S82.39[K,M,N,P,Q,R]: See S02.0[K]

    ● S82.391   Other fracture of lower end of right tibia B, C, K, M, N, P, Q, R 🝙, B, C 🝙

    ● S82.392   Other fracture of lower end of left tibia B, C, K, M, N, P, Q, R 🝙, B, C 🝙
       Coding Clinic: 2015, Q1, P25

    ● S82.399   Other fracture of lower end of unspecified tibia B, C, K, M, N, P, Q, R 🝙, B, C 🝙

● S82.4   Fracture of shaft of fibula

   Excludes2   fracture of lateral malleolus alone (S82.6-)
     Ⓔⓧ For category S82.4 CC codes S82.4[B,C]: See S82.101[B,C]
     For S82.4[K,M,N,P,Q,R]: See S02.0[K]

  ● S82.40   Unspecified fracture of shaft of fibula

    ● S82.401   Unspecified fracture of shaft of right fibula K, M, N, P, Q, R 🝙, B, C 🝙, B, C 🝙

    ● S82.402   Unspecified fracture of shaft of left fibula K, M, N, P, Q, R 🝙, B, C 🝙, B, C 🝙

    ● S82.409   Unspecified fracture of shaft of unspecified fibula K, M, N, P, Q, R 🝙, B, C 🝙, B, C 🝙

  ● S82.42   Transverse fracture of shaft of fibula

    ● S82.421   Displaced transverse fracture of shaft of right fibula K, M, N, P, Q, R 🝙, B, C 🝙, B, C 🝙

    ● S82.422   Displaced transverse fracture of shaft of left fibula K, M, N, P, Q, R 🝙, B, C 🝙, B, C 🝙

    ● S82.423   Displaced transverse fracture of shaft of unspecified fibula K, M, N, P, Q, R 🝙, B, C 🝙, B, C 🝙

    ● S82.424   Nondisplaced transverse fracture of shaft of right fibula K, M, N, P, Q, R 🝙, B, C 🝙, B, C 🝙

    ● S82.425   Nondisplaced transverse fracture of shaft of left fibula K, M, N, P, Q, R 🝙, B, C 🝙, B, C 🝙

    ● S82.426   Nondisplaced transverse fracture of shaft of unspecified fibula K, M, N, P, Q, R 🝙, B, C 🝙, B, C 🝙

  ● S82.43   Oblique fracture of shaft of fibula

    ● S82.431   Displaced oblique fracture of shaft of right fibula K, M, N, P, Q, R 🝙, B, C 🝙, B, C 🝙

    ● S82.432   Displaced oblique fracture of shaft of left fibula K, M, N, P, Q, R 🝙, B, C 🝙, B, C 🝙

    ● S82.433   Displaced oblique fracture of shaft of unspecified fibula K, M, N, P, Q, R 🝙, B, C 🝙, B, C 🝙

    ● S82.434   Nondisplaced oblique fracture of shaft of right fibula K, M, N, P, Q, R 🝙, B, C 🝙, B, C 🝙

    ● S82.435   Nondisplaced oblique fracture of shaft of left fibula K, M, N, P, Q, R 🝙, B, C 🝙, B, C 🝙

    ● S82.436   Nondisplaced oblique fracture of shaft of unspecified fibula K, M, N, P, Q, R 🝙, B, C 🝙, B, C 🝙

◀ New   ◀║ Revised   ~~deleted~~ Deleted   Excludes 1   Excludes 2   Includes   Use additional   Code first   Code also   Unspecified
OGCR Official Guidelines   ● Unacceptable Principal Diagnosis   X Assign placeholder X   ● Use Additional Character(s)   ▶ Manifestation Code   **Coding Clinic**

● **S82.44**   Spiral fracture of shaft of fibula

   ● **S82.441**   Displaced spiral fracture of shaft of right fibula K, M, N, P, Q, R 🝐, B, C 🝐, B, C 🝐

   ● **S82.442**   Displaced spiral fracture of shaft of left fibula K, M, N, P, Q, R 🝐, B, C 🝐, B, C 🝐

   ● **S82.443**   Displaced spiral fracture of shaft of unspecified fibula K, M, N, P, Q, R 🝐, B, C 🝐, B, C 🝐

   ● **S82.444**   Nondisplaced spiral fracture of shaft of right fibula K, M, N, P, Q, R 🝐, B, C 🝐, B, C 🝐

   ● **S82.445**   Nondisplaced spiral fracture of shaft of left fibula K, M, N, P, Q, R 🝐, B, C 🝐, B, C 🝐

   ● **S82.446**   Nondisplaced spiral fracture of shaft of unspecified fibula K, M, N, P, Q, R 🝐, B, C 🝐, B, C 🝐

● **S82.45**   Comminuted fracture of shaft of fibula

   ● **S82.451**   Displaced comminuted fracture of shaft of right fibula K, M, N, P, Q, R 🝐, B, C 🝐, B, C 🝐

   ● **S82.452**   Displaced comminuted fracture of shaft of left fibula K, M, N, P, Q, R 🝐, B, C 🝐, B, C 🝐

   ● **S82.453**   Displaced comminuted fracture of shaft of unspecified fibula K, M, N, P, Q, R 🝐, B, C 🝐, B, C 🝐

   ● **S82.454**   Nondisplaced comminuted fracture of shaft of right fibula K, M, N, P, Q, R 🝐, B, C 🝐, B, C 🝐

   ● **S82.455**   Nondisplaced comminuted fracture of shaft of left fibula K, M, N, P, Q, R 🝐, B, C 🝐, B, C 🝐

   ● **S82.456**   Nondisplaced comminuted fracture of shaft of unspecified fibula K, M, N, P, Q, R 🝐, B, C 🝐, B, C 🝐

● **S82.46**   Segmental fracture of shaft of fibula

   ● **S82.461**   Displaced segmental fracture of shaft of right fibula K, M, N, P, Q, R 🝐, B, C 🝐, B, C 🝐

   ● **S82.462**   Displaced segmental fracture of shaft of left fibula K, M, N, P, Q, R 🝐, B, C 🝐, B, C 🝐

   ● **S82.463**   Displaced segmental fracture of shaft of unspecified fibula K, M, N, P, Q, R 🝐, B, C 🝐, B, C 🝐

   ● **S82.464**   Nondisplaced segmental fracture of shaft of right fibula K, M, N, P, Q, R 🝐, B, C 🝐, B, C 🝐

   ● **S82.465**   Nondisplaced segmental fracture of shaft of left fibula K, M, N, P, Q, R 🝐, B, C 🝐, B, C 🝐

   ● **S82.466**   Nondisplaced segmental fracture of shaft of unspecified fibula K, M, N, P, Q, R 🝐, B, C 🝐, B, C 🝐

● **S82.49**   Other fracture of shaft of fibula

   ● **S82.491**   Other fracture of shaft of right fibula K, M, N, P, Q, R 🝐, B, C 🝐, B, C 🝐

   ● **S82.492**   Other fracture of shaft of left fibula K, M, N, P, Q, R 🝐, B, C 🝐, B, C 🝐

   ● **S82.499**   Other fracture of shaft of unspecified fibula K, M, N, P, Q, R 🝐, B, C 🝐, B, C 🝐

● **S82.5**   Fracture of medial malleolus

    Excludes1   pilon fracture of distal tibia (S82.87-)
        Salter-Harris type III of lower end of tibia (S89.13-)
        Salter-Harris type IV of lower end of tibia (S89.14-)

    (Ex:) For category S82.5 CC codes S82.5[B,C]: See S82.30[B,C]
       For S82.5[K,M,N,P,Q,R]: See S02.0[K]

    X ● **S82.51**   Displaced fracture of medial malleolus of right tibia B, C, K, M, N, P, Q, R 🝐, B, C 🝐

    X ● **S82.52**   Displaced fracture of medial malleolus of left tibia B, C, K, M, N, P, Q, R 🝐, B, C 🝐

    X ● **S82.53**   Displaced fracture of medial malleolus of unspecified tibia B, C, K, M, N, P, Q, R 🝐, B, C 🝐

    X ● **S82.54**   Nondisplaced fracture of medial malleolus of right tibia B, C, K, M, N, P, Q, R 🝐, B, C 🝐

    X ● **S82.55**   Nondisplaced fracture of medial malleolus of left tibia B, C, K, M, N, P, Q, R 🝐, B, C 🝐

    X ● **S82.56**   Nondisplaced fracture of medial malleolus of unspecified tibia B, C, K, M, N, P, Q, R 🝐, B, C 🝐

● **S82.6**   Fracture of lateral malleolus

    Excludes1   pilon fracture of distal tibia (S82.87-)

    (Ex:) For category S82.6 CC codes S82.6[B,C]: See S82.30[B,C]
       For S82.6[K,M,N,P,Q,R]: See S02.0[K]

    X ● **S82.61**   Displaced fracture of lateral malleolus of right fibula B, C, K, M, N, P, Q, R 🝐, B, C 🝐

    X ● **S82.62**   Displaced fracture of lateral malleolus of left fibula B, C, K, M, N, P, Q, R 🝐, B, C 🝐

    X ● **S82.63**   Displaced fracture of lateral malleolus of unspecified fibula B, C, K, M, N, P, Q, R 🝐, B, C 🝐

    X ● **S82.64**   Nondisplaced fracture of lateral malleolus of right fibula B, C, K, M, N, P, Q, R 🝐, B, C 🝐

    X ● **S82.65**   Nondisplaced fracture of lateral malleolus of left fibula B, C, K, M, N, P, Q, R 🝐, B, C 🝐

    X ● **S82.66**   Nondisplaced fracture of lateral malleolus of unspecified fibula B, C, K, M, N, P, Q, R 🝐, B, C 🝐

● **S82.8**   Other fractures of lower leg

   ● **S82.81**   Torus fracture of upper end of fibula

       The appropriate 7th character is to be added to all codes in subcategory S82.81

A	initial encounter for closed fracture
D	subsequent encounter for fracture with routine healing
G	subsequent encounter for fracture with delayed healing
K	subsequent encounter for fracture with nonunion
P	subsequent encounter for fracture with malunion
S	sequela

       (Ex:) For category S82.81 CC codes: See S02.0[K]

     ● **S82.811**   Torus fracture of upper end of right fibula K, P 🝐

     ● **S82.812**   Torus fracture of upper end of left fibula K, P 🝐

     ● **S82.819**   Torus fracture of upper end of unspecified fibula K, P 🝐

● **S82.82   Torus fracture of lower end of fibula**

The appropriate 7th character is to be added to all codes in subcategory S82.82

> A   initial encounter for closed fracture
> D   subsequent encounter for fracture with routine healing
> G   subsequent encounter for fracture with delayed healing
> K   subsequent encounter for fracture with nonunion
> P   subsequent encounter for fracture with malunion
> S   sequela

(Ex) For category S82.82 CC codes: See S02.0[K]

● **S82.821   Torus fracture of lower end of right fibula** K, P 🔗

● **S82.822   Torus fracture of lower end of left fibula** K, P 🔗

● **S82.829   Torus fracture of lower end of** unspecified **fibula** K, P 🔗

● **S82.83   Other fracture of upper and lower end of fibula**
(Ex) For category S82.83 CC codes S82.83[B,C]:
See S82.101[B,C] For S82.83[K,M,N,P,Q,R]: See S02.0[K]

● **S82.831   Other fracture of upper and lower end of right fibula** K, M, N, P, Q, R 🔗, B, C 🔗, B, C 🔗

● **S82.832   Other fracture of upper and lower end of left fibula** K, M, N, P, Q, R 🔗, B, C 🔗, B, C 🔗
Coding Clinic: 2015, Q1, P9-10

● **S82.839   Other fracture of upper and lower end of** unspecified **fibula** K, M, N, P, Q, R 🔗, B, C 🔗, B, C 🔗

● **S82.84   Bimalleolar fracture of lower leg**
(Ex) For category S82.84 CC codes S82.84[B,C]:
See S82.30[B,C] For S82.84[K,M,N,P,Q,R]: See S02.0[K]

● **S82.841   Displaced bimalleolar fracture of right lower leg** B, C, K, M, N, P, Q, R 🔗, B, C 🔗

● **S82.842   Displaced bimalleolar fracture of left lower leg** B, C, K, M, N, P, Q, R 🔗, B, C 🔗

● **S82.843   Displaced bimalleolar fracture of** unspecified **lower leg** B, C, K, M, N, P, Q, R 🔗, B, C 🔗

● **S82.844   Nondisplaced bimalleolar fracture of right lower leg** B, C, K, M, N, P, Q, R 🔗, B, C 🔗

● **S82.845   Nondisplaced bimalleolar fracture of left lower leg** B, C, K, M, N, P, Q, R 🔗, B, C 🔗

● **S82.846   Nondisplaced bimalleolar fracture of** unspecified **lower leg** B, C, K, M, N, P, Q, R 🔗, B, C 🔗

● **S82.85   Trimalleolar fracture of lower leg**
(Ex) For category S82.85 CC codes S82.85[B,C]:
See S82.30[B,C] For S82.85[K,M,N,P,Q,R]: See S02.0[K]

● **S82.851   Displaced trimalleolar fracture of right lower leg** B, C, K, M, N, P, Q, R 🔗, B, C 🔗

● **S82.852   Displaced trimalleolar fracture of left lower leg** B, C, K, M, N, P, Q, R 🔗, B, C 🔗

● **S82.853   Displaced trimalleolar fracture of** unspecified **lower leg** B, C, K, M, N, P, Q, R 🔗, B, C 🔗

● **S82.854   Nondisplaced trimalleolar fracture of right lower leg** B, C, K, M, N, P, Q, R 🔗, B, C 🔗

● **S82.855   Nondisplaced trimalleolar fracture of left lower leg** B, C, K, M, N, P, Q, R 🔗, B, C 🔗

● **S82.856   Nondisplaced trimalleolar fracture of** unspecified **lower leg** B, C, K, M, N, P, Q, R 🔗, B, C 🔗

● **S82.86   Maisonneuve's fracture**
(Ex) For category S82.86 CC codes S82.86[B,C]:
See S82.101[B,C] For S82.86[K,M,N,P,Q,R]: See S02.0[K]

● **S82.861   Displaced Maisonneuve's fracture of right leg** K, M, N, P, Q, R 🔗, B, C 🔗, B, C 🔗

● **S82.862   Displaced Maisonneuve's fracture of left leg** K, M, N, P, Q, R 🔗, B, C 🔗, B, C 🔗

● **S82.863   Displaced Maisonneuve's fracture of** unspecified **leg** K, M, N, P, Q, R 🔗, B, C 🔗, B, C 🔗

● **S82.864   Nondisplaced Maisonneuve's fracture of right leg** K, M, N, P, Q, R 🔗, B, C 🔗, B, C 🔗

● **S82.865   Nondisplaced Maisonneuve's fracture of left leg** K, M, N, P, Q, R 🔗, B, C 🔗, B, C 🔗

● **S82.866   Nondisplaced Maisonneuve's fracture of** unspecified **leg** K, M, N, P, Q, R 🔗, B, C 🔗, B, C 🔗

● **S82.87   Pilon fracture of tibia**
(Ex) For category S82.87 CC codes S82.87[B,C]:
See S82.30[B,C] For S82.87[K,M,N,P,Q,R]: See S02.0[K]

● **S82.871   Displaced pilon fracture of right tibia** B, C, K, M, N, P, Q, R 🔗, B, C 🔗

● **S82.872   Displaced pilon fracture of left tibia** B, C, K, M, N, P, Q, R 🔗, B, C 🔗

● **S82.873   Displaced pilon fracture of** unspecified **tibia** B, C, K, M, N, P, Q, R 🔗, B, C 🔗

● **S82.874   Nondisplaced pilon fracture of right tibia** B, C, K, M, N, P, Q, R 🔗, B, C 🔗

● **S82.875   Nondisplaced pilon fracture of left tibia** B, C, K, M, N, P, Q, R 🔗, B, C 🔗

● **S82.876   Nondisplaced pilon fracture of** unspecified **tibia** B, C, K, M, N, P, Q, R 🔗, B, C 🔗

● **S82.89   Other fractures of lower leg**
Fracture of ankle NOS
(Ex) For category S82.89 CC codes S82.89[B,C]: See S82.30[B,C] For S82.89[K,M,N,P,Q,R]: See S02.0[K]

● **S82.891   Other fracture of right lower leg** B, C, K, M, N, P, Q, R 🔗, B, C 🔗

● **S82.892   Other fracture of left lower leg** B, C, K, M, N, P, Q, R 🔗, B, C 🔗

● **S82.899   Other fracture of** unspecified **lower leg** B, C, K, M, N, P, Q, R 🔗, B, C 🔗

● **S82.9   Unspecified fracture of lower leg**
(Ex) For category S82.9 CC codes S82.9[B,C]: S72.001-S72.92X[A,B,C], S79.001-S79.199[A], S82.001-S82.156[A,B,C], S82.191-S82.309[A,B,C], S82.391-S82.66X[A,B,C], S82.831-S82.92X[A,B,C], S89.001-S89.399[A], S92.001-S92.599[A,B], S92.811-S92.919[A,B] For S82.9[K,M,N,P,Q,R]: See S02.0[K]

X ● **S82.90   Unspecified fracture of unspecified lower leg** A, K, M, N, P, Q, R 🔗, B, C 🔗

X ● **S82.91   Unspecified fracture of right lower leg** A, K, M, N, P, Q, R 🔗, B, C 🔗

X ● **S82.92   Unspecified fracture of left lower leg** A, K, M, N, P, Q, R 🔗, B, C 🔗

◀ New   ◀◀ Revised   ~~deleted~~ Deleted   Excludes 1   Excludes 2   Includes   Use additional   Code first   Code also   Unspecified
OGCR Official Guidelines   ● Unacceptable Principal Diagnosis   X Assign placeholder X   ● Use Additional Character(s)   🔗 Manifestation Code   **Coding Clinic**

● **S83**   **Dislocation and sprain of joints and ligaments of knee**

     Includes   avulsion of joint or ligament of knee
                 laceration of cartilage, joint or ligament of knee
                 sprain of cartilage, joint or ligament of knee
                 traumatic hemarthrosis of joint or ligament of
                     knee
                 traumatic rupture of joint or ligament of knee
                 traumatic subluxation of joint or ligament of knee
                 traumatic tear of joint or ligament of knee

     Code also any associated open wound

     Excludes1   derangement of patella (M22.0-M22.3)
                 injury of patellar ligament (tendon) (S76.1-)
                 internal derangement of knee (M23.-)
                 old dislocation of knee (M24.36)
                 pathological dislocation of knee (M24.36)
                 recurrent dislocation of knee (M22.0)

     Excludes2   strain of muscle, fascia and tendon of lower leg
                 (S86.-)

     The appropriate 7th character is to be added to each code from
     category S83

> A   initial encounter
> D   subsequent encounter
> S   sequela

● **S83.0**   **Subluxation and dislocation of patella**
   ● **S83.00**   **Unspecified subluxation and dislocation of patella**
     ● **S83.001**   Unspecified subluxation of right patella
     ● **S83.002**   Unspecified subluxation of left patella
     ● **S83.003**   Unspecified subluxation of unspecified patella
     ● **S83.004**   Unspecified dislocation of right patella
     ● **S83.005**   Unspecified dislocation of left patella
     ● **S83.006**   Unspecified dislocation of unspecified patella
   ● **S83.01**   **Lateral subluxation and dislocation of patella**
     ● **S83.011**   Lateral subluxation of right patella
     ● **S83.012**   Lateral subluxation of left patella
     ● **S83.013**   Lateral subluxation of unspecified patella
     ● **S83.014**   Lateral dislocation of right patella
     ● **S83.015**   Lateral dislocation of left patella
     ● **S83.016**   Lateral dislocation of unspecified patella
   ● **S83.09**   **Other subluxation and dislocation of patella**
     ● **S83.091**   Other subluxation of right patella
     ● **S83.092**   Other subluxation of left patella
     ● **S83.093**   Other subluxation of unspecified patella
     ● **S83.094**   Other dislocation of right patella
     ● **S83.095**   Other dislocation of left patella
     ● **S83.096**   Other dislocation of unspecified patella
● **S83.1**   **Subluxation and dislocation of knee**
     Excludes2   instability of knee prosthesis (T84.022, T84.023)
   ● **S83.10**   **Unspecified subluxation and dislocation of knee**
     ● **S83.101**   Unspecified subluxation of right knee
     ● **S83.102**   Unspecified subluxation of left knee
     ● **S83.103**   Unspecified subluxation of unspecified knee
     ● **S83.104**   Unspecified dislocation of right knee
     ● **S83.105**   Unspecified dislocation of left knee
     ● **S83.106**   Unspecified dislocation of unspecified knee

● **S83.11**   **Anterior subluxation and dislocation of proximal end of tibia**
     Posterior subluxation and dislocation of distal end of femur
   ● **S83.111**   Anterior subluxation of proximal end of tibia, right knee
   ● **S83.112**   Anterior subluxation of proximal end of tibia, left knee
   ● **S83.113**   Anterior subluxation of proximal end of tibia, unspecified knee
   ● **S83.114**   Anterior dislocation of proximal end of tibia, right knee
   ● **S83.115**   Anterior dislocation of proximal end of tibia, left knee
   ● **S83.116**   Anterior dislocation of proximal end of tibia, unspecified knee
● **S83.12**   **Posterior subluxation and dislocation of proximal end of tibia**
     Anterior dislocation of distal end of femur
   ● **S83.121**   Posterior subluxation of proximal end of tibia, right knee
   ● **S83.122**   Posterior subluxation of proximal end of tibia, left knee
   ● **S83.123**   Posterior subluxation of proximal end of tibia, unspecified knee
   ● **S83.124**   Posterior dislocation of proximal end of tibia, right knee
   ● **S83.125**   Posterior dislocation of proximal end of tibia, left knee
   ● **S83.126**   Posterior dislocation of proximal end of tibia, unspecified knee
● **S83.13**   **Medial subluxation and dislocation of proximal end of tibia**
   ● **S83.131**   Medial subluxation of proximal end of tibia, right knee
   ● **S83.132**   Medial subluxation of proximal end of tibia, left knee
   ● **S83.133**   Medial subluxation of proximal end of tibia, unspecified knee
   ● **S83.134**   Medial dislocation of proximal end of tibia, right knee
   ● **S83.135**   Medial dislocation of proximal end of tibia, left knee
   ● **S83.136**   Medial dislocation of proximal end of tibia, unspecified knee
● **S83.14**   **Lateral subluxation and dislocation of proximal end of tibia**
   ● **S83.141**   Lateral subluxation of proximal end of tibia, right knee
   ● **S83.142**   Lateral subluxation of proximal end of tibia, left knee
   ● **S83.143**   Lateral subluxation of proximal end of tibia, unspecified knee
   ● **S83.144**   Lateral dislocation of proximal end of tibia, right knee
   ● **S83.145**   Lateral dislocation of proximal end of tibia, left knee
   ● **S83.146**   Lateral dislocation of proximal end of tibia, unspecified knee
● **S83.19**   **Other subluxation and dislocation of knee**
   ● **S83.191**   Other subluxation of right knee
   ● **S83.192**   Other subluxation of left knee
   ● **S83.193**   Other subluxation of unspecified knee
   ● **S83.194**   Other dislocation of right knee
   ● **S83.195**   Other dislocation of left knee
   ● **S83.196**   Other dislocation of unspecified knee

N   Newborn Age: 0   **P**   Pediatric Age: 0–17   **M**   Maternity DX: 12–55   **A**   Adult Age: 15–124   ♀   Females Only   ♂   Males Only

🔖 Complication\Comorbidity   🔖 Major C\C   (Ex) CC/MCC Exclusions   🔖 Hospital-Acquired Condition   **1389**

● S83.2 Tear of meniscus, current injury
    Excludes1 old bucket-handle tear (M23.2)
● S83.20 Tear of unspecified meniscus, current injury
    Tear of meniscus of knee NOS
    ● S83.200 Bucket-handle tear of unspecified meniscus, current injury, right knee
    ● S83.201 Bucket-handle tear of unspecified meniscus, current injury, left knee
    ● S83.202 Bucket-handle tear of unspecified meniscus, current injury, unspecified knee
    ● S83.203 Other tear of unspecified meniscus, current injury, right knee
    ● S83.204 Other tear of unspecified meniscus, current injury, left knee
    ● S83.205 Other tear of unspecified meniscus, current injury, unspecified knee
    ● S83.206 Unspecified tear of unspecified meniscus, current injury, right knee
    ● S83.207 Unspecified tear of unspecified meniscus, current injury, left knee
    ● S83.209 Unspecified tear of unspecified meniscus, current injury, unspecified knee
● S83.21 Bucket-handle tear of medial meniscus, current injury
    ● S83.211 Bucket-handle tear of medial meniscus, current injury, right knee
    ● S83.212 Bucket-handle tear of medial meniscus, current injury, left knee
    ● S83.219 Bucket-handle tear of medial meniscus, current injury, unspecified knee
● S83.22 Peripheral tear of medial meniscus, current injury
    ● S83.221 Peripheral tear of medial meniscus, current injury, right knee
    ● S83.222 Peripheral tear of medial meniscus, current injury, left knee
    ● S83.229 Peripheral tear of medial meniscus, current injury, unspecified knee
● S83.23 Complex tear of medial meniscus, current injury
    ● S83.231 Complex tear of medial meniscus, current injury, right knee
    ● S83.232 Complex tear of medial meniscus, current injury, left knee
    ● S83.239 Complex tear of medial meniscus, current injury, unspecified knee
● S83.24 Other tear of medial meniscus, current injury
    ● S83.241 Other tear of medial meniscus, current injury, right knee
    ● S83.242 Other tear of medial meniscus, current injury, left knee
    ● S83.249 Other tear of medial meniscus, current injury, unspecified knee
● S83.25 Bucket-handle tear of lateral meniscus, current injury
    ● S83.251 Bucket-handle tear of lateral meniscus, current injury, right knee
    ● S83.252 Bucket-handle tear of lateral meniscus, current injury, left knee
    ● S83.259 Bucket-handle tear of lateral meniscus, current injury, unspecified knee

● S83.26 Peripheral tear of lateral meniscus, current injury
    ● S83.261 Peripheral tear of lateral meniscus, current injury, right knee
    ● S83.262 Peripheral tear of lateral meniscus, current injury, left knee
    ● S83.269 Peripheral tear of lateral meniscus, current injury, unspecified knee
● S83.27 Complex tear of lateral meniscus, current injury
    ● S83.271 Complex tear of lateral meniscus, current injury, right knee
    ● S83.272 Complex tear of lateral meniscus, current injury, left knee
    ● S83.279 Complex tear of lateral meniscus, current injury, unspecified knee
● S83.28 Other tear of lateral meniscus, current injury
    ● S83.281 Other tear of lateral meniscus, current injury, right knee
    ● S83.282 Other tear of lateral meniscus, current injury, left knee
    ● S83.289 Other tear of lateral meniscus, current injury, unspecified knee
● S83.3 Tear of articular cartilage of knee, current
  X ● S83.30 Tear of articular cartilage of unspecified knee, current
  X ● S83.31 Tear of articular cartilage of right knee, current
  X ● S83.32 Tear of articular cartilage of left knee, current
● S83.4 Sprain of collateral ligament of knee
    ● S83.40 Sprain of unspecified collateral ligament of knee
      ● S83.401 Sprain of unspecified collateral ligament of right knee
      ● S83.402 Sprain of unspecified collateral ligament of left knee
      ● S83.409 Sprain of unspecified collateral ligament of unspecified knee
    ● S83.41 Sprain of medial collateral ligament of knee
      Sprain of tibial collateral ligament
      ● S83.411 Sprain of medial collateral ligament of right knee
      ● S83.412 Sprain of medial collateral ligament of left knee
      ● S83.419 Sprain of medial collateral ligament of unspecified knee
    ● S83.42 Sprain of lateral collateral ligament of knee
      Sprain of fibular collateral ligament
      ● S83.421 Sprain of lateral collateral ligament of right knee
      ● S83.422 Sprain of lateral collateral ligament of left knee
      ● S83.429 Sprain of lateral collateral ligament of unspecified knee
● S83.5 Sprain of cruciate ligament of knee
    ● S83.50 Sprain of unspecified cruciate ligament of knee
      ● S83.501 Sprain of unspecified cruciate ligament of right knee
      ● S83.502 Sprain of unspecified cruciate ligament of left knee
      ● S83.509 Sprain of unspecified cruciate ligament of unspecified knee
    ● S83.51 Sprain of anterior cruciate ligament of knee
      ● S83.511 Sprain of anterior cruciate ligament of right knee
        Coding Clinic: 2016, Q2, P4
      ● S83.512 Sprain of anterior cruciate ligament of left knee
      ● S83.519 Sprain of anterior cruciate ligament of unspecified knee

◀ New　◀▬ Revised　~~deleted~~ Deleted　Excludes 1　Excludes 2　Includes　Use additional　Code first　Code also　Unspecified
OGCR Official Guidelines　● Unacceptable Principal Diagnosis　X Assign placeholder X　● Use Additional Character(s)　▶ Manifestation Code　**Coding Clinic**

● S83.52   Sprain of posterior cruciate ligament of knee
  ● S83.521   Sprain of posterior cruciate ligament of right knee
  ● S83.522   Sprain of posterior cruciate ligament of left knee
  ● S83.529   Sprain of posterior cruciate ligament of unspecified knee
● S83.6   Sprain of the superior tibiofibular joint and ligament
  X ● S83.60   Sprain of the superior tibiofibular joint and ligament, unspecified knee
  X ● S83.61   Sprain of the superior tibiofibular joint and ligament, right knee
  X ● S83.62   Sprain of the superior tibiofibular joint and ligament, left knee
● S83.8   Sprain of other specified parts of knee
  ● S83.8X   Sprain of other specified parts of knee
    ● S83.8X1   Sprain of other specified parts of right knee
    ● S83.8X2   Sprain of other specified parts of left knee
    ● S83.8X9   Sprain of other specified parts of unspecified knee
● S83.9   Sprain of unspecified site of knee
  X ● S83.90   Sprain of unspecified site of unspecified knee
  X ● S83.91   Sprain of unspecified site of right knee
  X ● S83.92   Sprain of unspecified site of left knee

● S84   Injury of nerves at lower leg level
  Code also any associated open wound (S81.-)
  Excludes2   injury of nerves at ankle and foot level (S94.-)
  The appropriate 7th character is to be added to each code from category S84

A	initial encounter
D	subsequent encounter
S	sequela

● S84.0   Injury of tibial nerve at lower leg level
  X ● S84.00   Injury of tibial nerve at lower leg level, unspecified leg
  X ● S84.01   Injury of tibial nerve at lower leg level, right leg
  X ● S84.02   Injury of tibial nerve at lower leg level, left leg
● S84.1   Injury of peroneal nerve at lower leg level
  X ● S84.10   Injury of peroneal nerve at lower leg level, unspecified leg
  X ● S84.11   Injury of peroneal nerve at lower leg level, right leg
  X ● S84.12   Injury of peroneal nerve at lower leg level, left leg
● S84.2   Injury of cutaneous sensory nerve at lower leg level
  X ● S84.20   Injury of cutaneous sensory nerve at lower leg level, unspecified leg
  X ● S84.21   Injury of cutaneous sensory nerve at lower leg level, right leg
  X ● S84.22   Injury of cutaneous sensory nerve at lower leg level, left leg
● S84.8   Injury of other nerves at lower leg level
  ● S84.80   Injury of other nerves at lower leg level
    ● S84.801   Injury of other nerves at lower leg level, right leg
    ● S84.802   Injury of other nerves at lower leg level, left leg
    ● S84.809   Injury of other nerves at lower leg level, unspecified leg

● S84.9   Injury of unspecified nerve at lower leg level
  X ● S84.90   Injury of unspecified nerve at lower leg level, unspecified leg
  X ● S84.91   Injury of unspecified nerve at lower leg level, right leg
  X ● S84.92   Injury of unspecified nerve at lower leg level, left leg

● S85   Injury of blood vessels at lower leg level
  Code also any associated open wound (S81.-)
  Excludes2   injury of blood vessels at ankle and foot level (S95.-)
  The appropriate 7th character is to be added to each code from category S85

A	initial encounter
D	subsequent encounter
S	sequela

● S85.0   Injury of popliteal artery
  ● S85.00   Unspecified injury of popliteal artery
    ● S85.001   Unspecified injury of popliteal artery, right leg A 🩺
      (Ex) S75.801[A], S75.809-S75.811[A], S75.819-S75.891[A], S75.899-S75.901[A], S75.909-S75.911[A], S75.919-S75.991[A], S75.999[A], S85.001[A], S85.009-S85.011[A], S85.019-S85.091[A], S85.099[A], S85.201[A], S85.209-S85.211[A], S85.219-S85.291[A], S85.299[A], S85.801[A], S85.809-S85.811[A], S85.819-S85.891[A], S85.899-S85.901[A], S85.909-S85.911[A], S85.919-S85.991[A], S85.999[A], S95.001[A], S95.009-S95.011[A], S95.019-S95.091[A], S95.099-S95.201[A], S95.209-S95.211[A], S95.219-S95.291[A], S95.299-S95.801[A], S95.809-S95.811[A], S95.819-S95.891[A], S95.899-S95.901[A], S95.909-S95.911[A], S95.919-S95.991[A], S95.999[A]
    ● S85.002   Unspecified injury of popliteal artery, left leg A 🩺
      (Ex) S75.802-S75.809[A], S75.812-S75.819[A], S75.892-S75.899[A], S75.902-S75.909[A], S75.912-S75.919[A], S75.992-S75.999[A], S85.002-S85.009[A], S85.012-S85.019[A], S85.092-S85.099[A], S85.202-S85.209[A], S85.212-S85.219[A], S85.292-S85.299[A], S85.802-S85.809[A], S85.812-S85.819[A], S85.892-S85.899[A], S85.902-S85.909[A], S85.912-S85.919[A], S85.992-S85.999[A], S95.002-S95.009[A], S95.012-S95.019[A], S95.092-S95.099[A], S95.202-S95.209[A], S95.212-S95.219[A], S95.292-S95.299[A], S95.802-S95.809[A], S95.812-S95.819[A], S95.892-S95.899[A], S95.902-S95.909[A], S95.912-S95.919[A], S95.992-S95.999[A]
    ● S85.009   Unspecified injury of popliteal artery, unspecified leg A 🩺
      (Ex) S75.802-S75.809[A], S75.812-S75.819[A], S75.892-S75.899[A], S75.902-S75.909[A], S75.912-S75.919[A], S75.992-S75.999[A], S85.162-S85.169[A], S85.172-S85.179[A], S85.182-S85.189[A], S85.202-S85.209[A], S85.212-S85.219[A], S85.292-S85.299[A], S85.802-S85.809[A], S85.812-S85.819[A], S85.892-S85.899[A], S85.902-S85.909[A], S85.912-S85.919[A], S85.992-S85.999[A], S95.002-S95.009[A], S95.012-S95.019[A], S95.092-S95.099[A], S95.202-S95.209[A], S95.212-S95.219[A], S95.292-S95.299[A], S95.802-S95.809[A], S95.812-S95.819[A], S95.892-S95.899[A], S95.902-S95.909[A], S95.912-S95.919[A], S95.992-S95.999[A]

N Newborn Age: 0   P Pediatric Age: 0–17   M Maternity DX: 12–55   A Adult Age: 15–124   ♀ Females Only   ♂ Males Only
🩺 Complication\Comorbidity   🩺 Major C\C   (Ex) CC/MCC Exclusions   🩺 Hospital-Acquired Condition

1391

CHAPTER 19 (S00-T88)

● **S85.01**   **Laceration of popliteal artery**
  ● **S85.011**   **Laceration of popliteal artery, right leg** A 🦟
    Ex: See S85.001
  ● **S85.012**   **Laceration of popliteal artery, left leg** A 🦟
    Ex: See S85.002
  ● **S85.019**   **Laceration of popliteal artery, unspecified leg** A 🦟
    Ex: See S85.009

● **S85.09**   **Other specified injury of popliteal artery**
  ● **S85.091**   **Other specified injury of popliteal artery, right leg** A 🦟
    Ex: See S85.001
  ● **S85.092**   **Other specified injury of popliteal artery, left leg** A 🦟
    Ex: See S85.002
  ● **S85.099**   **Other specified injury of popliteal artery, unspecified leg** A 🦟
    Ex: See S85.009

● **S85.1**   **Injury of tibial artery**
  ● **S85.10**   **Unspecified injury of unspecified tibial artery**
    Injury of tibial artery NOS
    ● **S85.101**   **Unspecified injury of unspecified tibial artery, right leg** A 🦟
      Ex: S75.801[A], S75.809-S75.811[A], S75.819-S75.891[A], S75.899-S75.901[A], S75.909-S75.911[A], S75.919-S75.991[A], S75.999[A], S85.101[A], S85.109-S85.111[A], S85.119-S85.121[A], S85.129[A], S85.201[A], S85.209-S85.211[A], S85.219-S85.291[A], S85.299[A], S85.801[A], S85.809-S85.811[A], S85.819-S85.891[A], S85.899-S85.901[A], S85.909-S85.911[A], S85.919-S85.991[A], S85.999[A], S95.001[A], S95.009-S95.011[A], S95.019-S95.091[A], S95.099-S95.201[A], S95.209-S95.211[A], S95.219-S95.291[A], S95.299-S95.801[A], S95.809-S95.811[A], S95.819-S95.891[A], S95.899-S95.901[A], S95.909-S95.911[A], S95.919-S95.991[A], S95.999[A]
    ● **S85.102**   **Unspecified injury of unspecified tibial artery, left leg** A 🦟
      Ex: S75.802-S75.809[A], S75.812-S75.819[A], S75.892-S75.899[A], S75.902-S75.909[A], S75.912-S75.919[A], S75.992-S75.999[A], S85.102-S85.109[A], S85.112-S85.119[A], S85.122-S85.129[A], S85.202-S85.209[A], S85.212-S85.219[A], S85.292-S85.299[A], S85.802-S85.809[A], S85.812-S85.819[A], S85.892-S85.899[A], S85.902-S85.909[A], S85.912-S85.919[A], S85.992-S85.999[A], S95.002-S95.009[A], S95.012-S95.019[A], S95.092-S95.099[A], S95.202-S95.209[A], S95.212-S95.219[A], S95.292-S95.299[A], S95.802-S95.809[A], S95.812-S95.819[A], S95.892-S95.899[A], S95.902-S95.909[A], S95.912-S95.919[A], S95.992-S95.999[A]
    ● **S85.109**   **Unspecified injury of unspecified tibial artery, unspecified leg** A 🦟
      Ex: S75.801-S75.999[A], S85.101-S85.129[A], S85.201-S85.299[A], S85.801-S85.999[A], S95.001-S95.099[A], S95.201-S95.999[A]

● **S85.11**   **Laceration of unspecified tibial artery**
  ● **S85.111**   **Laceration of unspecified tibial artery, right leg** A 🦟
    Ex: See S85.101
  ● **S85.112**   **Laceration of unspecified tibial artery, left leg** A 🦟
    Ex: See S85.102
  ● **S85.119**   **Laceration of unspecified tibial artery, unspecified leg** A 🦟
    Ex: See S85.109

● **S85.12**   **Other specified injury of unspecified tibial artery**
  ● **S85.121**   **Other specified injury of unspecified tibial artery, right leg** A 🦟
    Ex: See S85.101
  ● **S85.122**   **Other specified injury of unspecified tibial artery, left leg** A 🦟
    Ex: See S85.102
  ● **S85.129**   **Other specified injury of unspecified tibial artery, unspecified leg** A 🦟
    Ex: See S85.109

● **S85.13**   **Unspecified injury of anterior tibial artery**
  ● **S85.131**   **Unspecified injury of anterior tibial artery, right leg** A 🦟
    Ex: S75.801[A], S75.809-S75.811[A], S75.819-S75.891[A], S75.899-S75.901[A], S75.909-S75.911[A], S75.919-S75.991[A], S75.999[A], S85.131[A], S85.139-S85.141[A], S85.149-S85.151[A], S85.159[A], S85.201[A], S85.209-S85.211[A], S85.219-S85.291[A], S85.299[A], S85.801[A], S85.809-S85.811[A], S85.819-S85.891[A], S85.899-S85.901[A], S85.909-S85.911[A], S85.919-S85.991[A], S85.999[A], S95.001[A], S95.009-S95.011[A], S95.019-S95.091[A], S95.099-S95.201[A], S95.209-S95.211[A], S95.219-S95.291[A], S95.299-S95.801[A], S95.809-S95.811[A], S95.819-S95.891[A], S95.899-S95.901[A], S95.909-S95.911[A], S95.919-S95.991[A], S95.999[A]
  ● **S85.132**   **Unspecified injury of anterior tibial artery, left leg** A 🦟
    Ex: S75.802-S75.809[A], S75.812-S75.819[A], S75.892-S75.899[A], S75.902-S75.909[A], S75.912-S75.919[A], S75.992-S75.999[A], S85.132-S85.139[A], S85.142-S85.149[A], S85.152-S85.159[A], S85.202-S85.209[A], S85.212-S85.219[A], S85.292-S85.299[A], S85.802-S85.809[A], S85.812-S85.819[A], S85.892-S85.899[A], S85.902-S85.909[A], S85.912-S85.919[A], S85.992-S85.999[A], S95.002-S95.009[A], S95.012-S95.019[A], S95.092-S95.099[A], S95.202-S95.209[A], S95.212-S95.219[A], S95.292-S95.299[A], S95.802-S95.809[A], S95.812-S95.819[A], S95.892-S95.899[A], S95.902-S95.909[A], S95.912-S95.919[A], S95.992-S95.999[A]
  ● **S85.139**   **Unspecified injury of anterior tibial artery, unspecified leg** A 🦟
    Ex: S75.801-S75.999[A], S85.131-S85.159[A], S85.201-S85.299[A], S85.801-S85.999[A], S95.001-S95.099[A], S95.201-S95.999[A]

◄ New   ⬅ Revised   ~~deleted~~ Deleted   Excludes 1   Excludes 2   Includes   Use additional   Code first   Code also   Unspecified
OGCR Official Guidelines   ● Unacceptable Principal Diagnosis   X Assign placeholder X   ● Use Additional Character(s)   ▶ Manifestation Code   **Coding Clinic**

- S85.14   **Laceration of anterior tibial artery**
  - S85.141   **Laceration of anterior tibial artery, right leg** A
    - (Ex:) See S85.131
  - S85.142   **Laceration of anterior tibial artery, left leg** A
    - (Ex:) See S85.132
  - S85.149   **Laceration of anterior tibial artery, unspecified leg** A
    - (Ex:) See S85.139
- S85.15   **Other specified injury of anterior tibial artery**
  - S85.151   **Other specified injury of anterior tibial artery, right leg** A
    - (Ex:) See S85.131
  - S85.152   **Other specified injury of anterior tibial artery, left leg** A
    - (Ex:) See S85.132
  - S85.159   **Other specified injury of anterior tibial artery, unspecified leg** A
    - (Ex:) See S85.139
- S85.16   **Unspecified injury of posterior tibial artery**
  - S85.161   **Unspecified injury of posterior tibial artery, right leg** A
    - (Ex:) S75.801[A], S75.809-S75.811[A], S75.819-S75.891[A], S75.899-S75.901[A], S75.909-S75.911[A], S75.919-S75.991[A], S75.999[A], S85.161[A], S85.169-S85.171[A], S85.179-S85.181[A], S85.189-S85.201[A], S85.209-S85.211[A], S85.219-S85.291[A], S85.299[A], S85.801[A], S85.809-S85.811[A], S85.819-S85.891[A], S85.899-S85.901[A], S85.909-S85.911[A], S85.919-S85.991[A], S85.999[A], S95.001[A], S95.009-S95.011[A], S95.019-S95.091[A], S95.099-S95.201[A], S95.209-S95.211[A], S95.219-S95.291[A], S95.299-S95.801[A], S95.809-S95.811[A], S95.819-S95.891[A], S95.899-S95.901[A], S95.909-S95.911[A], S95.919-S95.991[A], S95.999[A]
  - S85.162   **Unspecified injury of posterior tibial artery, left leg** A
    - (Ex:) S75.802-S75.809[A], S75.812-S75.819[A], S75.892-S75.899[A], S75.902-S75.909[A], S75.912-S75.919[A], S75.992-S75.999[A], S85.162-S85.169[A], S85.172-S85.179[A], S85.182-S85.189[A], S85.202-S85.209[A], S85.212-S85.219[A], S85.292-S85.299[A], S85.802-S85.809[A], S85.812-S85.819[A], S85.892-S85.899[A], S85.902-S85.909[A], S85.912-S85.919[A], S85.992-S85.999[A], S95.002-S95.009[A], S95.012-S95.019[A], S95.092-S95.099[A], S95.202-S95.209[A], S95.212-S95.219[A], S95.292-S95.299[A], S95.802-S95.809[A], S95.812-S95.819[A], S95.892-S95.899[A], S95.902-S95.909[A], S95.912-S95.919[A], S95.992-S95.999[A]
  - S85.169   **Unspecified injury of posterior tibial artery, unspecified leg** A
    - (Ex:) S75.801-S75.999[A], S85.161-S85.189[A], S85.201-S85.299[A], S85.801-S85.999[A], S95.001-S95.099[A], S95.201-S95.999[A]
- S85.17   **Laceration of posterior tibial artery**
  - S85.171   **Laceration of posterior tibial artery, right leg** A
    - (Ex:) See S85.161
  - S85.172   **Laceration of posterior tibial artery, left leg** A
    - (Ex:) See S85.162
  - S85.179   **Laceration of posterior tibial artery, unspecified leg** A
    - (Ex:) See S85.169
- S85.18   **Other specified injury of posterior tibial artery**
  - S85.181   **Other specified injury of posterior tibial artery, right leg** A
    - (Ex:) See S85.161
  - S85.182   **Other specified injury of posterior tibial artery, left leg** A
    - (Ex:) See S85.162
  - S85.189   **Other specified injury of posterior tibial artery, unspecified leg** A
    - (Ex:) See S85.169
- S85.2   **Injury of peroneal artery**
  - S85.20   **Unspecified injury of peroneal artery**
    - S85.201   **Unspecified injury of peroneal artery, right leg** A
      - (Ex:) See S75.801
    - S85.202   **Unspecified injury of peroneal artery, left leg** A
      - (Ex:) See S75.802
    - S85.209   **Unspecified injury of peroneal artery, unspecified leg** A
      - (Ex:) See S75.809
  - S85.21   **Laceration of peroneal artery**
    - S85.211   **Laceration of peroneal artery, right leg** A
      - (Ex:) See S75.801
    - S85.212   **Laceration of peroneal artery, left leg** A
      - (Ex:) See S75.802
    - S85.219   **Laceration of peroneal artery, unspecified leg** A
      - (Ex:) See S75.809
  - S85.29   **Other specified injury of peroneal artery**
    - S85.291   **Other specified injury of peroneal artery, right leg** A
      - (Ex:) See S75.801
    - S85.292   **Other specified injury of peroneal artery, left leg** A
      - (Ex:) See S75.802
    - S85.299   **Other specified injury of peroneal artery, unspecified leg** A
      - (Ex:) See S75.809
- S85.3   **Injury of greater saphenous vein at lower leg level**
  - Injury of greater saphenous vein NOS
  - Injury of saphenous vein NOS
  - S85.30   **Unspecified injury of greater saphenous vein at lower leg level**
    - S85.301   **Unspecified injury of greater saphenous vein at lower leg level, right leg** A
      - (Ex:) See S75.201
    - S85.302   **Unspecified injury of greater saphenous vein at lower leg level, left leg** A
      - (Ex:) See S75.202
    - S85.309   **Unspecified injury of greater saphenous vein at lower leg level, unspecified leg** A
      - (Ex:) See S75.209
  - S85.31   **Laceration of greater saphenous vein at lower leg level**
    - S85.311   **Laceration of greater saphenous vein at lower leg level, right leg** A
      - (Ex:) See S75.201
    - S85.312   **Laceration of greater saphenous vein at lower leg level, left leg** A
      - (Ex:) See S75.202
    - S85.319   **Laceration of greater saphenous vein at lower leg level, unspecified leg** A
      - (Ex:) See S75.209

CHAPTER 19 (S00–T88)

● S85.39 Other specified injury of greater saphenous vein at lower leg level
  ● S85.391 Other specified injury of greater saphenous vein at lower leg level, right leg A ✎
    (Ex) See S75.201
  ● S85.392 Other specified injury of greater saphenous vein at lower leg level, left leg A ✎
    (Ex) See S75.202
  ● S85.399 Other specified injury of greater saphenous vein at lower leg level, unspecified leg A ✎
    (Ex) See S75.209

● S85.4 Injury of lesser saphenous vein at lower leg level
  ● S85.40 Unspecified injury of lesser saphenous vein at lower leg level
    ● S85.401 Unspecified injury of lesser saphenous vein at lower leg level, right leg A ✎
      (Ex) See S75.201
    ● S85.402 Unspecified injury of lesser saphenous vein at lower leg level, left leg A ✎
      (Ex) See S75.202
    ● S85.409 Unspecified injury of lesser saphenous vein at lower leg level, unspecified leg A ✎
      (Ex) See S75.209
  ● S85.41 Laceration of lesser saphenous vein at lower leg level
    ● S85.411 Laceration of lesser saphenous vein at lower leg level, right leg A ✎
      (Ex) See S75.201
    ● S85.412 Laceration of lesser saphenous vein at lower leg level, left leg A ✎
      (Ex) See S75.202
    ● S85.419 Laceration of lesser saphenous vein at lower leg level, unspecified leg A ✎
      (Ex) See S75.209
  ● S85.49 Other specified injury of lesser saphenous vein at lower leg level
    ● S85.491 Other specified injury of lesser saphenous vein at lower leg level, right leg A ✎
      (Ex) See S75.201
    ● S85.492 Other specified injury of lesser saphenous vein at lower leg level, left leg A ✎
      (Ex) See S75.202
    ● S85.499 Other specified injury of lesser saphenous vein at lower leg level, unspecified leg A ✎
      (Ex) See S75.209

● S85.5 Injury of popliteal vein
  ● S85.50 Unspecified injury of popliteal vein
    ● S85.501 Unspecified injury of popliteal vein, right leg A ✎
      (Ex) S75.801[A], S75.809-S75.811[A],
      S75.819-S75.891[A], S75.899-S75.901[A],
      S75.909-S75.911[A], S75.919-S75.991[A],
      S75.999[A], S85.201[A], S85.209-S85.211[A],
      S85.219-S85.291[A], S85.299[A], S85.501[A],
      S85.509-S85.511[A], S85.519-S85.591[A],
      S85.599[A], S85.801[A], S85.809-S85.811[A],
      S85.819-S85.891[A], S85.899-S85.901[A],
      S85.909-S85.911[A], S85.919-S85.991[A],
      S85.999[A], S95.001[A], S95.009-S95.011[A],
      S95.019-S95.091[A], S95.099-S95.201[A],
      S95.209-S95.211[A], S95.219-S95.291[A],
      S95.299-S95.801[A], S95.809-S95.811[A],
      S95.819-S95.891[A], S95.899-S95.901[A],
      S95.909-S95.911[A], S95.919-S95.991[A],
      S95.999[A]

● S85.502 Unspecified injury of popliteal vein, left leg A ✎
    (Ex) S75.802-S75.809[A], S75.812-S75.819[A],
    S75.892-S75.899[A], S75.902-S75.909[A],
    S75.912-S75.919[A], S75.992-S75.999[A],
    S85.202-S85.209[A], S85.212-S85.219[A],
    S85.292-S85.299[A], S85.502-S85.509[A],
    S85.512-S85.519[A], S85.592-S85.599[A],
    S85.802-S85.809[A], S85.812-S85.819[A],
    S85.892-S85.899[A], S85.902-S85.909[A],
    S85.912-S85.919[A], S85.992-S85.999[A],
    S95.002-S95.009[A], S95.012-S95.019[A],
    S95.092-S95.099[A], S95.202-S95.209[A],
    S95.212-S95.219[A], S95.292-S95.299[A],
    S95.802-S95.809[A], S95.812-S95.819[A],
    S95.892-S95.899[A], S95.902-S95.909[A],
    S95.912-S95.919[A], S95.992-S95.999[A]

  ● S85.509 Unspecified injury of popliteal vein, unspecified leg A ✎
    (Ex) S75.801-S75.999[A], S85.201-S85.299[A],
    S85.501-S85.599[A], S85.801-S85.999[A],
    S95.001-S95.099[A], S95.201-S95.999[A]

● S85.51 Laceration of popliteal vein
  ● S85.511 Laceration of popliteal vein, right leg A ✎
    (Ex) See S85.501
  ● S85.512 Laceration of popliteal vein, left leg A ✎
    (Ex) See S85.502
  ● S85.519 Laceration of popliteal vein, unspecified leg A ✎
    (Ex) See S85.509

● S85.59 Other specified injury of popliteal vein
  ● S85.591 Other specified injury of popliteal vein, right leg A ✎
    (Ex) See S85.501
  ● S85.592 Other specified injury of popliteal vein, left leg A ✎
    (Ex) See S85.502
  ● S85.599 Other specified injury of popliteal vein, unspecified leg A ✎
    (Ex) See S85.509

● S85.8 Injury of other blood vessels at lower leg level
  ● S85.80 Unspecified injury of other blood vessels at lower leg level
    ● S85.801 Unspecified injury of other blood vessels at lower leg level, right leg A ✎
      (Ex) See S75.801
    ● S85.802 Unspecified injury of other blood vessels at lower leg level, left leg A ✎
      (Ex) See S75.802
    ● S85.809 Unspecified injury of other blood vessels at lower leg level, unspecified leg A ✎
      (Ex) See S75.809
  ● S85.81 Laceration of other blood vessels at lower leg level
    ● S85.811 Laceration of other blood vessels at lower leg level, right leg A ✎
      (Ex) See S75.801
    ● S85.812 Laceration of other blood vessels at lower leg level, left leg A ✎
      (Ex) See S75.802
    ● S85.819 Laceration of other blood vessels at lower leg level, unspecified leg A ✎
      (Ex) See S75.809

◄ New ◀ Revised deleted Deleted Excludes 1 Excludes 2 Includes Use additional Code first Code also Unspecified
OGCR Official Guidelines ● Unacceptable Principal Diagnosis X Assign placeholder X ● Use Additional Character(s) ▶ Manifestation Code Coding Clinic

- **S85.89**   Other specified injury of other blood vessels at lower leg level
  - **S85.891**   Other specified injury of other blood vessels at lower leg level, right leg A ⓒ
    Ex: See S75.801
  - **S85.892**   Other specified injury of other blood vessels at lower leg level, left leg A ⓒ
    Ex: See S75.802
  - **S85.899**   Other specified injury of other blood vessels at lower leg level, unspecified leg A ⓒ
    Ex: See S75.809

- **S85.9**   Injury of unspecified blood vessel at lower leg level
  - **S85.90**   Unspecified injury of unspecified blood vessel at lower leg level
    - **S85.901**   Unspecified injury of unspecified blood vessel at lower leg level, right leg A ⓒ
      Ex: See S75.801
    - **S85.902**   Unspecified injury of unspecified blood vessel at lower leg level, left leg A ⓒ
      Ex: See S75.802
    - **S85.909**   Unspecified injury of unspecified blood vessel at lower leg level, unspecified leg A ⓒ
      Ex: See S75.809
  - **S85.91**   Laceration of unspecified blood vessel at lower leg level
    - **S85.911**   Laceration of unspecified blood vessel at lower leg level, right leg A ⓒ
      Ex: See S75.801
    - **S85.912**   Laceration of unspecified blood vessel at lower leg level, left leg A ⓒ
      Ex: See S75.802
    - **S85.919**   Laceration of unspecified blood vessel at lower leg level, unspecified leg A ⓒ
      Ex: See S75.809
  - **S85.99**   Other specified injury of unspecified blood vessel at lower leg level
    - **S85.991**   Other specified injury of unspecified blood vessel at lower leg level, right leg A ⓒ
      Ex: See S75.801
    - **S85.992**   Other specified injury of unspecified blood vessel at lower leg level, left leg A ⓒ
      Ex: See S75.802
    - **S85.999**   Other specified injury of unspecified blood vessel at lower leg level, unspecified leg A ⓒ
      Ex: See S75.809

- **S86**   Injury of muscle, fascia and tendon at lower leg level

  Code also any associated open wound (S81.-)

  Excludes2   injury of muscle, fascia and tendon at ankle (S96.-)
  injury of patellar ligament (tendon) (S76.1-)
  sprain of joints and ligaments of knee (S83.-)

  The appropriate 7th character is to be added to each code from category S86

A	initial encounter
D	subsequent encounter
S	sequela

  - **S86.0**   Injury of Achilles tendon
    - **S86.00**   Unspecified injury of Achilles tendon
      - **S86.001**   Unspecified injury of right Achilles tendon
      - **S86.002**   Unspecified injury of left Achilles tendon
      - **S86.009**   Unspecified injury of unspecified Achilles tendon
    - **S86.01**   Strain of Achilles tendon
      - **S86.011**   Strain of right Achilles tendon
      - **S86.012**   Strain of left Achilles tendon
      - **S86.019**   Strain of unspecified Achilles tendon
    - **S86.02**   Laceration of Achilles tendon
      - **S86.021**   Laceration of right Achilles tendon A ⓒ
        Ex: S81.001[A], S81.009-S81.011[A], S81.019-S81.021[A], S81.029-S81.031[A], S81.039-S81.041[A], S81.049-S81.051[A], S81.059-S81.801[A], S81.809-S81.811[A], S81.819-S81.821[A], S81.829-S81.831[A], S81.839-S81.841[A], S81.849-S81.851[A], S81.859[A], S86.021[A], S86.029[A], S86.121[A], S86.129[A], S86.221[A], S86.229[A], S86.321[A], S86.329[A], S86.821[A], S86.829-S86.921[A], S86.929[A], S91.001[A], S91.009[A], S91.011[A], S91.019-S91.021[A], S91.029-S91.031[A], S91.039-S91.041[A], S91.049-S91.051[A], S91.059[A], S96.021[A], S96.029[A], S96.121[A], S96.129[A], S96.221[A], S96.229[A], S96.821[A], S96.829[A], S96.921[A], S96.929[A]
      - **S86.022**   Laceration of left Achilles tendon A ⓒ
        Ex: S81.002-S81.009[A], S81.012-S81.019[A], S81.022-S81.029[A], S81.032-S81.039[A], S81.042-S81.049[A], S81.052-S81.059[A], S81.802-S81.809[A], S81.812-S81.819[A], S81.822-S81.829[A], S81.832-S81.839[A], S81.842-S81.849[A], S81.852-S81.859[A], S86.022-S86.029[A], S86.122-S86.129[A], S86.222-S86.229[A], S86.322-S86.329[A], S86.822-S86.829[A], S86.922-S86.929[A], S91.002-S91.009[A], S91.012-S91.019[A], S91.022-S91.029[A], S91.032-S91.039[A], S91.042-S91.049[A], S91.052-S91.059[A], S96.022-S96.029[A], S96.122-S96.129[A], S96.222-S96.229[A], S96.822-S96.829[A], S96.922-S96.929[A]
      - **S86.029**   Laceration of unspecified Achilles tendon A ⓒ
        Ex: S81.001-S81.859[A], S86.021-S86.029[A], S86.121-S86.129[A], S86.221-S86.229[A], S86.321-S86.329[A], S86.821-S86.829[A], S86.921-S86.929[A], S91.001-S91.059[A], S96.021-S96.029[A], S96.121-S96.129[A], S96.221-S96.229[A], S96.821-S96.829[A], S96.921-S96.929[A]
    - **S86.09**   Other specified injury of Achilles tendon
      - **S86.091**   Other specified injury of right Achilles tendon
      - **S86.092**   Other specified injury of left Achilles tendon
      - **S86.099**   Other specified injury of unspecified Achilles tendon
  - **S86.1**   Injury of other muscle(s) and tendon(s) of posterior muscle group at lower leg level
    - **S86.10**   Unspecified injury of other muscle(s) and tendon(s) of posterior muscle group at lower leg level
      - **S86.101**   Unspecified injury of other muscle(s) and tendon(s) of posterior muscle group at lower leg level, right leg
      - **S86.102**   Unspecified injury of other muscle(s) and tendon(s) of posterior muscle group at lower leg level, left leg
      - **S86.109**   Unspecified injury of other muscle(s) and tendon(s) of posterior muscle group at lower leg level, unspecified leg

● **S86.11** Strain of other muscle(s) and tendon(s) of posterior muscle group at lower leg level

  ● **S86.111** Strain of other muscle(s) and tendon(s) of posterior muscle group at lower leg level, right leg

  ● **S86.112** Strain of other muscle(s) and tendon(s) of posterior muscle group at lower leg level, left leg

  ● **S86.119** Strain of other muscle(s) and tendon(s) of posterior muscle group at lower leg level, unspecified leg

● **S86.12** Laceration of other muscle(s) and tendon(s) of posterior muscle group at lower leg level

  ● **S86.121** Laceration of other muscle(s) and tendon(s) of posterior muscle group at lower leg level, right leg A
    (Ex:) See S86.021

  ● **S86.122** Laceration of other muscle(s) and tendon(s) of posterior muscle group at lower leg level, left leg A
    (Ex:) See S86.022

  ● **S86.129** Laceration of other muscle(s) and tendon(s) of posterior muscle group at lower leg level, unspecified leg A
    (Ex:) See S86.029

● **S86.19** Other injury of other muscle(s) and tendon(s) of posterior muscle group at lower leg level

  ● **S86.191** Other injury of other muscle(s) and tendon(s) of posterior muscle group at lower leg level, right leg

  ● **S86.192** Other injury of other muscle(s) and tendon(s) of posterior muscle group at lower leg level, left leg

  ● **S86.199** Other injury of other muscle(s) and tendon(s) of posterior muscle group at lower leg level, unspecified leg

● **S86.2** Injury of muscle(s) and tendon(s) of anterior muscle group at lower leg level

  ● **S86.20** Unspecified injury of muscle(s) and tendon(s) of anterior muscle group at lower leg level

    ● **S86.201** Unspecified injury of muscle(s) and tendon(s) of anterior muscle group at lower leg level, right leg

    ● **S86.202** Unspecified injury of muscle(s) and tendon(s) of anterior muscle group at lower leg level, left leg

    ● **S86.209** Unspecified injury of muscle(s) and tendon(s) of anterior muscle group at lower leg level, unspecified leg

  ● **S86.21** Strain of muscle(s) and tendon(s) of anterior muscle group at lower leg level

    ● **S86.211** Strain of muscle(s) and tendon(s) of anterior muscle group at lower leg level, right leg

    ● **S86.212** Strain of muscle(s) and tendon(s) of anterior muscle group at lower leg level, left leg

    ● **S86.219** Strain of muscle(s) and tendon(s) of anterior muscle group at lower leg level, unspecified leg

● **S86.22** Laceration of muscle(s) and tendon(s) of anterior muscle group at lower leg level

  ● **S86.221** Laceration of muscle(s) and tendon(s) of anterior muscle group at lower leg level, right leg A
    (Ex:) See S86.021

  ● **S86.222** Laceration of muscle(s) and tendon(s) of anterior muscle group at lower leg level, left leg A
    (Ex:) See S86.022

  ● **S86.229** Laceration of muscle(s) and tendon(s) of anterior muscle group at lower leg level, unspecified leg A
    (Ex:) See S86.029

● **S86.29** Other injury of muscle(s) and tendon(s) of anterior muscle group at lower leg level

  ● **S86.291** Other injury of muscle(s) and tendon(s) of anterior muscle group at lower leg level, right leg

  ● **S86.292** Other injury of muscle(s) and tendon(s) of anterior muscle group at lower leg level, left leg

  ● **S86.299** Other injury of muscle(s) and tendon(s) of anterior muscle group at lower leg level, unspecified leg

● **S86.3** Injury of muscle(s) and tendon(s) of peroneal muscle group at lower leg level

  ● **S86.30** Unspecified injury of muscle(s) and tendon(s) of peroneal muscle group at lower leg level

    ● **S86.301** Unspecified injury of muscle(s) and tendon(s) of peroneal muscle group at lower leg level, right leg

    ● **S86.302** Unspecified injury of muscle(s) and tendon(s) of peroneal muscle group at lower leg level, left leg

    ● **S86.309** Unspecified injury of muscle(s) and tendon(s) of peroneal muscle group at lower leg level, unspecified leg

  ● **S86.31** Strain of muscle(s) and tendon(s) of peroneal muscle group at lower leg level

    ● **S86.311** Strain of muscle(s) and tendon(s) of peroneal muscle group at lower leg level, right leg

    ● **S86.312** Strain of muscle(s) and tendon(s) of peroneal muscle group at lower leg level, left leg

    ● **S86.319** Strain of muscle(s) and tendon(s) of peroneal muscle group at lower leg level, unspecified leg

  ● **S86.32** Laceration of muscle(s) and tendon(s) of peroneal muscle group at lower leg level

    ● **S86.321** Laceration of muscle(s) and tendon(s) of peroneal muscle group at lower leg level, right leg A
     (Ex:) See S86.021

    ● **S86.322** Laceration of muscle(s) and tendon(s) of peroneal muscle group at lower leg level, left leg A
     (Ex:) See S86.022

    ● **S86.329** Laceration of muscle(s) and tendon(s) of peroneal muscle group at lower leg level, unspecified leg A
     (Ex:) See S86.029

◄ New   ◄▥ Revised   ~~deleted~~ Deleted   Excludes 1   Excludes 2   Includes   Use additional   Code first   Code also   Unspecified

OGCR Official Guidelines   ● Unacceptable Principal Diagnosis   X Assign placeholder X   ● Use Additional Character(s)   ▶ Manifestation Code   **Coding Clinic**

- **S86.39**   Other injury of muscle(s) and tendon(s) of peroneal muscle group at lower leg level
  - **S86.391**   Other injury of muscle(s) and tendon(s) of peroneal muscle group at lower leg level, right leg
  - **S86.392**   Other injury of muscle(s) and tendon(s) of peroneal muscle group at lower leg level, left leg
  - **S86.399**   Other injury of muscle(s) and tendon(s) of peroneal muscle group at lower leg level, unspecified leg
- **S86.8**   Injury of other muscles and tendons at lower leg level
  - **S86.80**   Unspecified injury of other muscles and tendons at lower leg level
    - **S86.801**   Unspecified injury of other muscle(s) and tendon(s) at lower leg level, right leg
    - **S86.802**   Unspecified injury of other muscle(s) and tendon(s) at lower leg level, left leg
    - **S86.809**   Unspecified injury of other muscle(s) and tendon(s) at lower leg level, unspecified leg
  - **S86.81**   Strain of other muscles and tendons at lower leg level
    - **S86.811**   Strain of other muscle(s) and tendon(s) at lower leg level, right leg
    - **S86.812**   Strain of other muscle(s) and tendon(s) at lower leg level, left leg
    - **S86.819**   Strain of other muscle(s) and tendon(s) at lower leg level, unspecified leg
  - **S86.82**   Laceration of other muscles and tendons at lower leg level
    - **S86.821**   Laceration of other muscle(s) and tendon(s) at lower leg level, right leg A
      - (Ex:) See S86.021
    - **S86.822**   Laceration of other muscle(s) and tendon(s) at lower leg level, left leg A
      - (Ex:) See S86.022
    - **S86.829**   Laceration of other muscle(s) and tendon(s) at lower leg level, unspecified leg A
      - (Ex:) See S86.029
  - **S86.89**   Other injury of other muscles and tendons at lower leg level
    - **S86.891**   Other injury of other muscle(s) and tendon(s) at lower leg level, right leg
    - **S86.892**   Other injury of other muscle(s) and tendon(s) at lower leg level, left leg
    - **S86.899**   Other injury of other muscle(s) and tendon(s) at lower leg level, unspecified leg
- **S86.9**   Injury of unspecified muscle and tendon at lower leg level
  - **S86.90**   Unspecified injury of unspecified muscle and tendon at lower leg level
    - **S86.901**   Unspecified injury of unspecified muscle(s) and tendon(s) at lower leg level, right leg
    - **S86.902**   Unspecified injury of unspecified muscle(s) and tendon(s) at lower leg level, left leg
    - **S86.909**   Unspecified injury of unspecified muscle(s) and tendon(s) at lower leg level, unspecified leg

- **S86.91**   Strain of unspecified muscle and tendon at lower leg level
  - **S86.911**   Strain of unspecified muscle(s) and tendon(s) at lower leg level, right leg
  - **S86.912**   Strain of unspecified muscle(s) and tendon(s) at lower leg level, left leg
  - **S86.919**   Strain of unspecified muscle(s) and tendon(s) at lower leg level, unspecified leg
- **S86.92**   Laceration of unspecified muscle and tendon at lower leg level
  - **S86.921**   Laceration of unspecified muscle(s) and tendon(s) at lower leg level, right leg A
    - (Ex:) See S86.021
  - **S86.922**   Laceration of unspecified muscle(s) and tendon(s) at lower leg level, left leg A
    - (Ex:) See S86.022
  - **S86.929**   Laceration of unspecified muscle(s) and tendon(s) at lower leg level, unspecified leg A
    - (Ex:) See S86.029
- **S86.99**   Other injury of unspecified muscle and tendon at lower leg level
  - **S86.991**   Other injury of unspecified muscle(s) and tendon(s) at lower leg level, right leg
  - **S86.992**   Other injury of unspecified muscle(s) and tendon(s) at lower leg level, left leg
  - **S86.999**   Other injury of unspecified muscle(s) and tendon(s) at lower leg level, unspecified leg
- **S87**   Crushing injury of lower leg
  - Use additional code(s) for all associated injuries
  - **Excludes2**   crushing injury of ankle and foot (S97.-)
  - The appropriate 7th character is to be added to each code from category S87

A	initial encounter
D	subsequent encounter
S	sequela

  - **S87.0**   Crushing injury of knee
    - X **S87.00**   Crushing injury of unspecified knee
    - X **S87.01**   Crushing injury of right knee
    - X **S87.02**   Crushing injury of left knee
  - **S87.8**   Crushing injury of lower leg
    - X **S87.80**   Crushing injury of unspecified lower leg
    - X **S87.81**   Crushing injury of right lower leg
    - X **S87.82**   Crushing injury of left lower leg

CHAPTER 19 (S00-T88)

● **S88   Traumatic amputation of lower leg**
      An amputation not identified as partial or complete should be coded to complete

      Excludes1   traumatic amputation of ankle and foot (S98.-)

      The appropriate 7th character is to be added to each code from category S88

A	initial encounter
D	subsequent encounter
S	sequela

   ● **S88.0   Traumatic amputation at knee level**
     ● **S88.01   Complete traumatic amputation at knee level**
       ● **S88.011   Complete traumatic amputation at knee level, right lower leg** A 📞
           (Ex:) See S78.011
       ● **S88.012   Complete traumatic amputation at knee level, left lower leg** A 📞
           (Ex:) See S78.012
       ● **S88.019   Complete traumatic amputation at knee level, unspecified lower leg** A 📞
           (Ex:) See S78.019
     ● **S88.02   Partial traumatic amputation at knee level**
       ● **S88.021   Partial traumatic amputation at knee level, right lower leg** A 📞
           (Ex:) See S78.011
       ● **S88.022   Partial traumatic amputation at knee level, left lower leg** A 📞
           (Ex:) See S78.012
       ● **S88.029   Partial traumatic amputation at knee level, unspecified lower leg** A 📞
           (Ex:) See S78.019

   ● **S88.1   Traumatic amputation at level between knee and ankle**
     ● **S88.11   Complete traumatic amputation at level between knee and ankle**
       ● **S88.111   Complete traumatic amputation at level between knee and ankle, right lower leg** A 📞
           (Ex:) See S78.011
       ● **S88.112   Complete traumatic amputation at level between knee and ankle, left lower leg** A 📞
           (Ex:) See S78.012
       ● **S88.119   Complete traumatic amputation at level between knee and ankle, unspecified lower leg** A 📞
           (Ex:) See S78.019
     ● **S88.12   Partial traumatic amputation at level between knee and ankle**
       ● **S88.121   Partial traumatic amputation at level between knee and ankle, right lower leg** A 📞
           (Ex:) See S78.011
       ● **S88.122   Partial traumatic amputation at level between knee and ankle, left lower leg** A 📞
           (Ex:) See S78.012
       ● **S88.129   Partial traumatic amputation at level between knee and ankle, unspecified lower leg** A 📞
           (Ex:) See S78.019

   ● **S88.9   Traumatic amputation of lower leg, level unspecified**
     ● **S88.91   Complete traumatic amputation of lower leg, level unspecified**
       ● **S88.911   Complete traumatic amputation of right lower leg, level unspecified** A 📞
           (Ex:) See S78.011
       ● **S88.912   Complete traumatic amputation of left lower leg, level unspecified** A 📞
           (Ex:) See S78.012
       ● **S88.919   Complete traumatic amputation of unspecified lower leg, level unspecified** A 📞
           (Ex:) See S78.019

     ● **S88.92   Partial traumatic amputation of lower leg, level unspecified**
       ● **S88.921   Partial traumatic amputation of right lower leg, level unspecified** A 📞
           (Ex:) See S78.011
       ● **S88.922   Partial traumatic amputation of left lower leg, level unspecified** A 📞
           (Ex:) See S78.012
       ● **S88.929   Partial traumatic amputation of unspecified lower leg, level unspecified** A 📞
           (Ex:) See S78.019

● **S89   Other and unspecified injuries of lower leg**
      Note: A fracture not indicated as open or closed should be coded to closed

      Excludes2   other and unspecified injuries of ankle and foot (S99.-)

      The appropriate 7th character is to be added to each code from subcategories S89.0, S89.1, S89.2, and S89.3

A	initial encounter for closed fracture
D	subsequent encounter for fracture with routine healing
G	subsequent encounter for fracture with delayed healing
K	subsequent encounter for fracture with nonunion
P	subsequent encounter for fracture with malunion
S	sequela

   ● **S89.0   Physeal fracture of upper end of tibia**
     ● **S89.00   Unspecified physeal fracture of upper end of tibia**
       ● **S89.001   Unspecified physeal fracture of upper end of right tibia** A, K, P 📞, A 📞
           (Ex:) **For S89.001[A]:** See S82.101[A]
             For S89.001[K,P]: See S02.0[K]
       ● **S89.002   Unspecified physeal fracture of upper end of left tibia** A, K, P 📞, A 📞
           (Ex:) **For S89.002[A]:** See S82.102[A]
             For S89.002[K,P]: See S02.0[K]
       ● **S89.009   Unspecified physeal fracture of upper end of unspecified tibia** A, K, P 📞, A 📞
           (Ex:) **For S89.009[A]:** See S82.101[B,C]
             For S89.009[K,P]: See S02.0[K]
     ● **S89.01   Salter-Harris Type I physeal fracture of upper end of tibia**
       ● **S89.011   Salter-Harris Type I physeal fracture of upper end of right tibia** A, K, P 📞, A 📞
           (Ex:) **For S89.011[A]:** See S82.101[A]
             For S89.011[K,P]: See S02.0[K]
       ● **S89.012   Salter-Harris Type I physeal fracture of upper end of left tibia** A, K, P 📞, A 📞
           (Ex:) **For S89.012[A]:** See S82.102[A]
             For S89.012[K,P]: See S02.0[K]
       ● **S89.019   Salter-Harris Type I physeal fracture of upper end of unspecified tibia** A, K, P 📞, A 📞
           (Ex:) **For S89.019[A]:** See S82.101[B,C]
             For S89.019[K,P]: See S02.0[K]

◀ New   ◀══ Revised   ~~deleted~~ Deleted   Excludes 1   Excludes 2   Includes   Use additional   Code first   Code also   Unspecified

OGCR Official Guidelines   ● Unacceptable Principal Diagnosis   X Assign placeholder X   📞 Use Additional Character(s)   ▶ Manifestation Code   **Coding Clinic**

● **S89.02   Salter-Harris Type II physeal fracture of upper end of tibia**
  ● **S89.021   Salter-Harris Type II physeal fracture of upper end of right tibia** A, K, P 🐾, A 🐾
      (Ex:) For S89.021[A]: See S82.101[A]
           For S89.021[K,P]: See S02.0[K]
  ● **S89.022   Salter-Harris Type II physeal fracture of upper end of left tibia** A, K, P 🐾, A 🐾
      (Ex:) For S89.022[A]: See S82.102[A]
           For S89.022[K,P]: See S02.0[K]
  ● **S89.029   Salter-Harris Type II physeal fracture of upper end of unspecified tibia** A, K, P 🐾, A 🐾
      (Ex:) For S89.029[A]: See S82.101[B,C]
           For S89.029[K,P]: See S02.0[K]

● **S89.03   Salter-Harris Type III physeal fracture of upper end of tibia**
  ● **S89.031   Salter-Harris Type III physeal fracture of upper end of right tibia** A, K, P 🐾, A 🐾
      (Ex:) For S89.031[A]: See S82.101[A]
           For S89.031[K,P]: See S02.0[K]
  ● **S89.032   Salter-Harris Type III physeal fracture of upper end of left tibia** A, K, P 🐾, A 🐾
      (Ex:) For S89.032[A]: See S82.102[A]
           For S89.032[K,P]: See S02.0[K]
  ● **S89.039   Salter-Harris Type III physeal fracture of upper end of unspecified tibia** A, K, P 🐾, A 🐾
      (Ex:) For S89.039[A]: See S82.101[B,C]
           For S89.039[K,P]: See S02.0[K]

● **S89.04   Salter-Harris Type IV physeal fracture of upper end of tibia**
  ● **S89.041   Salter-Harris Type IV physeal fracture of upper end of right tibia** A, K, P 🐾, A 🐾
      (Ex:) For S89.041[A]: See S82.101[A]
           For S89.041[K,P]: See S02.0[K]
  ● **S89.042   Salter-Harris Type IV physeal fracture of upper end of left tibia** A, K, P 🐾, A 🐾
      (Ex:) For S89.042[A]: See S82.102[A]
           For S89.042[K,P]: See S02.0[K]
  ● **S89.049   Salter-Harris Type IV physeal fracture of upper end of unspecified tibia** A, K, P 🐾, A 🐾
      (Ex:) For S89.049[A]: See S82.101[B,C]
           For S89.049[K,P]: See S02.0[K]

● **S89.09   Other physeal fracture of upper end of tibia**
  ● **S89.091   Other physeal fracture of upper end of right tibia** A, K, P 🐾, A 🐾
      (Ex:) For S89.091[A]: See S82.101[A]
           For S89.091[K,P]: See S02.0[K]
  ● **S89.092   Other physeal fracture of upper end of left tibia** A, K, P 🐾, A 🐾
      (Ex:) For S89.092[A]: See S82.102[A]
           For S89.092[K,P]: See S02.0[K]
  ● **S89.099   Other physeal fracture of upper end of unspecified tibia** A, K, P 🐾, A 🐾
      (Ex:) For S89.099[A]: See S82.101[B,C]
           For S89.099[K,P]: See S02.0[K]

● **S89.1   Physeal fracture of lower end of tibia**
    (Ex:) For category S89.1 CC codes: See S02.0[K]
  ● **S89.10   Unspecified physeal fracture of lower end of tibia**
    ● **S89.101   Unspecified physeal fracture of lower end of right tibia** K, P 🐾
    ● **S89.102   Unspecified physeal fracture of lower end of left tibia** K, P 🐾
    ● **S89.109   Unspecified physeal fracture of lower end of unspecified tibia** K, P 🐾
  ● **S89.11   Salter-Harris Type I physeal fracture of lower end of tibia**
    ● **S89.111   Salter-Harris Type I physeal fracture of lower end of right tibia** K, P 🐾
    ● **S89.112   Salter-Harris Type I physeal fracture of lower end of left tibia** K, P 🐾
    ● **S89.119   Salter-Harris Type I physeal fracture of lower end of unspecified tibia** K, P 🐾
  ● **S89.12   Salter-Harris Type II physeal fracture of lower end of tibia**
    ● **S89.121   Salter-Harris Type II physeal fracture of lower end of right tibia** K, P 🐾
    ● **S89.122   Salter-Harris Type II physeal fracture of lower end of left tibia** K, P 🐾
    ● **S89.129   Salter-Harris Type II physeal fracture of lower end of unspecified tibia** K, P 🐾
  ● **S89.13   Salter-Harris Type III physeal fracture of lower end of tibia**
      Excludes1   fracture of medial malleolus (adult) (S82.5-)
    ● **S89.131   Salter-Harris Type III physeal fracture of lower end of right tibia** K, P 🐾
    ● **S89.132   Salter-Harris Type III physeal fracture of lower end of left tibia** K, P 🐾
    ● **S89.139   Salter-Harris Type III physeal fracture of lower end of unspecified tibia** K, P 🐾
  ● **S89.14   Salter-Harris Type IV physeal fracture of lower end of tibia**
      Excludes1   fracture of medial malleolus (adult) (S82.5-)
    ● **S89.141   Salter-Harris Type IV physeal fracture of lower end of right tibia** K, P 🐾
    ● **S89.142   Salter-Harris Type IV physeal fracture of lower end of left tibia** K, P 🐾
    ● **S89.149   Salter-Harris Type IV physeal fracture of lower end of unspecified tibia** K, P 🐾
  ● **S89.19   Other physeal fracture of lower end of tibia**
    ● **S89.191   Other physeal fracture of lower end of right tibia** K, P 🐾
    ● **S89.192   Other physeal fracture of lower end of left tibia** K, P 🐾
    ● **S89.199   Other physeal fracture of lower end of unspecified tibia** K, P 🐾

● **S89.2   Physeal fracture of upper end of fibula**
    (Ex:) For category S89.2 CC codes: See S02.0[K]
  ● **S89.20   Unspecified physeal fracture of upper end of fibula**
    ● **S89.201   Unspecified physeal fracture of upper end of right fibula** K, P 🐾
    ● **S89.202   Unspecified physeal fracture of upper end of left fibula** K, P 🐾
    ● **S89.209   Unspecified physeal fracture of upper end of unspecified fibula** K, P 🐾

CHAPTER 19 (S00-T88)

S89.21 Salter-Harris Type I physeal fracture of upper end of fibula

    S89.211 Salter-Harris Type I physeal fracture of upper end of right fibula K, P 🔖

    S89.212 Salter-Harris Type I physeal fracture of upper end of left fibula K, P 🔖

    S89.219 Salter-Harris Type I physeal fracture of upper end of unspecified fibula K, P 🔖

S89.22 Salter-Harris Type II physeal fracture of upper end of fibula

    S89.221 Salter-Harris Type II physeal fracture of upper end of right fibula K, P 🔖

    S89.222 Salter-Harris Type II physeal fracture of upper end of left fibula K, P 🔖

    S89.229 Salter-Harris Type II physeal fracture of upper end of unspecified fibula K, P 🔖

S89.29 Other physeal fracture of upper end of fibula

    S89.291 Other physeal fracture of upper end of right fibula K, P 🔖

    S89.292 Other physeal fracture of upper end of left fibula K, P 🔖

    S89.299 Other physeal fracture of upper end of unspecified fibula K, P 🔖

S89.3 Physeal fracture of lower end of fibula

    Ex: For category S89.3 CC codes: See S02.0[K]

    S89.30 Unspecified physeal fracture of lower end of fibula

        S89.301 Unspecified physeal fracture of lower end of right fibula K, P 🔖

        S89.302 Unspecified physeal fracture of lower end of left fibula K, P 🔖

        S89.309 Unspecified physeal fracture of lower end of unspecified fibula K, P 🔖

    S89.31 Salter-Harris Type I physeal fracture of lower end of fibula

        S89.311 Salter-Harris Type I physeal fracture of lower end of right fibula K, P 🔖

        S89.312 Salter-Harris Type I physeal fracture of lower end of left fibula K, P 🔖

        S89.319 Salter-Harris Type I physeal fracture of lower end of unspecified fibula K, P 🔖

    S89.32 Salter-Harris Type II physeal fracture of lower end of fibula

        S89.321 Salter-Harris Type II physeal fracture of lower end of right fibula K, P 🔖

        S89.322 Salter-Harris Type II physeal fracture of lower end of left fibula K, P 🔖

        S89.329 Salter-Harris Type II physeal fracture of lower end of unspecified fibula K, P 🔖

    S89.39 Other physeal fracture of lower end of fibula

        S89.391 Other physeal fracture of lower end of right fibula K, P 🔖

        S89.392 Other physeal fracture of lower end of left fibula K, P 🔖

        S89.399 Other physeal fracture of lower end of unspecified fibula K, P 🔖

S89.8 Other specified injuries of lower leg

The appropriate 7th character is to be added to each code in subcategory S89.8

A	initial encounter
D	subsequent encounter
S	sequela

X **S89.80** Other specified injuries of unspecified lower leg

X **S89.81** Other specified injuries of right lower leg

X **S89.82** Other specified injuries of left lower leg

S89.9 Unspecified injury of lower leg

The appropriate 7th character is to be added to each code in subcategory S89.9

A	initial encounter
D	subsequent encounter
S	sequela

X **S89.90** Unspecified injury of unspecified lower leg

X **S89.91** Unspecified injury of right lower leg

X **S89.92** Unspecified injury of left lower leg

INJURIES TO THE ANKLE AND FOOT (S90-S99)

Excludes2 burns and corrosions (T20-T32)
fracture of ankle and malleolus (S82.-)
frostbite (T33-T34)
insect bite or sting, venomous (T63.4)

S90 Superficial injury of ankle, foot and toes

The appropriate 7th character is to be added to each code from category S90

A	initial encounter
D	subsequent encounter
S	sequela

S90.0 Contusion of ankle

X **S90.00** Contusion of unspecified ankle

X **S90.01** Contusion of right ankle

X **S90.02** Contusion of left ankle

S90.1 Contusion of toe without damage to nail

    S90.11 Contusion of great toe without damage to nail

        S90.111 Contusion of right great toe without damage to nail

        S90.112 Contusion of left great toe without damage to nail

        S90.119 Contusion of unspecified great toe without damage to nail

    S90.12 Contusion of lesser toe without damage to nail

        S90.121 Contusion of right lesser toe(s) without damage to nail

        S90.122 Contusion of left lesser toe(s) without damage to nail

        S90.129 Contusion of unspecified lesser toe(s) without damage to nail

        Contusion of toe NOS

S90.2 Contusion of toe with damage to nail

    S90.21 Contusion of great toe with damage to nail

        S90.211 Contusion of right great toe with damage to nail

        S90.212 Contusion of left great toe with damage to nail

        S90.219 Contusion of unspecified great toe with damage to nail

◀ New   ◀ Revised   ~~deleted~~ Deleted   Excludes 1   Excludes 2   Includes   Use additional   Code first   Code also   Unspecified

OGCR Official Guidelines   ● Unacceptable Principal Diagnosis   X Assign placeholder X   ● Use Additional Character(s)   ▶ Manifestation Code   **Coding Clinic**

● **S90.22**   Contusion of lesser toe with damage to nail
   ● **S90.221**   Contusion of right lesser toe(s) with damage to nail
   ● **S90.222**   Contusion of left lesser toe(s) with damage to nail
   ● **S90.229**   Contusion of unspecified lesser toe(s) with damage to nail

● **S90.3**   Contusion of foot
   Excludes2   contusion of toes (S90.1-, S90.2-)
  X ● **S90.30**   Contusion of unspecified foot
        Contusion of foot NOS
  X ● **S90.31**   Contusion of right foot
  X ● **S90.32**   Contusion of left foot

● **S90.4**   Other superficial injuries of toe
   ● **S90.41**   Abrasion of toe
     ● **S90.411**   Abrasion, right great toe
     ● **S90.412**   Abrasion, left great toe
     ● **S90.413**   Abrasion, unspecified great toe
     ● **S90.414**   Abrasion, right lesser toe(s)
     ● **S90.415**   Abrasion, left lesser toe(s)
     ● **S90.416**   Abrasion, unspecified lesser toe(s)
   ● **S90.42**   Blister (nonthermal) of toe
     ● **S90.421**   Blister (nonthermal), right great toe
     ● **S90.422**   Blister (nonthermal), left great toe
     ● **S90.423**   Blister (nonthermal), unspecified great toe
     ● **S90.424**   Blister (nonthermal), right lesser toe(s)
     ● **S90.425**   Blister (nonthermal), left lesser toe(s)
     ● **S90.426**   Blister (nonthermal), unspecified lesser toe(s)
   ● **S90.44**   External constriction of toe
        Hair tourniquet syndrome of toe
     ● **S90.441**   External constriction, right great toe
     ● **S90.442**   External constriction, left great toe
     ● **S90.443**   External constriction, unspecified great toe
     ● **S90.444**   External constriction, right lesser toe(s)
     ● **S90.445**   External constriction, left lesser toe(s)
     ● **S90.446**   External constriction, unspecified lesser toe(s)
   ● **S90.45**   Superficial foreign body of toe
        Splinter in the toe
     ● **S90.451**   Superficial foreign body, right great toe
     ● **S90.452**   Superficial foreign body, left great toe
     ● **S90.453**   Superficial foreign body, unspecified great toe
     ● **S90.454**   Superficial foreign body, right lesser toe(s)
     ● **S90.455**   Superficial foreign body, left lesser toe(s)
     ● **S90.456**   Superficial foreign body, unspecified lesser toe(s)

● **S90.46**   Insect bite (nonvenomous) of toe
   ● **S90.461**   Insect bite (nonvenomous), right great toe
   ● **S90.462**   Insect bite (nonvenomous), left great toe
   ● **S90.463**   Insect bite (nonvenomous), unspecified great toe
   ● **S90.464**   Insect bite (nonvenomous), right lesser toe(s)
   ● **S90.465**   Insect bite (nonvenomous), left lesser toe(s)
   ● **S90.466**   Insect bite (nonvenomous), unspecified lesser toe(s)

● **S90.47**   Other superficial bite of toe
   Excludes1   open bite of toe (S91.15-, S91.25-)
   ● **S90.471**   Other superficial bite of right great toe
   ● **S90.472**   Other superficial bite of left great toe
   ● **S90.473**   Other superficial bite of unspecified great toe
   ● **S90.474**   Other superficial bite of right lesser toe(s)
   ● **S90.475**   Other superficial bite of left lesser toe(s)
   ● **S90.476**   Other superficial bite of unspecified lesser toe(s)

● **S90.5**   Other superficial injuries of ankle
   ● **S90.51**   Abrasion of ankle
     ● **S90.511**   Abrasion, right ankle
     ● **S90.512**   Abrasion, left ankle
     ● **S90.519**   Abrasion, unspecified ankle
   ● **S90.52**   Blister (nonthermal) of ankle
     ● **S90.521**   Blister (nonthermal), right ankle
     ● **S90.522**   Blister (nonthermal), left ankle
     ● **S90.529**   Blister (nonthermal), unspecified ankle
   ● **S90.54**   External constriction of ankle
     ● **S90.541**   External constriction, right ankle
     ● **S90.542**   External constriction, left ankle
     ● **S90.549**   External constriction, unspecified ankle
   ● **S90.55**   Superficial foreign body of ankle
        Splinter in the ankle
     ● **S90.551**   Superficial foreign body, right ankle
     ● **S90.552**   Superficial foreign body, left ankle
     ● **S90.559**   Superficial foreign body, unspecified ankle
   ● **S90.56**   Insect bite (nonvenomous) of ankle
     ● **S90.561**   Insect bite (nonvenomous), right ankle
     ● **S90.562**   Insect bite (nonvenomous), left ankle
     ● **S90.569**   Insect bite (nonvenomous), unspecified ankle
   ● **S90.57**   Other superficial bite of ankle
     Excludes1   open bite of ankle (S91.05-)
     ● **S90.571**   Other superficial bite of ankle, right ankle
     ● **S90.572**   Other superficial bite of ankle, left ankle
     ● **S90.579**   Other superficial bite of ankle, unspecified ankle

CHAPTER 19 (S00-T88)

N   Newborn Age: 0   **P**   Pediatric Age: 0–17   **M**   Maternity DX: 12–55   **A**   Adult Age: 15–124   ♀   Females Only   ♂   Males Only

🏵 Complication\Comorbidity   🏵 Major C\C   (Ex) CC/MCC Exclusions   🏵 Hospital-Acquired Condition   **1401**

CHAPTER 19 (S00-T88)

- ● S90.8 **Other superficial injuries of foot**
  - ● S90.81 **Abrasion of foot**
    - ● S90.811 **Abrasion, right foot**
    - ● S90.812 **Abrasion, left foot**
    - ● S90.819 **Abrasion, unspecified foot**
  - ● S90.82 **Blister (nonthermal) of foot**
    - ● S90.821 **Blister (nonthermal), right foot**
    - ● S90.822 **Blister (nonthermal), left foot**
    - ● S90.829 **Blister (nonthermal), unspecified foot**
  - ● S90.84 **External constriction of foot**
    - ● S90.841 **External constriction, right foot**
    - ● S90.842 **External constriction, left foot**
    - ● S90.849 **External constriction, unspecified foot**
  - ● S90.85 **Superficial foreign body of foot**
    Splinter in the foot
    - ● S90.851 **Superficial foreign body, right foot**
    - ● S90.852 **Superficial foreign body, left foot**
    - ● S90.859 **Superficial foreign body, unspecified foot**
  - ● S90.86 **Insect bite (nonvenomous) of foot**
    - ● S90.861 **Insect bite (nonvenomous), right foot**
    - ● S90.862 **Insect bite (nonvenomous), left foot**
    - ● S90.869 **Insect bite (nonvenomous), unspecified foot**
  - ● S90.87 **Other superficial bite of foot**
    Excludes1 open bite of foot (S91.35-)
    - ● S90.871 **Other superficial bite of right foot**
    - ● S90.872 **Other superficial bite of left foot**
    - ● S90.879 **Other superficial bite of unspecified foot**
- ● S90.9 **Unspecified superficial injury of ankle, foot and toe**
  - ● S90.91 **Unspecified superficial injury of ankle**
    - ● S90.911 **Unspecified superficial injury of right ankle**
    - ● S90.912 **Unspecified superficial injury of left ankle**
    - ● S90.919 **Unspecified superficial injury of unspecified ankle**
  - ● S90.92 **Unspecified superficial injury of foot**
    - ● S90.921 **Unspecified superficial injury of right foot**
    - ● S90.922 **Unspecified superficial injury of left foot**
    - ● S90.929 **Unspecified superficial injury of unspecified foot**
  - S90.93 **Unspecified superficial injury of toes**
    - ● S90.931 **Unspecified superficial injury of right great toe**
    - ● S90.932 **Unspecified superficial injury of left great toe**
    - ● S90.933 **Unspecified superficial injury of unspecified great toe**
    - ● S90.934 **Unspecified superficial injury of right lesser toe(s)**
    - ● S90.935 **Unspecified superficial injury of left lesser toe(s)**
    - ● S90.936 **Unspecified superficial injury of unspecified lesser toe(s)**

- ● S91 **Open wound of ankle, foot and toes**
  Code also any associated wound infection
  Excludes1 open fracture of ankle, foot and toes (S92.-with 7th character B)
  traumatic amputation of ankle and foot (S98.-)
  The appropriate 7th character is to be added to each code from category S91

A	initial encounter
D	subsequent encounter
S	sequela

  - ● S91.0 **Open wound of ankle**
    - ● S91.00 **Unspecified open wound of ankle**
      - ● S91.001 **Unspecified open wound, right ankle**
      - ● S91.002 **Unspecified open wound, left ankle**
      - ● S91.009 **Unspecified open wound, unspecified ankle**
    - ● S91.01 **Laceration without foreign body of ankle**
      - ● S91.011 **Laceration without foreign body, right ankle**
      - ● S91.012 **Laceration without foreign body, left ankle**
      - ● S91.019 **Laceration without foreign body, unspecified ankle**
    - ● S91.02 **Laceration with foreign body of ankle**
      - ● S91.021 **Laceration with foreign body, right ankle**
      - ● S91.022 **Laceration with foreign body, left ankle**
      - ● S91.029 **Laceration with foreign body, unspecified ankle**
    - ● S91.03 **Puncture wound without foreign body of ankle**
      - ● S91.031 **Puncture wound without foreign body, right ankle**
      - ● S91.032 **Puncture wound without foreign body, left ankle**
      - ● S91.039 **Puncture wound without foreign body, unspecified ankle**
    - ● S91.04 **Puncture wound with foreign body of ankle**
      - ● S91.041 **Puncture wound with foreign body, right ankle**
      - ● S91.042 **Puncture wound with foreign body, left ankle**
      - ● S91.049 **Puncture wound with foreign body, unspecified ankle**
    - ● S91.05 **Open bite of ankle**
      Excludes1 superficial bite of ankle (S90.56-, S90.57-)
      - ● S91.051 **Open bite, right ankle**
      - ● S91.052 **Open bite, left ankle**
      - ● S91.059 **Open bite, unspecified ankle**
  - ● S91.1 **Open wound of toe without damage to nail**
    - ● S91.10 **Unspecified open wound of toe without damage to nail**
      - ● S91.101 **Unspecified open wound of right great toe without damage to nail**
      - ● S91.102 **Unspecified open wound of left great toe without damage to nail**
      - ● S91.103 **Unspecified open wound of unspecified great toe without damage to nail**

◄ New ◄ Revised ~~deleted~~ Deleted | Excludes 1 | Excludes 2 | Includes | Use additional | Code first | Code also | Unspecified
OGCR Official Guidelines ● Unacceptable Principal Diagnosis X Assign placeholder X ● Use Additional Character(s) ▶ Manifestation Code **Coding Clinic**

● S91.104 Unspecified open wound of right lesser toe(s) without damage to nail

● S91.105 Unspecified open wound of left lesser toe(s) without damage to nail

● S91.106 Unspecified open wound of unspecified lesser toe(s) without damage to nail

● S91.109 Unspecified open wound of unspecified toe(s) without damage to nail

● S91.11 Laceration without foreign body of toe without damage to nail

● S91.111 Laceration without foreign body of right great toe without damage to nail

● S91.112 Laceration without foreign body of left great toe without damage to nail

● S91.113 Laceration without foreign body of unspecified great toe without damage to nail

● S91.114 Laceration without foreign body of right lesser toe(s) without damage to nail

● S91.115 Laceration without foreign body of left lesser toe(s) without damage to nail

● S91.116 Laceration without foreign body of unspecified lesser toe(s) without damage to nail

● S91.119 Laceration without foreign body of unspecified toe without damage to nail

● S91.12 Laceration with foreign body of toe without damage to nail

● S91.121 Laceration with foreign body of right great toe without damage to nail

● S91.122 Laceration with foreign body of left great toe without damage to nail

● S91.123 Laceration with foreign body of unspecified great toe without damage to nail

● S91.124 Laceration with foreign body of right lesser toe(s) without damage to nail

● S91.125 Laceration with foreign body of left lesser toe(s) without damage to nail

● S91.126 Laceration with foreign body of unspecified lesser toe(s) without damage to nail

● S91.129 Laceration with foreign body of unspecified toe(s) without damage to nail

● S91.13 Puncture wound without foreign body of toe without damage to nail

● S91.131 Puncture wound without foreign body of right great toe without damage to nail

● S91.132 Puncture wound without foreign body of left great toe without damage to nail

● S91.133 Puncture wound without foreign body of unspecified great toe without damage to nail

● S91.134 Puncture wound without foreign body of right lesser toe(s) without damage to nail

● S91.135 Puncture wound without foreign body of left lesser toe(s) without damage to nail

● S91.136 Puncture wound without foreign body of unspecified lesser toe(s) without damage to nail

● S91.139 Puncture wound without foreign body of unspecified toe(s) without damage to nail

● S91.14 Puncture wound with foreign body of toe without damage to nail

● S91.141 Puncture wound with foreign body of right great toe without damage to nail

● S91.142 Puncture wound with foreign body of left great toe without damage to nail

● S91.143 Puncture wound with foreign body of unspecified great toe without damage to nail

● S91.144 Puncture wound with foreign body of right lesser toe(s) without damage to nail

● S91.145 Puncture wound with foreign body of left lesser toe(s) without damage to nail

● S91.146 Puncture wound with foreign body of unspecified lesser toe(s) without damage to nail

● S91.149 Puncture wound with foreign body of unspecified toe(s) without damage to nail

● S91.15 Open bite of toe without damage to nail
Bite of toe NOS

Excludes1   superficial bite of toe (S90.46-, S90.47-)

● S91.151 Open bite of right great toe without damage to nail

● S91.152 Open bite of left great toe without damage to nail

● S91.153 Open bite of unspecified great toe without damage to nail

● S91.154 Open bite of right lesser toe(s) without damage to nail

● S91.155 Open bite of left lesser toe(s) without damage to nail

● S91.156 Open bite of unspecified lesser toe(s) without damage to nail

● S91.159 Open bite of unspecified toe(s) without damage to nail

● S91.2   Open wound of toe with damage to nail

● S91.20   Unspecified open wound of toe with damage to nail

● S91.201 Unspecified open wound of right great toe with damage to nail

● S91.202 Unspecified open wound of left great toe with damage to nail

● S91.203 Unspecified open wound of unspecified great toe with damage to nail

● S91.204 Unspecified open wound of right lesser toe(s) with damage to nail

● S91.205 Unspecified open wound of left lesser toe(s) with damage to nail

● S91.206 Unspecified open wound of unspecified lesser toe(s) with damage to nail

● S91.209 Unspecified open wound of unspecified toe(s) with damage to nail

N Newborn Age: 0   **P** Pediatric Age: 0–17   **M** Maternity DX: 12–55   **A** Adult Age: 15–124   ♀ Females Only   ♂ Males Only

🅒 Complication\Comorbidity   🅜 Major C\C   🄴🅇 CC/MCC Exclusions   🅗 Hospital-Acquired Condition

1403

● **S91.21** **Laceration without foreign body of toe with damage to nail**
- ● **S91.211** Laceration without foreign body of right great toe with damage to nail
- ● **S91.212** Laceration without foreign body of left great toe with damage to nail
- ● **S91.213** Laceration without foreign body of unspecified great toe with damage to nail
- ● **S91.214** Laceration without foreign body of right lesser toe(s) with damage to nail
- ● **S91.215** Laceration without foreign body of left lesser toe(s) with damage to nail
- ● **S91.216** Laceration without foreign body of unspecified lesser toe(s) with damage to nail
- ● **S91.219** Laceration without foreign body of unspecified toe(s) with damage to nail

● **S91.22** **Laceration with foreign body of toe with damage to nail**
- ● **S91.221** Laceration with foreign body of right great toe with damage to nail
- ● **S91.222** Laceration with foreign body of left great toe with damage to nail
- ● **S91.223** Laceration with foreign body of unspecified great toe with damage to nail
- ● **S91.224** Laceration with foreign body of right lesser toe(s) with damage to nail
- ● **S91.225** Laceration with foreign body of left lesser toe(s) with damage to nail
- ● **S91.226** Laceration with foreign body of unspecified lesser toe(s) with damage to nail
- ● **S91.229** Laceration with foreign body of unspecified toe(s) with damage to nail

● **S91.23** **Puncture wound without foreign body of toe with damage to nail**
- ● **S91.231** Puncture wound without foreign body of right great toe with damage to nail
- ● **S91.232** Puncture wound without foreign body of left great toe with damage to nail
- ● **S91.233** Puncture wound without foreign body of unspecified great toe with damage to nail
- ● **S91.234** Puncture wound without foreign body of right lesser toe(s) with damage to nail
- ● **S91.235** Puncture wound without foreign body of left lesser toe(s) with damage to nail
- ● **S91.236** Puncture wound without foreign body of unspecified lesser toe(s) with damage to nail
- ● **S91.239** Puncture wound without foreign body of unspecified toe(s) with damage to nail

● **S91.24** **Puncture wound with foreign body of toe with damage to nail**
- ● **S91.241** Puncture wound with foreign body of right great toe with damage to nail
- ● **S91.242** Puncture wound with foreign body of left great toe with damage to nail
- ● **S91.243** Puncture wound with foreign body of unspecified great toe with damage to nail
- ● **S91.244** Puncture wound with foreign body of right lesser toe(s) with damage to nail

● **S91.245** Puncture wound with foreign body of left lesser toe(s) with damage to nail
● **S91.246** Puncture wound with foreign body of unspecified lesser toe(s) with damage to nail
● **S91.249** Puncture wound with foreign body of unspecified toe(s) with damage to nail

● **S91.25** **Open bite of toe with damage to nail**
Bite of toe with damage to nail NOS
Excludes1   superficial bite of toe (S90.46-, S90.47-)
- ● **S91.251** Open bite of right great toe with damage to nail
- ● **S91.252** Open bite of left great toe with damage to nail
- ● **S91.253** Open bite of unspecified great toe with damage to nail
- ● **S91.254** Open bite of right lesser toe(s) with damage to nail
- ● **S91.255** Open bite of left lesser toe(s) with damage to nail
- ● **S91.256** Open bite of unspecified lesser toe(s) with damage to nail
- ● **S91.259** Open bite of unspecified toe(s) with damage to nail

● **S91.3** **Open wound of foot**
- ● **S91.30** **Unspecified open wound of foot**
  - ● **S91.301** Unspecified open wound, right foot
  - ● **S91.302** Unspecified open wound, left foot
  - ● **S91.309** Unspecified open wound, unspecified foot
- ● **S91.31** **Laceration without foreign body of foot**
  - ● **S91.311** Laceration without foreign body, right foot
  - ● **S91.312** Laceration without foreign body, left foot
  - ● **S91.319** Laceration without foreign body, unspecified foot
- ● **S91.32** **Laceration with foreign body of foot**
  - ● **S91.321** Laceration with foreign body, right foot
  - ● **S91.322** Laceration with foreign body, left foot
  - ● **S91.329** Laceration with foreign body, unspecified foot
- ● **S91.33** **Puncture wound without foreign body of foot**
  - ● **S91.331** Puncture wound without foreign body, right foot
  - ● **S91.332** Puncture wound without foreign body, left foot
  - ● **S91.339** Puncture wound without foreign body, unspecified foot
- ● **S91.34** **Puncture wound with foreign body of foot**
  - ● **S91.341** Puncture wound with foreign body, right foot
  - ● **S91.342** Puncture wound with foreign body, left foot
  - ● **S91.349** Puncture wound with foreign body, unspecified foot
- ● **S91.35** **Open bite of foot**
  Excludes1   superficial bite of foot (S90.86-, S90.87-)
  - ● **S91.351** Open bite, right foot
  - ● **S91.352** Open bite, left foot
  - ● **S91.359** Open bite, unspecified foot

◄ New   ◄▦ Revised   ~~deleted~~ Deleted   Excludes 1   Excludes 2   Includes   Use additional   Code first   Code also   Unspecified
OGCR Official Guidelines   ● Unacceptable Principal Diagnosis   X Assign placeholder X   ● Use Additional Character(s)   ▶ Manifestation Code   **Coding Clinic**

● S92 **Fracture of foot and toe, except ankle**

Note: A fracture not indicated as displaced or nondisplaced should be coded to displaced

A fracture not indicated as open or closed should be coded to closed

Excludes1   traumatic amputation of ankle and foot (S98.-)

Excludes2   fracture of ankle (S82.-)
fracture of malleolus (S82.-)

The appropriate 7th character is to be added to each code from category S92

> A   initial encounter for closed fracture
> B   initial encounter for open fracture
> D   subsequent encounter for fracture with routine healing
> G   subsequent encounter for fracture with delayed healing
> K   subsequent encounter for fracture with nonunion
> P   subsequent encounter for fracture with malunion
> S   sequela

● S92.0   **Fracture of calcaneus**
Heel bone   Os calcis

Excludes2   Physeal fracture of calcaneus (S99.0-) ◀

(Ex) **For category S92.0 CC codes S92.0[B]:** M80.00X-M80.019[A], M80.041-M80.049[A], M80.061-M80.819[A], M80.841-M80.849[A], M80.861-M80.879[A], M84.40X-M84.419[A], M84.441-M84.446[A], M84.454[A], M84.461-M84.519[A], M84.541-M84.550[A], M84.561-M84.576[A], M84.60X-M84.619[A], M84.641-M84.650[A], M84.661-M84.68X[A], S03.8XX-S03.9XX[A], S29.011-S29.019[A], S38.3XX[A], S39.011-S39.013[A], S73.101-S73.199[A], S76.001-S76.019[A], S76.091-S76.219[A], S76.291-S76.319[A], S76.391-S76.819[A], S76.891-S76.919[A], S76.991-S76.999[A], S79.811-S79.929[A], S82.90X-S82.92X[A,B,C], S92.001-S92.066[B], S92.101-S92.356[A,B], S92.811-S92.819[A,B], S92.901-S92.909[A,B], T14.90-T14.91, T79.A9X-T79.9XX[A] **For S92.0[K,P]:** See S02.0[K]

● S92.00   **Unspecified fracture of calcaneus**

● S92.001   Unspecified fracture of right calcaneus B, K, P 🔹, B 🔹

● S92.002   Unspecified fracture of left calcaneus B, K, P 🔹, B 🔹

● S92.009   Unspecified fracture of unspecified calcaneus B, K, P 🔹, B 🔹

● S92.01   **Fracture of body of calcaneus**

● S92.011   Displaced fracture of body of right calcaneus B, K, P 🔹, B 🔹

● S92.012   Displaced fracture of body of left calcaneus B, K, P 🔹, B 🔹

● S92.013   Displaced fracture of body of unspecified calcaneus B, K, P 🔹, B 🔹

● S92.014   Nondisplaced fracture of body of right calcaneus B, K, P 🔹, B 🔹

● S92.015   Nondisplaced fracture of body of left calcaneus B, K, P 🔹, B 🔹

● S92.016   Nondisplaced fracture of body of unspecified calcaneus B, K, P 🔹, B 🔹

● S92.02   **Fracture of anterior process of calcaneus**

● S92.021   Displaced fracture of anterior process of right calcaneus B, K, P 🔹, B 🔹

● S92.022   Displaced fracture of anterior process of left calcaneus B, K, P 🔹, B 🔹

● S92.023   Displaced fracture of anterior process of unspecified calcaneus B, K, P 🔹, B 🔹

● S92.024   Nondisplaced fracture of anterior process of right calcaneus B, K, P 🔹, B 🔹

● S92.025   Nondisplaced fracture of anterior process of left calcaneus B, K, P 🔹, B 🔹

● S92.026   Nondisplaced fracture of anterior process of unspecified calcaneus B, K, P 🔹, B 🔹

● S92.03   **Avulsion fracture of tuberosity of calcaneus**

● S92.031   Displaced avulsion fracture of tuberosity of right calcaneus B, K, P 🔹, B 🔹

● S92.032   Displaced avulsion fracture of tuberosity of left calcaneus B, K, P 🔹, B 🔹

● S92.033   Displaced avulsion fracture of tuberosity of unspecified calcaneus B, K, P 🔹, B 🔹

● S92.034   Nondisplaced avulsion fracture of tuberosity of right calcaneus B, K, P 🔹, B 🔹

● S92.035   Nondisplaced avulsion fracture of tuberosity of left calcaneus B, K, P 🔹, B 🔹

● S92.036   Nondisplaced avulsion fracture of tuberosity of unspecified calcaneus B, K, P 🔹, B 🔹

● S92.04   **Other fracture of tuberosity of calcaneus**

● S92.041   Displaced other fracture of tuberosity of right calcaneus B, K, P 🔹, B 🔹

● S92.042   Displaced other fracture of tuberosity of left calcaneus B, K, P 🔹, B 🔹

● S92.043   Displaced other fracture of tuberosity of unspecified calcaneus B, K, P 🔹, B 🔹

● S92.044   Nondisplaced other fracture of tuberosity of right calcaneus B, K, P 🔹, B 🔹

● S92.045   Nondisplaced other fracture of tuberosity of left calcaneus B, K, P 🔹, B 🔹

● S92.046   Nondisplaced other fracture of tuberosity of unspecified calcaneus B, K, P 🔹, B 🔹

● S92.05   **Other extraarticular fracture of calcaneus**

● S92.051   Displaced other extraarticular fracture of right calcaneus B, K, P 🔹, B 🔹

● S92.052   Displaced other extraarticular fracture of left calcaneus B, K, P 🔹, B 🔹

● S92.053   Displaced other extraarticular fracture of unspecified calcaneus B, K, P 🔹, B 🔹

● S92.054   Nondisplaced other extraarticular fracture of right calcaneus B, K, P 🔹, B 🔹

● S92.055   Nondisplaced other extraarticular fracture of left calcaneus B, K, P 🔹, B 🔹

● S92.056   Nondisplaced other extraarticular fracture of unspecified calcaneus B, K, P 🔹, B 🔹

● S92.06   **Intraarticular fracture of calcaneus**

● S92.061   Displaced intraarticular fracture of right calcaneus B, K, P 🔹, B 🔹

● S92.062   Displaced intraarticular fracture of left calcaneus B, K, P 🔹, B 🔹

● S92.063   Displaced intraarticular fracture of unspecified calcaneus B, K, P 🔹, B 🔹

● S92.064   Nondisplaced intraarticular fracture of right calcaneus B, K, P 🔹, B 🔹

● S92.065   Nondisplaced intraarticular fracture of left calcaneus B, K, P 🔹, B 🔹

● S92.066   Nondisplaced intraarticular fracture of unspecified calcaneus B, K, P 🔹, B 🔹

N Newborn Age: 0   **P** Pediatric Age: 0–17   **M** Maternity DX: 12–55   **A** Adult Age: 15–124   ♀ Females Only   ♂ Males Only
🔹 Complication\Comorbidity   🔹 Major C\C   (Ex) CC/MCC Exclusions   🔹 Hospital-Acquired Condition

1405

● S92.1   **Fracture of talus**
     Astragalus
     (Ex) For category S92.1 CC codes S92.1[B]: M80.00X-M80.019[A],
     M80.041-M80.049[A], M80.80X-M80.819[A], M80.841-M80.849[A],
     M84.40X-M84.419[A], M84.441-M84.446[A], M84.454[A],
     M84.474-M84.519[A], M84.541-M84.550[A], M84.574-M84.576[A],
     M84.60X-M84.619[A], M84.641-M84.650[A], M84.674-M84.68X[A],
     S03.8XX-S03.9XX[A], S29.011-S29.019[A], S38.3XX[A],
     S39.011-S39.013[A], S73.101-S73.199[A], S76.001-S76.019[A],
     S76.091-S76.219[A], S76.291-S76.319[A], S76.391-S76.819[A],
     S76.891-S76.919[A], S76.991-S76.999[A], S79.821-S79.929[A],
     S82.90X-S82.92X[A,B,C], S92.001-S92.066[B], S92.101-S92.356[A,B],
     S92.811-S92.819[A,B], S92.901-S92.909[A,B], T14.90-T14.91, T79.
     A9X-T79.9XX[A] **For S92.1[K,P]:** See S02.0[K]

  ● S92.10   Unspecified fracture of talus

    ● S92.101   Unspecified fracture of right talus
        B, K, P 🔒, B 🔒

    ● S92.102   Unspecified fracture of left talus
        B, K, P 🔒, B 🔒

    ● S92.109   Unspecified fracture of unspecified
        talus B, K, P 🔒, B 🔒

  ● S92.11   Fracture of neck of talus

    ● S92.111   Displaced fracture of neck of right
        talus B, K, P 🔒, B 🔒

    ● S92.112   Displaced fracture of neck of left
        talus B, K, P 🔒, B 🔒

    ● S92.113   Displaced fracture of neck of
        unspecified talus B, K, P 🔒, B 🔒

    ● S92.114   Nondisplaced fracture of neck of
        right talus B, K, P 🔒, B 🔒

    ● S92.115   Nondisplaced fracture of neck of left
        talus B, K, P 🔒, B 🔒

    ● S92.116   Nondisplaced fracture of neck of
        unspecified talus B, K, P 🔒, B 🔒

  ● S92.12   Fracture of body of talus

    ● S92.121   Displaced fracture of body of right
        talus B, K, P 🔒, B 🔒

    ● S92.122   Displaced fracture of body of left
        talus B, K, P 🔒, B 🔒

    ● S92.123   Displaced fracture of body of
        unspecified talus B, K, P 🔒, B 🔒

    ● S92.124   Nondisplaced fracture of body of
        right talus B, K, P 🔒, B 🔒

    ● S92.125   Nondisplaced fracture of body of left
        talus B, K, P 🔒, B 🔒

    ● S92.126   Nondisplaced fracture of body of
        unspecified talus B, K, P 🔒, B 🔒

  ● S92.13   Fracture of posterior process of talus

    ● S92.131   Displaced fracture of posterior
        process of right talus B, K, P 🔒, B 🔒

    ● S92.132   Displaced fracture of posterior
        process of left talus B, K, P 🔒, B 🔒

    ● S92.133   Displaced fracture of posterior
        process of unspecified talus B, K, P 🔒,
        B 🔒

    ● S92.134   Nondisplaced fracture of posterior
        process of right talus B, K, P 🔒, B 🔒

    ● S92.135   Nondisplaced fracture of posterior
        process of left talus B, K, P 🔒, B 🔒

    ● S92.136   Nondisplaced fracture of posterior
        process of unspecified talus B, K, P 🔒,
        B 🔒

  ● S92.14   Dome fracture of talus
     Excludes1   osteochondritis dissecans
                  (M93.2)

    ● S92.141   Displaced dome fracture of right talus
        B, K, P 🔒, B 🔒

    ● S92.142   Displaced dome fracture of left talus
        B, K, P 🔒, B 🔒

    ● S92.143   Displaced dome fracture of
        unspecified talus B, K, P 🔒, B 🔒

    ● S92.144   Nondisplaced dome fracture of right
        talus B, K, P 🔒, B 🔒

    ● S92.145   Nondisplaced dome fracture of left
        talus B, K, P 🔒, B 🔒

    ● S92.146   Nondisplaced dome fracture of
        unspecified talus B, K, P 🔒, B 🔒

  ● S92.15   Avulsion fracture (chip fracture) of talus

    ● S92.151   Displaced avulsion fracture (chip
        fracture) of right talus B, K, P 🔒, B 🔒

    ● S92.152   Displaced avulsion fracture (chip
        fracture) of left talus B, K, P 🔒, B 🔒

    ● S92.153   Displaced avulsion fracture (chip
        fracture) of unspecified talus
        B, K, P 🔒, B 🔒

    ● S92.154   Nondisplaced avulsion fracture (chip
        fracture) of right talus B, K, P 🔒, B 🔒

    ● S92.155   Nondisplaced avulsion fracture (chip
        fracture) of left talus B, K, P 🔒, B 🔒

    ● S92.156   Nondisplaced avulsion fracture (chip
        fracture) of unspecified talus
        B, K, P 🔒, B 🔒

  ● S92.19   Other fracture of talus

    ● S92.191   Other fracture of right talus B, K, P 🔒,
        B 🔒

    ● S92.192   Other fracture of left talus B, K, P 🔒,
        B 🔒

    ● S92.199   Other fracture of unspecified talus
        B, K, P 🔒, B 🔒

● S92.2   **Fracture of other and unspecified tarsal bone(s)**
     (Ex) For category S92.2 CC codes S92.2[B]: See S92.1[B] For S92.2[K,P]:
     See S02.0[K] unless otherwise indicated

  ● S92.20   Fracture of unspecified tarsal bone(s)
     (Ex) For category S92.20 CC codes S92.20[B]:
     S92.811-S92.819[A,B], S92.001-S92.919[A,B]
     For S92.20[K,P]: See S02.0[K]

    ● S92.201   Fracture of unspecified tarsal bone(s)
        of right foot B, K, P 🔒, B 🔒

    ● S92.202   Fracture of unspecified tarsal bone(s)
        of left foot B, K, P 🔒, B 🔒

    ● S92.209   Fracture of unspecified tarsal bone(s)
        of unspecified foot B, K, P 🔒, B 🔒

  ● S92.21   Fracture of cuboid bone

    ● S92.211   Displaced fracture of cuboid bone of
        right foot B, K, P 🔒, B 🔒

    ● S92.212   Displaced fracture of cuboid bone of
        left foot B, K, P 🔒, B 🔒

    ● S92.213   Displaced fracture of cuboid bone of
        unspecified foot B, K, P 🔒, B 🔒

    ● S92.214   Nondisplaced fracture of cuboid bone
        of right foot B, K, P 🔒, B 🔒

    ● S92.215   Nondisplaced fracture of cuboid bone
        of left foot B, K, P 🔒, B 🔒

    ● S92.216   Nondisplaced fracture of cuboid bone
        of unspecified foot B, K, P 🔒, B 🔒

◀ New   ◀◀◀ Revised   ~~deleted~~ Deleted   Excludes 1   Excludes 2   Includes   Use additional   Code first   Code also   Unspecified

OGCR Official Guidelines   ● Unacceptable Principal Diagnosis   **X** Assign placeholder X   ● Use Additional Character(s)   ▶ Manifestation Code   **Coding Clinic**

● S92.22   Fracture of lateral cuneiform
  ● S92.221   Displaced fracture of lateral cuneiform of right foot B, K, P 🔖, B 🔖
  ● S92.222   Displaced fracture of lateral cuneiform of left foot B, K, P 🔖, B 🔖
  ● S92.223   Displaced fracture of lateral cuneiform of unspecified foot B, K, P 🔖, B 🔖
  ● S92.224   Nondisplaced fracture of lateral cuneiform of right foot B, K, P 🔖, B 🔖
  ● S92.225   Nondisplaced fracture of lateral cuneiform of left foot B, K, P 🔖, B 🔖
  ● S92.226   Nondisplaced fracture of lateral cuneiform of unspecified foot B, K, P 🔖, B 🔖

● S92.23   Fracture of intermediate cuneiform
  ● S92.231   Displaced fracture of intermediate cuneiform of right foot B, K, P 🔖, B 🔖
  ● S92.232   Displaced fracture of intermediate cuneiform of left foot B, K, P 🔖, B 🔖
  ● S92.233   Displaced fracture of intermediate cuneiform of unspecified foot B, K, P 🔖, B 🔖
  ● S92.234   Nondisplaced fracture of intermediate cuneiform of right foot B, K, P 🔖, B 🔖
  ● S92.235   Nondisplaced fracture of intermediate cuneiform of left foot B, K, P 🔖, B 🔖
  ● S92.236   Nondisplaced fracture of intermediate cuneiform of unspecified foot B, K, P 🔖, B 🔖

● S92.24   Fracture of medial cuneiform
  ● S92.241   Displaced fracture of medial cuneiform of right foot B, K, P 🔖, B 🔖
  ● S92.242   Displaced fracture of medial cuneiform of left foot B, K, P 🔖, B 🔖
  ● S92.243   Displaced fracture of medial cuneiform of unspecified foot B, K, P 🔖, B 🔖
  ● S92.244   Nondisplaced fracture of medial cuneiform of right foot B, K, P 🔖, B 🔖
  ● S92.245   Nondisplaced fracture of medial cuneiform of left foot B, K, P 🔖, B 🔖
  ● S92.246   Nondisplaced fracture of medial cuneiform of unspecified foot B, K, P 🔖, B 🔖

● S92.25   Fracture of navicular [scaphoid] of foot
  ● S92.251   Displaced fracture of navicular [scaphoid] of right foot B, K, P 🔖, B 🔖
  ● S92.252   Displaced fracture of navicular [scaphoid] of left foot B, K, P 🔖, B 🔖
  ● S92.253   Displaced fracture of navicular [scaphoid] of unspecified foot B, K, P 🔖, B 🔖
  ● S92.254   Nondisplaced fracture of navicular [scaphoid] of right foot B, K, P 🔖, B 🔖
  ● S92.255   Nondisplaced fracture of navicular [scaphoid] of left foot B, K, P 🔖, B 🔖
  ● S92.256   Nondisplaced fracture of navicular [scaphoid] of unspecified foot B, K, P 🔖, B 🔖

● S92.3   Fracture of metatarsal bone(s)
  Excludes2   Physeal fracture of metatarsal (S99.1-) ◄
  (Ex) For category S92.3 CC codes S92.3[B]: See S92.1[B] For S92.3[K,P]: See S02.0[K]
  ● S92.30   Fracture of unspecified metatarsal bone(s)
    ● S92.301   Fracture of unspecified metatarsal bone(s), right foot B, K, P 🔖, B 🔖
    ● S92.302   Fracture of unspecified metatarsal bone(s), left foot B, K, P 🔖, B 🔖
    ● S92.309   Fracture of unspecified metatarsal bone(s), unspecified foot B, K, P 🔖, B 🔖
  ● S92.31   Fracture of first metatarsal bone
    ● S92.311   Displaced fracture of first metatarsal bone, right foot B, K, P 🔖, B 🔖
    ● S92.312   Displaced fracture of first metatarsal bone, left foot B, K, P 🔖, B 🔖
    ● S92.313   Displaced fracture of first metatarsal bone, unspecified foot B, K, P 🔖, B 🔖
    ● S92.314   Nondisplaced fracture of first metatarsal bone, right foot B, K, P 🔖, B 🔖
    ● S92.315   Nondisplaced fracture of first metatarsal bone, left foot B, K, P 🔖, B 🔖
    ● S92.316   Nondisplaced fracture of first metatarsal bone, unspecified foot B, K, P 🔖, B 🔖
  ● S92.32   Fracture of second metatarsal bone
    ● S92.321   Displaced fracture of second metatarsal bone, right foot B, K, P 🔖, B 🔖
    ● S92.322   Displaced fracture of second metatarsal bone, left foot B, K, P 🔖, B 🔖
    ● S92.323   Displaced fracture of second metatarsal bone, unspecified foot B, K, P 🔖, B 🔖
    ● S92.324   Nondisplaced fracture of second metatarsal bone, right foot B, K, P 🔖, B 🔖
    ● S92.325   Nondisplaced fracture of second metatarsal bone, left foot B, K, P 🔖, B 🔖
    ● S92.326   Nondisplaced fracture of second metatarsal bone, unspecified foot B, K, P 🔖, B 🔖
  ● S92.33   Fracture of third metatarsal bone
    ● S92.331   Displaced fracture of third metatarsal bone, right foot B, K, P 🔖, B 🔖
    ● S92.332   Displaced fracture of third metatarsal bone, left foot B, K, P 🔖, B 🔖
    ● S92.333   Displaced fracture of third metatarsal bone, unspecified foot B, K, P 🔖, B 🔖
    ● S92.334   Nondisplaced fracture of third metatarsal bone, right foot B, K, P 🔖, B 🔖
    ● S92.335   Nondisplaced fracture of third metatarsal bone, left foot B, K, P 🔖, B 🔖
    ● S92.336   Nondisplaced fracture of third metatarsal bone, unspecified foot B, K, P 🔖, B 🔖

- S92.34   Fracture of fourth metatarsal bone
  - S92.341   Displaced fracture of fourth metatarsal bone, right foot B, K, P 🜨, B 🜨
  - S92.342   Displaced fracture of fourth metatarsal bone, left foot B, K, P 🜨, B 🜨
  - S92.343   Displaced fracture of fourth metatarsal bone, unspecified foot B, K, P 🜨, B 🜨
  - S92.344   Nondisplaced fracture of fourth metatarsal bone, right foot B, K, P 🜨, B 🜨
  - S92.345   Nondisplaced fracture of fourth metatarsal bone, left foot B, K, P 🜨, B 🜨
  - S92.346   Nondisplaced fracture of fourth metatarsal bone, unspecified foot B, K, P 🜨, B 🜨
- S92.35   Fracture of fifth metatarsal bone
  - S92.351   Displaced fracture of fifth metatarsal bone, right foot B, K, P 🜨, B 🜨
  - S92.352   Displaced fracture of fifth metatarsal bone, left foot B, K, P 🜨, B 🜨
  - S92.353   Displaced fracture of fifth metatarsal bone, unspecified foot B, K, P 🜨, B 🜨
  - S92.354   Nondisplaced fracture of fifth metatarsal bone, right foot B, K, P 🜨, B 🜨
  - S92.355   Nondisplaced fracture of fifth metatarsal bone, left foot B, K, P 🜨, B 🜨
  - S92.356   Nondisplaced fracture of fifth metatarsal bone, unspecified foot B, K, P 🜨, B 🜨
- S92.4   Fracture of great toe

  Excludes2   Physeal fracture of phalanx of toe (S99.2-) ◀

  (Ex) **For category S92.4 CC codes:** See S02.0[K]

  - S92.40   Unspecified fracture of great toe
    - S92.401   Displaced unspecified fracture of right great toe K, P 🜨
    - S92.402   Displaced unspecified fracture of left great toe K, P 🜨
    - S92.403   Displaced unspecified fracture of unspecified great toe K, P 🜨
    - S92.404   Nondisplaced unspecified fracture of right great toe K, P 🜨
    - S92.405   Nondisplaced unspecified fracture of left great toe K, P 🜨
    - S92.406   Nondisplaced unspecified fracture of unspecified great toe K, P 🜨
  - S92.41   Fracture of proximal phalanx of great toe
    - S92.411   Displaced fracture of proximal phalanx of right great toe K, P 🜨
    - S92.412   Displaced fracture of proximal phalanx of left great toe K, P 🜨
    - S92.413   Displaced fracture of proximal phalanx of unspecified great toe K, P 🜨
    - S92.414   Nondisplaced fracture of proximal phalanx of right great toe K, P 🜨
    - S92.415   Nondisplaced fracture of proximal phalanx of left great toe K, P 🜨
    - S92.416   Nondisplaced fracture of proximal phalanx of unspecified great toe K, P 🜨

- S92.42   Fracture of distal phalanx of great toe
  - S92.421   Displaced fracture of distal phalanx of right great toe K, P 🜨
  - S92.422   Displaced fracture of distal phalanx of left great toe K, P 🜨
  - S92.423   Displaced fracture of distal phalanx of unspecified great toe K, P 🜨
  - S92.424   Nondisplaced fracture of distal phalanx of right great toe K, P 🜨
  - S92.425   Nondisplaced fracture of distal phalanx of left great toe K, P 🜨
  - S92.426   Nondisplaced fracture of distal phalanx of unspecified great toe K, P 🜨
- S92.49   Other fracture of great toe
  - S92.491   Other fracture of right great toe K, P 🜨
  - S92.492   Other fracture of left great toe K, P 🜨
  - S92.499   Other fracture of unspecified great toe K, P 🜨
- S92.5   Fracture of lesser toe(s)

  Excludes2   Physeal fracture of phalanx of toe (S99.2-) ◀

  (Ex) **For category S92.5 CC codes:** See S02.0[K]

  - S92.50   Unspecified fracture of lesser toe(s)
    - S92.501   Displaced unspecified fracture of right lesser toe(s) K, P 🜨
    - S92.502   Displaced unspecified fracture of left lesser toe(s) K, P 🜨
    - S92.503   Displaced unspecified fracture of unspecified lesser toe(s) K, P 🜨
    - S92.504   Nondisplaced unspecified fracture of right lesser toe(s) K, P 🜨
    - S92.505   Nondisplaced unspecified fracture of left lesser toe(s) K, P 🜨
    - S92.506   Nondisplaced unspecified fracture of unspecified lesser toe(s) K, P 🜨
  - S92.51   Fracture of proximal phalanx of lesser toe(s)
    - S92.511   Displaced fracture of proximal phalanx of right lesser toe(s) K, P 🜨
    - S92.512   Displaced fracture of proximal phalanx of left lesser toe(s) K, P 🜨
    - S92.513   Displaced fracture of proximal phalanx of unspecified lesser toe(s) K, P 🜨
    - S92.514   Nondisplaced fracture of proximal phalanx of right lesser toe(s) K, P 🜨
    - S92.515   Nondisplaced fracture of proximal phalanx of left lesser toe(s) K, P 🜨
    - S92.516   Nondisplaced fracture of proximal phalanx of unspecified lesser toe(s) K, P 🜨
  - S92.52   Fracture of medial phalanx of lesser toe(s)
    - S92.521   Displaced fracture of medial phalanx of right lesser toe(s) K, P 🜨
    - S92.522   Displaced fracture of medial phalanx of left lesser toe(s) K, P 🜨
    - S92.523   Displaced fracture of medial phalanx of unspecified lesser toe(s) K, P 🜨
    - S92.524   Nondisplaced fracture of medial phalanx of right lesser toe(s) K, P 🜨
    - S92.525   Nondisplaced fracture of medial phalanx of left lesser toe(s) K, P 🜨
    - S92.526   Nondisplaced fracture of medial phalanx of unspecified lesser toe(s) K, P 🜨

◀ New   ◀◀◀ Revised   ~~deleted~~ Deleted   Excludes 1   Excludes 2   Includes   Use additional   Code first   Code also   Unspecified

OGCR Official Guidelines   ● Unacceptable Principal Diagnosis   X Assign placeholder X   ● Use Additional Character(s)   🜨 Manifestation Code   **Coding Clinic**

- S92.53 **Fracture of distal phalanx of lesser toe(s)**
  - S92.531 **Displaced fracture of distal phalanx of right lesser toe(s)** K, P 🖐
  - S92.532 **Displaced fracture of distal phalanx of left lesser toe(s)** K, P 🖐
  - S92.533 **Displaced fracture of distal phalanx of unspecified lesser toe(s)** K, P 🖐
  - S92.534 **Nondisplaced fracture of distal phalanx of right lesser toe(s)** K, P 🖐
  - S92.535 **Nondisplaced fracture of distal phalanx of left lesser toe(s)** K, P 🖐
  - S92.536 **Nondisplaced fracture of distal phalanx of unspecified lesser toe(s)** K, P 🖐
  - S92.59 **Other fracture of lesser toe(s)**
    - S92.591 **Other fracture of right lesser toe(s)** K, P 🖐
    - S92.592 **Other fracture of left lesser toe(s)** K, P 🖐
    - S92.599 **Other fracture of unspecified lesser toe(s)** K, P 🖐
- S92.8 **Other fracture of foot, except ankle** ◀
  - Ⓔⅹ **For category S92.8 CC codes S92.8[B]:** S92.001-S92.919[A,B]
  For S92.90[K,P]: See S02.0[K]
  - S92.81 **Other fracture of foot** ◀
    Sesamoid fracture of foot
    - S92.811 **Other fracture of right foot** B, K, P 🖐, B 🖐 ◀
    - S92.812 **Other fracture of left foot** B, K, P 🖐, B 🖐 ◀
    - S92.819 **Other fracture of unspecified foot** B, K, P 🖐, B 🖐 ◀
  - S92.9 **Unspecified fracture of foot and toe**
    - S92.90 **Unspecified fracture of foot**
      - Ⓔⅹ **For category S92.90 CC codes S92.90[B]:** S92.811-S92.819[A,B], S92.001-S92.919[A,B]
      For S92.90[K,P]: See S02.0[K]
      - S92.901 **Unspecified fracture of right foot** B, K, P 🖐, B 🖐
      - S92.902 **Unspecified fracture of left foot** B, K, P 🖐, B 🖐
      - S92.909 **Unspecified fracture of unspecified foot** B, K, P 🖐, B 🖐
    - S92.91 **Unspecified fracture of toe**
      - Ⓔⅹ **For category S92.91 CC codes:** See S02.0[K]
      - S92.911 **Unspecified fracture of right toe(s)** K, P 🖐
      - S92.912 **Unspecified fracture of left toe(s)** K, P 🖐
      - S92.919 **Unspecified fracture of unspecified toe(s)** K, P 🖐

- S93 **Dislocation and sprain of joints and ligaments at ankle, foot and toe level**
  - **Includes** avulsion of joint or ligament of ankle, foot and toe
    laceration of cartilage, joint or ligament of ankle, foot and toe
    sprain of cartilage, joint or ligament of ankle, foot and toe
    traumatic hemarthrosis of joint or ligament of ankle, foot and toe
    traumatic rupture of joint or ligament of ankle, foot and toe
    traumatic subluxation of joint or ligament of ankle, foot and toe
    traumatic tear of joint or ligament of ankle, foot and toe
  - Code also any associated open wound
  - **Excludes2** strain of muscle and tendon of ankle and foot (S96.-)
  - The appropriate 7th character is to be added to each code from category S93

A	initial encounter
D	subsequent encounter
S	sequela

  - S93.0 **Subluxation and dislocation of ankle joint**
    Subluxation and dislocation of astragalus
    Subluxation and dislocation of fibula, lower end
    Subluxation and dislocation of talus
    Subluxation and dislocation of tibia, lower end
    - X ● S93.01 **Subluxation of right ankle joint**
    - X ● S93.02 **Subluxation of left ankle joint**
    - X ● S93.03 **Subluxation of unspecified ankle joint**
    - X ● S93.04 **Dislocation of right ankle joint**
    - X ● S93.05 **Dislocation of left ankle joint**
    - X ● S93.06 **Dislocation of unspecified ankle joint**
  - S93.1 **Subluxation and dislocation of toe**
    - S93.10 **Unspecified subluxation and dislocation of toe**
      Dislocation of toe NOS
      Subluxation of toe NOS
      - S93.101 **Unspecified subluxation of right toe(s)**
      - S93.102 **Unspecified subluxation of left toe(s)**
      - S93.103 **Unspecified subluxation of unspecified toe(s)**
      - S93.104 **Unspecified dislocation of right toe(s)**
      - S93.105 **Unspecified dislocation of left toe(s)**
      - S93.106 **Unspecified dislocation of unspecified toe(s)**
    - S93.11 **Dislocation of interphalangeal joint**
      - S93.111 **Dislocation of interphalangeal joint of right great toe**
      - S93.112 **Dislocation of interphalangeal joint of left great toe**
      - S93.113 **Dislocation of interphalangeal joint of unspecified great toe**
      - S93.114 **Dislocation of interphalangeal joint of right lesser toe(s)**
      - S93.115 **Dislocation of interphalangeal joint of left lesser toe(s)**
      - S93.116 **Dislocation of interphalangeal joint of unspecified lesser toe(s)**
      - S93.119 **Dislocation of interphalangeal joint of unspecified toe(s)**

CHAPTER 19 (S00-T88)

● S93.12　Dislocation of metatarsophalangeal joint
　　● S93.121　Dislocation of metatarsophalangeal joint of right great toe
　　● S93.122　Dislocation of metatarsophalangeal joint of left great toe
　　● S93.123　Dislocation of metatarsophalangeal joint of unspecified great toe
　　● S93.124　Dislocation of metatarsophalangeal joint of right lesser toe(s)
　　● S93.125　Dislocation of metatarsophalangeal joint of left lesser toe(s)
　　● S93.126　Dislocation of metatarsophalangeal joint of unspecified lesser toe(s)
　　● S93.129　Dislocation of metatarsophalangeal joint of unspecified toe(s)

● S93.13　Subluxation of interphalangeal joint
　　● S93.131　Subluxation of interphalangeal joint of right great toe
　　● S93.132　Subluxation of interphalangeal joint of left great toe
　　● S93.133　Subluxation of interphalangeal joint of unspecified great toe
　　● S93.134　Subluxation of interphalangeal joint of right lesser toe(s)
　　● S93.135　Subluxation of interphalangeal joint of left lesser toe(s)
　　● S93.136　Subluxation of interphalangeal joint of unspecified lesser toe(s)
　　● S93.139　Subluxation of interphalangeal joint of unspecified toe(s)

● S93.14　Subluxation of metatarsophalangeal joint
　　● S93.141　Subluxation of metatarsophalangeal joint of right great toe
　　● S93.142　Subluxation of metatarsophalangeal joint of left great toe
　　● S93.143　Subluxation of metatarsophalangeal joint of unspecified great toe
　　● S93.144　Subluxation of metatarsophalangeal joint of right lesser toe(s)
　　● S93.145　Subluxation of metatarsophalangeal joint of left lesser toe(s)
　　● S93.146　Subluxation of metatarsophalangeal joint of unspecified lesser toe(s)
　　● S93.149　Subluxation of metatarsophalangeal joint of unspecified toe(s)

● S93.3　Subluxation and dislocation of foot
　　Excludes2　dislocation of toe (S93.1-)

● S93.30　Unspecified subluxation and dislocation of foot
　　Dislocation of foot NOS
　　Subluxation of foot NOS
　　● S93.301　Unspecified subluxation of right foot
　　● S93.302　Unspecified subluxation of left foot
　　● S93.303　Unspecified subluxation of unspecified foot
　　● S93.304　Unspecified dislocation of right foot
　　● S93.305　Unspecified dislocation of left foot
　　● S93.306　Unspecified dislocation of unspecified foot

● S93.31　Subluxation and dislocation of tarsal joint
　　● S93.311　Subluxation of tarsal joint of right foot
　　● S93.312　Subluxation of tarsal joint of left foot
　　● S93.313　Subluxation of tarsal joint of unspecified foot
　　● S93.314　Dislocation of tarsal joint of right foot
　　● S93.315　Dislocation of tarsal joint of left foot
　　● S93.316　Dislocation of tarsal joint of unspecified foot

● S93.32　Subluxation and dislocation of tarsometatarsal joint
　　● S93.321　Subluxation of tarsometatarsal joint of right foot
　　● S93.322　Subluxation of tarsometatarsal joint of left foot
　　● S93.323　Subluxation of tarsometatarsal joint of unspecified foot
　　● S93.324　Dislocation of tarsometatarsal joint of right foot
　　● S93.325　Dislocation of tarsometatarsal joint of left foot
　　● S93.326　Dislocation of tarsometatarsal joint of unspecified foot

● S93.33　Other subluxation and dislocation of foot
　　● S93.331　Other subluxation of right foot
　　● S93.332　Other subluxation of left foot
　　● S93.333　Other subluxation of unspecified foot
　　● S93.334　Other dislocation of right foot
　　● S93.335　Other dislocation of left foot
　　● S93.336　Other dislocation of unspecified foot

● S93.4　Sprain of ankle
　　Injury to ligaments when one or more is stretched/torn
　　Excludes2　injury of Achilles tendon (S86.0-)

● S93.40　Sprain of unspecified ligament of ankle
　　Sprain of ankle NOS
　　Sprained ankle NOS
　　● S93.401　Sprain of unspecified ligament of right ankle
　　● S93.402　Sprain of unspecified ligament of left ankle
　　● S93.409　Sprain of unspecified ligament of unspecified ankle

● S93.41　Sprain of calcaneofibular ligament
　　● S93.411　Sprain of calcaneofibular ligament of right ankle
　　● S93.412　Sprain of calcaneofibular ligament of left ankle
　　● S93.419　Sprain of calcaneofibular ligament of unspecified ankle

● S93.42　Sprain of deltoid ligament
　　● S93.421　Sprain of deltoid ligament of right ankle
　　● S93.422　Sprain of deltoid ligament of left ankle
　　● S93.429　Sprain of deltoid ligament of unspecified ankle

● S93.43　Sprain of tibiofibular ligament
　　● S93.431　Sprain of tibiofibular ligament of right ankle
　　● S93.432　Sprain of tibiofibular ligament of left ankle
　　● S93.439　Sprain of tibiofibular ligament of unspecified ankle

● **S93.49**   Sprain of other ligament of ankle
       Sprain of internal collateral ligament
       Sprain of talofibular ligament
     ● **S93.491**   Sprain of other ligament of right ankle
     ● **S93.492**   Sprain of other ligament of left ankle
     ● **S93.499**   Sprain of other ligament of unspecified ankle

● **S93.5**   Sprain of toe
   ● **S93.50**   Unspecified sprain of toe
     ● **S93.501**   Unspecified sprain of right great toe
     ● **S93.502**   Unspecified sprain of left great toe
     ● **S93.503**   Unspecified sprain of unspecified great toe
     ● **S93.504**   Unspecified sprain of right lesser toe(s)
     ● **S93.505**   Unspecified sprain of left lesser toe(s)
     ● **S93.506**   Unspecified sprain of unspecified lesser toe(s)
     ● **S93.509**   Unspecified sprain of unspecified toe(s)
   ● **S93.51**   Sprain of interphalangeal joint of toe
     ● **S93.511**   Sprain of interphalangeal joint of right great toe
     ● **S93.512**   Sprain of interphalangeal joint of left great toe
     ● **S93.513**   Sprain of interphalangeal joint of unspecified great toe
     ● **S93.514**   Sprain of interphalangeal joint of right lesser toe(s)
     ● **S93.515**   Sprain of interphalangeal joint of left lesser toe(s)
     ● **S93.516**   Sprain of interphalangeal joint of unspecified lesser toe(s)
     ● **S93.519**   Sprain of interphalangeal joint of unspecified toe(s)
   ● **S93.52**   Sprain of metatarsophalangeal joint of toe
     ● **S93.521**   Sprain of metatarsophalangeal joint of right great toe
     ● **S93.522**   Sprain of metatarsophalangeal joint of left great toe
     ● **S93.523**   Sprain of metatarsophalangeal joint of unspecified great toe
     ● **S93.524**   Sprain of metatarsophalangeal joint of right lesser toe(s)
     ● **S93.525**   Sprain of metatarsophalangeal joint of left lesser toe(s)
     ● **S93.526**   Sprain of metatarsophalangeal joint of unspecified lesser toe(s)
     ● **S93.529**   Sprain of metatarsophalangeal joint of unspecified toe(s)

● **S93.6**   Sprain of foot
     Excludes2   sprain of metatarsophalangeal joint of toe (S93.52-)
                sprain of toe (S93.5-)
   ● **S93.60**   Unspecified sprain of foot
     ● **S93.601**   Unspecified sprain of right foot
     ● **S93.602**   Unspecified sprain of left foot
     ● **S93.609**   Unspecified sprain of unspecified foot
   ● **S93.61**   Sprain of tarsal ligament of foot
     ● **S93.611**   Sprain of tarsal ligament of right foot
     ● **S93.612**   Sprain of tarsal ligament of left foot
     ● **S93.619**   Sprain of tarsal ligament of unspecified foot

   ● **S93.62**   Sprain of tarsometatarsal ligament of foot
     ● **S93.621**   Sprain of tarsometatarsal ligament of right foot
     ● **S93.622**   Sprain of tarsometatarsal ligament of left foot
     ● **S93.629**   Sprain of tarsometatarsal ligament of unspecified foot
   ● **S93.69**   Other sprain of foot
     ● **S93.691**   Other sprain of right foot
     ● **S93.692**   Other sprain of left foot
     ● **S93.699**   Other sprain of unspecified foot

● **S94**   Injury of nerves at ankle and foot level
     The appropriate 7th character is to be added to each code from category S94

A	initial encounter
D	subsequent encounter
S	sequela

     Code also any associated open wound (S91.-)

● **S94.0**   Injury of lateral plantar nerve
   X ● **S94.00**   Injury of lateral plantar nerve, unspecified leg
   X ● **S94.01**   Injury of lateral plantar nerve, right leg
   X ● **S94.02**   Injury of lateral plantar nerve, left leg
● **S94.1**   Injury of medial plantar nerve
   X ● **S94.10**   Injury of medial plantar nerve, unspecified leg
   X ● **S94.11**   Injury of medial plantar nerve, right leg
   X ● **S94.12**   Injury of medial plantar nerve, left leg
● **S94.2**   Injury of deep peroneal nerve at ankle and foot level
     Injury of terminal, lateral branch of deep peroneal nerve
   X ● **S94.20**   Injury of deep peroneal nerve at ankle and foot level, unspecified leg
   X ● **S94.21**   Injury of deep peroneal nerve at ankle and foot level, right leg
   X ● **S94.22**   Injury of deep peroneal nerve at ankle and foot level, left leg
● **S94.3**   Injury of cutaneous sensory nerve at ankle and foot level
   X ● **S94.30**   Injury of cutaneous sensory nerve at ankle and foot level, unspecified leg
   X ● **S94.31**   Injury of cutaneous sensory nerve at ankle and foot level, right leg
   X ● **S94.32**   Injury of cutaneous sensory nerve at ankle and foot level, left leg
● **S94.8**   Injury of other nerves at ankle and foot level
   ● **S94.8X**   Injury of other nerves at ankle and foot level
     ● **S94.8X1**   Injury of other nerves at ankle and foot level, right leg
     ● **S94.8X2**   Injury of other nerves at ankle and foot level, left leg
     ● **S94.8X9**   Injury of other nerves at ankle and foot level, unspecified leg
● **S94.9**   Injury of unspecified nerve at ankle and foot level
   X ● **S94.90**   Injury of unspecified nerve at ankle and foot level, unspecified leg
   X ● **S94.91**   Injury of unspecified nerve at ankle and foot level, right leg
   X ● **S94.92**   Injury of unspecified nerve at ankle and foot level, left leg

CHAPTER 19 (S00-T88)

● S95   Injury of blood vessels at ankle and foot level
         Code also any associated open wound (S91.-)
         Excludes2 injury of posterior tibial artery and vein (S85.1-, S85.8-)

         The appropriate 7th character is to be added to each code from category S95

A	initial encounter
D	subsequent encounter
S	sequela

● S95.0   Injury of dorsal artery of foot
    ● S95.00   Unspecified injury of dorsal artery of foot
        ● S95.001   Unspecified injury of dorsal artery of right foot A 🐾
                     (Ex:) See S75.801
        ● S95.002   Unspecified injury of dorsal artery of left foot A 🐾
                     (Ex:) See S75.802
        ● S95.009   Unspecified injury of dorsal artery of unspecified foot A 🐾
                     (Ex:) See S75.809
    ● S95.01   Laceration of dorsal artery of foot
        ● S95.011   Laceration of dorsal artery of right foot A 🐾
                     (Ex:) See S75.801
        ● S95.012   Laceration of dorsal artery of left foot A 🐾
                     (Ex:) See S75.802
        ● S95.019   Laceration of dorsal artery of unspecified foot A 🐾
                     (Ex:) See S75.809
    ● S95.09   Other specified injury of dorsal artery of foot
        ● S95.091   Other specified injury of dorsal artery of right foot A 🐾
                     (Ex:) See S75.801
        ● S95.092   Other specified injury of dorsal artery of left foot A 🐾
                     (Ex:) See S75.802
        ● S95.099   Other specified injury of dorsal artery of unspecified foot A 🐾
                     (Ex:) See S75.809

● S95.1   Injury of plantar artery of foot
    ● S95.10   Unspecified injury of plantar artery of foot
        ● S95.101   Unspecified injury of plantar artery of right foot A 🐾
                     (Ex:) S75.801[A], S75.809-S75.811[A],
                     S75.819-S75.891[A], S75.899-S75.901[A],
                     S75.909-S75.911[A], S75.919-S75.991[A],
                     S75.999[A], S85.201[A], S85.209-S85.211[A],
                     S85.219-S85.291[A], S85.299[A], S85.801[A],
                     S85.809-S85.811[A], S85.819-S85.891[A],
                     S85.899-S85.901[A], S85.909-S85.911[A],
                     S85.919-S85.991[A], S85.999[A], S95.001[A],
                     S95.009-S95.011[A], S95.019-S95.091[A],
                     S95.099-S95.201[A], S95.209-S95.211[A],
                     S95.219-S95.291[A], S95.299-S95.801[A],
                     S95.809-S95.811[A], S95.819-S95.891[A],
                     S95.899-S95.901[A], S95.909-S95.911[A],
                     S95.919-S95.991[A], S95.999[A]

● S95.102   Unspecified injury of plantar artery of left foot A 🐾
             (Ex:) S75.802-S75.809[A], S75.812-S75.819[A],
             S75.892-S75.899[A], S75.902-S75.909[A],
             S75.912-S75.919[A], S75.992-S75.999[A],
             S85.202-S85.209[A], S85.212-S85.219[A],
             S85.292-S85.299[A], S85.802-S85.809[A],
             S85.812-S85.819[A], S85.892-S85.899[A],
             S85.902-S85.909[A], S85.912-S85.919[A],
             S85.992-S85.999[A], S95.002-S95.009[A],
             S95.012-S95.019[A], S95.092-S95.099[A],
             S95.102-S95.109[A], S95.112-S95.119[A],
             S95.192-S95.199[A], S95.202-S95.209[A],
             S95.212-S95.219[A], S95.292-S95.299[A],
             S95.802-S95.809[A], S95.812-S95.819[A],
             S95.892-S95.899[A], S95.902-S95.909[A],
             S95.912-S95.919[A], S95.992-S95.999[A]
    ● S95.109   Unspecified injury of plantar artery of unspecified foot A 🐾
                 (Ex:) S75.801-S75.999[A], S85.201-S85.299[A],
                 S85.801-S85.999[A], S95.001-S95.099[A],
                 S95.101-S95.999[A]
● S95.11   Laceration of plantar artery of foot
    ● S95.111   Laceration of plantar artery of right foot A 🐾
                 (Ex:) See S95.101
    ● S95.112   Laceration of plantar artery of left foot A 🐾
                 (Ex:) See S95.102
    ● S95.119   Laceration of plantar artery of unspecified foot A 🐾
                 (Ex:) See S95.109
● S95.19   Other specified injury of plantar artery of foot
    ● S95.191   Other specified injury of plantar artery of right foot A 🐾
                 (Ex:) See S95.101
    ● S95.192   Other specified injury of plantar artery of left foot A 🐾
                 (Ex:) See S95.102
    ● S95.199   Other specified injury of plantar artery of unspecified foot A 🐾
                 (Ex:) See S95.109

● S95.2   Injury of dorsal vein of foot
    ● S95.20   Unspecified injury of dorsal vein of foot
        ● S95.201   Unspecified injury of dorsal vein of right foot A 🐾
                     (Ex:) See S75.801
        ● S95.202   Unspecified injury of dorsal vein of left foot A 🐾
                     (Ex:) See S75.802
        ● S95.209   Unspecified injury of dorsal vein of unspecified foot A 🐾
                     (Ex:) See S75.809
    ● S95.21   Laceration of dorsal vein of foot
        ● S95.211   Laceration of dorsal vein of right foot A 🐾
                     (Ex:) See S75.801
        ● S95.212   Laceration of dorsal vein of left foot A 🐾
                     (Ex:) See S75.802
        ● S95.219   Laceration of dorsal vein of unspecified foot A 🐾
                     (Ex:) See S75.809
    ● S95.29   Other specified injury of dorsal vein of foot
        ● S95.291   Other specified injury of dorsal vein of right foot A 🐾
                     (Ex:) See S75.801
        ● S95.292   Other specified injury of dorsal vein of left foot A 🐾
                     (Ex:) See S75.802
        ● S95.299   Other specified injury of dorsal vein of unspecified foot A 🐾
                     (Ex:) See S75.809

◀ New   ◀▥ Revised   ~~deleted~~ Deleted   Excludes 1   Excludes 2   Includes   Use additional   Code first   Code also   Unspecified
OGCR Official Guidelines   ● Unacceptable Principal Diagnosis   X Assign placeholder X   ● Use Additional Character(s)   ▶ Manifestation Code   **Coding Clinic**

● **S95.8   Injury of other blood vessels at ankle and foot level**
  ● **S95.80   Unspecified injury of other blood vessels at ankle and foot level**
    ● **S95.801   Unspecified injury of other blood vessels at ankle and foot level, right leg** A 🔧
       Ⓔⓧ See S75.801
    ● **S95.802   Unspecified injury of other blood vessels at ankle and foot level, left leg** A 🔧
       Ⓔⓧ See S75.802
    ● **S95.809   Unspecified injury of other blood vessels at ankle and foot level, unspecified leg** A 🔧
       Ⓔⓧ See S75.809
  ● **S95.81   Laceration of other blood vessels at ankle and foot level**
    ● **S95.811   Laceration of other blood vessels at ankle and foot level, right leg** A 🔧
       Ⓔⓧ See S75.801
    ● **S95.812   Laceration of other blood vessels at ankle and foot level, left leg** A 🔧
       Ⓔⓧ See S75.802
    ● **S95.819   Laceration of other blood vessels at ankle and foot level, unspecified leg** A 🔧
       Ⓔⓧ See S75.809
  ● **S95.89   Other specified injury of other blood vessels at ankle and foot level**
    ● **S95.891   Other specified injury of other blood vessels at ankle and foot level, right leg** A 🔧
       Ⓔⓧ See S75.801
    ● **S95.892   Other specified injury of other blood vessels at ankle and foot level, left leg** A 🔧
       Ⓔⓧ See S75.802
    ● **S95.899   Other specified injury of other blood vessels at ankle and foot level, unspecified leg** A 🔧
       Ⓔⓧ See S75.809

● **S95.9   Injury of unspecified blood vessel at ankle and foot level**
  ● **S95.90   Unspecified injury of unspecified blood vessel at ankle and foot level**
    ● **S95.901   Unspecified injury of unspecified blood vessel at ankle and foot level, right leg** A 🔧
       Ⓔⓧ See S75.801
    ● **S95.902   Unspecified injury of unspecified blood vessel at ankle and foot level, left leg** A 🔧
       Ⓔⓧ See S75.802
    ● **S95.909   Unspecified injury of unspecified blood vessel at ankle and foot level, unspecified leg** A 🔧
       Ⓔⓧ See S75.809
  ● **S95.91   Laceration of unspecified blood vessel at ankle and foot level**
    ● **S95.911   Laceration of unspecified blood vessel at ankle and foot level, right leg** A 🔧
       Ⓔⓧ See S75.801
    ● **S95.912   Laceration of unspecified blood vessel at ankle and foot level, left leg** A 🔧
       Ⓔⓧ See S75.802
    ● **S95.919   Laceration of unspecified blood vessel at ankle and foot level, unspecified leg** A 🔧
       Ⓔⓧ See S75.809

● **S95.99   Other specified injury of unspecified blood vessel at ankle and foot level**
  ● **S95.991   Other specified injury of unspecified blood vessel at ankle and foot level, right leg** A 🔧
     Ⓔⓧ See S75.801
  ● **S95.992   Other specified injury of unspecified blood vessel at ankle and foot level, left leg** A 🔧
     Ⓔⓧ See S75.802
  ● **S95.999   Other specified injury of unspecified blood vessel at ankle and foot level, unspecified leg** A 🔧
     Ⓔⓧ See S75.809

● **S96   Injury of muscle and tendon at ankle and foot level**
   Code also any associated open wound (S91.-)
   Excludes2   injury of Achilles tendon (S86.0-)
           sprain of joints and ligaments of ankle and foot (S93.-)
   The appropriate 7th character is to be added to each code from category S96

A	initial encounter
D	subsequent encounter
S	sequela

  ● **S96.0   Injury of muscle and tendon of long flexor muscle of toe at ankle and foot level**
    ● **S96.00   Unspecified injury of muscle and tendon of long flexor muscle of toe at ankle and foot level**
      ● **S96.001   Unspecified injury of muscle and tendon of long flexor muscle of toe at ankle and foot level, right foot**
      ● **S96.002   Unspecified injury of muscle and tendon of long flexor muscle of toe at ankle and foot level, left foot**
      ● **S96.009   Unspecified injury of muscle and tendon of long flexor muscle of toe at ankle and foot level, unspecified foot**
    ● **S96.01   Strain of muscle and tendon of long flexor muscle of toe at ankle and foot level**
      ● **S96.011   Strain of muscle and tendon of long flexor muscle of toe at ankle and foot level, right foot**
      ● **S96.012   Strain of muscle and tendon of long flexor muscle of toe at ankle and foot level, left foot**
      ● **S96.019   Strain of muscle and tendon of long flexor muscle of toe at ankle and foot level, unspecified foot**
    ● **S96.02   Laceration of muscle and tendon of long flexor muscle of toe at ankle and foot level**
      ● **S96.021   Laceration of muscle and tendon of long flexor muscle of toe at ankle and foot level, right foot** A 🔧
         Ⓔⓧ See S86.021
      ● **S96.022   Laceration of muscle and tendon of long flexor muscle of toe at ankle and foot level, left foot** A 🔧
         Ⓔⓧ See S86.022
      ● **S96.029   Laceration of muscle and tendon of long flexor muscle of toe at ankle and foot level, unspecified foot** A 🔧
         Ⓔⓧ See S86.029

● S96.09   Other injury of muscle and tendon of long flexor muscle of toe at ankle and foot level

   ● S96.091   Other injury of muscle and tendon of long flexor muscle of toe at ankle and foot level, right foot

   ● S96.092   Other injury of muscle and tendon of long flexor muscle of toe at ankle and foot level, left foot

   ● S96.099   Other injury of muscle and tendon of long flexor muscle of toe at ankle and foot level, unspecified foot

● S96.1   Injury of muscle and tendon of long extensor muscle of toe at ankle and foot level

  ● S96.10   Unspecified injury of muscle and tendon of long extensor muscle of toe at ankle and foot level

   ● S96.101   Unspecified injury of muscle and tendon of long extensor muscle of toe at ankle and foot level, right foot

   ● S96.102   Unspecified injury of muscle and tendon of long extensor muscle of toe at ankle and foot level, left foot

   ● S96.109   Unspecified injury of muscle and tendon of long extensor muscle of toe at ankle and foot level, unspecified foot

  ● S96.11   Strain of muscle and tendon of long extensor muscle of toe at ankle and foot level

   ● S96.111   Strain of muscle and tendon of long extensor muscle of toe at ankle and foot level, right foot

   ● S96.112   Strain of muscle and tendon of long extensor muscle of toe at ankle and foot level, left foot

   ● S96.119   Strain of muscle and tendon of long extensor muscle of toe at ankle and foot level, unspecified foot

  ● S96.12   Laceration of muscle and tendon of long extensor muscle of toe at ankle and foot level

   ● S96.121   Laceration of muscle and tendon of long extensor muscle of toe at ankle and foot level, right foot A 🔗
       Ex: See S86.021

   ● S96.122   Laceration of muscle and tendon of long extensor muscle of toe at ankle and foot level, left foot A 🔗
       Ex: See S86.022

   ● S96.129   Laceration of muscle and tendon of long extensor muscle of toe at ankle and foot level, unspecified foot A 🔗
       Ex: See S86.029

  ● S96.19   Other specified injury of muscle and tendon of long extensor muscle of toe at ankle and foot level

   ● S96.191   Other specified injury of muscle and tendon of long extensor muscle of toe at ankle and foot level, right foot

   ● S96.192   Other specified injury of muscle and tendon of long extensor muscle of toe at ankle and foot level, left foot

   ● S96.199   Other specified injury of muscle and tendon of long extensor muscle of toe at ankle and foot level, unspecified foot

● S96.2   Injury of intrinsic muscle and tendon at ankle and foot level

  ● S96.20   Unspecified injury of intrinsic muscle and tendon at ankle and foot level

   ● S96.201   Unspecified injury of intrinsic muscle and tendon at ankle and foot level, right foot

   ● S96.202   Unspecified injury of intrinsic muscle and tendon at ankle and foot level, left foot

   ● S96.209   Unspecified injury of intrinsic muscle and tendon at ankle and foot level, unspecified foot

  ● S96.21   Strain of intrinsic muscle and tendon at ankle and foot level

   ● S96.211   Strain of intrinsic muscle and tendon at ankle and foot level, right foot

   ● S96.212   Strain of intrinsic muscle and tendon at ankle and foot level, left foot

   ● S96.219   Strain of intrinsic muscle and tendon at ankle and foot level, unspecified foot

  ● S96.22   Laceration of intrinsic muscle and tendon at ankle and foot level

   ● S96.221   Laceration of intrinsic muscle and tendon at ankle and foot level, right foot A 🔗
       Ex: See S86.021

   ● S96.222   Laceration of intrinsic muscle and tendon at left ankle and foot level, left foot A 🔗
       Ex: See S86.022

   ● S96.229   Laceration of intrinsic muscle and tendon at ankle and foot level, unspecified foot A 🔗
       Ex: See S86.029

  ● S96.29   Other specified injury of intrinsic muscle and tendon at ankle and foot level

   ● S96.291   Other specified injury of intrinsic muscle and tendon at ankle and foot level, right foot

   ● S96.292   Other specified injury of intrinsic muscle and tendon at ankle and foot level, left foot

   ● S96.299   Other specified injury of intrinsic muscle and tendon at ankle and foot level, unspecified foot

● S96.8   Injury of other specified muscles and tendons at ankle and foot level

  ● S96.80   Unspecified injury of other specified muscles and tendons at ankle and foot level

   ● S96.801   Unspecified injury of other specified muscles and tendons at ankle and foot level, right foot

   ● S96.802   Unspecified injury of other specified muscles and tendons at ankle and foot level, left foot

   ● S96.809   Unspecified injury of other specified muscles and tendons at ankle and foot level, unspecified foot

  ● S96.81   Strain of other specified muscles and tendons at ankle and foot level

   ● S96.811   Strain of other specified muscles and tendons at ankle and foot level, right foot

   ● S96.812   Strain of other specified muscles and tendons at ankle and foot level, left foot

   ● S96.819   Strain of other specified muscles and tendons at ankle and foot level, unspecified foot

◀ New   ◀▥ Revised   ~~deleted~~ Deleted   Excludes 1   Excludes 2   Includes   Use additional   Code first   Code also   Unspecified

OGCR Official Guidelines   ● Unacceptable Principal Diagnosis   X Assign placeholder X   ● Use Additional Character(s)   ▌ Manifestation Code   **Coding Clinic**

● **S96.82**   **Laceration of other specified muscles and tendons at ankle and foot level**
   ● **S96.821**   Laceration of other specified muscles and tendons at ankle and foot level, right foot A 🗲
      (Ex:) See S86.021
   ● **S96.822**   Laceration of other specified muscles and tendons at ankle and foot level, left foot A 🗲
      (Ex:) See S86.022
   ● **S96.829**   Laceration of other specified muscles and tendons at ankle and foot level, unspecified foot A 🗲
      (Ex:) See S86.029

● **S96.89**   **Other specified injury of other specified muscles and tendons at ankle and foot level**
   ● **S96.891**   Other specified injury of other specified muscles and tendons at ankle and foot level, right foot
   ● **S96.892**   Other specified injury of other specified muscles and tendons at ankle and foot level, left foot
   ● **S96.899**   Other specified injury of other specified muscles and tendons at ankle and foot level, unspecified foot

● **S96.9**   **Injury of unspecified muscle and tendon at ankle and foot level**
   ● **S96.90**   Unspecified injury of unspecified muscle and tendon at ankle and foot level
      ● **S96.901**   Unspecified injury of unspecified muscle and tendon at ankle and foot level, right foot
      ● **S96.902**   Unspecified injury of unspecified muscle and tendon at ankle and foot level, left foot
      ● **S96.909**   Unspecified injury of unspecified muscle and tendon at ankle and foot level, unspecified foot
   ● **S96.91**   Strain of unspecified muscle and tendon at ankle and foot level
      ● **S96.911**   Strain of unspecified muscle and tendon at ankle and foot level, right foot
      ● **S96.912**   Strain of unspecified muscle and tendon at ankle and foot level, left foot
      ● **S96.919**   Strain of unspecified muscle and tendon at ankle and foot level, unspecified foot
   ● **S96.92**   Laceration of unspecified muscle and tendon at ankle and foot level
      ● **S96.921**   Laceration of unspecified muscle and tendon at ankle and foot level, right foot A 🗲
         (Ex:) See S86.021
      ● **S96.922**   Laceration of unspecified muscle and tendon at ankle and foot level, left foot A 🗲
         (Ex:) See S86.022
      ● **S96.929**   Laceration of unspecified muscle and tendon at ankle and foot level, unspecified foot A 🗲
         (Ex:) See S86.029
   ● **S96.99**   Other specified injury of unspecified muscle and tendon at ankle and foot level
      ● **S96.991**   Other specified injury of unspecified muscle and tendon at ankle and foot level, right foot
      ● **S96.992**   Other specified injury of unspecified muscle and tendon at ankle and foot level, left foot
      ● **S96.999**   Other specified injury of unspecified muscle and tendon at ankle and foot level, unspecified foot

● **S97**   **Crushing injury of ankle and foot**
   Use additional code(s) for all associated injuries
   The appropriate 7th character is to be added to each code from category S97

A	initial encounter
D	subsequent encounter
S	sequela

   ● **S97.0**   **Crushing injury of ankle**
      X ● **S97.00**   Crushing injury of unspecified ankle
      X ● **S97.01**   Crushing injury of right ankle
      X ● **S97.02**   Crushing injury of left ankle
   ● **S97.1**   **Crushing injury of toe**
      ● **S97.10**   Crushing injury of unspecified toe(s)
         ● **S97.101**   Crushing injury of unspecified right toe(s)
         ● **S97.102**   Crushing injury of unspecified left toe(s)
         ● **S97.109**   Crushing injury of unspecified toe(s)
            Crushing injury of toe NOS
      ● **S97.11**   Crushing injury of great toe
         ● **S97.111**   Crushing injury of right great toe
         ● **S97.112**   Crushing injury of left great toe
         ● **S97.119**   Crushing injury of unspecified great toe
      ● **S97.12**   Crushing injury of lesser toe(s)
         ● **S97.121**   Crushing injury of right lesser toe(s)
         ● **S97.122**   Crushing injury of left lesser toe(s)
         ● **S97.129**   Crushing injury of lesser toe(s), unspecified toe(s)
   ● **S97.8**   **Crushing injury of foot**
      X ● **S97.80**   Crushing injury of foot, unspecified side
         Crushing injury of foot NOS
      X ● **S97.81**   Crushing injury of right foot
      X ● **S97.82**   Crushing injury of left foot

● **S98**   **Traumatic amputation of ankle and foot**
   An amputation not identified as partial or complete should be coded to complete
   The appropriate 7th character is to be added to each code from category S98

A	initial encounter
D	subsequent encounter
S	sequela

   ● **S98.0**   **Traumatic amputation of foot at ankle level**
      ● **S98.01**   Complete traumatic amputation of foot at ankle level
         ● **S98.011**   Complete traumatic amputation of right foot at ankle level A 🗲
            (Ex:) See S78.011
         ● **S98.012**   Complete traumatic amputation of left foot at ankle level A 🗲
            (Ex:) See S78.012
         ● **S98.019**   Complete traumatic amputation of unspecified foot at ankle level A 🗲
            (Ex:) See S78.019
      ● **S98.02**   Partial traumatic amputation of foot at ankle level
         ● **S98.021**   Partial traumatic amputation of right foot at ankle level A 🗲
            (Ex:) See S78.011
         ● **S98.022**   Partial traumatic amputation of left foot at ankle level A 🗲
            (Ex:) See S78.012
         ● **S98.029**   Partial traumatic amputation of unspecified foot at ankle level A 🗲
            (Ex:) See S78.019

CHAPTER 19 (S00-T88)

- S98.1   Traumatic amputation of one toe
  - S98.11   Complete traumatic amputation of great toe
    - S98.111   Complete traumatic amputation of right great toe
    - S98.112   Complete traumatic amputation of left great toe
    - S98.119   Complete traumatic amputation of unspecified great toe
  - S98.12   Partial traumatic amputation of great toe
    - S98.121   Partial traumatic amputation of right great toe
    - S98.122   Partial traumatic amputation of left great toe
    - S98.129   Partial traumatic amputation of unspecified great toe
  - S98.13   Complete traumatic amputation of one lesser toe
    - Traumatic amputation of toe NOS
    - S98.131   Complete traumatic amputation of one right lesser toe
    - S98.132   Complete traumatic amputation of one left lesser toe
    - S98.139   Complete traumatic amputation of one unspecified lesser toe
  - S98.14   Partial traumatic amputation of one lesser toe
    - S98.141   Partial traumatic amputation of one right lesser toe
    - S98.142   Partial traumatic amputation of one left lesser toe
    - S98.149   Partial traumatic amputation of one unspecified lesser toe
- S98.2   Traumatic amputation of two or more lesser toes
  - S98.21   Complete traumatic amputation of two or more lesser toes
    - S98.211   Complete traumatic amputation of two or more right lesser toes
    - S98.212   Complete traumatic amputation of two or more left lesser toes
    - S98.219   Complete traumatic amputation of two or more unspecified lesser toes
  - S98.22   Partial traumatic amputation of two or more lesser toes
    - S98.221   Partial traumatic amputation of two or more right lesser toes
    - S98.222   Partial traumatic amputation of two or more left lesser toes
    - S98.229   Partial traumatic amputation of two or more unspecified lesser toes
- S98.3   Traumatic amputation of midfoot
  - S98.31   Complete traumatic amputation of midfoot
    - S98.311   Complete traumatic amputation of right midfoot A
      - Ex: See S78.011
    - S98.312   Complete traumatic amputation of left midfoot A
      - Ex: See S78.012
    - S98.319   Complete traumatic amputation of unspecified midfoot A
      - Ex: See S78.019
  - S98.32   Partial traumatic amputation of midfoot
    - S98.321   Partial traumatic amputation of right midfoot A
      - Ex: See S78.011
    - S98.322   Partial traumatic amputation of left midfoot A
      - Ex: See S78.012
    - S98.329   Partial traumatic amputation of unspecified midfoot A
      - Ex: See S78.019

- S98.9   Traumatic amputation of foot, level unspecified
  - S98.91   Complete traumatic amputation of foot, level unspecified
    - S98.911   Complete traumatic amputation of right foot, level unspecified A
      - Ex: See S78.011
    - S98.912   Complete traumatic amputation of left foot, level unspecified A
      - Ex: See S78.012
    - S98.919   Complete traumatic amputation of unspecified foot, level unspecified A
      - Ex: See S78.019
  - S98.92   Partial traumatic amputation of foot, level unspecified
    - S98.921   Partial traumatic amputation of right foot, level unspecified A
      - Ex: See S78.011
    - S98.922   Partial traumatic amputation of left foot, level unspecified A
      - Ex: See S78.012
    - S98.929   Partial traumatic amputation of unspecified foot, level unspecified A
      - Ex: See S78.019
- S99   Other and unspecified injuries of ankle and foot
  - S99.0   Physeal fracture of calcaneus ◄
    - The appropriate 7th character is to be added to each code from subcategories S99.0 ◄

A	initial encounter for closed fracture ◄
B	initial encounter for open fracture ◄
D	subsequent encounter for fracture with routine healing ◄
G	subsequent encounter for fracture with delayed healing ◄
K	subsequent encounter for fracture with nonunion ◄
P	subsequent encounter for fracture with malunion ◄
S	sequela ◄

    - S99.00   Unspecified physeal fracture of calcaneus ◄
      - S99.001   Unspecified physeal fracture of right calcaneus ◄
      - S99.002   Unspecified physeal fracture of left calcaneus ◄
      - S99.009   Unspecified physeal fracture of unspecified calcaneus ◄
    - S99.01   Salter-Harris Type I physeal fracture of calcaneus ◄
      - S99.011   Salter-Harris Type I physeal fracture of right calcaneus ◄
      - S99.012   Salter-Harris Type I physeal fracture of left calcaneus ◄
      - S99.019   Salter-Harris Type I physeal fracture of unspecified calcaneus ◄
    - S99.02   Salter-Harris Type II physeal fracture of calcaneus ◄
      - S99.021   Salter-Harris Type II physeal fracture of right calcaneus ◄
      - S99.022   Salter-Harris Type II physeal fracture of left calcaneus ◄
      - S99.029   Salter-Harris Type II physeal fracture of unspecified calcaneus ◄

◄ New   ◄ Revised   ~~deleted~~ Deleted   Excludes 1   Excludes 2   Includes   Use additional   Code first   Code also   Unspecified

OGCR Official Guidelines   ● Unacceptable Principal Diagnosis   X Assign placeholder X   ● Use Additional Character(s)   ▶ Manifestation Code   **Coding Clinic**

● **S99.03**   Salter-Harris Type III physeal fracture of calcaneus ◄
- ● **S99.031**   Salter-Harris Type III physeal fracture of right calcaneus ◄
- ● **S99.032**   Salter-Harris Type III physeal fracture of left calcaneus ◄
- ● **S99.039**   Salter-Harris Type III physeal fracture of unspecified calcaneus ◄

● **S99.04**   Salter-Harris Type IV physeal fracture of calcaneus ◄
- ● **S99.041**   Salter-Harris Type IV physeal fracture of right calcaneus ◄
- ● **S99.042**   Salter-Harris Type IV physeal fracture of left calcaneus ◄
- ● **S99.049**   Salter-Harris Type IV physeal fracture of unspecified calcaneus ◄

● **S99.09**   Other physeal fracture of calcaneus ◄
- ● **S99.091**   Other physeal fracture of right calcaneus ◄
- ● **S99.092**   Other physeal fracture of left calcaneus ◄
- ● **S99.099**   Other physeal fracture of unspecified calcaneus ◄

● **S99.1**   Physeal fracture of metatarsal ◄

The appropriate 7th character is to be added to each code from subcategories S99.1 ◄

> A   initial encounter for closed fracture ◄
> B   initial encounter for open fracture ◄
> D   subsequent encounter for fracture with routine healing ◄
> G   subsequent encounter for fracture with delayed healing ◄
> K   subsequent encounter for fracture with nonunion ◄
> P   subsequent encounter for fracture with malunion ◄
> S   sequela ◄

● **S99.10**   Unspecified physeal fracture of metatarsal ◄
- ● **S99.101**   Unspecified physeal fracture of right metatarsal ◄
- ● **S99.102**   Unspecified physeal fracture of left metatarsal ◄
- ● **S99.109**   Unspecified physeal fracture of unspecified metatarsal ◄

● **S99.11**   Salter-Harris Type I physeal fracture of metatarsal ◄
- ● **S99.111**   Salter-Harris Type I physeal fracture of right metatarsal ◄
- ● **S99.112**   Salter-Harris Type I physeal fracture of left metatarsal ◄
- ● **S99.119**   Salter-Harris Type I physeal fracture of unspecified metatarsal ◄

● **S99.12**   Salter-Harris Type II physeal fracture of metatarsal ◄
- ● **S99.121**   Salter-Harris Type II physeal fracture of right metatarsal ◄
- ● **S99.122**   Salter-Harris Type II physeal fracture of left metatarsal ◄
- ● **S99.129**   Salter-Harris Type II physeal fracture of unspecified metatarsal ◄

● **S99.13**   Salter-Harris Type III physeal fracture of metatarsal ◄
- ● **S99.131**   Salter-Harris Type III physeal fracture of right metatarsal ◄
- ● **S99.132**   Salter-Harris Type III physeal fracture of left metatarsal ◄
- ● **S99.139**   Salter-Harris Type III physeal fracture of unspecified metatarsal ◄

● **S99.14**   Salter-Harris Type IV physeal fracture of metatarsal ◄
- ● **S99.141**   Salter-Harris Type IV physeal fracture of right metatarsal ◄
- ● **S99.142**   Salter-Harris Type IV physeal fracture of left metatarsal ◄
- ● **S99.149**   Salter-Harris Type IV physeal fracture of unspecified metatarsal ◄

● **S99.19**   Other physeal fracture of metatarsal ◄
- ● **S99.191**   Other physeal fracture of right metatarsal ◄
- ● **S99.192**   Other physeal fracture of left metatarsal ◄
- ● **S99.199**   Other physeal fracture of unspecified metatarsal ◄

● **S99.2**   Physeal fracture of phalanx of toe ◄

The appropriate 7th character is to be added to each code from subcategories S99.2 ◄

> A   initial encounter for closed fracture ◄
> B   initial encounter for open fracture ◄
> D   subsequent encounter for fracture with routine healing ◄
> G   subsequent encounter for fracture with delayed healing ◄
> K   subsequent encounter for fracture with nonunion ◄
> P   subsequent encounter for fracture with malunion ◄
> S   sequela ◄

● **S99.20**   Unspecified physeal fracture of phalanx of toe ◄
- ● **S99.201**   Unspecified physeal fracture of phalanx of right toe ◄
- ● **S99.202**   Unspecified physeal fracture of phalanx of right toe ◄
- ● **S99.209**   Unspecified physeal fracture of phalanx of unspecified toe ◄

● **S99.21**   Salter-Harris Type I physeal fracture of phalanx of toe ◄
- ● **S99.211**   Salter-Harris Type I physeal fracture of phalanx of right toe ◄
- ● **S99.212**   Salter-Harris Type I physeal fracture of phalanx of left toe ◄
- ● **S99.219**   Salter-Harris Type I physeal fracture of phalanx of unspecified toe ◄

● **S99.22**   Salter-Harris Type II physeal fracture of phalanx of toe ◄
- ● **S99.221**   Salter-Harris Type II physeal fracture of phalanx of right toe ◄
- ● **S99.222**   Salter-Harris Type II physeal fracture of phalanx of left toe ◄
- ● **S99.229**   Salter-Harris Type II physeal fracture of phalanx of unspecified toe ◄

CHAPTER 19 (S00-T88)

● S99.23　Salter-Harris Type III physeal fracture of phalanx of toe ◀
　　● S99.231　Salter-Harris Type III physeal fracture of phalanx of right toe ◀
　　● S99.232　Salter-Harris Type III physeal fracture of phalanx of left toe ◀
　　● S99.239　Salter-Harris Type III physeal fracture of phalanx of unspecified toe ◀
● S99.24　Salter-Harris Type IV physeal fracture of phalanx of toe ◀
　　● S99.241　Salter-Harris Type IV physeal fracture of phalanx of right toe ◀
　　● S99.242　Salter-Harris Type IV physeal fracture of phalanx of left toe ◀
　　● S99.249　Salter-Harris Type IV physeal fracture of phalanx of unspecified toe ◀
● S99.29　Other physeal fracture of phalanx of toe ◀
　　● S99.291　Other physeal fracture of phalanx of right toe ◀
　　● S99.292　Other physeal fracture of phalanx of left toe ◀
　　● S99.299　Other physeal fracture of phalanx of unspecified toe ◀

● S99.8　Other specified injuries of ankle and foot

The appropriate 7th character is to be added to each code from subcategory S99.8 ◀

A	initial encounter ◀
D	subsequent encounter ◀
S	sequela ◀

　● S99.81　Other specified injuries of ankle
　　● S99.811　Other specified injuries of right ankle
　　● S99.812　Other specified injuries of left ankle
　　● S99.819　Other specified injuries of unspecified ankle
　● S99.82　Other specified injuries of foot
　　● S99.821　Other specified injuries of right foot
　　● S99.822　Other specified injuries of left foot
　　● S99.829　Other specified injuries of unspecified foot

● S99.9　Unspecified injury of ankle and foot

The appropriate 7th character is to be added to each code from subcategory S99.9 ◀

A	initial encounter ◀
D	subsequent encounter ◀
S	sequela ◀

　● S99.91　Unspecified injury of ankle
　　● S99.911　Unspecified injury of right ankle
　　● S99.912　Unspecified injury of left ankle
　　● S99.919　Unspecified injury of unspecified ankle
　● S99.92　Unspecified injury of foot
　　● S99.921　Unspecified injury of right foot
　　● S99.922　Unspecified injury of left foot
　　● S99.929　Unspecified injury of unspecified foot

INJURY, POISONING AND CERTAIN OTHER CONSEQUENCES OF EXTERNAL CAUSES (T07-T88)

INJURIES INVOLVING MULTIPLE BODY REGIONS (T07)

Excludes1　burns and corrosions (T20-T32)
　　　　　　frostbite (T33-T34)
　　　　　　insect bite or sting, venomous (T63.4)
　　　　　　sunburn (L55.-)

T07　Unspecified multiple injuries
　　Excludes1　injury NOS (T14)

INJURY OF UNSPECIFIED BODY REGION (T14)

● T14　Injury of unspecified body region
　　Excludes1　multiple unspecified injuries (T07)
　　T14.8　Other injury of unspecified body region
　　　　Abrasion NOS　　　　　Fracture NOS
　　　　Contusion NOS　　　　 Skin injury NOS
　　　　Crush injury NOS　　　 Vascular injury NOS
　● T14.9　Unspecified injury
　　T14.90　Injury, unspecified
　　　　Injury NOS
　　T14.91　Suicide attempt
　　　　Attempted suicide NOS

EFFECTS OF FOREIGN BODY ENTERING THROUGH NATURAL ORIFICE (T15-T19)

Excludes2　foreign body accidentally left in operation wound (T81.5-)
　　　　　　foreign body in penetrating wound - see open wound by body region
　　　　　　residual foreign body in soft tissue (M79.5)
　　　　　　splinter, without open wound - see superficial injury by body region

● T15　Foreign body on external eye
　　Excludes2　foreign body in penetrating wound of orbit and eye ball (S05.4-, S05.5-)
　　　　　　open wound of eyelid and periocular area (S01.1-)
　　　　　　retained foreign body in eyelid (H02.8-)
　　　　　　retained (old) foreign body in penetrating wound of orbit and eye ball (H05.5-, H44.6-, H44.7-)
　　　　　　superficial foreign body of eyelid and periocular area (S00.25-)

The appropriate 7th character is to be added to each code from category T15

A	initial encounter
D	subsequent encounter
S	sequela

　● T15.0　Foreign body in cornea
　　X ● T15.00　Foreign body in cornea, unspecified eye
　　X ● T15.01　Foreign body in cornea, right eye
　　X ● T15.02　Foreign body in cornea, left eye
　● T15.1　Foreign body in conjunctival sac
　　X ● T15.10　Foreign body in conjunctival sac, unspecified eye
　　X ● T15.11　Foreign body in conjunctival sac, right eye
　　X ● T15.12　Foreign body in conjunctival sac, left eye
　● T15.8　Foreign body in other and multiple parts of external eye
　　　　Foreign body in lacrimal punctum
　　X ● T15.80　Foreign body in other and multiple parts of external eye, unspecified eye
　　X ● T15.81　Foreign body in other and multiple parts of external eye, right eye
　　X ● T15.82　Foreign body in other and multiple parts of external eye, left eye

◀ New　◀▥ Revised　d̶e̶l̶e̶t̶e̶d̶ Deleted　Excludes 1　Excludes 2　Includes　Use additional　Code first　Code also　Unspecified
OGCR Official Guidelines　● Unacceptable Principal Diagnosis　X Assign placeholder X　● Use Additional Character(s)　▮ Manifestation Code　Coding Clinic

● **T15.9**   Foreign body on external eye, part unspecified

X ● **T15.90**   Foreign body on external eye, part unspecified, unspecified eye

X ● **T15.91**   Foreign body on external eye, part unspecified, right eye

X ● **T15.92**   Foreign body on external eye, part unspecified, left eye

● **T16**   Foreign body in ear

   Includes   foreign body in auditory canal

   The appropriate 7th character is to be added to each code from category T16

A	initial encounter
D	subsequent encounter
S	sequela

X ● **T16.1**   Foreign body in right ear

X ● **T16.2**   Foreign body in left ear

X ● **T16.9**   Foreign body in ear, unspecified ear

● **T17**   Foreign body in respiratory tract

   The appropriate 7th character is to be added to each code from category T17

A	initial encounter
D	subsequent encounter
S	sequela

X ● **T17.0**   Foreign body in nasal sinus

X ● **T17.1**   Foreign body in nostril

   Foreign body in nose NOS

● **T17.2**   Foreign body in pharynx

   Foreign body in nasopharynx
   Foreign body in throat NOS

   ● **T17.20**   Unspecified foreign body in pharynx

   ● **T17.200**   Unspecified foreign body in pharynx causing asphyxiation

   ● **T17.208**   Unspecified foreign body in pharynx causing other injury

   ● **T17.21**   Gastric contents in pharynx

   Aspiration of gastric contents into pharynx
   Vomitus in pharynx

   ● **T17.210**   Gastric contents in pharynx causing asphyxiation

   ● **T17.218**   Gastric contents in pharynx causing other injury

   ● **T17.22**   Food in pharynx

   Bones in pharynx
   Seeds in pharynx

   ● **T17.220**   Food in pharynx causing asphyxiation

   ● **T17.228**   Food in pharynx causing other injury

   ● **T17.29**   Other foreign object in pharynx

   ● **T17.290**   Other foreign object in pharynx causing asphyxiation

   ● **T17.298**   Other foreign object in pharynx causing other injury

● **T17.3**   Foreign body in larynx

   ● **T17.30**   Unspecified foreign body in larynx

   ● **T17.300**   Unspecified foreign body in larynx causing asphyxiation

   ● **T17.308**   Unspecified foreign body in larynx causing other injury

   ● **T17.31**   Gastric contents in larynx

   Aspiration of gastric contents into larynx
   Vomitus in larynx

   ● **T17.310**   Gastric contents in larynx causing asphyxiation

   ● **T17.318**   Gastric contents in larynx causing other injury

● **T17.32**   Food in larynx

   Bones in larynx ◀▥
   Seeds in larynx

   ● **T17.320**   Food in larynx causing asphyxiation

   ● **T17.328**   Food in larynx causing other injury

● **T17.39**   Other foreign object in larynx

   ● **T17.390**   Other foreign object in larynx causing asphyxiation

   ● **T17.398**   Other foreign object in larynx causing other injury

● **T17.4**   Foreign body in trachea

   (Ex) For category **T17.4** CC codes: T17.400-T17.498[A]

   ● **T17.40**   Unspecified foreign body in trachea

   ● **T17.400**   Unspecified foreign body in trachea causing asphyxiation A 🝔

   ● **T17.408**   Unspecified foreign body in trachea causing other injury A 🝔

   ● **T17.41**   Gastric contents in trachea

   Aspiration of gastric contents into trachea
   Vomitus in trachea

   ● **T17.410**   Gastric contents in trachea causing asphyxiation A 🝔

   ● **T17.418**   Gastric contents in trachea causing other injury A 🝔

   ● **T17.42**   Food in trachea

   Bones in trachea
   Seeds in trachea

   ● **T17.420**   Food in trachea causing asphyxiation A 🝔

   ● **T17.428**   Food in trachea causing other injury A 🝔

   ● **T17.49**   Other foreign object in trachea

   ● **T17.490**   Other foreign object in trachea causing asphyxiation A 🝔

   ● **T17.498**   Other foreign object in trachea causing other injury A 🝔

● **T17.5**   Foreign body in bronchus

   (Ex) For category **T17.5** CC codes: T17.400-T17.998[A]

   ● **T17.50**   Unspecified foreign body in bronchus

   ● **T17.500**   Unspecified foreign body in bronchus causing asphyxiation A 🝔

   ● **T17.508**   Unspecified foreign body in bronchus causing other injury A 🝔

   ● **T17.51**   Gastric contents in bronchus

   Aspiration of gastric contents into bronchus
   Vomitus in bronchus

   ● **T17.510**   Gastric contents in bronchus causing asphyxiation A 🝔

   ● **T17.518**   Gastric contents in bronchus causing other injury A 🝔

   ● **T17.52**   Food in bronchus

   Bones in bronchus
   Seeds in bronchus

   ● **T17.520**   Food in bronchus causing asphyxiation A 🝔

   ● **T17.528**   Food in bronchus causing other injury A 🝔

   ● **T17.59**   Other foreign object in bronchus

   ● **T17.590**   Other foreign object in bronchus causing asphyxiation A 🝔

   ● **T17.598**   Other foreign object in bronchus causing other injury A 🝔

● **T17.8**   **Foreign body in other parts of respiratory tract**
Foreign body in bronchioles
Foreign body in lung
(Ex) For category T17.8 CC codes: T17.400-T17.998[A]

● **T17.80**   Unspecified foreign body in other parts of respiratory tract

● **T17.800**   Unspecified foreign body in other parts of respiratory tract causing asphyxiation A 🔊

● **T17.808**   Unspecified foreign body in other parts of respiratory tract causing other injury A 🔊

● **T17.81**   Gastric contents in other parts of respiratory tract
Aspiration of gastric contents into other parts of respiratory tract
Vomitus in other parts of respiratory tract

● **T17.810**   Gastric contents in other parts of respiratory tract causing asphyxiation A 🔊

● **T17.818**   Gastric contents in other parts of respiratory tract causing other injury A 🔊

● **T17.82**   Food in other parts of respiratory tract
Bones in other parts of respiratory tract
Seeds in other parts of respiratory tract

● **T17.820**   Food in other parts of respiratory tract causing asphyxiation A 🔊

● **T17.828**   Food in other parts of respiratory tract causing other injury A 🔊

● **T17.89**   Other foreign object in other parts of respiratory tract

● **T17.890**   Other foreign object in other parts of respiratory tract causing asphyxiation A 🔊

● **T17.898**   Other foreign object in other parts of respiratory tract causing other injury A 🔊

● **T17.9**   **Foreign body in respiratory tract, part unspecified**

● **T17.90**   Unspecified foreign body in respiratory tract, part unspecified

● **T17.900**   Unspecified foreign body in respiratory tract, part unspecified causing asphyxiation

● **T17.908**   Unspecified foreign body in respiratory tract, part unspecified causing other injury

● **T17.91**   Gastric contents in respiratory tract, part unspecified
Aspiration of gastric contents into respiratory tract, part unspecified
Vomitus in trachea respiratory tract, part unspecified

● **T17.910**   Gastric contents in respiratory tract, part unspecified causing asphyxiation

● **T17.918**   Gastric contents in respiratory tract, part unspecified causing other injury

● **T17.92**   Food in respiratory tract, part unspecified
Bones in respiratory tract, part unspecified
Seeds in respiratory tract, part unspecified

● **T17.920**   Food in respiratory tract, part unspecified causing asphyxiation

● **T17.928**   Food in respiratory tract, part unspecified causing other injury

● **T17.99**   Other foreign object in respiratory tract, part unspecified

● **T17.990**   Other foreign object in respiratory tract, part unspecified in causing asphyxiation

● **T17.998**   Other foreign object in respiratory tract, part unspecified causing other injury

● **T18**   **Foreign body in alimentary tract**
     Excludes2   foreign body in pharynx (T17.2-)
The appropriate 7th character is to be added to each code from category T18

A	initial encounter
D	subsequent encounter
S	sequela

X ● **T18.0**   **Foreign body in mouth**

X ● **T18.1**   **Foreign body in esophagus**
     Excludes2   foreign body in respiratory tract (T17.-)

● **T18.10**   Unspecified foreign body in esophagus

● **T18.100**   Unspecified foreign body in esophagus causing compression of trachea
Unspecified foreign body in esophagus causing obstruction of respiration

● **T18.108**   Unspecified foreign body in esophagus causing other injury

● **T18.11**   Gastric contents in esophagus
Vomitus in esophagus

● **T18.110**   Gastric contents in esophagus causing compression of trachea
Gastric contents in esophagus causing obstruction of respiration

● **T18.118**   Gastric contents in esophagus causing other injury

● **T18.12**   Food in esophagus
Bones in esophagus
Seeds in esophagus

● **T18.120**   Food in esophagus causing compression of trachea
Food in esophagus causing obstruction of respiration

● **T18.128**   Food in esophagus causing other injury

● **T18.19**   Other foreign object in esophagus

● **T18.190**   Other foreign object in esophagus causing compression of trachea
Other foreign body in esophagus causing obstruction of respiration
Coding Clinic: 2015, Q1, P24

● **T18.198**   Other foreign object in esophagus causing other injury
Coding Clinic: 2015, Q1, P24

X ● **T18.2**   **Foreign body in stomach**

X ● **T18.3**   **Foreign body in small intestine**

X ● **T18.4**   **Foreign body in colon**

X ● **T18.5**   **Foreign body in anus and rectum**
Foreign body in rectosigmoid (junction)

X ● **T18.8**   **Foreign body in other parts of alimentary tract**

X ● **T18.9**   **Foreign body of alimentary tract, part unspecified**
Foreign body in digestive system NOS
Swallowed foreign body NOS

◄ New   ◄▦ Revised   ~~deleted~~ Deleted   Excludes 1   Excludes 2   Includes   Use additional   Code first   Code also   Unspecified

1420   OGCR Official Guidelines   ● Unacceptable Principal Diagnosis   X Assign placeholder X   ● Use Additional Character(s)   ▶ Manifestation Code   **Coding Clinic**

● **T19 Foreign body in genitourinary tract**

    Excludes2 complications due to implanted mesh (T83.7-)
                mechanical complications of contraceptive device
                    (intrauterine) (vaginal) (T83.3-)
                presence of contraceptive device (intrauterine)
                    (vaginal) (Z97.5)

The appropriate 7th character is to be added to each code from category T19

> A   initial encounter
> D   subsequent encounter
> S   sequela

X● **T19.0 Foreign body in urethra**
X● **T19.1 Foreign body in bladder**
X● **T19.2 Foreign body in vulva and vagina ♀**
X● **T19.3 Foreign body in uterus ♀**
X● **T19.4 Foreign body in penis ♂**
X● **T19.8 Foreign body in other parts of genitourinary tract**
X● **T19.9 Foreign body in genitourinary tract, part unspecified**

BURNS AND CORROSIONS (T20-T32)

    Includes burns (thermal) from electrical heating appliances
                 burns (thermal) from electricity
                 burns (thermal) from flame
                 burns (thermal) from friction
                 burns (thermal) from hot air and hot gases
                 burns (thermal) from hot objects
                 burns (thermal) from lightning
                 burns (thermal) from radiation chemical
                 burn [corrosion] (external) (internal) scalds

    Excludes2 erythema [dermatitis] ab igne (L59.0)
                radiation-related disorders of the skin and
                    subcutaneous tissue (L55-L59)
                sunburn (L55.-)

OGCR Section I.C.19.d.

> Burns and Corrosions
>
> The ICD-10-CM makes a distinction between burn and corrosions. The burn codes are for thermal burns, except sunburns, that come from a heat source, such as a fire or hot appliance. The burn codes are also for burns resulting from electricity and radiation. Corrosions are burns due to chemicals. The guidelines for burns and corrosions are the same.
>
> Current burns (T20-T25) are classified by depth, extent and by agent (X code). Burns are classified by depth as first degree (erythema), second degree (blistering), and third degree (full-thickness involvement). Burns of the eye and internal organs (T26-T28) are classified by site, but not by degree.
>
> 1) Sequencing of burn and related condition codes
>
> Sequence first the code that reflects the highest degree of burn when more than one burn is present.
>
> a. When the reason for the admission or encounter is for treatment of external multiple burns, sequence first the code that reflects the burn of the highest degree.
>
> b. When a patient has both internal and external burns, the circumstances of admission govern the selection of the principal diagnosis or first-listed diagnosis.
>
> c. When a patient is admitted for burn injuries and other related conditions such as smoke inhalation and/or respiratory failure, the circumstances of admission govern the selection of the principal or first-listed diagnosis.
>
> 2) Burns of the same local site
>
> Classify burns of the same local site (three-character category level, T20-T28) but of different degrees to the subcategory identifying the highest degree recorded in the diagnosis.

Figure 19-15 A. Second-degree burn. **B.** Third-degree burn. (From Cummings: Otolaryngology: Head & Neck Surgery, ed 4, Mosby, 2005)

BURNS AND CORROSIONS OF EXTERNAL BODY SURFACE, SPECIFIED BY SITE (T20-T25)

    Includes burns and corrosions of first degree [erythema]
                 burns and corrosions of second degree [blisters]
                    [epidermal loss]
                 burns and corrosions of third degree [deep
                    necrosis of underlying tissue] [full-thickness
                    skin loss]

Use additional code from category T31 or T32 to identify extent of body surface involved

● **T20 Burn and corrosion of head, face, and neck**

    Excludes2 burn and corrosion of ear drum (T28.41, T28.91)
                burn and corrosion of eye and adnexa (T26.-)
                burn and corrosion of mouth and pharynx (T28.0)

The appropriate 7th character is to be added to each code from category T20

> A   initial encounter
> D   subsequent encounter
> S   sequela

● **T20.0 Burn of unspecified degree of head, face, and neck**

    Use additional external cause code to identify the source, place and intent of the burn (X00-X19, X75-X77, X96-X98, Y92)

X● **T20.00 Burn of unspecified degree of head, face, and neck, unspecified site**

● **T20.01 Burn of unspecified degree of ear [any part, except ear drum]**

    Excludes2 burn of ear drum (T28.41-)

    ● **T20.011 Burn of unspecified degree of right ear [any part, except ear drum]**
    ● **T20.012 Burn of unspecified degree of left ear [any part, except ear drum]**
    ● **T20.019 Burn of unspecified degree of unspecified ear [any part, except ear drum]**

X● **T20.02 Burn of unspecified degree of lip(s)**
X● **T20.03 Burn of unspecified degree of chin**
X● **T20.04 Burn of unspecified degree of nose (septum)**
X● **T20.05 Burn of unspecified degree of scalp [any part]**
X● **T20.06 Burn of unspecified degree of forehead and cheek**
X● **T20.07 Burn of unspecified degree of neck**
X● **T20.09 Burn of unspecified degree of multiple sites of head, face, and neck**

N Newborn Age: 0   **P** Pediatric Age: 0–17   **M** Maternity DX: 12–55   **A** Adult Age: 15–124   ♀ Females Only   ♂ Males Only

 Complication\Comorbidity   Major C\C   (Ex) CC/MCC Exclusions   Hospital-Acquired Condition

1421

● **T20.1   Burn of first degree of head, face, and neck**

Use additional external cause code to identify the source, place and intent of the burn (X00-X19, X75-X77, X96-X98, Y92)

X ● **T20.10   Burn of first degree of head, face, and neck, unspecified site**

● **T20.11   Burn of first degree of ear [any part, except ear drum]**

Excludes2   burn of ear drum (T28.41-)

● **T20.111   Burn of first degree of right ear [any part, except ear drum]**

● **T20.112   Burn of first degree of left ear [any part, except ear drum]**

● **T20.119   Burn of first degree of unspecified ear [any part, except ear drum]**

X ● **T20.12   Burn of first degree of lip(s)**

X ● **T20.13   Burn of first degree of chin**

X ● **T20.14   Burn of first degree of nose (septum)**

X ● **T20.15   Burn of first degree of scalp [any part]**

X ● **T20.16   Burn of first degree of forehead and cheek**

X ● **T20.17   Burn of first degree of neck**

X ● **T20.19   Burn of first degree of multiple sites of head, face, and neck**

● **T20.2   Burn of second degree of head, face, and neck**

Use additional external cause code to identify the source, place and intent of the burn (X00-X19, X75-X77, X96-X98, Y92)

X ● **T20.20   Burn of second degree of head, face, and neck, unspecified site**

● **T20.21   Burn of second degree of ear [any part, except ear drum]**

Excludes2   burn of ear drum (T28.41-)

● **T20.211   Burn of second degree of right ear [any part, except ear drum]**

● **T20.212   Burn of second degree of left ear [any part, except ear drum]**

● **T20.219   Burn of second degree of unspecified ear [any part, except ear drum]**

X ● **T20.22   Burn of second degree of lip(s)**

X ● **T20.23   Burn of second degree of chin**

X ● **T20.24   Burn of second degree of nose (septum)**

X ● **T20.25   Burn of second degree of scalp [any part]**
Coding Clinic: 2015, Q1, P19

X ● **T20.26   Burn of second degree of forehead and cheek**

X ● **T20.27   Burn of second degree of neck**

X ● **T20.29   Burn of second degree of multiple sites of head, face, and neck**

● **T20.3   Burn of third degree of head, face, and neck**

Use additional external cause code to identify the source, place and intent of the burn (X00-X19, X75-X77, X96-X98, Y92)

X ● **T20.30   Burn of third degree of head, face, and neck, unspecified site** A 🐾, A 🐾
Ⓔx T20.30X[A], T20.39X[A], T20.70X[A], T20.79X[A]

● **T20.31   Burn of third degree of ear [any part, except ear drum]**

Excludes2   burn of ear drum (T28.41-)

Ⓔx For category T20.31 CC codes: T20.311-T20.319[A], T20.39X[A], T20.711-T20.719[A], T20.79X[A]

● **T20.311   Burn of third degree of right ear [any part, except ear drum]** A 🐾, A 🐾

● **T20.312   Burn of third degree of left ear [any part, except ear drum]** A 🐾, A 🐾
Coding Clinic: 2015, Q1, P18

● **T20.319   Burn of third degree of unspecified ear [any part, except ear drum]** A 🐾, A 🐾

X ● **T20.32   Burn of third degree of lip(s)** A 🐾, A 🐾
Ⓔx T20.32X[A], T20.39X[A], T20.72X[A], T20.79X[A]

X ● **T20.33   Burn of third degree of chin** A 🐾, A 🐾
Ⓔx T20.33X[A], T20.39X[A], T20.73X[A], T20.79X[A]

X ● **T20.34   Burn of third degree of nose (septum)** A 🐾, A 🐾
Ⓔx T20.34X[A], T20.39X[A], T20.74X[A], T20.79X[A]

X ● **T20.35   Burn of third degree of scalp [any part]** A 🐾, A 🐾
Ⓔx T20.35X[A], T20.39X[A], T20.75X[A], T20.79X[A]

X ● **T20.36   Burn of third degree of forehead and cheek** A 🐾, A 🐾
Ⓔx T20.36X[A], T20.39X[A], T20.76X[A], T20.79X[A]

X ● **T20.37   Burn of third degree of neck** A 🐾, A 🐾
Ⓔx T20.37X-T20.39X[A], T20.77X-T20.79X[A]

X ● **T20.39   Burn of third degree of multiple sites of head, face, and neck** A 🐾, A 🐾
Ⓔx T20.30X-T20.39X[A], T20.70X-T20.79X[A]

● **T20.4   Corrosion of unspecified degree of head, face, and neck**

Code first (T51-T65) to identify chemical and intent

Use additional external cause code to identify place (Y92)

X ● **T20.40   Corrosion of unspecified degree of head, face, and neck, unspecified site**

● **T20.41   Corrosion of unspecified degree of ear [any part, except ear drum]**

Excludes2   corrosion of ear drum (T28.91-)

● **T20.411   Corrosion of unspecified degree of right ear [any part, except ear drum]**

● **T20.412   Corrosion of unspecified degree of left ear [any part, except ear drum]**

● **T20.419   Corrosion of unspecified degree of unspecified ear [any part, except ear drum]**

X ● **T20.42   Corrosion of unspecified degree of lip(s)**

X ● **T20.43   Corrosion of unspecified degree of chin**

X ● **T20.44   Corrosion of unspecified degree of nose (septum)**

X ● **T20.45   Corrosion of unspecified degree of scalp [any part]**

X ● **T20.46   Corrosion of unspecified degree of forehead and cheek**

X ● **T20.47   Corrosion of unspecified degree of neck**

X ● **T20.49   Corrosion of unspecified degree of multiple sites of head, face, and neck**

● **T20.5   Corrosion of first degree of head, face, and neck**

Code first (T51-T65) to identify chemical and intent

Use additional external cause code to identify place (Y92)

X ● **T20.50   Corrosion of first degree of head, face, and neck, unspecified site**

● **T20.51   Corrosion of first degree of ear [any part, except ear drum]**

Excludes2   corrosion of ear drum (T28.91-)

● **T20.511   Corrosion of first degree of right ear [any part, except ear drum]**

● **T20.512   Corrosion of first degree of left ear [any part, except ear drum]**

● **T20.519   Corrosion of first degree of unspecified ear [any part, except ear drum]**

X ● **T20.52   Corrosion of first degree of lip(s)**

X ● **T20.53   Corrosion of first degree of chin**

X ● **T20.54   Corrosion of first degree of nose (septum)**

X ● **T20.55   Corrosion of first degree of scalp [any part]**

X ● **T20.56   Corrosion of first degree of forehead and cheek**

X ● **T20.57   Corrosion of first degree of neck**

X ● **T20.59   Corrosion of first degree of multiple sites of head, face, and neck**

◀ New   ◀◀ Revised   ~~deleted~~ Deleted   Excludes 1   Excludes 2   Includes   Use additional   Code first   Code also   Unspecified

OGCR Official Guidelines   ● Unacceptable Principal Diagnosis   X Assign placeholder X   ● Use Additional Character(s)   ▶ Manifestation Code   Coding Clinic

1422

● **T20.6**   **Corrosion of second degree of head, face, and neck**

Code first (T51-T65) to identify chemical and intent

Use additional external cause code to identify place (Y92)

X ● **T20.60**   **Corrosion of second degree of head, face, and neck, unspecified site**

● **T20.61**   **Corrosion of second degree of ear [any part, except ear drum]**

Excludes2   corrosion of ear drum (T28.91-)

● **T20.611**   **Corrosion of second degree of right ear [any part, except ear drum]**

● **T20.612**   **Corrosion of second degree of left ear [any part, except ear drum]**

● **T20.619**   **Corrosion of second degree of unspecified ear [any part, except ear drum]**

X ● **T20.62**   **Corrosion of second degree of lip(s)**

X ● **T20.63**   **Corrosion of second degree of chin**

X ● **T20.64**   **Corrosion of second degree of nose (septum)**

X ● **T20.65**   **Corrosion of second degree of scalp [any part]**

X ● **T20.66**   **Corrosion of second degree of forehead and cheek**

X ● **T20.67**   **Corrosion of second degree of neck**

X ● **T20.69**   **Corrosion of second degree of multiple sites of head, face, and neck**

● **T20.7**   **Corrosion of third degree of head, face, and neck**

Code first (T51-T65) to identify chemical and intent

Use additional external cause code to identify place (Y92)

X ● **T20.70**   **Corrosion of third degree of head, face, and neck, unspecified site** A 🅖, A 🅜
    (Ex) See T20.30

● **T20.71**   **Corrosion of third degree of ear [any part, except ear drum]**

Excludes2   corrosion of ear drum (T28.91-)

(Ex) For category T20.71 CC codes: See T20.31

● **T20.711**   **Corrosion of third degree of right ear [any part, except ear drum]** A 🅖, A 🅜

● **T20.712**   **Corrosion of third degree of left ear [any part, except ear drum]** A 🅖, A 🅜

● **T20.719**   **Corrosion of third degree of unspecified ear [any part, except ear drum]** A 🅖, A 🅜

X ● **T20.72**   **Corrosion of third degree of lip(s)** A 🅖, A 🅜
    (Ex) See T20.32

X ● **T20.73**   **Corrosion of third degree of chin** A 🅖, A 🅜
    (Ex) See T20.33

X ● **T20.74**   **Corrosion of third degree of nose (septum)** A 🅖, A 🅜
    (Ex) See T20.34

X ● **T20.75**   **Corrosion of third degree of scalp [any part]** A 🅖, A 🅜
    (Ex) See T20.35

X ● **T20.76**   **Corrosion of third degree of forehead and cheek** A 🅖, A 🅜
    (Ex) See T20.36

X ● **T20.77**   **Corrosion of third degree of neck** A 🅖, A 🅜
    (Ex) See T20.37

X ● **T20.79**   **Corrosion of third degree of multiple sites of head, face, and neck** A 🅖, A 🅜
    (Ex) See T20.39

● **T21**   **Burn and corrosion of trunk**

Includes   burns and corrosion of hip region

Excludes2   burns and corrosion of axilla (T22.- with fifth character 4)

burns and corrosion of scapular region (T22.- with fifth character 6)

burns and corrosion of shoulder (T22.- with fifth character 5)

The appropriate 7th character is to be added to each code from category T21

A	initial encounter
D	subsequent encounter
S	sequela

● **T21.0**   **Burn of unspecified degree of trunk**

Use additional external cause code to identify the source, place and intent of the burn (X00-X19, X75-X77, X96-X98, Y92)

X ● **T21.00**   **Burn of unspecified degree of trunk, unspecified site**

X ● **T21.01**   **Burn of unspecified degree of chest wall**
Burn of of unspecified degree of breast

X ● **T21.02**   **Burn of unspecified degree of abdominal wall**
Burn of unspecified degree of flank
Burn of unspecified degree of groin

X ● **T21.03**   **Burn of unspecified degree of upper back**
Burn of unspecified degree of interscapular region

X ● **T21.04**   **Burn of unspecified degree of lower back**

X ● **T21.05**   **Burn of unspecified degree of buttock**
Burn of unspecified degree of anus

X ● **T21.06**   **Burn of unspecified degree of male genital region** ♂
Burn of unspecified degree of penis
Burn of unspecified degree of scrotum
Burn of unspecified degree of testis

X ● **T21.07**   **Burn of unspecified degree of female genital region** ♀
Burn of unspecified degree of labium (majus) (minus)
Burn of unspecified degree of perineum
Burn of unspecified degree of vulva

Excludes2   burn of vagina (T28.3)

X ● **T21.09**   **Burn of unspecified degree of other site of trunk**

● **T21.1**   **Burn of first degree of trunk**

Use additional external cause code to identify the source, place and intent of the burn (X00-X19, X75-X77, X96-X98, Y92)

X ● **T21.10**   **Burn of first degree of trunk, unspecified site**

X ● **T21.11**   **Burn of first degree of chest wall**
Burn of first degree of breast

X ● **T21.12**   **Burn of first degree of abdominal wall**
Burn of first degree of flank
Burn of first degree of groin

X ● **T21.13**   **Burn of first degree of upper back**
Burn of first degree of interscapular region

X ● **T21.14**   **Burn of first degree of lower back**

X ● **T21.15**   **Burn of first degree of buttock**
Burn of first degree of anus

X ● **T21.16**   **Burn of first degree of male genital region** ♂
Burn of first degree of penis
Burn of first degree of scrotum
Burn of first degree of testis

N Newborn Age: 0   **P** Pediatric Age: 0–17   **M** Maternity DX: 12–55   **A** Adult Age: 15–124   ♀ Females Only   ♂ Males Only

🅖 Complication\Comorbidity   🅜 Major C\C   (Ex) CC/MCC Exclusions   🅗 Hospital-Acquired Condition

X ● **T21.17**   **Burn of first degree of female genital region** ♀
  Burn of first degree of labium (majus) (minus)
  Burn of first degree of perineum
  Burn of first degree of vulva
  Excludes2   burn of vagina (T28.3)

X ● **T21.19**   **Burn of first degree of other site of trunk**

● **T21.2**   **Burn of second degree of trunk**
  Use additional external cause code to identify the
    source, place and intent of the burn (X00-X19,
    X75-X77, X96-X98, Y92)

X ● **T21.20**   **Burn of second degree of trunk, unspecified site**

X ● **T21.21**   **Burn of second degree of chest wall**
  Burn of second degree of breast

X ● **T21.22**   **Burn of second degree of abdominal wall**
  Burn of second degree of flank
  Burn of second degree of groin

X ● **T21.23**   **Burn of second degree of upper back**
  Burn of second degree of interscapular region

X ● **T21.24**   **Burn of second degree of lower back**

X ● **T21.25**   **Burn of second degree of buttock**
  Burn of second degree of anus

X ● **T21.26**   **Burn of second degree of male genital region** ♂
  Burn of second degree of penis
  Burn of second degree of scrotum
  Burn of second degree of testis

X ● **T21.27**   **Burn of second degree of female genital region** ♀
  Burn of second degree of labium (majus) (minus)
  Burn of second degree of perineum
  Burn of second degree of vulva
  Excludes2   burn of vagina (T28.3)

X ● **T21.29**   **Burn of second degree of other site of trunk**

● **T21.3**   **Burn of third degree of trunk**
  Use additional external cause code to identify the
    source, place and intent of the burn (X00-X19,
    X75-X77, X96-X98, Y92)

X ● **T21.30**   **Burn of third degree of trunk, unspecified site**
  A 🔖, A 🔖
  (Ex:) T21.30X[A], T21.39X[A], T21.70X[A], T21.79X[A]

X ● **T21.31**   **Burn of third degree of chest wall** A 🔖, A 🔖
  Burn of third degree of breast
  (Ex:) T21.30X-T21.31X[A], T21.39X[A], T21.70X-T21.71X[A],
    T21.79X[A]
  Coding Clinic: 2016, Q2, P6

X ● **T21.32**   **Burn of third degree of abdominal wall** A 🔖,
  A 🔖
  Burn of third degree of flank
  Burn of third degree of groin
  (Ex:) T21.30X[A], T21.32X[A], T21.39X[A], T21.70X[A], T21.72X[A],
    T21.79X[A]

X ● **T21.33**   **Burn of third degree of upper back** A 🔖, A 🔖
  Burn of third degree of interscapular region
  (Ex:) T21.30X[A], T21.33X-T21.35X[A], T21.39X[A], T21.70X[A],
    T21.73X-T21.75X[A], T21.79X[A]

X ● **T21.34**   **Burn of third degree of lower back** A 🔖, A 🔖
  (Ex:) See T21.33

X ● **T21.35**   **Burn of third degree of buttock** A 🔖, A 🔖
  Burn of third degree of anus
  (Ex:) See T21.33

X ● **T21.36**   **Burn of third degree of male genital region** ♂
  A 🔖, A 🔖
  Burn of third degree of penis
  Burn of third degree of scrotum
  Burn of third degree of testis
  (Ex:) T21.30X[A], T21.36X-T21.39X[A], T21.70X[A],
    T21.76X-T21.79X[A]

X ● **T21.37**   **Burn of third degree of female genital region** ♀
  A 🔖, A 🔖
  Burn of third degree of labium (majus) (minus)
  Burn of third degree of perineum
  Burn of third degree of vulva
  Excludes2   burn of vagina (T28.3)
  (Ex:) See T21.36

X ● **T21.39**   **Burn of third degree of other site of trunk** A 🔖,
  A 🔖
  (Ex:) See T21.30

● **T21.4**   **Corrosion of unspecified degree of trunk**
  Code first (T51-T65) to identify chemical and intent
  Use additional external cause code to identify
    place (Y92)

X ● **T21.40**   **Corrosion of unspecified degree of trunk, unspecified site**

X ● **T21.41**   **Corrosion of unspecified degree of chest wall**
  Corrosion of unspecified degree of breast

X ● **T21.42**   **Corrosion of unspecified degree of abdominal wall**
  Corrosion of unspecified degree of flank
  Corrosion of unspecified degree of groin

X ● **T21.43**   **Corrosion of unspecified degree of upper back**
  Corrosion of unspecified degree of
    interscapular region

X ● **T21.44**   **Corrosion of unspecified degree of lower back**

X ● **T21.45**   **Corrosion of unspecified degree of buttock**
  Corrosion of unspecified degree of anus

X ● **T21.46**   **Corrosion of unspecified degree of male genital region** ♂
  Corrosion of unspecified degree of penis
  Corrosion of unspecified degree of scrotum
  Corrosion of unspecified degree of testis

X ● **T21.47**   **Corrosion of unspecified degree of female genital region** ♀
  Corrosion of unspecified degree of labium
    (majus) (minus)
  Corrosion of unspecified degree of perineum
  Corrosion of unspecified degree of vulva
  Excludes2   corrosion of vagina (T28.8)

X ● **T21.49**   **Corrosion of unspecified degree of other site of trunk**

● **T21.5**   **Corrosion of first degree of trunk**
  Code first (T51-T65) to identify chemical and intent
  Use additional external cause code to identify
    place (Y92)

X ● **T21.50**   **Corrosion of first degree of trunk, unspecified site**

X ● **T21.51**   **Corrosion of first degree of chest wall**
  Corrosion of first degree of breast

X ● **T21.52**   **Corrosion of first degree of abdominal wall**
  Corrosion of first degree of flank
  Corrosion of first degree of groin

X ● **T21.53**   **Corrosion of first degree of upper back**
  Corrosion of first degree of interscapular
    region

X ● **T21.54**   **Corrosion of first degree of lower back**

X ● **T21.55**   **Corrosion of first degree of buttock**
  Corrosion of first degree of anus

X ● **T21.56**   **Corrosion of first degree of male genital region** ♂
  Corrosion of first degree of penis
  Corrosion of first degree of scrotum
  Corrosion of first degree of testis

X ● **T21.57**   **Corrosion of first degree of female genital region ♀**
    Corrosion of first degree of labium (majus) (minus)
    Corrosion of first degree of perineum
    Corrosion of first degree of vulva
    Excludes2   corrosion of vagina (T28.8)

X ● **T21.59**   **Corrosion of first degree of other site of trunk**

● **T21.6**   **Corrosion of second degree of trunk**
    Code first (T51-T65) *to identify chemical and intent*
    Use additional external cause code to identify place (Y92)

X ● **T21.60**   **Corrosion of second degree of trunk, unspecified site**

X ● **T21.61**   **Corrosion of second degree of chest wall**
    Corrosion of second degree of breast

X ● **T21.62**   **Corrosion of second degree of abdominal wall**
    Corrosion of second degree of flank
    Corrosion of second degree of groin

X ● **T21.63**   **Corrosion of second degree of upper back**
    Corrosion of second degree of interscapular region

X ● **T21.64**   **Corrosion of second degree of lower back**

X ● **T21.65**   **Corrosion of second degree of buttock**
    Corrosion of second degree of anus

X ● **T21.66**   **Corrosion of second degree of male genital region ♂**
    Corrosion of second degree of penis
    Corrosion of second degree of scrotum
    Corrosion of second degree of testis

X ● **T21.67**   **Corrosion of second degree of female genital region ♀**
    Corrosion of second degree of labium (majus) (minus)
    Corrosion of second degree of perineum
    Corrosion of second degree of vulva
    Excludes2   corrosion of vagina (T28.8)

X ● **T21.69**   **Corrosion of second degree of other site of trunk**

● **T21.7**   **Corrosion of third degree of trunk**
    Code first (T51-T65) *to identify chemical and intent*
    Use additional external cause code to identify place (Y92)

X ● **T21.70**   **Corrosion of third degree of trunk, unspecified site** A 🔵, A 🔷
    (Ex:) See T21.30

X ● **T21.71**   **Corrosion of third degree of chest wall** A 🔵, A 🔷
    Corrosion of third degree of breast
    (Ex:) See T21.31

X ● **T21.72**   **Corrosion of third degree of abdominal wall** A 🔵, A 🔷
    Corrosion of third degree of flank
    Corrosion of third degree of groin
    (Ex:) See T21.32

X ● **T21.73**   **Corrosion of third degree of upper back** A 🔵, A 🔷
    Corrosion of third degree of interscapular region
    (Ex:) See T21.33

X ● **T21.74**   **Corrosion of third degree of lower back** A 🔵, A 🔷
    (Ex:) See T21.33

X ● **T21.75**   **Corrosion of third degree of buttock** A 🔵, A 🔷
    Corrosion of third degree of anus
    (Ex:) See T21.33

X ● **T21.76**   **Corrosion of third degree of male genital region ♂** A 🔵, A 🔷
    Corrosion of third degree of penis
    Corrosion of third degree of scrotum
    Corrosion of third degree of testis
    (Ex:) See T21.36

X ● **T21.77**   **Corrosion of third degree of female genital region ♀** A 🔵, A 🔷
    Corrosion of third degree of labium (majus) (minus)
    Corrosion of third degree of perineum
    Corrosion of third degree of vulva
    Excludes2   corrosion of vagina (T28.8)
    (Ex:) See T21.36

X ● **T21.79**   **Corrosion of third degree of other site of trunk** A 🔵, A 🔷
    (Ex:) See T21.30

● **T22**   **Burn and corrosion of shoulder and upper limb, except wrist and hand**
    Excludes2   burn and corrosion of interscapular region (T21.-)
                burn and corrosion of wrist and hand (T23.-)
    The appropriate 7th character is to be added to each code from category T22

A	initial encounter
D	subsequent encounter
S	sequela

● **T22.0**   **Burn of unspecified degree of shoulder and upper limb, except wrist and hand**
    Use additional external cause code to identify the source, place and intent of the burn (X00-X19, X75-X77, X96-X98, Y92)

X ● **T22.00**   **Burn of unspecified degree of shoulder and upper limb, except wrist and hand, unspecified site**

● **T22.01**   **Burn of unspecified degree of forearm**
    ● **T22.011**   **Burn of unspecified degree of right forearm**
    ● **T22.012**   **Burn of unspecified degree of left forearm**
    ● **T22.019**   **Burn of unspecified degree of unspecified forearm**

● **T22.02**   **Burn of unspecified degree of elbow**
    ● **T22.021**   **Burn of unspecified degree of right elbow**
    ● **T22.022**   **Burn of unspecified degree of left elbow**
    ● **T22.029**   **Burn of unspecified degree of unspecified elbow**

● **T22.03**   **Burn of unspecified degree of upper arm**
    ● **T22.031**   **Burn of unspecified degree of right upper arm**
    ● **T22.032**   **Burn of unspecified degree of left upper arm**
    ● **T22.039**   **Burn of unspecified degree of unspecified upper arm**

● **T22.04**   **Burn of unspecified degree of axilla**
    ● **T22.041**   **Burn of unspecified degree of right axilla**
    ● **T22.042**   **Burn of unspecified degree of left axilla**
    ● **T22.049**   **Burn of unspecified degree of unspecified axilla**

N Newborn Age: 0   **P** Pediatric Age: 0–17   **M** Maternity DX: 12–55   **A** Adult Age: 15–124   ♀ Females Only   ♂ Males Only

🔵 Complication\Comorbidity   🔷 Major C\C   (Ex:) CC/MCC Exclusions   🔶 Hospital-Acquired Condition   **1425**

CHAPTER 19 (S00-T88)

CHAPTER 19 (S00-T88)

● T22.05   Burn of unspecified degree of shoulder
- ● T22.051   Burn of <mark>unspecified</mark> degree of right shoulder
- ● T22.052   Burn of <mark>unspecified</mark> degree of left shoulder
- ● T22.059   Burn of <mark>unspecified</mark> degree of unspecified shoulder

● T22.06   Burn of unspecified degree of scapular region
- ● T22.061   Burn of <mark>unspecified</mark> degree of right scapular region
- ● T22.062   Burn of <mark>unspecified</mark> degree of left scapular region
- ● T22.069   Burn of <mark>unspecified</mark> degree of unspecified scapular region

● T22.09   Burn of unspecified degree of multiple sites of shoulder and upper limb, except wrist and hand
- ● T22.091   Burn of <mark>unspecified</mark> degree of multiple sites of right shoulder and upper limb, except wrist and hand
- ● T22.092   Burn of <mark>unspecified</mark> degree of multiple sites of left shoulder and upper limb, except wrist and hand
- ● T22.099   Burn of <mark>unspecified</mark> degree of multiple sites of unspecified shoulder and upper limb, except wrist and hand

● T22.1   Burn of first degree of shoulder and upper limb, except wrist and hand

    Use additional external cause code to identify the source, place and intent of the burn (X00-X19, X75-X77, X96-X98, Y92)

X ● T22.10   Burn of first degree of shoulder and upper limb, except wrist and hand, <mark>unspecified</mark> site

● T22.11   Burn of first degree of forearm
- ● T22.111   Burn of first degree of right forearm
- ● T22.112   Burn of first degree of left forearm
- ● T22.119   Burn of first degree of <mark>unspecified</mark> forearm

● T22.12   Burn of first degree of elbow
- ● T22.121   Burn of first degree of right elbow
- ● T22.122   Burn of first degree of left elbow
- ● T22.129   Burn of first degree of <mark>unspecified</mark> elbow

● T22.13   Burn of first degree of upper arm
- ● T22.131   Burn of first degree of right upper arm
- ● T22.132   Burn of first degree of left upper arm
- ● T22.139   Burn of first degree of <mark>unspecified</mark> upper arm

● T22.14   Burn of first degree of axilla
- ● T22.141   Burn of first degree of right axilla
- ● T22.142   Burn of first degree of left axilla
- ● T22.149   Burn of first degree of <mark>unspecified</mark> axilla

● T22.15   Burn of first degree of shoulder
- ● T22.151   Burn of first degree of right shoulder
- ● T22.152   Burn of first degree of left shoulder
- ● T22.159   Burn of first degree of <mark>unspecified</mark> shoulder

● T22.16   Burn of first degree of scapular region
- ● T22.161   Burn of first degree of right scapular region
- ● T22.162   Burn of first degree of left scapular region
- ● T22.169   Burn of first degree of <mark>unspecified</mark> scapular region

● T22.19   Burn of first degree of multiple sites of shoulder and upper limb, except wrist and hand
- ● T22.191   Burn of first degree of multiple sites of right shoulder and upper limb, except wrist and hand
- ● T22.192   Burn of first degree of multiple sites of left shoulder and upper limb, except wrist and hand
- ● T22.199   Burn of first degree of multiple sites of <mark>unspecified</mark> shoulder and upper limb, except wrist and hand

● T22.2   Burn of second degree of shoulder and upper limb, except wrist and hand

    Use additional external cause code to identify the source, place and intent of the burn (X00-X19, X75-X77, X96-X98, Y92)

X ● T22.20   Burn of second degree of shoulder and upper limb, except wrist and hand, <mark>unspecified</mark> site

● T22.21   Burn of second degree of forearm
- ● T22.211   Burn of second degree of right forearm
- ● T22.212   Burn of second degree of left forearm
- ● T22.219   Burn of second degree of <mark>unspecified</mark> forearm

● T22.22   Burn of second degree of elbow
- ● T22.221   Burn of second degree of right elbow
- ● T22.222   Burn of second degree of left elbow
- ● T22.229   Burn of second degree of <mark>unspecified</mark> elbow

● T22.23   Burn of second degree of upper arm
- ● T22.231   Burn of second degree of right upper arm
- ● T22.232   Burn of second degree of left upper arm
- ● T22.239   Burn of second degree of <mark>unspecified</mark> upper arm

● T22.24   Burn of second degree of axilla
- ● T22.241   Burn of second degree of right axilla
- ● T22.242   Burn of second degree of left axilla
- ● T22.249   Burn of second degree of <mark>unspecified</mark> axilla

● T22.25   Burn of second degree of shoulder
- ● T22.251   Burn of second degree of right shoulder
- ● T22.252   Burn of second degree of left shoulder
- ● T22.259   Burn of second degree of <mark>unspecified</mark> shoulder

● T22.26   Burn of second degree of scapular region
- ● T22.261   Burn of second degree of right scapular region
- ● T22.262   Burn of second degree of left scapular region
- ● T22.269   Burn of second degree of <mark>unspecified</mark> scapular region

● T22.29   Burn of second degree of multiple sites of shoulder and upper limb, except wrist and hand
- ● T22.291   Burn of second degree of multiple sites of right shoulder and upper limb, except wrist and hand
- ● T22.292   Burn of second degree of multiple sites of left shoulder and upper limb, except wrist and hand
- ● T22.299   Burn of second degree of multiple sites of <mark>unspecified</mark> shoulder and upper limb, except wrist and hand

◄ New   ◄▬ Revised   ~~deleted~~ Deleted   Excludes 1   Excludes 2   Includes   Use additional   Code first   Code also   <mark>Unspecified</mark>

OGCR Official Guidelines   ● Unacceptable Principal Diagnosis   X Assign placeholder X   ● Use Additional Character(s)   ▶ Manifestation Code   **Coding Clinic**

● **T22.3**   **Burn of third degree of shoulder and upper limb, except wrist and hand**

> Use additional external cause code to identify the source, place and intent of the burn (X00-X19, X75-X77, X96-X98, Y92)

X● **T22.30**   **Burn of third degree of shoulder and upper limb, except wrist and hand, unspecified site** A 🔵, A 🔵
> (Ex) T22.30X[A], T22.391-T22.399[A], T22.70X[A], T22.791-T22.799[A]

● **T22.31**   **Burn of third degree of forearm**
> (Ex) For category T22.31 CC codes: T22.30X-T22.319[A], T22.391-T22.399[A], T22.70X-T22.719[A], T22.791-T22.799[A]

  ● **T22.311**   **Burn of third degree of right forearm** A 🔵, A 🔵

  ● **T22.312**   **Burn of third degree of left forearm** A 🔵, A 🔵

  ● **T22.319**   **Burn of third degree of unspecified forearm** A 🔵, A 🔵

● **T22.32**   **Burn of third degree of elbow**
> (Ex) For category T22.32 CC codes: T22.30X[A], T22.321-T22.329[A], T22.391-T22.399[A], T22.70X[A], T22.721-T22.729[A], T22.791-T22.799[A]

  ● **T22.321**   **Burn of third degree of right elbow** A 🔵, A 🔵

  ● **T22.322**   **Burn of third degree of left elbow** A 🔵, A 🔵

  ● **T22.329**   **Burn of third degree of unspecified elbow** A 🔵, A 🔵

● **T22.33**   **Burn of third degree of upper arm**
> (Ex) For category T22.33 CC codes: T22.30X[A], T22.331-T22.339[A], T22.391-T22.399[A], T22.70X[A], T22.731-T22.739[A], T22.791-T22.799[A]

  ● **T22.331**   **Burn of third degree of right upper arm** A 🔵, A 🔵

  ● **T22.332**   **Burn of third degree of left upper arm** A 🔵, A 🔵

  ● **T22.339**   **Burn of third degree of unspecified upper arm** A 🔵, A 🔵

● **T22.34**   **Burn of third degree of axilla**
> (Ex) For category T22.34 CC codes: T22.30X[A], T22.341-T22.349[A], .T22.391-T22.399[A], T22.70X[A], T22.741-T22.749[A], T22.791-T22.799[A]

  ● **T22.341**   **Burn of third degree of right axilla** A 🔵, A 🔵

  ● **T22.342**   **Burn of third degree of left axilla** A 🔵, A 🔵

  ● **T22.349**   **Burn of third degree of unspecified axilla** A 🔵, A 🔵

● **T22.35**   **Burn of third degree of shoulder**
> (Ex) For category T22.35 CC codes: T22.30X[A], T22.351-T22.359[A], T22.391-T22.399[A], T22.70X[A], T22.751-T22.759[A], T22.791-T22.799[A]

  ● **T22.351**   **Burn of third degree of right shoulder** A 🔵, A 🔵

  ● **T22.352**   **Burn of third degree of left shoulder** A 🔵, A 🔵

  ● **T22.359**   **Burn of third degree of unspecified shoulder** A 🔵, A 🔵

● **T22.36**   **Burn of third degree of scapular region**
> (Ex) For category T22.36 CC codes: T22.30X[A], T22.361-T22.369[A], T22.391-T22.399[A], T22.70X[A], T22.761-T22.769[A], T22.791-T22.799[A]

  ● **T22.361**   **Burn of third degree of right scapular region** A 🔵, A 🔵

  ● **T22.362**   **Burn of third degree of left scapular region** A 🔵, A 🔵

  ● **T22.369**   **Burn of third degree of unspecified scapular region** A 🔵, A 🔵

● **T22.39**   **Burn of third degree of multiple sites of shoulder and upper limb, except wrist and hand**
> (Ex) For category T22.39 CC codes: See T22.30

  ● **T22.391**   **Burn of third degree of multiple sites of right shoulder and upper limb, except wrist and hand** A 🔵, A 🔵

  ● **T22.392**   **Burn of third degree of multiple sites of left shoulder and upper limb, except wrist and hand** A 🔵, A 🔵

  ● **T22.399**   **Burn of third degree of multiple sites of unspecified shoulder and upper limb, except wrist and hand** A 🔵, A 🔵

● **T22.4**   **Corrosion of unspecified degree of shoulder and upper limb, except wrist and hand**

> *Code first* (T51-T65) *to identify chemical and intent*
> Use additional external cause code to identify place (Y92)

X● **T22.40**   **Corrosion of unspecified degree of shoulder and upper limb, except wrist and hand, unspecified site**

● **T22.41**   **Corrosion of unspecified degree of forearm**

  ● **T22.411**   **Corrosion of unspecified degree of right forearm**

  ● **T22.412**   **Corrosion of unspecified degree of left forearm**

  ● **T22.419**   **Corrosion of unspecified degree of unspecified forearm**

● **T22.42**   **Corrosion of unspecified degree of elbow**

  ● **T22.421**   **Corrosion of unspecified degree of right elbow**

  ● **T22.422**   **Corrosion of unspecified degree of left elbow**

  ● **T22.429**   **Corrosion of unspecified degree of unspecified elbow**

● **T22.43**   **Corrosion of unspecified degree of upper arm**

  ● **T22.431**   **Corrosion of unspecified degree of right upper arm**

  ● **T22.432**   **Corrosion of unspecified degree of left upper arm**

  ● **T22.439**   **Corrosion of unspecified degree of unspecified upper arm**

● **T22.44**   **Corrosion of unspecified degree of axilla**

  ● **T22.441**   **Corrosion of unspecified degree of right axilla**

  ● **T22.442**   **Corrosion of unspecified degree of left axilla**

  ● **T22.449**   **Corrosion of unspecified degree of unspecified axilla**

● **T22.45**   **Corrosion of unspecified degree of shoulder**

  ● **T22.451**   **Corrosion of unspecified degree of right shoulder**

  ● **T22.452**   **Corrosion of unspecified degree of left shoulder**

  ● **T22.459**   **Corrosion of unspecified degree of unspecified shoulder**

● **T22.46**   **Corrosion of unspecified degree of scapular region**

  ● **T22.461**   **Corrosion of unspecified degree of right scapular region**

  ● **T22.462**   **Corrosion of unspecified degree of left scapular region**

  ● **T22.469**   **Corrosion of unspecified degree of unspecified scapular region**

N Newborn Age: 0   P Pediatric Age: 0–17   M Maternity DX: 12–55   A Adult Age: 15–124   ♀ Females Only   ♂ Males Only
🔵 Complication\Comorbidity   🔵 Major C\C   (Ex) CC/MCC Exclusions   🔵 Hospital-Acquired Condition
1427

- **T22.49** Corrosion of unspecified degree of multiple sites of shoulder and upper limb, except wrist and hand
  - **T22.491** Corrosion of unspecified degree of multiple sites of right shoulder and upper limb, except wrist and hand
  - **T22.492** Corrosion of unspecified degree of multiple sites of left shoulder and upper limb, except wrist and hand
  - **T22.499** Corrosion of unspecified degree of multiple sites of unspecified shoulder and upper limb, except wrist and hand
- **T22.5** Corrosion of first degree of shoulder and upper limb, except wrist and hand

  Code first (T51-T65) to identify chemical and intent

  Use additional external cause code to identify place (Y92)
  - X **T22.50** Corrosion of first degree of shoulder and upper limb, except wrist and hand unspecified site
  - **T22.51** Corrosion of first degree of forearm
    - **T22.511** Corrosion of first degree of right forearm
    - **T22.512** Corrosion of first degree of left forearm
    - **T22.519** Corrosion of first degree of unspecified forearm
  - **T22.52** Corrosion of first degree of elbow
    - **T22.521** Corrosion of first degree of right elbow
    - **T22.522** Corrosion of first degree of left elbow
    - **T22.529** Corrosion of first degree of unspecified elbow
  - **T22.53** Corrosion of first degree of upper arm
    - **T22.531** Corrosion of first degree of right upper arm
    - **T22.532** Corrosion of first degree of left upper arm
    - **T22.539** Corrosion of first degree of unspecified upper arm
  - **T22.54** Corrosion of first degree of axilla
    - **T22.541** Corrosion of first degree of right axilla
    - **T22.542** Corrosion of first degree of left axilla
    - **T22.549** Corrosion of first degree of unspecified axilla
  - **T22.55** Corrosion of first degree of shoulder
    - **T22.551** Corrosion of first degree of right shoulder
    - **T22.552** Corrosion of first degree of left shoulder
    - **T22.559** Corrosion of first degree of unspecified shoulder
  - **T22.56** Corrosion of first degree of scapular region
    - **T22.561** Corrosion of first degree of right scapular region
    - **T22.562** Corrosion of first degree of left scapular region
    - **T22.569** Corrosion of first degree of unspecified scapular region

- **T22.59** Corrosion of first degree of multiple sites of shoulder and upper limb, except wrist and hand
  - **T22.591** Corrosion of first degree of multiple sites of right shoulder and upper limb, except wrist and hand
  - **T22.592** Corrosion of first degree of multiple sites of left shoulder and upper limb, except wrist and hand
  - **T22.599** Corrosion of first degree of multiple sites of unspecified shoulder and upper limb, except wrist and hand
- **T22.6** Corrosion of second degree of shoulder and upper limb, except wrist and hand

  Code first (T51-T65) to identify chemical and intent

  Use additional external cause code to identify place (Y92)
  - X **T22.60** Corrosion of second degree of shoulder and upper limb, except wrist and hand, unspecified site
  - **T22.61** Corrosion of second degree of forearm
    - **T22.611** Corrosion of second degree of right forearm
    - **T22.612** Corrosion of second degree of left forearm
    - **T22.619** Corrosion of second degree of unspecified forearm
  - **T22.62** Corrosion of second degree of elbow
    - **T22.621** Corrosion of second degree of right elbow
    - **T22.622** Corrosion of second degree of left elbow
    - **T22.629** Corrosion of second degree of unspecified elbow
  - **T22.63** Corrosion of second degree of upper arm
    - **T22.631** Corrosion of second degree of right upper arm
    - **T22.632** Corrosion of second degree of left upper arm
    - **T22.639** Corrosion of second degree of unspecified upper arm
  - **T22.64** Corrosion of second degree of axilla
    - **T22.641** Corrosion of second degree of right axilla
    - **T22.642** Corrosion of second degree of left axilla
    - **T22.649** Corrosion of second degree of unspecified axilla
  - **T22.65** Corrosion of second degree of shoulder
    - **T22.651** Corrosion of second degree of right shoulder
    - **T22.652** Corrosion of second degree of left shoulder
    - **T22.659** Corrosion of second degree of unspecified shoulder
  - **T22.66** Corrosion of second degree of scapular region
    - **T22.661** Corrosion of second degree of right scapular region
    - **T22.662** Corrosion of second degree of left scapular region
    - **T22.669** Corrosion of second degree of unspecified scapular region

◀ New   ◀ Revised   ~~deleted~~ Deleted   Excludes 1   Excludes 2   Includes   Use additional   Code first   Code also   Unspecified

OGCR Official Guidelines   ● Unacceptable Principal Diagnosis   X Assign placeholder X   ● Use Additional Character(s)   ▶ Manifestation Code   **Coding Clinic**

- **T22.69** Corrosion of second degree of multiple sites of shoulder and upper limb, except wrist and hand
  - **T22.691** Corrosion of second degree of multiple sites of right shoulder and upper limb, except wrist and hand
  - **T22.692** Corrosion of second degree of multiple sites of left shoulder and upper limb, except wrist and hand
  - **T22.699** Corrosion of second degree of multiple sites of unspecified shoulder and upper limb, except wrist and hand
- **T22.7** Corrosion of third degree of shoulder and upper limb, except wrist and hand
  - *Code first (T51-T65) to identify chemical and intent*
  - Use additional external cause code to identify place (Y92)
  - X **T22.70** Corrosion of third degree of shoulder and upper limb, except wrist and hand, unspecified site A 🦠, A 🦠
    - (Ex) See T22.30
  - **T22.71** Corrosion of third degree of forearm
    - (Ex) For category T22.71 CC codes: See T22.31
    - **T22.711** Corrosion of third degree of right forearm A 🦠, A 🦠
    - **T22.712** Corrosion of third degree of left forearm A 🦠, A 🦠
    - **T22.719** Corrosion of third degree of unspecified forearm A 🦠, A 🦠
  - **T22.72** Corrosion of third degree of elbow
    - (Ex) For category T22.72 CC codes: See T22.32
    - **T22.721** Corrosion of third degree of right elbow A 🦠, A 🦠
    - **T22.722** Corrosion of third degree of left elbow A 🦠, A 🦠
    - **T22.729** Corrosion of third degree of unspecified elbow A 🦠, A 🦠
  - **T22.73** Corrosion of third degree of upper arm
    - (Ex) For category T22.73 CC codes: T22.33
    - **T22.731** Corrosion of third degree of right upper arm A 🦠, A 🦠
    - **T22.732** Corrosion of third degree of left upper arm A 🦠, A 🦠
    - **T22.739** Corrosion of third degree of unspecified upper arm A 🦠, A 🦠
  - **T22.74** Corrosion of third degree of axilla
    - (Ex) For category T22.74 CC codes: T22.34
    - **T22.741** Corrosion of third degree of right axilla A 🦠, A 🦠
    - **T22.742** Corrosion of third degree of left axilla A 🦠, A 🦠
    - **T22.749** Corrosion of third degree of unspecified axilla A 🦠, A 🦠
  - **T22.75** Corrosion of third degree of shoulder
    - (Ex) For category T22.75 CC codes: T22.35
    - **T22.751** Corrosion of third degree of right shoulder A 🦠, A 🦠
    - **T22.752** Corrosion of third degree of left shoulder A 🦠, A 🦠
    - **T22.759** Corrosion of third degree of unspecified shoulder A 🦠, A 🦠
- **T22.76** Corrosion of third degree of scapular region
  - (Ex) For category T22.76 CC codes: T22.36
  - **T22.761** Corrosion of third degree of right scapular region A 🦠, A 🦠
  - **T22.762** Corrosion of third degree of left scapular region A 🦠, A 🦠
  - **T22.769** Corrosion of third degree of unspecified scapular region A 🦠, A 🦠
- **T22.79** Corrosion of third degree of multiple sites of shoulder and upper limb, except wrist and hand
  - (Ex) For category T22.79 CC codes: See T22.30
  - **T22.791** Corrosion of third degree of multiple sites of right shoulder and upper limb, except wrist and hand A 🦠, A 🦠
  - **T22.792** Corrosion of third degree of multiple sites of left shoulder and upper limb, except wrist and hand A 🦠, A 🦠
  - **T22.799** Corrosion of third degree of multiple sites of unspecified shoulder and upper limb, except wrist and hand A 🦠, A 🦠
- **T23** Burn and corrosion of wrist and hand
  - The appropriate 7th character is to be added to each code from category T23

A	initial encounter
D	subsequent encounter
S	sequela

  - **T23.0** Burn of unspecified degree of wrist and hand
    - Use additional external cause code to identify the source, place and intent of the burn (X00-X19, X75-X77, X96-X98, Y92)
    - **T23.00** Burn of unspecified degree of hand, unspecified site
      - **T23.001** Burn of unspecified degree of right hand, unspecified site
      - **T23.002** Burn of unspecified degree of left hand, unspecified site
      - **T23.009** Burn of unspecified degree of unspecified hand, unspecified site
    - **T23.01** Burn of unspecified degree of thumb (nail)
      - **T23.011** Burn of unspecified degree of right thumb (nail)
      - **T23.012** Burn of unspecified degree of left thumb (nail)
      - **T23.019** Burn of unspecified degree of unspecified thumb (nail)
    - **T23.02** Burn of unspecified degree of single finger (nail) except thumb
      - **T23.021** Burn of unspecified degree of single right finger (nail) except thumb
      - **T23.022** Burn of unspecified degree of single left finger (nail) except thumb
      - **T23.029** Burn of unspecified degree of unspecified single finger (nail) except thumb
    - **T23.03** Burn of unspecified degree of multiple fingers (nail), not including thumb
      - **T23.031** Burn of unspecified degree of multiple right fingers (nail), not including thumb
      - **T23.032** Burn of unspecified degree of multiple left fingers (nail), not including thumb
      - **T23.039** Burn of unspecified degree of unspecified multiple fingers (nail), not including thumb

CHAPTER 19 (S00-T88)

N Newborn Age: 0   **P** Pediatric Age: 0–17   **M** Maternity DX: 12–55   **A** Adult Age: 15–124   ♀ Females Only   ♂ Males Only

🦠 Complication\Comorbidity   🦠 Major C\C   (Ex) CC/MCC Exclusions   🦠 Hospital-Acquired Condition   **1429**

● T23.04   Burn of unspecified degree of multiple fingers (nail), including thumb
    ● T23.041   Burn of unspecified degree of multiple right fingers (nail), including thumb
    ● T23.042   Burn of unspecified degree of multiple left fingers (nail), including thumb
    ● T23.049   Burn of unspecified degree of unspecified multiple fingers (nail), including thumb
● T23.05   Burn of unspecified degree of palm
    ● T23.051   Burn of unspecified degree of right palm
    ● T23.052   Burn of unspecified degree of left palm
    ● T23.059   Burn of unspecified degree of unspecified palm
● T23.06   Burn of unspecified degree of back of hand
    ● T23.061   Burn of unspecified degree of back of right hand
    ● T23.062   Burn of unspecified degree of back of left hand
    ● T23.069   Burn of unspecified degree of back of unspecified hand
● T23.07   Burn of unspecified degree of wrist
    ● T23.071   Burn of unspecified degree of right wrist
    ● T23.072   Burn of unspecified degree of left wrist
    ● T23.079   Burn of unspecified degree of unspecified wrist
● T23.09   Burn of unspecified degree of multiple sites of wrist and hand
    ● T23.091   Burn of unspecified degree of multiple sites of right wrist and hand
    ● T23.092   Burn of unspecified degree of multiple sites of left wrist and hand
    ● T23.099   Burn of unspecified degree of multiple sites of unspecified wrist and hand

● T23.1   Burn of first degree of wrist and hand
    Use additional external cause code to identify the source, place and intent of the burn (X00-X19, X75-X77, X96-X98, Y92)
  ● T23.10   Burn of first degree of hand, unspecified site
    ● T23.101   Burn of first degree of right hand, unspecified site
    ● T23.102   Burn of first degree of left hand, unspecified site
    ● T23.109   Burn of first degree of unspecified hand, unspecified site
  ● T23.11   Burn of first degree of thumb (nail)
    ● T23.111   Burn of first degree of right thumb (nail)
    ● T23.112   Burn of first degree of left thumb (nail)
    ● T23.119   Burn of first degree of unspecified thumb (nail)
  ● T23.12   Burn of first degree of single finger (nail) except thumb
    ● T23.121   Burn of first degree of single right finger (nail) except thumb
    ● T23.122   Burn of first degree of single left finger (nail) except thumb
    ● T23.129   Burn of first degree of unspecified single finger (nail) except thumb

● T23.13   Burn of first degree of multiple fingers (nail), not including thumb
    ● T23.131   Burn of first degree of multiple right fingers (nail), not including thumb
    ● T23.132   Burn of first degree of multiple left fingers (nail), not including thumb
    ● T23.139   Burn of first degree of unspecified multiple fingers (nail), not including thumb
● T23.14   Burn of first degree of multiple fingers (nail), including thumb
    ● T23.141   Burn of first degree of multiple right fingers (nail), including thumb
    ● T23.142   Burn of first degree of multiple left fingers (nail), including thumb
    ● T23.149   Burn of first degree of unspecified multiple fingers (nail), including thumb
● T23.15   Burn of first degree of palm
    ● T23.151   Burn of first degree of right palm
    ● T23.152   Burn of first degree of left palm
    ● T23.159   Burn of first degree of unspecified palm
● T23.16   Burn of first degree of back of hand
    ● T23.161   Burn of first degree of back of right hand
    ● T23.162   Burn of first degree of back of left hand
    ● T23.169   Burn of first degree of back of unspecified hand
● T23.17   Burn of first degree of wrist
    ● T23.171   Burn of first degree of right wrist
    ● T23.172   Burn of first degree of left wrist
    ● T23.179   Burn of first degree of unspecified wrist
● T23.19   Burn of first degree of multiple sites of wrist and hand
    ● T23.191   Burn of first degree of multiple sites of right wrist and hand
    ● T23.192   Burn of first degree of multiple sites of left wrist and hand
    ● T23.199   Burn of first degree of multiple sites of unspecified wrist and hand

● T23.2   Burn of second degree of wrist and hand
    Use additional external cause code to identify the source, place and intent of the burn (X00-X19, X75-X77, X96-X98, Y92)
  ● T23.20   Burn of second degree of hand, unspecified site
    ● T23.201   Burn of second degree of right hand, unspecified site
    ● T23.202   Burn of second degree of left hand, unspecified site
    ● T23.209   Burn of second degree of unspecified hand, unspecified site
  ● T23.21   Burn of second degree of thumb (nail)
    ● T23.211   Burn of second degree of right thumb (nail)
    ● T23.212   Burn of second degree of left thumb (nail)
    ● T23.219   Burn of second degree of unspecified thumb (nail)

◄ New   ◄ Revised   ~~deleted~~ Deleted   Excludes 1   Excludes 2   Includes   Use additional   Code first   Code also   Unspecified
OGCR Official Guidelines   ● Unacceptable Principal Diagnosis   X Assign placeholder X   ● Use Additional Character(s)   ▶ Manifestation Code   **Coding Clinic**

● **T23.22**   Burn of second degree of single finger (nail) except thumb

    ● **T23.221**   Burn of second degree of single right finger (nail) except thumb

    ● **T23.222**   Burn of second degree of single left finger (nail) except thumb

    ● **T23.229**   Burn of second degree of unspecified single finger (nail) except thumb

● **T23.23**   Burn of second degree of multiple fingers (nail), not including thumb

    ● **T23.231**   Burn of second degree of multiple right fingers (nail), not including thumb

    ● **T23.232**   Burn of second degree of multiple left fingers (nail), not including thumb

    ● **T23.239**   Burn of second degree of unspecified multiple fingers (nail), not including thumb

● **T23.24**   Burn of second degree of multiple fingers (nail), including thumb

    ● **T23.241**   Burn of second degree of multiple right fingers (nail), including thumb

    ● **T23.242**   Burn of second degree of multiple left fingers (nail), including thumb

    ● **T23.249**   Burn of second degree of unspecified multiple fingers (nail), including thumb

● **T23.25**   Burn of second degree of palm

    ● **T23.251**   Burn of second degree of right palm

    ● **T23.252**   Burn of second degree of left palm

    ● **T23.259**   Burn of second degree of unspecified palm

● **T23.26**   Burn of second degree of back of hand

    ● **T23.261**   Burn of second degree of back of right hand

    ● **T23.262**   Burn of second degree of back of left hand

    ● **T23.269**   Burn of second degree of back of unspecified hand

● **T23.27**   Burn of second degree of wrist

    ● **T23.271**   Burn of second degree of right wrist

    ● **T23.272**   Burn of second degree of left wrist

    ● **T23.279**   Burn of second degree of unspecified wrist

● **T23.29**   Burn of second degree of multiple sites of wrist and hand

    ● **T23.291**   Burn of second degree of multiple sites of right wrist and hand

    ● **T23.292**   Burn of second degree of multiple sites of left wrist and hand

    ● **T23.299**   Burn of second degree of multiple sites of unspecified wrist and hand

● **T23.3**   Burn of third degree of wrist and hand

    Use additional external cause code to identify the source, place and intent of the burn (X00-X19, X75-X77, X96-X98, Y92)

● **T23.30**   Burn of third degree of hand, unspecified site

    (Ex) **For category T23.30 CC codes:** T23.301-T23.309[A], T23.391-T23.399[A], T23.701-T23.709[A], T23.791-T23.799[A]

    ● **T23.301**   Burn of third degree of right hand, unspecified site A 🪙, A 🪙

      Coding Clinic: 2015, Q1, P19

    ● **T23.302**   Burn of third degree of left hand, unspecified site A 🪙, A 🪙

      Coding Clinic: 2016, Q2, P5

    ● **T23.309**   Burn of third degree of unspecified hand, unspecified site A 🪙, A 🪙

● **T23.31**   Burn of third degree of thumb (nail)

    (Ex) **For category T23.31 CC codes:** T23.301-T23.319[A], T23.391-T23.399[A], T23.701-T23.719[A], T23.791-T23.799[A]

    ● **T23.311**   Burn of third degree of right thumb (nail) A 🪙, A 🪙

    ● **T23.312**   Burn of third degree of left thumb (nail) A 🪙, A 🪙

    ● **T23.319**   Burn of third degree of unspecified thumb (nail) A 🪙, A 🪙

● **T23.32**   Burn of third degree of single finger (nail) except thumb

    (Ex) **For category T23.32 CC codes:** T23.301-T23.309[A], T23.321-T23.329[A], T23.391-T23.399[A], T23.701-T23.709[A], T23.721-T23.729[A], T23.791-T23.799[A]

    ● **T23.321**   Burn of third degree of single right finger (nail) except thumb A 🪙, A 🪙

    ● **T23.322**   Burn of third degree of single left finger (nail) except thumb A 🪙, A 🪙

    ● **T23.329**   Burn of third degree of unspecified single finger (nail) except thumb A 🪙, A 🪙

● **T23.33**   Burn of third degree of multiple fingers (nail), not including thumb

    (Ex) **For category T23.33 CC codes:** T23.301-T23.309[A], T23.331-T23.339[A], T23.391-T23.399[A], T23.701-709[A], T23.731-T23.739[A], T23.791-T23.799[A]

    ● **T23.331**   Burn of third degree of multiple right fingers (nail), not including thumb A 🪙, A 🪙

    ● **T23.332**   Burn of third degree of multiple left fingers (nail), not including thumb A 🪙, A 🪙

    ● **T23.339**   Burn of third degree of unspecified multiple fingers (nail), not including thumb A 🪙, A 🪙

● **T23.34**   Burn of third degree of multiple fingers (nail), including thumb

    (Ex) **For category T23.34 CC codes:** T23.301-T23.309[A], T23.341-T23.349[A], T23.391-T23.399[A], T23.701-T23.709[A], T23.741-T23.749[A], T23.791-T23.799[A]

    ● **T23.341**   Burn of third degree of multiple right fingers (nail), including thumb A 🪙, A 🪙

    ● **T23.342**   Burn of third degree of multiple left fingers (nail), including thumb A 🪙, A 🪙

    ● **T23.349**   Burn of third degree of unspecified multiple fingers (nail), including thumb A 🪙, A 🪙

● **T23.35**   Burn of third degree of palm

    (Ex) **For category T23.35 CC codes:** T23.301-T23.309[A], T23.351-T23.359[A], T23.391-T23.399[A], T23.701-T23.709[A], T23.751-T23.759[A], T23.791-T23.799[A]

    ● **T23.351**   Burn of third degree of right palm A 🪙, A 🪙

    ● **T23.352**   Burn of third degree of left palm A 🪙, A 🪙

    ● **T23.359**   Burn of third degree of unspecified palm A 🪙, A 🪙

● **T23.36**   Burn of third degree of back of hand

    (Ex) **For category T23.36 CC codes:** T23.301-T23.309[A], T23.361-T23.369[A], T23.391-T23.399[A], T23.701-T23.709[A], T23.761-T23.769[A], T23.791-T23.799[A]

    ● **T23.361**   Burn of third degree of back of right hand A 🪙, A 🪙

    ● **T23.362**   Burn of third degree of back of left hand A 🪙, A 🪙

    ● **T23.369**   Burn of third degree of back of unspecified hand A 🪙, A 🪙

CHAPTER 19 (S00-T88)

N Newborn Age: 0   **P** Pediatric Age: 0–17   **M** Maternity DX: 12–55   **A** Adult Age: 15–124   ♀ Females Only   ♂ Males Only

🪙 Complication\Comorbidity   🪙 Major C\C   (Ex) CC/MCC Exclusions   🪙 Hospital-Acquired Condition   **1431**

- **T23.37** **Burn of third degree of wrist**
  - Ⓔⓧ **For category T23.37 CC codes:** T23.301-T23.309[A], T23.371-T23.379[A], T23.391-T23.399[A], T23.701-T23.709[A], T23.771-T23.779[A], T23.791-T23.799[A]
  - **T23.371** **Burn of third degree of right wrist** A 🪙, A 🪙
  - **T23.372** **Burn of third degree of left wrist** A 🪙, A 🪙
  - **T23.379** **Burn of third degree of unspecified wrist** A 🪙, A 🪙
- **T23.39** **Burn of third degree of multiple sites of wrist and hand**
  - Ⓔⓧ **For category T23.39 CC codes:** T23.30
  - **T23.391** **Burn of third degree of multiple sites of right wrist and hand** A 🪙, A 🪙
  - **T23.392** **Burn of third degree of multiple sites of left wrist and hand** A 🪙, A 🪙
  - **T23.399** **Burn of third degree of multiple sites of unspecified wrist and hand** A 🪙, A 🪙
- **T23.4** **Corrosion of unspecified degree of wrist and hand**
  - *Code first* (T51-T65) *to identify chemical and intent*
  - Use additional external cause code to identify place (Y92)
  - **T23.40** **Corrosion of unspecified degree of hand, unspecified site**
    - **T23.401** **Corrosion of unspecified degree of right hand, unspecified site**
    - **T23.402** **Corrosion of unspecified degree of left hand, unspecified site**
    - **T23.409** **Corrosion of unspecified degree of unspecified hand, unspecified site**
  - **T23.41** **Corrosion of unspecified degree of thumb (nail)**
    - **T23.411** **Corrosion of unspecified degree of right thumb (nail)**
    - **T23.412** **Corrosion of unspecified degree of left thumb (nail)**
    - **T23.419** **Corrosion of unspecified degree of unspecified thumb (nail)**
  - **T23.42** **Corrosion of unspecified degree of single finger (nail) except thumb**
    - **T23.421** **Corrosion of unspecified degree of single right finger (nail) except thumb**
    - **T23.422** **Corrosion of unspecified degree of single left finger (nail) except thumb**
    - **T23.429** **Corrosion of unspecified degree of unspecified single finger (nail) except thumb**
  - **T23.43** **Corrosion of unspecified degree of multiple fingers (nail), not including thumb**
    - **T23.431** **Corrosion of unspecified degree of multiple right fingers (nail), not including thumb**
    - **T23.432** **Corrosion of unspecified degree of multiple left fingers (nail), not including thumb**
    - **T23.439** **Corrosion of unspecified degree of unspecified multiple fingers (nail), not including thumb**
  - **T23.44** **Corrosion of unspecified degree of multiple fingers (nail), including thumb**
    - **T23.441** **Corrosion of unspecified degree of multiple right fingers (nail), including thumb**
    - **T23.442** **Corrosion of unspecified degree of multiple left fingers (nail), including thumb**
    - **T23.449** **Corrosion of unspecified degree of unspecified multiple fingers (nail), including thumb**

- **T23.45** **Corrosion of unspecified degree of palm**
  - **T23.451** **Corrosion of unspecified degree of right palm**
  - **T23.452** **Corrosion of unspecified degree of left palm**
  - **T23.459** **Corrosion of unspecified degree of unspecified palm**
- **T23.46** **Corrosion of unspecified degree of back of hand**
  - **T23.461** **Corrosion of unspecified degree of back of right hand**
  - **T23.462** **Corrosion of unspecified degree of back of left hand**
  - **T23.469** **Corrosion of unspecified degree of back of unspecified hand**
- **T23.47** **Corrosion of unspecified degree of wrist**
  - **T23.471** **Corrosion of unspecified degree of right wrist**
  - **T23.472** **Corrosion of unspecified degree of left wrist**
  - **T23.479** **Corrosion of unspecified degree of unspecified wrist**
- **T23.49** **Corrosion of unspecified degree of multiple sites of wrist and hand**
  - **T23.491** **Corrosion of unspecified degree of multiple sites of right wrist and hand**
  - **T23.492** **Corrosion of unspecified degree of multiple sites of left wrist and hand**
  - **T23.499** **Corrosion of unspecified degree of multiple sites of unspecified wrist and hand**
- **T23.5** **Corrosion of first degree of wrist and hand**
  - *Code first* (T51-T65) *to identify chemical and intent*
  - Use additional external cause code to identify place (Y92)
  - **T23.50** **Corrosion of first degree of hand, unspecified site**
    - **T23.501** **Corrosion of first degree of right hand, unspecified site**
    - **T23.502** **Corrosion of first degree of left hand, unspecified site**
    - **T23.509** **Corrosion of first degree of unspecified hand, unspecified site**
  - **T23.51** **Corrosion of first degree of thumb (nail)**
    - **T23.511** **Corrosion of first degree of right thumb (nail)**
    - **T23.512** **Corrosion of first degree of left thumb (nail)**
    - **T23.519** **Corrosion of first degree of unspecified thumb (nail)**
  - **T23.52** **Corrosion of first degree of single finger (nail) except thumb**
    - **T23.521** **Corrosion of first degree of single right finger (nail) except thumb**
    - **T23.522** **Corrosion of first degree of single left finger (nail) except thumb**
    - **T23.529** **Corrosion of first degree of unspecified single finger (nail) except thumb**

● T23.53   Corrosion of first degree of multiple fingers (nail), not including thumb

   ● T23.531   Corrosion of first degree of multiple right fingers (nail), not including thumb

   ● T23.532   Corrosion of first degree of multiple left fingers (nail), not including thumb

   ● T23.539   Corrosion of first degree of unspecified multiple fingers (nail), not including thumb

● T23.54   Corrosion of first degree of multiple fingers (nail), including thumb

   ● T23.541   Corrosion of first degree of multiple right fingers (nail), including thumb

   ● T23.542   Corrosion of first degree of multiple left fingers (nail), including thumb

   ● T23.549   Corrosion of first degree of unspecified multiple fingers (nail), including thumb

● T23.55   Corrosion of first degree of palm

   ● T23.551   Corrosion of first degree of right palm

   ● T23.552   Corrosion of first degree of left palm

   ● T23.559   Corrosion of first degree of unspecified palm

● T23.56   Corrosion of first degree of back of hand

   ● T23.561   Corrosion of first degree of back of right hand

   ● T23.562   Corrosion of first degree of back of left hand

   ● T23.569   Corrosion of first degree of back of unspecified hand

● T23.57   Corrosion of first degree of wrist

   ● T23.571   Corrosion of first degree of right wrist

   ● T23.572   Corrosion of first degree of left wrist

   ● T23.579   Corrosion of first degree of unspecified wrist

● T23.59   Corrosion of first degree of multiple sites of wrist and hand

   ● T23.591   Corrosion of first degree of multiple sites of right wrist and hand

   ● T23.592   Corrosion of first degree of multiple sites of left wrist and hand

   ● T23.599   Corrosion of first degree of multiple sites of unspecified wrist and hand

● T23.6   Corrosion of second degree of wrist and hand

   Code first (T51-T65) to identify chemical and intent

   Use additional external cause code to identify place (Y92)

   ● T23.60   Corrosion of second degree of hand, unspecified site

      ● T23.601   Corrosion of second degree of right hand, unspecified site

      ● T23.602   Corrosion of second degree of left hand, unspecified site

      ● T23.609   Corrosion of second degree of unspecified hand, unspecified site

   ● T23.61   Corrosion of second degree of thumb (nail)

      ● T23.611   Corrosion of second degree of right thumb (nail)

      ● T23.612   Corrosion of second degree of left thumb (nail)

      ● T23.619   Corrosion of second degree of unspecified thumb (nail)

● T23.62   Corrosion of second degree of single finger (nail) except thumb

   ● T23.621   Corrosion of second degree of single right finger (nail) except thumb

   ● T23.622   Corrosion of second degree of single left finger (nail) except thumb

   ● T23.629   Corrosion of second degree of unspecified single finger (nail) except thumb

● T23.63   Corrosion of second degree of multiple fingers (nail), not including thumb

   ● T23.631   Corrosion of second degree of multiple right fingers (nail), not including thumb

   ● T23.632   Corrosion of second degree of multiple left fingers (nail), not including thumb

   ● T23.639   Corrosion of second degree of unspecified multiple fingers (nail), not including thumb

● T23.64   Corrosion of second degree of multiple fingers (nail), including thumb

   ● T23.641   Corrosion of second degree of multiple right fingers (nail), including thumb

   ● T23.642   Corrosion of second degree of multiple left fingers (nail), including thumb

   ● T23.649   Corrosion of second degree of unspecified multiple fingers (nail), including thumb

● T23.65   Corrosion of second degree of palm

   ● T23.651   Corrosion of second degree of right palm

   ● T23.652   Corrosion of second degree of left palm

   ● T23.659   Corrosion of second degree of unspecified palm

● T23.66   Corrosion of second degree of back of hand

   ● T23.661   Corrosion of second degree back of right hand

   ● T23.662   Corrosion of second degree back of left hand

   ● T23.669   Corrosion of second degree back of unspecified hand

● T23.67   Corrosion of second degree of wrist

   ● T23.671   Corrosion of second degree of right wrist

   ● T23.672   Corrosion of second degree of left wrist

   ● T23.679   Corrosion of second degree of unspecified wrist

● T23.69   Corrosion of second degree of multiple sites of wrist and hand

   ● T23.691   Corrosion of second degree of multiple sites of right wrist and hand

   ● T23.692   Corrosion of second degree of multiple sites of left wrist and hand

   ● T23.699   Corrosion of second degree of multiple sites of unspecified wrist and hand

CHAPTER 19 (S00-T88)

● **T23.7** **Corrosion of third degree of wrist and hand**
　　Code first (T51-T65) *to identify chemical and intent*
　　Use additional external cause code to identify
　　　　place (Y92)

　● **T23.70** **Corrosion of third degree of hand, unspecified
　　　　site**
　　　Ⓔⓧ For category T23.70 CC codes: T23.30

　　● **T23.701** Corrosion of third degree of right
　　　　hand, unspecified site A Ⓒ, A Ⓠ

　　● **T23.702** Corrosion of third degree of left hand,
　　　　unspecified site A Ⓒ, A Ⓠ

　　● **T23.709** Corrosion of third degree of
　　　　unspecified hand, unspecified site
　　　　A Ⓒ, A Ⓠ

　● **T23.71** **Corrosion of third degree of thumb (nail)**
　　　Ⓔⓧ For category T23.71 CC codes: See T23.31

　　● **T23.711** Corrosion of third degree of right
　　　　thumb (nail) A Ⓒ, A Ⓠ

　　● **T23.712** Corrosion of third degree of left
　　　　thumb (nail) A Ⓒ, A Ⓠ

　　● **T23.719** Corrosion of third degree of
　　　　unspecified thumb (nail) A Ⓒ, A Ⓠ

　● **T23.72** **Corrosion of third degree of single finger (nail)
　　　　except thumb**
　　　Ⓔⓧ For category T23.72 CC codes: See T23.32

　　● **T23.721** Corrosion of third degree of single
　　　　right finger (nail) except thumb A Ⓒ,
　　　　A Ⓠ

　　● **T23.722** Corrosion of third degree of single
　　　　left finger (nail) except thumb A Ⓒ,
　　　　A Ⓠ

　　● **T23.729** Corrosion of third degree of
　　　　unspecified single finger (nail) except
　　　　thumb A Ⓒ, A Ⓠ

　● **T23.73** **Corrosion of third degree of multiple fingers
　　　　(nail), not including thumb**
　　　Ⓔⓧ For category T23.73 CC codes: See T23.33

　　● **T23.731** Corrosion of third degree of multiple
　　　　right fingers (nail), not including
　　　　thumb A Ⓒ, A Ⓠ

　　● **T23.732** Corrosion of third degree of multiple
　　　　left fingers (nail), not including
　　　　thumb A Ⓒ, A Ⓠ

　　● **T23.739** Corrosion of third degree of
　　　　unspecified multiple fingers (nail),
　　　　not including thumb A Ⓒ, A Ⓠ

　● **T23.74** **Corrosion of third degree of multiple fingers
　　　　(nail), including thumb**
　　　Ⓔⓧ For category T23.74 CC codes: See T23.34

　　● **T23.741** Corrosion of third degree of multiple
　　　　right fingers (nail), including thumb
　　　　A Ⓒ, A Ⓠ

　　● **T23.742** Corrosion of third degree of multiple
　　　　left fingers (nail), including thumb
　　　　A Ⓒ, A Ⓠ

　　● **T23.749** Corrosion of third degree of
　　　　unspecified multiple fingers (nail),
　　　　including thumb A Ⓒ, A Ⓠ

　● **T23.75** **Corrosion of third degree of palm**
　　　Ⓔⓧ For category T23.75 CC codes: See T23.35

　　● **T23.751** Corrosion of third degree of right
　　　　palm A Ⓒ, A Ⓠ

　　● **T23.752** Corrosion of third degree of left palm
　　　　A Ⓒ, A Ⓠ

　　● **T23.759** Corrosion of third degree of
　　　　unspecified palm A Ⓒ, A Ⓠ

　● **T23.76** **Corrosion of third degree of back of hand**
　　　Ⓔⓧ For category T23.76 CC codes: See T23.36

　　● **T23.761** Corrosion of third degree of back of
　　　　right hand A Ⓒ, A Ⓠ

　　● **T23.762** Corrosion of third degree of back of
　　　　left hand A Ⓒ, A Ⓠ

　　● **T23.769** Corrosion of third degree of back of
　　　　unspecified hand A Ⓒ, A Ⓠ

　● **T23.77** **Corrosion of third degree of wrist**
　　　Ⓔⓧ For category T23.77 CC codes: See T23.37

　　● **T23.771** Corrosion of third degree of right
　　　　wrist A Ⓒ, A Ⓠ

　　● **T23.772** Corrosion of third degree of left wrist
　　　　A Ⓒ, A Ⓠ

　　● **T23.779** Corrosion of third degree of
　　　　unspecified wrist A Ⓒ, A Ⓠ

　● **T23.79** **Corrosion of third degree of multiple sites of
　　　　wrist and hand**
　　　Ⓔⓧ For category T23.79 CC codes: T23.30

　　● **T23.791** Corrosion of third degree of multiple
　　　　sites of right wrist and hand A Ⓒ,
　　　　A Ⓠ

　　● **T23.792** Corrosion of third degree of multiple
　　　　sites of left wrist and hand A Ⓒ, A Ⓠ

　　● **T23.799** Corrosion of third degree of multiple
　　　　sites of unspecified wrist and hand
　　　　A Ⓒ, A Ⓠ

● **T24** **Burn and corrosion of lower limb, except ankle and foot**
　　Excludes2 burn and corrosion of ankle and foot (T25.-)
　　　　　　　burn and corrosion of hip region (T21.-)
　　The appropriate 7th character is to be added to each code from
　　　category T24

A	initial encounter
D	subsequent encounter
S	sequela

　● **T24.0** **Burn of unspecified degree of lower limb, except ankle
　　　　and foot**
　　　Use additional external cause code to identify the
　　　　source, place and intent of the burn (X00-X19,
　　　　X75-X77, X96-X98, Y92)

　　● **T24.00** **Burn of unspecified degree of unspecified site
　　　　of lower limb, except ankle and foot**

　　　● **T24.001** Burn of unspecified degree of
　　　　unspecified site of right lower limb,
　　　　except ankle and foot

　　　● **T24.002** Burn of unspecified degree of
　　　　unspecified site of left lower limb,
　　　　except ankle and foot

　　　● **T24.009** Burn of unspecified degree of
　　　　unspecified site of unspecified lower
　　　　limb, except ankle and foot

　　● **T24.01** **Burn of unspecified degree of thigh**

　　　● **T24.011** Burn of unspecified degree of right
　　　　thigh

　　　● **T24.012** Burn of unspecified degree of left
　　　　thigh

　　　● **T24.019** Burn of unspecified degree of
　　　　unspecified thigh

　　● **T24.02** **Burn of unspecified degree of knee**

　　　● **T24.021** Burn of unspecified degree of right
　　　　knee

　　　● **T24.022** Burn of unspecified degree of left
　　　　knee

　　　● **T24.029** Burn of unspecified degree of
　　　　unspecified knee

◀ New　◀▥ Revised　~~deleted~~ Deleted　Excludes 1　Excludes 2　Includes　Use additional　Code first　Code also　Unspecified
OGCR Official Guidelines　● Unacceptable Principal Diagnosis　X Assign placeholder X　● Use Additional Character(s)　▷ Manifestation Code　**Coding Clinic**

● **T24.03**   **Burn of unspecified degree of lower leg**
  ● T24.031   Burn of <mark>unspecified</mark> degree of right lower leg
  ● T24.032   Burn of <mark>unspecified</mark> degree of left lower leg
  ● T24.039   Burn of <mark>unspecified</mark> degree of unspecified lower leg

● **T24.09**   **Burn of unspecified degree of multiple sites of lower limb, except ankle and foot**
  ● T24.091   Burn of <mark>unspecified</mark> degree of multiple sites of right lower limb, except ankle and foot
  ● T24.092   Burn of <mark>unspecified</mark> degree of multiple sites of left lower limb, except ankle and foot
  ● T24.099   Burn of <mark>unspecified</mark> degree of multiple sites of unspecified lower limb, except ankle and foot

● **T24.1**   **Burn of first degree of lower limb, except ankle and foot**
   Use additional external cause code to identify the source, place and intent of the burn (X00-X19, X75-X77, X96-X98, Y92)

  ● **T24.10**   **Burn of first degree of unspecified site of lower limb, except ankle and foot**
    ● T24.101   Burn of first degree of <mark>unspecified</mark> site of right lower limb, except ankle and foot
    ● T24.102   Burn of first degree of <mark>unspecified</mark> site of left lower limb, except ankle and foot
    ● T24.109   Burn of first degree of <mark>unspecified</mark> site of unspecified lower limb, except ankle and foot

  ● **T24.11**   **Burn of first degree of thigh**
    ● T24.111   Burn of first degree of right thigh
    ● T24.112   Burn of first degree of left thigh
    ● T24.119   Burn of first degree of <mark>unspecified</mark> thigh

  ● **T24.12**   **Burn of first degree of knee**
    ● T24.121   Burn of first degree of right knee
    ● T24.122   Burn of first degree of left knee
    ● T24.129   Burn of first degree of <mark>unspecified</mark> knee

  ● **T24.13**   **Burn of first degree of lower leg**
    ● T24.131   Burn of first degree of right lower leg
    ● T24.132   Burn of first degree of left lower leg
    ● T24.139   Burn of first degree of <mark>unspecified</mark> lower leg

  ● **T24.19**   **Burn of first degree of multiple sites of lower limb, except ankle and foot**
    ● T24.191   Burn of first degree of multiple sites of right lower limb, except ankle and foot
    ● T24.192   Burn of first degree of multiple sites of left lower limb, except ankle and foot
    ● T24.199   Burn of first degree of multiple sites of <mark>unspecified</mark> lower limb, except ankle and foot

● **T24.2**   **Burn of second degree of lower limb, except ankle and foot**
   Use additional external cause code to identify the source, place and intent of the burn (X00-X19, X75-X77, X96-X98, Y92)

  ● **T24.20**   **Burn of second degree of unspecified site of lower limb, except ankle and foot**
    ● T24.201   Burn of second degree of <mark>unspecified</mark> site of right lower limb, except ankle and foot
    ● T24.202   Burn of second degree of <mark>unspecified</mark> site of left lower limb, except ankle and foot
    ● T24.209   Burn of second degree of <mark>unspecified</mark> site of unspecified lower limb, except ankle and foot

  ● **T24.21**   **Burn of second degree of thigh**
    ● T24.211   Burn of second degree of right thigh
    ● T24.212   Burn of second degree of left thigh
    ● T24.219   Burn of second degree of <mark>unspecified</mark> thigh

  ● **T24.22**   **Burn of second degree of knee**
    ● T24.221   Burn of second degree of right knee
    ● T24.222   Burn of second degree of left knee
    ● T24.229   Burn of second degree of <mark>unspecified</mark> knee

  ● **T24.23**   **Burn of second degree of lower leg**
    ● T24.231   Burn of second degree of right lower leg
    ● T24.232   Burn of second degree of left lower leg
    ● T24.239   Burn of second degree of <mark>unspecified</mark> lower leg

  ● **T24.29**   **Burn of second degree of multiple sites of lower limb, except ankle and foot**
    ● T24.291   Burn of second degree of multiple sites of right lower limb, except ankle and foot
    ● T24.292   Burn of second degree of multiple sites of left lower limb, except ankle and foot
    ● T24.299   Burn of second degree of multiple sites of <mark>unspecified</mark> lower limb, except ankle and foot

● **T24.3**   **Burn of third degree of lower limb, except ankle and foot**
   Use additional external cause code to identify the source, place and intent of the burn (X00-X19, X75-X77, X96-X98, Y92)

  ● **T24.30**   **Burn of third degree of unspecified site of lower limb, except ankle and foot**
    (Ex) For category **T24.30 CC codes:** T24.301-T24.309[A], T24.391-T24.399[A], T24.701-T24.709[A], T24.791-T24.799[A], T25.391-T25.399[A], T25.791-T25.799[A]
    ● T24.301   Burn of third degree of <mark>unspecified</mark> site of right lower limb, except ankle and foot A 🖱, A 🖱
    ● T24.302   Burn of third degree of <mark>unspecified</mark> site of left lower limb, except ankle and foot A 🖱, A 🖱
    ● T24.309   Burn of third degree of <mark>unspecified</mark> site of unspecified lower limb, except ankle and foot A 🖱, A 🖱

N Newborn Age: 0   **P** Pediatric Age: 0–17   **M** Maternity DX: 12–55   **A** Adult Age: 15–124   ♀ Females Only   ♂ Males Only
🖱 Complication\Comorbidity   🖱 Major C\C   (Ex) CC/MCC Exclusions   🖱 Hospital-Acquired Condition

1435

CHAPTER 19 (S00-T88)

● **T24.31**   Burn of third degree of thigh
Ⓔⓧ For category T24.31 CC codes: T24.301-T24.309[A],
T24.311-T24.319[A], T24.391-T24.399[A],
T24.701-T24.709-T24.719[A], T24.791-T24.799[A],
T25.391-T25.399[A], T25.791-T25.799[A]

● **T24.311**   Burn of third degree of right thigh
A 🪙, A 🪙

● **T24.312**   Burn of third degree of left thigh
A 🪙, A 🪙

● **T24.319**   Burn of third degree of unspecified
thigh A 🪙, A 🪙

● **T24.32**   Burn of third degree of knee
Ⓔⓧ For category T24.32 CC codes: T24.301-T24.309[A],
T24.321-T24.329[A], T24.391-T24.399[A],
T24.701-T24.709[A], T24.721-T24.729[A],
T24.791-T24.799[A], T25.391-T25.399[A], T25.791-T25.799[A]

● **T24.321**   Burn of third degree of right knee
A 🪙, A 🪙

● **T24.322**   Burn of third degree of left knee A 🪙,
A 🪙

● **T24.329**   Burn of third degree of unspecified
knee A 🪙, A 🪙

● **T24.33**   Burn of third degree of lower leg
Ⓔⓧ For category T24.33 CC codes: T24.301-T24.309[A],
T24.331-T24.339[A], T24.391-T24.399[A],
T24.701-T24.709[A], T24.731-T24.739[A],
T24.791-T24.799[A], T25.391-T25.399[A], T25.791-T25.799[A]

● **T24.331**   Burn of third degree of right lower
leg A 🪙, A 🪙

● **T24.332**   Burn of third degree of left lower leg
A 🪙, A 🪙

● **T24.339**   Burn of third degree of unspecified
lower leg A 🪙, A 🪙

● **T24.39**   Burn of third degree of multiple sites of lower
limb, except ankle and foot
Ⓔⓧ For category T24.39 CC codes: See T24.30

● **T24.391**   Burn of third degree of multiple sites
of right lower limb, except ankle and
foot A 🪙, A 🪙
Coding Clinic: 2016, Q2, P5

● **T24.392**   Burn of third degree of multiple sites
of left lower limb, except ankle and
foot A 🪙, A 🪙

● **T24.399**   Burn of third degree of multiple sites
of unspecified lower limb, except
ankle and foot A 🪙, A 🪙

● **T24.4**   Corrosion of unspecified degree of lower limb, except
ankle and foot
Code first (T51-T65) to identify chemical and intent
Use additional external cause code to identify
place (Y92)

● **T24.40**   Corrosion of unspecified degree of unspecified
site of lower limb, except ankle and foot

● **T24.401**   Corrosion of unspecified degree of
unspecified site of right lower limb,
except ankle and foot

● **T24.402**   Corrosion of unspecified degree of
unspecified site of left lower limb,
except ankle and foot

● **T24.409**   Corrosion of unspecified degree of
unspecified site of unspecified lower
limb, except ankle and foot

● **T24.41**   Corrosion of unspecified degree of thigh

● **T24.411**   Corrosion of unspecified degree of
right thigh

● **T24.412**   Corrosion of unspecified degree of
left thigh

● **T24.419**   Corrosion of unspecified degree of
unspecified thigh

● **T24.42**   Corrosion of unspecified degree of knee

● **T24.421**   Corrosion of unspecified degree of
right knee

● **T24.422**   Corrosion of unspecified degree of
left knee

● **T24.429**   Corrosion of unspecified degree of
unspecified knee

● **T24.43**   Corrosion of unspecified degree of lower leg

● **T24.431**   Corrosion of unspecified degree of
right lower leg

● **T24.432**   Corrosion of unspecified degree of
left lower leg

● **T24.439**   Corrosion of unspecified degree of
unspecified lower leg

● **T24.49**   Corrosion of unspecified degree of multiple
sites of lower limb, except ankle and foot

● **T24.491**   Corrosion of unspecified degree of
multiple sites of right lower limb,
except ankle and foot

● **T24.492**   Corrosion of unspecified degree of
multiple sites of left lower limb,
except ankle and foot

● **T24.499**   Corrosion of unspecified degree of
multiple sites of unspecified lower
limb, except ankle and foot

● **T24.5**   Corrosion of first degree of lower limb, except ankle and
foot
Code first (T51-T65) to identify chemical and intent
Use additional external cause code to identify
place (Y92)

● **T24.50**   Corrosion of first degree of unspecified site of
lower limb, except ankle and foot

● **T24.501**   Corrosion of first degree of
unspecified site of right lower limb,
except ankle and foot

● **T24.502**   Corrosion of first degree of
unspecified site of left lower limb,
except ankle and foot

● **T24.509**   Corrosion of first degree of
unspecified site of unspecified lower
limb, except ankle and foot

● **T24.51**   Corrosion of first degree of thigh

● **T24.511**   Corrosion of first degree of right thigh

● **T24.512**   Corrosion of first degree of left thigh

● **T24.519**   Corrosion of first degree of
unspecified thigh

● **T24.52**   Corrosion of first degree of knee

● **T24.521**   Corrosion of first degree of right knee

● **T24.522**   Corrosion of first degree of left knee

● **T24.529**   Corrosion of first degree of
unspecified knee

● **T24.53**   Corrosion of first degree of lower leg

● **T24.531**   Corrosion of first degree of right
lower leg

● **T24.532**   Corrosion of first degree of left lower
leg

● **T24.539**   Corrosion of first degree of
unspecified lower leg

● **T24.59**   Corrosion of first degree of multiple sites of
lower limb, except ankle and foot

● **T24.591**   Corrosion of first degree of multiple
sites of right lower limb, except ankle
and foot

● **T24.592**   Corrosion of first degree of multiple
sites of left lower limb, except ankle
and foot

● **T24.599**   Corrosion of first degree of multiple
sites of unspecified lower limb, except
ankle and foot

◀ New   ◀▦ Revised   d̶e̶l̶e̶t̶e̶d̶ Deleted   Excludes 1   Excludes 2   Includes   Use additional   Code first   Code also   Unspecified
OGCR Official Guidelines   ● Unacceptable Principal Diagnosis   ✗ Assign placeholder X   ● Use Additional Character(s)   ▸ Manifestation Code   **Coding Clinic**

● **T24.6 Corrosion of second degree of lower limb, except ankle and foot**

    Code first (T51-T65) *to identify chemical and intent*

    Use additional external cause code to identify place (Y92)

● **T24.60 Corrosion of second degree of unspecified site of lower limb, except ankle and foot**

  ● **T24.601 Corrosion of second degree of** unspecified **site of right lower limb, except ankle and foot**

  ● **T24.602 Corrosion of second degree of** unspecified **site of left lower limb, except ankle and foot**

  ● **T24.609 Corrosion of second degree of** unspecified **site of unspecified lower limb, except ankle and foot**

● **T24.61 Corrosion of second degree of thigh**

  ● **T24.611 Corrosion of second degree of right thigh**

  ● **T24.612 Corrosion of second degree of left thigh**

  ● **T24.619 Corrosion of second degree of** unspecified **thigh**

● **T24.62 Corrosion of second degree of knee**

  ● **T24.621 Corrosion of second degree of right knee**

  ● **T24.622 Corrosion of second degree of left knee**

  ● **T24.629 Corrosion of second degree of** unspecified **knee**

● **T24.63 Corrosion of second degree of lower leg**

  ● **T24.631 Corrosion of second degree of right lower leg**

  ● **T24.632 Corrosion of second degree of left lower leg**

  ● **T24.639 Corrosion of second degree of** unspecified **lower leg**

● **T24.69 Corrosion of second degree of multiple sites of lower limb, except ankle and foot**

  ● **T24.691 Corrosion of second degree of multiple sites of right lower limb, except ankle and foot**

  ● **T24.692 Corrosion of second degree of multiple sites of left lower limb, except ankle and foot**

  ● **T24.699 Corrosion of second degree of multiple sites of** unspecified **lower limb, except ankle and foot**

● **T24.7 Corrosion of third degree of lower limb, except ankle and foot**

    Code first (T51-T65) *to identify chemical and intent*

    Use additional external cause code to identify place (Y92)

● **T24.70 Corrosion of third degree of unspecified site of lower limb, except ankle and foot**

    (Ex) For category T24.70 CC codes: See T24.30

  ● **T24.701 Corrosion of third degree of** unspecified **site of right lower limb, except ankle and foot** A 🔖, A 🔖

  ● **T24.702 Corrosion of third degree of** unspecified **site of left lower limb, except ankle and foot** A 🔖, A 🔖

  ● **T24.709 Corrosion of third degree of** unspecified **site of unspecified lower limb, except ankle and foot** A 🔖, A 🔖

● **T24.71 Corrosion of third degree of thigh**

    (Ex) For category T24.71 CC codes: See T24.31

  ● **T24.711 Corrosion of third degree of right thigh** A 🔖, A 🔖

  ● **T24.712 Corrosion of third degree of left thigh** A 🔖, A 🔖

  ● **T24.719 Corrosion of third degree of** unspecified **thigh** A 🔖, A 🔖

● **T24.72 Corrosion of third degree of knee**

    (Ex) For category T24.72 CC codes: See T24.32

  ● **T24.721 Corrosion of third degree of right knee** A 🔖, A 🔖

  ● **T24.722 Corrosion of third degree of left knee** A 🔖, A 🔖

  ● **T24.729 Corrosion of third degree of** unspecified **knee** A 🔖, A 🔖

● **T24.73 Corrosion of third degree of lower leg**

    (Ex) For category T24.73 CC codes: See T24.33

  ● **T24.731 Corrosion of third degree of right lower leg** A 🔖, A 🔖

  ● **T24.732 Corrosion of third degree of left lower leg** A 🔖, A 🔖

  ● **T24.739 Corrosion of third degree of** unspecified **lower leg** A 🔖, A 🔖

● **T24.79 Corrosion of third degree of multiple sites of lower limb, except ankle and foot**

    (Ex) For category T24.79 CC codes: See T24.30

  ● **T24.791 Corrosion of third degree of multiple sites of right lower limb, except ankle and foot** A 🔖, A 🔖

  ● **T24.792 Corrosion of third degree of multiple sites of left lower limb, except ankle and foot** A 🔖, A 🔖

  ● **T24.799 Corrosion of third degree of multiple sites of** unspecified **lower limb, except ankle and foot** A 🔖, A 🔖

● **T25 Burn and corrosion of ankle and foot**

    The appropriate 7th character is to be added to each code from category T25

    | A | initial encounter |
    | D | subsequent encounter |
    | S | sequela |

● **T25.0 Burn of unspecified degree of ankle and foot**

    Use additional external cause code to identify the source, place and intent of the burn (X00-X19, X75-X77, X96-X98, Y92)

  ● **T25.01 Burn of unspecified degree of ankle**

    ● **T25.011 Burn of** unspecified **degree of right ankle**

    ● **T25.012 Burn of** unspecified **degree of left ankle**

    ● **T25.019 Burn of** unspecified **degree of unspecified ankle**

  ● **T25.02 Burn of unspecified degree of foot**

    Excludes2 burn of unspecified degree of toe(s) (nail) (T25.03-)

    ● **T25.021 Burn of** unspecified **degree of right foot**

    ● **T25.022 Burn of** unspecified **degree of left foot**

    ● **T25.029 Burn of** unspecified **degree of unspecified foot**

CHAPTER 19 (S00-T88)

● T25.03   Burn of unspecified degree of toe(s) (nail)
- ● T25.031   Burn of unspecified degree of right toe(s) (nail)
- ● T25.032   Burn of unspecified degree of left toe(s) (nail)
- ● T25.039   Burn of unspecified degree of unspecified toe(s) (nail)

● T25.09   Burn of unspecified degree of multiple sites of ankle and foot
- ● T25.091   Burn of unspecified degree of multiple sites of right ankle and foot
- ● T25.092   Burn of unspecified degree of multiple sites of left ankle and foot
- ● T25.099   Burn of unspecified degree of multiple sites of unspecified ankle and foot

● T25.1   Burn of first degree of ankle and foot

Use additional external cause code to identify the source, place and intent of the burn (X00-X19, X75-X77, X96-X98, Y92)

● T25.11   Burn of first degree of ankle
- ● T25.111   Burn of first degree of right ankle
- ● T25.112   Burn of first degree of left ankle
- ● T25.119   Burn of first degree of unspecified ankle

● T25.12   Burn of first degree of foot

Excludes2   burn of first degree of toe(s) (nail) (T25.13-)
- ● T25.121   Burn of first degree of right foot
- ● T25.122   Burn of first degree of left foot
- ● T25.129   Burn of first degree of unspecified foot

● T25.13   Burn of first degree of toe(s) (nail)
- ● T25.131   Burn of first degree of right toe(s) (nail)
- ● T25.132   Burn of first degree of left toe(s) (nail)
- ● T25.139   Burn of first degree of unspecified toe(s) (nail)

● T25.19   Burn of first degree of multiple sites of ankle and foot
- ● T25.191   Burn of first degree of multiple sites of right ankle and foot
- ● T25.192   Burn of first degree of multiple sites of left ankle and foot
- ● T25.199   Burn of first degree of multiple sites of unspecified ankle and foot

● T25.2   Burn of second degree of ankle and foot

Use additional external cause code to identify the source, place and intent of the burn (X00-X19, X75-X77, X96-X98, Y92)

● T25.21   Burn of second degree of ankle
- ● T25.211   Burn of second degree of right ankle
- ● T25.212   Burn of second degree of left ankle
- ● T25.219   Burn of second degree of unspecified ankle

● T25.22   Burn of second degree of foot

Excludes2   burn of second degree of toe(s) (nail) (T25.23-)
- ● T25.221   Burn of second degree of right foot
- ● T25.222   Burn of second degree of left foot
- ● T25.229   Burn of second degree of unspecified foot

● T25.23   Burn of second degree of toe(s) (nail)
- ● T25.231   Burn of second degree of right toe(s) (nail)
- ● T25.232   Burn of second degree of left toe(s) (nail)
- ● T25.239   Burn of second degree of unspecified toe(s) (nail)

● T25.29   Burn of second degree of multiple sites of ankle and foot
- ● T25.291   Burn of second degree of multiple sites of right ankle and foot
- ● T25.292   Burn of second degree of multiple sites of left ankle and foot
- ● T25.299   Burn of second degree of multiple sites of unspecified ankle and foot

● T25.3   Burn of third degree of ankle and foot

Use additional external cause code to identify the source, place and intent of the burn (X00-X19, X75-X77, X96-X98, Y92)

● T25.31   Burn of third degree of ankle

(Ex) For category **T25.31** CC codes: T24.301-T24.309[A], T24.391-T24.399[A], T24.701-T24.709[A], T24.791-T24.799[A], T25.311-T25.319[A], T25.391-T25.399[A], T25.711-T25.719[A], T25.791-T25.799[A]
- ● T25.311   Burn of third degree of right ankle A 🐾, A 🐾
- ● T25.312   Burn of third degree of left ankle A 🐾, A 🐾
- ● T25.319   Burn of third degree of unspecified ankle A 🐾, A 🐾

● T25.32   Burn of third degree of foot

Excludes2   burn of third degree of toe(s) (nail) (T25.33-)

(Ex) For category **T25.32** CC codes: T24.301-T24.309[A], T24.391-T24.399[A], T24.701-T24.709[A], T24.791-T24.799[A], T25.321-T25.329[A], T25.391-T25.399[A], T25.721-T25.729[A], T25.791-T25.799[A]
- ● T25.321   Burn of third degree of right foot A 🐾, A 🐾
- ● T25.322   Burn of third degree of left foot A 🐾, A 🐾
- ● T25.329   Burn of third degree of unspecified foot A 🐾, A 🐾

● T25.33   Burn of third degree of toe(s) (nail)

(Ex) For category **T25.33** CC codes: T24.301-T24.309[A], T24.391-T24.399[A], T24.701-T24.709[A], T24.791-T24.799[A], T25.331-T25.339[A], T25.391-T25.399[A], T25.731-T25.739[A], T25.791-T25.799[A]
- ● T25.331   Burn of third degree of right toe(s) (nail) A 🐾, A 🐾
- ● T25.332   Burn of third degree of left toe(s) (nail) A 🐾, A 🐾
- ● T25.339   Burn of third degree of unspecified toe(s) (nail) A 🐾, A 🐾

● T25.39   Burn of third degree of multiple sites of ankle and foot

(Ex) For category **T25.39** CC codes: See T24.30
- ● T25.391   Burn of third degree of multiple sites of right ankle and foot A 🐾, A 🐾
- ● T25.392   Burn of third degree of multiple sites of left ankle and foot A 🐾, A 🐾
- ● T25.399   Burn of third degree of multiple sites of unspecified ankle and foot A 🐾, A 🐾

● **T25.4**   **Corrosion of unspecified degree of ankle and foot**
  Code first (T51-T65) *to identify chemical and intent*
  Use additional external cause code to identify place (Y92)

  ● **T25.41**   **Corrosion of unspecified degree of ankle**

    ● **T25.411**   Corrosion of unspecified degree of right ankle

    ● **T25.412**   Corrosion of unspecified degree of left ankle

    ● **T25.419**   Corrosion of unspecified degree of unspecified ankle

  ● **T25.42**   **Corrosion of unspecified degree of foot**

    Excludes2   corrosion of unspecified degree of toe(s) (nail) (T25.43-)

    ● **T25.421**   Corrosion of unspecified degree of right foot

    ● **T25.422**   Corrosion of unspecified degree of left foot

    ● **T25.429**   Corrosion of unspecified degree of unspecified foot

  ● **T25.43**   **Corrosion of unspecified degree of toe(s) (nail)**

    ● **T25.431**   Corrosion of unspecified degree of right toe(s) (nail)

    ● **T25.432**   Corrosion of unspecified degree of left toe(s) (nail)

    ● **T25.439**   Corrosion of unspecified degree of unspecified toe(s) (nail)

  ● **T25.49**   **Corrosion of unspecified degree of multiple sites of ankle and foot**

    ● **T25.491**   Corrosion of unspecified degree of multiple sites of right ankle and foot

    ● **T25.492**   Corrosion of unspecified degree of multiple sites of left ankle and foot

    ● **T25.499**   Corrosion of unspecified degree of multiple sites of unspecified ankle and foot

● **T25.5**   **Corrosion of first degree of ankle and foot**
  Code first (T51-T65) *to identify chemical and intent*
  Use additional external cause code to identify place (Y92)

  ● **T25.51**   **Corrosion of first degree of ankle**

    ● **T25.511**   Corrosion of first degree of right ankle

    ● **T25.512**   Corrosion of first degree of left ankle

    ● **T25.519**   Corrosion of first degree of unspecified ankle

  ● **T25.52**   **Corrosion of first degree of foot**

    Excludes2   corrosion of first degree of toe(s) (nail) (T25.53-)

    ● **T25.521**   Corrosion of first degree of right foot

    ● **T25.522**   Corrosion of first degree of left foot

    ● **T25.529**   Corrosion of first degree of unspecified foot

  ● **T25.53**   **Corrosion of first degree of toe(s) (nail)**

    ● **T25.531**   Corrosion of first degree of right toe(s) (nail)

    ● **T25.532**   Corrosion of first degree of left toe(s) (nail)

    ● **T25.539**   Corrosion of first degree of unspecified toe(s) (nail)

  ● **T25.59**   **Corrosion of first degree of multiple sites of ankle and foot**

    ● **T25.591**   Corrosion of first degree of multiple sites of right ankle and foot

    ● **T25.592**   Corrosion of first degree of multiple sites of left ankle and foot

    ● **T25.599**   Corrosion of first degree of multiple sites of unspecified ankle and foot

● **T25.6**   **Corrosion of second degree of ankle and foot**
  Code first (T51-T65) *to identify chemical and intent*
  Use additional external cause code to identify place (Y92)

  ● **T25.61**   **Corrosion of second degree of ankle**

    ● **T25.611**   Corrosion of second degree of right ankle

    ● **T25.612**   Corrosion of second degree of left ankle

    ● **T25.619**   Corrosion of second degree of unspecified ankle

  ● **T25.62**   **Corrosion of second degree of foot**

    Excludes2   corrosion of second degree of toe(s) (nail) (T25.63-)

    ● **T25.621**   Corrosion of second degree of right foot

    ● **T25.622**   Corrosion of second degree of left foot

    ● **T25.629**   Corrosion of second degree of unspecified foot

  ● **T25.63**   **Corrosion of second degree of toe(s) (nail)**

    ● **T25.631**   Corrosion of second degree of right toe(s) (nail)

    ● **T25.632**   Corrosion of second degree of left toe(s) (nail)

    ● **T25.639**   Corrosion of second degree of unspecified toe(s) (nail)

  ● **T25.69**   **Corrosion of second degree of multiple sites of ankle and foot**

    ● **T25.691**   Corrosion of second degree of right ankle and foot

    ● **T25.692**   Corrosion of second degree of left ankle and foot

    ● **T25.699**   Corrosion of second degree of unspecified ankle and foot

● **T25.7**   **Corrosion of third degree of ankle and foot**
  Code first (T51-T65) *to identify chemical and intent*
  Use additional external cause code to identify place (Y92)

  ● **T25.71**   **Corrosion of third degree of ankle**
  Ⓔⓧ **For category T25.71 CC codes:** See T25.31

    ● **T25.711**   Corrosion of third degree of right ankle A 🦠, A 🦠

    ● **T25.712**   Corrosion of third degree of left ankle A 🦠, A 🦠

    ● **T25.719**   Corrosion of third degree of unspecified ankle A 🦠, A 🦠

  ● **T25.72**   **Corrosion of third degree of foot**

    Excludes2   corrosion of third degree of toe(s) (nail) (T25.73-)
  Ⓔⓧ **For category T25.72 CC codes:** See T25.32

    ● **T25.721**   Corrosion of third degree of right foot A 🦠, A 🦠

    ● **T25.722**   Corrosion of third degree of left foot A 🦠, A 🦠

    ● **T25.729**   Corrosion of third degree of unspecified foot A 🦠, A 🦠

  ● **T25.73**   **Corrosion of third degree of toe(s) (nail)**
  Ⓔⓧ **For category T25.73 CC codes:** See T25.33

    ● **T25.731**   Corrosion of third degree of right toe(s) (nail) A 🦠, A 🦠

    ● **T25.732**   Corrosion of third degree of left toe(s) (nail) A 🦠, A 🦠

    ● **T25.739**   Corrosion of third degree of unspecified toe(s) (nail) A 🦠, A 🦠

N Newborn Age: Ø   **P** Pediatric Age: Ø–17   **M** Maternity DX: 12–55   **A** Adult Age: 15–124   ♀ Females Only   ♂ Males Only

🦠 Complication\Comorbidity   🦠 Major C\C   Ⓔⓧ CC/MCC Exclusions   🦠 Hospital-Acquired Condition

1439

● T25.79 Corrosion of third degree of multiple sites of ankle and foot
(Ex) For category T25.79 CC codes: See T24.30

  ● T25.791 Corrosion of third degree of multiple sites of right ankle and foot A 🐾, A 🐾
  ● T25.792 Corrosion of third degree of multiple sites of left ankle and foot A 🐾, A 🐾
  ● T25.799 Corrosion of third degree of multiple sites of unspecified ankle and foot A 🐾, A 🐾

BURNS AND CORROSIONS CONFINED TO EYE AND INTERNAL ORGANS (T26-T28)

● T26 Burn and corrosion confined to eye and adnexa

The appropriate 7th character is to be added to each code from category T26

A	initial encounter
D	subsequent encounter
S	sequela

● T26.0 Burn of eyelid and periocular area
Use additional external cause code to identify the source, place and intent of the burn (X00-X19, X75-X77, X96-X98, Y92)

  X ● T26.00 Burn of unspecified eyelid and periocular area
  X ● T26.01 Burn of right eyelid and periocular area
  X ● T26.02 Burn of left eyelid and periocular area

● T26.1 Burn of cornea and conjunctival sac
Use additional external cause code to identify the source, place and intent of the burn (X00-X19, X75-X77, X96-X98, Y92)

  X ● T26.10 Burn of cornea and conjunctival sac, unspecified eye
  X ● T26.11 Burn of cornea and conjunctival sac, right eye
  X ● T26.12 Burn of cornea and conjunctival sac, left eye

● T26.2 Burn with resulting rupture and destruction of eyeball
Use additional external cause code to identify the source, place and intent of the burn (X00-X19, X75-X77, X96-X98, Y92)
(Ex) For category T26.2 CC codes: No exclusions

  X ● T26.20 Burn with resulting rupture and destruction of unspecified eyeball A 🐾, A 🐾
  X ● T26.21 Burn with resulting rupture and destruction of right eyeball A 🐾, A 🐾
  X ● T26.22 Burn with resulting rupture and destruction of left eyeball A 🐾, A 🐾

● T26.3 Burns of other specified parts of eye and adnexa
Use additional external cause code to identify the source, place and intent of the burn (X00-X19, X75-X77, X96-X98, Y92)

  X ● T26.30 Burns of other specified parts of unspecified eye and adnexa
  X ● T26.31 Burns of other specified parts of right eye and adnexa
  X ● T26.32 Burns of other specified parts of left eye and adnexa

● T26.4 Burn of eye and adnexa, part unspecified
Use additional external cause code to identify the source, place and intent of the burn (X00-X19, X75-X77, X96-X98, Y92)

  X ● T26.40 Burn of unspecified eye and adnexa, part unspecified
  X ● T26.41 Burn of right eye and adnexa, part unspecified
  X ● T26.42 Burn of left eye and adnexa, part unspecified

● T26.5 Corrosion of eyelid and periocular area
Code first (T51-T65) to identify chemical and intent
Use additional external cause code to identify place (Y92)

  X ● T26.50 Corrosion of unspecified eyelid and periocular area
  X ● T26.51 Corrosion of right eyelid and periocular area
  X ● T26.52 Corrosion of left eyelid and periocular area

● T26.6 Corrosion of cornea and conjunctival sac
Code first (T51-T65) to identify chemical and intent
Use additional external cause code to identify place (Y92)

  X ● T26.60 Corrosion of cornea and conjunctival sac, unspecified eye
  X ● T26.61 Corrosion of cornea and conjunctival sac, right eye
  X ● T26.62 Corrosion of cornea and conjunctival sac, left eye

● T26.7 Corrosion with resulting rupture and destruction of eyeball
Code first (T51-T65) to identify chemical and intent
Use additional external cause code to identify place (Y92)
(Ex) For category T26.7 CC codes: No exclusions

  X ● T26.70 Corrosion with resulting rupture and destruction of unspecified eyeball A 🐾, A 🐾
  X ● T26.71 Corrosion with resulting rupture and destruction of right eyeball A 🐾, A 🐾
  X ● T26.72 Corrosion with resulting rupture and destruction of left eyeball A 🐾, A 🐾

● T26.8 Corrosions of other specified parts of eye and adnexa
Code first (T51-T65) to identify chemical and intent
Use additional external cause code to identify place (Y92)

  X ● T26.80 Corrosions of other specified parts of unspecified eye and adnexa
  X ● T26.81 Corrosions of other specified parts of right eye and adnexa
  X ● T26.82 Corrosions of other specified parts of left eye and adnexa

● T26.9 Corrosion of eye and adnexa, part unspecified
Code first (T51-T65) to identify chemical and intent
Use additional external cause code to identify place (Y92)

  X ● T26.90 Corrosion of unspecified eye and adnexa, part unspecified
  X ● T26.91 Corrosion of right eye and adnexa, part unspecified
  X ● T26.92 Corrosion of left eye and adnexa, part unspecified

● T27 Burn and corrosion of respiratory tract
Use additional external cause code to identify the source and intent of the burn (X00-X19, X75-X77, X96-X98)
Use additional external cause code to identify place (Y92)
The appropriate 7th character is to be added to each code from category T27

A	initial encounter
D	subsequent encounter
S	sequela

(Ex) For category T27 CC codes: T27.0XX-T27.7XX[A], T28.3XX-T28.49X[A], T28.8XX-T28.99X[A]

  X ● T27.0 Burn of larynx and trachea A 🐾, A 🐾
  X ● T27.1 Burn involving larynx and trachea with lung A 🐾, A 🐾
  X ● T27.2 Burn of other parts of respiratory tract A 🐾, A 🐾
       Burn of thoracic cavity

◄ New   ◄▥ Revised   ~~deleted~~ Deleted   Excludes 1   Excludes 2   Includes   Use additional   Code first   Code also   Unspecified
OGCR Official Guidelines   ● Unacceptable Principal Diagnosis   X Assign placeholder X   ● Use Additional Character(s)   ▶ Manifestation Code   Coding Clinic

X ● **T27.3**   **Burn of respiratory tract, part unspecified** A 🔹, A 🔹
     Code first (T51-T65) to identify chemical and intent for codes
     T27.4-T27.7

X ● **T27.4**   **Corrosion of larynx and trachea** A 🔹, A 🔹

X ● **T27.5**   **Corrosion involving larynx and trachea with lung** A 🔹, A 🔹

X ● **T27.6**   **Corrosion of other parts of respiratory tract** A 🔹, A 🔹

X ● **T27.7**   **Corrosion of respiratory tract, part unspecified** A 🔹, A 🔹

● **T28**   **Burn and corrosion of other internal organs**
     Use additional external cause code to identify the source and
     intent of the burn (X00-X19, X75-X77, X96-X98)
     Use additional external cause code to identify place (Y92)
     The appropriate 7th character is to be added to each code from
     category T28

> A   initial encounter
> D   subsequent encounter
> S   sequela

X ● **T28.0**   **Burn of mouth and pharynx**

X ● **T28.1**   **Burn of esophagus** A 🔹, A 🔹
     Ex: T28.1XX[A], T28.3XX-T28.49X[A], T28.6XX[A], T28.8XX-T28.99X[A]

X ● **T28.2**   **Burn of other parts of alimentary tract** A 🔹, A 🔹
     Ex: T28.2XX-T28.49X[A], T28.7XX-T28.99X[A]

X ● **T28.3**   **Burn of internal genitourinary organs**

X ● **T28.4**   **Burns of other and unspecified internal organs**

     X ● **T28.40**   **Burn of unspecified internal organ**

     ● **T28.41**   **Burn of ear drum**

         ● **T28.411**   **Burn of right ear drum**

         ● **T28.412**   **Burn of left ear drum**

         ● **T28.419**   **Burn of unspecified ear drum**

     X ● **T28.49**   **Burn of other internal organ**
         Code first (T51-T65) to identify chemical and
         intent for T28.5-T28.9-

X ● **T28.5**   **Corrosion of mouth and pharynx**

X ● **T28.6**   **Corrosion of esophagus** A 🔹, A 🔹
     Ex: See T28.1

X ● **T28.7**   **Corrosion of other parts of alimentary tract** A 🔹, A 🔹
     Ex: See T28.2

X ● **T28.8**   **Corrosion of internal genitourinary organs**

● **T28.9**   **Corrosions of other and unspecified internal organs**

     X ● **T28.90**   **Corrosions of unspecified internal organs**

     ● **T28.91**   **Corrosions of ear drum**

         ● **T28.911**   **Corrosions of right ear drum**

         ● **T28.912**   **Corrosions of left ear drum**

         ● **T28.919**   **Corrosions of unspecified ear drum**

     X ● **T28.99**   **Corrosions of other internal organs**

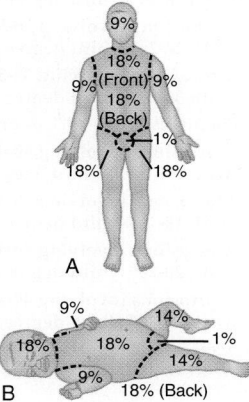

Figure 19-16   Rule of nines: percentages of total body area. (From Marx: Rosen's Emergency Medicine: Concepts and Clinical Practice, ed 6, Mosby, 2006)

OGCR Section I.C.19.d.5.

Assign separate code for each burn site
When coding burns, assign separate codes for each burn site. Category T30, Burn and corrosion, body region unspecified is extremely vague and should rarely be used.

BURNS AND CORROSIONS OF MULTIPLE AND UNSPECIFIED BODY REGIONS (T30-T32)

● **T30**   **Burn and corrosion, body region unspecified**

     T30.0   **Burn of unspecified body region, unspecified degree**
         This code is not for inpatient use. Code to specified site
         and degree of burns
         Burn NOS
         Multiple burns NOS

     T30.4   **Corrosion of unspecified body region, unspecified degree**
         This code is not for inpatient use. Code to specified site
         and degree of corrosion
         Corrosion NOS
         Multiple corrosion NOS

● **T31**   **Burns classified according to extent of body surface involved**
     Note: This category is to be used as the primary code only
         when the site of the burn is unspecified. It should be used
         as a supplementary code with categories T20-T25 when the
         site is specified.
     Ex: For category T31 CC codes: T31.0-T32.99

     T31.0   **Burns involving less than 10% of body surface**

     ● **T31.1**   **Burns involving 10-19% of body surface**

         T31.10   **Burns involving 10-19% of body surface with 0% to 9% third degree burns** 🔹 🔹
             Burns involving 10-19% of body surface NOS

         T31.11   **Burns involving 10-19% of body surface with 10-19% third degree burns** 🔹 🔹

     ● **T31.2**   **Burns involving 20-29% of body surface**

         T31.20   **Burns involving 20-29% of body surface with 0% to 9% third degree burns** 🔹 🔹
             Burns involving 20-29% of body surface NOS

         T31.21   **Burns involving 20-29% of body surface with 10-19% third degree burns** 🔹 🔹

         T31.22   **Burns involving 20-29% of body surface with 20-29% third degree burns** 🔹 🔹

     ● **T31.3**   **Burns involving 30-39% of body surface**

         T31.30   **Burns involving 30-39% of body surface with 0% to 9% third degree burns** 🔹 🔹
             Burns involving 30-39% of body surface NOS

         T31.31   **Burns involving 30-39% of body surface with 10-19% third degree burns** 🔹 🔹

         T31.32   **Burns involving 30-39% of body surface with 20-29% third degree burns** 🔹 🔹

         T31.33   **Burns involving 30-39% of body surface with 30-39% third degree burns** 🔹 🔹

     ● **T31.4**   **Burns involving 40-49% of body surface**

         T31.40   **Burns involving 40-49% of body surface with 0% to 9% third degree burns** 🔹 🔹
             Burns involving 40-49% of body surface NOS

         T31.41   **Burns involving 40-49% of body surface with 10-19% third degree burns** 🔹 🔹

         T31.42   **Burns involving 40-49% of body surface with 20-29% third degree burns** 🔹 🔹

         T31.43   **Burns involving 40-49% of body surface with 30-39% third degree burns** 🔹 🔹

         T31.44   **Burns involving 40-49% of body surface with 40-49% third degree burns** 🔹 🔹

● **T31.5**   **Burns involving 50-59% of body surface**

    T31.50   **Burns involving 50-59% of body surface with 0% to 9% third degree burns** 🔖 🔖
         Burns involving 50-59% of body surface NOS

    T31.51   **Burns involving 50-59% of body surface with 10-19% third degree burns** 🔖 🔖

    T31.52   **Burns involving 50-59% of body surface with 20-29% third degree burns** 🔖 🔖

    T31.53   **Burns involving 50-59% of body surface with 30-39% third degree burns** 🔖 🔖

    T31.54   **Burns involving 50-59% of body surface with 40-49% third degree burns** 🔖 🔖

    T31.55   **Burns involving 50-59% of body surface with 50-59% third degree burns** 🔖 🔖

● **T31.6**   **Burns involving 60-69% of body surface**

    T31.60   **Burns involving 60-69% of body surface with 0% to 9% third degree burns** 🔖 🔖
         Burns involving 60-69% of body surface NOS

    T31.61   **Burns involving 60-69% of body surface with 10-19% third degree burns** 🔖 🔖

    T31.62   **Burns involving 60-69% of body surface with 20-29% third degree burns** 🔖 🔖

    T31.63   **Burns involving 60-69% of body surface with 30-39% third degree burns** 🔖 🔖

    T31.64   **Burns involving 60-69% of body surface with 40-49% third degree burns** 🔖 🔖

    T31.65   **Burns involving 60-69% of body surface with 50-59% third degree burns** 🔖 🔖

    T31.66   **Burns involving 60-69% of body surface with 60-69% third degree burns** 🔖 🔖

● **T31.7**   **Burns involving 70-79% of body surface**

    T31.70   **Burns involving 70-79% of body surface with 0% to 9% third degree burns** 🔖 🔖
         Burns involving 70-79% of body surface NOS

    T31.71   **Burns involving 70-79% of body surface with 10-19% third degree burns** 🔖 🔖

    T31.72   **Burns involving 70-79% of body surface with 20-29% third degree burns** 🔖 🔖

    T31.73   **Burns involving 70-79% of body surface with 30-39% third degree burns** 🔖 🔖

    T31.74   **Burns involving 70-79% of body surface with 40-49% third degree burns** 🔖 🔖

    T31.75   **Burns involving 70-79% of body surface with 50-59% third degree burns** 🔖 🔖

    T31.76   **Burns involving 70-79% of body surface with 60-69% third degree burns** 🔖 🔖

    T31.77   **Burns involving 70-79% of body surface with 70-79% third degree burns** 🔖 🔖

● **T31.8**   **Burns involving 80-89% of body surface**

    T31.80   **Burns involving 80-89% of body surface with 0% to 9% third degree burns** 🔖 🔖
         Burns involving 80-89% of body surface NOS

    T31.81   **Burns involving 80-89% of body surface with 10-19% third degree burns** 🔖 🔖

    T31.82   **Burns involving 80-89% of body surface with 20-29% third degree burns** 🔖 🔖

    T31.83   **Burns involving 80-89% of body surface with 30-39% third degree burns** 🔖 🔖

    T31.84   **Burns involving 80-89% of body surface with 40-49% third degree burns** 🔖 🔖

    T31.85   **Burns involving 80-89% of body surface with 50-59% third degree burns** 🔖 🔖

    T31.86   **Burns involving 80-89% of body surface with 60-69% third degree burns** 🔖 🔖

    T31.87   **Burns involving 80-89% of body surface with 70-79% third degree burns** 🔖 🔖

    T31.88   **Burns involving 80-89% of body surface with 80-89% third degree burns** 🔖 🔖

● **T31.9**   **Burns involving 90% or more of body surface**

    T31.90   **Burns involving 90% or more of body surface with 0% to 9% third degree burns** 🔖 🔖
         Burns involving 90% or more of body surface NOS

    T31.91   **Burns involving 90% or more of body surface with 10-19% third degree burns** 🔖 🔖

    T31.92   **Burns involving 90% or more of body surface with 20-29% third degree burns** 🔖 🔖

    T31.93   **Burns involving 90% or more of body surface with 30-39% third degree burns** 🔖 🔖

    T31.94   **Burns involving 90% or more of body surface with 40-49% third degree burns** 🔖 🔖

    T31.95   **Burns involving 90% or more of body surface with 50-59% third degree burns** 🔖 🔖

    T31.96   **Burns involving 90% or more of body surface with 60-69% third degree burns** 🔖 🔖

    T31.97   **Burns involving 90% or more of body surface with 70-79% third degree burns** 🔖 🔖

    T31.98   **Burns involving 90% or more of body surface with 80-89% third degree burns** 🔖 🔖

    T31.99   **Burns involving 90% or more of body surface with 90% or more third degree burns** 🔖 🔖

● **T32**   **Corrosions classified according to extent of body surface involved**

    Note: This category is to be used as the primary code only when the site of the corrosion is unspecified. It may be used as a supplementary code with categories T20-T25 when the site is specified.
    (Ex) **For category T32 CC codes:** T31.0-T32.99

    T32.0   **Corrosions involving less than 10% of body surface**

● **T32.1**   **Corrosions involving 10-19% of body surface**

    T32.10   **Corrosions involving 10-19% of body surface with 0% to 9% third degree corrosion** 🔖 🔖
         Corrosions involving 10-19% of body surface NOS

    T32.11   **Corrosions involving 10-19% of body surface with 10-19% third degree corrosion** 🔖 🔖

● **T32.2**   **Corrosions involving 20-29% of body surface**

    T32.20   **Corrosions involving 20-29% of body surface with 0% to 9% third degree corrosion** 🔖 🔖

    T32.21   **Corrosions involving 20-29% of body surface with 10-19% third degree corrosion** 🔖 🔖

    T32.22   **Corrosions involving 20-29% of body surface with 20-29% third degree corrosion** 🔖 🔖

● **T32.3**   **Corrosions involving 30-39% of body surface**

    T32.30   **Corrosions involving 30-39% of body surface with 0% to 9% third degree corrosion** 🔖 🔖

    T32.31   **Corrosions involving 30-39% of body surface with 10-19% third degree corrosion** 🔖 🔖

    T32.32   **Corrosions involving 30-39% of body surface with 20-29% third degree corrosion** 🔖 🔖

    T32.33   **Corrosions involving 30-39% of body surface with 30-39% third degree corrosion** 🔖 🔖

● **T32.4**   **Corrosions involving 40-49% of body surface**

    T32.40   **Corrosions involving 40-49% of body surface with 0% to 9% third degree corrosion** 🔖 🔖

    T32.41   **Corrosions involving 40-49% of body surface with 10-19% third degree corrosion** 🔖 🔖

    T32.42   **Corrosions involving 40-49% of body surface with 20-29% third degree corrosion** 🔖 🔖

    T32.43   **Corrosions involving 40-49% of body surface with 30-39% third degree corrosion** 🔖 🔖

    T32.44   **Corrosions involving 40-49% of body surface with 40-49% third degree corrosion** 🔖 🔖

◄ New   ◄║║ Revised   ~~deleted~~ Deleted   Excludes 1   Excludes 2   Includes   Use additional   Code first   Code also   Unspecified

1442   OGCR Official Guidelines   ● Unacceptable Principal Diagnosis   X Assign placeholder X   ● Use Additional Character(s)   ▶ Manifestation Code   **Coding Clinic**

● **T32.5**   Corrosions involving 50-59% of body surface

   T32.50   Corrosions involving 50-59% of body surface with 0% to 9% third degree corrosion 🗇 🗇

   T32.51   Corrosions involving 50-59% of body surface with 10-19% third degree corrosion 🗇 🗇

   T32.52   Corrosions involving 50-59% of body surface with 20-29% third degree corrosion 🗇 🗇

   T32.53   Corrosions involving 50-59% of body surface with 30-39% third degree corrosion 🗇 🗇

   T32.54   Corrosions involving 50-59% of body surface with 40-49% third degree corrosion 🗇 🗇

   T32.55   Corrosions involving 50-59% of body surface with 50-59% third degree corrosion 🗇 🗇

● **T32.6**   Corrosions involving 60-69% of body surface

   T32.60   Corrosions involving 60-69% of body surface with 0% to 9% third degree corrosion 🗇 🗇

   T32.61   Corrosions involving 60-69% of body surface with 10-19% third degree corrosion 🗇 🗇

   T32.62   Corrosions involving 60-69% of body surface with 20-29% third degree corrosion 🗇 🗇

   T32.63   Corrosions involving 60-69% of body surface with 30-39% third degree corrosion 🗇 🗇

   T32.64   Corrosions involving 60-69% of body surface with 40-49% third degree corrosion 🗇 🗇

   T32.65   Corrosions involving 60-69% of body surface with 50-59% third degree corrosion 🗇 🗇

   T32.66   Corrosions involving 60-69% of body surface with 60-69% third degree corrosion 🗇 🗇

● **T32.7**   Corrosions involving 70-79% of body surface

   T32.70   Corrosions involving 70-79% of body surface with 0% to 9% third degree corrosion 🗇 🗇

   T32.71   Corrosions involving 70-79% of body surface with 10-19% third degree corrosion 🗇 🗇

   T32.72   Corrosions involving 70-79% of body surface with 20-29% third degree corrosion 🗇 🗇

   T32.73   Corrosions involving 70-79% of body surface with 30-39% third degree corrosion 🗇 🗇

   T32.74   Corrosions involving 70-79% of body surface with 40-49% third degree corrosion 🗇 🗇

   T32.75   Corrosions involving 70-79% of body surface with 50-59% third degree corrosion 🗇 🗇

   T32.76   Corrosions involving 70-79% of body surface with 60-69% third degree corrosion 🗇 🗇

   T32.77   Corrosions involving 70-79% of body surface with 70-79% third degree corrosion 🗇 🗇

● **T32.8**   Corrosions involving 80-89% of body surface

   T32.80   Corrosions involving 80-89% of body surface with 0% to 9% third degree corrosion 🗇 🗇

   T32.81   Corrosions involving 80-89% of body surface with 10-19% third degree corrosion 🗇 🗇

   T32.82   Corrosions involving 80-89% of body surface with 20-29% third degree corrosion 🗇 🗇

   T32.83   Corrosions involving 80-89% of body surface with 30-39% third degree corrosion 🗇 🗇

   T32.84   Corrosions involving 80-89% of body surface with 40-49% third degree corrosion 🗇 🗇

   T32.85   Corrosions involving 80-89% of body surface with 50-59% third degree corrosion 🗇 🗇

   T32.86   Corrosions involving 80-89% of body surface with 60-69% third degree corrosion 🗇 🗇

   T32.87   Corrosions involving 80-89% of body surface with 70-79% third degree corrosion 🗇 🗇

   T32.88   Corrosions involving 80-89% of body surface with 80-89% third degree corrosion 🗇 🗇

● **T32.9**   Corrosions involving 90% or more of body surface

   T32.90   Corrosions involving 90% or more of body surface with 0% to 9% third degree corrosion 🗇 🗇

   T32.91   Corrosions involving 90% or more of body surface with 10-19% third degree corrosion 🗇 🗇

   T32.92   Corrosions involving 90% or more of body surface with 20-29% third degree corrosion 🗇 🗇

   T32.93   Corrosions involving 90% or more of body surface with 30-39% third degree corrosion 🗇 🗇

   T32.94   Corrosions involving 90% or more of body surface with 40-49% third degree corrosion 🗇 🗇

   T32.95   Corrosions involving 90% or more of body surface with 50-59% third degree corrosion 🗇 🗇

   T32.96   Corrosions involving 90% or more of body surface with 60-69% third degree corrosion 🗇 🗇

   T32.97   Corrosions involving 90% or more of body surface with 70-79% third degree corrosion 🗇 🗇

   T32.98   Corrosions involving 90% or more of body surface with 80-89% third degree corrosion 🗇 🗇

   T32.99   Corrosions involving 90% or more of body surface with 90% or more third degree corrosion 🗇 🗇

FROSTBITE (T33-T34)

Excludes2   hypothermia and other effects of reduced temperature (T68, T69.-)

● **T33**   **Superficial frostbite**

   Includes   frostbite with partial thickness skin loss

   The appropriate 7th character is to be added to each code from category T33

> A   initial encounter
> D   subsequent encounter
> S   sequela

● **T33.0**   **Superficial frostbite of head**
Ex: **For category T33.0 CC codes:** T33.011-T33.42X[A], T33.60X-T33.72X[A], T33.90X-T34.42X[A], T34.60X-T34.72X[A], T34.90X-T34.99X[A]

   ● **T33.01**   **Superficial frostbite of ear**

     ● **T33.011**   **Superficial frostbite of right ear** A 🗇, A 🗇

     ● **T33.012**   **Superficial frostbite of left ear** A 🗇, A 🗇

     ● **T33.019**   **Superficial frostbite of unspecified ear** A 🗇, A 🗇

   X ● **T33.02**   **Superficial frostbite of nose** A 🗇, A 🗇

   X ● **T33.09**   **Superficial frostbite of other part of head** A 🗇, A 🗇

X ● **T33.1**   **Superficial frostbite of neck** A 🗇, A 🗇
Ex: See T33.0

X ● **T33.2**   **Superficial frostbite of thorax** A 🗇, A 🗇
Ex: T33.011-T34.99X[A], T69.021-T69.029[A]

X ● **T33.3**   **Superficial frostbite of abdominal wall, lower back and pelvis** A 🗇, A 🗇
Ex: See T33.2

N   Newborn Age: 0   P   Pediatric Age: 0–17   M   Maternity DX: 12–55   A   Adult Age: 15–124   ♀ Females Only   ♂ Males Only
🗇 Complication\Comorbidity   🗇 Major C\C   Ex: CC/MCC Exclusions   🗇 Hospital-Acquired Condition

1443

● **T33.4** **Superficial frostbite of arm**
  Excludes2 superficial frostbite of wrist and hand (T33.5-)
  (Ex:) **For category T33.4 CC codes:** See T33.2

  X● **T33.40** **Superficial frostbite of** unspecified **arm** A 🖐, A 👣

  X● **T33.41** **Superficial frostbite of right arm** A 🖐, A 👣

  X● **T33.42** **Superficial frostbite of left arm** A 🖐, A 👣

● **T33.5** **Superficial frostbite of wrist, hand, and fingers**
  (Ex:) **For category T33.5 CC codes:** T33.2XX-T33.72X[A], T33.90X-T33.99X[A], T34.2XX-T34.72X[A], T34.90X-T34.99X[A]

  ● **T33.51** **Superficial frostbite of wrist**

    ● **T33.511** **Superficial frostbite of right wrist** A 🖐, A 👣

    ● **T33.512** **Superficial frostbite of left wrist** A 🖐, A 👣

    ● **T33.519** **Superficial frostbite of** unspecified **wrist** A 🖐, A 👣

  ● **T33.52** **Superficial frostbite of hand**
    Excludes2 superficial frostbite of fingers (T33.53-)

    ● **T33.521** **Superficial frostbite of right hand** A 🖐, A 👣

    ● **T33.522** **Superficial frostbite of left hand** A 🖐, A 👣

    ● **T33.529** **Superficial frostbite of** unspecified **hand** A 🖐, A 👣

  ● **T33.53** **Superficial frostbite of finger(s)**

    ● **T33.531** **Superficial frostbite of right finger(s)** A 🖐, A 👣

    ● **T33.532** **Superficial frostbite of left finger(s)** A 🖐, A 👣

    ● **T33.539** **Superficial frostbite of** unspecified **finger(s)** A 🖐, A 👣

● **T33.6** **Superficial frostbite of hip and thigh**
  (Ex:) **For category T33.6 CC codes:** See T33.2

  X● **T33.60** **Superficial frostbite of** unspecified **hip and thigh** A 🖐, A 👣

  X● **T33.61** **Superficial frostbite of right hip and thigh** A 🖐, A 👣

  X● **T33.62** **Superficial frostbite of left hip and thigh** A 🖐, A 👣

● **T33.7** **Superficial frostbite of knee and lower leg**
  Excludes2 superficial frostbite of ankle and foot (T33.8-)
  (Ex:) **For category T33.7 CC codes:** See T33.2

  X● **T33.70** **Superficial frostbite of** unspecified **knee and lower leg** A 🖐, A 👣

  X● **T33.71** **Superficial frostbite of right knee and lower leg** A 🖐, A 👣

  X● **T33.72** **Superficial frostbite of left knee and lower leg** A 🖐, A 👣

● **T33.8** **Superficial frostbite of ankle, foot, and toe(s)**
  (Ex:) **For category T33.8 CC codes:** T33.2XX-T33.42X[A], T33.60X-T33.99X[A], T34.2XX-T34.42X[A], T34.60X-T34.99X[A]

  ● **T33.81** **Superficial frostbite of ankle**

    ● **T33.811** **Superficial frostbite of right ankle** A 🖐, A 👣

    ● **T33.812** **Superficial frostbite of left ankle** A 🖐, A 👣

    ● **T33.819** **Superficial frostbite of** unspecified **ankle** A 🖐, A 👣

● **T33.82** **Superficial frostbite of foot**

  ● **T33.821** **Superficial frostbite of right foot** A 🖐, A 👣

  ● **T33.822** **Superficial frostbite of left foot** A 🖐, A 👣

  ● **T33.829** **Superficial frostbite of** unspecified **foot** A 🖐, A 👣

● **T33.83** **Superficial frostbite of toe(s)**

  ● **T33.831** **Superficial frostbite of right toe(s)** A 🖐, A 👣

  ● **T33.832** **Superficial frostbite of left toe(s)** A 🖐, A 👣

  ● **T33.839** **Superficial frostbite of** unspecified **toe(s)** A 🖐, A 👣

● **T33.9** **Superficial frostbite of other and unspecified sites**
  (Ex:) **For category T33.9 CC codes:** See T33.2

  X● **T33.90** **Superficial frostbite of** unspecified **sites** A 🖐, A 👣
    Superficial frostbite NOS

  X● **T33.99** **Superficial frostbite of other sites** A 🖐, A 👣
    Superficial frostbite of leg NOS
    Superficial frostbite of trunk NOS

● **T34** **Frostbite with tissue necrosis**
  The appropriate 7th character is to be added to each code from category T34

  > A   initial encounter
  > D   subsequent encounter
  > S   sequela

● **T34.0** **Frostbite with tissue necrosis of head**
  (Ex:) **For category T34.0 CC codes:** See T33.0

  ● **T34.01** **Frostbite with tissue necrosis of ear**

    ● **T34.011** **Frostbite with tissue necrosis of right ear** A 🖐, A 👣

    ● **T34.012** **Frostbite with tissue necrosis of left ear** A 🖐, A 👣

    ● **T34.019** **Frostbite with tissue necrosis of** unspecified **ear** A 🖐, A 👣

  X● **T34.02** **Frostbite with tissue necrosis of nose** A 🖐, A 👣

  X● **T34.09** **Frostbite with tissue necrosis of other part of head** A 🖐, A 👣

● **T34.1** **Frostbite with tissue necrosis of neck** A 🖐, A 👣
  (Ex:) See T33.0

● **T34.2** **Frostbite with tissue necrosis of thorax** A 🖐, A 👣
  (Ex:) See T33.2

● **T34.3** **Frostbite with tissue necrosis of abdominal wall, lower back and pelvis** A 🖐, A 👣
  (Ex:) See T33.2

● **T34.4** **Frostbite with tissue necrosis of arm**
  Excludes2 frostbite with tissue necrosis of wrist and hand (T34.5-)
  (Ex:) **For category T34.4 CC codes:** See T33.2

  X● **T34.40** **Frostbite with tissue necrosis of** unspecified **arm** A 🖐, A 👣

  X● **T34.41** **Frostbite with tissue necrosis of right arm** A 🖐, A 👣

  X● **T34.42** **Frostbite with tissue necrosis of left arm** A 🖐, A 👣

● **T34.5** **Frostbite with tissue necrosis of wrist, hand, and finger(s)**
  (Ex:) **For category T34.5 CC codes:** See T33.5

  ● **T34.51** **Frostbite with tissue necrosis of wrist**

    ● **T34.511** **Frostbite with tissue necrosis of right wrist** A 🖐, A 👣

    ● **T34.512** **Frostbite with tissue necrosis of left wrist** A 🖐, A 👣

    ● **T34.519** **Frostbite with tissue necrosis of** unspecified **wrist** A 🖐, A 👣

◄ New   ◄ Revised   ̶d̶e̶l̶e̶t̶e̶d̶ Deleted   Excludes 1   Excludes 2   Includes   Use additional   Code first   Code also   Unspecified
OGCR Official Guidelines   ● Unacceptable Principal Diagnosis   X Assign placeholder X   ● Use Additional Character(s)   ▶ Manifestation Code   **Coding Clinic**

● **T34.52**   **Frostbite with tissue necrosis of hand**

     Excludes2   frostbite with tissue necrosis of finger(s) (T34.53-)

    ● **T34.521**   **Frostbite with tissue necrosis of right hand** A 🏥, A 🏥

    ● **T34.522**   **Frostbite with tissue necrosis of left hand** A 🏥, A 🏥

    ● **T34.529**   **Frostbite with tissue necrosis of unspecified hand** A 🏥, A 🏥

● **T34.53**   **Frostbite with tissue necrosis of finger(s)**

    ● **T34.531**   **Frostbite with tissue necrosis of right finger(s)** A 🏥, A 🏥

    ● **T34.532**   **Frostbite with tissue necrosis of left finger(s)** A 🏥, A 🏥

    ● **T34.539**   **Frostbite with tissue necrosis of unspecified finger(s)** A 🏥, A 🏥

● **T34.6**   **Frostbite with tissue necrosis of hip and thigh**

    (Ex) For category T34.6 CC codes: See T33.2

X ● **T34.60**   **Frostbite with tissue necrosis of unspecified hip and thigh** A 🏥, A 🏥

X ● **T34.61**   **Frostbite with tissue necrosis of right hip and thigh** A 🏥, A 🏥

X ● **T34.62**   **Frostbite with tissue necrosis of left hip and thigh** A 🏥, A 🏥

● **T34.7**   **Frostbite with tissue necrosis of knee and lower leg**

     Excludes2   frostbite with tissue necrosis of ankle and foot (T34.8-)

    (Ex) For category T34.7 CC codes: See T33.2

X ● **T34.70**   **Frostbite with tissue necrosis of unspecified knee and lower leg** A 🏥, A 🏥

X ● **T34.71**   **Frostbite with tissue necrosis of right knee and lower leg** A 🏥, A 🏥

X ● **T34.72**   **Frostbite with tissue necrosis of left knee and lower leg** A 🏥, A 🏥

● **T34.8**   **Frostbite with tissue necrosis of ankle, foot, and toe(s)**

    (Ex) For category T34.8 CC codes: See T33.8

    ● **T34.81**   **Frostbite with tissue necrosis of ankle**

        ● **T34.811**   **Frostbite with tissue necrosis of right ankle** A 🏥, A 🏥

        ● **T34.812**   **Frostbite with tissue necrosis of left ankle** A 🏥, A 🏥

        ● **T34.819**   **Frostbite with tissue necrosis of unspecified ankle** A 🏥, A 🏥

    ● **T34.82**   **Frostbite with tissue necrosis of foot**

        ● **T34.821**   **Frostbite with tissue necrosis of right foot** A 🏥, A 🏥

        ● **T34.822**   **Frostbite with tissue necrosis of left foot** A 🏥, A 🏥

        ● **T34.829**   **Frostbite with tissue necrosis of unspecified foot** A 🏥, A 🏥

    ● **T34.83**   **Frostbite with tissue necrosis of toe(s)**

        ● **T34.831**   **Frostbite with tissue necrosis of right toe(s)** A 🏥, A 🏥

        ● **T34.832**   **Frostbite with tissue necrosis of left toe(s)** A 🏥, A 🏥

        ● **T34.839**   **Frostbite with tissue necrosis of unspecified toe(s)** A 🏥, A 🏥

● **T34.9**   **Frostbite with tissue necrosis of other and unspecified sites**

    (Ex) For category T34.9 CC codes: See T33.2

X ● **T34.90**   **Frostbite with tissue necrosis of unspecified sites** A 🏥, A 🏥

     Frostbite with tissue necrosis NOS

X ● **T34.99**   **Frostbite with tissue necrosis of other sites** A 🏥, A 🏥

     Frostbite with tissue necrosis of leg NOS

     Frostbite with tissue necrosis of trunk NOS

OGCR   See Section I.C.19.e.

Adverse Effects, Poisoning , Underdosing and Toxic Effects

Codes in categories T36-T65 are combination codes that include the substance that was taken as well as the intent. No additional external cause code is required for poisonings, toxic effects, adverse effects and underdosing codes.

POISONING BY, ADVERSE EFFECTS OF AND UNDERDOSING OF DRUGS MEDICAMENTS AND BIOLOGICAL SUBSTANCES (T36-T50)

Includes   adverse effect of correct substance properly administered
poisoning by overdose of substance
poisoning by wrong substance given or taken in error
underdosing by (inadvertently) (deliberately) taking less substance than prescribed or instructed

Code first, for adverse effects, the nature of the adverse effect, such as:
adverse effect NOS (T88.7)
aspirin gastritis (K29.-)
blood disorders (D56-D76)
contact dermatitis (L23-L25)
dermatitis due to substances taken internally (L27.-)
nephropathy (N14.0-N14.2)

Note: The drug giving rise to the adverse effect should be identified by use of codes from categories T36-T50 with fifth or sixth character 5.

Use additional code(s) to specify:
manifestations of poisoning
underdosing or failure in dosage during medical and surgical care (Y63.6, Y63.8-Y63.9)
underdosing of medication regimen (Z91.12-, Z91.13-)

Excludes1   toxic reaction to local anesthesia in pregnancy (O29.3-)

Excludes2   abuse and dependence of psychoactive substances (F10-F19)
abuse of non-dependence-producing substances (F55.-)
drug reaction and poisoning affecting newborn (P00-P96)
pathological drug intoxication (inebriation) (F10-F19)

● **T36**   **Poisoning by, adverse effect of and underdosing of systemic antibiotics**

     Excludes1   antineoplastic antibiotics (T45.1-)
locally applied antibiotic NEC (T49.0)
topically used antibiotic for ear, nose and throat (T49.6)
topically used antibiotic for eye (T49.5)

The appropriate 7th character is to be added to each code from category T36

A	initial encounter
D	subsequent encounter
S	sequela

    ● **T36.0**   **Poisoning by, adverse effect of and underdosing of penicillins**

        ● **T36.0X**   **Poisoning by, adverse effect of and underdosing of penicillins**

            ● **T36.0X1**   **Poisoning by penicillins, accidental (unintentional)**

             Poisoning by penicillins NOS

            ● **T36.0X2**   **Poisoning by penicillins, intentional self-harm**

            ● **T36.0X3**   **Poisoning by penicillins, assault**

            ● **T36.0X4**   **Poisoning by penicillins, undetermined**

            ● **T36.0X5**   **Adverse effect of penicillins**

            ● **T36.0X6**   **Underdosing of penicillins**

CHAPTER 19 (S00-T88)

● **T36.1**   **Poisoning by, adverse effect of and underdosing of cephalosporins and other betalactam antibiotics**

   ● **T36.1X**   Poisoning by, adverse effect of and underdosing of cephalosporins and other beta-lactam antibiotics

     ● **T36.1X1**   Poisoning by cephalosporins and other beta-lactam antibiotics, accidental (unintentional)

        Poisoning by cephalosporins and other beta-lactam antibiotics NOS

     ● **T36.1X2**   Poisoning by cephalosporins and other beta-lactam antibiotics, intentional self-harm

     ● **T36.1X3**   Poisoning by cephalosporins and other beta-lactam antibiotics, assault

     ● **T36.1X4**   Poisoning by cephalosporins and other beta-lactam antibiotics, undetermined

     ● **T36.1X5**   Adverse effect of cephalosporins and other beta-lactam antibiotics

     ● **T36.1X6**   Underdosing of cephalosporins and other beta-lactam antibiotics

● **T36.2**   **Poisoning by, adverse effect of and underdosing of chloramphenicol group**

   ● **T36.2X**   Poisoning by, adverse effect of and underdosing of chloramphenicol group

     ● **T36.2X1**   Poisoning by chloramphenicol group, accidental (unintentional)

        Poisoning by chloramphenicol group NOS

     ● **T36.2X2**   Poisoning by chloramphenicol group, intentional self-harm

     ● **T36.2X3**   Poisoning by chloramphenicol group, assault

     ● **T36.2X4**   Poisoning by chloramphenicol group, undetermined

     ● **T36.2X5**   Adverse effect of chloramphenicol group

     ● **T36.2X6**   Underdosing of chloramphenicol group

● **T36.3**   **Poisoning by, adverse effect of and underdosing of macrolides**

   ● **T36.3X**   Poisoning by, adverse effect of and underdosing of macrolides

     ● **T36.3X1**   Poisoning by macrolides, accidental (unintentional)

        Poisoning by macrolides NOS

     ● **T36.3X2**   Poisoning by macrolides, intentional self-harm

     ● **T36.3X3**   Poisoning by macrolides, assault

     ● **T36.3X4**   Poisoning by macrolides, undetermined

     ● **T36.3X5**   Adverse effect of macrolides

     ● **T36.3X6**   Underdosing of macrolides

● **T36.4**   **Poisoning by, adverse effect of and underdosing of tetracyclines**

   ● **T36.4X**   Poisoning by, adverse effect of and underdosing of tetracyclines

     ● **T36.4X1**   Poisoning by tetracyclines, accidental (unintentional)

        Poisoning by tetracyclines NOS

     ● **T36.4X2**   Poisoning by tetracyclines, intentional self-harm

     ● **T36.4X3**   Poisoning by tetracyclines, assault

     ● **T36.4X4**   Poisoning by tetracyclines, undetermined

     ● **T36.4X5**   Adverse effect of tetracyclines

     ● **T36.4X6**   Underdosing of tetracyclines

● **T36.5**   **Poisoning by, adverse effect of and underdosing of aminoglycosides**

     Poisoning by, adverse effect of and underdosing of streptomycin

   ● **T36.5X**   Poisoning by, adverse effect of and underdosing of aminoglycosides

     ● **T36.5X1**   Poisoning by aminoglycosides, accidental (unintentional)

        Poisoning by aminoglycosides NOS

     ● **T36.5X2**   Poisoning by aminoglycosides, intentional self-harm

     ● **T36.5X3**   Poisoning by aminoglycosides, assault

     ● **T36.5X4**   Poisoning by aminoglycosides, undetermined

     ● **T36.5X5**   Adverse effect of aminoglycosides

     ● **T36.5X6**   Underdosing of aminoglycosides

● **T36.6**   **Poisoning by, adverse effect of and underdosing of rifampicins**

   ● **T36.6X**   Poisoning by, adverse effect of and underdosing of rifampicins

     ● **T36.6X1**   Poisoning by rifampicins, accidental (unintentional)

        Poisoning by rifampicins NOS

     ● **T36.6X2**   Poisoning by rifampicins, intentional self-harm

     ● **T36.6X3**   Poisoning by rifampicins, assault

     ● **T36.6X4**   Poisoning by rifampicins, undetermined

     ● **T36.6X5**   Adverse effect of rifampicins

     ● **T36.6X6**   Underdosing of rifampicins

● **T36.7**   **Poisoning by, adverse effect of and underdosing of antifungal antibiotics, systemically used**

   ● **T36.7X**   Poisoning by, adverse effect of and underdosing of antifungal antibiotics, systemically used

     ● **T36.7X1**   Poisoning by antifungal antibiotics, systemically used, accidental (unintentional)

        Poisoning by antifungal antibiotics, systemically used NOS

     ● **T36.7X2**   Poisoning by antifungal antibiotics, systemically used, intentional self-harm

     ● **T36.7X3**   Poisoning by antifungal antibiotics, systemically used, assault

     ● **T36.7X4**   Poisoning by antifungal antibiotics, systemically used, undetermined

     ● **T36.7X5**   Adverse effect of antifungal antibiotics, systemically used

     ● **T36.7X6**   Underdosing of antifungal antibiotics, systemically used

● **T36.8**   **Poisoning by, adverse effect of and underdosing of other systemic antibiotics**

   ● **T36.8X**   Poisoning by, adverse effect of and underdosing of other systemic antibiotics

     ● **T36.8X1**   Poisoning by other systemic antibiotics, accidental (unintentional)

        Poisoning by other systemic antibiotics NOS

     ● **T36.8X2**   Poisoning by other systemic antibiotics, intentional self-harm

     ● **T36.8X3**   Poisoning by other systemic antibiotics, assault

     ● **T36.8X4**   Poisoning by other systemic antibiotics, undetermined

     ● **T36.8X5**   Adverse effect of other systemic antibiotics

     ● **T36.8X6**   Underdosing of other systemic antibiotics

◀ New   ◀▥ Revised   ~~deleted~~ Deleted   Excludes 1   Excludes 2   Includes   Use additional   Code first   Code also   Unspecified

OGCR Official Guidelines   ● Unacceptable Principal Diagnosis   X Assign placeholder X   ● Use Additional Character(s)   ▶ Manifestation Code   **Coding Clinic**

● **T36.9** **Poisoning by, adverse effect of and underdosing of unspecified systemic antibiotic**

X ● **T36.91** **Poisoning by unspecified systemic antibiotic, accidental (unintentional)**
Poisoning by systemic antibiotic NOS

X ● **T36.92** **Poisoning by unspecified systemic antibiotic, intentional self-harm**

X ● **T36.93** **Poisoning by unspecified systemic antibiotic, assault**

X ● **T36.94** **Poisoning by unspecified systemic antibiotic, undetermined**

X ● **T36.95** **Adverse effect of unspecified systemic antibiotic**

X ● **T36.96** **Underdosing of unspecified systemic antibiotic**

● **T37** **Poisoning by, adverse effect of and underdosing of other systemic anti-infectives and antiparasitics**

Excludes1   anti-infectives topically used for ear, nose and throat (T49.6-)
anti-infectives topically used for eye (T49.5-)
locally applied anti-infectives NEC (T49.0-)

The appropriate 7th character is to be added to each code from category T37

A	initial encounter
D	subsequent encounter
S	sequela

● **T37.0** **Poisoning by, adverse effect of and underdosing of sulfonamides**

● **T37.0X** **Poisoning by, adverse effect of and underdosing of sulfonamides**

● **T37.0X1** **Poisoning by sulfonamides, accidental (unintentional)**
Poisoning by sulfonamides NOS

● **T37.0X2** **Poisoning by sulfonamides, intentional self-harm**

● **T37.0X3** **Poisoning by sulfonamides, assault**

● **T37.0X4** **Poisoning by sulfonamides, undetermined**

● **T37.0X5** **Adverse effect of sulfonamides**

● **T37.0X6** **Underdosing of sulfonamides**

● **T37.1** **Poisoning by, adverse effect of and underdosing of antimycobacterial drugs**

Excludes1   rifampicins (T36.6-) streptomycin (T36.5-)

● **T37.1X** **Poisoning by, adverse effect of and underdosing of antimycobacterial drugs**

● **T37.1X1** **Poisoning by antimycobacterial drugs, accidental (unintentional)**
Poisoning by antimycobacterial drugs NOS

● **T37.1X2** **Poisoning by antimycobacterial drugs, intentional self-harm**

● **T37.1X3** **Poisoning by antimycobacterial drugs, assault**

● **T37.1X4** **Poisoning by antimycobacterial drugs, undetermined**

● **T37.1X5** **Adverse effect of antimycobacterial drugs**

● **T37.1X6** **Underdosing of antimycobacterial drugs**

● **T37.2** **Poisoning by, adverse effect of and underdosing of antimalarials and drugs acting on other blood protozoa**

Excludes1   hydroxyquinoline derivatives (T37.8-)

● **T37.2X** **Poisoning by, adverse effect of and underdosing of antimalarials and drugs acting on other blood protozoa**

● **T37.2X1** **Poisoning by antimalarials and drugs acting on other blood protozoa, accidental (unintentional)**
Poisoning by antimalarials and drugs acting on other blood protozoa NOS

● **T37.2X2** **Poisoning by antimalarials and drugs acting on other blood protozoa, intentional self-harm**

● **T37.2X3** **Poisoning by antimalarials and drugs acting on other blood protozoa, assault**

● **T37.2X4** **Poisoning by antimalarials and drugs acting on other blood protozoa, undetermined**

● **T37.2X5** **Adverse effect of antimalarials and drugs acting on other blood protozoa**

● **T37.2X6** **Underdosing of antimalarials and drugs acting on other blood protozoa**

● **T37.3** **Poisoning by, adverse effect of and underdosing of other antiprotozoal drugs**

● **T37.3X** **Poisoning by, adverse effect of and underdosing of other antiprotozoal drugs**

● **T37.3X1** **Poisoning by other antiprotozoal drugs, accidental (unintentional)**
Poisoning by other antiprotozoal drugs NOS

● **T37.3X2** **Poisoning by other antiprotozoal drugs, intentional self-harm**

● **T37.3X3** **Poisoning by other antiprotozoal drugs, assault**

● **T37.3X4** **Poisoning by other antiprotozoal drugs, undetermined**

● **T37.3X5** **Adverse effect of other antiprotozoal drugs**

● **T37.3X6** **Underdosing of other antiprotozoal drugs**

● **T37.4** **Poisoning by, adverse effect of and underdosing of anthelminthics**

● **T37.4X** **Poisoning by, adverse effect of and underdosing of anthelminthics**

● **T37.4X1** **Poisoning by anthelminthics, accidental (unintentional)**
Poisoning by anthelminthics NOS

● **T37.4X2** **Poisoning by anthelminthics, intentional self-harm**

● **T37.4X3** **Poisoning by anthelminthics, assault**

● **T37.4X4** **Poisoning by anthelminthics, undetermined**

● **T37.4X5** **Adverse effect of anthelminthics**

● **T37.4X6** **Underdosing of anthelminthics**

CHAPTER 19 (S00-T88)

● **T37.5** **Poisoning by, adverse effect of and underdosing of antiviral drugs**

> **Excludes1**   amantadine (T42.8-)
> cytarabine (T45.1-)

    ● **T37.5X** **Poisoning by, adverse effect of and underdosing of antiviral drugs**

       ● **T37.5X1** **Poisoning by antiviral drugs, accidental (unintentional)**
> Poisoning by antiviral drugs NOS

       ● **T37.5X2** **Poisoning by antiviral drugs, intentional self-harm**

       ● **T37.5X3** **Poisoning by antiviral drugs, assault**

       ● **T37.5X4** **Poisoning by antiviral drugs, undetermined**

       ● **T37.5X5** **Adverse effect of antiviral drugs**

       ● **T37.5X6** **Underdosing of antiviral drugs**

● **T37.8** **Poisoning by, adverse effect of and underdosing of other specified systemic anti-infectives and antiparasitics**
> Poisoning by, adverse effect of and underdosing of hydroxyquinoline derivatives

> **Excludes1**   antimalarial drugs (T37.2-)

    ● **T37.8X** **Poisoning by, adverse effect of and underdosing of other specified systemic anti-infectives and antiparasitics**

       ● **T37.8X1** **Poisoning by other specified systemic anti-infectives and antiparasitics, accidental (unintentional)**
> Poisoning by other specified systemic anti-infectives and antiparasitics NOS

       ● **T37.8X2** **Poisoning by other specified systemic anti-infectives and antiparasitics, intentional self-harm**

       ● **T37.8X3** **Poisoning by other specified systemic anti-infectives and antiparasitics, assault**

       ● **T37.8X4** **Poisoning by other specified systemic anti-infectives and antiparasitics, undetermined**

       ● **T37.8X5** **Adverse effect of other specified systemic anti-infectives and antiparasitics**

       ● **T37.8X6** **Underdosing of other specified systemic anti-infectives and antiparasitics**

● **T37.9** **Poisoning by, adverse effect of and underdosing of unspecified systemic anti-infective and antiparasitics**

    X ● **T37.91** **Poisoning by unspecified systemic anti-infective and antiparasitics, accidental (unintentional)**
> Poisoning by, adverse effect of and underdosing of systemic anti-infective and antiparasitics NOS

    X ● **T37.92** **Poisoning by unspecified systemic anti-infective and antiparasitics, intentional self-harm**

    X ● **T37.93** **Poisoning by unspecified systemic anti-infective and antiparasitics, assault**

    X ● **T37.94** **Poisoning by unspecified systemic anti-infective and antiparasitics, undetermined**

    X ● **T37.95** **Adverse effect of unspecified systemic anti-infective and antiparasitic**

    X ● **T37.96** **Underdosing of unspecified systemic anti-infectives and antiparasitics**

● **T38** **Poisoning by, adverse effect of and underdosing of hormones and their synthetic substitutes and antagonists, not elsewhere classified**

> **Excludes1**   mineralocorticoids and their antagonists (T50.0-)
> oxytocic hormones (T48.0-)
> parathyroid hormones and derivatives (T50.9-)

The appropriate 7th character is to be added to each code from category T38

> A   initial encounter
> D   subsequent encounter
> S   sequela

● **T38.0** **Poisoning by, adverse effect of and underdosing of glucocorticoids and synthetic analogues**

> **Excludes1**   glucocorticoids, topically used (T49.-)

    ● **T38.0X** **Poisoning by, adverse effect of and underdosing of glucocorticoids and synthetic analogues**

       ● **T38.0X1** **Poisoning by glucocorticoids and synthetic analogues, accidental (unintentional)**
> Poisoning by glucocorticoids and synthetic analogues NOS

       ● **T38.0X2** **Poisoning by glucocorticoids and synthetic analogues, intentional self-harm**

       ● **T38.0X3** **Poisoning by glucocorticoids and synthetic analogues, assault**

       ● **T38.0X4** **Poisoning by glucocorticoids and synthetic analogues, undetermined**

       ● **T38.0X5** **Adverse effect of glucocorticoids and synthetic analogues**

       ● **T38.0X6** **Underdosing of glucocorticoids and synthetic analogues**

● **T38.1** **Poisoning by, adverse effect of and underdosing of thyroid hormones and substitutes**

    ● **T38.1X** **Poisoning by, adverse effect of and underdosing of thyroid hormones and substitutes**

       ● **T38.1X1** **Poisoning by thyroid hormones and substitutes, accidental (unintentional)**
> Poisoning by thyroid hormones and substitutes NOS

       ● **T38.1X2** **Poisoning by thyroid hormones and substitutes, intentional self-harm**

       ● **T38.1X3** **Poisoning by thyroid hormones and substitutes, assault**

       ● **T38.1X4** **Poisoning by thyroid hormones and substitutes, undetermined**

       ● **T38.1X5** **Adverse effect of thyroid hormones and substitutes**

       ● **T38.1X6** **Underdosing of thyroid hormones and substitutes**

● **T38.2** **Poisoning by, adverse effect of and underdosing of antithyroid drugs**

    ● **T38.2X** **Poisoning by, adverse effect of and underdosing of antithyroid drugs**

       ● **T38.2X1** **Poisoning by antithyroid drugs, accidental (unintentional)**
> Poisoning by antithyroid drugs NOS

       ● **T38.2X2** **Poisoning by antithyroid drugs, intentional self-harm**

       ● **T38.2X3** **Poisoning by antithyroid drugs, assault**

       ● **T38.2X4** **Poisoning by antithyroid drugs, undetermined**

       ● **T38.2X5** **Adverse effect of antithyroid drugs**

       ● **T38.2X6** **Underdosing of antithyroid drugs**

◀ New   ◀ Revised   ~~deleted~~ Deleted   Excludes 1   Excludes 2   Includes   Use additional   Code first   Code also   Unspecified

OGCR Official Guidelines   ● Unacceptable Principal Diagnosis   X Assign placeholder X   ● Use Additional Character(s)   ▶ Manifestation Code   **Coding Clinic**

- **T38.3 Poisoning by, adverse effect of and underdosing of insulin and oral hypoglycemic [antidiabetic] drugs**
  - **T38.3X Poisoning by, adverse effect of and underdosing of insulin and oral hypoglycemic [antidiabetic] drugs**
    - **T38.3X1 Poisoning by insulin and oral hypoglycemic [antidiabetic] drugs, accidental (unintentional)**
      Poisoning by insulin and oral hypoglycemic [antidiabetic] drugs NOS
    - **T38.3X2 Poisoning by insulin and oral hypoglycemic [antidiabetic] drugs, intentional self-harm**
    - **T38.3X3 Poisoning by insulin and oral hypoglycemic [antidiabetic] drugs, assault**
    - **T38.3X4 Poisoning by insulin and oral hypoglycemic [antidiabetic] drugs, undetermined**
    - **T38.3X5 Adverse effect of insulin and oral hypoglycemic [antidiabetic] drugs**
    - **T38.3X6 Underdosing of insulin and oral hypoglycemic [antidiabetic] drugs**
- **T38.4 Poisoning by, adverse effect of and underdosing of oral contraceptives**
  Poisoning by, adverse effect of and underdosing of multiple- and single-ingredient oral contraceptive preparations
  - **T38.4X Poisoning by, adverse effect of and underdosing of oral contraceptives**
    - **T38.4X1 Poisoning by oral contraceptives, accidental (unintentional)**
      Poisoning by oral contraceptives NOS
    - **T38.4X2 Poisoning by oral contraceptives, intentional self-harm**
    - **T38.4X3 Poisoning by oral contraceptives, assault**
    - **T38.4X4 Poisoning by oral contraceptives, undetermined**
    - **T38.4X5 Adverse effect of oral contraceptives**
    - **T38.4X6 Underdosing of oral contraceptives**
- **T38.5 Poisoning by, adverse effect of and underdosing of other estrogens and progestogens**
  Poisoning by, adverse effect of and underdosing of estrogens and progestogens mixtures and substitutes
  - **T38.5X Poisoning by, adverse effect of and underdosing of other estrogens and progestogens**
    - **T38.5X1 Poisoning by other estrogens and progestogens, accidental (unintentional)**
      Poisoning by other estrogens and progestogens NOS
    - **T38.5X2 Poisoning by other estrogens and progestogens, intentional self-harm**
    - **T38.5X3 Poisoning by other estrogens and progestogens, assault**
    - **T38.5X4 Poisoning by other estrogens and progestogens, undetermined**
    - **T38.5X5 Adverse effect of other estrogens and progestogens**
    - **T38.5X6 Underdosing of other estrogens and progestogens**

- **T38.6 Poisoning by, adverse effect of and underdosing of antigonadotrophins, antiestrogens, antiandrogens, not elsewhere classified**
  Poisoning by, adverse effect of and underdosing of tamoxifen
  - **T38.6X Poisoning by, adverse effect of and underdosing of antigonadotrophins, antiestrogens, antiandrogens, not elsewhere classified**
    - **T38.6X1 Poisoning by antigonadotrophins, antiestrogens, antiandrogens, not elsewhere classified, accidental (unintentional)**
      Poisoning by antigonadotrophins, antiestrogens, antiandrogens, not elsewhere classified NOS
    - **T38.6X2 Poisoning by antigonadotrophins, antiestrogens, antiandrogens, not elsewhere classified, intentional self-harm**
    - **T38.6X3 Poisoning by antigonadotrophins, antiestrogens, antiandrogens, not elsewhere classified, assault**
    - **T38.6X4 Poisoning by antigonadotrophins, antiestrogens, antiandrogens, not elsewhere classified, undetermined**
    - **T38.6X5 Adverse effect of antigonadotrophins, antiestrogens, antiandrogens, not elsewhere classified**
    - **T38.6X6 Underdosing of antigonadotrophins, antiestrogens, antiandrogens, not elsewhere classified**
- **T38.7 Poisoning by, adverse effect of and underdosing of androgens and anabolic congeners**
  - **T38.7X Poisoning by, adverse effect of and underdosing of androgens and anabolic congeners**
    - **T38.7X1 Poisoning by androgens and anabolic congeners, accidental (unintentional)**
      Poisoning by androgens and anabolic congeners NOS
    - **T38.7X2 Poisoning by androgens and anabolic congeners, intentional self-harm**
    - **T38.7X3 Poisoning by androgens and anabolic congeners, assault**
    - **T38.7X4 Poisoning by androgens and anabolic congeners, undetermined**
    - **T38.7X5 Adverse effect of androgens and anabolic congeners**
    - **T38.7X6 Underdosing of androgens and anabolic congeners**
- **T38.8 Poisoning by, adverse effect of and underdosing of other and unspecified hormones and synthetic substitutes**
  - **T38.80 Poisoning by, adverse effect of and underdosing of unspecified hormones and synthetic substitutes**
    - **T38.801 Poisoning by unspecified hormones and synthetic substitutes, accidental (unintentional)**
      Poisoning by unspecified hormones and synthetic substitutes NOS
    - **T38.802 Poisoning by unspecified hormones and synthetic substitutes, intentional self-harm**
    - **T38.803 Poisoning by unspecified hormones and synthetic substitutes, assault**
    - **T38.804 Poisoning by unspecified hormones and synthetic substitutes, undetermined**
    - **T38.805 Adverse effect of unspecified hormones and synthetic substitutes**
    - **T38.806 Underdosing of unspecified hormones and synthetic substitutes**

CHAPTER 19 (S00-T88)

● **T38.81**   **Poisoning by, adverse effect of and underdosing of anterior pituitary [adenohypophyseal] hormones**

    ● **T38.811**   **Poisoning by anterior pituitary [adenohypophyseal] hormones, accidental (unintentional)**
         Poisoning by anterior pituitary [adenohypophyseal] hormones NOS

    ● **T38.812**   **Poisoning by anterior pituitary [adenohypophyseal] hormones, intentional self-harm**

    ● **T38.813**   **Poisoning by anterior pituitary [adenohypophyseal] hormones, assault**

    ● **T38.814**   **Poisoning by anterior pituitary [adenohypophyseal] hormones, undetermined**

    ● **T38.815**   **Adverse effect of anterior pituitary [adenohypophyseal] hormones**

    ● **T38.816**   **Underdosing of anterior pituitary [adenohypophyseal] hormones**

● **T38.89**   **Poisoning by, adverse effect of and underdosing of other hormones and synthetic substitutes**

    ● **T38.891**   **Poisoning by other hormones and synthetic substitutes, accidental (unintentional)**
         Poisoning by other hormones and synthetic substitutes NOS

    ● **T38.892**   **Poisoning by other hormones and synthetic substitutes, intentional self-harm**

    ● **T38.893**   **Poisoning by other hormones and synthetic substitutes, assault**

    ● **T38.894**   **Poisoning by other hormones and synthetic substitutes, undetermined**

    ● **T38.895**   **Adverse effect of other hormones and synthetic substitutes**

    ● **T38.896**   **Underdosing of other hormones and synthetic substitutes**

● **T38.9**   **Poisoning by, adverse effect of and underdosing of other and unspecified hormone antagonists**

    ● **T38.90**   **Poisoning by, adverse effect of and underdosing of unspecified hormone antagonists**

       ● **T38.901**   **Poisoning by unspecified hormone antagonists, accidental (unintentional)**
           Poisoning by unspecified hormone antagonists NOS

       ● **T38.902**   **Poisoning by unspecified hormone antagonists, intentional self-harm**

       ● **T38.903**   **Poisoning by unspecified hormone antagonists, assault**

       ● **T38.904**   **Poisoning by unspecified hormone antagonists, undetermined**

       ● **T38.905**   **Adverse effect of unspecified hormone antagonists**

       ● **T38.906**   **Underdosing of unspecified hormone antagonists**

● **T38.99**   **Poisoning by, adverse effect of and underdosing of other hormone antagonists**

    ● **T38.991**   **Poisoning by other hormone antagonists, accidental (unintentional)**
         Poisoning by other hormone antagonists NOS

    ● **T38.992**   **Poisoning by other hormone antagonists, intentional self-harm**

    ● **T38.993**   **Poisoning by other hormone antagonists, assault**

    ● **T38.994**   **Poisoning by other hormone antagonists, undetermined**

    ● **T38.995**   **Adverse effect of other hormone antagonists**

    ● **T38.996**   **Underdosing of other hormone antagonists**

● **T39**   **Poisoning by, adverse effect of and underdosing of nonopioid analgesics, antipyretics and antirheumatics**

   The appropriate 7th character is to be added to each code from category T39

> A   initial encounter
> D   subsequent encounter
> S   sequela

● **T39.0**   **Poisoning by, adverse effect of and underdosing of salicylates**

    ● **T39.01**   **Poisoning by, adverse effect of and underdosing of aspirin**
       Poisoning by, adverse effect of and underdosing of acetylsalicylic acid

       ● **T39.011**   **Poisoning by aspirin, accidental (unintentional)**

       ● **T39.012**   **Poisoning by aspirin, intentional self-harm**

       ● **T39.013**   **Poisoning by aspirin, assault**

       ● **T39.014**   **Poisoning by aspirin, undetermined**

       ● **T39.015**   **Adverse effect of aspirin**
         Coding Clinic: 2016, Q1, P15

       ● **T39.016**   **Underdosing of aspirin**

    ● **T39.09**   **Poisoning by, adverse effect of and underdosing of other salicylates**

       ● **T39.091**   **Poisoning by salicylates, accidental (unintentional)**
           Poisoning by salicylates NOS

       ● **T39.092**   **Poisoning by salicylates, intentional self-harm**

       ● **T39.093**   **Poisoning by salicylates, assault**

       ● **T39.094**   **Poisoning by salicylates, undetermined**

       ● **T39.095**   **Adverse effect of salicylates**

       ● **T39.096**   **Underdosing of salicylates**

● **T39.1**   **Poisoning by, adverse effect of and underdosing of 4-Aminophenol derivatives**

    ● **T39.1X**   **Poisoning by, adverse effect of and underdosing of 4-Aminophenol derivatives**

       ● **T39.1X1**   **Poisoning by 4-Aminophenol derivatives, accidental (unintentional)**
           Poisoning by 4-Aminophenol derivatives NOS

       ● **T39.1X2**   **Poisoning by 4-Aminophenol derivatives, intentional self-harm**

       ● **T39.1X3**   **Poisoning by 4-Aminophenol derivatives, assault**

       ● **T39.1X4**   **Poisoning by 4-Aminophenol derivatives, undetermined**

       ● **T39.1X5**   **Adverse effect of 4-Aminophenol derivatives**

       ● **T39.1X6**   **Underdosing of 4-Aminophenol derivatives**

◀ New   ◀▥ Revised   ~~deleted~~ Deleted   Excludes 1   Excludes 2   Includes   Use additional   Code first   Code also   Unspecified

OGCR Official Guidelines   ● Unacceptable Principal Diagnosis   X Assign placeholder X   ● Use Additional Character(s)   ▸ Manifestation Code   **Coding Clinic**

- T39.2　Poisoning by, adverse effect of and underdosing of pyrazolone derivatives
  - T39.2X　Poisoning by, adverse effect of and underdosing of pyrazolone derivatives
    - T39.2X1　Poisoning by pyrazolone derivatives, accidental (unintentional)
      Poisoning by pyrazolone derivatives NOS
    - T39.2X2　Poisoning by pyrazolone derivatives, intentional self-harm
    - T39.2X3　Poisoning by pyrazolone derivatives, assault
    - T39.2X4　Poisoning by pyrazolone derivatives, undetermined
    - T39.2X5　Adverse effect of pyrazolone derivatives
    - T39.2X6　Underdosing of pyrazolone derivatives
- T39.3　Poisoning by, adverse effect of and underdosing of other nonsteroidal anti-inflammatory drugs [NSAID]
  - T39.31　Poisoning by, adverse effect of and underdosing of propionic acid derivatives
    Poisoning by, adverse effect of and underdosing of fenoprofen
    Poisoning by, adverse effect of and underdosing of flurbiprofen
    Poisoning by, adverse effect of and underdosing of ibuprofen
    Poisoning by, adverse effect of and underdosing of ketoprofen
    Poisoning by, adverse effect of and underdosing of naproxen
    Poisoning by, adverse effect of and underdosing of oxaprozin
    - T39.311　Poisoning by propionic acid derivatives, accidental (unintentional)
    - T39.312　Poisoning by propionic acid derivatives, intentional self-harm
    - T39.313　Poisoning by propionic acid derivatives, assault
    - T39.314　Poisoning by propionic acid derivatives, undetermined
    - T39.315　Adverse effect of propionic acid derivatives
    - T39.316　Underdosing of propionic acid derivatives
  - T39.39　Poisoning by, adverse effect of and underdosing of other nonsteroidal anti-inflammatory drugs [NSAID]
    - T39.391　Poisoning by other nonsteroidal anti-inflammatory drugs [NSAID], accidental (unintentional)
      Poisoning by other nonsteroidal anti-inflammatory drugs NOS
    - T39.392　Poisoning by other nonsteroidal anti-inflammatory drugs [NSAID], intentional self-harm
    - T39.393　Poisoning by other nonsteroidal anti-inflammatory drugs [NSAID], assault
    - T39.394　Poisoning by other nonsteroidal anti-inflammatory drugs [NSAID], undetermined
    - T39.395　Adverse effect of other nonsteroidal anti-inflammatory drugs [NSAID]
    - T39.396　Underdosing of other nonsteroidal anti-inflammatory drugs [NSAID]

- T39.4　Poisoning by, adverse effect of and underdosing of antirheumatics, not elsewhere classified
  - **Excludes1**　poisoning by, adverse effect of and underdosing of glucocorticoids (T38.Ø-)
    poisoning by, adverse effect of and underdosing of salicylates (T39.Ø-)
  - T39.4X　Poisoning by, adverse effect of and underdosing of antirheumatics, not elsewhere classified
    - T39.4X1　Poisoning by antirheumatics, not elsewhere classified, accidental (unintentional)
      Poisoning by antirheumatics, not elsewhere classified NOS
    - T39.4X2　Poisoning by antirheumatics, not elsewhere classified, intentional self-harm
    - T39.4X3　Poisoning by antirheumatics, not elsewhere classified, assault
    - T39.4X4　Poisoning by antirheumatics, not elsewhere classified, undetermined
    - T39.4X5　Adverse effect of antirheumatics, not elsewhere classified
    - T39.4X6　Underdosing of antirheumatics, not elsewhere classified
- T39.8　Poisoning by, adverse effect of and underdosing of other nonopioid analgesics and antipyretics, not elsewhere classified
  - T39.8X　Poisoning by, adverse effect of and underdosing of other nonopioid analgesics and antipyretics, not elsewhere classified
    - T39.8X1　Poisoning by other nonopioid analgesics and antipyretics, not elsewhere classified, accidental (unintentional)
      Poisoning by other nonopioid analgesics and antipyretics, not elsewhere classified NOS
    - T39.8X2　Poisoning by other nonopioid analgesics and antipyretics, not elsewhere classified, intentional self-harm
    - T39.8X3　Poisoning by other nonopioid analgesics and antipyretics, not elsewhere classified, assault
    - T39.8X4　Poisoning by other nonopioid analgesics and antipyretics, not elsewhere classified, undetermined
    - T39.8X5　Adverse effect of other nonopioid analgesics and antipyretics, not elsewhere classified
    - T39.8X6　Underdosing of other nonopioid analgesics and antipyretics, not elsewhere classified
- T39.9　Poisoning by, adverse effect of and underdosing of unspecified nonopioid analgesic, antipyretic and antirheumatic
  - X● T39.91　Poisoning by unspecified nonopioid analgesic, antipyretic and antirheumatic, accidental (unintentional)
    Poisoning by nonopioid analgesic, antipyretic and antirheumatic NOS
  - X● T39.92　Poisoning by unspecified nonopioid analgesic, antipyretic and antirheumatic, intentional self-harm
  - X● T39.93　Poisoning by unspecified nonopioid analgesic, antipyretic and antirheumatic, assault
  - X● T39.94　Poisoning by unspecified nonopioid analgesic, antipyretic and antirheumatic, undetermined
  - X● T39.95　Adverse effect of unspecified nonopioid analgesic, antipyretic and antirheumatic
  - X● T39.96　Underdosing of unspecified nonopioid analgesic, antipyretic and antirheumatic

CHAPTER 19 (SØØ-T88)

- **T40** **Poisoning by, adverse effect of and underdosing of narcotics and psychodysleptics [hallucinogens]**

  Excludes2   drug dependence and related mental and behavioral disorders due to psychoactive substance use (F10.-F19.-)

  The appropriate 7th character is to be added to each code from category T40

A	initial encounter
D	subsequent encounter
S	sequela

  - **T40.0** **Poisoning by, adverse effect of and underdosing of opium**
    - **T40.0X** **Poisoning by, adverse effect of and underdosing of opium**
      - **T40.0X1** **Poisoning by opium, accidental (unintentional)**
        Poisoning by opium NOS
      - **T40.0X2** **Poisoning by opium, intentional self-harm**
      - **T40.0X3** **Poisoning by opium, assault**
      - **T40.0X4** **Poisoning by opium, undetermined**
      - **T40.0X5** **Adverse effect of opium**
      - **T40.0X6** **Underdosing of opium**
  - **T40.1** **Poisoning by and adverse effect of heroin**
    - **T40.1X** **Poisoning by and adverse effect of heroin**
      - **T40.1X1** **Poisoning by heroin, accidental (unintentional)**
        Poisoning by heroin NOS
      - **T40.1X2** **Poisoning by heroin, intentional self-harm**
      - **T40.1X3** **Poisoning by heroin, assault**
      - **T40.1X4** **Poisoning by heroin, undetermined**
  - **T40.2** **Poisoning by, adverse effect of and underdosing of other opioids**
    - **T40.2X** **Poisoning by, adverse effect of and underdosing of other opioids**
      - **T40.2X1** **Poisoning by other opioids, accidental (unintentional)**
        Poisoning by other opioids NOS
      - **T40.2X2** **Poisoning by other opioids, intentional self-harm**
      - **T40.2X3** **Poisoning by other opioids, assault**
      - **T40.2X4** **Poisoning by other opioids, undetermined**
      - **T40.2X5** **Adverse effect of other opioids**
      - **T40.2X6** **Underdosing of other opioids**
  - **T40.3** **Poisoning by, adverse effect of and underdosing of methadone**
    - **T40.3X** **Poisoning by, adverse effect of and underdosing of methadone**
      - **T40.3X1** **Poisoning by methadone, accidental (unintentional)**
        Poisoning by methadone NOS
      - **T40.3X2** **Poisoning by methadone, intentional self-harm**
      - **T40.3X3** **Poisoning by methadone, assault**
      - **T40.3X4** **Poisoning by methadone, undetermined**
      - **T40.3X5** **Adverse effect of methadone**
      - **T40.3X6** **Underdosing of methadone**

- **T40.4** **Poisoning by, adverse effect of and underdosing of other synthetic narcotics**
  - **T40.4X** **Poisoning by, adverse effect of and underdosing of other synthetic narcotics**
    - **T40.4X1** **Poisoning by other synthetic narcotics, accidental (unintentional)**
      Poisoning by other synthetic narcotics NOS
    - **T40.4X2** **Poisoning by other synthetic narcotics, intentional self-harm**
    - **T40.4X3** **Poisoning by other synthetic narcotics, assault**
    - **T40.4X4** **Poisoning by other synthetic narcotics, undetermined**
    - **T40.4X5** **Adverse effect of other synthetic narcotics**
    - **T40.4X6** **Underdosing of other synthetic narcotics**
- **T40.5** **Poisoning by, adverse effect of and underdosing of cocaine**
  - **T40.5X** **Poisoning by, adverse effect of and underdosing of cocaine**
    - **T40.5X1** **Poisoning by cocaine, accidental (unintentional)**
      Poisoning by cocaine NOS
      Coding Clinic: 2016, Q2, P9
    - **T40.5X2** **Poisoning by cocaine, intentional self-harm**
    - **T40.5X3** **Poisoning by cocaine, assault**
    - **T40.5X4** **Poisoning by cocaine, undetermined**
    - **T40.5X5** **Adverse effect of cocaine**
    - **T40.5X6** **Underdosing of cocaine**
- **T40.6** **Poisoning by, adverse effect of and underdosing of other and unspecified narcotics**
  - **T40.60** **Poisoning by, adverse effect of and underdosing of unspecified narcotics**
    - **T40.601** **Poisoning by unspecified narcotics, accidental (unintentional)**
      Poisoning by narcotics NOS
    - **T40.602** **Poisoning by unspecified narcotics, intentional self-harm**
    - **T40.603** **Poisoning by unspecified narcotics, assault**
    - **T40.604** **Poisoning by unspecified narcotics, undetermined**
    - **T40.605** **Adverse effect of unspecified narcotics**
    - **T40.606** **Underdosing of unspecified narcotics**
  - **T40.69** **Poisoning by, adverse effect of and underdosing of other narcotics**
    - **T40.691** **Poisoning by other narcotics, accidental (unintentional)**
      Poisoning by other narcotics NOS
    - **T40.692** **Poisoning by other narcotics, intentional self-harm**
    - **T40.693** **Poisoning by other narcotics, assault**
    - **T40.694** **Poisoning by other narcotics, undetermined**
    - **T40.695** **Adverse effect of other narcotics**
    - **T40.696** **Underdosing of other narcotics**

- **T40.7** Poisoning by, adverse effect of and underdosing of cannabis (derivatives)
  - **T40.7X** Poisoning by, adverse effect of and underdosing of cannabis (derivatives)
    - **T40.7X1** Poisoning by cannabis (derivatives), accidental (unintentional)
      Poisoning by cannabis NOS
    - **T40.7X2** Poisoning by cannabis (derivatives), intentional self-harm
    - **T40.7X3** Poisoning by cannabis (derivatives), assault
    - **T40.7X4** Poisoning by cannabis (derivatives), undetermined
    - **T40.7X5** Adverse effect of cannabis (derivatives)
    - **T40.7X6** Underdosing of cannabis (derivatives)
- **T40.8** Poisoning by and adverse effect of lysergide [LSD]
  - **T40.8X** Poisoning by and adverse effect of lysergide [LSD]
    - **T40.8X1** Poisoning by lysergide [LSD], accidental (unintentional)
      Poisoning by lysergide [LSD] NOS
    - **T40.8X2** Poisoning by lysergide [LSD], intentional self-harm
    - **T40.8X3** Poisoning by lysergide [LSD], assault
    - **T40.8X4** Poisoning by lysergide [LSD], undetermined
- **T40.9** Poisoning by, adverse effect of and underdosing of other and unspecified psychodysleptics [hallucinogens]
  - **T40.90** Poisoning by, adverse effect of and underdosing of unspecified psychodysleptics [hallucinogens]
    - **T40.901** Poisoning by unspecified psychodysleptics [hallucinogens], accidental (unintentional)
    - **T40.902** Poisoning by unspecified psychodysleptics [hallucinogens], intentional self-harm
    - **T40.903** Poisoning by unspecified psychodysleptics [hallucinogens], assault
    - **T40.904** Poisoning by unspecified psychodysleptics [hallucinogens], undetermined
    - **T40.905** Adverse effect of unspecified psychodysleptics [hallucinogens]
    - **T40.906** Underdosing of unspecified psychodysleptics
  - **T40.99** Poisoning by, adverse effect of and underdosing of other psychodysleptics [hallucinogens]
    - **T40.991** Poisoning by other psychodysleptics [hallucinogens], accidental (unintentional)
      Poisoning by other psychodysleptics [hallucinogens] NOS
    - **T40.992** Poisoning by other psychodysleptics [hallucinogens], intentional self-harm
    - **T40.993** Poisoning by other psychodysleptics [hallucinogens], assault
    - **T40.994** Poisoning by other psychodysleptics [hallucinogens], undetermined
    - **T40.995** Adverse effect of other psychodysleptics [hallucinogens]
    - **T40.996** Underdosing of other psychodysleptics

- **T41** Poisoning by, adverse effect of and underdosing of anesthetics and therapeutic gases
  - **Excludes1** benzodiazepines (T42.4-)
    cocaine (T40.5-)
    complications of anesthesia during pregnancy (O29.-)
    complications of anesthesia during labor and delivery (O74.-)
    complications of anesthesia during the puerperium (O89.-) opioids (T40.0-T40.2-)

  The appropriate 7th character is to be added to each code from category T41

A	initial encounter
D	subsequent encounter
S	sequela

  - **T41.0** Poisoning by, adverse effect of and underdosing of inhaled anesthetics
    - **Excludes1** oxygen (T41.5-)
    - **T41.0X** Poisoning by, adverse effect of and underdosing of inhaled anesthetics
      - **T41.0X1** Poisoning by inhaled anesthetics, accidental (unintentional)
        Poisoning by inhaled anesthetics NOS
      - **T41.0X2** Poisoning by inhaled anesthetics, intentional self-harm
      - **T41.0X3** Poisoning by inhaled anesthetics, assault
      - **T41.0X4** Poisoning by inhaled anesthetics, undetermined
      - **T41.0X5** Adverse effect of inhaled anesthetics
      - **T41.0X6** Underdosing of inhaled anesthetics
  - **T41.1** Poisoning by, adverse effect of and underdosing of intravenous anesthetics
    Poisoning by, adverse effect of and underdosing of thiobarbiturates
    - **T41.1X** Poisoning by, adverse effect of and underdosing of intravenous anesthetics
      - **T41.1X1** Poisoning by intravenous anesthetics, accidental (unintentional)
        Poisoning by intravenous anesthetics NOS
      - **T41.1X2** Poisoning by intravenous anesthetics, intentional self-harm
      - **T41.1X3** Poisoning by intravenous anesthetics, assault
      - **T41.1X4** Poisoning by intravenous anesthetics, undetermined
      - **T41.1X5** Adverse effect of intravenous anesthetics
      - **T41.1X6** Underdosing of intravenous anesthetics
  - **T41.2** Poisoning by, adverse effect of and underdosing of other and unspecified general anesthetics
    - **T41.20** Poisoning by, adverse effect of and underdosing of unspecified general anesthetics
      - **T41.201** Poisoning by unspecified general anesthetics, accidental (unintentional)
        Poisoning by general anesthetics NOS
      - **T41.202** Poisoning by unspecified general anesthetics, intentional self-harm
      - **T41.203** Poisoning by unspecified general anesthetics, assault
      - **T41.204** Poisoning by unspecified general anesthetics, undetermined
      - **T41.205** Adverse effect of unspecified general anesthetics
      - **T41.206** Underdosing of unspecified general anesthetics

N Newborn Age: 0　　**P** Pediatric Age: 0–17　　**M** Maternity DX: 12–55　　**A** Adult Age: 15–124　　♀ Females Only　　♂ Males Only

Complication\Comorbidity　　Major C\C　　(Ex) CC/MCC Exclusions　　Hospital-Acquired Condition

1453

CHAPTER 19 (S00-T88)

● T41.29   **Poisoning by, adverse effect of and underdosing of other general anesthetics**

   ● T41.291   **Poisoning by other general anesthetics, accidental (unintentional)**
         Poisoning by other general anesthetics NOS

   ● T41.292   **Poisoning by other general anesthetics, intentional self-harm**

   ● T41.293   **Poisoning by other general anesthetics, assault**

   ● T41.294   **Poisoning by other general anesthetics, undetermined**

   ● T41.295   **Adverse effect of other general anesthetics**

   ● T41.296   **Underdosing of other general anesthetics**

● T41.3   **Poisoning by, adverse effect of and underdosing of local anesthetics**
   Cocaine (topical)

   Excludes2   poisoning by cocaine used as a central nervous system stimulant (T40.5X1-T40.5X4)

  ● T41.3X   **Poisoning by, adverse effect of and underdosing of local anesthetics**

   ● T41.3X1   **Poisoning by local anesthetics, accidental (unintentional)**
         Poisoning by local anesthetics NOS

   ● T41.3X2   **Poisoning by local anesthetics, intentional self-harm**

   ● T41.3X3   **Poisoning by local anesthetics, assault**

   ● T41.3X4   **Poisoning by local anesthetics, undetermined**

   ● T41.3X5   **Adverse effect of local anesthetics**

   ● T41.3X6   **Underdosing of local anesthetics**

● T41.4   **Poisoning by, adverse effect of and underdosing of unspecified anesthetic**

X● T41.41   **Poisoning by unspecified anesthetic, accidental (unintentional)**
      Poisoning by anesthetic NOS

X● T41.42   **Poisoning by unspecified anesthetic, intentional self-harm**

X● T41.43   **Poisoning by unspecified anesthetic, assault**

X● T41.44   **Poisoning by unspecified anesthetic, undetermined**

X● T41.45   **Adverse effect of unspecified anesthetic**

X● T41.46   **Underdosing of unspecified anesthetics**

● T41.5   **Poisoning by, adverse effect of and underdosing of therapeutic gases**

  ● T41.5X   **Poisoning by, adverse effect of and underdosing of therapeutic gases**

   ● T41.5X1   **Poisoning by therapeutic gases, accidental (unintentional)**
         Poisoning by therapeutic gases NOS

   ● T41.5X2   **Poisoning by therapeutic gases, intentional self-harm**

   ● T41.5X3   **Poisoning by therapeutic gases, assault**

   ● T41.5X4   **Poisoning by therapeutic gases, undetermined**

   ● T41.5X5   **Adverse effect of therapeutic gases**

   ● T41.5X6   **Underdosing of therapeutic gases**

● T42   **Poisoning by, adverse effect of and underdosing of antiepileptic, sedative-hypnotic and antiparkinsonism drugs**

  Excludes2   drug dependence and related mental and behavioral disorders due to psychoactive substance use (F10.--F19.-)

  The appropriate 7th character is to be added to each code from category T42

     A   initial encounter
     D   subsequent encounter
     S   sequela

● T42.0   **Poisoning by, adverse effect of and underdosing of hydantoin derivatives**

  ● T42.0X   **Poisoning by, adverse effect of and underdosing of hydantoin derivatives**

   ● T42.0X1   **Poisoning by hydantoin derivatives, accidental (unintentional)**
         Poisoning by hydantoin derivatives NOS

   ● T42.0X2   **Poisoning by hydantoin derivatives, intentional self-harm**

   ● T42.0X3   **Poisoning by hydantoin derivatives, assault**

   ● T42.0X4   **Poisoning by hydantoin derivatives, undetermined**

   ● T42.0X5   **Adverse effect of hydantoin derivatives**

   ● T42.0X6   **Underdosing of hydantoin derivatives**

● T42.1   **Poisoning by, adverse effect of and underdosing of iminostilbenes**
   Poisoning by, adverse effect of and underdosing of carbamazepine

  ● T42.1X   **Poisoning by, adverse effect of and underdosing of iminostilbenes**

   ● T42.1X1   **Poisoning by iminostilbenes, accidental (unintentional)**
         Poisoning by iminostilbenes NOS

   ● T42.1X2   **Poisoning by iminostilbenes, intentional self-harm**

   ● T42.1X3   **Poisoning by iminostilbenes, assault**

   ● T42.1X4   **Poisoning by iminostilbenes, undetermined**

   ● T42.1X5   **Adverse effect of iminostilbenes**

   ● T42.1X6   **Underdosing of iminostilbenes**

● T42.2   **Poisoning by, adverse effect of and underdosing of succinimides and oxazolidinediones**

  ● T42.2X   **Poisoning by, adverse effect of and underdosing of succinimides and oxazolidinediones**

   ● T42.2X1   **Poisoning by succinimides and oxazolidinediones, accidental (unintentional)**
         Poisoning by succinimides and oxazolidinediones NOS

   ● T42.2X2   **Poisoning by succinimides and oxazolidinediones, intentional self-harm**

   ● T42.2X3   **Poisoning by succinimides and oxazolidinediones, assault**

   ● T42.2X4   **Poisoning by succinimides and oxazolidinediones, undetermined**

   ● T42.2X5   **Adverse effect of succinimides and oxazolidinediones**

   ● T42.2X6   **Underdosing of succinimides and oxazolidinediones**

● **T42.3** **Poisoning by, adverse effect of and underdosing of barbiturates**

   Excludes1   poisoning by, adverse effect of and underdosing of thiobarbiturates (T41.1-)

  ● **T42.3X** **Poisoning by, adverse effect of and underdosing of barbiturates**

    ● **T42.3X1** **Poisoning by barbiturates, accidental (unintentional)**
       Poisoning by barbiturates NOS

    ● **T42.3X2** **Poisoning by barbiturates, intentional self-harm**

    ● **T42.3X3** **Poisoning by barbiturates, assault**

    ● **T42.3X4** **Poisoning by barbiturates, undetermined**

    ● **T42.3X5** **Adverse effect of barbiturates**

    ● **T42.3X6** **Underdosing of barbiturates**

● **T42.4** **Poisoning by, adverse effect of and underdosing of benzodiazepines**

  ● **T42.4X** **Poisoning by, adverse effect of and underdosing of benzodiazepines**

    ● **T42.4X1** **Poisoning by benzodiazepines, accidental (unintentional)**
       Poisoning by benzodiazepines NOS

    ● **T42.4X2** **Poisoning by benzodiazepines, intentional self-harm**

    ● **T42.4X3** **Poisoning by benzodiazepines, assault**

    ● **T42.4X4** **Poisoning by benzodiazepines, undetermined**

    ● **T42.4X5** **Adverse effect of benzodiazepines**

    ● **T42.4X6** **Underdosing of benzodiazepines**

● **T42.5** **Poisoning by, adverse effect of and underdosing of mixed antiepileptics**

  ● **T42.5X** **Poisoning by, adverse effect of and underdosing of antiepileptics**

    ● **T42.5X1** **Poisoning by mixed antiepileptics, accidental (unintentional)**
       Poisoning by mixed antiepileptics NOS

    ● **T42.5X2** **Poisoning by mixed antiepileptics, intentional self-harm**

    ● **T42.5X3** **Poisoning by mixed antiepileptics, assault**

    ● **T42.5X4** **Poisoning by mixed antiepileptics, undetermined**

    ● **T42.5X5** **Adverse effect of mixed antiepileptics**

    ● **T42.5X6** **Underdosing of mixed antiepileptics**

● **T42.6** **Poisoning by, adverse effect of and underdosing of other antiepileptic and sedative-hypnotic drugs**
    Poisoning by, adverse effect of and underdosing of methaqualone
    Poisoning by, adverse effect of and underdosing of valproic acid

   Excludes1   poisoning by, adverse effect of and underdosing of carbamazepine (T42.1-)

● **T42.6X** **Poisoning by, adverse effect of and underdosing of other antiepileptic and sedative-hypnotic drugs**

  ● **T42.6X1** **Poisoning by other antiepileptic and sedative-hypnotic drugs, accidental (unintentional)**
     Poisoning by other antiepileptic and sedative-hypnotic drugs NOS

  ● **T42.6X2** **Poisoning by other antiepileptic and sedative-hypnotic drugs, intentional self-harm**

  ● **T42.6X3** **Poisoning by other antiepileptic and sedative-hypnotic drugs, assault**

  ● **T42.6X4** **Poisoning by other antiepileptic and sedative-hypnotic drugs, undetermined**

  ● **T42.6X5** **Adverse effect of other antiepileptic and sedative-hypnotic drugs**

  ● **T42.6X6** **Underdosing of other antiepileptic and sedative-hypnotic drugs**

● **T42.7** **Poisoning by, adverse effect of and underdosing of unspecified antiepileptic and sedative-hypnotic drugs**

  X ● **T42.71** **Poisoning by unspecified antiepileptic and sedative-hypnotic drugs, accidental (unintentional)**
     Poisoning by antiepileptic and sedative-hypnotic drugs NOS

  X ● **T42.72** **Poisoning by unspecified antiepileptic and sedative-hypnotic drugs, intentional self-harm**

  X ● **T42.73** **Poisoning by unspecified antiepileptic and sedative-hypnotic drugs, assault**

  X ● **T42.74** **Poisoning by unspecified antiepileptic and sedative-hypnotic drugs, undetermined**

  X ● **T42.75** **Adverse effect of unspecified antiepileptic and sedative-hypnotic drugs**

  X ● **T42.76** **Underdosing of unspecified antiepileptic and sedative-hypnotic drugs**

● **T42.8** **Poisoning by, adverse effect of and underdosing of antiparkinsonism drugs and other central muscle-tone depressants**
    Poisoning by, adverse effect of and underdosing of amantadine

  ● **T42.8X** **Poisoning by, adverse effect of and underdosing of antiparkinsonism drugs and other central muscle-tone depressants**

    ● **T42.8X1** **Poisoning by antiparkinsonism drugs and other central muscle-tone depressants, accidental (unintentional)**
       Poisoning by antiparkinsonism drugs and other central muscle-tone depressants NOS

    ● **T42.8X2** **Poisoning by antiparkinsonism drugs and other central muscle-tone depressants, intentional self-harm**

    ● **T42.8X3** **Poisoning by antiparkinsonism drugs and other central muscle-tone depressants, assault**

    ● **T42.8X4** **Poisoning by antiparkinsonism drugs and other central muscle-tone depressants, undetermined**

    ● **T42.8X5** **Adverse effect of antiparkinsonism drugs and other central muscle-tone depressants**

    ● **T42.8X6** **Underdosing of antiparkinsonism drugs and other central muscle-tone depressants**

CHAPTER 19 (S00-T88)

N   Newborn Age: 0   **P**   Pediatric Age: 0–17   **M**   Maternity DX: 12–55   **A**   Adult Age: 15–124   ♀   Females Only   ♂   Males Only

   Complication\Comorbidity   Major C\C   (Ex)   CC/MCC Exclusions   Hospital-Acquired Condition

1455

● **T43**   **Poisoning by, adverse effect of and underdosing of psychotropic drugs, not elsewhere classified**

     Excludes1   appetite depressants (T50.5-)
                  barbiturates (T42.3-)
                  benzodiazepines (T42.4-)
                  methaqualone (T42.6-)
                  psychodysleptics [hallucinogens] (T40.7-T40.9-)

     Excludes2   drug dependence and related mental and behavioral disorders due to psychoactive substance use (F10.--F19.-)

The appropriate 7th character is to be added to each code from category T43

> A   initial encounter
> D   subsequent encounter
> S   sequela

● **T43.0**   Poisoning by, adverse effect of and underdosing of tricyclic and tetracyclic antidepressants

    ● **T43.01**   Poisoning by, adverse effect of and underdosing of tricyclic antidepressants

       ● **T43.011**   Poisoning by tricyclic antidepressants, accidental (unintentional)
                 Poisoning by tricyclic antidepressants NOS

       ● **T43.012**   Poisoning by tricyclic antidepressants, intentional self-harm

       ● **T43.013**   Poisoning by tricyclic antidepressants, assault

       ● **T43.014**   Poisoning by tricyclic antidepressants, undetermined

       ● **T43.015**   Adverse effect of tricyclic antidepressants

       ● **T43.016**   Underdosing of tricyclic antidepressants

    ● **T43.02**   Poisoning by, adverse effect of and underdosing of tetracyclic antidepressants

       ● **T43.021**   Poisoning by tetracyclic antidepressants, accidental (unintentional)
                 Poisoning by tetracyclic antidepressants NOS

       ● **T43.022**   Poisoning by tetracyclic antidepressants, intentional self-harm

       ● **T43.023**   Poisoning by tetracyclic antidepressants, assault

       ● **T43.024**   Poisoning by tetracyclic antidepressants, undetermined

       ● **T43.025**   Adverse effect of tetracyclic antidepressants

       ● **T43.026**   Underdosing of tetracyclic antidepressants

● **T43.1**   Poisoning by, adverse effect of and underdosing of monoamine-oxidase-inhibitor antidepressants

    ● **T43.1X**   Poisoning by, adverse effect of and underdosing of monoamine-oxidase-inhibitor antidepressants

       ● **T43.1X1**   Poisoning by monoamine-oxidase-inhibitor antidepressants, accidental (unintentional)
                 Poisoning by monoamine-oxidase-inhibitor antidepressants NOS

       ● **T43.1X2**   Poisoning by monoamine-oxidase-inhibitor antidepressants, intentional self-harm

       ● **T43.1X3**   Poisoning by monoamine-oxidase-inhibitor antidepressants, assault

       ● **T43.1X4**   Poisoning by monoamine-oxidase-inhibitor antidepressants, undetermined

       ● **T43.1X5**   Adverse effect of monoamine-oxidase-inhibitor antidepressants

       ● **T43.1X6**   Underdosing of monoamine-oxidase-inhibitor antidepressants

● **T43.2**   Poisoning by, adverse effect of and underdosing of other and unspecified antidepressants

    ● **T43.20**   Poisoning by, adverse effect of and underdosing of unspecified antidepressants

       ● **T43.201**   Poisoning by unspecified antidepressants, accidental (unintentional)
                 Poisoning by antidepressants NOS

       ● **T43.202**   Poisoning by unspecified antidepressants, intentional self-harm

       ● **T43.203**   Poisoning by unspecified antidepressants, assault

       ● **T43.204**   Poisoning by unspecified antidepressants, undetermined

       ● **T43.205**   Adverse effect of unspecified antidepressants

       ● **T43.206**   Underdosing of unspecified antidepressants

    ● **T43.21**   Poisoning by, adverse effect of and underdosing of selective serotonin and norepinephrine reuptake inhibitors
          Poisoning by, adverse effect of and underdosing of SSNRI antidepressants

       ● **T43.211**   Poisoning by selective serotonin and norepinephrine reuptake inhibitors, accidental (unintentional)

       ● **T43.212**   Poisoning by selective serotonin and norepinephrine reuptake inhibitors, intentional self-harm

       ● **T43.213**   Poisoning by selective serotonin and norepinephrine reuptake inhibitors, assault

       ● **T43.214**   Poisoning by selective serotonin and norepinephrine reuptake inhibitors, undetermined

       ● **T43.215**   Adverse effect of selective serotonin and norepinephrine reuptake inhibitors

       ● **T43.216**   Underdosing of selective serotonin and norepinephrine reuptake inhibitors

    ● **T43.22**   Poisoning by, adverse effect of and underdosing of selective serotonin reuptake inhibitors
          Poisoning by, adverse effect of and underdosing of SSRI antidepressants

       ● **T43.221**   Poisoning by selective serotonin reuptake inhibitors, accidental (unintentional)

       ● **T43.222**   Poisoning by selective serotonin reuptake inhibitors, intentional self-harm

       ● **T43.223**   Poisoning by selective serotonin reuptake inhibitors, assault

       ● **T43.224**   Poisoning by selective serotonin reuptake inhibitors, undetermined

       ● **T43.225**   Adverse effect of selective serotonin reuptake inhibitors

       ● **T43.226**   Underdosing of selective serotonin reuptake inhibitors

◄ New   ◄◄ Revised   ~~deleted~~ Deleted   Excludes 1   Excludes 2   Includes   Use additional   Code first   Code also   Unspecified
OGCR Official Guidelines   ● Unacceptable Principal Diagnosis   X Assign placeholder X   ● Use Additional Character(s)   ▶ Manifestation Code   **Coding Clinic**

- T43.29   **Poisoning by, adverse effect of and underdosing of other antidepressants**
  - T43.291   **Poisoning by other antidepressants, accidental (unintentional)**
    Poisoning by other antidepressants NOS
  - T43.292   **Poisoning by other antidepressants, intentional self-harm**
  - T43.293   **Poisoning by other antidepressants, assault**
  - T43.294   **Poisoning by other antidepressants, undetermined**
  - T43.295   **Adverse effect of other antidepressants**
  - T43.296   **Underdosing of other antidepressants**
- T43.3   **Poisoning by, adverse effect of and underdosing of phenothiazine antipsychotics and neuroleptics**
  - T43.3X   **Poisoning by, adverse effect of and underdosing of phenothiazine antipsychotics and neuroleptics**
    - T43.3X1   **Poisoning by phenothiazine antipsychotics and neuroleptics, accidental (unintentional)**
      Poisoning by phenothiazine antipsychotics and neuroleptics NOS
    - T43.3X2   **Poisoning by phenothiazine antipsychotics and neuroleptics, intentional self-harm**
    - T43.3X3   **Poisoning by phenothiazine antipsychotics and neuroleptics, assault**
    - T43.3X4   **Poisoning by phenothiazine antipsychotics and neuroleptics, undetermined**
    - T43.3X5   **Adverse effect of phenothiazine antipsychotics and neuroleptics**
    - T43.3X6   **Underdosing of phenothiazine antipsychotics and neuroleptics**
- T43.4   **Poisoning by, adverse effect of and underdosing of butyrophenone and thiothixene neuroleptics**
  - T43.4X   **Poisoning by, adverse effect of and underdosing of butyrophenone and thiothixene neuroleptics**
    - T43.4X1   **Poisoning by butyrophenone and thiothixene neuroleptics, accidental (unintentional)**
      Poisoning by butyrophenone and thiothixene neuroleptics NOS
    - T43.4X2   **Poisoning by butyrophenone and thiothixene neuroleptics, intentional self-harm**
    - T43.4X3   **Poisoning by butyrophenone and thiothixene neuroleptics, assault**
    - T43.4X4   **Poisoning by butyrophenone and thiothixene neuroleptics, undetermined**
    - T43.4X5   **Adverse effect of butyrophenone and thiothixene neuroleptics**
    - T43.4X6   **Underdosing of butyrophenone and thiothixene neuroleptics**

- T43.5   **Poisoning by, adverse effect of and underdosing of other and unspecified antipsychotics and neuroleptics**
  > **Excludes1**   poisoning by, adverse effect of and underdosing of rauwolfia (T46.5-)
  - T43.50   **Poisoning by, adverse effect of and underdosing of unspecified antipsychotics and neuroleptics**
    - T43.501   **Poisoning by unspecified antipsychotics and neuroleptics, accidental (unintentional)**
      Poisoning by antipsychotics and neuroleptics NOS
    - T43.502   **Poisoning by unspecified antipsychotics and neuroleptics, intentional self-harm**
    - T43.503   **Poisoning by unspecified antipsychotics and neuroleptics, assault**
    - T43.504   **Poisoning by unspecified antipsychotics and neuroleptics, undetermined**
    - T43.505   **Adverse effect of unspecified antipsychotics and neuroleptics**
    - T43.506   **Underdosing of unspecified antipsychotics and neuroleptics**
  - T43.59   **Poisoning by, adverse effect of and underdosing of other antipsychotics and neuroleptics**
    - T43.591   **Poisoning by other antipsychotics and neuroleptics, accidental (unintentional)**
      Poisoning by other antipsychotics and neuroleptics NOS
    - T43.592   **Poisoning by other antipsychotics and neuroleptics, intentional self-harm**
    - T43.593   **Poisoning by other antipsychotics and neuroleptics, assault**
    - T43.594   **Poisoning by other antipsychotics and neuroleptics, undetermined**
    - T43.595   **Adverse effect of other antipsychotics and neuroleptics**
    - T43.596   **Underdosing of other antipsychotics and neuroleptics**
- T43.6   **Poisoning by, adverse effect of and underdosing of psychostimulants**
  > **Excludes1**   poisoning by, adverse effect of and underdosing of cocaine (T40.5-)
  - T43.60   **Poisoning by, adverse effect of and underdosing of unspecified psychostimulant**
    - T43.601   **Poisoning by unspecified psychostimulants, accidental (unintentional)**
      Poisoning by psychostimulants NOS
    - T43.602   **Poisoning by unspecified psychostimulants, intentional self-harm**
    - T43.603   **Poisoning by unspecified psychostimulants, assault**
    - T43.604   **Poisoning by unspecified psychostimulants, undetermined**
    - T43.605   **Adverse effect of unspecified psychostimulants**
    - T43.606   **Underdosing of unspecified psychostimulants**

N Newborn Age: 0   **P** Pediatric Age: 0–17   **M** Maternity DX: 12–55   **A** Adult Age: 15–124   ♀ Females Only   ♂ Males Only

Complication\Comorbidity   Major C\C   Ⓔˣ CC/MCC Exclusions   Hospital-Acquired Condition

1457

CHAPTER 19 (S00-T88)

● **T43.61** Poisoning by, adverse effect of and underdosing of caffeine
- ● **T43.611** Poisoning by caffeine, accidental (unintentional)
  - Poisoning by caffeine NOS
- ● **T43.612** Poisoning by caffeine, intentional self-harm
- ● **T43.613** Poisoning by caffeine, assault
- ● **T43.614** Poisoning by caffeine, undetermined
- ● **T43.615** Adverse effect of caffeine
- ● **T43.616** Underdosing of caffeine

● **T43.62** Poisoning by, adverse effect of and underdosing of amphetamines
- Poisoning by, adverse effect of and underdosing of methamphetamines
- ● **T43.621** Poisoning by amphetamines, accidental (unintentional)
  - Poisoning by amphetamines NOS
- ● **T43.622** Poisoning by amphetamines, intentional self-harm
- ● **T43.623** Poisoning by amphetamines, assault
- ● **T43.624** Poisoning by amphetamines, undetermined
- ● **T43.625** Adverse effect of amphetamines
- ● **T43.626** Underdosing of amphetamines

● **T43.63** Poisoning by, adverse effect of and underdosing of methylphenidate
- ● **T43.631** Poisoning by methylphenidate, accidental (unintentional)
  - Poisoning by methylphenidate NOS
- ● **T43.632** Poisoning by methylphenidate, intentional self-harm
- ● **T43.633** Poisoning by methylphenidate, assault
- ● **T43.634** Poisoning by methylphenidate, undetermined
- ● **T43.635** Adverse effect of methylphenidate
- ● **T43.636** Underdosing of methylphenidate

● **T43.69** Poisoning by, adverse effect of and underdosing of other psychostimulants
- ● **T43.691** Poisoning by other psychostimulants, accidental (unintentional)
  - Poisoning by other psychostimulants NOS
- ● **T43.692** Poisoning by other psychostimulants, intentional self-harm
- ● **T43.693** Poisoning by other psychostimulants, assault
- ● **T43.694** Poisoning by other psychostimulants, undetermined
- ● **T43.695** Adverse effect of other psychostimulants
- ● **T43.696** Underdosing of other psychostimulants

● **T43.8** Poisoning by, adverse effect of and underdosing of other psychotropic drugs
- ● **T43.8X** Poisoning by, adverse effect of and underdosing of other psychotropic drugs
  - ● **T43.8X1** Poisoning by other psychotropic drugs, accidental (unintentional)
    - Poisoning by other psychotropic drugs NOS
  - ● **T43.8X2** Poisoning by other psychotropic drugs, intentional self-harm
  - ● **T43.8X3** Poisoning by other psychotropic drugs, assault

- ● **T43.8X4** Poisoning by other psychotropic drugs, undetermined
- ● **T43.8X5** Adverse effect of other psychotropic drugs
- ● **T43.8X6** Underdosing of other psychotropic drugs

● **T43.9** Poisoning by, adverse effect of and underdosing of unspecified psychotropic drug
- X ● **T43.91** Poisoning by unspecified psychotropic drug, accidental (unintentional)
  - Poisoning by psychotropic drug NOS
- X ● **T43.92** Poisoning by unspecified psychotropic drug, intentional self-harm
- X ● **T43.93** Poisoning by unspecified psychotropic drug, assault
- X ● **T43.94** Poisoning by unspecified psychotropic drug, undetermined
- X ● **T43.95** Adverse effect of unspecified psychotropic drug
- X ● **T43.96** Underdosing of unspecified psychotropic drug

● **T44** Poisoning by, adverse effect of and underdosing of drugs primarily affecting the autonomic nervous system

The appropriate 7th character is to be added to each code from category T44

A	initial encounter
D	subsequent encounter
S	sequela

● **T44.0** Poisoning by, adverse effect of and underdosing of anticholinesterase agents
- ● **T44.0X** Poisoning by, adverse effect of and underdosing of anticholinesterase agents
  - ● **T44.0X1** Poisoning by anticholinesterase agents, accidental (unintentional)
    - Poisoning by anticholinesterase agents NOS
  - ● **T44.0X2** Poisoning by anticholinesterase agents, intentional self-harm
  - ● **T44.0X3** Poisoning by anticholinesterase agents, assault
  - ● **T44.0X4** Poisoning by anticholinesterase agents, undetermined
  - ● **T44.0X5** Adverse effect of anticholinesterase agents
  - ● **T44.0X6** Underdosing of anticholinesterase agents

● **T44.1** Poisoning by, adverse effect of and underdosing of other parasympathomimetics [cholinergics]
- ● **T44.1X** Poisoning by, adverse effect of and underdosing of other parasympathomimetics [cholinergics]
  - ● **T44.1X1** Poisoning by other parasympathomimetics [cholinergics], accidental (unintentional)
    - Poisoning by other parasympathomimetics [cholinergics] NOS
  - ● **T44.1X2** Poisoning by other parasympathomimetics [cholinergics], intentional self-harm
  - ● **T44.1X3** Poisoning by other parasympathomimetics [cholinergics], assault
  - ● **T44.1X4** Poisoning by other parasympathomimetics [cholinergics], undetermined
  - ● **T44.1X5** Adverse effect of other parasympathomimetics [cholinergics]
  - ● **T44.1X6** Underdosing of other parasympathomimetics

◀ New   ◀▥ Revised   ~~deleted~~ Deleted   Excludes 1   Excludes 2   Includes   Use additional   Code first   Code also   Unspecified

OGCR Official Guidelines   ● Unacceptable Principal Diagnosis   X Assign placeholder X   ● Use Additional Character(s)   ▶ Manifestation Code   **Coding Clinic**

● T44.2   Poisoning by, adverse effect of and underdosing of
           ganglionic blocking drugs
     ● T44.2X   Poisoning by, adverse effect of and
                underdosing of ganglionic blocking drugs
          ● T44.2X1   Poisoning by ganglionic blocking
                      drugs, accidental (unintentional)
                          Poisoning by ganglionic blocking
                              drugs NOS
          ● T44.2X2   Poisoning by ganglionic blocking
                      drugs, intentional self-harm
          ● T44.2X3   Poisoning by ganglionic blocking
                      drugs, assault
          ● T44.2X4   Poisoning by ganglionic blocking
                      drugs, undetermined
          ● T44.2X5   Adverse effect of ganglionic blocking
                      drugs
          ● T44.2X6   Underdosing of ganglionic blocking
                      drugs
● T44.3   Poisoning by, adverse effect of and underdosing
           of other parasympatholytics [anticholinergics and
           antimuscarinics] and spasmolytics
                Poisoning by, adverse effect of and underdosing of
                papaverine
     ● T44.3X   Poisoning by, adverse effect of and
                underdosing of other parasympatholytics
                [anticholinergics and antimuscarinics] and
                spasmolytics
          ● T44.3X1   Poisoning by other
                      parasympatholytics [anticholinergics
                      and antimuscarinics] and
                      spasmolytics, accidental
                      (unintentional)
                          Poisoning by other
                              parasympatholytics
                              [anticholinergics and
                              antimuscarinics] and
                              spasmolytics NOS
          ● T44.3X2   Poisoning by other
                      parasympatholytics [anticholinergics
                      and antimuscarinics] and
                      spasmolytics, intentional self-harm
          ● T44.3X3   Poisoning by other
                      parasympatholytics [anticholinergics
                      and antimuscarinics] and
                      spasmolytics, assault
          ● T44.3X4   Poisoning by other
                      parasympatholytics [anticholinergics
                      and antimuscarinics] and
                      spasmolytics, undetermined
          ● T44.3X5   Adverse effect of other
                      parasympatholytics [anticholinergics
                      and antimuscarinics] and
                      spasmolytics
          ● T44.3X6   Underdosing of other
                      parasympatholytics [anticholinergics
                      and antimuscarinics] and
                      spasmolytics

● T44.4   Poisoning by, adverse effect of and underdosing of
           predominantly alpha-adrenoreceptor agonists
                Poisoning by, adverse effect of and underdosing of
                metaraminol
     ● T44.4X   Poisoning by, adverse effect of and underdosing
                of predominantly alpha-adrenoreceptor agonists
          ● T44.4X1   Poisoning by predominantly alpha-
                      adrenoreceptor agonists, accidental
                      (unintentional)
                          Poisoning by predominantly alpha-
                              adrenoreceptor agonists NOS
          ● T44.4X2   Poisoning by predominantly alpha-
                      adrenoreceptor agonists, intentional
                      self-harm
          ● T44.4X3   Poisoning by predominantly alpha-
                      adrenoreceptor agonists, assault
          ● T44.4X4   Poisoning by predominantly
                      alpha-adrenoreceptor agonists,
                      undetermined
          ● T44.4X5   Adverse effect of predominantly
                      alpha-adrenoreceptor agonists
          ● T44.4X6   Underdosing of predominantly alpha-
                      adrenoreceptor agonists
● T44.5   Poisoning by, adverse effect of and underdosing of
           predominantly beta-adrenoreceptor agonists
                Excludes 1   poisoning by, adverse effect of and
                                  underdosing of beta-adrenoreceptor
                                  agonists used in asthma therapy
                                  (T48.6-)
     ● T44.5X   Poisoning by, adverse effect of and underdosing
                of predominantly beta-adrenoreceptor agonists
          ● T44.5X1   Poisoning by predominantly beta-
                      adrenoreceptor agonists, accidental
                      (unintentional)
                          Poisoning by predominantly beta-
                              adrenoreceptor agonists NOS
          ● T44.5X2   Poisoning by predominantly beta-
                      adrenoreceptor agonists, intentional
                      self-harm
          ● T44.5X3   Poisoning by predominantly beta-
                      adrenoreceptor agonists, assault
          ● T44.5X4   Poisoning by predominantly
                      beta-adrenoreceptor agonists,
                      undetermined
          ● T44.5X5   Adverse effect of predominantly beta-
                      adrenoreceptor agonists
          ● T44.5X6   Underdosing of predominantly beta-
                      adrenoreceptor agonists
● T44.6   Poisoning by, adverse effect of and underdosing of
           alpha-adrenoreceptor antagonists
                Excludes 1   poisoning by, adverse effect of and
                                  underdosing of ergot alkaloids
                                  (T48.0)
     ● T44.6X   Poisoning by, adverse effect of and underdosing
                of alpha-adrenoreceptor antagonists
          ● T44.6X1   Poisoning by alpha-adrenoreceptor
                      antagonists, accidental
                      (unintentional)
                          Poisoning by alpha-adrenoreceptor
                              antagonists NOS
          ● T44.6X2   Poisoning by alpha-adrenoreceptor
                      antagonists, intentional self-harm
          ● T44.6X3   Poisoning by alpha-adrenoreceptor
                      antagonists, assault
          ● T44.6X4   Poisoning by alpha-adrenoreceptor
                      antagonists, undetermined
          ● T44.6X5   Adverse effect of alpha-
                      adrenoreceptor antagonists
          ● T44.6X6   Underdosing of alpha-adrenoreceptor
                      antagonists

CHAPTER 19 (S00-T88)

● **T44.7** **Poisoning by, adverse effect of and underdosing of beta-adrenoreceptor antagonists**

  ● **T44.7X** Poisoning by, adverse effect of and underdosing of beta-adrenoreceptor antagonists

    ● **T44.7X1** **Poisoning by beta-adrenoreceptor antagonists, accidental (unintentional)**
         Poisoning by beta-adrenoreceptor antagonists NOS

    ● **T44.7X2** **Poisoning by beta-adrenoreceptor antagonists, intentional self-harm**

    ● **T44.7X3** **Poisoning by beta-adrenoreceptor antagonists, assault**

    ● **T44.7X4** **Poisoning by beta-adrenoreceptor antagonists, undetermined**

    ● **T44.7X5** **Adverse effect of beta-adrenoreceptor antagonists**

    ● **T44.7X6** **Underdosing of beta-adrenoreceptor antagonists**

● **T44.8** **Poisoning by, adverse effect of and underdosing of centrally-acting and adrenergic-neuron-blocking agents**

  Excludes1   poisoning by, adverse effect of and underdosing of clonidine (T46.5)
           poisoning by, adverse effect of and underdosing of guanethidine (T46.5)

  ● **T44.8X** Poisoning by, adverse effect of and underdosing of centrally-acting and adrenergic-neuron-blocking agents

    ● **T44.8X1** **Poisoning by centrally-acting and adrenergic-neuron-blocking agents, accidental (unintentional)**
         Poisoning by centrally-acting and adrenergic-neuron-blocking agents NOS

    ● **T44.8X2** **Poisoning by centrally-acting and adrenergic-neuron-blocking agents, intentional self-harm**

    ● **T44.8X3** **Poisoning by centrally-acting and adrenergic-neuron-blocking agents, assault**

    ● **T44.8X4** **Poisoning by centrally-acting and adrenergic-neuron-blocking agents, undetermined**

    ● **T44.8X5** **Adverse effect of centrally-acting and adrenergic-neuron-blocking agents**

    ● **T44.8X6** **Underdosing of centrally-acting and adrenergic-neuron-blocking agents**

● **T44.9** **Poisoning by, adverse effect of and underdosing of other and unspecified drugs primarily affecting the autonomic nervous system**
   Poisoning by, adverse effect of and underdosing of drug stimulating both alpha and beta-adrenoreceptors

  ● **T44.90** **Poisoning by, adverse effect of and underdosing of unspecified drugs primarily affecting the autonomic nervous system**

    ● **T44.901** **Poisoning by unspecified drugs primarily affecting the autonomic nervous system, accidental (unintentional)**
         Poisoning by unspecified drugs primarily affecting the autonomic nervous system NOS

    ● **T44.902** **Poisoning by unspecified drugs primarily affecting the autonomic nervous system, intentional self-harm**

    ● **T44.903** **Poisoning by unspecified drugs primarily affecting the autonomic nervous system, assault**

    ● **T44.904** **Poisoning by unspecified drugs primarily affecting the autonomic nervous system, undetermined**

    ● **T44.905** **Adverse effect of unspecified drugs primarily affecting the autonomic nervous system**

    ● **T44.906** **Underdosing of unspecified drugs primarily affecting the autonomic nervous system**

  ● **T44.99** **Poisoning by, adverse effect of and underdosing of other drugs primarily affecting the autonomic nervous system**

    ● **T44.991** **Poisoning by other drug primarily affecting the autonomic nervous system, accidental (unintentional)**
         Poisoning by other drugs primarily affecting the autonomic nervous system NOS

    ● **T44.992** **Poisoning by other drug primarily affecting the autonomic nervous system, intentional self-harm**

    ● **T44.993** **Poisoning by other drug primarily affecting the autonomic nervous system, assault**

    ● **T44.994** **Poisoning by other drug primarily affecting the autonomic nervous system, undetermined**

    ● **T44.995** **Adverse effect of other drug primarily affecting the autonomic nervous system**

    ● **T44.996** **Underdosing of other drug primarily affecting the autonomic nervous system**

● **T45** **Poisoning by, adverse effect of and underdosing of primarily systemic and hematological agents, not elsewhere classified**

   The appropriate 7th character is to be added to each code from category T45

A	initial encounter
D	subsequent encounter
S	sequela

  ● **T45.0** **Poisoning by, adverse effect of and underdosing of antiallergic and antiemetic drugs**

    Excludes1   poisoning by, adverse effect of and underdosing of phenothiazine-based neuroleptics (T43.3)

  ● **T45.0X** Poisoning by, adverse effect of and underdosing of antiallergic and antiemetic drugs

    ● **T45.0X1** **Poisoning by antiallergic and antiemetic drugs, accidental (unintentional)**
         Poisoning by antiallergic and antiemetic drugs NOS

    ● **T45.0X2** **Poisoning by antiallergic and antiemetic drugs, intentional self-harm**

    ● **T45.0X3** **Poisoning by antiallergic and antiemetic drugs, assault**

    ● **T45.0X4** **Poisoning by antiallergic and antiemetic drugs, undetermined**

    ● **T45.0X5** **Adverse effect of antiallergic and antiemetic drugs**

    ● **T45.0X6** **Underdosing of antiallergic and antiemetic drugs**

● **T45.1**   **Poisoning by, adverse effect of and underdosing of antineoplastic and immunosuppressive drugs**

    Excludes1   poisoning by, adverse effect of and underdosing of tamoxifen (T38.6)

   ● **T45.1X**   **Poisoning by, adverse effect of and underdosing of antineoplastic and immunosuppressive drugs**

     ● **T45.1X1**   **Poisoning by antineoplastic and immunosuppressive drugs, accidental (unintentional)**
        Poisoning by antineoplastic and immunosuppressive drugs NOS

     ● **T45.1X2**   **Poisoning by antineoplastic and immunosuppressive drugs, intentional self-harm**

     ● **T45.1X3**   **Poisoning by antineoplastic and immunosuppressive drugs, assault**

     ● **T45.1X4**   **Poisoning by antineoplastic and immunosuppressive drugs, undetermined**

     ● **T45.1X5**   **Adverse effect of antineoplastic and immunosuppressive drugs**

     ● **T45.1X6**   **Underdosing of antineoplastic and immunosuppressive drugs**

● **T45.2**   **Poisoning by, adverse effect of and underdosing of vitamins**

    Excludes2   poisoning by, adverse effect of and underdosing of nicotinic acid (derivatives) (T46.7)
         poisoning by, adverse effect of and underdosing of iron (T45.4)
         poisoning by, adverse effect of and underdosing of vitamin K (T45.7)

   ● **T45.2X**   **Poisoning by, adverse effect of and underdosing of vitamins**

     ● **T45.2X1**   **Poisoning by vitamins, accidental (unintentional)**
        Poisoning by vitamins NOS

     ● **T45.2X2**   **Poisoning by vitamins, intentional self-harm**

     ● **T45.2X3**   **Poisoning by vitamins, assault**

     ● **T45.2X4**   **Poisoning by vitamins, undetermined**

     ● **T45.2X5**   **Adverse effect of vitamins**

     ● **T45.2X6**   **Underdosing of vitamins**

        Excludes1   vitamin deficiencies (E50-E56)

● **T45.3**   **Poisoning by, adverse effect of and underdosing of enzymes**

   ● **T45.3X**   **Poisoning by, adverse effect of and underdosing of enzymes**

     ● **T45.3X1**   **Poisoning by enzymes, accidental (unintentional)**
        Poisoning by enzymes NOS

     ● **T45.3X2**   **Poisoning by enzymes, intentional self-harm**

     ● **T45.3X3**   **Poisoning by enzymes, assault**

     ● **T45.3X4**   **Poisoning by enzymes, undetermined**

     ● **T45.3X5**   **Adverse effect of enzymes**

     ● **T45.3X6**   **Underdosing of enzymes**

● **T45.4**   **Poisoning by, adverse effect of and underdosing of iron and its compounds**

   ● **T45.4X**   **Poisoning by, adverse effect of and underdosing of iron and its compounds**

     ● **T45.4X1**   **Poisoning by iron and its compounds, accidental (unintentional)**
        Poisoning by iron and its compounds NOS

     ● **T45.4X2**   **Poisoning by iron and its compounds, intentional self-harm**

     ● **T45.4X3**   **Poisoning by iron and its compounds, assault**

     ● **T45.4X4**   **Poisoning by iron and its compounds, undetermined**

     ● **T45.4X5**   **Adverse effect of iron and its compounds**

     ● **T45.4X6**   **Underdosing of iron and its compounds**

        Excludes1   iron deficiency (E61.1)

● **T45.5**   **Poisoning by, adverse effect of and underdosing of anticoagulants and antithrombotic drugs**

   ● **T45.51**   **Poisoning by, adverse effect of and underdosing of anticoagulants**

     T45.511   **Poisoning by anticoagulants, accidental (unintentional)**
        Poisoning by anticoagulants NOS

     ● **T45.512**   **Poisoning by anticoagulants, intentional self-harm**

     ● **T45.513**   **Poisoning by anticoagulants, assault**

     ● **T45.514**   **Poisoning by anticoagulants, undetermined**

     ● **T45.515**   **Adverse effect of anticoagulants**
        Coding Clinic: 2016, Q1, P14; 2013, Q2, P35

     ● **T45.516**   **Underdosing of anticoagulants**

   ● **T45.52**   **Poisoning by, adverse effect of and underdosing of antithrombotic drugs**
     Poisoning by, adverse effect of and underdosing of antiplatelet drugs

     Excludes2   poisoning by, adverse effect of and underdosing of aspirin (T39.01-)
         poisoning by, adverse effect of and underdosing of acetylsalicylic acid (T39.01-)

     ● **T45.521**   **Poisoning by antithrombotic drugs, accidental (unintentional)**
        Poisoning by antithrombotic drug NOS

     ● **T45.522**   **Poisoning by antithrombotic drugs, intentional self-harm**

     ● **T45.523**   **Poisoning by antithrombotic drugs, assault**

     ● **T45.524**   **Poisoning by antithrombotic drugs, undetermined**

     ● **T45.525**   **Adverse effect of antithrombotic drugs**
        Coding Clinic: 2016, Q1, P15

     ● **T45.526**   **Underdosing of antithrombotic drugs**

● **T45.6**   **Poisoning by, adverse effect of and underdosing of fibrinolysis-affecting drugs**

   ● **T45.60**   **Poisoning by, adverse effect of and underdosing of unspecified fibrinolysis-affecting drugs**

     ● **T45.601**   **Poisoning by unspecified fibrinolysis-affecting drugs, accidental (unintentional)**
        Poisoning by fibrinolysis-affecting drug NOS

     ● **T45.602**   **Poisoning by unspecified fibrinolysis-affecting drugs, intentional self-harm**

     ● **T45.603**   **Poisoning by unspecified fibrinolysis-affecting drugs, assault**

     ● **T45.604**   **Poisoning by unspecified fibrinolysis-affecting drugs, undetermined**

     ● **T45.605**   **Adverse effect of unspecified fibrinolysis-affecting drugs**

     ● **T45.606**   **Underdosing of unspecified fibrinolysis-affecting drugs**

CHAPTER 19 (S00-T88)

CHAPTER 19 (S00-T88)

● T45.61   **Poisoning by, adverse effect of and underdosing of thrombolytic drugs**
- ● T45.611   **Poisoning by thrombolytic drug, accidental (unintentional)**
  - Poisoning by thrombolytic drug NOS
- ● T45.612   **Poisoning by thrombolytic drug, intentional self-harm**
- ● T45.613   **Poisoning by thrombolytic drug, assault**
- ● T45.614   **Poisoning by thrombolytic drug, undetermined**
- ● T45.615   **Adverse effect of thrombolytic drugs**
- ● T45.616   **Underdosing of thrombolytic drugs**

● T45.62   **Poisoning by, adverse effect of and underdosing of hemostatic drugs**
- ● T45.621   **Poisoning by hemostatic drug, accidental (unintentional)**
  - Poisoning by hemostatic drug NOS
- ● T45.622   **Poisoning by hemostatic drug, intentional self-harm**
- ● T45.623   **Poisoning by hemostatic drug, assault**
- ● T45.624   **Poisoning by hemostatic drug, undetermined**
- ● T45.625   **Adverse effect of hemostatic drug**
- ● T45.626   **Underdosing of hemostatic drugs**

● T45.69   **Poisoning by, adverse effect of and underdosing of other fibrinolysis-affecting drugs**
- ● T45.691   **Poisoning by other fibrinolysis-affecting drugs, accidental (unintentional)**
  - Poisoning by other fibrinolysis-affecting drug NOS
- ● T45.692   **Poisoning by other fibrinolysis-affecting drugs, intentional self-harm**
- ● T45.693   **Poisoning by other fibrinolysis-affecting drugs, assault**
- ● T45.694   **Poisoning by other fibrinolysis-affecting drugs, undetermined**
- ● T45.695   **Adverse effect of other fibrinolysis-affecting drugs**
- ● T45.696   **Underdosing of other fibrinolysis-affecting drugs**

● T45.7   **Poisoning by, adverse effect of and underdosing of anticoagulant antagonists, vitamin K and other coagulants**
- ● T45.7X   **Poisoning by, adverse effect of and underdosing of anticoagulant antagonists, vitamin K and other coagulants**
  - ● T45.7X1   **Poisoning by anticoagulant antagonists, vitamin K and other coagulants, accidental (unintentional)**
    - Poisoning by anticoagulant antagonists, vitamin K and other coagulants NOS
  - ● T45.7X2   **Poisoning by anticoagulant antagonists, vitamin K and other coagulants, intentional self-harm**
  - ● T45.7X3   **Poisoning by anticoagulant antagonists, vitamin K and other coagulants, assault**

● T45.7X4   **Poisoning by anticoagulant antagonists, vitamin K and other coagulants, undetermined**
● T45.7X5   **Adverse effect of anticoagulant antagonists, vitamin K and other coagulants**
● T45.7X6   **Underdosing of anticoagulant antagonist, vitamin K and other coagulants**
> **Excludes1**   vitamin K deficiency (E56.1)

● T45.8   **Poisoning by, adverse effect of and underdosing of other primarily systemic and hematological agents**
- Poisoning by, adverse effect of and underdosing of liver preparations and other antianemic agents
- Poisoning by, adverse effect of and underdosing of natural blood and blood products
- Poisoning by, adverse effect of and underdosing of plasma substitute
> **Excludes2**   poisoning by, adverse effect of and underdosing of immunoglobulin (T50.Z1)
> poisoning by, adverse effect of and underdosing of iron (T45.4)
> transfusion reactions (T80.-)

- ● T45.8X   **Poisoning by, adverse effect of and underdosing of other primarily systemic and hematological agents**
  - ● T45.8X1   **Poisoning by other primarily systemic and hematological agents, accidental (unintentional)**
    - Poisoning by other primarily systemic and hematological agents NOS
  - ● T45.8X2   **Poisoning by other primarily systemic and hematological agents, intentional self-harm**
  - ● T45.8X3   **Poisoning by other primarily systemic and hematological agents, assault**
  - ● T45.8X4   **Poisoning by other primarily systemic and hematological agents, undetermined**
  - ● T45.8X5   **Adverse effect of other primarily systemic and hematological agents**
  - ● T45.8X6   **Underdosing of other primarily systemic and hematological agents**

● T45.9   **Poisoning by, adverse effect of and underdosing of unspecified primarily systemic and hematological agent**
- X ● T45.91   **Poisoning by unspecified primarily systemic and hematological agent, accidental (unintentional)**
  - Poisoning by primarily systemic and hematological agent NOS
- X ● T45.92   **Poisoning by unspecified primarily systemic and hematological agent, intentional self-harm**
- X ● T45.93   **Poisoning by unspecified primarily systemic and hematological agent, assault**
- X ● T45.94   **Poisoning by unspecified primarily systemic and hematological agent, undetermined**
- X ● T45.95   **Adverse effect of unspecified primarily systemic and hematological agent**
- X ● T45.96   **Underdosing of unspecified primarily systemic and hematological agent**

◀ New   ◀ Revised   ~~deleted~~ Deleted   Excludes 1   Excludes 2   Includes   Use additional   Code first   Code also   Unspecified
OGCR Official Guidelines   ● Unacceptable Principal Diagnosis   X Assign placeholder X   ● Use Additional Character(s)   ▶ Manifestation Code   **Coding Clinic**

T46 **Poisoning by, adverse effect of and underdosing of agents primarily affecting the cardiovascular system**

Excludes1 poisoning by, adverse effect of and underdosing of metaraminol (T44.4)

The appropriate 7th character is to be added to each code from category T46

A	initial encounter
D	subsequent encounter
S	sequela

T46.0 **Poisoning by, adverse effect of and underdosing of cardiac-stimulant glycosides and drugs of similar action**

T46.0X **Poisoning by, adverse effect of and underdosing of cardiac-stimulant glycosides and drugs of similar action**

T46.0X1 **Poisoning by cardiac-stimulant glycosides and drugs of similar action, accidental (unintentional)**
Poisoning by cardiac-stimulant glycosides and drugs of similar action NOS

T46.0X2 **Poisoning by cardiac-stimulant glycosides and drugs of similar action, intentional self-harm**

T46.0X3 **Poisoning by cardiac-stimulant glycosides and drugs of similar action, assault**

T46.0X4 **Poisoning by cardiac-stimulant glycosides and drugs of similar action, undetermined**

T46.0X5 **Adverse effect of cardiac-stimulant glycosides and drugs of similar action**

T46.0X6 **Underdosing of cardiac-stimulant glycosides and drugs of similar action**

T46.1 **Poisoning by, adverse effect of and underdosing of calcium-channel blockers**

T46.1X **Poisoning by, adverse effect of and underdosing of calcium-channel blockers**

T46.1X1 **Poisoning by calcium-channel blockers, accidental (unintentional)**
Poisoning by calcium-channel blockers NOS

T46.1X2 **Poisoning by calcium-channel blockers, intentional self-harm**

T46.1X3 **Poisoning by calcium-channel blockers, assault**

T46.1X4 **Poisoning by calcium-channel blockers, undetermined**

T46.1X5 **Adverse effect of calcium-channel blockers**

T46.1X6 **Underdosing of calcium-channel blockers**

T46.2 **Poisoning by, adverse effect of and underdosing of other antidysrhythmic drugs, not elsewhere classified**

Excludes1 poisoning by, adverse effect of and underdosing of beta-adrenoreceptor antagonists (T44.7-)

T46.2X **Poisoning by, adverse effect of and underdosing of other antidysrhythmic drugs**

T46.2X1 **Poisoning by other antidysrhythmic drugs, accidental (unintentional)**
Poisoning by other antidysrhythmic drugs NOS

T46.2X2 **Poisoning by other antidysrhythmic drugs, intentional self-harm**

T46.2X3 **Poisoning by other antidysrhythmic drugs, assault**

T46.2X4 **Poisoning by other antidysrhythmic drugs, undetermined**

T46.2X5 **Adverse effect of other antidysrhythmic drugs**

T46.2X6 **Underdosing of other antidysrhythmic drugs**

T46.3 **Poisoning by, adverse effect of and underdosing of coronary vasodilators**
Poisoning by, adverse effect of and underdosing of dipyridamole

Excludes1 poisoning by, adverse effect of and underdosing of calcium-channel blockers (T46.1)

T46.3X **Poisoning by, adverse effect of and underdosing of coronary vasodilators**

T46.3X1 **Poisoning by coronary vasodilators, accidental (unintentional)**
Poisoning by coronary vasodilators NOS

T46.3X2 **Poisoning by coronary vasodilators, intentional self-harm**

T46.3X3 **Poisoning by coronary vasodilators, assault**

T46.3X4 **Poisoning by coronary vasodilators, undetermined**

T46.3X5 **Adverse effect of coronary vasodilators**

T46.3X6 **Underdosing of coronary vasodilators**

T46.4 **Poisoning by, adverse effect of and underdosing of angiotensin-converting-enzyme inhibitors**

T46.4X **Poisoning by, adverse effect of and underdosing of angiotensin-converting-enzyme inhibitors**

T46.4X1 **Poisoning by angiotensin-converting-enzyme inhibitors, accidental (unintentional)**
Poisoning by angiotensin-converting-enzyme inhibitors NOS

T46.4X2 **Poisoning by angiotensin-converting-enzyme inhibitors, intentional self-harm**

T46.4X3 **Poisoning by angiotensin-converting-enzyme inhibitors, assault**

T46.4X4 **Poisoning by angiotensin-converting-enzyme inhibitors, undetermined**

T46.4X5 **Adverse effect of angiotensin-converting-enzyme inhibitors**

T46.4X6 **Underdosing of angiotensin-converting-enzyme inhibitors**

CHAPTER 19 (S00-T88)

N Newborn Age: 0 P Pediatric Age: 0–17 M Maternity DX: 12–55 A Adult Age: 15–124 ♀ Females Only ♂ Males Only
 Complication\Comorbidity Major C\C (Ex) CC/MCC Exclusions Hospital-Acquired Condition

1463

● **T46.5**   **Poisoning by, adverse effect of and underdosing of other antihypertensive drugs**

     Excludes2   poisoning by, adverse effect of and underdosing of beta-adrenoreceptor antagonists (T44.7)

                poisoning by, adverse effect of and underdosing of calcium-channel blockers (T46.1)

                poisoning by, adverse effect of and underdosing of diuretics (T50.0-T50.2)

   ● **T46.5X**   **Poisoning by, adverse effect of and underdosing of other antihypertensive drugs**

     ● **T46.5X1**   **Poisoning by other antihypertensive drugs, accidental (unintentional)**

          Poisoning by other antihypertensive drugs NOS

     ● **T46.5X2**   **Poisoning by other antihypertensive drugs, intentional self-harm**

     ● **T46.5X3**   **Poisoning by other antihypertensive drugs, assault**

     ● **T46.5X4**   **Poisoning by other antihypertensive drugs, undetermined**

     ● **T46.5X5**   **Adverse effect of other antihypertensive drugs**

     ● **T46.5X6**   **Underdosing of other antihypertensive drugs**

● **T46.6**   **Poisoning by, adverse effect of and underdosing of antihyperlipidemic and antiarteriosclerotic drugs**

   ● **T46.6X**   **Poisoning by, adverse effect of and underdosing of antihyperlipidemic and antiarteriosclerotic drugs**

     ● **T46.6X1**   **Poisoning by antihyperlipidemic and antiarteriosclerotic drugs, accidental (unintentional)**

          Poisoning by antihyperlipidemic and antiarteriosclerotic drugs NOS

     ● **T46.6X2**   **Poisoning by antihyperlipidemic and antiarteriosclerotic drugs, intentional self-harm**

     ● **T46.6X3**   **Poisoning by antihyperlipidemic and antiarteriosclerotic drugs, assault**

     ● **T46.6X4**   **Poisoning by antihyperlipidemic and antiarteriosclerotic drugs, undetermined**

     ● **T46.6X5**   **Adverse effect of antihyperlipidemic and antiarteriosclerotic drugs**

     ● **T46.6X6**   **Underdosing of antihyperlipidemic and antiarteriosclerotic drugs**

● **T46.7**   **Poisoning by, adverse effect of and underdosing of peripheral vasodilators**

     Poisoning by, adverse effect of and underdosing of nicotinic acid (derivatives)

     Excludes1   poisoning by, adverse effect of and underdosing of papaverine (T44.3)

   ● **T46.7X**   **Poisoning by, adverse effect of and underdosing of peripheral vasodilators**

     ● **T46.7X1**   **Poisoning by peripheral vasodilators, accidental (unintentional)**

          Poisoning by peripheral vasodilators NOS

     ● **T46.7X2**   **Poisoning by peripheral vasodilators, intentional self-harm**

     ● **T46.7X3**   **Poisoning by peripheral vasodilators, assault**

     ● **T46.7X4**   **Poisoning by peripheral vasodilators, undetermined**

     ● **T46.7X5**   **Adverse effect of peripheral vasodilators**

     ● **T46.7X6**   **Underdosing of peripheral vasodilators**

● **T46.8**   **Poisoning by, adverse effect of and underdosing of antivaricose drugs, including sclerosing agents**

   ● **T46.8X**   **Poisoning by, adverse effect of and underdosing of antivaricose drugs, including sclerosing agents**

     ● **T46.8X1**   **Poisoning by antivaricose drugs, including sclerosing agents, accidental (unintentional)**

          Poisoning by antivaricose drugs, including sclerosing agents NOS

     ● **T46.8X2**   **Poisoning by antivaricose drugs, including sclerosing agents, intentional self-harm**

     ● **T46.8X3**   **Poisoning by antivaricose drugs, including sclerosing agents, assault**

     ● **T46.8X4**   **Poisoning by antivaricose drugs, including sclerosing agents, undetermined**

     ● **T46.8X5**   **Adverse effect of antivaricose drugs, including sclerosing agents**

     ● **T46.8X6**   **Underdosing of antivaricose drugs, including sclerosing agents**

● **T46.9**   **Poisoning by, adverse effect of and underdosing of other and unspecified agents primarily affecting the cardiovascular system**

   ● **T46.90**   **Poisoning by, adverse effect of and underdosing of unspecified agents primarily affecting the cardiovascular system**

     ● **T46.901**   **Poisoning by unspecified agents primarily affecting the cardiovascular system, accidental (unintentional)**

     ● **T46.902**   **Poisoning by unspecified agents primarily affecting the cardiovascular system, intentional self-harm**

     ● **T46.903**   **Poisoning by unspecified agents primarily affecting the cardiovascular system, assault**

     ● **T46.904**   **Poisoning by unspecified agents primarily affecting the cardiovascular system, undetermined**

     ● **T46.905**   **Adverse effect of unspecified agents primarily affecting the cardiovascular system**

     ● **T46.906**   **Underdosing of unspecified agents primarily affecting the cardiovascular system**

   ● **T46.99**   **Poisoning by, adverse effect of and underdosing of other agents primarily affecting the cardiovascular system**

     ● **T46.991**   **Poisoning by other agents primarily affecting the cardiovascular system, accidental (unintentional)**

     ● **T46.992**   **Poisoning by other agents primarily affecting the cardiovascular system, intentional self-harm**

     ● **T46.993**   **Poisoning by other agents primarily affecting the cardiovascular system, assault**

     ● **T46.994**   **Poisoning by other agents primarily affecting the cardiovascular system, undetermined**

     ● **T46.995**   **Adverse effect of other agents primarily affecting the cardiovascular system**

     ● **T46.996**   **Underdosing of other agents primarily affecting the cardiovascular system**

◀ New   ◀ Revised   ~~deleted~~ Deleted   Excludes 1   Excludes 2   Includes   Use additional   Code first   Code also   Unspecified

OGCR Official Guidelines   ● Unacceptable Principal Diagnosis   X Assign placeholder X   ● Use Additional Character(s)   ▌ Manifestation Code   **Coding Clinic**

● **T47 Poisoning by, adverse effect of and underdosing of agents primarily affecting the gastrointestinal system**

The appropriate 7th character is to be added to each code from category T47

A	initial encounter
D	subsequent encounter
S	sequela

● **T47.0 Poisoning by, adverse effect of and underdosing of histamine H2-receptor blockers**

  ● **T47.0X Poisoning by, adverse effect of and underdosing of histamine H2-receptor blockers**

    ● **T47.0X1 Poisoning by histamine H2-receptor blockers, accidental (unintentional)**
      Poisoning by histamine H2-receptor blockers NOS

    ● **T47.0X2 Poisoning by histamine H2-receptor blockers, intentional self-harm**

    ● **T47.0X3 Poisoning by histamine H2-receptor blockers, assault**

    ● **T47.0X4 Poisoning by histamine H2-receptor blockers, undetermined**

    ● **T47.0X5 Adverse effect of histamine H2-receptor blockers**

    ● **T47.0X6 Underdosing of histamine H2-receptor blockers**

● **T47.1 Poisoning by, adverse effect of and underdosing of other antacids and anti-gastric-secretion drugs**

  ● **T47.1X Poisoning by, adverse effect of and underdosing of other antacids and anti-gastric-secretion drugs**

    ● **T47.1X1 Poisoning by other antacids and anti-gastric-secretion drugs, accidental (unintentional)**
      Poisoning by other antacids and anti-gastric-secretion drugs NOS

    ● **T47.1X2 Poisoning by other antacids and anti-gastric-secretion drugs, intentional self-harm**

    ● **T47.1X3 Poisoning by other antacids and anti-gastric-secretion drugs, assault**

    ● **T47.1X4 Poisoning by other antacids and anti-gastric-secretion drugs, undetermined**

    ● **T47.1X5 Adverse effect of other antacids and anti-gastric-secretion drugs**

    ● **T47.1X6 Underdosing of other antacids and anti-gastric-secretion drugs**

● **T47.2 Poisoning by, adverse effect of and underdosing of stimulant laxatives**

  ● **T47.2X Poisoning by, adverse effect of and underdosing of stimulant laxatives**

    ● **T47.2X1 Poisoning by stimulant laxatives, accidental (unintentional)**
      Poisoning by stimulant laxatives NOS

    ● **T47.2X2 Poisoning by stimulant laxatives, intentional self-harm**

    ● **T47.2X3 Poisoning by stimulant laxatives, assault**

    ● **T47.2X4 Poisoning by stimulant laxatives, undetermined**

    ● **T47.2X5 Adverse effect of stimulant laxatives**

    ● **T47.2X6 Underdosing of stimulant laxatives**

● **T47.3 Poisoning by, adverse effect of and underdosing of saline and osmotic laxatives**

  ● **T47.3X Poisoning by and adverse effect of saline and osmotic laxatives**

    ● **T47.3X1 Poisoning by saline and osmotic laxatives, accidental (unintentional)**
      Poisoning by saline and osmotic laxatives NOS

    ● **T47.3X2 Poisoning by saline and osmotic laxatives, intentional self-harm**

    ● **T47.3X3 Poisoning by saline and osmotic laxatives, assault**

    ● **T47.3X4 Poisoning by saline and osmotic laxatives, undetermined**

    ● **T47.3X5 Adverse effect of saline and osmotic laxatives**

    ● **T47.3X6 Underdosing of saline and osmotic laxatives**

● **T47.4 Poisoning by, adverse effect of and underdosing of other laxatives**

  ● **T47.4X Poisoning by, adverse effect of and underdosing of other laxatives**

    ● **T47.4X1 Poisoning by other laxatives, accidental (unintentional)**
      Poisoning by other laxatives NOS

    ● **T47.4X2 Poisoning by other laxatives, intentional self-harm**

    ● **T47.4X3 Poisoning by other laxatives, assault**

    ● **T47.4X4 Poisoning by other laxatives, undetermined**

    ● **T47.4X5 Adverse effect of other laxatives**

    ● **T47.4X6 Underdosing of other laxatives**

● **T47.5 Poisoning by, adverse effect of and underdosing of digestants**

  ● **T47.5X Poisoning by, adverse effect of and underdosing of digestants**

    ● **T47.5X1 Poisoning by digestants, accidental (unintentional)**
      Poisoning by digestants NOS

    ● **T47.5X2 Poisoning by digestants, intentional self-harm**

    ● **T47.5X3 Poisoning by digestants, assault**

    ● **T47.5X4 Poisoning by digestants, undetermined**

    ● **T47.5X5 Adverse effect of digestants**

    ● **T47.5X6 Underdosing of digestants**

● **T47.6 Poisoning by, adverse effect of and underdosing of antidiarrheal drugs**

  Excludes2   poisoning by, adverse effect of and underdosing of systemic antibiotics and other anti-infectives (T36-T37)

  ● **T47.6X Poisoning by, adverse effect of and underdosing of antidiarrheal drugs**

    ● **T47.6X1 Poisoning by antidiarrheal drugs, accidental (unintentional)**
      Poisoning by antidiarrheal drugs NOS

    ● **T47.6X2 Poisoning by antidiarrheal drugs, intentional self-harm**

    ● **T47.6X3 Poisoning by antidiarrheal drugs, assault**

    ● **T47.6X4 Poisoning by antidiarrheal drugs, undetermined**

    ● **T47.6X5 Adverse effect of antidiarrheal drugs**

    ● **T47.6X6 Underdosing of antidiarrheal drugs**

CHAPTER 19 (S00-T88)

● T47.7 Poisoning by, adverse effect of and underdosing of emetics

  ● T47.7X Poisoning by, adverse effect of and underdosing of emetics

    ● T47.7X1 Poisoning by emetics, accidental (unintentional)
      Poisoning by emetics NOS

    ● T47.7X2 Poisoning by emetics, intentional self-harm

    ● T47.7X3 Poisoning by emetics, assault

    ● T47.7X4 Poisoning by emetics, undetermined

    ● T47.7X5 Adverse effect of emetics

    ● T47.7X6 Underdosing of emetics

● T47.8 Poisoning by, adverse effect of and underdosing of other agents primarily affecting gastrointestinal system

  ● T47.8X Poisoning by, adverse effect of and underdosing of other agents primarily affecting gastrointestinal system

    ● T47.8X1 Poisoning by other agents primarily affecting gastrointestinal system, accidental (unintentional)
      Poisoning by other agents primarily affecting gastrointestinal system NOS

    ● T47.8X2 Poisoning by other agents primarily affecting gastrointestinal system, intentional self-harm

    ● T47.8X3 Poisoning by other agents primarily affecting gastrointestinal system, assault

    ● T47.8X4 Poisoning by other agents primarily affecting gastrointestinal system, undetermined

    ● T47.8X5 Adverse effect of other agents primarily affecting gastrointestinal system

    ● T47.8X6 Underdosing of other agents primarily affecting gastrointestinal system

● T47.9 Poisoning by, adverse effect of and underdosing of unspecified agents primarily affecting the gastrointestinal system

  X ● T47.91 Poisoning by unspecified agents primarily affecting the gastrointestinal system, accidental (unintentional)
    Poisoning by agents primarily affecting the gastrointestinal system NOS

  X ● T47.92 Poisoning by unspecified agents primarily affecting the gastrointestinal system, intentional self-harm

  X ● T47.93 Poisoning by unspecified agents primarily affecting the gastrointestinal system, assault

  X ● T47.94 Poisoning by unspecified agents primarily affecting the gastrointestinal system, undetermined

  X ● T47.95 Adverse effect of unspecified agents primarily affecting the gastrointestinal system

  X ● T47.96 Underdosing of unspecified agents primarily affecting the gastrointestinal system

● T48 Poisoning by, adverse effect of and underdosing of agents primarily acting on smooth and skeletal muscles and the respiratory system

  The appropriate 7th character is to be added to each code from category T48

A	initial encounter
D	subsequent encounter
S	sequela

● T48.0 Poisoning by, adverse effect of and underdosing of oxytocic drugs

  Excludes1   poisoning by, adverse effect of and underdosing of estrogens, progestogens and antagonists (T38.4-T38.6)

  ● T48.0X Poisoning by, adverse effect of and underdosing of oxytocic drugs

    ● T48.0X1 Poisoning by oxytocic drugs, accidental (unintentional)
      Poisoning by oxytocic drugs NOS

    ● T48.0X2 Poisoning by oxytocic drugs, intentional self-harm

    ● T48.0X3 Poisoning by oxytocic drugs, assault

    ● T48.0X4 Poisoning by oxytocic drugs, undetermined

    ● T48.0X5 Adverse effect of oxytocic drugs

    ● T48.0X6 Underdosing of oxytocic drugs

● T48.1 Poisoning by, adverse effect of and underdosing of skeletal muscle relaxants [neuromuscular blocking agents]

  ● T48.1X Poisoning by, adverse effect of and underdosing of skeletal muscle relaxants [neuromuscular blocking agents]

    ● T48.1X1 Poisoning by skeletal muscle relaxants [neuromuscular blocking agents], accidental (unintentional)
      Poisoning by skeletal muscle relaxants [neuromuscular blocking agents] NOS

    ● T48.1X2 Poisoning by skeletal muscle relaxants [neuromuscular blocking agents], intentional self-harm

    ● T48.1X3 Poisoning by skeletal muscle relaxants [neuromuscular blocking agents], assault

    ● T48.1X4 Poisoning by skeletal muscle relaxants [neuromuscular blocking agents], undetermined

    ● T48.1X5 Adverse effect of skeletal muscle relaxants [neuromuscular blocking agents]

    ● T48.1X6 Underdosing of skeletal muscle relaxants [neuromuscular blocking agents]

● T48.2 Poisoning by, adverse effect of and underdosing of other and unspecified drugs acting on muscles

  ● T48.20 Poisoning by, adverse effect of and underdosing of unspecified drugs acting on muscles

    ● T48.201 Poisoning by unspecified drugs acting on muscles, accidental (unintentional)
      Poisoning by unspecified drugs acting on muscles NOS

    ● T48.202 Poisoning by unspecified drugs acting on muscles, intentional self-harm

    ● T48.203 Poisoning by unspecified drugs acting on muscles, assault

    ● T48.204 Poisoning by unspecified drugs acting on muscles, undetermined

    ● T48.205 Adverse effect of unspecified drugs acting on muscles

    ● T48.206 Underdosing of unspecified drugs acting on muscles

CHAPTER 19 (S00-T88)

◀ New   ◀ Revised   ~~deleted~~ Deleted   Excludes 1   Excludes 2   Includes   Use additional   Code first   Code also   Unspecified

OGCR Official Guidelines   ● Unacceptable Principal Diagnosis   X Assign placeholder X   ● Use Additional Character(s)   ▌ Manifestation Code   **Coding Clinic**

- **T48.29** Poisoning by, adverse effect of and underdosing of other drugs acting on muscles
  - **T48.291** Poisoning by other drugs acting on muscles, accidental (unintentional)
    Poisoning by other drugs acting on muscles NOS
  - **T48.292** Poisoning by other drugs acting on muscles, intentional self-harm
  - **T48.293** Poisoning by other drugs acting on muscles, assault
  - **T48.294** Poisoning by other drugs acting on muscles, undetermined
  - **T48.295** Adverse effect of other drugs acting on muscles
  - **T48.296** Underdosing of other drugs acting on muscles
- **T48.3** Poisoning by, adverse effect of and underdosing of antitussives
  - **T48.3X** Poisoning by, adverse effect of and underdosing of antitussives
    - **T48.3X1** Poisoning by antitussives, accidental (unintentional)
      Poisoning by antitussives NOS
    - **T48.3X2** Poisoning by antitussives, intentional self-harm
    - **T48.3X3** Poisoning by antitussives, assault
    - **T48.3X4** Poisoning by antitussives, undetermined
    - **T48.3X5** Adverse effect of antitussives
    - **T48.3X6** Underdosing of antitussives
- **T48.4** Poisoning by, adverse effect of and underdosing of expectorants
  - **T48.4X** Poisoning by, adverse effect of and underdosing of expectorants
    - **T48.4X1** Poisoning by expectorants, accidental (unintentional)
      Poisoning by expectorants NOS
    - **T48.4X2** Poisoning by expectorants, intentional self-harm
    - **T48.4X3** Poisoning by expectorants, assault
    - **T48.4X4** Poisoning by expectorants, undetermined
    - **T48.4X5** Adverse effect of expectorants
    - **T48.4X6** Underdosing of expectorants
- **T48.5** Poisoning by, adverse effect of and underdosing of other anti-common-cold drugs
  Poisoning by, adverse effect of and underdosing of decongestants
  > **Excludes2**   poisoning by, adverse effect of and underdosing of antipyretics, NEC (T39.9-)
  > poisoning by, adverse effect of and underdosing of non-steroidal antiinflammatory drugs (T39.3-)
  > poisoning by, adverse effect of and underdosing of salicylates (T39.0-)
  - **T48.5X** Poisoning by, adverse effect of and underdosing of other anti-common-cold drugs
    - **T48.5X1** Poisoning by other anti-common-cold drugs, accidental (unintentional)
      Poisoning by other anti-common-cold drugs NOS
    - **T48.5X2** Poisoning by other anti-common-cold drugs, intentional self-harm
    - **T48.5X3** Poisoning by other anti-common-cold drugs, assault
    - **T48.5X4** Poisoning by other anti-common-cold drugs, undetermined
    - **T48.5X5** Adverse effect of other anti-common-cold drugs
    - **T48.5X6** Underdosing of other anti-common-cold drugs

- **T48.6** Poisoning by, adverse effect of and underdosing of antiasthmatics, not elsewhere classified
  Poisoning by, adverse effect of and underdosing of beta-adrenoreceptor agonists used in asthma therapy
  > **Excludes1**   poisoning by, adverse effect of and underdosing of beta-adrenoreceptor agonists not used in asthma therapy (T44.5)
  > poisoning by, adverse effect of and underdosing of anterior pituitary [adenohypophyseal] hormones (T38.8)
  - **T48.6X** Poisoning by, adverse effect of and underdosing of antiasthmatics
    - **T48.6X1** Poisoning by antiasthmatics, accidental (unintentional)
      Poisoning by antiasthmatics NOS
    - **T48.6X2** Poisoning by antiasthmatics, intentional self-harm
    - **T48.6X3** Poisoning by antiasthmatics, assault
    - **T48.6X4** Poisoning by antiasthmatics, undetermined
    - **T48.6X5** Adverse effect of antiasthmatics
    - **T48.6X6** Underdosing of antiasthmatics
- **T48.9** Poisoning by, adverse effect of and underdosing of other and unspecified agents primarily acting on the respiratory system
  - **T48.90** Poisoning by, adverse effect of and underdosing of unspecified agents primarily acting on the respiratory system
    - **T48.901** Poisoning by unspecified agents primarily acting on the respiratory system, accidental (unintentional)
    - **T48.902** Poisoning by unspecified agents primarily acting on the respiratory system, intentional self-harm
    - **T48.903** Poisoning by unspecified agents primarily acting on the respiratory system, assault
    - **T48.904** Poisoning by unspecified agents primarily acting on the respiratory system, undetermined
    - **T48.905** Adverse effect of unspecified agents primarily acting on the respiratory system
    - **T48.906** Underdosing of unspecified agents primarily acting on the respiratory system
  - **T48.99** Poisoning by, adverse effect of and underdosing of other agents primarily acting on the respiratory system
    - **T48.991** Poisoning by other agents primarily acting on the respiratory system, accidental (unintentional)
    - **T48.992** Poisoning by other agents primarily acting on the respiratory system, intentional self-harm
    - **T48.993** Poisoning by other agents primarily acting on the respiratory system, assault
    - **T48.994** Poisoning by other agents primarily acting on the respiratory system, undetermined
    - **T48.995** Adverse effect of other agents primarily acting on the respiratory system
    - **T48.996** Underdosing of other agents primarily acting on the respiratory system

CHAPTER 19 (S00-T88)

N Newborn Age: 0   **P** Pediatric Age: 0–17   **M** Maternity DX: 12–55   **A** Adult Age: 15–124   ♀ Females Only   ♂ Males Only

 Complication\Comorbidity   Major C\C   CC/MCC Exclusions   Hospital-Acquired Condition

1467

CHAPTER 19 (S00-T88)

● **T49**   **Poisoning by, adverse effect of and underdosing of topical agents primarily affecting skin and mucous membrane and by ophthalmological, otorhinorlaryngological and dental drugs**

    Includes   poisoning by, adverse effect of and underdosing of glucocorticoids, topically used

    The appropriate 7th character is to be added to each code from category T49

A	initial encounter
D	subsequent encounter
S	sequela

● **T49.0**   **Poisoning by, adverse effect of and underdosing of local antifungal, anti-infective and anti-inflammatory drugs**

  ● **T49.0X**   **Poisoning by, adverse effect of and underdosing of local antifungal, anti-infective and anti-inflammatory drugs**

    ● **T49.0X1**   **Poisoning by local antifungal, anti-infective and anti-inflammatory drugs, accidental (unintentional)**

        Poisoning by local antifungal, anti-infective and anti-inflammatory drugs NOS

    ● **T49.0X2**   **Poisoning by local antifungal, anti-infective and anti-inflammatory drugs, intentional self-harm**

    ● **T49.0X3**   **Poisoning by local antifungal, anti-infective and anti-inflammatory drugs, assault**

    ● **T49.0X4**   **Poisoning by local antifungal, anti-infective and anti-inflammatory drugs, undetermined**

    ● **T49.0X5**   **Adverse effect of local antifungal, anti-infective and anti-inflammatory drugs**

    ● **T49.0X6**   **Underdosing of local antifungal, anti-infective and anti-inflammatory drugs**

● **T49.1**   **Poisoning by, adverse effect of and underdosing of antipruritics**

  ● **T49.1X**   **Poisoning by, adverse effect of and underdosing of antipruritics**

    ● **T49.1X1**   **Poisoning by antipruritics, accidental (unintentional)**

        Poisoning by antipruritics NOS

    ● **T49.1X2**   **Poisoning by antipruritics, intentional self-harm**

    ● **T49.1X3**   **Poisoning by antipruritics, assault**

    ● **T49.1X4**   **Poisoning by antipruritics, undetermined**

    ● **T49.1X5**   **Adverse effect of antipruritics**

    ● **T49.1X6**   **Underdosing of antipruritics**

● **T49.2**   **Poisoning by, adverse effect of and underdosing of local astringents and local detergents**

  ● **T49.2X**   **Poisoning by, adverse effect of and underdosing of local astringents and local detergents**

    ● **T49.2X1**   **Poisoning by local astringents and local detergents, accidental (unintentional)**

        Poisoning by local astringents and local detergents NOS

    ● **T49.2X2**   **Poisoning by local astringents and local detergents, intentional self-harm**

    ● **T49.2X3**   **Poisoning by local astringents and local detergents, assault**

    ● **T49.2X4**   **Poisoning by local astringents and local detergents, undetermined**

    ● **T49.2X5**   **Adverse effect of local astringents and local detergents**

    ● **T49.2X6**   **Underdosing of local astringents and local detergents**

● **T49.3**   **Poisoning by, adverse effect of and underdosing of emollients, demulcents and protectants**

  ● **T49.3X**   **Poisoning by, adverse effect of and underdosing of emollients, demulcents and protectants**

    ● **T49.3X1**   **Poisoning by emollients, demulcents and protectants, accidental (unintentional)**

        Poisoning by emollients, demulcents and protectants NOS

    ● **T49.3X2**   **Poisoning by emollients, demulcents and protectants, intentional self-harm**

    ● **T49.3X3**   **Poisoning by emollients, demulcents and protectants, assault**

    ● **T49.3X4**   **Poisoning by emollients, demulcents and protectants, undetermined**

    ● **T49.3X5**   **Adverse effect of emollients, demulcents and protectants**

    ● **T49.3X6**   **Underdosing of emollients, demulcents and protectants**

● **T49.4**   **Poisoning by, adverse effect of and underdosing of keratolytics, keratoplastics, and other hair treatment drugs and preparations**

  ● **T49.4X**   **Poisoning by, adverse effect of and underdosing of keratolytics, keratoplastics, and other hair treatment drugs and preparations**

    ● **T49.4X1**   **Poisoning by keratolytics, keratoplastics, and other hair treatment drugs and preparations, accidental (unintentional)**

        Poisoning by keratolytics, keratoplastics, and other hair treatment drugs and preparations NOS

    ● **T49.4X2**   **Poisoning by keratolytics, keratoplastics, and other hair treatment drugs and preparations, intentional self-harm**

    ● **T49.4X3**   **Poisoning by keratolytics, keratoplastics, and other hair treatment drugs and preparations, assault**

    ● **T49.4X4**   **Poisoning by keratolytics, keratoplastics, and other hair treatment drugs and preparations, undetermined**

    ● **T49.4X5**   **Adverse effect of keratolytics, keratoplastics, and other hair treatment drugs and preparations**

    ● **T49.4X6**   **Underdosing of keratolytics, keratoplastics, and other hair treatment drugs and preparations**

● **T49.5**   **Poisoning by, adverse effect of and underdosing of ophthalmological drugs and preparations**

  ● **T49.5X**   **Poisoning by, adverse effect of and underdosing of ophthalmological drugs and preparations**

    ● **T49.5X1**   **Poisoning by ophthalmological drugs and preparations, accidental (unintentional)**

        Poisoning by ophthalmological drugs and preparations NOS

    ● **T49.5X2**   **Poisoning by ophthalmological drugs and preparations, intentional self-harm**

    ● **T49.5X3**   **Poisoning by ophthalmological drugs and preparations, assault**

    ● **T49.5X4**   **Poisoning by ophthalmological drugs and preparations, undetermined**

    ● **T49.5X5**   **Adverse effect of ophthalmological drugs and preparations**

    ● **T49.5X6**   **Underdosing of ophthalmological drugs and preparations**

◄ New   ⬅ Revised   ~~deleted~~ Deleted   Excludes 1   Excludes 2   Includes   Use additional   Code first   Code also   Unspecified

OGCR Official Guidelines   ● Unacceptable Principal Diagnosis   X Assign placeholder X   ● Use Additional Character(s)   ▶ Manifestation Code   **Coding Clinic**

● **T49.6 Poisoning by, adverse effect of and underdosing of otorhinolaryngological drugs and preparations**

  ● **T49.6X Poisoning by, adverse effect of and underdosing of otorhinolaryngological drugs and preparations**

    ● **T49.6X1 Poisoning by otorhinolaryngological drugs and preparations, accidental (unintentional)**
         Poisoning by otorhinolaryngological drugs and preparations NOS

    ● **T49.6X2 Poisoning by otorhinolaryngological drugs and preparations, intentional self-harm**

    ● **T49.6X3 Poisoning by otorhinolaryngological drugs and preparations, assault**

    ● **T49.6X4 Poisoning by otorhinolaryngological drugs and preparations, undetermined**

    ● **T49.6X5 Adverse effect of otorhinolaryngological drugs and preparations**

    ● **T49.6X6 Underdosing of otorhinolaryngological drugs and preparations**

● **T49.7 Poisoning by, adverse effect of and underdosing of dental drugs, topically applied**

  ● **T49.7X Poisoning by, adverse effect of and underdosing of dental drugs, topically applied**

    ● **T49.7X1 Poisoning by dental drugs, topically applied, accidental (unintentional)**
         Poisoning by dental drugs, topically applied NOS

    ● **T49.7X2 Poisoning by dental drugs, topically applied, intentional self-harm**

    ● **T49.7X3 Poisoning by dental drugs, topically applied, assault**

    ● **T49.7X4 Poisoning by dental drugs, topically applied, undetermined**

    ● **T49.7X5 Adverse effect of dental drugs, topically applied**

    ● **T49.7X6 Underdosing of dental drugs, topically applied**

● **T49.8 Poisoning by, adverse effect of and underdosing of other topical agents**
     Poisoning by, adverse effect of and underdosing of spermicides

  ● **T49.8X Poisoning by, adverse effect of and underdosing of other topical agents**

    ● **T49.8X1 Poisoning by other topical agents, accidental (unintentional)**
         Poisoning by other topical agents NOS

    ● **T49.8X2 Poisoning by other topical agents, intentional self-harm**

    ● **T49.8X3 Poisoning by other topical agents, assault**

    ● **T49.8X4 Poisoning by other topical agents, undetermined**

    ● **T49.8X5 Adverse effect of other topical agents**

    ● **T49.8X6 Underdosing of other topical agents**

● **T49.9 Poisoning by, adverse effect of and underdosing of unspecified topical agent**

  X ● **T49.91 Poisoning by unspecified topical agent, accidental (unintentional)**

  X ● **T49.92 Poisoning by unspecified topical agent, intentional self-harm**

  X ● **T49.93 Poisoning by unspecified topical agent, assault**

  X ● **T49.94 Poisoning by unspecified topical agent, undetermined**

  X ● **T49.95 Adverse effect of unspecified topical agent**

  X ● **T49.96 Underdosing of unspecified topical agent**

● **T50 Poisoning by, adverse effect of and underdosing of diuretics and other and unspecified drugs, medicaments and biological substances**
     The appropriate 7th character is to be added to each code from category T50

A	initial encounter
D	subsequent encounter
S	sequela

● **T50.0 Poisoning by, adverse effect of and underdosing of mineralocorticoids and their antagonists**

  ● **T50.0X Poisoning by, adverse effect of and underdosing of mineralocorticoids and their antagonists**

    ● **T50.0X1 Poisoning by mineralocorticoids and their antagonists, accidental (unintentional)**
         Poisoning by mineralocorticoids and their antagonists NOS

    ● **T50.0X2 Poisoning by mineralocorticoids and their antagonists, intentional self-harm**

    ● **T50.0X3 Poisoning by mineralocorticoids and their antagonists, assault**

    ● **T50.0X4 Poisoning by mineralocorticoids and their antagonists, undetermined**

    ● **T50.0X5 Adverse effect of mineralocorticoids and their antagonists**

    ● **T50.0X6 Underdosing of mineralocorticoids and their antagonists**

● **T50.1 Poisoning by, adverse effect of and underdosing of loop [high-ceiling] diuretics**

  ● **T50.1X Poisoning by, adverse effect of and underdosing of loop [high-ceiling] diuretics**

    ● **T50.1X1 Poisoning by loop [high-ceiling] diuretics, accidental (unintentional)**
         Poisoning by loop [high-ceiling] diuretics NOS

    ● **T50.1X2 Poisoning by loop [high-ceiling] diuretics, intentional self-harm**

    ● **T50.1X3 Poisoning by loop [high-ceiling] diuretics, assault**

    ● **T50.1X4 Poisoning by loop [high-ceiling] diuretics, undetermined**

    ● **T50.1X5 Adverse effect of loop [high-ceiling] diuretics**

    ● **T50.1X6 Underdosing of loop [high-ceiling] diuretics**

CHAPTER 19 (S00-T88)

N Newborn Age: 0   **P** Pediatric Age: 0–17   **M** Maternity DX: 12–55   **A** Adult Age: 15–124   ♀ Females Only   ♂ Males Only

   Complication\Comorbidity   Major C\C   (Ex.) CC/MCC Exclusions   Hospital-Acquired Condition

1469

● **T50.2** **Poisoning by, adverse effect of and underdosing of carbonic-anhydrase inhibitors, benzothiadiazides and other diuretics**
> Poisoning by, adverse effect of and underdosing of acetazolamide

● **T50.2X** **Poisoning by, adverse effect of and underdosing of carbonic-anhydrase inhibitors, benzothiadiazides and other diuretics**

● **T50.2X1** **Poisoning by carbonic-anhydrase inhibitors, benzothiadiazides and other diuretics, accidental (unintentional)**
> Poisoning by carbonic-anhydrase inhibitors, benzothiadiazides and other diuretics NOS

● **T50.2X2** **Poisoning by carbonic-anhydrase inhibitors, benzothiadiazides and other diuretics, intentional self-harm**

● **T50.2X3** **Poisoning by carbonic-anhydrase inhibitors, benzothiadiazides and other diuretics, assault**

● **T50.2X4** **Poisoning by carbonic-anhydrase inhibitors, benzothiadiazides and other diuretics, undetermined**

● **T50.2X5** **Adverse effect of carbonic-anhydrase inhibitors, benzothiadiazides and other diuretics**

● **T50.2X6** **Underdosing of carbonic-anhydrase inhibitors, benzothiadiazides and other diuretics**

● **T50.3** **Poisoning by, adverse effect of and underdosing of electrolytic, caloric and water-balance agents**
> Poisoning by, adverse effect of and underdosing of oral rehydration salts

● **T50.3X** **Poisoning by, adverse effect of and underdosing of electrolytic, caloric and water-balance agents**

● **T50.3X1** **Poisoning by electrolytic, caloric and water-balance agents, accidental (unintentional)**
> Poisoning by electrolytic, caloric and water-balance agents NOS

● **T50.3X2** **Poisoning by electrolytic, caloric and water-balance agents, intentional self-harm**

● **T50.3X3** **Poisoning by electrolytic, caloric and water-balance agents, assault**

● **T50.3X4** **Poisoning by electrolytic, caloric and water-balance agents, undetermined**

● **T50.3X5** **Adverse effect of electrolytic, caloric and water-balance agents**

● **T50.3X6** **Underdosing of electrolytic, caloric and water-balance agents**

● **T50.4** **Poisoning by, adverse effect of and underdosing of drugs affecting uric acid metabolism**

● **T50.4X** **Poisoning by, adverse effect of and underdosing of drugs affecting uric acid metabolism**

● **T50.4X1** **Poisoning by drugs affecting uric acid metabolism, accidental (unintentional)**
> Poisoning by drugs affecting uric acid metabolism NOS

● **T50.4X2** **Poisoning by drugs affecting uric acid metabolism, intentional self-harm**

● **T50.4X3** **Poisoning by drugs affecting uric acid metabolism, assault**

● **T50.4X4** **Poisoning by drugs affecting uric acid metabolism, undetermined**

● **T50.4X5** **Adverse effect of drugs affecting uric acid metabolism**

● **T50.4X6** **Underdosing of drugs affecting uric acid metabolism**

● **T50.5** **Poisoning by, adverse effect of and underdosing of appetite depressants**

● **T50.5X** **Poisoning by, adverse effect of and underdosing of appetite depressants**

● **T50.5X1** **Poisoning by appetite depressants, accidental (unintentional)**
> Poisoning by appetite depressants NOS

● **T50.5X2** **Poisoning by appetite depressants, intentional self-harm**

● **T50.5X3** **Poisoning by appetite depressants, assault**

● **T50.5X4** **Poisoning by appetite depressants, undetermined**

● **T50.5X5** **Adverse effect of appetite depressants**

● **T50.5X6** **Underdosing of appetite depressants**

● **T50.6** **Poisoning by, adverse effect of and underdosing of antidotes and chelating agents**
> Poisoning by, adverse effect of and underdosing of alcohol deterrents

● **T50.6X** **Poisoning by, adverse effect of and underdosing of antidotes and chelating agents**

● **T50.6X1** **Poisoning by antidotes and chelating agents, accidental (unintentional)**
> Poisoning by antidotes and chelating agents NOS

● **T50.6X2** **Poisoning by antidotes and chelating agents, intentional self-harm**

● **T50.6X3** **Poisoning by antidotes and chelating agents, assault**

● **T50.6X4** **Poisoning by antidotes and chelating agents, undetermined**

● **T50.6X5** **Adverse effect of antidotes and chelating agents**

● **T50.6X6** **Underdosing of antidotes and chelating agents**

● **T50.7** **Poisoning by, adverse effect of and underdosing of analeptics and opioid receptor antagonists**

● **T50.7X** **Poisoning by, adverse effect of and underdosing of analeptics and opioid receptor antagonists**

● **T50.7X1** **Poisoning by analeptics and opioid receptor antagonists, accidental (unintentional)**
> Poisoning by analeptics and opioid receptor antagonists NOS

● **T50.7X2** **Poisoning by analeptics and opioid receptor antagonists, intentional self-harm**

● **T50.7X3** **Poisoning by analeptics and opioid receptor antagonists, assault**

● **T50.7X4** **Poisoning by analeptics and opioid receptor antagonists, undetermined**

● **T50.7X5** **Adverse effect of analeptics and opioid receptor antagonists**

● **T50.7X6** **Underdosing of analeptics and opioid receptor antagonists**

◀ New   ◀▥ Revised   ~~deleted~~ Deleted   Excludes 1   Excludes 2   Includes   Use additional   Code first   Code also   Unspecified

OGCR Official Guidelines   ● Unacceptable Principal Diagnosis   X Assign placeholder X   ● Use Additional Character(s)   ▶ Manifestation Code   **Coding Clinic**

1470

● **T50.8** Poisoning by, adverse effect of and underdosing of diagnostic agents
  ● **T50.8X** Poisoning by, adverse effect of and underdosing of diagnostic agents
    ● **T50.8X1** Poisoning by diagnostic agents, accidental (unintentional)
         Poisoning by diagnostic agents NOS
    ● **T50.8X2** Poisoning by diagnostic agents, intentional self-harm
    ● **T50.8X3** Poisoning by diagnostic agents, assault
    ● **T50.8X4** Poisoning by diagnostic agents, undetermined
    ● **T50.8X5** Adverse effect of diagnostic agents
    ● **T50.8X6** Underdosing of diagnostic agents
● **T50.A** Poisoning by, adverse effect of and underdosing of bacterial vaccines
  ● **T50.A1** Poisoning by, adverse effect of and underdosing of pertussis vaccine, including combinations with a pertussis component
    ● **T50.A11** Poisoning by pertussis vaccine, including combinations with a pertussis component, accidental (unintentional)
    ● **T50.A12** Poisoning by pertussis vaccine, including combinations with a pertussis component, intentional self-harm
    ● **T50.A13** Poisoning by pertussis vaccine, including combinations with a pertussis component, assault
    ● **T50.A14** Poisoning by pertussis vaccine, including combinations with a pertussis component, undetermined
    ● **T50.A15** Adverse effect of pertussis vaccine, including combinations with a pertussis component
    ● **T50.A16** Underdosing of pertussis vaccine, including combinations with a pertussis component
  ● **T50.A2** Poisoning by, adverse effect of and underdosing of mixed bacterial vaccines without a pertussis component
    ● **T50.A21** Poisoning by mixed bacterial vaccines without a pertussis component, accidental (unintentional)
    ● **T50.A22** Poisoning by mixed bacterial vaccines without a pertussis component, intentional self-harm
    ● **T50.A23** Poisoning by mixed bacterial vaccines without a pertussis component, assault
    ● **T50.A24** Poisoning by mixed bacterial vaccines without a pertussis component, undetermined
    ● **T50.A25** Adverse effect of mixed bacterial vaccines without a pertussis component
    ● **T50.A26** Underdosing of mixed bacterial vaccines without a pertussis component

● **T50.A9** Poisoning by, adverse effect of and underdosing of other bacterial vaccines
    ● **T50.A91** Poisoning by other bacterial vaccines, accidental (unintentional)
    ● **T50.A92** Poisoning by other bacterial vaccines, intentional self-harm
    ● **T50.A93** Poisoning by other bacterial vaccines, assault
    ● **T50.A94** Poisoning by other bacterial vaccines, undetermined
    ● **T50.A95** Adverse effect of other bacterial vaccines
    ● **T50.A96** Underdosing of other bacterial vaccines
● **T50.B** Poisoning by, adverse effect of and underdosing of viral vaccines
  ● **T50.B1** Poisoning by, adverse effect of and underdosing of smallpox vaccines
    ● **T50.B11** Poisoning by smallpox vaccines, accidental (unintentional)
    ● **T50.B12** Poisoning by smallpox vaccines, intentional self-harm
    ● **T50.B13** Poisoning by smallpox vaccines, assault
    ● **T50.B14** Poisoning by smallpox vaccines, undetermined
    ● **T50.B15** Adverse effect of smallpox vaccines
    ● **T50.B16** Underdosing of smallpox vaccines
  ● **T50.B9** Poisoning by, adverse effect of and underdosing of other viral vaccines
    ● **T50.B91** Poisoning by other viral vaccines, accidental (unintentional)
    ● **T50.B92** Poisoning by other viral vaccines, intentional self-harm
    ● **T50.B93** Poisoning by other viral vaccines, assault
    ● **T50.B94** Poisoning by other viral vaccines, undetermined
    ● **T50.B95** Adverse effect of other viral vaccines
    ● **T50.B96** Underdosing of other viral vaccines
● **T50.Z** Poisoning by, adverse effect of and underdosing of other vaccines and biological substances
  ● **T50.Z1** Poisoning by, adverse effect of and underdosing of immunoglobulin
    ● **T50.Z11** Poisoning by immunoglobulin, accidental (unintentional)
    ● **T50.Z12** Poisoning by immunoglobulin, intentional self-harm
    ● **T50.Z13** Poisoning by immunoglobulin, assault
    ● **T50.Z14** Poisoning by immunoglobulin, undetermined
    ● **T50.Z15** Adverse effect of immunoglobulin
    ● **T50.Z16** Underdosing of immunoglobulin

CHAPTER 19 (S00–T88)

N Newborn Age: 0   **P** Pediatric Age: 0–17   **M** Maternity DX: 12–55   **A** Adult Age: 15–124   ♀ Females Only   ♂ Males Only

 Complication\Comorbidity   Major C\C   (Ex) CC/MCC Exclusions   Hospital-Acquired Condition

1471

● T50.Z9   Poisoning by, adverse effect of and underdosing of other vaccines and biological substances

   ● T50.Z91   Poisoning by other vaccines and biological substances, accidental (unintentional)

   ● T50.Z92   Poisoning by other vaccines and biological substances, intentional self-harm

   ● T50.Z93   Poisoning by other vaccines and biological substances, assault

   ● T50.Z94   Poisoning by other vaccines and biological substances, undetermined

   ● T50.Z95   Adverse effect of other vaccines and biological substances

   ● T50.Z96   Underdosing of other vaccines and biological substances

● T50.9   Poisoning by, adverse effect of and underdosing of other and unspecified drugs, medicaments and biological substances

   ● T50.90   Poisoning by, adverse effect of and underdosing of unspecified drugs, medicaments and biological substances

     ● T50.901   Poisoning by unspecified drugs, medicaments and biological substances, accidental (unintentional)
         Coding Clinic: 2015, Q1, P21

     ● T50.902   Poisoning by unspecified drugs, medicaments and biological substances, intentional self-harm

     ● T50.903   Poisoning by unspecified drugs, medicaments and biological substances, assault

     ● T50.904   Poisoning by unspecified drugs, medicaments and biological substances, undetermined

     ● T50.905   Adverse effect of unspecified drugs, medicaments and biological substances

     ● T50.906   Underdosing of unspecified drugs, medicaments and biological substances

   ● T50.99   Poisoning by, adverse effect of and underdosing of other drugs, medicaments and biological substances

     ● T50.991   Poisoning by other drugs, medicaments and biological substances, accidental (unintentional)

     ● T50.992   Poisoning by other drugs, medicaments and biological substances, intentional self-harm

     ● T50.993   Poisoning by other drugs, medicaments and biological substances, assault

     ● T50.994   Poisoning by other drugs, medicaments and biological substances, undetermined

     ● T50.995   Adverse effect of other drugs, medicaments and biological substances

     ● T50.996   Underdosing of other drugs, medicaments and biological substances

TOXIC EFFECTS OF SUBSTANCES CHIEFLY NONMEDICINAL AS TO SOURCE (T51-T65)

Note: When no intent is indicated code to accidental. Undetermined intent is only for use when there is specific documentation in the record that the intent of the toxic effect cannot be determined.

Use additional code(s): for all associated manifestations of toxic effect, such as:
respiratory conditions due to external agents (J60-J70)
personal history of foreign body fully removed (Z87.821)
to identify any retained foreign body, if applicable (Z18.-)

Excludes1   contact with and (suspected) exposure to toxic substances (Z77.-)

● T51   Toxic effect of alcohol

The appropriate 7th character is to be added to each code from category T51

A	initial encounter
D	subsequent encounter
S	sequela

   ● T51.0   Toxic effect of ethanol
     Toxic effect of ethyl alcohol

     Excludes2   acute alcohol intoxication or 'hangover' effects (F10.129, F10.229, F10.929)
       drunkenness (F10.129, F10.229, F10.929)
       pathological alcohol intoxication (F10.129, F10.229, F10.929)

     ● T51.0X   Toxic effect of ethanol

       ● T51.0X1   Toxic effect of ethanol, accidental (unintentional)
         Toxic effect of ethanol NOS

       ● T51.0X2   Toxic effect of ethanol, intentional self-harm

       ● T51.0X3   Toxic effect of ethanol, assault

       ● T51.0X4   Toxic effect of ethanol, undetermined

   ● T51.1   Toxic effect of methanol
     Toxic effect of methyl alcohol

     ● T51.1X   Toxic effect of methanol

       ● T51.1X1   Toxic effect of methanol, accidental (unintentional)
         Toxic effect of methanol NOS

       ● T51.1X2   Toxic effect of methanol, intentional self-harm

       ● T51.1X3   Toxic effect of methanol, assault

       ● T51.1X4   Toxic effect of methanol, undetermined

   ● T51.2   Toxic effect of 2-Propanol
     Toxic effect of isopropyl alcohol

     ● T51.2X   Toxic effect of 2-Propanol

       ● T51.2X1   Toxic effect of 2-Propanol, accidental (unintentional)
         Toxic effect of 2-Propanol NOS

       ● T51.2X2   Toxic effect of 2-Propanol, intentional self-harm

       ● T51.2X3   Toxic effect of 2-Propanol, assault

       ● T51.2X4   Toxic effect of 2-Propanol, undetermined

   ● T51.3   Toxic effect of fusel oil
     Toxic effect of amyl alcohol
     Toxic effect of butyl [1-butanol] alcohol
     Toxic effect of propyl [1-propanol] alcohol

     ● T51.3X   Toxic effect of fusel oil

       ● T51.3X1   Toxic effect of fusel oil, accidental (unintentional)
         Toxic effect of fusel oil NOS

       ● T51.3X2   Toxic effect of fusel oil, intentional self-harm

       ● T51.3X3   Toxic effect of fusel oil, assault

       ● T51.3X4   Toxic effect of fusel oil, undetermined

● **T51.8   Toxic effect of other alcohols**
    ● **T51.8X   Toxic effect of other alcohols**
        ● **T51.8X1   Toxic effect of other alcohols,
                        accidental (unintentional)**
                        Toxic effect of other alcohols NOS
        ● **T51.8X2   Toxic effect of other alcohols,
                        intentional self-harm**
        ● **T51.8X3   Toxic effect of other alcohols, assault**
        ● **T51.8X4   Toxic effect of other alcohols,
                        undetermined**
● **T51.9   Toxic effect of unspecified alcohol**
    X● **T51.91   Toxic effect of unspecified alcohol, accidental
                    (unintentional)**
    X● **T51.92   Toxic effect of unspecified alcohol, intentional
                    self-harm**
    X● **T51.93   Toxic effect of unspecified alcohol, assault**
    X● **T51.94   Toxic effect of unspecified alcohol,
                    undetermined**
● **T52   Toxic effect of organic solvents**

> **Excludes1**   halogen derivatives of aliphatic and aromatic
>   hydrocarbons (T53.-)

> The appropriate 7th character is to be added to each code from
> category T52

> | A | initial encounter |
> |---|---|
> | D | subsequent encounter |
> | S | sequela |

● **T52.0   Toxic effects of petroleum products**
            Toxic effects of gasoline [petrol]
            Toxic effects of kerosene [paraffin oil]
            Toxic effects of paraffin wax
            Toxic effects of ether petroleum
            Toxic effects of naphtha petroleum
            Toxic effects of spirit petroleum
    ● **T52.0X   Toxic effects of petroleum products**
        ● **T52.0X1   Toxic effect of petroleum products,
                        accidental (unintentional)**
                        Toxic effects of petroleum products
                        NOS
        ● **T52.0X2   Toxic effect of petroleum products,
                        intentional self-harm**
        ● **T52.0X3   Toxic effect of petroleum products,
                        assault**
        ● **T52.0X4   Toxic effect of petroleum products,
                        undetermined**
● **T52.1   Toxic effects of benzene**

> **Excludes1**   homologues of benzene (T52.2)
>   nitroderivatives and aminoderivatives of
>   benzene and its homologues (T65.3)

    ● **T52.1X   Toxic effects of benzene**
        ● **T52.1X1   Toxic effect of benzene, accidental
                        (unintentional)**
                        Toxic effects of benzene NOS
        ● **T52.1X2   Toxic effect of benzene, intentional
                        self-harm**
        ● **T52.1X3   Toxic effect of benzene, assault**
        ● **T52.1X4   Toxic effect of benzene, undetermined**
● **T52.2   Toxic effects of homologues of benzene**
            Toxic effects of toluene [methylbenzene]
            Toxic effects of xylene [dimethylbenzene]
    ● **T52.2X   Toxic effects of homologues of benzene**
        ● **T52.2X1   Toxic effect of homologues of
                        benzene, accidental (unintentional)**
                        Toxic effects of homologues of
                        benzene NOS
        ● **T52.2X2   Toxic effect of homologues of
                        benzene, intentional self-harm**
        ● **T52.2X3   Toxic effect of homologues of
                        benzene, assault**
        ● **T52.2X4   Toxic effect of homologues of
                        benzene, undetermined**

● **T52.3   Toxic effects of glycols**
    ● **T52.3X   Toxic effects of glycols**
        ● **T52.3X1   Toxic effect of glycols, accidental
                        (unintentional)**
                        Toxic effects of glycols NOS
        ● **T52.3X2   Toxic effect of glycols, intentional
                        self-harm**
        ● **T52.3X3   Toxic effect of glycols, assault**
        ● **T52.3X4   Toxic effect of glycols, undetermined**
● **T52.4   Toxic effects of ketones**
    ● **T52.4X   Toxic effects of ketones**
        ● **T52.4X1   Toxic effect of ketones, accidental
                        (unintentional)**
                        Toxic effects of ketones NOS
        ● **T52.4X2   Toxic effect of ketones, intentional
                        self-harm**
        ● **T52.4X3   Toxic effect of ketones, assault**
        ● **T52.4X4   Toxic effect of ketones, undetermined**
● **T52.8   Toxic effects of other organic solvents**
    ● **T52.8X   Toxic effects of other organic solvents**
        ● **T52.8X1   Toxic effect of other organic solvents,
                        accidental (unintentional)**
                        Toxic effects of other organic
                        solvents NOS
        ● **T52.8X2   Toxic effect of other organic solvents,
                        intentional self-harm**
        ● **T52.8X3   Toxic effect of other organic solvents,
                        assault**
        ● **T52.8X4   Toxic effect of other organic solvents,
                        undetermined**
● **T52.9   Toxic effects of unspecified organic solvent**
    X● **T52.91   Toxic effect of unspecified organic solvent,
                    accidental (unintentional)**
    X● **T52.92   Toxic effect of unspecified organic solvent,
                    intentional self-harm**
    X● **T52.93   Toxic effect of unspecified organic solvent,
                    assault**
    X● **T52.94   Toxic effect of unspecified organic solvent,
                    undetermined**
● **T53   Toxic effect of halogen derivatives of aliphatic and aromatic
            hydrocarbons**

> The appropriate 7th character is to be added to each code from
> category T53

> | A | initial encounter |
> |---|---|
> | D | subsequent encounter |
> | S | sequela |

● **T53.0   Toxic effects of carbon tetrachloride**
            Toxic effects of tetrachloromethane
    ● **T53.0X   Toxic effects of carbon tetrachloride**
        ● **T53.0X1   Toxic effect of carbon tetrachloride,
                        accidental (unintentional)**
                        Toxic effects of carbon tetrachloride
                        NOS
        ● **T53.0X2   Toxic effect of carbon tetrachloride,
                        intentional self-harm**
        ● **T53.0X3   Toxic effect of carbon tetrachloride,
                        assault**
        ● **T53.0X4   Toxic effect of carbon tetrachloride,
                        undetermined**

CHAPTER 19 (S00-T88)

N Newborn Age: 0   **P** Pediatric Age: 0–17   **M** Maternity DX: 12–55   **A** Adult Age: 15–124   ♀ Females Only   ♂ Males Only

🐱 Complication\Comorbidity   🐱 Major C\C   (Ex) CC/MCC Exclusions   🐱 Hospital-Acquired Condition

1473

● **T53.1   Toxic effects of chloroform**
  Toxic effects of trichloromethane
  ● **T53.1X   Toxic effects of chloroform**
    ● **T53.1X1   Toxic effect of chloroform, accidental (unintentional)**
      Toxic effects of chloroform NOS
    ● **T53.1X2   Toxic effect of chloroform, intentional self-harm**
    ● **T53.1X3   Toxic effect of chloroform, assault**
    ● **T53.1X4   Toxic effect of chloroform, undetermined**
● **T53.2   Toxic effects of trichloroethylene**
  Toxic effects of trichloroethene
  ● **T53.2X   Toxic effects of trichloroethylene**
    ● **T53.2X1   Toxic effect of trichloroethylene, accidental (unintentional)**
      Toxic effects of trichloroethylene NOS
    ● **T53.2X2   Toxic effect of trichloroethylene, intentional self-harm**
    ● **T53.2X3   Toxic effect of trichloroethylene, assault**
    ● **T53.2X4   Toxic effect of trichloroethylene, undetermined**
● **T53.3   Toxic effects of tetrachloroethylene**
  Toxic effects of perchloroethylene
  Toxic effect of tetrachloroethene
  ● **T53.3X   Toxic effects of tetrachloroethylene**
    ● **T53.3X1   Toxic effect of tetrachloroethylene, accidental (unintentional)**
      Toxic effects of tetrachloroethylene NOS
    ● **T53.3X2   Toxic effect of tetrachloroethylene, intentional self-harm**
    ● **T53.3X3   Toxic effect of tetrachloroethylene, assault**
    ● **T53.3X4   Toxic effect of tetrachloroethylene, undetermined**
● **T53.4   Toxic effects of dichloromethane**
  Toxic effects of methylene chloride
  ● **T53.4X   Toxic effects of dichloromethane**
    ● **T53.4X1   Toxic effect of dichloromethane, accidental (unintentional)**
      Toxic effects of dichloromethane NOS
    ● **T53.4X2   Toxic effect of dichloromethane, intentional self-harm**
    ● **T53.4X3   Toxic effect of dichloromethane, assault**
    ● **T53.4X4   Toxic effect of dichloromethane, undetermined**
● **T53.5   Toxic effects of chlorofluorocarbons**
  ● **T53.5X   Toxic effects of chlorofluorocarbons**
    ● **T53.5X1   Toxic effect of chlorofluorocarbons, accidental (unintentional)**
      Toxic effects of chlorofluorocarbons NOS
    ● **T53.5X2   Toxic effect of chlorofluorocarbons, intentional self-harm**
    ● **T53.5X3   Toxic effect of chlorofluorocarbons, assault**
    ● **T53.5X4   Toxic effect of chlorofluorocarbons, undetermined**

● **T53.6   Toxic effects of other halogen derivatives of aliphatic hydrocarbons**
  ● **T53.6X   Toxic effects of other halogen derivatives of aliphatic hydrocarbons**
    ● **T53.6X1   Toxic effect of other halogen derivatives of aliphatic hydrocarbons, accidental (unintentional)**
      Toxic effects of other halogen derivatives of aliphatic hydrocarbons NOS
    ● **T53.6X2   Toxic effect of other halogen derivatives of aliphatic hydrocarbons, intentional self-harm**
    ● **T53.6X3   Toxic effect of other halogen derivatives of aliphatic hydrocarbons, assault**
    ● **T53.6X4   Toxic effect of other halogen derivatives of aliphatic hydrocarbons, undetermined**
● **T53.7   Toxic effects of other halogen derivatives of aromatic hydrocarbons**
  ● **T53.7X   Toxic effects of other halogen derivatives of aromatic hydrocarbons**
    ● **T53.7X1   Toxic effect of other halogen derivatives of aromatic hydrocarbons, accidental (unintentional)**
      Toxic effects of other halogen derivatives of aromatic hydrocarbons NOS
    ● **T53.7X2   Toxic effect of other halogen derivatives of aromatic hydrocarbons, intentional self-harm**
    ● **T53.7X3   Toxic effect of other halogen derivatives of aromatic hydrocarbons, assault**
    ● **T53.7X4   Toxic effect of other halogen derivatives of aromatic hydrocarbons, undetermined**
● **T53.9   Toxic effects of unspecified halogen derivatives of aliphatic and aromatic hydrocarbons**
  X ● **T53.91   Toxic effect of unspecified halogen derivatives of aliphatic and aromatic hydrocarbons, accidental (unintentional)**
  X ● **T53.92   Toxic effect of unspecified halogen derivatives of aliphatic and aromatic hydrocarbons, intentional self-harm**
  X ● **T53.93   Toxic effect of unspecified halogen derivatives of aliphatic and aromatic hydrocarbons, assault**
  X ● **T53.94   Toxic effect of unspecified halogen derivatives of aliphatic and aromatic hydrocarbons, undetermined**

● **T54   Toxic effect of corrosive substances**
  The appropriate 7th character is to be added to each code from category T54

A	initial encounter
D	subsequent encounter
S	sequela

  ● **T54.0   Toxic effects of phenol and phenol homologues**
    ● **T54.0X   Toxic effects of phenol and phenol homologues**
      ● **T54.0X1   Toxic effect of phenol and phenol homologues, accidental (unintentional)**
        Toxic effects of phenol and phenol homologues NOS
      ● **T54.0X2   Toxic effect of phenol and phenol homologues, intentional self-harm**
      ● **T54.0X3   Toxic effect of phenol and phenol homologues, assault**
      ● **T54.0X4   Toxic effect of phenol and phenol homologues, undetermined**

● **T54.1**   **Toxic effects of other corrosive organic compounds**
- ● **T54.1X**   **Toxic effects of other corrosive organic compounds**
  - ● **T54.1X1**   **Toxic effect of other corrosive organic compounds, accidental (unintentional)**
    Toxic effects of other corrosive organic compounds NOS
  - ● **T54.1X2**   **Toxic effect of other corrosive organic compounds, intentional self-harm**
  - ● **T54.1X3**   **Toxic effect of other corrosive organic compounds, assault**
  - ● **T54.1X4**   **Toxic effect of other corrosive organic compounds, undetermined**

● **T54.2**   **Toxic effects of corrosive acids and acid-like substances**
Toxic effects of hydrochloric acid
Toxic effects of sulfuric acid
- ● **T54.2X**   **Toxic effects of corrosive acids and acid-like substances**
  - ● **T54.2X1**   **Toxic effect of corrosive acids and acid-like substances, accidental (unintentional)**
    Toxic effects of corrosive acids and acid-like substances NOS
  - ● **T54.2X2**   **Toxic effect of corrosive acids and acid-like substances, intentional self-harm**
  - ● **T54.2X3**   **Toxic effect of corrosive acids and acid-like substances, assault**
  - ● **T54.2X4**   **Toxic effect of corrosive acids and acid-like substances, undetermined**

● **T54.3**   **Toxic effects of corrosive alkalis and alkali-like substances**
Toxic effects of potassium hydroxide
Toxic effects of sodium hydroxide
- ● **T54.3X**   **Toxic effects of corrosive alkalis and alkali-like substances**
  - ● **T54.3X1**   **Toxic effect of corrosive alkalis and alkali-like substances, accidental (unintentional)**
    Toxic effects of corrosive alkalis and alkali-like substances NOS
  - ● **T54.3X2**   **Toxic effect of corrosive alkalis and alkali-like substances, intentional self-harm**
  - ● **T54.3X3**   **Toxic effect of corrosive alkalis and alkali-like substances, assault**
  - ● **T54.3X4**   **Toxic effect of corrosive alkalis and alkali-like substances, undetermined**

● **T54.9**   **Toxic effects of unspecified corrosive substance**
- X● **T54.91**   **Toxic effect of unspecified corrosive substance, accidental (unintentional)**
- X● **T54.92**   **Toxic effect of unspecified corrosive substance, intentional self-harm**
- X● **T54.93**   **Toxic effect of unspecified corrosive substance, assault**
- X● **T54.94**   **Toxic effect of unspecified corrosive substance, undetermined**

● **T55**   **Toxic effect of soaps and detergents**
The appropriate 7th character is to be added to each code from category T55

> | A | initial encounter |
> | D | subsequent encounter |
> | S | sequela |

- ● **T55.0**   **Toxic effect of soaps**
  - ● **T55.0X**   **Toxic effect of soaps**
    - ● **T55.0X1**   **Toxic effect of soaps, accidental (unintentional)**
      Toxic effect of soaps NOS
    - ● **T55.0X2**   **Toxic effect of soaps, intentional self-harm**
    - ● **T55.0X3**   **Toxic effect of soaps, assault**
    - ● **T55.0X4**   **Toxic effect of soaps, undetermined**
- ● **T55.1**   **Toxic effect of detergents**
  - ● **T55.1X**   **Toxic effect of detergents**
    - ● **T55.1X1**   **Toxic effect of detergents, accidental (unintentional)**
      Toxic effect of detergents NOS
    - ● **T55.1X2**   **Toxic effect of detergents, intentional self-harm**
    - ● **T55.1X3**   **Toxic effect of detergents, assault**
    - ● **T55.1X4**   **Toxic effect of detergents, undetermined**

● **T56**   **Toxic effect of metals**

Includes   toxic effects of fumes and vapors of metals
         toxic effects of metals from all sources, except medicinal substances

Use additional code to identify any retained metal foreign body, if applicable (Z18.0-, T18.1-)

Excludes1   arsenic and its compounds (T57.0)
         manganese and its compounds (T57.2)

The appropriate 7th character is to be added to each code from category T56

> | A | initial encounter |
> | D | subsequent encounter |
> | S | sequela |

- ● **T56.0**   **Toxic effects of lead and its compounds**
  - ● **T56.0X**   **Toxic effects of lead and its compounds**
    - ● **T56.0X1**   **Toxic effect of lead and its compounds, accidental (unintentional)**
      Toxic effects of lead and its compounds NOS
    - ● **T56.0X2**   **Toxic effect of lead and its compounds, intentional self-harm**
    - ● **T56.0X3**   **Toxic effect of lead and its compounds, assault**
    - ● **T56.0X4**   **Toxic effect of lead and its compounds, undetermined**
- ● **T56.1**   **Toxic effects of mercury and its compounds**
  - ● **T56.1X**   **Toxic effects of mercury and its compounds**
    - ● **T56.1X1**   **Toxic effect of mercury and its compounds, accidental (unintentional)**
      Toxic effects of mercury and its compounds NOS
    - ● **T56.1X2**   **Toxic effect of mercury and its compounds, intentional self-harm**
    - ● **T56.1X3**   **Toxic effect of mercury and its compounds, assault**
    - ● **T56.1X4**   **Toxic effect of mercury and its compounds, undetermined**

CHAPTER 19 (S00-T88)

N Newborn Age: 0   **P** Pediatric Age: 0–17   **M** Maternity DX: 12–55   **A** Adult Age: 15–124   ♀ Females Only   ♂ Males Only

🐾 Complication\Comorbidity   🐾 Major C\C   (Ex) CC/MCC Exclusions   🐾 Hospital-Acquired Condition

1475

● **T56.2**   Toxic effects of chromium and its compounds
  ● **T56.2X**   Toxic effects of chromium and its compounds
    ● **T56.2X1**   **Toxic effect of chromium and its compounds, accidental (unintentional)**
       Toxic effects of chromium and its compounds NOS
    ● **T56.2X2**   **Toxic effect of chromium and its compounds, intentional self-harm**
    ● **T56.2X3**   **Toxic effect of chromium and its compounds, assault**
    ● **T56.2X4**   **Toxic effect of chromium and its compounds, undetermined**

● **T56.3**   Toxic effects of cadmium and its compounds
  ● **T56.3X**   Toxic effects of cadmium and its compounds
    ● **T56.3X1**   **Toxic effect of cadmium and its compounds, accidental (unintentional)**
       Toxic effects of cadmium and its compounds NOS
    ● **T56.3X2**   **Toxic effect of cadmium and its compounds, intentional self-harm**
    ● **T56.3X3**   **Toxic effect of cadmium and its compounds, assault**
    ● **T56.3X4**   **Toxic effect of cadmium and its compounds, undetermined**

● **T56.4**   Toxic effects of copper and its compounds
  ● **T56.4X**   Toxic effects of copper and its compounds
    ● **T56.4X1**   **Toxic effect of copper and its compounds, accidental (unintentional)**
       Toxic effects of copper and its compounds NOS
    ● **T56.4X2**   **Toxic effect of copper and its compounds, intentional self-harm**
    ● **T56.4X3**   **Toxic effect of copper and its compounds, assault**
    ● **T56.4X4**   **Toxic effect of copper and its compounds, undetermined**

● **T56.5**   Toxic effects of zinc and its compounds
  ● **T56.5X**   Toxic effects of zinc and its compounds
    ● **T56.5X1**   **Toxic effect of zinc and its compounds, accidental (unintentional)**
       Toxic effects of zinc and its compounds NOS
    ● **T56.5X2**   **Toxic effect of zinc and its compounds, intentional self-harm**
    ● **T56.5X3**   **Toxic effect of zinc and its compounds, assault**
    ● **T56.5X4**   **Toxic effect of zinc and its compounds, undetermined**

● **T56.6**   Toxic effects of tin and its compounds
  ● **T56.6X**   Toxic effects of tin and its compounds
    ● **T56.6X1**   **Toxic effect of tin and its compounds, accidental (unintentional)**
       Toxic effects of tin and its compounds NOS
    ● **T56.6X2**   **Toxic effect of tin and its compounds, intentional self-harm**
    ● **T56.6X3**   **Toxic effect of tin and its compounds, assault**
    ● **T56.6X4**   **Toxic effect of tin and its compounds, undetermined**

● **T56.7**   Toxic effects of beryllium and its compounds
  ● **T56.7X**   Toxic effects of beryllium and its compounds
    ● **T56.7X1**   **Toxic effect of beryllium and its compounds, accidental (unintentional)**
       Toxic effects of beryllium and its compounds NOS
    ● **T56.7X2**   **Toxic effect of beryllium and its compounds, intentional self-harm**
    ● **T56.7X3**   **Toxic effect of beryllium and its compounds, assault**
    ● **T56.7X4**   **Toxic effect of beryllium and its compounds, undetermined**

● **T56.8**   Toxic effects of other metals
  ● **T56.81**   Toxic effect of thallium
    ● **T56.811**   **Toxic effect of thallium, accidental (unintentional)**
       Toxic effect of thallium NOS
    ● **T56.812**   **Toxic effect of thallium, intentional self-harm**
    ● **T56.813**   **Toxic effect of thallium, assault**
    ● **T56.814**   **Toxic effect of thallium, undetermined**
  ● **T56.89**   Toxic effects of other metals
    ● **T56.891**   **Toxic effect of other metals, accidental (unintentional)**
       Toxic effects of other metals NOS
    ● **T56.892**   **Toxic effect of other metals, intentional self-harm**
    ● **T56.893**   **Toxic effect of other metals, assault**
    ● **T56.894**   **Toxic effect of other metals, undetermined**

● **T56.9**   Toxic effects of unspecified metal
  X ● **T56.91**   **Toxic effect of unspecified metal, accidental (unintentional)**
  X ● **T56.92**   **Toxic effect of unspecified metal, intentional self-harm**
  X ● **T56.93**   **Toxic effect of unspecified metal, assault**
  X ● **T56.94**   **Toxic effect of unspecified metal, undetermined**

● **T57**   Toxic effect of other inorganic substances
   The appropriate 7th character is to be added to each code from category T57

A	initial encounter
D	subsequent encounter
S	sequela

● **T57.0**   Toxic effect of arsenic and its compounds
  ● **T57.0X**   Toxic effect of arsenic and its compounds
    ● **T57.0X1**   **Toxic effect of arsenic and its compounds, accidental (unintentional)**
       Toxic effect of arsenic and its compounds NOS
    ● **T57.0X2**   **Toxic effect of arsenic and its compounds, intentional self-harm**
    ● **T57.0X3**   **Toxic effect of arsenic and its compounds, assault**
    ● **T57.0X4**   **Toxic effect of arsenic and its compounds, undetermined**

◄ New   ◄ Revised   ~~deleted~~ Deleted   Excludes 1   Excludes 2   Includes   Use additional   Code first   Code also   Unspecified
OGCR Official Guidelines   ● Unacceptable Principal Diagnosis   X Assign placeholder X   ● Use Additional Character(s)   ▶ Manifestation Code   **Coding Clinic**

● **T57.1**   **Toxic effect of phosphorus and its compounds**
    Excludes1   organophosphate insecticides (T60.0)
  ● **T57.1X**   **Toxic effect of phosphorus and its compounds**
    ● **T57.1X1**   **Toxic effect of phosphorus and its compounds, accidental (unintentional)**
      Toxic effect of phosphorus and its compounds NOS
    ● **T57.1X2**   **Toxic effect of phosphorus and its compounds, intentional self-harm**
    ● **T57.1X3**   **Toxic effect of phosphorus and its compounds, assault**
    ● **T57.1X4**   **Toxic effect of phosphorus and its compounds, undetermined**
● **T57.2**   **Toxic effect of manganese and its compounds**
  ● **T57.2X**   **Toxic effect of manganese and its compounds**
    ● **T57.2X1**   **Toxic effect of manganese and its compounds, accidental (unintentional)**
      Toxic effect of manganese and its compounds NOS
    ● **T57.2X2**   **Toxic effect of manganese and its compounds, intentional self-harm**
    ● **T57.2X3**   **Toxic effect of manganese and its compounds, assault**
    ● **T57.2X4**   **Toxic effect of manganese and its compounds, undetermined**
● **T57.3**   **Toxic effect of hydrogen cyanide**
  ● **T57.3X**   **Toxic effect of hydrogen cyanide**
    ● **T57.3X1**   **Toxic effect of hydrogen cyanide, accidental (unintentional)**
      Toxic effect of hydrogen cyanide NOS
    ● **T57.3X2**   **Toxic effect of hydrogen cyanide, intentional self-harm**
    ● **T57.3X3**   **Toxic effect of hydrogen cyanide, assault**
    ● **T57.3X4**   **Toxic effect of hydrogen cyanide, undetermined**
● **T57.8**   **Toxic effect of other specified inorganic substances**
  ● **T57.8X**   **Toxic effect of other specified inorganic substances**
    ● **T57.8X1**   **Toxic effect of other specified inorganic substances, accidental (unintentional)**
      Toxic effect of other specified inorganic substances NOS
    ● **T57.8X2**   **Toxic effect of other specified inorganic substances, intentional self-harm**
    ● **T57.8X3**   **Toxic effect of other specified inorganic substances, assault**
    ● **T57.8X4**   **Toxic effect of other specified inorganic substances, undetermined**
● **T57.9**   **Toxic effect of unspecified inorganic substance**
  X● **T57.91**   **Toxic effect of unspecified inorganic substance, accidental (unintentional)**
  X● **T57.92**   **Toxic effect of unspecified inorganic substance, intentional self-harm**
  X● **T57.93**   **Toxic effect of unspecified inorganic substance, assault**
  X● **T57.94**   **Toxic effect of unspecified inorganic substance, undetermined**

● **T58**   **Toxic effect of carbon monoxide**
    Includes   asphyxiation from carbon monoxide
      toxic effect of carbon monoxide from all sources
  The appropriate 7th character is to be added to each code from category T58

A	initial encounter
D	subsequent encounter
S	sequela

● **T58.0**   **Toxic effect of carbon monoxide from motor vehicle exhaust**
    Toxic effect of exhaust gas from gas engine
    Toxic effect of exhaust gas from motor pump
  X● **T58.01**   **Toxic effect of carbon monoxide from motor vehicle exhaust, accidental (unintentional)**
  X● **T58.02**   **Toxic effect of carbon monoxide from motor vehicle exhaust, intentional self-harm**
  X● **T58.03**   **Toxic effect of carbon monoxide from motor vehicle exhaust, assault**
  X● **T58.04**   **Toxic effect of carbon monoxide from motor vehicle exhaust, undetermined**
● **T58.1**   **Toxic effect of carbon monoxide from utility gas**
    Toxic effect of acetylene
    Toxic effect of gas NOS used for lighting, heating, cooking
    Toxic effect of water gas
  X● **T58.11**   **Toxic effect of carbon monoxide from utility gas, accidental (unintentional)**
  X● **T58.12**   **Toxic effect of carbon monoxide from utility gas, intentional self-harm**
  X● **T58.13**   **Toxic effect of carbon monoxide from utility gas, assault**
  X● **T58.14**   **Toxic effect of carbon monoxide from utility gas, undetermined**
● **T58.2**   **Toxic effect of carbon monoxide from incomplete combustion of other domestic fuels**
    Toxic effect of carbon monoxide from incomplete combustion of coal, coke, kerosene, wood
  ● **T58.2X**   **Toxic effect of carbon monoxide from incomplete combustion of other domestic fuels**
    ● **T58.2X1**   **Toxic effect of carbon monoxide from incomplete combustion of other domestic fuels, accidental (unintentional)**
    ● **T58.2X2**   **Toxic effect of carbon monoxide from incomplete combustion of other domestic fuels, intentional self-harm**
    ● **T58.2X3**   **Toxic effect of carbon monoxide from incomplete combustion of other domestic fuels, assault**
    ● **T58.2X4**   **Toxic effect of carbon monoxide from incomplete combustion of other domestic fuels, undetermined**
● **T58.8**   **Toxic effect of carbon monoxide from other source**
    Toxic effect of carbon monoxide from blast furnace gas
    Toxic effect of carbon monoxide from fuels in industrial use
    Toxic effect of carbon monoxide from kiln vapor
  ● **T58.8X**   **Toxic effect of carbon monoxide from other source**
    ● **T58.8X1**   **Toxic effect of carbon monoxide from other source, accidental (unintentional)**
    ● **T58.8X2**   **Toxic effect of carbon monoxide from other source, intentional self-harm**
    ● **T58.8X3**   **Toxic effect of carbon monoxide from other source, assault**
    ● **T58.8X4**   **Toxic effect of carbon monoxide from other source, undetermined**

CHAPTER 19 (S00-T88)

● **T58.9**   Toxic effect of carbon monoxide from unspecified source

   X● **T58.91**   Toxic effect of carbon monoxide from unspecified source, accidental (unintentional)

   X● **T58.92**   Toxic effect of carbon monoxide from unspecified source, intentional self-harm

   X● **T58.93**   Toxic effect of carbon monoxide from unspecified source, assault

   X● **T58.94**   Toxic effect of carbon monoxide from unspecified source, undetermined

● **T59**   Toxic effect of other gases, fumes and vapors

     | **Includes** | aerosol propellants |
     | **Excludes1** | chlorofluorocarbons (T53.5) |

   The appropriate 7th character is to be added to each code from category T59

     A   initial encounter
     D   subsequent encounter
     S   sequela

   ● **T59.Ø**   Toxic effect of nitrogen oxides

     ● **T59.ØX**   Toxic effect of nitrogen oxides

       ● **T59.ØX1**   Toxic effect of nitrogen oxides, accidental (unintentional)
         Toxic effect of nitrogen oxides NOS

       ● **T59.ØX2**   Toxic effect of nitrogen oxides, intentional self-harm

       ● **T59.ØX3**   Toxic effect of nitrogen oxides, assault

       ● **T59.ØX4**   Toxic effect of nitrogen oxides, undetermined

   ● **T59.1**   Toxic effect of sulfur dioxide

     ● **T59.1X**   Toxic effect of sulfur dioxide

       ● **T59.1X1**   Toxic effect of sulfur dioxide, accidental (unintentional)
         Toxic effect of sulfur dioxide NOS

       ● **T59.1X2**   Toxic effect of sulfur dioxide, intentional self-harm

       ● **T59.1X3**   Toxic effect of sulfur dioxide, assault

       ● **T59.1X4**   Toxic effect of sulfur dioxide, undetermined

   ● **T59.2**   Toxic effect of formaldehyde

     ● **T59.2X**   Toxic effect of formaldehyde

       ● **T59.2X1**   Toxic effect of formaldehyde, accidental (unintentional)
         Toxic effect of formaldehyde NOS

       ● **T59.2X2**   Toxic effect of formaldehyde, intentional self-harm

       ● **T59.2X3**   Toxic effect of formaldehyde, assault

       ● **T59.2X4**   Toxic effect of formaldehyde, undetermined

   ● **T59.3**   Toxic effect of lacrimogenic gas
     Toxic effect of tear gas

     ● **T59.3X**   Toxic effect of lacrimogenic gas

       ● **T59.3X1**   Toxic effect of lacrimogenic gas, accidental (unintentional)
         Toxic effect of lacrimogenic gas NOS

       ● **T59.3X2**   Toxic effect of lacrimogenic gas, intentional self-harm

       ● **T59.3X3**   Toxic effect of lacrimogenic gas, assault

       ● **T59.3X4**   Toxic effect of lacrimogenic gas, undetermined

● **T59.4**   Toxic effect of chlorine gas

   ● **T59.4X**   Toxic effect of chlorine gas

     ● **T59.4X1**   Toxic effect of chlorine gas, accidental (unintentional)
       Toxic effect of chlorine gas NOS

     ● **T59.4X2**   Toxic effect of chlorine gas, intentional self-harm

     ● **T59.4X3**   Toxic effect of chlorine gas, assault

     ● **T59.4X4**   Toxic effect of chlorine gas, undetermined

● **T59.5**   Toxic effect of fluorine gas and hydrogen fluoride

   ● **T59.5X**   Toxic effect of fluorine gas and hydrogen fluoride

     ● **T59.5X1**   Toxic effect of fluorine gas and hydrogen fluoride, accidental (unintentional)
       Toxic effect of fluorine gas and hydrogen fluoride NOS

     ● **T59.5X2**   Toxic effect of fluorine gas and hydrogen fluoride, intentional self-harm

     ● **T59.5X3**   Toxic effect of fluorine gas and hydrogen fluoride, assault

     ● **T59.5X4**   Toxic effect of fluorine gas and hydrogen fluoride, undetermined

● **T59.6**   Toxic effect of hydrogen sulfide

   ● **T59.6X**   Toxic effect of hydrogen sulfide

     ● **T59.6X1**   Toxic effect of hydrogen sulfide, accidental (unintentional)
       Toxic effect of hydrogen sulfide NOS

     ● **T59.6X2**   Toxic effect of hydrogen sulfide, intentional self-harm

     ● **T59.6X3**   Toxic effect of hydrogen sulfide, assault

     ● **T59.6X4**   Toxic effect of hydrogen sulfide, undetermined

● **T59.7**   Toxic effect of carbon dioxide

   ● **T59.7X**   Toxic effect of carbon dioxide

     ● **T59.7X1**   Toxic effect of carbon dioxide, accidental (unintentional)
       Toxic effect of carbon dioxide NOS

     ● **T59.7X2**   Toxic effect of carbon dioxide, intentional self-harm

     ● **T59.7X3**   Toxic effect of carbon dioxide, assault

     ● **T59.7X4**   Toxic effect of carbon dioxide, undetermined

● **T59.8**   Toxic effect of other specified gases, fumes and vapors

   ● **T59.81**   Toxic effect of smoke
     Smoke inhalation

     | **Excludes2** | toxic effect of cigarette (tobacco) smoke (T65.22-) |

     ● **T59.811**   Toxic effect of smoke, accidental (unintentional)
       Toxic effect of smoke NOS

     ● **T59.812**   Toxic effect of smoke, intentional self-harm

     ● **T59.813**   Toxic effect of smoke, assault

     ● **T59.814**   Toxic effect of smoke, undetermined

   ● **T59.89**   Toxic effect of other specified gases, fumes and vapors

     ● **T59.891**   Toxic effect of other specified gases, fumes and vapors, accidental (unintentional)

     ● **T59.892**   Toxic effect of other specified gases, fumes and vapors, intentional self-harm

     ● **T59.893**   Toxic effect of other specified gases, fumes and vapors, assault

     ● **T59.894**   Toxic effect of other specified gases, fumes and vapors, undetermined

◀ New   ◀▦ Revised   ~~deleted~~ Deleted   Excludes 1   Excludes 2   Includes   Use additional   Code first   Code also   Unspecified

OGCR Official Guidelines   ● Unacceptable Principal Diagnosis   X Assign placeholder X   ● Use Additional Character(s)   ▶ Manifestation Code   **Coding Clinic**

- **T59.9**   Toxic effect of unspecified gases, fumes and vapors
  - X ● **T59.91**   Toxic effect of unspecified gases, fumes and vapors, accidental (unintentional)
  - X ● **T59.92**   Toxic effect of unspecified gases, fumes and vapors, intentional self-harm
  - X ● **T59.93**   Toxic effect of unspecified gases, fumes and vapors, assault
  - X ● **T59.94**   Toxic effect of unspecified gases, fumes and vapors, undetermined

- ● **T60**   Toxic effect of pesticides

  Includes   toxic effect of wood preservatives

  The appropriate 7th character is to be added to each code from category T60

A	initial encounter
D	subsequent encounter
S	sequela

  - ● **T60.0**   Toxic effect of organophosphate and carbamate insecticides
    - ● **T60.0X**   Toxic effect of organophosphate and carbamate insecticides
      - ● **T60.0X1**   Toxic effect of organophosphate and carbamate insecticides, accidental (unintentional)
        Toxic effect of organophosphate and carbamate insecticides NOS
      - ● **T60.0X2**   Toxic effect of organophosphate and carbamate insecticides, intentional self-harm
      - ● **T60.0X3**   Toxic effect of organophosphate and carbamate insecticides, assault
      - ● **T60.0X4**   Toxic effect of organophosphate and carbamate insecticides, undetermined
  - ● **T60.1**   Toxic effect of halogenated insecticides

    Excludes1   chlorinated hydrocarbon (T53.-)
    - ● **T60.1X**   Toxic effect of halogenated insecticides
      - ● **T60.1X1**   Toxic effect of halogenated insecticides, accidental (unintentional)
        Toxic effect of halogenated insecticides NOS
      - ● **T60.1X2**   Toxic effect of halogenated insecticides, intentional self-harm
      - ● **T60.1X3**   Toxic effect of halogenated insecticides, assault
      - ● **T60.1X4**   Toxic effect of halogenated insecticides, undetermined
  - ● **T60.2**   Toxic effect of other insecticides
    - ● **T60.2X**   Toxic effect of other insecticides
      - ● **T60.2X1**   Toxic effect of other insecticides, accidental (unintentional)
        Toxic effect of other insecticides NOS
      - ● **T60.2X2**   Toxic effect of other insecticides, intentional self-harm
      - ● **T60.2X3**   Toxic effect of other insecticides, assault
      - ● **T60.2X4**   Toxic effect of other insecticides, undetermined
  - ● **T60.3**   Toxic effect of herbicides and fungicides
    - ● **T60.3X**   Toxic effect of herbicides and fungicides
      - ● **T60.3X1**   Toxic effect of herbicides and fungicides, accidental (unintentional)
        Toxic effect of herbicides and fungicides NOS
      - ● **T60.3X2**   Toxic effect of herbicides and fungicides, intentional self-harm
      - ● **T60.3X3**   Toxic effect of herbicides and fungicides, assault
      - ● **T60.3X4**   Toxic effect of herbicides and fungicides, undetermined

- ● **T60.4**   Toxic effect of rodenticides

  Excludes1   strychnine and its salts (T65.1)
  thallium (T56.81-)
  - ● **T60.4X**   Toxic effect of rodenticides
    - ● **T60.4X1**   Toxic effect of rodenticides, accidental (unintentional)
      Toxic effect of rodenticides NOS
    - ● **T60.4X2**   Toxic effect of rodenticides, intentional self-harm
    - ● **T60.4X3**   Toxic effect of rodenticides, assault
    - ● **T60.4X4**   Toxic effect of rodenticides, undetermined
- ● **T60.8**   Toxic effect of other pesticides
  - ● **T60.8X**   Toxic effect of other pesticides
    - ● **T60.8X1**   Toxic effect of other pesticides, accidental (unintentional)
      Toxic effect of other pesticides NOS
    - ● **T60.8X2**   Toxic effect of other pesticides, intentional self-harm
    - ● **T60.8X3**   Toxic effect of other pesticides, assault
    - ● **T60.8X4**   Toxic effect of other pesticides, undetermined
- ● **T60.9**   Toxic effect of unspecified pesticide
  - X ● **T60.91**   Toxic effect of unspecified pesticide, accidental (unintentional)
  - X ● **T60.92**   Toxic effect of unspecified pesticide, intentional self-harm
  - X ● **T60.93**   Toxic effect of unspecified pesticide, assault
  - X ● **T60.94**   Toxic effect of unspecified pesticide, undetermined

- ● **T61**   Toxic effect of noxious substances eaten as seafood

  Excludes1   allergic reaction to food, such as:
  anaphylactic reaction or shock due to adverse food reaction (T78.0-)
  bacterial foodborne intoxications (A05.-)
  dermatitis (L23.6, L25.4, L27.2)
  food protein-induced enterocolitis syndrome (K52.21) ◀
  food protein-induced enteropathy (K52.22) ◀
  gastroenteritis (noninfective) (K52.29) ◀
  toxic effect of aflatoxin and other mycotoxins (T64)
  toxic effect of cyanides (T65.0-)
  toxic effect of harmful algae bloom (T65.82-)
  toxic effect of hydrogen cyanide (T57.3-)
  toxic effect of mercury (T56.1-)
  toxic effect of red tide (T65.82-)

  The appropriate 7th character is to be added to each code from category T61

A	initial encounter
D	subsequent encounter
S	sequela

  - ● **T61.0**   Ciguatera fish poisoning
    - X ● **T61.01**   Ciguatera fish poisoning, accidental (unintentional)
    - X ● **T61.02**   Ciguatera fish poisoning, intentional self-harm
    - X ● **T61.03**   Ciguatera fish poisoning, assault
    - X ● **T61.04**   Ciguatera fish poisoning, undetermined
  - ● **T61.1**   Scombroid fish poisoning
    Histamine-like syndrome
    - X ● **T61.11**   Scombroid fish poisoning, accidental (unintentional)
    - X ● **T61.12**   Scombroid fish poisoning, intentional self-harm
    - X ● **T61.13**   Scombroid fish poisoning, assault
    - X ● **T61.14**   Scombroid fish poisoning, undetermined

CHAPTER 19 (S00-T88)

N Newborn Age: 0   **P** Pediatric Age: 0–17   **M** Maternity DX: 12–55   **A** Adult Age: 15–124   ♀ Females Only   ♂ Males Only

🖢 Complication\Comorbidity   🖢 Major C\C   (Ex) CC/MCC Exclusions   🖢 Hospital-Acquired Condition

1479

- ● T61.7   Other fish and shellfish poisoning
  - ● T61.77   Other fish poisoning
    - ● T61.771   Other fish poisoning, accidental (unintentional)
    - ● T61.772   Other fish poisoning, intentional self-harm
    - ● T61.773   Other fish poisoning, assault
    - ● T61.774   Other fish poisoning, undetermined
  - ● T61.78   Other shellfish poisoning
    - ● T61.781   Other shellfish poisoning, accidental (unintentional)
    - ● T61.782   Other shellfish poisoning, intentional self-harm
    - ● T61.783   Other shellfish poisoning, assault
    - ● T61.784   Other shellfish poisoning, undetermined
- ● T61.8   Toxic effect of other seafood
  - ● T61.8X   Toxic effect of other seafood
    - ● T61.8X1   Toxic effect of other seafood, accidental (unintentional)
    - ● T61.8X2   Toxic effect of other seafood, intentional self-harm
    - ● T61.8X3   Toxic effect of other seafood, assault
    - ● T61.8X4   Toxic effect of other seafood, undetermined
- ● T61.9   Toxic effect of unspecified seafood
  - X ● T61.91   Toxic effect of unspecified seafood, accidental (unintentional)
  - X ● T61.92   Toxic effect of unspecified seafood, intentional self-harm
  - X ● T61.93   Toxic effect of unspecified seafood, assault
  - X ● T61.94   Toxic effect of unspecified seafood, undetermined

- ● T62   Toxic effect of other noxious substances eaten as food

  Excludes1   allergic reaction to food, such as:
  anaphylactic shock (reaction) due to adverse food reaction (T78.0-)
  dermatitis (L23.6, L25.4, L27.2)
  food protein-induced enterocolitis syndrome (K52.21) ◀
  food protein-induced enteropathy (K52.22) ◀
  gastroenteritis (noninfective) (K52.29) ◀
  bacterial food borne intoxications (A05.-)
  toxic effect of aflatoxin and other mycotoxins (T64)
  toxic effect of cyanides (T65.0-)
  toxic effect of hydrogen cyanide (T57.3-)
  toxic effect of mercury (T56.1-)

  The appropriate 7th character is to be added to each code from category T62

A	initial encounter
D	subsequent encounter
S	sequela

- ● T62.0   Toxic effect of ingested mushrooms
  - ● T62.0X   Toxic effect of ingested mushrooms
    - ● T62.0X1   Toxic effect of ingested mushrooms, accidental (unintentional)
      Toxic effect of ingested mushrooms NOS
    - ● T62.0X2   Toxic effect of ingested mushrooms, intentional self-harm
    - ● T62.0X3   Toxic effect of ingested mushrooms, assault
    - ● T62.0X4   Toxic effect of ingested mushrooms, undetermined

- ● T62.1   Toxic effect of ingested berries
  - ● T62.1X   Toxic effect of ingested berries
    - ● T62.1X1   Toxic effect of ingested berries, accidental (unintentional)
      Toxic effect of ingested berries NOS
    - ● T62.1X2   Toxic effect of ingested berries, intentional self-harm
    - ● T62.1X3   Toxic effect of ingested berries, assault
    - ● T62.1X4   Toxic effect of ingested berries, undetermined
- ● T62.2   Toxic effect of other ingested (parts of) plant(s)
  - ● T62.2X   Toxic effect of other ingested (parts of) plant(s)
    - ● T62.2X1   Toxic effect of other ingested (parts of) plant(s), accidental (unintentional)
      Toxic effect of other ingested (parts of) plant(s) NOS
    - ● T62.2X2   Toxic effect of other ingested (parts of) plant(s), intentional self-harm
    - ● T62.2X3   Toxic effect of other ingested (parts of) plant(s), assault
    - ● T62.2X4   Toxic effect of other ingested (parts of) plant(s), undetermined
- ● T62.8   Toxic effect of other specified noxious substances eaten as food
  - ● T62.8X   Toxic effect of other specified noxious substances eaten as food
    - ● T62.8X1   Toxic effect of other specified noxious substances eaten as food, accidental (unintentional)
      Toxic effect of other specified noxious substances eaten as food NOS
    - ● T62.8X2   Toxic effect of other specified noxious substances eaten as food, intentional self-harm
    - ● T62.8X3   Toxic effect of other specified noxious substances eaten as food, assault
    - ● T62.8X4   Toxic effect of other specified noxious substances eaten as food, undetermined
- ● T62.9   Toxic effect of unspecified noxious substance eaten as food
  - X ● T62.91   Toxic effect of unspecified noxious substance eaten as food, accidental (unintentional)
    Toxic effect of unspecified noxious substance eaten as food NOS
  - X ● T62.92   Toxic effect of unspecified noxious substance eaten as food, intentional self-harm
  - X ● T62.93   Toxic effect of unspecified noxious substance eaten as food, assault
  - X ● T62.94   Toxic effect of unspecified noxious substance eaten as food, undetermined

- ● T63   Toxic effect of contact with venomous animals and plants

  Includes   bite or touch of venomous animal
  pricked or stuck by thorn or leaf

  Excludes2   ingestion of toxic animal or plant (T61.-, T62.-)

  The appropriate 7th character is to be added to each code from category T63

A	initial encounter
D	subsequent encounter
S	sequela

- ● T63.0   Toxic effect of snake venom
  - ● T63.00   Toxic effect of unspecified snake venom
    - ● T63.001   Toxic effect of unspecified snake venom, accidental (unintentional)
      Toxic effect of unspecified snake venom NOS
    - ● T63.002   Toxic effect of unspecified snake venom, intentional self-harm

◀ New   ◀▥ Revised   deleted Deleted   Excludes 1   Excludes 2   Includes   Use additional   Code first   Code also   Unspecified

OGCR Official Guidelines   ● Unacceptable Principal Diagnosis   X Assign placeholder X   ● Use Additional Character(s)   ▶ Manifestation Code   **Coding Clinic**

●　**T63.003**   Toxic effect of unspecified snake venom, assault

●　**T63.004**   Toxic effect of unspecified snake venom, undetermined

●　**T63.01**   Toxic effect of rattlesnake venom

   ●　**T63.011**   Toxic effect of rattlesnake venom, accidental (unintentional)
       Toxic effect of rattlesnake venom NOS

   ●　**T63.012**   Toxic effect of rattlesnake venom, intentional self-harm

   ●　**T63.013**   Toxic effect of rattlesnake venom, assault

   ●　**T63.014**   Toxic effect of rattlesnake venom, undetermined

●　**T63.02**   Toxic effect of coral snake venom

   ●　**T63.021**   Toxic effect of coral snake venom, accidental (unintentional)
       Toxic effect of coral snake venom NOS

   ●　**T63.022**   Toxic effect of coral snake venom, intentional self-harm

   ●　**T63.023**   Toxic effect of coral snake venom, assault

   ●　**T63.024**   Toxic effect of coral snake venom, undetermined

●　**T63.03**   Toxic effect of taipan venom

   ●　**T63.031**   Toxic effect of taipan venom, accidental (unintentional)
       Toxic effect of taipan venom NOS

   ●　**T63.032**   Toxic effect of taipan venom, intentional self-harm

   ●　**T63.033**   Toxic effect of taipan venom, assault

   ●　**T63.034**   Toxic effect of taipan venom, undetermined

●　**T63.04**   Toxic effect of cobra venom

   ●　**T63.041**   Toxic effect of cobra venom, accidental (unintentional)
       Toxic effect of cobra venom NOS

   ●　**T63.042**   Toxic effect of cobra venom, intentional self-harm

   ●　**T63.043**   Toxic effect of cobra venom, assault

   ●　**T63.044**   Toxic effect of cobra venom, undetermined

●　**T63.06**   Toxic effect of venom of other North and South American snake

   ●　**T63.061**   Toxic effect of venom of other North and South American snake, accidental (unintentional)
       Toxic effect of venom of other North and South American snake NOS

   ●　**T63.062**   Toxic effect of venom of other North and South American snake, intentional self-harm

   ●　**T63.063**   Toxic effect of venom of other North and South American snake, assault

   ●　**T63.064**   Toxic effect of venom of other North and South American snake, undetermined

●　**T63.07**   Toxic effect of venom of other Australian snake

   ●　**T63.071**   Toxic effect of venom of other Australian snake, accidental (unintentional)
       Toxic effect of venom of other Australian snake NOS

   ●　**T63.072**   Toxic effect of venom of other Australian snake, intentional self-harm

   ●　**T63.073**   Toxic effect of venom of other Australian snake, assault

   ●　**T63.074**   Toxic effect of venom of other Australian snake, undetermined

●　**T63.08**   Toxic effect of venom of other African and Asian snake

   ●　**T63.081**   Toxic effect of venom of other African and Asian snake, accidental (unintentional)
       Toxic effect of venom of other African and Asian snake NOS

   ●　**T63.082**   Toxic effect of venom of other African and Asian snake, intentional self-harm

   ●　**T63.083**   Toxic effect of venom of other African and Asian snake, assault

   ●　**T63.084**   Toxic effect of venom of other African and Asian snake, undetermined

●　**T63.09**   Toxic effect of venom of other snake

   ●　**T63.091**   Toxic effect of venom of other snake, accidental (unintentional)
       Toxic effect of venom of other snake NOS

   ●　**T63.092**   Toxic effect of venom of other snake, intentional self-harm

   ●　**T63.093**   Toxic effect of venom of other snake, assault

   ●　**T63.094**   Toxic effect of venom of other snake, undetermined

●　**T63.1**   Toxic effect of venom of other reptiles

   ●　**T63.11**   Toxic effect of venom of gila monster

      ●　**T63.111**   Toxic effect of venom of gila monster, accidental (unintentional)
          Toxic effect of venom of gila monster NOS

      ●　**T63.112**   Toxic effect of venom of gila monster, intentional self-harm

      ●　**T63.113**   Toxic effect of venom of gila monster, assault

      ●　**T63.114**   Toxic effect of venom of gila monster, undetermined

   ●　**T63.12**   Toxic effect of venom of other venomous lizard

      ●　**T63.121**   Toxic effect of venom of other venomous lizard, accidental (unintentional)
          Toxic effect of venom of other venomous lizard NOS

      ●　**T63.122**   Toxic effect of venom of other venomous lizard, intentional self-harm

      ●　**T63.123**   Toxic effect of venom of other venomous lizard, assault

      ●　**T63.124**   Toxic effect of venom of other venomous lizard, undetermined

CHAPTER 19 (S00–T88)

N Newborn Age: 0   **P** Pediatric Age: 0–17   **M** Maternity DX: 12–55   **A** Adult Age: 15–124   ♀ Females Only   ♂ Males Only

 Complication\Comorbidity   Major C\C   (Ex) CC/MCC Exclusions   Hospital-Acquired Condition

1481

- ● T63.19 Toxic effect of venom of other reptiles
  - ● T63.191 Toxic effect of venom of other reptiles, accidental (unintentional)
    Toxic effect of venom of other reptiles NOS
  - ● T63.192 Toxic effect of venom of other reptiles, intentional self-harm
  - ● T63.193 Toxic effect of venom of other reptiles, assault
  - ● T63.194 Toxic effect of venom of other reptiles, undetermined
- ● T63.2 Toxic effect of venom of scorpion
  - ● T63.2X Toxic effect of venom of scorpion
    - ● T63.2X1 Toxic effect of venom of scorpion, accidental (unintentional)
      Toxic effect of venom of scorpion NOS
    - ● T63.2X2 Toxic effect of venom of scorpion, intentional self-harm
    - ● T63.2X3 Toxic effect of venom of scorpion, assault
    - ● T63.2X4 Toxic effect of venom of scorpion, undetermined
- ● T63.3 Toxic effect of venom of spider
  - ● T63.30 Toxic effect of unspecified spider venom
    - ● T63.301 Toxic effect of unspecified spider venom, accidental (unintentional)
    - ● T63.302 Toxic effect of unspecified spider venom, intentional self-harm
    - ● T63.303 Toxic effect of unspecified spider venom, assault
    - ● T63.304 Toxic effect of unspecified spider venom, undetermined
  - ● T63.31 Toxic effect of venom of black widow spider
    - ● T63.311 Toxic effect of venom of black widow spider, accidental (unintentional)
    - ● T63.312 Toxic effect of venom of black widow spider, intentional self-harm
    - ● T63.313 Toxic effect of venom of black widow spider, assault
    - ● T63.314 Toxic effect of venom of black widow spider, undetermined
  - ● T63.32 Toxic effect of venom of tarantula
    - ● T63.321 Toxic effect of venom of tarantula, accidental (unintentional)
    - ● T63.322 Toxic effect of venom of tarantula, intentional self-harm
    - ● T63.323 Toxic effect of venom of tarantula, assault
    - ● T63.324 Toxic effect of venom of tarantula, undetermined
  - ● T63.33 Toxic effect of venom of brown recluse spider
    - ● T63.331 Toxic effect of venom of brown recluse spider, accidental (unintentional)
    - ● T63.332 Toxic effect of venom of brown recluse spider, intentional self-harm
    - ● T63.333 Toxic effect of venom of brown recluse spider, assault
    - ● T63.334 Toxic effect of venom of brown recluse spider, undetermined

- ● T63.39 Toxic effect of venom of other spider
  - ● T63.391 Toxic effect of venom of other spider, accidental (unintentional)
  - ● T63.392 Toxic effect of venom of other spider, intentional self-harm
  - ● T63.393 Toxic effect of venom of other spider, assault
  - ● T63.394 Toxic effect of venom of other spider, undetermined
- ● T63.4 Toxic effect of venom of other arthropods
  - ● T63.41 Toxic effect of venom of centipedes and venomous millipedes
    - ● T63.411 Toxic effect of venom of centipedes and venomous millipedes, accidental (unintentional)
    - ● T63.412 Toxic effect of venom of centipedes and venomous millipedes, intentional self-harm
    - ● T63.413 Toxic effect of venom of centipedes and venomous millipedes, assault
    - ● T63.414 Toxic effect of venom of centipedes and venomous millipedes, undetermined
  - ● T63.42 Toxic effect of venom of ants
    - ● T63.421 Toxic effect of venom of ants, accidental (unintentional)
    - ● T63.422 Toxic effect of venom of ants, intentional self-harm
    - ● T63.423 Toxic effect of venom of ants, assault
    - ● T63.424 Toxic effect of venom of ants, undetermined
  - ● T63.43 Toxic effect of venom of caterpillars
    - ● T63.431 Toxic effect of venom of caterpillars, accidental (unintentional)
    - ● T63.432 Toxic effect of venom of caterpillars, intentional self-harm
    - ● T63.433 Toxic effect of venom of caterpillars, assault
    - ● T63.434 Toxic effect of venom of caterpillars, undetermined
  - ● T63.44 Toxic effect of venom of bees
    - ● T63.441 Toxic effect of venom of bees, accidental (unintentional)
    - ● T63.442 Toxic effect of venom of bees, intentional self-harm
    - ● T63.443 Toxic effect of venom of bees, assault
    - ● T63.444 Toxic effect of venom of bees, undetermined
  - ● T63.45 Toxic effect of venom of hornets
    - ● T63.451 Toxic effect of venom of hornets, accidental (unintentional)
    - ● T63.452 Toxic effect of venom of hornets, intentional self-harm
    - ● T63.453 Toxic effect of venom of hornets, assault
    - ● T63.454 Toxic effect of venom of hornets, undetermined
  - ● T63.46 Toxic effect of venom of wasps
    Toxic effect of yellow jacket
    - ● T63.461 Toxic effect of venom of wasps, accidental (unintentional)
    - ● T63.462 Toxic effect of venom of wasps, intentional self-harm
    - ● T63.463 Toxic effect of venom of wasps, assault
    - ● T63.464 Toxic effect of venom of wasps, undetermined

◀ New   ◀▥ Revised   ~~deleted~~ Deleted   Excludes 1   Excludes 2   Includes   Use additional   Code first   Code also   Unspecified

OGCR Official Guidelines   ● Unacceptable Principal Diagnosis   X Assign placeholder X   ● Use Additional Character(s)   ▶ Manifestation Code   **Coding Clinic**

● **T63.48**   Toxic effect of venom of other arthropod
  ● **T63.481**   Toxic effect of venom of other arthropod, accidental (unintentional)
  ● **T63.482**   Toxic effect of venom of other arthropod, intentional self-harm
  ● **T63.483**   Toxic effect of venom of other arthropod, assault
  ● **T63.484**   Toxic effect of venom of other arthropod, undetermined
● **T63.5**   Toxic effect of contact with venomous fish
  Excludes2   poisoning by ingestion of fish (T61.-)
  ● **T63.51**   Toxic effect of contact with stingray
    ● **T63.511**   Toxic effect of contact with stingray, accidental (unintentional)
    ● **T63.512**   Toxic effect of contact with stingray, intentional self-harm
    ● **T63.513**   Toxic effect of contact with stingray, assault
    ● **T63.514**   Toxic effect of contact with stingray, undetermined
  ● **T63.59**   Toxic effect of contact with other venomous fish
    ● **T63.591**   Toxic effect of contact with other venomous fish, accidental (unintentional)
    ● **T63.592**   Toxic effect of contact with other venomous fish, intentional self-harm
    ● **T63.593**   Toxic effect of contact with other venomous fish, assault
    ● **T63.594**   Toxic effect of contact with other venomous fish, undetermined
● **T63.6**   Toxic effect of contact with other venomous marine animals
  Excludes1   sea-snake venom (T63.09)
  Excludes2   poisoning by ingestion of shellfish (T61.78-)
  ● **T63.61**   Toxic effect of contact with Portugese Man-o-war
    Toxic effect of contact with bluebottle
    ● **T63.611**   Toxic effect of contact with Portugese Man-o-war, accidental (unintentional)
    ● **T63.612**   Toxic effect of contact with Portugese Man-o-war, intentional self-harm
    ● **T63.613**   Toxic effect of contact with Portugese Man-o-war, assault
    ● **T63.614**   Toxic effect of contact with Portugese Man-o-war, undetermined
  ● **T63.62**   Toxic effect of contact with other jellyfish
    ● **T63.621**   Toxic effect of contact with other jellyfish, accidental (unintentional)
    ● **T63.622**   Toxic effect of contact with other jellyfish, intentional self-harm
    ● **T63.623**   Toxic effect of contact with other jellyfish, assault
    ● **T63.624**   Toxic effect of contact with other jellyfish, undetermined
  ● **T63.63**   Toxic effect of contact with sea anemone
    ● **T63.631**   Toxic effect of contact with sea anemone, accidental (unintentional)
    ● **T63.632**   Toxic effect of contact with sea anemone, intentional self-harm
    ● **T63.633**   Toxic effect of contact with sea anemone, assault
    ● **T63.634**   Toxic effect of contact with sea anemone, undetermined

● **T63.69**   Toxic effect of contact with other venomous marine animals
  ● **T63.691**   Toxic effect of contact with other venomous marine animals, accidental (unintentional)
  ● **T63.692**   Toxic effect of contact with other venomous marine animals, intentional self-harm
  ● **T63.693**   Toxic effect of contact with other venomous marine animals, assault
  ● **T63.694**   Toxic effect of contact with other venomous marine animals, undetermined
● **T63.7**   Toxic effect of contact with venomous plant
  ● **T63.71**   Toxic effect of contact with venomous marine plant
    ● **T63.711**   Toxic effect of contact with venomous marine plant, accidental (unintentional)
    ● **T63.712**   Toxic effect of contact with venomous marine plant, intentional self-harm
    ● **T63.713**   Toxic effect of contact with venomous marine plant, assault
    ● **T63.714**   Toxic effect of contact with venomous marine plant, undetermined
  ● **T63.79**   Toxic effect of contact with other venomous plant
    ● **T63.791**   Toxic effect of contact with other venomous plant, accidental (unintentional)
    ● **T63.792**   Toxic effect of contact with other venomous plant, intentional self-harm
    ● **T63.793**   Toxic effect of contact with other venomous plant, assault
    ● **T63.794**   Toxic effect of contact with other venomous plant, undetermined
● **T63.8**   Toxic effect of contact with other venomous animals
  ● **T63.81**   Toxic effect of contact with venomous frog
    Excludes1   contact with nonvenomous frog (W62.0)
    ● **T63.811**   Toxic effect of contact with venomous frog, accidental (unintentional)
    ● **T63.812**   Toxic effect of contact with venomous frog, intentional self-harm
    ● **T63.813**   Toxic effect of contact with venomous frog, assault
    ● **T63.814**   Toxic effect of contact with venomous frog, undetermined
  ● **T63.82**   Toxic effect of contact with venomous toad
    Excludes1   contact with nonvenomous toad (W62.1)
    ● **T63.821**   Toxic effect of contact with venomous toad, accidental (unintentional)
    ● **T63.822**   Toxic effect of contact with venomous toad, intentional self-harm
    ● **T63.823**   Toxic effect of contact with venomous toad, assault
    ● **T63.824**   Toxic effect of contact with venomous toad, undetermined

CHAPTER 19 (S00-T88)

N Newborn Age: 0   **P** Pediatric Age: 0–17   **M** Maternity DX: 12–55   **A** Adult Age: 15–124   ♀ Females Only   ♂ Males Only
  Complication\Comorbidity   Major C\C   (Ex) CC/MCC Exclusions   Hospital-Acquired Condition

● **T63.83**   **Toxic effect of contact with other venomous amphibian**

     Excludes1   contact with nonvenomous amphibian (W62.9)

  ● **T63.831**   Toxic effect of contact with other venomous amphibian, accidental (unintentional)

  ● **T63.832**   Toxic effect of contact with other venomous amphibian, intentional self-harm

  ● **T63.833**   Toxic effect of contact with other venomous amphibian, assault

  ● **T63.834**   Toxic effect of contact with other venomous amphibian, undetermined

● **T63.89**   **Toxic effect of contact with other venomous animals**

  ● **T63.891**   Toxic effect of contact with other venomous animals, accidental (unintentional)

  ● **T63.892**   Toxic effect of contact with other venomous animals, intentional self-harm

  ● **T63.893**   Toxic effect of contact with other venomous animals, assault

  ● **T63.894**   Toxic effect of contact with other venomous animals, undetermined

● **T63.9**   **Toxic effect of contact with unspecified venomous animal**

X ● **T63.91**   Toxic effect of contact with unspecified venomous animal, accidental (unintentional)

X ● **T63.92**   Toxic effect of contact with unspecified venomous animal, intentional self-harm

X ● **T63.93**   Toxic effect of contact with unspecified venomous animal, assault

X ● **T63.94**   Toxic effect of contact with unspecified venomous animal, undetermined

● **T64**   **Toxic effect of aflatoxin and other mycotoxin food contaminants**

The appropriate 7th character is to be added to each code from category T64

A	initial encounter
D	subsequent encounter
S	sequela

● **T64.0**   **Toxic effect of aflatoxin**

X ● **T64.01**   Toxic effect of aflatoxin, accidental (unintentional)

X ● **T64.02**   Toxic effect of aflatoxin, intentional self-harm

X ● **T64.03**   Toxic effect of aflatoxin, assault

X ● **T64.04**   Toxic effect of aflatoxin, undetermined

● **T64.8**   **Toxic effect of other mycotoxin food contaminants**

X ● **T64.81**   Toxic effect of other mycotoxin food contaminants, accidental (unintentional)

X ● **T64.82**   Toxic effect of other mycotoxin food contaminants, intentional self-harm

X ● **T64.83**   Toxic effect of other mycotoxin food contaminants, assault

X ● **T64.84**   Toxic effect of other mycotoxin food contaminants, undetermined

● **T65**   **Toxic effect of other and unspecified substances**

The appropriate 7th character is to be added to each code from category T65

A	initial encounter
D	subsequent encounter
S	sequela

● **T65.0**   **Toxic effect of cyanides**

     Excludes1   hydrogen cyanide (T57.3-)

● **T65.0X**   **Toxic effect of cyanides**

  ● **T65.0X1**   Toxic effect of cyanides, accidental (unintentional)
      Toxic effect of cyanides NOS

  ● **T65.0X2**   Toxic effect of cyanides, intentional self-harm

  ● **T65.0X3**   Toxic effect of cyanides, assault

  ● **T65.0X4**   Toxic effect of cyanides, undetermined

● **T65.1**   **Toxic effect of strychnine and its salts**

● **T65.1X**   **Toxic effect of strychnine and its salts**

  ● **T65.1X1**   Toxic effect of strychnine and its salts, accidental (unintentional)
      Toxic effect of strychnine and its salts NOS

  ● **T65.1X2**   Toxic effect of strychnine and its salts, intentional self-harm

  ● **T65.1X3**   Toxic effect of strychnine and its salts, assault

  ● **T65.1X4**   Toxic effect of strychnine and its salts, undetermined

● **T65.2**   **Toxic effect of tobacco and nicotine**

     Excludes2   nicotine dependence (F17.-)

● **T65.21**   **Toxic effect of chewing tobacco**

  ● **T65.211**   Toxic effect of chewing tobacco, accidental (unintentional)
      Toxic effect of chewing tobacco NOS

  ● **T65.212**   Toxic effect of chewing tobacco, intentional self-harm

  ● **T65.213**   Toxic effect of chewing tobacco, assault

  ● **T65.214**   Toxic effect of chewing tobacco, undetermined

● **T65.22**   **Toxic effect of tobacco cigarettes**
     Toxic effect of tobacco smoke

     Use additional code for exposure to second hand tobacco smoke (Z57.31, Z77.22)

  ● **T65.221**   Toxic effect of tobacco cigarettes, accidental (unintentional)
      Toxic effect of tobacco cigarettes NOS

  ● **T65.222**   Toxic effect of tobacco cigarettes, intentional self-harm

  ● **T65.223**   Toxic effect of tobacco cigarettes, assault

  ● **T65.224**   Toxic effect of tobacco cigarettes, undetermined

● **T65.29**   **Toxic effect of other tobacco and nicotine**

  ● **T65.291**   Toxic effect of other tobacco and nicotine, accidental (unintentional)
      Toxic effect of other tobacco and nicotine NOS

  ● **T65.292**   Toxic effect of other tobacco and nicotine, intentional self-harm

  ● **T65.293**   Toxic effect of other tobacco and nicotine, assault

  ● **T65.294**   Toxic effect of other tobacco and nicotine, undetermined

◀ New   ◀ Revised   ~~deleted~~ Deleted   Excludes 1   Excludes 2   Includes   Use additional   Code first   Code also   Unspecified

OGCR Official Guidelines   ● Unacceptable Principal Diagnosis   X Assign placeholder X   ● Use Additional Character(s)   ● Manifestation Code   **Coding Clinic**

● **T65.3** **Toxic effect of nitroderivatives and aminoderivatives of benzene and its homologues**
     Toxic effect of anilin [benzenamine]
     Toxic effect of nitrobenzene
     Toxic effect of trinitrotoluene
   ● **T65.3X** **Toxic effect of nitroderivatives and aminoderivatives of benzene and its homologues**
     ● **T65.3X1** **Toxic effect of nitroderivatives and aminoderivatives of benzene and its homologues, accidental (unintentional)**
       Toxic effect of nitroderivatives and aminoderivatives of benzene and its homologues NOS
     ● **T65.3X2** **Toxic effect of nitroderivatives and aminoderivatives of benzene and its homologues, intentional self-harm**
     ● **T65.3X3** **Toxic effect of nitroderivatives and aminoderivatives of benzene and its homologues, assault**
     ● **T65.3X4** **Toxic effect of nitroderivatives and aminoderivatives of benzene and its homologues, undetermined**

● **T65.4** **Toxic effect of carbon disulfide**
   ● **T65.4X** **Toxic effect of carbon disulfide**
     ● **T65.4X1** **Toxic effect of carbon disulfide, accidental (unintentional)**
       Toxic effect of carbon disulfide NOS
     ● **T65.4X2** **Toxic effect of carbon disulfide, intentional self-harm**
     ● **T65.4X3** **Toxic effect of carbon disulfide, assault**
     ● **T65.4X4** **Toxic effect of carbon disulfide, undetermined**

● **T65.5** **Toxic effect of nitroglycerin and other nitric acids and esters**
     Toxic effect of 1,2,3-Propanetriol trinitrate
   ● **T65.5X** **Toxic effect of nitroglycerin and other nitric acids and esters**
     ● **T65.5X1** **Toxic effect of nitroglycerin and other nitric acids and esters, accidental (unintentional)**
       Toxic effect of nitroglycerin and other nitric acids and esters NOS
     ● **T65.5X2** **Toxic effect of nitroglycerin and other nitric acids and esters, intentional self-harm**
     ● **T65.5X3** **Toxic effect of nitroglycerin and other nitric acids and esters, assault**
     ● **T65.5X4** **Toxic effect of nitroglycerin and other nitric acids and esters, undetermined**

● **T65.6** **Toxic effect of paints and dyes, not elsewhere classified**
   ● **T65.6X** **Toxic effect of paints and dyes, not elsewhere classified**
     ● **T65.6X1** **Toxic effect of paints and dyes, not elsewhere classified, accidental (unintentional)**
       Toxic effect of paints and dyes NOS
     ● **T65.6X2** **Toxic effect of paints and dyes, not elsewhere classified, intentional self-harm**
     ● **T65.6X3** **Toxic effect of paints and dyes, not elsewhere classified, assault**
     ● **T65.6X4** **Toxic effect of paints and dyes, not elsewhere classified, undetermined**

● **T65.8** **Toxic effect of other specified substances**
   ● **T65.81** **Toxic effect of latex**
     ● **T65.811** **Toxic effect of latex, accidental (unintentional)**
       Toxic effect of latex NOS
     ● **T65.812** **Toxic effect of latex, intentional self-harm**
     ● **T65.813** **Toxic effect of latex, assault**
     ● **T65.814** **Toxic effect of latex, undetermined**
   ● **T65.82** **Toxic effect of harmful algae and algae toxins**
     Toxic effect of (harmful) algae bloom NOS
     Toxic effect of blue-green algae bloom
     Toxic effect of brown tide
     Toxic effect of cyanobacteria bloom
     Toxic effect of Florida red tide
     Toxic effect of pfiesteria piscicida
     Toxic effect of red tide
     ● **T65.821** **Toxic effect of harmful algae and algae toxins, accidental (unintentional)**
       Toxic effect of harmful algae and algae toxins NOS
     ● **T65.822** **Toxic effect of harmful algae and algae toxins, intentional self-harm**
     ● **T65.823** **Toxic effect of harmful algae and algae toxins, assault**
     ● **T65.824** **Toxic effect of harmful algae and algae toxins, undetermined**
   ● **T65.83** **Toxic effect of fiberglass**
     ● **T65.831** **Toxic effect of fiberglass, accidental (unintentional)**
       Toxic effect of fiberglass NOS
     ● **T65.832** **Toxic effect of fiberglass, intentional self-harm**
     ● **T65.833** **Toxic effect of fiberglass, assault**
     ● **T65.834** **Toxic effect of fiberglass, undetermined**
   ● **T65.89** **Toxic effect of other specified substances**
     ● **T65.891** **Toxic effect of other specified substances, accidental (unintentional)**
       Toxic effect of other specified substances NOS
     ● **T65.892** **Toxic effect of other specified substances, intentional self-harm**
     ● **T65.893** **Toxic effect of other specified substances, assault**
     ● **T65.894** **Toxic effect of other specified substances, undetermined**

● **T65.9** **Toxic effect of unspecified substance**
   X ● **T65.91** **Toxic effect of unspecified substance, accidental (unintentional)**
     Poisoning NOS
   X ● **T65.92** **Toxic effect of unspecified substance, intentional self-harm**
   X ● **T65.93** **Toxic effect of unspecified substance, assault**
   X ● **T65.94** **Toxic effect of unspecified substance, undetermined**

N Newborn Age: 0   **P** Pediatric Age: 0–17   **M** Maternity DX: 12–55   **A** Adult Age: 15–124   ♀ Females Only   ♂ Males Only
     🅫 Complication\Comorbidity   🅫 Major C\C   (Ex) CC/MCC Exclusions   🅗 Hospital-Acquired Condition

1485

CHAPTER 19 (S00-T88)

OTHER AND UNSPECIFIED EFFECTS OF EXTERNAL CAUSES (T66-T78)

● **T66**   **Radiation sickness, unspecified**

     Excludes1   specified adverse effects of radiation, such as:
             burns (T20-T31)
             leukemia (C91-C95)
             radiation gastroenteritis and colitis (K52.0)
             radiation pneumonitis (J70.0)
             radiation related disorders of the skin and
               subcutaneous tissue (L55-L59)
             sunburn (L55.-)

     The appropriate 7th character is to be added to code T66

       A   initial encounter
       D   subsequent encounter
       S   sequela

● **T67**   **Effects of heat and light**

     Excludes1   erythema [dermatitis] ab igne (L59.0)
             malignant hyperpyrexia due to anesthesia (T88.3)
             radiation-related disorders of the skin and
               subcutaneous tissue (L55-L59)

     Excludes2   burns (T20-T31)
             sunburn (L55.-)
             sweat disorder due to heat (L74-L75)

     The appropriate 7th character is to be added to each code from
     category T67

       A   initial encounter
       D   subsequent encounter
       S   sequela

X ● **T67.0**   **Heatstroke and sunstroke** A 🔵, A 🔵
         Heat apoplexy
         Heat pyrexia
         Siriasis
         Thermoplegia
         Use additional code(s) to identify any associated
             complications of heatstroke, such as:
             coma and stupor (R40.-)
             systemic inflammatory response syndrome (R65.1-)
         (Ex) T67.0XX-T67.9XX[A]

X ● **T67.1**   **Heat syncope**
         Heat collapse

X ● **T67.2**   **Heat cramp**

X ● **T67.3**   **Heat exhaustion, anhydrotic**
         Heat prostration due to water depletion
         Excludes1   heat exhaustion due to salt depletion
                   (T67.4)

X ● **T67.4**   **Heat exhaustion due to salt depletion**
         Heat prostration due to salt (and water) depletion

X ● **T67.5**   **Heat exhaustion, unspecified**
         Heat prostration NOS

X ● **T67.6**   **Heat fatigue, transient**

X ● **T67.7**   **Heat edema**

X ● **T67.8**   **Other effects of heat and light**

X ● **T67.9**   **Effect of heat and light, unspecified**

X ● **T68**   **Hypothermia**
     Accidental hypothermia
     Hypothermia NOS
     Use additional code to identify source of exposure:
       Exposure to excessive cold of man-made origin (W93)
       Exposure to excessive cold of natural origin (X31)
     Excludes1   hypothermia following anesthesia (T88.51)
             hypothermia not associated with low
               environmental temperature (R68.0)
             hypothermia of newborn (P80.-)
     Excludes2   frostbite (T33-T34)
     The appropriate 7th character is to be added to code T68

       A   initial encounter
       D   subsequent encounter
       S   sequela

● **T69**   **Other effects of reduced temperature**
     Use additional code to identify source of exposure:
       Exposure to excessive cold of man-made origin (W93)
       Exposure to excessive cold of natural origin (X31)
     Excludes2   frostbite (T33-T34)
     The appropriate 7th character is to be added to each code from
     category T69

       A   initial encounter
       D   subsequent encounter
       S   sequela

● **T69.0**   **Immersion hand and foot**

   ● **T69.01**   **Immersion hand**

     ● **T69.011**   **Immersion hand, right hand**

     ● **T69.012**   **Immersion hand, left hand**

     ● **T69.019**   **Immersion hand, unspecified hand**

   ● **T69.02**   **Immersion foot**
         Trench foot
         (Ex) **For category T69.02 CC codes:** T33.2XX-T33.42X[A],
           T33.60X-T33.72X[A], T33.90X-T33.99X[A],
           T34.2XX-T34.42X[A], T34.60X-T34.72X[A],
           T34.90X-T34.99X[A], T69.021-T69.029[A]

     ● **T69.021**   **Immersion foot, right foot** A 🔵, A 🔵

     ● **T69.022**   **Immersion foot, left foot** A 🔵, A 🔵

     ● **T69.029**   **Immersion foot, unspecified foot** A 🔵, A 🔵

X ● **T69.1**   **Chilblains**

X ● **T69.8**   **Other specified effects of reduced temperature**

X ● **T69.9**   **Effect of reduced temperature, unspecified**

● **T70**   **Effects of air pressure and water pressure**
     The appropriate 7th character is to be added to each code from
     category T70

       A   initial encounter
       D   subsequent encounter
       S   sequela

X ● **T70.0**   **Otitic barotrauma**
         Aero-otitis media
         Effects of change in ambient atmospheric pressure or
             water pressure on ears

X ● **T70.1**   **Sinus barotrauma**
         Aerosinusitis
         Effects of change in ambient atmospheric pressure on
             sinuses

● **T70.2**   **Other and unspecified effects of high altitude**
     Excludes2   polycythemia due to high altitude (D75.1)

X ● **T70.20**   **Unspecified effects of high altitude**

X ● **T70.29**   **Other effects of high altitude**
         Alpine sickness
         Anoxia due to high altitude
         Barotrauma NOS
         Hypobaropathy
         Mountain sickness

X ● **T70.3**   **Caisson disease [decompression sickness]** A 🔵, A 🔵
         Compressed-air disease
         Diver's palsy or paralysis
         (Ex) T70.3XX-T70.9XX[A]

X ● **T70.4**   **Effects of high-pressure fluids**
         Hydraulic jet injection (industrial)
         Pneumatic jet injection (industrial)
         Traumatic jet injection (industrial)

X ● **T70.8**   **Other effects of air pressure and water pressure**

X ● **T70.9**   **Effect of air pressure and water pressure, unspecified**

◀ New   ◀◀◀ Revised   ~~deleted~~ Deleted   Excludes 1   Excludes 2   Includes   Use additional   Code first   Code also   Unspecified

OGCR Official Guidelines   ● Unacceptable Principal Diagnosis   X Assign placeholder X   ● Use Additional Character(s)   ▶ Manifestation Code   **Coding Clinic**

● **T71 Asphyxiation**
　　Mechanical suffocation
　　Traumatic suffocation
　　Excludes1 acute respiratory distress (syndrome) (J80)
　　　　　anoxia due to high altitude (T70.2)
　　　　　asphyxia NOS (R09.01)
　　　　　asphyxia from carbon monoxide (T58.-)
　　　　　asphyxia from inhalation of food or foreign body
　　　　　　(T17.-)
　　　　　asphyxia from other gases, fumes and vapors
　　　　　　(T59.-)
　　　　　respiratory distress (syndrome) in newborn
　　　　　　(P22.-)
　　The appropriate 7th character is to be added to each code from
　　　category T71

A	initial encounter
D	subsequent encounter
S	sequela

　　(Ex) **For category T71 CC codes:** T71.111-T71.9XX[A]

● **T71.1 Asphyxiation due to mechanical threat to breathing**
　　Suffocation due to mechanical threat to breathing
　　● **T71.11 Asphyxiation due to smothering under pillow**
　　　　● **T71.111 Asphyxiation due to smothering
　　　　　　under pillow, accidental** A 🐷, A 🐷
　　　　　　Asphyxiation due to smothering
　　　　　　　under pillow NOS
　　　　● **T71.112 Asphyxiation due to smothering
　　　　　　under pillow, intentional self-harm**
　　　　　　A 🐷, A 🐷
　　　　● **T71.113 Asphyxiation due to smothering
　　　　　　under pillow, assault** A 🐷, A 🐷
　　　　● **T71.114 Asphyxiation due to smothering
　　　　　　under pillow, undetermined** A 🐷,
　　　　　　A 🐷
　　● **T71.12 Asphyxiation due to plastic bag**
　　　　● **T71.121 Asphyxiation due to plastic bag,
　　　　　　accidental** A 🐷, A 🐷
　　　　　　Asphyxiation due to plastic bag
　　　　　　　NOS
　　　　● **T71.122 Asphyxiation due to plastic bag,
　　　　　　intentional self-harm** A 🐷, A 🐷
　　　　● **T71.123 Asphyxiation due to plastic bag,
　　　　　　assault** A 🐷, A 🐷
　　　　● **T71.124 Asphyxiation due to plastic bag,
　　　　　　undetermined** A 🐷, A 🐷
　　● **T71.13 Asphyxiation due to being trapped in bed
　　　　linens**
　　　　● **T71.131 Asphyxiation due to being trapped in
　　　　　　bed linens, accidental** A 🐷, A 🐷
　　　　　　Asphyxiation due to being trapped
　　　　　　　in bed linens NOS
　　　　● **T71.132 Asphyxiation due to being trapped in
　　　　　　bed linens, intentional self-harm**
　　　　　　A 🐷, A 🐷
　　　　● **T71.133 Asphyxiation due to being trapped in
　　　　　　bed linens, assault** A 🐷, A 🐷
　　　　● **T71.134 Asphyxiation due to being trapped in
　　　　　　bed linens, undetermined** A 🐷, A 🐷

● **T71.14 Asphyxiation due to smothering under another
　　person's body (in bed)**
　　● **T71.141 Asphyxiation due to smothering
　　　　under another person's body (in bed),
　　　　accidental** A 🐷, A 🐷
　　　　Asphyxiation due to smothering
　　　　　under another person's body
　　　　　(in bed) NOS
　　● **T71.143 Asphyxiation due to smothering
　　　　under another person's body (in bed),
　　　　assault** A 🐷, A 🐷
　　● **T71.144 Asphyxiation due to smothering
　　　　under another person's body (in bed),
　　　　undetermined** A 🐷, A 🐷
● **T71.15 Asphyxiation due to smothering in furniture**
　　● **T71.151 Asphyxiation due to smothering in
　　　　furniture, accidental** A 🐷, A 🐷
　　　　Asphyxiation due to smothering in
　　　　　furniture NOS
　　● **T71.152 Asphyxiation due to smothering in
　　　　furniture, intentional self-harm** A 🐷,
　　　　A 🐷
　　● **T71.153 Asphyxiation due to smothering in
　　　　furniture, assault** A 🐷, A 🐷
　　● **T71.154 Asphyxiation due to smothering in
　　　　furniture, undetermined** A 🐷, A 🐷
● **T71.16 Asphyxiation due to hanging**
　　Hanging by window shade cord
　　Use additional code for any associated injuries,
　　　such as:
　　　crushing injury of neck (S17.-)
　　　fracture of cervical vertebrae (S12.0-S12.2-)
　　　open wound of neck (S11.-)
　　● **T71.161 Asphyxiation due to hanging,
　　　　accidental** A 🐷, A 🐷
　　　　Asphyxiation due to hanging NOS
　　　　Hanging NOS
　　● **T71.162 Asphyxiation due to hanging,
　　　　intentional self-harm** A 🐷, A 🐷
　　● **T71.163 Asphyxiation due to hanging, assault**
　　　　A 🐷, A 🐷
　　● **T71.164 Asphyxiation due to hanging,
　　　　undetermined** A 🐷, A 🐷
● **T71.19 Asphyxiation due to mechanical**
　　Threat to breathing due to other causes
　　● **T71.191 Asphyxiation due to mechanical
　　　　threat to breathing due to other
　　　　causes, accidental** A 🐷, A 🐷
　　　　Asphyxiation due to other causes
　　　　　NOS
　　● **T71.192 Asphyxiation due to mechanical
　　　　threat to breathing due to other
　　　　causes, intentional self-harm** A 🐷,
　　　　A 🐷
　　● **T71.193 Asphyxiation due to mechanical
　　　　threat to breathing due to other
　　　　causes, assault** A 🐷, A 🐷
　　● **T71.194 Asphyxiation due to mechanical
　　　　threat to breathing due to other
　　　　causes, undetermined** A 🐷, A 🐷

CHAPTER 19 (S00-T88)

N Newborn Age: 0　　**P** Pediatric Age: 0–17　　**M** Maternity DX: 12–55　　**A** Adult Age: 15–124　　♀ Females Only　　♂ Males Only

🐷 Complication\Comorbidity　　🐷 Major C\C　　(Ex) CC/MCC Exclusions　　🐷 Hospital-Acquired Condition

1487

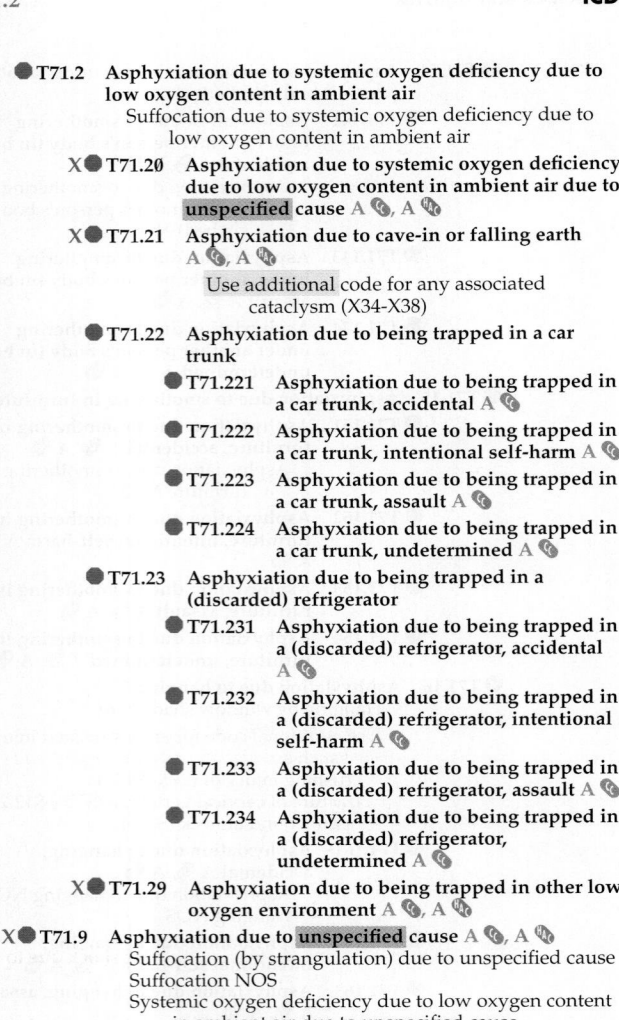

● **T71.2** **Asphyxiation due to systemic oxygen deficiency due to low oxygen content in ambient air**
Suffocation due to systemic oxygen deficiency due to low oxygen content in ambient air

X ● **T71.20** **Asphyxiation due to systemic oxygen deficiency due to low oxygen content in ambient air due to** unspecified **cause** A 🔲, A 🔲

X ● **T71.21** **Asphyxiation due to cave-in or falling earth** A 🔲, A 🔲
Use additional code for any associated cataclysm (X34-X38)

● **T71.22** **Asphyxiation due to being trapped in a car trunk**

  ● **T71.221** **Asphyxiation due to being trapped in a car trunk, accidental** A 🔲

  ● **T71.222** **Asphyxiation due to being trapped in a car trunk, intentional self-harm** A 🔲

  ● **T71.223** **Asphyxiation due to being trapped in a car trunk, assault** A 🔲

  ● **T71.224** **Asphyxiation due to being trapped in a car trunk, undetermined** A 🔲

● **T71.23** **Asphyxiation due to being trapped in a (discarded) refrigerator**

  ● **T71.231** **Asphyxiation due to being trapped in a (discarded) refrigerator, accidental** A 🔲

  ● **T71.232** **Asphyxiation due to being trapped in a (discarded) refrigerator, intentional self-harm** A 🔲

  ● **T71.233** **Asphyxiation due to being trapped in a (discarded) refrigerator, assault** A 🔲

  ● **T71.234** **Asphyxiation due to being trapped in a (discarded) refrigerator, undetermined** A 🔲

X ● **T71.29** **Asphyxiation due to being trapped in other low oxygen environment** A 🔲, A 🔲

X ● **T71.9** **Asphyxiation due to** unspecified **cause** A 🔲, A 🔲
Suffocation (by strangulation) due to unspecified cause
Suffocation NOS
Systemic oxygen deficiency due to low oxygen content in ambient air due to unspecified cause
Systemic oxygen deficiency due to mechanical threat to breathing due to unspecified cause
Traumatic asphyxia NOS

● **T73** **Effects of other deprivation**
The appropriate 7th character is to be added to each code from category T73

A	initial encounter
D	subsequent encounter
S	sequela

X ● **T73.Ø** **Starvation**
Deprivation of food

X ● **T73.1** **Deprivation of water**

X ● **T73.2** **Exhaustion due to exposure**

X ● **T73.3** **Exhaustion due to excessive exertion**
Exhaustion due to overexertion

X ● **T73.8** **Other effects of deprivation**

X ● **T73.9** **Effect of deprivation,** unspecified

● **T74** **Adult and child abuse, neglect and other maltreatment, confirmed**
Use additional code, if applicable, to identify any associated current injury
Use additional external cause code to identify perpetrator, if known (YØ7.-)

Excludes1 abuse and maltreatment in pregnancy (O9A.3-, O9A.4-, O9A.5-)
adult and child maltreatment, suspected (T76.-)

The appropriate 7th character is to be added to each code from category T74

A	initial encounter
D	subsequent encounter
S	sequela

(Ex) For category T74 CC codes unless otherwise indicated: T74.Ø1X-T74.92X[A], T76.Ø1X-T76.92X[A]

● **T74.Ø** **Neglect or abandonment, confirmed**

X ● **T74.Ø1** **Adult neglect or abandonment, confirmed** A 🔲   A

X ● **T74.Ø2** **Child neglect or abandonment, confirmed** A 🔲   P

● **T74.1** **Physical abuse, confirmed**
Excludes2 sexual abuse (T74.2-)

X ● **T74.11** **Adult physical abuse, confirmed** A 🔲   A

X ● **T74.12** **Child physical abuse, confirmed** A 🔲   P
Excludes2 shaken infant syndrome (T74.4)

● **T74.2** **Sexual abuse, confirmed**
Rape, confirmed
Sexual assault, confirmed

X ● **T74.21** **Adult sexual abuse, confirmed** A 🔲   A

X ● **T74.22** **Child sexual abuse, confirmed** A 🔲   P

● **T74.3** **Psychological abuse, confirmed**

X ● **T74.31** **Adult psychological abuse, confirmed**   A

X ● **T74.32** **Child psychological abuse, confirmed** A 🔲   P

X ● **T74.4** **Shaken infant syndrome** A 🔲   P

● **T74.9** **Unspecified maltreatment, confirmed**

X ● **T74.91** Unspecified **adult maltreatment, confirmed** A 🔲   A
(Ex) T74.91X[A], T76.91X[A]

X ● **T74.92** Unspecified **child maltreatment, confirmed** A 🔲   P

● **T75** **Other and unspecified effects of other external causes**
Excludes1 adverse effects NEC (T78.-)
Excludes2 burns (electric) (T2Ø-T31)

The appropriate 7th character is to be added to each code from category T75

A	initial encounter
D	subsequent encounter
S	sequela

● **T75.Ø** **Effects of lightning**
Struck by lightning

X ● **T75.ØØ** Unspecified **effects of lightning**
Struck by lightning NOS

X ● **T75.Ø1** **Shock due to being struck by lightning**

X ● **T75.Ø9** **Other effects of lightning**
Use additional code for other effects of lightning

X ● **T75.1** Unspecified **effects of drowning and nonfatal submersion** A 🔲, A 🔲
Immersion
Excludes1 specified effects of drowning code to effects
(Ex) T75.1XX[A]

● **T75.2 Effects of vibration**
   X● **T75.20** Unspecified **effects of vibration**
   X● **T75.21** **Pneumatic hammer syndrome**
   X● **T75.22** **Traumatic vasospastic syndrome**
   X● **T75.23** **Vertigo from infrasound**
      Excludes1 vertigo NOS (R42)
   X● **T75.29** **Other effects of vibration**
X● **T75.3 Motion sickness**
   Airsickness   Travel sickness
   Seasickness
   Use additional external cause code to identify vehicle or type of motion (Y92.81-, Y93.5-)
X● **T75.4 Electrocution**
   Shock from electric current
   Shock from electroshock gun (taser)
● **T75.8 Other specified effects of external causes**
   X● **T75.81** **Effects of abnormal gravitation [G] forces**
   X● **T75.82** **Effects of weightlessness**
   X● **T75.89** **Other specified effects of external causes**

● **T76 Adult and child abuse, neglect and other maltreatment, suspected**
   Use additional code, if applicable, to identify any associated current injury
   Excludes1 adult and child maltreatment, confirmed (T74.-)
      suspected abuse and maltreatment in pregnancy (O9A.3-, O9A.4-, O9A.5-)
      suspected adult physical abuse, ruled out (Z04.71)
      suspected adult sexual abuse, ruled out (Z04.41)
      suspected child physical abuse, ruled out (Z04.72)
      suspected child sexual abuse, ruled out (Z04.42)
   The appropriate 7th character is to be added to each code from category T76

    | A | initial encounter |
    | D | subsequent encounter |
    | S | sequela |

   (Ex) For category T76 CC codes unless otherwise indicated: T74.01X-T74.92X[A], T76.01X-T76.92X[A]

● **T76.0 Neglect or abandonment, suspected**
   X● **T76.01** **Adult neglect or abandonment, suspected** A 🦠   A
   X● **T76.02** **Child neglect or abandonment, suspected** A 🦠   P
● **T76.1 Physical abuse, suspected**
   X● **T76.11** **Adult physical abuse, suspected** A 🦠   A
   X● **T76.12** **Child physical abuse, suspected** A 🦠   P
● **T76.2 Sexual abuse, suspected**
   Rape, suspected
   Sexual abuse, suspected
      Excludes1 alleged abuse, ruled out (Z04.7)
   X● **T76.21** **Adult sexual abuse, suspected** A 🦠   A
   X● **T76.22** **Child sexual abuse, suspected** A 🦠   P
● **T76.3 Psychological abuse, suspected**
   X● **T76.31** **Adult psychological abuse, suspected** A   A
   X● **T76.32** **Child psychological abuse, suspected** A 🦠   P
● **T76.9 Unspecified maltreatment, suspected**
   X● **T76.91** Unspecified **adult maltreatment, suspected** A 🦠   A
      (Ex) T74.91X[A], T76.91X[A]
   X● **T76.92** Unspecified **child maltreatment, suspected** A 🦠   P

● **T78 Adverse effects, not elsewhere classified**
   Excludes2 complications of surgical and medical care NEC (T80-T88)
   The appropriate 7th character is to be added to each code from category T78

    | A | initial encounter |
    | D | subsequent encounter |
    | S | sequela |

   (Ex) For category T78 CC codes: T78.00X-T78.09X[A]
● **T78.0 Anaphylactic reaction due to food**
   Anaphylactic reaction due to adverse food reaction
   Anaphylactic shock or reaction due to nonpoisonous foods
   Anaphylactoid reaction due to food
   X● **T78.00** **Anaphylactic reaction due to** unspecified **food** A 🦠
   X● **T78.01** **Anaphylactic reaction due to peanuts** A 🦠
   X● **T78.02** **Anaphylactic reaction due to shellfish (crustaceans)** A 🦠
   X● **T78.03** **Anaphylactic reaction due to other fish** A 🦠
   X● **T78.04** **Anaphylactic reaction due to fruits and vegetables** A 🦠
   X● **T78.05** **Anaphylactic reaction due to tree nuts and seeds** A 🦠
      Excludes2 anaphylactic reaction due to peanuts (T78.01) ◄
   X● **T78.06** **Anaphylactic reaction due to food additives** A 🦠
   X● **T78.07** **Anaphylactic reaction due to milk and dairy products** A 🦠
   X● **T78.08** **Anaphylactic reaction due to eggs** A 🦠
   X● **T78.09** **Anaphylactic reaction due to other food products** A 🦠
X● **T78.1 Other adverse food reactions, not elsewhere classified**
   Use additional code to identify the type of reaction, if applicable ◄▥
      Excludes1 anaphylactic reaction or shock due to adverse food reaction (T78.0-)
       anaphylactic reaction due to food (T78.0-)
       bacterial food borne intoxications (A05.-)
      Excludes2 allergic and dietetic gastroenteritis and colitis (K52.29) ◄▥
       allergic rhinitis due to food (J30.5)
       dermatitis due to food in contact with skin (L23.6, L24.6, L25.4)
       dermatitis due to ingested food (L27.2)
       food protein-induced enterocolitis syndrome (K52.21) ◄
       food protein-induced enteropathy (K52.22) ◄
X● **T78.2 Anaphylactic shock,** unspecified A 🦠
   Occurs when allergic response triggers large quantities of histamines, prostaglandins, leukotrienes resulting in systemic vasodilation
   Allergic shock
   Anaphylactic reaction
   Anaphylaxis
      Excludes1 anaphylactic reaction or shock due to adverse effect of correct medicinal substance properly administered (T88.6)
       anaphylactic reaction or shock due to adverse food reaction (T78.0-)
       anaphylactic reaction or shock due to serum (T80.5-)
X● **T78.3 Angioneurotic edema**
   Allergic angioedema
   Giant urticaria
   Vascular disorder resulting from abnormalities of autonomic nervous system fibers supplying blood vessels
   Quincke's edema
      Excludes1 serum urticaria (T80.6-)
       urticaria (L50.-)

CHAPTER 19 (S00-T88)

● **T78.4**   **Other and unspecified allergy**

Excludes1   specified types of allergic reaction such
as:
    allergic diarrhea (K52.29) ◄▦
    allergic gastroenteritis and colitis
       (K52.29) ◄▦
    dermatitis (L23-L25, L27.-)
    food protein-induced enterocolitis
       syndrome (K52.21) ◄
    food protein-induced enteropathy
       (K52.22) ◄
    hay fever (J30.1)

X● **T78.40**   **Allergy, unspecified**
    Allergic reaction NOS
    Hypersensitivity NOS

X● **T78.41**   **Arthus phenomenon**
    Arthus reaction

X● **T78.49**   **Other allergy**

X● **T78.8**   **Other adverse effects, not elsewhere classified**

CERTAIN EARLY COMPLICATIONS OF TRAUMA (T79)

● **T79**   **Certain early complications of trauma, not elsewhere classified**

Excludes2   acute respiratory distress syndrome (J80)
complications occurring during or following
    medical procedures (T80-T88)
complications of surgical and medical care NEC
    (T80-T88)
newborn respiratory distress syndrome (P22.0)

The appropriate 7th character is to be added to each code from
category T79

A	initial encounter	
D	subsequent encounter	
S	sequela	

X● **T79.0**   **Air embolism (traumatic)** A 🔖

Excludes1   air embolism complicating abortion
    or ectopic or molar pregnancy
    (O00-O07, O08.2)
air embolism complicating pregnancy,
    childbirth and the puerperium
    (O88.0)
air embolism following infusion,
    transfusion, and therapeutic injection
    (T80.0)
air embolism following procedure NEC
    (T81.7-)

(Ex) D78.81-D78.89, E36.8, E89.810-E89.89, H59.011-H59.019,
H59.031-H59.039, H59.091-H59.099, H59.811-H59.89, H95.811-H95.89,
I97.3, L76.81-L76.82, M96.89, N98.1-N98.9, T14.90-T14.91, T79.0XX[A],
T79.A0X- T79.9XX[A], T80.0XX[A], T81.82X[A], T81.89X-T81.9XX[A]

X● **T79.1**   **Fat embolism (traumatic)** A 🔖

Excludes1   fat embolism complicating:
      abortion or ectopic or molar pregnancy
        (O00-O07, O08.2)
      pregnancy, childbirth and the
        puerperium (O88.8)

(Ex) D78.81-D78.89, E36.8, E89.810-E89.89, H59.011-H59.019,
H59.031-H59.039, H59.091-H59.099, H59.811-H59.89, H95.811-H95.89,
I97.3, L76.81-L76.82, M96.89, N98.1-N98.9, T14.90-T14.91, T79.0XX[A],
T79.A0X- T79.9XX[A], T81.82X[A], T81.89X-T81.9XX[A]

X● **T79.2**   **Traumatic secondary and recurrent hemorrhage and seroma** A 🔖

(Ex) D78.81-D78.89, E36.8, E89.810-E89.89, H59.011-H59.019,
H59.031-H59.039, H59.091-H59.099, H59.811-H59.89, H95.811-H95.89,
I97.3, L76.81-L76.82, M96.89, N98.1-N98.9, T14.90-T14.91, 79.2XX[A],
T79.A0X-T79.9XX[A], T81.82X-T81.9XX[A]

X● **T79.4**   **Traumatic shock** A 🔖
    Shock (immediate) (delayed) following injury

Excludes1   anaphylactic shock due to adverse food
    reaction (T78.0-)
anaphylactic shock due to correct
    medicinal substance properly
    administered (T88.6)
anaphylactic shock due to serum (T80.5-)
anaphylactic shock NOS (T78.2)
anesthetic shock (T88.2)
electric shock (T75.4)
nontraumatic shock NEC (R57.-)
obstetric shock (O75.1)
postprocedural shock (T81.1-)
septic shock (R65.21)
shock complicating abortion or ectopic or
    molar pregnancy (O00-O07, O08.3)
shock due to lightning (T75.01)
shock NOS (R57.9)

(Ex) D78.81-D78.89, E36.8, E89.810-E89.89, H59.011-H59.019,
H59.031-H59.039, H59.091-H59.099, H59.811-H59.89, H95.811-H95.89,
I97.3, L76.81-L76.82, M96.89, N98.1-N98.9, T14.90-T14.91, T79.4XX[A],
T79.A0X-T79.9XX[A], T81.82X-T81.9XX[A]

X● **T79.5**   **Traumatic anuria** A 🔖
    Crush syndrome
    Renal failure following crushing

(Ex) D78.01-D78.02, D78.21-D78.22, D78.31-D78.34, D78.81-D78.89, E36.01-E36.02,
E36.8, E89.810-E89.89, G97.51-G97.52, G97.61-G97.64, H59.011-H59.019,
H59.031-H59.039, H59.091-H59.099, H59.111-H59.129, H59.311-H59.329,
H59.331-H59.369, H59.811-H59.819, H59.88-H59.89, H95.21-H95.22,
H95.41-H95.42, H95.51-H92.52, H95.551-H95.554, H95.811-H95.819,
H95.88-H95.89, I97.3-I97.42, I97.610-I97.648, J95.61-J95.62, J95.830-J95.831,
J95.860-J95.863, K91.61-K91.62, K91.840-K91.841, K91.870-K91.873,
L76.01-L76.02, L76.21-L76.22, L76.31-L76.34, L76.81-L76.82,
M96.810-M96.811, M96.830-M96.89, N98.1-N98.9, N99.61-N99.62,
N99.820-N99.821, N99.840-N99.843, T14.90-T14.91, T79.5XX[A], T79.
A0X-T79.9XX[A], T81.10X-T81.19X[A], T81.82X-T81.9XX[A], T88.2XX[A]

X● **T79.6**   **Traumatic ischemia of muscle**
    Traumatic rhabdomyolysis
    Volkmann's ischemic contracture

Excludes2   anterior tibial syndrome (M76.8)
compartment syndrome (traumatic)
    (T79.A-)
nontraumatic ischemia of muscle (M62.2-)

X● **T79.7**   **Traumatic subcutaneous emphysema** A 🔖

Excludes1   emphysema NOS (J43)
emphysema (subcutaneous) resulting
    from a procedure (T81.82)

(Ex) D78.81-D78.89, E36.8, E89.810-E89.89, H59.011-H59.019, H59.031-H59.039,
H59.091-H59.099, H59.811-H59.89, H95.811-H95.89, I97.3, L76.81-L76.82,
M96.89, N98.1-N98.9, S21.101-S21.159[A], S21.301-S21.459[A],
S21.90X-S21.95X[A], S27.0XX-S27.399[A], S27.50X-S27.809[A], S27.892—
S27.9XX[A], S28.1XX[A], S29.021-S29.029[A], T14.90-T14.91,
T79.7XX-T79.9XX[A], T81.82X-T81.9XX[A]

● **T79.A**   **Traumatic compartment syndrome**

Excludes1   fibromyalgia (M79.7)
nontraumatic compartment syndrome
    (M79.A-)
traumatic ischemic infarction of muscle
    (T79.6)

(Ex) **For category T79.A CC codes unless otherwise indicated:**
M70.80-M70.99, M79.81-M79.9, R29.898

X● **T79.A0**   **Compartment syndrome, unspecified** A 🔖
    Compartment syndrome NOS

(Ex) S31.001[A], S31.011[A], S31.021[A], S31.031[A], S31.041[A],
S31.051[A], S31.600-S31.659[A], S36.81X-S36.899[A]

● **T79.A1**   **Traumatic compartment syndrome of upper extremity**
    Traumatic compartment syndrome of shoulder,
    arm, forearm, wrist, hand, and fingers

● **T79.A11**   **Traumatic compartment syndrome of right upper extremity** A 🔖

● **T79.A12**   **Traumatic compartment syndrome of left upper extremity** A 🔖

● **T79.A19**   **Traumatic compartment syndrome of unspecified upper extremity** A 🔖

◄ New   ◄▦ Revised   ~~deleted~~ Deleted   Excludes 1   Excludes 2   Includes   Use additional   Code first   Code also   Unspecified

OGCR Official Guidelines   ● Unacceptable Principal Diagnosis   X Assign placeholder X   ● Use Additional Character(s)   🔖 Manifestation Code   **Coding Clinic**

1490

● **T79.A2 Traumatic compartment syndrome of lower extremity**
    Traumatic compartment syndrome of hip, buttock, thigh, leg, foot, and toes

  ● **T79.A21 Traumatic compartment syndrome of right lower extremity** A 🏥

  ● **T79.A22 Traumatic compartment syndrome of left lower extremity** A 🏥

  ● **T79.A29 Traumatic compartment syndrome of unspecified lower extremity** A 🏥

X ● **T79.A3 Traumatic compartment syndrome of abdomen** A 🏥
    (Ex) S31.001[A], S31.011[A], S31.021[A], S31.031[A], S31.041[A], S31.051[A], S31.100-S31.159[A], S31.600-S31.659[A], S31.831-S31.839[A], S36.00X-S37.599[A], S37.812-S37.99X[A], S38.3XX[A], S39.021-S39.023[A], T14.90-T14.91, T79.8XX-T79.9XX[A]

X ● **T79.A9 Traumatic compartment syndrome of other sites** A 🏥
    (Ex) See T79.A0

X ● **T79.8 Other early complications of trauma**

X ● **T79.9 Unspecified early complication of trauma**

COMPLICATIONS OF SURGICAL AND MEDICAL CARE NOT ELSEWHERE CLASSIFIED (T80-T88)

Use additional code for adverse effect, if applicable, to identify drug (T36-T50 with fifth or sixth character 5)

Use additional code(s) to identify the specified condition resulting from the complication.

Use additional code to identify devices involved and details of circumstances (Y62-Y82)

Excludes2   any encounters with medical care for postprocedural conditions in which no complications are present, such as:
    artificial opening status (Z93.-)
    closure of external stoma (Z43.-)
    fitting and adjustment of external prosthetic device (Z44.-)
  burns and corrosions from local applications and irradiation (T20-T32)
  complications of surgical procedures during pregnancy, childbirth and the puerperium (O00-O9A)
  mechanical complication of respirator [ventilator] (J95.850)
  poisoning and toxic effects of drugs and chemicals (T36-T65 with fifth or sixth character 1-4 or 6)
  postprocedural fever (R50.82)
  specified complications classified elsewhere, such as:
    cerebrospinal fluid leak from spinal puncture (G97.0)
    colostomy malfunction (K94.0-)
    disorders of fluid and electrolyte imbalance (E86-E87)
    functional disturbances following cardiac surgery (I97.0-I97.1)
    intraoperative and postprocedural complications of specified body systems (D78.-, E36.-, E89.-, G97.3-, G97.4, H59.3-, H59.-, H95.2-, H95.3, I97.4-, I97.5, J95.6-, J95.7, K91.6-, L76.-, M96.-, N99.-)
    ostomy complications (J95.0-, K94.-, N99.5-)
    postgastric surgery syndromes (K91.1)
    postlaminectomy syndrome NEC (M96.1)
    postmastectomy lymphedema syndrome (I97.2)
    postsurgical blind-loop syndrome (K91.2)
    ventilator associated pneumonia (J95.851)

● **T80 Complications following infusion, transfusion and therapeutic injection**

  Includes   complications following perfusion

  Excludes2   bone marrow transplant rejection (T86.01)
    febrile nonhemolytic transfusion reaction (R50.84)
    fluid overload due to transfusion (E87.71)
    posttransfusion purpura (D69.51)
    transfusion associated circulatory overload (TACO) (E87.71)
    transfusion (red blood cell) associated hemochromatosis (E83.111)
    transfusion related acute lung injury (TRALI) (J95.84)

The appropriate 7th character is to be added to each code from category T80

A	initial encounter
D	subsequent encounter
S	sequela

X ● **T80.0 Air embolism following infusion, transfusion and therapeutic injection** A 🏥, A 🏥
    (Ex) T79.0XX[A], T80.0XX[A]

X ● **T80.1 Vascular complications following infusion, transfusion and therapeutic injection** A 🏥
  Use additional code to identify the vascular complication

  Excludes2   extravasation of vesicant agent (T80.81-)
    infiltration of vesicant agent (T80.81-)
    vascular complications specified as due to prosthetic devices, implants and grafts (T82.8- T83.8-, T84.8-, T85.8-) ◄▥
    postprocedural vascular complications (T81.7-)
    (Ex) T80.1XX[A], T80.810-T80.818[A], T80.90X[A]

● **T80.2 Infections following infusion, transfusion and therapeutic injection**
  Use additional code to identify the specific infection, such as:
    sepsis (A41.9)

  Use additional code (R65.2-) to identify severe sepsis, if applicable

  Excludes2   infections specified as due to prosthetic devices, implants and grafts (T82.6-T82.7, T83.5-T83.6, T84.5-T84.7, T85.7)
    postprocedural infections (T81.4-) ◄▥
    (Ex) **For category T80.2 CC codes:** Ex: N98.0, T80.211-T80.29X[A], T82.7XX[A], T88.0XX[A]

  ● **T80.21 Infection due to central venous catheter**
    Infection due to pulmonary artery catheter (Swan-Ganz catheter) ◄

    ● **T80.211 Bloodstream infection due to central venous catheter** A 🏥, A 🏥
      Catheter-related bloodstream infection (CRBSI) NOS
      Central line-associated bloodstream infection (CLABSI)
      Bloodstream infection due to Hickman catheter
      Bloodstream infection due to peripherally inserted central catheter (PICC)
      Bloodstream infection due to portacath (port-a-cath)
      Bloodstream infection due to pulmonary artery catheter ◄
      Bloodstream infection due to triple lumen catheter
      Bloodstream infection due to umbilical venous catheter

N Newborn Age: 0   **P** Pediatric Age: 0–17   **M** Maternity DX: 12–55   **A** Adult Age: 15–124   ♀ Females Only   ♂ Males Only
🏥 Complication\Comorbidity   🏥 Major C\C   (Ex) CC/MCC Exclusions   🏥 Hospital-Acquired Condition
1491

CHAPTER 19 (S00-T88)

● **T80.212**   **Local infection due to central venous catheter** A 🝉, A 🝉
  Exit or insertion site infection
  Local infection due to Hickman catheter
  Local infection due to peripherally inserted central catheter (PICC)
  Local infection due to portacath (port-a-cath)
  Local infection due to pulmonary artery catheter ◄
  Local infection due to triple lumen catheter
  Local infection due to umbilical venous catheter
  Port or reservoir infection
  Tunnel infection

● **T80.218**   **Other infection due to central venous catheter** A 🝉, A 🝉
  Other central line-associated infection
  Other infection due to Hickman catheter
  Other infection due to peripherally inserted central catheter (PICC)
  Other infection due to portacath (port-a-cath)
  Other infection due to pulmonary artery catheter ◄
  Other infection due to triple lumen catheter
  Other infection due to umbilical venous catheter

● **T80.219**   **Unspecified infection due to central venous catheter** A 🝉, A 🝉
  Central line-associated infection NOS
  Unspecified infection due to Hickman catheter
  Unspecified infection due to peripherally inserted central catheter (PICC)
  Unspecified infection due to portacath (port-a-cath)
  Unspecified infection due to pulmonary artery catheter ◄
  Unspecified infection due to triple lumen catheter
  Unspecified infection due to umbilical venous catheter

X ● **T80.22**   **Acute infection following transfusion, infusion, or injection of blood and blood products** A 🝉

X ● **T80.29**   **Infection following other infusion, transfusion and therapeutic injection** A 🝉

● **T80.3**   **ABO incompatibility reaction due to transfusion of blood or blood products**
  Excludes1   minor blood group antigens reactions (Duffy) (E) (K(ell)) (Kidd) (Lewis) (M) (N) (P) (S) (T80.A)
  (Ex:) **For category T80.3 CC codes unless otherwise indicated:** T80.30X-T80.A9X[A], T80.910-T80.92X[A]

X ● **T80.30**   **ABO incompatibility reaction due to transfusion of blood or blood products, unspecified** A 🝉, A 🝉
  ABO incompatibility blood transfusion NOS
  Reaction to ABO incompatibility from transfusion NOS

● **T80.31**   **ABO incompatibility with hemolytic transfusion reaction**

  ● **T80.310**   **ABO incompatibility with acute hemolytic transfusion reaction** A 🝉, A 🝉
    ABO incompatibility with hemolytic transfusion reaction less than 24 hours after transfusion
    Acute hemolytic transfusion reaction (AHTR) due to ABO incompatibility

  ● **T80.311**   **ABO incompatibility with delayed hemolytic transfusion reaction** A 🝉, A 🝉
    ABO incompatibility with hemolytic transfusion reaction 24 hours or more after transfusion
    Delayed hemolytic transfusion reaction (DHTR) due to ABO incompatibility

  ● **T80.319**   **ABO incompatibility with hemolytic transfusion reaction, unspecified** A 🝉, A 🝉
    ABO incompatibility with hemolytic transfusion reaction at unspecified time after transfusion
    Hemolytic transfusion reaction (HTR) due to ABO incompatibility NOS

X ● **T80.39**   **Other ABO incompatibility reaction due to transfusion of blood or blood products** A 🝉, A 🝉
  Delayed serologic transfusion reaction (DSTR) from ABO incompatibility
  Other ABO incompatible blood transfusion
  Other reaction to ABO incompatible blood transfusion

● **T80.4**   **Rh incompatibility reaction due to transfusion of blood or blood products**
  Reaction due to incompatibility of Rh antigens (C) (c) (D) (E) (e)
  (Ex:) **For category T80.4 CC codes unless otherwise indicated:** See T80.3

X ● **T80.40**   **Rh incompatibility reaction due to transfusion of blood or blood products, unspecified** A 🝉
  Reaction due to Rh factor in transfusion NOS
  Rh incompatible blood transfusion NOS

● **T80.41**   **Rh incompatibility with hemolytic transfusion reaction**

  ● **T80.410**   **Rh incompatibility with acute hemolytic transfusion reaction** A 🝉
    Acute hemolytic transfusion reaction (AHTR) due to Rh incompatibility
    Rh incompatibility with hemolytic transfusion reaction less than 24 hours after transfusion

  ● **T80.411**   **Rh incompatibility with delayed hemolytic transfusion reaction** A 🝉
    Delayed hemolytic transfusion reaction (DHTR) due to Rh incompatibility
    Rh incompatibility with hemolytic transfusion reaction 24 hours or more after transfusion

  ● **T80.419**   **Rh incompatibility with hemolytic transfusion reaction, unspecified** A 🝉
    Rh incompatibility with hemolytic transfusion reaction at unspecified time after transfusion
    Hemolytic transfusion reaction (HTR) due to Rh incompatibility NOS

X ● **T80.49**   **Other Rh incompatibility reaction due to transfusion of blood or blood products** A 🝉
  Delayed serologic transfusion reaction (DSTR) from Rh incompatibility
  Other reaction to Rh incompatible blood transfusion
  (Ex:) T80.30X-T80.419[A], T80.910-T80.92X[A], T80.A9X[A]

◄ New   ◄▥ Revised   ~~deleted~~ Deleted   Excludes 1   Excludes 2   Includes   Use additional   Code first   Code also   Unspecified
OGCR Official Guidelines   ● Unacceptable Principal Diagnosis   X Assign placeholder X   🝉 Use Additional Character(s)   ▸ Manifestation Code   **Coding Clinic**

● **T80.A**   **Non-ABO incompatibility reaction due to transfusion of blood or blood products**
Reaction due to incompatibility of minor antigens (Duffy) (Kell) (Kidd) (Lewis) (M) (N) (P) (S)
(Ex:) For category T80.A CC codes unless otherwise indicated: See T80.49

X● **T80.A0**   **Non-ABO incompatibility reaction due to transfusion of blood or blood products, unspecified** A 🦠
Non-ABO antigen incompatibility reaction from transfusion NOS

● **T80.A1**   **Non-ABO incompatibility with hemolytic transfusion reaction**

● **T80.A10**   **Non-ABO incompatibility with acute hemolytic transfusion reaction** A 🦠
Acute hemolytic transfusion reaction (AHTR) due to non-ABO incompatibility
Non-ABO incompatibility with hemolytic transfusion reaction less than 24 hours after transfusion

● **T80.A11**   **Non-ABO incompatibility with delayed hemolytic transfusion reaction** A 🦠
Delayed hemolytic transfusion reaction (DHTR) due to non-ABO incompatibility
Non-ABO incompatibility with hemolytic transfusion reaction 24 or more hours after transfusion

● **T80.A19**   **Non-ABO incompatibility with hemolytic transfusion reaction, unspecified** A 🦠
Hemolytic transfusion reaction (HTR) due to non-ABO incompatibility NOS
Non-ABO incompatibility with hemolytic transfusion reaction at unspecified time after transfusion

X● **T80.A9**   **Other non-ABO incompatibility reaction due to transfusion of blood or blood products** A 🦠
Delayed serologic transfusion reaction (DSTR) from non-ABO incompatibility
Other reaction to non-ABO incompatible blood transfusion
(Ex:) See T80.3

● **T80.5**   **Anaphylactic reaction due to serum**
Allergic reaction due to serum
Anaphylactic shock due to serum
Anaphylactoid reaction due to serum
Anaphylaxis due to serum

     Excludes1   ABO incompatibility reaction due to transfusion of blood or blood products (T80.3-)
allergic reaction or shock NOS (T78.2)
anaphylactic reaction or shock NOS (T78.2)
anaphylactic reaction or shock due to adverse effect of correct medicinal substance properly administered (T88.6)
other serum reaction (T80.6-)
(Ex:) For category T80.5 CC codes: T80.51X-T80.69X[A]

X● **T80.51**   **Anaphylactic reaction due to administration of blood and blood products** A 🦠

X● **T80.52**   **Anaphylactic reaction due to vaccination** A 🦠

X● **T80.59**   **Anaphylactic reaction due to other serum** A 🦠

● **T80.6**   **Other serum reactions**
Intoxication by serum   Serum sickness
Protein sickness   Serum urticaria
Serum rash

     Excludes2   serum hepatitis (B16-B19) ◄▦
(Ex:) For category T80.6 CC codes unless otherwise indicated:
T80.51X-T80.69X[A]

X● **T80.61**   **Other serum reaction due to administration of blood and blood products** A 🦠

X● **T80.62**   **Other serum reaction due to vaccination** A 🦠

X● **T80.69**   **Other serum reaction due to other serum** A 🦠
(Ex:) T80.61X-T80.69X[A]

● **T80.8**   **Other complications following infusion, transfusion and therapeutic injection**

● **T80.81**   **Extravasation of vesicant agent**
Infiltration of vesicant agent
(Ex:) For category T80.81 CC codes: T80.1XX[A], T80.810-T80.818[A], T80.90X[A]

● **T80.810**   **Extravasation of vesicant antineoplastic chemotherapy** A 🦠
Infiltration of vesicant antineoplastic chemotherapy

● **T80.818**   **Extravasation of other vesicant agent** A 🦠
Infiltration of other vesicant agent

X● **T80.89**   **Other complications following infusion, transfusion and therapeutic injection**
Delayed serologic transfusion reaction (DSTR), unspecified incompatibility
Use additional code to identify graft-versus-host reaction, if applicable, (D89.81-)

● **T80.9**   **Unspecified complication following infusion, transfusion and therapeutic injection**

X● **T80.90**   **Unspecified complication following infusion and therapeutic injection**

● **T80.91**   **Hemolytic transfusion reaction, unspecified incompatibility**

     Excludes1   ABO incompatibility with hemolytic transfusion reaction (T80.31-)
Non-ABO incompatibility with hemolytic transfusion reaction (T80.A1-)
Rh incompatibility with hemolytic transfusion reaction (T80.41-)
(Ex:) For category T80.91 CC codes unless otherwise indicated: See T80.3

● **T80.910**   **Acute hemolytic transfusion reaction, unspecified incompatibility** A 🦠

● **T80.911**   **Delayed hemolytic transfusion reaction, unspecified incompatibility** A 🦠

● **T80.919**   **Hemolytic transfusion reaction, unspecified incompatibility, unspecified as acute or delayed** A 🦠
Hemolytic transfusion reaction NOS

X● **T80.92**   **Unspecified transfusion reaction**
Transfusion reaction NOS

N   Newborn Age: 0   **P**   Pediatric Age: 0–17   **M**   Maternity DX: 12–55   **A**   Adult Age: 15–124   ♀   Females Only   ♂   Males Only

🦠   Complication\Comorbidity   🦠   Major C\C   (Ex:)   CC/MCC Exclusions   🦠   Hospital-Acquired Condition

1493

CHAPTER 19 (S00-T88)

● **T81** **Complications of procedures, not elsewhere classified**

Use additional code for adverse effect, if applicable, to identify drug (T36-T50 with fifth or sixth character 5)

Excludes2 complications following immunization (T88.0-T88.1)

complications following infusion, transfusion and therapeutic injection (T80.-)

complications of transplanted organs and tissue (T86.-)

poisoning and toxic effects of drugs and chemicals (T36-T65 with fifth or sixth character 1-4 or 6)

specified complications classified elsewhere, such as:

complication of prosthetic devices, implants and grafts (T82-T85)

dermatitis due to drugs and medicaments (L23.3, L24.4, L25.1, L27.0-L27.1)

endosseous dental implant failure (M27.6-)

floppy iris syndrome (IFIS) (intraoperative) H21.81

intraoperative and postprocedural complications of specific body system (D78.-, E36.-, E89.-, G97.3-, G97.4, H59.3-, H59.-, H95.2-, H95.3, I97.4-, I97.5, J95, K91.-, L76.-, M96.-, N99.-)

ostomy complications (J95.0-, K94.-, N99.5-)

plateau iris syndrome (post-iridectomy) (postprocedural) H21.82

The appropriate 7th character is to be added to each code from category T81

A	initial encounter
D	subsequent encounter
S	sequela

● **T81.1** **Postprocedural shock**

Shock during or resulting from a procedure, not elsewhere classified

Excludes1 anaphylactic shock NOS (T78.2)

anaphylactic shock due to correct substance properly administered (T88.6)

anaphylactic shock due to serum (T80.5-)

anesthetic shock (T88.2)

electric shock (T75.4)

obstetric shock (O75.1)

septic shock (R65.21)

shock following abortion or ectopic or molar pregnancy (O00-O07, O08.3)

traumatic shock (T79.4)

(Ex) For category T81.1 CC codes: D78.01-D78.02, D78.21-D78.22, D78.31-D78.34, D78.81-D78.89, E36.01-E36.02, E36.8, E89.810-E89.89, G97.51-G97.52, G97.61-G97.64, H59.011-H59.019, H59.031-H59.039, H59.091-H59.099, H59.111-H59.129, H59.311-H59.369, H59.331-H59.349, H59.811-H59.819, H59.88-H59.89, H95.21-H95.22, H95.41-H95.42, H59.51-H59.54, H95.811-H95.819, H95.88-H95.89, I97.3-I97.42, I97.610-I97.648, J95.61-J95.62, J95.830-J95.831, J95.860-J95.863, K91.61-K91.62, K91.840-K91.841, K91.870-K91.873, L76.01-L76.02, L76.21-L76.22, L76.31-L76.34, L76.81-L76.82, M96.810-M96.811, M96.830-M96.89, N98.1-N98.9, N99.61-N99.62, N99.820-N99.821, N99.840-N99.843, T79.4XX[A], T81.10X-T81.19X[A], T81.82X-T81.9XX[A], T88.2XX[A]

X ● **T81.10** **Postprocedural shock unspecified** A 🔖

Collapse NOS during or resulting from a procedure, not elsewhere classified

Postprocedural failure of peripheral circulation

Postprocedural shock NOS

X ● **T81.11** **Postprocedural cardiogenic shock** A 🔖

A ● X ● **T81.12** **Postprocedural septic shock** A 🔖

Postprocedural endotoxic shock resulting from a procedure, not elsewhere classified ◀▥

Postprocedural gram-negative shock resulting from a procedure, not elsewhere classified ◀▥

Code first underlying infection

Use additional code, to identify any associated acute organ dysfunction, if applicable

X ● **T81.19** **Other postprocedural shock** A 🔖

Postprocedural hypovolemic shock

● **T81.3** **Disruption of wound, not elsewhere classified**

Disruption of any suture materials or other closure methods

Excludes1 breakdown (mechanical) of permanent sutures (T85.612)

displacement of permanent sutures (T85.622)

disruption of cesarean delivery wound (O90.0)

disruption of perineal obstetric wound (O90.1)

mechanical complication of permanent sutures NEC (T85.692)

(Ex) For category T81.3 CC codes: D78.81-D78.89, E36.8, E89.810-E89.89, H59.011-H59.019, H59.031-H59.039, H59.091-H59.099, H59.811-H59.89, H95.811-H95.89, I97.3, L76.81-L76.82, M96.89, N98.1-N98.9, T81.30X-T81.33X[A], T81.82X-T81.9XX[A]

X ● **T81.30** **Disruption of wound, unspecified** A 🔖

Disruption of wound NOS

X ● **T81.31** **Disruption of external operation (surgical) wound, not elsewhere classified** A 🔖

Excludes1 dehiscence of amputation stump (T87.81)

Dehiscence of operation wound NOS

Disruption of operation wound NOS

Disruption or dehiscence of closure of cornea

Disruption or dehiscence of closure of mucosa

Disruption or dehiscence of closure of skin and subcutaneous tissue

Full-thickness skin disruption or dehiscence

Superficial disruption or dehiscence of operation wound

Coding Clinic: 2015, Q1, P20

X ● **T81.32** **Disruption of internal operation (surgical) wound, not elsewhere classified** A 🔖

Deep disruption or dehiscence of operation wound NOS

Disruption or dehiscence of closure of internal organ or other internal tissue

Disruption or dehiscence of closure of muscle or muscle flap

Disruption or dehiscence of closure of ribs or rib cage

Disruption or dehiscence of closure of skull or craniotomy

Disruption or dehiscence of closure of sternum or sternotomy

Disruption or dehiscence of closure of tendon or ligament

Disruption or dehiscence of closure of superficial or muscular fascia

X ● **T81.33** **Disruption of traumatic injury wound repair** A 🔖

Disruption or dehiscence of closure of traumatic laceration (external) (internal)

X● **T81.4** **Infection following a procedure** A 🝝, A 🝝
  Intra-abdominal abscess following a procedure
  Postprocedural infection, not elsewhere classified
  Sepsis following a procedure
  Stitch abscess following a procedure
  Subphrenic abscess following a procedure
  Wound abscess following a procedure
  Use additional code to identify infection
  Use additional code (R65.2-) to identify severe sepsis, if applicable

  Excludes1 obstetric surgical wound infection (O86.0)
      postprocedural fever NOS (R50.82)
      postprocedural retroperitoneal abscess (K68.11)

  Excludes2 bleb associated endophthalmitis (H59.4-)
      infection due to infusion, transfusion and therapeutic injection (T80.2-)
      infection due to prosthetic devices, implants and grafts (T82.6-T82.7, T83.5-T83.6, T84.5-T84.7, T85.7)

  (Ex) D78.81-D78.89, E36.8, E89.810-E89.89, H59.011-H59.019, H59.031-H59.099, H59.811-H59.89, H95.811-H95.89, I97.3, K68.11, L76.81-L76.82, M96.89, N98.1-N98.9, T81.4XX[A], T81.82X[A], T81.89X-T81.9XX[A]

  Coding Clinic: 2015, Q4, P37

● **T81.5** **Complications of foreign body accidentally left in body following procedure**
  (Ex) For category T81.5 CC codes: D78.81-D78.89, E36.8, E89.810-E89.89, H59.011-H59.019, H59.031-H59.039, H59.091-H59.099, H59.811-H59.89, H95.811-H95.89, I97.3, L76.81-L76.82, M96.89, N98.1-N98.9, T81.500-T81.599[A], T81.82X-T81.9XX[A]

 ● **T81.50** **Unspecified complication of foreign body accidentally left in body following procedure**
  ● **T81.500** **Unspecified complication of foreign body accidentally left in body following surgical operation** A 🝝, A 🝝
  ● **T81.501** **Unspecified complication of foreign body accidentally left in body following infusion or transfusion** A 🝝, A 🝝
  ● **T81.502** **Unspecified complication of foreign body accidentally left in body following kidney dialysis** A 🝝, A 🝝
  ● **T81.503** **Unspecified complication of foreign body accidentally left in body following injection or immunization** A 🝝, A 🝝
  ● **T81.504** **Unspecified complication of foreign body accidentally left in body following endoscopic examination** A 🝝, A 🝝
  ● **T81.505** **Unspecified complication of foreign body accidentally left in body following heart catheterization** A 🝝, A 🝝
  ● **T81.506** **Unspecified complication of foreign body accidentally left in body following aspiration, puncture or other catheterization** A 🝝, A 🝝
  ● **T81.507** **Unspecified complication of foreign body accidentally left in body following removal of catheter or packing** A 🝝, A 🝝
  ● **T81.508** **Unspecified complication of foreign body accidentally left in body following other procedure** A 🝝, A 🝝
  ● **T81.509** **Unspecified complication of foreign body accidentally left in body following unspecified procedure** A 🝝, A 🝝

 ● **T81.51** **Adhesions due to foreign body accidentally left in body following procedure**
  ● **T81.510** **Adhesions due to foreign body accidentally left in body following surgical operation** A 🝝, A 🝝
  ● **T81.511** **Adhesions due to foreign body accidentally left in body following infusion or transfusion** A 🝝, A 🝝
  ● **T81.512** **Adhesions due to foreign body accidentally left in body following kidney dialysis** A 🝝, A 🝝
  ● **T81.513** **Adhesions due to foreign body accidentally left in body following injection or immunization** A 🝝, A 🝝
  ● **T81.514** **Adhesions due to foreign body accidentally left in body following endoscopic examination** A 🝝, A 🝝
  ● **T81.515** **Adhesions due to foreign body accidentally left in body following heart catheterization** A 🝝, A 🝝
  ● **T81.516** **Adhesions due to foreign body accidentally left in body following aspiration, puncture or other catheterization** A 🝝, A 🝝
  ● **T81.517** **Adhesions due to foreign body accidentally left in body following removal of catheter or packing** A 🝝, A 🝝
  ● **T81.518** **Adhesions due to foreign body accidentally left in body following other procedure** A 🝝, A 🝝
  ● **T81.519** **Adhesions due to foreign body accidentally left in body following unspecified procedure** A 🝝, A 🝝

 ● **T81.52** **Obstruction due to foreign body accidentally left in body following procedure**
  ● **T81.520** **Obstruction due to foreign body accidentally left in body following surgical operation** A 🝝, A 🝝
  ● **T81.521** **Obstruction due to foreign body accidentally left in body following infusion or transfusion** A 🝝, A 🝝
  ● **T81.522** **Obstruction due to foreign body accidentally left in body following kidney dialysis** A 🝝, A 🝝
  ● **T81.523** **Obstruction due to foreign body accidentally left in body following injection or immunization** A 🝝, A 🝝
  ● **T81.524** **Obstruction due to foreign body accidentally left in body following endoscopic examination** A 🝝, A 🝝
  ● **T81.525** **Obstruction due to foreign body accidentally left in body following heart catheterization** A 🝝, A 🝝
  ● **T81.526** **Obstruction due to foreign body accidentally left in body following aspiration, puncture or other catheterization** A 🝝, A 🝝
  ● **T81.527** **Obstruction due to foreign body accidentally left in body following removal of catheter or packing** A 🝝, A 🝝
  ● **T81.528** **Obstruction due to foreign body accidentally left in body following other procedure** A 🝝, A 🝝
  ● **T81.529** **Obstruction due to foreign body accidentally left in body following unspecified procedure** A 🝝, A 🝝

N Newborn Age: 0 **P** Pediatric Age: 0–17 **M** Maternity DX: 12–55 **A** Adult Age: 15–124 ♀ Females Only ♂ Males Only

🝝 Complication\Comorbidity 🝝 Major C\C (Ex) CC/MCC Exclusions 🝝 Hospital-Acquired Condition

1495

● **T81.53**   **Perforation due to foreign body accidentally left in body following procedure**
- ● **T81.530**   **Perforation due to foreign body accidentally left in body following surgical operation** A 🔵, A 🔵
- ● **T81.531**   **Perforation due to foreign body accidentally left in body following infusion or transfusion** A 🔵, A 🔵
- ● **T81.532**   **Perforation due to foreign body accidentally left in body following kidney dialysis** A 🔵, A 🔵
- ● **T81.533**   **Perforation due to foreign body accidentally left in body following injection or immunization** A 🔵, A 🔵
- ● **T81.534**   **Perforation due to foreign body accidentally left in body following endoscopic examination** A 🔵, A 🔵
- ● **T81.535**   **Perforation due to foreign body accidentally left in body following heart catheterization** A 🔵, A 🔵
- ● **T81.536**   **Perforation due to foreign body accidentally left in body following aspiration, puncture or other catheterization** A 🔵, A 🔵
- ● **T81.537**   **Perforation due to foreign body accidentally left in body following removal of catheter or packing** A 🔵, A 🔵
- ● **T81.538**   **Perforation due to foreign body accidentally left in body following other procedure** A 🔵, A 🔵
- ● **T81.539**   **Perforation due to foreign body accidentally left in body following unspecified procedure** A 🔵, A 🔵

● **T81.59**   **Other complications of foreign body accidentally left in body following procedure**

> **Excludes2**   obstruction or perforation due to prosthetic devices and implants intentionally left in body (T82.0-T82.5, T83.0-T83.4, T83.7, T84.0-T84.4, T85.0-T85.6)

- ● **T81.590**   **Other complications of foreign body accidentally left in body following surgical operation** A 🔵, A 🔵
- ● **T81.591**   **Other complications of foreign body accidentally left in body following infusion or transfusion** A 🔵, A 🔵
- ● **T81.592**   **Other complications of foreign body accidentally left in body following kidney dialysis** A 🔵, A 🔵
- ● **T81.593**   **Other complications of foreign body accidentally left in body following injection or immunization** A 🔵, A 🔵
- ● **T81.594**   **Other complications of foreign body accidentally left in body following endoscopic examination** A 🔵, A 🔵
- ● **T81.595**   **Other complications of foreign body accidentally left in body following heart catheterization** A 🔵, A 🔵
- ● **T81.596**   **Other complications of foreign body accidentally left in body following aspiration, puncture or other catheterization** A 🔵, A 🔵
- ● **T81.597**   **Other complications of foreign body accidentally left in body following removal of catheter or packing** A 🔵, A 🔵

- ● **T81.598**   **Other complications of foreign body accidentally left in body following other procedure** A 🔵, A 🔵
- ● **T81.599**   **Other complications of foreign body accidentally left in body following unspecified procedure** A 🔵, A 🔵

● **T81.6**   **Acute reaction to foreign substance accidentally left during a procedure**

> **Excludes2**   complications of foreign body accidentally left in body cavity or operation wound following procedure (T81.5-)

> (Ex) **For category T81.6 CC codes:** D78.81-D78.89, E36.8, E89.810-E89.89, H59.011-H59.019, H59.031-H59.039, H59.091-H59.099, H59.811-H59.89, H95.811-H95.89, I97.3, L76.81-L76.82, M96.89, N98.1-N98.9, T81.60X-T81.69X[A], T81.82X-T81.9XX[A]

X ● **T81.60**   **Unspecified acute reaction to foreign substance accidentally left during a procedure** A 🔵, A 🔵

X ● **T81.61**   **Aseptic peritonitis due to foreign substance accidentally left during a procedure** A 🔵, A 🔵
     Chemical peritonitis

X ● **T81.69**   **Other acute reaction to foreign substance accidentally left during a procedure** A 🔵, A 🔵

● **T81.7**   **Vascular complications following a procedure, not elsewhere classified**
     Air embolism following procedure NEC
     Phlebitis or thrombophlebitis resulting from a procedure

> **Excludes1**   embolism complicating abortion or ectopic or molar pregnancy (O00-O07, O08.2)
> embolism complicating pregnancy, childbirth and the puerperium (O88.-)
> traumatic embolism (T79.0)

> **Excludes2**   embolism due to prosthetic devices, implants and grafts (T82.8, T83.81, T84.8-, T85.1-) ◀▥
> embolism following infusion, transfusion and therapeutic injection (T80.0)

● **T81.71**   **Complication of artery following a procedure, not elsewhere classified**

> (Ex) **For category T81.71 CC codes T81.710-T81.711:** D78.81-D78.89, E36.8, E89.810-E89.89, H59.011-H59.019, H59.031-H59.039, H59.091-H59.099, H59.811-H59.89, H95.811-H95.89, I97.3, L76.81-L76.82, M96.89, N98.1-N98.9, T81.710-T81.72X[A], T81.82X-T81.9XX[A]
> **For T81.718-T81.719:** D78.81-D78.89, E36.8, E89.810-E89.89, H59.011-H59.019, H59.031-H59.039, H59.091-H59.099, H59.811-H59.89, H95.811-H95.89, I97.3, L76.81-L76.82, M96.89, N98.1-N98.9, T81.718-T81.72X[A], T81.82X-T81.9XX[A]

- ● **T81.710**   **Complication of mesenteric artery following a procedure, not elsewhere classified** A 🔵
- ● **T81.711**   **Complication of renal artery following a procedure, not elsewhere classified** A 🔵
- ● **T81.718**   **Complication of other artery following a procedure, not elsewhere classified** A 🔵
- ● **T81.719**   **Complication of unspecified artery following a procedure, not elsewhere classified** A 🔵

X ● **T81.72**   **Complication of vein following a procedure, not elsewhere classified** A 🔵
> (Ex) See T81.718-T81.719

● **T81.8** **Other complications of procedures, not elsewhere classified**

　　Excludes2　hypothermia following anesthesia (T88.51)
　　　　　　　　malignant hyperpyrexia due to anesthesia (T88.3)

X ● **T81.81** **Complication of inhalation therapy**

X ● **T81.82** **Emphysema (subcutaneous) resulting from a procedure**

X ● **T81.83** **Persistent postprocedural fistula** A 🔾
　　Ⓔⓧ D78.81-D78.89, E36.8, E89.810-E89.89, H59.011-H59.019,
　　H59.031-H59.039, H59.091-H59.099, H59.811-H59.89,
　　H95.811-H95.89, I97.3, L76.81-L76.82, M96.89, N98.1-N98.9,
　　T81.82X-T81.9XX[A]

X ● **T81.89** **Other complications of procedures, not elsewhere classified**
　　　　Use additional code to specify complication, such as:
　　　　　postprocedural delirium (F05)

X ● **T81.9** **Unspecified complication of procedure**

● **T82** **Complications of cardiac and vascular prosthetic devices, implants and grafts**

　　Excludes2　failure and rejection of transplanted organs and tissue (T86.-)

　　The appropriate 7th character is to be added to each code from category T82

　　┌─────────────────────────────┐
　　│ A　initial encounter   │
　　│ D　subsequent encounter   │
　　│ S　sequela   │
　　└─────────────────────────────┘

● **T82.0** **Mechanical complication of heart valve prosthesis**
　　Mechanical complication of artificial heart valve

　　Excludes1　mechanical complication of biological heart valve graft (T82.22-)
　　Ⓔⓧ **For category T82.0 CC codes:** D78.81-D78.89, E36.8, E89.810-E89.89,
　　H59.011-H59.019, H59.031-H59.039, H59.091-H59.099, H59.811-H59.89,
　　H95.811-H95.89, I97.3, L76.81-L76.82, M96.89, N98.1-N98.9,
　　T81.82X-T81.9XX[A], T82.01X-T82.09X[A]

X ● **T82.01** **Breakdown (mechanical) of heart valve prosthesis** A 🔾

X ● **T82.02** **Displacement of heart valve prosthesis** A 🔾
　　　　Malposition of heart valve prosthesis

X ● **T82.03** **Leakage of heart valve prosthesis** A 🔾

X ● **T82.09** **Other mechanical complication of heart valve prosthesis** A 🔾
　　　　Obstruction (mechanical) of heart valve prosthesis
　　　　Perforation of heart valve prosthesis
　　　　Protrusion of heart valve prosthesis

● **T82.1** **Mechanical complication of cardiac electronic device**
　　Ⓔⓧ **For category T82.1 CC codes:** D78.81-D78.89, E36.8, E89.810-E89.89,
　　H59.011-H59.019, H59.031-H59.039, H59.091-H59.099, H59.811-H59.89,
　　H95.811-H95.89, I97.3, L76.81-L76.82, M96.89, N98.1-N98.9,
　　T81.82X-T81.9XX[A], T82.110-T82.111[A], T82.120-T82.121[A],
　　T82.190-T82.191[A]

● **T82.11** **Breakdown (mechanical) of cardiac electronic device**

　● **T82.110** **Breakdown (mechanical) of cardiac electrode** A 🔾

　● **T82.111** **Breakdown (mechanical) of cardiac pulse generator (battery)** A 🔾

　● **T82.118** **Breakdown (mechanical) of other cardiac electronic device** A 🔾
　　　Ⓔⓧ D78.81-D78.89, E36.8, E89.810-E89.89,
　　　H59.011-H59.019, H59.031-H59.039,
　　　H59.091-H59.099, H59.811-H59.89,
　　　H95.811-H95.89, I97.3, L76.81-L76.82, M96.89,
　　　N98.1-N98.9, T81.82X-T81.9XX[A], T82.118[A],
　　　T82.128[A], T82.198[A], T82.221-T82.228[A],
　　　T82.512[A], T82.522[A], T82.532[A],
　　　T82.592[A], T82.594[A], T82.598[A]

● **T82.119** **Breakdown (mechanical) of unspecified cardiac electronic device** A 🔾
　　　Ⓔⓧ No Exclusions

● **T82.12** **Displacement of cardiac electronic device**
　　Malposition of cardiac electronic device

　● **T82.120** **Displacement of cardiac electrode** A 🔾

　● **T82.121** **Displacement of cardiac pulse generator (battery)** A 🔾

　● **T82.128** **Displacement of other cardiac electronic device** A 🔾
　　　Ⓔⓧ See T82.118A

　● **T82.129** **Displacement of unspecified cardiac electronic device** A 🔾
　　　Ⓔⓧ No Exclusions

● **T82.19** **Other mechanical complication of cardiac electronic device**
　　Leakage of cardiac electronic device
　　Obstruction of cardiac electronic device
　　Perforation of cardiac electronic device
　　Protrusion of cardiac electronic device

　● **T82.190** **Other mechanical complication of cardiac electrode** A 🔾

　● **T82.191** **Other mechanical complication of cardiac pulse generator (battery)** A 🔾

　● **T82.198** **Other mechanical complication of other cardiac electronic device** A 🔾
　　　Ⓔⓧ See T82.118A

　● **T82.199** **Other mechanical complication of unspecified cardiac device** A 🔾
　　　Ⓔⓧ No Exclusions

● **T82.2** **Mechanical complication of coronary artery bypass graft and biological heart valve graft**

　　Excludes1　mechanical complication of artificial heart valve prosthesis (T82.0-)

● **T82.21** **Mechanical complication of coronary artery bypass graft**
　　Ⓔⓧ **For category T82.21 CC codes:** D78.81-D78.89, E36.8,
　　E89.810-E89.89, H59.011-H59.019, H59.031-H59.039,
　　H59.091-H59.099, H59.811-H59.89, H95.811-H95.89, I97.3,
　　L76.81-L76.82, M96.89, N98.1-N98.9, T81.82X-T81.9XX[A],
　　T82.211-T82.218[A]

　● **T82.211** **Breakdown (mechanical) of coronary artery bypass graft** A 🔾

　● **T82.212** **Displacement of coronary artery bypass graft** A 🔾
　　　Malposition of coronary artery bypass graft

　● **T82.213** **Leakage of coronary artery bypass graft** A 🔾

　● **T82.218** **Other mechanical complication of coronary artery bypass graft** A 🔾
　　　Obstruction, mechanical of coronary artery bypass graft
　　　Perforation of coronary artery bypass graft
　　　Protrusion of coronary artery bypass graft

● **T82.22** **Mechanical complication of biological heart valve graft**
　　Ⓔⓧ **For category T82.22 CC codes:** See T82.118A

　● **T82.221** **Breakdown (mechanical) of biological heart valve graft** A 🔾

　● **T82.222** **Displacement of biological heart valve graft** A 🔾
　　　Malposition of biological heart valve graft

N Newborn Age: 0　　**P** Pediatric Age: 0–17　　**M** Maternity DX: 12–55　　**A** Adult Age: 15–124　　♀ Females Only　　♂ Males Only
🔾 Complication\Comorbidity　　🔾 Major C\C　　Ⓔⓧ CC/MCC Exclusions　　🔾 Hospital-Acquired Condition

1497

CHAPTER 19 (S00-T88)

● T82.223   **Leakage of biological heart valve graft** A 🐾

● T82.228   **Other mechanical complication of biological heart valve graft** A 🐾
　　Obstruction of biological heart valve graft
　　Perforation of biological heart valve graft
　　Protrusion of biological heart valve graft

● T82.3   **Mechanical complication of other vascular grafts**
　(Ex:) **For category T82.3 CC codes:** D78.81-D78.89, E36.8, E89.810-E89.89, H59.011-H59.019, H59.031-H59.039, H59.091-H59.099, H59.811-H59.89, H95.811-H95.89, I97.3, L76.81-L76.82, M96.89, N98.1-N98.9, T81.82X-T81.9XX[A], T82.310-T82.538[A], T82.590-T82.595[A]

　● T82.31   **Breakdown (mechanical) of other vascular grafts**

　　● T82.310   **Breakdown (mechanical) of aortic (bifurcation) graft (replacement)** A 🐾

　　● T82.311   **Breakdown (mechanical) of carotid arterial graft (bypass)** A 🐾

　　● T82.312   **Breakdown (mechanical) of femoral arterial graft (bypass)** A 🐾

　　● T82.318   **Breakdown (mechanical) of other vascular grafts** A 🐾

　　● T82.319   **Breakdown (mechanical) of unspecified vascular grafts** A 🐾

　● T82.32   **Displacement of other vascular grafts**
　　Malposition of other vascular grafts

　　● T82.320   **Displacement of aortic (bifurcation) graft (replacement)** A 🐾

　　● T82.321   **Displacement of carotid arterial graft (bypass)** A 🐾

　　● T82.322   **Displacement of femoral arterial graft (bypass)** A 🐾

　　● T82.328   **Displacement of other vascular grafts** A 🐾

　　● T82.329   **Displacement of unspecified vascular grafts** A 🐾

　● T82.33   **Leakage of other vascular grafts**

　　● T82.330   **Leakage of aortic (bifurcation) graft (replacement)** A 🐾

　　● T82.331   **Leakage of carotid arterial graft (bypass)** A 🐾

　　● T82.332   **Leakage of femoral arterial graft (bypass)** A 🐾

　　● T82.338   **Leakage of other vascular grafts** A 🐾

　　● T82.339   **Leakage of unspecified vascular graft** A 🐾

　● T82.39   **Other mechanical complication of other vascular grafts**
　　Obstruction (mechanical) of other vascular grafts
　　Perforation of other vascular grafts
　　Protrusion of other vascular grafts

　　● T82.390   **Other mechanical complication of aortic (bifurcation) graft (replacement)** A 🐾

　　● T82.391   **Other mechanical complication of carotid arterial graft (bypass)** A 🐾

　　● T82.392   **Other mechanical complication of femoral arterial graft (bypass)** A 🐾

　　● T82.398   **Other mechanical complication of other vascular grafts** A 🐾

　　● T82.399   **Other mechanical complication of unspecified vascular grafts** A 🐾

● T82.4   **Mechanical complication of vascular dialysis catheter**
　Mechanical complication of hemodialysis catheter
　Excludes1   mechanical complication of intraperitoneal dialysis catheter (T85.62)
　(Ex:) **For category T82.4 CC codes:** See T82.3

　X ● T82.41   **Breakdown (mechanical) of vascular dialysis catheter** A 🐾

　X ● T82.42   **Displacement of vascular dialysis catheter** A 🐾
　　Malposition of vascular dialysis catheter

　X ● T82.43   **Leakage of vascular dialysis catheter** A 🐾

　X ● T82.49   **Other complication of vascular dialysis catheter** A 🐾
　　Obstruction (mechanical) of vascular dialysis catheter
　　Perforation of vascular dialysis catheter
　　Protrusion of vascular dialysis catheter

● T82.5   **Mechanical complication of other cardiac and vascular devices and implants**
　Excludes2   mechanical complication of epidural and subdural infusion catheter (T85.61)
　(Ex:) **For category T82.5 CC codes unless otherwise indicated:** See T82.3

　● T82.51   **Breakdown (mechanical) of other cardiac and vascular devices and implants**

　　● T82.510   **Breakdown (mechanical) of surgically created arteriovenous fistula** A 🐾

　　● T82.511   **Breakdown (mechanical) of surgically created arteriovenous shunt** A 🐾

　　● T82.512   **Breakdown (mechanical) of artificial heart** A 🐾
　　　(Ex:) See T82.118A

　　● T82.513   **Breakdown (mechanical) of balloon (counterpulsation) device** A 🐾

　　● T82.514   **Breakdown (mechanical) of infusion catheter** A 🐾

　　● T82.515   **Breakdown (mechanical) of umbrella device** A 🐾

　　● T82.518   **Breakdown (mechanical) of other cardiac and vascular devices and implants** A 🐾

　　● T82.519   **Breakdown (mechanical) of unspecified cardiac and vascular devices and implants** A 🐾
　　　(Ex:) D78.81-D78.89, E36.8, E89.810-E89.89, H59.011-H59.019, H59.031-H59.039, H59.091-H59.099, H59.811-H59.89, H95.811-H95.89, I97.3, L76.81-L76.82, M96.89, N98.1-N98.9, T81.82X-T81.9XX[A], T82.519[A], T82.539[A], T82.599-T82.9XX[A], T85.9XX[A]

　● T82.52   **Displacement of other cardiac and vascular devices and implants**
　　Malposition of other cardiac and vascular devices and implants

　　● T82.520   **Displacement of surgically created arteriovenous fistula** A 🐾

　　● T82.521   **Displacement of surgically created arteriovenous shunt** A 🐾

　　● T82.522   **Displacement of artificial heart** A 🐾
　　　(Ex:) See T82.118A

　　● T82.523   **Displacement of balloon (counterpulsation) device** A 🐾

　　● T82.524   **Displacement of infusion catheter** A 🐾

　　● T82.525   **Displacement of umbrella device** A 🐾

　　● T82.528   **Displacement of other cardiac and vascular devices and implants** A 🐾

　　● T82.529   **Displacement of unspecified cardiac and vascular devices and implants** A 🐾

◀ New   ◀━ Revised   ~~deleted~~ Deleted   Excludes 1   Excludes 2   Includes   Use additional   Code first   Code also   Unspecified
OGCR Official Guidelines   ● Unacceptable Principal Diagnosis   X Assign placeholder X   ● Use Additional Character(s)   ▶ Manifestation Code   **Coding Clinic**

● **T82.53**   **Leakage of other cardiac and vascular devices and implants**

   ● **T82.530**   **Leakage of surgically created arteriovenous fistula** A 🏷

   ● **T82.531**   **Leakage of surgically created shunt** A 🏷

   ● **T82.532**   **Leakage of artificial heart** A 🏷
      Ⓔx See T82.118A

   ● **T82.533**   **Leakage of balloon (counterpulsation) device** A 🏷

   ● **T82.534**   **Leakage of infusion catheter** A 🏷

   ● **T82.535**   **Leakage of umbrella device** A 🏷

   ● **T82.538**   **Leakage of other cardiac and vascular devices and implants** A 🏷

   ● **T82.539**   **Leakage of unspecified cardiac and vascular devices and implants** A 🏷
      Ⓔx See T82.519

● **T82.59**   **Other mechanical complication of other cardiac and vascular devices and implants**
    Obstruction (mechanical) of other cardiac and vascular devices and implants
    Perforation of other cardiac and vascular devices and implants
    Protrusion of other cardiac and vascular devices and implants

   ● **T82.590**   **Other mechanical complication of surgically created arteriovenous fistula** A 🏷

   ● **T82.591**   **Other mechanical complication of surgically created arteriovenous shunt** A 🏷

   ● **T82.592**   **Other mechanical complication of artificial heart** A 🏷
      Ⓔx See T82.118A

   ● **T82.593**   **Other mechanical complication of balloon (counterpulsation) device** A 🏷

   ● **T82.594**   **Other mechanical complication of infusion catheter** A 🏷
      Ⓔx See T82.118A

   ● **T82.595**   **Other mechanical complication of umbrella device** A 🏷

   ● **T82.598**   **Other mechanical complication of other cardiac and vascular devices and implants** A 🏷
      Ⓔx See T82.118A

   ● **T82.599**   **Other mechanical complication of unspecified cardiac and vascular devices and implants** A 🏷
      Ⓔx See T82.519

X ● **T82.6**   **Infection and inflammatory reaction due to cardiac valve prosthesis** A 🏷, A 🏷
   Use additional code to identify infection
   Ⓔx D78.81-D78.89, E36.8, E89.810-E89.89, H59.011-H59.019, H59.031-H59.039, H59.091-H59.099, H59.811-H59.89, H95.811-H95.89, I97.3, L76.81-L76.82, M96.89, N98.1-N98.9, T81.82X-T81.9XX[A], T82.01X-T82.118[A], T82.120-T82.128[A], T82.190-T82.198[A], T82.211-T82.9XX[A], T85.310-T85.311[A], T85.320-T85.321[A], T85.390-T85.391[A], T85.510-T85.738[A], T85.7XX[A], T85.810[A,D], T85.820[A,D], T85.830[A,D], T85.840[A,D], T85.850[A,D], T85.860[A,D], T85.890[A,D], T86.820-T86.829, T86.842-T86.849

X ● **T82.7**   **Infection and inflammatory reaction due to other cardiac and vascular devices, implants and grafts** A 🏷, A 🏷
   Use additional code to identify infection
   Ⓔx See T82.6

● **T82.8**   **Other specified complications of cardiac and vascular prosthetic devices, implants and grafts**

● **T82.81**   **Embolism due to cardiac and vascular prosthetic devices, implants and grafts** ◀▥

   ● **T82.817**   **Embolism due to cardiac prosthetic devices, implants and grafts** A 🏷 ◀▥
      Ⓔx D78.81-D78.89, E36.8, E89.810-E89.89, H59.011-H59.019, H59.031-H59.039, H59.091-H59.099, H59.811-H59.89, H95.811-H95.89, I97.3, L76.81-L76.82, M96.89, N98.1-N98.9, T81.82X-T81.9XX[A], T82.01X-T82.118[A], T82.120-T82.128[A], T82.190-T82.198[A], T82.221-T82.9XX[A], T85.310-T85.311[A], T85.320-T85.321[A], T85.390-T85.391[A], T85.510-T85.738[A], T85.79XA, T85.810[A,D], T85.820[A,D], T85.830[A,D], T85.840[A,D], T85.850[A,D], T85.860[A,D], T85.890[A,D], T85.9XX[A], T86.820-T86.829, T86.842-T86.849

      Coding Clinic: 2015, Q1, P20

   ● **T82.818**   **Embolism due to vascular prosthetic devices, implants and grafts** A 🏷 ◀▥
      Ⓔx See T82.6

● **T82.82**   **Fibrosis due to cardiac and vascular prosthetic devices, implants and grafts** ◀▥

   ● **T82.827**   **Fibrosis due to cardiac prosthetic devices, implants and grafts** A 🏷 ◀▥
      Ⓔx See T82.817

   ● **T82.828**   **Fibrosis due to vascular prosthetic devices, implants and grafts** A 🏷 ◀▥
      Ⓔx See T82.6

● **T82.83**   **Hemorrhage due to cardiac and vascular prosthetic devices, implants and grafts** ◀▥

   ● **T82.837**   **Hemorrhage due to cardiac prosthetic devices, implants and grafts** A 🏷 ◀▥
      Ⓔx See T82.817

   ● **T82.838**   **Hemorrhage due to vascular prosthetic devices, implants and grafts** A 🏷 ◀▥
      Ⓔx See T82.6

● **T82.84**   **Pain due to cardiac and vascular prosthetic devices, implants and grafts** ◀▥

   ● **T82.847**   **Pain due to cardiac prosthetic devices, implants and grafts** A 🏷 ◀▥
      Ⓔx See T82.817

   ● **T82.848**   **Pain due to vascular prosthetic devices, implants and grafts** A 🏷 ◀▥
      Ⓔx See T82.6

● **T82.85**   **Stenosis due to cardiac and vascular prosthetic devices, implants and grafts** ◀▥

   ● **T82.855**   **Stenosis of coronary artery stent** A 🏷 ◀
      In-stent stenosis (restenosis) of coronary artery stent ◀
      Restenosis of coronary artery stent ◀
      Ⓔx D78.81-D78.89, E36.8, E89.810-E89.89, H59.011-H59.019, H59.031-H59.039, H59.091-H59.099, H59.811-H59.89, H95.811-H95.89, I60.2, I97.3, L76.81-L76.82, M96.89, N98.1-N98.9, S02.101-S02.82X[A,B], T81.82X-T81.9XX[A], T82.01X-T82.118[A], T82.120-T82.128[A], T82.190-T82.198[A], T82.221-T82.9XX[A], T85.310-T85.311[A], T85.320-T85.321[A], T85.390-T85.391[A], T85.510-T85.79X[A], T85.9XX[A], T86.820-T86.829, T86.842-T86.849

● **T82.856　Stenosis of peripheral vascular stent** A ◄
　　In-stent stenosis (restenosis) of peripheral vascular stent ◄
　　Restenosis of peripheral vascular stent ◄
　　(Ex:) D78.81-D78.89, E36.8, E89.810-E89.89,
　　H59.011-H59.019, H59.031-H59.039,
　　H59.091-H59.099, H59.811-H59.89,
　　H95.811-H95.89, I60.2, I97.3, L76.81-L76.82,
　　M96.89, N98.1-N98.9, S02.101-S02.82X[A,B],
　　T81.82X-T81.9XX[A], T82.01X-T82.118[A],
　　T82.120-T82.128[A], T82.190-T82.198[A],
　　T82.221-T82.9XX[A], T85.310-T85.311[A],
　　T85.320-T85.321[A], T85.390-T85.391[A],
　　T85.510-T85.79X[A], T85.9XX[A],
　　T86.820-T86.829, T86.842-T86.849

● **T82.857　Stenosis of other cardiac prosthetic devices, implants and grafts** A ◄
　　(Ex:) See T82.817

● **T82.858　Stenosis of other vascular prosthetic devices, implants and grafts** A ◄
　　(Ex:) See T82.6

● **T82.86　Thrombosis of cardiac and vascular prosthetic devices, implants and grafts**

● **T82.867　Thrombosis due to cardiac prosthetic devices, implants and grafts** A ◄
　　(Ex:) See T82.817

● **T82.868　Thrombosis due to vascular prosthetic devices, implants and grafts** A ◄
　　(Ex:) See T82.6

● **T82.89　Other specified complication of cardiac and vascular prosthetic devices, implants and grafts**

● **T82.897　Other specified complication of cardiac prosthetic devices, implants and grafts** A
　　(Ex:) See T82.817

● **T82.898　Other specified complication of vascular prosthetic devices, implants and grafts** A
　　(Ex:) See T82.6

X ● **T82.9　Unspecified complication of cardiac and vascular prosthetic device, implant and graft** A
　　(Ex:) See T82.817

● **T83　Complications of genitourinary prosthetic devices, implants and grafts**

　Excludes2　failure and rejection of transplanted organs and tissue (T86.-)

　The appropriate 7th character is to be added to each code from category T83

A	initial encounter
D	subsequent encounter
S	sequela

　(Ex:) For category T83 CC codes unless otherwise indicated: D78.81-D78.89, E36.8, E89.810-E89.89, H59.011-H59.019, H59.031-H59.039, H59.091-H59.099, H59.811-H59.89, H95.811-H95.89, I97.3, L76.81-L76.82, M96.89, N98.1-N98.9, N99.510-N99.518, T81.82[A], T81.89-T81.9[A], T83.010[A], T83.020[A], T83.030[A], T83.090[A], T83.110-T83.29X[A], T83.410-T83.69[A], T83.712-T83.714[A], T83.718[A], T83.719A, T83.722-T83.724[A], T83.728-T83.9XX[A]

● **T83.0　Mechanical complication of urinary catheter** ◄▦

　Excludes2　complications of stoma of urinary tract (N99.5-)

● **T83.01　Breakdown (mechanical) of urinary catheter** ◄▦

● **T83.010　Breakdown (mechanical) of cystostomy catheter** A

● **T83.011　Breakdown (mechanical) of indwelling urethral catheter** ◄

● **T83.012　Breakdown (mechanical) of nephrostomy catheter** ◄

● **T83.018　Breakdown (mechanical) of other urinary catheter** ◄▦
　　Breakdown (mechanical) of Hopkins catheter ◄
　　Breakdown (mechanical) of ileostomy catheter ◄
　　Breakdown (mechanical) urostomy catheter ◄

● **T83.02　Displacement of urinary catheter** ◄▦
　　Malposition of urinary catheter ◄▦

● **T83.020　Displacement of cystostomy catheter** A

● **T83.021　Displacement of indwelling urethral catheter** ◄

● **T83.022　Displacement of nephrostomy catheter** ◄

● **T83.028　Displacement of other urinary catheter** ◄▦
　　Displacement of Hopkins catheter ◄
　　Displacement of ileostomy catheter ◄
　　Displacement of urostomy catheter ◄

● **T83.03　Leakage of urinary catheter** ◄▦

● **T83.030　Leakage of cystostomy catheter** A

● **T83.031　Leakage of indwelling urethral catheter** ◄

● **T83.032　Leakage of nephrostomy catheter** ◄

● **T83.038　Leakage of other urinary catheter** ◄▦
　　Leakage of Hopkins catheter ◄
　　Leakage of ileostomy catheter ◄
　　Leakage of urostomy catheter ◄

● **T83.09　Other mechanical complication of urinary catheter** ◄▦
　　Obstruction (mechanical) of urinary catheter ◄▦
　　Perforation of urinary catheter ◄▦
　　Protrusion of urinary catheter ◄▦

● **T83.090　Other mechanical complication of cystostomy catheter** A

● **T83.091　Other mechanical complication of indwelling urethral catheter** ◄

● **T83.092　Other mechanical complication of nephrostomy catheter** ◄

● **T83.098　Other mechanical complication of other urinary catheter** ◄▦
　　Other mechanical complication of Hopkins catheter ◄
　　Other mechanical complication of ileostomy catheter ◄
　　Other mechanical complication of urostomy catheter ◄

● **T83.1　Mechanical complication of other urinary devices and implants**

● **T83.11　Breakdown (mechanical) of other urinary devices and implants**

● **T83.110　Breakdown (mechanical) of urinary electronic stimulator device** A

　Excludes2　Breakdown (mechanical) of electrode (lead) for sacral nerve neurostimulator (T85.111) ◄
　　Breakdown (mechanical) of implanted electronic sacral neurostimulator, pulse generator or receiver (T85.113) ◄

● **T83.111　Breakdown (mechanical) of implanted urinary sphincter** A ◄▦

◄ New　◄▦ Revised　~~deleted~~ Deleted　Excludes 1　Excludes 2　Includes　Use additional　Code first　Code also　Unspecified

OGCR Official Guidelines　● Unacceptable Principal Diagnosis　X Assign placeholder X　● Use Additional Character(s)　▶ Manifestation Code　**Coding Clinic**

● **T83.112** **Breakdown (mechanical) of indwelling ureteral stent** A 🦠 ◄▥

● **T83.113** **Breakdown (mechanical) of other urinary stents** A 🦠 ◄

    Breakdown (mechanical) of ileal conduit stent ◄

    Breakdown (mechanical) of nephroureteral stent ◄

    Ⓔ𝕩 D78.81-D78.89, E36.8, E89.810-E89.89, H59.011-H59.019, H59.031-H59.039, H59.091-H59.099, H59.811-H59.89, H95.811-H95.89, I60.2, I97.3, K55.011-K55.069, K55.30-K55.33, L76.81-76.82, M96.89, N98.1-N98.9, N99.510-N99.518, S02.101-S02.82X[A,B], T81.82[A], T81.89-T81.9[A], T83.010[A], T83.020[A], T83.030[A], T83.090[A], T83.110-T83.29X[A], T83.410-T83.498[A], T83.718[A], T83.728-T83.9XX[A]

● **T83.118** **Breakdown (mechanical) of other urinary devices and implants** A 🦠

● **T83.12** **Displacement of other urinary devices and implants**

    Malposition of other urinary devices and implants

● **T83.120** **Displacement of urinary electronic stimulator device** A 🦠

    Excludes2 Displacement of electrode (lead) for sacral nerve neurostimulator (T85.121) ◄

             Displacement of implanted electronic sacral neurostimulator, pulse generator or receiver (T85.123) ◄

● **T83.121** **Displacement of implanted urinary sphincter** A 🦠 ◄▥

● **T83.122** **Displacement of indwelling ureteral stent** A 🦠 ◄▥

● **T83.123** **Displacement of other urinary stents** A 🦠 ◄

    Displacement of ileal conduit stent ◄

    Displacement of nephroureteral stent ◄

    Ⓔ𝕩 See T83.113A

● **T83.128** **Displacement of other urinary devices and implants** A 🦠

● **T83.19** **Other mechanical complication of other urinary devices and implants**

    Leakage of other urinary devices and implants

    Obstruction (mechanical) of other urinary devices and implants

    Perforation of other urinary devices and implants

    Protrusion of other urinary devices and implants

● **T83.190** **Other mechanical complication of urinary electronic stimulator device** A 🦠

    Excludes2 Other mechanical complication of electrode (lead) for sacral nerve neurostimulator (T85.191) ◄

             Other mechanical complication of implanted electronic sacral neurostimulator, pulse generator or receiver (T85.193) ◄

● **T83.191** **Other mechanical complication of implanted urinary sphincter** A 🦠 ◄▥

● **T83.192** **Other mechanical complication of indwelling ureteral stent** A 🦠 ◄▥

● **T83.193** **Other mechanical complication of other urinary stent** A 🦠 ◄

    Other mechanical complication of ileal conduit stent ◄

    Other mechanical complication of nephroureteral stent ◄

    Ⓔ𝕩 See T83.113A

● **T83.198** **Other mechanical complication of other urinary devices and implants** A 🦠

● **T83.2** **Mechanical complication of graft of urinary organ**

X ● **T83.21** **Breakdown (mechanical) of graft of urinary organ** A 🦠

X ● **T83.22** **Displacement of graft of urinary organ** A 🦠

    Malposition of graft of urinary organ

X ● **T83.23** **Leakage of graft of urinary organ** A 🦠

X ● **T83.24** **Erosion of graft of urinary organ** A 🦠 ◄

    Ⓔ𝕩 See T83.113A

X ● **T83.25** **Exposure of graft of urinary organ** A 🦠 ◄

    Ⓔ𝕩 See T83.113A

X ● **T83.29** **Other mechanical complication of graft of urinary organ** A 🦠

    Obstruction (mechanical) of graft of urinary organ

    Perforation of graft of urinary organ

    Protrusion of graft of urinary organ

● **T83.3** **Mechanical complication of intrauterine contraceptive device**

X ● **T83.31** **Breakdown (mechanical) of intrauterine contraceptive device** ♀

X ● **T83.32** **Displacement of intrauterine contraceptive device** ♀

    Malposition of intrauterine contraceptive device

    Missing string of intrauterine contraceptive device

X ● **T83.39** **Other mechanical complication of intrauterine contraceptive device** ♀

    Leakage of intrauterine contraceptive device

    Obstruction (mechanical) of intrauterine contraceptive device

    Perforation of intrauterine contraceptive device

    Protrusion of intrauterine contraceptive device

● **T83.4** **Mechanical complication of other prosthetic devices, implants and grafts of genital tract**

● **T83.41** **Breakdown (mechanical) of other prosthetic devices, implants and grafts of genital tract**

● **T83.410** **Breakdown (mechanical) of implanted penile prosthesis** ♂ A 🦠 ◄▥

    Breakdown (mechanical) of penile prosthesis cylinder ◄

    Breakdown (mechanical) of penile prosthesis pump ◄

    Breakdown (mechanical) of penile prosthesis reservoir ◄

● **T83.411** **Breakdown (mechanical) of implanted testicular prosthesis** A 🦠 ◄

    Ⓔ𝕩 See T83.113A

● **T83.418** **Breakdown (mechanical) of other prosthetic devices, implants and grafts of genital tract** A 🦠

N Newborn Age: 0　　**P** Pediatric Age: 0–17　　**M** Maternity DX: 12–55　　**A** Adult Age: 15–124　　♀ Females Only　　♂ Males Only

🦠 Complication\Comorbidity　　🦠 Major C\C　　Ⓔ𝕩 CC/MCC Exclusions　　🦠 Hospital-Acquired Condition

1501

T83.42 **Displacement of other prosthetic devices, implants and grafts of genital tract**
Malposition of other prosthetic devices, implants and grafts of genital tract

● T83.420 **Displacement of implanted penile prosthesis** ♂ A ◐ ◀▥
Displacement of penile prosthesis cylinder ◀
Displacement of penile prosthesis pump ◀
Displacement of penile prosthesis reservoir ◀

● T83.421 **Displacement of implanted testicular prosthesis** A ◐ ◀
Ⓔⓧ See T83.113A

● T83.428 **Displacement of other prosthetic devices, implants and grafts of genital tract** A ◐

T83.49 **Other mechanical complication of other prosthetic devices, implants and grafts of genital tract**
Leakage of other prosthetic devices, implants and grafts of genital tract
Obstruction, mechanical of other prosthetic devices, implants and grafts of genital tract
Perforation of other prosthetic devices, implants and grafts of genital tract
Protrusion of other prosthetic devices, implants and grafts of genital tract

● T83.490 **Other mechanical complication of implanted penile prosthesis** ♂ A ◐ ◀▥
Other mechanical complication of penile prosthesis cylinder ◀
Other mechanical complication of penile prosthesis pump ◀
Other mechanical complication of penile prosthesis reservoir ◀

● T83.491 **Other mechanical complication of implanted testicular prosthesis** A ◐ ◀

● T83.498 **Other mechanical complication of other prosthetic devices, implants and grafts of genital tract** A ◐

● T83.5 **Infection and inflammatory reaction due to prosthetic device, implant and graft in urinary system**
Use additional code to identify infection
Ⓔⓧ For category T83.5 CC codes unless otherwise indicated:
D78.81-D78.89, E36.8, E89.810-E89.89, H59.011-H59.019,
H59.031-H59.039, H59.091-H59.099, H59.811-H59.89, H95.811-H95.89,
I97.3, L76.81-L76.82, M96.89, N39.0, N98.1-N98.9, N99.510-N99.518,
T81.82X-T81.9XX[A], T83.010[A], T83.020[A], T83.030[A], T83.090[A],
T83.110-T83.29X[A], T83.410-T83.498[A], T83.510-T83.518[A],
T83.590-T83.598[A], T83.61X-T83.69X[A], T83.712-T83.719[A],
T83.722-T83.729[A], T83.79XA, T83.81X-T83.9XX[A], T85.310-T85.738[A],
T85.79XA, T85.810[A,D], T85.820[A,D], T85.830[A,D], T85.840[A,D],
T85.850[A,D], T85.860[A,D], T850.890[A,D], T85.9XX[A], T86.820-T86.849

● T83.51 **Infection and inflammatory reaction due to urinary catheter** ◀▥

Excludes2 complications of stoma of urinary tract (N99.5-)

● T83.510 **Infection and inflammatory reaction due to cystostomy catheter** A ◐ ◀

● T83.511 **Infection and inflammatory reaction due to indwelling urethral catheter** A ◐ ◑ ◀
Ⓔⓧ D78.81-D78.89, E36.8, E89.810-E89.89,
H59.011-H59.019, H59.031-H59.039,
H59.091-H59.099, H59.811-H59.89,
H95.811-H95.89, I97.3, L76.81-L76.82,
M96.89, N98.1-N98.9, N99.510-N99.518,
R82.71, T81.82X-T81.9XX[A], T83.010[A],
T83.020[A], T83.030[A], T83.090[A],
T83.110-T83.29X[A], T83.410-T83.498[A],
T83.510-T83.518[A], T83.590-T83.598[A],
T83.61X-T83.69X[A], T83.712-T83.719[A],
T83.722-T83.729[A], T83.79XA,
T83.81X-T83.9XX[A], T85.310-T85.311[A],
T85.320-T85.321[A], T85.390-T85.391[A],
T85.510-T85.79X[A], T85.810[A,D],
T85.820[A,D], T85.830[A,D], T85.840[A,D],
T85.850[A,D], T85.860[A,D], T850.890[A,D],
T85.9XXA, T86.842-T86.849

● T83.512 **Infection and inflammatory reaction due to nephrostomy catheter** A ◐ ◀

● T83.518 **Infection and inflammatory reaction due to other urinary catheter** A ◐ ◑ ◀
Infection and inflammatory reaction due to Hopkins catheter ◀
Infection and inflammatory reaction due to ileostomy catheter ◀
Infection and inflammatory reaction due to urostomy catheter ◀

● T83.59 **Infection and inflammatory reaction due to prosthetic device, implant and graft in urinary system**

● T83.590 **Infection and inflammatory reaction due to implanted urinary neurostimulation device** A ◐ ◀

Excludes2 Infection and inflammatory reaction due to electrode lead of sacral nerve neurostimulator (T85.732) ◀
Infection and inflammatory reaction due to pulse generator or receiver of sacral nerve neurostimulator (T85.734) ◀

● T83.591 **Infection and inflammatory reaction due to implanted urinary sphincter** A ◐ ◀

● T83.592 **Infection and inflammatory reaction due to indwelling ureteral stent** A ◐ ◀

● T83.593 **Infection and inflammatory reaction due to other urinary stents** A ◐ ◀
Infection and inflammatory reaction due to ileal conduit stents ◀
Infection and inflammatory reaction due to nephroureteral stent ◀

● T83.598 **Infection and inflammatory reaction due to other prosthetic device, implant and graft in urinary system** A ◐ ◀

● **T83.6** **Infection and inflammatory reaction due to prosthetic device, implant and graft in genital tract**
    Use additional code to identify infection
    (Ex) For category T83.6: See T83.5

  ● **T83.61** **Infection and inflammatory reaction due to implanted penile prosthesis** A 🦠 ◄
    Infection and inflammatory reaction due to penile prosthesis cylinder ◄
    Infection and inflammatory reaction due to penile prosthesis pump ◄
    Infection and inflammatory reaction due to penile prosthesis reservoir ◄

  ● **T83.62** **Infection and inflammatory reaction due to implanted testicular prosthesis** A 🦠 ◄

  ● **T83.69** **Infection and inflammatory reaction due to other prosthetic device, implant and graft in genital tract** A 🦠 ◄

● **T83.7** **Complications due to implanted mesh and other prosthetic materials**
    (Ex) For Category T83.7 CC codes unless otherwise indicated: See T83.510A

  ● **T83.71** **Erosion of implanted mesh and other prosthetic materials to surrounding organ or tissue**

    ● **T83.711** **Erosion of implanted vaginal mesh to surrounding organ or tissue** ♀ ◄▥
      Erosion of implanted vaginal mesh into pelvic floor muscles ◄▥

    ● **T83.712** **Erosion of implanted urethral mesh to surrounding organ or tissue** A 🦠 ◄
      Erosion of implanted female urethral sling ◄
      Erosion of implanted male urethral sling ◄
      Erosion of implanted urethral mesh into pelvic floor muscles ◄

    ● **T83.713** **Erosion of implanted urethral bulking agent to surrounding organ or tissue** A 🦠 ◄

    ● **T83.714** **Erosion of implanted ureteral bulking agent to surrounding organ or tissue** A 🦠 ◄

    ● **T83.718** **Erosion of other implanted mesh to organ or tissue** A 🦠 ◄▥

    ● **T83.719** **Erosion of other prosthetic materials to surrounding organ or tissue** A 🦠 ◄

  ● **T83.72** **Exposure of implanted mesh and other prosthetic materials into surrounding organ or tissue**
    Extrusion of implanted mesh ◄

    ● **T83.721** **Exposure of implanted vaginal mesh into vagina** ♀ ◄▥
      Exposure of implanted vaginal mesh through vaginal wall ◄▥

    ● **T83.722** **Exposure of implanted urethral mesh into urethra** A 🦠 ◄
      Exposure of implanted female urethral sling ◄
      Exposure of implanted male urethral sling ◄
      Exposure of implanted urethral mesh through urethral wall ◄

    ● **T83.723** **Exposure of implanted urethral bulking agent into urethra** A 🦠 ◄

    ● **T83.724** **Exposure of implanted ureteral bulking agent into ureter** A 🦠 ◄

    ● **T83.728** **Exposure of other implanted mesh into organ or tissue** A 🦠 ◄▥

    ● **T83.729** **Exposure of other prosthetic materials into organ or tissue** A 🦠 ◄

  X ● **T83.79** **Other specified complications due to other genitourinary prosthetic materials** A 🦠 ◄
    (Ex) See T83.5

● **T83.8** **Other specified complications of genitourinary prosthetic devices, implants and grafts**
    (Ex) For category T83.8 CC codes: See T83.5

  X ● **T83.81** **Embolism due to genitourinary prosthetic devices, implants and grafts** A 🦠 ◄▥

  X ● **T83.82** **Fibrosis due to genitourinary prosthetic devices, implants and grafts** A 🦠 ◄▥

  X ● **T83.83** **Hemorrhage due to genitourinary prosthetic devices, implants and grafts** A 🦠 ◄▥

  X ● **T83.84** **Pain due to genitourinary prosthetic devices, implants and grafts** A ◄▥

  X ● **T83.85** **Stenosis due to genitourinary prosthetic devices, implants and grafts** A 🦠 ◄▥

  X ● **T83.86** **Thrombosis due to genitourinary prosthetic devices, implants and grafts** A 🦠 ◄▥

  X ● **T83.89** **Other specified complication of genitourinary prosthetic devices, implants and grafts** A 🦠

X ● **T83.9** **Unspecified complication of genitourinary prosthetic device, implant and graft** A 🦠
    (Ex) See T83.5

● **T84** **Complications of internal orthopedic prosthetic devices, implants and grafts**
    Excludes2   failure and rejection of transplanted organs and tissues (T86.-)
       fracture of bone following insertion of orthopedic implant, joint prosthesis or bone plate (M96.6)

The appropriate 7th character is to be added to each code from category T84

A	initial encounter
D	subsequent encounter
S	sequela

  (Ex) D78.81, D78.89, E36.8, E89.810-E89.89, H59.011-H59.019, H59.031-H59.819, H59.88-H59.89, H95.811-H95.89, I97.3, L76.81-L76.82, M96.621-M96.69, M96.89, M97.01X-M97.9XX[A], N98.1-N98.9, T81.82X[A], T81.89X-T81.9XX[A], T84.010-T84.9XX[A]

● **T84.0** **Mechanical complication of internal joint prosthesis**

  ● **T84.01** **Broken internal joint prosthesis**
    Breakage (fracture) of prosthetic joint
    Broken prosthetic joint implant

    Excludes1   periprosthetic joint implant fracture (T84.04)

    ● **T84.010** **Broken internal right hip prosthesis** A 🦠

    ● **T84.011** **Broken internal left hip prosthesis** A 🦠

    ● **T84.012** **Broken internal right knee prosthesis** A 🦠

    ● **T84.013** **Broken internal left knee prosthesis** A 🦠

    ● **T84.018** **Broken internal joint prosthesis, other site** A 🦠
      Use additional code to identify the joint (Z96.6-)

    ● **T84.019** **Broken internal joint prosthesis, unspecified site** A 🦠

  ● **T84.02** **Dislocation of internal joint prosthesis**
    Instability of internal joint prosthesis
    Subluxation of internal joint prosthesis

    ● **T84.020** **Dislocation of internal right hip prosthesis** A 🦠

    ● **T84.021** **Dislocation of internal left hip prosthesis** A 🦠

    ● **T84.022** **Instability of internal right knee prosthesis** A 🦠

    ● **T84.023** **Instability of internal left knee prosthesis** A 🦠

    ● **T84.028** **Dislocation of other internal joint prosthesis** A 🦠
      Use additional code to identify the joint (Z96.6-)

    ● **T84.029** **Dislocation of unspecified internal joint prosthesis** A 🦠

- ● **T84.03** **Mechanical loosening of internal prosthetic joint**
  Aseptic loosening of prosthetic joint
  - ● **T84.030** Mechanical loosening of internal right hip prosthetic joint A
  - ● **T84.031** Mechanical loosening of internal left hip prosthetic joint A
  - ● **T84.032** Mechanical loosening of internal right knee prosthetic joint A
  - ● **T84.033** Mechanical loosening of internal left knee prosthetic joint A
  - ● **T84.038** Mechanical loosening of other internal prosthetic joint A
    Use additional code to identify the joint (Z96.6-)
  - ● **T84.039** Mechanical loosening of ==unspecified== internal prosthetic joint A
  - ~~T84.04~~ ~~Periprosthetic fracture around internal prosthetic joint~~
    - ~~T84.040~~ ~~Periprosthetic fracture around internal prosthetic right hip joint~~
    - ~~T84.041~~ ~~Periprosthetic fracture around internal prosthetic left hip joint~~
    - ~~T84.042~~ ~~Periprosthetic fracture around internal prosthetic right knee joint~~
    - ~~T84.043~~ ~~Periprosthetic fracture around internal prosthetic left knee joint~~
    - ~~T84.048~~ ~~Periprosthetic fracture around other internal prosthetic joint~~
    - ~~T84.049~~ ~~Periprosthetic fracture around unspecified internal prosthetic joint~~
- ● **T84.05** **Periprosthetic osteolysis of internal prosthetic joint**
  Use additional code to identify major osseous defect, if applicable (M89.7-)
  - ● **T84.050** Periprosthetic osteolysis of internal prosthetic right hip joint A
  - ● **T84.051** Periprosthetic osteolysis of internal prosthetic left hip joint A
  - ● **T84.052** Periprosthetic osteolysis of internal prosthetic right knee joint A
  - ● **T84.053** Periprosthetic osteolysis of internal prosthetic left knee joint A
  - ● **T84.058** Periprosthetic osteolysis of other internal prosthetic joint A
    Use additional code to identify the joint (Z96.6-)
  - ● **T84.059** Periprosthetic osteolysis of ==unspecified== internal prosthetic joint A
- ● **T84.06** **Wear of articular bearing surface of internal prosthetic joint**
  - ● **T84.060** Wear of articular bearing surface of internal prosthetic right hip joint A
  - ● **T84.061** Wear of articular bearing surface of internal prosthetic left hip joint A
  - ● **T84.062** Wear of articular bearing surface of internal prosthetic right knee joint A
  - ● **T84.063** Wear of articular bearing surface of internal prosthetic left knee joint A
  - ● **T84.068** Wear of articular bearing surface of other internal prosthetic joint A
    Use additional code to identify the joint (Z96.6-)
  - ● **T84.069** Wear of articular bearing surface of ==unspecified== internal prosthetic joint A

- ● **T84.09** **Other mechanical complication of internal joint prosthesis**
  Prosthetic joint implant failure NOS
  - ● **T84.090** Other mechanical complication of internal right hip prosthesis A
  - ● **T84.091** Other mechanical complication of internal left hip prosthesis A
  - ● **T84.092** Other mechanical complication of internal right knee prosthesis A
  - ● **T84.093** Other mechanical complication of internal left knee prosthesis A
  - ● **T84.098** Other mechanical complication of other internal joint prosthesis A
    Use additional code to identify the joint (Z96.6-)
  - ● **T84.099** Other mechanical complication of ==unspecified== internal joint prosthesis A
- ● **T84.1** **Mechanical complication of internal fixation device of bones of limb**
  Excludes2   mechanical complication of internal fixation device of bones of feet (T84.2-)
      mechanical complication of internal fixation device of bones of fingers (T84.2-)
      mechanical complication of internal fixation device of bones of hands (T84.2-)
      mechanical complication of internal fixation device of bones of toes (T84.2-)
- ● **T84.11** **Breakdown (mechanical) of internal fixation device of bones of limb**
  - ● **T84.110** Breakdown (mechanical) of internal fixation device of right humerus A
  - ● **T84.111** Breakdown (mechanical) of internal fixation device of left humerus A
  - ● **T84.112** Breakdown (mechanical) of internal fixation device of bone of right forearm A
  - ● **T84.113** Breakdown (mechanical) of internal fixation device of bone of left forearm A
  - ● **T84.114** Breakdown (mechanical) of internal fixation device of right femur A
  - ● **T84.115** Breakdown (mechanical) of internal fixation device of left femur A
  - ● **T84.116** Breakdown (mechanical) of internal fixation device of bone of right lower leg A
  - ● **T84.117** Breakdown (mechanical) of internal fixation device of bone of left lower leg A
  - ● **T84.119** Breakdown (mechanical) of internal fixation device of ==unspecified== bone of limb A
- ● **T84.12** **Displacement of internal fixation device of bones of limb**
  Malposition of internal fixation device of bones of limb
  - ● **T84.120** Displacement of internal fixation device of right humerus A
  - ● **T84.121** Displacement of internal fixation device of left humerus A
  - ● **T84.122** Displacement of internal fixation device of bone of right forearm A
  - ● **T84.123** Displacement of internal fixation device of bone of left forearm A
  - ● **T84.124** Displacement of internal fixation device of right femur A

● **T84.125**   Displacement of internal fixation device of left femur A 🦠

● **T84.126**   Displacement of internal fixation device of bone of right lower leg A 🦠

● **T84.127**   Displacement of internal fixation device of bone of left lower leg A 🦠

● **T84.129**   Displacement of internal fixation device of unspecified bone of limb A 🦠

● **T84.19**   Other mechanical complication of internal fixation device of bones of limb

Obstruction (mechanical) of internal fixation device of bones of limb

Perforation of internal fixation device of bones of limb

Protrusion of internal fixation device of bones of limb

● **T84.190**   Other mechanical complication of internal fixation device of right humerus A 🦠

● **T84.191**   Other mechanical complication of internal fixation device of left humerus A 🦠

● **T84.192**   Other mechanical complication of internal fixation device of bone of right forearm A 🦠

● **T84.193**   Other mechanical complication of internal fixation device of bone of left forearm A 🦠

● **T84.194**   Other mechanical complication of internal fixation device of right femur A 🦠

● **T84.195**   Other mechanical complication of internal fixation device of left femur A 🦠

● **T84.196**   Other mechanical complication of internal fixation device of bone of right lower leg A 🦠

● **T84.197**   Other mechanical complication of internal fixation device of bone of left lower leg A 🦠

● **T84.199**   Other mechanical complication of internal fixation device of unspecified bone of limb A 🦠

● **T84.2**   Mechanical complication of internal fixation device of other bones

● **T84.21**   Breakdown (mechanical) of internal fixation device of other bones

● **T84.210**   Breakdown (mechanical) of internal fixation device of bones of hand and fingers A 🦠

● **T84.213**   Breakdown (mechanical) of internal fixation device of bones of foot and toes A 🦠

● **T84.216**   Breakdown (mechanical) of internal fixation device of vertebrae A 🦠

● **T84.218**   Breakdown (mechanical) of internal fixation device of other bones A 🦠

● **T84.22**   Displacement of internal fixation device of other bones

Malposition of internal fixation device of other bones

● **T84.220**   Displacement of internal fixation device of bones of hand and fingers A 🦠

● **T84.223**   Displacement of internal fixation device of bones of foot and toes A 🦠

● **T84.226**   Displacement of internal fixation device of vertebrae A 🦠

● **T84.228**   Displacement of internal fixation device of other bones A 🦠

● **T84.29**   Other mechanical complication of internal fixation device of other bones

Obstruction (mechanical) of internal fixation device of other bones

Perforation of internal fixation device of other bones

Protrusion of internal fixation device of other bones

● **T84.290**   Other mechanical complication of internal fixation device of bones of hand and fingers A 🦠

● **T84.293**   Other mechanical complication of internal fixation device of bones of foot and toes A 🦠

● **T84.296**   Other mechanical complication of internal fixation device of vertebrae A 🦠

● **T84.298**   Other mechanical complication of internal fixation device of other bones A 🦠

● **T84.3**   Mechanical complication of other bone devices, implants and grafts

    Excludes2   other complications of bone graft (T86.83-)

● **T84.31**   Breakdown (mechanical) of other bone devices, implants and grafts

● **T84.310**   Breakdown (mechanical) of electronic bone stimulator A 🦠

● **T84.318**   Breakdown (mechanical) of other bone devices, implants and grafts A 🦠

● **T84.32**   Displacement of other bone devices, implants and grafts

Malposition of other bone devices, implants and grafts

● **T84.320**   Displacement of electronic bone stimulator A 🦠

● **T84.328**   Displacement of other bone devices, implants and grafts A 🦠

● **T84.39**   Other mechanical complication of other bone devices, implants and grafts

Obstruction (mechanical) of other bone devices, implants and grafts

Perforation of other bone devices, implants and grafts

Protrusion of other bone devices, implants and grafts

● **T84.390**   Other mechanical complication of electronic bone stimulator A 🦠

● **T84.398**   Other mechanical complication of other bone devices, implants and grafts A 🦠

● **T84.4**   Mechanical complication of other internal orthopedic devices, implants and grafts

● **T84.41**   Breakdown (mechanical) of other internal orthopedic devices, implants and grafts

● **T84.410**   Breakdown (mechanical) of muscle and tendon graft A 🦠

● **T84.418**   Breakdown (mechanical) of other internal orthopedic devices, implants and grafts A 🦠

● **T84.42**   Displacement of other internal orthopedic devices, implants and grafts

Malposition of other internal orthopedic devices, implants and grafts

● **T84.420**   Displacement of muscle and tendon graft A 🦠

● **T84.428**   Displacement of other internal orthopedic devices, implants and grafts A 🦠

CHAPTER 19 (S00-T88)

CHAPTER 19 (S00-T88)

● T84.49   **Other mechanical complication of other internal orthopedic devices, implants and grafts**
Mechanical complication of other internal orthopedic devices, implants and grafts NOS
Obstruction (mechanical) of other internal orthopedic devices, implants and grafts
Perforation of other internal orthopedic devices, implants and grafts
Protrusion of other internal orthopedic devices, implants and grafts

   ● T84.490   **Other mechanical complication of muscle and tendon graft** A 🔵

   ● T84.498   **Other mechanical complication of other internal orthopedic devices, implants and grafts** A 🔵

● T84.5   **Infection and inflammatory reaction due to internal joint prosthesis**

Use additional code to identify infection

(Ex:) **For category T84.5 CC codes:** D78.81-D78.89, E36.8, E89.810-E89.89, H59.011-H59.019, H59.031-H59.039, H59.091-H59.099, H59.811-H59.89, H95.811-H95.89, I97.3, L76.81-L76.82, M96.621-M96.69, M96.89, M97.01X-M97.02X[A], M97.11X-M97.12X[A], M97.21X-M97.22X[A], M97.31X-M97.32X[A], M97.41X-M97.42X[A], M97.8XXA, M97.9XXA, N98.1-N98.9, T81.82X-T81.9XX[A], T84.010-T84.039[A], T84.050-T84.9XX[A], T85.310-T85.311[A], T85.320-T85.321[A], T85.390-T85.391[A], T85.510-T85.738[A], T85.79XA, T85.810[A,D], T85.820[A,D], T85.830[A,D], T85.840[A,D], T85.850[A,D], T85.860[A,D], T85.890[A,D],T85.9XX[A], T86.820-T86.829, T86.842-T86.849

Coding Clinic: 2015, Q1, P16

X ● T84.50   **Infection and inflammatory reaction due to unspecified internal joint prosthesis** A 🔵
Coding Clinic: 2015, Q1, P3

X ● T84.51   **Infection and inflammatory reaction due to internal right hip prosthesis** A 🔵
Coding Clinic: 2015, Q4, P36

X ● T84.52   **Infection and inflammatory reaction due to internal left hip prosthesis** A 🔵
Coding Clinic: 2015, Q1, P16-17

X ● T84.53   **Infection and inflammatory reaction due to internal right knee prosthesis** A 🔵

X ● T84.54   **Infection and inflammatory reaction due to internal left knee prosthesis** A 🔵

X ● T84.59   **Infection and inflammatory reaction due to other internal joint prosthesis** A 🔵

● T84.6   **Infection and inflammatory reaction due to internal fixation device**

Use additional code to identify infection

(Ex:) **For category T84.6 CC codes:** See T84.5

X ● T84.60   **Infection and inflammatory reaction due to internal fixation device of unspecified site** A 🔵, A 🔵

● T84.61   **Infection and inflammatory reaction due to internal fixation device of arm**

   ● T84.610   **Infection and inflammatory reaction due to internal fixation device of right humerus** A 🔵, A 🔵

   ● T84.611   **Infection and inflammatory reaction due to internal fixation device of left humerus** A 🔵, A 🔵

   ● T84.612   **Infection and inflammatory reaction due to internal fixation device of right radius** A 🔵, A 🔵

   ● T84.613   **Infection and inflammatory reaction due to internal fixation device of left radius** A 🔵, A 🔵

   ● T84.614   **Infection and inflammatory reaction due to internal fixation device of right ulna** A 🔵, A 🔵

   ● T84.615   **Infection and inflammatory reaction due to internal fixation device of left ulna** A 🔵, A 🔵

   ● T84.619   **Infection and inflammatory reaction due to internal fixation device of unspecified bone of arm** A 🔵, A 🔵

● T84.62   **Infection and inflammatory reaction due to internal fixation device of leg**

   ● T84.620   **Infection and inflammatory reaction due to internal fixation device of right femur** A 🔵

   ● T84.621   **Infection and inflammatory reaction due to internal fixation device of left femur** A 🔵

   ● T84.622   **Infection and inflammatory reaction due to internal fixation device of right tibia** A 🔵

   ● T84.623   **Infection and inflammatory reaction due to internal fixation device of left tibia** A 🔵

   ● T84.624   **Infection and inflammatory reaction due to internal fixation device of right fibula** A 🔵

   ● T84.625   **Infection and inflammatory reaction due to internal fixation device of left fibula** A 🔵

   ● T84.629   **Infection and inflammatory reaction due to internal fixation device of unspecified bone of leg** A 🔵

X ● T84.63   **Infection and inflammatory reaction due to internal fixation device of spine** A 🔵, A 🔵

X ● T84.69   **Infection and inflammatory reaction due to internal fixation device of other site** A 🔵, A 🔵

● T84.7   **Infection and inflammatory reaction due to other internal orthopedic prosthetic devices, implants and grafts** A 🔵, A 🔵

Use additional code to identify infection

(Ex:) See T84.5

● T84.8   **Other specified complications of internal orthopedic prosthetic devices, implants and grafts**

(Ex:) **For category T84.8 CC codes:** See T84.5

X ● T84.81   **Embolism due to internal orthopedic prosthetic devices, implants and grafts** A 🔵

X ● T84.82   **Fibrosis due to internal orthopedic prosthetic devices, implants and grafts** A 🔵

X ● T84.83   **Hemorrhage due to internal orthopedic prosthetic devices, implants and grafts** A 🔵

X ● T84.84   **Pain due to internal orthopedic prosthetic devices, implants and grafts** A 🔵

X ● T84.85   **Stenosis due to internal orthopedic prosthetic devices, implants and grafts** A 🔵

X ● T84.86   **Thrombosis due to internal orthopedic prosthetic devices, implants and grafts** A 🔵

X ● T84.89   **Other specified complication of internal orthopedic prosthetic devices, implants and grafts** A 🔵

X ● T84.9   **Unspecified complication of internal orthopedic prosthetic device, implant and graft** A 🔵

(Ex:) See T84.5

◀ New   ◀▥ Revised   ~~deleted~~ Deleted   Excludes 1   Excludes 2   Includes   Use additional   Code first   Code also   Unspecified
OGCR Official Guidelines   ● Unacceptable Principal Diagnosis   X Assign placeholder X   ● Use Additional Character(s)   ▶ Manifestation Code   **Coding Clinic**

● **T85**   **Complications of other internal prosthetic devices, implants and grafts**

     Excludes2   failure and rejection of transplanted organs and tissue (T86.-)

     The appropriate 7th character is to be added to each code from category T85

A	initial encounter
D	subsequent encounter
S	sequela

● **T85.0**   **Mechanical complication of ventricular intracranial (communicating) shunt**

     (Ex) **For category T85.0 CC codes:** D78.81-D78.89, E36.8, E89.810-E89.89, H59.011-H59.019, H59.031-H59.039, H59.091-H59.099, H59.811-H59.89, H95.811-H95.89, I97.3, L76.81-L76.82, M96.89, N98.1-N98.9, T81.82X-T81.9XX[A], T85.01X-T85.199[A]

   X ● **T85.01**   **Breakdown (mechanical) of ventricular intracranial (communicating) shunt** A 🦠

   X ● **T85.02**   **Displacement of ventricular intracranial (communicating) shunt** A 🦠

       Malposition of ventricular intracranial (communicating) shunt

   X ● **T85.03**   **Leakage of ventricular intracranial (communicating) shunt** A 🦠

   X ● **T85.09**   **Other mechanical complication of ventricular intracranial (communicating) shunt** A 🦠

       Obstruction (mechanical) of ventricular intracranial (communicating) shunt

       Perforation of ventricular intracranial (communicating) shunt

       Protrusion of ventricular intracranial (communicating) shunt

● **T85.1**   **Mechanical complication of implanted electronic stimulator of nervous system**

     (Ex) **For category T85.1 CC codes:** See T85.0

   ● **T85.11**   **Breakdown (mechanical) of implanted electronic stimulator of nervous system**

     ● **T85.110**   **Breakdown (mechanical) of implanted electronic neurostimulator of brain electrode (lead)** A 🦠 ◀▦

     ● **T85.111**   **Breakdown (mechanical) of implanted electronic neurostimulator of peripheral nerve electrode (lead)** A 🦠 ◀▦

         Breakdown of electrode (lead) for cranial nerve neurostimulators ◀

         Breakdown of electrode (lead) for gastric neurostimulator ◀

         Breakdown of electrode (lead) for sacral nerve neurostimulator ◀

         Breakdown of electrode (lead) for vagal nerve neurostimulators ◀

     ● **T85.112**   **Breakdown (mechanical) of implanted electronic neurostimulator of spinal cord electrode (lead)** A 🦠 ◀▦

     ● **T85.113**   **Breakdown (mechanical) of implanted electronic neurostimulator, generator** A 🦠 ◀

         Breakdown (mechanical) of implanted electronic neurostimuator generator, brain, peripheral, gastric, spinal ◀

         Breakdown (mechanical) of implanted electronic sacral neurostimulator, pulse generator or receiver ◀

     ● **T85.118**   **Breakdown (mechanical) of other implanted electronic stimulator of nervous system** A 🦠

   ● **T85.12**   **Displacement of implanted electronic stimulator of nervous system**

       Malposition of implanted electronic stimulator of nervous system

     ● **T85.120**   **Displacement of implanted electronic neurostimulator of brain electrode (lead)** A 🦠 ◀▦

     ● **T85.121**   **Displacement of implanted electronic neurostimulator of peripheral nerve electrode (lead)** A 🦠 ◀▦

         Displacement of electrode (lead) for cranial nerve neurostimulators ◀

         Displacement of electrode (lead) for gastric neurostimulator ◀

         Displacement of electrode (lead) for sacral nerve neurostimulator ◀

         Displacement of electrode (lead) for vagal nerve neurostimulators ◀

     ● **T85.122**   **Displacement of implanted electronic neurostimulator of spinal cord electrode (lead)** A 🦠 ◀▦

     ● **T85.123**   **Displacement of implanted electronic neurostimulator, generator** A 🦠 ◀

         Displacement of implanted electronic neurostimulator generator, brain, peripheral, gastric, spinal ◀

         Displacement of implanted electronic sacral neurostimulator, pulse generator or receiver ◀

     ● **T85.128**   **Displacement of other implanted electronic stimulator of nervous system** A 🦠

N   Newborn Age: 0   **P**   Pediatric Age: 0–17   **M**   Maternity DX: 12–55   **A**   Adult Age: 15–124   ♀   Females Only   ♂   Males Only

🦠   Complication\Comorbidity   🦠   Major C\C   (Ex)   CC/MCC Exclusions   🦠   Hospital-Acquired Condition

1507

CHAPTER 19 (S00-T88)

● **T85.19** **Other mechanical complication of implanted electronic stimulator of nervous system**
Leakage of implanted electronic stimulator of nervous system
Obstruction (mechanical) of implanted electronic stimulator of nervous system
Perforation of implanted electronic stimulator of nervous system
Protrusion of implanted electronic stimulator of nervous system

● **T85.190** **Other mechanical complication of implanted electronic neurostimulator of brain electrode (lead)** A ◐ ◀▥

● **T85.191** **Other mechanical complication of implanted electronic neurostimulator of peripheral nerve electrode (lead)** A ◐ ◀▥
Other mechanical complication of electrode (lead) for cranial nerve neurostimulators ◀
Other mechanical complication of electrode (lead) for gastric neurostimulator ◀
Other mechanical complication of electrode (lead) for sacral nerve neurostimulator ◀
Other mechanical complication of electrode (lead) for vagal nerve neurostimulators ◀

● **T85.192** **Other mechanical complication of implanted electronic neurostimulator of spinal cord electrode (lead)** A ◐ ◀▥

● **T85.193** **Other mechanical complication of implanted electronic neurostimulator, generator** A ◐ ◀
Other mechanical complication of implanted electronic neurostimulator generator, brain, peripheral, gastric, spinal ◀
Other mechanical complication of implanted electronic sacral neurostimulator, pulse generator or receiver ◀
(Ex) See T85.113A

● **T85.199** **Other mechanical complication of other implanted electronic stimulator of nervous system** A ◐

● **T85.2** **Mechanical complication of intraocular lens**
(Ex) For category T85.2 CC codes: D78.81-D78.89, E89.810-E89.89, H59.011-H59.019, H59.031-H59.039, H59.091-H59.099, H59.811-H59.89, H95.811-H95.89, I97.3, M96.89, N98.1-N98.9, T85.21X-T85.29X[A]

X ● **T85.21** **Breakdown (mechanical) of intraocular lens** A ◐

X ● **T85.22** **Displacement of intraocular lens** A ◐
Malposition of intraocular lens

X ● **T85.29** **Other mechanical complication of intraocular lens** A ◐
Obstruction (mechanical) of intraocular lens
Perforation of intraocular lens
Protrusion of intraocular lens

● **T85.3** **Mechanical complication of other ocular prosthetic devices, implants and grafts**
Excludes2 other complications of corneal graft (T86.84-)
(Ex) For category T85.3 CC codes: H59.011-H59.019, H59.031-H59.819, H59.88-H59.89, H95.811-H95.89, I97.3, M96.89, N98.1-N98.9, T85.310-T85.311[A], T85.320-T85.321[A], T85.390-T85.391[A], T85.612A, T85.615A, T85.618A, T85.622A, T85.625A, T85.628A, T85.635A, T85.638A, T85.692A, T85.695A, T85.698-T85.738[A], T85.79XA, T85.810[A,D], T85.820[A,D], T85.830[A,D], T85.840[A,D], T85.850[A,D], T85.860[A,D], T85.890[A,D], T85.9XX[A], T86.842-T86.849

● **T85.31** **Breakdown (mechanical) of other ocular prosthetic devices, implants and grafts**

● **T85.310** **Breakdown (mechanical) of prosthetic orbit of right eye** A ◐

● **T85.311** **Breakdown (mechanical) of prosthetic orbit of left eye** A ◐

● **T85.318** **Breakdown (mechanical) of other ocular prosthetic devices, implants and grafts**

● **T85.32** **Displacement of other ocular prosthetic devices, implants and grafts**
Malposition of other ocular prosthetic devices, implants and grafts

● **T85.320** **Displacement of prosthetic orbit of right eye** A ◐

● **T85.321** **Displacement of prosthetic orbit of left eye** A ◐

● **T85.328** **Displacement of other ocular prosthetic devices, implants and grafts**

● **T85.39** **Other mechanical complication of other ocular prosthetic devices, implants and grafts**
Obstruction (mechanical) of other ocular prosthetic devices, implants and grafts
Perforation of other ocular prosthetic devices, implants and grafts
Protrusion of other ocular prosthetic devices, implants and grafts

● **T85.390** **Other mechanical complication of prosthetic orbit of right eye** A ◐

● **T85.391** **Other mechanical complication of prosthetic orbit of left eye** A ◐

● **T85.398** **Other mechanical complication of other ocular prosthetic devices, implants and grafts**

● **T85.4** **Mechanical complication of breast prosthesis and implant**
(Ex) For category T85.4 CC codes: D78.81-D78.89, E89.810-E89.89, H59.011-H59.019, H59.031-H59.039, H59.091-H59.099, H59.811-H59.89, H95.811-H95.89, I97.3, M96.89, N98.1-N98.9, T85.41X-T85.49X[A]

X ● **T85.41** **Breakdown (mechanical) of breast prosthesis and implant** A ◐

X ● **T85.42** **Displacement of breast prosthesis and implant** A ◐
Malposition of breast prosthesis and implant

X ● **T85.43** **Leakage of breast prosthesis and implant** A ◐

X ● **T85.44** **Capsular contracture of breast implant** A ◐

X ● **T85.49** **Other mechanical complication of breast prosthesis and implant** A ◐
Obstruction (mechanical) of breast prosthesis and implant
Perforation of breast prosthesis and implant
Protrusion of breast prosthesis and implant

◀ New   ◀▥ Revised   ~~deleted~~ Deleted   Excludes 1   Excludes 2   Includes   Use additional   Code first   Code also   Unspecified
OGCR Official Guidelines   ● Unacceptable Principal Diagnosis   X Assign placeholder X   ● Use Additional Character(s)   ▷ Manifestation Code   **Coding Clinic**

● **T85.5　Mechanical complication of gastrointestinal prosthetic devices, implants and grafts**

(Ex) **For category T85.5 CC codes:** H95.811-H95.89, I97.3, M96.89, N98.1-N98.9, T85.510-T85.598[A], T85.612A, T85.615A, T85.618A, T85.622A, T85.625A, T85.628A, T85.635A, T85.638A, T85.692A, T85.695A, T85.698-T85.738[A], T85.79XA, T85.810[A,D], T85.820[A,D], T85.830[A,D], T85.840[A,D], T85.850[A,D], T85.860[A,D], T85.890[A,D], T85.9XXA

● **T85.51　Breakdown (mechanical) of gastrointestinal prosthetic devices, implants and grafts**

● **T85.510　Breakdown (mechanical) of bile duct prosthesis** A 🔖

● **T85.511　Breakdown (mechanical) of esophageal anti-reflux device** A 🔖

● **T85.518　Breakdown (mechanical) of other gastrointestinal prosthetic devices, implants and grafts** A 🔖

● **T85.52　Displacement of gastrointestinal prosthetic devices, implants and grafts**

Malposition of gastrointestinal prosthetic devices, implants and grafts

● **T85.520　Displacement of bile duct prosthesis** A 🔖

● **T85.521　Displacement of esophageal anti-reflux device** A 🔖

● **T85.528　Displacement of other gastrointestinal prosthetic devices, implants and grafts** A 🔖

● **T85.59　Other mechanical complication of gastrointestinal prosthetic devices, implants and**

Obstruction, mechanical of gastrointestinal prosthetic devices, implants and grafts

Perforation of gastrointestinal prosthetic devices, implants and grafts

Protrusion of gastrointestinal prosthetic devices, implants and grafts

● **T85.590　Other mechanical complication of bile duct prosthesis** A 🔖

● **T85.591　Other mechanical complication of esophageal anti-reflux device** A 🔖

● **T85.598　Other mechanical complication of other gastrointestinal prosthetic devices, implants and grafts** A 🔖

● **T85.6　Mechanical complication of other specified internal and external prosthetic devices, implants and grafts**

● **T85.61　Breakdown (mechanical) of other specified internal prosthetic devices, implants and grafts**

● **T85.610　Breakdown (mechanical) of cranial or spinal infusion catheter** A 🔖 ◀▥

Breakdown (mechanical) of epidural infusion catheter ◀

Breakdown (mechanical) of intrathecal infusion catheter ◀

Breakdown (mechanical) of subarachnoid infusion catheter ◀

Breakdown (mechanical) of subdural infusion catheter ◀

(Ex) H95.811-H95.89, I97.3, M96.89, N98.1-N98.9, T85.610A, T85.612A, T85.615A, T85.618-T85.620A, T85.622A, T85.625A, T85.628-T85.630A, T85.635A, T85.638-T85.690[A], T85.692A, T85.695A, T85.698-T85.738[A], T85.79XA, T85.810[A,D], T85.820[A,D], T85.830[A,D], T85.840[A,D], T85.850[A,D], T85.860[A,D], T85.890[A,D], T85.9XXA

● **T85.611　Breakdown (mechanical) of intraperitoneal dialysis catheter** A 🔖

Excludes1　mechanical complication of vascular dialysis catheter (T82.4-)

(Ex) H95.811-H95.89, I97.3, M96.89, N98.1-N98.9, T85.611-T85.612[A], T85.614-T85.618[A], T85.621-T85.622[A], T85.624-T85.628[A], T85.631-T85.638[A], T85.691-T85.692[A], T85.694-T85.738[A], T85.79XA, T85.810[A,D], T85.820[A,D], T85.830[A,D], T85.840[A,D], T85.850[A,D], T85.860[A,D], T85.890[A,D], T85.9XXA

● **T85.612　Breakdown (mechanical) of permanent sutures** A 🔖

Excludes1　mechanical complication of permanent (wire) suture used in bone repair (T84.1-T84.2)

(Ex) D78.81-D78.89, E89.810-E89.89, H59.011-H59.019, H59.031-H59.039, H59.091-H59.099, H59.811-H59.89, H95.811-H95.89, I97.3, M96.89, N98.1-N98.9, T85.310-T85.311[A], T85.320-T85.321[A], T85.390-T85.391[A], T85.510-T85.738A, T85.79XA, T85.810[A,D], T85.820[A,D], T85.830[A,D], T85.840[A,D], T85.850[A,D], T85.860[A,D], T85.890[A,D], T85.9XXA, T86.842-T86.849

● **T85.613　Breakdown (mechanical) of artificial skin graft and decellularized allodermis** A 🔖

Failure of artificial skin graft and decellularized allodermis

Non-adherence of artificial skin graft and decellularized allodermis

Poor incorporation of artificial skin graft and decellularized allodermis

Shearing of artificial skin graft and decellularized allodermis

(Ex) H95.811-H95.89, I97.3, M96.89, N98.1-N98.9, T85.612-T85.613[A], T85.615A, T85.618[A], T85.622-T85.623[A], T85.625A, T85.628[A], T85.635A, T85.638[A], T85.692-T85.693[A], T85.695A, T85.698-T85.738[A], T85.79XA, T85.810[A,D], T85.820[A,D], T85.830[A,D], T85.840[A,D], T85.850[A,D], T85.860[A,D], T85.890[A,D], T85.9XXA, T86.820-T86.829

● **T85.614　Breakdown (mechanical) of insulin pump** A 🔖

(Ex) H95.811-H95.89, I97.3, M96.621-M96.89, M97.01X-M97.9XX[A], N98.1-N98.9, N99.510-N99.518, T81.82X-T81.9XX[A], T82.01X-T82.118[A], T82.120-T82.128[A], T82.192-T82.198[A], T82.211-T83.010[A], T83.020[A], T83.030[A], T83.090[A], T83.110-T83.29X[A], T83.410-T83.69X[A], T83.712A-T83.714[A], T83.718[A], T83.719A, T83.722-T83.724[A], T83.728-T83.9XX[A], T84.010-T84.039[A], T84.050-T85.29X[A], T85.41X-T85.49X[A], T85.611-T85.618[A], T85.621-T85.622[A], T85.624-T85.628[A], T85.631-T85.638[A], T85.691-T85.692[A], T85.694-T85.738[A], T85.79XA, T85.810[A,D], T85.820[A,D], T85.830[A,D], T85.840[A,D], T85.850[A,D], T85.860[A,D], T85.890[A,D], T85.9XXA, T86.820-T86.829

CHAPTER 19 (S00-T88)

● **T85.615** **Breakdown (mechanical) of other nervous system device, implant or graft** A 🐾 ◀
　　　　Breakdown (mechanical) of intrathecal infusion pump ◀
　　　　(Ex:) See T85.612

● **T85.618** **Breakdown (mechanical) of other specified internal prosthetic devices, implants and grafts** A 🐾
　　　　(Ex:) See T85.612

● **T85.62** **Displacement of other specified internal prosthetic devices, implants and grafts**
　　　Malposition of other specified internal prosthetic devices, implants and grafts

● **T85.620** **Displacement of cranial or spinal infusion catheter** A 🐾 ◀▥
　　　　Displacement of epidural infusion catheter ◀
　　　　Displacement of intrathecal infusion catheter ◀
　　　　Displacement of subarachnoid infusion catheter ◀
　　　　Displacement of subdural infusion catheter ◀
　　　　(Ex:) See T85.610

● **T85.621** **Displacement of intraperitoneal dialysis catheter** A 🐾
　　　　Excludes1　mechanical complication of vascular dialysis catheter (T82.4-)
　　　　(Ex:) See T85.611

● **T85.622** **Displacement of permanent sutures** A 🐾
　　　　Excludes1　mechanical complication of permanent (wire) suture used in bone repair (T84.1-T84.2)
　　　　(Ex:) See T85.612

● **T85.623** **Displacement of artificial skin graft and decellularized allodermis** A 🐾
　　　　Dislodgement of artificial skin graft and decellularized allodermis
　　　　Displacement of artificial skin graft and decellularized allodermis
　　　　(Ex:) See T85.613

● **T85.624** **Displacement of insulin pump** A 🐾
　　　　(Ex:) See T85.614

● **T85.625** **Displacement of other nervous system device, implant or graft** A 🐾 ◀
　　　　Displacement of intrathecal infusion pump ◀
　　　　(Ex:) See T85.612

● **T85.628** **Displacement of other specified internal prosthetic devices, implants and grafts** A 🐾
　　　　(Ex:) See T85.612
　　　　Coding Clinic: 2015, Q1, P15

● **T85.63** **Leakage of other specified internal prosthetic devices, implants and grafts**

● **T85.630** **Leakage of cranial or spinal infusion catheter** A 🐾 ◀▥
　　　　Leakage of epidural infusion catheter ◀
　　　　Leakage of intrathecal infusion catheter ◀
　　　　Leakage of subdural infusion catheter ◀
　　　　Leakage of subarachnoid infusion catheter ◀
　　　　(Ex:) See T85.610

● **T85.631** **Leakage of intraperitoneal dialysis catheter** A 🐾
　　　　Excludes1　mechanical complication of vascular dialysis catheter (T82.4)
　　　　(Ex:) See T85.611

● **T85.633** **Leakage of insulin pump** A 🐾
　　　　(Ex:) See T85.614

● **T85.635** **Leakage of other nervous system device, implant or graft** A 🐾 ◀
　　　　Leakage of intrathecal infusion pump ◀
　　　　(Ex:) See T85.612

● **T85.638** **Leakage of other specified internal prosthetic devices, implants and grafts** A 🐾
　　　　(Ex:) See T85.612

● **T85.69** **Other mechanical complication of other specified internal prosthetic devices, implants and grafts**
　　　Obstruction, mechanical of other specified internal prosthetic devices, implants and grafts
　　　Perforation of other specified internal prosthetic devices, implants and grafts
　　　Protrusion of other specified internal prosthetic devices, implants and grafts

● **T85.690** **Other mechanical complication of cranial or spinal infusion catheter** A 🐾 ◀▥
　　　　Other mechanical complication of epidural infusion catheter ◀
　　　　Other mechanical complication of intrathecal infusion catheter ◀
　　　　Other mechanical complication of subarachnoid infusion catheter ◀
　　　　Other mechanical complication of subdural infusion catheter ◀
　　　　(Ex:) See T85.610

● **T85.691** **Other mechanical complication of intraperitoneal dialysis catheter** A 🐾
　　　　Excludes1　mechanical complication of vascular dialysis catheter (T82.4)
　　　　(Ex:) See T85.611

● **T85.692** **Other mechanical complication of permanent sutures** A 🐾
　　　　Excludes1　mechanical complication of permanent (wire) suture used in bone repair (T84.1-T84.2)
　　　　(Ex:) See T85.612

◀ New　◀▥ Revised　~~deleted~~ Deleted　Excludes 1　Excludes 2　Includes　Use additional　Code first　Code also　Unspecified
OGCR Official Guidelines　● Unacceptable Principal Diagnosis　X Assign placeholder X　● Use Additional Character(s)　▌ Manifestation Code　**Coding Clinic**

● T85.693 **Other mechanical complication of artificial skin graft and decellularized allodermis** A 🐾
　　　(Ex:) See T85.613

● T85.694 **Other mechanical complication of insulin pump** A 🐾
　　　(Ex:) See T85.614

● T85.695 **Other mechanical complication of other nervous system device, implant or graft** A 🐾 ◄
　　Other mechanical complication of intrathecal infusion pump ◄
　　　(Ex:) See T85.612

● T85.698 **Other mechanical complication of other specified internal prosthetic devices, implants and grafts** A 🐾
　　Mechanical complication of nonabsorbable surgical material NOS
　　　(Ex:) See T85.612

● T85.7 **Infection and inflammatory reaction due to other internal prosthetic devices, implants and grafts**
　　Use additional code to identify infection
　　(Ex:) **For category T85.7 CC codes unless otherwise indicated:**
　　D78.81-D78.89, E36.8, E89.810-E89.89, H59.011-H59.019,
　　H59.031-H59.039, H59.091-H59.099, H59.811-H59.89, H95.811-H95.89,
　　I97.3, L76.81-L76.82, M96.621-M96.89, M97.01X-M97.9XX[A],
　　N98.1-N98.9, N99.510-N99.518, T81.82X-T81.9XX[A], T82.01X-T82.118[A],
　　T82.120-T82.128[A], T82.192-T82.198[A], T82.211-T83.29X[A],
　　T83.410-T83.69X[A], T83.712-T83.714[A], T83.718A, T83.719A,
　　T83.722-T83.724[A], T83.728-T83.9XX[A], T84.010-T84.039[A],
　　T84.050-T85.738[A], T85.79XA, T85.810[A,D], T85.820[A,D], T85.830[A,D],
　　T85.840[A,D], T85.850[A,D], T85.860[A,D], T85.890[A,D], T85.9XX[A],
　　T86.820-T86.849

X ● T85.71 **Infection and inflammatory reaction due to peritoneal dialysis catheter** A 🐾
　　　(Ex:) See T85.612

X ● T85.72 **Infection and inflammatory reaction due to insulin pump** A 🐾

● T85.73 **Infection and inflammatory reaction due to nervous system devices, implants and graft** ◄

● T85.730 **Infection and inflammatory reaction due to ventricular intracranial (communicating) shunt** A 🐾 ◄

● T85.731 **Infection and inflammatory reaction due to implanted electronic neurostimulator of brain, electrode (lead)** A 🐾 ◄

● T85.732 **Infection and inflammatory reaction due to implanted electronic neurostimulator of peripheral nerve, electrode (lead)** A 🐾 ◄
　　Infection and inflammatory reaction due to electrode (lead) for cranial nerve neurostimulators
　　Infection and inflammatory reaction due to electrode (lead) for gastric neurostimulator ◄
　　Infection and inflammatory reaction due to electrode (lead) for sacral nerve neurostimulator ◄
　　Infection and inflammatory reaction due to electrode (lead) for vagal nerve neurostimulators ◄

● T85.733 **Infection and inflammatory reaction due to implanted electronic neurostimulator of spinal cord, electrode (lead)** A 🐾 ◄

● T85.734 **Infection and inflammatory reaction due to implanted electronic neurostimulator, generator** A 🐾 ◄
　　Generator pocket infection ◄

● T85.735 **Infection and inflammatory reaction due to cranial or spinal infusion catheter** A 🐾 ◄
　　Infection and inflammatory reaction due to epidural catheter ◄
　　Infection and inflammatory reaction due to intrathecal infusion catheter ◄
　　Infection and inflammatory reaction due to subarachnoid catheter ◄
　　Infection and inflammatory reaction due to subdural catheter ◄

● T85.738 **Infection and inflammatory reaction due to other nervous system device, implant or graft** A 🐾 ◄
　　Infection and inflammatory reaction due to intrathecal infusion pump ◄

X ● T85.79 **Infection and inflammatory reaction due to other internal prosthetic devices, implants and grafts** A 🐾

● T85.8 **Other specified complications of internal prosthetic devices, implants and grafts, not elsewhere classified**
　　(Ex:) **For category T85.8 CC codes:** See T85.7

● T85.81 **Embolism due to internal prosthetic devices, implants and grafts, not elsewhere classified**

● T85.810 **Embolism due to nervous system prosthetic devices, implants and grafts** A, D 🐾

● T85.818 **Embolism due to other internal prosthetic devices, implants and grafts** ◄

● T85.82 **Fibrosis due to internal prosthetic devices, implants and grafts, not elsewhere classified**

● T85.820 **Fibrosis due to nervous system prosthetic devices, implants and grafts** A, D 🐾 ◄

● T85.828 **Fibrosis due to other internal prosthetic devices, implants and grafts** ◄

● T85.83 **Hemorrhage due to internal prosthetic devices, implants and grafts, not elsewhere classified**

● T85.830 **Hemorrhage due to nervous system prosthetic devices, implants and grafts** A, D 🐾 ◄

● T85.838 **Hemorrhage due to other internal prosthetic devices, implants and grafts** ◄

● T85.84 **Pain due to internal prosthetic devices, implants and grafts, not elsewhere classified**

● T85.840 **Pain due to nervous system prosthetic devices, implants and grafts** A, D 🐾 ◄

● T85.848 **Pain due to other internal prosthetic devices, implants and grafts** ◄

● T85.85 **Stenosis due to internal prosthetic devices, implants and grafts, not elsewhere classified**

● T85.850 **Stenosis due to nervous system prosthetic devices, implants and grafts** A, D 🐾 ◄

● T85.858 **Stenosis due to other internal prosthetic devices, implants and grafts** ◄

CHAPTER 19 (S00-T88)

N Newborn Age: 0　　**P** Pediatric Age: 0–17　　**M** Maternity DX: 12–55　　**A** Adult Age: 15–124　　♀ Females Only　　♂ Males Only

🐾 Complication\Comorbidity　　🐾 Major C\C　　(Ex:) CC/MCC Exclusions　　🐾 Hospital-Acquired Condition

1511

CHAPTER 19 (S00-T88)

● T85.86   **Thrombosis due to internal prosthetic devices, implants and grafts, not elsewhere classified**

   ● T85.860   **Thrombosis due to nervous system prosthetic devices, implants and grafts** A, D 🜲 ◀

   ● T85.868   **Thrombosis due to other internal prosthetic devices, implants and grafts** ◀

● T85.89   **Other specified complication of internal prosthetic devices, implants and grafts, not elsewhere classified**

   ● T85.890   **Other specified complication of nervous system prosthetic devices, implants and grafts** A, D 🜲 ◀

   ● T85.898   **Other specified complication of other internal prosthetic devices, implants and grafts** ◀

X ● T85.9   **Unspecified** **complication of internal prosthetic device, implant and graft**

    Complication of internal prosthetic device, implant and graft NOS

● T86   **Complications of transplanted organs and tissue**

   Use additional code to identify other transplant complications, such as:

    graft-versus-host disease (D89.81-)

    malignancy associated with organ transplant (C80.2)

    post-transplant lymphoproliferative disorders (PTLD) (D47.Z1)

  ● T86.0   **Complications of bone marrow transplant**

    (Ex:) For category T86.0 CC codes: D78.81-D78.89, D89.810-D89.813, E89.810-E89.89, H59.011-H59.019, H59.031-H59.099, H59.811-H59.89, H95.811-H95.89, I97.3, M96.89, N98.1-N98.9, T86.00-T86.09

   T86.00   **Unspecified** **complication of bone marrow transplant**

   T86.01   **Bone marrow transplant rejection** 🜲

   T86.02   **Bone marrow transplant failure** 🜲

   T86.03   **Bone marrow transplant infection** 🜲

   T86.09   **Other complications of bone marrow transplant** 🜲

  ● T86.1   **Complications of kidney transplant**

    (Ex:) For category T86.1 CC codes: D78.81-D78.89, E89.810-E89.89, H59.011-H59.019, H59.031-H59.099, H59.091-H59.099, H59.811-H59.89, H95.811-H95.89, I97.3, M96.89, N98.1-N98.9, T86.10-T86.19

   T86.10   **Unspecified** **complication of kidney transplant** 🜲

   T86.11   **Kidney transplant rejection** 🜲

   T86.12   **Kidney transplant failure** 🜲
     Coding Clinic: 2013, Q1, P24

   T86.13   **Kidney transplant infection** 🜲

    Use additional code to specify infection

   T86.19   **Other complication of kidney transplant** 🜲

OGCR Section I.C.19.g.3.

Organ Transplant Complications

Transplant Complications

(a) Transplant complications other than kidney

Codes under category T86, Complications of transplanted organs and tissues, are for use for both complications and rejection of transplanted organs. A transplant complication code is only assigned if the complication affects the function of the transplanted organ. Two codes are required to fully describe a transplant complication: the appropriate code from category T86 and a secondary code that identifies the complication.

Pre-existing conditions or conditions that develop after the transplant are not coded as complications unless they affect the function of the transplanted organ.

See I.C.21 for transplant organ removal status

See I.C.2 for malignant neoplasm associated with transplanted organ.

● T86.2   **Complications of heart transplant**

   Excludes1   complication of:
     artificial heart device (T82.5)
     heart-lung transplant (T86.3)

   (Ex:) For category T86.2 CC codes: D78.81-D78.89, E89.810-E89.89, H59.011-H59.019, H59.031-H59.039, H59.091-H59.099, H59.811-H59.89, H95.811-H95.89, I97.3, M96.89, N98.1-N98.9, T86.20-T86.39

   T86.20   **Unspecified** **complication of heart transplant** 🜲

   T86.21   **Heart transplant rejection** 🜲

   T86.22   **Heart transplant failure** 🜲

   T86.23   **Heart transplant infection** 🜲

    Use additional code to specify infection

  ● T86.29   **Other complications of heart transplant**

   T86.290   **Cardiac allograft vasculopathy** 🜲

     Excludes1   atherosclerosis of coronary arteries (I25.75-, I25.76-, I25.81-)

   T86.298   **Other complications of heart transplant** 🜲

● T86.3   **Complications of heart-lung transplant**

   (Ex:) For category T86.3 CC codes: See T86.2

   T86.30   **Unspecified** **complication of heart-lung transplant** 🜲
    CC when PDx is its own CC

   T86.31   **Heart-lung transplant rejection** 🜲
    CC when PDx is its own CC

   T86.32   **Heart-lung transplant failure** 🜲
    CC when PDx is its own CC

   T86.33   **Heart-lung transplant infection** 🜲
    Use additional code to specify infection
    CC when PDx is its own CC

   T86.39   **Other complications of heart-lung transplant** 🜲
    CC when PDx is its own CC

● T86.4   **Complications of liver transplant**

   (Ex:) For category T86.4 CC codes: D78.81-D78.89, E89.810-E89.89, H59.011-H59.019, H59.031-H59.039, H59.091-H59.099, H59.811-H59.89, H95.811-H95.89, I97.3, M96.89, N98.1-N98.9, T86.40-T86.49

   T86.40   **Unspecified** **complication of liver transplant** 🜲

   T86.41   **Liver transplant rejection** 🜲

   T86.42   **Liver transplant failure** 🜲

   T86.43   **Liver transplant infection** 🜲

    Use additional code to identify infection, such as:
     Cytomegalovirus (CMV) infection (B25.-)

   T86.49   **Other complications of liver transplant** 🜲

● T86.5   **Complications of stem cell transplant** 🜲
   Complications from stem cells from peripheral blood
   Complications from stem cells from umbilical cord

   (Ex:) D78.81-D78.89, E89.810-E89.89, H59.011-H59.019, H59.031-H59.039, H59.091-H59.099, H59.811-H59.89, H95.811-H95.89, I97.3, M96.89, N98.1-N98.9, T86.5, T86.830-T86.839

● T86.8   **Complications of other transplanted organs and tissues**

  ● T86.81   **Complications of lung transplant**

   Excludes1   complication of heart-lung transplant (T86.3-)

   (Ex:) For category T86.81 CC codes: D78.81-D78.89, E89.810-E89.89, H59.011-H59.019, H59.031-H59.039, H59.091-H59.099, H59.811-H59.89, H95.811-H95.89, I97.3, M96.89, N98.1-N98.9, T86.810-T86.819

   T86.810   **Lung transplant rejection** 🜲

   T86.811   **Lung transplant failure** 🜲

   T86.812   **Lung transplant infection** 🜲
    Use additional code to specify infection

   T86.818   **Other complications of lung transplant** 🜲

   T86.819   **Unspecified** **complication of lung transplant** 🜲

◀ New   ◀▥ Revised   ~~deleted~~ Deleted   Excludes 1   Excludes 2   Includes   Use additional   Code first   Code also   Unspecified

OGCR Official Guidelines   ● Unacceptable Principal Diagnosis   X Assign placeholder X   ● Use Additional Character(s)   ▮ Manifestation Code   **Coding Clinic**

● **T86.82** **Complications of skin graft (allograft) (autograft)**

> **Excludes2**   complication of artificial skin graft (T85.693)
> (Ex) **For category T86.82 CC codes:** D78.81-D78.89, E89.810-E89.89, H59.011-H59.019, H59.031-H59.039, H59.091-H59.099, H59.811-H59.89, H95.811-H95.89, I97.3, M96.89, N98.1-N98.9, T85.613[A], T85.623[A], T85.693[A], T86.820-T86.829

     T86.820   Skin graft (allograft) rejection🔗

     T86.821   Skin graft (allograft) (autograft) failure🔗

     T86.822   Skin graft (allograft) (autograft) infection🔗

>   Use additional code to specify infection

     T86.828   Other complications of skin graft (allograft) (autograft)🔗

     T86.829   Unspecified complication of skin graft (allograft) (autograft)🔗

● **T86.83** **Complications of bone graft**

> **Excludes2**   mechanical complications of bone graft (T84.3-)
> (Ex) **For category T86.83 CC codes:** H95.811-H95.89, I97.3, M96.89, N98.1-N98.9, T86.5, T86.830-T86.839

     T86.830   Bone graft rejection🔗

     T86.831   Bone graft failure🔗

     T86.832   Bone graft infection🔗

>   Use additional code to specify infection

     T86.838   Other complications of bone graft🔗

     T86.839   Unspecified complication of bone graft🔗

● **T86.84** **Complications of corneal transplant**

> **Excludes2**   mechanical complications of corneal graft (T85.3-)
> (Ex) **For category T86.84 CC codes unless otherwise indicated:** H59.011-H59.019, H59.031-H59.039, H59.091-H59.099, H59.811-H59.89, H95.811-H95.89, I97.3, M96.621-M96.89, M97.01X-M97.9XX[A], N98.1-N98.9, N99.510-N99.518, T81.82X[A], T81.89X-T81.9XX[A], T82.01X-T82.118[A], T82.120-T82.128[A], T82.192-T82.198[A], T82.211-T83.010[A], T83.020[A], T83.030[A], T83.090[A], T83.110-T83.29X[A], T83.410-T83.69X[A], T83.712A-T83.714A, T83.718A, T83.719[A], T83.722-T83.724[A], T83.728-T84.039[A], T84.050-T85.49X[A], T85.612[A], T85.615[A], T85.618[A], T85.622[A], T85.625[A], T85.628[A], T85.635A, T85.638[A], T85.692[A], T85.695A, T85.698, T85.738[A], T85.79XA, T85.810[A,D], T85.820[A,D], T85.830[A,D], T85.840[A,D], T85.850[A,D], T85.860[A,D], T85.890[A,D], T85.9XX[A], T86.820-T86.829, T86.840-T86.849

     T86.840   Corneal transplant rejection🔗
> (Ex) H59.031-H59.039, H59.091-H59.099, H59.811-H59.89, H95.811-H95.89, I97.3, M96.89, N98.1-N98.9, T85.318[A], T85.328[A], T85.398[A], T85.810[A,D], T85.820[A,D], T85.830[A,D], T85.840[A,D], T85.850[A,D], T85.860[A,D], T85.890[A,D], T86.840-T86.841

     T86.841   Corneal transplant failure🔗
> (Ex) See T86.840

     T86.842   Corneal transplant infection🔗

>   Use additional code to specify infection

     T86.848   Other complications of corneal transplant🔗

     T86.849   Unspecified complication of corneal transplant🔗

● **T86.85** **Complication of intestine transplant**

> (Ex) **For category T86.85 CC codes:** D47.Z1, D78.81-D78.89, E89.810-E89.89, H59.011-H59.019, H59.031-H59.099, H59.811-H59.89, H95.811-H95.89, I97.3, M96.89, N98.1-N98.9, T86.850-T86.99

     T86.850   Intestine transplant rejection🔗

     T86.851   Intestine transplant failure🔗

     T86.852   Intestine transplant infection🔗

>   Use additional code to specify infection

     T86.858   Other complications of intestine transplant🔗

     T86.859   Unspecified complication of intestine transplant🔗

● **T86.89** **Complications of other transplanted tissue**

> Transplant failure or rejection of pancreas
> (Ex) **For category T86.89 CC codes:** D78.81-D78.89, E89.810-E89.89, H59.011-H59.019, H59.031-H59.039, H59.091-H59.099, H59.811-H59.89, H95.811-H95.89, I97.3, M96.89, N98.1-N98.9, T86.890-T86.899

     T86.890   Other transplanted tissue rejection🔗

     T86.891   Other transplanted tissue failure🔗

     T86.892   Other transplanted tissue infection🔗

>   Use additional code to specify infection

     T86.898   Other complications of other transplanted tissue🔗

     T86.899   Unspecified complication of other transplanted tissue🔗

● **T86.9** **Complication of unspecified transplanted organ and tissue**

> (Ex) **For category T86.9 CC codes:** See T86.85

   T86.90   Unspecified complication of unspecified transplanted organ and tissue🔗

   T86.91   Unspecified transplanted organ and tissue rejection🔗

   T86.92   Unspecified transplanted organ and tissue failure🔗

   T86.93   Unspecified transplanted organ and tissue infection🔗

>   Use additional code to specify infection

   T86.99   Other complications of unspecified transplanted organ and tissue🔗

● **T87** **Complications peculiar to reattachment and amputation**

● **T87.0** **Complications of reattached (part of) upper extremity**

> (Ex) **For category T87.0 CC codes:** D78.81-D78.89, E36.8, E89.810-E89.89, H59.011-H59.019, H59.031-H59.039, H59.091-H59.099, H59.811-H59.89, H95.811-H95.89, I97.3, L76.81-L76.82, M96.89, N98.1-N98.9, T81.82X-T81.9XX[A], T87.0X1-T87.0X9

● **T87.0X** **Complications of reattached (part of) upper extremity**

     T87.0X1   Complications of reattached (part of) right upper extremity🔗

     T87.0X2   Complications of reattached (part of) left upper extremity🔗

     T87.0X9   Complications of reattached (part of) unspecified upper extremity🔗

● **T87.1** **Complications of reattached (part of) lower extremity**

> (Ex) **For category T87.1 CC codes:** D78.81-D78.89, E36.8, E89.810-E89.89, H59.011-H59.019, H59.031-H59.039, H59.091-H59.099, H59.811-H59.89, H95.811-H95.89, I97.3, L76.81-L76.82, M96.89, N98.1-N98.9, T81.82X-T81.9XX[A], T87.1X1-T87.1X9

● **T87.1X** **Complications of reattached (part of) lower extremity**

     T87.1X1   Complications of reattached (part of) right lower extremity🔗

     T87.1X2   Complications of reattached (part of) left lower extremity🔗

     T87.1X9   Complications of reattached (part of) unspecified lower extremity🔗

CHAPTER 19 (S00-T88)

N Newborn Age: 0   **P** Pediatric Age: 0–17   **M** Maternity DX: 12–55   **A** Adult Age: 15–124   ♀ Females Only   ♂ Males Only

 Complication\Comorbidity   Major C\C   (Ex) CC/MCC Exclusions   🔗 Hospital-Acquired Condition

1513

CHAPTER 19 (S00-T88)

T87.2 **Complications of other reattached body part** 🔵
Ex: D78.81-D78.89, E36.8, E89.810-E89.89, H59.011-H59.019,
H59.031-H59.039, H59.091-H59.099, H59.811-H59.89, H95.811-H95.89,
I97.3, L76.81-L76.82, M96.89, N98.1-N98.9, T81.82X-T81.9XX[A], T87.2

● T87.3 **Neuroma of amputation stump**

T87.30 **Neuroma of amputation stump, unspecified extremity**

T87.31 **Neuroma of amputation stump, right upper extremity**

T87.32 **Neuroma of amputation stump, left upper extremity**

T87.33 **Neuroma of amputation stump, right lower extremity**

T87.34 **Neuroma of amputation stump, left lower extremity**

● T87.4 **Infection of amputation stump**
Ex: **For category T87.4 CC codes:** D78.81-D78.89, E36.8, E89.810-E89.89,
H59.011-H59.019, H59.031-H59.039, H59.091-H59.099, H59.811-H59.89,
H95.811-H95.89, I97.3, L76.81-L76.82, M96.89, N98.1-N98.9,
T81.82X-T81.9XX[A], T87.40-T87.9

T87.40 **Infection of amputation stump, unspecified extremity** 🔵

T87.41 **Infection of amputation stump, right upper extremity** 🔵

T87.42 **Infection of amputation stump, left upper extremity** 🔵

T87.43 **Infection of amputation stump, right lower extremity** 🔵

T87.44 **Infection of amputation stump, left lower extremity** 🔵

● T87.5 **Necrosis of amputation stump**

T87.50 **Necrosis of amputation stump, unspecified extremity**

T87.51 **Necrosis of amputation stump, right upper extremity**

T87.52 **Necrosis of amputation stump, left upper extremity**

T87.53 **Necrosis of amputation stump, right lower extremity**

T87.54 **Necrosis of amputation stump, left lower extremity**

● T87.8 **Other complications of amputation stump**

T87.81 **Dehiscence of amputation stump**

T87.89 **Other complications of amputation stump**
Amputation stump contracture
Amputation stump contracture of next proximal joint
Amputation stump flexion
Amputation stump edema
Amputation stump hematoma

Excludes2 phantom limb syndrome (G54.6-G54.7)

● T87.9 **Unspecified complications of amputation stump**

● T88 **Other complications of surgical and medical care, not elsewhere classified**

Excludes2 complication following infusion, transfusion and therapeutic injection (T80.-)
complication following procedure NEC (T81.-)
complications of anesthesia in labor and delivery (O74.-)
complications of anesthesia in pregnancy (O29.-)
complications of anesthesia in puerperium (O89.-)
complications of devices, implants and grafts (T82-T85)
complications of obstetric surgery and procedure (O75.4)
dermatitis due to drugs and medicaments (L23.3, L24.4, L25.1, L27.0-L27.1)
poisoning and toxic effects of drugs and chemicals (T36-T65 with fifth or sixth character 1-4 or 6)
specified complications classified elsewhere

The appropriate 7th character is to be added to each code from category T88

A	initial encounter
D	subsequent encounter
S	sequela

X ● T88.0 **Infection following immunization** A 🔵
Sepsis following immunization
Ex: N98.0, T80.211-T80.29X[A], T82.7XX[A], T88.0XX[A]

X ● T88.1 **Other complications following immunization, not elsewhere classified** A 🔵
Generalized vaccinia
Rash following immunization

Excludes1 vaccinia not from vaccine (B08.011)

Excludes2 anaphylactic shock due to serum (T80.5-)
other serum reactions (T80.6-)
postimmunization arthropathy (M02.2)
postimmunization encephalitis (G04.02)
postimmunization fever (R50.83)

Ex: T88.1XX[A]

X ● T88.2 **Shock due to anesthesia** A 🔵
Use additional code for adverse effect, if applicable, to identify drug (T41.- with fifth or sixth character 5)

Excludes1 complications of anesthesia (in):
labor and delivery (O74.-)
pregnancy (O29.-)
puerperium (O89.-)
postprocedural shock NOS (T81.1-)

Ex: See T81.1

X ● T88.3 **Malignant hyperthermia due to anesthesia** A 🔵
Use additional code for adverse effect, if applicable, to identify drug (T41.- with fifth or sixth character 5)
Ex: D78.01-D78.02, D78.21-D78.89, E36.01-E36.02, E36.8, E89.810-E89.89,
G97.51-G97.52, G97.61-G97.64, H59.011-H59.019, H59.031-H59.039,
H59.091-H59.099, H59.111-H59.129, H59.311-H59.329, H59.331-H59.369,
H59.811-H59.89, H95.21-H95.22, H95.41-H95.42, H95.51-H95.54,
H95.811-H95.89, I97.3-I97.42, I97.610-I97.648, J95.61-J95.62,
J95.830-J95.831, J95.860-J95.863, K91.61-K91.62, K91.840-K91.841,
K91.870-K91.873, L76.01-L76.02, L76.21-L76.22, L76.31-L76.34,
L76.81-L76.82, M96.810-M96.811, M96.830-M96.89, N98.1-N98.9,
N99.61-N99.62, N99.820-N99.821, T79.4XX[A], T81.10X-T81.19X[A],
T81.82X[A], T81.89X-T81.9XX[A], T88.2XX-T88.3XX[A]

X● **T88.4** **Failed or difficult intubation**

X● **T88.5** **Other complications of anesthesia**

    Use additional code for adverse effect, if applicable, to identify drug (T41.- with fifth or sixth character 5)

  X● **T88.51** **Hypothermia following anesthesia**

  X● **T88.52** **Failed moderate sedation during procedure**

      Failed conscious sedation during procedure

      Excludes2 personal history of failed moderate sedation (Z92.83)

  X● **T88.53** **Unintended awareness under general anesthesia during procedure** ◀

      Excludes2 personal history of unintended awareness under general anesthesia (Z92.84) ◀

  X● **T88.59** **Other complications of anesthesia**

X● **T88.6** **Anaphylactic reaction due to adverse effect of correct drug or medicament properly administered** A 🐾

    Anaphylactic shock due to adverse effect of correct drug or medicament properly administered

    Anaphylactoid reaction NOS

    Use additional code for adverse effect, if applicable, to identify drug (T36-T50 with fifth or sixth character 5)

    Excludes1 anaphylactic reaction due to serum (T80.5-)

             anaphylactic shock or reaction due to adverse food reaction (T78.0-)

    (Ex.) T78.00X-T78.09X[A]

X● **T88.7** **Unspecified adverse effect of drug or medicament**

    Drug hypersensitivity NOS

    Drug reaction NOS

    Use additional code for adverse effect, if applicable, to identify drug (T36-T50 with fifth or sixth character 5)

    Excludes1 specified adverse effects of drugs and medicaments (A00-R94 and T80-T88.6, T88.8)

X● **T88.8** **Other specified complications of surgical and medical care, not elsewhere classified**

    Use additional code to identify the complication

X● **T88.9** **Complication of surgical and medical care, unspecified**

N Newborn Age: 0   **P** Pediatric Age: 0–17   **M** Maternity DX: 12–55   **A** Adult Age: 15–124   ♀ Females Only   ♂ Males Only

🐾 Complication\Comorbidity   🐾 Major C\C   (Ex.) CC/MCC Exclusions   🐾 Hospital-Acquired Condition

CHAPTER 19 (S00-T88)

1515

CHAPTER 20

EXTERNAL CAUSES OF MORBIDITY (V00-Y99)

OGCR Chapter-Specific Coding Guidelines

20. **Chapter 20: External Causes of Morbidity (V00-Y99)**
The external causes of morbidity codes should never be sequenced as the first-listed or principal diagnosis.

External cause codes are intended to provide data for injury research and evaluation of injury prevention strategies. These codes capture how the injury or health condition happened (cause), the intent (unintentional or accidental; or intentional, such as suicide or assault), the place where the event occurred the activity of the patient at the time of the event, and the person's status (e.g., civilian, military).

There is no national requirement for mandatory ICD-10-CM external cause code reporting. Unless a provider is subject to a state-based external cause code reporting mandate or these codes are required by a particular payer, reporting of ICD-10-CM codes in Chapter 20, External Causes of Morbidity, is not required. In the absence of a mandatory reporting requirement, providers are encouraged to voluntarily report external cause codes, as they provide valuable data for injury research and evaluation of injury prevention strategies.

a. General External Cause Coding Guidelines

1) Used with any code in the range of A00.0-T88.9, Z00-Z99
An external cause code may be used with any code in the range of A00.0-T88.9, Z00-Z99, classification that is a health condition due to an external cause. Though they are most applicable to injuries, they are also valid for use with such things as infections or diseases due to an external source, and other health conditions, such as a heart attack that occurs during strenuous physical activity.

2) External cause code used for length of treatment
Assign the external cause code, with the appropriate 7th character (initial encounter, subsequent encounter or sequela) for each encounter for which the injury or condition is being treated.

Most categories in chapter 20 have a 7th character requirement for each applicable code. Most categories in this chapter have three 7th character values: A, initial encounter, D, subsequent encounter and S, sequela. While the patient may be seen by a new or different provider over the course of treatment for an injury or condition, assignment of the 7th character for external cause should match the 7th character of the code assigned for the associated injury or condition for the encounter.

3) Use the full range of external cause codes
Use the full range of external cause codes to completely describe the cause, the intent, the place of occurrence and if applicable, the activity of the patient at the time of the event, and the patient's status, for all injuries, and other health conditions due to an external cause.

4) Assign as many external cause codes as necessary
Assign as many external cause codes as necessary to fully explain each cause. If only one external code can be recorded, assign the code most related to the principal diagnosis.

5) The selection of the appropriate external cause code
The selection of the appropriate external cause code is guided by the Alphabetic Index of External Causes and by Inclusion and Exclusion notes in the Tabular List.

6) External cause code can never be a principal diagnosis
An external cause code can never be a principal (first-listed) diagnosis.

7) Combination external cause codes
Certain of the external cause codes are combination codes that identify sequential events that result in an injury, such as a fall which results in striking against an object. The injury may be due to either event or both. The combination external cause code used should correspond to the sequence of events regardless of which caused the most serious injury.

8) No external cause code needed in certain circumstances
No external cause code from Chapter 20 is needed if the external cause and intent are included in a code from another chapter (e.g. T36.0X1- Poisoning by penicillins, accidental (unintentional)).

b. Place of Occurrence Guideline
Codes from category Y92, Place of occurrence of the external cause, are secondary codes for use after other external cause codes to identify the location of the patient at the time of injury or other condition.

Generally, a place of occurrence code is **assigned** only once, at the initial encounter for treatment. **However, in the rare instance that a new injury occurs during hospitalization, an additional place of occurrence code may be assigned.** No 7th characters are used for Y92. Only one code from Y92 should be recorded on a medical record.

Do not use place of occurrence code Y92.9 if the place is not stated or is not applicable.

c. Activity Code
Assign a code from category Y93, Activity code, to describe the activity of the patient at the time the injury or other health condition occurred.

An activity code is used only once, at the initial encounter for treatment. Only one code from Y93 should be recorded on a medical record.

The activity codes are not applicable to poisonings, adverse effects, misadventures or sequela.

Do not assign Y93.9, Unspecified activity, if the activity is not stated.

A code from category Y93 is appropriate for use with external cause and intent codes if identifying the activity provides additional information about the event.

d. Place of Occurrence, Activity, and Status Codes Used with other External Cause Code
When applicable, place of occurrence, activity, and external cause status codes are sequenced after the main external cause code(s). Regardless of the number of external cause codes assigned, there should be only one place of occurrence code, one activity code, and one external cause status code assigned to an encounter.

◀ New ◀═ Revised ~~deleted~~ Deleted | Excludes 1 | Excludes 2 | Includes | Use additional | Code first | Code also | Unspecified

OGCR Official Guidelines ● Unacceptable Principal Diagnosis X Assign placeholder X ● Use Additional Character(s) ▶ Manifestation Code **Coding Clinic**

e. If the Reporting Format Limits the Number of External Cause Codes

If the reporting format limits the number of external cause codes that can be used in reporting clinical data, report the code for the cause/intent most related to the principal diagnosis. If the format permits capture of additional external cause codes, the cause/intent, including medical misadventures, of the additional events should be reported rather than the codes for place, activity, or external status.

f. Multiple External Cause Coding Guidelines

More than one external cause code is required to fully describe the external cause of an illness or injury. The assignment of external cause codes should be sequenced in the following priority:

If two or more events cause separate injuries, an external cause code should be assigned for each cause. The first-listed external cause code will be selected in the following order:

External codes for child and adult abuse take priority over all other external cause codes.

See Section I.C.19., Child and Adult abuse guidelines.

External codes for terrorism events take priority over all other external cause codes except child and adult abuse.

External cause codes for cataclysmic events take priority over all other external cause codes except child and adult abuse and terrorism.

External cause codes for transport accidents take priority over all other external cause codes except cataclysmic events, child and adult abuse and terrorism.

Activity and external cause status codes are assigned following all causal (intent) external cause codes.

The first-listed external cause code should correspond to the cause of the most serious diagnosis due to an assault, accident, or self-harm, following the order of hierarchy listed above.

g. Child and Adult Abuse Guideline

Adult and child abuse, neglect and maltreatment are classified as assault. Any of the assault codes may be used to indicate the external cause of any injury resulting from the confirmed abuse.

For confirmed cases of abuse, neglect and maltreatment, when the perpetrator is known, a code from Y07, Perpetrator of maltreatment and neglect, should accompany any other assault codes.

See Section I.C.19. Adult and child abuse, neglect and other maltreatment

h. Unknown or Undetermined Intent Guideline

If the intent (accident, self-harm, assault) of the cause of an injury or other condition is unknown or unspecified, code the intent as accidental intent. All transport accident categories assume accidental intent.

1) Use of undetermined intent

External cause codes for events of undetermined intent are only for use if the documentation in the record specifies that the intent cannot be determined.

i. Sequelae (Late Effects) of External Cause Guidelines

1) Sequelae external cause codes

Sequela are reported using the external cause code with the 7th character "S" for sequela. These codes should be used with any report of a late effect or sequela resulting from a previous injury.

See Section I.B.10. Sequela, (Late Effects)

2) Sequela external cause code with a related current injury

A sequela external cause code should never be used with a related current nature of injury code.

3) Use of sequela external cause codes for subsequent visits

Use a late effect external cause code for subsequent visits when a late effect of the initial injury is being treated. Do not use a late effect external cause code for subsequent visits for follow-up care (e.g., to assess healing, to receive rehabilitative therapy) of the injury when no late effect of the injury has been documented.

j. Terrorism Guidelines

1) Cause of injury identified by the Federal Government (FBI) as terrorism

When the cause of an injury is identified by the Federal Government (FBI) as terrorism, the first-listed external cause code should be a code from category Y38, Terrorism. The definition of terrorism employed by the FBI is found at the inclusion note at the beginning of category Y38. Use additional code for place of occurrence (Y92.-). More than one Y38 code may be assigned if the injury is the result of more than one mechanism of terrorism.

2) Cause of an injury is suspected to be the result of terrorism

When the cause of an injury is suspected to be the result of terrorism a code from category Y38 should not be assigned. Suspected cases should be classified as assault.

3) Code Y38.9, Terrorism, secondary effects

Assign code Y38.9, Terrorism, secondary effects, for conditions occurring subsequent to the terrorist event. This code should not be assigned for conditions that are due to the initial terrorist act.

It is acceptable to assign code Y38.9 with another code from Y38 if there is an injury due to the initial terrorist event and an injury that is a subsequent result of the terrorist event.

k. External cause status

A code from category Y99, External cause status, should be assigned whenever any other external cause code is assigned for an encounter, including an Activity code, except for the events noted below. Assign a code from category Y99, External cause status, to indicate the work status of the person at the time the event occurred. The status code indicates whether the event occurred during military activity, whether a non-military person was at work, whether an individual including a student or volunteer was involved in a non-work activity at the time of the causal event.

A code from Y99, External cause status, should be assigned, when applicable, with other external cause codes, such as transport accidents and falls. The external cause status codes are not applicable to poisonings, adverse effects, misadventures or late effects.

Do not assign a code from category Y99 if no other external cause codes (cause, activity) are applicable for the encounter.

An external cause status code is used only once, at the initial encounter for treatment. Only one code from Y99 should be recorded on a medical record.

Do not assign code Y99.9, Unspecified external cause status, if the status is not stated.

CHAPTER 20 (V01-Y99)

N Newborn Age: 0   **P** Pediatric Age: 0–17   **M** Maternity DX: 12–55   **A** Adult Age: 15–124   ♀ Females Only   ♂ Males Only

Complication\Comorbidity   Major C\C   Ⓔ CC/MCC Exclusions   Hospital-Acquired Condition

1517

CHAPTER 20

EXTERNAL CAUSES OF MORBIDITY (V00-Y99)

Note: This chapter permits the classification of environmental events and circumstances as the cause of injury, and other adverse effects. Where a code from this section is applicable, it is intended that it shall be used secondary to a code from another chapter of the Classification indicating the nature of the condition. Most often, the condition will be classifiable to Chapter 19, Injury, poisoning and certain other consequences of external causes (S00-T88). Other conditions that may be stated to be due to external causes are classified in Chapters I to XVIII. For these conditions, codes from Chapter 20 should be used to provide additional information as to the cause of the condition.

This chapter contains the following blocks:

V00-X58	Accidents
V00-V99	Transport accidents
V00-V09	Pedestrian injured in transport accident
V10-V19	Pedal cycle rider injured in transport accident
V20-V29	Motorcycle rider injured in transport accident
V30-V39	Occupant of three-wheeled motor vehicle injured in transport accident
V40-V49	Car occupant injured in transport accident
V50-V59	Occupant of pick-up truck or van injured in transport accident
V60-V69	Occupant of heavy transport vehicle injured in transport accident
V70-V79	Bus occupant injured in transport accident
V80-V89	Other land transport accidents
V90-V94	Water transport accidents
V95-V97	Air and space transport accidents
V98-V99	Other and unspecified transport accidents
W00-X58	Other external causes of accidental injury
W00-W19	Slipping, tripping, stumbling and falls
W20-W49	Exposure to inanimate mechanical forces
W50-W64	Exposure to animate mechanical forces
W65-W74	Accidental non-transport drowning and submersion
W85-W99	Exposure to electric current, radiation and extreme ambient air temperature and pressure
X00-X08	Exposure to smoke, fire and flames
X10-X19	Contact with heat and hot substances
X30-X39	Exposure to forces of nature
X50	Overexertion and strenuous or repetitive movements ◄
X52, X58	Accidental exposure to other specified factors
X71-X83	Intentional self-harm
X92-Y09 ◄	Assault
Y21-Y33	Event of undetermined intent
Y35-Y38	Legal intervention, operations of war, military operations, and terrorism
Y62-Y84	Complications of medical and surgical care
Y62-Y69	Misadventures to patients during surgical and medical care
Y70-Y82	Medical devices associated with adverse incidents in diagnostic and therapeutic use
Y83-Y84	Surgical and other medical procedures as the cause of abnormal reaction of the patient, or of later complication, without mention of misadventure at the time of the procedure
Y90-Y99	Supplementary factors related to causes of morbidity classified elsewhere

ACCIDENTS (V00-X58)

TRANSPORT ACCIDENTS (V00-V99)

Note: This section is structured in 12 groups. Those relating to land transport accidents (V00-V89) reflect the victim's mode of transport and are subdivided to identify the victim's 'counterpart' or the type of event. The vehicle of which the injured person is an occupant is identified in the first two characters since it is seen as the most important factor to identify for prevention purposes. A transport accident is one in which the vehicle involved must be moving or running or in use for transport purposes at the time of the accident. ◄

Use additional code to identify:
Airbag injury (W22.1)
Type of street or road (Y92.4-)
Use of cellular telephone and other electronic equipment at the time of the transport accident (Y93.C-)

Excludes1 agricultural vehicles in stationary use or maintenance (W31.-)
assault by crashing of motor vehicle (Y03.-)
automobile or motor cycle in stationary use or maintenance - code to type of accident
crashing of motor vehicle, undetermined intent (Y32)
intentional self-harm by crashing of motor vehicle (X82)

Excludes2 transport accidents due to cataclysm (X34-X38)

Note: Definitions related to transport accidents: ◄

(a) A transport accident (V00-V99) is any accident involving a device designed primarily for, or used at the time primarily for, conveying persons or good from one place to another. ◄

(b) A public highway [trafficway] or street is the entire width between property lines (or other boundary lines) of land open to the public as a matter of right or custom for purposes of moving persons or property from one place to another. A roadway is that part of the public highway designed, improved and customarily used for vehicular traffic.

(c) A traffic accident is any vehicle accident occurring on the public highway [i.e., originating on, terminating on, or involving a vehicle partially on the highway]. A vehicle accident is assumed to have occurred on the public highway unless another place is specified, except in the case of accidents involving only off-road motor vehicles, which are classified as nontraffic accidents unless the contrary is stated.

(d) A nontraffic accident is any vehicle accident that occurs entirely in any place other than a public highway.

(e) A pedestrian is any person involved in an accident who was not at the time of the accident riding in or on a motor vehicle, railway train, streetcar or animal-drawn or other vehicle, or on a pedal cycle or animal. This includes, a person changing a tire, working on a parked car, or a person on foot. It also includes the user of a pedestrian conveyance such as a baby-stroller, ice-skates, skis, sled, roller skates, a skateboard, nonmotorized or motorized wheelchair, motorized mobility scooter, or nonmotorized scooter. ◄

(f) A driver is an occupant of a transport vehicle who is operating or intending to operate it.

(g) A passenger is any occupant of a transport vehicle other than the driver, except a person traveling on the outside of the vehicle.

(h) A person on the outside of a vehicle is any person being transported by a vehicle but not occupying the space normally reserved for the driver or passengers, or the space intended for the transport of property. This includes a person travelling on the bodywork, bumper, fender, roof, running board or step of a vehicle, as well as, hanging on the outside of the vehicle. ◄

(i) A pedal cycle is any land transport vehicle operated solely by nonmotorized pedals including a bicycle or tricycle.

(j) A pedal cyclist is any person riding a pedal cycle or in a sidecar or trailer attached to a pedal cycle.

◄ New   ◄▬ Revised   ~~deleted~~ Deleted   Excludes 1   Excludes 2   Includes   Use additional   Code first   Code also   Unspecified

OGCR Official Guidelines   ● Unacceptable Principal Diagnosis   X Assign placeholder X   ● Use Additional Character(s)   ▶ Manifestation Code   **Coding Clinic**

(k) A motorcycle is a two-wheeled motor vehicle with one or two riding saddles and sometimes with a third wheel for the support of a sidecar. The sidecar is considered part of the motorcycle. This includes a moped, motor scooter, or motorized bicycle. ◄▥

(l) A motorcycle rider is any person riding a motorcycle or in a sidecar or trailer attached to the motorcycle.

(m) A three-wheeled motor vehicle is a motorized tricycle designed primarily for on-road use. This includes a motor-driven tricycle, a motorized rickshaw, or a three-wheeled motor car.

(n) A car [automobile] is a four-wheeled motor vehicle designed primarily for carrying up to 7 persons. A trailer being towed by the car is considered part of the car. It does not include a van or minivan—see definition (o) ◄▥

(o) A pick-up truck or van is a four or six-wheeled motor vehicle designed for carrying passengers as well as property or cargo weighing less than the local limit for classification as a heavy goods vehicle, and not requiring a special driver's license. This includes a minivan and a sport-utility vehicle (SUV).

(p) A heavy transport vehicle is a motor vehicle designed primarily for carrying property, meeting local criteria for classification as a heavy goods vehicle in terms of weight and requiring a special driver's license.

(q) A bus (coach) is a motor vehicle designed or adapted primarily for carrying more than 10 passengers, and requiring a special driver's license.

(r) A railway train or railway vehicle is any device, with or without freight or passenger cars coupled to it, designed for traffic on a railway track. This includes subterranean (subways) or elevated trains.

(s) A streetcar is a device designed and used primarily for transporting passengers within a municipality, running on rails, usually subject to normal traffic control signals, and operated principally on a right-of-way that forms part of the roadway. This includes a tram or trolley that runs on rails. A trailer being towed by a streetcar is considered part of the streetcar.

(t) A special vehicle mainly used on industrial premises is a motor vehicle designed primarily for use within the buildings and premises of industrial or commercial establishments. This includes battery-powered airport passenger vehicles or baggage/mail trucks, forklifts, coal-cars in a coal mine, logging cars and trucks used in mines or quarries. ◄▥

(u) A special vehicle mainly used in agriculture is a motor vehicle designed specifically for use in farming and agriculture (horticulture), to work the land, tend and harvest crops and transport materials on the farm. This includes harvesters, farm machinery and tractor and trailers.

(v) A special construction vehicle is a motor vehicle designed specifically for use on construction and demolition sites. This includes bulldozers, diggers, earth levellers, dump trucks, backhoes, front-end loaders, pavers, and mechanical shovels.

(w) A special all-terrain vehicle is a motor vehicle of special design to enable it to negotiate over rough or soft terrain, snow or sand. Examples of special design are high construction, special wheels and tires, tracks, and support on a cushion of air. This includes snow mobiles, all-terrain vehicles (ATV), and dune buggies. It does not include passenger vehicle designated as sport utility vehicles (SUV). ◄▥

(x) A watercraft is any device designed for transporting passengers or goods on water. This includes motor or sail boats, ships, and hovercraft.

(y) An aircraft is any device for transporting passengers or goods in the air. This includes hot-air balloons, gliders, helicopters and airplanes.

(z) A military vehicle is any motorized vehicle operating on a public roadway owned by the military and being operated by a member of the military.

PEDESTRIAN INJURED IN TRANSPORT ACCIDENT (V00-V09)

Includes	person changing tire on transport vehicle
	person examining engine of vehicle broken down in (on side of) road

Excludes1	fall due to non-transport collision with other person (W03)
	pedestrian on foot falling (slipping) on ice and snow (W00.-)
	struck or bumped by another person (W51)

● **V00 Pedestrian conveyance accident**

Use additional place of occurrence and activity external cause codes, if known (Y92.-, Y93.-)

Excludes1	collision with another person without fall (W51)
	fall due to person on foot colliding with another person on foot (W03)
	fall from non-moving wheelchair, nonmotorized scooter and motorized mobility scooter without collision (W05.-)
	pedestrian (conveyance) collision with other land transport vehicle (V01-V09)
	pedestrian on foot falling (slipping) on ice and snow (W00.-)

The appropriate 7th character is to be added to each code from category V00

A	initial encounter
D	subsequent encounter
S	sequela

● **V00.0 Pedestrian on foot injured in collision with pedestrian conveyance**

X● **V00.01 Pedestrian on foot injured in collision with roller-skater**

X● **V00.02 Pedestrian on foot injured in collision with skateboarder**

X● **V00.09 Pedestrian on foot injured in collision with other pedestrian conveyance**

● **V00.1 Rolling-type pedestrian conveyance accident**

Excludes1	accident with babystroller (V00.82-)
	accident with wheelchair (powered) (V00.81-)
	accident with motorized mobility scooter (V00.83-)

● **V00.11 In-line roller-skate accident**

● **V00.111 Fall from in-line roller-skates**

● **V00.112 In-line roller-skater colliding with stationary object**

● **V00.118 Other in-line roller-skate accident**

Excludes1	roller-skater collision with other land transport vehicle (V01-V09 with 5th character 1)

● **V00.12 Non-in-line roller-skate accident**

● **V00.121 Fall from non-in-line roller-skates**

● **V00.122 Non-in-line roller-skater colliding with stationary object**

● **V00.128 Other non-in-line roller-skating accident**

Excludes1	roller-skater collision with other land transport vehicle (V01-V09 with 5th character 1)

CHAPTER 20 (V01-Y99)

● **V00.13   Skateboard accident**
  ● **V00.131   Fall from skateboard**
  ● **V00.132   Skateboarder colliding with stationary object**
  ● **V00.138   Other skateboard accident**
    Excludes1   skateboarder collision with other land transport vehicle (V01-V09 with 5th character 2)

● **V00.14   Scooter (nonmotorized) accident**
  Excludes1   motorscooter accident (V20-V29)
  ● **V00.141   Fall from scooter (nonmotorized)**
  ● **V00.142   Scooter (nonmotorized) colliding with stationary object**
  ● **V00.148   Other scooter (nonmotorized) accident**
    Excludes1   scooter (non-motorized) collision with other land transport vehicle (V01-V09 with fifth character 9)

● **V00.15   Heelies accident**
  Rolling shoe
  Wheeled shoe
  Wheelies accident
  ● **V00.151   Fall from heelies**
  ● **V00.152   Heelies colliding with stationary object**
  ● **V00.158   Other heelies accident**

● **V00.18   Accident on other rolling-type pedestrian conveyance**
  ● **V00.181   Fall from other rolling-type pedestrian conveyance**
  ● **V00.182   Pedestrian on other rolling-type pedestrian conveyance colliding with stationary object**
  ● **V00.188   Other accident on other rolling-type pedestrian conveyance**

● **V00.2   Gliding-type pedestrian conveyance accident**
  ● **V00.21   Ice-skates accident**
    ● **V00.211   Fall from ice-skates**
    ● **V00.212   Ice-skater colliding with stationary object**
    ● **V00.218   Other ice-skates accident**
      Excludes1   ice-skater collision with other land transport vehicle (V01-V09 with 5th digit 9)

  ● **V00.22   Sled accident**
    ● **V00.221   Fall from sled**
    ● **V00.222   Sledder colliding with stationary object**
    ● **V00.228   Other sled accident**
      Excludes1   sled collision with other land transport vehicle (V01-V09 with 5th digit 9)

● **V00.28   Other gliding-type pedestrian conveyance accident**
  ● **V00.281   Fall from other gliding-type pedestrian conveyance**
  ● **V00.282   Pedestrian on other gliding-type pedestrian conveyance colliding with stationary object**
  ● **V00.288   Other accident on other gliding-type pedestrian conveyance**
    Excludes1   gliding-type pedestrian conveyance collision with other land transport vehicle (V01-V09 with 5th digit 9)

● **V00.3   Flat-bottomed pedestrian conveyance accident**
  ● **V00.31   Snowboard accident**
    ● **V00.311   Fall from snowboard**
    ● **V00.312   Snowboarder colliding with stationary object**
    ● **V00.318   Other snowboard accident**
      Excludes1   snowboarder collision with other land transport vehicle (V01-V09 with 5th digit 9)

  ● **V00.32   Snow-ski accident**
    ● **V00.321   Fall from snow-skis**
      Coding Clinic: 2015, Q1, P12
    ● **V00.322   Snow-skier colliding with stationary object**
    ● **V00.328   Other snow-ski accident**
      Excludes1   snow-skier collision with other land transport vehicle (V01-V09 with 5th digit 9)

  ● **V00.38   Other flat-bottomed pedestrian conveyance accident**
    ● **V00.381   Fall from other flat-bottomed pedestrian conveyance**
    ● **V00.382   Pedestrian on other flat-bottomed pedestrian conveyance colliding with stationary object**
    ● **V00.388   Other accident on other flat-bottomed pedestrian conveyance**

● **V00.8   Accident on other pedestrian conveyance**
  ● **V00.81   Accident with wheelchair (powered)**
    ● **V00.811   Fall from moving wheelchair (powered)**
      Excludes1   fall from non-moving wheelchair (W05.0)
    ● **V00.812   Wheelchair (powered) colliding with stationary object**
    ● **V00.818   Other accident with wheelchair (powered)**
  ● **V00.82   Accident with babystroller**
    ● **V00.821   Fall from babystroller**
    ● **V00.822   Babystroller colliding with stationary object**
    ● **V00.828   Other accident with babystroller**

◄ New   ◄━ Revised   ~~deleted~~ Deleted   Excludes 1   Excludes 2   Includes   Use additional   Code first   Code also   Unspecified
OGCR Official Guidelines   ● Unacceptable Principal Diagnosis   X Assign placeholder X   ● Use Additional Character(s)   ▶ Manifestation Code   **Coding Clinic**

● V00.83   Accident with motorized mobility scooter
 ● V00.831   Fall from motorized mobility scooter
  Excludes1   fall from non-moving motorized mobility scooter (W05.2)
 ● V00.832   Motorized mobility scooter colliding with stationary object
 ● V00.838   Other accident with motorized mobility scooter
● V00.89   Accident on other pedestrian conveyance
 ● V00.891   Fall from other pedestrian conveyance
 ● V00.892   Pedestrian on other pedestrian conveyance colliding with stationary object
 ● V00.898   Other accident on other pedestrian conveyance
  Excludes1   other pedestrian (conveyance) collision with other land transport vehicle (V01-V09 with 5th digit 9)

● V01   Pedestrian injured in collision with pedal cycle

The appropriate 7th character is to be added to each code from category V01

A	initial encounter
D	subsequent encounter
S	sequela

● V01.0   Pedestrian injured in collision with pedal cycle in nontraffic accident
 X● V01.00   Pedestrian on foot injured in collision with pedal cycle in nontraffic accident
  Pedestrian NOS injured in collision with pedal cycle in nontraffic accident
 X● V01.01   Pedestrian on roller-skates injured in collision with pedal cycle in nontraffic accident
 X● V01.02   Pedestrian on skateboard injured in collision with pedal cycle in nontraffic accident
 X● V01.09   Pedestrian with other conveyance injured in collision with pedal cycle in nontraffic accident
  Pedestrian with babystroller injured in collision with pedal cycle in nontraffic accident
  Pedestrian in wheelchair (powered) injured in collision with pedal cycle in nontraffic accident
  Pedestrian in motorized mobility scooter injured in collision with pedal cycle in nontraffic accident
  Pedestrian on ice-skates injured in collision with pedal cycle in nontraffic accident
  Pedestrian on nonmotorized scooter injured in collision with pedal cycle in nontraffic accident
  Pedestrian on sled injured in collision with pedal cycle in nontraffic accident
  Pedestrian on snowboard injured in collision with pedal cycle in nontraffic accident
  Pedestrian on snow-skis injured in collision with pedal cycle in nontraffic accident

● V01.1   Pedestrian injured in collision with pedal cycle in traffic accident
 X● V01.10   Pedestrian on foot injured in collision with pedal cycle in traffic accident
  Pedestrian NOS injured in collision with pedal cycle in traffic accident
 X● V01.11   Pedestrian on roller-skates injured in collision with pedal cycle in traffic accident
 X● V01.12   Pedestrian on skateboard injured in collision with pedal cycle in traffic accident
 X● V01.19   Pedestrian with other conveyance injured in collision with pedal cycle in traffic accident
  Pedestrian with babystroller injured in collision with pedal cycle in traffic accident
  Pedestrian in wheelchair (powered) injured in collision with pedal cycle in traffic accident
  Pedestrian in motorized mobility scooter injured in collision with pedal cycle in traffic accident
  Pedestrian on ice-skates injured in collision with pedal cycle in traffic accident
  Pedestrian on nonmotorized scooter injured in collision with pedal cycle in traffic accident
  Pedestrian on sled injured in collision with pedal cycle in traffic accident
  Pedestrian on snowboard injured in collision with pedal cycle in traffic accident
  Pedestrian on snow-skis injured in collision with pedal cycle in traffic accident

● V01.9   Pedestrian injured in collision with pedal cycle, unspecified whether traffic or nontraffic accident
 X● V01.90   Pedestrian on foot injured in collision with pedal cycle, unspecified whether traffic or nontraffic accident
  Pedestrian NOS injured in collision with pedal cycle, unspecified whether traffic or nontraffic accident
 X● V01.91   Pedestrian on roller-skates injured in collision with pedal cycle, unspecified whether traffic or nontraffic accident
 X● V01.92   Pedestrian on skateboard injured in collision with pedal cycle, unspecified whether traffic or nontraffic accident
 X● V01.99   Pedestrian with other conveyance injured in collision with pedal cycle, unspecified whether traffic or nontraffic accident
  Pedestrian with babystroller injured in collision with pedal cycle, unspecified whether traffic or nontraffic accident
  Pedestrian in wheelchair (powered) injured in collision with pedal cycle, unspecified whether traffic or nontraffic accident
  Pedestrian in motorized mobility scooter injured in collision with pedal cycle, unspecified whether traffic or nontraffic accident
  Pedestrian on ice-skates injured in collision with pedal cycle unspecified, whether traffic or nontraffic accident
  Pedestrian on nonmotorized scooter injured in collision with pedal cycle, unspecified whether traffic or nontraffic accident
  Pedestrian on sled injured in collision with pedal cycle unspecified, whether traffic or nontraffic accident
  Pedestrian on snowboard injured in collision with pedal cycle, unspecified whether traffic or nontraffic accident
  Pedestrian on snow-skis injured in collision with pedal cycle, unspecified whether traffic or nontraffic accident

● **V02**   **Pedestrian injured in collision with two- or three-wheeled motor vehicle**

The appropriate 7th character is to be added to each code from category V02

> A   initial encounter
> D   subsequent encounter
> S   sequela

● **V02.0**   **Pedestrian injured in collision with two- or three-wheeled motor vehicle in nontraffic accident**

X● **V02.00**   **Pedestrian on foot injured in collision with two- or three-wheeled motor vehicle in nontraffic accident**
> Pedestrian NOS injured in collision with two- or three-wheeled motor vehicle in nontraffic accident

X● **V02.01**   **Pedestrian on roller-skates injured in collision with two- or three-wheeled motor vehicle in nontraffic accident**

X● **V02.02**   **Pedestrian on skateboard injured in collision with two- or three-wheeled motor vehicle in nontraffic accident**

X● **V02.09**   **Pedestrian with other conveyance injured in collision with two- or three-wheeled motor vehicle in nontraffic accident**
> Pedestrian with babystroller injured in collision with two- or three-wheeled motor vehicle in nontraffic accident
> Pedestrian on ice-skates injured in collision with two- or three-wheeled motor vehicle in nontraffic accident
> Pedestrian in wheelchair (powered) injured in collision with two- or three-wheeled motor vehicle in nontraffic accident
> Pedestrian in motorized mobility scooter injured in collision with two- or three-wheeled motor vehicle in nontraffic accident
> Pedestrian on nonmotorized scooter injured in collision with two- or three-wheeled motor vehicle in nontraffic accident
> Pedestrian on sled injured in collision with two- or three-wheeled motor vehicle in nontraffic accident
> Pedestrian on snowboard injured in collision with two- or three-wheeled motor vehicle in nontraffic accident
> Pedestrian on snow-skis injured in collision with two- or three-wheeled motor vehicle in nontraffic accident

● **V02.1**   **Pedestrian injured in collision with two- or three-wheeled motor vehicle in traffic accident**

X● **V02.10**   **Pedestrian on foot injured in collision with two- or three-wheeled motor vehicle in traffic accident**
> Pedestrian NOS injured in collision with two- or three-wheeled motor vehicle in traffic accident

X● **V02.11**   **Pedestrian on roller-skates injured in collision with two- or three-wheeled motor vehicle in traffic accident**

X● **V02.12**   **Pedestrian on skateboard injured in collision with two- or three-wheeled motor vehicle in traffic accident**

X● **V02.19**   **Pedestrian with other conveyance injured in collision with two- or three-wheeled motor vehicle in traffic accident**
> Pedestrian with babystroller injured in collision with two- or three-wheeled motor vehicle in traffic accident
> Pedestrian in wheelchair (powered) injured in collision with two- or three-wheeled motor vehicle in traffic accident
> Pedestrian in motorized mobility scooter injured in collision with two- or three-wheeled motor vehicle in traffic accident
> Pedestrian on ice-skates injured in collision with two- or three-wheeled motor vehicle in traffic accident
> Pedestrian on nonmotorized scooter injured in collision with two- or three-wheeled motor vehicle in traffic accident
> Pedestrian on sled injured in collision with two- or three-wheeled motor vehicle in traffic accident
> Pedestrian on snowboard injured in collision with two- or three-wheeled motor vehicle in traffic accident
> Pedestrian on snow-skis injured in collision with two- or three-wheeled motor vehicle in traffic accident

● **V02.9**   **Pedestrian injured in collision with two- or three-wheeled motor vehicle, unspecified whether traffic or nontraffic accident**

X● **V02.90**   **Pedestrian on foot injured in collision with two- or three-wheeled motor vehicle, unspecified whether traffic or nontraffic accident**
> Pedestrian NOS injured in collision with two- or three-wheeled motor vehicle, unspecified whether traffic or nontraffic accident

X● **V02.91**   **Pedestrian on roller-skates injured in collision with two- or three-wheeled motor vehicle, unspecified whether traffic or nontraffic accident**

X● **V02.92**   **Pedestrian on skateboard injured in collision with two- or three-wheeled motor vehicle, unspecified whether traffic or nontraffic accident**

◀ New   ◀ Revised   ~~deleted~~ Deleted   Excludes 1   Excludes 2   Includes   Use additional   Code first   Code also   Unspecified
OGCR Official Guidelines   ● Unacceptable Principal Diagnosis   X Assign placeholder X   ● Use Additional Character(s)   ▌ Manifestation Code   **Coding Clinic**

X● **V02.99 Pedestrian with other conveyance injured in collision with two- or three-wheeled motor vehicle, unspecified whether traffic or nontraffic accident**

Pedestrian with babystroller injured in collision with two- or three-wheeled motor vehicle, unspecified whether traffic or nontraffic accident

Pedestrian in wheelchair (powered) injured in collision with two- or three-wheeled motor vehicle, unspecified whether traffic or nontraffic accident

Pedestrian in motorized mobility scooter injured in collision with two- or three-wheeled motor vehicle, unspecified whether traffic or nontraffic accident

Pedestrian on ice-skates injured in collision with two- or three-wheeled motor vehicle, unspecified whether traffic or nontraffic accident

Pedestrian on nonmotorized scooter injured in collision with two- or three-wheeled motor vehicle, unspecified whether traffic or nontraffic accident

Pedestrian on sled injured in collision with two- or three-wheeled motor vehicle, unspecified whether traffic or nontraffic accident

Pedestrian on snowboard injured in collision with two- or three-wheeled motor vehicle, unspecified whether traffic or nontraffic accident

Pedestrian on snow-skis injured in collision with two- or three-wheeled motor vehicle, unspecified whether traffic or nontraffic accident

● **V03 Pedestrian injured in collision with car, pick-up truck or van**

The appropriate 7th character is to be added to each code from category V03

A	initial encounter
D	subsequent encounter
S	sequela

● **V03.0 Pedestrian injured in collision with car, pick-up truck or van in nontraffic accident**

X● **V03.00 Pedestrian on foot injured in collision with car, pick-up truck or van in nontraffic accident**

Pedestrian NOS injured in collision with car, pick-up truck or van in nontraffic accident

X● **V03.01 Pedestrian on roller-skates injured in collision with car, pick-up truck or van in nontraffic accident**

X● **V03.02 Pedestrian on skateboard injured in collision with car, pick-up truck or van in nontraffic accident**

X● **V03.09 Pedestrian with other conveyance injured in collision with car, pick-up truck or van in nontraffic accident**

Pedestrian with babystroller injured in collision with car, pick-up truck or van in nontraffic accident

Pedestrian in wheelchair (powered) injured in collision with car, pick-up truck or van in nontraffic accident

Pedestrian in motorized mobility scooter injured in collision with car, pick-up truck or van in nontraffic accident

Pedestrian on ice-skates injured in collision with car, pick-up truck or van in nontraffic accident

Pedestrian on nonmotorized scooter injured in collision with car, pick-up truck or van in nontraffic accident

Pedestrian on sled injured in collision with car, pick-up truck or van in nontraffic accident

Pedestrian on snowboard injured in collision with car, pick-up truck or van in nontraffic accident

Pedestrian on snow-skis injured in collision with car, pick-up truck or van in nontraffic accident

● **V03.1 Pedestrian injured in collision with car, pick-up truck or van in traffic accident**

X● **V03.10 Pedestrian on foot injured in collision with car, pick-up truck or van in traffic accident**

Pedestrian NOS injured in collision with car, pick-up truck or van in traffic accident

X● **V03.11 Pedestrian on roller-skates injured in collision with car, pick-up truck or van in traffic accident**

X● **V03.12 Pedestrian on skateboard injured in collision with car, pick-up truck or van in traffic accident**

X● **V03.19 Pedestrian with other conveyance injured in collision with car, pick-up truck or van in traffic accident**

Pedestrian with babystroller injured in collision with car, pick-up truck or van in traffic accident

Pedestrian in wheelchair (powered) injured in collision with car, pick-up truck or van in traffic accident

Pedestrian in motorized mobility scooter injured in collision with car, pick-up truck or van in traffic accident

Pedestrian on ice-skates injured in collision with car, pick-up truck or van in traffic accident

Pedestrian on nonmotorized scooter injured in collision with car, pick-up truck or van in traffic accident

Pedestrian on sled injured in collision with car, pick-up truck or van in traffic accident

Pedestrian on snowboard injured in collision with car, pick-up truck or van in traffic accident

Pedestrian on snow-skis injured in collision with car, pick-up truck or van in traffic accident

CHAPTER 20 (V01–Y99)

CHAPTER 20 (V01-Y99)

X● **V03.9** Pedestrian injured in collision with car, pick-up truck or van, unspecified whether traffic or nontraffic accident

X● **V03.90** Pedestrian on foot injured in collision with car, pick-up truck or van, unspecified whether traffic or nontraffic accident

Pedestrian NOS injured in collision with car, pick-up truck or van, unspecified whether traffic or nontraffic accident

X● **V03.91** Pedestrian on roller-skates injured in collision with car, pick-up truck or van, unspecified whether traffic or nontraffic accident

X● **V03.92** Pedestrian on skateboard injured in collision with car, pick-up truck or van, unspecified whether traffic or nontraffic accident

X● **V03.99** Pedestrian with other conveyance injured in collision with car, pick-up truck or van, unspecified whether traffic or nontraffic accident

Pedestrian with babystroller injured in collision with car, pick-up truck or van, unspecified whether traffic or nontraffic accident

Pedestrian in wheelchair (powered) injured in collision with car, pick-up truck or van, unspecified whether traffic or nontraffic accident

Pedestrian in motorized mobility scooter injured in collision with car, pick-up truck or van, unspecified whether traffic or nontraffic accident

Pedestrian on ice-skates injured in collision with car, pick-up truck or van, unspecified whether traffic or nontraffic accident

Pedestrian on nonmotorized scooter injured in collision with car, pick-up truck or van, unspecified whether traffic or nontraffic accident

Pedestrian on sled injured in collision with car, pick-up truck or van in nontraffic accident

Pedestrian on snowboard injured in collision with car, pick-up truck or van, unspecified whether traffic or nontraffic accident

Pedestrian on snow-skis injured in collision with car, pick-up truck or van, unspecified whether traffic or nontraffic accident

● **V04** Pedestrian injured in collision with heavy transport vehicle or bus

Excludes1 pedestrian injured in collision with military vehicle (V09.01, V09.21)

The appropriate 7th character is to be added to each code from category V04

A	initial encounter
D	subsequent encounter
S	sequela

● **V04.0** Pedestrian injured in collision with heavy transport vehicle or bus in nontraffic accident

X● **V04.00** Pedestrian on foot injured in collision with heavy transport vehicle or bus in nontraffic accident

Pedestrian NOS injured in collision with heavy transport vehicle or bus in nontraffic accident

X● **V04.01** Pedestrian on roller-skates injured in collision with heavy transport vehicle or bus in nontraffic accident

X● **V04.02** Pedestrian on skateboard injured in collision with heavy transport vehicle or bus in nontraffic accident

X● **V04.09** Pedestrian with other conveyance injured in collision with heavy transport vehicle or bus in nontraffic accident

Pedestrian with babystroller injured in collision with heavy transport vehicle or bus in nontraffic accident

Pedestrian in wheelchair (powered) injured in collision with heavy transport vehicle or bus in nontraffic accident

Pedestrian in motorized mobility scooter injured in collision with heavy transport vehicle or bus in nontraffic accident

Pedestrian on ice-skates injured in collision with heavy transport vehicle or bus in nontraffic accident

Pedestrian on nonmotorized scooter injured in collision with heavy transport vehicle or bus in nontraffic accident

Pedestrian on sled injured in collision with heavy transport vehicle or bus in nontraffic accident

Pedestrian on snowboard injured in collision with heavy transport vehicle or bus in nontraffic accident

Pedestrian on snow-skis injured in collision with heavy transport vehicle or bus in nontraffic accident

● **V04.1** Pedestrian injured in collision with heavy transport vehicle or bus in traffic accident

X● **V04.10** Pedestrian on foot injured in collision with heavy transport vehicle or bus in traffic accident

Pedestrian NOS injured in collision with heavy transport vehicle or bus in traffic accident

X● **V04.11** Pedestrian on roller-skates injured in collision with heavy transport vehicle or bus in traffic accident

X● **V04.12** Pedestrian on skateboard injured in collision with heavy transport vehicle or bus in traffic accident

X● **V04.19** Pedestrian with other conveyance injured in collision with heavy transport vehicle or bus in traffic accident

Pedestrian with babystroller injured in collision with heavy transport vehicle or bus in traffic accident

Pedestrian in wheelchair (powered) injured in collision with heavy transport vehicle or bus in traffic accident

Pedestrian in motorized mobility scooter injured in collision with heavy transport vehicle or bus in traffic accident

Pedestrian on ice-skates injured in collision with heavy transport vehicle or bus in traffic accident

Pedestrian on nonmotorized scooter injured in collision with heavy transport vehicle or bus in traffic accident

Pedestrian on sled injured in collision with heavy transport vehicle or bus in traffic accident

Pedestrian on snowboard injured in collision with heavy transport vehicle or bus in traffic accident

Pedestrian on snow-skis injured in collision with heavy transport vehicle or bus in traffic accident

◀ New　　⬅ Revised　　~~deleted~~ Deleted　　Excludes 1　　Excludes 2　　Includes　　Use additional　　Code first　　Code also　　Unspecified

OGCR Official Guidelines　　● Unacceptable Principal Diagnosis　　X Assign placeholder X　　● Use Additional Character(s)　　▶ Manifestation Code　　Coding Clinic

● **V04.9**　**Pedestrian injured in collision with heavy transport vehicle or bus, unspecified whether traffic or nontraffic accident**

　　X ● **V04.90**　**Pedestrian on foot injured in collision with heavy transport vehicle or bus, unspecified whether traffic or nontraffic accident**
　　　　　Pedestrian NOS injured in collision with heavy transport vehicle or bus, unspecified whether traffic or nontraffic accident

　　X ● **V04.91**　**Pedestrian on roller-skates injured in collision with heavy transport vehicle or bus, unspecified whether traffic or nontraffic accident**

　　X ● **V04.92**　**Pedestrian on skateboard injured in collision with heavy transport vehicle or bus, unspecified whether traffic or nontraffic accident**

　　X ● **V04.99**　**Pedestrian with other conveyance injured in collision with heavy transport vehicle or bus, unspecified whether traffic or nontraffic accident**
　　　　　Pedestrian with babystroller injured in collision with heavy transport vehicle or bus, unspecified whether traffic or nontraffic accident
　　　　　Pedestrian in wheelchair (powered) injured in collision with heavy transport vehicle or bus, unspecified whether traffic or nontraffic accident
　　　　　Pedestrian in motorized mobility scooter injured in collision with heavy transport vehicle or bus, unspecified whether traffic or nontraffic accident
　　　　　Pedestrian on ice-skates injured in collision with heavy transport vehicle or bus, unspecified whether traffic or nontraffic accident
　　　　　Pedestrian on nonmotorized scooter injured in collision with heavy transport vehicle or bus, unspecified whether traffic or nontraffic accident
　　　　　Pedestrian on sled injured in collision with heavy transport vehicle or bus, unspecified whether traffic or nontraffic accident
　　　　　Pedestrian on snowboard injured in collision with heavy transport vehicle or bus, unspecified whether traffic or nontraffic accident
　　　　　Pedestrian on snow-skis injured in collision with heavy transport vehicle or bus, unspecified whether traffic or nontraffic accident

● **V05**　**Pedestrian injured in collision with railway train or railway vehicle**

　　The appropriate 7th character is to be added to each code from category V05

　　┌─────────────────────────┐
　　│ A　initial encounter　　　│
　　│ D　subsequent encounter　│
　　│ S　sequela　　　　　　　　│
　　└─────────────────────────┘

　● **V05.0**　**Pedestrian injured in collision with railway train or railway vehicle in nontraffic accident**

　　X ● **V05.00**　**Pedestrian on foot injured in collision with railway train or railway vehicle in nontraffic accident**
　　　　　Pedestrian NOS injured in collision with railway train or railway vehicle in nontraffic accident

　　X ● **V05.01**　**Pedestrian on roller-skates injured in collision with railway train or railway vehicle in nontraffic accident**

　　X ● **V05.02**　**Pedestrian on skateboard injured in collision with railway train or railway vehicle in nontraffic accident**

　　X ● **V05.09**　**Pedestrian with other conveyance injured in collision with railway train or railway vehicle in nontraffic accident**
　　　　　Pedestrian with babystroller injured in collision with railway train or railway vehicle in nontraffic accident
　　　　　Pedestrian in wheelchair (powered) injured in collision with railway train or railway vehicle in nontraffic accident
　　　　　Pedestrian in motorized mobility scooter injured in collision with railway train or railway vehicle in nontraffic accident
　　　　　Pedestrian on ice-skates injured in collision with railway train or railway vehicle in nontraffic accident
　　　　　Pedestrian on nonmotorized scooter injured in collision with railway train or railway vehicle in nontraffic accident
　　　　　Pedestrian on sled injured in collision with railway train or railway vehicle in nontraffic accident
　　　　　Pedestrian on snowboard injured in collision with railway train or railway vehicle in nontraffic accident
　　　　　Pedestrian on snow-skis injured in collision with railway train or railway vehicle in nontraffic accident

　● **V05.1**　**Pedestrian injured in collision with railway train or railway vehicle in traffic accident**

　　X ● **V05.10**　**Pedestrian on foot injured in collision with railway train or railway vehicle in traffic accident**
　　　　　Pedestrian NOS injured in collision with railway train or railway vehicle in traffic accident

　　X ● **V05.11**　**Pedestrian on roller-skates injured in collision with railway train or railway vehicle in traffic accident**

　　X ● **V05.12**　**Pedestrian on skateboard injured in collision with railway train or railway vehicle in traffic accident**

　　X ● **V05.19**　**Pedestrian with other conveyance injured in collision with railway train or railway vehicle in traffic accident**
　　　　　Pedestrian with babystroller injured in collision with railway train or railway vehicle in traffic accident
　　　　　Pedestrian in wheelchair (powered) injured in collision with railway train or railway vehicle in traffic accident
　　　　　Pedestrian in motorized mobility scooter injured in collision with railway train or railway vehicle in traffic accident
　　　　　Pedestrian on ice-skates injured in collision with railway train or railway vehicle in traffic accident
　　　　　Pedestrian on nonmotorized scooter injured in collision with railway train or railway vehicle in traffic accident
　　　　　Pedestrian on sled injured in collision with railway train or railway vehicle in traffic accident
　　　　　Pedestrian on snowboard injured in collision with railway train or railway vehicle in traffic accident
　　　　　Pedestrian on snow-skis injured in collision with railway train or railway vehicle in traffic accident

● **V05.9**   **Pedestrian injured in collision with railway train or railway vehicle, unspecified whether traffic or nontraffic accident**

   X● **V05.90**   **Pedestrian on foot injured in collision with railway train or railway vehicle, unspecified whether traffic or nontraffic accident**

       Pedestrian NOS injured in collision with railway train or railway vehicle, unspecified whether traffic or nontraffic accident

   X● **V05.91**   **Pedestrian on roller-skates injured in collision with railway train or railway vehicle, unspecified whether traffic or nontraffic accident**

   X● **V05.92**   **Pedestrian on skateboard injured in collision with railway train or railway vehicle, unspecified whether traffic or nontraffic accident**

   X● **V05.99**   **Pedestrian with other conveyance injured in collision with railway train or railway vehicle, unspecified whether traffic or nontraffic accident**

       Pedestrian with babystroller injured in collision with railway train or railway vehicle, unspecified whether traffic or nontraffic

       Pedestrian in wheelchair (powered) injured in collision with railway train or railway vehicle, unspecified whether traffic or nontraffic

       Pedestrian in motorized mobility scooter injured in collision with railway train or railway vehicle, unspecified whether traffic or nontraffic

       Pedestrian on ice-skates injured in collision with railway train or railway vehicle, unspecified whether traffic or nontraffic

       Pedestrian on nonmotorized scooter injured in collision with railway train or railway vehicle, unspecified whether traffic or nontraffic

       Pedestrian on sled injured in collision with railway train or railway vehicle, unspecified whether traffic or nontraffic

       Pedestrian on snowboard injured in collision with railway train or railway vehicle, unspecified whether traffic or nontraffic

       Pedestrian on snow-skis injured in collision with railway train or railway vehicle, unspecified whether traffic or nontraffic

● **V06**   **Pedestrian injured in collision with other nonmotor vehicle**

   Includes   collision with animal-drawn vehicle, animal being ridden, nonpowered streetcar

   Excludes1   pedestrian injured in collision with pedestrian conveyance (V00.0-)

   The appropriate 7th character is to be added to each code from category V06

     | | |
     A   initial encounter
     D   subsequent encounter
     S   sequela

● **V06.0**   **Pedestrian injured in collision with other nonmotor vehicle in nontraffic accident**

   X● **V06.00**   **Pedestrian on foot injured in collision with other nonmotor vehicle in nontraffic accident**

       Pedestrian NOS injured in collision with other nonmotor vehicle in nontraffic accident

   X● **V06.01**   **Pedestrian on roller-skates injured in collision with other nonmotor vehicle in nontraffic accident**

   X● **V06.02**   **Pedestrian on skateboard injured in collision with other nonmotor vehicle in nontraffic accident**

   X● **V06.09**   **Pedestrian with other conveyance injured in collision with other nonmotor vehicle in nontraffic accident**

       Pedestrian with babystroller injured in collision with other nonmotor vehicle in nontraffic accident

       Pedestrian in wheelchair (powered) injured in collision with other nonmotor vehicle in nontraffic accident

       Pedestrian in motorized mobility scooter injured in collision with other nonmotor vehicle in nontraffic accident

       Pedestrian on ice-skates injured in collision with other nonmotor vehicle in nontraffic accident

       Pedestrian on nonmotorized scooter injured in collision with other nonmotor vehicle in nontraffic accident

       Pedestrian on sled injured in collision with other nonmotor vehicle in nontraffic accident

       Pedestrian on snowboard injured in collision with other nonmotor vehicle in nontraffic accident

       Pedestrian on snow-skis injured in collision with other nonmotor vehicle in nontraffic accident

● **V06.1**   **Pedestrian injured in collision with other nonmotor vehicle in traffic accident**

   X● **V06.10**   **Pedestrian on foot injured in collision with other nonmotor vehicle in traffic accident**

       Pedestrian NOS injured in collision with other nonmotor vehicle in traffic accident

   X● **V06.11**   **Pedestrian on roller-skates injured in collision with other nonmotor vehicle in traffic accident**

   X● **V06.12**   **Pedestrian on skateboard injured in collision with other nonmotor vehicle in traffic accident**

   X● **V06.19**   **Pedestrian with other conveyance injured in collision with other nonmotor vehicle in traffic accident**

       Pedestrian with babystroller injured in collision with other nonmotor vehicle in nontraffic accident

       Pedestrian in wheelchair (powered) injured in collision with other nonmotor vehicle in traffic accident

       Pedestrian in motorized mobility scooter injured in collision with other nonmotor vehicle in traffic accident

       Pedestrian on ice-skates injured in collision with other nonmotor vehicle in traffic accident

       Pedestrian on nonmotorized scooter injured in collision with other nonmotor vehicle in traffic accident

       Pedestrian on sled injured in collision with other nonmotor vehicle in traffic accident

       Pedestrian on snowboard injured in collision with other nonmotor vehicle in traffic accident

       Pedestrian on snow-skis injured in collision with other nonmotor vehicle in traffic accident

● **V06.9**   **Pedestrian injured in collision with other nonmotor vehicle, unspecified whether traffic or nontraffic accident**

   X● **V06.90**   **Pedestrian on foot injured in collision with other nonmotor vehicle, unspecified whether traffic or nontraffic accident**

       Pedestrian NOS injured in collision with other nonmotor vehicle, unspecified whether traffic or nontraffic accident

   X● **V06.91**   **Pedestrian on roller-skates injured in collision with other nonmotor vehicle, unspecified whether traffic or nontraffic accident**

X● **V06.92** Pedestrian on skateboard injured in collision with other nonmotor vehicle, unspecified whether traffic or nontraffic accident

X● **V06.99** Pedestrian with other conveyance injured in collision with other nonmotor vehicle, unspecified whether traffic or nontraffic accident

> Pedestrian with babystroller injured in collision with other nonmotor vehicle, unspecified whether traffic or nontraffic accident
>
> Pedestrian in wheelchair (powered) injured in collision with other nonmotor vehicle, unspecified whether traffic or nontraffic accident
>
> Pedestrian in motorized mobility scooter injured in collision with other nonmotor vehicle, unspecified whether traffic or nontraffic accident
>
> Pedestrian on ice-skates injured in collision with other nonmotor vehicle, unspecified whether traffic or nontraffic accident
>
> Pedestrian on nonmotorized scooter injured in collision with other nonmotor vehicle, unspecified whether traffic or nontraffic accident
>
> Pedestrian on sled injured in collision with other nonmotor vehicle, unspecified whether traffic or nontraffic accident
>
> Pedestrian on snowboard injured in collision with other nonmotor vehicle, unspecified whether traffic or nontraffic accident
>
> Pedestrian on snow-skis injured in collision with other nonmotor vehicle, unspecified whether traffic or nontraffic accident

●**V09** Pedestrian injured in other and unspecified transport accidents

The appropriate 7th character is to be added to each code from category V09

A	initial encounter
D	subsequent encounter
S	sequela

●**V09.0** Pedestrian injured in nontraffic accident involving other and unspecified motor vehicles

X● **V09.00** Pedestrian injured in nontraffic accident involving unspecified motor vehicles

X● **V09.01** Pedestrian injured in nontraffic accident involving military vehicle

X● **V09.09** Pedestrian injured in nontraffic accident involving other motor vehicles

> Pedestrian injured in nontraffic accident by special vehicle

X● **V09.1** Pedestrian injured in unspecified nontraffic accident

●**V09.2** Pedestrian injured in traffic accident involving other and unspecified motor vehicles

X● **V09.20** Pedestrian injured in traffic accident involving unspecified motor vehicles

X● **V09.21** Pedestrian injured in traffic accident involving military vehicle

X● **V09.29** Pedestrian injured in traffic accident involving other motor vehicles

X● **V09.3** Pedestrian injured in unspecified traffic accident

X● **V09.9** Pedestrian injured in unspecified transport accident

---

PEDAL CYCLE RIDER INJURED IN TRANSPORT ACCIDENT (V10-V19)

Includes	any non-motorized vehicle, excluding an animal-drawn vehicle, or a sidecar or trailer attached to the pedal cycle
Excludes2	rupture of pedal cycle tire (W37.0)

●**V10** Pedal cycle rider injured in collision with pedestrian or animal

Excludes1	pedal cycle rider collision with animal-drawn vehicle or animal being ridden (V16.-)

The appropriate 7th character is to be added to each code from category V10

A	initial encounter
D	subsequent encounter
S	sequela

X● **V10.0** Pedal cycle driver injured in collision with pedestrian or animal in nontraffic accident

X● **V10.1** Pedal cycle passenger injured in collision with pedestrian or animal in nontraffic accident

X● **V10.2** Unspecified pedal cyclist injured in collision with pedestrian or animal in nontraffic accident

X● **V10.3** Person boarding or alighting a pedal cycle injured in collision with pedestrian or animal

X● **V10.4** Pedal cycle driver injured in collision with pedestrian or animal in traffic accident

X● **V10.5** Pedal cycle passenger injured in collision with pedestrian or animal in traffic accident

X● **V10.9** Unspecified pedal cyclist injured in collision with pedestrian or animal in traffic accident

●**V11** Pedal cycle rider injured in collision with other pedal cycle

The appropriate 7th character is to be added to each code from category V11

A	initial encounter
D	subsequent encounter
S	sequela

X● **V11.0** Pedal cycle driver injured in collision with other pedal cycle in nontraffic accident

X● **V11.1** Pedal cycle passenger injured in collision with other pedal cycle in nontraffic accident

X● **V11.2** Unspecified pedal cyclist injured in collision with other pedal cycle in nontraffic accident

X● **V11.3** Person boarding or alighting a pedal cycle injured in collision with other pedal cycle

X● **V11.4** Pedal cycle driver injured in collision with other pedal cycle in traffic accident

X● **V11.5** Pedal cycle passenger injured in collision with other pedal cycle in traffic accident

X● **V11.9** Unspecified pedal cyclist injured in collision with other pedal cycle in traffic accident

N Newborn Age: 0   **P** Pediatric Age: 0–17   **M** Maternity DX: 12–55   **A** Adult Age: 15–124   ♀ Females Only   ♂ Males Only

🅒 Complication\Comorbidity   🅜 Major C\C   ⒺⓍ CC/MCC Exclusions   🅗 Hospital-Acquired Condition

1527

● **V12   Pedal cycle rider injured in collision with two- or three-wheeled motor vehicle**

The appropriate 7th character is to be added to each code from category V12

A	initial encounter
D	subsequent encounter
S	sequela

X ● **V12.0   Pedal cycle driver injured in collision with two- or three-wheeled motor vehicle in nontraffic accident**

X ● **V12.1   Pedal cycle passenger injured in collision with two- or three-wheeled motor vehicle in nontraffic accident**

X ● **V12.2   Unspecified pedal cyclist injured in collision with two- or three-wheeled motor vehicle in nontraffic accident**

X ● **V12.3   Person boarding or alighting a pedal cycle injured in collision with two- or three-wheeled motor vehicle**

X ● **V12.4   Pedal cycle driver injured in collision with two- or three-wheeled motor vehicle in traffic accident**

X ● **V12.5   Pedal cycle passenger injured in collision with two- or three-wheeled motor vehicle in traffic accident**

X ● **V12.9   Unspecified pedal cyclist injured in collision with two- or three-wheeled motor vehicle in traffic accident**

● **V13   Pedal cycle rider injured in collision with car, pick-up truck or van**

The appropriate 7th character is to be added to each code from category V13

A	initial encounter
D	subsequent encounter
S	sequela

X ● **V13.0   Pedal cycle driver injured in collision with car, pick-up truck or van in nontraffic accident**

X ● **V13.1   Pedal cycle passenger injured in collision with car, pick-up truck or van in nontraffic accident**

X ● **V13.2   Unspecified pedal cyclist injured in collision with car, pick-up truck or van in nontraffic accident**

X ● **V13.3   Person boarding or alighting a pedal cycle injured in collision with car, pick-up truck or van**

X ● **V13.4   Pedal cycle driver injured in collision with car, pick-up truck or van in traffic accident**

X ● **V13.5   Pedal cycle passenger injured in collision with car, pick-up truck or van in traffic accident**

X ● **V13.9   Unspecified pedal cyclist injured in collision with car, pick-up truck or van in traffic accident**

● **V14   Pedal cycle rider injured in collision with heavy transport vehicle or bus**

> **Excludes1**   pedal cycle rider injured in collision with military vehicle (V19.81)

The appropriate 7th character is to be added to each code from category V14

A	initial encounter
D	subsequent encounter
S	sequela

X ● **V14.0   Pedal cycle driver injured in collision with heavy transport vehicle or bus in nontraffic accident**

X ● **V14.1   Pedal cycle passenger injured in collision with heavy transport vehicle or bus in nontraffic accident**

X ● **V14.2   Unspecified pedal cyclist injured in collision with heavy transport vehicle or bus in nontraffic accident**

X ● **V14.3   Person boarding or alighting a pedal cycle injured in collision with heavy transport vehicle or bus**

X ● **V14.4   Pedal cycle driver injured in collision with heavy transport vehicle or bus in traffic accident**

X ● **V14.5   Pedal cycle passenger injured in collision with heavy transport vehicle or bus in traffic accident**

X ● **V14.9   Unspecified pedal cyclist injured in collision with heavy transport vehicle or bus in traffic accident**

● **V15   Pedal cycle rider injured in collision with railway train or railway vehicle**

The appropriate 7th character is to be added to each code from category V15

A	initial encounter
D	subsequent encounter
S	sequela

X ● **V15.0   Pedal cycle driver injured in collision with railway train or railway vehicle in nontraffic accident**

X ● **V15.1   Pedal cycle passenger injured in collision with railway train or railway vehicle in nontraffic accident**

X ● **V15.2   Unspecified pedal cyclist injured in collision with railway train or railway vehicle in nontraffic accident**

X ● **V15.3   Person boarding or alighting a pedal cycle injured in collision with railway train or railway vehicle**

X ● **V15.4   Pedal cycle driver injured in collision with railway train or railway vehicle in traffic accident**

X ● **V15.5   Pedal cycle passenger injured in collision with railway train or railway vehicle in traffic accident**

X ● **V15.9   Unspecified pedal cyclist injured in collision with railway train or railway vehicle in traffic accident**

● **V16   Pedal cycle rider injured in collision with other nonmotor vehicle**

> **Includes**   collision with animal-drawn vehicle, animal being ridden, streetcar

The appropriate 7th character is to be added to each code from category V16

A	initial encounter
D	subsequent encounter
S	sequela

X ● **V16.0   Pedal cycle driver injured in collision with other nonmotor vehicle in nontraffic accident**

X ● **V16.1   Pedal cycle passenger injured in collision with other nonmotor vehicle in nontraffic accident**

X ● **V16.2   Unspecified pedal cyclist injured in collision with other nonmotor vehicle in nontraffic accident**

X ● **V16.3   Person boarding or alighting a pedal cycle injured in collision with other nonmotor vehicle in nontraffic accident**

X ● **V16.4   Pedal cycle driver injured in collision with other nonmotor vehicle in traffic accident**

X ● **V16.5   Pedal cycle passenger injured in collision with other nonmotor vehicle in traffic accident**

X ● **V16.9   Unspecified pedal cyclist injured in collision with other nonmotor vehicle in traffic accident**

● **V17   Pedal cycle rider injured in collision with fixed or stationary object**

The appropriate 7th character is to be added to each code from category V17

A	initial encounter
D	subsequent encounter
S	sequela

X ● **V17.0   Pedal cycle driver injured in collision with fixed or stationary object in nontraffic accident**

X ● **V17.1   Pedal cycle passenger injured in collision with fixed or stationary object in nontraffic accident**

X ● **V17.2   Unspecified pedal cyclist injured in collision with fixed or stationary object in nontraffic accident**

X ● **V17.3   Person boarding or alighting a pedal cycle injured in collision with fixed or stationary object**

X ● **V17.4   Pedal cycle driver injured in collision with fixed or stationary object in traffic accident**

X ● **V17.5   Pedal cycle passenger injured in collision with fixed or stationary object in traffic accident**

X ● **V17.9   Unspecified pedal cyclist injured in collision with fixed or stationary object in traffic accident**

◄ New   ◄ Revised   ~~deleted~~ Deleted   Excludes 1   Excludes 2   Includes   Use additional   Code first   Code also   Unspecified

OGCR Official Guidelines   ● Unacceptable Principal Diagnosis   X Assign placeholder X   ● Use Additional Character(s)   ▶ Manifestation Code   **Coding Clinic**

● **V18**   **Pedal cycle rider injured in noncollision transport accident**

     Includes   fall or thrown from pedal cycle (without antecedent collision)
                    overturning pedal cycle NOS
                    overturning pedal cycle without collision

     The appropriate 7th character is to be added to each code from category V18

         A   initial encounter
         D   subsequent encounter
         S   sequela

X● **V18.0**   **Pedal cycle driver injured in noncollision transport accident in nontraffic accident**

X● **V18.1**   **Pedal cycle passenger injured in noncollision transport accident in nontraffic accident**

X● **V18.2**   Unspecified **pedal cyclist injured in noncollision transport accident in nontraffic accident**

X● **V18.3**   **Person boarding or alighting a pedal cycle injured in noncollision transport accident**

X● **V18.4**   **Pedal cycle driver injured in noncollision transport accident in traffic accident**

X● **V18.5**   **Pedal cycle passenger injured in noncollision transport accident in traffic accident**

X● **V18.9**   Unspecified **pedal cyclist injured in noncollision transport accident in traffic accident**

● **V19**   **Pedal cycle rider injured in other and unspecified transport accidents**

     The appropriate 7th character is to be added to each code from category V19

         A   initial encounter
         D   subsequent encounter
         S   sequela

● **V19.0**   **Pedal cycle driver injured in collision with other and unspecified motor vehicles in nontraffic accident**

   X● **V19.00**   **Pedal cycle driver injured in collision with** unspecified **motor vehicles in nontraffic accident**

   X● **V19.09**   **Pedal cycle driver injured in collision with other motor vehicles in nontraffic accident**

● **V19.1**   **Pedal cycle passenger injured in collision with other and unspecified motor vehicles in nontraffic accident**

   X● **V19.10**   **Pedal cycle passenger injured in collision with** unspecified **motor vehicles in nontraffic accident**

   X● **V19.19**   **Pedal cycle passenger injured in collision with other motor vehicles in nontraffic accident**

● **V19.2**   **Unspecified pedal cyclist injured in collision with other and unspecified motor vehicles in nontraffic accident**

   X● **V19.20**   Unspecified **pedal cyclist injured in collision with unspecified motor vehicles in nontraffic accident**

       Pedal cycle collision NOS, nontraffic

   X● **V19.29**   Unspecified **pedal cyclist injured in collision with other motor vehicles in nontraffic accident**

X● **V19.3**   **Pedal cyclist (driver) (passenger) injured in** unspecified **nontraffic accident**

     Pedal cycle accident NOS, nontraffic
     Pedal cyclist injured in nontraffic accident NOS

● **V19.4**   **Pedal cycle driver injured in collision with other and unspecified motor vehicles in traffic accident**

   X● **V19.40**   **Pedal cycle driver injured in collision with** unspecified **motor vehicles in traffic accident**

   X● **V19.49**   **Pedal cycle driver injured in collision with other motor vehicles in traffic accident**

● **V19.5**   **Pedal cycle passenger injured in collision with other and unspecified motor vehicles in traffic accident**

   X● **V19.50**   **Pedal cycle passenger injured in collision with** unspecified **motor vehicles in traffic accident**

   X● **V19.59**   **Pedal cycle passenger injured in collision with other motor vehicles in traffic accident**

● **V19.6**   **Unspecified pedal cyclist injured in collision with other and unspecified motor vehicles in traffic accident**

   X● **V19.60**   Unspecified **pedal cyclist injured in collision with unspecified motor vehicles in traffic accident**

       Pedal cycle collision NOS (traffic)

   X● **V19.69**   Unspecified **pedal cyclist injured in collision with other motor vehicles in traffic accident**

● **V19.8**   **Pedal cyclist (driver) (passenger) injured in other specified transport accidents**

   X● **V19.81**   **Pedal cyclist (driver) (passenger) injured in transport accident with military vehicle**

   X● **V19.88**   **Pedal cyclist (driver) (passenger) injured in other specified transport accidents**

X● **V19.9**   **Pedal cyclist (driver) (passenger) injured in** unspecified **traffic accident**

     Pedal cycle accident NOS

MOTORCYCLE RIDER INJURED IN TRANSPORT ACCIDENT (V20-V29)

     Includes   moped motorcycle with sidecar motorized bicycle motor scooter

     Excludes1   three-wheeled motor vehicle (V30-V39)

● **V20**   **Motorcycle rider injured in collision with pedestrian or animal**

     Excludes1   motorcycle rider collision with animal-drawn vehicle or animal being ridden (V26.-)

     The appropriate 7th character is to be added to each code from category V20

         A   initial encounter
         D   subsequent encounter
         S   sequela

X● **V20.0**   **Motorcycle driver injured in collision with pedestrian or animal in nontraffic accident**

X● **V20.1**   **Motorcycle passenger injured in collision with pedestrian or animal in nontraffic accident**

X● **V20.2**   Unspecified **motorcycle rider injured in collision with pedestrian or animal in nontraffic accident**

X● **V20.3**   **Person boarding or alighting a motorcycle injured in collision with pedestrian or animal**

X● **V20.4**   **Motorcycle driver injured in collision with pedestrian or animal in traffic accident**

X● **V20.5**   **Motorcycle passenger injured in collision with pedestrian or animal in traffic accident**

X● **V20.9**   Unspecified **motorcycle rider injured in collision with pedestrian or animal in traffic accident**

● **V21**   **Motorcycle rider injured in collision with pedal cycle**

     The appropriate 7th character is to be added to each code from category V21

         A   initial encounter
         D   subsequent encounter
         S   sequela

X● **V21.0**   **Motorcycle driver injured in collision with pedal cycle in nontraffic accident**

X● **V21.1**   **Motorcycle passenger injured in collision with pedal cycle in nontraffic accident**

X● **V21.2**   Unspecified **motorcycle rider injured in collision with pedal cycle in nontraffic accident**

X● **V21.3**   **Person boarding or alighting a motorcycle injured in collision with pedal cycle**

X● **V21.4**   **Motorcycle driver injured in collision with pedal cycle in traffic accident**

X● **V21.5**   **Motorcycle passenger injured in collision with pedal cycle in traffic accident**

X● **V21.9**   Unspecified **motorcycle rider injured in collision with pedal cycle in traffic accident**

CHAPTER 20 (V01-Y99)

N Newborn Age: 0   **P** Pediatric Age: 0–17   **M** Maternity DX: 12–55   **A** Adult Age: 15–124   ♀ Females Only   ♂ Males Only

     Complication\Comorbidity   Major C\C   (Ex) CC/MCC Exclusions   Hospital-Acquired Condition   **1529**

● **V22**   **Motorcycle rider injured in collision with two- or three-wheeled motor vehicle**

> The appropriate 7th character is to be added to each code from category V22

> | | |
> |---|---|
> | A | initial encounter |
> | D | subsequent encounter |
> | S | sequela |

X● **V22.0**   Motorcycle driver injured in collision with two- or three-wheeled motor vehicle in nontraffic accident

X● **V22.1**   Motorcycle passenger injured in collision with two- or three-wheeled motor vehicle in nontraffic accident

X● **V22.2**   Unspecified motorcycle rider injured in collision with two- or three-wheeled motor vehicle in nontraffic accident

X● **V22.3**   Person boarding or alighting a motorcycle injured in collision with two- or three-wheeled motor vehicle

X● **V22.4**   Motorcycle driver injured in collision with two- or three-wheeled motor vehicle in traffic accident

X● **V22.5**   Motorcycle passenger injured in collision with two- or three-wheeled motor vehicle in traffic accident

X● **V22.9**   Unspecified motorcycle rider injured in collision with two- or three-wheeled motor vehicle in traffic accident

● **V23**   **Motorcycle rider injured in collision with car, pick-up truck or van**

> The appropriate 7th character is to be added to each code from category V23

> | | |
> |---|---|
> | A | initial encounter |
> | D | subsequent encounter |
> | S | sequela |

X● **V23.0**   Motorcycle driver injured in collision with car, pick-up truck or van in nontraffic accident

X● **V23.1**   Motorcycle passenger injured in collision with car, pick-up truck or van in nontraffic accident

X● **V23.2**   Unspecified motorcycle rider injured in collision with car, pick-up truck or van in nontraffic accident

X● **V23.3**   Person boarding or alighting a motorcycle injured in collision with car, pick-up truck or van

X● **V23.4**   Motorcycle driver injured in collision with car, pick-up truck or van in traffic accident

X● **V23.5**   Motorcycle passenger injured in collision with car, pick-up truck or van in traffic accident

X● **V23.9**   Unspecified motorcycle rider injured in collision with car, pick-up truck or van in traffic accident

● **V24**   **Motorcycle rider injured in collision with heavy transport vehicle or bus**

> **Excludes1**   motorcycle rider injured in collision with military vehicle (V29.81)

> The appropriate 7th character is to be added to each code from category V24

> | | |
> |---|---|
> | A | initial encounter |
> | D | subsequent encounter |
> | S | sequela |

X● **V24.0**   Motorcycle driver injured in collision with heavy transport vehicle or bus in nontraffic accident

X● **V24.1**   Motorcycle passenger injured in collision with heavy transport vehicle or bus in nontraffic accident

X● **V24.2**   Unspecified motorcycle rider injured in collision with heavy transport vehicle or bus in nontraffic accident

X● **V24.3**   Person boarding or alighting a motorcycle injured in collision with heavy transport vehicle or bus

X● **V24.4**   Motorcycle driver injured in collision with heavy transport vehicle or bus in traffic accident

X● **V24.5**   Motorcycle passenger injured in collision with heavy transport vehicle or bus in traffic accident

X● **V24.9**   Unspecified motorcycle rider injured in collision with heavy transport vehicle or bus in traffic accident

● **V25**   **Motorcycle rider injured in collision with railway train or railway vehicle**

> The appropriate 7th character is to be added to each code from category V25

> | | |
> |---|---|
> | A | initial encounter |
> | D | subsequent encounter |
> | S | sequela |

X● **V25.0**   Motorcycle driver injured in collision with railway train or railway vehicle in nontraffic accident

X● **V25.1**   Motorcycle passenger injured in collision with railway train or railway vehicle in nontraffic accident

X● **V25.2**   Unspecified motorcycle rider injured in collision with railway train or railway vehicle in nontraffic accident

X● **V25.3**   Person boarding or alighting a motorcycle injured in collision with railway train or railway vehicle

X● **V25.4**   Motorcycle driver injured in collision with railway train or railway vehicle in traffic accident

X● **V25.5**   Motorcycle passenger injured in collision with railway train or railway vehicle in traffic accident

X● **V25.9**   Unspecified motorcycle rider injured in collision with railway train or railway vehicle in traffic accident

● **V26**   **Motorcycle rider injured in collision with other nonmotor vehicle**

> **Includes**   collision with animal-drawn vehicle, animal being ridden, streetcar

> The appropriate 7th character is to be added to each code from category V26

> | | |
> |---|---|
> | A | initial encounter |
> | D | subsequent encounter |
> | S | sequela |

X● **V26.0**   Motorcycle driver injured in collision with other nonmotor vehicle in nontraffic accident

X● **V26.1**   Motorcycle passenger injured in collision with other nonmotor vehicle in nontraffic accident

X● **V26.2**   Unspecified motorcycle rider injured in collision with other nonmotor vehicle in nontraffic accident

X● **V26.3**   Person boarding or alighting a motorcycle injured in collision with other nonmotor vehicle

X● **V26.4**   Motorcycle driver injured in collision with other nonmotor vehicle in traffic accident

X● **V26.5**   Motorcycle passenger injured in collision with other nonmotor vehicle in traffic accident

X● **V26.9**   Unspecified motorcycle rider injured in collision with other nonmotor vehicle in traffic accident

● **V27**   **Motorcycle rider injured in collision with fixed or stationary object**

> The appropriate 7th character is to be added to each code from category V27

> | | |
> |---|---|
> | A | initial encounter |
> | D | subsequent encounter |
> | S | sequela |

X● **V27.0**   Motorcycle driver injured in collision with fixed or stationary object in nontraffic accident

X● **V27.1**   Motorcycle passenger injured in collision with fixed or stationary object in nontraffic accident

X● **V27.2**   Unspecified motorcycle rider injured in collision with fixed or stationary object in nontraffic accident

X● **V27.3**   Person boarding or alighting a motorcycle injured in collision with fixed or stationary object

X● **V27.4**   Motorcycle driver injured in collision with fixed or stationary object in traffic accident

X● **V27.5**   Motorcycle passenger injured in collision with fixed or stationary object in traffic accident

X● **V27.9**   Unspecified motorcycle rider injured in collision with fixed or stationary object in traffic accident

◀ New   ◀ Revised   ~~deleted~~ Deleted   Excludes 1   Excludes 2   Includes   Use additional   Code first   Code also   Unspecified

1530   OGCR Official Guidelines   ● Unacceptable Principal Diagnosis   X Assign placeholder X   ● Use Additional Character(s)   ▶ Manifestation Code   **Coding Clinic**

● **V28** **Motorcycle rider injured in noncollision transport accident**

    Includes   fall or thrown from motorcycle (without antecedent collision)
                      overturning motorcycle NOS
                      overturning motorcycle without collision

    The appropriate 7th character is to be added to each code from category V28

    A   initial encounter
    D   subsequent encounter
    S   sequela

X● **V28.0** Motorcycle driver injured in noncollision transport accident in nontraffic accident

X● **V28.1** Motorcycle passenger injured in noncollision transport accident in nontraffic accident

X● **V28.2** Unspecified motorcycle rider injured in noncollision transport accident in nontraffic accident

X● **V28.3** Person boarding or alighting a motorcycle injured in noncollision transport accident

X● **V28.4** Motorcycle driver injured in noncollision transport accident in traffic accident

X● **V28.5** Motorcycle passenger injured in noncollision transport accident in traffic accident

X● **V28.9** Unspecified motorcycle rider injured in noncollision transport accident in traffic accident

● **V29** **Motorcycle rider injured in other and unspecified transport accidents**

    The appropriate 7th character is to be added to each code from category V29

    A   initial encounter
    D   subsequent encounter
    S   sequela

    Coding Clinic: 2015, Q3, P20

● **V29.0** Motorcycle driver injured in collision with other and unspecified motor vehicles in nontraffic accident

  X● **V29.00** Motorcycle driver injured in collision with unspecified motor vehicles in nontraffic accident

  X● **V29.09** Motorcycle driver injured in collision with other motor vehicles in nontraffic accident

● **V29.1** Motorcycle passenger injured in collision with other and unspecified motor vehicles in nontraffic accident

  X● **V29.10** Motorcycle passenger injured in collision with unspecified motor vehicles in nontraffic accident

  X● **V29.19** Motorcycle passenger injured in collision with other motor vehicles in nontraffic accident

● **V29.2** Unspecified motorcycle rider injured in collision with other and unspecified motor vehicles in nontraffic accident

  X● **V29.20** Unspecified motorcycle rider injured in collision with unspecified motor vehicles in nontraffic accident
        Motorcycle collision NOS, nontraffic

  X● **V29.29** Unspecified motorcycle rider injured in collision with other motor vehicles in nontraffic accident

X● **V29.3** Motorcycle rider (driver) (passenger) injured in unspecified nontraffic accident
    Motorcycle accident NOS, nontraffic
    Motorcycle rider injured in nontraffic accident NOS

● **V29.4** Motorcycle driver injured in collision with other and unspecified motor vehicles in traffic accident

  X● **V29.40** Motorcycle driver injured in collision with unspecified motor vehicles in traffic accident

  X● **V29.49** Motorcycle driver injured in collision with other motor vehicles in traffic accident

● **V29.5** Motorcycle passenger injured in collision with other and unspecified motor vehicles in traffic accident

  X● **V29.50** Motorcycle passenger injured in collision with unspecified motor vehicles in traffic accident

  X● **V29.59** Motorcycle passenger injured in collision with other motor vehicles in traffic accident

● **V29.6** Unspecified motorcycle rider injured in collision with other and unspecified motor vehicles in traffic accident

  X● **V29.60** Unspecified motorcycle rider injured in collision with unspecified motor vehicles in traffic accident
        Motorcycle collision NOS (traffic)

  X● **V29.69** Unspecified motorcycle rider injured in collision with other motor vehicles in traffic accident

● **V29.8** Motorcycle rider (driver) (passenger) injured in other specified transport accidents

  X● **V29.81** Motorcycle rider (driver) (passenger) injured in transport accident with military vehicle

  X● **V29.88** Motorcycle rider (driver) (passenger) injured in other specified transport accidents

X● **V29.9** Motorcycle rider (driver) (passenger) injured in unspecified traffic accident
    Motorcycle accident NOS

OCCUPANT OF THREE-WHEELED MOTOR VEHICLE INJURED IN TRANSPORT ACCIDENT (V30-V39)

    Includes   motorized tricycle
                      motorized rickshaw
                      three-wheeled motor car

    Excludes1   all-terrain vehicles (V86.-)
                      motorcycle with sidecar (V20-V29)
                      vehicle designed primarily for off-road use (V86.-)

● **V30** **Occupant of three-wheeled motor vehicle injured in collision with pedestrian or animal**

    Excludes1   three-wheeled motor vehicle collision with animal-drawn vehicle or animal being ridden (V36.-)

    The appropriate 7th character is to be added to each code from category V30

    A   initial encounter
    D   subsequent encounter
    S   sequela

X● **V30.0** Driver of three-wheeled motor vehicle injured in collision with pedestrian or animal in nontraffic accident

X● **V30.1** Passenger in three-wheeled motor vehicle injured in collision with pedestrian or animal in nontraffic accident

X● **V30.2** Person on outside of three-wheeled motor vehicle injured in collision with pedestrian or animal in nontraffic accident

X● **V30.3** Unspecified occupant of three-wheeled motor vehicle injured in collision with pedestrian or animal in nontraffic accident

X● **V30.4** Person boarding or alighting a three-wheeled motor vehicle injured in collision with pedestrian or animal

X● **V30.5** Driver of three-wheeled motor vehicle injured in collision with pedestrian or animal in traffic accident

X● **V30.6** Passenger in three-wheeled motor vehicle injured in collision with pedestrian or animal in traffic accident

X● **V30.7** Person on outside of three-wheeled motor vehicle injured in collision with pedestrian or animal in traffic accident

X● **V30.9** Unspecified occupant of three-wheeled motor vehicle injured in collision with pedestrian or animal in traffic accident

CHAPTER 20 (V01-Y99)

● **V31 Occupant of three-wheeled motor vehicle injured in collision with pedal cycle**

The appropriate 7th character is to be added to each code from category V31

A	initial encounter
D	subsequent encounter
S	sequela

X ● **V31.0** Driver of three-wheeled motor vehicle injured in collision with pedal cycle in nontraffic accident

X ● **V31.1** Passenger in three-wheeled motor vehicle injured in collision with pedal cycle in nontraffic accident

X ● **V31.2** Person on outside of three-wheeled motor vehicle injured in collision with pedal cycle in nontraffic accident

X ● **V31.3** Unspecified occupant of three-wheeled motor vehicle injured in collision with pedal cycle in nontraffic accident

X ● **V31.4** Person boarding or alighting a three-wheeled motor vehicle injured in collision with pedal cycle

X ● **V31.5** Driver of three-wheeled motor vehicle injured in collision with pedal cycle in traffic accident

X ● **V31.6** Passenger in three-wheeled motor vehicle injured in collision with pedal cycle in traffic accident

X ● **V31.7** Person on outside of three-wheeled motor vehicle injured in collision with pedal cycle in traffic accident

X ● **V31.9** Unspecified occupant of three-wheeled motor vehicle injured in collision with pedal cycle in traffic accident

● **V32 Occupant of three-wheeled motor vehicle injured in collision with two- or three-wheeled motor vehicle**

The appropriate 7th character is to be added to each code from category V32

A	initial encounter
D	subsequent encounter
S	sequela

X ● **V32.0** Driver of three-wheeled motor vehicle injured in collision with two- or three-wheeled motor vehicle in nontraffic accident

X ● **V32.1** Passenger in three-wheeled motor vehicle injured in collision with two- or three-wheeled motor vehicle in nontraffic accident

X ● **V32.2** Person on outside of three-wheeled motor vehicle injured in collision with two- or three-wheeled motor vehicle in nontraffic accident

X ● **V32.3** Unspecified occupant of three-wheeled motor vehicle injured in collision with two- or three-wheeled motor vehicle in nontraffic accident

X ● **V32.4** Person boarding or alighting a three-wheeled motor vehicle injured in collision with two- or three-wheeled motor vehicle

X ● **V32.5** Driver of three-wheeled motor vehicle injured in collision with two- or three-wheeled motor vehicle in traffic accident

X ● **V32.6** Passenger in three-wheeled motor vehicle injured in collision with two- or three-wheeled motor vehicle in traffic accident

X ● **V32.7** Person on outside of three-wheeled motor vehicle injured in collision with two- or three-wheeled motor vehicle in traffic accident

X ● **V32.9** Unspecified occupant of three-wheeled motor vehicle injured in collision with two- or three-wheeled motor vehicle in traffic accident

● **V33 Occupant of three-wheeled motor vehicle injured in collision with car, pick-up truck or van**

The appropriate 7th character is to be added to each code from category V33

A	initial encounter
D	subsequent encounter
S	sequela

X ● **V33.0** Driver of three-wheeled motor vehicle injured in collision with car, pick-up truck or van in nontraffic accident

X ● **V33.1** Passenger in three-wheeled motor vehicle injured in collision with car, pick-up truck or van in nontraffic accident

X ● **V33.2** Person on outside of three-wheeled motor vehicle injured in collision with car, pick-up truck or van in nontraffic accident

X ● **V33.3** Unspecified occupant of three-wheeled motor vehicle injured in collision with car, pick-up truck or van in nontraffic accident

X ● **V33.4** Person boarding or alighting a three-wheeled motor vehicle injured in collision with car, pick-up truck or van

X ● **V33.5** Driver of three-wheeled motor vehicle injured in collision with car, pick-up truck or van in traffic accident

X ● **V33.6** Passenger in three-wheeled motor vehicle injured in collision with car, pick-up truck or van in traffic accident

X ● **V33.7** Person on outside of three-wheeled motor vehicle injured in collision with car, pick-up truck or van in traffic accident

X ● **V33.9** Unspecified occupant of three-wheeled motor vehicle injured in collision with car, pick-up truck or van in traffic accident

● **V34 Occupant of three-wheeled motor vehicle injured in collision with heavy transport vehicle or bus**

Excludes1 occupant of three-wheeled motor vehicle injured in collision with military vehicle (V39.81)

The appropriate 7th character is to be added to each code from category V34

A	initial encounter
D	subsequent encounter
S	sequela

X ● **V34.0** Driver of three-wheeled motor vehicle injured in collision with heavy transport vehicle or bus in nontraffic accident

X ● **V34.1** Passenger in three-wheeled motor vehicle injured in collision with heavy transport vehicle or bus in nontraffic accident

X ● **V34.2** Person on outside of three-wheeled motor vehicle injured in collision with heavy transport vehicle or bus in nontraffic accident

X ● **V34.3** Unspecified occupant of three-wheeled motor vehicle injured in collision with heavy transport vehicle or bus in nontraffic accident

X ● **V34.4** Person boarding or alighting a three-wheeled motor vehicle injured in collision with heavy transport vehicle or bus

X ● **V34.5** Driver of three-wheeled motor vehicle injured in collision with heavy transport vehicle or bus in traffic accident

X ● **V34.6** Passenger in three-wheeled motor vehicle injured in collision with heavy transport vehicle or bus in traffic accident

X ● **V34.7** Person on outside of three-wheeled motor vehicle injured in collision with heavy transport vehicle or bus in traffic accident

X ● **V34.9** Unspecified occupant of three-wheeled motor vehicle injured in collision with heavy transport vehicle or bus in traffic accident

◀ New   ◀■ Revised   ~~deleted~~ Deleted   Excludes 1   Excludes 2   Includes   Use additional   Code first   Code also   Unspecified

OGCR Official Guidelines   ● Unacceptable Principal Diagnosis   X Assign placeholder X   ● Use Additional Character(s)   ▶ Manifestation Code   **Coding Clinic**

● **V35 Occupant of three-wheeled motor vehicle injured in collision with railway train or railway vehicle**

The appropriate 7th character is to be added to each code from category V35

A	initial encounter
D	subsequent encounter
S	sequela

X● **V35.0 Driver of three-wheeled motor vehicle injured in collision with railway train or railway vehicle in nontraffic accident**

X● **V35.1 Passenger in three-wheeled motor vehicle injured in collision with railway train or railway vehicle in nontraffic accident**

X● **V35.2 Person on outside of three-wheeled motor vehicle injured in collision with railway train or railway vehicle in nontraffic accident**

X● **V35.3 Unspecified occupant of three-wheeled motor vehicle injured in collision with railway train or railway vehicle in nontraffic accident**

X● **V35.4 Person boarding or alighting a three-wheeled motor vehicle injured in collision with railway train or railway vehicle**

X● **V35.5 Driver of three-wheeled motor vehicle injured in collision with railway train or railway vehicle in traffic accident**

X● **V35.6 Passenger in three-wheeled motor vehicle injured in collision with railway train or railway vehicle in traffic accident**

X● **V35.7 Person on outside of three-wheeled motor vehicle injured in collision with railway train or railway vehicle in traffic accident**

X● **V35.9 Unspecified occupant of three-wheeled motor vehicle injured in collision with railway train or railway vehicle in traffic accident**

● **V36 Occupant of three-wheeled motor vehicle injured in collision with other nonmotor vehicle**

Includes collision with animal-drawn vehicle, animal being ridden, streetcar

The appropriate 7th character is to be added to each code from category V36

A	initial encounter
D	subsequent encounter
S	sequela

X● **V36.0 Driver of three-wheeled motor vehicle injured in collision with other nonmotor vehicle in nontraffic accident**

X● **V36.1 Passenger in three-wheeled motor vehicle injured in collision with other nonmotor vehicle in nontraffic accident**

X● **V36.2 Person on outside of three-wheeled motor vehicle injured in collision with other nonmotor vehicle in nontraffic accident**

X● **V36.3 Unspecified occupant of three-wheeled motor vehicle injured in collision with other nonmotor vehicle in nontraffic accident**

X● **V36.4 Person boarding or alighting a three-wheeled motor vehicle injured in collision with other nonmotor vehicle**

X● **V36.5 Driver of three-wheeled motor vehicle injured in collision with other nonmotor vehicle in traffic accident**

X● **V36.6 Passenger in three-wheeled motor vehicle injured in collision with other nonmotor vehicle in traffic accident**

X● **V36.7 Person on outside of three-wheeled motor vehicle injured in collision with other nonmotor vehicle in traffic accident**

X● **V36.9 Unspecified occupant of three-wheeled motor vehicle injured in collision with other nonmotor vehicle in traffic accident**

● **V37 Occupant of three-wheeled motor vehicle injured in collision with fixed or stationary object**

The appropriate 7th character is to be added to each code from category V37

A	initial encounter
D	subsequent encounter
S	sequela

X● **V37.0 Driver of three-wheeled motor vehicle injured in collision with fixed or stationary object in nontraffic accident**

X● **V37.1 Passenger in three-wheeled motor vehicle injured in collision with fixed or stationary object in nontraffic accident**

X● **V37.2 Person on outside of three-wheeled motor vehicle injured in collision with fixed or stationary object in nontraffic accident**

X● **V37.3 Unspecified occupant of three-wheeled motor vehicle injured in collision with fixed or stationary object in nontraffic accident**

X● **V37.4 Person boarding or alighting a three-wheeled motor vehicle injured in collision with fixed or stationary object**

X● **V37.5 Driver of three-wheeled motor vehicle injured in collision with fixed or stationary object in traffic accident**

X● **V37.6 Passenger in three-wheeled motor vehicle injured in collision with fixed or stationary object in traffic accident**

X● **V37.7 Person on outside of three-wheeled motor vehicle injured in collision with fixed or stationary object in traffic accident**

X● **V37.9 Unspecified occupant of three-wheeled motor vehicle injured in collision with fixed or stationary object in traffic accident**

● **V38 Occupant of three-wheeled motor vehicle injured in noncollision transport accident**

Includes fall or thrown from three-wheeled motor vehicle overturning of three-wheeled motor vehicle NOS overturning of three-wheeled motor vehicle without collision

The appropriate 7th character is to be added to each code from category V38

A	initial encounter
D	subsequent encounter
S	sequela

X● **V38.0 Driver of three-wheeled motor vehicle injured in noncollision transport accident in nontraffic accident**

X● **V38.1 Passenger in three-wheeled motor vehicle injured in noncollision transport accident in nontraffic accident**

X● **V38.2 Person on outside of three-wheeled motor vehicle injured in noncollision transport accident in nontraffic accident**

X● **V38.3 Unspecified occupant of three-wheeled motor vehicle injured in noncollision transport accident in nontraffic accident**

X● **V38.4 Person boarding or alighting a three-wheeled motor vehicle injured in noncollision transport accident**

X● **V38.5 Driver of three-wheeled motor vehicle injured in noncollision transport accident in traffic accident**

X● **V38.6 Passenger in three-wheeled motor vehicle injured in noncollision transport accident in traffic accident**

X● **V38.7 Person on outside of three-wheeled motor vehicle injured in noncollision transport accident in traffic accident**

X● **V38.9 Unspecified occupant of three-wheeled motor vehicle injured in noncollision transport accident in traffic accident**

CHAPTER 20 (V01-Y99)

●**V39** **Occupant of three-wheeled motor vehicle injured in other and unspecified transport accidents**

The appropriate 7th character is to be added to each code from category V39

A	initial encounter
D	subsequent encounter
S	sequela

●**V39.0** **Driver of three-wheeled motor vehicle injured in collision with other and unspecified motor vehicles in nontraffic accident**

X● **V39.00** Driver of three-wheeled motor vehicle injured in collision with unspecified motor vehicles in nontraffic accident

X● **V39.09** Driver of three-wheeled motor vehicle injured in collision with other motor vehicles in nontraffic accident

●**V39.1** **Passenger in three-wheeled motor vehicle injured in collision with other and unspecified motor vehicles in nontraffic accident**

X● **V39.10** Passenger in three-wheeled motor vehicle injured in collision with unspecified motor vehicles in nontraffic accident

X● **V39.19** Passenger in three-wheeled motor vehicle injured in collision with other motor vehicles in nontraffic accident

●**V39.2** **Unspecified occupant of three-wheeled motor vehicle injured in collision with other and unspecified motor vehicles in nontraffic accident**

X● **V39.20** Unspecified occupant of three-wheeled motor vehicle injured in collision with unspecified motor vehicles in nontraffic accident

Collision NOS involving three-wheeled motor vehicle, nontraffic

X● **V39.29** Unspecified occupant of three-wheeled motor vehicle injured in collision with other motor vehicles in nontraffic accident

X● **V39.3** Occupant (driver) (passenger) of three-wheeled motor vehicle injured in unspecified nontraffic accident

Accident NOS involving three-wheeled motor vehicle, nontraffic

Occupant of three-wheeled motor vehicle injured in nontraffic accident NOS

●**V39.4** **Driver of three-wheeled motor vehicle injured in collision with other and unspecified motor vehicles in traffic accident**

X● **V39.40** Driver of three-wheeled motor vehicle injured in collision with unspecified motor vehicles in traffic accident

X● **V39.49** Driver of three-wheeled motor vehicle injured in collision with other motor vehicles in traffic accident

●**V39.5** **Passenger in three-wheeled motor vehicle injured in collision with other and unspecified motor vehicles in traffic accident**

X● **V39.50** Passenger in three-wheeled motor vehicle injured in collision with unspecified motor vehicles in traffic accident

X● **V39.59** Passenger in three-wheeled motor vehicle injured in collision with other motor vehicles in traffic accident

●**V39.6** **Unspecified occupant of three-wheeled motor vehicle injured in collision with other and unspecified motor vehicles in traffic accident**

X● **V39.60** Unspecified occupant of three-wheeled motor vehicle injured in collision with unspecified motor vehicles in traffic accident

Collision NOS involving three-wheeled motor vehicle (traffic)

X● **V39.69** Unspecified occupant of three-wheeled motor vehicle injured in collision with other motor vehicles in traffic accident

●**V39.8** **Occupant (driver) (passenger) of three-wheeled motor vehicle injured in other specified transport accidents**

X● **V39.81** Occupant (driver) (passenger) of three-wheeled motor vehicle injured in transport accident with military vehicle

X● **V39.89** Occupant (driver) (passenger) of three-wheeled motor vehicle injured in other specified transport accidents

X● **V39.9** Occupant (driver) (passenger) of three-wheeled motor vehicle injured in unspecified traffic accident

Accident NOS involving three-wheeled motor vehicle

CAR OCCUPANT INJURED IN TRANSPORT ACCIDENT (V40-V49)

Includes	a four-wheeled motor vehicle designed primarily for carrying passengers
	automobile (pulling a trailer or camper)

Excludes1	bus (V50-V59)
	minibus (V50-V59)
	minivan (V50-V59)
	motorcoach (V70-V79)
	pick-up truck (V50-V59)
	sport utility vehicle (SUV) (V50-V59)

●**V40** **Car occupant injured in collision with pedestrian or animal**

Excludes1	car collision with animal-drawn vehicle or animal being ridden (V46.-)

The appropriate 7th character is to be added to each code from category V40

A	initial encounter
D	subsequent encounter
S	sequela

X● **V40.0** Car driver injured in collision with pedestrian or animal in nontraffic accident

X● **V40.1** Car passenger injured in collision with pedestrian or animal in nontraffic accident

X● **V40.2** Person on outside of car injured in collision with pedestrian or animal in nontraffic accident

X● **V40.3** Unspecified car occupant injured in collision with pedestrian or animal in nontraffic accident

X● **V40.4** Person boarding or alighting a car injured in collision with pedestrian or animal

X● **V40.5** Car driver injured in collision with pedestrian or animal in traffic accident

X● **V40.6** Car passenger injured in collision with pedestrian or animal in traffic accident

X● **V40.7** Person on outside of car injured in collision with pedestrian or animal in traffic accident

X● **V40.9** Unspecified car occupant injured in collision with pedestrian or animal in traffic accident

●**V41** **Car occupant injured in collision with pedal cycle**

The appropriate 7th character is to be added to each code from category V41

A	initial encounter
D	subsequent encounter
S	sequela

X● **V41.0** Car driver injured in collision with pedal cycle in nontraffic accident

X● **V41.1** Car passenger injured in collision with pedal cycle in nontraffic accident

X● **V41.2** Person on outside of car injured in collision with pedal cycle in nontraffic accident

X● **V41.3** Unspecified car occupant injured in collision with pedal cycle in nontraffic accident

X● **V41.4** Person boarding or alighting a car injured in collision with pedal cycle

X● **V41.5** Car driver injured in collision with pedal cycle in traffic accident

X● **V41.6** Car passenger injured in collision with pedal cycle in traffic accident

◄ New   ◄ Revised   ~~deleted~~ Deleted   Excludes 1   Excludes 2   Includes   Use additional   Code first   Code also   Unspecified

OGCR Official Guidelines   ● Unacceptable Principal Diagnosis   X Assign placeholder X   ● Use Additional Character(s)   ▶ Manifestation Code   **Coding Clinic**

X ● **V41.7**   Person on outside of car injured in collision with pedal cycle in traffic accident

X ● **V41.9**   Unspecified car occupant injured in collision with pedal cycle in traffic accident

● **V42**   Car occupant injured in collision with two- or three-wheeled motor vehicle

> The appropriate 7th character is to be added to each code from category V42

> | | |
> |---|---|
> | A | initial encounter |
> | D | subsequent encounter |
> | S | sequela |

X ● **V42.0**   Car driver injured in collision with two- or three-wheeled motor vehicle in nontraffic accident

X ● **V42.1**   Car passenger injured in collision with two- or three-wheeled motor vehicle in nontraffic accident

X ● **V42.2**   Person on outside of car injured in collision with two- or three-wheeled motor vehicle in nontraffic accident

X ● **V42.3**   Unspecified car occupant injured in collision with two- or three-wheeled motor vehicle in nontraffic accident

X ● **V42.4**   Person boarding or alighting a car injured in collision with two- or three-wheeled motor vehicle

X ● **V42.5**   Car driver injured in collision with two- or three-wheeled motor vehicle in traffic accident

X ● **V42.6**   Car passenger injured in collision with two- or three-wheeled motor vehicle in traffic accident

X ● **V42.7**   Person on outside of car injured in collision with two- or three-wheeled motor vehicle in traffic accident

X ● **V42.9**   Unspecified car occupant injured in collision with two- or three-wheeled motor vehicle in traffic accident

● **V43**   Car occupant injured in collision with car, pick-up truck or van

> The appropriate 7th character is to be added to each code from category V43

> | | |
> |---|---|
> | A | initial encounter |
> | D | subsequent encounter |
> | S | sequela |

● **V43.0**   Car driver injured in collision with car, pick-up truck or van in nontraffic accident

   X ● **V43.01**   Car driver injured in collision with sport utility vehicle in nontraffic accident

   X ● **V43.02**   Car driver injured in collision with other type car in nontraffic accident

   X ● **V43.03**   Car driver injured in collision with pick-up truck in nontraffic accident

   X ● **V43.04**   Car driver injured in collision with van in nontraffic accident

● **V43.1**   Car passenger injured in collision with car, pick-up truck or van in nontraffic accident

   X ● **V43.11**   Car passenger injured in collision with sport utility vehicle in nontraffic accident

   X ● **V43.12**   Car passenger injured in collision with other type car in nontraffic accident

   X ● **V43.13**   Car passenger injured in collision with pick-up in nontraffic accident

   X ● **V43.14**   Car passenger injured in collision with van in nontraffic accident

● **V43.2**   Person on outside of car injured in collision with car, pick-up truck or van in nontraffic accident

   X ● **V43.21**   Person on outside of car injured in collision with sport utility vehicle in nontraffic accident

   X ● **V43.22**   Person on outside of car injured in collision with other type car in nontraffic accident

   X ● **V43.23**   Person on outside of car injured in collision with pick-up truck in nontraffic accident

   X ● **V43.24**   Person on outside of car injured in collision with van in nontraffic accident

● **V43.3**   Unspecified car occupant injured in collision with car, pick-up truck or van in nontraffic accident

   X ● **V43.31**   Unspecified car occupant injured in collision with sport utility vehicle in nontraffic accident

   X ● **V43.32**   Unspecified car occupant injured in collision with other type car in nontraffic accident

   X ● **V43.33**   Unspecified car occupant injured in collision with pick-up truck in nontraffic accident

   X ● **V43.34**   Unspecified car occupant injured in collision with van in nontraffic accident

● **V43.4**   Person boarding or alighting a car injured in collision with car, pick-up truck or van

   X ● **V43.41**   Person boarding or alighting a car injured in collision with sport utility vehicle

   X ● **V43.42**   Person boarding or alighting a car injured in collision with other type car

   X ● **V43.43**   Person boarding or alighting a car injured in collision with pick-up truck

   X ● **V43.44**   Person boarding or alighting a car injured in collision with van

● **V43.5**   Car driver injured in collision with car, pick-up truck or van in traffic accident

   X ● **V43.51**   Car driver injured in collision with sport utility vehicle in traffic accident

   X ● **V43.52**   Car driver injured in collision with other type car in traffic accident

   X ● **V43.53**   Car driver injured in collision with pick-up truck in traffic accident

   X ● **V43.54**   Car driver injured in collision with van in traffic accident

● **V43.6**   Car passenger injured in collision with car, pick-up truck or van in traffic accident

   X ● **V43.61**   Car passenger injured in collision with sport utility vehicle in traffic accident
     Coding Clinic: 2015, Q1, P5-7

   X ● **V43.62**   Car passenger injured in collision with other type car in traffic accident

   X ● **V43.63**   Car passenger injured in collision with pick-up truck in traffic accident

   X ● **V43.64**   Car passenger injured in collision with van in traffic accident

● **V43.7**   Person on outside of car injured in collision with car, pick-up truck or van in traffic accident

   X ● **V43.71**   Person on outside of car injured in collision with sport utility vehicle in traffic accident

   X ● **V43.72**   Person on outside of car injured in collision with other type car in traffic accident

   X ● **V43.73**   Person on outside of car injured in collision with pick-up truck in traffic accident

   X ● **V43.74**   Person on outside of car injured in collision with van in traffic accident

● **V43.9**   Unspecified car occupant injured in collision with car, pick-up truck or van in traffic accident

   X ● **V43.91**   Unspecified car occupant injured in collision with sport utility vehicle in traffic accident

   X ● **V43.92**   Unspecified car occupant injured in collision with other type car in traffic accident

   X ● **V43.93**   Unspecified car occupant injured in collision with pick-up truck in traffic accident

   X ● **V43.94**   Unspecified car occupant injured in collision with van in traffic accident

● **V44**   **Car occupant injured in collision with heavy transport vehicle or bus**

     Excludes1   car occupant injured in collision with military vehicle (V49.81)

     The appropriate 7th character is to be added to each code from category V44

> A   initial encounter
> D   subsequent encounter
> S   sequela

X● **V44.0**   Car driver injured in collision with heavy transport vehicle or bus in nontraffic accident

X● **V44.1**   Car passenger injured in collision with heavy transport vehicle or bus in nontraffic accident

X● **V44.2**   Person on outside of car injured in collision with heavy transport vehicle or bus in nontraffic accident

X● **V44.3**   Unspecified car occupant injured in collision with heavy transport vehicle or bus in nontraffic accident

X● **V44.4**   Person boarding or alighting a car injured in collision with heavy transport vehicle or bus

X● **V44.5**   Car driver injured in collision with heavy transport vehicle or bus in traffic accident

X● **V44.6**   Car passenger injured in collision with heavy transport vehicle or bus in traffic accident

X● **V44.7**   Person on outside of car injured in collision with heavy transport vehicle or bus in traffic accident

X● **V44.9**   Unspecified car occupant injured in collision with heavy transport vehicle or bus in traffic accident

● **V45**   **Car occupant injured in collision with railway train or railway vehicle**

     The appropriate 7th character is to be added to each code from category V45

> A   initial encounter
> D   subsequent encounter
> S   sequela

X● **V45.0**   Car driver injured in collision with railway train or railway vehicle in nontraffic accident

X● **V45.1**   Car passenger injured in collision with railway train or railway vehicle in nontraffic accident

X● **V45.2**   Person on outside of car injured in collision with railway train or railway vehicle in nontraffic accident

X● **V45.3**   Unspecified car occupant injured in collision with railway train or railway vehicle in nontraffic accident

X● **V45.4**   Person boarding or alighting a car injured in collision with railway train or railway vehicle

X● **V45.5**   Car driver injured in collision with railway train or railway vehicle in traffic accident

X● **V45.6**   Car passenger injured in collision with railway train or railway vehicle in traffic accident

X● **V45.7**   Person on outside of car injured in collision with railway train or railway vehicle in traffic accident

X● **V45.9**   Unspecified car occupant injured in collision with railway train or railway vehicle in traffic accident

● **V46**   **Car occupant injured in collision with other nonmotor vehicle**

     Includes   collision with animal-drawn vehicle, animal being ridden, streetcar

     The appropriate 7th character is to be added to each code from category V46

> A   initial encounter
> D   subsequent encounter
> S   sequela

X● **V46.0**   Car driver injured in collision with other nonmotor vehicle in nontraffic accident

X● **V46.1**   Car passenger injured in collision with other nonmotor vehicle in nontraffic accident

X● **V46.2**   Person on outside of car injured in collision with other nonmotor vehicle in nontraffic accident

X● **V46.3**   Unspecified car occupant injured in collision with other nonmotor vehicle in nontraffic accident

X● **V46.4**   Person boarding or alighting a car injured in collision with other nonmotor vehicle

X● **V46.5**   Car driver injured in collision with other nonmotor vehicle in traffic accident

X● **V46.6**   Car passenger injured in collision with other nonmotor vehicle in traffic accident

X● **V46.7**   Person on outside of car injured in collision with other nonmotor vehicle in traffic accident

X● **V46.9**   Unspecified car occupant injured in collision with other nonmotor vehicle in traffic accident

● **V47**   **Car occupant injured in collision with fixed or stationary object**

     The appropriate 7th character is to be added to each code from category V47

> A   initial encounter
> D   subsequent encounter
> S   sequela

X● **V47.0**   Car driver injured in collision with fixed or stationary object in nontraffic accident

     ~~V47.01   Driver of sport utility vehicle injured in collision with fixed or stationary object in nontraffic accident~~

     ~~V47.02   Driver of other type car injured in collision with fixed or stationary object in nontraffic accident~~

X● **V47.1**   Car passenger injured in collision with fixed or stationary object in nontraffic accident

     ~~V47.11   Passenger of sport utility vehicle injured in collision with fixed or stationary object in nontraffic accident~~

     ~~V47.12   Passenger of other type car injured in collision with fixed or stationary object in nontraffic accident~~

X● **V47.2**   Person on outside of car injured in collision with fixed or stationary object in nontraffic accident

X● **V47.3**   Unspecified car occupant injured in collision with fixed or stationary object in nontraffic accident

     ~~V47.31   Unspecified occupant of sport utility vehicle injured in collision with fixed or stationary object in nontraffic accident~~

     ~~V47.32   Unspecified occupant of other type car injured in collision with fixed or stationary object in nontraffic accident~~

X● **V47.4**   Person boarding or alighting a car injured in collision with fixed or stationary object

X● **V47.5**   Car driver injured in collision with fixed or stationary object in traffic accident

     ~~V47.51   Driver of sport utility vehicle injured in collision with fixed or stationary object in traffic accident~~

     ~~V47.52   Driver of other type car injured in collision with fixed or stationary object in traffic accident~~

X● **V47.6**   Car passenger injured in collision with fixed or stationary object in traffic accident

     ~~V47.61   Passenger of sport utility vehicle injured in collision with fixed or stationary object in traffic accident~~

     ~~V47.62   Passenger of other type car injured in collision with fixed or stationary object in traffic accident~~

X● **V47.7**   Person on outside of car injured in collision with fixed or stationary object in traffic accident

X● **V47.9**   Unspecified car occupant injured in collision with fixed or stationary object in traffic accident

     ~~V47.91   Unspecified occupant of sport utility vehicle injured in collision with fixed or stationary object in traffic accident~~

     ~~V47.92   Unspecified occupant of other type car injured in collision with fixed or stationary object in traffic accident~~

◀ New   ◀ Revised   ~~deleted~~ Deleted   Excludes 1   Excludes 2   Includes   Use additional   Code first   Code also   Unspecified

OGCR Official Guidelines   ● Unacceptable Principal Diagnosis   X Assign placeholder X   ● Use Additional Character(s)   ▶ Manifestation Code   **Coding Clinic**

● **V48**   **Car occupant injured in noncollision transport accident**

> **Includes**   overturning car NOS
> overturning car without collision

The appropriate 7th character is to be added to each code from category V48

> A   initial encounter
> D   subsequent encounter
> S   sequela

X● **V48.0**   Car driver injured in noncollision transport accident in nontraffic accident

X● **V48.1**   Car passenger injured in noncollision transport accident in nontraffic accident

X● **V48.2**   Person on outside of car injured in noncollision transport accident in nontraffic accident

X● **V48.3**   Unspecified car occupant injured in noncollision transport accident in nontraffic accident

X● **V48.4**   Person boarding or alighting a car injured in noncollision transport accident

X● **V48.5**   Car driver injured in noncollision transport accident in traffic accident

X● **V48.6**   Car passenger injured in noncollision transport accident in traffic accident

X● **V48.7**   Person on outside of car injured in noncollision transport accident in traffic accident

X● **V48.9**   Unspecified car occupant injured in noncollision transport accident in traffic accident

● **V49**   **Car occupant injured in other and unspecified transport accidents**

The appropriate 7th character is to be added to each code from category V49

> A   initial encounter
> D   subsequent encounter
> S   sequela

● **V49.0**   Driver injured in collision with other and unspecified motor vehicles in nontraffic accident

   X● **V49.00**   Driver injured in collision with unspecified motor vehicles in nontraffic accident

   X● **V49.09**   Driver injured in collision with other motor vehicles in nontraffic accident

● **V49.1**   Passenger injured in collision with other and unspecified motor vehicles in nontraffic accident

   X● **V49.10**   Passenger injured in collision with unspecified motor vehicles in nontraffic accident

   X● **V49.19**   Passenger injured in collision with other motor vehicles in nontraffic accident

● **V49.2**   Unspecified car occupant injured in collision with other and unspecified motor vehicles in nontraffic accident

   X● **V49.20**   Unspecified car occupant injured in collision with unspecified motor vehicles in nontraffic accident
     Car collision NOS, nontraffic

   X● **V49.29**   Unspecified car occupant injured in collision with other motor vehicles in nontraffic accident

X● **V49.3**   Car occupant (driver) (passenger) injured in unspecified nontraffic accident
   Car accident NOS, nontraffic
   Car occupant injured in nontraffic accident NOS

● **V49.4**   Driver injured in collision with other and unspecified motor vehicles in traffic accident

   X● **V49.40**   Driver injured in collision with unspecified motor vehicles in traffic accident

   X● **V49.49**   Driver injured in collision with other motor vehicles in traffic accident

● **V49.5**   Passenger injured in collision with other and unspecified motor vehicles in traffic accident

   X● **V49.50**   Passenger injured in collision with unspecified motor vehicles in traffic accident

   X● **V49.59**   Passenger injured in collision with other motor vehicles in traffic accident

● **V49.6**   Unspecified car occupant injured in collision with other and unspecified motor vehicles in traffic accident

   X● **V49.60**   Unspecified car occupant injured in collision with unspecified motor vehicles in traffic accident
     Car collision NOS (traffic)

   X● **V49.69**   Unspecified car occupant injured in collision with other motor vehicles in traffic accident

● **V49.8**   Car occupant (driver) (passenger) injured in other specified transport accidents

   X● **V49.81**   Car occupant (driver) (passenger) injured in transport accident with military vehicle

   X● **V49.88**   Car occupant (driver) (passenger) injured in other specified transport accidents

X● **V49.9**   Car occupant (driver) (passenger) injured in unspecified traffic accident
   Car accident NOS
   Coding Clinic: 2015, Q1, P11

OCCUPANT OF PICK-UP TRUCK OR VAN INJURED IN TRANSPORT ACCIDENT (V50-V59)

> **Includes**   a four- or six-wheel motor vehicle designed primarily for carrying passengers and property but weighing less than the local limit for classification as a heavy goods vehicle
> minibus
> minivan
> sport utility vehicle (SUV)
> truck
> van

> **Excludes1**   heavy transport vehicle (V60-V69)

● **V50**   **Occupant of pick-up truck or van injured in collision with pedestrian or animal**

> **Excludes1**   pick-up truck or van collision with animal-drawn vehicle or animal being ridden (V56.-)

The appropriate 7th character is to be added to each code from category V50

> A   initial encounter
> D   subsequent encounter
> S   sequela

X● **V50.0**   Driver of pick-up truck or van injured in collision with pedestrian or animal in nontraffic accident

X● **V50.1**   Passenger in pick-up truck or van injured in collision with pedestrian or animal in nontraffic accident

X● **V50.2**   Person on outside of pick-up truck or van injured in collision with pedestrian or animal in nontraffic accident

X● **V50.3**   Unspecified occupant of pick-up truck or van injured in collision with pedestrian or animal in nontraffic accident

X● **V50.4**   Person boarding or alighting a pick-up truck or van injured in collision with pedestrian or animal

X● **V50.5**   Driver of pick-up truck or van injured in collision with pedestrian or animal in traffic accident

X● **V50.6**   Passenger in pick-up truck or van injured in collision with pedestrian or animal in traffic accident

X● **V50.7**   Person on outside of pick-up truck or van injured in collision with pedestrian or animal in traffic accident

X● **V50.9**   Unspecified occupant of pick-up truck or van injured in collision with pedestrian or animal in traffic accident

● **V51**   **Occupant of pick-up truck or van injured in collision with pedal cycle**

The appropriate 7th character is to be added to each code from category V51

A	initial encounter
D	subsequent encounter
S	sequela

X● **V51.0**   Driver of pick-up truck or van injured in collision with pedal cycle in nontraffic accident

X● **V51.1**   Passenger in pick-up truck or van injured in collision with pedal cycle in nontraffic accident

X● **V51.2**   Person on outside of pick-up truck or van injured in collision with pedal cycle in nontraffic accident

X● **V51.3**   Unspecified occupant of pick-up truck or van injured in collision with pedal cycle in nontraffic accident

X● **V51.4**   Person boarding or alighting a pick-up truck or van injured in collision with pedal cycle

X● **V51.5**   Driver of pick-up truck or van injured in collision with pedal cycle in traffic accident

X● **V51.6**   Passenger in pick-up truck or van injured in collision with pedal cycle in traffic accident

X● **V51.7**   Person on outside of pick-up truck or van injured in collision with pedal cycle in traffic accident

X● **V51.9**   Unspecified occupant of pick-up truck or van injured in collision with pedal cycle in traffic accident

● **V52**   **Occupant of pick-up truck or van injured in collision with two- or three-wheeled motor vehicle**

The appropriate 7th character is to be added to each code from category V52

A	initial encounter
D	subsequent encounter
S	sequela

X● **V52.0**   Driver of pick-up truck or van injured in collision with two- or three-wheeled motor vehicle in nontraffic accident

X● **V52.1**   Passenger in pick-up truck or van injured in collision with two- or three-wheeled motor vehicle in nontraffic accident

X● **V52.2**   Person on outside of pick-up truck or van injured in collision with two- or three-wheeled motor vehicle in nontraffic accident

X● **V52.3**   Unspecified occupant of pick-up truck or van injured in collision with two- or three-wheeled motor vehicle in nontraffic accident

X● **V52.4**   Person boarding or alighting a pick-up truck or van injured in collision with two- or three-wheeled motor vehicle

X● **V52.5**   Driver of pick-up truck or van injured in collision with two- or three-wheeled motor vehicle in traffic accident

X● **V52.6**   Passenger in pick-up truck or van injured in collision with two- or three-wheeled motor vehicle in traffic accident

X● **V52.7**   Person on outside of pick-up truck or van injured in collision with two- or three-wheeled motor vehicle in traffic accident

X● **V52.9**   Unspecified occupant of pick-up truck or van injured in collision with two- or three-wheeled motor vehicle in traffic accident

● **V53**   **Occupant of pick-up truck or van injured in collision with car, pick-up truck or van**

The appropriate 7th character is to be added to each code from category V53

A	initial encounter
D	subsequent encounter
S	sequela

X● **V53.0**   Driver of pick-up truck or van injured in collision with car, pick-up truck or van in nontraffic accident

X● **V53.1**   Passenger in pick-up truck or van injured in collision with car, pick-up truck or van in nontraffic accident

X● **V53.2**   Person on outside of pick-up truck or van injured in collision with car, pick-up truck or van in nontraffic accident

X● **V53.3**   Unspecified occupant of pick-up truck or van injured in collision with car, pick-up truck or van in nontraffic accident

X● **V53.4**   Person boarding or alighting a pick-up truck or van injured in collision with car, pick-up truck or van

X● **V53.5**   Driver of pick-up truck or van injured in collision with car, pick-up truck or van in traffic accident

X● **V53.6**   Passenger in pick-up truck or van injured in collision with car, pick-up truck or van in traffic accident

X● **V53.7**   Person on outside of pick-up truck or van injured in collision with car, pick-up truck or van in traffic accident

X● **V53.9**   Unspecified occupant of pick-up truck or van injured in collision with car, pick-up truck or van in traffic accident

● **V54**   **Occupant of pick-up truck or van injured in collision with heavy transport vehicle or bus**

> **Excludes1**   occupant of pick-up truck or van injured in collision with military vehicle (V59.81)

The appropriate 7th character is to be added to each code from category V54

A	initial encounter
D	subsequent encounter
S	sequela

X● **V54.0**   Driver of pick-up truck or van injured in collision with heavy transport vehicle or bus in nontraffic accident

X● **V54.1**   Passenger in pick-up truck or van injured in collision with heavy transport vehicle or bus in nontraffic accident

X● **V54.2**   Person on outside of pick-up truck or van injured in collision with heavy transport vehicle or bus in nontraffic accident

X● **V54.3**   Unspecified occupant of pick-up truck or van injured in collision with heavy transport vehicle or bus in nontraffic accident

X● **V54.4**   Person boarding or alighting a pick-up truck or van injured in collision with heavy transport vehicle or bus

X● **V54.5**   Driver of pick-up truck or van injured in collision with heavy transport vehicle or bus in traffic accident

X● **V54.6**   Passenger in pick-up truck or van injured in collision with heavy transport vehicle or bus in traffic accident

X● **V54.7**   Person on outside of pick-up truck or van injured in collision with heavy transport vehicle or bus in traffic accident

X● **V54.9**   Unspecified occupant of pick-up truck or van injured in collision with heavy transport vehicle or bus in traffic accident

CHAPTER 20 (V01-Y99)

◄ New   ◄█ Revised   ~~deleted~~ Deleted   Excludes 1   Excludes 2   Includes   Use additional   Code first   Code also   Unspecified

OGCR Official Guidelines   ● Unacceptable Principal Diagnosis   X Assign placeholder X   ● Use Additional Character(s)   ▶ Manifestation Code   Coding Clinic

● **V55 Occupant of pick-up truck or van injured in collision with railway train or railway vehicle**

The appropriate 7th character is to be added to each code from category V55

> A   initial encounter
> D   subsequent encounter
> S   sequela

X ● **V55.0** Driver of pick-up truck or van injured in collision with railway train or railway vehicle in nontraffic accident

X ● **V55.1** Passenger in pick-up truck or van injured in collision with railway train or railway vehicle in nontraffic accident

X ● **V55.2** Person on outside of pick-up truck or van injured in collision with railway train or railway vehicle in nontraffic accident

X ● **V55.3** Unspecified occupant of pick-up truck or van injured in collision with railway train or railway vehicle in nontraffic accident

X ● **V55.4** Person boarding or alighting a pick-up truck or van injured in collision with railway train or railway vehicle

X ● **V55.5** Driver of pick-up truck or van injured in collision with railway train or railway vehicle in traffic accident

X ● **V55.6** Passenger in pick-up truck or van injured in collision with railway train or railway vehicle in traffic accident

X ● **V55.7** Person on outside of pick-up truck or van injured in collision with railway train or railway vehicle in traffic accident

X ● **V55.9** Unspecified occupant of pick-up truck or van injured in collision with railway train or railway vehicle in traffic accident

● **V56 Occupant of pick-up truck or van injured in collision with other nonmotor vehicle**

> **Includes**   collision with animal-drawn vehicle, animal being ridden, streetcar

The appropriate 7th character is to be added to each code from category V56

> A   initial encounter
> D   subsequent encounter
> S   sequela

X ● **V56.0** Driver of pick-up truck or van injured in collision with other nonmotor vehicle in nontraffic accident

X ● **V56.1** Passenger in pick-up truck or van injured in collision with other nonmotor vehicle in nontraffic accident

X ● **V56.2** Person on outside of pick-up truck or van injured in collision with other nonmotor vehicle in nontraffic accident

X ● **V56.3** Unspecified occupant of pick-up truck or van injured in collision with other nonmotor vehicle in nontraffic accident

X ● **V56.4** Person boarding or alighting a pick-up truck or van injured in collision with other nonmotor vehicle

X ● **V56.5** Driver of pick-up truck or van injured in collision with other nonmotor vehicle in traffic accident

X ● **V56.6** Passenger in pick-up truck or van injured in collision with other nonmotor vehicle in traffic accident

X ● **V56.7** Person on outside of pick-up truck or van injured in collision with other nonmotor vehicle in traffic accident

X ● **V56.9** Unspecified occupant of pick-up truck or van injured in collision with other nonmotor vehicle in traffic accident

● **V57 Occupant of pick-up truck or van injured in collision with fixed or stationary object**

The appropriate 7th character is to be added to each code from category V57

> A   initial encounter
> D   subsequent encounter
> S   sequela

X ● **V57.0** Driver of pick-up truck or van injured in collision with fixed or stationary object in nontraffic accident

X ● **V57.1** Passenger in pick-up truck or van injured in collision with fixed or stationary object in nontraffic accident

X ● **V57.2** Person on outside of pick-up truck or van injured in collision with fixed or stationary object in nontraffic accident

X ● **V57.3** Unspecified occupant of pick-up truck or van injured in collision with fixed or stationary object in nontraffic accident

X ● **V57.4** Person boarding or alighting a pick-up truck or van injured in collision with fixed or stationary object

X ● **V57.5** Driver of pick-up truck or van injured in collision with fixed or stationary object in traffic accident

X ● **V57.6** Passenger in pick-up truck or van injured in collision with fixed or stationary object in traffic accident

X ● **V57.7** Person on outside of pick-up truck or van injured in collision with fixed or stationary object in traffic accident

X ● **V57.9** Unspecified occupant of pick-up truck or van injured in collision with fixed or stationary object in traffic accident

● **V58 Occupant of pick-up truck or van injured in noncollision transport accident**

> **Includes**   overturning pick-up truck or van NOS
> overturning pick-up truck or van without collision

The appropriate 7th character is to be added to each code from category V58

> A   initial encounter
> D   subsequent encounter
> S   sequela

X ● **V58.0** Driver of pick-up truck or van injured in noncollision transport accident in nontraffic accident

X ● **V58.1** Passenger in pick-up truck or van injured in noncollision transport accident in nontraffic accident

X ● **V58.2** Person on outside of pick-up truck or van injured in noncollision transport accident in nontraffic accident

X ● **V58.3** Unspecified occupant of pick-up truck or van injured in noncollision transport accident in nontraffic accident

X ● **V58.4** Person boarding or alighting a pick-up truck or van injured in noncollision transport accident

X ● **V58.5** Driver of pick-up truck or van injured in noncollision transport accident in traffic accident

X ● **V58.6** Passenger in pick-up truck or van injured in noncollision transport accident in traffic accident

X ● **V58.7** Person on outside of pick-up truck or van injured in noncollision transport accident in traffic accident

X ● **V58.9** Unspecified occupant of pick-up truck or van injured in noncollision transport accident in traffic accident

CHAPTER 20 (V01-Y99)

● **V59**   **Occupant of pick-up truck or van injured in other and unspecified transport accidents**

> The appropriate 7th character is to be added to each code from category V59

> | A | initial encounter |
> |---|---|
> | D | subsequent encounter |
> | S | sequela |

● **V59.0**   Driver of pick-up truck or van injured in collision with other and unspecified motor vehicles in nontraffic accident

X● **V59.00**   Driver of pick-up truck or van injured in collision with unspecified motor vehicles in nontraffic accident

X● **V59.09**   Driver of pick-up truck or van injured in collision with other motor vehicles in nontraffic accident

● **V59.1**   Passenger in pick-up truck or van injured in collision with other and unspecified motor vehicles in nontraffic accident

X● **V59.10**   Passenger in pick-up truck or van injured in collision with unspecified motor vehicles in nontraffic accident

X● **V59.19**   Passenger in pick-up truck or van injured in collision with other motor vehicles in nontraffic accident

● **V59.2**   Unspecified occupant of pick-up truck or van injured in collision with other and unspecified motor vehicles in nontraffic accident

X● **V59.20**   Unspecified occupant of pick-up truck or van injured in collision with unspecified motor vehicles in nontraffic accident
> Collision NOS involving pick-up truck or van, nontraffic

X● **V59.29**   Unspecified occupant of pick-up truck or van injured in collision with other motor vehicles in nontraffic accident

X● **V59.3**   Occupant (driver) (passenger) of pick-up truck or van injured in unspecified nontraffic accident
> Accident NOS involving pick-up truck or van, nontraffic
> Occupant of pick-up truck or van injured in nontraffic accident NOS

● **V59.4**   Driver of pick-up truck or van injured in collision with other and unspecified motor vehicles in traffic accident

X● **V59.40**   Driver of pick-up truck or van injured in collision with unspecified motor vehicles in traffic accident

X● **V59.49**   Driver of pick-up truck or van injured in collision with other motor vehicles in traffic accident

● **V59.5**   Passenger in pick-up truck or van injured in collision with other and unspecified motor vehicles in traffic accident

X● **V59.50**   Passenger in pick-up truck or van injured in collision with unspecified motor vehicles in traffic accident

X● **V59.59**   Passenger in pick-up truck or van injured in collision with other motor vehicles in traffic accident

● **V59.6**   Unspecified occupant of pick-up truck or van injured in collision with other and unspecified motor vehicles in traffic accident

X● **V59.60**   Unspecified occupant of pick-up truck or van injured in collision with unspecified motor vehicles in traffic accident
> Collision NOS involving pick-up truck or van (traffic)

X● **V59.69**   Unspecified occupant of pick-up truck or van injured in collision with other motor vehicles in traffic accident

● **V59.8**   Occupant (driver) (passenger) of pick-up truck or van injured in other specified transport accidents

X● **V59.81**   Occupant (driver) (passenger) of pick-up truck or van injured in transport accident with military vehicle

X● **V59.88**   Occupant (driver) (passenger) of pick-up truck or van injured in other specified transport accidents

X● **V59.9**   Occupant (driver) (passenger) of pick-up truck or van injured in unspecified traffic accident
> Accident NOS involving pick-up truck or van

OCCUPANT OF HEAVY TRANSPORT VEHICLE INJURED IN TRANSPORT ACCIDENT (V60-V69)

> **Includes**   18 wheeler
> armored car
> panel truck

> **Excludes 1**   bus
> motorcoach

● **V60**   **Occupant of heavy transport vehicle injured in collision with pedestrian or animal**

> **Excludes 1**   heavy transport vehicle collision with animal-drawn vehicle or animal being ridden (V66.-)

> The appropriate 7th character is to be added to each code from category V60

> | A | initial encounter |
> |---|---|
> | D | subsequent encounter |
> | S | sequela |

X● **V60.0**   Driver of heavy transport vehicle injured in collision with pedestrian or animal in nontraffic accident

X● **V60.1**   Passenger in heavy transport vehicle injured in collision with pedestrian or animal in nontraffic accident

X● **V60.2**   Person on outside of heavy transport vehicle injured in collision with pedestrian or animal in nontraffic accident

X● **V60.3**   Unspecified occupant of heavy transport vehicle injured in collision with pedestrian or animal in nontraffic accident

X● **V60.4**   Person boarding or alighting a heavy transport vehicle injured in collision with pedestrian or animal

X● **V60.5**   Driver of heavy transport vehicle injured in collision with pedestrian or animal in traffic accident

X● **V60.6**   Passenger in heavy transport vehicle injured in collision with pedestrian or animal in traffic accident

X● **V60.7**   Person on outside of heavy transport vehicle injured in collision with pedestrian or animal in traffic accident

X● **V60.9**   Unspecified occupant of heavy transport vehicle injured in collision with pedestrian or animal in traffic accident

● **V61**   **Occupant of heavy transport vehicle injured in collision with pedal cycle**

> The appropriate 7th character is to be added to each code from category V61

> | A | initial encounter |
> |---|---|
> | D | subsequent encounter |
> | S | sequela |

X● **V61.0**   Driver of heavy transport vehicle injured in collision with pedal cycle in nontraffic accident

X● **V61.1**   Passenger in heavy transport vehicle injured in collision with pedal cycle in nontraffic accident

X● **V61.2**   Person on outside of heavy transport vehicle injured in collision with pedal cycle in nontraffic accident

X● **V61.3**   Unspecified occupant of heavy transport vehicle injured in collision with pedal cycle in nontraffic accident

X● **V61.4**   Person boarding or alighting a heavy transport vehicle injured in collision with pedal cycle while boarding or alighting

X● **V61.5**   Driver of heavy transport vehicle injured in collision with pedal cycle in traffic accident

◀ New   ◀══ Revised   ~~deleted~~ Deleted   Excludes 1   Excludes 2   Includes   Use additional   Code first   Code also   Unspecified

OGCR Official Guidelines   ● Unacceptable Principal Diagnosis   X Assign placeholder X   ● Use Additional Character(s)   ▶ Manifestation Code   **Coding Clinic**

X● **V61.6** Passenger in heavy transport vehicle injured in collision with pedal cycle in traffic accident

X● **V61.7** Person on outside of heavy transport vehicle injured in collision with pedal cycle in traffic accident

X● **V61.9** Unspecified occupant of heavy transport vehicle injured in collision with pedal cycle in traffic accident

●**V62** Occupant of heavy transport vehicle injured in collision with two- or three-wheeled motor vehicle

The appropriate 7th character is to be added to each code from category V62

A	initial encounter
D	subsequent encounter
S	sequela

X● **V62.0** Driver of heavy transport vehicle injured in collision with two- or three-wheeled motor vehicle in nontraffic accident

X● **V62.1** Passenger in heavy transport vehicle injured in collision with two- or three-wheeled motor vehicle in nontraffic accident

X● **V62.2** Person on outside of heavy transport vehicle injured in collision with two- or three-wheeled motor vehicle in nontraffic accident

X● **V62.3** Unspecified occupant of heavy transport vehicle injured in collision with two- or three-wheeled motor vehicle in nontraffic accident

X● **V62.4** Person boarding or alighting a heavy transport vehicle injured in collision with two- or three-wheeled motor vehicle

X● **V62.5** Driver of heavy transport vehicle injured in collision with two- or three-wheeled motor vehicle in traffic accident

X● **V62.6** Passenger in heavy transport vehicle injured in collision with two- or three-wheeled motor vehicle in traffic accident

X● **V62.7** Person on outside of heavy transport vehicle injured in collision with two- or three-wheeled motor vehicle in traffic accident

X● **V62.9** Unspecified occupant of heavy transport vehicle injured in collision with two- or three-wheeled motor vehicle in traffic accident

●**V63** Occupant of heavy transport vehicle injured in collision with car, pick-up truck or van

The appropriate 7th character is to be added to each code from category V63

A	initial encounter
D	subsequent encounter
S	sequela

X● **V63.0** Driver of heavy transport vehicle injured in collision with car, pick-up truck or van in nontraffic accident

X● **V63.1** Passenger in heavy transport vehicle injured in collision with car, pick-up truck or van in nontraffic accident

X● **V63.2** Person on outside of heavy transport vehicle injured in collision with car, pick-up truck or van in nontraffic accident

X● **V63.3** Unspecified occupant of heavy transport vehicle injured in collision with car, pick-up truck or van in nontraffic accident

X● **V63.4** Person boarding or alighting a heavy transport vehicle injured in collision with car, pick-up truck or van

X● **V63.5** Driver of heavy transport vehicle injured in collision with car, pick-up truck or van in traffic accident

X● **V63.6** Passenger in heavy transport vehicle injured in collision with car, pick-up truck or van in traffic accident

X● **V63.7** Person on outside of heavy transport vehicle injured in collision with car, pick-up truck or van in traffic accident

X● **V63.9** Unspecified occupant of heavy transport vehicle injured in collision with car, pick-up truck or van in traffic accident

●**V64** Occupant of heavy transport vehicle injured in collision with heavy transport vehicle or bus

　　Excludes1　occupant of heavy transport vehicle injured in collision with military vehicle (V69.81)

The appropriate 7th character is to be added to each code from category V64

A	initial encounter
D	subsequent encounter
S	sequela

X● **V64.0** Driver of heavy transport vehicle injured in collision with heavy transport vehicle or bus in nontraffic accident

X● **V64.1** Passenger in heavy transport vehicle injured in collision with heavy transport vehicle or bus in nontraffic accident

X● **V64.2** Person on outside of heavy transport vehicle injured in collision with heavy transport vehicle or bus in nontraffic accident

X● **V64.3** Unspecified occupant of heavy transport vehicle injured in collision with heavy transport vehicle or bus in nontraffic accident

X● **V64.4** Person boarding or alighting a heavy transport vehicle injured in collision with heavy transport vehicle or bus while boarding or alighting

X● **V64.5** Driver of heavy transport vehicle injured in collision with heavy transport vehicle or bus in traffic accident

X● **V64.6** Passenger in heavy transport vehicle injured in collision with heavy transport vehicle or bus in traffic accident

X● **V64.7** Person on outside of heavy transport vehicle injured in collision with heavy transport vehicle or bus in traffic accident

X● **V64.9** Unspecified occupant of heavy transport vehicle injured in collision with heavy transport vehicle or bus in traffic accident

●**V65** Occupant of heavy transport vehicle injured in collision with railway train or railway vehicle

The appropriate 7th character is to be added to each code from category V65

A	initial encounter
D	subsequent encounter
S	sequela

X● **V65.0** Driver of heavy transport vehicle injured in collision with railway train or railway vehicle in nontraffic accident

X● **V65.1** Passenger in heavy transport vehicle injured in collision with railway train or railway vehicle in nontraffic accident

X● **V65.2** Person on outside of heavy transport vehicle injured in collision with railway train or railway vehicle in nontraffic accident

X● **V65.3** Unspecified occupant of heavy transport vehicle injured in collision with railway train or railway vehicle in nontraffic accident

X● **V65.4** Person boarding or alighting a heavy transport vehicle injured in collision with railway train or railway vehicle

X● **V65.5** Driver of heavy transport vehicle injured in collision with railway train or railway vehicle in traffic accident

X● **V65.6** Passenger in heavy transport vehicle injured in collision with railway train or railway vehicle in traffic accident

X● **V65.7** Person on outside of heavy transport vehicle injured in collision with railway train or railway vehicle in traffic accident

X● **V65.9** Unspecified occupant of heavy transport vehicle injured in collision with railway train or railway vehicle in traffic accident

N Newborn Age: Ø　　**P** Pediatric Age: Ø–17　　**M** Maternity DX: 12–55　　**A** Adult Age: 15–124　　♀ Females Only　　♂ Males Only

🅒 Complication\Comorbidity　　🅜 Major C\C　　(Ex) CC/MCC Exclusions　　🅗 Hospital-Acquired Condition

1541

● **V66**   **Occupant of heavy transport vehicle injured in collision with other nonmotor vehicle**

     Includes   collision with animal-drawn vehicle, animal being ridden, streetcar

     The appropriate 7th character is to be added to each code from category V66

A	initial encounter
D	subsequent encounter
S	sequela

X● **V66.0**   Driver of heavy transport vehicle injured in collision with other nonmotor vehicle in nontraffic accident

X● **V66.1**   Passenger in heavy transport vehicle injured in collision with other nonmotor vehicle in nontraffic accident

X● **V66.2**   Person on outside of heavy transport vehicle injured in collision with other nonmotor vehicle in nontraffic accident

X● **V66.3**   Unspecified occupant of heavy transport vehicle injured in collision with other nonmotor vehicle in nontraffic accident

X● **V66.4**   Person boarding or alighting a heavy transport vehicle injured in collision with other nonmotor vehicle

X● **V66.5**   Driver of heavy transport vehicle injured in collision with other nonmotor vehicle in traffic accident

X● **V66.6**   Passenger in heavy transport vehicle injured in collision with other nonmotor vehicle in traffic accident

X● **V66.7**   Person on outside of heavy transport vehicle injured in collision with other nonmotor vehicle in traffic accident

X● **V66.9**   Unspecified occupant of heavy transport vehicle injured in collision with other nonmotor vehicle in traffic accident

● **V67**   **Occupant of heavy transport vehicle injured in collision with fixed or stationary object**

     The appropriate 7th character is to be added to each code from category V67

A	initial encounter
D	subsequent encounter
S	sequela

X● **V67.0**   Driver of heavy transport vehicle injured in collision with fixed or stationary object in nontraffic accident

X● **V67.1**   Passenger in heavy transport vehicle injured in collision with fixed or stationary object in nontraffic accident

X● **V67.2**   Person on outside of heavy transport vehicle injured in collision with fixed or stationary object in nontraffic accident

X● **V67.3**   Unspecified occupant of heavy transport vehicle injured in collision with fixed or stationary object in nontraffic accident

X● **V67.4**   Person boarding or alighting a heavy transport vehicle injured in collision with fixed or stationary object

X● **V67.5**   Driver of heavy transport vehicle injured in collision with fixed or stationary object in traffic accident

X● **V67.6**   Passenger in heavy transport vehicle injured in collision with fixed or stationary object in traffic accident

X● **V67.7**   Person on outside of heavy transport vehicle injured in collision with fixed or stationary object in traffic accident

X● **V67.9**   Unspecified occupant of heavy transport vehicle injured in collision with fixed or stationary object in traffic accident

● **V68**   **Occupant of heavy transport vehicle injured in noncollision transport accident**

     Includes   overturning heavy transport vehicle NOS

                overturning heavy transport vehicle without collision

     The appropriate 7th character is to be added to each code from category V68

A	initial encounter
D	subsequent encounter
S	sequela

X● **V68.0**   Driver of heavy transport vehicle injured in noncollision transport accident in nontraffic accident

X● **V68.1**   Passenger in heavy transport vehicle injured in noncollision transport accident in nontraffic accident

X● **V68.2**   Person on outside of heavy transport vehicle injured in noncollision transport accident in nontraffic accident

X● **V68.3**   Unspecified occupant of heavy transport vehicle injured in noncollision transport accident in nontraffic accident

X● **V68.4**   Person boarding or alighting a heavy transport vehicle injured in noncollision transport accident

X● **V68.5**   Driver of heavy transport vehicle injured in noncollision transport accident in traffic accident

X● **V68.6**   Passenger in heavy transport vehicle injured in noncollision transport accident in traffic accident

X● **V68.7**   Person on outside of heavy transport vehicle injured in noncollision transport accident in traffic accident

X● **V68.9**   Unspecified occupant of heavy transport vehicle injured in noncollision transport accident in traffic accident

● **V69**   **Occupant of heavy transport vehicle injured in other and unspecified transport accidents**

     The appropriate 7th character is to be added to each code from category V69

A	initial encounter
D	subsequent encounter
S	sequela

● **V69.0**   Driver of heavy transport vehicle injured in collision with other and unspecified motor vehicles in nontraffic accident

     X● **V69.00**   Driver of heavy transport vehicle injured in collision with unspecified motor vehicles in nontraffic accident

     X● **V69.09**   Driver of heavy transport vehicle injured in collision with other motor vehicles in nontraffic accident

● **V69.1**   Passenger in heavy transport vehicle injured in collision with other and unspecified motor vehicles in nontraffic accident

     X● **V69.10**   Passenger in heavy transport vehicle injured in collision with unspecified motor vehicles in nontraffic accident

     X● **V69.19**   Passenger in heavy transport vehicle injured in collision with other motor vehicles in nontraffic accident

● **V69.2**   Unspecified occupant of heavy transport vehicle injured in collision with other and unspecified motor vehicles in nontraffic accident

     X● **V69.20**   Unspecified occupant of heavy transport vehicle injured in collision with unspecified motor vehicles in nontraffic accident

          Collision NOS involving heavy transport vehicle, nontraffic

     X● **V69.29**   Unspecified occupant of heavy transport vehicle injured in collision with other motor vehicles in nontraffic accident

◀ New   ◀▥ Revised   ~~deleted~~ Deleted   Excludes 1   Excludes 2   Includes   Use additional   Code first   Code also   Unspecified

OGCR Official Guidelines   ● Unacceptable Principal Diagnosis   X Assign placeholder X   ● Use Additional Character(s)   ▶ Manifestation Code   **Coding Clinic**

X ● **V69.3**   **Occupant (driver) (passenger) of heavy transport vehicle injured in unspecified nontraffic accident**
     Accident NOS involving heavy transport vehicle, nontraffic
     Occupant of heavy transport vehicle injured in nontraffic accident NOS

● **V69.4**   **Driver of heavy transport vehicle injured in collision with other and unspecified motor vehicles in traffic accident**

   X ● **V69.40**   **Driver of heavy transport vehicle injured in collision with unspecified motor vehicles in traffic accident**

   X ● **V69.49**   **Driver of heavy transport vehicle injured in collision with other motor vehicles in traffic accident**

● **V69.5**   **Passenger in heavy transport vehicle injured in collision with other and unspecified motor vehicles in traffic accident**

   X ● **V69.50**   **Passenger in heavy transport vehicle injured in collision with unspecified motor vehicles in traffic accident**

   X ● **V69.59**   **Passenger in heavy transport vehicle injured in collision with other motor vehicles in traffic accident**

● **V69.6**   **Unspecified occupant of heavy transport vehicle injured in collision with other and unspecified motor vehicles in traffic accident**

   X ● **V69.60**   **Unspecified occupant of heavy transport vehicle injured in collision with unspecified motor vehicles in traffic accident**
       Collision NOS involving heavy transport vehicle (traffic)

   X ● **V69.69**   **Unspecified occupant of heavy transport vehicle injured in collision with other motor vehicles in traffic accident**

● **V69.8**   **Occupant (driver) (passenger) of heavy transport vehicle injured in other specified transport accidents**

   X ● **V69.81**   **Occupant (driver) (passenger) of heavy transport vehicle injured in transport accidents with military vehicle**

   X ● **V69.88**   **Occupant (driver) (passenger) of heavy transport vehicle injured in other specified transport accidents**

X ● **V69.9**   **Occupant (driver) (passenger) of heavy transport vehicle injured in unspecified traffic accident**
     Accident NOS involving heavy transport vehicle

BUS OCCUPANT INJURED IN TRANSPORT ACCIDENT (V70-V79)

Includes   motorcoach
Excludes1   minibus (V50-V59)

● **V70**   **Bus occupant injured in collision with pedestrian or animal**
     Excludes1   bus collision with animal-drawn vehicle or animal being ridden (V76.-)

     The appropriate 7th character is to be added to each code from category V70

     | A | initial encounter |
     | D | subsequent encounter |
     | S | sequela |

X ● **V70.0**   **Driver of bus injured in collision with pedestrian or animal in nontraffic accident**

X ● **V70.1**   **Passenger on bus injured in collision with pedestrian or animal in nontraffic accident**

X ● **V70.2**   **Person on outside of bus injured in collision with pedestrian or animal in nontraffic accident**

X ● **V70.3**   **Unspecified occupant of bus injured in collision with pedestrian or animal in nontraffic accident**

X ● **V70.4**   **Person boarding or alighting from bus injured in collision with pedestrian or animal**

X ● **V70.5**   **Driver of bus injured in collision with pedestrian or animal in traffic accident**

X ● **V70.6**   **Passenger on bus injured in collision with pedestrian or animal in traffic accident**

X ● **V70.7**   **Person on outside of bus injured in collision with pedestrian or animal in traffic accident**

X ● **V70.9**   **Unspecified occupant of bus injured in collision with pedestrian or animal in traffic accident**

● **V71**   **Bus occupant injured in collision with pedal cycle**
     The appropriate 7th character is to be added to each code from category V71

     | A | initial encounter |
     | D | subsequent encounter |
     | S | sequela |

X ● **V71.0**   **Driver of bus injured in collision with pedal cycle in nontraffic accident**

X ● **V71.1**   **Passenger on bus injured in collision with pedal cycle in nontraffic accident**

X ● **V71.2**   **Person on outside of bus injured in collision with pedal cycle in nontraffic accident**

X ● **V71.3**   **Unspecified occupant of bus injured in collision with pedal cycle in nontraffic accident**

X ● **V71.4**   **Person boarding or alighting from bus injured in collision with pedal cycle**

X ● **V71.5**   **Driver of bus injured in collision with pedal cycle in traffic accident**

X ● **V71.6**   **Passenger on bus injured in collision with pedal cycle in traffic accident**

X ● **V71.7**   **Person on outside of bus injured in collision with pedal cycle in traffic accident**

X ● **V71.9**   **Unspecified occupant of bus injured in collision with pedal cycle in traffic accident**

● **V72**   **Bus occupant injured in collision with two- or three-wheeled motor vehicle**
     The appropriate 7th character is to be added to each code from category V72

     | A | initial encounter |
     | D | subsequent encounter |
     | S | sequela |

X ● **V72.0**   **Driver of bus injured in collision with two- or three-wheeled motor vehicle in nontraffic accident**

X ● **V72.1**   **Passenger on bus injured in collision with two- or three-wheeled motor vehicle in nontraffic accident**

X ● **V72.2**   **Person on outside of bus injured in collision with two- or three-wheeled motor vehicle in nontraffic accident**

X ● **V72.3**   **Unspecified occupant of bus injured in collision with two- or three-wheeled motor vehicle in nontraffic accident**

X ● **V72.4**   **Person boarding or alighting from bus injured in collision with two- or three-wheeled motor vehicle**

X ● **V72.5**   **Driver of bus injured in collision with two- or three-wheeled motor vehicle in traffic accident**

X ● **V72.6**   **Passenger on bus injured in collision with two- or three-wheeled motor vehicle in traffic accident**

X ● **V72.7**   **Person on outside of bus injured in collision with two- or three-wheeled motor vehicle in traffic accident**

X ● **V72.9**   **Unspecified occupant of bus injured in collision with two- or three-wheeled motor vehicle in traffic accident**

CHAPTER 20 (V01-Y99)

● **V73** **Bus occupant injured in collision with car, pick-up truck or van**

The appropriate 7th character is to be added to each code from category V73

A	initial encounter
D	subsequent encounter
S	sequela

X● **V73.0** Driver of bus injured in collision with car, pick-up truck or van in nontraffic accident

X● **V73.1** Passenger on bus injured in collision with car, pick-up truck or van in nontraffic accident

X● **V73.2** Person on outside of bus injured in collision with car, pick-up truck or van in nontraffic accident

X● **V73.3** Unspecified occupant of bus injured in collision with car, pick-up truck or van in nontraffic accident

X● **V73.4** Person boarding or alighting from bus injured in collision with car, pick-up truck or van

X● **V73.5** Driver of bus injured in collision with car, pick-up truck or van in traffic accident

X● **V73.6** Passenger on bus injured in collision with car, pick-up truck or van in traffic accident

X● **V73.7** Person on outside of bus injured in collision with car, pick-up truck or van in traffic accident

X● **V73.9** Unspecified occupant of bus injured in collision with car, pick-up truck or van in traffic accident

● **V74** **Bus occupant injured in collision with heavy transport vehicle or bus**

Excludes1 bus occupant injured in collision with military vehicle (V79.81)

The appropriate 7th character is to be added to each code from category V74

A	initial encounter
D	subsequent encounter
S	sequela

X● **V74.0** Driver of bus injured in collision with heavy transport vehicle or bus in nontraffic accident

X● **V74.1** Passenger on bus injured in collision with heavy transport vehicle or bus in nontraffic accident

X● **V74.2** Person on outside of bus injured in collision with heavy transport vehicle or bus in nontraffic accident

X● **V74.3** Unspecified occupant of bus injured in collision with heavy transport vehicle or bus in nontraffic accident

X● **V74.4** Person boarding or alighting from bus injured in collision with heavy transport vehicle or bus

X● **V74.5** Driver of bus injured in collision with heavy transport vehicle or bus in traffic accident

X● **V74.6** Passenger on bus injured in collision with heavy transport vehicle or bus in traffic accident

X● **V74.7** Person on outside of bus injured in collision with heavy transport vehicle or bus in traffic accident

X● **V74.9** Unspecified occupant of bus injured in collision with heavy transport vehicle or bus in traffic accident

● **V75** **Bus occupant injured in collision with railway train or railway vehicle**

The appropriate 7th character is to be added to each code from category V75

A	initial encounter
D	subsequent encounter
S	sequela

X● **V75.0** Driver of bus injured in collision with railway train or railway vehicle in nontraffic accident

X● **V75.1** Passenger on bus injured in collision with railway train or railway vehicle in nontraffic accident

X● **V75.2** Person on outside of bus injured in collision with railway train or railway vehicle in nontraffic accident

X● **V75.3** Unspecified occupant of bus injured in collision with railway train or railway vehicle in nontraffic accident

X● **V75.4** Person boarding or alighting from bus injured in collision with railway train or railway vehicle

X● **V75.5** Driver of bus injured in collision with railway train or railway vehicle in traffic accident

X● **V75.6** Passenger on bus injured in collision with railway train or railway vehicle in traffic accident

X● **V75.7** Person on outside of bus injured in collision with railway train or railway vehicle in traffic accident

X● **V75.9** Unspecified occupant of bus injured in collision with railway train or railway vehicle in traffic accident

● **V76** **Bus occupant injured in collision with other nonmotor vehicle**

Includes collision with animal-drawn vehicle, animal being ridden, streetcar

The appropriate 7th character is to be added to each code from category V76

A	initial encounter
D	subsequent encounter
S	sequela

X● **V76.0** Driver of bus injured in collision with other nonmotor vehicle in nontraffic accident

X● **V76.1** Passenger on bus injured in collision with other nonmotor vehicle in nontraffic accident

X● **V76.2** Person on outside of bus injured in collision with other nonmotor vehicle in nontraffic accident

X● **V76.3** Unspecified occupant of bus injured in collision with other nonmotor vehicle in nontraffic accident

X● **V76.4** Person boarding or alighting from bus injured in collision with other nonmotor vehicle

X● **V76.5** Driver of bus injured in collision with other nonmotor vehicle in traffic accident

X● **V76.6** Passenger on bus injured in collision with other nonmotor vehicle in traffic accident

X● **V76.7** Person on outside of bus injured in collision with other nonmotor vehicle in traffic accident

X● **V76.9** Unspecified occupant of bus injured in collision with other nonmotor vehicle in traffic accident

● **V77** **Bus occupant injured in collision with fixed or stationary object**

The appropriate 7th character is to be added to each code from category V77

A	initial encounter
D	subsequent encounter
S	sequela

X● **V77.0** Driver of bus injured in collision with fixed or stationary object in nontraffic accident

X● **V77.1** Passenger on bus injured in collision with fixed or stationary object in nontraffic accident

X● **V77.2** Person on outside of bus injured in collision with fixed or stationary object in nontraffic accident

X● **V77.3** Unspecified occupant of bus injured in collision with fixed or stationary object in nontraffic accident

X● **V77.4** Person boarding or alighting from bus injured in collision with fixed or stationary object

X● **V77.5** Driver of bus injured in collision with fixed or stationary object in traffic accident

X● **V77.6** Passenger on bus injured in collision with fixed or stationary object in traffic accident

X● **V77.7** Person on outside of bus injured in collision with fixed or stationary object in traffic accident

X● **V77.9** Unspecified occupant of bus injured in collision with fixed or stationary object in traffic accident

◀ New ◀ Revised ~~deleted~~ Deleted | Excludes 1 | Excludes 2 | Includes | Use additional | Code first | Code also | Unspecified

OGCR Official Guidelines ● Unacceptable Principal Diagnosis X Assign placeholder X ● Use Additional Character(s) ▶ Manifestation Code **Coding Clinic**

X ● **V78** **Bus occupant injured in noncollision transport accident**

 Includes overturning bus NOS
     overturning bus without collision

 The appropriate 7th character is to be added to each code from category V78

A	initial encounter
D	subsequent encounter
S	sequela

X ● **V78.0** **Driver of bus injured in noncollision transport accident in nontraffic accident**

X ● **V78.1** **Passenger on bus injured in noncollision transport accident in nontraffic accident**

X ● **V78.2** **Person on outside of bus injured in noncollision transport accident in nontraffic accident**

X ● **V78.3** Unspecified **occupant of bus injured in noncollision transport accident in nontraffic accident**

X ● **V78.4** **Person boarding or alighting from bus injured in noncollision transport accident**

X ● **V78.5** **Driver of bus injured in noncollision transport accident in traffic accident**

X ● **V78.6** **Passenger on bus injured in noncollision transport accident in traffic accident**

X ● **V78.7** **Person on outside of bus injured in noncollision transport accident in traffic accident**

X ● **V78.9** Unspecified **occupant of bus injured in noncollision transport accident in traffic accident**

● **V79** **Bus occupant injured in other and unspecified transport accidents**

 The appropriate 7th character is to be added to each code from category V79

A	initial encounter
D	subsequent encounter
S	sequela

● **V79.0** **Driver of bus injured in collision with other and unspecified motor vehicles in nontraffic accident**

 X ● **V79.00** **Driver of bus injured in collision with** unspecified **motor vehicles in nontraffic accident**

 X ● **V79.09** **Driver of bus injured in collision with other motor vehicles in nontraffic accident**

● **V79.1** **Passenger on bus injured in collision with other and unspecified motor vehicles in nontraffic accident**

 X ● **V79.10** **Passenger on bus injured in collision with** unspecified **motor vehicles in nontraffic accident**

 X ● **V79.19** **Passenger on bus injured in collision with other motor vehicles in nontraffic accident**

● **V79.2** **Unspecified bus occupant injured in collision with other and unspecified motor vehicles in nontraffic accident**

 X ● **V79.20** Unspecified **bus occupant injured in collision with unspecified motor vehicles in nontraffic accident**

   Bus collision NOS, nontraffic

 X ● **V79.29** Unspecified **bus occupant injured in collision with other motor vehicles in nontraffic accident**

X ● **V79.3** **Bus occupant (driver) (passenger) injured in** unspecified **nontraffic accident**

  Bus accident NOS, nontraffic
  Bus occupant injured in nontraffic accident NOS

● **V79.4** **Driver of bus injured in collision with other and unspecified motor vehicles in traffic accident**

 X ● **V79.40** **Driver of bus injured in collision with** unspecified **motor vehicles in traffic accident**

 X ● **V79.49** **Driver of bus injured in collision with other motor vehicles in traffic accident**

● **V79.5** **Passenger on bus injured in collision with other and unspecified motor vehicles in traffic accident**

 X ● **V79.50** **Passenger on bus injured in collision with** unspecified **motor vehicles in traffic accident**

 X ● **V79.59** **Passenger on bus injured in collision with other motor vehicles in traffic accident**

● **V79.6** **Unspecified bus occupant injured in collision with other and unspecified motor vehicles in traffic accident**

 X ● **V79.60** Unspecified **bus occupant injured in collision with unspecified motor vehicles in traffic accident**

   Bus collision NOS (traffic)

 X ● **V79.69** Unspecified **bus occupant injured in collision with other motor vehicles in traffic accident**

● **V79.8** **Bus occupant (driver) (passenger) injured in other specified transport accidents**

 X ● **V79.81** **Bus occupant (driver) (passenger) injured in transport accidents with military vehicle**

 X ● **V79.88** **Bus occupant (driver) (passenger) injured in other specified transport accidents**

X ● **V79.9** **Bus occupant (driver) (passenger) injured in** unspecified **traffic accident**

  Bus accident NOS

OTHER LAND TRANSPORT ACCIDENTS (V80-V89)

● **V80** **Animal-rider or occupant of animal-drawn vehicle injured in transport accident**

 The appropriate 7th character is to be added to each code from category V80

A	initial encounter
D	subsequent encounter
S	sequela

● **V80.0** **Animal-rider or occupant of animal drawn vehicle injured by fall from or being thrown from animal or animal-drawn vehicle in noncollision accident**

 ● **V80.01** **Animal-rider injured by fall from or being thrown from animal in noncollision accident**

  ● **V80.010** **Animal-rider injured by fall from or being thrown from horse in noncollision accident**

  ● **V80.018** **Animal-rider injured by fall from or being thrown from other animal in noncollision accident**

 X ● **V80.02** **Occupant of animal-drawn vehicle injured by fall from or being thrown from animal-drawn vehicle in noncollision accident**

  Overturning animal-drawn vehicle NOS
  Overturning animal-drawn vehicle without collision

● **V80.1** **Animal-rider or occupant of animal-drawn vehicle injured in collision with pedestrian or animal**

 Excludes1 animal-rider or animal-drawn vehicle collision with animal-drawn vehicle or animal being ridden (V80.7)

 X ● **V80.11** **Animal-rider injured in collision with pedestrian or animal**

 X ● **V80.12** **Occupant of animal-drawn vehicle injured in collision with pedestrian or animal**

● **V80.2** **Animal-rider or occupant of animal-drawn vehicle injured in collision with pedal cycle**

 X ● **V80.21** **Animal-rider injured in collision with pedal cycle**

 X ● **V80.22** **Occupant of animal-drawn vehicle injured in collision with pedal cycle**

N Newborn Age: 0 P Pediatric Age: 0–17 M Maternity DX: 12–55 A Adult Age: 15–124 ♀ Females Only ♂ Males Only

  Complication\Comorbidity Major C\C (Ex) CC/MCC Exclusions Hospital-Acquired Condition   **1545**

● **V80.3** **Animal-rider or occupant of animal-drawn vehicle injured in collision with two- or three-wheeled motor vehicle**

X● **V80.31** Animal-rider injured in collision with two- or three-wheeled motor vehicle

X● **V80.32** Occupant of animal-drawn vehicle injured in collision with two- or three-wheeled motor vehicle

● **V80.4** **Animal-rider or occupant of animal-drawn vehicle injured in collision with car, pick-up truck, van, heavy transport vehicle or bus**

> **Excludes1**   animal-rider injured in collision with military vehicle (V80.910)
> occupant of animal-drawn vehicle injured in collision with military vehicle (V80.920)

X● **V80.41** Animal-rider injured in collision with car, pick-up truck, van, heavy transport vehicle or bus

X● **V80.42** Occupant of animal-drawn vehicle injured in collision with car, pick-up truck, van, heavy transport vehicle or bus

● **V80.5** **Animal-rider or occupant of animal-drawn vehicle injured in collision with other specified motor vehicle**

X● **V80.51** Animal-rider injured in collision with other specified motor vehicle

X● **V80.52** Occupant of animal-drawn vehicle injured in collision with other specified motor vehicle

● **V80.6** **Animal-rider or occupant of animal-drawn vehicle injured in collision with railway train or railway vehicle**

X● **V80.61** Animal-rider injured in collision with railway train or railway vehicle

X● **V80.62** Occupant of animal-drawn vehicle injured in collision with railway train or railway vehicle

● **V80.7** **Animal-rider or occupant of animal-drawn vehicle injured in collision with other nonmotor vehicles**

● **V80.71** Animal-rider or occupant of animal-drawn vehicle injured in collision with animal being ridden

    ● **V80.710** Animal-rider injured in collision with other animal being ridden

    ● **V80.711** Occupant of animal-drawn vehicle injured in collision with animal being ridden

● **V80.72** Animal-rider or occupant of animal-drawn vehicle injured in collision with other animal-drawn vehicle

    ● **V80.720** Animal-rider injured in collision with animal-drawn vehicle

    ● **V80.721** Occupant of animal-drawn vehicle injured in collision with other animal-drawn vehicle

● **V80.73** Animal-rider or occupant of animal-drawn vehicle injured in collision with streetcar

    ● **V80.730** Animal-rider injured in collision with streetcar

    ● **V80.731** Occupant of animal-drawn vehicle injured in collision with streetcar

● **V80.79** Animal-rider or occupant of animal-drawn vehicle injured in collision with other nonmotor vehicles

    ● **V80.790** Animal-rider injured in collision with other nonmotor vehicles

    ● **V80.791** Occupant of animal-drawn vehicle injured in collision with other nonmotor vehicles

● **V80.8** **Animal-rider or occupant of animal-drawn vehicle injured in collision with fixed or stationary object**

X● **V80.81** Animal-rider injured in collision with fixed or stationary object

X● **V80.82** Occupant of animal-drawn vehicle injured in collision with fixed or stationary object

● **V80.9** **Animal-rider or occupant of animal-drawn vehicle injured in other and unspecified transport accidents**

● **V80.91** Animal-rider injured in other and unspecified transport accidents

    ● **V80.910** Animal-rider injured in transport accident with military vehicle

    ● **V80.918** Animal-rider injured in other transport accident

    ● **V80.919** Animal-rider injured in <mark>unspecified</mark> transport accident
        Animal rider accident NOS

● **V80.92** Occupant of animal-drawn vehicle injured in other and unspecified transport accidents

    ● **V80.920** Occupant of animal-drawn vehicle injured in transport accident with military vehicle

    ● **V80.928** Occupant of animal-drawn vehicle injured in other transport accident

    ● **V80.929** Occupant of animal-drawn vehicle injured in <mark>unspecified</mark> transport accident
        Animal-drawn vehicle accident NOS

● **V81** **Occupant of railway train or railway vehicle injured in transport accident**

> **Includes**   derailment of railway train or railway vehicle
> person on outside of train

> **Excludes1**   streetcar (V82.-)

The appropriate 7th character is to be added to each code from category V81

A	initial encounter
D	subsequent encounter
S	sequela

X● **V81.0** **Occupant of railway train or railway vehicle injured in collision with motor vehicle in nontraffic accident**

> **Excludes1**   occupant of railway train or railway vehicle injured due to collision with military vehicle (V81.83)

X● **V81.1** **Occupant of railway train or railway vehicle injured in collision with motor vehicle in traffic accident**

> **Excludes1**   occupant of railway train or railway vehicle injured due to collision with military vehicle (V81.83)

X● **V81.2** **Occupant of railway train or railway vehicle injured in collision with or hit by rolling stock**

X● **V81.3** **Occupant of railway train or railway vehicle injured in collision with other object**
    Railway collision NOS

X● **V81.4** **Person injured while boarding or alighting from railway train or railway vehicle**

X● **V81.5** **Occupant of railway train or railway vehicle injured by fall in railway train or railway vehicle**

X● **V81.6** **Occupant of railway train or railway vehicle injured by fall from railway train or railway vehicle**

X● **V81.7** **Occupant of railway train or railway vehicle injured in derailment without antecedent collision**

◀ New   ◀▪▪ Revised   ~~deleted~~ Deleted   Excludes 1   Excludes 2   Includes   Use additional   Code first   Code also   Unspecified

OGCR Official Guidelines   ● Unacceptable Principal Diagnosis   X Assign placeholder X   ● Use Additional Character(s)   ▸ Manifestation Code   **Coding Clinic**

● **V81.8**   **Occupant of railway train or railway vehicle injured in other specified railway accidents**

   X● **V81.81**   **Occupant of railway train or railway vehicle injured due to explosion or fire on train**

   X● **V81.82**   **Occupant of railway train or railway vehicle injured due to object falling onto train**

     Occupant of railway train or railway vehicle injured due to falling earth onto train

     Occupant of railway train or railway vehicle injured due to falling rocks onto train

     Occupant of railway train or railway vehicle injured due to falling snow onto train

     Occupant of railway train or railway vehicle injured due to falling trees onto train

   X● **V81.83**   **Occupant of railway train or railway vehicle injured due to collision with military vehicle**

   X● **V81.89**   **Occupant of railway train or railway vehicle injured due to other specified railway accident**

  X● **V81.9**   **Occupant of railway train or railway vehicle injured in** unspecified **railway accident**

     Railway accident NOS

● **V82**   **Occupant of powered streetcar injured in transport accident**

    Includes   interurban electric car
          person on outside of streetcar
          tram (car)
          trolley (car)

    Excludes1   bus (V70-V79)
          motorcoach (V70-V79)
          nonpowered streetcar (V76.-)
          train (V81.-)

The appropriate 7th character is to be added to each code from category V82

A	initial encounter
D	subsequent encounter
S	sequela

  X● **V82.0**   **Occupant of streetcar injured in collision with motor vehicle in nontraffic accident**

  X● **V82.1**   **Occupant of streetcar injured in collision with motor vehicle in traffic accident**

  X● **V82.2**   **Occupant of streetcar injured in collision with or hit by rolling stock**

  X● **V82.3**   **Occupant of streetcar injured in collision with other object**

    Excludes1   collision with animal-drawn vehicle or animal being ridden (V82.8)

  X● **V82.4**   **Person injured while boarding or alighting from streetcar**

  X● **V82.5**   **Occupant of streetcar injured by fall in streetcar**

    Excludes1   fall in streetcar:
          while boarding or alighting (V82.4)
          with antecedent collision (V82.0-V82.3)

  X● **V82.6**   **Occupant of streetcar injured by fall from streetcar**

    Excludes1   fall from streetcar:
          while boarding or alighting (V82.4)
          with antecedent collision (V82.0-V82.3)

  X● **V82.7**   **Occupant of streetcar injured in derailment without antecedent collision**

    Excludes1   occupant of streetcar injured in derailment with antecedent collision (V82.0-V82.3)

  X● **V82.8**   **Occupant of streetcar injured in other specified transport accidents**

     Streetcar collision with military vehicle
     Streetcar collision with train or nonmotor vehicles

  X● **V82.9**   **Occupant of streetcar injured in** unspecified **traffic accident**

     Streetcar accident NOS

● **V83**   **Occupant of special vehicle mainly used on industrial premises injured in transport accident**

    Includes   battery-powered airport passenger vehicle
          battery-powered truck (baggage) (mail)
          coal-car in mine
          forklift (truck)
          logging car
          self-propelled industrial truck
          station baggage truck (powered)
          tram, truck, or tub (powered) in mine or quarry

    Excludes1   special construction vehicles (V85.-)
          special industrial vehicle in stationary use or maintenance (W31.-)

The appropriate 7th character is to be added to each code from category V83

A	initial encounter
D	subsequent encounter
S	sequela

  X● **V83.0**   **Driver of special industrial vehicle injured in traffic accident**

  X● **V83.1**   **Passenger of special industrial vehicle injured in traffic accident**

  X● **V83.2**   **Person on outside of special industrial vehicle injured in traffic accident**

  X● **V83.3**   Unspecified **occupant of special industrial vehicle injured in traffic accident**

  X● **V83.4**   **Person injured while boarding or alighting from special industrial vehicle**

  X● **V83.5**   **Driver of special industrial vehicle injured in nontraffic accident**

  X● **V83.6**   **Passenger of special industrial vehicle injured in nontraffic accident**

  X● **V83.7**   **Person on outside of special industrial vehicle injured in nontraffic accident**

  X● **V83.9**   Unspecified **occupant of special industrial vehicle injured in nontraffic accident**

     Special-industrial-vehicle accident NOS

● **V84**   **Occupant of special vehicle mainly used in agriculture injured in transport accident**

    Includes   self-propelled farm machinery
          tractor (and trailer)

    Excludes1   animal-powered farm machinery accident (W30.8-)
          contact with combine harvester (W30.0)
          special agricultural vehicle in stationary use or maintenance (W30.-)

The appropriate 7th character is to be added to each code from category V84

A	initial encounter
D	subsequent encounter
S	sequela

  X● **V84.0**   **Driver of special agricultural vehicle injured in traffic accident**

  X● **V84.1**   **Passenger of special agricultural vehicle injured in traffic accident**

  X● **V84.2**   **Person on outside of special agricultural vehicle injured in traffic accident**

  X● **V84.3**   Unspecified **occupant of special agricultural vehicle injured in traffic accident**

  X● **V84.4**   **Person injured while boarding or alighting from special agricultural vehicle**

  X● **V84.5**   **Driver of special agricultural vehicle injured in nontraffic accident**

  X● **V84.6**   **Passenger of special agricultural vehicle injured in nontraffic accident**

  X● **V84.7**   **Person on outside of special agricultural vehicle injured in nontraffic accident**

  X● **V84.9**   Unspecified **occupant of special agricultural vehicle injured in nontraffic accident**

     Special-agricultural vehicle accident NOS

CHAPTER 20 (V01-Y99)

● **V85 Occupant of special construction vehicle injured in transport accident**

> **Includes**   bulldozer
> digger
> dump truck
> earth-leveller
> mechanical shovel
> road-roller

> **Excludes1**   special industrial vehicle (V83.-)
> special construction vehicle in stationary use or maintenance (W31.-)

The appropriate 7th character is to be added to each code from category V85

> A   initial encounter
> D   subsequent encounter
> S   sequela

X● **V85.0 Driver of special construction vehicle injured in traffic accident**

X● **V85.1 Passenger of special construction vehicle injured in traffic accident**

X● **V85.2 Person on outside of special construction vehicle injured in traffic accident**

X● **V85.3 Unspecified occupant of special construction vehicle injured in traffic accident**

X● **V85.4 Person injured while boarding or alighting from special construction vehicle**

X● **V85.5 Driver of special construction vehicle injured in nontraffic accident**

X● **V85.6 Passenger of special construction vehicle injured in nontraffic accident**

X● **V85.7 Person on outside of special construction vehicle injured in nontraffic accident**

X● **V85.9 Unspecified occupant of special construction vehicle injured in nontraffic accident**
> Special-construction-vehicle accident NOS

● **V86 Occupant of special all-terrain or other off-road motor vehicle, injured in transport accident**

> **Excludes1**   special all-terrain vehicle in stationary use or maintenance (W31.-)
> sport-utility vehicle (V50-V59)
> three-wheeled motor vehicle designed for on-road use (V30-V39)

The appropriate 7th character is to be added to each code from category V86

> A   initial encounter
> D   subsequent encounter
> S   sequela

● **V86.0 Driver of special all-terrain or other off-road motor vehicle injured in traffic accident**

X● **V86.01 Driver of ambulance or fire engine injured in traffic accident**

X● **V86.02 Driver of snowmobile injured in traffic accident**

X● **V86.03 Driver of dune buggy injured in traffic accident**

X● **V86.04 Driver of military vehicle injured in traffic accident**

X● **V86.09 Driver of other off-road special all-terrain or other off-road vehicle injured in traffic accident**
> Driver of dirt bike injured in traffic accident
> Driver of go cart injured in traffic accident
> Driver of golf cart injured in traffic accident

● **V86.1 Passenger of special all-terrain or other off-road motor vehicle injured in traffic accident**

X● **V86.11 Passenger of ambulance or fire engine injured in traffic accident**

X● **V86.12 Passenger of snowmobile injured in traffic accident**

X● **V86.13 Passenger of dune buggy injured in traffic accident**

X● **V86.14 Passenger of military vehicle injured in traffic accident**

X● **V86.19 Passenger of other off-road special all-terrain or other off-road off-road motor vehicle injured in traffic accident**
> Passenger of dirt bike injured in traffic accident
> Passenger of go cart injured in traffic accident
> Passenger of golf cart injured in traffic accident

● **V86.2 Person on outside of special all-terrain or other off-road motor vehicle injured in traffic accident**

X● **V86.21 Person on outside of ambulance or fire engine injured in traffic accident**

X● **V86.22 Person on outside of snowmobile injured in traffic accident**

X● **V86.23 Person on outside of dune buggy injured in traffic accident**

X● **V86.24 Person on outside of military vehicle injured in traffic accident**

X● **V86.29 Person on outside of other special all-terrain or other off-road motor vehicle injured in traffic accident**
> Person on outside of dirt bike injured in traffic accident
> Person on outside of go cart in traffic accident
> Person on outside of golf cart injured in traffic accident

● **V86.3 Unspecified occupant of special all-terrain or other off-road motor vehicle injured in traffic accident**

X● **V86.31 Unspecified occupant of ambulance or fire engine injured in traffic accident**

X● **V86.32 Unspecified occupant of snowmobile injured in traffic accident**

X● **V86.33 Unspecified occupant of dune buggy injured in traffic accident**

X● **V86.34 Unspecified occupant of military vehicle injured in traffic accident**

X● **V86.39 Unspecified occupant of other special all-terrain or other off-road motor vehicle injured in traffic accident**
> Unspecified occupant of dirt bike injured in traffic accident
> Unspecified occupant of go cart injured in traffic accident
> Unspecified occupant of golf cart injured in traffic accident

● **V86.4 Person injured while boarding or alighting from special all-terrain or other off-road motor vehicle**

X● **V86.41 Person injured while boarding or alighting from ambulance or fire engine**

X● **V86.42 Person injured while boarding or alighting from snowmobile**

X● **V86.43 Person injured while boarding or alighting from dune buggy**

X● **V86.44 Person injured while boarding or alighting from military vehicle**

X● **V86.49 Person injured while boarding or alighting from other special all-terrain or other off-road motor vehicle**
> Person injured while boarding or alighting from dirt bike
> Person injured while boarding or alighting from go cart
> Person injured while boarding or alighting from golf cart

◀ New   ◀▥ Revised   ~~deleted~~ Deleted   Excludes 1   Excludes 2   Includes   Use additional   Code first   Code also   Unspecified

OGCR Official Guidelines   ● Unacceptable Principal Diagnosis   X Assign placeholder X   ● Use Additional Character(s)   ▶ Manifestation Code   **Coding Clinic**

● **V86.5**   **Driver of special all-terrain or other off-road motor vehicle injured in nontraffic accident**

   X● **V86.51**   Driver of ambulance or fire engine injured in nontraffic accident

   X● **V86.52**   Driver of snowmobile injured in nontraffic accident

   X● **V86.53**   Driver of dune buggy injured in nontraffic accident

   X● **V86.54**   Driver of military vehicle injured in nontraffic accident

   X● **V86.59**   Driver of other off-road special all-terrain or other off-road motor vehicle injured in nontraffic accident

       Driver of dirt bike injured in nontraffic accident

       Driver of go cart injured in nontraffic accident

       Driver of golf cart injured in nontraffic accident

● **V86.6**   **Passenger of special all-terrain or other off-road motor vehicle injured in nontraffic accident**

   X● **V86.61**   Passenger of ambulance or fire engine injured in nontraffic accident

   X● **V86.62**   Passenger of snowmobile injured in nontraffic accident

   X● **V86.63**   Passenger of dune buggy injured in nontraffic accident

   X● **V86.64**   Passenger of military vehicle injured in nontraffic accident

   X● **V86.69**   Passenger of other special all-terrain or other off-road vehicle injured in nontraffic accident

       Passenger of dirt bike injured in nontraffic accident

       Passenger of go cart injured in nontraffic accident

       Passenger of golf cart injured in nontraffic accident

● **V86.7**   **Person on outside of special all-terrain or other off-road motor vehicle injured in nontraffic accident**

   X● **V86.71**   Person on outside of ambulance or fire engine injured in nontraffic accident

   X● **V86.72**   Person on outside of snowmobile injured in nontraffic accident

   X● **V86.73**   Person on outside of dune buggy injured in nontraffic accident

   X● **V86.74**   Person on outside of military vehicle injured in nontraffic accident

   X● **V86.79**   Person on outside of other special all-terrain or other off-road motor vehicles injured in nontraffic accident

       Person on outside of dirt bike injured in nontraffic accident

       Person on outside of go cart injured in nontraffic accident

       Person on outside of golf cart injured in nontraffic accident

● **V86.9**   **Unspecified occupant of special all-terrain or other off-road motor vehicle injured in nontraffic accident**

   X● **V86.91**   Unspecified occupant of ambulance or fire engine injured in nontraffic accident

   X● **V86.92**   Unspecified occupant of snowmobile injured in nontraffic accident

   X● **V86.93**   Unspecified occupant of dune buggy injured in nontraffic accident

   X● **V86.94**   Unspecified occupant of military vehicle injured in nontraffic accident

   X● **V86.99**   Unspecified occupant of other off-road special all-terrain or other off-road motor vehicle injured in nontraffic accident

       All-terrain motor-vehicle accident NOS

       Off-road motor-vehicle accident NOS

       Other motor-vehicle accident NOS

       Unspecified occupant of dirt bike injured in nontraffic accident

       Unspecified occupant of go cart injured in nontraffic accident

       Unspecified occupant of golf cart injured in nontraffic accident

       Unspecified occupant of race car injured in nontraffic accident

● **V87**   **Traffic accident of specified type but victim's mode of transport unknown**

   Excludes1   collision involving:
         pedal cycle (V10-V19)
         pedestrian (V01-V09)

   The appropriate 7th character is to be added to each code from category V87

A	initial encounter
D	subsequent encounter
S	sequela

   X● **V87.0**   Person injured in collision between car and two- or three-wheeled powered vehicle (traffic)

   X● **V87.1**   Person injured in collision between other motor vehicle and two- or three-wheeled motor vehicle (traffic)

   X● **V87.2**   Person injured in collision between car and pick-up truck or van (traffic)

   X● **V87.3**   Person injured in collision between car and bus (traffic)

   X● **V87.4**   Person injured in collision between car and heavy transport vehicle (traffic)

   X● **V87.5**   Person injured in collision between heavy transport vehicle and bus (traffic)

   X● **V87.6**   Person injured in collision between railway train or railway vehicle and car (traffic)

   X● **V87.7**   Person injured in collision between other specified motor vehicles (traffic)

   X● **V87.8**   Person injured in other specified noncollision transport accidents involving motor vehicle (traffic)

   X● **V87.9**   Person injured in other specified (collision) (noncollision) transport accidents involving nonmotor vehicle (traffic)

● **V88**   **Nontraffic accident of specified type but victim's mode of transport unknown**

   Excludes1   collision involving:
         pedal cycle (V10-V19)
         pedestrian (V01-V09)

   The appropriate 7th character is to be added to each code from category V88

A	initial encounter
D	subsequent encounter
S	sequela

   X● **V88.0**   Person injured in collision between car and two- or three-wheeled motor vehicle, nontraffic

   X● **V88.1**   Person injured in collision between other motor vehicle and two- or three-wheeled motor vehicle, nontraffic

   X● **V88.2**   Person injured in collision between car and pick-up truck or van, nontraffic

CHAPTER 20 (V01-Y99)

X⬤ **V88.3** **Person injured in collision between car and bus, nontraffic**

X⬤ **V88.4** **Person injured in collision between car and heavy transport vehicle, nontraffic**

X⬤ **V88.5** **Person injured in collision between heavy transport vehicle and bus, nontraffic**

X⬤ **V88.6** **Person injured in collision between railway train or railway vehicle and car, nontraffic**

X⬤ **V88.7** **Person injured in collision between other specified motor vehicle, nontraffic**

X⬤ **V88.8** **Person injured in other specified noncollision transport accidents involving motor vehicle, nontraffic**

X⬤ **V88.9** **Person injured in other specified (collision) (noncollision) transport accidents involving nonmotor vehicle, nontraffic**

⬤ **V89** **Motor- or nonmotor-vehicle accident, type of vehicle unspecified**

The appropriate 7th character is to be added to each code from category V89

> A   initial encounter
> D   subsequent encounter
> S   sequela

X⬤ **V89.0** **Person injured in unspecified motor-vehicle accident, nontraffic**
Motor-vehicle accident NOS, nontraffic

X⬤ **V89.1** **Person injured in unspecified nonmotor-vehicle accident, nontraffic**
Nonmotor-vehicle accident NOS (nontraffic)

X⬤ **V89.2** **Person injured in unspecified motor-vehicle accident, traffic**
Motor-vehicle accident [MVA] NOS
Road (traffic) accident [RTA] NOS

X⬤ **V89.3** **Person injured in unspecified nonmotor-vehicle accident, traffic**
Nonmotor-vehicle traffic accident NOS

X⬤ **V89.9** **Person injured in unspecified vehicle accident**
Collision NOS

WATER TRANSPORT ACCIDENTS (V90-V94)

⬤ **V90** **Drowning and submersion due to accident to watercraft**

> **Excludes1**   civilian water transport accident involving military watercraft (V94.81-)
> fall into water not from watercraft (W16.-)
> military watercraft accident in military or war operations (Y36.0-, Y37.0-)
> water-transport–related drowning or submersion without accident to watercraft (V92.-)

The appropriate 7th character is to be added to each code from category V90

> A   initial encounter
> D   subsequent encounter
> S   sequela

⬤ **V90.0** **Drowning and submersion due to watercraft overturning**

X⬤ **V90.00** **Drowning and submersion due to merchant ship overturning**

X⬤ **V90.01** **Drowning and submersion due to passenger ship overturning**
Drowning and submersion due to ferry-boat overturning
Drowning and submersion due to liner overturning

X⬤ **V90.02** **Drowning and submersion due to fishing boat overturning**

X⬤ **V90.03** **Drowning and submersion due to other powered watercraft overturning**
Drowning and submersion due to hovercraft (on open water) overturning
Drowning and submersion due to jet ski overturning

X⬤ **V90.04** **Drowning and submersion due to sailboat overturning**

X⬤ **V90.05** **Drowning and submersion due to canoe or kayak overturning**

X⬤ **V90.06** **Drowning and submersion due to (nonpowered) inflatable craft overturning**

X⬤ **V90.08** **Drowning and submersion due to other unpowered watercraft overturning**
Drowning and submersion due to windsurfer overturning

X⬤ **V90.09** **Drowning and submersion due to unspecified watercraft overturning**
Drowning and submersion due to boat NOS overturning
Drowning and submersion due to ship NOS overturning
Drowning and submersion due to watercraft NOS overturning

⬤ **V90.1** **Drowning and submersion due to watercraft sinking**

X⬤ **V90.10** **Drowning and submersion due to merchant ship sinking**

X⬤ **V90.11** **Drowning and submersion due to passenger ship sinking**
Drowning and submersion due to ferry-boat sinking
Drowning and submersion due to liner sinking

X⬤ **V90.12** **Drowning and submersion due to fishing boat sinking**

X⬤ **V90.13** **Drowning and submersion due to other powered watercraft sinking**
Drowning and submersion due to hovercraft (on open water) sinking
Drowning and submersion due to jet ski sinking

X⬤ **V90.14** **Drowning and submersion due to sailboat sinking**

X⬤ **V90.15** **Drowning and submersion due to canoe or kayak sinking**

X⬤ **V90.16** **Drowning and submersion due to (nonpowered) inflatable craft sinking**

X⬤ **V90.18** **Drowning and submersion due to other unpowered watercraft sinking**

X⬤ **V90.19** **Drowning and submersion due to unspecified watercraft sinking**
Drowning and submersion due to boat NOS sinking
Drowning and submersion due to ship NOS sinking
Drowning and submersion due to watercraft NOS sinking

⬤ **V90.2** **Drowning and submersion due to falling or jumping from burning watercraft**

X⬤ **V90.20** **Drowning and submersion due to falling or jumping from burning merchant ship**

X⬤ **V90.21** **Drowning and submersion due to falling or jumping from burning passenger ship**
Drowning and submersion due to falling or jumping from burning ferry-boat
Drowning and submersion due to falling or jumping from burning liner

X⬤ **V90.22** **Drowning and submersion due to falling or jumping from burning fishing boat**

X⬤ **V90.23** **Drowning and submersion due to falling or jumping from other burning powered watercraft**
Drowning and submersion due to falling and jumping from burning hovercraft (on open water)
Drowning and submersion due to falling and jumping from burning jet ski

X⬤ **V90.24** **Drowning and submersion due to falling or jumping from burning sailboat**

X⬤ **V90.25** **Drowning and submersion due to falling or jumping from burning canoe or kayak**

◀ New   ◀▥ Revised   ~~deleted~~ Deleted   Excludes 1   Excludes 2   Includes   Use additional   Code first   Code also   Unspecified

OGCR Official Guidelines   ⬤ Unacceptable Principal Diagnosis   X Assign placeholder X   ⬤ Use Additional Character(s)   ▶ Manifestation Code   **Coding Clinic**

X● **V90.26**   **Drowning and submersion due to falling or jumping from burning (nonpowered) inflatable craft**

X● **V90.27**   **Drowning and submersion due to falling or jumping from burning water-skis**

X● **V90.28**   **Drowning and submersion due to falling or jumping from other burning unpowered watercraft**
     Drowning and submersion due to falling and jumping from burning surf-board
     Drowning and submersion due to falling and jumping from burning windsurfer

X● **V90.29**   **Drowning and submersion due to falling or jumping from unspecified burning watercraft**
     Drowning and submersion due to falling or jumping from burning boat NOS
     Drowning and submersion due to falling or jumping from burning ship NOS
     Drowning and submersion due to falling or jumping from burning watercraft NOS

● **V90.3**   **Drowning and submersion due to falling or jumping from crushed watercraft**

X● **V90.30**   **Drowning and submersion due to falling or jumping from crushed merchant ship**

X● **V90.31**   **Drowning and submersion due to falling or jumping from crushed passenger ship**
     Drowning and submersion due to falling and jumping from crushed ferry-boat
     Drowning and submersion due to falling and jumping from crushed liner

X● **V90.32**   **Drowning and submersion due to falling or jumping from crushed fishing boat**

X● **V90.33**   **Drowning and submersion due to falling or jumping from other crushed powered watercraft**
     Drowning and submersion due to falling and jumping from crushed hovercraft
     Drowning and submersion due to falling and jumping from crushed jet ski

X● **V90.34**   **Drowning and submersion due to falling or jumping from crushed sailboat**

X● **V90.35**   **Drowning and submersion due to falling or jumping from crushed canoe or kayak**

X● **V90.36**   **Drowning and submersion due to falling or jumping from crushed (nonpowered) inflatable craft**

X● **V90.37**   **Drowning and submersion due to falling or jumping from crushed water-skis**

X● **V90.38**   **Drowning and submersion due to falling or jumping from other crushed unpowered watercraft**
     Drowning and submersion due to falling and jumping from crushed surf-board
     Drowning and submersion due to falling and jumping from crushed windsurfer

X● **V90.39**   **Drowning and submersion due to falling or jumping from crushed unspecified watercraft**
     Drowning and submersion due to falling and jumping from crushed boat NOS
     Drowning and submersion due to falling and jumping from crushed ship NOS
     Drowning and submersion due to falling and jumping from crushed watercraft NOS

● **V90.8**   **Drowning and submersion due to other accident to watercraft**

X● **V90.80**   **Drowning and submersion due to other accident to merchant ship**

X● **V90.81**   **Drowning and submersion due to other accident to passenger ship**
     Drowning and submersion due to other accident to ferry-boat
     Drowning and submersion due to other accident to liner

X● **V90.82**   **Drowning and submersion due to other accident to fishing boat**

X● **V90.83**   **Drowning and submersion due to other accident to other powered watercraft**
     Drowning and submersion due to other accident to hovercraft (on open water)
     Drowning and submersion due to other accident to jet ski

X● **V90.84**   **Drowning and submersion due to other accident to sailboat**

X● **V90.85**   **Drowning and submersion due to other accident to canoe or kayak**

X● **V90.86**   **Drowning and submersion due to other accident to (nonpowered) inflatable craft**

X● **V90.87**   **Drowning and submersion due to other accident to water-skis**

X● **V90.88**   **Drowning and submersion due to other accident to other unpowered watercraft**
     Drowning and submersion due to other accident to surf-board
     Drowning and submersion due to other accident to windsurfer

X● **V90.89**   **Drowning and submersion due to other accident to unspecified watercraft**
     Drowning and submersion due to other accident to boat NOS
     Drowning and submersion due to other accident to ship NOS
     Drowning and submersion due to other accident to watercraft NOS

● **V91**   **Other injury due to accident to watercraft**

   Includes   any injury except drowning and submersion as a result of an accident to watercraft

   Excludes1   civilian water transport accident involving military watercraft (V94.81-)
     military watercraft accident in military or war operations (Y36, Y37.-)

   Excludes2   drowning and submersion due to accident to watercraft (V90.-)

The appropriate 7th character is to be added to each code from category V91

A	initial encounter
D	subsequent encounter
S	sequela

● **V91.0**   **Burn due to watercraft on fire**

   Excludes1   burn from localized fire or explosion on board ship without accident to watercraft (V93.-)

X● **V91.00**   **Burn due to merchant ship on fire**

X● **V91.01**   **Burn due to passenger ship on fire**
     Burn due to ferry-boat on fire
     Burn due to liner on fire

X● **V91.02**   **Burn due to fishing boat on fire**

X● **V91.03**   **Burn due to other powered watercraft on fire**
     Burn due to hovercraft (on open water) on fire
     Burn due to jet ski on fire

X● **V91.04**   **Burn due to sailboat on fire**

X● **V91.05**   **Burn due to canoe or kayak on fire**

X● **V91.06**   **Burn due to (nonpowered) inflatable craft on fire**

X● **V91.07**   **Burn due to water-skis on fire**

X● **V91.08**   **Burn due to other unpowered watercraft on fire**

X● **V91.09**   **Burn due to unspecified watercraft on fire**
     Burn due to boat NOS on fire
     Burn due to ship NOS on fire
     Burn due to watercraft NOS on fire

● **V91.1   Crushed between watercraft and other watercraft or other object due to collision**

     Crushed by lifeboat after abandoning ship in a collision

     Note: Select the specified type of watercraft that the victim was on at the time of the collision.

X ● **V91.10   Crushed between merchant ship and other watercraft or other object due to collision**

X ● **V91.11   Crushed between passenger ship and other watercraft or other object due to collision**

     Crushed between ferry-boat and other watercraft or other object due to collision

     Crushed between liner and other watercraft or other object due to collision

X ● **V91.12   Crushed between fishing boat and other watercraft or other object due to collision**

X ● **V91.13   Crushed between other powered watercraft and other watercraft or other object due to collision**

     Crushed between hovercraft (on open water) and other watercraft or other object due to collision

     Crushed between jet ski and other watercraft or other object due to collision

X ● **V91.14   Crushed between sailboat and other watercraft or other object due to collision**

X ● **V91.15   Crushed between canoe or kayak and other watercraft or other object due to collision**

X ● **V91.16   Crushed between (nonpowered) inflatable craft and other watercraft or other object due to collision**

X ● **V91.18   Crushed between other unpowered watercraft and other watercraft or other object due to collision**

     Crushed between surfboard and other watercraft or other object due to collision

     Crushed between windsurfer and other watercraft or other object due to collision

X ● **V91.19   Crushed between unspecified watercraft and other watercraft or other object due to collision**

     Crushed between boat NOS and other watercraft or other object due to collision

     Crushed between ship NOS and other watercraft or other object due to collision

     Crushed between watercraft NOS and other watercraft or other object due to collision

● **V91.2   Fall due to collision between watercraft and other watercraft or other object**

     Fall while remaining on watercraft after collision

     Note: Select the specified type of watercraft that the victim was on at the time of the collision.

     Excludes1   crushed between watercraft and other watercraft and other object due to collision (V91.1-)

            drowning and submersion due to falling from crushed watercraft (V90.3-)

X ● **V91.20   Fall due to collision between merchant ship and other watercraft or other object**

X ● **V91.21   Fall due to collision between passenger ship and other watercraft or other object**

     Fall due to collision between ferry-boat and other watercraft or other object

     Fall due to collision between liner and other watercraft or other object

X ● **V91.22   Fall due to collision between fishing boat and other watercraft or other object**

X ● **V91.23   Fall due to collision between other powered watercraft and other watercraft or other object**

     Fall due to collision between hovercraft (on open water) and other watercraft or other object

     Fall due to collision between jet ski and other watercraft or other object

X ● **V91.24   Fall due to collision between sailboat and other watercraft or other object**

X ● **V91.25   Fall due to collision between canoe or kayak and other watercraft or other object**

X ● **V91.26   Fall due to collision between (nonpowered) inflatable craft and other watercraft or other object**

X ● **V91.29   Fall due to collision between unspecified watercraft and other watercraft or other object**

     Fall due to collision between boat NOS and other watercraft or other object

     Fall due to collision between ship NOS and other watercraft or other object

     Fall due to collision between watercraft NOS and other watercraft or other object

● **V91.3   Hit or struck by falling object due to accident to watercraft**

     Hit or struck by falling object (part of damaged watercraft or other object) after falling or jumping from damaged watercraft

     Excludes2   drowning or submersion due to fall or jumping from damaged watercraft (V90.2-, V90.3-)

X ● **V91.30   Hit or struck by falling object due to accident to merchant ship**

X ● **V91.31   Hit or struck by falling object due to accident to passenger ship**

     Hit or struck by falling object due to accident to ferry-boat

     Hit or struck by falling object due to accident to liner

X ● **V91.32   Hit or struck by falling object due to accident to fishing boat**

X ● **V91.33   Hit or struck by falling object due to accident to other powered watercraft**

     Hit or struck by falling object due to accident to hovercraft (on open water)

     Hit or struck by falling object due to accident to jet ski

X ● **V91.34   Hit or struck by falling object due to accident to sailboat**

X ● **V91.35   Hit or struck by falling object due to accident to canoe or kayak**

X ● **V91.36   Hit or struck by falling object due to accident to (nonpowered) inflatable craft**

X ● **V91.37   Hit or struck by falling object due to accident to water-skis**

     Hit by water-skis after jumping off of waterskis

X ● **V91.38   Hit or struck by falling object due to accident to other unpowered watercraft**

     Hit or struck by surf-board after falling off damaged surf-board

     Hit or struck by object after falling off damaged windsurfer

X ● **V91.39   Hit or struck by falling object due to accident to unspecified watercraft**

     Hit or struck by falling object due to accident to boat NOS

     Hit or struck by falling object due to accident to ship NOS

     Hit or struck by falling object due to accident to watercraft NOS

◀ New   ◀◀◀ Revised   ~~deleted~~ Deleted   Excludes 1   Excludes 2   Includes   Use additional   Code first   Code also   Unspecified

OGCR Official Guidelines   ● Unacceptable Principal Diagnosis   X Assign placeholder X   ● Use Additional Character(s)   ▶ Manifestation Code   **Coding Clinic**

● **V91.8   Other injury due to other accident to watercraft**

X● **V91.80   Other injury due to other accident to merchant ship**

X● **V91.81   Other injury due to other accident to passenger ship**

Other injury due to other accident to ferry-boat
Other injury due to other accident to liner

X● **V91.82   Other injury due to other accident to fishing boat**

X● **V91.83   Other injury due to other accident to other powered watercraft**

Other injury due to other accident to hovercraft (on open water)
Other injury due to other accident to jet ski

X● **V91.84   Other injury due to other accident to sailboat**

X● **V91.85   Other injury due to other accident to canoe or kayak**

X● **V91.86   Other injury due to other accident to (nonpowered) inflatable craft**

X● **V91.87   Other injury due to other accident to water-skis**

X● **V91.88   Other injury due to other accident to other unpowered watercraft**

Other injury due to other accident to surf-board
Other injury due to other accident to windsurfer

X● **V91.89   Other injury due to other accident to** unspecified **watercraft**

Other injury due to other accident to boat NOS
Other injury due to other accident to ship NOS
Other injury due to other accident to watercraft NOS

● **V92   Drowning and submersion due to accident on board watercraft, without accident to watercraft**

Excludes1   civilian water transport accident involving military watercraft (V94.81-)
drowning or submersion due to accident to watercraft (V90-V91)
drowning or submersion of diver who voluntarily jumps from boat not involved in an accident (W16.711, W16.721)
fall into water without watercraft (W16.-)
military watercraft accident in military or war operations (Y36, Y37)

The appropriate 7th character is to be added to each code from category V92

A   initial encounter
D   subsequent encounter
S   sequela

● **V92.0   Drowning and submersion due to fall off watercraft**

Drowning and submersion due to fall from gangplank of watercraft
Drowning and submersion due to fall overboard watercraft

Excludes2   hitting head on object or bottom of body of water due to fall from watercraft (V94.0-)

X● **V92.00   Drowning and submersion due to fall off merchant ship**

X● **V92.01   Drowning and submersion due to fall off passenger ship**

Drowning and submersion due to fall off ferry-boat
Drowning and submersion due to fall off liner

X● **V92.02   Drowning and submersion due to fall off fishing boat**

X● **V92.03   Drowning and submersion due to fall off other powered watercraft**

Drowning and submersion due to fall off hovercraft (on open water)
Drowning and submersion due to fall off jet ski

X● **V92.04   Drowning and submersion due to fall off sailboat**

X● **V92.05   Drowning and submersion due to fall off canoe or kayak**

X● **V92.06   Drowning and submersion due to fall off (nonpowered) inflatable craft**

X● **V92.07   Drowning and submersion due to fall off water-skis**

Excludes1   drowning and submersion due to falling off burning water-skis (V90.27)
drowning and submersion due to falling off crushed water-skis (V90.37)
hit by boat while water-skiing NOS (V94.X)

X● **V92.08   Drowning and submersion due to fall off other unpowered watercraft**

Drowning and submersion due to fall off surf-board
Drowning and submersion due to fall off windsurfer

Excludes1   drowning and submersion due to fall off burning unpowered watercraft (V90.28)
drowning and submersion due to fall off crushed unpowered watercraft (V90.38)
drowning and submersion due to fall off damaged unpowered watercraft (V90.88)
drowning and submersion due to rider of nonpowered watercraft being hit by other watercraft (V94.-)
other injury due to rider of nonpowered watercraft being hit by other watercraft (V94.-)

X● **V92.09   Drowning and submersion due to fall off** unspecified **watercraft**

Drowning and submersion due to fall off boat NOS
Drowning and submersion due to fall off ship NOS
Drowning and submersion due to fall off watercraft NOS

● **V92.1   Drowning and submersion due to being thrown overboard by motion of watercraft**

Excludes1   drowning and submersion due to fall off surf-board (V92.08)
drowning and submersion due to fall off water-skis (V92.07)
drowning and submersion due to fall off windsurfer (V92.08)

X● **V92.10   Drowning and submersion due to being thrown overboard by motion of merchant ship**

X● **V92.11   Drowning and submersion due to being thrown overboard by motion of passenger ship**

Drowning and submersion due to being thrown overboard by motion of ferry-boat
Drowning and submersion due to being thrown overboard by motion of liner

X● **V92.12** **Drowning and submersion due to being thrown overboard by motion of fishing boat**

X● **V92.13** **Drowning and submersion due to being thrown overboard by motion of other powered watercraft**
    Drowning and submersion due to being thrown overboard by motion of hovercraft

X● **V92.14** **Drowning and submersion due to being thrown overboard by motion of sailboat**

X● **V92.15** **Drowning and submersion due to being thrown overboard by motion of canoe or kayak**

X● **V92.16** **Drowning and submersion due to being thrown overboard by motion of (nonpowered) inflatable craft**

X● **V92.19** **Drowning and submersion due to being thrown overboard by motion of** unspecified **watercraft**
    Drowning and submersion due to being thrown overboard by motion of boat NOS
    Drowning and submersion due to being thrown overboard by motion of ship NOS
    Drowning and submersion due to being thrown overboard by motion of watercraft NOS

● **V92.2** **Drowning and submersion due to being washed overboard from watercraft**
    Code first any associated cataclysm (X37.0-)

X● **V92.20** **Drowning and submersion due to being washed overboard from merchant ship**

X● **V92.21** **Drowning and submersion due to being washed overboard from passenger ship**
    Drowning and submersion due to being washed overboard from ferry-boat
    Drowning and submersion due to being washed overboard from liner

X● **V92.22** **Drowning and submersion due to being washed overboard from fishing boat**

X● **V92.23** **Drowning and submersion due to being washed overboard from other powered watercraft**
    Drowning and submersion due to being washed overboard from hovercraft (on open water)
    Drowning and submersion due to being washed overboard from jet ski

X● **V92.24** **Drowning and submersion due to being washed overboard from sailboat**

X● **V92.25** **Drowning and submersion due to being washed overboard from canoe or kayak**

X● **V92.26** **Drowning and submersion due to being washed overboard from (nonpowered) inflatable craft**

X● **V92.27** **Drowning and submersion due to being washed overboard from water-skis**
    Excludes1   drowning and submersion due to fall off water-skis (V92.07)

X● **V92.28** **Drowning and submersion due to being washed overboard from other unpowered watercraft**
    Drowning and submersion due to being washed overboard from surf-board
    Drowning and submersion due to being washed overboard from windsurfer

X● **V92.29** **Drowning and submersion due to being washed overboard from** unspecified **watercraft**
    Drowning and submersion due to being washed overboard from boat NOS
    Drowning and submersion due to being washed overboard from ship NOS
    Drowning and submersion due to being washed overboard from watercraft NOS

● **V93** **Other injury due to accident on board watercraft, without accident to watercraft**
    Excludes1   civilian water transport accident involving military watercraft (V94.81-)
        other injury due to accident to watercraft (V91.-)
        military watercraft accident in military or war operations (Y36, Y37.-)
    Excludes2   drowning and submersion due to accident on board watercraft, without accident to watercraft (V92.-)

The appropriate 7th character is to be added to each code from category V93

> A   initial encounter
> D   subsequent encounter
> S   sequela

● **V93.0** **Burn due to localized fire on board watercraft**
    Excludes1   burn due to watercraft on fire (V91.0-)

X● **V93.00** **Burn due to localized fire on board merchant vessel**

X● **V93.01** **Burn due to localized fire on board passenger vessel**
    Burn due to localized fire on board ferry-boat
    Burn due to localized fire on board liner

X● **V93.02** **Burn due to localized fire on board fishing boat**

X● **V93.03** **Burn due to localized fire on board other powered watercraft**
    Burn due to localized fire on board hovercraft
    Burn due to localized fire on board jet ski

X● **V93.04** **Burn due to localized fire on board sailboat**

X● **V93.09** **Burn due to localized fire on board** unspecified **watercraft**
    Burn due to localized fire on board boat NOS
    Burn due to localized fire on board ship NOS
    Burn due to localized fire on board watercraft NOS

● **V93.1** **Other burn on board watercraft**
    Burn due to source other than fire on board watercraft
    Excludes1   burn due to watercraft on fire (V91.0-)

X● **V93.10** **Other burn on board merchant vessel**

X● **V93.11** **Other burn on board passenger vessel**
    Other burn on board ferry-boat
    Other burn on board liner

X● **V93.12** **Other burn on board fishing boat**

X● **V93.13** **Other burn on board other powered watercraft**
    Other burn on board hovercraft
    Other burn on board jet ski

X● **V93.14** **Other burn on board sailboat**

X● **V93.19** **Other burn on board** unspecified **watercraft**
    Other burn on board boat NOS
    Other burn on board ship NOS
    Other burn on board watercraft NOS

● **V93.2** **Heat exposure on board watercraft**
    Excludes1   exposure to man-made heat not aboard watercraft (W92)
        exposure to natural heat while on board watercraft (X30)
        exposure to sunlight while on board watercraft (X32)
    Excludes2   burn due to fire on board watercraft (V93.0-)

X● **V93.20** **Heat exposure on board merchant ship**

X● **V93.21** **Heat exposure on board passenger ship**
    Heat exposure on board ferry-boat
    Heat exposure on board liner

X● **V93.22** **Heat exposure on board fishing boat**

X● **V93.23** **Heat exposure on board other powered watercraft**
    Heat exposure on board hovercraft

◀ New   ◀▥ Revised   ~~deleted~~ Deleted   Excludes 1   Excludes 2   Includes   Use additional   Code first   Code also   Unspecified

OGCR Official Guidelines   ● Unacceptable Principal Diagnosis   X Assign placeholder X   ● Use Additional Character(s)   ▶ Manifestation Code   **Coding Clinic**

X ● **V93.24**   **Heat exposure on board sailboat**
X ● **V93.29**   **Heat exposure on board** unspecified **watercraft**
       Heat exposure on board boat NOS
       Heat exposure on board ship NOS
       Heat exposure on board watercraft NOS

● **V93.3**   **Fall on board watercraft**
     Excludes1   fall due to collision of watercraft (V91.2-)

X ● **V93.30**   **Fall on board merchant ship**
X ● **V93.31**   **Fall on board passenger ship**
       Fall on board ferry-boat
       Fall on board liner
X ● **V93.32**   **Fall on board fishing boat**
X ● **V93.33**   **Fall on board other powered watercraft**
       Fall on board hovercraft (on open water)
       Fall on board jet ski
X ● **V93.34**   **Fall on board sailboat**
X ● **V93.35**   **Fall on board canoe or kayak**
X ● **V93.36**   **Fall on board (nonpowered) inflatable craft**
X ● **V93.38**   **Fall on board other unpowered watercraft**
X ● **V93.39**   **Fall on board** unspecified **watercraft**
       Fall on board boat NOS
       Fall on board ship NOS
       Fall on board watercraft NOS

● **V93.4**   **Struck by falling object on board watercraft**
       Hit by falling object on board watercraft
     Excludes1   struck by falling object due to accident to watercraft (V91.3)

X ● **V93.40**   **Struck by falling object on merchant ship**
X ● **V93.41**   **Struck by falling object on passenger ship**
       Struck by falling object on ferry-boat
       Struck by falling object on liner
X ● **V93.42**   **Struck by falling object on fishing boat**
X ● **V93.43**   **Struck by falling object on other powered watercraft**
       Struck by falling object on hovercraft
X ● **V93.44**   **Struck by falling object on sailboat**
X ● **V93.48**   **Struck by falling object on other unpowered watercraft**
X ● **V93.49**   **Struck by falling object on** unspecified **watercraft**

● **V93.5**   **Explosion on board watercraft**
       Boiler explosion on steamship
     Excludes2   fire on board watercraft (V93.0-)

X ● **V93.50**   **Explosion on board merchant ship**
X ● **V93.51**   **Explosion on board passenger ship**
       Explosion on board ferry-boat
       Explosion on board liner
X ● **V93.52**   **Explosion on board fishing boat**
X ● **V93.53**   **Explosion on board other powered watercraft**
       Explosion on board hovercraft
       Explosion on board jet ski
X ● **V93.54**   **Explosion on board sailboat**
X ● **V93.59**   **Explosion on board** unspecified **watercraft**
       Explosion on board boat NOS
       Explosion on board ship NOS
       Explosion on board watercraft NOS

● **V93.6**   **Machinery accident on board watercraft**
     Excludes1   machinery explosion on board watercraft (V93.4-)
                 machinery fire on board watercraft (V93.0-)

X ● **V93.60**   **Machinery accident on board merchant ship**
X ● **V93.61**   **Machinery accident on board passenger ship**
       Machinery accident on board ferry-boat
       Machinery accident on board liner
X ● **V93.62**   **Machinery accident on board fishing boat**

X ● **V93.63**   **Machinery accident on board other powered watercraft**
       Machinery accident on board hovercraft
X ● **V93.64**   **Machinery accident on board sailboat**
X ● **V93.69**   **Machinery accident on board** unspecified **watercraft**
       Machinery accident on board boat NOS
       Machinery accident on board ship NOS
       Machinery accident on board watercraft NOS

● **V93.8**   **Other injury due to other accident on board watercraft**
       Accidental poisoning by gases or fumes on watercraft

X ● **V93.80**   **Other injury due to other accident on board merchant ship**
X ● **V93.81**   **Other injury due to other accident on board passenger ship**
       Other injury due to other accident on board ferry-boat
       Other injury due to other accident on board liner
X ● **V93.82**   **Other injury due to other accident on board fishing boat**
X ● **V93.83**   **Other injury due to other accident on board other powered watercraft**
       Other injury due to other accident on board hovercraft
       Other injury due to other accident on board jet ski
X ● **V93.84**   **Other injury due to other accident on board sailboat**
X ● **V93.85**   **Other injury due to other accident on board canoe or kayak**
X ● **V93.86**   **Other injury due to other accident on board (nonpowered) inflatable craft**
X ● **V93.87**   **Other injury due to other accident on board water-skis**
       Hit or struck by object while waterskiing
X ● **V93.88**   **Other injury due to other accident on board other unpowered watercraft**
       Hit or struck by object while surfing
       Hit or struck by object while on board windsurfer
X ● **V93.89**   **Other injury due to other accident on board** unspecified **watercraft**
       Other injury due to other accident on board boat NOS
       Other injury due to other accident on board ship NOS
       Other injury due to other accident on board watercraft NOS

● **V94**   **Other and unspecified water transport accidents**
     Excludes1   military watercraft accidents in military or war operations (Y36, Y37)

     The appropriate 7th character is to be added to each code from category V94

A	initial encounter
D	subsequent encounter
S	sequela

X ● **V94.0**   **Hitting object or bottom of body of water due to fall from watercraft**
     Excludes2   drowning and submersion due to fall from watercraft (V92.0-)

● **V94.1**   **Bather struck by watercraft**
       Swimmer hit by watercraft
X ● **V94.11**   **Bather struck by powered watercraft**
X ● **V94.12**   **Bather struck by nonpowered watercraft**

CHAPTER 20 (V01-Y99)

● **V94.2** **Rider of nonpowered watercraft struck by other watercraft**

X● **V94.21** **Rider of nonpowered watercraft struck by other nonpowered watercraft**
Canoer hit by other nonpowered watercraft
Surfer hit by other nonpowered watercraft
Windsurfer hit by other nonpowered watercraft

X● **V94.22** **Rider of nonpowered watercraft struck by powered watercraft**
Canoer hit by motorboat
Surfer hit by motorboat
Windsurfer hit by motorboat

● **V94.3** **Injury to rider of (inflatable) watercraft being pulled behind other watercraft**

X● **V94.31** **Injury to rider of (inflatable) recreational watercraft being pulled behind other watercraft**
Injury to rider of inner-tube pulled behind motor boat

X● **V94.32** **Injury to rider of non-recreational watercraft being pulled behind other watercraft**
Injury to occupant of dingy being pulled behind boat or ship
Injury to occupant of life-raft being pulled behind boat or ship

X● **V94.4** **Injury to barefoot water-skier**
Injury to person being pulled behind boat or ship

● **V94.8** **Other water transport accident**

● **V94.81** **Water transport accident involving military watercraft**

● **V94.810** **Civilian watercraft involved in water transport accident with military watercraft**
Passenger on civilian watercraft injured due to accident with military watercraft

● **V94.811** **Civilian in water injured by military watercraft**

● **V94.818** **Other water transport accident involving military watercraft**

X● **V94.89** **Other water transport accident**

X● **V94.9** **Unspecified water transport accident**
Water transport accident NOS

AIR AND SPACE TRANSPORT ACCIDENTS (V95-V97)

Excludes1 military aircraft accidents in military or war operations (Y36, Y37)

● **V95** **Accident to powered aircraft causing injury to occupant**
The appropriate 7th character is to be added to each code from category V95

A	initial encounter
D	subsequent encounter
S	sequela

● **V95.0** **Helicopter accident injuring occupant**

X● **V95.00** **Unspecified helicopter accident injuring occupant**

X● **V95.01** **Helicopter crash injuring occupant**

X● **V95.02** **Forced landing of helicopter injuring occupant**

X● **V95.03** **Helicopter collision injuring occupant**
Helicopter collision with any object, fixed, movable or moving

X● **V95.04** **Helicopter fire injuring occupant**

X● **V95.05** **Helicopter explosion injuring occupant**

X● **V95.09** **Other helicopter accident injuring occupant**

● **V95.1** **Ultralight, microlight or powered-glider accident injuring occupant**

X● **V95.10** **Unspecified ultralight, microlight or powered-glider accident injuring occupant**

X● **V95.11** **Ultralight, microlight or powered-glider crash injuring occupant**

X● **V95.12** **Forced landing of ultralight, microlight or powered-glider injuring occupant**

X● **V95.13** **Ultralight, microlight or powered-glider collision injuring occupant**
Ultralight, microlight or powered-glider collision with any object, fixed, movable or moving

X● **V95.14** **Ultralight, microlight or powered-glider fire injuring occupant**

X● **V95.15** **Ultralight, microlight or powered-glider explosion injuring occupant**

X● **V95.19** **Other ultralight, microlight or powered-glider accident injuring occupant**

● **V95.2** **Other private fixed-wing aircraft accident injuring occupant**

X● **V95.20** **Unspecified accident to other private fixed-wing aircraft, injuring occupant**

X● **V95.21** **Other private fixed-wing aircraft crash injuring occupant**

X● **V95.22** **Forced landing of other private fixed-wing aircraft injuring occupant**

X● **V95.23** **Other private fixed-wing aircraft collision injuring occupant**
Other private fixed-wing aircraft collision with any object, fixed, movable or moving

X● **V95.24** **Other private fixed-wing aircraft fire injuring occupant**

X● **V95.25** **Other private fixed-wing aircraft explosion injuring occupant**

X● **V95.29** **Other accident to other private fixed-wing aircraft injuring occupant**

● **V95.3** **Commercial fixed-wing aircraft accident injuring occupant**

X● **V95.30** **Unspecified accident to commercial fixed-wing aircraft injuring occupant**

X● **V95.31** **Commercial fixed-wing aircraft crash injuring occupant**

X● **V95.32** **Forced landing of commercial fixed-wing aircraft injuring occupant**

X● **V95.33** **Commercial fixed-wing aircraft collision injuring occupant**
Commercial fixed-wing aircraft collision with any object, fixed, movable or moving

X● **V95.34** **Commercial fixed-wing aircraft fire injuring occupant**

X● **V95.35** **Commercial fixed-wing aircraft explosion injuring occupant**

X● **V95.39** **Other accident to commercial fixed-wing aircraft injuring occupant**

● **V95.4** **Spacecraft accident injuring occupant**

X● **V95.40** **Unspecified spacecraft accident injuring occupant**

X● **V95.41** **Spacecraft crash injuring occupant**

X● **V95.42** **Forced landing of spacecraft injuring occupant**

X● **V95.43** **Spacecraft collision injuring occupant**
Spacecraft collision with any object, fixed, moveable or moving

X● **V95.44** **Spacecraft fire injuring occupant**

X● **V95.45** **Spacecraft explosion injuring occupant**

X● **V95.49** **Other spacecraft accident injuring occupant**

X● **V95.8** **Other powered aircraft accidents injuring occupant**

X● **V95.9** **Unspecified aircraft accident injuring occupant**
Aircraft accident NOS
Air transport accident NOS

◀ New   ◀▥ Revised   ~~deleted~~ Deleted   Excludes 1   Excludes 2   Includes   Use additional   Code first   Code also   Unspecified
OGCR Official Guidelines   ● Unacceptable Principal Diagnosis   X Assign placeholder X   ● Use Additional Character(s)   ▶ Manifestation Code   **Coding Clinic**

● **V96   Accident to nonpowered aircraft causing injury to occupant**

     The appropriate 7th character is to be added to each code from category V96

     | | |
     A   initial encounter
     D   subsequent encounter
     S   sequela

   ● **V96.0   Balloon accident injuring occupant**

     X● **V96.00   Unspecified balloon accident injuring occupant**

     X● **V96.01   Balloon crash injuring occupant**

     X● **V96.02   Forced landing of balloon injuring occupant**

     X● **V96.03   Balloon collision injuring occupant**

         Balloon collision with any object, fixed, moveable or moving

     X● **V96.04   Balloon fire injuring occupant**

     X● **V96.05   Balloon explosion injuring occupant**

     X● **V96.09   Other balloon accident injuring occupant**

   ● **V96.1   Hang-glider accident injuring occupant**

     X● **V96.10   Unspecified hang-glider accident injuring occupant**

     X● **V96.11   Hang-glider crash injuring occupant**

     X● **V96.12   Forced landing of hang-glider injuring occupant**

     X● **V96.13   Hang-glider collision injuring occupant**

         Hang-glider collision with any object, fixed, moveable or moving

     X● **V96.14   Hang-glider fire injuring occupant**

     X● **V96.15   Hang-glider explosion injuring occupant**

     X● **V96.19   Other hang-glider accident injuring occupant**

   ● **V96.2   Glider (nonpowered) accident injuring occupant**

     X● **V96.20   Unspecified glider (nonpowered) accident injuring occupant**

     X● **V96.21   Glider (nonpowered) crash injuring occupant**

     X● **V96.22   Forced landing of glider (nonpowered) injuring occupant**

     X● **V96.23   Glider (nonpowered) collision injuring occupant**

         Glider (nonpowered) collision with any object, fixed, moveable or moving

     X● **V96.24   Glider (nonpowered) fire injuring occupant**

     X● **V96.25   Glider (nonpowered) explosion injuring occupant**

     X● **V96.29   Other glider (nonpowered) accident injuring occupant**

   X● **V96.8   Other nonpowered-aircraft accidents injuring occupant**

     Kite carrying a person accident injuring occupant

   X● **V96.9   Unspecified nonpowered-aircraft accident injuring occupant**

     Nonpowered-aircraft accident NOS

● **V97   Other specified air transport accidents**

     The appropriate 7th character is to be added to each code from category V97

     | | |
     A   initial encounter
     D   subsequent encounter
     S   sequela

   X● **V97.0   Occupant of aircraft injured in other specified air transport accidents**

     Fall in, on or from aircraft in air transport accident

     Excludes1   accident while boarding or alighting aircraft (V97.1)

   X● **V97.1   Person injured while boarding or alighting from aircraft**

   ● **V97.2   Parachutist accident**

     X● **V97.21   Parachutist entangled in object**

         Parachutist landing in tree

     X● **V97.22   Parachutist injured on landing**

     X● **V97.29   Other parachutist accident**

   ● **V97.3   Person on ground injured in air transport accident**

     X● **V97.31   Hit by object falling from aircraft**

         Hit by crashing aircraft

         Injured by aircraft hitting house

         Injured by aircraft hitting car

     X● **V97.32   Injured by rotating propeller**

     X● **V97.33   Sucked into jet engine**

     X● **V97.39   Other injury to person on ground due to air transport accident**

   ● **V97.8   Other air transport accidents, not elsewhere classified**

     Excludes1   aircraft accident NOS (V95.9)

         exposure to changes in air pressure during ascent or descent (W94.-)

     ● **V97.81   Air transport accident involving military aircraft**

       ● **V97.810   Civilian aircraft involved in air transport accident with military aircraft**

         Passenger in civilian aircraft injured due to accident with military aircraft

       ● **V97.811   Civilian injured by military aircraft**

       ● **V97.818   Other air transport accident involving military aircraft**

     X● **V97.89   Other air transport accidents, not elsewhere classified**

         Injury from machinery on aircraft

OTHER AND UNSPECIFIED TRANSPORT ACCIDENTS (V98-V99)

     Excludes1   vehicle accident, type of vehicle unspecified (V89.-)

● **V98   Other specified transport accidents**

     The appropriate 7th character is to be added to each code from category V98

     | | |
     A   initial encounter
     D   subsequent encounter
     S   sequela

   X● **V98.0   Accident to, on or involving cable-car, not on rails**

     Caught or dragged by cable-car, not on rails

     Fall or jump from cable-car, not on rails

     Object thrown from or in cable-car, not on rails

   X● **V98.1   Accident to, on or involving land-yacht**

   X● **V98.2   Accident to, on or involving ice yacht**

   X● **V98.3   Accident to, on or involving ski lift**

     Accident to, on or involving ski chair-lift

     Accident to, on or involving ski-lift with gondola

   X● **V98.8   Other specified transport accidents**

X● **V99   Unspecified transport accident**

     The appropriate 7th character is to be added to code V99

     | | |
     A   initial encounter
     D   subsequent encounter
     S   sequela

OTHER EXTERNAL CAUSES OF ACCIDENTAL INJURY (W00-X58)

SLIPPING, TRIPPING, STUMBLING AND FALLS (W00-W19)

Excludes1   assault involving a fall (Y01-Y02)
fall from animal (V80.-)
fall (in) (from) machinery (in operation) (W28-W31)
fall (in) (from) transport vehicle (V01-V99)
intentional self-harm involving a fall (X80-X81)

Excludes2   at risk for fall (history of fall) Z91.81
fall (in) (from) burning building (X00.-)
fall into fire (X00-X04, X08-X09)

● **W00   Fall due to ice and snow**

Includes   pedestrian on foot falling (slipping) on ice and snow

Excludes1   fall on (from) ice and snow involving pedestrian conveyance (V00.-)
fall from stairs and steps not due to ice and snow (W10.-)

The appropriate 7th character is to be added to each code from category W00

A	initial encounter
D	subsequent encounter
S	sequela

X● **W00.0   Fall on same level due to ice and snow**
Coding Clinic: 2016, Q2, P5

X● **W00.1   Fall from stairs and steps due to ice and snow**

X● **W00.2   Other fall from one level to another due to ice and snow**

X● **W00.9   Unspecified fall due to ice and snow**

● **W01   Fall on same level from slipping, tripping and stumbling**

Includes   fall on moving sidewalk

Excludes1   fall due to bumping (striking) against object (W18.0-)
fall in shower or bathtub (W18.2-)
fall on same level NOS (W18.30)
fall on same level from slipping, tripping and stumbling due to ice or snow (W00.0)
fall off or from toilet (W18.1-)
slipping, tripping and stumbling NOS (W18.40)
slipping, tripping and stumbling without falling (W18.4-)

The appropriate 7th character is to be added to each code from category W01

A	initial encounter
D	subsequent encounter
S	sequela

X● **W01.0   Fall on same level from slipping, tripping and stumbling without subsequent striking against object**
Falling over animal

● **W01.1   Fall on same level from slipping, tripping and stumbling with subsequent striking against object**

X● **W01.10   Fall on same level from slipping, tripping and stumbling with subsequent striking against unspecified object**

● **W01.11   Fall on same level from slipping, tripping and stumbling with subsequent striking against sharp object**

● **W01.110   Fall on same level from slipping, tripping and stumbling with subsequent striking against sharp glass**

● **W01.111   Fall on same level from slipping, tripping and stumbling with subsequent striking against power tool or machine**

● **W01.118   Fall on same level from slipping, tripping and stumbling with subsequent striking against other sharp object**

● **W01.119   Fall on same level from slipping, tripping and stumbling with subsequent striking against unspecified sharp object**

● **W01.19   Fall on same level from slipping, tripping and stumbling with subsequent striking against other object**

● **W01.190   Fall on same level from slipping, tripping and stumbling with subsequent striking against furniture**

● **W01.198   Fall on same level from slipping, tripping and stumbling with subsequent striking against other object**

X● **W03   Other fall on same level due to collision with another person**
Fall due to non-transport collision with other person

Excludes1   collision with another person without fall (W51)
crushed or pushed by a crowd or human stampede (W52)
fall involving pedestrian conveyance (V00-V09)
fall due to ice or snow (W00)
fall on same level NOS (W18.30)

The appropriate 7th character is to be added to code W03

A	initial encounter
D	subsequent encounter
S	sequela

Coding Clinic: 2015, Q1, P9-10; 2012, Q4, P108

X● **W04   Fall while being carried or supported by other persons**
Accidentally dropped while being carried

The appropriate 7th character is to be added to code W04

A	initial encounter
D	subsequent encounter
S	sequel

● **W05   Fall from non-moving wheelchair, nonmotorized scooter and motorized mobility scooter**

Excludes1   fall from moving wheelchair (powered) (V00.811)
fall from moving motorized mobility scooter (V00.831)
fall from nonmotorized scooter (V00.141)

The appropriate 7th character is to be added to each code from category W05

A	initial encounter
D	subsequent encounter
S	sequela

X● **W05.0   Fall from non-moving wheelchair**

X● **W05.1   Fall from non-moving nonmotorized scooter**

X● **W05.2   Fall from non-moving motorized mobility scooter**

CHAPTER 20 (V01-Y99)

◀ New   ◀ Revised   ~~deleted~~ Deleted   Excludes 1   Excludes 2   Includes   Use additional   Code first   Code also   Unspecified
OGCR Official Guidelines   ● Unacceptable Principal Diagnosis   X Assign placeholder X   ● Use Additional Character(s)   ▌ Manifestation Code   Coding Clinic

X● **W06   Fall from bed**

     The appropriate 7th character is to be added to code W06

A	initial encounter
D	subsequent encounter
S	sequela

X● **W07   Fall from chair**

     The appropriate 7th character is to be added to code W07

A	initial encounter
D	subsequent encounter
S	sequela

X● **W08   Fall from other furniture**

     The appropriate 7th character is to be added to code W08

A	initial encounter
D	subsequent encounter
S	sequela

● **W09   Fall on and from playground equipment**

     Excludes1   fall involving recreational machinery (W31)

     The appropriate 7th character is to be added to each code from category W09

A	initial encounter
D	subsequent encounter
S	sequela

   X● **W09.0   Fall on or from playground slide**

   X● **W09.1   Fall from playground swing**

   X● **W09.2   Fall on or from jungle gym**

   X● **W09.8   Fall on or from other playground equipment**

● **W10   Fall on and from stairs and steps**

     Excludes1   fall from stairs and steps due to ice and snow (W00.1)

     The appropriate 7th character is to be added to each code from category W10

A	initial encounter
D	subsequent encounter
S	sequela

   X● **W10.0   Fall (on) (from) escalator**

   X● **W10.1   Fall (on) (from) sidewalk curb**

   X● **W10.2   Fall (on) (from) incline**

        Fall (on) (from) ramp

   X● **W10.8   Fall (on) (from) other stairs and steps**

   X● **W10.9   Fall (on) (from) unspecified stairs and steps**

X● **W11   Fall on and from ladder**

     The appropriate 7th character is to be added to code W11

A	initial encounter
D	subsequent encounter
S	sequela

X● **W12   Fall on and from scaffolding**

     The appropriate 7th character is to be added to code W12

A	initial encounter
D	subsequent encounter
S	sequela

● **W13   Fall from, out of or through building or structure**

     The appropriate 7th character is to be added to each code from category W13

A	initial encounter
D	subsequent encounter
S	sequela

   X● **W13.0   Fall from, out of or through balcony**

        Fall from, out of or through railing

   X● **W13.1   Fall from, out of or through bridge**

   X● **W13.2   Fall from, out of or through roof**

   X● **W13.3   Fall through floor**

   X● **W13.4   Fall from, out of or through window**

        Excludes2   fall with subsequent striking against sharp glass (W01.110)

   X● **W13.8   Fall from, out of or through other building or structure**

        Fall from, out of or through viaduct

        Fall from, out of or through wall

        Fall from, out of or through flag-pole

   X● **W13.9   Fall from, out of or through building, not otherwise specified**

        Excludes1   collapse of a building or structure (W20.-)

                     fall or jump from burning building or structure (X00.-)

X● **W14   Fall from tree**

     The appropriate 7th character is to be added to code W14

A	initial encounter
D	subsequent encounter
S	sequela

X● **W15   Fall from cliff**

     The appropriate 7th character is to be added to code W15

A	initial encounter
D	subsequent encounter
S	sequela

● **W16   Fall, jump or diving into water**

     Excludes1   accidental non-watercraft drowning and submersion not involving fall (W65-W74)

                     effects of air pressure from diving (W94.-)

                     fall into water from watercraft (V90-V94)

                     hitting an object or against bottom when falling from watercraft (V94.0)

     Excludes2   striking or hitting diving board (W21.4)

     The appropriate 7th character is to be added to each code from category W16

A	initial encounter
D	subsequent encounter
S	sequela

   ● **W16.0   Fall into swimming pool**

        Fall into swimming pool NOS

        Excludes1   fall into empty swimming pool (W17.3)

     ● **W16.01   Fall into swimming pool striking water surface**

       ● **W16.011   Fall into swimming pool striking water surface causing drowning and submersion**

            Excludes1   drowning and submersion while in swimming pool without fall (W67)

       ● **W16.012   Fall into swimming pool striking water surface causing other injury**

N   Newborn Age: 0   **P**   Pediatric Age: 0–17   **M**   Maternity DX: 12–55   **A**   Adult Age: 15–124   ♀   Females Only   ♂   Males Only

🔖 Complication\Comorbidity   🔖 Major C\C   (Ex) CC/MCC Exclusions   🔖 Hospital-Acquired Condition

1559

CHAPTER 20 (V01-Y99)

●W16.02 **Fall into swimming pool striking bottom**
    ●W16.021 **Fall into swimming pool striking bottom causing drowning and submersion**
        Excludes1 drowning and submersion while in swimming pool without fall (W67)
    ●W16.022 **Fall into swimming pool striking bottom causing other injury**
●W16.03 **Fall into swimming pool striking wall**
    ●W16.031 **Fall into swimming pool striking wall causing drowning and submersion**
        Excludes1 drowning and submersion while in swimming pool without fall (W67)
    ●W16.032 **Fall into swimming pool striking wall causing other injury**
●W16.1 **Fall into natural body of water**
    Fall into lake
    Fall into open sea
    Fall into river
    Fall into stream
  ●W16.11 **Fall into natural body of water striking water surface**
    ●W16.111 **Fall into natural body of water striking water surface causing drowning and submersion**
        Excludes1 drowning and submersion while in natural body of water without fall (W69)
    ●W16.112 **Fall into natural body of water striking water surface causing other injury**
  ●W16.12 **Fall into natural body of water striking bottom**
    ●W16.121 **Fall into natural body of water striking bottom causing drowning and submersion**
        Excludes1 drowning and submersion while in natural body of water without fall (W69)
    ●W16.122 **Fall into natural body of water striking bottom causing other injury**
  ●W16.13 **Fall into natural body of water striking side**
    ●W16.131 **Fall into natural body of water striking side causing drowning and submersion**
        Excludes1 drowning and submersion while in natural body of water without fall (W69)
    ●W16.132 **Fall into natural body of water striking side causing other injury**
●W16.2 **Fall in (into) filled bathtub or bucket of water**
  ●W16.21 **Fall in (into) filled bathtub**
    Excludes1 fall into empty bathtub (W18.2)
    ●W16.211 **Fall in (into) filled bathtub causing drowning and submersion**
        Excludes1 drowning and submersion while in filled bathtub without fall (W65)
    ●W16.212 **Fall in (into) filled bathtub causing other injury**

  ●W16.22 **Fall in (into) bucket of water**
    ●W16.221 **Fall in (into) bucket of water causing drowning and submersion**
    ●W16.222 **Fall in (into) bucket of water causing other injury**
●W16.3 **Fall into other water**
    Fall into fountain
    Fall into reservoir
  ●W16.31 **Fall into other water striking water surface**
    ●W16.311 **Fall into other water striking water surface causing drowning and submersion**
        Excludes1 drowning and submersion while in other water without fall (W73)
    ●W16.312 **Fall into other water striking water surface causing other injury**
  ●W16.32 **Fall into other water striking bottom**
    ●W16.321 **Fall into other water striking bottom causing drowning and submersion**
        Excludes1 drowning and submersion while in other water without fall (W73)
    ●W16.322 **Fall into other water striking bottom causing other injury**
  ●W16.33 **Fall into other water striking wall**
    ●W16.331 **Fall into other water striking wall causing drowning and submersion**
        Excludes1 drowning and submersion while in other water without fall (W73)
    ●W16.332 **Fall into other water striking wall causing other injury**
●W16.4 **Fall into unspecified water**
  X●W16.41 **Fall into unspecified water causing drowning and submersion**
  X●W16.42 **Fall into unspecified water causing other injury**
●W16.5 **Jumping or diving into swimming pool**
  ●W16.51 **Jumping or diving into swimming pool striking water surface**
    ●W16.511 **Jumping or diving into swimming pool striking water surface causing drowning and submersion**
        Excludes1 drowning and submersion while in swimming pool without jumping or diving (W67)
    ●W16.512 **Jumping or diving into swimming pool striking water surface causing other injury**
  ●W16.52 **Jumping or diving into swimming pool striking bottom**
    ●W16.521 **Jumping or diving into swimming pool striking bottom causing drowning and submersion**
        Excludes1 drowning and submersion while in swimming pool without jumping or diving (W67)
    ●W16.522 **Jumping or diving into swimming pool striking bottom causing other injury**

◀ New ◀ Revised ~~deleted~~ Deleted Excludes 1 Excludes 2 Includes Use additional Code first Code also Unspecified
OGCR Official Guidelines ● Unacceptable Principal Diagnosis X Assign placeholder X ● Use Additional Character(s) ❱ Manifestation Code **Coding Clinic**

- **W16.53** **Jumping or diving into swimming pool striking wall**
  - **W16.531** **Jumping or diving into swimming pool striking wall causing drowning and submersion**
    - **Excludes1**   drowning and submersion while in swimming pool without jumping or diving (W67)
  - **W16.532** **Jumping or diving into swimming pool striking wall causing other injury**
- **W16.6** **Jumping or diving into natural body of water**

  Jumping or diving into lake
  Jumping or diving into open sea
  Jumping or diving into river
  Jumping or diving into stream
  - **W16.61** **Jumping or diving into natural body of water striking water surface**
    - **W16.611** **Jumping or diving into natural body of water striking water surface causing drowning and submersion**
      - **Excludes1**   drowning and submersion while in natural body of water without jumping or diving (W69)
    - **W16.612** **Jumping or diving into natural body of water striking water surface causing other injury**
  - **W16.62** **Jumping or diving into natural body of water striking bottom**
    - **W16.621** **Jumping or diving into natural body of water striking bottom causing drowning and submersion**
      - **Excludes1**   drowning and submersion while in natural body of water without jumping or diving (W69)
    - **W16.622** **Jumping or diving into natural body of water striking bottom causing other injury**
- **W16.7** **Jumping or diving from boat**
  - **Excludes1**   fall from boat into water - see watercraft accident (V90-V94)
  - **W16.71** **Jumping or diving from boat striking water surface**
    - **W16.711** **Jumping or diving from boat striking water surface causing drowning and submersion**
    - **W16.712** **Jumping or diving from boat striking water surface causing other injury**
  - **W16.72** **Jumping or diving from boat striking bottom**
    - **W16.721** **Jumping or diving from boat striking bottom causing drowning and submersion**
    - **W16.722** **Jumping or diving from boat striking bottom causing other injury**

- **W16.8** **Jumping or diving into other water**

  Jumping or diving into fountain
  Jumping or diving into reservoir
  - **W16.81** **Jumping or diving into other water striking water surface**
    - **W16.811** **Jumping or diving into other water striking water surface causing drowning and submersion**
      - **Excludes1**   drowning and submersion while in other water without jumping or diving (W73)
    - **W16.812** **Jumping or diving into other water striking water surface causing other injury**
  - **W16.82** **Jumping or diving into other water striking bottom**
    - **W16.821** **Jumping or diving into other water striking bottom causing drowning and submersion**
      - **Excludes1**   drowning and submersion while in other water without jumping or diving (W73)
    - **W16.822** **Jumping or diving into other water striking bottom causing other injury**
  - **W16.83** **Jumping or diving into other water striking wall**
    - **W16.831** **Jumping or diving into other water striking wall causing drowning and submersion**
      - **Excludes1**   drowning and submersion while in other water without jumping or diving (W73)
    - **W16.832** **Jumping or diving into other water striking wall causing other injury**
- **W16.9** **Jumping or diving into unspecified water**
  - X **W16.91** **Jumping or diving into unspecified water causing drowning and submersion**
  - X **W16.92** **Jumping or diving into unspecified water causing other injury**
- **W17** **Other fall from one level to another**

  The appropriate 7th character is to be added to each code from category W17

A	initial encounter
D	subsequent encounter
S	sequela

  - X **W17.0** **Fall into well**
  - X **W17.1** **Fall into storm drain or manhole**
  - X **W17.2** **Fall into hole**

    Fall into pit
  - X **W17.3** **Fall into empty swimming pool**
    - **Excludes1**   fall into filled swimming pool (W16.0-)
  - X **W17.4** **Fall from dock**
  - **W17.8** **Other fall from one level to another**
    - X **W17.81** **Fall down embankment (hill)**
    - X **W17.82** **Fall from (out of) grocery cart**

      Fall due to grocery cart tipping over
    - X **W17.89** **Other fall from one level to another**

      Fall from cherry picker
      Fall from lifting device
      Fall from mobile elevated work platform [MEWP]
      Fall from sky lift
      Coding Clinic: 2015, Q2, P6

N Newborn Age: Ø   **P** Pediatric Age: Ø–17   **M** Maternity DX: 12–55   **A** Adult Age: 15–124   ♀ Females Only   ♂ Males Only

 Complication\Comorbidity   Major C\C   (Ex) CC/MCC Exclusions   Hospital-Acquired Condition

1561

CHAPTER 20 (V01-Y99)

● **W18**   **Other slipping, tripping and stumbling and falls**

> The appropriate 7th character is to be added to each code from category W18

A	initial encounter
D	subsequent encounter
S	sequela

● **W18.0**   **Fall due to bumping against object**
> Striking against object with subsequent fall
>> **Excludes1**   fall on same level due to slipping, tripping, or stumbling with subsequent striking against object (W01.1-)

X ● **W18.00**   **Striking against unspecified object with subsequent fall**

X ● **W18.01**   **Striking against sports equipment with subsequent fall**

X ● **W18.02**   **Striking against glass with subsequent fall**

X ● **W18.09**   **Striking against other object with subsequent fall**

● **W18.1**   **Fall from or off toilet**

X ● **W18.11**   **Fall from or off toilet without subsequent striking against object**
> Fall from (off) toilet NOS

X ● **W18.12**   **Fall from or off toilet with subsequent striking against object**

X ● **W18.2**   **Fall in (into) shower or empty bathtub**
>> **Excludes1**   fall in full bathtub causing drowning or submersion (W16.21-)

● **W18.3**   **Other and unspecified fall on same level**

X ● **W18.30**   **Fall on same level, unspecified**

X ● **W18.31**   **Fall on same level due to stepping on an object**
> Fall on same level due to stepping on an animal
>> **Excludes1**   slipping, tripping and stumbling without fall due to stepping on animal (W18.41)

X ● **W18.39**   **Other fall on same level**

● **W18.4**   **Slipping, tripping and stumbling without falling**
>> **Excludes1**   collision with another person without fall (W51)

X ● **W18.40**   **Slipping, tripping and stumbling without falling, unspecified**

X ● **W18.41**   **Slipping, tripping and stumbling without falling due to stepping on object**
> Slipping, tripping and stumbling without falling due to stepping on animal
>> **Excludes1**   slipping, tripping and stumbling with fall due to stepping on animal (W18.31)

X ● **W18.42**   **Slipping, tripping and stumbling without falling due to stepping into hole or opening**

X ● **W18.43**   **Slipping, tripping and stumbling without falling due to stepping from one level to another**

X ● **W18.49**   **Other slipping, tripping and stumbling without falling**

X ● **W19**   **Unspecified fall**
> Accidental fall NOS
> The appropriate 7th character is to be added to code W19

A	initial encounter
D	subsequent encounter
S	sequela

Coding Clinic: 2012, Q4, P95

EXPOSURE TO INANIMATE MECHANICAL FORCES (W20-W49)

> **Excludes1**   assault (X92-Y09) ◄▥
>> contact or collision with animals or persons (W50-W64)
>> exposure to inanimate mechanical forces involving military or war operations (Y36.-, Y37.-)
>> intentional self-harm (X71-X83)

● **W20**   **Struck by thrown, projected or falling object**
> *Code first any associated:*
> cataclysm (X34-X39)
> lightning strike (T75.00)
>> **Excludes1**   falling object in machinery accident (W24, W28-W31)
>> falling object in transport accident (V01-V99)
>> object set in motion by explosion (W35-W40)
>> object set in motion by firearm (W32-W34)
>> struck by thrown sports equipment (W21.-)

> The appropriate 7th character is to be added to each code from category W20

A	initial encounter
D	subsequent encounter
S	sequela

X ● **W20.0**   **Struck by falling object in cave-in**
>> **Excludes2**   asphyxiation due to cave-in (T71.21)

X ● **W20.1**   **Struck by object due to collapse of building**
>> **Excludes1**   struck by object due to collapse of burning building (X00.2, X02.2)

X ● **W20.8**   **Other cause of strike by thrown, projected or falling object**
>> **Excludes1**   struck by thrown sports equipment (W21.-)

● **W21**   **Striking against or struck by sports equipment**
>> **Excludes1**   assault with sports equipment (Y08.0-)
>> striking against or struck by sports equipment with subsequent fall (W18.01)

> The appropriate 7th character is to be added to each code from category W21

A	initial encounter
D	subsequent encounter
S	sequela

● **W21.0**   **Struck by hit or thrown ball**

X ● **W21.00**   **Struck by hit or thrown ball, unspecified type**

X ● **W21.01**   **Struck by football**

X ● **W21.02**   **Struck by soccer ball**

X ● **W21.03**   **Struck by baseball**

X ● **W21.04**   **Struck by golf ball**

X ● **W21.05**   **Struck by basketball**

X ● **W21.06**   **Struck by volleyball**

X ● **W21.07**   **Struck by softball**

X ● **W21.09**   **Struck by other hit or thrown ball**

● **W21.1**   **Struck by bat, racquet or club**

X ● **W21.11**   **Struck by baseball bat**

X ● **W21.12**   **Struck by tennis racquet**

X ● **W21.13**   **Struck by golf club**

X ● **W21.19**   **Struck by other bat, racquet or club**

◄ New   ◄▥ Revised   ~~deleted~~ Deleted   Excludes 1   Excludes 2   Includes   Use additional   Code first   Code also   Unspecified

OGCR Official Guidelines   ● Unacceptable Principal Diagnosis   X Assign placeholder X   ● Use Additional Character(s)   ▸ Manifestation Code   Coding Clinic

● **W21.2 Struck by hockey stick or puck**
    ● **W21.21 Struck by hockey stick**
        ● **W21.210 Struck by ice hockey stick**
        ● **W21.211 Struck by field hockey stick**
    ● **W21.22 Struck by hockey puck**
        ● **W21.220 Struck by ice hockey puck**
        ● **W21.221 Struck by field hockey puck**
● **W21.3 Struck by sports foot wear**
    X ● **W21.31 Struck by shoe cleats**
        Stepped on by shoe cleats
    X ● **W21.32 Struck by skate blades**
        Skated over by skate blades
    X ● **W21.39 Struck by other sports foot wear**
X ● **W21.4 Striking against diving board**
       Use additional code for subsequent falling into water, if applicable (W16.-)
● **W21.8 Striking against or struck by other sports equipment**
    X ● **W21.81 Striking against or struck by football helmet**
    X ● **W21.89 Striking against or struck by other sports equipment**
X ● **W21.9 Striking against or struck by unspecified sports equipment**

● **W22 Striking against or struck by other objects**
    Excludes1 striking against or struck by object with subsequent fall (W18.09)
    The appropriate 7th character is to be added to each code from category W22

A	initial encounter
D	subsequent encounter
S	sequela

    ● **W22.0 Striking against stationary object**
        Excludes1 striking against stationary sports equipment (W21.8)
    X ● **W22.01 Walked into wall**
    X ● **W22.02 Walked into lamppost**
    X ● **W22.03 Walked into furniture**
    ● **W22.04 Striking against wall of swimming pool**
        ● **W22.041 Striking against wall of swimming pool causing drowning and submersion**
            Excludes1 drowning and submersion while swimming without striking against wall (W67)
        ● **W22.042 Striking against wall of swimming pool causing other injury**
    X ● **W22.09 Striking against other stationary object**
● **W22.1 Striking against or struck by automobile airbag**
    X ● **W22.10 Striking against or struck by unspecified automobile airbag**
    X ● **W22.11 Striking against or struck by driver side automobile airbag**
    X ● **W22.12 Striking against or struck by front passenger side automobile airbag**
    X ● **W22.19 Striking against or struck by other automobile airbag**
X ● **W22.8 Striking against or struck by other objects**
    Striking against or struck by object NOS
        Excludes1 struck by thrown, projected or falling object (W20.-)

● **W23 Caught, crushed, jammed or pinched in or between objects**
    Excludes1 injury caused by cutting or piercing instruments (W25-W27)
        injury caused by firearms malfunction (W32.1, W33.1-, W34.1-)
        injury caused by lifting and transmission devices (W24.-)
        injury caused by machinery (W28-W31)
        injury caused by nonpowered hand tools (W27.-)
        injury caused by transport vehicle being used as a means of transportation (V01-V99)
        injury caused by struck by thrown, projected or falling object (W20.-)
    The appropriate 7th character is to be added to each code from category W23

A	initial encounter
D	subsequent encounter
S	sequela

    X ● **W23.0 Caught, crushed, jammed, or pinched between moving objects**
    X ● **W23.1 Caught, crushed, jammed, or pinched between stationary objects**

● **W24 Contact with lifting and transmission devices, not elsewhere classified**
    Excludes1 transport accidents (V01-V99)
    The appropriate 7th character is to be added to each code from category W24

A	initial encounter
D	subsequent encounter
S	sequela

    X ● **W24.0 Contact with lifting devices, not elsewhere classified**
        Contact with chain hoist
        Contact with drive belt
        Contact with pulley (block)
    X ● **W24.1 Contact with transmission devices, not elsewhere classified**
        Contact with transmission belt or cable

X ● **W25 Contact with sharp glass**
    Code first any associated:
        injury due to flying glass from explosion or firearm discharge (W32-W40)
        transport accident (V00-V99)
    Excludes1 fall on same level due to slipping, tripping and stumbling with subsequent striking against sharp glass (W01.10)
        striking against sharp glass with subsequent fall (W18.02)
    Excludes2 glass embedded in skin (W45) ◄
    The appropriate 7th character is to be added to code W25

A	initial encounter
D	subsequent encounter
S	sequela

● **W26 Contact with other sharp objects** ◄▥
    Excludes2 sharp object(s) embedded in skin (W45) ◄
    The appropriate 7th character is to be added to each code from category W26

A	initial encounter
D	subsequent encounter
S	sequela

    X ● **W26.0 Contact with knife**
        Excludes1 contact with electric knife (W29.1)
    X ● **W26.1 Contact with sword or dagger**
    X ● **W26.2 Contact with edge of stiff paper** ◄
        Paper cut ◄
    X ● **W26.8 Contact with other sharp object(s), not elsewhere classified** ◄
        Contact with tin can lid ◄
    X ● **W26.9 Contact with unspecified sharp object(s)** ◄

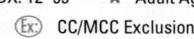

CHAPTER 20 (V01-Y99)

● **W27   Contact with nonpowered hand tool**

The appropriate 7th character is to be added to each code from category W27

> A   initial encounter
> D   subsequent encounter
> S   sequela

X● **W27.0   Contact with workbench tool**
Contact with auger
Contact with axe
Contact with chisel
Contact with handsaw
Contact with screwdriver

X● **W27.1   Contact with garden tool**
Contact with hoe
Contact with nonpowered lawn mower
Contact with pitchfork
Contact with rake

X● **W27.2   Contact with scissors**

X● **W27.3   Contact with needle (sewing)**

> **Excludes1**   contact with hypodermic needle (W46.-)

X● **W27.4   Contact with kitchen utensil**
Contact with fork
Contact with ice-pick
Contact with can-opener NOS

X● **W27.5   Contact with paper-cutter**

X● **W27.8   Contact with other nonpowered hand tool**
Contact with nonpowered sewing machine
Contact with shovel

X● **W28   Contact with powered lawn mower**
Powered lawn mower (commercial) (residential)

> **Excludes1**   contact with nonpowered lawn mower (W27.1)
> **Excludes2**   exposure to electric current (W86.-)

The appropriate 7th character is to be added to code W28

> A   initial encounter
> D   subsequent encounter
> S   sequela

● **W29   Contact with other powered hand tools and household machinery**

> **Excludes1**   contact with commercial machinery (W31.82)
> contact with hot household appliance (X15)
> contact with nonpowered hand tool (W27.-)
> exposure to electric current (W86)

The appropriate 7th character is to be added to each code from category W29

> A   initial encounter
> D   subsequent encounter
> S   sequela

X● **W29.0   Contact with powered kitchen appliance**
Contact with blender
Contact with can-opener
Contact with garbage disposal
Contact with mixer

X● **W29.1   Contact with electric knife**

X● **W29.2   Contact with other powered household machinery**
Contact with electric fan
Contact with powered dryer (clothes) (powered) (spin)
Contact with washing-machine
Contact with sewing machine

X● **W29.3   Contact with powered garden and outdoor hand tools and machinery**
Contact with chainsaw
Contact with edger
Contact with garden cultivator (tiller)
Contact with hedge trimmer
Contact with other powered garden tool

> **Excludes1**   contact with powered lawn mower (W28)

X● **W29.4   Contact with nail gun**

X● **W29.8   Contact with other powered powered hand tools and household machinery**
Contact with do-it-yourself tool NOS

● **W30   Contact with agricultural machinery**

> **Includes**   animal-powered farm machine
> **Excludes1**   agricultural transport vehicle accident (V01-V99)
> explosion of grain store (W40.8)
> exposure to electric current (W86.-)

The appropriate 7th character is to be added to each code from category W30

> A   initial encounter
> D   subsequent encounter
> S   sequela

X● **W30.0   Contact with combine harvester**
Contact with reaper
Contact with thresher

X● **W30.1   Contact with power take-off devices (PTO)**

X● **W30.2   Contact with hay derrick**

X● **W30.3   Contact with grain storage elevator**

> **Excludes1**   explosion of grain store (W40.8)

● **W30.8   Contact with other specified agricultural machinery**

X● **W30.81   Contact with agricultural transport vehicle in stationary use**
Contact with agricultural transport vehicle under repair, not on public roadway

> **Excludes1**   agricultural transport vehicle accident (V01-V99)

X● **W30.89   Contact with other specified agricultural machinery**

X● **W30.9   Contact with unspecified agricultural machinery**
Contact with farm machinery NOS

● **W31   Contact with other and unspecified machinery**

> **Excludes1**   contact with agricultural machinery (W30.-)
> contact with machinery in transport under own power or being towed by a vehicle (V01-V99)
> exposure to electric current (W86)

The appropriate 7th character is to be added to each code from category W31

> A   initial encounter
> D   subsequent encounter
> S   sequela

X● **W31.0   Contact with mining and earth-drilling machinery**
Contact with bore or drill (land) (seabed)
Contact with shaft hoist
Contact with shaft lift
Contact with undercutter

X● **W31.1   Contact with metalworking machines**
Contact with abrasive wheel
Contact with forging machine
Contact with lathe
Contact with mechanical shears
Contact with metal drilling machine
Contact with milling machine
Contact with power press
Contact with rolling-mill
Contact with metal sawing machine

X● **W31.2   Contact with powered woodworking and forming machines**
Contact with band saw
Contact with bench saw
Contact with circular saw
Contact with molding machine
Contact with overhead plane
Contact with powered saw
Contact with radial saw
Contact with sander

> **Excludes1**   nonpowered woodworking tools (W27.0)

◀ New   ◀▬ Revised   ~~deleted~~ Deleted   Excludes 1   Excludes 2   Includes   Use additional   Code first   Code also   Unspecified
OGCR Official Guidelines   ● Unacceptable Principal Diagnosis   X Assign placeholder X   ● Use Additional Character(s)   ◣ Manifestation Code   **Coding Clinic**

X● **W31.3**   **Contact with prime movers**
     Contact with gas turbine
     Contact with internal combustion engine
     Contact with steam engine
     Contact with water driven turbine

● **W31.8**   **Contact with other specified machinery**

X● **W31.81**   **Contact with recreational machinery**
     Contact with roller-coaster

X● **W31.82**   **Contact with other commercial machinery**
     Contact with commercial electric fan
     Contact with commercial kitchen appliances
     Contact with commercial powered dryer
       (clothes) (powered) (spin)
     Contact with commercial washing-machine
     Contact with commercial sewing machine

> **Excludes1**   contact with household
>   machinery (W29.-)
>   contact with powered lawn
>   mower (W28)

X● **W31.83**   **Contact with special construction vehicle in stationary use**
     Contact with special construction vehicle
       under repair, not on public roadway

> **Excludes1**   special construction vehicle
>   accident (V01-V99)

X● **W31.89**   **Contact with other specified machinery**

X● **W31.9**   **Contact with unspecified machinery**
     Contact with machinery NOS

● **W32**   **Accidental handgun discharge and malfunction**

> **Includes**   accidental discharge and malfunction of gun for
>   single hand use
>   accidental discharge and malfunction of pistol
>   accidental discharge and malfunction of revolver
>   handgun discharge and malfunction NOS

> **Excludes1**   accidental airgun discharge and malfunction
>   (W34.010, W34.110)
>   accidental BB gun discharge and malfunction
>   (W34.010, W34.110)
>   accidental pellet gun discharge and malfunction
>   (W34.010, W34.110)
>   accidental shotgun discharge and malfunction
>   (W33.01, W33.11)
>   assault by handgun discharge (X93)
>   handgun discharge involving legal intervention
>   (Y35.0-)
>   handgun discharge involving military or war
>   operations (Y36.4-)
>   intentional self-harm by handgun discharge (X72)
>   Very pistol discharge and malfunction (W34.09,
>   W34.19)

The appropriate 7th character is to be added to each code from
category W32

A	initial encounter
D	subsequent encounter
S	sequela

X● **W32.0**   **Accidental handgun discharge**

X● **W32.1**   **Accidental handgun malfunction**
     Injury due to explosion of handgun (parts)
     Injury due to malfunction of mechanism or component
       of handgun
     Injury due to recoil of handgun
     Powder burn from handgun

● **W33**   **Accidental rifle, shotgun and larger firearm discharge and malfunction**

> **Includes**   rifle, shotgun and larger firearm discharge and
>   malfunction NOS

> **Excludes1**   accidental airgun discharge and malfunction
>   (W34.010, W34.110)
>   accidental BB gun discharge and malfunction
>   (W34.010, W34.110)
>   accidental handgun discharge and malfunction
>   (W32.-)
>   accidental pellet gun discharge and malfunction
>   (W34.010, W34.110)
>   assault by rifle, shotgun and larger firearm
>   discharge (X94)
>   firearm discharge involving legal intervention
>   (Y35.0-)
>   firearm discharge involving military or war
>   operations (Y36.4-)
>   intentional self-harm by rifle, shotgun and larger
>   firearm discharge (X73)

The appropriate 7th character is to be added to each code from
category W33

A	initial encounter
D	subsequent encounter
S	sequela

● **W33.0**   **Accidental rifle, shotgun and larger firearm discharge**

X● **W33.00**   **Accidental discharge of unspecified larger firearm**
     Discharge of unspecified larger firearm NOS

X● **W33.01**   **Accidental discharge of shotgun**
     Discharge of shotgun NOS

X● **W33.02**   **Accidental discharge of hunting rifle**
     Discharge of hunting rifle NOS

X● **W33.03**   **Accidental discharge of machine gun**
     Discharge of machine gun NOS

X● **W33.09**   **Accidental discharge of other larger firearm**
     Discharge of other larger firearm NOS

● **W33.1**   **Accidental rifle, shotgun and larger firearm malfunction**
     Injury due to explosion of rifle, shotgun and larger
       firearm (parts)
     Injury due to malfunction of mechanism or component
       of rifle, shotgun and larger firearm
     Injury due to piercing, cutting, crushing or pinching
       due to (by) slide trigger mechanism, scope or other
       gun part
     Injury due to recoil of rifle, shotgun and larger firearm
     Powder burn from rifle, shotgun and larger firearm

X● **W33.10**   **Accidental malfunction of unspecified larger firearm**
     Malfunction of unspecified larger firearm NOS

X● **W33.11**   **Accidental malfunction of shotgun**
     Malfunction of shotgun NOS

X● **W33.12**   **Accidental malfunction of hunting rifle**
     Malfunction of hunting rifle NOS

X● **W33.13**   **Accidental malfunction of machine gun**
     Malfunction of machine gun NOS

X● **W33.19**   **Accidental malfunction of other larger firearm**
     Malfunction of other larger firearm NOS

CHAPTER 20 (V01-Y99)

● **W34   Accidental discharge and malfunction from other and unspecified firearms and guns**

> The appropriate 7th character is to be added to each code from category W34

> | A | initial encounter |
> |---|---|
> | D | subsequent encounter |
> | S | sequela |

● **W34.0   Accidental discharge from other and unspecified firearms and guns**

X ● **W34.00   Accidental discharge from unspecified firearms or gun**

> Discharge from firearm NOS
> Gunshot wound NOS
> Shot NOS
> **Coding Clinic: 2015, Q1, P17**

● **W34.01   Accidental discharge of gas, air or spring-operated guns**

● **W34.010   Accidental discharge of airgun**
> Accidental discharge of BB gun
> Accidental discharge of pellet gun

● **W34.011   Accidental discharge of paintball gun**
> Accidental injury due to paintball discharge

● **W34.018   Accidental discharge of other gas, air or spring-operated gun**

X ● **W34.09   Accidental discharge from other specified firearms**
> Accidental discharge from Very pistol [flare]

● **W34.1   Accidental malfunction from other and unspecified firearms and guns**

X ● **W34.10   Accidental malfunction from unspecified firearms or gun**
> Firearm malfunction NOS

● **W34.11   Accidental malfunction of gas, air or spring-operated guns**

● **W34.110   Accidental malfunction of airgun**
> Accidental malfunction of BB gun
> Accidental malfunction of pellet gun

● **W34.111   Accidental malfunction of paintball gun**
> Accidental injury due to paintball gun malfunction

● **W34.118   Accidental malfunction of other gas, air or spring-operated gun**

X ● **W34.19   Accidental malfunction from other specified firearms**
> Accidental malfunction from Very pistol [flare]

X ● **W35   Explosion and rupture of boiler**

> **Excludes1**   explosion and rupture of boiler on watercraft (V93.4)

> The appropriate 7th character is to be added to code W35

> | A | initial encounter |
> |---|---|
> | D | subsequent encounter |
> | S | sequela |

● **W36   Explosion and rupture of gas cylinder**

> The appropriate 7th character is to be added to each code from category W36

> | A | initial encounter |
> |---|---|
> | D | subsequent encounter |
> | S | sequela |

X ● **W36.1   Explosion and rupture of aerosol can**

X ● **W36.2   Explosion and rupture of air tank**

X ● **W36.3   Explosion and rupture of pressurized-gas tank**

X ● **W36.8   Explosion and rupture of other gas cylinder**

X ● **W36.9   Explosion and rupture of unspecified gas cylinder**

● **W37   Explosion and rupture of pressurized tire, pipe or hose**

> The appropriate 7th character is to be added to each code from category W37

> | A | initial encounter |
> |---|---|
> | D | subsequent encounter |
> | S | sequela |

X ● **W37.0   Explosion of bicycle tire**

X ● **W37.8   Explosion and rupture of other pressurized tire, pipe or hose**

X ● **W38   Explosion and rupture of other specified pressurized devices**

> The appropriate 7th character is to be added to code W38

> | A | initial encounter |
> |---|---|
> | D | subsequent encounter |
> | S | sequela |

X ● **W39   Discharge of firework**

> The appropriate 7th character is to be added to code W39

> | A | initial encounter |
> |---|---|
> | D | subsequent encounter |
> | S | sequela |

● **W40   Explosion of other materials**

> **Excludes1**   assault by explosive material (X96)
> explosion involving legal intervention (Y35.1-)
> explosion involving military or war operations (Y36.0-, Y36.2-)
> intentional self-harm by explosive material (X75)

> The appropriate 7th character is to be added to each code from category W40

> | A | initial encounter |
> |---|---|
> | D | subsequent encounter |
> | S | sequela |

X ● **W40.0   Explosion of blasting material**
> Explosion of blasting cap
> Explosion of detonator
> Explosion of dynamite
> Explosion of explosive (any) used in blasting operations

X ● **W40.1   Explosion of explosive gases**
> Explosion of acetylene
> Explosion of butane
> Explosion of coal gas
> Explosion in mine NOS
> Explosion of explosive gas
> Explosion of fire damp
> Explosion of gasoline fumes
> Explosion of methane
> Explosion of propane

X ● **W40.8   Explosion of other specified explosive materials**
> Explosion in dump NOS
> Explosion in factory NOS
> Explosion in grain store
> Explosion in munitions

> > **Excludes1**   explosion involving legal intervention (Y35.1-)
> > explosion involving military or war operations (Y36.0-, Y36.2-)

X ● **W40.9   Explosion of unspecified explosive materials**
> Explosion NOS

● **W42   Exposure to noise**

> The appropriate 7th character is to be added to each code from category W42

> | A | initial encounter |
> |---|---|
> | D | subsequent encounter |
> | S | sequela |

X ● **W42.0   Exposure to supersonic waves**

X ● **W42.9   Exposure to other noise**
> Exposure to sound waves NOS

◄ New   ◄▥▥ Revised   ~~deleted~~ Deleted   Excludes 1   Excludes 2   Includes   Use additional   Code first   Code also   Unspecified

1566   OGCR Official Guidelines   ● Unacceptable Principal Diagnosis   X Assign placeholder X   ● Use Additional Character(s)   ▮ Manifestation Code   **Coding Clinic**

● **W45** **Foreign body or object entering through skin**

Includes	foreign body or object embedded in skin ◄
	nail embedded in skin ◄
Excludes2	contact with hand tools (nonpowered) (powered) (W27-W29)
	contact with other sharp object(s) (W26.-) ◄▦
	contact with sharp glass (W25.-)
	struck by objects (W20-W22)

The appropriate 7th character is to be added to each code from category W45

A	initial encounter
D	subsequent encounter
S	sequela

X● **W45.0** **Nail entering through skin**

~~W45.1~~ ~~Paper entering through skin~~
~~Paper cut~~

~~W45.2~~ ~~Lid of can entering through skin~~

X● **W45.8** **Other foreign body or object entering through skin**
Splinter in skin NOS

● **W46** **Contact with hypodermic needle**

The appropriate 7th character is to be added to each code from category W46

A	initial encounter
D	subsequent encounter
S	sequela

X● **W46.0** **Contact with hypodermic needle**
Hypodermic needle stick NOS

X● **W46.1** **Contact with contaminated hypodermic needle**

● **W49** **Exposure to other inanimate mechanical forces**

Includes	exposure to abnormal gravitational [G] forces
	exposure to inanimate mechanical forces NEC
Excludes1	exposure to inanimate mechanical forces involving military or war operations (Y36.-, Y37.-)

The appropriate 7th character is to be added to each code from category W49

A	initial encounter
D	subsequent encounter
S	sequela

● **W49.0** **Item causing external constriction**

X● **W49.01** **Hair causing external constriction**

X● **W49.02** **String or thread causing external constriction**

X● **W49.03** **Rubber band causing external constriction**

X● **W49.04** **Ring or other jewelry causing external constriction**

X● **W49.09** **Other item causing external constriction**

X● **W49.9** **Exposure to other inanimate mechanical forces**

EXPOSURE TO ANIMATE MECHANICAL FORCES (W50-W64)

| **Excludes1** | toxic effect of contact with venomous animals and plants (T63.-) |

● **W50** **Accidental hit, strike, kick, twist, bite or scratch by another person**

Includes	hit, strike, kick, twist, bite, or scratch by another person NOS
Excludes1	assault by bodily force (Y04)
	struck by objects (W20-W22)

The appropriate 7th character is to be added to each code from category W50

A	initial encounter
D	subsequent encounter
S	sequela

X● **W50.0** **Accidental hit or strike by another person**
Hit or strike by another person NOS

X● **W50.1** **Accidental kick by another person**
Kick by another person NOS

X● **W50.2** **Accidental twist by another person**
Twist by another person NOS
Coding Clinic: 2015, Q1, P8

X● **W50.3** **Accidental bite by another person**
Human bite
Bite by another person NOS

X● **W50.4** **Accidental scratch by another person**
Scratch by another person NOS

X● **W51** **Accidental striking against or bumped into by another person**

| **Excludes1** | assault by striking against or bumping into by another person (Y04.2) |
| | fall due to collision with another person (W03) |

The appropriate 7th character is to be added to code W51

A	initial encounter
D	subsequent encounter
S	sequela

X● **W52** **Crushed, pushed or stepped on by crowd or human stampede**
Crushed, pushed or stepped on by crowd or human stampede with or without fall

The appropriate 7th character is to be added to code W52

A	initial encounter
D	subsequent encounter
S	sequela

● **W53** **Contact with rodent**

| **Includes** | contact with saliva, feces or urine of rodent |

The appropriate 7th character is to be added to each code from category W53

A	initial encounter
D	subsequent encounter
S	sequela

● **W53.0** **Contact with mouse**

X● **W53.01** **Bitten by mouse**

X● **W53.09** **Other contact with mouse**

● **W53.1** **Contact with rat**

X● **W53.11** **Bitten by rat**

X● **W53.19** **Other contact with rat**

● **W53.2** **Contact with squirrel**

X● **W53.21** **Bitten by squirrel**

X● **W53.29** **Other contact with squirrel**

● **W53.8** **Contact with other rodent**

X● **W53.81** **Bitten by other rodent**

X● **W53.89** **Other contact with other rodent**

● **W54** **Contact with dog**

| **Includes** | contact with saliva, feces or urine of dog |

The appropriate 7th character is to be added to each code from category W54

A	initial encounter
D	subsequent encounter
S	sequela

X● **W54.0** **Bitten by dog**

X● **W54.1** **Struck by dog**
Knocked over by dog

X● **W54.8** **Other contact with dog**

CHAPTER 20 (V01-Y99)

● W55   **Contact with other mammals**

    | Includes | contact with saliva, feces or urine of mammal |
    | Excludes1 | animal being ridden - see transport accidents |

               bitten or struck by dog (W54)
               bitten or struck by rodent (W53.-)
               contact with marine mammals (W56.X-)

    The appropriate 7th character is to be added to each code from category W55

> A   initial encounter
> D   subsequent encounter
> S   sequela

   ● **W55.0**   **Contact with cat**
     X● **W55.01**   **Bitten by cat**
     X● **W55.03**   **Scratched by cat**
     X● **W55.09**   **Other contact with cat**

   ● **W55.1**   **Contact with horse**
     X● **W55.11**   **Bitten by horse**
     X● **W55.12**   **Struck by horse**
     X● **W55.19**   **Other contact with horse**

   ● **W55.2**   **Contact with cow**
         Contact with bull
     X● **W55.21**   **Bitten by cow**
     X● **W55.22**   **Struck by cow**
           Gored by bull
     X● **W55.29**   **Other contact with cow**

   ● **W55.3**   **Contact with other hoof stock**
         Contact with goats
         Contact with sheep
     X● **W55.31**   **Bitten by other hoof stock**
     X● **W55.32**   **Struck by other hoof stock**
           Gored by goat
           Gored by ram
     X● **W55.39**   **Other contact with other hoof stock**

   ● **W55.4**   **Contact with pig**
     X● **W55.41**   **Bitten by pig**
     X● **W55.42**   **Struck by pig**
     X● **W55.49**   **Other contact with pig**

   ● **W55.5**   **Contact with raccoon**
     X● **W55.51**   **Bitten by raccoon**
     X● **W55.52**   **Struck by raccoon**
     X● **W55.59**   **Other contact with raccoon**

   ● **W55.8**   **Contact with other mammals**
     X● **W55.81**   **Bitten by other mammals**
     X● **W55.82**   **Struck by other mammals**
     X● **W55.89**   **Other contact with other mammals**

● W56   **Contact with nonvenomous marine animal**

    | Excludes1 | contact with venomous marine animal (T63.-) |

    The appropriate 7th character is to be added to each code from category W56

> A   initial encounter
> D   subsequent encounter
> S   sequela

   ● **W56.0**   **Contact with dolphin**
     X● **W56.01**   **Bitten by dolphin**
     X● **W56.02**   **Struck by dolphin**
     X● **W56.09**   **Other contact with dolphin**

   ● **W56.1**   **Contact with sea lion**
     X● **W56.11**   **Bitten by sea lion**
     X● **W56.12**   **Struck by sea lion**
     X● **W56.19**   **Other contact with sea lion**

   ● **W56.2**   **Contact with orca**
         Contact with killer whale
     X● **W56.21**   **Bitten by orca**
     X● **W56.22**   **Struck by orca**
     X● **W56.29**   **Other contact with orca**

   ● **W56.3**   **Contact with other marine mammals**
     X● **W56.31**   **Bitten by other marine mammals**
     X● **W56.32**   **Struck by other marine mammals**
     X● **W56.39**   **Other contact with other marine mammals**

   ● **W56.4**   **Contact with shark**
     X● **W56.41**   **Bitten by shark**
     X● **W56.42**   **Struck by shark**
     X● **W56.49**   **Other contact with shark**

   ● **W56.5**   **Contact with other fish**
     X● **W56.51**   **Bitten by other fish**
     X● **W56.52**   **Struck by other fish**
     X● **W56.59**   **Other contact with other fish**

   ● **W56.8**   **Contact with other nonvenomous marine animals**
     X● **W56.81**   **Bitten by other nonvenomous marine animals**
     X● **W56.82**   **Struck by other nonvenomous marine animals**
     X● **W56.89**   **Other contact with other nonvenomous marine animals**

X● W57   **Bitten or stung by nonvenomous insect and other nonvenomous arthropods**

    | Excludes1 | contact with venomous insects and arthropods (T63.2-, T63.3-, T63.4-) |

    The appropriate 7th character is to be added to code W57

> A   initial encounter
> D   subsequent encounter
> S   sequela

● W58   **Contact with crocodile or alligator**

    The appropriate 7th character is to be added to each code from category W58

> A   initial encounter
> D   subsequent encounter
> S   sequela

   ● **W58.0**   **Contact with alligator**
     X● **W58.01**   **Bitten by alligator**
     X● **W58.02**   **Struck by alligator**
     X● **W58.03**   **Crushed by alligator**
     X● **W58.09**   **Other contact with alligator**

   ● **W58.1**   **Contact with crocodile**
     X● **W58.11**   **Bitten by crocodile**
     X● **W58.12**   **Struck by crocodile**
     X● **W58.13**   **Crushed by crocodile**
     X● **W58.19**   **Other contact with crocodile**

● W59   **Contact with other nonvenomous reptiles**

    | Excludes1 | contact with venomous reptile (T63.0-, T63.1-) |

    The appropriate 7th character is to be added to each code from category W59

> A   initial encounter
> D   subsequent encounter
> S   sequela

   ● **W59.0**   **Contact with nonvenomous lizards**
     X● **W59.01**   **Bitten by nonvenomous lizards**
     X● **W59.02**   **Struck by nonvenomous lizards**
     X● **W59.09**   **Other contact with nonvenomous lizards**
           Exposure to nonvenomous lizards

◀ New   ◀■ Revised   ~~deleted~~ Deleted   Excludes 1   Excludes 2   Includes   Use additional   Code first   Code also   Unspecified

OGCR Official Guidelines   ● Unacceptable Principal Diagnosis   X Assign placeholder X   ● Use Additional Character(s)   ▶ Manifestation Code   Coding Clinic

- W59.1 **Contact with nonvenomous snakes**
  - X● W59.11 **Bitten by nonvenomous snake**
  - X● W59.12 **Struck by nonvenomous snake**
  - X● W59.13 **Crushed by nonvenomous snake**
  - X● W59.19 **Other contact with nonvenomous snake**
- W59.2 **Contact with turtles**

  Excludes1   contact with tortoises (W59.8-)
  - X● W59.21 **Bitten by turtle**
  - X● W59.22 **Struck by turtle**
  - X● W59.29 **Other contact with turtle**
    Exposure to turtles
- W59.8 **Contact with other nonvenomous reptiles**
  - X● W59.81 **Bitten by other nonvenomous reptiles**
  - X● W59.82 **Struck by other nonvenomous reptiles**
  - X● W59.83 **Crushed by other nonvenomous reptiles**
  - X● W59.89 **Other contact with other nonvenomous reptiles**

X● W60 **Contact with nonvenomous plant thorns and spines and sharp leaves**

Excludes1   contact with venomous plants (T63.X7-)

The appropriate 7th character is to be added to code W60

A	initial encounter
D	subsequent encounter
S	sequela

● W61 **Contact with birds (domestic) (wild)**

Includes   contact with excreta of birds

The appropriate 7th character is to be added to each code from category W61

A	initial encounter
D	subsequent encounter
S	sequela

- W61.0 **Contact with parrot**
  - X● W61.01 **Bitten by parrot**
  - X● W61.02 **Struck by parrot**
  - X● W61.09 **Other contact with parrot**
    Exposure to parrots
- W61.1 **Contact with macaw**
  - X● W61.11 **Bitten by macaw**
  - X● W61.12 **Struck by macaw**
  - X● W61.19 **Other contact with macaw**
    Exposure to macaws
- W61.2 **Contact with other psittacines**
  - X● W61.21 **Bitten by other psittacines**
  - X● W61.22 **Struck by other psittacines**
  - X● W61.29 **Other contact with other psittacines**
    Exposure to other psittacines
- W61.3 **Contact with chicken**
  - X● W61.32 **Struck by chicken**
  - X● W61.33 **Pecked by chicken**
  - X● W61.39 **Other contact with chicken**
    Exposure to chickens
- W61.4 **Contact with turkey**
  - X● W61.42 **Struck by turkey**
  - X● W61.43 **Pecked by turkey**
  - X● W61.49 **Other contact with turkey**
- W61.5 **Contact with goose**
  - X● W61.51 **Bitten by goose**
  - X● W61.52 **Struck by goose**
  - X● W61.59 **Other contact with goose**
- W61.6 **Contact with duck**
  - X● W61.61 **Bitten by duck**
  - X● W61.62 **Struck by duck**
  - X● W61.69 **Other contact with duck**

- W61.9 **Contact with other birds**
  - X● W61.91 **Bitten by other birds**
  - X● W61.92 **Struck by other birds**
  - X● W61.99 **Other contact with other birds**
    Contact with bird NOS

● W62 **Contact with nonvenomous amphibians**

Excludes1   contact with venomous amphibians (T63.81-R63.83)

The appropriate 7th character is to be added to each code from category W62

A	initial encounter
D	subsequent encounter
S	sequela

- X● W62.0 **Contact with nonvenomous frogs**
- X● W62.1 **Contact with nonvenomous toads**
- X● W62.9 **Contact with other nonvenomous amphibians**

X● W64 **Exposure to other animate mechanical forces**

Includes   exposure to nonvenomous animal NOS

Excludes1   contact with venomous animal (T63.-)

The appropriate 7th character is to be added to code W64

A	initial encounter
D	subsequent encounter
S	sequela

ACCIDENTAL NON-TRANSPORT DROWNING AND SUBMERSION (W65-W74)

Excludes1   accidental drowning and submersion due to fall into water (W16.-)

accidental drowning and submersion due to water transport accident (V90.-, V92.-)

Excludes2   accidental drowning and submersion due to cataclysm (X34-X39)

X● W65 **Accidental drowning and submersion while in bathtub**

Excludes1   accidental drowning and submersion due to fall in (into) bathtub (W16.211)

The appropriate 7th character is to be added to code W65

A	initial encounter
D	subsequent encounter
S	sequela

X● W67 **Accidental drowning and submersion while in swimming pool**

Excludes1   accidental drowning and submersion due to fall into swimming pool (W16.011, W16.021, W16.031)

accidental drowning and submersion due to striking into wall of swimming pool (W22.041)

The appropriate 7th character is to be added to code W67

A	initial encounter
D	subsequent encounter
S	sequela

X● W69 **Accidental drowning and submersion while in natural water**

Accidental drowning and submersion while in lake
Accidental drowning and submersion while in open sea
Accidental drowning and submersion while in river
Accidental drowning and submersion while in stream

Excludes1   accidental drowning and submersion due to fall into natural body of water (W16.111, W16.121, W16.131)

The appropriate 7th character is to be added to code W69

A	initial encounter
D	subsequent encounter
S	sequela

N Newborn Age: 0   **P** Pediatric Age: 0–17   **M** Maternity DX: 12–55   **A** Adult Age: 15–124   ♀ Females Only   ♂ Males Only

🔗 Complication\Comorbidity   🔗 Major C\C   ⒺⓍ CC/MCC Exclusions   🔗 Hospital-Acquired Condition   **1569**

X● **W73** **Other specified cause of accidental non-transport drowning and submersion**
     Accidental drowning and submersion while in quenching tank
     Accidental drowning and submersion while in reservoir

     Excludes1   accidental drowning and submersion due to
                 fall into other water (W16.311, W16.321,
                 W16.331)

     The appropriate 7th character is to be added to code W73

A	initial encounter
D	subsequent encounter
S	sequela

X● **W74** **Unspecified cause of accidental drowning and submersion**
     Drowning NOS

     The appropriate 7th character is to be added to code W74

A	initial encounter
D	subsequent encounter
S	sequela

EXPOSURE TO ELECTRIC CURRENT, RADIATION AND EXTREME AMBIENT AIR TEMPERATURE AND PRESSURE (W85-W99)

     Excludes1   exposure to:
                 failure in dosage of radiation or temperature
                     during surgical and medical care
                     (Y63.2-Y63.5)
                 lightning (T75.Ø-)
                 natural cold (X31)
                 natural heat (X3Ø)
                 natural radiation NOS (X39)
                 radiological procedure and radiotherapy
                     (Y84.2)
                 sunlight (X32)

X● **W85** **Exposure to electric transmission lines**
     Broken power line

     The appropriate 7th character is to be added to code W85

A	initial encounter
D	subsequent encounter
S	sequela

● **W86** **Exposure to other specified electric current**

     The appropriate 7th character is to be added to each code from
     category W86

A	initial encounter
D	subsequent encounter
S	sequela

X● **W86.Ø** **Exposure to domestic wiring and appliances**

X● **W86.1** **Exposure to industrial wiring, appliances and electrical machinery**
     Exposure to conductors
     Exposure to control apparatus
     Exposure to electrical equipment and machinery
     Exposure to transformers

X● **W86.8** **Exposure to other electric current**
     Exposure to wiring and appliances in or on farm (not
         farmhouse)
     Exposure to wiring and appliances outdoors
     Exposure to wiring and appliances in or on public
         building
     Exposure to wiring and appliances in or on residential
         institutions
     Exposure to wiring and appliances in or on schools

● **W88** **Exposure to ionizing radiation**
     Excludes1   exposure to sunlight (X32)

     The appropriate 7th character is to be added to each code from
     category W88

A	initial encounter
D	subsequent encounter
S	sequela

X● **W88.Ø** **Exposure to X-rays**

X● **W88.1** **Exposure to radioactive isotopes**

X● **W88.8** **Exposure to other ionizing radiation**

● **W89** **Exposure to man-made visible and ultraviolet light**
     Includes   exposure to welding light (arc)
     Excludes1   exposure to sunlight (X32) ◀

     The appropriate 7th character is to be added to each code from
     category W89

A	initial encounter
D	subsequent encounter
S	sequela

X● **W89.Ø** **Exposure to welding light (arc)**

X● **W89.1** **Exposure to tanning bed**

X● **W89.8** **Exposure to other man-made visible and ultraviolet light**

X● **W89.9** **Exposure to unspecified man-made visible and ultraviolet light**

● **W9Ø** **Exposure to other nonionizing radiation**
     Excludes1   exposure to sunlight (X32)

     The appropriate 7th character is to be added to each code from
     category W9Ø

A	initial encounter
D	subsequent encounter
S	sequela

X● **W9Ø.Ø** **Exposure to radiofrequency**

X● **W9Ø.1** **Exposure to infrared radiation**

X● **W9Ø.2** **Exposure to laser radiation**

X● **W9Ø.8** **Exposure to other nonionizing radiation**

X● **W92** **Exposure to excessive heat of man-made origin**
     The appropriate 7th character is to be added to code W92

A	initial encounter
D	subsequent encounter
S	sequela

● **W93** **Exposure to excessive cold of man-made origin**
     The appropriate 7th character is to be added to each code from
     category W93

A	initial encounter
D	subsequent encounter
S	sequela

● **W93.Ø** **Contact with or inhalation of dry ice**

X● **W93.Ø1** **Contact with dry ice**

X● **W93.Ø2** **Inhalation of dry ice**

● **W93.1** **Contact with or inhalation of liquid air**

X● **W93.11** **Contact with liquid air**
     Contact with liquid hydrogen
     Contact with liquid nitrogen

X● **W93.12** **Inhalation of liquid air**
     Inhalation of liquid hydrogen
     Inhalation of liquid nitrogen

X● **W93.2** **Prolonged exposure in deep freeze unit or refrigerator**

X● **W93.8** **Exposure to other excessive cold of man-made origin**

◀ New   ⬅ Revised   ~~deleted~~ Deleted   Excludes 1   Excludes 2   Includes   Use additional   Code first   Code also   Unspecified

1570   OGCR Official Guidelines   ● Unacceptable Principal Diagnosis   X Assign placeholder X   ● Use Additional Character(s)   ▶ Manifestation Code   Coding Clinic

● **W94**   **Exposure to high and low air pressure and changes in air pressure**

> The appropriate 7th character is to be added to each code from category W94

> | | |
> |---|---|
> | A | initial encounter |
> | D | subsequent encounter |
> | S | sequela |

X● **W94.0**   **Exposure to prolonged high air pressure**

● **W94.1**   **Exposure to prolonged low air pressure**

   X● **W94.11**   **Exposure to residence or prolonged visit at high altitude**

   X● **W94.12**   **Exposure to other prolonged low air pressure**

● **W94.2**   **Exposure to rapid changes in air pressure during ascent**

   X● **W94.21**   **Exposure to reduction in atmospheric pressure while surfacing from deep-water diving**

   X● **W94.22**   **Exposure to reduction in atmospheric pressure while surfacing from underground**

   X● **W94.23**   **Exposure to sudden change in air pressure in aircraft during ascent**

   X● **W94.29**   **Exposure to other rapid changes in air pressure during ascent**

● **W94.3**   **Exposure to rapid changes in air pressure during descent**

   X● **W94.31**   **Exposure to sudden change in air pressure in aircraft during descent**

   X● **W94.32**   **Exposure to high air pressure from rapid descent in water**

   X● **W94.39**   **Exposure to other rapid changes in air pressure during descent**

X● **W99**   **Exposure to other man-made environmental factors**

> The appropriate 7th character is to be added to code W99

> | | |
> |---|---|
> | A | initial encounter |
> | D | subsequent encounter |
> | S | sequela |

EXPOSURE TO SMOKE, FIRE AND FLAMES (X00-X08)

Excludes1   arson (X97)

Excludes2   explosions (W35-W40)
lightning (T75.0-)
transport accident (V01-V99)

● **X00**   **Exposure to uncontrolled fire in building or structure**

> **Includes**   conflagration in building or structure

> *Code first any associated cataclysm*

> **Excludes2**   exposure to ignition or melting of nightwear (X05)
> exposure to ignition or melting of other clothing and apparel (X06.-)
> exposure to other specified smoke, fire and flames (X08.-)

> The appropriate 7th character is to be added to each code from category X00

> | | |
> |---|---|
> | A | initial encounter |
> | D | subsequent encounter |
> | S | sequela |

X● **X00.0**   **Exposure to flames in uncontrolled fire in building or structure**
     Coding Clinic: 2016, Q2, P5-6; 2015, Q1, P19

X● **X00.1**   **Exposure to smoke in uncontrolled fire in building or structure**

X● **X00.2**   **Injury due to collapse of burning building or structure in uncontrolled fire**
> **Excludes1**   injury due to collapse of building not on fire (W20.1)

X● **X00.3**   **Fall from burning building or structure in uncontrolled fire**

X● **X00.4**   **Hit by object from burning building or structure in uncontrolled fire**

X● **X00.5**   **Jump from burning building or structure in uncontrolled fire**

X● **X00.8**   **Other exposure to uncontrolled fire in building or structure**

● **X01**   **Exposure to uncontrolled fire, not in building or structure**

> **Includes**   exposure to forest fire

> The appropriate 7th character is to be added to each code from category X01

> | | |
> |---|---|
> | A | initial encounter |
> | D | subsequent encounter |
> | S | sequela |

X● **X01.0**   **Exposure to flames in uncontrolled fire, not in building or structure**

X● **X01.1**   **Exposure to smoke in uncontrolled fire, not in building or structure**

X● **X01.3**   **Fall due to uncontrolled fire, not in building or structure**

X● **X01.4**   **Hit by object due to uncontrolled fire, not in building or structure**

X● **X01.8**   **Other exposure to uncontrolled fire, not in building or structure**

● **X02**   **Exposure to controlled fire in building or structure**

> **Includes**   exposure to fire in fireplace exposure to fire in stove

> The appropriate 7th character is to be added to each code from category X02

> | | |
> |---|---|
> | A | initial encounter |
> | D | subsequent encounter |
> | S | sequela |

X● **X02.0**   **Exposure to flames in controlled fire in building or structure**

X● **X02.1**   **Exposure to smoke in controlled fire in building or structure**

X● **X02.2**   **Injury due to collapse of burning building or structure in controlled fire**
> **Excludes1**   injury due to collapse of building not on fire (W20.1)

X● **X02.3**   **Fall from burning building or structure in controlled fire**

X● **X02.4**   **Hit by object from burning building or structure in controlled fire**

X● **X02.5**   **Jump from burning building or structure in controlled fire**

X● **X02.8**   **Other exposure to controlled fire in building or structure**

● **X03**   **Exposure to controlled fire, not in building or structure**

> **Includes**   exposure to bon fire exposure to camp fire exposure to trash fire

> The appropriate 7th character is to be added to each code from category X03

> | | |
> |---|---|
> | A | initial encounter |
> | D | subsequent encounter |
> | S | sequela |

X● **X03.0**   **Exposure to flames in controlled fire, not in building or structure**
     Coding Clinic: 2015, Q1, P19

X● **X03.1**   **Exposure to smoke in controlled fire, not in building or structure**

X● **X03.3**   **Fall due to controlled fire, not in building or structure**

X● **X03.4**   **Hit by object due to controlled fire, not in building or structure**

X● **X03.8**   **Other exposure to controlled fire, not in building or structure**

N Newborn Age: 0   **P** Pediatric Age: 0–17   **M** Maternity DX: 12–55   **A** Adult Age: 15–124   ♀ Females Only   ♂ Males Only

🔷 Complication\Comorbidity   🔶 Major C\C   ⒺⓍ CC/MCC Exclusions   🔷 Hospital-Acquired Condition

X ● **X04**   **Exposure to ignition of highly flammable material**
Exposure to ignition of gasoline
Exposure to ignition of kerosene
Exposure to ignition of petrol

> **Excludes2**   exposure to ignition or melting of nightwear (X05)
> exposure to ignition or melting of other clothing and apparel (X06)

The appropriate 7th character is to be added to code X04

A	initial encounter
D	subsequent encounter
S	sequela

Coding Clinic: 2016, Q2, P4

X ● **X05**   **Exposure to ignition or melting of nightwear**

> **Excludes2**   exposure to uncontrolled fire in building or structure (X00.-)
> exposure to uncontrolled fire, not in building or structure (X01.-)
> exposure to controlled fire in building or structure (X02.-)
> exposure to controlled fire, not in building or structure (X03.-)
> exposure to ignition of highly flammable materials (X04.-)

The appropriate 7th character is to be added to code X05

A	initial encounter
D	subsequent encounter
S	sequela

● **X06**   **Exposure to ignition or melting of other clothing and apparel**

> **Excludes2**   exposure to uncontrolled fire in building or structure (X00.-)
> exposure to uncontrolled fire, not in building or structure (X01.-)
> exposure to controlled fire in building or structure (X02.-)
> exposure to controlled fire, not in building or structure (X03.-)
> exposure to ignition of highly flammable materials (X04.-)

The appropriate 7th character is to be added to each code from category X06

A	initial encounter
D	subsequent encounter
S	sequela

X ● **X06.0**   **Exposure to ignition of plastic jewelry**
X ● **X06.1**   **Exposure to melting of plastic jewelry**
X ● **X06.2**   **Exposure to ignition of other clothing and apparel**
X ● **X06.3**   **Exposure to melting of other clothing and apparel**

● **X08**   **Exposure to other specified smoke, fire and flames**
The appropriate 7th character is to be added to each code from category X08

A	initial encounter
D	subsequent encounter
S	sequela

● **X08.0**   **Exposure to bed fire**
Exposure to mattress fire

X ● **X08.00**   **Exposure to bed fire due to unspecified burning material**
X ● **X08.01**   **Exposure to bed fire due to burning cigarette**
     Coding Clinic: 2015, Q1, P19
X ● **X08.09**   **Exposure to bed fire due to other burning material**

● **X08.1**   **Exposure to sofa fire**

X ● **X08.10**   **Exposure to sofa fire due to unspecified burning material**
X ● **X08.11**   **Exposure to sofa fire due to burning cigarette**
X ● **X08.19**   **Exposure to sofa fire due to other burning material**

● **X08.2**   **Exposure to other furniture fire**

X ● **X08.20**   **Exposure to other furniture fire due to unspecified burning material**
X ● **X08.21**   **Exposure to other furniture fire due to burning cigarette**
X ● **X08.29**   **Exposure to other furniture fire due to other burning material**

X ● **X08.8**   **Exposure to other specified smoke, fire and flames**

CONTACT WITH HEAT AND HOT SUBSTANCES (X10-X19)

> **Excludes1**   exposure to excessive natural heat (X30)
> exposure to fire and flames (X00-X09)

● **X10**   **Contact with hot drinks, food, fats and cooking oils**
The appropriate 7th character is to be added to each code from category X10

A	initial encounter
D	subsequent encounter
S	sequela

X ● **X10.0**   **Contact with hot drinks**
X ● **X10.1**   **Contact with hot food**
X ● **X10.2**   **Contact with fats and cooking oils**

● **X11**   **Contact with hot tap-water**

> **Includes**   contact with boiling tap-water
> contact with boiling water NOS

> **Excludes1**   contact with water heated on stove (X12)

The appropriate 7th character is to be added to each code from category X11

A	initial encounter
D	subsequent encounter
S	sequela

X ● **X11.0**   **Contact with hot water in bath or tub**

> **Excludes1**   contact with running hot water in bath or tub (X11.1)

X ● **X11.1**   **Contact with running hot water**
Contact with hot water running out of hose
Contact with hot water running out of tap

X ● **X11.8**   **Contact with other hot tap-water**
Contact with hot water in bucket
Contact with hot tap-water NOS

X ● **X12**   **Contact with other hot fluids**
Contact with water heated on stove

> **Excludes1**   hot (liquid) metals (X18)

The appropriate 7th character is to be added to code X12

A	initial encounter
D	subsequent encounter
S	sequela

● **X13**   **Contact with steam and other hot vapors**
The appropriate 7th character is to be added to each code from category X13

A	initial encounter
D	subsequent encounter
S	sequela

X ● **X13.0**   **Inhalation of steam and other hot vapors**
X ● **X13.1**   **Other contact with steam and other hot vapors**

◀ New   ◀━ Revised   ~~deleted~~ Deleted   Excludes 1   Excludes 2   Includes   Use additional   Code first   Code also   Unspecified
OGCR Official Guidelines   ● Unacceptable Principal Diagnosis   X Assign placeholder X   ● Use Additional Character(s)   ▷ Manifestation Code   Coding Clinic

● **X14** **Contact with hot air and other hot gases**

The appropriate 7th character is to be added to each code from category X14

> A   initial encounter
> D   subsequent encounter
> S   sequela

X● **X14.0** **Inhalation of hot air and gases**

X● **X14.1** **Other contact with hot air and other hot gases**

● **X15** **Contact with hot household appliances**

> **Excludes1**   contact with heating appliances (X16)
> contact with powered household appliances (W29.-)
> exposure to controlled fire in building or structure due to household appliance (X02.8)
> exposure to household appliances electrical current (W86.0)

The appropriate 7th character is to be added to each code from category X15

> A   initial encounter
> D   subsequent encounter
> S   sequela

X● **X15.0** **Contact with hot stove (kitchen)**

X● **X15.1** **Contact with hot toaster**

X● **X15.2** **Contact with hotplate**

X● **X15.3** **Contact with hot saucepan or skillet**

X● **X15.8** **Contact with other hot household appliances**
> Contact with cooker
> Contact with kettle
> Contact with light bulbs

X● **X16** **Contact with hot heating appliances, radiators and pipes**

> **Excludes1**   contact with powered appliances (W29.-)
> exposure to controlled fire in building or structure due to appliance (X02.8)
> exposure to industrial appliances electrical current (W86.1)

The appropriate 7th character is to be added to code X16

> A   initial encounter
> D   subsequent encounter
> S   sequela

X● **X17** **Contact with hot engines, machinery and tools**

> **Excludes1**   contact with hot heating appliances, radiators and pipes (X16)
> contact with hot household appliances (X15)

The appropriate 7th character is to be added to code X17

> A   initial encounter
> D   subsequent encounter
> S   sequela

X● **X18** **Contact with other hot metals**
> Contact with liquid metal

The appropriate 7th character is to be added to code X18

> A   initial encounter
> D   subsequent encounter
> S   sequela

X● **X19** **Contact with other heat and hot substances**

> **Excludes1**   objects that are not normally hot, e.g., an object made hot by a house fire (X00-X09)

The appropriate 7th character is to be added to code X19

> A   initial encounter
> D   subsequent encounter
> S   sequela

EXPOSURE TO FORCES OF NATURE (X30-X39)

X● **X30** **Exposure to excessive natural heat**
> Exposure to excessive heat as the cause of sunstroke
> Exposure to heat NOS

> **Excludes1**   excessive heat of man-made origin (W92)
> exposure to man-made radiation (W89)
> exposure to sunlight (X32)
> exposure to tanning bed (W89)

The appropriate 7th character is to be added to code X30

> A   initial encounter
> D   subsequent encounter
> S   sequela

X● **X31** **Exposure to excessive natural cold**
> Excessive cold as the cause of chilblains NOS
> Excessive cold as the cause of immersion foot or hand
> Exposure to cold NOS
> Exposure to weather conditions

> **Excludes1**   cold of man-made origin (W93.-)
> contact with or inhalation of dry ice (W93.-)
> contact with or inhalation of liquefied gas (W93.-)

The appropriate 7th character is to be added to code X31

> A   initial encounter
> D   subsequent encounter
> S   sequela

X● **X32** **Exposure to sunlight**

> **Excludes1**   ~~radiation-related disorders of the skin and subcutaneous tissue (L55-L59)~~
> man-made radiation (tanning bed) (W89)

The appropriate 7th character is to be added to code X32

> A   initial encounter
> D   subsequent encounter
> S   sequela

X● **X34** **Earthquake**

> **Excludes2**   tidal wave (tsunami) due to earthquake (X37.41)

The appropriate 7th character is to be added to code X34

> A   initial encounter
> D   subsequent encounter
> S   sequela

X● **X35** **Volcanic eruption**

> **Excludes2**   tidal wave (tsunami) due to volcanic eruption (X37.41)

The appropriate 7th character is to be added to code X35

> A   initial encounter
> D   subsequent encounter
> S   sequela

● **X36** **Avalanche, landslide and other earth movements**

> **Includes**   victim of mudslide of cataclysmic nature
> **Excludes1**   earthquake (X34)
> **Excludes2**   transport accident involving collision with avalanche or landslide not in motion (V01-V99)

The appropriate 7th character is to be added to each code from category X36

> A   initial encounter
> D   subsequent encounter
> S   sequela

X● **X36.0** **Collapse of dam or man-made structure causing earth movement**

X● **X36.1** **Avalanche, landslide, or mudslide**

CHAPTER 20 (V01-Y99)

CHAPTER 20 (V01-Y99)

● **X37**   **Cataclysmic storm**

The appropriate 7th character is to be added to each code from category X37

> A   initial encounter
> D   subsequent encounter
> S   sequela

X● **X37.0**   **Hurricane**
Storm surge   Typhoon

X● **X37.1**   **Tornado**
Cyclone   Twister

X● **X37.2**   **Blizzard (snow) (ice)**

X● **X37.3**   **Dust storm**

● **X37.4**   **Tidalwave**

     X● **X37.41**   **Tidal wave due to earthquake or volcanic eruption**
         Tidal wave NOS
         Tsunami

     X● **X37.42**   **Tidal wave due to storm**

     X● **X37.43**   **Tidal wave due to landslide**

X● **X37.8**   **Other cataclysmic storms**
Cloudburst
Torrential rain
> **Excludes2**   flood (X38)

X● **X37.9**   **Unspecified cataclysmic storm**
Storm NOS
> **Excludes1**   collapse of dam or man-made structure causing earth movement (X39.0)

X● **X38**   **Flood**
Flood arising from remote storm
Flood of cataclysmic nature arising from melting snow
Flood resulting directly from storm
> **Excludes1**   collapse of dam or man-made structure causing earth movement (X39.0)
>   tidal wave NOS (X37.41)
>   tidal wave caused by storm (X37.2)

The appropriate 7th character is to be added to code X38

> A   initial encounter
> D   subsequent encounter
> S   sequela

● **X39**   **Exposure to other forces of nature**

The appropriate 7th character is to be added to each code from category X39

> A   initial encounter
> D   subsequent encounter
> S   sequela

   ● **X39.0**   **Exposure to natural radiation**
> **Excludes1**   contact with and (suspected) exposure to radon and other naturally occuring radiation (Z77.123) ◀▥
>   exposure to man-made radiation (W88-W90)
>   exposure to sunlight (X32)

     X● **X39.01**   **Exposure to radon**

     X● **X39.08**   **Exposure to other natural radiation**

X● **X39.8**   **Other exposure to forces of nature**

OVEREXERTION AND STRENUOUS OR REPETITIVE MOVEMENTS (X50) ◀

●**X50**   **Overexertion and strenuous or repetitive movements** ◀

The appropriate 7th character is to be added to each code from category X50 ◀

> A   initial encounter ◀
> D   subsequent encounter ◀
> S   sequela ◀

X● **X50.0**   **Overexertion from strenuous movement or load** ◀
Lifting heavy objects ◀
Lifting weights ◀

X● **X50.1**   **Overexertion from prolonged static or awkward postures** ◀
Prolonged bending ◀
Prolonged kneeling ◀
Prolonged reaching ◀
Prolonged sitting ◀
Prolonged standing ◀
Prolonged twisting ◀
Static bending ◀
Static kneeling ◀
Static reaching ◀
Static sitting ◀
Static standing ◀
Static twisting ◀

X● **X50.3**   **Overexertion from repetitive movements** ◀
Use of hand as hammer ◀
> **Excludes2**   Overuse from prolonged static or awkward postures (X50.1) ◀

X● **X50.9**   **Other and unspecified overexertion or strenuous movements or postures** ◀
Contact pressure ◀
Contact stress ◀

ACCIDENTAL EXPOSURE TO OTHER SPECIFIED FACTORS (X52, X58)

X● **X52**   **Prolonged stay in weightless environment**
Weightlessness in spacecraft (simulator)

The appropriate 7th character is to be added to code X52

> A   initial encounter
> D   subsequent encounter
> S   sequela

X● **X58**   **Exposure to other specified factors**
Accident NOS
Exposure NOS

The appropriate 7th character is to be added to code X58

> A   initial encounter
> D   subsequent encounter
> S   sequela

INTENTIONAL SELF-HARM (X71-X83)

Purposely self-inflicted injury
Suicide (attempted)

●**X71**   **Intentional self-harm by drowning and submersion**

The appropriate 7th character is to be added to each code from category X71

> A   initial encounter
> D   subsequent encounter
> S   sequela

X● **X71.0**   **Intentional self-harm by drowning and submersion while in bathtub**

X● **X71.1**   **Intentional self-harm by drowning and submersion while in swimming pool**

X● **X71.2**   **Intentional self-harm by drowning and submersion after jump into swimming pool**

◀ New   ◀▥ Revised   ~~deleted~~ Deleted   Excludes 1   Excludes 2   Includes   Use additional   Code first   Code also   Unspecified

OGCR Official Guidelines   ● Unacceptable Principal Diagnosis   X Assign placeholder X   ● Use Additional Character(s)   ▶ Manifestation Code   Coding Clinic

X● **X71.3**   **Intentional self-harm by drowning and submersion in natural water**

X● **X71.8**   **Other intentional self-harm by drowning and submersion**

X● **X71.9**   **Intentional self-harm by drowning and submersion, unspecified**

X●**X72**   **Intentional self-harm by handgun discharge**
Intentional self-harm by gun for single hand use
Intentional self-harm by pistol
Intentional self-harm by revolver

Excludes1   Very pistol (X74.8)

The appropriate 7th character is to be added to code X72

A	initial encounter
D	subsequent encounter
S	sequela

●**X73**   **Intentional self-harm by rifle, shotgun and larger firearm discharge**

Excludes1   airgun (X74.01)

The appropriate 7th character is to be added to each code from category X73

A	initial encounter
D	subsequent encounter
S	sequela

X● **X73.0**   **Intentional self-harm by shotgun discharge**

X● **X73.1**   **Intentional self-harm by hunting rifle discharge**

X● **X73.2**   **Intentional self-harm by machine gun discharge**

X● **X73.8**   **Intentional self-harm by other larger firearm discharge**

X● **X73.9**   **Intentional self-harm by unspecified larger firearm discharge**

●**X74**   **Intentional self-harm by other and unspecified firearm and gun discharge**

The appropriate 7th character is to be added to each code from category X74

A	initial encounter
D	subsequent encounter
S	sequela

● **X74.0**   **Intentional self-harm by gas, air or spring-operated guns**

X● **X74.01**   **Intentional self-harm by airgun**
Intentional self-harm by BB gun discharge
Intentional self-harm by pellet gun discharge

X● **X74.02**   **Intentional self-harm by paintball gun**

X● **X74.09**   **Intentional self-harm by other gas, air or spring-operated gun**

X● **X74.8**   **Intentional self-harm by other firearm discharge**
Intentional self-harm by Very pistol [flare] discharge

X● **X74.9**   **Intentional self-harm by unspecified firearm discharge**

X●**X75**   **Intentional self-harm by explosive material**

The appropriate 7th character is to be added to code X75

A	initial encounter
D	subsequent encounter
S	sequela

X●**X76**   **Intentional self-harm by smoke, fire and flames**

The appropriate 7th character is to be added to code X76

A	initial encounter
D	subsequent encounter
S	sequela

●**X77**   **Intentional self-harm by steam, hot vapors and hot objects**

The appropriate 7th character is to be added to each code from category X77

A	initial encounter
D	subsequent encounter
S	sequela

X● **X77.0**   **Intentional self-harm by steam or hot vapors**

X● **X77.1**   **Intentional self-harm by hot tap water**

X● **X77.2**   **Intentional self-harm by other hot fluids**

X● **X77.3**   **Intentional self-harm by hot household appliances**

X● **X77.8**   **Intentional self-harm by other hot objects**

X● **X77.9**   **Intentional self-harm by unspecified hot objects**

●**X78**   **Intentional self-harm by sharp object**

The appropriate 7th character is to be added to each code from category X78

A	initial encounter
D	subsequent encounter
S	sequela

X● **X78.0**   **Intentional self-harm by sharp glass**

X● **X78.1**   **Intentional self-harm by knife**

X● **X78.2**   **Intentional self-harm by sword or dagger**

X● **X78.8**   **Intentional self-harm by other sharp object**

X● **X78.9**   **Intentional self-harm by unspecified sharp object**

X●**X79**   **Intentional self-harm by blunt object**

The appropriate 7th character is to be added to code X79

A	initial encounter
D	subsequent encounter
S	sequela

X●**X80**   **Intentional self-harm by jumping from a high place**
Intentional fall from one level to another

The appropriate 7th character is to be added to code X80

A	initial encounter
D	subsequent encounter
S	sequela

●**X81**   **Intentional self-harm by jumping or lying in front of moving object**

The appropriate 7th character is to be added to each code from category X81

A	initial encounter
D	subsequent encounter
S	sequela

X● **X81.0**   **Intentional self-harm by jumping or lying in front of motor vehicle**

X● **X81.1**   **Intentional self-harm by jumping or lying in front of (subway) train**

X● **X81.8**   **Intentional self-harm by jumping or lying in front of other moving object**

●**X82**   **Intentional self-harm by crashing of motor vehicle**

The appropriate 7th character is to be added to each code from category X82

A	initial encounter
D	subsequent encounter
S	sequela

X● **X82.0**   **Intentional collision of motor vehicle with other motor vehicle**

X● **X82.1**   **Intentional collision of motor vehicle with train**

X● **X82.2**   **Intentional collision of motor vehicle with tree**

X● **X82.8**   **Other intentional self-harm by crashing of motor vehicle**

CHAPTER 20 (V01-Y99)

N Newborn Age: 0   **P** Pediatric Age: 0–17   **M** Maternity DX: 12–55   **A** Adult Age: 15–124   ♀ Females Only   ♂ Males Only

 Complication\Comorbidity   Major C\C   Ⓔ CC/MCC Exclusions   Hospital-Acquired Condition

1575

● X83   **Intentional self-harm by other specified means**

> **Excludes1**   intentional self-harm by poisoning or contact with toxic substance - see Table of Drugs and Chemicals
>
> The appropriate 7th character is to be added to each code from category X83

> | | |
> |---|---|
> | A | initial encounter |
> | D | subsequent encounter |
> | S | sequela |

X ● X83.0   **Intentional self-harm by crashing of aircraft**
X ● X83.1   **Intentional self-harm by electrocution**
X ● X83.2   **Intentional self-harm by exposure to extremes of cold**
X ● X83.8   **Intentional self-harm by other specified means**

ASSAULT (X92-Y09) ◀▥▥

> **Includes**   homicide injuries inflicted by another person with intent to injure or kill, by any means
>
> **Excludes1**   injuries due to legal intervention (Y35.-)
> injuries due to operations of war (Y36.-)
> injuries due to terrorism (Y38.-)

● X92   **Assault by drowning and submersion**

> The appropriate 7th character is to be added to each code from category X92

> | | |
> |---|---|
> | A | initial encounter |
> | D | subsequent encounter |
> | S | sequela |

X ● X92.0   **Assault by drowning and submersion while in bathtub**
X ● X92.1   **Assault by drowning and submersion while in swimming pool**
X ● X92.2   **Assault by drowning and submersion after push into swimming pool**
X ● X92.3   **Assault by drowning and submersion in natural water**
X ● X92.8   **Other assault by drowning and submersion**
X ● X92.9   **Assault by drowning and submersion, unspecified**

X ● X93   **Assault by handgun discharge**
Assault by discharge of gun for single hand use
Assault by discharge of pistol
Assault by discharge of revolver

> **Excludes1**   Very pistol (X95.8)
>
> The appropriate 7th character is to be added to code X93

> | | |
> |---|---|
> | A | initial encounter |
> | D | subsequent encounter |
> | S | sequela |

● X94   **Assault by rifle, shotgun and larger firearm discharge**

> **Excludes1**   airgun (X95.01)
>
> The appropriate 7th character is to be added to each code from category X94

> | | |
> |---|---|
> | A | initial encounter |
> | D | subsequent encounter |
> | S | sequela |

X ● X94.0   **Assault by shotgun**
X ● X94.1   **Assault by hunting rifle**
X ● X94.2   **Assault by machine gun**
X ● X94.8   **Assault by other larger firearm discharge**
X ● X94.9   **Assault by unspecified larger firearm discharge**

● X95   **Assault by other and unspecified firearm and gun discharge**

> The appropriate 7th character is to be added to each code from category X95

> | | |
> |---|---|
> | A | initial encounter |
> | D | subsequent encounter |
> | S | sequela |

● X95.0   **Assault by gas, air or spring-operated guns**

X ● X95.01   **Assault by airgun discharge**
Assault by BB gun discharge
Assault by pellet gun discharge

X ● X95.02   **Assault by paintball gun discharge**

X ● X95.09   **Assault by other gas, air or spring-operated gun**

X ● X95.8   **Assault by other firearm discharge**
Assault by very pistol [flare] discharge

X ● X95.9   **Assault by unspecified firearm discharge**

● X96   **Assault by explosive material**

> **Excludes1**   incendiary device (X97)
> terrorism involving explosive material (Y38.2-)
>
> The appropriate 7th character is to be added to each code from category X96

> | | |
> |---|---|
> | A | initial encounter |
> | D | subsequent encounter |
> | S | sequela |

X ● X96.0   **Assault by antipersonnel bomb**

> **Excludes1**   antipersonnel bomb use in military or war (Y36.2-)

X ● X96.1   **Assault by gasoline bomb**
X ● X96.2   **Assault by letter bomb**
X ● X96.3   **Assault by fertilizer bomb**
X ● X96.4   **Assault by pipe bomb**
X ● X96.8   **Assault by other specified explosive**
X ● X96.9   **Assault by unspecified explosive**

X ● X97   **Assault by smoke, fire and flames**
Assault by arson
Assault by cigarettes
Assault by incendiary device

> The appropriate 7th character is to be added to code X97

> | | |
> |---|---|
> | A | initial encounter |
> | D | subsequent encounter |
> | S | sequela |

● X98   **Assault by steam, hot vapors and hot objects**

> The appropriate 7th character is to be added to each code from category X98

> | | |
> |---|---|
> | A | initial encounter |
> | D | subsequent encounter |
> | S | sequela |

X ● X98.0   **Assault by steam or hot vapors**
X ● X98.1   **Assault by hot tap water**
X ● X98.2   **Assault by hot fluids**
X ● X98.3   **Assault by hot household appliances**
X ● X98.8   **Assault by other hot objects**
X ● X98.9   **Assault by unspecified hot objects**

◀ New   ◀▥▥ Revised   ~~deleted~~ Deleted   Excludes 1   Excludes 2   Includes   Use additional   Code first   Code also   Unspecified

OGCR Official Guidelines   ● Unacceptable Principal Diagnosis   X Assign placeholder X   ● Use Additional Character(s)   ▶ Manifestation Code   **Coding Clinic**

● X99 **Assault by sharp object**

> **Excludes1** assault by strike by sports equipment (Y08.0-)

The appropriate 7th character is to be added to each code from category X99

> A initial encounter
> D subsequent encounter
> S sequela

X ● X99.0 **Assault by sharp glass**
X ● X99.1 **Assault by knife**
X ● X99.2 **Assault by sword or dagger**
X ● X99.8 **Assault by other sharp object**
X ● X99.9 **Assault by unspecified sharp object**
  Assault by stabbing NOS

X ● Y00 **Assault by blunt object**

> **Excludes1** assault by strike by sports equipment (Y08.0)

The appropriate 7th character is to be added to code Y00

> A initial encounter
> D subsequent encounter
> S sequela

X ● Y01 **Assault by pushing from high place**

The appropriate 7th character is to be added to code Y01

> A initial encounter
> D subsequent encounter
> S sequela

● Y02 **Assault by pushing or placing victim in front of moving object**

The appropriate 7th character is to be added to each code from category Y02

> A initial encounter
> D subsequent encounter
> S sequela

X ● Y02.0 **Assault by pushing or placing victim in front of motor vehicle**
X ● Y02.1 **Assault by pushing or placing victim in front of (subway) train**
X ● Y02.8 **Assault by pushing or placing victim in front of other moving object**

● Y03 **Assault by crashing of motor vehicle**

The appropriate 7th character is to be added to each code from category Y03

> A initial encounter
> D subsequent encounter
> S sequela

X ● Y03.0 **Assault by being hit or run over by motor vehicle**
X ● Y03.8 **Other assault by crashing of motor vehicle**

● Y04 **Assault by bodily force**

> **Excludes1** assault by:
>   submersion (X92.-)
>   use of weapon (X93-X95, X99, Y00)

The appropriate 7th character is to be added to each code from category Y04

> A initial encounter
> D subsequent encounter
> S sequela

X ● Y04.0 **Assault by unarmed brawl or fight**
X ● Y04.1 **Assault by human bite**
X ● Y04.2 **Assault by strike against or bumped into by another person**
X ● Y04.8 **Assault by other bodily force**
  Assault by bodily force NOS

OGCR Section I.C.19.f.

Adult and child abuse, neglect and other maltreatment

Sequence first the appropriate code from categories T74.- or T76.- for abuse, neglect and other maltreatment, followed by any accompanying mental health or injury code(s).

If the documentation in the medical record states abuse or neglect it is coded as confirmed. It is coded as suspected if it is documented as suspected.

For cases of confirmed abuse or neglect an external cause code from the assault section (X92-Y08) should be added to identify the cause of any physical injuries. A perpetrator code (Y07) should be added when the perpetrator of the abuse is known. For suspected cases of abuse or neglect, do not report external cause or perpetrator code.

If a suspected case of abuse, neglect or mistreatment is ruled out during an encounter code Z04.71, Encounter for examination and observation following alleged physical adult abuse, ruled out, or code Z04.72, Encounter for examination and observation following alleged child physical abuse, ruled out, should be used, not a code from T76.

If a suspected case of alleged rape or sexual abuse is ruled out during an encounter code Z04.41, Encounter for examination and observation following alleged physical adult abuse, ruled out, or code Z04.42, Encounter for examination and observation following alleged rape or sexual abuse, ruled out, should be used, not a code from T76.

● Y07 **Perpetrator of assault, maltreatment and neglect**

> **Note:** Codes from this category are for use only in cases of confirmed abuse (T74.-)
>
> Selection of the correct perpetrator code is based on the relationship between the perpetrator and the victim
>
> **Includes** perpetrator of abandonment
>   perpetrator of emotional neglect
>   perpetrator of mental cruelty
>   perpetrator of physical abuse
>   perpetrator of physical neglect
>   perpetrator of sexual abuse
>   perpetrator of torture

● Y07.0 **Spouse or partner, perpetrator of maltreatment and neglect**
  Spouse or partner, perpetrator of maltreatment and neglect against spouse or partner

  Y07.01 **Husband, perpetrator of maltreatment and neglect**
  Y07.02 **Wife, perpetrator of maltreatment and neglect**
  Y07.03 **Male partner, perpetrator of maltreatment and neglect**
  Y07.04 **Female partner, perpetrator of maltreatment and neglect**

● Y07.1 **Parent (adoptive) (biological), perpetrator of maltreatment and neglect**
  Y07.11 **Biological father, perpetrator of maltreatment and neglect**
  Y07.12 **Biological mother, perpetrator of maltreatment and neglect**
  Y07.13 **Adoptive father, perpetrator of maltreatment and neglect**
  Y07.14 **Adoptive mother, perpetrator of maltreatment and neglect**

● Y07.4 **Other family member, perpetrator of maltreatment and neglect**
  ● Y07.41 **Sibling, perpetrator of maltreatment and neglect**

  > **Excludes1** stepsibling, perpetrator of maltreatment and neglect (Y07.435, Y07.436)

    Y07.410 **Brother, perpetrator of maltreatment and neglect**
    Y07.411 **Sister, perpetrator of maltreatment and neglect**

● Y07.42 Foster parent, perpetrator of maltreatment and neglect

  Y07.420 Foster father, perpetrator of maltreatment and neglect

  Y07.421 Foster mother, perpetrator of maltreatment and neglect

● Y07.43 Stepparent or stepsibling, perpetrator of maltreatment and neglect

  Y07.430 Stepfather, perpetrator of maltreatment and neglect

  Y07.432 Male friend of parent (co-residing in household), perpetrator of maltreatment and neglect

  Y07.433 Stepmother, perpetrator of maltreatment and neglect

  Y07.434 Female friend of parent (co-residing in household), perpetrator of maltreatment and neglect

  Y07.435 Stepbrother, perpetrator or maltreatment and neglect

  Y07.436 Stepsister, perpetrator of maltreatment and neglect

● Y07.49 Other family member, perpetrator of maltreatment and neglect

  Y07.490 Male cousin, perpetrator of maltreatment and neglect

  Y07.491 Female cousin, perpetrator of maltreatment and neglect

  Y07.499 Other family member, perpetrator of maltreatment and neglect

● Y07.5 Non-family member, perpetrator of maltreatment and neglect

  Y07.50 Unspecified non-family member, perpetrator of maltreatment and neglect

● Y07.51 Daycare provider, perpetrator of maltreatment and neglect

  Y07.510 At-home childcare provider, perpetrator of maltreatment and neglect

  Y07.511 Daycare center childcare provider, perpetrator of maltreatment and neglect

  Y07.512 At-home adultcare provider, perpetrator of maltreatment and neglect

  Y07.513 Adultcare center provider, perpetrator of maltreatment and neglect

  Y07.519 Unspecified daycare provider, perpetrator of maltreatment and neglect

● Y07.52 Healthcare provider, perpetrator of maltreatment and neglect

  Y07.521 Mental health provider, perpetrator of maltreatment and neglect

  Y07.528 Other therapist or healthcare provider, perpetrator of maltreatment and neglect

    Nurse perpetrator of maltreatment and neglect

    Occupational therapist perpetrator of maltreatment and neglect

    Physical therapist perpetrator of maltreatment and neglect

    Speech therapist perpetrator of maltreatment and neglect

  Y07.529 Unspecified healthcare provider, perpetrator of maltreatment and neglect

  Y07.53 Teacher or instructor, perpetrator of maltreatment and neglect

    Coach, perpetrator of maltreatment and neglect

  Y07.59 Other non-family member, perpetrator of maltreatment and neglect

  Y07.9 Unspecified perpetrator of maltreatment and neglect

● Y08 Assault by other specified means

  The appropriate 7th character is to be added to each code from category Y08

A	initial encounter
D	subsequent encounter
S	sequela

● Y08.0 Assault by strike by sport equipment

 X ● Y08.01 Assault by strike by hockey stick

 X ● Y08.02 Assault by strike by baseball bat

 X ● Y08.09 Assault by strike by other specified type of sport equipment

● Y08.8 Assault by other specified means

 X ● Y08.81 Assault by crashing of aircraft

 X ● Y08.89 Assault by other specified means

● Y09 Assault by unspecified means

  Assassination (attempted) NOS

  Homicide (attempted) NOS

  Manslaughter (attempted) NOS

  Murder (attempted) NOS

EVENT OF UNDETERMINED INTENT (Y21-Y33)

Undetermined intent is only for use when there is specific documentation in the record that the intent of the injury cannot be determined. If no such documentation is present, code to accidental (unintentional)

● Y21 Drowning and submersion, undetermined intent

  The appropriate 7th character is to be added to each code from category Y21

A	initial encounter
D	subsequent encounter
S	sequela

 X ● Y21.0 Drowning and submersion while in bathtub, undetermined intent

 X ● Y21.1 Drowning and submersion after fall into bathtub, undetermined intent

 X ● Y21.2 Drowning and submersion while in swimming pool, undetermined intent

 X ● Y21.3 Drowning and submersion after fall into swimming pool, undetermined intent

 X ● Y21.4 Drowning and submersion in natural water, undetermined intent

 X ● Y21.8 Other drowning and submersion, undetermined intent

 X ● Y21.9 Unspecified drowning and submersion, undetermined intent

X ● Y22 Handgun discharge, undetermined intent

  Discharge of gun for single hand use, undetermined intent

  Discharge of pistol, undetermined intent

  Discharge of revolver, undetermined intent

  Excludes2 very pistol (Y24.8)

  The appropriate 7th character is to be added to code Y22

A	initial encounter
D	subsequent encounter
S	sequela

◀ New ◀▥ Revised ~~deleted~~ Deleted Excludes 1 Excludes 2 Includes Use additional Code first Code also Unspecified

OGCR Official Guidelines ● Unacceptable Principal Diagnosis X Assign placeholder X ● Use Additional Character(s) ▶ Manifestation Code **Coding Clinic**

● **Y23** Rifle, shotgun and larger firearm discharge, undetermined intent

Excludes2 airgun (Y24.0)

The appropriate 7th character is to be added to each code from category Y23

A	initial encounter
D	subsequent encounter
S	sequela

X ● **Y23.0** Shotgun discharge, undetermined intent
X ● **Y23.1** Hunting rifle discharge, undetermined intent
X ● **Y23.2** Military firearm discharge, undetermined intent
X ● **Y23.3** Machine gun discharge, undetermined intent
X ● **Y23.8** Other larger firearm discharge, undetermined intent
X ● **Y23.9** Unspecified larger firearm discharge, undetermined intent

● **Y24** Other and unspecified firearm discharge, undetermined intent

The appropriate 7th character is to be added to each code from category Y24

A	initial encounter
D	subsequent encounter
S	sequela

X ● **Y24.0** Airgun discharge, undetermined intent
BB gun discharge, undetermined intent
Pellet gun discharge, undetermined intent
X ● **Y24.8** Other firearm discharge, undetermined intent
Paintball gun discharge, undetermined intent
Very pistol [flare] discharge, undetermined intent
X ● **Y24.9** Unspecified firearm discharge, undetermined intent

X ● **Y25** Contact with explosive material, undetermined intent

The appropriate 7th character is to be added to code Y25

A	initial encounter
D	subsequent encounter
S	sequela

X ● **Y26** Exposure to smoke, fire and flames, undetermined intent

The appropriate 7th character is to be added to code Y26

A	initial encounter
D	subsequent encounter
S	sequela

● **Y27** Contact with steam, hot vapors and hot objects, undetermined intent

The appropriate 7th character is to be added to each code from category Y27

A	initial encounter
D	subsequent encounter
S	sequela

X ● **Y27.0** Contact with steam and hot vapors, undetermined intent
X ● **Y27.1** Contact with hot tap water, undetermined intent
X ● **Y27.2** Contact with hot fluids, undetermined intent
X ● **Y27.3** Contact with hot household appliance, undetermined intent
X ● **Y27.8** Contact with other hot objects, undetermined intent
X ● **Y27.9** Contact with unspecified hot objects, undetermined intent

● **Y28** Contact with sharp object, undetermined intent

The appropriate 7th character is to be added to each code from category Y28

A	initial encounter
D	subsequent encounter
S	sequela

X ● **Y28.0** Contact with sharp glass, undetermined intent
X ● **Y28.1** Contact with knife, undetermined intent
X ● **Y28.2** Contact with sword or dagger, undetermined intent
X ● **Y28.8** Contact with other sharp object, undetermined intent
X ● **Y28.9** Contact with unspecified sharp object, undetermined intent

X ● **Y29** Contact with blunt object, undetermined intent

The appropriate 7th character is to be added to code Y29

A	initial encounter
D	subsequent encounter
S	sequela

X ● **Y30** Falling, jumping or pushed from a high place, undetermined intent

Victim falling from one level to another, undetermined intent

The appropriate 7th character is to be added to code Y30

A	initial encounter
D	subsequent encounter
S	sequela

X ● **Y31** Falling, lying or running before or into moving object, undetermined intent

The appropriate 7th character is to be added to code Y31

A	initial encounter
D	subsequent encounter
S	sequela

X ● **Y32** Crashing of motor vehicle, undetermined intent

The appropriate 7th character is to be added to code Y32

A	initial encounter
D	subsequent encounter
S	sequela

X ● **Y33** Other specified events, undetermined intent

The appropriate 7th character is to be added to code Y33

A	initial encounter
D	subsequent encounter
S	sequela

LEGAL INTERVENTION, OPERATIONS OF WAR, MILITARY OPERATIONS, AND TERRORISM (Y35-Y38)

● Y35 **Legal intervention**

Includes   any injury sustained as a result of an encounter with any law enforcement official, serving in any capacity at the time of the encounter, whether on-duty or off-duty. Includes: injury to law enforcement official, suspect and bystander

The appropriate 7th character is to be added to each code from category Y35

A	initial encounter
D	subsequent encounter
S	sequela

● Y35.0   **Legal intervention involving firearm discharge**

● Y35.00   **Legal intervention involving unspecified firearm discharge**
Legal intervention involving gunshot wound
Legal intervention involving shot NOS

◀ Y35.001   **Legal intervention involving unspecified firearm discharge, law enforcement official injured**

◀ Y35.002   **Legal intervention involving unspecified firearm discharge, bystander injured**

◀ Y35.003   **Legal intervention involving unspecified firearm discharge, suspect injured**

● Y35.01   **Legal intervention involving injury by machine gun**

◀ Y35.011   **Legal intervention involving injury by machine gun, law enforcement official injured**

◀ Y35.012   **Legal intervention involving injury by machine gun, bystander injured**

◀ Y35.013   **Legal intervention involving injury by machine gun, suspect injured**

● Y35.02   **Legal intervention involving injury by handgun**

◀ Y35.021   **Legal intervention involving injury by handgun, law enforcement official injured**

◀ Y35.022   **Legal intervention involving injury by handgun, bystander injured**

◀ Y35.023   **Legal intervention involving injury by handgun, suspect injured**

● Y35.03   **Legal intervention involving injury by rifle pellet**

◀ Y35.031   **Legal intervention involving injury by rifle pellet, law enforcement official injured**

◀ Y35.032   **Legal intervention involving injury by rifle pellet, bystander injured**

◀ Y35.033   **Legal intervention involving injury by rifle pellet, suspect injured**

● Y35.04   **Legal intervention involving injury by rubber bullet**

◀ Y35.041   **Legal intervention involving injury by rubber bullet, law enforcement official injured**

◀ Y35.042   **Legal intervention involving injury by rubber bullet, bystander injured**

◀ Y35.043   **Legal intervention involving injury by rubber bullet, suspect injured**

● Y35.09   **Legal intervention involving other firearm discharge**

● Y35.091   **Legal intervention involving other firearm discharge, law enforcement official injured**

● Y35.092   **Legal intervention involving other firearm discharge, bystander injured**

● Y35.093   **Legal intervention involving other firearm discharge, suspect injured**

● Y35.1   **Legal intervention involving explosives**

● Y35.10   **Legal intervention involving unspecified explosives**

● Y35.101   **Legal intervention involving unspecified explosives, law enforcement official injured**

● Y35.102   **Legal intervention involving unspecified explosives, bystander injured**

● Y35.103   **Legal intervention involving unspecified explosives, suspect injured**

● Y35.11   **Legal intervention involving injury by dynamite**

● Y35.111   **Legal intervention involving injury by dynamite, law enforcement official injured**

● Y35.112   **Legal intervention involving injury by dynamite, bystander injured**

● Y35.113   **Legal intervention involving injury by dynamite, suspect injured**

● Y35.12   **Legal intervention involving injury by explosive shell**

● Y35.121   **Legal intervention involving injury by explosive shell, law enforcement official injured**

● Y35.122   **Legal intervention involving injury by explosive shell, bystander injured**

● Y35.123   **Legal intervention involving injury by explosive shell, suspect injured**

● Y35.19   **Legal intervention involving other explosives**
Legal intervention involving injury by grenade
Legal intervention involving injury by mortar bomb

● Y35.191   **Legal intervention involving other explosives, law enforcement official injured**

● Y35.192   **Legal intervention involving other explosives, bystander injured**

● Y35.193   **Legal intervention involving other explosives, suspect injured**

● Y35.2   **Legal intervention involving gas**
Legal intervention involving asphyxiation by gas
Legal intervention involving poisoning by gas

● Y35.20   **Legal intervention involving unspecified gas**

● Y35.201   **Legal intervention involving unspecified gas, law enforcement official injured**

● Y35.202   **Legal intervention involving unspecified gas, bystander injured**

● Y35.203   **Legal intervention involving unspecified gas, suspect injured**

◀ New   ◀ Revised   ~~deleted~~ Deleted   Excludes 1   Excludes 2   Includes   Use additional   Code first   Code also   Unspecified

OGCR Official Guidelines   ● Unacceptable Principal Diagnosis   X Assign placeholder X   ● Use Additional Character(s)   ▶ Manifestation Code   **Coding Clinic**

- **Y35.21**   Legal intervention involving injury by tear gas
  - **Y35.211**   Legal intervention involving injury by tear gas, law enforcement official injured
  - **Y35.212**   Legal intervention involving injury by tear gas, bystander injured
  - **Y35.213**   Legal intervention involving injury by tear gas, suspect injured
- **Y35.29**   Legal intervention involving other gas
  - **Y35.291**   Legal intervention involving other gas, law enforcement official injured
  - **Y35.292**   Legal intervention involving other gas, bystander injured
  - **Y35.293**   Legal intervention involving other gas, suspect injured
- **Y35.3**   Legal intervention involving blunt objects
  Legal intervention involving being hit or struck by blunt object
  - **Y35.30**   Legal intervention involving unspecified blunt objects
    - **Y35.301**   Legal intervention involving unspecified blunt objects, law enforcement official injured
    - **Y35.302**   Legal intervention involving unspecified blunt objects, bystander injured
    - **Y35.303**   Legal intervention involving unspecified blunt objects, suspect injured
  - **Y35.31**   Legal intervention involving baton
    - **Y35.311**   Legal intervention involving baton, law enforcement official injured
    - **Y35.312**   Legal intervention involving baton, bystander injured
    - **Y35.313**   Legal intervention involving baton, suspect injured
  - **Y35.39**   Legal intervention involving other blunt objects
    - **Y35.391**   Legal intervention involving other blunt objects, law enforcement official injured
    - **Y35.392**   Legal intervention involving other blunt objects, bystander injured
    - **Y35.393**   Legal intervention involving other blunt objects, suspect injured
- **Y35.4**   Legal intervention involving sharp objects
  Legal intervention involving being cut by sharp objects
  Legal intervention involving being stabbed by sharp objects
  - **Y35.40**   Legal intervention involving unspecified sharp objects
    - **Y35.401**   Legal intervention involving unspecified sharp objects, law enforcement official injured
    - **Y35.402**   Legal intervention involving unspecified sharp objects, bystander injured
    - **Y35.403**   Legal intervention involving unspecified sharp objects, suspect injured
  - **Y35.41**   Legal intervention involving bayonet
    - **Y35.411**   Legal intervention involving bayonet, law enforcement official injured
    - **Y35.412**   Legal intervention involving bayonet, bystander injured
    - **Y35.413**   Legal intervention involving bayonet, suspect injured
- **Y35.49**   Legal intervention involving other sharp objects
  - **Y35.491**   Legal intervention involving other sharp objects, law enforcement official injured
  - **Y35.492**   Legal intervention involving other sharp objects, bystander injured
  - **Y35.493**   Legal intervention involving other sharp objects, suspect injured
- **Y35.8**   Legal intervention involving other specified means
  - **Y35.81**   Legal intervention involving manhandling
    - **Y35.811**   Legal intervention involving manhandling, law enforcement official injured
    - **Y35.812**   Legal intervention involving manhandling, bystander injured
    - **Y35.813**   Legal intervention involving manhandling, suspect injured
  - **Y35.89**   Legal intervention involving other specified means
    - **Y35.891**   Legal intervention involving other specified means, law enforcement official injured
    - **Y35.892**   Legal intervention involving other specified means, bystander injured
    - **Y35.893**   Legal intervention involving other specified means, suspect injured
- **Y35.9**   Legal intervention, means unspecified
  - X **Y35.91**   Legal intervention, means unspecified, law enforcement official injured
  - X **Y35.92**   Legal intervention, means unspecified, bystander injured
  - X **Y35.93**   Legal intervention, means unspecified, suspect injured
- **Y36**   Operations of war

Includes	injuries to military personnel and civilians caused by war, civil insurrection, and peacekeeping missions
Excludes1	injury to military personnel occurring during peacetime military operations (Y37.-) military vehicles involved in transport accidents with non-military vehicle during peacetime (VØ9.Ø1, VØ9.21, V19.81, V29.81, V39.81, V49.81, V59.81, V69.81, V79.81)

  The appropriate 7th character is to be added to each code from category Y36

A	initial encounter
D	subsequent encounter
S	sequela

  - **Y36.Ø**   War operations involving explosion of marine weapons
    Weapons and military watercraft
    - **Y36.ØØ**   War operations involving explosion of unspecified marine weapon
      War operations involving underwater blast NOS
      - **Y36.ØØØ**   War operations involving explosion of unspecified marine weapon, military personnel
      - **Y36.ØØ1**   War operations involving explosion of unspecified marine weapon, civilian
    - **Y36.Ø1**   War operations involving explosion of depth-charge
      - **Y36.Ø1Ø**   War operations involving explosion of depth-charge, military personnel
      - **Y36.Ø11**   War operations involving explosion of depth-charge, civilian

CHAPTER 2Ø (VØ1-Y99)

N Newborn Age: Ø   **P** Pediatric Age: Ø–17   **M** Maternity DX: 12–55   **A** Adult Age: 15–124   ♀ Females Only   ♂ Males Only

Complication\Comorbidity   Major C\C   (Ex) CC/MCC Exclusions   Hospital-Acquired Condition

1581

- Y36.02 **War operations involving explosion of marine mine**
  - War operations involving explosion of marine mine, at sea or in harbor
  - Y36.020 **War operations involving explosion of marine mine, military personnel**
  - Y36.021 **War operations involving explosion of marine mine, civilian**
- Y36.03 **War operations involving explosion of sea-based artillery shell**
  - Y36.030 **War operations involving explosion of sea-based artillery shell, military personnel**
  - Y36.031 **War operations involving explosion of sea-based artillery shell, civilian**
- Y36.04 **War operations involving explosion of torpedo**
  - Y36.040 **War operations involving explosion of torpedo, military personnel**
  - Y36.041 **War operations involving explosion of torpedo, civilian**
- Y36.05 **War operations involving accidental detonation of onboard marine weapons**
  - Y36.050 **War operations involving accidental detonation of onboard marine weapons, military personnel**
  - Y36.051 **War operations involving accidental detonation of onboard marine weapons, civilian**
- Y36.09 **War operations involving explosion of other marine weapons**
  - Y36.090 **War operations involving explosion of other marine weapons, military personnel**
  - Y36.091 **War operations involving explosion of other marine weapons, civilian**
- Y36.1 **War operations involving destruction of aircraft**
  - Y36.10 **War operations involving unspecified destruction of aircraft**
    - Y36.100 **War operations involving** unspecified **destruction of aircraft, military personnel**
    - Y36.101 **War operations involving** unspecified **destruction of aircraft, civilian**
  - Y36.11 **War operations involving destruction of aircraft due to enemy fire or explosives**
    - War operations involving destruction of aircraft due to air to air missile
    - War operations involving destruction of aircraft due to explosive placed on aircraft
    - War operations involving destruction of aircraft due to rocket propelled grenade [RPG]
    - War operations involving destruction of aircraft due to small arms fire
    - War operations involving destruction of aircraft due to surface to air missile
    - Y36.110 **War operations involving destruction of aircraft due to enemy fire or explosives, military personnel**
    - Y36.111 **War operations involving destruction of aircraft due to enemy fire or explosives, civilian**
  - Y36.12 **War operations involving destruction of aircraft due to collision with other aircraft**
    - Y36.120 **War operations involving destruction of aircraft due to collision with other aircraft, military personnel**
    - Y36.121 **War operations involving destruction of aircraft due to collision with other aircraft, civilian**

- Y36.13 **War operations involving destruction of aircraft due to onboard fire**
  - Y36.130 **War operations involving destruction of aircraft due to onboard fire, military personnel**
  - Y36.131 **War operations involving destruction of aircraft due to onboard fire, civilian**
- Y36.14 **War operations involving destruction of aircraft due to accidental detonation of onboard munitions and explosives**
  - Y36.140 **War operations involving destruction of aircraft due to accidental detonation of onboard munitions and explosives, military personnel**
  - Y36.141 **War operations involving destruction of aircraft due to accidental detonation of onboard munitions and explosives, civilian**
- Y36.19 **War operations involving other destruction of aircraft**
  - Y36.190 **War operations involving other destruction of aircraft, military personnel**
  - Y36.191 **War operations involving other destruction of aircraft, civilian**
- Y36.2 **War operations involving other explosions and fragments**

  Excludes1   war operations involving explosion of aircraft (Y36.1-)
  war operations involving explosion of marine weapons (Y36.0-)
  war operations involving explosion of nuclear weapons (Y36.5-)
  war operations involving explosion occurring after cessation of hostilities (Y36.8-)

  - Y36.20 **War operations involving unspecified explosion and fragments**
    - War operations involving air blast NOS
    - War operations involving blast NOS
    - War operations involving blast fragments NOS
    - War operations involving blast wave NOS
    - War operations involving blast wind NOS
    - War operations involving explosion NOS
    - War operations involving explosion of bomb NOS
    - Y36.200 **War operations involving** unspecified **explosion and fragments, military personnel**
    - Y36.201 **War operations involving** unspecified **explosion and fragments, civilian**
  - Y36.21 **War operations involving explosion of aerial bomb**
    - Y36.210 **War operations involving explosion of aerial bomb, military personnel**
    - Y36.211 **War operations involving explosion of aerial bomb, civilian**
  - Y36.22 **War operations involving explosion of guided missile**
    - Y36.220 **War operations involving explosion of guided missile, military personnel**
    - Y36.221 **War operations involving explosion of guided missile, civilian**

◀ New   ◀|||| Revised   ~~deleted~~ Deleted   Excludes 1   Excludes 2   Includes   Use additional   Code first   Code also   Unspecified

OGCR Official Guidelines   ● Unacceptable Principal Diagnosis   X Assign placeholder X   ● Use Additional Character(s)   ▶ Manifestation Code   **Coding Clinic**

● **Y36.23**   **War operations involving explosion of improvised explosive device [IED]**
     War operations involving explosion of person-borne improvised explosive device [IED]
     War operations involving explosion of vehicle-borne improvised explosive device [IED]
     War operations involving explosion of roadside improvised explosive device [IED]

   ● **Y36.230**   **War operations involving explosion of improvised explosive device [IED], military personnel**

   ● **Y36.231**   **War operations involving explosion of improvised explosive device [IED], civilian**

● **Y36.24**   **War operations involving explosion due to accidental detonation and discharge of own munitions or munitions launch device**

   ● **Y36.240**   **War operations involving explosion due to accidental detonation and discharge of own munitions or munitions launch device, military personnel**

   ● **Y36.241**   **War operations involving explosion due to accidental detonation and discharge of own munitions or munitions launch device, civilian**

● **Y36.25**   **War operations involving fragments from munitions**

   ● **Y36.250**   **War operations involving fragments from munitions, military personnel**

   ● **Y36.251**   **War operations involving fragments from munitions, civilian**

● **Y36.26**   **War operations involving fragments of improvised explosive device [IED]**
     War operations involving fragments of person-borne improvised explosive device [IED]
     War operations involving fragments of vehicle-borne improvised explosive device [IED]
     War operations involving fragments of roadside improvised explosive device [IED]

   ● **Y36.260**   **War operations involving fragments of improvised explosive device [IED], military personnel**

   ● **Y36.261**   **War operations involving fragments of improvised explosive device [IED], civilian**

● **Y36.27**   **War operations involving fragments from weapons**

   ● **Y36.270**   **War operations involving fragments from weapons, military personnel**

   ● **Y36.271**   **War operations involving fragments from weapons, civilian**

● **Y36.29**   **War operations involving other explosions and fragments**
     War operations involving explosion of grenade
     War operations involving explosions of land mine
     War operations involving shrapnel NOS

   ● **Y36.290**   **War operations involving other explosions and fragments, military personnel**

   ● **Y36.291**   **War operations involving other explosions and fragments, civilian**

● **Y36.3**   **War operations involving fires, conflagrations and hot substances**
     War operations involving smoke, fumes, and heat from fires, conflagrations and hot substances

   Excludes1   war operations involving fires and conflagrations aboard military aircraft (Y36.1-)
       war operations involving fires and conflagrations aboard military watercraft (Y36.0-)
       war operations involving fires and conflagrations caused indirectly by conventional weapons (Y36.2-)
       war operations involving fires and thermal effects of nuclear weapons (Y36.53-)

● **Y36.30**   **War operations involving unspecified fire, conflagration and hot substance**

   ● **Y36.300**   **War operations involving unspecified fire, conflagration and hot substance, military personnel**

   ● **Y36.301**   **War operations involving unspecified fire, conflagration and hot substance, civilian**

● **Y36.31**   **War operations involving gasoline bomb**
     War operations involving incendiary bomb
     War operations involving petrol bomb

   ● **Y36.310**   **War operations involving gasoline bomb, military personnel**

   ● **Y36.311**   **War operations involving gasoline bomb, civilian**

● **Y36.32**   **War operations involving incendiary bullet**

   ● **Y36.320**   **War operations involving incendiary bullet, military personnel**

   ● **Y36.321**   **War operations involving incendiary bullet, civilian**

● **Y36.33**   **War operations involving flamethrower**

   ● **Y36.330**   **War operations involving flamethrower, military personnel**

   ● **Y36.331**   **War operations involving flamethrower, civilian**

● **Y36.39**   **War operations involving other fires, conflagrations and hot substances**

   ● **Y36.390**   **War operations involving other fires, conflagrations and hot substances, military personnel**

   ● **Y36.391**   **War operations involving other fires, conflagrations and hot substances, civilian**

● **Y36.4**   **War operations involving firearm discharge and other forms of conventional warfare**

   ● **Y36.41**   **War operations involving rubber bullets**

     ● **Y36.410**   **War operations involving rubber bullets, military personnel**

     ● **Y36.411**   **War operations involving rubber bullets, civilian**

   ● **Y36.42**   **War operations involving firearms pellets**

     ● **Y36.420**   **War operations involving firearms pellets, military personnel**

     ● **Y36.421**   **War operations involving firearms pellets, civilian**

CHAPTER 20 (V01–Y99)

● **Y36.43** **War operations involving other firearms discharge**
　　　War operations involving bullets NOS
　　　Excludes1 war operations involving munitions fragments (Y36.25-)
　　　　　　war operations involving incendiary bullets (Y36.32-)

　● **Y36.430** **War operations involving other firearms discharge, military personnel**

　● **Y36.431** **War operations involving other firearms discharge, civilian**

● **Y36.44** **War operations involving unarmed hand to hand combat**
　　　Excludes1 war operations involving combat using blunt or piercing object (Y36.45-)
　　　　　　war operations involving intentional restriction of air and airway (Y36.46-)
　　　　　　war operations involving unintentional restriction of air and airway (Y36.47-)

　● **Y36.440** **War operations involving unarmed hand to hand combat, military personnel**

　● **Y36.441** **War operations involving unarmed hand to hand combat, civilian**

● **Y36.45** **War operations involving combat using blunt or piercing object**

　● **Y36.450** **War operations involving combat using blunt or piercing object, military personnel**

　● **Y36.451** **War operations involving combat using blunt or piercing object, civilian**

● **Y36.46** **War operations involving intentional restriction of air and airway**

　● **Y36.460** **War operations involving intentional restriction of air and airway, military personnel**

　● **Y36.461** **War operations involving intentional restriction of air and airway, civilian**

● **Y36.47** **War operations involving unintentional restriction of air and airway**

　● **Y36.470** **War operations involving unintentional restriction of air and airway, military personnel**

　● **Y36.471** **War operations involving unintentional restriction of air and airway, civilian**

● **Y36.49** **War operations involving other forms of conventional warfare**

　● **Y36.490** **War operations involving other forms of conventional warfare, military personnel**

　● **Y36.491** **War operations involving other forms of conventional warfare, civilian**

● **Y36.5** **War operations involving nuclear weapons**
　　　War operations involving dirty bomb NOS

　● **Y36.50** **War operations involving unspecified effect of nuclear weapon**

　　● **Y36.500** **War operations involving** unspecified **effect of nuclear weapon, military personnel**

　　● **Y36.501** **War operations involving** unspecified **effect of nuclear weapon, civilian**

● **Y36.51** **War operations involving direct blast effect of nuclear weapon**
　　　War operations involving blast pressure of nuclear weapon

　● **Y36.510** **War operations involving direct blast effect of nuclear weapon, military personnel**

　● **Y36.511** **War operations involving direct blast effect of nuclear weapon, civilian**

● **Y36.52** **War operations involving indirect blast effect of nuclear weapon**
　　　War operations involving being thrown by blast of nuclear weapon
　　　War operations involving being struck or crushed by blast debris of nuclear weapon

　● **Y36.520** **War operations involving indirect blast effect of nuclear weapon, military personnel**

　● **Y36.521** **War operations involving indirect blast effect of nuclear weapon, civilian**

● **Y36.53** **War operations involving thermal radiation effect of nuclear weapon**
　　　War operations involving direct heat from nuclear weapon
　　　War operation involving fireball effects from nuclear weapon

　● **Y36.530** **War operations involving thermal radiation effect of nuclear weapon, military personnel**

　● **Y36.531** **War operations involving thermal radiation effect of nuclear weapon, civilian**

● **Y36.54** **War operation involving nuclear radiation effects of nuclear weapon**
　　　War operation involving acute radiation exposure from nuclear weapon
　　　War operation involving exposure to immediate ionizing radiation from nuclear weapon
　　　War operation involving fallout exposure from nuclear weapon
　　　War operation involving secondary effects of nuclear weapons

　● **Y36.540** **War operation involving nuclear radiation effects of nuclear weapon, military personnel**

　● **Y36.541** **War operation involving nuclear radiation effects of nuclear weapon, civilian**

● **Y36.59** **War operation involving other effects of nuclear weapons**

　● **Y36.590** **War operation involving other effects of nuclear weapons, military personnel**

　● **Y36.591** **War operation involving other effects of nuclear weapons, civilian**

● **Y36.6** **War operations involving biological weapons**

　● **Y36.6X** **War operations involving biological weapons**

　　● **Y36.6X0** **War operations involving biological weapons, military personnel**

　　● **Y36.6X1** **War operations involving biological weapons, civilian**

◄ New　◄▥ Revised　~~deleted~~ Deleted　Excludes 1　Excludes 2　Includes　Use additional　Code first　Code also　Unspecified
OGCR Official Guidelines　● Unacceptable Principal Diagnosis　X Assign placeholder X　● Use Additional Character(s)　▷ Manifestation Code　Coding Clinic

● **Y36.7 War operations involving chemical weapons and other forms of unconventional warfare**

     Excludes1   war operations involving incendiary devices (Y36.3-, Y36.5-)

   ● **Y36.7X War operations involving chemical weapons and other forms of unconventional warfare**

     ● **Y36.7X0 War operations involving chemical weapons and other forms of unconventional warfare, military personnel**

     ● **Y36.7X1 War operations involving chemical weapons and other forms of unconventional warfare, civilian**

● **Y36.8 War operations occurring after cessation of hostilities**

     War operations classifiable to categories Y36.0-Y36.8 but occurring after cessation of hostilities

   ● **Y36.81 Explosion of mine placed during war operations but exploding after cessation of hostilities**

     ● **Y36.810 Explosion of mine placed during war operations but exploding after cessation of hostilities, military personnel**

     ● **Y36.811 Explosion of mine placed during war operations but exploding after cessation of hostilities, civilian**

   ● **Y36.82 Explosion of bomb placed during war operations but exploding after cessation of hostilities**

     ● **Y36.820 Explosion of bomb placed during war operations but exploding after cessation of hostilities, military personnel**

     ● **Y36.821 Explosion of bomb placed during war operations but exploding after cessation of hostilities, civilian**

   ● **Y36.88 Other war operations occurring after cessation of hostilities**

     ● **Y36.880 Other war operations occurring after cessation of hostilities, military personnel**

     ● **Y36.881 Other war operations occurring after cessation of hostilities, civilian**

   ● **Y36.89 Unspecified war operations occurring after cessation of hostilities**

     ● **Y36.890 Unspecified war operations occurring after cessation of hostilities, military personnel**

     ● **Y36.891 Unspecified war operations occurring after cessation of hostilities, civilian**

● **Y36.9 Other and unspecified war operations**

   X ● **Y36.90 War operations, unspecified**

   X ● **Y36.91 War operations involving unspecified weapon of mass destruction [WMD]**

   X ● **Y36.92 War operations involving friendly fire**

● **Y37 Military operations**

   Includes   Injuries to military personnel and civilians occurring during peacetime on military property and during routine military exercises and operations

   Excludes1   military aircraft involved in aircraft accident with civilian aircraft (V97.81-)

     military vehicles involved in transport accident with civilian vehicle (V09.01, V09.21, V19.81, V29.81, V39.81, V49.81, V59.81, V69.81, V79.81)

     military watercraft involved in water transport accident with civilian watercraft (V94.81-)

     war operations (Y36.-)

The appropriate 7th character is to be added to each code from category Y37

     A   initial encounter
     D   subsequent encounter
     S   sequela

● **Y37.0 Military operations involving explosion of marine weapons**

   ● **Y37.00 Military operations involving explosion of unspecified marine weapon**

     Military operations involving underwater blast NOS

     ● **Y37.000 Military operations involving explosion of unspecified marine weapon, military personnel**

     ● **Y37.001 Military operations involving explosion of unspecified marine weapon, civilian**

   ● **Y37.01 Military operations involving explosion of depth-charge**

     ● **Y37.010 Military operations involving explosion of depth-charge, military personnel**

     ● **Y37.011 Military operations involving explosion of depth-charge, civilian**

   ● **Y37.02 Military operations involving explosion of marine mine**

     Military operations involving explosion of marine mine, at sea or in harbor

     ● **Y37.020 Military operations involving explosion of marine mine, military personnel**

     ● **Y37.021 Military operations involving explosion of marine mine, civilian**

   ● **Y37.03 Military operations involving explosion of sea-based artillery shell**

     ● **Y37.030 Military operations involving explosion of sea-based artillery shell, military personnel**

     ● **Y37.031 Military operations involving explosion of sea-based artillery shell, civilian**

   ● **Y37.04 Military operations involving explosion of torpedo**

     ● **Y37.040 Military operations involving explosion of torpedo, military personnel**

     ● **Y37.041 Military operations involving explosion of torpedo, civilian**

   ● **Y37.05 Military operations involving accidental detonation of onboard marine weapons**

     ● **Y37.050 Military operations involving accidental detonation of onboard marine weapons, military personnel**

     ● **Y37.051 Military operations involving accidental detonation of onboard marine weapons, civilian**

- Y37.09   Military operations involving explosion of other marine weapons
  - Y37.090   Military operations involving explosion of other marine weapons, military personnel
  - Y37.091   Military operations involving explosion of other marine weapons, civilian
- Y37.1   Military operations involving destruction of aircraft
  - Y37.10   Military operations involving unspecified destruction of aircraft
    - Y37.100   Military operations involving unspecified destruction of aircraft, military personnel
    - Y37.101   Military operations involving unspecified destruction of aircraft, civilian
  - Y37.11   Military operations involving destruction of aircraft due to enemy fire or explosives
    Military operations involving destruction of aircraft due to air to air missile
    Military operations involving destruction of aircraft due to explosive placed on aircraft
    Military operations involving destruction of aircraft due to rocket propelled grenade [RPG]
    Military operations involving destruction of aircraft due to small arms fire
    Military operations involving destruction of aircraft due to surface to air missile
    - Y37.110   Military operations involving destruction of aircraft due to enemy fire or explosives, military personnel
    - Y37.111   Military operations involving destruction of aircraft due to enemy fire or explosives, civilian
  - Y37.12   Military operations involving destruction of aircraft due to collision with other aircraft
    - Y37.120   Military operations involving destruction of aircraft due to collision with other aircraft, military personnel
    - Y37.121   Military operations involving destruction of aircraft due to collision with other aircraft, civilian
  - Y37.13   Military operations involving destruction of aircraft due to onboard fire
    - Y37.130   Military operations involving destruction of aircraft due to onboard fire, military personnel
    - Y37.131   Military operations involving destruction of aircraft due to onboard fire, civilian
  - Y37.14   Military operations involving destruction of aircraft due to accidental detonation of onboard munitions and explosives
    - Y37.140   Military operations involving destruction of aircraft due to accidental detonation of onboard munitions and explosives, military personnel
    - Y37.141   Military operations involving destruction of aircraft due to accidental detonation of onboard munitions and explosives, civilian
  - Y37.19   Military operations involving other destruction of aircraft
    - Y37.190   Military operations involving other destruction of aircraft, military personnel
    - Y37.191   Military operations involving other destruction of aircraft, civilian

- Y37.2   Military operations involving other explosions and fragments
  - **Excludes1**   military operations involving explosion of aircraft (Y37.1-)
    military operations involving explosion of marine weapons (Y37.0-)
    military operations involving explosion of nuclear weapons (Y37.5-)
  - Y37.20   Military operations involving unspecified explosion and fragments
    Military operations involving air blast NOS
    Military operations involving blast NOS
    Military operations involving blast fragments NOS
    Military operations involving blast wave NOS
    Military operations involving blast wind NOS
    Military operations involving explosion NOS
    Military operations involving explosion of bomb NOS
    - Y37.200   Military operations involving unspecified explosion and fragments, military personnel
    - Y37.201   Military operations involving unspecified explosion and fragments, civilian
  - Y37.21   Military operations involving explosion of aerial bomb
    - Y37.210   Military operations involving explosion of aerial bomb, military personnel
    - Y37.211   Military operations involving explosion of aerial bomb, civilian
  - Y37.22   Military operations involving explosion of guided missile
    - Y37.220   Military operations involving explosion of guided missile, military personnel
    - Y37.221   Military operations involving explosion of guided missile, civilian
  - Y37.23   Military operations involving explosion of improvised explosive device [IED]
    Military operations involving explosion of person-borne improvised explosive device [IED]
    Military operations involving explosion of vehicle-borne improvised explosive device [IED]
    Military operations involving explosion of roadside improvised explosive device [IED]
    - Y37.230   Military operations involving explosion of improvised explosive device [IED], military personnel
    - Y37.231   Military operations involving explosion of improvised explosive device [IED], civilian
  - Y37.24   Military operations involving explosion due to accidental detonation and discharge of own munitions or munitions launch device
    - Y37.240   Military operations involving explosion due to accidental detonation and discharge of own munitions or munitions launch device, military personnel
    - Y37.241   Military operations involving explosion due to accidental detonation and discharge of own munitions or munitions launch device, civilian

◄ New   ◄|||| Revised   ~~deleted~~ Deleted   Excludes 1   Excludes 2   Includes   Use additional   Code first   Code also   Unspecified
OGCR Official Guidelines   ● Unacceptable Principal Diagnosis   X Assign placeholder X   ● Use Additional Character(s)   ▶ Manifestation Code   **Coding Clinic**

● **Y37.25   Military operations involving fragments from munitions**

　　● **Y37.250   Military operations involving fragments from munitions, military personnel**

　　● **Y37.251   Military operations involving fragments from munitions, civilian**

● **Y37.26   Military operations involving fragments of improvised explosive device [IED]**

　　Military operations involving fragments of person-borne improvised explosive device [IED]

　　Military operations involving fragments of vehicle-borne improvised explosive device [IED]

　　Military operations involving fragments of roadside improvised explosive device [IED]

　　● **Y37.260   Military operations involving fragments of improvised explosive device [IED], military personnel**

　　● **Y37.261   Military operations involving fragments of improvised explosive device [IED], civilian**

● **Y37.27   Military operations involving fragments from weapons**

　　● **Y37.270   Military operations involving fragments from weapons, military personnel**

　　● **Y37.271   Military operations involving fragments from weapons, civilian**

● **Y37.29   Military operations involving other explosions and fragments**

　　Military operations involving explosion of grenade

　　Military operations involving explosions of land mine

　　Military operations involving shrapnel NOS

　　● **Y37.290   Military operations involving other explosions and fragments, military personnel**

　　● **Y37.291   Military operations involving other explosions and fragments, civilian**

● **Y37.3   Military operations involving fires, conflagrations and hot substances**

　　Military operations involving smoke, fumes, and heat from fires, conflagrations and hot substances

　　Excludes 1   military operations involving fires and conflagrations aboard military aircraft (Y37.1-)

　　　　military operations involving fires and conflagrations aboard military watercraft (Y37.0-)

　　　　military operations involving fires and conflagrations caused indirectly by conventional weapons (Y37.2-)

　　　　military operations involving fires and thermal effects of nuclear weapons (Y36.53-)

　　● **Y37.30   Military operations involving unspecified fire, conflagration and hot substance**

　　　　● **Y37.300   Military operations involving unspecified fire, conflagration and hot substance, military personnel**

　　　　● **Y37.301   Military operations involving unspecified fire, conflagration and hot substance, civilian**

　　● **Y37.31   Military operations involving gasoline bomb**

　　　　Military operations involving incendiary bomb

　　　　Military operations involving petrol bomb

　　　　● **Y37.310   Military operations involving gasoline bomb, military personnel**

　　　　● **Y37.311   Military operations involving gasoline bomb, civilian**

● **Y37.32   Military operations involving incendiary bullet**

　　● **Y37.320   Military operations involving incendiary bullet, military personnel**

　　● **Y37.321   Military operations involving incendiary bullet, civilian**

● **Y37.33   Military operations involving flamethrower**

　　● **Y37.330   Military operations involving flamethrower, military personnel**

　　● **Y37.331   Military operations involving flamethrower, civilian**

● **Y37.39   Military operations involving other fires, conflagrations and hot substances**

　　● **Y37.390   Military operations involving other fires, conflagrations and hot substances, military personnel**

　　● **Y37.391   Military operations involving other fires, conflagrations and hot substances, civilian**

● **Y37.4   Military operations involving firearm discharge and other forms of conventional warfare**

　　● **Y37.41   Military operations involving rubber bullets**

　　　　● **Y37.410   Military operations involving rubber bullets, military personnel**

　　　　● **Y37.411   Military operations involving rubber bullets, civilian**

　　● **Y37.42   Military operations involving firearms pellets**

　　　　● **Y37.420   Military operations involving firearms pellets, military personnel**

　　　　● **Y37.421   Military operations involving firearms pellets, civilian**

　　● **Y37.43   Military operations involving other firearms discharge**

　　　　Military operations involving bullets NOS

　　　　Excludes 1   military operations involving munitions fragments (Y37.25-)

　　　　　　military operations involving incendiary bullets (Y37.32-)

　　　　● **Y37.430   Military operations involving other firearms discharge, military personnel**

　　　　● **Y37.431   Military operations involving other firearms discharge, civilian**

　　● **Y37.44   Military operations involving unarmed hand to hand combat**

　　　　Excludes 1   military operations involving combat using blunt or piercing object (Y37.45-)

　　　　　　military operations involving intentional restriction of air and airway (Y37.46-)

　　　　　　military operations involving unintentional restriction of air and airway (Y37.47-)

　　　　● **Y37.440   Military operations involving unarmed hand to hand combat, military personnel**

　　　　● **Y37.441   Military operations involving unarmed hand to hand combat, civilian**

　　● **Y37.45   Military operations involving combat using blunt or piercing object**

　　　　● **Y37.450   Military operations involving combat using blunt or piercing object, military personnel**

　　　　● **Y37.451   Military operations involving combat using blunt or piercing object, civilian**

CHAPTER 20 (V01-Y99)

N Newborn Age: 0   **P** Pediatric Age: 0–17   **M** Maternity DX: 12–55   **A** Adult Age: 15–124   ♀ Females Only   ♂ Males Only

 Complication\Comorbidity   ◈ Major C\C   (Ex) CC/MCC Exclusions   ◈ Hospital-Acquired Condition

1587

● Y37.46   **Military operations involving intentional restriction of air and airway**
- ● Y37.460   **Military operations involving intentional restriction of air and airway, military personnel**
- ● Y37.461   **Military operations involving intentional restriction of air and airway, civilian**

● Y37.47   **Military operations involving unintentional restriction of air and airway**
- ● Y37.470   **Military operations involving unintentional restriction of air and airway, military personnel**
- ● Y37.471   **Military operations involving unintentional restriction of air and airway, civilian**

● Y37.49   **Military operations involving other forms of conventional warfare**
- ● Y37.490   **Military operations involving other forms of conventional warfare, military personnel**
- ● Y37.491   **Military operations involving other forms of conventional warfare, civilian**

● Y37.5   **Military operations involving nuclear weapons**
Military operation involving dirty bomb NOS

● Y37.50   **Military operations involving unspecified effect of nuclear weapon**
- ● Y37.500   **Military operations involving unspecified effect of nuclear weapon, military personnel**
- ● Y37.501   **Military operations involving unspecified effect of nuclear weapon, civilian**

● Y37.51   **Military operations involving direct blast effect of nuclear weapon**
Military operations involving blast pressure of nuclear weapon
- ● Y37.510   **Military operations involving direct blast effect of nuclear weapon, military personnel**
- ● Y37.511   **Military operations involving direct blast effect of nuclear weapon, civilian**

● Y37.52   **Military operations involving indirect blast effect of nuclear weapon**
Military operations involving being thrown by blast of nuclear weapon
Military operations involving being struck or crushed by blast debris of nuclear weapon
- ● Y37.520   **Military operations involving indirect blast effect of nuclear weapon, military personnel**
- ● Y37.521   **Military operations involving indirect blast effect of nuclear weapon, civilian**

● Y37.53   **Military operations involving thermal radiation effect of nuclear weapon**
Military operations involving direct heat from nuclear weapon
Military operation involving fireball effects from nuclear weapon
- ● Y37.530   **Military operations involving thermal radiation effect of nuclear weapon, military personnel**
- ● Y37.531   **Military operations involving thermal radiation effect of nuclear weapon, civilian**

● Y37.54   **Military operation involving nuclear radiation effects of nuclear weapon**
Military operation involving acute radiation exposure from nuclear weapon
Military operation involving exposure to immediate ionizing radiation from nuclear weapon
Military operation involving fallout exposure from nuclear weapon
Military operation involving secondary effects of nuclear weapons
- ● Y37.540   **Military operation involving nuclear radiation effects of nuclear weapon, military personnel**
- ● Y37.541   **Military operation involving nuclear radiation effects of nuclear weapon, civilian**

● Y37.59   **Military operation involving other effects of nuclear weapons**
- ● Y37.590   **Military operation involving other effects of nuclear weapons, military personnel**
- ● Y37.591   **Military operation involving other effects of nuclear weapons, civilian**

● Y37.6   **Military operations involving biological weapons**
● Y37.6X   **Military operations involving biological weapons**
- ● Y37.6X0   **Military operations involving biological weapons, military personnel**
- ● Y37.6X1   **Military operations involving biological weapons, civilian**

● Y37.7   **Military operations involving chemical weapons and other forms of unconventional warfare**
   Excludes1   military operations involving incendiary devices (Y36.3-, Y36.5-)
● Y37.7X   **Military operations involving chemical weapons and other forms of unconventional warfare**
- ● Y37.7X0   **Military operations involving chemical weapons and other forms of unconventional warfare, military personnel**
- ● Y37.7X1   **Military operations involving chemical weapons and other forms of unconventional warfare, civilian**

● Y37.9   **Other and unspecified military operations**
- X ● Y37.90   **Military operations, unspecified**
- X ● Y37.91   **Military operations involving unspecified weapon of mass destruction [WMD]**
- X ● Y37.92   **Military operations involving friendly fire**

◄ New   ◄█ Revised   ~~deleted~~ Deleted   Excludes 1   Excludes 2   Includes   Use additional   Code first   Code also   Unspecified
OGCR Official Guidelines   ● Unacceptable Principal Diagnosis   X Assign placeholder X   ◆ Use Additional Character(s)   ■ Manifestation Code   Coding Clinic

● **Y38   Terrorism**

These codes are for use to identify injuries resulting from the unlawful use of force or violence against persons or property to intimidate or coerce a government, the civilian population, or any segment thereof, in furtherance of political or social objective

Use additional code for place of occurrence (Y92.-)

The appropriate 7th character is to be added to each code from category Y38

A	initial encounter
D	subsequent encounter
S	sequela

● **Y38.0   Terrorism involving explosion of marine weapons**
Terrorism involving depth-charge
Terrorism involving marine mine
Terrorism involving mine NOS, at sea or in harbor
Terrorism involving sea-based artillery shell
Terrorism involving torpedo
Terrorism involving underwater blast

  ● **Y38.0X   Terrorism involving explosion of marine weapons**

    ● **Y38.0X1   Terrorism involving explosion of marine weapons, public safety official injured**

    ● **Y38.0X2   Terrorism involving explosion of marine weapons, civilian injured**

    ● **Y38.0X3   Terrorism involving explosion of marine weapons, terrorist injured**

● **Y38.1   Terrorism involving destruction of aircraft**
Terrorism involving aircraft burned
Terrorism involving aircraft exploded
Terrorism involving aircraft being shot down
Terrorism involving aircraft used as a weapon

  ● **Y38.1X   Terrorism involving destruction of aircraft**

    ● **Y38.1X1   Terrorism involving destruction of aircraft, public safety official injured**

    ● **Y38.1X2   Terrorism involving destruction of aircraft, civilian injured**

    ● **Y38.1X3   Terrorism involving destruction of aircraft, terrorist injured**

● **Y38.2   Terrorism involving other explosions and fragments**
Terrorism involving antipersonnel (fragments) bomb
Terrorism involving blast NOS
Terrorism involving explosion NOS
Terrorism involving explosion of breech block
Terrorism involving explosion of cannon block
Terrorism involving explosion (fragments) of artillery shell
Terrorism involving explosion (fragments) of bomb
Terrorism involving explosion (fragments) of grenade
Terrorism involving explosion (fragments) of guided missile
Terrorism involving explosion (fragments) of land mine
Terrorism involving explosion of mortar bomb
Terrorism involving explosion of munitions
Terrorism involving explosion (fragments) of rocket
Terrorism involving explosion (fragments) of shell
Terrorism involving shrapnel
Terrorism involving mine NOS, on land

  Excludes1   terrorism involving explosion of nuclear weapon (Y38.5)
               terrorism involving suicide bomber (Y38.81)

  ● **Y38.2X   Terrorism involving other explosions and fragments**

    ● **Y38.2X1   Terrorism involving other explosions and fragments, public safety official injured**

    ● **Y38.2X2   Terrorism involving other explosions and fragments, civilian injured**

    ● **Y38.2X3   Terrorism involving other explosions and fragments, terrorist injured**

● **Y38.3   Terrorism involving fires, conflagration and hot substances**
Terrorism involving conflagration NOS
Terrorism involving fire NOS
Terrorism involving petrol bomb

  Excludes1   terrorism involving fire or heat of nuclear weapon (Y38.5)

  ● **Y38.3X   Terrorism involving fires, conflagration and hot substances**

    ● **Y38.3X1   Terrorism involving fires, conflagration and hot substances, public safety official injured**

    ● **Y38.3X2   Terrorism involving fires, conflagration and hot substances, civilian injured**

    ● **Y38.3X3   Terrorism involving fires, conflagration and hot substances, terrorist injured**

● **Y38.4   Terrorism involving firearms**
Terrorism involving carbine bullet
Terrorism involving machine gun bullet
Terrorism involving pellets (shotgun)
Terrorism involving pistol bullet
Terrorism involving rifle bullet
Terrorism involving rubber (rifle) bullet

  ● **Y38.4X   Terrorism involving firearms**

    ● **Y38.4X1   Terrorism involving firearms, public safety official injured**

    ● **Y38.4X2   Terrorism involving firearms, civilian injured**

    ● **Y38.4X3   Terrorism involving firearms, terrorist injured**

● **Y38.5   Terrorism involving nuclear weapons**
Terrorism involving blast effects of nuclear weapon
Terrorism involving exposure to ionizing radiation from nuclear weapon
Terrorism involving fireball effect of nuclear weapon
Terrorism involving heat from nuclear weapon

  ● **Y38.5X   Terrorism involving nuclear weapons**

    ● **Y38.5X1   Terrorism involving nuclear weapons, public safety official injured**

    ● **Y38.5X2   Terrorism involving nuclear weapons, civilian injured**

    ● **Y38.5X3   Terrorism involving nuclear weapons, terrorist injured**

● **Y38.6   Terrorism involving biological weapons**
Terrorism involving anthrax
Terrorism involving cholera
A serious, often deadly, infectious disease of small intestine
Terrorism involving smallpox

  ● **Y38.6X   Terrorism involving biological weapons**

    ● **Y38.6X1   Terrorism involving biological weapons, public safety official injured**

    ● **Y38.6X2   Terrorism involving biological weapons, civilian injured**

    ● **Y38.6X3   Terrorism involving biological weapons, terrorist injured**

● **Y38.7   Terrorism involving chemical weapons**
Terrorism involving gases, fumes, chemicals
Terrorism involving hydrogen cyanide
Terrorism involving phosgene
Terrorism involving sarin

  ● **Y38.7X   Terrorism involving chemical weapons**

    ● **Y38.7X1   Terrorism involving chemical weapons, public safety official injured**

    ● **Y38.7X2   Terrorism involving chemical weapons, civilian injured**

    ● **Y38.7X3   Terrorism involving chemical weapons, terrorist injured**

CHAPTER 20 (V01-Y99)

N Newborn Age: 0   P Pediatric Age: 0–17   M Maternity DX: 12–55   A Adult Age: 15–124   ♀ Females Only   ♂ Males Only

 Complication\Comorbidity   Major C\C   Ⓔⓧ CC/MCC Exclusions   Hospital-Acquired Condition

● **Y38.8   Terrorism involving other and unspecified means**
  ● **Y38.80   Terrorism involving unspecified means**
             Terrorism NOS
  ● **Y38.81   Terrorism involving suicide bomber**
    ● **Y38.811   Terrorism involving suicide bomber, public safety official injured**
    ● **Y38.812   Terrorism involving suicide bomber, civilian injured**
  ● **Y38.89   Terrorism involving other means**
             Terrorism involving drowning and submersion
             Terrorism involving lasers
             Terrorism involving piercing or stabbing instruments
    ● **Y38.891   Terrorism involving other means, public safety official injured**
    ● **Y38.892   Terrorism involving other means, civilian injured**
    ● **Y38.893   Terrorism involving other means, terrorist injured**

● **Y38.9   Terrorism, secondary effects**
        Note: This code is for use to identify conditions occurring subsequent to a terrorist attack not those that are due to the initial terrorist attack.
  ● **Y38.9X   Terrorism, secondary effects**
    ● **Y38.9X1   Terrorism, secondary effects, public safety official injured**
    ● **Y38.9X2   Terrorism, secondary effects, civilian injured categories**

COMPLICATIONS OF MEDICAL AND SURGICAL CARE (Y62–Y84)

> **Includes**   complications of medical devices surgical and medical procedures as the cause of abnormal reaction of the patient, or of later complication, without mention of misadventure at the time of the procedure

MISADVENTURES TO PATIENTS DURING SURGICAL AND MEDICAL CARE (Y62–Y69)

> **Excludes1**   surgical and medical procedures as the cause of abnormal reaction of the patient, without mention of misadventure at the time of the procedure (Y83–Y84) ◄
>
> **Excludes2**   breakdown or malfunctioning of medical device (during procedure) (after implantation) (ongoing use) (Y70–Y82)

● **Y62   Failure of sterile precautions during surgical and medical care**
   Y62.0   Failure of sterile precautions during surgical operation
   Y62.1   Failure of sterile precautions during infusion or transfusion
   Y62.2   Failure of sterile precautions during kidney dialysis and other perfusion
   Y62.3   Failure of sterile precautions during injection or immunization
   Y62.4   Failure of sterile precautions during endoscopic examination
   Y62.5   Failure of sterile precautions during heart catheterization
   Y62.6   Failure of sterile precautions during aspiration, puncture and other catheterization
   Y62.8   Failure of sterile precautions during other surgical and medical care
   Y62.9   Failure of sterile precautions during unspecified surgical and medical care

● **Y63   Failure in dosage during surgical and medical care**
> **Excludes2**   accidental overdose of drug or wrong drug given in error (T36–T50)

   Y63.0   Excessive amount of blood or other fluid given during transfusion or infusion
   Y63.1   Incorrect dilution of fluid used during infusion
   Y63.2   Overdose of radiation given during therapy
   Y63.3   Inadvertent exposure of patient to radiation during medical care
   Y63.4   Failure in dosage in electroshock or insulin-shock therapy
   Y63.5   Inappropriate temperature in local application and packing
   Y63.6   Underdosing and nonadministration of necessary drug, medicament or biological substance
   Y63.8   Failure in dosage during other surgical and medical care
   Y63.9   Failure in dosage during unspecified surgical and medical care

● **Y64   Contaminated medical or biological substances**
   Y64.0   Contaminated medical or biological substance, transfused or infused
   Y64.1   Contaminated medical or biological substance, injected or used for immunization
   Y64.8   Contaminated medical or biological substance administered by other means
   Y64.9   Contaminated medical or biological substance administered by unspecified means
          Administered contaminated medical or biological substance NOS

● **Y65   Other misadventures during surgical and medical care**
   Y65.0   Mismatched blood in transfusion
   Y65.1   Wrong fluid used in infusion
   Y65.2   Failure in suture or ligature during surgical operation
   Y65.3   Endotracheal tube wrongly placed during anesthetic procedure
   Y65.4   Failure to introduce or to remove other tube or instrument
  ● **Y65.5   Performance of wrong procedure (operation)**
    ● **Y65.51   Performance of wrong procedure (operation) on correct patient**
             Wrong device implanted into correct surgical site
>   **Excludes1**   performance of correct procedure (operation) on wrong side or body part (Y65.53)

             MCE: Wrong procedure performed
    ● **Y65.52   Performance of procedure (operation) on patient not scheduled for surgery**
             Performance of procedure (operation) intended for another patient
             Performance of procedure (operation) on wrong patient
             MCE: Wrong procedure performed
    ● **Y65.53   Performance of correct procedure (operation) on wrong side or body part**
             Performance of correct procedure (operation) on wrong side
             Performance of correct procedure (operation) on wrong site
             MCE: Wrong procedure performed
   Y65.8   Other specified misadventures during surgical and medical care

   Y66   Nonadministration of surgical and medical care
             Premature cessation of surgical and medical care
>   **Excludes1**   DNR status (Z66)
>   palliative care (Z51.5)

   Y69   Unspecified misadventure during surgical and medical care

◄ New   ◄◄ Revised   ~~deleted~~ Deleted   Excludes 1   Excludes 2   Includes   Use additional   Code first   Code also   Unspecified

OGCR Official Guidelines   ● Unacceptable Principal Diagnosis   X Assign placeholder X   ● Use Additional Character(s)   ▌ Manifestation Code   **Coding Clinic**

MEDICAL DEVICES ASSOCIATED WITH ADVERSE INCIDENTS IN DIAGNOSTIC AND THERAPEUTIC USE (Y70-Y82)

Includes   breakdown or malfunction of medical devices (during use) (after implantation) (ongoing use)

Excludes2   breakdown or malfunctioning of medical device (after implantation) (during procedure) (ongoing use) (Y70-Y82) ◄

later complications following use of medical devices without breakdown or malfunctioning of device (Y83-Y84) ◄

misadventure to patients during surgical and medical care, classifiable to (Y62-Y69) ◄

surgical and other medical procedures as the cause of abnormal reaction of the patient, or of later complication, without mention of misadventure at the time of the procedure (Y83-Y84) ◄

● **Y70**   Anesthesiology devices associated with adverse incidents

   Y70.0   Diagnostic and monitoring anesthesiology devices associated with adverse incidents

   Y70.1   Therapeutic (nonsurgical) and rehabilitative anesthesiology devices associated with adverse incidents

   Y70.2   Prosthetic and other implants, materials and accessory anesthesiology devices associated with adverse incidents

   Y70.3   Surgical instruments, materials and anesthesiology devices (including sutures) associated with adverse incidents

   Y70.8   Miscellaneous anesthesiology devices associated with adverse incidents, not elsewhere classified

● **Y71**   Cardiovascular devices associated with adverse incidents

   Y71.0   Diagnostic and monitoring cardiovascular devices associated with adverse incidents

   Y71.1   Therapeutic (nonsurgical) and rehabilitative cardiovascular devices associated with adverse incidents

   Y71.2   Prosthetic and other implants, materials and accessory cardiovascular devices associated with adverse incidents

   Y71.3   Surgical instruments, materials and cardiovascular devices (including sutures) associated with adverse incidents

   Y71.8   Miscellaneous cardiovascular devices associated with adverse incidents, not elsewhere classified

● **Y72**   Otorhinolaryngological devices associated with adverse incidents

   Y72.0   Diagnostic and monitoring otorhinolaryngological devices associated with adverse incidents

   Y72.1   Therapeutic (nonsurgical) and rehabilitative otorhinolaryngological devices associated with adverse incidents

   Y72.2   Prosthetic and other implants, materials and accessory otorhinolaryngological devices associated with adverse incidents

   Y72.3   Surgical instruments, materials and otorhinolaryngological devices (including sutures) associated with adverse incidents

   Y72.8   Miscellaneous otorhinolaryngological devices associated with adverse incidents, not elsewhere classified

● **Y73**   Gastroenterology and urology devices associated with adverse incidents

   Y73.0   Diagnostic and monitoring gastroenterology and urology devices associated with adverse incidents

   Y73.1   Therapeutic (nonsurgical) and rehabilitative gastroenterology and urology devices associated with adverse incidents

   Y73.2   Prosthetic and other implants, materials and accessory gastroenterology and urology devices associated with adverse incidents

   Y73.3   Surgical instruments, materials and gastroenterology and urology devices (including sutures) associated with adverse incidents

   Y73.8   Miscellaneous gastroenterology and urology devices associated with adverse incidents, not elsewhere classified

● **Y74**   General hospital and personal-use devices associated with adverse incidents

   Y74.0   Diagnostic and monitoring general hospital and personal-use devices associated with adverse incidents

   Y74.1   Therapeutic (nonsurgical) and rehabilitative general hospital and personal-use devices associated with adverse incidents

   Y74.2   Prosthetic and other implants, materials and accessory general hospital and personal-use devices associated with adverse incidents

   Y74.3   Surgical instruments, materials and general hospital and personal-use devices (including sutures) associated with adverse incidents

   Y74.8   Miscellaneous general hospital and personal-use devices associated with adverse incidents, not elsewhere classified

● **Y75**   Neurological devices associated with adverse incidents

   Y75.0   Diagnostic and monitoring neurological devices associated with adverse incidents

   Y75.1   Therapeutic (nonsurgical) and rehabilitative neurological devices associated with adverse incidents

   Y75.2   Prosthetic and other implants, materials and neurological devices associated with adverse incidents

   Y75.3   Surgical instruments, materials and neurological devices (including sutures) associated with adverse incidents

   Y75.8   Miscellaneous neurological devices associated with adverse incidents, not elsewhere classified

● **Y76**   Obstetric and gynecological devices associated with adverse incidents

   Y76.0   Diagnostic and monitoring obstetric and gynecological devices associated with adverse incidents ♀

   Y76.1   Therapeutic (nonsurgical) and rehabilitative obstetric and gynecological devices associated with adverse incidents ♀

   Y76.2   Prosthetic and other implants, materials and accessory obstetric and gynecological devices associated with adverse incidents ♀

   Y76.3   Surgical instruments, materials and obstetric and gynecological devices (including sutures) associated with adverse incidents ♀

   Y76.8   Miscellaneous obstetric and gynecological devices associated with adverse incidents, not elsewhere classified ♀

CHAPTER 20 (V01-Y99)

N Newborn Age: 0   **P** Pediatric Age: 0–17   **M** Maternity DX: 12–55   **A** Adult Age: 15–124   ♀ Females Only   ♂ Males Only

🔗 Complication\Comorbidity   🔗 Major C\C   (Ex) CC/MCC Exclusions   🔗 Hospital-Acquired Condition   **1591**

CHAPTER 20 (V01-Y99)

- Y77　Ophthalmic devices associated with adverse incidents
  - Y77.0　Diagnostic and monitoring ophthalmic devices associated with adverse incidents
  - Y77.1　Therapeutic (nonsurgical) and rehabilitative ophthalmic devices associated with adverse incidents
  - Y77.2　Prosthetic and other implants, materials and accessory ophthalmic devices associated with adverse incidents
  - Y77.3　Surgical instruments, materials and ophthalmic devices (including sutures) associated with adverse incidents
  - Y77.8　Miscellaneous ophthalmic devices associated with adverse incidents, not elsewhere classified

- Y78　Radiological devices associated with adverse incidents
  - Y78.0　Diagnostic and monitoring radiological devices associated with adverse incidents
  - Y78.1　Therapeutic (nonsurgical) and rehabilitative radiological devices associated with adverse incidents
  - Y78.2　Prosthetic and other implants, materials and accessory radiological devices associated with adverse incidents
  - Y78.3　Surgical instruments, materials and radiological devices (including sutures) associated with adverse incidents
  - Y78.8　Miscellaneous radiological devices associated with adverse incidents, not elsewhere classified

- Y79　Orthopedic devices associated with adverse incidents
  - Y79.0　Diagnostic and monitoring orthopedic devices associated with adverse incidents
  - Y79.1　Therapeutic (nonsurgical) and rehabilitative orthopedic devices associated with adverse incidents
  - Y79.2　Prosthetic and other implants, materials and accessory orthopedic devices associated with adverse incidents
  - Y79.3　Surgical instruments, materials and orthopedic devices (including sutures) associated with adverse incidents
  - Y79.8　Miscellaneous orthopedic devices associated with adverse incidents, not elsewhere classified

- Y80　Physical medicine devices associated with adverse incidents
  - Y80.0　Diagnostic and monitoring physical medicine devices associated with adverse incidents
  - Y80.1　Therapeutic (nonsurgical) and rehabilitative physical medicine devices associated with adverse incidents
  - Y80.2　Prosthetic and other implants, materials and accessory physical medicine devices associated with adverse incidents
  - Y80.3　Surgical instruments, materials and physical medicine devices (including sutures) associated with adverse incidents
  - Y80.8　Miscellaneous physical medicine devices associated with adverse incidents, not elsewhere classified

- Y81　General- and plastic-surgery devices associated with adverse incidents
  - Y81.0　Diagnostic and monitoring general- and plastic-surgery devices associated with adverse incidents
  - Y81.1　Therapeutic (nonsurgical) and rehabilitative general- and plastic-surgery devices associated with adverse incidents
  - Y81.2　Prosthetic and other implants, materials and accessory general- and plastic-surgery devices associated with adverse incidents
  - Y81.3　Surgical instruments, materials and general- and plastic-surgery devices (including sutures) associated with adverse incidents
  - Y81.8　Miscellaneous general- and plastic-surgery devices associated with adverse incidents, not elsewhere classified

- Y82　Other and unspecified medical devices associated with adverse incidents
  - Y82.8　Other medical devices associated with adverse incidents
  - Y82.9　Unspecified medical devices associated with adverse incidents

SURGICAL AND OTHER MEDICAL PROCEDURES AS THE CAUSE OF ABNORMAL REACTION OF THE PATIENT, OR OF LATER COMPLICATION, WITHOUT MENTION OF MISADVENTURE AT THE TIME OF THE PROCEDURE (Y83-Y84)

> **Excludes1** misadventures to patients during surgical and medical care, classifiable to (Y62-Y69)
>
> **Excludes2** breakdown or malfunctioning of medical device (after implantation) (during procedure) (ongoing use) (Y70-Y82) ◄

- Y83　Surgical operation and other surgical procedures as the cause of abnormal reaction of the patient, or of later complication, without mention of misadventure at the time of the procedure
  - Y83.0　Surgical operation with transplant of whole organ as the cause of abnormal reaction of the patient, or of later complication, without mention of misadventure at the time of the procedure
  - Y83.1　Surgical operation with implant of artificial internal device as the cause of abnormal reaction of the patient, or of later complication, without mention of misadventure at the time of the procedure
  - Y83.2　Surgical operation with anastomosis, bypass or graft as the cause of abnormal reaction of the patient, or of later complication, without mention of misadventure at the time of the procedure
  - Y83.3　Surgical operation with formation of external stoma as the cause of abnormal reaction of the patient, or of later complication, without mention of misadventure at the time of the procedure
  - Y83.4　Other reconstructive surgery as the cause of abnormal reaction of the patient, or of later complication, without mention of misadventure at the time of the procedure
  - Y83.5　Amputation of limb(s) as the cause of abnormal reaction of the patient, or of later complication, without mention of misadventure at the time of the procedure
  - Y83.6　Removal of other organ (partial) (total) as the cause of abnormal reaction of the patient, or of later complication, without mention of misadventure at the time of the procedure
  - Y83.8　Other surgical procedures as the cause of abnormal reaction of the patient, or of later complication, without mention of misadventure at the time of the procedure
  - Y83.9　Surgical procedure, unspecified as the cause of abnormal reaction of the patient, or of later complication, without mention of misadventure at the time of the procedure

- Y84　Other medical procedures as the cause of abnormal reaction of the patient, or of later complication, without mention of misadventure at the time of the procedure
  - Y84.0　Cardiac catheterization as the cause of abnormal reaction of the patient, or of later complication, without mention of misadventure at the time of the procedure
  - Y84.1　Kidney dialysis as the cause of abnormal reaction of the patient, or of later complication, without mention of misadventure at the time of the procedure
  - Y84.2　Radiological procedure and radiotherapy as the cause of abnormal reaction of the patient, or of later complication, without mention of misadventure at the time of the procedure
  - Y84.3　Shock therapy as the cause of abnormal reaction of the patient, or of later complication, without mention of misadventure at the time of the procedure
  - Y84.4　Aspiration of fluid as the cause of abnormal reaction of the patient, or of later complication, without mention of misadventure at the time of the procedure
  - Y84.5　Insertion of gastric or duodenal sound as the cause of abnormal reaction of the patient, or of later complication, without mention of misadventure at the time of the procedure
  - Y84.6　Urinary catheterization as the cause of abnormal reaction of the patient, or of later complication, without mention of misadventure at the time of the procedure
  - Y84.7　Blood-sampling as the cause of abnormal reaction of the patient, or of later complication, without mention of misadventure at the time of the procedure

◄ New　◄▬ Revised　~~deleted~~ Deleted　Excludes 1　Excludes 2　Includes　Use additional　Code first　Code also　Unspecified
OGCR Official Guidelines　● Unacceptable Principal Diagnosis　X Assign placeholder X　● Use Additional Character(s)　▶ Manifestation Code　**Coding Clinic**

Y84.8   Other medical procedures as the cause of abnormal reaction of the patient, or of later complication, without mention of misadventure at the time of the procedure

Y84.9   Medical procedure, unspecified as the cause of abnormal reaction of the patient, or of later complication, without mention of misadventure at the time of the procedure

SUPPLEMENTARY FACTORS RELATED TO CAUSES OF MORBIDITY CLASSIFIED ELSEWHERE (Y90-Y99)

Note: These categories may be used to provide supplementary information concerning causes of morbidity. They are not to be used for single-condition coding.

● Y90   **Evidence of alcohol involvement determined by blood alcohol level**

Code first any associated alcohol related disorders (F10)

Y90.0   Blood alcohol level of less than 20 mg/100 ml

Y90.1   Blood alcohol level of 20-39 mg/100 ml

Y90.2   Blood alcohol level of 40-59 mg/100 ml

Y90.3   Blood alcohol level of 60-79 mg/100 ml

Y90.4   Blood alcohol level of 80-99 mg/100 ml

Y90.5   Blood alcohol level of 100-119 mg/100 ml

Y90.6   Blood alcohol level of 120-199 mg/100 ml

Y90.7   Blood alcohol level of 200-239 mg/100 ml

Y90.8   Blood alcohol level of 240 mg/100 ml or more

Y90.9   Presence of alcohol in blood, level not specified

OGCR   Section I.C.20.b.

> Place of Occurrence Guideline
>
> Codes from category Y92, Place of occurrence of the external cause, are secondary codes for use after other external cause codes to identify the location of the patient at the time of injury or other condition.
>
> Generally, a place of occurrence code is assigned only once, at the initial encounter for treatment. However, in the rare instance that a new injury occurs during hospitalization, an additional place of occurrence code may be assigned. No 7th characters are used for Y92. Only one code from Y92 should be recorded on a medical record. A place of occurrence code should be used in conjunction with an activity code, Y93.
>
> Do not use place of occurrence code Y92.9 if the place is not stated or is not applicable.

● Y92   **Place of occurrence of the external cause**

The following category is for use, when relevant, to identify the place of the external cause. Use in conjunction with an activity code.

Place of occurrence should be recorded only at the initial encounter for treatment

● Y92.0   **Non-institutional (private) residence as the place of occurrence of the external cause**

    Excludes1   abandoned or derelict house (Y92.89)
home under construction but not yet occupied (Y92.6-)
institutional place of residence (Y92.1-)

    ● Y92.00   **Unspecified non-institutional (private) residence as the place of occurrence of the external cause**

       Y92.000   Kitchen of unspecified non-institutional (private) residence as the place of occurrence of the external cause

       Y92.001   Dining room of unspecified non-institutional (private) residence as the place of occurrence of the external cause

       Y92.002   Bathroom of unspecified non-institutional (private) residence single-family (private) house as the place of occurrence of the external cause

       Y92.003   Bedroom of unspecified non-institutional (private) residence as the place of occurrence of the external cause

       Y92.007   Garden or yard of unspecified non-institutional (private) residence as the place of occurrence of the external cause

       Y92.008   Other place in unspecified non-institutional (private) residence as the place of occurrence of the external cause

       Y92.009   Unspecified place in unspecified non-institutional (private) residence as the place of occurrence of the external cause

         Home (NOS) as the place of occurrence of the external cause

● Y92.01   **Single-family non-institutional (private) house as the place of occurrence of the external cause**

Farmhouse as the place of occurrence of the external cause

    Excludes1   barn (Y92.71)
chicken coop or hen house (Y92.72)
farm field (Y92.73)
orchard (Y92.74)
single family mobile home or trailer (Y92.02-)
slaughter house (Y92.86)

    Y92.010   Kitchen of single-family (private) house as the place of occurrence of the external cause

    Y92.011   Dining room of single-family (private) house as the place of occurrence of the external cause

    Y92.012   Bathroom of single-family (private) house as the place of occurrence of the external cause

    Y92.013   Bedroom of single-family (private) house as the place of occurrence of the external cause

    Y92.014   Private driveway to single-family (private) house as the place of occurrence of the external cause

    Y92.015   Private garage of single-family (private) house as the place of occurrence of the external cause

    Y92.016   Swimming pool in single-family (private) house or garden as the place of occurrence of the external cause

    Y92.017   Garden or yard in single-family (private) house as the place of occurrence of the external cause

    Y92.018   Other place in single-family (private) house as the place of occurrence of the external cause

    Y92.019   Unspecified place in single-family (private) house as the place of occurrence of the external cause

CHAPTER 20 (V01-Y99)

● **Y92.02** Mobile home as the place of occurrence of the external cause

Y92.020 Kitchen in mobile home as the place of occurrence of the external cause

Y92.021 Dining room in mobile home as the place of occurrence of the external cause

Y92.022 Bathroom in mobile home as the place of occurrence of the external cause

Y92.023 Bedroom in mobile home as the place of occurrence of the external cause

Y92.024 Driveway of mobile home as the place of occurrence of the external cause

Y92.025 Garage of mobile home as the place of occurrence of the external cause

Y92.026 Swimming pool of mobile home as the place of occurrence of the external cause

Y92.027 Garden or yard of mobile home as the place of occurrence of the external cause

Y92.028 Other place in mobile home as the place of occurrence of the external cause

Y92.029 Unspecified place in mobile home as the place of occurrence of the external cause

● **Y92.03** Apartment as the place of occurrence of the external cause

Condominium as the place of occurrence of the external cause

Co-op apartment as the place of occurrence of the external cause

Y92.030 Kitchen in apartment as the place of occurrence of the external cause

Y92.031 Bathroom in apartment as the place of occurrence of the external cause

Y92.032 Bedroom in apartment as the place of occurrence of the external cause

Y92.038 Other place in apartment as the place of occurrence of the external cause

Y92.039 Unspecified place in apartment as the place of occurrence of the external cause

● **Y92.04** Boarding-house as the place of occurrence of the external cause

Y92.040 Kitchen in boarding-house as the place of occurrence of the external cause

Y92.041 Bathroom in boarding-house as the place of occurrence of the external cause

Y92.042 Bedroom in boarding-house as the place of occurrence of the external cause

Y92.043 Driveway of boarding-house as the place of occurrence of the external cause

Y92.044 Garage of boarding-house as the place of occurrence of the external cause

Y92.045 Swimming pool of boarding-house as the place of occurrence of the external cause

Y92.046 Garden or yard of boarding-house as the place of occurrence of the external cause

Y92.048 Other place in boarding-house as the place of occurrence of the external cause

Y92.049 Unspecified place in boarding-house as the place of occurrence of the external cause

● **Y92.09** Other non-institutional residence as the place of occurrence of the external cause

Y92.090 Kitchen in other non-institutional residence as the place of occurrence of the external cause

Y92.091 Bathroom in other non-institutional residence as the place of occurrence of the external cause

Y92.092 Bedroom in other non-institutional residence as the place of occurrence of the external cause

Y92.093 Driveway of other non-institutional residence as the place of occurrence of the external cause

Y92.094 Garage of other non-institutional residence as the place of occurrence of the external cause

Y92.095 Swimming pool of other non-institutional residence as the place of occurrence of the external cause

Y92.096 Garden or yard of other non-institutional residence as the place of occurrence of the external cause

Y92.098 Other place in other non-institutional residence as the place of occurrence of the external cause

Y92.099 Unspecified place in other non-institutional residence as the place of occurrence of the external cause

● **Y92.1** Institutional (nonprivate) residence as the place of occurrence of the external cause

Y92.10 Unspecified residential institution as the place of occurrence of the external cause

● **Y92.11** Children's home and orphanage as the place of occurrence of the external cause

Y92.110 Kitchen in children's home and orphanage as the place of occurrence of the external cause

Y92.111 Bathroom in children's home and orphanage as the place of occurrence of the external cause

Y92.112 Bedroom in children's home and orphanage as the place of occurrence of the external cause

Y92.113 Driveway of children's home and orphanage as the place of occurrence of the external cause

Y92.114 Garage of children's home and orphanage as the place of occurrence of the external cause

Y92.115 Swimming pool of children's home and orphanage as the place of occurrence of the external cause

Y92.116 Garden or yard of children's home and orphanage as the place of occurrence of the external cause

Y92.118 Other place in children's home and orphanage as the place of occurrence of the external cause

Y92.119 Unspecified place in children's home and orphanage as the place of occurrence of the external cause

● **Y92.12** Nursing home as the place of occurrence of the external cause

Home for the sick as the place of occurrence of the external cause

Hospice as the place of occurrence of the external cause

Y92.120   Kitchen in nursing home as the place of occurrence of the external cause

Y92.121   Bathroom in nursing home as the place of occurrence of the external cause

Y92.122   Bedroom in nursing home as the place of occurrence of the external cause

Y92.123   Driveway of nursing home as the place of occurrence of the external cause

Y92.124   Garage of nursing home as the place of occurrence of the external cause

Y92.125   Swimming pool of nursing home as the place of occurrence of the external cause

Y92.126   Garden or yard of nursing home as the place of occurrence of the external cause

Y92.128   Other place in nursing home as the place of occurrence of the external cause

Y92.129   Unspecified place in nursing home as the place of occurrence of the external cause

● **Y92.13** Military base as the place of occurrence of the external cause

> Excludes1   military training grounds (Y92.83)

Y92.130   Kitchen on military base as the place of occurrence of the external cause

Y92.131   Mess hall on military base as the place of occurrence of the external cause

Y92.133   Barracks on military base as the place of occurrence of the external cause

Y92.135   Garage on military base as the place of occurrence of the external cause

Y92.136   Swimming pool on military base as the place of occurrence of the external cause

Y92.137   Garden or yard on military base as the place of occurrence of the external cause

Y92.138   Other place on military base as the place of occurrence of the external cause

Y92.139   Unspecified place military base as the place of occurrence of the external cause

● **Y92.14** Prison as the place of occurrence of the external cause

Y92.140   Kitchen in prison as the place of occurrence of the external cause

Y92.141   Dining room in prison as the place of occurrence of the external cause

Y92.142   Bathroom in prison as the place of occurrence of the external cause

Y92.143   Cell of prison as the place of occurrence of the external cause

Y92.146   Swimming pool of prison as the place of occurrence of the external cause

Y92.147   Courtyard of prison as the place of occurrence of the external cause

Y92.148   Other place in prison as the place of occurrence of the external cause

Y92.149   Unspecified place in prison as the place of occurrence of the external cause

● **Y92.15** Reform school as the place of occurrence of the external cause

Y92.150   Kitchen in reform school as the place of occurrence of the external cause

Y92.151   Dining room in reform school as the place of occurrence of the external cause

Y92.152   Bathroom in reform school as the place of occurrence of the external cause

Y92.153   Bedroom in reform school as the place of occurrence of the external cause

Y92.154   Driveway of reform school as the place of occurrence of the external cause

Y92.155   Garage of reform school as the place of occurrence of the external cause

Y92.156   Swimming pool of reform school as the place of occurrence of the external cause

Y92.157   Garden or yard of reform school as the place of occurrence of the external cause

Y92.158   Other place in reform school as the place of occurrence of the external cause

Y92.159   Unspecified place in reform school as the place of occurrence of the external cause

● **Y92.16** School dormitory as the place of occurrence of the external cause

> Excludes1   reform school as the place of occurrence of the external cause (Y92.15-)
> school buildings and grounds as the place of occurrence of the external cause (Y92.2-)
> school sports and athletic areas as the place of occurrence of the external cause (Y92.3-)

Y92.160   Kitchen in school dormitory as the place of occurrence of the external cause

Y92.161   Dining room in school dormitory as the place of occurrence of the external cause

Y92.162   Bathroom in school dormitory as the place of occurrence of the external cause

Y92.163   Bedroom in school dormitory as the place of occurrence of the external cause

Y92.168   Other place in school dormitory as the place of occurrence of the external cause

Y92.169   Unspecified place in school dormitory as the place of occurrence of the external cause

● **Y92.19** Other specified residential institution as the place of occurrence of the external cause

Y92.190 Kitchen in other specified residential institution as the place of occurrence of the external cause

Y92.191 Dining room in other specified residential institution as the place of occurrence of the external cause

Y92.192 Bathroom in other specified residential institution as the place of occurrence of the external cause

Y92.193 Bedroom in other specified residential institution as the place of occurrence of the external cause

Y92.194 Driveway of other specified residential institution as the place of occurrence of the external cause

Y92.195 Garage of other specified residential institution as the place of occurrence of the external cause

Y92.196 Pool of other specified residential institution as the place of occurrence of the external cause

Y92.197 Garden or yard of other specified residential institution as the place of occurrence of the external cause

Y92.198 Other place in other specified residential institution as the place of occurrence of the external cause

Y92.199 Unspecified place in other specified residential institution as the place of occurrence of the external cause

● **Y92.2** School, other institution and public administrative area as the place of occurrence of the external cause

Building and adjacent grounds used by the general public or by a particular group of the public

Excludes1 building under construction as the place of occurrence of the external cause (Y92.6)

residential institution as the place of occurrence of the external cause (Y92.1)

school dormitory as the place of occurrence of the external cause (Y92.16-)

sports and athletics area of schools as the place of occurrence of the external cause (Y92.3-)

● **Y92.21** School (private) (public) (state) as the place of occurrence of the external cause

Y92.210 Daycare center as the place of occurrence of the external cause

Y92.211 Elementary school as the place of occurrence of the external cause
　Kindergarten as the place of occurrence of the external cause

Y92.212 Middle school as the place of occurrence of the external cause

Y92.213 High school as the place of occurrence of the external cause
　Coding Clinic: 2012, Q4, P108

Y92.214 College as the place of occurrence of the external cause
　University as the place of occurrence of the external cause

Y92.215 Trade school as the place of occurrence of the external cause

Y92.218 Other school as the place of occurrence of the external cause

Y92.219 Unspecified school as the place of occurrence of the external cause

Y92.22 Religious institution as the place of occurrence of the external cause
　Church as the place of occurrence of the external cause
　Mosque as the place of occurrence of the external cause
　Synagogue as the place of occurrence of the external cause

● **Y92.23** Hospital as the place of occurrence of the external cause

Excludes1 ambulatory (outpatient) health services establishments (Y92.53-)

home for the sick as the place of occurrence of the external cause (Y92.12-)

hospice as the place of occurrence of the external cause (Y92.12-)

nursing home as the place of occurrence of the external cause (Y92.12-)

Y92.230 Patient room in hospital as the place of occurrence of the external cause

Y92.231 Patient bathroom in hospital as the place of occurrence of the external cause

Y92.232 Corridor of hospital as the place of occurrence of the external cause

Y92.233 Cafeteria of hospital as the place of occurrence of the external cause

Y92.234 Operating room of hospital as the place of occurrence of the external cause

Y92.238 Other place in hospital as the place of occurrence of the external cause

Y92.239 Unspecified place in hospital as the place of occurrence of the external cause

● **Y92.24** Public administrative building as the place of occurrence of the external cause

Y92.240 Courthouse as the place of occurrence of the external cause

Y92.241 Library as the place of occurrence of the external cause

Y92.242 Post office as the place of occurrence of the external cause

Y92.243 City hall as the place of occurrence of the external cause

Y92.248 Other public administrative building as the place of occurrence of the external cause

● **Y92.25** Cultural building as the place of occurrence of the external cause

Y92.250 Art gallery as the place of occurrence of the external cause

Y92.251 Museum as the place of occurrence of the external cause

Y92.252 Music hall as the place of occurrence of the external cause

Y92.253 Opera house as the place of occurrence of the external cause

Y92.254 Theater (live) as the place of occurrence of the external cause

Y92.258 Other cultural public building as the place of occurrence of the external cause

Y92.26 Movie house or cinema as the place of occurrence of the external cause

Y92.29 Other specified public building as the place of occurrence of the external cause
　Assembly hall as the place of occurrence of the external cause
　Clubhouse as the place of occurrence of the external cause

◀ New　　◀══ Revised　　~~deleted~~ Deleted　　Excludes 1　　Excludes 2　　Includes　　Use additional　　Code first　　Code also　　Unspecified

OGCR Official Guidelines　　● Unacceptable Principal Diagnosis　　X Assign placeholder X　　● Use Additional Character(s)　　▶ Manifestation Code　　**Coding Clinic**

- ● Y92.3   **Sports and athletics area as the place of occurrence of the external cause**
  - ● Y92.31   **Athletic court as the place of occurrence of the external cause**
    - **Excludes1**   tennis court in private home or garden (Y92.09)
    - Y92.310   **Basketball court as the place of occurrence of the external cause**
    - Y92.311   **Squash court as the place of occurrence of the external cause**
    - Y92.312   **Tennis court as the place of occurrence of the external cause**
    - Y92.318   **Other athletic court as the place of occurrence of the external cause**
  - ● Y92.32   **Athletic field as the place of occurrence of the external cause**
    - Y92.320   **Baseball field as the place of occurrence of the external cause**
    - Y92.321   **Football field as the place of occurrence of the external cause**
    - Y92.322   **Soccer field as the place of occurrence of the external cause**
    - Y92.328   **Other athletic field as the place of occurrence of the external cause**
      Cricket field as the place of occurrence of the external cause
      Hockey field as the place of occurrence of the external cause
  - ● Y92.33   **Skating rink as the place of occurrence of the external cause**
    - Y92.330   **Ice skating rink (indoor) (outdoor) as the place of occurrence of the external cause**
    - Y92.331   **Roller skating rink as the place of occurrence of the external cause**
  - Y92.34   **Swimming pool (public) as the place of occurrence of the external cause**
    - **Excludes1**   swimming pool in private home or garden (Y92.016)
  - Y92.39   **Other specified sports and athletic area as the place of occurrence of the external cause**
    Golf-course as the place of occurrence of the external cause
    Gymnasium as the place of occurrence of the external cause
    Riding-school as the place of occurrence of the external cause
    Stadium as the place of occurrence of the external cause
- ● Y92.4   **Street, highway and other paved roadways as the place of occurrence of the external cause** ◀
  - **Excludes1**   private driveway of residence (Y92.014, Y92.024, Y92.043, Y92.093, Y92.113, Y92.123, Y92.154, Y92.194)
  - ● Y92.41   **Street and highway as the place of occurrence of the external cause**
    - Y92.410   **Unspecified street and highway as the place of occurrence of the external cause**
      Road NOS as the place of occurrence of the external cause
    - Y92.411   **Interstate highway as the place of occurrence of the external cause**
      Freeway as the place of occurrence of the external cause
      Motorway as the place of occurrence of the external cause
    - Y92.412   **Parkway as the place of occurrence of the external cause**
    - Y92.413   **State road as the place of occurrence of the external cause**
    - Y92.414   **Local residential or business street as the place of occurrence of the external cause**
    - Y92.415   **Exit ramp or entrance ramp of street or highway as the place of occurrence of the external cause**
  - ● Y92.48   **Other paved roadways as the place of occurrence of the external cause**
    - Y92.480   **Sidewalk as the place of occurrence of the external cause**
    - Y92.481   **Parking lot as the place of occurrence of the external cause**
    - Y92.482   **Bike path as the place of occurrence of the external cause**
    - Y92.488   **Other paved roadways as the place of occurrence of the external cause**
- ● Y92.5   **Trade and service area as the place of occurrence of the external cause**
  - **Excludes1**   garage in private home (Y92.015)
    schools and other public administration buildings (Y92.2-)
  - ● Y92.51   **Private commercial establishments as the place of occurrence of the external cause**
    - Y92.510   **Bank as the place of occurrence of the external cause**
    - Y92.511   **Restaurant or café as the place of occurrence of the external cause**
    - Y92.512   **Supermarket, store or market as the place of occurrence of the external cause**
    - Y92.513   **Shop (commercial) as the place of occurrence of the external cause**
  - ● Y92.52   **Service areas as the place of occurrence of the external cause**
    - Y92.520   **Airport as the place of occurrence of the external cause**
    - Y92.521   **Bus station as the place of occurrence of the external cause**
    - Y92.522   **Railway station as the place of occurrence of the external cause**
    - Y92.523   **Highway rest stop as the place of occurrence of the external cause**
    - Y92.524   **Gas station as the place of occurrence of the external cause**
      Petroleum station as the place of occurrence of the external cause
      Service station as the place of occurrence of the external cause
  - ● Y92.53   **Ambulatory health services establishments as the place of occurrence of the external cause**
    - Y92.530   **Ambulatory surgery center as the place of occurrence of the external cause**
      Outpatient surgery center, including that connected with a hospital as the place of occurrence of the external cause
      Same day surgery center, including that connected with a hospital as the place of occurrence of the external cause
    - Y92.531   **Health care provider office as the place of occurrence of the external cause**
      Physician office as the place of occurrence of the external cause
    - Y92.532   **Urgent care center as the place of occurrence of the external cause**
    - Y92.538   **Other ambulatory health services establishments as the place of occurrence of the external cause**

CHAPTER 20 (V01-Y99)

N Newborn Age: 0   **P** Pediatric Age: 0–17   **M** Maternity DX: 12–55   **A** Adult Age: 15–124   ♀ Females Only   ♂ Males Only

🔗 Complication\Comorbidity   🔗 Major C\C   (EX) CC/MCC Exclusions   🔗 Hospital-Acquired Condition   **1597**

Y92.59 **Other trade areas as the place of occurrence of the external cause**
Office building as the place of occurrence of the external cause
Casino as the place of occurrence of the external cause
Garage (commercial) as the place of occurrence of the external cause
Hotel as the place of occurrence of the external cause
Radio or television station as the place of occurrence of the external cause
Shopping mall as the place of occurrence of the external cause
Warehouse as the place of occurrence of the external cause

● **Y92.6** **Industrial and construction area as the place of occurrence of the external cause**

Y92.61 **Building [any] under construction as the place of occurrence of the external cause**

Y92.62 **Dock or shipyard as the place of occurrence of the external cause**
Dockyard as the place of occurrence of the external cause
Dry dock as the place of occurrence of the external cause
Shipyard as the place of occurrence of the external cause

Y92.63 **Factory as the place of occurrence of the external cause**
Factory building as the place of occurrence of the external cause
Factory premises as the place of occurrence of the external cause
Industrial yard as the place of occurrence of the external cause

Y92.64 **Mine or pit as the place of occurrence of the external cause**
Mine as the place of occurrence of the external cause

Y92.65 **Oil rig as the place of occurrence of the external cause**
Pit (coal) (gravel) (sand) as the place of occurrence of the external cause

Y92.69 **Other specified industrial and construction area as the place of occurrence of the external cause**
Gasworks as the place of occurrence of the external cause
Power-station (coal) (nuclear) (oil) as the place of occurrence of the external cause
Tunnel under construction as the place of occurrence of the external cause
Workshop as the place of occurrence of the external cause

● **Y92.7** **Farm as the place of occurrence of the external cause**
Ranch as the place of occurrence of the external cause
Excludes1 farmhouse and home premises of farm (Y92.01-)

Y92.71 **Barn as the place of occurrence of the external cause**

Y92.72 **Chicken coop as the place of occurrence of the external cause**
Hen house as the place of occurrence of the external cause

Y92.73 **Farm field as the place of occurrence of the external cause**

Y92.74 **Orchard as the place of occurrence of the external cause**

Y92.79 **Other farm location as the place of occurrence of the external cause**

● **Y92.8** **Other places as the place of occurrence of the external cause**

● **Y92.81** **Transport vehicle as the place of occurrence of the external cause**
Excludes1 transport accidents (V00-V99)

Y92.810 **Car as the place of occurrence of the external cause**

Y92.811 **Bus as the place of occurrence of the external cause**

Y92.812 **Truck as the place of occurrence of the external cause**

Y92.813 **Airplane as the place of occurrence of the external cause**

Y92.814 **Boat as the place of occurrence of the external cause**

Y92.815 **Train as the place of occurrence of the external cause**

Y92.816 **Subway car as the place of occurrence of the external cause**

Y92.818 **Other transport vehicle as the place of occurrence of the external cause**

● **Y92.82** **Wilderness area**

Y92.820 **Desert as the place of occurrence of the external cause**

Y92.821 **Forest as the place of occurrence of the external cause**

Y92.828 **Other wilderness area as the place of occurrence of the external cause**
Swamp as the place of occurrence of the external cause
Mountain as the place of occurrence of the external cause
Marsh as the place of occurrence of the external cause
Prairie as the place of occurrence of the external cause

● **Y92.83** **Recreation area as the place of occurrence of the external cause**

Y92.830 **Public park as the place of occurrence of the external cause**

Y92.831 **Amusement park as the place of occurrence of the external cause**

Y92.832 **Beach as the place of occurrence of the external cause**
Seashore as the place of occurrence of the external cause

Y92.833 **Campsite as the place of occurrence of the external cause**

Y92.834 **Zoological garden (zoo) as the place of occurrence of the external cause**

Y92.838 **Other recreation area as the place of occurrence of the external cause**

Y92.84 **Military training ground as the place of occurrence of the external cause**

Y92.85 **Railroad track as the place of occurrence of the external cause**

Y92.86 **Slaughter house as the place of occurrence of the external cause**

Y92.89 **Other specified places as the place of occurrence of the external cause**
Derelict house as the place of occurrence of the external cause

OGCR Section I.C.20.b.

Do not use place of occurrence code Y92.9 if the place is not stated or is not applicable.

● **Y92.9** **Unspecified place or not applicable**

◀ New　◀◀◀ Revised　̶d̶e̶l̶e̶t̶e̶d̶ Deleted　Excludes 1　Excludes 2　Includes　Use additional　Code first　Code also　Unspecified

OGCR Official Guidelines　● Unacceptable Principal Diagnosis　X Assign placeholder X　● Use Additional Character(s)　▶ Manifestation Code　**Coding Clinic**

OGCR See Section I.C.20.c.

> Activity Code
>
> Assign a code from category Y93, Activity code, to describe the activity of the patient at the time the injury or other health condition occurred.
>
> An activity code is used only once, at the initial encounter for treatment. Only one code from Y93 should be recorded on a medical record.
>
> The activity codes are not applicable to poisonings, adverse effects, misadventures or sequela.
>
> Do not assign Y93.9, Unspecified activity, if the activity is not stated.
>
> A code from category Y93 is appropriate for use with external cause and intent codes if identifying the activity provides additional information about the event.

● **Y93   Activity codes**

Note: Category Y93 is provided for use to indicate the activity of the person seeking healthcare for an injury or health condition, such as a heart attack while shoveling snow, which resulted from, or was contributed to, by the activity. These codes are appropriate for use for both acute injuries, such as those from chapter 19, and conditions that are due to the long-term, cumulative effects of an activity, such as those from chapter 13. They are also appropriate for use with external cause codes for cause and intent if identifying the activity provides additional information on the event. These codes should be used in conjunction with codes for external cause status (Y99) and place of occurrence (Y92).

This section contains the following broad activity categories:

Y93.0   Activities involving walking and running

Y93.1   Activities involving water and water craft

Y93.2   Activities involving ice and snow

Y93.3   Activities involving climbing, rappelling, and jumping off

Y93.4   Activities involving dancing and other rhythmic movement

Y93.5   Activities involving other sports and athletics played individually

Y93.6   Activities involving other sports and athletics played as a team or group

Y93.7   Activities involving other specified sports and athletics

Y93.A   Activities involving other cardiorespiratory exercise

Y93.B   Activities involving other muscle strengthening exercises

Y93.C   Activities involving computer technology and electronic devices

Y93.D   Activities involving arts and handcrafts

Y93.E   Activities involving personal hygiene and interior property and clothing maintenance

Y93.F   Activities involving caregiving

Y93.G   Activities involving food preparation, cooking and grilling

Y93.H   Activities involving exterior property and land maintenance, building and construction

Y93.I   Activities involving roller coasters and other types of external motion

Y93.J   Activities involving playing musical instrument

Y93.K   Activities involving animal care

Y93.8   Activities, other specified

Y93.9   Activity, unspecified

● **Y93.0   Activities involving walking and running**

> **Excludes1**   Activity, walking an animal (Y93.K1)
> Activity, walking or running on a treadmill (Y93.A1)

Y93.01   Activity, walking, marching and hiking
Activity, walking, marching and hiking on level or elevated terrain

> **Excludes1**   activity, mountain climbing (Y93.31)

Y93.02   Activity, running

● **Y93.1   Activities involving water and water craft**

> **Excludes1**   activities involving ice (Y93.2-)

Y93.11   Activity, swimming

Y93.12   Activity, springboard and platform diving

Y93.13   Activity, water polo

Y93.14   Activity, water aerobics and water exercise

Y93.15   Activity, underwater diving and snorkeling
Activity, SCUBA diving

Y93.16   Activity, rowing, canoeing, kayaking, rafting and tubing
Activity, canoeing, kayaking, rafting and tubing in calm and turbulent water

Y93.17   Activity, water skiing and wake boarding

Y93.18   Activity, surfing, windsurfing and boogie boarding
Activity, water sliding

Y93.19   Activity, other involving water and watercraft
Activity involving water NOS
Activity, parasailing
Activity, water survival training and testing

● **Y93.2   Activities involving ice and snow**

> **Excludes1**   activity, shoveling ice and snow (Y93.H1)

Y93.21   Activity, ice skating
Activity, figure skating (singles) (pairs)
Activity, ice dancing

> **Excludes1**   activity, ice hockey (Y93.22)

Y93.22   Activity, ice hockey

Y93.23   Activity, snow (alpine) (downhill) skiing, snow boarding, sledding, tobogganing and snow tubing

> **Excludes1**   activity, cross country skiing (Y93.24)

Y93.24   Activity, cross country skiing
Activity, nordic skiing

Y93.29   Activity, other activity involving ice and snow
Activity, activity involving ice and snow NOS

● **Y93.3   Activities involving climbing, rappelling and jumping off**

> **Excludes1**   activity, hiking on level or elevated terrain (Y93.01)
> activity, jumping rope (Y93.56)
> activity, trampoline jumping (Y93.44)

Y93.31   Activity, mountain climbing, rock climbing and wall climbing

Y93.32   Activity, rappelling

Y93.33   Activity, BASE jumping
Activity, building, Antenna, Span, Earth jumping

Y93.34   Activity, bungee jumping

Y93.35   Activity, hang gliding

Y93.39   Activity, other activity involving climbing, rappelling and jumping off

● **Y93.4   Activities involving dancing and other rhythmic movement**

> **Excludes1**   activity, martial arts (Y93.75)

Y93.41   Activity, dancing
Coding Clinic: 2012, Q4, P108

Y93.42   Activity, yoga

Y93.43   Activity, gymnastics
Activity, rhythmic gymnastics

> **Excludes1**   activity, trampolining (Y93.44)

Y93.44   Activity, trampolining

Y93.45   Activity, cheerleading

Y93.49   Activity, other involving dancing and other rhythmic movements

CHAPTER 20 (V01-Y99)

CHAPTER 20 (V01-Y99)

● **Y93.5 Activities involving other sports and athletics played individually**

     Excludes1   activity, dancing (Y93.41)
                         activity, gymnastic (Y93.43)
                         activity, trampolining (Y93.44)
                         activity, yoga (Y93.42)

Y93.51 Activity, roller skating (inline) and skateboarding

Y93.52 Activity, horseback riding

Y93.53 Activity, golf

Y93.54 Activity, bowling

Y93.55 Activity, bike riding

Y93.56 Activity, jumping rope

Y93.57 Activity, non-running track and field events

     Excludes1   activity, running (any form) (Y93.02)

Y93.59 Activity, other involving other sports and athletics played individually

     Excludes1   activities involving climbing, rappelling, and jumping (Y93.3-)
                         activities involving ice and snow (Y93.2-)
                         activities involving walking and running (Y93.0-)
                         activities involving water and watercraft (Y93.1-)

● **Y93.6 Activities involving other sports and athletics played as a team or group**

     Excludes1   activity, ice hockey (Y93.22)
                         activity, water polo (Y93.13)

Y93.61 Activity, American tackle football
     Activity, football NOS

Y93.62 Activity, American flag or touch football

Y93.63 Activity, rugby

Y93.64 Activity, baseball
     Activity, softball

Y93.65 Activity, lacrosse and field hockey
     Coding Clinic: 2015, Q1, P9

Y93.66 Activity, soccer

Y93.67 Activity, basketball

Y93.68 Activity, volleyball (beach) (court)

Y93.6A Activity, physical games generally associated with school recess, summer camp and children
     Activity, capture the flag
     Activity, dodge ball
     Activity, four square
     Activity, kickball

Y93.69 Activity, other involving other sports and athletics played as a team or group
     Cricket

● **Y93.7 Activities involving other specified sports and athletics**

Y93.71 Activity, boxing

Y93.72 Activity, wrestling

Y93.73 Activity, racquet and hand sports
     Activity, handball
     Activity, racquetball
     Activity, squash
     Activity, tennis

Y93.74 Activity, frisbee
     Activity, ultimate frisbee

Y93.75 Activity, martial arts
     Activity, combatives

Y93.79 Activity, other specified sports and athletics

     Excludes1   sports and athletics activities specified in categories Y93.0-Y93.6

● **Y93.A Activities involving other cardiorespiratory exercise**
     Activities involving physical training

Y93.A1 Activity, exercise machines primarily for cardiorespiratory conditioning
     Activity, elliptical and stepper machines
     Activity, stationary bike
     Activity, treadmill

Y93.A2 Activity, calisthenics
     Activity, jumping jacks
     Activity, warm up and cool down

Y93.A3 Activity, aerobic and step exercise

Y93.A4 Activity, circuit training

Y93.A5 Activity, obstacle course
     Activity, challenge course
     Activity, confidence course

Y93.A6 Activity, grass drills
     Activity, guerilla drills

Y93.A9 Activity, other involving other cardiorespiratory exercise

     Excludes1   activities involving cardiorespiratory exercise specified in categories Y93.0-Y93.7

● **Y93.B Activity involving other muscle strengthening exercises**

Y93.B1 Activity, exercise machines primarily for muscle strengthening

Y93.B2 Activity, push-ups, pull-ups, sit-ups

Y93.B3 Activity, free weights
     Activity, barbells
     Activity, dumbbells

Y93.B4 Activity, pilates

Y93.B9 Activity, other involving other muscle strengthening exercises

     Excludes1   activities involving muscle strengthening specified in categories Y93.0-Y93.A

● **Y93.C Activities involving computer technology and electronic devices**

     Excludes1   activity, electronic musical keyboard or instruments (Y93.J-)

Y93.C1 Activity, computer keyboarding
     Activity, electronic game playing using keyboard or other stationary device

Y93.C2 Activity, hand held interactive electronic device
     Activity, cellular telephone and communication device
     Activity, electronic game playing using interactive device

       Excludes1   activity, electronic game playing using keyboard or other stationary device (Y93.C1)

Y93.C9 Activity, other involving computer technology and electronic devices

● **Y93.D Activities involving arts and handcrafts**

     Excludes1   activities involving playing musical instrument (Y93.J-)

Y93.D1 Knitting and crocheting

Y93.D2 Sewing

Y93.D3 Furniture building and finishing
     Furniture repair

Y93.D9 Activity, other involving arts and handcrafts

◄ New   ◄ Revised   ~~deleted~~ Deleted   Excludes 1   Excludes 2   Includes   Use additional   Code first   Code also   Unspecified

OGCR Official Guidelines   ● Unacceptable Principal Diagnosis   X Assign placeholder X   ● Use Additional Character(s)   ▶ Manifestation Code   **Coding Clinic**

● **Y93.E Activities involving personal hygiene and interior property and clothing maintenance**

> **Excludes1** activities involving cooking and grilling (Y93.G-)
> activities involving exterior property and land maintenance, building and construction (Y93.H-)
> activity involving caregiving (Y93.F-)
> activity, dishwashing (Y93.G1)
> activity, food preparation (Y93.G1)
> activity, gardening (Y93.H2)

   Y93.E1 **Activity, personal bathing and showering**

   Y93.E2 **Activity, laundry**

   Y93.E3 **Activity, vacuuming**

   Y93.E4 **Activity, ironing**

   Y93.E5 **Activity, floor mopping and cleaning**

   Y93.E6 **Activity, residential relocation**
> Activity, packing up and unpacking involved in moving to a new residence

   Y93.E8 **Activity, other personal hygiene activity**

   Y93.E9 **Activity, other household maintenance**

● **Y93.F Activities involving person providing caregiving**
> Activity involving the provider of caregiving

   Y93.F1 **Activity, caregiving involving bathing**

   Y93.F2 **Activity, caregiving involving lifting**

   Y93.F9 **Activity, other caregiving**

● **Y93.G Activities involving food preparation, cooking and grilling**

   Y93.G1 **Activity, food preparation and clean up**
> Activity, dishwashing

   Y93.G2 **Activity, grilling and smoking food**

   Y93.G3 **Activity, cooking and baking**
> Activity, use of stove, oven and microwave oven

   Y93.G9 **Activity, other activity involving cooking and grilling**

● **Y93.H Activities involving property and land maintenance, building and construction**

   Y93.H1 **Activity, digging, shoveling and raking**
> Activity, dirt digging
> Activity, raking leaves
> Activity, snow shoveling

   Y93.H2 **Activity, gardening and landscaping**
> Activity, pruning, trimming shrubs, weeding

   Y93.H3 **Activity, building and construction**

   Y93.H9 **Activity, other activity involving property and land maintenance, building and construction**

● **Y93.I Activities involving roller coasters and other types of external motion**

   Y93.I1 **Activity, rollercoaster riding**

   Y93.I9 **Activity, other involving external motion**

● **Y93.J Activities involving playing musical instrument**
> Activity involving playing electric musical instrument

   Y93.J1 **Activity, piano playing**
> Activity, musical keyboard (electronic) playing

   Y93.J2 **Activity, drum and other percussion instrument playing**

   Y93.J3 **Activity, string instrument playing**

   Y93.J4 **Activity, winds and brass instrument playing**

● **Y93.K Activities involving animal care**

> **Excludes1** activity, horseback riding (Y93.52)

   Y93.K1 **Activity, walking an animal**

   Y93.K2 **Activity, milking an animal**

   Y93.K3 **Activity, grooming and shearing an animal**

   Y93.K9 **Activity, other activity involving animal care**

● **Y93.8 Other activity**

   Y93.81 **Activity, refereeing a sports activity**

   Y93.82 **Activity, spectator at an event**

   Y93.83 **Activity, rough housing and horseplay**
> **Coding Clinic: 2015, Q1, P8**

   Y93.84 **Activity, sleeping**

   Y93.85 **Activity, choking game** ◄
> Activity, blackout game ◄
> Activity, fainting game ◄
> Activity, pass out game ◄

   Y93.89 **Activity, other specified**

OGCR See Section I.C.20.c.

> Do not assign Y93.9, Unspecified activity, if the activity is not stated.

● **Y93.9 Activity, unspecified**

Y95 Nosocomial condition

● **Y99 External cause status**

> **Note:** A single code from category Y99 should be used in conjunction with the external cause code(s) assigned to a record to indicate the status of the person at the time the event occurred.

   Y99.0 **Civilian activity done for income or pay**
> Civilian activity done for financial or other compensation

> **Excludes1** military activity (Y99.1)
> volunteer activity (Y99.2)

   Y99.1 **Military activity**

> **Excludes1** activity of off duty military personnel (Y99.8)

   Y99.2 **Volunteer activity**

> **Excludes1** activity of child or other family member assisting in compensated work of other family member (Y99.8)

   Y99.8 **Other external cause status**
> Activity NEC
> Activity of child or other family member assisting in compensated work of other family member
> Hobby not done for income
> Leisure activity
> Off-duty activity of military personnel
> Recreation or sport not for income or while a student
> Student activity

> **Excludes1** civilian activity done for income or compensation (Y99.0)
> military activity (Y99.1)
> **Coding Clinic: 2012, Q4, P108**

   Y99.9 **Unspecified external cause status**

N Newborn Age: 0   **P** Pediatric Age: 0–17   **M** Maternity DX: 12–55   **A** Adult Age: 15–124   ♀ Females Only   ♂ Males Only

🔹 Complication\Comorbidity   🔹 Major C\C   (Ex) CC/MCC Exclusions   🔹 Hospital-Acquired Condition

CHAPTER 21

FACTORS INFLUENCING HEALTH STATUS AND CONTACT WITH HEALTH SERVICES (Z00-Z99)

OGCR Chapter-Specific Coding Guidelines

21. **Chapter 21: Factors influencing health status and contact with health services (Z00-Z99)**
Note: The chapter specific guidelines provide additional information about the use of Z codes for specified encounters.

a. Use of Z codes in any healthcare setting
Z codes are for use in any healthcare setting. Z codes may be used as either a first-listed (principal diagnosis code in the inpatient setting) or secondary code, depending on the circumstances of the encounter. Certain Z codes may only be used as first-listed or principal diagnosis.

b. Z Codes indicate a reason for an encounter
Z codes are not procedure codes. A corresponding procedure code must accompany a Z code to describe any procedure performed.

c. Categories of Z Codes
1) Contact/Exposure
Category Z20 indicates contact with, and suspected exposure to, communicable diseases. These codes are for patients who do not show any sign or symptom of a disease but are suspected to have been exposed to it by close personal contact with an infected individual or are in an area where a disease is epidemic.

Category Z77, **Other contact with and (suspected) exposures hazardous to health,** indicates contact with and suspected exposures hazardous to health.

Contact/exposure codes may be used as a first-listed code to explain an encounter for testing, or, more commonly, as a secondary code to identify a potential risk.

2) Inoculations and vaccinations
Code Z23 is for encounters for inoculations and vaccinations. It indicates that a patient is being seen to receive a prophylactic inoculation against a disease. Procedure codes are required to identify the actual administration of the injection and the type(s) of immunizations given. Code Z23 may be used as a secondary code if the inoculation is given as a routine part of preventive health care, such as a well-baby visit.

3) Status
Status codes indicate that a patient is either a carrier of a disease or has the sequelae or residual of a past disease or condition. This includes such things as the presence of prosthetic or mechanical devices resulting from past treatment. A status code is informative, because the status may affect the course of treatment and its outcome. A status code is distinct from a history code. The history code indicates that the patient no longer has the condition.

A status code should not be used with a diagnosis code from one of the body system chapters, if the diagnosis code includes the information provided by the status code. For example, code Z94.1, Heart transplant status, should not be used with a code from subcategory T86.2, Complications of heart transplant. The status code does not provide additional information. The complication code indicates that the patient is a heart transplant patient.

For encounters for weaning from a mechanical ventilator, assign a code from subcategory J96.1, Chronic respiratory failure, followed by code Z99.11, Dependence on respirator [ventilator] status.

The status Z codes/categories are:

Z14   Genetic carrier
Genetic carrier status indicates that a person carries a gene, associated with a particular disease, which may be passed to offspring who may develop that disease. The person does not have the disease and is not at risk of developing the disease.

Z15   Genetic susceptibility to disease Genetic susceptibility indicates that a person has a gene that increases the risk of that person developing the disease.

Codes from category Z15 should not be used as principal or first-listed codes. If the patient has the condition to which he/she is susceptible, and that condition is the reason for the encounter, the code for the current condition should be sequenced first. If the patient is being seen for follow-up after completed treatment for this condition, and the condition no longer exists, a follow-up

code should be sequenced first, followed by the appropriate personal history and genetic susceptibility codes. If the purpose of the encounter is genetic counseling associated with procreative management, code Z31.5, Encounter for genetic counseling, should be assigned as the first-listed code, followed by a code from category Z15. Additional codes should be assigned for any applicable family or personal history.

Z16   Resistance to antimicrobial drugs
This code indicates that a patient has a condition that is resistant to antimicrobial drug treatment. Sequence the infection code first.

Z17   Estrogen receptor status

Z18   Retained foreign body fragments

Z19   **Hormone sensitivity malignancy status**

Z21   Asymptomatic HIV infection status This code indicates that a patient has tested positive for HIV but has manifested no signs or symptoms of the disease.

Z22   Carrier of infectious disease Carrier status indicates that a person harbors the specific organisms of a disease without manifest symptoms and is capable of transmitting the infection.

Z28.3   Underimmunization status

Z33.1   Pregnant state, incidental This code is a secondary code only for use when the pregnancy is in no way complicating the reason for visit. Otherwise, a code from the obstetric chapter is required.

Z66   Do not resuscitate
This code may be used when it is documented by the provider that a patient is on do not resuscitate status at any time during the stay.

Z67   Blood type

Z68   Body mass index (BMI)
As with all other secondary diagnosis codes, the BMI codes should only be assigned when they meet the definition of a reportable diagnosis (see Section III, Reporting Additional Diagnoses).

Z74.01   Bed confinement status

Z76.82   Awaiting organ transplant status

Z78   Other specified health status
Code Z78.1, Physical restraint status, may be used when it is documented by the provider that a patient has been put in restraints during the current encounter. Please note that this code should not be reported when it is documented by the provider that a patient is temporarily restrained during a procedure.

Z79   Long-term (current) drug therapy
Codes from this category indicate a patient's continuous use of a prescribed drug (including such things as aspirin therapy) for the long-term treatment of a condition or for prophylactic use. It is not for use for patients who have addictions to drugs. This subcategory is not for use of medications for detoxification or maintenance programs to prevent withdrawal symptoms in patients with drug dependence (e.g., methadone maintenance for opiate dependence). Assign the appropriate code for the drug dependence instead.

Assign a code from Z79 if the patient is receiving a medication for an extended period as a prophylactic measure (such as for the prevention of deep vein thrombosis) or as treatment of a chronic condition (such as arthritis) or a disease requiring a lengthy course of treatment (such as cancer). Do not assign a code from category Z79 for medication being administered for a brief period of time to treat an acute illness or injury (such as a course of antibiotics to treat acute bronchitis).

Z88   Allergy status to drugs, medicaments and biological substances Except: Z88.9, Allergy status to unspecified drugs, medicaments and biological substances status

Z89   Acquired absence of limb

Z90   Acquired absence of organs, not elsewhere classified

Z91.0-   Allergy status, other than to drugs and biological substances

Z92.82   Status post administration of tPA (rtPA) in a different facility within the last 24 hours prior to admission to a current facility Assign code Z92.82, Status post administration of tPA (rtPA) in a different facility within the last 24 hours prior to admission to current facility, as a secondary diagnosis when a patient is received by transfer into a facility and documentation indicates they were administered tissue plasminogen activator (tPA) within the last 24 hours prior to admission to the current facility. This guideline applies even if the patient is still receiving the tPA at the time they are received into the current facility. The appropriate code for the condition for which the tPA was administered (such as cerebrovascular disease or myocardial infarction) should be assigned first. Code Z92.82 is only applicable to the receiving facility record and not to the transferring facility record.

Z93	Artificial opening status
Z94	Transplanted organ and tissue status
Z95	Presence of cardiac and vascular implants and grafts
Z96	Presence of other functional implants
Z97	Presence of other devices
Z98	Other postprocedural states

Assign code Z98.85, Transplanted organ removal status, to indicate that a transplanted organ has been previously removed. This code should not be assigned for the encounter in which the transplanted organ is removed. The complication necessitating removal of the transplant organ should be assigned for that encounter.

See section I.C.19. for information on the coding of organ transplant complications.

Z99	Dependence on enabling machines and devices, not elsewhere classified

Note: Categories Z89-Z90 and Z93-Z99 are for use only if there are no complications or malfunctions of the organ or tissue replaced, the amputation site or the equipment on which the patient is dependent.

4) History (of)

There are two types of history Z codes, personal and family. Personal history codes explain a patient's past medical condition that no longer exists and is not receiving any treatment, but that has the potential for recurrence, and therefore may require continued monitoring.

Family history codes are for use when a patient has a family member(s) who has had a particular disease that causes the patient to be at higher risk of also contracting the disease.

Personal history codes may be used in conjunction with follow-up codes and family history codes may be used in conjunction with screening codes to explain the need for a test or procedure. History codes are also acceptable on any medical record regardless of the reason for visit. A history of an illness, even if no longer present, is important information that may alter the type of treatment ordered.

The history Z code categories are:

Z80	Family history of primary malignant neoplasm
Z81	Family history of mental and behavioral disorders
Z82	Family history of certain disabilities and chronic diseases (leading to disablement)
Z83	Family history of other specific disorders
Z84	Family history of other conditions
Z85	Personal history of malignant neoplasm
Z86	Personal history of certain other diseases
Z87	Personal history of other diseases and conditions
Z91.4-	Personal history of psychological trauma, not elsewhere classified
Z91.5	Personal history of self-harm
Z91.8-	Other specified personal risk factors, not elsewhere classified Exception: Z91.83, Wandering in diseases classified elsewhere
Z92	Personal history of medical treatment Except: Z92.0, Personal history of contraception Except: Z92.82, Status post administration of tPA (rtPA) in a different facility within the last 24 hours prior to admission to a current facility

5) Screening

Screening is the testing for disease or disease precursors in seemingly well individuals so that early detection and treatment can be provided for those who test positive for the disease (e.g., screening mammogram).

The testing of a person to rule out or confirm a suspected diagnosis because the patient has some sign or symptom is a diagnostic examination, not a screening. In these cases, the sign or symptom is used to explain the reason for the test.

A screening code may be a first-listed code if the reason for the visit is specifically the screening exam. It may also be used as an additional code if the screening is done during

an office visit for other health problems. A screening code is not necessary if the screening is inherent to a routine examination, such as a pap smear done during a routine pelvic examination.

Should a condition be discovered during the screening then the code for the condition may be assigned as an additional diagnosis.

The Z code indicates that a screening exam is planned. A procedure code is required to confirm that the screening was performed.

The screening Z codes/categories:

Z11	Encounter for screening for infectious and parasitic diseases
Z12	Encounter for screening for malignant neoplasms
Z13	Encounter for screening for other diseases and disorders Except: Z13.9, Encounter for screening, unspecified
Z36	Encounter for antenatal screening for mother

6) Observation

There are **three** observation Z code categories. They are for use in very limited circumstances when a person is being observed for a suspected condition that is ruled out. The observation codes are not for use if an injury or illness or any signs or symptoms related to the suspected condition are present. In such cases the diagnosis/symptom code is used with the corresponding external cause code.

The observation codes are to be used as principal diagnosis only. **The only exception to this is when the principal diagnosis is required to be a code from category Z38, Liveborn infants according to place of birth and type of delivery. Then a code from category Z05, Encounter for observation and evaluation of newborn for suspected diseases and conditions ruled out, is sequenced after the Z38 code.** Additional codes may be used in addition to the observation code but only if they are unrelated to the suspected condition being observed.

Codes from subcategory Z03.7 Encounter for suspected maternal and fetal conditions ruled out, may either be used as a first-listed or as an additional code assignment depending on the case. They are for use in very limited circumstances on a maternal record when an encounter is for a suspected maternal or fetal condition that is ruled out during that encounter (for example, a maternal or fetal condition may be suspected due to an abnormal test result). These codes should not be used when the condition is confirmed. In those cases, the confirmed condition should be coded. In addition, these codes are not for use if an illness or any signs or symptoms related to the suspected condition or problem are present. In such cases the diagnosis/symptom code is used.

Additional codes may be used in addition to the code from subcategory Z03.7, but only if they are unrelated to the suspected condition being evaluated.

Codes from subcategory Z03.7 may not be used for encounters for antenatal screening of mother. *See Section I.C.21. Screening.*

For encounters for suspected fetal condition that are inconclusive following testing and evaluation, assign the appropriate code from category O35, O36, O40 or O41.

The observation Z code categories:

Z03	Encounter for medical observation for suspected diseases and conditions ruled out
Z04	Encounter for examination and observation for other reasons Except: Z04.9, Encounter for examination and observation for unspecified reason
Z05	**Encounter for observation and evaluation of newborn for suspected diseases and conditions ruled out**

7) Aftercare

Aftercare visit codes cover situations when the initial treatment of a disease has been performed and the patient requires continued care during the healing or recovery phase, or for the long-term consequences of the disease. The aftercare Z code should not be used if treatment is directed at a current, acute disease. The diagnosis code is to be used in these cases.

Exceptions to this rule are codes Z51.0, Encounter for antineoplastic radiation therapy, and codes from subcategory Z51.1, Encounter for antineoplastic chemotherapy and immunotherapy. These codes are to be first-listed, followed by the diagnosis code when a patient's encounter is solely to receive radiation therapy, chemotherapy, or immunotherapy for the treatment of a neoplasm. If the reason for the encounter is more than one type of antineoplastic therapy, code Z51.0 and a code from subcategory Z51.1 may be assigned together, in which case one of these codes would be reported as a secondary diagnosis.

The aftercare Z codes should also not be used for aftercare for injuries. For aftercare of an injury, assign the acute injury code with the appropriate 7th character (for subsequent encounter).

The aftercare codes are generally first-listed to explain the specific reason for the encounter. An aftercare code may be used as an additional code when some type of aftercare is provided in addition to the reason for admission and no diagnosis code is applicable. An example of this would be the closure of a colostomy during an encounter for treatment of another condition.

Aftercare codes should be used in conjunction with other aftercare codes or diagnosis codes to provide better detail on the specifics of an aftercare encounter visit, unless otherwise directed by the classification. Should a patient receive multiple types of antineoplastic therapy during the same encounter, code Z51.0, Encounter for antineoplastic radiation therapy, and codes from subcategory Z51.1, Encounter for antineoplastic chemotherapy and immunotherapy, may be used together on a record. The sequencing of multiple aftercare codes depends on the circumstances of the encounter.

Certain aftercare Z code categories need a secondary diagnosis code to describe the resolving condition or sequelae. For others, the condition is included in the code title.

Additional Z code aftercare category terms include fitting and adjustment, and attention to artificial openings.

Status Z codes may be used with aftercare Z codes to indicate the nature of the aftercare. For example code Z95.1, Presence of aortocoronary bypass graft, may be used with code Z48.812, Encounter for surgical aftercare following surgery on the circulatory system, to indicate the surgery for which the aftercare is being performed. A status code should not be used when the aftercare code indicates the type of status, such as using Z43.0, Encounter for attention to tracheostomy, with Z93.0, Tracheostomy status.

The aftercare Z category/codes:

Z42	Encounter for plastic and reconstructive surgery following medical procedure or healed injury
Z43	Encounter for attention to artificial openings
Z44	Encounter for fitting and adjustment of external prosthetic device
Z45	Encounter for adjustment and management of implanted device
Z46	Encounter for fitting and adjustment of other devices
Z47	Orthopedic aftercare
Z48	Encounter for other postprocedural aftercare
Z49	Encounter for care involving renal dialysis
Z51	Encounter for other aftercare **and medical care**

8) Follow-up

The follow-up codes are used to explain continuing surveillance following completed treatment of a disease, condition, or injury. They imply that the condition has been fully treated and no longer exists. They should not be confused with aftercare codes, or injury codes with a 7th character for subsequent encounter, that explain ongoing care of a healing condition or its sequelae. Follow-up codes may be used in conjunction with history codes to provide the full picture of the healed condition and its treatment. The follow-up code is sequenced first, followed by the history code.

A follow-up code may be used to explain multiple visits. Should a condition be found to have recurred on the follow-up visit, then the diagnosis code for the condition should be assigned in place of the follow-up code.

The follow-up Z code categories:

Z08	Encounter for follow-up examination after completed treatment for malignant neoplasm
Z09	Encounter for follow-up examination after completed treatment for conditions other than malignant neoplasm
Z39	Encounter for maternal postpartum care and examination

9) Donor

Codes in category Z52, Donors of organs and tissues, are used for living individuals who are donating blood or other body tissue.

These codes are only for individuals donating for others, not for self-donations. They are not used to identify cadaveric donations.

10) Counseling

Counseling Z codes are used when a patient or family member receives assistance in the aftermath of an illness or injury, or when support is required in coping with family or social problems. They are not used in conjunction with a diagnosis code when the counseling component of care is considered integral to standard treatment.

The counseling Z codes/categories:

Z30.0-	Encounter for general counseling and advice on contraception
Z31.5	Encounter for genetic counseling
Z31.6-	Encounter for general counseling and advice on procreation
Z32.2	Encounter for childbirth instruction
Z32.3	Encounter for childcare instruction
Z69	Encounter for mental health services for victim and perpetrator of abuse
Z70	Counseling related to sexual attitude, behavior and orientation
Z71	Persons encountering health services for other counseling and medical advice, not elsewhere classified
Z76.81	Expectant mother prebirth pediatrician visit

11) Encounters for Obstetrical and Reproductive Services

See Section I.C.15. Pregnancy, Childbirth, and the Puerperium, for further instruction on the use of these codes.

Z codes for pregnancy are for use in those circumstances when none of the problems or complications included in the codes from the Obstetrics chapter exist (a routine prenatal visit or postpartum care). Codes in category Z34, Encounter for supervision of normal pregnancy, are always first listed and are not to be used with any other code from the OB chapter.

Codes in category Z3A, Weeks of gestation, may be assigned to provide additional information about the pregnancy. **Category Z3A codes should not be assigned for pregnancies with abortive outcomes (categories O00-O08), elective termination of pregnancy (code Z33.32), nor for postpartum conditions, as category Z3A is not applicable to these conditions.** The date of the admission should be used to determine weeks of gestation for inpatient admissions that encompass more than one gestational week.

The outcome of delivery, category Z37, should be included on all maternal delivery records. It is always a secondary code. Codes in category Z37 should not be used on the newborn record.

Z codes for family planning (contraceptive) or procreative management and counseling should be included on an obstetric record either during the pregnancy or the postpartum stage, if applicable.

Z codes/categories for obstetrical and reproductive services:

Z30	Encounter for contraceptive management
Z31	Encounter for procreative management
Z32.2	Encounter for childbirth instruction
Z32.3	Encounter for childcare instruction
Z33	Pregnant state
Z34	Encounter for supervision of normal pregnancy
Z36	Encounter for antenatal screening of mother
Z3A	Weeks of gestation
Z37	Outcome of delivery
Z39	Encounter for maternal postpartum care and examination
Z76.81	Expectant mother prebirth pediatrician visit

12) Newborns and Infants

See Section I.C.16. Newborn (Perinatal) Guidelines, for further instruction on the use of these codes.

Newborn Z codes/categories:

Z76.1	Encounter for health supervision and care of foundling
Z00.1-	Encounter for routine child health examination
Z38	Liveborn infants according to place of birth and type of delivery

13) Routine and administrative examinations

The Z codes allow for the description of encounters for routine examinations, such as, a general check-up, or, examinations for administrative purposes, such as, a pre-employment physical. The codes are not to be used if the examination is for diagnosis of a suspected condition or for treatment purposes. In such cases the diagnosis code is used. During a routine exam, should a diagnosis or condition be discovered, it should be coded as an additional code. Pre-existing and chronic conditions and history codes may also be included as additional codes as long as the examination is for administrative purposes and not focused on any particular condition.

Some of the codes for routine health examinations distinguish between "with" and "without" abnormal findings. Code assignment depends on the information that is known at the time the encounter is being coded. For example, if no abnormal findings were found during the examination, but the encounter is being coded before test results are back, it is acceptable to assign the code for "without abnormal findings." When assigning a code for "with abnormal findings," additional code(s) should be assigned to identify the specific abnormal finding(s).

Pre-operative examination and pre-procedural laboratory examination Z codes are for use only in those situations when a patient is being cleared for a procedure or surgery and no treatment is given.

The Z codes/categories for routine and administrative examinations:

Z00	Encounter for general examination without complaint, suspected or reported diagnosis
Z01	Encounter for other special examination without complaint, suspected or reported diagnosis
Z02	Encounter for administrative examination Except: Z02.9, Encounter for administrative examinations, unspecified
Z32.0-	Encounter for pregnancy test

14) Miscellaneous Z codes

The miscellaneous Z codes capture a number of other health care encounters that do not fall into one of the other categories. Certain of these codes identify the reason for the encounter; others are for use as additional codes that provide useful information on circumstances that may affect a patient's care and treatment.

Prophylactic Organ Removal

For encounters specifically for prophylactic removal of an organ (such as prophylactic removal of breasts due to a genetic susceptibility to cancer or a family history of cancer), the principal or first-listed code should be a code from category Z40, Encounter for prophylactic surgery, followed by the appropriate codes to identify the associated risk factor (such as genetic susceptibility or family history).

If the patient has a malignancy of one site and is having prophylactic removal at another site to prevent either a new primary malignancy or metastatic disease, a code for the malignancy should also be assigned in addition to a code from subcategory Z40.0, Encounter for prophylactic surgery for risk factors related to malignant neoplasms. A Z40.0 code should not be assigned if the patient is having organ removal for treatment of a malignancy, such as the removal of the testes for the treatment of prostate cancer.

Miscellaneous Z codes/categories:

Z28	Immunization not carried out Except: Z28.3, Underimmunization status
Z29	**Encounter for other prophylactic measures**
Z40	Encounter for prophylactic surgery
Z41	Encounter for procedures for purposes other than remedying health state Except: Z41.9, Encounter for procedure for purposes other than remedying health state, unspecified
Z53	Persons encountering health services for specific procedures and treatment, not carried out
Z55	Problems related to education and literacy
Z56	Problems related to employment and unemployment
Z57	Occupational exposure to risk factors
Z58	Problems related to physical environment
Z59	Problems related to housing and economic circumstances
Z60	Problems related to social environment
Z62	Problems related to upbringing
Z63	Other problems related to primary support group, including family circumstances
Z64	Problems related to certain psychosocial circumstances
Z65	Problems related to other psychosocial circumstances

Z72	Problems related to lifestyle Note: These codes should be assigned only when the documentation specifies that the patient has an associated problem
Z73	Problems related to life management difficulty
Z74	Problems related to care provider dependency Except: Z74.01, Bed confinement status
Z75	Problems related to medical facilities and other health care
Z76.0	Encounter for issue of repeat prescription
Z76.3	Healthy person accompanying sick person
Z76.4	Other boarder to healthcare facility
Z76.5	Malingerer [conscious simulation]
Z91.1-	Patient's noncompliance with medical treatment and regimen
Z91.83	Wandering in diseases classified elsewhere
Z91.89	Other specified personal risk factors, not elsewhere classified

15) Nonspecific Z codes

Certain Z codes are so non-specific, or potentially redundant with other codes in the classification, that there can be little justification for their use in the inpatient setting. Their use in the outpatient setting should be limited to those instances when there is no further documentation to permit more precise coding. Otherwise, any sign or symptom or any other reason for visit that is captured in another code should be used.

Nonspecific Z codes/categories:

Z02.9	Encounter for administrative examinations, unspecified
Z04.9	Encounter for examination and observation for unspecified reason
Z13.9	Encounter for screening, unspecified
Z41.9	Encounter for procedure for purposes other than remedying health state, unspecified
Z52.9	Donor of unspecified organ or tissue
Z86.59	Personal history of other mental and behavioral disorders
Z88.9	Allergy status to unspecified drugs, medicaments and biological substances status
Z92.0	Personal history of contraception

16) Z Codes That May Only be Principal/First-Listed Diagnosis

The following Z codes/categories may only be reported as the principal/first-listed diagnosis, except when there are multiple encounters on the same day and the medical records for the encounters are combined:

Z00	Encounter for general examination without complaint, suspected or reported diagnosis Except: Z00.6
Z01	Encounter for other special examination without complaint, suspected or reported diagnosis
Z02	Encounter for administrative examination
Z03	Encounter for medical observation for suspected diseases and conditions ruled out
Z04	Encounter for examination and observation for other reasons
Z33.2	Encounter for elective termination of pregnancy
Z31.81	Encounter for male factor infertility in female patient
Z31.83	Encounter for assisted reproductive fertility procedure cycle
Z31.84	Encounter for fertility preservation procedure
Z34	Encounter for supervision of normal pregnancy
Z39	Encounter for maternal postpartum care and examination
Z38	Liveborn infants according to place of birth and type of delivery
Z42	Encounter for plastic and reconstructive surgery following medical procedure or healed injury
Z51.0	Encounter for antineoplastic radiation therapy
Z51.1-	Encounter for antineoplastic chemotherapy and immunotherapy
Z52	Donors of organs and tissues Except: Z52.9, Donor of unspecified organ or tissue
Z76.1	Encounter for health supervision and care of foundling
Z76.2	Encounter for health supervision and care of other healthy infant and child
Z99.12	Encounter for respirator [ventilator] dependence during power failure

CHAPTER 21

FACTORS INFLUENCING HEALTH STATUS AND CONTACT WITH HEALTH SERVICES (ZØØ-Z99)

Note: Z codes represent reasons for encounters. A corresponding procedure code must accompany a Z code if a procedure is performed. Categories ZØØ-Z99 are provided for occasions when circumstances other than a disease, injury or external cause classifiable to categories AØØ-Y89 are recorded as 'diagnoses' or 'problems.' This can arise in two main ways:

(a) When a person who may or may not be sick encounters the health services for some specific purpose, such as to receive limited care or service for a current condition, to donate an organ or tissue, to receive prophylactic vaccination (immunization), or to discuss a problem which is in itself not a disease or injury.

(b) When some circumstance or problem is present which influences the person's health status but is not in itself a current illness or injury.

This chapter contains the following blocks:

ZØØ-Z13	Persons encountering health services for examination
Z14-Z15	Genetic carrier and genetic susceptibility to disease
Z16	Resistance to antimicrobial drugs
Z17	Estrogen receptor status
Z18	Retained foreign body fragments
Z19	Hormone sensitivity malignancy status ◄
Z20-Z29	Persons with potential health hazards related to communicable diseases ◄
Z30-Z39	Persons encountering health services in circumstances related to reproduction
Z40-Z53	Encounters for other specific health care
Z55-Z65	Persons with potential health hazards related to socioeconomic and psychosocial circumstances
Z66	Do not resuscitate status
Z67	Blood type
Z68	Body mass index (BMI)
Z69-Z76	Persons encountering health services in other circumstances
Z77-Z99	Persons with potential health hazards related to family and personal history and certain conditions influencing health status

PERSONS ENCOUNTERING HEALTH SERVICES FOR EXAMINATIONS (ZØØ-Z13)

Note: Nonspecific abnormal findings disclosed at the time of these examinations are classified to categories R70-R94.

Excludes1 examinations related to pregnancy and reproduction (Z30-Z36, Z39.-)

● **ZØØ Encounter for general examination without complaint, suspected or reported diagnosis**

Excludes1 encounter for examination for administrative purposes (ZØ2.-)

Excludes2 encounter for pre-procedural examinations (ZØ1.81-)
special screening examinations (Z11-Z13)

● **ZØØ.Ø Encounter for general adult medical examination**
Encounter for adult periodic examination (annual) (physical) and any associated laboratory and radiologic examinations

Excludes1 encounter for examination of sign or symptom - code to sign or symptom general health check-up of infant or child (ZØØ.12.-)

● **ZØØ.ØØ Encounter for general adult medical examination without abnormal findings** A
Encounter for adult health check-up NOS
Coding Clinic: 2016, Q1, P37

● **ZØØ.Ø1 Encounter for general adult medical examination with abnormal findings** A
Use additional code to identify abnormal findings
Coding Clinic: 2016, Q1, P36

● **ZØØ.1 Encounter for newborn, infant and child health examinations**

● **ZØØ.11 Newborn health examination**
Health check for child under 29 days old
Use additional code to identify any abnormal findings

Excludes1 health check for child over 28 days old (ZØØ.12-)

● **ZØØ.110 Health examination for newborn under 8 days old** N
Health check for newborn under 8 days old

● **ZØØ.111 Health examination for newborn 8 to 28 days old** N
Health check for newborn 8 to 28 days old
Newborn weight check

● **ZØØ.12 Encounter for routine child health examination**
Encounter for development testing of infant or child
Health check (routine) for child over 28 days old

Excludes1 health check for child under 29 days old (ZØØ.11-)
health supervision of foundling or other healthy infant or child (Z76.1-Z76.2)
newborn health examination (ZØØ.11-)

● **ZØØ.121 Encounter for routine child health examination with abnormal findings** P
Use additional code to identify abnormal findings
Coding Clinic: 2016, Q1, P34-35

● **ZØØ.129 Encounter for routine child health examination without abnormal findings** P
Encounter for routine child health examination NOS
Coding Clinic: 2016, Q1, P34

● **ZØØ.2 Encounter for examination for period of rapid growth in childhood** P

● **ZØØ.3 Encounter for examination for adolescent development state** P
Encounter for puberty development state

● **ZØØ.5 Encounter for examination of potential donor of organ and tissue** P

ZØØ.6 Encounter for examination for normal comparison and control in clinical research program
Examination of participant or control in clinical research program

● **ZØØ.7 Encounter for examination for period of delayed growth in childhood**

● **ZØØ.70 Encounter for examination for period of delayed growth in childhood without abnormal findings** P

● **ZØØ.71 Encounter for examination for period of delayed growth in childhood with abnormal findings** P
Use additional code to identify abnormal findings

● **ZØØ.8 Encounter for other general examination**
Encounter for health examination in population surveys

◄ New ◄▓ Revised ~~deleted~~ Deleted | Excludes 1 | Excludes 2 | Includes | Use additional | Code first | Code also | Unspecified
OGCR Official Guidelines ● Unacceptable Principal Diagnosis X Assign placeholder X ● Use Additional Character(s) ▶ Manifestation Code **Coding Clinic**

● **Z01**   **Encounter for other special examination without complaint, suspected or reported diagnosis**

> **Includes**   routine examination of specific system

> **Note:** Codes from category Z01 represent the reason for the encounter. A separate procedure code is required to identify any examinations or procedures performed.

> **Excludes1**   encounter for examination for administrative purposes (Z02.-)
> encounter for examination for suspected conditions, proven not to exist (Z03.-)
> encounter for laboratory and radiologic examinations as a component of general medical examinations (Z00.0-)
> encounter for laboratory, radiologic and imaging examinations for sign(s) and symptom(s) - code to the sign(s) or symptom(s)

> **Excludes2**   screening examinations (Z11-Z13)

● **Z01.0**   **Encounter for examination of eyes and vision**

> **Excludes1**   examination for driving license (Z02.4)

Z01.00   **Encounter for examination of eyes and vision without abnormal findings**
> Encounter for examination of eyes and vision NOS

Z01.01   **Encounter for examination of eyes and vision with abnormal findings**
> Use additional code to identify abnormal findings

● **Z01.1**   **Encounter for examination of ears and hearing**

● **Z01.10**   **Encounter for examination of ears and hearing without abnormal findings**
> Encounter for examination of ears and hearing NOS

● **Z01.11**   **Encounter for examination of ears and hearing with abnormal findings**

> ● **Z01.110**   **Encounter for hearing examination following failed hearing screening**

> ● **Z01.118**   **Encounter for examination of ears and hearing with other abnormal findings**
> > Use additional code to identify abnormal findings

● **Z01.12**   **Encounter for hearing conservation and treatment**

● **Z01.2**   **Encounter for dental examination and cleaning**

● **Z01.20**   **Encounter for dental examination and cleaning without abnormal findings**
> Encounter for dental examination and cleaning NOS

● **Z01.21**   **Encounter for dental examination and cleaning with abnormal findings**
> Use additional code to identify abnormal findings

● **Z01.3**   **Encounter for examination of blood pressure**

● **Z01.30**   **Encounter for examination of blood pressure without abnormal findings**
> Encounter for examination of blood pressure NOS

● **Z01.31**   **Encounter for examination of blood pressure with abnormal findings**
> Use additional code to identify abnormal findings

● **Z01.4**   **Encounter for gynecological examination**

> **Excludes2**   pregnancy examination or test (Z32.0-)
> routine examination for contraceptive maintenance (Z30.4-)

● **Z01.41**   **Encounter for routine gynecological examination**
> Encounter for general gynecological examination with or without cervical smear
> Encounter for gynecological examination (general) (routine) NOS
> Encounter for pelvic examination (annual) (periodic)

> Use additional code:
> > for screening for human papillomavirus, if applicable (Z11.51)
> > for screening vaginal pap smear, if applicable (Z12.72)
> > to identify acquired absence of uterus, if applicable (Z90.71-)

> **Excludes1**   gynecologic examination status-post hysterectomy for malignant condition (Z08)
> screening cervical pap smear not a part of a routine gynecological examination (Z12.4)

Z01.411   **Encounter for gynecological examination (general) (routine) with abnormal findings ♀**
> Use additional code to identify any abnormal findings ◀

Z01.419   **Encounter for gynecological examination (general) (routine) without abnormal findings ♀**

Z01.42   **Encounter for cervical smear to confirm findings of recent normal smear following initial abnormal smear ♀**

● **Z01.8**   **Encounter for other specified special examinations**

● **Z01.81**   **Encounter for preprocedural examinations**
> Encounter for preoperative examinations
> Encounter for radiological and imaging examinations as part of preprocedural examination

Z01.810   **Encounter for preprocedural cardiovascular examination**

Z01.811   **Encounter for preprocedural respiratory examination**

● **Z01.812**   **Encounter for preprocedural laboratory examination**
> Blood and urine tests prior to treatment or procedure

● **Z01.818**   **Encounter for other preprocedural examination**
> Encounter for preprocedural examination NOS
> Encounter for examinations prior to antineoplastic chemotherapy

● **Z01.82**   **Encounter for allergy testing**
> **Excludes1**   encounter for antibody response examination (Z01.84)

● **Z01.83**   **Encounter for blood typing**
> Encounter for Rh typing

● **Z01.84**   **Encounter for antibody response examination**
> Encounter for immunity status testing
> **Excludes1**   encounter for allergy testing (Z01.82)

● **Z01.89**   **Encounter for other specified special examinations**

N Newborn Age: 0   **P** Pediatric Age: 0–17   **M** Maternity DX: 12–55   **A** Adult Age: 15–124   ♀ Females Only   ♂ Males Only

🔖 Complication\Comorbidity   🔖 Major C\C   Ⓔₓ CC/MCC Exclusions   🔖 Hospital-Acquired Condition

● **Z02**   **Encounter for administrative examination**
    ● **Z02.0**   **Encounter for examination for admission to educational institution**
         Encounter for examination for admission to preschool (education)
         Encounter for examination for re-admission to school following illness or medical treatment
    Z02.1   **Encounter for pre-employment examination**
    ● **Z02.2**   **Encounter for examination for admission to residential institution**
         Excludes1   examination for admission to prison (Z02.89)
    Z02.3   **Encounter for examination for recruitment to armed forces**
    ● **Z02.4**   **Encounter for examination for driving license**
    ● **Z02.5**   **Encounter for examination for participation in sport**
         Excludes1   blood-alcohol and blood-drug test (Z02.83)
    ● **Z02.6**   **Encounter for examination for insurance purposes**
    ● **Z02.7**   **Encounter for issue of medical certificate**
         Excludes1   encounter for general medical examination (Z00-Z01, Z02.0-Z02.6, Z02.8-Z02.9)
       ● **Z02.71**   **Encounter for disability determination**
           Encounter for issue of medical certificate of incapacity
           Encounter for issue of medical certificate of invalidity
       ● **Z02.79**   **Encounter for issue of other medical certificate**
    ● **Z02.8**   **Encounter for other administrative examinations**
       Z02.81   **Encounter for paternity testing**
       ● **Z02.82**   **Encounter for adoption services**
       Z02.83   **Encounter for blood-alcohol and blood-drug test**
           Use additional code for findings of alcohol or drugs in blood (R78.-)
       ● **Z02.89**   **Encounter for other administrative examinations**
           Encounter for examination for admission to prison
           Encounter for examination for admission to summer camp
           Encounter for immigration examination
           Encounter for naturalization examination
           Encounter for premarital examination
           Excludes1   health supervision of foundling or other healthy infant or child (Z76.1-Z76.2)
    ● **Z02.9**   **Encounter for administrative examinations, unspecified**

OGCR Section II.C.21.c.6.

Observation

There are **three** observation Z code categories. They are for use in very limited circumstances when a person is being observed for a suspected condition that is ruled out. The observation codes are not for use if an injury or illnesses or any signs or symptoms related to the suspected condition are present. In such cases the diagnosis/symptom code is used with the corresponding external cause code.

The observation codes are to be used as principal diagnosis only. **The only exception to this is when the principal diagnosis is required to be a code from category Z38, Liveborn infants according to place of birth and type of delivery. Then a code from category Z05, Encounter for observation and evaluation of newborn for suspected diseases and conditions ruled out, is sequenced after the Z38 code.** Additional codes may be used in addition to the observation code but only if they are unrelated to the suspected condition being observed.

Codes from subcategory Z03.7 Encounter for suspected maternal and fetal conditions ruled out, may either be used as a first listed or as an additional code assignment depending on the case. They are for use in very limited circumstances on a maternal record when an encounter is for a suspected maternal or fetal condition that is ruled out during that encounter (for example, a maternal or fetal condition may be suspected due to an abnormal test result). These codes should not be used when the condition is confirmed. In those cases, the confirmed condition should be coded. In addition, these codes are not for use if an illness or any signs or symptoms related to the suspected condition or problem are present. In such cases the diagnosis/symptom code is used.

Additional codes may be used in addition to the code from subcategory Z03.7, but only if they are unrelated to the suspected condition being evaluated.

Codes from subcategory Z03.7 may not be used for encounters for antenatal screening of mother. *See Section I.C.21. Screening.*

For encounters for suspected fetal condition that are inconclusive following testing and evaluation, assign the appropriate code from category O35, O36, O40 or O41.

The observation Z code categories:

Z03   Encounter for medical observation for suspected diseases and conditions ruled out

Z04   Encounter for examination and observation for other reasons
      Except: Z04.9, Encounter for examination and observation for unspecified reason

Z05   **Encounter for observation and evaluation of newborn for suspected diseases and conditions ruled out**

● **Z03**   **Encounter for medical observation for suspected diseases and conditions ruled out**
       This category is to be used when a person without a diagnosis is suspected of having an abnormal condition, without signs or symptoms, which requires study, but after examination and observation, is ruled out. This category is also for use for administrative and legal observation status.
       Excludes1   contact with and (suspected) exposures hazardous to health (Z77.-)
           newborn observation for suspected condition, ruled out (P00-P04)
           person with feared complaint in whom no diagnosis is made (Z71.1)
           signs or symptoms under study - code to signs or symptoms
    Z03.6   **Encounter for observation for suspected toxic effect from ingested substance ruled out**
         Encounter for observation for suspected adverse effect from drug
         Encounter for observation for suspected poisoning

◄ New   ◄▥▥ Revised   ~~deleted~~ Deleted   Excludes 1   Excludes 2   Includes   Use additional   Code first   Code also   Unspecified

OGCR Official Guidelines   ● Unacceptable Principal Diagnosis   X Assign placeholder X   ● Use Additional Character(s)   ▶ Manifestation Code   **Coding Clinic**

● **Z03.7**   **Encounter for suspected maternal and fetal conditions ruled out**
Encounter for suspected maternal and fetal conditions not found

> **Excludes1**   known or suspected fetal anomalies affecting management of mother, not ruled out (O26.-, O35.-, O36.-, O40.-, O41.-)

● **Z03.71**   **Encounter for suspected problem with amniotic cavity and membrane ruled out ♀**   **M**
Encounter for suspected oligohydramnios ruled out
Encounter for suspected polyhydramnios ruled out

● **Z03.72**   **Encounter for suspected placental problem ruled out ♀**   **M**

● **Z03.73**   **Encounter for suspected fetal anomaly ruled out ♀**   **M**

● **Z03.74**   **Encounter for suspected problem with fetal growth ruled out ♀**   **M**

● **Z03.75**   **Encounter for suspected cervical shortening ruled out ♀**   **M**

● **Z03.79**   **Encounter for other suspected maternal and fetal conditions ruled out ♀**   **M**

● **Z03.8**   **Encounter for observation for other suspected diseases and conditions ruled out**

● **Z03.81**   **Encounter for observation for suspected exposure to biological agents ruled out**

    Z03.810   **Encounter for observation for suspected exposure to anthrax ruled out**

    Z03.818   **Encounter for observation for suspected exposure to other biological agents ruled out**

    Z03.89   **Encounter for observation for other suspected diseases and conditions ruled out**

● **Z04**   **Encounter for examination and observation for other reasons**

> **Includes**   encounter for examination for medicolegal reasons
This category is to be used when a person without a diagnosis is suspected of having an abnormal condition, without signs or symptoms, which requires study, but after examination and observation, is ruled-out. This category is also for use for administrative and legal observation status.

    Z04.1   **Encounter for examination and observation following transport accident**

> **Excludes1**   encounter for examination and observation following work accident (Z04.2)

    Z04.2   **Encounter for examination and observation following work accident**

    Z04.3   **Encounter for examination and observation following other accident**

● **Z04.4**   **Encounter for examination and observation following alleged rape**
Encounter for examination and observation of victim following alleged rape
Encounter for examination and observation of victim following alleged sexual abuse

    Z04.41   **Encounter for examination and observation following alleged adult rape**   **A**
Suspected adult rape, ruled out
Suspected adult sexual abuse, ruled out

    Z04.42   **Encounter for examination and observation following alleged child rape**   **P**
Suspected child rape, ruled out
Suspected child sexual abuse, ruled out

    Z04.6   **Encounter for general psychiatric examination, requested by authority**

● **Z04.7**   **Encounter for examination and observation following alleged physical abuse**

    Z04.71   **Encounter for examination and observation following alleged adult physical abuse**   **A**
Suspected adult physical abuse, ruled out

> **Excludes1**   confirmed case of adult physical abuse (T74.-)
encounter for examination and observation following alleged adult sexual abuse (Z04.41)
suspected case of adult physical abuse, not ruled out (T76.-)

    Z04.72   **Encounter for examination and observation following alleged child physical abuse**   **P**
Suspected child physical abuse, ruled out

> **Excludes1**   confirmed case of child physical abuse (T74.-)
encounter for examination and observation following alleged child sexual abuse (Z04.42)
suspected case of child physical abuse, not ruled out (T76.-)

● **Z04.8**   **Encounter for examination and observation for other specified reasons**
Encounter for examination and observation for request for expert evidence

● **Z04.9**   **Encounter for examination and observation for unspecified reason**
Encounter for observation NOS

● **Z05**   **Encounter for observation and evaluation of newborn for suspected diseases and conditions ruled out ◄**
This category is to be used for newborns, within the neonatal period (the first 28 days of life), who are suspected of having an abnormal condition unrelated to exposure from the mother or the birth process, but without signs or symptoms, and which, after examination and observation, is ruled out. ◄

> **Excludes2**   newborn observation for suspected condition, related to exposure from the mother or birth process (P00-P04) ◄

● **Z05.0**   **Observation and evaluation of newborn for suspected cardiac condition ruled out ◄**

● **Z05.1**   **Observation and evaluation of newborn for suspected infectious condition ruled out ◄**

● **Z05.2**   **Observation and evaluation of newborn for suspected neurological condition ruled out ◄**

● **Z05.3**   **Observation and evaluation of newborn for suspected respiratory condition ruled out ◄**

● **Z05.4**   **Observation and evaluation of newborn for suspected genetic, metabolic or immunologic condition ruled out ◄**

● **Z05.41**   **Observation and evaluation of newborn for suspected genetic condition ruled out ◄**

● **Z05.42**   **Observation and evaluation of newborn for suspected metabolic condition ruled out ◄**

● **Z05.43**   **Observation and evaluation of newborn for suspected immunologic condition ruled out ◄**

● **Z05.5**   **Observation and evaluation of newborn for suspected gastrointestinal condition ruled out ◄**

● **Z05.6**   **Observation and evaluation of newborn for suspected genitourinary condition ruled out ◄**

● **Z05.7**   **Observation and evaluation of newborn for suspected skin, subcutaneous, musculoskeletal and connective tissue condition ruled out ◄**

● **Z05.71**   **Observation and evaluation of newborn for suspected skin and subcutaneous tissue condition ruled out ◄**

● **Z05.72**   **Observation and evaluation of newborn for suspected musculoskeletal condition ruled out ◄**

● **Z05.73**   **Observation and evaluation of newborn for suspected connective tissue condition ruled out ◄**

CHAPTER 21 (Z00-Z99)

N Newborn Age: 0   **P** Pediatric Age: 0–17   **M** Maternity DX: 12–55   **A** Adult Age: 15–124   ♀ Females Only   ♂ Males Only

🔖 Complication\Comorbidity   🔖 Major C\C   ⓍⓍ CC/MCC Exclusions   🔖 Hospital-Acquired Condition

CHAPTER 21 (Z00–Z99)

● **Z05.8** **Observation and evaluation of newborn for other specified suspected condition ruled out** ◀

● **Z05.9** **Observation and evaluation of newborn for** unspecified **suspected condition ruled out** ◀

OGCR See Section II.C.21.c.8.

> The follow-up codes are used to explain continuing surveillance following completed treatment of a disease, condition, or injury. They imply that the condition has been fully treated and no longer exists. They should not be confused with aftercare codes, or injury codes with 7th character "D," that explain ongoing care of a healing condition or its sequelae. Follow-up codes may be used in conjunction with history codes to provide the full picture of the healed condition and its treatment. The follow-up code is sequenced first, followed by the history code.
>
> A follow-up code may be used to explain multiple visits. Should a condition be found to have recurred on the follow-up visit, then the diagnosis code for the condition should be assigned in place of the follow-up code.
>
> The follow-up Z code categories:
>
> Z08 Encounter for follow-up examination after completed treatment for malignant neoplasm
>
> Z09 Encounter for follow-up examination after completed treatment for conditions other than malignant neoplasm
>
> Z39 Encounter for maternal postpartum care and examination

● **Z08** **Encounter for follow-up examination after completed treatment for malignant neoplasm**
    Medical surveillance following completed treatment
    Use additional code to identify any acquired absence of organs (Z90.-)
    Use additional code to identify the personal history of malignant neoplasm (Z85.-)
    Excludes1 aftercare following medical care (Z43-Z49, Z51)

● **Z09** **Encounter for follow-up examination after completed treatment for conditions other than malignant neoplasm**
    Medical surveillance following completed treatment
    Use additional code to identify any applicable history of disease code (Z86.-. Z87.-)
    Excludes1 aftercare following medical care (Z43-Z49, Z51)
                    surveillance of contraception (Z30.4-)
                    surveillance of prosthetic and other medical devices (Z44-Z46)
    Coding Clinic: 2015, Q1, P8

OGCR Section II.C.21.c.5.

> Screening
>
> Screening is the testing for disease or disease precursors in seemingly well individuals so that early detection and treatment can be provided for those who test positive for the disease (e.g., screening mammogram).
>
> The testing of a person to rule out or confirm a suspected diagnosis because the patient has some sign or symptom is a diagnostic examination, not a screening. In these cases, the sign or symptom is used to explain the reason for the test.
>
> A screening code may be a first listed code if the reason for the visit is specifically the screening exam. It may also be used as an additional code if the screening is done during an office visit for other health problems. A screening code is not necessary if the screening is inherent to a routine examination, such as a pap smear done during a routine pelvic examination.
>
> Should a condition be discovered during the screening then the code for the condition may be assigned as an additional diagnosis.
>
> The Z code indicates that a screening exam is planned. A procedure code is required to confirm that the screening was performed.
>
> The screening Z codes /categories:
>
> Z11 Encounter for screening for infectious and parasitic diseases
>
> Z12 Encounter for screening for malignant neoplasms
>
> Z13 Encounter for screening for other diseases and disorders
>   Except: Z13.9, Encounter for screening, unspecified
>
> Z36 Encounter for antenatal screening for mother

● **Z11** **Encounter for screening for infectious and parasitic diseases**
    Screening is the testing for disease or disease precursors in asymptomatic individuals so that early detection and treatment can be provided for those who test positive for the disease.
    Excludes1 encounter for diagnostic examination - code to sign or symptom

● **Z11.0** **Encounter for screening for intestinal infectious diseases**

● **Z11.1** **Encounter for screening for respiratory tuberculosis**

● **Z11.2** **Encounter for screening for other bacterial diseases**

● **Z11.3** **Encounter for screening for infections with a predominantly sexual mode of transmission**
    Excludes2 encounter for screening for human immunodeficiency virus [HIV] (Z11.4)
                    encounter for screening for human papillomavirus (Z11.51)

● **Z11.4** **Encounter for screening for human immunodeficiency virus [HIV]**

● **Z11.5** **Encounter for screening for other viral diseases**
    Excludes2 encounter for screening for viral intestinal disease (Z11.0)

  ● **Z11.51** **Encounter for screening for human papillomavirus (HPV)**

  ● **Z11.59** **Encounter for screening for other viral diseases**

● **Z11.6** **Encounter for screening for other protozoal diseases and helminthiases**
    Diseases or infestations caused by parasitic worms
    Excludes2 encounter for screening for protozoal intestinal disease (Z11.0)

● **Z11.8** **Encounter for screening for other infectious and parasitic diseases**
    Encounter for screening for chlamydia
    Encounter for screening for rickettsial
    Encounter for screening for spirochetal
    Encounter for screening for mycoses

● **Z11.9** **Encounter for screening for infectious and parasitic diseases,** unspecified

● **Z12** **Encounter for screening for malignant neoplasms**
    Screening is the testing for disease or disease precursors in asymptomatic individuals so that early detection and treatment can be provided for those who test positive for the disease.
    Use additional code to identify any family history of malignant neoplasm (Z80.-)
    Excludes1 encounter for diagnostic examination - code to sign or symptom

● **Z12.0** **Encounter for screening for malignant neoplasm of stomach**

● **Z12.1** **Encounter for screening for malignant neoplasm of intestinal tract**

  ● **Z12.10** **Encounter for screening for malignant neoplasm of intestinal tract,** unspecified

  ● **Z12.11** **Encounter for screening for malignant neoplasm of colon**
        Encounter for screening colonoscopy NOS

  ● **Z12.12** **Encounter for screening for malignant neoplasm of rectum**

  ● **Z12.13** **Encounter for screening for malignant neoplasm of small intestine**

● **Z12.2** **Encounter for screening for malignant neoplasm of respiratory organs**

● **Z12.3** **Encounter for screening for malignant neoplasm of breast**

  ● **Z12.31** **Encounter for screening mammogram for malignant neoplasm of breast**
        Excludes1 inconclusive mammogram (R92.2)
        Coding Clinic: 2015, Q1, P24

  ● **Z12.39** **Encounter for other screening for malignant neoplasm of breast**

◀ New   ◀▦ Revised   deleted Deleted   Excludes 1   Excludes 2   Includes   Use additional   Code first   Code also   Unspecified

OGCR Official Guidelines   ● Unacceptable Principal Diagnosis   X Assign placeholder X   ● Use Additional Character(s)   ▶ Manifestation Code   **Coding Clinic**

● **Z12.4** **Encounter for screening for malignant neoplasm of cervix** ♀

    Encounter for screening pap smear for malignant neoplasm of cervix

    Excludes1 when screening is part of general gynecological examination (Z01.4-)

    Excludes2 encounter for screening for human papillomavirus (Z11.51) ◀

Z12.5 **Encounter for screening for malignant neoplasm of prostate** ♂

● **Z12.6** **Encounter for screening for malignant neoplasm of bladder**

● **Z12.7** **Encounter for screening for malignant neoplasm of other genitourinary organs**

    ● **Z12.71** **Encounter for screening for malignant neoplasm of testis** ♂

    ● **Z12.72** **Encounter for screening for malignant neoplasm of vagina** ♀

        Vaginal pap smear status - post hysterectomy for non-malignant condition

        Use additional code to identify acquired absence of uterus (Z90.71-)

        Excludes1 vaginal pap smear status - post hysterectomy for malignant conditions (Z08)

    ● **Z12.73** **Encounter for screening for malignant neoplasm of ovary** ♀

    ● **Z12.79** **Encounter for screening for malignant neoplasm of other genitourinary organs**

● **Z12.8** **Encounter for screening for malignant neoplasm of other sites**

    ● **Z12.81** **Encounter for screening for malignant neoplasm of oral cavity**

    ● **Z12.82** **Encounter for screening for malignant neoplasm of nervous system**

    ● **Z12.83** **Encounter for screening for malignant neoplasm of skin**

    ● **Z12.89** **Encounter for screening for malignant neoplasm of other sites**

● **Z12.9** **Encounter for screening for malignant neoplasm, site unspecified**

● **Z13** **Encounter for screening for other diseases and disorders**

    Screening is the testing for disease or disease precursors in asymptomatic individuals so that early detection and treatment can be provided for those who test positive for the disease.

    Excludes1 encounter for diagnostic examination - code to sign or symptom

● **Z13.0** **Encounter for screening for diseases of the blood and blood-forming organs and certain disorders involving the immune mechanism**

● **Z13.1** **Encounter for screening for diabetes mellitus**

● **Z13.2** **Encounter for screening for nutritional, metabolic and other endocrine disorders**

    ● **Z13.21** **Encounter for screening for nutritional disorder**

    ● **Z13.22** **Encounter for screening for metabolic disorder**

        ● **Z13.220** **Encounter for screening for lipoid disorders**

            Encounter for screening for cholesterol level

            Encounter for screening for hypercholesterolemia

            Encounter for screening for hyperlipidemia

        ● **Z13.228** **Encounter for screening for other metabolic disorders**

    ● **Z13.29** **Encounter for screening for other suspected endocrine disorder**

        Excludes1 encounter for screening for diabetes mellitus (Z13.1)

● **Z13.4** **Encounter for screening for certain developmental disorders in childhood** P

    Encounter for screening for developmental handicaps in early childhood

    Excludes1 routine development testing of infant or child (Z00.1-)

● **Z13.5** **Encounter for screening for eye and ear disorders**

    Excludes2 encounter for general hearing examination (Z01.1-)

        encounter for general vision examination (Z01.0-)

● **Z13.6** **Encounter for screening for cardiovascular disorders**

● **Z13.7** **Encounter for screening for genetic and chromosomal anomalies**

    Excludes1 genetic testing for procreative management (Z31.4-)

    ● **Z13.71** **Encounter for nonprocreative screening for genetic disease carrier status**

    ● **Z13.79** **Encounter for other screening for genetic and chromosomal anomalies**

● **Z13.8** **Encounter for screening for other specified diseases and disorders**

    Excludes2 screening for malignant neoplasms (Z12.-)

    ● **Z13.81** **Encounter for screening for digestive system disorders**

        ● **Z13.810** **Encounter for screening for upper gastrointestinal disorder**

        ● **Z13.811** **Encounter for screening for lower gastrointestinal disorder**

            Excludes1 encounter for screening for intestinal infectious disease (Z11.0)

        ● **Z13.818** **Encounter for screening for other digestive system disorders**

    ● **Z13.82** **Encounter for screening for musculoskeletal disorder**

        ● **Z13.820** **Encounter for screening for osteoporosis**

        ● **Z13.828** **Encounter for screening for other musculoskeletal disorder**

    ● **Z13.83** **Encounter for screening for respiratory disorder NEC**

        Excludes1 encounter for screening for respiratory tuberculosis (Z11.1)

    ● **Z13.84** **Encounter for screening for dental disorders**

    ● **Z13.85** **Encounter for screening for nervous system disorders**

        ● **Z13.850** **Encounter for screening for traumatic brain injury**

        ● **Z13.858** **Encounter for screening for other nervous system disorders**

    ● **Z13.88** **Encounter for screening for disorder due to exposure to contaminants**

        Excludes1 those exposed to contaminants without suspected disorders (Z57-Z77.-)

    ● **Z13.89** **Encounter for screening for other disorder**

        Encounter for screening for genitourinary disorders

● **Z13.9** **Encounter for screening, unspecified**

CHAPTER 21 (Z00-Z99)

N Newborn Age: 0   **P** Pediatric Age: 0–17   **M** Maternity DX: 12–55   **A** Adult Age: 15–124   ♀ Females Only   ♂ Males Only

🐾 Complication\Comorbidity   🐾 Major C\C   (Exc) CC/MCC Exclusions   🐾 Hospital-Acquired Condition

1611

GENETIC CARRIER AND GENETIC SUSCEPTIBILITY TO DISEASE (Z14-Z15)

● **Z14**   **Genetic carrier**
- ● **Z14.0**   **Hemophilia A carrier**
  - ● **Z14.01**   **Asymptomatic hemophilia A carrier**
  - ● **Z14.02**   **Symptomatic hemophilia A carrier**
- ● **Z14.1**   **Cystic fibrosis carrier**
- ● **Z14.8**   **Genetic carrier of other disease**

● **Z15**   **Genetic susceptibility to disease**
> **Excludes1**   chromosomal anomalies (Q90-Q99)
>
> **Includes**   confirmed abnormal gene
>
> Use additional code, if applicable, for any associated family history of the disease (Z80-Z84)

- ● **Z15.0**   **Genetic susceptibility to malignant neoplasm**
  > *Code first if applicable, any current malignant neoplasm (C00-C75, C81-C96)*
  >
  > Use additional code, if applicable, for any personal history of malignant neoplasm (Z85.-)
  - ● **Z15.01**   **Genetic susceptibility to malignant neoplasm of breast**
  - ● **Z15.02**   **Genetic susceptibility to malignant neoplasm of ovary ♀**
  - ● **Z15.03**   **Genetic susceptibility to malignant neoplasm of prostate ♂**
  - ● **Z15.04**   **Genetic susceptibility to malignant neoplasm of endometrium ♀**
  - ● **Z15.09**   **Genetic susceptibility to other malignant neoplasm**
- ● **Z15.8**   **Genetic susceptibility to other disease**
  - ● **Z15.81**   **Genetic susceptibility to multiple endocrine neoplasia [MEN]**
    > **Excludes1**   multiple endocrine neoplasia [MEN] syndromes (E31.2-)
  - ● **Z15.89**   **Genetic susceptibility to other disease**

RESISTANCE TO ANTIMICROBIAL DRUGS (Z16)

● **Z16**   **Resistance to antimicrobial drugs**
> **Note:** The codes in this category are provided for use as additional codes to identify the resistance and non-responsiveness of a condition to antimicrobial drugs.
>
> *Code first the infection*
>
> **Excludes1**   Methicillin resistant Staphylococcus aureus infection (A49.02)
> Methicillin resistant Staphylococcus aureus infection in diseases classified elsewhere (B95.62)
> Methicillin resistant Staphylococcus aureus pneumonia (J15.212)
> Sepsis due to Methicillin resistant Staphylococcus aureus (A41.02)

- ● **Z16.1**   **Resistance to beta lactam antibiotics**
  - ● **Z16.10**   **Resistance to unspecified beta lactam antibiotics**
  - ● **Z16.11**   **Resistance to penicillins**
    Resistance to amoxicillin
    Resistance to ampicillin
  - ● **Z16.12**   **Extended spectrum beta lactamase (ESBL) resistance**
  - ● **Z16.19**   **Resistance to other specified beta lactam antibiotics**
    Resistance to cephalosporins
- ● **Z16.2**   **Resistance to other antibiotics**
  - ● **Z16.20**   **Resistance to unspecified antibiotic**
    Resistance to antibiotics NOS
  - ● **Z16.21**   **Resistance to vancomycin**
  - ● **Z16.22**   **Resistance to vancomycin related antibiotics**
  - ● **Z16.23**   **Resistance to quinolones and fluoroquinolones**
  - ● **Z16.24**   **Resistance to multiple antibiotics**

- ● **Z16.29**   **Resistance to other single specified antibiotic**
  Resistance to aminoglycosides
  Resistance to macrolides
  Resistance to sulfonamides
  Resistance to tetracyclines
- ● **Z16.3**   **Resistance to other antimicrobial drugs**
  > **Excludes1**   resistance to antibiotics (Z16.1-, Z16.2-)
  - ● **Z16.30**   **Resistance to unspecified antimicrobial drugs**
    Drug resistance NOS
  - ● **Z16.31**   **Resistance to antiparasitic drug(s)**
    Resistance to quinine and related compounds
  - ● **Z16.32**   **Resistance to antifungal drug(s)**
  - ● **Z16.33**   **Resistance to antiviral drug(s)**
  - ● **Z16.34**   **Resistance to antimycobacterial drug(s)**
    Resistance to tuberculostatics
    - ● **Z16.341**   **Resistance to single antimycobacterial drug**
      Resistance to antimycobacterial drug NOS
    - ● **Z16.342**   **Resistance to multiple antimycobacterial drugs**
  - ● **Z16.35**   **Resistance to multiple antimicrobial drugs**
    > **Excludes1**   Resistance to multiple antibiotics only (Z16.24)
  - ● **Z16.39**   **Resistance to other specified antimicrobial drug**

ESTROGEN RECEPTOR STATUS (Z17)

● **Z17**   **Estrogen receptor status**
> *Code first malignant neoplasm of breast (C50.-)*
- ● **Z17.0**   **Estrogen receptor positive status [ER+]**
- ● **Z17.1**   **Estrogen receptor negative status [ER-]**

RETAINED FOREIGN BODY FRAGMENTS (Z18)

● **Z18**   **Retained foreign body fragments**
> **Includes**   embedded fragment (status)
> embedded splinter (status)
> retained foreign body status
>
> **Excludes1**   artificial joint prosthesis status (Z96.6-)
> foreign body accidentally left during a procedure (T81.5-)
> foreign body entering through orifice (T15-T19)
> in situ cardiac device (Z95.-)
> organ or tissue replaced by means other than transplant (Z96.-, Z97.-)
> organ or tissue replaced by transplant (Z94.-)
> personal history of retained foreign body fully removed Z87.821
> superficial foreign body (non-embedded splinter) - code to superficial foreign body, by site

- ● **Z18.0**   **Retained radioactive fragments**
  - ● **Z18.01**   **Retained depleted uranium fragments**
  - ● **Z18.09**   **Other retained radioactive fragments**
    Other retained depleted isotope fragments
    Retained nontherapeutic radioactive fragments
- ● **Z18.1**   **Retained metal fragments**
  > **Excludes1**   retained radioactive metal fragments (Z18.01-Z18.09)
  - ● **Z18.10**   **Retained metal fragments, unspecified**
    Retained metal fragment NOS
  - ● **Z18.11**   **Retained magnetic metal fragments**
  - ● **Z18.12**   **Retained nonmagnetic metal fragments**
- ● **Z18.2**   **Retained plastic fragments**
  Acrylics fragments
  Diethylhexylphthalates fragments
  Isocyanate fragments
- ● **Z18.3**   **Retained organic fragments**
  - ● **Z18.31**   **Retained animal quills or spines**
  - ● **Z18.32**   **Retained tooth**
  - ● **Z18.33**   **Retained wood fragments**
  - ● **Z18.39**   **Other retained organic fragments**

- **Z18.8** Other specified retained foreign body
  - **Z18.81** Retained glass fragments
  - **Z18.83** Retained stone or crystalline fragments
    Retained concrete or cement fragments
  - **Z18.89** Other specified retained foreign body fragments
- **Z18.9** Retained foreign body fragments, unspecified material

---

HORMONE SENSITIVITY MALIGNANCY STATUS (Z19) ◄

- **Z19** Hormone sensitivity malignancy status ◄
  Code first malignant neoplasm —*see* Table of Neoplasms, by site, malignant ◄
  - **Z19.1** Hormone sensitive malignancy status ◄
  - **Z19.2** Hormone resistant malignancy status ◄
    Castrate resistant prostate malignancy status ◄

PERSONS WITH POTENTIAL HEALTH HAZARDS RELATED TO COMMUNICABLE DISEASES (Z20-Z29) ◄◄◄

- **Z20** Contact with and (suspected) exposure to communicable diseases
  Excludes1 carrier of infectious disease (Z22.-)
    diagnosed current infectious or parasitic disease - see Alphabetic Index
  Excludes2 personal history of infectious and parasitic diseases (Z86.1-)
  - **Z20.0** Contact with and (suspected) exposure to intestinal infectious diseases
    - **Z20.01** Contact with and (suspected) exposure to intestinal infectious diseases due to Escherichia coli (E. coli)
    - **Z20.09** Contact with and (suspected) exposure to other intestinal infectious diseases
  - **Z20.1** Contact with and (suspected) exposure to tuberculosis
  - **Z20.2** Contact with and (suspected) exposure to infections with a predominantly sexual mode of transmission
  - **Z20.3** Contact with and (suspected) exposure to rabies
  - **Z20.4** Contact with and (suspected) exposure to rubella
  - **Z20.5** Contact with and (suspected) exposure to viral hepatitis
  - **Z20.6** Contact with and (suspected) exposure to human immunodeficiency virus [HIV]
    Excludes1 asymptomatic human immunodeficiency virus [HIV]
      HIV infection status (Z21)
  - **Z20.7** Contact with and (suspected) exposure to pediculosis, acariasis and other infestations
  - **Z20.8** Contact with and (suspected) exposure to other communicable diseases
    - **Z20.81** Contact with and (suspected) exposure to other bacterial communicable diseases
      - **Z20.810** Contact with and (suspected) exposure to anthrax
      - **Z20.811** Contact with and (suspected) exposure to meningococcus
      - **Z20.818** Contact with and (suspected) exposure to other bacterial communicable diseases
    - **Z20.82** Contact with and (suspected) exposure to other viral communicable diseases
      - **Z20.820** Contact with and (suspected) exposure to varicella
      - **Z20.828** Contact with and (suspected) exposure to other viral communicable diseases
    - **Z20.89** Contact with and (suspected) exposure to other communicable diseases
  - **Z20.9** Contact with and (suspected) exposure to unspecified communicable disease

- **Z21** Asymptomatic human immunodeficiency virus [HIV] infection status
  HIV positive NOS
  Code first Human immunodeficiency virus [HIV] disease complicating pregnancy, childbirth and the puerperium, if applicable (O98.7-)
  Excludes1 acquired immunodeficiency syndrome (B20)
    contact with human immunodeficiency virus [HIV] (Z20.6)
    exposure to human immunodeficiency virus [HIV] (Z20.6)
    human immunodeficiency virus [HIV] disease (B20)
    inconclusive laboratory evidence of human immunodeficiency virus [HIV] (R75)
  MCE: Questionable admission when principal dx

- **Z22** Carrier of infectious disease
  Includes colonization status
    suspected carrier
  Excludes2 carrier of viral hepatitis (B18.-) ◄
  - **Z22.0** Carrier of typhoid
  - **Z22.1** Carrier of other intestinal infectious diseases
  - **Z22.2** Carrier of diphtheria
  - **Z22.3** Carrier of other specified bacterial diseases
    - **Z22.31** Carrier of bacterial disease due to meningococci
    - **Z22.32** Carrier of bacterial disease due to staphylococci
      - **Z22.321** Carrier or suspected carrier of Methicillin susceptible Staphylococcus aureus
        MSSA colonization
      - **Z22.322** Carrier or suspected carrier of Methicillin resistant Staphylococcus aureus
        MRSA colonization
    - **Z22.33** Carrier of bacterial disease due to streptococci
      - **Z22.330** Carrier of Group B streptococcus
        Excludes1 Carrier of streptococcus group B (GBS) complicating pregnancy, childbirth and the puerperium (O99.82-) ◄
      - **Z22.338** Carrier of other streptococcus
    - **Z22.39** Carrier of other specified bacterial diseases
  - **Z22.4** Carrier of infections with a predominantly sexual mode of transmission
  - ~~**Z22.5** Carrier of viral hepatitis~~
    - ~~**Z22.50** Carrier of unspecified viral hepatitis~~
    - ~~**Z22.51** Carrier of viral hepatitis B~~
      ~~Hepatitis B surface antigen [HBsAg] carrier~~
    - ~~**Z22.52** Carrier of viral hepatitis C~~
    - ~~**Z22.59** Carrier of other viral hepatitis~~
  - **Z22.6** Carrier of human T-lymphotropic virus type-1 [HTLV-1] infection
  - **Z22.8** Carrier of other infectious diseases
  - **Z22.9** Carrier of infectious disease, unspecified

- **Z23** Encounter for immunization
  Code first any routine childhood examination
  Note: Procedure codes are required to identify the types of immunizations given.

CHAPTER 21 (Z00-Z99)

● **Z28   Immunization not carried out and underimmunization status**
    Includes   vaccination not carried out

● **Z28.0   Immunization not carried out because of contraindication**

   ● Z28.01   Immunization not carried out because of acute illness of patient

   ● Z28.02   Immunization not carried out because of chronic illness or condition of patient

   ● Z28.03   Immunization not carried out because of immune compromised state of patient

   ● Z28.04   Immunization not carried out because of patient allergy to vaccine or component

   ● Z28.09   Immunization not carried out because of other contraindication

● **Z28.1   Immunization not carried out because of patient decision for reasons of belief or group pressure**
    Immunization not carried out because of religious belief

● **Z28.2   Immunization not carried out because of patient decision for other and unspecified reason**

   ● Z28.20   Immunization not carried out because of patient decision for unspecified reason

   ● Z28.21   Immunization not carried out because of patient refusal

   ● Z28.29   Immunization not carried out because of patient decision for other reason

● **Z28.3   Underimmunization status**
    Delinquent immunization status
    Lapsed immunization schedule status

● **Z28.8   Immunization not carried out for other reason**

   ● Z28.81   Immunization not carried out due to patient having had the disease

   ● Z28.82   Immunization not carried out because of caregiver refusal
      Immunization not carried out because of guardian refusal
      Immunization not carried out because of parent refusal
      Excludes1   immunization not carried out because of caregiver refusal because of religious belief (Z28.1)

   ● Z28.89   Immunization not carried out for other reason

● **Z28.9   Immunization not carried out for unspecified reason**

● **Z29   Encounter for other prophylactic measures** ◄
    Excludes1   desensitization to allergens (Z51.6) ◄
                 prophylactic surgery (Z40.-) ◄

● **Z29.1   Encounter for prophylactic immunotherapy** ◄
    Encounter for administration of immunoglobulin ◄

   ● Z29.11   Encounter for prophylactic immunotherapy for respiratory syncytial virus (RSV) ◄

   ● Z29.12   Encounter for prophylactic antivenin ◄

   ● Z29.13   Encounter for prophylactic Rho(D) immune globulin ◄

   ● Z29.14   Encounter for prophylactic rabies immune globin ◄

● **Z29.3   Encounter for prophylactic fluoride administration** ◄

● **Z29.8   Encounter for other specified prophylactic measures** ◄

● **Z29.9   Encounter for prophylactic measures, unspecified** ◄

PERSONS ENCOUNTERING HEALTH SERVICES IN CIRCUMSTANCES RELATED TO REPRODUCTION (Z30-Z39)

● **Z30   Encounter for contraceptive management**

● **Z30.0   Encounter for general counseling and advice on contraception**

   ● **Z30.01   Encounter for initial prescription of contraceptives**
      Excludes1   encounter for surveillance of contraceptives (Z30.4-)

     ● Z30.011   Encounter for initial prescription of contraceptive pills ♀

     ● Z30.012   Encounter for prescription of emergency contraception ♀
        Encounter for postcoital contraception

     ● Z30.013   Encounter for initial prescription of injectable contraceptive ♀

     ● Z30.014   Encounter for initial prescription of intrauterine contraceptive device ♀
        Excludes1   encounter for insertion of intrauterine contraceptive device (Z30.430, Z30.432)

     ● Z30.015   Encounter for initial prescription of vaginal ring hormonal contraceptive ♀ ◄

     ● Z30.016   Encounter for initial prescription of transdermal patch hormonal contraceptive device ◄

     ● Z30.017   Encounter for initial prescription of implantable subdermal contraceptive ◄

     ● Z30.018   Encounter for initial prescription of other contraceptives ♀
        Encounter for initial prescription of barrier contraception ◄
        Encounter for initial prescription of diaphragm ◄

     ● Z30.019   Encounter for initial prescription of contraceptives, unspecified ♀

   ● Z30.02   Counseling and instruction in natural family planning to avoid pregnancy

   ● Z30.09   Encounter for other general counseling and advice on contraception
      Encounter for family planning advice NOS

● **Z30.2   Encounter for sterilization**

● **Z30.4   Encounter for surveillance of contraceptives**

   ● Z30.40   Encounter for surveillance of contraceptives, unspecified

   ● Z30.41   Encounter for surveillance of contraceptive pills ♀
      Encounter for repeat prescription for contraceptive pill

   ● Z30.42   Encounter for surveillance of injectable contraceptive ♀

   ● **Z30.43   Encounter for surveillance of intrauterine contraceptive device**

     ● Z30.430   Encounter for insertion of intrauterine contraceptive device ♀

     ● Z30.431   Encounter for routine checking of intrauterine contraceptive device ♀

     ● Z30.432   Encounter for removal of intrauterine contraceptive device ♀

     ● Z30.433   Encounter for removal and reinsertion of intrauterine contraceptive device ♀
        Encounter for replacement of intrauterine contraceptive device

◄ New   ◄▬ Revised   ~~deleted~~ Deleted   Excludes 1   Excludes 2   Includes   Use additional   Code first   Code also   Unspecified

OGCR Official Guidelines   ● Unacceptable Principal Diagnosis   X Assign placeholder X   ● Use Additional Character(s)   ▶ Manifestation Code   **Coding Clinic**

- **Z30.44** Encounter for surveillance of vaginal ring hormonal contraceptive device ♀ ◀
- **Z30.45** Encounter for surveillance of transdermal patch hormonal contraceptive device ♀ ◀
- **Z30.46** Encounter for surveillance of implantable subdermal contraceptive ♀ ◀
  Encounter for checking, reinsertion or removal of implantable subdermal contraceptive ◀
- **Z30.49** Encounter for surveillance of other contraceptives ♀ ◀
  Encounter for surveillance of barrier contraception ◀
  Encounter for surveillance of diaphragm ◀
- **Z30.8** Encounter for other contraceptive management
  Encounter for postvasectomy sperm count
  Encounter for routine examination for contraceptive maintenance
  > **Excludes1**   sperm count following sterilization reversal (Z31.42)
  > sperm count for fertility testing (Z31.41)
- **Z30.9** Encounter for contraceptive management, unspecified

- **Z31** Encounter for procreative management
  > **Excludes1**   complications associated with artificial fertilization (N98.-)
  > female infertility (N97.-)
  > male infertility (N46.-)

  Z31.0 Encounter for reversal of previous sterilization
- **Z31.4** Encounter for procreative investigation and testing
  > **Excludes1**   postvasectomy sperm count (Z30.8)
  - **Z31.41** Encounter for fertility testing
    Encounter for fallopian tube patency testing
    Encounter for sperm count for fertility testing
  - **Z31.42** Aftercare following sterilization reversal
    Sperm count following sterilization reversal
  - **Z31.43** Encounter for genetic testing of female for procreative management
    Use additional code for recurrent pregnancy loss, if applicable (N96, O26.2-)
    > **Excludes1**   nonprocreative genetic testing (Z13.7-)
    - **Z31.430** Encounter of female for testing for genetic disease carrier status for procreative management ♀
    - **Z31.438** Encounter for other genetic testing of female for procreative management ♀
  - **Z31.44** Encounter for genetic testing of male for procreative management
    > **Excludes1**   nonprocreative genetic testing (Z13.7-)
    - **Z31.440** Encounter of male for testing for genetic disease carrier status for procreative management ♂
    - **Z31.441** Encounter for testing of male partner of patient with recurrent pregnancy loss ♂   A
    - **Z31.448** Encounter for other genetic testing of male for procreative management ♂ A
  - **Z31.49** Encounter for other procreative investigation and testing
- **Z31.5** Encounter for genetic counseling
- **Z31.6** Encounter for general counseling and advice on procreation
  - **Z31.61** Procreative counseling and advice using natural family planning
  - **Z31.62** Encounter for fertility preservation counseling
    Encounter for fertility preservation counseling prior to cancer therapy
    Encounter for fertility preservation counseling prior to surgical removal of gonads
  - **Z31.69** Encounter for other general counseling and advice on procreation

- **Z31.7** Encounter for procreative management and counseling for gestational carrier ◀
  > **Excludes1**   pregnant state, gestational carrier (Z33.3) ◀
- **Z31.8** Encounter for other procreative management
  - **Z31.81** Encounter for male factor infertility in female patient ♀
  - **Z31.82** Encounter for Rh incompatibility status ♀
    Coding Clinic: 2015, Q3, P40
  - **Z31.83** Encounter for assisted reproductive fertility procedure cycle ♀
    Patient undergoing in vitro fertilization cycle
    Use additional code to identify the type of infertility
    > **Excludes1**   pre-cycle diagnosis and testing - code to reason for encounter
  - **Z31.84** Encounter for fertility preservation procedure
    Encounter for fertility preservation procedure prior to cancer therapy
    Encounter for fertility preservation procedure prior to surgical removal of gonads
  - **Z31.89** Encounter for other procreative management
- **Z31.9** Encounter for procreative management, unspecified

- **Z32** Encounter for pregnancy test and childbirth and childcare instruction
- **Z32.0** Encounter for pregnancy test
  - **Z32.00** Encounter for pregnancy test, result unknown ♀
    Encounter for pregnancy test NOS
  - **Z32.01** Encounter for pregnancy test, result positive ♀   M
  - **Z32.02** Encounter for pregnancy test, result negative ♀   M
- **Z32.2** Encounter for childbirth instruction
- **Z32.3** Encounter for childcare instruction
  Encounter for prenatal or postpartum childcare instruction

- **Z33** Pregnant state
- **Z33.1** Pregnant state, incidental ♀   M
  Pregnant state NOS
  > **Excludes1**   complications of pregnancy (O00-O9A)
  > pregnant state, gestational carrier (Z33.3) ◀
- **Z33.2** Encounter for elective termination of pregnancy ♀   M
  > **Excludes1**   early fetal death with retention of dead fetus (O02.1)
  > late fetal death (O36.4)
  > spontaneous abortion (O03)
- **Z33.3** Pregnant state, gestational carrier ♀ ◀
  > **Excludes1**   encounter for procreative management and counseling for gestational carrier (Z31.7) ◀

- **Z34** Encounter for supervision of normal pregnancy
  > **Excludes1**   any complication of pregnancy (O00-O9A)
  > encounter for pregnancy test (Z32.0-)
  > encounter for supervision of high risk pregnancy (O09.-)
- **Z34.0** Encounter for supervision of normal first pregnancy
  - **Z34.00** Encounter for supervision of normal first pregnancy, unspecified trimester ♀   M
  - **Z34.01** Encounter for supervision of normal first pregnancy, first trimester ♀   M
  - **Z34.02** Encounter for supervision of normal first pregnancy, second trimester ♀   M
  - **Z34.03** Encounter for supervision of normal first pregnancy, third trimester ♀   M

N Newborn Age: 0   **P** Pediatric Age: 0–17   **M** Maternity DX: 12–55   **A** Adult Age: 15–124   ♀ Females Only   ♂ Males Only

Complication\Comorbidity   Major C\C   (Ex) CC/MCC Exclusions   Hospital-Acquired Condition

CHAPTER 21 (Z00-Z99)

1615

| First trimester (0 to 14 weeks) | Second trimester (14 to 28 weeks) | Third trimester (28 weeks to delivery) |

Figure 21-1 Trimesters. (From Shiland, Betsy J. Medical Terminology & Anatomy for ICD-10 Coding, ed 2, Mosby, 2015)

- **Z34.8 Encounter for supervision of other normal pregnancy**
  - **Z34.80 Encounter for supervision of other normal pregnancy, unspecified trimester** ♀   M
  - **Z34.81 Encounter for supervision of other normal pregnancy, first trimester** ♀   M
  - **Z34.82 Encounter for supervision of other normal pregnancy, second trimester** ♀   M
  - **Z34.83 Encounter for supervision of other normal pregnancy, third trimester** ♀   M
- **Z34.9 Encounter for supervision of normal pregnancy, unspecified**
  - **Z34.90 Encounter for supervision of normal pregnancy, unspecified, unspecified trimester** ♀   M
  - **Z34.91 Encounter for supervision of normal pregnancy, unspecified, first trimester** ♀   M
  - **Z34.92 Encounter for supervision of normal pregnancy, unspecified, second trimester** ♀   M
  - **Z34.93 Encounter for supervision of normal pregnancy, unspecified, third trimester** ♀   M

- **Z36 Encounter for antenatal screening of mother** ♀   M
  - **Excludes1**   abnormal findings on antenatal screening of mother (O28.-)
    diagnostic examination - code to sign or symptom
    encounter for suspected maternal and fetal conditions ruled out (Z03.7-)
    suspected fetal condition affecting management of pregnancy - code to condition in Chapter 15
  - **Excludes2**   genetic counseling and testing (Z31.43-, Z31.5)
    routine prenatal care (Z34)

- **Z3A Weeks of gestation**
  - **Note:** Codes from category Z3A are for use, only on the maternal record, to indicate the weeks of gestation of the pregnancy, if known.
  - *Code first complications of pregnancy, childbirth and the puerperium (O00-O9A)*
  - Coding Clinic: 2013, Q2, P33
  - **Z3A.0 Weeks of gestation of pregnancy, unspecified or less than 10 weeks**
    - **Z3A.00 Weeks of gestation of pregnancy not specified** ♀   M
    - **Z3A.01 Less than 8 weeks gestation of pregnancy** ♀   M
    - **Z3A.08 8 weeks gestation of pregnancy** ♀   M
    - **Z3A.09 9 weeks gestation of pregnancy** ♀   M

- **Z3A.1 Weeks of gestation of pregnancy, weeks 10-19**
  - **Z3A.10 10 weeks gestation of pregnancy** ♀   M
  - **Z3A.11 11 weeks gestation of pregnancy** ♀   M
  - **Z3A.12 12 weeks gestation of pregnancy** ♀   M
  - **Z3A.13 13 weeks gestation of pregnancy** ♀   M
  - **Z3A.14 14 weeks gestation of pregnancy** ♀   M
  - **Z3A.15 15 weeks gestation of pregnancy** ♀   M
  - **Z3A.16 16 weeks gestation of pregnancy** ♀   M
  - **Z3A.17 17 weeks gestation of pregnancy** ♀   M
  - **Z3A.18 18 weeks gestation of pregnancy** ♀   M
  - **Z3A.19 19 weeks gestation of pregnancy** ♀   M
- **Z3A.2 Weeks of gestation of pregnancy, weeks 20-29**
  - **Z3A.20 20 weeks gestation of pregnancy** ♀   M
  - **Z3A.21 21 weeks gestation of pregnancy** ♀   M
  - **Z3A.22 22 weeks gestation of pregnancy** ♀   M
  - **Z3A.23 23 weeks gestation of pregnancy** ♀   M
  - **Z3A.24 24 weeks gestation of pregnancy** ♀   M
  - **Z3A.25 25 weeks gestation of pregnancy** ♀   M
  - **Z3A.26 26 weeks gestation of pregnancy** ♀   M
  - **Z3A.27 27 weeks gestation of pregnancy** ♀   M
  - **Z3A.28 28 weeks gestation of pregnancy** ♀   M
  - **Z3A.29 29 weeks gestation of pregnancy** ♀   M
- **Z3A.3 Weeks of gestation of pregnancy, weeks 30-39**
  - **Z3A.30 30 weeks gestation of pregnancy** ♀   M
  - **Z3A.31 31 weeks gestation of pregnancy** ♀   M
  - **Z3A.32 32 weeks gestation of pregnancy** ♀   M
  - **Z3A.33 33 weeks gestation of pregnancy** ♀   M
  - **Z3A.34 34 weeks gestation of pregnancy** ♀   M
  - **Z3A.35 35 weeks gestation of pregnancy** ♀   M
  - **Z3A.36 36 weeks gestation of pregnancy** ♀   M
  - **Z3A.37 37 weeks gestation of pregnancy** ♀   M
  - **Z3A.38 38 weeks gestation of pregnancy** ♀   M
  - Coding Clinic: 2016, Q2, P34
  - **Z3A.39 39 weeks gestation of pregnancy** ♀   M
- **Z3A.4 Weeks of gestation of pregnancy, weeks 40 or greater**
  - **Z3A.40 40 weeks gestation of pregnancy** ♀   M
  - **Z3A.41 41 weeks gestation of pregnancy** ♀   M
  - **Z3A.42 42 weeks gestation of pregnancy** ♀   M
  - **Z3A.49 Greater than 42 weeks gestation of pregnancy** ♀   M

- **Z37 Outcome of delivery**
  - This category is intended for use as an additional code to identify the outcome of delivery on the mother's record. It is not for use on the newborn record.
  - **Excludes1**   stillbirth (P95)
  - **Z37.0 Single live birth** ♀   M
    - Coding Clinic: 2016, Q2, P34
  - **Z37.1 Single stillbirth** ♀   M
  - **Z37.2 Twins, both liveborn** ♀   M
  - **Z37.3 Twins, one liveborn and one stillborn** ♀   M
  - **Z37.4 Twins, both stillborn** ♀   M
  - **Z37.5 Other multiple births, all liveborn**
    - **Z37.50 Multiple births, unspecified, all liveborn** ♀   M
    - **Z37.51 Triplets, all liveborn** ♀   M
    - **Z37.52 Quadruplets, all liveborn** ♀   M
    - **Z37.53 Quintuplets, all liveborn** ♀   M
    - **Z37.54 Sextuplets, all liveborn** ♀   M
    - **Z37.59 Other multiple births, all liveborn** ♀   M

◀ New   ⬅ Revised   ~~deleted~~ Deleted   Excludes 1   Excludes 2   Includes   Use additional   Code first   Code also   Unspecified
OGCR Official Guidelines   ● Unacceptable Principal Diagnosis   X Assign placeholder X   ● Use Additional Character(s)   ▮ Manifestation Code   **Coding Clinic**

- **Z37.6** Other multiple births, some liveborn
  - **Z37.60** Multiple births, unspecified, some liveborn ♀ M
  - **Z37.61** Triplets, some liveborn ♀ M
  - **Z37.62** Quadruplets, some liveborn ♀ M
  - **Z37.63** Quintuplets, some liveborn ♀ M
  - **Z37.64** Sextuplets, some liveborn ♀ M
  - **Z37.69** Other multiple births, some liveborn ♀ M
- **Z37.7** Other multiple births, all stillborn ♀ M
- **Z37.9** Outcome of delivery, unspecified ♀ M
  Multiple birth NOS
  Single birth NOS

- **Z38** Liveborn infants according to place of birth and type of delivery
  This category is for use as the principal code on the initial record of a newborn baby. It is to be used for the initial birth record only. It is not to be used on the mother's record.
  Coding Clinic: 2015, Q2, P15
  - **Z38.0** Single liveborn infant, born in hospital
    Single liveborn infant, born in birthing center or other health care facility
    - **Z38.00** Single liveborn infant, delivered vaginally N
    - **Z38.01** Single liveborn infant, delivered by cesarean N
  - **Z38.1** Single liveborn infant, born outside hospital N
  - **Z38.2** Single liveborn infant, unspecified as to place of birth N
    Single liveborn infant NOS
  - **Z38.3** Twin liveborn infant, born in hospital
    - **Z38.30** Twin liveborn infant, delivered vaginally N
    - **Z38.31** Twin liveborn infant, delivered by cesarean N
  - **Z38.4** Twin liveborn infant, born outside hospital N
  - **Z38.5** Twin liveborn infant, unspecified as to place of birth N
  - **Z38.6** Other multiple liveborn infant, born in hospital
    - **Z38.61** Triplet liveborn infant, delivered vaginally N
    - **Z38.62** Triplet liveborn infant, delivered by cesarean N
    - **Z38.63** Quadruplet liveborn infant, delivered vaginally N
    - **Z38.64** Quadruplet liveborn infant, delivered by cesarean N
    - **Z38.65** Quintuplet liveborn infant, delivered vaginally N
    - **Z38.66** Quintuplet liveborn infant, delivered by cesarean N
    - **Z38.68** Other multiple liveborn infant, delivered vaginally N
    - **Z38.69** Other multiple liveborn infant, delivered by cesarean N
  - **Z38.7** Other multiple liveborn infant, born outside hospital N
  - **Z38.8** Other multiple liveborn infant, unspecified as to place of birth N

- **Z39** Encounter for maternal postpartum care and examination
  - **Z39.0** Encounter for care and examination of mother immediately after delivery ♀ M
    Care and observation in uncomplicated cases when the delivery occurs outside a healthcare facility
    Excludes1 care for postpartum complication - see Alphabetic index
  - **Z39.1** Encounter for care and examination of lactating mother ♀ M
    Encounter for supervision of lactation
    Excludes1 disorders of lactation (O92.-)
  - **Z39.2** Encounter for routine postpartum follow-up ♀ M

ENCOUNTERS FOR OTHER SPECIFIC HEALTH CARE (Z40-Z53)

Categories Z40-Z53 are intended for use to indicate a reason for care. They may be used for patients who have already been treated for a disease or injury, but who are receiving aftercare or prophylactic care, or care to consolidate the treatment, or to deal with a residual state

Excludes2 follow-up examination for medical surveillance after treatment (Z08-Z09)

- **Z40** Encounter for prophylactic surgery
  Excludes1 organ donations (Z52.-)
  therapeutic organ removal - code to condition
  - **Z40.0** Encounter for prophylactic surgery for risk factors related to malignant neoplasms
    Admission for prophylactic organ removal
    Use additional code to identify risk factor
    - **Z40.00** Encounter for prophylactic removal of unspecified organ
    - **Z40.01** Encounter for prophylactic removal of breast
    - **Z40.02** Encounter for prophylactic removal of ovary ♀
    - **Z40.09** Encounter for prophylactic removal of other organ
  - **Z40.8** Encounter for other prophylactic surgery
  - **Z40.9** Encounter for prophylactic surgery, unspecified

- **Z41** Encounter for procedures for purposes other than remedying health state
  - **Z41.1** Encounter for cosmetic surgery
    Encounter for cosmetic breast implant
    Encounter for cosmetic procedure
    Excludes1 encounter for plastic and reconstructive surgery following medical procedure or healed injury (Z42.-)
    encounter for post-mastectomy breast implantation (Z42.1)
  - **Z41.2** Encounter for routine and ritual male circumcision ♂
  - **Z41.3** Encounter for ear piercing
  - **Z41.8** Encounter for other procedures for purposes other than remedying health state
  - **Z41.9** Encounter for procedure for purposes other than remedying health state, unspecified

- **Z42** Encounter for plastic and reconstructive surgery following medical procedure or healed injury
  Excludes1 encounter for cosmetic plastic surgery (Z41.1)
  encounter for plastic surgery for treatment of current injury - code to relevent injury
  - **Z42.1** Encounter for breast reconstruction following mastectomy A
    Excludes1 deformity and disproportion of reconstructed breast (N65.1-)
  - **Z42.8** Encounter for other plastic and reconstructive surgery following medical procedure or healed injury

CHAPTER 21 (Z00-Z99)

N Newborn Age: 0   P Pediatric Age: 0–17   M Maternity DX: 12–55   A Adult Age: 15–124   ♀ Females Only   ♂ Males Only
⬥ Complication\Comorbidity   ⬥ Major C\C   (Ex) CC/MCC Exclusions   ⬥ Hospital-Acquired Condition

1617

● Z43   Encounter for attention to artificial openings

Includes   closure of artificial openings
passage of sounds or bougies through artificial
openings
reforming artificial openings
removal of catheter from artificial openings
toilet or cleansing of artificial openings

Excludes1   artificial opening status only, without need for
care (Z93.-)
complications of external stoma (J95.0-, K94.-,
N99.5-)

Excludes2   fitting and adjustment of prosthetic and other
devices (Z44-Z46)

Z43.0   Encounter for attention to tracheostomy

Z43.1   Encounter for attention to gastrostomy 🔖
Ⓔ⨯ Z43.1

Z43.2   Encounter for attention to ileostomy

Z43.3   Encounter for attention to colostomy

**Z43.4   Encounter for attention to other artificial openings of
digestive tract**

Z43.5   Encounter for attention to cystostomy

**Z43.6   Encounter for attention to other artificial openings of
urinary tract**
Encounter for attention to nephrostomy
Encounter for attention to ureterostomy
Encounter for attention to urethrostomy

Z43.7   Encounter for attention to artificial vagina

Z43.8   Encounter for attention to other artificial openings

● Z43.9   Encounter for attention to unspecified artificial opening

**● Z44   Encounter for fitting and adjustment of external prosthetic
device**

Includes   removal or replacement of external prosthetic
device

Excludes1   malfunction or other complications of device - see
Alphabetical Index presence of prosthetic
device (Z97.-)

● Z44.0   Encounter for fitting and adjustment of artificial arm

**● Z44.00   Encounter for fitting and adjustment of
unspecified artificial arm**

**Z44.001   Encounter for fitting and adjustment
of unspecified right artificial arm**

**Z44.002   Encounter for fitting and adjustment
of unspecified left artificial arm**

**Z44.009   Encounter for fitting and adjustment
of unspecified artificial arm,
unspecified arm**

**● Z44.01   Encounter for fitting and adjustment of
complete artificial arm**

**Z44.011   Encounter for fitting and adjustment
of complete right artificial arm**

**Z44.012   Encounter for fitting and adjustment
of complete left artificial arm**

**Z44.019   Encounter for fitting and adjustment
of complete artificial arm, unspecified
arm**

**● Z44.02   Encounter for fitting and adjustment of partial
artificial arm**

**Z44.021   Encounter for fitting and adjustment
of partial artificial right arm**

**Z44.022   Encounter for fitting and adjustment
of partial artificial left arm**

**Z44.029   Encounter for fitting and adjustment
of partial artificial arm, unspecified
arm**

● Z44.1   Encounter for fitting and adjustment of artificial leg

**● Z44.10   Encounter for fitting and adjustment of
unspecified artificial leg**

**Z44.101   Encounter for fitting and adjustment
of unspecified right artificial leg**

**Z44.102   Encounter for fitting and adjustment
of unspecified left artificial leg**

**Z44.109   Encounter for fitting and adjustment
of unspecified artificial leg,
unspecified leg**

**● Z44.11   Encounter for fitting and adjustment of
complete artificial leg**

**Z44.111   Encounter for fitting and adjustment
of complete right artificial leg**

**Z44.112   Encounter for fitting and adjustment
of complete left artificial leg**

**Z44.119   Encounter for fitting and adjustment
of complete artificial leg, unspecified
leg**

**● Z44.12   Encounter for fitting and adjustment of partial
artificial leg**

**Z44.121   Encounter for fitting and adjustment
of partial artificial right leg**

**Z44.122   Encounter for fitting and adjustment
of partial artificial left leg**

**Z44.129   Encounter for fitting and adjustment
of partial artificial leg, unspecified leg**

● Z44.2   Encounter for fitting and adjustment of artificial eye

Excludes1   mechanical complication of ocular
prosthesis (T85.3)

**Z44.20   Encounter for fitting and adjustment of artificial
eye, unspecified**

**Z44.21   Encounter for fitting and adjustment of artificial
right eye**

**Z44.22   Encounter for fitting and adjustment of artificial
left eye**

**● Z44.3   Encounter for fitting and adjustment of external breast
prosthesis**

Excludes1   complications of breast implant (T85.4-)
encounter for adjustment or removal of
breast implant (Z45.81-)
encounter for initial breast implant
insertion for cosmetic breast
augmentation (Z41.1)
encounter for breast reconstruction
following mastectomy (Z42.1)

**Z44.30   Encounter for fitting and adjustment of external
breast prosthesis, unspecified breast**

**Z44.31   Encounter for fitting and adjustment of external
right breast prosthesis**

**Z44.32   Encounter for fitting and adjustment of external
left breast prosthesis**

**Z44.8   Encounter for fitting and adjustment of other external
prosthetic devices**

**● Z44.9   Encounter for fitting and adjustment of unspecified
external prosthetic device**

◀ New   ◀▥ Revised   ~~deleted~~ Deleted   Excludes 1   Excludes 2   Includes   Use additional   Code first   Code also   Unspecified
OGCR Official Guidelines   ● Unacceptable Principal Diagnosis   X Assign placeholder X   ▶ Use Additional Character(s)   ▶ Manifestation Code   Coding Clinic

● **Z45 Encounter for adjustment and management of implanted device**

Includes   removal or replacement of implanted device

Excludes1   malfunction or other complications of device - see Alphabetical Index

presence of prosthetic and other devices (Z95-Z97)

Excludes2   encounter for fitting and adjustment of non-implanted device (Z46.-)

● **Z45.0 Encounter for adjustment and management of cardiac device**

   ● **Z45.01 Encounter for adjustment and management of cardiac pacemaker**

     Encounter for adjustment and management of cardiac resynchronization therapy pacemaker (CRT-P) ◄

     Excludes1   encounter for adjustment and management of automatic implantable cardiac defibrillator with synchronous cardiac pacemaker (Z45.02)

     Z45.010 Encounter for checking and testing of cardiac pacemaker pulse generator [battery]

       Encounter for replacing cardiac pacemaker pulse generator [battery]

       MCE: Questionable admission when principal dx

     Z45.018 Encounter for adjustment and management of other part of cardiac pacemaker

       MCE: Questionable admission when principal dx

   Z45.02 Encounter for adjustment and management of automatic implantable cardiac defibrillator

     Encounter for adjustment and management of automatic implantable cardiac defibrillator with synchronous cardiac pacemaker

     Encounter for adjustment and management of cardiac resynchronization therapy defibrillator (CRT-D) ◄

     MCE: Questionable admission when principal dx

   Z45.09 Encounter for adjustment and management of other cardiac device

     MCE: Questionable admission when principal dx

● **Z45.1 Encounter for adjustment and management of infusion pump**

● **Z45.2 Encounter for adjustment and management of vascular access device**

   Encounter for adjustment and management of vascular catheters

   Excludes1   encounter for adjustment and management of renal dialysis catheter (Z49.01)

● **Z45.3 Encounter for adjustment and management of implanted devices of the special senses**

   Z45.31 Encounter for adjustment and management of implanted visual substitution device

   ● **Z45.32 Encounter for adjustment and management of implanted hearing device**

     Excludes1   encounter for fitting and adjustment of hearing aide (Z46.1)

     Z45.320 Encounter for adjustment and management of bone conduction device

     Z45.321 Encounter for adjustment and management of cochlear device

     Z45.328 Encounter for adjustment and management of other implanted hearing device

● **Z45.4 Encounter for adjustment and management of implanted nervous system device**

   Z45.41 Encounter for adjustment and management of cerebrospinal fluid drainage device

     Encounter for adjustment and management of cerebral ventricular (communicating) shunt

   Z45.42 Encounter for adjustment and management of neuropacemaker (brain) (peripheral nerve) (spinal cord)

   Z45.49 Encounter for adjustment and management of other implanted nervous system device

● **Z45.8 Encounter for adjustment and management of other implanted devices**

   ● **Z45.81 Encounter for adjustment or removal of breast implant**

     Encounter for elective implant exchange (different material) (different size)

     Encounter removal of tissue expander without synchronous insertion of permanent implant

     Excludes1   complications of breast implant (T85.4-)

       encounter for initial breast implant insertion for cosmetic breast augmentation (Z41.1)

       encounter for breast reconstruction following mastectomy (Z42.1)

     Z45.811 Encounter for adjustment or removal of right breast implant

     Z45.812 Encounter for adjustment or removal of left breast implant

     Z45.819 Encounter for adjustment or removal of unspecified breast implant

   ● **Z45.82 Encounter for adjustment or removal of myringotomy device (stent) (tube)**

   ● **Z45.89 Encounter for adjustment and management of other implanted devices**

● **Z45.9 Encounter for adjustment and management of unspecified implanted device**

● **Z46 Encounter for fitting and adjustment of other devices**

Includes   removal or replacement of other device

Excludes1   malfunction or other complications of device - see Alphabetical Index

Excludes2   encounter for fitting and management of implanted devices (Z45.-)

   issue of repeat prescription only (Z76.0)

   presence of prosthetic and other devices (Z95-Z97)

● **Z46.0 Encounter for fitting and adjustment of spectacles and contact lenses**

● **Z46.1 Encounter for fitting and adjustment of hearing aid**

   Excludes1   encounter for adjustment and management of implanted hearing device (Z45.32-)

● **Z46.2 Encounter for fitting and adjustment of other devices related to nervous system and special senses**

   Excludes2   encounter for adjustment and management of implanted nervous system device (Z45.4-)

     encounter for adjustment and management of implanted visual substitution device (Z45.31)

● **Z46.3 Encounter for fitting and adjustment of dental prosthetic device**

   Encounter for fitting and adjustment of dentures

● **Z46.4 Encounter for fitting and adjustment of orthodontic device**

CHAPTER 21 (Z00-Z99)

● **Z46.5**   **Encounter for fitting and adjustment of other gastrointestinal appliance and device**

> **Excludes1**   encounter for attention to artificial openings of digestive tract (Z43.1-Z43.4)

  ● **Z46.51**   **Encounter for fitting and adjustment of gastric lap band**

  ● **Z46.59**   **Encounter for fitting and adjustment of other gastrointestinal appliance and device**

● **Z46.6**   **Encounter for fitting and adjustment of urinary device**

> **Excludes2**   attention to artificial openings of urinary tract (Z43.5, Z43.6)

● **Z46.8**   **Encounter for fitting and adjustment of other specified devices**

  ● **Z46.81**   **Encounter for fitting and adjustment of insulin pump**
> Encounter for insulin pump instruction and training
> Encounter for insulin pump titration

  Z46.82   **Encounter for fitting and adjustment of non-vascular catheter**

  ● **Z46.89**   **Encounter for fitting and adjustment of other specified devices**
> Encounter for fitting and adjustment of wheelchair

● **Z46.9**   **Encounter for fitting and adjustment of unspecified device**

● **Z47**   **Orthopedic aftercare**

> **Excludes1**   aftercare for healing fracture - code to fracture with 7th character D

  Z47.1   **Aftercare following joint replacement surgery**
> Use additional code to identify the joint (Z96.6-)

  Z47.2   **Encounter for removal of internal fixation device**

> **Excludes1**   encounter for adjustment of internal fixation device for fracture treatment - code to fracture with appropriate 7th character
> encounter for removal of external fixation device - code to fracture with 7th character D
> infection or inflammatory reaction to internal fixation device (T84.6-)
> mechanical complication of internal fixation device (T84.1-)

● **Z47.3**   **Aftercare following explantation of joint prosthesis**
> Aftercare following explantation of joint prosthesis, staged procedure
> Encounter for joint prosthesis insertion following prior explantation of joint prosthesis
> **Coding Clinic: 2015, Q1, P17**

  Z47.31   **Aftercare following explantation of shoulder joint prosthesis**

> **Excludes1**   acquired absence of shoulder joint following prior explantation of shoulder joint prosthesis (Z89.23-)
> shoulder joint prosthesis explantation status (Z89.23-)

  Z47.32   **Aftercare following explantation of hip joint prosthesis**

> **Excludes1**   acquired absence of hip joint following prior explantation of hip joint prosthesis (Z89.62-)
> hip joint prosthesis explantation status (Z89.62-)
> **Coding Clinic: 2015, Q1, P17**

  Z47.33   **Aftercare following explantation of knee joint prosthesis**

> **Excludes1**   acquired absence of knee joint following prior explantation of knee prosthesis (Z89.52-)
> knee joint prosthesis explantation status (Z89.52-)

  Z47.8   **Encounter for other orthopedic aftercare**

  Z47.81   **Encounter for orthopedic aftercare following surgical amputation**
> Use additional code to identify the limb amputated (Z89.-)

  Z47.82   **Encounter for orthopedic aftercare following scoliosis surgery**

  Z47.89   **Encounter for other orthopedic aftercare**
> **Coding Clinic: 2015, Q1, P8**

● **Z48**   **Encounter for other postprocedural aftercare**

> **Excludes1**   encounter for follow-up examination after completed treatment (Z08-Z09)

> **Excludes2**   encounter for attention to artificial openings (Z43.-)
> encounter for fitting and adjustment of prosthetic and other devices (Z44-Z46)

● **Z48.0**   **Encounter for attention to dressings, sutures and drains**

> **Excludes1**   encounter for planned postprocedural wound closure (Z48.1)

  ● **Z48.00**   **Encounter for change or removal of nonsurgical wound dressing**
> Encounter for change or removal of wound dressing NOS

  ● **Z48.01**   **Encounter for change or removal of surgical wound dressing**
> **Coding Clinic: 2015, Q4, P38**

  ● **Z48.02**   **Encounter for removal of sutures**
> Encounter for removal of staples
> **Coding Clinic: 2015, Q1, P6**

  Z48.03   **Encounter for change or removal of drains**

  Z48.1   **Encounter for planned postprocedural wound closure**

> **Excludes1**   encounter for attention to dressings and sutures (Z48.0-)

● **Z48.2**   **Encounter for aftercare following organ transplant**

  Z48.21   **Encounter for aftercare following heart transplant** 🔖
> CC when PDx is its own CC
> ⓔⅹ D47.Z1, T86.20-T86.39, T86.850-T86.859, T86.90-T86.99, Z94.1, Z94.3, Z94.89-Z94.9

  Z48.22   **Encounter for aftercare following kidney transplant** 🔖
> CC when PDx is its own CC
> ⓔⅹ D47.Z1, T86.10-T86.19, T86.850-T86.859, T86.90-T86.99, Z94.0, Z94.89-Z94.9

  Z48.23   **Encounter for aftercare following liver transplant** 🔖
> CC when PDx is its own CC
> ⓔⅹ D47.Z1, T86.40-T86.49, T86.850-T86.859, T86.90-T86.99, Z94.4, Z94.89, Z94.9

  Z48.24   **Encounter for aftercare following lung transplant** 🔖
> CC when PDx is its own CC
> ⓔⅹ D47.Z1, T86.810-T86.819, T86.850-T86.859, T86.90-T86.99, Z94.2, Z94.89-Z94.9

  ● **Z48.28**   **Encounter for aftercare following multiple organ transplant**

    Z48.280   **Encounter for aftercare following heart-lung transplant** 🔖
> CC when PDx is its own CC
> ⓔⅹ See Z48.21

    Z48.288   **Encounter for aftercare following multiple organ transplant**

  ● **Z48.29**   **Encounter for aftercare following other organ transplant**

    Z48.290   **Encounter for aftercare following bone marrow transplant** 🔖
> CC when PDx is its own CC
> ⓔⅹ D47.Z1, D89.810-D89.813, T86.00-T86.09, T86.850-T86.859, T86.90-T86.99, Z94.9

    Z48.298   **Encounter for aftercare following other organ transplant**

Z48.3   Aftercare following surgery for neoplasm
>   Use additional code to identify the neoplasm

● **Z48.8   Encounter for other specified postprocedural aftercare**

●   **Z48.81   Encounter for surgical aftercare following surgery on specified body systems**
>   These codes identify the body system requiring aftercare. They are for use in conjunction with other aftercare codes to fully explain the aftercare encounter. The condition treated should also be coded if still present.
>
>   **Excludes1**   aftercare for injury - code the injury with 7th character D
>   aftercare following surgery for neoplasm (Z48.3)
>
>   **Excludes2**   aftercare following organ transplant (Z48.2-)
>   orthopedic aftercare (Z47.-)

   Z48.810   Encounter for surgical aftercare following surgery on the sense organs

   Z48.811   Encounter for surgical aftercare following surgery on the nervous system
>   **Excludes2**   encounter for surgical aftercare following surgery on the sense organs (Z48.810)

   Z48.812   Encounter for surgical aftercare following surgery on the circulatory system
>   Coding Clinic: 2012, Q4, P96

   Z48.813   Encounter for surgical aftercare following surgery on the respiratory system

   Z48.814   Encounter for surgical aftercare following surgery on the teeth or oral cavity

   Z48.815   Encounter for surgical aftercare following surgery on the digestive system
>   Coding Clinic: 2015, Q4, P38

   Z48.816   Encounter for surgical aftercare following surgery on the genitourinary system
>   **Excludes1**   encounter for aftercare following sterilization reversal (Z31.42)

   Z48.817   Encounter for surgical aftercare following surgery on the skin and subcutaneous tissue
>   Coding Clinic: 2015, Q1, P6

   Z48.89   Encounter for other specified surgical aftercare

● **Z49   Encounter for care involving renal dialysis**
>   Code also associated end stage renal disease (N18.6)

●   **Z49.0   Preparatory care for renal dialysis**
>   Encounter for dialysis instruction and training

   Z49.01   Encounter for fitting and adjustment of extracorporeal dialysis catheter
>   Removal or replacement of renal dialysis catheter
>   Toilet or cleansing of renal dialysis catheter

●   **Z49.02   Encounter for fitting and adjustment of peritoneal dialysis catheter**

●   **Z49.3   Encounter for adequacy testing for dialysis**

●   **Z49.31   Encounter for adequacy testing for hemodialysis**

●   **Z49.32   Encounter for adequacy testing for peritoneal dialysis**
>   Encounter for peritoneal equilibration test

● **Z51   Encounter for other aftercare and medical care** ◀▥
>   Code also condition requiring care
>   **Excludes1**   follow-up examination after treatment (Z08-Z09)

   Z51.0   Encounter for antineoplastic radiation therapy

● **Z51.1   Encounter for antineoplastic chemotherapy and immunotherapy**
>   **Excludes2**   encounter for chemotherapy and immunotherapy for nonneoplastic condition-code to condition

   Z51.11   Encounter for antineoplastic chemotherapy
>   Coding Clinic: 2015, Q3, P19

   Z51.12   Encounter for antineoplastic immunotherapy

● **Z51.5   Encounter for palliative care**

● **Z51.6   Encounter for desensitization to allergens** ◀

● **Z51.8   Encounter for other specified aftercare**
>   **Excludes1**   holiday relief care (Z75.5)

   Z51.81   Encounter for therapeutic drug level monitoring
>   Code also any long-term (current) drug therapy (Z79.-)
>   **Excludes1**   encounter for blood-drug test for administrative or medicolegal reasons (Z02.83)

●   **Z51.89   Encounter for other specified aftercare**
>   MCE: This code may be considered "acceptable" when a secondary diagnosis is also coded on the record.
>   Coding Clinic: 2012, Q4, P96-97

● **Z52   Donors of organs and tissues**
>   **Includes**   autologous and other living donors
>   **Excludes1**   cadaveric donor - omit code
>   examination of potential donor (Z00.5)
>   Coding Clinic: 2012, Q4, P100

● **Z52.0   Blood donor**

●   **Z52.00   Unspecified blood donor**

   ● **Z52.000   Unspecified donor, whole blood**
   ● **Z52.001   Unspecified donor, stem cells**
   ● **Z52.008   Unspecified donor, other blood**

●   **Z52.01   Autologous blood donor**
   ● **Z52.010   Autologous donor, whole blood**
   ● **Z52.011   Autologous donor, stem cells**
   ● **Z52.018   Autologous donor, other blood**

●   **Z52.09   Other blood donor**
>   Volunteer donor
   ● **Z52.090   Other blood donor, whole blood**
   ● **Z52.091   Other blood donor, stem cells**
   ● **Z52.098   Other blood donor, other blood**

● **Z52.1   Skin donor**
   Z52.10   Skin donor, unspecified
   Z52.11   Skin donor, autologous
   Z52.19   Skin donor, other

● **Z52.2   Bone donor**
   Z52.20   Bone donor, unspecified
   Z52.21   Bone donor, autologous
   Z52.29   Bone donor, other

   Z52.3   Bone marrow donor
   Z52.4   Kidney donor
   Z52.5   Cornea donor
   Z52.6   Liver donor
>   Coding Clinic: 2012, Q4, P100

N Newborn Age: 0   **P** Pediatric Age: 0-17   **M** Maternity DX: 12-55   **A** Adult Age: 15-124   ♀ Females Only   ♂ Males Only

🔖 Complication\Comorbidity   🔖 Major C\C   (Ex.) CC/MCC Exclusions   🔖 Hospital-Acquired Condition

● **Z52.8** Donor of other specified organs or tissues
  ● **Z52.81** Egg (Oocyte) donor
    ● **Z52.810** Egg (Oocyte) donor under age 35, anonymous recipient ♀
      Egg donor under age 35 NOS
    ● **Z52.811** Egg (Oocyte) donor under age 35, designated recipient ♀
    ● **Z52.812** Egg (Oocyte) donor age 35 and over, anonymous recipient ♀
      Egg donor age 35 and over NOS
    ● **Z52.813** Egg (Oocyte) donor age 35 and over, designated recipient ♀
    ● **Z52.819** Egg (Oocyte) donor, unspecified ♀
  Z52.89 Donor of other specified organs or tissues
Z52.9 Donor of unspecified organ or tissue
  Donor NOS

● **Z53** Persons encountering health services for specific procedures and treatment, not carried out
  ● **Z53.0** Procedure and treatment not carried out because of contraindication
    ● **Z53.01** Procedure and treatment not carried out due to patient smoking
    ● **Z53.09** Procedure and treatment not carried out because of other contraindication
  ● **Z53.1** Procedure and treatment not carried out because of patient's decision for reasons of belief and group pressure
  ● **Z53.2** Procedure and treatment not carried out because of patient's decision for other and unspecified reasons
    ● **Z53.20** Procedure and treatment not carried out because of patient's decision for unspecified reasons
    ● **Z53.21** Procedure and treatment not carried out due to patient leaving prior to being seen by health care provider
    ● **Z53.29** Procedure and treatment not carried out because of patient's decision for other reasons
  ● **Z53.3** Procedure converted to open procedure ◀
    ● **Z53.31** Laparoscopic surgical procedure converted to open procedure ◀
    ● **Z53.32** Thoracoscopic surgical procedure converted to open procedure ◀
    ● **Z53.33** Arthroscopic surgical procedure converted to open procedure ◀
    ● **Z53.39** Other specified procedure converted to open procedure ◀
  ● **Z53.8** Procedure and treatment not carried out for other reasons
  ● **Z53.9** Procedure and treatment not carried out, unspecified reason

PERSONS WITH POTENTIAL HEALTH HAZARDS RELATED TO SOCIOECONOMIC AND PSYCHOSOCIAL CIRCUMSTANCES (Z55-Z65)

● **Z55** Problems related to education and literacy
  Excludes1 disorders of psychological development (F80-F89)
  ● **Z55.0** Illiteracy and low-level literacy
  ● **Z55.1** Schooling unavailable and unattainable
  ● **Z55.2** Failed school examinations
  ● **Z55.3** Underachievement in school
  ● **Z55.4** Educational maladjustment and discord with teachers and classmates
  ● **Z55.8** Other problems related to education and literacy
    Problems related to inadequate teaching
  ● **Z55.9** Problems related to education and literacy, unspecified
    Academic problems NOS

● **Z56** Problems related to employment and unemployment
  Excludes2 occupational exposure to risk factors (Z57.-)
    problems related to housing and economic circumstances (Z59.-)
  ● **Z56.0** Unemployment, unspecified
  ● **Z56.1** Change of job
  ● **Z56.2** Threat of job loss
  ● **Z56.3** Stressful work schedule
  ● **Z56.4** Discord with boss and workmates
  ● **Z56.5** Uncongenial work environment
    Difficult conditions at work
  ● **Z56.6** Other physical and mental strain related to work
  ● **Z56.8** Other problems related to employment
    ● **Z56.81** Sexual harassment on the job
    ● **Z56.82** Military deployment status
      Individual (civilian or military) currently deployed in theater or in support of military war, peacekeeping and humanitarian operations
    ● **Z56.89** Other problems related to employment
  ● **Z56.9** Unspecified problems related to employment
    Occupational problems NOS

● **Z57** Occupational exposure to risk factors
  ● **Z57.0** Occupational exposure to noise
  ● **Z57.1** Occupational exposure to radiation
  ● **Z57.2** Occupational exposure to dust
  ● **Z57.3** Occupational exposure to other air contaminants
    ● **Z57.31** Occupational exposure to environmental tobacco smoke
      Excludes2 exposure to environmental tobacco smoke (Z77.22)
    ● **Z57.39** Occupational exposure to other air contaminants
  ● **Z57.4** Occupational exposure to toxic agents in agriculture
    Occupational exposure to solids, liquids, gases or vapors in agriculture
  ● **Z57.5** Occupational exposure to toxic agents in other industries
    Occupational exposure to solids, liquids, gases or vapors in other industries
  ● **Z57.6** Occupational exposure to extreme temperature
  ● **Z57.7** Occupational exposure to vibration
  ● **Z57.8** Occupational exposure to other risk factors
  ● **Z57.9** Occupational exposure to unspecified risk factor

● **Z59** Problems related to housing and economic circumstances
  Excludes2 problems related to upbringing (Z62.-)
  ● **Z59.0** Homelessness
  ● **Z59.1** Inadequate housing
    Lack of heating
    Restriction of space
    Technical defects in home preventing adequate care
    Unsatisfactory surroundings
    Excludes1 problems related to the natural and physical environment (Z77.1-)
  ● **Z59.2** Discord with neighbors, lodgers and landlord
  ● **Z59.3** Problems related to living in residential institution
    Boarding-school resident
    Excludes1 institutional upbringing (Z62.2)
  ● **Z59.4** Lack of adequate food and safe drinking water
    Inadequate drinking water supply
    Excludes1 effects of hunger (T73.0)
      inappropriate diet or eating habits (Z72.4)
      malnutrition (E40-E46)
  ● **Z59.5** Extreme poverty
  ● **Z59.6** Low income
  ● **Z59.7** Insufficient social insurance and welfare support

A

◀ New   ⬅ Revised   ~~deleted~~ Deleted   Excludes 1   Excludes 2   Includes   Use additional   Code first   Code also   Unspecified
OGCR Official Guidelines   ● Unacceptable Principal Diagnosis   X Assign placeholder X   ● Use Additional Character(s)   ▶ Manifestation Code   **Coding Clinic**

● **Z59.8**   **Other problems related to housing and economic circumstances**
     Foreclosure on loan
     Isolated dwelling
     Problems with creditors

● **Z59.9**   **Problem related to housing and economic circumstances, unspecified**

● **Z60**   **Problems related to social environment**

● **Z60.0**   **Problems of adjustment to life-cycle transitions**
     Empty nest syndrome
     Phase of life problem
     Problem with adjustment to retirement [pension]

● **Z60.2**   **Problems related to living alone**

● **Z60.3**   **Acculturation difficulty**
     Problem with migration
     Problem with social transplantation

● **Z60.4**   **Social exclusion and rejection**
     Exclusion and rejection on the basis of personal characteristics, such as unusual physical appearance, illness or behavior.
     Excludes1   target of adverse discrimination such as for racial or religious reasons (Z60.5)

● **Z60.5**   **Target of (perceived) adverse discrimination and persecution**
     Excludes1   social exclusion and rejection (Z60.4)

● **Z60.8**   **Other problems related to social environment**

● **Z60.9**   **Problem related to social environment, unspecified**

● **Z62**   **Problems related to upbringing**
     Includes   current and past negative life events in childhood
       current and past problems of a child related to upbringing
     Excludes2   maltreatment syndrome (T74.-)
       problems related to housing and economic circumstances (Z59.-)

● **Z62.0**   **Inadequate parental supervision and control**

● **Z62.1**   **Parental overprotection**

● **Z62.2**   **Upbringing away from parents**
     Excludes1   problems with boarding school (Z59.3)

   ● **Z62.21**   **Child in welfare custody**   P
       Child in care of non-parental family member
       Child in foster care
       Excludes2   problem for parent due to child in welfare custody (Z63.5)

   ● **Z62.22**   **Institutional upbringing**
       Child living in orphanage or group home

   ● **Z62.29**   **Other upbringing away from parents**

● **Z62.3**   **Hostility towards and scapegoating of child**   P

● **Z62.6**   **Inappropriate (excessive) parental pressure**

● **Z62.8**   **Other specified problems related to upbringing**

   ● **Z62.81**   **Personal history of abuse in childhood**

     ● **Z62.810**   **Personal history of physical and sexual abuse in childhood**
       Excludes1   current child physical abuse (T74.12, T76.12)
       current child sexual abuse (T74.22, T76.22)

     ● **Z62.811**   **Personal history of psychological abuse in childhood**
       Excludes1   current child psychological abuse (T74.32, T76.32)

     ● **Z62.812**   **Personal history of neglect in childhood**
       Excludes1   current child neglect (T74.02, T76.02)

     ● **Z62.819**   **Personal history of unspecified abuse in childhood**
       Excludes1   current child abuse NOS (T74.92, T76.92)

   ● **Z62.82**   **Parent-child conflict**

     ● **Z62.820**   **Parent-biological child conflict**
       Parent-child problem NOS

     ● **Z62.821**   **Parent-adopted child conflict**

     ● **Z62.822**   **Parent-foster child conflict**

   ● **Z62.89**   **Other specified problems related to upbringing**

     ● **Z62.890**   **Parent-child estrangement NEC**

     ● **Z62.891**   **Sibling rivalry**

     ● **Z62.898**   **Other specified problems related to upbringing**

● **Z62.9**   **Problem related to upbringing, unspecified**

● **Z63**   **Other problems related to primary support group, including family circumstances**
     Excludes2   maltreatment syndrome (T74.-, T76)
       parent-child problems (Z62.-)
       problems related to negative life events in childhood (Z62.-)
       problems related to upbringing (Z62.-)

● **Z63.0**   **Problems in relationship with spouse or partner**
     Excludes1   counseling for spousal or partner abuse problems (Z69.1)
       counseling related to sexual attitude, behavior, and orientation (Z70.-)

● **Z63.1**   **Problems in relationship with in-laws**

● **Z63.3**   **Absence of family member**
     Excludes1   absence of family member due to disappearance and death (Z63.4)
       absence of family member due to separation and divorce (Z63.5)

   ● **Z63.31**   **Absence of family member due to military deployment**
       Individual or family affected by other family member being on military deployment
       Excludes1   family disruption due to return of family member from military deployment (Z63.71)

   ● **Z63.32**   **Other absence of family member**

● **Z63.4**   **Disappearance and death of family member**
     Assumed death of family member
     Bereavement

● **Z63.5**   **Disruption of family by separation and divorce**
     Marital estrangement

● **Z63.6**   **Dependent relative needing care at home**

● **Z63.7**   **Other stressful life events affecting family and household**

   ● **Z63.71**   **Stress on family due to return of family member from military deployment**
       Individual or family affected by family member having returned from military deployment (current or past conflict)

   ● **Z63.72**   **Alcoholism and drug addiction in family**

   ● **Z63.79**   **Other stressful life events affecting family and household**
       Anxiety (normal) about sick person in family
       Health problems within family
       Ill or disturbed family member
       Isolated family

CHAPTER 21 (Z00-Z99)

● **Z63.8**   **Other specified problems related to primary support group**
     Family discord NOS
     Family estrangement NOS
     High expressed emotional level within family
     Inadequate family support NOS
     Inadequate or distorted communication within family

● **Z63.9**   **Problem related to primary support group, unspecified**
     Relationship disorder NOS

● **Z64**   **Problems related to certain psychosocial circumstances**

   ● **Z64.0**   **Problems related to unwanted pregnancy** ♀

   ● **Z64.1**   **Problems related to multiparity** ♀

   ● **Z64.4**   **Discord with counselors**
       Discord with probation officer
       Discord with social worker

● **Z65**   **Problems related to other psychosocial circumstances**

   ● **Z65.0**   **Conviction in civil and criminal proceedings without imprisonment**

   ● **Z65.1**   **Imprisonment and other incarceration**

   ● **Z65.2**   **Problems related to release from prison**

   ● **Z65.3**   **Problems related to other legal circumstances**
       Arrest
       Child custody or support proceedings
       Litigation
       Prosecution

   ● **Z65.4**   **Victim of crime and terrorism**
       Victim of torture

   ● **Z65.5**   **Exposure to disaster, war and other hostilities**
       Excludes1   target of perceived discrimination or persecution (Z60.5)

   ● **Z65.8**   **Other specified problems related to psychosocial circumstances**

   ● **Z65.9**   **Problem related to unspecified psychosocial circumstances**

DO NOT RESUSCITATE STATUS (Z66)

● **Z66**   **Do not resuscitate**
     DNR status

BLOOD TYPE (Z67)

● **Z67**   **Blood type**
     Coding Clinic: 2015, Q3, P40

   ● **Z67.1**   **Type A blood**
     ● **Z67.10**   Type A blood, Rh positive
     ● **Z67.11**   Type A blood, Rh negative

   ● **Z67.2**   **Type B blood**
     ● **Z67.20**   Type B blood, Rh positive
     ● **Z67.21**   Type B blood, Rh negative

   ● **Z67.3**   **Type AB blood**
     ● **Z67.30**   Type AB blood, Rh positive
     ● **Z67.31**   Type AB blood, Rh negative

   ● **Z67.4**   **Type O blood**
     ● **Z67.40**   Type O blood, Rh positive
     ● **Z67.41**   Type O blood, Rh negative

   ● **Z67.9**   **Unspecified blood type**
     ● **Z67.90**   Unspecified blood type, Rh positive
     ● **Z67.91**   Unspecified blood type, Rh negative
       Coding Clinic: 2015, Q3, P40

BODY MASS INDEX [BMI] (Z68)

OGCR **Section I.B.14.**

General Coding Guidelines

14. Documentation for BMI, *Depth of* Non-pressure ulcers, Pressure Ulcer Stages, **Coma Scale,** *and NIH Stroke Scale*

For the Body Mass Index (BMI), depth of non-pressure chronic ulcers, pressure ulcer stage, **coma scale, and NIH stroke scale (NIHSS) codes,** code assignment may be based on medical record documentation from clinicians who are not the patient's provider (i.e., physician or other qualified healthcare practitioner legally accountable for establishing the patient's diagnosis), since this information is typically documented by other clinicians involved in the care of the patient (e.g., a dietitian often documents the BMI, a nurse often documents the pressure ulcer stages, **and an emergency medical technician often documents the coma scale).** However, the associated diagnosis (such as overweight, obesity, **acute stroke,** or pressure ulcer) must be documented by the patient's provider. If there is conflicting medical record documentation, either from the same clinician or different clinicians, the patient's attending provider should be queried for clarification.

The BMI, **coma scale, and NIHSS** codes should only be reported as secondary diagnoses.

● **Z68**   **Body mass index [BMI]**
     Kilograms per meters squared
     Note: BMI adult codes are for use for persons 21 years of age or older.
       BMI pediatric codes are for use for persons 2-20 years of age. These percentiles are based on the growth charts published by the Centers for Disease Control and Prevention (CDC)

   ● **Z68.1**   **Body mass index (BMI) 19 or less, adult**   A
     (Ex) E66.01-E66.1, E66.8-E66.9, Z68.1-Z68.54

   ● **Z68.2**   **Body mass index (BMI) 20-29, adult**
     ● **Z68.20**   Body mass index (BMI) 20.0-20.9, adult   A
     ● **Z68.21**   Body mass index (BMI) 21.0-21.9, adult   A
     ● **Z68.22**   Body mass index (BMI) 22.0-22.9, adult   A
     ● **Z68.23**   Body mass index (BMI) 23.0-23.9, adult   A
     ● **Z68.24**   Body mass index (BMI) 24.0-24.9, adult   A
     ● **Z68.25**   Body mass index (BMI) 25.0-25.9, adult   A
     ● **Z68.26**   Body mass index (BMI) 26.0-26.9, adult   A
     ● **Z68.27**   Body mass index (BMI) 27.0-27.9, adult   A
     ● **Z68.28**   Body mass index (BMI) 28.0-28.9, adult   A
     ● **Z68.29**   Body mass index (BMI) 29.0-29.9, adult   A

   ● **Z68.3**   **Body mass index (BMI) 30-39, adult**
     ● **Z68.30**   Body mass index (BMI) 30.0-30.9, adult   A
     ● **Z68.31**   Body mass index (BMI) 31.0-31.9, adult   A
     ● **Z68.32**   Body mass index (BMI) 32.0-32.9, adult   A
     ● **Z68.33**   Body mass index (BMI) 33.0-33.9, adult   A
     ● **Z68.34**   Body mass index (BMI) 34.0-34.9, adult   A
     ● **Z68.35**   Body mass index (BMI) 35.0-35.9, adult   A
     ● **Z68.36**   Body mass index (BMI) 36.0-36.9, adult   A
     ● **Z68.37**   Body mass index (BMI) 37.0-37.9, adult   A
     ● **Z68.38**   Body mass index (BMI) 38.0-38.9, adult   A
     ● **Z68.39**   Body mass index (BMI) 39.0-39.9, adult   A

   ● **Z68.4**   **Body mass index (BMI) 40 or greater, adult**
     (Ex) For category Z68.4 CC codes: E65-E66.1, E66.8-E66.9, Z68.1-Z68.54
     ● **Z68.41** Body mass index (BMI) 40.0-44.9, adult   A
     ● **Z68.42** Body mass index (BMI) 45.0-49.9, adult   A
     ● **Z68.43** Body mass index (BMI) 50-59.9, adult   A
     ● **Z68.44** Body mass index (BMI) 60.0-69.9, adult   A
     ● **Z68.45** Body mass index (BMI) 70 or greater, adult   A

◄ New   ◄ Revised   ~~deleted~~ Deleted   Excludes 1   Excludes 2   Includes   Use additional   Code first   Code also   Unspecified

OGCR Official Guidelines   ● Unacceptable Principal Diagnosis   X Assign placeholder X   ● Use Additional Character(s)   ▶ Manifestation Code   Coding Clinic

● **Z68.5**   **Body mass index (BMI) pediatric**
     ● **Z68.51**   **Body mass index (BMI) pediatric, less than 5th percentile for age**
     ● **Z68.52**   **Body mass index (BMI) pediatric, 5th percentile to less than 85th percentile for age**
     ● **Z68.53**   **Body mass index (BMI) pediatric, 85th percentile to less than 95th percentile for age**
     ● **Z68.54**   **Body mass index (BMI) pediatric, greater than or equal to 95th percentile for age**

PERSONS ENCOUNTERING HEALTH SERVICES IN OTHER CIRCUMSTANCES (Z69-Z76)

● **Z69**   **Encounter for mental health services for victim and perpetrator of abuse**
     Includes   counseling for victims and perpetrators of abuse
● **Z69.0**   **Encounter for mental health services for child abuse problems**
     ● **Z69.01**   **Encounter for mental health services for parental child abuse**
         Z69.010   **Encounter for mental health services for victim of parental child abuse**   P
         ● **Z69.011**   **Encounter for mental health services for perpetrator of parental child abuse**
             Excludes1   encounter for mental health services for non-parental child abuse (Z69.02-)
     ● **Z69.02**   **Encounter for mental health services for non-parental child abuse**
         Z69.020   **Encounter for mental health services for victim of non-parental child abuse**   P
         ● **Z69.021**   **Encounter for mental health services for perpetrator of non- parental child abuse**
● **Z69.1**   **Encounter for mental health services for spousal or partner abuse problems**
     ● **Z69.11**   **Encounter for mental health services for victim of spousal or partner abuse**
     ● **Z69.12**   **Encounter for mental health services for perpetrator of spousal or partner abuse**
● **Z69.8**   **Encounter for mental health services for victim or perpetrator of other abuse**
     ● **Z69.81**   **Encounter for mental health services for victim of other abuse**
         Encounter for rape victim counseling
     ● **Z69.82**   **Encounter for mental health services for perpetrator of other abuse**

● **Z70**   **Counseling related to sexual attitude, behavior and orientation**
     Includes   encounter for mental health services for sexual attitude, behavior and orientation
     Excludes2   contraceptive or procreative counseling (Z30-Z31)
● **Z70.0**   **Counseling related to sexual attitude**
● **Z70.1**   **Counseling related to patient's sexual behavior and orientation**
     Patient concerned regarding impotence
     Patient concerned regarding non-responsiveness
     Patient concerned regarding promiscuity
     Patient concerned regarding sexual orientation
● **Z70.2**   **Counseling related to sexual behavior and orientation of third party**
     Advice sought regarding sexual behavior and orientation of child
     Advice sought regarding sexual behavior and orientation of partner
     Advice sought regarding sexual behavior and orientation of spouse
● **Z70.3**   **Counseling related to combined concerns regarding sexual attitude, behavior and orientation**
● **Z70.8**   **Other sex counseling**
     Encounter for sex education
● **Z70.9**   **Sex counseling, unspecified**

● **Z71**   **Persons encountering health services for other counseling and medical advice, not elsewhere classified**
     Excludes2   contraceptive or procreation counseling (Z30-Z31)
         sex counseling (Z70.-)
● **Z71.0**   **Person encountering health services to consult on behalf of another person**
     Person encountering health services to seek advice or treatment for non-attending third party
     Excludes2   anxiety (normal) about sick person in family (Z63.7)
         expectant (adoptive) parent(s) pre-birth pediatrician visit (Z76.81)
● **Z71.1**   **Person with feared health complaint in whom no diagnosis is made**
     Person encountering health services with feared condition which was not demonstrated
     Person encountering health services in which problem was normal state
     'Worried well'
     Excludes1   medical observation for suspected diseases and conditions proven not to exist (Z03.-)
● **Z71.2**   **Person consulting for explanation of examination or test findings**
● **Z71.3**   **Dietary counseling and surveillance**
     Use additional code for any associated underlying medical condition
     Use additional code to identify body mass index (BMI), if known (Z68.-)
● **Z71.4**   **Alcohol abuse counseling and surveillance**
     Use additional code for alcohol abuse or dependence (F10.-)
     ● **Z71.41**   **Alcohol abuse counseling and surveillance of alcoholic**
     ● **Z71.42**   **Counseling for family member of alcoholic**
         Counseling for significant other, partner, or friend of alcoholic
● **Z71.5**   **Drug abuse counseling and surveillance**
     Use additional code for drug abuse or dependence (F11-F16, F18-F19)
     ● **Z71.51**   **Drug abuse counseling and surveillance of drug abuser**
     ● **Z71.52**   **Counseling for family member of drug abuser**
         Counseling for significant other, partner, or friend of drug abuser
● **Z71.6**   **Tobacco abuse counseling**
     Use additional code for nicotine dependence (F17.-)
● **Z71.7**   **Human immunodeficiency virus [HIV] counseling**
● **Z71.8**   **Other specified counseling**
     Excludes2   counseling for contraception (Z30.0-)
         counseling for genetics (Z31.5)
         counseling for procreative management (Z31.6-)
     ● **Z71.81**   **Spiritual or religious counseling**
     ● **Z71.89**   **Other specified counseling**
● **Z71.9**   **Counseling, unspecified**
     Encounter for medical advice NOS

● **Z72   Problems related to lifestyle**
   Excludes2   problems related to life-management difficulty (Z73.-)
   problems related to socioeconomic and psychosocial circumstances (Z55-Z65)

● **Z72.0   Tobacco use**
   Tobacco use NOS
   Excludes1   history of tobacco dependence (Z87.891)
   nicotine dependence (F17.2-)
   tobacco dependence (F17.2-)
   tobacco use during pregnancy (O99.33-)

● **Z72.3   Lack of physical exercise**

● **Z72.4   Inappropriate diet and eating habits**
   Excludes1   behavioral eating disorders of infancy or childhood (F98.2.-F98.3)
   eating disorders (F50.-)
   lack of adequate food (Z59.4)
   malnutrition and other nutritional deficiencies (E40-E64)

● **Z72.5   High risk sexual behavior**
   Promiscuity
   Excludes1   paraphilias (F65)

   ● **Z72.51   High risk heterosexual behavior**

   ● **Z72.52   High risk homosexual behavior**

   ● **Z72.53   High risk bisexual behavior**

● **Z72.6   Gambling and betting**
   Excludes1   compulsive or pathological gambling (F63.0)

● **Z72.8   Other problems related to lifestyle**

   ● **Z72.81   Antisocial behavior**
      Excludes1   conduct disorders (F91.-)

      Z72.810   Child and adolescent antisocial behavior   P
         Antisocial behavior (child) (adolescent) without manifest psychiatric disorder
         Delinquency NOS
         Group delinquency
         Offenses in the context of gang membership
         Stealing in company with others
         Truancy from school

      Z72.811   Adult antisocial behavior   A
         Adult antisocial behavior without manifest psychiatric disorder

   ● **Z72.82   Problems related to sleep**
      Z72.820   Sleep deprivation
         Lack of adequate sleep
         Excludes1   insomnia (G47.0-)

      ● **Z72.821   Inadequate sleep hygiene**
         Bad sleep habits
         Irregular sleep habits
         Unhealthy sleep wake schedule
         Excludes1   insomnia (F51.0-, G47.0-)

   ● **Z72.89   Other problems related to lifestyle**
      Self-damaging behavior

● **Z72.9   Problem related to lifestyle, unspecified**

● **Z73   Problems related to life management difficulty**
   Excludes2   problems related to socioeconomic and psychosocial circumstances (Z55-Z65)

● **Z73.0   Burn-out**

● **Z73.1   Type A behavior pattern**

● **Z73.2   Lack of relaxation and leisure**

● **Z73.3   Stress, not elsewhere classified**
   Physical and mental strain NOS
   Excludes1   stress related to employment or unemployment (Z56.-)

● **Z73.4   Inadequate social skills, not elsewhere classified**

● **Z73.5   Social role conflict, not elsewhere classified**

● **Z73.6   Limitation of activities due to disability**
   Excludes1   care-provider dependency (Z74.-)

● **Z73.8   Other problems related to life management difficulty**

   ● **Z73.81   Behavioral insomnia of childhood**
      ● **Z73.810   Behavioral insomnia of childhood, sleep-onset association type**   P

      ● **Z73.811   Behavioral insomnia of childhood, limit setting type**   P

      ● **Z73.812   Behavioral insomnia of childhood, combined type**   P

      ● **Z73.819   Behavioral insomnia of childhood, unspecified type**   P

   ● **Z73.82   Dual sensory impairment**

   ● **Z73.89   Other problems related to life management difficulty**

● **Z73.9   Problem related to life management difficulty, unspecified**

● **Z74   Problems related to care provider dependency**
   Excludes2   dependence on enabling machines or devices NEC (Z99.-)

● **Z74.0   Reduced mobility**

   ● **Z74.01   Bed confinement status**
      Bedridden

   ● **Z74.09   Other reduced mobility**
      Chairridden
      Reduced mobility NOS
      Excludes2   wheelchair dependence (Z99.3)

● **Z74.1   Need for assistance with personal care**

● **Z74.2   Need for assistance at home and no other household member able to render care**

● **Z74.3   Need for continuous supervision**

● **Z74.8   Other problems related to care provider dependency**

● **Z74.9   Problem related to care provider dependency, unspecified**

● **Z75   Problems related to medical facilities and other health care**

● **Z75.0   Medical services not available in home**
   Excludes1   no other household member able to render care (Z74.2)

● **Z75.1   Person awaiting admission to adequate facility elsewhere**

● **Z75.2   Other waiting period for investigation and treatment**

● **Z75.3   Unavailability and inaccessibility of health care facilities**
   Excludes1   bed unavailable (Z75.1)

● **Z75.4   Unavailability and inaccessibility of other helping agencies**

● **Z75.5   Holiday relief care**

● **Z75.8   Other problems related to medical facilities and other health care**

● **Z75.9   Unspecified problem related to medical facilities and other health care**

◄ New   ◄▦ Revised   ~~deleted~~ Deleted   Excludes 1   Excludes 2   Includes   Use additional   Code first   Code also   Unspecified
OGCR Official Guidelines   ● Unacceptable Principal Diagnosis   X Assign placeholder X   ● Use Additional Character(s)   ▶ Manifestation Code   **Coding Clinic**

- **Z76** **Persons encountering health services in other circumstances**
  - **Z76.0** **Encounter for issue of repeat prescription**
    - Encounter for issue of repeat prescription for appliance
    - Encounter for issue of repeat prescription for medicaments
    - Encounter for issue of repeat prescription for spectacles
    - **Excludes2** issue of medical certificate (Z02.7)
      - repeat prescription for contraceptive (Z30.4-)
  - **Z76.1** **Encounter for health supervision and care of foundling**
  - **Z76.2** **Encounter for health supervision and care of other healthy infant and child**   P
    - Encounter for medical or nursing care or supervision of healthy infant under circumstances such as adverse socioeconomic conditions at home
    - Encounter for medical or nursing care or supervision of healthy infant under circumstances such as awaiting foster or adoptive placement
    - Encounter for medical or nursing care or supervision of healthy infant under circumstances such as maternal illness
    - Encounter for medical or nursing care or supervision of healthy infant under circumstances such as number of children at home preventing or interfering with normal care
  - **Z76.3** **Healthy person accompanying sick person**
  - **Z76.4** **Other boarder to healthcare facility**
    - **Excludes1** homelessness (Z59.0)
  - **Z76.5** **Malingerer [conscious simulation]**
    - Person feigning illness (with obvious motivation)
    - **Excludes1** factitious disorder (F68.1-)
      - peregrinating patient (F68.1-)
  - **Z76.8** **Persons encountering health services in other specified circumstances**
    - **Z76.81** **Expectant parent(s) prebirth pediatrician visit**
      - Pre-adoption pediatrician visit for adoptive parent(s)
    - **Z76.82** **Awaiting organ transplant status**
      - Patient waiting for organ availability
    - **Z76.89** **Persons encountering health services in other specified circumstances**
      - Persons encountering health services NOS

PERSONS WITH POTENTIAL HEALTH HAZARDS RELATED TO FAMILY AND PERSONAL HISTORY AND CERTAIN CONDITIONS INFLUENCING HEALTH STATUS (Z77-Z99)

Code also any follow-up examination (Z08-Z09)

- **Z77** **Other contact with and (suspected) exposures hazardous to health**
  - **Includes** contact with and (suspected) exposures to potential hazards to health
  - **Excludes2** contact with and (suspected) exposure to communicable diseases (Z20.-)
    - exposure to (parental) (environmental) tobacco smoke in the perinatal period (P96.81)
    - newborn affected by noxious substances transmitted via placenta or breast milk (P04.-) ◀▥
    - occupational exposure to risk factors (Z57.-)
    - retained foreign body (Z18.-)
    - retained foreign body fully removed (Z87.821)
    - toxic effects of substances chiefly nonmedicinal as to source (T51-T65)
  - **Z77.0** **Contact with and (suspected) exposure to hazardous, chiefly nonmedicinal, chemicals**
    - **Z77.01** **Contact with and (suspected) exposure to hazardous metals**
      - **Z77.010** **Contact with and (suspected) exposure to arsenic**
      - **Z77.011** **Contact with and (suspected) exposure to lead**

- **Z77.012** **Contact with and (suspected) exposure to uranium**
  - **Excludes1** retained depleted uranium fragments (Z18.01)
- **Z77.018** **Contact with and (suspected) exposure to other hazardous metals**
  - Contact with and (suspected) exposure to chromium compounds
  - Contact with and (suspected) exposure to nickel dust
  - **Z77.02** **Contact with and (suspected) exposure to hazardous aromatic compounds**
    - **Z77.020** **Contact with and (suspected) exposure to aromatic amines**
    - **Z77.021** **Contact with and (suspected) exposure to benzene**
    - **Z77.028** **Contact with and (suspected) exposure to other hazardous aromatic compounds**
      - Aromatic dyes NOS
      - Polycyclic aromatic hydrocarbons
  - **Z77.09** **Contact with and (suspected) exposure to other hazardous, chiefly nonmedicinal, chemicals**
    - **Z77.090** **Contact with and (suspected) exposure to asbestos**
    - **Z77.098** **Contact with and (suspected) exposure to other hazardous, chiefly nonmedicinal, chemicals**
      - Dyes NOS
- **Z77.1** **Contact with and (suspected) exposure to environmental pollution and hazards in the physical environment**
  - **Z77.11** **Contact with and (suspected) exposure to environmental pollution**
    - **Z77.110** **Contact with and (suspected) exposure to air pollution**
    - **Z77.111** **Contact with and (suspected) exposure to water pollution**
    - **Z77.112** **Contact with and (suspected) exposure to soil pollution**
    - **Z77.118** **Contact with and (suspected) exposure to other environmental pollution**
  - **Z77.12** **Contact with and (suspected) exposure to hazards in the physical environment**
    - **Z77.120** **Contact with and (suspected) exposure to mold (toxic)**
    - **Z77.121** **Contact with and (suspected) exposure to harmful algae and algae toxins**
      - Contact with and (suspected) exposure to (harmful) algae bloom NOS
      - Contact with and (suspected) exposure to blue-green algae bloom
      - Contact with and (suspected) exposure to brown tide
      - Contact with and (suspected) exposure to cyanobacteria bloom
      - Contact with and (suspected) exposure to Florida red tide
      - Contact with and (suspected) exposure to pfiesteria piscicida
      - Contact with and (suspected) exposure to red tide
    - **Z77.122** **Contact with and (suspected) exposure to noise**

N Newborn Age: 0   **P** Pediatric Age: 0–17   **M** Maternity DX: 12–55   **A** Adult Age: 15–124   ♀ Females Only   ♂ Males Only

🔗 Complication\Comorbidity   🔗 Major C\C   (Ex) CC/MCC Exclusions   🔗 Hospital-Acquired Condition

1627

● **Z77.123**   **Contact with and (suspected) exposure to radon and other naturally occuring radiation**

     Excludes2   radiation exposure as the cause of a confirmed condition (W88-W90, X39.0-)
                 radiation sickness NOS (T66)

● **Z77.128**   **Contact with and (suspected) exposure to other hazards in the physical environment**

● **Z77.2**   **Contact with and (suspected) exposure to other hazardous substances**

    ● **Z77.21**   **Contact with and (suspected) exposure to potentially hazardous body fluids**

    ● **Z77.22**   **Contact with and (suspected) exposure to environmental tobacco smoke (acute) (chronic)**
        Exposure to second hand tobacco smoke (acute) (chronic)
        Passive smoking (acute) (chronic)

         Excludes1   nicotine dependence (F17.-)
                    tobacco use (Z72.0)

         Excludes2   occupational exposure to environmental tobacco smoke (Z57.31)

    ● **Z77.29**   **Contact with and (suspected) exposure to other hazardous substances**
        Coding Clinic: 2016, Q2, P34

● **Z77.9**   **Other contact with and (suspected) exposures hazardous to health**

● **Z78**   **Other specified health status**
    Excludes2   asymptomatic human immunodeficiency virus [HIV] infection status (Z21)
                 postprocedural status (Z93-Z99)
                 sex reassignment status (Z87.890)

● **Z78.0**   **Asymptomatic menopausal state ♀**   A
        Menopausal state NOS
        Postmenopausal status NOS

     Excludes2   symptomatic menopausal state (N95.1)

● **Z78.1**   **Physical restraint status**
     Excludes1   physical restraint due to a procedure - omit code

● **Z78.9**   **Other specified health status**

● **Z79**   **Long term (current) drug therapy**
    Includes   long term (current) drug use for prophylactic purposes
    Code also any therapeutic drug level monitoring (Z51.81)
    Excludes2   drug abuse and dependence (F11-F19)
                 drug use complicating pregnancy, childbirth, and the puerperium (O99.32-)
                 long term (current) use of oral antidiabetic drugs (Z79.84) ◀
                 long term (current) use of oral hypoglycemic drugs (Z79.84) ◀

● **Z79.0**   **Long term (current) use of anticoagulants and antithrombotics/antiplatelets**
     Excludes2   long term (current) use of aspirin (Z79.82)

    Z79.01   **Long term (current) use of anticoagulants**

    ● **Z79.02**   **Long term (current) use of antithrombotics/antiplatelets**

● **Z79.1**   **Long term (current) use of non-steroidal anti-inflammatories (NSAID)**
     Excludes2   long term (current) use of aspirin (Z79.82)

● **Z79.2**   **Long term (current) use of antibiotics**

    Z79.3   **Long term (current) use of hormonal contraceptives**
        Long term (current) use of birth control pill or patch

    Z79.4   **Long term (current) use of insulin**

● **Z79.5**   **Long term (current) use of steroids**
    ● **Z79.51**   **Long term (current) use of inhaled steroids**
    ● **Z79.52**   **Long term (current) use of systemic steroids**

● **Z79.8**   **Other long term (current) drug therapy**
    ● **Z79.81 Long term (current) use of agents affecting estrogen receptors and estrogen levels**
        Code first, if applicable:
        malignant neoplasm of breast (C50.-)
        malignant neoplasm of prostate (C61)
        Use additional code, if applicable, to identify:
        estrogen receptor positive status (Z17.0)
        family history of breast cancer (Z80.3)
        genetic susceptibility to malignant neoplasm (cancer) (Z15.0-)
        personal history of breast cancer (Z85.3)
        personal history of prostate cancer (Z85.46)
        postmenopausal status (Z78.0)

       Excludes1   hormone replacement therapy (postmenopausal) (Z79.890)

    ● **Z79.810**   **Long term (current) use of selective estrogen receptor modulators (SERMs)**
        Long term (current) use of raloxifene (Evista)
        Long term (current) use of tamoxifen (Nolvadex)
        Long term (current) use of toremifene (Fareston)

    ● **Z79.811**   **Long term (current) use of aromatase inhibitors**
        Long term (current) use of anastrozole (Arimidex)
        Long term (current) use of exemestane (Aromasin)
        Long term (current) use of letrozole (Femara)

    ● **Z79.818**   **Long term (current) use of other agents affecting estrogen receptors and estrogen levels**
        Long term (current) use of estrogen receptor downregulators
        Long term (current) use of fulvestrant (Faslodex)
        Long term (current) use of gonadotropin-releasing hormone (GnRH) agonist
        Long term (current) use of goserelin acetate (Zoladex)
        Long term (current) use of leuprolide acetate (leuprorelin) (Lupron)
        Long term (current) use of megestrol acetate (Megace)

    Z79.82   **Long term (current) use of aspirin**

    ● **Z79.83**   **Long term (current) use of bisphosphonates**

    ● **Z79.84**   **Long term (current) use of oral hypoglycemic drugs** ◀
        Long term (current) use of oral antidiabetic drugs ◀

       Excludes2   long term (current) use of insulin (Z79.4) ◀

● **Z79.89**   **Other long term (current) drug therapy**
    ● **Z79.890**   **Hormone replacement therapy (postmenopausal)**

    Z79.891   **Long term (current) use of opiate analgesic**
        Long term (current) use of methadone for pain management

       Excludes1   methadone use NOS (F11.9-) ◀⫿
                 use of methadone for treatment of heroin addiction (F11.2-)

    Z79.899   **Other long term (current) drug therapy**
        Coding Clinic: 2015, Q4, P34, Q3, P21

◀ New   ◀⫿ Revised   ~~deleted~~ Deleted   Excludes 1   Excludes 2   Includes   Use additional   Code first   Code also   Unspecified

1628   OGCR Official Guidelines   ● Unacceptable Principal Diagnosis   X Assign placeholder X   ● Use Additional Character(s)   ▶ Manifestation Code   **Coding Clinic**

● **Z80　Family history of primary malignant neoplasm**
　● **Z80.0　Family history of malignant neoplasm of digestive organs**
　　　Conditions classifiable to C15-C26
　● **Z80.1　Family history of malignant neoplasm of trachea, bronchus and lung**
　　　Conditions classifiable to C33-C34
　● **Z80.2　Family history of malignant neoplasm of other respiratory and intrathoracic organs**
　　　Conditions classifiable to C30-C32, C37-C39
　● **Z80.3　Family history of malignant neoplasm of breast**
　　　Conditions classifiable to C50.-
　● **Z80.4　Family history of malignant neoplasm of genital organs**
　　　Conditions classifiable to C51-C63
　　● **Z80.41　Family history of malignant neoplasm of ovary**
　　● **Z80.42　Family history of malignant neoplasm of prostate**
　　● **Z80.43　Family history of malignant neoplasm of testis**
　　● **Z80.49　Family history of malignant neoplasm of other genital organs**
　● **Z80.5　Family history of malignant neoplasm of urinary tract**
　　　Conditions classifiable to C64-C68
　　● **Z80.51　Family history of malignant neoplasm of kidney**
　　● **Z80.52　Family history of malignant neoplasm of bladder**
　　● **Z80.59　Family history of malignant neoplasm of other urinary tract organ**
　● **Z80.6　Family history of leukemia**
　　　Conditions classifiable to C91-C95
　● **Z80.7　Family history of other malignant neoplasms of lymphoid, hematopoietic and related tissues**
　　　Conditions classifiable to C81-C90, C96.-
　● **Z80.8　Family history of malignant neoplasm of other organs or systems**
　　　Conditions classifiable to C00-C14, C40-C49, C69-C79
　● **Z80.9　Family history of malignant neoplasm, unspecified**
　　　Conditions classifiable to C80.1

● **Z81　Family history of mental and behavioral disorders**
　● **Z81.0　Family history of intellectual disabilities**
　　　Conditions classifiable to F70-F79
　● **Z81.1　Family history of alcohol abuse and dependence**
　　　Conditions classifiable to F10.-
　● **Z81.2　Family history of tobacco abuse and dependence**
　　　Conditions classifiable to F17.-
　● **Z81.3　Family history of other psychoactive substance abuse and dependence**
　　　Conditions classifiable to F11-F16, F18-F19
　● **Z81.4　Family history of other substance abuse and dependence**
　　　Conditions classifiable to F55
　● **Z81.8　Family history of other mental and behavioral disorders**
　　　Conditions classifiable elsewhere in F01-F99

● **Z82　Family history of certain disabilities and chronic diseases (leading to disablement)**
　● **Z82.0　Family history of epilepsy and other diseases of the nervous system**
　　　Conditions classifiable to G00-G99
　● **Z82.1　Family history of blindness and visual loss**
　　　Conditions classifiable to H54.-
　● **Z82.2　Family history of deafness and hearing loss**
　　　Conditions classifiable to H90-H91
　● **Z82.3　Family history of stroke**
　　　Conditions classifiable to I60-I64

● **Z82.4　Family history of ischemic heart disease and other diseases of the circulatory system**
　　　Conditions classifiable to I00-I52, I65-I99
　　● **Z82.41　Family history of sudden cardiac death**
　　● **Z82.49　Family history of ischemic heart disease and other diseases of the circulatory system**
　● **Z82.5　Family history of asthma and other chronic lower respiratory diseases**
　　　Conditions classifiable to J40-J47
　　　Excludes2　family history of other diseases of the respiratory system (Z83.6)
　● **Z82.6　Family history of arthritis and other diseases of the musculoskeletal system and connective tissue**
　　　Conditions classifiable to M00-M99
　　● **Z82.61　Family history of arthritis**
　　● **Z82.62　Family history of osteoporosis**
　　● **Z82.69　Family history of other diseases of the musculoskeletal system and connective tissue**
　● **Z82.7　Family history of congenital malformations, deformations and chromosomal abnormalities**
　　　Conditions classifiable to Q00-Q99
　　● **Z82.71　Family history of polycystic kidney**
　　● **Z82.79　Family history of other congenital malformations, deformations and chromosomal abnormalities**
　● **Z82.8　Family history of other disabilities and chronic diseases leading to disablement, not elsewhere classified**

● **Z83　Family history of other specific disorders**
　　　Excludes2　contact with and (suspected) exposure to communicable disease in the family (Z20.-)
　● **Z83.0　Family history of human immunodeficiency virus [HIV] disease**
　　　Conditions classifiable to B20
　● **Z83.1　Family history of other infectious and parasitic diseases**
　　　Conditions classifiable to A00-B19, B25-B94, B99
　● **Z83.2　Family history of diseases of the blood and blood-forming organs and certain disorders involving the immune mechanism**
　　　Conditions classifiable to D50-D89
　● **Z83.3　Family history of diabetes mellitus**
　　　Conditions classifiable to E08-E13
　● **Z83.4　Family history of other endocrine, nutritional and metabolic diseases**
　　　Conditions classifiable to E00-E07, E15-E88
　　● **Z83.41　Family history of multiple endocrine neoplasia [MEN] syndrome**
　　● **Z83.42　Family history of familial hypercholesterolemia** ◀
　　● **Z83.49　Family history of other endocrine, nutritional and metabolic diseases**
　● **Z83.5　Family history of eye and ear disorders**
　　● **Z83.51　Family history of eye disorders**
　　　　Conditions classifiable to H00-H53, H55-H59
　　　　Excludes2　family history of blindness and visual loss (Z82.1)
　　　● **Z83.511　Family history of glaucoma**
　　　● **Z83.518　Family history of other specified eye disorder**
　　● **Z83.52　Family history of ear disorders**
　　　　Conditions classifiable to H60-H83, H92-H95
　　　　Excludes2　family history of deafness and hearing loss (Z82.2)
　● **Z83.6　Family history of other diseases of the respiratory system**
　　　Conditions classifiable to J00-J39, J60-J99
　　　Excludes2　family history of asthma and other chronic lower respiratory diseases (Z82.5)

N Newborn Age: 0　　**P** Pediatric Age: 0–17　　**M** Maternity DX: 12–55　　**A** Adult Age: 15–124　　♀ Females Only　　♂ Males Only
🔧 Complication\Comorbidity　　🔧 Major C\C　　(Ex) CC/MCC Exclusions　　🔧 Hospital-Acquired Condition

● **Z83.7   Family history of diseases of the digestive system**
Conditions classifiable to K00-K93

  ● **Z83.71   Family history of colonic polyps**
Excludes1   family history of malignant neoplasm of digestive organs (Z80.0)

  ● **Z83.79   Family history of other diseases of the digestive system**

● **Z84   Family history of other conditions**

  ● **Z84.0   Family history of diseases of the skin and subcutaneous tissue**
Conditions classifiable to L00-L99

  ● **Z84.1   Family history of disorders of kidney and ureter**
Conditions classifiable to N00-N29

  ● **Z84.2   Family history of other diseases of the genitourinary system**
Conditions classifiable to N30-N99

  ● **Z84.3   Family history of consanguinity**

  ● **Z84.8   Family history of other specified conditions**

    ● **Z84.81   Family history of carrier of genetic disease**

    ● **Z84.82   Family history of sudden infant death syndrome ◄**
Family history of SIDS ◄

    ● **Z84.89   Family history of other specified conditions**

● **Z85   Personal history of malignant neoplasm**
Code first any follow-up examination after treatment of malignant neoplasm (Z08)

Use additional code to identify:
alcohol use and dependence (F10.-)
exposure to environmental tobacco smoke (Z77.22)
history of tobacco dependence (Z87.891) ◄▥
occupational exposure to environmental tobacco smoke (Z57.31)
tobacco dependence (F17.-)
tobacco use (Z72.0)

Excludes2   personal history of benign neoplasm (Z86.01-)
personal history of carcinoma-in-situ (Z86.00-)

  ● **Z85.0   Personal history of malignant neoplasm of digestive organs**

    ● **Z85.00   Personal history of malignant neoplasm of unspecified digestive organ**

    ● **Z85.01   Personal history of malignant neoplasm of esophagus**
Conditions classifiable to C15

    ● **Z85.02   Personal history of malignant neoplasm of stomach**

      ● **Z85.020   Personal history of malignant carcinoid tumor of stomach**
Conditions classifiable to C7A.092

      ● **Z85.028   Personal history of other malignant neoplasm of stomach**
Conditions classifiable to C16

    ● **Z85.03   Personal history of malignant neoplasm of large intestine**

      ● **Z85.030   Personal history of malignant carcinoid tumor of large intestine**
Conditions classifiable to C7A.022-C7A.025, C7A.029

      ● **Z85.038   Personal history of other malignant neoplasm of large intestine**
Conditions classifiable to C18

    ● **Z85.04   Personal history of malignant neoplasm of rectum, rectosigmoid junction, and anus**

      ● **Z85.040   Personal history of malignant carcinoid tumor of rectum**
Conditions classifiable to C7A.026

      ● **Z85.048   Personal history of other malignant neoplasm of rectum, rectosigmoid junction, and anus**
Conditions classifiable to C19-C21

  ● **Z85.05   Personal history of malignant neoplasm of liver**
Conditions classifiable to C22

  ● **Z85.06   Personal history of malignant neoplasm of small intestine**

    ● **Z85.060   Personal history of malignant carcinoid tumor of small intestine**
Conditions classifiable to C7A.01-

    ● **Z85.068   Personal history of other malignant neoplasm of small intestine**
Conditions classifiable to C17

  ● **Z85.07   Personal history of malignant neoplasm of pancreas**
Conditions classifiable to C25

  ● **Z85.09   Personal history of malignant neoplasm of other digestive organs**

● **Z85.1   Personal history of malignant neoplasm of trachea, bronchus and lung**

  ● **Z85.11   Personal history of malignant neoplasm of bronchus and lung**

    ● **Z85.110   Personal history of malignant carcinoid tumor of bronchus and lung**
Conditions classifiable to C7A.090

    ● **Z85.118   Personal history of other malignant neoplasm of bronchus and lung**
Conditions classifiable to C34

  ● **Z85.12   Personal history of malignant neoplasm of trachea**
Conditions classifiable to C33

● **Z85.2   Personal history of malignant neoplasm of other respiratory and intrathoracic organs**

  ● **Z85.20   Personal history of malignant neoplasm of unspecified respiratory organ**

  ● **Z85.21   Personal history of malignant neoplasm of larynx**
Conditions classifiable to C32

  ● **Z85.22   Personal history of malignant neoplasm of nasal cavities, middle ear, and accessory sinuses**
Conditions classifiable to C30-C31

  ● **Z85.23   Personal history of malignant neoplasm of thymus**

    ● **Z85.230   Personal history of malignant carcinoid tumor of thymus**
Conditions classifiable to C7A.091

    ● **Z85.238   Personal history of other malignant neoplasm of thymus**
Conditions classifiable to C37

  ● **Z85.29   Personal history of malignant neoplasm of other respiratory and intrathoracic organs**

● **Z85.3   Personal history of malignant neoplasm of breast**
Conditions classifiable to C50.-

● **Z85.4   Personal history of malignant neoplasm of genital organs**
Conditions classifiable to C51-C63

  ● **Z85.40   Personal history of malignant neoplasm of unspecified female genital organ ♀**

  ● **Z85.41   Personal history of malignant neoplasm of cervix uteri ♀**

  ● **Z85.42   Personal history of malignant neoplasm of other parts of uterus ♀**

  ● **Z85.43   Personal history of malignant neoplasm of ovary ♀**

  ● **Z85.44   Personal history of malignant neoplasm of other female genital organs ♀**

  ● **Z85.45   Personal history of malignant neoplasm of unspecified male genital organ ♂**

  ● **Z85.46   Personal history of malignant neoplasm of prostate ♂**

  ● **Z85.47   Personal history of malignant neoplasm of testis ♂**

◄ New   ◄▥ Revised   ~~deleted~~ Deleted   Excludes 1   Excludes 2   Includes   Use additional   Code first   Code also   Unspecified

OGCR Official Guidelines   ● Unacceptable Principal Diagnosis   X Assign placeholder X   ● Use Additional Character(s)   ▌ Manifestation Code   **Coding Clinic**

● **Z85.48　Personal history of malignant neoplasm of epididymis** ♂

● **Z85.49　Personal history of malignant neoplasm of other male genital organs** ♂

● **Z85.5　Personal history of malignant neoplasm of urinary tract**
  Conditions classifiable to C64-C68

  ● **Z85.50　Personal history of malignant neoplasm of unspecified urinary tract organ**

  ● **Z85.51　Personal history of malignant neoplasm of bladder**

  ● **Z85.52　Personal history of malignant neoplasm of kidney**

  > **Excludes1**　personal history of malignant neoplasm of renal pelvis (Z85.53)

    ● **Z85.520　Personal history of malignant carcinoid tumor of kidney**
      Conditions classifiable to C7A.093

    ● **Z85.528　Personal history of other malignant neoplasm of kidney**
      Conditions classifiable to C64

  ● **Z85.53　Personal history of malignant neoplasm of renal pelvis**

  ● **Z85.54　Personal history of malignant neoplasm of ureter**

  ● **Z85.59　Personal history of malignant neoplasm of other urinary tract organ**

● **Z85.6　Personal history of leukemia**
  Conditions classifiable to C91-C95

  > **Excludes1**　leukemia in remission C91.0-C95.9 with 5th character 1

● **Z85.7　Personal history of other malignant neoplasms of lymphoid, hematopoietic and related tissues**

  ● **Z85.71　Personal history of Hodgkin lymphoma**
    Conditions classifiable to C81

  ● **Z85.72　Personal history of non-Hodgkin lymphomas**
    Conditions classifiable to C82-C85

  ● **Z85.79　Personal history of other malignant neoplasms of lymphoid, hematopoietic and related tissues**
    Conditions classifiable to C88-C90, C96

  > **Excludes1**　multiple myeloma in remission (C90.01)
  > plasma cell leukemia in remission (C90.11)
  > plasmacytoma in remission (C90.21)

● **Z85.8　Personal history of malignant neoplasms of other organs and systems**
  Conditions classifiable to C00-C14, C40-C49, C69-C75, C7A.098, C76-C79 ◀▥▥

  ● **Z85.81　Personal history of malignant neoplasm of lip, oral cavity, and pharynx**

    ● **Z85.810　Personal history of malignant neoplasm of tongue**

    ● **Z85.818　Personal history of malignant neoplasm of other sites of lip, oral cavity, and pharynx**

    ● **Z85.819　Personal history of malignant neoplasm of unspecified site of lip, oral cavity, and pharynx**

  ● **Z85.82　Personal history of malignant neoplasm of skin**

    ● **Z85.820　Personal history of malignant melanoma of skin**
      Conditions classifiable to C43

    ● **Z85.821　Personal history of Merkel cell carcinoma**
      Conditions classifiable to C4A

    ● **Z85.828　Personal history of other malignant neoplasm of skin**
      Conditions classifiable to C44

● **Z85.83　Personal history of malignant neoplasm of bone and soft tissue**

  ● **Z85.830　Personal history of malignant neoplasm of bone**

  ● **Z85.831　Personal history of malignant neoplasm of soft tissue**

    > **Excludes2**　personal history of malignant neoplasm of skin (Z85.82-)

● **Z85.84　Personal history of malignant neoplasm of eye and nervous tissue**

  ● **Z85.840　Personal history of malignant neoplasm of eye**

  ● **Z85.841　Personal history of malignant neoplasm of brain**

  ● **Z85.848　Personal history of malignant neoplasm of other parts of nervous tissue**

● **Z85.85　Personal history of malignant neoplasm of endocrine glands**

  ● **Z85.850　Personal history of malignant neoplasm of thyroid**

  ● **Z85.858　Personal history of malignant neoplasm of other endocrine glands**

● **Z85.89　Personal history of malignant neoplasm of other organs and systems**

● **Z85.9　Personal history of malignant neoplasm, unspecified**
  Conditions classifiable to C7A.00, C80.1

● **Z86　Personal history of certain other diseases**
  Code first any follow-up examination after treatment (Z09)

  ● **Z86.0　Personal history of in-situ and benign neoplasms and neoplasms of uncertain behavior**

    > **Excludes2**　personal history of malignant neoplasms (Z85.-)

    ● **Z86.00　Personal history of in-situ neoplasm**
      Conditions classifiable to D00-D09 ◀

      ● **Z86.000　Personal history of in-situ neoplasm of breast**

      ● **Z86.001　Personal history of in-situ neoplasm of cervix uteri** ♀
        Personal history of cervical intraepithelial neoplasia III [CIN III] ◀

      ● **Z86.008　Personal history of in-situ neoplasm of other site**
        Personal history of vaginal intraepithelial neoplasia III [VAIN III] ◀
        Personal history of vulvar intraepithelial neoplasia III [VIN III] ◀

    ● **Z86.01　Personal history of benign neoplasm**

      ● **Z86.010　Personal history of colonic polyps**

      ● **Z86.011　Personal history of benign neoplasm of the brain**

      ● **Z86.012　Personal history of benign carcinoid tumor**

      ● **Z86.018　Personal history of other benign neoplasm**

    ● **Z86.03　Personal history of neoplasm of uncertain behavior**

- **Z86.1 Personal history of infectious and parasitic diseases**
  Conditions classifiable to A00-B89, B99

  Excludes1 personal history of infectious diseases specific to a body system sequelae of infectious and parasitic diseases (B90-B94)

  - **Z86.11 Personal history of tuberculosis**
  - **Z86.12 Personal history of poliomyelitis**
  - **Z86.13 Personal history of malaria**
  - **Z86.14 Personal history of Methicillin resistant Staphylococcus aureus infection**
    Personal history of MRSA infection
  - **Z86.19 Personal history of other infectious and parasitic diseases**

- **Z86.2 Personal history of diseases of the blood and blood-forming organs and certain disorders involving the immune mechanism**
  Conditions classifiable to D50-D89

- **Z86.3 Personal history of endocrine, nutritional and metabolic diseases**
  Conditions classifiable to E00-E88

  - **Z86.31 Personal history of diabetic foot ulcer**

    Excludes2 current diabetic foot ulcer (E08.621, E09.621, E10.621, E11.621, E13.621)

  - **Z86.32 Personal history of gestational diabetes ♀**
    Personal history of conditions classifiable to O24.4-

    Excludes1 gestational diabetes mellitus in current pregnancy (O24.4-)

  - **Z86.39 Personal history of other endocrine, nutritional and metabolic disease**

- **Z86.5 Personal history of mental and behavioral disorders**
  Conditions classifiable to F40-F59

  - **Z86.51 Personal history of combat and operational stress reaction**
  - **Z86.59 Personal history of other mental and behavioral disorders** A

- **Z86.6 Personal history of diseases of the nervous system and sense organs**
  Conditions classifiable to G00-G99, H00-H95

  - **Z86.61 Personal history of infections of the central nervous system**
    Personal history of encephalitis
    Personal history of meningitis
  - **Z86.69 Personal history of other diseases of the nervous system and sense organs**

- **Z86.7 Personal history of diseases of the circulatory system**
  Conditions classifiable to I00-I99

  Excludes2 old myocardial infarction (I25.2)
  personal history of anaphylactic shock (Z87.892)
  postmyocardial infarction syndrome (I24.1)

  - **Z86.71 Personal history of venous thrombosis and embolism**
    - **Z86.711 Personal history of pulmonary embolism**
    - **Z86.718 Personal history of other venous thrombosis and embolism**

- **Z86.72 Personal history of thrombophlebitis**
- **Z86.73 Personal history of transient ischemic attack (TIA), and cerebral infarction without residual deficits**
  Personal history of prolonged reversible ischemic neurological deficit (PRIND)
  Personal history of stroke NOS without residual deficits

  Excludes1 personal history of traumatic brain injury (Z87.820)
  sequelae of cerebrovascular disease (I69.-)

  Coding Clinic: 2012, Q4, P3

- **Z86.74 Personal history of sudden cardiac arrest**
  Personal history of sudden cardiac death successfully resuscitated
- **Z86.79 Personal history of other diseases of the circulatory system**

- **Z87 Personal history of other diseases and conditions**
  Code first any follow-up examination after treatment (Z09)

  - **Z87.0 Personal history of diseases of the respiratory system**
    Conditions classifiable to J00-J99

    - **Z87.01 Personal history of pneumonia (recurrent)**
    - **Z87.09 Personal history of other diseases of the respiratory system**

  - **Z87.1 Personal history of diseases of the digestive system**
    Conditions classifiable to K00-K93

    - **Z87.11 Personal history of peptic ulcer disease**
    - **Z87.19 Personal history of other diseases of the digestive system**

  - **Z87.2 Personal history of diseases of the skin and subcutaneous tissue**
    Conditions classifiable to L00-L99

    Excludes2 personal history of diabetic foot ulcer (Z86.31)

  - **Z87.3 Personal history of diseases of the musculoskeletal system and connective tissue**
    Conditions classifiable to M00-M99

    Excludes2 personal history of (healed) traumatic fracture (Z87.81)

    - **Z87.31 Personal history of (healed) nontraumatic fracture**
      - **Z87.310 Personal history of (healed) osteoporosis fracture**
        Personal history of (healed) fragility fracture
        Personal history of (healed) collapsed vertebra due to osteoporosis
      - **Z87.311 Personal history of (healed) other pathological fracture**
        Personal history of (healed) collapsed vertebra NOS

        Excludes2 personal history of osteoporosis fracture (Z87.310)

      - **Z87.312 Personal history of (healed) stress fracture**
        Personal history of (healed) fatigue fracture

    - **Z87.39 Personal history of other diseases of the musculoskeletal system and connective tissue**

● **Z87.4 Personal history of diseases of genitourinary system**
Conditions classifiable to N00-N99

  ● **Z87.41 Personal history of dysplasia of the female genital tract**

     Excludes1   personal history of intraepithelial neoplasia III of female genital tract (Z87.001, Z87.008) ◄
personal history of malignant neoplasm of female genital tract (Z85.40-Z85.44)

    ● **Z87.410 Personal history of cervical dysplasia** ♀

    ● **Z87.411 Personal history of vaginal dysplasia** ♀

    ● **Z87.412 Personal history of vulvar dysplasia** ♀

  ● **Z87.42 Personal history of other diseases of the female genital tract** ♀

  ● **Z87.43 Personal history of diseases of male genital organs**

    ● **Z87.430 Personal history of prostatic dysplasia** ♂

       Excludes1   personal history of malignant neoplasm of prostate (Z85.46)

    ● **Z87.438 Personal history of other diseases of male genital organs** ♂

  ● **Z87.44 Personal history of diseases of urinary system**

     Excludes1   personal history of malignant neoplasm of cervix uteri (Z85.41)

    ● **Z87.440 Personal history of urinary (tract) infections**

    ● **Z87.441 Personal history of nephrotic syndrome**

    ● **Z87.442 Personal history of urinary calculi**
Personal history of kidney stones

    ● **Z87.448 Personal history of other diseases of urinary system**

● **Z87.5 Personal history of complications of pregnancy, childbirth and the puerperium**
Conditions classifiable to O00-O9A

   Excludes2   recurrent pregnancy loss (N96)

  ● **Z87.51 Personal history of pre-term labor** ♀

     Excludes1   current pregnancy with history of pre-term labor (O09.21-)

  ● **Z87.59 Personal history of other complications of pregnancy, childbirth and the puerperium** ♀
Personal history of trophoblastic disease

● **Z87.7 Personal history of (corrected) congenital malformations**
Conditions classifiable to Q00-Q89 that have been repaired or corrected

   Excludes1   congenital malformations that have been partially corrected or repair but which still require medical treatment - code to condition

   Excludes2   other postprocedural states (Z98.-)
personal history of medical treatment (Z92.-)
presence of cardiac and vascular implants and grafts (Z95.-)
presence of other devices (Z97.-)
presence of other functional implants (Z96.-)
transplanted organ and tissue status (Z94.-)

  ● **Z87.71 Personal history of (corrected) congenital malformations of genitourinary system**

    ● **Z87.710 Personal history of (corrected) hypospadias** ♂

    ● **Z87.718 Personal history of other specified (corrected) congenital malformations of genitourinary system**

  ● **Z87.72 Personal history of (corrected) congenital malformations of nervous system and sense organs**

    ● **Z87.720 Personal history of (corrected) congenital malformations of eye**

    ● **Z87.721 Personal history of (corrected) congenital malformations of ear**

    ● **Z87.728 Personal history of other specified (corrected) congenital malformations of nervous system and sense organs**

  ● **Z87.73 Personal history of (corrected) congenital malformations of digestive system**

    ● **Z87.730 Personal history of (corrected) cleft lip and palate**

    ● **Z87.738 Personal history of other specified (corrected) congenital malformations of digestive system**

  ● **Z87.74 Personal history of (corrected) congenital malformations of heart and circulatory system**

  ● **Z87.75 Personal history of (corrected) congenital malformations of respiratory system**

  ● **Z87.76 Personal history of (corrected) congenital malformations of integument, limbs and musculoskeletal system**

  ● **Z87.79 Personal history of other (corrected) congenital malformations**

    ● **Z87.790 Personal history of (corrected) congenital malformations of face and neck**

    ● **Z87.798 Personal history of other (corrected) congenital malformations**

● **Z87.8 Personal history of other specified conditions**

   Excludes2   personal history of self harm (Z91.5)

  ● **Z87.81 Personal history of (healed) traumatic fracture**

     Excludes2   personal history of (healed) nontraumatic fracture (Z87.31-)

  ● **Z87.82 Personal history of other (healed) physical injury and trauma**
Conditions classifiable to S00-T88, except traumatic fractures

    ● **Z87.820 Personal history of traumatic brain injury**

       Excludes1   personal history of transient ischemic attack (TIA), and cerebral infarction without residual deficits (Z86.73)

    ● **Z87.821 Personal history of retained foreign body fully removed**

    ● **Z87.828 Personal history of other (healed) physical injury and trauma**

● **Z87.89 Personal history of other specified conditions**

     Z87.890 Personal history of sex reassignment

  ● **Z87.891 Personal history of nicotine dependence**

     Excludes1   current nicotine dependence (F17.2-)

  ● **Z87.892 Personal history of anaphylaxis**
Code also allergy status such as:
allergy status to drugs, medicaments and biological substances (Z88.-)
allergy status, other than to drugs and biological substances (Z91.0-)

  ● **Z87.898 Personal history of other specified conditions**
Coding Clinic: 2013, Q1, P21

CHAPTER 21 (Z00-Z99)

● Z88   Allergy status to drugs, medicaments and biological substances

     Excludes2   allergy status, other than to drugs and biological substances (Z91.0-)

   ● **Z88.0**   Allergy status to penicillin

   ● **Z88.1**   Allergy status to other antibiotic agents status

   ● **Z88.2**   Allergy status to sulfonamides status
         Coding Clinic: 2015, Q3, P23

   ● **Z88.3**   Allergy status to other anti-infective agents status

   ● **Z88.4**   Allergy status to anesthetic agent status

   ● **Z88.5**   Allergy status to narcotic agent status

   ● **Z88.6**   Allergy status to analgesic agent status

   ● **Z88.7**   Allergy status to serum and vaccine status

   ● **Z88.8**   Allergy status to other drugs, medicaments and biological substances status

   ● **Z88.9**   Allergy status to unspecified drugs, medicaments and biological substances status

● Z89   Acquired absence of limb

     Includes   amputation status
               postprocedural loss of limb
               post-traumatic loss of limb

     Excludes1   acquired deformities of limbs (M20-M21)
                congenital absence of limbs (Q71-Q73)

   ● **Z89.0**   Acquired absence of thumb and other finger(s)

     ● **Z89.01**   Acquired absence of thumb

       ● **Z89.011**   Acquired absence of right thumb

       ● **Z89.012**   Acquired absence of left thumb

       ● **Z89.019**   Acquired absence of unspecified thumb

     ● **Z89.02**   Acquired absence of other finger(s)

         Excludes2   acquired absence of thumb (Z89.01-)

       ● **Z89.021**   Acquired absence of right finger(s)

       ● **Z89.022**   Acquired absence of left finger(s)

       ● **Z89.029**   Acquired absence of unspecified finger(s)

   ● **Z89.1**   Acquired absence of hand and wrist

     ● **Z89.11**   Acquired absence of hand

       ● **Z89.111**   Acquired absence of right hand

       ● **Z89.112**   Acquired absence of left hand

       ● **Z89.119**   Acquired absence of unspecified hand

     ● **Z89.12**   Acquired absence of wrist
           Disarticulation at wrist

       ● **Z89.121**   Acquired absence of right wrist

       ● **Z89.122**   Acquired absence of left wrist

       ● **Z89.129**   Acquired absence of unspecified wrist

   ● **Z89.2**   Acquired absence of upper limb above wrist

     ● **Z89.20**   Acquired absence of upper limb, unspecified level

       ● **Z89.201**   Acquired absence of right upper limb, unspecified level

       ● **Z89.202**   Acquired absence of left upper limb, unspecified level

       ● **Z89.209**   Acquired absence of unspecified upper limb, unspecified level
            Acquired absence of arm NOS

     ● **Z89.21**   Acquired absence of upper limb below elbow

       ● **Z89.211**   Acquired absence of right upper limb below elbow

       ● **Z89.212**   Acquired absence of left upper limb below elbow

       ● **Z89.219**   Acquired absence of unspecified upper limb below elbow

   ● **Z89.22**   Acquired absence of upper limb above elbow
          Disarticulation at elbow

     ● **Z89.221**   Acquired absence of right upper limb above elbow

     ● **Z89.222**   Acquired absence of left upper limb above elbow

     ● **Z89.229**   Acquired absence of unspecified upper limb above elbow

   ● **Z89.23**   Acquired absence of shoulder
         Acquired absence of shoulder joint following explantation of shoulder joint prosthesis, with or without presence of antibiotic-impregnated cement spacer

     ● **Z89.231**   Acquired absence of right shoulder

     ● **Z89.232**   Acquired absence of left shoulder

     ● **Z89.239**   Acquired absence of unspecified shoulder

   ● **Z89.4**   Acquired absence of toe(s), foot, and ankle

     ● **Z89.41**   Acquired absence of great toe

       ● **Z89.411**   Acquired absence of right great toe

       ● **Z89.412**   Acquired absence of left great toe

       ● **Z89.419**   Acquired absence of unspecified great toe

     ● **Z89.42**   Acquired absence of other toe(s)

         Excludes2   acquired absence of great toe (Z89.41-)

       ● **Z89.421**   Acquired absence of other right toe(s)

       ● **Z89.422**   Acquired absence of other left toe(s)

       ● **Z89.429**   Acquired absence of other toe(s), unspecified side

     ● **Z89.43**   Acquired absence of foot

       ● **Z89.431**   Acquired absence of right foot

       ● **Z89.432**   Acquired absence of left foot

       ● **Z89.439**   Acquired absence of unspecified foot

     ● **Z89.44**   Acquired absence of ankle
          Disarticulation of ankle

       ● **Z89.441**   Acquired absence of right ankle

       ● **Z89.442**   Acquired absence of left ankle

       ● **Z89.449**   Acquired absence of unspecified ankle

   ● **Z89.5**   Acquired absence of leg below knee

     ● **Z89.51**   Acquired absence of leg below knee

       ● **Z89.511**   Acquired absence of right leg below knee

       ● **Z89.512**   Acquired absence of left leg below knee

       ● **Z89.519**   Acquired absence of unspecified leg below knee

     ● **Z89.52**   Acquired absence of knee
         Acquired absence of knee joint following explantation of knee joint prosthesis, with or without presence of antibiotic-impregnated cement spacer

       ● **Z89.521**   Acquired absence of right knee

       ● **Z89.522**   Acquired absence of left knee

       ● **Z89.529**   Acquired absence of unspecified knee

◀ New   ◀= Revised   ~~deleted~~ Deleted   Excludes 1   Excludes 2   Includes   Use additional   Code first   Code also   Unspecified

OGCR Official Guidelines   ● Unacceptable Principal Diagnosis   X Assign placeholder X   ● Use Additional Character(s)   ▶ Manifestation Code   **Coding Clinic**

- **Z89.6** Acquired absence of leg above knee
  - **Z89.61** Acquired absence of leg above knee
    Acquired absence of leg NOS
    Disarticulation at knee
    - **Z89.611** Acquired absence of right leg above knee
    - **Z89.612** Acquired absence of left leg above knee
    - **Z89.619** Acquired absence of unspecified leg above knee
  - **Z89.62** Acquired absence of hip
    Acquired absence of hip joint following explantation of hip joint prosthesis, with or without presence of antibiotic-impregnated cement spacer
    Disarticulation at hip
    - **Z89.621** Acquired absence of right hip joint
    - **Z89.622** Acquired absence of left hip joint
    - **Z89.629** Acquired absence of unspecified hip joint
- **Z89.9** Acquired absence of limb, unspecified
- **Z90** Acquired absence of organs, not elsewhere classified
  - **Includes** postprocedural or post-traumatic loss of body part NEC
  - **Excludes1** congenital absence - see Alphabetical Index
  - **Excludes2** postprocedural absence of endocrine glands (E89.-)
  - **Z90.0** Acquired absence of part of head and neck
    - **Z90.01** Acquired absence of eye
    - **Z90.02** Acquired absence of larynx
    - **Z90.09** Acquired absence of other part of head and neck
      Acquired absence of nose
      - **Excludes2** teeth (K08.1)
  - **Z90.1** Acquired absence of breast and nipple
    - **Z90.10** Acquired absence of unspecified breast and nipple
    - **Z90.11** Acquired absence of right breast and nipple
    - **Z90.12** Acquired absence of left breast and nipple
    - **Z90.13** Acquired absence of bilateral breasts and nipples
  - **Z90.2** Acquired absence of lung [part of]
  - **Z90.3** Acquired absence of stomach [part of]
  - **Z90.4** Acquired absence of other specified parts of digestive tract
    - **Z90.41** Acquired absence of pancreas
      Code also exocrine pancreatic insufficiency (K86.81) ◄
      Use additional code to identify any associated:
      insulin use (Z79.4)
      diabetes mellitus, postpancreatectomy (E13.-)
      - **Z90.410** Acquired total absence of pancreas
        Acquired absence of pancreas NOS
      - **Z90.411** Acquired partial absence of pancreas
    - **Z90.49** Acquired absence of other specified parts of digestive tract
  - **Z90.5** Acquired absence of kidney
  - **Z90.6** Acquired absence of other parts of urinary tract
    Acquired absence of bladder

- **Z90.7** Acquired absence of genital organ(s)
  - **Excludes1** personal history of sex reassignment (Z87.890)
  - **Excludes2** female genital mutilation status (N90.81-)
  - **Z90.71** Acquired absence of cervix and uterus
    - **Z90.710** Acquired absence of both cervix and uterus ♀
      Acquired absence of uterus NOS
      Status post total hysterectomy
    - **Z90.711** Acquired absence of uterus with remaining cervical stump ♀
      Status post partial hysterectomy with remaining cervical stump
    - **Z90.712** Acquired absence of cervix with remaining uterus ♀
  - **Z90.72** Acquired absence of ovaries
    - **Z90.721** Acquired absence of ovaries, unilateral ♀
    - **Z90.722** Acquired absence of ovaries, bilateral ♀
  - **Z90.79** Acquired absence of other genital organ(s)
- **Z90.8** Acquired absence of other organs
  - **Z90.81** Acquired absence of spleen
  - **Z90.89** Acquired absence of other organs
- **Z91** Personal risk factors, not elsewhere classified
  - **Excludes2** contact with and (suspected) exposures hazardous to health (Z77.-)
    exposure to pollution and other problems related to physical environment (Z77.1-)
    occupational exposure to risk factors (Z57.-)
    personal history of physical injury and trauma (Z87.81, Z87.82)
  - **Z91.0** Allergy status, other than to drugs and biological substances
    - **Excludes2** allergy status to drugs, medicaments, and biological substances (Z88.-)
    - **Z91.01** Food allergy status
      - **Excludes2** food additives allergy status (Z91.02)
      - **Z91.010** Allergy to peanuts
      - **Z91.011** Allergy to milk products
        - **Excludes1** lactose intolerance (E73.-)
      - **Z91.012** Allergy to eggs
      - **Z91.013** Allergy to seafood
        Allergy to shellfish
        Allergy to octopus or squid ink
      - **Z91.018** Allergy to other foods
        Allergy to nuts other than peanuts
    - **Z91.02** Food additives allergy status
    - **Z91.03** Insect allergy status
      - **Z91.030** Bee allergy status
      - **Z91.038** Other insect allergy status
    - **Z91.04** Nonmedicinal substance allergy status
      - **Z91.040** Latex allergy status
        Latex sensitivity status
      - **Z91.041** Radiographic dye allergy status
        Allergy status to contrast media used for diagnostic X-ray procedure
      - **Z91.048** Other nonmedicinal substance allergy status
    - **Z91.09** Other allergy status, other than to drugs and biological substances

CHAPTER 21 (Z00-Z99)

● **Z91.1   Patient's noncompliance with medical treatment and regimen**

    ● **Z91.11   Patient's noncompliance with dietary regimen**

    ● **Z91.12   Patient's intentional underdosing of medication regimen**

        Code first underdosing of medication (T36-T50) with fifth or sixth character 6

        Excludes1   adverse effect of prescribed drug taken as directed - code to adverse effect

                    poisoning (overdose) - code to poisoning

      ● **Z91.120   Patient's intentional underdosing of medication regimen due to financial hardship**

      ● **Z91.128   Patient's intentional underdosing of medication regimen for other reason**

    ● **Z91.13   Patient's unintentional underdosing of medication regimen**

        Code first underdosing of medication (T36-T50) with fifth or sixth character 6

        Excludes1   adverse effect of prescribed drug taken as directed - code to adverse effect

                    poisoning (overdose) - code to poisoning

      ● **Z91.130   Patient's unintentional underdosing of medication regimen due to age-related debility**

      ● **Z91.138   Patient's unintentional underdosing of medication regimen for other reason**

    ● **Z91.14   Patient's other noncompliance with medication regimen**

        Patient's underdosing of medication NOS

    ● **Z91.15   Patient's noncompliance with renal dialysis**

    ● **Z91.19   Patient's noncompliance with other medical treatment and regimen**

● **Z91.4   Personal history of psychological trauma, not elsewhere classified**

    ● **Z91.41   Personal history of adult abuse**

        Excludes2   personal history of abuse in childhood (Z62.81-)

      ● **Z91.410   Personal history of adult physical and sexual abuse   A**

          Excludes1   current adult physical abuse (T74.11, T76.11)

                    current adult sexual abuse (T74.21, T76.11)

      ● **Z91.411   Personal history of adult psychological abuse   A**

      ● **Z91.412   Personal history of adult neglect   A**

          Excludes1   current adult neglect (T74.01, T76.01)

      ● **Z91.419   Personal history of unspecified adult abuse   A**

    ● **Z91.49   Other personal history of psychological trauma, not elsewhere classified**

● **Z91.5   Personal history of self-harm**

    Personal history of parasuicide

    Personal history of self-poisoning

    Personal history of suicide attempt

● **Z91.8   Other specified personal risk factors, not elsewhere classified**

    ● **Z91.81   History of falling**

        At risk for falling

    ● **Z91.82   Personal history of military deployment   A**

        Individual (civilian or military) with past history of military war, peacekeeping and humanitarian deployment (current or past conflict)

        Returned from military deployment

    ▷ **Z91.83   *Wandering in diseases classified elsewhere***

        Code first underlying disorder such as:

          Alzheimer's disease (G30.-)

          autism or pervasive developmental disorder (F84.-)

          intellectual disabilities (F70-F79)

          unspecified dementia with behavioral disturbance (F03.9-)

    ● **Z91.89   Other specified personal risk factors, not elsewhere classified**

● **Z92   Personal history of medical treatment**

    Excludes2   postprocedural states (Z98.-)

    ● **Z92.0   Personal history of contraception**

        Excludes1   counseling or management of current contraceptive practices (Z30.-)

                   long term (current) use of contraception (Z79.3)

                   presence of (intrauterine) contraceptive device (Z97.5)

    ● **Z92.2   Personal history of drug therapy**

        Excludes2   long term (current) drug therapy (Z79.-)

      ● **Z92.21   Personal history of antineoplastic chemotherapy**

      ● **Z92.22   Personal history of monoclonal drug therapy**

      ● **Z92.23   Personal history of estrogen therapy**

      ● **Z92.24   Personal history of steroid therapy**

        ● **Z92.240   Personal history of inhaled steroid therapy**

        ● **Z92.241   Personal history of systemic steroid therapy**

          Personal history of steroid therapy NOS

      ● **Z92.25   Personal history of immunosupression therapy**

        Excludes2   personal history of steroid therapy (Z92.24)

      ● **Z92.29   Personal history of other drug therapy**

    ● **Z92.3   Personal history of irradiation**

        Personal history of exposure to therapeutic radiation

        Excludes1   exposure to radiation in the physical environment (Z77.12)

                   occupational exposure to radiation (Z57.1)

    ● **Z92.8   Personal history of other medical treatment**

      ● **Z92.81   Personal history of extracorporeal membrane oxygenation (ECMO)**

      ● **Z92.82   Status post administration of tPA (rtPA) in a different facility within the last 24 hours prior to admission to current facility**

        Code first condition requiring tPA administration, such as:

          acute cerebral infarction (I63.-)

          acute myocardial infarction (I21.-, I22.-)

      ● **Z92.83   Personal history of failed moderate sedation**

        Personal history of failed conscious sedation

        Excludes2   failed moderate sedation during procedure (T88.52)

◀ New   ◀▬ Revised   ~~deleted~~ Deleted   Excludes 1   Excludes 2   Includes   Use additional   Code first   Code also   Unspecified

1636   OGCR Official Guidelines   ● Unacceptable Principal Diagnosis   X Assign placeholder X   ● Use Additional Character(s)   ▷ Manifestation Code   **Coding Clinic**

- **Z92.84** **Personal history of unintended awareness under general anesthesia ◀**

  Excludes2   unintended awareness under general anesthesia during procedure (T88.53) ◀

- **Z92.89** **Personal history of other medical treatment**

- **Z93** **Artificial opening status**

  Excludes1   artificial openings requiring attention or management (Z43.-)

  complications of external stoma (J95.0-, K94.-, N99.5-)

  - **Z93.0** **Tracheostomy status**
  - **Z93.1** **Gastrostomy status**
  - **Z93.2** **Ileostomy status**
  - **Z93.3** **Colostomy status**
  - **Z93.4** **Other artificial openings of gastrointestinal tract status**
  - **Z93.5** **Cystostomy status**
    - **Z93.50** **Unspecified cystostomy status**
    - **Z93.51** **Cutaneous-vesicostomy status**
    - **Z93.52** **Appendico-vesicostomy status**
    - **Z93.59** **Other cystostomy status**
  - **Z93.6** **Other artificial openings of urinary tract status**

    Nephrostomy status

    Ureterostomy status

    Urethrostomy status
  - **Z93.8** **Other artificial opening status**
  - **Z93.9** **Artificial opening status, unspecified**

- **Z94** **Transplanted organ and tissue status**

  Includes   organ or tissue replaced by heterogenous or homogenous transplant

  Excludes1   complications of transplanted organ or tissue - see Alphabetical Index

  Excludes2   presence of vascular grafts (Z95.-)

  - **Z94.0** **Kidney transplant status** 🅒

    (Ex:) D47.Z1, T86.10-T86.19, T86.850-T86.859, T86.90-T86.99, Z94.0, Z94.89-Z94.9

  - **Z94.1** **Heart transplant status** 🅒

    Excludes1   artificial heart status (Z95.812)

    heart-valve replacement status (Z95.2-Z95.4)

    (Ex:) D47.Z1, T86.20-T86.39, T86.850-T86.859, T86.90-T86.99, Z94.1, Z94.3, Z94.89-Z94.9

  - **Z94.2** **Lung transplant status** 🅒

    (Ex:) D47.Z1, T86.810-T86.819, T86.850-T86.859, T86.90-T86.99, Z94.2, Z94.89-Z94.9

  - **Z94.3** **Heart and lungs transplant status** 🅒

    CC when PDx is its own CC

    (Ex:) See Z94.1

  - **Z94.4** **Liver transplant status** 🅒

    (Ex:) D47.Z1, T86.40-T86.49, T86.850-T86.859, T86.90-T86.99, Z94.4, Z94.89, Z94.9

  - **Z94.5** **Skin transplant status**

    Autogenous skin transplant status

  - **Z94.6** **Bone transplant status**
  - **Z94.7** **Corneal transplant status**
  - **Z94.8** **Other transplanted organ and tissue status**
    - **Z94.81** **Bone marrow transplant status** 🅒

      (Ex:) D47.Z1, D89.810-D89.813, T86.00-T86.09, T86.850-T86.859, T86.90-T86.99, Z94.9

    - **Z94.82** **Intestine transplant status** 🅒

      (Ex:) D47.Z1, T86.830-T86.839, T86.90-T86.99, Z94.82, Z94.89-Z94.9

    - **Z94.83** **Pancreas transplant status** 🅒

      (Ex:) D47.Z1, T86.850-T86.859, T86.890-T86.99, Z94.83, Z94.9

    - **Z94.84** **Stem cells transplant status** 🅒

      (Ex:) D47.Z1, T86.850-T86.859, T86.90-T86.99, Z94.9

    - **Z94.89** **Other transplanted organ and tissue status**
  - **Z94.9** **Transplanted organ and tissue status, unspecified**

- **Z95** **Presence of cardiac and vascular implants and grafts**

  Excludes1   complications of cardiac and vascular devices, implants and grafts (T82.-)

  - **Z95.0** **Presence of cardiac pacemaker**

    Presence of cardiac resynchronization therapy (CRT-P) pacemaker ◀

    Excludes1   adjustment or management of cardiac device (Z45.0-) ◀

    adjustment or management of cardiac pacemaker (Z45.0)

    presence of automatic (implantable) cardiac defibrillator with synchronous cardiac pacemaker (Z95.810)

  - **Z95.1** **Presence of aortocoronary bypass graft**

    Presence of coronary artery bypass graft ◀

  - **Z95.2** **Presence of prosthetic heart valve**

    Presence of heart valve NOS

  - **Z95.3** **Presence of xenogenic heart valve**
  - **Z95.4** **Presence of other heart-valve replacement**
  - **Z95.5** **Presence of coronary angioplasty implant and graft**

    Excludes1   coronary angioplasty status without implant and graft (Z98.61)

  - **Z95.8** **Presence of other cardiac and vascular implants and grafts**
    - **Z95.81** **Presence of other cardiac implants and grafts**

      (Ex:) For category **Z95.81** CC codes: D47.Z1, T86.20-T86.39, T86.850-T86.99, Z94.1, Z94.3, Z95.811-Z95.812

      - **Z95.810** **Presence of automatic (implantable) cardiac defibrillator**

        Presence of automatic (implantable) cardiac defibrillator with synchronous cardiac pacemaker

        Presence of cardiac resynchronization therapy defibrillator (CRT-D) ◀

        Presence of cardioverter-defibrillator (ICD) ◀

      - **Z95.811** **Presence of heart assist device** 🅒
      - **Z95.812** **Presence of fully implantable artificial heart** 🅒
      - **Z95.818** **Presence of other cardiac implants and grafts**
    - **Z95.82** **Presence of other vascular implants and grafts**
      - **Z95.820** **Peripheral vascular angioplasty status with implants and grafts**

        Excludes1   peripheral vascular angioplasty without implant and graft (Z98.62)

      - **Z95.828** **Presence of other vascular implants and grafts**

        Presence of intravascular prosthesis NEC

  - **Z95.9** **Presence of cardiac and vascular implant and graft, unspecified**

● **Z96   Presence of other functional implants**

Excludes2   complications of internal prosthetic devices, implants and grafts (T82-T85)
fitting and adjustment of prosthetic and other devices (Z44-Z46)

● **Z96.0   Presence of urogenital implants**

● **Z96.1   Presence of intraocular lens**
Presence of pseudophakia

● **Z96.2   Presence of otological and audiological implants**

　● **Z96.20   Presence of otological and audiological implant, unspecified**

　● **Z96.21   Cochlear implant status**

　● **Z96.22   Myringotomy tube(s) status**

　● **Z96.29   Presence of other otological and audiological implants**
Presence of bone-conduction hearing device
Presence of eustachian tube stent
Stapes replacement

● **Z96.3   Presence of artificial larynx**

● **Z96.4   Presence of endocrine implants**

　● **Z96.41   Presence of insulin pump (external) (internal)**

　● **Z96.49   Presence of other endocrine implants**

● **Z96.5   Presence of tooth-root and mandibular implants**

● **Z96.6   Presence of orthopedic joint implants**

　● **Z96.60   Presence of unspecified orthopedic joint implant**

　● **Z96.61   Presence of artificial shoulder joint**

　　● **Z96.611   Presence of right artificial shoulder joint**

　　● **Z96.612   Presence of left artificial shoulder joint**

　　● **Z96.619   Presence of unspecified artificial shoulder joint**

　● **Z96.62   Presence of artificial elbow joint**

　　● **Z96.621   Presence of right artificial elbow joint**

　　● **Z96.622   Presence of left artificial elbow joint**

　　● **Z96.629   Presence of unspecified artificial elbow joint**

　● **Z96.63   Presence of artificial wrist joint**

　　● **Z96.631   Presence of right artificial wrist joint**

　　● **Z96.632   Presence of left artificial wrist joint**

　　● **Z96.639   Presence of unspecified artificial wrist joint**

　● **Z96.64   Presence of artificial hip joint**
Hip-joint replacement (partial) (total)

　　● **Z96.641   Presence of right artificial hip joint**

　　● **Z96.642   Presence of left artificial hip joint**
Coding Clinic: 2015, Q1, P16

　　● **Z96.643   Presence of artificial hip joint, bilateral**

　　● **Z96.649   Presence of unspecified artificial hip joint**

　● **Z96.65   Presence of artificial knee joint**

　　● **Z96.651   Presence of right artificial knee joint**

　　● **Z96.652   Presence of left artificial knee joint**

　　● **Z96.653   Presence of artificial knee joint, bilateral**

　　● **Z96.659   Presence of unspecified artificial knee joint**

　● **Z96.66   Presence of artificial ankle joint**

　　● **Z96.661   Presence of right artificial ankle joint**

　　● **Z96.662   Presence of left artificial ankle joint**

　　● **Z96.669   Presence of unspecified artificial ankle joint**

　● **Z96.69   Presence of other orthopedic joint implants**

　　● **Z96.691   Finger-joint replacement of right hand**

　　● **Z96.692   Finger-joint replacement of left hand**

　　● **Z96.693   Finger-joint replacement, bilateral**

　　● **Z96.698   Presence of other orthopedic joint implants**

● **Z96.7   Presence of other bone and tendon implants**
Presence of skull plate

● **Z96.8   Presence of other specified functional implants**

　● **Z96.81   Presence of artificial skin**

　● **Z96.89   Presence of other specified functional implants**

● **Z96.9   Presence of functional implant, unspecified**

● **Z97   Presence of other devices**

Excludes1   complications of internal prosthetic devices, implants and grafts (T82-T85)
fitting and adjustment of prosthetic and other devices (Z44-Z46)

Excludes2   presence of cerebrospinal fluid drainage device (Z98.2)

● **Z97.0   Presence of artificial eye**

● **Z97.1   Presence of artificial limb (complete) (partial)**

　● **Z97.10   Presence of artificial limb (complete) (partial), unspecified**

　● **Z97.11   Presence of artificial right arm (complete) (partial)**

　● **Z97.12   Presence of artificial left arm (complete) (partial)**

　● **Z97.13   Presence of artificial right leg (complete) (partial)**

　● **Z97.14   Presence of artificial left leg (complete) (partial)**

　● **Z97.15   Presence of artificial arms, bilateral (complete) (partial)**

　● **Z97.16   Presence of artificial legs, bilateral (complete) (partial)**

● **Z97.2   Presence of dental prosthetic device (complete) (partial)**
Presence of dentures (complete) (partial)

● **Z97.3   Presence of spectacles and contact lenses**

● **Z97.4   Presence of external hearing-aid**

● **Z97.5   Presence of (intrauterine) contraceptive device ♀**

Excludes1   checking, reinsertion or removal of implantable subdermal contraceptive (Z30.46) ◀▥
checking, reinsertion or removal of intrauterine contraceptive device (Z30.43-) ◀

● **Z97.8   Presence of other specified devices**

● **Z98   Other postprocedural states**

Excludes2   aftercare (Z43-Z49, Z51)
follow-up medical care (Z08-Z09)
postprocedural complication - see Alphabetical Index

● **Z98.0   Intestinal bypass and anastomosis status**

Excludes2   bariatric surgery status (Z98.84)
gastric bypass status (Z98.84)
obesity surgery status (Z98.84)

● **Z98.1   Arthrodesis status**

● **Z98.2   Presence of cerebrospinal fluid drainage device**
Presence of CSF shunt

● **Z98.3   Post therapeutic collapse of lung status**
Code first underlying disease

● **Z98.4   Cataract extraction status**
Use additional code to identify intraocular lens implant status (Z96.1)

Excludes1   aphakia (H27.0)

　● **Z98.41   Cataract extraction status, right eye**

　● **Z98.42   Cataract extraction status, left eye**

　● **Z98.49   Cataract extraction status, unspecified eye**

◀ New   ◀▥ Revised   ~~deleted~~ Deleted   Excludes 1   Excludes 2   Includes   Use additional   Code first   Code also   Unspecified
OGCR Official Guidelines   ● Unacceptable Principal Diagnosis   X Assign placeholder X   ● Use Additional Character(s)   ▶ Manifestation Code   **Coding Clinic**

- Z98.5   **Sterilization status**
  - **Excludes1**   female infertility (N97.-)
                 male infertility (N46.-)
  - Z98.51   **Tubal ligation status** ♀
  - Z98.52   **Vasectomy status** ♂   A
- Z98.6   **Angioplasty status**
  - Z98.61   **Coronary angioplasty status**
    - **Excludes1**   coronary angioplasty status with implant and graft (Z95.5)
  - Z98.62   **Peripheral vascular angioplasty status**
    - **Excludes1**   peripheral vascular angioplasty status with implant and graft (Z95.820)
- Z98.8   **Other specified postprocedural states**
  - Z98.81   **Dental procedure status**
    - Z98.810   **Dental sealant status**
    - Z98.811   **Dental restoration status**
      Dental crown status
      Dental fillings status
    - Z98.818   **Other dental procedure status**
  - Z98.82   **Breast implant status**
    - **Excludes1**   breast implant removal status (Z98.86)
  - Z98.83   **Filtering (vitreous) bleb after glaucoma surgery status**
    - **Excludes1**   inflammation (infection) of postprocedural bleb (H59.4-)
  - Z98.84   **Bariatric surgery status**
    Gastric banding status
    Gastric bypass status for obesity
    Obesity surgery status
    - **Excludes1**   bariatric surgery status complicating pregnancy, childbirth, or the puerperium (O99.84)
    - **Excludes2**   intestinal bypass and anastomosis status (Z98.0)
  - Z98.85   **Transplanted organ removal status**
    Transplanted organ previously removed due to complication, failure, rejection or infection
    - **Excludes1**   encounter for removal of transplanted organ -code to complication of transplanted organ (T86.-)
  - Z98.86   **Personal history of breast implant removal**
  - Z98.87   **Personal history of in utero procedure**
    - Z98.870   **Personal history of in utero procedure during pregnancy** ♀
      - **Excludes2**   complications from in utero procedure for current pregnancy (O35.7)
        supervision of current pregnancy with history of in utero procedure during previous pregnancy (O09.82-)
    - Z98.871   **Personal history of in utero procedure while a fetus**
- Z98.89   **Other specified postprocedural states**
  - Z98.890   **Other specified postprocedural states** ◄
    Personal history of surgery, not elsewhere classified ◄
  - Z98.891   **History of uterine scar from previous surgery** ◄
    - **Excludes1**   Maternal care due to uterine scar from previous surgery (O34.2-) ◄
- Z99   **Dependence on enabling machines and devices, not elsewhere classified**
  - **Excludes1**   cardiac pacemaker status (Z95.0)
  - Z99.0   **Dependence on aspirator**
  - Z99.1   **Dependence on respirator**
    Dependence on ventilator
    Ⓔⓧ **For category Z99.1 CC codes:** J95.850, Z99.0-Z99.12, Z99.81-Z99.89
    - Z99.11   **Dependence on respirator [ventilator] status** 🏥
      Coding Clinic: 2015, Q1, P21
    - Z99.12   **Encounter for respirator [ventilator] dependence during power failure** 🏥
      - **Excludes1**   mechanical complication of respirator [ventilator] (J95.850)
  - Z99.2   **Dependence on renal dialysis**
    Hemodialysis status
    Peritoneal dialysis status
    Presence of arteriovenous shunt for dialysis
    Renal dialysis status NOS
    - **Excludes1**   encounter for fitting and adjustment of dialysis catheter (Z49.0-)
    - **Excludes2**   noncompliance with renal dialysis (Z91.15) ◄
    Coding Clinic: 2016, Q1, P13
  - Z99.3   **Dependence on wheelchair**
    Wheelchair confinement status
    Code first cause of dependence, such as:
    muscular dystrophy (G71.0)
    obesity (E66.-)
  - Z99.8   **Dependence on other enabling machines and devices**
    - Z99.81   **Dependence on supplemental oxygen**
      Dependence on long-term oxygen
    - Z99.89   **Dependence on other enabling machines and devices**
      Dependence on machine or device NOS

CHAPTER 21 (Z00-Z99)

N   Newborn Age: 0   **P**   Pediatric Age: 0–17   **M**   Maternity DX: 12–55   **A**   Adult Age: 15–124   ♀   Females Only   ♂   Males Only

🏥   Complication\Comorbidity   Major C\C   Ⓔⓧ   CC/MCC Exclusions   Hospital-Acquired Condition   **1639**

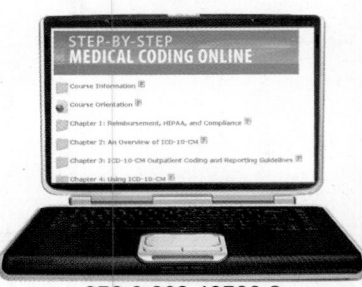